*Brenner & Rector's*

# THE KIDNEY

*Brenner & Rector's*

VOLUME II

# THE KIDNEY

Fifth Edition

*Edited by*

## Barry M. Brenner, M.D.

Samuel A. Levine Professor of Medicine
Harvard Medical School
Director, Renal Division, Brigham and Women's Hospital
Boston, Massachusetts

**W.B. SAUNDERS COMPANY**
*A Division of Harcourt Brace & Company*
Philadelphia London Toronto Montreal Sydney Tokyo

**W.B. SAUNDERS COMPANY**
*A Division of Harcourt Brace & Company*

The Curtis Center
Independence Square West
Philadelphia, Pennsylvania 19106

### Library of Congress Cataloging-in-Publication Data

Brenner and Rector's the kidney / edited by Barry M. Brenner. — 5th ed.

p.    cm.

Rev. ed. of: The kidney / edited by Barry M. Brenner, Floyd C. Rector, Jr. 4th ed. 1991.

Includes bibliographical references and index.

ISBN 0–7216–5075–9

1. Kidneys—Diseases.    2. Kidneys.    I. Brenner, Barry M.
II. Rector, Floyd C.    III. Title: Kidney.    [DNLM: 1. Kidney
Diseases. 2. Kidney—physiology. 3. Kidney—
physiopathology.    WJ 300   B8375   1996]

RC902.K53 1996

616.6′1—dc20

DNLM/DLC                                             95–3459

Volume 1 ISBN 0–7216–5073–2
Volume 2 ISBN 0–7216–5074–0

BRENNER AND RECTOR'S THE KIDNEY, 5th ed.    Two-Volume Set ISBN 0–7216–5075–9

Printed in the United States of America.

Last digit is the print number:    9    8    7    6    5    4    3    2    1

# Tribute to Floyd C. Rector, Jr.

Floyd Rector served as coeditor of this work from its inception in 1973 to the fourth edition, published in 1991. A towering figure in renal physiology for four decades, Dr. Rector was educated at Texas Tech University, University of Texas Southwestern Medical School and its affiliate, Parkland Hospital, in Dallas, and studied renal physiology in the Berliner-Orloff program at the National Institutes of Health. But it was the close association with his long-time mentor and colleague in Dallas, Dr. Donald W. Seldin, that defined his unrelenting interests in acid-base and volume homeostasis, tubule ion transport, and the intricacies of urinary concentration and dilution. Himself mentor to many of today's leading workers in nephrology, Dr. Rector has held positions successively as Professor of Medicine in Dallas, and Director, Division of Nephrology, and Professor and Chairman, Department of Medicine, University of California, San Francisco.

Dr. Rector's contributions to the initial design and organization of *The Kidney* and the subsequent periodic revisions of content through four editions have helped to secure a special role for this book in the education of students, residents, fellows, and practitioners of nephrology, urology, internal medicine, and pediatrics. For Floyd Rector's vision, guidance, and encouragement over the years, I extend heartfelt appreciation and warmly dedicate this fifth edition.

BARRY M. BRENNER, M.D.

# Contributors

**Sharon G. Adler, M.D.**
Associate Professor of Medicine, UCLA School of Medicine, Los Angeles; Associate Chief, Division of Nephrology, Harbor-UCLA Medical Center, Torrance, California
*Primary Glomerular Diseases; Secondary Glomerular Diseases*

**Stephen Adler, M.D.**
Associate Professor of Medicine, New York Medical College and Westchester County Medical Center, Valhalla, New York
*Cell-Cell and Cell-Matrix Interactions*

**Rajiv Agarwal, M.B.B.S., M.D., D.N.B.**
Chief Resident and Nephrologist, Presbyterian Hospital of Dallas, Dallas, Texas
*Hypophosphatemia and Hyperphosphatemia*

**R. Wayne Alexander, M.D., Ph.D.**
R. Bruce Logue Professor of Medicine, Emory University School of Medicine; Director, Division of Cardiology, Emory University Hospital, Atlanta, Georgia
*Biology of the Vascular Wall in Hypertension*

**Robert J. Alpern, M.D.**
Professor of Internal Medicine, Chief of Nephrology, and Ruth W. and Milton P. Levy, Senior Chair in Molecular Nephrology, University of Texas Southwestern Medical Center; Chief of Nephrology, Parkland Memorial Hospital and Zale Lipshy University Medical Center, Dallas, Texas
*Renal Acidification Mechanisms*

**Pamela W. Anderson, M.D.**
Assistant Professor of Medicine, University of Southern California Medical School, Los Angeles, California
*Diabetic Nephropathy*

**Sharon Anderson, M.D.**
Associate Professor of Medicine, Oregon Health Sciences University, Portland, Oregon
*Renal and Systemic Manifestations of Glomerular Disease*

**Anita C. Aperia, M.D.**
Professor of Pediatrics, Karolinska Institute, St. Goran's Hospital, Stockholm, Sweden
*Development and Maturation of the Kidney*

**Raymond Ardaillou, M.D.**
Professor of Physiology, Faculty of Medicine, Saint-Antoine; Department of Biology, Hôpital Tenon, Paris, France
*Biology of Renal Cells in Culture*

**John R. Asplin, M.D.**
Assistant Professor of Medicine, University of Chicago, Chicago, Illinois
*Nephrolithiasis*

**Keshwar Baboolal**
Fellow in Nephrology, Stanford University School of Medicine, Palo Alto, California
*Nephron Adaptation to Renal Injury*

**Kamal F. Badr, M.D.**
Professor of Medicine, Emory University School of Medicine; Chief, Renal Division, Atlanta Veterans Affairs Medical Center, Attending Physician, Emory University Hospital, Atlanta, Georgia
*Arachidonic Acid Metabolites and the Kidney; Microvascular Diseases of the Kidney*

**Lise Bankir, D.Sc.**
Directeur de Recherche, INSERM, Unit 90, Hôpital Necker, Paris, France
*Urea and the Kidney*

**John H. Bauer, M.D.**
Professor of Medicine and Associate Chairman, Department of Internal Medicine, University of Missouri; Chief, Medical Service, Harry S. Truman Memorial Veterans Hospital, Columbia, Missouri
*Antihypertensive Drugs*

**William M. Bennett, M.D.**
Professor of Medicine and Pharmacology, Oregon Health Sciences University, Portland, Oregon
*Prescribing Drugs in Renal Disease*

**Bradford C. Berk, M.D., Ph.D.**
Associate Professor of Medicine and Director, Cardiovascular Research, University of Washington, Seattle, Washington
*Biology of the Vascular Wall in Hypertension*

**Tomas Berl, M.D.**
Professor of Medicine and Head, Division of Renal Diseases and Hypertension, University of Colorado

School of Medicine; Staff, University Hospital, Denver, Colorado
*Pathophysiology of Water Metabolism*

**Robert W. Berliner, M.D.**
Professor Emeritus, Yale University School of Medicine, New Haven, Connecticut
*Control of Renal Potassium Excretion*

**Christine A. Berry, Ph.D.**
Professor of Physiology and Medicine, University of California, San Francisco, School of Medicine, San Francisco, California
*Renal Transport of Glucose, Amino Acids, Sodium, Chloride, and Water*

**Jon D. Blumenfeld, M.D.**
Associate Professor of Medicine, Cornell University Medical College; Assistant Attending in Medicine, The New York Hospital–Cornell Medical Center, New York, New York
*Essential Hypertension; Renovascular Hypertension and Ischemic Nephropathy*

**Jordi Bover, M.D.**
Attending Physician, Hospital de Bellvitge, Barcelona, Spain
*Renal Osteodystrophy*

**Hugh R. Brady, M.D., Ph.D., F.R.C.P.I.**
Associate Professor of Medicine, Harvard Medical School; Chief, Renal Section, Brockton–West Roxbury Veterans Affairs Medical Center, and Physician, Brigham and Women's Hospital, Boston, Massachusetts
*Cell-Cell and Cell-Matrix Interactions; Acute Renal Failure*

**Barry M. Brenner, M.D.**
Samuel A. Levine Professor of Medicine, Harvard Medical School; Director, Renal Division, Brigham and Women's Hospital, Boston, Massachusetts
*Development and Maturation of the Kidney; The Renal Circulations; Glomerular Ultrafiltration; Vasoactive Peptides and the Kidney; Reactive Nitrogen and Oxygen Intermediates and the Kidney; Acute Renal Failure; Renal and Systemic Manifestations of Glomerular Disease; Nephron Adaptation to Renal Injury*

**Matthew D. Breyer, M.D.**
Associate Professor of Medicine and Molecular Physiology and Biophysics, Vanderbilt University Nashville, Tennessee
*Arachidonic Acid Metabolites and the Kidney*

**John M. Burkart, M.D.**
Associate Professor of Medicine/Nephrology, Bowman Gray School of Medicine, Winston-Salem, North Carolina
*Peritoneal Dialysis*

**Orville C. Campbell, M.D.**
Nephrology Fellow, Emory University School of Medicine, Atlanta, Georgia
*Microvascular Diseases of the Kidney*

**Charles B. Carpenter, M.D.**
Professor of Medicine, Harvard Medical School; Senior Physician, Brigham and Women's Hospital, Boston, Massachusetts
*Immunobiology of Transplantation*

**Fredric L. Coe, M.D.**
Professor of Medicine and Physiology and Chief, Section of Nephrology, University of Chicago, Chicago, Illinois
*Nephrolithiasis*

**Martin G. Cogan, M.D.**
Professor of Medicine, University of California, San Francisco, School of Medicine; Chief, Nephrology Section, San Francisco Veterans Administration Medical Center, San Francisco, California
*Acid-Base Disorders*

**Arthur H. Cohen, M.D.**
Professor of Pathology and Medicine, UCLA School of Medicine; Attending Pathologist, Cedars-Sinai Medical Center, Los Angeles, California
*Primary Glomerular Diseases; Secondary Glomerular Diseases*

**Ramzi S. Cotran, M.D.**
F. B. Mallory Professor of Pathology, Harvard Medical School; Chairman, Department of Pathology, Brigham and Women's Hospital and Children's Hospital, Boston, Massachusetts
*Urinary Tract Infection, Pyelonephritis, and Reflux Nephropathy*

**Robert E. Cronin, M.D.**
Professor of Internal Medicine, University of Texas Southwestern Medical Center; Chief of Staff, Veterans Affairs Medical Center, Dallas, Texas
*Toxic Nephropathy*

**Gary C. Curhan, M.D., M.S.**
Instructor in Medicine, Harvard Medical School, Boston; Chief, Clinical Nephrology, West Roxbury Veterans Affairs Medical Center, West Roxbury, Massachusetts
*Urinary Tract Obstruction*

**Bradley M. Denker, M.D.**
Assistant Professor of Medicine, Harvard Medical School; Associate Physician, Brigham and Women's Hospital, Boston, Massachusetts
*Hemodialysis*

**Gerald F. DiBona, M.D.**
Professor and Vice-Chairman of Internal Medicine, University of Iowa College of Medicine; Chief,

Medical Service, Department of Veterans Affairs
Medical Center, Iowa City, Iowa
*Effects of Renal Nerves and Neurotransmitters on
Renal Function*

**John H. Dirks, M.D.**
Dean and Acting Rector, Aga Khan University,
Karachi, Pakistan
*Disturbances of Calcium and Magnesium Metabolism*

**Thomas D. DuBose, Jr., M.D.**
Professor of Internal Medicine, Physiology, and Cell
Biology and Director, Division of Nephrology,
University of Texas Medical School–Houston; Chief,
Nephrology Section, M. D. Anderson Cancer Center,
Medical Director, Nephrology Unit and Acute Dialysis
Unit, Hermann Hospital, and Medical Director,
University Kidney Centers, Houston, Texas
*Acid-Base Disorders*

**Lance D. Dworkin, M.D.**
Associate Professor of Medicine and Director, Division
of Renal Diseases, Brown University; Director,
Division of Renal Diseases, Rhode Island Hospital,
Providence, Rhode Island
*The Renal Circulations*

**Mark D. Faber, M.D.**
Clinical Instructor of Medicine, University of Michigan
Medical School, Ann Arbor; Director, Peritoneal
Dialysis, and Senior Staff Physician, Henry Ford
Hospital, Detroit, Michigan
*Disorders of Potassium Balance*

**Murray J. Favus, M.D.**
Professor of Medicine, University of Chicago, Chicago,
Illinois
*Nephrolithiasis*

**Thomas F. Ferris, M.D.**
Professor and Chairman of Medicine, University of
Minnesota, Minneapolis, Minnesota
*The Kidney and Hypertension in Pregnancy*

**John H. Galla, M.D.**
Professor of Medicine and Director, Division of
Nephrology and Hypertension, University of Cincinnati
College of Medicine, Cincinnati, Ohio
*Hypertension in Renal Parenchymal Disease*

**Marc B. Garnick, M.D.**
Associate Professor of Medicine, Dana-Farber Cancer
Institute, Harvard Medical School, Boston,
Massachusetts
*Renal Neoplasia*

**Gerhard Giebisch, M.D.**
Sterling Professor of Cellular and Molecular
Physiology, Yale University School of Medicine, New
Haven, Connecticut
*Control of Renal Potassium Excretion*

**Thomas A. Golper, M.D.**
Professor of Medicine, Nephrology, and Director of
Clinical Research, University of Arkansas for Medical
Sciences; Director of Dialysis, John McClellan Veterans
Affairs Hospital, Little Rock, Arkansas
*Prescribing Drugs in Renal Disease*

**Richard J. Glassock, M.D.**
Professor, University of Kentucky College of Medicine;
Chairman, Department of Internal Medicine, Chandler
Medical Center, University of Kentucky, Lexington,
Kentucky
*Primary Glomerular Diseases; Secondary Glomerular
Diseases*

**Jared J. Grantham, M.D.**
Professor of Medicine and Director of Nephrology and
Hypertension, University of Kansas Medical Center,
Kansas City, Kansas
*Cystic and Developmental Diseases of the Kidney*

**Steven R. Gullans, Ph.D.**
Associate Professor of Medicine, Harvard Medical
School; Staff, Brigham and Women's Hospital, Boston,
Massachusetts
*Metabolic Basis of Ion Transport*

**Mark E. Gunning, M.D., M.R.C.P.**
Assistant Professor of Medicine, Harvard Medical
School; Staff Physician/Nephrologist, Division of
Nephrology, New England Deaconess Hospital, Joslin
Diabetes Center, Boston, Massachusetts
*Vasoactive Peptides and the Kidney*

**Anne V. Hall, M.D.**
Post-doctoral Fellow of Medicine, Division of
Nephrology, University of Toronto School of Medicine,
Toronto, Ontario, Canada
*Reactive Nitrogen and Oxygen Intermediates and the
Kidney*

**Mitchell L. Halperin, M.D.**
Professor of Medicine, University of Toronto School of
Medicine; Attending Staff, Renal Division, St.
Michael's Hospital, Toronto, Ontario, Canada
*Disorders of Potassium Balance*

**H. William Harris, Jr., M.D., Ph.D.**
Associate Professor of Pediatrics, Harvard Medical
School; Associate in Medicine, Children's Hospital,
Boston, Massachusetts
*Cell Biology of Vasopressin*

**Steven C. Hebert, M.D.**
Professor of Medicine (Physiology), Harvard Medical
School; Physician, Brigham and Women's Hospital,
Boston, Massachusetts
*Metabolic Basis of Ion Transport*

**Charles W. Heilig, M.D.**
Assistant Professor of Medicine, Case Western Reserve University School of Medicine, Cleveland, Ohio; Senior Staff Physician, Henry Ford Hospital, Detroit, Michigan
*Disorders of Potassium Balance*

**William L. Henrich, M.D.**
Professor of Internal Medicine, University of Texas Southwestern Medical Center; ACOS for Research and Development, Veterans Affairs Medical Center, Dallas, Texas
*Toxic Nephropathy*

**Hedvig Hricak, M.D., Ph.D.**
Professor of Radiology, Urology, and Radiation Oncology, University of California, San Francisco, School of Medicine, San Francisco, California
*Radiologic Assessment of the Kidney*

**Willa A. Hsueh, M.D.**
Professor of Medicine and Chief, Division of Endocrinology, Diabetes, and Hypertension, University of Southern California Medical School, Los Angeles, California
*Diabetic Nephropathy*

**Julie R. Ingelfinger, M.D.**
Associate Professor of Pediatrics, Harvard Medical School; Chief, Pediatric Nephrology, Massachusetts General Hospital, Boston, Massachusetts
*Vasoactive Peptides and the Kidney*

**Harlan E. Ives, M.D., Ph.D.**
Professor of Medicine and Pharmacology, Director, Division of Nephrology, and Senior Scientist, Cardiovascular Research Institute, University of California, San Francisco, School of Medicine; Attending Physician, Moffitt Hospital, San Francisco, California
*Renal Transport of Glucose, Amino Acids, Sodium, Chloride, and Water; Inherited Disorders of the Renal Tubule*

**Kamel S. Kamel, M.D.**
Assistant Professor, University of Toronto School of Medicine; Attending Staff, Renal Division, St. Michael's Hospital, Toronto, Ontario, Canada
*Disorders of Potassium Balance*

**Bertram L. Kasiske, M.D.**
Professor of Medicine, University of Minnesota; Staff Physician, Hennepin County Medical Center, Minneapolis, Minnesota
*Laboratory Assessment of Renal Disease: Clearance, Urinalysis, and Renal Biopsy*

**William F. Keane, M.D.**
Professor of Medicine, University of Minnesota; Staff Physician, Hennepin County Medical Center, Minneapolis, Minnesota
*Laboratory Assessment of Renal Disease: Clearance, Urinalysis, and Renal Biopsy*

**Carolyn J. Kelly, M.D.**
Associate Professor of Medicine, University of California, San Diego, School of Medicine, San Diego; Staff Physician, Veterans Affairs Medical Center, La Jolla, California
*Tubulointerstitial Diseases*

**Thomas M. Kennefick, M.D.**
Research Fellow in Nephrology, Oregon Health Sciences University, Portland, Oregon
*Renal and Systemic Manifestations of Glomerular Disease*

**Andrew J. King, M.D.**
Assistant Professor of Medicine, Tufts University Medical School; Assistant Physician, Division of Nephrology, New England Medical Center, Boston, Massachusetts
*Vasoactive Peptides and the Kidney*

**Mark A. Knepper, M.D., Ph.D.**
Chief, Renal Mechanisms Section, Laboratory of Kidney and Electrolyte Metabolism, National Heart, Lung, and Blood Institute, National Institutes of Health, Bethesda, Maryland
*Urine Concentration and Dilution*

**James P. Knochel, M.D., F.A.C.P.**
Clinical Professor, University of Texas Southwestern Medical Center at Dallas; Chairman of Internal Medicine, Presbyterian Hospital of Dallas, Dallas, Texas
*Hypophosphatemia and Hyperphosphatemia*

**Ulla C. Kopp, Ph.D.**
Assistant Professor of Internal Medicine, University of Iowa College of Medicine; Research Health Science Specialist, Department of Veterans Affairs Medical Center, Iowa City, Iowa
*Effects of Renal Nerves and Neurotransmitters on Renal Function*

**Fadi G. Lakkis, M.D.**
Assistant Professor of Medicine, Emory University School of Medicine; Attending Physician, Emory University Hospital and Veterans Affairs Medical Center, Atlanta, Georgia
*Microvascular Diseases of the Kidney*

**John H. Laragh, M.D.**
Master Professor of Medicine, Director, Cardiovascular Center, and Chief, Cardiology Division, The New York Hospital–Cornell Medical Center, New York, New York
*Essential Hypertension; Renovascular Hypertension and Ischemic Nephropathy*

**J. Michael Lazarus, M.D.**
Associate Professor of Medicine, Harvard Medical School; Director of Clinical Services, Division of

Nephrology, Brigham and Women's Hospital, Boston, Massachusetts
*Hemodialysis*

**Moshe Levi, M.D.**
Associate Professor of Internal Medicine, University of Texas Southwestern Medical Center; Chief, Nephrology Section, Department of Veterans Affairs Medical Center, Dallas, Texas
*Effect of Aging on Renal Function and Disease*

**Wilfred Lieberthal, M.D.**
Associate Professor of Medicine, Boston University Medical Center, Boston, Massachusetts
*Acute Renal Failure*

**Francisco Llach, M.D.**
Professor of Medicine, University of New Jersey Medical School; Director of Nephrology, Newark Beth Israel Medical Center, Newark, New Jersey
*Renal Osteodystrophy*

**Robert G. Luke, M.D.**
Taylor Professor of Medicine and Director, Department of Internal Medicine, University of Cincinnati Medical School; Director, Department of Internal Medicine, University of Cincinnati Medical Center, Cincinnati, Ohio
*Hypertension in Renal Parenchymal Disease*

**David A. Maddox, Ph.D.**
Research Associate Professor, College of Medicine, University of Vermont, Burlington, Vermont
*Glomerular Ultrafiltration*

**Kirsten M. Madsen, M.D., Ph.D.**
Associate Professor of Medicine, University of Florida College of Medicine, Gainesville, Florida
*Anatomy of the Kidney*

**Gerhard Malnic, M.D.**
Professor, Departmento de Fisiologia, Universidade de Sao Paulo Instituto de Ciencias Biomedicas, Sao Paulo, Brazil
*Control of Renal Potassium Excretion*

**Philip A. Marsden, M.D.**
Assistant Professor of Medicine, University of Toronto School of Medicine; Physician, Division of Nephrology, St. Michael's Hospital, Toronto, Ontario, Canada
*Reactive Nitrogen and Oxygen Intermediates and the Kidney*

**Robert C. May, M.D.**
Attending Physician, St. Joseph Mercy Hospital, Ann Arbor, Michigan
*Pathophysiology of Uremia*

**Dianne B. McKay, M.D.**
Assistant Professor of Medicine, Harvard Medical School; Associate Director, Renal Transplantation, Brigham and Women's Hospital, Boston, Massachusetts
*Clinical Aspects of Renal Transplantation*

**Timothy W. Meyer, M.D.**
Associate Professor of Medicine, Stanford University School of Medicine, Palo Alto, California
*Nephron Adaptation to Renal Injury*

**Edgar L. Milford, M.D.**
Associate Professor of Medicine, Harvard Medical School; Director, Renal Transplantation, Brigham and Women's Hospital, Boston, Massachusetts
*Clinical Aspects of Renal Transplantation*

**Judith A. Miller, M.Sc., M.D., F.R.C.P.(C.)**
Assistant Professor of Medicine, University of Toronto School of Medicine; Staff Nephrologist, Women's College Hospital and Toronto Hospital, Toronto, Ontario, Canada
*Control of Extracellular Fluid Volume and the Pathophysiology of Edema Formation*

**William E. Mitch, M.D.**
Garland Herndon Professor of Medicine and Director of Nephrology, Emory University School of Medicine, Atlanta, Georgia
*Pathophysiology of Uremia; Nutritional Therapy for the Uremic Patient*

**R. Curtis Morris, Jr., M.D.**
Professor of Medicine, Pediatrics, and Radiology and Director, General Clinical Research Center, University of California, San Francisco, School of Medicine, San Francisco, California
*Inherited Disorders of the Renal Tubule*

**Robert G. Narins, M.D.**
Professor of Medicine, Case Western Reserve University, Cleveland, Ohio; Head, Division of Nephrology and Hypertension, Henry Ford Hospital, Detroit, Michigan
*Disorders of Potassium Balance*

**Eric G. Neilson, M.D.**
C. Mahlon Kline Professor of Medicine and Pediatrics, University of Pennsylvania School of Medicine; Chief, Renal-Electrolyte and Hypertension Division, Hospital of the University of Pennsylvania, Philadelphia, Pennsylvania
*Tubulointerstitial Diseases*

**Sanjay K. Nigam, M.D.**
Associate Professor of Medicine, Harvard Medical School; Physician, Brigham and Women's Hospital, Boston, Massachusetts
*Development and Maturation of the Kidney*

**Karl D. Nolph, M.D.**
Professor of Internal Medicine, University of Missouri;
Director of Nephrology, University of Missouri Health
Sciences Center, Columbia, Missouri
*Peritoneal Dialysis*

**Ruth Østerby, M.D.**
Associate Professor, Aarhus University School of
Medicine and University Institute of Pathology,
Research Laboratory for Electron Microscopy, Aarhus
Kommunehospital, Aarhus, Denmark
*Diabetic Nephropathy*

**William F. Owen, Jr., M.D.**
Assistant Professor of Medicine, Harvard Medical
School; Associate Director of Dialysis Services,
Brigham and Women's Hospital, Boston, Massachusetts
*Hemodialysis*

**Mark S. Paller, M.D.**
Associate Professor of Medicine, University of
Minnesota, Minneapolis, Minnesota
*The Kidney and Hypertension in Pregnancy*

**Biff F. Palmer, M.D.**
Associate Professor of Internal Medicine, Division of
Nephrology, University of Texas Southwestern Medical
Center; Director of Outpatient Hemodialysis and
Peritoneal Dialysis Programs, Parkland Memorial
Hospital, Dallas, Texas
*Effect of Aging on Renal Function and Disease*

**Hans-Henrik Parving, M.D., D.M.Sc.**
Chief Physician, Steno Diabetes Center, Gentofte,
Denmark
*Diabetic Nephropathy*

**David L. Perkins, M.D., Ph.D.**
Assistant Professor of Medicine, Harvard Medical
School; Associate Physician, Brigham and Women's
Hospital, Boston, Massachusetts
*Immunobiology of Transplantation*

**Thomas G. Pickering, M.D., D.Phil.**
Professor of Medicine, Cornell University Medical
College; Attending Physician, The New York Hospital
New York, New York
*Renovascular Hypertension and Ischemic Nephropathy*

**Garry P. Reams, M.D.**
Associate Professor of Internal Medicine, University of
Missouri; Chief, Renal Section, Harry S. Truman
Memorial Veterans Hospital, Columbia, Missouri
*Antihypertensive Drugs*

**Floyd C. Rector, Jr., M.D.**
Professor and Chair of Medicine, University of
California, San Francisco, School of Medicine; Senior
Scientist, Cardiovascular Research Institute, University
of California, San Francisco, California

*Renal Transport of Glucose, Amino Acids, Sodium,
Chloride, and Water; Renal Acidification Mechanisms;
Urine Concentration and Dilution; Acid-Base Disorders*

**Giuseppe Remuzzi, M.D.**
Director, Negri Bergamo Laboratories, and Associate
Professor, Ospedale Riuniti di Bergamo, Bergamo, Italy
*Hematologic Consequences of Renal Failure*

**Jerome P. Richie, M.D.**
Elliott Carr Cutler Professor of Urological Surgery,
Harvard Medical School; Chief of Urology, Brigham
and Women's Hospital, Boston, Massachusetts
*Renal Neoplasia*

**Gary L. Robertson, M.D.**
Professor of Medicine and Neurology, Northwestern
University Medical School; Program Director, Clinical
Research Center, Northwestern Memorial Hospital,
Chicago, Illinois
*Pathophysiology of Water Metabolism*

**Pierre Ronco, M.D.**
Professor of Nephrology, Pierre et Marie Curie
University; Department of Nephrology, Hôpital Tenon,
Paris, France
*Biology of Renal Cells in Culture*

**Eric Rondeau, M.D.**
Professor of Nephrology, Faculty of Medicine, Saint-
Antoine; Department of Nephrology, Hôpital Tenon,
Paris, France
*Biology of Renal Cells in Culture*

**Ennio C. Rossi, M.D.**
Professor of Medicine, Northwestern University
Medical School; Medical Director, Apheresis Center,
Northwestern Memorial Hospital, Chicago, Illinois
*Hematologic Consequences of Renal Failure*

**Diane Rouse, Ph.D.**
Assistant Professor of Medicine and of Physiology and
Molecular Biophysics, Baylor College of Medicine,
Houston, Texas
*Renal Transport of Calcium, Magnesium, and
Phosphate*

**Robert H. Rubin, M.D.**
Director, Center for Experimental Pharmacology and
Therapeutics, Harvard–M.I.T. Division of Health
Sciences and Technology; Associate Professor of
Medicine, Harvard Medical School; Chief of
Transplantation Infectious Disease, Massachusetts
General Hospital, Boston, Massachusetts
*Urinary Tract Infection, Pyelonephritis, and Reflux
Nephropathy*

**Mohamed H. Sayegh, M.D.**
Assistant Professor of Medicine, Harvard Medical
School; Associate Physician, Brigham and Women's
Hospital, Boston, Massachusetts
*Clinical Aspects of Renal Transplantation*

*Anton C. Schoolwerth, M.D.*
Professor of Medicine and Physiology, Medical College of Virginia, Virginia Commonwealth University, Richmond, Virginia
*Renal Handling of Organic Anions and Cations and Renal Excretion of Uric Acid*

*Cathryn Shuler, M.D.*
Assistant Professor of Medicine, Oregon Health Sciences University, Portland, Oregon
*Prescribing Drugs in Renal Disease*

*Domenic A. Sica, M.D.*
Professor of Medicine and Chairman, Clinical Pharmacology and Hypertension, Medical College of Virginia, Virginia Commonwealth University, Richmond, Virginia
*Renal Handling of Organic Anions and Cations and Renal Excretion of Uric Acid*

*Karl L. Skorecki, M.D., F.R.C.P.(C.)*
Professor of Medicine, Pediatrics, and Clinical Biochemistry, University of Toronto School of Medicine; Chief, Division of Nephrology, Hospital for Sick Children, and Staff Nephrologist, Toronto Hospital, Toronto, Ontario, Canada
*Control of Extracellular Fluid Volume and the Pathophysiology of Edema Formation*

*Susan P. Steigerwalt, M.D.*
Clinical Instructor, University of Michigan; Acting Section Chief, Hypertension Section, Division of Nephrology and Hypertension, Henry Ford Hospital, Detroit, Michigan
*Disorders of Potassium Balance*

*Wadi N. Suki, M.D.*
Professor of Medicine and of Physiology and Molecular Biophysics, Baylor College of Medicine; Senior Attending Physician and Chief, Renal Service, The Methodist Hospital, Houston, Texas
*Renal Transport of Calcium, Magnesium, and Phosphate*

*Roger A. L. Sutton, D.M., F.R.C.P., F.R.C.P.(C.)*
Professor and Chairman of Medicine, Aga Khan University, Karachi, Pakistan
*Disturbances of Calcium and Magnesium Metabolism*

*C. Craig Tisher, M.D.*
Professor of Medicine and Pathology and Chief, Division of Nephrology, Hypertension, and

Transplantation, University of Florida College of Medicine; Staff, Shands Hospital, Gainesville, Florida
*Anatomy of the Kidney*

*Sheldon W. Tobe, B.Sc., M.D., F.R.C.P.(C.)*
Assistant Professor of Medicine, University of Toronto School of Medicine; Staff Nephrologist, Sunnybrook Health Sciences Centre, Toronto, Ontario, Canada
*Control of Extracellular Fluid Volume and the Pathophysiology of Edema Formation*

*Nina E. Tolkoff-Rubin, M.D.*
Associate Professor of Medicine, Harvard Medical School; Director of Hemodialysis and CAPD Units, Massachusetts General Hospital, Boston, Massachusetts
*Urinary Tract Infection, Pyelonephritis, and Reflux Nephropathy*

*Mackenzie Walser, M.D.*
Professor of Pharmacology and Molecular Sciences and of Medicine, Johns Hopkins University School of Medicine, Baltimore, Maryland
*Nutritional Therapy for the Uremic Patient*

*Larry W. Welling, M.D., Ph.D.*
Professor of Pathology, University of Kansas Medical Center; Staff Pathologist, Department of Veterans Affairs Medical Center, Kansas City, Missouri
*Cystic and Developmental Diseases of the Kidney*

*Scott S. White, M.D.*
Director of Body MRI, St. Anthony's Hospital, Rockford, Illinois
*Radiologic Assessment of the Kidney*

*Christopher S. Wilcox, M.D., Ph.D.*
George E. Schreiner Professor of Medicine and Chief, Division of Nephrology and Hypertension, Georgetown University Medical Center, Washington, DC
*Diuretics*

*Curtis B. Wilson, M.D.*
Member, Department of Immunology, The Scripps Research Institute, La Jolla, California
*Renal Response to Immunologic Glomerular Injury*

*Mark L. Zeidel, M.D.*
Associate Professor of Medicine and Director, Renal-Electrolyte Division, University of Pittsburgh School of Medicine, Pittsburgh, Pennsylvania
*Cell Biology of Vasopressin; Urinary Tract Obstruction*

# Preface

When the first edition of this book appeared in 1976, Floyd Rector and I came away from the 3-year task of formulating and implementing an ambitious first-stage synthesis of knowledge in nephrology with a sense that a major change in the renal sciences would soon be upon us. In particular, we came to view the traditional separation of physiologists, biochemists, pharmacologists, geneticists, and cell biologists as arbitrary and inefficient, especially because each group was beginning to characterize proteins in terms of commonly studied functions—ion transport across membranes, metabolic transformation of substrates to free energy, and intracellular signaling, to name a few. Now, two decades later, we marvel not that the reductionist approach based on the tools of modern molecular biology and genetics has become so entrenched but rather at the pervasiveness of the transformation from descriptive renal science and medicine to the current high level of comprehension of molecular process and pathology. Furthermore, the rate of acquisition of new knowledge—whether derived from cloning and sequencing complementary DNA constructs encoding various transporters; from defining the complex interplay of second messengers, G proteins, and intracellular calcium transients; or from linking genomic abnormalities with phenotype as in Alport syndrome, autosomal dominant polycystic kidney disease, or the various oncogene-associated renal neoplasms—continues to accelerate as more and more scientists and clinicians adopt the new biology and expand the effort to define the molecular basis of kidney function and dysfunction.

The resulting progress again compels a major revision of this work even though it was extensively updated in 1991. In fact, assembly of this fifth edition was initiated in 1993, with liberal additions and revisions to text and references made not only in manuscript but also continued in galley and page proof stages, even to the inclusion of numerous references to literature published in 1995. As our readers have come to expect, an extremely current and complete list of references for each chapter continues to be a major distinguishing feature of *The Kidney,* which has been enlarged to include nearly 35,000 references and more than 1200 illustrations and tables, many of them likewise new to this edition.

In this edition we continue our commitment to keep serious students of nephrology apace of the explosion in new knowledge via the basic five-part organizational format employed successfully in previous editions. Of necessity, the fifth edition has been enlarged by the addition of seven new chapters in areas deserving of particular emphasis, namely, renal development and maturation, cell-cell and cell-matrix interactions, the increasingly important role of urea in kidney function, neural influences on renal function, biochemistry and actions of reactive oxygen and nitrogen intermediates (e.g., nitric oxide), cellular biology of the blood vessel wall, and gerontologic aspects of renal function in health and disease. Furthermore, 12 major chapters have been written entirely anew by leading authorities to bring a fresh perspective to areas of rapid progress and expansion. The remaining 41 chapters have once again undergone extensive revision and updating, often with complete rewriting of the text and accompanying reference lists.

Credit for past and any current success this work might enjoy rightfully belongs to the many dedicated scholars who have enriched this endeavor by their commitments to excellence in research, teaching, and writing. To all I express my deepest gratitude and respect. To colleagues and close associates too numerous to acknowledge individually, I extend warm appreciation for their invaluable criticisms and suggestions. I also offer special thanks to Mss. Michelle Deraney, Lee Riley, and Julia Troy for their day-to-day assistance and support. Likewise, to the many professionals at W.B. Saunders Company who labored to ensure the best book possible, I extend heartfelt gratitude. I especially thank Mss. Kathleen Fisher, Judith Gandy, Linda R. Garber, Hazel Hacker, and Karen O'Keefe for their unfailing expertise and good-humored efficiency throughout the design and production process and to Mr. Richard Zorab, Senior Medical Editor, and Mr. Lewis Reines, President, W.B. Saunders Company, for their sound guidance and advice.

Editorial undertakings of this scale and duration, when combined with already demanding research, clinical, teaching, and administrative responsibilities, inevitably detract from other vital sectors of a busy life. Fearing that the sacrifice is forced on those who deserve it least, namely my devoted wife Jane and dearest children Rob, Jen, and Ron, I can only beg forgiveness and express loving thanks for their patience, forbearance, and unwavering support.

BARRY M. BRENNER, M.D.

# Contents

## *IV* PATHOPHYSIOLOGY OF RENAL DISEASE, 1979

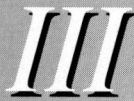

# III

# PATHOGENESIS OF RENAL DISEASE

# 26

# Laboratory Assessment of Renal Disease: Clearance, Urinalysis, and Renal Biopsy

*Bertram L. Kasiske*
*William F. Keane*

## DETECTION AND DIAGNOSIS OF RENAL DISEASE

Because patients destined to develop end-stage renal failure often exhibit few signs and symptoms early in their course of disease, tests for screening and diagnosis are of critical importance in nephrology. Directly, or indirectly, these tests measure renal structure and function. Ideally, they should detect abnormalities early enough to alert patients and physicians to the potential need for therapy that may prevent morbidity and mortality associated with renal disease. In addition, tests can help establish a specific diagnosis that will suggest the correct therapy and the likelihood of response to treatment. Even in the absence of effective therapy, accurate diagnosis of renal disease helps determine prognosis, which often serves a useful purpose in its own right. Tests to determine renal structure and function can also be important for measuring disease progression. Once disease has been detected and therapy begun, it is desirable to determine whether the therapy has been effective so that ineffective therapy can be discontinued or altered. Even in the absence of effective therapy, it is important to predict the clinical course of disease to better inform patients and to help determine when renal replacement therapy may be appropriate.

Tests that best detect abnormalities in renal function are those that measure glomerular filtration rate. However, measurements of glomerular filtration rate may not be useful for screening purposes in many clinical settings. Patients with early renal disease may have a normal or even increased glomerular filtration rate. Because there is a large amount of physiologic variability among normal individuals, it is virtually impossible to define limits for a normal glomerular filtration rate. Indeed, patients who have identical glomerular filtration rates can have substantial differences in the amount of structural renal damage. Furthermore, measuring glomerular filtration rate is of little value in establishing a diagnosis once renal abnormalities have been detected. On the other hand, an accurate determination of glomerular filtration rate may provide useful prognostic information and may be particularly helpful in following the clinical course.

Examining the microscopic structure of renal tissue is invaluable in detecting and diagnosing renal disease. However, major limitations of renal biopsy include the risk and inconvenience of the procedure as well as the potential for sampling errors. The careful selection of patients who undergo biopsy can be aided by measurements in urine samples that help screen for renal injury. Indeed, urinalysis is often the most useful test available for detecting early renal abnormalities. Measuring urinary protein level or examining the urinary sediment can also help in establishing a diagnosis or in deciding which patients should be subjected to biopsy.

Glomerular filtration rate measurement, renal biopsy, and urinalysis serve complementary roles in the detection and diagnosis of renal disease. However, the relative usefulness of these tests is, in large part, determined by their sensitivity and specificity. Sensitivity and specificity are, in turn, dependent on accuracy and precision. Moreover, the prevalence of abnormalities in the population of individuals being tested will also affect the clinical utility of each of these tests. To judge their utility, it is helpful to understand a few basic principles concerning the diagnostic discrimination of tests in general.

The sensitivity, or true-positive rate, for a test is the proportion of test results that are positive in patients known to have disease (Table 26–1). The specificity is the proportion of test results that are negative in disease-free individuals. The false-positive rate is the proportion of positive test results in individuals without disease, and the false-negative rate is the proportion of negative test results in individuals with disease. The positive predictive value of a test is the proportion of individuals with a positive test result who have disease, or the likelihood of disease if the test result is positive. The negative predictive value is the proportion of individuals with a negative test result who are disease free.

The sensitivity and specificity of any test are ultimately dictated by its accuracy (determined by comparison with a "gold standard") and precision (determined by comparing repeated measurements with the same test). The accuracy and precision of a test that yields values on a continuum are also dependent on the cutoff values used to define what is abnormal. Often the utility of a test can be determined by examining receiver-operating characteristic (ROC) curves generated for each test. ROC curves are plots of the true-positive rate (sensitivity) on the y axis with the false-positive rate (1 − specificity) on the x axis.[1, 2] A perfect test is one in which the ROC is described by a line on which all values for y are between 0 and 100 when x is 0, and y is 100 when x is greater than 0. A worthless test is one in which the ROC is described by a line on which y is equal to x for all values of x and y. The extent to which a ROC resembles that of a perfect or a worthless test is indicative of its utility.

Finally, the number of true- and false-positive results as well as the number of true- and false-negative results ultimately depends on the prevalence of dysfunction in the population being screened. Some simple algebraic calculations can easily demonstrate how the prevalence of a disease will influence the diagnostic discrimination of a test (Table 26–2). Take the case of a hypothetic test evaluated in 100 individuals known to have a high prevalence (30%) of disease. The test would appear to be reasonable with a sensitivity of 0.90 and specificity of 0.90. Among the 100

patients tested, a positive test result would indicate a 79% likelihood that disease was present, whereas a negative test result would indicate a 95% likelihood that disease was absent. If the same test were then applied to a general population of 10,000 individuals where the prevalence of disease was 0.3%, the sensitivity and specificity of the test would be unchanged. However, in this population, a positive test result would indicate only a 2.6% likelihood of disease, and the number of false-positive results would greatly exceed the number of true-positive results (see Table 26–2).

In this chapter, we review the usefulness and limitations of currently available techniques for measuring glomerular filtration rate, examining urine constituents, and assessing renal structure. In reality, precise data on the sensitivity and specificity of tests of renal structure and function are often not available. Even when these data are available, the prevalence (prior probability) of the outcome being measured can be only crudely estimated. Nevertheless, data on sensitivity and specificity are discussed when these data are available. An empirical estimation of the effect of differences in the underlying prevalence of abnormalities on the diagnostic discrimination of the test is made where possible.

# CLEARANCE

## Historical Perspective

The modern era for measuring renal function began with the measurement of urea. Urea was first isolated from human urine by Rouelle in 1773.[3] In the early 1800s, Fourcroy coined the term "urée," carefully choosing a name that would avoid confusion with "urique," or uric acid. In 1827, Richard Bright observed that urea accumulated in the blood of patients with dropsy, and he linked this phenomenon to decreased urinary urea concentration, proteinuria, and diseased kidneys. One year later, Wöhler synthesized urea from ammonium cyanate, and in so doing helped discredit the doctrines of vitalism that were then prevalent. In 1842, Dumas and Cahours demonstrated that urea was a product of dietary protein catabolism. In 1903, Strauss introduced blood urea as a diagnostic test for renal disease.

Homer Smith[3] credited Ambard and Weill with one of the first attempts to measure renal function with a "dynamic" test in 1912. They characterized renal function (K) as blood urea concentration (B) divided by the product of the square root of the rate of urea excretion (D) times the square root of urinary urea concentration (U):

$$K = B/(\sqrt{D} \cdot \sqrt{U})$$

In 1928, Addis described renal function as a urea excretion ratio, or the quantity of urea excreted divided by the concentration in blood.[3] One year later, the concept of clearance as a measure of renal function was described in detail by Möller, McIntosh, and Van Slyke for urea.[4] In 1931, Jolliffe and Smith extended the concept of clearance to creatinine.[3]

**TABLE 26–1. Definitions of Parameters Commonly Used to Assess the Diagnostic Discrimination of a Clinical Test**

| | Disease (Total = a + c) | No Disease (Total = b + d) |
|---|---|---|
| Test result positive (Total = a + b) | a | b |
| Test result negative (Total = c + d) | c | d |

Sensitivity = a/(a + c)
Specificity = d/(b + d)
False-positive rate = 1 − specificity = b/(b + d)
False-negative rate = 1 − sensitivity = c/(a + c)
Positive predictive value = a/(a + b)
Negative predictive value = d/(c + d)

**TABLE 26–2. Influence of Disease Prevalence on the Diagnostic Discrimination of a Hypothetic Clinical Test**

| Population | 100 Test Patients with 30% Disease Prevalence | | 10,000 Screened Patients with 0.3% Disease Prevalence | |
|---|---|---|---|---|
| | *Disease* | *No Disease* | *Disease* | *No Disease* |
| Number with positive test result | 27 | 7 | 27 | 997 |
| Number with negative test result | 3 | 63 | 3 | 8973 |
| | Sensitivity = 0.90 | | Sensitivity = 0.90 | |
| | Specificity = 0.90 | | Specificity = 0.90 | |
| | Disease likelihood if result is positive = 0.79 | | Disease likelihood if result is positive = 0.0264 | |
| | Disease likelihood if result is negative = 0.05 | | Disease likelihood if result is negative = 0.0003 | |

## Overview

Glomerular filtration rate is traditionally measured as the renal clearance of a particular substance or marker from plasma. The clearance of an indicator substance is the amount removed from plasma divided by the average plasma concentration over the time of measurement. Clearance is expressed in moles or weight of the indicator per volume per time. It can be thought of as the volume of plasma that can be completely cleared of the indicator in a unit of time.

Under the right conditions, measuring the amount of an indicator in both plasma and urine can allow the accurate calculation of glomerular filtration rate (Fig. 26–1). Indeed, if we assume that there is no extrarenal elimination, tubule reabsorption, or tubule secretion of the marker, then

Glomerular filtration rate = UV/PT

where U is the urinary marker concentration, V is the urine volume, and P is the average plasma concentration of the marker over the time (T) of the urine collection. Unfortunately, tubule secretion or tubule reabsorption of the indicator can cause renal clearance measurements to give, respectively, falsely high or falsely low estimates of the glomerular filtration rate.

Under the right conditions, plasma concentrations of an indicator substance can be completely dependent on renal clearance and can accurately reflect glomerular filtration rate. When the amount of an indicator added to the plasma from an exogenous or endogenous source is constant, and when there is no extrarenal elimination, tubule secretion, or tubule reabsorption, then the glomerular filtration rate is equal to the inverse plasma concentration of the indicator multiplied by a constant. That constant is the amount excreted by glomerular filtration, which, under steady-state conditions, must equal the amount added to the plasma (see Fig. 26–1). In other words, under these conditions, UV/T is equal to a constant (C) so that glomerular filtration rate equals C/P, and changes in glomerular filtration rate must be inversely proportional to changes in P.

We can use this information to define the characteristics of an ideal indicator for measuring glomerular filtration rate (Table 26–3). Although such an indicator does not exist, its definition can serve as a useful benchmark for comparing

the advantages and disadvantages of tests designed to measure glomerular filtration rate. The ideal endogenous indicator should be produced at the same constant rate under all conditions so that changes in the plasma levels would be inversely proportional to changes in glomerular filtration rate multiplied by a constant. This constant would be uniquely determined for an individual patient by measuring the urinary excretion rate of the marker (glomerular filtration rate equals the urinary excretion rate divided by the plasma concentration). Thereafter, only a single plasma determination would be needed to accurately assess glomerular filtration rate in that patient, unless the renal function is

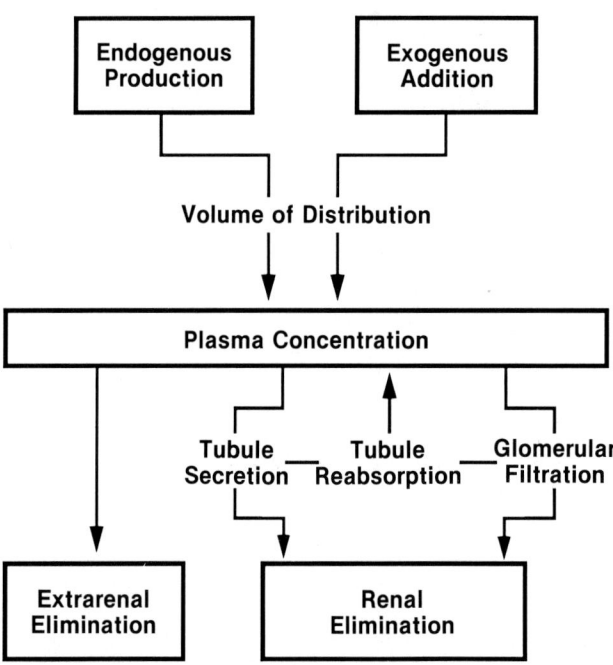

**Figure 26–1.** Factors influencing the relationship between an indicator used to measure renal function and true glomerular filtration rate. When tubule secretion and reabsorption of the indicator are nil and plasma concentration is constant, then glomerular filtration rate is equal to renal elimination divided by plasma concentration. If, in addition, the sum of endogenous production and exogenous addition minus extrarenal elimination is constant, then renal elimination is constant and the glomerular filtration rate is inversely proportional to plasma concentration.

**TABLE 26–3. Characteristics of an Ideal Endogenous or Exogenous Marker for Measuring Glomerular Filtration Rate**

Constant production
Safe
Convenient
Readily diffusible in extracellular space
No protein binding and freely filterable
No tubule reabsorption
No tubule secretion
No extrarenal elimination or degradation
Accurate and reproducible assay
No compounds interfere
Inexpensive

changing so rapidly that a steady state cannot be achieved. An ideal exogenous indicator should have all of these same characteristics but should also be safe, easy to administer, and inexpensive.

Whether endogenous or exogenous, an ideal indicator should distribute freely and instantaneously throughout the extracellular space. It should not bind to plasma proteins and should be freely filtered at the glomerulus. It should be subject to neither secretion nor reabsorption in the tubules or urinary collecting system. It should be completely resistant to degradation, and its elimination should be entirely dependent on glomerular filtration. It should be easy to measure in plasma and in urine, and nothing should interfere with the assay. Ideally, the interpatient and intrapatient coefficient of variation should be low.

Obviously, the ideal marker for measuring glomerular filtration rate has yet to be discovered. Nevertheless, a mythic gold standard obeys principles that should be considered in any discussion of methods used to measure glomerular filtration rate. Actual methods violate these principles in different ways and with different tradeoffs of accuracy and practicality. In the end, these tradeoffs can be tailored to the clinical situation, taking into account estimated prior probabilities, to achieve a maximal amount of information for a minimal cost. The question is not which test is best, but which test is best suited for the clinical situation at hand.

## Plasma Urea

Urea was one of the first indicators used to measure glomerular filtration rate.[4] Unfortunately, it shares few of the attributes of an ideal marker, and plasma urea has been shown to be a poor measure of glomerular filtration rate.[5] Urea production is variable and is largely dependent on protein intake. Although one quarter of the urea produced is metabolized in the intestine, the ammonia produced is reconverted to urea. Thus, most of the urea is ultimately excreted by the kidneys. Urea (molecular mass 60 daltons) is freely filtered at the glomerulus. However, it can be readily reabsorbed, and the amount of tubule reabsorption is variable.[6, 7] Indeed, medullary collecting duct urea reabsorption is functionally linked to water reabsorption. In

states of diuresis and low levels of antidiuretic hormone, the medullary collecting duct is relatively impermeable to urea. However, in states of decreased effective intravascular volume, low tubule fluid flow, and increased antidiuretic hormone, urea reabsorption can be substantial.[6, 7]

Plasma urea, or blood urea nitrogen, is affected by a number of factors other than alterations in glomerular filtration rate. As indicated before, increased plasma urea levels accompany decreased urine flow in patients with intravascular volume depletion, for example, after the administration of diuretics.[8] Congestive heart failure also raises the plasma urea level, probably by similar mechanisms.[9] Increased plasma urea levels that are probably caused by increased production are seen with elevated dietary protein intake,[10–12] gastrointestinal bleeding,[10] and tetracycline.[13] On the other hand, reduced levels of plasma urea can be seen in patients with alcohol abuse and chronic liver disease.[14]

Some substances may interfere with the laboratory determination of urea. Substances that may give falsely high urea levels include acetohexamide, allantoin, aminosalicylic acid, bilirubin (very high levels), chloral hydrate, dextran, free hemoglobin, hydantoin derivatives, lipids (lipemia), sulfonamides, tetracycline, thiourea, and uric acid.[15] Substances that may give falsely low analytic values of urea include ascorbic acid, levodopa, lipids (lipemia), and streptomycin.[16]

## Urea Clearance

Because of tubule urea reabsorption, renal urea clearance usually underestimates glomerular filtration rate. Urea clearance may be as little as one half or less of the glomerular filtration rate measured by other techniques.[6, 7] As with plasma urea, the state of hydration can markedly influence urea clearance. However, the degree of underestimation of glomerular filtration and the tendency for urea clearance to vary with the state of hydration are both less in patients with markedly reduced renal function.[6] Moreover, because creatinine clearance overestimates glomerular filtration rate, some investigators have suggested that the mean of creatinine and urea clearance would be a reasonable estimate of glomerular filtration rate, at least in patients with low levels of renal function.[17, 18] In a large enough sample of patients, errors from tubule reabsorption of urea may negate errors from tubule secretion of creatinine, so that mean urea and creatinine clearances may better approximate the true glomerular filtration rate. However, the factors that affect tubule creatinine secretion and urea reabsorption are different, and any tendency for "two wrongs to make a right" would probably be coincidental and infrequent in an individual patient.

Urea clearance determinations are made by measuring renal urea excretion. The accuracy of any clearance technique that relies on urinary excretion measurements is compromised by problems associated with obtaining accurate urine collections. The 24-hour collection is inconvenient and difficult for most patients to complete accurately. Patients should be instructed to empty the bladder, note the time, and save all subsequent urine, including urine voided at exactly the same time 24 hours from the time of initiation. They should be warned to empty the bladder before defecation to avoid inadvertent loss of urine. The completeness of 24-hour urine collections can be examined by measuring creatinine excretion (see following). Shorter collection times enhance compliance of patients but sample only a portion of the day during which glomerular filtration rate varies in a diurnal pattern. Incomplete bladder emptying may also reduce the accuracy of timed urine collections. The shorter the collection interval and smaller the volume, the greater the potential for a significant portion of the collection to be left behind in the bladder. Incomplete bladder emptying can be obviated by catheterization, but the discomfort, risk, and inconvenience of this procedure often make it unacceptable.

## Serum Creatinine

Creatinine is a metabolic product of creatine and phosphocreatine, which are both found almost exclusively in muscle. Thus, creatinine production is proportional to muscle mass and varies little from day to day.[19] However, production may change over longer periods if there are changes in muscle mass.[20–23] Age- and sex-associated differences in creatinine production among individuals are also largely attributable to differences in muscle mass.[24, 25] Although diet is ordinarily the source of a relatively small proportion of overall creatinine excretion, it is another source of variability in serum creatinine levels. Creatine from ingested meat is converted to creatinine and can be the source for up to 30% of total creatinine excretion.[26–30] Thus, variability in meat intake can also contribute to variability in serum creatinine levels. The conversion of creatine to creatinine can occur with cooking. Because creatinine is readily absorbed from the gastrointestinal tract, ingesting cooked meat can lead to a rapid increase in serum creatinine levels.[31, 32]

Creatinine is small (molecular mass 113 daltons), does not bind to plasma proteins, and is freely filtered by the renal glomerulus. However, it has long been appreciated that creatinine is also secreted by the renal tubule.[33] Secretion is a saturable process that probably occurs through the organic cation pathway and is blocked by some commonly used medications, including cimetidine, trimethoprim, pyrimethamine, and dapsone.[34–39] If tubule secretion of creatinine were constant, differences in serum creatinine and renal clearance should still reflect differences in glomerular filtration rate. However, evidence suggests that the secretion of creatinine varies substantially both in the same individuals over time and between different individuals.[7, 40, 41] Particularly troublesome is that the proportion of total renal creatinine excretion due to tubule secretion increases with decreasing renal function.[41, 42] This could have a dampening effect on serial measurements in individuals, in whom glomerular filtration rate could fall more rapidly than indicated by either serum creatinine or creatinine clearance.

Whereas proportional tubule secretion of creatinine increases with decreasing glomerular filtration rate, total urinary creatinine excretion actually declines.[41] This is because extrarenal creatinine degradation increases with declining renal function.[43–46] Indeed, it has been shown that increased

extrarenal creatinine degradation may be sufficient to entirely account for the decrease in urinary creatinine excretion associated with declining glomerular filtration rate.[43] The extrarenal degradation of creatinine has been attributed to its conversion to carbon dioxide and methylamine by bacteria in the intestine. The increase in extrarenal creatinine degradation with declining renal function can be expected to cause plasma creatinine to underestimate declines in glomerular filtration rate.

A number of methods are used to measure creatinine.[47–51] The original Folin-Wu method used the Jaffé reaction,[52, 53] and the Jaffé reaction has been used with various modifications since. The method of Hare[47] involved the isolation of creatinine by absorption on Lloyd reagent. More recently, the direct alkaline picrate method of Bonsnes and Taussky[48] has been used. This method involves the complexing of creatinine with alkaline picrate and measurement by a colorimetric technique. The Jaffé reaction has also been adapted for use on autoanalyzers. Other methods currently in use employ *o*-nitrobenzaldehyde (Sakaguchi reaction) and imidohydrolase.[51]

There is probably more variation in what laboratories report as the upper limit of normal for serum creatinine than for any other standard chemistry value.[54] In the absence of procedures to remove noncreatinine chromogens, the upper limit of the normal measured by the Jaffé reaction may be as high as 1.6 to 1.9 mg/dL for adults (to convert milligrams per deciliter to millimoles per liter, multiply by 88). The upper limit of normal for serum creatinine measured by autoanalyzer or the imidohydrolase methods is usually 1.2 to 1.4 mg/dL. Some laboratories report separate normal ranges for men and women and for adults and children.

A number of normal plasma constituents may interfere with some laboratory methods used to measure creatinine. Glucose, fructose, pyruvate, acetoacetate, uric acid, ascorbic acid, and plasma proteins may all cause the Jaffé colorimetric assay to yield falsely high creatinine values.[55–58] The low levels of these substances generally do not interfere with the Jaffé assay of creatinine in urine. Normally, interfering chromogens increase the creatinine result by about 20%, but in some disease states, the interference can be much greater. In diabetic ketoacidosis, for example, spurious elevations in serum creatinine can be significant. Cephalosprin antibiotics can also interfere with the Jaffé reaction.[58–62] In marked renal insufficiency, serum creatinine increases and noncreatinine chromogens contribute proportionally less to the total reaction.[63] In individuals with normal renal function, it was found that noncreatinine chromogens made up 14% (range, 4.5% to 22.3%) of the total; in individuals with serum creatinine levels of 5.6 to 29.4 mg/dL, noncreatinine chromogens contributed only 5% (range, 0% to 14.6%) to the total measured level.[63] This same study found no effect of the noncreatinine chromogens on the variability of plasma values.

Several modifications in the classic Jaffé assay have been designed to remove interfering chromogens before analysis.[50] These have included deproteinization with specific adsorption of creatinine by use of Fuller earth and ion exchange resins, the measurement of Jaffé-positive chromogens before and after the destruction of creatinine with bacteria, and dialysis separation. These methods have largely been replaced by less costly and more convenient autoanalyzer techniques. Autoanalyzer methods use the Jaffé reaction but separate creatinine from noncreatinine chromogens by the rate of color development.[50] This avoids most of the interference seen with the standard Jaffé method.[55] However, high serum bilirubin levels can cause falsely low creatinine levels.[64] Newer techniques measuring true serum creatinine give plasma levels that are slightly lower than those from the Jaffé assay method.[50] The imidohydrolase method can be perturbed by extremely high glucose levels[51, 65] and by the antifungal agent flucytosine.[66–68]

Serum creatinine level is probably the most widely used indirect measure of glomerular filtration rate. Its popularity is attributable to convenience and low cost. Unfortunately, the correct interpretation of serum creatinine in the clinical setting is a problem. Failure to consider variation in creatinine production from differences in muscle mass frequently leads to an erroneous misinterpretation of serum creatinine. This confusion may be compounded by the use of standard normal ranges for creatinine levels that appear on routine laboratory reports. For example, a serum creatinine level that falls in the normal range may indicate a normal glomerular filtration rate in a young, healthy individual. However, the same serum creatinine level in an elderly individual could indicate a twofold reduction in glomerular filtration rate as a result of a comparable reduction in muscle mass.[24]

Muscle mass may also decline over a relatively short time. For example, significant declines in creatinine excretion were seen in kidney transplant patients, especially patients who had long-term declines in allograft function.[69] The decline in creatinine excretion was probably due to decreases in muscle mass from multiple causes, including the effects of corticosteroids.[22] As a result of this decline in muscle mass, changes in serum creatinine underestimated the amount of decline in renal function.

Failure to remember the potential effects of tubule secretion on serum creatinine, especially in patients with reduced renal function, may lead the clinician to believe that renal function is better than it actually is. Moreover, the potential for interference from plasma constituents and medications requires the clinician to know what assay is being used to measure serum creatinine. On the basis of whether the reported upper limit of normal for adults is high (1.4 to 1.9 mg/dL) or low (1.2 to 1.4 mg/dL), it may sometimes be possible to correctly surmise whether an unmodified alkaline picrate–Jaffé reaction (higher normal limits) or a newer method that removes interference with chromogens (lower normal limits) is being used. The clinician should also be aware of the precision of the assay. Precision is commonly measured by the coefficient of variation, which is the mean of replicate samples divided by the standard deviation.

## Creatinine Clearance

Measuring creatinine clearance obviates some of the problems of using serum creatinine as a marker of glomerular filtration rate but creates others. Differences in steady-state creatinine production due to differences in muscle mass that affect serum creatinine should not affect creatinine clearance. Extrarenal elimination of creatinine should also have little influence on the ability of creatinine clearance to estimate glomerular filtration rate. However, the reliability of creatinine clearance is greatly diminished by variability in tubule secretion of creatinine and by the inability of most patients to accurately collect timed urine samples. Indeed, some have argued that creatinine clearance is a less reliable measure of glomerular filtration rate than is serum creatinine and that the use of the creatinine clearance should be abandoned.[70–73]

Tubule secretion of creatinine causes creatinine clearance to overestimate true glomerular filtration rate. The overestimation is reduced somewhat if serum and urinary creatinine levels are both measured by the Jaffé method.[74] As discussed before, plasma constituents tend to falsely raise the serum creatinine level measured by the Jaffé assay, whereas urinary creatinine levels are largely unaffected. Thus, creatinine clearance determinations, calculated from serum and urinary creatinine levels measured with the Jaffé assay, tend to be falsely low. In a population of patients, this error tends to cancel the error introduced by tubule creatinine secretion, and the creatinine clearance more closely resembles true glomerular filtration rate.[74–76] However, the two errors are independent, and the occurrence of opposing errors of the same magnitude in the same patient is largely a result of chance. Thus, variability in the precision of creatinine clearance as an estimate of true glomerular filtration rate is not reduced and may be increased by this fortuitous combination of errors. Indeed, the creatinine clearance determined in 30 patients with a total chromogen method was only 9% higher than inulin clearance, whereas the true creatinine clearance was 31% higher.[77] However, the correlation coefficient with inulin clearance compared with the true creatinine clearance was much better (.96) than that of inulin clearance compared with the total chromogen creatinine clearance (.86), which suggests that the latter technique was more accurate but less precise.

Prolonged storage of the urine can introduce error in the creatinine clearance determination by perturbing urinary creatinine levels. High temperature and low pH of urine enhance the conversion of creatine to creatinine in urine.[78] Indeed, storing urine under adverse conditions for 24 hours was shown to cause a 20% increase in the amount of measured urinary creatinine.[78] This problem can be obviated by refrigerating urine samples and by measuring the creatinine level without undue delay.

Tubule secretion of creatinine would cause little difficulty if it were constant, and a constant correction factor could be subtracted from creatinine clearance determinations to yield a more accurate estimate of glomerular filtration rate. Unfortunately, interpatient and intrapatient variability in tubule creatinine secretion makes this impossible. The tendency for tubule secretion to increase proportionally with declining levels of renal function, for example, decreases the usefulness of creatinine clearance determinations to accurately reflect glomerular filtration rate in patients with renal disease.[42, 79]

As discussed before, all renal clearance techniques that rely on measuring a marker of glomerular filtration rate in the urine are subject to the vagaries of urine collection.

Variability in the adequacy of timed urine samples can introduce substantial error in the clearance determination. Carrying out collections under direct supervision can enhance the accuracy of timed collections. However, decreasing the collection time may increase the contribution of errors because of incomplete bladder emptying, especially if urine volumes are not increased with water loading. In addition, short-interval urine collections negate the advantages of time-averaged glomerular filtration rate estimates made from 24-hour urine collection. The cost of the procedure can also be substantially higher if trained personnel are used to directly supervise urine collections in a clinical setting.

In principle, the renal clearance of creatinine is the urinary creatinine excretion divided by the area under the plasma creatinine concentration-time curve over the period in which the urine was sampled. In practice, creatinine clearance is usually measured by determining the urinary creatinine excretion and sampling a single plasma creatinine value. It is then assumed that the plasma creatinine was constant over the time of the urine collection. Plasma creatinine remains relatively constant over 24 hours if food intake and activity are also constant.[80] However, in a 24-hour period, there may be substantial variability in plasma creatinine levels,[81] largely owing to effects of diet.[82] Thus, under usual clinical conditions, the assumption that plasma creatinine levels are constant during the period of urine collection may not be valid and may be a source of error.

The day-to-day coefficient of variation for serum creatinine is approximately 8%.[71, 83] Because two creatinine determinations must be made to calculate a creatinine clearance, the coefficient of variation of the creatinine clearance should be higher than that of serum creatinine. Indeed, the coefficient of variation of creatinine clearance could be expected to be at least 11.3% (the square root of 2 times the square of 8%). This is in fact similar to the coefficient of variation for creatinine clearance reported in at least one investigation.[83] Others have reported a day-to-day coefficient of variation for creatinine clearance, when carried out in the routine clinical setting, as high as 27%.[84]

## Cimetidine-Enhanced Creatinine Clearance

Because tubule secretion of creatinine is a major limitation of the creatinine clearance, several investigators have tried to enhance the accuracy of creatinine clearance by blocking tubule creatinine secretion with the histamine H$_2$-receptor antagonist cimetidine.[85–89] In these studies, cimetidine substantially improved the creatinine clearance estimate of glomerular filtration rate in patients with mild to moderate renal impairment. However, in many patients, tubule secretion of creatinine was not completely blocked, and the cimetidine-enhanced creatinine clearance still overestimated glomerular filtration rate in these individuals. Moreover, only a limited number of patients have been studied so far, and the optimal dosing schedule for cimetidine has not yet been worked out.

A cimetidine-enhanced creatinine clearance measurement requires little more cooperation from the patient than for a standard creatinine clearance determination. Cimetidine is safe. Indeed, it was reported that the incidence of adverse reactions during prolonged treatment of 622 patients with cimetidine (10.9%) was similar to that seen during treatment of 516 patients with placebo (10.1%).[90] Moreover, the cimetidine-enhanced creatinine clearance can be measured in most clinical laboratories. Thus, the technique may be especially useful for patients who live in areas where more expensive glomerular filtration rate measurement techniques are not readily available. Although it will not replace other more accurate methods for measuring glomerular filtration rate, the cimetidine-enhanced creatinine clearance could prove to be a cost-effective alternative suitable in many clinical situations.

## Serum Creatinine Formulas to Estimate Renal Function

The need to collect a urine sample remains a major limitation of the creatinine clearance technique, with or without enhancement using cimetidine. Therefore, many have attempted to mathematically transform or correct serum creatinine so that it may more accurately reflect glomerular filtration rate.[70, 91–102] Under ideal conditions, glomerular filtration rate, as measured by a marker such as creatinine, should be equal to the inverse of the serum creatinine value multiplied by a constant rate of creatinine excretion. Thus, in an ideal situation, changes in the inverse serum creatinine value should be directly proportional to changes in glomerular filtration rate. However, the ideal situation is rarely applicable. Changes in creatinine production, extrarenal elimination, and tubule secretion of creatinine can all create errors in the use of the inverse serum creatinine value to measure changes in glomerular filtration rate. Indeed, none of the shortcomings of using serum creatinine as a marker of glomerular filtration rate is avoided by using the inverse serum creatinine value.[103]

One of the problems with using serum creatinine or its inverse value as a measure of glomerular filtration rate is that interpatient and intrapatient differences in creatinine production often occur. Variations in creatinine production due to age- and sex-related differences in muscle mass have been measured and have been incorporated in formulas to improve the ability of serum creatinine to estimate glomerular filtration rate. The most widely used formula is that of Cockcroft and Gault[91]:

$$\text{Creatinine clearance} = (140 - \text{age})(\text{wt})/72P_{cr}$$

where age is age in years, wt is body weight in kilograms, and $P_{cr}$ is plasma creatinine concentration in milligrams per deciliter. This formula applies to men and should be multiplied by 0.85 for women. The formula reduces the variability of serum creatinine estimates of glomerular filtration measured in a population of men and women of different ages. However, the formula does not take into account differences in creatinine production between individuals of the same age and sex or even in the same individual over time.[98, 101] The formula systematically overestimates glomerular filtration rate in individuals who are obese or edematous.[101] Moreover, the formula does not take into account extrarenal elimination, tubule handling, or inaccuracies in the laboratory measurement of creatinine, each of which contributes to the error in the serum creatinine estimate of glomerular filtration rate.

It cannot be assumed that formulas to predict renal function derived from data in one population of patients will be valid when applied to a second population. For example, few diabetic individuals were included in some of the original studies that examined formulas for predicting glomerular filtration rate. When these formulas were subsequently tested in diabetic patients, they were found by some investigators to be inaccurate.[103, 104]

## Inulin

Inulin has long been considered the gold standard of exogenously administered markers of glomerular filtration rate. However, scarcity and high cost have greatly diminished the usefulness of inulin as a marker for glomerular filtration rate. Inulin (molecular mass 5200 daltons) is a polymer of fructose found in tubers such as the dahlia, the Jerusalem artichoke, and chicory. Inulin is inert and does not bind to plasma proteins. It distributes in extracellular fluid, is freely filtered at the glomerulus, and is neither reabsorbed nor secreted by renal tubules.[105] Inulin is readily measured in plasma and urine by one of several colorimetric assays. These assays are time-consuming but can be adapted for use on an autoanalyzer. Glucose is also detected in most inulin assays and must, therefore, be either removed beforehand or measured independently in the sample and subtracted. In any case, appropriate care must be taken in patients with high plasma or urinary glucose levels, especially if the levels fluctuate during the glomerular filtration rate determination.

The renal clearance method for using inulin to measure glomerular filtration rate was originally developed and championed by Homer Smith.[106] Over the years, this technique has been used by clinical investigators and has been modified little. Generally, measurements are made under standardized conditions. Patients are typically studied in the morning, after an overnight fast. An oral water load of 10 to 15 mL/kg body weight is given before inulin is infused. Additional water is administered throughout the test to ensure a constant urine flow rate of at least 4 mL/min. When a good urine flow has been established, a loading dose of inulin is given. This is then followed by a constant infusion to maintain plasma levels. Once a steady state has been achieved, several timed (generally 30-minute) urine collections are carried out. Ideally, a bladder catheter is used to ensure the accuracy of the timed urine collections. Serial plasma levels of inulin are also measured.

Inulin clearance is calculated from the plasma inulin level (time-averaged), urinary inulin concentration, and urine flow rate. Usually an average of three to five separate determinations is made. Each of these measurements is subject to inaccuracies. Indeed, the coefficient of variation between clearance periods is 10%.[107] The coefficient of variation of inulin clearance measured on different days in the same individual is approximately 7.5%.[107] Some of the variability in inulin clearance determinations made in the

same individual is no doubt due to error in measurement, and some is due to true fluctuation in glomerular filtration rate (see later). It has been estimated that a difference of 20 mL/1.73 m$^2$/min in the values of inulin clearances measured in the same individual on two separate days predicts a real difference in glomerular filtration rate at $P$ less than .05.[108] A difference of 27 mL/1.73 m$^2$/min between measurements predicts a real difference at $P$ less than .01.[108]

The renal inulin clearance method has a number of drawbacks that limit its widespread use in a clinical setting. Bladder catheterization is associated with some risk and is not readily accepted by many patients. Although inulin clearance measurements can be carried out with use of spontaneous voiding, incomplete bladder emptying may introduce additional variability. Unfortunately, no studies have compared inulin clearance results obtained by use of bladder catheterization with those obtained by use of spontaneous voiding. Problems with residual urine will most likely occur in individuals with prostatism and in patients with neurogenic bladder dysfunction. Large urine volumes probably help reduce the effect of incomplete bladder emptying, but water loading is itself uncomfortable for many patients. It has been noted that inulin clearance tends to decline during serial urine collections, and this decline may be due, in part, to the difficulty patients have in maintaining a high water intake throughout the procedure. An intravenous cannula and a constant infusion are other sources of discomfort and inconveniences. Thus, despite its accuracy, the renal inulin clearance technique is cumbersome and inconvenient.

To avoid problems related to urine collection, many investigators have turned to plasma clearance techniques. Plasma clearance can be measured by use of either a constant infusion or a bolus injection.[109] If, during a constant infusion, both the distribution space and the plasma level of inulin are constant, the rate of infusion will be equal to the rate of elimination. The inulin clearance then becomes the rate of infusion divided by the plasma concentration. There is a high degree of correlation between results from this technique and those from the renal clearance method.[109] However, maintaining constant plasma concentrations is difficult, and the constant infusion technique is rarely used. The bolus injection technique is discussed in greater detail in the section on radionuclide markers.

As previously noted, a number of problems limit the usefulness of inulin as a marker of glomerular filtration rate. Although most data suggest that inulin is freely filtered and is not handled by the renal tubules, this may not be true in all clinical situtations. For example, it has been suggested that impaired filtration or back-diffusion of inulin may limit its usefulness in kidney transplant recipients.[110] However, the decline in the use of inulin as a marker of glomerular filtration rate has largely been due to its scarcity and cost.

## Radionuclide Markers

Any of the radionuclide-labeled markers of glomerular filtration rate may be used in either renal or plasma clearance studies. Estimating glomerular filtration rate by plasma clearance of an intravenous bolus injection of an indicator

is convenient and has been used more often than constant infusion or renal clearance techniques. The assumptions underlying the measurement of renal clearance by use of a single-injection technique are of critical importance. Basically, renal clearance is measured as the plasma clearance, or the amount of indicator injected divided by the integrated area of the plasma concentration curve over time.[111] Because it is not possible to measure enough samples to accurately determine the area under the plasma concentration-time curve, estimation of this area is based on mathematic formulations that describe the decline in plasma levels over time.

Models used to estimate plasma clearance assume that the volume of distribution and renal excretion are constant over time. A constant renal excretion has been demonstrated for at least two indicators, [125]I-labeled iothalamate and [51]Cr-labeled ethylenediaminetetraacetic acid (EDTA). However, underestimation of glomerular filtration rate with use of [125m]Tc-labeled diethylenetriaminepentaacetic acid (DTPA) may be due to plasma protein binding and decreasing renal clearance over time.[113, 114]

The indicator is eliminated directly from the arterial circulation. However, the indicator is injected intravenously, and blood samples for measurement of the plasma clearance are drawn from the venous compartment. The assumption that there is instantaneous equilibration between the arterial and venous circulations is incorrect.[115, 116] Thus, any method used to calculate renal clearance must correct for inaccuracies due to delayed equilibration between the venous and arterial compartments.

Because it is not possible to measure the entire plasma concentration-time curve, a limited number of samples must be measured, and an appropriate curve fitted to these points must be used to measure the plasma clearance. Both one- and two-compartment models have been used to measure plasma clearance (Fig. 26–2). In the two-compartment model, the first compartment can be thought of as corresponding to plasma and the second to extracellular fluid.[117] Two slopes and two intercepts are derived from plotting plasma values over time after injection.[118, 119] One slope and intercept are derived from the initial data that fit a straight line when plotted on a logarithmic scale. The other slope and intercept are derived from a line that fits data of the terminal elimination phase.

Unfortunately, the two-compartment method requires frequent plasma samples. Therefore, most now use a one-compartment model whereby only values measured during the terminal elimination phase (generally commencing 90 to 120 minutes after injection) are sampled.[120–123] In this model, the slope and intercept of a line plotted on a logarithmic scale are used to calculate clearance by the formula

$$\text{Clearance} = V_0(\ln(2))/t_{1/2}$$

where $V_0$ is the volume of distribution and $t_{1/2}$ is the half-time for decay in plasma levels. The value derived from this relationship is multiplied by a constant to correct for systematic errors attributable to overestimation of $V_0$ and a higher concentration of marker in venous compared with arterial blood.[115, 116, 122, 124] The clearance calculated by this simple monoexponential model is surprisingly accurate.[122, 124] Also surprising is the fact that as few as two samples yield results that seem to be as accurate as results of multiple samples.[120–122, 124–126]

Single-sample techniques have also been used to estimate plasma clearance.[127, 128] One such method was based on the use of different sampling times dictated on the predicted glomerular filtration rate.[128] Tepe and co-workers[129] compared different sampling times using monoexponential models for glomerular filtration rate determinations in 139 individuals. They found that a single-sample method was accurate and that sampling between 60 and 240 minutes after injection was optimal.

Whether a single sample or multiple samples are used with a monoexponential model, it is probably important that the sampling time be adjusted to the level of renal function.[111] To sample after only 2 hours may be too short for patients with normal to moderately decreased renal function.[112] In such a patient, a sampling time 4 to 5 hours after injection is probably more appropriate.[111] However, this interval may be too short in individuals with more marked declines in renal function or in patients with ascites. In such patients, sampling times up to 24 hours may be appropriate.[111]

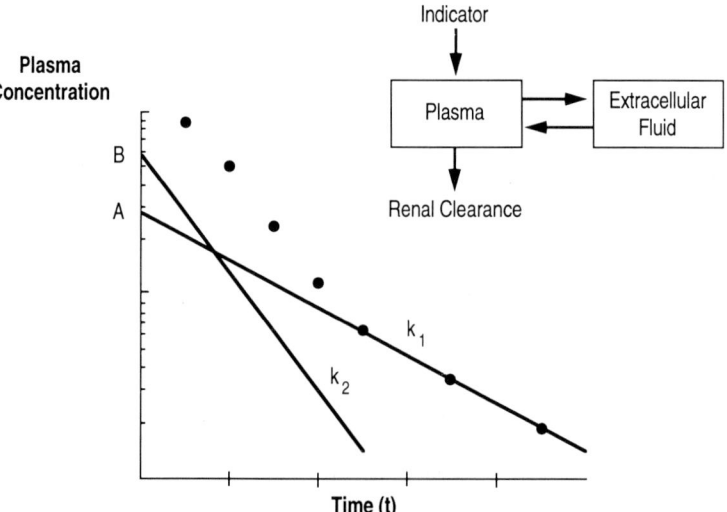

**Figure 26–2.** Plasma disappearance curve for the indicator of glomerular filtration rate after bolus intravenous administration. Dots represent measured concentrations. The line with slope $k_1$ and intercept A is the least-squares best fit of the terminal elimination phase. The line with slope $k_2$ and intercept B represents best fit of the difference between actual values and values calculated from the line fitted to the terminal elimination phase. Glomerular filtration rate (one-compartment method) is calculated as $Qk_1/A$, where Q is the quantity of indicator administered. Glomerular filtration rate (two-compartment method) is calculated as $Qk_1k_2/(Ak_2 + Bk_1)$.

The use of radiolabeling has reduced the amount of marker that needs to be administered, and this, in turn, has permitted subcutaneous administration.[130, 131] It has been shown that reasonably predictable plasma concentrations can be achieved after subcutaneous injection of a radiolabeled marker such as [125]I-iothalamate. Thus, the renal clearance of such a marker can be measured after subcutaneous injection.

The measurement of plasma clearance need not require plasma sampling at all. A gamma camera positioned over the kidneys can be used to measure renal elimination of a radioactive indicator.[132] Quantitative renal imaging most commonly uses [99m]Tc-DTPA, radioiodinated Hippuran, [123]I–o-iodohippuran, or [99m]Tc-mercaptoacetyltriglycine.[132] In general, glomerular filtration rate determination with quantitative renal imaging is not as precise as that obtained with plasma sampling.[133, 134] The advantage of quantitative renal imaging is that additional information pertaining to the anatomy of renal function can be obtained. Indeed, the "split function," or relative contribution to total glomerular filtration rate from each kidney, can be calculated. This can provide important information in the evaluation of some patients with renal vascular disease and may be crucial, for example, in deciding whether to carry out a unilateral nephrectomy.

Finally, it is assumed that the marker used to measure plasma clearance is not extensively protein bound, is freely filtered, is neither secreted nor reabsorbed by the tubules, and is eliminated only by the kidneys. A number of radionuclide markers have been developed to measure glomerular filtration rate. In general, they share most of the characteristics of inulin that made it a good indicator of glomerular filtration rate. The popularity of these radionuclide-labeled agents is attributable to their ready availability, ease of administration, relatively low cost, and accuracy of laboratory assay.

Probably the most extensively investigated radionuclide-bound indicator of glomerular filtration rate has been [51]Cr-EDTA.[120, 122, 124, 135–139] It is small (molecular mass 292 daltons), appears to have little binding to plasma proteins, and is freely filtered by the glomerulus. Studies in humans have reported that the renal clearance of [51]Cr-EDTA was about 10% lower than that of inulin when both were measured simultaneously. Although the reason for these lower values is not known, it could be due to plasma protein binding, tubule reabsorption, or in vivo dissociation of the nuclide from EDTA.

Sodium iothalamate (Conray) is a derivative of triiodobenzoic acid and is a high-osmolar, ionic radiocontrast agent. It is small (molecular mass 614 daltons) and appears to be only slightly bound to plasma proteins.[140, 141] Several studies in humans have found that simultaneously measured renal clearances of [125]I-iothalamate and inulin are similar.[142, 143] These studies could not discern whether this resulted from similar renal handling of inulin and iothalamate or whether there was a fortuitous cancellation of errors due, for example, to plasma protein binding that countered the effects of tubule secretion. The use of [125]I-iothalamate to measure renal function is generally considered safe, although there are virtually no long-term follow-up data. The potential problem of thyroid uptake and concentration of

the radionuclide can be avoided by administering a large dose of oral iodine (Lugol solution) before the procedure. The half-life of [125]I is approximately 60 days.

DTPA (molecular mass 393 daltons) has frequently been chelated to radionuclides for use in renal imaging.[132, 144] The compound used most commonly to measure glomerular filtration rate is [99m]Tc-DTPA.[145, 146] The radiolabeling of DTPA with [99m]Tc must be carried out immediately before use because of the chelate's instability. The half-life of [99m]Tc is only 6 hours, so samples must be counted soon after the procedure.[132] Protein binding of [99m]Tc-DTPA may be a significant source of error in some patients.[113, 114] A comparison of clearance determinations based on whole plasma and protein-free, ultrafiltered plasma found measurements to be significantly different, especially in patients taking multiple medications.[134]

All radionuclide markers are radioactive. This fact has begun to erode their acceptance by patients, and they have been subjected to close monitoring by regulatory agencies. In the United States, the storage and disposal of all radioactive waste have come under growing scrutiny and regulation, and the use of isotopes now requires that a number of conditions be met. The actual amount of radiation delivered is generally considered less than the amount patients receive while undergoing most standard radiologic procedures.[142] However, the isotope is concentrated in the urine, so exposure of the urinary system may be greater.[132, 142, 147, 148] To alleviate this potential problem, patients are advised to maintain a high fluid intake and urine volume after the procedure. There are no long-term follow-up studies to assess the risk of this exposure of the collecting system to radiation.

## Radiocontrast Agents

In an effort to avoid use of radiolabeled compounds, techniques have been developed to measure low levels of iodine in urine and plasma. These techniques permit the use of unlabeled radiocontrast agents, which are inherently rich in iodine, to measure glomerular filtration rate. A high-performance liquid chromatography assay has been used to measure renal clearance of iothalamate (Conray) and diatrizoate meglumine (Hypaque).[149] The sensitivity of the assay allows the use of as little as 1 mL of radiocontrast agent, which can be injected subcutaneously. However, the main disadvantage of this technique is the expense, time, and labor needed to carry out the high-performance liquid chromatography assay.

A rapid and convenient method was developed to measure low concentrations of iodine.[150, 151] This method has been applied to the measurement of the plasma clearance of the low-osmolality, nonionic radiocontrast agent iohexol (Omnipaque). Clearance determinations using this method appear to be comparable to those made with use of other radionuclide-labeled markers and to inulin.[152–157] Up to 30 mL may be required, but the amount administered is reduced in patients with decreased renal function. The technique appears to be safe. This is not surprising, because even in high-risk diabetic patients with markedly reduced renal function, nephrotoxic effects from radiocontrast

agents occurred only at doses higher than those used by others to measure renal function.[158] The incidence of extrarenal adverse reactions from higher doses of nonionic radiocontrast agents used in radiographic procedures is low.[159] All of the methods that use labeled or unlabeled radiocontrast agents share the risk of allergic reactions. Although this risk is small, none of these agents should be administered to patients who are allergic to iodine.

## Normalizing Glomerular Filtration Rate

The measurement of glomerular filtration rate is usually better suited for monitoring disease progression than for detection of disease or diagnosis. This is true not only because of cost and inconvenience but also because it is difficult to define what a normal glomerular filtration rate should be for an individual patient. The difficulty in defining a reasonably narrow range of normal is in large part due to the enormous physiologic variability of glomerular filtration rate in healthy individuals.[160] An understanding of the factors that contribute to this normal variability is essential in interpreting any test of glomerular filtration rate.

A number of investigators have attempted to normalize glomerular filtration rate in populations of humans who have no known renal disease. For years, body surface area has been used to normalize glomerular filtration rate.[161, 162] The rationale has been that the weight of the kidney and the basal metabolic rate are proportional to body surface area in normal individuals of different age and body size.[162] Generally, the Du Bois formula for calculating body surface area using power functions of height and weight has been used to estimate body surface area.[163] This formula is less accurate at extremes of age.

It has also been suggested that extracellular fluid volume be used to normalize glomerular filtration rate.[164] The argument was made that extracellular fluid volume should be used to normalize glomerular filtration rate because the purpose of the kidney is to maintain the composition of the extracellular fluid.[164] A comparison of the use of extracellular volume with calculated body surface area to normalize glomerular filtration rate found that the two methods yielded similar results.[165] Like extracellular fluid volume, blood volume is also closely correlated to calculated body surface area in adult men and women.[166-168] In addition, both kidney and glomerulus correlate in size to body surface area.[169, 170] Thus, to the extent that glomular filtration rate may be expected to correlate to the size of the kidney and glomerulus, the use of body surface area to normalize glomerular filtration rate seems to be sound.

Blood volume, extracellular fluid volume, and basal metabolic rate can be more accurately predicted by use of indices of lean body mass than by calculated body surface area alone.[168, 171-173] Thus, measures of lean body mass could theoretically be better predictors of normal glomerular filtration rate, at least in adults. However, until this is clearly demonstrated to be the case, the more convenient, calculated body surface area will, no doubt, continue to be the standard for normalizing glomerular filtration rate.

Although the variability in glomerular filtration rate measurements in normal individuals can be reduced by taking body surface area differences into account, the residual variability is substantial. A number of factors may contribute to this variability.[160] Glomerular filtration rate normally declines with age but does so to a variable degree.[24] It is well known that dietary protein intake can affect glomerular filtration rate.[174] Similarly, salt intake, water consumption, posture, and normal diurnal variation can all affect glomerular filtration rate determinations in normal individuals.[160]

The concept of "renal functional reserve" was introduced in studies that demonstrated increased glomerular filtration rate after an oral protein load.[175] This concept led to an unfortunate confusion between increased function due to structural changes after a reduction in renal mass and short-term increases in glomerular filtration rate of a functional nature, for example, after an oral protein load.[175] In theory, the normal intraindividual physiologic variability in glomerular filtration rate could be reduced if the measurement was made after a short-term maneuver that maximized renal function. By use of oral protein loading or other maneuvers to maximize glomerular filtration rate, it could be possible to reduce variability due to fluctuations in physiologic variables that normally modulate renal function. However, there are inadequate data to determine whether this is the case. Moreover, such maneuvers substantially increase the complexity and expense of the measurement.

## Applications

A number of factors should be considered in selecting a clinical test to measure glomerular filtration rate. Unfortunately, the necessary information on accuracy, precision, and expected prevalence of abnormal results is usually not available for each test of glomerular filtration rate in each specific clinical situation. However, recognition of how these factors affect the utility of a test along with crude estimations of these critical parameters can provide guidance in test selection. Finally, the usefulness of a test to measure glomerular filtration rate is dictated not only by issues of accuracy and precision but also by cost, safety, and convenience. In general, the tests that are most accurate and precise are also those that are most costly and inconvenient (Fig. 26–3).

No single test of glomerular filtration rate is ideally suited for every clinical and research application. Rather, the goal should be to select the most accurate and precise test to answer the question being addressed in the safest, most cost-effective, and most convenient manner possible in the population being studied. In clinical practice, tests of glomerular filtration rate are most commonly used for 1) screening for the presence of renal disease, 2) measuring disease progression to determine prognosis and effects of therapy, 3) confirming the need for treatment of end-stage renal disease with dialysis or transplantation, and 4) estimating renal clearance of drugs to guide dosing. For research purposes, tests of glomerular filtration rate are most commonly used to distinguish differences in the rate of change between two or more experimental groups.

Although precise data do not exist, it is probable that none of the currently available tests of renal function is

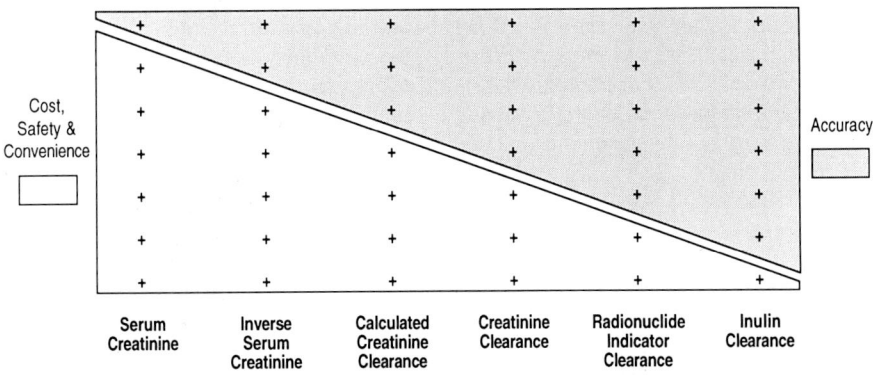

**Figure 26–3.** Conflict between practicality (cost, safety, and convenience) and accuracy of methods to estimate glomerular filtration rate. On one end of the spectrum, serum creatinine is most practical but least accurate. On the other end of the spectrum, inulin clearance is most accurate but least practical.

well suited for detecting early or mild renal disease in the general population. Nevertheless, there is a legitimate need for tests to identify patients with moderate or marked declines in renal function in high-risk situations. The cost and inconvenience of creatinine clearance and radionuclide measurements of glomerular filtration rate ordinarily preclude their use for these screening purposes. Therefore, serum creatinine has most often been used to screen for the presence of significant renal impairment. For example, serum creatinine is commonly used to screen for impaired renal function to identify patients who are at increased risk for radiocontrast-induced acute renal failure. Serum creatinine has been shown to be useful in this situation.[176, 177] Clearly, the number of patients who receive radiocontrast agents would preclude the use of other more expensive and inconvenient tests in this instance. Similarly, the high prevalence of essential hypertension in the Western world would generally make radionuclide determinations of glomerular filtration rate impractical as a first-line screening procedure for a renal cause of hypertension in low-risk individuals.

In contrast to the situation for individuals who are unlikely to have renal disease, the use of more expensive but more accurate measures of glomerular filtration rate may be warranted in patients at high risk for renal functional impairment. For example, the prevalence of renal dysfunction in patients with systemic lupus erythematosus and low serum complement levels may be high enough to justify the use of a radionuclide determination of glomerular filtration rate to screen for renal dysfunction that could suggest a need for therapy or additional diagnostic tests. Similarly, the high incidence of both acute and chronic renal allograft rejection could make the use of relatively complex tests of renal function cost-effective.

Much effort has been devoted to defining methods for measuring renal disease progression. It as been noted that plots of inverse serum creatinine values over time can often be closely fitted (by least squares) to a straight line.[178–184] The use of the inverse creatinine value has generally been found to provide fits of the data as good as or better than those obtained by plots of logarithmically transformed serum creatinine values.[179, 182, 183] Serial inverse serum creatinine values can be corrected for changes in creatinine excretion (measured less frequently than serum creatinine)

to reduce error attributable to changes in muscle mass over time.[185–187] Because changes in the rate of decline in inverse creatinine values may indicate an effect of therapeutic intervention, a method developed to determine whether there is a "break point" of two hinged regression lines has been applied to plots of inverse serum creatinine values.[184, 188–190]

Changes in renal function estimated by plots of serial inverse serum creatinine values can vary substantially from changes estimated by radionuclide-determined glomerular filtration rate.[185, 186, 191] Correlation between radionuclide measurements of glomerular filtration rate and changes in creatinine clearance is no better or is even worse than that for inverse creatinine.[186, 192] Spontaneous changes in the slope of inverse creatinine are frequent.[184, 187, 189, 193, 194] As a result, inverse serum creatinine plots are not reliable predictors of the time remaining to dialysis or transplantation or of changes in the rate of functional decline attributable to therapy.

Estimating renal clearance of drugs that are predominantly eliminated by glomerular filtration, in the absence of tubule secretion and reabsorption, is yet another potential application for tests of renal function.[195, 196] In principle, the rate of drug elimination is often proportional to the glomerular filtration rate. However, because most drugs are either weak acids or weak bases, changes in urine pH can alter tubule handling and affect the relationship between glomerular filtration rate and renal elimination. Competition of drugs for the same secretory pathway can also perturb renal elimination. Nevertheless, impaired renal function is the most common way in which the kidney affects drug levels, and glomerular filtration rate can approximate renal excretion of many drugs. Cost, convenience, and timeliness make creatinine clearance and radionuclide determination of glomerular filtration rate impractical for guiding drug dosing. Most investigators have used formulas to calculate glomerular filtration rate from age, sex, and serum creatinine to adjust doses of drugs that are excreted primarily by the kidney.[97, 197–199] Although the accuracy of these calculated clearances has been studied with use of other measures of renal function as a gold standard, the ability of these formulas to predict pharmacokinetic profiles has not been determined for most therapeutic agents.

Obtaining serial renal biopsies in clinical trials is difficult and is rarely carried out. Many studies have attempted to

examine changes in the rate of decline in glomerular filtration rate, determined by inverse creatinine plots or other techniques, to assess the effectiveness of therapeutic interventions. However, measuring changes in the rate of decline is a problem, as discussed before. Moreover, it has also been shown that in groups of patients, a substantial proportion of apparent amelioration in functional declines measured by inverse creatinine or radionuclide-determined glomerular filtration rate can be attributed to regression to the mean.[192] Therefore, comparing the rate of change in glomerular filtration rate between two or more experimental groups has become the most reliable method for studying interventions designed to delay or prevent renal disease progression.[105, 200, 201] Generally, cost and inconvenience are subordinated to the increased accuracy and precision of radionuclide measurements of glomerular filtration rate in a clinical trial, and these tests are routinely used in that setting.

## URINALYSIS

### Historical Background

In common English usage, urinalysis is the "chemical analysis of urine."[202] However, analysis is "the identification or separation of ingredients of a substance," and as such, urinalysis can take on a much broader meaning.[202] Historically, inspection of the urine for diagnosis is virtually as old as medicine itself. The connection between sweet-tasting urine and diabetes was made as early as 600 BC. Hippocrates used the appearance, color, and consistency of urine to diagnose disease and predict outcome. In the Middle Ages, prognostication from the examination of urine was raised to an art by the "Pisse Prophets."

### Overview

There are three ways to obtain a urine specimen: spontaneous voiding, urethral catheterization, and percutaneous bladder puncture. Although the safety and utility of suprapubic needle aspiration of the bladder have been demonstrated, this technique is generally reserved for situations in which urine cannot be easily obtained by other means. It may be particularly useful in infants, for example. Once a specimen is obtained, there are countless techniques for examining the urine and its contents.

In this section, we review only those analytic techniques that are readily available and in common use. We focus on three broad areas: 1) chemical content, 2) protein composition, and 3) formed elements. The discussion of chemical content is limited to tests readily available through the use of reagent strips, such as specific gravity, pH, bilirubin, urobilinogen, nitrite, leukocyte esterase, glucose, ketoacetate, hemoglobin, and myoglobin. More specific chemical tests (e.g., tests to diagnose metabolic disorders) are not discussed. Similarly, the measurement and interpretation of urinary electrolyte composition are excluded from this section. The discussion on protein composition focuses on

proteins from both tubule and glomerular sources. Formed elements include commonly encountered cells and casts.

As with all laboratory procedures and clinical tests, the usefulness of urinalysis techniques depends not only on accuracy and precision but also on prior probabilities of the occurrence of positive results. Studies have found that routine hospital admission or preoperative urinalysis that includes both reagent strip testing and microscopic examination rarely leads to better outcomes for patients and is generally not cost-effective.[203–208] As a result, most have concluded that routine urinalysis should be abandoned in this setting. Whether a more limited approach to routine screening that relies on reagent strip testing without microscopy will be more effective remains to be determined.[209, 210]

The probability of a positive result on urinalysis is no doubt greater for patients who are already known to have proteinuria than for otherwise normal patients routinely admitted to a medical ward. Therefore, reason would suggest that the utility of examining the urine sediment may be different in patients with proteinuria from that in patients routinely admitted to the hospital. Indeed, in patients who were thought to have renal disease and therefore underwent biopsy, microscopic examination of the urine was highly predictive of abnormal renal histology.[211] Data such as these have led to the suggestion that examining the urine sediment is of critical importance in assessing the implications of proteinuria.[212] Although accurate data on the sensitivity and specificity of urinalysis techniques are not available for most clinical conditions, an awareness of how individual tests are influenced by the underlying likelihood of diseases can be helpful in determining the appropriate use of urinalysis and in assessing the implications of the results.

### Chemical Content

#### COLOR

The color of urine is determined by chemical content, concentration, and pH. Urine may be almost colorless if the output is high and the concentration is low. Cloudy urine is generally the result of phosphates (usually normal) or leukocytes and bacteria (usually abnormal). Black urine is seen in alkaptonuria.[213] Acute intermittent porphyria frequently causes dark urine. A number of exogenous chemicals and drugs can make urine green, but green urine may also be associated with *Pseudomonas* bacteriuria and urinary bile pigments. The most common cause of red urine is hemoglobin.[214] Red urine in the absence of red blood cells usually indicates either free hemoglobin or myoglobin. Red urine and red plasma indicate hemoglobin. Red urine and clear plasma are most often the result of myoglobin but may also be seen in some porphyrias. Among endogenous sources, bile pigments are the most common cause of orange urine.

#### SPECIFIC GRAVITY

The measurement of the specific gravity is usually included as part of the standard urinalysis. Specific gravity is a convenient and rapidly obtained indicator of urine osmolality. It can be measured accurately with a refractometer or with a hygrometer or estimated with a dipstick. The accuracy and usefulness of the reagent strip method have been debated.[215, 216] Measurement of specific gravity by dipstick is dependent on the ionic strength of the urine and the fact that there is generally a linear relationship between ionic strength and osmolality in urine. The strip contains a poly-ionic polymer with binding sites saturated with $H^+$. The release of $H^+$ when competitively replaced with urinary cations causes a change in the pH-sensitive indicator dye.[217] Specific gravity measured by dipstick tends to be falsely high at urine pH less than 6 and falsely low if the pH is greater than 7.[218] Effects of albumin, glucose, and urea on osmolality are not reflected by changes in the dipstick specific gravity.[215] In newborn infants, specific gravity measurement with either a refractometer or a reagent strip is inaccurate.[219, 220]

The specific gravity of urine reflects the relative proportion of dissolved solutes to total volume. As such, specific gravity is a measure of urine concentration. The normal range for specific gravity is 1.003 to 1.030,[217, 221] but values decrease with age as the kidney's ability to concentrate urine decreases. Specific gravity can be used to rudely estimate how the concentration of other urine constituents may reflect total excretion of those constituents,[222, 223] because specific gravity correlates inversely with 24-hour urine volume.[224] Self-monitoring of urine specific gravity may be useful for stone-forming patients who benefit from maintaining a dilute urine.[216, 224] Most clinical decisions should be based only on more accurate determinations of urine osmolality.

## URINE pH

Urine pH is usually measured with a reagent test strip. Most commonly, the double indicators methyl red and bromthymol blue are used in the reagent strips to give a broad range of colors at different pH values. In conjunction with other specific urine and plasma measurements, urine pH is often invaluable in diagnosing systemic acid-base disorders. By itself, however, urine pH provides little useful diagnostic information. The normal range for urine pH is 4.5 to 7.8. An alkaline urine (pH $\geq$ 7.0) can be suggestive of infection with a urea-splitting organism. Prolonged storage can lead to overgrowth of urea-splitting bacteria and a high urine pH. However, diet (vegetarian), diuretic therapy, vomiting, gastric suction, and alkali therapy can also cause a high urine pH. Low urine pH (pH $\leq$ 5.0) is seen most commonly in metabolic acidosis. An acid urine is also associated with the ingestion of large amounts of meat.

## BILIRUBIN AND UROBILINOGEN

Only conjugated bilirubin is passed into the urine. Thus, a reagent test response for bilirubin is typically positive in patients with obstructive jaundice or jaundice due to hepatocellular injury, whereas the response for urinary bilirubin is usually negative in patients with jaundice due to hemolysis. In patients with hemolysis, however, the test result for urinary urobilinogen is often positive. Reagent test strips are sensitive to bilirubin, detecting as little as 0.05 mg/dL. However, the detection of bilirubin in the urine is not sen-

sitive for detecting liver disease.[225] False-positive results for urinary bilirubin can occur if the urine is contaminated with stool. Prolonged storage and exposure to light can lead to false-negative results.[226]

## LEUKOCYTE ESTERASE AND NITRITES

Dipstick screening for urinary tract infection has been recommended for high-risk individuals. Indeed, an expert panel recommended screening for asymptomatic bacteriuria in persons with diabetes, in pregnant women, and possibly in preschool children.[227] The esterase method relies on the fact that esterases are released from lysed urinary granulocytes. These esterases liberate 3-hydroxy-5-phenyl pyrrole after substrate hydrolysis. The pyrrole reacts with a diazonium salt, which results in a pink to purple color.[228] The result is usually interpreted as negative, trace, small, moderate, or large. Urine that is allowed to stand results in a greater lysis of leukocytes and a more intense reaction. False-positive results may occur with vaginal contamination. High levels of glucose, albumin, ascorbic acid, tetracycline, cephalexin, or cephalothin or large amounts of oxalic acid may inhibit the reaction.[229]

Urinary bacteria convert nitrates to nitrites. In the reagent strip test, nitrite reacts with a $p$-arsanilic acid to form a diazonium compound, which after further reaction with 1,2,3,4-tetrahydrobenzo(h)quinolin-3-ol results in a pink end point.[228, 230] Results are usually interpreted as positive or negative. High specific gravity and ascorbic acid may interfere with the test. False-positive results are common and may be due to low urinary nitrate levels resulting from low dietary intake. It may take up to 4 hours to convert nitrate to nitrite, so inadequate bladder retention time can also give false-negative results.[230] Prolonged storage of the sample can lead to degradation of nitrites and be another source of false-negative results. Finally, several potential urinary pathogens (such as *Streptococcus faecalis*) other gram-positive organisms, *Neisseria gonorrheae,* and *Mycobacterium tuberculosis* do not convert nitrate to nitrite.[230]

Studies have examined the sensitivity and specificity of reagent strip tests for urinary tract infection in different clinical settings. For example, these screening tests have been evaluated in patients attending a general medicine clinic,[231] in patients visiting an emergency department because of abdominal pain,[232] in children with neurogenic bladders,[233] in children attending a general medical outpatient clinic,[228, 234, 235] in men being screened for sexually transmitted disease,[236] and in women.[237] A meta-analysis of the results of 51 relevant studies compared the use of nitrite alone, leukocyte estrerase alone, dysjunctive pairing (result of either test positive), and conjunctive pairing (result of both tests positive).[238] ROC curves were fitted to the data by use of logistic transformations and weighted linear regression. This analysis indicated that the dysjunctive pairing of both tests is the most accurate approach to screening for infection. However, when the likelihood of infection is high (e.g., when signs and symptoms are present), a negative result of both tests is still inadequate to exclude infection. These tests, in combination with other clinical information, may be more useful in situations in which the likelihood of infection is low.

## GLUCOSE

Glucose testing is generally included with routine urinalysis reagent strips. The measurement of urinary glucose level, once used to monitor diabetic therapy, has been almost completely replaced by more reliable finger-stick methods that measure blood glucose. Urinary glucose is less quantitative than blood glucose, and the appearance of glucose in the urine always occurs later than blood glucose elevations do. Thus, the value of the reagent strip test for glucose is limited almost entirely to screening purposes.

Most reagent strips use a glucose oxidase/peroxidase method. This method generally detects levels of glucose as low as 50 mg/dL.[221, 239] Because the renal threshold for glucose is generally 160 to 180 mg/dL, the presence of a detectable urinary glucose level generally indicates blood glucose in excess of 210 mg/dL. Large quantities of ketones, ascorbate, and phenazopyridine (Pyridium) metabolites may interfere with the color reaction.[239, 240] Urinary peroxide contamination may cause false-positive results. Nevertheless, the appearance of glucose in the urine is a specific indicator of high serum glucose levels. Glucosuria due to a low renal threshold for glucose reabsorption is rare. As a screening test for diabetes, fasting urinary glucose testing has a specificity of 98% but a sensitivity of only 17%.[241]

## KETONES

Ketones (acetoacetate and acetone) are generally detected with the nitroprusside reaction.[242] Ascorbic acid and phenazopyridine can give false-positive reactions. β-Hydroxybutyrate (often 80% of total serum ketones in ketosis) is not normally detected by the nitroprusside reaction. Ketones may appear in the urine, but not in serum, with prolonged fasting or starvation. Ketones may also be measured in the urine in alcoholic or diabetic ketoacidosis.

## HEMOGLOBIN AND MYOGLOBIN

Reagent strips use the peroxidase-like activity of hemoglobin to catalyze the reaction of cumene hydroperoxide and 3,3′,5,5′-tetramethylbenzidine. Hematuria, or contamination of the urine with menstrual blood, produces a positive reaction. Oxidizing contaminants and povidone-iodine (Betadine) cause false-positive reactions.[239] Myoglobin also reacts positively.

Free hemoglobin is filtered at the renal glomerulus and thus appears in the urine when the capacity for plasma protein binding with haptoglobin is exceeded. Some of the hemoglobin is catabolized by the proximal tubules. The principal cause of increased serum and urinary free hemoglobin is hemolysis. Rhabdomyolysis, on the other hand, gives rise to myoglobin. A positive dipstick test result for hemoglobin in the absence of red blood cells in the urine sediment may suggest either hemolysis or rhabdomyolysis. The clinical history often provides important differential diagnostic information. Hemolysis can usually be diag-

nosed by examining the peripheral blood smear and measuring levels of lactate dehydrogenase, haptoglobin, and serum free hemoglobin. Rhabdomyolysis is accompanied by increased levels of serum creatine kinase. In the end, specific assays for hemoglobin and myoglobin can be used to measure urinary levels.

## Protein Content

### NORMAL PHYSIOLOGY

Normally, large quantities of high-molecular-weight plasma proteins traverse the glomerular capillaries or mesangium without entering the urinary space. Both charge- and size-selective properties of the capillary wall prevent all but a tiny fraction of albumin, globulin, and other large plasma proteins from crossing.[243, 244] Smaller proteins (less than 20,000 daltons) pass readily across the capillary wall.[245, 246] However, the plasma concentration of these proteins is much less than that of albumin and globulins, so that the filtered load is small. Moreover, low-molecular-weight proteins are normally reabsorbed by the proximal tubule. Thus, proteins such as $\beta_2$-microglobulin, apoproteins, enzymes, and peptide hormones are normally excreted in only small amounts in the urine.[245, 246] Most healthy individuals excrete between 30 and 130 mg/d of protein, and the upper limit of normal total urinary protein excretion is generally given as 150 to 200 mg/d for adults.[247–249] Most normal urinary protein is albumin, but the upper limit of normal albumin excretion is usually given as 30 mg/d.[249]

A small amount of protein that normally appears in the urine is the result of normal tubule secretion. Tamm-Horsfall protein is a large molecular mass glycoprotein (23 × $10^6$ daltons) that is formed on the epithelial surface of the thick ascending limb of the loop of Henle and early distal convoluted tubule.[250, 251] Interestingly, Tamm-Horsfall protein, also known as uromodulin, binds and inactivates the cytokines interleukin-1 and tumor necrosis factor.[252, 253] Immunoglobulin A and urokinase are also secreted by the renal tubule and appear in the urine in small amounts.[254]

From a consideration of normal physiology, it is apparent that abnormal amounts of protein may appear in the urine as the result of three mechanisms. First, a disruption of the capillary wall barrier may lead to a large amount of high-molecular-weight plasma proteins that overwhelm the limited capacity of tubule reabsorption and cause protein to appear in the urine. The resulting proteinuria can be classified as glomerular in origin. Second, tubule damage or dysfunction can inhibit the normal absorptive capacity of the proximal tubule and result in increased amounts of mostly low-molecular-weight protein to appear in the urine. Such proteinuria can be classified as tubule proteinuria. Third, increased production of normal or abnormal plasma proteins can be filtered at the glomerulus and overwhelm the absorptive capacity of the proximal tubule. The amount of these proteins filtered may be especially large if their size is small or if they are positively charged. Finally, although increased urinary protein excretion could also result from increased tubule production of protein, this is rarely the case.

## TECHNIQUES TO MEASURE URINARY PROTEIN

Protein can be measured in random samples, in timed or untimed overnight samples, or in 24-hour collections. Inaccurate urine collection is probably the greatest source of error in quantifying protein excretion in timed collections, and this is particularly true in 24-hour collections. However, urinary creatinine excretion can be measured to judge the adequacy of the 24-hour collection. If creatinine excretion is similar to what has been measured in previous 24-hour samples, the collection is likely to be reasonably accurate. If no other collections are available for comparison, the adequacy of collection can be judged from the expected normal range of creatinine excretion. For hospitalized men of ages 20 to 50 years, this was found to be 18.5 to 25.0 mg/kg body weight per day; for women of the same age, it was 16.5 to 22.4 mg/kg/d[92] (Fig. 26–4). These values declined with age, so that for men of ages 50 to 70 years, creatinine excretion was 15.7 to 20.2 mg/kg/d; for women, it was 11.8 to 16.1 mg/kg/d (see Fig. 26–4). Patients who are malnourished or who may have reduced muscle mass for other reasons can be expected to have lower than normal creatinine excretion rates.

Tests to accurately measure total protein concentration in urine rely on precipitation. In the commonly used sulfosalicylic acid method, sulfosalicylic acid is added to a sample of urine, and the turbidity is measured with a photometer or a nephelometer. Protein is quantified by comparing the turbidity of the sample to that of a standard. This method lacks precision, and the coefficient of variation is as high as 20%.[255] A number of proteins are detected with this method, including gamma globulin light chains and albumin. The method is more sensitive to albumin than to globulins. Trichloroacetic acid can be used in place of sulfosalicylic acid to increase the sensitivity to gamma globulin. False-positive results may be caused by high levels of tolmetin (Tolectin), tolbutamide, antibiotics, and radiocontrast agents.[15, 256, 257] Total protein can be more accurately quantified by use of several monospecific antibodies to different types of urinary protein.[258] However, this method is somewhat cumbersome and is seldom used in clinical laboratories.

Total protein concentration in urine can be estimated at the bedside with use of chemically impregnated plastic strips. Most dipstick reagents contain a pH-sensitive colorimetric indicator that changes color when negatively charged proteins bind.[259] However, positively charged proteins are less readily detected. Positively charged immunoglobulin light chains, for example, may escape dipstick detection even when there are large amounts of light chains in the urine.[260] A high urine pH (greater than 7.0) can also give false-positive results. In addition, contamination of the urine with blood may give false-positive results. The dipstick technique is sensitive to low urinary protein concentrations (the lower limit of detection is 10 to 20 mg/dL).[261] However, at these low levels, the major constituent of urinary protein may be Tamm-Horsfall protein, and, thus, a positive test result may not reflect renal injury. This is especially likely to occur when the urine volume is low and the concentration is high. On the other hand, when urine volume is high and the urine is maximally dilute, a relatively large amount of protein may go undetected. Indeed, total protein excretion approaching 1 g/d may not be detected if urine output is high. If, for example, urine output is 10 L/d, the concentration of 1 g of protein would be 10 mg/dL, or below the limit of detection for most reagent strip tests of total protein.

The consistency of results with the same sample assessed repeatedly or the precision of reagent strip tests of urinary total protein concentration is generally poor.[261, 262] Variability in interpretation both within and between technologists has been examined and has been found to be relatively high. For example, at low levels of urinary protein concentration (e.g., 6 to 39 mg/dL), inconsistent results between different technologists were seen in 19% to 56% of the determinations.[261] At higher concentrations (e.g., 196 to 328 mg/dL), inconsistencies were seen in 19% to 44%.[261] Similar findings were reported in a study that also found that inconsistencies were somewhat dependent on the experience of the operator and the type of reagent strip. Inconsistencies were found among experienced technologists in up to 33% and among inexperienced technologists in up to 93%.[262]

The sensitivity and specificity of reagent strip protein tests have also been assessed by use of more accurate quantitative determinations as gold standards. Interestingly, the sensitivity of these tests appears to be higher when it is

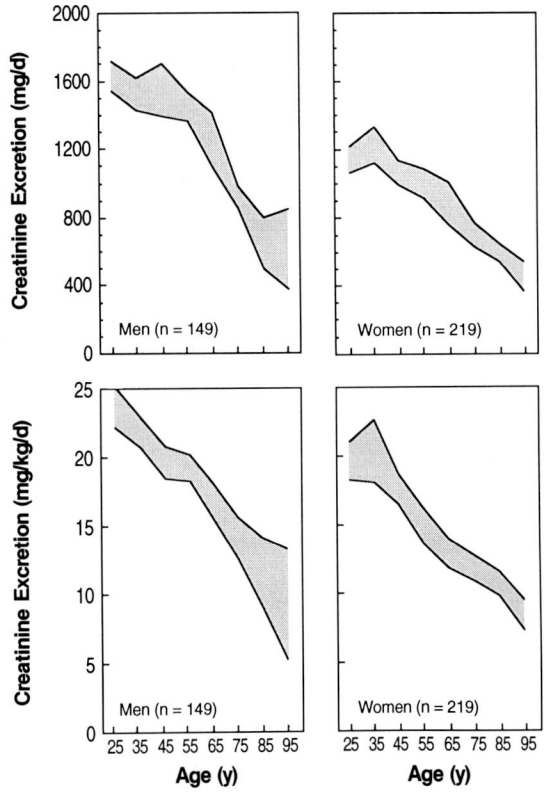

**Figure 26–4.** Age-related differences in urinary creatinine excretion in normal men *(left)* and women *(right).* Shaded areas represent 95% confidence intervals calculated from the data of Kampmann and co-workers.[92] Values in the upper panels are milligrams per day; values in the lower panels are milligrams per kilogram of body weight per day.

assessed with use of samples prepared by adding albumin and globulin to normal, protein-free urine than when it is assessed by use of actual specimens from patients.[261, 262] This no doubt reflects the inability of reagent strips to react to many of the heterogeneous proteins found in human urine. When 20 to 25 mg/dL is used as the limit of detection in clinical specimens, the sensitivity of reagent strips has been found to be only 32% to 46%, whereas the specificity was 97% to 100%.[261, 262] The effect of the sensitivity and specificity on the utility of these reagent strip tests is, of course, also dependent on the prevalence of proteinuria in the population being screened. In a population with a low prevalence of disease, the low sensitivity of the reagent strip tests suggests that the majority of individuals with proteinuria would be missed.[262]

Urinary albumin concentrations can be quantified by a number of techniques. The most commonly used include 1) radioimmunoassay, which can be carried out by a double-antibody technique. Albumin in a urine sample competes with a known amount of radiolabeled albumin for fixed binding sites of antibodies. Free albumin can be separated from bound albumin by immunoabsorption of the (albumin-bound) antibody. Albumin concentration in the sample is inversely proportional to the radioactivity.[263–265] 2) The immunoturbidimetric technique depends on the turbidity of a solution when albumin in a sample of urine reacts with a specific antibody. The turbidity is measured with a spectrophotometer, and the absorbance is proportional to the albumin concentration.[266, 267] 3) Albumin in the urine sample forms light-scattering antigen-antibody complexes when it reacts with a specific antibody. This can be measured with a laser nephelometer. The amount of albumin is proportional to scatter in the signal.[268, 269] 4) The competitive enzyme-linked immunosorbent assay has also been used to measure urinary albumin level.[270]

The correlation between most of these quantitative techniques is high. For example, the correlation coefficients ($r$ values) between radioimmunoassay and immunoturbidimetry and between radioimmunoassay and nephelometry were both .98.[271] Intra-assay coefficients of variation for immunoturbidimetry and nephelometry, respectively, were found to be 6.6% and 11.5% at low concentrations and 11.1% and 4.1% at high concentrations.[271] Interassay coefficients of variation were 11.4% and 11.5% at low concentrations and 5.4% and 1.4% at high concentrations for these two techniques, respectively.[271] In another study, the intra-assay coefficients of variation for radioimmunoassay and nephelometry were, respectively, 1.7% and 7.7% at low albumin concentrations and 3.7% and 6.3% at high albumin concentrations. Corresponding values for interassay coefficients of variation were 6.7% and 8.9%, and 8.1% and 11.0%.[272] The within-run coefficient of variation for an immunoturbidimetric method was found to be 3.5% at low and 2.4% at high albumin concentrations.[273] The day-to-day coefficient of variation for the same assay was 5.1% at low or high albumin concentrations.[273] These results are similar to those reported by others for the intra-assay and interassay coefficients of variation for nephelometric urinary albumin determinations.[274] Thus, the precision of these different methods appears to be similar, and choosing between them is largely determined by issues of accuracy, cost, and convenience.

Reagent strip methods have been developed to qualitatively screen for urinary albumin excretion. The Albustix (Bayer Diagnostik, Munich, Germany) reagent strip uses a protein error of indicators method that causes color changes in the presence of albumin.[272] Trace reactions indicate urinary albumin concentrations between 50 and 200 mg/L. Thus, more positive reactions can be used to indicate albumin concentrations higher than those generally found in patients with microalbuminuria. In one study,[272] the sensitivity and specificity of the Albustix were found to be only 81% and 55%, respectively. Thus, there was almost a 50% chance of a false-negative result with the Albustix method.

Screening methods have been developed to measure albumin concentrations low enough to detect albumin excretion rates that are abnormal but below the level of detection with standard reagent strips (i.e., in the microalbuminuria range).[271, 275–289] One of the most extensively investigated methods to screen for microalbuminuria is the immunometric dipstick Micral-Test (Boehringer Mannheim, Mannheim, Germany).[271, 276] The strip is made up of a series of reagent pads through which the urine sample passes sequentially. Urine is first drawn into a wick fleece and then passes into a buffer fleece that adjusts the sample pH. Next, it passes into a third pad where albumin in the sample is bound by a soluble conjugate of antibodies linked to the enzyme β-galactosidase. Excess antibody is then adsorbed on immobilized albumin in the next pad so that only albumin bound to antibody and enzyme reaches the color pad. There the β-galactosidase reacts with a chemical substrate to produce a red dye, the intensity of which is proportional to the bound albumin concentration. The test strip must be read at precisely 5 minutes.[271, 276]

Another qualitative test that has been examined in several investigations is the Micro-Bumintest (Ames, Miles Diagnostics Division, Elkhart, IN). This test uses a reagent tablet containing the indicator dye bromphenol blue. The intensity of the bluish green color produced after a drop of urine is placed on the surface of the tablet is proportional to the concentration of albumin.[271] A latex agglutination method, Albusure (Cambridge Life Sciences, Cambridge, UK), binds albumin in the urine sample to latex.[272] Agglutination occurs when the sample is mixed with sheep antihuman antibody. When urinary albumin concentrations are greater than 20 mg/L, agglutination is inhibited (antigen excess). Thus, agglutination indicates urinary albumin concentration below 20 mg/L.

A number of studies have examined the sensitivity and specificity of screening methods designed to detect low levels of albumin in urine.[271, 275–289] Because these tests are only semiquantitative (i.e., nonparametric), a true coefficient of variation cannot be determined. Nevertheless, in one evaluation of the Micral-Test method, an estimated coefficient of variation of the same sample interpreted by different technicians was 12.4%.[275] Experience in reading the Micral-Test was shown to be important.[288] Observer concordance for the Micro-Bumintest was found to be 95% in one study.[285]

Several studies have examined the sensitivity and specificity of the newer reagent strips that measure low concentrations of urinary albumin. Most of these investigations studied patients with diabetes, and most examined the Mi-

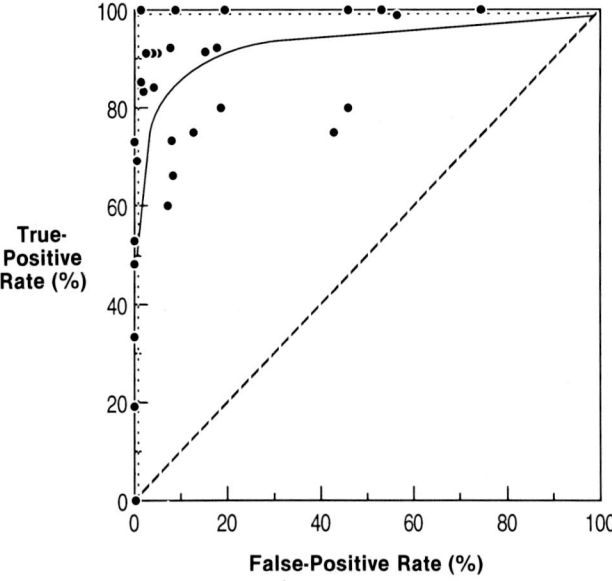

**Figure 26–5.** ROC curve for Micral-Test screening of urinary albumin concentrations generated by combining results from different studies of Albustix-negative diabetics. Each point represents data from a single study group using a different test cutoff (10 to 100 mg/L) for detecting an albumin concentration (20 to 50 mg/L) determined by radioimmunoassay in timed or untimed urine samples.[271, 276–280, 288] All points would be on the dotted line if the test were perfect, or on the dashed line if the test were worthless.

cral-Test,[271, 276–280, 288] the Micro-Bumintest,[271, 281–285, 287] or both. ROC curves were generated from the unweighted results of these investigations (Figs. 26–5 and 26–6) by use of the method of Hurlbut and Littenberg.[238] In general, these newer albumin reagent strip tests were more sensitive than standard dipsticks but also appeared to have a relatively high rate of false-positive results. Moreover, it should be remembered that these reagent strips were tested in populations of diabetic patients with a high prior probability of a positive result. The number of false-positive results would be expected to be much higher in populations where the prevalence of albuminuria was lower.

All of the qualitative or semiquantitative urinary protein and albumin screening tests discussed so far measure only total protein concentration or albumin concentration. The sensitivity and specificity of these tests can be markedly influenced by fluid intake, the state of diuresis, and the resulting urinary concentration. Indeed, in one study,[290] albumin concentration had a low discriminant value for detecting increased albumin excretion in a 12-hour timed urine sample (Fig. 26–7). In an effort to correct for problems arising out of variability in urine volume and concentration, many investigators have used the protein/creatinine or albumin/creatinine ratio in random or timed urine collections. There is a high degree of correlation between 24-hour urinary protein excretion and protein/creatinine ratios in random, single-voided urine samples in patients with a variety of renal disease.[291, 292] It has been suggested that a protein/creatinine ratio of greater than 3.0 or 3.5 mg/mg or less than 0.2 mg/mg indicates protein excretion rates of

greater than 3.0 or 3.5 g/24 h or less than 0.2 g/24 h, respectively.[291, 292] However, few studies have systematically examined the sensitivity and specificity or defined optimal levels of detection for protein/creatinine ratios in large numbers of patients in different clinical settings.

Many of the data on the usefulness of albumin/creatinine ratios have been derived from studies of patients with diabetes.[282, 290, 293–304] In most of these investigations, the sensitivity and specificity of albumin/creatinine ratios were determined with use of albumin excretion rates from timed urine collections as a standard. Data from several studies were combined to examine the true- and false-positive rates for albumin/creatinine ratios to detect albuminuria (greater than 30 μg/min) in overnight urine[295, 300–304] (Fig. 26–8). Independent of the albumin/creatinine ratio cutoff used, the sensitivities and specificities appeared to be reasonable (see Fig. 26–8). Altogether, these data suggest that albumin/creatinine ratios may be useful as a screening test for renal disease in populations where the expected prevalence of disease is high, such as in diabetes. Less clear is the potential usefulness of albumin/creatinine ratios in other populations of patients where the prior probability of disease may be different.[305]

Although protein/creatinine or albumin/creatinine ratios may be more quantitative than a simple dipstick screening procedure, their use has a number of limitations. For example, obtaining protein/creatinine or albumin/creatinine ratios on morning, first-void samples may underestimate 24-hour protein excretion because of the reduction in proteinuria that normally occurs at night. The fact that urinary creatinine level must be measured in addition to albumin

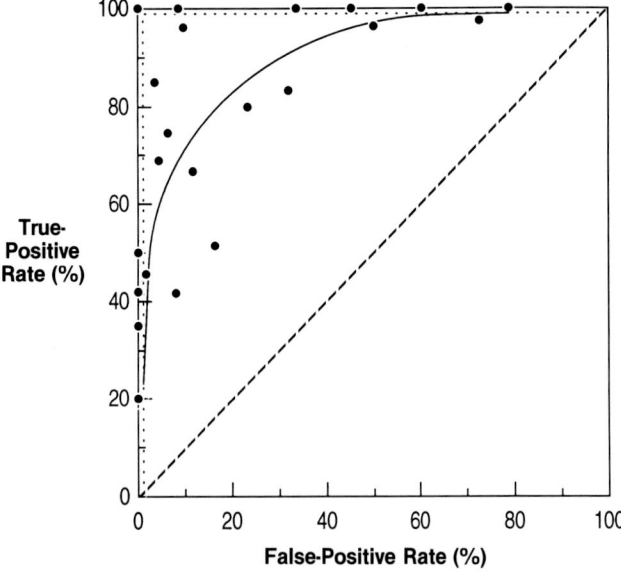

**Figure 26–6.** ROC curve for Micro-Bumintest screening of urinary albumin concentrations generated by combining results of different studies of Albustix-negative diabetics. Each point represents data from a single study group using a different test cutoff (1+ or 2+) for detecting an albumin concentration (20 to 50 mg/L) determined by radioimmunoassay in timed or untimed urine samples.[271, 281–285, 287] All points would be on the dotted line if the test were perfect, or on the dashed line if the test were worthless.

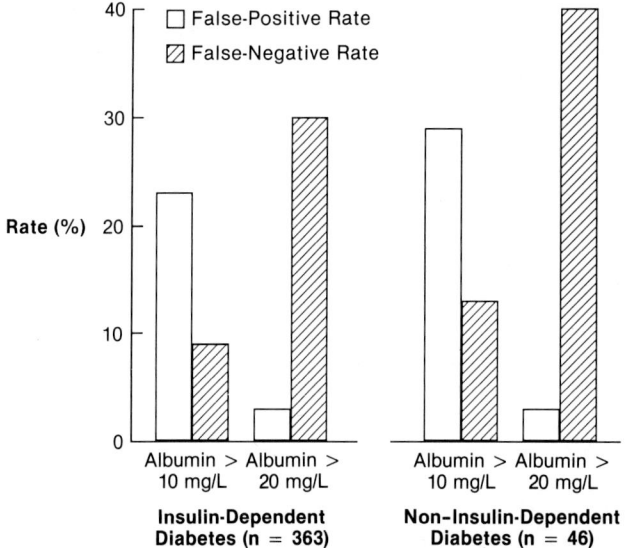

**Figure 26–7.** Comparison of false-positive and false-negative rates when urinary albumin concentration was used to predict 12-hour (overnight) excretion greater than 15 μg/min in diabetics. At a concentration cutoff greater than 10 mg/L, the false-positive rate is high. At a concentration cutoff greater than 20 mg/L, the false-positive rate is reduced, but the false-negative rate is high. (Data from Kouri TT, Viikari JSA, Mattila KS, Irjala KMA: Invalidity of simple concentration-based screening tests for early nephropathy due to urinary volumes of diabetic patients. Diabetes Care 14:591, 1991.)

introduces another source of error. Indeed, the errors of two measurements combined will be greater than the error of either one alone (the coefficient of variation is the square root of the sum of the two coefficients of variations, each squared). Urinary creatinine concentration is extremely variable, so different ratios can be obtained in individuals with similar protein excretion rates. Moreover, a number of variables that may interfere with creatinine determinations may affect the ratios.[306] Despite these limitations, the urinary protein/creatinine or albumin/creatinine ratio may be useful,

especially in individuals in whom urine collection is difficult or impossible.

A number of analytic tools have been developed to separate and identify individual urinary proteins.[307] These techniques include agarose gel electrophoresis, column gel chromatography, polyacrylamide gel electrophoresis, immunoelectrophoresis, and isoelectric focusing. Each of these techniques is generally designed to identify, but not accurately measure, urinary proteins. Some of the techniques have been used in clinical laboratories to determine the selectivity of urinary protein or to identify monoclonal immunoglobulin heavy and light chains. Otherwise, they have been largely confined to research applications.

## APPLICATIONS

### Screening for Renal Disease

Although measuring urinary protein level can be used to assist in the diagnosis of renal disease and to assess progression and response to therapy (discussed later), it is most commonly used as a screening test. Screening tests are generally applied to relatively large numbers of patients, so convenience and cost are major considerations. To make screening more convenient, a number of methods have been developed to measure urinary protein in a single-voided, or "spot," urine sample so that timed urine collections can be avoided.

Several questions regarding the use of urinary protein screening tests should be kept in mind. Are tests that measure albumin concentration more reliable than tests that measure urinary total protein, or is the greater sensitivity of albumin measurements matched by higher false-positive rates? Is the measurement of urinary albumin concentration in a single-voided sample, rather than in timed collections, sufficiently reliable to justify the reduced cost and enhanced convenience? Can protein/creatinine or albumin/creatinine ratios better estimate urinary protein excretion rate? Ideally, all screening tests should be judged by their ability to predict clinical outcomes and not by their ability to replace or

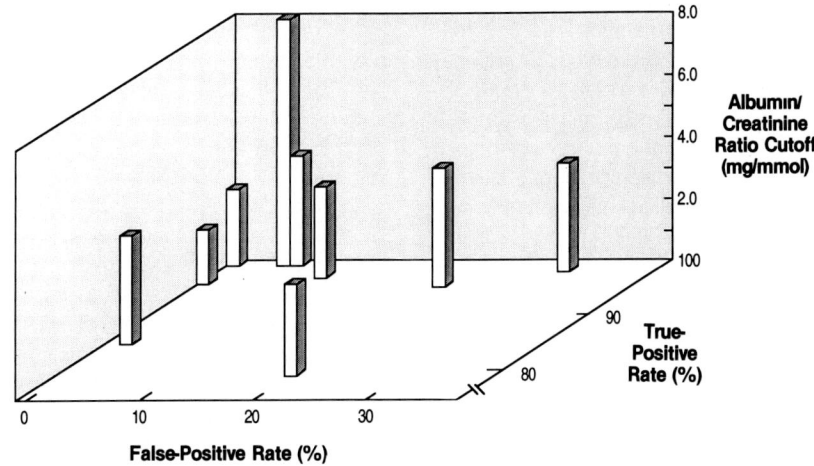

**Figure 26–8.** Relationship between true-positive rate (sensitivity), false-positive rate (1 − specificity), and albumin/creatinine ratio cutoff values used in different studies[295, 300–304] that each defined microalbuminuria as an albumin excretion rate of 30 μg/min in a timed overnight urine sample.

correlate with the results of other laboratory tests. However, most clinical studies examining the relationship between albuminuria and outcome have used radioimmunoassay to assess urinary albumin excretion. Thus, judging the potential usefulness of other screening tests requires their direct comparison with radioimmunoassay and inferring that their relationship to outcome will be similar.

In 1982, Viberti and co-workers[308] reported that clinical (Albustix-positive) proteinuria subsequently developed in patients with insulin-dependent diabetes who had albumin excretion rates of 30 to 140 μg/min measured by radioimmunoassay in timed overnight urine collections. In contrast, patients with rates less than 30 μg/min did not develop overt proteinuria.[308] Viberti[308] coined the term "microalbuminuria" to indicate increased urinary albumin excretion rates in patients with normal urinary total protein. A follow-up of the original cohort confirmed that the patients with microalbuminuria had not only a higher risk of developing overt proteinuria but also a greater risk of dying from cardiovascular disease.[309] Similar findings have been reported by others in patients with insulin-dependent and non–insulin-dependent diabetes.[310–314] Some investigators have used 15 to 150 μg/min,[314] whereas others have used 20 to 200 μg/min to define microalbuminuria.[310, 315] Microalbuminuria has also been defined as urinary albumin excretion of 30 to 300 mg/d.[249] Whatever definition is used, microalbuminuria appears to be an important risk factor for end-organ damage in patients with diabetes.

Most studies showing a relationship between microalbuminuria and end-organ damage have used quantitative techniques to measure urinary albumin excretion. Although few studies have examined whether other screening techniques predict outcome, there is no reason to believe that the results cannot be extrapolated to other screening tests, taking differences in sensitivity and specificity into account. Indeed, albumin/creatinine ratios have been shown to predict the subsequent development of overt renal disease. In a population of diabetic southwestern Native Americans, albumin/creatinine ratios of 0.03 to 0.30 mg/mg (microalbuminuria range) were a strong predictor of diabetic nephropathy.[293]

The recognition that microalbuminuria identifies diabetic patients at risk for subsequent renal and cardiovascular disease complications has given great impetus to the development of effective screening tools. Borch-Johnsen and co-workers,[315] using published data, carried out a critical appraisal of screening for microalbuminuria in patients with diabetes. Making a number of assumptions, they performed a cost-benefit analysis of the impact of screening and antihypertensive treatment. They concluded that screening and intervention programs are likely to lead to considerable reductions in cost and mortality.[315] Ultimately, the effects of such screening and intervention programs will need to be evaluated in actual clinical trials.

The use of dipstick tests for total protein excretion and microalbuminuria to screen for renal disease has not been rigorously examined in populations of nondiabetic patients. Epidemiologic data suggest that even in nondiabetic patients, proteinuria is a risk factor for cardiovascular disease,[316–320] perhaps because proteinuria is a sensitive indicator of renal damage. However strong these correlations

are statistically (low P value), the amount of unexplained variability (low r value) is great. This suggests that the sensitivity and specificity for proteinuria detection of renal injury in the general population could be too low to make this a useful screening tool in an individual patient. Nevertheless, data to assess this are generally not available for individuals who are not diabetic. Whether or not measuring urinary protein excretion in the general population is a cost-effective approach to the early detection of renal disease, such screening may be useful, combined with other clinical parameters, to estimate vascular disease risk. However, the prospective data needed to assess the utility of this application of urinary protein excretion are also incomplete.

The appropriate manner in which to use various tests to screen for renal disease has not been extensively investigated. Because the number of false-positive dipstick test results of protein excretion is high, a positive test result should probably be followed by tests designed to more accurately measure urinary protein excretion. However, in some clinical circumstances, the likelihood that a positive dipstick test result for urinary protein excretion indicates chronic renal disease is so low that the screening test should be repeated at a later date before more costly quantitation procedures are undertaken. A positive dipstick test result for protein in a patient with a urinary tract infection, for example, could be dismissed if subsequent results are negative when the infection has been treated. Fever can cause tubule and glomerular proteinuria that most often disappears when the fever resolves.[321–323] Congestive heart failure and seizures can also cause transient proteinuria.[324] Light or strenuous exercise is often associated with urinary protein excretion that resolves spontaneously.[325, 326]

It seems clear that even in the absence of identifiable causes of transient proteinuria, some individuals have increases in urinary protein excretion that are not associated with renal disease.[327] This proteinuria can be classified in two categories, intermittent and postural. Several dipstick measurements of urinary protein over time can be made to determine whether an individual patient fits in either of these two distinct patterns. Intermittent proteinuria is less well characterized than postural proteinuria, but it apears to be relatively benign in otherwise normal individuals. It has been shown, for example, that mortality after more than 40 years of follow-up of college students with intermittently positive results of urinary protein screens was no different from that of normal individuals.[328] However, few histologic studies including sufficiently large numbers of patients have been carried out to precisely characterize intermittent proteinuria.[329]

Posture can cause an increase in urinary protein excretion in otherwise normal individuals.[327, 330] This postural proteinuria should be distinguished from the increase in proteinuria seen in patients with renal disease who assume an upright posture. Postural proteinuria usually does not exceed 1 g/24 h. It is usually diagnosed by detecting protein excretion during the day that is absent at night while the patient is recumbent. Renal histology in patients with postural proteinuria is generally normal or nonspecific.[331–333] Patients with postural proteinuria have been shown to have an excellent long-term prognosis.[334] Indeed, six patients diagnosed by Thomas Addis had no evidence of renal disease after 42 to 50 years of follow-up.[335] Even in individuals without postural proteinuria or renal disease, levels of urinary protein excretion are lower at night than during the day.[336] Thus, the timing of urine collection is likely to influence the sensitivity and specificity of screening tests for urinary protein excretion.

### Diagnosis and Prognosis

Once proteinuria has been detected by screening, it is important not only to confirm the results of screening but also to precisely measure the amount of protein excretion in a timed urine collection. Quantifying urinary protein excretion may help distinguish glomerular from tubule proteinuria. If it is found, for example, that protein excretion is in the nephrotic range (e.g., greater than 3 g/24 h), a glomerular source is almost certain. Quantitation of urinary protein excretion may also provide useful prognostic information and assist in monitoring the response to therapy.

After detection and quantification, determining the composition of urinary protein may provide diagnostic information. An increased amount of albumin and high-molecular-weight proteins suggests glomerular proteinuria, whereas isolated increases in low-molecular-weight protein fractions are more suggestive of tubule proteinuria. It is unusual for tubule proteinuria to exceed 1 to 2 g/d, and only a small fraction of protein excretion due to tubule damage should be albumin. Tubule proteins are heterogeneous; however, $\beta_2$-microglobulin is often a major constituent.

$\beta_2$-Microglobulin is a small (molecular mass 11,800 daltons) protein that has been identified as the light chain of class I major histocompatibility antigens (e.g., human leukocyte antigens A, B, and C).[337] $\beta_2$-Microglobulin is most commonly measured in urine by radioimmunoassay or enzyme-linked immunosorbent assay. $\beta_2$-Microglobulin is freely filtered at the glomerulus and is avidly taken up and catabolized by the proximal tubule. Not surprisingly, therefore, urinary $\beta_2$-microglobulin levels have been associated with many pathologic conditions involving the proximal tubule. Aminoglycoside-induced kidney damage, Balkan endemic nephropathy, heavy metal nephropathies, radiocontrast nephropathy, and kidney transplant rejection are among the many acute and chronic tubulointerstitial nephropathies that are associated with increased urinary $\beta_2$-microglobulin levels.[338–343] $\beta_2$-Microglobulin has also been found to be useful in distinguishing upper from lower urinary tract infection.[344] Because urinary $\beta_2$-microglobulin is a nonspecific marker of renal tubule injury, it is not useful in differentiating among different causes of renal disease. However, when the likely cause is already known, measurement of $\beta_2$-microglobulin may be useful in detecting and monitoring injury. Nevertheless, the sensitivity and specificity for this test of tubule injury have generally not been established in different clinical situations where prior probabilities of various renal disorders may strongly influence its usefulness. Thus, the test may be useful in monitoring factory workers exposed to heavy metals when other causes of tubule injury could be expected to be uncommon. On the other hand, measuring $\beta_2$-microglobulin may be of limited value in diagnosing kidney transplant rejection when other causes of tubule injury are frequent.

Glomerular proteinuria can be further characterized as selective or nonselective.[345, 346] Patients with a clearance ratio of immunoglobulin G (a high-molecular-weight protein) to albumin that is less than 0.10 are said to have a selective glomerular proteinuria. Patients with immunoglobulin G/albumin clearance ratios of greater than 0.50 have a nonselective pattern. In general, selective proteinuria is more often seen in patients with minimal-change disease and suggests a good response to treatment with corticosteroids.[345, 346] The sensitivity and specificity of determining the selectivity of glomerular proteinuria have not been systematically examined in large numbers of patients with different renal disease. Moreover, the cost of the protein separation procedures has limited their widespread clinical use.

Plasma cell dyscrasias may produce monoclonal proteins, immunoglobulin, or free light chains. Light chains are filtered at the glomerulus and may appear in the urine as Bence Jones protein. The detection of urinary immunoglobulin light chains can be the first clue to a number of important clinical syndromes associated with plasma cell dyscrasias that involve the kidney.[347–349] Unfortunately, urinary immunoglobulin light chains may not be detected by reagent strip tests for protein. However, plasma cell dyscrasias may also present with proteinuria, or albuminuria, when the glomerular deposition of light chains causes disruption of the normally impermeable capillary wall.[350–353] The diagnosis of a plasma cell dyscrasia can be suspected when a tall, narrow band on electrophoresis suggests the presence of a monoclonal gamma globulin or immunoglobulin light chain.[354] However, monoclonal proteins are best detected by immunoelectrophoresis of serum and urine.[354]

Once patients have been screened and a diagnosis of renal disease has been established, measuring the amount of urinary protein excretion can provide additional prognostic information and can be used to monitor the response to therapy. The amount of urinary protein excretion has consistently been shown to predict subsequent disease progression in different clinical settings. For example, protein excretion correlated with progression in patients presenting with the nephrotic syndrome[355] and in patients with mild renal insufficiency of various causes.[356] Similar findings have been reported in patients with immunoglobulin A nephropathy,[357–360] membranous nephropathy,[357, 361, 362] and type I membranoproliferative glomerulonephritis.[357] The clinical course and effect of immunosuppressive therapy can also be monitored with sequential quantitation of urinary protein excretion.[363]

## Formed Elements

### MICROSCOPY METHODS

The examination of the urine by microscopy remains a useful qualitative and semiquantitative procedure. Efforts to measure formed elements in the urine more accurately have been made over the years.[364–368] For example, Addis[364, 369] measured excretion rates of erythrocytes using timed urine collections. However, formed elements can quickly deteriorate in the urine, and timed collections are difficult for most patients to carry out with accuracy. Moreover, the excretion rate of many formed elements correlates with urine concentration, so that often little additional information is gained from the effort made to collect timed specimens.[365] For all of these reasons, the use of timed collections to obtain excretion rates of formed elements has not gained widespread acceptance. Quantifying the number of formed elements can still be carried out with use of untimed specimens and a counting chamber.

A number of conditions affect formed elements in the urine, and when possible, these conditions should be optimized. Contamination with bacteria can be minimized with careful attention to collection technique. A midstream, ''clean-catch'' specimen should be collected when possible. Foreskin and labia should be retracted. A high urine concentration and a low urine pH help preserve formed elements.[369, 370] Thus, a first-void morning urine specimen, which is most likely to be acid and concentrated, should be used whenever possible. Strenuous exercise and bladder catheterization can cause hematuria, and urine specimens collected to detect hematuria should not be obtained under these conditions. Urine should be examined as soon as possible after collection to avoid lysis of the formed elements and bacterial overgrowth. The specimen should not be refrigerated because lowering the temperature causes the precipitation of phosphates and urates.

It is helpful to first measure the urine specific gravity and pH to judge the density of formed elements according to the concentration and acidity of the specimen. A greater density of formed elements may be expected in specimens from concentrated and acid urine than in dilute and alkaline specimens from the same patients. Urine should be centrifuged at approximately 2000 rpm for 5 to 10 minutes. The supernatant should be carefully poured off, the pellet resuspended by gentle agitation, and a drop placed on a slide under a coverslip.

Most commonly, urine is examined under an ordinary bright-field microscope. However, polarized light can be used to identify anisotropic crystals, and phase-contrast microscopy can enhance the contrast of cell membranes. The urine should first be examined under low power ($\times$ 100) to best judge the number of formed elements. These elements can then be examined in detail under high power ($\times$ 400). Generally, the urine is examined unstained. Stains can occasionally be helpful in distinguishing cell types.

## HEMATURIA

Gross hematuria may first be detected by a change in urine color. Microscopic hematuria can be detected by the dipstick method or microscopic examination. These methods may be applied as diagnostic tests in patients with known renal disease or as screening tools in normal or high-risk individuals. The sensitivity and specificity of screening tests for hematuria have not been thoroughly examined in many pertinent populations of patients. Moreover, the cost/benefit ratio of screening is often unclear.

The most cogent reason to screen for occult hematuria may be to facilitate the early and potentially life-saving detection of urologic malignant neoplasms. A dipstick test in more than 10,000 adult men undergoing health screening was found to give a positive result in about 2.5%.[371] About one fourth of those who were investigated had cystoscopic abnormalities, including bladder neoplasms in two. However, more than one third of those found to have occult hematuria in this retrospective study had not been investigated further. In a study of more than 2000 men, 4% were found to have occult hematuria. One of these patients was found to have bladder carcinoma.[372] Higher detection rates have been reported by others.[373, 374] On the basis of data such as these, the U.S. Preventive Services Task Force has recommended screening for occult hematuria for individuals older than 60 years to detect urologic malignant neoplasms.[227] The value of screening for occult hematuria in other populations is questionable,[375] and the role for occult hematuria screening to detect parenchymal renal disease is unclear.

Even when the urine is red, or when a dipstick screening test result is positive, the sediment should be examined to determine whether red blood cells are present. Other pigments, such as free hemoglobin and myoglobin, can masquerade as hematuria. In addition, red blood cells can be detected in the urine sediment when screening test results are negative. An occasional red blood cell can be seen in normal individuals, but generally only one or two per high-power field.

The differential diagnosis of hematuria is broad, but for practical purposes, hematuria can be categorized as originating in the upper or lower urinary tract. Hematuria that is accompanied by red blood cell casts or marked proteinuria is most likely to be glomerular in origin. In the absence of these important findings, distinguishing glomerular from postglomerular bleeding can be difficult. It has been reported that red blood cells originating in glomeruli have a distinctive dysmorphic appearance that is most readily appreciated by use of phase-contrast microscopy.[376–378] Automated blood cell analysis has also been used to determine the number of dysmorphic red blood cells in urine.[379–382] In vitro studies suggest that pH and osmolality changes found in the distal tubule could explain the increased number of dysmorphic red blood cells in patients with glomerular disease.[382–384]

The clinical utility of tests to distinguish dysmorphic red blood cells in the urine has been examined in several studies.[382, 385–393] Most investigators concluded that detecting dysmorphic red blood cells reliably predicted patients with glomerular disease; however, one investigator-blinded, controlled trial found unacceptable interobserver variability.[385] A meta-analysis of 21 published studies using predetermined criteria for evaluation of dysmorphic red blood cells in urine was carried out.[394] All studies originated in referral centers. The weighted average sensitivity and specificity for dysmorphic red blood cell test detection of glomerular disease were (with 95% confidence intervals) 88% (86% to 91%) and 95% (93% to 97%), respectively. The sensitivity and specificity for the use of abnormal (automated) red blood cell volumes to detect glomerular disease were 100% (98% to 100%) and 87% (80% to 91%). These authors concluded that the negative predictive value of these tests were probably not sufficient to rule out important urologic lesions, especially in a referral setting where the prevalence of urologic disease may be relatively high. The sensitivity and specificity of these tests in primary care patients with low-grade hematuria have not been assessed. The use of automated determinations of cell size in individuals with low-grade hematuria may be particularly unreliable because of interference from cell debris.

## LEUKOCYTURIA

The number of white blood cells that can normally be found in the urine is controversial. A conservative approach is to consider more than one per high-power field to be abnormal. The differential diagnosis of leukocyturia is broad. White blood cells can enter the urine from anywhere along the excretory system. The presence of proteinuria and casts may suggest a glomerular source. In the absence of proteinuria and casts, the clinician must look beyond the urine sediment for additional clues to find the origin of leukocytes in the urine. There are no effective methods to identify the origin of white blood cells found in the urine. Contamination is a common cause of leukocyturia that should always be considered in the absence of other suggestive clinical findings.

Most often, leukocytes in the urine are polymorphonuclear. However, it should not be assumed that all urinary leukocytes are neutrophils. The presence of non-neutrophil white blood cells in the urine, for example, eosinophils, can sometimes be an important diagnostic clue. The association between eosinophiluria and drug-induced hypersensitivity reactions was first reported by Eisenstaedt[395] in 1951. Since then, a number of investigators have reported the association between eosinophiluria and renal disease.[396–402] The Wright stain can be used to detect urinary eosinophils, but a urine pH less than 7 inhibits this stain.[403] The use of the Hansel stain improves the sensitivity of urinary eosinophil detection over the standard Wright stain.[397, 402] In one retrospective investigation, the use of the Hansel stain compared with the Wright stain improved the sensitivity of using the presence of any urinary eosinophils for detecting acute interstitial nephritis from 25% to 63%.[402] The positive predictive value was improved from 25% to 50%.[402] However, not all patients in this study underwent renal biopsy to establish the diagnosis of interstitial nephritis, and the retrospective inclusion of only patients in whom urinary eosinophils were sought by clinicians makes interpretation of these data difficult. The true sensitivity and specificity of urinary eosinophils for detecting different clinical renal diseases are unclear. Indeed, the list of diseases that may be associated with eosinophiluria is long and continues to grow (Table 26–4). Moreover, the sensitivity and specificity of eosinophiluria in detecting renal disease can be expected to vary with the threshold value used.[399] The ROC curves for different numbers or percentages of white blood cells that are eosinophils have not been examined.

## OTHER CELLS

It is difficult to identify the origin of cells that are neither leukocytes nor red blood cells without special stains. Most common are probably squamous epithelial cells. They shed

**TABLE 26–4. Diseases Associated with Eosinophiluria**

**Common**
Acute allergic interstitial nephritis[395, 397, 398, 402, 404, 405]
Urinary tract infection (upper and lower tract)[399]

**Unusual**
Acute tubule necrosis[399]
Diabetic nephropathy[399]
Focal segmental glomerulosclerosis[399]
Polycystic kidney disease[399]
Obstruction[399]
Rapidly progressive glomerulonephritis[397]
Postinfectious glomerulonephritis[397, 399]
Immunoglobulin nephropathy[399]
Acute cystitis[397]
Acute prostatitis[397]
Atheroembolic renal disease[400]
Kidney transplant rejection[406, 407]

from the bladder or urethra and are rarely pathologic. Renal tubule cells may appear whenever there has been tubule damage. Transitional epithelial cells are rare but may be seen with collecting system infection or neoplasias.

## FAT

In the absence of contamination, urinary lipids almost always indicate a pathologic condition.[408, 409] On the other hand, lipids are not usually seen as an isolated finding, and the presence of urinary lipid is rarely diagnostic. Lipids usually appear as free fat droplets or oval fat bodies. They have a distinctive appearance but are most readily seen under polarized light as doubly refractile Maltese crosses. The Maltese cross is indicative of cholesterol and cholesterol esters. Maltese crosses can also be seen with some crystals and with starch granules.[410] Neutral fat can be identified with special lipid stains. Urinary lipids are most commonly associated with proteinuria and are particularly common in patients with the nephrotic syndrome. However, urinary lipids may also occur in the absence of heavy proteinuria.[411] Urinary lipids can also be seen in bone marrow or fat embolization syndromes.

## CASTS

Casts are cylindric bodies severalfold larger than leukocytes and red blood cells. They form in distal tubules and collecting ducts where Tamm-Horsfall glycoprotein precipitates and entraps cells present in the urinary space.[412] Dehydration and the resulting increased tubule fluid concentration favor the formation of casts. An acid urine is also conducive to cast formation. Observing casts in the urine sediment often provides helpful diagnostic information. The differential diagnosis of cast formation is aided by first considering the type of cast found. A number of different types can be readily distinguished (Fig. 26–9).

Hyaline or finely granular casts can be seen in normal individuals and provide little useful diagnostic information. Cellular casts are generally more helpful. Red blood cell casts, for example, are distinctive and most often indicate glomerular disease. White blood cell casts are most com-

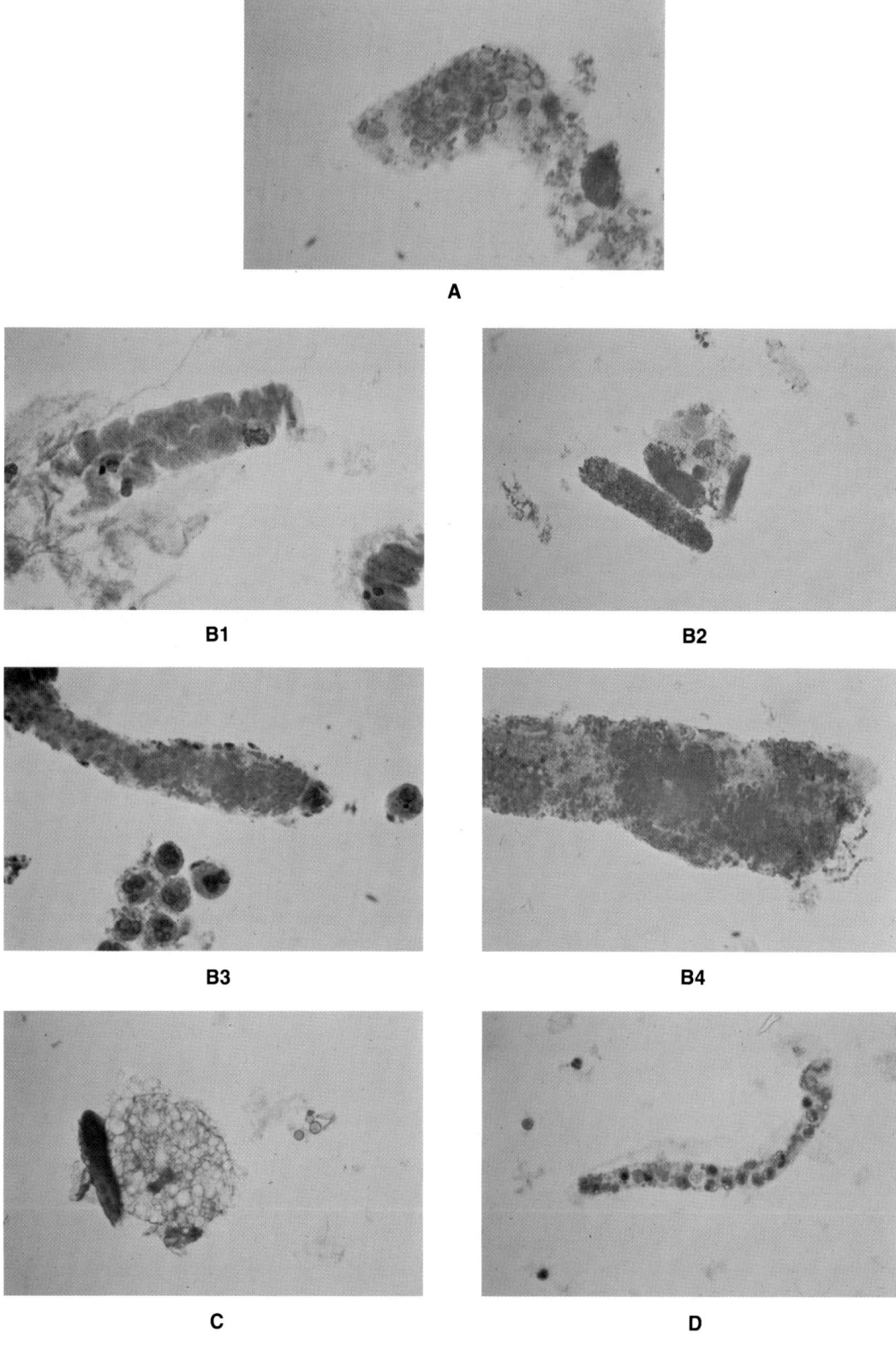

**Figure 26–9.** Abnormalities in urine sediment stained to enhance detail. *A.* Red blood cell cast (× 900). *B.* Hyaline cast (× 900). *C.* Hyaline and granular casts (× 400). *D.* Coarse granular cast with adjacent white blood cells (× 750). *E.* Fine and coarse granular cast (× 900). *F.* Oval fat body with adjacent hyaline cast (× 400). *G.* White blood cell cast (× 400).

monly associated with interstitial nephritis. However, white blood cell casts can also be seen in glomerulonephritis. Casts made up of renal tubule epithelial cells are always indicative of tubule damage. Coarsely granular casts often result from the degeneration of different cellular casts. They also contain protein aggregates. Thus, the presence of granular casts is usually pathologic but nonspecific. Waxy casts are also nonspecific. They are thought to result from the degeneration of cellular casts and, thus, can be seen in a variety of renal diseases. Pigmented casts usually derive their distinctive color from bilirubin or hemoglobin. They are found in hyperbilirubinemia and hemoglobinuria, respectively. Fatty casts contain lipid and oval fat bodies (see earlier).

## CRYSTALS AND OTHER ELEMENTS

A large variety of crystals can be seen in the urine sediment. Most result from urine concentration, acidification, and ex vivo cooling of the sample and have little pathologic significance. However, an experienced observer can gain useful information in patients with microhematuria, nephrolithiasis, or toxin ingestion by examining a freshly voided, warm specimen.[413] For example, a large number of calcium oxalate crystals may suggest toxic effects of ethylene glycol in the right clinical setting. Calcium oxalate crystals are uniform, small, double pyramids that often appear as crosses in a square. Calcium phosphate crystals, on the other hand, are usually narrow rectangular needles, often clumped in a flower-like configuration. Uric acid crystals are reddish brown, rectangular or rhomboid, and also frequently seen in flower-like clumps. Calcium magnesium ammonium pyrophosphate (so-called triple phosphate) crystals form domed rectangles that take on the appearance of coffin lids.

## MICROORGANISMS

The most common cause of bacteria in the urine is contamination. This is particularly true of specimens that have been improperly collected. The concomitant presence of leukocytes, however, suggests infection. Fungal elements can also be seen, especially in women. Like bacteria, fungi can be contaminants or pathogens. The most common protozoan seen in the urine is *Trichomonas vaginalis*. Urinary parasites are generally not seen in the urine sediment. In Africa and the Middle East, however, *Schistosoma haematobium* is common.

## RENAL BIOPSY

### Overview

Percutaneous renal biopsy was first performed by Ball[414] in 1934 using an aspiration technique. The next consistent attempt at biopsy of the kidney appears to be that of Alwall[415] in 1944, although his results were not reported until 1952. The biggest impetus to the use of renal biopsy came from reports of Perez-Ara[416] in 1950 followed shortly thereafter by Iversen and Brun,[417] which showed that per-

cutaneous renal biopsy can be safe and useful. The technique described by Kark and Muehrcke[418] in 1954 is similar to that commonly used today. The introduction of the Franklin modified Vim-Silverman needle and the initial localization of the kidney with a small atraumatic needle resulted in a better core of tissue and an improved success rate.[419] Since these initial reports, the major advances that have occurred center around improved localization of the kidney by use of ultrasound technology[420] and the introduction of more automated and smaller biopsy needles. Improved methods of tissue processing and staining and the correlation of the light microscopic studies with those of electron microscopy[421] and immunofluorescence techniques[422] have led to dramatic increases in our knowledge of renal disease.

A renal biopsy may be performed to help establish the diagnosis, suggest prognosis, or direct therapy. The information obtained from a biopsy is mostly qualitative. Although morphometric techniques have been developed to quantify histopathologic alterations, these techniques have been used almost exclusively in research. Even in this setting, there are few data comparing the reproducibility of different techniques to quantify renal biopsy results. The reliability of the National Institutes of Health histologic scoring system for lupus nephritis was shown to be only moderately reproducible in a nonreferral setting.[423] Probably as important, there are virtually no data that clearly indicate which specific renal histopathologic finding predicts progression of structural injury. In general, the relationship between the extent of tubulointerstitial and vascular damage is better correlated with the level of renal function than is the extent of glomerular injury. A number of studies have inversely correlated the extent of tubulointerstitial damage and fibrosis with renal function in a variety of renal diseases.[424–426] Because biopsy results are largely qualitative, the sensitivity and specificity of biopsy findings are often unclear.

In this section, we discuss the technical aspects of the renal biopsy, what information can be gained from a detailed histopathologic study of the biopsy specimen, and the current indications for renal biopsy.

## Specific Indications

During the past 40 years, the renal biopsy has been most instrumental in the development of our understanding of the various types of renal histopathologic abnormalities that contribute to abnormalities of the urine sediment. The use of this technique not only has improved our diagnostic acumen but also has given new insights into the pathogenesis of human renal disease. However, as our sophistication and knowledge of the various forms of renal disease have expanded, questions regarding the routine use of renal biopsy in all patients with clinical evidence of kidney disease have been articulated. In one study by Paone and Meyer,[427] a retrospective evaluation of whether the biopsy result influenced therapeutic judgments was performed. Although a definite or probable diagnosis was ascertained in 77% of patients, therapy was modified in only 19%. In large part, changes in therapy were confined to patients with proteinuria, with little influence on therapy in those who had hematuria. Although therapy was also unaltered in those who had acute or chronic renal disease, it should be underscored that therapy for these indications is relatively nonspecific. Similarly, Cohen and associates[428] and Turner and colleagues[429] reported the influence of the renal histopathologic results on physicians' judgments regarding diagnosis, prognosis, and treatment in patients with diverse types of renal disease. They reported changes in judgments for more than half of patients as a result of information gained directly from the biopsy results. In contrast, Whiting-O'Keefe and co-workers[430] retrospectively analyzed the case histories of 30 patients who underwent renal biopsy for severe lupus nephritis. Knowledge of the renal biopsy results failed to improve predictive accuracy scores of estimates of future serum creatinine levels, urinary protein levels, renal death, and long-term immunosuppressive therapy.

Questions about the role of renal biopsy in patients with idiopathic nephrotic syndrome have also emerged.[431–434] Levey and colleagues,[434] using decision analysis, concluded that initial therapy based on clinical data alone could avoid the use of renal biopsy in all patients. However, this technique has not been uniformly embraced, and additional studies detailing outcomes for patients, quality of life, and complications of therapeutic misadventures are needed before universal application of decision analysis. It is also important to recognize that the technique of renal biopsy in today's environment is relatively safe and inexpensive; it provides a specific diagnosis and is an efficient way to define a therapeutic strategy. At present, there are no specific clinical indications that mandate the use of renal biopsy, and its utility must be taken in the context of the patient's needs in terms of diagnosis, prognosis, and therapy. Nonetheless, there are clinical settings in which renal biopsy seems more valuable than not. In the following, we provide some guidelines that may be used in defining the relative clinical value of a renal biopsy.

## NEPHROTIC SYNDROME

The causes of the nephrotic syndrome are many, and the laboratory parameters consistent with this diagnosis are discussed elsewhere. The nephrotic syndrome is either primary or secondary; the secondary forms reflect either a systemic disease or a toxic drug effect. Once the secondary forms of the nephrotic syndrome are excluded by appropriate clinical or laboratory data, there remains a group of patients with idiopathic nephrotic syndrome who can be precisely differentiated only by renal biopsy. This category includes minimal-change glomerulopathy, focal glomerulosclerosis, and membranous nephropathy. In the adult, the distribution of these entities is different from that in the pediatric age group, and different approaches have emerged as a result. In children with the idiopathic nephrotic syndrome, a renal biopsy is generally not performed initially, and empirical steroid therapy is initiated. This is in large part due to the fact that minimal-change glomerulopathy, which is sensitive to steroid therapy, accounts for nearly 80% of cases in children.[435–437] However, in children who fail to respond to an appropriate course of steroids or have frequent relapses during a period of a year, a renal biopsy may become

indicated. This would allow specific diagnosis and the potential for tailoring therapy with more potent immunosuppressive therapy. In the adult patient, minimal-change disease is responsible for 20% to 25% of cases; thus, a propensity for performance of a renal biopsy has traditionally been followed.[427, 438] The goals for therapy as well as disease-specific protocols have evolved in the past few years and have made the rationale for an initial biopsy more compelling.

In patients with elevated levels of circulating or urinary light chains in association with nephrotic range proteinuria, a renal biopsy is frequently of use in distinguishing between amyloid and light chain glomerulopathy. In the presence or absence of multiple myeloma, the detection of light chain deposits in the renal biopsy specimen appears to have prognostic and therapeutic implications.[439]

## SYSTEMIC LUPUS ERYTHEMATOSUS

The diagnosis of systemic lupus erythematosus is generally established by a variety of clinical and laboratory criteria. Rarely may the diagnosis first be suggested by the biopsy,[440, 441] particularly when the result of laboratory testing is negative.[442–444] However, the yield of renal biopsy in this clinical situation is low, and the amount of information obtained that would have an impact on therapy is relatively small.[443] Renal involvement in systemic lupus erythematosus correlates with overall prognosis: the more severe the renal involvement, the worse the prognosis.[445, 446] In systemic lupus erythematosus, the principal glomerular lesion is cellular proliferation, which is variably present in amount and distribution. These changes have most frequently formed the basis for a number of histologic classifications,[447–450] the World Health Organization classification representing the most commonly used today. The World Health Organization classification is correlated with clinical features such as hypertension, urine sediment, degree of proteinuria, and reduction in glomerular filtration rate as well as with prognosis. In this system, patients with minimal proliferative glomerular changes have the best prognosis, whereas those with diffuse proliferative changes have the worst prognosis.[445, 451, 452] In patients with diffuse proliferative glomerular changes, immunosuppressive therapy with high-dose prednisone has consistently demonstrated improved survival of the kidney and the patient, although no prospective trial has been performed.[450, 453–455] It has been proposed that the biopsy results in this form of systemic lupus erythematosus may help in the selection of the dose and route of administration of steroids as well as the selection of other immunosuppressive drugs. However, this has not been proved in controlled trials. Some investigators,[430, 447, 456–459] but not others,[423, 460, 461] have found the morphologic findings of activity or chronicity of glomerular and interstitial lesions are related to the risk of subsequent progression of renal disease independent of their correlation with clinical indicators of severity of renal disease. In addition, the intraobserver variability when these approaches are used in routine clinical settings makes their utility marginal at best.[423] Currently, it appears that the addition of more sophisticated quantitative analysis adds little to selection of therapy or prognostication of outcomes. Chagnac and co-workers[462] have performed morphometric studies of glomerular capillary surface area on serial biopsy specimens obtained from patients with systemic lupus erythematosus. They reported evidence of progressive loss of glomerular capillary surface area with no change or minimal changes in proteinuria, glomerular filtration rate, or serum creatinine. These studies would suggest that the renal biopsy findings may be a more sensitive index of progression than clinical features alone are. However, the lack of standardization of morphometric analysis and the time required to perform these studies do not allow their routine histopathologic use.

## RAPIDLY PROGRESSIVE GLOMERULONEPHRITIS

In patients with abnormalities of the urine sediment consistent with a nephritic syndrome and rapidly progressive loss of renal function, a renal biopsy may provide invaluable information. Frequently, patients with this syndrome demonstrate the histologic presence of crescents. Ellis[463] is credited with first noting the relationship between the loss of renal function and the presence of glomerular crescents. Although the number of glomeruli with crescents is variable, most clinical studies that have evaluated outcomes report a poor renal prognosis when the proportion of glomeruli with circumferential crescents exceeds 50%.[464, 465] The pathogenesis of rapidly progressive–crescenteric glomerulonephritis is diverse and is most commonly seen with three types of immunologic injury: anti–glomerular basement membrane antibody with or without pulmonary hemorrhage (Goodpasture syndrome), immune complex disease, and the so-called pauci-immune glomerulonephritis. This last entity is the most frequently diagnosed disease, particularly when systemic illnesses are excluded. The recognition of the association between antineutrophilic cytoplasmic antibodies, systemic vasculitic syndromes, and pauci-immune crescenteric glomerulonephritis has provided new and important insights into the understanding of the pathogenesis of this disease as well as therapeutic strategies that are clinically useful.[466] Nonetheless, the renal biopsy may still provide important information regarding the severity of disease and, thus, has clinical management implications.

## POST-TRANSPLANTATION BIOPSY

The biopsy of the transplanted kidney has been established as an important diagnostic and therapeutic technique in the management of patients in whom rejection of the renal allograft is suspected. This has become particularly important in the era in which cyclosporine is commonly used.[467–469] Although a variety of histologic techniques including fine-needle aspiration cytology and monoclonal antibody staining of needle core biopsies have been suggested, the standard needle core biopsy processed for conventional histology remains the most reliable biopsy technique for the diagnosis of rejection of renal allografts.[470] Recurrence of the original glomerulopathy in the transplanted kidney has been observed with a variety of renal diseases.[471–474] Other than focal glomerulosclerosis, most of the other recurrent glomerulopathies appear to have little functional impact on the renal allograft.[471–474]

## Possible Indications

### ASYMPTOMATIC URINARY ABNORMALITIES

The finding of low levels of isolated proteinuria is a common clinical problem. In a survey of 68,000 army recruits without a history of hypertension or renal disease, 1% were found to have isolated proteinuria.[331] Of the 45 patients who had a biopsy, 33 (73%) had mild mesangial proliferation with or without glomerulosclerosis. If the proteinuria was intermittent or postural, notable glomerular lesions were infrequent. No lesion was serious enough to warrant therapy. Although no changes in renal function were noted during a 3-year interval, longer term follow-up has not been reported. At present, there is no evidence that a renal biopsy provides better prognostication than evaluating the pattern of proteinuria and routine clinical follow-up do.

Isolated hematuria is a frequent clinical problem that occurs as commonly as isolated proteinuria.[475] Frequently, routine evaluation of the urinary tract will indicate the nonrenal source of the hematuria, and renal biopsy is not an issue. However, as an alternative to a long and involved invasive radiologic evaluation and even surgery, a renal biopsy has been proposed as an accurate and direct way of identifying a diagnosis.[476] Renal biopsy is abnormal in more than 75% of patients with hematuria in whom proteinuria or reduced renal function is present.[476–478] In this setting, immunoglobulin A nephropathy is the most common diagnosis, although hereditary nephritis or thinning of the glomerular basement membrane is also seen.[476, 477] Proven, effective, and specific therapy for such entities as immunoglobulin A nephropathy has not as yet been developed; thus, the utility of the biopsy to guide therapy has not been shown. Although a number of histopathologic changes predict renal outcomes, several clinical features, such as reduced renal function, proteinuria, and hypertension, accurately predict a poor prognosis.[478–483] Thus, at present, additional therapeutic or prognostic information is not gained from a renal biopsy.

### OTHER INDICATIONS

There does not appear to be any indication for a renal biopsy in patients with chronic, end-stage renal failure, and they are at risk for considerable morbidity.[484] In patients with acute renal failure in whom no obvious cause for rapid deterioration in renal function can be found, a case for renal biopsy has been made.[485] In our experience, the value in this setting appears to be mostly for those few patients with acute allergic interstitial nephritis in whom a course of corticosteroids may be of benefit. Cholesterol embolic acute renal failure without the typical clinical presentation has been observed more frequently in older patients with atherosclerotic disease and presents a diagnostic challenge. Because some of these patients may regain renal function after prolonged intervals, closer attention to renal function while they are undergoing dialysis is appropriate. However, a clear-cut case for the utility of a renal biopsy for diagnosis, prognosis, or therapy has not been made in patients with acute renal failure.

Patients with diabetes mellitus may occasionally be considered for renal biopsy, particularly when they present with severe proteinuria in the absence of other manifestations of diabetic microvascular disease or when the duration of the disease is short. In this setting, the idiopathic nephrotic syndrome has usually been observed.[486, 487]

## Percutaneous Procedure

### PREPARATION OF THE PATIENT

Before biopsy, the patient should be evaluated for conditions that may increase the risk for or consequences of complications. Because postbiopsy bleeding can necessitate nephrectomy, the consequences of this complication are greater in patients with only one functioning kidney. In addition, it is often ill-advised to perform biopsy of a small, shrunken kidney. Therefore, it is useful to use one or more radiologic procedures to assess the functional renal anatomy of a biopsy candidate. This can be accomplished with either a radionuclide scan or ultrasonography.

Because bleeding is the major complication of biopsy, most clinicians obtain a coagulation profile. A platelet count, prothrombin time, partial thromboplastin time, and bleeding time can be used to screen for bleeding tendencies. Although the exact correlation between abnormalities in these coagulation screening tests and postbiopsy bleeding is not known, prudence would dictate that biopsies should be carried out with great reluctance in patients with coagulation abnormalities. Probably the most frequently encountered abnormality is a prolonged bleeding time caused by platelet dysfunction in patients who are uremic. A number of steps can be taken to correct the prolonged bleeding time associated with uremia. These include the use of fresh frozen plasma, arginine vasopressin, and estrogens.[488–491] If the patient is acutely uremic, hemodialysis is usually of value in improving the coagulopathy. A low hemoglobin level that would substantially increase the risk of bleeding should also be corrected before a renal biopsy is undertaken.

Uncontrolled hypertension may also increase the risk of biopsy. Therefore, it is advisable to control blood pressure before the procedure is undertaken. Some investigators believe that the presence of a nontransplanted solitary kidney is only a relative contraindication to renal biopsy,[429, 493] but most consider it an absolute contraindication.[494] Voiding immediately before the biopsy may help reduce the risk of inadvertently puncturing the bladder. Because a major complication of biopsy may require surgical intervention, it may be advisable to carry out the procedure with the patient fasting to reduce the potential risks of vomiting and aspiration during anesthesia induction. However, these risks must be weighed against the risk of hypoglycemia in patients with diabetes.

### LOCALIZATION

There are no controlled studies comparing the use of different radiographic localization techniques for percutaneous renal biopsy. Indeed, there are insufficient objective data to conclude that any localization technique reduces the risk of complications or increases the likelihood of success. Therefore, empirical logic must be used to justify the additional expense and inconvenience of a radiographic procedure to guide renal biopsy.

X-ray fluoroscopy can be used, but adequate imaging of the kidneys often requires intravenous administration of contrast media, which can be nephrotoxic. Computed tomography can be used, but the inability to guide the biopsy needle in ''real time'' makes the procedure somewhat cumbersome.[495, 496] Ultrasonography with continuous visualization of the biopsy needle usually provides adequate imaging.[420, 497, 498] A renal biopsy using ultrasound visualization can be done efficiently and is less costly than computed tomography.

### NEEDLE SELECTION

In the past, the Tru-Cut (Travenol) needle and the Franklin modified Vim-Silverman needle were most commonly used to perform percutaneous renal biopsies. More recently, automatic, spring-loaded biopsy devices have been developed.[499–505] There have not been any large, prospective studies comparing the use of different biopsy needles. However, uncontrolled data suggest that the new automated devices may reduce the occurrence of postbiopsy bleeding without reducing the chances of obtaining adequate tissue.[499, 500]

### PROCESSING OF THE SPECIMEN

Proper interpretation of a renal biopsy specimen optimally requires examination by light, immunofluorescence, and electron microscopy. Placement of tissue in appropriate fixatives immediately is important for obtaining the best histologically stained material. The availability of a pathologist experienced in processing renal specimens is particularly helpful in preparing adequate renal tissue. In general, obtaining two cores of cortical tissue usually provides sufficient material for all examinations. Each core is divided longitudinally with a razor blade to obtain glomeruli in each section. The majority of the tissue is processed for light microscopy and the remainder for immunofluorescence and electron microscopy.

There are numerous fixatives for histologic preparation, and tissue for light microscopy is usually fixed in paraffin or plastic and cut in 2-µm-thick sections, which are routinely stained with hematoxylin and eosin, a silver methenamine stain, and a periodic acid–Schiff or trichrome stain. If amyloidosis is suspected, Congo red and thioflavine T stains are performed.

Tissue for immunofluorescence microscopy is placed in precooled isopentane and snap frozen in liquid nitrogen. Frozen sections are cut 4 µm in thickness and typically stained with fluoresceinated antisera against immunoglobulin G, immunoglobulin M, immunoglobulin A, C3, C4, fibrin/fibrinogen, and albumin. When indicated, antibodies for specific immunoglobulin light chains or specific cell surface markers can be used.

For electron microscopic studies, small (1-mm) pieces of the biopsy specimen are fixed in buffered glutaraldehyde or other suitable fixatives, dehydrated in graded alcohols, embedded in plastic, and sectioned. Ultrathin sections are stained with uranyl acetate and lead citrate and examined with a transmission electron microscope.

## Complications

The most common complication of a renal biopsy is hematuria.[494] Microscopic hematuria occurs in virtually all patients, whereas gross hematuria occurs in 5% to 9% of patients. Gross hematuria has also been associated with intrarenal arteriovenous fistulas.[506] The presence of uncontrolled hypertension or azotemia increases the risk for hematuria.[494, 506, 507] Hematuria usually resolves spontaneously in 48 to 72 hours, although in approximately 0.5% of patients, it persists for 2 to 3 weeks.[494, 506] Occasionally, gross hematuria occurs days after the biopsy, but it usually resolves within a few days with rest.[494] Transfusions are necessary in 0.1% to 3% of patients.[494, 507] Surgery for persistent bleeding is required in less than 0.3% of patients.[494, 506–509]

Perinephric hematomas occur commonly. In patients evaluated immediately after renal biopsy by computed tomography, hematomas were detected in 57% to 85% of patients.[510–512] Most of these are clinically occult and may be associated only with a fall in hemoglobin level.[494, 507] In 1% to 2% of patients, perinephric hematoma is manifested by flank pain and swelling associated with signs of volume contraction and a decrease in hematocrit. Rarely, these hematomas can become infected and require antibiotic therapy and surgical drainage.[506]

Less common complications of renal biopsy include arteriovenous fistulas, aneurysms, and infections. Arteriovenous fistulas can be demonstrated by arteriography in 15% to 18% of patients.[513–519] They are usually clinically silent, and the majority spontaneously resolve in 2 years.[513] Postbiopsy aneurysms have been reported in less than 1% of patients.[494] Infections are unusual except in the presence of pyelonephritis. The development of sepsis and bacteremia after renal biopsy has been reported.[520] A number of unusual complications of renal biopsy have been reported, including ileus, lacerations of other abdominal organs, pneumothorax, ureteral obstruction, and dissemination of carcinoma.[508, 509, 521, 522] The mortality associated with 14,492 reported renal biopsies is 0.12%.[506]

## REFERENCES

1. Peirce JC, Cornell RG: Integrating stratum-specific likelihood ratios with the analysis of ROC curves. Med Decis Making 13:141, 1993.
2. Centor RM: Signal detectability: The use of ROC curves and their analyses. Med Decis Making 11:102, 1991.
3. Smith HW: The Kidney: Structure and Function in Health and Disease. Oxford University Press, New York, 1951, pp 63–66.
4. Möller E, McIntosh JF, Van Slyke DD: Studies of urea excretion. II. Relationship between urine volume and the rate of urea excretion by normal adults. J Clin Invest 6:427, 1929.
5. Rickers H, Brøchner-Mortensen J, Rødbro P: The diagnostic value of plasma urea for assessment of renal function. Scand J Urol Nephrol 12:39, 1978.
6. Chasis H, Smith WH: The excretion of urea in normal man and in subjects with glomerulonephritis. J Clin Invest 17:347, 1938.
7. Steinitz K, Türkand H: The determination of the glomerular filtration by the endogenous creatinine clearance. J Clin Invest 19:285, 1940.
8. Veterans Administration Cooperative Study Group on Antihypertensive Agents: Comparison of propranolol and hydrochlorothiazide treatment in hypertension: I. Results of short-term titration with emphasis on racial differences in response. JAMA 248:1996, 1982.
9. Thomas RD, Newill A, Morgan DB: The cause of the raised plasma urea of acute heart failure. Postgrad Med J 55:10, 1979.
10. Cohn TD, Lane M, Zuckerman S, et al: Induced azotemia in humans following massive protein and blood ingestion and the mechanism of azotemia in gastrointestinal hemorrhage. Am J Med Sci 231:394, 1956.
11. Cottini EP, Gallina DL, Dominguez JM: Urea excretion in adult humans with varying degrees of kidney malfunction fed milk, egg or amino acid mixture: Assessment of nitrogen balance. J Nutr 103:11, 1973.
12. Maroni BJ, Steinman TI, Mitch WE: A method for estimating nitrogen intake of patients with chronic renal failure. Kidney Int 27:58, 1985.
13. Shils ME: Renal disease and the metabolic effects of tetracycline. Ann Intern Med 58:389, 1963.
14. Shaper AG, Popcock SJ, Ashby D, et al: Biochemical and haematological response to alcohol intake. Ann Clin Biochem 22:50, 1985.
15. Young DS: Effects of Drugs on Clinical Laboratory Tests, 3rd ed. American Association for Clinical Chemistry Press, Washington, DC, 1990, pp 3-356–3-357.
16. Young DS: Effects of Drugs on Clinical Laboratory Tests, 3rd ed. American Association for Clinical Chemistry Press, Washington, DC, 1990, p 3-359.
17. Lubowitz H, Slatopolsky E, Shankel S, et al: Glomerular filtration rate: Determination in patients with chronic renal disease. JAMA 199:252, 1967.
18. Lavender S, Hilton PJ, Jones NF: The measurement of glomerular filtration rate in renal disease. Lancet 2:1216, 1969.
19. Heymsfield SB, Arteaga C, McManus C, et al: Measurement of muscle mass in humans: Validity of the 24-hour urinary creatinine method. Am J Clin Nutr 37:478, 1983.
20. Kaw DG, Levy E, Kahn T: Decrease of urine creatinine in vitro in spinal cord injury patients. Clin Nephrol 30:216, 1988.
21. Fitch CD, Sinton DW: A study of creatine metabolism in diseases causing muscle wasting. J Clin Invest 43:444, 1964.
22. Horber FF, Scheidegger J, Frey FJ: Overestimation of renal function in glucocorticoid treated patients. Eur J Clin Pharmacol 28:537, 1985.
23. Cocchetto DM, Tschanz C, Bjornsson TD: Decreased rate of creatinine production in patients with hepatic disease: Implications for estimation of creatinine clearance. Ther Drug Monit 5:161, 1983.
24. Rowe JW, Andres R, Tobin JD, et al: The effect of age on creatinine clearance in men: A cross-sectional and longitudinal study. J Gerontol 31:155, 1976.
25. James GD, Sealey JE, Alderman M, et al: A longitudinal study of urinary creatinine and creatinine clearance in normal subjects: Race, sex, and age differences. Am J Hypertens 1:124, 1988.
26. Walser M: Creatinine excretion as a measure of protein nutrition in adults of varying age. JPEN 11:73S, 1987.
27. Bleiler RE, Schendl HP: Creatinine excretion: Variability and relationships to diet and body size. J Lab Clin Med 59:945, 1962.
28. Crim MC, Calloway DH, Margen S: Creatine metabolism in men: Creatine pool size and turnover in relation to creatine intake. J Nutr 106:371, 1976.
29. Lew SQ, Bosch JP: Effect of diet on creatinine clearance and excretion in young and elderly healthy subjects and in patients with renal disease. J Am Soc Nephrol 2:856, 1991.
30. Hoogwerf BJ, Laine DC, Greene E: Urine C-peptide and creatinine (Jaffe method) excretion in healthy young adults on varied diets: Sustained effects of varied carbohydrate, protein, and meat content. Am J Clin Nutr 43:350, 1986.
31. Jacobsen FK, Christensen CK, Mogensen CE, et al: Pronounced increase in serum creatinine concentration after eating cooked meat. Br Med J 1:1049, 1979.

32. Mayersohn M, Conrad KA, Achari R: The influence of a cooked meat meal on creatinine plasma concentration and creatinine clearance. Br J Clin Pharmacol 15:227, 1983.

33. Shannon JA: The renal excretion of creatinine in man. J Clin Invest 14:403, 1935.

34. Olsen NV, Ladefoged SD, Feldt-Rasmussen B, et al: The effects of cimetidine on creatinine excretion, glomerular filtration rate and tubular function in renal transplant recipients. Scand J Clin Lab Invest 49:155, 1989.

35. Dubb JW, Stote RM, Familiar RG, et al: Effect of cimetidine on renal function in normal man. Clin Pharmacol Ther 24:76, 1978.

36. Burgess E, Blair A, Krichman K, Cutler RE: Inhibition of renal creatinine secretion by cimetidine in humans. Renal Physiol 5:27, 1982.

37. Berglund F, Killander J, Pompeius R: Effect of trimethoprim-sulfamethoxazole on the renal excretion of creatinine in man. J Urol 114:802, 1975.

38. Myre SA, McCann J, First MR, Cluxton RJ Jr: Effect of trimethoprim on serum creatinine in healthy and chronic renal failure volunteers. Ther Drug Monit 9:161, 1987.

39. Opravil M, Keusch G, Lüthy R: Pyrimethamine inhibits renal secretion of creatinine. Antimicrob Agents Chemother 37:1056, 1993.

40. Sjöström PA, Odlind BG, Wolgast M: Extensive tubular secretion and reabsorption of creatinine in humans. Scand J Urol Nephrol 22:129, 1988.

41. Levey AS, Berg RL, Gassman JJ, et al: Creatinine filtration, secretion and excretion during progressive renal disease. Kidney Int 36(suppl 27):S-73, 1989.

42. Shemesh O, Golbetz H, Kriss JP, Myers BD: Limitations of creatinine as a filtration marker in glomerulopathic patients. Kidney Int 28:830, 1985.

43. Mitch WE, Collier VU, Walser M: Creatinine metabolism in chronic renal failure. Clin Sci 58:327, 1980.

44. Mitch WE, Walser M: A proposed mechanism for reduced creatinine excretion in severe chronic renal failure. Nephron 21:248, 1978.

45. Jones JD, Burnett PC: Creatinine metabolism in humans with decreased renal function: Creatinine deficit. Clin Chem 20:1204, 1974.

46. Hankins DA, Babb AL, Uvelli DA, Scribner BH: Creatinine degradation: I: The kinetics of creatinine removal in patients with chronic kidney disease. Int J Artif Organs 4:35, 1981.

47. Hare RS: Endogenous creatinine in serum and urine. Proc Soc Exp Biol Med 74:148, 1950.

48. Bonsnes RW, Taussky HH: On the colorimetric determination of creatinine by Jaffé reaction. J Biol Chem 158:581, 1945.

49. Mandel EE, Jones FL: Studies in nonprotein nitrogen: III. Evaluation of methods measuring creatinine. J Lab Clin Med 41:323, 1953.

50. Fabiny DL, Ertingshausen G: Automated reaction-rate method for determination of serum creatinine with the Centritichem. Clin Chem 17:696, 1971.

51. Toffaletti J, Blosser N, Hall T, et al: An automated dry-slide enzymatic method evaluated for measurement of creatinine in serum. Clin Chem 29:684, 1983.

52. Folin O, Wu H: A system of blood analysis. J Biol Chem 38:81, 1919.

53. Jaffé M: Über den Niederschlag welchen Pikrinsaure in normalen Harn erzeugt und über eine neue Reaction des Kreatinins. Z Physiol Chem 10:391, 1886.

54. Jacobs DS, De Mott WR, Strobel SL, Fody EP: Chemistry. In Jacobs DS, Kasten BL, De Mott WR, Wolfson WL (eds): Laboratory Test Handbook, 2nd ed. Williams & Wilkins, Baltimore, 1990, pp 171–172.

55. Gerard SK, Khayam-Bashi H: Characterization of creatinine error in ketotic patients: A prospective comparison of alkaline picrate methods with an enzymatic method. Am J Clin Pathol 84:659, 1985.

56. Mascioli SR, Bantle JP, Freier EF, Hoogwerf BJ: Artifactual elevation of serum creatinine level due to fasting. Arch Intern Med 144:1575, 1984.

57. Mali B, Nicholas PC: Jaffes' reaction for creatinine: Kinetic study and spectrophotometric characteristics of the product of the reactions of creatinine, acetoacetate and creatinine and acetoacetate with alkaline picrate. Biochem Soc Trans 16:549, 1988.

58. Young DS: Effects of Drugs on Clinical Laboratory Tests, 3rd ed. American Association of Clinical Chemistry Press, Washington, DC, 1990, p 3-128.

59. Kroll MH, Hagengruber C, Elin RJ: Reaction of picrate with creatinine and cepha antibiotics. Clin Chem 30:1664, 1984.

60. Saah AJ, Koch TR, Drusano GL: Cefoxitin falsely elevates creatinine levels. JAMA 247:205, 1982.

61. Swain RR, Briggs SL: Positive interference with the Jaffé reaction by cephalosporin antibiotics. Clin Chem 23:1340, 1977.

62. Durham SR, Bignell AHC, Wise R: Interference of cefoxitin in the creatinine estimation and its clinical relevance. J Clin Pathol 32:1148, 1979.

63. Doolan PD, Alpen EL, Theil GB: A clinical appraisal of the plasma concentration and endogenous clearance of creatinine. Am J Med 32:65, 1962.

64. Osberg IM, Hammond KB: A solution to the problem of bilirubin interference with the kinetic Jaffé method for serum creatinine. Clin Chem 24:1196, 1978.

65. Gerard S, Khayam-Bashi H: Negative interference with the Ektachem (Kodak) enzymic assay for creatinine by high serum glucose. Clin Chem 30:1884, 1984. Letter.

66. Kennedy CA, Goetz MB, Mathisen G: Artifactual elevation of the serum creatinine in patients receiving flucytosine for cryptococcal meningitis. J Infect Dis 160:1090, 1989.

67. Noble MA, Harper B, Grant AG, Bernstein M: Rapid determination of 5-fluorocytosine levels in blood. J Clin Microbiol 20:996, 1984.

68. Herrington D, Drusano GL, Smalls U, Standiford HC: False elevation in serum creatinine levels. JAMA 252:2962, 1984. Letter.

69. Kasiske BL: Creatinine excretion after renal transplantation. Transplantation 48:424, 1989.

70. DeSanto NG, Coppola S, Anastasio P, et al: Predicted creatinine clearance to assess glomerular filtration rate in chronic renal disease in humans. Am J Nephrol 11:181, 1991.

71. Morgan DB, Dillon S, Payne RB: The assessment of glomerular function: Creatinine clearance or plasma creatinine? Postgrad Med J 54:302, 1978.

72. Dodge WF, Travis LB, Daeschner CW: Comparison of endogenous creatinine clearance with inulin clearance. Am J Dis Child 113:683, 1967.

73. Payne RB: Creatinine clearance: A redundant clinical investigation. Ann Clin Biochem 23:243, 1986.

74. Brod J, Sirota JH: The renal clearance of endogenous "creatinine" in man. J Clin Invest 27:645, 1948.

75. Rapoport A, Husdan H: Endogenous creatinine clearance and serum creatinine in the clinical assessment of kidney function. Can Med Assoc J 99:149, 1968.

76. Bauer JH, Brooks CS, Burch RN: Renal function studies in man with advanced renal insufficiency. Am J Kidney Dis 2:30, 1982.

77. Healy JK: Clinical assessment of glomerular filtration rate by different forms of creatinine clearance and a modified urinary phenolsulphonphthalein excretion test. Am J Med 44:348, 1968.

78. Fuller NJ, Elia M: Factors influencing the production of creatinine: Implications for the determination and interpretation of urinary creatinine and creatine in man. Clin Chim Acta 175:199, 1988.

79. Carrie BJ, Golbetz HV, Michaels AS, Myers BD: Creatinine: An inadequate filtration marker in glomerular diseases. Am J Med 69:177, 1980.

80. van Acker BAC, Koomen GCM, Koopman MG, et al: Discrepancy between circadian rhythms of inulin and creatinine clearance. J Lab Clin Med 120:400, 1992.

81. Sirota JH, Baldwin DS, Villarreal H: Diurnal variations of renal function in man. J Clin Invest 29:187, 1950.

82. Pasternack A, Kuhlbäck B: Diurnal variations of serum and urine creatine and creatinine. Scand J Clin Lab Invest 27:1, 1971.

83. Rosano TG, Brown HH: Analytical and biological variability of serum creatinine and creatinine clearance: Implications for clinical interpretation. Clin Chem 28:2330, 1982.

84. Bröchner-Mortensen J, Rödbro P: Selection of routine method for determination of glomerular filtration rate in adult patients. Scand J Clin Lab Invest 36:35, 1976.

85. van Acker BAC, Koomen GCM, Koopman MG, et al: Creatinine clearance during cimetidine administration for measurement of glomerular filtration rate. Lancet 340:1326, 1992.

86. Roubenoff R, Drew H, Moyer M, et al: Oral cimetidine improves the accuracy and precision of creatinine clearance in lupus nephritis. Ann Intern Med 113:501, 1990.

87. Hilbrands LB, Artz MA, Wetzels JFM, Koene RAP: Cimetidine improves the reliability of creatinine as a marker of glomerular filtration. Kidney Int 40:1171, 1991.

88. Hellerstein S, Alon U, Blowey D, et al: Use of serum creatinine

KASISKE and KEANE • LABORATORY ASSESSMENT OF RENAL DISEASE 1167

concentration for estimation of glomerular filtration rate. Am J Dis Child 147:719, 1993.

89. Hirata-Dulas CAI, Halstenson CE, Kasiske BL: Improvement in the accuracy and precision of creatinine clearance as a measure of glomerular filtration rate with oral cimetidine in renal transplant recipients. Clin Transpl 7:552, 1993.

90. Richter JM, Colditz GA, Huse DM, et al: Cimetidine and adverse reactions: A meta-analysis of randomized clinical trials of short-term therapy. Am J Med 87:278, 1989.

91. Cockcroft DW, Gault MH: Prediction of creatinine clearance from serum creatinine. Nephron 16:31, 1976.

92. Kampmann J, Siersbæk-Nielson K, Kristensen M, Mølholm-Hansen J: Rapid evaluation of creatinine clearance. Acta Med Scand 196:517, 1974.

93. Sinton TJ, De Leacy EA, Cowley DM: Comparison of $^{51}$Cr EDTA clearance with formulae in the measurement of glomerular filtration rate. Pathology 18:445, 1986.

94. Gault MH, Longerich LL, Harnett JD, Wesolowski C: Predicting glomerular function from adjusted serum creatinine. Nephron 62:249, 1992.

95. Sawyer WT, Canaday BR, Poe TE, et al: A multicenter evaluation of variables affecting the predictability of creatinine clearance. Am J Clin Pathol 78:832, 1982.

96. Trollfors B, Alestig K, Jagenburg R: Prediction of glomerular filtration rate from serum creatinine, age, sex and body weight. Acta Med Scand 221:495, 1987.

97. Bjornsson TD, Cocchetto DM, McGowan FX, et al: Nomogram for estimating creatinine clearance. Clin Pharmacokinet 8:365, 1983.

98. Taylor GO, Bamgboye EA, Oyediran ABOO, Longe O: Serum creatinine and prediction formulae for creatinine clearance. Afr J Med Sci 11:175, 1982.

99. Gates GF: Creatinine clearance estimation from serum creatinine values: An analysis of three mathematical models of glomerular function. Am J Kidney Dis 5:199, 1985.

100. Jelliffe RW: Creatinine clearance: Bedside estimate. Ann Intern Med 79:604, 1973.

101. Rolin HA III, Hall PM, Wei R: Inaccuracy of estimated creatinine clearance for prediction of iothalamate glomerular filtration rate. Am J Kidney Dis 4:48, 1984.

102. Walser M, Drew HH, Guldan JL: Prediction of glomerular filtration rate from serum creatinine concentration in advanced chronic renal failure. Kidney Int 44:1145, 1993.

103. Norden G, Björck S, Granerus G, Nyberg G: Estimation of renal function in diabetic nephropathy—comparison of five methods. Nephron 47:36, 1987.

104. Waz WR, Feld LG, Quattrin T: Serum creatinine, height, and weight do not predict glomerular filtration rate in children with IDDM. Diabetes Care 16:1067, 1993.

105. Levey AS: Measurement of renal function in chronic renal disease. Kidney Int 38:167, 1990.

106. Smith HW, Goldring W, Chasis H: The measurement of tubular excretory mass, effective blood flow and filtration rate in the normal human kidney. J Clin Invest 17:263, 1938.

107. Levey AS: Use of glomerular filtration rate measurements to assess the progression of renal disease. Semin Nephrol 9:370, 1989.

108. Davies DF, Shock NW: The variability of measurement of inulin and Diodrast tests of kidney function. J Clin Invest 29:491, 1950.

109. Schnurr E, Lahme W, Küppers H: Measurement of renal clearance of inulin and PAH in the steady state without urine collection. Clin Nephrol 13:26, 1980.

110. Rosenbaum RW, Hruska KA, Anderson C, et al: Inulin: An inadequate marker of glomerular filtration rate in kidney donors and transplant recipients? Kidney Int 16:179, 1979.

111. Brøchner-Mortensen J: Current status on assessment and measurement of glomerular filtration rate. Clin Physiol 5:1, 1984.

112. Pihl B: The single injection technique for determination of renal clearance. V. A comparison with the continuous infusion technique in the dog and in man. Scand J Urol Nephrol 8:147, 1974.

113. Russell CD, Bischoff PG, Rowell KL, et al: Quality control of Tc-99m DTPA for measurement of glomerular filtration: Concise communication. J Nucl Med 24:722, 1983.

114. Carlsen JE, Moller ML, Lund JO, Trap-Jensen J: Comparison of four commercial Tc-99m(Sn)DTPA preparations used for the measurement of glomerular filtration rate: Concise communication. J Nucl Med 21:126, 1980.

115. Brun C, Hilden T, Raaschou F: The significance of the difference in systemic arterial and venous plasma concentrations in renal clearance methods. J Clin Invest 28:144, 1949.

116. Robson JS, Ferguson MH, Olbrich O, Stewart CP: The determination of the renal clearance of inulin in man. Q J Exp Physiol 35:111, 1949.

117. Sapirstein LA, Vidt DG, Mandel MJ, Hanusek G: Volumes of distribution and clearance of intravenously injected creatinine in the dog. Am J Physiol 181:330, 1955.

118. Bianchi C, Donadio C, Tramonti G: Noninvasive methods for the measurement of total renal function. Nephron 28:53, 1981.

119. Farmer CD, Tauxe WN, Maher FT, Hunt JC: Measurement of renal function with radioiodinate diatrizoate and o-iodohippurate. Am J Clin Pathol 467:9, 1967.

120. Ditzel J, Vestergaard P, Brinkløv M: Glomerular filtration rate determined by $^{51}$Cr-EDTA-complex. Scand J Urol Nephrol 6:166, 1972.

121. Garnett ES, Parsons V, Veall N: Measurement of glomerular filtration rate in man using a $^{51}$Cr–edetic-acid complex. Lancet 1:818, 1967.

122. Chantler C, Garnett ES, Parsons V, Veall N: Glomerular filtration rate measurement in man by the single injection method using $^{51}$Cr-EDTA. Clin Sci 37:169, 1969.

123. Hagstam KE, Nordenfelt I, Svensson L, Svensson SE: Comparison of different methods for determination of glomerular filtration rate in renal disease. Scand J Clin Lab Med 34:31, 1974.

124. Chantler C, Barratt TM: Estimation of glomerular filtration rate from plasma clearance of 51-chromium edetic acid. Arch Dis Child 47:613, 1972.

125. Gaspari F, Mosconi L, Viganò G, et al: Measurement of GFR with a single intravenous injection of nonradioactive iothalamate. Kidney Int 41:1081, 1992.

126. Russell CD, Bischoff PG, Kontzen FN et al: Measurement of glomerular filtration rate: Single injection plasma clearance method without urine collection. J Nucl Med 26:1243, 1985.

127. Groth T, Tengström B: A simple method for the determination of glomerular filtration rate. Scand J Clin Lab Invest 37:39, 1977.

128. Tauxe WN: Determination of glomerular filtration rate by single sample technique following injection of radioiodinated diatrizoate. J Nucl Med 27:45, 1986.

129. Tepe PG, Tauxe WN, Bagchi A, et al: Comparison of measurement of glomerular filtration rate by single sample, plasma disappearance slope/intercept and other methods. Eur J Nucl Med 13:28, 1987.

130. Al-Uzri A, Holliday MA, Gambertoglio JG, et al: An accurate practical method for estimating GFR in clinical studies using a constant subcutaneous infusion. Kidney Int 41:1701, 1992.

131. Barbour G, Crumb CK, Boyd CM, et al: Comparison of inulin, iothalamate, and $^{99m}$Tc-DTPA for measurement of glomerular filtration rate. J Nucl Med 17:317, 1976.

132. Sanger JJ, Kramer EL: Radionuclide quantitation of renal function. Urol Radiol 14:69, 1992.

133. Russell CD, Bischoff PG, Kontzen F, et al: Measurement of glomerular filtration rate using $^{99m}$Tc-DTPA and the gamma camera: A comparison of methods. Eur J Nucl Med 10:519, 1985.

134. Goates JJ, Morton KA, Whooten WW, et al: Comparison of methods for calculating glomerular filtration rate: Technetium-99m–DTPA scintigraphic analysis, protein-free and whole-plasma clearance of technetium-99m–DTPA and iodine-125–iothalamate clearance. J Nucl Med 31:424, 1990.

135. Mak RHK, Dahhan JA, Azzopardi D, et al: Measurement of glomerular filtration rate in children after renal transplantation. Kidney Int 23:410, 1983.

136. Brøchner-Mortensen J: Routine methods and their reliability for assessment of glomerular filtration rate in adults. Dan Med Bull 25:181, 1978.

137. Bailey RR, Rogers TGH, Tait JJ: Measurement of glomerular filtration rate using a single injection of $^{51}$Cr-edetic acid. Australas Ann Med 3:255, 1970.

138. Lingårdh G: Renal clearance investigations with $^{51}$Cr-EDTA and $^{125}$I-Hippuran. Scand J Urol Nephrol 6:63, 1972.

139. Brøchner-Mortensen J, Giese J, Rossing J: Renal inulin clearance versus total plasma clearance of $^{51}$Cr-EDTA. Scand J Clin Lab Invest 23:301, 1969.

140. Griep RJ, Nelp WB: Mechanism of excretion of radioiodinated sodium iothalamate. Radiology 93:807, 1969.

141. Anderson CF, Sawyer TK, Cutler RE: Iothalamate sodium I-125 vs

cyanocobalamin Co-57 as a measure of glomerular filtration rate in man. JAMA 204:105, 1968.

142. Cohen ML, Smith FG Jr, Mindell RS, Vernier RL: A simple reliable method of measuring glomerular filtration rate using single, low-dose sodium iothalamate I[131]. Pediatrics 43:407, 1969.

143. Elwood CM, Sigman EM, Treger C: The measurement of glomerular filtration rate with [125]I–sodium iothalamate (Conray). Br J Radiol 40:581, 1967.

144. Hauser W, Atkins HL, Nelson KG, Richards P: Technetium-99m DTPA: A new radiopharmaceutical for brain and kidney scanning. Radiology 94:679, 1970.

145. Dubovsky EV, Russell CD: Quantitation of renal function with glomerular and tubular agents. Semin Nucl Med 12:308, 1982.

146. Bianchi C, Bonadio M, Donadio C, et al: Measurement of glomerular filtration rate in man using DTPA-[99m]Tc. Nephron 24:174, 1979.

147. Stabin M, Taylor A Jr, Eshima D, Wooter W: Radiation dosimetry for technetium-99m–MAG3, technetium-99m DTPA, and iodine-131–OIH based on human biodistribution studies. J Nucl Med 33:33, 1992.

148. Smith T, Veall N, Altman DG: Dosimetry of renal radio pharmaceuticals: The importance of bladder radioactivity and a simple aid for its estimation. Br J Radiol 54:961, 1981.

149. Prueksaritanont T, Chen ML, Chiou WL: Simple and micro high-performance liquid chromatographic method for simultaneous determination of p-aminohippuric acid and iothalamate in biological fluids. J Chromatogr 306:89, 1984.

150. O'Reilly PH, Brooman PJC, Martin PJ, et al: Accuracy and reproducibility of a new contrast clearance method for the determination of glomerular filtration rate. BMJ 293:234, 1986.

151. O'Reilly PH, Jones DA, Farah NB: Measurement of the plasma clearance of urographic contrast media for the determination of glomerular filtration rate. J Urol 139:9, 1988.

152. Stake G, Monclair T: A single plasma sample method for estimation of the glomerular filtration rate in infants and children using iohexol, I: Establishment of a body weight–related formula for the distribution volume of iohexol. Scand J Clin Lab Invest 51:335, 1991.

153. Stake G, Monn E, Rootwelt K, Monclair T: A single plasma sample method for estimation of the glomerular filtration rate in infants and children using iohexol, II: Establishment of the optimal plasma sampling time and a comparison with the [99]Tc[m]-DTPA method. Scand J Clin Lab Invest 51:343, 1991.

154. Stake G, Monn E, Rootwelt K, Monclair T: The clearance of iohexol as a measure of the glomerular filtration rate in children with chronic renal failure. Scand J Clin Lab Invest 51:729, 1991.

155. Stake G, Monn E, Rootwelt K, et al: Glomerular filtration rate estimated by X-ray fluorescence technique in children: Comparison between the plasma disappearance of [99]Tc[m]-DTPA in iohexol after urography. Scand J Clin Lab Invest 50:161, 1990.

156. Brown SCW, O'Reilly PH: Iohexol clearance for the determination of glomerular filtration rate in clinical practice: Evidence for a new gold standard. J Urol 146:675, 1991.

157. Lewis R, Kerr N, Van Buren C, et al: Comparative evaluation of urographic contrast media, inulin, and [99m]Tc-DTPA clearance methods for determination of glomerular filtration rate in clinical transplantation. Transplantation 48:790, 1989.

158. Manske CL, Sprafka JM, Strony JT, Wang Y: Contrast nephropathy in azotemic diabetic patients undergoing coronary angiography. Am J Med 89:615, 1990.

159. Schrott VKM, Behrends B, Clauss W, et al: Iohexol in der Ausscheidungsurographie. Fortsch Med 104:153, 1986.

160. Wesson LG Jr: Renal hemodynamics in physiological states. In Wesson LG Jr (ed): Physiology of the Human Kidney. Grune & Stratton, New York, 1969, pp 96–154.

161. MacKay EM: Kidney weight, body size and renal function. Arch Intern Med 50:590, 1932.

162. McCance RA, Widdowson EM: The correct physiological basis on which to compare infant and adult renal function. Lancet 2:860, 1952.

163. Du Bois D, Du Bois EF: A formula to estimate the approximate surface area if height and weight are known. Arch Intern Med 17:863, 1916.

164. Newman EV, Bordley J, Winternitz J: The interrelationships of glomerular filtration rate (mannitol clearance), extracellular fluid volume, surface area of the body, and plasma concentration of mannitol. Johns Hopkins Med J 75:253, 1944.

165. White AJ, Strydom WJ: Normalisation of glomerular filtration rate measurements. Eur J Nucl Med 18:385, 1991.

166. Feldschuh J, Enson Y: Prediction of the normal blood volume. Circulation 56:605, 1977.

167. Brown BE, Hopper J Jr, Hodges JL Jr, et al: Red cell, plasma, and blood volume in healthy women measured by radiochromium cell-labeling and hematocrit. J Clin Invest 41:2182, 1962.

168. Wennesland R, Brown E, Hopper J Jr, et al: Red cell, plasma and blood volume in healthy men measured by radiochromium (Cr[51]) cell tagging and hematocrit: Influence of age, somatotype and habits of physical activity on the variance after regression of volumes to height and weight combined. J Clin Invest 38:1065, 1959.

169. Nyengaard JR, Bendtsen TF: Glomerular number and size in relation to age, kidney weight, and body surface in normal man. Anat Rec 232:194, 1992.

170. Kasiske BL, Umen AJ: The influence of age, sex, race, and body habitus on kidney weight in humans. Arch Pathol Lab Med 110:55, 1986.

171. Boer P: Estimated lean body mass as an index for normalization of body fluid volumes in humans. Am J Physiol 247:F632, 1984.

172. Bogardus C, Lillioja S, Ravussin E, et al: Familial dependence of the resting metabolic rate. N Engl J Med 315:96, 1986.

173. Ford LE: Some consequences of body size. Am J Physiol 247:H495, 1984.

174. King AJ, Levey AS: Dietary protein and renal function. J Am Soc Nephrol 3:1723, 1993.

175. Zuccalá A, Zucchelli P: Use and misuse of the renal functional reserve concept in clinical nephrology. Nephrol Dial Transplant 5:410, 1990.

176. D'Elia JA, Gleason RE, Alday M, et al: Nephrotoxicity from angiographic contrast material. Am J Med 72:719, 1982.

177. Lautin EM, Freeman NJ, Schoenfeld AH, et al: Radiocontrast-associated renal dysfunction: Incidence and risk factors. AJR 157:49, 1991.

178. Mitch WE, Walser M, Buffington GA, Lemann J: A simple method of estimating progression of chronic renal failure. Lancet 2:1326, 1976.

179. Rutherford WE, Blondin J, Miller JP, et al: Chronic progressive renal disease: Rate of change of serum creatinine concentration. Kidney Int 11:62, 1977.

180. Jones RH, Hayakawa H, MacKay JD, et al: Progression of diabetic nephropathy. Lancet 1:1105, 1979.

181. Arbus GS, Bacheyie GS: Method for predicting when children with progressive renal disease may reach serum creatinine levels. Pediatrics 67:871, 1981.

182. Reimold EW: Chronic progressive renal failure—rate of progression monitored by change of serum creatinine concentration. Am J Dis Child 135:1039, 1981.

183. Oksa H, Pasternack A, Luomala M, Sirviö M: Progression of chronic renal failure. Nephron 35:31, 1983.

184. Kirschbaum BB: Analysis of reciprocal creatinine plots in renal failure. Am J Med Sci 29:401, 1986.

185. Walser M, Drew HH, LaFrance ND: Reciprocal creatinine slopes often give erroneous estimates of progression of chronic renal failure. Kidney Int 36(suppl 27):S-81, 1989.

186. Walser M, Drew HH, LaFrance ND: Creatinine measurements often yield false estimates of progression in chronic renal failure. Kidney Int 34:412, 1988.

187. Kasiske BL, Heim-Duthoy KL, Tortorice KL, Rao KV: The variable nature of chronic declines in renal allograft function. Transplantation 51:330, 1991.

188. Jones RH, Molitoris BA: A statistical method for determining the breakpoint of two lines. Anal Biochem 141:287, 1984.

189. Bergström J, Alvestrand A, Bucht H, Gutierrez A: Progression of chronic renal failure is retarded with more frequent clinical follow-up. Proc Eur Dial Transplant Assoc Eur Ren Assoc 22:1153, 1985.

190. Wright JP, Salzano S, Brown CB, El Nahas AM: Natural history of chronic renal failure: A reappraisal. Nephrol Dial Transplant 7:379, 1992.

191. Viberti GC, Bilous RW, Mackintosh D, Keen H: Monitoring glomerular function in diabetic nephropathy. Am J Med 74:256, 1983.

192. Levey AS, Gassman JJ, Hall PM, Walker WG: Assessing the progression of renal disease in clinical studies: Effects of duration of follow-up and regression to the mean. J Am Soc Nephrol 1:1087, 1991.

193. Shah BV, Levey AS: Spontaneous changes in the rate of decline in reciprocal serum creatinine: Errors in predicting the progression of renal disease from extrapolation of the slope. J Am Soc Nephrol 2:1186, 1992.

194. Gretz N, Manz F, Strauch M: Predictability of the progression of chronic renal failure. Kidney Int 24(suppl 15):S2, 1983.

195. Dettli L: Drug dosage in renal disease. Clin Pharmacokinet 1:126, 1983.

196. Reidenberg MM: Kidney function and drug action. N Engl J Med 313:816, 1985.

197. Chennavasin P, Brater DC: Nomograms for drug use in renal disease. Clin Pharmacokinet 6:193, 1981.

198. Bennett WM: Update on drugs in renal failure. In Grünfeld J-P, Bach J-F, Crosnier J, et al (eds): Advances in Nephrology. Year Book Medical Publishers, Chicago, 1986, pp 379–395.

199. Maderazo EG, Sun H, Jay GT: Simplification of antibiotic dose adjustments in renal insufficiency: The DREM system. Lancet 340:767, 1992.

200. Walser M: Progression of chronic renal failure in man. Kidney Int 37:1195, 1990.

201. Beck GJ, Berg RL, Coggins CH, et al: Design and statistical issues of the modification of diet in renal disease trial. Controlled Clin Trials 12:566, 1991.

202. Webster's Ninth New Collegiate Dictionary. Merriam-Webster, Springfield, MA, 1986.

203. Akin BV, Hubbell FA, Frye EB, et al: Efficacy of the routine admission urinalysis. Am J Med 82:719, 1987.

204. Johnson H Jr, Knee-Ioli S, Butler TA, et al: Are routine preoperative laboratory screening tests necessary to evaluate ambulatory surgical patients? Surgery 104:639, 1988.

205. Kroenke K, Hanley JF, Copley JB, et al: The admission urinalysis: Impact on patient care. J Gen Intern Med 1:238, 1986.

206. Berber MJ, McFeely N: Efficacy of routine admission urinalyses in psychiatric hospitals. Can J Psychiatry 36:190, 1991.

207. Mitchell N, Stapleton FB: Routine admission urinalysis examination in pediatric patients: A poor value. Pediatrics 86:345, 1990.

208. Lawrence VA, Kroenke K: The unproven utility of preoperative urinalysis. Clinical use. Arch Intern Med 148:1370, 1988.

209. Schumann GB, Greenberg NF: Usefulness of macroscopic urinalysis as a screening procedure. Am J Clin Pathol 71:452, 1979.

210. Is routine urinalysis worthwhile? Lancet 1:747, 1988.

211. Györy AZ, Hadfield C, Lauer CS: Value of urine microscopy in predicting histological changes in the kidney: Double blind comparison. BMJ 288:819, 1984.

212. Morrin PAF: Urinary sediment in the interpretation of proteinuria. Ann Intern Med 98:254, 1983.

213. Gaines JJ: The pathology of alkaptonuric ochronosis. Hum Pathol 20:40, 1989.

214. Berman LB: When the urine is red. JAMA 237:2753, 1977.

215. Assadi FK, Fornell L: Estimation of urine specific gravity in neonates with a reagent strip. J Pediatr 108:995, 1986.

216. Siegrist D, Hess B, Montandon M, et al: Spezifisches Gewicht des Urinsvergleichende Messungen mit Teststreifen und Refraktometer bei 340 Morgenurinproben. Schweiz Rundsch Med Prax 82:112, 1993.

217. Jacobs DS, De Mott WR, Willie GR: Urinalysis and clinical microscopy. In Jacobs DS, Kasten BL, De Mott WR, Wolfson WL (eds): Laboratory Test Handbook, 2nd ed. Williams & Wilkins, Baltimore, 1990, pp 933–934.

218. Adams LJ: Evaluation of Ames Multistix SG for urine specific gravity versus refractometer specific gravity. Am J Pathol 80:871, 1983.

219. Benitez OA, Benitez M, Stijnen T, et al: Inaccuracy of neonatal measurement of urine concentration with a refractometer. J Pediatr 108:613, 1986.

220. Gouyon JB, Houchan N: Assessment of urine specific gravity by reagent strip test in newborn infants. Pediatr Nephrol 7:77, 1993.

221. Sheets C, Lyman JL: Urinalysis. Emerg Med Clin North Am 4:263, 1986.

222. Murakami T, Kawakami H: Urine concentration adjustment with a dipstick is dispensable for urinary beta 2–microglobulin screening in children. Nippon Jinzo Gakkai Shi 34:993, 1992.

223. Jung K: Enzyme activities in urine: How should we express their excretion? A critical literature review. Eur J Clin Chem Clin Biochem 29:725, 1991.

224. McCormack M, Dessureault J, Guitard M: The urine specific gravity dipstick: A useful tool to increase fluid intake in stone forming patients. J Urol 146:1475, 1991.

225. Binder L, Smith D, Kupka T, et al: Failure of prediction of liver function test abnormalities with the urine urobilinogen and urine bilirubin assays. Arch Pathol Lab Med 113:73, 1989.

226. Jacobs DS, De Mott WR, Willie GR: Urinalysis and clinical microscopy. In Jacobs DS, Kasten BL, De Mott WR, Wolfson WL (eds): Laboratory Test Handbook, 2nd ed. Williams & Wilkins, Baltimore, 1990, pp 898–899.

227. Screening for asymptomatic bacteriuria, hematuria and proteinuria. The U.S. Preventive Services Task Force. Am Fam Physician 42:389, 1990.

228. Goldsmith BM, Campos JM: Comparison of urine dipstick, microscopy, and culture for the detection of bacteriuria in children. Clin Pediatr (Phila) 29:214, 1990.

229. Jacobs DS, De Mott WR, Willie GR: Urinalysis and clinical microscopy. In Jacobs DS, Kasten BL, De Mott WR, Wolfson WL (eds): Laboratory Test Handbook, 2nd ed. Williams & Wilkins, Baltimore, 1990, pp 914–915.

230. Jacobs DS, De Mott WR, Willie GR: Urinalysis and clinical microscopy. In Jacobs DS, Kasten BL, De Mott WR, Wolfson WL (eds): Laboratory Test Handbook, 2nd ed. Williams & Wilkins, Baltimore, 1990, p 919.

231. Ditchburn RK, Ditchburn JS: A study of microscopical and chemical tests for the rapid diagnosis of urinary tract infections in general practice [see comments]. Br J Gen Pract 40:406, 1990.

232. McGlone R, Lambert M, Clancy M, Hawkey PM: Use of Ames SG10 Urine Dipstick for diagnosis of abdominal pain in the accident and emergency department. Arch Emerg Med 7:42, 1990.

233. Liptak GS, Campbell J, Stewart R, Hulbert WC Jr: Screening for urinary tract infection in children with neurogenic bladders. Am J Phys Med Rehabil 72:122, 1993.

234. Lohr JA, Portilla MG, Geuder TG, et al: Making a presumptive diagnosis of urinary tract infection by using a urinalysis performed in an on-site laboratory. J Pediatr 122:22, 1993.

235. Weinberg AG, Gan VN: Urine screen for bacteriuria in symptomatic pediatric outpatients [see comments]. Pediatr Infect Dis J 10:651, 1991.

236. McNagny SE, Parker RM, Zenilman JM, Lewis JS: Urinary leukocyte esterase test: A screening method for the detection of asymptomatic chlamydial and gonococcal infections in men. J Infect Dis 165:573, 1992.

237. Blum RN, Wright RA: Detection of pyuria and bacteriuria in symptomatic ambulatory women. J Gen Intern Med 7:140, 1992.

238. Hurlbut TA III, Littenberg B: The diagnostic accuracy of rapid dipstick tests to predict urinary tract infection. Am J Clin Pathol 96:582, 1991.

239. Jacobs DS, De Mott WR, Willie GR: Urinalysis and clinical microscopy. In Jacobs DS, Kasten BL, De Mott WR, Wolfson WL (eds): Laboratory Test Handbook, 2nd ed. Williams & Wilkins, Baltimore, 1990, pp 906–909.

240. Brigden ML, Edgell D, McPherson M, et al: High incidence of significant urinary ascorbic acid concentrations in a west coast population—implications for routine urinalysis. Clin Chem 38:426, 1992.

241. Singer DE, Coley CM, Samet JH, Nathan DM: Tests of glycemia in diabetes mellitus: Their use in establishing a diagnosis and in treatment. Ann Intern Med 110:125, 1989.

242. Jacobs DS, De Mott WR, Willie GR: Urinalysis and clinical microscopy. In Jacobs DS, Kasten BL, De Mott WR, Wolfson WL (eds): Laboratory Test Handbook, 2nd ed. Williams & Wilkins, Baltimore, 1990, p 912.

243. Brenner BM, Hostetter TH, Humes HD: Molecular basis of proteinuria of glomerular origin. N Engl J Med 298:826, 1978.

244. Rennke HG, Olson JL, Venkatachalam MA: Glomerular filtration of macromolecules: Normal mechanisms and the pathogenesis of proteinuria. Contrib Nephrol 24:30, 1981.

245. Maack T, Johnson V, Kau ST, et al: Renal filtration, transport, and metabolism of low-molecular-weight proteins: A review. Kidney Int 16:251, 1979.

246. Waldmann TA, Strober W, Mogielnicki RP: The renal handling of low molecular weight proteins. J Clin Invest 51:2162, 1972.

247. McGarry E, Sehon AH, Rose B: The isolation and electrophoretic characterization of the proteins in the urine of normal subjects. J Clin Invest 34:832, 1955.

248. Abuelo JG: Proteinuria: Diagnostic principles and procedures. Ann Intern Med 98:186, 1983.
249. Shihabi ZK, Konen JC, O'Connor ML: Albuminuria vs urinary total protein for detecting chronic renal disorders. Clin Chem 37:621, 1991.
250. Tamm I, Horsfall FL Jr: A mucoprotein derived from human urine which reacts with influenza, mumps and Newcastle disease viruses. J Exp Med 95:71, 1952.
251. Hoyer JR, Seiler MW: Pathophysiology of Tamm-Horsfall protein. Kidney Int 16:279, 1979.
252. Hession C, Decker JM, Sherblom AP, et al: Uromodulin (Tamm-Horsfall glycoprotein): A renal ligand for lymphokines. Science 237:1479, 1987.
253. Pennica D, Kohr WJ, Kuang W-J, et al: Identification of human uromodulin as the Tamm-Horsfall urinary glycoprotein. Science 236:83, 1987.
254. Bienenstock J, Tomasi TB Jr: Secretory IgA in normal urine. J Clin Invest 47:1162, 1968.
255. Henry RJ, Sorbe C, Segalove M: Turbidometric determination of urine proteins with sulfosalicyclic and trichloroacetic acids. Proc Soc Exp Biol Med 92:748, 1956.
256. Line DE, Adler S, Fraley DS, Burns FJ: Massive pseudoproteinuria caused by nafcillin. JAMA 235:1259, 1976.
257. Tejler L, Almén T, Holtås S: Proteinuria following nephroangiography. I. Clinical experiences. Acta Radiol 18:634, 1977.
258. Killingsworth LM, Savory J: Nephelometric methods for the determination of urinary albumin, transferrin, and alpha-2 macroglobulin. Ann Clin Lab Sci 4:46, 1974.
259. Bowie L, Smith S, Gochman N: Characteristics of binding between reagent-strip indicators and urinary proteins. Clin Chem 23:128, 1977.
260. Gyure WL: Comparison of several methods for semiquantitative determination of urinary protein. Clin Chem 23:876, 1977.
261. James GP, Bee DE, Fuller JB: Proteinuria: Accuracy and precision of laboratory diagnosis by dip-stick analysis. Clin Chem 24:1934, 1978.
262. Allen JK, Krauss EA, Deeter RG: Dipstick analysis of urinary protein. A comparison of Chemstrip-9 and Multistix-10SG. Arch Pathol Lab Med 115:34, 1991.
263. Keen H, Chlouverakis C: An immunoassay for urinary albumin at low concentrations. Lancet 2:913, 1963.
264. Miles DW, Mogensen CE, Gundersen HJG: Radioimmunoassay for urinary albumin using a single antibody. Scand J Clin Lab Invest 26:5, 1970.
265. Rowe DJF, Dawnay A, Watts GF: Microalbuminuria in diabetes mellitus: Review and recommendations for the measurement of albumin in urine. Ann Clin Biochem 27:297, 1990.
266. Harmoinen A, Vuorinen P, Jokela H: Turbidimetric measurement of microalbuminuria. Clin Chim Acta 166:85, 1987.
267. Lloyd DR, Hindle EJ, Marples J, Gatt JA: Urinary albumin measurement by immunoturbidimetry. Ann Clin Biochem 24:209, 1987.
268. Ellis D, Buffone GJ: New approach to evaluation of proteinuric states. Clin Chem 23:666, 1977.
269. Stamp RJ: Measurement of albumin in urine by end-point immunonephelometry. Ann Clin Biochem 25:442, 1988.
270. Neuman RG, Cohen MP: Improved competitive enzyme-linked immunoassay (ELISA) for albuminuria. Clin Chim Acta 179:229, 1989.
271. Tiu SC, Lee SS, Cheng MW: Comparison of six commercial techniques in the measurement of microalbuminuria in diabetic patients [see comments]. Diabetes Care 16:616, 1993.
272. Sawicki PT, Heinemann L, Berger M: Comparison of methods for determination of microalbuminuria in diabetic patients. Diabetic Med 6:412, 1989.
273. Ballantyne FC, Gibbons J, O'Reilly DS: Urine albumin should replace total protein for the assessment of glomerular proteinuria. Ann Clin Biochem 30(pt 1):101, 1993.
274. Coonrod BA, Ellis D, Becker DJ, et al: Predictors of microalbuminuria in individuals with IDDM. Diabetes Care 16:1376, 1993.
275. Schaufelberger H, Caduff F, Engler H, Spinas GA: Evaluation eines Streifentests (Micral-Test) zur semiquantitativen Erfassung der Mikroalbinurie in der Praxis. Schweiz Med Wochenschr 122:576, 1992.
276. Marshall SM, Schearing PA, Alberti KG: Micral-test strips evaluated for screening for albuminuria. Clin Chem 38:588, 1992.
277. Bangstad HJ, Try K, Dahl-Jørgensen K, Hanssen KF: New semiquantitative dipstick test for microalbuminuria. Diabetes Care 14:1094, 1991.

278. Jury DR, Mikkelsen DJ, Glen D, Dunn PJ: Assessment of Micral-test microalbuminuria test strip in the laboratory and in diabetic outpatients. Ann Clin Biochem 29(pt 1):96, 1992.
279. Spooren PF, Lekkerkerker JF, Vermes I: Micral-test: A qualitative dipstick test for micro-albuminuria. Diabetes Res 18:83, 1992.
280. Gilbert RE, Akdeniz A, Jerums G: Semi-quantitative determination of microalbuminuria by urinary dipstick. Aust N Z J Med 22:334, 1992.
281. Bashyam MM, O'Sullivan NJ, Baker HH, et al: Microalbuminuria in NIDDM. Diabetes Care 16:634, 1993.
282. Kruseman AC, van den Berg BW, Degenaar CP, Wolfenbuttel BHR: Screening for micro-albuminuria with Micro-Bumintest tablets and albumin/creatinine ratio. Horm Metab Res Suppl 26:71, 1992.
283. Vernetta i Porta MA, Berenguìe i Iglesias MD, Alvarez i Funes V, et al: Detección de microalbuminuria mediante tabletas reactivas en la DMND: Validación de la técnica en atención primaria. Aten Primaria 7:482, 1990.
284. Williams BT, Ketchum CH, Robinson CA, Bell DS: Screening for slight albuminuria: A comparison of selected commercially available methods. South Med J 83:1447, 1990.
285. Tai J, Tze WJ: Evaluation of Micro-Bumintest reagent tablets for screening of microalbuminuria. Diabetes Res Clin Pract 9:137, 1990.
286. Collins V, Zimmet P, Dowse GK, et al: Performance of ''Micro-Bumintest'' tablets for detection of microalbuminuria in Nauruans. Diabetes Res Clin Pract 15:271, 1989.
287. Colwell M, Halsey JF: High incidence of false-positive albuminuria results with the Micro-Bumintest. Clin Chem 35:1252, 1989.
288. Poulsen PL, Hansen B, Amby T, et al: Evaluation of a dipstick test for microalbuminuria in three different clinical settings, including the correlation with urinary albumin excretion rate. Diabete Metab 18:395, 1992.
289. Schwab SJ, Dunn FL, Feinglos MN: Screening for microalbuminuria. Diabetes Care 15:1581, 1992.
290. Kouri TT, Viikari JSA, Mattila KS, Irjala KMA: Invalidity of simple concentration-based screening tests for early nephropathy due to urinary volumes of diabetic patients. Diabetes Care 14:591, 1991.
291. Ginsberg JM, Chang BS, Matarese RA, Garella S: Use of single voided urine samples to estimate quantitative proteinuria. N Engl J Med 309:1543, 1983.
292. Schwab SJ, Christensen L, Dougherty K, Klahr S: Quantitation of proteinuria by the use of protein-to-creatinine ratios in single urine samples. Arch Intern Med 147:943, 1987.
293. Nelson RG, Knowler WC, Pettitt DJ, et al: Assessment of risk of overt nephropathy in diabetic patients from albumin excretion in untimed urine specimens. Arch Intern Med 151:1761, 1991.
294. McHardy KC, Gann ME, Ross IS, Pearson DW: A simple approach to screening for microalbuminuria in a type 1 (insulin-dependent) diabetic population. Ann Clin Biochem 28(pt 5):450, 1991.
295. Gatling W, Knight C, Mullee MA, Hill RD: Microalbuminuria in diabetes: A population study of the prevalence and an assessment of three screening tests. Diabetic Med 5:343, 1988.
296. Dunn PJ, Jury DR: Random urine albumin: creatinine ratio measurements as a screening test for diabetic microalbuminuria—a five year follow up. N Z Med J 103:562, 1990.
297. Sochett E, Daneman D: Screening tests to detect microalbuminuria in children with diabetes. J Pediatr 112:744, 1988.
298. Stehouwer CDA, Fischer HRA, Hackeng WHL, Den Ottolander GJH: Identifying patients with incipient diabetic nephropathy: Should 24-hour urine collections be used? Arch Intern Med 150:373, 1990.
299. Ellis D, Coonrad BA, Dorman JS, et al: Choice of urine sample predictive of microalbuminuria in patients with insulin-dependent diabetes mellitus. Am J Kidney Dis 13:321, 1989.
300. Gatling W, Knight C, Hill RD: Screening for early diabetic nephropathy: Which sample to detect microalbuminuria? Diabetic Med 2:451, 1985.
301. Watts GF, Shaw KM, Polak A: The use of random urine samples to screen for microalbuminuria in the diabetic clinic. Practical Diabetes 3:86, 1986.
302. Marshall SM, Alberti KGMM: Screening for early diabetic nephropathy. Ann Clin Biochem 23:195, 1986.
303. Hutchison AS, O'Reilly D St J, MacCuish AC: Albumin excretion rate, albumin concentration, and albumin creatinine ratio compared for screening diabetics for slight albuminuria. Clin Chem 34:2019, 1988.

304. Cohen DL, Close CF, Viberti GC: The variability of overnight urinary albumin excretion in insulin-dependent diabetic and normal subjects. Diabetic Med 4:437, 1987.
305. Sessoms S, Mehta K, Kovarsky J: Quantitation of proteinuria in systemic lupus erythematosus by use of a random, spot urine collection. Arthritis Rheum 26:918, 1983.
306. Watts GF, Pillay D: Effect of ketones and glucose on the estimation of urinary creatinine: Implications for microalbuminuria screening. Diabetic Med 7:263, 1990.
307. Weber MH: Urinary protein analysis. J Chromatogr 429:315, 1988.
308. Viberti GC, Jarrett RJ, Mahmud U, et al: Microalbuminuria as a predictor of clinical nephropathy in insulin-dependent diabetes mellitus. Lancet 1:1430, 1982.
309. Messent JWC, Elliott TG, Hill RD, et al: Prognostic significance of microalbuminuria in insulin-dependent diabetes mellitus: A twenty-three year follow-up study. Kidney Int 41:836, 1992.
310. Mattock MB, Morrish NJ, Viberti G, et al: Prospective study of microalbuminuria as predictor of mortality in NIDDM. Diabetes 41:736, 1992.
311. Mogensen CE: Microalbuminuria predicts clinical proteinuria and early mortality in maturity-onset diabetes. N Engl J Med 310:356, 1984.
312. Jarrett RJ, Viberti CG, Argyropoulos A, et al: Microalbuminuria predicts mortality in non–insulin-dependent diabetes. Diabetic Med 1:17, 1984.
313. Schmitz A, Vaeth M: Microalbuminuria: A major risk factor in non–insulin-dependent diabetes. A 10-year follow-up study of 503 patients. Diabetic Med 5:126, 1988.
314. Morgensen CE, Christensen CK: Predicting diabetic nephropathy in insulin-dependent patients. N Engl J Med 311:89, 1984.
315. Borch-Johnsen K, Wenzel H, Viberti GC, Morgensen CE: Is screening and intervention for microalbuminuria worthwhile in patients with insulin dependent diabetes? Br Med J 306:1722, 1993.
316. Kannel WB, Stampfer MJ, Castelli WP, Verter J: The prognostic significance of proteinuria: The Framingham study. Am Heart J 108:1347, 1984.
317. Samuelsson O, Wilhelmsen L, Elmfeldt D, et al: Predictors of cardiovascular morbidity in treated hypertension: Results from the primary preventive trial in Goteborg, Sweden. J Hypertens 3:167, 1985.
318. Bulpitt CJ, Beevers DG, Butler A, et al: The survival of treated hypertensive patients and their causes of death: A report from the DHSS hypertensive care computing project (DHCCP). J Hypertens 4:93, 1986.
319. Kaplan NM: Microalbuminuria: A risk factor for vascular and renal complications of hypertension. Am J Med 92(4B):8S, 1992.
320. Haffner SM, Stern MP, Gruber KK, et al: Microalbuminuria: Potential markers for increased cardiovascular risk factors in nondiabetic subject? Arteriosclerosis 10:727, 1990.
321. Welty JW: Febrile albuminuria. Am J Med Sci 194:70, 1937.
322. Marks MI, McLaine PN, Drummond KN: Proteinuria in children with febrile illnesses. Arch Dis Child 45:250, 1970.
323. Hemmingsen L, Skaarup P: Urinary excretion of ten plasma proteins in patients with febrile diseases. Acta Med Scand 201:359, 1977.
324. Reuben DB, Wachtel TJ, Brown PC, Driscoll JL: Transient proteinuria in emergency medical admissions. N Engl J Med 306:1031, 1982.
325. Poortmans JR: Postexercise proteinuria in humans: Facts and mechanisms. JAMA 253:236, 1985.
326. Krämer BK, Kernz M, Ress KM, et al: Influence of strenuous exercise on albumin excretion. Clin Chem 34:2516, 1988.
327. Robinson RR: Nephrology Forum: Isolated proteinuria in asymptomatic patients. Kidney Int 18:395, 1980.
328. Levitt JI: The prognostic significance of proteinuria in young college students. Ann Intern Med 66:685, 1967.
329. Muth RG: Asymptomatic mild intermittent proteinuria. Arch Intern Med 115:569, 1965.
330. Glassock RJ: Postural (orthostatic) proteinuria: No cause for concern. N Engl J Med 305:639, 1981. Editorial.
331. Sinniah R, Law CH, Pwee HS: Glomerular lesions in patients with asymptomatic persistent and orthostatic proteinuria discovered on routine medical examination. Clin Nephrol 7:1, 1977.
332. Robinson RR: Isolated proteinuria. Contrib Nephrol 24:53, 1981.
333. von Bonsdorff M, Koskenvuo K, Salmi HA, Pasternack A: Prevalence and causes of proteinuria in 20-year-old Finnish men. Scand J Urol Nephrol 15:285, 1981.

334. Springberg PD, Garrett LE Jr, Thompson AL Jr, et al: Fixed and reproducible orthostatic proteinuria: Results of a 20-year follow-up. Ann Intern Med 97:516, 1982.
335. Rytand DA, Spreiter S: Prognosis in postural (orthostatic) proteinuria. N Engl J Med 305:618, 1981.
336. Houser MT: Characterization of recumbent, ambulatory, and postexercise proteinuria in the adolescent. Pediatr Res 21:442, 1987.
337. Schardijn GHC, Statius van Eps LW: $\beta_2$-Microglobulin: Its significance in the evaluation of renal function. Kidney Int 32:635, 1987.
338. Schentag JJ, Sutfin TA, Plaut ME, Jusko WJ: Early detection of aminoglycoside nephrotoxicity with urinary $\beta$-2 microglobulin. J Med 9:201, 1978.
339. Hall PW III, Dammin GJ: Balkan nephropathy. Nephron 22:281, 1978.
340. Taniguchi N, Tanaka M, Kishihara C, et al: Determination of carbonic anhydrase C and $\beta_2$-microglobulin by radioimmunoassay in urine of heavy-metal–exposed subjects and patients with renal tubular acidosis. Environ Res 20:154, 1979.
341. Statius van Eps LW, Schardijn GHC: Value of determination of $\beta_2$-microglobulin in toxic nephropathy and interstitial nephritis. Klin Wochenschr 18:673, 1984.
342. Bäckman L, Ringdén O, Björkhem I, Lindbäck B: Increased serum $\beta_2$-microglobulin during rejection, cyclosporine-induced nephrotoxicity and cytomegalovirus infection in renal transplant recipients. Transplantation 42:368, 1986.
343. Roxe DM, Siddiqui F, Santhanam S, et al: Rationale and application of $\beta_2$-microglobulin measurements to detect acute transplant rejection. Nephron 27:260, 1981.
344. Schardijn GHC, Statius van Eps LW, Pauw W, et al: Comparison of reliability of tests to distinguish upper from lower urinary tract infections. Br Med J 289:284, 1984.
345. Joachim GR, Cameron JS, Schwartz M, Becker EL: Selectivity of protein excretion in patients with the nephrotic syndrome. J Clin Invest 43:2332, 1964.
346. Ghiggeri GM, Candiano G, Ginevri F, et al: Renal selectivity properties towards endogenous albumin in minimal change nephropathy. Kidney Int 32:69, 1987.
347. Kyle RA: Monoclonal gammopathies and the kidney. Annu Rev Med 40:53, 1989.
348. Pascali E, Pezzoli A: The clinical spectrum of pure Bence Jones proteinuria: A study of 66 patients. Cancer 62:2408, 1988.
349. Pasquali S, Zucchelli P, Casanova S, et al: Renal histological lesions and clinical syndromes in multiple myeloma. Clin Nephrol 27:222, 1987.
350. Isobe T, Osserman EF: Patterns of amyloidosis and their association with plasma-cell dyscrasia, monoclonal immunoglobulins and Bence-Jones proteins. N Engl J Med 290:473, 1974.
351. Smithline N, Kassirer JP, Cohen JJ: Light-chain nephropathy. Renal tubular dysfunction associated with light-chain proteinuria. N Engl J Med 294:71, 1976.
352. Buxbaum JN, Chuba JV, Hellman GC, et al: Monoclonal immunoglobulin deposition disease: Light chain and light and heavy chain deposition diseases and their relation to light chain amyloidosis. Ann Intern Med 112:455, 1990.
353. Venkataseshan VS, Faraggiana T, Hughson MD, et al: Morphologic variants of light-chain deposition disease in the kidney. Am J Nephrol 8:272, 1988.
354. Kyle RA, Greipp PR: Laboratory Medicine Series on Clinical Testing. 3. The laboratory investigation of monoclonal gammopathies. Mayo Clin Proc 53:719, 1978.
355. Hunt LP, Short CD, Mallick NP: Prognostic indicators in patients presenting with the nephrotic syndrome. Kidney Int 34:382, 1988.
356. Williams PS, Fass G, Bone JM: Renal pathology and proteinuria determine progression in untreated mild/moderate chronic renal failure. Q J Med 67:343, 1988.
357. D'Amico G: Influence of clinical and histological features on actuarial renal survival in adult patients with idiopathic IgA nephropathy, membranous nephropathy, and membranoproliferative glomerulonephritis: Survey of the recent literature. Am J Kidney Dis 20:315, 1992.
358. Lai KN, HO CP, Chan KW, et al: Nephrotic range proteinuria—a good predictive index of disease in IgA nephropathy? Q J Med 57:677, 1985.
359. Neelakantappa K, Gallo GAR, Baldwin DS: Proteinuria in IgA nephropathy. Kidney Int 33:716, 1988.

360. Alamartine E, Sabatier J-C, Guerin C, et al: Prognostic factors in mesangial IgA glomerulonephritis: An extensive study with univariate and multivariate analyses. Am J Kidney Dis 18:12, 1991.

361. Donadio JV Jr, Torres VE, Velosa JA, et al: Idiopathic membranous nephropathy: The natural history of untreated patients. Kidney Int 33:708, 1988.

362. Cattran DC, Pei Y, Greenwood C: Predicting progression in membranous glomerulonephritis. Nephrol Dial Transplant Suppl 1:48, 1992.

363. Brahm M, Brammer M, Balsløv JT, et al: Prognosis in glomerulonephritis. III. A longitudinal analysis of changes in serum creatinine and proteinuria during the course of disease: Effect of immunosuppressive treatment. Report from Copenhagen Study Group of Renal Diseases. J Intern Med 231:339, 1992.

364. Addis T: The number of formed elements in the urinary sediment of normal individuals. J Clin Invest 2:409, 1926.

365. Gadeholt H: Quantitative estimation of cells in urine. Acta Med Scand 183:369, 1968.

366. Gadeholt H: Quantitative estimation of urinary sediment, with special regard to sources of error. Br Med J 1:1547, 1964.

367. Stamm WE: Measurement of pyuria and its relation to bacteriuria. Am J Med 75(suppl):53, 1983.

368. Kesson AM, Talbott JM, Gyory AZ: Microscopic examination of urine. Lancet 2:809, 1978.

369. Addis T: A clinical classification of Bright's diseases. JAMA 85:163, 1925.

370. Burton JR, Rowe JW, Hill RN: Quantitation of casts in urine sediment. Ann Intern Med 83:518, 1975.

371. Ritchie CD, Bevan EA, Collier SJ: Importance of occult haematuria found at screening. Br Med J 292:681, 1986.

372. Thompson IM: The evaluation of microscopic hematuria: A population-based study. J Urol 138:1189, 1987.

373. Messing EM, Vaillancourt A: Hematuria screening for bladder cancer. J Occup Med 32:838, 1990.

374. Britton JP, Dowell AC, Whelan P, Harris CM: A community study of bladder cancer screening by the detection of occult urinary bleeding. J Urol 148:788, 1992.

375. Lieu TA, Grasmeder HM III, Kaplan BS: An approach to the evaluation and treatment of microscopic hematuria. Pediatr Clin North Am 38:579, 1991.

376. Fairley KF, Birch DF: Hematuria: A simple method for identifying glomerular bleeding. Kidney Int 21:105, 1982.

377. Fassett RG, Horgan BA, Mathew TH: Detection of glomerular bleeding by phase-contrast microscopy. Lancet 1:1432, 1982.

378. Van Iseghem PH, Hauglastaine D, Bollens W, Michielsen P: Urinary erythrocyte morphology in acute glomerulonephritis. BMJ 287:1183, 1983.

379. Shichiri M, Nishio Y, Suenaga M, et al: Red-cell volume distribution curves in diagnosis of glomerular and non-glomerular haematuria. Lancet 1:908, 1988.

380. Naicker S, Poovalingam V, Mlisana K, et al: Comparative assessment of phase contrast microscopy and Coulter counter measurements in localising the site of haematuria. S Afr Med J 82:183, 1992.

381. de Metz M, Schiphorst PP, Go RI: The analysis of erythrocyte morphologic characteristics in urine using a hematologic flow cytometer and microscopic methods. Am J Clin Pathol 95:257, 1991.

382. Goldwasser P, Antignani A, Mittman N, et al: Urinary red cell size: Diagnostic value and determinants. Am J Nephrol 10:148, 1990.

383. Schramek P, Moritsch A, Haschkowitz H, et al: In vitro generation of dysmorphic erythrocytes. Kidney Int 36:72, 1989.

384. Kitamoto Y, Yide C, Tomita M, Sato T: The mechanism of glomerular dysmorphic red cell formation in the kidney. Tohoku J Exp Med 167:93, 1992.

385. Raman GV, Pead L, Lee HA, Maskell R: A blind controlled trial of phase-contrast microscopy by two observers for evaluating the source of hematuria. Nephron 44:304, 1986.

386. Crompton CH, Ward PB, Hewitt IK: The use of urinary red cell morphology to determine the source of hematuria in children. Clin Nephrol 39:44, 1993.

387. Köhler H, Wandel E, Brunck B: Acanthocyturia—a characteristic marker for glomerular bleeding. Kidney Int 40:115, 1991.

388. Roth S, Renner E, Rathert P: Microscopic hematuria: Advances in identification of glomerular dysmorphic erythrocytes. J Urol 146:680, 1991.

389. Sayer J, McCarthy MP, Schmidt JD: Identification and significance of dysmorphic versus isomorphic hematuria. J Urol 143:545, 1990.

390. Pollock C, Pei-Ling L, Györy AZ, et al: Dysmorphism of urinary red blood cells—value in diagnosis. Kidney Int 36:1045, 1989.

391. Pillsworth TJ Jr, Haver VM, Abrass CK, Delaney CJ: Differentiation of renal from non-renal hematuria by microscopic examination of erythrocytes. Clin Chem 33:1791, 1987.

392. Thal SM, DeBellis CC, Iverson SA, Schumann GB: Comparison of dysmorphic erythrocytes with other urinary sediment parameters of renal bleeding. Am J Clin Pathol 86:784, 1986.

393. Marcussen N, Schumann JL, Schumann GB, et al: Analysis of cytodiagnostic urinalysis findings in 77 patients with concurrent renal biopsies. Am J Kidney Dis 20:618, 1992.

394. Offringa M, Benbassat J: The value of urinary red cell shape in the diagnosis of glomerular and post-glomerular haematuria. A meta-analysis. Postgrad Med J 68:648, 1992.

395. Eisenstaedt JS: Allergy and drug hypersensitivity of the urinary tract. J Urol 65:154, 1951.

396. Helgason S, Lindqvist B: Eosinophiluria. Scand J Urol Nephrol 6:257, 1972.

397. Nolan CR III, Anger MS, Kelleher SP: Eosinophiluria—a new method of detection and definition of the clinical spectrum. N Engl J Med 315:1516, 1986.

398. Galpin JE, Shinaberger JH, Stanley TM, et al: Acute interstitial nephritis due to methicillin. Am J Med 65:756, 1978.

399. Corwin HL, Korbet SM, Schwartz MM: Clinical correlates of eosinophiluria. Arch Intern Med 145:1097, 1985.

400. Wilson DM, Salazer TL, Farkouh ME: Eosinophiluria in atheroembolic renal disease. Am J Med 91:186, 1991.

401. Corwin HL, Haber MH: The clinical significance of eosinophiluria. Am J Clin Pathol 88:520, 1987.

402. Corwin HL, Bray RA, Haber MH: The detection and interpretation of urinary eosinophils. Arch Pathol Lab Med 113:1256, 1989.

403. Jacobs DS, De Mott WR, Willie GR: Urinalysis and clinical microscopy. In Jacobs DS, Kasten BL, De Mott WR, Wolfson WL (eds): Laboratory Test Handbook, 2nd ed. Williams & Wilkins, Baltimore, 1990, pp 903–904.

404. Ditlove J, Weidmann P, Bernstein M, Massry SG: Methicillin nephritis. Medicine (Baltimore) 56:483, 1977.

405. Linton AL, Clark WF, Driedger AA, et al: Acute interstitial nephritis due to drugs: Review of the literature with a report of nine cases. Ann Intern Med 93:735, 1980.

406. Weir MR, Hall-Craggs M, Shen SY, et al: The prognostic value of the eosinophil in acute renal allograft rejection. Transplantation 41:709, 1986.

407. Spencer ES, Peterson VP: The urinary sediment after renal transplantation. Quantitative changes as an index of the activity of the renal allograft reaction. Acta Med Scand 182:73, 1967.

408. Miloslavich E: Occurrence of lipoids in urine and their diagnostic importance. J Lab Clin Med 13:542, 1928.

409. Neuman M, West M, Zimmerman HJ: The relationship between proteinuria and fatty elements in the urine sediment. Am J Med Sci 241:617, 1961.

410. Senécal PE, Rochette J: Misidentification of urine lipid bodies owing to use of starch-powdered gloves. Clin Chem 34:1926, 1988.

411. Braden GL, Sanchez PG, Fitzgibbons JP, et al: Urinary doubly refractile lipid bodies in nonglomerular diseases. Am J Kidney Dis 11:332, 1988.

412. McQueen EG: The nature of urinary casts. J Clin Pathol 15:367, 1962.

413. Jacobs DS, De Mott WR, Willie GR: Urinalysis and clinical microscopy. In Jacobs DS, Kasten BL, De Mott WR, Wolfson WL (eds): Laboratory Test Handbook, 2nd ed. Williams & Wilkins, Baltimore, 1990, pp 938.

414. Ball RP: Needle (aspiration) biopsy. J Tenn Med Assoc 27:203, 1934.

415. Alwall N: Aspiration biopsy of the kidney. Acta Med Scand 143:430, 1952.

416. Perez-Ara A: La biopsie-punctural del rinon no megalico—consid-erationes generales y aportacion de un nuevo metodo. Bol Liga Contra Cancer 25:121, 1950.

417. Iverson P, Brun C: Aspiration biopsy of kidney. Am J Med 11:324, 1951.

418. Kark RM, Muehrcke RC: Biopsy of kidney in prone position. Lancet 1:1047, 1954.

419. Muehrcke RC, Kark RM, Pirani CL: Biopsy of the kidney in the diagnosis and management of renal disease. N Engl J Med 253:537, 1955.

420. Arenson AM: Ultrasound guided percutaneous renal biopsy. Australas Radiol 35:38, 1991.

421. Farquhar MG, Vernier RL, Good RA: An electron microscopy study of the glomerulus in nephrosis, glomerulonephritis and lupus erythematosus. J Exp Med 106:649, 1957.

422. Mellors RC, Ortega LG: Analytical pathology. III. New observations on pathogenesis of glomerulonephritis, lipid nephrosis, periarteritis nodosa and secondary amyloidosis in man. Am J Pathol 32:455, 1956.

423. Wernick RM, Smith DL, Houghton DC, et al: Reliability of histologic scoring for lupus nephritis: A community-based evaluation. Ann Intern Med 119:805, 1993.

424. Schainuck LI, Striker GE, Cutler RE, Benditt EP: Structural-functional correlations in renal diseases: II. The correlations. Hum Pathol 1:631, 1970.

425. Striker GE, Schainuck LI, Cutler RE, Benditt EP: Structural-functional correlations in renal diseases: I. A method for assaying and classifying histopathologic changes in renal biopsies. Hum Pathol 1:615, 1970.

426. Striker LJ: Modern renal biopsy interpretation: Can we predict glomerulosclerosis? Semin Nephrol 13:508, 1993.

427. Paone DB, Meyer LE: The effect of biopsy on therapy in renal disease. Arch Intern Med 141:1039, 1981.

428. Cohen AH, Nast CC, Adler SG, Kopple JD: The clinical usefulness of kidney biopsies in the diagnosis and management of renal disease. Kidney Int 27:135, 1985. Abstract.

429. Turner MW, Hutchinson TA, Barré PE, et al: A prospective study on the impact of the renal biopsy in clinical management. Clin Nephrol 26:217, 1986.

430. Whiting-O'Keefe Q, Riccardi PJ, Henke JE, et al: Recognition of information in renal biopsies of patients with lupus nephritis. Ann Intern Med 96(pt 1):723, 1982.

431. Hlatky MA: Is renal biopsy necessary in adults with nephrotic syndrome? Lancet 2:1264, 1982.

432. Kassirer JP: Is renal biopsy necessary for optimal management of the idiopathic nephrotic syndrome? Kidney Int 24:561, 1983.

433. Primack WA, Schulman SL, Kaplan BS: An analysis of the approach to management of childhood nephrotic syndrome by pediatric nephrologists. Am J Kidney Dis 23:524, 1994.

434. Levey AS, Lau J, Pauker SG, Kassirer JP: Idiopathic nephrotic syndrome: Puncturing the biopsy myth. Ann Intern Med 107:697, 1987.

435. Churg J, Habib R, White RHR: Pathology of the nephrotic syndrome in children. Lancet 1:1299, 1970.

436. International Study of Kidney Disease in Children: Primary nephrotic syndrome in children: Clinical significance of histopathologic variants of minimal change and of diffuse mesangial hypercellularity. Kidney Int 20:765, 1981.

437. White RHR, Glasgow EF, Mills RJ: Clinicopathological study of nephrotic syndrome in childhood. Lancet 1:1353, 1970.

438. Tomura S, Tsutani K, Sakuma A, Takeuchi J: Discriminant analysis in renal histological diagnosis of primary glomerular diseases. Clin Nephrol 23:55, 1985.

439. Ganeval D, Noel L-H, Preud'homme J-L, et al: Light-chain deposition disease: Its relation with AL-type amyloidosis. Kidney Int 26:1, 1984.

440. Lynn RI, Siegel NJ, Hayslett JP: Lupus nephropathy as the initial manifestation of systemic lupus erythematosus. Yale J Biol Med 53:353, 1980.

441. Eiser AR, Katz SM, Swartz C: Clinically occult diffuse proliferative lupus nephritis: An age-related phenomenon. Arch Intern Med 139:1022, 1979.

442. Mahajan SK, Ordóñez NG, Feitelson PJ, et al: Lupus nephropathy without clinical renal involvement. Medicine (Baltimore) 56:493, 1977.

443. Font J, Torras A, Cervera R, et al: Silent renal disease in systemic lupus erythematosus. Clin Nephrol 27:283, 1987.

444. Woolf A, Croker B, Osofsky SG, Kredich DW: Nephritis in children and young adults with systemic lupus erythematosus and normal urinary sediment. Pediatrics 64:678, 1979.

445. Esdaile JM, Levinton C, Federgreen W, et al: The clinical and renal biopsy predictors of long-term outcome in lupus nephritis: A study of 87 patients and review of the literature. Q J Med 72:779, 1989.

446. Hill GS, Hinglais N, Tron F, Bach J: Systemic lupus erythematosus. Morphologic correlations with immunologic and clinical data at the time of biopsy. Am J Med 64:61, 1978.

447. Whiting-O'Keefe Q, Henke JE, Shearn MA, et al: The information content from renal biopsy in systemic lupus erythematosus. Ann Intern Med 96(pt 1):718, 1982.

448. Muehrcke RC, Kark RM, Pirani CL, Pollak VE: Lupus nephritis: A clinical and pathologic study based on renal biopsies. Medicine (Baltimore) 36:1, 1957.

449. Baldwin DS, Lowenstein J, Rothfield NF, et al: The clinical course of the proliferative and membranous forms of lupus nephritis. Ann Intern Med 73:929, 1970.

450. Baldwin DS, Gluck MC, Lowenstein J, Gallo G: Lupus nephritis. Clinical course as related to morphologic forms and their transitions. Am J Med 62:12, 1977.

451. Schwartz MM, Kawala KS, Corwin HL, Lewis EJ: The prognosis of segmental glomerulonephritis in systemic lupus erythematosus. Kidney Int 32:274, 1987.

452. Schwartz MM, Lan SP, Bonsib SM, et al: Clinical outcome of 3 discrete glomerular lesions in severe lupus glomerulonephritis. The Lupus Nephritis Collaborative Study Group. Am J Kidney Dis 13:273, 1989.

453. Austin HA III, Klippel JH, Balow JE, et al: Therapy of lupus nephritis: Controlled trial of prednisone and cytotoxic drugs. N Engl J Med 314:614, 1986.

454. Pollak VE, Pirani CL, Kark RM: Effect of large doses of prednisone on the renal lesions and life span of patients with lupus glomerulonephritis. J Lab Clin Med 57:495, 1961.

455. Pollak VE, Pirani CL, Schwartz F: The natural history of the renal manifestations of systemic lupus erythematosus. J Lab Clin Med 63:537, 1964.

456. Austin HA III, Muenz LR, Joyce KM, et al: Prognostic factors in lupus nephritis: Contribution of renal histologic data. Am J Med 75:382, 1983.

457. Austin HA III, Muenz LR, Joyce KM, et al: Diffuse proliferative lupus nephritis: Identification of specific pathologic features affecting renal outcome. Kidney Int 25:689, 1984.

458. Fries JF, Porta J, Liang MH: Marginal benefit of renal biopsy in systemic lupus erythematosus. Arch Intern Med 138:1386, 1978.

459. Nossent HC, Henzen-Logmans SC, Vroom TM, et al: Contribution of renal biopsy data in predicting outcome in lupus nephritis: Analysis of 116 patients. Arthritis Rheum 33:970, 1990.

460. Schwartz MM, Bernstein J, Hill GS, et al: Predictive value of renal pathology in diffuse proliferative lupus glomerulonephritis. Kidney Int 36:891, 1989.

461. Schwartz MM, Lan SP, Bernstein J, et al: Role of pathology indices in the management of severe lupus glomerulonephritis. Lupus Nephritis Collaborative Study Group. Kidney Int 42:743, 1992.

462. Chagnac A, Kiberd BA, Farinas MC, et al: Outcome of acute glomerular injury in proliferative lupus nephritis. J Clin Invest 84:922, 1989.

463. Ellis A: Natural history of Bright's disease: Clinical and experimental observations. Lancet 1:1, 1942.

464. Schwartz MM, Korbet SM: Crescentic glomerulonephritis. Prog Reprod Urinary Tract Pathol 1:163, 1989.

465. Morrin PAF, Hinglais N, Nabarra B, Kreis H: Rapidly progressive glomerulonephritis: A clinical and pathologic study. Am J Med 65:446, 1978.

466. Falk RJ: ANCA-associated renal disease. Kidney Int 38:998, 1990.

467. Strom TB, Loertscher R: Cyclosporine-induced nephrotoxicity, inevitable and intractable? N Engl J Med 311:728, 1984.

468. Klintmalm G, Bergstrand A, Ringden O, et al: Graft biopsy for the differentiation between nephrotoxicity and rejection in cyclosporin-A treated renal transplant recipients. Transplant Proc 15:493, 1983.

469. Sibley RK, Rynasiewicz J, Ferguson RM, et al: Morphology of cyclosporine nephrotoxicity and acute rejection in patients immunosuppressed with cyclosporine and prednisone. Surgery 15:493, 1983.

470. Gray DWR, Richardson A, Hughes D, et al: A prospective, randomized, blind comparison of three biopsy techniques in the management of patients after renal transplantation. Transplantation 53:1226, 1992.

471. Hamburger J, Crosnier J, Noel LH: Recurrent glomerulonephritis after renal transplantation. Annu Rev Med 29:67, 1978.

472. McClean RH, Geigler H, Burke B, et al: Recurrence of membranoproliferative glomerulonephritis following kidney transplantation. Am J Med 60:60, 1976.

473. Leumann EP, Briner J, Donckerwolcke R, et al: Recurrence of focal segmental glomerulosclerosis in the transplanted kidney. Nephron 25:65, 1980.

474. Zimmerman CE: Renal transplantation for focal segmental glomerulosclerosis. Transplantation 29:172, 1980.

475. Sinniah R, Pwee HS, Lim CM: Glomerular lesions in asymptomatic microscopic hematuria discovered on routine medical examinations. Clin Nephrol 5:216, 1976.

476. Michael J, Jones NF, Davies DR, Tighe TR: Recurrent hematuria: Role of renal biopsy and investigative radiology. Br Med J 1:686, 1976.

477. Copley JB, Hasbargen JA: Idiopathic hematuria: A prospective evaluation. Arch Intern Med 147:434, 1987.

478. Trachtman H, Weiss RA, Bennett B, Greifer I: Isolated hematuria in children: Indications for a renal biopsy. Kidney Int 25:94, 1984.

479. Nomoto Y, Endoh M, Suga T, et al: Minimum requirements for renal biopsy size for patients with IgA nephropathy. Nephron 60:171, 1992.

480. Clarkson AR, Seymour AE, Thomson AJ, et al: IgA nephropathy: A syndrome of uniform morphology, diverse clinical features and uncertain prognosis. Clin Nephrol 8:459, 1977.

481. Van der Peet J, Arisz L, Brentjens JRH, et al: The clinical course of IgA nephropathy in adults. Clin Nephrol 8:335, 1977.

482. Hood SA, Velosa JA, Holley KE, Donadio JV: IgA-IgG nephropathy: Predictive indices of progressive disease. Clin Nephrol 16:55, 1981.

483. D'Amico G, Ferrario F, Colasanti G, et al: Ig-A–mesangial nephropathy (Berger's disease) with rapid decline in renal function. Clin Nephrol 16:251, 1981.

484. Kropp KA, Shapiro RS, Jhunjhunwala JS: Role of renal biopsy in end-stage renal failure. Urology 12:631, 1978.

485. Beaufils M: Glomerular disease complicating abdominal sepsis. Kidney Int 19:609, 1981.

486. Urizar RE, Schwarty A, Top F, Vernier RL: The nephrotic syndrome in children with diabetes mellitus of recent onset. N Engl J Med 281:173, 1969.

487. Rao KV, Crosson JT: Idiopathic membranous glomerulonephritis in diabetic patients. Report of three cases and review of the literature. Arch Intern Med 140:624, 1980.

488. Deykin D: Uremic bleeding. Kidney Int 24:698, 1983.

489. Mannucci PM, Remuzzi G, Pusineri F, et al: Deamino-8-D-arginine vasopressin shortens the bleeding time in uremia. N Engl J Med 308:8, 1983.

490. Liu YK, Kosfeld RE, Marcum SG: Treatment of uraemic bleeding with conjugated oestrogen. Lancet 2:887, 1984.

491. Shemin D, Elnour M, Amarantes B, et al: Oral estrogens decrease bleeding time and improve clinical bleeding in patients with renal failure. Am J Med 89:436, 1990.

492. Schow DA, Vinson RK, Morrisseau PM: Percutaneous renal biopsy of the solitary kidney: A contradiction? J Urol 147:1235, 1992.

493. Takacs FJ, Dodd JB, Zinman L: The liberal approach to renal biopsy. Lahey Clin Found Bull 18:1, 1969.

494. Wickre CG, Golper TA: Complications of percutaneous needle biopsy of the kidney. Am J Nephrol 2:173, 1982.

495. Sateriale M, Cronan JJ, Savadier LD: A 5-year experience with 307 CT-guided biopsies: Results and complications. J Vasc Interv Radiol 2:401, 1991.

496. Saghafi D: Kidney biopsy under CT guidance. Clin Nephrol 39:356, 1993.

497. Burstein DM, Schwartz MM, Korbet SM: Percutaneous renal biopsy with the use of real-time ultrasound. Am J Nephrol 11:195, 1991.

498. Saitoh M: Color doppler flow imaging in interventional ultrasound of the kidney. Scand J Urol Nephrol Suppl 137:59, 1991.

499. Tung KT, Downes MO, O'Donnell PJ: Renal biopsy in diffuse renal diseases—experience with a 14-gauge automated biopsy gun. Clin Radiol 46:111, 1992.

500. Donovan KL, Thomas DM, Wheeler DC, et al: Experience with a new method for percutaneous renal biopsy. Nephrol Dial Transplant 6:731, 1991.

501. Bogan ML, Kopecky KK, Kraft JL, et al: Needle biopsy of renal allografts: Comparison of two techniques. Radiology 174:273, 1990.

502. Belitsky P, Gupta R: Minicore needle biopsy of kidney transplants: A safer sampling method. J Urol 144:310, 1990.

503. Dixon TK, Bowman JS, Sago AL, Jaffers G: A safer renal allograft needle biopsy. Clin Transplant 5:126, 1991.

504. Newstead CG, Brown JH: The safety of automated "Biopty" renal transplant biopsies. Transplantation 53:954, 1992.

505. Calconi G, Maresca MC, Amici G, et al: Core biopsy of the transplanted kidney using 1.1-mm needles: Results and comparisons with the Tru-Cut technique. Nephron 61:487, 1992.

506. Parrish AE: Complications of percutaneous renal biopsy: A review of 37 years' experience. Clin Nephrol 38:135, 1992.

507. Diaz-Buxo JA, Donadio JV Jr: Complications of percutaneous renal biopsy: An analysis of 1,000 consecutive biopsies. Clin Nephrol 4:223, 1975.

508. Slotkin EA, Madsen PO: Complications of renal biopsy: Incidence in 5,000 reported cases. J Urol 87:13, 1962.

509. Muth RG: The safety of percutaneous renal biopsy: An analysis of 500 consecutive cases. J Urol 94:1, 1965.

510. Ginsburg JC, Fransman SL, Singer MA, et al: Use of computerized tomography (CT) to evaluate bleeding after renal biopsy. Nephron 26:240, 1980.

511. Rosenbaum R, Hoffsten PE, Stanley RJ, Klahr S: Use of computerized tomography to diagnose complications of percutaneous renal biopsy. Kidney Int 14:87, 1978.

512. Alter AJ, Zimmerman S, Kirachaiwanich C: Computerized tomographic assessment of retroperitoneal hemorrhage after percutaneous renal biopsy. Arch Intern Med 140:1323, 1980.

513. Bennett AR, Wiener SN: Intrarenal arteriovenous fistula and aneurysm: A complication of percutaneous renal biopsy. Am J Roentgenol 95:372, 1965.

514. Ekelund L, Lindholm T: Arteriovenous fistulae following percutaneous renal biopsy. Acta Radiol 11:38, 1971.

515. Grau JH, Gonick P, Wilson A: Post-biopsy intrarenal arteriovenous fistula. J Urol 122:233, 1979.

516. Blake S, Heffernan S, McCann P: Renal arteriovenous fistula after percutaneous renal biopsy. Br Med J 1:1458, 1963.

517. O'Brien DP III, Parrott TS, Walton KN, Lewis EL: Renal arteriovenous fistulas. Surg Gynecol Obstet 139:739, 1974.

518. Leiter E, Gribetz D, Cohen S: Arteriovenous fistula after percutaneous needle biopsy: Surgical repair with preservation of renal function. N Engl J Med 287:971, 1972.

519. Merkus JWS, Zeebregts CJAM, Hoitsma AJ, et al: High incidence of arteriovenous fistula after biopsy of kidney allografts. Br J Surg 80:310, 1993.

520. Jackson GG, Poirier KP, Grieble HG: Concepts of pyelonephritis: Experience with renal biopsies and long-term clinical observations. Ann Intern Med 47:1165, 1957.

521. Figueroa TE, Frentz GD: Anuria secondary to percutaneous needle biopsy of a transplant kidney: A case report. J Urol 140:355, 1988.

522. River GL, Dovenbarger WV, Nikolai TF, Moffat NA: Unusual complications of kidney biopsy. J Urol 103:15, 1970.

# 27

# Radiologic Assessment of the Kidney

*Hedvig Hricak*
*Scott S. White*

In the last decade, imaging of the kidneys has undergone significant changes spurred by the explosive growth of technology. Gray-scale digital ultrasonography (US), high-resolution and rapid computed tomography (CT), and the development of magnetic resonance imaging (MRI) have all contributed to advances in diagnostic evaluation of the kidneys. Even selective angiography has been made safer and faster with the advent of computerized digital subtraction methods. All of these developments have improved renal diagnostic evaluation, facilitated interventional approaches for diagnosis and treatment, and refined the assessment of therapeutic results. To derive the most benefit from this vast array of imaging options, to avoid duplication, and to achieve the best results efficiently, it is necessary to understand the advantages and limitations of each of these modalities.

## TECHNICAL CONSIDERATIONS

### Conventional Radiology

X-rays were discovered by Wilhelm Konrad Röntgen in 1895, and although the proliferation of new, highly technologic imaging modalities has been fascinating, conventional radiographic methods still have their place in modern imaging evaluation of the kidney. Plain films of the abdomen (kidney, ureter, and bladder, or KUB), intravenous urogram (IVU; intravenous pyelogram, IVP, is an old but still often used term), and angiography all rely on tissue absorption of x-rays to produce an image.

X-rays are generated when high-energy electrons in a vacuum tube strike a tungsten anode, producing photons of energy as high as 140 kV. The x-rays, which emanate from the anode, pass through a port in the housing holding the x-ray tube and are restricted to a region of interest within the patient by lead collimators. As the x-ray beam passes through the patient, the x-rays are attenuated differentially, primarily depending on tissue density. The beam emerging from the patient is absorbed by fluorescent screens that sandwich the x-ray film. The x-ray energy is then converted to visible light energy, exposing the film and producing a shadowgraph of tissue density. With dense structures, such as bone, the x-ray beam is greatly attenuated, and these structures appear light on the film. Low-density tissues, such as fat, attenuate the beam to a far lesser extent and therefore appear dark.[1]

### KIDNEY, URETER, AND BLADDER FILMS

Plain films of the kidneys (which depend on the difference in x-ray attenuation between the kidneys and the enveloping perirenal fat) provide a crude index of renal anatomy and pathologic change. Except for the detection of calcifications and abnormalities of renal contour, plain films do not provide sufficient information for evaluation of renal status, which requires opacification by intravenous injection of iodinated contrast medium.

### INTRAVENOUS UROGRAPHY

IVU is used to evaluate kidney size, shape, and orientation; the appearance and homogeneity of the nephrogram phase; symmetric excretion; and the appearance of the calyces, pelves, and ureters. Assessment of the urinary bladder by IVU is global, but it can be informative. Although IVU provides useful information about renal status, it is hampered by some significant drawbacks. The reported mortality during excretory urography ranges from 1 in 17,000 to 1 in 75,000.[2, 3] The use of contrast media is known to produce reactions that may be minor (nausea, vomiting, urticaria, itching, and sneezing), moderate (nephrotoxic effects, congestive heart failure, pulmonary edema), or severe (bronchospasm, anaphylaxis, and even death). Although the occurrence of minor and moderate reactions to contrast media has been significantly reduced by the introduction of nonionic contrast media, reduction in the number of severe reactions has not been definitely established.[4]

The timing of film sequence during IVU is governed by the rate of injection (infusion versus bolus) of the contrast medium. With the bolus method, a high plasma concentration of contrast media is reached, which provides an excellent nephrogram. Because the volume of contrast media is relatively small, however, visualization of the renal calyces, pelves, and ureters requires abdominal compression. The infusion method results in a lower peak concentration of contrast media, but the average level is maintained over a longer period. Because a larger volume of contrast media is injected with this method, calyces are routinely distended and ureters are visualized.

## ANGIOGRAPHY

Angiographic procedures use the same radiographic approach, but a lower dose of contrast media, with intravenous or direct selective intra-arterial injections.

## Diagnostic Ultrasonography

In B-mode US, an ultrasonic pulse is generated by a piezoelectric transducer that converts a short electric energizing pulse into ultrasound waves, which propagate coherently directly away from the transducer.[5] Because interfaces between tissues have different acoustic impedances, part of the energy in the ultrasonic pulse is reflected toward the transducer, which converts this reflected sound intensity into an electrical signal. Because the velocity of sound in soft tissue is constant (1540 m/s), depth information is obtained by determining the time between the emission of a sound pulse and the detection of a reflected signal.[5] A cross-sectional image is obtained by rapidly sweeping the sound beam through a layer of the body. The US image is digital, with picture element (pixel) values assigned light intensity levels (a gray shade) proportional to the intensity of the reflected sound beam. Newer ultrasound devices are also equipped with Doppler, which can demonstrate the patency of arteries and veins as well as the direction, amount, and speed of flow.

Sonograms are primarily used to assess kidney size, cortical thickness and echogenicity, corticomedullary differentiation, and status of the pelvicalyceal system (Fig. 27–1). Ultrasound imaging of the kidneys is routinely performed in both longitudinal and transverse planes. The right kidney is normally viewed in a parasagittal plane, with the liver used as an acoustic window. The best images of the left kidney are obtained from a slightly posterior approach, usually near the midaxillary line, which avoids interference from bowel gas in the left colon.[6]

Although it is nonspecific, increased renal echogenicity is a uniformly abnormal finding.[7] Renal echogenicity is a subjective visual assessment that should be made in relation to the echogenicity of adjacent structures—the liver on the right and the spleen on the left.[6, 7] In adults, the normal renal cortex appears less echogenic than the adjacent liver. When renal echogenicity is evaluated, however, it must be remembered that the assessment is not reliable if the internal standard (i.e., the liver) is altered by primary disease (such as fatty infiltration, which is associated with increased hepatic echogenicity). The echogenicity of the left kidney is compared with that of the spleen. Because the spleen is normally more echogenic than the liver, it is more difficult to detect mild abnormalities in the echogenicity of the left

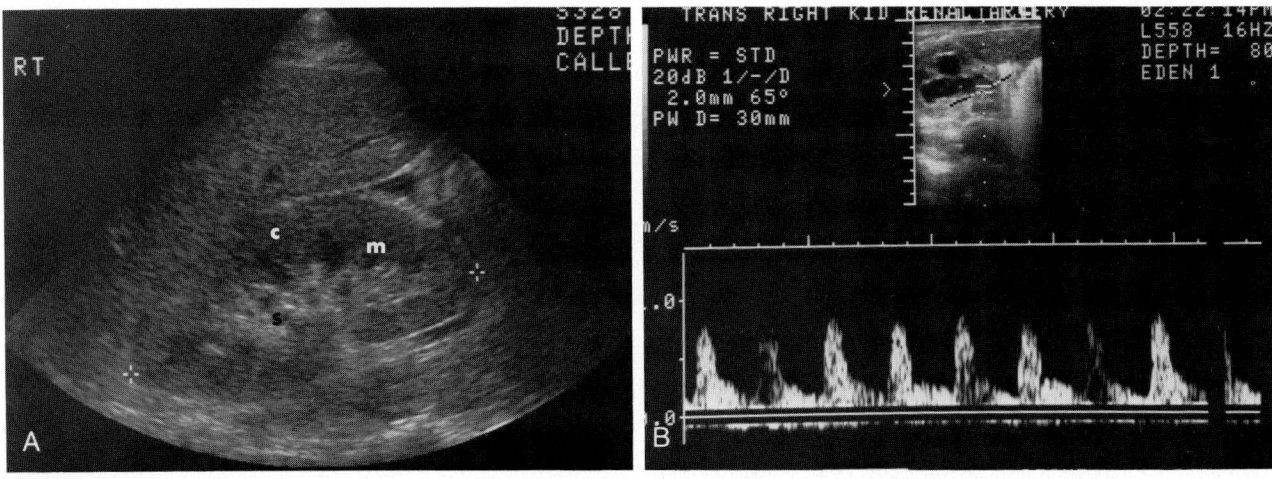

**Figure 27–1.** Normal right kidney, sonogram. *A.* Longitudinal (sagittal) plane demonstrating renal size and, within the renal parenchyma, differentiation between higher echogenicity renal cortex (c) and lower echogenicity renal medulla (m). High-intensity renal sinus echoes (s). *B.* Doppler ultrasound study through the right renal artery showing normal flow.

kidney, but medical renal disease is bilateral, so this is rarely a significant drawback.

The normal medullary pyramids appear hypoechoic relative to the renal cortex, and in the majority of normal persons (especially in young patients), the cortex and medulla can be differentiated on a sonogram.[6] The hypoechogenic pyramids should not be mistaken for the echolucent, dilated, fluid-filled calyces seen in hydronephrosis. On real-time imaging, the pyramids can be recognized by their regularly spaced anatomic distribution, by their continuity with the peripheral cortical parenchyma, and by demonstration of a bright reflection from the arcuate artery at the corticomedullary junction. In addition, the normal renal sinus can be identified because it demonstrates echogenic and compact echo patterns generated by sinus adipose tissue, pelvic blood vessels, and collapsed collecting structures. The renal arteries and veins can be visualized extending from the renal hilum to the aorta and inferior vena cava, respectively. The ureters can be seen only when they are distended. When the kidney is assessed for congenital anomalies or acute renal failure, examination of the pelvis is essential. The fluid-filled urinary bladder is easily identified and, when distended, the ureter at the ureterovesical junction can be demonstrated.

Color Doppler US provides visualization of flowing blood and has proved valuable in evaluating both the native and allograft kidney in the diagnosis of renal arterial and venous thrombosis, stenosis, pseudoaneurysms, and arteriovenous fistulas.[8]

## Computed Tomography

CT is a digital, x-ray–based, cross-sectional imaging modality. A computer is used to reconstruct images from hundreds of thousands of x-ray data samples, each of which is a measure of the x-ray attenuation along an x-ray beam through a given cross section of the body.[9] The samples are obtained by moving the x-ray source around the patient during the x-ray exposure. An image is formed by the computer by dividing the cross-sectional area through the patient into pixels and using the data samples to calculate the x-ray attenuation occurring within the tissue represented by each pixel. The resulting numbers (the pixel values) are scaled to the x-ray attenuation of pure water, which is assigned a CT number of zero. Tissues less dense than water, such as fat, have negative CT numbers. Denser structures, such as most soft tissues, have positive CT numbers. Images are viewed by converting the pixel values to light intensity values on a cathode ray tube, from which hard copy film can also be made. Newer CT devices offer high spatial resolution (from 6 to 20 line pairs per centimeter), high speed (from 100 milliseconds to 4 seconds per scan), fast patient "throughput," and a wide range of software options.

The principal advantages offered by CT lie in its ability to detect subtle differences in the x-ray attenuation properties of various tissues and in its generation of cross-sectional images.[9] These features provide detailed demonstration of anatomy in all parts of the body and have been useful in the previously difficult evaluation of retroperito-

neum. The superior soft tissue contrast resolution is obtained by technical features of scanner design, including a sophisticated x-ray detection system (which allows higher signal/noise ratios than can be produced with conventional radiographic methods), narrow and precise collimation of the x-ray beam (which decreases scattered radiation), and methods of image reconstruction (which eliminate the visual effects of structures lying outside the desired imaging plane). CT scanners presently in clinical use are capable of resolving x-ray attenuation differences of as little as 0.3% and of providing spatial resolution of 0.5 to 1 mm.[9]

CT evaluation of renal anatomy and pathologic change generally requires intravenous injection of iodinated contrast media. Only when renal or perirenal calcification, intrarenal and perirenal hemorrhage, or urine extravasation is suspected are nonenhanced scans recommended.[10] In these situations, scans obtained after the administration of contrast media may mask abnormalities. Nonenhanced scans are also helpful in characterizing renal masses.[10]

As with IVU studies, contrast medium may be administered either as a rapid intravenous bolus or by infusion techniques. The bolus technique is preferred for assessment of renal anatomy or measurement of aortorenal transit time. Infusion methods may facilitate evaluation of inferior vena cava patency.[11] With use of a bolus injection and rapid sequence scanning, renal arterial opacification is followed immediately by enhancement of the renal cortex. A nephrogram phase with medullary enhancement is reached within 60 seconds (Fig. 27–2). Excretion of contrast material into the collecting structures can be expected within 2 to 3 minutes after it is injected.

The intrarenal calyces are rarely visible unless they are dilated, but infundibula and renal pelves are well delineated, particularly after contrast medium is excreted. Even without contrast material, it is usually possible to distinguish the renal pelves and the ureters. The renal pelvis is thin walled and saccular, whereas the ureter, viewed in cross section, is circular. The ureters lie lateral to the aorta on the left and the inferior vena cava on the right and course inferiorly anterior to the psoas muscles. Distal to the aortic bifurcation, the ureters run ventral to the iliac vessels and into the pelvis.

Because much of the diagnostic information available from CT depends on patterns of contrast enhancement, the evaluation of patients with renal failure is difficult. Carefully tailored examinations can allow use of minimal amounts of contrast material to reduce osmotic loads and iodine doses.

## Magnetic Resonance Imaging

MRI requires a large and powerful magnet into which the patient can fit. Systems with permanent, resistive, or superconducting magnets are available. The method is based on the fact that in a strong external magnetic field, nuclei with an uneven number of particles have a magnetic moment and align with the external field.[12] Theoretically, imaging can be carried out with any atom that has a magnetic moment, but because $H^+$ is abundant in the human body and has a high gyromagnetic ratio (causing nuclei to

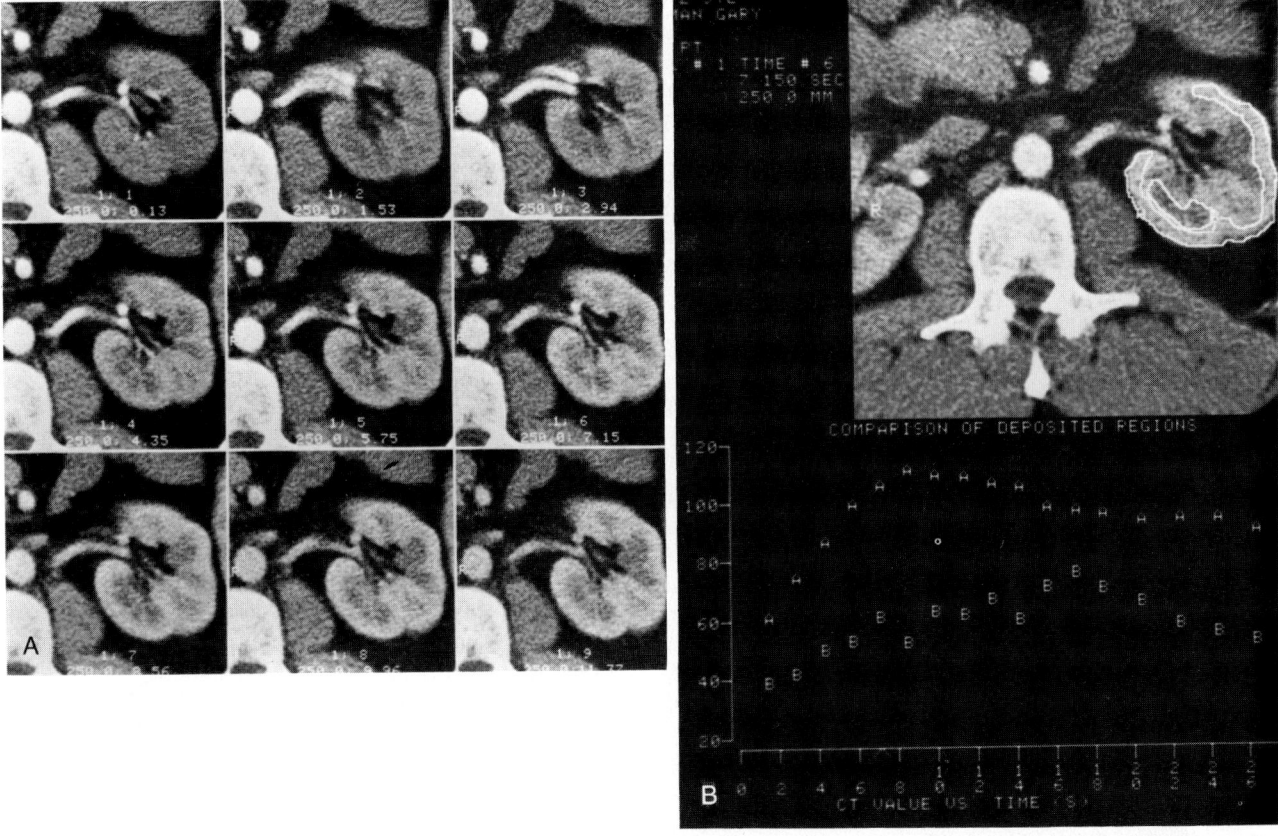

**Figure 27–2.** CT appearance of normal left kidney after bolus injection. *A.* Serial images are obtained every 1.5 seconds on the first image. Opacification of the aorta and of the left renal artery at the left upper corner is followed by opacification of the renal cortex, rendering excellent corticomedullary contrast. *B.* Serial density measurements plotted against time showing enhancement pattern of the cortex (A) and the medulla (B).

precess at a relatively high rate), MRI is at present carried out almost exclusively with $H^+$ nuclei (protons). By bombarding the aligned $H^+$ with a specific (Larmor) radio frequency (RF), the magnetic moment can be flipped out of alignment. After the RF pulse is turned off, the $H^+$ ions gradually realign with the external magnetic field, and to do so, they emit signals of the same RF as the one absorbed. Because the Larmor frequency is directly related to the strength of the magnetic field, spatial information can be obtained by shaping the main magnetic field with relatively small gradient fields in a known way so that a given frequency can be equated with $H^+$ at a given point in space.

MRI produces an image by applying many sets of RF pulses over several minutes.[12] These pulses flip the aligned $H^+$ through a known angle relative to the direction of the main magnetic field (e.g., a 90-degree pulse flips the $H^+$ to right angles with the main field). The time between the sets of RF pulses is called the repetition time (TR). The period between the initial pulse in a sequence and the time that the signal is acquired from the sample is called the echo delay time (TE).

The intensity of the signal depends on the $H^+$ density and on tissue contrast determinants (T1 and T2 relaxation times). T1 relaxation time represents the time needed for $H^+$ to realign with the external magnetic field after having been tilted or flipped by an RF pulse. T2 relaxation time

represents the time needed for $H^+$ ions to misalign with one another after cessation of an RF pulse.[12]

By altering the TR and TE parameters, it is possible to accentuate differences in the T1 and T2 relaxation times of different tissues, producing contrast between these tissues (Fig. 27–3). This is referred to as T1 weighting or T2 weighting of images. With conventional spin-echo techniques (each RF pulse set consists of a 90-degree pulse followed by a 180-degree pulse), T1-weighted images have short TR and TE intervals (TR is typically 200 to 600 milliseconds and TE is typically 15 to 30 milliseconds), whereas T2-weighted images have long TR and TE intervals (typically at least 2000 and 60 milliseconds, respectively). T1 and T2 weighting for new fast-imaging (gradient-echo) techniques is achieved to some extent by variations in the flip angles (<90 degrees) induced in the direction of $H^+$ spin by the initial RF pulse. These techniques permit effective T1 and T2 weighting with shorter imaging times than are needed with conventional techniques.[13] MRI allows direct imaging in any plane desired, but the three orthogonal planes—transverse, sagittal, and coronal—are most commonly used (see Fig. 27–3).

MRI consistently delineates the internal architecture of the normal kidney. The appearance of the normal kidney, however, varies with the type of MRI technique used. With T1-weighted spin-echo imaging, the renal cortex demon-

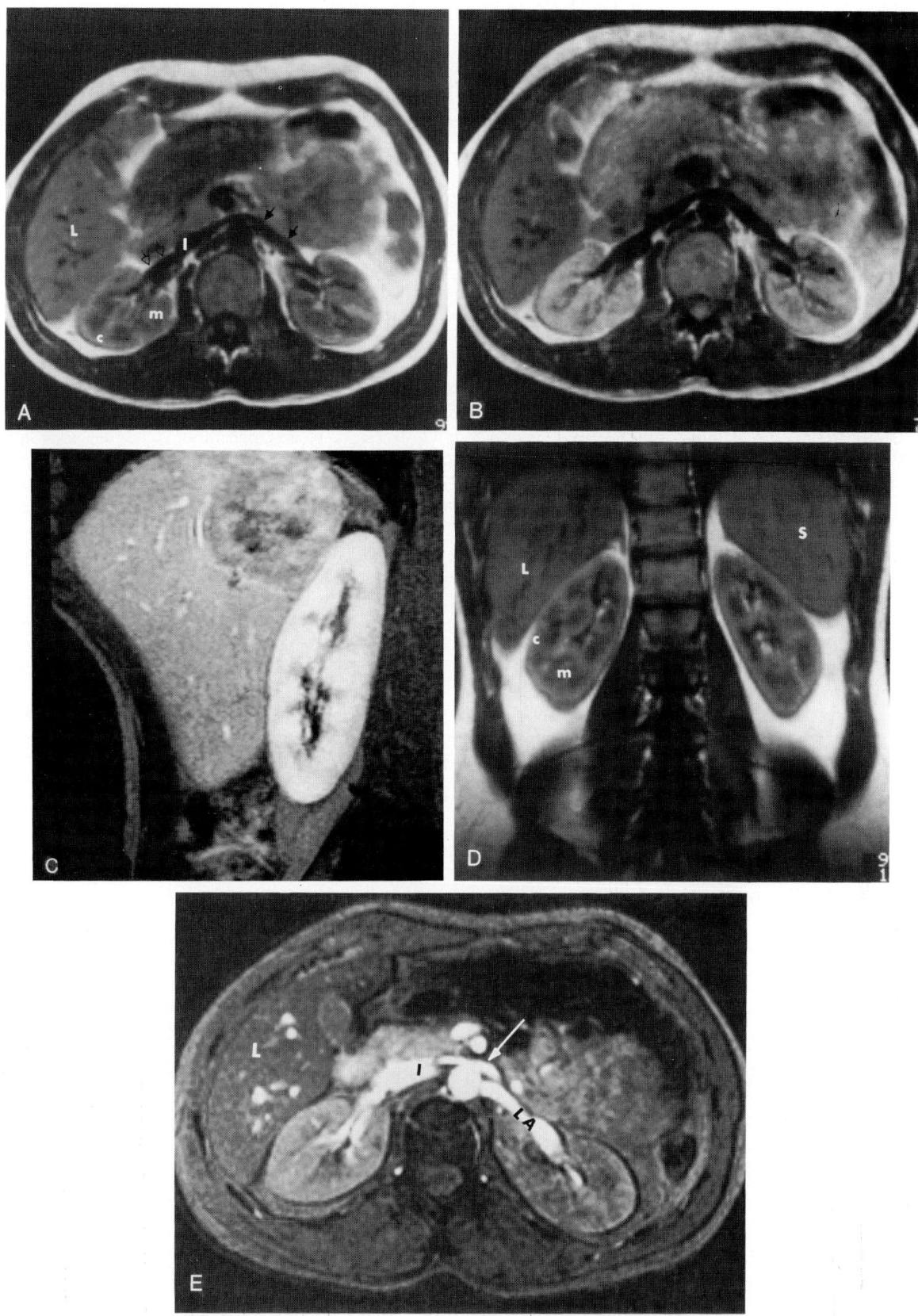

**Figure 27–3.** Normal kidney on MRI scan. *A.* Spin-echo T1-weighted transverse image. *B.* Spin-echo T2-weighted transverse image. *C.* Contrast-enhanced T1-weighted sagittal image. *D.* Spin-echo T1-weighted coronal image. *E.* Gradient-echo transverse image. Normal renal anatomy with differentiation between high-intensity cortex (c) and low-intensity medulla (m) is well appreciated on a T1-weighted image. There is also excellent demonstration of the left renal vein *(black arrows)*, the inferior vena cava (I), and the right renal vein *(open black arrows)*. On the T2-weighted image, the vascular anatomy is well seen, but the corticomedullary differentiation is not appreciated. With the gradient-echo image, all the vessels including left renal artery (LA), left renal vein *(white arrow)*, and inferior vena cava (I) are of high signal intensity. Because all flowing blood will emit high signal intensity, this sequence is particularly well suited for the evaluation of the intravascular thrombus. L = liver; S = spleen.

**1179**

strates higher signal intensity than the lower intensity medulla (see Fig. 27–3A). The cortex, however, is not as bright as either the hilar or perirenal adipose tissue. On T2-weighted images, the corticomedullary differentiation is diminished. The renal hilum is imaged with high signal intensity because of the hilar adipose tissue. Because normally flowing blood does not produce a magnetic resonance signal, the renal veins and arteries appear as tubular or round structures of signal void coursing through the hilar region. When slightly distended with urine, the pelvicalyceal systems and proximal ureters are imaged with low signal intensity on T1-weighted images and with increased signal intensity on T2-weighted images. Perirenal fat is imaged with high signal intensity, and Gerota fascia (dividing the perirenal from the pararenal spaces) is depicted with low signal intensity (see Fig. 27–3). A T1-weighted pulse sequence is best for demonstrating the anatomy of the kidney; however, both T1- and T2-weighted images are essential for tissue characterization in pathologic states.

The new advance in renal MRI is the use of contrast media. With gadolinium contrast medium, bolus injection, and rapid sequence imaging, both renal anatomy and function can be assessed[14] (Fig. 27–4).

Gadolinium, similar to iodine, is an intravascular, extracellular tissue contrast agent primarily excreted by glomerular filtration. Whereas iodinated contrast agents uniformly enhance the tissue density on x-ray or CT images, the effect of gadolinium on the signal intensity on magnetic resonance images depends on its concentration. The relationship between signal intensity and the concentration of the paramagnetic contrast media, such as gadolinium, is nonlinear. At lower concentrations, gadolinium causes an increase in signal intensity (predominantly because of shortening of the T1 relaxation time), whereas at higher concentrations, signal intensity decreases (owing to intervening shortening of the T2 relaxation time). Dynamic postcontrast images of the kidney demonstrate four phases of contrast enhancement: 1) A cortical enhancement phase is seen 0.5 minute

after injection; both the cortex and the medulla demonstrate signal enhancement, but the signal intensity of the cortex is greater than the signal intensity of the medulla, which results in excellent corticomedullary differentiation. 2) An early tubule phase (see Fig. 27–4B) is apparent at 1 minute after injection; the signal intensity of the cortex remains similar to that in the cortical enhancement phase, but there is interval increase in the enhancement of the medulla, which decreases or obliterates corticomedullary differentiation. 3) A ductal phase (see Fig. 27–4C) seen at 1.5 minutes after injection demonstrates a slight decrease in the signal intensity of the cortex with marked decrease in the signal intensity of the medulla, once more accentuating corticomedullary differentiation. This is due to high concentration of gadolinium within collecting ducts and indicates the concentrating ability of the renal tubules (see Fig. 27–4C). 4) An excretory phase appears at 2 minutes after injection. Low-intensity urine is seen in the collecting system (see Fig. 27–4D). Gadolinium, therefore, reflects not only glomerular filtration but also the tubule concentration function. Gadolinium has shown good renal tolerance in patients with pre-existing renal failure,[15, 16] and there is effective hemodialysis of gadolinium in the clinical setting.[17]

Magnetic resonance angiography has quickly proved its utility for a variety of applications, including detection of venous tumor or thrombus and evaluation of renal transplant vasculature.[18–20] With use of newer techniques such as contrast-enhanced dynamic imaging and diffusion weighted imaging, magnetic resonance is showing potential for quantitative evaluation of the glomerular filtration rate,[21] for evaluation of renal blood flow and function,[22] and for screening of microvascular disease.[23]

## Magnetic Resonance Spectroscopy

Magnetic resonance spectroscopy is the newest addition to the noninvasive diagnostic armamentarium in nephrol-

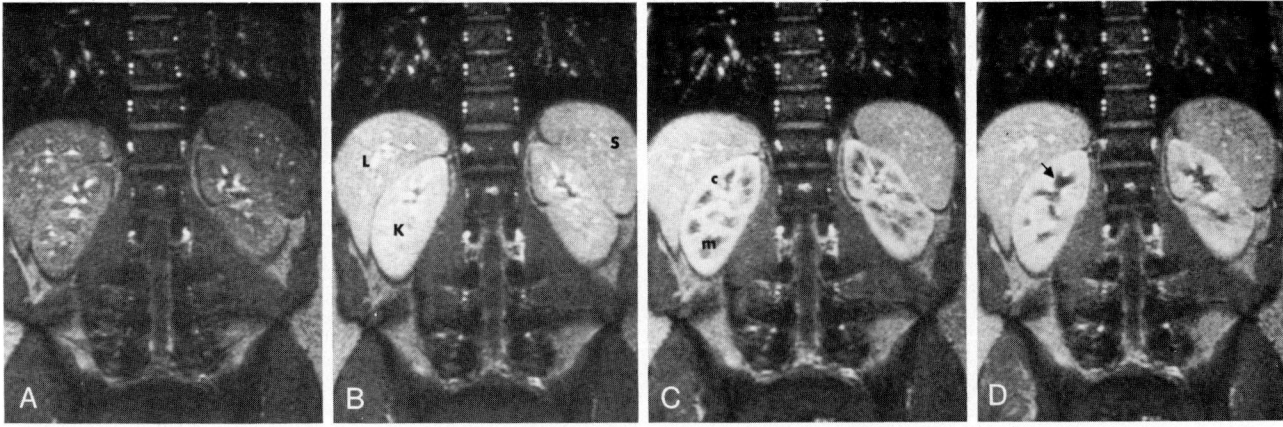

**Figure 27–4.** Serial gradient-echo images after gadolinium injection. *A.* Before injection of contrast medium. *B.* One minute after injection of contrast medium. *C.* One and one-half minutes after injection of contrast medium. *D.* Three minutes after injection of contrast medium. There is marked enhancement of the liver (L), spleen (S), and renal parenchyma (K) on the image obtained 1 minute after gadolinium injection *(B).* Corticomedullary differentiation is not seen. At 1.5 minutes after gadolinium injection *(C),* there is excellent contrast between high-intensity cortex (c) and low-intensity medulla (m). The reason for low intensity of the medulla is higher concentration of the gadolinium within collecting ducts. On film obtained at 3 minutes after gadolinium injection *(D),* excretion is evident by low-intensity urine seen within nondilated collecting system *(arrow).*

ogy. It uses the same instrument as MRI, but the magnet must be superconducting with the magnetic field strength of at least 1.5 T, and the field homogeneity over the volume studied must be less than 0.5 ppm. (For imaging, field homogeneity of 50 ppm is sufficient.) Spectroscopy permits the noninvasive analysis of metabolism at the molecular level.[24] At present, the nuclei used in spectroscopy are phosphorus ($^{31}$P), carbon ($^{13}$C), hydrogen ($^{1}$H), and fluorine ($^{19}$F). The most experience today has been gathered with $^{31}$P to study energy transfer metabolism[24] and ATP hydrolysis and to determine intracellular pH. It is the easiest to use because of the availability of the nuclei and their relatively high sensitivity. $^{1}$H, however, is even more abundant and sensitive, but at present, owing to the technical difficulties (the large water and fat peaks need to be suppressed to be able to study the fatty acid, lactate, and other peaks), its use is limited. $^{13}$C, which can be used in studying glucose metabolism, is naturally found in small quantities. This, combined with its low sensitivity, limits its use at present. It can be used as an administered tracer to enrich metabolites that can be observed dynamically, and a technique of decoupling can significantly increase the sensitivity of $^{13}$C.

Although magnetic resonance spectroscopy is promising in the study of kidney disease, it suffers currently from disadvantages that need to be corrected. The relatively large size of the voxel (2 to 3 cm$^3$ for $^{31}$P, and 1 to 5 mm$^3$ for $^{1}$H) is a problem. Localization methods to define these volumes from images also beg for improvement and new approaches. Localization of the signal from depths beyond 10 cm is frought with problems. Motion compensation methods to ensure obtaining the signal from the same volume during respiration have not yet been worked out.

## ACUTE RENAL FAILURE

The causes of acute renal failure are usually categorized as prerenal (renal hypoperfusion), intrinsic (renal medical disease), or postrenal (urinary obstruction). The prerenal causes of acute renal failure (e.g., hypotension, congestive heart failure, shock) are best evaluated and treated clinically, and radiologic evaluation is seldom requested. With intrinsic causes of renal failure, both clinical and radiologic characterizations of renal medical disease are nonspecific. Diagnosis requires renal biopsy, after which treatment can be initiated. Because renal biopsy is invasive, the evaluation of renal medical disease is usually deferred until prerenal and postrenal causes of renal failure have been excluded.

Although renal obstruction, the postrenal cause of acute renal failure, is the least common of the three (1% to 10%), it is potentially curable and can be surgically corrected if it is diagnosed early.[25] It is difficult to identify urinary obstruction clinically, and radiologic evaluation is necessary. High-dose contrast urography has for years been the initial method of examination, but decreased renal function, which causes poor renal opacification and excretion during IVU, has often resulted in nondiagnostic studies. Consequently, US has now replaced excretory urography as the initial radiologic method for evaluating suspected urinary obstruction. With US, there is no need for contrast medium, and the display of renal morphologic features is independent of renal function.

## Ultrasonography

US is accurate in detecting hydronephrosis; its sensitivity is estimated between 90% and 100%.[26] Hydronephrosis is diagnosed when the compact sinus complex echo is separated by branching nonechoing (fluid-filled) calyces, infundibula, and pelves (Fig. 27–5). The blunted configuration of the dilated calyx may also be discerned. The degree of dilatation is judged subjectively. Mild hydronephrosis is characterized by fluid-filled intrarenal collecting structures that are not significantly distorted but are slightly separate from the sinus fat (see Fig. 27–5). In moderate hydronephrosis, there is obvious distention and rounding of the intrarenal collecting structures, with well-preserved cortical thickness (Fig. 27–6). The diagnosis of severe hydronephrosis is usually reserved for those cases in which the sinus fat is virtually replaced by rounded and dilated infundibulae and calyces in a kidney in which there is significant cortical thinning[7] (Fig. 27–7).

Although the morphologic display by US is excellent, the detection of hydronephrosis is not peculiar to urinary tract obstruction, and the severity of hydronephrosis does not correlate with the degree of renal failure. Hydronephrosis is a descriptive term that denotes dilatation of the collecting system. It may be caused by obstruction; high-output urine flow; or nonobstructive entities, such as vesicoureteral reflux, postobstructive renal atrophy, or congenital megacalyces. Renal Doppler US examination may be of some assistance in the evaluation of acute obstruction, before onset of hydronephrosis.[27, 28] Hydronephrosis demonstrated by sonography should be correlated with the clinical findings and previous radiographs, if available. If there is suspicion that the hydronephrosis is due to urinary obstruction, the diagnosis needs to be confirmed by contrast studies, such as IVU or antegrade or retrograde pyelography (see Fig. 27–6B).

If both kidneys are functioning, obstruction must be bilateral to cause renal failure. In such cases, the obstruction

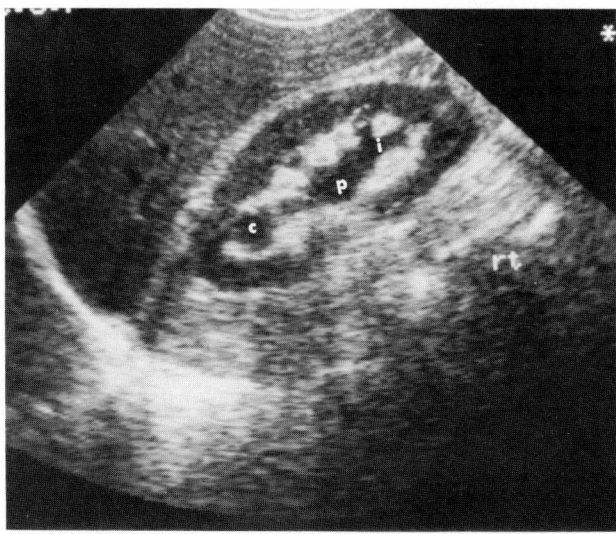

**Figure 27–5.** Mild hydronephrosis, right kidney, sonogram. The calyces (c), infundibula (i), and pelvis (p) are slightly dilated as demonstrated by the widening of the high-amplitude sinus echoes.

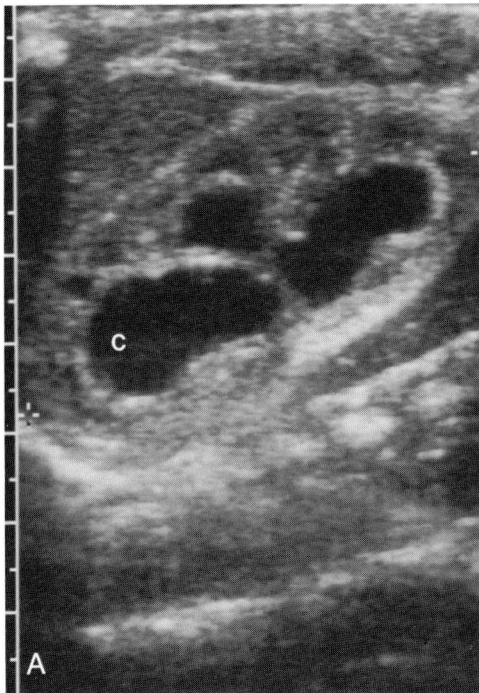

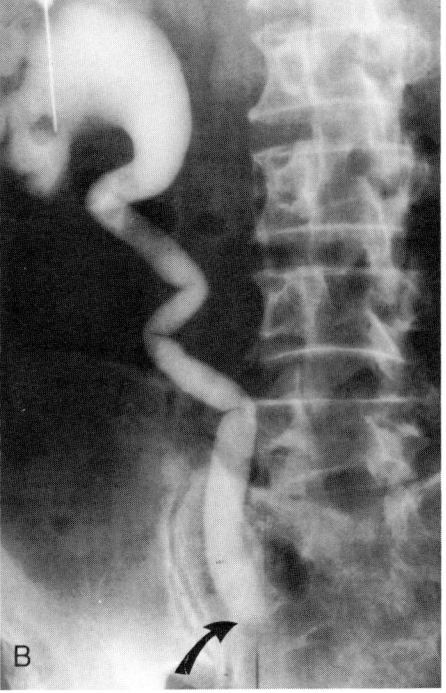

**Figure 27–6.** Moderate to severe hydronephrosis due to tumor obstruction in the distal ureter. *A.* Longitudinal sonogram showing dilatation and blunting (rounding) of the renal calyces (c). A small amount of residual bright renal sinus echoes can be seen. *B.* Antegrade pyelogram demonstrating severe hydronephrosis, hydroureter, and obstruction in distal ureter *(arrow)*.

is usually at the level of the bladder or pelvic inlet, and careful scanning of the pelvis and bladder is mandatory once hydronephrosis is detected. Frequently, dilated hydroureters can be followed into the pelvis to the level of an obstructing mass. Scanning of the pelvis and examination of the architecture of the distal ureters and bladder are optimally performed through the acoustic window of a filled bladder.

## Computed Tomography

Although sonography is the principal approach to the evaluation of obstructive nephropathy, CT may be advantageous when sonography is technically limited. The dilated, fluid-filled renal pelvis and proximal ureter are clearly demonstrated even in nonenhanced CT images, and scrutiny of sequential transverse sections allows location of

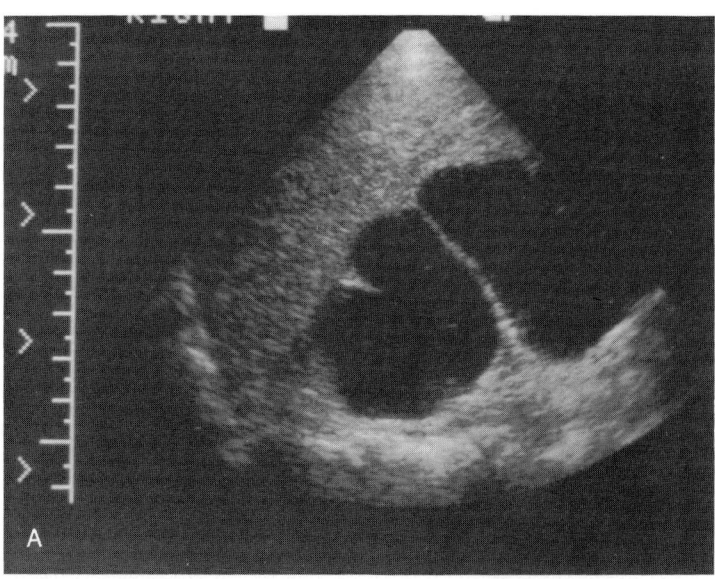

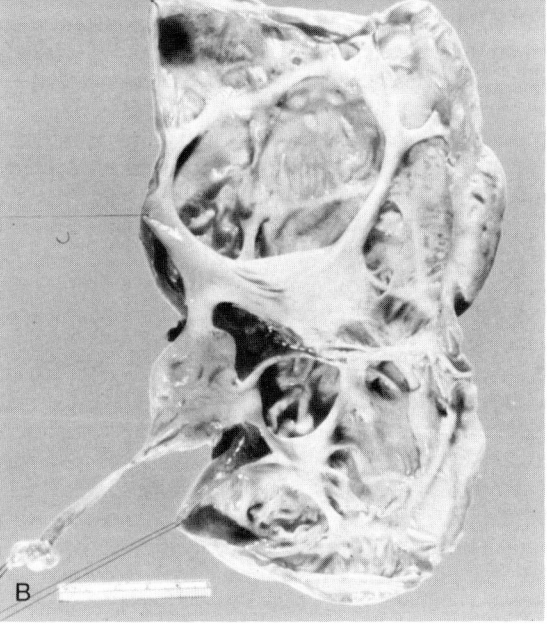

**Figure 27–7.** Severe hydronephrosis with marked thinning of the renal parenchyma. *A.* Sonogram. *B.* Gross specimen.

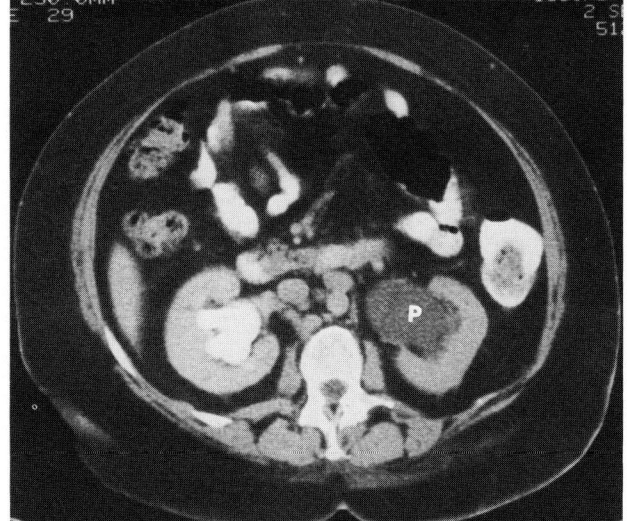

**Figure 27–8.** Bilateral renal obstruction, CT scan. The right kidney shows excretion, whereas no excretion is seen in the left renal pelvis (P), indicating severe high-grade obstruction.

the site of ureteral obstruction. Retroperitoneal or pelvic tumors and ureteral calculi are reliably demonstrated on CT scans. If residual renal function is present, contrast-enhanced images show the pattern of a delayed and prolonged nephrogram familiar from conventional urography (Fig. 27–8).

## Magnetic Resonance Imaging

The MRI appearance of renal obstruction has been studied extensively. Because urine demonstrates low signal intensity on T1-weighted images, ureteral dilatation and renal pelvic dilatation are most readily appreciated on these images (Fig. 27–9). The distended ureter can be differentiated from other structures, and the site of the obstruction can be located by evaluating sequential contiguous images. In addition, it is possible to detect infected urine within the dilated collecting system.[29] The presence of pus changes urine characteristics; on T1-weighted images, infected urine is of higher signal intensity than normal.[29] The cause of an

obstruction, such as pelvic tumors, lymphadenopathy, or retroperitoneal fibrosis, can also be identified (Fig. 27–10). In a case of retroperitoneal fibrosis, MRI, unlike US or CT, can differentiate malignant from benign causes in a large number of patients.[30] The appearance of the obstructed kidney varies, depending on the "age" of the obstruction. In acute and subacute obstruction, the kidney may appear normal, or the tissue contrast between the cortex and medulla on T1-weighted images may decrease.[29] With chronic obstruction, however, it is no longer possible to differentiate the cortex from the medulla. The kidney is often smaller, and the cortex demonstrates a decrease in signal intensity on T2-weighted images (see Fig. 27–9).

The role of gadolinium in the assessment of renal obstruction relative to the degree of renal damage and likelihood of functional recovery is currently being investigated. It is already established that with loss of the kidney's ability to concentrate, as seen during obstruction, the renal medulla does not show the normal decrease in signal intensity 90 seconds after injection (see Fig. 27–11), and in the renal pelvis, the dilute urine demonstrates high signal intensity.[14]

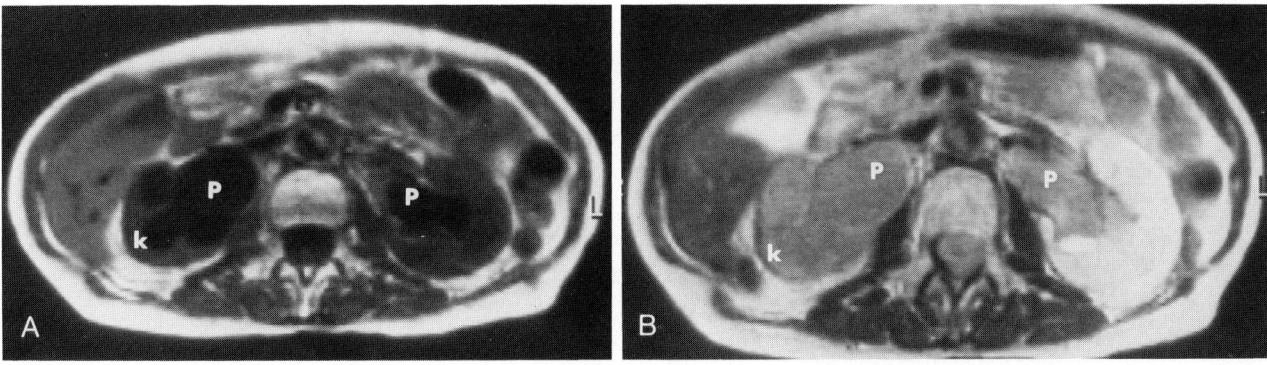

**Figure 27–9.** Bilateral renal obstruction, MRI scan. *A.* T1-weighted scan. *B.* T2-weighted scan. On the T1-weighted image, calyces and pelvis (P) of both right and left kidney are dilated. There is thinning of the kidney parenchyma (k) on the right. On the T2-weighted image, the renal parenchyma on the right demonstrates a low signal intensity indicating presence of ischemia or fibrosis. On the left side, however, the renal parenchyma shows normal increase in signal intensity.

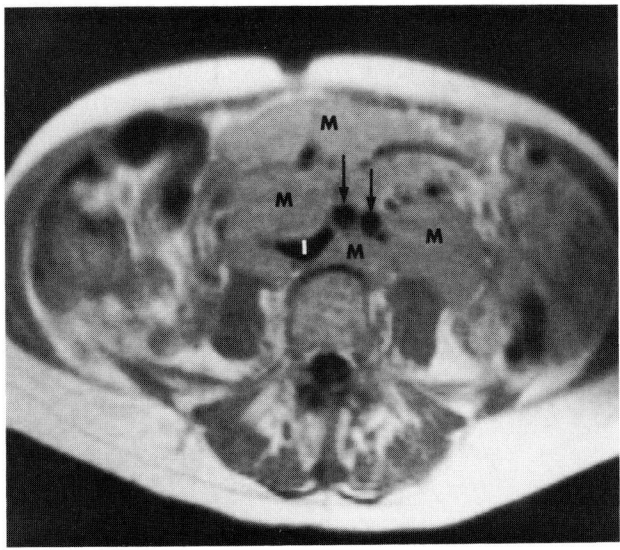

**Figure 27–10.** Large adenopathy encompassing the common iliac arteries *(arrows)* and distorting the outline of the inferior vena cava (I). The numerous enlarged lymph nodes (M) are causing bilateral renal obstruction.

## MEDICAL RENAL DISEASE

The role of radiology in diagnosing medical renal disease is limited. Because IVU studies are compromised by poor renal function and subsequent insufficient excretion, they have only a limited role in the evaluation of a patient with renal failure. US and CT are helpful to the extent that they demonstrate morphologic findings, such as symmetrically small kidneys or altered echogenicity (on US), both of which indicate pathologic changes.[6, 7] MRI consistently demonstrates loss of corticomedullary differentiation as an indicator of renal disease, but this finding, too, is nonspecific.

### Ultrasonography

Diagnostic US allows assessment of kidney size and cortical thickness and evaluation of cortical echogenicity.[7] Cortical echogenicity can be graded as normal (0) when the echo amplitude of the renal cortex is less than that of the adjacent liver (see Fig. 27–1). It is judged as grade I when the amplitude of the cortical echoes equals that of the liver; grade II when it is greater than that of the liver but less than that of the renal sinus; and grade III when the echogenicity of the renal parenchyma is markedly increased,

approaching that of renal sinus fat[7] (Fig. 27–12). A significant correlation has been found between cortical echogenicity and the prevalence of global sclerosis, focal tubule atrophy, and the number of hyaline casts per glomerulus.[7] Although cortical echogenicity corresponds to the severity of histopathologic changes, it does not allow specific diagnosis.[7] There are no distinct sonographic features that enable diagnosis of specific renal medical disease, and renal biopsy remains essential.[7] US does have a role in guiding the renal biopsy and, if needed, in the evaluation of possible complications due to biopsy. Furthermore, after the initial histopathologic diagnosis has been obtained, US can be used to monitor the progression of disease by assessing renal size and echogenicity on sequential films.[6]

### Computed Tomography

Similar to US, the role of CT in the evaluation of medical renal disease is limited to the demonstration of morphologic findings, including symmetrically small kidneys, often with abundant amounts of hilar fat. CT is helpful in the evaluation of patients with medical renal disease who routinely receive hemodialysis and are therefore at increased risk for both benign (cystic metaplasia) and malignant renal neoplasm.[31] Poor renal function hampers CT diagnosis by denying the benefit of contrast enhancement.

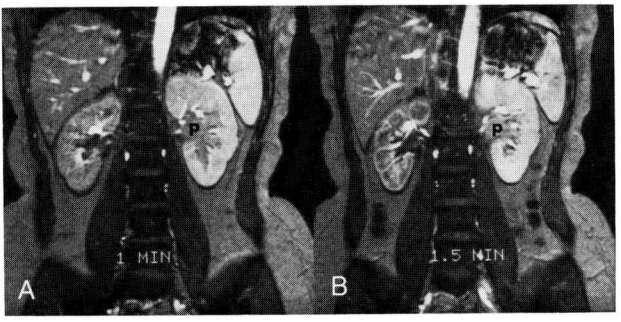

**Figure 27–11.** Left-sided acute renal obstruction. Gradient-echo MRI scans *(A)* 1 minute and *(B)* 1.5 minutes after gadolinium injection. The right kidney shows normal enhancement pattern. In the left kidney, the pelvis (P) is dilated, and there is a persistently high signal intensity of the renal parenchyma indicating prolonged nephrogram phase.

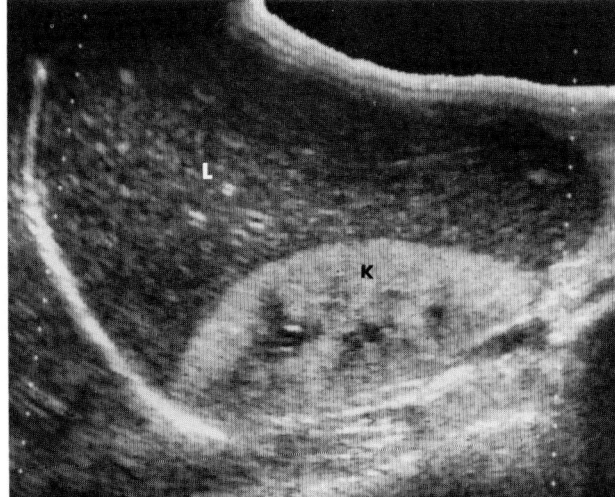

**Figure 27–12.** US scan, heroin-induced nephropathy. The right kidney (k) is enlarged and demonstrates marked increase in echogenicity compared with adjacent liver (L).

## Magnetic Resonance Imaging

MRI may be useful in the evaluation of a variety of medical renal diseases.[32] A moderately to severely damaged kidney, regardless of the cause, demonstrates loss of the corticomedullary boundary. The loss of corticomedullary differentiation is believed to be due to a reduction in the T1 relaxation time of the renal cortex resulting from relative ischemia, glomerular atrophy, or interstitial infiltration (Fig.

27–13). Although loss of corticomedullary differentiation is a sensitive indicator of renal disease, it is nonspecific and provides no information as to the cause of the renal damage.[32] In addition to renal parenchymal disease, conditions such as renal vein thrombosis, diffuse infiltrative involvement in leukemia, or, rarely, lymphoma may cause loss of the corticomedullary boundary; histologic diagnosis remains essential. In chronic renal failure, MRI, similar to CT, can demonstrate associated cortical cysts or tumors.[33]

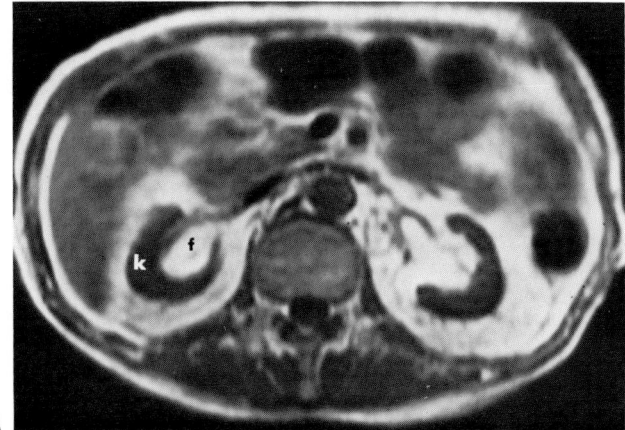
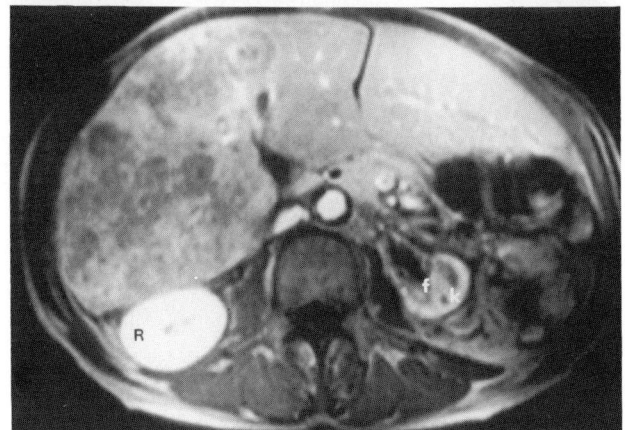

**Figure 27–13.** *A.* Chronic glomerular nephritis, MRI scan. Both kidneys show thinning of the renal parenchyma (k) with increased hilar fat (f). Renal parenchyma is of abnormally low signal intensity, and corticomedullary differentiation is not seen. *B.* Chronic ischemia, left kidney, MRI scan. Gadolinium-enhanced scan shows thinning of the left renal parenchyma (k) with increased hilar fat (f). Decreased brightness of the left renal parenchyma relative to the right (R) is due to diminished function and therefore decreased excretion of contrast medium.

## RENAL VEIN THROMBOSIS

Renal vein thrombosis is a recognized but often silent complication of nephrotic syndrome. The diagnosis of renal vein thrombosis in patients with nephrotic syndrome is a challenging clinical problem. IVU is often unremarkable and has been reported to be normal in 25% of patients with renal vein thrombosis.[34] Renal venography remains the most definitive study in the diagnosis of renal vein thrombosis. Selective renal venography, however, is an invasive and costly procedure not suitable for screening an asymptomatic population at high risk for renal vein thrombosis. Cross-sectional imaging modalities—Doppler US, contrast-enhanced CT, and MRI—have replaced the invasive venogram. With cross-sectional imaging modalities, the diagnosis of this condition relies on the demonstration of a widened renal vein containing the thrombus, thrombus extension into the inferior vena cava, renal enlargement, thickened Gerota fascia, and formation of pericapsular venous collaterals (Figs. 27–14 and 27–15). On CT scans after injection of the contrast media, there is an abnormal renal parenchymal enhancement pattern consisting of prolonged corticomedullary differentiation, delayed or persistent parenchymal opacification, and delay in visualizing or failure to visualize pyelocalyces. The accuracy of CT in diagnosing renal vein thrombosis is excellent,[35] but because it requires an injection of contrast medium, Doppler US and MRI are being explored to replace it. On US scans, the involved kidney appears swollen and relatively echolucent compared with the normal renal parenchyma (see Fig. 27–15B). On MRI scans, it is swollen, and the corticomedullary differentiation is not seen. Both US and MRI are excellent in displaying the renal vein and detecting thrombus.

## RENAL HYPERTENSION

For many years, hypertensive IVU has been considered the screening modality for renovascular hypertension. In hypertensive urography, a bolus of contrast medium is injected, and a rapid sequence of films is made—one each minute for the first 3 minutes, followed by films at 5, 10, 15, and 30 minutes. Findings indicative of renovascular hypertension include a difference in kidney length of 1.5 cm or greater, a delay in the appearance of the collecting system, and hyperconcentration of the contrast medium in the collecting system on the delayed films. In the last several years, however, numerous studies from different investigators have demonstrated the inadequacy of IVU as a screening modality for renovascular hypertension. In a se-

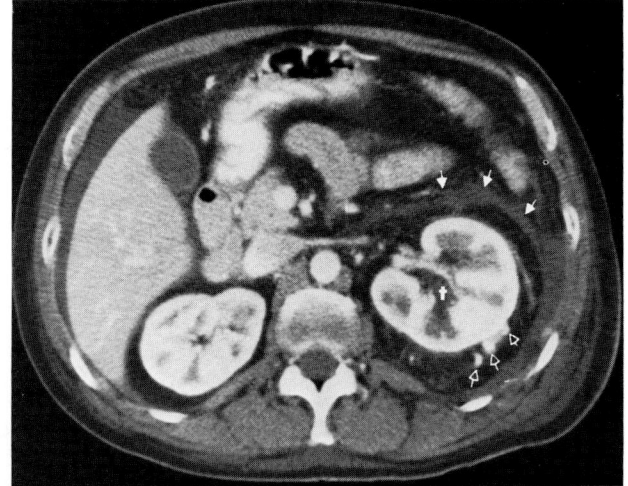

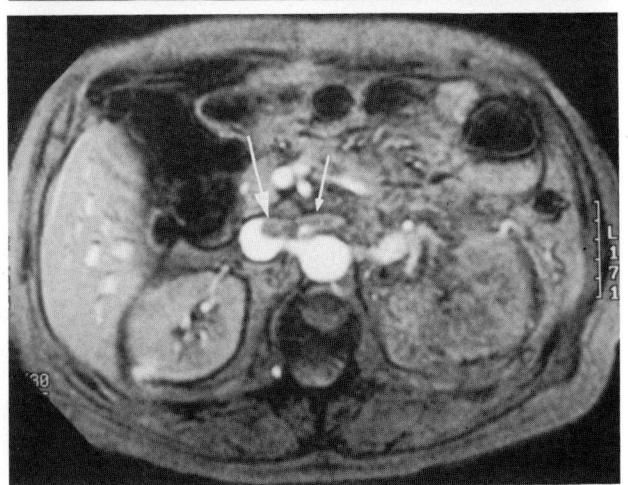

**Figure 27–14.** *A.* Renal vein thrombosis, left kidney, MRI scan. The left kidney is enlarged. There are numerous venous collaterals *(open arrows)*; Gerota fascia *(white arrows)* is thickened. Thrombus (t) is seen within the veins of the renal hilum. *B.* Left renal vein thrombosis extending into the inferior vena cava. A flow-sensitive gradient-echo MRI scan shows low-intensity thrombus within the left renal vein *(small arrow)* extending into the inferior vena cava *(large arrow)*.

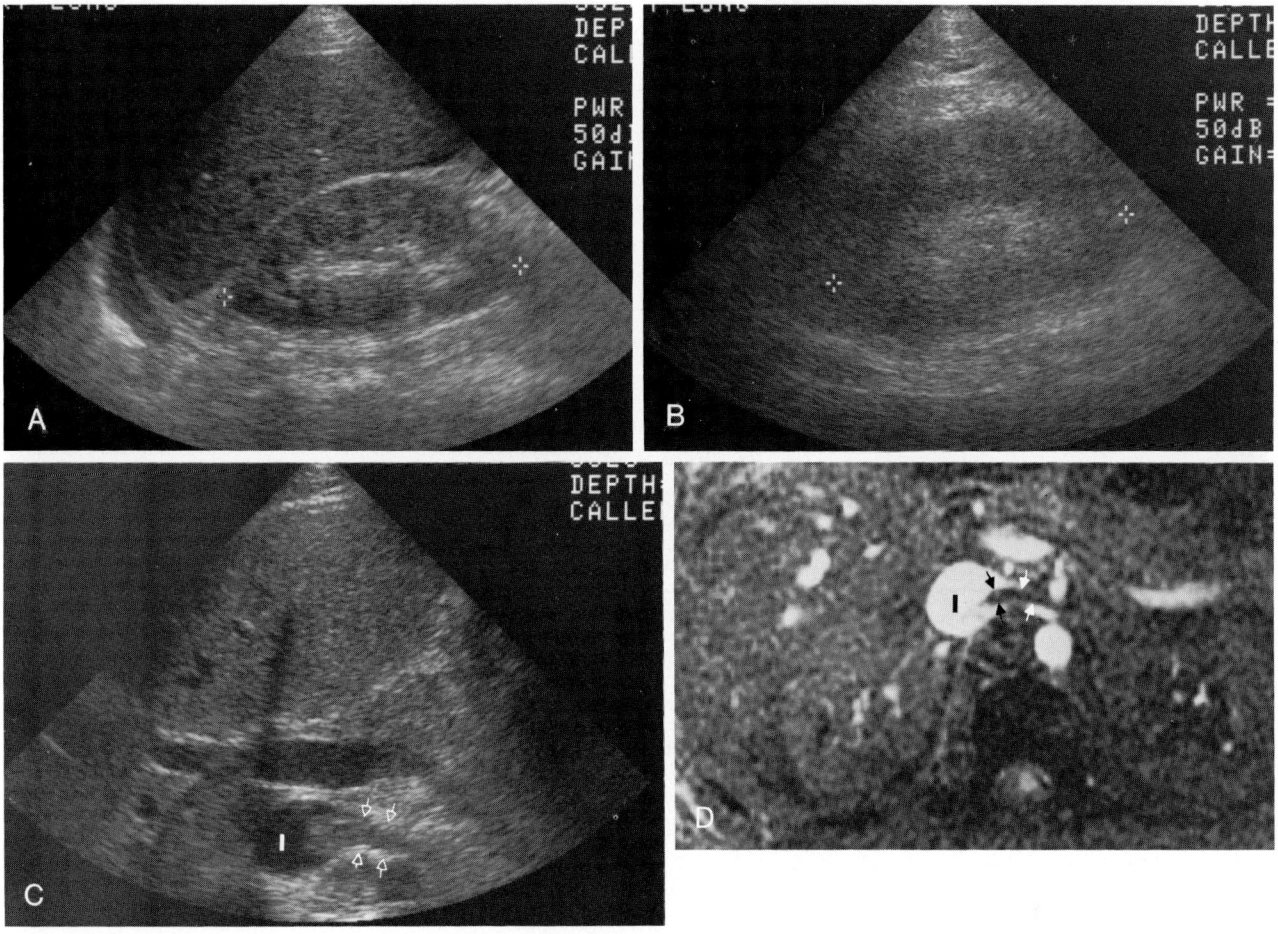

**Figure 27–15.** Nephrotic syndrome with left-sided renal vein thrombosis. *A.* Sonographic appearance, normal right kidney. *B.* The left kidney is enlarged, and corticomedullary differentiation cannot be seen. *C.* The thrombus *(arrows)* is seen in the left renal vein extending into the inferior vena cava (I). *D.* MRI scan showing thrombus *(arrows)* extending from the left renal vein into the inferior vena cava (I).

ries of 416 patients with proven renovascular hypertension and renal artery stenosis greater than 50%, results of IVU studies were positive in 59% of cases and falsely negative in 41%.[36] Similar results were reported by Thornbury and co-workers.[37] They found that IVU examinations failed to confirm the diagnosis in 41.6% of patients with a high degree of arterial stenosis. They also stressed that only 0.8% of all patients with hypertension had a positive urogram finding and that only 24% of these were candidates for surgery.[37] Results from a study at the Mayo Clinic[38] indicated that only 0.18% of patients with renal hypertension detected by IVU had surgically correctable disease. Because of these drawbacks, IVU can no longer be considered an adequate test for renovascular hypertension.

The role of US in renovascular hypertension is limited to evaluation of kidney size. The introduction of Doppler US initiated many investigations into its use in renal artery stenosis, with varying results. At present, however, it appears that US has limited value in the screening of hypertensive patients for renal artery stenosis.[39] Spiral CT angiography has shown promise in this application.[40]

MRI is well suited to the evaluation of vascular anomalies, but the oblique course and small size of the renal arteries are, at present, limiting factors in the evaluation of renovascular hypertension. The effect of long-standing renal hypertension on the kidneys can be depicted. On T1-weighted images, such kidneys are small, with indistinct corticomedullary differentiation and decreased signal intensity of the cortex. Acute unilateral arterial occlusion produced loss of corticomedullary differentiation on T1-weighted images and a decrease in signal intensity on T2-weighted images.[33] Magnetic resonance angiography may prove useful in screening patients for renovascular disease in the setting of renal impairment.[23]

Captopril renography can detect renal artery stenoses greater than 50% with sensitivities and specificities as high as 90% in screened populations of hypertensive patients.[41] This method employs computer-assisted quantitative evaluation of a technetium Tc 99m renogram augmented by administration of 25 to 50 mg of oral captopril. Captopril, an angiotensin-converting enzyme inhibitor, can pharmacologically unmask renal artery stenosis, which may appear normal by standard renography. For further discussion, see Chapter 47.

The diagnostic procedure of choice for patients with renal hypertension is intra-arterial digital subtraction angiography, with assays of venous renin (Fig. 27–16) when appropriate.

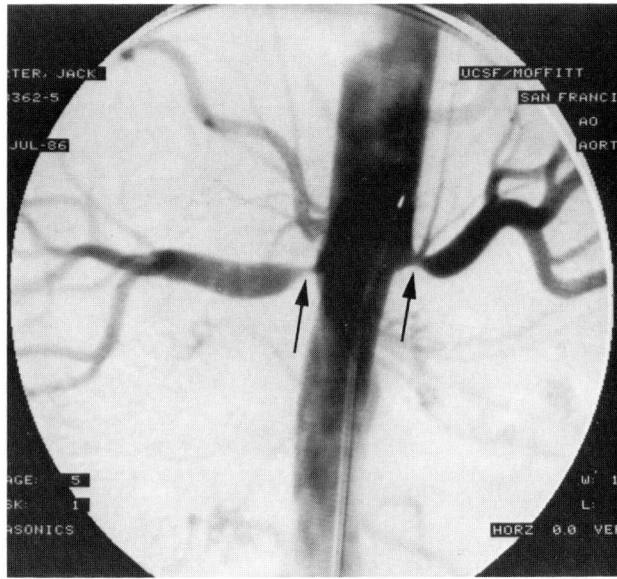

**Figure 27–16.** Midstream digital subtraction aortogram using dilute contrast medium shows significant bilateral renal artery stenosis *(arrows)*.

When digital subtraction arteriography was introduced, there was an attempt to simplify the procedure by obtaining arterial assessment by intravenous injection. Limitations in spatial resolution made this approach inadequate for the diagnosis of many lesions. Today, intravenous digital subtraction arteriography is practically abandoned. Arterial digital subtraction angiography has been perfected and is performed as an outpatient procedure with smaller catheters and half the dose of contrast material used in conventional angiography, which makes the procedure safer and less painful. Furthermore, selective renal artery injection allows demonstration of better detail. When the stenosis is deemed to be significant, angioplasty can be performed during the same procedure.[42]

## INFECTIONS

Renal infection may be localized, or it may involve the entire kidney and prerenal fossa. IVU is not particularly helpful in the evaluation of renal infections, and CT has now replaced it as the preferred diagnostic approach. Although US and MRI findings in renal inflammatory disease have been described, CT is the single most helpful modality for initial evaluation and follow-up of patients with renal inflammatory disease.[43] In patients with acquired immunodeficiency syndrome and suspected renal dysfunction, US is a useful screening study. CT or MRI may be necessary to identify focal infectious, ischemic, and neoplastic processes.[44]

### Intravenous Urography

IVU findings in renal infection may include enlargement of the kidney, striated nephrogram, delayed excretion of contrast material, and either a spidery appearance of the

collecting system (due to interstitial edema) or a dilated collecting system (when a concomitant urinary obstruction is present). Calyceal distortion due to stricture has been reported in 68% of cases of renal tuberculosis. Despite these findings, IVU is not a sensitive modality for the evaluation of renal infection, and a normal IVU has been reported in 75% of patients with proven renal infection.[45]

## Ultrasonography

The sonographic appearance of renal inflammatory disease is not specific; it varies with the type of infection. Renal enlargement with relatively echolucent parenchyma has been reported in acute pyelonephritis. In focal bacterial nephritis, the sonogram may demonstrate localized areas of decreased or heterogeneous echogenicity indistinguishable from tumor (Fig. 27–17). A perinephric abscess may be seen as an anechoic or hypoechoic region with or without internal echoes, but US cannot consistently distinguish between sterile and pyogenic perinephric fluid collections. In addition, the sonogram may remain normal even in the presence of disease[43] (Fig. 27–18). Renal US in patients with acquired immunodeficiency syndrome may show increased cortical echogenicity, hydronephrosis, nephromegaly, and focal abnormalities due to infection, neoplasm, or infarct.[44]

## Computed Tomography

The presence and extent of parenchymal or perinephric infection are detected most accurately with contrast-enhanced CT. CT is helpful in the detection of intrarenal abscess or phlegmon and in the assessment of the presence and extent of perinephric effusion or abscess.[43, 45, 46] Diffuse interstitial nephritis, focal bacterial nephritis, and renal ab-

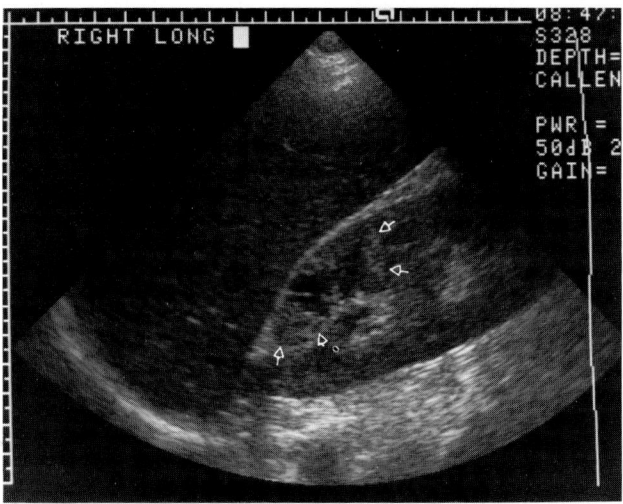

**Figure 27–17.** Lobar nephronia, right kidney. On this longitudinal sonogram of the right kidney, there is ill-defined focus of heterogeneous echogenicity *(arrows)*. The area of low echogenicity may represent liquefaction, but this patient responded to intravenous antibiotic therapy. In view of the clinical findings, this was consistent with lobar nephronia.

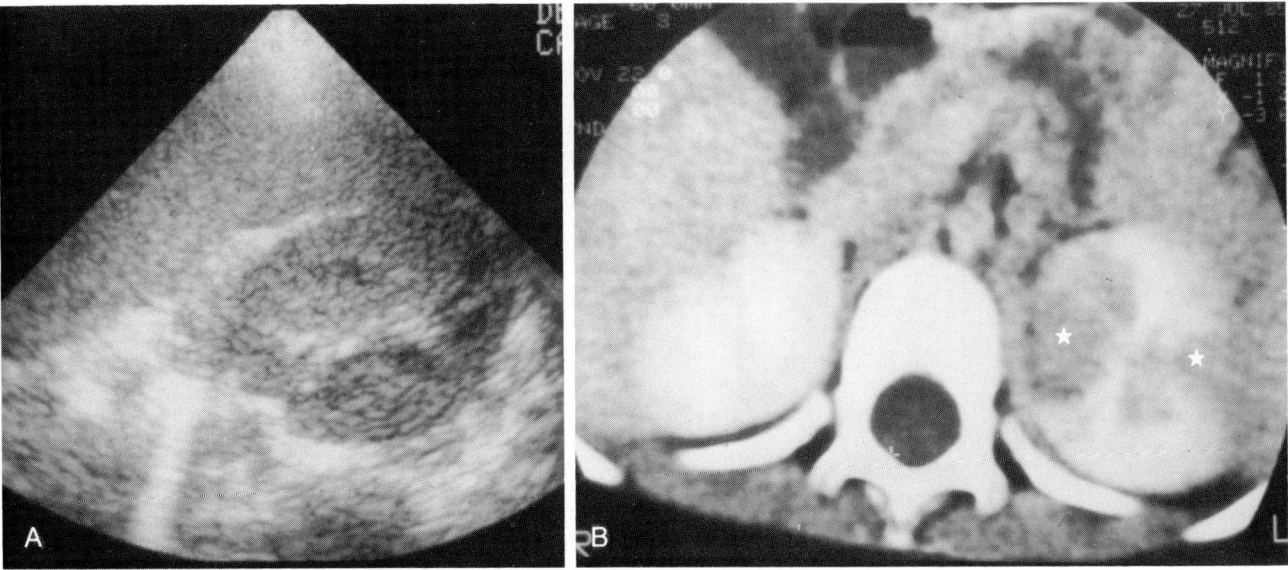

**Figure 27–18.** Severe bacterial infection, left kidney. *A.* On this sonogram, the left kidney shows an indistinct corticomedullary boundary but is otherwise unremarkable. *B.* On the CT scan, however, in the left kidney, there are wedge-shaped, poorly marginated, low-density lesions lobar in distribution and consistent with infection *(asterisk).*

scesses produce a spectrum of CT abnormalities related to the extent of parenchymal edema, distribution of inflammation, and severity of functional impairment. Interstitial nephritis produces renal enlargement, inhomogeneous enhancement, and delayed excretion of contrast material (see Fig. 27–18). Striated collections of gas may be seen in the renal parenchyma, and perinephric fluid collections may be detected. Focal bacterial nephritis produces wedge-shaped areas of low attenuation in both nonenhanced and enhanced images (see Fig. 27–18*B*). These wedge-shaped lesions are poorly marginated, lobar in distribution, and typically unilateral (see Fig. 27–18*B*). Renal abscesses appear as irregularly shaped focal masses that are thick walled and of heterogeneous attenuation with central low-density fluid and gas collections. Penetration of the renal capsule with formation of a perinephric abscess is manifested on CT scans by the appearance of a collection of mixed fluid density and soft tissue density that surrounds and sometimes deforms the kidney. The detection of gas within a perinephric collection indicates bacterial infection, extensive tissue necrosis, or previous diagnostic instrumentation. Perinephric fluid may be seen to be confined by bridging septa within the perinephric fascia. In this situation, CT images can be employed to facilitate correct percutaneous positioning of drainage catheters. Inflammatory tissue may contact and thicken perinephric fascia and may penetrate this fascia to extend into the anterior or posterior pararenal spaces.

## Magnetic Resonance Imaging

In infectious processes, the MRI appearance of the kidney is determined by the amount and distribution of renal edema.[32] In severe pyelonephritis, the kidney is swollen and the corticomedullary differentiation is no longer visible (Fig. 27–19). In focal pyelonephritis, lobar areas of lower

signal intensity may be seen extending through the medulla to the cortex and obscuring corticomedullary contrast (Fig. 27–20). In sequential scans, portions of the unaffected kidney will appear relatively normal. Renal abscesses appear as somewhat ill-defined masses, usually of low signal intensity on T1-weighted images, but signal intensity can vary, depending on the underlying pathologic processes. Because the MRI appearance of abscesses may be indistinguishable

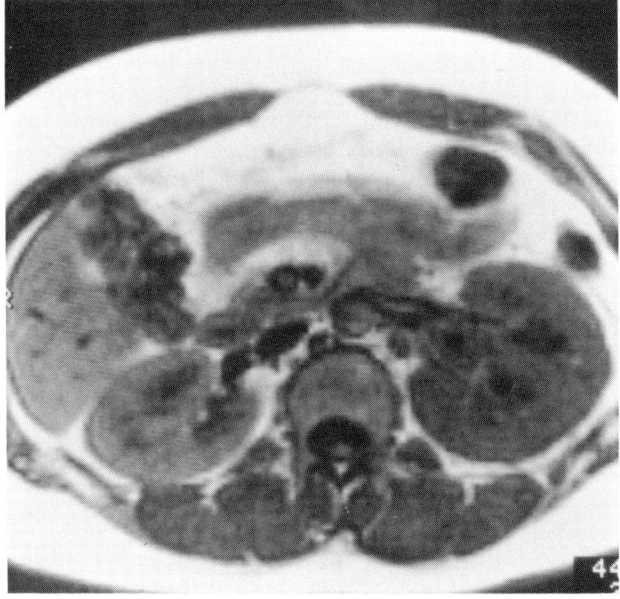

**Figure 27–19.** Acute bacterial infection, left kidney, MRI scan, T1-weighted image. The left kidney is enlarged. The corticomedullary differentiation is obliterated, and the signal intensity of the left kidney is lower compared with the normal right kidney, indicating edema. Findings are consistent with acute pyelonephritis.

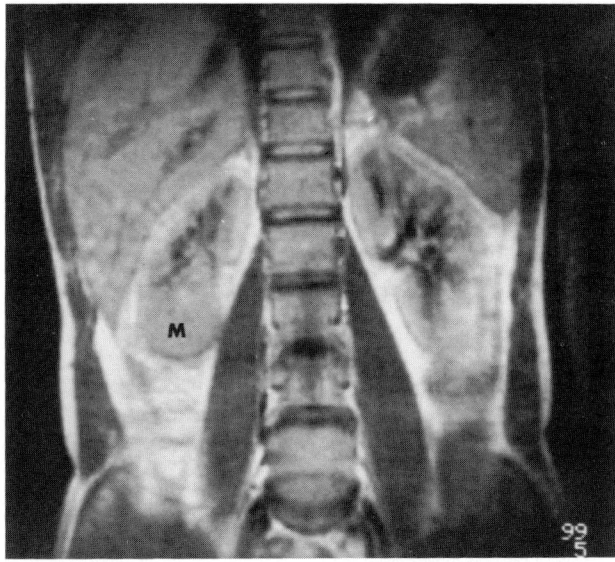

**Figure 27–20.** Lobar nephronia of the right kidney, coronal MRI scan. There is a localized mass effect (M) with indistinct corticomedullary differentiation in the lower pole of the right kidney. Differential diagnosis includes tumor or infection. In this clinical setting, this represented lobar nephronia.

from complicated cysts or from solid neoplasms, the specific diagnosis depends on clinical criteria and biopsy.

## CALCULI

### Plain Film and Intravenous Urography

In the routine workup of a patient with renal colic, a plain film of the abdomen (kidney, ureter, and bladder) is the initial examination of choice. About 85% of urinary calculi contain calcium and are, therefore, visualized on plain films. Depending on the plain film findings and the clinical symptoms, the next step in the diagnostic workup has traditionally been the excretory urogram. In obstruction, IVU findings consist of a prolonged nephrogram, delayed excretion of contrast medium, and pelvocalyceal and ureteral dilatation. Because the concentrating ability of the kidneys is diminished, the excreted contrast medium is less radiopaque, and it becomes even more so as it is further diluted by the urine in the dilated collecting system. Whereas IVU still remains the most accurate modality for the diagnosis of obstruction by urinary calculus, owing to the potential risk from injection of contrast medium US is now being advocated as an initial examination of choice.

### Ultrasonography

In obstructive uropathy, US studies demonstrate hydronephrosis and may display the calculus itself (Figs. 27–21 and 27–22). Obstructive calculi are most commonly located at the ureteropelvic or ureterovesical junction, however, and assessment of these two locations by US requires experience and expertise (see Fig. 27–21). When US is used in

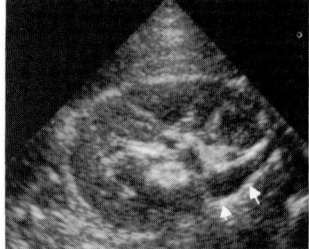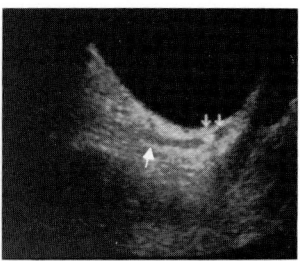

**Figure 27–21.** Acute obstruction caused by a calculus at the right ureterovesical junction. *Left.* An oblique scan through the right kidney shows minor hydronephrosis with dilatation of the right proximal ureter *(arrows)*. *Right.* The dilated ureter *(large arrow)* can be seen posterior to the urinary bladder, with a calculus causing acoustic shadowing in its distal portion *(small arrows)*.

the diagnosis of renal calculi, it is important to remember that findings may be misleading if there is obstruction without hydronephrosis. For example, hydronephrosis may be absent if the obstruction is partial or there has been forniceal rupture resulting in urinary decompression. So negative US findings in the presence of clinical symptoms that suggest calculous obstruction should not preclude further evaluation by IVU.[47] Color flow Doppler US of the arcuate and interlobar arteries may be of assistance in detecting acute obstruction (>6 hours' duration) in the absence of hydronephrosis.[27] US may be helpful in detecting concomitant pyonephrosis (Fig. 27–23).

### Computed Tomography

Because the majority of renal and ureteral calculi appear dense on CT images, CT may be used to detect stones that are not evident on conventional radiographs.[48] In this situation, scanning before administration of intravenous contrast material is essential, because dense stones can be obscured by opacified urine.[48]

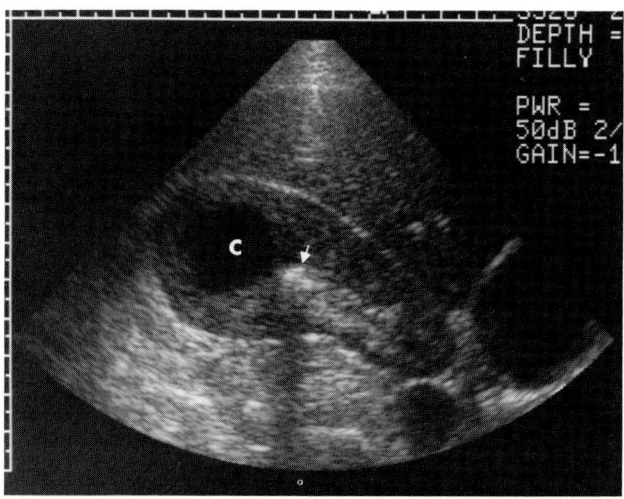

**Figure 27–22.** Calculus *(arrow)* in the infundibulum of the right kidney causing a localized dilatation of the proximal calyx (c).

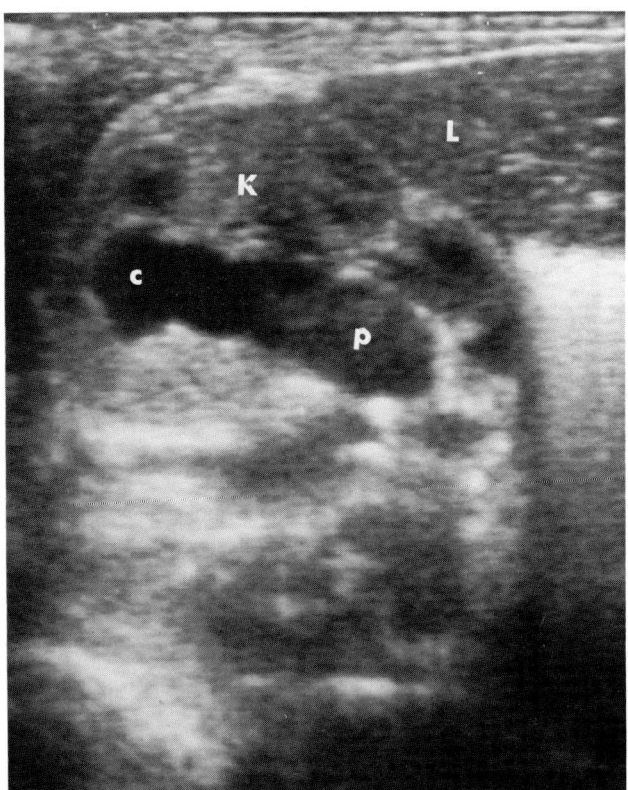

**Figure 27–23.** Pyonephrosis, sonogram. The collecting system is dilated. The calyces (c) are clubbed, and there are numerous echoes in the dependent portion of the pelvis (p). In view of the clinical findings, this is consistent with pyonephrosis. K = kidney; L = liver.

## Magnetic Resonance Imaging

MRI is of little help in the evaluation of nephrolithiasis. Calculi do not contain mobile H$^+$ and, so, do not emit signals for MRI. Calculi may be evident if their foci of signal void are sufficiently large or if they lie adjacent to tissue of relatively high signal intensity. Both conventional urography and CT are superior to MRI in this setting.

## RENAL MASSES

IVU is still considered the best initial study in the search for renal masses, but in the presence of a renal mass confirmed by CT, the detection demonstrated by IVU is only 10% when the lesion is less than 1 cm in diameter, 21% when it is between 1 and 2 cm, 52% when the lesion is between 2 and 3 cm, and 85% when it is 3 cm or more.[49] Therefore, a normal IVU does not exclude the presence of a renal mass. Furthermore, when a mass is detected, it is not possible to differentiate between cystic and solid lesions with IVU.[49, 50] Even when a mass appears unchanged on sequential IVUs, it is risky to assume that it represents a simple cyst, because renal cell carcinomas, particularly of the cystic type, may be growing slowly. Further studies, such as US, CT, or MRI, are necessary to determine the character of the mass.[51] If IVU findings suggest a cystic mass, US is the next imaging examination of choice; if a solid lesion is suspected, the examination should be CT.

## Renal Cysts

Benign cortical cysts are the most frequently encountered renal masses. They may be solitary or numerous, and although they are often asymptomatic, they may cause pain by stretching the renal capsule. Intracystic hemorrhage or infection can also lead to symptoms of pain or fever.

### ULTRASONOGRAPHY

A lesion is considered a benign simple cyst if the following sonographic criteria are present: 1) absence of internal echoes (a single septum can be accepted); 2) all the walls of the cyst are smooth and sharply defined; 3) acoustic enhancement beyond the posterior wall of the cyst is proportional to the fluid content (this is the single most important finding); and 4) a narrow band of acoustic shadowing is seen beyond the outer margin (Fig. 27–24). If these criteria are met, no further studies are necessary to characterize the mass. If, however, US is technically suboptimal or if the mass is characterized as intermediate or has the characteristics of a solid lesion, further diagnostic tests are required.[51] At present, CT is the best choice for the next study.

### COMPUTED TOMOGRAPHY

A renal mass can be confidently called a simple cyst when it meets the following CT criteria[48, 51]: 1) it has a homogeneous attenuation value near that of water; 2) its wall is so thin that it is nearly indiscernible; 3) it is sharply delineated from surrounding renal parenchyma; and 4) its fluid contents do not increase in attenuation value after intravenous infusion of contrast medium (Fig. 27–25). If the fluid contents of the cyst are of higher density, or if the cyst is irregularly shaped with thickened or calcified walls, it may be a complicated renal cyst or a solid tumor. Such lesions require further diagnostic evaluation,[51] especially when clinical symptoms such as pain or hemorrhage raise the possibility of renal tumor. Percutaneous cyst aspiration and biopsy may be performed with CT guidance, and if a

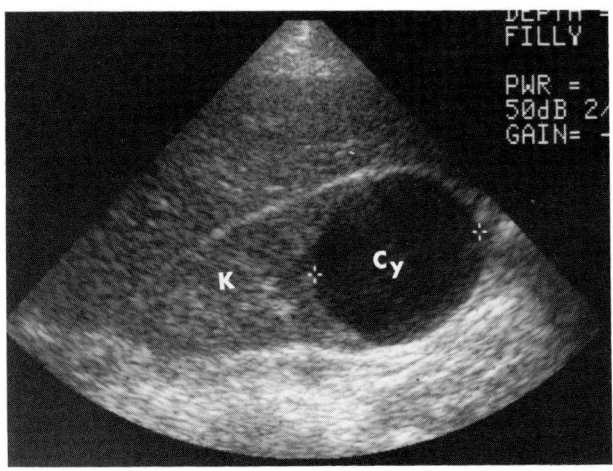

**Figure 27–24.** Simple renal cyst (Cy), lower pole of the right kidney (K), sonogram.

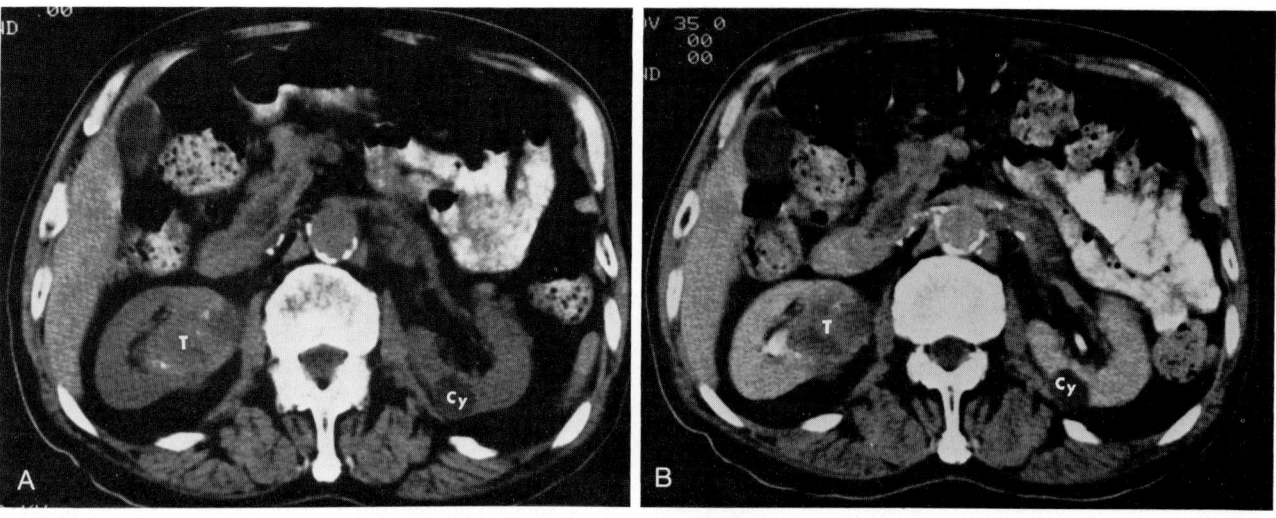

**Figure 27–25.** CT scan before *(A)* and after *(B)* contrast enhancement demonstrating a simple renal cyst (Cy) in the left kidney. The solid heterogeneous tumor (T) with punctate calcification is seen in the right kidney. After injection of the contrast medium, the tumor shows heterogeneous enhancement, but predominantly it is less dense compared with adjacent renal parenchyma.

solid renal mass is detected, CT is helpful in evaluating the anatomic extent of disease. CT is not helpful in the assessment of possible cyst infection.

### MAGNETIC RESONANCE IMAGING

On MRI scans, simple renal cysts (i.e., the composition of the fluid within them is similar to urine) appear as clearly defined, rounded masses of homogeneous signal intensity, low on T1-weighted images and increasing on T2-weighted images. Once a cyst is complicated by either hemorrhage or infection, the magnetic resonance signal usually becomes heterogeneous and nonspecific. Calcification within the walls of a complicated cyst may cause wall thickening, but unlike findings with CT, MRI findings are nonspecific and do not clearly identify calcifications. In complicated cysts, benign disease cannot be differentiated from malignant disease, and differentiation between cystic and solid lesions is not possible.[33]

## Polycystic Kidney Disease

The radiologic evaluation of adult-type polycystic kidney disease can be obtained by IVU, US, CT, or MRI. The IVU finding of bilateral enlarged kidneys with spidery appearance of the infundibula and calyces is well known but nonspecific. US is an excellent modality for evaluating polycystic kidney disease. Kidney size and presence of cysts are accurately evaluated. The CT presentation of polycystic kidney disease demonstrates variation in cyst size. Because of variation in cyst size and contents and in residual renal function, CT presentation is variable[48] (Fig. 27–26). Generally, the kidneys are enlarged by multiple cysts, which may differ from one another in density. Hemorrhage may produce fluid-fluid levels within individual cysts, and debris may cause heterogeneous attenuation in others. Renal tissue with residual function is enhanced after injec-

tion of contrast material, and excretion into the collecting system may be apparent. Calcification in cyst walls is more readily appreciated in nonenhanced images. Associated hepatic, splenic, and pancreatic cysts produce rounded visceral masses of low attenuation.

The MRI appearance of the kidneys in polycystic disease depends on the size and number of cysts; the kidneys often display marked enlargement and replacement of the renal parenchyma by cysts of various sizes. Intracystic hemorrhage, a common occurrence in this condition, usually results in cysts with a range of signal intensities. Hemorrhagic cysts can demonstrate homogeneous, medium to high signal intensity, and, in some cases, fluid-iron levels are indicated by layering within the cysts.[52] Some cysts demonstrate heterogeneous signal intensity.[33, 52] Although differentiation between uncomplicated and complicated (hemorrhagic) cysts is possible with MRI, it does not offer much advantage over CT or US in reliably detecting either neoplasms or infections in such cysts.

## Solid Renal Masses

For the detection of solid renal masses, IVU, US, CT, or MRI can be used. The limitations of IVU have already been discussed. Although US is an excellent modality for detecting renal cysts, it is considerably less accurate in detecting solid lesions. Compared with CT, US allowed detection of 26% of CT-confirmed lesions less than 1 cm in diameter, 60% of lesions of at least 1 but less than 2 cm, 82% of lesions at least 2 but less than 3 cm, and 85% of lesions 3 cm or larger.[49] It is certainly insufficient to recommend US as a modality for the detection of solid renal lesions; the best modality is CT.[49, 53] MRI is reserved for patients with impaired renal function, for patients with a history of allergy to iodinated intravenous contrast material, or for those in whom contrast material is otherwise contraindicated.[54] MRI is also useful when the results of CT or US are

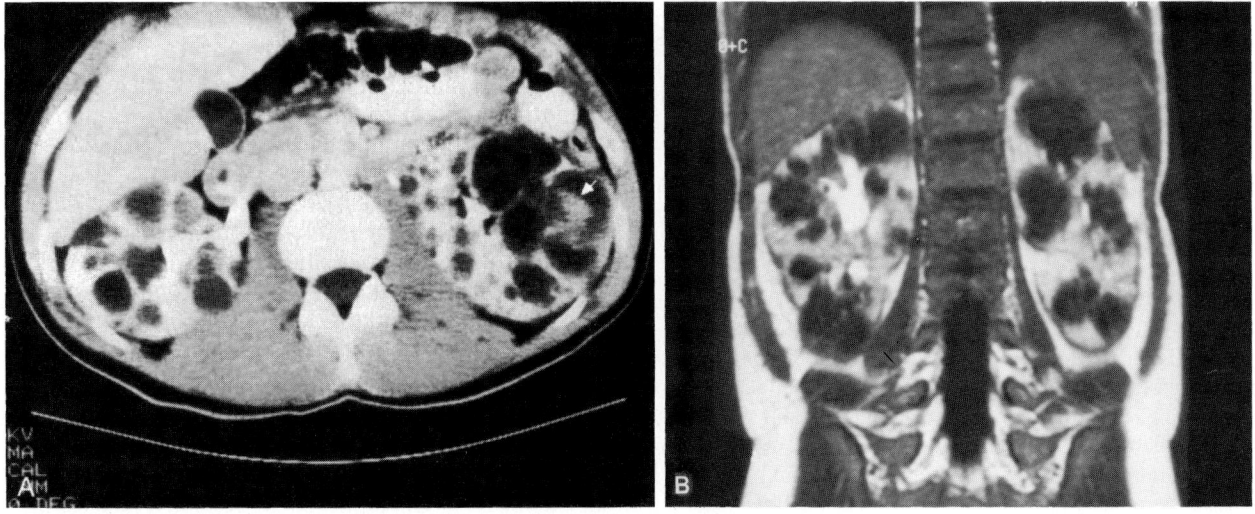

**Figure 27–26.** CT *(A)* and MRI *(B)* scans of polycystic disease showing bilateral renal enlargement with numerous cysts of various sizes and density (for CT) or signal intensity (for MRI). The lesion in the left kidney *(arrow)* at surgery represented a blood clot, but by either CT or MRI criteria, tumor within the cyst cannot be excluded.

indeterminate and further lesion characterization is desired.[55] When gadolinium is used, the accuracy of contrast-enhanced MRI for tumor diagnosis is slightly above that of CT.[56, 57]

With use of conventional spin-echo T1- and T2-weighted images, the accuracy of MRI in depicting solid renal lesions smaller than 3 cm is only 65%,[34] which is significantly below the 95% to 99% accuracy of CT. This low detection rate by MRI is due to the lack of signal intensity difference between tumor and normal kidney regardless of the technique used. Early reports on the use of gadolinium for tumor diagnosis are encouraging. When gadolinium is used, the accuracy of this contrast-enhanced MRI matches that of CT.[14]

## BENIGN TUMORS

Benign mesenchymal tumors of the kidney, including leiomyomas, fibromas, lipomas, oncocytomas, and hamartomas, are relatively unusual lesions. Sonographic evaluation is limited to the differentiation of solid and cystic lesions. For that purpose, US has an accuracy of 94%.[58] For solid lesions smaller than 2 cm, however, US is not useful, and it is necessary to use CT to clarify the diagnosis of a space-occupying renal lesion.[49] CT is the most useful radiologic modality in the assessment of a hamartoma or angiomyolipoma when its appearance is characteristic enough to allow noninvasive diagnosis[59] (Fig. 27–27). Angiomyolipomas contain vascular, smooth muscle, and fatty tissue in

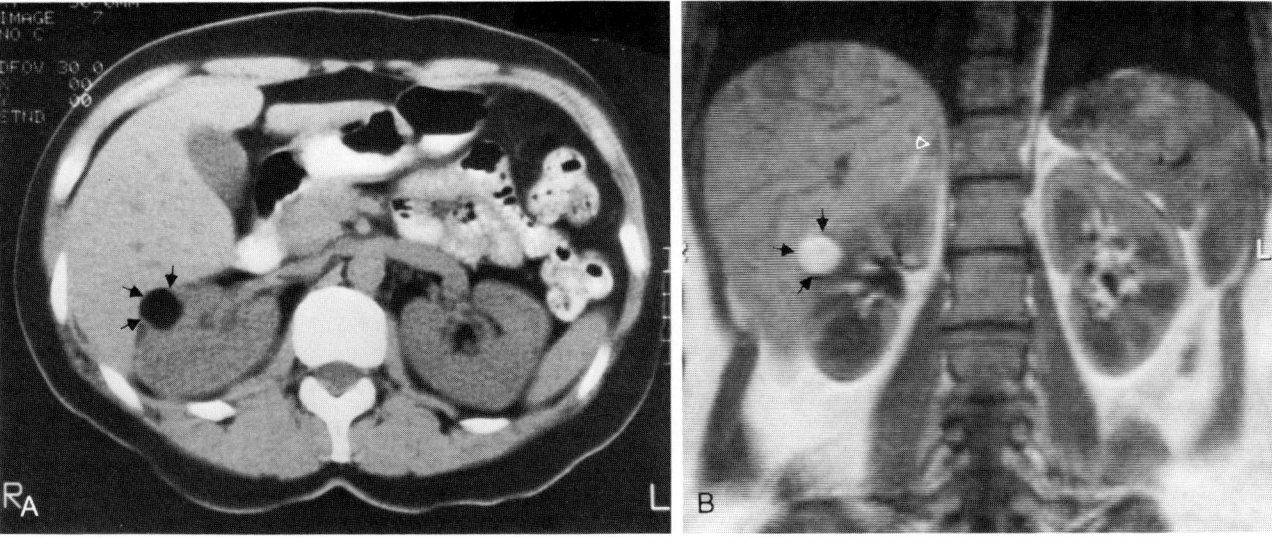

**Figure 27–27.** *A.* CT scan demonstrating angiomyolipoma *(arrows)* of the right kidney. The negative attenuation value of the lesion is specific for the diagnosis. *B.* Angiomyolipoma *(arrows)* on MRI scan (T1-weighted gradient recall acquisition in steady state) in the same patient. The right adrenal gland *(arrowhead)* is normal. At present, MRI is inferior to CT for the specific diagnosis of angiomyolipoma.

varying proportions. If fatty tissue predominates, a diagnosis can be made by measuring CT attenuation.[59] If there is intralesional hemorrhage or a predominance of vascular tissue or muscle tissue, however, the fatty component may be obscured and the diagnosis complicated. Other benign solid renal neoplasms are typically isodense with renal parenchyma on nonenhanced scans and less dense than enhanced renal parenchyma. Precise diagnosis requires histologic examination.

## RENAL CELL CARCINOMA

The CT appearance of renal cell carcinoma varies with tumor size and vascularity.[60, 61] When large enough, these tumors appear as masses that alter renal contour or intrarenal architecture. Detection of small lesions is facilitated by rapid sequence scanning techniques during administration of contrast material because abnormal enhancement may be evident even when renal contours are normal. Heterogeneous enhancement is characteristic, but after administration of the contrast medium, renal cell carcinomas typically appear less dense than surrounding renal tissue (see Fig. 27–25). Large intralesional vascular channels and retroperitoneal collateral vessels may also be present.

Renal cell carcinoma can be staged according to the classifications described by Robson and Churchill.[53] According to these criteria, tumors confined by the renal capsule are classified as stage 1, and lesions confined by perirenal fascia are stage 2. Stage 3 lesions are subdivided into three categories. Stage 3A tumors extend to the renal vein or inferior vena cava; stage 3B lesions extend to retroperitoneal lymph nodes; and stage 3C lesions involve both draining vessels and retroperitoneal lymph nodes. Tumors that have invaded adjacent viscera or muscle structures are classified as stage 4A, and lesions that have metastasized distantly are considered stage 4B. Metastases to the lungs, the mediastinum, and the liver are readily appreciated, but demonstration of renal vein and inferior vena cava tumor thrombus requires administration of contrast material. Typically, tumor thrombi enlarge the renal vein and inferior vena cava and cause the density of these vessels to be heterogeneous[35, 53, 60] (Fig. 27–28). Care must be taken to avoid confusing artifacts caused by laminar flow of intravascular contrast material with intraluminal thrombi. Such artifacts may be seen after injections of either the arm or foot vein and may be eliminated by use of both rapid sequence scanning during injection of contrast material and delayed scanning in the region of the suprarenal inferior vena cava. The accuracy of CT in staging renal cell carcinoma exceeds 80% in many series.[53]

With MRI, renal cell carcinomas demonstrate a spectrum of findings.[33, 34] On spin-echo T1-weighted images, the intensity of tumors ranges from intermediate to high. On spin-echo T2-weighted images, a tumor pseudocapsule can sometimes be detected as a line of lower intensity interposed between the tumor and the normal renal parenchyma. On gadolinium contrast–enhanced MRI scans, tumors generally enhance to a lesser degree than the surrounding renal parenchyma. Lesion sensitivity is increased when dynamic postcontrast scanning is employed.[57]

At present, MRI is used mostly in the staging of renal cell carcinomas and is reported to have an accuracy rate of 82% to 93%.[34, 57] Combined transverse and sagittal MRI planes are optimal for the evaluation of venous anatomy and the normal tissue-tumor interfaces. The particular advantages of MRI staging include the determination of the origin of the mass, the evaluation of vascular patency, the detection of perihilar lymph node metastases, and the eval-

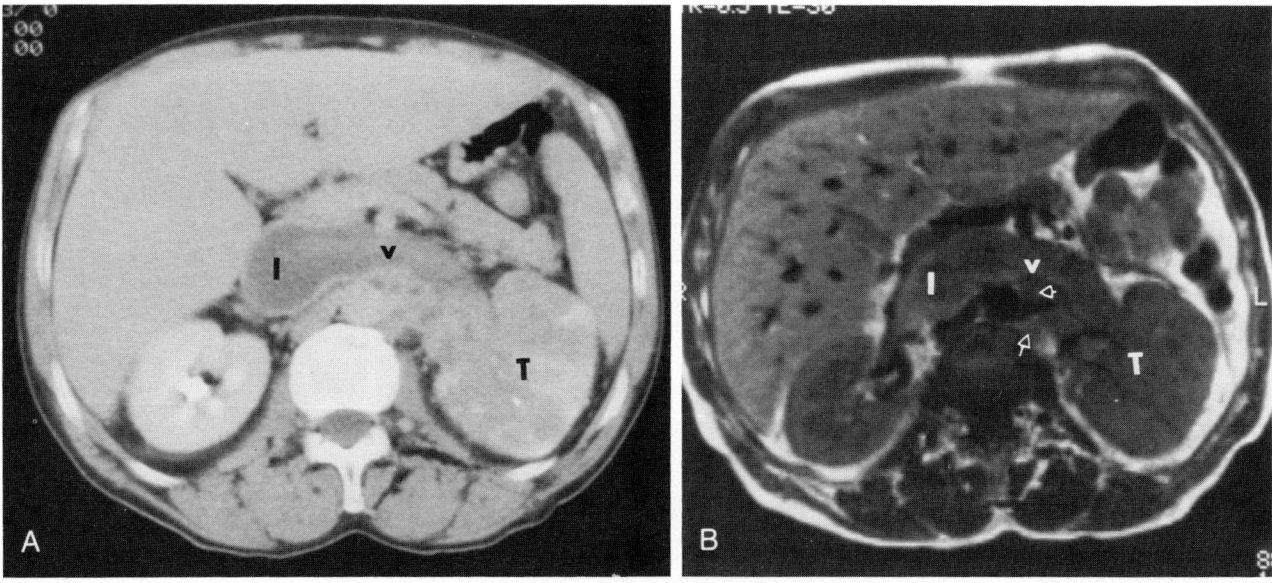

**Figure 27–28.** Left-sided renal cell carcinoma with tumor extension in the left renal vein (v) and inferior vena cava (I). *A.* A CT scan demonstrates enlargement of diffusely infiltrative tumor (T) in the left kidney with widening and heterogeneous density of the left renal vein and tumor extension into the enlarged inferior vena cava. *B.* Corresponding MRI scan B shows similar findings. Also note numerous lymph nodes *(arrows)* surrounding the left renal artery.

uation of direct tumor invasion to adjacent organs. MRI is also a sensitive tool for determining the extent of tumor thrombus (seen as abnormal signal intensity within the renal vein or inferior vena cava) and for demonstrating invasion of the wall of the inferior vena cava (Fig. 27–29). In the assessment of thrombus extension into the renal vein or inferior vena cava, MRI has replaced venography (Fig. 27–30).

## EVALUATION OF THE RENAL TRANSPLANT

MRI, renal scintigraphy, conventional and color Doppler US, and fine-needle aspiration biopsy are used in the evaluation of renal graft complications and failure. MRI, renal scintigraphy, and US are sensitive in detecting acute failure and acute tubule necrosis but cannot reliably differentiate between these two entities (Fig. 27–31). When there is doubt about the diagnosis, US-guided biopsy should be performed. Conventional US is essential for characterization and management of perinephric fluid collections and ureteric obstruction. Color Doppler US has been shown to be valuable in evaluating post-transplant renal artery stenosis, with a sensitivity of 100% and specificity of 86%,[62] and therefore spares the need for angiography in most patients. Serial US scanning of renal transplants and aggressive use of interventional radiologic techniques can lead to preservation of graft function and improvement in graft survival figures.[63] Initially, there was enthusiasm for MRI in the evaluation of graft failure and complications. Although MRI is helpful, the high cost of MRI combined with excellent performance of US has diminished enthusiasm for MRI. MRI is reserved primarily for detection of thrombus and angiographic applications.

## ³¹P MAGNETIC RESONANCE SPECTROSCOPY OF THE KIDNEY

Kidney spectra show a characteristic fingerprint of six peaks that correspond to phosphomonoester; inorganic phosphate ($P_i$); phosphodiester; and β-, α- and γ-phosphates of ATP.[64-68] The amplitude of the phosphomonoester peak varies between immature and fully developed kidneys, being larger in fetal than in adult kidneys. No phosphocreatine has been detected within the kidney spectrum.

Presently, the ³¹P magnetic resonance spectra are obtained from a large voxel, and therefore the peaks from the cortex, medulla, and papilla are averaged. It is known that the spectra from the three ATP areas, the $P_i$, and the phosphomonoester as well as intracellular pH are different when isolated renal tubules from the cortex, medulla, and papilla are studied separately.[64]

Although the amplitude of the peaks is related to the concentration, absolute values are presently not quantifiable, and the results are usually expressed in ratios. Different ratios have been proposed. ATP/$P_i$ ratios have been used in the assessment of renal damage due to ischemia, hypoxia, or urinary obstruction, but in studying renal preservation, ATP levels in a stored kidney declined rapidly. Therefore, the phosphomonoester/$P_i$ ratios have been chosen as predictors of renal viability.

During renal failure caused by different mechanisms (hypoxia, ischemia, acidosis, obstruction), ³¹P magnetic resonance spectra demonstrate rapid loss of high-energy phosphate (depletion of ATP) with progressive increase in $P_i$ and decline of intracellular pH. Whereas the changes in ³¹P magnetic resonance spectroscopy are nonspecific, the severity of renal failure correlates with the severity of the metabolic disturbance.[64] For example, partial ureteral obstruction, even 3 weeks after its occurrence, causes only minor changes in the ³¹P spectra, whereas complete obstruction

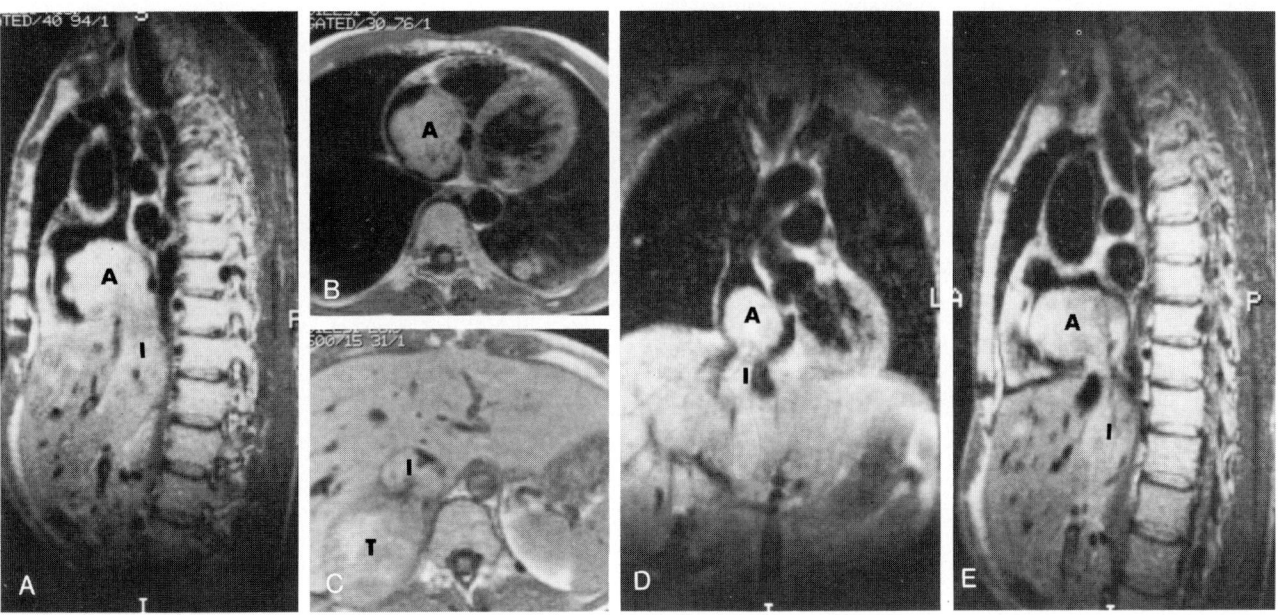

**Figure 27–29.** A large right-sided renal cell carcinoma (T) with direct tumor extension into the inferior vena cava (I). The tumor extends to the right atrium (A). This finding is appreciated on sagittal *(A, E)*, transverse *(B, C)*, and coronal *(D)* MRI scans.

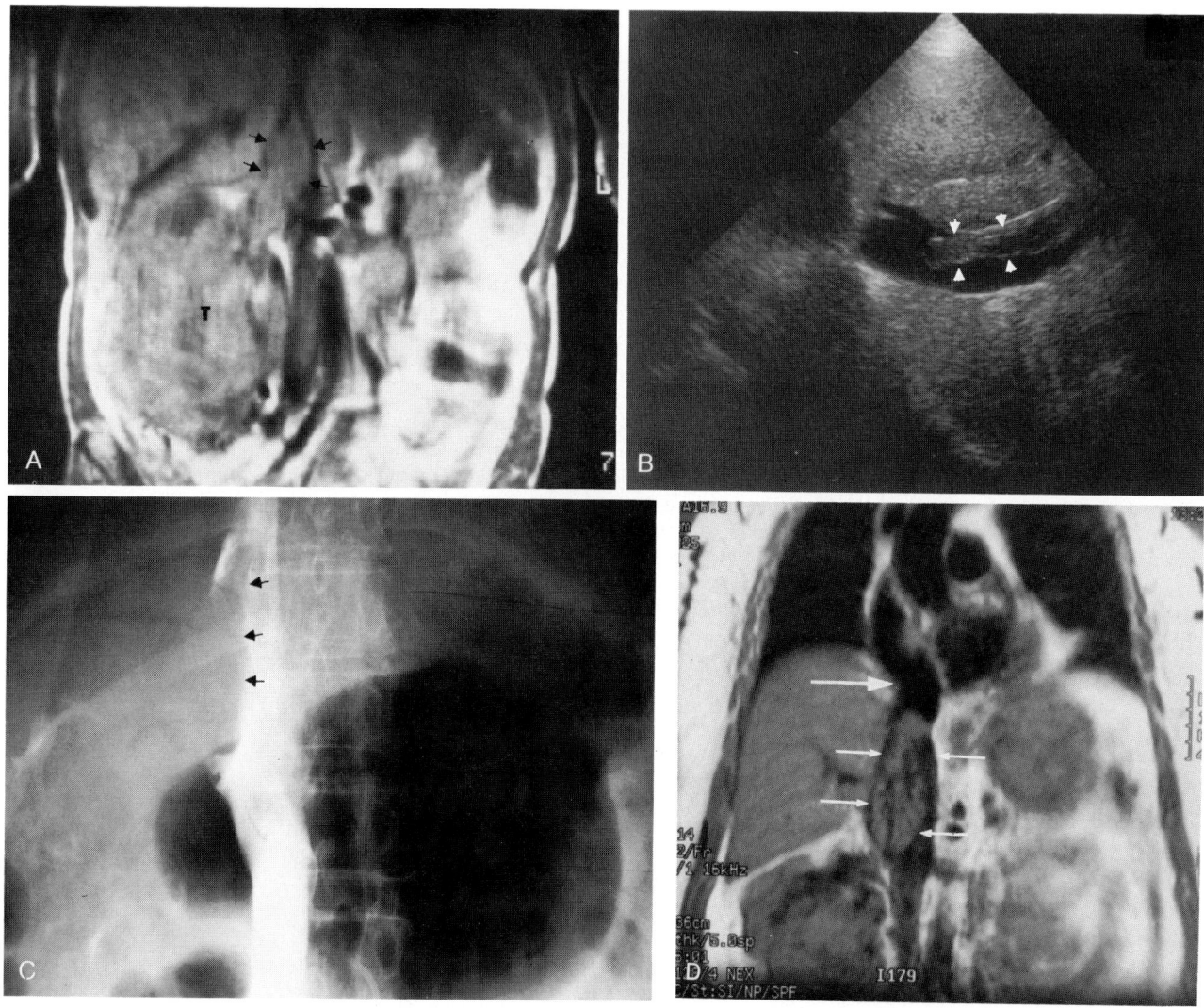

**Figure 27–30.** Renal cell carcinoma (T) with tumor extension into the right renal vein and inferior vena cava *(arrows)*. Findings are demonstrated on MRI scan *(A)*, US image *(B)*, and inferior venacavogram *(C)*. Because the accuracy of MRI in detection of tumor thrombus is similar to that of venography, the noninvasive nature of MRI prevails in the decision. US is accurate but often highly operator dependent. *D.* Tumor extension into the inferior vena cava in another patient. A coronal MRI scan demonstrates tumor extending into the intrahepatic portion of the inferior vena cava *(small arrows)*; however, the right atrium *(large arrow)* is free of tumor.

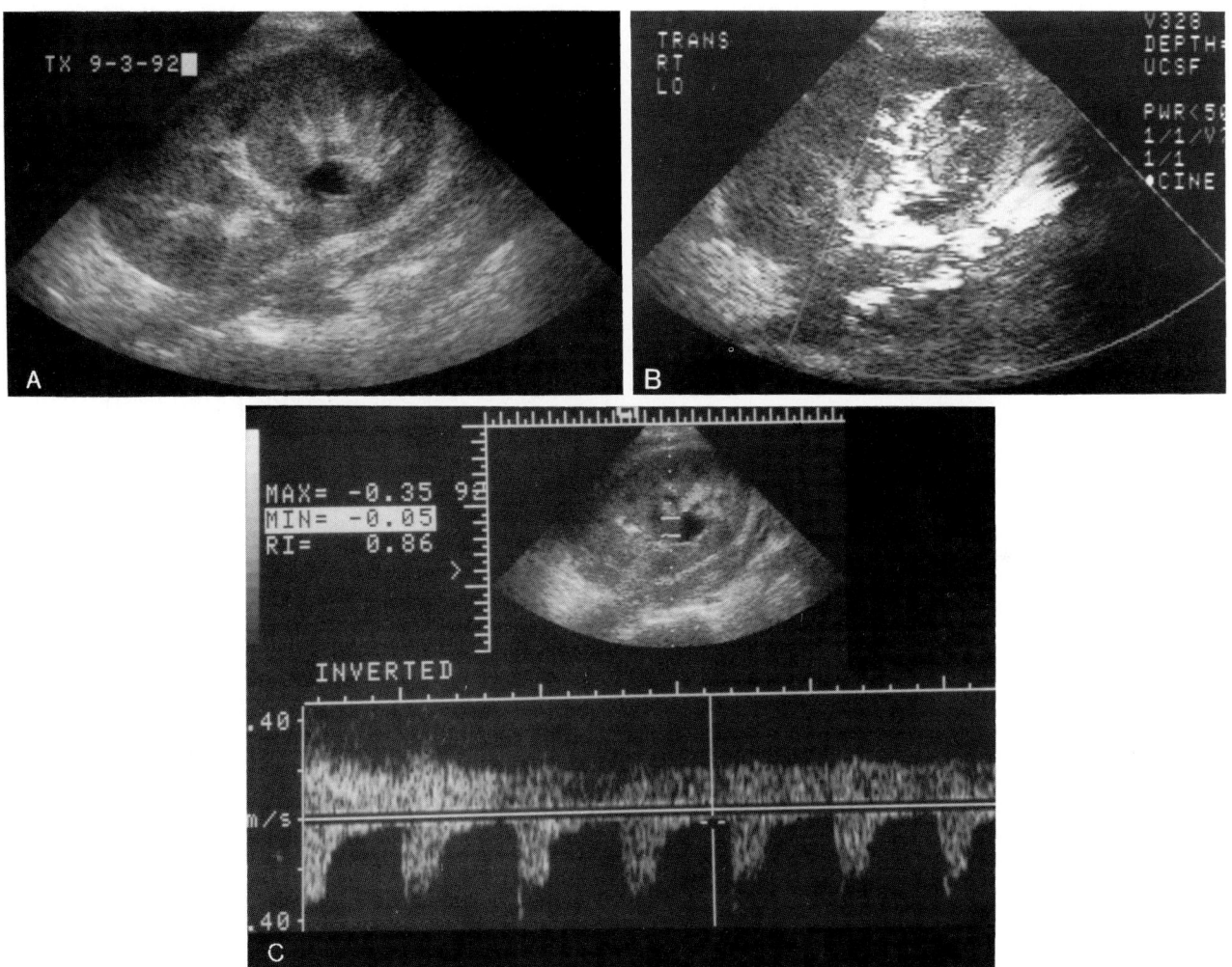

**Figure 27–31.** Acute rejection in a kidney transplant. *A.* Conventional US image shows loss of the corticomedullary differentiation and a small fluid collection within the renal pelvis. *B.* Color Doppler image shows flow within the native external iliac artery and the graft renal and interlobar arteries. *C.* Spectral Doppler analysis shows an elevated resistive index of 0.86. These findings are compatible with but not specific for acute rejection.

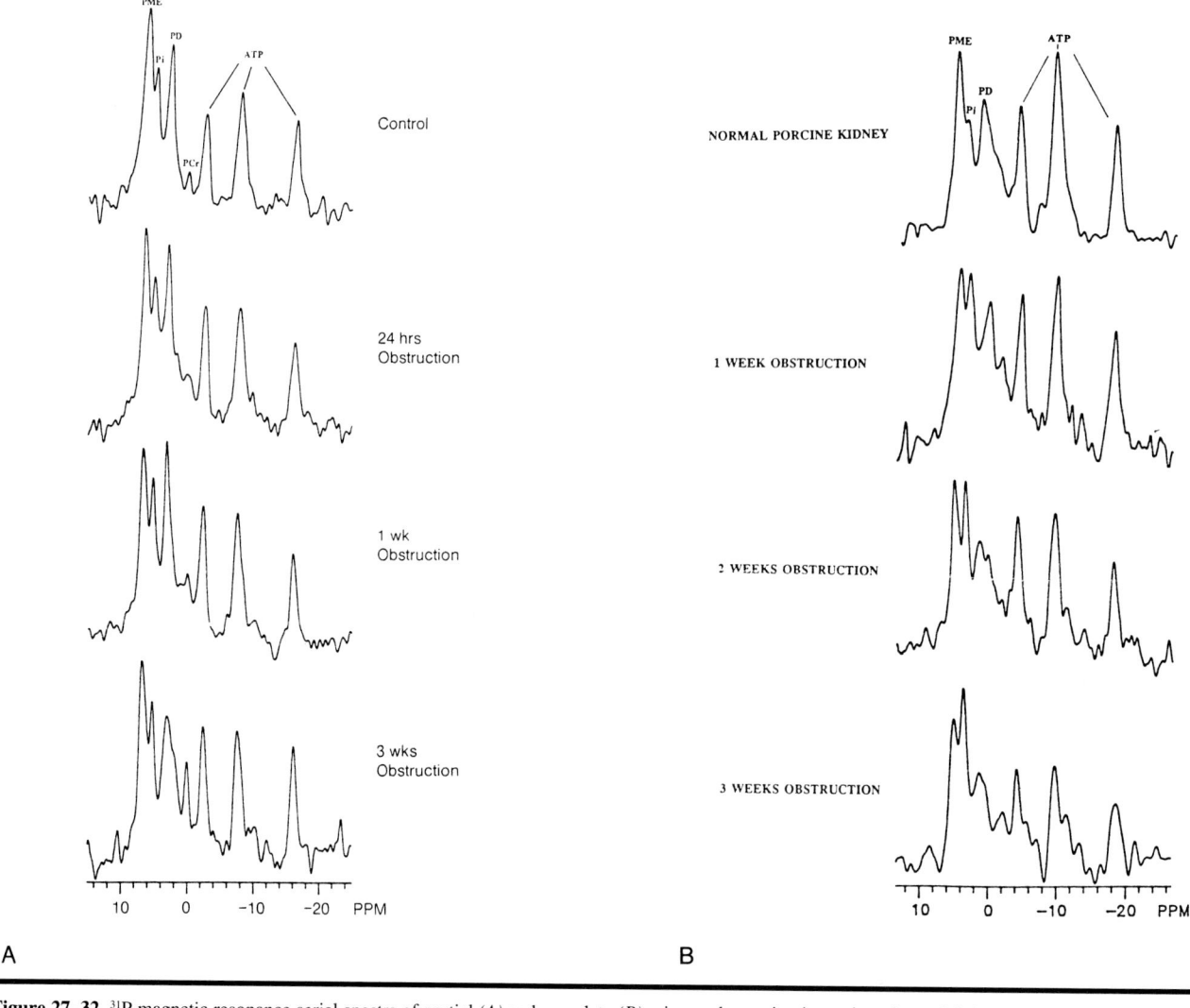

**Figure 27–32.** [31]P magnetic resonance serial spectra of partial *(A)* and complete *(B)* urinary obstruction in a micropig model demonstrating the differences in spectral changes (ATP/P$_i$ reduction) between the two entities. PME = phosphomonoester; PD = phosphodiester; PCr = phosphocreatine.

produces a significant reduction of the ATP/P$_i$ ratio at 2 weeks after ureteral ligation[66] (Fig. 27–32). Although these findings are nonspecific as to the cause, they may, as further knowledge is gathered, permit prediction of recovery of renal function. The use of [31]P magnetic resonance spectroscopy has also been extended to the assessment of methods for renal preservation and to the study of renal viability and function after transplantation.[67, 68]

## REFERENCES

1. Curry TS, Dowdey JE, Murry RC: Christensen's Introduction to the Physics of Diagnostic Radiology. Lea & Febiger, Philadelphia, 1984.
2. Hattery RR, Williamson B Jr, Hartman FQ, et al: Intravenous urographic technique. Radiology 167:593–599, 1988.
3. Hartman GW, Hattery RR, Witten DM, Williamson B Jr: Mortality during excretory urography: Mayo Clinic experience. AJR 139:919–922, 1982.
4. Jacobson BF, Jorulf H, Kalantar MS, Narasimham DL: Nonionic versus ionic contrast media in intravenous urography: Clinical trial in 1,000 consecutive patients. Radiology 167:601–605, 1988.
5. Price RR, Jones T, Fleischer AC, James AE: Ultrasound: Basic principles. *In* Coulam GM (ed): The Physical Basis of Medical Imaging. Appleton-Century-Crofts, New York, 1981, p 155.
6. Hricak H: Renal ultrasound. *In* Sarti DA (ed): Diagnostic Ultrasound. Text and Cases, 2nd ed. Year Book Medical Publishers, Chicago, 1987, pp 350–364.
7. Hricak H, Cruz C, Romanski R, et al: Renal parenchymal disease: Sonographic-histologic correlation. Radiology 144:141–147, 1982.
8. Jafri SZ, Madrazo BL, Miller JH: Color Doppler ultrasound of the genitourinary tract. Curr Opin Radiol 4:16–23, 1992.
9. Hounsfield GN: Computerized transverse axial scanning (tomography). Br J Radiol 46:1016, 1973.
10. Engelstad BE, McClennan BL, Levitt RG: The role of pre-contrast images in CT of the kidney. Radiology 136:153, 1980.
11. Didier D, Racle A, Etievent JP, Weill F: Tumor thrombus of the inferior vena cava secondary to malignant abdominal neoplasms: US and CT evaluation. Radiology 162:83–89, 1987.
12. Pykett IL, Newhouse JH, Buonanno FS, et al: Principles of nuclear magnetic resonance imaging. Radiology 143:157, 1982.
13. Wehrli FW: Introduction to fast-scan magnetic resonance. General Electric Publication No. 7299, Milwaukee 1986.
14. von Schulthess GK: Morphology and Function in MRI Cardiovascular and Renal Systems. Springer-Verlag, Berlin, Germany, 1989.
15. Haustein J, Neindorf HP, Krestin G, et al: Renal tolerance of gadolinium-DTPA/dimeglumine in patients with chronic renal failure. Invest Radiol 27:153–156, 1992.
16. Bellin MF, Deray G, Assogba U, et al: Gd DOTA: Evaluation of its renal tolerance in patients with chronic renal failure. Magn Reson Imaging 10:115–118, 1992.

17. Haustern J, Schumann-Giampieri G: Elimination of Gd-DTPA by means of hemodialysis. Eur J Radiol 11:227–229, 1990.
18. Gedroyc WM, Negus R, al-Kutoubi A, et al: Magnetic resonance angiography of renal transplants. Lancet 339:789–791, 1992.
19. Kallman DA, King BF, Hattery RR, et al: Renal vein and inferior vena cava tumor thrombus in renal cell carcinoma: CT, US, MRI, and venacavography. J Comput Assist Tomogr 16:240–247, 1992.
20. Rubidoux MA, Donnick NR, Sostman HD, Leder RA: Renal carcinoma: Detection of venous extension with gradient echo MR imaging. Radiology 182:269–272, 1992.
21. Schad LR, Semmler W, Knopp MV, et al: Preliminary evaluation: Magnetic resonance of urography using a saturation inversion projection spin-echo sequence. Magn Reson Imaging 11:319–327, 1993.
22. Lorenz CH, Powers TA, Partain CC: Quantitative imaging of renal blood flow and function. Invest Radiol 2(suppl):5109–5114, 1992.
23. Farrugia E, King BF, Larson TS: Magnetic resonance angiography and detection of renal artery stenosis in a patient with impaired renal function. Mayo Clin Proc 68:157–160, 1993.
24. Weiner MW: The promise of magnetic resonance spectroscopy for medical diagnosis. Invest Radiol 23:253–261, 1988.
25. Anderson RJ, Schrier RW: Acute renal failure. In Braunwald E, Isselbacher KJ, Petersdoorf RG, et al (eds): Harrison's Principles of Internal Medicine, 11th ed. McGraw-Hill, New York, 1987, pp 1149–1155.
26. Lee JKT, Baron RL, Melson GL, et al: Can real-time ultrasonography replace static B-scanning in the diagnosis of renal obstruction? Radiology 139:161, 1981.
27. Platt JF, Rubin JM, Ellis JH: Acute renal obstruction: Evaluation with intrarenal duplex Doppler and conventional ultrasound. Radiology 186:685–688, 1993.
28. Rodger PM, Bates JA, Irving HC: Intrarenal Doppler ultrasound studies in normal and acutely obstructed kidneys. Br J Radiol 65:207–212, 1992.
29. Thurnher S, Tzika AA, Hricak H, et al: Noncontrast and contrast enhanced MR imaging in the evaluation of partial ureteral obstruction: An experimental study in the micropig. Invest Radiol 24:544–554, 1989.
30. Arrive L, Hricak H, Tavares NJ, Miller TR: Malignant versus nonmalignant retroperitoneal fibrosis: Differentiation with MR imaging. Radiology 172:139–143, 1989.
31. Jabour BA, Ralls PW, Tang WW, et al: Acquired cystic disease of the kidneys. Computed tomography and ultrasonography appraisal in patients on peritoneal and hemodialysis. Invest Radiol 22:728–732, 1987.
32. Marotti M, Hricak H, Terrier F, et al: MR in renal disease: Importance of cortical-medullary distinction. Magn Reson Med 5:160, 1987.
33. Demas B, Thurnher S, Hricak H: The kidney, adrenal gland, and retroperitoneum. In Higgins CB, Hricak H (eds): Magnetic Resonance Imaging of the Body. Raven Press, New York, 1987, pp 373–401.
34. Hricak H, Thoeni RF, Carroll P, et al: MRI in the detection and staging of renal neoplasms: A reassessment. Radiology 135:479–482, 1988.
35. Gatewood OMB, Fishman EK, Burrow CR, et al: Renal vein thrombosis in patients with nephrotic syndrome: CT diagnosis. Radiology 159:117–122, 1986.
36. Kaufman JJ: Renovascular hypertension: The UCLA experience. J Urol 121:139–144, 1979.
37. Thornbury JR, Stanley JC, Fryback DG: Hypertensive urogram: A non-discriminatory test for renovascular hypertension. AJR 138:43–49, 1982.
38. Tucker RM, Labarthe DR: Frequency of surgical treatment for hypertension in adults at the Mayo Clinic for 1973 through 1975. Mayo Clin Proc 52:549–555, 1977.
39. Postman CT, van Aalen J, de Boo T, et al: Doppler ultrasound scanning in the detection of renal artery stenosis in hypertensive patients. Br J Radiol 65:857–860, 1992.
40. Galanski M, Prokop M, Chavan A, et al: Renal artery stenosis: Spinal CT angiography. Radiology 189:185–192, 1993.
41. Palmer E, Scott J, Strauss H: Practical Nuclear Medicine. WB Saunders, Philadelphia, 1992, pp 254–258.
42. Gattoni F, Avogadro A, Baldini U, et al: Digital subtraction angiography of the kidney. Br J Urol 62:214–218, 1988.
43. Hoddick W, Jeffrey RB, Goldberg HI, et al: CT and sonography of severe renal and perirenal infections. AJR 140:517, 1983.
44. Miller FH, Parikh S, Gore RM, et al: Renal manifestations of AIDS. Radiographics 13:587–596, 1993.
45. Wicks JD, Thornbury JR: Acute renal infections in adults. Radiol Clin North Am 17:245, 1979.
46. Goldman SM, Hartman DS, Fishman EK, et al: CT of xanthogranulomatous pyelonephritis: Radiologic-pathologic correlation. AJR 142:963, 1984.
47. Middleton WD, Dodds WJ, Lawson TL, Foley WD: Renal calculi: Sensitivity for detection with US. Radiology 167:239–244, 1988.
48. McClennan BL, Rabin DN: Kidney. In Lee JKT, Sagel SS, Stanley RJ (eds): Computed Body Tomography with MRI Correlation, 2nd ed. Raven Press, New York, 1989, pp 755–826.
49. Warshauer DM, McCarthy SM, Street L, et al: Detection of renal masses: Sensitivities and specificities of excretory urography/linear tomography, US, and CT. Radiology 169:363–365, 1988.
50. Kass DA, Hricak H, Davidson AJ: Renal malignancies with normal excretory urograms. AJR 141:731–734, 1983.
51. Bosniak MA: Current radiological approach to renal cysts. Radiology 158:1, 1986.
52. Hilpert PL, Friedman AC, Radecki PD, et al: MRI of hemorrhagic renal cysts in polycystic kidney disease. AJR 146:1167–1172, 1986.
53. Johnson CD, Dunnick NR, Cohan RH, Illescas FF: Renal adenocarcinoma: CT staging of 100 tumors. AJR 148:59–63, 1987.
54. Rofsky NM, Weinreb JC, Bosniak MA, et al: Renal lesion characterization with gadolinium enhanced MR imaging: Efficacy and safety in patients with renal insufficiency. Radiology 180:85–89, 1991.
55. Rominger MB, Kenney PJ, Morgan DE, et al: Gadolinium-enhanced MR imaging of renal masses. Radiographics 12:1097, 1992.
56. Semelka RC, Shoenut JP, Kroeker MA, et al: Renal lesions: Controlled comparison between CT and 1.5-T MR imaging with nonenhanced and gadolinium-enhanced fat-suppressed spin-echo and breath-hold FLASH techniques. Radiology 1982:425–430, 1992.
57. Semelka RC, Shoenut JP, Magro CM, et al: Renal cancer staging: Comparison of contrast-enhanced fat-suppressed spin-echo and gradient-echo MR imaging. J Magn Reson Imaging 3:597–602, 1993.
58. Pollack HM, Bamier MP, Arges PH, et al: The accuracy of grey-scale renal ultrasonography in differentiating cystic neoplasm from benign cysts. Radiology 143:741–745, 1982.
59. Bosniak MA, Megibow AJ, Hulnick DH, et al: CT diagnosis of renal angiomyolipoma: The importance of detecting small amounts of fat. AJR 151:497–501, 1988.
60. Zeman RK, Cronan JJ, Rosenfield AT, et al: Renal cell carcinoma: Dynamic thin-section CT assessment of vascular invasion and tumor vascularity. Radiology 167:393–396, 1988.
61. Siegel SC, Sandler MA, Alpern MB, Pearlberg JL: CT of renal cell carcinoma in patients on chronic hemodialysis. AJR 150:583–585, 1988.
62. Duda SH, Erley CM, Wakat JP, et al: Post transplant renal artery stenosis—outpatient intraarterial DSA versus color aided duplex Doppler sonography. Eur J Radiol 16:95–101, 1993.
63. Irving HC, Kashi SH: Complications of renal transplantation and the role of interventional radiology. J Clin Ultrasound 20:545–552, 1992.
64. Wong GG, Ross BD: Application of phosphorus nuclear magnetic resonance to problems of renal physiology and metabolism. Miner Electrolyte Metab 9:282–289, 1983.
65. Radda GK, Ackerman JJH, Bore P, et al: P-31 NMR studies on kidney intracellular pH in acute renal acidosis. Int J Biochem 12:277–281, 1980.
66. Vigneron DB, Tzika AA, Hricak H, et al: Complete and partial ureteral obstruction: Evaluation of renal effects with P-31 MR spectroscopy and Tc-DMSA scintigraphy. Radiology 168:645–650, 1988.
67. Bretan PN Jr, Vigneron DB, James TL, et al: Assessment of renal viability by 31-phosphorus magnetic resonance spectroscopy. J Urol 135:866–871, 1986.
68. Bretan PN Jr, Vigernon DB, Hricak H, et al: Assessment of clinical renal preservation by phosphorus-31 magnetic resonance spectroscopy. J Urol 137:146–150, 1987.

# Acute Renal Failure

*Hugh R. Brady*
*Barry M. Brenner*
*Wilfred Lieberthal*

## DEFINITIONS, INCIDENCE, AND CLASSIFICATION

Acute renal failure (ARF) is a syndrome characterized by rapid (hours to weeks) decline in glomerular filtration rate (GFR) and retention of nitrogenous waste products such as blood urea nitrogen (BUN) and creatinine.[1] ARF complicates approximately 5% of hospital admissions and up to 30% of admissions to intensive care units.[2] ARF is usually asymptomatic and diagnosed when routine biochemical screening of hospitalized patients reveals a recent increase in BUN and serum creatinine level. Oliguria (urine output < 400 mL/d) is a frequent (~50%) but not invariable clinical feature.[3-8] The kidney is remarkable among organs of the body in its ability to recover from almost complete loss of function, and most ARF is reversible. Nevertheless, ARF is a major cause of in-hospital morbidity and mortality because of the serious nature of the underlying illnesses and the high incidence of complications. ARF may complicate a host of diseases that for purposes of diagnosis and management are conveniently divided into three categories: 1) diseases characterized by renal hypoperfusion in which the integrity of renal parenchymal tissue is preserved (prerenal azotemia, prerenal ARF) (~55% to 60%); 2) diseases involving renal parenchymal tissue (renal azotemia, intrinsic renal ARF) (~35% to 40%); and 3) diseases associated with acute obstruction of the urinary tract (postrenal azotemia, postrenal ARF) (≤5%) (Table 28–1). Most acute intrinsic renal azotemia is caused by ischemia or nephrotoxins and is classically associated with acute

tubule necrosis (ATN). Thus, the term ATN is commonly used to denote ischemic or nephrotoxic ARF in clinical practice.

The diagnosis of ARF usually hinges on serial analysis of BUN and serum creatinine, and it should be noted that these are relatively insensitive indices of glomerular function and several caveats must be entertained when extrapolating their levels to GFR (Fig. 28–1). GFR may fall by 50% before the serum creatinine value rises because the initial decrement in creatinine filtration is matched by enhanced creatinine secretion by proximal tubule cells.[9, 10] Conversely, a relatively large increment in the serum creatinine value reflects a relatively small decrement in GFR in patients with pre-existing chronic renal insufficiency. GFR may fall without a marked elevation in creatinine or BUN level in patients with reduced muscle mass (such as the elderly) or urea generation (e.g., malnutrition, liver disease), respectively. Furthermore, BUN or serum creatinine values may rise without an acute decline in GFR in patients with pre-existing chronic renal insufficiency and enhanced urea or creatinine production, inhibition of proximal tubule creatinine secretion, or circulating substances that cross-react with creatinine in laboratory assays[11-20] (see Fig. 28–1, *inset*). Under the latter circumstances, BUN and serum creatinine values seldom rise above 30 mg/dL and 2.0 mg/dL, respectively, and simultaneous elevation of both parameters is rare. Despite these limitations, measurements of BUN and serum creatinine are likely to remain the principal method for diagnosis of ARF in the foreseeable future.

This chapter focuses on the clinical features, pathophys-

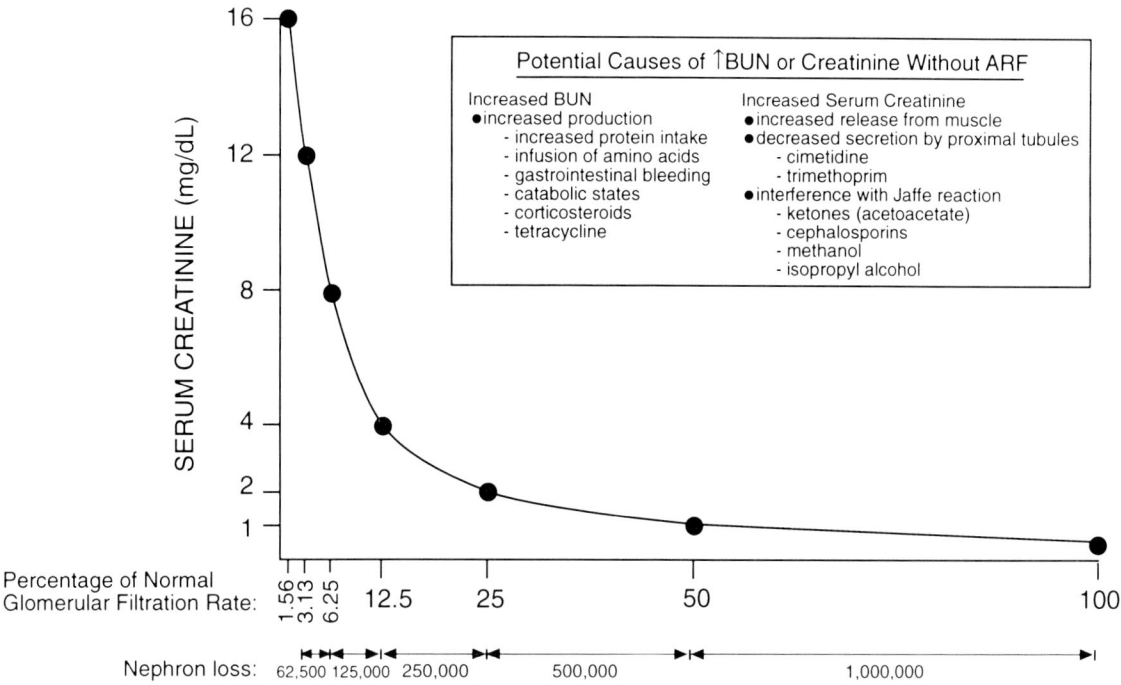

**Figure 28–1.** Relationship between serum creatinine and glomerular filtration rate (GFR) illustrating the relative lack of sensitivity of the former parameter as an index of renal function. GFR may fall by more than 50% before the serum creatinine value rises because the fall in glomerular filtration of creatinine is balanced by increased creatinine secretion by proximal tubule cells. In contrast, loss of a relatively small number of nephrons is associated with a relatively dramatic rise in serum creatinine level in patients with severe renal insufficiency. The inset lists some circumstances in which BUN or serum creatinine may be elevated without an acute decline in GFR. This phenomenon is probably limited to patients with pre-existing chronic subclinical impairment of GFR. (Modified from Faber MD, Kupin WL, Krishna G, Nairns RG: The differential diagnosis of acute renal failure. *In* Lazarus JM, Brenner BM [eds]: Acute Renal Failure, 3rd ed. Churchill Livingstone, New York, 1993, p 133.)

iology, and treatment of prerenal azotemia and ischemic ATN. Special emphasis is placed on changing concepts and new research. Extensive discussions of other causes of intrinsic renal azotemia and postrenal azotemia are included in other chapters of this book. Readers are also referred to a textbook devoted entirely to the syndrome of ARF.[21]

**TABLE 28–1. Classification and Major Disease Categories Causing Acute Renal Failure**

| Disease Category | % of Patients with Acute Renal Failure |
| --- | --- |
| Prerenal azotemia caused by acute renal hypoperfusion | 55–60 |
| Intrinsic renal azotemia caused by acute diseases of renal parenchyma | 35–40 |
| Diseases involving large renal vessels | |
| Diseases of small renal vessels and glomeruli | |
| Acute injury to renal tubules mediated by ischemia or toxins* | |
| Acute diseases of the tubulointerstitium | |
| Postrenal azotemia caused by acute obstruction of urinary collecting system | ≤5 |

*Accounts for more than 90% of cases in the intrinsic renal azotemia category in most series.

# ETIOLOGY OF ACUTE RENAL FAILURE

## Prerenal Azotemia

Prerenal azotemia is the most common cause of ARF and is an appropriate physiologic response to renal hypoperfusion.[2, 22] By definition, the integrity of renal parenchymal tissue is maintained and GFR is corrected rapidly on restoration of renal perfusion and glomerular ultrafiltration pressure. Indeed, kidneys from individuals with prerenal azotemia function satisfactorily when transplanted into recipients with normal cardiovascular function. Severe or prolonged renal hypoperfusion may lead to ischemic ATN. Thus, prerenal azotemia and ischemic ATN are part of a spectrum of manifestations of renal hypoperfusion.

Prerenal azotemia can complicate any disease characterized by hypovolemia, low cardiac output, systemic vasodilatation, or intrarenal vasoconstriction (Table 28–2). True or "effective" hypovolemia leads to a fall in mean systemic arterial pressure, which in turn triggers arterial (e.g., carotid sinus) and cardiac baroreceptors and initiates a series of neural and humoral responses that include activation of the sympathetic nervous system and renin-angiotensin-aldosterone system and release of antidiuretic hormone [23–26] (Fig. 28–2). Norepinephrine, angiotensin II, and antidiuretic hormone act in concert in an attempt to preserve cardiac and

**TABLE 28–2. Major Causes of Prerenal Azotemia**

Intravascular volume depletion
  Hemorrhage: traumatic, surgical, gastrointestinal, post partum
  Gastrointestinal losses: vomiting, nasogastric suction, diarrhea
  Renal losses: drug-induced or osmotic diuresis, diabetes insipidus, adrenal insufficiency
  Skin and mucous membrane losses: burns, hyperthermia, and other causes of increased insensible losses
  "Third-space" losses: pancreatitis, crush syndrome, hypoalbuminemia
Decreased cardiac output
  Diseases of myocardium, valves, pericardium, or conducting system
  Pulmonary hypertension, pulmonary embolism, positive-pressure mechanical ventilation
Systemic vasodilatation
  Drugs: antihypertensives, afterload reduction, anesthetics, drug overdoses
  Sepsis, liver failure, anaphylaxis
Renal vasoconstriction
  Norepinephrine, ergotamine, liver disease, sepsis, hypercalcemia
Pharmacologic agents that acutely impair autoregulation and GFR in specific settings
  Angiotensin-converting enzyme inhibitors in renal artery stenosis or severe renal hypoperfusion
  Inhibition of prostaglandin synthesis by nonsteroidal anti-inflammatory drugs during renal hypoperfusion

cerebral perfusion by stimulating vasoconstriction in relatively nonessential vascular beds such as the musculocutaneous and splanchnic circulations, inhibiting salt loss through sweat glands, stimulating thirst and salt appetite, and promoting renal salt and water retention. Glomerular perfusion, ultrafiltration pressure, and filtration rate are preserved during mild hypoperfusion through several compensatory mechanisms.[27] Stretch receptors in afferent arterioles,

in response to a reduction in perfusion pressure, trigger relaxation of afferent arteriolar smooth muscle cells and vasodilation (autoregulation). Intrarenal biosynthesis of vasodilator prostaglandins (e.g, prostacyclin, prostaglandin $E_2$), kallikrein and kinins, and possibly nitric oxide (NO) is enhanced.[28–33] Angiotensin II may induce preferential constriction of efferent arterioles, possibly by virtue of the increased density of angiotensin II receptors at this location.[34] As a result, intraglomerular pressure is preserved, the fraction of renal plasma that is filtered by glomeruli (filtration fraction) is increased, and GFR is maintained.

These compensatory renal responses are overwhelmed during states of severe hypoperfusion and ARF ensues.[27] Autoregulatory dilatation of afferent arterioles is maximal at a mean systemic arterial blood pressure of about 80 mm Hg and hypotension below this level is associated with a precipitous decline in glomerular ultrafiltration pressure and GFR. Lesser degrees of hypotension may provoke prerenal azotemia in the elderly and in patients with diseases affecting the integrity of afferent arterioles (e.g., hypertensive nephrosclerosis, diabetic nephropathy). In addition, high levels of angiotensin II, as are found in patients with marked circulatory failure, provoke constriction of both afferent and efferent arterioles, thus negating the relatively selective effect of low levels of this peptide on efferent arteriolar resistance.[24] Several classes of commonly used drugs impair renal adaptive responses and convert compensated renal hypoperfusion to overt prerenal azotemia or trigger progression of prerenal azotemia to intrinsic ischemic renal azotemia. Nonsteroidal anti-inflammatory drugs (NSAIDs), inhibitors of renal prostaglandin biosynthesis, do not affect GFR in normal individuals but may precipitate prerenal azotemia in subjects with true or effective volume depletion or patients with chronic renal insufficiency in whom GFR is maintained in part by prostaglandin-mediated

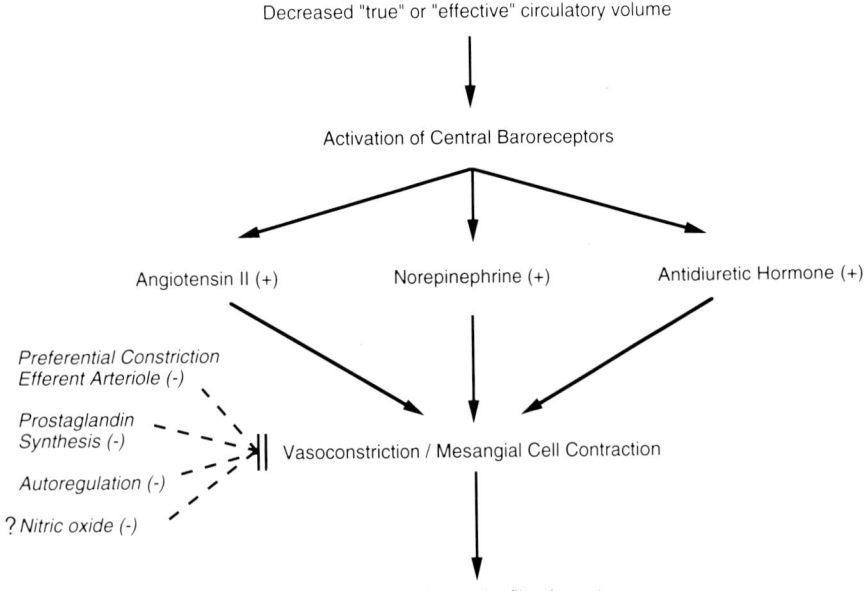

**Figure 28–2.** Pathophysiology of prerenal azotemia: an appropriate physiologic response to renal hypoperfusion. In response to a fall in systemic arterial blood pressure, carotid artery baroreceptors are activated and trigger activation of the the renin-angiotensin and sympathetic nervous systems and secretion of vasopressin. Angiotensin II, norepinephrine, and vasopressin act in concert to restore intravascular volume and blood pressure in an attempt to preserve perfusion of "essential" organs such as heart and brain at the expense of perfusion of "nonessential" organs such as skin, muscle, and gut. Glomerular filtration is preserved in the context of mild to moderate renal hypoperfusion because of 1) autoregulation of afferent arteriolar tone probably through an intrinsic baroreceptor pathway within the vessel wall, 2) the relatively selective action of angiotensin II on efferent arteriolar resistance, and 3) stimulation of intrarenal production of vasodilator prostaglandins. ARF may supervene if these compensatory responses are impaired (e.g., with administration of ACE inhibitors or NSAIDs or arterio-

sclerosis or other diseases affecting the integrity of afferent arterioles) or overwhelmed (as in severe renal hypoperfusion). See text for explanation. (Adapted from Brady HR, Brenner BM: Acute renal failure. *In* Isselbacher K , Braunwald EB, Wilson JD, et al [eds]: Harrison's Principles of Internal Medicine, 13th ed. McGraw-Hill, New York, 1994, p 1265. Reproduced with permission of McGraw-Hill Inc.)

hyperfiltration through remnant nephrons.[35–64] Similarly, inhibitors of angiotensin-converting enzyme (ACE) may trigger prerenal azotemia in individuals in whom intraglomerular pressure and GFR are dependent on angiotensin II.[65–76] This complication is classically seen in patients with bilateral renal artery stenosis or unilateral stenosis in a solitary functioning kidney.[66, 68] Here, angiotensin II preserves glomerular filtration pressure distal to renal arterial stenosis by increasing systemic arterial pressure and by triggering selective constriction of efferent arterioles. ACE inhibitors blunt these compensatory responses and precipitate reversible ARF in approximately 30% of patients. ACE inhibitors, like NSAIDs, may also precipitate prerenal azotemia in patients with compensated renal hypoperfusion of other causes, mandating close monitoring of the serum creatinine level when these drugs are administered to high-risk individuals.[65–76]

The classic urinary and biochemical sequelae of prerenal azotemia may be predicted from the stimulatory actions of norepinephrine, angiotensin II, antidiuretic hormone, and low urine flow rate on salt and water reabsorption from urine and include a concentrated urine (specific gravity > 1.018, osmolality > 500 mOsm/kg $H_2O$), low urinary $Na^+$ concentration, and benign urine sediment. Some vasoactive mediators, drugs, and diagnostic agents stimulate intense intrarenal vasoconstriction and induce glomerular hypoperfusion and ARF with many of the functional, clinical, and biochemical features of prerenal azotemia. Examples include hypercalcemia, endotoxin, radiocontrast agents, cyclosporine, amphotericin B, epinephrine and norepinephrine (e.g., theraputic, pheochromocytoma, brain damage), ergotamine, and high doses of dopamine. Because many of these agents also induce injury to renal tubules, they are usually categorized as causes of acute intrinsic renal azotemia and are discussed in subsequent sections.

## Intrinsic Renal Azotemia

From a clinicopathologic viewpoint, it is helpful to categorize the causes of acute intrinsic renal azotemia into 1) diseases involving large renal vessels, 2) diseases of the renal microvasculature and glomeruli, 3) ischemic and nephrotoxic ATN, and 4) other acute processes involving the tubulointerstitium (Table 28–3). Ischemic ATN and toxic ATN, as already discussed, account for about 90% of acute intrinsic renal azotemia.[2, 77, 78]

### DISEASES OF LARGE RENAL VESSELS, MICROVASCULATURE, AND TUBULOINTERSTITIUM

Occlusion of large renal vessels, either arteries or veins, is an uncommon cause of ARF. To affect BUN and serum creatinine, occlusion must be either bilateral or unilateral in patients with underlying chronic renal insufficiency or a solitary functioning kidney. Renal arteries may be occluded acutely by atheroemboli, thromboemboli, thrombosis, dissection of an aortic aneurysm, or, rarely, vasculitis. Atheroemboli are the most common culprits and are usually dislodged from an atheromatous aorta during arteriography,

---

**TABLE 28–3. Major Causes of Acute Intrinsic Renal Azotemia**

Diseases involving large renal vessels
  Renal arteries:* thrombosis, atheroembolism, thromboembolism, dissection, vasculitis (e.g., Takayasu)
  Renal veins:* thrombosis, compression
Diseases of glomeruli and the renal microvasculature (see Table 28–4)
  Inflammatory: acute or rapidly progressive glomerulonephritis, vasculitis, allograft rejection, radiation
  Vasospastic: malignant hypertension, toxemia of pregnancy, scleroderma, hypercalcemia, drugs, radiocontrast agents
  Hematologic: hemolytic-uremic syndrome or thrombotic thrombocytopenic purpura, disseminated intravascular coagulation, hyperviscosity syndromes
Diseases characterized by prominent injury to renal tubules often with ATN†‡
  Ischemia caused by renal hypoperfusion (see Table 28–2)
  Exogenous toxins (e.g., antibiotics, anticancer agents, radiocontrast agents, poisons; see Table 28–6)
  Endogenous toxins (e.g., myoglobin, hemoglobin, myeloma light chains, uric acid, tumor lysis; see Table 28–7)
Acute diseases of the tubulointerstitium (see Table 28–5)
  Allergic interstitial nephritis (e.g., antibiotics, NSAIDs)
  Infectious (viral, bacterial, fungal)
  Acute cellular allograft rejection
  Infiltration§ (e.g., lymphoma, leukemia, sarcoid)

*ARF in this context usually implies bilateral disease or unilateral disease in a solitary functioning kidney.
†The majority of cases of acute intrinsic renal azotemia fall into this category.
‡Although frank necrosis of renal tubules is not invariably present, the term ATN is used by convention to denote ARF related to tubule injury by either ischemia or nephrotoxins (see section on pathophysiology of ischemic ATN).
§Although infiltration of renal parenchyma is common, renal failure rarely occurs.

---

angioplasty, or aortic surgery.[79–85] Cholesterol emboli lodge in medium or small renal arteries, where they incite an inflammatory reaction characterized classically by intimal proliferation, infiltration of vessel wall by macrophages and giant cells, fibrosis, and irreversible occlusion of the vessel lumen.[84] Thromboemboli arise most commonly from the heart in patients with atrial arrhythmias or mural thrombi and produce acute infarction of renal tissue.[86–88] Renal artery thrombosis is usually superimposed on an atheromatous plaque but may also complicate traumatic intimal tears or the site of surgical anastomosis after renal transplantation. Renal vein thrombosis is an exceedingly rare cause of ARF and is usually encountered as a complication of the nephrotic syndrome in adults or of severe dehydration in children.[89–91]

Virtually all diseases that compromise blood flow within the renal microvasculature may induce ARF. These include inflammatory (e.g., glomerulonephritis or vasculitis) and noninflamatory (e.g., malignant hypertension) diseases of the vessel wall, thrombotic microangiopathies, and hyperviscosity syndromes (Table 28–4). Indeed, the decrement in renal perfusion in these settings may be severe enough to trigger superimposed ischemic ATN.[91, 92] In general, these disorders can be distinguished from prerenal azotemia and ischemic or nephrotoxic ATN by clinical or laboratory criteria; however, a renal biopsy may be required for definitive diagnosis (see later section on differential diagnosis). Disorders of the tubulointerstitium that induce ARF, other than

**TABLE 28–4. Some Diseases of Glomeruli and the Renal Microvasculature Associated with Acute Intrinsic Renal Azotemia**

Glomerulonephritis or vasculitis
  Associated with anti–glomerular basement membrane antibody*
    (anti-GBM Ab)
    (Goodpasture syndrome if associated with lung hemorrhage)
  Associated with antineutrophil cytoplasmic antibodies* (ANCA)
    Wegener granulomatosis
    Microscopic or Churg-Strauss variant of polyarteritis nodosa
    Renal-limited crescentic glomerulonephritis
  Associated with glomerular immune complexes and
    hypocomplementemia
    Acute diffuse proliferative glomerulonephritis (postinfectious)
    Membranoproliferative glomerulonephritis
    Subacute bacterial endocarditis
    Cryoglobulinemia
    Systemic lupus erythematosus (SLE)
  Associated with absence of hypocomplementemia, ANCA, and
    anti-GBM Ab
    Immunoglobulin A nephropathy
    Schönlein-Henoch purpura
    Classic polyarteritis nodosa
    Radiation injury
    Abdominal abscess
Hyperviscosity syndromes
  Multiple myeloma
  Waldenström macroglobulinemia
  Polycythemia

Hemolytic-uremic syndrome or thrombotic thrombocytopenic purpura
  Infections
    Viral (e.g., enterovirus, coxsackievirus, influenza virus, hepatitis
      A virus, human immunodeficiency virus)
    Bacterial (e.g., *Escherichia coli, Shigella, Salmonella, Yersinia,*
      *Campylobacter*)
  Chemotherapeutic agents and other drugs
    Chemotherapeutic agents (mitomycin C, cisplatin + bleomycin)
    Cyclosporine, oral contraceptives
  Immunologic diseases
    SLE, rheumatoid arthritis, Sjögren, ankylosing spondylitis
  Other: Idiopathic, familial, pregnancy and puerperium, after renal or
    bone marrow transplantation
Miscellaneous
  Accelerated hypertension
  Scleroderma crisis
  Toxemia of pregnancy
  Drugs
    Cyclosporine
    Amphotericin B
    Radiocontrast agents

*Serum complement levels are usually normal in these diseases.

ischemia or tubule cell toxins, include allergic interstitial nephritis, severe infections, allograft rejection, and, rarely, infiltrative disorders such as sarcoid, lymphoma, or leukemia (Table 28–5). A comprehensive discussion of these diseases is beyond the scope of this chapter and is presented elsewhere in this book.

## ACUTE TUBULE NECROSIS

Although the pathologic term ATN and the clinical term ARF are often used interchangeably when referring to is-

chemic and nephrotoxic renal injury, evidence of frank necrosis of renal tubules is sparse or absent in most cases (see later section on pathology). Prerenal azotemia and ischemic ATN are part of a spectrum of manifestations of renal hypoperfusion, prerenal azotemia being a response to mild or moderate hypoperfusion and ischemic ATN being the result of more severe or prolonged hypoperfusion, often coexistent with other renal insults (e.g., nephrotoxins or sepsis). They differ in that ischemic ATN, unlike prerenal azotemia, is associated with injury to renal parenchyma and does not resolve immediately on restoration of renal perfu-

**TABLE 28–5. Diseases of the Tubulointerstitium Associated with Acute Intrinsic Renal Azotemia***

| **Drug-Induced Allergic Interstitial Nephritis** | | | | | | |
|---|---|---|---|---|---|---|
| *β-Lactams* | *Other Antibiotics* | *NSAIDs* | *Diuretics* | *Other* | **Infections** | **Miscellaneous** |
| Ampicillin | Ethambutol | Aspirin | Chlorthalidone | α-Methyldopa | Bacterial | Systemic diseases |
| Amoxicillin | *p*-Aminosalicylate | Diflunisal | Furosemide | Allopurinol | Acute pyelonephritis† | Systemic lupus |
| Carbenicillin | Rifampin | Fenoprofen | Thiazides | Azathioprine | Leptospirosis | erythematosus |
| Methicillin | Sulfonamides | Glafenine | Ticrynafen | Carbamazepine | Scarlet fever | Sjögren syndrome |
| Nafcillin | Trimethoprim- | Ibuprofen | | Cimetidine | Typhoid fever | Renal ocular syndrome |
| Oxacillin | sulfamethoxazole | Indomethacin | | Clofibrate | Legionnaire disease | Cancer |
| Penicillin G | Ciprofloxacin | Meclofenamate | | Diphenylhydantoin | Viral | Lymphoma |
| Cephalexin | | Mefenamic acid | | Interferon alfa | Cytomegalovirus infection | Leukemia |
| Cephalothin | | Naproxen | | Phenindione | Measles | Myeloma |
| Cephradine | | Phenazone | | Phenobarbital | Infectious mononucleosis | |
| Cefotaxime | | Phenylbutazone | | Phenylpropanolamine | Rocky Mountain spotted | |
| | | Tolmetin | | Sulfinpyrazone | fever | |
| | | | | | Other | |
| | | | | | Candidiasis, other fungi‡ | |
| | | | | | Toxoplasmosis | |

*See Chapters 33 and 34 for more extensive discussion.
†Rare to get ARF unless bilateral disease in diabetic patients.
‡May cause ARF by obstruction of tubules (fungus balls), in addition to causing acute interstitial nephritis.

sion. In its more extreme form, renal hypoperfusion may result in bilateral renal cortical necrosis and irreversible renal failure. Ischemic ATN is observed most frequently in patients who have major surgery, trauma, severe hypovolemia, overwhelming sepsis, and burns.[2, 78, 92–94] The risk of ischemic ATN after cardiac surgery correlates directly with the duration of cardiopulmonary bypass and the degree of postoperative cardiac impairment.[95–100] ATN most commonly complicates aortic surgery in patients undergoing emergency repair of ruptured abdominal aneurysms or after complicated elective procedures requiring prolonged (>60 minutes) clamping of the aorta above the origin of the renal arteries.[101–103] However, 50% of cases of postsurgical ATN occur in the absence of documented hypotension.[2] ATN complicating trauma is frequently multifactorial in origin and due to the combined effects of hypovolemia and myoglobin or other toxins released by damaged tissue. ATN occurs in 20% to 40% of patients who suffer burns involving more than 15% of their surface area and, again, is frequently multifactorial and due to the combined effects of hypovolemia, rhabdomyolysis, sepsis, and nephrotoxic antibiotics.[104–106] Sepsis induces renal hypoperfusion by provoking a combination of systemic vasodilatation and intrarenal vasoconstriction.[107–112] In addition, endotoxin sensitizes renal tissue to the deleterious effects of ischemia.[107–112] The pathophysiology, pathology, management, and clinical course of ischemic ATN are discussed in detail later in this chapter.

Nephrotoxic ATN complicates the administration of many structurally diverse pharmacologic agents and poisons.[113] In addition, some endogenous compounds provoke ARF when present in the circulation at high concentrations. In general, nephrotoxins cause renal injury by inducing a varying combination of intrarenal vasoconstriction, direct tubule toxicity, and/or intratubular obstruction. The kidney is particularly vulnerable to nephrotoxic renal injury by virtue of its rich blood supply (25% of cardiac output) and its ability to concentrate toxins to high levels within the medullary interstitium (via the renal countercurrent mechanisms) and renal epithelial cells (via specific transporters).[113] In addition, the kidney is an important site for xenobiotic metabolism and may transform relatively harmless parent compounds into toxic metabolites.[113] The nephrotoxic potential of most agents is dramatically increased in the presence of borderline or overt renal ischemia, sepsis, or other renal insults. A detailed description of the pathophysiology and clinical features of drug-induced toxic nephropathies is presented in Chapter 34 and only a brief review of some common nephrotoxic syndromes is included here.

Tables 28–6 and 28–7 list the toxins that are most frequently associated with ATN. Acute intrarenal vasoconstriction is an important pathophysiologic event in ARF associated with radiocontrast agents (contrast nephropathy) and cyclosporine. Contrast nephropathy typically presents as an acute decline in GFR within 24 to 48 hours of administration, a peak in serum creatinine value after 3 to 5 days, and return of the serum creatinine value to the ''normal'' range within 1 week.[114–135] Individuals with chronic renal insufficiency (serum creatinine > 2.0 mg/dL), diabetic nephropathy, severe cardiac failure, volume depletion, and

multiple myeloma appear particularly vulnerable. Patients usually present with a benign urine sediment, concentrated urine, and low fractional excretion of $Na^+$ and thus have many features of prerenal azotemia; however, in severe cases there may be evidence of tubule cell injury. The newer nonionic low-osmolality contrast agents do not differ dramatically in their nephrotoxic potential from conventional ionic high-osmolality agents and most authorities agree that this marginal advantage does not outweigh their prohibitive cost, except perhaps for high-risk patients.[135] Postulated mechanisms of contrast agent–induced renal injury include intrarenal vasoconstriction and ischemia, possibly triggered by endothelin release from endothelial cells and/or suppression of intrarenal NO production, direct tubule toxicity, intraluminal precipitation of protein or uric acid or contrast agent crystals, and congestion of medullary blood vessels.[136–149] Cyclosporine also precipitates ARF by inducing intrarenal vasoconstriction and hypoperfusion, and by stimulating mesangial cell contraction and a fall in glomerular filtration surface area.[150–164] Frank tubule necrosis is rare in this setting, although long-term cyclosporine therapy may lead to irreversible renal impairment, probably as a consequence of obliterative arteriolopathy and chronic medullary ischemia.[164] As with contrast nephropathy, endothelin has been implicated as an important mediator of intrarenal vasoconstriction in cyclosporine nephrotoxicity and patients often present with urinary findings similar to those in prerenal azotemia.[148, 149] Intrarenal vasoconstriction is also a central component of ARF complicating hypercalcemia and, in addition, contributes to the nephrotoxicity of myoglobin and hemoglobin. Interestingly, hemoglobin and myoglobin may promote vasoconstriction, at least in part by scavenging the vasodilator NO and thereby disrupting the balance between vasodilators and vasoconstrictors that is critical for maintenance of normal renal perfusion.

Therapeutic agents that are directly toxic to renal tubule epithelium include antimicrobials such as aminoglycosides, amphotericin B, acyclovir, pentamidine, and foscarnet and chemotherapeutic agents such as cisplatin and ifosfamide. Nonoliguric ATN complicates 10% to 30% of courses of aminoglycoside antibiotics, even when blood levels are in the therapeutic range.[165–179] Aminoglycosides are polycations and are freely filtered across the glomerular filtration

**TABLE 28–6. Some Exogenous Nephrotoxins That Are Common Causes of Acute Intrinsic Renal Azotemia with Acute Tubule Necrosis\***

| | |
|---|---|
| Antibiotics | Chemotherapeutic agents |
|   Acyclovir |   Cisplatin |
|   Aminoglycosides |   Ifosfamide |
|   Amphotericin B | Anti-inflammatory and immunosuppressive |
|   Foscarnet |   agents |
|   Pentamidine |   NSAIDs |
| Organic solvents |   Cyclosporine |
|   Ethylene glycol | Radiocontrast agents |
|   Toluene | Bacterial toxins |
| Poisons | |
|   Paraquat | |
|   Snake bites | |

\*For more extensive list, see Chapter 34.

**TABLE 28–7. Some Sources of Endogenous Nephrotoxins That Cause Acute Intrinsic Renal Azotemia with Acute Tubule Necrosis***

| | |
|---|---|
| Rhabdomyolysis with myoglobinuria† | |
| Muscle injury | Trauma,‡ electric shock, hypothermia, hyperthermia (e.g., malignant hyperpyrexia) |
| Extreme muscular exertion | Seizures,‡ delirium tremens,‡ physical exercise |
| Muscle ischemia | Prolonged compression‡ (e.g., coma), compromise of major vessels (e.g., thrombosis, embolism, dissection) |
| Metabolic disorders | Hypokalemia, hypophosphatemia, hypo- and hypernatremia, diabetic ketoacidosis, and hyperosmolar states |
| Infections | Influenza, infectious mononucleosis, legionnaire disease, tetanus |
| Toxins | Ethanol,‡ isopropyl alcohol, ethylene glycol, toluene, snake and insect bites |
| Drugs | Amphetamines, phencyclidine, lysergic acid diethylamide, heroin, methadone, salicylate overdose, succinylcholine |
| Immunologic diseases | Polymyositis, dermatomyositis |
| Inherited diseases | Myophosphorylase, phosphofructokinase, carnitine palmityltransferase, or myoadenylate deaminase deficiency |
| Hemolysis with hemoglobinuria† | |
| Immunologic | Transfusion reactions‡ |
| Infections and venoms | Malaria,‡ clostridia, spider bite (e.g., tarantula, brown recluse), snake bite‡ (e.g., rattlesnake, copperhead) |
| Drugs and chemicals | Aniline, arsine, benzene, cresol, fava beans, glycerol, hydralazine, phenol, quinidine |
| Genetic diseases | Glucose 6-phosphate deficiency, paroxysmal nocturnal hemoglobinuria, march hemoglobinuria |
| Mechanical | Valvular prosthesis, extracorporeal circulation, microangiopathic hemolytic anemias, distilled water (intravenous dialysis, transurethral prostatectomy) |
| Increased uric acid production with hyperuricosuria | |
| Primary increase in uric acid production | Hypoxanthine-guanine phosphoribosyltransferase deficiency |
| Secondary increase in uric acid production | Treatment of malignancies‡ (especially lymphoproliferative or myeloproliferative) |
| Miscellaneous | Myeloma light chains,‡ oxalate‡ (e.g., ethylene glycol toxicity), products of tumor lysis other than uric acid |

*All of these diseases are sources of potential nephrotoxins, but not all have been definitively associated with ARF.
†Hemoglobin and myoglobin cause little compromise of glomerular filtration when administered to experimental animals. Thus, it remains to be determined whether ARF in these settings is due to hemoglobin or myoglobin, metabolites of these compounds, or other toxic species released from red blood cells or muscle, or requires the coexistence of other renal insults (e.g., hypoperfusion).
‡Denotes most common causes of ARF. Renal failure is rare in other circumstances.

barrier and accumulated by proximal tubule cells after interaction with negatively charged phospholipid residues on brush border membranes. Important risk factors for aminoglycoside nephrotoxicity include use of high or repeated doses or prolonged therapy, pre-existing renal insufficiency, advanced age, volume depletion, and the coexistence of renal ischemia or other nephrotoxins.[180–184] Although the precise cellular mechanisms by which aminoglycosides perturb renal function has not been elucidated, these agents appear to disrupt normal processing of membrane phospholipids by proximal tubule lysosomes.[185–199] Hypomagnesemia is a relatively common additional finding in patients with aminoglycoside-induced ATN and suggests coexistent injury to the thick ascending limb of the loop of Henle, the major site of $Mg^{2+}$ reabsorption.[171, 175] ARF is usually detected during the second week of therapy, probably reflecting a requirement for accumulation within epithelial cells, but may be manifest earlier in the presence of ischemia or other nephrotoxins.[165–179, 200–202] ATN is almost invariable in patients receiving cumulative doses of amphotericin B of more than 1 g and is a common complication even with lower doses.[203–209] Amphotericin B perturbs the function of many nephron segments and has been reported to cause intrarenal vasoconstriction, ATN, hypomagnesemia, and renal tubular acidosis due to back-leakage of secreted $H^+$ in the distal cortical nephron.[203–209] Acyclovir causes ARF

within 24 to 48 hours in 10% to 30% of patients, particularly if they are volume depleted or if the drug is administered as a bolus.[210–215] ARF is usually nonoliguric, frequently associated with colic, nausea, and vomiting, and appears to be induced by intratubular precipitation of acyclovir crystals.[210–215] Pentamidine induces ARF in 25% to 95% of patients, usually during the second week of therapy and frequently in association with hypomagnesemia, hypo- or hyperkalemia, and a distal renal tubular acidosis.[216–220] The mechanism of injury is unclear but may involve an immune process, as ARF does not appear to be dose dependent and is often associated with pyuria, hematuria, proteinuria, and casts.[216–220] Foscarnet causes a distinct pattern of renal injury characterized by nonoliguric, often polyuric, ARF within 7 days, hyperphosphatemia, ATN, interstitial fibrosis, and a slow recovery that may take months.[221–226] ATN complicates up to 70% of courses of cisplatin and ifosfamide, two commonly used chemotherapeutic agents.[221–226] Cisplatin is accumulated by proximal tubule cells and induces mitochondrial injury, inhibition of ATPase activity and solute transport, and free radical-mediated injury to cell membranes.[227–230] In addition, cisplatin may cause severe hypomagnesemia, even in the absence of ARF, which may persist long after therapy has been stopped. Ifosfamide-induced ATN is being recognized increasingly and is often associated with Fanconi syndrome, an unusual complication of proximal tubule injury by other agents.[231–233] The mechanism of proximal tubule injury in this setting is unknown.

Myoglobin, hemoglobin, uric acid, and myeloma light chains are the endogenous toxins that are most commonly associated with ATN. Renal dysfunction complicates approximately 30% of cases of rhabdomyolysis, the most common causes of which are listed in Table 28–7.[234–261] Hemoglobin-induced ATN is rare and is most commonly encountered after blood transfusion reactions (see Table 28–7). The precise mechanisms by which rhabdomyolysis and hemolysis impair GFR are unclear, but intrarenal vasoconstriction, intratubular obstruction, and tubule injury have been well documented as contributory pathophysiologic events in experimental animals.[236, 238, 245, 257, 258–261] Neither myoglobin nor hemoglobin is markedly nephrotoxic when injected in vivo. Both pigments induce intrarenal vasoconstriction, probably by scavenging the vasodilator NO in the renal microcirculation.[236, 238, 245, 257, 258–261] At acid pH, myoglobin and hemoglobin are also sources of ferrihemate, a substance that is a potent inhibitor of tubule transport.[260, 261] In this regard, it is noteworthy that hypovolemia and acidosis predispose experimental animals and humans to pigment-induced ATN.[249] Finally, both pigments, being ferrous iron compounds, may potentially induce tubule injury by stimulating local production of $OH^-$.[260, 261]

Intratubular obstruction has been implicated as a central event in the pathophysiology of ATN induced by some other endogenous (e.g., myeloma light chains, uric acid) and exogenous (ethylene glycol) nephrotoxins. Casts, composed of filtered immunoglobulin light chains and other urinary proteins such as Tamm-Horsfall protein, induce ARF in patients with multiple myeloma (myeloma-cast nephropathy).[262–270] High urinary salt concentrations and low urine pH promote this process.[270] The correlation between cast formation and renal insufficiency is relatively weak, however, suggesting that light chains may be directly toxic to tubule epithelial cells.[262–270] Acute uric acid nephropathy typically complicates treatment of lymphoproliferative or myeloproliferative disorders and is usually associated with other biochemical evidence of tumor lysis such as hyper-

kalemia, hyperphosphatemia, and hypocalcemia.[271–276] Acute uric acid nephropathy is rare when plasma concentrations are less than 15 to 20 mg/dL but may be precipitated at relatively low levels by volume depletion or low urine pH.[271–276] Both myeloma cast nephropathy and acute urate nephropathy are usually encountered in the setting of widespread malignancy and/or massive tumor destruction, and other potential contributory toxins in these clinical settings include hypercalcemia, hyperphosphatemia, and other products of tumor lysis[277–289] (see later discussion of ARF in the cancer patient). Oxalate-induced ARF is usually encountered as a complication of ethylene glycol toxicity but occasionally complicates primary defects in oxalate metabolism (primary hyperoxaluria) or other secondary forms of hyperoxaluria (e.g., malabsorption, massive vitamin C ingestion, methoxyflurane anesthesia).[290–297]

## Postrenal Azotemia

Urinary tract obstruction accounts for less than 5% of cases of ARF. Because one kidney has sufficient clearance capacity to excrete the nitrogenous waste products generated daily, ARF resulting from obstruction requires either obstruction of urine flow between the external urethral meatus and bladder neck, bilateral ureteric obstruction, or unilateral ureteric obstruction in a patient with one functioning kidney or underlying chronic renal insufficiency (Table 28–8). Obstruction of the bladder neck is the most common cause of postrenal azotemia and may complicate prostatic disease (e.g., hypertrophy, neoplasia, or infection), neurogenic bladder, or therapy with anticholinergic drugs. Less common causes of acute lower urinary tract obstruction include blood clots, calculi, and urethritis with spasm. Ureteric obstruction may result from intraluminal obstruction (e.g., calculi, blood clots, sloughed renal papillae), infiltration of the ureteric wall (e.g., neoplasia), or external compression (e.g., retroperitoneal fibrosis, neoplasia or abscess, inadvertent surgical ligature). During the early stages of obstruction (hours to days) continued glomerular filtration leads to increased intraluminal pressure upstream of the site of obstruction. This results in gradual distention of proximal ureter, renal pelvis, and calyces and a fall in GFR. Although acute obstruction may lead to an initial modest increase in renal blood flow, arterial vasoconstriction soon supervenes, leading to a further decline in glomerular filtration. The pathophysiology and treatment of obstructive uropathy are discussed extensively in Chapter 41.

## TABLE 28–8. Causes of Acute Postrenal Azotemia

Ureteric obstruction*
  Intraluminal: stones, blood clot, sloughed renal papillae, uric acid or sulfonamide crystals, fungus balls
  Intramural: postoperative edema after ureteric surgery
  Extraureteric: iatrogenic (ligation during pelvic surgery)
  Periureteric: hemorrhage, tumor, or fibrosis†
Bladder neck obstruction
  Intraluminal: stones, blood clots, sloughed papillae
  Intramural: bladder carcinoma, bladder infection with mural edema, neurogenic, drugs (e.g., tricyclic antidepressants, ganglion blockers)
  Extramural: prostatic hypertrophy, prostatic carcinoma
Urethral obstruction†
  Phimosis, congenital valves, stricture, tumor

*ARF in this setting implies bilateral ureteric obstruction or unilateral obstruction in a patient with a solitary functioning kidney (e.g., renal allograft) or chronic renal insufficiency.
†More commonly causes chronic obstruction.

# PATHOLOGY AND PATHOPHYSIOLOGY OF ISCHEMIC ACUTE TUBULE NECROSIS

The proximal tubule is the predominant site of injury after renal ischemia in humans, experimental animals, and isolated kidneys perfused with an erythrocyte-containing buffer. Injury to the distal tubule and particularly the medullary thick ascending limb (mTAL) of the loop of Henle has also been described in some cases of ATN in humans.

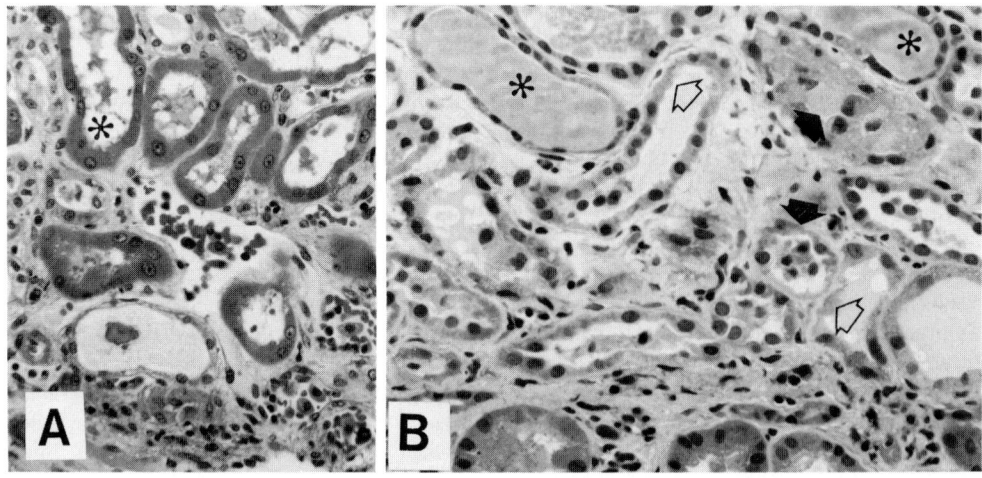

**Figure 28–3.** Morphology of human ATN. Micrographs of histologic sections of biopsy specimens from patients with ischemic ATN. *A.* Focal areas of proximal tubule vacuolization, flattening of proximal tubule cells, and tubule dilatation. There is marked brush border loss; brush border debris and blebs are present in the lumen of some tubules *(asterisks).* (Magnification × 250.) *B.* Tubule cell detachment and the presence of cells in the tubule lumen *(solid arrows),* focal areas of denuded basement membrane *(open arrows),* and the presence of intralumenal casts *(asterisks).* (Magnification × 250.) (Courtesy of LC Racusen.)

Here we review the pathology of ischemic ATN and current concepts regarding the mechanisms of cellular injury and reduction in GFR after oxygen deprivation injury. These concepts are derived predominantly from studies in experimental animals and in vitro systems such as isolated perfused kidneys, isolated proximal tubules in suspension, and renal cells in culture. The value of these models lies in defining the multiple factors that may potentially contribute to the pathophysiology of ischemic renal injury. However, it is important to appreciate that no experimental model faithfully replicates the process of renal injury in humans, and the conclusions drawn from these studies should be extrapolated to the pathophysiology of human ATN with appropriate caution. Furthermore, because ATN in humans can occur in a large spectrum of clinical situations (see Tables 28–3, 28–6, and 28–7), it is likely that several different pathophysiologic mechanisms, acting alone or in combination, lead to renal insufficiency in individual patients with ATN.

## Morphology of Ischemic Acute Tubule Necrosis

### MORPHOLOGY OF ATN IN HUMANS

In 1946, Lucke[298] reported that tubule injury in humans with ATN largely involved the loop of Henle and distal nephron segments and coined the term "lower nephron nephrosis" to describe this disorder. However, multiple subsequent analyses of biopsy and autopsy materials, beginning in 1951 with the classic microdissection studies of Oliver and colleagues,[299] clearly demonstrated that the predominant site of injury in ATN is the straight segment of the proximal tubule (S₃ segment, pars recta),[299–304] as has been reported for most experimental models of ATN. Thus, the term lower nephron nephrosis has been abandoned by the majority of investigators. Despite the term ATN, frank

necrosis is usually inconspicuous or absent in human disease.[304] The major abnormality is usually patchy and focal loss of individual or clusters of cells from tubule epithelium with resultant gaps and exposure of areas of denuded basement membrane[302, 305, 306] (Fig. 28–3). Diffuse effacement and thinning of the proximal tubular brush border are also common features of human ATN[302, 303] (see Fig. 28–3), a finding that has also been consistently described in experimental models of ischemic renal injury.[307] The pars recta is the most severely affected segment in ATN, but injury is usually also observed to some extent in more distal nephron segments[299, 301–303] including the mTAL.[308]

The presence of casts in the lumen of distal nephron segments is another characteristic morphologic feature of ischemic ATN in humans[299, 302] (see Fig. 28–3). These casts are believed to be composed of protein (predominantly Tamm-Horsfall glycoprotein), as well as cells, remnants of shed brush border, and other cellular debris. Although the mechanism of cast formation remains uncertain, there is compelling evidence for involvement of cell adhesion molecules in this process[309–311] (vide infra).

Evidence of cellular regeneration, specifically basophilic cytoplasm, large hyperchromatic nuclei, and occasional mitoses, is seen in many biopsy specimens and is most common in areas of greatest cell loss and necrosis. Indeed, regenerative changes and signs of fresh epithelial injury are often observed together in the same biopsy specimen.[302] These observations support the contention that repeated episodes of renal ischemia commonly occur during the maintenance phase of ATN and result in repeated cycles of necrosis, exfoliation, and regeneration of epithelial cells.[302]

The morphologic characteristics of the common forms of toxic ATN in the current era, particularly nephrotoxicity induced by aminoglycosides, are similar to those seen in ischemic ATN and are characterized by scattered foci of patchy necrosis and cell loss in both proximal and distal nephron segments.[302, 312, 313] The extensive necrosis involving much of the proximal tubule that was reported in the past in nephrotoxic ATN induced by heavy metals and carbon tetrachloride poisoning is rarely seen today.[312]

A marked clinicopathologic disparity between the severity of impairment of GFR and the relatively subtle histologic lesions on biopsy specimens is a well-recognized paradox of ATN.[304–306] Because each individual nephron segment functions as a morphologically and functionally discrete entity acting in series with other segments, subtle focal areas of necrosis and cast formation seen histologically may theoretically severely compromise the function of the whole nephron by causing tubule back-leakage or obstruction. However, insights from experimental models suggest that sublethal injury to renal epithelial cells may also contribute to severe impairment of renal function in the absence of pronounced histologic changes.[305, 306]

## EXPERIMENTAL MODELS

Studies of experimental animals have proved useful in documenting the temporal sequence of morphologic injury in ischemic ATN and defining the functional consequences of these changes at the whole kidney, single nephron, and cell level. Although renal hypoperfusion caused by hemorrhagic shock is the most common cause of ATN in humans, the effects of hypoperfusion have not been extensively studied in experimental models. Rats, the most common species studied, are relatively resistant to oxygen deprivation induced by hypoperfusion and, unlike humans, do not develop ARF unless renal perfusion pressures are reduced to low levels (15 to 20 mm Hg).[314–316] Indeed, 1 to 2 hours of moderate hypotension does not usually result in ARF in rats, despite development of necrosis of the straight portion (pars recta) of the proximal tubule.[314, 315]

Renal ischemia induced by total cessation of renal blood flow (typically in renal artery clamping) is the most extensively studied experimental model of ischemic ATN. As in humans with ATN, the proximal tubule, predominantly the pars recta, is the segment most severely affected. However, unlike the situation in ATN, injury to the pars recta is typically diffuse rather than focal and distal tubule injury is unusual in experimental models of ischemia.[299–304] Brief ischemia (25 minutes) induces necrosis of cells in the straight portion of the proximal tubule with relative sparing of proximal tubule cells in the cortex and mild renal failure. More prolonged ischemia (60 minutes) is associated with more extensive necrosis involving the entire proximal tubule and severe renal failure.[299–304]

As in humans with ATN, disruption of the proximal tubule brush border is a characteristic feature of experimental renal ischemia. Swelling and blebbing of the plasma membrane are early morphologic changes in this setting.[307–317] Microvilli are shed into the tubule lumen and/or internalized into proximal tubule cells.[307, 317] Blebs of brush border shed into the lumen continue to swell during their transit down the tubules and are packed in large numbers within the straight segments of the proximal tubules as well as in more distal segments. These morphologic changes not only are found in experimental ischemia in vivo but also are characteristic of ischemia in the isolated erythrocyte-perfused kidney model.[318] A striking feature of these brush border changes is their rapid reversibility. Microvilli typically regenerate within 30 to 60 minutes of reflow. Indeed, the rapidity of regeneration of the brush border suggests that damaged membranes, which have been internalized into the cytoplasm during ischemia, are recycled during recovery.[307, 317] These histologic and ultramicroscopic changes in the brush border correlate temporally with the striking alterations observed in brush border actin, leading to the hypothesis that injury to the actin cytoskeleton is an important factor in the causation of the brush border injury.[318, 319]

Studies of oxygen deprivation injury in isolated perfused kidneys have yielded conflicting results. The isolated kidney perfused by a conventional, erythrocyte-free buffer develops severe ischemic injury in the absence of renal artery occlusion. The morphologic pattern of injury in this model is characterized by necrosis of the cells of the mTAL segment with relative sparing of proximal tubule cells.[320, 321] This morphologic pattern of injury is probably related to the absence of red cells in the perfusate. When isolated kidneys are perfused with a more physiologic erythrocyte-containing buffer, the proximal tubule segment and not the mTAL is injured in response to ischemia[318] and hypoxia (low oxygen tensions).[322] The profound mTAL necrosis characteristic of the erythrocyte-free isolated kidney is probably related in part to increased countercurrent loss of oxygen in the vasa recta of the medulla because of the absence of erythrocytes.[322] Addition of erythrocytes to the perfusate (even at a hematocrit as low as 2%) prevents mTAL injury, presumably by facilitating delivery of oxygen to the mTAL segments in the outer medulla.[318, 322] Furthermore, the erythrocyte-free isolated kidney model is characterized by a relatively high GFR, which imposes large transport and energy requirements on the nephron that are highly atypical of other experimental models of ischemic injury or of ATN in humans. When transport demands are reduced in the erythrocyte-free isolated kidney by decreasing GFR, mTAL injury is markedly ameliorated.[323]

## Pathophysiology of Ischemic Injury

Intrarenal vasoconstriction and tubule dysfunction have been clearly defined as the two major mechanisms for the profound reduction in GFR after renal ischemia (Fig. 28–4). The consensus view is that epithelial cell injury compromises GFR by promoting back-leakage of glomerular filtrate and by obstruction of tubules. As already discussed, the pars recta of the proximal tubule and, to a lesser degree, the mTAL of the loop of Henle, both situated in the outer medulla, are the nephron segments that are most susceptible to ischemic injury, probably because of their high ATP requirements for active solute transport and the regional differences in renal blood flow that render the outer medulla more hypoxic than other regions of the kidney.

This section reviews current concepts of the relative contributions of derangements in renal hemodynamics and epithelial cell dysfunction to impairment of GFR in ischemic ATN and focuses particularly on the cellular events that subserve these abnormalities.

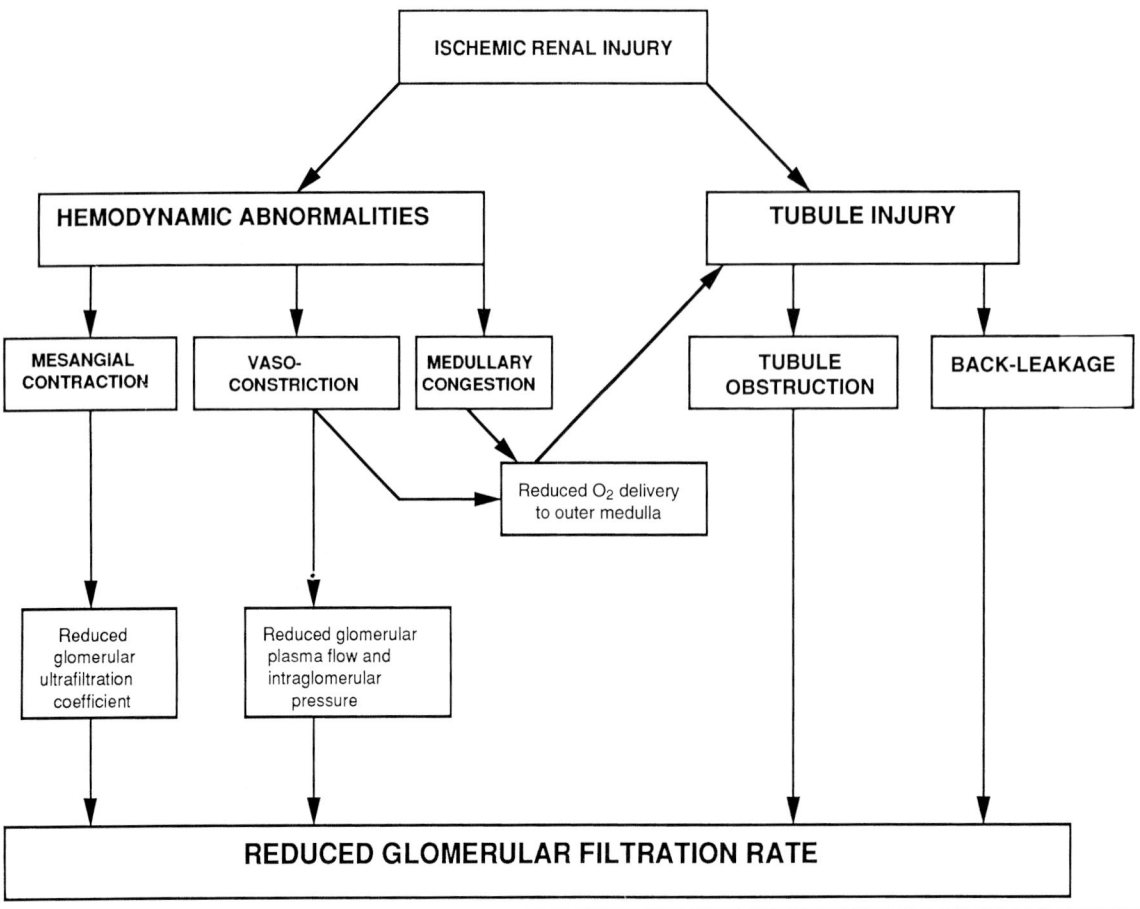

**Figure 28–4.** Pathophysiology of ischemic renal failure. The profound reduction in GFR associated with renal ischemia is due to a combination of intrarenal hemodynamic alterations and renal tubule epithelial injury leading to back-leakage of glomerular ultrafiltrate and tubule obstruction.

## HEMODYNAMIC ALTERATIONS IN ATN

A reduction in total renal blood flow to 40% to 50% of normal has been consistently reported after renal ischemia in experimental models[324–326] and humans.[327, 328] Formerly, many investigators had concluded that these hemodynamic alterations were relatively unimportant in the maintenance phase of ischemic ATN. This conclusion was based on a number of observations. The reduction in renal blood flow observed during the maintenance phase of experimental and human ischemic ATN is clearly not sufficient to account for the profound reduction in GFR. Although a decrease in glomerular ultrafiltration coefficient ($K_f$) has been demonstrated in some models of toxic ATN, $K_f$ has been reported to be unchanged[329] or only modestly reduced[330] in ischemic renal injury. Furthermore, augmentation of total renal blood flow by volume expansion or administration of vasodilators such as dopamine or acetylcholine does not substantially improve GFR. However, newer evidence suggests that persistent and severe regional disturbances in renal blood flow and oxygen supply, affecting predominantly the outer medulla of the kidney, may indeed contribute to the maintenance phase of ATN. Oxygen tensions are low in the outer medulla of normally perfused kidneys, presumably because of countercurrent exchange and shunting of oxygen.[331, 332]

The outer medulla remains profoundly hypoxic on restoration of blood flow after renal ischemia, while oxygen tension in the cortex and papilla improve.[333–335] This outer medullary hypoxia would be expected to prolong cellular injury in tubule segments with high energy requirements in this region, namely the straight segment of the proximal tubule and mTAL, even after renal blood flow has been restored (Fig. 28–5).

The mechanisms responsible for intrarenal vasoconstriction and outer medullary hypoperfusion remain incompletely defined and probably involve multiple factors. There is persuasive evidence that endothelin is an important mediator of vasoconstriction[336] as well as tubule injury and renal insufficiency[337] in the reflow period. Postischemic intrarenal vasoconstriction is ameliorated by intrarenal infusion of antibodies to endothelin.[336] Furthermore, blockade of endothelin action using an endothelin receptor antagonist has been shown to ameliorate the functional and histologic abnormalities associated with renal ischemia.[337] There is also evidence that ischemia reduces the constitutive release of NO by endothelial cells in the kidney.[338] A deficiency in NO production would be expected to cause vasoconstriction, because NO normally plays an important role in regulating systemic and renal vascular tone by maintaining basal renal arterial vasodilatation. Thus, endothelial injury, leading to an imbalance in the production of endothelin and

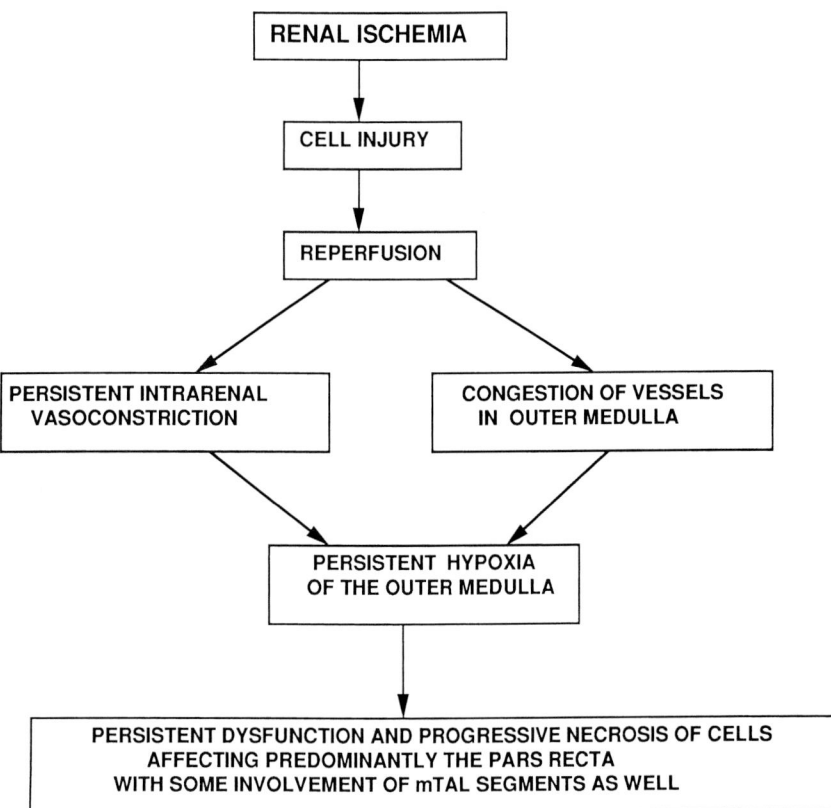

**Figure 28–5.** Role of persistent hypoxia of the outer medulla in the pathophysiology of ATN. Persistent hypoxia after reflow, caused by vasoconstriction and outer medullary congestion, results in continued injury to renal tubule cells (involving the pars recta of the proximal tubule and mTAL segments) after blood flow is restored to the kidney.

NO, has emerged as an important cause of intrarenal vasoconstriction after ischemia (Fig. 28–6).

Several other factors have been identified as potential contributors to persistent regional hypoxia in the outer medulla after renal ischemia and reperfusion. Congestion of medullary vessels by trapping of red blood cells is commonly observed in this setting[335] (see Fig. 28–5). However, evidence supporting a pathogenetic link between medullary

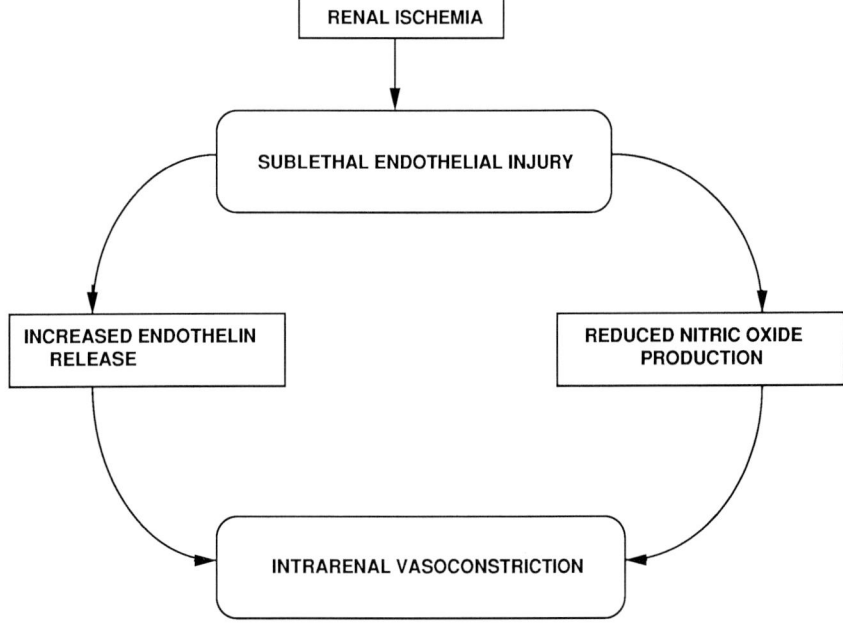

**Figure 28–6.** Role of sublethal endothelial injury in the intrarenal vasoconstriction after ischemia and reflow. Endothelin-1, a peptide hormone synthesized by endothelial cells and other cell types, is a potent stimulus for intrarenal vasoconstriction. Endothelin-1 release from cultured endothelial cells is increased under hypoxic conditions in vitro and circulating levels of endothelin-1 are elevated in several experimental models of acute renal failure (e.g., cyclosporine nephrotoxicity, contrast nephropathy) and in human hepatorenal syndrome. Intriguingly, antiendothelin antibodies and endothelin-1 receptor antagonists attenuate functional and/or morphologic abnormalities in experimental ischemic ARF. In contrast, NO is a potent vasodilator released by endothelial cells whose production appears blunted under hypoxic conditions in vivo and in vitro. Together, these observations suggest that sublethal endothelial cell injury may induce vasodilator-vasoconstrictor imbalance within the kidney that contributes to renal hypoperfusion (see text for further discussion and references).

congestion and renal injury is indirect; reduction in the systemic hematocrit greatly reduces medullary congestion and ameliorates ischemic injury, and increases in hematocrit have the opposite effect.[339]

Abnormalities in proximal tubule reabsorption of Na[+] and water have been proposed to stimulate the tubuloglomerular feedback system through activation of the macula densa and cause afferent arteriolar vasoconstriction.[340] However, the relative pathophysiologic importance of increased tubuloglomerular feedback in the causation of postischemic vasoconstriction has been difficult to evaluate.[340]

Despite extensive experimental investigation, there is little convincing evidence to support a role for vasoconstrictors such as angiotensin, arachidonic acid metabolities, vasopressin, catecholamines, or renal nerves in the hemodynamic changes after renal ischemia.[341]

## TUBULE DYSFUNCTION IN ATN

Experimental studies in animals have clearly established that tubule injury plays a central role in the reduction in GFR in ischemic ATN (see Fig. 28–4). Two major tubule abnormalities have been demonstrated: obstruction and back-leakage of glomerular filtrate. There is general agreement that tubules are obstructed by detached tubule epithelial cells and debris after renal arterial occlusion and reperfusion.[317, 342–345] Elevated proximal and distal intratubular pressures have been demonstrated by micropuncture in this model. Although tubule pressures tend to fall toward normal after 24 hours, the presence of persistent obstruction can be revealed by extracellular volume expansion, which again elevates pressures. Conclusive evidence for the presence of tubule leakiness in renal artery occlusion models of ischemic injury has been derived from studies of the fate of molecular markers injected into tubule fluid by micropuncture. A variable fraction of inulin injected into proximal or distal tubules of ischemic kidneys leaks into the circulation and appears in the urine of the contralateral uninjured kidney.[317, 342, 343] The extent of the tubule leakiness correlates with the duration of ischemia[317] and is greater in oliguric than nonoliguric failure.[342]

The tubule abnormalities demonstrated in experimental ischemic injury also appear to be important in the pathophysiology of human ATN. The presence of areas of tubule cell loss, focal areas of tubule necrosis, and distal tubule casts on biopsy and autopsy specimens from patients with ATN clearly provide a morphologic basis for tubule backleakage and obstruction (see earlier section on morphology).[299–306] In addition, Moran and Myers,[346, 347] in a series of innovative clinical studies, have provided more direct evidence that back-leakage of glomerular filtrate and intratubular obstruction contribute to renal insufficiency in patients with ischemic ATN after cardiac or aortic surgery.

## Cell Biology of Ischemic Injury

The abnormalities in tubule epithelial cell function that ultimately lead to obstruction and back-leakage of ultrafiltrate can be understood only by defining the alterations in cell biology that result from oxygen deprivation. A decrease in cellular ATP stores is the proximate event in ischemic injury and is responsible for initiating a cascade of biochemical events that lead to cellular dysfunction, sublethal injury, and eventually cell death.[348–350] Some major consequences of cell ATP depletion include inhibition of ATP-dependent transport pumps with loss of the ion gradients that are normally maintained across cell membranes and polarized epithelia, unregulated activation of injurious enzyme systems such as phospholipases and proteases, oxidant injury caused by generation of reactive oxygen species, and alterations in the cytoskeleton (Table 28–9). There is compelling evidence that these events act in concert to perturb epithelial cell function in ischemic ATN.

## ATP DEPLETION

A fall in cell ATP levels is an early event after oxygen deprivation resulting from ischemia, hypoperfusion, or hypoxia. Oxygen deprivation results in rapid degradation of ATP to ADP and AMP. Epithelial cell membranes are relatively impermeable to these nucleotides and, as a result, they are not lost from the cell. Restoration of oxygen availability results in rapid resynthesis of ATP from these nucleotides. If ischemia is prolonged, however, AMP is metabolized further to nucleosides (adenosine and inosine) and to hypoxanthine. These purine metabolites are able to diffuse from the cell. As a result, there is loss of the metabolites that serve as a reservoir for the rapid resynthesis of ATP during reperfusion.[348–350] De novo synthesis of ATP from nonpurine precursors is complex, energetically unfavorable, and probably plays little role in the recovery of ATP after ischemia.[349] Prolonged ischemia also ultimately results in irreversible loss of mitochondrial function, which further impairs rapid regeneration of ATP after reperfusion. Thus, cell ATP levels rise rapidly to near-baseline levels after short periods of ischemia, but ATP recovery during reperfusion is limited after prolonged periods of ischemia. The rate of cell ATP recovery after reperfusion and the ability of the cell to survive ischemia are therefore dependent on the duration of the ischemic period.[348–350]

The central and proximate role played by ATP depletion in ischemic injury has been established in studies in which

---

**TABLE 28–9. Potential Mechanisms of Cell Injury After Ischemia**

Depletion of cellular energy (ATP) stores
Disruption of the actin cytoskeleton and cell adhesion molecules
Impaired function of plasma and microsomal membrane pumps
    Alterations in cell electrolyte content
    Cell swelling
    Increase in cytosolic free $Ca^{2+}$
    Intracellular acidosis
Enzyme activation
    Phospholipases
    Proteases
Reperfusion injury after reflow
    Persistent hypoxia of the outer medulla (see Fig. 28–5)
    Generation of reactive oxygen species (see Fig. 28–7)
    Reversal of intracellular acidosis
    Leukocyte-induced injury

ATP levels were manipulated during ischemia or after reperfusion. Hypothermia during ischemia markedly reduces cellular injury by preserving cell ATP levels,[318] but hypothermia is of no benefit when limited to the reperfusion period.[348] The importance of the adenine nucleotide pool to the recovery of sublethally injured cells after ischemia has been demonstrated by Siegel and colleagues[351] and subsequently confirmed by other investigators.[348–350, 352–354] Provision of adenosine, inosine, and exogenous adenine nucleotides (AMP, ADP, and ATP) accelerates recovery of cellular ATP and lessens cellular injury after ischemic injury in vivo or hypoxia in vitro.[348–354] The beneficial effects of these exogenous adenine nucleotides are mediated through their breakdown to adenosine and subsequent cellular uptake of adenosine and conversion of adenosine to AMP via adenosine kinase.[355] Additional proof of the benefit of maintaining cell nucleotide levels during ischemia has been derived from studies in which inhibitors of 5'-nucleotidase (which catalyzes the dephosphorylation of AMP to adenosine) and adenosine deaminase preserved cell ATP levels and cellular function after ischemia.[348–350, 356]

Cellular ATP is produced by oxidative phosphorylation by mitochondria as well as by glycolysis. Because oxygen deprivation reduces ATP production by mitochondria without affecting glycolysis, it is not surprising that the proximal tubule, which depends predominantly on mitochondria for its ATP production, is generally more susceptible to ATP depletion and ischemic renal injury than other nephron segments.[299–306, 348–350] However, the medullary straight portion of the proximal tubule appears to be more sensitive to ischemic injury in vivo than cortical segments of the proximal tubule, despite the fact that the straight portion (pars recta) has enhanced glycolytic capacity compared with the cortical segments and is more resistant than cortical segments to the injurious effects of ischemia in vitro.[350] These observations support the contention that differences in susceptibility of different regions of the kidney to oxygen deprivation are related to regional differences in oxygen supply after reperfusion, in addition to differences in ATP requirements. Thus, the more prominent injury to the pars recta compared with other proximal tubule segments with lower glycolytic capacity, is probably due to the combined effects of persistent medullary hypoperfusion and hypoxia and the high metabolic requirements of this tubule segment.[348–350] In keeping with this interpretation, the mTAL has been demonstrated to be highly susceptible to ischemic injury in the isolated kidney perfused in the absence of red blood cells, despite substantial glycolytic capacity.[320, 321]

Finally, it should be emphasized that oxygen delivery and the ATP content of cells are not the only factors that determine susceptibility to injury. Balance between energy availability and oxygen demand has also been shown to influence the extent to which oxygen deprivation causes injury to renal epithelial cells. Studies of the isolated kidney perfused by an erythrocyte-free buffer have shown that interventions that reduce Na+ transport and therefore oxygen demand ameliorate the severe hypoxic injury that is expressed predominantly in the mTAL segments in this experimental model.[323]

## CELL SWELLING

Immediate effects of cellular ATP depletion are reduction of plasma membrane ATPase activity, loss of the normal Na+ and K+ concentrations in the cytosol, and cell swelling.[348] Cytoskeletal injury may also contribute to cell swelling.[357] Cell swelling has been proposed to contribute to renal dysfunction after ischemic injury by contributing to obstruction of the tubule lumen and to the vascular congestion in the outer medulla.[349] The beneficial effects of impermeable solutes such as mannitol in vivo may be mediated in part by protecting the kidney against the effects of epithelial and endothelial cell swelling and by reducing outer medullary congestion.[349] However, solutes such as mannitol have not been consistently found to be cytoprotective in experiments in vitro.[348] It is therefore likely that the protective effect of mannitol in ischemia in vivo results predominantly from mechanisms independent of effects on cell swelling, including hemodynamic alterations, osmotic diuresis, and scavenging of $OH^-$.[349]

## INCREASED INTRACELLULAR FREE $Ca^{2+}$

An early rise in the concentration of intracellular free $Ca^{2+}$ after ATP depletion has the potential to cause cell injury and death. However, despite extensive investigation the role of $Ca^{2+}$ in ischemic injury remains uncertain. The cytosolic and organellar $Ca^{2+}$ concentration within cells requires tight regulation by active transport because the concentration of $Ca^{2+}$ in extracellular fluid exceeds the intracellular concentration (of approximately 100 nM) approximately 10,000-fold. This gradient is maintained by plasma membrane and endoplasmic reticulum $Ca^{2+}$-ATPases and a plasma membrane $Na^+/Ca^{2+}$ exchanger.[348–350, 358] With ATP depletion, inhibition of $Ca^{2+}$-ATPases impairs active extrusion of $Ca^{2+}$ from the cell and sequestration of $Ca^{2+}$ in endoplasmic reticulum.[348–350] In addition, the rise in intracellular Na+ associated with inhibition of Na+,K+-ATPase activity potentiates $Ca^{2+}$ entry into the cell via the $Na^+/Ca^{2+}$ exchanger.[349] Under normal conditions, the endoplasmic reticulum plays a more important role than mitochondria in acting as a sink for $Ca^{2+}$ and buffering increases in cytosolic $Ca^{2+}$.[350] Uptake of $Ca^{2+}$ by mitochondria becomes substantial only when cytosolic levels of free $Ca^{2+}$ exceed 500 nM, as may occur during cellular injury. Pronounced $Ca^{2+}$ uptake by mitochondria can cause mitochondrial swelling[349, 350, 358] and activation of mitochondrial phospholipases with release of toxic fatty acids that uncouple oxidative phosphorylation and thus compound the primary effect of hypoxia on cell energetics.[349, 350]

$Ca^{2+}$ overload is characteristic in renal tissue with lethally injured cells after toxic or ischemic injury. More relevant to the question of the pathophysiologic role of $Ca^{2+}$ in ischemic ATN is whether cytosolic free $Ca^{2+}$ or mitochondrial $Ca^{2+}$ increases before lethal or sublethal cell injury. Several investigators, using cells in culture, have shown that cytosolic free $Ca^{2+}$ concentrations increase rapidly during ATP depletion.[359,360] In one study this rise in cytosolic $Ca^{2+}$ was shown to be due to a combination of

Ca$^{2+}$ entry across the plasma membrane and release of Ca$^{2+}$ from the endoplasmic reticulum.[360] The increase in Ca$^{2+}$ during ATP depletion is usually modest and in the range reported after hormonal stimulation.[348,349] This has led some investigators to argue that the rise in Ca$^{2+}$ may be relatively unimportant.[349] However, unlike the physiologic increases in cell Ca$^{2+}$, which are generally transient, the increase in Ca$^{2+}$ in response to ATP depletion is persistent, increases progressively with time,[360] and may therefore lead to unregulated activation of injurious enzymes.

Increases in serum Ca$^{2+}$ in vivo[361] and in the perfusate of the isolated kidney[362] exacerbate ischemic and hypoxic injury. Also, removal of extracellular Ca$^{2+}$ from the media ameliorates anoxic injury in freshly isolated proximal tubules[363] and in cultured renal tubule cells.[364] However, interpretation of studies using low-Ca$^{2+}$ conditions can be complicated by other effects of Ca$^{2+}$ removal on cellular function.[350]

The effect of Ca$^{2+}$ channel blockers has provided additional suggestive evidence of a pathogenetic role for Ca$^{2+}$ in ischemia. These agents have been shown to ameliorate injury in experimental ischemic injury in vivo[348-350,365,366] and in vitro.[350,367] Furthermore, Ca$^{2+}$ channel blockers are among the few pharmacologic agents with demonstrated efficacy in ameliorating ARF in humans. In clinical studies, the administration of Ca$^{2+}$ channel blockers, in particular diltiazem and verapamil, has been demonstrated to reduce the incidence of ARF immediately after cadaveric kidney transplantation when given to both recipient and donor.[368] However, the mechanism of protection of Ca$^{2+}$ channel blockers is uncertain and not clearly related to reducing cytosolic levels of Ca$^{2+}$ in renal epithelial cels.[348-350,369] Ca$^{2+}$ channel blockers may ameliorate ischemic injury in the kidney by improving renal hemodynamics. In addition, these agents may directly affect tubule epithelial cell function by many mechanisms other than blocking Ca$^{2+}$ entry into cells. Ca$^{2+}$ channel blockers antagonize calmodulin action as well as phosphodiesterases and have "membrane-stabilizing" effects that may contribute to their beneficial effects in ischemic injury.[348-350,369]

Although the precise role of Ca$^{2+}$ in the pathophysiology of ischemic ATN is still being evaluated, these studies, when taken in aggregate, suggest that increased intracellular Ca$^{2+}$ is an important event in the evolution of hypoxic renal cell injury. Ca$^{2+}$ has been proposed to result in cell injury by disrupting cytoskeletal microfilaments, activating Ca$^{2+}$-dependent phospholipases, facilitating the generation of reactive oxygen species by accelerating the conversion of xanthine dehydrogenase to xanthine oxidase (Fig. 28–7), and uncoupling oxidative phosphorylation.[348-350,358]

## INTRACELLULAR ACIDOSIS

A fall in intracellular pH occurs in most cells exposed to oxygen deprivation. In glycolytic cells the fall in pH is partly due to increased lactate production. However, intracellular acidosis occurs even in cells with relatively low glycolytic capacity such as proximal tubule cells.[350] Hydrolysis of ATP to its breakdown products results in the release of acidic metabolites,[370] while ATP depletion impedes the transport processes that normally maintain intracellular

acid-base balance. Although severe intracellular acidosis can clearly contribute to ischemic cell injury, there is convincing evidence that a decrease in cellular pH in the range observed during ischemia in vivo is more likely to protect cells from the damaging effects of oxygen deprivation.[370-373] If intracellular acidosis is important in ameliorating cell injury during ischemia, the rapid correction of intracellular pH associated with return of oxygen supply to ischemic renal tissue could potentially contribute to the development of reperfusion injury (see Table 28–9).

The mechanisms responsible for the protective effect of acidosis are not known but are probably multifactorial. Inhibition of 5'-nucleotidase by acidosis may reduce AMP metabolism and preserve the intracellular nucleotide pool.[374] Intracellular acidosis would be expected to reduce the activity of some isoforms of phospholipase A$_2$ (PLA$_2$) that act optimally at physiologic pH.[349,350] The affinity of Ca$^{2+}$ for calmodulin is also reduced by a decrease in pH so that intracellular acidosis may also impair multiple Ca$^{2+}$-calmodulin–regulated events that are potential contributors to ischemic injury, including the conversion of xanthine dehydrogenase to xanthine oxidase and calpain activation[350,357,375] (see Fig. 28–7).

## PHOSPHOLIPASE ACTIVATION

Activation of phospholipases and consequent alterations in the composition and functional properties of lipid bilayers of the plasma membrane and subcellular organelles (e.g., mitochondria) are well-documented consequences of ischemic injury in many organs, including the heart, liver, and kidney.[348-350,376] Characteristic changes include marked loss of phospholipid mass and intracellular accumulation of free fatty acids, lysophospholipids, diacylglycerol, acyl-coenzyme A, acyl carnitine esters, and inositol phosphates. These metabolic events are probably exacerbated by reduced reacylation into phospholipid and de novo phospholipid synthesis,[350] other functional consequences of cell ATP depletion. Ischemic cell injury is characterized by activation of multiple phospholipases. Increased cell diacylglycerol and phosphatidic acid levels are compatible with activation of phospholipases C and D,[377] and elevated levels of all classes of free fatty acids[378] are consistent with generalized disruption of lipid metabolism. However, the lipid metabolites released in largest amount with fatty acids after ischemia are lysophospholipids, suggesting that PLA$_2$ activation (which releases fatty acids and lysophospholipid in equimolar amounts) accounts for the major release of fatty acids.[349,378] Protein kinase C activation may enhance PLA$_2$ activity by phosphorylating one isoform of this enzyme, thereby acting as a positive feedback loop for enhanced PLA$_2$ activity.[349,379]

Several isoforms of Ca$^{2+}$-dependent PLA$_2$ activity have been demonstrated in the cytosol and mitochondrial and microsomal fractions of rat kidneys.[349,380] Ischemia and reperfusion result in stable activation of soluble and membrane-bound forms of these Ca$^{2+}$-dependent PLA$_2$ isoforms, an observation that may explain the continued phospholipid degradation that occurs after reflow is established.[349,381] A novel class of intracellular Ca$^{2+}$-independent isoform of PLA$_2$ has been identified in myocardium, brain, and kid-

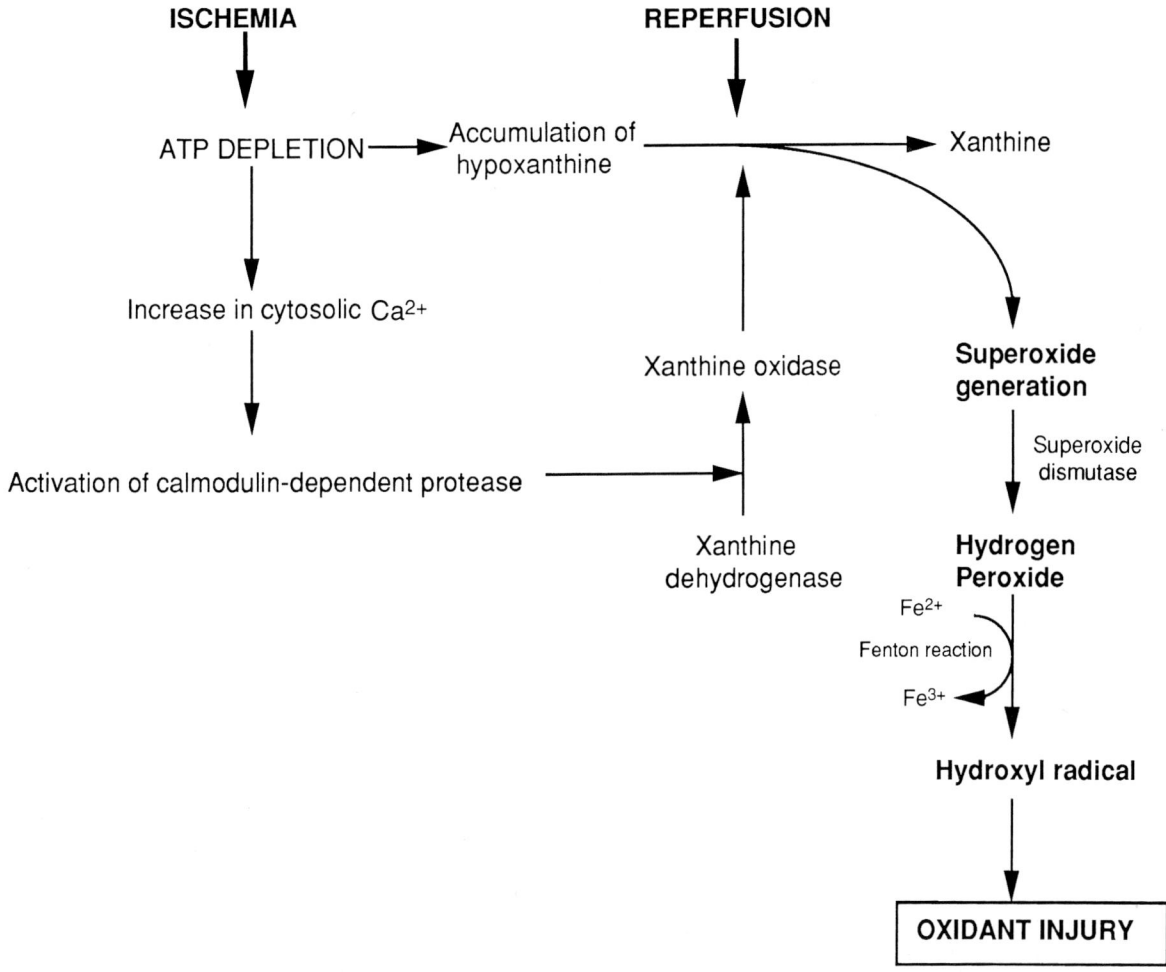

**Figure 28–7.** Potential role of ROS in reperfusion injury after ischemia. During ischemia and ATP depletion, xanthine dehydrogenase is converted to xanthine oxidase by a calmodulin-dependent protease. At the same time, ATP is metabolized to hypoxanthine. During reperfusion and reoxygenation, the conversion of hypoxanthine to xanthine by xanthine oxidase generates superoxide. Superoxide is converted to OH⁻ by a two-step reaction referred to as the Haber-Weiss reaction. Superoxide is first converted to hydrogen peroxide, a reaction catalyzed by superoxide dismutase. Then hydrogen peroxide is converted to OH⁻ by the iron-catalyzed Fenton reaction. Resultant oxidant injury to cell membrane, protein, and DNA contributes to cellular injury, dysfunction, and necrosis. See text for further details.

ney.[382–384] This isoform of PLA$_2$ acts selectively on plasmalogens, a subclass of phospholipids characterized by a vinyl ether linkage (instead of a fatty acid) at the sn-1 position. Plasmalogens are an important constituent of renal cortex membranes.[385] Portilla and colleagues[384] provided evidence that a substantial fraction of PLA$_2$ activity in proximal tubules is Ca$^{2+}$ independent and that activation of this enzyme also plays a role in the pathogenesis of hypoxic injury in the proximal tubule.

Although PLA$_2$ activation and release of free fatty acids and lysophospholipid have been invoked as important mediators of myocardial, intestinal, and renal ischemic injury,[349, 350] the evidence supporting this hypothesis remains largely indirect because specific inhibitors of PLA$_2$ are not yet available. Mepacrine and dibucaine, putative inhibitors of the Ca$^{2+}$-dependent PLA$_2$, were protective against ischemic injury to heart[349] and intestine[349] in some studies, as well as in renal cells in culture.[386] An inhibitor of the Ca$^{2+}$-independent isoform of PLA$_2$ has also been reported to ameliorate hypoxic injury in proximal tubules.[384] Albumin, which effectively binds free fatty acids, reduces the accumulation of fatty acid in isolated renal tubules exposed to PLA$_2$[387] and in renal cells in culture subjected to ATP depletion[386] and ameliorates cellular injury in both situations. PLA$_2$ activation and free fatty acid accumulation may also contribute to mitochondrial injury and further aggravate cell ATP depletion. Ca$^{2+}$ uptake by isolated mitochondria is associated with functional deterioration that leads, in turn, to release of free fatty acids. This deterioration in mitochondrial function can be blocked by phospholipase inhibitors or by trapping of free fatty acids with albumin.[388, 389]

High levels of free fatty acids are toxic to most cells. Addition of exogenous fatty acids or PLA$_2$ to hypoxic proximal tubules results in severe cellular injury and uncoupling of oxidative phosphorylation.[349] However, the mechanism by which fatty acids mediate cellular toxicity has not been established. It is commonly stated that fatty acids have a detergent-like effect on cellular membranes.[349, 350] However, this conventional wisdom is an unlikely mechanism of fatty acid toxicity, because fatty acids have little detergent activity at physiologic pH.[390] The cytotoxic role of lysophospholipid, which does have weak detergent properties and is released together with fatty acids after PLA$_2$ action, has not been determined.

## PROTEASE ACTIVATION

There is little evidence to suggest a pathogenetic role for lysozomal hydrolases in ischemic injury. However, activation of calpain, a neutral cysteine protease, may be important.[350, 391–393] This cytosolic and membrane-associated enzyme regulates multiple intracellular events including the activity of membrane channels, receptor function, kinase activation (including protein kinase C), and interactions between cytoskeletal proteins.[391–393] Insufficient information is available to assess the importance of calpain activation in ischemia. However, in some preliminary reports, a cysteine protease inhibitor active against calpain ameliorated ischemic injury in isolated segments of proximal tubules[394] and in proximal tubule cells in culture.[395]

## OXIDANT INJURY

Reactive oxygen species (ROS) have been implicated as important effectors of cell injury in both ischemic and toxic ATN. ROS have numerous deleterious effects on cells, including lipid peroxidation, oxidation of cell proteins, and damage to DNA.[396] These effects, in turn, can result in loss of plasma membrane and mitochondrial membrane integrity, impairment of protein function, and inhibition of cell repair and proliferation.[397–399] The three primary ROS incriminated in the causation of ischemic renal injury are superoxide anion, hydrogen peroxide, and OH$^-$. The last is the most reactive of all ROS and is generated from superoxide by a three-step process known as the Haber-Weiss reaction[396] (see Fig. 28–7). Cells are protected from the injurious effects of ROS, generated under physiologic and pathophysiologic situations, by specific scavenging systems.[350, 396] Superoxide dismutase, a cytosolic and mitochondrial metalloenzyme, catalyzes the conversion of superoxide to hydrogen peroxide. Catalase, a peroxisomal enzyme, and glutathione peroxidase, a cytosolic and mitochondrial enzyme, catalyze conversion of hydrogen peroxide to water. These enzymes and antioxidants represent the major defenses against ROS production within the proximal tubule cell. Oxidant injury occurs when these defenses are overwhelmed by massive production of ROS.[348–350, 396]

In ischemic injury, ROS are formed when oxygen is delivered to tissue during reperfusion. During ischemia, the stage is set for ROS generation. ATP is metabolized to hypoxanthine. Intracellular Ca$^{2+}$ increases and activates a Ca$^{2+}$-calmodulin–dependent protease that converts xanthine dehydrogenase (the normal form of this enzyme) to xanthine oxidase[400, 401] (see Fig. 28–7). The xanthine oxidase–catalyzed conversion of hypoxanthine to xanthine during reperfusion is believed to be the major source of superoxide after ischemia.[400, 401] Superoxide dismutase then converts superoxide to hydrogen peroxide, which can then be converted to the highly reactive OH$^-$ by the iron-requiring Fenton reaction[400, 401] (see Fig. 28–7).

Two lines of evidence have suggested a role for ROS in ischemic renal injury. First, cellular markers suggesting ROS generation and lipid peroxidation have been detected during ischemia reperfusion injury. These include the production of malondialdehyde[402, 403] and ethane,[404] increased ratios of oxidized to reduced glutathione,[405] and consumption of dimethylthiourea.[406] Second, Paller and colleagues[403, 407] as well as other investigators[406, 408–412] have reported in a series of studies that inhibitors of ROS production as well as ROS scavengers ameliorate renal ischemic injury.[369] Allopurinol, which acts as both an inhibitor of xanthine oxidase and a scavenger of OH$^-$, and deferoxamine, which inhibits the Fenton reaction by binding free iron, have both been shown to reduce the severity of ischemia-induced renal dysfunction.[406, 408] Administration of superoxide dismutase and other ROS scavengers[403, 407, 409–418] and interventions that increase the levels of glutathione in the kidney have all been shown to ameliorate ischemic injury in some studies.[415]

It should be noted, however, that a number of studies of experimental models of renal ischemia have not demonstrated protection by agents that scavenge or prevent the production of ROS.[419–423] Also, in two studies in humans receiving cadaveric renal transplants, administration of allopurinol[424] and superoxide dismutase[425] to the perfusate during kidney preservation also conferred no benefit. Furthermore, the significance of lipid peroxidation detected in ischemic kidneys has been questioned by other studies showing that malondialdehyde content was not increased after ischemia and reflow when contamination of tissue samples by hemoglobin was avoided before malondialdehyde assay.[419, 421] Other observations also raise concerns regarding the role of oxidant injury after ischemia. Proximal tubule cells, as compared with other cell types, are resistant to oxidants, presumably because of high endogenous levels of glutathione.[420] Species differences and the rate at which xanthine dehydrogenase is converted to xanthine oxidase also determine whether oxidants play a role in the pathophysiology of renal ischemia. There are large differences in xanthine oxidase content of rabbit, rat, and human tissue, with the rabbit and human samples having low levels.[348, 426] The conversion of xanthine dehydrogenase to xanthine oxidase may also not occur within the time period available for xanthine oxidase to play a role in ROS generation during early reperfusion.[427] Thus, although the role of oxidant injury in myocardial and intestinal injury seems well established, the importance of this mechanism in ischemic injury to the kidney remains controversial. The extent to which generation of ROS contributes to ischemic injury may depend on many variables, such as the species studied, the period of ischemia, and the redox state of the kidney at the time of reflow.

### OXIDANT INJURY INDUCED BY NEUTROPHILS

There is compelling evidence that neutrophils play a central role in ischemia-reperfusion injury in many organ systems, including the heart, splanchnic circulation, and muscle. In contrast, the contribution of neutrophils to the pathogenesis of renal ischemic injury remains controversial. Neutrophils have been shown to contribute to renal injury in some studies[428–430] but not in others.[430, 431] The identification of leukocyte adhesion molecules as potential targets for therapeutic intervention in this setting has renewed interest in the role of neutrophils in ATN (see Chapter 4). Leukocyte adhesion to endothelium is initiated by interaction of leukocyte or endothelial selection adhesion molecules with their carbohydrate-containing ligands and facilitates subsequent interactions of leukocyte $\beta_2$-integrins with immunoglobulin-like endothelial cell adhesion molecules such as intercellular adhesion molecule type 1 (ICAM-1).[432] In one study, monoclonal antibodies against $\beta_2$-integrins and ICAM-1 did not confer protection against renal ischemia-reperfusion injury in rabbits[433] despite inhibiting leukocyte trafficking in other vascular beds.[432] In contrast, in one other report, monoclonal antibody active against ICAM-1 dramatically attenuated neutrophil recruitment and functional renal impairment in rats subjected to renal ischemia.[434] It remains to be determined which model most closely reflects the role of neutrophils and adhesion molecules in the pathogenesis of ATN in humans.

It is important to appreciate that oxidant injury is not the only mechanism that may account for "reperfusion injury," the well-described phenomenon that cellular injury is often aggravated by reflow after a period of ischemia. Other potential factors that may contribute are listed in Table 28–9.

## Cytoskeletal Injury: A Potentially Pivotal Event in Ischemic Acute Tubule Necrosis

The actin cytoskeleton plays an important role in a number of aspects of epithelial cell function, including the maintenance of cellular polarity, the barrier function of the junctional complex, the structure of the microvilli that constitute the proximal tubule brush border, and adhesion of epithelial cells to the tubule basement membrane matrix proteins[435] (Fig. 28–8). The alterations in the structure of the actin cytoskeleton that precede lethal cell injury after ischemia may contribute to cell dysfunction by causing loss of cell polarity, by leading to loss of the proximal tubule brush border, by impairing the function of the junctional complex, and by disrupting normal cell-cell and cell-substrate adhesion[435] (see Fig. 28–8).

### INFLUENCE OF ATP DEPLETION ON THE ACTIN CYTOSKELETON

The actin cytoskeleton is composed of bundles of microfilaments formed by the assembly of monomers of globular actin (G-actin) monomers into polymers of filamentous actin (F-actin).[435] ATP is required for regulation and maintenance of the cell cytoskeleton,[435–438] and depletion of cell ATP results in profound alterations in actin ultrastructure. Studies of cells in culture using immunofluorescence microscopy indicate that ATP depletion induces progressive disassembly of actin bundles and microfilaments.[439–441] Transmission electron microscopy of the actin cytoskeleton in ATP-depleted cells reveals destruction of stress fibers and the simultaneous appearance of shorter and wider "cigar-shaped" fragments of F-actin bundles in the predominantly perinuclear distribution within the cytosol.[442] These changes are not due to complete depolymerization of F-actin to G-actin monomers but rather to severing of the F-actin bundles into shorter fragments. In fact, quantitative assay of G-actin has shown that the G-actin pool falls with ATP depletion, suggesting that net polymerization of actin occurs during this period.[438] Under normal circumstances, distribution between pools of G- and F-actin is tightly regulated by other actin-associated proteins, intracellular divalent cation concentration, and the composition of cell phospholipids.[435, 438] The precise mechanisms responsible for this rapid conversion of G- to F-actin during ATP depletion and its pathologic significance remain unexplained.

The effect of ischemia on the actin cytoskeleton has also been studied in the intact kidney in vivo.[319, 443] Immunofluorescence of normal proximal tubule cells reveals that the majority of actin staining is associated with the apical pole, where actin forms a circumferential terminal web with extension of individual microfilaments into the microvilli.[319, 443] Ischemia results in disruption of the actin cytoskeleton with loss of actin staining in the area of the microvilli and redistribution of stainable actin from the apical domain and

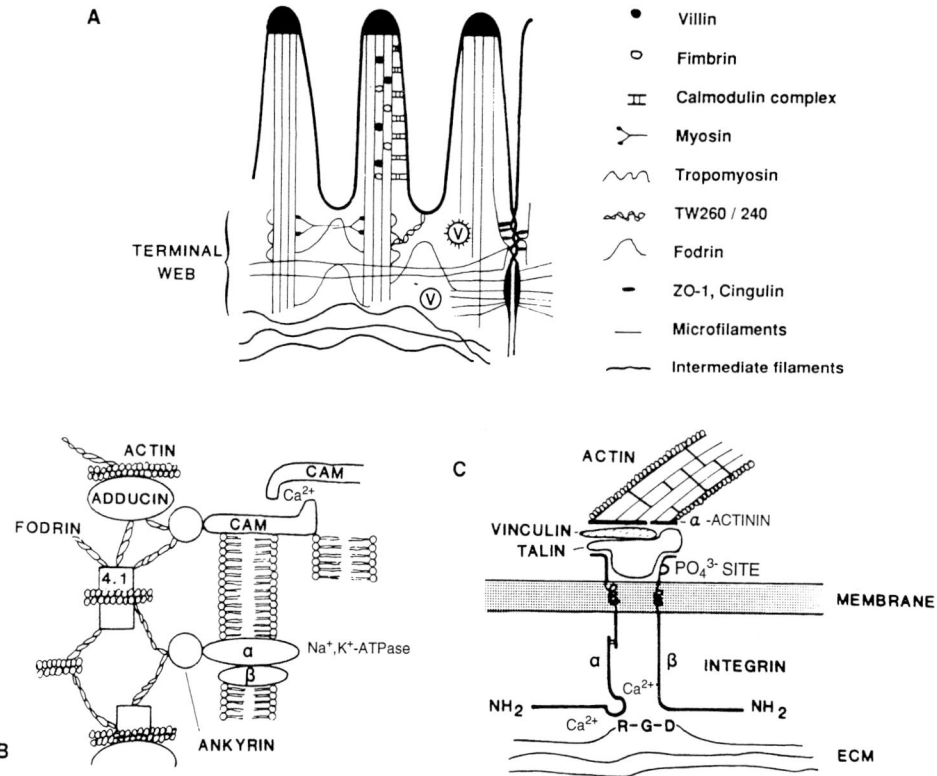

**Figure 28–8.** Functions of the actin cytoskeleton and associated cell adhesion molecules. *A.* Actin microfilaments extend from the terminal web into individual microvilli, which interact with the suface membrane via a calmodulin-protein complex. These actin filaments provide structural stability to the proximal tubule brush border. Microfilaments of actin also interact with the tight junction and zonula adherens and regulate the function of the junctional complex. *B.* The actin cytoskeleton maintains polarity by anchoring the Na⁺,K⁺-ATPase and other basolaterally located proteins to the cell membrane via interactions with ankyrin. Uvomorulin (cell adhesion molecule or CAM) mediates cell-cell adhesion via homophilic interactions between the uvomorulin molecules. Ankyrin attaches to the cytoplasmic domain of uvomorulin. *C.* The actin cytoskeleton (via interaction with the actin-binding proteins vinculin, talin, and α-actinin) attaches to and anchors the intracellular domain of the integrin that mediates cell-substrate adhesion to the basolateral membrane. (Adapted from Molitoris BA: Cellular basis of ischemic acute renal failure. *In* Lazarus JM, Brenner BM [eds]: Acute Renal Failure, 3rd ed. Churchill Livingstone, New York, 1993, p 1.)

microvilli into the cytoplasmic domain. After reflow, F-actin moves back from the cytoplasm to the apical membrane.[319, 443] These changes may underlie the ultrastructural alterations in proximal tubule brush border after ischemic injury[307, 317] (refer to the earlier section on morphology for further details).

Alterations in the actin cytoskeletal changes are markers of reversible sublethal cell injury. If cell ATP levels are restored before cell death supervenes, the normal actin cytoskeletal architecture recovers within 30 minutes and the cell survives.[441] Thus, the disruption of the actin is clearly a preterminal event and not merely a manifestation of cell death, and it probably accounts for many of the functional abnormalities of sublethally injured renal epithelial cells.[309–311, 435, 441, 444]

## CYTOSKELETAL INJURY AND LOSS OF CELL POLARITY

In an elegant series of studies, Molitoris[435] and collaborators[445–450] made the seminal observation that ATP depletion in renal epithelial cells causes loss of epithelial cell polarity, a process that is reversible when cells recover from ATP depletion. These investigators showed that the Na⁺,K⁺-ATPase, which is normally restricted to the basolateral surface, is rapidly redistributed to the apical membrane during chemical anoxia.[445, 446] These biochemical studies were subsequently confirmed by histochemical and immunocytochemical techniques.[446, 447] Apical redistribution occurred in all segments of the proximal tubule but not in cells of the distal nephron.[447] The apically expressed Na⁺,K⁺-ATPase has been shown to remain functional.[448] During ATP depletion, redistribution of Na⁺,K⁺-ATPase occurs in parallel with substantial redistribution of lipids from the basolateral to the apical membrane, specifically a marked increase in apical sphingomyelin, cholesterol, phosphatidylcholine, and phosphatidylinositol content.[445–447] These changes are consistent with increased lateral mobility of phospholipids within the lipid bilayer of the cell membrane and are probably due to disruption of the actin cytoskeleton and consequent loss of the fence function of the junctional complex.[445, 446] The polar distribution within the lipid bilayer of proteins such as Na⁺,K⁺-ATPase and other basolateral proteins such as the β₁-integrins also depends on anchoring to an intact cell cytoskeleton (see Fig. 28–8). Thus, although causality remains to be proved, disruption of the actin cytoskeleton probably contributes to the loss of cell polarity after ATP depletion.[435]

Several lines of evidence suggest that this loss of cell membrane polarity could account for many of the abnormalities in proximal tubule epithelial cell function associated with ischemic ATN.[435] The loss of polarity of the $Na^+,K^+$-ATPase would be expected to result in impairment of unidirectional transport of solutes from tubule fluid to

blood[435] (Fig. 28–9). Normalization of both $Na^+$ and $Li^+$ reabsorption after renal ischemia has been shown to depend on the re-establishment of surface membrane polarity in proximal tubule cells.[450] These data are consistent with the hypothesis that normal reabsorption of $Na^+$, water, and other solutes by the proximal tubule depends on the establishment and maintenance of cell polarity and that this polarity is lost after ischemic injury.[435]

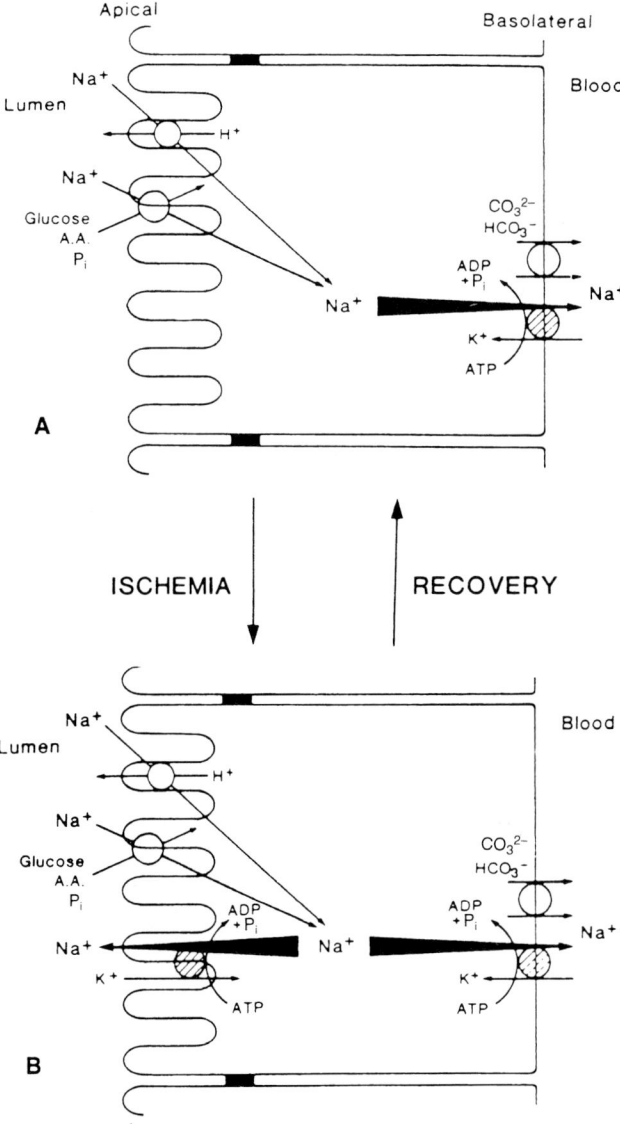

**Figure 28–9.** Effects of ischemia on $Na^+,K^+$-ATPase polarity and $Na^+$ transport. *A.* In a normally polarized epithelium, $Na^+$ enters the apical membrane down an electrochemical gradient and is pumped out of the basal aspect of the cell by the energy-requiring $Na^+,K^+$-ATPase, which is localized to the basolateral membrane. *B.* Ischemia results in loss of polarity of $Na^+,K^+$-ATPase, which becomes expressed on both apical and basolateral domains of the cell. The apically expressed $Na^+,K^+$-ATPase maintains its functional activity and is therefore able to compete with the basolaterally located pump for intracellular $Na^+$. This sequence of events impairs unidirectional $Na^+$ and water transport. The continued activity of the apical $Na^+,K^+$-ATPase utilizes ATP and promotes ATP depletion. (Adapted from Molitoris BA: Cellular basis of ischemic acute renal failure. *In* Lazarus JM, Brenner BM [eds]: Acute Renal Failure, 3rd ed. Churchill Livingstone, New York, 1993, p 1.)

## LOSS OF STRUCTURAL INTEGRITY OF BRUSH BORDER

Disruption of the proximal tubular brush border is a consistent and striking ultrastructural event in experimental models of ischemic injury[307, 317] and in humans with ATN.[302, 303] Because the structural integrity of microvilli depends on the actin core bundle (see Fig. 28–8) and ATP depletion causes rapid loss of actin within this bundle,[319, 443] it has been postulated that the disruption of the actin cytoskeleton is a central event in the evolution of these morphologic alterations.[435] Thus, alterations in the cytoskeleton associated with sublethal injury may theoretically contribute to renal dysfunction by causing tubule obstruction by impaction of fragments of proximal tubule brush border in the lumens of more distal segments (Fig. 28–10).

## IMPAIRED FUNCTION OF THE TIGHT JUNCTION

The actin cytoskeleton plays an important role in maintaining the gate and fence function of the junction complex and thus limiting paracellular reabsorption of glomerular filtrate. Using in vivo microperfusion of early loops of proximal tubules, Molitoris and colleagues[445] showed that ischemia is associated with a time-dependent increase in the permeability of tight junctions. In studies of cells in culture, ATP depletion induced by chemical anoxia has also been shown to impair the gate function of tight junctions, resulting in abnormal paracellular flux of molecules such as mannitol across renal epithelium between cells.[435, 437, 441, 445] These changes are reversible if cell ATP levels are allowed to rise before lethal cell injury supervenes.[441, 445] Loss of the gate function of proximal tubule tight junctions[435, 437, 441, 445] may explain, at least in part, the back-leakage of glomerular filtrate and decline in GFR that occur in ischemic ATN despite the subtle histologic abnormalities seen in this disease.[304–306]

## LOSS OF CELL-CELL AND CELL-SUBSTRATE ADHESION

Sublethal injury to renal cells in culture leads to loss of the normal adherence of cells to their substrate.[309–311, 441] The molecular events responsible for this loss of cell adherence are still being elucidated but may include loss of polarity of the $\beta_1$-integrins, transmembrane proteins that normally mediate cell-substrate adhesion[435] (see Fig. 28–8). The extracellular domain of these proteins attaches to lig-

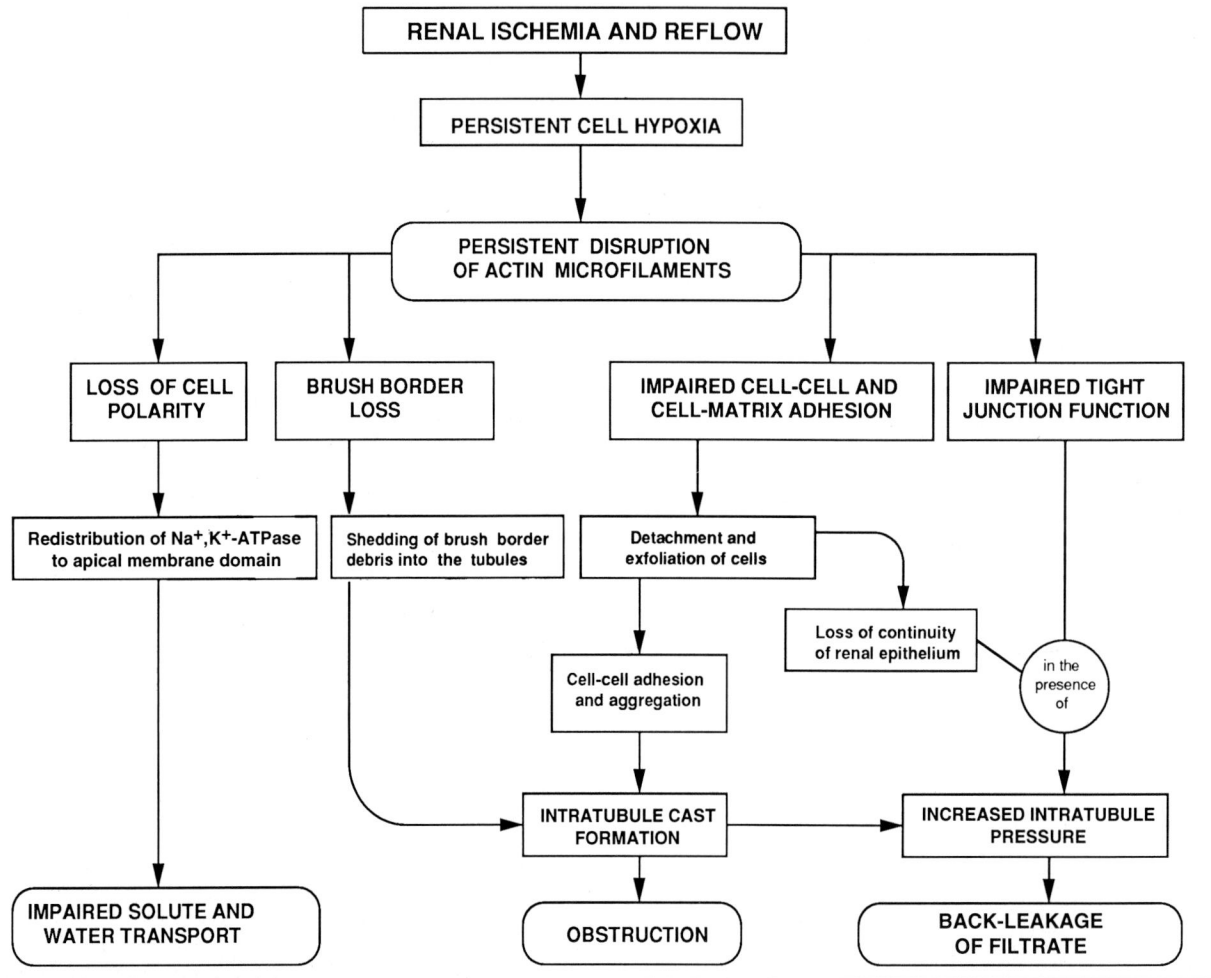

**Figure 28–10.** Potential mechanisms leading to tubule dysfunction and reduced GFR after sublethal cell injury: a hypothetic schema demonstrating the potential functional consequences of sublethal injury. Disruption of the actin cytoskeleton is an early event after ischemia and ATP depletion. The major consequences of cytoskeletal disruption are loss of cell polarity, brush border injury, loss of cell adhesion, and impaired formation of the intercellular junctional complex. The potential pathways leading from these abnormalities to the alterations in transport, back-leakage of glomerular filtrate, and tubule obstruction are outlined.

ands on matrix proteins, and the intracellular domain is tethered to the actin cytoskeleton via a complex of protein molecules referred to collectively as the focal adhesion plaque.[309, 435] Injury to epithelial cells in culture results in loss of focal contacts[309, 310] and redistribution of the $\alpha_3$-subunit[310] and $\beta_1$-subunit[451] of the $\alpha_3\beta_1$-integrin heterodimer from its physiologic location in the basal membrane to the apical membrane and eventual detachment of viable cells from their matrix. Disrupted cell-substrate attachment in sublethal injury in vitro may be extremely relevant to the pathophysiology of human ATN, in which detachment of renal epithelial cells from basement membrane has been documented repeatedly by renal biopsy[302, 305, 306] (see Fig. 28–3). Additional evidence of the pathogenetic significance of loss of cell adhesion in the pathophysiology of ATN has been provided by studies showing that viable renal tubule cells are excreted in urine in increased amounts in experimental models of ischemic injury and in patients with ATN.[452–454] Detachment of viable cells from the epithelium would provide another mechanism for back-leakage of glomerular filtrate, in addition to loss of junctional complex function and frank cell necrosis (see Fig. 28–10).

## ABNORMAL ADHESION BETWEEN SUBLETHALLY INJURED RENAL TUBULE CELLS LEADING TO CELLULAR CAST FORMATION AND OBSTRUCTION

Goligorsky and colleagues[309] have postulated that adhesion of detached renal epithelial cells to sublethally injured cells that remain attached to the basement membrane as well as the aggregation of detached cells within the lumen of renal epithelial cells may contribute to intraluminal cast formation and obstruction in ATN (Fig. 28–11). This hypothesis is supported by evidence that sublethal injury to renal epithelial cells in culture increases their adhesiveness for epithelial cells added in suspension.[309, 451] Although there are many potential explanations for these interactions,[309] there is compelling evidence that abnormal cell-cell adhesion may be mediated, at least in part, by binding of $\beta_1$-integrins expressed apically on injured cells to their receptors on fragments of matrix proteins present on exfoliated renal cells.[310, 451] An intriguing study by Goligorsky and DiBona[311] suggested that these integrin-receptor interactions may contribute to the pathogenesis of cast formation and tubule obstruction after ischemic injury in vivo. They have demonstrated that short peptides bearing the Arg-Gly-Asp (RGD) amino acid motif of integrin receptors (see Fig. 28–8) inhibit cast formation and functional renal impairment in experimental ATN, probably by competing with other epithelial cells for binding to $\beta_1$-integrins[311] (see Fig. 28–11).

In summary, morphologic studies of ATN in humans as well as experimental studies with in vivo and in vitro models of ischemia support the hypothesis that sublethal cell injury and disruption of the actin cytoskeleton may play an important role in the tubule leakiness and obstruction that lead to the profound impairment of GFR characteristic of ATN (see Figs. 28–3, 28–10, and 28–11).

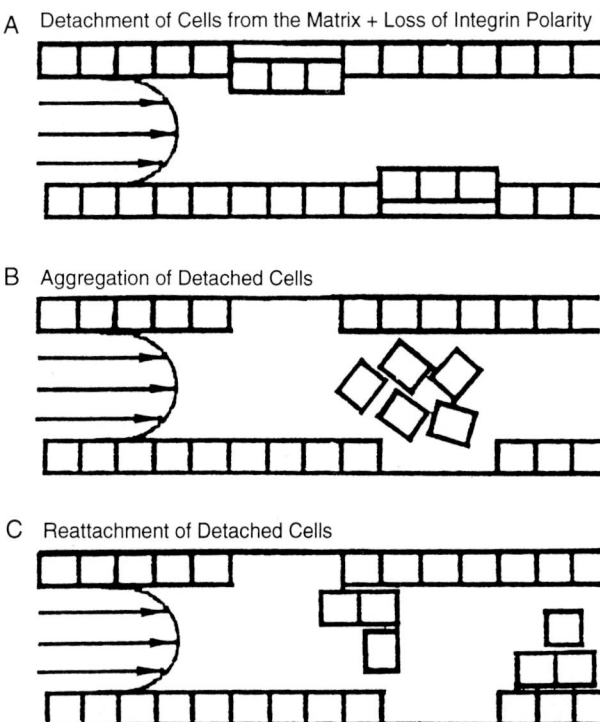

**A** Detachment of Cells from the Matrix + Loss of Integrin Polarity

**B** Aggregation of Detached Cells

**C** Reattachment of Detached Cells

**Figure 28–11.** Potential role of loss of renal cell detachment and abnormal cell-cell aggregation in the pathogenesis of cast formation. A hypothetic schema of events leading to back-leakage of filtrate and tubule obstruction. *A.* Cell-matrix adhesion and cell-cell adhesion are disrupted with resultant detachment of cells from the underlying matrix proteins. *B.* Tubule cells exfoliate into tubule lumen, leaving behind areas of denuded basement mambrane. *C.* Abnormal adhesion of exfoliated cells to sublethally injured but still adherent cells and aggregation of cells within the tubule lumen lead to intratubule obstruction. The abnormal cell-cell adhesion and aggregation may be mediated, in part, by interactions between the $\beta_1$-integrin and its matrix protein ligands, particularly the Arg-Gly-Asp (RGD) receptor. (Adapted from Goligorsky MS, Lieberthal W, Racusen LC, Simon EE: Integrin receptors in renal tubular epithelium: New insights into pathophysiology of acute renal failure. Am J Physiol 264:F1–F8, 1993. Editorial.)

## Recovery, Regeneration, and Repair After Ischemic Injury

A striking characteristic of ischemic and toxic ATN is that patients usually regain sufficient renal function for normal life (see later section on outcome). This process depends on recovery of sublethally injured cells, removal of necrotic cells and intratubular casts, and regeneration of renal cells to restore the normal continuity and function of the tubule epithelium. Replacement of cells lost by exfoliation and necrosis requires replication and regeneration of renal epithelial cells. The factors that induce normally quiescent renal tubule cells to enter the growth cycle and undergo mitosis are still being elucidated. Interestingly, the alterations in gene expression induced by ischemia are similar to those induced by growth fators in cells in culture.[455] Expression of the early immediate response genes such as *FOS* and *EGR1* increases almost immediately after renal ischemia and precedes increased protein or DNA synthesis.[456–458] These genes probably regulate the transcription of

**TABLE 28–10. Clinical Approach to the Diagnosis of Acute Renal Failure**

History, physical examination (including funduscopy and weight), detailed review of hospital chart, previous records, and drug history
Urinalysis including specific gravity, dipstick, sulfosalicylic acid, microscopy, and staining for eosinophils
Flowchart of serial blood pressures, weights, BUN, serum creatinine, major clinical events, interventions, and therapies
Routine blood chemistry assays (BUN, creatinine, $Na^+$, $K^+$, $Ca^{2+}$, $HCO_3^-$, $Cl^-$, $PO_4^{3-}$) and hematologic tests (complete blood count and differential white blood cell count)
Selected special investigations:
  Urine chemistry, eosinophils, and/or immunoelectrophoresis
  Serologic tests: anti–glomerular basement membrane antibodies, antineutrophil cytoplasmic antibodies, complement, antinuclear antibodies, cryoglobulins, serum protein electrophoresis, anti–streptolysin O or anti-DNase titers
  Radiologic evaluation: plain abdominal film, renal ultrasonography, intravenous pyelography, renal angiography
Renal biopsy

the many other genes that ultimately mediate cell division.[455]

The molecules that mediate this growth response have not been defined, and the role of known proximal tubule cell mitogens such as epidermal growth factor, transforming growth factor-α, insulin-like growth factor, and hepatocyte growth factor remains uncertain.[455] However, it has been clearly demonstrated that the pharmacologic administration of epidermal growth factor,[459] transforming growth factor-α,[460] or insulin-like growth factor[461] accelerates cellular regeneration and hastens recovery of renal function in experimental models of ischemic and toxic renal injury. Defining the molecular mechanisms underlying recovery from ATN and testing the efficacy of growth factors in humans with ATN remain exciting and potentially rewarding goals for future research.

## COURSE OF ACUTE TUBULE NECROSIS

The clinical course of ATN can be divided into three phases: the initiation phase, the maintenance phase, and the recovery phase. The initiation phase is the period when patients are exposed to the ischemic or toxic insults and parenchymal renal injury is evolving but not yet established. ATN is potentially preventable during this period, which may last hours to days. The initiation phase is followed by a maintenance phase during which parenchymal injury is established and GFR stabilizes at a value of 5 to 10 mL/min. Urine output is usually lowest during this period.[3–8, 462–470] The maintenance phase typically lasts 1 to 2 weeks but may be prolonged for 1 to 11 months before recovery.[465–468] A reassessment of the likely causes of ARF is warranted if recovery has not begun after 4 to 6 weeks to exclude other possible etiologic diseases. In general, severe oliguria and a prolonged maintenance phase are associated with a slower recovery and a greater chance of permanent renal impairment.[4–8, 462–470] Uremic complications

usually arise during the maintenance phase. The recovery phase is the period during which patients recover renal function through repair and regeneration of renal tissue. Its onset is typically heralded by a gradual increase in urine output and fall in serum creatinine, although the latter may lag behind the onset of diuresis by several days. This "post-ATN" diuresis may reflect appropriate excretion of salt and water accumulated during the maintenance phase, osmotic diuresis induced by filtered urea and other retained solutes, and/or the actions of diuretics administered to hasten salt and water excretion. Occasionally, diuresis may be inappropriate and excessive if recovery of tubule reabsorptive processes lags behind glomerular filtration, although this phenomenon is more common after relief of urinary tract obstruction.[4–8, 462–471]

## DIFFERENTIATION OF ACUTE TUBULE NECROSIS FROM OTHER CAUSES OF ACUTE RENAL FAILURE

### Clinical Features, Urinary Findings, and Confirmatory Tests

The assessment of patients with ARF requires a meticulous history, physical examination and urinalysis, in-depth review of previous records and recent drug history, discriminating utilization of laboratory tests, renal imaging, and occasionally renal biopsy (Table 28–10). A graph of remote and recent serum creatinine levels versus time, incorporating drug therapy and interventions, is invaluable for differentiation of acute and chronic renal failure and the identification of the cause of ARF. An acute process is easily established if review of laboratory records reveals a recent rise in BUN and serum creatinine levels. Spurious causes of increased BUN or serum creatinine values should be excluded (see Fig. 28–1). When previous measurements are not available, anemia, hyperphosphatemia, hypocalcemia, neuropathy, band keratopathy, and radiologic evidence of renal osteodystrophy or small scarred kidneys are useful pointers to a chronic process. However, it should be noted that anemia, hyperphosphatemia, and hypocalcemia may also complicate ARF and that renal size can be normal or increased in a variety of chronic renal diseases (e.g., diabetic nephropathy, amyloid, polycystic kidney disease). Once a diagnosis of ARF is established, attention should focus on the differentiation between prerenal, intrinsic renal, and postrenal azotemia, and the identification of the specific causative disease. Table 28–11 summarizes some clinical features, urinary findings, and confirmatory tests that are useful for diagnosis of the most common causes of ARF.

#### CLINICAL ASSESSMENT

Prerenal azotemia should be suspected when the serum creatinine value rises after hemorrhage; excessive gastrointestinal, urinary, or insensible fluid losses; or extensive burns, particularly if access to fluids is restricted (e.g., comatose, sedated, or obtunded patients). Supportive findings

**TABLE 28–11. Useful Clinical Features, Urinary Findings, and Confirmatory Tests in the Differential Diagnosis of Major Causes of Acute Azotemia**

| Cause of Acute Renal Failure | Some Suggestive Clinical Features | Typical Urinalysis* | Some Confirmatory Tests |
|---|---|---|---|
| Prerenal azotemia | Evidence of true volume depletion (thirst, postural or absolute hypotension and tachycardia, low jugular vein pressure, dry mucous membranes and axillae, weight loss, fluid output > input) or decreased effective circulatory volume (e.g., heart failure, liver failure), treatment with NSAIDs or ACE inhibitor | Hyaline casts $FE_{Na} < 1\%$ $U_{Na} < 10$ mEq/L $SG > 1.018$ | Occasionally requires invasive hemodynamic monitoring; rapid resolution of ARF on restoration of renal perfusion |
| Intrinsic renal azotemia | | | |
| Diseases involving large renal vessels | | | |
| Renal artery thrombosis | History of atrial fibrillation or recent myocardial infarct, nausea, vomiting, flank or abdominal pain | Mild proteinuria Occasionally red blood cells | Elevated lactate dehydrogenase with normal transaminases, renal arteriogram |
| Atheroembolism | Usually > 50 y, recent manipulation of aorta, retinal plaques, subcutaneous nodules, palpable purpura, livedo reticularis, vasculopathy, hypertension | Often normal, eosinophiluria, rarely casts | Eosinophilia, hypocomplementemia, skin biopsy, renal biopsy |
| Renal vein thrombosis | Evidence of nephrotic syndrome or pulmonary embolism, flank pain | Proteinuria, hematuria | Inferior venacavogram and selective renal venogram; Doppler flow studies; MRI |
| Diseases of small vessels and glomeruli | | | |
| Glomerulonephritis or vasculitis | Compatible clinical history (e.g., recent infection) sinusitis, lung hemorrhage, rash or skin ulcers, arthralgias, hypertension, edema | Red blood cell or granular casts, red blood cells, white blood cells, mild proteinuria | Low C3, antineutrophil cytoplasmic antibodies, anti–glomerular basement membrane antibodies, antinuclear antibodies, anti–streptolysin O, anti-DNase, cryoglobulins, renal biopsy |
| HUS or TTP | Compatible clinical history (e.g., recent gastrointestinal infection, cyclosporine, anovulants), fever, pallor, ecchymoses, neurologic abnormalities | May be normal, red blood cells, mild proteinuria, rarely red blood cell or granular casts | Anemia, thrombocytopenia, schistocytes on blood smear, increased lactate dehydrogenase, renal biopsy |
| Malignant hypertension | Severe hypertension with headaches, cardiac failure, retinopathy, neurologic dysfunction, papilledema | Red blood cells, red blood cell casts, proteinuria | LVH by echocardiography or electrocardiography, resolution of ARF with control of blood pressure |
| ARF mediated by ischemia or toxins (ATN) | | | |
| Ischemia | Recent hemorrhage, hypotension (e.g., cardiac arrest), surgery | Muddy brown granular or tubule epithelial cell casts, $FE_{Na} > 1\%$, $U_{Na} > 20$ mEq/L, $SG = 1.010$ | Clinical assessment and urinalysis usually sufficient for diagnosis |

*Table continued on following page*

on clinical assessment include symptoms of thirst or orthostatic dizziness and objective evidence of orthostatic hypotension (fall in diastolic pressure greater than 10 mm Hg) and tachycardia (increase of more than 10 beats/min), reduced jugular venous pressure, decreased skin turgor, dry mucous membranes, and reduced axillary sweating. However, florid symptoms or signs of hypovolemia are usually not manifest until extracellular fluid volume has fallen by 10% to 20%. Nursing and pharmacy records should be reviewed for evidence of a progressive fall in urine output and body weight and recent use of cyclooxygenase or ACE inhibitors. Careful clinical examination may reveal stigmata of chronic liver disease and portal hypertension (e.g., palmar erythema, jaundice, telangiectasia, caput medusae, splenomegaly, ascites), advanced cardiac failure (e.g., peripheral edema, hepatic congestion, ascites, elevated jugular venous pressure, bibasilar lung crackles, pleural effusion,

cardiomegaly, gallop rhythm, cold extremities), or other causes of effective hypovolemia. Although clinical assessment provides a satisfactory index of cardiac output and tissue perfusion in most patients, invasive hemodynamic monitoring (central venous and/or Swan-Ganz catheterization) is often necessary in complicated cases.[472] Definitive diagnosis of prerenal azotemia hinges on prompt resolution of ARF after restoration of renal perfusion.

There is a high likelihood of ischemic ATN if ARF follows a period of prolonged or severe renal hypoperfusion and if ARF persists despite restoration of renal perfusion. It should be noted, however, that significant hypotension is recorded in less than 50% of patients with postsurgical ATN. Diagnosis of nephrotoxic ARF requires scouring of clinical, pharmacy, nursing, and radiology records for evidence of recent administration of nephrotoxic medications or radiocontrast agents. ARF after cancer chemotherapy

**TABLE 28–11.** Useful Clinical Features, Urinary Findings, and Confirmatory Tests in the Differential Diagnosis of Major Causes of Acute Azotemia *Continued*

| Cause of Acute Renal Failure | Some Suggestive Clinical Features | Typical Urinalysis* | Some Confirmatory Tests |
|---|---|---|---|
| Exogenous toxins | Recent radiocontrast study, nephrotoxic antibiotics or anticancer agents often coexistent with volume depletion, sepsis, or chronic renal insufficiency | Muddy brown granular or tubule epithelial cell casts, $FE_{Na} >$ 1%, $U_{Na} > 20$ mEq/L, SG = 1.010 | Clinical assessment and urinalysis usually sufficient for diagnosis |
| Endogenous toxins | History suggestive of rhabdomyolysis (seizures, coma, ethanol abuse, trauma) | Urine supernatant tests positive for heme | Hyperkalemia, hyperphosphatemia, hypocalcemia, increased circulating myoglobin, creatine kinase MM, uric acid |
| | History suggestive of hemolysis (blood transfusion) | Urine supernatant pink and positive for heme | Hyperkalemia, hyperphosphatemia, hypocalcemia, hyperuricemia, pink plasma positive for hemoglobin |
| | History suggestive of tumor lysis (recent chemotherapy), myeloma (bone pain), or ethylene glycol ingestion | Urate crystals, dipstick-negative proteinuria, oxalate crystals, respectively | Hyperuricemia, hyperkalemia, hyperphosphatemia (for tumor lysis); circulating or urinary monoclonal spike (for myeloma); toxicology screen, acidosis, osmolal gap (for ethylene glycol) |
| Acute diseases of the tubulointerstitium | | | |
| Allergic interstitial nephritis | Recent ingestion of drug and fever, rash, or arthralgias | White blood cell casts, white blood cells (frequently eosinphiluria), red blood cells, rarely red blood cell casts, proteinuria (occasionally nephrotic) | Systemic eosinophilia, skin biopsy of rash area (leukocytoclastic vasculitis), renal biopsy |
| Acute bilateral pyelonephritis | Flank pain and tenderness, toxic state, febrile | Leukocytes, proteinuria, red blood cells, bacteria | Urine and blood cultures |
| Postrenal azotemia | Abdominal or flank pain, palpable bladder | Frequently normal, hematuria if stones, hemorrhage, malignancy or prostatic hypertrophy | Plain film, renal ultrasonography, intravenous pyelography, retrograde or anterograde pyelography, computed tomography |

*$U_{Na}$ = urine $Na^+$ concentration; SG = specific gravity.

suggests a diagnosis of tumor lysis syndrome and acute urate nephropathy, although other diagnoses must be considered (see later section on differential diagnosis in specific settings). Pigment-induced ATN may be suspected if the clinical assessment reveals clues to rhabdomyolysis (e.g., seizures, excessive exercise, alcohol or drug abuse, muscle tenderness, limb ischemia) or hemolysis (e.g., recent transfusion).

Although most ARF is prerenal or due to ischemic and nephrotoxic ATN, patients should be assessed carefully for evidence of other renal parenchymal diseases, because many of the latter are treatable and their diagnosis alters management and prognosis. Flank pain may be a prominent symptom of acute renal artery or vein occlusion, acute pyelonephritis, and occasionally necrotizing glomerulonephritis. Close examination of the skin may reveal the subcutaneous nodules, livido reticularis, digital ischemia, and/or palpable purpura of atheroembolism or vasculitis, the butterfly rash of systemic lupus erythematosus (SLE), impetigo in patients with postinfectious glomerulonephritis, a maculopapular rash suggestive of allergic interstitial nephri-

tis, the yellow hue of liver disease or phenazopyridine (Pyridium) toxicity,[473] telltale puncture marks of intravenous drug abuse, or the scarletiniform eruption of staphylococcal toxic shock syndrome.[474] The eyes should be assessed for the bright orange retinal arteriolar stigmata of atheroembolism; hypertensive or diabetic retinopathy; the keratitis, scleritis, uveitis, and iritis of autoimmune vasculitides; icterus; and the rare but nevertheless pathognomonic band keratopathy of hypercalcemia and flecked retina of hyperoxalemia. Examination of the ears, nose, and throat may reveal conductive deafness and mucosal inflammation or ulceration suggestive of Wegener granulomatosis (conductive deficit) or the nerve deafness caused by aminoglycoside toxicity (neural deficit). Respiratory difficulty or the stigmata of chronic liver disease should immediately suggest a pulmonary-renal or hepatorenal syndrome, respectively. Cardiovascular assessment may be notable for marked elevation in systemic blood pressure and suggest malignant hypertension or scleroderma, or it may reveal a new arrhythmia or murmur that is a potential source of thromboemboli or subacute bacterial endocarditis (acute glomerulonephritis), respectively. Chest or abdominal pain and reduced pulses in the lower limbs should suggest aortic dissection or rarely Takayasu arteritis, and widespread atheromatous disease increases the likelihood of atheroembolic disease. Pallor and recent bruising are important clues to the thrombotic microangiopathies, and the combination of bleeding and fever should raise the possibility of ARF in association with viral hemorrhagic fevers. A recent jejunoileal bypass may be a vital clue to a rare but reversible cause of ARF in obese patients.[475, 476]

Postrenal azotemia may be asymptomatic if obstruction develops relatively slowly. Alternatively, patients may present with suprapubic or flank pain if there is acute distention of the bladder or renal collecting system and capsule, respectively. Colicky flank pain radiating to the groin suggests acute ureteric obstruction. Prostatic disease should be suspected in patients with a history of nocturia, frequency, and hesitancy and an enlarged or indurated prostate gland on rectal examination. Similarly, a rectal and/or pelvic examination may reveal obstructing tumors in female patients. Neurogenic bladder is a likely diagnosis in patients receiving anticholinergic medications (e.g., tricyclic antidepressants) or with physical evidence of neurologic disease and autonomic insufficiency (e.g., paralysis, abnormal rectal sphincter tone, postvoid urine volume more than 200 to 300 mL). Bladder distention may be evident on abdominal percussion and palpation in patients with bladder neck or urethral obstruction. Definitive diagnosis of postrenal azotemia usually relies on judicious use of radiologic investigations and rapid improvement in renal function after relief of obstruction.

## URINALYSIS

Assessment of the urine is a mandatory and inexpensive tool in the evaluation of ARF. Urine volume is a relatively unhelpful parameter in differential diagnosis. Anuria suggests complete urinary tract obstruction but may be a complication of severe prerenal or intrinsic renal azotemia (e.g., renal artery occlusion, severe proliferative glomerulonephritis or vasculitis, bilateral cortical necrosis). Wide fluctuations in urine output suggest intermittent obstruction. Patients with partial urinary tract obstruction may present with polyuria caused by secondary impairment of urine concentrating mechanisms. In contrast, analysis of the sediment and supernatant of a centrifuged urine specimen is valuable for distinguishing between prerenal, intrinsic renal, and postrenal azotemia and elucidating the precise etiology of intrinsic renal azotemia (Table 28–12). Urine sediment should be inspected for the presence of cells, casts, and crystals. The sediment is typically acellular in prerenal azotemia and may contain transparent hyaline casts ("bland," "benign," "inactive" urine sediment). Hyaline casts are formed in concentrated urine from normal constituents of urine, principally Tamm-Horsfall protein secreted by epithelial cells of the loop of Henle. Postrenal azotemia may also present with a benign sediment, although hematuria and pyuria are common in patients with intraluminal obstruction (e.g., stones, sloughed papilla, blood clot) or prostatic disease. Pigmented "muddy brown" granular casts and tubule epithelial cell casts are characteristic of ischemic

### TABLE 28–12. Urine Sediment in the Differential Diagnosis of Acute Renal Failure

Normal or few red blood cells or white blood cells
    Prerenal azotemia
    Arterial thrombosis or embolism
    Preglomerular vasculitis
    HUS or TTP
    Scleroderma crisis
    Postrenal azotemia
Granular casts
    ATN (muddy brown)
    Glomerulonephritis or vasculitis
    Interstitial nephritis
Red blood cell casts
    Glomerulonephritis or vasculitis
    Malignant hypertension
    Rarely interstitial nephritis
White blood cell casts
    Acute interstitial nephritis or exudative glomerulonephritis
    Severe pyelonephritis
    Marked leukemic or lymphomatous infiltration
Eosinophiluria (>5%)
    Allergic interstitial nephritis (antibiotics > NSAIDs)
    Atheroembolic disease
Crystalluria
    Acute urate nephropathy
    Calcium oxalate (ethylene glycol toxicity)
    Acyclovir
    Sulfonamides
    Radiocontrast agents

or nephrotoxic ATN.[477] They are usually found in association with microscopic hematuria and mild "tubule" proteinuria (<1 g/d). Casts may be absent, however, in approximately 20% to 30% of patients with ischemic or nephrotoxic ATN and are not a requisite for diagnosis.[477] Indeed, there is generally a poor correlation between the severity of renal failure and the amount of debris in the urine sediment in these conditions (see section on pathology and pathophysiology of ischemic ATN). Red blood cell casts almost always indicate acute glomerular injury but may also be observed, albeit rarely, in acute interstitial nephritis. Dysmorphic red blood cells are a more common urinary finding in patients with glomerular injury but are a significantly less specific finding than red blood cell casts. Urine sediment abnormalities vary in diseases involving preglomerular blood vessels, such as hemolytic-uremic syndrome (HUS), thrombotic thrombocytopenic purpura (TTP), atheroembolic disease, and vasculitis involving medium-sized or large vessels, and range from benign to frankly nephritic. White blood cell casts and nonpigmented granular casts suggest interstitial nephritis, and broad granular casts are characteristic of chronic renal disease and probably reflect interstitial fibrosis and dilatation of tubules. Plasma cells are occasionally found in multiple myeloma.[478] Eosinophiluria (between 1% and 50% of urine leukocytes) is a common finding (~90%) in drug-induced allergic interstitial nephritis when studies are done with Hansel stain.[479, 480] The traditional Wright stain is significantly less sensitive (~20%) in this regard. However, eosinophiluria is only 85% specific for allergic interstitial nephritis, and eosinophiluria of 1% to 5% can occur in a variety of other diseases including atheroembolization, ischemic and nephrotoxic ARF, proliferative glomerulonephritis, pyelonephritis, cystitis, and prostatitis.[479, 480] Uric acid crystals (pleomorphic) may be seen in urine in prerenal azotemia but should raise the possibility of acute urate nephropathy if seen in abundance. Oxalate (envelope shaped) and hippurate (needle shaped) crystals suggest a diagnosis of ethylene glycol toxicity.

Increased urinary protein excretion, characteristically less than 1 g/d, is a common finding in ischemic or nephrotoxic ARF and reflects both failure of injured proximal tubule cells to reabsorb normally filtered protein and excretion of cellular debris (tubule proteinuria). Proteinuria greater than 1 g/d suggests injury to the glomerular ultrafiltration barrier (glomerular proteinuria) or excretion of myeloma light chains. The latter are not detected by conventional dipsticks (which detect albumin) and must be sought by other means (e.g., sulfosalicylic acid test, immunoelectrophoresis). Heavy proteinuria is also a frequent finding (~80%) in patients with allergic interstitial nephritis triggered by cyclooxygenase inhibitors. These patients have a glomerular lesion that is almost identical to minimal-change glomerulonephritis, in addition to acute interstitial inflammation. A similar syndrome has been reported in patients receiving other agents such as ampicillin, rifampin, or interferon alfa. Hemoglobinuria or myoglobinuria should be suspected if urine is strongly positive for hemoglobin by dipstick but contains few red blood cells and if the supernatant of centrifuged urine is pink and also positive for free hemoglobin. Hemolysis and rhabdomyolysis can usually be differentiated by inspection of plasma. The latter is usually pink in hemolysis, but not in rhabdomyolysis, as free hemoglobin (65,000 daltons) is a larger molecule than myoglobin (17,000 daltons) that is heavily protein bound and filtered slowly by the kidney. Bilirubinuria may provide a clue to the presence of hepatorenal syndrome.

## CONFIRMATORY TESTS

The pattern of change in serum creatinine value often provides clues to the cause of ARF. Prerenal azotemia is typified by rapid fluctuations in creatinine that parallel changes in hemodynamic function and renal perfusion. The serum creatinine level begins to rise within 24 to 48 hours in patients with ARF after renal ischemia, atheroembolization, and radiocontrast exposure, three major diagnostic possibilities in patients undergoing emergency cardiac or aortic angiography and surgery. Creatinine levels, as already discussed, usually peak after 3 to 5 days in contrast nephropathy and return to the normal range within 5 to 7 days. In contrast, creatinine levels typically peak later (7 to 10 days) in ischemic ATN and atheroembolic disease. ARF usually resolves in the next 7 to 14 days in ischemic ATN but is frequently irreversible in atheroembolic disease. These rapid changes are in marked contrast to the delayed elevation in serum creatinine levels (7 to 10 days) that is characteristic of many tubule epithelial cell toxins (e.g., aminoglycosides, cisplatin).

Additional diagnostic clues can be gleaned from routine biochemical and hematologic tests. Hyperkalemia, hyperphosphatemia, hypocalcemia, and elevated serum uric acid and creatine kinase ($CK_3$ [MM] isoenzyme) levels suggest a diagnosis of rhabdomyolysis. A similar biochemical profile in association with ARF after cancer chemotherapy, but with higher levels of uric acid and normal or marginally elevated creatine kinase, is typical of acute urate nephropathy and tumor lysis syndrome. Severe hypercalcemia of any cause can induce ARF. Widening of the serum anion $[Na^+ - (HCO_3^- + Cl^-)]$ and osmolal (measured serum osmolality minus calculated osmolality) gaps is a clue to diagnosis of ethylene glycol toxicity and should prompt a search for urine oxalate crystals. Severe anemia in the absence of hemorrhage may reflect the presence of hemolysis, multiple myeloma, or thrombotic microangiopathy (e.g., HUS, TTP, toxemia, disseminated intravascular coagulation, accelerated hypertension, SLE, scleroderma, radiation injury). Other laboratory findings suggestive of thrombotic microangiopathy include thrombocytopenia, dysmorphic red blood cells on a peripheral blood smear, and elevated circulating levels of lactate dehydrogenase. Systemic eosinophilia suggests allergic interstitial nephritis but may also be a prominent feature in other diseases such as atheroembolic disease and polyarteritis nodosa, particularly the Churg-Strauss variant. Depressed complement levels and high titers of anti–glomerular basement membrane antibodies, antineutrophil cytoplasmic antibodies, antinuclear antibodies, circulating immune complexes, or cryoglobulins are useful diagnostic tools in patients with suspected glomerulonephritis or vasculitis (see Table 28–4).

Imaging of the urinary tract by plain film of the abdomen, ultrasonography, computed tomography, or magnetic resonance is recommended for most patients with ARF to distinguish between acute and chronic renal failure and exclude acute obstructive uropathy.[481–486] The plain film of the abdomen, with tomography if necessary, usually provides a reliable index of kidney size and may detect $Ca^{2+}$-containing kidney stones. However, the capacity of ultrasonography to determine cortical thickness, differences in cortical and medullary density, and the integrity of the collecting system, in addition to kidney size, makes it the screening modality of choice in most cases of ARF.[481, 482] Although pelvicalyceal dilatation is usual in cases of urinary tract obstruction (98% sensitivity), dilatation may not be observed during the initial period after obstruction or in patients with obstruction caused by ureteric encasement or infiltration (e.g., retroperitoneal fibrosis, neoplasia).[483] Retrograde pyelography via cystography or percutaneous anterograde pyelography is used for definitive diagnosis when these conditions are considered likely, and these tools are useful for precise localization of the site of obstruction in other cases.[484] There is a general consensus that intravenous pyelography is best avoided in patients with ARF to avoid adding contrast nephropathy to already compromised renal function. Radionuclide scans have been touted as useful for assessing renal blood flow, glomerular filtration, tubule function, and infiltration by inflammatory cells in ARF; however, these tests generally lack specificity or yield conflicting or poor results in controlled studies.[487] Doppler ultrasonography, magnetic resonance flow imaging, and spiral computed tomography appear promising for assessment of patency of renal arteries and veins in patients with suspected vascular obstruction; however, contrast angiography is still usually required for definitive diagnosis.

Renal biopsy is usually reserved for patients in whom prerenal and postrenal failure have been excluded and the cause of intrinsic renal azotemia is unclear. Renal biopsy is particularly useful when clinical assessment, urinalysis, and laboratory investigation suggest diagnoses other than ischemic or nephrotoxic injury that may respond to specific therapy. Examples include anti–glomerular basement membrane disease and other forms of necrotizing glomerulonephritis, vasculitis, HUS and TTP, allergic interstitial nephritis, and acute allograft rejection.

## Renal Failure Indices for Differentiation of Prerenal Azotemia and Ischemic Acute Tubule Necrosis

Analysis of urine and blood biochemistry is useful for discriminating between the major categories of ARF, namely prerenal azotemia and intrinsic renal azotemia caused by ischemia or nephrotoxins (Table 28–13). The fractional excretion of $Na^+$ ($FE_{Na}$) is the most sensitive index for this purpose.[488-504] The $FE_{Na}$ relates $Na^+$ clearance to creatinine clearance. $Na^+$ is reabsorbed avidly from glomerular filtrate in patients with prerenal azotemia as a consequence of suppression of atrial natriuretic peptide secretion, activation of renal nerves and the renin-angiotensin-aldosterone axis, and local changes in peritubular hemodynamics. In contrast, $Na^+$ reabsorption is inhibited in ATN as a result of tubule cell injury. Creatinine is reabsorbed to a much smaller extent than $Na^+$ in both conditions. Consequently, patients with prerenal azotemia typically have an $FE_{Na}$ of less than 1.0% (frequently <0.01%), whereas the $FE_{Na}$ is usually greater than 1.0% in patients with ischemic or nephrotoxic ARF.[488, 489] The renal failure index (see Table 28–13) provides comparable information, because clinical variations in serum $Na^+$ concentration are relatively

small. Urinary $Na^+$ concentration is a less sensitive index for distinguishing prerenal azotemia from ATN. Similarly, indices of urinary concentrating ability such as urine specific gravity, urine osmolality, urine/plasma creatinine or urea ratios, and serum urea nitrogen/creatinine ratio are of limited value in differential diagnosis.[488-504] This is particularly true for elderly subjects, in whom urine concentrating mechanisms are frequently impaired while mechanisms for $Na^+$ reabsorption are preserved.[503]

Although beloved by textbooks and clinical teachers, the $FE_{Na}$ is only of limited discriminatory value.[490-504] The $FE_{Na}$ is frequently greater than 1.0% in prerenal azotemia in patients receiving diuretics or with bicarbonaturia (when $HCO_3^-$ is excreted with $Na^+$ to maintain electroneutrality), underlying chronic renal failure complicated by salt wasting, or adrenal insufficiency.[502] On the other hand, approximately 15% of patients with nonoliguric ischemic or nephrotoxic ARF have an $FE_{Na}$ less than 1.0%, which probably reflects a milder form of renal injury (sometimes termed the intermediate syndrome).[489-501] The latter has been described in patients with ATN of a variety of causes, including ischemia, aminoglycosides, radiocontrast agents, rhabdomyolysis, hemolysis, burns, sepsis, and hepatorenal syndrome.[489-501] Under these circumstances, epithelial cell damage is probably localized to the corticomedullary junction and outer medulla with relative preservation of function in other $Na^+$ transporting segments. The apparent increase in frequency of the intermediate syndrome may reflect increasing attention by physicians to volume status and drug therapy in high-risk patients. It should be noted that the $FE_{Na}$ is usually less than 1.0% in ARF caused by urinary tract obstruction, glomerulonephritis, and diseases of the renal vasculature, and other parameters must be employed to distinguish these conditions from prerenal azotemia.[504]

## Differential Diagnosis of Acute Renal Failure in Specific Clinical Settings

### ARF IN A CANCER PATIENT

The differential diagnosis of ARF in several common clinical situations warrants special mention (Table 28–14). Most ARF in patients with cancer is due to either prerenal azotemia induced by vomiting or intrinsic renal azotemia triggered by chemotherapeutic drugs or products of tumor lysis.[271-289] Rarer causes include hypercalcemia of malignancy, tumor-associated glomerulonephritis, HUS or TTP induced by drugs or irradiation, and infiltration of kidney or urinary collecting system by tumor (see Table 28–14). ARF in association with multiple myeloma carries a wide differential diagnosis that includes hypovolemia, hyperproteinemia, hypercalcemia, cryoglobulinemia, hyperviscosity syndrome, contrast nephropathy, myeloma cast nephropathy, light chain deposition disease, plasma cell infiltration, vascular amyloidosis, sepsis caused by immunocompromise, and ATN induced by drugs or tumor lysis during therapy.[262-269]

### ARF IN PREGNANCY

The incidence of ARF in pregnancy is declining as a result of improved prenatal care and obstetric practice.[505-512]

**TABLE 28–13. Urine Indices Used in the Differential Diagnosis of Prerenal and Ischemic Intrinsic Renal Azotemia**

| Diagnostic Index | Prerenal Azotemia | Ischemic Intrinsic Azotemia |
|---|---|---|
| Fractional excretion of $Na^+$ (%),* $\frac{U_{Na} \times P_{cr}}{P_{Na} \times U_{cr}} \times 100$ | <1 | >1 |
| Urinary $Na^+$ concentration (mEq/L) | <10 | >20 |
| Urinary creatinine/plasma creatinine ratio | >40 | <20 |
| Urinary urea nitrogen/plasma urea nitrogen ratio | >8 | <3 |
| Urine specific gravity | >1.018 | <1.012 |
| Urine osmolality (mOsm/kg $H_2O$) | >500 | <250 |
| Plasma BUN/creatinine ratio | >20 | <10–15 |
| Renal failure index,* $U_{Na}/U_{cr}/P_{cr}$ | <1 | >1 |
| Urine sediment | Hyaline casts | Muddy brown granular casts |

*Most sensitive indices. $U_{Na}$ = urine $Na^+$ concentration; $U_{cr}$ = urine creatinine concentration; $P_{Na}$ = plasma $Na^+$ concentration; $P_{cr}$ = plasma creatinine concentration.

**TABLE 28–14. Major Causes of Acute Renal Failure in Specific Clinical Settings**

ARF in the cancer patient
  Prerenal azotemia
    Hypovolemia (e.g., poor intake, vomiting, diarrhea)
  Intrinsic renal azotemia
    Exogenous nephrotoxins: chemotherapy, antibiotics, radiocontrast
      agents
    Endogenous toxins: hyperuricemia, hypercalcemia, tumor lysis, light
      chains
    Other: radiation, HUS, TTP, glomerulonephritis, amyloid, infiltration
  Postrenal azotemia
    Ureteric or bladder neck obstruction
ARF after cardiac surgery
  Prerenal azotemia
    Hypovolemia (surgical losses, diuretics), cardiac failure, vasodilators
  Intrinsic renal azotemia
    Ischemic renal failure with ATN (even in absence of documented
      hypotension)
    Atheroembolic renal disease after aortic manipulation
    Pre- or perioperative administration of radiocontrast agent
    Allergic interstitial nephritis induced by perioperative antibiotics
  Postrenal azotemia
    Blocked urinary catheter
ARF in pregnancy
  Intrinsic renal azotemia
    Preeclampsia or eclampsia
    Ischemia: postpartum hemorrhage, abruptio placentae, amniotic fluid
      embolus
    Direct toxicity of illegal abortifacients
    Postpartum HUS or TTP
    Acute fatty liver of pregnancy
  Postrenal
    Obstruction with pyelonephritis
ARF after renal transplantation
  Prerenal azotemia
    Intravascular volume depletion (e.g., diuretic therapy, diuretic phase
      of ATN)
  Intrinsic renal azotemia
    Large renal vessels: arterial or venous thrombosis
    Microvasculature: vascular rejection, cyclosporine, de novo or
      glomerulonephritis, HUS, TTP
    ATN: ischemia, cyclosporine, aminoglycosides
    Tubulointerstitial nephritis: cellular rejection, drugs, infection
      (e.g., cytomegalovirus), OKT3
  Postrenal azotemia
    Ureteric obstruction (clot, ureteral stenosis, lymphocoele, hematoma)
      or urine leakage

ARF and pulmonary disease (pulmonary-renal syndrome)
  Vasculitis: Goodpasture syndrome, Wegener syndrome, SLE, Churg-
    Strauss syndrome, or classic polyarteritis nodosa, cryoglobulinemia,
    right-sided endocarditis, lymphomatoid granulomatosis, sarcoidosis,
    scleroderma
  Toxins: ingestion of paraquat or diquat
  Infections: legionnaire disease, mycoplasma infection, tuberculosis,
    disseminated viral or fungal infection
  Acute renal azotemia from any cause with hypervolemia and
    pulmonary edema
  Prerenal azotemia caused by diminished cardiac output complicating
    pulmonary embolism, severe pulmonary hypertension, or positive-
    pressure mechanical ventilation.
  Lung cancer with hypercalcemia, tumor lysis, or glomerulonephritis
ARF and liver disease
  Prerenal azotemia
    Primary liver disease with secondary renal failure caused by reduced
      effective (hypoalbuminemia, splanchnic vasodilatation) or true
      (gastrointestinal hemorrhage, diuretics) circulatory volume
    Right-sided heart failure with liver and renal failure
  Intrinsic renal azotemia
    Ischemia (severe hypoperfusion—see above) or direct nephrotoxicity
      and hepatotoxicity of drugs or toxins (e.g., carbon tetrachloride,
      acetaminophen, tetracyclines, methoxyfluorane)
    Tubulointerstitial nephritis + hepatitis caused by drugs (e.g.,
      sulfonamides, rifampin, phenytoin, allopurinol, phenindione),
      infections (leptospirosis, brucellosis, Epstein-Barr virus infection,
      cytomegalovirus infection), malignant infiltration (lymphoma,
      leukemia), or sarcoidosis
    Glomerulonephritis or vasculitis (e.g., polyarteritis nodosa, Wegener
      syndrome, cryoglobulinemia, SLE, postinfectious hepatitis or liver
      abscess)
ARF and nephrotic syndrome
  Prerenal azotemia
    Intravascular volume depletion (diuretic therapy, hypoalbuminemia)
  Intrinsic renal azotemia
    Manifestation of primary glomerular disease
    Associated interstitial nephritis (NSAIDs), rifampin, interferon alfa)
    Myeloma cast nephropathy or light chain deposition disease
    Renal vein thrombosis
    Severe interstital edema

ATN induced by nephrotoxic abortifacients is still a relatively common cause of ARF in developing countries but is rarely seen in the developed world.[505–507] Ischemic ATN, severe toxemia of pregnancy, and postpartum HUS and TTP are the most common causes later in pregnancy[506–512] (see Table 28–14). Ischemic ATN is usually provoked by postpartum hemorrhage or abruptio placentae and less commonly by amniotic fluid embolism or sepsis. Glomerular filtration is usually normal in mild or moderate preeclampsia; however, ARF may complicate severe disease.[508, 509] In this setting, ARF is typically transient and found in association with intrarenal vasospasm, marked hypertension, neurologic abnormalities, and laboratory evidence of disseminated intravascular coagulation. This presentation contrasts with that of postpartum HUS or TTP, which typically occurs against a background of normal pregnancy; is characterized by thrombocytopenia, microangiopathic anemia, and normal prothrombin and partial thromboplastin times; and

frequently causes long-term impairment of renal function.[512] Acute fatty liver of pregnancy is a rare condition that induces acute renal impairment probably by triggering intrarenal vasoconstriction, as in other hepatorenal syndromes.[510] The disease may be idiopathic or associated with diverse insults such as viral hepatitis or tetracycline administration and frequently requires termination of pregnancy.[510] Acute bilateral pyelonephritis may also precipitate ARF in pregnancy and should be obvious from clinical assessment (fever, flank pain) and routine urinalysis (bacteria, leukocytes) and laboratory tests (leukocytosis, increase in serum creatinine from basal levels).[511]

## ARF AFTER CARDIOVASCULAR SURGERY

ARF in this setting can usually be attributed to prerenal azotemia, ischemic ATN, atheroembolic disease, or the effects of radiocontrast material administered perioperatively[78-85, 93-103, 114-135] (see Table 28–14). The pattern of rise in serum creatinine may be extremely helpful in the differential diagnosis of ARF in this setting. As noted earlier, prerenal azotemia is typified by rapid fluctuations in serum creatinine values that usually precede surgery and mirror changes in systemic hemodynamics and renal perfusion. Overzealous use of diuretics or afterload-reducing agents is a frequent cause of prerenal azotemia postoperatively, particularly in elderly patients in whom renal autoregulation is frequently reduced secondary to hypertensive, atherosclerotic, or diabetic vasculopathy. The serum creatinine value characteristically rises for 3 to 4 days after the administration of contrast agent and returns rapidly to the normal range within 1 week. This pattern contrasts with those observed with ischemic ATN and atheroembolic disease, in which the serum creatinine value also rises progressively after surgery but typically takes 7 to 14 days before recovery begins (ATN) or fails to resolve (atheroemboli). Rarer but nevertheless important causes include allergic tubulo-interstitial nephritis induced by antibiotics administered perioperatively and obstruction of urine drainage.

## ARF IN A RENAL ALLOGRAFT

The causes of ARF after renal transplantation can be conveniently categorized into 1) complications of any major surgical procedure (e.g., prerenal azotemia, ischemic ATN), 2) technical complications affecting surgical anastamoses (e.g., thrombosis of the renal artery or vein; ureteric dehiscence, obstruction, or leak), 3) allograft rejection or the side effects of immunosuppressive therapy (cyclosporine nephrotoxicity), and 4) rapid recurrence of the primary renal disease (see Table 28–14). The differential diagnosis of renal impairment in this setting is discussed in detail in Chapter 59 and elsewhere.[513] ARF is also a common complication of bone marrow transplantation (>50%).[514] ARF is usually multifactorial in origin and often preceded by either hepatic dysfunction, often related to hepatic veno-occlusive disease, weight gain, use of amphotericin B, septicemia, and/or hypotension. The prognosis is grave, particularly for patients requiring dialysis (>80% mortality).[514]

## ARF IN ASSOCIATION WITH PULMONARY DISEASE

The coexistence of ARF and pulmonary disease (pulmonary-renal syndrome) classically suggests a diagnosis of Goodpasture syndrome, Wegener granulomatosis, or other vasculitides. The detection of circulating antineutrophil cytoplasmic antibodies, anti–glomerular basement membrane antibodies, or hypocomplementemia can be useful in the differentiation of these diseases (see Tables 28–4 and 28–14), although the urgent need for definitive diagnosis and treatment may mandate a lung or renal biopsy. Several toxic ingestions and infections may also cause simultaneous pulmonary and renal injury that mimics a vasculitic process[515, 516] (see Table 28–14). Furthermore, intrinsic renal or postrenal azotemia of any cause may be complicated by secondary hypervolemia and pulmonary

edema, and severe lung diseases may compromise cardiac output and induce prerenal azotemia (see Table 28–14).

## ARF IN ASSOCIATION WITH LIVER DISEASE

The differential diagnosis for ARF in association with liver disease is similarly large.[517-537] The term "hepatorenal syndrome" is usually reserved for a syndrome of irreversible ARF that usually complicates advanced liver disease and is characterized by intense intrarenal vasoconstriction and hypoperfusion, decreased effective systemic circulatory volume despite an expanded total extracellular fluid volume as a result of splanchnic pooling, a benign urine sediment, concentrated urine, a low $FE_{Na}$, and progressive renal failure in the absence of other causes of renal disease.[517-530] Most patients have clinical evidence of cirrhosis; however, this syndrome has been described in association with fulminant hepatitis, hepatic tumors, and other liver diseases.[517-530] BUN and serum creatinine values are characteristically deceptively low, despite marked impairment of GFR, because of impaired urea generation and coexisting muscle wasting. The hepatorenal syndrome almost certainly represents the terminal stage of a hypoperfusion state that begins early in the course of liver diseases. The pathogenetic mechanisms for the dramatic hemodynamic alterations are incompletely understood. Potential contributors include liver-derived circulatory or neural stimuli, gut-derived endotoxin, and alterations in systemic and/or intrarenal levels of angiotensin II, aldosterone, vasoactive intestinal polypeptide, adenosine, endothelin, NO, kallikrein and kinins, prostaglandins, and inactive amines.[517] Patients are exquisitely sensitive to relatively small changes in extracellular fluid volume or vascular resistance. Common precipitants of the hepatorenal syndrome in patients with compensated cirrhosis include vigorous diuresis or paracentesis, gastrointestinal bleeding, infections, minor surgery, or the use of NSAIDs and other drugs.[517] Other diagnoses that must be excluded in patients with hepatorenal syndrome include toxic ingestions, combined hepatitis and tubulointerstitial nephritis induced by drugs or infectious agents, and multiorgan involvement in vasculitides (see Table 28–14). Death is almost invariable in true hepatorenal syndrome and is usually due to hepatic failure, infection, hemorrhage, or circulatory failure.[517]

### ARF AND NEPHROTIC SYNDROME

ARF in the context of the nephrotic syndrome presents a unique array of potential diagnoses. These include prerenal azotemia complicating diuretic therapy for mobilization of edema, combined allergic interstitial nephritis and minimal-change disease induced by drugs, myeloma kidney with massive excretion of light chain protein, or a manifestation of the primary glomerular disease.[90, 538-541]

## COMPLICATIONS OF ACUTE RENAL FAILURE

ARF impairs renal excretion of $Na^+$, $K^+$, and water; divalent cation homeostasis; and urinary acidification mechanisms. As a result, ARF is frequently complicated by intravascular volume overload, hyperkalemia, hyponatremia, hyperphosphatemia, hypocalcemia, hypermagnesemia, and metabolic acidosis (Table 28–15). In addition, patients are unable to excrete nitrogenous waste products and may develop the uremic syndrome. In general, the severity of these complications mirrors the severity of renal injury and the catabolic state of the patient.[3, 542–544] For example, the average daily increases in BUN and serum creatinine values in patients with nonoliguric, noncatabolic renal failure range from 10 to 20 mg/dL and 0.5 to 1.0 mg/dL, respectively. Comparable increments in BUN and creatinine levels in oliguric, catabolic patients typically range from 20 to 100 mg/dL and 2 to 3 mg/dL, respectively.[3, 542–544] Not surprisingly, therefore, the latter group is at significantly higher risk for life-threatening metabolic complications and has a worse prognosis (see later).

Intravascular volume overload is an almost inevitable consequence of diminished salt and water excretion in ARF and may present clinically as mild hypertension, increased jugular venous pressure, bibasilar lung crackles, pleural effusions or ascites, peripheral edema, increased body weight, and life-threatening pulmonary edema.[542–545] Hypervolemia may be particularly troublesome in patients receiving multiple intravenous medications, sodium bicarbonate for correction of acidosis, or enteral or parenteral nutrition. Moderate or severe hypertension is unusual in ATN and should suggest other diagnoses such as hypertensive nephrosclerosis, glomerulonephritis, renal artery stenosis, and other diseases of the renal vasculature. Excessive water ingestion or administration of hypotonic saline or isotonic dextrose solutions can trigger hyponatremia, which, if severe, may cause cerebral edema, seizures, and other neurologic abnormalities.[546]

Hyperkalemia is a common and potentially life-threatening complication of ARF.[5, 542, 547–549] Serum K$^+$ typically rises by 0.5 mEq/L/d in oligoanuric patients and reflects impaired excretion of K$^+$ derived from diet, K$^+$-containing solutions, drugs administered as potassium salts (e.g., penicillin V), and K$^+$ released from injured tubule epithelium. Hyperkalemia may be compounded by coexistent metabolic acidosis that promotes K$^+$ efflux from cells. Severe hyperkalemia or hyperkalemia present at the time of diagnosis of ARF suggests massive tissue destruction such as rhabdomyolysis, hemolysis, or tumor lysis. Mild hyperkalemia (<6.0 mEq/L) is usually asymptomatic. Higher levels are frequently associated with electrocardiographic abnormalities, typically peaked T waves, prolongation of the PR

interval, flattening of P waves, widening of the QRS complex, and left axis deviation. These changes may antecede the onset of life-threatening cardiac arrhythmias such as bradycardia, heart block, ventricular tachycardia or fibrillation, and asystole. In addition, hyperkalemia may induce neuromuscular abnormalities such as paresthesias, hyporeflexia, weakness, ascending flaccid paralysis, and respiratory failure. Hypokalemia is unusual in ARF but may complicate nonoliguric ATN caused by aminoglycosides, cisplatin, or amphotericin B, presumably by causing epithelial cell injury in the thick ascending limb of the loop of Henle, the last major site of K$^+$ reabsorption.

Normal metabolism of dietary protein yields between 50 and 100 mmol/d of fixed nonvolatile acids (principally sulfuric and phosphoric acid), which must be excreted by the kidneys for preservation of acid-base homeostasis. Predictably, ARF is commonly complicated by metabolic acidosis, typically with a widening of the serum anion gap.[542, 550] Acidosis may be severe (daily fall in plasma HCO$_3^-$ > 2 mEq/L) when the generation of H$^+$ is increased by additional mechanisms (e.g., diabetic or fasting ketoacidosis; lactic acidosis complicating generalized tissue hypoperfusion, liver disease, or sepsis; metabolism of ethylene glycol). In contrast, metabolic alkalosis is an infrequent finding but may complicate overzealous correction of acidosis with HCO$_3^-$ or loss of gastric acid by vomiting or nasogastric aspiration.

Uric acid is cleared from blood by glomerular filtration and secretion by proximal tubule cells, and mild asymptomatic hyperuricemia (12 to 15 mg/dL) is typical in established ARF.[542] Higher levels suggest increased production of uric acid and should suggest a diagnosis of acute urate nephropathy. In borderline cases, measurement of the urinary urate/creatinine ratio on a random specimen may help distinguish between hyperuricemia caused by overproduction and impaired excretion.[274] This ratio is typically greater than 1.0 when uric acid production is increased and less than 0.75 in normal individuals and patients with renal failure.[274]

Mild hyperphosphatemia (5 to 10 mg/dL) is a common consequence of ARF and hyperphosphatemia may be severe (10 to 20 mg/dL) in highly catabolic patients or when ARF is associated with rapid cell death as in rhabdomyolysis, hemolysis, or tumor lysis.[542, 551, 552] Metastatic deposition of calcium phosphate can lead to hypocalcemia, particularly when the product of serum Ca$^{2+}$ (mg/dL) and PO$_4^{3-}$ (mg/dL) concentrations exceeds 70.[542, 553, 554] Other factors that potentially contribute to hypocalcemia include

**TABLE 28–15. Common Complications of Acute Renal Failure**

| Metabolic | Cardiovascular | Gastrointestinal | Neurologic | Hematologic | Infectious | Other |
|---|---|---|---|---|---|---|
| Hyperkalemia | Pulmonary edema | Nausea | Neuromuscular | Anemia | Pneumonia | Hiccups |
| Metabolic acidosis | Arrhythmias | Vomiting |   irritability | Bleeding | Wound infections | Decreased insulin catabolism |
| Hyponatremia | Pericarditis | Malnutrition | Asterixis | | Intravenous line | Mild insulin resistance |
| Hypocalcemia | Pericardial effusion | Gastritis | Seizures | |   infections | Elevated parathyroid hormone |
| Hyperphosphatemia | Hypertension | Gastrointestinal ulcers | Mental status changes | | Septicemia | Reduced 1,25-dihydroxy- and |
| Hypermagnesemia | Myocardial infarction | Gastrointestinal bleeding | Somnolence | | Urinary tract |   25-hydroxyvitamin D |
| Hyperuricemia | Pulmonary embolism | Stomatitis or gingivitis | Coma | |   infection | Low total triiodothyronine and |
| | Pneumonitis | Parotitis or pancreatitis | | | |   thyroxine |
| | | | | | | Normal free thyroxine |

skeletal resistance to the actions of parathyroid hormone, reduced levels of 1,25-dihydroxyvitamin D, and $Ca^{2+}$ sequestration in injured tissues.[542, 553, 554] Hypocalcemia is usually asymptomatic, possibly because of the counterbalancing effects of acidosis on neuromuscular excitability. However, symptomatic hypocalcemia can occur in patients with rhabdomyolysis or acute pancreatitis or after treatment of acidosis with $HCO_3^-$. Clinical manifestations of hypocalcemia include perioral paresthesias, muscle cramps, seizures, hallucinations and confusion, and prolongation of the QT interval and nonspecific T wave changes on an electrocardiogram. The Chvostek sign (contraction of facial muscles on tapping of the jaw over the facial nerve) and the Trousseau sign (carpopedal spasm after occlusion of arterial blood supply to the arm for 3 minutes with a blood pressure cuff) are useful indicators of latent tetany in high-risk patients. Mild asymptomatic hypermagnesemia is usual in oliguric ARF and reflects impaired excretion of ingested magnesium (dietary magnesium, magnesium-containing laxatives, or antacids).[542, 555] Hypomagnesemia occasionally complicates nonoliguric ATN associated with cisplatin or amphotericin B and, as with hypokalemia, probably reflects injury to the thick ascending limb of loop of Henle, the principal site for $Mg^{2+}$ reabsorption.[161, 171, 556] Hypomagnesemia is usually asymptomatic but may occasionally be manifest as neuromuscular instability, cramps, seizures, cardiac arrhythmias, or resistant hypokalemia or hypocalcemia.

Anemia develops rapidly in ARF and is usually mild and multifactorial in origin. Contributing factors include inhibition of erythropoiesis, hemolysis, bleeding, hemodilution, and reduced red blood cell survival time.[557, 558] Prolongation of the bleeding time and leukocytosis are also common.[559–564] The former may result from mild thrombocytopenia, platelet dysfunction, and/or clotting factor abnormalities (e.g., factor VIII dysfunction) and the complementary actions of administered drugs (e.g., penicillins), and leukocytosis usually reflects sepsis, stress response, and/or other concurrent illness.[561–564] Infection is the most common and serious complication of ARF, occurring in 50% to 90% of cases and accounting for up to 75% of deaths.[5, 7, 22, 102, 565–573] It is unclear whether this high incidence of infection is due to a defect in host immune responses or repeated breaches of mucocutaneous barriers (e.g., intravenous cannula, mechanical ventilation, bladder catheterization).

Cardiac complications include arrhythmias, myocardial infarction, and pulmonary embolism.[567] Although these events may reflect primary cardiac disease, abnormalities in myocardial contractility and excitability may be triggered or compounded by hypervolemia, acidosis, hyperkalemia, and other metabolic sequelae of acute azotemia. The increased incidence of pulmonary embolism probably reflects protracted periods of immobilization. Mild gastrointestinal bleeding is common (10% to 30%) and is usually due to stress ulceration of gastric or small intestinal mucosa.[574, 575] Alterations in neurologic function may reflect the onset of the uremic syndrome, metabolic complications of ARF, impaired excretion of prescribed neuropsychiatric medications, or primary neurologic disease.[576–581]

Malnutrition remains one of the most frustrating and troublesome complications of ARF.[542, 582] The majority of patients have net protein breakdown, which may exceed 200 g/d in catabolic subjects. Malnutrition is usually multifactorial in origin and may reflect 1) inability to eat or loss of appetite; 2) the catabolic nature of the underlying medical disorder (e.g., sepsis, rhabdomyolysis, trauma); 3) nutrient losses in drainage fluids or dialysate; 4) increased breakdown and reduced synthesis of muscle protein and increased hepatic gluconeogenesis, probably through the actions of toxins, hormones (e.g., glucagon, parathyroid hormone), or other substances (e.g., proteases) that are accumulated in ARF; and 5) inadequate nutritional support.[542]

Protracted periods of severe ARF or short periods of catabolic, anuric azotemia often lead to the development of the uremic syndrome.[542, 583, 584] Clinical manifestations of the uremic syndrome, in addition to those already listed, include pericarditis, pericardial effusion, and cardiac tamponade; gastrointestinal complications such as anorexia, nausea, vomiting, and ileus; and neuropsychiatric disturbances including lethargy, confusion, stupor, coma, agitation, psychosis, asterixis, myoclonus, hyperreflexia, restless leg syndrome, focal neurologic deficit, or seizures (see Table 28–15). The uremic toxin (or toxins) responsible for this syndrome has yet to be defined. Candidate molecules include 1) urea and its breakdown products, 2) other products of nitrogen metabolism such as guanidino compounds, 3) products of bacterial metabolism such as aromatic amines and skatoles, and 4) other compounds that are inappropriately retained in the circulation in ARF,[542] or are underproduced, such as NO.[542a]

A vigorous diuresis may complicate the recovery phase of ARF and precipitate intravascular volume depletion and a delay in recovery of renal function. This diuretic response probably reflects the combined effects of an osmotic diuresis induced by retained urea and other waste products and delayed recovery of tubule function relative to glomerular filtration. Hypernatremia may also complicate this recovery phase if free water losses are not replenished or are inappropriately replaced by relatively hypertonic saline solutions. Hypokalemia, hypomagnesemia, hypophosphatemia, and hypocalcemia are rarer metabolic complications during recovery from ARF. Mild transient hypercalcemia is relatively frequent during recovery and appears to be a consequence of hyperparathyroidism. In addition, hypercalcemia may complicate recovery from rhabdomyolysis because of mobilization of sequestered $Ca^{2+}$ from injured muscle.

# MANAGEMENT OF ACUTE RENAL FAILURE

## Prerenal Azotemia

By definition, prerenal azotemia is rapidly reversible on restoration of renal perfusion. The composition of replacement fluids for treatment of hypovolemia varies depending on the source of fluid loss. Hypovolemia caused by hemorrhage is ideally corrected with packed red blood cells in saline, and isotonic saline is usually appropriate replacement for plasma losses (e.g., burns, pancreatitis). Urinary or gastrointestinal fluids vary greatly in composition but are usually hypotonic. Accordingly, initial replacement is best achieved with hypotonic solutions (e.g., 0.45% saline), and subsequent therapy should be based on measurements of the volume and ionic content of excreted or drained fluids. Serum $K^+$ and acid-base status should be monitored in all subjects. $K^+$ supplementation of replacement fluids is rarely required unless sodium bicarbonate induces hypokalemia during treatment of metabolic acidosis. Cardiac failure may require aggressive management with antiarrhythmic drugs, positive inotropes, preload- and/or afterload-reducing agents, and mechanical aids such as intra-aortic balloon pumps. Invasive hemodynamic monitoring is invaluable for guiding therapy in complicated patients in whom clinical assessment of cardiovascular function and intravascular volume may be difficult and unreliable.

Fluid management may be particularly challenging in patients with ARF and cirrhosis.[517, 531–534] Although these subjects typically have intense intrarenal vasoconstriction and expanded total plasma volume because of pooling of blood in the splanchnic circulation, true or effective systemic arterial hypovolemia may be an important contributory factor to ARF. The relative contribution of hypovolemia to ARF in this setting can be determined only by administration of a fluid challenge, often with invasive monitoring of systemic hemodynamics. Fluids should be administered slowly, as nonresponders may suffer an increase in ascites formation and/or pulmonary edema. Paracentesis can be employed to remove large volumes of ascitic fluid without deterioration in renal function if albumin is administered simultaneously. Indeed, large-volume paracentesis may occasionally improve GFR, possibly by lowering intra-abdominal pressure and promoting blood flow in renal veins. Shunting of ascitic fluid from the peritoneum to a central vein (peritoneojugular shunt, LeVeen or Denver shunt) is an alternative approach in refractory cases.[517, 531–534] This maneuver may also cause a transient improvement in GFR and $Na^+$ excretion, probably because the increase in central blood volume stimulates release of atrial natriuretic peptides and inhibits aldosterone and norepinephrine secretion.

## Intrinsic Renal Azotemia

### PREVENTION

Optimization of cardiovascular function and intravascular volume is the single most important maneuver in the management of acute intrinsic azotemia. There is compelling evidence that aggressive restoration of intravascular volume dramatically reduces the incidence of ATN after major surgery or trauma, burns, and cholera.[585–589] Volume depletion has been identified as a risk factor for nephrotoxic ATN induced by radiocontrast material, acyclovir, aminoglycosides, amphotericin B, cisplatin, acute urate nephropathy, rhabdomyolysis, hemolysis, multiple myeloma, hypercalcemia, and numerous other nephrotoxins.[585–590] Restoration of volume prevents the development of experimental and human ATN in many of these settings. The importance of maintaining euvolemia in high-risk clinical situations has been demonstrated most convincingly with

contrast nephropathy, in which close attention to intravascular volume status ensures a low frequency of ARF[134] and prophylactic infusion of half-normal saline appears more effective in preventing ARF than are other commonly used agents such as mannitol and furosemide.[590a] Diuretics, cyclooxygenase inhibitors, ACE inhibitors, and other vasodilators should be used with caution in patients with suspected true or effective hypovolemia or renovascular disease, as they may convert prerenal azotemia to ischemic ATN and sensitize such patients to the actions of nephrotoxins. Careful monitoring of circulating drug levels appears to reduce the incidence of ARF associated with aminoglycoside antibiotics or cyclosporine. Interestingly, the antimicrobial efficacy of aminoglycosides appears to persist in tissues even after the drug has been cleared from the circulation and there is convincing evidence that once-daily dosing with these agents affords equal antimicrobial activity and less nephrotoxicity than conventional regimens.[200, 201] Several other agents are commonly employed to prevent ARF in specific clinical settings. Allopurinol is useful for limiting uric acid generation in patients at high risk for acute urate nephropathy; however, occasional patients receiving allopurinol still develop ARF, probably through the toxic actions of hypoxanthine crystals on tubule function. Forced diuresis and alkalinization of urine may attenuate renal injury caused by uric acid or methotrexate and after rhabdomyolysis. N-Acetylcysteine limits acetaminophen-induced renal injury if given within 24 hours of ingestion and dimercaprol, a chelating agent, may prevent heavy metal nephrotoxicity. Ethanol inhibits ethylene glycol metabolism to oxalic acid and other toxic metabolites and is an important adjunct to hemodialysis in the emergency management of this intoxication.

### SPECIFIC THERAPIES

A variety of agents have been tested for their ability to attenuate injury or hasten recovery in ischemic and nephrotoxic ATN; however, none has consistently been shown to be of benefit. Tables 28–16 and 28–17 summarize the strategies that have been tried to alter the course of experimental and clinical ARF, respectively.[591–761] A more extensive discussion of these issues is given by Conger.[762] The strategies include maneuvers to increase renal blood flow and urine flow (e.g., low-dose dopamine, atrial natriuretic peptide, mannitol, loop diuretics), relieve tubule obstruction (e.g., mannitol, loop diuretics, RGD peptides), reduce epithelial cell swelling (e.g., mannitol), lower epithelial cell ATP and oxygen requirements by inhibiting ion transport (e.g., loop diuretics), replenish cell ATP levels (MgATP), scavenge oxygen free radicals (e.g., superoxide dismutase, catalase, mannitol), prevent accumulation of intracellular $Ca^{2+}$ ($Ca^{2+}$ channel blockers), inhibit leukocyte–endothelial cell adhesion during reperfusion (e.g., anti-CD18 and anti–ICAM-1 monoclonal antibodies), and stimulate cellular regeneration (e.g., amino acid infusions). Although many of these and other agents (e.g., glycine infusion, epidermal growth factor, growth hormone) afford some benefit in experimental models of ischemic or nephrotoxic ARF, they either have failed to confer consistent clinically significant benefit or are too toxic for use in humans.

**TABLE 28–16. Drugs Used to Alter the Course of Experimental Ischemic and Nephrotoxic Acute Renal Failure**

| Class and Specific Drug | Cause of Acute Renal Failure | Time of Administration | Observed Effect | References |
|---|---|---|---|---|
| Vasoactive agents | | | | |
| Propranolol | Ischemic | Before, during, after | ↓ BUN and SeCr* if before or during | 591–593 |
| Phenoxybenzamine | Toxic | Before, during, after | Prevented fall in RBF* | 594 |
| Clonidine | Ischemic | After | ↓ BUN and SeCr | 595 |
| Bradykinin | Ischemic | Before, during | ↑ RBF and GFR | 596 |
| Acetylcholine | Ischemic | Before, after | ↑ RBF, no change in GFR | 597 |
| Prostaglandin E$_1$ | Ischemic | After | ↑ RBF, no change in GFR | 598 |
| Prostaglandin E$_2$ | Ischemic, toxic | Before, during | ↑ GFR | 599 |
| Prostacyclin | Ischemic | Before, during, after | ↑ GFR | 600–603 |
| Saralasin | Ischemic, toxic | Before | ↑ RBF, no change in SeCr or BUN | 604, 605 |
| Captopril | Ischemic, toxic | Before | ↑ RBF, no change in SeCr or BUN | 605 |
| Verapamil | Ischemic, toxic | Before, during, after | ↑ RBF and GFR in most studies | 606–608 |
| Nifedipine | Ischemic | Before | ↑ GFR | 609 |
| Nitrendipine | Toxic | Before, during | ↑ GFR | 610 |
| Diltiazem | Toxic | Before, during, after | ↑ GFR and ↓ recovery time | 611 |
| Chlorpromazine | Toxic | Before | ↑ GFR and ↓ recovery time | 612 |
| Atrial natriuretic peptide | Ischemic, toxic | After | ↑ GFR and GFR | 613–623 |
| Theophylline | Ischemic | Before or after | ↑ RBF and GFR, or no change | 624–627 |
| Antiendothelin antibody | Ischemic | After | ↑ RBF and GFR | 628, 629 |
| Dopamine | Ischemic, toxic | Before or after | ↑ RBF and GFR or no change | 762b |
| Diuretics | | | | |
| Mannitol | Ischemic, toxic | Before | ↑ RBF and GFR | 630–641 |
| Furosemide | Ischemic, toxic | Before, during, after | Consistent ↑ GFR only if before | 642–647 |
| Inhibitors or scavengers of ROS | | | | |
| Allopurinol | Ischemic | Before | ↓ SeCr or no effect | 648–652 |
| Oxypurinol | Ischemic | Before | No effect of BUN or SeCr | 651, 652 |
| Deferoxamine | Ischemic | Reperfusion | ↑ GFR | 260, 653–657 |
| Dimethylthiourea | Ischemic | Before, reperfusion | ↑ GFR if short-term ischemia | 260, 640, 650–659 |
| Dimethyl sulfoxide | Ischemic | Before, reperfusion | ↑ GFR if short-term ischemia | 648, 659 |
| Superoxide dismutase | Ischemic | Before, reperfusion | ↓ SeCr or no change | 650, 660 |
| Catalase | Ischemic, toxic | Before, reperfusion | ↓ SeCr or no change | 260, 648 |
| Glutathione | Ischemic | Before | Further decrease in GFR | 652 |
| Probucol | Ischemic | Before | No change in GFR | 661, 662 |
| Diethylthiocarbamate | Toxic | Before | ↓ SeCr | 757 |
| Neutrophil depletion or inhibition or leukocyte adhesion | | | | |
| Antineutrophil serum | Ischemic | Before | ↑ GFR or no change | 663, 664 |
| Nitrogen mustard | Ischemic | Before | No change in GFR | 663 |
| Anti-CD18 antibody | Ischemic | Before, reperfusion | No change in BUN and SeCr | 665, 666 |
| Anti–ICAM-1 antibody | Ischemic | Before, reperfusion | ↓ BUN and SeCr, or no change | 666, 667 |
| Elastase cathepsin inhibitors | | | | |
| Elgin C | Ischemic | Reperfusion | Mixed effects on GFR and BUN | 668, 669 |
| Agents to restore cell energetics | | | | |
| ATP-MgCl$_2$ | Ischemic | After | ↑ GFR | 670–676 |
| Thyroxine | Ischemic, toxic | After | ↑ GFR | 677–681 |
| Glycine | Ischemic | Before | ↑ GFR | 682–685 |
| Anticoagulants and antiplatelet agents | | | | |
| Pentoxifyline | Toxic | After | ↑ GFR | 686 |
| Dipyridamole | Ischemic | Before | No change or further ↓ in GFR | 687 |
| Heparin | Ischemic | Before | No change in GFR | 688 |
| Aspirin | Ischemic | Before | No change in GFR | 688 |
| Growth factors | | | | |
| Epidermal growth factor | Ischemic | After | ↑ GFR | 689, 690, 765a |
| Insulin-like growth factor-1 | Ischemic | After | ↑ GFR | 461, 765a |
| Inhibitors of cast formation | | | | |
| RGD peptides | Ischemic | Before | ↑ GFR | 311 |
| Alkalinizing agents | | | | |
| Tris(hydroxymethyl) aminomethane | Ischemic | After | ↑ RBF, minimal effect on GFR | 691 |

*RBF = renal blood flow; SeCr = serum creatinine.

Modified from Conger JD: Drug therapy in acute renal failure. *In* Lazarus JM, Brenner BM (eds): Acute Renal Failure, 3rd ed. Churchill Livingstone, New York, 1993, p 529.

**TABLE 28–17. Drugs Used to Alter the Course of Clinical Ischemic or Toxic Acute Renal Failure**

| Class and Specific Drug | Cause of Acute Renal Failure | Observed Effect* | Remarks | References |
|---|---|---|---|---|
| Vasoactive agents | | | | |
| Dopamine | Ischemic, toxic | No change or improved $\dot{V}$, SeCr if used early | Combined with furosemide | 692–698, 514, 762a, 762b |
| Phenoxybenzamine | Ischemic, toxic | No change in $\dot{V}$, RBF | | 699 |
| Phentolamine | Ischemic, toxic | No change in $\dot{V}$, RBF | | 700 |
| Prostaglandin A₁ | Ischemic | No change in $\dot{V}$, SeCr | Used with dopamine | 701 |
| Prostaglandin E₁ | Ischemic | ↑ RBF, no change $\dot{V}$, Clcr | Used with norepinephrine | 702 |
| Verapamil | Ischemic | ↑ Clcr or no effect | | 703, 704 |
| Diltiazem | Transplantation, toxic | ↑ Clcr or no effect | Prophylactic use | 705, 706 |
| Nifedipine | Radiocontrast agent | No effect | | 707 |
| Atrial natriuretic peptide | Ischemic, toxic | No change in Clcr | | 708, 709 |
| Diuretics | | | | |
| Mannitol | Ischemic, toxic, transplantation | ↑ $\dot{V}$ if used early, variable ↑ GFR | Prophylactic use may be beneficial used alone or with dopamine or CCB | 710–725 |
| Furosemide | Ischemic, toxic | ↑ $\dot{V}$ if used early, variable ↑ GFR | | 726–729, 731–737 |
| Ethacrynic acid | Ischemic, toxic | ↑ $\dot{V}$ if used early, no ↑ in GFR | | 726, 730 |
| Toxin chelators, scavengers, or inhibitors | | | | |
| Dimercaprol | Mercury, arsenic, gold | ↓ ARF if given early | Prophylactic use | 736–739 |
| Edetate calcium disodium | Lead | ↓ ARF if given early | Prophylactic use | 740–743 |
| Penicillamine | Lead, mercury | ↓ ARF if given early | Prophylactic use | 744, 745 |
| N-Acetylcysteine | Acetaminophen | ↓ ARF if given early | Prophylactic use | 746, 747 |
| Leucovorin | Methotrexate | ↓ ARF in adequate doses | Prophylactic use | 748, 749 |
| Allopurinol | Uric acid | ↓ ARF if given early | Prophylactic use | 750–754 |
| Haptoglobin | Hemoglobinuria, burns | ↓ ARF if given early | Prophylactic use | 755, 756 |
| Sodium thiosulfate | Cisplatin | ↓ ARF if given before cisplatin | Prophylactic use | 757 |
| Ethanol | Ethylene glycol | ↓ ARF if given early | Prophylactic use | 758–760 |
| 4-Methylpyrazole | Ethylene glycol | ↓ ARF if given early | Prophylactic use | 761 |
| Alkalinizing agents | | | | |
| Sodium bicarbonate | Toxic, rhabdomyolysis | Promotes toxin removal | Prophylactic use | 247, 259, 808 |

*Clcr = creatinine clearance; RBF = renal blood flow; SeCr = serum creatinine; $\dot{V}$ = urine flow rate; CCB = $Ca^{2+}$ channel blockers.
Modified from Conger JD: Drug therapy in acute renal failure. *In* Lazarus JM, Brenner BM (eds): Acute Renal Failure, 3rd ed. Churchill Livingstone, New York, 1993, p 529.

ARF caused by other intrinsic renal diseases such as acute glomerulonephritis or vasculitis may respond to corticosteroids, alkylating agents, and/or plasmapheresis, depending on the primary disease. Corticosteroids appear to hasten remission in some cases of allergic interstitial nephritis. Antiplatelet agents, plasma exchange, and plasma infusion are useful in treatment of HUS and TTP. Aggressive control of systemic arterial pressure is of paramount importance in limiting renal injury in malignant hypertensive nephrosclerosis, toxemia of pregnancy, and other vascular diseases. Hypertension and ARF associated with scleroderma may be exquisitely sensitive to treatment with ACE inhibitors. The specifics of treatment strategies for these disorders are discussed in other chapters.

## MANAGEMENT OF COMPLICATIONS

Metabolic complications such as intravascular volume overload, hyperkalemia, hyperphosphatemia, and metabolic acidosis are almost invariable in oliguric ARF, and preventive measures should be taken from the time of diagnosis (Table 28–18). Prescription of nutrition should be designed to meet caloric requirements and minimize catabolism. In addition, doses of drugs excreted via the kidney must be adjusted for the degree of renal impairment.

After correction of intravascular volume deficits, salt and water intake should be adjusted to match losses (urinary, gastrointestinal, drainage sites, insensible losses). Intravas-

cular volume overload can usually be managed by restriction of salt and water intake and by use of diuretics. Indeed, there is as yet no proven rationale for routine administration of diuretics to patients with ARF other than to treat this complication. High doses of loop diuretics such as furosemide (up to 400 mg intravenously) or bumetanide (up to 10 mg intravenously) may be required in patients who fail to respond to conventional doses. Diuretic therapy should be discontinued in resistant patients to avoid complications such as deafness. Continuous intravenous infusion of low doses of dopamine (2 to 5 µg/kg/min) may promote salt and water excretion by increasing renal blood flow and GFR and inhibiting tubule $Na^+$ reabsorption.[762a] However, the role of dopamine in the management of ARF remains to be definitively established and renal responses are variable under these circumstances.[762a, 762b] Ultrafiltration or dialysis may be required for removal of volume when conservative measures fail. Hyponatremia associated with a fall in effective serum osmolality can usually be corrected by restriction of water intake. Conversely, hypernatremia is treated by administration of water, hypotonic saline solutions, or isotonic dextrose-containing solutions (the latter are effectively hypotonic as dextrose is rapidly metabolized).

Mild hyperkalemia (<5.5 mEq/L) should be managed initially by restriction of dietary potassium intake and elimination of potassium supplements and potassium-sparing diuretics. Moderate hyperkalemia (5.5 to 6.5 mEq/L) in patients without clinical or electrocardiographic evidence of

**TABLE 28–18. Supportive Management of Intrinsic Acute Renal Failure**

| Complication | Treatment |
|---|---|
| Intravascular volume overload | Restriction of salt (1–2 g/d) and water (usually < 1 L/d)<br>Diuretics (usually loop blockers ± thiazide)<br>Ultrafiltration or dialysis |
| Hyponatremia | Restriction of free water intake (oral and dextrose-containing solutions) |
| Hyperkalemia | Restriction of dietary potassium intake<br>Eliminate $K^+$ supplements and $K^+$-sparing diuretics<br>$K^+$-binding ion exchange resins (see text)<br>Glucose (50 mL of 50% dextrose) and insulin (10 U regular)<br>Sodium bicarbonate (usually 50–100 mEq)<br>Calcium gluconate (10 mL of 10% solution over 5 min)<br>Dialysis |
| Metabolic acidosis | Restriction of dietary protein<br>Sodium bicarbonate (maintain serum $HCO_3^-$ > 15 mEq/L)<br>Dialysis |
| Hyperphosphatemia | Restriction of dietary phosphate intake<br>$PO_4^{3-}$-binding agents (calcium carbonate, aluminum hydroxide) |
| Hypocalcemia | Calcium carbonate (if symptomatic or if sodium bicarbonate to be administered)<br>Calcium gluconate (10–20 mL of 10% solution) |
| Hypermagnesemia | Discontinue $Mg^{2+}$-containing antacids |
| Hyperuricemia | Treatment usually not necessary (if < 15 mg/dL) |
| Nutrition | Restriction of dietary protein (~0.5 g/kg/d)<br>Carbohydrate (~100 g/d)<br>Enteral or parenteral nutrition (if recovery prolonged) |
| Drug dosage | Adjust doses for degree of renal impairment |
| Indications for dialysis | Clinical evidence (symptoms or signs) of uremia<br>Intractable intravascular volume overload<br>Hyperkalemia or severe acidosis resistant to conservative measures<br>? Prophylactic dialysis when BUN > 100–150 mg/dL or creatinine > 8–10 mg/dL |

hyperkalemia can usually be controlled by administration of $K^+$-binding ion exchange resins such as sodium polystyrene sulfonate (15 to 30 g every 3 or 4 hours) with sorbitol (50 to 100 mL of 20% solution) by mouth or as a retention enema. Loop diuretics also increase $K^+$ excretion in diuretic-responsive patients. Emergency measures should be employed for patients with serum $K^+$ values greater than 6.5 mEq/L and all patients with electrocardiographic abnor-

malities or clinical features of hyperkalemia. Intravenous insulin (10 U of regular insulin) and glucose (50 mL of 50% dextrose) promote $K^+$ shift into cells within 30 to 60 minutes, a benefit that lasts for several hours. Sodium bicarbonate (1 ampule, 44.6 mEq intravenously over 5 min) also promotes rapid (onset <15 minutes, duration 1 to 2 hours) shift of $K^+$ into the intracellular space. Sodium polysterene sulfonate and sodium bicarbonate have an obligatory sodium load; these compounds should be used judiciously for oliguric patients to avoid intravascular volume overload and life-threatening pulmonary edema. Calcium gluconate (10 mL of 10% solution intravenously over 5 minutes) antagonizes the cardiac and neuromuscular effects of hyperkalemia and is a valuable emergency temporizing measure while other agents reduce serum $K^+$ concentration. Dialysis is indicated if hyperkalemia is resistant to these measures.

Metabolic acidosis does not require treatment unless the serum $HCO_3^-$ concentration falls below 15 mEq/L. More severe acidosis can be corrected by either oral or intravenous bicarbonate administration. Initial rates of replacement should be based on estimates of $HCO_3^-$ deficit and adjusted thereafter according to serum levels. Patients should be monitored for complications of bicarbonate administration including metabolic alkalosis, hypocalcemia, hypokalemia, volume overload, and pulmonary edema. Hyperphosphatemia can usually be controlled by restriction of dietary phosphate intake and oral administration of agents (e.g., aluminum hydroxide or calcium carbonate) that reduce absorption of $PO_4^{3-}$ from the gastrointestinal tract. Hypocalcemia does not usually require treatment unless it is severe, as may occur in patients with rhabdomyolysis or pancreatitis or after administration of bicarbonate. Hyperuricemia is usually mild in ARF (<15 mg/dL) and does not require specific intervention.

Nutritional management in patients with ARF requires close collaboration between physicians, nurses, and dietitians.[582, 763–765a] The objective of dietary modification during the maintenance phase of ARF is to provide sufficient calories to avoid catabolism and starvation ketoacidosis, while minimizing production of nitrogenous waste. This is best achieved by restricting dietary protein intake to protein of high biologic value (i.e., rich in essential amino acids) at approximately 0.5 g/kg/d and providing most calories in the form of carbohydrate (approximately 100 g/d). Management of nutrition is easier in nonoliguric patients and after institution of dialysis. Vigorous parenteral hyperalimentation has been claimed to improve prognosis in ARF; however, a consistent benefit has yet to be demonstrated in this regard.

Anemia may necessitate blood transfusion or administration of recombinant human erythropoietin if severe or if recovery is delayed. Uremic bleeding usually responds to desmopressin, correction of anemia, estrogens, or dialysis.[542, 560] Doses of drugs that are excreted by the kidney must be adjusted for the degree of renal impairment. Regular doses of antacids appear to reduce significantly the incidence of gastrointestinal hemorrhage and may be more potent than histamine $H_2$ antagonists in this regard.[575] Febrile patients must be investigated aggressively for infection and may require treatment with broad-spectrum antibiotics while awaiting identification of specific organisms.

### TABLE 28–19. Dialytic Modalities in Acute Renal Failure

| Modality | Dialyzer | Physical Principle |
|---|---|---|
| **Hemodialysis** | | |
| Conventional | Hemodialyzer | Intermittent diffusive clearance and ultrafiltration (UF) concurrently |
| Sequential ultrafiltration and clearance | Hemodialyzer | Intermittent UF followed by diffusive clearance |
| Continuous arteriovenous hemodialysis (CAVHD) | Hemodialyzer | Slow diffusive clearance and UF concurrently without blood pump |
| Continuous venovenous hemodialysis (CVVHD) | Hemodialyzer | Slow diffusive clearance and UF concurrently with blood pump |
| **Hemofiltration*** | | |
| Continuous arteriovenous hemofiltration (CAVHF) | Hemofilter | Continuous convective clearance without a blood pump |
| Continuous venovenous hemofiltration (CVVHF) | Hemofilter | Continuous convective clearance with a blood pump |
| **Hemodialysis plus hemofiltration†** | | |
| Continuous arteriovenous hemodialysis plus hemofiltration (CAVHDF) | Hemofilter | Continuous convective plus diffusive clearance without a blood pump |
| Continuous venovenous hemodialysis plus hemofiltration (CVVHDH) | Hemofilter | Continuous convective plus diffusive clearance with a blood pump |
| **UF** | | |
| Isolated UF | Hemodialyzer | Intermittent UF alone without diffusive or convective clearance |
| Slow continuous UF (SCUF) | Hemofilter | Continuous arteriovenous (no pump) or venovenous (pump) UF alone without diffusive or convective clearance |
| **Peritoneal dialysis** | | |
| Continuous | Peritoneum | Continuous clearance and UF via exchanges performed at varying intervals |
| Intermittent | Peritoneum | Intermittent clearance and UF via exchanges performed for 10–12 h every 2–3 d |

*Filtrate generated across dialysis membrane is replaced with a physiologic replacement solution

†The most efficient form of continuous dialysis. The use of biocompatible dialysis membranes (e.g., polyacrylonitrile, polysulfone, polymethylmethacrylate) appears to be associated with a shorter maintenance phase of ATN and improved survival when compared with conventional cuprophane or cellulose acetate membranes.[590a, 775a]

Adapted from Owen WF Jr, Lazarus JM: Dialytic management of acute renal failure. *In* Lazarus JM, Brenner BM (eds): Acute Renal Failure, 3rd ed. Churchill Livingstone, New York, 1993, p 495.

---

Meticulous care of intravenous cannulas, Foley catheters, and other invasive devices is mandatory. Unfortunately, prophylactic antibiotics have not been shown to reduce the incidence of infection in these high-risk patients.

### INDICATIONS AND MODALITIES OF DIALYSIS

Dialysis does not appear to hasten recovery in ARF. Initial studies suggesting that early dialysis therapy im-

### TABLE 28–20. Causes of Death in Patients with Acute Renal Failure

| | % of patients | | | |
|---|---|---|---|---|
| | 1956–1959 | 1960–1969 | 1970–1979 | 1980–1989 |
| Underlying disorder | 50.0 | 59.6 | 68.4 | 69.6 |
| Infection | 42.9 | 38.2 | 50.0 | 43.9 |
| Cardiovascular | 20.0 | 22.8 | 19.4 | 36.0 |
| Treatment withdrawn | 5.7 | 5.5 | 13.3 | 15.5 |
| Neurologic | 2.9 | 5.1 | 5.1 | 2.8 |
| Hemorrhage | 5.7 | 5.5 | 4.1 | 2.3 |
| Nonrecovery (renal) | 18.6 | 18.5 | 5.1 | 2.3 |
| Other | | | | 1.0 |

From Finn WF. Recovery from acute renal failure. *In* Lazarus JM, Brenner BM (eds): Acute Renal Failure, 3rd ed. Churchill Livingstone, New York, 1993, p 555.

proved prognosis for patients with ARF have not been confirmed.[766–774] Similarly, it is unclear whether the intensity of dialysis favorably affects outcome. Indeed, hemodialysis may potentially exacerbate renal hypoperfusion, as transient hypotension is a common complication of this treatment modality and leukocytes activated on exposure to dialysis membranes may potentially aggravate ischemic renal injury.[773–775] Along these lines, two randomized controlled trials[775a, 775b] indicate that the maintenance phase of ATN is significantly shorter with use of biocompatible dialysis membranes than with conventional cuprophane or cellulose acetate membranes, probably because of less activation of complement, leukocytes, and other mediator systems. Accordingly, dialysis is reserved for treatment of symptoms or signs of uremia and management of volume overload, hyperkalemia, or acidosis that is refractory to conservative therapy. The type of dialysis (peritoneal dialysis, hemodialysis) and prescription must be individualized for the patient (Table 28–19). Peritoneal dialysis is effected through a temporary intraperitoneal catheter, whereas vascular access for short-term hemodialysis is usually achieved using a double-lumen catheter inserted into the subclavian, internal jugular, or femoral vein.[766] Slow continuous arteriovenous or venovenous hemofiltration or dialysis is an alternative modality for patients who do not tolerate conventional short-term dialysis and in whom peritoneal dialysis is not possible (e.g., after abdominal surgery).[766] An advan-

**TABLE 28–21. Clinical Features, Renal Failure Indices, Morbidity, and Mortality in Patients with Acute Renal Failure: Comparison of Oliguric and Nonoliguric Acute Renal Failure**

| Clinical or Biochemical Parameter | Oliguric Patients (n = 38) | Nonoliguric Patients (n = 54) | P Value |
|---|---|---|---|
| Mean maximal serum creatinine (mg/dL) | $9.0 \pm 0.5$ | $6.0 \pm 0.3$ | <.001 |
| Mean maximal BUN (mg/dL) | $114 \pm 5$ | $95 \pm 5$ | <.02 |
| BUN/serum creatinine > 50/5 mg/dL (d) | $18.0 \pm 2.0$ | $8.0 \pm 0.8$ | <.001 |
| Fractional excretion of $Na^+$ (%) | $6.8 \pm 1.4$ | $3.1 \pm 0.5$ | <.05 |
| Urinary $Na^+$ (mEq/dL) | $68 \pm 6$ | $50 \pm 5$ | <.05 |
| Urinary osmolality (mOsm/kg) | $369 \pm 22$ | $343 \pm 17$ | NS* |
| Urinary BUN/plasma BUN | $3.3 \pm 0.5$ | $7.4 \pm 1.1$ | <.02 |
| Urinary creatinine/plasma creatinine | $16.5 \pm 3.0$ | $17.2 \pm 2.1$ | NS |
| Hospitalization (d) | $31 \pm 3$ | $22 \pm 21$ | <.01 |
| % of patients requiring dialysis | 84 | 28 | <.001 |
| Morbidity (% of patients) | | | |
|   Hyperkalemia | 58 | 46 | NS |
|   Metabolic acidemia | 45 | 20 | <.025 |
|   Neurologic abnormalities | 50 | 30 | <.05 |
|   Septicemia | 42 | 20 | <.05 |
|   Gastrointestinal bleeding | 39 | 19 | <.025 |
|   Pulmonary infiltrates | 34 | 24 | NS |
| Mortality (% of patients) | 50 | 26 | <.05 |

*NS = not significant; d = days.
Adapted with permission from Anderson RJ, Linas SL, Berns AS, et al: Non-oliguric acute renal failure. N Engl J Med 1977; 296:1134–1138. Copyright 1977. Massachusetts Medical Society. All rights reserved.

tage of these newer continuous forms of hemodialysis over conventional intermittent dialysis has yet to be demonstrated. Ultrafiltration of plasma, without dialysis, may be used to treat intractable volume overload in patients without symptomatic uremia. Although most patients recover from ARF, a few (<5%) require long-term renal replacement therapy. With this in mind, every effort should be made to preserve veins (i.e., avoid venipuncture) on the nondominant arm of patients with severe ARF, as these veins may

**TABLE 28–22. Residual Defects in Renal Structure and Function After Acute Renal Failure**

Glomerular abnormalities
  Thickening and/or splitting of glomerular basement membrane
  Glomerular hyalinosis or sclerosis
  Decrease in GFR
  Hyperfiltration through remnant nephrons
  Decrease in inulin clearance
  Elevation in serum creatinine
  Decrease in urea clearance
  Decrease in p-aminohippurate clearance
  Increase in filtration fraction
Tubule abnormalities
  Tubule atrophy
  Interstitial fibrosis
  Decrease in phenolsulfonphthalein excretion
  Concentrating defects
  Urinary acidification defects
Other
  Proteinuria
  Decrease in renal size
  Predisposition to further episodes of ARF
  Occasionally progression to chronic renal failure

Adapted from Finn WF: Recovery from acute renal failure. In Lazarus JM, Brenner BM (eds): Acute Renal Failure, 3rd ed. Churchill Livingstone, New York, 1993, p 553.

be required for chronic hemodialysis access (arteriovenous fistula) at a later date.

## Postrenal Azotemia

Management of postrenal azotemia usually involves a multidisciplinary approach and requires close collaboration among nephrologist, urologist, and radiologist. This topic is reviewed extensively in Chapter 41. Urethral or bladder neck obstruction is usually relieved temporarily by transurethral or suprapubic placement of a bladder catheter, thereby providing a window for identification and treatment of the obstructing lesion. Similarly, ureteric obstruction may be treated initially by percutaneous catheterization of the dilated ureteric pelvis or ureter. Indeed, obstructing lesions can often be removed percutaneously (e.g., calculus, sloughed papilla) or bypassed by insertion of a ureteric stent (e.g., carcinoma). Most patients experience an appropriate diuresis for several days after relief of obstruction; however, approximately 5% develop a transient salt-wasting syndrome, because of delayed recovery of tubule function relative to GFR, that may require intravenous fluid replacement to maintain blood pressure.

## OUTCOME

The mortality rate for acute intrinsic renal azotemia approximates 50% and has changed little in the past three decades[776–795] (Table 28–20). This lack of improvement in outcome, despite significant advances in supportive care, may be more apparent than real and reflect a tendency for more aggressive surgical and medical intervention in an aging population. Mortality rates differ markedly depending on the cause of ARF: approximately 15% in obstetric patients, 30% in toxin-related ARF, and 60% after trauma or major surgery.[776–791] Oliguria (<400 mL/d) at time of presentation before administration of diuretics and a rise in the serum creatinine value of greater than 3 mg/dL are associated with a poor prognosis and probably reflect more severe renal injury and/or underlying disease[3] (Table 28–21). Mortality rates are higher in older debilitated patients and those with multiple organ failure.[794, 795] Indeed, death is almost universal if ARF is associated with failure of more than three other organ systems.[794, 795] With appropriate supportive management of ARF, death is usually a consequence of the primary disease (see Table 28–20) and rarely of a direct complication of uremia per se.

Most patients who survive an episode of ARF recover sufficient renal function to live normal lives. However, 50% have subclinical functional defects in glomerular filtration, tubule solute transport, H+ secretion, and urinary concentrating mechanisms, and glomerular or tubulointerstitial scarring on renal biopsy[796–807] (Table 28–22). ARF is irreversible in approximately 5% of patients, usually as a consequence of complete cortical necrosis, and requires long-term renal replacement therapy with dialysis or transplantation.[796–807] An additional 5% of patients suffer progressive deterioration in renal function after an initial recovery phase, probably because of hyperfiltration and subsequent sclerosis of remnant glomeruli. In addition, experimental animals and humans who experience one episode of ARF are at increased risk of additional episodes of ARF on subsequent exposure to ischemia or nephrotoxins. It is possible that the latter predisposition to acute and chronic renal failure may become increasingly relevant as human life expectancy increases.

# REFERENCES

1. Anderson RJ, Schrier RW: Clinical spectrum of oliguric and non-oliguric acute renal failure. *In* Brenner BM, Stein JH (eds): Acute Renal Failure. Contemporary Issues in Nephrology, Vol 6. Churchill Livingstone, New York, 1980.
2. Hou SH, Bushinsky DA, Wish JB, et al: Hospital acquired renal insufficiency: A prospective study. Am J Med 74:243, 1983.
3. Anderson RJ, Linas SL, Berns AS, et al: Nonoliguric acute renal failure. N Engl J Med 296:1134, 1977.
4. Danovitch G, Carvounis C, Weinstein E, Levenson S: Non-oliguric acute renal failure. J Med Sci 15:5, 1979.
5. Lordon RE, Burton JR: Post-traumatic renal failure in military personnel in Southeast Asia. Am J Med 53:137, 1972.
6. Meyers CD, Roxe DM, Hano JE: The clinical course of nonoliguric acute renal failure. Cardiovasc Med 2:669, 1977.
7. Swann RC, Merrill JP: The clinical course of acute renal failure. Medicine (Baltimore) 32:215, 1953.
8. Vertel RM, Knochel JP: Non-oliguric acute renal failure. JAMA 200:598, 1967.
9. Doolan PD, Alpen EL, Theil GB: A clinical appraisal of the plasma concentration and endogenous clearance of creatinine. Am J Med 32:65, 1962.
10. Bennett WM, Porter GA: Endogenous creatinine clearance as a clinical measure of glomerular filtration rate. Br Med J 4:84, 1971.
11. Hamilton RW, Gardner LB, Penn AS, Goldberg M: Acute tubular necrosis caused by exercise-induced myoglobinuria. Ann Intern Med 77:77, 1972.
12. Jacobsen KF, Christensen CK, Mogensen CE, et al: Pronounced increase in serum creatinine after eating cooked meat. Br Med J 1:1049, 1979.
13. Berglund F, Killander J, Pompeius R: Effect of trimethoprim-sulfamethoxazole on the renal excretion of creatinine in man. J Urol 114:802, 1975.
14. Burgess E, Blair A, Krichman K, Cutler R: Inhibition of renal creatinine by cimetidine in humans. Renal Physiol 5:27, 1982.
15. Dubb JW, Stote RM, Familiar RG, et al: Effect of cimetidine on renal function in normal man. Clin Pharmacol Ther 24:76, 1978.
16. Faloon WW, Downs JJ, Duggan K, Prior JT: Nitrogen and electrolyte metabolism and hepatic function and histology in patients receiving tetracycline. Am J Med Sci 233:563, 1957.
17. Shils ME: Renal disease and metabolic effects of tetracycline. Ann Intern Med 58:389, 1963.
18. Molitch ME, Rodman E, Hirsch CA, Dubinsky E: Spurious serum creatinine elevations in ketoacidosis. Ann Intern Med 93:280, 1980.
19. Saah AJ, Koch TR, Drusano GL: Cefoxitin falsely elevates serum creatinine. JAMA 247:205, 1982.
20. Swain RR, Briggs SL: Positive interference with the Jaffe reaction by cephalosporin. Clin Chem 23:1340, 1977.
21. Lazarus JM, Brenner BM (eds): Acute Renal Failure, 3rd ed. Churchill Livingstone, New York, 1993.
22. Baslov JT, Jorgensen HE: A survey of 499 patients with acute anuric renal insufficiency: Causes, treatment, complications and mortality. Am J Med 34:753, 1963.
23. Kon V, Yared A, Ishikawa I: Role of renal sympathetic nerves in mediating hypoperfusion of renal cortical microcirculation in experimental congestive heart failure and acute extracellular fluid volume depletion. J Clin Invest 76:1913, 1985.
24. Ishikawa I, Pfeffer JM, Pfeffer MA, et al: Role of angiotensin II in the altered renal function of congestive heart failure. Circ Res 55:669, 1984.
25. Posternak L, Brunner HR, Gavras H, Brunner DB: Angiotensin II blockade in normal man: Interaction of renin and sodium in maintaining blood pressure. Kidney Int 11:197, 1977.
26. Aisenberry GA, Handleman WA, Arnold P, et al: Vascular effects of arginine vasopressin during fluid deprivation in the rat. J Clin Invest 67:961, 1981.
27. Badr KF, Ishikawa I: Prerenal failure: A deleterious shift from renal compensation to decompensation. N Engl J Med 319:623, 1988.
28. Arendshorst WJ, Finn WF, Gottschalk CW: Autoregulation of blood flow in the rat kidney. Am J Physiol 228:127, 1975.
29. Baylis C, Brenner BM: Modulation by prostaglandin synthesis inhibitors of the action of exogenous angiotensin II on glomerular ultrafiltration in the rat. Circ Res 43:889, 1978.
30. Dzau VJ, Colucci WS, Williams GH, et al: Prostaglandins in severe congestive heart failure. Relation to activation of the renin-angiotensin system and hyponatremia. N Engl J Med 310:347, 1984.
31. Oliver JA, Sciacci RR, Pinto J, Cannon PJ: Participation of the prostaglandins in the control of renal blood flow during acute reduction of cardiac output in the dog. J Clin Invest 67:229, 1981.
32. Yared A, Kon V, Ichikawa I: Mechanisms of preservation of renal perfusion and filtration during acute extracellular fluid volume depletion. Importance of intrarenal vasopressin-prostaglandin interaction for protecting kidneys from constrictor action of vasopressin. J Clin Invest 75:1477, 1985.
33. Johnston PA, Bernard DB, Perrin NS, et al: Control of the rat renal vascular resistance during alterations in sodium balance. Circ Res 48:728, 1981.
34. Hall JE, Guyton AC, Jackson TE, et al: Control of glomerular filtration rate by the renin-angiotensin system. Am J Physiol 233:F366, 1977.
35. Schor N, Ichikawa I, Brenner BM: Glomerular adaptations to chronic dietary salt restriction or excess. Am J Physiol 238:F428, 1980.
36. Zipsner RD, Hoefs JC, Speekan P, et al: Prostaglandins: Modulators of renal function and pressor resistance in chronic liver disease. J Clin Endocrinol Metab 48:895, 1975.
37. Arisz L, Donker AJM, Brentjens JRH, van der Hem GK: The effect of indomethacin on proteinuria and kidney function in the nephrotic syndrome. Acta Med Scand 199:121, 1976.
38. Kimberly RP, Plotz PH: Aspirin induced depression of renal function. N Engl J Med 296:418, 1977.
39. Berg KJ: Acute effects of acetylsalicylic acid in patients with chronic renal insufficiency. Eur J Clin Pharmacol 11:111, 1977.
40. Brandstetter RD, Mar DD: Reversible oliguric renal failure associated with ibuprofen treatment. Br Med J 2:1194, 1978.
41. Kimberly RP, Gill JR Jr, Bowden RE, et al: Elevated urinary prostaglandins and the effects of aspirin on renal function in lupus erythematosus. Ann Intern Med 89:336, 1978.

42. Kimberly RP, Bowden RE, Keiser HR, Plotz PH: Reduction of renal function by newer nonsteroidal anti-inflammatory drugs. Am J Med 64:804, 1978.
43. Brandstetter RD, Mar DD: Reversible oliguric renal failure associated with ibuprofen treatment. Br Med J 2:1194, 1978.
44. Tan SY, Shapiro R, Kish MA: Reversible acute renal failure induced by indomethacin. JAMA 291:2732, 1979.
45. Walshe JJ, Venuto RC: Acute oliguric renal failure induced by indomethacin: Possible mechanisms. Ann Intern Med 91:47, 1979.
46. Boyer TD, Zia P, Reynolds TB: Effect of indomethacin and prostaglandin A₁ on renal function and plasma renin activity in alcoholic liver disease. Gastroenterology 77:215, 1979.
47. Kimberly RP, Sherman RL, Mouradian J, Lockshin MD: Apparent acute renal failure associated with therapeutic aspirin and ibuprofen administration. Arthritis Rheum 22:281, 1979.
48. Kleinkneeht C, Broyer M, Gubler MC, Palcoux JB: Irreversible renal failure after indomethacin in steroid resistant nephrosis. N Engl J Med 302:691, 1980.
49. Dunn MJ, Zambraski EJ: Renal effects of drugs that inhibit prostaglandin synthesis. Kidney Int 18:609, 1980.
50. O'Meara ME, Eknoyan G: Acute renal failure associated with indomethacin administration. South Med J 73:587, 1980.
51. Fawaz-Estrup F, Ho G Jr: Reversible renal failure induced by indomethacin. Arch Intern Med 141:1670, 1981.
52. Galler M, Folkert VW, Schlondorff D: Reversible acute renal insufficiency and hyperkalemia following indomethacin therapy. JAMA 246:154, 1981.
53. Muther RS, Potter DM, Bennett WM: Aspirin induced depression of glomerular filtration rate in normal humans—role of sodium balance. Ann Intern Med 94:317, 1981.
54. McCarthy JT, Torres VE, Romero JC, et al: Acute intrinsic renal failure induced by indomethacin: Role of prostaglandin synthetase inhibition. Mayo Clin Proc 57:289, 1982.
55. Favre L, Glasson P, Vallotton MB: Reversible acute renal failure from combined triamterene and indomethacin. A study in healthy subjects. Ann Intern Med 96:317, 1982.
56. Cinotti GA, Manzi M, Mene P, et al: Prostaglandin dependence of renal function in chronic glomerular disease. Clin Res 30:445A, 1982.
57. Fong HJ, Cohen AH: Ibuprofen-induced acute renal failure with acute tubular necrosis. Am J Nephrol 2:28, 1982.
58. Levenson DJ, Simmons CE Jr, Brenner BM: Arachidonic acid metabolism, prostaglandins and the kidney. Am J Med 72:354, 1982.
59. Patrono C, Pugliese F, Ciabattoni C, et al: Evidence for a direct stimulatory effect of prostacyclin in renin release in man. J Clin Invest 69:231, 1982.
60. Bunning RD, Barh WF: Sulindac: A potential renal sparing nonsteroidal anti-inflammatory drug. JAMA 248:2864, 1982.
61. Whelton A, Bender W, Vaghaiwalla F, et al: Sulindac and renal impairment. JAMA 249:2892, 1983.
62. Blackshear JL, Davidman M, Stillman MT: Identification of risk for renal insufficiency from non-steroidal anti-inflammatory drugs. Arch Intern Med 143:1130, 1983.
63. Ciabattoni G, Cinotti GA, Pierucci A, et al: Effects of sulindac and ibuprofen in patients with chronic glomerular disease: Evidence for dependence of renal function on prostacyclin. N Engl J Med 310:279, 1984.
64. Clive DM, Stoff JS: Renal syndromes associated with nonsteroidal anti-inflammatory drugs. N Engl J Med 310:563, 1984.
65. Luderer JR, Schoolwerth AC, Sinicrope RA, et al: Acute renal failure, hemolytic anemia and skin rash associated with captopril therapy. Am J Med 71:493, 1981.
66. Kawamura J, Okada Y, Nishibuchi S, Yoshida O: Transient anuria following administration of angiotensin I–converting enzyme inhibitor (SQ 14225) in a patient with renal artery stenosis of the solitary kidney successfully treated with renal autotransplantation. J Urol 127:111, 1982.
67. Colavita RD, Gaudio KM, Siegel NJ: Reversible reduction in renal function during treatment with captopril. Pediatrics 71:839, 1983.
68. Hricik DE, Browning PJ, Kopelman R, et al: Captopril-induced functional renal insufficiency in patients with bilateral renal-artery stenoses or renal-artery stenosis in a solitary kidney. N Engl J Med 308:373, 1983.
69. Chrysant SG, Dunn M, Marples D, Demasters K: Severe reversible azotemia from captopril therapy. Report of three cases and review of the literature. Arch Intern Med 143:437, 1983.
70. Fotino S, Sporn P: Non-oliguric acute renal failure after captopril therapy. Arch Intern Med 143:1252, 1983.
71. Curtis JJ, Luke RG, Whelchel JD, et al: Inhibition of angiotensin-converting enzyme in renal-transplant recipients with hypertension. N Engl J Med 308:377, 1983.
72. Hays R, Aquinu A, Lee BB, et al: Captopril-induced acute renal failure in a kidney transplant recipient. Clin Nephrol 19:320, 1983.
73. Mason JC, Hilton PJ: Reversible renal failure due to captopril in a patient with transplant artery stenosis. Case report. Hypertension 5:623, 1983.
74. Blythe WB: Captopril and renal autoregulation. N Engl J Med 308:390, 1983. Editorial.
75. Steinman TI, Silva P: Acute renal failure, skin rash and eosinophilia associated with captopril therapy. Am J Med 75:154, 1983.
76. Packer M: Why do the kidneys release renin in patients with congestive heart failure? A nephrocentric view of converting enzyme inhibition. Am J Cardiol 60:179, 1987.
77. Rasmussen HH, Ibels LS: Acute renal failure. Multivariate analysis of causes and risk factors. Am J Med 73:211, 1982.
78. Lunding M, Steiness I, Thaysen JH: Acute renal failure due to tubular necrosis. Immediate prognosis and complications. Acta Med Scand 176:103, 1964.
79. Retan JW, Miller RW: Microembolic complications of atherosclerosis: Literature review and report of a patient. Arch Intern Med 118:534, 1966.
80. Thurlbeck WM, Castleman B: Atheromatous emboli to the kidneys after aortic surgery. N Engl J Med 138:1430, 1978.
81. Ramirez G, O'Neill WW Jr, Lambert R, Bloomer A: Cholesterol embolization: A complication of angiography. Arch Intern Med 138:1430, 1978.
82. Harrington JT, Sommers SC, Kassirer JP: Atheromatous emboli with progressive renal failure: Renal anteriography as the possible inciting factor. Ann Intern Med 68:152, 1968.
83. Sieniewicz DJ, Moore S, Moir FD, McDade DF: Atheromatous emboli in the kidneys. Radiology 92:1231, 1969.
84. Handler FD: Clinical and pathologic significance of atheromatous embolization with emphasis on the etiology of renal hypertension. Am J Med 20:366, 1956.
85. Kassirer JP: Atheroembolic renal disease. N Engl J Med 280:812, 1969.
86. Hoxie HJ, Coggins CB: Renal infarction: Statistical study of two hundred and five cases and detailed report of an unusual case. Arch Intern Med 65:587, 1940.
87. Peterson NE, McDonald DF: Renal embolization. J Urol 100:140, 1968.
88. Lessman RK, Johnson SF, Coburn JW, Kaufman JJ: Renal artery embolism: Clinical features and longterm follow-up of 17 cases. Ann Intern Med 89:477, 1978.
89. Llach F, Papper S, Massry SG: The clinical spectrum of renal vein thrombosis: Acute and chronic. Am J Med 69:819, 1980.
90. Llach F: Hypercoagulability, renal vein thrombosis, and other thrombotic complications of nephrotic syndrome. Kidney Int 28:429, 1985.
91. Cohen AH, Wang H, Bider WA, Glassock RJ: Acute renal failure due to acute tubular necrosis in lupus nephritis. Proc Am Soc Nephrol 15:26A, 1982. Abstract.
92. Kincaid-Smith P, Bennett WM, Dowling JP, Ryan GB: Acute renal failure and tubular necrosis associated with hematuria due to glomerulonephritis. Clin Nephrol 19:206, 1983.
92a. Miller PD, Krebs RA, Neal BJ, McIntyre DO: Polyuric prerenal failure. Arch Intern Med 140:907, 1980.
93. McMurray SD, Luft FC, Maxwell DR, et al: Prevailing patterns and predictor variables in patients with acute tubular necrosis. Arch Intern Med 138:950, 1978.
94. Wilkins RG, Faragher EB: Acute renal failure in an intensive care unit: Incidence, prediction and outcome. Anesthesia 38:628, 1983.
95. Abel RM, Buckley MJ, Austen WB, et al: Etiology, incidence and prognosis of renal failure following cardiac operations. Results of a prospective analysis of 500 consecutive patients. J Thorac Cardiovasc Surg 71:323, 1976.
96. Bhat JG, Gluck MC, Lowenstein J, Baldwin DS: Renal failure after open heart surgery. Ann Intern Med 84:677, 1976.
97. Hilberman M, Myers BD, Carrie BJ, et al: Acute renal failure following cardiac surgery. J Thorac Cardiovasc Surg 77:880, 1979.
98. Kron IL, Joob AW, Meter CV: Acute renal failure in the cardiovascular surgical patient. Ann Surg 39:590, 1985.

99. Yeboah ED, Petrie A, Pead JL: Acute renal failure and open heart surgery. Br Med J 1:415, 1972.

100. Myers BD, Moran SM: Hemodynamically mediated acute renal failure. N Engl J Med 314:97, 1986.

101. Abbott WM, Abel RM, Beck CHJ, Fischer JE: Renal failure after ruptured aneurysm. Arch Surg 110:1110, 1975.

102. Gornick CCJ, Kjellstrand CM: Acute renal failure complicating aortic aneurysm surgery. Nephron 35:145, 1983.

103. Myers BD, Miller DC, Mehigan JT, et al: Nature of the renal injury following total renal ischemia in man. J Clin Invest 73:329, 1984.

104. Cameron JS, Miller-Jones CMH: Renal function and renal failure in badly burned children. Br J Surg 54:132, 1967.

105. Clarkson P, Cameron JS: Disturbances of renal function in burned patients. Proc R Soc Med 62:49, 1969.

106. Planas M, Wachtel T, Frank H, Henderson LW: Characterization of acute renal failure in the burned patient. Arch Intern Med 142:2087, 1982.

107. Zager RA: *Escherichia coli* endotoxin injections potentiate experimental ischemic renal injury. Am J Physiol 251:F988, 1986.

108. Zager RA, Prior RB: Gentamicin and gram negative bacteremia. A synergism for the development of experimental nephrotoxic acute renal failure. J Clin Invest 78:196, 1986.

109. Badr KF, Kelley VE, Rennke HG, Brenner BM: Roles for thromboxane A$_2$ and leukotrienes in endotoxin-induced acute renal failure. Kidney Int 30:474, 1986.

110. Stone AM, Stein T, Lafortune J, Wise L: Changes in intrarenal blood flow during sepsis. Surg Gynecol Obstet 148:731, 1979.

111. Auguste LJ, Stone AM, Wise L: The effects of *Escherichia coli* bacteremia on in vitro perfused kidneys. Ann Surg 192:65, 1980.

112. Bourgoignie JJ, Valle GA: Endotoxin and renal dysfunction in liver diseases. *In* Epstein M (ed): The Kidney in Liver Disease, 3rd ed. Williams & Wilkins, Baltimore, 1988, p 486.

113. Bennett WM, Porter GA: Nephrotoxic acute renal failure due to common drugs. Am J Physiol 241:F1, 1981.

114. Canales CO, Smith GH, Robinson JC, et al: Acute renal failure after administration of iopanoic acid. N Engl J Med 281:89, 1969.

115. Weinrauch LA, Healy RW, Leland OS Jr, et al: Coronary angiography and acute renal failure in diabetic azotemic nephropathy. Ann Intern Med 86:56, 1977.

116. Harkonen S, Kjellstrand CM: Exacerbation of diabetic renal failure following intravenous pyelography. Am J Med 63:939, 1977.

117. Vanzee BE, Hoy WE, Talley TE, Jaenike JR: Renal injury associated with intravenous pyelography in nondiabetic and diabetic patients. Ann Intern Med 89:51, 1978.

118. Krumlovsky FA, Simon N, Santhanam S, et al: Acute renal failure: Association with administration of radiographic contrast material. JAMA 239:125, 1978.

119. Swartz RD, Rubin JE, Leeming BW, Silva P: Renal failure following major angiography. Am J Med 65:31, 1978.

120. Harkmen S, Kjellstrand CM: Intravenous pyelography in nonuremic diabetic patients. Nephron 24:268, 1979.

121. Byrd L, Sherman RL: Radiocontrast-induced acute renal failure: A clinical and pathophysiologic review. Medicine (Baltimore) 58:270, 1979.

122. Becker JA: Prevention of radiocontrast induced acute renal failure with mannitol. Lancet 1:1147, 1980. Letter.

123. Old CW, Lehrner LM: Prevention of radiocontrast induced acute renal failure with mannitol. Lancet 1:885, 1980. Letter.

124. Teruel JL, Marcen R, Onaindia JM, et al: Renal function impairment caused by intravenous urography. A prospective study. Arch Intern Med 141:1271, 1981.

125. Lang EK, Foreman J, Schlegel JU, et al: The incidence of contrast medium induced acute tubular necrosis following arteriography. Radiology 138:203, 1981.

126. Anto HR, Chou SY, Porush JG, Shapiro WB: Infusion intravenous pyelography and renal function. Effect of hypertonic mannitol in patients with chronic renal insufficiency. Arch Intern Med 141:1652, 1981.

127. Eisenberg RL, Bank WO, Hedgock MW: Renal failure after major angiography can be avoided with hydration. AJR 136:859, 1981.

128. Talner LB: Does hydration prevent contrast material renal injury? AJR 136:1021, 1981. Editorial.

129. Levitz CS, Friedman EA: Failure of protective measures to prevent contrast media–induced renal failure. Arch Intern Med 142:642, 1982.

130. D'Elia JA, Gleason RE, Alday M, et al: Nephrotoxicity from angiographic contrast material. A prospective study. Am J Med 72:719, 1982.

131. Cramer BC, Parfrey PS, Hutchinson TA, et al: Renal function following infusion of radiologic contrast material. A prospective controlled study. Arch Intern Med 145:87, 1985.

132. Taliercio CP, Vlietstra RE, Fisher LD, Burnett JC: Risks for renal dysfunction with cardiac angiography. Ann Intern Med 104:501, 1986.

133. Davidson CJ, Hlatky M, Morris KG, et al: Cardiovascular and renal toxicity of nonionic radiographic contrast agent after cardiac catheterization. A prospective trial. Ann Intern Med 110:119, 1989.

134. Parfrey PS, Griffiths SM, Barrett BJ, et al: Contrast material–induced renal failure in patients with diabetes mellitus, renal insufficiency or both. N Engl J Med 320:143, 1989.

135. Schwab SJ, Hlatky MA, Pieper KS, et al: Contrast nephrotoxicity: A randomized controlled trial of a nonionic and an ionic radiographic contrast agent. N Engl J Med 320:149, 1989.

136. Schwartz RH, Berdon WE, Wagner HE, et al: Tamm-Horsfall urinary mucoprotein precipitation by urographic contrast agents. Am J Roentgenol 100:698, 1970.

137. Lasser EC: Contrast material-red blood cell reactions. Invest Radiol 8:189, 1973. Editorial.

138. Kleinknecht D, Deloux J, Hornberg JC: Acute renal failure after intravenous urography: Detection of antibodies against contrast media. Clin Nephrol 2:116, 1974.

139. Ziegler TW, Ludens JH, Fanestil DD: Inhibition of active sodium transport by radiographic contrast media. Kidney Int 7:68, 1975.

140. Gelman LM, Rowe JW, Coggins CH: Effects of an angiographic contrast agent on renal function. Cardiovasc Med 4:313, 1978.

141. Fang LS, Sirota RA, Ebert TH, Lichtenstein NS: Low fractional excretion of sodium with contrast media–induced acute renal failure. Arch Intern Med 140:531, 1980.

142. Rao VM, Rao AK, Steiner RM, et al: The effect of ionic and nonionic contrast media on the sickling phenomenon. Radiology 144:291, 1982.

143. Freyria AM, Pinet A, Belleville J, et al: Effects of five different contrast agents on serum complement and calcium levels after excretory urography. J Allergy Clin Immunol 69:397, 1982.

144. Heyman SN, Brezis M, Reubinoff CA, et al: Acute renal failure with selective medullary injury in the rat. J Clin Invest 82:401, 1988.

145. Brezis M, Epstein FH: A closer look at radiocontrast-induced nephropathy. N Engl J Med 320:179, 1989.

146. Margulies KB, Schirger J, Burnett JC Jr: Radiocontrast-induced nephropathy: Current status and future prospects. Int Angiol 11:20, 1991.

147. Heyman SN, Clark BA, Kaiser N, et al: Radiocontrast agents induce endothelin release in vivo and in vitro. J Am Soc Nephrol 3:58, 1992.

148. Clavell AL, Burnett JC: Physiologic and pathophysiologic roles of endothelin in the kidney. Curr Opin Nephrol Hypertens 3:66, 1994.

149. Kon V, Awazu M: Endothelin and cyclosporine nephrotoxicity. Ren Fail 14:345, 1992.

150. Shulman H, Striker G, Deeg HJ, et al: Nephrotoxicity of cyclosporin A after allogeneic marrow transplantation: Glomerular thromboses and tubular injury. N Engl J Med 305:1392, 1981.

151. Hows JM, Palmer S, Want S, et al: Serum levels of cyclosporin A and nephrotoxicity in bone marrow transplant patients. Lancet 1:145, 1981.

152. Klintmalm GBV, Iwatsuki S, Starzl TE: Nephrotoxicity of cyclosporin A in liver and kidney transplant patients. Lancet 1:470, 1981.

153. Starzl TE, Klintmalm GB, Weil R 3rd, et al: Cyclosporin A and steroid therapy in sixty-six cadaver kidney recipients. Surg Gynecol Obstet 153:486, 1981.

154. Klintmalm GB, Klingensmith WC 3rd, Iwatsuki S, et al: $^{99m}$Tc-DTPA and $^{131}$I-hippuran findings in liver transplant recipients treated with cyclosporin A. Radiology 142:199, 1982.

155. Sibley RK, Burchanowski B, Fryd D, Ferguson R: Histopathology of cyclosporin A nephrotoxicity and of acute rejection in cyclosporin A prednisone immunosuppressed renal allograft recipients. Lab Invest 48:77A, 1983.

156. Bennett WM, Pulliam JP: Cyclosporine nephrotoxicity. Ann Intern Med 99:851, 1983.

157. The Canadian Multicentre Transplant Study Group: A randomized clinical trial of cyclosporine in cadaveric renal transplantation. N Engl J Med 309:809, 1983.

158. Neild GH, Reuben R, Hanley RB, et al: Glomerular thrombi in renal allografts associated with cyclosporine treatment. J Clin Pathol 38:253, 1985.
159. VanBuren D, VanBuren CT, Fiechner SM, et al: De novo hemolytic uremic syndrome in renal transplant recipients immunosuppressed with cyclosporine. Surgery 98:54, 1985.
160. Experimental cyclosporine A nephrotoxicity: An international workshop, Basel, April 24–26, 1985. Clin Nephrol (suppl I):S1–S210, 1986.
161. Myers BD: Cyclosporine nephrotoxicity. Kidney Int 30:964, 1986.
162. Jackson NM, Hsu CH, Visscher GE, et al: Alterations in renal structure and function in a rat model of cyclosporine nephrotoxicity. J Pharmacol Exp Ther 242:749, 1987.
163. Mihatsch MJ, Steiner K, Abeywickrama KH, et al: Risk factors for the development of chronic cyclosporine nephrotoxicity. Clin Nephrol 29:165, 1988.
164. Myers B, Sibley R, Newton L, et al: The long-term course of cyclosporine-associated chronic nephropathy. Kidney Int 33:590, 1988.
165. Gary NE, Buzzeo L, Salaki J, Eisinger RP: Gentamicin-associated acute renal failure. Arch Intern Med 136:1101, 1976.
166. Ginsberg DS, Quintanilla A, Levin M: Renal glycosuria due to gentamicin in rabbits. J Infect Dis 134:119, 1976.
167. Keating MJ, Sethi MR, Bodey GP, Samaan NA: Hypocalcemia with hypoparathyroidism and renal tubular dysfunction associated with aminoglycoside therapy. Cancer 39:1410, 1977.
168. Bennett WM, Plamp C, Reger K, et al: The concentrating defect in experimental gentamicin nephrotoxicity. Clin Res 26:540A, 1978. Abstract.
169. Bennett WM, Plamp CE, Gilbert DN, et al: The influence of dosage regimen on experimental gentamicin nephrotoxicity: Dissociation of peak serum levels from renal failure. J Infect Dis 140:576, 1979.
170. Plamp CE, Roger K, Bennett WM, et al: Vasopressin resistant polyuria in gentamicin nephrotoxicity. Clin Res 26:151A, 1979. Abstract.
171. Patel R, Savage A: Symptomatic hypomagnesemia associated with gentamicin therapy. Nephron 23:50, 1979.
172. Cronin RE, Bulger RE, Southern P, et al: Natural history of aminoglycoside nephrotoxicity in the dog. J Lab Clin Med 95:463, 1980.
173. Russo JC, Adelman RD: Gentamicin-induced Fanconi syndrome. J Pediatr 96:151, 1980.
174. Keys TF, Kurtz SB, Jones JD, Muller SM: Renal toxicity during therapy with gentamicin or tobramycin. Mayo Clin Proc 56:556, 1981.
175. Smith P, Guntupalli J, Eby B, et al: Evidence that gentamicin produces tubular wastage of K⁺ and Mg⁺⁺ independent of reduced GFR and aldosterone. Clin Res 29:475A, 1981. Abstract.
176. Humes HD, Weinberg JM, Knauss TC: Clinical and pathophysiological aspects of aminoglycoside nephrotoxicity. Am J Kidney Dis 2:5, 1982.
177. Schentag JJ, Cerra FB, Plaut ME: Clinical and pharmacokinetic characteristics of aminoglycoside nephrotoxicity in 201 critically ill patients. Antimicrob Agents Chemother 21:721, 1982.
178. Safirstein R, Miller P, Kahn T: Cortical and papillary absorptive defects in gentamicin nephrotoxicity. Kidney Int 24:526, 1983.
179. Edson RS, Keys TF: The aminoglycosides. Streptomycin, kanamycin, gentamicin, tobramycin, amikacin, netilmicin, sisomicin. Mayo Clin Proc 58:99, 1983.
180. Bennett WM, Hartnett MN, Gilbert D, et al: Effect of sodium intake on gentamicin nephrotoxicity in the rat. Proc Soc Exp Biol Med 151:736, 1976.
181. Riviere JE: A possible mechanism for increased susceptibility to aminoglycoside nephrotoxicity in chronic renal disease. N Engl J Med 307:252, 1982.
182. Browning MC, Hsu CY, Wang PL, Tune BM: Interaction of ischemic and antibiotic-induced injury in the rabbit kidney. J Infect Dis 147:341, 1983.
183. Zager RA, Sharma HM: Gentamicin increases renal susceptibility to an acute ischemic insult. J Lab Clin Med 101:670, 1983.
184. Moore RD, Smith CR, Lipsky JJ, et al: Risk factors for nephrotoxicity in patients treated with aminoglycosides. Ann Intern Med 100:352, 1984.
185. Fabre J, Rudhardt M, Blanchard P, Regamey C: Persistence of sisomicin and gentamicin in renal cortex and medulla compared with other organs and serum of rats. Kidney Int 10:444, 1976.
186. Houghton DC, Hartnett MN, Campbell-Boswell M, et al: A light and electron microscopic analysis of gentamicin nephrotoxicity in rats. Am J Pathol 82:589, 1976.

187. Luft FC, Yum MN, Walker PD, et al: Gentamicin gradient patterns and morphological change in human kidneys. Nephron 18:167, 1977.
188. Baylis C, Rennke HG, Brenner BM: Mechanisms of the defect in glomerular ultrafiltration associated with gentamicin administration. Kidney Int 12:344, 1977.
189. Kaloyanides GJ, Pastoriza-Munor E: Aminoglycoside nephrotoxicity. Kidney Int 18:571, 1980.
190. Schentag JJ, Plaut ME, Cerra FB: Comparative nephrotoxicity of gentamicin and tobramycin: Pharmacokinetic and clinical studies in 201 patients. Antimicrob Agents Chemother 19:859, 1981.
191. Fong IW, Fenton RS, Bird R: Comparative toxicity of gentamicin versus tobramycin. A randomized prospective study. J Antimicrob Chemother 7:81, 1981.
192. Schor N, Ichikawa I, Rennke HG, et al: Pathophysiology of altered glomerular function in aminoglycoside treated rats. Kidney Int 19:288, 1981.
193. Lipsky JJ, Lietman PS: Aminoglycoside inhibition of a renal phosphatidylinositol phospholipase C. J Pharmacol Exp Ther 220:287, 1982.
194. Feldman S, Wang MY, Kaloyanides GJ: Aminoglycosides induce a phospholipidosis in the renal cortex of the rat: An early manifestation of nephrotoxicity. J Pharmacol Exp Ther 220:514, 1982.
195. Hostetler KY, Hall LB: Inhibition of kidney lysosomal phospholipases A and C by aminoglycoside antibiotics: Possible mechanism of aminoglycoside toxicity. Proc Natl Acad Sci USA 79:1663, 1982.
196. Lipsky JJ, Lietman PS: Aminoglycoside inhibition of a renal phosphatidylinositol phospholipase C. J Pharmacol Exp Ther 220:287, 1982.
197. Luft FC, Aronoff GR, Evan AP, et al: The renin-angiotensin system in aminoglycoside-induced acute renal failure. J Pharmacol Exp Ther 220:433, 1982.
198. Matzke GR, Lucarotti RL, Shapiro HS: Controlled comparison of gentamicin and tobramycin nephrotoxicity. Am J Nephrol 3:11, 1983.
199. Neugarten J, Aynedjian HS, Bank N: Role of tubular obstruction in acute renal failure due to gentamicin. Kidney Int 24:330, 1983.
200. Prins JM, Buller HR, Kuijper EG, et al: Once versus thrice daily gentamicin in patients with serious infections. Lancet 341:35, 1993.
201. Gilbert DM: Once-daily aminoglycoside therapy. Antimicrob Agents Chemother 35:399, 1991.
202. Mattie H, Craig WA, Pechere JC: Determinants of efficacy and toxicity of aminoglycosides. J Antimicrob Chemother 24:291, 1989.
203. Butler WT, Bennett JE, Alling DW, et al: Nephrotoxicity of amphotericin B: Early and late effects in 81 patients. Ann Intern Med 61:175, 1964.
204. Olivero JJ, Lozano-Mendez J, Ghafary EM, et al: Mitigation of amphotericin B nephrotoxicity by mannitol. Br J Med 1:550, 1975.
205. Gerkens JF, Branch RA: The influence of sodium status and furosemide on canine acute amphotericin B nephrotoxicity. J Pharmacol Exp Ther 214:306, 1980.
206. Heideman HT, Gerkens JF, Spickard WA, et al: Amphotericin nephrotoxicity decreased by salt repletion. Am J Med 75:476, 1983.
207. Dismukes WE, Stamm AM, Graybill JR, et al: Treatment of systemic mycoses with ketoconazole: Emphasis on toxicity and clinical response in 52 patients. National Institute of Allergy and Infectious Diseases Collaborative Antifungal Study. Ann Intern Med 98:13, 1983.
208. Brezis M, Rosen S, Silva P, et al: Polyene toxicity in renal medulla: Injury mediated by transport activity. Science 224:66, 1984.
209. Swan SK, Bennett WM: Nephrotoxic acute renal failure. In Brenner BM, Lazarus JM (eds): Acute Renal Failure, 3rd ed. Churchill Livingstone, New York, 1993, p 357.
210. Brigden D, Rosling AE, Woods NC: Renal function after acyclovir intravenous injection. Am J Med 73(suppl 1A):182, 1982.
211. Kenney RF, Kirk LE, Brigden D: Acyclovir tolerance in humans. Am J Med 73(suppl 1A):171, 1982.
212. Peterslund NA, Beach FT, Tauris T: Impaired renal function after bolus injections of acyclovir. Lancet 1:243, 1983.
213. Spiegel D, Lau K: Acute renal failure and coma secondary to acyclovir therapy. JAMA 255:1882, 1986. Letter.
214. Sawyer MH, Webb DF, Balow JE, Strauss SE: Acyclovir-induced renal failure: Clinical course and histology. Am J Med 84:1067, 1988.
215. Giustma A, Romanelli G, Cimino A, Brunon G: Low dose acyclovir and acute renal failure. Ann Intern Med 108:312, 1988. Letter.

216. Sands M, Kron M, Brown R: Pentamidine: A review. Rev Infect Dis 7:625, 1985.
217. Andersen R, Boedicker M, Ma M, et al: Adverse reactions associated with pentamidine isethionate in AIDS patients. Recommendations for monitoring therapy. Drug Intell Clin Pharmacol 20:862, 1986.
218. Lachaal M, Venuto R: Nephrotoxicity and hyperkalemia in patients with AIDS treated with pentamidine. Am J Med 87:260, 1989.
219. Chapelon C, Raguin G, DeGennes C: Renal insufficiency with nebulised pentamidine. Lancet 2:1045, 1989. Letter.
220. Miller RF, Delaney S, Semple SJ: Acute renal failure after nebulised pentamidine. Lancet 1:1271, 1989. Letter.
221. Cacoub P, Deray G, Baumelou A, et al: Acute renal failure induced by foscarnet: 4 cases. Clin Nephrol 29:315, 1988.
222. Ringden O, Lonnquist B, Paulin T, et al: Pharmacokinetics, safety and preliminary clinical experiences using foscarnet in the treatment of CMV infections in bone marrow and renal transplant recipients. J Antimicrob Chemother 17:373, 1986.
223. Deray G, Martinez F, Katlama C, et al: Foscarnet nephrotoxicity: Mechanism, incidence and prevention. Am J Nephrol 9:316, 1989.
224. Deray G, Katlama C, Dohin E: Prevention of foscarnet nephrotoxicity. Ann Intern Med 113:332, 1990. Letter.
225. Farese RV, Schambelan M, Hollander H, et al: Nephrogenic diabetes insipidus associated with foscarnet treatment of cytomegalovirus retinitis. Ann Intern Med 112:955, 1990.
226. Beaufils H, Deray G, Katlama C, et al: Foscarnet and crystals in glomerular capillary lumens. Lancet 336:755, 1990. Letter.
227. Safirstein R, Winston J, Golstein M, et al: Cisplatin nephrotoxicity. Am J Kidney Dis 8:356, 1986.
228. Hannemann J, Baumann K: Nephrotoxicity of cisplatin, carboplatin, and transplatin. Arch Toxicol 64:393, 1990.
229. Brady HR, Kone BC, Stromski ME, et al: Mitochondrial injury: An early event in cisplatin toxicity to renal proximal tubules. Am J Physiol 258:F1181, 1990.
230. Brady HR, Zeidel ML, Kone BC, et al: Differential actions of cisplatin on renal proximal tubule and inner medullary collecting duct cells. J Pharmacol Exp Ther 265:1421, 1993.
231. Smeitink J, Verreussel M, Schroder C, Lippens R: Nephrotoxicity associated with ifosfamide. Eur J Pediatr 148:164, 1988.
232. Patterson WP, Khojasteh A: Ifosfamide-induced renal tubular defects. Cancer 63:649, 1989.
233. Skinner R, Pearson A, Price L, et al: Nephrotoxicity after ifosfamide. Arch Dis Child 65:132, 1990.
234. Bywaters EGL, Beall D: Crush injuries with impairment of renal function. Br Med J 1:427, 1941.
235. Perri GC, Gorini P: Uraemia in the rabbit after injection of crystalline myoglobin. Br J Exp Pathol 33:440, 1952.
236. Finckh ES: Experimental acute tubular necrosis following subcutaneous injection of glycerol. J Pathol 73:69, 1957.
237. Perkoff GT, Dioso MM, Bleisch V, Klinkerfuss G: A spectrum of myopathy associated with alcoholism. 1. Clinical and laboratory features. Ann Intern Med 67:481, 1967.
238. Braun SR, Weiss FR, Keller AI, et al: Evaluation of the renal toxicity of heme proteins and their derivatives: A role in genesis of acute tubular necrosis. J Exp Med 131:443, 1970.
239. Richter RW, Challenor YB, Pearson J, et al: Acute myoglobinuria associated with heroin addiction. JAMA 216:1172, 1971.
240. Penn AS, Rowland LP, Fraser DW: Drugs, coma and myoglobinuria. Arch Neurol 26:336, 1972.
241. Knochel JP, Schlein EM: On the mechanism of rhabdomyolysis in potassium depletion. J Clin Invest 51:1750, 1972.
242. Grossman RA, Hamilton RW, Morse BM, et al: Nontraumatic rhabdomyolysis and acute renal failure. N Engl J Med 291:807, 1974.
243. Hibrawi H, Blaker RG: Improved estimation of urinary myoglobin by counterimmunoelectrophoresis, as compared with double immunodiffusion technique. Clin Chem 21:765, 1975.
244. Koffler A, Friedler RM, Massry SG: Acute renal failure due to nontraumatic rhabdomyolysis. Ann Intern Med 85:23, 1976.
245. Mason J, Olbricht C, Takabatake T, Thurau K: The early phase of experimental acute renal failure. I. Intratubular pressure and obstruction. Pflugers Arch 370:155, 1977.
246. Knochel JP, Barcenas C, Cotton JR, et al: Hypophosphatemia and rhabdomyolysis. J Clin Invest 62:1240, 1978.
247. Eneas JF, Schoenfeld PY, Humphreys MH: The effect of infusion of mannitol–sodium bicarbonate on the clinical course of myoglobinuria. Arch Intern Med 139:801, 1979.
248. Chugh KS, Nath IVS, Ubroi HS, et al: Acute renal failure due to non-traumatic rhabdomyolysis. Postgrad Med J 55:386, 1979.
249. Garcia G, Snider T, Feldman C, Clyne DH: Nephrotoxicity of myoglobin in the rat: Relative importance of urine pH and prior dehydration. Kidney Int 19:200, 1981. Abstract.
250. Knochel JP: Rhabdomyolysis and myoglobinuria. Semin Nephrol 1:75, 1981.
251. Gabow PA, Kaehn WP, Kelleher SP: The spectrum of rhabdomyolysis. Medicine (Baltimore) 61:141, 1982.
252. Honda N, Kurokawa K: Acute renal failure and rhabdomyolysis. Kidney Int 23:888, 1983.
253. Saltissi D, Parfrey PS, Curtis JR, et al: Rhabdomyolysis and acute renal failure in chronic alcoholics with myopathy, unrelated to acute alcohol ingestion. Clin Nephrol 21:294, 1984.
254. Ron D, Traitelman U, Michaelson M, et al: Prevention of acute renal failure in traumatic rhabdomyolysis. Arch Intern Med 144:277, 1984.
255. Roth D, Alarcon FJ, Fernandez JA, et al: Acute rhabdomyolysis associated with cocaine intoxication. N Engl J Med 319:673, 1988.
256. Lowenstein J, Faulstick DA, Yiengst MJ, Shock NW: The glomerular clearance and renal transport of hemoglobin in adult males. J Clin Invest 40:1172, 1961.
257. Jaenike JR: The renal lesion associated with hemoglobinemia. 1. Its production and functional evolution in the rat. J Exp Med 123:523, 1966.
258. Edwards DH, Griffith TM, Rylev HC, Hendersen AH: Haptoglobin-hemoglobin complex in human plasma inhibits endothelium-dependent relaxation: Evidence that endothelium-derived relaxing factor acts as a local autocoid. Cardiovasc Res 20:549, 1986.
259. Flamenbaum W, Dubrow A: Acute renal failure associated with myoglobinuria and hemoglobinuria. In Brenner BM, Lazarus JM (eds): Acute Renal Failure, 2nd ed. Churchill Livingstone, New York, 1988, p 351.
260. Zager RA, Gamelin LM: Pathogenetic mechanisms in experimental hemoglobinuric acute renal failure. Am J Physiol 256:F446, 1989.
261. Zager RA, Foerder CA: Effects of inorganic iron and myoglobin on in vitro proximal tubule lipid peroxidation and cytoxicity. J Clin Invest 89:989, 1992.
262. Border WA, Cohen AH: Renal biopsy diagnosis of clinically silent multiple myeloma. Ann Intern Med 93:283, 1983.
263. Booth LJ, Minielly JA, Smith EKM: Acute renal failure in multiple myeloma. Can Med Assoc J 111:334, 1974.
264. Healy JK: Acute oliguric renal failure associated with multiple myeloma. Br Med J 1:1126, 1964.
265. Kjeldsberg CR, Holman RE: Acute renal failure in multiple myeloma. J Urol 105:21, 1971.
266. Bardana EJ, Bennett WM, Porter GA: Multiple myeloma presenting as acute renal failure. Problems encountered in diagnosis. Northwest Med 67:965, 1968.
267. Smolens P, Venkatachalam M, Stein JH: Myeloma kidney cast nephropathy in a rat model of multiple myeloma. Kidney Int 24:192, 1983.
268. Cohen DJ, Sherman WH, Osserman EF, Appel GB: Acute renal failure in patients with multiple myeloma. Am J Med 76:247, 1984.
269. Lazarus HM, Adelstein DJ, Herzig RH, Smith MC: Long-term survival of patients with multiple myeloma and acute renal failure at presentation. Am J Kidney Dis 2:521, 1983.
270. Sanders PW, Booker BB: Pathobiology of cast nephropathy from human Bence Jones proteins. J Clin Invest 89:630, 1992.
271. Conger JD, Falk SA, Guggenheim SJ, Burke TJ: A micropuncture study of the early phase of acute urate nephropathy. J Clin Invest 58:681, 1976.
272. Conger JD, Falk SA: Intrarenal dynamics in the pathogenesis and prevention of acute urate nephropathy. J Clin Invest 59:786, 1977.
273. Warren DJ, Leitch AG, Leggett RJ: Hyperuricaemic acute renal failure after epileptic seizures. Lancet 2:385, 1975.
274. Kelton J, Kelley WN, Holms EW: A rapid method of diagnosis of acute uric acid nephropathy. Arch Intern Med 138:612, 1978.
275. Conger JD: Acute uric acid nephropathy. Semin Nephrol 1:69, 1981.
276. Robinson RR, Yarger WE: Acute uric acid nephropathy. Arch Intern Med 137:839, 1977. Editorial.
277. Lins LE: Reversible renal failure caused by hypercalcemia. A retrospective study. Acta Med Scand 203:309, 1978.
278. Humes HD, Ichikawa I, Troy JL, Brenner BM: Evidence for parathyroid hormone–dependent influence of calcium as the glomerular ultrafiltration coefficient. J Clin Invest 61:32, 1978.

279. Fems R, Kashgarian M, Levitan H, et al: Renal tubular acidosis and renal potassium wasting acquired as a result of hypercalcemic nephropathy. N Engl J Med 265:924, 1961.
280. Benabe JE, Martinez-Maldonado M: Hypercalcemic nephropathy. Arch Intern Med 138:777, 1978.
281. Ganote CE, Philipsborn DS, Chen E, et al: Acute calcium nephrotoxicity: An electron microscopical and semiquantitative light microscopical study. Arch Pathol Lab Med 99:650, 1975.
282. Tsokos GC, Balow JE, Spiegel RJ, Magrath IT, et al: Renal and metabolic complications of undifferentiated and lymphoblastic lymphomas. Medicine (Baltimore) 60:218, 1981.
283. Cohen LE, Balow JE, Magrath IT, et al: Acute tumor lysis syndrome: A review of 37 patients with Burkitt's lymphoma. Am J Med 68:486, 1980.
284. Kaplan BS, Hebert D, Morrell RE: Acute renal failure induced by hyperphosphatemia in acute lymphoblastic leukemia. Can Med Assoc J 124:429, 1981.
285. Ettinger DS, Harker WG, Gerry HW, et al: Hyperphosphatemia hypocalcemia and transient renal failure: Result of cytotoxic treatment of acute lymphoblastic leukemia. JAMA 239:2472, 1978.
286. Kanfer A, Roland J, Chatelet RF, Richet G: Hyperphosphatemic acute renal failure following therapy of lymphosarcoma. Kidney Int 15:450A, 1979.
287. Boles JM, Putel JL, Briere J, et al: Acute renal failure caused by extreme hyperphosphatemia after chemotherapy of an acute lymphoblastic leukemia. Cancer 53:2425, 1984.
288. Webster D, Zager RA, Resnick M: Black urinary granules and hyperphosphatemic renal failure. Ann Intern Med 99:283, 1983.
289. Hobbs JR, Evans DJ, Wrong GM: Renal tubular obstruction by microproteins from adenocarcinoma of the pancreas. Br Med J 2:87, 1974.
290. Berman LB, Schreiner GE, Feys J: The nephrotoxic lesion of ethylene glycol. Ann Intern Med 46:611, 1957.
291. Friedman EA, Greenberg JB, Merrill JP, Dammin GJ: Consequences of ethylene glycol poisoning. Report of four cases and review of the literature. Am J Med 32:891, 1962.
292. Wacker WEC, Haynes H, Druyan R, et al: Treatment of ethylene glycol poisoning with ethyl alcohol. JAMA 194:173, 1965.
293. Gilboa N, Largent JA, Unzar RE: Primary oxalosis presenting as anuric renal failure in infancy: Diagnosis by x-ray diffraction of kidney tissue. J Pediatr 103:88, 1983.
294. Ehlers SM, Posalaky Z, Strate RG, Quattlebaum FW: Acute reversible renal failure following jejunoileal bypass for morbid obesity: A clinical and pathological (EM) study of a case. Surgery 82:629, 1977.
295. Mandell I, Krauss E, Milian JC: Oxalate-induced acute renal failure in Crohn's disease. Am J Med 69:628, 1980.
296. Frommer JP, Ayus JC: Acute ethylene glycol intoxication. Am J Nephrol 2:1, 1982.
297. Gabow PA, Clay K, Sullivan JB, Lepoff R: Organic acids in ethylene glycol intoxication. Ann Intern Med 105:16, 1986.
298. Lucke B: Lower nephron nephrosis. (The renal lesions of the crush syndrome of burns, transfusion, and other conditions affecting the lower segments of the nephron.) Mil Surg 99:371, 1946.
299. Oliver J, MacDowell M, Tracy A: The pathogenesis of acute renal failure associated with traumatic and toxic injury. Renal ischemia, nephrotic damage and the ischemuric episode. J Clin Invest 30:1307, 1951.
300. Bohle A, Jahnecke J, Meyer D, Schubert GE: Morphology of acute renal failure: Comparative data from biopsy and autopsy. Kidney Int 10:S9, 1976.
301. Dunnill MS: A review of the pathology and pathogenesis of acute renal failure due to acute tubular necrosis. J Clin Invest 27:2, 1974.
302. Solez K, Morel-Maroger L, Straer JD: The morphology of "acute tubular necrosis" in man: Analysis of 57 renal biopsies and a comparison with glycerol model. Medicine (Baltimore) 58:362, 1979.
303. Jones DB: Ultrastructure of human acute renal failure. Lab Invest 46:254, 1982.
304. Solez K: The morphology of acute renal failure in acute renal failure. In Lazarus JM, Brenner BM (eds): Acute Renal Failure, 3rd ed. Churchill Livingstone, New York, 1993, p 33.
305. Racusen LC, Fivush BA, Li Y-L, et al: Dissociation of tubular cell detachment and tubular cell death in clinical and experimental "acute tubular necrosis." Lab Invest 64:546, 1991.
306. Racusen LC: Alterations in tubular epithelial cell adhesion and mechanisms of acute renal failure. Lab Invest 67:158, 1992.
307. Venkatachalam MA, Bernard DB, Donohoe JF, Levinsky NG: Ischemic damage and repair in the rat proximal tubule. Differences among $S_1$, $S_2$ and $S_3$ segments. Kidney Int 14:13, 1978.
308. Olsen TS, Hansen HE: Ultrastructure of medullary tubules in ischemic acute tubular necrosis and interstitial nephritis in man. APMIS 98:1139, 1990.
309. Gailit J, Colflesh D, Rabiner I, et al: Redistribution and dysfunction of integrins in cultured renal epithelial cells exposed to oxidative stress. Am J Physiol 264:F149, 1993.
310. Goligorsky MS, Lieberthal W, Racusen LC, Simon EE: Integrin receptors in renal tubular epithelium: New insights into pathophysiology of acute renal failure. Am J Physiol 264:F1, 1993. Editorial.
311. Goligorsky MS, DiBona GF: Pathogenetic role of Arg-Gly-Asp–recognizing integrins in acute renal failure. Proc Natl Acad Sci USA 90:5700, 1993.
312. Schriener GE, Maher JF: Toxic nephropathy. Am J Med 38:409, 1965.
313. Humes HD, Weinberg JM, Knauss TC: Clinical and pathophysiologic aspects of aminoglycoside nephrotoxicity. Am J Kidney Dis 2:5, 1983.
314. Kreisberg JI, Bulger RE, Trump GF, Nagle RB: Effects of transient hypotension on the structure and function of rat kidney. Virchows Arch 22:121, 1976.
315. Dobyan DC, Nagle RB, Bulger RE: Acute tubular necrosis in the rat kidney following sustained hypotension. Lab Invest 36:411, 1977.
316. Zager RA: Partial aortic ligation: A hypoperfusion model of ischemic acute renal failure and a comparison with renal artery occlusion. J Lab Clin Med 110:396, 1987.
317. Donohoe JF, Venkatachalam MA, Bernard DB, Levinsky NG: Tubular leakage and obstruction in acute ischemic renal failure. Kidney Int 13:208, 1978.
318. Lieberthal W, Rennke HG, Sandock KM, et al: Ischemia in the isolated erythrocyte-perfused rat kidney. Protective effect of hypothermia. Renal Physiol Biochem 11:60, 1988.
319. Kellerman PS, Clark RAF, Linas SL, Molitoris BA: Role of microfilaments in maintenance of proximal tubule structural and functional integrity. Am J Physiol 259:F279, 1990.
320. Alcorn D, Emslie KR, Ross BD, et al: Selective distal nephron damage during isolated kidney perfusion. Kidney Int 19:638, 1981.
321. Brezis M, Rosen S, Silva P, Epstein FH: Selective vulnerability of the medullary thick ascending limb to anoxia in the isolated perfused rat kidney. J Clin Invest 73:182, 1984.
322. Endre ZH, Ratcliffe PJ, Tange JD, et al: Erythrocytes alter the pattern of renal hypoxic injury: Predominance of proximal tubular injury with moderate hypoxia. Clin Sci 76:19, 1989.
323. Brezis M, Rosen S, Spokes K, et al: Transport-dependent anoxic cell injury in the isolated perfused rat kidney. Am J Pathol 116:327, 1984.
324. Kashgarian M, Siegel NJ, Ries AL, et al: Hemodynamic aspects in development and recovery phases of experimental postischemic acute renal failure. Kidney Int 10:S160, 1976.
325. Axelsen RA, Cartwright VE: Renal function, cortical blood flow and morphometry in ischaemic acute renal failure in the rat. Pathology 11:629, 1979.
326. Finn WF, Chevalier RL: Recovery from postischemic acute renal failure in the rat. Kidney Int 16:113, 1979.
327. Brun C, Crone C, Davidsen HG, et al: Renal blood flow in anuric human subject determined by use of radioactive krypton. Proc Soc Exp Biol Med 89:687, 1955.
328. Reubi FC, Vorburger C: Renal hemodynamics in acute renal failure after shock in man. Kidney Int 10:S137, 1976.
329. Daugharty TM, Ueki IF, Mercer PF, Brenner BM: Dynamics of glomerular ultrafiltration in the rat. V. Response to ischemic injury. J Clin Invest 53:105, 1974.
330. Williams RH, Thomas CE, Navar LG, Evan AP: Hemodynamic and single nephron function. Kidney Int 19:503, 1981.
331. Levy MN, Imperial ES: Oxygen shunting in renal cortical and medullary capillaries. Am J Physiol 200:159, 1961.
332. Leichtweiss H-P, Lubbers DW, Weiss C, et al: The oxygen supply of the rat kidney: Measurement of the intra-renal $pO_2$. Pflugers Arch 309:328, 1969.
333. Vetterlein F, Petho A, Schmidt G: Distribution of capillary blood flow in rat kidney during postischemic renal failure. Am J Physiol 251:H510, 1986.
334. Hellberg POA, Kallskog O, Wolgast M: Red cell trapping and post-

ischemic renal blood flow. Differences between the cortex, outer and inner medulla. Kidney Int 40:625, 1991.

335. Mason J: The pathophysiology of ischemic acute renal failure. A new hypothesis about the initiation phase. Renal Physiol 9:129, 1986.

336. Kon V, Yuoshioka T, Fogo A, Ichikawa I: Glomerular actions of endothelin in vivo. J Clin Invest 83:1762, 1989.

337. Chan L, Chittinandana A, Shapiro JI, et al: Effect of an endothelin-receptor antagonist on ischemic acute renal failure. Am J Physiol 266:F135, 1994.

338. Lieberthal W, Wolf EF, Rennke HG, et al: Renal ischemia and reperfusion impair endothelium-dependent vascular relaxation. Am J Physiol 256:F894, 1989.

339. Hellbert POA, Bayati A, Kallskog O, Wolgast M: Red cell trapping after ischemia and long-term kidney damage. Influence of hematocrit. Kidney Int 37:1240, 1990.

340. Beck F, Thurau K, Getraunthaler G: Pathophysiology and pathobiochemistry of acute renal failure. In Soldin DW, Giebisch G (eds): The Kidney: Physiology and Pathophysiology, 2nd ed. Raven Press, New York, 1992, p 3157.

341. Collins D, Klotman PE: Renin-angiotensin system and arachidonic acid metabolites in acute renal failure. In Lazarus JM, Brenner BM (eds): Acute Renal Failure, 3rd ed. Churchill Livingstone, New York, 1993, p 53.

342. Eisenbach GM, Steinhausen M: Micropuncture studies after temporary ischemia of rat kidneys. Pflugers Arch 343:11, 1973.

343. Tanner GA, Sloan KL, Sophasan S: Effects of renal artery occlusion on kidney function in the rat. Kidney Int 4:377, 1973.

344. Arendshorst WJ, Finn WF, Gottschalk CW: Pathogenesis of acute renal failure following temporary renal ischemia in the rat. Circ Res 37:558, 1975.

345. Tanner GA, Steinhausen M: Tubular obstruction in ischemia-induced acute renal failure in the rat. Kidney Int 10:S65, 1976.

346. Moran SM, Myers BD: Pathophysiology of protracted acute renal failure in man. J Clin Invest 76:1440, 1985.

347. Myers BD, Moran SM: Hemodynamically mediated acute renal failure. N Engl J Med 314:97, 1986.

348. Molitoris BA: Cellular basis of ischemic acute renal failure. In Lazarus JM, Brenner BM (eds): Acute Renal Failure, 3rd ed. Churchill-Livingstone, New York, 1993, p 1.

349. Bonventre JV: Mechanisms of ischemic acute renal failure. Kidney Int 43:1160, 1993.

350. Weinberg JM: The cell biology of ischemic renal injury. Kidney Int 39:476, 1991.

351. Siegel NJ, Glazier WB, Chaudry IH, et al: Enhanced recovery from acute renal failure by the postischemic infusion of adenine nucleotides and magnesium chloride in rats. Kidney Int 17:338, 1980.

352. Andrews PM, Coffey AK: Protection of kidney from acute renal failure resulting from normothermic ischemia. Lab Invest 49:87, 1983.

353. Gaudio KM, Ardito TA, Reilly HF, et al: Accelerated cellular recovery after an ischemic renal injury. Am J Pathol 112:338, 1983.

354. Sumpio BE, Chaudry IH, Clemens MG, Baue AE: Accelerated functional recovery of isolated rat kidney with ATP-MgCl$_2$ after warm ischemia. Am J Physiol 247:R1047, 1984.

355. Stomski ME, Cooper K, Thulin G, et al: Postischemic ATP-MgCl$_2$ provides precursors for resynthesis of cellular ATP in rats. Am J Physiol 250:F834, 1986.

356. Van Waarde A, Stromski ME, Thulin G, et al: Protection of the kidney against ischemic injury by inhibition of 5'-nucleotidase. Am J Physiol 256:F298, 1989.

357. Linshaw MA, MacAlister T, Welling LW: Importance of the cytoskeleton in stabilizing cell volume of proximal convoluted tubules. Kidney Int 37:226, 1990. Abstract.

358. Humes HD, Weinberg JM: Alterations of renal tubular cell metabolism in acute renal failure. Miner Electrolyte Metab 9:290, 1983.

359. Snowdowne KW, Freudenrich C, Borle AB: The effects of anoxia on cytosolic free calcium, calcium fluxes, and cellular ATP levels in cultured kidney cells. Am J Physiol 260:11619, 1985.

360. McCoy CE, Selvaggio AM, Alexander EA, Schwartz JH: Adenosine triphosphate depletion induced a rise in cytosolic free calcium in canine renal epithelial cells. J Clin Invest 82:1326, 1988.

361. Levi M, Molitoris BA, Burke TJ, et al: Effects of vitamin D–induced chronic hypercalcemia on rat renal cortical plasma membranes and mitochondria. Am J Physiol 252:F267, 1987.

362. Brezis M, Shina A, Kidroni G, et al: Calcium and hypoxic injury in the renal medulla of the perfused rat kidney. Kidney Int 34:186, 1988.

363. Takano T, Soltoff SP, Murdaugh S, Mande LJ: Intracellular respiratory dysfunction and cell injury in short-term anoxia of rabbits renal proximal tubules. J Clin Invest 76:2377, 1985.

364. Wilson PD, Schrier RW: Nephron segment and calcium as determinants of anoxic cell death in renal cultures. Kidney Int 29:1172, 1986.

365. Goldfarb D, Iaina A, Serban I, et al: Beneficial effect of verapamil in ischemic acute renal failure in the rat. Proc Soc Exp Biol Med 172:389, 1983.

366. Burke TJ, Arnold PE, Gordon JA, et al: Protective effect of intrarenal calcium membrane blockers before or after renal ischemia. Functional, morphological, and mitrochondrial studies. J Clin Invest 74:1830, 1984.

367. Schwertschlag U, Schrier RW, Wilson P: Beneficial effects of calcium channel blockers and calmodulin binding drugs on in vitro renal cell anoxia. J Pharmacol Exp Ther 238:119, 1986.

368. Wagner K, Albrecht S, Neumayer H-H: Prevention of posttransplant acute tubular necrosis by the calcium antagonist diltiazem: A prospective randomized study. Am J Nephrol 7:287, 1987.

369. Lieberthal W, Levinsky NG: Treatment of acute tubular necrosis. Semin Nephrol 10:571, 1990.

370. Hochachka PW, Mommsen TP: Protons and anaerobiosis. Science 219:1391, 1983.

371. Pentilla A, Trump BF: Extracellular acidosis protects Ehrlich ascites tumor cells and rat renal cortex against anoxic injury. Science 185:277, 1974.

372. Bore PJ, Sehr PA, Chan L, et al: The importance of pH in renal preservation. Transplant Proc 3:707, 1981.

373. Shanley PF, Shapiro JI, Chan L, et al: Acidosis and hypoxic medullary injury in the isolated perfused kidney. Kidney Int 34:791, 1988.

374. Weinberg JM: Oxygen deprivation–induced injury to isolated rabbit kidney tubules. J Clin Invest 76:1193, 1985.

375. Trachuk VA, Menshikov MY: Effect of pH on calcium binding properties of calmodulin and on its interaction with Ca$^{2+}$-dependent cyclic nucleotide phosphodiesterase. Biokhimia 46:965, 1981.

376. Chien KR, Abrams J, Serroni A, et al: Accelerated phospholipid degradation and associated membrane dysfunction in irreversible, ischemic liver cell injury. J Biol Chem 253:4809, 1978.

377. Chien KR, Reeves JP, Buja CM, et al: Phospholipid alterations in canine ischemic myocardium. Circ Res 48:711, 1981.

378. Matthys E, Patel Y, Kreisberg J, et al: Lipid alterations induced by renal ischemia: Pathogenic factor in membrane damage. Kidney Int 26:153, 1984.

379. Nemenoff RA, Winitz S, Qian N-X, et al: Phosphorylation and activation of a high molecular weight form of phospholipase A$_2$ by p42 microtubule-associated protein 2 kinase and protein kinase C. J Biol Chem 268:1960, 1993.

380. Gronich JH, Bonventre JV, Nemenoff RA: Purification of a high molecular mass phospholipase A$_2$ from rat kidney activated at physiological calcium concentrations. Biochem J 271:37, 1990.

381. Nakamura H, Nemenoff RA, Gronich JH, Bonventre JV: Subcellular characteristics of phospholipase A$_2$ activity in rat kidney. Enhanced cytosolic, mitochondrial, and microsomal phospholipase A$_2$ enzymatic activity after renal ischemia and reperfusion. J Clin Invest 87:1810, 1990.

382. Hazen SL, Stuppy RJ, Gross RW: Purification and characterization of canine myocardial cystosolic phospholipase A$_2$. A calcium-independent phospholipase with absolute sn-2 regiospecificity for diradylglycerophopholipids. J Biol Chem 265:10622, 1990.

383. Hirashima Y, Mills JS, Yates AJ, Horrocks LA: Phospholipase A$_2$ activities with a plasmalogen substrate in brain and in neural tumor cells: A sensitive and specific assay using pyrenesulfonyl-labeled plasmenylethanolamine. Biochim Biophys Acta 1047:35, 1990.

384. Portilla D, Shah SV, Lehman PA, Creer MH: Role of cytosolic calcium-independent plasmalogen-selective phospholipase A$_2$ in hypoxic injury to rabbit proximal tubules. J Clin Invest 93:1609, 1994.

385. Molitoris BA, Simon FR: Renal cortical brush border and basolateral membranes: Cholesterol and phospholipid composition and relative turnover. J Membr Biol 83:207, 1985.

386. Sheridan AM, Schwartz JH, Kroshian VM, et al: Renal mouse proximal tubular cells are more susceptible than MDCK cells to chemical anoxia. Am J Physiol 265:F342, 1993.

387. Nguyen VD, Cieslinski DA, Humes HD: Importance of adenosine triphosphate in phospholipase $A_2$-induced rabbit renal proximal tubule injury. J Clin Invest 82:1098, 1988.

388. Weinberg JM, Humes HD: Calcium transport and inner mitochondrial membrane damage in renal cortical mitochondria. Am J Physiol 248:F876, 1985.

389. Pfeiffer DR, Schmid PC, Beatrice MC, Schmid HMO: Intramitochondrial phospholipase activity and the effects of $Ca^{2+}$ plus N-ethylmaleimide on mitochondrial function. J Biol Chem 254:11485, 1979.

390. Cistola DP, Hamilton JA, Jackson D, Small DM: Ionization and phase behavior of fatty acids in water: Application of the Gibbs phase rule. Biochemistry 27:1881, 1988.

391. Suzuki K, Imajoh S, Emori Y, et al: Calcium-activated neutral protease and its endogenous inhibitor activation at the cell membrane and biological function. FEBS Lett 220:271, 1987.

392. Mellgren RL: Calcium-dependent proteases: An enzyme system active at cellular membranes. FASEB J 1:110, 1987.

393. Cong J, Goll DE, Peterson AM, Kapprell H-P: The role of autolysis in activity of the $Ca^{2+}$-dependent proteinases ($\mu$-calpain and m-calpain). J Biol Chem 264:10096, 1989.

394. Edelstein CL, Wieder ED, Gengaro PE, et al: The role of cysteine proteases in hypoxia induced renal proximal tubular injury. Clin Res 42:220A, 1994. Abstract.

395. Hreniuk D, Guerra E, Wilson PD: A common final pathway of renal tubule cell killing by toxins and anoxia (AN): Attenuation by protease inhibition. Kidney Int 35:408, 1989. Abstract.

396. Ichikawa I, Kiyama S, Yoshioka T: Renal antioxidant enzymes: Their regulation and function. Kidney Int 45:1, 1994.

397. Davies KJA, Lin SW, Pacific RE: Protein damage and degradation by oxygen radicals. IV. Degradation of denatured proteins. J Biol Chem 262:9914, 1987.

398. Aruoma OI, Halliwells B, Dizdaroglus M: Iron ion–dependent modification of bases in DNA by the superoxide radical–generating system hypoxanthine/xanthine oxidase. J Biol Chem 264:13024, 1989.

399. Schraufstatter IU, Hyslop PA, Hinshaw DB: Hydrogen peroxide–induced injury of cells and its prevention by inhibitors of poly(ADP-ribose) polymerase. Proc Natl Acad Sci USA 83:4908, 1986.

400. McCord JM: Oxygen-derived free radicals in postischemic tissue injury. N Engl J Med 312:159, 1985.

401. Granger DN: Role of xanthine oxidase and granulocytes in ischemia-reperfusion injury. Am J Physiol 255:H1269, 1988.

402. Joannidis M, Bonn G, Pfaller W: Lipid peroxidation—an initial event in experimental acute renal failure. Renal Physiol Biochem 12:47, 1989.

403. Paller MS, Hoidal JR, Ferris TF: Oxygen free radicals in ischemic acute renal ischemia. J Clin Invest 74:1156, 1984.

404. Paller MS, Hebbel RP: Ethane production as a measure of lipid peroxidation after renal ischemia. Am J Physiol 251:F839, 1986.

405. McCoy RN, Hillk KE, Ayonk MA: Oxidant stress following renal ischemia: Changes in the glutathione redox ratio. Kidney Int 33:812, 1988.

406. Linas SL, Shanley PF, White CW: $O_2$ metabolite–mediated injury in perfused kidney is reflected by consumption of DMTU and glutathione. Am J Physiol 253:F692, 1987.

407. Paller MS, Hedlund BE, Sikora JJ: Role of iron in postischemic renal injury in the rat. Kidney Int 34:474, 1988.

408. Das DK, Engleman RM, Clement R: Role for xanthine oxidase inhibitor as free radical scavenger: A novel mechanism of action of allopurinol and oxypurinol in myocardial salvage. Biochem Biophys Res Commun 148:314, 1987.

409. Hansson R, Jonsson O, Lundstam S: Effects of free radical scavengers on renal circulation after ischaemia in the rabbit. Clin Sci 65:605, 1983.

410. Baker GL, Corry RJ, Autor AP: Oxygen free radical induced damage in kidneys subjected to warm ischemia and reperfusion. Ann Surg 202:628, 1985.

411. Bayati A, Hellberg O, Odlind B: Prevention of ischaemic acute renal failure with superoxide dismutase and sucrose. Acta Physiol Scand 130:367, 1987.

412. Ouriel KI, Smedira NG, Ricott JJ: Protection of the kidney after temporary ischemia: Free radical scavengers. J Vasc Surg 2:49–53, 1985.

413. Vasko KA, Dewall RA, Riley AM: Effect of allopurinol in renal ischemia. Surgery 71:787, 1972.

414. Kedar I, Jacob ET, Bar-Natan N, Ravid M: Dimethyl sulfoxide in acute ischemia of the kidney. Ann N Y Acad Sci 411:131, 1983.

415. Paller MS, Sikora JJ: Renal work, glutathione and susceptibility to free radical–mediated postischemic injury. Kidney Int 33:843, 1988.

416. Linas SL, Whittenburg D, Repine JE: Role of xanthine oxidase in ischemia/reperfusion injury. Am J Physiol 258:F711, 1990.

417. Greene EL, Paller MS: Calcium and free radicals in hypoxia/reoxygenation injury of renal epithelial cells. Am J Physiol 266:F13, 1994.

418. Paller MS, Neumann TV: Reactive oxygen species and rat renal epithelial cells during hypoxia and reoxygenation. Kidney Int 40:1041, 1991.

419. Gamelin LM, Zager RA: Evidence against oxidant injury in a critical mediator of postischemic acute renal failure. Am J Physiol 257:F114, 1991.

420. Borkan SC, Schwartz JH: Role of oxygen free radical species in in vitro models of proximal tubular ischemia. Am J Physiol 257:F114, 1989.

421. Zager RA, Gmur DJ: Effect of xanthine oxidase inhibition on ischemic acute renal failure in the rat. Am J Physiol 257:F953, 1989.

422. Joannidis M, Gstraunthaler G, Pfaller W: Evidence against a causative role in renal reperfusion injury. Am J Physiol 258:F232, 1990.

423. Doctor RB, Mandel LJ: Minimal role of xanthine oxidase in cellular injury in isolated rat proximal tubules during anoxia and reoxygenation. Kidney Int 37:480, 1990.

424. Toled-Pereyra JH, Simmons RL, Olson LC: Clinical effect of allopurinol on preserved kidneys: A randomized double-blind study. Ann Surg 185:128, 1977.

425. Schneeberger H, Illner WD, Abendroth D: First clinical experiences with superoxide disumutase in kidney transplantation—results of a double-blind randomized study. Transplant Proc 21:1245, 1989.

426. Grum CM, Gallagher KP, Kirsh MM, Shlafer M: Absence of detectable xanthine oxidase in human myocardium. J Mol Cell Cardiol 21:263, 1989.

427. Engerson TD, McKelvey TG, Rhyne DB: Conversion of xanthine dehydrogenase to oxidase in ischemic rat tissue. J Clin Invest 79:1564, 1987.

428. Hellberg POA, Kallskog TOK: Neutrophil-mediated post-ischemic tubular leakage in the rat kidney. Kidney Int 36:555, 1989.

429. Klausner JM, Paterson IS, Goldman G: Postischemic renal injury is mediated by neutrophils and leukotrienes. Am J Physiol 256:F794, 1989.

430. Hellberg POA, Kallskog O, Wolgost M, Ojteg A: Effects of neutrophil granulocytes on the inulin barrier of renal tubular epithelium after ischemic damage. Acta Physiol Scand 134:313, 1988.

431. Paller MS: Effect of neutrophil depletion on ischemic injury in the rat. J Lab Clin Med 113:379, 1989.

432. Brady HR: Leukocyte adhesion molecules and kidney diseases. Kidney Int 45:1285, 1994.

433. Thornton MN, Winn R, Alpers CE, Zager R: An evaluation of neutrophils as a mediator of in vivo ischemia in renal injury. Am J Pathol 135:509, 1989.

434. Kelly KJ, Williams WW Jr, Colvin RB, Bonventre JV: Antibody to intercellular adhesion molecule 1 protects the kidney against ischemic injury. Proc Natl Acad Sci USA 91:812, 1994.

435. Molitoris BA: Ischemia-induced loss of epithelial polarity: Potential role of the actin cytoskeleton. Am J Physiol 260:F769, 1991.

436. Kellerman PS, Clark RAF, Hoilien CA, et al: Role of microfilaments in the maintenance of proximal tubule structural and functional integrity. Am J Physiol 259:F279, 1990.

437. Canfield PE, Geerdes AE, Molitoris BA: Effect of reversible ATP depletion on tight junction integrity. Am J Physiol 261:F1038, 1991.

438. Molitoris BA, Geerdes AE, McIntosh JR: Dissociation and redistribution of $Na^+,K^+$-ATPase from its surface membrane actin cytoskeleton complex during cellular ATP depletion. J Clin Invest 88:462, 1991.

439. Bershadsky AD, Gelfand VI: Role of ATP in the regulation of stability of cytoskeletal structures. Cell Biol Int Rep 7:173, 1983.

440. Sanger JW, Sanger JM: Differential response of three types of actin filament bundles to depletion of cellular ATP levels. Eur J Cell Biol 31:197, 1983.

441. Kroshian VM, Sheridan AM, Lieberthal W: Functional and cytoskeletal changes induced by sublethal injury in epithelial cells. Am J Physiol 266:F21, 1994.

442. Hinshaw DB, Armstrong BC, Beals TF, Hyslop PA: A cellular model of endothelial cell ischemia. J Surg Res 44:527, 1988.

443. Kellerman PS, Bogusky RT: Microfilament disruption occurs very early in ischemic proximal tubular cell injury. Kidney Int 42:896, 1992.

444. Racusen LC: Alterations in human proximal tubule cell attachment in response to hypoxia: Role of microfilaments. J Lab Clin Med 123:357, 1994.

445. Molitoris BA, Dahl RH, Falk SA: Ischemic-induced loss of epithelial polarity. Role of the tight junction. J Clin Invest 1334: 1339, 1984.

446. Molitoris BA, Hoilin CA, Dahl RH, et al: Characterization of ischemia-induced loss of epithelial polarity. J Membr Biol 106:233, 1988.

447. Molitoris BA, Dahl R, Geerdes A: Cytoskeleton disruption and apical redistribution of proximal tubule Na$^+$-K$^+$-ATPase during ischemia. Am J Physiol 263:F488, 1992.

448. Molitoris BA: Na$^+$-K$^+$-ATPase that redistributes to apical membrane during ATP depletion remains functional. Am J Physiol 265:F693, 1993.

449. Molitoris BA, Chan LK, Shapiro JL, et al: Loss of epithelial polarity: A novel hypothesis for reduced proximal tubule Na$^+$ transport following ischemic injury. J Membr Biol 107:119, 1989.

450. Spiegel DM, Wilson PD, Molitoris BA: Epithelial polarity following ischemia: A requirement for normal cell function. Am J Physiol 256:F430, 1989.

451. Kroshian VM, Tannatt D, Lieberthal W: Sublethal injury to renal epithelial cells causes abnormal but reversible cell-cell interactions. Clin Res 42:220A, 1994. Abstract.

452. Mandal AK, Sklar AH, Hudson JB: Transmission electron microscopy of urinary sediment in human acute renal failure. Kidney Int 28:58, 1985.

453. Graber M, Lane B, Lamia R, Pastoriza-Munox E: Bubble cells: Renal tubular cells in the urinary sediment with characteristics of viability. J Am Soc Nephrol 1:999, 1991.

454. Racusen LC, Fivush BA, Li YL, et al: Dissociation of tubular cell detachment and tubular cell death in clinical and experimental "acute tubular necrosis." Lab Invest 64:546, 1991.

455. Safirstein R: Gene expression in nephrotoxic and ischemic acute renal failure. J Am Soc Nephrol 4:1387, 1994.

456. Ouellete AJ, Malt RA, Sukhatme VP, Bonventre JV: Expression of two immediate early genes, Egr-1 and c-fos, in response to renal ischemia and during renal hypertrophy in mice. J Clin Invest 85:776, 1990.

457. Safirstein R, Price PM, Saggi SJ, Harris RC: Changes in gene expression after temporary renal ischemia. Kidney Int 37:1515, 1990.

458. Rosenberg ME, Paller MS: Differential gene expression in the recovery from ischemic renal injury. Kidney Int 39:1156, 1991.

459. Humes HD, Cieslinski DA, Coimbra T, et al: Epidermal growth factor enhances renal tubule cell regeneration and repair and accelerates the recovery of renal function in postischemic acute renal failure. J Clin Invest 84:1757, 1989.

460. Reiss R, Cieslinski DA, Humes HD: Transforming growth factor-alpha accelerates renal repair and recovery following ischemic injury. Kidney Int 37:492, 1990.

461. Miller SB, Martin DR, Kissane J, Hammerman MR: Insulin-like growth factor I accelerates recovery from ischemic acute tubular necrosis in the rat. Proc Natl Acad Sci USA 89:11876, 1992.

462. Bull GM, Joekes AM, Lowe KG: Renal function studies in acute tubular necrosis. Clin Sci 9:379, 1950.

463. Kirkland K, Edwards KDG, Whyte HM: Oliguric renal failure: A report of 400 cases including the classification, survival and response to dialysis. Aust Ann Med 14:275, 1965.

464. Platts MM: Electrolyte excretion in uremia. Clin Sci 30:453, 1966.

465. Ward EE, Richards P, Wrong OM: Urine concentration after acute renal failure. Nephron 3:289, 1966.

466. Hall JW, Johnson WI, Maher FT, Hunt IC: Immediate and longterm prognosis in acute renal failure. Ann Intern Med 73:515, 1970.

467. Siegler RL, Bloomer HA: Acute renal failure with prolonged oliguria. An account of five cases. JAMA 225:133, 1973.

468. Belizon IJ, Chou S, Porush JG, et al: Recovery without a diuresis after protracted acute tubular necrosis. Arch Intern Med 140:133, 1980.

469. Baek S, Makabali GG, Shoemaker WC: Clinical determinants of survival from post-operative acute renal failure. Surg Gynecol Obstet 140:685, 1975.

470. Loughridge LW, Milne MD, Shackman R, Wootton IDP: Clinical course of uncomplicated acute tubular necrosis. Lancet 1:351, 1960.

471. Yarger WE, Buerket J: Effect of urinary tract obstruction on renal tubular function. Semin Nephrol 2:17, 1982.

472. Chung HM, Kluge R, Schrier RW, Anderson RJ: Clinical assessment of extracellular fluid in hyponatremia. Am J Med 83:905, 1987.

473. Alano FA Jr, Webster GD Jr: Acute renal failure and pigmentation due to phenazopyridine (Pyridium). Ann Intern Med 72:89, 1970.

474. Chesney RW, Chesney PJ, Davis JP, Segar WT: Renal manifestation of the staphylococcal toxic shock syndrome. Am J Med 71:583, 1981.

475. Shah GM, Winer RL: Reversible acute renal failure after jejunoileal bypass for obesity. South Med J 74:1535, 1981.

476. Zsigmond GL, Verrier E, Way LW: Sudden reversal of renal failure after take-down of a jejunoileal bypass. Report of a case involving hemorrhagic proctocolitis, and renal and hepatic failure late after jejunoileal bypass for obesity. Am J Gastroenterol 77:216, 1982.

477. Levinsky NG, Alexander EA, Venkatachalam MA: Acute renal failure. In Brenner BM, Rector FC Jr (eds): The Kidney, 2nd ed. WB Saunders, Philadelphia, 1981, p 1185.

478. Riggs SA, Minuth AN, Nottebohm GA, et al: Plasma cells in urine, occurrence in multiple myeloma. Arch Intern Med 135:1245, 1975.

479. Corwin HL, Korbet SM, Schwartz MM: Clinical correlates of eosinophiluria. Arch Intern Med 145:1097, 1985.

480. Nolan CR, Anger MS, Kelleher SP: Eosinophiluria—a new method for detection and definition of the clinical spectrum. N Engl J Med 315:1516, 1986.

481. Witten DM, Myers GH Jr, Utz DC: Emmett's Clinical Urography. WB Saunders, Philadelphia, 1977.

482. Ellenbogen PH, Scheible FW, Talner LB, Leopold GR: Sensitivity of grey scale ultrasound in detecting urinary tract obstruction. AJR 130:731, 1978.

483. Rascoff JH, Golden RA, Spinowitz BS, Charytan C: Non-dilated obstructive uropathy. Arch Intern Med 143:696, 1983.

484. Pollack HM, Banner MP: Commentary: Percutaneous nephrostomy and related pyelo-ureteral manipulative techniques. Urol Radiol 2:147, 1981.

485. Vandenbroucke JM, Gibeaux JP, van Ypersele de Strihou C: Excretion urography in acute renal failure. Br Med J 4:291, 1973.

486. Sherwood T, Doyle FH, Boultan-Jones M, et al: The intravenous urogram in acute renal failure. Br J Radiol 43:368, 1974.

487. Sherman RA, Byun KJ: Nuclear medicine in acute and chronic renal failure. Semin Nucl Med 12:265, 1982.

488. Espinel, CH: The FE$_{Na}$ test: Use in the differential diagnosis of acute renal failure. JAMA 236:579, 1976.

489. Miller TR, Anderson RJ, Linas SL, et al: Urinary diagnostic indices in acute renal failure: A prospective study. Ann Intern Med 89:47, 1978.

490. Baldus WP, Feichter RN, Summerskill WH: The kidney in cirrhosis. 1. Clinical and biochemical features of azotemia in hepatic failure. Ann Intern Med 60:353, 1964.

491. Vencl RM, Knochel JP: Non-oliguric acute renal failure. JAMA 200:598, 1967.

492. Counahan R, Cameron JS, Ogg CS, et al: Presentation, management, complications, and outcome of acute renal failure in childhood: Five years' experience. Br Med J 1:599, 1977.

493. Danovitch G, Carvounis C, Weinstein E, Levenson S: Non-oliguric acute renal failure. Isr J Med Sci 15:5, 1979.

494. Fang LST, Sirota RA, Ebert TH, Lichenstein NS: Low fractional excretion of sodium with contrast media–induced acute renal failure. Arch Intern Med 140:531, 1980.

495. Oken DE: On the differential diagnosis of acute renal failure. Am J Med 71:916, 1981.

496. Planas M, Wachtel T, Frank H, Henderson LW: Characterization of acute renal failure in the burned patient. Arch Intern Med 142:2087, 1982.

497. Diamond IR, Yoburn DC: Nonoliguric acute renal failure associated with a low fractional excretion of sodium. Ann Intern Med 96:597, 1982.

498. Steiner RW: Low fractional excretion of sodium in myoglobinuric acute renal failure. Arch Intern Med 142:1216, 1982.

499. Vaz AJ: Low fractional excretion of urine sodium in acute renal failure due to sepsis. Arch Intern Med 143:738, 1983.

500. Corwin HL, Schreiber MJ, Fang LST: Low fractional excretion of sodium. Occurrence with hemoglobinuric and myoglobinuric acute renal failure. Arch Intern Med 144:981, 1984.

501. Zarich S, Fang LST, Diamond JR: Fractional excretion of sodium. Exceptions to its diagnostic value. Arch Intern Med 145:108, 1985.

502. Nanji AJ: Increased fractional excretion of sodium in prerenal azotemia: Need for careful interpretation. Clin Chem 27:1314, 1981.

503. Sporn IN, Lancestremere RG, Papper S: Differential diagnosis of oliguria in aged patients. N Engl J Med 267:130, 1961.
504. Hilton PJ, Barraclough MA, Jones NF, Lloyd-Davies RW: Urinary osmolality in acute renal failure due to glomerulonephritis. Lancet 2:655, 1969.
505. Chugh KS, Singhal PC, Kher VK, et al: Spectrum of acute cortical necrosis in Indian patients. Am J Med Sci 286:10, 1983.
506. Lindheimer MD, Katz AI, Ganeval D, Grunfeld J-P: Acute renal failure in pregnancy. In Lazarus JM, Brenner BM (eds): Acute Renal Failure, 3rd ed. Churchill Livingstone, New York, 1993, p 417.
507. Grunfeld JP, Ganeval D, Bournerias F: Acute renal failure in pregnancy. Kidney Int 18:179, 1980.
508. Conger JD, Falk SA, Guggenheim SJ: Glomerular dynamics and morphologic changes in the generalized Shwartzman reaction in postpartum rats. J Clin Invest 67:1334, 1981.
509. Ferris TF, Weir EK: Effect of captopril on uterine blood flow and prostaglandin E synthesis in the pregnant rabbit. J Clin Invest 71:809, 1983.
510. Davies MH, Wilkinson SP, Hanid MA, et al: Acute liver disease with encephalopathy and renal failure in late pregnancy and the early puerperium: A study of fourteen patients. Br J Obstet Gynaecol 87:1005, 1980.
511. D'Elia FL, Brenner RE, Brownstein PK: Acute renal failure secondary to ureteral obstruction by a gravid uterus. J Urol 128:803, 1982.
512. Hayslett JP: Postpartum renal failure. N Engl J Med 312:1556, 1985.
513. Ramos EL, Ravenscraft MD: Acute renal failure in renal transplantation. In Lazarus JM, Brenner BM (eds): Acute Renal Failure, 3rd ed. Churchill Livingstone, New York, 1993, p 441.
514. Zager RA, O'Quigley J, Zager BK, et al: Acute renal failure following bone marrow transplantation: A retrospective study of 272 patients. Am J Kidney Dis 13:210–216, 1989.
515. Mathay RA, Bromberg SI, Putman CE: Pulmonary renal syndromes: A review. Yale J Biol Med 53:497, 1980.
516. Levine JS, Lieberthal W, Bernard DB, Salant J: Acute renal failure associated with renal vascular disease, vasculitis, glomerulonephritis and nephrotic syndrome. In Lazarus JM, Brenner BM (eds): Acute Renal Failure, 3rd ed. Churchill Livingstone, New York, 1993, p 247.
517. Epstein M (ed): The Kidney in Liver Disease, 3rd ed. Williams & Wilkins, Baltimore, 1988.
518. Wilkinson SP, Davies MH, Portmann B, Williams R: Renal failure in otherwise uncomplicated acute viral hepatitis: Report of 12 cases. Br J Med 2:338, 1978.
519. Better OS: Acute renal failure complicating obstructive jaundice. In Lazarus JM, Brenner BM (eds): Acute Renal Failure. Churchill Livingstone, New York, 1980, p 108.
520. Rosansky SJ, Mullens CC: The hepatorenal syndrome associated with metastatic angiosarcoma of the gallbladder. Ann Intern Med 96:191, 1980.
521. Epstein M, Oster JR, de Velasco RE: Hepatorenal syndrome following hepatectomy. Clin Nephrol 5:128, 1976.
522. Said SI, Hirose, T., Kitamura S, Siegel SR: Vasoactive intestinal peptide (VIP): Mediator of hemodynamic and respiratory changes in cirrhosis? J Clin Invest 50:80a, 1971.
523. Fischer JE, Baldessarini RJ: False neurotransmitters and hepatic failure. Lancet 2:75, 1971.
524. Bloom DS, McCalden TA, Rosendorff C: Effects of jaundiced plasma on vascular sensitivity to noradrenaline. Kidney Int 8:149, 1975.
525. Schroeder ET, Anderson GH, Goldman SH, Streeten DD: Effect of blockade of angiotensin II on blood pressure renin and aldosterone in cirrhosis. Kidney Int 9:511, 1976.
526. Wong PT, Tolamo RC, Williams GH: Kallikrein-kinin and renin-angiotensin systems in functional renal failure and cirrhosis of the liver. Gastroenterology 73:1114, 1977.
527. Bichet D, Szatalowicz V, Chaimovitz C, Schrier RW: Role of vasopressin in abnormal water excretion in cirrhotic patients. Ann Intern Med 96:413, 1982.
528. Bichet DG, Van Putten VJ, Schrier RW: Potential role of increased sympathetic activity in impaired sodium and water excretion in cirrhotic patients. N Engl J Med 307:1552, 1982.
529. Unikowsky B, Wexler MJ, Levy M: Dogs with experimental cirrhosis of the liver but without intrahepatic hypertension do not retain sodium or form ascites. J Clin Invest 72:1594, 1983.
530. Zipser RD, Radvan GH, Kronborg IJ et al: Urinary thromboxane B and prostaglandin E in the hepatorenal syndrome: Evidence for increased vasoconstrictor and decreased vasodilator factors. Gastroenterology 84:697, 1983.
531. Levinsky NG, Bernard DB: The LeVeen shunt. In Isselbacher KJ, Braunwald E, Wilson JD, et al (eds): Update II, Harrison's Principles of Internal Medicine. McGraw-Hill, New York, 1982, p 147.
532. Epstein M: Peritoneovenous shunt in the management of ascites and the hepatorenal syndrome. Gastroenterology 82:790, 1982.
533. Smadja C, Franco D: The LeVeen shunt in the elective treatment of ascites in cirrhosis. A prospective study of 140 patients. Ann Surg 201:488, 1985.
534. Wilkinson SP, Weston MJ, Parsons V: Dialysis in the treatment of renal failure in patients with liver disease. Clin Nephrol 8:287, 1977.
535. Wilkinson SP, Hirst D, Day DW, Williams R: The spectrum of renal tubular damage in renal failure secondary to cirrhosis and fulminant hepatic failure. J Clin Pathol 31:101, 1978.
536. Koppel MH, Coburn JW, Mims MM, et al: Transplantation of cadaveric kidneys from patients with hepatorenal syndrome: Evidence for the functional nature of renal failure in advanced liver disease. N Engl J Med 280:1367, 1969.
537. Iwatsuki S, Popovtzer MM, Corman JL, et al.: Recovery from "hepatorenal syndrome" after orthotopic liver transplantation. N Engl J Med 289:1155, 1973.
538. Lowenstein J, Schacht RG, Baldwin DS: Renal failure in minimal change nephrotic syndrome. Am J Med 70:227, 1981.
539. Rennke HG, Roos PC, Wall SG: Drug-induced interstitial nephritis with heavy glomerular proteinuria. N Engl J Med 302:691, 1980. Letter.
540. Neugarten J, Gallo GR, Baldwin DS: Rifampin-induced nephrotic syndrome and acute interstitial nephritis. Am J Nephrol 3:38, 1983.
541. Averbuch SD, Austen HA III, Sherwin T, et al: Acute interstitial nephritis with the nephrotic syndrome following recombinant leukocyte α interferon therapy for mycosis fungoides. N Engl J Med 310:32, 1984.
542. May RC, Stivelman JC, Maroni BJ: Metabolic and electrolyte disturbances in acute renal failure. In Lazarus JM, Brenner BM (eds): Acute Renal Failure, 3rd ed. Churchill Livingstone, New York, 1993, p 107.
542a. Yu A, Brenner BM, Yu ASL: Uremic syndrome revisited: A pathogenetic role for retained endogenous inhibitors of nitric oxide synthesis. Curr Opin Nephrol Hypertens 1:3–7, 1992.
543. Cameron JS, Ogg C, Trounce JR: Peritoneal dialysis in hypercatabolic acute renal failure. Lancet 1:1188, 1967.
544. Silva H, Pomeroy J, Rae AI, et al: Haemodialysis in "hypercatabolic" acute renal failure. Br Med J 2:407, 1964.
545. Bluemle LW Jr, Porter HP, Elkinton JR: Changes in body composition in acute renal failure. J Clin Invest 35:1094, 1951.
546. Anderson RJ, Chung HM, Kluge R, et al: Hyponatremia: A study of its incidence and pathogenic role of vasopressin. Ann Intern Med 102:164, 1985.
547. Bluemle LW, Webster GD, Elkinton JR: Acute tubular necrosis. Arch Intern Med 104:180, 1959.
548. Teschan PE, Post R, Smith L Jr, et al.: Post-traumatic renal insufficiency in military casualties. 1. Clinical characteristics. Am J Med 18:172, 1955.
549. Maher JF, Schreiner GE: Cause of death in acute renal failure. Arch Intern Med 110:493, 1962.
550. Relman AS: Renal acidosis and renal excretion of acid health and disease. Adv Intern Med 12:295, 1964.
551. Massry SG, Arieff AI, Coburn JW, et al: Divalent ion metabolism in patients with acute renal failure. Studies on the mechanism of hypocalcemia. Kidney Int 5:437, 1974.
552. Llach F, Felsenfeld AJ, Haussler MR: The pathophysiology of altered calcium metabolism in rhabdomyolysis-induced acute renal failure. Interactions of parathyroid hormone, 25-hydroxycholecalciferol and 1,25-dihydroxycholecalciferol. N Engl J Med 305:117, 1981.
553. de Torrente A, Berl T, Cohn PD, et al: Hypercalcemia of acute renal failure: Clinical significance and pathogenesis. Am J Med 61:119, 1976.
554. Pietrek J, Kokot F, Kuska J: Serum 25-hydroxyvitamin D and parathyroid hormone in patients with acute renal failure. Kidney Int 13:178, 1978.
555. Arieff AI, Massry SG: Effects of uremia, hemodialysis, and parathyroid hormone. J Clin Invest 53:387, 1974.

556. Blachley JD, Hill IB: Renal and electrolyte disturbances associated with cisplatin. Ann Intern Med 95:628, 1981.
557. Radtke HW, Claussner A, Erbes PM, et al: Serum erythropoietin concentration in chronic renal failure: Relationship to degree of anemia and excretory renal function. Blood 54:877, 1979.
558. Radtke HW, Rege AB, LaMarche MB, et al: Identification of spermine as an inhibitor of erythropoiesis in patients with chronic renal failure. J Clin Invest 67:1623, 1981.
559. Eknoyan G, Wacksman SJ, Glueck HL, Will JJ: Platelet function in renal failure. N Engl J Med 280:677, 1969.
560. Mannucci PM, Remuzzi G, Pusineri F, et al: Deamino-8-D-arginine vasopressin shortens the bleeding time in uremia. N Engl J Med 308:8, 1983.
561. Andrassy K, Llach FV, Ritz E: Penicillin induced hemorrhage: A common complication of acute renal failure. Proc Am Soc Nephrol 15:107A, 1982.
562. Andrassy K, Ritz E, Haspcr B, et al: Penicillin-induced coagulation disorder. Lancet 2:1039, 1976.
563. Shattil SJ, Bennett JS, McDonough M, Turnbull J: Carbenicillin and penicillin G inhibit platelet function in vitro by impairing the interaction of agonists with the platelet surface. J Clin Invest 65:329, 1980.
564. Brown CH 3rd, Bradshaw MJ, Natelson EA, et al: Defective platelet function following the administration of penicillin compounds. Blood 47:949, 1976.
565. Montgomerie JZ, Kalmanson GM, Guze LB.: Renal failure and infection. Medicine (Baltimore) 47:1, 1968.
566. Stott RB, Cameron JS, Ogg CS, Bewick M: Why the persistently high mortality in acute renal failure? Lancet 2:75, 1972.
567. Kennedy AC, Burton JA, Luke RG, et al: Factors affecting the prognosis in acute renal failure. Q J Med 42:73, 1973.
568. Baek SM, Makabali GG, Shoemaker WC: Clinical determinants of survival from postoperative renal failure. Surg Gynecol Obstet 140:685, 1975.
569. McMurray SD, Luft FC, Maxwell DR, et al: Prevailing patterns and predictor variables in patients with acute tubular necrosis. Arch Intern Med 138:950, 1978.
570. Bullock ML, Umen AJ, Finkelstein M, Keane WF: The assessment of risk factors in 462 patients with acute renal failure. Am J Kidney Dis 5:97, 1985.
571. Rasmussen HH, Pitt EA, Ibels LS, McNeil DR: Prediction of outcome in acute renal failure by discriminant analysis of clinical variables. Arch Intern Med 145:2015, 1985.
572. Lien J, Chan V: Risk factors influencing survival in acute renal failure treated by hemodialysis. Arch Intern Med 145:2067, 1985.
573. Cameron JS: Acute renal failure: The continuing challenge. Q J Med 59:337, 1986.
574. Kleinknecht D, Jungers P, Chanard J, et al: Uremic and non-uremic complications in acute renal failure: Evaluation of early and frequent dialysis on prognosis. Kidney Int 1:190, 1972.
575. Priebe HJ, Skillman JJ, Bushnell LS, et al: Antacid versus cimetidine in preventing acute gastrointestinal bleeding. A randomized trial in 75 critically ill patients. N Engl J Med 302:426, 1980.
576. Locke S, Merrill JP, Tyler HR: Neurologic considerations of acute uremia. Arch Intern Med 108:75, 1961.
577. Tyler HR: Neurological disorders in renal failure. Am J Med 44:734, 1968.
578. Raskin NH, Fishman RA: Neurologic disorders in renal failure (first of two parts). N Engl J Med 294:143–148, 1976.
579. Raskin NM, Fishman RA: Neurologic disorders in renal failure (second of two parts). N Engl J Med 294:204–210, 1976.
580. Arieff AI, Massry SG: Calcium metabolism of brain in acute renal failure. Effects of uremia. Hemodialysis and parathyroid hormone. J Clin Invest 53:387, 1974.
581. Guisado R, Arieff AI, Massry SG: Changes in the electroencephalogram in acute uremia. J Clin Invest 55:738, 1975.
582. Wolfson M, Kopple JD: Nutritional management of acute renal failure. In Lazarus JM, Brenner BM (eds): Acute Renal Failure, 3rd ed. Churchill Livingstone, New York, 1993, p 267.
583. Schreiner GE, Maher JF: Uremia: Biochemistry, Pathogenesis and Treatment. Charles C Thomas, Springfield, IL, 1961.
584. Bergstrom J, Furst P: Uremic toxins. In Drukker W, Parson FM, Maher JF (eds): Replacement of Renal Function by Dialysis. Martinus Nijhoff, Boston, 1983, p 354.
585. Carpenter CCJ, Mondal A, Sack RB, et al: Clinical studies in Asiatic cholera. II. Development of 2:1 saline:lactate regimen. Comparison of this regimen with traditional methods of treatment. Bull Johns Hopkins Hosp 118:174, 1966.
586. Carpenter CCJ, Mitra PP, Sack RB: Clinical studies in Asiatic cholera. I. Preliminary observations. Bull Johns Hopkins Hosp 118:165, 1966.
587. Carpenter CCJ, Mitra PP, Sack RB, et al: Clinical studies in Asiatic cholera. III. Physiologic studies during treatment of the acute cholera patient: Comparison of lactate and bicarbonate in correction of acidosis; effects of potassium depletion. Bull Johns Hopkins Hosp 118:197, 1966.
588. Whelton A, Donadio JV: Post-traumatic acute renal failure in Vietnam. Johns Hopkins Med J 124:95, 1969.
589. Bush HL, Huse JB, Johnson WC, et al: Prevention of renal insufficiency after abdominal aortic aneurysm resection by optimal volume loading. Arch Surg 116:1517, 1981.
590. Ozols RF, Corden BJ, Jacob J, et al: High-dose cisplatin in hypertonic saline. Ann Intern Med 100:19, 1984.
590a. Solomon R, Werner C, Mann D, et al: Effects of saline, mannitol and furosemide on acute decreases in renal function induced by radiocontrast agents. N Engl J Med 331:1416, 1994.
591. Solez K, Freshwater MF, Su C-T: The effect of propranolol on postischemic acute renal failure in the rat. Transplantation 24:148, 1977.
592. Iaina A, Solomon S, Eliahou HE: Reduction in severity of acute renal failure in rats by beta-adrenergic blockade. Lancet 2:158, 1975.
593. Eliahou HE, Solomon S, Iaina A, et al: Alleviation of acute anoxic renal failure in rats by $\beta_1$-adrenergic blockade with practolol. Isr J Med Sci 14:274, 1978.
594. Solomon HS, Hollenberg NK: Catecholamine release: Mechanism of mercury-induced vascular smooth muscle contraction. Am J Physiol 229:8, 1975.
595. Solez K, Ideura T, Silva CB, et al: Clonidine after renal ischemia to lessen acute renal failure and microvascular damage. Kidney Int 18:309, 1980.
596. Patak RV, Fadem SZ, Lifschitz MD, Stein JH: Study of the factors which modify the development of norepinephrine-induced acute renal failure in the dog. Kidney Int 15:227, 1979.
597. Conger JD, Robinette JB, Guggenheim SJ: Effect of acetylcholine on the early phase of reversible norepinephrine-induced acute renal failure. Kidney Int 19:399, 1981.
598. Moskowitz PS, Korobkin M, Rambo ON: Diuresis and improved renal hemodynamics produced by prostaglandin E in the dog with norepinephrine-induced acute renal failure. Invest Radiol 10:284, 1975.
599. Mauk RH, Patak RV, Fadem SZ, et al: Effect of prostaglandin E administration in a nephrotoxic and a vasoconstrictor model of acute renal failure. Kidney Int 12:122, 1977.
600. Lifschitz MD, Barnes JL: Prostaglandin $I_2$ attenuates ischemic acute renal failure in the rat. Am J Physiol 247:F714, 1984.
601. Finn WF, Hak LJ, Grossman SH: Protective effect of prostacyclin on postischemic acute renal failure in the rat. Kidney Int 32:479, 1987.
602. Tobimatsu M, Ueda Y, Saito S, et al: Effects of a stable prostacyclin analog on experimental ischemic acute renal failure. Ann Surg 208:65, 1988.
603. Neumayer HH, Wagner K, Preuschof L, et al: Amelioration of postischemic acute renal failure by prostacyclin analogue (iloprost): Long-term studies with chronically instrumented conscious dogs. J Cardiovasc Pharmacol 8:785, 1986.
604. Ishikawa I, Hollenberg NK: Pharmacological interruption of the renin-angiotensin system in myohemoglobinuric acute renal failure. Kidney Int 10:S183, 1976.
605. Bauereiss K, Hofbauer KG, Konrads A, Gross F: Effect of saralasin and serum in myohemoglobinuric acute renal failure of rats. Clin Sci Mol Med 54:555, 1978.
606. Malis CD, Cheung JY, Leaf A, Bonventre JV: Effects of verapamil in models of ischemic acute renal failure in the rat. Am J Physiol 245:F735, 1983.
607. Burke TJ, Arnold PE, Gordon JA, et al: Protective effect of intrarenal calcium membrane blockers before or after renal ischemia. J Clin Invest 74:1830, 1984.
608. Watson AJ, Gimenez LF, Klassen DK, et al: Calcium channel blockade in experimental aminoglycoside nephrotoxicity. J Clin Pharmacol 27:625, 1987.

609. Deray G, Dubois M, Beaufils H, et al: Effects of nifedipine on cisplatin-induced nephrotoxicity in rats. Clin Nephrol 30:146, 1988.

610. Lee SM, Michael UF: The protective effect of nitrendipine on gentamicin acute renal failure in rats. Exp Mol Pathol 43:107, 1985.

611. Wagner K, Schultze G, Molzahn M, Neumayer HH: The influence of long-term infusion of the calcium antagonist diltiazem on postischemic acute renal failure in conscious dogs. Klin Wochenschr 64:P135, 1986.

612. Dobyan DC, Bulger RE: Partial protection by chlorpromazine in mercuric chloride–induced acute renal failure in rats. Lab Invest 40:578, 1984.

613. Schafferhans K, Heidbreder E, Grimm D, Heidland A: Norepinephrine-induced acute renal failure: Beneficial effects of atrial natriuretic factor. Nephron 44:240, 1986.

614. Shaw SG, Weidemann P, Hodler J, et al: Atrial natriuretic peptide protects against acute ischemic renal failure in the rat. J Clin Invest 80:1232, 1987.

615. Nakamota M, Shapiro JI, Shanley PF, et al: In vitro and in vivo protective effect of atriopeptin III on ischemic acute renal failure. J Clin Invest 80:698, 1987.

616. Neumayer HH, Blossei N, Seherr-Thots U, Wagner K: Amelioration of postischaemic acute renal failure in conscious dogs by human atrial natriuretic peptide. Nephrol Dial Transplant 5:32, 1990.

617. Lieberthal W, Sheridan AM, Valeri CR: Protective effect of atrial natriuretic factor and mannitol following renal ischemia. Am J Physiol 258:F1266, 1990.

618. Pollock DM, Opgenorth TJ: Beneficial effect of the atrial natriuretic factor analog A68828 in postischemic acute renal failure. J Pharmacol Exp Ther 255:1166, 1990.

619. Conger JD, Falk SA, Yuan BH, Schrier RW: Atrial natriuretic peptide and dopamine in a rat model of ischemic acute renal failure. Kidney Int 35:1126, 1989.

620. Conger JD, Falk SA, Hammond WS: Atrial natriuretic peptide and dopamine in established acute renal failure in the rat. Kidney Int 10:21, 1991.

621. Schafferhans K, Heidbreder E, Sperber S, et al: Atrial natriuretic peptide in gentamicin-induced acute renal failure. Kidney Int Suppl 25:S101, 1988.

622. Heidbreder E, Schafferhans K, Heyd A, et al: Uranyl nitrate–induced acute renal failure in rats: Effect of atrial natriuretic peptide on renal function. Kidney Int Suppl 3:S79, 1988.

623. Capasso G, Anastasio P, Giordano D, et al: Beneficial effects of atrial natriuretic factor on cisplatin-induced acute renal failure in the rat. Am J Nephrol 7:228, 1987.

624. Lin JJ, Churchill PC, Bidani AK: The effect of theophylline on the initiation phase of post-ischemic acute renal failure in rats. J Lab Clin Med 108:150, 1986.

625. Lin JJ, Churchill PC, Bidani AK: Theophylline in rats during maintenance phase of post-ischemic acute renal failure. Kidney Int 33:24, 1988.

626. Bowmer CJ, Collis MG, Yates MS: Amelioration of glycerol-induced acute renal failure in the rat with 8-phenyltheophylline: Timing of intervention. J Pharm Pharmacol 40:733, 1988.

627. Boumer CJ, Collis MG, Yates MS: Effect of alkylxanthines on gentamicin-induced acute renal failure in rats. J Pharm Pharmacol 40:849, 1988.

628. Kon VT, Yoshioka T, Fogo A, Ichikawa I: Glomerular actions of endothelin in vivo. J Clin Invest 83:1762, 1989.

629. Kon V, Sugiura A, Inagamli T, et al: Role of endothelin in cyclosporin-induced glomerular dysfunction. Kidney Int 37:1487, 1990.

630. Selkurt EE: Changes in renal clearance following complete ischemia of the kidney. Am J Physiol 144:395, 1945.

631. Flores J, DiBona DR, Beck CH. Leaf A: The role of cell swelling in ischemic renal damage and the protective effect of hypertonic solute. J Clin Invest 51:118, 1972.

632. Hanley MJ, Davidson K: Prior mannitol infusion in a model of ischemic renal failure. Am J Physiol 241:F556, 1981.

633. Hatcher CR, Gagnon JA, Clarke RW: The effects of hydration on epinephrine-induced renal shutdown in dogs. Surg Forum 9:106, 1958.

634. Cronin RE, de Torrente A, Miller PD, et al: Pathogenic mechanisms in early norepinephrine-induced acute renal failure. Functional and histologic correlates of protection. Kidney Int 14:115, 1978.

635. Burke TJ, Cronin RE, Duchen KL, et al: Ischemia and tubule obstruction during acute renal failure in dogs: Mannitol in protection. Am J Physiol 238:F305, 1980.

636. Mason J, Jolris B, Welsch J, Kriz W: Vascular congestion in ischemic renal failure: The role of cell swelling. Miner Electrolyte Metab 15:114, 1989.

637. Wilson DR, Thiel G, Arce ML, Oken DE: Glycerol induced hemoglobinuric acute renal failure in the rat. III. Micropuncture study of the effects of mannitol and isotonic saline on individual nephron function. Nephron 4:377, 1967.

638. Parry WL, Schaffer JA, Mueller CB: Experimental studies of acute renal failure. I. The protective effect of mannitol. J Urol 89:1, 1963.

639. Teschan PE, Lawson NL: Studies in acute renal failure. Prevention by osmotic diuresis, and observations on the effect of plasma and extracellular volume expansion. Nephron 3:1, 1966.

640. Pera MF, Zook BC, Harder HC: Effects of mannitol or furosemide diuresis on the nephrotoxicity and physiological disposition of cis-dichlorodiammineplatinum (II) in rats. Cancer Res 39:1269, 1979.

641. Hellebusch AA, Salama F, Eadie E: The use of mannitol to reduce the nephrotoxicity of amphotericin B. Surg Gynecol Obstet 134:241, 1973.

642. Kramer HJ, Schuurmann J, Wasserman C, Dusing R: Prostaglandin-independent protection by furosemide from oliguric ischemic renal failure in conscious rats. Kidney Int 17:455, 1980.

643. Papadimitriou M, Milionis A, Sakellariou G, Metaxas P: Effect of furosemide on acute ischemic renal failure in the dog. Nephron 20:157, 1978.

644. Bailey RR, Natale R, Turnbull DI, Linton AL: Protective effect of furosemide in acute tubular necrosis and acute renal failure. Clin Sci Mol Med 45:1, 1973.

645. Ufferman RC, Jaenike JR, Freeman RB, Pabico RC: Effects of furosemide on low-dose mercuric chloride acute renal failure in the rat. Kidney Int 8:362, 1975.

646. Lindner A, Cutler RE, Goodman WG: Synergism of dopamine plus furosemide in preventing acute renal failure in the dog. Kidney Int 16:158, 1979.

647. Greven J, Klein H: Renal effects of furosemide in glycerol-induced acute renal failure of the rat. Pflugers Arch 365:81, 1976.

648. Paller MS, Hoidal JR, Ferris TF: Oxygen free radicals in ischemic acute renal failure in the rat. J Clin Invest 74:1156, 1984.

649. Hansson RB, Gustafsson D, Jonsson S, et al: Effect of xanthine oxidase inhibition on renal circulation after ischemia. Transplant Proc 14:51, 1982.

650. Gamelin LM, Zager RA: Evidence against oxidant injury as a critical mediator of postischemic acute renal failure. Am J Physiol 255:F450, 1988.

651. Zager RA, Gmur DJ: Effect of xanthine oxidase inhibition on ischemic acute renal failure in the rat. Am J Physiol 257:F953, 1989.

652. Zager RA: Hypoperfusion induced acute renal failure in the rat: An evaluation of oxidant tissue injury. Circ Res 62:430, 1988.

653. Paller MS, Hedlund BE: Role of iron in postischemic renal injury in the rat. Kidney Int 34:474, 1988.

654. Paller MS: Hemoglobin and myoglobin induced renal failure in the rats: Role of iron in nephrotoxicity. Am J Physiol 255:F539, 1988.

655. Shah SV, Walker PD: Evidence suggesting a role for hydroxyl radical in glycerol-induced acute renal failure. Am J Physiol 255:F438, 1988.

656. Walker PD, Shah SV: Evidence suggestive for a role for hydroxyl radical in gentamicin-induced acute renal failure in rats. J Clin Invest 81:334, 1988.

657. Walker PD, Shah SV: Reactive oxygen metabolites in endotoxin-induced acute renal failure in rats. Kidney Int 38:1125, 1990.

658. Borch RF, Katz JC, Lieder PH, et al: Effect of diethyldithiocarbamate rescue on tumor response to cisplatinum in a rat model. Proc Natl Acad Sci USA 77:5441, 1980.

659. Linas SL, Whittenburg D, Repine JE: O₂ metabolites cause reperfusion injury after short but not prolonged renal ischemia. Am J Physiol 253:F685, 1987.

660. Bayati A, Kallskog O, Wolgast M: The long-term outcome of postischaemic acute renal failure. 1. A functional study after treatment with SOD and sucrose. Acta Physiol Scand 138:25, 1990.

661. Bird JE, Milhoan K, Wilson CB, et al: Ischemic acute renal failure and antioxidant therapy in the rat. The relation between glomerular and tubular dysfunction. J Clin Invest 81:1630, 1988.

662. Bird JE, Evans AP, Peterson OW, Blantz RC: Early events in ischemic renal failure in the rat: Effects of antioxidant therapy. Kidney Int 35:1282, 1985.

663. Paller MS: Effect of neutrophil depletion on ischemic renal injury in the rat. J Lab Clin Med 113:379, 1989.

664. Hellberg POA, Kallskog TOK: Neutrophil-mediated post-ischemic tubular leakage in the rat kidney. Kidney Int 36:555, 1989.

665. Thornton MN, Winn R, Alpers CE, Zager R: An evaluation of the neutrophil as a mediator of in vivo renal ischemia-reperfusion injury. Am J Pathol 135:509, 1988.

666. Brady HR: Leukocyte adhesion molecules and kidney diseases. Kidney Int 45:1285, 1994.

667. Kelly KJ, Williams WW, Colvin RB, Bonventre JV: Antibody to intercellular adhesion molecule-1 protects the kidney against ischemic injury. Proc Natl Acad Sci USA 91:812, 1994.

668. Teschner M, Schaefer RM, Rudolf C, et al: Eglin C fails to reduce catabolism in acutely uremic rats. Adv Exp Med Biol 240:331, 1988.

669. Linas SL, Whittenburg D, Repine JE: Role of neutrophil-derived oxidants and elastase in lipopolysaccharide-mediated renal injury. Kidney Int 39:618, 1991.

670. Osias MB, Siegel NJ, Chaudry IH, et al: Post-ischaemic acute renal failure. Arch Surg 112:729, 1977.

671. Siegel NJ, Glazier WB, Chaudry IH, et al: Enhanced recovery from acute renal failure by the postischemic infusion of adenine nucleotides and magnesium chloride in rats. Kidney Int 17:338, 1980.

672. Siegel NJ, Taylor M, Gaudio KM, Kashgarian M: Ischemic acute renal failure: Delayed infusion of ATP-MgCl$_2$. Pediatr Res 14:1017, 1980.

673. Sumpio BE, Chaudry IH, Clemens MG, Baue AE: Accelerated functional recovery of isolated rat kidney with ATP-MgCl$_2$ after warm ischemia. Am J Physiol 247:1047, 1984.

674. Gaudio KM, Siegel NJ, Chaudry IH, Kashgarian M: Diminished tubular backleak by the post-ischemic infusion of ATP-MgCl$_2$. Kidney Int 19:200, 1981.

675. Gaudio KM, Ardito TA, Reilly HF, et al: Accelerated cellular recovery after an ischemic renal injury. Am J Pathol 112:338, 1983.

676. Glaumann B, Trump B: Studies on the pathogenesis of ischemic cell injury. III. Morphological changes of the proximal pars recta tubules (P3) of the rat kidney made ischemic in vivo. Virchows Arch B 19:303, 1975.

677. Schulte-Wissermann H, Straub E, Funke PJ: Influence of L-thyroxine upon enzymatic activity in the renal tubular epithelium of the rat under normal conditions and in mercury-induced lesions. I. Histochemical studies of alkaline phosphatase, acid phosphatase, adenosine-triphosphatase and leucine-aminopeptidase. Virchows Arch B 23:163, 1977.

678. Schulte-Wissermann H, Straub E, Funke PJ: Influence of L-thyroxine upon enzymatic activity in the renal tubular epithelium of the rat under normal conditions and in mercury-induced lesions. II. Histochemical studies of lactate dehydrogenase, malate dehydrogenase, unspecific esterase, and glucose-6-phosphate dehydrogenase. Virchows Arch B 23:175, 1977.

679. Cronin RE, Newman JA: Protective effect of thyroxine but not parathyroidectomy on gentamicin nephrotoxicity. Am J Physiol 248:F332, 1985.

680. Siegel NJ, Gaudio KM, Katz LA, et al: Beneficial effect of thyroxin on recovery from toxic acute renal failure. Kidney Int 25:906, 1984.

681. Sutter PM, Thulin G, Stromski M, et al: Beneficial effect of thyroxin in the treatment of ischemic acute renal failure. Pediatr Nephrol 20:1, 1988.

682. Heyman SN, Rosen S, Silva P, et al: Protective action of glycine in cisplatin nephrotoxicity. Kidney Int 40:273, 1991.

683. Zager RA, Johannes G, Tuttle SE, Sharma HM: Acute amino acid nephrotoxicity. J Lab Clin Med 101:130, 1983.

684. Zager RA, Venkatachalam MA: Potentiation of ischemic renal injury by amino acid infusion. Kidney Int 24:620, 1983.

685. Racusen LC, Whelton A, Solez K: Effects of lysine and other amino acids on kidney structure and function in the rat. Am J Pathol 120:436, 1985.

686. Vadiei K, Brunner LJ, Luke DR: Effects of pentoxifylline in experimental acute renal failure. Kidney Int 36:466, 1989.

687. Paterson AR: Adenosine transport. In Baer HP, Drummond GI (eds): Physiological and Regulatory Functions of Adenosine and Adenine Nucleotides. Raven Press, New York, 1979, p 305.

688. Mason J, Welsch J, Terhorst J: The contribution of vascular congestion to the functional defect that follows renal ischemia. Kidney Int 31:65, 1987.

689. Humes HD, Cieslinski DA, Coimbra TM, et al: Epidermal growth factor enhances renal tubule cell regeneration and repair and accelerates the recovery of renal function in postischemic acute renal failure. J Clin Invest 84:1757, 1989.

690. Norman J, Tsau YK, Bacay A, Fine LG: Epidermal growth factor accelerates functional recovery from ischaemic acute tubular necrosis in the rat: Role of the epidermal growth factor receptor. Clin Sci 78:445, 1990.

691. Jacobs RP, Korobkin M, Lieberman RS, et al: Reversal of oliguric and renal cortical ischemia of hemorrhagic shock in the dog with tris(hydroxymethyl)aminomethane (THAM). Invest Radiol 10:273, 1975.

692. Henderson B, Beattie TJ, Kennedy AC: Dopamine hydrochloride in oliguric states. Lancet 18:827, 1980.

693. Parker S, Carlon GC, Isaacs M, et al: Dopamine administration in oliguric and nonoliguric renal failure. Crit Care Med 9:630, 1981.

694. Davis RF, Demitrios GL, Kirklin JK, et al: Acute oliguria after cardiopulmonary bypass: Functional improvement with low dose dopamine infusion. Crit Care Med 10:852, 1982.

695. Graziani G, Casati S, Cantaluppi A, et al: Dopamine-frusemide therapy in acute renal failure. Proc Eur Dial Transpl Assoc 19:319, 1983.

696. Lindner A: A synergism of dopamine and furosemide in diuretic resistant oliguruc acute renal failure. Nephron 33:121, 1983.

697. Lumlertgul D, Keopling M, Sitprija V, et al: Furosemide and dopamine in malaria acute renal failure. Nephron 52:40, 1989.

698. Baldwin L, Henderson A, Hickman P: Effect of post-operative low-dose dopamine on renal function after elective major vascular surgery. Ann Intern Med 120:744, 1994.

699. Thompson AE, Fung HYM: Adrenergic and cholinergic mechanisms in acute renal failure in the dog and in man. In Friedman EA, Eliahou HE (eds): Proceedings: Conference on Acute Renal Failure. Government Printing Office, Washington, DC, 1974, p 293. DHEW Pub No. (NIH) 74-608.

700. Reubi FC, Vorberger C: Renal hemodynamics after acute renal failure after shock in man. Kidney Int 10:S137, 1976.

701. Vincenti F, Goldberg LI: Combined use of dopamine and prostaglandin A$_1$ in patients with acute renal failure and hepatorenal syndrome. Prostaglandins 15:463, 1978.

702. Ladefoged J, Winkler K: Hemodynamics in acute renal failure. Scand J Clin Lab Invest 26:83, 1970.

703. Lumlertgul D, Hutdagoon P, Sirivanichai C, et al: Beneficial effect of intrarenal verapamil in human acute renal failure. Ren Fail 11:201, 1989–90.

704. Duggan KA, MacDonald GJ, Charlesworth JA: Verapamil prevents post-transplant oliguric renal failure. Clin Nephrol 24:289, 1985.

705. Wagner K, Albrecht S, Neumayer HH: Prevention of posttransplant acute tubular necrosis by the calcium antagonist diltiazem: A prospective randomized study. Am J Nephrol 7:287, 1987.

706. Deray G, Khayat D, Cacoub P, et al: The effects of diltiazem on methotrexate induced nephrotoxicity. Eur J Clin Pharmacol 37:377, 1989.

707. Cacoub P, Baumelou A, Jacobs C: No evidence for protective effects of nifedipine against contrast-induced acute renal failure. Clin Nephrol 29:215, 1988.

708. Gotz R, Bausewein K, Heidbreder E, et al: Acute renal failure in the intensive care unit: Are there benefits of atrial natriuretic factor for dopamine/furosemide resistant acute renal failure? Kidney Int 35:282, 1989.

709. Bozkurt F, Kirste G, Leipziger J, et al: Effects of human atrial natriuretic peptide on diuresis and hemodynamics in oligoanuric renal transplant recipients. Transplant Proc 19:4192, 1987.

710. Berman LM, Smith LL, Chisolm GD, Weston RE: Mannitol and renal function in cardiovascular surgery. Arch Surg 88:239, 1964.

711. Barry KG, Cohen A, Knochel JP, et al: Mannitol infusion. II. The prevention of acute functional failure during resection of an aneurysm of the abdominal aorta. N Engl J Med 264:967, 1961.

712. Baird RJ, Firor WB, Barr HWK: Protection of renal function during surgery of the abdominal aorta. Can Med Assoc J 89:705, 1963.

713. Beall AC, Holman RM, Morris CC, DeBakey ME: Mannitol induced osmotic diuresis during vascular surgery. Arch Surg 86:34, 1963.

714. Kahn DR, Cerny JC, Lee RWS, Sloan H: The effect of dextran and mannitol on renal function during cardiovascular surgery. Surgery 5:676, 1965.

715. Smith LL, Berman LB, Chisolm GD: Effect of mannitol on renal function during cardiovascular surgery. Surg Forum 14:103, 1963.

716. Gubern JM, Sancho JJ, Simo J, Sitges-Serra A: A randomized trial on the effect of mannitol on postoperative renal function in patients with obstructive jaundice. Surgery 103:39, 1988.

717. Dawson JL: Post-operative renal function in obstructive jaundice. Effect of a mannitol diuresis. Br Med J 1:82, 1965.

718. Untura A: Incidence and prophylaxis of acute post-operative renal failure in obstructive jaundice. Rev Med Chir Soc Med Nat Iasi 83:249, 1979.

719. Olivero JJ, Lozano-Mendez J, Ghafary EM, et al: Mitigation of amphotericin B nephrotoxicity by mannitol. Br Med J 1:550, 1975.

720. Hayes DM, Cvitkovic E, Golbey RB, et al: High dose *cis*-platinum diammine dichloride. Amelioration of renal toxicity by mannitol diuresis. Cancer 39:1372, 1977.

721. Anto HR, Chou SY, Porush JG, Shapiro WB: Mannitol prevention of acute renal failure associated with infusion intravenous pyelography. Clin Res 27:407A, 1979.

722. Old CW, Lehrner LM: Prevention of radiocontrast induced acute renal failure with mannitol. Lancet 2:885, 1980. Letter.

723. van Valenberg PLJ, Hoitsma AJ, Tiggeler RGWL, et al: Mannitol as an indispensable constituent of an intraoperative hydration protocol for the prevention of acute renal failure after renal cadaveric transplantation. Transplantation 44:784, 1987.

724. Grino JM, Miravitlles R, Castelao AM, et al: Flush solution with mannitol in the prevention of post-transplant renal failure. Transplant Proc 19:4140, 1987.

725. Conger JD: Acute renal failure: Diagnosis, management, complications and prognosis in a war zone setting. Pres Concepts Int Med 4:739, 1971.

726. Stone AM, Sahl WM: Effects of ethacrynic acid and furosemide on renal function in hypovolemia. Ann Surg 174:1, 1971.

727. Nuutinen LS, Kairaluoma M, Tuononen S, Larmi TKI: The effect of furosemide on renal function in open heart surgery. J Cardiovasc Surg 19:471, 1978.

728. Lucas CE, Zito JG, Carter KM, et al: Questionable value of furosemide in preventing renal failure. Surgery 82:314, 1977.

729. Oguagha C, Porush JG, Chou SY, et al: Prevention of acute renal failure following infusion intravenous pyelography in patients with chronic renal insufficiency by furosemide. *In* Zurukzoglu W, et al (eds): Advances in Basic and Clinical Nephrology: Proceedings of the 8th International Congress of Nephrology, Athens, Greece. S Karger, Basel, 1981, p 290.

730. Kjellstrand CM: Ethacrynic acid in acute tubular necrosis. Indications and effect on the natural course. Nephron 9:337, 1972.

731. Muth RG: Furosemide in acute renal failure. Symposium on Acute Renal Failure, National Institutes of Health, Bethesda, MD, 1973, p 245.

732. Cantarovich F, Locatelli A, Fernandez JC, et al: Furosemide in high doses in the treatment of acute renal failure. Postgrad Med 47(suppl):13, 1971.

733. Cantarovich F, Galli C, Benedetti L, et al: High dose furosemide in established acute renal failure. Br Med J 4:449, 1973.

734. Kleinknecht D, Ganeval D, Gonzalez-Duque LA, Fermanian J: Furosemide in acute oliguric renal failure: A controlled trial. Nephron 17:51, 1976.

735. Brown CB, Ogg CS, Cameron JS: High dose furosemide in acute renal failure. A controlled trial. Clin Nephrol 15:90, 1986.

736. Schreiner GE, Maher JF: Toxic nephropathy. Am J Med 38:409, 1965.

737. Jaffe KM, Shurtleff DB, Robertson WO: Survival after acute mercury vapor poisoning. Am J Chest Dis 137:749, 1983.

738. Murray KM, Hedgepeth JC: Intravenous self-administration of elemental mercury: Efficacy of dimercaprol therapy. Drug Intell Clin Pharm 22:972, 1988.

739. Doolan PD, Hess WC, Kyle LH: Acute renal insufficiency due to bichloride of mercury. Observations on gastrointestinal hemorrhage and BAL therapy. N Engl J Med 249:273, 1953.

740. Emmerson BT: Chronic lead nephropathy: The diagnostic use of calcium EDTA and the association with gout. Aust Ann Med 12:310, 1963.

741. Batuman VB, Maesaka JK, Haddad B, et al: The role of lead in gout nephropathy. N Engl J Med 304:520, 1981.

742. Wedeen RP, Maesaka JK, Weiner B, et al: Occupational lead nephropathy. Am J Med 59:630, 1975.

743. Morgan JM: Chelation therapy in lead nephropathy. South Med J 68:1001, 1975.

744. Swaiman KF, Flayler DG: Mercury poisoning with central and peripheral nervous system involvement treated with penicillamine. Pediatrics 48:639, 1971.

745. Chisolm JJ: Poisoning from heavy metals (mercury, lead, cadmium). Pediatr Ann 9:458, 1980.

746. Prescott LF, Illingsworth RN, Critchley JA, et al: Intravenous *N*-acetylcysteine: The treatment of choice for paracetamol poisoning. Br J Med 2:1097, 1979.

747. Smilkstein MJ, Knapp GL, Kulig KW, Rumack BH: Efficacy of oral *N*-acetylcysteine in the treatment of acetaminophen overdose. N Engl J Med 319:1557, 1988.

748. Tattersall MHN, Brown B, Frei E III: The reversal of methotrexate toxicity by thymidine with maintenance of tumour effects. Nature 253:198, 1975.

749. Stoller RG, Hande KR, Jacobs SA, et al: Use of plasma pharmacokinetics to predict and prevent methotrexate toxicity. N Engl J Med 297:630, 1977.

750. Andreoli SP, Clark JH, McGuire WA, et al: Purine excretion during tumor-lysis in children with acute lymphocytic leukemia receiving allopurinol: Relationship to acute renal failure. J Pediatr 109:292, 1986.

751. Krakoff IH: Use of allopurinol in preventing hyperuricemia in leukemia and lymphoma. Cancer 19:1489, 1966.

752. DeConti RC, Calabresi P: Use of allopurinol and control of hyperuricemia in patients with neoplastic disease. N Engl J Med 274:481, 1966.

753. Cohen LF, Balow JE, Magrath IT, et al: Acute tumor lysis: A review of 37 patients with Burkitt's lymphoma. Am J Med 68:486, 1980.

754. Wats RWE, Watkins PJ, Mattias JQ, et al: Allopurinol and uric acid nephropathy. Br Med J 1:205, 1966.

755. Ito M, Imoto S, Nakagawa T, et al: Administration of haptoglobin in ABO incompatible bone marrow transplantation. Rinsho Ketsueki 31:1716, 1990.

756. Aikawa N, Wakabayashi G, Ueda M, Shinozawa Y: Regulation of renal function in thermal injury. J Trauma 30(12 suppl):S174, 1990.

757. Howell SB, Pfeifle CL, Wung WE, et al: Intraperitoneal cisplatin with systemic thiosulfate protection. Ann Intern Med 97:845, 1982.

758. Peterson CD: Ethylene glycol poisoning: Pharmacokinetics during therapy with ethanol and hemodialysis. N Engl J Med 304:21, 1981.

759. Frommer JP: Acute ethylene glycol intoxication. Am J Nephrol 2:1, 1982.

760. Clay KL, Murphy RC: On the metabolic acidosis of ethylene glycol intoxication. Toxicol Appl Pharmacol 39:39, 1977.

761. Baud FJ, Galliott M, Astier A, et al: Treatment of ethylene glycol poisoning with intravenous 4-methylpyrazole. N Engl J Med 319:97, 1988.

762. Conger JD: Drug therapy in acute renal failure. *In* Lazaraus JM, Brenner BM (eds): Acute Renal Failure, 3rd ed. Churchill Livingstone, New York, 1993, p 527.

762a. Baldwin L, Henderson A, Hickman P: Effect of postoperative low-dose dopamine on renal function after elective major vascular surgery. Ann Intern Med 120:744, 1994.

762b. Denton ME, Chertow G, Brady HR: Renal-dose dopamine for the treatment of acute renal failure: A review of the rationale and results of experimental and human studies. Ann Intern Med (in press).

763. Schrimshaw NS: An analysis of past and present recommended dietary allowances for protein in health and disease. N Engl J Med 294:136, 1976.

764. Borah MF, Schoenfeld PY, Gotch FA, et al: Nitrogen balance during intermittent dialysis therapy of uremia. Kidney Int 14:491, 1978.

765. Wesson DE, Mitch WE, Wilmore DW: Nutritional considerations in the treatment of acute renal failure. *In* Brenner BM, Lazarus JM (eds): Acute Renal Failure. WB Saunders, Philadelphia, 1983, p 618.

765a. Hammerman MR, Miller SB: Therapeutic use of growth factors in renal failure. J Am Soc Nephrol 5:11, 1994.

766. Owen WF Jr, Lazarus JM: Dialytic management of acute renal failure. *In* Lazarus JM, Brenner BM (eds): Acute Renal Failure, 3rd ed. Churchill Livingstone, New York, 1993, p 487.

767. Teschan PE, Baxter CR, O'Brien TF, et al: Prophylactic hemodialysis in the treatment of acute renal failure. Ann Intern Med 53:992, 1960.

768. Fischer RP, Griffin WO, Resiser M, Clark DS: Early dialysis in the treatment of acute renal failure. Surg Gynecol Obstet 123:1019, 1966.

769. Conger JD: A controlled evaluation of prophylactic dialysis in post-traumatic acute renal failure. J Trauma 15:1056, 1975.

770. Mentzer SJ, Fryd DS, Kjellstrand CM: Why do patients with post-surgical acute renal failure die? Arch Surg 120:907, 1985.

771. Gillum DM, Dixon BS, Yanover MJ, et al: The role of intensive dialysis in acute renal failure. Clin Nephrol 25:249, 1986.

772. Mault JR, Dechert RE, Lees P, et al: Continuous arteriovenous filtration: An effective treatment for surgical acute renal failure. Surgery 101:478, 1987.
773. Conger JD: Does hemodialysis delay recovery from acute renal failure? Semin Dial 3:146, 1990.
774. Schulman G, Hakim R: Differences in vascular reactivity in models of ischemic renal failure. Kidney Int 39:1087, 1991.
775. Hakim RM: Clinical implications of hemodialysis membrane biocompatibility. Kidney Int 44:484, 1993.
775a. Schiffl H, Lang SM, Konig A, et al: Biocompatible membranes in acute renal failure: Prospective case-controlled study. Lancet 344:570, 1994.
775b. Hakim RM, Wingard R, Parker RA: Effect of the dialysis membrane in the treatment of patients with acute renal failure. N Engl J Med 331:1338, 1994.
776. Finn WF: Recovery from acute renal failure. In Lazarus JM, Brenner BM (eds): Acute Renal Failure, 3rd ed. Churchill Livingstone, New York, 1993, p 553.
777. Kiley JE, Powers SR, Beebe RT: Acute renal failure. Eighty cases of renal tubular necrosis. N Engl J Med 262:481, 1960.
778. Shackman R, Perkash I: Gastrointestinal bleeding in acute renal failure. Proc Eur Dial Transplant Assoc 1:15, 1964.
779. Lunding M, Steiness IB, Thaysen JH: Acute renal failure due to tubular necrosis. Acta Med Scand 176:103, 1964.
780. Blagg RC: The management of acute reversible intrinsic renal failure. Postgrad Med J 43:290, 1967.
781. Smith K, Browne JCM, Shackman R, Wrong OM: Renal failure of obstetric origin. Br Med Bull 24:49, 1968.
782. Domcott NJ, Dawson-Dewards P, Blainey JE: Surgical disasters and renal failure. Proc R Soc Med 61:215, 1968.
783. Flynn CT: Post-traumatic renal failure, including the use of the mobile artificial kidney. Proc R Soc Med 63:563, 1970.
784. Whelton A: Post-traumatic acute renal failure in Vietnam combat injuries: Incidence, morbidity and mortality. In Friedman EA, Eliahou HE (eds): Proceedings: Conference on Acute Renal Failure. Government Printing Office, Washington, DC, 1973, p 125. DHEW Publ. No. (NIH) 74-608.
785. Ireland GW, Kass AS: Post-traumatic acute renal failure. J Urol 111:425, 1974.
786. Stone WJ, Knepshield JH: Post-traumatic acute renal insufficiency in Vietnam. Clin Nephrol 2:186, 1974.
787. Merino GE, Buselmier TJ, Kjellstrand CM: Postoperative chronic renal failure: A new syndrome? Ann Surg 182:37 1975.
788. Alderson T, Meredith WT, Bubeck R, Weber H: Acute renal failure: An analysis of 80 patients requiring hemodialysis. J Kans Med Soc 77:481, 1976.
789. Minuth AN, Terrell JB, Suki, WN: Acute renal failure: A study of the course and prognosis of 104 patients and of the rule of furosemide. Am J Med Sci 271:317, 1976.
790. Karatson A, Juhasz J, Hubler J, et al: Factors influencing the prognosis of acute renal failure (analysis of 228 cases). Int Urol Nephrol 10:321, 1978.
791. Frankel MC, Weinstein AM, Stenzel KH: Prognostic patterns in acute renal failure: The New York Hospital, 1981–1982. Clin Exp Dial Apheresis 7:145, 1983.
792. Butkus DE: Persistent high mortality in acute renal failure. Are we asking the right question? Arch Intern Med 143:209, 1983.
793. Abreo K, Moorthy AV, Osborne M: Changing patterns and outcome of acute renal failure requiring hemodialysis. Arch Intern Med 146:1338, 1981.
794. Bullock ML, Umen AJ, Finkelstein M, Keane WF: The assessment of risk factors of 462 patients with acute renal failure. Am J Kidney Dis 5:97, 1985.
795. Rasmussen HH, Pitt EA, Ibels LS, McNeil DR: Prediction of outcome in acute renal failure by discriminant analysis of clinical variables. Arch Intern Med 145:2015, 1985.
796. Edwards KDG: Recovery of renal function after acute renal failure. Aust Ann Med 8:195, 1959.
797. Price JDE, Palmer RA: A functional and morphological follow-up study of acute renal failure. Arch Intern Med 105:114, 1960.
798. Morrin PAF, Gedney WB, Barth W, Heptinstall RH: Acute tubular necrosis. Ann Intern Med 56:925, 1962.
799. Muehrcke RC, Rasen S, Pirani CL, Kark RM: Renal lesions in patients recovering from acute renal failure. J Lab Clin Med 54:888, 1964.
800. Briggs JD, Kennedy AC, Young LN, et al: Renal function after acute tubular necrosis. Br J Med 3:513, 1967.
801. Muehrcke RC, Pirani CL: Arsine-induced anuria. A correlative clinicopathological study with electron microscopic observations. Ann Intern Med 68:853, 1968.
802. Pasternack A, Tallqvist G, Kuhlback B: Occurrence of interstitial nephritis in acute renal failure. Acta Med Scand 187:27, 1970.
803. Lewers DT, Mathew TH, Maher JF, Schreiner GE: Long term follow-up of renal function and history after acute tubular necrosis. Ann Intern Med 73:523, 1970.
804. Ameno A, Vercellone A, Benedictis G, et al: Longterm prognosis in acute renal failure of primarily tubular origin. Minerva Nephrol 19:7, 1972.
805. Levin ML, Simon NM, Herdson PB, del Greco F: Acute renal failure followed by protracted slowly resolving chronic uremia. J Chronic Dis 25:645, 1972.
806. Harvig B, Engberg A, Ezicsson JLE: Effects of cold ischemia on the preserved and transplanted rat kidney. Structural changes in the proximal tubules. Virchows Arch B 34:153, 1980.
807. Pru C, Ebben J, Kjellstrand CM: Chronic renal failure after acute tubular necrosis. Proc Am Soc Nephrol 14:49A, 1981.
808. Better OS, Stein JH: Early management of shock and prophylaxis of acute renal failure in traumatic rhabdomyolysis. N Engl J Med 322:825–829, 1990.

# Renal Response to Immunologic Glomerular Injury

*Curtis B. Wilson*

## OVERVIEW OF HUMORAL AND CELLULAR IMMUNE MECHANISMS

Immune mechanisms are clearly responsible for virtually all forms of glomerulonephritis (GN) seen in animals, as shown by experimental studies dating to the turn of the century, and similar mechanisms are being identified as the predominant cause of this disease in humans.[1,*][2,*][3,*][4] The immune mechanisms continue to be under scrutiny, with rearrangement of views an expected evolution.[3,5–16] Investigations of the immunopathogenesis of renal disease, initially of GN and then of tubulointerstitial nephritis (TIN),[3] have established the principal humoral mechanisms leading to immunologic renal injury, with more attention turning to cellular immune processes. The importance of antibodies (Abs) and their associated mediator mechanisms is emphasized by the ability to reproduce renal injury in passive transfer experiments. The explosion of information in the past few years is related directly to the application of cell culture and molecular methods including transgenic and "knockout" alterations in in vivo gene expression, and successful gene transfer to glomerular or tubule cells ensures continued progress and manipulation.[17,18]

*To abide by space limitations, many reference citations included in the previous editions of this chapter are omitted and simply noted as being available in the second (1), third (2), or fourth (3) edition. The chapter has also been further oriented to immunologic mechanisms exemplified in experimental models, with much of the information on human immune renal disease deleted to avoid overlap with other chapters. In this edition, information on immune tubulointerstitial injury is covered in Chapter 33.

## Humoral Mechanisms of Glomerular Injury

The two major humoral mechanisms leading to deposition of Abs within renal tissue are outlined in Table 29–1 in terms of the location of the antigen (Ag), that is, fixed within the kidney or present in soluble form in the vascular compartment (or other body fluids). Ab reactions with either type of Ag can lead to immune deposit formation; however, the dynamics of the Ag-Ab reaction are different because the soluble Ag is free to diffuse away but the tissue-fixed one is not. In the first humoral mechanism involving fixed Ags, Abs have specificity for an Ag present within the kidney either as a natural structural element or as a material trapped or "planted" there for a variety of physiologic, immunologic, or physicochemical reasons. Best known among the nephritogenic structural antigenic constituents would be the glomerular basement membranes (GBM) or tubule basement membrane (TBM). The Ab reaction with the evenly distributed GBM Ag results in characteristic linear immunoglobulin G (IgG) deposition in glomeruli by immunofluorescence study (Fig. 29–1). The immune deposit leads to mediator activation and subsequent rather nonselective injury to tissue in the vicinity. In contrast, renal cell surface Ags have been shown to serve as targets for often selective immune injury that may be confined to a single renal cell type. This type of immune reaction can lead to either Ab-induced cell injury or immune deposit formation through a capping and shedding mechanism.[6,19] Ab reactions with trapped Ags generally lead to immune deposit formation, with the pattern of im-

**Humoral Immune Mechanisms***
Direct antibody reactions with tissue-fixed antigens
  Antibody reactions with native renal antigens
    Basement membrane and extracellular matrix antigens
      Glomerular basement membrane, tubule basement membrane components, ? tubule basement membrane–drug conjugates, and others
  Antibody reactions with renal cell antigens†
    Cell surface and other antigens such as Fx1A, gp330, angiotensin-converting enzyme, Thy-1.1, Tamm-Horsfall protein, infectious agents, phagocytosed materials, other monoclonal antibody–reactive antigens
  Antibody reactions with antigens trapped or "planted" in the kidney
    Charged or lectin-like molecules, DNA, immune deposit components, ? infectious products
Antibody reactions with soluble antigens to form immune complexes‡
  Exogenous antigens
    Drugs, microbial antigens, and so on
  Endogenous antigens
    Nuclear and cellular materials, tumor antigens, thyroglobulin, and others

**Cellular Immune Mechanisms**
Glomerular injury—role as yet unquantified, good evidence in chicken and rat models
Tubulointerstitial renal injury—prominent role in some forms
?? Cellular immune contribution to minimal-change nephrotic syndrome

**? Activation of Mediator Pathways**
? Immune or nonimmune
  Glomerular or tubule mediator deposition
    Complement proteins, coagulation proteins, and others
  ?? Antibody-induced activation of neutrophils (disease associated with antineutrophil cytoplasmic antibodies)

*Antibody reactions typically result in formation of immune deposits (with mediator activation) in glomeruli or tubulointerstitial renal structures. Antibody reactions (local or systemic) without renal immune deposit formation need to be considered as well and could involve mediator activation or release or other mechanisms yet to be defined.

†Antibody reactions with cell surface antigens can lead to immune deposit formation and can also induce cell injury with destruction or proliferation.

‡Immune complex formation can occur in the vascular compartment or in extravascular sites depending on systemic or local release of antigen.

munoglobulin (Ig) deposition corresponding to the site and pattern of Ag binding. Such reactions could result in direct cellular injury, depending on the extent and site of Ag localization.

In the second humoral mechanism, Abs interact in dynamic equilibrium with soluble Ags, present in the circulation or other body fluids, to form immune complexes (ICs). The ICs (and their components), which escape clearance by the mononuclear phagocytic system, circulate and can accumulate primarily in the glomeruli, GBM, and mesangium as well as in vessels, TBM, and interstitium. Because the Ag is soluble, it can diffuse away from the site during the continual IC rearrangement that goes on to maintain the dynamic equilibrium between varying concentrations of Ag and Ab. ICs may also form locally when the soluble Ag is in extravascular fluids of the interstitial tissue or vessel walls of an organ, resulting in a type of Arthus phenomenon. The pattern of Ig deposition seen in IC disease is typically granular and irregular (see Fig. 29–1).

Once Abs combine with Ag and deposit in the kidney or other tissue, interrelated mediator pathways are activated.[20–23] The understanding of these mediator pathways continues to evolve, and the renal cells themselves have become a focus of study because these cells are capable of supplying a rather large number of mediators including cytokines, arachidonic acid metabolites, and enzymes capable of contributing to the evolution of the lesion. The mediator pathways are those normally associated with the body's defense system, in which Abs recognize an invader or an altered portion of "self" leading to the destruction of either. These systems include complement (C), leukocytes and their products, and coagulation proteins, which when directed by nephritogenic Ab reactions can injure renal tissue as well. A section of this chapter is devoted to a discussion of the potential mediation systems.

A third potential mechanism of humoral immune injury needs to be considered (see Table 29–1). Glomerular injury sometimes occurs in the absence of detected Ab deposition, identified as Ig deposition, but with striking glomerular C accumulation and depressions in serum C levels as in patients with hypocomplementemic membranoproliferative GN. Autoantibodies are often present and can cause activation of the alternative C pathway (see later). These observations suggest that immune mediator activation unrelated to immune deposit formation may also be involved in the development of inflammatory glomerular lesions.

In the so-called pauci-immune necrotizing and crescentic rapidly progressive GN it is suggested that Abs may contribute directly to mediator activation. These diseases, such as Wegener granulomatosis and some other forms of microvasculitis, have a conspicuous morphologic GN with little or no evidence of glomerular immune deposits, leading to the term pauci-immune. In these diseases, circulating Abs, termed antineutrophil cytoplasmic antibodies (ANCAs), reactive with Ag in the cytoplasm of neutrophils and monocytes have been recognized.[24–32] Two types of ANCA are separated by their staining pattern on ethanol-fixed neutrophils. In one, the reaction is found in a diffuse granular cytoplasmic pattern, which is termed C-ANCA, with the reaction directed mainly to proteinase 3.[33–38] In the other, the staining pattern is perinuclear and termed P-ANCA, with a major reactivity to myeloperoxidase (MPO).[26] The MPO present in the primary granules is a basic protein and redistributes to the negatively charged nucleus during fixation. The C-ANCA reaction is quite specific for Wegener granulomatosis, and levels of ANCA can be used as guides for treatment; in contrast, P-ANCAs, which may resemble antinuclear Abs, occur in a variety of diseases.[39] When coupled with a specific assay for MPO, these Abs aid in the diagnosis of pauci-immune necrotizing-crescentic GN.[40] The affinity of the IgG anti-MPO Ab falls with treatment, and although the levels of IgG anti-MPO Ab increase with relapse, the affinity remains low.[41] In this study, IgM anti-MPO Ab, when present, is usually seen early in the course of disease. IgM ANCA is reported to be seen in patients presenting with pulmonary hemorrhage.[42, 43] P-ANCAs are also found in some patients presenting with anti-GBM Abs with and without pulmonary hemorrhage[44] (see later). False-positive reactions can occur, for example, when lactoferrin is detected in MPO enzyme-linked immunosorbent

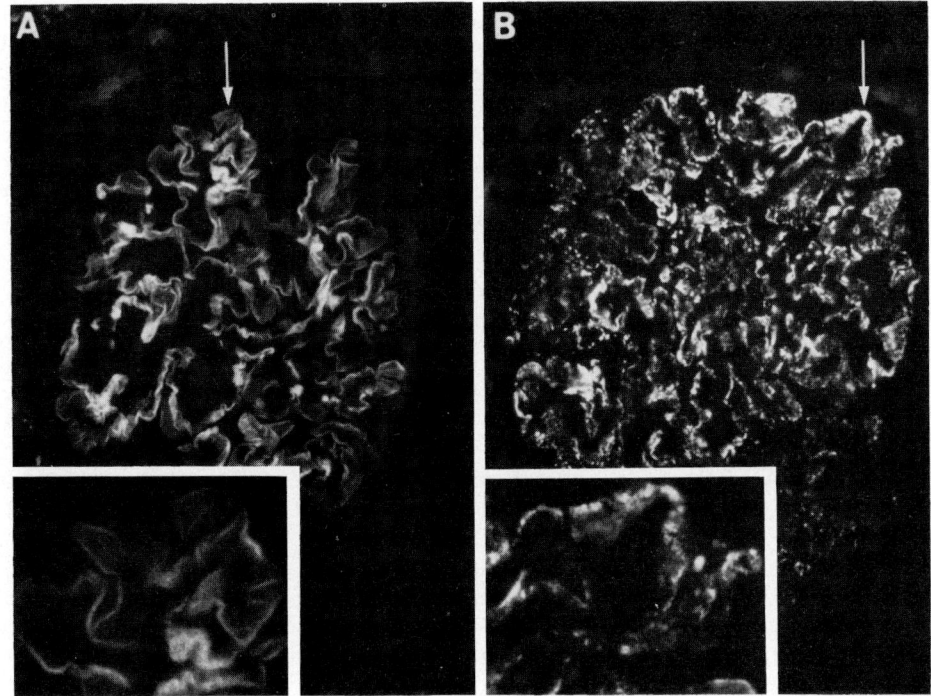

**Figure 29–1.** Immunofluorescence comparison of anti-GBM and IC deposits in human GN. *A.* Smooth linear deposits of anti-GBM Ab are present uniformly along the GBM of a patient with Goodpasture syndrome. The continuity of the deposit even at high magnification of the capillary loop *(arrow)* is evident in the inset. *B.* Irregular granular deposits of Ig in randomly deposited presumed IC deposits are present in the GBM and mesangium. The granular nature of the deposit in the GBM *(arrow)* is evident at high magnification in the inset. (Fluorescein isothiocyanate–conjugated antihuman IgG; original magnification in *A* and *B* × 250; insets × 630.)

assay in patients with antinuclear reactivity.[45] Of interest, the brown Norway (BN) rat, which develops a number of autoantibodies including anti-GBM Abs after exposure to mercuric chloride, also develops anti-MPO Abs after such treatment.[46–49] The time courses of the development of the two Abs appear to be independent.

The immunopathogenic role (if any) of these Abs is not yet defined; however, if the Abs are more than an epiphenomenon, their role would be expected to be different from that of Abs leading to immune deposit formation and may involve neutrophil activation.[50] For example, the Abs could be involved in disrupting some element of neutrophil physiology, which in turn may be phlogogenic to the glomerular capillary wall or other vessel walls, perhaps by mediator release, activation, or compromise of control mechanisms.[51] Indeed, both forms of ANCA are capable of inducing an oxidative burst and degranulation in neutrophils in vitro.[52, 53] Neutrophils activated with tumor necrosis factor (TNF) in the presence of endotoxin can be induced to damage endothelial cell cultures in a dose-response fashion when exposed to anti-MPO ANCA.[54] MPO can bind to the GBM and be active in oxidative reactions in vivo.[55] Immune responses can be induced to MPO.[56] MPO binding in rats previously immunized against MPO can induce glomerular injury and MPO binding from neutrophil lysosomal enzymes, and hydrogen peroxide production in the presence of anti-MPO Ab enhances glomerular damage (see later in trapped Ag section).[57] ANCA can interfere with signal transduction pathways and $Ca^{2+}$ mobilization, possibly via a reduction of platelet-activating factor (PAF) synthesis.[58] Activated neutrophils are found in glomeruli of patients with ANCA and Wegener granulomatosis.[59] TNF-α, interleukin-1β (IL-1β), and IL-2 receptor–positive cells are found in periglomerular and interstitial sites.[60] Injury resulting from antiendothelial Abs sometimes found in such sera

(see later) is also to be considered, as is the role of cell adhesion molecules and other endothelial components.[61]

The relationship between the control of the immune response and genes linked with the major histocompatibility complex (MHC) in animal studies has focused attention on the possible relationship of immune forms of GN with the human leukocyte antigen (HLA) system in humans. The interplay between the MHC, Ag-derived peptide, and the T cell receptor is central to the immune response. The HLA gene complex resides on chromosome 6 in humans, and genes in this region code for the HLA products (class I [A, B, and C loci] and class II [DR, DQ, and DP loci]). In the same region, HLA class III genes for a number of C components are situated between those for HLA class I and class II genes.

The MHC gene products are essential for proper communication between Ag-presenting cells (APCs), B cells, and T cell subsets and in turn offer a site for immune intervention.[62–66] The class I protein is a noncovalently linked dimer of a polymorphic α-chain encoded by the A, B, or C locus and a smaller polypeptide called $β_2$-microglobulin. The structure of the class I protein provides a groove in the molecule for presenting a bound peptide to a $CD8^+$ T cell. Each allelic form of class I protein has specificity for a particular peptide of 8 to 10 amino acids. The peptides that bind class I molecules are derived endogenously from proteins synthesized in the cell, that is, viral proteins. The class II proteins are also noncovalently linked dimers, but both the α- and β-chains are encoded by genes in the HLA complex. The peptide binding site is similar to the class I molecule and is composed of the $NH_2$-terminal α1 and β1 regions of the two chains, each containing a helical segment, and β-sheet structures that form one wall and half the floor of the groove produced by the chains. The peptides that bind are 10 to 18 amino acids in length and the peptides for presentation to CD4$^+$ T cells are derived from exogenous proteins that have been taken in by the APCs. The diversity of the MHC then functions to determine which peptide Ags can be presented to the immune cells.

The results of several sometimes conflicting studies of different populations of patients with identifiable forms of GN have been reviewed and indicate that HLA as well as C factors, Ig genes, and T cell receptors may be related to the immunogenetics of GN.[67–81] Anti-GBM Ab disease (see later), membranous nephropathy, IgA nephropathy, and systemic lupus erythematosus (SLE) all have associations with various DR Ags and in some cases with HLA-A and -B Ags that are in linkage disequilibrium with them.

## Cellular Immunity and Glomerular Injury

Ab alone is adequate to induce glomerular injury rapidly (within minutes for anti-GBM Ab), as evidenced by passive transfer studies. These studies exclude any role for induced cellular immunity in this acute experimental situation. In active immunization models and in human immune-related renal diseases associated with immune deposit formation, it appears that in most instances Ab is also of major importance; however, it is likely that cellular immune processes are stimulated and may contribute in varying ways in different situations.[3, 82–93] For example, in experimental anti-TBM Ab–associated TIN in rats, striking mononuclear infiltrates with large numbers of T cells develop after an initial invasion of neutrophils, which accompany Ab and C deposition.[3, 94] Some models of TIN, particularly those in mice, are the clearest examples of cellular immune renal injury.[3, 95–99] The cellular immune responses in TIN are described in Chapter 33.

Models of cellular immune glomerular injury are evolving. Transfer of sensitized cells specific for a planted Ag in anti-GBM or IC GN leads to accumulation of low numbers of mononuclear cells in glomeruli.[100, 101] Systemic cell-mediated reactions could also lead to accumulation of mononuclear cells in the lungs and glomeruli.[102] A role for T cells was suggested in a model of glomerular injury induced using cationized conjugates of trinitrophenol and bovine serum albumin (BSA) planted in the kidneys of rats previously sensitized to trinitrophenol.[103] These rats immunized to trinitrophenol manifested contact sensitivity to the immunogen. In autoimmune GN in chickens, there is good evidence for a prominent role for cellular immunity because the glomerular lesion (which is accompanied by production of anti-GBM Ab) has been induced in chickens that have undergone ablation of their humoral immune system by cyclophosphamide-induced bursectomy.[104–106] In addition, the nephritic lesion can be transferred with sensitized lymphoid cells in syngeneic chickens.[107] Models of autoimmune GN in BN or Wistar-Kyoto rats immunized with GBM Ags have been described, similar in concept to that originally described in sheep by Steblay[1837] for induction of anti-GBM Ab (see later).[108, 109] In these BN models, transfer of T cells is able to prime the immune response of naive recipients to the GBM Ags. Ab to CD4$^+$ T cells reduced

circulating anti-GBM Ab and largely prevented disease.[110] Azobenzenearsonate, a hapten that directly modifies surface-expressed proteins and induces delayed hypersensitivity, was used to induce a severe cellular glomerular injury by infusion into one kidney of previously sensitized BN rats.[111] The lesion can be reproduced in naive rats by adoptive transfer of T cells but not by passive Ab. A model of acute cell-mediated glomerular injury has been described by Andres and colleagues[112] in which rats receiving renal allografts were injected with phytohemagglutinin shortly after transplantation. Phytohemagglutin, as well as IL-1β and TNF-α, enhances the severity of lymphocyte infiltration in acute serum sickness in rabbits.[113]

A role for lymphocytes in the early infiltration of glomeruli after anti-GBM Ab in rats was suggested on morphologic grounds in 1979 by Kreisberg and colleagues.[114] Studies with monoclonal Abs have reported on average about one T cell per glomerular cross section in saline-perfused normal rat kidneys (T helper/T suppressor ratio, 2:1).[115] The T cell subsets found in glomerular disease have been the subject of review.[116] T cells consisting mainly of helper T cells (one or two per glomerular cross section) were noted (using monoclonal Abs) in an augmented autologous phase anti-GBM Ab lesion in rats.[117] In this model, suppression of T cell function with cyclosporine impaired T cell accumulation and subsequent macrophage influx. Lymphokine production by glomerular T cells was reported in this situation as well.[118] Nonetheless, humoral mechanisms related to the magnitude of Ab response in the autologous phase of injury appear to have much more significance than the presence of delayed-type hypersensitivity.[119] Activated T cells and MHC class I and II proteins were found in glomeruli of rabbits with anti-GBM GN.[120] T cells were also reported early in acute serum sickness.[121] A role for activated T cells has been suggested in the development of glomerular crescents associated with rupture of the Bowman capsule.[122] T cell infiltration has been reported in anti-GBM Ab–induced lung injury in rats with onset by 3 days.[123] T cells and monocytes also occur as interstitial infiltrates in anti-GBM GN.[124] The increase in T cells in lymph nodes draining the kidney correlates with the interstitial infiltrate and the autologous Ab response to the heterologous anti-GBM Ab Ig.[125] Aleutian mink disease has an IC type of GN with interstitial infiltrates in which tubule cell expression of the Aleutian mink disease parvovirus is associated with T cell accumulation, suggesting the contribution of T cells to the lesion.[126]

Anti-CD4 Ab reduced immune deposits and proteinuria in Heymann nephritis (HN) and anti-CD8 AG reduced proteinuria without any effect on immune deposits.[127] CD4$^+$ T cell depletion prevents anti-DNA Ab with increased survival in the (NZB × NZW)F$_1$, MRL-*lpr/lpr,* and BXSB murine lupus models.[128–130] The autosomal recessive lymphoproliferation (*lpr*) gene identified as the *Fas* Ag gene involved in apoptosis[131] causes a massive proliferation of abnormal T cells with disease induction modulated by measures that abrogate the proliferation of these cells. The development of murine lupus was suppressed using a graft-versus-host reaction with CD8$^+$ T cells.[132] CD4$^+$ donor cells in chronic graft-versus-host disease have defects including overproduction of IL-4 and IL-10, with anti–IL-4 Ab delaying development of the glomerular lesion.[133–135] In graft-versus-host disease, CD4[+] T cell depletion prevents the associated autoimmune disease.[136, 137] The alloreactive host CD4[+] cells have a T helper type 2 (Th2) phenotype, producing little IL-2 or interferon-γ (IFN-γ) but secreting IL-4 and IL-10.[138–140] A Th2 response is also suggested in mercuric chloride-induced disease in the BN rat in studies using anti–IL-4 Ab.[141, 142] Depletion of CD8[+] T cells prevented the induction of crescentic GN produced with small doses of anti-GBM Ab in the Wistar-Kyoto rat.[143] Optimal T cell activation after T cell receptor–MHC class II interaction requires costimulatory signals including CD28 (CTLA-4) on T cells and B7 molecules on APCs. CTLA-4 administration reduced the severity of the anti-GBM Ab GN model in the Wistar-Kyoto rat.[144] Neonatal thymectomy in ddY mice (which spontaneously develop a form of IgA nephropathy) modulated the glomerular IgA deposition somewhat without changing serum IgA or macromolecular IgA levels.[145]

In patients, cellular sensitivity usually accompanies a nephritogenic humoral immune response and was identified years ago using in vitro techniques, particularly those in which renal basement membrane materials are used to stimulate lymphoid cells.[3] For example, a cellular response to proteinase-3 in C-ANCA disease has been reported.[146] The phenotypic characteristics of circulating lymphoid cells have been studied in a number of laboratories and groups of patients with varying results. Increased ratios of CD4[+] to CD8[+] T cells were revealed in patients with membranous GN, IgA nephropathy, and mesangial cell proliferative GN in some[147–150] but not other[151–153] studies. In IgA nephropathy, with its increased levels of circulating IgA, there was evidence of increased T helper activity; use of IL-2 and IFN-γ as markers of Th1 and IL-4 and IL-5 to distinguish Th2 in the CD4[+] population showed that both Th1 and Th2 were activated.[154] IL-4 is also overproduced in IgA nephropathy patients.[155] Abnormalities in T cell (as well as B cell) function are present in uremia and can be found in many types of GN, with alterations in SLE and membranous GN.[3] Autoantigen-specific T helper cells are thought to drive the production of autoantibodies by B cells.[156]

Monoclonal Abs reactive with phenotypic markers unique to T cell subsets, with some Ags persisting for detection in paraffin-embedded tissues as well as lectins specific for certain mononuclear cell types, are being used to identify these cells in tissue sections.[157–159] Dendritic cells positive for CD1b and HLA-DR are found in glomeruli in GN.[160] T cells are prominent in both experimental and human TIN.[94, 161–163] In glomerular lesions, T cells are identified in only small numbers in some but not all studies.[86] A fraction of 1% of the glomerular cells in poststreptococcal GN are T cells, with CD4[+] cells early and CD8[+] cells later.[164] Increased T cells are found in proliferative histologic forms of GN, with a scattering of numbers among individual cases; in IgA nephropathy there were few glomerular leukocytes.[165, 166] Other studies using similar techniques have identified few if any T cells in glomeruli in any form of GN but have defined large numbers of such cells in accompanying tubulointerstitial infiltrates.[167] The reason for the differences in these studies is unclear; however, the numbers of T cells are small at most and their role

in directly damaging the glomerular wall or more likely being involved in monocyte accumulation (see later) remains to be defined and quantitated.

An important step in the immune response is the presentation of Ag via the MHC molecule to the T cell receptor. This characteristically occurs when Ag fragments are processed by the APC and then are presented on its surface bound in a groove present in an MHC Ag molecule (see earlier). The evaluation of the T cell response induced by the MHC and T cell receptor interaction is profoundly affected by the cytokine environment during T cell differentiation.[168] Class II MHC Ag presentation causes CD4[+] cells to proliferate, and class I presentation leads to cell death via CD8[+] T cells. Endothelial cells can present alloantigens to circulating T cells.[169] There has been interest in the possible role of renal cells, initially renal tubule epithelial cells, functioning as APCs. MHC class I and particularly class II (Ia in mice and rats, DR in humans) expression is modulated in tubule epithelial cells by rejection and during autoimmune reactions in the kidney.[3] A murine proximal tubule cell line that produces the 3M-1 target Ag of murine autoimmune TIN has class II MHC Ags recognized by cloned L3T4[+] helper T cells specific for 3M-1.[170–172] The cultured tubule cell supported the growth of the T cell line and probably functions as an APC of its own Ag. Steroids reduce Ia expression and GN in autoimmune lupus mice.[173] Studies by Rubin-Kelley and co-workers[174–177] have shown that cloned tubule epithelial cells can present Ag and that in murine lupus autoreactive, kidney-infiltrating T cells of the same phenotype as the T cells regulated by the *lpr* gene proliferate to tubule epithelial cells and mesangial cells. T cell clones from the interstitial T cells express α/β T cell receptor and β cell markers but not CD4 or CD8. They proliferate to renal tubule cells, but not other cells, and they secrete IFN-γ, which induces MHC class II Ags and intercellular adhesion molecule-1 (ICAM-1) on renal tubule cells.[178] Transgenic tubule cell expression of class II Ag alone is insufficient to induce immune renal injury.[179] Ag processing and presentation by glomerular visceral epithelial cells are also reported.[180] The mesangial cell expressed class II MHC Ags, ICAM, a variety of cytokines, and T cell or monocyte chemoattractants and is also a candidate for Ag presentation.[181] Studies suggest that IFN-γ stimulated both class I and class II MHC on cultured mesangial cells, whereas TNF-α induced only class I and IL-1 had little effect.[182] The mouse mesangial cell is effective in inducing syngeneic T helper lymphocytes to proliferate, as are allogenic mesangial cells.[183] Increased MHC class II expression is observed in human glomerular inflammation and correlates with IFN-γ levels.[184]

The MHC is involved in yet another type of reaction that has been hypothesized to be related to autoimmune responses.[185, 186] Microbial superantigens that can bind directly to MHC class II molecules activate a large number of T cells through the variable region of the T cell receptor β-chain.[187] Superantigens can induce rheumatoid factors[188] and have been reported to reduce lupus nephritis in MRL/*lpr* mice in association with a reduction in T cell receptor Vβ8op[+], CD4[-]CD8[-] peripheral T cells.[189]

The glomerular lesion of minimal-change nephrotic syndrome (MCNS) and the sometimes associated focal and segmental glomerulosclerosis (FSGS) lesion can be differentiated from mesangial disorders such as IgM mesangial proliferative GN.[190, 191] In both MCNS and FSGS, there are decreased anionic sites and epithelial cell vacuolization may be a feature of FSGS.[192, 193] MCNS has been postulated to be related to abnormal T cell function, and some of the older information including MHC associations has been summarized.[194–196] Serum from patients with MCNS inhibits blastogenesis of normal lymphocytes in response to mitogens, although the finding may be present in other forms of nephrotic syndrome.[197] Lymphocytes recovered from patients with MCNS may also exhibit impaired blastogenesis in nephrotic or normal sera. The function of the peripheral cells can be increased with recombinant granulocyte-macrophage colony-stimulating factors.[198] CD8$^+$ cells are increased and histamine H$_2$-receptor–bearing T cells are decreased.[199, 200] The role of factors related to nephrotic syndrome (such as hyperlipidemia) that have known effects on normal lymphocytes needs to be considered, as does the role of decreased transferrin levels.[197, 201, 202] The observation of decreased lymphokine production associated with measles infection and remission in MCNS also spurs interest in a possible T cell relationship in this disease.

Studies of patients with MCNS have shown impaired T colony-forming capacity and T colony-stimulating factor that could be enhanced with IL-2.[203, 204] IL-2 production by T cells from patients with MCNS is decreased.[205] The T cell abnormalities in one study were related to lowering of the blood zinc level.[206] Impaired delayed-type hypersensitivity reactions and local graft-versus-host reaction are also noted.[207–209] Serum IgE levels may be increased; however, the increase is not confined to nephrotic syndrome of MCNS.[210, 211] Increased concanavalin A (Con A)–induced suppressor cell activity is noted in MCNS but is not confined to it and is not consistently found.[212–216] A factor is present in the urine and serum of patients with MCNS and some, but not all, nephrotic urines that suppresses polyclonal plaque-forming cell responses.[217] The factor disappeared with a response of the nephrotic syndrome to steroids.[218] It has been shown that a CD4$^+$ inducer T cell from patients with steroid-responsive nephrotic syndrome secretes a protein that causes CD8$^+$ suppressor T cells to produce this inhibitor.[219] A study using serum, urine, and culture supernatants of mitogen-stimulated peripheral blood mononuclear cells found that among IL-1β, IL-2, IFN-α, IFN-γ, and TNF-α, only TNF-α was elevated in FSGS compared with normal individuals and MCNS patients, although the latter had increased TNF-α in cell supernatants.[220] Increased IL-1 and IL-2 from mitogen-stimulated lymphocyte cultures were found in another study.[221]

A factor released from lymphocytes in patients with MCNS, but not confined to this disease, increases permeability of capillaries and is reported to produce alteration in the glomerular epithelial cell foot processes after infusion into the renal artery.[222] This lymphocyte product tested by cutaneous permeability assays or injection into rats can alter the appearance of glomerular epithelial cells and is related to the CD4$^+$ T cell population.[223–227] It is reported to be a small molecule, 12 kd, distinct from IL-2.[228] Its production is inhibited by cyclosporine and FK 506.[229, 230] This T cell factor is different from the 34- to 43-kd dimeric vascular permeability factor/vascular endothelial cell growth factor

that is synthesized and secreted by a variety of tumor cells as well as normal cells including glomerular cells. Several different molecular species arise from alternative splicing of the vascular endothelial cell growth factor messenger RNA (mRNA).[231, 232] The factor is active in maintaining the vascular endothelium and in promoting tumor angiogenesis. It has been found in glomerular epithelial, mesangial, and endothelial cells.[233–236] It is an autocrine factor in glomerular endothelial cells. It increases production of collagenase by endothelial cells and may contribute to proteinuria by proteolytic effects on the GBM in addition to its permeability effects.[237]

A vascular reactivity factor may be present in the serum of patients with active MCNS.[238] Infused serum from patients with MCNS reduced glomerular anionic sites and was found to contain a cationic protein.[239, 240] The frequent recurrence of nephrotic syndrome in patients with corticosteroid resistance and focal glomerulosclerosis who require renal transplantation has led to the use of plasmapheresis and plasma protein adsorption on protein A–Sepharose to remove a protein and reduce protein excretion by the patients.[241, 242] The material recovered induced proteinuria in in vitro and in vivo testing.

IFN may induce nephrotic syndrome and is suggested as a candidate lymphokine that is elevated in some MCNS patients.[243, 244] IL-2 is not usually associated with increased permeability of the glomerular capillary wall.[245, 246] Serum and urine soluble IL-2 receptor is increased in MCNS, and the IL-2 receptor may represent one of the serum inhibitory factors.[247, 248] These multiple bits of information just reviewed provide a tantalizing, but as yet uncertain, basis for a role for cellular immunity in MCNS.

## MEDIATORS OF IMMUNOLOGICALLY INDUCED RENAL INJURY

After deposition of Ab in tissue, either during reactions directed to specific fixed antigenic sites or by random accumulation of ICs, multifaceted mediation pathways are brought into play, resulting in tissue injury. The several mediator systems overlap, making it difficult to assign the precise contribution of each to the varied histologic and functional parameters of glomerular damage. The contribution of each mediator also varies with the model used and the severity and stage of injury. The effects of these various systems have been studied, most often in models of GN induced by anti-GBM Abs (see later). Anti-GBM Ab–induced GN occurs in two distinct phases, an acute or heterologous phase, occurring within minutes to hours after sufficient quantities of Ab are administered, and a delayed or autologous phase that develops when the host's immune system reacts to the glomerulus-bound Ig from the heterologous anti-GBM Ab. C activation, with subsequent neutrophil-induced enzymatic damage to the glomerular capillary wall, is a well-documented mediation mechanism in the acute phase. The terminal C components, C5b-9, which make up the membrane attack complex (MAC), are important mediators, and the C effect is altered by plasma and membrane-bound inhibitors of both the early and terminal C components. The involvement of monocyte/macrophages is important, particularly in the later, more chronic stages of injury. Platelets and PAF contribute as well. The fibrin and fibrinolytic systems, perhaps triggered by tissue factor–related procoagulant activity of infiltrating cells, are implicated in crescent formation. Eicosanoids, reactive oxygen species (ROS), and mediator molecules produced by both infiltrating and intrinsic glomerular cells, particularly the glomerular mesangium, are also involved. Processes leading to sclerosis of the glomerulus eventuate in progressive damage and loss of renal function. There is a certain redundancy in the multiple interacting mediation systems, so inhibition of a single factor even at its point of maximal effect may produce only a partial amelioration. Studies are now being focused on the control elements that affect the expression of multiple proinflammatory molecules as a means of increasing therapeutic effect. For example, nuclear factor-κB, a transcription regulatory factor responsible for expression of several proinflammatory molecules, and the mechanism controlling mRNA stability of labile proinflammatory mRNAs that have multiple AUUUA motifs in their 3'-untranslated regions could be useful therapeutic targets. Interventions that modulate mediation have the value of not needing to confront the difficulties inherent in attempting to identify and specifically manipulate the precise immune mechanism responsible.

## Complement and the C5b-9 Membrane Attack Complex

When Abs react with their specific Ags, either in tissues or in circulating ICs, the C sequence may be activated.[3, 14, 23, 249–256] C deficiencies may predispose to the development of GN.[257] Renal C activation via ammonia interactions also needs to be considered, especially in tubule C deposits.[258]

The C system is composed of multiple plasma and membrane proteins having enzymatic, membrane-binding, and regulatory properties. Five of the components (C1r, C1s, C2, factor B, and factor D) are serine proteases. Activation of the C system through C3 can occur by the classic or alternative pathway and leads to release of several biologically active factors during the assembly of a common terminal C5b-9 pathway called the MAC.[259–261] The components are capable of transferring themselves from solution to form a solid-phase enzyme system by activation of binding sites that are revealed transiently by activating enzymes. The C5b-9 or MAC assembly, in addition to forming a transmembrane channel that functions in lysing cells, can stimulate glomerular epithelial and mesangial cells to express a number of inflammation-related molecules (see later). The classic pathway is activated by aggregated or IC IgG (subclasses IgG1, IgG2, and IgG3, not IgG4) and IgM. C1 can also be activated directly by RNA tumor viruses, vesicular stomatitis virus, certain endotoxins, and monosodium urate crystals. C1, a reversible $Ca^{2+}$-dependent complex of C1q, C1r, and C1s, binds to the Fc region of complexed Ig via the C1q subunit. C1r and C1s are cleaved, catalyzing the formation of the classic pathway C3 convertase from C2 and C4, in the presence of $Mg^{2+}$. First, C4 is cleaved into a and b fragments, and the larger C4b fragment binds to the IC. The breakdown product of C4b, namely C4d, can be used as a monitor of classic pathway activation.[3, 262–264] The cleavage of C4b to C4d by its inhibitor, factor I (C3b inactivator), and a cofactor, the C4b-binding protein, can be studied in glomeruli using immunofluorescence and can also identify activation of the classic pathway.[3] Two C4 molecules (C4A, C4B) are found as products of closely spaced genes on chromosome 6.[265] They differ in their ability to bind to substrates, thereby broadening the range of host defense. Next, C2 is cleaved with the larger bound C2a fragment, forming classic pathway C3 convertase. This cleaves the α-chain of C3, exposing a binding site through which C3b can bind to the IC. The C3a fragment formed is an anaphylatoxin and has been suggested to suppress specific and nonspecific immune responses.[3] C3 activation is also involved in B cell activation via CR2 receptors that bind iC3b, C3dg, and C3d and perhaps also CR1 receptors that bind C3b, iC3b, and C4b.[266, 267] The C fragments may also be mitogenic.[268]

The C4b,2a3b complex, in turn, cleaves C5, initiating the assembly of the C5b-9 MAC and releasing C5a, an anaphylatoxin that is also a chemotaxin. Regulatory proteins control the anaphylatoxin and chemotaxin properties and may be altered during hemodialysis.[3] The conversion of C5a to C5a des Arg by removal of its terminal arginine alters its anaphylatoxin properties, but does not destroy its inflammatory mediation properties, while slowing its clearance from the circulation.[3]

A variety of circulating and cell-bound C regulatory proteins modulate the amount of C activation and its consequences.[269–271] In addition to spatial and decay constraints, control is achieved by C1 inhibitor, which binds to activated C1r and C1s, and by C4-binding protein (C4bp), factor H, and factor I, which cleaves C3b and C4b in the presence of cofactor activity. The membrane proteins decay-accelerating factor (CD55) and complement receptor type 1 (CR1, CD35) inhibit the stability of the C3 and C5 convertase.[272, 273] CR1 and membrane cofactor protein (MCP, CD46) act indirectly as cofactors in the enzymatic degradation of C3b and C4b by factor I.[274] C regulatory factors are recovered from glomerular epithelial cells and CD35 is released from these cells.[275, 276] CD46 was identified in human kidneys and glomeruli and was found to be up-regulated in glomerulonephritic kidneys.[277–279] Decay-accelerating factor has been found to increase on glomerular mesangial cells in response to IC formation and the increase may be related to terminal C component activation.[280] CR1 is found on rat glomerular epithelial cells, but not rat glomeruli, in contrast to human glomeruli.[281] CR1 mRNA is found only in glomerular differentiation, suggesting slow or intermittent expression.[282]

The self-assembly of the MAC results in the generation of high-affinity phospholipid binding sites and overcomes the charge in the hydrophobic barrier of the cell membrane, producing lesions that resemble transmembrane channels. The channels result from the assembly or polymerization of C9 (poly C9) to C5b-8, which is only weakly lytic on red blood cells. In addition to lysis of cells (more difficult in nucleated cells than in red blood cells because of self-repair), the MAC has other effects on intracellular events.

The MAC channels are different from those produced by perforin in lymphocyte-mediated cytolysis.[283]

In addition to control of lysis via the inhibition of the C3 and C5 convertase in forming the MAC, the MAC is inhibited by a serum constituent called the S protein as well as the glycosylphosphatidylinositol (GPI)-anchored CD59 (membrane inhibitor of reactive lysis, protectin) and C8-binding protein, also called homologous restriction factor.[284–288] These molecules interfere with assembly of the terminal components of the MAC.[289, 290] The acquired mutation that leads to the inability of cells to synthesize GPI anchors to retain decay-accelerating factor C8bp (homologous restriction factor), and CD59, among other proteins, renders red blood cells susceptible to C lysis in paroxysmal nocturnal hemoglobinuria. Genetic deficiencies of C proteins not only increase susceptibility to infections but also increase the occurrence of autoimmune disease, including GN.[1, 3, 257, 291, 292]

The alternative C pathway evolved to provide an immediate response to infecting organisms.[293] The interplay of C and cytokine release in sepsis has been reviewed.[294] The alternative pathway is viewed as a system in which slow, continued, and controlled activation of C3 (C3b-dependent positive feedback mechanism) may be rapidly expanded by alterations of control mechanisms by certain activator substances.[1] These materials include particulate plant, fungal, and bacterial polysaccharides and lipopolysaccharides such as inulin, zymosan, and certain gram-negative bacteria. Human lymphoblastoid cells, rabbit erythrocytes, and neuraminidase-treated sheep erythrocytes can also be involved. In addition, in certain situations, the pathway can be activated by Abs including guinea pig $\gamma$-1 and aggregates of human IgA or IgE. The pathway is also reported to be activated by monoclonal $\lambda$ light chains in membranoproliferative GN.[295] Human IgG antiviral Abs reacting with virally infected cells can also activate the pathway.

The alternative pathway utilizes C3, B (factor B), D (factor D), H ($\beta$-1H), factor I, and P (properdin).[3] Small amounts of C3b are continually formed in the serum and can complex with B in the presence of $Mg^{2+}$, rendering B susceptible to cleavage and activation by D and leading to the formation of the alternative pathway C3 convertase known as C3bBb. C3bBb would lead to formation of more molecules of C3b, generating more and more enzyme in the presence of unlimited amounts of B (D is not consumed and is used over and over). Control is achieved by regulatory proteins H and I. H binds to C3b and enhances its degradation by I. Once the C3b is inactivated to C3bi, H and I are released and continue their action on other molecules, thereby controlling the reaction. It is thought that the controlled production of C3b that initiates this system results from weak binding of native C3 to B in the presence of D and $Mg^{2+}$ to generate a weak C3 convertase activity. Alteration in levels of the inactivators has been correlated with disease exacerbation in SLE.[3]

Activators of the alternative pathway do so by their ability to interfere with the control of the feedback reactions.[1, 296] That is, when C3b deposits on the surface of an activator, binding of H is greatly reduced, in turn rendering I inefficient. The bound C3b remains active and interacts with more B, which on cleavage by D forms more

and more C3bBb, and, in turn, more C3b. This leads to C5 convertase activity as well as to opsonic activity. C3 and C5 convertase activity of the complex is stabilized by P. The cleavage subunits of B have biologic activity, with Ba chemotactic for neutrophils and Bb influencing the spreading behavior of macrophages and monocytes.[1] The control proteins for both C pathways can be altered in patients with GN.[297–299] Control is achieved at the C3b level using the same serum and membrane factors described for the classic C pathway.

The material termed nephritic factor (C3NeF) isolated from the sera of some patients with partial lipodystrophy and with hypocomplementemic membranoproliferative GN[300–304] is an IgG with reactivity for the alternative C pathway C3 convertase C3bBb, enhancing its activity. The lipodystrophy may be related to dysregulated C activation at the adipocyte plasma membrane.[305] The anti-idiotypic response as a means of control has been studied.[306] A 2:1 relative risk of developing C3NeF is reported in patients with the C3F allele of C3.[307] At least two types are now recognized related to properdin (P), C3bBb or C3bBbP.[308, 309] Variations in C3NeF activity and other C-activating factors are also present in sera from patients with GN.[310, 311] C3NeF has been recovered from Epstein-Barr virus–transformed B cell lines from patients with membranoproliferative GN.[312, 313] A clinical condition similar to that seen with C3NeF has been noted in two kindreds with hypocomplementemic GN in which the alternative pathway convertase, C3bBb, is resistant to control by factor H.[314, 315] H deficiency itself can rarely occur and has been associated with atypical intramembranous dense deposit disease.[316] Autoantibodies to other C components such as C1q in SLE are suggested to contribute to disease pathogenesis.[317] Reactions to C1q, which has a collagen-like domain, are observed in anti-GBM Ab disease as well; however, the two reactions are separable by inhibition studies.[318]

C activation leads to the generation of several biologically active products derived from C molecules including anaphylatoxins, other vasoactive fragments and factors promoting leukocytosis, chemotaxins for neutrophils, and stimulatory agents of monocyte and macrophage function.[3] Systemic C activation induced by infusion of cobra venom factor (CVF) leads to acute lung injury involving neutrophils and ROS, and a glomerular lesion can be induced by infusing CVF.[319] Systemic administration of C5a induces vascular changes via cyclooxygenase (COX) products.[320] C5a infusion in the renal artery induced glomerular hemodynamic changes in the absence of involvement of neutrophils, with a decrease in glomerular plasma flow caused by increased efferent resistance.[321, 322] Dialysis membranes can activate the C system, releasing C3a and C5a into the circulation, with chemotactic unresponsiveness of neutrophils unrelated to C5a receptor binding.[3] C3a and C5a plasma levels are elevated in active SLE.[323] C5a can be generated by hydrogen peroxide such as that generated by neutrophils during the respiratory burst, coupling the C and neutrophil mediator systems in yet another way.[324] C-related reactions may also release vasoactive amines from mast cells and platelets, and factors such as C1q may interact in the Hageman factor–dependent systems.[1] These vasoactive materials, which can enhance vascular permeability and subsequent proteinuria,[1] may contribute to the deposition of IC in vessel walls.

C3 and C3d can bind to laminin in the GBM.[325] C3d, a breakdown product of C3, may be detected in glomeruli when C3 cannot and may also be found as an isolated deposit.[326, 327] C3c deposits in glomeruli are cleared within 24 hours of cessation of C activation.[328] Vimentin filaments of glomerular epithelial cells can activate the classic C pathway.[329] Heat-killed human kidney cells can bind C3 in the presence of factors B and D, a process stabilized by C3NeF.[330] The C4A and C4B isotypes are detected in the mesangium of normal human glomeruli.[331]

Studies demonstrate that C3 is transcribed and secreted by glomerular epithelial cells, mesangial cells, and renal tubule cells as well as vascular endothelial cells in culture with regulation by IL-1 and IFN-$\gamma$.[332–337] Local glomerular production is enhanced in vivo during inflammation and can be modulated by proinflammatory cytokines.[338–340]

The role of C as a mediator in immune renal disease generally involves interaction with other mediator systems such as neutrophils and is described later in conjunction with these cells. Of interest, studies suggest that C in the absence of neutrophils or other inflammatory cells may cause injury to the glomerular filtration barrier, and the MAC has come under consideration as a noninflammatory mediator of glomerular damage leading to proteinuria in some model systems and perhaps in humans as well.[13, 14, 21, 341–344] C5b-9 can increase albumin permeability in isolated glomeruli in vitro.[345] In a model of anti-GBM Ab GN in the isolated perfused kidney, proteinuria occurred after C fixation in a situation in which neutrophils are not present to contribute.[346] In planted Ag GN induced with cationic Ag, both C and inflammatory cells are needed for full development of injury.[347] In models of experimental membranous GN, proteinuria appeared only with an intact C system and when C-fixing Ab reactions were used and was unaffected by neutrophil or leukocyte depletion.[348, 349] In this model, Ab fragments also caused proteinuria.[350]

A role for the MAC in experimental GN is indicated in C6-deficient rabbits with experimental membranous nephropathy, acute serum sickness, or anti-GBM nephritis.[351–354] In studies using Ab-induced C6 depletion in rats, proteinuria was modulated in passive Heymann nephritis (PHN) and other experimental GN models.[355, 356] When the PHN studies were extended to the isolated perfused kidney and C sources deficient in C6 or C8, the necessity of the MAC for induction of proteinuria in this noninflammatory membranous nephritis model was well documented.[357]

The HN Ag-Ab reaction takes place on the surface of the glomerular epithelial podocyte, and electron microscopic studies done in PHN in the isolated perfused kidney in the presence of C8-deficient and replenished C sources detected epithelial cell injury.[358] In vitro studies with this Ab system and cultured epithelial cells provide additional evidence for epithelial cell damage related to the formation of the MAC as well as alternative C pathway activation by anti-Fx1A Ab.[359, 360] The MAC components appear to become inserted into the glomerular epithelial cell membrane and are endocytosed in the PHN model.[361]

In a rat model of C-dependent Ab-induced mesangial cell lysis, MAC lesions were demonstrated morphologically on the mesangial cell surface in vitro, and ongoing studies of the isolated perfused kidney support a role for the MAC in mesangial cell lysis in vivo in this model.[362] The MAC was capable of stimulating cultured mesangial cells to release vasodilatory prostaglandin and IL-1.[363] Experimental anti–alveolar basement membrane Abs, when reacted with alveolar basement membrane (ABM), consumed C9 and produced electron microscopic lesions similar to those caused by C in erythrocyte membranes.[364] C5b-9 is reported to induce $Ca^{2+}$ influx and to activate phospholipase C, whose products down-regulate glomerular epithelial cell injury.[365, 366] Protein kinase C activation also protects via a diacylglycerol mechanism.[367]

The C5b-9 can induce proinflammatory responses including IL-1, TNF, and eicosanoid release.[368–370] The C5b-9 complex can also cause translocation of P-selectin (granule membrane protein-140, CD62P, PADGEM [platelet activation–dependent granule-external membrane protein]) to the endothelial surface—an important early step in inducing leukocyte rolling.[371] Sublytic C5b-9 did not increase extracellular matrix (ECM) synthesis or gene expression in glomerular epithelial cells in vitro in one study but did in another.[372, 373] C5b-9 also releases basic fibroblast growth factor (bFGF) and platelet-derived growth factor (PDGF) from vascular endothelial cells.[374] There is some evidence of alterations in glomerular epithelial cell antiadhesive protein in response to C5b-9, as suggested by an increase in secreted protein, acidic and rich in cysteine (SPARC; osteonectin, BM-40).[375, 376] It is possible that the antiadhesive effect of SPARC could contribute to injury-associated detachment of glomerular epithelial cells. The MAC also may contribute to GBM and glomerular capillary wall injury via oxidant production[377, 378] and by interaction with platelets.[379]

The MAC deposits seen in a number of experimental models of GN correlate with the appearance of proteinuria[3]; the MAC deposits appear to be associated with glomerular structures and do not elute as do most immune deposits. A correlation between MAC deposits and C dependence of the lesion based on CVF treatment is reported.[3] Studies have demonstrated MAC components, neoantigens, and poly C9 in human SLE GN and skin lesions, in poststreptococcal GN, in IgA nephropathy, and in various other forms of GN.[3] Of interest, elements of the MAC are found in normal kidney tissue and also in kidneys with nonnephritic conditions such as diabetes, hypertension, and obstructive uropathy.[380, 381] The deposits appear to be associated with membrane and vesicular structures. In de novo membranous GN occurring in renal transplants, MAC neoantigens were found above background only in more advanced lesions with large immune deposits of IgG, C3d, and factor H.[382] In the models of membranous GN as well as in humans, C5b-9 is found in the urine, where it may serve as a marker of disease activity and correlate with glomerular MAC localization.[328, 383–388]

As already noted, control of the MAC is provided by CD59, C8bp, and other molecules, including S protein and clusterin, and alterations in these inhibitors could be involved in glomerular injury. C8bp is up-regulated by IL-1, endotoxin, and IFN-$\gamma$.[389] A monoclonal Ab reactive with C9 neoantigen associated with C5b-9 in plasma was used to detect the MAC in the circulation of patients with SLE, where it correlated with disease activity[340]; the S protein binds to C5b-9 in the circulation, preventing the MAC from attacking target membranes. The S protein colocalized with C5b-9 in immune deposits in glomeruli.[391-395]

The regulation of the C inhibitory molecules, at least in part, may be through cytokine expression,[396] with evidence that CD59 is regulated at the level of transcription.[397] The rat homologue of CD59 has been reported.[398] The GPI-anchored CD59 is found in abundance in glomeruli, collecting ducts, and distal tubules and can be removed with GPI-specific phospholipase C.[399] The molecule is found on glomerular epithelial cells.[400] In humans, the CD59 on the glomerular capillary wall is enhanced in SLE with subendothelial deposits.[401] The mouse CD59 homologue Ly-6 present in glomeruli is enhanced in murine lupus and mercuric chloride nephropathy.[402] CD59 on endothelial cells is thought to contribute to protection against C injury.[403] Ab to rat CD59 to inhibit the protective effect of the CD59 molecule worsens a lectin-antilectin Ab GN.[404] Glomerular cells also synthesize and secrete a chondroitin sulfate B proteoglycan that is C inhibitory.[405] Clusterin (serum protein-40,40), a heterodimeric multifunctional protein with some properties similar to those of S protein, can also interact with C9 and participate in control of lytic activity.[406] The pattern of glomerular clusterin deposition in GN has been reported.[407-411] Clusterin depletion enhances immune glomerular injury in the isolated perfused kidney, indicating a potential value in MAC inhibition.[412] Clusterin is also said to enhance formation of insoluble IC[413] and to play a role in apoptosis.

The exact contribution of the MAC, among the other recognized mediator systems known to provide additively to the phlogogenic stimulus directed by specific Ab binding or passive IC accumulation, remains to be quantitated; however, current evidence suggests that in some model systems the MAC is an important element in producing alterations leading to proteinuria as in PHN. Even in this model, however, other factors probably also contribute, because C depletion did not prevent some of the associated glomerular hemodynamic changes even though proteinuria was modulated.[414] In the future, drugs effecting C activation may have therapeutic evaluation based on initial studies in hypocomplementemic and IC GN.[415-417]

## Neutrophils and Monocyte-Macrophages

### LEUKOCYTE ATTRACTION

Neutrophils are drawn to and accumulate in sites of Ag-Ab-C localization in glomeruli through a combination of chemoattractants including cytokine release, eicosanoids, chemokines, PAF, C-induced chemotaxis, and immune adherence (C3b receptors, CR1) as well as the potential interaction of Fc receptors. A series of interactions involving a number of cell adhesion molecules with their cell surface ligands contribute to glomerular inflammation.[418-432]

The interactions between the selectins and their sialyl carbohydrate ligands result in rolling of leukocytes along the vascular endothelium, particularly in the venules. The selectin family of adhesion molecules have $Ca^{2+}$-dependent

lectins at the $NH_2$ terminus.[433] P-selectin (CD62P, PAD-GEM, granule membrane protein-140) is found stored in Weibel-Palade bodies in endothelial cells and in platelet granules, from which it can be moved to the cell membrane. P-selectin is also expressed in response to C5a.[434] P-selectin–deficient mice have defects in leukocyte rolling and extravasation.[435] For example, P-selectin can be translocated to the cell surface in response to C5b-9 assembly.[371] Anti–P-selectin Ab modulates C-independent glomerular injury in mice induced by anti-GBM Ab.[436] L-selectin (CD62L, Mel-14, LAM-1) is present on circulating leukocytes and is shed rapidly on cell activation.[437, 438] It is required for CD18-mediated neutrophil adhesion at physiologic shear rates in vivo.[439] E-selectin (CD62E, endothelial leukocyte adhesion molecule-1) is induced on endothelial cells in response to IL-1 or TNF, requiring mRNA and protein synthesis. The selectins react with sialylated carbohydrate related to sialyl Lewis x and sialyl Lewis a (AM6). A search is on to find carbohydrate ligands that may offer anti-inflammatory activity.[440]

Subsequent adhesiveness of the leukocytes induced to roll by the selectins involves interactions with integrins and their ligands. The integrins are composed of noncovalently linked α- and β-subunits. The integrin-ligand reaction results in more firm, but reversible, binding than the selectin interactions and leads to subsequent extravasation as appropriate to the stimulus. The integrins and their ligands are transiently activated in response to chemoattractants that provide a directionality to leukocyte adhesion. The integrin $α_Lβ_2$ (lymphocyte function–associated antigen-1 [LFA-1], CD11a/CD18) on neutrophils and monocytes binds the ligands ICAM-1, ICAM-2, and ICAM-3. ICAM-1 can also interact at a different site with the integrin $α_Mβ_2$ (MAC-1, CR3, CD11b/CD19) present on neutrophils and monocytes. Both $α_Mβ_2$ and $α_Lβ_2$ are activated by the chemokine IL-8, which may impart a conformational change in a portion of the molecules.[441-443] Other integrins involved in lymphocyte binding include $α_4β_1$ (very late antigen-4, CD49d/CD29), which binds to vascular cell adhesion molecule-1 (VCAM-1), with the latter also binding weakly to $α_4β_7$ (lymphocyte Peyer patch adhesion molecule-1, CD49d/CD).[426, 429, 444-448] The platelet/endothelial cell adhesion molecule-1 (CD31) present on platelets and at intercellular junctions of vascular endothelial cells has been implicated in transendothelial migration of leukocytes at a point distal to the integrin-mediated adhesion.[449] The distribution of the ligands varies among specific endothelial cell populations.[450]

In a study using an anti–L-selectin Ab and L-selectin, transfected glomerular endothelial cells with TNF activation indicated a role for L-selectin in leukocyte binding.[451] Monoclonal anti–L-selectin inhibits mononuclear cell extravasation.[452] Adhesion of neutrophils and monocyte-macrophages to human mesangial cells involved ICAM-1 and CD11/CD18.[453] ICAM-1 is regulated by shear stress on vascular endothelial cells.[454] ICAM-1 and VCAM-1 are expressed on glomerular epithelial cells.[455] VCAM-1 is expressed in murine lupus and in renal allografts.[456-458] ICAM is up-regulated on mesangial cells and may function in Ag presentation.[459] ICAM-1 expression is up-regulated in autoimmune lupus nephritis in mice[460] and has been reported to be increased in various forms of human GN.[461-464] ICAM and LFA-1 are increased in experimental anti-GBM Ab–induced lung injury.[465] ICAM-1 is also reported to play a role in interstitial leukocyte accumulation.[466] Renal tubule cells also express adhesion molecules.[467, 468]

Studies have begun to show the protective role of Abs to these adhesion molecules in inflammation, including that in the kidney. Abs to TNF-α or CD18 diminished neutrophil accumulation in anti–GBM Ab GN, whereas anti–E-selectin or CD11b was ineffective.[469] In another study using this model, anti-CD11b Ab decreased proteinuria but did not alter neutrophil influx or eicosanoid production.[470] In anti–GBM Ab GN it has been reported that TNF-α (but not IL-1), CD11b, and very late antigen-4 (but not E-selectin) are required for full accumulation of neutrophils and full development of proteinuria.[471] We found that IL-1 receptor antagonist decreased neutrophil accumulation and ICAM-1 expression in the same model.[472] This was confirmed in another study.[473] The pattern of IL-1 receptor antagonist expression in anti–GBM Ab GN is limited to individual but unidentified cells by in situ hybridization.[474] Abs reactive with ICAM-1 or LFA-1α reduced injury in anti–GBM Ab GN in the Wistar-Kyoto rat.[475, 476] Inflammatory responses are impaired in ICAM-1–deficient mice.[477]

Leukocyte migration from blood into tissue then depends on a cascade of events including chemoattractants and selectin- and integrin-mediated adhesion of cells to the endothelium. Adhesion requires not only integrin and selectin interaction with their ligands but also activation signals provided by chemoattractants including the chemokine superfamily.[478] For example, C5a- and leukotriene B$_4$ (LTB$_4$)-induced adhesion of monocytes to human mesangial cells could be partially inhibited by Abs reactive with the common β CD18 subunit of CD11/CD18[479]; of interest, anti–L-selectin Ab had no effect.

Members of the chemokine superfamily are being associated with glomerular injury.[480] This superfamily of basic, heparin-binding molecules of molecular mass 8 to 10 kd with chemotactic and inflammatory properties has been termed intercrines, small cytokines, and by the recommended nomenclature, chemokines.[481] The superfamily is characterized by four conserved cysteines with two disulfide bridges and is subdivided into the α-subfamily, in which the first two cysteines are separated by another amino acid, and the β-subfamily, in which the cysteines are adjacent.[482, 483]

The α-subfamily includes platelet factor-4, interleukin-8 (IL-8, neutrophil-activating protein-1), GRO or melanoma growth-stimulatory activity, KC, interferon-inducible protein-10 (IP-10), and macrophage inflammatory protein-2 (MIP-2), which are neutrophil chemoattractants and activators. The β-subfamily includes RANTES (regulated on activation, normal T cell expressed and secreted), MIP-1, and monocyte chemoattractant protein-1 (MCP-1)/JE and are monocyte/macrophage chemoattractants. MIP-1α is found in synovial fluid.[484] Of interest, both IL-8 and MCP-1 also appear to function as T cell chemoattractants and, in turn, could contribute to the influx of the large number of bystander T cells that accompany an Ag-specific T cell infiltrate.[485, 486] The two subfamilies represent two gene clusters on two different chromosomes. A new class of chemokine termed lymphotactin, which is a lymphocyte

chemoattractant, has just been described.[486a] The renal isoform of the erythrocyte chemokine receptor is under study.[487]

In the rat, IL-8, which is a major neutrophil chemoattractant in humans, has not been identified with certainty, and KC/cytokine-induced neutrophil chemoattractant and MIP-2 may provide this function.[488] These two chemokines are presumed to be homologues of the human GRO α, β, and γ genes.[489–491] The rat cytokine-induced neutrophil chemoattractant was isolated from the rat kidney epithelioid cell line NRK-52E, has been cloned, and is most closely related to human GRO γ.[492, 493] Previous studies in the mouse showed that anti–MIP-2 Ab delayed, but did not prevent, inflammation produced by intracisternal challenge of pneumococci[494]; however, it did reduce, by about 40%, the influx of neutrophils in a model of *Mycobacterium bovis* bacille Calmette-Guérin–induced peritonitis.[495] Pulmonary instillation of lipopolysaccharide in rats produced a rapid and marked increase in MIP-2 and KC levels,[496] and a marked induction of both KC and MIP-2 was observed in the alveolar macrophages of hamsters after injection of opsonized particles.[497] KC is expressed by glomerular mesangial cells in response to IL-1β with induction inhibited by dexamethasone.[498] Studies in our laboratory using an Ab to MIP-2 strongly suggest that MIP-2 contributes to neutrophil infiltration in the early hours of anti–GBM Ab GN in rats.[499] Abs to cytokine-induced neutrophil chemoattractant also modulate this model.[500] IL-8 has been identified in glomeruli from patients with IgA GN[501] and is found in the urine of patients with glomerular disease including hemolytic-uremic syndrome.[502, 503] IL-8 can be induced in mesangial cells and renal epithelial cells by cytokines including IL-1.[504–508] Its synthesis in monocytes can be induced with C5a.[509] The neutrophil itself can be a source of IL-8 in response to TNF-α or IL-1β.[510] IL-8 can stimulate PAF expression.[511] Although a chemokine, IL-8 can also inhibit neutrophil adherence via receptor desensitization.[512–514] Neutrophil migration is impaired in mice overexpressing human IL-8.[515] MCP-1 also has been found in mesangial cells,[507, 516–521] as has IP-10.[522] MCP-1 (as well as IL-8) expression is inhibited by the IL-1 receptor antagonist.[523] IL-4 induces synthesis and secretion of MCP-1 in human endothelial cells.[524] MCP-1 in human renal cortical epithelial cells is regulated by IFN-γ.[525] In endothelial cells or fibroblasts IL-1, TNF, or IL-6 enhances expression of MCP-1.[526] RANTES has been found in renal tubule epithelium[527] and is up-regulated in mouse mesangial cells by TNF-α.[528, 529]

## NEUTROPHILS

Neutrophils, once attracted to a site, can actually displace the endothelial lining of the glomerular capillary and come to lie in close contact with the GBM[1] (Fig. 29–2) or even penetrate the GBM, events that have been documented in humans.[1] Gaps then appear in the GBM,[1] and its permeability to lanthanum increases, as visualized by electron microscopy.[1] Morphologic and filtration properties of proteinase-treated GBM are altered.[3] Differences in susceptibility to enzyme treatment have been reported for GBM and TBM.[3] Neutrophils produce ROS and eicosanoids and in-

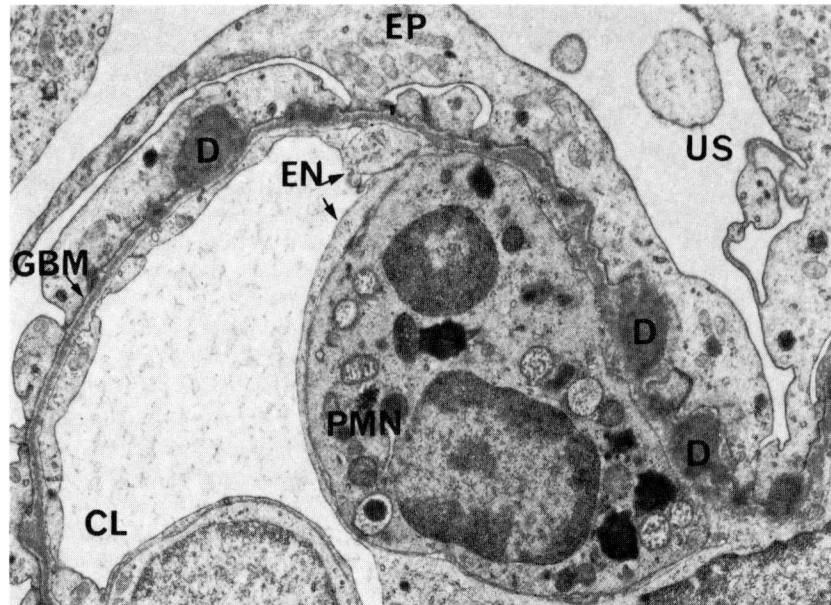

**Figure 29–2.** A polymorphonuclear leukocyte (PMN) is seen closely approximated along the glomerular basement membrane (GBM) in proximity to subepithelial (EP) electron-dense deposits (D) in a rabbit with chronic serum sickness GN. The endothelial cell (EN) has been displaced. CL = capillary lumen; US = urinary space.

teract with platelets. In turn, leukotrienes can stimulate neutrophil adhesion to mesangial cells via a CD18 mechanism.[530] Platelets precede neutrophils in the planted Ag (Con A) model in rats and augment injury but are not involved in the actual neutrophil influx.[531] A number of neutrophil-platelet interactions are involved in the genesis of inflammation.[532] Neutrophils also possess clot-promoting properties, and fibrinogen mediates platelet and neutrophil cooperation in IC GN in rats.[533]

The neutrophil provides a variety of phlogistons, acid mucopolysaccharides, acid cathepsins, and numerous neutral proteases including fibrinolysins, collagenase, elastase, and other enzymes.[1, 534] The neutrophils store their contents in azurophil granules (MPO, lysozyme, elastase, cathepsin G, acid hydrolases), in specific granules (lysozyme, collagenase, lactoferrin, vitamin $B_{12}$–binding protein), and in smaller storage organelles (proteinase-3, gelatinase, plasminogen activator, acid hydrolases) for selective release.[3, 535, 536] Neutrophils can then destroy glomerular tissue by releasing lysosomal materials much as they do in other sites, including producing injury to endothelium.[537–541] The potential role of ANCA reactions with activated neutrophils has been considered in vasculitis (see earlier). Endothelial cell killing by neutrophils can occur via oxidant mechanisms.[542, 543]

The proteinase activity can take place in the presence of powerful circulating inhibitors, because the neutrophil is in direct contact with the GBM.[3] Neutrophil metalloproteinase can inactivate $\alpha_1$-antiproteinase.[544] Deficiency of $\alpha_1$-antitrypsin, a potential inhibitor of neutral proteases from neutrophils, has been linked to a number of immune disorders including some instances of GN.[545, 546] The events associated with neutrophil activation have been the subject of review.[547–551]

The neutrophil enzymes can fragment type IV collagen[552] and renal basement membrane in vitro,[1] and particles of the GBM have been identified in the urine of animals with experimentally induced glomerular injury.[1] Infusion of neutrophil elastase and cathepsin is associated with glomerular injury.[553] GBM degradation by neutrophils is modulated in vitro by nonsteroidal anti-inflammatory drugs that inhibit degranulation.[554] Neutrophil heparanase activity facilitated by serine proteases can degrade heparan sulfate.[555] The degradation of endothelial cell heparan sulfate matrix by elastase and that by MPO, hydrogen peroxide, and chloride are additive if elastase is used first.[556] Inhibition of ROS reduces the elastase effect on GBM.[557] Anti-GBM Ab injury in beige mice that lack the leukocyte neutral proteinases elastase and cathepsin G produces little proteinuria compared with that in mice reconstructed with normal cells.[558] The contribution of renal and glomerular cell lysosomal enzymes in degradation of GBM also needs to be considered.[559–564] A neutral metalloproteinase present in normal rat glomeruli can degrade GBM, indicating an intrinsic pathway for damage as well.[565] Lysosomal enzymes are also reported to be present in normal GBM matrix.[566] Cationic proteins from neutrophils (and platelets) are localized in glomeruli of rabbits with experimental serum sickness and have been found in patients with SLE.[567, 568]

Urinary proteinase activity and GBM components increase in anti-GBM Ab GN.[569] In addition, urinary proteinase activity and GBM fragments correlate with glomerular neutrophil infiltration in patients with proliferative GN.[570] Glycosaminoglycans and heparan sulfate are also increased in glomerular injury.[571] Finally, 3-hydroxyproline, prominent in type IV collagen of the GBM, is also increased in the urine of patients with acute glomerular disease.[572] The source of urinary proteinase activity and excretion of laminin and type IV collagen is not clear because inflammatory lesions such as anti-GBM Ab GN and noninflammatory aminonucleoside nephrosis have similar levels related to levels of proteinuria.[573]

Proteinase inhibition reduces proteinuria in anti-GBM Ab GN.[574, 575] Synthetic protease inhibitors reduce glomerular necrosis, but not IC localization or leukocyte influx, in the apoferritin model of IC GN in mice.[576] Synthetic protease

inhibitors also reduce glomerular injury in (NZB ×
NZW)F$_1$ SLE GN.[577]

The neutrophil-dependent mechanisms have been defined
by experiments in which anti-GBM Abs are given to animals depleted of either C or neutrophils.[1] Depletion of
neutrophils by nitrogen mustard or specific antineutrophil
Ab, leaving C levels intact, prevents neutrophil-dependent
forms of acute (heterologous-phase) anti-GBM Ab GN in
rats and rabbits.[1] A monoclonal antineutrophil Ab selectively reduces neutrophils in anti-GBM Ab GN without
altering proteinuria, malondialdehyde, or superoxide dismutase (SOD) activities.[578]

In addition to inhibition of changes such as proteinuria,
measures of glomerular hemodynamic alterations of function induced by anti-GBM, such as the normally observed
decrease in glomerular capillary ultrafiltration coefficient
(K$_f$) and single-nephron glomerular filtration rate (SNGFR),
are returned to normal by leukocyte depletion.[579, 580]

After C depletion, neutrophils fail to accumulate in
glomeruli[1] during the heterologous phase of anti-GBM Ab
GN, indicating the central role of C in attracting neutrophils
to the site during the acute stage of injury. The C depletion
does not attenuate subsequent monocyte migration into glomeruli.[581] Glomerular neutrophil accumulation in heterologous-phase anti-GBM Ab GN in the mouse can occur in C-
deficient or depleted mice and is suggested to be Fc
dependent.[3, 582] Fcα receptor and ROS production by neutrophils is reported in patients with IgA nephropathy.[583–585]

C depletion during the autologous phase of anti-GBM
Ab injury neither affects the number of neutrophils found
nor modifies the injury in this more complex stage of disease.[1] By using F(ab')$_2$ Ab fragments, neutrophil localization during the autologous phase is suggested to be via Fc
receptors.[1] The induction of anti-GBM GN in C5-deficient
mice or C6-deficient rabbits and the spontaneous occurrence of IC GN in C5-deficient NZB mice indicate the
importance of the first four C components (C1, C2, C4,
C3).[1, 586, 587] C5 deficiency is also said to reduce glomerular
IC localization in the apoferritin model in mice.[588] K-76
monocarboxylic acid, an anticomplementary agent, affecting C5 in particular, is noted to reduce proteinuria in anti-
GBM GN, (NZB × NZW)F$_1$ SLE mice, and early stages
of chronic serum sickness.[589, 590] Studies in C6-deficient
rabbits suggest a role for the terminal C cascade and the
MAC in the acute phases of anti-GBM Ab GN.[352, 353]

C can bind in glomeruli without attracting neutrophils or
causing damage,[1] and in later stages of acute IC disease
amounts of C may actually increase during a time when the
lesion is healing.[1] In IC GN of the acute serum sickness
type, C and neutrophils are not essential to induction of the
severe but transient glomerular injury that is observed;
however, C and neutrophils do appear to be involved in
mediating the arteritic lesions also induced by IC deposition
in acute serum sickness.[1] The acute serum sickness lesion
relies more on monocytes than on neutrophils.

Neutrophil-independent mediation is a factor in renal disease, because avian anti-GBM Abs instigate injury in the
absence of overt neutrophil (and C) participation.[1] An interesting mammalian (sheep) anti-GBM Ab contains two
classes of Ig that mediate glomerular injury differently.[1, 591]
An IgG1 fraction activates C and attracts neutrophils, pro-

ducing injury with relatively low amounts of Ab bound in
glomeruli. The neutrophil dependence of this fraction can
be overcome by using two to three times as much Ab in
rabbits that have been depleted of neutrophils. A comparably large amount of an IgG2 fraction from the same antiserum causes injury equally well in normal and neutrophil-
depleted rabbits. However, larger amounts of another IgG2
fraction from the same antiserum bound, but did not induce,
proteinuria.

## MONOCYTE-MACROPHAGES

In addition to neutrophils, monocyte-macrophages are
often attracted to renal sites of immune injury via the general mechanics already described. Monocytes and macrophages are prominent in glomeruli during the height of
acute serum sickness and in chronic serum sickness (Fig.
29–3). Macrophage depletion with an antimacrophage Ab
can prevent the glomerular injury of acute serum sickness
to a large degree.[3, 592]

The attraction and activation of monocyte-macrophages,
the role of their Fc receptors in phagocytosis, and the reciprocal interaction of the class II MHC antigen (Ia Ag–positive) subset of macrophages with T cells via soluble mediators have been the subject of review.[593, 594] In acute serum
sickness, for example, T cells and monocyte-macrophages
increase in glomeruli at or slightly before immune elimination, suggesting a possible contribution to the lesion.[121] In
addition to lymphocyte factors, Fc receptors and recognition of C products, fibronectin fragments, and factors extracted from sites of delayed hypersensitivity are under
study as macrophage chemoattractants.[3] The macrophages
can serve as immunoregulatory cells or as effector cells. As
effector cells, they are involved in many networks through
their production of enzymes and their inhibitors, C components, chemokines, reactive oxygen metabolites, bioactive
lipids, and growth-promoting and -inhibiting factors.[3, 595]
These cells can also produce procoagulant activity (PCA).
Although glomerular mesangial cells and other cells produce proinflammatory cytokines, monocyte-macrophages
are also a major source of IL-1 and TNF but not transforming growth factor-β (TGF-β).[596–600] Basement membrane
containing ICs stimulates IL-1 and TNF production in
monocytes.[601] Colony-stimulating factor-1 produced in glomeruli and their mesangial cells has been shown to correlate with monocyte-macrophage differentiation in murine
lupus.[602–604] Glomerular macrophages secrete IL-1.[605] C activation during hemodialysis may stimulate transcription of
IL-1β in peripheral monocytes.[606] In anti–Thy-1 Ab–induced mesangial cell injury, MCP-1 is increased while colony-stimulating factor-1 remains unchanged.[518] Macrophage secretory products stimulated by Fc receptor–
mediated endocytosis induce mesangial cell proliferation.[607]

A molecule of considerable interest associated with both
monocyte-macrophages and intrinsic glomerular cells is nitric oxide (NO), which is the reactive element of the so-
called endothelium-derived relaxing factor[605–614] (see also
Chapter 17). NO is an active biologic messenger and activates soluble guanylate cyclase. For example, NO produced
by glomerular endothelial cells increases cyclic GMP in

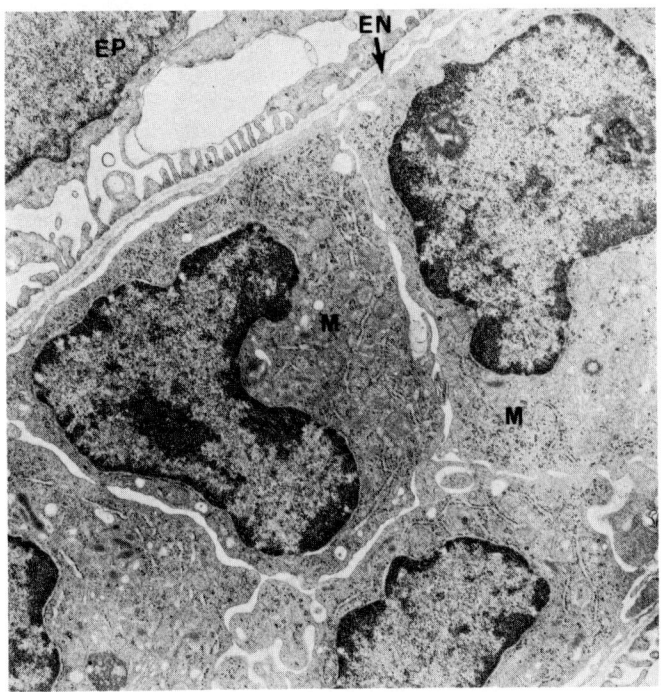

**Figure 29–3.** Mononuclear cells (M) are packed within the lumen of a glomerular capillary from a rabbit with acute serum sickness. Epithelial (EP) cell foot processes and endothelium (EN) remain largely intact.

mesangial cells.[615] Subsequent alterations in mesangial cell contractility may contribute to alterations in glomerular function.[616]

NO is derived from the terminal guanidino nitrogen of L-arginine with L-citrulline as a coproduct through the action of nitric oxide synthase (NOS). The alternative metabolism of L-arginine via arginase produces urea and ornithine. At least three NOS isozymes have been identified and cloned.[617, 618] One isoform is found in neuronal and epithelial cells. The gene for this isoform resides on human chromosome 12. This isoform has been located in the kidney macula densa cells[619, 620] and, using reverse transcription–polymerase chain reaction, in renal tubule segments.[621] A second isoform is found in vascular endothelial cells, where it is constitutively expressed and often referred to as constitutive NOS (cNOS). Its gene is located on human chromosome 7. It functions to keep blood vessels dilated (endothelium-derived relaxing factor), counteracting the vasoconstrictive effects of angiotensin II (AII). For example, PAF's vasodilatory effect is suggested to be via NO production.[622] It also prevents adhesion of platelets and leukocytes to the endothelial cells through effects on adhesion molecules.[623–626]

The third isoform of NOS is usually not constitutively expressed but is induced in macrophages and many other cells including mesangial glomerular cells[616, 627–632] by proinflammatory stimuli such as endotoxin and cytokines. The NOS mRNA induced by IL-1β has a shorter half-life than that expressed in response to cAMP-elevating agents.[633] Human mesangial cells require multiple cytokines (IL-1β, IFN-γ, and TNF-α) to produce an NOS response.[634] More than one inducible NOS (iNOS) isoform is reported in the kidney.[635] Its gene is located on human chromosome 17. A number of cytokines and growth factors including TGF-β, IL-4, IL-10, and PDGF can inhibit the endotoxin and IL-1– or TNF-induced NO synthesis.[636–640] NO can also

inhibit superoxide generation as well as interacting with ROS.[641] The combination of NO with ROS in neutrophils can lead to the formation of the toxic peroxynitrite anion.[642, 643] iNOS mRNA has been shown to be present in the outer medullary strip as well as in glomeruli in the rat kidney.[644] In contrast to the physiologic levels of NO produced by cNOS, the induction of iNOS results in large amounts of NO that serve in the cytotoxic functions of macrophages and presumably in other cell types that express iNOS. The brain NOS and cNOS are regulated by $Ca^{2+}$ and calmodulin, whereas calmodulin appears to be in tight association with iNOS almost as a subunit.[645] iNOS regulation is largely at the transcriptional level. Measurement of nitrite and nitrate is used to monitor NO production. Structural analogues of L-arginine such as $N^G$-monomethyl-L-arginine that block NO production have been used to demonstrate a role for NO in various inflammatory situations including glomerular injury.

It is difficult to establish the differential contribution of infiltrating monocyte-macrophages in terms of NO production from that of other inflammatory cells and the intrinsic glomerular cells in immune glomerular injury. In a series of studies, Cattell and co-workers[646–648] as well as others have shown increased nitrite synthesis in several models of experimental glomerular injury with a relationship to monocyte-macrophage infiltration. Differential expression of NO in the anti–Thy-1 model of mesangial cell injury correlated with the proliferative mesangial cell response, which has been shown to be related to PDGF, a molecule noted to suppress cytokine-induced NO formation.[649] The same workers have also shown the presence of arginase activity in glomeruli of nephritic rats, which could alter the L-arginine substrate availability for NOS-induced NO production.[650] iNOS has been shown in immune glomerular injury to be in intraglomerular mononuclear cells, in cells in the Bowman space, and in interstitial infiltrates.[651]

Administration of $N^G$-monomethyl-L-arginine reduced arthritis and GN without altering circulating anti-DNA Ab levels.[652] In ongoing short-term studies in our laboratory, $N^G$-monomethyl-L-arginine appears to enhance glomerular accumulation of neutrophils and worsen the anti-GBM Ab lesion. NO inhibition caused an increase in proteinuria in this model.[653] $N^G$-Nitro-L-arginine methyl ester enhanced glomerular thrombosis in endotoxin injury, an effect that could be reduced by giving an NO donor.[654] In the unilateral obstructed hydronephrotic kidney, NO release from iNOS activates inducible cyclooxygenase-2 (COX-2) with a marked increase in proinflammatory prostaglandins.[655]

As already noted, monocytes are important in the autologous phase of anti-GBM Ab–induced GN and in acute serum sickness GN (see Fig. 29–3).[3, 592, 656–658] The monocyte accumulation has been correlated with migration inhibitory factor.[659] Monocyte-macrophages were also identified in other experimental models of IC GN including murine SLE,[3] in chronic serum sickness in rabbits[658, 660] and rats,[3] in *Trypanosoma rhodesiense* infection in rabbits,[3] and in passive serum sickness clearly defined by the presence of the lysosomal abnormality used to identify monocytes in Chédiak-Higashi mice.[661] Glomerular IgA deposits induced in rats are associated with an influx in macrophages.[662] IC degradation by macrophages was reported to be enhanced by the supernatant of the human T cell line HUT102.[663] Urinary IL-1 excretion was reported to correlate with T cell and monocyte-macrophage accumulation in the glomeruli.[664]

The transient neutrophil accumulation observed in the heterologous phase of anti-GBM Ab–induced GN was replaced by an influx of monocytes that were presumably active in phagocytosis. Glomerular macrophage phagocytic activity declines over time in chronic serum sickness.[665] Both mononuclear cells and neutrophils appeared in the renal lymph after anti-GBM Ab.[666] Macrophage trafficking to the draining lymph nodes detected in anti-GBM Ab GN in the rat led the authors to suggest that the macrophage may present nephritogenic Ags to T and B lymphocytes and thereby amplify the immune response.[667] Products derived from collagen breakdown, as might occur in acute GBM damage, were suggested to be chemotactic for blood monocytes.[668] In the accelerated autologous phase of anti-GBM Ab–induced GN of rats preimmunized to the heterologous Ig, monocytes and macrophages identifiable by electron microscopy were observed after 48 to 96 hours, when the neutrophils had essentially disappeared.[656] In addition, monocytes were observed in glomeruli of rats that received subnephritic injections of heterologous anti-GBM Ab and transfers of lymph node cells sensitized to heterologous Ig.[100] The effects of leukocyte depletion in blocking anti-GBM Ab–induced injury were reconstituted with intravenous administration of peritoneal mononuclear inflammatory cells.[669] Steroid treatment induces a monocytopenia and reduction in glomerular macrophage accumulation.[670, 671] Monocyte-macrophages were also suggested to contribute to the development of PHN in studies using antimacrophage Abs.[672] Monocyte-macrophages are observed in the focal glomerulosclerosis of the Zucker rat.[673] Macrophage depletion using irradiation slowed progression of glomerular injury in renal ablation.[674] Similar depletion

in puromycin nephrosis was also beneficial in the progressive phase of injury.[675] Other studies have also suggested that macrophages are involved in glomerular sclerosis. The monocyte-macrophage has been studied and identified as a major contributor to the lung injury induced in rats with a passive accelerated anti-GBM Ab disease.[123]

Monocyte-macrophages are also identified as a component of glomerular crescents, where they presumably functioned in part to phagocytose products of coagulation and were prevented by defibrination.[3, 676] In addition, macrophages were suggested to be at least in part responsible for the fibrin accumulation related to their PCA activity.[677]

The in vivo kinetics of monocyte migration have been studied in the skin but not extensively in the kidney, where some relationship to increased glomerular cell [³H]thymidine incorporation is reported.[3] Bone marrow–derived monocytes have also been shown to be involved in the clearance of preformed ICs from glomeruli.[3] Monocyte-macrophages were perhaps more effective than neutrophils at degrading GBM via neutral proteinase[595]; however, it was suggested that neutrophils degrade GBM more rapidly via the action of serine proteinases.[678] Macrophages may bind to the GBM via receptors with preferential binding to laminin (compared to type I or type IV collagen).[679] Macrophage adherence to cultured endothelial cells is enhanced by β-very low density lipoproteins.[680]

Monocyte-macrophages are detected by a number of methods in human GN including focal glomerular sclerosis.[3, 681, 682] The extrarenal origin of the crescentic cells is suggested by detection of Y bodies in cells in this site in female-to-male human renal transplants.[683] The contribution of monocytes to glomerular hypercellularity is variable but has a loose correlation with immune deposits and some evidence of phagocytosis of the deposits.[3] Tissue culture, histochemical, and monoclonal Ab techniques also suggest a prominent role for monocyte-macrophages in glomerular crescent formation in humans.[3, 162, 684, 685] The proportion of monocytes and cells of epithelial origin in crescent formation varies among patients and is also influenced by the integrity of the Bowman capsule, which, if disrupted, appears to increase the number of monocytes and lymphoid cells present (the latter appearing to be activated T cells).[686–691] Activated IL-2 receptor–positive mononuclear cells were associated with active crescent formation in IgA nephropathy and other crescentic lesions.[692–694] The relationship of the monocyte-macrophages to T cells and T cell subsets in glomeruli has already been discussed.

A cell resembling the mononuclear phagocyte is present in the normal glomerular mesangium, representing about 2% of the total cell content in rats.[695] The cell is Ia-positive, can present Ag in a genetically restricted manner to syngeneic lymphocytes, and can selectively stimulate allogeneic lymphocytes. On electron microscopic study, the cells appear to be in the mesangium, phagocytic in vivo, and distinct from the contractile smooth muscle–like mesangial cell.[696] Local amplification of the mesangial macrophage in experimental IC glomerular injury has been suggested.[697] These cells can increase in numbers in response to materials such as polyvinyl alcohol and, minimally, to ferritin lodged in glomeruli.[698, 699]

Another role for monocyte-macrophages in GN has come under study. Apoptosis or programmed cell death can involve phagocytosis of the dying cells by other cells including macrophages.[700, 701] The apoptotic cells have a characteristic breakdown of DNA that produces a laddering effect when analyzed by electrophoresis.[702, 703] Activation of the *BCL2* gene can regulate apoptosis as that in immune cells.[704, 705] Indeed, enforced *BCL2* expression can prolong Ab responses and may elicit autoimmune disease.[706] *BCL2*-deficient mice develop polycystic kidneys.[707] Clusterin, a protein observed in tissues undergoing programmed cell death, is increased in renal tubule cells after ureteral obstruction.[708] Clusterin is also found in association with C5b-9, the MAC, in glomerular deposits and is an inhibitor of C hemolysis.[408–410] Clusterin depletion of serum used in a PHN injury model in an isolated perfused kidney enhanced injury.[412] The role of clusterin in death or survival of cells is being studied.[709–713]

Regression of mitogen-induced renal hyperplasia or glomerular disease may display features of apoptitic changes.[714, 715] IgG anti–double-stranded DNA Ab from patients with SLE is reported to be cytotoxic to rat mesangial cells.[716] The *lpr* mutation of lupus mice is suggested to be in the *Fas* apoptosis gene.[717] The mutations of the *Fas* receptor (apoptosis-1) or its putative ligand defined in lupus mice are being studied in human SLE, and an increase in apoptosis-1 is seen in T and B cells; however, no consistent defect in its function could be detected.[718] Neutrophils in inflammatory glomerular disease undergo apoptosis and are taken up by macrophages and by glomerular mesangial cells.[719] The vitronectin receptor integrin $\alpha_v\beta_3$ on the macrophages may contribute.[720] Apoptotic cells within mesangial cells were noted in a patient with hemolytic-uremic syndrome.[721] Removal of neutrophils is an important step in resolution of acute inflammation.

## Reactive Oxygen Species
(see also Chapter 17)

Studies of the role of ROS in the mediation of immune-initiated glomerular disease[722, 723] include the role of ROS released by the respiratory burst of neutrophils and macrophages into the immediate environment of the cell without cell lysis, as well as the production of ROS by glomerular cells themselves.[3, 724–730] For example, macrophages isolated from glomeruli after immune renal injury exhibit enhanced ROS production.[731–733] When the ROS exceed the amounts of antioxidants that normally detoxify them, oxidative injury to proteins, membrane lipids, and nucleic acids can occur. ROS also interact with other inflammatory mediator systems and can be involved in cell signaling pathways. For example, DNA synthesis can be stimulated in cultured mesangial cells by ROS, and we have just found that ROS can induce COX-2 in these cells as well as protein tyrosine phosphatase (PTPase).[734–736]

The ROS include superoxide anion, hydrogen peroxide, hydroxyl radical, and hypochlorous acid.[737, 738] The respiratory burst responsible for their generation is believed to be related to a plasma membrane oxidase that catalyzes the one-electron reduction of oxygen to superoxide anion at the expense of NADPH,[739] a mechanism defective in chronic granulomatous disease.[740] Dismutation of the superoxide

anion spontaneously or by the enzyme SOD leads to the relatively weak oxidant hydrogen peroxide and, subsequently, to the more toxic hydroxyl radical formed by interaction of iron or copper with hydrogen peroxide (Haber-Weiss reactions) or with hydrogen peroxidase and iron (Fenton reaction).[741, 742] The reaction of hydrogen peroxide with halides leads to hypohalides, particularly hypochlorite, through the activity of MPO found in the neutrophil's azurophilic granules. The interaction of hypochlorite with ammonia or amines leads to the formation of chloramines. The inflammatory cell system functions to destroy phagocytosed bacteria but can contribute to inflammatory tissue injury and the interplay of protective enzymes and scavengers such as SOD, glutathione peroxidase, glutathione, vitamin E, and ascorbic acid.[743] The levels of antioxidant enzymes CuZnSOD, MnSOD, and catalase vary with time in glomerular culture; catalase activity was low and rapidly declined.[744] Oxidants induce transcriptional activation of MnSOD in glomerular cells.[745] Methylprednisolone induces cellular MnSOD in glomerular endothelial cells.[746] Mice transgenic for MnSOD express it in mitochondria of the kidney interstitium and glomeruli.[747]

In addition to the production of ROS by inflammatory cells, renal and glomerular cells, particularly mesangial cells, can generate ROS independently of infiltrating cells and these ROS may serve an autacoid role in glomerular injury.[728] The MAC of C as well as both IL-1 and TNF can induce superoxide and hydrogen peroxide in cultured mesangial cells, with the production by the latter increasing through 90 minutes.[748, 749] The oxidative burst in mesangial cells stimulated by phagocytosis may be related to stimulation of the lipoxygenase pathway.[750, 751] Membrane-bound NADPH-dependent oxidase components have been identified on human mesangial cells and have been suggested as a source for generation of ROS by these cells just as in neutrophils.[752–754]

In turn, ROS can be shown to be toxic to mesangial cells.[730] Mesangial cells can be killed by activated neutrophils in a manner in which catalase is highly protective and SOD less so.[755] The ROS produced by mesangial cells are thought to play a role in oxidative modification of low-density lipoproteins, which have mitogenic effects on the cells.[756] Glomerular epithelial cells have been shown to contain the neutrophil respiratory burst cytochrome $b_{558}$, a material that is increased in glomeruli during PHN.[378] Renal tubule epithelial cells have also been shown to produce ROS.[757]

ROS can modulate enzymes and enzyme inhibitors, chemotaxis, and arachidonic acid metabolism, thereby widely influencing many aspects of an inflammatory process. For example, ROS can increase endothelial ICAM's ability to bind neutrophils.[758] Oxidants from neutrophils are suggested to enhance glomerular thrombus formation via a decrease in glomerular ADPase activity.[759] Ab-dependent cellular cytotoxicity and chemiluminescence induced in vitro with anti-GBM Abs were shown to be dependent on ROS.[760] Degradation of human GBM by stimulated neutrophils is thought to be due to activation of a latent metalloproteinase by an oxidant generated by the MPO–hydrogen peroxidase–halide system.[761] Neutrophils can circumvent the protective effects of $\alpha_1$-proteinase inhibitor by a hydrogen peroxide–dependent (catalase-inhibited) process.[762]

ROS are also reported to decrease glomerular synthesis of the nascent core peptide of heparan sulfate proteoglycan.[763]

A respiratory burst was detected as chemiluminescence in neutrophils exposed to GBM–anti-GBM Ab IC; associated selective release of lysosomal enzymes was also found.[764] Studies suggest that GBM collagen is made more digestible by MPO-derived oxidants.[765]

A role for ROS in experimental renal injury is suggested from studies using SOD, an inhibitor of superoxide anion, in IC types of GN in mice and in primate pyelonephritis.[3] Catalase, an inhibitor of hydrogen peroxide, has been reported to inhibit proteinuria induced by injection of phorbol myristate acetate (a potent activator of neutrophils and macrophages to generate oxygen species) into the renal artery.[766] Catalase also inhibited proteinuria induced by infusion of CVF into the renal artery; however, SOD and hydroxyl radical scavengers were not effective.[319] Glomerular injury can be induced by exposure to singlet oxygen produced by a photodynamic reaction from pheophorbide a.[767] Exposure to superoxide and its products via infusion of xanthine oxidase and xanthine can cause glomerular endothelial and mesangial cell damage.[768] Infusion of low concentrations of hydrogen peroxide is reported to induce proteinuria without causing histologic changes.[769] In the isolated glomerulus, exposure to superoxide via xanthine and xanthine oxidase increased albumin permeability.[770] In this study, activated macrophages were shown to enhance albumin permeability as well, an effect blocked by SOD. In glomerular culture, ROS, of which hydrogen peroxide was most potent, were suggested to modulate the surface area of mesangial cells and, in turn, the ultrafiltration coefficient with a decrease in glomerular filtration rate (GFR)[771]; PAF was perhaps involved in the effect.

Anti-GBM Ab–induced GN in rats was modulated by catalase but not by SOD or dimethyl sulfoxide, suggesting that hydrogen peroxide, but not superoxide or hydroxyl radical, was important in mediation.[772, 773] In contrast, superoxide was shown by administration of SOD to play a role in this model in another study.[774] Deferoxamine, an iron chelator, and dimethythiourea, a hydroxyl radical scavenger, were effective in preventing proteinuria in anti-GBM Ab GN.[775] Quantitative features may be responsible for the disparate results regarding hydroxyl radicals in the two studies. Autologous-phase anti–GMB Ab GN was modulated with SOD, and the increase of renal malondialdehyde seen in control subjects was suppressed.[776] Dimethyl sulfoxide treatment of PHN reduced proteinuria associated with fewer glomerular immune deposits, particularly C3, making interpretation of the result difficult[777]; the effect was blocked by low, but not high, doses of indomethacin.[778] Dimethylthiourea was reported to improve proteinuria in PHN without changing the immune deposits.[779] Dimethylthiourea was also effective in IC GN in the rat.[780] NZB/W $F_1$ female mice treated with dimethyl sulfoxide had less proteinuria without differences in antinuclear Ab levels or IgG deposits in glomeruli.[781] SOD is also said to improve this model with an influence on antinuclear Ab.[782] In contrast to the use of inhibitors, selenium-deficient diets that reduce levels of glutathione peroxidase, a major defense against oxidative injury, worsened PHN.[783] Studies suggest that glucocorticoids may act to enhance glomerular antioxidant enzyme activities.[784, 785]

The MPO–hydrogen peroxide–halide formation of oxidants was suggested to play a role in a model of planted Ag GN in rats in which neutrophil depletion prevented injury.[786] MPO was implicated when radiolabeled iodine was incorporated in the glomeruli and GBM. The contribution of MPO had been suggested by an experiment in which MPO was infused into the renal artery, followed by hydrogen peroxidase in a chloride-containing solution, which induced endothelial and mesangial cell injury.[55, 787] MPO was localized along the GBM, probably on the basis of charge interaction. Proteinuria, endothelial cell swelling, and epithelial cell foot process effacement were induced, and radiolabeled iodine was incorporated in the GBM and mesangium. A planted Ag form of glomerular injury has been reported in rats immunized against MPO.[57] Of interest, autoantibodies reactive with neutrophil Ags including MPO obtained from patients with vasculitis are capable of inducing release of oxygen radicals from neutrophils in vitro.[52]

In aminonucleoside of puromycin nephrosis in rats, ROS presumably generated by xanthine oxidase from hypoxanthine, a breakdown product of aminonucleoside, appear to be responsible and are blocked by SOD or allopurinol.[788] Catalase coupled to polyethylene glycol to extend its half-life in the circulation was also able to modify the aminonucleoside-induced lesion.[789] SOD was able to reduce proteinuria in doxorubicin (Adriamycin) nephropathy.[790] Reperfusion injury, as in acute ischemic renal failure, has been related to oxygen free radicals with lipid peroxidation.[791] The antioxidant probucol improved glomerular function after ischemic injury, but this improvement appeared to worsen overall tubule damage, perhaps through increased work generated by the improved GFR.[792]

## Eicosanoids

Eicosanoids are derived from arachidonic acid and are involved in several aspects of immune glomerular injury, including that related to the contribution of intrinsic glomerular cells themselves.[793–795] The multiple biologically reactive eicosanoids include the prostaglandins and the thromboxanes generated by the COX (prostaglandin G/H synthase) pathway, and the leukotrienes and hydroxy fatty acids (hydroxyeicosatetraenoic acids, HETEs) produced by three major lipoxygenase metabolic pathways.[796–805] Lipoxygenase products in glomeruli of various species include 12-HETE, 15-HETE, $LTB_4$, $LTC_4$, and $LTE_4$. Cytochrome P-450 epoxygenase oxygenates arachidonic acid to epoxyeicosatrienoic acid, which is acted on by COX to produce mitogens for glomerular mesangial cells.[806, 807]

Arachidonic acid release in response to a number of vasoactive hormones and cytokines occurs via phospholipase $A_2$ ($PLA_2$). Another product of this reaction is a precursor of PAF. The $PLA_2$ lipolytic enzymes include a low-molecular-mass (14 kd) group of secretory molocules and a higher molecular mass (60 to 110 kd) group of cytosolic enzymes. Several of the $PLA_2$ enzymes have been cloned, including cytosolic $PLA_2$.[808–814] Soluble $PLA_2$ is present in inflammatory sites, as during peritoneal exudation, or in inflammatory synovial fluid and is a potential target for anti-inflammatory therapy.[815] Multiple types of $PLA_2$ are active in the kidney and in mesangial cells.[816, 817]

Secretion of $PLA_2$ from mesangial cells in response to IL-1 or TNF is reported and can be blocked by dexamethasone.[818–821] The $PLA_2$ from mesangial cells can stimulate arachidonic acid release and prostaglandin $E_2$ ($PGE_2$) synthesis in cultured glomerular epithelial and endothelial cells, with endothelial cells being particularly sensitive. Cytosolic $PLA_2$ is also activated by cytokines in mesangial cells.[822–825] IL-4 antagonizes the IL-1 and TNF induction of $PGE_2$ synthesis.[826] Coculture of glomerular endothelial cells with mesangial cells increases mesangial cell $PGE_2$ synthesis dependent on endothelium-derived endothelin.[827] Protein kinase C signaling in early diabetes enhances $PLA_2$ and $PGE_2$, $PGI_2$, and thromboxane $A_2$ ($TXA_2$).[828]

Mesangial cell COX is inducible.[829, 830] A constitutively expressed COX-1 and a mitogen-inducible COX-2 have been discerned, and we have cloned the rat counterpart and shown that it is induced by IL-1 in vitro and in the kidney by endotoxin in vivo.[831] Its expression in mesangial cells in response to IL-1 is inhibited by dexamethasone and cyclosporine.[832, 833] IL-1–induced COX-2 expression in rat mesangial cells is in part dependent on ROS.[735] The inducible COX-2 is related to inflammation, and selective inhibition of COX-2 would be suggested to involve fewer side effects than are associated with standard COX inhibitors, which have variable effects on both COX enzymes.[834–836] These products are coming under study as mediators in renal injury in addition to their role in the immune process, in renal physiology, and in the renin-angiotensin system.[3] For example, the control of glomerular blood flow and filtration occurs in part through the interactions between the vasoconstrictor AII and the glomerular production of vasodilatory prostaglandins, $PGE_2$ and $PGI_2$,[837, 838] with a role in mesangial contractility.[839, 840] In a general way, increased amounts of the E series prostaglandins appear to be beneficial in immune renal injury via effects on renal hemodynamics, inflammatory cells, membrane function, and immune suppression. Inhibition of thromboxane and leukotriene production or binding is also helpful. Essential fatty acid deficiency inhibits both PGE and thromboxane production, eliminating both pro and con effects on inflammatory injury.

Isolated glomeruli, glomerular epithelial cells, and mesangial cells produce several COX metabolites including $PGE_2$, prostacyclin ($PGI_2$), thromboxane, and lipoxygenase products.[3] Activated T cells are reported to induce $PGE_2$ release from syngeneic mesangial cells with growth inhibition.[841] Thrombin induces $PGE_2$ production by mesangial cells.[842] Proximal tubule fluid obtained by micropuncture techniques or study of isolated nephron segments can also be used to assess glomerular and tubule prostaglandin and thromboxane production.[843, 844] Immunohistochemical localization studies show that Abs to COX react with the glomerular mesangium.[845]

Modulation of inflammatory reactions or other factors such as nephritogenic Ab production and IC localization is reported after administration of PGE and its stable analogues in the Arthus reaction, spontaneous and experimental IC GN, and nephrotoxic serum nephritis.[3, 846–850] $PGE_1$ reduces infiltrating macrophages in accelerated anti-GBM

GN.[851] Dietary enrichment with linoleic acid, a major substrate for the formation of arachidonic acid, is reported to have a protective effect in experimental IC GN.[852] $PGE_1$ with cyclophosphamide improves the outcome in murine lupus and corrects the T-to-B lymphocyte ratios.[853] Indomethacin and the thromboxane receptor antagonist L-670,596 improve the lupus of the MRL-*lpr/lpr* mouse.[854] Short-term infusion of $PGE_1$ in humans with chronic GN is said to decrease plasma creatinine.[855] Intravenous $PGE_1$ may also improve steroid- and immunosuppressive drug–resistant SLE.[856] Glomeruli of diabetic rats and mesangial cells derived from them exhibit enhanced prostaglandin synthesis, and the glomerular hemodynamic compensation of such rats is altered by indomethacin.[857–859] COX inhibition with indomethacin enhances IL-1–stimulated mesangial cell growth.[860]

Thromboxane synthase has been cloned[861–863] and glomerular and mesangial receptors have been characterized.[864, 865] In nephrotoxic nephritis in rats, $TXB_2$, the stable degradation product of vasoconstrictive $TXA_2$, is increased in isolated glomeruli within 2 hours after Ab administration, with the suggestion that its effects may subsequently be offset by increases in the vasodilatory prostaglandins ($PGE_2$ and $PGI_2$).[3] COX, thromboxane synthetase, and 5-lipoxygenase activities increase, and the last two are decreased with depletion of neutrophils or platelets.[866] The associated decrease in GFR is partially prevented by administration of thromboxane synthetase inhibitors, with the effects varying with the stage of disease.[3] Enhanced $TXA_2$ can be inhibited with a PAF antagonist.[867] A role for AII along with the vasodilatory prostaglandins is also suggested in this model.[868] In the late autologous phase of anti-GBM GN (14 days), the alteration in glomerular ultrafiltration coefficient was controlled by both prostaglandins and $TXA_2$.[869]

1-Benzylimidazole, a $TXA_2$ synthetase inhibitor, lessened neutrophil infiltration, mononuclear cell infiltration, and fibrin deposition in a form of acute serum sickness in rabbits.[870] The thromboxane synthetase inhibitor OKY-046 decreased immunoreactive urinary $TXB_2$ and worsened anti-GBM Ab GN in rabbits.[871] The thromboxane synthetase inhibitor CGS 12970 improved a Con A planted Ag model of GN in beagle dogs.[872] The thromboxane synthetase inhibitor dazmegrel did not inhibit proteinuria or glomerular hypercellularity in a unilateral cationic Ag model of GN in rats,[873] and the thromboxane synthetase inhibitor UK-38,485 was ineffective in another cationic Ag Ig model.[874]

The increase in glomerular $PGE_2$ and $TXB_2$ production associated with proteinuria in PHN is lacking in rats given CVF, which prevents proteinuria in this model.[875] In this study, UK-38,485, which lowered $TXB_2$ production, did not affect the development of proteinuria. In contrast, in a study using the isolated perfused kidney in which a C-fixing Ab reaction to planted anti-Fx1A Ab was used, proteinuria was modulated with the thromboxane synthetase inhibitor OKY-046.[876] In Ab-induced mesangial cell injury, leukocytes and platelets contribute to functional changes via thromboxane, $LTB_4$, and 12-HETE.[877] In the cationic bovine gamma globulin model, proteinuria and elevation in glomerular $TXB_2$ production were independent of C and leukocytes.[878] Ab-induced mesangial cell injury is associated with increased $TXB_2$, which can be inhibited with CVF to block the lesion.[879] In anti-GBM, CVF blocked the fall in GRF without changing $TXB_2$ elevation; however, $PGE_2$ was elevated in comparison to the non–CVF-treated contact.[880]

In lupus mice, an increase in $TXB_2$ production occurred in preparations of cortical glomeruli, an effect inhibited by prevention of disease with $PGE_2$.[881] In this study, ibuprofen, which inhibited platelet $TXB_2$ but not intrarenal levels, did not retard progression of renal damage. $TXA_2$ and sulfido-peptide leukotrienes are suggested to play a role in endotoxin-induced renal injury.[882] Glomerular $TXB_2$ production is enhanced in Adriamycin-induced nephrosis, and proteinuria is reduced by treatment with UK-38,485.[883] Fawn-hooded rats that develop segmental glomerulosclerosis have increased GFR and elevated urinary $TXB_2$, 6-keto-$PGF_{1\alpha}$, and $PGE_2$.[884] Thromboxane can enhance production of ECM and eicosanoids enhance the epidermal growth factor (EGF) receptor activation of glomerular epithelial cells.[885, 886] Administration of thromboxane receptor blockers and synthetase inhibitors reduces glomerular sclerotic mesangial damage.[887]

Indomethacin reduces protein excretion in active HN (AHN)[888] and in PHN; however, the thromboxane synthetase inhibitor UK-38,485 did not.[889] In a model of chronic cationized Ag GN, rats receiving high-protein diets had an increase in their depressed GFR after thromboxane receptor blockers and an even greater decrease in GFR after indomethacin.[890] Low doses of indomethacin interfere with the proteinuria-sparing effect of dimethyl sulfoxide (perhaps C related) noted in PHN.[778] Indomethacin is noted to accelerate damage in aminonucleoside nephrosis and to enhance leukocyte influx in mild anti-GBM GN.[3, 891] Aspirin, at a dosage that inhibited both circulating cell and renal arachidonic acid metabolites, worsened the morphologic findings in anti-GBM Ab GN in rabbits, in contrast to the beneficial effect of sulindac at a dose that suppressed platelet COX activity but only partially suppressed renal prostaglandin synthesis.[892] A similar effect on renal function is suggested in humans with impaired renal function.[893]

The lipoxygenase products of arachidonic acid metabolites are gaining increased attention.[894–896] Serial studies showed enhanced glomerular arachidonate 12-lipoxygenation in experimental anti-GBM Ab GN in rats and suggested a possible mediating role for 12-HETE via its effects on leukocyte function.[897] The 5-lipoxygenase pathway leads to the formation of leukotrienes. $LTB_4$ synthesis is reported in glomeruli recovered from rats with cationic bovine gamma globulin–induced GN in anti-GBM GN and PHN.[898–900] $LTB_4$ stimulates neutrophil adhesion to vascular endothelial cells and can cause monocyte transendothelial migration.[901, 902] C depletion (more effectively than neutrophil depletion) in anti-GBM Ab GN significantly decreased glomerular 12-HETE, 5-HETE, and $LTB_4$ production, which occurred within 15 minutes of Ab administration,[903] and the glomerular leukocyte is thought to be a major source of the $LTB_4$.[904] Administration of $LTB_4$ to rats with mild anti-GBM GN increased glomerular neutrophil infiltration.[905] $LTB_4$ and $LTD_4$ enhanced neutrophil adhesion to mesangial cells.[906]

A glomerular $LTC_4$ receptor has been described, and $LTC_4$ has been noted to bind to glomerular epithelial cells and induce proliferation.[907, 908] $LTC_4$ decreases perfusion rate in the isolated kidney in experimental anaphylactic reactions.[909] In addition, glomerular lipoxygenase products enhance adhesion of macrophages to glomeruli and stimulate prostaglandin synthesis by macrophages.[910] Rat glomeruli can convert exogenously added $LTC_4$ to $LTD_4$ and $LTE_4$.[911] $LTD_4$ induces an increase in efferent arteriolar resistance in studies of glomerular hemodynamics.[912] $LTE_4$ induces gaps in endothelium.[913] Antagonism of $LTD_4$ receptors preserved the SNGFR by abrogating changes in the ultrafiltration coefficient.[914] The $LTD_4$ receptor antagonist SK&F 104353 blocked glomerular hemodynamic changes in the autologous phase of PHN.[915] Macrophage depletion abolished leukotriene synthesis in this model.

Inhibitors of 12-lipoxygenase and/or 5-lipoxygenase improved the decrease in GFR and renal blood flow of anti-GBM GN.[916, 917] Glomerular cell proliferation assessed by studying proliferating cell nuclear antigen was also depressed by a 5-lipoxygenase inhibitor in this model.[918] Studies suggest that the 15-lipoxygenase 15-(S)-HETE, a precursor of lipoxin biosynthesis, may counteract the initial effects of 5-lipoxygenase leukotriene products.[919] IL-4 may enhance the production of the 12/15-lipoxygenase products that counteract the leukotrienes.[920] Patients with GN, particularly with lower GFR values, had increased 5-lipoxygenase and 5-lipoxygenase–activating protein in their renal tissue as assessed by polymerase chain reaction.[921]

Dietary manipulation to increase or decrease arachidonic acid and other fatty acids to alter prostaglandin synthesis and subsequent experimental glomerular injury potentially has multiple effects not only on possible mediating systems but also on the underlying immune response, clouding interpretation of beneficial outcomes.[922–924] Alterations in fat intake including the arachidonic acid analogue eicosapentaenoic acid, an n-3 fatty acid contained in fish oil, alters prostaglandin production and is capable of modulating human and murine lupus GN (decreasing proteinuria and histologic change) as well as cationic Ag-induced membranous GN and glomerulosclerosis in Zucker rats.[925–931] Diets with increased n-3 fatty acids or linoleic acid reduced proteinuria in apoferritin-induced IC GN in mice and severity of disease in mercuric chloride nephritis in rats.[932, 933]

Essential fatty acid deficiency reduces glomerular (and renal cortical) macrophage numbers and glomerular eicosanoid production, an effect reversed by supplementation with n-6 but not n-3 fatty acids.[934] The effect is suggested to be related to inhibition of glomeruli to produce a specific lipid monocyte chemoattractant that is normally induced by the response to anti-GBM GN.[935, 936] The histologic improvement in anti-GBM GN associated with essential fatty acid deficiency is noted to be particularly striking at 2 weeks.[937] Also, the lipid carried by albumin that is released by tubule catabolism during proteinuria may contribute to the decline in renal function.[938] Diets deficient in n-6 fatty acids markedly attenuate the ability of glomeruli to synthesize $LTB_4$.[939] The n-3 fatty acids also inhibit endothelial cell production of PDGF.[940] It would be of interest to explore the clinical features of GN in societies with altered lipid composition associated with marine diets.

Experimentally, urinary assessment of thromboxane and LTB$_4$ may reflect glomerular inflammation.[941] Measurement of urinary excretion of prostaglandins in patients with GN gives varied results.[942–944] Urinary PGE$_2$ excretion is reported to be reduced in acute poststreptococcal GN.[945] Clinical use of prostaglandin inhibitors such as indomethacin also has led to unclear results over the years.[3] An increase in creatinine clearance has been found in patients with chronic renal disease and in one patient with rapidly progressive GN after PGE$_2$ administration, possibly for hemodynamic reasons.[946, 947] Thromboxane receptor antagonists improve renal hemodynamics in SLE.[948, 949]

## Platelets and Platelet-Activating Factor

Other cellular elements, such as platelets and their products, have drawn attention as mediators[950–953] and as contributors to glomerular thrombotic elements in conditions such as hemolytic-uremic syndrome and thrombotic thrombocytopenic purpura, which may involve the metabolism of PGI$_2$.[3] PGI$_2$ generation is also reported to be impaired in SLE.[3] The possible role of platelets and in particular their polycationic mediators in glomerular injury has been noted.[954] Thrombin-stimulated platelets can injure vascular endothelium,[955] and platelet factors influence the growth of mesangial cells in culture.[956] Thrombospondin, a major $\alpha$ platelet granule protein, has been identified in the mesangium and can advance monocyte adhesion.[957, 958] It is increased in glomerular inflammation in human kidneys.[959] Antiplatelet Abs may play a role in SLE.[960] C depletion decreases platelet accumulation in antimesangial Ab GN.[961] Experimental studies using Ab-induced platelet depletion resulted in a significant reduction in albuminuria in a planted Ag form of GN in rats.[962] Antiplatelet Abs also decrease the number of proliferating cells detected by cyclin staining in anti–mesangial cell Ab GN.[963] Antiplatelet drugs and adenine nucleotides also modulate this model.[964, 965] Depletion of platelets in anti-GBM GN or in anti–mesangial cell Ab GN attenuated increased glomerular eicosanoid synthesis.[866, 877] In serum sickness, antiplatelet Ab also reduced glomerular injury.[966]

In GN, in vivo platelet activation has been suggested by monitoring platelet aggregation and plasma serotonin concentrations, PAF, $\beta$-thromboglobulin, and platelet factor-4,[3] which might contribute to mediation of hypercoagulability. Platelet factor-4 localized in the glomerular capillary walls concomitant with a decrease in glomerular polyanion in hyperimmune rabbits infused with Ag[967] or in rats given habu snake venom.[968] Platelet Ags have also been localized in glomeruli,[3] although, of interest, human GBM is reported not to aggregate platelets, an effect that may be modified by changing its composition of adenosine diphosphatase.[3, 969]

PDGF, besides being a potent mesenchymal mitogen, has several other biologic properties, and its isoforms bind to two cell surface receptors.[970–973] Its role in glomerular injury has been reviewed[974] and expression of its receptors studied in human GN.[975] PDGF chemotaxis for neutrophils and monocytes approaches that of C5a,[976] and PDGF also activates these cells,[977, 978] among its broad range of mitogenic actions.[979] This cationic protein can activate and cause syn-

thesis of COX[980] and could contribute to glomerular inflammation. Its role in the evolution of injury and sclerosis is discussed later. Platelet-derived heparitinase can degrade sulfated proteoglycans in the subendothelial ECM.[981] Glomerular mesangial cells migrate in response to PDGF and also to platelet-released fibronectin; the latter response is inhibited by an RGDS (Arg-Gly-Asp-Ser) peptide.[982]

Serotonin levels in the blood are increased in both experimental IC and anti-GBM nephritis.[3] Inhibition of histamine and serotonin release from rabbit platelets has been suggested to modify IC localization in rabbits, thereby altering acute serum sickness.[1] Serotonin also has direct nephrotoxic effects[3]; however, antiplatelet drug effects in experimental models have been partial, with some benefit to proteinuria and glomerular IC localization in serum sickness GN in rats and rabbits or anti-GBM GN in rats.[983–986] Some benefit of antiplatelet drugs in human membranoproliferative GN, but not IgA nephropathy, was reported.[987, 988]

Another platelet protein, platelet factor-4, a member of the chemokine family, has been shown to interact with the glomerular capillary wall because of charge differences.[989] The interaction is suggested to be with heparan sulfate anionic sites.[990] Plasma clearances are rapid, modulated by heparin,[991] and the protein binds strongly to N-sulfated glycosaminoglycans. Its binding to the glomeruli can be blocked by prior exposure to polyethyleneimine. The latter factor, however, can interact with inflammatory cells in addition to binding to glomerular polyanions.[954] Platelet factor-4 and activated platelets are reported in the kidneys and urine of patients with IgA nephropathy,[992, 993] and platelets and PDGF are also found in glomeruli of a portion of such patients.[994]

PAF, a phospholipid (1-$O$-alkyl-2-acetyl-$sn$-glycero-3-phosphocholine), is a substance released by basophils and many other cells including neutrophils, monocytes, and platelets that has platelet- as well as neutrophil- and monocyte-activating properties, is spasmogenic and hypotensive, and causes increased vascular permeability in nanomolar quantities.[995–1001]

The cellular receptors (extra- and intracellular) for PAF have been the subject of review.[1002, 1003] Specific PAF receptor complementary DNAs have been cloned from guinea pig lung and other cell types and by sequence analysis were found to belong to the superfamily of G protein–coupled receptors.[1004–1006] In the G protein–coupled rhodopsin family receptors, replacement of a highly conserved asparagine residue in the seventh membrane-spanning region by aspartic acid is seen in the TXA$_2$ receptor, another lipid receptor.[1007] The PAF signal transduction pathways, including those in the glomerular mesangial cell, have been the subject of review.[1008, 1009]

PAF plays a role in kidney injury and in GN.[1010, 1011] There is a close relationship between PAF action and arachidonic acid metabolism through protein kinase C and phospholipase pathways, and both are released from the same precursor. Many cell types release arachidonic acid metabolites in response to PAF with PGE$_2$ production in glomerular mesangial cells.[1012] Numerous studies indicate that one of the key events in PAF-mediated signaling is phosphoinositide turnover, including that in mesangial cells[1013, 1014] and in inflammatory cells including macrophages.[1015, 1016]

PAF increases cytosolic free $Ca^{2+}$ in various cell types including mesangial and endothelial cells.[1013, 1017] PAF also stimulates tyrosine phosphorylation of cellular proteins in platelets, neutrophils, and macrophages.[1018–1022] PAF plays a role in gene expression because it can induce transcription of *FOS* and *JUN* in B cells, astroglial cells, and A-431 cells (epidermoid carcinoma cells), an effect blocked by PAF antagonists.[1023–1025] This enhanced transcription is an effect shared by growth factors important in evolution of glomerular and renal injury such as EGF.[1026]

PAF also rapidly induced *FOS* and *JUN* in corneal epithelial cells, followed by increased expression of collagenase type I.[1027] The delayed expression of the collagenase gene is inhibited by cycloheximide (which superinduces *FOS* and *JUN*), suggesting that a transcriptional factor is involved between the two expressions. The expression of all three genes is blocked by PAF antagonists of intracellular PAF-binding sites. These findings may link PAF's early proinflammatory role with the tissue repair process that involves growth factors. Platelet supernatants cause mesangial cells to contract, and PAF was suggested to be responsible.[1028] Of interest in this regard, the PAF- and EGF-induced expression of *FOS* in A-431 cells has been shown to involve two distinct mechanisms, with PAF receptor activation mediated via tyrosine kinase and protein kinase C.[1029] The EGF signaling pathway involves transcription factor p91, which is activated by tyrosine phosphorylation and is a component of the DNA-binding factor that recognizes SIE (*SIS*-inducible element) in the *FOS* gene promoter.[1030]

PAF, along with slow-reacting substances (LTC and LTD) and vasoactive substances, can be released from the isolated kidney.[1031] PAF can also be released from the isolated kidney by IgE-induced immune reactions.[1032] PAF is reported to alter vascular permeability with proteinuria (prevented by PAF antagonists) in the isolated perfused rat kidney[1033–1036] and to decrease vascular resistance in spontaneously hypertensive rats.[1037] Its production and degradation by glomeruli and cultured mesangial cells have been reported,[1038–1043] and it can stimulate renal prostaglandin synthesis in the isolated kidney[1044] with a spectrum of renal pathophysiologic effects.[1045, 1046] Studies using PAF antagonists suggest that PAF may have an intermediary role in glomerular hemodynamic effects of ROS, cyclosporine, and endothelin via effects on mesangial cells.[771, 1047, 1048] Of interest, AII can cause cultured rat mesangial cells to produce PAF.[1049] Mesangial cell biosynthesis of PAF is modulated by proteinase inhibitors.[1050]

In experimental GN, a C-dependent increase in PAF levels was found that may be related in part to platelets, as shown by the use of antiplatelet Ab.[1051] PAF presumably of renal origin is increased in murine lupus and in the urine of patients with membranous nephropathy.[1052–1054]

PAF was long ago implicated in glomerular IC deposition in acute serum sickness,[1055] and later in IC localization.[1056, 1057] Localization of cationic proteins from platelets and neutrophils with loss of anionic sites was reported in acute serum sickness in rabbits.[1058] Administered platelet cationic proteins, as well as PAF-induced in vivo release of such materials, can result in glomerular binding and can induce loss of glomerular anionic charges.[1059, 1060] Cationic platelet proteins have been seen in glomerular deposits in patients with SLE GN.[1061]

A number of studies have shown beneficial effects of PAF antagonists in immune and toxic glomerular injury. A PAF antagonist, L-652,731, decreased glomerular damage in anti-GBM Ab GN in rabbits, with early reduction in proteinuria. The early change was accompanied by a lessening of fibrin deposits during the autologous phase of injury.[1062] The benefit has been supported in other studies of this model and may include an effect on $TXA_2$ as well.[867, 1063–1065] PAF receptor antagonists improve GFR and reduce neutrophil infiltration in anti–mesangial cell Ab GN.[1066]

Benefits of PAF antagonists are also reported in models of lupus nephritis.[1067, 1068] However, antagonists were not effective in PHN, a relatively noninflammatory, immune deposit disease involving glomerular epithelial cell Ags.[1069] Platelet receptor antagonists were beneficial in a unilateral cationic Ag form of GN in rats, although quantitative comparisons of glomerular immune deposits were not presented.[1070] PAF release has been reported in hyperacute renal allograft rejection in association with glomerular platelet and neutrophil cationic protein deposits.[1071] PAF inhibitors are also reported as beneficial in puromycin as well as Adriamycin nephropathy in rats,[1072–1075] a condition that damages glomerular epithelial cells.[1076, 1077] PAF and TNF participate in the induction of glomerular epithelial cell injury in this lesion.[1078] PAF has been suggested to have a direct cytotoxic effect on cultured rat glomerular cells.[1011] PAF antagonists also decrease the interstitial inflammation that is associated with puromycin or Adriamycin nephropathy.[1079, 1080]

## Coagulation and Tissue Factor Procoagulant Activity

The extrinsic and intrinsic coagulation pathways and the factor XII (Hageman factor)–related contact system with activation of kinin, coagulation, and fibrinolysis pathways are possible candidates for the mediators of immune glomerular injury.[1081–1084] In addition, coagulation and thromboembolism may be complications of nephrotic syndrome.[1085–1088]

Accumulation of fibrin and associated cleavage neoantigens is a feature in certain types of human glomerular lesions and can be prominent in areas of crescent formation. Cross-linked fibrin, detected by monoclonal Abs, is present in areas containing fibrinogen-related Ags and is associated with electron-dense deposits but may be discordant from platelet membrane Ag and von Willebrand factor Ag.[1089] Factor XII deposits can be identified in areas of fibrinogen-related Ag deposits.[1090] Fibronectin staining extends past its normal mesangial location and accompanies fibrin, $\alpha_2$-plasmin inhibitor, and plasminogen deposits.[1091–1094] Thrombin has been shown to stimulate proliferation of glomerular epithelial cells via specific membrane receptors while decreasing their fibrinolytic activity.[1095] Factor XII recovered from the urine of guinea pigs with anti-GBM Ab GN had undergone proteolysis compatible with its activation possibly in the Bowman space.[1096]

Fibrin deposits are often not striking in the early stages of immune glomerular injury or in the milder forms of this disorder; however, with an active fibrinolytic system, such deposits may be removed rapidly and go undetected. The possible effects of the fibrinogen peptides on vascular permeability and chemotaxis must also be considered. Fibrin is more involved in severe proliferative and crescentic forms of GN, and its accumulation in glomerular capillaries and Bowman space does seem to be related to crescent formation and eventual glomerular scarring. There are suggestions that fibrin fibers may hinder outgrowth of glomerular epithelial cells but not mesangial cells.[1097]

The role of accumulated fibrin in glomeruli has been studied in experiments using anticoagulants, but these studies must be interpreted in the light of varying severities of the immunologic insult as well as the type and adequacy of anticoagulation. In early studies in which heparin and warfarin anticoagulation was used for relatively mild anti-GBM GN, the treatment seemed to be beneficial. However, large amounts of heparin were shown to have little or no effect on fibrin accumulation in severe heterologous forms of anti-GBM GN,[1098] suggesting that other than heparin-sensitive coagulation pathways were involved. Variable results have also been seen in experimental IC-induced injury. Heparin can have an effect on removal of cationic Ags from glomeruli in IC GN independent of its anticoagulant properties. Of interest, fibrin accumulations in glomeruli and areas of crescent formation in humans with GN have had no identifiable antihemophilic factor (factor VIII),[1099] again suggesting fibrin accumulation from other than the usual systemic coagulation pathways. Factor VIII, fibrinogen, and fibrin degradation products were found in thrombotic microangiopathy and less frequently in other glomerular lesions.[1100] Factor VIII has also been used to study endothelial cell abnormalities in GN.[3]

Ancrod, a material obtained from Malaysian pit viper venom, can cleave fibrinogen and remove clottable fibrinogen before immune glomerular injury begins. The removal of the fibrin products, presumably by mononuclear phagocyte systems, does not seem to impair clearance of IC.[3] Ancrod treatment has little effect on the induction of proteinuria or on glomerular hypercellularity in anti-GBM Ab GN but does seem to diminish fibrin accumulation in glomeruli, lessen crescent formation, and preserve renal function, as determined by measuring serum creatinine concentration during the later and more chronic stages of injury.[3] As with anticoagulation, the effects of ancrod are related to the severity of the immune insult, being effective in mild anti-GBM Ab GN and ineffective in severe disease.[1101] Ancrod delays the development of glomerular fibrin deposits in BXSB lupus mice and lowers plasma procoagulant activity (PCA).[1102] Leukocyte depletion diminishes fibrin deposition, perhaps related to the interplay of monocyte PCA.[677] Fibrinolytic treatment with streptokinase can be effective after established fibrin deposition.[1103, 1104] Defibrination has been used with limited success in the treatment of coagulation-related glomerular complications in SLE as well.[1105–1108] The role of the lupus anticoagulant, an antiphospholipid Ab that has been associated with venous and arterial thrombosis, is unclear in glomerular injury.[1109–1111]

A relationship between fibrinolysis and fibrin-induced

glomerular injury would be suspected.[3] In early studies, glomerular fibrinolytic activity increased as fibrin deposition and crescent formation occurred in experimental anti-GBM GN; in other studies an inverse correlation was found.[3] Urinary fibrinolytic activity was decreased in human GN.[1112] Tissue-type plasminogen activator (t-PA) is identified in glomerular endothelium with urokinase-type plasminogen activator (u-PA) found in the glomerular epithelium,[1113, 1114] and an assay for glomerular plasminogen activator activity is described.[1115] The glomerular fibrinolytic activity is enhanced by polyunsaturated fatty acids.[1116] A decline in urinary t-PA and u-PA was reported in glomerular disease.[1117] TNF infusion in rabbits decreased glomerular fibrinolytic activity.[1118] Plasminogen activator inhibitor-1 (PAI-1) was reported in human glomeruli associated with fibrin deposits.[1119] Plasminogen receptors on glomerular epithelial cells and autocrine saturation of u-PA receptors provide a complete membrane-bound plasminogen-activating system.[1120]

Thrombin has been shown to increase both t-PA and PAI-1 production by human mesangial cells with PAI-1 release, which may inhibit fibrinolysis.[1121] A decrease in plasminogen activator was reported in IC disease in rabbits; however, this did not correlate with the type or severity of GN.[1122] In augmented anti-GBM Ab GN in rats, t-PA and u-PA remain unchanged or decrease, but glomerular PAI-1 mRNA and bioactivity increase at 6 hours and peak at 1 day.[1123] In this study, the PAI-1 increase correlated with maximal glomerular capillary fibrin accumulations, which recanalized as the PAI-1 mRNA and bioactivity declined during the subsequent 2 weeks. The initial PAI-1 increase correlated with an increase in IL-1 and later TGF-β mRNA. TNF enhanced PAI-1 activity in another anti-GBM Ab GN study.[1124] In rabbits a reduction in glomerular fibrinolytic activity, predominantly t-PA, along with an increase in PAI-1 correlated with macrophage influx and fibrin deposition.[1125] IL-1 and TNF increase PAI-1 mRNA and protein in cultured human endothelial cells,[1126, 1127] as do EGF and TGF-β.[1128–1130] PAI-1 is deposited in the ECM of cultured human mesangial cells.[1131] PAI-1 is increased in vivo by TGF-β and TNF-α.[1132] The PAI-1 deposition in the glomeruli can be blocked with anti–TGF-β Ab.[1133] In experimental HN the autoantibody reactive with the epithelial cell Ag glycoprotein gp330 has been reported also to bind plasminogen and, in turn, can act as a competitive inhibitor of urokinase.[1134]

Urokinase therapy is reported to enhance fibrinolysis and decrease glomerular fibrin deposits but does not alter proteinuria.[1135] Urokinase improved, and an inhibitor of fibrinolysis worsened, anti-GBM Ab GN.[1136] Recombinant t-PA was reported to protect rabbits with anti-GBM Ab GN from crescent formation.[1137, 1138] When evaluated in relation to severity of disease, it was partially effective in mild, but not severe, anti-GBM Ab GN.[1101] Urokinase combined with prednisolone, antiplatelet drugs, and heparin was said in a case report to diminish hematuria and increase renal function in a patient with IgA nephropathy.[1139]

Numerous studies demonstrate fibrin degradation products in serum or urine, and the presence of such products has been correlated with the activity of glomerulonephritic processes and glomerular fibrin deposition. Levels of fibrin degradation products are modified as the disease is treated; however, the usefulness of these assays remains unclear.[3, 1140–1145] Fibrin fragments have vasoactive and vascular permeability effects and, in addition, cause chemotaxis of neutrophils.[3, 1146, 1147] The fragments have also been shown to be immunosuppressive,[3] and the D fragment has been reported to have an effect on vascular endothelial cells in culture.[1148] Fibrin peptides can cause vascular endothelial cells to retract.[1149]

Thrombomodulin and the vitamin K–dependent protein C and protein S are produced by endothelial cells[1150, 1151] and provide anticoagulant action at the site of thrombin formation. Thrombomodulin alters the substrate specificity of thrombin, changing it from a procoagulant enzyme to an anticoagulant. Thrombin activates protein C, which is a potent inhibitor of factors Va and VIIIa.[1152, 1153] Protein S combines with the activated protein C and accelerates its activity.[1154] Thrombomodulin bound to thrombin is endocytosed, in part controlled by protein C.[1155] Activated protein C is inactivated by protein C inhibitor and $\alpha_1$-antitrypsin.[1156, 1157] Thrombin can cleave protein S and prothrombin can competitively inhibit its cofactor activity.[1158, 1159] Protein S is also limited by complexing with the C regulatory protein C4b-binding protein. Preliminary studies in our laboratory have shown protein C inhibitor in a population of proximal tubules and protein C in glomerular endothelium and possibly epithelium, with protein S associated with connective tissue.[1160, 1161] Hancock and colleagues[1162, 1163] have reported decreased immunostaining for thrombomodulin and decreased plasma protein C and free protein S Ag in experimental anti-GBM GN or transplant rejection.[1162, 1163] Thrombomodulin has also been found in rabbit and human glomeruli by immunohistochemistry and activity shown in detergent-solubilized rat and human glomeruli.[1164–1167] Both TNF-α and bacterial lipopolysaccharide (LPS) depress thrombomodulin activity, and its localization is increased in human GN. Glomerular endothelial cells show the least thrombomodulin activity of many organ endothelia studied.[1164] Serum protein C and S activities found in patients with nephrotic syndrome, a hypercoagulable state, vary among studies, being most often increased and correlating with proteinuria in some studies and with type of glomerular disease in others; elevated protein S Ag and decreased activity were due to loss of free protein S and binding to elevated C4b-binding protein.[1168–1175] Levels of plasma antithrombin III decrease or remain unchanged in patients with proteinuria and nephrotic syndrome or increase in patients with IgA nephropathy.[1168, 1170, 1173, 1176]

The factor XII intrinsic coagulation and related kinin-forming system, with its products such as kallikrein, bradykinin, fibrinogen fragments, plasma, and activated C proteins, is a candidate for mediation in immunologic renal injury.[1177] The products can cause vascular permeability changes, pain, smooth muscle contraction, chemotaxis of leukocytes, and coagulation. Factor XII binds to negatively charged surfaces and, after autoactivation of its catalytic site, the serine protease can act on factor XI to form factor XIa of the intrinsic coagulation system. It can also activate plasma kallikrein. The plasma and tissue kallikreins can release the vasodilatory bradykinin.[1178] At least two kallikrein gene family members have been noted in rat kidney, and two distinct bradykinin receptors are found on rat mesangial cells.[1179, 1180]

Urinary kallikrein is impaired at the gene transcription level in immune glomerular injury and nephrotic syndrome in rats and is normalized by treatment with converting enzyme inhibition, which reduces urinary protein excretion.[1181] Kallikrein is also present in the distal nephron.[1182] Urinary kallikrein has been noted to decrease in association with proteinuria induced by experimental anti-GBM Ab[1] and after renal transplantation.[1183]

Coagulation within the glomeruli may be induced in situ by inflammatory cells or intrinsic glomerular cells. Monocytes can produce PCA (tissue factor, factor VII/VIIa) in collaboration with lymphocytes when exposed to ICs, endotoxin, and cytokines.[3, 1184] Coagulation products including thrombin are chemoattractants for monocytes,[1185] and in turn monocytes can be induced to produce PCA that stimulates coagulation locally[1186] and in glomeruli.[1187, 1188] Wiggins and colleagues[1189] correlated PCA in sieved glomeruli with fibrin deposits in augmented anti-GBM nephritis in rabbits, and PCA also appeared in the urine. The forms of glomerular and urine PCA were complex. They seemed to be driven primarily by thromboplastin (tissue factor) but also appeared to require the presence of the intrinsic coagulation pathway for full expression. PCA in normal urine has been suggested by others to be thromboplastin-like, and this molecule has been localized in the luminal and intercellular borders as well as in the cytoplasm of epithelial cells in the loop of Henle and distal convoluted tubule.[3] The PCA in the urine of rabbits with anti-GBM Ab nephritis is associated with microvesicles.[3] Tipping and colleagues[1190, 1191] showed a correlation with monocyte infiltration, fibrin deposition, and increased PCA in the anti-GBM and acute serum sickness models, and von Willebrand factor deposits occurred at later stages.[1190, 1192] The glomerular PCA in the anti-GBM model was tissue factor–like and derived in part from glomerular macrophages.[1193] Cole and associates[1194] found that splenic macrophage PCA rose with age and correlated with the development of GN in BXSB lupus mice. Macrophages of 1-month-old mice could be induced to express PCA when incubated with lymphocytes, lymphocyte supernatants, or plasma from 5-month-old mice. PCA in circulating mononuclear cells of patients with SLE was found to be a direct prothrombinase whose presence seemed to correlate with endocapillary proliferative forms of glomerular injury.[1195] The activity was not neutralized with anti–factor X antisera. The monocyte PCA is independent of the lupus anticoagulant in SLE patients.[1196] Tissue factor–like PCA has been recovered from glomeruli of patients with proliferative GN, and a monoclonal anti–tissue factor Ab was noted to react with the glomeruli of these patients.[1197] Urinary PCA was somewhat, but not significantly, increased in patients with GN compared with control subjects, in contrast to finding significantly decreased t-PA and u-PA.[1112] Glomerular PCA was shown to correlate with fibrin formation in the mercuric chloride model of autoimmune nephritis in rats and was not correlated with the number of monocyte-macrophages or Ia-positive cells in the glomeruli.[1198] Kidney PCA increased after systemic endotoxin injection in rabbits, with activity in glomeruli and cortex greater than that in medulla.[1199]

Of interest, PCA also develops on endothelial cells,[3, 1200] and tissue factor production has been reported after IC or anti–endothelial cell Ab stimulation of umbilical venous endothelial cells.[3] IL-1 was reported to induce a tissue factor–like PCA in human vascular endothelial cells,[1201, 1202] and IL-1 containing supernatants from thrombin-stimulated endothelial cells can induce tissue factor PCA in fresh endothelial cultures.[1203] Another macrophage product, TNF-α, can induce tissue factor–like PCA in endothelium as well as suppressing the protein C pathway, an antithrombotic mechanism.[1204]

Tissue factor was found to be associated with monocyte-macrophages in glomerular crescents using immunoperoxidase-Ab techniques[1205] and is correlated with T cells and macrophages.[1206] The specificity of the monoclonal Ab used for tissue factor per se remains to be defined. Other monoclonal Abs have been used to analyze and inhibit the activity of cell-associated tissue factor.[1207] These Abs localize tissue factor in normal glomeruli.[1208] Tissue factor activity has been demonstrated in isolated glomeruli as well, pointing to one or another of the glomerular cell populations as an intrinsic initiator of coagulation.[1209] Tissue factor is also produced by rat mesangial cells in response to TNF-α and LPS,[1210] and it is produced by rat glomerular epithelial cells.[1211] The glomerular tissue factor can stimulate thromboxane synthesis in human platelets in a process mediated by thrombin.[1212] Tissue factor has been cloned, providing more opportunities to study more precisely its effects in glomeruli.[1213–1215]

## Contributions of Glomerular Cells, Proinflammatory Cytokines, and Other Molecules

It has become apparent that intrinsic glomerular cells, including epithelial,[1216–1219] mesangial,[20, 1220–1229] endothelial,[1230–1241] and peripolar[1095, 1242] cells, produce physiologic as well as proinflammatory molecules that play a central role in mediating glomerular inflammation as well as contributing to ECM production and sclerosis via both paracrine and autocrine effects (see next section).[20, 1220] Glomerular culture is useful for identifying and quantitating glomerular elements in the inflammatory process.[1232, 1243–1246] The numbers of the various glomerular cells have been quantitated in the rat and the in vivo turnover of glomerular cells is determined to be less than about 1%/d for endothelial and mesangial cells, with little evidence of proliferation in glomerular epithelial cells.[1247–1249] The use of cultured glomerular cells[1250] to show the possible roles played by these intrinsic cells in glomerular inflammation has been discussed as it applies to each of the preceding sections and will be addressed in the next section on progression and sclerosis as well. In this section, areas that pertain more to acute inflammation that are not adequately covered elsewhere are mentioned.

Anatomically, the mesangial cell has similarities to vascular smooth muscle cells and its location and contractility contribute to glomerular function.[3, 1251] Mesangial cells have a large number of inflammation-related responses, includ-

ing production of IL-1, IL-6, IL-8, TNF-α, PAF, PDGF, bFGF, TGF-β, tissue factor, ROS, thrombospondin, NO, endothelin, renin, and arachidonic acid metabolites as well as ECM components and the proteases that remodel ECM[3, 1252–1254] (also see individual sections). The proinflammatory cytokines contribute to chemotaxis, activation, and margination of leukocytes and production of PCA and vascular endothelial fibrinolytic activities.[3]

These functions of mesangial cells in culture can be stimulated by such diverse inflammatory stimuli as IC, the MAC of the C system, bacterial LPS, fibrinogen degradation products, and histamine.[3, 1255] ROS stimulate at low doses and inhibit at higher doses the mesangial cell production of $PGE_2$ and $TXB_2$.[1256] We have found that COX-2 expression in mesangial cells is at least in part induced by ROS.[735]

ROS also cause the expression of PTPase in cultured mesangial cells and in nephritic glomeruli.[736] The mouse PTPase homologue 3CH134 can be induced in vascular smooth muscle cells by AII.[1257] The PTPase may function to help control the effects of mitogen-activated protein kinases. The mitogen-activated protein kinases are part of the intracellular signaling apparatus between the membrane and the nucleus.[1258] IL-1 is reported to induce p42 mitogen-activated protein kinases in glomerular mesangial cells.[1259] IL-1 functions in part by activation of mesangial cell plasma membrane protein kinases.[1260] Cell signaling via protein tyrosine kinases is the subject of review.[1261, 1262] The protein tyrosine kinase inhibitor genistein blocks IL-1–stimulated $PGE_2$ production in mesangial cells.[1263] A membrane PTPase has also been reported to be present in glomerular epithelial foot processes, with the suggestion that it is involved in the maintenance of structure-function relations in the foot processes.[1264] For example, the CD45 PTPase of the leukocyte cell surface is an extremely important element in lymphocyte activation and development.[1265–1267] IL-1 most commonly increases cellular metabolism and expression of biologically active molecules and stimulates production of arachidonic acid metabolites as well. It acts synergistically with other cytokines, particularly TNF. Signal transduction used by mesangial cells has been reviewed.[1268–1271]

The mesangium and its cells are a focal point for the accumulation of IC and the initiation of glomerular inflammation.[3] Fc binding can activate mesangial cells including IL-1 production.[1272] Macrophages attach and enhance proliferation of mesangial cells.[1273] A specific 60-kd IgA receptor has been reported on mesangial cells that can bind IgA with high affinity.[1274] A functional C1q receptor has also been reported on rat mesangial cells.[1275] The role of cultured mesangial cells in degradation of ICs has been studied.[1276] Lectins, such as gliadin (a lectinic component of gluten), which binds polymeric IgA, can stimulate cytokine expression in mesangial cells.[1277] Mesangiolysis may also be a factor in some renal lesions.[3]

The mesangial cell can respond to cytokines in macrophage supernatants and can, in addition, produce and respond to IL-1 by proliferating.[3, 1278–1282] The effect of IL-1 on mesangial cells is enhanced by β-endorphin, which may play a role in mesangial expansion in opiate addicts.[1283–1285] IL-1 can stimulate mesangial cells to produce neutral proteinase as well as punctuated (putative) metalloproteinase-1 (PUMP-1)[1286] and other metalloproteinases, which may contribute to acute tissue injury. If protease proenzymes are not activated or are inhibited by an overabundance of inhibitors such as PAI-1 or tissue inhibitor of metalloproteinase (TIMP), it could contribute to defective remodeling of excess ECM and thereby contribute to sclerosis.[561, 1287–1289]

The proinflammatory response to cytokines, growth factors, and proteinases released from the glomerular and infiltrating inflammatory cells is countered by a series of receptor antagonists, soluble receptors, and other binding proteins including $\alpha_2$-macroglobulin, $\alpha_1$-antitrypsin, and other acute-phase proteins that probably affect the outcome of the glomerular inflammation.[1290] For example, proteases are held in the $\alpha_2$-macroglobulin molecule until endocytosis by an $\alpha_2$-macroglobulin receptor–bearing cell such as a macrophage or hepatocyte. The $\alpha_2$-macroglobulin receptor is in the same receptor family as the gp330 molecule, a receptor complex that recognizes many of the same molecules as the $\alpha_2$-macroglobulin receptor.[1291] The gp330 and the $\alpha_2$-macroglobulin receptor–associated protein that co-purifies with both $\alpha_2$-macroglobulin and gp330 are distributed in coated pits on glomerular epithelial cells and in the proximal tubule brush border.[1292] The gp330 is an Ag involved in the HN model of membranous nephropathy in rats. The tissue distribution of gp330 is more restricted than that of the $\alpha_2$-macroglobulin receptor.[1293] $\alpha_2$-Macroglobulin, $\alpha_1$-antitrypsin, $\alpha_1$-antichymotrypsin, and C-reactive protein are all acute-phase proteins that are elevated in the kidney and urine of patients with inflammatory renal injury.[1294–1298] Soluble cytokine receptors are found in serum and urine.[1299, 1300] The urinary Tamm-Horsfall protein, also called uromodulin, can bind cytokines.

TNF can be produced by mesangial cells and is a potent inflammatory mediator whose possible role in glomerular injury has been the subject of review.[1254, 1301–1309] TNF infusion, which produces many of the deleterious effects of LPS, induces glomerular neutrophil influx and fibrin deposits.[1309] TNF-$\alpha$ is noted to have a cytocidal effect on mesangial cells in culture.[1310] The Shwartzman-like toxicity of TNF is synergistic with IFN-$\gamma$ and is reduced with COX inhibitors.[1311] TNF-$\alpha$ can increase antifibrinolytic activity in cultured human mesangial cells by enhancing production of PAI-1.[1312] In addition to glomerular cells, renal tubule cells are reported to produce TNF-$\alpha$, which, with monocyte-produced TNF-$\alpha$, may contribute to interstitial inflammation.[1313, 1314]

IL-1 and TNF are potent effectors of inflammatory injury.[1315, 1316] IL-1 is produced during glomerular inflammation including that produced by anti-GBM Ab, IC GN, and murine SLE.[3, 1123, 1317–1322] In addition to glomerular cell production, inflammatory cells, primarily monocyte-macrophages, can be major sources of IL-1 in immune glomerular injury.[1272, 1323–1325] IL-1$\alpha$ and IL-1$\beta$ can each bind to two different IL-1 receptors, and the IL-1 receptor antagonist is often expressed with IL-1 but can be differentially expressed.[1326] The IL-1 receptor antagonist can interfere with IL-1–regulated mesangial cytokine gene expression in vitro and is able to modulate anti-GBM Ab GN in vivo.[472, 1327] LPS can enhance development of murine lupus, and LPS, IL-1, and/or TNF can worsen anti-GBM Ab GN.[1328, 1329]

Administration of recombinant TNF-$\alpha$ or recombinant IL-1$\alpha$ accelerated renal disease in MRL-*lpr/lpr* lupus mice if begun at 4 months of age.[1330] In another study, recombinant TNF-$\alpha$ was reported to improve survival in the (NZB × NZW)F$_1$ lupus model.[1331] Passive immunization against TNF-$\alpha$ and IL-1$\beta$ protected against the augmentation of anti-GBM Ab GN produced by exposure to LPS.[1332] Anti-TNF Ab and the amidine-type protease inhibitor bis(5-amidino-2-benzimidazolyl)methane (BABIM) benefited accelerated autologous-phase anti-GBM Ab GN.[1333] IL-1$\beta$–converting enzyme processes the 33-kd inactive precursor of IL-1$\beta$ to the active 17-kd inflammatory cytokine and thus is another potential target for anti-inflammatory intervention.[1334, 1335]

IL-6, initially described as a B cell growth and differentiation factor, is induced by IL-1 or LPS in mesangial cells and in vivo.[1336] In addition to IL-6, MCP-1 and IL-8 are produced in human mesangial cells in response to IL-1$\beta$, TNF-$\alpha$, PDGF, and endotoxin. The IL-1–induced IL-8 and IL-6 expression is inhibited by the IL-1 receptor antagonist.[1337, 1338] INF is reported to induce IL-1 but not IL-6 expression in mesangial cells.[1339] IL-6 is also an autocrine growth factor for mesangial cells.[1340–1343] However, IL-1 and IL-6 are noted to inhibit mitogenesis in serum-stimulated mesangial cells probably via a PGE$_2$ mechanism.[1344–1346] Repeated oxidant stress enhances the mesangial proliferative response of IL-6.[1347] Leukemia inhibitory factor, a member of the pleiotropic factor group with Il-6, IL-1, and so forth, has been identified in mesangial cells.[1348] PDGF BB or AB enhanced prostanoid production in mesangial cells in response to IL-6.[1349] Vascular endothelial cells also express IL-6 in response to IL-1 and TNF-$\alpha$.[1350] Aggregated IgG as well as dimeric and polymeric IgA binds to mesangial cells and enhances the release of IL-6.[1351, 1352] IL-6 exacerbated GN in (NZB × NZW)F$_1$ lupus mice and anti–IL-6 Ab reduced development of anti–double-stranded DNA Ab, reduced proteinuria, and prolonged life in these mice.[1353, 1354] Ab to the IL-6 receptor preserved glomerular function in MRL-*lpr/lpr* mice.[1355] In contrast, IL-6 was reported to reduce IL-1$\beta$ and TNF expression and to have anti-inflammatory properties in anti-GBM Ab GN in rats.[1356] IL-6 distribution in diseased human kidneys correlated with the number of glomerular cells.[1357] Urinary IL-6 is increased in IgA nephropathy patients with more active disease.[1358, 1359] The contribution of IL-6 to glomerular cell proliferation and sclerosis is outlined in the next section.

IL-13 was cloned from renal cortical RNA after induction of anti-GBM Ab GN and the IL-13 was found to be increased for 48 hours in this model.[1360] Mesangial cells produce colony-stimulating factor-1 in response to IFN-$\gamma$.[1361] Mesangial cells in culture also secrete granulocyte-macrophage colony-stimulating factor.[1362]

In human GN, cytokine and growth factors were demonstrated with the findings related to the course, degree of inflammation, and progression.[60, 1363, 1364] That is, in extracapillary GN infiltrating and glomerular cells were positive for IL-1$\beta$, TNF-$\alpha$, IL-1, IFN-$\gamma$, PDGF, and TGF-$\beta$. In contrast, in mesangial IgA nephropathy IL-1$\beta$, TNF-$\alpha$, IFN-$\gamma$, and IL-2 were absent; however, the mesangial expansion expressed PDGF, PDGF-$\beta$ receptor, TGF-$\beta$, and

IL-6. These patterns are consistent with the findings outlined in this section and in the next on progression and sclerosis. The EGF receptor has been reported to be increased in IgA nephropathy.[1365]

Reviews have outlined cellular signaling by endothelin peptides,[1366] the interactions of NO and endothelin effects related to roles of endothelin in the kidney, and the roles of endothelin in glomerular injury.[1367–1370] Endothelin is produced and released by glomerular mesangial cells and is regulated in part by TNF and TGF-β.[1371–1373] Glomerular epithelial cells also produce endothelin-1.[1374, 1375] Endothelin, as shown by anti–endothelin-1 Ab or a selective A-type endothelin receptor antagonist, modulates the mitogenic effect of PDGF AB or BB.[1376] Endothelin peptides are mitogenic, with studies suggesting cross-talk between the G protein–coupled endothelin receptors and protein tyrosine kinase activity.[1377] Heparin inhibits endothelin-1 production in cultured rat mesangial cells stimulated with PDGF or arginine vasopressin.[1378] Endothelin-1 can increase mitogen-activated protein kinase p42 in rat mesangial cells via phosphorylation rather than by transcriptional or translational induction.[1379] Endothelin activates expression of the urokinase receptor on glomerular epithelial cells.[1380] Endothelin receptors are present on mesangial and epithelial cells and have been characterized.[1381, 1382] An endothelin subtype A receptor antagonist is suggested to protect against progression in experimental reduction of renal mass.[1383] Endothelin mRNA and receptors are increased in NZB/W mice.[1384]

AII also induces proliferation of mesangial cells, an effect inhibited by atrial natriuretic peptide (ANP).[1385] We have shown that the ANP A receptor present on glomerular epithelial cells and collecting duct cells is the major biologically active receptor.[1386] ANP inhibits endothelin-induced activation of mitogen-activated protein kinase in glomerular mesangial cells.[1387] ANP is suggested to increase permeability of the GBM to protein in GN.[1388, 1389] ANP and endothelin levels are reported to increase in the plasma of patients with acute poststreptococcal GN.[1390]

Immediate early gene expression (*FOS, MYC, JUN,* and/or *EGR1*) is seen in immune glomerular as well as tubule injury[1391] and in unilateral ureteral obstruction or unilateral nephrectomy as well as nephrotoxic and ischemic injury.[1392–1394] Immediate early gene induction in mesangial cells is inhibited by polyamine depletion.[1395]

The mesangial AII receptors provide a means for functional hemodynamic contraction of the cell that may vary with the culture conditions.[3] AII induces phosphoinositide metabolism in cultured mesangial cells via a G protein.[3] The arachidonic acid metabolites are important in effecting mesangial cell contractility.[3] Numerous attachments exist between mesangial cells and the GBM, with the points of contact particularly prominent at the mesangial angles.[1396] In addition, this physical arrangement of contractile elements within the mesangial cell suggests its contribution to controlling glomerular function.[1397] AII has been suggested to have an effect on mesangial localization of potentially phlogogenic macromolecules.[1398]

The precursor of EGF has been demonstrated in kidney by in situ hybridization and EGF and TGF-α are found in distal tubules and collecting ducts.[3, 1399] Mesangial cells have receptors for EGF and its infusion in vivo produces glomerular hemodynamic changes.[1400] The potent glomerular cell mitogen heparin-binding EGF (HB-EGF) is increased in glomerular epithelial cells by PAF via PAF receptors and in glomeruli in anti-GBM Ab GN.[1401] When infused into the renal parenchyma, heparin-binding EGF has an effect on glomerular hemodynamics similar to that found in anti-GBM Ab GN.[1402]

The glomerular epithelial cell contributes to the hydraulic and macromolecular permeability of the glomerular capillary wall.[1403, 1404] Glomerular epithelial cells have also become available through culture techniques, including transformed lines.[1216–1219, 1405–1408] The identity of the cells and differention as to parietal or visceral are needed to provide useful systems.[1219] The use of these cells has been referred to throughout the individual sections of this chapter when indicated.

Glomerular epithelial cells proliferate in response to EGF.[1409] TNF stimulates glomerular epithelial growth via an EGF effect and IL-1 is growth inhibitory.[1410] Eicosanoids enhance EGF receptor activation and proliferation in glomerular epithelial cells.[886] Glomerular epithelial cells are not affected by the cytolytic effects of TNF under conditions that produce such effects in mesangial cells.[1310] Glomerular cells proliferate in response to PDGF.[1411] IL-6 and IL-6 receptors are expressed on glomerular epithelial cells.[1412] Glomerular epithelial cells express ICAM-1 and VCAM-1.[455] Thrombin stimulates glomerular epithelial cell growth and decreases fibrinolytic activity.[1095] Plasminogen or plasmin receptors are found on human glomerular epithelial cells.[1120] u-PA is synthesized by human epithelial cells.[1114] Glomerular epithelial cells produce ECM.[1218] Proteoglycan synthesis by glomerular epithelial cells reveals heparan sulfate proteoglycan.[1413, 1414] TGF-β increases proteoglycan synthesis by glomerular epithelial cells.[1415, 1416] Heparin inhibits glomerular epithelial cell growth via an EGF mechanism.[1417] Glomerular epithelial cells secrete a gelatinase.[1418, 1419]

Control of epithelial cell growth is influenced by the surrounding ECM and action of integrins.[1420–1422] This activity is in part related to the EGF receptor tyrosine kinase.[1423] Glomerular epithelial cells in culture produce inhibitors and stimulators of mesangial cell growth.[1424] Approximately half of the inhibitory activity in the culture medium can be blocked with purified heparinase (the remaining portion is sensitive to trypsin).

Neutralization of the surface charge of cultured glomerular epithelial cells increases prostanoid synthesis.[1425] The glomerular epithelial effects of the aminonucleoside of puromycin have been suggested to be mediated by reactive oxygen metabolites.[788] Glomerular epithelial cells process ICs formed on their surface; rapid endocytosis occurs with slow and inefficient lysosomal processing and discharge of free Ab into the medium.[1426] The dipeptidylpeptidase IV expression on human epithelial cells is induced by IFN-γ.[1427] This enzyme is linked to the HN model in rats.

Glomerular endothelial cells play a central role in glomerular physiology and inflammation, and cultures of these cells are the most difficult to establish of the three main glomerular cell types.[1230–1241] The use of fractionation of endothelial cells by fluorescence-activated cell sorting, heparin-binding fibroblast growth factors (acidic and basic FGFs), and suppression of mesangial cell growth was successful.[1233] The cultured cells were characterized by expression of angiotensin-converting enzyme, factor VIII, and acetylated low-density lipoprotein uptake. A transformed rat endothelial line has been described.[1240] Glomerular endothelial cells have also been grown from human and baboon kidneys,[1428] and human immunodeficiency virus is reported to infect glomerular endothelial cells and a small percentage of mesangial cells but not epithelial cells.[1429]

Endothelial cells, located at the interface between the blood and the tissues, respond to cytokines and mechanical stress.[1430, 1431] Much of the information about the potential role of the glomerular endothelial cells in inflammation has been extrapolated from the vast number of studies done with vascular endothelial cells such as those from the umbilical vein.[431, 1241] The roles of the endothelium and its factors in infiltration of leukocytes and in the production of NO (endothelium-derived relaxing factor) and endothelin have already been addressed. In studies using glomerular endothelial cells, the adhesion molecule activation necessary for leukocyte attraction is similar to that in other endothelia.[431, 451, 1432] Glomerular endothelial cells have manganese SOD,[746] produce vascular endothelial growth factor,[236] and release prostaglandins in response to mesangial cell $PLA_2$.[819] Integrin receptors influence the growth of cultured endothelial cells,[1239] and the role of integrins is addressed further in the next section.[1433] The expression of proteoglycans by glomerular endothelial cells is regulated by TGF-β. Vascular endothelial cells in coculture with mesangial cells initially inhibited mesangial cell growth (days 0 to 3) and later stimulated growth (days 3 to 5).[1434] The role of the glomerular endothelium and its relationship to other glomerular cells have been reviewed.[1236]

Cultured glomerular endothelial cells take up and process insulin.[1238] Insulin-like growth factor-1 (IGF-1) affects renal function and utilizes eicosanoids.[1435] IGF-1 receptors can be identified on human glomerular endothelial cells.[1436] IGF-1 and EGF have been suggested as therapeutic growth factors in acute renal failure.[1437, 1438] Mesangial cells also have specific receptors for IGF-1, and IGF-1 is a progression factor in the cell cycle.[1439]

The use of cultured glomerular cells has rapidly expanded knowledge regarding the physiologic and pathophysiologic roles of the individual cells. The lessons learned from tissue culture, however, provide information about what can be expected from a particular cell in specific culture situations and must be used in that context when expanding the ideas generated in vitro to the in vivo situation. Some of the correlations and the inconsistencies in these extrapolations have been reviewed.[1246]

## Glomerular Cells, Growth Factors, and Sclerosis

The focus of this chapter is to review the immune events that initiate renal injury through the contribution of Abs, Ags, immune cells, and associated mediator systems. This focus puts most of the emphasis on the events at or near the onset of the lesion. The initial events are often followed

by glomerular cellular events that can lead to scarring and influence the long-term outcome of the disease process both in models and in humans.[3, 1440–1446] Continued immunologic stimuli, repeated episodes of injury, chronic mediator activation, glomerular epithelial and mesangial hyperplasia and/or dysfunction, altered responses to lipids, vascular and hypertensive changes, and glomerular hyperfiltration may contribute in interrelated ways to make the lesion become progressive.[1444, 1447–1449] Tubulointerstitial injury that may be associated with the glomerular lesions and proteinuria is also an important sequela leading to loss of renal function.[1450–1457] In SLE, interstitial lymphocytes, monocyte-macrophages, and immune deposits are suggested to be associated with more proliferative forms of injury.[1458] Osteopontin (uropontin), an acidic phosphorylated, secreted cell attachment glycoprotein, is up-regulated in the proximal and distal tubules in models of GN and may contribute to accumulation of monocyte-macrophages.[1459, 1460] Striking changes in ECM components occur in autoimmune tubulointerstitial injury.[1461] Oxidants may contribute to the tubule injury.[1462] The contribution of "secondary" and perhaps largely cellular immune responses needs to be assessed. Genetic[3] and other nonimmunologic events appear to play a role and are addressed in more detail in other chapters. Primary focal segmental glomerulosclerosis (FSGS) shares some of the same events associated with progression of inflammatory damage discussed herein.[1463]

The hallmark of the progressive glomerular damage is sclerosis and expansion of ECM. Numerous studies at the mRNA and protein levels have focused on the characteristics of increasing, decreasing, and remodeling of ECM components at different stages of injury in models and in patients.[1464–1478] In general, an increase in glomerular cell products including collagen types IV, V, and VI, laminin, fibronectin, tenascin, and heparan sulfate proteoglycan is noted, whereas the interstitial collagen types I and III are less often found and then more often in crescents. Distribution of the GBM-associated Goodpasture Ag also varies with the histologic change.[1473, 1479, 1480] Fibronectin increases in glomerular cells in response to macrophages in anti-GBM Ab GN.[1481] Embryonic fibronectin, as a result of alternative splicing that changes during development and in response to injury,[1482, 1483] may also appear during immune renal injury.[1484]

The stimulus for glomerular cell proliferation and excess ECM production by cytokines and growth factors has been outlined in previous sections and is the subject of review.[1252, 1485] Although cytokines (such as IL-1, IL-6, and TNF) and growth factors (PDGF, TGF-β, EGF, and bFGF) are involved in regulation of ECM, the interrelationship between the ECM and the glomerular cell is also important for growth and contractility.[1486–1488] Collagen production includes types I, III, IV, and V.[1489] IFN is reported to inhibit fibroblast collagen synthesis.[1490] Type IV collagen or laminin secreted by mesangial cells has an autocrine function in production of other ECM components.[1491] ECM modulates EGF receptor activities on glomerular epithelial cells, and EGF can modify ECM production by kidney epithelioid cells.[1423, 1492] The mesangial cell migratory or contractility responses are inhibited by heparan-like glycosaminoglycan ECM components.[1493, 1494] $PGE_2$ reduced mRNA levels for interstitial collagens but not for type IV collagen or fibronectin.[1495] Glutathione, which is involved in the cellular redox state and influences the activity of transcription factors, enhances transcription of collagen in mesangial cells.[1496]

A granulocyte inhibitory protein that regulates IL-6 was reported in chronic renal disease, and IL-8 increases transcription and expression of IL-6 and IL-8 in human mesangial cells.[1497] IL-6 overexpression is associated with the development of mesangial cell proliferation and glomerular sclerosis in mice transgenic for IL-6 as well as in patients.[1498, 1499]

The interaction of glomerular cells and ECM components may contribute to the ECM changes.[1486] The binding or adhesion of glomerular cells to the ECM of the glomerulus and GBM involves integrins,[1500] with the epithelial and mesangial cells contributing most of the GBM synthesis during adult life.[376, 1501, 1502] Human mesangial cells express $\alpha_1$-, $\alpha_2$-, $\alpha_3$-, $\alpha_5$-, and $\beta_1$-integrins, with the rat also expressing $\alpha_6\beta_1$.[1503, 1504] Mesangial cells use a number of integrins, including $\alpha_1\beta_1$ for binding on collagen and laminin, $\alpha_2\beta_1$ on collagen, $\alpha_5\beta_1$ on fibronectin, and $\alpha_v\beta_1$ on vitronectin, with $\alpha_3\beta_1$ at focal contacts on fibronectin, collagen, and laminin.[1505] Rat glomerular epithelial cells express $\alpha_2$-, $\alpha_3$-, and $\beta_1$-integrin.[1421, 1422] Rat glomerular epithelial cells express the $\alpha_2\beta_1$-integrin receptor very late antigen-2 after a few days in culture and use this receptor to attach to collagen.[1506] Better understanding of these cell-matrix interactions can be expected to provide targets for manipulation of altered responses.

Anti-Fx1A Ab is reported to recognize a $\beta_1$-integrin on glomerular epithelial cells and to inhibit adhesion and growth of these cells.[1507] Ab to glomerular lysates reacts with a $\beta_1$-integrin on rat glomerular epithelial cells and significantly inhibits epithelial cell adhesion and spreading on type I and type IV collagen.[1508] A $\beta_1$-integrin related to the fibronectin receptor is reported in normal and diseased glomeruli.[1509] Integrins on renal tubule cells are also being characterized with a focus on detachment during acute renal failure.[1510, 1511] Human umbilical endothelial cell attachment, spreading, and migration on collagen and vitronectin are mediated by $\alpha_2\beta_1$- and $\alpha_v\beta_3$-integrins.[1512]

Rats provide a useful model system because they exhibit an accelerated glomerular sclerosing process with age that varies somewhat among strains and is manifest as abnormal proteinuria of varying intensity among strains.[3, 1513] Fawn-hooded rats develop systemic hypertension, proteinuria, and glomerular sclerosis at a young age.[3, 1514–1516] The mouse FGS/Nga strain has also been suggested as a model of FSGS with immune deposits.[1517] The PVG/c strain is resistant to sclerosis even after unilateral nephrectomy; the Lewis and Milan hypertensive strains are also relatively resistant.[3]

An immunologic event in the age-related sclerosis of rat glomeruli is suggested based on the frequent findings of IgM and sometimes other Igs and C3 in the sclerotic mesangial lesions.[3] Elution studies, however, do not suggest any direct glomerular Ab reaction of the Ig.[3] The identification of the MAC components both early and late in the sclerosis of PHN[1466, 1518] suggests a possible etiologic role for this mediator of glomerular capillary wall dysfunc-

tion.[348, 357, 358] The mesangial overload mechanism has been suggested by the presence of mesangial IgM deposits with increased uptake of exogenous macromolecules in the mesangium and in areas of sclerosis in models of reduced renal mass and toxic glomerular cell injury.[3] Mesangial accumulation of lipids and increased mesangial uptake of the marker colloidal carbon correlated with sclerosis after aminonucleoside.[3] These findings suggest that altered mesangial function may lead to increased matrix production and eventually sclerosis.

The development of sclerosis is then related to a sequential evolution of the multiple inflammatory stimuli outlined in previous sections, including oxidant and cytokine release and subsequent activation of growth factors, which in turn leads to cell proliferation and overproduction of ECM. The excess ECM may not be successfully remodeled because of imbalances in the expression of proteinases and their inhibitors. A number of confounding influences have been noted that contribute to the rapidity of progression.

FSGS has been suggested to involve features or mechanisms common to the smooth muscle–like glomerular mesangial cells and vascular smooth muscle cells in atherosclerosis, with a role for lipids in each.[1519] Mesangial proliferation in the remnant kidney precedes glomerular sclerosis.[1520] In habu snake venom injury, mesangial cell migration precedes proliferation.[1521] A relationship has been reported between increased intraglomerular pressure, mesangial stretching, and ECM formation.[1522–1525] The production of ECM by glomerular and mesangial cells contributes to glomerular sclerosis, including induction of TGF-β.[1526–1532]

In extending the relationship between mesangial cells and smooth muscle cells, the growth of smooth muscle cells is inhibited in vivo and in vitro by anticoagulant and nonanticoagulant heparin.[3] Both forms of heparin have been reported to decrease habu snake venom–induced mesangial proliferation.[1533] Both heparins inhibited [³H]thymidine uptake and mesangial cell proliferation in culture.[1424] Other classes of glycosaminoglycans (hyaluronic acid, chondroitin sulfate, and dermatan sulfate) were ineffective. The inhibition varied with the heparin source.[1424] Previous studies had shown a beneficial effect of anticoagulant heparin on the hypertension, albuminuria, and glomerular damage with mesangial cell proliferation that is associated with five-sixths renal infarction.[3] In the latter model, heparin may reduce some of the glomerular hemodynamics (hyperfiltration) postulated to be responsible through its antihypertensive effects and inhibition of renal kallikrein, a serine protease that interacts with renal prostaglandins.[3] The effect on albuminuria may include restoration of negative charge to the filtration barrier by the polyanionic heparin molecule.[3] Decreasing mesangial proliferation with heparin after anti–Thy-1 Ab injury reduces glomerular sclerosis[1534, 1535]; heparin may also influence ECM synthesis.[1536]

TGF-β has multiple effects on the inflammatory and healing process and the anti–Thy-1 Ab model has also been used to demonstrate a role for TGF-β using anti–TGF-β Ab or the proteoglycan decorin, which binds and neutralizes TGF-β.[1537–1542] In anti-GBM Ab GN, TGF-β expression is suggested to be macrophage dependent.[1543] TGF-β receptors are present on mesangial cells and mesangial cell hypertrophy can be induced by chronic TGF-β exposure.[1544] AII stimulates mesangial cells to produce ECM via TGF-β expression.[1545] TGF-β inhibits mesangial cell growth in vitro.[1546] Sustained TGF-β1 activity is implicated in interstitial fibrosis that occurs after repeated administration of anti–Thy-1 Ab.[1547] Protein restriction reduces TGF-β in anti–Thy-1 Ab–induced mesangial cell injury and interstitial fibrosis in puromycin aminonucleoside injury.[1548, 1549] The study of TGF-β is complicated by the relative amounts of active and latent TGF-β that may be present.[1550, 1551] In Adriamycin nephropathy with glomerular and interstitial fibrosis it was found that although TGF-β mRNA was high, the amount of latent TGF-β increased progressively.[1552] An increase in TGF-β receptors was also found, correlating with an increase in fibronectin expression. The latent TGF-β–binding protein increased in parallel. Increased urinary TGF-β was reported in patients with focal glomerular sclerosis.[1553] TGF-β knockout mice, generated by gene targeting embryonic stem cells for subsequent chimera construction and selection of the trait, have a multifocal inflammatory disease caused by the abrogation of anti-inflammatory and immunosuppressive effects of TGF-β.[1554–1556] TGF-β is suspected to be responsible for the neutrophil phagocytosis defect seen in MRL/*lpr* lupus mice.[1557]

Glomerular proliferation and PDGF expression precede the development of glomerular sclerosis in the Thy-1 Ab model in which the mesangial cell changes phenotype, expressing α-smooth muscle actin and type I collagen, and anti-PDGF Ab can reduce these effects.[1520, 1558–1566] Cultured rat mesangial cells express α-smooth muscle actin not present normally in vivo.[1567] The roles of the PDGF homodimers or heterodimers in mesangial cells were examined and PDGF BB and AB were found to be most active.[1568] Both PDGF A chain and B chain can be induced in mesangial cells by PDGF BB homodimer.[1569] The PDGF mitogenic effect on mesangial cells is suggested to involve protein kinase C-α.[1570] The response of mesangial cells to PDGF varies with the culture situation, with the cells unresponsive in a gel-type "three-dimensional" culture.[1571]

A low-protein diet decreases the glomerular sclerosis, and TGF-β attenuates the increased gene expression of PDGF A and B chains.[1572] Glomerular PDGF B chain expression (as well as IL-1 expression) is increased in IC-mediated GN.[1573] The PDGF A chain is also increased in anti–GBM Ab GN.[1565] Both PDGF A and B chain mRNAs increase in lupus mice.[1574] The developmental aspects of PDGF and its receptors have been studied, and an autocrine function in development of the glomerulus has been suggested with a correlation with the appearance of α-smooth muscle actin.[1575] In humans and primates, the PDGF receptor binding the PDGF B chain was found on mesangial, parietal epithelial, and interstitial cells.[1576] The PDGF receptor and PDGF are up-regulated during glomerular inflammation.[1577] The antagonist effects of modified PDGF molecules that can bind PDGF receptors offer a possible beneficial manipulative avenue.[1578–1581] The extracellular glycoprotein SPARC, which binds PDGF AB and PDGF BB dimers, is up-regulated after injury and may serve as a regulatory activity.[1411, 1582] The mitogenic effects of PDGF were modulated in mesangial cell cultures by inflammatory cytokines and in turn modulated IL-1–induced expres-

sion.[1583, 1584] Thrombospondin, an ECM glycoprotein involved in mesangial cell adhesion and migration, induces EGF and PDGF secretion by mesangial cells, and its effects on mesangial cell growth are inhibited by anti-PDGF Ab.[1585]

Another growth factor that influences glomerular mesangial expansion is bFGF. Mesangial cells release bFGF, and a decrease in bFGF in glomeruli after anti–Thy-1 Ab–induced mesangial cell lysis suggests its release.[1586] During repair, glomeruli bFGF produced and bFGF administration increased the proliferation of glomerular cells. The response was less than that observed after PDGF infusion.[1587] FGF receptor expression and alternative splicing vary during development in the kidney.[1588]

Abnormal lipid metabolism can alter progression of renal damage via a number of interactions, including macrophage function, alteration of mesangial and vascular function, mediator alterations, and membrane changes.[1558, 1589] Low-density lipoproteins stimulate growth-related genes in mesangial cells,[1590] and lipids from mesangial cells are chemotactic for monocyte-macrophages.[1591] Glomerular monocyte-macrophages and foam cells (monocytes-macrophages containing lipids) are frequently found in focal glomerular sclerosis.[1592, 1593] A paracrine role for monocyte-macrophages on mesangial cells is suggested in aminonucleoside nephrosis–associated glomerular sclerosis,[1594] and monocyte-macrophage depletion reduces the sclerosis.[674] Hypercholesterolemia increases macrophages that produce TGF-β in the mesangial matrix expansion induced by aminonucleoside.[1595] Perhaps related to the lipid metabolic changes, thromboxane synthesis inhibition increases PGI$_2$ and decreases glomerular sclerosis in the remnant kidney.[1596]

A role for epithelial cells in some forms of injury leading to glomerular sclerosis is under study.[1597–1601] Glomerular epithelial cells normally contribute to the glomerular filtration barrier. Functionally, EGF[1602] and heparin-binding EGF can decrease GFR.[1402] EGF is also a growth factor for glomerular epithelial cells, and EGF receptors are identified on glomerular epithelial cells.[886, 1409, 1603] The growth of glomerular epithelial cells is inhibited by heparin, which alters the uptake and degradation of EGF.[1417, 1604] Glomerular and epithelial cell hypertrophy is thought to contribute to the generation of glomerular sclerosis as shown in the study of the remnant kidney or FSGS, particularly that associated with hypertension.[1597, 1598, 1605–1608] Glomerular epithelial cells produce ECM in response to TGF-β1 and proliferate and synthesize PDGF B chain.[1411, 1416]

A number of observations suggest that an inappropriate imbalance of proteinases and their inhibitors may contribute to the sclerotic lesions that follow glomerular injury.[1123, 1609, 1610] Cytokines and growth factors alter the production of proteases and protease inhibitors, which are important regulators of ECM remodeling and normal cellular proliferation.[1611, 1612] The proteases include the serine proteinases and the matrix metalloproteinases (MMPs). Proteinases such as elastase are also effective in degrading type IV basement membrane collagen.[1613] Of the former, plasmin is activated by plasminogen activators (u-PA, t-PA), which in turn are inhibited by PAI-1.[1614, 1615] Plasminogen can bind to the α1(IV) and α2(IV) chains of type IV collagen.[1616] PAI-1 serves to control fibrinolysis, and there appears to be an overlap between glomerular fibrin deposition associated with increased PAI-1 and glomerular sclerosis in experimental anti-GBM Ab–induced GN.[1123] The MMPs include type I collagenase (MMP-1) and 72-kd (MMP-2, gelatinase A) and 92-kd (MMP-9, gelatinase B) type IV collagenases, transin/stromelysin (MMP-3), transin-2 (MMP-10), and PUMP-1 (MMP-7). Neutrophils have a 72-kd collagenase (MMP-8) that is stored in granules until the neutrophil is stimulated to exocytosis; the activities of the MMPs are inhibited by a family of tissue inhibitors of metalloproteinase (TIMPs).[1617–1621] For example, human glomeruli with glomerular sclerosis express TIMP-1 and TIMP-2.[1622] Additional control is achieved because the MMPs are secreted as zymogens and are then activated by several mechanisms including proteolysis by plasmin and by other MMPs.[1623, 1624]

The serine proteinases, MMPs, and their inhibitors may interact in an autocrine or paracrine fashion within the glomerulus, because glomerular and kidney cells can synthesize some of them.[1610, 1622, 1625] Mesangial cells produce transin,[1626] types I[1627] and IV[1628] collagenase, TIMP,[1626, 1629, 1630] and PAI-1[1631]; glomerular epithelial cells produce u-PA[1632] and collagenases.[1418, 1419, 1628] The mesangial cell constitutive neutral proteinase is identified as MMP-2 and there is induced expression of MMP-9.[1633] In mesangial cells in culture, plasmin produced from plasminogen by mesangial cell plasminogen activators degrades ECM as well as activating a mesangial cell metalloproteinase.[1634] Activation of MMP-2 is linked to cytoskeletal reorganization.[1635] Type IV collagenase is also found in renal tubules.[1636] Transfection of mesangial cells with transin alters shape and growth characteristics.[1637] In addition, infiltrating monocytes can produce u-PA,[1638] transin, types I and IV collagenase,[1639] and TIMP,[1640] and neutrophils can produce type IV collagenase,[1641] resulting in complex interactions. The complexity of the interacting systems is increased by the capacity of mesangial cells and monocytes to produce TNF-α,[1210] IL-1,[1642] and IL-6.[1643] IL-1β and TNF-α can synergistically induce MMPs without affecting TIMP expression.[1644] By comparison, IL-6 selectively increases the expression of TIMP,[1645] which may contribute to the glomerular sclerosis seen in mice transgenic for IL-6.[1646] IL-1β and TNF-α inhibit u-PA and increase PAI-1,[1127] favoring ECM accumulation. Growth factors also contribute. TGF-β may favor ECM accumulation by decreasing expression of transin[1647] and type I collagenase[1648] and increasing that of PAI-1[1649] and TIMP.[1648] TGF-β1 does stimulate synthesis of a 72-kd type IV collagenase in glomerular mesangial cells.[1289] By comparison, the effects of bFGF and EGF are difficult to delineate because they increase the expression of u-PA, PAI-1, transin, type I collagenase, and TIMP.[1612, 1618] Heparin inhibits the induction of three MMPs without altering TIMP.[1650] The relationships in vivo may differ from those in the cell culture studies, and the temporal and/or spatial expression of the proteinases, their subsequent activation, and their inhibitors may determine the aggregate effect on ECM accumulation.

Hypertension is a common sequela of renal damage.[3] Hypertension can produce vascular changes and sclerosis, which appear to increase the rate of decline in renal function in patients related to age.[1651] Hypertension is also re-

ported to accelerate sclerosis in experimental GN.[1651–1654] AII-mediated hypertension increases expression of α-smooth muscle actin in mesangial cells and desmin in visceral glomerular epithelial cells.[1655] Rats transgenic for the mouse renin gene develop hypertension, proteinuria, and glomerular sclerosis.[1656] In our studies of anti-GBM Ab GN, the focal and mesangial sclerosis associated with hypertension appeared only to be additive to the more diffuse glomerular capillary wall change of the experimental GN lesion.[1657] Antihypertensive treatment, particularly angiotensin-converting enzyme (ACE) inhibition, can have a beneficial effect on progression of glomerular damage including sclerosis associated with severe reduction in renal mass.[1658–1661] When the glomeruli are protected from increased pressure by preglomerular vasoconstriction, as in the spontaneously hypertensive rat, the hypertensive effects on experimental GN are less evident or are prevented.[1662, 1663] Lowering systemic blood pressure and, in turn, normalizing glomerular capillary hydraulic pressure with ACE inhibition inhibit or lessen later development of glomerular sclerosis in aminonucleoside nephrosis.[1664, 1665] Comparison of ACE inhibitors with AII receptor antagonists shows the need for reduction in AII.[1666] Captopril is said to inhibit the 72- and 92-kd MMPs by interacting with the zinc ion at their active center.[1667] The structural and functional effects of ACE inhibition are separable; the effects on early proteinuria do not correlate with the late effects on glomerular sclerosis.[1668, 1669] $Ca^{2+}$ entry blockers inhibit compensatory kidney growth.[1670, 1671] The benefit appears to represent a combination of hemodynamic effects and potentially the participation of a variety of growth factors interacting with AII that can lead to overproduction of ECM.[1672, 1673] The mechanisms whereby ACE inhibition ameliorates glomerular sclerosis are then complex. The glomerular effects of AII are mediated via the AII AT-1 receptor.[1674–1676] Our studies show that anti–GBM Ab GN produces diffuse thickening or sclerosis of the GBM, suggesting a role for cells (endothelial, epithelial) closely associated with the GBM. When hypertension is added, a form of focal segmental or mesangial sclerosis is superimposed on the diffuse process, suggesting that the mesangial cell may be the major focus of excess ECM production. ACE inhibition prevents, to a degree, both forms of glomerular sclerosis but especially the form induced by hypertension.[1677] ACE inhibition independent of AII can cause prolongation of the half-life of bradykinin and the secondary increase in NO in tissue,[1678] which may be anti-inflammatory. Other reports suggest that AII may contribute to cell hypertrophy (including mesangial cells) and increased protein and ECM synthesis and PDGF production,[1679–1684] all factors involved in enhancement of glomerular sclerosis. Arginine vasopressin also alters ECM production, induces proliferation of mesangial cells, and can induce *EGR1* in a protein kinase C–dependent fashion.[1685]

There is significant interaction between NO and AII.[1686] Several laboratories have demonstrated that administration of $N^G$-monomethyl-L-arginine, a competitive inhibitor of NO synthase (NOS), produces glomerular hemodynamic changes strikingly similar to those observed after the infusion or endogenous generation of AII.[1687–1689] NO is among several factors including $PGI_2$ and endothelin produced by endothelium that contributes to the control of blood flow.[1690] Its production in vascular endothelial cells is stimulated by proinflammatory mediators such as TNF-α, an effect inhibited by IFN-γ.[1691, 1692]

Stimulation of AII may produce effects similar to those of reductions in NO generation. This antagonism may also hold for the process of glomerular sclerosis because studies by Zatz and Baylis and co-workers[1689, 1693] have suggested that inhibition of NOS via administration of $N^G$-monomethyl-L-arginine accelerates the process of glomerular ischemia or sclerosis in nonimmune renal models.[1694, 1695] Na$^+$ excess aggravates the hypertension as well as the interstitial expansion.[1696] In vitro studies have also suggested that inhibition of NO generation with $N^G$-monomethyl-L-arginine enhances the protein synthesis induced by AII in vascular smooth muscle.[1681] As noted before, hypertension can accelerate the development of glomerular sclerosis in immune models of renal disease, and there is evidence that in several hypertension models there is diminished generation of NO.[1697–1699] It is possible that hypertension may accelerate glomerular sclerosis by mechanisms that are independent of its glomerular hemodynamic effects via diminished generation of NO and the acceleration of glomerular sclerosis by the actions of AII. Supplementation with L-arginine, the precursor of NO, counteracts the glomerular hemodynamic effects of cyclosporine, which may contribute to its nephrotoxicity with sclerosis.[1700] Cyclosporine also inhibits IL-1β–induced NOS mRNA in mesangial cells.[1701] L-Arginine also prevents glomerular hyperfiltration and decreases proteinuria in diabetic rats.[1702] Cytokines, TGF-β, and PDGF may alter L-arginine as well.[1703]

The sclerosing process is greatly accelerated by ablation of renal mass and attendant changes in glomerular hemodynamics in the remaining nephrons.[1672, 1704–1709] Reduction in nephrons, whether by disease, age, or surgical removal, subjects the residual glomeruli to hypertrophy with increased perfusion and filtration.[1710, 1711] The contribution of hypertrophy has been reviewed.[1712] Sclerosis is rapid after severe reduction of the renal mass (one and five sixths) in rats. Epithelial cell protein reabsorption, detachment of epithelial and endothelial cells, mesangial expansion, and increased mesangial uptake of markers are found with increased production of mesangial matrix thought to lead to sclerosis.[1705, 1708, 1713] Studies suggest that the epithelial cell detachment and cell damage related to compensatory glomerular hypertrophy may be of focal importance in creating the sclerotic lesions.[1597] An early increase in glomerular leukocytes follows reduction of renal mass and the cells could contribute as in immune lesions.[1714] Heparin devoid of anticoagulant activity can abrogate the sclerotic process and also alters mesangial cell responses in other experimental models including Ab-induced mesangial cell injury complicated by sclerosis.[1534, 1715, 1716]

The suspected hemodynamic lesion can be altered by reducing protein intake or caloric intake,[1717–1721] which is successful for lesions in cats as well as in rats.[1722] Caloric restriction decreased autoantibody formation and sclerosis in NZB × NZW mice,[1723] and long-term benefit has been suggested in immune models.[1724] Of some interest, caloric restriction can modify a number of immunologic parameters including the onset of spontaneous murine lupus GN.[1725, 1726]

The similarity in mechanisms between glomerular sclerosis and atherosclerosis extends to lipids, and glomerular mesangial cells and macrophages can take up lipoproteins.[1558, 1727–1731] Hypercholesterolemia enhances glomerular macrophages containing lipids (foam cells) in anti-GBM Ab GN and enhances glomerular sclerosis as well.[1732] Low-density and very low density lipoproteins with evidence of oxidative modification by mesangial cells are noted in various glomerular injury models and in patients.[756, 1733–1737] Glomerular epithelial cells from nephrotic patients are also involved in low-density lipoprotein uptake via receptors.[1738] Apolipoproteins are recognized in glomerular epithelial cells and mesangial cells in nephritis.[1739] The protective effect of synthesis inhibitors such as hydroxymethylglutaryl coenzyme A may include nonsteroid products of hydroxymethylglutaryl-CoA reductase that modulate glomerular cellular function.[1740]

Renal function and pathology are being reexamined in humans after unilateral nephrectomy or unilateral agenesis.[3, 1741] A mild increase in protein excretion and sclerosis was found in biopsy specimens from four patients undergoing unilateral nephrectomy as with transplant donation.[3, 1742]

The use of transgenic mice in the study of kidney disease is growing, particularly in the area of glomerular sclerosis, because a number of transgenes have been associated with this lesion. Initial findings of glomerular sclerosis were made in mice transgenic for diverse molecules including growth hormone,[1743, 1744] the large simian virus 40 T Ag,[1745] IL-6,[1646] and transgenes that interrupt endogenous genes.[1746] Mice transgenic for bovine growth hormone have hypertrophic glomeruli and increased type I and type IV collagen, laminin, and heparan sulfate proteoglycan in their glomeruli.[1747] The effects of overexpression of native or mutated bovine growth factor with type IV collagen mRNA overproduction in these mice have been delineated.[1748–1751] IL-6 transgenic mice generated with the metallothionein-I gene promoter developed progressive renal damage; the initial membranous GN was followed by focal glomerular sclerosis and later extensive tubule damage and a myeloma-like kidney.[1752] Mice transgenic for copies of a defective human immunodeficiency virus provirus developed proteinuria and focal glomerular sclerosis with features similar to those of human immunodeficiency virus nephropathy in humans; the mice had increased laminin, type IV collagen, and heparan sulfate in their glomeruli along with human immunodeficiency virus protein.[1753, 1754] Mice of the MPV17 strain[1746] have been studied to identify the defective gene caused by the integration. An MPV17 human homologue has been identified that is a membrane-associated protein mapping to chromosome 2, and studies of its possible contribution to congenital nephrotic syndrome are under way.[1755] Studies have excluded the *PAX2* gene in this disease even though mice transgenic for this family of transcription factors active during embryonic development have histologic abnormalities and dysfunctional renal epithelium with properties similar to those of congenital nephrotic syndrome.[1756, 1757] Glomerular ultrafiltration coefficients are elevated in hypertensive rats transgenic for the mouse renin gene and the incidence of glomerular sclerosis is increased.[1656] Glomerular sclerosis is induced in mice transgenic for TGF-β or PDGF B chain, with the TGF-β affecting ECM accumulation and the PDGF affecting cell proliferation.[1758] Ectopic expression of Thy-1 in podocytes of transgenic mice resulted in severe proteinuria and sudden death in the founders; when the Thy-1 was expressed in the tubule epithelium, cystic dilatation and in situ tumors were found.[1759] Mice transgenic for the class II HLA-DRA gene had expression in the glomerular capillaries.[1760] The genes necessary to induce severe lupus nephritis are under study with transgenic mice.[1761] A line of mice with a recessive defect in lymphocyte or granulocyte function resulting from an insertional mutation developed granulocyte and mononuclear infiltrates in several organs and Ig deposits in the kidney.[1762] A number of lipoprotein transport genes have been added to the germline of mice by transgenic techniques or knocked out by homologous recombination in embryonic stem cells for use in the study of atherosclerosis and potentially in assessing lipid-related problems in glomerular sclerosis.[1763]

## NEPHRITOGENIC IMMUNE REACTIONS INVOLVING TISSUE-FIXED ANTIGENS

### Experimental Anti–Glomerular Basement Membrane Antibody–Induced Glomerulonephritis

In 1900, Lindemann demonstrated that injection of heterologous antikidney Ab caused rabbits to develop proteinuria and uremia.[1] The pathology of nephrotoxic nephritis was studied extensively in the 1930s by Masugi. Later, the GBM was shown to be the source of the nephritogenic Ags[1] and the major site of reactivity. The earlier terms "nephrotoxic nephritis" and "Masugi nephritis" have been superseded by the more precise term "anti-GBM GN." One would expect that as the biochemical and antigenic structure of the GBM and adjacent glomerular capillary wall becomes further defined the true complexity of heterologous anti-"GBM" Abs will be understood and the designation of the disease further refined. Abs reactive with Ags in or of the GBM bind to the glomerular capillary wall in a linear pattern conforming to the distribution of the GBM. This contrasts with the irregular, often granular reaction of Ig seen with Abs that react with discontinuously distributed Ags, including cell surface Ags (see next section).

### GLOMERULAR INJURY PRODUCED BY ANTI-GBM AB

#### Heterologous Phase of Anti-GBM Ab-Induced Injury

Renal damage induced by heterologous anti-GBM Abs is assessed by examining the acute (heterologous) and delayed (autologous) phases of injury. The heterologous phase (usually defined as abnormal proteinuria within the first 24 hours) occurs only when sufficient amounts of Ab are administered for the species under study. Intravenous administration results in maximal binding of Ab to the kidney.

Intramuscular and intraperitoneal routes are less effective, presumably because of local absorption by vascular structures.[1] By using paired label isotope techniques, it is possible to quantitate the amounts of Ab bound in the kidney and to relate this directly to the renal injury that is produced. Species vary in susceptibility: 75 μg of kidney-fixing Ab per gram of kidney is required to produce heterologous-phase injury in the rat,[1764] 5 μg/g is required in the sheep,[1765] and rabbits require 15 μg/g.[1766] It can be calculated that acute (heterologous-phase) proteinuria is induced in the rat when $1.2 \times 10^{10}$ molecules of Ab per glomerulus are fixed or one Ab molecule for every 26 μm$^2$ of glomerular capillary filtering surface area (about half the filtering surface would be covered by Ab molecules).[1764] Immunogold electron microscopic techniques can provide quantitation at the GBM level.[1767] The bulk of nephrotoxic Abs bind rapidly to the kidney after intravenous injection, with maximal binding observed at 1 hour; 63% to 79% is bound in a single pass.[1] Disease induction is enhanced by rate of Ab binding when similar amounts of Ab are delivered by bolus or prolonged infusion.[1768] Some basement membrane Ags appear to be unique to the GBM, and others are shared by other basement membranes. Krakower and Greenspon[1769, 1770] showed that the "nephritogenic Ag" content of an organ was related to its content of vascular tissue, so that after the kidney, the lung and placenta were the best sources of this Ag. Heterologous anti-GBM Abs react by direct immunofluorescence with most basement membranes in the kidney as well as in other visceral organs, including lung, liver, spleen, and choroid plexus. Species cross-reactivity is also apparent. There is considerable variation in the type and severity of GN induced by the Ab in different species. Ags are present for binding of heterologous anti-GBM Abs at birth in the rat, and clearance of bound Ab is prolonged.[1, 1771]

The GBM is composed of collagenous and noncollagenous proteins. Abs to interstitial collagen appear to have little or no nephrotoxicity, and absorption of anti-GBM serum with interstitial collagen does not diminish its nephrotoxicity.[1] Abs reactive with both collagenous and noncollagenous proteins develop in guinea pigs after immunization with heterologous renal basement membranes, although the anti-interstitial collagen Abs that react with the GBM are not associated with injury.[1] As the biochemical structure of the GBM has unfolded, attempts have been made to define the nephritogenic potential of some of its subunits. The renal distributions of type IV collagen, laminin, and entactin are being defined with changes in chemical structure and assembly suggested during development.[1772–1783] Administration of antiserum reactive with type IV collagen causes respiratory distress in mice and mild histologic changes in the lungs and glomeruli.[1784, 1785] The same authors found that antilaminin Abs were less nephritogenic. Quantitative binding studies[1785] suggest less tissue binding at low doses of antilaminin Abs compared with anti–type IV collagen Abs. The immunofluorescence of antilaminin Ab was linear, whereas the anti–type IV collagen Ab was noted to bind to the mesangium as well. Antilaminin Ab in large amounts can cause proteinuria in rats after 3 to 6 weeks without evidence of an autologous-phase injury.[1786] Type IV collagen and laminin have been used to induce delayed-type hypersensitivity in mice.[1787–1789] Of interest, antilaminin Abs have been found in subhuman primates infected with *Trypanosoma cruzi*.[1790] Abs reactive with type IV collagen and laminin are also noted in *Trypanosoma brucei* infection in rats.[1791] Heterologous antilaminin Ab has been used as a planted Ag to produce GN in a kidney transplanted to a host immunized against the heterologous Ig.[1792] Mild nephritogenicity of anti–heparan sulfate proteoglycan Ab has also been reported.[1793, 1794] The lesion varies among rat strains.[1795] Administration of anti–heparan sulfate proteoglycan Abs to rat presensitized to the heterologous Ab Ig produced a proliferative GN with electron-dense subepithelial deposits.[1796, 1797] A monoclonal anti–rat GBM heparan sulfate Ab is reported to induce proteinuria.[1798] It will become increasingly important to integrate information about the nature of previously reported nephritogenic GBM fractions[1, 1799] into the growing knowledge of GBM biochemistry. For example, we have found that collagenous extracts of GBM retain their nephritogenic potential; elastase extracts are also reported to be nephritogenic.[1800]

## Autologous Phase of Anti-GBM Ab–Induced Injury

The host's immune response to heterologous Ig bound to the GBM is the determining factor in the autologous phase of anti-GBM Ab–induced injury. Abs to the foreign Ig can be demonstrated in the circulation and bound to the kidney. Amounts of heterologous anti-GBM Ab easily visible by immunofluorescence (5 μg/g), when insufficient to induce acute (heterologous-phase) injury, can eventually result in damage when host Ig is deposited.[1801] The autologous phase can be induced passively by administering Ab to the foreign Ig. Autologous-phase injury can also be enhanced (rapidity of onset and severity) by preimmunization with the foreign Ig[1] or impaired by immunosuppression.[1802–1804] Studies of nude rats with impaired but not absent Ab response to the heterologous IgG showed little difference in severity of GN compared with their heterozygous littermates.[1805] Preformed complexes of anti-GBM Ab with Ab to the heterologous Ig are also acutely nephritogenic.[1] There is little evidence to support a role of autoantibodies in the autologous phase of injury. The freedom from anti-GBM Ab–induced injury in a kidney clamped during administration of an Ab in the maturing glomerulus of an animal injected as a newborn, or in a kidney transplanted into a nephritic host, is evidence against an induced autoimmune pathogenesis.[1806]

## Pathophysiology of Experimental Anti-GBM GN

The glomerular lesions induced by anti-GBM Abs vary depending on the species and, to a lesser extent, the age and sex of the recipient, the quantities and type of Ab used, and the intensity of the heterologous and autologous phases as well as the duration of the disease, as previously reviewed.[1] For example, crescentic GN is common in rabbits after anti-GBM Ab administration but is more difficult to induce in rats.[1807] As noted earlier, the Wistar-Kyoto rat is susceptible to induction of a crescentic GN with small doses of heterologous anti-GBM Ab.[1808] The lesion is characterized by an early mononuclear cell infiltrate, and the rat strain has increased activity of natural killer cells and antibody-dependent cell-mediated cytotoxicity. The lesion is modulated by depletion of CD8+ cells, which includes the natural killer cell population.[143] The lesion can also be modified by Abs against ICAM-1 and LFA-1.[475] ICAM expression in glomerular endothelial cells is increased after anti-GBM Ab in rats.[1809] The initial neutrophils expressed CD18 and the subsequent monocyte-macrophages had CD11a/CD18, suggesting that LFA-1 was the major counter-receptor.

Heterogeneous anti-GBM Ab injury is induced slowly in mice[1810] and occurs in spite of cyclophosphamide-associated alterations by the autologous phase.[1811] A crescentic model in mice is described.[1812] The lesion also develops in nude (*nu/nu*) mice deficient in T cells.[1813, 1814] Although induction of heterologous-phase anti-GBM Ab disease in the mouse has been difficult, success with heterologous Ab to homologous GBM or TBM has been suggested.[1815]

As noted in an earlier section on immune mediation, heterologous-phase anti-GBM Ab–induced injury is usually mediated by C fixation, followed by a transient influx of polymorphonuclear leukocytes (PMNs) within minutes after injecting sufficient PMN-dependent GBM Ab[1, 1816] (Fig. 29–4A). The PMN accumulation peaks during the first few hours, and monocytes have been noted when the PMNs are decreasing.[1] Interruption of the GBM, probably in part caused by lysosomal enzymes in PMNs, allows fragments of the GBM to enter the urine, particularly in the autologous phase.[1] Studies of beige mice with defective leukocyte neutral proteinases support the role of PMN enzymes.[1817] Gaps in the GBM may be responsible for hematuria.[1818] Injury (monitored by proteinuria) may occur with only C fixation or from Ab binding alone, with the latter effect most clearly demonstrated by studies of the isolated perfused kidney.[1819–1821] The predominant lesion is that of proliferative GN with variable degrees of crescent formation[1] (Fig. 29–4B to D), and rabbits are more susceptible than rats to the latter.[1807] The severity of involvement may vary slightly from glomerulus to glomerulus, possibly reflecting quantitative differences in the amounts of bound Ab caused by the unequal distribution of blood flow; however, overall all levels of the cortex are quite uniform.[1822]

By means of immunofluorescence, the heterologous (anti-GBM Ab) and later autologous (anti-Ig Ab) Igs are observed in a smooth, continuous linear pattern along the GBM (Fig. 29–5A). The initial smooth Ig deposits become increasingly distorted as the GBM becomes damaged, deformed, corrugated, and interrupted (Fig. 29–5B). Binding is usually restricted to the glomeruli, even with anti-GBM sera that have striking in vitro TBM reactivity; however, TBM fixation is occasionally seen (Fig. 29–5C), and interstitial injury may accompany the anti-GBM Ab–induced injury.[124, 1823] The Ig is usually accompanied by C, particularly during the autologous phase. Fibrin, if sought, is often prominent in areas of crescent formation.

By using electron microscopy, wispy material may be noted along the endothelial aspect of the GBM shortly after injection (as the endothelium separates), after which PMNs may further displace the endothelium to approximate them-

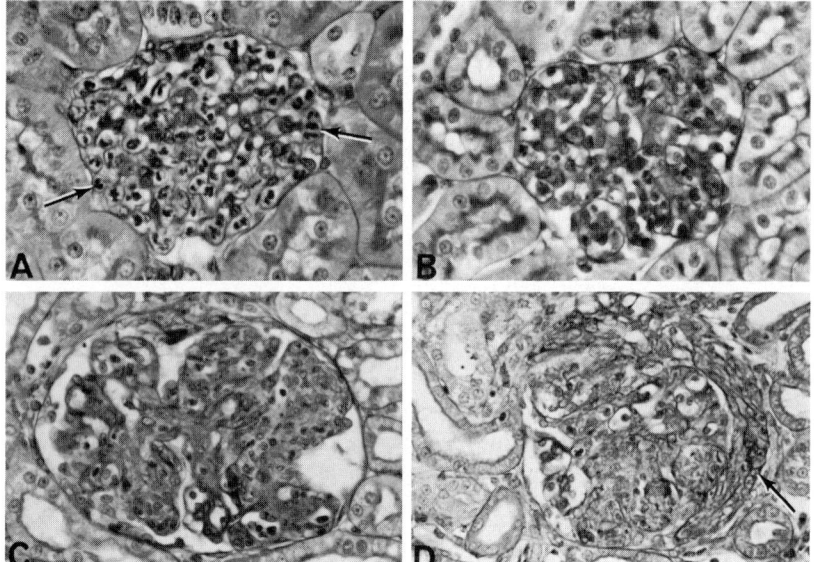

**Figure 29–4.** Histologic changes in rabbit kidneys after administration of horse antirabbit GBM Ab. *A.* Two hours after administration, numerous polymorphonuclear leukocytes *(arrows)* are evident in the glomerular capillary lumens. *B.* Proliferative changes are apparent within 2 days. *C.* The proliferation progresses and may be accompanied by crescent formation *(arrow)* as seen in *D.* (Original magnification × 215.)

selves on the Ab-coated GBM.[1] The GBM is more permeable to albumin in the areas of endothelial separation.[1] Electron-dense deposits have been observed in experimental anti-GBM glomerular injury, which, late in the disease, resemble accretions thought to be characteristic of IC deposits.[1] The composition of these deposits has not been defined, but they could represent Ag-Ab ICs from the circulation or aggregations of basement membrane Ag, nephrotoxic Ig, and autologous Ab to the nephrotoxic protein.

Electron microscopy studies have also been used to visualize binding of anti-GBM Ab to the GBM; however, the exact site of binding varies somewhat with the technique employed.[1] In vivo fixed anti-GBM Abs are found localized primarily at inner and outer aspects of the GBM.[1]

Micropuncture physiology studies after anti-GBM Ab administration have demonstrated an immediate decrease in

SNGFR secondary to a decrease in glomerular ultrafiltration coefficient ($K_f$) and an increase in hydraulic pressure gradient (which minimizes the effect of the reduced $K_f$ on SNGFR).[1824] The decreased $K_f$ is the result of decreased membrane hydraulic conductivity and/or membrane area caused by inflammatory cells and endothelial abnormalities. Leukocyte depletion minimizes the effect of anti-GBM Ab on $K_f$.[579] With some anti-GBM Abs, an associated C-dependent decrease in glomerular plasma flow is seen.[1] The acute effects of C5a infusions on glomerular functions have had preliminary evaluation.[321] C activation with cobra venom factor (CVF) is said to enhance proteinuria in anti-GBM GN.[1825] Some hemodynamic changes appear to be related to Ab binding alone, as shown by studies using the isolated perfused kidney.[1826] In later stages of the disease, glomerular filtration may be obtained owing to a compensating

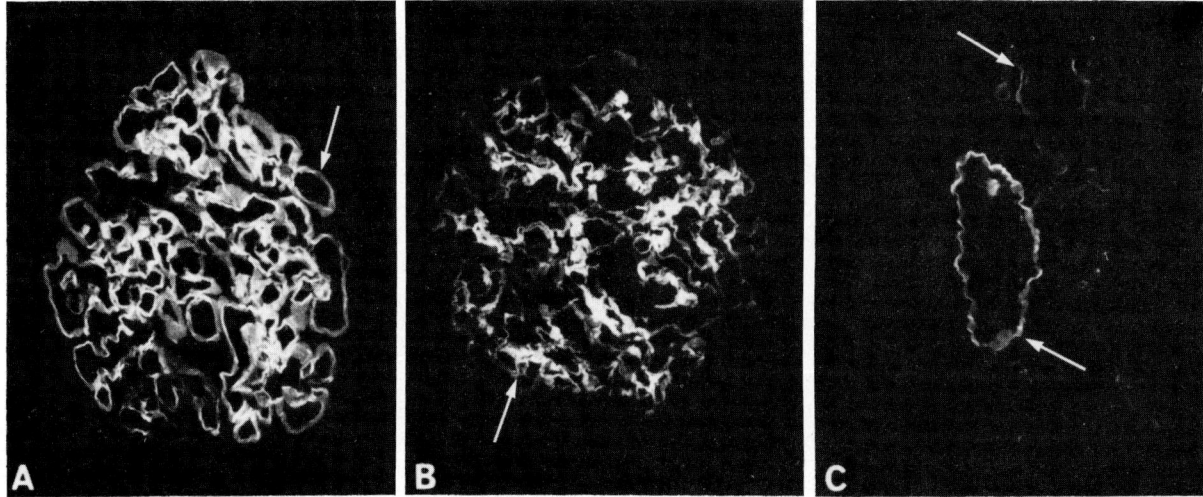

**Figure 29–5.** Immunofluorescence findings in experimental anti-GBM GN induced in rabbits with horse antirabbit GBM Ab. *A.* Smooth linear deposits *(arrow)* are present 1 hour after intravenous administration of the anti-GBM Ab. *B.* Three days later, sufficient GBM damage has occurred to make the deposition irregular *(arrow)* although still generally linear. *C.* Linear TBM deposits *(arrows)* are also present surrounding isolated renal tubules. (Fluorescein isothiocyanate–conjugated antihorse Ig; original magnification in *A* and *B* × 250, in *C* × 400.)

effect of increased transcapillary hydraulic pressure.[1] Glomeruli isolated from rats with anti-GBM nephritis have been shown to produce increased amounts of $TXA_2$ and $PGE_2$. The latter was suggested by inhibitors to help maintain SNGFR on day 14. Glomerular AII receptors are down-regulated within 16 hours of anti-GBM Ab.[1827] As the disease progresses, considerable heterogeneity of the SNGFR has been noted, and functional changes correlate with the degree of glomerular hypercellularity and overall architectural derangement.[1] Of interest, glomerulotubular balance is maintained despite markedly different filtration rates in single nephrons. Urinary protein loss also increases during a time when glomerular filtration of water and small molecules is decreasing. Phentolamine, an $\alpha$-receptor blocking agent, may lessen acute changes in glomerular hemodynamics, whereas Sar[1]-Ala[8]-AII, an AII receptor antagonist, enhances them.[1828] Histamine was found to have a major role.[1829] Long-term size-selective dysfunction of the glomerular filtration barrier is diminished with antihypertension treatment.[1830]

For the most part, injury induced by heterologous anti-GBM Abs is confined to the kidney, probably related to the quantitatively poor fixation in and more rapid disappearance of this Ab from other organs. Occasionally, pulmonary edema and hemorrhage have been noted after administration of nephrotoxic Ab.[1] Heterologous antilung Abs also produce lung lesions and can induce glomerular injury as well.[1, 1831, 1832] A model of lung involvement in augmented anti-GBM Ab disease in rats has been described with a transient influx of PMNs during the first 12 hours, followed immediately by Ed-1[+] macrophages and 3 days later by T cells.[123] A role for alterations in permeability of the alveolar capillary wall (produced by oxygen toxicity) in the ability of heterologous antilung basement membrane Abs to bind to the alveolar basement membrane (ABM) has been reported.[1833, 1834] In this situation, oxygen toxicity was associated with a rapidly repairable alteration in permeability to the heterologous Ab, and oxygen toxicity could be repeated to allow fixation of autologous Ab to the previously fixed heterologous IgG. Gasoline-induced pulmonary injury also allows pulmonary fixation of anti-GBM Ab containing antilung reactivity that does not normally bind to lung after in vivo administration,[1835] although another study trying to demonstrate this effect was unsuccessful.[1836] Cytokine infusion also can alter lung binding of anti-GBM Ab (see ahead).

## INDUCTION OF AUTOIMMUNE ANTI-GBM AB RESPONSES

In 1962, Steblay[1837] reported the induction of proliferative and crescentic GN in sheep injected with heterologous or homologous GBM in complete Freund adjuvant, but induction was not observed with autologous GBM.[1838] The lesion was characterized by linear deposits of Ig and C along the GBM and TBM revealed by immunofluorescence studies. Electron microscopic examination revealed increased electron density of the GBM with substantial breaks in its continuity.[1] Immunizations with GBM from humans, dogs, rabbits, or rats were effective, as was human lung.[1]

Circulating Abs that are both reactive and absorbable with the GBM can transfer the GN to normal sheep by cross-circulating plasma transfusions.[1] Even better, circulating Abs recovered from nephrectomized nephritic sheep transfer nephritis to unilaterally nephrectomized lambs.[1] The disease also recurs in renal allografts.[1839] Quantitative studies of sheep indicate that the autologous anti-GBM autoantibody is only 1/15 as nephrotoxic as heterologous anti-GBM Ab.[1] The reactivity of the renal-bound anti-GBM Ab from sheep immunized with human GBM was shown to be directed toward the same monomer subunit of the collagenase-resistant globular domain of type IV collagen, termed the NC1 domain, that is thought to be the major reactive site in human anti-GBM Ab disease.[1840]

Immunization with various basement membrane preparations produces anti-GBM and anti-TBM Ab–induced lesions in several species.[1841] Anti-GBM Abs and GN have been reported in chickens immunized with bovine GBM,[104] although this lesion is thought to have a major cellular immune component.[105] Although severe glomerular and tubulointerstitial lesions can be induced, severe lung hemorrhage, as seen in anti-GBM Ab–induced Goodpasture syndrome, has not yet been produced in this manner. For example, in sheep immunized with either human GBM or ABM Ags sufficient to produce severe GN, lung lesions do not develop and lung fixation of Ab is not demonstrated in vivo or in vitro, even though fixation to human lung in vitro is striking.[1840, 1842] Minimal pulmonary lesions were reported in rabbits immunized with choroid plexus.[1] Feeding the proline analogue 2,3-dehydroproline was reported to alter GBM structure and induce antibody reactive with altered but not with normal GBM.[1843] Immunization of mice with the NC1 of type IV collagen from the murine Engelbreth-Holm-Swarm tumor induced Abs that bound to the GBM and ABM with some evidence of histologic changes in both organs.[1844] Immunization of rats with cells of this tumor induce an HN-like disease (see next section).[1845] Mice immunized with laminin from the tumor developed dense deposits in subendothelial positions along the GBM and mouse IgG along the GBM without detected circulating Ab.[1846] In another study, mice repeatedly given human GBM developed subepithelial extensions composed of laminin but not type IV collagen, raising the question of overproduction of laminin by the epithelial cells.[1847] A mild nonproteinuric glomerular lesion has been induced in rats by immunization with heparan sulfate.[1848] Abs against GBM, TBM, and ABM have been induced in rats by immunization with homologous renal basement membrane Ags.[1849, 1850] Immunization of rats with trypsin-solubilized and additionally purified bovine GBM induced Abs reactive with the GBM, GN, and some pulmonary hemorrhage, but no detected ABM fixation of Ab.[1851–1854] The bovine Ag is suggested to be similar to the human $\alpha3(IV)$ NC1 Ag responsible for human anti-GBM disease.[1855] The lesion is transferable with Ab recovered from the urine of affected rats,[1856] or with isologous monoclonal Ab from hybridomas derived from immunized rat spleen cells.[1857] Cyclosporine can modulate the induction of autoimmune anti-GBM Ab GN in rats.[1850] This model in the Wistar-Kyoto rat has been used to demonstrate the protective effects of Abs reactive with ICAM-1 and LFA-1 as well as the possible role of hyaluronate in glomerular crescent formation.[476, 1858] The Ag recovered from bovine GBM, as well as the rat strain, is important in the successful injection of this lesion with acid-treated, collagenase-digested GBM in the Wistar-Kyoto rat.[109] In this study, delayed-type hypersensitivity was present, and the T cells were induced to incorporate thymidine in response to the acid-treated Ag. In an interesting variation of this model, homologous GBM from rats with Masugi nephritis, but not from normal rats, was successful in inducing disease.[1859] The bovine homologue of the human GBM antigen, the α3(IV) NC1 dimer, has been used to induce Abs in rabbits that bound to the GBM and ABM and were associated with evidence of inflammatory cells in glomeruli and of pulmonary hemorrhage.[1860]

It has been observed that urine of normal subjects contains Ags that are cross-reactive with the GBM and capable of inducing anti-GBM GN when reintroduced into rabbits.[1] The importance of the anti-GBM Ab in this model can be shown by transfer of GN by injecting eluted Ab fractions. The urinary GBM Ags, which change qualitatively and quantitatively in association with nephrotoxic glomerular injury, can also be detected in the circulation of nephrectomized animals, suggesting that these Ags are part of basement membrane breakdown throughout the body and are normally excreted into the urine.[1] The relative contribution of catabolism of the GBM per se versus nonrenal basement membrane to the total urinary basement membrane Ag is unknown.

Polyclonal B cell activation in response to renal toxins such as mercuric chloride or associated with exposure to endotoxin or graft-versus-host reactions can lead to induction of autoantibodies including anti-GBM Ab reactions.[1861–1863] Anti-GBM Abs as well as other autoantibodies including anti-DNA Abs have been induced transiently in brown Norway (BN) rats by mercuric chloride administration or exposure to mercury vapor.[1, 1864–1873] The MAXX rat may also be susceptible[1874] and the DZB strain has anti-GBM reactivity with the glomerular histologic lesion resembling membranous glomerulopathy.[1875]

The immune response to basement membrane components includes laminin, noncollagenase elements of type IV collagen, and fibronectin.[1876, 1877] These Abs could be detected in our radioimmunoassay for human anti-GBM Abs and have been noted by others to cross-react with human GBM.[1878]

The anti-GBM Abs are part of a polyclonal Ab response that includes anti-DNA Ab and elevated IgE levels.[1879–1882] The ability to respond was transferable with immunocompetent cells from susceptible F₁ hybrids to their nonsusceptible parent.[1883] Monoclonal Abs derived from spleen cells from mercuric chloride–treated BN rats can transfer enough disease to produce mild proteinuria in naive BN rats.[1884] The mercuric chloride appears to induce autoreactive T cells related to MHC.[1885–1887] In some studies of polyclonal B cell activation in mice, the *H-2s* haplotype encodes susceptibility and the *H-2d* resistance and in others no relationship is found.[1888, 1889] The disease can be suppressed with cyclosporine[1890–1893] or administration of polyspecific human Ig.[1894] Suppressor T cells and auto-anti-idiotypic Abs are suggested to play a role in control of this autoimmune response.[1895–1899] IL-2 production is decreased in vivo by mercuric chloride and, of interest, the compound impairs

development of active HN in Lewis rats.[1900, 1901] Susceptible strains of mice also develop a glomerular lesion after mercuric chloride, with immune deposits present in the mesangium.[1902, 1903] The mercuric chloride–induced alterations in the immune response can be modulated by PGs of the E series.[1904, 1905] Other toxins, sodium aurothiopropanol sulfonate, or D-penicillamine can induce anti-GBM Abs that share idiotypes with those induced by graft-versus-host disease.[1906, 1907] Cadmium toxicity can cause GN and B cell proliferation in rats.[1908]

Mercuric chloride also induces a granular form of immune deposit GN somewhat after the decline of anti-GBM reactivity.[1909] Abs eluted from the kidneys of mercuric chloride–treated rats react with laminin and type VI collagen synthesized by cultured rat glomerular visceral epithelial cells, which may help explain the formation of the granular immune deposits.[1910] A disseminated intravascular coagulopathy may also occur in some mercuric chloride–treated rats.[1911] Rabbits given mercuric chloride develop Abs reactive with the GBM as well as with an extracellular collagen matrix. The Abs are not nephritogenic; however, the rabbits eventually develop apparent IC glomerular injury postulated to involve soluble collagen polysaccharides.[1912]

Graft-versus-host disease using transfer of DBA/2 donor lymphocytes into (C57BL/10 × DBA/2)F₁ hybrids induces Abs to nuclear Ags and to GBM components including laminin as well as to glomerular dipeptidyl peptidase IV.[1913, 1914] Graft-versus-host disease in BALB/c mice given (A/J × BALB/c)F₁ hybrid spleen cells at birth also develop anti-GBM Abs as well as antitubule epithelial antibodies as part of their polyclonal B cell activation.[1915]

Spontaneous development of anti-GBM Abs is not frequently recognized in animals. Three horses were found to have linear deposits of Ig along the GBM.[1] Eluates from the isolated glomeruli of one of these horses contained Abs reactive with GBM. We have detected anti-GBM and anti-GBM Abs in 9- to 12-month-old mice of several strains, and although these Abs were elutable, their exact role in producing injury is not clear.[1]

## Experimental Nephritogenic Antibody Responses Involving Other Antigens in or of the Glomerulus

Nephritogenic immune responses to endogenous or exogenous non–basement membrane renal Ags have been identified in a variety of animal models of renal disease. These Ags may be normal constituents of the glomerulus, such as glomerular cell surface Ags (distinct from classic GBM Ags). Model systems involving cell surface Ags have now been described for each of the major glomerular cell types and may involve cytolytic cell injury or cross-linking and shedding of surface Ag to form immune deposits.[6, 19, 1916–1918] Other renal cell surface Ags are known to be involved in tubulointerstitial nephritis (TIN) (see Chapter 33). Alternatively, foreign Ags may become trapped or planted in glomeruli for subsequent interaction with Ab.[2, 3, 1841, 1919–1921] The classic example of a planted Ag would be the heterologous anti-GBM Ab Ig bound in the glomerulus

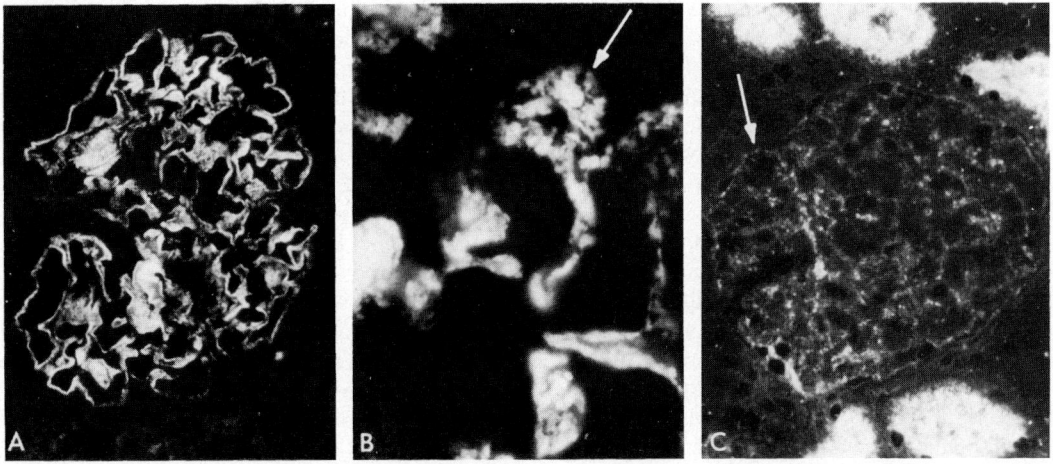

**Figure 29–6.** Immunopathologic findings in HN. *A.* Striking finely granular irregular deposits of IgG are present in the GBM of a rat several months after immunization with Fx1A. *B.* On high-power examination, the IgG deposit appears in a geographic irregular distribution along the GBM. *C.* Concentrated IgG eluted from kidneys of rats with HN is seen binding intensely to the brush border of proximal renal tubules and in a finely granular irregular pattern *(arrow)* along the GBM. (Fluorescein isothiocyanate–labeled antirat IgG; original magnification in *A* and *C* × 250, in *B* × 640.)

that serves as an Ag in the autologous phase of anti-GBM Ab–induced GN (described in the preceding section). Any Ag that can selectively bind to the glomerulus for any of a number of physicochemical reasons becomes a candidate for subsequent Ab binding. Because these Ags reach the kidney through the circulation, an overlap with the IC mechanism of glomerular immune deposit formation is inevitable.

## NEPHRITOGENIC AB REACTIONS WITH GLOMERULAR CELL AGS

### Epithelial Cell Ags

The glomerular epithelial cells' foot processes are involved in multiple ways in glomerular disease.[1922] HN, in its active (AHN) and passive (PHN) forms[1923, 1924] in rats, is an extensively studied model of immune glomerular injury that is now thought to exemplify anti–glomerular epithelial cell Ab–induced injury. The HN model has immunofluorescence and electron microscopic features of human membranous GN as well as lipid abnormalities associated with nephrotic syndrome including defective lipolysis.[1925, 1926] Selective transcriptional augmentation of hepatic albumin and fibrinogen gene expression has also been demonstrated.[1927] The Ab response needed for either form of HN is typically induced with Fx1A in complete Freund adjuvant. The Fx1A is an ultracentrifugation-derived sediment of the "soluble" supernatant remaining after low-speed centrifugation of rat cortex that has been pressed through a stainless steel screen[1928]; the glomerular and tubule fragments are removed by the initial low-speed centrifugation. Other preparations of homologous or heterologous renal tubule elements can also induce nephritogenic antisera.[1929–1931] Immunization of rabbits with Freund adjuvant alone is reported to induce Abs capable of producing glomerular immune deposits typical of those seen in PHN.[1932] It should be remembered that the heterologous Abs induced by immunization with the crude Fx1A Ags are complex, containing Abs to such

diverse sites as the glomerular endothelium, GBM components, and T cells.[1933–1935] The latter reactivity is said to be involved in glomerular binding of the Ab using absorption studies.[1936] Rat strain variation in susceptibility to induction of AHN is reported to be related in part to T cell regulation of the autoimmune response.[1937]

In studies beginning in 1967, Edgington and associates[1938, 1939] demonstrated that a subfraction of Fx1A termed RTE-α-5 could induce AHN and that as little as 3 μg of the material was sufficient to produce disease. Reactive Ag was not then demonstrated in the glomerulus, and the disease mechanism was thought to involve ICs, with renal tubule Ags responsible for the IC formation. Circulating ICs have been reported in HN,[1940] although similar evaluations in our laboratory and by others have been negative.[1941–1943] A 60/65 kd tubule antigen present in circulating IC in one study was reported to induce AHN.[1944] The difference may be related in part to the diversity of Ab responses generated by different Fx1A preparations. Binding of injected Fx1A Ag to glomeruli has been reported,[1945] and increases or decreases in the mononuclear phagocyte system function had an inverse relationship with the formation of glomerular Ig deposits in AHN.[1946]

It now appears that HN is caused by direct binding of Ab to Ag normally present in the glomerulus and now known to be present on the epithelial cell podocyte. In the PHN model, direct glomerular binding was shown by in vivo or in vitro perfusion experiments using heterologous anti-Fx1A Ab.[1947, 1948] The Ab localized at subepithelial sites where the reactive Ag is now known to reside. Heterologous RTE-α-5 Abs from the original study[1938] were shown to react weakly with irregularly distributed glomerular capillary wall Ags by improved indirect immunofluorescence studies.[1943] We were able to show that concentrated glomerular eluates from a large number of rats with AHN reacted with the glomerular capillary wall in vitro but in lower dilutions than Abs in the eluate that were reactive with the proximal renal tubule brush border[1943] (Fig. 29–6). The reaction was with Ags distributed in punctate foci at the junction of the epithelial cell foot processes and the GBM.[1943, 1949] Infusion of the AHN eluates into isolated perfused kidneys demonstrated binding[1950] that could be competitively inhibited with heterologous anti-Fx1A Abs.[1951] The perfusion model has been reported to enhance binding.[1952] In vivo binding of cationic, compared with anionic, fractions of the Ig eluted from AHN kidneys was favored.[1953] The demonstrated direct glomerular binding found in both AHN and PHN suggested strongly that Abs reactive with the glomerular capillary wall were responsible for the lesion, leaving any additional contribution of ICs open to question.

The rather slow glomerular uptake of the passively administered anti-Fx1A Ab has been quantitated, with 12 μg bound in glomeruli at 4 hours and 48 μg bound at 5 days after 10 mg of immune IgG was administered.[1954] Binding of 38 μg on day 3 increased to 52 μg per $7.7 \times 10^4$ glomeruli at onset of proteinuria on day 5 and correlated with increasing electron-dense subepithelial deposits and effacement of the foot processes.[1955] Previous studies of PHN demonstrated that glomerular deposits of Ig were reduced by aminonucleoside of puromycin or anti-GBM Ab injury[1956, 1957] but not after Adriamycin administration, which also diminished the polyanion detected by colloidal iron stain.[1958] Glomerular sialic acid remains unchanged in AHN.[1959] Aminonucleoside also alters glomerular accumulation of Ig deposits in AHN.[1960, 1961] These findings are probably related to changes in the reactive glomerular Ags that are rendered undetectable in sections from aminonucleoside-treated kidneys studied by indirect immunofluorescence using eluates from kidneys with AHN.[1943] The reactive glomerular Ag is present for reaction as blood flow into developing glomeruli allows in pre- and postnatal rats.[1962] The glomerular binding of Ab in PHN has a sequential localization.[1963]

As with heterologous anti-GBM Ab GN, PHN has an autologous phase of injury.[1964] Passive transfer of homologous or isologous anti-Fx1A Ab is reported to induce circulating IC and glomerular Fx1A Ag accumulation, with later appearance of autologous antiglomerular Ab, leading the authors to suggest that both the IC and direct binding mechanisms may play a role.[1965] The appearance of autoantibody to tubule Ag after passive Ab administration has been suggested in other studies.[1966–1968] Anti-idiotypic Abs are also suggested to contribute to the glomerular deposit in AHN.[1969] Monoclonal Abs reactive with brush border Ags have been recovered from hybridomas produced from rats with AHN[1970] and used to study idiotype reactivity.[1971]

In addition to RTE-α-5, other solubilized fractions of renal tubules have been shown to induce AHN.[1929, 1972] A glycoprotein of 330 kd from the brush border area can induce an AHN-like lesion,[1973] and Abs to this Ag are reactive with coated pits on the glomerular epithelial cell surface.[1974] The gp330 Ag is reported to be present in the microvilli of rat embryonic visceral yolk sac.[1977] Another 280-kd protein found in the intermicrovillar domain of the renal tubule brush border and yolk sac is a teratogenic Ag when reacted with monoclonal Abs.[1978, 1979] The 280-kd protein present in coated pits of the brush border of the proximal tubule has similarities to gp330 on a peptide and limited immunologic cross-reactivity basis but has asyn-

chronous expression during ontogenesis.[1980, 1981] Studies using monoclonal Abs, heterologous anti–RTE-α-5 Abs, and eluted Abs from AHN kidneys confirm the importance of gp330 as a reactive Ag in HN.[1982–1986] An Ag of apparent molecular mass 400 kd that is cross-reactive with rat gp330 is present in human kidney proximal tubules but is absent from glomeruli, and the 440-kd molecule was not detected in 30 biopsy specimens of membranous GN.[1987] HN in rats is said to be induced with human gp440.[1988] An Ag reactive with Abs from rats with HN has been reported in human kidney.[1989] Impairment of glomerular epithelial cell endocytosis in HN has been suggested as a factor in deposit accumulations.[1990, 1991] Comparisons of Fx1A and gp330 in terms of AHN induction have shown that Fx1A induces a more severe form of AHN and induces Abs to gp330 as well as another glomerular Ag of 94 kd.[1992] Monoclonal Abs derived from mice immunized with Fx1A or whole glomeruli react with gp330 and a 110-kd Ag present in normal glomeruli and in the deposits of AHN, the latter only equivocally.[1993] Monoclonal Abs have been developed that react with gp330 and gp90, the latter being a tubule and glomerular Ag with a diffuse glomerular distribution on epithelial and endothelial cells as well as other organ sites,[1994–1996] and immune deposits formed by it after in vivo administration are transient.[1997] When in vivo comparisons are made in rats and mice, coarse irregular glomerular binding in rats was related to gp330 and in mice to gp90.[1998, 1999] Monoclonal Abs indicate that the gp90 is also found on the surface of T and B cells.[2000] Other Ags have been reported, including gp600.[2001–2004] A related 70-kd Ag is localized at the endothelium-GBM interface and is reported in normal rat serum.[2005–2007] Still others, such as Ags gp108 (similar to the 90-kd Ag dipeptidyl peptidase IV), are reported to induce PHN.[2008] The F344 rat, which is deficient in the 90-kd Ag, is susceptible to induction of PHN with rabbit anti–F344 Fx1A Abs.[2009] A 460 kd molecule reactive with anti-gp330 that is present in the dog is resistant to an HN-like lesion.[2010] Abs raised to cultured glomerular epithelial cells react with gp330 and other brush border Ags and can induce immune deposit formation on systemic administration.[2011]

Advances in determining the nature of the Ags involved have included the isolation of complementary DNA for gp330 by screening a rat kidney λgt11 expression library with a polyclonal rabbit antirat gp300 antiserum.[2012] The deduced amino acid sequence predicted a large extracellular domain, a 29–amino acid transmembrane sequence, and a 188–amino acid cytoplasmic region at the COOH terminus. Homology with the human low-density lipoprotein receptor (also called the $\alpha_2$-macroglobulin receptor) suggested that gp330 was in the same receptor family. The presence of gp330 in coated pits would be consistent with a receptor function. Subsequently, a similar library was screened with anti-gp330 antibody eluted from the kidneys of rats with PHN that recovered a complementary DNA thought to code for the COOH-terminal 319 amino acids of gp330.[2013] Antibodies raised to the fusion protein from the complementary DNA were reported to produce immune deposits after injection in normal rats, and the protein could be used to induce subepithelial deposits thought to be similar to those of AHN. This clone, called C14, was subsequently shown to be a separate protein of 39 to 44 kd that complexes to gp330 and has 73% sequence homology with the human $\alpha_2$-macroglobulin receptor–associated protein as well as homology with the mouse heparin-binding protein termed HBP-44.[2014] The 39-kd receptor–associated protein binds to both $\alpha_2$-macroglobulin and gp330 and appears to inhibit ligand binding.[2015, 2016] The 44-kd C14 protein was found to form heterodimeric associations with gp330, and the complex was reactive with Abs eluted from rats with HN and those made to C14.[2017] The authors suggested the possibility of multiple pathogenic epitopes, cross-reactive epitopes, or pathogenic and nonpathogenic epitopes to explain why the 44-kd protein was apparently not antigenic when associated with $\alpha_2$-macroglobulin receptor. The 44-kd component of complex (now referred to by the authors as the HN antigenic complex) was truncated, and an 86–amino acid fusion protein was shown to induce smaller immune deposits than those induced with poly-epitope–specific anti-gp330 Abs, suggesting the role of additional epitopes in disease generation.[2018] A similar 45-kd protein was reported by others.[2019]

The biosynthesis of the gp330–44-kd antigenic complex takes place in the endoplasmic reticulum,[2020] and a rat yolk sac cell line is reported to be a useful experimental source.[2021, 2022] The $Ca^{2+}$-binding receptor function of gp330 is under study with binding of plasminogen, plasminogen activator-inhibitor complexes, lipoprotein lipase, and other ligands.[2023–2028] The affinity of gp330 for fibronectin, laminin, and type I collagen has been reported.[2029] Anti-Fx1A Abs recognize a $\beta_1$-integrin on glomerular epithelial cells and in turn inhibit adhesion of the cells.[1507] Two forms of gp330 (extracellular, cytoplasmic) with somewhat different distributions in the apical region of the proximal tubule are identified with Abs to the extracellular epitopes reactive with HN deposits.[2030] A particular fragment-specific subset of Abs to gp330 is believed to be involved in proteinuric glomerular damage in AHN.[2031]

The relative roles of the receptor-associated protein and gp330 in HN remain unsettled, and studies suggest that in vivo the two proteins may not be colocalized.[1292] That is, studies using fixation to immobilize the two proteins show that the $\alpha_2$-macroglobulin receptor–associated protein was confined to the rough endoplasmic reticulum. In contrast to the studies of fixed tissue when frozen sections were used, the receptor-associated protein was able to move from the cytoplasm and combine with the cell surface gp330. Exogenous receptor-associated protein was also shown to bind to the cell surface gp330.

The mechanism by which anti-Fx1A or anti-gp330 Abs induce HN now appears to be via a reaction of these Abs with Ags present on the epithelial cell surfaces in the area of the foot processes. The reaction leads to cross-linking of the Ag sites, leading to shedding of the resultant Ag-Ab complex as an immune deposit adjacent to the subepithelial aspect of the GBM.[2032–2036] The cross-linking converts the reactive Ag from a detergent-soluble, membrane-associated form to an insoluble form bound to the cytoskeleton mediated by microfilaments.[2037] Studies have demonstrated rapid binding of anti-gp330 Ab to the coated pits on epithelial cell foot processes, with larger electron-dense deposits often located under the slit diaphragms after 1 day.[2038] These deposits coisolate with the GBM, and serial section-

ing indicates that the deposits maintain contact with the coated pits as well. Studies of human and monkey kidneys indicate the potential for redistribution of glomerular Ags in these species as well as in the rat.[2039]

Epithelial cell loss is not a prominent feature of HN, although there is a correlation between the degree of epithelial cell podocyte effacement and the onset of proteinuria between days 3 and 5 after administration of heterologous anti-Fx1A Ab.[1955] Anti-Fx1A Ab can induce C-dependent and MAC-related lysis of cultured epithelial cells,[359] so the possibility of altered epithelial cell function or even death must be considered in evaluating the possible pathophysiologic consequences of this type of Ab reaction. The induction of proteinuria in the PHN model is C dependent and requires the MAC (see earlier C mediator section).[348, 357, 358, 2040] A study suggests that an Ab reactive with a glycolipid Ag(s) is present in the anti-Fx1A in addition to anti-gp330 Ab and that the former rather than the latter is responsible for C activation.[2041] C depletion with CVF does not prevent all effects of passive anti-Fx1A Ab, as monitored by glomerular micropuncture studies,[414] and additional factors may be involved. ROS and neutrophil respiratory burst cytochrome $b_{558}$ are produced by glomerular epithelial cells and could contribute to the injury.[378]

AHN can be modified by impairing Ab formation with immunosuppressive agents,[2042] including FK 506 and cyclosporine,[2043, 2044] or by inducing suppressor mechanisms by prior immunization with Fx1A in incomplete Freund adjuvant.[2045, 2046] The latter effect is inhibited by anti-CD4 Ab.[2047] In vitro Ab production using draining lymph node cells in AHN has been reported, and the response has been suggested to be modulated by a suppressor mechanism.[2048–2050] Reimmunization in standard AHN causes a second wave of Ab fixation and injury with differences in IgG subclass restriction and C deposition in resistant rats.[2051, 2052] The AHN lesion is made worse by concomitant induction of hypertension,[2053] streptozocin-induced diabetes,[2054] and five-sixths nephrectomy.[2055] Colchicine reduces proteinuria in PHN, an effect blocked by indomethacin.[2056] A study has found that intraperitoneal injection of protease causes some decrease in the amount of Ig deposited in glomeruli and abnormal proteinuria depending on the dose of anti-Fx1A Ab used and the timing of protease treatment.[2057]

The glomerular lesion in AHN is one of membranous GN with thickened GBM, minimal infiltration or proliferation, and diffuse subepithelial deposits of Ig and C with subepithelial electron-dense deposits.[1822] The alterations in GBM structure occurred without detected changes in the synthetic rate of type IV collagen, laminin, or fibronectin.[1474] The importance of C and the MAC as a mediator of HN has already been discussed, and studies suggest a role for monocytes as well.[648, 672, 2058] Fibronectin deposits have been reported along the GBM in AHN,[2059] as has clusterin.[409]

In micropuncture studies, the active and passive models differ with regard to time course and the degree of heterogeneity of glomerular and tubule abnormalities among nephrons. Both active and passive lesions are characterized by reduction in $K_f$ and increase in hydraulic pressure gra-

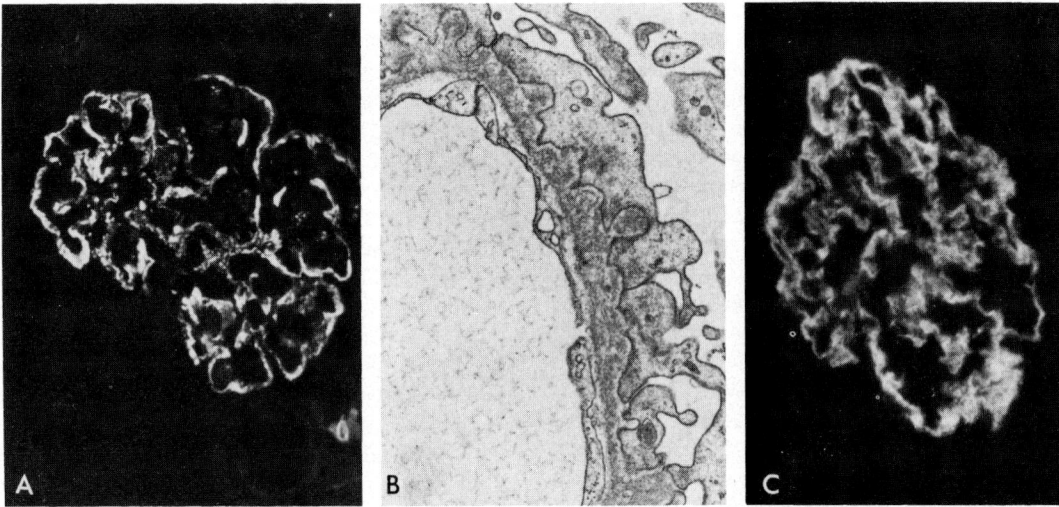

**Figure 29–7.** Immunopathologic findings in New Zealand White rabbits developing spontaneous GN are illustrated. *A.* Irregular granular and segmental deposits of IgG are observed along the GBM. *B.* Electron-dense deposits are observed irregularly and nearly confluently along the subepithelial aspect of the GBM. *C.* Concentrated eluates recovered from kidneys of rabbits with spontaneous GN react in an irregular pattern with the glomerular capillary wall. The reaction appears fuzzy owing to projections of reactive material on the epithelial aspect of the GBM.

dient.[2060] The glomerular permselectivity defect of PHN is noted to be due to impaired size selectivity related to the prevailing increase in hydraulic pressure gradient.[2061] In the passive model, homogeneous involvement of all glomeruli is found.[2060] Glomerular hemodynamics are maintained at 3 days after anti-Fx1A Ab administration, but as the deposits increase at day 5, whole kidney GFR and SNGFR decrease, with an increase in hydraulic pressure gradient and an increase in $K_f$ correlating with increasing epithelial cell foot process effacement.[1955] In the slowly developing (3 to 4 months) AHN, internephronal heterogeneity is found functionally and morphologically with maintenance of glomerular tubule balance.[1822, 2060, 2062] Proximal tubule damage parallels the glomerular leak of Ab into the proximal tubule fluid, where it can react with the tubule brush border Ag.[1822, 2063, 2064] The tubule injury is associated with tubule dysfunction.[2065] A C-independent increase in $LTB_4$ synthesis occurs within the first hour of PHN.[900] $LTD_4$ is implicated as a mediator of proteinuria and the glomerular hemodynamic changes of PHN,[915] and C5a and the α-adrenergic nervous system are also suggested to be involved.[322, 2066] Altered renal kallikrein and renin gene expression that can be modulated by converting enzyme inhibitors is also reported.[1181] ACE inhibition also reduces proteinuria.[2067] The effects of brush border Ag are separable from those of basolateral membrane Ag in terms of brush border damage, even though both Ags induced similar AHN glomerular lesions.[2068] Detection of brush border Ag in urine of humans is suggested to correlate with toxic tubule injury.[2069]

Rats with long-standing AHN have evidence of Abs (presumably filtered through the glomerulus) reacting with brush border Ags, as well as a variety of immune deposits in and around proximal tubule cells.[2070] An associated stripping of brush border material by mononuclear cells, which then tend to surround the brush border material and form rosettes within the tubule lumen, has been observed.[1822] This type of tubule injury has been studied in detail and the

tubule brush border IgG deposits correlate with anti–brush border Ab titer and glomerular leak of Abs into the tubule lumen.[2063, 2071] Ab fixation is associated with extensive loss of microvilli and degeneration and proliferation of the proximal tubule epithelium. Deposits of IgG are also found near the TBM. The lesions are C independent, as shown in studies using CVF.[2064] The associated interstitial cellular infiltration is dominated by $Ia^+$ and $ED-1^+$ macrophages.[2072] The mechanism of deposit formation is assumed to be similar to that described earlier for the formation of glomerular immune deposits in HN through a process that includes reactions of cell surface Ags with shedding of the reactants. Studies supporting this concept indicate that divalent Abs capable of cross-linking the Ag are required.[2073] Immunohistochemical studies reveal a decrease in gp330, clathrin, and $H^+$-pumping ATPase in AHN associated with a decrease in endocytotic uptake of intravenously injected macromolecules.[2074] Disruption of microtubules with colchicine alters the distribution of gp330 on the tubule cells from the normal apical plasma membrane location to a dispersion of vesicles with gp330 throughout the cytoplasm.[2075]

The immunized rabbit producing the anti-Fx1A Ab may also develop GN[2076] but usually has deposits only in the tubulointerstitial tissues. Anti-Fx1A Ab or Abs to other tubule Ag induce a glomerular lesion in rabbits of somewhat different course and epitope reactivity than in the rat.[2077, 2078] A passive form of glomerular disease can be produced in rabbits given heterologous anti-Fx1A Ab.[2078] Mice also develop immune deposits after being given heterologous Ab to mouse Fx1A.[2079]

We have evaluated rabbits with a spontaneously occurring form of GN[1] that seems to be induced by antibodies reactive with non–basement membrane Ags located in the vicinity of the epithelial cell foot processes.[2080, 2081] Immunofluorescence reveals that these rabbits have segmental irregular IgG and C3 deposits along their GBMs (Fig. 29–7A). By electron microscopy, the subepithelial aspect of the

GBM contains an irregular accumulation of electron-dense materials scattered in a less circumscribed manner than is the deposit typical of HN or human membranous GN (Fig. 29–7*B*). Abs eluted from the glomeruli of involved rabbit kidneys react by immunofluorescence with an irregularly distributed glomerular capillary wall Ag and, to a lesser extent, of the arteriole wall (Fig. 29–7*C*). Immunoelectron microscopy techniques place the site of reaction of these Abs in the area where epithelial cell foot processes attach to the GBM.[2081] It is suspected that the immunopathogenesis of this spontaneous form of GN involves the direct binding of Abs that are reactive with Ags, which may be on the epithelial cell foot processes as in HN or in the immediate vicinity. Of interest, the human glomerulus reacts strongly with the eluted Ig from the spontaneous rabbit GN, suggesting that a similar and potentially nephritogenic Ag system is present.[2081]

## Endothelial Cell Ags

The endothelial cell has been a focus of study in the production of arterial lesions[169, 418–420] and contributes to hemodynamic, adhesion, and inflammatory responses in immune glomerular injury.[1234] ACE present on endothelium has been used as a target Ag for Ab interaction in the lung, producing severe injury, with evidence that the reactive Ag can be modulated with the Ab.[2082–2084] Injections of Ab reactive with ACE into the aorta above the renal artery resulted in binding to the endothelium as small aggregates on the plasma membrane.[2085] Systemic administration resulted in fine granular deposits on the glomerular endothelium accompanied by C by day 2. By day 3 to 5, the immunofluorescent deposit appeared almost linear, and the deposit was localized to the base of the foot processes and filtration slits. The endothelium was swollen and contained numerous blebs. From day 8 onward, the deposit was an interrupted linear, occasionally finely granular one with immunoelectron microscopic localization of the material to the filtration slits. Captopril, which increases the expression of ACE, had no effect on the glomerular lesion. Overall, the amounts of Ab bound were relatively small, being about 33 µg. The endothelial reaction presumably led to shedding of the surface complexes, which were moved through the GBM to be retained by the filtration slits. The authors postulated that the movement may have been facilitated by potent vasoactive polar lipids such as PAF released from PMNs or stimulated endothelial cells that would alter vascular permeability.[2086–2088] Injection of an IgG anti–von Willebrand factor Ab reactive with endothelium resulted in endothelial and mesangial deposits, C3, and a few electron-dense deposits with a mild leukocyte influx.[2089] A number of examples of anti–endothelial cell Abs are known in humans. Increasingly successful culture of glomerular endothelial cells should allow more direct study of this particular endothelium.[1230–1233, 1240]

## Mesangial Cell Ags

The mesangial cell, a smooth muscle–like cell, is the third major cell type in the glomerulus. Its central location and accessibility to the circulation via the fenestrated endothelial cell lining of the glomerular capillary make it especially vulnerable to several forms of injury. Models of mesangial cell damage include the use of snake venom,[2090–2092] as well as injury caused by Ab attack directed against materials previously taken up by the mesangium.[2093] Abs reactive with rat mesangium have been reported after immunization with porcine lung,[2094] and anti-Forssman Abs have been noted to bind to guinea pig mesangium, with subsequent increased cellularity.[2095] A monoclonal Ab reactive in vivo with mesangial matrix, which can induce immune deposits, has also been reported.[2096] Abs to double-stranded DNA from patients with SLE have been reported to cause cytotoxic effects on cultured rat mesangial cells.[2097] In the same study, anticardiolipin Abs were also inhibitory to mesangial cell growth.

A model of Ab-induced mesangial cell injury that differs from those described for epithelial and endothelial cells involves C-dependent mesangial cell lysis as a prominent feature of the initial phases of the disease (Fig. 29–8*A*). The lytic phase is followed by a phase of marked glomerular hypercellularity and mesangial cell proliferation (Fig. 29–8*C*). We have used polyclonal anti–rat thymus serum (ATS) reactive with a Thy-1.1–like mesangial cell surface Ag to injure the mesangial cells[2098, 2099] (Fig. 29–8*B*); others have used ATS[2100] or monoclonal anti–Thy-1.1 monoclonal Abs[2101, 2102] to induce similar lesions.

Thy-1 is a phosphatidylinositol-anchored glycoprotein located on the surface of certain cells, particularly those of the thymus and brain. Its relative molecular mass is 18 kd (one third is carbohydrate), and its complementary DNA indicates 143 amino acids with a hydrophobic domain for insertion into cell membranes.[2103, 2104] Anti–Thy-1.1 Abs react with brain, thymocytes, B cell precursors, bone marrow cells, fibroblasts, and rat kidney cells.[2105] Glomerular reactivity is striking in the rat using either monoclonal anti–Thy-1.1 Abs or ATS,[2106–2108] with the reaction localized to the cell membrane on electron microscopic study.[2109–2111] In humans, the Thy-1 glycoprotein has been reported in proximal tubular epithelial cells and in the Bowman capsule.[2112]

Intravenously administered ATS binds rapidly to the mesangial cells and causes a C-dependent mesangial cell lysis, as demonstrated by prevention of lysis in experiments in which C depletion was produced by administration of CVF.[362, 2113] Induction of lesions was also not possible with anti–Thy 1.1 monoclonal Abs that did not fix C, providing further evidence of the C dependence of the lesion.[2101]

Only 11 µg of Ab bound in the total glomerular mass was needed to cause the lesion.[2099] This contrasted with the 150 to 175 µg of Ab per two kidneys needed to induce immune deposit injury with anti-GBM Abs or anti–Con A Abs in the rat.[2114, 2115] Extrarenal binding of the ATS was low, with 0.38 µg/g dry weight in the liver at 6 hours and only minimal binding to lungs, hearts, spleens, brains, or thymuses. The maximal observed binding to thymus was only 0.01 µg/g dry weight at 24 hours. Ab deposits disappeared over several days; however, autologous-phase reactions have been reported.[2116]

The early lytic lesion is associated with glomerular deposits of C components C3, C5, C6, C7, C9, and C5b-9.[2113] This suggests that the MAC was involved in the degeneration of the mesangial cells. Cultured mesangial cells treated

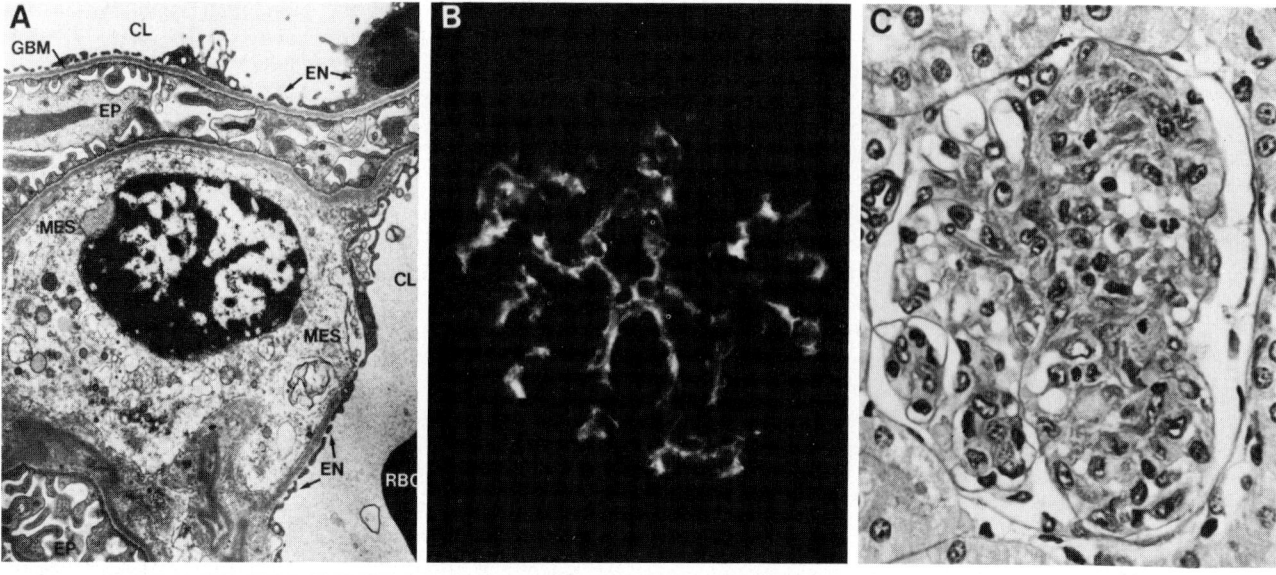

**Figure 29–8.** Ab-induced C-dependent mesangial cell injury in the rat. *A.* One hour after administration of rabbit antirat thymocyte serum, which reacts with a Thy-1.1–like Ag on the mesangial cell surface, acute mesangial cell (MES) injury was found without involvement of epithelial (EP) or endothelial (EN) cells. Other abbreviations: GBM = glomerular basement membrane; CL = capillary lumen; RBC = red blood cell. *B.* The fixation of the rabbit antithymocyte Ab monitored as rabbit IgG deposits was confined to the mesangial area. *C.* Glomerular hypercellularity follows the initial mesangial cell injury phase by day 4, the majority of the cells having characteristics of mesangial cells.

in vitro with ATS were lysed as monitored by $^{51}$Cr release within 30 minutes in the presence, but not the absence, of C. By using electron microscopy with negative staining to study cultured mesangial cells treated with ATS and C in vitro, doughnut-shaped lesions of about 90 Å were found[362] and were typical of those associated with MAC lesions seen in other nucleated cells.[2117–2120] Our ongoing studies using ATS and C sources lacking in terminal C components in the isolated perfused kidney support a role for the MAC in lysis of mesangial cells "in vivo."

The almost immediate mesangial cell lysis (1 hour through 2 days) was followed by a mesangial hypercellularity that was marked by day 4. The majority of cells in the expanded mesangial areas had characteristics of mesangial cells by electron microscopy. Phenotypic characterization of the hypercellular lesion revealed that most of the cells reacted by immunofluorescence with the anti–Thy 1.1 Abs, although a few cells had leukocyte common Ag or Ia Ags on their surfaces. A contribution of monocyte-macrophages is suggested by depletion studies.[2121, 2122] Monocyte-macrophages recovered from glomeruli of the ATS lesion produce superoxide and LTB$_4$.[733] Many of the cells reacted with Ab against proliferating cell nuclear Ag,[2123, 2124] and frequent mitotic figures were present. The proliferative lesion was prevented if the initial lysis was inhibited by C depletion using CVF but not by leukocyte depletion using irradiation or anti-PMN Abs, suggesting the mesangial origin of the cells.[2098, 2113] The number of cells was decreased slightly by leukocyte depletion, suggesting that a minor population of the total cells was infiltrative in nature. Platelet depletion also modulates the lesion.[952] Nucleotidases are reported to have an anti-inflammatory effect.[964] The injured mesangial cells express α-actin, suggesting their derivation from smooth muscle cells and expression of this phenotype

during proliferation.[2125] Muscle-specific actins are also increased in human GN.[2126]

Very large initial doses of ATS prevented or greatly delayed the proliferative phase of the injury; this was probably related to more complete initial killing of the mesangial cells, preventing their subsequent expansion. Readministration of ATS during the hypercellular phase of the injury results in a second lytic effect, although to a lesser degree than in the initial insult. Perhaps this is due in part to alterations in expression of the target Ag. Repeated administration increases the degree of mesangial sclerosis that occurs, particularly with uninephrectomy.[2127] Inhibitors of the thromboxane receptor and thromboxane synthesis improve the outcome of the repeated-injection ATS model in uninephrectomized rats.[887]

As already outlined, the model has been used to study the mechanisms for increase in mesangial matrix. Heparin decreases mesangial proliferation and in turn the amount of focal mesangial matrix increase without altering the initial mesangiolysis.[1534] Several other growth factors including TGF-β and PDGF have been implicated in the accumulation of excess matrix.[1520, 1538, 1526] Neutralizing Abs to TGF-β and PDGF decrease the focal increase in mesangial matrix, as does decorin, a natural regulator of TGF-β.[1537, 1540, 1561] The chemokine MCP-1 is increased early in the ATS lesion.[518]

The ATS-induced mesangial lesion caused a striking (almost 50-fold) increase in the glomerular uptake of macromolecular test aggregates (heat-aggregated human IgG) when administered 4 hours after ATS. The uptake of aggregated BSA and preformed IC also increased.[2099] The test aggregates rapidly disappeared from the glomeruli even though the mesangial cells were probably no longer functional. The hypercellular lesion slowly resolved with a residual increase in mesangial matrix and focal glomerulosclerosis. Development of proteinuria associated with the lesion varied with the rat strain used and presumably with the severity of the injury.

Glomerular hemodynamic studies in the initial lytic phases of this mesangial lesion demonstrated that 24 hours after the intravenous administration of ATS, major glomerular hemodynamic abnormalities occurred.[2128] The rate of glomerular plasma flow increased and glomerular capillary pressure rose significantly, but so did the Bowman space pressure, resulting in only a modest elevation in the hydraulic pressure gradient. SNGFR fell, however, compared with that of normal animals, primarily, if not solely, as a result of a large decrease in $K_f$ to approximately 35% of the normal values. On day 6 during the hypercellular phase of injury, glomerular plasma flow was decreased with a further decrease in SNGFR. The hydraulic pressure gradient did not increase and $K_f$ remained diminished. These findings suggest that the Ab induced injury with mesangial cell lysis and opened up the mesangial spaces with shunting of a portion of the plasma flow away from the usual filtration surface. During the hypercellular phase, with its severe architectural disruption, plasma flow decreased and the glomerulus did not compensate for the decrease in SNGFR by raising its filtration pressure, the hydraulic pressure gradient, suggesting that intact and properly organized mesangial cells may be needed to contribute to this expected response. Studies using this model also suggest a role of the mesangial cell in tubuloglomerular feedback.[2129]

The nephritogenicity of ATS outlined in this section indicates the need to include such reactivity among the complications to be considered with the clinical use of ATS.[2130] Anti-GBM Abs, for example, well documented in some ATS preparations, are probably related to inclusion of connective tissue in the crude lymphoid inoculum.[2131] The Thy-1.1 cross-reactivity between thymocytes and glomerular mesangial cells suggests that even pure T cell immunogens have the potential to induce Abs with antiglomerular reactivity, at least in rats. A monoclonal Ab capable of eliciting a lesion similar to that elicited by ATS or anti–Thy-1.1 monoclonal Ab is reported.[2132] Heavy proteinuria is a feature of the Ag-induced mesangial injury. Subtle differences in binding pattern led the investigator to suggest that an epitope different from that seen by OX7 on Thy-1.1 may be involved.

## OTHER NEPHRITOGENIC GLOMERULAR AGS

In addition to the structural and cellular Ags recognized and outlined in some detail earlier, a number of other potential nephritogenic Ag-Ab systems have been suggested. For example, a model under study with apparent antiglomerular Abs is that of experimentally induced penicillamine toxicity.[2133] Renal eluates contain Abs reactive with normal glomeruli in a linear pattern, although the precise nature of the Ag remains to be defined.

There are potentially many more Ag-Ab systems that could be involved, as recognized years ago.[2134, 2135] For example, fibronectin could serve as a nephritogenic Ag[2136] and

heterologous antifibronectin Abs could accumulate in the mesangial area after in vivo administration.[2137] Immunization of rabbits with human plasma fibronectin induced Abs reactive with a 27-kd fragment of rabbit fibronectin and caused dense deposits in the GBM.[2138] Fibronectin can also trap Ags for subsequent nephritogenic immune reaction. The nephritogenic glycopeptide studies over the years by Shibata and colleagues[2139, 2140] remain to be integrated into the model nephritogenic systems. This Ag has been sequenced and is a glycopeptide reactive with Con A.[2141] Many Ags are present in both animal and human kidneys and are known to be important in allograft rejection,[2142–2147] to be involved in teratogenesis,[2148] or to be present in the urine.[2149] The possible nephritogenic role of other glomerular components such as podocalyxin of visceral epithelial cell and endothelial cell surfaces,[2150–2152] as well as intermediate filament proteins,[2153, 2154] remains to be defined, although these components can bind to glomeruli after injection.[2155, 2156] The same is true of tumor-associated proteins such as villin and epithelial membrane Ag.[2157–2159] Monoclonal Abs reactive with podocalyxin are reported to bind to neuraminidase-infused rat kidneys.[2160]

Increasing numbers of monoclonal Abs are being prepared that are reactive with a wide variety of defined and undefined glomerular (and tubule) renal Ags, including components of the GBM such as type IV collagen,[1775, 2161–2176] and human Ags are being sought with a similar approach.[2177, 2178] Ags present in renal tumors and their distribution in normal renal tissue are also being studied.[2179–2181] Many in vivo administrations of monoclonal Abs have not been very nephritogenic.[1997, 2096, 2182, 2183] A monoclonal Ab, 1G10, recognizes a mesangial Ag that can be used to detect mesangial hypercellularity in human kidneys.[2184] A study using a monoclonal Ab reactive with podocytes and slit diaphragms was capable of inducing rather severe proteinuria on in vivo administration to rats.[2185] The relationship of this reaction to better-defined elements of the podocytes, including podocalyxin and podoendin, remains to be defined.[2186–2190] In studies using the monoclonal Ab reactive with the podocytes and slit diaphragms, SNGFR and plasma flow were unchanged 2 hours after the Ab; however, the glomerular hydraulic pressure gradient and glomerular capillary hydraulic pressure were increased, with a 50% decrease in the glomerular ultrafiltration coefficient without proteinuria.[2191] By 24 hours, when increased proteinuria was found, there was an increase in SNGFR and plasma flow and the glomerular ultrafiltration coefficient had returned to normal. The increase in GFR and plasma flow was blocked by meclofenamate. The studies suggest that barriers controlling hydraulic conductivity and protein excretion reside in the region of the slit diaphragm and that these factors can be affected individually. Chlorpromazine, which inhibits cytoskeletal movement, was not effective in altering the lesion, in contrast to its modulation of PHN.[2192] A monoclonal Ab reactive with mouse aminopeptidase A induces proteinuria after intravenous injection in mice.[2193] The Ab reacts with the visceral glomerular epithelial cell membranes, and the Ag is also present in the brush border of the proximal tubules as a 140-kd protein with aminopeptidase activity.

## Nephritogenic Antibody Reactions with Trapped or Planted Antigens

The in situ formation of ICs in glomeruli by the interaction of Ab with foreign Ags that were previously trapped or planted in a glomerulus is yet another immune mechanism of GN. In addition to heterologous anti-GBM Abs, which serve as planted Ags in autologous phases of nephrotoxic renal injury, aggregated Ig trapped in the mesangium can serve as a planted Ag when such a kidney is exposed to circulating anti-Ig Ab.[2093] Izui and colleagues[2194, 2195] suggested that DNA can bind to the GBM and serve as a planted Ag for reaction with anti-DNA Abs in the SLE of New Zealand mice. Double-stranded DNA can bind to fibronectin, a component of the glomerulus,[2196] and DNA–anti-DNA IC binding to fibronectin is increased by C1q.[2197] The binding of DNA to the GBM is diminished when basic proteins such as lysozyme or other polycations such as hexadimethrine are present.[2198]

Histone-DNA complexes bind to the endothelium and GBM and serve as target Ags for anti-DNA Abs as a potential contributor to immune deposit formation in SLE and in its murine models.[2199–2202] The reaction with DNA has been suggested to explain the cross-reactivity of some purified and monoclonal anti-DNA Abs reported to react with some glomerular components.[2203] DNA released during the hybridoma production is thought also to become complexed with the anti-DNA Ab, which in turn could complex with glomerulus-bound histone. Models to produce DNA–anti-DNA IC in situ have been unsuccessful using monoclonal anti-DNA Abs in situations in which endotoxin-induced DNA deposits or passively administered DNA was used[2204, 2205]; however, when large amounts of ultraviolet light–treated DNA were infused into the renal artery, anti-DNA Ab was able to bind with the production of mesangial Ig deposits and minimal histologic change.[2206]

In addition to DNA binding other Ags to fibronectin, phenylated gelatin (dinitrophenol [DNP]-GL), which binds to fibronectin in the mesangium, has been used as a planted Ag to be the target of administered anti-DNP Ab.[2207] Precipitating rather than nonprecipitating Ab is retained longer in this model.[2208] DNP bound to F(ab′)$_2$ anti–Thy 1 monoclonal Ab has been used to direct the DNP to rat mesangial cells for subsequent nephritogenic reaction with polymeric monoclonal IgA Ab.[2209]

We used lectins to demonstrate that foreign substances binding to the glomerular capillary wall for physicochemical reasons can serve as nephritogenic planted Ags.[2115] Lectins are proteins with carbohydrate-binding properties that can bind to the GBM and serve as planted Ags for subsequent nephritogenic interaction with specific antilectin Ab. Con A, a glucose- and mannose-binding lectin, binds to glomerular endothelium and subendothelial aspects of the GBM.[2210] In rats, unilateral renal artery perfusion of 500 μg of Con A resulted in the fixation of 75 μg of Con A along the glomerular capillary wall (Fig. 29–9A and B). The nonperfused right kidney served as a "negative" control. Clinically overt GN developed with binding of about 70 μg of heterologous anti–Con A Ab per gram of kidney, a value similar to that necessary to induce heterologous anti-GBM Ab–induced GN. It was also possible to induce GN by

perfusing Con A into the renal artery of a rat previously immunized with Con A, resulting in direct fixation of the circulating Ab to the planted Con A. The Con A can be removed from the glomeruli by administration of its competitive inhibitor, α-methyl-mannoside.[2115] The Con A model, which has a severe PMN-dominated early inflammatory phase, has been used with success to demonstrate the role of PMNs and their myeloperoxidase (MPO)–hydrogen peroxide system for generating ROS in glomerular injury.[786] Fixation of Con A in the glomeruli of preimmunized beagles has been used to produce GN and to show that inhibition of thromboxane synthetase may have benefit.[872] Con A binding to glomerular structures in rats has been used to evaluate the role of polymeric or secretory IgA–Con A complexes versus monomeric IgA–Con A complexes in the generation of glomerular inflammation.[2211, 2212] Five hundred micrograms of the polymeric IgA–Con A complex produced a focal and segmental proliferative GN within 1 hour, with rat C3 and fibrin deposits and infiltration of PMNs. The lectin *Helix pomatia* agglutinin was planted (by perfusion of the isolated kidney with neuraminidase) along the glomerular endothelial cell and subsequently reacted with Ab to the lectin.[2213] The initial formation of granular deposits in the subendothelial space was followed in 2 days by the appearance of subendothelial deposits. The mechanisms for the apparent movement of the deposits include possible podocyte binding of this lectin.[2214] Lectin binding sites in glomeruli have been found to change in response to different histologic lesions in GN.[2215] A similar model using the lectin *Lens culinaris* hemagglutinin, which binds to glomerular endothelial cells, has been described.[2216]

Many lectins can bind to renal structures.[2217] Lectin-like materials, as well as materials that can bind to glomerular capillary walls for other physicochemical reasons, are present in infectious organisms pathogenic for experimental animals as well as humans, suggesting the possibility of similar mechanisms in the production of human GN.[2218] It has been suggested that Ags from *Dirofilaria immitis* (canine heartworm disease) bind to the GBM for subsequent linear fixation of anti-worm Ab.[2219] Purposeful infusion of *D. immitis* extract into the renal artery of hyperimmunized dogs resulted in a glomerular lesion.[2220] *D. immitis* Ags are found in glomeruli and sera of infected dogs by using monoclonal Abs.[2221] Circulating IC levels were inconsistent.[2222] *Schistosoma* Ags may also bind in experimental models in baboons.[2223] Intact *Escherichia coli* can localize, at least transiently, on glomerular endothelium.[2224] Some features of poststreptococcal GN, for example, suggest direct glomerular binding of Ag, as streptococcal Ags have been identified that are bound in the glomeruli early in the course of disease.[1, 2225, 2226] Endostreptosin, an Ag from nephritogenic group A streptococci, injected intravenously in rats binds to rat basement membranes and after 8 days is associated with rat IgG and C3 with circulating Abs to the Ag.[2227] Even if this sequence plays a role in this disease, other features of poststreptococcal GN, including potentially nephritogenic mechanisms such as circulating ICs, cryoglobulins, and peculiarities in C deposition and perhaps activation, also need to be considered. The so-called preabsorbing Ag from nephritogenic streptococci found in the

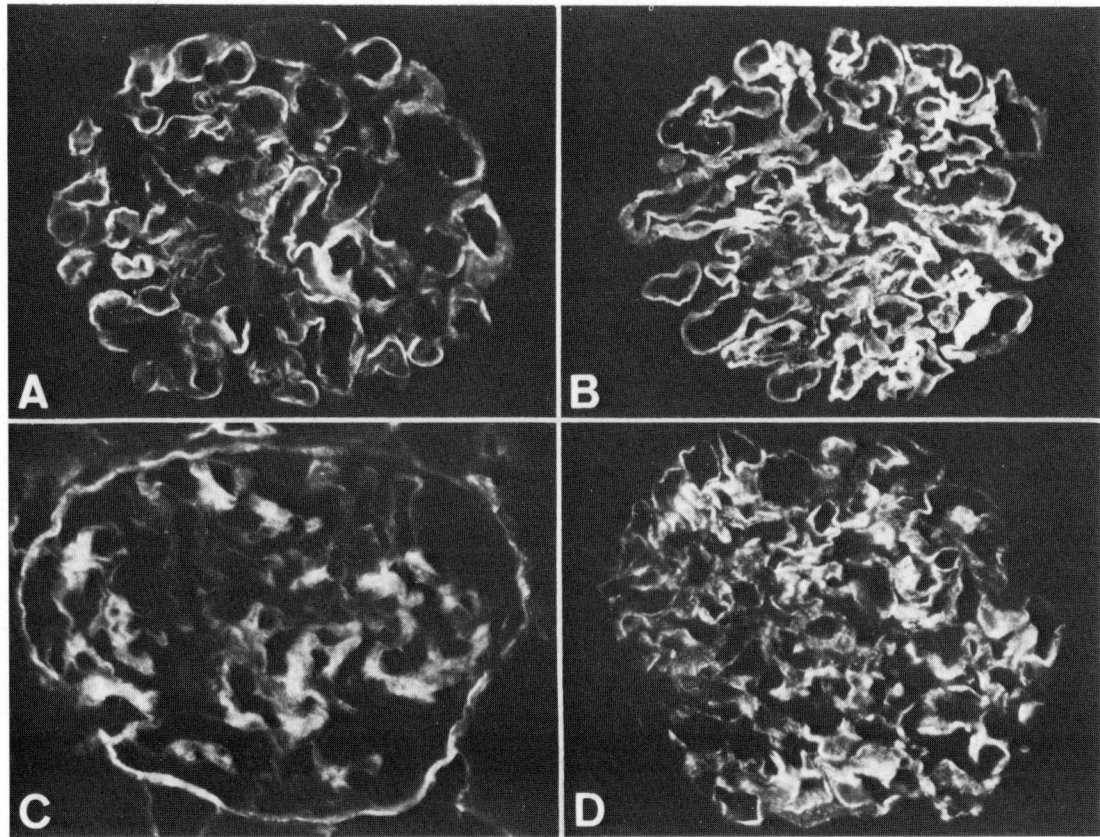

**Figure 29–9.** Immunofluorescence patterns of planted Ag depositions and subsequent Ab interactions are demonstrated. In *A*, the nearly continuous deposit of Con A is demonstrated in glomerular capillary loops 24 hours after intrarenal artery infusion and systemic administration of anti–Con A Ab. In *B*, nearly linear deposition of the heterologous anti–Con A Ab is seen in another glomerulus from the animal depicted in *A* also at 24 hours. In *C*, the fixation of cationic BSA as an Ag to glomerular capillary wall, mesangium, and focally in peritubular capillary structures and Bowman capsule is demonstrated 4 hours after systemic administration of this charge-altered material. In *D*, the finely granular, nearly continuous deposition of anti-BSA Ab is seen in an animal similar to that in *C* 24 hours after Ab administration. (Original magnification × 400.)

glomeruli early in poststreptococcal GN activates the alternative C pathway.[2228] Components of human GBM have been reported[2229] to have lectin-like activity, suggesting a physicochemical way, in addition to charge, by which foreign materials might become trapped in the glomerulus.

Another physicochemical feature of the glomerular capillary wall that makes it a potential site of Ag trapping is its polyanionic charge characteristics.[3, 1921, 2230, 2231] This concept is also considered later during the discussion of physicochemical interactions that influence the dynamic interchange of Ag and Ab in nephritogenic IC accumulation and rearrangement. In terms of a planted Ag mechanism, the polyanionic charge of the glomerular capillary wall has been used to bind cationized ferritin, human IgG, human IgM, ovalbumin, and serum albumin to the GBM, where they rather rapidly become concentrated in subepithelial positions (Fig. 29–9*C* and *D*). Native cationic avidin can also be used.[2232] Ab fixation to the planted Ag can induce proteinuria.[2233–2238] Using cationic ferritin, initial subendothelial deposits move to subepithelial locations.[2239] Anionic sites on the epithelial cells are most altered by administration of cationic Ag.[2240] Variations in binding of cationized proteins to different rat strains are noted, suggesting some genetic variation in anionic sites.[2241] Epitope density of sub-

stituted cationic carrier molecules may influence the severity of the lesion.[2242] Replacing native BSA with cationized BSA in a chronic serum sickness injection protocol in rabbits produced much more rapid capillary wall IC accumulation, and the cationized BSA was shown to bind directly to the glomerulus.[2243] The injury increases in relation to epitope density on the cationic Ag in a trinitrophenol-cationic human IgG model.[2244] Mice are also susceptible to rapid development of GN, glomerular capillary thrombosis, and crescent formation after immunization with and administration of cationic bovine gamma globulin.[2245] Cationized Ag can also be used to induce IC deposits in the choroid plexus.[2246] A study suggests that highly anionic BSA or bovine gamma globulin can also bind to the glomerular capillary wall,[2247] and both cationic and anionic Abs have been recovered from glomeruli with HN.[1953] Glomerular binding of cationic Ab has usually been favored; the location of the Ag plays a role (enhanced binding of cationic Ab to subepithelial Ag) and the charge of the Ag itself is also a factor.[2248, 2249] Naturally occurring charged molecules such as MPO can also induce a planted Ag form of glomerular injury.[55–57, 2249a]

Polycation administration increases glomerular capillary permeability with inhibition of binding of additional cationic materials to the glomerular capillary wall, and at high doses such treatment may alter podocyte structure.[2250–2256] Neutralization of glomerular polycation enhances the deposition and alters the distribution of preformed ICs in glomeruli.[2257] Heparin can enhance removal of cationic BSA glomerular deposits.[2258] Heparitinase-induced alterations in the heparan sulfate proteoglycan–rich anionic sites alter binding of cationic IC to the glomerular capillary wall.[2259] Collagenase also alters glomerular permeability to anionic ferritin.[2260] Binding of cationized Ag can be modified competitively by injection of protamine sulfate, a polycation, but this is less effective in established lesions.[2261, 2262] The amount of Ab present is thought to govern the ability of protamine to displace cationic glomerular IC deposits.[2263] In another version of the in situ IC formation model, alternate renal perfusion of BSA and anti-BSA or lysozyme and antilysozyme resulted in detectable glomerular IC deposits.[2264] Cationic phlogogenic materials from cells such as platelets or leukocytes can bind to the glomerular capillary wall as well.[567, 568, 954, 1061] The cationic bovine gamma globulin model of GN in rats has been used to demonstrate the enhanced role of targeting proteases to the glomerulus as a means of decreasing glomerular immune deposits and urinary protein excretion.[2265] Another consideration is that anionic sites in the glomerulus are decreased in IC GN.[2266]

Other examples of possible planted Ags in human GN might be the reaction of anti-idiotypic Abs or rheumatoid factors with previously deposited IC.[2267–2270] For example, we have shown the presence of auto-anti-idiotypic Abs in the glomerular IC deposits in chronic serum sickness in rabbits,[2271] and similar findings have been reported in glomerular ICs occurring after polyclonal B cell activation in mice.[2272, 2273] Auto-anti-idiotypic Ab production increases in old mice.[2274] Circulating ICs contain idiotypic–anti-idiotypic Abs in antiphosphorylcholine immune responses and during the polyclonal B cell activation induced by African trypanosomes.[2275, 2276] Immunoconglutinins such as C3NeF[2277] could conceivably also interact with glomerular C component deposits, which would serve as a type of planted Ag. In addition, as discussed in more detail in a subsequent section, ICs localized in the glomerulus are in dynamic equilibrium with Ag and Ab from the circulation, serving as a nidus for continual local in situ interaction.

IgG3 rheumatoid factors derived from MRL-*lpr/lpr* lupus mice react with IgG2a and can form cryoglobulins via IgG3 Fc-Fc interactions and also induce glomerular lesions.[2278–2280] The cryoglobulin induction is associated with glomerular "wire loop" formation as subendothelial deposits occurred 5 to 8 days after intraperitoneal transfer of hybridoma cells producing the IgG3.[2281] The development of skin lesions and glomerular lesions could be dissociated by depleting the rheumatoid factor activity of the IgG3.[2282] An anti-idiotypic Ab to the IgG3 prevented the skin and glomerular lesion and noncryogenerating IgG3 may interact with the pathogenic cryoglobulins and be protective.[2283, 2284] IgG3 antitrinitrophenol monoclonal Abs derived from nonlupus mice were able to induce glomerular lesions in mice as cryoglobulins, with cryoprecipitation prevented by keeping the mice at 37°C.[2285]

Ags derived from infectious agents that can replicate in glomerular structures could also be considered a form of trapped glomerular Ag. The cytomegalovirus replication in human glomerular mesangial cells serves as a possible prototype of this kind of local Ag production, which in turn could be a target for Ab reaction in selective induction of glomerular injury.[2286]

## Anti–Basement Membrane Antibody– Induced Disease in Humans

The lessons derived from the study of animal models of anti-GBM Ab GN and other types of direct Ab binding to glomerular Ags provide a background for understanding the factors affecting the pathogenicity of nephritogenic Ab reactions with glomerular Ags in humans. In the models and presumably in humans, the induction and severity of glomerular damage are greatly influenced by the quantitative aspects of Ab binding. This includes the amounts of Ab bound as well as the tempo of binding and, to some extent, the location of binding, which is related to the distribution of the reactive Ag in addition to such things as charge interactions between Ab and Ag and background charge of the glomerular capillary wall.[3, 2287–2289] The quantities of Ab needed for induction of injury are also related in part to the ability of the Ab to enlist mediators of inflammation. For example, C-fixing anti-GBM Ab is able to initiate injury in lower amounts than its non–C-fixing counterpart. Adequate amounts of C-fixing anti-GBM Ab can induce infiltration of PMNs and endothelial cell damage within 15 minutes of administration in rats.[2114] The accessibility of the Ag to the circulating Ab is also an important feature and may explain the comparatively slow binding of anti-TBM Ab to TBM Ag (peaking only after 6 days).[2290] The accessibility issue (and events that alter it) also appears to be central to the development of lung lesions in model systems and in humans exposed to circulating anti-GBM Ab reactive with ABM.

Anti-GBM Ab GN is the best example of Ab-induced glomerular disease in humans, and its study has set the standards whereby the immunopathogenesis of a human form of GN can be clearly defined. This was done in 1967 by Lerner and associates[2291] using four approaches. First, they demonstrated the Abs bound to the GBM as linear deposits of IgG and C3 indistinguishable from those of known anti-GBM Ab model systems (Figs. 29–10 and 29–11). Second, anti-GBM Ab could be demonstrated in the circulation and could be recovered from renal eluates. Third, GN and linear deposits of IgG could be transferred to nonhuman primates with the recovered Abs. And fourth, anti-GBM Ab GN was shown to recur after renal transplantation when anti-GBM Ab persisted in the circulation. Several additional examples in which anti-GBM Ab GN have been transferred to transplant recipients are known; however, the recurrence is not always severe enough to cause graft failure and is probably modified by the concomitant immunosuppression given the transplant recipient.[1, 2292, 2293]

Anti–basement membrane Abs (e.g., anti-GBM, anti-TBM, anti-ABM) are associated with a variety of clinical presentations in humans (Table 29–2) and have been the subject of review.[1, 9, 2294–2302] The clinical, diagnostic, and therapeutic features of this group of diseases are addressed in Chapters 30 and 31. It is to

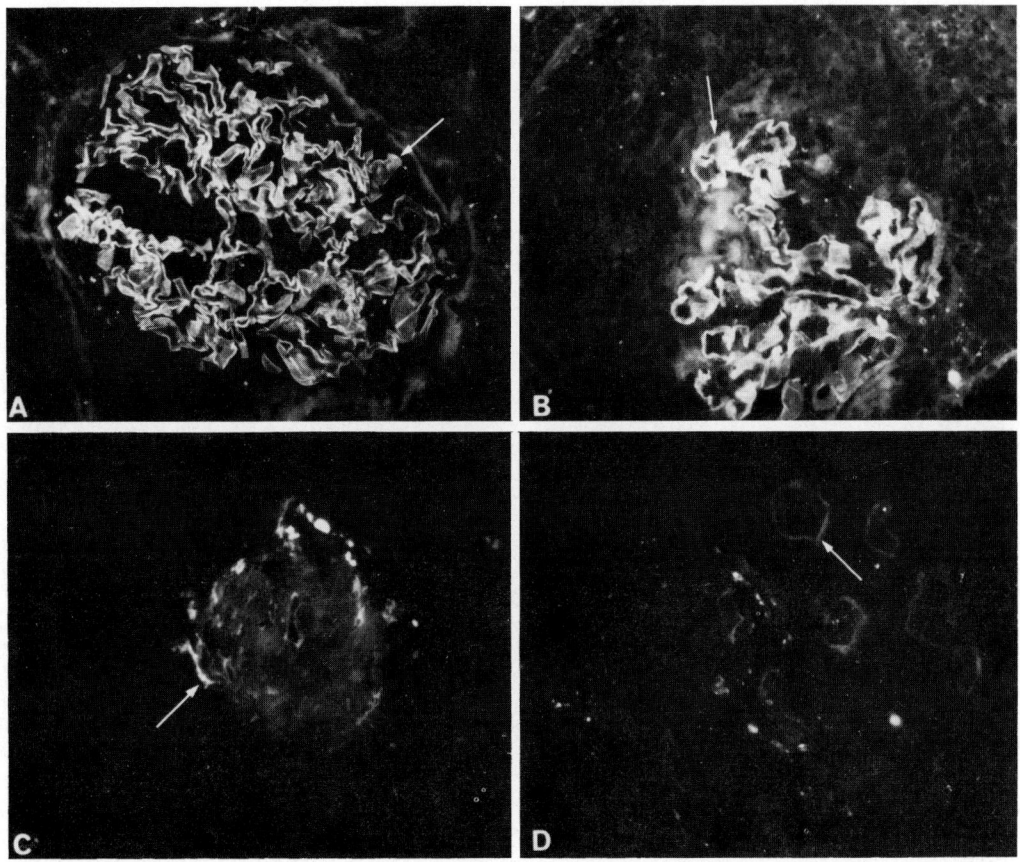

**Figure 29–10.** Immunofluorescence findings in anti-GBM GN. *A,* Smooth linear deposits of Ig are present along the GBM of a patient with early anti-GBM GN. *B,* Irregular linear deposits of Ig are noted along the corrugated and compressed GBM of a glomerulus with severe crescent formation. *C,* Little Ig remains in a hyalinized glomerulus from a patient with elution-confirmed end-stage anti-GBM GN. *D,* Faint focal linear deposits of Ig along the TBM of the kidney shown in *C* suggested the diagnosis of anti–basement membrane Abs. (Fluorescein isothiocyanate–conjugated antihuman IgG; original magnification × 250.)

be expected that the descriptive terms anti–basement membrane, anti-GBM, and anti-TBM Abs will eventually be replaced by precise biochemical definitions of the antigenic epitopes involved. Indeed, because regions of the type IV collagen molecule appear to be the major antigen(s) in this disease, a designation of anti–type IV collagen disease might be the first step in this process.

### TABLE 29–2. Anti–Basement Membrane Diseases

Combined pulmonary hemorrhage and GN (Goodpasture syndrome)
Severe, often rapidly progressive GN
Occasionally milder, sometimes remitting forms of GN
Pulmonary hemorrhage presenting as idiopathic pulmonary
  hemosiderosis
Tubulointerstitial nephritis
  Complicating anti-GBM GN
  Complicating IC GN
  Drug-associated TIN
  Rarely primary TIN
Other basement membranes
  ? Choroid plexus
  ? Intestinal
Transplantation
  Recurrent or de novo GN or TIN

The demographics of the clinicopathologic features of anti–basement membrane Ab disease are changing, and roughly half of the patients present with Goodpasture syndrome and half have their disease confined to the kidneys. A few (1% to 2%) have clinical involvement only in the lung.[1, 2303, 2304] Even though individuals in the 15- to 40-year-old age groups (males more commonly than females) still predominate, an increasing number of individuals, particularly with kidney involvement only, are found in the group older than 50 years (females most commonly involved).

Although anti-GBM Abs are probably the most common cause of GN and pulmonary hemorrhage in the absence of systemic vasculitic disease, other conditions need to be considered.[1, 2305–2318] In addition, the presence of vasculitis or thrombotic microangiopathy may not exclude the diagnosis of anti-GBM Ab GN; clinical features of Wegener granulomatosis and anti-GBM Ab may coexist.[1, 2319–2321] The description of Abs, termed antineutrophil cytoplasmic antibodies (ANCAs), reactive with PMNs and monocyte cytoplasmic Ags in some patients with anti-GBM Ab disease* is of interest in this regard because these Abs are associated with Wegener granulomatosis and microvasculitis at least

*References 40, 44, 2298, 2299, 2322–2327.

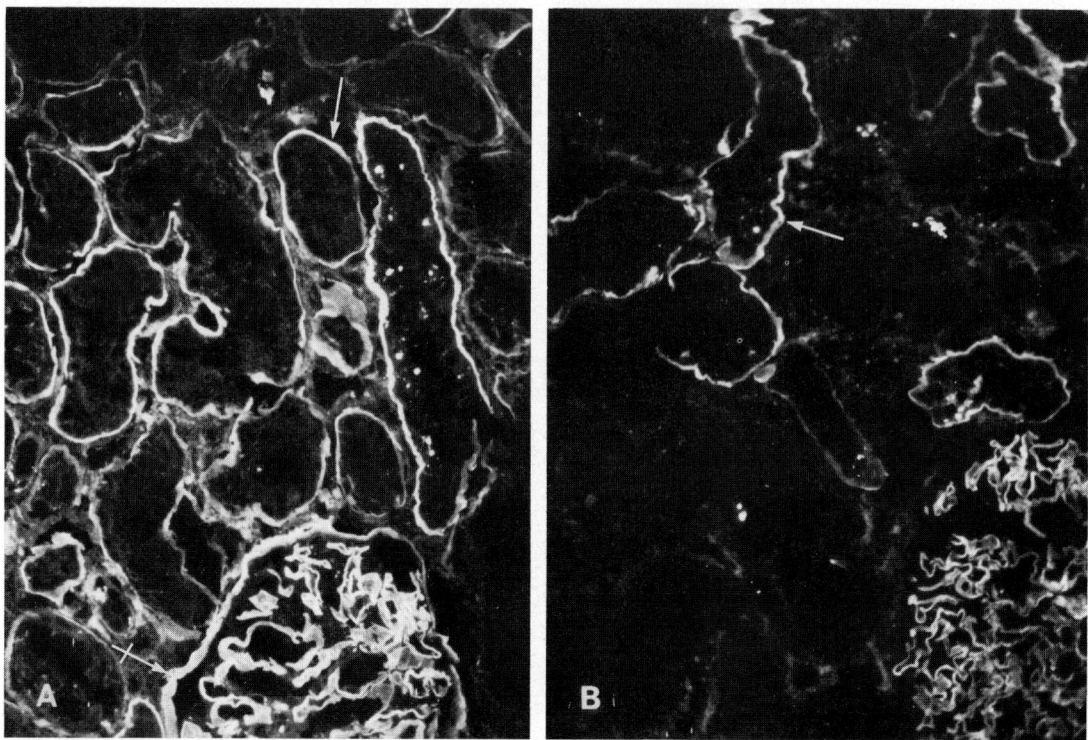

**Figure 29–11.** Varied anti-TBM reactivity in IgG eluted from kidneys of patients with anti-GBM GN. The two IgG eluates were tested on the same normal human kidney. Both eluates contained anti-GBM Ab. *A,* Generalized staining of TBM *(arrow)* and Bowman capsule *(hatched arrow)* are seen in one eluate. *B,* In another eluate only focal TBM reactivity was noted *(arrow).* (Indirect immunofluorescence, second antibody fluorescein isothiocyanate–conjugated antihuman IgG; original magnification × 160.)

as markers (if not involved in immunopathogenesis perhaps via activation of neutrophils). The ANCA associated with anti-GBM Abs is almost always of the P-ANCA or anti-MPO type. Some of the studies have shown a correlation between the presence of P-ANCA and extraglomerular vasculitis as well as with improved response to immunosuppression. IgM ANCAs have been associated with systemic vasculitis and pulmonary hemorrhage.[42, 43] Of interest, the mercuric chloride model of autoantibody induction in BN rats that develop anti-GBM Abs is also reported to develop an anti-MPO form of ANCA.[48]

Anti–basement membrane Abs (anti-GBM, anti-TBM, anti-ABM) produce linear IgG deposits along the respective basement membranes. IgG1 and IgG4 are relatively over-represented.[2328–2331] Although IgG1 predominates, a group consisting of predominantly females had high titers of IgG4 Abs reactive with the α3-chain of type IV collagen. Non-specific linear background accumulations of Ig must be excluded and may involve negatively charged Ig subclasses.[1, 2332] Elution studies to determine the specificity of any detected Ig are obvious adjuncts.[1] Rarely, IgA or IgM anti-GBM Abs are reported[1, 2333] and light chains with anti-GBM reactivity have been reported.[2334] Radioimmunoassay or enzyme immunoassays for circulating (or eluted) anti-GBM Abs have largely replaced indirect immunofluorescence assays.[1, 2335–2340] The relationship, if any, between anti-GBM Ab and the anti–epidermal basement membrane zone Ab seen in bullous pemphigoid is unclear[2341–2343]; however, localization of the pemphigoid Ags to chromosomes 6 and 10 instead of chromosome 2 would seem to separate

the two conditions.[2344–2346] Several assays have been devised for anti-GBM Ab, and the nephrologist needs to become acquainted with the sensitivity and specificity of the particular test being used to ensure needed reliability.

## NATURE OF GBM AGS INVOLVED IN ANTI-GBM AB–ASSOCIATED GN

Basement membranes lie adjacent to the cells that secrete them, providing support as well as contributing to function, with the GBM an integral portion of the glomerular filtration barrier.[3] In situ reverse transcription studies of the rat suggest that heparan sulfate proteoglycan and laminin S chain are produced by epithelial cells, and α1(IV) and α2(IV) collagen are present in endothelial cells.[2347] In this study, entactin and laminin A and B2 chains were found in all three glomerular cells and laminin B1 and fibronectin were present in mesangial cells. The GBM and adjacent glomerular capillary wall is a complex biochemical and antigenic structure.[3] It contains several collagenous and noncollagenous components, including type IV and type V collagen, laminin, heparan sulfate proteoglycan, entactin/nidogen, and amyloid P component.[3, 2348–2352] Indirect immunofluorescence studies using human anti-GBM Abs suggest a band of reactivity on the inner aspect of the membrane at a site also reactive with the Ab from sheep with Steblay nephritis,[2353, 2354] although Abs to both collagenous and noncollagenous Ags are reported in the sheep model.[2355] A similar localization was demonstrated using immunoelectron microscopy.[2356] The distribution of the reactive GBM Ag is altered by morphologic change in the glomerular capillary wall.[1479]

Using pepsin digests of basement membranes, Kefalides[2357] identified a type of collagen with a molecular weight greater than that found for interstitial collagens. This collagen, designated type IV,[2358] is thought to resemble in many respects a procollagen molecule that does not undergo conversion to collagen but interacts with matrix glycoproteins by means of hydrogen disulfide– and aldehyde-derived cross-links. The type IV collagen molecule is a triple helix composed of three $\alpha$-chains[2359] (Fig. 29–12). The individual $\alpha$-chains have a long collagenous domain of about 1400 residues of Gyl-Xaa-Yaa repeats. The collagenous domain is interrupted by 21 to 23 conserved short noncollagenous regions that may confer flexibility to the molecule. The $NH_2$-terminal region of the type IV molecule joins with three other type IV molecules via their 7S domains to form a tetramer.[2360] The 7S is a heavily cross-linked collagenous region that is resistant to collagenase. The COOH terminus is a noncollagenous region (approximately 230 residues) called the NC1 domain.[2361, 2362] It joins with the NC1 of another type IV molecule to form a dimer.[2363] The NC1 domain is highly conserved with retention of 12 cysteine residues among each of its six $\alpha$-chains. The overall structure is suggested to be a chicken wire–like mesh with additional interactions.[2364] The chains are glycosylated with hydroxylysine-linked disaccharide units along the collagenous region and with an asparagine-linked oligosaccharide unit near the $NH_2$ terminus.[2365–2367]

Currently, six type IV collagen $\alpha$-chains ($\alpha$1–6) with different tissue distributions and presumably functions have been identified. The most common type IV collagen isoform is $(\alpha 1)_2(\alpha 2)$ in its $\alpha$-chain composition. Complete sequences of the human as well as other species of $\alpha$1 and $\alpha$2 are available.[2368–2370] The genes for $\alpha$1 and $\alpha$2 are located head to head on chromosome 13, where they utilize a bidirectional promoter.[2371] This arrangement is not universal, because *Caenorhabditis elegans* has homologues present on different chromosomes.[2372] Two additional sets of paired $\alpha$-chain genes for $\alpha$3[2373–2376] and $\alpha$4 on chromosome 2[2377, 2378] and for $\alpha$5[2370, 2379–2381] and $\alpha$6 in the middle (Xq22 region) of the long arm of the X chromosome[2378] are arranged in a similar head-to-head fashion. This suggests that the genes evolved via duplication and inversion of the ancestral gene with subsequent divergence of $\alpha$1 and $\alpha$2, which in turn duplicated, leading to the three pairs currently identified. The chains fall into two classes of $\alpha$1-like ($\alpha$1, $\alpha$3, $\alpha$5) and $\alpha$2-like ($\alpha$2, $\alpha$4, $\alpha$6) subsets. With six $\alpha$-chains available, many possible arrangements of individual chains within the triple helix are possible. In addition to the usual $(\alpha 1)_2(\alpha 2)$ arrangement, $(\alpha 3)_2(\alpha 4)$ and homodimers $(\alpha 1)_3$ and $(\alpha 3)_3$ have been reported.[2349, 2382–2384] The distribution of the newly identified $\alpha$-chains is different from that of the ubiquitous $\alpha$1 and $\alpha$2 chains, with $\alpha$3, $\alpha$4, and $\alpha$5 chains more confined to GBM and segments of the TBM.[2380, 2385]

That nephritogenic Ags are evident in the glycoproteins remaining after collagenase digestion of the GBM has been shown by the ability of such extracts to absorb and block the indirect immunofluorescence reactivity of spontaneously occurring human anti-GBM Abs.[1, 2386] Similar Ags can be shown to react with human anti-GBM Abs by radioimmunoassay or immunoprecipitation in gel.[1, 2335, 2336] The collagenase digests of GBM also induce anti-GBM Abs; the nephrotoxic antigenicity of the digest is lost after pronase digestion.[1] The murine Engelbreth-Holm-Swarm sarcoma, which produces extracellular material resembling basement membrane collagen, reacts with human anti-GBM Abs[1, 2387, 2388]; however, a study did not find such reactivity and in addition noted that only $\alpha$1- and $\alpha$2-chains were present in the tumor.[2389]

In the late 1970s, we used immunoabsorbent techniques to recover two major Ag species that react with human anti-GBM Abs. These Ags are in the range of 54 and 27 kd, with some larger materials not well resolved on the gels used.[2390–2392] Peptide maps indicated a high degree of homology between the two major Ags, and amino acid analysis indicated absence of amino acids associated with collagen. These Ags have been recognized as monomers and dimers of the noncollagenous NC1 terminal region of type IV collagen.[2393, 2394] Subsequently, a 25-kd Ag was noted by others.[2395, 2396] An Ag recovered from collagenase-extracted GBM reacted with anti-GBM Abs from patients with Goodpasture syndrome, and guanidine hydrochloride produced Ags reactive with sera representing a variety of nephritides including IgA nephropathy and SLE.[2337] The reactive Ag in the collagenase extract was again found to be 26 kd.[2397] By immunoblotting, cationic 25- and 45-kd materials reactive with human anti-GBM Abs have also been found in collagenase digests of GBM, and heterogeneity in Ags reactive with human anti-GBM Abs was suggested.[2398] The development of a monoclonal Ab reactive with the same Ag that is detected by immunoblotting using human anti-GBM Abs suggests that commonality in Ags between patients is likely.[2166, 2399] Our own experiences with several hundred different human anti-GBM Abs and our immunopurified GBM Ags indicate that at least the approximately 54- and

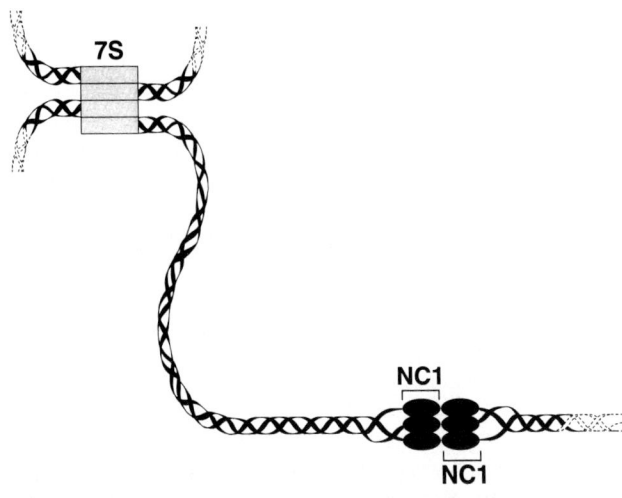

**Figure 29–12.** This schematic representation of the type IV collagen molecule depicts the triple-helical structure of the $\alpha$ chains, $\alpha$1 to 6(IV), in the long collagenous portion of the molecule with the 7S region near the $NH_2$ terminus involved in joining four similar molecules together. The noncollagenous NC1 region at the COOH terminus of the molecule is involved in joining with the NC1 region of another type IV collagen $\alpha$-chain. The NC1 domain of the $\alpha$3(IV) chain is the site of a major Ag in human anti-GBM Ab disease.

27-kd fractions carry Ag sites with common reactivity, although somewhat varying relative binding preference, in all patients studied.

Studies in the past several years have shown that the Ags reactive with anti-GBM antibodies reside in the NC1 domain of α3[2383, 2400-2402] and, to a lesser extent, α1 and α4, and that the reactive Ags may be absent from the GBM of individuals with Alport syndrome. Initially, as the structure of the GBM became better understood, the NC1 region of the type IV collagen was shown to harbor Ag reactive with human anti-GBM Abs,[2403, 2404] and it was suggested that the site may be localized in a novel chain of basement membrane collagen.[2405] The reactive site in the hexamer is reversibly dissociated by denaturation in 6 M guanidine or in acidic solutions, and, under these conditions, there is enhanced reactivity with ''Goodpasture Ab.''[2406] The density of the reactive epitopes in human NC1 exceeds that from the Engelbreth-Holm-Swarm tumor[2407] and is present in glomerular, lung, and placental basement membrane.[2408, 2409] The NC1 reactivity has been associated with experimentally induced anti-GBM Ab models.[1840, 1844] A radioimmunoassay for NC1 in body fluids has been described[2410] and Ab assay systems using NC1 are coming into use clinically.[2411] Some differences in the degree of cationic charge have been reported between the reactive 28-kd monomer recovered from human GBM and that from sheep GBM.[2412]

With denaturing polyacrylamide gel electrophoresis, monomers from 24 to 28 kd named M24, M26, M28+++, and M28+ (the last two 28-kd monomers separated by two-dimensional gel electrophoresis) were found corresponding to the NC1 regions of α2(IV), α1(IV), α3(IV), and α4(IV).[2412, 2413] The NC1 monomer most reactive with human anti-GBM Ab is M28+++ from α3(IV).[2394, 2405, 2414] Synthetic peptides constructed from the deduced amino acid sequence of the α3(IV) NC1 domain suggest that a region near the COOH terminus is a major epitope.[2415] Expression of the NC1 domains of human α1 to α5(IV) in *E. coli* was used to demonstrate strong reactivity of anti-GBM Abs with α3(IV) and to a lesser extent with α4(IV) and other NC1s.[2416] A reactive α3(IV) recombinant protein has been produced using the baculovirus expression system in Sf9 cells.[2417] Reactivity with the 7S domain of type IV collagen has also been suggested in occasional patients.[2418-2421] The exact clinical immunopathogenic potential of antibodies reactive with various regions has not yet been defined; however, one patient with a monoclonal Ab reactive with the α1(IV) had only mild disease, suggesting that differences may be found.[2422] Bovine ABM contains α3(IV) chains reactive with anti-GBM Abs, suggesting that the same Ag systems are present in the lung as well as in the kidney,[2423] a point confirmed by studies with human GBM and ABM.[2424] Serum NC1 levels are increased in some patients with nephritis, including one with Goodpasture syndrome.[2425] Sera from 57 patients positive for anti-GBM Ab as detected in our anti-GBM Ab radioimmunoassay were also studied collaboratively with a panel of the six bovine and recombinant human α(IV) chains. All samples positive by radioimmunoassay were also reactive with α3(IV). In 85% of the patients this was the sole reactivity and in the others 15% also reacted with α1(IV) and 3% with α4(IV).

The human α3(IV) gene has been cloned, and we and

others have shown that the mRNAs from the gene are alternatively spliced.[2376, 2426, 2427] While cloning the α3(IV) complementary DNA by polymerase chain reaction, we found one major (Q1) and two more minor (L5 and V) α3(IV) mRNAs in kidney RNA.[2428] Based on our genomic structure, L5 resulted from the deletion of exon 4 and V from the deletion of exon 2. L5 lacked a 183-residue segment that contained 11 of the 12 evolutionarily conserved cysteine residues, and the 11 carboxyl amino acid residues became a unique L5 peptide. The expected 27 carboxyl amino acid residues of V were substituted by a novel peptide of 51 residues. Bernal and colleagues[2426] reported that alternative splicing of this gene produced a product similar to our L5 and another spliced form lacking two exons. Our screening indicates developmental alterations in the ratios of our alternatively spliced mRNAs. The alternative splicing could control the amount of mature type IV collagen produced, as well as its interaction with normal molecules, because the conserved cysteine residues used for interchain interactions are altered. There is no direct evidence as yet that L5 and V are found in collagen molecules; however, if translated, they could contribute to the variable basement membrane antigenic expression found over the years in ''normal'' kidneys and lungs of humans and to the possible susceptibility to the autoimmune anti-GBM Ab response, as well as to some of the antigenic losses of patients with defective GBMs in Alport syndrome.

Differences in GBM (and TBM) Ags are present among individuals.[2429] For example, anti-TBM Ab can form after transplantation with a TBM Ag–negative kidney[2430] and also when no Ag differences are detected.[3] Lewis rats that carry Fischer 344 renal allografts produce Abs against one or more novel Ags of donor GBM and TBM.[2431] Some variation in GBM Ags (and biochemical structures) have been suggested during development.[2398, 2432-2435] Certain human anti-GBM Abs do not react with fetal kidney; however, the reactive Ag can be demonstrated after enzyme treatment.[2436-2438] Alport syndrome, a form of hereditary nephritis, involves defects in the type IV collagen chain.[2439] The Alport type of hereditary nephritis involves morphologic abnormalities in the GBM.[2440-2443] Some patients in certain kindreds with the disease lack the GBM Ags that typically react with human anti-GBM Abs.[2444-2448] In one large series, altered or absent α3 NC1 staining was found in 47 of 70 patients with Alport syndrome.[2449] The serum amyloid P component normally present in human GBM was also reported to be lacking in these patients.[2450] The GBMs of these patients stained normally with heterologous anti-GBM Abs, indicating the presence of many normal GBM components in spite of the probable selective lack of the novel α-chains reactive with anti-GBM antibodies, mainly α3 and α4. Certain monoclonal Abs reactive with Ags detected by anti-GBM Abs can be used to detect the missing GBM elements as well.[2451-2454] A monoclonal Ab, Mab A7, which reacts with α5(IV), does not react with GBM of patients in whom *COL4A5* mutations prevent incorporation of α5(IV) in the GBM.[2455] Transplantation-induced anti-GBM Abs reactive with a 26-kd NC1 peptide were also useful for detecting Ag defects.[2456, 2457] This antibody identified two of three families with Alport syndrome mapping to the Xq21-q22 region of the long arm of the X chromosome.[2458] Identification of reactive Ags in acid-urea–treated skin may be useful for screening family members in Alport-type familial nephritis in which a defect in NC1 is suspected.[2459] As glomeruli sclerose in Alport syndrome, they accumulate larger amounts of types V and VI collagen than do kidneys in those without Alport disease.[2460]

Two-dimensional gels have shown some heterogeneity of NC1 reactions, and anti-GBM Abs induced in familial nephritis by transplantation are less reactive with cationic fragments.[2398] The normal 28-kd NC1 monomers of GBM were absent in three males with Alport-type familial nephritis.[2461] Basement membrane defects may extend to the lens capsule.[2462] Studies indicate that the NC1 regions of α3(IV) and α4(IV) as well as α5(IV) chains are missing in collagenase-digested renal basement membranes from some patients with Alport syndrome,[2461, 2463] as well as exhibit different banding patterns.[2464] The transplantation-induced Abs are noted to react with a 26-kd Ag that may be the α5(IV) NC1[2465] and with α3(IV).[2466–2468]

Multiple mutations in type IV collagen α5 and α6 chain genes, *COL4A5* and *COL4A6*, have been found in X-linked forms of Alport syndrome.[2378, 2469–2488] These include major rearrangements and deletions as well as single-base mutations. The gene defect in the less frequent autosomal form of the disease is being sought and defects in the genes for α3 and α4 chains are likely candidates. The relationship between mutations in α5(IV) and absence of α3 or α4(IV), when detected, is unclear and could involve alterations in synthesis, abnormalities in assembly, or antigenic epitope masking or cleavage. Detection of α3 NC1 in DNA from six Alport syndrome patients (two had developed anti-GBM after transplantation) using a 75–base pair probe indicated that the gene was at least relatively intact.[2489] The hereditary nephritis of the Samoyed dog also lacks the Goodpasture Ag and may prove to be a useful model for study.[2490, 2491] A number of less well characterized forms of hereditary nephritis are found in various breeds of dogs.[2492] Other inherited diseases have defects in the GBM including thin basement membrane disease(s) and nail-patella syndrome. In thin basement membrane disease,[2493] the antigens reactive with anti-GBM sera are present but may be diminished.[2449, 2494, 2495] No defects in α1(IV), α2(IV), α3(IV), or α4(IV), B1e, B2e, or B2t chains of laminin or heparan sulfate proteoglycan core protein were found in congenital nephrotic syndrome of the Finnish type.[2496] Chemical toxicity may also affect renal basement membrane structure and can lead to renal cysts with changes in basement membrane component distribution.[2497, 2498]

The differences in GBM Ag content in patients with Alport syndrome can serve as alloantigens in renal transplantation.[2429, 2447, 2499–2501] As experience increases, it is clear that only a small minority (0% to 50%) of patients with Alport syndrome develop circulating or kidney-bound anti-GBM Abs after renal transplantation.[2502–2507] The true incidence of anti-GBM Ab in Alport syndrome induction by transplantation cannot be determined without information about the Ag defects in the native basement membrane, which vary among kindreds. In some instances the Abs are sufficient to induce rapidly progressive nephritis in the graft, resulting in its loss and problems of recurrence with subsequent transplantation attempts.[2508–2511] The Ab response is probably related in part to the degree and location of the defect in the genetically altered collagen and its relationship to α3 and α4 NC1, as well as the degree of immune presentation of the defects and ability of the individual to mount an immune response to the defective collagen, which may require a certain HLA makeup, as appears to be the case with spontaneous anti-GBM antibody formation.

## THE ANTI-GBM AB RESPONSE

Although a good deal is known about the participation of anti-GBM Abs in GN, we know little about the events that induce the anti-GBM Ab response. Its generally transient nature suggests that the stimuli may also be short-lived. Recurrence of the anti-GBM Ab response is infrequent.[1, 2, 2512–2514] Even after transplantation, recurrent anti-GBM Ab responses are unusual if transplantation is delayed until circulating Ab has disappeared. Three-year cadaveric graft survival, however, is among the lowest of all groups in one study.[2515] Post-transplantation immunosuppression may contribute, because at least one recurrence was seen in an immunosuppressed recipient of a kidney from an identical twin.[2293] Re-exposure to Ags identical to those in the native kidneys may also have contributed.

Genetic factors in anti-GBM antibody disease may be important, with a high frequency of HLA-DR2 found in such patients.[2516–2520] Severity is noted to be related to HLA-linked genes, particularly the HLA-B7 gene, and Ig Gm allotype associations and Ig subclass restrictions are also noted.[2328, 2329, 2518, 2521] Reports of the development of anti-GBM Ab–induced Goodpasture syndrome in identical twins are also of interest in this regard.[1, 2]

The association of anti-GBM Ab disease and HLA-DR2 has been dissected using DNA-HLA typing by restriction fragment length polymorphisms to split DR2 into DR15 and DR16, of which DR15 was found to be associated.[69] Using sequence-specific oligonucleotide probes, we found that all DR2 anti-GBM Ab disease patients were restricted to DRB1-1501 and DQB1-0602 alleles.[2522] We also found a highly significant association between the disease and the alleles of DRB1-0301 and DQB1-0201. The association of an aspartic acid at position 57 of the NQ β-chain suggested by Burns and colleagues[2519] was not confirmed in this study. The increase in the DR15, B1-1501 allele with some increase in B1-1502 was subsequently confirmed.[81] Susceptibility may be related to differential abilities of various HLA molecules to present self-Ags. Alternatively, the difference may serve only as a linked genetic marker to the true disease gene located in or near the MHC.

Several bits of information generate speculations about endogenous and exogenous factors that could be responsible for the induction of the anti-GBM response. Goodpasture's original description of pulmonary hemorrhage and GN developing after influenza suggests a possible causal relationship. However, evidence of concomitant influenza A2 viral infections is rare in a patient with anti-GBM Ab–induced Goodpasture syndrome.[1] Of interest, however, we have identified an area of linear amino acid sequence homology of SEGTGQA between the α3-chain NC1 domain and the influenza A hemagglutinin,[2427] suggesting a possible example of molecular mimicry in the disease induction.[2523, 2524] Cross-reactivity between human GBM or human urinary Ags and streptococci has been reported; however, there is little evidence to associate streptococcal infection with induction of anti-GBM Abs.[1, 2525] The cross-reactivity may be related in some manner to poststreptococcal GN and other GBM Ags.

Environmental exposures, particularly to hydrocarbons, are being examined in regard to their possible association with induction of anti-GBM Ab or other GN in some but not all studies.[1, 2, 2526-2528] For example, exposure to hydrocarbons such as perchloroethylene, used by dry cleaners, can produce renal abnormalities.[2529] In our own series, histories of extensive hydrocarbon exposure are infrequent (less than 5%), although detailed toxicologic surveys are not available. Case reports have coupled anti-GBM disease with trichloromethane, carbon tetrachloride, herbicides and insecticides, hard metal dust, and toluene sniffing with renal damage, with improvement sometimes related to avoidance.[2, 2530-2533]

Little good experimental evidence is available on hydrocarbon exposure; benzene and $N,N'$-diacetylbenzidine have been reported to induce glomerular injury, but anti-GBM Abs were not identified.[1] Carbon tetrachloride administration to rats and petroleum middle distillates given to mice caused renal injury but no report of anti-GBM Abs.[2] In studies in our laboratory, short-term (6-week) exposure to gasoline vapors did not induce anti-GBM Abs in rats or rabbits. Long-term gasoline vapor exposure of mice and rats has not caused anti-GBM Ab formation, even though renal tubule abnormalities and carcinogenesis were observed.[2534] If important, the noxious effects of chemical agents might be to expose or alter self-Ags, rendering them immunogenic. Alternatively, the environmental factors might act by altering the anatomic integrity of the basement membrane structures, particularly in the lung, so that circulating anti-GBM Abs induced by some unrelated event could then react with normally sequestered Ags, leading to immune injury. Drugs, notably methicillin and phenytoin, have been infrequently associated with development of anti–basement membrane Abs, particularly those reactive with the TBM.[1] An allergic rash after antibiotic treatment was seen in four of six cases of anti-GBM Ab diseases.[2535] Clinical Goodpasture syndrome has also been associated with penicillamine; however, anti-GBM Abs have been infrequently identified.[1, 2, 2536] Mercury toxicity in rats and rabbits has been associated with the development of antibodies having GBM reactivity.* The antigenic stimulus responsible for anti-GBM Ab production might also originate from the host, because endogenous cross-reactive GBM Ags are present in the circulation, urine, and tissues.[2] These Ags might be altered or reintroduced in such a way as to render them immunogenic, particularly if augmented by the adjuvant effects of a concurrent infection, terminating the normal state of immunologic unresponsiveness.

Physical injury to the GBM might also lead to anti-GBM Ab formation, as suggested by its development in patients with renal failure secondary to trauma-associated renal cortical necrosis, hydronephrosis, rejection, or lithotripsy or

---

*References 1864, 1867, 1876, 1910, 2537.

after IC GN, particularly membranous GN.[1, 2538-2544] The physical injury could expose the immune system to potentially immunogenic basement membrane fragments in the serum or urine.[2410, 2545] The observation that urine concentrates can be used experimentally to induce anti-GBM Abs in rabbits supports the possibility.[2546] A few patients who have anti-GBM Abs have had Hodgkin disease or another lymphoma.[1] A connection between lymphoid stroma and induction of anti-GBM Abs in clinical preparations of anti-lymphocyte globulin was previously noted.[1] As work progresses toward isolation, purification, and characterization of specifically involved basement membrane Ags, the mechanisms responsible for the induction of the anti-GBM Ab response should become clearer.

## PULMONARY INJURY IN ANTI-GBM AB–INDUCED GN

The association of pulmonary hemorrhage[2547] with anti-GBM Ab–induced glomerular disease (Goodpasture syndrome) and the fixation of IgG along the ABM with anti-GBM Abs elutable from the lung[1] suggest a common immunopathogenic mechanism. There is no clear-cut relationship between the level of circulating anti-GBM Ab detected by radioimmunoassay and the episodes of pulmonary hemorrhage, although hemorrhage does not usually recur after circulating anti-GBM Ab has disappeared. There is a greater tendency for circulating anti-GBM Abs from patients with Goodpasture syndrome to react in vitro with ABM Ags than with Abs recovered from patients with kidney involvement only (Wilson CB, unpublished observations). Studies suggest a variation in the NC1 monomer-dimer composition of the ABM as another possible explanation for the variable lung involvement in patients with anti-GBM Ab disease.[2548] The clinical episodes of pulmonary hemorrhage associated with anti-GBM Ab (with or without overt GN) often seem to be precipitated by some infectious or physiologic disturbance.[1, 2297, 2549-2552] Such events should be carefully sought and corrected for good treatment of patients.

It is currently thought that the events just noted may act to compromise the normal limited accessibility of the ABM Ag to the circulation and allow circulating anti-GBM Ab the opportunity to bind. This idea would help explain the episodic nature of pulmonary hemorrhage in anti-GBM Ab Goodpasture syndrome. These ideas are based on studies of animals in which circulating anti-GBM Ab that was capable of binding to ABM in vitro did not bind in vivo unless lung alterations were induced with oxygen toxicity, hydrocarbon-related injury, or cytokine infusions (IL-1 and IFN-$\alpha$).[1833-1835, 2553] An augmenting effect of cigarette smoke was less clear.[2554]

It has been hard to develop models of anti–basement membrane Ab forms of lung injury that mimic the severity of the pulmonary hemorrhage in Goodpasture syndrome. Broader (organ and species) basement membrane reactivity had been noted with anti-GBM Abs eluted from patients with Goodpasture syndrome than with GN alone; however, the Abs failed to bind to monkey lung when injected in vivo.[1] Anti-GBM Abs, however, were detected in patients whose clinical manifestations of anti–basement membrane disease were confined to the lung with a clinical presentation of pulmonary hemosiderosis.[1, 2297]

## Nephritogenic Immune Reactions in Humans Involving Other Glomerular Antigens

### AB REACTIVE WITH GLOMERULAR AGS

It is not clear how frequently reactions with glomerular Ags (structural or planted), other than the classic GBM Ag(s), will be identified in humans to parallel the model systems being defined in animals (see previous section). We have found one or possibly two human GN eluates that appear to react with glomeruli in normal kidney sections in an irregular nonlinear pattern, suggesting that such reactions may occur. Circulating antimesangial Abs have been reported in patients free of renal disease.[2555] Antimesangial Ab was also reported in the renal eluate of a patient with IgA nephropathy[2556] but not in others.[2557] Two Ags expressed on cultured mesangial cells were reported to react with IgG Abs in the serum of patients with IgA nephropathy as well as Schönlein-Henoch purpura.[2558] A number of antikidney, but not antiglomerular, Abs were described in eluates from cadaver renal allografts.[2559] Autoantibodies reactive with glomerular Ags were reported in mixed cryoglobulins from patients with renal involvement.[2560]

Antiendothelial Abs have been suggested in some patients with SLE.[2561, 2562] Glomerular endothelial damage was suggested to be the primary pathologic change in the renal lesion of Crow-Fukase syndrome (polyneuropathy, organomegaly, endocrinopathy, M protein, and skin changes [POEMS] syndrome).[2563] C-fixing anti–endothelial cell Abs have been found in patients with SLE, rheumatoid arthritis, mixed connective tissue disease, and hemolytic-uremic syndrome.[2561, 2564–2569] Antiendothelial Abs were also found in patients with diabetes mellitus, with the finding increasing with disease duration.[2570] The endothelium is also rich in HLA Ags as well as other Ags that can be involved in injury, particularly those associated with renal allograft rejection.[2571–2575] Anti–vascular endothelial cell Abs of the IgA class have also been identified in patients with IgA nephropathy.[2576, 2577] Autoantibodies reactive with Ags in or on cultured glomerular cells have been reported in sera from patients with Wegener granulomatosis.[2578] These Abs are associated with those reactive with Ags present in the cytoplasm of PMNs and monocytes.

Anti–tubule brush border Abs suggestive of those reactive with epithelial cell surface Ags in HN have infrequently been suggested in the circulation or renal eluates of nephritic patients or allograft recipients.[1, 2, 2579–2581] There is also little evidence to support a role for HN-associated brush border Ags in most patients with membranous GN.[1, 2579–2583] Kidney BE Ag was reported in a patient with membranous GN; however, antisera to this renal tubule Ag failed to stain glomeruli.[2584] Renal eluates containing brush border–reactive Abs have been reported,[2] in addition to direct staining of glomerular deposits[2] with heterologous

Abs prepared by immunization with crude Fx1A-type Ags. In our experience, the latter techniques can produce false-positive reactions if care is not taken to remove anti–serum protein Abs usually present in the heterologous anti-Fx1A Ab mixtures that can react with Ig or other IC-associated proteins. Renal lesions characterized by severe arteriolar endothelial swelling have been associated with IgM Abs reactive with the A549 epithelial cell line.[2585] Antiepithelial Abs detected using the A549 line have also been reported in pediatric transplant recipients.[2586] A patient with circulating Abs reactive with renal tubule brush border and small intestinal epithelial cells had enteropathy and membranous glomerulopathy.[2587] ICs containing human renal tubule epithelial Ags were reported to cause IL-1 release from peripheral monocytes taken from patients with GN.[2588] Monoclonal Abs prepared against glomerular Ags are being studied to help define possible nephritogenic Ags.[2177, 2178] The spontaneous rabbit GN Ag system, which is shared by human glomeruli, is also a candidate for this sort of study.

Patients with IgA nephropathy were reported to have circulating anti–basement membrane Abs reactive with structures located in the triple-helical part of type IV collagen.[2589] This reactivity has been ascribed to a fibronectin-IgA complex in the serum that binds to collagen via the collagen binding site of fibronectin.[2590] Abs reactive with laminin were also reported in IgA nephropathy.[2591] Entactin/nidogen has been suggested to be an Ag in certain patients with granular Ig deposits along their GBM.[2592, 2593] The role of antilaminin Ab noted in such diverse conditions as Chagas disease and preeclampsia remains to be defined.[1790, 2594] Similar Abs have been reported in systemic sclerosis.[2595]

### CROSS-REACTIVITY, MOLECULAR MIMICRY, AND AUTOIMMUNITY

Monoclonal Abs reactive with human glomeruli were reported to cross-react with streptococcal M protein,[2596] and Abs to laminin, type IV collagen, and glomerular heparan sulfate proteoglycan were noted in patients with poststreptococcal GN.[2597, 2598] A common amino acid sequence has also been reported to occur between a portion of the M protein of certain streptococci and human GBM.[2599] Monoclonal Abs raised to kidney tissue react with glomeruli and M proteins.[2596] The reactive Ag is a 43-kd protein present in mesangial cells and myocardium.[2600] Monoclonal Abs to group A type 12 streptococcal cell membrane react with both the streptococcal Ag and GBM Ag.[2601] Different M proteins were found to share epitopes with vimentin in glomerular mesangial cells.[2602, 2603] The possible role of streptococcal superantigen as well as cross-reactive streptococcal Ag in rheumatic disease and autoimmunity or connective tissue disease has been the subject of review.[2524, 2604, 2605] These findings of molecular mimicry suggest yet another possible manner in which Abs might form and react with glomerular Ags. The concept of molecular mimicry,[2606–2609] a definition of cross-reactivity of Ab based on sharing epitopes of amino acid sequence homology between two disparate molecules, needs to be considered as a mechanism of Ab reaction with glomerular Ags. For example, Candida albicans shares an epitope with adhesive epitopes on neutrophil CD11b/CD18.[2610] We have also noted a homologous area of seven amino acids in the primary structure of the α3(IV) chain of human GBM and a segment of the hemagglutinin of the influenza A virus, an infectious agent possibly associated with the onset of human anti–GBM Ab disease.[2427]

Autoantibodies in serum[2611–2614] and isolated from murine and human Ab-forming cells[2615–2617] have cross-reactivity (possibly molecular mimicry) with the glomerulus. In murine SLE, certain monoclonal anti-DNA Abs derived from MRL-*lpr/lpr* mice can bind directly to non-DNA Ags in the glomerulus.[2618–2620] Binding of this Ab appears to be directed to laminin.[2621] In humans with SLE, anti-DNA Abs have been shown to be cross-reactive with molecules containing backbones with diester-linked phosphate groups, including polynucleotides and cardiolipin; reactions of anti-DNA Abs with glomerular Ags such as proteoglycans and vimentin, as well as cell surface Ags on glomerular cells, have been reported.[2622–2627] Abs reactive with both DNA and heparan sulfate proteoglycan, a major GBM constituent, have been recovered by elution from kidneys of humans or mice with SLE.[2628] Infusion of mouse and human anti-DNA Ab into the isolated perfused rat kidney induces proteinuria; the effect is blocked by preabsorption of the Ab with DNA.[2629] Different patterns of immune deposit formation and glomerular response are seen with various monoclonal anti-DNA Abs, including mesangial immune deposit formation.[2630] Eluates from murine lupus and graft-versus-host diseased kidneys contain anti-DNA, histone, and laminin Abs with in vivo binding of the Abs from the eluates.[2631] The patterns of binding vary with the Ab composition. The exact contribution of these cross-reactive Abs to the immunopathogenesis of SLE remains to be defined. The binding of anti-DNA monoclonal Abs to cells may be related in part to cell-associated DNA.[2201, 2632, 2633] Abs to nucleosomal Ags become DNA reactive when complexed to nucleosomes, and these complexes can bind to GBM in part via heparan sulfate.[2634] In another study, monoclonal anti-DNA complexed to small DNA bound poorly to the glomeruli unless first complexed with core histones.[2635]

Anti–double-stranded DNA Ab from patients' sera as well as anticardiolipin Abs can inhibit proliferation of rat mesangial cells.[2097] Anti-C1q Abs purified from sera of patients with SLE react with human C1q that has been purposely localized in mouse glomeruli.[2636] Antithrombomodulin Abs in SLE patients were reported to correlate with serum creatinine levels and in turn might reflect renal endothelial cell damage.[2637] Anticollagen (types IV and V) Abs were reported in SLE sera.[2638]

The induction of autoantibodies in graft-versus-host disease may extend to human bone marrow transplants, in which membranous glomerulopathy has been associated with antinuclear Abs.[2639]

## TRAPPED AGS

The possibility of trapping Ags in glomeruli for subsequent nephritogenic reaction was discussed in an earlier section, and it was suggested that streptococcal or other infectious products as well as DNA might act in this way in model systems and perhaps also in humans.[1, 2194, 2219, 2223] For example, cationic streptococcal products have been reported in glomeruli early in poststreptococcal GN associated with Ig.[2225, 2226] Cationic materials derived from platelets and leukocytes have also been demonstrated to bind to glomeruli.[567, 954, 1061] Glycosylated collagen, as found in diabetes mellitus, has been reported to attract proteins that retain immunologic reactivity.[2640] The potential phlogogenic role of continued interaction of immune deposits with rheumatoid factors, anti-idiotypic Abs, and other ''secondary'' reactions must also be kept in mind.[1, 2270–2276] Anti-idiotypic Abs have been used to demonstrate cross-reactive idiotypes on mesangial Ig deposits and ICs in IgA nephropathy.[2641] Rheumatoid factors were suggested to play a role in lupus nephritis and perhaps in the mesangiopathic glomerular lesion of rheumatoid arthritis as well.[2642, 2643]

## NEPHRITOGENIC IMMUNE REACTIONS INVOLVING SOLUBLE ANTIGENS

### Experimental Immune Complex Glomerulonephritis

The previous section dealt with nephritogenic immune reactions in which Abs reacted with Ags expressed or otherwise fixed in the kidney. This section deals with nephritogenic immune reactions in which the Ag is present in the circulation, where it can interact with Ab to form an IC before reaching the kidney. Even in models in which good evidence exists for Ab binding directly to glomerular Ags, such as in AHN, a possible role for circulating ICs is also suggested.[1944]

In 1911, von Pirquet recognized the relationship between the host's immune response to foreign serum protein and the development of serum sickness.[1] During the 1950s, ICs in glomerular deposits and in the circulation were identified by the work of Germuth and associates and Dixon and colleagues as the toxic products of the immune response envisioned many years earlier by von Pirquet.[1] As noted earlier, the concepts of IC disease have been the focus of reevaluation and modification of thinking, particularly in the areas of dynamics of IC formation, factors that influence tissue accumulation, and continuing in situ modification, which may be influenced by properties of the Ag or Ab that may include some selectivity for localization in the glomerular capillary wall or blood vessels.*

When soluble Ags gain access to the vascular compartment they can combine with circulating Ab to form ICs, which may escape clearance by the mononuclear phagocyte system and then accumulate in vascular structures including the glomerulus (or tubulointerstitial tissues). The immune deposits can incite an inflammatory response utilizing the general mediation pathways described earlier that are activated when Ab reacts with a structural or planted glomerular Ag. The nephritogenic IC is in dynamic equilibrium with its Ag and Ab components and is constantly changing with the concentrations of each component in its immediate locale (either in the circulation or in tissue deposits).[1, 2, 2134, 2651] The dynamic interchange is compounded by the

---

*References 1, 2, 11, 12, 15, 16, 2644–2650.

presence of multiple Abs, often of different classes or subclasses, with different binding strengths (or affinities). The individual Abs react with one or more of the multiple different antigenic sites (or epitopes) present on most Ag molecules. The solubility of the Ag and its ability to diffuse away from the IC deposits change the dynamics of the local immune reaction compared with the situation with structural or other fixed Ags. It is apparent that overlap between the soluble IC mechanisms and the planted Ag mechanisms is influenced by the physicochemical attraction of the Ag (or Ab) for glomerular structures. No experiments have yet been devised to quantitate accurately the individual contributions of circulating IC deposition, dynamic interchange, and in situ formation of IC when circulating Ags with affinity for the glomerular capillary wall are involved.

## EXPERIMENTAL MODELS OF SERUM SICKNESS

### Acute (One-Shot) Serum Sickness

This classic model is the basis for the idea that circulating ICs can induce tissue injury. During the first 24 hours after the injection of a large amount of radiolabeled BSA into rabbits, about three fourths of the injected dose leaves the vascular compartment during equilibration with intra- and extravascular fluids[1] (Fig. 29–13). The circulating BSA then is lost, with a half-disappearance time of about 4 days. Anti-BSA Ab is detectable by day 4 to 5 and is completely complexed to the circulating excess BSA. The initial BSA–anti-BSA ICs formed in the presence of great Ag excess

are small, are not easily phagocytosed, and continue to circulate. As Ab production increases, the Ag/Ab ratio decreases and the circulating ICs increase to sufficient size by day 10 or so to be eliminated from the circulation by the mononuclear phagocytic system. During this immune elimination phase, small amounts of IC deposit within glomeruli and vascular structures to initiate GN, arteritis, endocarditis, and synovitis; ICs can also deposit in the choroid plexus.[1] A portion of the circulating ICs at immune elimination are cold insoluble.[2] Glomerular deposition is presumably related to IC size, possibly to characteristics of the Ab response, and potentially to vascular permeability induced by vasoactive substances released in conjunction with the immune reaction.[1] C fixation occurs concomitantly with the immune elimination phase; however, the glomerular inflammation in the rabbit (but not the vasculitic lesion) is C and PMN independent, as shown in depletion studies.[1] Instead, monocyte-macrophages are the major infiltrating cells, and the glomerular lesion can be blocked with an antimacrophage serum.[1, 592] A role for T cells has been suggested,[2652] and migration inhibition factor, a lymphokine involved in monocyte-macrophage accumulation, has been found in supernatants of glomeruli from rabbits with acute serum sickness.[659] Activation of leukocytes and perhaps glomerular cells via systemic administration of phytohemagglutinin enhances the glomerular lesion in acute serum sickness.[113]

Quantitative studies of acute serum sickness show that about 20 μg of IC BSA ($4.4 \times 10^8$ molecules per glomerulus) deposits in the kidneys of rabbits with the most rapid immune elimination; the half-disappearance time of the bound BSA from the kidney is about 10 days.[2653] The glo-

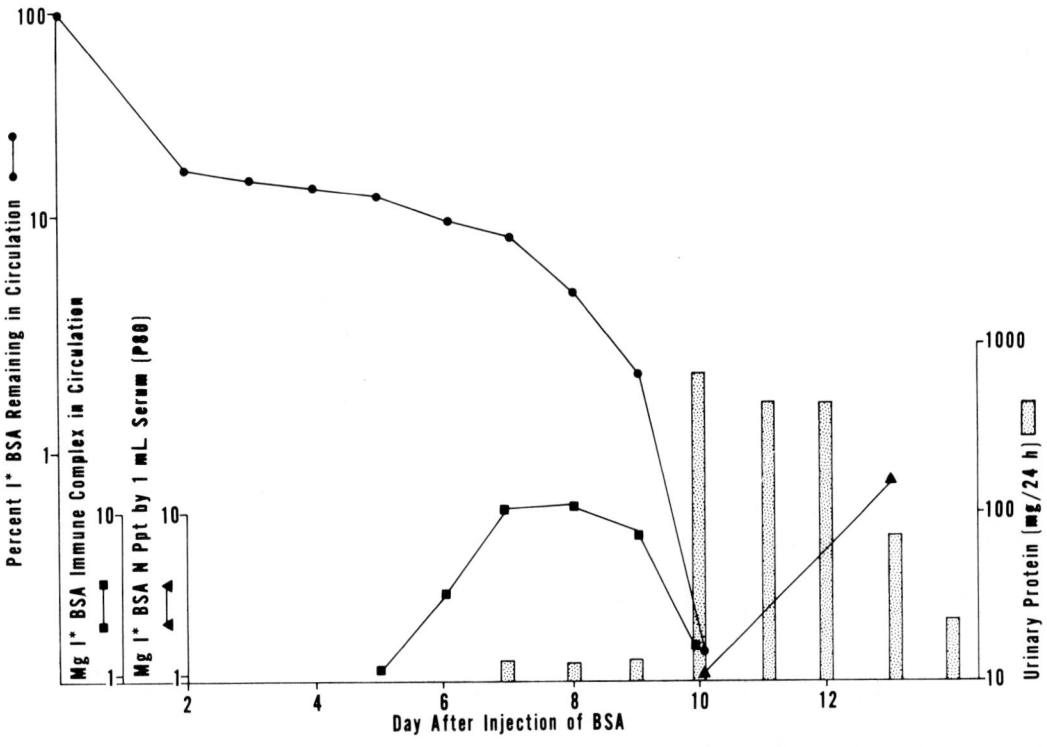

**Figure 29–13.** The fate of 750 mg of radioiodine (I*)-labeled BSA is shown after intravenous administration in a 3-kg rabbit. The I* BSA (●—●) rapidly equilibrates with the intra- and extravascular fluids and then disappears at its catabolic rate until eliminated in conjunction with IC formation (■—■) about day 10. Transient proteinuria commences with immune elimination, the latter followed by the appearance of free circulating anti-BSA Ab (▲—▲).

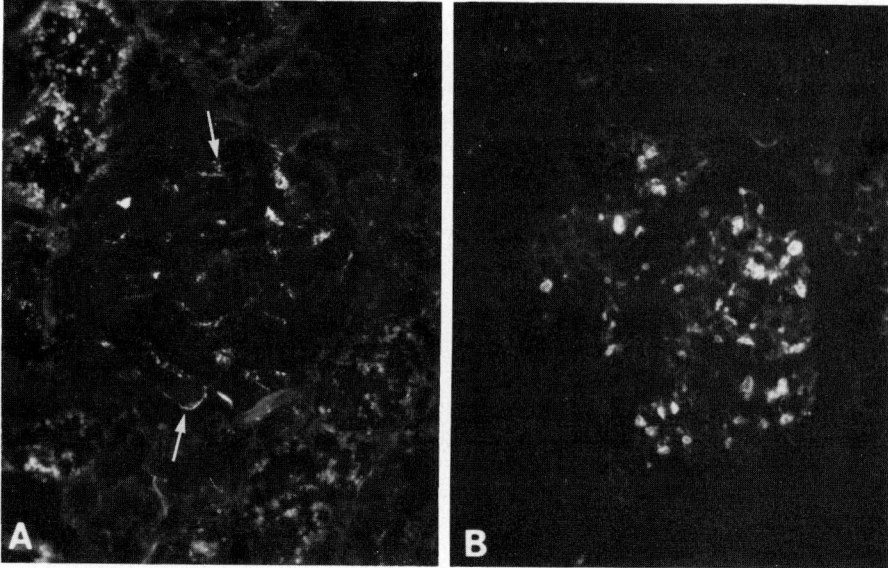

**Figure 29–14.** Glomerular IC deposits in BSA-induced acute serum sickness in rabbits. *A.* Fine granular deposits of IgG *(arrows)* are seen along the GBM at the time of immune elimination when proteinuria begins and is most severe. *B.* Seven days later in the same rabbit the IgG deposits have become more prominent as circulating anti-BSA Ab continues to accumulate on the previously deposited IC. (Fluorescein isothiocyanate–conjugated antirabbit IgG Ab; original magnification × 250.)

merular IC accumulations are seen by immunofluorescence as fine granular deposits of Ig, C, and BSA (Fig. 29–14*A*). Free anti-BSA Ab that appears in the circulation after immune elimination can bind to the glomerular IC deposits, and the IgG and C3 in the IC deposits can be detected by immunofluorescence increase for a few days after immune elimination of the Ag[1] (Fig. 29–14*B*). This increasing accumulation of Ig renders the persisting BSA less detectable by immunofluorescence.[1] Such a reaction demonstrates that IC deposits are not static but are continually modified by Ab (or Ag) from the circulation. Of interest, the increasing Ig and C accumulation occurs during the time the short-lived inflammation is resolving.[1]

### Chronic (Daily Injection) Serum Sickness

Rabbits immunized daily with foreign serum proteins (most often BSA) for periods of 5 to 8 weeks develop GN similar in many respects to human GN.[1] Rabbits with poor immune responses or given inadequate amounts of Ag to balance active Ab responses do not develop GN. Nephritogenic ICs form only in rabbits given sufficient amounts of Ag to balance their individual level of Ab production. The ratio between amounts of Ag and Ab, not the absolute amount of either, determines the formation of nephritogenic IC. Alterations in Ab response induced by immunosuppression would be expected to affect nephritogenicity, depending on the relative levels of Ab and Ag dose.[2654]

During daily injection before the onset of proteinuria, a mean of about 50 μg or about 0.04% of the daily dose of 50 to 200 mg of BSA deposits in the kidney. Concomitant with and after the onset of proteinuria, the deposition increases to a mean of about 600 μg, representing about 0.5% of a similar daily dose.[2655] The half-disappearance time of the glomerular BSA deposits is about 5 days and can be hastened by administration of Ag excess to dissolve the glomerular IC deposits.[2655] By immunofluorescence, the quantitative increase in deposition at or near the onset of proteinuria can be correlated with a shift in the location of IC deposits from the mesangium to the glomerular capillary

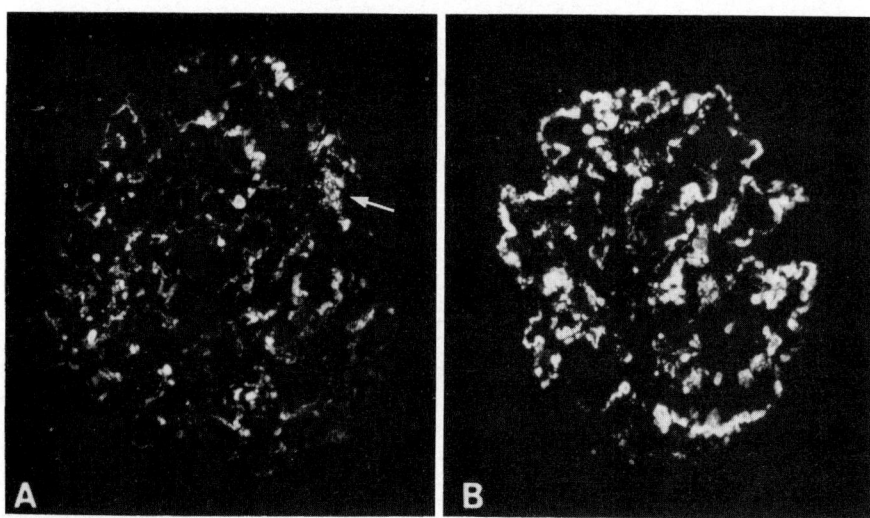

**Figure 29–15.** Glomerular IC deposits of BSA develop slowly in a rabbit with BSA-induced chronic serum sickness. *A.* During the 6 to 8 weeks of daily injection required for induction of GN, the deposition of IC is largely confined to the mesangium *(arrow).* *B.* One week later, during which proteinuria developed, the IC deposition has shifted to the GBM. IgG, BSA, and C3 are present in identical patterns. (Fluorescein isothiocyanate–conjugated anti-BSA; original magnification × 250.)

wall (Fig. 29–15). The histologic lesions of chronic serum sickness are varied (Fig. 29–16), resembling different forms of human GN, and may change during the course of the lesion.[1, 2656] The lesion often leads to progressive glomerular changes including sclerosis, with death resulting from renal failure. The granular IC (Ab, Ag, C) deposits seen by immunofluorescence are also detectable as electron-dense deposits by electron microscopy.[1] With newer electron microscopic techniques, the deposits can be seen among the fibrils of the GBM and the mesangial matrix structure.[2657] Glomerular epithelial cells can endocytose the IC material in models and in humans.[2658–2660]

The majority of the IC deposits occur in the glomerulus; however, in some rabbits, particularly those with active immune responses given correspondingly large amounts of Ag, extraglomerular (TBM and interstitium) and extrarenal (including lungs, spleen, serous membranes, and ciliary body) IC deposits may occur as well[1] (Fig. 29–17). These observations are similar to those in humans with SLE who develop interstitial and tubule immunologic renal injury associated with IC deposits in the tubulointerstitial area. These extrarenal deposits have also been quantitated.[2661] A model using a trapped Ag, Con A, has been suggested as useful for the study of the clearance of immune deposits from the peritubular capillaries.[2662] Clearance studies of interstitial deposits have also been done using the Tamm-Horsfall model in rats.[2663]

Although many of the chronic serum sickness experiments have been performed in rabbits, repeated injections of foreign proteins also induce GN in rats and mice,[1, 2664–2670] as well as in chickens and cats.[2671–2673] The chronic serum sickness model has also been duplicated in

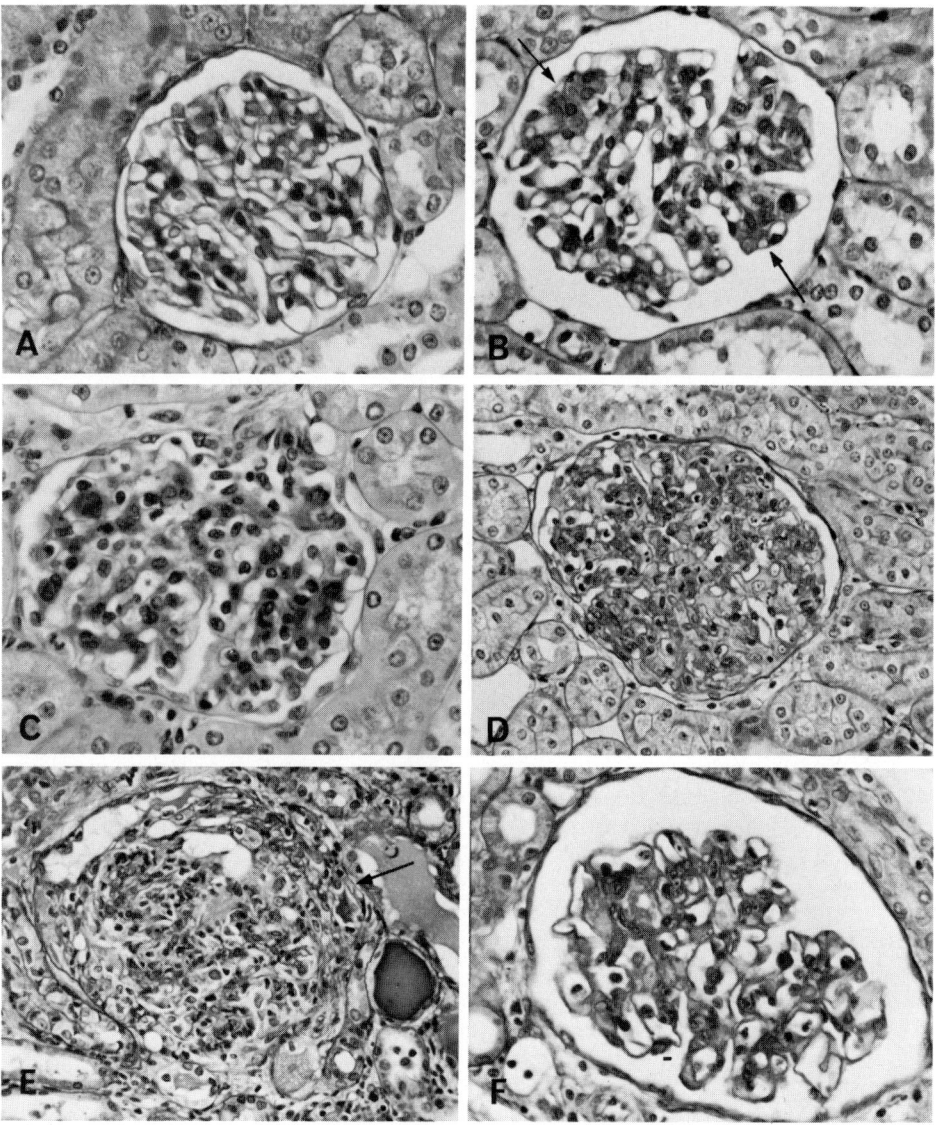

**Figure 29–16.** A wide variety of histologic forms of GN are observed in BSA-induced chronic serum sickness in rabbits. *A.* A normal glomerulus is shown. *B.* Focal mesangial hypertrophy *(arrows)* is the first abnormality encountered. *C* and *D.* Proliferative GN of varying severity is the most common lesion. *E.* Rapidly progressive proliferative crescent-forming *(arrow)* GN is also frequently found. *F.* Purely membranous GN is also seen in some chronic serum sickness rabbits. (Original magnification × 215.)

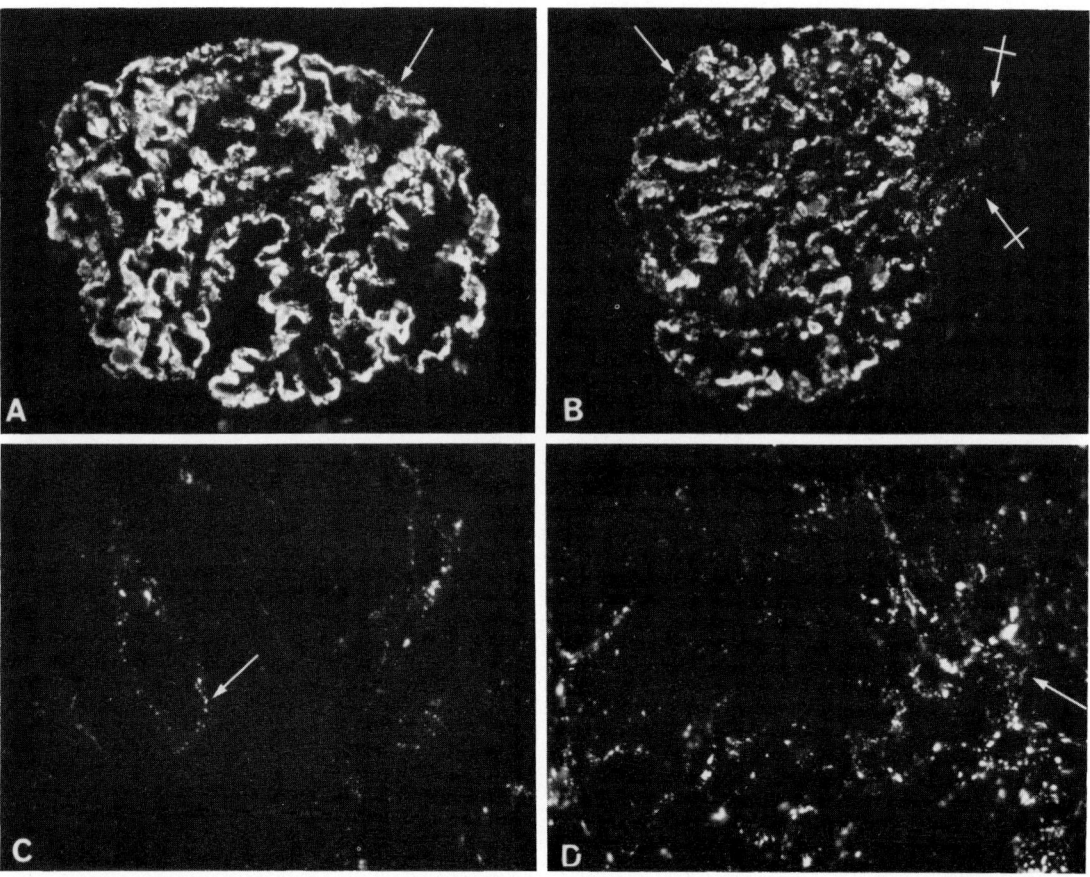

**Figure 29–17.** Renal and extrarenal IC deposits in BSA-induced chronic serum sickness. *A.* Heavy coarse granular deposits *(arrow)* are present along the GBM. *B.* Granular deposits *(arrow)* are seen along the GBM with slight but definite granular deposits seen in the afferent arteriole *(hatched arrows). C.* Fine granular deposits are also seen along the TBM *(arrow)* of rabbits with active immune responses requiring large amounts of daily BSA to balance Ab production. *D.* Extrarenal IC deposits can also be found as seen here in the splenic pulp. IgG, BSA, and C3 are present in identical patterns. (Fluorescein isothiocyanate–conjugated anti-BSA; original magnification × 250.)

the cynomolgus monkey.[2674, 2675] Progressive glomerulosclerosis has been described in chronic serum sickness in the rat.[2676] The uptake of BSA has been quantitated in rats.[2677] The clearance of macromolecules decreased during immunization, and PMNs were suggested to play a role in handling complexed Ag, particularly in the lung.[2678–2680] The onset of proteinuria in the rat model was noted to occur with the disappearance of precipitating Ab from the circulation.[2681] Proximal tubule dysfunction has been noted in the rat model.[2682] Using large Ags such as thyroglobulin to cause serum sickness results in predominantly mesangial lesions in rabbits; however, small Ags such as ovalbumin induce glomerular dysfunction without evidence of IC localization.[1, 2683] In addition, DNA treated with ultraviolet light has been used as an Ag and increased nephritogenicity if it was sonicated to reduce its size.[2684, 2685] Ferritin, another large Ag, also causes a predominantly mesangial lesion after prolonged administration in mice.[1, 2686] In mice, apoferritin administration leads to GN, with the histologic pattern related to the dose and immune response of the strain used.[2687–2690] Therapeutic benefits reported after treatment with PGE$_1$ or PGE$_2$ in serum sickness in mice were related to alteration in Ab production.[2691–2693]

Infusion of ICs performed in vitro usually causes only

mild and transient glomerular injury in mice and rats.[1] The major criticisms of the preformed IC models have been of their variable reproducibility and the different glomerular sites of IC localization (predominantly mesangial) compared with the active models. Some studies, however, have suggested greater glomerular capillary wall localization and more severe and characteristic histologic lesions of serum sickness.[2694–2696] Care must be taken in analyzing the results of experiments using preformed ICs because the contribution of dynamic interchange is largely lacking in this situation. In addition, any physicochemical interactions of the Ag (or Ab), such as charge differences, with the glomerular capillary wall would alter the kinetics and possibly the location of in vivo deposition.

### IgA Models of IC GN

IgA nephropathy, characterized by mesangial IgA, C3, and often IgG deposits, is one of the most common forms of human GN. The immunopathogenesis of human IgA nephropathy is incompletely understood[2697–2708] and is addressed in detail in Chapter 31. Major features include abnormalities in the control of IgA production, with increases in polymeric IgA predominantly of bone marrow and tonsillar rather than mucosal origin. The material accumulates in the mesangium and may represent ICs, other macromolecular species, rheumatoid factors, and complexes with fibronectin. Ags from food and mucosal infectious agents as well as glomerular structures are suspected but infrequently proved in individual patients.

Active and passive models of glomerular IgA deposition as models of human IgA nephropathy have been developed and the possible IC mechanisms reviewed.[2709–2714] IC formed in vitro or in vivo using DNP-conjugated BSA and IgA MOPC-315 myeloma anti-DNP Ab deposits in glomeruli when the IgA is polymeric.[2715–2717] Monomeric IgA is normally removed more slowly from the circulation.[2718] The glomerular deposits of polymeric IgA and Ag were able to react with monomeric IgA from the circulation.[2719] C activation by the glomerular IC was suggested to relate at least in part to the nature of the Ag used to produce the IC.[2720] In mice given IgA, anti-DNP Ab and DNP conjugated with IgA antiphosphorylcholine Ab glomerular deposits could be made more phlogogenic by administration of phosphorylcholine-conjugated molecules as a way of trapping the molecules in the glomerulus.[2721] Phosphorylcholine-conjugated pneumococcal C polysaccharide was more phlogogenic than either Ficoll or BSA. Mesangial deposits of IgA after administration of TEPC-15 hybridoma–derived IgA antiphosphorylcholine and phosphorylcholine conjugated to different molecules were enhanced by maneuvers to induce proteinuria.[2722]

The hematuria associated with IgA nephropathy induced by oral immunization is thought to be C dependent.[2723] Systemic administration of dextran (a carbohydrate Ag) produced a proliferative mesangial lesion with IgA deposition.[2724, 2725] Oral dextran administration is also effective.[2726] Polycationic diethylaminoethyl dextran and myeloma-derived murine IgA antidextran Ab produced ICs that localized in mesangial areas.[2727] In a passive model of dextran sulfate and monoclonal antidextran IgA or IgM nephropathy, dextranase treatment reduced mesangial Ig or dextran deposits.[2728] In the same study, in the active dextran immunization model, dextranase and protease attenuated the glomerular lesion.

Oral administration of protein Ags results in an IgA immune response and glomerular deposition without morphologic changes.[2729] Oral immunization with ferritin was suggested to cause a nonspecific increase in circulating IgA and glomerular deposition without detected Ag.[2730] Oral immunization with gluten or its lectin-like fraction, gliadin, in addition to ovalbumin or human gamma globulin, induced mesangial IgA deposits in mice.[2731] Antigliadin IgA Abs were found in renal eluates of gluten-immunized mice but were also found in control mice, apparently related to gluten in regular mouse chow. Addition of colloidal carbon to impair mononuclear phagocytic function enhances the development of glomerular deposits after oral administration of lactalbumin.[2732] Clearance of IgA aggregates from the glomerulus is more prolonged than that of IgG aggregates in spite of similar initial uptakes, a finding that should be given consideration in weighing the phlogogenic contributions of IC deposits based on residual glomerular findings.[2733] Injections of N-nitrosodimethylamine or D-galactosamine increase serum IgA levels in rats and are associated with glomerular IgA deposits.[2734]

Extended oral exposure to trichothecene vomitoxin (deoxynivalenol), a fungal contaminant of cereal grains, induces increased serum IgA levels, Abs to bacterial and self-antigens, and mesangial IgA deposits without C3 in the B6C3F1 mouse.[2735, 2736] Strain and sex differences were reported.[2737] Hybridoma clones from Peyer patches of vomitoxin-fed BALB/c mice react with a variety of self- and nonself Ags.[2738] IgA eluted from glomeruli of the vomitoxin-fed mice reacted with inulin, DNA, and casein.[2739] Spontaneous glomerular deposition of IgA has been described in aging ddY mice that also have mammary and/or lymphoid neoplasia.[2740] The glomerular deposit correlates with increasing serum IgA levels. The more acidic IgA among the polyclonally expanded IgAs in the old ddY mice, as well as the polymeric form, is suggested to lead to glomerular mesangial deposits in studies of glomerular eluates.[2741] Glomerular complexes composed of retroviral gp70 as well as histones have been reported in separate studies of these mice.[2742, 2743] The antihistone reaction is similar to that seen in murine lupus nephropathy, but in the ddY mouse it occurs in the absence of anti-DNA Ab. The presence or absence of gp70 is said to vary with the substrain of the ddY mouse and is not essential for IgA deposition.[2744] The glomerular mesangial deposition of IgA in the ddY mouse was accelerated by injection of sheep anti–type IV collagen antiserum, which was reported to delay mesangial transport of heterologous IgA.[2745]

Morphometric studies indicate a progressive increase in glomerular extracellular matrices in ddY mice without a decrease in glomerular anionic sites.[2746] The steady-state mRNA for α1(IV); laminin A, B1, and B2; and heparan sulfate proteoglycan increased with age and IgA deposition in the ddY mouse.[2747] In this study, the authors noted no increase in T cells or macrophages in glomeruli of the mice. The PDGF A and B chain mRNA expression in the ddY mice increased only slightly with age, compared with a large increase in murine lupus nephropathy.[1574] A rat anti–murine CD4 monoclonal Ab was reported to reduce glomerular IgA deposits in the ddY mouse without affecting serum IgA levels.[2748] In spite of somewhat lower glomerular IgA deposits, no changes in the rate of ECM accumulation were noted after the anti-CD4 Ab treatment of ddY mice.[2749] Neonatal thymectomy was also noted to lessen glomerular IgA deposition without altering serum IgA levels.[145] Spontaneous IgA nephropathy has also been reported in dogs.[2750]

A model of IgA nephropathy in response to Sendai virus infection has characteristics resembling the exacerbations of IgA GN seen in humans in association with respiratory infections.[2751] Natural infection or mucosal immunization with Sendai virus and intravenous challenge with various virus preparations induced glomerular IgA, IgG, IgM, and Sendai virus deposits.[2752] The physical form of the viral Ag used to challenge the mice was related to functional changes in the model.

Normal hepatic clearance of IgA ICs with transport into the bile[2753, 2754] may be related to glomerular accumulation of IgA in experimental carbon tetrachloride–induced liver damage[2755–2757] and after bile duct ligation.[2758] Rats with liver damage induced with lipotrope-deficient and oral alcohol have IgA in their hepatic sinusoids, suggesting impaired transport from blood to bile, and also have mesangial IgA deposits.[2759] In the latter model, the glomerular deposits were characterized by the presence of secretory component. Bile duct ligation enhances glomerular localization of IgA ICs, again with secretory component, after oral administration of protein Ags.[2760, 2761] These observations may help explain the glomerular IgA deposits in patients with alcoholic cirrhosis and in biliary atresia, in which secretory IgA is present in glomerular deposits.[2762]

## FACTORS INFLUENCING ACCUMULATION, REARRANGEMENT, AND REMOVAL OF GLOMERULAR IC DEPOSITS

Multiple interrelated factors appear to be responsible for localization of ICs in the glomerulus,[1] which is a large-volume ultrafilter that seems particularly predisposed to deposition of ICs even when they are present in low levels in the circulation. Delivery of ICs to the glomeruli is influenced by blood flow and the efficiency of systemic mononuclear phagocytic clearance versus the rate of IC production. Hydraulic pressure, glomerular permeability, IC size, Ab affinity, preceding glomerular damage, and clearance by the mesangial region contribute in varying degrees. As noted earlier, continuing intrarenal modification of IC deposits takes place in situ by interaction with Ag, Ab, or additional IC from the circulation. To illustrate the importance of these intrarenal features, we transplanted normal kidneys alongside nephritic kidneys in rabbits with ongoing chronic serum sickness GN. Using quantitative methods, we found only minimal uptake of IC by each normal kidney at a time when IC accumulation in the nephritic kidney was nearly maximal.[2763]

The in situ interaction of ICs with their individual components was found in experiments mentioned earlier, in which glomerular IC deposits in rabbits with acute serum sickness were shown to accumulate Ig (and C) and then enlarge after immune elimination.[1] In chronic serum sickness, free BSA binds to the glomerular IC deposits. To demonstrate this, the IC-containing kidney was first transplanted into a nonimmune host to exclude circulating anti-BSA Abs that could lead to further IC formation.[2763] Alternatively, an in situ perfusion model was used to exclude formation of additional ICs; in this perfusion model the interchange of Ag (or Ab) was related to the relative Ab (or Ag) "excess" of the glomerular IC deposits (Wilson CB, unpublished observations). Similar results are found in rat chronic serum sickness kidneys during isolated perfusion ex vivo to exclude additional IC formation.[2764]

Administration of a huge excess of Ag results in dissolution of glomerular deposits in rabbits with chronic serum sickness.[1] Amounts of BSA greater than 1 g/d cause a fivefold increase in the disappearance rate of glomerulus-bound IC Ag.[2655] Administration of an Ag excess to rabbits with chronic serum sickness has been reported to be beneficial[1] and, if given in proper regimens, Ag excess dissolves IC deposits, as demonstrable by both immunofluorescence and electron microscopy. Histologic and functional abnormalities of GN subsequently disappear. In addition to dissolving glomerular IC deposits, Ag excess

therapy also inhibits further Ab production, thereby reducing any additional IC formation (Wilson CB, unpublished observation). The effects of Ag excess in removing glomerular IC deposits have also been shown in passive and active IC disease in mice.[2765, 2766] The interaction of glomerular IC with circulating IC components, enhancing glomerular IC accumulation, has also been reported using a planted Ag aggregate type of model.[2767-2769] The dissolution of IC by Ag excess treatment can be shown to be Ag specific in multiple Ag IC models.[2770] Periods of Ag excess were suggested to correlate with improvement in renal function in a patient with IC nephritis associated with hepatitis B surface Ag.[2771]

It has been shown that covalently cross-linked ICs that cannot rearrange do not persist in the glomerular capillary wall, in comparison with their dissociable counterparts.[2772] In contrast, hapten-substituted covalent ICs of 550 kd do bind, perhaps because of hapten interaction with the glomerular capillary wall.[2773] Continued interaction or "condensation" of the IC into progressively larger deposits was also suggested to be involved in the retention of IC in the glomerulus.[2774] Precipitating Ag-Ab systems are thought to foster this condensation, particularly in the subepithelial region, although the highly substituted Ags employed may have contributed via selective binding.[2775]

In an extension of the in situ modification concept, glomerular IC in the circulation or in deposits can be a target for anti-idiotypic Ab or rheumatoid factor, which in turn can bind more ICs from the circulation.[2271, 2643, 2776-2782] Abs reactive with C, such as C3NeF, could also contribute.[309] Autoantibodies to human C1q are observed in systemic and renal diseases and such Abs purified from the serum of patients with SLE bind to human C1q-containing IC placed in mouse glomeruli.[2636, 2783] These types of secondary Ab interactions might also be important in changing the dynamic interchange of the glomerular IC deposit by cross-linking individual Ab molecules, by steric hindrance, or by other physical effects. For example, rheumatoid factor can bind to glomerular IC deposits in murine models and may retard Ag-induced, in vitro dissolution of IC deposits with Ig in kidneys from patients with SLE.[2779, 2784-2786] Purposeful immunizations of rabbits with physicochemically altered homologous IgG of defined allotype induced antiallotypic as well as rheumatoid-like factor activity and glomerular immune deposits of autologous IgG.[2787]

The in situ interaction and modification of glomerular ICs would be influenced by a number of features that have not yet been studied in quantitative detail. The affinity of the Ag-Ab reaction in the IC would influence the degree to which interchange could proceed. The location of the IC and the concomitant inflammatory response, including morphologic, hemodynamic, and physiologic disturbances in its microenvironment, would also be expected to alter interchange. Physicochemical properties, such as charge of the IC components, which might contribute to glomerular capillary wall binding, would affect the diffusion of the IC components away from the glomerular capillary wall. The charge interaction concept transcends Ab formation because injection of two non-Ab charged molecules that can interact can cause a glomerular lesion.[2788]

The finding that infusion of proteolytic enzymes enhanced cationic bovine gamma globulin IC disappearance suggests a role for enzymes released as part of the mediation of inflammation.[2789] When the enzymes are targeted to the GBM, the ameliorative effects appear to be enhanced.[2265] PMN elastase was also reported to alter IC structure.[2790]

As noted earlier in the discussion of planted nephritogenic Ags, the charge interaction of cationic Ags (or Abs) with the polyanionic glomerular capillary wall has drawn considerable interest (see Fig. 29–9). The model systems have employed cationized Ags* for reaction with actively formed or passively administered Ab or to produce preformed IC for study in vivo. Cationic Ags may lead to somewhat different Ab responses and IC characteristics than their native counterparts.[2792–2795] For example, cationic BSA is reported to have a 50% reduction in $\alpha$-helical content compared with the native molecule.[2796] A cationic region in a molecule with net anionic charge may be sufficient to bind to the glomeruli.[2797]

Cationic Ag containing preformed IC can bind to subepithelial and subendothelial anionic sites.[2798, 2799] The removal rates are more rapid from subendothelial than subepithelial sites.[2800, 2801] As might be expected, passive Ab or stimulation of the immune response to the cationic Ag slows its removal from the GBM.[2802, 2803] The site of binding can have a substantial effect on the subsequent inflammatory response.[2804] Translocation of Ag across the GBM occurs in close association with Ab.[2805] Cationization shifted low-molecular-weight dextran IC deposits from mesangium to glomerular capillary wall.[2727] The possibility of dissociation and local glomerular reformation of the passive IC was addressed by demonstrating glomerular binding of nondissociating cationic IC.[2806] ICs containing cationized Ab, when in a large lattice, bind and persist in glomeruli in subepithelial locations.[2807] Studies have suggested that a small proportion of cationic Abs in ICs is sufficient to cause binding to the glomeruli.[2808] The enhanced subendothelial and subepithelial deposition of cationic Ag-containing ICs was shown to be independent of Fc binding by using Ab fragments.[2809] Anionized Abs in preformed ICs bound in the mesangial areas; ICs containing cationized Ags bound to endothelial areas, moving later to mesangium and subepithelial positions.[2810] Precipitating IC systems are required to cause deposits to exceed those of cationized Ag alone.[2775] It can also be shown that ICs containing cationized Abs deposit in the glomerulus much more easily than the cationized Abs alone.[2811] Only the initial binding of cationic ICs is mediated by charge interactions, with the IC interacting to form larger aggregates that are difficult to displace by administration of other cations.[2774] Cationized Ags lead to the development of glomerular IC deposits in mice with poor immune responses inadequate to form IC deposits with native Ag molecules.[2812]

It has been shown that anti-DNA Abs recovered from the kidneys of mice with SLE are more cationic than Abs of similar reactivity recovered from the circulation.[2813, 2814] In the (NZB $\times$ SWR)$F_1$ mouse, which is prone to a severe form of murine SLE, Abs eluted from the kidneys are

cationic and share idiotypes with the non–SLE-prone parental SWR.[2815–2817] Cationic fractions of anti-DNA Abs recovered from aging (NZB $\times$ NZW)$F_1$ mice showed preferential binding to glomeruli when administered in vivo or when reacted with isolated nephritic glomeruli in vitro.[2818] A shift to cationic autoantibody production in murine SLE was said to coincide with the onset of glomerular abnormalities.[2819]

The anionic charge contributed to the glomerular capillary wall by heparan sulfate proteoglycan can be altered by heparitinase and, in turn, the binding of cationic Ag–containing IC decreases.[2259] Heparin was reported to enhance removal of glomerular cationic BSA IC in rats.[2258, 2820] Neutralization of polyanions with the polycation polyethyleneimine shifted the localization of 40-fold Ag excess (native BSA) IC from the mesangium to the peripheral capillary wall.[2257] Administration of the polyanionic protamine sulfate with cationic BSA reduces glomerular IC deposits.[2261]

A change in anionic groups measured by decreased binding of cationic ferritin was said to correlate with the early phases of IC localization in murine SLE.[2821] Anionic sites also become masked in egg albumin–induced serum sickness.[2822] Cationic molecules bound to the glomerular capillary wall enhance subsequent binding of anionic macromolecules and anionic ICs.[2823] Cationic Abs bound to the glomerular capillary wall can interact with circulating Ags and may have importance in glomerular IC formation, because anionic Ags normally induce cationic Abs.[2824] Cationic IgM rheumatoid factor can also be localized in the glomerulus and, in turn, can bind IC.[2825] Cationic Ag has been shown to be more effective than its anionic counterpart in removal of cationic IC deposits.[2826]

Cationized Ags have also been compared with their native and anionic counterparts for induction of active models of IC disease. A difficulty with these studies is in trying to differentiate in situ IC formation from circulating IC localization enhanced for reasons of charge. The in vivo uptake of cationized and native molecules such as ferritin by the mononuclear phagocytic system is different, with the cationized molecules persisting longer in the circulation.[2827] Immunization with cationic BSA in rabbits and cationic bovine gamma globulin in mice results in GBM deposits, whereas with their anionic counterparts ICs accumulate in the mesangium.[2243, 2828] The more cationic molecules are present in subepithelial locations. An opposite localization (GBM versus mesangium) of cationic and anionic BSA–induced IC was reported in rats.[2829] Dextrans of various sizes and charges can induce an IC type of GN in which IgA is the prominent Ig found in deposits.[2830] A cationic Ag model has been described in dogs as well as in cats.[2831, 2832] The cationic Ag models in rats lead to progressive glomerular injury.[2833]

From the foregoing, it can be seen that the physicochemical properties of IC components can influence glomerular localization and presumably subsequent dynamic rearrangement and must be considered with other factors that affect glomerular IC accumulation. The cationic BSA model in rabbits, with its relatively rapid subepithelial accumulation of ICs, contrasts with classic native (largely anionic) BSA–induced chronic serum sickness, which takes several weeks

---

*References 2230, 2231, 2233–2239, 2243, 2245, 2260, 2261, 2264, 2791.

of injection to produce a natural sequence of mesangial to subepithelial IC localization.[2655]

The effects of C on modification of IC must also be considered, and C deficiencies are associated with IC disease.[1, 2, 291, 2834, 2835] ICs are exposed to the effects of C in the circulation, and studies suggest that intrinsic glomerular cells can synthesize C components in culture or in vivo in response to IC injury.[332–340, 2836] C3 activation via the alternative C pathway (accelerated by the classic C pathway) can lead to the dissolution of IC.[2837–2839] The early C components including C3 also have the ability to inhibit precipitation of IC.[2840–2842] Potential in vivo importance of C interaction was suggested when C depletion via CVF given to rabbits with acute serum sickness delayed the dissolution of glomerular IC deposits.[2843, 2844] Systemic clearance of C-solubilized IC was similar to that of Ag-solubilized IC; however, the spleen took up more of the C-solubilized variety.[2845] Dissolution of cationic BSA IC deposits was also slowed after CVF treatment.[2846] In addition, the solubilization of test IC by serum is reduced in SLE and other IC diseases.[2847–2850]

C3b (and C4b) on IC can interact with C receptors (CR1) on human erythrocytes and leukocytes, with subsequent release and modification in size of the IC as C3b is degraded by CR1 together with I (C3b/C4b inactivator).[2851–2856] The CR1 are present in clusters on the erythrocyte surface.[2857, 2858] CR1 on lymphocytes can also degrade C3b, which if on ICs may protect the cell from lysis by preventing formation of the MAC after IC binding.[2859] In vivo, the erythrocyte C3b receptors (of humans and primates) were suggested to bind and transport ICs to the liver.[2860–2864] The number of CR1 is decreased on erythrocytes in patients with IC diseases such as SLE and in rheumatoid arthritis.[2865–2869] The role of autoantibodies to CR1 reported in patients with SLE is not yet defined.[2870, 2871] Studies using C3b-coated erythrocytes or bacteria, and specific Abs to the CR1 of erythrocytes and leukocytes,[2872, 2873] demonstrate C3b (and C4b) receptors on human glomerular epithelial cell podocytes in culture and in vivo.[1, 282, 2874, 2875] Clearance studies of baboons using IC (including human anti-DNA–DNA IC) suggest that erythrocytes transport IC to the liver and spleen for removal.[2876–2878] Erythrocyte CR1 levels can be increased by phlebotomy[2879] and are decreased in experimental serum sickness in nonhuman primates.[2880, 2881] Purposeful alteration of erythrocyte CR1 levels by exchange transfusion of erythrocytes with high or low CR1 expression provided no protection against glomerular IC accumulation in a chronic serum sickness model in nonhuman primates.[2882] The authors argued that the large amounts of IC formed from the daily injection of Ag provided an unphysiologic overload for the erythrocyte-CR1-IC clearing mechanism, making the study uninterpretable. In humans, a decrease in C3b receptors was noted in glomerular damage of some IC and non-IC types.[1, 2872, 2873, 2883] Use of Abs reactive with the CR1 receptor has shown no relationship between the presence of the receptor and C3 deposits. Rheumatoid factor was reported to inhibit binding of C3 to marker erythrocytes, thereby interfering with glomerular C3b receptor binding.[2884] Until 1986,[2885] a similar receptor had been controversial in animals used for IC models of GN. CR1 and receptors for other C proteins, or

the Fc portion of IgG, could alter the dynamics of IC accumulation and rearrangement in the glomerular capillary wall. Studies to evaluate interaction of IC with cultured glomerular cells have begun.[848, 2886]

Alterations in permeability of the glomerular capillary wall would be expected to influence IC deposition. Vasoactive substances released in conjunction with immune reactions influence IC deposition.[1] PAF released in rabbits from IgE-sensitized basophils liberates vasoactive amines from platelets and is believed to favor glomerular IC localization during acute serum sickness.[1056] In a more chronic serum sickness in the rat, a role for a PAF from monocyte-macrophages was also suggested and the contribution of histamine release from mast cells was considered.[2887] Platelets may play a role in mesangial localization of carbon particles.[2888] Antagonists of histamine and serotonin have also been effective in reducing the severity of acute serum sickness in rabbits.[1] Experimental depletion of platelets, a major source of immune release of vasoactive substances in rabbits, decreases the deposition of ICs in glomerular lesions during serum sickness.[1, 966] Because infusion of histamine and bradykinin may induce proteinuria,[1] the vasoactive substances may serve as mediators of immunologic glomerular injury as well as predisposing to IC deposition.

Depending on its Ag/Ab ratio, the size of an IC seems to be of great importance in determining its rate of disappearance from circulation and its site of tissue deposition. Large ICs formed near equivalence are eliminated much more rapidly than smaller Ag-excess ICs, with the major site of deposition being the mononuclear phagocytic cells in organs such as the spleen and liver, at which sites the complex material is rapidly catabolized. ICs formed with hapten-protein conjugates of limited valence demonstrate that $Ag_2Ab_5$ ICs greater than 19S are removed rapidly, whereas smaller $Ag_1Ab_2$ or $Ag_1Ab_1$ ICs persist in the circulation.[2889] ICs of $Ag_2Ab_2$ or larger result in glomerular localization in mice.[2890] Covalently cross-linked ICs of known lattice and Ag valence have been used for such studies.[2891, 2892] The physical character of circulating ICs may be important in determining their fate, because ICs made with reduced and alkylated Abs are also eliminated slowly.[1]

In the serum sickness models of GN in rabbits, IC size seems to be important in determining IC deposition. The ICs represent a mixture of sizes varying from 7S to a small fraction heavier than 19S, and it is difficult to assign a nephritogenicity index, especially when the dynamics of IC re-formation are considered. Small ICs less than 19S in size do not seem to be nephritogenic in rabbits with one-shot serum sickness, whereas rabbits with 19S or larger ICs develop glomerular IC deposits and injury.[2893] Similarly, rabbits with chronic serum sickness purposely kept in considerable Ag excess, or those having trivial immune responses, form only small ICs and have much less glomerular injury than rabbits immunized in such a way as to generate a portion of soluble complexes that are 19S or larger.[1] If the rabbits are given inadequate amounts of radiolabeled BSA to produce soluble IC, so that circulating Ab is in excess, large aggregates form that disappear from the circulation with a half-time of minutes. Even when deposited within the glomerular capillary lumina, and probably to some extent within the mesangium, the aggregates disappear with a half-time of hours rather than days, as is true of the nephritogenic variety of ICs referred to earlier (Wilson CB, unpublished observations). A similar effect has been induced by infusing ferritin into the renal artery of a previously immunized recipient.[1, 2894]

A mesangiopathic lesion with focal glomerulosclerosis has been reported to develop in swine after intrarenal "insoluble" IC formation.[2895] DNP-ovalbumin–anti-DNP ICs (<200 kd) have been reported to be excreted into the milk of lactating mice.[2896] The possible role of insoluble ICs in GN has been reviewed, with speculations based on "reinterpretation" of published works.[2897]

The size of the Ag or the number of epitopes on the Ag would also influence the size of the IC formed. Large Ags or heavily substituted hapten carriers form ICs that favor mesangial localization.[1, 2898] It must be kept in mind that substitution may alter the binding of the Ag to the glomerular capillary wall, as discussed previously when addressing physicochemical features of IC accumulation. In addition, consideration must be given to differences in Ab production and relative Ag/Ab ratios, which make comparison based on size alone difficult. Studies using mixtures of monoclonal Abs suggest that Ab heterogeneity is an important factor in determining IC size.[2899] Studies with monoclonal Abs would be expected to vary from those using polyclonal Abs because of limitations of epitope density on the Ag, resulting in decreased cross-linking.

The affinity of Abs governs the strength of the Ag-Ab bond that establishes the stability of the IC. Indeed, in rabbits undergoing daily injections of BSA to induce chronic serum sickness, we have found that Ab affinity progressively increases, with glomerular IC deposits becoming striking only after 5 to 6 weeks of daily immunization and coinciding temporally with an increase in Ab affinity.[1] In acute serum sickness, higher Ab affinity was also reported to enhance glomerular injury.[1] Ab affinity increases after immune elimination.[2900] Some investigators believe that poor immune responses with Abs of low affinity might result in impaired elimination of Ag and lead to increased exposure of the kidney to ICs and potentially greater nephritogenicity.[1] Indeed, rabbits known to have poor Ab responses have been reported to develop chronic serum sickness after immunization for periods of 14 to 18 weeks, during which Ab with little precipitating capability was observed.[2901] In contrast, rabbits with active Ab responses have large amounts of precipitating Ab and can be made to develop severe and rapidly fatal chronic serum sickness GN after only 6 to 8 weeks of immunization. Because Abs with the greatest affinity are preferentially removed from the circulation, measuring the affinity of residual circulating Abs may not give a true picture of the composition of the glomerular IC.[1] In a chronic serum sickness type of model in inbred mice with either high- or low-affinity Ab to human serum albumin, more severe nephritis with subepithelial IC deposits was found in the low-affinity group.[2902–2904] It is not clear, however, that comparable Ag/Ab ratios were maintained throughout. Ag feeding decreased IC deposition in the low-affinity Ab mice.[2905] Glomerular capillary localization of small, low-affinity Ab–containing ICs was suggested to act as a focus for subsequent localization of larger, high-affinity Ab–containing

ICs.[2906] Cyclosporine treatment alters the pattern of immune deposit formation (mesangial > loop) in these low-affinity Ab mice without affecting serum Ab levels.[2907] By using hapten-substituted Ags and monoclonal Abs of different affinities, low-affinity Abs were suggested to be associated with glomerular capillary wall IC localization.[2908, 2909] Employment of monoclonal Ab produced by class-switch variants of the same affinity demonstrated no influence of Ig isotype on glomerular localization of ICs containing IgE or IgG2A.[2910] Protein deficiency, which can modify the immune response, reduced the lesions of the low-affinity mice.[2911] Circulating Ab in an apoferritin model of IC GN in mice was of greater affinity in animals with mesangial deposits than in those with capillary wall deposits.[2912] Preformed ICs of higher affinity Abs clear more rapidly from the circulation than their low-affinity counterparts.[2913] Greater capillary wall localization was observed with preformed low-affinity ICs, whereas ICs made with high-affinity Abs localized in the mesangial areas, a factor probably related to IC size.[1]

The deposition of ICs in glomeruli is influenced by the rate at which the mononuclear phagocytic system clears the IC from the circulation.[2914] Considerable interest, both experimentally and clinically, has focused on the role of cell surface receptors for the Fc portion IgG (Fcγ), as well as receptors for C fragments, particularly C3b, in the clearance and metabolism of ICs.[2915–2918] Fc receptors (R) are members of the Ig superfamily, and three distinct classes of IgG Fc receptors, FcγRI (CD64), FcγRII (CD32), and FcγRIII (CD16), as well as multiple isoforms, exist, as do receptors for other Ig classes all having various patterns of tissue distribution.[2919–2923] In addition to phagocytosis, occupation of the receptors leads to release of proinflammatory mediators, Ab-dependent cellular cytotoxicity responses, and enhancement of Ag presentation. Patients with autoimmune disease produce Abs reactive with Fcγ receptors.[2924] Soluble Fcγ receptors are also present in the circulation.[2925] A monoclonal Ab reactive with the Fc receptor profoundly prolonged in vivo clearance of model IC in chimpanzees.[2926] FcγRII on platelets are involved in IC clearance in serum sickness in cynomolgus monkeys.[2927] In addition to phagocytosis, the interaction of ICs with Fcγ receptors modulates cellular function and receptor number and location, enhancing or inhibiting immune function as well as mediator function.[2928–2935] Apoptosis of neutrophils was reported to be associated with a reduction of FcγRIII.[2936] Fcγ receptor–mediated cell signaling includes tyrosine phosphorylation and the aspects of Fc receptor-mediated signal transduction have been reviewed.[2937–2939] For example, Fc receptor activation of mesangial cells leads to production of MCP-1 and colony-stimulating factor-1.[516] Bispecific Abs reactive with Fcγ receptor and a target Ag are being evaluated as a means of targeting cellular immune defense mechanisms.[2940]

The function of the mononuclear phagocytic system of mice was found to be depressed in autoimmune murine strains with IC disease.[2941–2946] Macrophage Fc receptor–mediated phagocytosis is impaired in streptozocin-induced diabetes.[2947] Carbohydrate receptors may contribute to hepatic uptake of certain types of ICs with exposed carbohydrate groups.[2948–2950] Such a mechanism has been suggested to be important in clearing IgM ICs.[2951] The nature of the Ag may contribute to the clearance of ICs, because the clearance of DNA that is rapidly removed by the liver is little affected when coupled with Ab to form ICs.[2952, 2953] Aggregated IgG is cleared more slowly in rats depleted of Kupffer cells; however, endothelial cell uptake persists.[2954] Splenic function detected by the clearance of altered erythrocytes is impaired in rabbits after administration of IC.[2955] Activation of the mononuclear phagocytic system enhances IC removal from the circulation and reduces glomerular deposition.[2956, 2957] PGE[1] was reported to increase the function of the mononuclear phagocytic system with serum sickness GN.[2958] Immunization with bacille Calmette-Guérin was also suggested to enhance mononuclear phagocyte clearance and decrease immune deposits in chronic serum sickness in rabbits.[2959] Staphylococcal protein A, which can bind to IgG, enhances IC uptake by PMNs and inhibits uptake by macrophages; however, the contribution to IC disease is unclear.[2960] Fibronectin administration has been reported to decrease glomerular deposits in ovalbumin-induced chronic serum sickness in rats through a mechanism suggested to involve increased clearance and renal processing of ICs.[2961] Fibronectin-Ig complexes were reported in some forms of human IC GN.[2962] Glomerular fibronectin was also reported to bind Ags and induce GN as a trapped Ag mechanism.[2207]

In humans, markers of mononuclear phagocytic system clearance are altered in patients with IC disease, especially in SLE patients with active GN.[2963-2969] The clearance defect that is not always correlated with circulating ICs appears to be influenced genetically.[2970, 2971] In vitro function of monocyte-macrophages and PMNs can be increased[2972, 2973] or decreased.[2974, 2975] The presence of Fcγ receptors in glomeruli has been controversial, although their presence there and in the renal interstitium was reported.[2976-2979] Fcγ receptors are also found on cultured glomerular mesangial cells.[751, 1255, 2980] The FcγRIII expression is stimulated in human glomerular mesangial cells by LPS and IFN-γ.[2981]

The role of the mononuclear phagocyte system locally within the glomerulus also needs to be considered, because monocyte-macrophages are prominent infiltrative mediator cells in these models. The monocyte-macrophage is the major mediator cell in acute serum sickness in rabbits[592] and these cells are prominent infiltrative cells in chronic serum sickness as well.[664] Glomerular macrophage proliferation was also reported in this model.[697] The Fcγ receptor–mediated phagocytic capacity of the glomerular macrophages increased during the early stages and decreased as the lesion progressed.[665] The monocyte-macrophage increase in chronic serum sickness was reported to occur in two phases, an early T cell–independent and a later T cell–independent phase, as suggested by the use of cyclosporine, which has multiple potential effects.[2982] Neutrophils were also suggested to contribute to the kinetics of IC accumulation in chronic serum sickness in rats.[2678-2680] A neutralizing Ab against IL-8 decreased neutrophil infiltration and effacement of glomerular epithelial cell foot processes in a chronic serum sickness model in rats.[2983]

Properties of the glomerular mesangium, including movement of fluid through it, may also influence the glomerular deposition and potential nephritogenicity of

ICs.[1398, 2984-2986] Macromolecular materials reach the mesangium via the endothelial fenestrae, pass through the mesangial matrix channels, and may be variably phagocytosed or eventually reach the vascular pole and the renal lymph.[2987-2989] Monocytes are suggested to play a small role in uptake when ferritin is the macromolecule used but are thought to be of major importance when polyvinyl alcohol is used.[698, 699, 2990, 2991] In proliferative GN, such as that induced with anti-GBM Ab, a portion of the glomerular uptake of test macromolecules (aggregated Ig) is by the infiltrating mononuclear cells.[2992] In malarial GN in rats, mesangial accumulation of IC deposits was reported with some editorial reservations, largely in the absence of monocytes.[2993, 2994]

Mesangial localization appears to be the first site of IC deposition in rabbits with chronic serum sickness[2655] and in other animals with experimental or spontaneous IC lesions. As just noted for macromolecular markers, the role of the mesangial cell versus resident or infiltrating monocyte-macrophages in the uptake of IC varies in different systems.[661, 2995] In tissue culture, the mesangial cell can degrade soluble but not insoluble IC, in contrast to macrophages, which bind and degrade both.[2996] ICs do interact and activate mesangial cells, even IgA ICs.[2997, 2998] Histologically, mesangial prominence may be the only finding in early or mild GN. In chronic serum sickness, the initial and relatively minimal mesangial IC localization is followed by quantitatively greater deposition of IC in glomerular capillary walls, leading to overt glomerular injury and functional abnormalities. The shift can be visualized dramatically by immunofluorescence (see Fig. 29–15A and B) and correlates with quantitative IC deposition.[2655] In this model, function of the mononuclear phagocytic system, as measured by the clearance of radiolabeled, heat-aggregated rabbit serum albumin, seems to be lowest after 6 to 8 weeks of injections, corresponding to enhanced glomerular localization.[2655] Clearance of polyvinylpyrrolidone from plasma is also depressed in New Zealand hybrid mice with SLE-like IC disease.[1] Similarly, uptake of aggregated human Ig is impaired in rats with pre-existing ferritin-antiferritin IC in the mesangium.[2999] Systemic mononuclear phagocytic function is reported to be retarded before the onset of proteinuria in rats developing chronic serum sickness.[2679]

Glomerular localization of preformed IC or aggregated Ig is largely in the mesangial region and is inversely related to the rate of clearance of the test material from the plasma.[1] Corticosteroid administration enhances glomerular uptake and persistence, as do reduction and alkylation of the Ab used to form the IC.[1] Studies using heat-denatured DNA and ultraviolet-irradiated DNA, generating IgM and IgG Abs, respectively, showed similar mesangial localization of deposits.[3000] Uptake by the mesangial region of the glomerulus can be estimated by the localization of colloidal carbon or quantitated by measuring the deposition of radiolabeled aggregates of Ig.[1] Competitive inhibition of clearance of aggregated Ig by administration of dextran increased Ig deposits in glomeruli.[3001] Studies using two macromolecules taken up by the mesangium demonstrated little competitive impairment of mesangial uptake or clearance of the molecules.[3002] In other studies, prior uptake actually enhanced uptake of a second marker and was related to increased monocytes responding to the initial polyvinyl alcohol stimulus.[3003] Administration of aminonucleoside of puromycin or polyvinyl alcohol to enhance activity of glomerular macrophages caused no change in the removal rate of cationic BSA IC.[3004] Enhanced glomerular uptake and degradation of aggregated Ig begin early in the course of immunization that incites chronic serum sickness and persist until the animal is moribund.[1] Similar findings have been reported in IC GN after lymphocytic choriomeningitis virus (LCMV) infection in mice and in aminonucleoside nephrosis and anti-GBM Ab nephritis in rats.[1, 3005]

Possible toxic effects of the macromolecular marker on subsequent mesangial function need to be considered in interpretation of mesangial uptake data.[3006, 3007] Impaired mesangial uptake has been noted in relation to snake venom–induced mesangiolysis.[1, 3008] In addition, in contrast to serum sickness, no infiltrating mononuclear cells accompany snake venom–induced mesangiolysis.[1] C-dependent mesangial cell injury induced by administration of an Ab reactive with the mesangial cell surface caused a striking increase in uptake of macromolecular markers in the damaged mesangial areas.[2128] The damaged glomerulus was able to clear the trapped material, suggesting the mesangial cells themselves, which were no longer functional, played little role in the clearance.

In all probability, mesangial dysfunction is not a major factor in glomerular IC accumulation, although in spontaneously hypertensive rats mesangial ''overloading'' with polyvinyl alcohol was reported to worsen chronic IC nephritis.[3009] Mesangial injury may hasten hypertension in Dahl rats.[3010] Studies suggest that ICs that can interact with fibronectin have enhanced mesangial uptake.[3011]

Other features of the host or glomerulus may influence IC deposition. For example, the severity of serum sickness is increased in the presence of hypertension, and vascular depositions of horseradish peroxidase and ferritin are enhanced in hypertensive animals.[1] Hemodynamic factors also play a role because 1) vascular lesions are most severe at bifurcations or at inferior surfaces of induced coarctations of the aorta and 2) impairment of glomerular filtration decreases glomerular IC deposition.[1] Cytoplasmic ridges on endothelial cells have been suggested as sites where ICs lodge.[3012] Renal vein constriction was reported to reduce GN in acute serum sickness.[3013] We have observed enhanced deposition of ICs in the kidneys of rabbits with serum sickness and partial renal vein obstructions when calculated in terms of the diminished renal blood flow present after ligation (Henderson LW, Wilson CB, unpublished observations).

## OTHER IC GN IN ANIMALS

It can be seen from the foregoing discussion that the term IC GN refers to the complicated and dynamic interaction of Abs with soluble Ags in the circulation and continuing within tissue deposits. The dynamics of glomerular localization are affected to varying extents by factors including physicochemical interaction of Ag (or Ab) with the glomerular capillary wall. The numerous examples of presumed IC GN in animals can be viewed in terms of the probable Ag source, either exogenous or endogenous.

### Exogenous Ags

The exogenous Ags used to cause serum sickness GN have been discussed and immunization with other exogenous Ags has been referred to in earlier sections. Naturally occurring Ags associated with infectious agents are those most commonly identified in IC GN of experimental animals; of these, viruses have been studied in greatest detail. Many of the viral infections implicated as sources of Ag for nephritogenic IC formation are not particularly cytopathic and do not cause significant tissue injury in the absence of a host immune response.[1] However, when the immune response does take place, even though the result may not be elimination of the viral agent, immune damage to virally infected cells as well as formation of ICs can cause vascular and glomerular injury. Viral infections in humans carry the same IC GN risks as do those in animals.[3014]

Chronic LCMV-related GN has been studied extensively and serves as an excellent prototype for understanding the various viral-associated GNs. When mice are infected neonatally or transplacentally, a persistent (lifelong) infection develops, with the level of viral growth and viremia determined by the mouse strain.[1] Circulating anti-LCMV Abs reactive with LCMV structural polypeptides in addition to C1q-reactive material are detected, varying among strains in part with the I region of the H-2 complex.[3015, 3016] Circulating anti-LCMV–LCMV virus ICs can be demonstrated by immune precipitation of either Ig or C3, with a striking loss of infectivity of the serum.[1] A similar immunoprecipitation technique has been employed for demonstration of circulating ICs in lactate dehydrogenase virus infection.[1] ICs containing LCMV Ag, Ab, and C deposit in the glomeruli and are seen with immunofluorescence[1] (Fig. 29–18A). IgG (60 μg per kidney), about half of which is anti-LCMV Ab, can be eluted from the glomeruli, further supporting the role of ICs in the causation of this glomerular lesion.[1] IFN, which can alter glomerular development, has been suggested to contribute to some of the morphologic aspects of LCMV-associated GN changes that can be blocked with anti-IFN Ab.[2]

Numerous other viruses have been implicated as etiologic agents in nephritogenic IC formation leading to spontaneous or experimental GN in animals[2] (Fig. 29–18B to E). Circulating ICs containing viral Ags can be found in hosts of virus infections.[3017, 3018] The glomerular immune deposits in Aleutian disease virus infection of mink have been reported to be predominantly IgA.[3019] The mink lesion also includes a possible cell-mediated interstitial nephritis.[126] Structural polypeptides of the virion are reported to vary between glomerular and vascular deposits, suggesting that the IC formation at these sites may be different.[3020] Electron-dense deposits containing viral particles have been identified in and along the GBM,[1, 3021] although it is most likely that glomerular IC deposits are composed of viral products rather than intact virions. In chickens, viral infection is suspected to damage tubule epithelium directly and produce nephritis without a defined immune component.[2]

Bacterial infections, other than streptococcal, have not been extensively studied. Exposure to streptococci or their products, even in combination with renal tissue, has led to

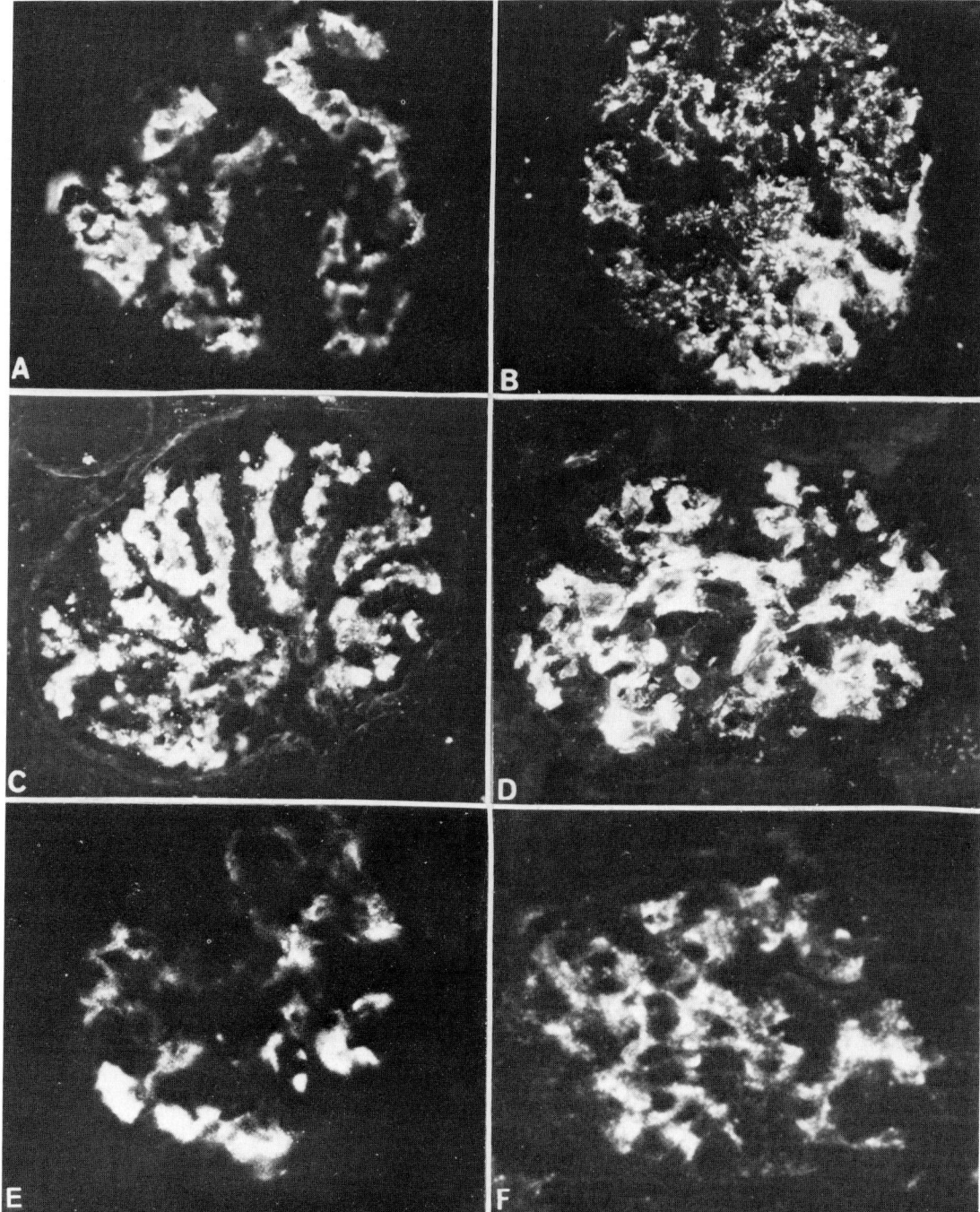

**Figure 29–18.** In animals, similarities are apparent in presumed glomerular IC deposits caused by a wide variety of Ags. *A.* IC GN in mice with chronic lymphocytic choriomeningitis virus infection. *B.* Glomerular IC deposits in mink with Aleutian disease virus–induced GN. (*B* from Porter DD, Larsen AE, Porter HG: The pathogenesis of Aleutian disease of mink. I. In vivo viral replication and the host antibody response to viral antigen. J Exp Med 130:575–593, 1969.) *C.* Granular IC deposits in GN in horses with infectious equine anemia virus GN. (*C* courtesy of K Banks.) *D.* IC GN in mice with spontaneous murine leukemia virus infection. (*D* from Porter DD, Porter HG, Cox NA: Immune complex glomerulonephritis in one-year-old C57BL-6 mice induced by endogenous murine leukemia virus and erythrocyte antigens. J Immunol 111:1626–1633, 1973.) *E.* IC GN in mice infected with CMV. (*E* courtesy of M Oldstone.) *F.* Granular IC deposits in the spontaneous SLE-like GN of New Zealand mice.

conflicting results.[1] Granular deposits of Ig and streptococcal M protein have been identified in glomeruli, and anti-streptococcal M protein Abs have been eluted from the kidneys, suggesting an IC-induced glomerular lesion.[1] Repeated nephritogenic streptococcal infections in rabbits also resulted in striking glomerular lesions, with Ig deposits identified in some glomeruli.[1] Streptococcal growth in chambers has been reported to induce glomerular Ig and C deposits in rabbits, and the lesion was prevented by antibiotic treatment early in the course.[3022, 3023] Rhesus monkeys immunized with soluble streptococcal protoplasmic membrane precipitated with alum were reported to develop irregular granular deposits of Ig and C predominantly in mesangial areas of the glomeruli.[1] Streptococcal vaccine has been suggested to produce glomerular C3 deposits in the absence of Ig.[1]

Disrupted *Streptococcus mutans,* a pathogen in dental caries, produces glomerular immune deposits with streptococcal Ag and also induces antitissue Abs.[3024, 3025] Circulating IC and glomerular septic emboli, as well as immune deposits, are found in *Streptococcus sanguis*–associated experimental bacterial endocarditis.[3026] Attention has been drawn to the cross-reactivity of certain streptococcal extracts with portions of the GBM and transplantation Ags.[1] The relationship between glomerular leptospiral Ag and Ig deposits in experimental leptospirosis-associated renal injury is unclear; most Ags were found in the tubulointerstitial regions.[3027]

Ag-Ab systems induced by other infectious agents can cause nephritogenic ICs in animals. Studies of experimental hemosporidian infection have demonstrated glomerular IC deposits containing plasmodial or babesial Ag or Ab with decline in renal function.[1, 2, 3028] Lipoprotein deposits in glomeruli were also suggested in mice infected with *Plasmodium chabaudi.*[3029] *Opisthorchis viverrini* infection in Syrian golden hamsters results in tegumental-antitegumental IC deposits and amyloid AA fibrils.[3030] Experimental schistosomal infections are also complicated by IC GN.[1, 2] Schistosomal Ags including circulating anodic Ag are found in glomeruli and IgA deposits may predominate in *Schistosoma mansoni* infection in mice or Syrian golden hamsters.[3031–3034] *Toxoplasma* Ag has been found in glomerular IC deposits in experimental toxoplasmosis.[1] *Trypanosoma* infection has also been associated with experimental IC GN.[1, 2, 3035] *Leishmania* infection in hamsters produces IC GN and *Leishmania donovani* Ags have been found in the glomerular deposits.[2, 3036–3040] *D. immitis* (canine heartworm disease) causes nephritis with glomerular deposits containing antiworm Abs and Ags.[2219, 2221] In some of these *D. immitis*–infected dogs, a linear Ig deposit has led to the speculation that worm Ags bind to the GBM in a manner similar to the lectin model of nephritis. Hydatid disease (*Echinococcus granulosus*) in sheep is associated with an IC GN with hydatid Ag detected using a human Ab from a patient with the disease.[3041] *Ehrlichia canis* induces proteinuria and Ig deposits with minimal histologic change or demonstration of Ag.[3042] *Renibacterium salmoninarum* infection in rainbow trout leads to an IC form of GN.[3043]

### Endogenous Ags

The lupus-like syndrome of mice (Fig. 29–18*F*) is characterized by the production of numerous autoantibodies and the development of glomerular immune deposits that appear to form via accumulation of ICs as well as direct reactions of autoantibodies with native and trapped glomerular Ags.[1–3, 3044–3046]

The immunopathogenesis of murine SLE involves the spontaneous production of autoantibodies much as in the human counterpart of this disease.[2620, 3047–3056] In addition to their immunopathogenic role, autoantibodies have served as

reagents to explore cellular function with respect to nuclear Ags.[3057, 3058] The first discernible immunologic abnormality is a polyclonal hyperactivity of B cells detectable as early as 2 weeks to 2 months of age, with evidence also suggesting autoantigen-driven production of autoantibodies.[1, 3059–3065] The polyclonal activation can be accelerated by giving LPS.[1329, 3066] This results in a polyclonal increase of serum Ig with the spontaneous appearance of Ig reactive with many Ags including host nuclear Ags and retroviral gp70. The autoantibodies participate in the formation of ICs as well as the immune deposits that accumulate in glomeruli, causing activation and consumption of C and the production of GN.[3046, 3067] The structure-function aspects of the murine lupus GN lesion have been considered.[3068] Lupus mice, particularly MRL-*lpr/lpr,* also often have prominent arthritis, degenerative vascular disease with myocardial infarction, and vasculitis and can serve as models for study of these conditions.[3069–3073] The MRL-*lpr/lpr* strain produces antinuclear glycoprotein SM Ab as seen in human SLE.[3074] Analysis of Ig eluted from the glomeruli of these SLE mice indicates that it contains a variety of autoantibodies including antinuclear Ab as well as Ab to retroviral Ag gp70 (also called SU).[1–3] Retroviral gp70 and DNA can both be identified by immunofluorescence in the diseased glomeruli.[1, 2] In addition, gp70-Ab IC can be found both in the renal eluates and in the circulation at the time of active disease.[1, 3075–3077] Other Ag-Ab systems also contribute, including anti–RNA polymerase I and antichromatin.[3078–3080] The gp70 molecule is not essential for the development of GN in the MRL-*lpr/lpr* mouse, in which backcrosses to the low-gp70 BALB/c strain virtually eliminated the gp70–anti-gp70 system without materially affecting the outcome of the GN.[3081] The possible role of retroviral proteins in immune activation in lupus mice as well as in human SLE is the subject of study and review.[3082–3084]

Genetic factors including MHC are implicated in SLE in humans as well as in lupus mice.[1761, 3085–3089] The murine lupus-prone genetic backgrounds include the multigenic NZB and single-locus mutations that include the two alleles of *lpr* (lymphoproliferation) and *lpr*cg as well as *gld* (generalized lymphoproliferative disease) and the *Yaa* (Y-chromosome linked autoimmune accelerator) gene of the BXSB male that accelerates rather than induces autoimmune disease.[3046, 3090–3094] Formerly, none of the gene products were available for study; however, the *lpr* and *lpr*cg mutations have now been found in genetic and molecular genetic studies to represent defects in the *Fas* gene, which normally mediates a pathway of apoptosis.[717, 3095] Fas is a 45-kd cell surface protein with a cytoplasmic anchor belonging to the TNF receptor family that is expressed on lymphoid as well as other tissues. In *lpr* an insertion has occurred in intron 2 of the *Fas* gene that causes premature termination and aberrant splicing of the *Fas* transcript, whereas *lpr*cg has a point mutation resulting in replacement of isoleucine with asparagine that abolishes the ability of *Fas* to transduce the apoptotic signal.[131, 3096–3099] Replacement of the mutated *lpr* gene with a normal *Fas* apoptosis gene in T cells of transgenic MRL-*lpr/lpr* mice eliminated GN and lymphadenopathy and decreased the autoantibody levels.[3100] The *gld* mutation is now believed to involve the *Fas* ligand gene and exhibits a point mutation in the COOH-terminal region of the molecule, an area highly conserved among members of the TNF family.[3101–3103] Identification of these specific genetic defects should allow understanding of the causes of the autoimmune responses in these lupus-prone strains.[3104–3108] The more general role of apoptosis in disease including autoimmune disease has also been reviewed.[3109, 3110]

The molecular genetics of the B and T cell immune response in murine models of SLE as well as in human SLE patients have been studied in detail.[3052, 3111–3120] The variable region gene usage suggests somatic mutations, with evidence that the mutations are being driven by DNA or a structurally homologous molecule or through selection by idiotype.[3121] There is no disease-associated polymorphism and there is no evidence that the somatic mutations differ in autoimmune and normal Ab responses. The recurrent usage of particular variable region genes that would be likely to promote protein binding to DNA, particularly arginine rich, supports the idea that DNA may be the Ag stimulating the response. Several monoclonal anti-DNA and other Abs associated with nephritis have been characterized.[3122–3127] Autoreactive T cells are involved in the control of the autoimmune response and studies of their receptor genes have suggested clonal restriction.[3128–3132] Purposeful alterations in T cell function using such diverse measures as IL-2–vaccinia recombinant viruses, Ab to IFN-γ or T cell Ags, or administration of bacterial superantigen reduce the autoimmune response and lupus nephritis.[128, 130, 189, 3133–3139] The reduction in Vβ8+ T cells using specific Ab has had variable results.[3140, 3141]

Idiotypes represent unique antigenic determinants related to the hypervariable regions (V gene sequences) unique to a particular Ab or group of Abs.[3142] As such, they serve as phenotypic markers of the variable Ig genes.[3117, 3127, 3143] Based on the view developed initially by Jerne, the idiotypic network included a system of stimulatory and inhibitory elements with Abs (idiotypes), anti-idiotypic Abs, and idiotype-specific B and T cells. Many idiotypes are common or public, shared among groups of Abs from individuals (even between species), whereas some are private. The frequent occurrence of public idiotypes among anti-DNA Abs has been a point of interest and review.[2620, 3144–3148] Auto-anti-idiotypes also develop in lupus mice and human SLE patients and are structurally diverse.[3149] Of the 20 or so anti-DNA Ab idiotypes identified, only some are associated with active disease and GN. Public idiotypes are recovered from glomerular eluates of murine and human SLE patients.[3052, 3150–3154]

Dysregulation of the idiotype–anti-idiotype network is also reported to play a role in SLE.[3155] Mice of certain strains immunized with monoclonal (or polyclonal) Abs carrying the 16/6 idiotype or murine monoclonal anti-idiotypic 16/6 develop autoantibodies, including anti-DNA Ab and glomerular immune deposits in some but not all studies.[3155–3160] Transfer of spleen cells from murine donors producing high titers of Ab to the 16/6 idiotype to severe combined immunodeficiency mice resulted in glomerular immune deposits.[3161] The immunization-induced anti-idiotypic 16/6 Ab was blunted by preimmunization with single-stranded DNA; however, the glomerular deposits were not altered.[3162] The 16/6 idiotype was found in 54% of SLE patients.[3163] Immunization of rabbits with human or murine

anti-DNA Abs resulted in production of typical lupus autoantibodies against multiple autoantigens, presumably via immune network interactions.[3164, 3165]

The potential role of idiotypic manipulation in therapy of autoimmune processes is the subject of review.[3166–3168] Monoclonal anti-DNA Abs were used to immunize (NZB × NZW)F₁ female mice with therapeutic benefit by a process suspected to involve anti-idiotypic Ab.[3169, 3170] Administration of monoclonal anti-idiotypes to major anti-DNA Ab idiotypes was also effective in activating anti-DNA Ab production and noted to result in the emergence of other idiotypes of anti-DNA Abs in these mice.[3171–3173] Immunization with double-stranded DNA and polyclonal anti-DNA Ab to boost anti-idiotypic Ab production in MRL/MpJ-*lpr/lpr* mice also improved survival.[3174] Immunization with monoclonal anti-DNA Ab derived from fetal or adult MRL/Mp-*lpr/lpr* mice induced lupus and heterogeneous anti-idiotype suppressed progression.[3175] Administration of anti-Id^LN^F₁ Ab reactive with a nephritic non–anti-DNA Ab in (SWR × NZB)F₁ was reported to delay onset of GN without altering anti-DNA Ab production.[3176] Anti-idiotypic Abs conjugated with the cytotoxic agent neocarzinostatin were beneficial in female (NZB × NZW)F₁ mice.[3177] Anti-idiotypic suppression of anti-DNA Ab responses was also suggested in humans.[3178] The beneficial effect of intravenous immune globulin in some instances of autoimmune and vasculitic disorders and its variable effects in SLE may include stimulation of anti-idiotypic autoantibodies.[3179–3181]

Although SLE has long been considered an example of IC disease,[1, 3, 3182] the mechanisms of immune deposit formation in the murine lupus models and in humans with SLE appear to involve varying participation of all the major concepts defined in previous sections of this chapter: direct Ab binding, trapped Ag mechanisms, and IC accumulation with dynamic interchange of the IC components. The contribution of each mechanism presumably varies with the nature and complexity of the individual autoimmune response over time, as well as factors that may alter Ag availability. The precise division of the immune deposit mechanisms may also include semantics, because an Ag capable of directly binding to a glomerular site as a trapped Ag may not reach the binding site in the form of a single molecule but rather as an IC, if Ag and Ab are present simultaneously in the circulation. The multiplicity of circulating Abs in the lupus mouse (or human patient) makes it unlikely that any nephritogenic Ag of nonrenal origin can reach the glomerulus without first encountering Ab in the circulation. Also, Abs involved in reactions or cross-reactions with native glomerular components may encounter soluble Ags before reaching the kidney, where dynamic interchange could contribute to the deposition. The multiple potential immune deposit possibilities may affect the site, tempo, and quantity of Ig and C accumulations, which in turn generate the phlogogenic immune mediator response and the pathologic and clinical manifestations of the lesion. In efforts to quantitate the contribution of the individual mechanisms, studies of renal eluates rather than Ab remaining in the circulation are most relevant; however, elution may not provide truly representative sampling because of differences in the avidity of the various Ag-Ab systems and denaturing effects of the harsher elution procedures needed to recover the more tightly bound Abs.

The serum of lupus mice or patients with active SLE contains large amounts of material consistent with ICs as determined by various assays.[2] Studies continue to better delineate the role of circulating ICs in renal immune deposits. For example, circulating anti-DNA ICs expressing the 0-81 idiotype were associated with active lupus nephritis,[3152, 3183] and absorption studies suggested that ICs as well as GBM-reactive anti-DNA Abs were present in renal eluates.[3184] DNA deposits in glomerular immune deposits have been reported[3185, 3186] and defined with immunogold techniques.[3187] Extrinsic DNA has also been suggested in circulating ICs and bacterial DNA can induce anti–double-stranded DNA responses.[3188–3191] By using an enzyme-linked immunosorbent assay with whole intact glomeruli as substrates, binding has been found in the serum of lupus mice; binding was diminished by DNAse treatment but not by DNA absorption, suggesting that ICs containing DNA were involved.[3192, 3193]

The role of Fc and C receptor activity in IC localization was considered earlier. An age-related impairment of macromolecular test aggregate clearance from the circulation is observed in MRL-*lpr/lpr* mice.[3194–3196] Age is a dependent variable in hepatic reticuloendothelial system activation in MRL-*lpr/lpr* mice, correlating with delayed clearance of test aggregates.[3197] The macrophages in the lupus mice have features of selective activation, defective Fc receptor–mediated phagocytosis, and impaired degradation of IC.[663, 3198, 3199] Defects in CR1 and Fc clearance are also found in human SLE patients.[1, 2, 3200, 3201]

Izui and colleagues[2194, 2195] have suggested that DNA can bind to glomeruli and serve as trapped Ags in SLE. Binding of DNA to GBM can be diminished when basic proteins or polycations are present.[2198] DNA or DNA–anti-DNA ICs may also bind to fibronectin, a component of the glomerulus.[2196, 2197]

Nucleosomes, the fundamental repeating units of the chromatin fiber, are formed of complexes of histone and DNA; they are being recognized as major Ags in SLE.[3202] DNA in the circulation in SLE was found to be present in multimeric complexes bound to histone resembling a 200–base pair "ladder."[3203] Abs to nucleosomal Ags become DNA reactive when complexed to nucleosomes, and these complexes can bind to GBM in part via heparan sulfate.[2634] In another study, monoclonal anti-DNA complexed to small DNA bound poorly to the glomerulus unless first complexed to core histones.[2635] An autoantibody specific for nucleosome core particles has been recovered from the MRL/Mp-*lpr/lpr* mouse.[3204] Histone-DNA complexes were suggested to bind to the endothelium and GBM, thereby serving as Ags for anti-DNA Abs in immune deposit formation in human and murine lupus.[2199–2202] Histone peptides are identified in glomerular deposits of (NZB × NZW)F₁ mice.[3205] The contribution of histones and other cationic molecules to immune deposit formation has been extensively reviewed.[2230, 2791] Production of cationic anti-DNA Abs was observed corresponding to the onset of lupus GN in humans as well as in murine lupus and were recovered from renal eluates.* Circulating antihistone Abs are found in SLE patients.[3210–3212] Some of the antihistone reactivities

are reported to be acquired when anti-DNA Ab is complexed to DNA.[3213, 3214] Native and ubiquitinated forms of histones can be identified in certain renal biopsy specimens from SLE patients.[3215, 3216] The reactivity of some SLE Abs with heparan sulfate was suggested to involve bound complexes of DNA and histones.[3217, 3218] Administration of Abs to heparan sulfate proteoglycan accentuates the glomerular injury in (NZB × NZW)F₁ mice.[3219]

The possible role of autoantibodies, particularly anti-DNA Ab, reacting or cross-reacting directly with glomerular Ag was introduced earlier in the section on nephritogenic immune reactions involving glomerular Ags.* Reactions of anti-DNA Abs with proteoglycans, vimentin, and cell surface Ags have been reported.[2624–2628, 2631] Administration of monoclonal anti-DNA Abs that cross-react with glomerular structures results in different patterns of immune deposit formation in glomeruli depending on the monoclonal Ab used.[2619, 2621, 2630] Eluates of MRL or graft-versus-host mice react with DNA, histones, and laminin and bind to glomeruli when given in vivo.[2631] In the isolated perfused kidney, mouse and human anti-DNA Abs can induce proteinuria, an effect that is blocked by prior absorption of the Ab with DNA.[2629] The binding of anti-DNA Ab to cells including other glomerular structures may be related in part to cell-associated DNA.[2201, 2203, 2632, 2633] Anti–endothelial cell Abs have been identified and may contribute to the renal and vascular injury in SLE.†

The cross-reactivity of anti-DNA Abs may include both polynucleotide and cardiolipin-phospholipid reactions characteristic of the lupus anticoagulant and the "antiphospholipid Ab syndrome," in which thrombotic problems may be encountered, although the contribution to glomerular damage is unclear.[2622, 2623, 3224–3228] Histones may bind to cardiolipin and need to be considered in evaluating antihistone reactions.[3229]

Other mouse strains and dogs develop lupus-like disease[1, 2]; however, these conditions have not been extensively studied. Dogs owned by SLE patients are said to have anti-DNA Ab more often than other dogs.[3230] Immunization with mitogens such as bacterial LPS can induce polyclonal B cell activation and autoantibody formation with anti-DNA Abs and GN.[2194, 2195, 3066] Injections of *E. coli, Corynebacterium parvum,* and *S. mansoni* can induce anti-DNA Abs that may be accompanied by GN.[2] DNA released by some of these mitogenic events has been suggested to bind to the GBM for subsequent in situ IC formation. Bacterial DNA can be used to induce anti-DNA Ab and glomerular immune deposits in normal mice.[3231, 3232] Expression of transgenes in mice encoding anti-DNA Ab is also associated with evidence of GN.[3233] Transfer of human peripheral blood lymphocytes from patients with SLE to severe combined immunodeficiency mice results in transfer of anti-DNA Ab production to these normally immunodeficient animals and some evidence of glomerular immune deposit formation.[3234–3236]

Other forms of experimental polyclonal B cell activation can also lead to the formation of anti-DNA Abs. As noted earlier, graft-versus-host disease is associated with devel-

---

*References 2813, 2819, 3052, 3206–3209.

*References 2203, 2618–2621, 3220–3222.
†References 1175, 2561, 2562, 2567–2569, 2577, 2632, 2633, 3223.

opment of anti-DNA and other autoantibodies that react with autoantigens such as laminin, histones, and dipeptidyl peptidase IV.[1, 2, 1913, 1914, 3237–3241] The use of this model for the study of lupus nephritis has been reviewed.[3242] Dipeptidyl peptidase IV, also called CD26, is a serine proteinase expressed on activated T cells including T cells form MRL/Mp-*lpr/lpr* mice.[3243] Mercuric chloride and other mercury-containing pharmaceutical products induce tubule injury and a form of presumed IC GN in some strains of rats.[1, 2] A polyclonal Ab response with anti-DNA Abs occurs in the affected rats, and in some strains the apparent IC disease occurs after initial anti-GBM Ab production. SJL mice also develop antinuclear Abs and glomerular immune deposits containing antinuclear Abs after mercuric chloride treatment.[3244, 3245] Cadmium toxicity also causes GN and B cell proliferation in rats.[1908]

The IC GN of experimental thyroiditis has a human counterpart and is induced in rabbits by injection of heterologous or chemically altered homologous thyroglobulin.[1] Circulating and antithyroglobulin Abs appear to be important in the genesis of this lesion, which can be passively transferred by Ab alone in rabbits, guinea pigs, and mice.[1] The thyroid lesion in mice is caused, at least in part, by antithyroglobulin Abs reacting with thyroglobulin as it emerges from the thyroid follicular cell to form ICs between the thyroid follicular basement membrane and the plasma membrane of the thyroid follicular cell in an Arthus-like reaction.[3246] Nephritogenic IC formation is enhanced by thyroid injury such as that induced by radioactive iodine, presumably by releasing thyroglobulin to form quantitatively large amounts of ICs as well as shifting Ag/Ab ratios, potentially favoring formation of circulating ICs.[1] Thyroglobulin-containing ICs have also been reported in glomeruli of obese chickens that spontaneously develop autoimmune thyroiditis.[2]

Erythrocyte Ags may also be involved in IC formation contributing to the GN that occurs spontaneously in NZB mice and is associated with murine leukemia and GN that occurs in mice.[1] Immunization of rabbits with physicochemically altered homologous IgG can induce immune responses to autologous IgG and histones with glomerular deposits.[2787] Neoplasia can also be accompanied by presumed IC GN.[1, 2] Insulin-containing deposits and elutable anti-insulin Abs characterize glomerular immune deposits in mice with inherited diabetes.[3247] Circulating ICs and glomerular Ig deposits are observed in streptozocin-induced diabetes in rats.[3248] An autoimmune disease with antinuclear and antierythrocyte Abs and glomerular immune deposits has been reported in the Afghan pika.[2]

Human cryoglobulins from patients with GN (IgMκ-IgG complexes that dissociate at 37°C) can induce GN when infused into mice; however, the glomerular binding may involve an in situ mechanism in which the IgMκ has an affinity for glomerular structures.[3249] Glomerular reactivity has been suggested in the IgG fraction of patients with mixed cryoglobulinemia as well.[2560] The contribution of IgG3 rheumatoid factor cryoglobulins in lupus and other mice was discussed earlier.[2278, 2285, 3250–3253] Glomerular immune deposits in lupus mice can be dissociated with Ig, suggesting that rheumatoid factor is present.[1, 3, 3254] In humans, cryoglobulins are more closely correlated with lupus nephritis than are rheumatoid factors.[3255]

## SPONTANEOUS PRESUMED IC GN IN ANIMALS

Laboratory animals commonly have a history of glomerular lesions associated with granular glomerular deposits of Ig and C. In mice, IC formation is most likely associated with endogenous murine leukemia infections.[1] In guinea pigs,[1] subhuman primates,[1, 3256–3258] and rats,[1, 2] no etiologic agents are yet apparent. A genetic model resembling focal glomerulosclerosis with glomerular IgM deposits has been reported in rats[3259] and, as noted earlier, rats have a tendency for IgM glomerular deposits and sclerosis. Mastomys (*Praomys [Mastomys] natalensis*) have a high incidence of GN with presumed IC deposits, suggested to be caused by retroviral IC.[1] Dogs and cats frequently have GN and/or TIN and, when examined closely, often have granular glomerular deposits of Ig and C.[1, 2, 3260–3262] The relationship between these cases and canine SLE[1] is not clear. Ampicillin, commonly used in therapy, was suggested to contribute to glomerular Ig deposits in dogs.[3263] An IC GN is also found in cats with lymphosarcoma.[3264] Horses have been shown to have ICs as well as anti-GBM Ab–associated GN.[1, 3265] Sheep and other ruminants have an unusually high incidence of presumed IC GN,[1] and the histologic lesion in Finnish Landrace lambs resembles hypocomplementemic membranoproliferative GN in humans.[1, 2, 3266] GN associated with C3 deficiency in dogs or levan (high-molecular-weight polyfructosan) in rabbits may have usefulness for study of C-related GN.[3267–3269] A porcine model of hypocomplementemic membranoproliferative GN was also described.[3270] No glomerular lesions were found in a group of C4 deficient guinea pigs.[3271] The frequent observation of IC-induced glomerular injury in common laboratory and domestic animals points out the need for careful controls when inducing experimental glomerular injury, particularly when the lesion under study is of a chronic nature.

## Immune Complex Glomerulonephritis in Humans

Most human GN appears to be caused by accumulation of IC-containing exogenous or endogenous Ags in glomeruli. Based on animal models of IC disease, immunofluorescence studies demonstrating granular deposits of Ig and C present in different distributions in most cases of human GN have been used to establish a presumptive diagnosis of IC GN.[1] The distribution and the quantitative and temporal features of IC accumulation and subsequent mediator response in turn influence the histologic response and clinical presentation of the nephritic process.[2] It is currently not possible to quantitate the contribution of direct deposition of IC in the glomerulus, dynamic rearrangement of IC components within the glomerular capillary, and in situ IC formation with planted Ags. From the information presented in the foregoing sections of this chapter, it is unlikely that these mechanisms are exclusive and any or all could result in a granular immune deposit detected by immunofluorescence study.

Ab reactions with glomerular Ags that are distributed in an irregular fashion, such as those on the epithelial podocyte in experimental HN, can also lead to irregular granular deposits. It is not unreasonable to expect human counterparts of this type of direct binding mechanism to be defined, making the interpretation of a granular deposit even more unclear without additional study. This needed study focuses on defining the nature of the Ag-Ab system(s) involved.

Ever-increasing numbers of nephritogenic Ag-Ab systems are being identified and/or implicated in patients with granular, presumably IC, deposits in glomeruli. Any chronic Ag exposure carries with it the risk of potentially nephritogenic IC formation. The Ags can be broadly divided into exogenous, or foreign, and endogenous, or self, Ags for ease of description. Although many different Ag-Ab systems have now been found in different iatrogenic, infectious, or autoimmune illnesses, the number of individual patients in whom successful detection of Ag-Ab systems has been achieved is small. Direct Ag identification, elution to recover and identify glomerulus-bound Abs, and work on the makeup of circulating ICs have been the mainstays for this type of study.[2] The low success rate in identifying glomerulus-bound Abs may include hiding of reactive sites with time because of progressive Ab binding, as evidenced by animal experiments in which antigenic sites become hidden.[2655] Ag (or Ab) epitopes (or binding sites) may decay with time; in addition, the deposition may be intermittent and perhaps of varying Ag and Ab content over the course of the nephritic process. Other factors, such as limited sample size and insufficient sampling at appropriate times, compound the technical problems. Numerous techniques for detection and isolation of circulating ICs have been described and used in the study of human IC GN.[2] Identification of an Ag or Ab in a circulating IC does not prove that such ICs are in the kidney, although such findings raise a reasonable level of suspicion in relation to patients with immune deposits and can be strengthened, for example, by showing the presence of a similar idiotype in both locations. Identification of Ag in glomerular immune deposits is strong evidence and elution of Ab from glomeruli, if it can be shown to be specifically concentrated over what would be expected from serum contamination, is equally useful.[2] Taken together, as has been done in SLE, these techniques leave little doubt about the Ag-Ab nature of the immune deposit, although the exact mechanism of accumulation may still be open to debate.

Many of the nephritogenic Ag-Ab systems in humans are similar to those already outlined in animal models of nephritis associated with administration of exogenous Ag, establishment of infection, or occurring spontaneously as part of an autoimmune reaction. A table provided in the previous edition of this chapter gave many of the Ag-Ab systems that have been identified with varying certainty in glomeruli (or circulating ICs) and are associated with apparent IC GN in humans.[3] Also listed were a number of other disease-related forms of GN in which Ag identification would be expected.[1, 2] The majority of Ags that have been identified are from infectious agents that would be expected in infective processes known to be a compounding feature of the particular GN under study. The other large category consists of Ags known from Ab measurements to be associated with a number of autoimmune diseases. As noted earlier, the majority of patients with presumed IC GN

do not have these clues to aid in the search for Ag-Ab systems in glomerular deposits and often remain idiopathic. For additional discussion of the various nephritogenic Ag-Ab systems in human IC GN and other forms of GN of presumed IC origin, the reader is referred to the previous edition of this chapter.[2]

Chapters 30 and 31 of this book are devoted to detailed descriptions of the pathogenic, diagnostic, clinical, and therapeutic aspects of the various morphologic forms and associated clinical presentations of human IC-related GN. Most of these are thought to be produced by the accumulation of immune deposits within glomeruli via the various IC mechanisms that have been outlined herein.

## CONCLUSIONS

The immunopathologic and molecular concepts presented herein implicate humoral and cellular immune mechanisms as well as activation of mediator systems in most cases of GN. Molecular studies have focused on such things as the genetics of the immune response, glomerular components such as $\alpha5(IV)$ collagen in Alport syndrome, and autoimmune responses such as the *Fas* apoptosis gene defect in murine lupus. Molecular immunopathologic approaches have also advanced our knowledge of mediator systems including cytokines, chemokines, and growth factors, which are in large part responsible for the often rather nonselective inflammatory responses induced by specific or nonspecific Ab localization in the kidney. The studies include the role of glomerular cells as contributors to the mediation of injury via production and release of mediator molecules and, just as important, their subsequent role in the response to the injury and its resolution, which often leads to sclerosis with loss of renal function. The study of mediators is being directed to better understanding of the cellular signaling pathways responsible for their activation as well as for their control. The immune mechanisms involve specific humoral and cellular reactions that focus on the action of multiple, often overlapping, and perhaps redundant mediator pathways that cause damage with varying degrees of cellular influx and inflammation. Abs can react directly with structural Ags, such as the GBM, or with planted antigenic components within the glomerulus. In addition, glomerular (and tubule) cells have been shown to be targets of rather selective Ab-induced injury. Glomerular cell surface Ags can be targets for Ab and C attack, sometimes with lysis, or for immune deposit formation. Alternatively, Abs can react with soluble Ags to form ICs that can accumulate in the kidney in dynamic equilibrium with their counterparts in the circulation. The IC localization may be enhanced by physicochemical features of the Ag (or Ab) that favor binding to the glomerulus and, in turn, alter dynamic interchange within the IC. The cellular limb of the immune system, a participant in experimental tubule injury, is being given increasing attention in glomerular injury, in which some models show convincing evidence of a cellular mechanism. Unfortunately, the knowledge about immune mechanisms of renal injury gained from the study of model systems continues to outdistance its translation to the understanding of human counterparts. The immunopathologic tools, including the molecular biologic approaches necessary for identifying the immune mechanisms and overlapping mediator systems responsible for renal injury, are at hand and must be applied vigorously to the evaluation of patients with renal problems. Interruption of ongoing humoral or cellular immune mechanisms, of their mediator systems, and of the factors contributing to sclerosis would be expected to have considerable therapeutic impact.

### *Acknowledgments*

The author gratefully acknowledges the contributions of Ms. Pauline Pess in preparation of the manuscript and the indispensable assistance of Ms. Coyla Wilson in compilation of the references.

### REFERENCES

1. Wilson CB, Dixon FJ: The renal response to immunological injury. *In* Brenner BM, Rector FC Jr (eds): The Kidney, 2nd ed. WB Saunders, Philadelphia, 1981, pp 1237–1350.
2. Wilson CB, Dixon FJ: The renal response to immunological injury. *In* Brenner BM, Rector FC Jr (eds): The Kidney, 3rd ed. WB Saunders, Philadelphia, 1986, pp 800–889.
3. Wilson CB: The renal response to immunological injury. *In* Brenner BM, Rector FC Jr (eds): The Kidney, 4th ed. WB Saunders, Philadelphia, 1991, pp 1062–1181.
4. Dixon FJ, Wilson CB: The development of immunopathologic investigation of kidney disease. Am J Kidney Dis 16:574–578, 1990.
5. Salant DJ, Cybulsky AV: Experimental glomerulonephritis. Methods Enzymol 162:421–461, 1988.
6. Wilson CB: Antibody reactions with native or planted glomerular antigens producing nephritogenic immune deposits or selective glomerular cell injury. *In* Wilson CB, Brenner BM, Stein JH (eds): Contemporary Issues in Nephrology, Vol 18. Churchill Livingstone, New York, 1988, pp 1–34.
7. Hoedemaeker PJ, Weening JJ: Relevance of experimental models for human nephropathology. Kidney Int 35:1015–1025, 1989.
8. Bruijn JA, Hoedemaeker PJ, Fleuren GJ: Pathogenesis of anti–basement membrane glomerulopathy and immune-complex glomerulonephritis: Dichotomy dissolved. Lab Invest 61:480–488, 1989.
9. Wilson CB: Nephritogenic immune reactions involving glomerular basement membrane and other structural renal antigens. *In* Massry SG, Glassock RJ (eds): Textbook of Nephrology, 2nd ed, Vol 1. Williams & Wilkins, Baltimore, 1989, pp 555–559.
10. Hoedemaeker PJ, Aten J, Hogendoorn PC, et al: Pathogenesis of glomerulonephritis: Experimental models revisited. Adv Nephrol Necker Hosp 20:73–90, 1991.
11. Wilson CB: Immunologic aspects of renal diseases. JAMA 268:2904–2909, 1992.
12. Wilson CB: Autoimmune renal disease. *In* Bona C, Siminovitch K, Zanetti M, Theofilopoulos A (eds): The Molecular Pathology of Autoimmune Diseases. Harwood Academic Publishers, Langhorne, PA, 1993, pp 673–704.
13. Couser WG: Pathogenesis of glomerulonephritis. Kidney Int 44(suppl 42):S19–S26, 1993.
14. Couser WG: New insights into mechanisms of immune glomerular injury. West J Med 160:440–446, 1994.
15. Wilson CB, Tang WW, Feng L, et al: Renal diseases. *In* Stites DP, Terr A, Parslow TG (eds): Basic and Clinical Immunology, 8th ed. Appleton & Lange, Norwalk, CT, 1994, pp 478–491.
16. Wilson CB, Tang WW: Immunological renal diseases. *In* Frank MM, Austin KF, Claman HN, Unanue ER (eds): Samter's Immunological Diseases, 5th ed, Vol II. Little, Brown, Boston, 1994, pp 1033–1060.
17. Kitamura M, Taylor S, Unwin R, et al: Gene transfer into the rat renal glomerulus via a mesangial cell vector: Site-specific delivery, in situ amplification, and sustained expression of an exogenous gene in vivo. J Clin Invest 94:497–505, 1994.
18. Moullier P, Friedlander G, Calise D, et al: Adenoviral-mediated gene transfer to renal tubular cells in vivo. Kidney Int 45:1220–1225, 1994.
19. Andres G, Brentjens JR, Caldwell PRB, et al: Formation of immune deposits and disease. Lab Invest 55:510–520, 1986.
20. Sterzel RB, Lovett DH: Interactions of inflammatory and glomerular cells in the response to glomerular injury. *In* Wilson CB, Brenner BM, Stein JH (eds): Contemporary Issues in Nephrology, Vol 18. Churchill Livingstone, New York, 1988, pp 137–173.
21. Couser WG: Mediation of immune glomerular injury. J Am Soc Nephrol 1:13–29, 1990.
22. Makker SP: Mediators of immune glomerular injury. Am J Nephrol 13:324–336, 1993.
23. Couser WG: Mediation of immune glomerular injury. Clin Investig 71:808–811, 1993.
24. van der Woude FJ, Rasmussen N, Lobatto S, et al: Autoantibodies against neutrophils and monocytes: Tool for diagnosis and marker of disease activity in Wegener's granulomatosis. Lancet 1:425–429, 1985.
25. Lockwood CM, Bakes D, Jones S, et al: Association of alkaline phosphatase with an autoantigen recognised by circulating antineutrophil antibodies in systemic vasculitis. Lancet 1:716–719, 1987.
26. Falk RJ, Jennette JC: Anti-neutrophil cytoplasmic autoantibodies with specificity for myeloperoxidase in patients with systemic vasculitis and idiopathic necrotizing and crescentic glomerulonephritis. N Engl J Med 318:1651–1657, 1988.
27. Falk RJ: ANCA-associated renal disease. Kidney Int 38:998–1010, 1990.
28. Jennette JC, Falk RJ: Antineutrophil cytoplasmic autoantibodies and associated disease: A review. Am J Kidney Dis 15:517–529, 1990.
29. Jennette JC: Antineutrophil cytoplasmic autoantibody-associated diseases: A pathologist's perspective. Am J Kidney Dis 18:164–170, 1991.
30. Wieslander J: How are antineutrophil cytoplasmic autoantibodies detected? Am J Kidney Dis 18:154–158, 1991.
31. Niles JL, Pan G, Collins AB, et al: Antigen-specific radioimmunoassays for anti-neutrophil cytoplasmic antibodies in the diagnosis of rapidly progressive glomerulonephritis. J Am Soc Nephrol 2:27–36, 1991.
32. Kallenberg CGM, Brouwer E, Weening JJ, Cohen Tervaert JW: Anti-neutrophil cytoplasmic antibodies: Current diagnostic and pathophysiological potential. Kidney Int 46:1–15, 1994.
33. Goldschmeding R, van der Schoot CE, Ten Bokkel Huinink D, et al: Wegener's granulomatosis autoantibodies identify a novel diisopropylfluorophosphate-binding protein in the lysosomes of normal human neutrophils. J Clin Invest 84:1577–1587, 1989.
34. Niles JL, McCluskey RT, Ahmed MF, Arnaout MA: Wegener's granulomatosis autoantigen is a novel neutrophil serine proteinase. Blood 74:1888–1893, 1989.
35. Ludemann J, Utecht B, Gross WL: Antineutrophil cytoplasm antibodies in Wegener's granulomatosis recognize an elastinolytic enzyme. J Exp Med 171:357–362, 1990.
36. Csernok E, Lüdemann J, Gross WL, Bainton DF: Ultrastructural localization of proteinase 3, the target antigen of anti-cytoplasmic antibodies circulating in Wegener's granulomatosis. Am J Pathol 137:1113–1120, 1990.
37. Braun MG, Csernok E, Gross WL, Müller-Hermelink H-K: Proteinase 3, the target antigen of anticytoplasmic antibodies circulating in Wegener's granulomatosis. Immunolocalization in normal and pathologic tissues. Am J Pathol 139:831–838, 1991.
38. Bini P, Gabay JE, Teitel A, et al: Antineutrophil cytoplasmic autoantibodies in Wegener's granulomatosis recognize conformational epitope(s) on proteinase 3. J Immunol 149:1409–1415, 1992.
39. Kallenberg CGM, Mulder AHL, Tervaert JWC: Antineutrophil cytoplasmic antibodies: A still-growing class of autoantibodies in inflammatory disorders. Am J Med 93:675–682, 1992.
40. Velosa JA, Homburger HA, Holley KE: Prospective study of antineutrophil cytoplasmic autoantibody tests in the diagnosis of idiopathic necrotizing-crescentic glomerulonephritis and renal vasculitis. Mayo Clin Proc 68:561–565, 1993.
41. Kokolina E, Noel L-H, Nusbaum P, et al: Isotype and affinity of anti-myeloperoxidase autoantibodies in systemic vasculitis. Kidney Int 46:177–184, 1994.

42. Esnault VLM, Soleimani B, Keogan MT, et al: Association of IgM with IgG ANCA in patients presenting with pulmonary hemorrhage. Kidney Int 41:1304–1310, 1992.
43. Thomas DM, Moore R, Donovan K, et al: Pulmonary-renal syndrome in association with anti-GBM and IgM ANCA. Lancet 339:1304, 1992.
44. Weber MFA, Andrassy K, Pullig O, et al: Antineutrophil-cytoplasmic antibodies and antiglomerular basement membrane antibodies in Goodpasture's syndrome and in Wegener's granulomatosis. J Am Soc Nephrol 2:1227–1234, 1992.
45. Esnault VLM, Short AK, Audrain MAP, et al: Autoantibodies to lactoferrin and histone in systemic vasculitis identified by anti-myeloperoxidase solid phase assays. Kidney Int 46:153–160, 1994.
46. Pusey CD, Holland MJ, Cashman SJ, et al: Experimental autoimmune glomerulonephritis induced by homologous and isologous glomerular basement membrane in Brown-Norway rats. Nephrol Dial Transplant 6:457–465, 1991.
47. Mathieson PW, Thiru S, Oliveira DBG: Mercuric chloride–treated brown Norway rats develop widespread tissue injury including necrotizing vasculitis. Lab Invest 67:121–129, 1992.
48. Esnault VLM, Mathieson PW, Thiru S, et al: Autoantibodies to myeloperoxidase in brown Norway rats treated with mercuric chloride. Lab Invest 67:114–120, 1992.
49. Qasim FJ, Mathieson PW, Thiru S, et al: Further characterization of an animal model of systemic vasculitis. Adv Exp Med Biol 336:133–137, 1993.
50. Jennette JC: Pathogenic potential of anti-neutrophil cytoplasmic autoantibodies. Lab Invest 70:135–137, 1994.
51. Ewert BH, Jennette JC, Falk RJ: The pathogenic role of antineutrophil cytoplasmic autoantibodies. Am J Kidney Dis 18:188–195, 1991.
52. Falk RJ, Terrell RA, Charles LA, Jennette JC: Anti-neutrophil cytoplasmic autoantibodies induce neutrophils to degranulate and produce oxygen radicals in vitro. Proc Natl Acad Sci USA 87:4115–4119, 1990.
53. Charles LA, Caldas MLR, Falk RJ, et al: Antibodies against granule proteins activate neutrophils in vitro. J Leukoc Biol 50:539–546, 1991.
54. Ewert BH, Jennette JC, Falk RJ: Antimyeloperoxidase antibodies stimulate neutrophils to damage human endothelial cells. Kidney Int 41:375–383, 1992.
55. Johnson RJ, Couser WG, Chi EY, et al: New mechanism for glomerular injury. Myeloperoxidase–hydrogen peroxide–halide system. J Clin Invest 79:1379–1387, 1987.
56. Brouwer E, Weening JJ, Klok PA, et al: Induction of an humoral and cellular (auto) immune response to human and rat myeloperoxidase (MPO) in Brown-Norway (BN), Lewis and Wistar Kyoto (WKY) rat strains. Adv Exp Med Biol 336:139–142, 1993.
57. Brouwer E, Huitema MG, Klok PA, et al: Antimyeloperoxidase-associated proliferative glomerulonephritis: An animal model. J Exp Med 177:905–914, 1993.
58. Lai KN, Leung JCK, Rifkin I, Lockwood CM: Effect of anti–neutrophil cytoplasm autoantibodies on the intracellular calcium concentration of human neutrophils. Lab Invest 70:152–162, 1994.
59. Brouwer E, Huitema MG, Leontine Mulder AH, et al: Neutrophil activation in vitro and in vivo in Wegener's granulomatosis. Kidney Int 45:1120–1131, 1994.
60. Noronha IL, Krüger C, Andrassy K, et al: In situ production of TNF-α, IL-1β and IL-2R in ANCA-positive glomerulonephritis. Kidney Int 43:682–692, 1993.
61. Pall AA, Savage COS: Mechanisms of endothelial cell injury in vasculitis. Springer Semin Immunopathol 16:23–37, 1994.
62. De Vries RRP: HLA and disease: From epidemiology to immunotherapy. Eur J Clin Invest 22:1–8, 1992.
63. Guery JC, Adorini L: Selective immunosuppression of class II–restricted T cells by MHC class II–binding peptides. Crit Rev Immunol 13:195–206, 1993.
64. Engelhard VH: Structure of peptides associated with class I and class II MHC molecules. Annu Rev Immunol 12:181–207, 1994.
65. Raulet DH: MHC class I–deficient mice. Adv Immunol 55:381–423, 1994.
66. Cardell S, Merkenschlager M, Bodmer H, et al: The immune system of mice lacking conventional MHC class II molecules. Adv Immunol 55:424–440, 1994.
67. Oliveira DB, Peters DK: The immunogenetic basis of autoimmunity. Autoimmunity 5:293–306, 1990.
68. Reveille JD: The molecular genetics of systemic lupus erythematosus and Sjögren's syndrome. Curr Opin Rheumatol 3:722–730, 1991.
69. Dunckley H, Chapman JR, Burke J, et al: HLA-DR and -DQ genotyping in anti-GBM disease. Dis Markers 9:249–256, 1991.
70. Ogahara S, Naito S, Abe K, et al: Analysis of HLA class II genes in Japanese patients with idiopathic membranous glomerulonephritis. Kidney Int 41:175–182, 1992.
71. Levy M, Lesavre P: Genetic factors in IgA nephropathy (Berger's disease). Adv Nephrol 21:23–52, 1992.
72. Sacks SH, Warner C, Campbell RD, Dunham I: Molecular mapping of the HLA class II region in HLA-DR3 associated idiopathic membranous nephropathy. Kidney Int 43(suppl 39):S13–S19, 1993.
73. Rambausek MH, Waldherr R, Ritz E: Immunogenetic findings in glomerulonephritis. Kidney Int 43(suppl 39):S3–S8, 1993.
74. Muller GA, Muller CA: Immunogenetics of glomerulonephritis. Clin Invest 71:822–824, 1993.
75. Moore R: MHC gene polymorphism in primary IgA nephropathy. Kidney Int 43(suppl 39):S9–S12, 1993.
76. Wyatt RJ: The complement system in IgA nephropathy and Henoch-Schönlein purpura: Functional and genetic aspects. Contrib Nephrol 104:82–91, 1993.
77. Berthoux FC, Alamartine E, Laurent B, et al: Primary IgA glomerulonephritis and MHC revisited. Contrib Nephrol 104:54–60, 1993.
78. Abe J, Kohsaka T, Tanaka M, Kobayashi N: Genetic study on HLA class II and class III region in the disease associated with IgA nephropathy. Nephron 65:17–22, 1993.
79. Freedman BI, Spray BJ, Heise ER: HLA associations in IgA nephropathy and focal segmental glomerulosclerosis. Am J Kidney Dis 23:352–357, 1994.
80. Freedman BI, Spray BJ, Dunston GM, Heise ER: HLA associations in end-stage renal disease due to membranous glomerulonephritis: HLA-DR3 associations with progressive renal injury. Am J Kidney Dis 23:797–802, 1994.
81. Rees AJ: The immunogenetics of glomerulonephritis. Kidney Int 45:377–383, 1994.
82. McCluskey RT, Bhan AK: Cell-mediated mechanisms in renal diseases. Kidney Int 21(suppl 11):S6, 1982.
83. Fillit HM, Zabriskie JB: Cellular immunity in glomerulonephritis. Am J Pathol 109:227–243, 1982.
84. Williams RC Jr: Cellular mechanism of tissue injury and immune derangement in systemic lupus erythematosus. Arthritis Rheum 25:810–813, 1982.
85. Neilson EG, Clayman MD, Haverty T, et al: Experimental strategies for the study of cellular immunity in renal disease. Kidney Int 30:264–279, 1986.
86. Atkins RC, Holdsworth SR: Cellular mechanisms of immune glomerular injury. In Wilson CB, Brenner BM, Stein JH (eds): Contemporary Issues in Nephrology, Vol 18. Churchill Livingstone, New York, 1988, pp 111–135.
87. Peters DK: Autoimmunity and nephritis. Contrib Nephrol 70:128–134, 1989.
88. Oliveira DBG, Peters DK: Autoimmunity and the pathogenesis of glomerulonephritis. Pediatr Nephrol 4:185–192, 1990.
89. Bolton WK: Mechanisms of glomerular injury: Injury mediated by sensitized lymphocytes. Semin Nephrol 11:285–293, 1991.
90. Rovin BH, Schreiner GF: Cell-mediated immunity in glomerular disease. Annu Rev Med 42:25–33, 1991.
91. Main IW, Nikolic-Paterson DJ, Atkins RC: T cells and macrophages and their role in renal injury. Semin Nephrol 12:395–407, 1992.
92. Lai KN: The cellular immunity and nature of IgA molecules in IgA nephropathy. Contrib Nephrol 104:99–111, 1993.
93. Remuzzi G, Zoja C, Perico N: Proinflammatory mediators of glomerular injury and mechanisms of activation of autoreactive T cells. Kidney Int 45(suppl 44):S-8–S-16, 1994.
94. Mamposo FM, Wilson CB: Characterization of inflammatory cells in autoimmune tubulointerstitial nephritis in rats. Kidney Int 23:448–457, 1983.
95. Meyers CM, Kelly CJ: Effector mechanisms in organ-specific autoimmunity. 1. Characterization of a CD8+ T cell line that mediates murine interstitial nephritis. J Clin Invest 88:408–416, 1991.
96. Kelly CJ, Roth DA, Meyers CM: Immune recognition and response to the renal interstitium. Kidney Int 31:518–530, 1991.
97. Kelly CJ: T cell regulation of autoimmune interstitial nephritis. J Am Soc Nephrol 1:140–149, 1990.

98. Wilson CB: Study of the immunopathogenesis of tubulointerstitial nephritis using model systems. Kidney Int 35:938–953, 1989.

99. Wilson CB: Nephritogenic tubulointerstitial antigens. Kidney Int 39:501–517, 1991.

100. Bhan AK, Schneeberger EE, Collins AB, McCluskey RT: Evidence for a pathogenic role of a cell-mediated immune mechanism in experimental glomerulonephritis. J Exp Med 148:246–260, 1978.

101. Bhan AK, Collins AB, Schneeberger EE, McCluskey RT: A cell-mediated reaction against glomerular-bound immune complexes. J Exp Med 150:1410–1420, 1979.

102. Bhan AK, Schneeberger EE, Collins AB, McCluskey RT: Systemic cell-mediated reactions in vivo. Effect of the interaction of circulating antigen with sensitized lymphocytes on glomeruli and pulmonary alveoli. Am J Pathol 116:77–84, 1984.

103. Oite T, Shimizu F, Kagami S, Morioka T: Hapten-specific cellular immune response producing glomerular injury. Clin Exp Immunol 76:463–468, 1989.

104. Bolton WK, Tucker FL, Sturgill BC: Experimental autoimmune glomerulonephritis in chickens. J Clin Lab Immunol 3:179–184, 1980.

105. Bolton WK, Tucker FL, Sturgill BC: New avian model of experimental glomerulonephritis consistent with mediation by cellular immunity. Nonhumorally mediated glomerulonephritis in chickens. J Clin Invest 73:1263–1276, 1984.

106. Tucker FL, Sturgill BC, Bolton WK: Ultrastructural studies of experimental autoimmune glomerulonephritis in normal and bursectomized chickens. Lab Invest 53:563–570, 1985.

107. Bolton WK, Chandra M, Tyson TM, et al: Transfer of experimental glomerulonephritis in chickens by mononuclear cells. Kidney Int 34:598–610, 1988.

108. Reynolds J, Sallie BA, Syrganis C, Pusey CD: The role of T-helper lymphocytes in priming for experimental autoimmune glomerulonephritis in the BN rat. J Autoimmun 6:571–585, 1993.

109. Bolton WK, May WJ, Sturgill BC: Proliferative autoimmune glomerulonephritis in rats: A model for autoimmune glomerulonephritis in humans. Kidney Int 44:294–306, 1993.

110. Reynolds J, Pusey CD: In vivo treatment with a monoclonal antibody to T helper cells in experimental autoimmune glomerulonephritis in the BN rat. Clin Exp Immunol 95:122–127, 1994.

111. Rennke HG, Klein PS, Sandstrom DJ, Mendrick DL: Cell-mediated immune injury in the kidney: Acute nephritis induced in the rat by azobenzenearsonate. Kidney Int 45:1044–1056, 1994.

112. Andres GA, Cerra F, Elti G, et al: Lymphocyte and blast cell glomerulonephritis in renal allografts of rats injected with phytohaemagglutinin. Cell Immunol 13:146–163, 1974.

113. Camussi G, Tetta C, Bussolino F, et al: Effect of leukocyte stimulation on rabbit immune complex glomerulonephritis. Kidney Int 38:1047–1055, 1990.

114. Kreisberg JI, Wayne DB, Karnovsky MJ: Rapid and focal loss of negative charge associated with mononuclear cell infiltration early in nephrotoxic serum sickness. Kidney Int 16:290–300, 1979.

115. Eddy AA, Crary GS, Michael AF: Identification of lymphohemopoietic cells in the kidneys of normal rats. Am J Pathol 124:335–342, 1986.

116. Florquin S, Goldman M: T cell subsets in glomerular diseases. Springer Semin Immunopathol 16:71–80, 1994.

117. Tipping PG, Neale TJ, Holdsworth SR: T lymphocyte participation in antibody-induced experimental glomerulonephritis. Kidney Int 27:530–537, 1985.

118. Boyce NW, Tipping PG, Holdsworth SR: Lymphokine (MIF) production by glomerular T-lymphocytes in experimental glomerulonephritis. Kidney Int 30:673–677, 1986.

119. Lowry RP, Clarke Forbes RD, Blackburn JH: Immune reactivity and immunosuppressive intervention (TLI) in experimental nephritis. I. Immunopathologic correlates in the accelerated autologous form of nephrotoxic serum nephritis. J Immunol 132:1001–1006, 1984.

120. Eldredge C, Merritt S, Goyal M, et al: Analysis of T cells and major histocompatibility complex class I and class II mRNA and protein content and distribution in antiglomerular basement membrane disease in the rabbit. Am J Pathol 139:1021–1035, 1991.

121. Lowe MG, Holdsworth SR, Tipping PG: T lymphocyte participation in acute serum sickness glomerulonephritis in rabbits. Immunol Cell Biol 69:81–87, 1991.

122. Lan HY, Nikolic-Paterson DJ, Atkins RC: Involvement of activated periglomerular leukocytes in the rupture of Bowman's capsule and glomerular crescent progression in experimental glomerulonephritis. Lab Invest 67:743–751, 1992.

123. Lan HY, Paterson DJ, Hutchinson P, Atkins RC: Leukocyte involvement in the pathogenesis of pulmonary injury in experimental Goodpasture's syndrome. Lab Invest 64:330–338, 1991.

124. Lan HY, Paterson DJ, Atkins RC: Initiation and evolution of interstitial leukocytic infiltration in experimental glomerulonephritis. Kidney Int 40:425–433, 1991.

125. Lan HY, Nikolic-Paterson DJ, Atkins RC: Immune events in lymphoid tissues during experimental glomerulonephritis. Pathology 25:159–166, 1993.

126. Mori S, Nose M, Miyazawa M, et al: Interstitial nephritis in Aleutian mink disease. Possible role of cell-mediated immunity against virus-infected tubular epithelial cells. Am J Pathol 144:1326–1333, 1994.

127. Quiza CG, Leenaerts PL, Hall BM: The role of T cells in the mediation of glomerular injury in Heymann's nephritis in the rat. Int Immunol 4:423–432, 1992.

128. Wofsy D, Seaman W: Successful treatment of autoimmunity in NZB/NZW F$_1$ mice with monoclonal antibody to L3T4. J Exp Med 161:378–391, 1985.

129. Wofsy D: Administration of monoclonal anti–T cell antibodies retards murine lupus in BXSB mice. J Immunol 136:4554–4560, 1986.

130. Santoro T, Portanova J, Kotzin B: The contribution of L3T4$^+$ T cells to lymphoproliferation and autoantibody production in MRL-*lpr/lpr* mice. J Exp Med 167:1713–1718, 1988.

131. Watanabe-Fukunaga R, Brannan CI, Copeland NG, et al: Lymphoproliferation in mice explained by defects in Fas antigen that mediates apoptosis. Nature 356:314–317, 1992.

132. Ito S, Ueno M, Nishi S, et al: Suppression of spontaneous murine lupus by inducing graft-versus-host reaction with CD8$^+$ cells. Clin Exp Immunol 90:260–265, 1992.

133. Doutrelepont J, Moser M, Leo O, et al: Hyper IgE in stimulatory graft-versus-host disease: Role of interleukin-4. Clin Exp Immunol 83:133–136, 1991.

134. Umland S, Razac S, Nahrebne DK, Seymour B: Effects of in vivo administration of interferon (IFN)-γ, anti–IFN-γ, or anti–interleukin-4 monoclonal antibodies in chronic autoimmune graft-versus-host disease. Clin Immunol Immunopathol 63:66–73, 1992.

135. De Wit D, Van Mechelen M, Zanin C, et al: Preferential activation of Th2 cells in chronic graft-versus-host reaction. J Immunol 150:361–366, 1993.

136. Merino J, Schurmans S, Luzuy S, et al: Autoimmune syndrome after induction of neonatal tolerance to alloantigens: Effects of in vivo treatment with anti–T cell subset monoclonal antibodies. J Immunol 139:1426–1431, 1987.

137. Schurmans S, Heusser C, Qin H, et al: In vivo effects of anti–IL-4 monoclonal antibody on neonatal induction of tolerance and on an associated autoimmune syndrome. J Immunol 145:2465–2473, 1990.

138. Feng H, Glasebrook A, Engers H, Louis J: Clonal analysis of T cell unresponsiveness to alloantigens induced by neonatal injection of F1 spleen cells into parental mice. J Immunol 131:2165–2169, 1983.

139. Abramowicz D, Doutrelepont J, Lambert P, et al: Increased expression of Ia antigens on B cells after neonatal induction of lymphoid chimerism in mice: Role of interleukin 4. Eur J Immunol 20:469–476, 1990.

140. Abramowicz D, Durez P, Gérard C, et al: Neonatal induction of transplantation tolerance in mice is associated with in vivo expression of IL-4 and 10 mRNAs. Transplant Proc 25:312–313, 1993.

141. Ochel M, Vohr H, Pfeiffer C, Gleichmann E: IL-4 is required for the IgE and IgG1 increase of IgG1 autoantibody formation in mice treated with mercuric chloride. J Immunol 146:3006–3011, 1991.

142. Goldman M, Druet P, Gleichmann E: T$_H$2 cells in systemic autoimmunity: Insights from allogeneic diseases and chemically-induced autoimmunity. Immunol Today 12:223–227, 1991.

143. Kawasaki K, Yaoita E, Yamamoto T, Kihara I: Depletion of CD8 positive cells in nephrotoxic serum nephritis of WKY rats. Kidney Int 41:1517–1526, 1992.

144. Nishikawa K, Linsley PS, Collins AB, et al: Effect of CTLA-4 chimeric protein on rat autoimmune anti–glomerular basement membrane glomerulonephritis. Eur J Immunol 24:1249–1254, 1994.

145. Nagasawa R, Mitarai T, Utsunomiya Y, et al: Neonatal thymectomy diminishes renal IgA deposition in IgA nephropathy–prone ddY mice. Nephron 66:326–332, 1994.
146. Rasmussen N, Petersen J: Cellular immune responses and pathogenesis in c-ANCA positive vasculitides. J Autoimmun 6:227–236, 1993.
147. Chatenoud L, Bach MA: Abnormalities of T-cell subsets in glomerulonephritis and systemic lupus erythematosus. Kidney Int 20:267–274, 1981.
148. Fornasieri A, Sinico RA, Goldaniga D, et al: B lymphocyte subpopulations and T-cell subsets in primary chronic glomerulonephritis. Clin Nephrol 20:267–268, 1983.
149. Lin CY, Yang YM, Fu YK: T cell subsets in glomerulonephritis. Int J Pediatr Nephrol 7:63–68, 1986.
150. Patel R, Connor G, Patel DR, et al: T cell subsets in idiopathic glomerulonephritis. Int Arch Allergy Appl Immunol 79:182–187, 1986.
151. Haworth SJ, Mundin J, Borysiewicz LK, Sissons JGP: T-cell subsets in glomerulonephritis. Clin Nephrol 21:248–249, 1984.
152. Sengar DPS, Acharya CD, Wolfish NM: HLA specificities, lymphocyte subsets, and mitogenic response in Henoch-Schönlein purpura nephritis. Int J Pediatr Nephrol 5:197–200, 1984.
153. Pettersson E, von Willebrand E, Honkanen E: Immunological mechanisms in glomerulonephritis. A short review and analysis of peripheral mononuclear cell subsets in IgA nephropathy and membranous glomerulonephritis. Scand J Urol Nephrol Suppl 90:29–34, 1985.
154. Lai KN, Ho RTH, Lai CKW, et al: Increase of both circulating Th1 and Th2 T lymphocyte subsets in IgA nephropathy. Clin Exp Immunol 96:116–121, 1994.
155. Scivittaro V, Gesualdo L, Ranieri E, et al: Profiles of immunoregulatory cytokine production in vitro in patients with IgA nephropathy and their kindred. Clin Exp Immunol 96:311–316, 1994.
156. Crow MK, DelGiudice-Asch G, Zehetbauer JB, et al: Autoantigen-specific T cell proliferation induced by the ribosomal P2 protein in patients with systemic lupus erythematosus. J Clin Invest 94:345–352, 1994.
157. Holthöfer H, Virtanen I, Törnroth T, Miettinen A: Lectins as markers for cells infiltrating human renal glomeruli. Virchows Arch B 46:119–126, 1984.
158. Linder J, Yuling Y, Harrington DS, et al: Monoclonal antibodies marking T lymphocytes in paraffin-embedded tissue. Am J Pathol 127:1–8, 1987.
159. Poppema S, Hollema H, Visser L, Vos H: Monoclonal antibodies (MT1, MT2, MB1, MB2, MB3) reactive with leukocyte subsets in paraffin-embedded tissue sections. Am J Pathol 127:418–429, 1987.
160. Cuzic S, Ritz E, Waldherr R: Dendritic cells in glomerulonephritis. Virchows Arch B 62:357–363, 1992.
161. Husby G, Tung KSK, Williams RC Jr: Characterization of renal tissue lymphocytes in patients with interstitial nephritis. Am J Med 70:31–38, 1981.
162. Atkins RC, Holdsworth SR, Hancock WW, et al: Cellular immune mechanisms in human glomerulonephritis: The role of mononuclear leucocytes. Springer Semin Immunopathol 5:269–296, 1982.
163. Arrizabalaga P, Mirapeix E, Darnell A, et al: Cellular immunity analysis using monoclonal antibodies in human glomerulonephritis. Nephron 53:41–49, 1989.
164. Parra G, Platt JL, Falk RJ, et al: Cell populations and membrane attack complex in glomeruli of patients with post-streptococcal glomerulonephritis: Identification using monoclonal antibodies by indirect immunofluorescence. Clin Immunol Immunopathol 33:324–332, 1984.
165. Stachura I, Si L, Madan E, Whiteside T: Mononuclear cell subsets in human renal disease. Enumeration in tissue sections with monoclonal antibodies. Clin Immunol Immunopathol 30:362–373, 1984.
166. Nolasco FEB, Cameron JS, Hartley B, et al: Intraglomerular T cells and monocytes in nephritis: study with monoclonal antibodies. Kidney Int 31:1160–1166, 1987.
167. Hooke DH, Gee DC, Atkins RC: Leukocyte analysis using monoclonal antibodies in human glomerulonephritis. Kidney Int 31:964–972, 1987.
168. Del Prete G, Maggi E, Romagnani S: Human Th1 and Th2 cells: Functional properties, mechanisms of regulation, and role in disease. Lab Invest 70:299–306, 1994.
169. Pober JS, Cotran RS: Immunologic interactions of T lymphocytes with vascular endothelium. Adv Immunol 50:261–302, 1991.
170. Hines WH, Kelly CJ, Haverty TP, Neilson EG: Recognition of antigen (Ag)-secreting renal epithelial cells by Ag-specific helper T cells. Kidney Int 33:317, 1988. Abstract.
171. Haverty TP, Kelly CJ, Hines WH, et al: Characterization of a renal tubular epithelial cell line which secretes the autologous target antigen of autoimmune experimental interstitial nephritis. J Cell Biol 107:1359–1368, 1988.
172. Wuthrich RP, Yui MA, Mazoujian G, et al: Enhanced MHC class II expression in renal proximal tubules precedes loss of renal function in MRL/lpr mice with lupus nephritis. Am J Pathol 134:45–51, 1989.
173. Jevnikar AM, Singer GG, Brennan DC, et al: Dexamethasone prevents autoimmune nephritis and reduces renal expression of Ia but not costimulatory signals. Am J Pathol 141:743–751, 1992.
174. Wuthrich RP, Glimcher LH, Yui MA, et al: MHC class II, antigen presentation and tumor necrosis factor in renal tubular epithelial cells. Kidney Int 37:783–792, 1990.
175. Rubin-Kelley VE, Jevnikar AM: Antigen presentation by renal tubular epithelial cells. J Am Soc Nephrol 2:13–26, 1991.
176. Diaz Gallo C, Jevnikar AM, Brennan DC, et al: Autoreactive kidney-infiltrating T-cell clones in murine lupus nephritis. Kidney Int 42:851–859, 1992.
177. Rubin-Kelley VE, Jevnikar AM, Brennan DC, Diaz-Gallo C: Autoreactive kidney-specific T cell clones captured from renal interstitium of MRL-lpr mice induce class II and intercellular adhesion molecule-1 (ICAM-1) on tubular epithelial cells (TECs). J Am Soc Nephrol 2:559, 1991.
178. Rubin Kelley VR, Diaz-Gallo C, Jevnikar AM, Singer GG: Renal tubular epithelial and T cell interactions in autoimmune renal disease. Kidney Int 43(suppl 39):S-108–S-115, 1993.
179. Jevnikar AM, Singer GG, Coffman T, et al: Transgenic tubular cell expression of class II is insufficient to initiate immune renal injury. J Am Soc Nephrol 3:1972–1977, 1993.
180. Mendrick DL, Kelly DM, Rennke HG: Antigen processing and presentation by glomerular visceral epithelium in vitro. Kidney Int 39:71–78, 1991.
181. Radeke HH, Resch K: The inflammatory function of renal glomerular mesangial cells and their interaction with the cellular immune system. Clin Investig 70:825–842, 1992.
182. Hawkins NJ, Ward RL, Wakefield D: Cytokine-mediated induction of HLA antigen expression on human glomerular mesangial cells. Cell Immunol 155:493–500, 1994.
183. Radeke HH, Emmendörffer A, Uciechowski P, et al: Activation of autoreactive T-lymphocytes by cultured syngeneic glomerular mesangial cells. Kidney Int 45:763–774, 1994.
184. Yokoyama H, Takabatake T, Takaeda M, et al: Up-regulated MHC-class II expression and γ-IFN and soluble IL-2R in lupus nephritis. Kidney Int 42:755–763, 1992.
185. Chatila T, Geha RS: Superantigens. Curr Opin Immunol 4:74–78, 1992.
186. Friedman SM, Tumang JR, Crow MK: Microbial superantigens as etiopathogenic agents in autoimmunity. Rheum Dis Clin North Am 19:207–222, 1993.
187. Irwin MJ, Gascoigne NR: Interplay between superantigens and the immune system. J Leukoc Biol 54:495–503, 1993.
188. He X, Goronzy J, Weyand C: Selective induction of rheumatoid factors by superantigens and human helper T cells. J Clin Invest 89:673–680, 1992.
189. Kim C, Siminovitch KA, Ochi A: Reduction of lupus nephritis in MRL/lpr mice by a bacterial superantigen treatment. J Exp Med 174:1431–1437, 1991.
190. Border WA: Distinguishing minimal-change disease from mesangial disorders. Kidney Int 34:419–434, 1988.
191. Garcia del Moral R, Gomez-Morales M, Cortes V, et al: Mononuclear cell subsets in IgM mesangial proliferative glomerulonephritis. Nephron 65:215–221, 1993.
192. Chiang ML, Hawkins EP, Berry PL, et al: Diagnostic and prognostic significance of glomerular epithelial cell vacuolization and podocyte effacement in children with minimal lesion nephrotic syndrome and focal segmental glomerulosclerosis: An ultrastructural study. Clin Nephrol 30:8–14, 1988.
193. Kitano Y, Yoshikawa N, Nakamura H: Glomerular anionic sites in minimal change nephrotic syndrome and focal segmental glomerulosclerosis. Clin Nephrol 40:199–204, 1993.
194. Hoyer JR: Idiopathic nephrotic syndrome with minimal glomerular

changes. *In* Brenner BM, Stein JH (eds): Nephrotic Syndrome. Contemporary Issues in Nephrology, Vol 9. Churchill Livingstone, New York, 1982, pp 145–174.

195. Schnaper HW: The immune system in minimal change nephrotic syndrome. Pediatr Nephrol 3:101–110, 1989.

196. Lagueruela CC, Buettner TL, Cole BR, et al: HLA extended haplotypes in steroid-sensitive nephrotic syndrome of childhood. Kidney Int 38:145–150, 1990.

197. Thomson NM, Kraft N: Normal human serum also contains the lymphotoxin found in minimal change nephropathy. Kidney Int 31:1186–1193, 1987.

198. Matsumoto K, Yasugi T: Recombinant granulocyte-macrophage colony-stimulating factor modulates in vitro function of the peripheral blood mononuclear cells in lipoid nephrosis. Am J Nephrol 13:100–106, 1993.

199. Inage Z, Wada N, Kikkawa Y, et al: Suppressor T-lymphocyte dysfunction in MCNS: Role of the $H_2$ histamine receptor–bearing suppressor T lymphocytes. Clin Nephrol 33:20–24, 1990.

200. Fiser RT, Arnold WC, Charlton RK, et al: T-lymphocyte subsets in nephrotic syndrome. Kidney Int 40:913–916, 1991.

201. Lenarsky C, Jordan SC, Ladisch S: Plasma inhibition of lymphocyte proliferation in nephrotic syndrome: Correlation with hyperlipidemia. J Clin Immunol 2:276–281, 1982.

202. Warshaw BL, Check IJ, Hymes LC, DiRusso SC: Decreased serum transferrin concentration in children with the nephrotic syndrome: Effect on lymphocyte proliferation and correlation with serum immunoglobulin levels. Clin Immunol Immunopathol 33:210–219, 1984.

203. Matsumoto K, Okano K, Yoshizawa N, et al: Impaired T-lymphocyte colony formation in lipoid nephrosis. Clin Nephrol 24:279–284, 1985.

204. Matsumoto K, Okano K, Hatano M: Evaluation of T colony-stimulating factor in patients with lipoid nephrosis. Nephron 42:87–88, 1986.

205. Hinoshita F, Noma T, Tomura S, et al: Decreased production and responsiveness of interleukin 2 in lymphocytes of patients with nephrotic syndrome. Nephron 54:122–126, 1990.

206. Bensman A, Dardenne M, Murnaghan K, et al: Decreased biological activity of serum thymic hormone (thymulin) in children with nephrotic syndrome. Int J Pediatr Nephrol 5:201–204, 1984.

207. Fodor P, Saitua MT, Rodriguez E, et al: T-cell dysfunction in minimal-change nephrotic syndrome of childhood. Am J Dis Child 136:713–717, 1982.

208. Matsumoto K, Osakabe K, Katayama H, et al: Impaired delayed hypersensitivity in lipoid nephrosis. Nephron 37:273–275, 1984.

209. Matsumoto K, Hatano M: Depression of local graft-versus-host reaction in patients with lipoid nephrosis. J Clin Lab Immunol 17:137–141, 1985.

210. Lagrue G, Laurent J, Hirbec G, et al: Serum IgE in primary glomerular diseases. Nephron 36:5–9, 1984.

211. Yokoyama H, Kida H, Tani Y, et al: Immunodynamics of minimal change nephrotic syndrome in adults T and B lymphocyte subsets and serum immunoglobulin levels. Clin Exp Immunol 61:601–607, 1985.

212. Matsumoto K, Osakabe K, Katayama H, et al: Defective cell-mediated immunity in lipoid nephrosis. Int Arch Allergy Appl Immunol 73:370–372, 1984.

213. Taube D, Brown Z, Williams DG: Impaired lymphocyte and suppressor cell function in minimal change nephropathy, membranous nephropathy and focal glomerulosclerosis. Clin Nephrol 22:176–182, 1984.

214. Gupta S, Yuceoglu AM: Immunological profile in children with minimal change nephrotic syndrome. Acta Paediatr Scand 74:726–732, 1985.

215. Mirapeix E, Montolin J, Suárez C, Revert L: Normal ConA induced suppressor cell function in minimal change nephrotic syndrome. Clin Nephrol 23:156–157, 1985.

216. Chen CH, Hsieh KH, Lee PP: Enhanced suppressor T cell activity resulting in increased IgM and decreased IgG productions in children with minimal change nephrotic syndrome. Int J Pediatr Nephrol 8:75–80, 1987.

217. Schnaper HW, Aune TM: Identification of the lymphokine soluble immune response suppressor in urine of nephrotic children. J Clin Invest 76:341–349, 1985.

218. Schnaper HW, Aune TM: Steroid-sensitive mechanism of soluble immune response suppressor production in steroid-responsive nephrotic syndrome. J Clin Invest 79:257–264, 1987.

219. Schnaper HW: A regulatory system for soluble immune response suppressor production in steroid-responsive nephrotic syndrome. Kidney Int 38:151–159, 1990.

220. Suranyi MG, Guasch A, Hall BM, Myers BD: Elevated levels of tumor necrosis factor-α in the nephrotic syndrome in humans. Am J Kidney Dis 21:251–259, 1993.

221. Saxena S, Mittal A, Andal A: Pattern of interleukins in minimal-change nephrotic syndrome of childhood. Nephron 65:56–61, 1993.

222. Boulton Jones JM, Tulloch I, Dore B, McLay A: Changes in the glomerular capillary wall induced by lymphocyte products and serum of nephrotic patients. Clin Nephrol 20:72–77, 1983.

223. Heslan JM, Branelles A, Laurent J, Lagrue G: The vascular permeability factor is a T lymphocyte product. Nephron 42:187–188, 1986.

224. Maruyama K, Tomizawa S, Shimabukuro N, et al: Effect of supernatants derived from T lymphocyte culture in minimal change nephrotic syndrome on rat kidney capillaries. Nephron 51:73–76, 1989.

225. Yoshizawa N, Kusumi Y, Matsumoto K, et al: Studies of a glomerular permeability factor in patients with minimal-change nephrotic syndrome. Nephron 51:370–376, 1989.

226. Tomizawa S, Nagasawa N, Maruyama K, et al: Release of the vascular permeability factor in minimal change nephrotic syndrome is related to $CD4^+$ lymphocytes. Nephron 56:341–342, 1990.

227. Tanaka R, Yoshikawa N, Nakamura H, Ito H: Infusion of peripheral blood mononuclear cell products from nephrotic children increases albuminuria in rats. Nephron 60:35–41, 1992.

228. Heslan J-MJ, Branellec AI, Pilatte Y, et al: Differentiation between vascular permeability factor and IL-2 in lymphocyte supernatants from patients with minimal-change nephrotic syndrome. Clin Exp Immunol 86:157–162, 1991.

229. Maruyama K, Tomizawa S, Seki Y, et al: Inhibition of vascular permeability factor production by ciclosporin in minimal change nephrotic syndrome. Nephron 62:27–30, 1992.

230. Maruyama K, Tomizawa S, Seki Y, et al: FK 506 for vascular permeability factor production in minimal change nephrotic syndrome. Nephron 66:486–487, 1994.

231. Tischer E, Mitchell R, Hartman T, et al: The human gene for vascular endothelial growth factor. J Biol Chem 266:11947–11954, 1991.

232. Houck KA, Ferrara N, Winer J, et al: The vascular endothelial growth factor family: Identification of a fourth molecular species and characterization of alternative splicing of RNA. Mol Endocrinol 5:1806–1814, 1991.

233. Brown LF, Berse B, Tognazzi K, et al: Vascular permeability factor mRNA and protein expression in human kidney. Kidney Int 42:1457–1461, 1992.

234. Iijima K, Yoshikawa N, Connolly DT, Nakamura H: Human mesangial cells and peripheral blood mononuclear cells produce vascular permeability factor. Kidney Int 44:959–966, 1993.

235. Monacci WT, Merrill MJ, Oldfield EH: Expression of vascular permeability factor/vascular endothelial growth factor in normal rat tissues. Am J Physiol 264:C995–C1002, 1993.

236. Uchida K, Uchida K, Nitta K, et al: Glomerular endothelial cells in culture express and secrete vascular endothelial growth factor. Am J Physiol 266:F81–F88, 1994.

237. Unemori EN, Ferrara N, Bauer EA, Amento EP: Vascular endothelial growth factor induces interstitial collagenase expression in human endothelial cells. J Cell Physiol 153:557–562, 1992.

238. Bakker WW, Baller JFW, van Luijk WHJ: A kallikrein-like molecule and plasma vasoactivity in minimal change disease. Increased turnover in relapse versus remission. Contrib Nephrol 67:31–36, 1988.

239. Wilkinson AH, Gillespie C, Hartley B, Williams DG: Increase in proteinuria and reduction in number of anionic sites on the glomerular basement membrane in rabbits by infusion of human nephrotic plasma in vivo. Clin Sci 77:43–48, 1989.

240. Levin M, Gascoine P, Turner MW, Barratt TM: A highly cationic protein in plasma and urine of children with steroid-responsive nephrotic syndrome. Kidney Int 36:867–877, 1989.

241. Dantal J, Bigot E, Bogers W, et al: Effect of plasma protein adsorption on protein excretion in kidney-transplant recipients with recurrent nephrotic syndrome. N Engl J Med 300:7–14, 1994.

242. Artero ML, Sharma R, Savin VJ, Vincenti F: Plasmapheresis reduces proteinuria and serum capacity to injure glomeruli in patients with recurrent focal glomerulosclerosis. Am J Kidney Dis 23:574–581, 1994.

243. Selby P, Kohn J, Raymond J, et al: Nephrotic syndrome during treatment with interferon. Br Med J 290:1180, 1985.

244. Schattner A, Wallach D, Revel M: Interferon and lipoid nephrosis. Am J Med 85:457–458, 1988.

245. Lotze MT, Frana LW, Sharrow SO, et al: In vivo administration of purified human interleukin 2. I. Half-life and immunologic effects of the Jurkat cell line–derived interleukin 2. J Immunol 134:157–166, 1985.

246. Moullier P, Altman A, Wilson CB: Recombinant human interleukin-2 (rIL2) increases glomerular filtration rate (GFR) in the isolated erythrocyte-perfused rat kidney (IEPK). Kidney Int 35:356, 1989. Abstract.

247. Mandreoli M, Beltrandi E, Casadei-Maldini M, et al: Lymphocyte release of soluble IL-2 receptors in patients with minimal change nephropathy. Clin Nephrol 37:177–182, 1992.

248. Bock GH, Ongkingco JR, Patterson LT, et al: Serum and urine soluble interleukin-2 receptor in idiopathic nephrotic syndrome. Pediatr Nephrol 7:523–528, 1993.

249. Kinoshita T: Biology of complement: The overture. Immunol Today 12:291–295, 1991.

250. Fishelson Z: Complement C3: A molecule mosaic of binding sites. Mol Immunol 28:545–552, 1991.

251. Sim RB, Reid KBM: C1: Molecular interactions with activating systems. Immunol Today 12:307–311, 1991.

252. Hebert LA, Cosio FG, Neff JC: Diagnostic significance of hypocomplementemia. Kidney Int 39:811–821, 1991.

253. Rother K, Hänsch GM, Rauterberg EW: Complement in inflammation: Induction of nephritides and progress to chronicity. Int Arch Allergy Appl Immunol 94:23–37, 1991.

254. Parker CJ: Regulation of complement by membrane proteins. An overview. Curr Top Microbiol Immunol 178:1–6, 1992.

255. Hostetter MK: The third component of complement: New functions for an old friend. J Lab Clin Med 122:491–496, 1993.

256. Liszewski MK, Atkinson JP: The complement system. In Paul WE (ed): Fundamental Immunology, 3rd ed. Raven Press, New York, 1993, pp 917–939.

257. Mathieson PW, Peters DK: Deficiency and depletion of complement in the pathogenesis of nephritis and vasculitis. Kidney Int 44(suppl 42):S-13–S-18, 1993.

258. Nath KA, Hostetter MK, Hostetter TH: Ammonia-complement interaction in the pathogenesis of progressive renal injury. Kidney Int 36(suppl 27):S-52–S-54, 1989.

259. Müller-Eberhard HJ: The membrane attack complex. Springer Semin Immunopathol 7:93–141, 1984.

260. Sodetz JM: Structure and function of C8 in the membrane attack sequence of complement. Curr Top Microbiol Immunol 140:19–31, 1989.

261. Morgan BP: Effects of the membrane attack complex of complement on nucleated cells. Curr Top Microbiol Immunol 178:115–140, 1992.

262. Milgrom H, Curd JG, Kaplan RA, et al: Activation of the fourth component of complement (C4): Assessment by rocket immunoelectrophoresis and correlation with the metabolism of C4. J Immunol 124:2780–2785, 1980.

263. Zwirner J, Felber E, Herzog V, et al: Classical pathway of complement activation in normal and diseased human glomeruli. Kidney Int 36:1069–1077, 1989.

264. Zwirner J, Felber E, Burger R, et al: Classical pathway of complement activation in mammalian kidneys. Immunology 80:162–167, 1993.

265. Schifferli JA, Paccaud JP: Two isotypes of human C4, C4A and C4B, have different structure and function. Complement Inflamm 6:19–26, 1989.

266. Klaus GGB, Humphrey JH: A re-evaluation of the role of C3 in B-cell activation. Immunol Today 7:163–167, 1986.

267. Erdei A, Füst G, Gergely J: The role of C3 in the immune response. Immunol Today 12:332–337, 1991.

268. Lévesque J-P, Hatzfeld A, Hatzfeld J: Mitogenic properties of major extracellular proteins. Immunol Today 12:258–262, 1991.

269. Hourcade D, Holers VM, Atkinson JP: The regulators of complement activation (RCA) gene cluster. Adv Immunol 45:381–416, 1989.

270. Hebert LA, Cosio FG, Birmingham DJ: The role of the complement system in renal injury. Semin Nephrol 12:408–427, 1992.

271. Morgan BP: Membrane regulators of complement. In Nariuchi H, et al (eds): The Molecular Basis of Immune Responses. Academic Press, Tokyo, 1993, pp 259–281.

272. Nicholson-Weller A: Decay accelerating factor (CD55). Curr Top Microbiol Immunol 178:8–30, 1992.

273. Ross GD: Complement receptor type 1. Curr Top Microbiol Immunol 178:31–43, 1992.

274. Liszewski MK, Atkinson JP: Membrane cofactor protein. Curr Top Microbiol Immunol 178:45–60, 1992.

275. Quigg RJ: Isolation of a novel complement regulatory factor (GCRF) from glomerular epithelial cells. Kidney Int 40:668–676, 1991.

276. Pascual M, Steiger G, Sadallah S, et al: Identification of membrane-bound CR1 (CD35) in human urine: Evidence for its release by glomerular podocytes. J Exp Med 179:889–899, 1994.

277. Endoh M, Yamashina M, Ohi H, et al: Immunohistochemical demonstration of membrane cofactor protein (MCP) of complement in normal and diseased kidney tissue. Clin Exp Immunol 94:182–188, 1993.

278. Johnstone RW, Loveland BE, McKenzie IFC: Identification and quantification of complement regulator CD46 on normal human tissues. Immunology 79:341–347, 1993.

279. Nakanishi I, Moutabarrik A, Hara T, et al: Identification and characterization of membrane cofactor protein (CD46) in the human kidneys. Eur J Immunol 24:1529–1535, 1994.

280. Shibata T, Cosio FG, Birmingham DJ: Complement activation induces the expression of decay-accelerating factor on human mesangial cells. J Immunol 147:3901–3908, 1991.

281. Quigg RJ, Galishoff ML, Sneed AE 3rd, Kim D: Isolation and characterization of complement receptor type 1 from rat glomerular epithelial cells. Kidney Int 43:730–736, 1993.

282. Appay M-D, Kazatchkine MD, Levi-Strauss M, et al: Expression of CR1 (CD35) mRNA in podocytes from adult and fetal human kidneys. Kidney Int 38:289–293, 1990.

283. Podack ER: Perforin: Structure, function, and regulation. Curr Top Microbiol Immunol 178:175–184, 1992.

284. Lachmann PJ: The control of homologous lysis. Immunol Today 12:312–315, 1991.

285. Hänsch GM: The complement attack phase: Control of lysis and non-lethal effects of C5b-9. Immunopharmacology 24:107–117, 1992.

286. Holguin MH, Parker CJ: Membrane inhibitor of reactive lysis. Curr Top Microbiol Immunol 178:61–85, 1992.

287. Zalman LS: Homologous restriction factor. Curr Top Microbiol Immunol 178:87–99, 1992.

288. Davies A, Lachmann PJ: Membrane defence against complement lysis: The structure and biological properties of CD59. Immunol Res 12:258–275, 1993.

289. Meri S, Morgan BP, Davies A, et al: Human protectin (CD59), an 18,000–20,000 MW complement lysis restricting factor, inhibits C5b-8 catalysed insertion of C9 into lipid bilayers. Immunology 71:1–9, 1990.

290. Lehto T, Meri S: Interactions of soluble CD59 with the terminal complement complexes. CD59 and C9 compete for a nascent epitope on C8. J Immunol 151:4941–4949, 1993.

291. Morgan BP, Walport MJ: Complement deficiency and disease. Immunol Today 12:301–306, 1991.

292. Lhotta K, Thoenes W, Glatzl J, et al: Hereditary complete deficiency of the fourth component of complement: Effects on the kidney. Clin Nephrol 39:117–124, 1993.

293. Farries TC, Atkinson JP: Evolution of the complement system. Immunol Today 12:295–300, 1991.

294. de Boer JP, Wolbink G-J, Thijs LG, et al: Interplay of complement and cytokines in the pathogenesis of septic shock. Immunopharmacology 24:135–148, 1992.

295. Meri S, Koistinen V, Miettinen A, et al: Activation of the alternative pathway of complement by monoclonal λ light chains in membranoproliferative glomerulonephritis. J Exp Med 175:939–950, 1992.

296. Müller-Eberhard HJ, Schreiber RD: Molecular biology and chemistry of the alternative pathway of complement. Adv Immunol 29:1–53, 1980.

297. Schena FP, Pertosa G, Stanziale P, et al: Serum profiles of the

regulatory complement proteins during the progression of renal damage in human glomerulonephritis. Nephron 44:272–276, 1986.

298. Strife CF, Jackson EC, Forristal J, West CD: Effect of the nephrotic syndrome on the concentration of serum complement components. Am J Kidney Dis 8:37–42, 1986.

299. Waldo FB, West CD: Quantitation of (C1INH)₂ C1r-C1s complexes in glomerulonephritis as an indicator of C1 activation. Clin Immunol Immunopathol 42:239–249, 1987.

300. McEnery PT: Membranoproliferative glomerulonephritis: The Cincinnati experience—cumulative renal survival from 1957–1989. J Pediatr 116:S109–S114, 1990.

301. Power DA, Ng YC, Simpson JG: Familial incidence of C3 nephritic factor, partial lipodystrophy and membranoproliferative glomerulonephritis. Q J Med 75:387–398, 1990.

302. Varade WS, Forristal J, West CD: Patterns of complement activation in idiopathic membranoproliferative glomerulonephritis, types I, II, and III. Am J Kidney Dis 16:196–206, 1990.

303. D'Amico G, Ferrario F: Mesangiocapillary glomerulonephritis. J Am Soc Nephrol 2:S159–S166, 1992.

304. Ohi H, Watanabe S, Fujita T, Yasugi T: Significance of C3 nephritic factor (C3NeF) in non-hypocomplementaemic serum with membranoproliferative glomerulonephritis (MPGN). Clin Exp Immunol 89:479–484, 1992.

305. Mathieson PW, Wurzner R, Oliveira DB, et al: Complement-mediated adipocyte lysis by nephritic factor sera. J Exp Med 177:1827–1831, 1993.

306. Spitzer RE, Stitzel AE, Tsokos GC: Study of the idiotypic response to autoantibody to the alternative pathway C3/C5 convertase in normal individuals, patients with membranoproliferative glomerulonephritis, and experimental animals. Clin Immunol Immunopathol 62:291–294, 1992.

307. Finn JE, Mathieson PW: Molecular analysis of C3 allotypes in patients with nephritic factor. Clin Exp Immunol 91:410–414, 1993.

308. Tanuma Y, Ohi H, Hatano M: Two types of C3 nephritic factor: Properdin-dependent C3NeF and properdin independent C3NeF. Clin Immunol Immunopathol 56:226–238, 1990.

309. Strife CF, Prada AL, Clardy CW, et al: Autoantibody to complement neoantigens in membranoproliferative glomerulonephritis. J Pediatr 116:S98–102, 1990.

310. Meri S: Complement activation by circulating serum factors in human glomerulonephritis. Clin Exp Immunol 59:276–284, 1985.

311. Ng YC, Peters DK: C3 nephritic factor (C3NeF): Dissociation of cell-bound and fluid phase stabilization of alternative pathway C3 convertase. Clin Exp Immunol 65:450–457, 1986.

312. Hiramatsu M, Balow JE, Tsokos GC: Production of nephritic factor of the alternative complement pathway by Epstein Barr virus–transformed B cell lines derived from a patient with membranoproliferative glomerulonephritis. J Immunol 136:4451–4455, 1986.

313. Marin MA, Fontan G, Lopez-Trascasa M: Requirements for the production of high-titre C3 nephritic factor (NEF) antibody in vitro. Immunology 76:318–323, 1992.

314. Marder HK, Coleman TH, Forristal J, et al: An inherited defect in the C3 convertase, C3b,Bb, associated with glomerulonephritis. Kidney Int 23:749–758, 1983.

315. Linshaw MA, Stapleton FB, Cuppage FE, et al: Hypocomplementemic glomerulonephritis in an infant and mother. Evidence for an abnormal form of C3. Am J Nephrol 7:470–477, 1987.

316. Levy M, Halbwachs-Mecarelli L, Gubler M-C, et al: H deficiency in two brothers with atypical dense intramembranous deposit disease. Kidney Int 30:949–956, 1986.

317. Siegert CEH, Daha MR, Tseng CMES, et al: Predictive value of IgG autoantibodies against C1q for nephritis in systemic lupus erythematosus. Ann Rheum Dis 52:851–856, 1993.

318. Coremans IEM, Daha MR, Van Der Voort EAM, et al: Antibodies against C1q in anti-glomerular basement membrane nephritis. Clin Exp Immunol 87:256–260, 1992.

319. Rehan A, Wiggins RC, Kunkel RG, et al: Glomerular injury and proteinuria in rats after intrarenal injection of cobra venom factor. Evidence for the role of neutrophil-derived oxygen free radicals. Am J Pathol 123:57–66, 1986.

320. Lundberg C, Marceau F, Hugli TE: C5a-induced hemodynamic and hematologic changes in the rabbit. Role of cyclooxygenase products and polymorphonuclear leukocytes. Am J Pathol 128:471–483, 1987.

321. Pelayo JC, Chenoweth DE, Hugli TE, et al: Effects of the anaphylatoxin, C5a, on renal and glomerular hemodynamics in the rat. Kidney Int 30:62–67, 1986.

322. Sekse I, Iversen BM, Daha MR, Ofstad J: Acute effect of passive Heymann nephritis on renal blood flow and glomerular filtration rate in the rat: Role of the anaphylatoxin C5a and the alpha-adrenergic nervous system. Nephron 60:453–459, 1992.

323. Belmont HM, Hopkins P, Edelson HS, et al: Complement activation during systemic lupus erythematosus. C3a and C5a anaphylatoxins circulate during exacerbations of disease. Arthritis Rheum 29:1085–1089, 1986.

324. Shingu M, Nobunaga M: Chemotactic activity generated in human serum from the fifth component of complement by hydrogen peroxide. Am J Pathol 117:201–206, 1984.

325. Leivo I, Engvall E: C3d fragment of complement interacts with laminin and binds to basement membranes of glomerulus and trophoblast. J Cell Biol 103:1091–1100, 1986.

326. Doi T, Kanatsu K, Nagai H, et al: Demonstration of C3d deposits in membranous nephropathy. Nephron 37:232–235, 1984.

327. Doi T, Kanatsu K, Suehiro F, et al: Clinicopathological study of patients with mesangial isolated C3d deposition in various glomerular diseases. Nephron 46:188–193, 1987.

328. Schulze M, Pruchno CJ, Burns M, et al: Glomerular C3c localization indicates ongoing immune deposit formation and complement activation in experimental glomerulonephritis. Am J Pathol 142:179–187, 1993.

329. Linder E, Helin H, Rantala I: Activation of complement by intermediate filaments of glomerular epithelial cells. Clin Immunol Immunopathol 40:265–275, 1986.

330. Baker PJ, Adler S, Yang Y, Couser WG: Complement activation by heat-killed human kidney cells: Formation, activity, and stabilization of cell-bound C3 convertases. J Immunol 133:877–881, 1984.

331. Feucht HE, Jung CM, Gokel MJ, et al: Detection of both isotypes of complement C4, C4A and C4B, in normal human glomeruli. Kidney Int 30:932–936, 1986.

332. Warren HB, Pantazis P, Davies PF: The third component of complement is transcribed and secreted by cultured human endothelial cells. Am J Pathol 129:9–13, 1987.

333. Zhou W, Campbell RD, Martin J, Sacks SH: Interferon-γ regulation of C4 gene expression in cultured human glomerular epithelial cells. Eur J Immunol 23:2477–2481, 1993.

334. Sacks S, Zhou W, Campbell RD, Martin J: C3 and C4 gene expression and interferon-gamma–mediated regulation in human glomerular mesangial cells. Clin Exp Immunol 93:411–417, 1993.

335. Sacks SH, Zhou W, Pani A, et al: Complement C3 gene expression and regulation in human glomerular epithelial cells. Immunology 79:348–354, 1993.

336. Seelen MAJ, Brooimans RA, van der Woude FJ, et al: IFN-γ mediates stimulation of complement C4 biosynthesis in human proximal tubular epithelial cells. Kidney Int 44:50–57, 1993.

337. van den Dobbelsteen MEA, Verhasselt V, Kaashoek JGJ, et al: Regulation of C3 and factor H synthesis of human glomerular mesangial cells by IL-1 and interferon-gamma. Clin Exp Immunol 95:173–180, 1994.

338. Sacks SH, Zhou W, Andrews PA, Hartley B: Endogenous complement C3 synthesis in immune complex nephritis. Lancet 342:1273–1274, 1993.

339. Montinaro V, Di Cillo M, Perissutti S, et al: Modulation of renal production of C3 by proinflammatory cytokines. Kidney Int 43(suppl 39):S-37–S-40, 1993.

340. Ravnskov U: Renal complement synthesis in glomerulonephritis. Lancet 343:235–236, 1994.

341. Biesecker G: Membrane attack complex of complement as a pathologic mediator. Lab Invest 49:237–249, 1983.

342. Couser WG, Baker PJ, Adler S: Complement and the direct mediation of immune glomerular injury: A new perspective. Kidney Int 28:879–890, 1985.

343. Quigg RJ: Mediation of glomerular injury. Glomerular injury induced by antibody and complement. Semin Nephrol 11:259–267, 1991.

344. McLean RH: Complement and glomerulonephritis—an update. Pediatr Nephrol 7:226–232, 1993.

345. Savin VJ, Johnson RJ, Couser WG: C5b-9 increases albumin permeability of isolated glomeruli in vitro. Kidney Int 46:382–387, 1994.

346. Boyce NW, Holdsworth SR: Evidence for direct renal injury as a consequence of glomerular complement activation. J Immunol 136:2421–2425, 1986.

347. Thaiss F, Batsford S, Mihatsch MJ, et al: Mediator systems in a passive model of in situ immune complex glomerulonephritis. Role for complement, polymorphonuclear granulocytes and monocytes. Lab Invest 54:624–635, 1986.

348. Salant DJ, Belok S, Madaio MP, Couser WG: A new role for complement in experimental membranous nephropathy in rats. J Clin Invest 66:1339–1350, 1980.

349. Adler S, Salant DJ, Dittmer JE, et al: Mediation of proteinuria in membranous nephropathy due to a planted glomerular antigen. Kidney Int 23:807–815, 1983.

350. Salant DJ, Madaio MP, Adler S, et al: Altered glomerular permeability induced by F(ab′)$_2$ and Fab′ antibodies to rat renal tubular epithelial antigen. Kidney Int 21:36–43, 1981.

351. Groggel GC, Adler S, Rennke HG, et al: Role of the terminal complement pathway in experimental membranous nephropathy in the rabbit. J Clin Invest 72:1948–1957, 1983.

352. Groggel GC, Salant DJ, Darby C, et al: Role of terminal complement pathway in the heterologous phase of antiglomerular basement membrane nephritis. Kidney Int 27:643–651, 1985.

353. Groggel GC, Terreros DA: Role of the terminal complement pathway in accelerated autologous anti–glomerular basement membrane nephritis. Am J Pathol 136:533–540, 1990.

354. Parra G, Takekoshi Y, Striegel J, et al: Acute serum sickness in normal and C6 deficient rabbits: Role of membrane attack complex. Int J Exp Pathol 73:299–312, 1992.

355. Baker PJ, Ochi RF, Schulze M, et al: Depletion of C6 prevents development of proteinuria in experimental membranous nephropathy in rats. Am J Pathol 135:185–194, 1989.

356. Couser WG, Ochi RF, Baker PJ, et al: C6 depletion reduces proteinuria in experimental nephropathy induced by a nonglomerular antigen. J Am Soc Nephrol 2:894–901, 1991.

357. Cybulsky AV, Quigg RJ, Salant DJ: The membrane attack complex in complement-mediated glomerular epithelial cell injury: Formation and stability of C5b-9 and C5b-7 in rat membranous nephropathy. J Immunol 137:1511–1516, 1986.

358. Cybulsky AV, Rennke HG, Feintzeig ID, Salant DJ: Complement-induced glomerular epithelial cell injury. Role of the membrane attack complex in rat membranous nephropathy. J Clin Invest 77:1096–1107, 1986.

359. Quigg RJ, Cybulsky AV, Jacobs JB, Salant DJ: Anti-Fx1A produces complement-dependent cytotoxicity of glomerular epithelial cells. Kidney Int 34:43–52, 1988.

360. Quigg RJ, Cybulsky AV, Salant DJ: Effect of nephritogenic antibody on complement regulation in cultured rat glomerular epithelial cells. J Immunol 147:838–845, 1991.

361. Kerjaschki D, Schulze M, Binder S, et al: Transcellular transport and membrane insertion of the C5b-9 membrane attack complex of complement by glomerular epithelial cells in experimental membranous nephropathy. J Immunol 143:546–552, 1989.

362. Yamamoto T, Wilson CB: Mesangial cell (MC) injury and proliferation produced by antibody: A role for the membrane attack complex (MAC). Kidney Int 31:333, 1987. Abstract.

363. Lovett DH, Haensch G-M, Goppelt M, et al: Activation of glomerular mesangial cells by the terminal membrane attack complex of complement. J Immunol 138:2473–2480, 1987.

364. Kopp WC, Burrell R: Evidence for antibody-dependent binding of the terminal complement component to alveolar basement membrane. Clin Immunol Immunopathol 23:10–21, 1982.

365. Cybulsky AV, Salant DJ, Quigg RJ, et al: Complement C5b-9 complex activates phospholipases in glomerular epithelial cells. Am J Physiol 257:F826–F836, 1989.

366. Cybulsky AV, Cyr M-D: Phosphatidylcholine-directed phospholipase C: Activation by complement C5b-9. Am J Physiol 265:F551–F560, 1993.

367. Cybulsky AV, Bonventre JV, Quigg RJ, et al: Cytosolic calcium and protein kinase C reduce complement-mediated glomerular epithelial injury. Kidney Int 38:803–811, 1990.

368. Schönermark M, Deppisch R, Riedasch G, et al: Induction of mediator release from human glomerular mesangial cells by the terminal complement components C5b-9. Int Arch Allergy Appl Immunol 96:331–337, 1991.

369. Cybulsky AV: Release of arachidonic acid by complement C5b-9 complex in glomerular epithelial cells. Am J Physiol 261:F427–F436, 1991.

370. Lianos EA, Zanglis A: Effects of complement activation on platelet-activating factor and eicosanoid synthesis in rat mesangial cells. J Lab Clin Med 120:459–464, 1992.

371. Hattori R, Hamilton KK, McEver RP, Sims PJ: Complement proteins C5b-9 induce secretion of high molecular weight multimers of endothelial von Willebrand factor and translocation of granule membrane protein GMP-140 to the cell surface. J Biol Chem 264:9053–9060, 1989.

372. Torbohm I, Schönermark M, Wingen A-M, et al: C5b-8 and C5b-9 modulate the collagen release of human glomerular epithelial cells. Kidney Int 37:1098–1104, 1990.

373. Floege J, Johnson RJ, Gordon K, et al: Altered glomerular extracellular matrix synthesis in experimental membranous nephropathy. Kidney Int 42:573–585, 1992.

374. Benzaquen LR, Nicholson-Weller A, Halperin JA: Terminal complement proteins C5b-9 release basic fibroblast growth factor and platelet-derived growth factor from endothelial cells. J Exp Med 179:985–992, 1994.

375. Floege J, Alpers CE, Sage EH, et al: Markers of complement-dependent and complement-independent glomerular visceral epithelial cell injury in vivo. Expression of anti-adhesive proteins and cytoskeletal changes. Lab Invest 67:486–497, 1992.

376. Adler S: Integrin matrix receptors in renal injury. Kidney Int 45(suppl 45):S-86–S-89, 1994.

377. Shah SV: Evidence suggesting a role for hydroxyl radical in passive Heymann nephritis in rats. Am J Physiol 254:F337–F344, 1988.

378. Neale TJ, Ullrich R, Ojha P, et al: Reactive oxygen species and neutrophil respiratory burst cytochrome $b_{558}$ are produced by kidney glomerular cells in passive Heymann nephritis. Proc Natl Acad Sci USA 90:3645–3649, 1993.

379. Sims PJ, Wiedmer T: The response of human platelets to activated components of the complement system. Immunol Today 12:338–342, 1991.

380. Falk RJ, Dalmasso AP, Kim Y, et al: Neoantigen of the polymerized ninth component of complement. Characterization of a monoclonal antibody and immunohistochemical localization in renal disease. J Clin Invest 72:560–573, 1983.

381. Hinglais N, Kazatchkine MD, Bhakdi S, et al: Immunohistochemical study of the C5b-9 complex of complement in human kidneys. Kidney Int 30:399–410, 1986.

382. Cosyns JP, Kazatchkine MD, Bhakdi S, et al: Immunohistochemical analysis of C3 cleavage fragments, factor H, and the C5b-9 terminal complex of complement in de novo membranous glomerulonephritis occurring in patients with renal transplant. Clin Nephrol 26:203–208, 1986.

383. Pruchno CJ, Burns MW, Schulze M, et al: Urinary excretion of C5b-9 reflects disease activity in passive Heymann nephritis. Kidney Int 36:65–71, 1989.

384. Pruchno CJ, Burns MM, Schulze M, et al: Urinary excretion of the C5b-9 membrane attack complex of complement is a marker of immune disease activity in autologous immune complex nephritis. Am J Pathol 138:203–211, 1991.

385. Schultze M, Donadio JV Jr, Pruchno CJ, et al: Elevated urinary excretion of C5b-9 in membranous nephropathy. Kidney Int 40:533–538, 1991.

386. Kusunoki Y, Akutsu Y, Itami N, et al: Urinary excretion of terminal complement complexes in glomerular disease. Nephron 59:27–32, 1991.

387. Ogrodowski JL, Hebert LA, Sedmak D, et al: Measurement of SC5b-9 in urine in patients with the nephrotic syndrome. Kidney Int 40:1141–1147, 1991.

388. Brenchley PE, Coupes B, Short CD, et al: Urinary C3dg and C5b-9 indicate active immune disease in human membranous nephropathy. Kidney Int 41:933–937, 1992.

389. Schieren G, Janssen O, Hänsch GM: Enhanced expression of the complement-regulatory factor C8 binding protein (C8bp) on U937 cells after stimulation with IL-1β, endotoxin, IFN-γ, or phorbol ester. J Immunol 148:3183–3188, 1992.

390. Falk RJ, Dalmasso AP, Kim Y, et al: Radioimmunoassay of the attack complex of complement in serum from patients with systemic lupus erythematosus. N Engl J Med 312:1594–1599, 1985.

391. Rauterberg EW, Lieberknecht HM, Wingen AM, Ritz E: Complement membrane attack (MAC) in idiopathic IgA-glomerulonephritis. Kidney Int 31:820–829, 1987.

392. Falk RJ, Podack E, Dalmasso AP, Jennette JC: Localization of S protein and its relationship to the membrane attack complex of complement in renal tissue. Am J Pathol 127:182–190, 1987.

393. Bariety J, Hinglais N, Bhakdi S: Immunohistochemical study of complement S protein (Vitronectin) in normal and diseased human kidneys: Relationship to neoantigens of the C5b-9 terminal complex. Clin Exp Immunol 75:76–81, 1989.

394. Lai KN, Lo STH, Lai FM-M: Immunohistochemical study of the membrane attack complex of complement and S-protein in idiopathic and secondary membranous nephropathy. Am J Pathol 135:469–476, 1989.

395. Okada M, Yoshioka K, Takemura T, et al: Immunohistochemical localization of C3d fragment of complement and S-protein (vitronectin) in normal and diseased human kidneys: Association with the C5b-9 complex and vitronectin receptor. Virchows Arch A 422:367–373, 1993.

396. Moutabarrik A, Nakanishi I, Namiki M, et al: Cytokine-mediated regulation of the surface expression of complement regulatory proteins, CD46(MCP), CD55(DAF), and CD59 on human vascular endothelial cells. Lymphokine Cytokine Res 12:167–172, 1993.

397. Holquin MH, Martin CB, Weis JH, Parker CJ: Enhanced expression of the complement regulatory protein, membrane inhibitor of reactive lysis (CD59), is regulated at the level of transcription. Blood 82:968–977, 1993.

398. Hughes TR, Piddlesden SJ, Williams JD, et al: Isolation and characterization of a membrane protein from rat erythrocytes which inhibits lysis by the membrane attack complex of rat complement. Biochem J 284:169–176, 1992.

399. Hughes TR, Meri S, Davies M, et al: Immunolocalization and characterization of the rat analogue of human CD59 in kidney and glomerular cells. Immunology 80:439–444, 1993.

400. Rooney IA, Davies A, Griffiths D, et al: The complement-inhibiting protein, protectin (CD59 antigen), is present and functionally active on glomerular epithelial cells. Clin Exp Immunol 83:251–256, 1991.

401. Tamai H, Matsuo S, Fukatsu A, et al: Localization of 20-kD homologous restriction factor (HRF20) in diseased human glomeruli. An immunofluorescence study. Clin Exp Immunol 84:256–262, 1991.

402. Blake PG, Madrenas J, Halloran PF: Ly-6 in kidney is widely expressed on tubular epithelium and vascular endothelium and is up-regulated by interferon gamma. J Am Soc Nephrol 4:1140–1150, 1993.

403. Brooimans RA, Van der Ark AA, Tomita M, et al: CD59 expressed by human endothelial cells functions as a protective molecule against complement-mediated lysis. Eur J Immunol 22:791–797, 1992.

404. Matsuo S, Nishikage H, Yoshida F, et al: Role of CD59 in experimental glomerulonephritis in rats. Kidney Int 46:191–200, 1994.

405. Quigg RJ: Inhibition of the alternative pathway of complement by glomerular chondroitin sulphate proteoglycan. Immunology 76:373–377, 1992.

406. Tschopp J, Chonn A, Hertig S, French LE: Clusterin, the human apolipoprotein and complement inhibitor, binds to complement C7, C8 beta, and the b domain of C9. J Immunol 151:2159–2165, 1993.

407. Murphy BF, Kirszbaum L, Walker ID, d'Apice AJF: SP-40,40, a newly identified normal human serum protein found in the SC5b-9 complex of complement and in the immune deposits in glomerulonephritis. J Clin Invest 81:1858–1864, 1988.

408. Murphy BF, Davies DJ, Morrow W, D'Apice AJF: Localisation of terminal complement components, S-protein and SP-40,40 in renal biopsies. Pathology 21:275–278, 1988.

409. Eddy AA, Fritz IB: Localization of clusterin in the epimembranous deposits of passive Heymann nephritis. Kidney Int 39:247–252, 1991.

410. French LE, Tschopp J, Schifferli JA: Clusterin in renal tissue: Preferential localization with the terminal complement complex and immunoglobulin deposits in glomeruli. Clin Exp Immunol 88:389–393, 1992.

411. Correa-Rotter R, Hostetter TH, Nath KA, et al: Interaction of complement and clusterin in renal injury. J Am Soc Nephrol 3:1172–1179, 1992.

412. Saunders JR, Aminian A, McRae JL, et al: Clusterin depletion enhances immune glomerular injury in the isolated perfused kidney. Kidney Int 45:817–827, 1994.

413. Wilson MR, Roeth PJ, Easterbrook-Smith SB: Clusterin enhances the formation of insoluble immune complexes. Biochem Biophys Res Commun 177:985–990, 1991.

414. Gabbai FB, Mundy C, Wilson CB, Blantz RC: An evaluation of the role of complement depletion in experimental membranous nephropathy in the rat. Lab Invest 58:539–544, 1988.

415. Bone RC: Inhibitors of complement and neutrophils: A critical evaluation of their role in the treatment of sepsis. Crit Care Med 20:891–898, 1992.

416. Fujita Y, Inoue I, Inagi R, et al: Inhibitory effect of FUT-175 on complement activation and its application for glomerulonephritis with hypocomplementemia. Nippon Jinzo Gakkai Shi 35:393–397, 1993.

417. Miyata T, Fujita Y, Inagi R, et al: Effectiveness of nafamostat mesilate on glomerulonephritis in immune-complex diseases. Lancet 341:1353, 1993. Letter.

418. Pober JS, Cotran RS: Cytokines and endothelial cell biology. Physiol Rev 70:427–451, 1990.

419. Osborn L: Leukocyte adhesion to endothelium in inflammation. Cell 62:3–6, 1990.

420. Cotran RS, Pober JS: Cytokine-endothelial interactions in inflammation, immunity, and vascular injury. J Am Soc Nephrol 1:225–235, 1990.

421. Butcher EC: Cellular and molecular mechanisms that direct leukocyte traffic. Am J Pathol 136:3–11, 1990.

422. Lawrence MB, Springer TA: Leukocytes roll on a selectin at physiologic flow rates: Distinction from and prerequisite for adhesion through integrins. Cell 65:859–873, 1991.

423. Albelda SM: Endothelial and epithelial cell adhesion molecules. Am J Respir Cell Mol Biol 4:195–203, 1991.

424. Butcher EC: Leukocyte–endothelial cell recognition: Three (or more) steps to specificity and diversity. Cell 67:1033–1036, 1991.

425. Zimmerman GA, Prescott SM, McIntyre TM: Endothelial cell interactions with granulocytes: Tethering and signaling molecules. Immunol Today 13:93–100, 1992.

426. Rosen SD: Cell surface lectins in the immune system. Semin Immunol 5:237–247, 1993.

427. Bevilacqua MP: Endothelial-leukocyte adhesion molecules. Annu Rev Immunol 11:767–804, 1993.

428. Briscoe DM, Cotran RS: Role of leukocyte–endothelial cell adhesion molecules in renal inflammation: In vitro and in vivo studies. Kidney Int 44 (suppl 42):S-27–S-34, 1993. (Erratum in Kidney Int 44:658, 1993.)

429. Springer TA: Traffic signals for lymphocyte recirculation and leukocyte emigration: Multistep paradigm. Cell 76:301–314, 1994.

430. Nikolic-Paterson DJ, Main IW, Lan HY, et al: Adhesion molecules in glomerulonephritis. Springer Semin Immunopathol 16:3–22, 1994.

431. Stewart RJ, Marsden PA: Vascular endothelial cell activation in models of vascular and glomerular injury. Kidney Int 45(suppl 45):S-37–S-44, 1994.

432. Brady HR: Leukocyte adhesion molecules and kidney diseases. Kidney Int 45:1285–1300, 1994.

433. Lasky LA: Selectins: Interpreters of cell-specific carbohydrate information during inflammation. Science 258:964–969, 1992.

434. Foreman KE, Vaporciyan AA, Bonish BK, et al: C5a-induced expression of P-selectin in endothelial cells. J Clin Invest 94:1147–1155, 1994.

435. Mayadas TN, Johnson RC, Rayburn H, et al: Leukocyte rolling and extravasation are severely compromised in P selectin–deficient mice. Cell 74:541–554, 1993.

436. Tipping PG, Huang XR, Berndt MC, Holdsworth SR: A role for P selectin in complement-independent neutrophil-mediated glomerular injury. Kidney Int 46:79–88, 1994.

437. Kishimoto TK, Jutila MA, Berg EL, Butcher EC: Neutrophil Mac-1 and MEL-14 adhesion proteins inversely regulated by chemotactic factors. Science 245:1238–1241, 1989.

438. Rot A: Endothelial cell binding of NAP-1/IL-8: Role in neutrophil emigration. Immunol Today 13:291–294, 1992.

439. Von Andrian UH, Hansell P, Chambers JD, et al: L-selectin function is required for β₂-integrin–mediated neutrophil adhesion at physiological shear rates in vivo. Am J Physiol 263:H1034–H1044, 1992.

440. Narasinga Rao BN, Anderson MB, Musser JH, et al: Sialyl Lewis X mimics derived from a pharmacophore search are selectin inhib-

itors with anti-inflammatory activity. J Biol Chem 269:19663–19666, 1994.

441. Larson RS, Springer TA: Structure and function of leukocyte integrins. Immunol Rev 114:181–217, 1990.

442. Diamond MS, Springer TA: A subpopulation of Mac-1 (CD11b/CD18) molecules mediates neutrophil adhesion to ICAM-1 and fibrinogen. J Cell Biol 120:545–556, 1993.

443. Pavalko FM, LaRoche SM: Activation of human neutrophils induces an interaction between the integrin $\beta_2$-subunit (CD18) and the actin binding protein $\alpha$-actinin. J Immunol 151:3795–3807, 1993.

444. Hemler ME: VLA proteins in the integrin family: Structures, functions, and their role on leukocytes. Annu Rev Immunol 8:365–400, 1990.

445. Picker LJ: Physiological and molecular mechanisms of lymphocyte homing. Annu Rev Immunol 10:561–591, 1992.

446. Mackay CR: Migration pathways and immunologic memory among T lymphocytes. Semin Immunol 4:51–58, 1992.

447. Berlin C, Berg EL, Briskin MJ, et al: $\alpha4\beta7$ integrin mediates lymphocyte binding to the mucosal vascular addressin MAdCAM-1. Cell 74:185–195, 1993.

448. Jutila MA: Function and regulation of leukocyte homing receptors. J Leukoc Biol 55:133–140, 1994.

449. Muller WA, Weigl SA, Deng X, Phillips DM: PECAM-1 is required for transendothelial migration of leukocytes. J Exp Med 178:449–460, 1993.

450. Page C, Rose M, Yacoub M, Pigott R: Antigenic heterogeneity of vascular endothelium. Am J Pathol 141:673–683, 1992.

451. Brady HR, Spertini O, Jimenez W, et al: Neutrophils, monocytes, and lymphocytes bind to cytokine-activated kidney glomerular endothelial cells through L-selectin (LAM-1) in vitro. J Immunol 149:2437–2444, 1992.

452. Pizcueta P, Luscinskas FW: Monoclonal antibody blockade of L-selectin inhibits mononuclear leukocyte recruitment to inflammatory sites in vivo. Am J Pathol 145:461–469, 1994.

453. Denton MD, Marsden PA, Luscinskas FW, et al: Cytokine-induced phagocyte adhesion to human mesangial cells: Role of CD11/CD18 integrins and ICAM-1. Am J Physiol 261:F1071–F1079, 1991.

454. Nagel T, Resnick N, Atkinson WJ, et al: Shear stress selectively upregulates intercellular adhesion molecule-1 expression in cultured human vascular endothelial cells. J Clin Invest 94:885–891, 1994.

455. Garner CM, Richards GM, Adu D, et al: Intercellular adhesion molecule-1 (ICAM-1) and vascular cell adhesion molecule-1 (VCAM-1) expression and function on cultured human glomerular epithelial cells. Clin Exp Immunol 95:322–326, 1994.

456. Briscoe DM, Pober JSS, Harmon WE, Cotran RS: Expression of vascular cell adhesion molecule-1 in human renal allografts. J Am Soc Nephrol 3:1180–1185, 1992.

457. Wuthrich RP: Vascular cell adhesion molecule-1 (VCAM-1) expression in murine lupus nephritis. Kidney Int 42:903–914, 1992.

458. Alpers CE, Hudkins KL, Davis CL, et al: Expression of vascular cell adhesion molecule-1 in kidney allograft rejection. Kidney Int 44:805–816, 1993.

459. Brennan DC, Jevnikar AM, Takei F, Reubin-Kelley VE: Mesangial cell accessory functions: Mediation by intercellular adhesion molecule-1. Kidney Int 38:1039–1046, 1990.

460. Wuthrich RP, Jevnikar AM, Takei F, et al: Intercellular adhesion molecule-1 (ICAM-1) expression is upregulated in autoimmune murine lupus nephritis. Am J Pathol 136:441–450, 1990.

461. Lhotta K, Neumayer HP, Joannidis M, et al: Renal expression of intercellular adhesion molecule-1 in different forms of glomerulonephritis. Clin Sci 81:477–481, 1991.

462. Müller GA, Markovic-Lipkovski J, Müller CA: Intercellular adhesion molecule-1 expression in human kidneys with glomerulonephritis. Clin Nephrol 36:203–208, 1991.

463. Waldherr R, Eberlein-Gonska M, Noronha IL, et al: TNF-$\alpha$ and ICAM-1 expression in renal disease. J Am Soc Nephrol 1:544, 1991.

464. Chow J, Hartley RB, Jagger C, Dilly SA: ICAM-1 expression in renal disease. J Clin Pathol 45:880–884, 1992.

465. Hill PA, Lan HY, Nikolic-Paterson DJ, Atkins RC: Pulmonary expression of ICAM-1 and LFA-1 in experimental Goodpasture's syndrome. Am J Pathol 145:220–227, 1994.

466. Hill PA, Lan HY, Nikolic-Paterson DJ, Atkins RC: ICAM-1 directs

migration and localization of interstitial leukocytes in experimental glomerulonephritis. Kidney Int 45:32–42, 1994.

467. Bishop A, Suranyi MG, Waugh J, Hall BM: Expression of adhesion molecules by human renal tubular cells in culture and binding of activated lymphocytes. Transplant Proc 21:314–315, 1989.

468. Jevnikar AM, Wuthrich RP, Takei F, et al: Differing regulation and function of ICAM-1 and class II antigens on renal tubular cells. Kidney Int 38:417–425, 1990.

469. Mulligan MS, Johnson KJ, Smith CW, et al: Nephrotoxic nephritis: Role of TNF$\alpha$ and adhesion molecules. J Am Soc Nephrol 2:555, 1991.

470. Wu X, Pippin J, Lefkowith JB: Attenuation of immune-mediated glomerulonephritis with an anti-CD11b monoclonal antibody. Am J Physiol 264:F715–F721, 1993.

471. Mulligan MS, Johnson KJ, Todd RF III, et al: Requirements for leukocyte adhesion molecules in nephrotoxic nephritis. J Clin Invest 91:577–587, 1993.

472. Tang WW, Feng L, Vannice JL, Wilson CB: Interleukin-1 receptor antagonist ameliorates experimental anti–glomerular basement membrane antibody–associated glomerulonephritis. J Clin Invest 93:273–279, 1994.

473. Nikolic-Paterson DJ, Lan HY, Hill PA, et al: Suppression of experimental glomerulonephritis by the interleukin-1 receptor antagonist: Inhibition of intercellular adhesion molecule-1 expression. J Am Soc Nephrol 4:1695–1700, 1994.

474. Tam FWK, Smith J, Cashman SJ, et al: Glomerular expression of interleukin-1 receptor antagonist and interleukin-1$\beta$ genes in antibody-mediated glomerulonephritis. Am J Pathol 145:126–136, 1994.

475. Kawasaki K, Yaoita E, Yamamoto T, et al: Antibodies against intercellular adhesion molecule-1 and lymphocyte function–associated antigen-1 prevent glomerular injury in rat experimental crescentic glomerulonephritis. J Immunol 150:1074–1083, 1993.

476. Nishikawa K, Guo YJ, Miyasaka M, et al: Antibodies to intercellular adhesion molecule 1/lymphocyte function–associated antigen 1 prevent crescent formation in rat autoimmune glomerulonephritis. J Exp Med 177:667–677, 1993.

477. Sligh JE Jr, Ballantyne CM, Rich SS, et al: Inflammatory and immune responses are impaired in mice deficient in intercellular adhesion molecule 1. Proc Natl Acad Sci USA 90:8529–8533, 1993.

478. Huber AR, Kunkel SL, Todd RF III, Weiss SJ: Regulation of transendothelial neutrophil migration by endogenous interleukin-8. Science 254:99–102, 1991.

479. Brady HR, Denton MD, Jimenez W, et al: Chemoattractants provoke monocyte adhesion to human mesangial cells and mesangial cell injury. Kidney Int 42:480–487, 1992.

480. Gómez-Chiarri M, Ortíz A, Serón D, et al: The intercrine superfamily and renal disease. Kidney Int 43(suppl 39):S-81–S-85, 1993.

481. Lindley IJD, Westwick J, Kunkel SL: Nomenclature announcement—the chemokines. Immunol Today 14:24, 1993.

482. Oppenheim JJ, Zachariae COC, Mukaida N, Matsushima K: Properties of the novel proinflammatory supergene "intercrine" cytokine family. Annu Rev Immunol 9:617–648, 1991.

483. Miller MD, Krangel MS: Biology and biochemistry of the chemokines: A family of chemotactic and inflammatory cytokines. Crit Rev Immunol 12:17–46, 1992.

484. Koch AE, Kunkel SL, Harlow LA, et al: Macrophage inflammatory protein-1$\alpha$. A novel chemotactic cytokine for macrophages in rheumatoid arthritis. J Clin Invest 93:921–928, 1994.

485. Larsen CG, Anderson AO, Appella E, et al: The neutrophil-activating protein (NAP-1) is also chemotactic for T lymphocytes. Science 243:1464–1466, 1989.

486. Carr MW, Roth SJ, Luther E, et al: Monocyte chemoattractant protein 1 acts as a T-lymphocyte chemoattractant. Immunology 91:3652–3656, 1994.

486a. Kelner GS, Kennedy J, Bacon KB, et al: Lymphotactin: A cytokine that represents a new class of chemokine. Science 266:1395–1399, 1994.

487. Hadley TJ, Lu Z, Wasniowska K, et al: Postcapillary venule endothelial cells in kidney express a multispecific chemokine receptor that is structurally and functionally identical to the erythroid isoform, which is the Duffy blood group antigen. J Clin Invest 94:985–991, 1994.

488. Watanabe K, Iida M, Takaishi K, et al: Chemoattractants for neu-

trophils in lipopolysaccharide-induced inflammatory exudate from rats are not interleukin-8 counterparts but gro-gene-product/melanoma-growth-stimulating-activity–related factors. Eur J Biochem 214:267–270, 1993.

489. Tekamp-Olson P, Gallegos C, Bauer D, et al: Cloning and characterization of cDNAs for murine macrophage inflammatory protein 2 and its human homologues. J Exp Med 172:911–919, 1990.

490. Iida N, Grotendorst GR: Cloning and sequencing of a new gro transcript from activated human monocytes: Expression in leukocytes and wound tissue. Mol Cell Biol 10:5596–5599, 1990.

491. Haskill S, Peace A, Morris J, et al: Identification of three related human GRO genes encoding cytokine functions. Proc Natl Acad Sci USA 87:7732–7736, 1990.

492. Watanabe K, Konishi K, Fujioka M, et al: The neutrophil chemoattractant produced by the rat kidney epithelioid cell line NRK-52E is a protein related to the KC/gro protein. J Biol Chem 264:19559–19563, 1989.

493. Konishi K, Takata Y, Yamamoto M, et al: Structure of the gene encoding rat neutrophil chemo-attractant Gro. Gene 126:285–286, 1993.

494. Saukkonen K, Sande S, Cioffe C, et al: The role of cytokines in the generation of inflammation and tissue damage in experimental gram-positive meningitis. J Exp Med 171:439–448, 1990.

495. Appelberg R: Macrophage inflammatory proteins MIP-1 and MIP-2 are involved in T cell–mediated neutrophil recruitment. J Leukoc Biol 52:303–306, 1992.

496. Huang S, Paulauskis JD, Godleski JJ, Kobzik L: Expression of macrophage inflammatory protein-2 and KC mRNA in pulmonary inflammation. Am J Pathol 141:981–988, 1992.

497. Kobzik L, Huang S, Paulauskis JD, Godleski JJ: Particle opsonization and lung macrophage cytokine response. J Immunol 151:2753–2759, 1993.

498. Feng L, Xia Y, Kreisberg JI, Wilson CB: Interleukin-1 alpha stimulates KC synthesis in rat mesangial cells: Glucocorticoids inhibit KC induction by IL-1, Am J Physiol 266:F713–F722, 1994.

499. Feng L, Xia Y, Yoshimura T, Wilson CB: Modulation of neutrophil influx in glomerulonephritis in the rat with anti-macrophage inflammatory protein-2 (MIP-2) antibody. J Clin Invest 95:1009–1017, 1995.

500. Wu X, Wittwer AJ, Carr LS, et al: Cytokine-induced neutrophil chemoattractant mediates neutrophil influx in immune complex glomerulonephritis in rat. J Clin Invest 94:337–344, 1994.

501. Yoshioka K, Takemura T, Murakami K, et al: In situ expression of cytokines in IgA nephritis. Kidney Int 44:825–833, 1993.

502. Wada T, Yokoyama H, Tomosugi N, et al: Detection of urinary interleukin-8 in glomerular diseases. Kidney Int 46:455–460, 1994.

503. Fitzpatrick MM, Shah V, Trompeter RS, et al: Interleukin-8 and polymorphoneutrophil leucocyte activation in hemolytic uremic syndrome of childhood. Kidney Int 42:951–956, 1992.

504. Brown Z, Strieter RM, Chensue SW, et al: Cytokine-activated human mesangial cells generate the neutrophil chemoattractant, interleukin 8. Kidney Int 40:86–90, 1991.

505. Kusner DJ, Luebbers EL, Nowinski RJ, et al: Cytokine- and LPS-induced synthesis of interleukin-8 from human mesangial cells. Kidney Int 39:1240–1248, 1991.

506. Abbott F, Ryan JJ, Ceska M, et al: Interleukin-1β stimulates human mesangial cells to synthesize and release interleukins-6 and -8. Kidney Int 40:597–605, 1991.

507. Zoja C, Wang JM, Bettoni S, et al: Interleukin-1β and tumor necrosis factor-α induce gene expression and production of leukocyte chemotactic factors, colony-stimulating factors, and interleukin-6 in human mesangial cells. Am J Pathol 138:991–1003, 1991.

508. Schmouder RL, Strieter RM, Wiggins RC, et al: In vitro and in vivo interleukin-8 production in human renal cortical epithelia. Kidney Int 41:191–198, 1992.

509. Ember JA, Sanderson SD, Hugli TE, Morgan EL: Induction of interleukin-8 synthesis from monocytes by human C5a anaphylatoxin. Am J Pathol 144:393–403, 1994.

510. Strieter RM, Kasahara K, Allen RM, et al: Cytokine-induced neutrophil-derived interleukin-8. Am J Pathol 141:397–407, 1992.

511. Bussolino F, Sironi M, Bocchietto E, Mantovani A: Synthesis of platelet-activating factor by polymorphonuclear neutrophils stimulated with interleukin-8. J Biol Chem 267:14598–14603, 1992.

512. Hetchman DH, Cybulsky MI, Fuchs HJ, et al: Intravascular IL-8. Inhibitor of polymorphonuclear leukocyte accumulation at sites of acute inflammation. J Immunol 147:883–892, 1991.

513. Luscinskas FW, Kiely J-M, Ding H, et al: In vitro inhibitory effect of IL-8 and other chemoattractants on neutrophil-endothelial adhesive interactions. J Immunol 149:2163–2171, 1992.

514. Baggiolini M, Clark-Lewis I: Interleukin-8, a chemotactic and inflammatory cytokine. FEBS Lett 307:97–101, 1992.

515. Simonet WS, Hughes TM, Nguyen HQ, et al: Long-term impaired neutrophil migration in mice overexpressing human interleukin-8. J Clin Invest 94:1310–1319, 1994.

516. Hora K, Satriano JA, Santiago A, et al: Receptors for IgG complexes activate synthesis of monocyte chemoattractant peptide 1 and colony-stimulating factor 1. Proc Natl Acad Sci USA 89:1745–1749, 1992.

517. Rovin BH, Yoshiumura T, Tan L: Cytokine-induced production of monocyte chemoattractant protein-1 by cultured human mesangial cells. J Immunol 148:2148–2153, 1992.

518. Stahl RAK, Thaiss F, Disser M, et al: Increased expression of monocyte chemoattractant protein-1 in anti-thymocyte antibody–induced glomerulonephritis. Kidney Int 44:1036–1047, 1993.

519. Satriano JA, Hora K, Shan Z, et al: Regulation of monocyte chemoattractant protein-1 and macrophage colony-stimulating factor-1 by IFN-γ, tumor necrosis factor-α, IgG aggregates, and cAMP in mouse mesangial cells. J Immunol 150:1971–1978, 1993.

520. Grandaliano G, Valente AJ, Rozek MM, Abboud HE: Gamma interferon stimulates monocyte chemotactic protein (MCP-1) in human mesangial cells. J Lab Clin Med 123:282–289, 1994.

521. Grande JP, Jones ML, Swenson CL, et al: Lipopolysaccharide induces monocyte chemoattractant protein production by rat mesangial cells. J Lab Clin Med 124:112–117, 1994.

522. Gomez-Chiarri M, Hamilton TA, Egido J, Emancipator SN: Expression of IP-10, a lipopolysaccharide- and interferon-gamma-inducible protein, in murine mesangial cells in culture. Am J Pathol 142:433–439, 1993.

523. Brown Z, Strieter RM, Neild GH, et al: IL-1 receptor antagonist inhibits monocyte chemotactic peptide 1 generation by human mesangial cells. Kidney Int 42:95–101, 1992.

524. Rollins BJ, Pober JS: Interleukin-4 induces the synthesis and secretion of MCP-1/JE by human endothelial cells. Am J Pathol 138:1315–1319, 1991.

525. Schmouder RL, Strieter RM, Kunkel SL: Interferon-γ regulation of human renal cortical epithelial cell-derived monocyte chemotactic peptide-1. Kidney Int 44:43–49, 1993.

526. Strieter RM, Wiggins R, Phan SH, et al: Monocyte chemotactic protein gene expression by cytokine-treated human fibroblasts and endothelial cells. Biochem Biophys Res Commun 162:694–700, 1989.

527. Heeger P, Wolf G, Meyers C, et al: Isolation and characterization of cDNA from renal tubular epithelium encoding murine Rantes. Kidney Int 41:220–225, 1992.

528. Wolf G, Aberle S, Thaiss F, et al: TNF alpha induces expression of the chemoattractant cytokine RANTES in cultured mouse mesangial cells. Kidney Int 44:795–804, 1993.

529. Nelson PJ, Kim HT, Manning WC, et al: Genomic organization and transcriptional regulation of the RANTES chemokine gene. J Immunol 151:2601–2612, 1993.

530. Brady HR, Persson U, Ballermann BJ, et al: Leukotrienes stimulate neutrophil adhesion to mesangial cells: Modulation with lipoxins. Am J Physiol 259:F809–F815, 1990.

531. Johnson RJ, Alpers CE, Pruchno C, et al: Mechanisms and kinetics for platelet and neutrophil localization in immune complex nephritis. Kidney Int 36:780–789, 1989.

532. Faint RW: Platelet-neutrophil interactions: Their significance. Blood Rev 6:83–91, 1992.

533. Wu X, Helfrich MH, Horton MA, et al: Fibrinogen mediates platelet–polymorphonuclear leukocyte cooperation during immune-complex glomerulonephritis in rats. J Clin Invest 94:928–936, 1994.

534. Jennette JC, Falk RJ: Acute renal failure secondary to leukocyte-mediated acute glomerular injury. Ren Fail 14:395–399, 1992.

535. Hasty KA, Pourmotabbed TF, Goldberg GI, et al: Human neutrophil collagenase. A distinct gene product with homology to other matrix metalloproteinases. J Biol Chem 265:11421–11424, 1990.

536. Ward PA: Mechanisms of endothelial cell injury. J Lab Clin Med 118:421–426, 1991.

537. Issekutz AC: Role of polymorphonuclear leukocytes in the vascular responses of acute inflammation. Lab Invest 50:605–607, 1984.

538. Movat HZ, Wasi S: Severe microvascular injury induced by lyso-

somal releasates of human polymorphonuclear leukocytes. Increase in vasopermeability, hemorrhage, and microthrombosis due to degradation of subendothelial and perivascular matrices. Am J Pathol 121:404–417, 1985.

539. Simon RH, DeHart PD, Todd RF III: Neutrophil-induced injury of rat pulmonary alveolar epithelial cells. J Clin Invest 78:1375–1386, 1986.

540. Morganroth ML, Till GO, Kunkel RG, Ward PA: Complement and neutrophil-mediated injury of perfused rat lungs. Lab Invest 54:507–514, 1986.

541. Baricos WH, Shah SV: Proteolytic enzymes as mediators of glomerular injury. Kidney Int 40:161–173, 1991.

542. Varani J, Ginsburg I, Schuger L, et al: Endothelial cell killing by neutrophils. Synergistic interaction of oxygen products and proteases. Am J Pathol 135:435–438, 1989.

543. Varani J, Dame MK, Gibbs DF, et al: Human umbilical vein endothelial cell killing by activated neutrophils. Loss of sensitivity to injury is accompanied by decreased iron content during in vitro culture and is restored with exogenous iron. Lab Invest 66:708–714, 1992.

544. Desrochers PE, Mookhtiar K, Van Wart HE, et al: Proteolytic inactivation of alpha 1-proteinase inhibitor and alpha 1-antichymotrypsin by oxidatively activated human neutrophil metalloproteinases. J Biol Chem 267:5005–5012, 1992.

545. Breit SN, Wakefield D, Robinson JP, et al: The role of alpha₁-antitrypsin deficiency in the pathogenesis of immune disorders. Clin Immunol Immunopathol 35:363–380, 1985.

546. Levy M: Severe deficiency of alpha₁-antitrypsin associated with cutaneous vasculitis, rapidly progressive glomerulonephritis, and colitis. Am J Med 81:363, 1986.

547. Sandborg RR, Smolen JE: Early biochemical events in leukocyte activation. Lab Invest 59:300–320, 1988.

548. Steinbeck MJ, Roth JA: Neutrophil activation by recombinant cytokines. Rev Infect Dis 11:549–568, 1989.

549. Weiss SJ: Tissue destruction by neutrophils. N Engl J Med 320:365–376, 1989.

550. De Nicola L, Gabbai FB, Feng L, et al: Inflammatory mediators in glomerular injury. Ren Fail 14:401–405, 1992.

551. Benigni A, Remuzzi G: Inflammation and glomerular injury. Springer Semin Immunopathol 16:39–51, 1994.

552. Mainardi CL, Dixit SN, Kang AH: Degradation of type IV (basement membrane) collagen by a proteinase isolated from human polymorphonuclear leukocyte granules. J Biol Chem 255:5435–5441, 1980.

553. Johnson RJ, Couser WG, Alpers CE, et al: The human neutrophil serine proteinases, elastase and cathepsin G, can mediate glomerular injury in vivo. J Exp Med 168:1169–1174, 1988.

554. Neal TM, Vissers MCM, Winterbourn CC: Inhibition of neutrophil-mediated degradation of isolated basement membrane collagen by nonsteroidal antiinflammatory drugs that inhibit degranulation. Arthritis Rheum 30:908–913, 1987.

555. Matzner Y, Bar-Ner M, Yahalom J, et al: Degradation of heparan sulfate in the subendothelial extracellular matrix by a readily released heparanase from human neutrophils. Possible role in invasion through basement membranes. J Clin Invest 76:1306–1313, 1985.

556. Klebanoff SJ, Kinsella MG, Wight TN: Degradation of endothelial cell matrix heparan sulfate proteoglycan by elastase and the myeloperoxidase-H₂O₂-chloride system. Am J Pathol 143:907–917, 1993.

557. Donovan KL, Davies M, Coles GA, Williams JD: Relative roles of elastase and reactive oxygen species in the degradation of human glomerular basement membrane by intact human neutrophils. Kidney Int 45:1555–1561, 1994.

558. Feith GW, Assmann KJ, Bogman MJ, et al: Lack of albuminuria in the early heterologous phase of anti-GBM nephritis in beige mice. Kidney Int 43:824–827, 1993.

559. Davies M, Hughes KT, Thomas GJ: Evidence that kidney lysosomal proteinases degrade the collagen of glomerular basement membrane. Renal Physiol 3:116–119, 1980.

560. Lovett DH, Ryan JL, Kashgarian M, Sterzel RB: Lysosomal enzymes in glomerular cells of the rat. Am J Pathol 107:161–166, 1982.

561. Lovett DH, Sterzel RB, Kashgarian M, Ryan JL: Neutral proteinase activity produced in vitro by cells of the glomerular mesangium. Kidney Int 23:342–349, 1983.

562. Bray J, Hume DA, Robinson GB: Degradation of rat or sheep glomerular basement membrane by rabbit neutrophils in vitro. The roles of proteinases, complement and oxygen-derived radicals. Mol Biol Med 1:253–269, 1983.

563. Vissers MCM, Winterbourn CC, Hunt JS: Degradation of glomerular basement membrane by human neutrophils in vitro. Biochim Biophys Acta 804:154–160, 1984.

564. Johnson RJ, Yamabe H, Chen Y-P, et al: Glomerular epithelial cells release a glomerular basement membrane degrading metalloprotease. J Am Soc Nephrol 2:1388–1397, 1992.

565. Nguyen HH, Baricos WH, Shah, SV: Degradation of glomerular basement membrane by a neutral metalloproteinase(s) present in glomeruli isolated from normal rat kidney. Biochem Biophys Res Commun 141:898–903, 1986.

566. Singh AK: Presence of lysosomal enzymes in the normal glomerular basement membrane matrix. Histochem J 25:562–568, 1993.

567. Camussi G, Tetta C, Segoloni G, et al: Localization of neutrophil cationic proteins and loss of anionic charges in glomeruli of patients with systemic lupus erythematosus glomerulonephritis. Clin Immunol Immunopathol 24:299–314, 1982.

568. Camussi G, Tetta C, Meroni M, et al: Localization of cationic proteins derived from platelets and polymorphonuclear neutrophils and local loss of anionic sites in glomeruli of rabbits with experimentally induced acute serum sickness. Lab Invest 55:56–62, 1986.

569. Davin J-C, Davies M, Foidart J-M, et al: Relation between urinary proteinases and proteinuria in rats with a glomerular disease. Adv Exp Med Biol 240:267–273, 1988.

570. Sanders E, Davies M, Coles GA: On the pathogenesis of glomerulonephritis. A clinico-pathological study indicating that neutrophils attack and degrade glomerular basement membrane. Renal Physiol 3:355–359, 1980.

571. Mitsuhashi H, Tsukada Y, Ono K, et al: Urine glycosaminoglycans and heparan sulfate excretions in adult patients with glomerular diseases. Clin Nephrol 39:231–238, 1993.

572. Chanard J, Szymanowicz A, Brunois J-P, et al: Increased renal excretion of 3 hydroxyproline in patients with active glomerular nephropathies and with polycystic renal disease. Clin Nephrol 17:64–69, 1982.

573. Davin J-C, Davies M, Foidart J-M, et al: Urinary excretion of neutral proteinases in nephrotic rats with a glomerular disease. Kidney Int 31:32–40, 1987.

574. Baricos WH, Shah SV: Role of cathepsin B and L in anti–glomerular basement membrane nephritis in rats. Renal Physiol Biochem 12:400–405, 1989.

575. Baricos WH, Cortez SL, Le QC, et al: Evidence suggesting a role for cathepsin L in an experimental model of glomerulonephritis. Arch Biochem Biophys 288:468–472, 1991.

576. Jennette JC, Tidwell RR, Geratz JD, et al: Amelioration of immune complex-mediated glomerulonephritis by synthetic protease inhibitors. Am J Pathol 127:499–506, 1987.

577. Ikehara S, Shimamura K, Aoyama T, et al: Effect of FUT-175, a new synthetic protease inhibitor, on the development of lupus nephritis in (NZB × NZW) F₁ mice. Immunology 55:595–600, 1985.

578. Yaguchi Y, Tomino Y, Ozaki T, et al: Correlation between reduction of polymorphonuclear leucocytes in glomeruli injected with a newly developed monoclonal antineutrophil antibody and proteinuria in Masugi nephritis. Nephron 62:444–448, 1992.

579. Tucker BJ, Gushwa LC, Wilson CB, Blantz RC: Effect of leukocyte depletion on glomerular dynamics during acute glomerular immune injury. Kidney Int 28:28–35, 1985.

580. Gabbai F, Wilson CB, Blantz RC: Glomerular hemodynamic consequences of immune injury. Semin Nephrol 11:367–372, 1991.

581. Eddy AA, McCulloch LM, Adams JA: Intraglomerular leukocyte recruitment during nephrotoxic serum nephritis in rats. Clin Immunol Immunopathol 57:441–458, 1990.

582. Schrijver G, Bogman MJ, Assmann KJ, et al: Anti-GBM nephritis in the mouse: Role of granulocytes in the heterologous phase. Kidney Int 38:86–95, 1990.

583. Chen HC, Tomino Y, Yaguchi Y, et al: Detection of polymorphonuclear cells, superoxide dismutase and poly C9 in glomeruli of patients with IgA nephropathy. Nephron 59:338, 1991.

584. Chen HC, Tomino Y, Yaguchi Y, et al: Oxidative metabolism of polymorphonuclear leukocytes (PMN) in patients with IgA nephropathy. J Clin Lab Anal 6:35–39, 1992.

585. Kashem A, Endoh M, Nomoto Y, et al: Fc alpha R expression on

polymorphonuclear leukocyte and superoxide generation in IgA nephropathy. Kidney Int 45:868–875, 1994.

586. Rother K, Rother U, Vassalli P, McCluskey RT: Nephrotoxic serum nephritis in C′6-deficient rabbits. I. Study of the second phase of the disease. J Immunol 98:965–971, 1967.

587. Sawtell NM, Hartman AL, Weiss MA, et al: C3 dependent, C5 independent immune complex glomerulopathy in the mouse. Lab Invest 58:287–293, 1988.

588. Falk RJ, Jennette JC: Immune complex induced glomerular lesions in C5 sufficient and deficient mice. Kidney Int 30:678–686, 1986.

589. Miyazaki W, Izawa T, Nakano Y, et al: Effects of K-76 monocarboxylic acid, an anticomplementary agent, on various in vivo immunological reactions and on experimental glomerulonephritis. Complement 1:134–146, 1984.

590. Iida H, Izumino K, Asaka M, et al: Effect of the anticomplementary agent, K-76 monocarboxylic acid, on experimental immune complex glomerulonephritis in rats. Clin Exp Immunol 67:130–134, 1987.

591. Cochrane CG: Mediation systems in neutrophil-independent immunologic injury of the glomerulus. In Wilson CB, Brenner BM, Stein JH (eds): Contemporary Issues in Nephrology, Vol 3. Churchill Livingstone, New York, 1979, pp 106–121.

592. Holdsworth SR, Neale TJ, Wilson CB: Abrogation of macrophage-dependent injury in experimental glomerulonephritis in the rabbit. Use of an antimacrophage serum. J Clin Invest 68:686–698, 1981.

593. Cattell V: Macrophages in acute glomerular inflammation. Kidney Int 45:945–952, 1994.

594. Nikolic-Paterson DJ, Lan HY, Hill PA, Atkins RC: Macrophages in renal injury. Kidney Int 45(suppl 45):S-79–S-82, 1994.

595. Davies M, Coles GA, Hughes KT: Glomerular basement membrane injury by neutrophil and monocyte neutral proteinases. Renal Physiol 3:106–111, 1980.

596. Matsumoto K: Production of interleukin-1 by glomerular macrophages in nephrotoxic serum nephritis. Am J Nephrol 10:502–506, 1990.

597. Tipping PG, Leong TW, Holdsworth SR: Tumor necrosis factor production by glomerular macrophages in anti–glomerular basement membrane glomerulonephritis in rabbits. Lab Invest 65:272–279, 1991.

598. Tipping PG, Lowe MG, Holdsworth SR: Glomerular interleukin 1 production is dependent on macrophage infiltration in anti-GBM glomerulonephritis. Kidney Int 39:103–110, 1991.

599. Matsumoto K: Production of tumor necrosis factor-α by glomerular macrophages in nephrotoxic serum nephritis. Clin Nephrol 38:237–238, 1992.

600. Oguchi S, Yamada S, Oguchi H, Nakane PK: In situ localization of transforming growth factor-β1 mRNA in the rat kidney with Masugi nephritis. J Clin Lab Anal 8:99–104, 1994.

601. Vissers MCM, Fantone JC, Wiggins R, Kunkel SL: Glomerular basement membrane–containing immune complexes stimulate tumor necrosis factor and interleukin-1 production by human monocytes. Am J Pathol 134:1–6, 1989.

602. Bloom RD, Florquin S, Singer GG, et al: Colony stimulating factor-1 in the induction of lupus nephritis. Kidney Int 43:1000–1009, 1993.

603. Kelley VR, Bloom RD, Yui MA, et al: Pivotal role of colony stimulating factor-1 in lupus nephritis. Kidney Int 45(suppl 45):S-83–S-85, 1994.

604. Yui MA, Brissette WH, Brennan DC, et al: Increased macrophage colony-stimulating factor in neonatal and adult autoimmune MRL-lpr mice. Am J Pathol 139:255–261, 1991.

605. Mampaso F, Bricio T, Martin A, Molina A: Production of interleukin-1-like cytokine by cultured rat glomerular macrophages. Immunology 76:408–412, 1992.

606. Schindler R, Lonnemann G, Shaldon S, et al: Transcription, not synthesis, of interleukin-1 and tumor necrosis factor by complement. Kidney Int 37:85–93, 1990.

607. Mattana J, Singhal PC: Macrophage Fc receptor activity modulates mesangial cell proliferation and matrix synthesis. Am J Physiol 266:F568–F575, 1994.

608. Ding AH, Nathan CF, Stuehr DJ: Release of reactive nitrogen intermediates and reactive oxygen intermediates from mouse peritoneal macrophages. Comparison of activating cytokines and evidence for independent production. J Immunol 141:2407–2412, 1988.

609. Kolb H, Kolb-Bachofen V: Nitric oxide: A pathogenetic factor in autoimmunity. Immunol Today 13:157–160, 1992.

610. Nathan C: Nitric acid as a secretory product of mammalian cells. FASEB J 6:3051–3064, 1992.

611. Nussler AK, Billiar TR: Inflammation, immunoregulation, and inducible nitric oxide synthase. J Leukoc Biol 54:171–178, 1993.

612. Cattell V, Cook HT: Nitric oxide: role in the physiology and pathology of the glomerulus. Exp Nephrol 1:265–280, 1993.

613. Moncada S, Higgs A: The L-arginine–nitric oxide pathway. N Engl J Med 329:2002–2012, 1993.

614. Langrehr JM, Hoffman RA, Lancaster JR Jr, Simmons RL: Nitric oxide—a new endogenous immunomodulator. Transplantation 55:1205–1212, 1993.

615. Shultz PJ, Schorer AE, Raij L: Effects of endothelium-derived relaxing factor and nitric oxide on rat mesangial cells. Am J Physiol 258:F162–F167, 1990.

616. Pfeilschifter J, Rob P, Mülsch A, et al: Interleukin 1β and tumour necrosis factor α induce a macrophage-type of nitric oxide synthase in rat renal mesangial cells. Eur J Biochem 203:251–255, 1992.

617. Geller DA, Billiar TR: Should surgeons clone genes? The strategy behind the cloning of the human inducible nitric oxide synthase gene. Arch Surg 128:1212–1220, 1993.

618. Förstermann U, Closs EI, Pollock JS, et al: Nitric oxide synthase isozymes. Characterization, purification, molecular cloning, and functions. Hypertension 23:1121–1131, 1994.

619. Schmidt HHHW, Gagne GD, Nakane M, et al: Mapping of neural nitric oxide synthase in the rat suggests frequent colocalization with NADPH diaphorase but not with soluble guanylyl cyclase, and novel paraneural functions for nitrinergic signal transduction. J Histochem Cytochem 40:1439–1456, 1992.

620. Tojo A, Gross SS, Zhang L, et al: Immunocytochemical localization of distinct isoforms of nitric oxide synthase in the juxtaglomerular apparatus of normal rat kidney. J Am Soc Nephrol 4:1438–1447, 1994.

621. Terada Y, Tomita K, Nonoguchi H, Marumo F: Polymerase chain reaction localization of constitutive nitric oxide synthase and soluble guanylate cyclase messenger RNAs in microdissected rat nephron segments. J Clin Invest 90:659–665, 1992.

622. Juncos LA, Ren Y, Arima S, Ito S: Vasodilator and constrictor actions of platelet-activating factor in the isolated microperfused afferent arteriole of the rabbit kidney. Role of endothelium-derived relaxing factor/nitric oxide and cyclooxygenase products. J Clin Invest 91:1374–1379, 1993.

623. Kubes P, Suzuki M, Granger DN: Nitric oxide: an endogenous modulator of leukocyte adhesion. Proc Natl Acad Sci USA 88:4651–4655, 1991.

624. Bienvenu K, Hernandez L, Granger DN: Leukocyte adhesion and emigration in inflammation. Ann N Y Acad Sci 664:388–399, 1992.

625. Arndt H, Smith CW, Granger DN: Leukocyte–endothelial cell adhesion in spontaneously hypertensive and normotensive rats. Hypertension 21:667–673, 1993.

626. Kurose I, Kubes P, Wolf R, et al: Inhibition of nitric oxide production. Mechanisms of vascular albumin leakage. Circ Res 73:164–171, 1993.

627. Marsden PA, Ballermann BJ: Tumor necrosis factor α activates soluble guanylate cyclase in bovine glomerular mesangial cells via an L-arginine–dependent mechanism. J Exp Med 172:1843–1852, 1990.

628. Shultz PJ, Tayeh MA, Marletta MA, Raij L: Synthesis and action of nitric oxide in rat glomerular mesangial cells. Am J Physiol 261:F600–F606, 1991.

629. Nicolson AG, Haites NE, McKay NG, et al: Induction of nitric oxide synthase in human mesangial cells. Biochem Biophys Res Commun 193:1269–1274, 1993.

630. Raij L, Shultz PJ: Endothelium-derived relaxing factor, nitric oxide: Effects on and production by mesangial cells and the glomerulus. J Am Soc Nephrol 3:1435–1441, 1993.

631. Pfeilschifter J, Kunz D, Mühl H: Nitric oxide: An inflammatory mediator of glomerular mesangial cells. Nephron 64:518–525, 1993.

632. Schultz PJ, Archer SL, Rosenberg ME: Inducible nitric oxide synthase mRNA and activity in glomerular mesangial cells. Kidney Int 46:683–689, 1994.

633. Kunz D, Muhl H, Walker G, Pfeilschifter J: Two distinct signaling pathways trigger the expression of inducible nitric oxide synthase

in rat renal mesangial cells. Proc Natl Acad Sci USA 91:5387–5391, 1994.

634. Rosenblum ND, Briscoe DM, Karnovsky MJ, Olsen BR: Alpha 1-VIII collagen is expressed in the rat glomerulus and in resident glomerular cells. Am J Physiol 264:F1003–F1010, 1993.

635. Mohaupt MG, Elzie JL, Ahn KY, et al: Differential expression and induction of mRNAs encoding two inducible nitric oxide synthases in rat kidney. Kidney Int 46:653–665, 1994.

636. Ding A, Nathan CF, Graycar J, et al: Macrophage deactivating factor and transforming growth factors-$\beta_1$, -$\beta_2$ and -$\beta_3$ inhibit induction of macrophage nitrogen oxide synthesis by IFN$\gamma$. J Immunol 145:940–944, 1990.

637. Pfeilschifter J, Vosbeck K: Transforming growth factor $\beta_2$ inhibits interleukin 1$\beta$- and tumour necrosis factor $\alpha$-induction of nitric oxide synthase in rat renal mesangial cells. Biochem Biophys Res Commun 175:372–379, 1991.

638. Pfeilschifter J: Platelet-derived growth factor inhibits cytokine induction of nitric oxide synthase in rat renal mesangial cells. Eur J Pharmacol Mol Pharmacol 208:339–340, 1991.

639. Oswald IP, Gazzinelli RT, Sher A, James SL: Il-10 synergizes with IL-4 and transforming growth factor-$\beta$ to inhibit macrophage cytotoxic activity. J Immunol 148:3578–3582, 1992.

640. Cunha FQ, Moncada S, Liew FY: Interleukin-10 (IL-10) inhibits the induction of nitric oxide synthase by interferon-$\gamma$ in murine macrophages. Biochem Biophys Res Commun 182:1155–1159, 1992.

641. Clancy RM, Leszczynska-Piziak J, Abramson SB: Nitric oxide, an endothelial cell relaxation factor, inhibits neutrophil superoxide anion production via a direct action on the NADPH oxidase. J Clin Invest 90:1116–1121, 1992.

642. Beckman JS, Beckman TW, Chen J, et al: Apparent hydroxyl radical production by peroxynitrite: Implications for endothelial injury from nitric oxide and superoxide. Proc Natl Acad Sci USA 87:1620–1624, 1990.

643. Hogg N, Darley-Usmar VM, Wilsohn MT, Moncada S: Production of hydroxyl radicals from the simultaneous generation of superoxide and nitric oxide. J Biochem 281:419–424, 1992.

644. Morrissey JJ, McCracken R, Kaneto H, et al: Location of an inducible nitric oxide synthase mRNA in the normal kidney. Kidney Int 45:998–1005, 1994.

645. Cho HJ, Xie QW, Calaycay J, et al: Calmodulin is a subunit of nitric oxide synthase from macrophages. J Exp Med 176:599–604, 1992.

646. Cattell V, Cook T, Moncada S: Glomeruli synthesize nitrite in experimental nephrotoxic nephritis. Kidney Int 38:1056–1060, 1990.

647. Cook HT, Sullivan R: Glomerular nitrite synthesis in in situ immune complex glomerulonephritis in the rat. Am J Pathol 139:1047–1052, 1991.

648. Cattell V, Largen P, De Heer E, Cook T: Glomeruli synthesize nitrite in active Heymann nephritis; the source is infiltrating macrophages. Kidney Int 40:847–851, 1991.

649. Cattell V, Lianos E, Largen P, Cook T: Glomerular NO synthase activity in mesangial cell immune injury. Exp Nephrol 1:36–40, 1993.

650. Jansen A, Lewis S, Cattell V, Cook HT: Arginase is a major pathway of L-arginine metabolism in nephritic glomeruli. Kidney Int 42:1107–1112, 1992.

651. Jansen A, Cook T, Taylor GM, et al: Induction of nitric oxide synthase in rat immune complex glomerulonephritis. Kidney Int 45:1215–1219, 1994.

652. Weinberg JB, Granger DL, Pisetsky DS, et al: The role of nitric oxide in the pathogenesis of spontaneous murine autoimmune disease: Increased nitric oxide production and nitric oxide synthase expression in MRL-lpr/lpr mice, and reduction of spontaneous glomerulonephritis and arthritis by orally administered $N^G$-monomethyl-L-arginine. J Exp Med 179:651–660, 1994.

653. Ferrario R, Takahashi K, Fogo A, Badr KF, Munger KA: Consequences of acute nitric oxide synthesis inhibition in experimental glomerulonephritis. J Am Soc Nephrol 4:1847–1854, 1994.

654. Westberg G, Shultz PJ, Raij L: Exogenous nitric oxide prevents endotoxin-induced glomerular thrombosis in rats. Kidney Int 46:711–716, 1994.

655. Salvemini D, Seibert K, Masferrer JL, et al: Endogenous nitric oxide enhances prostaglandin production in a model of renal inflammation. J Clin Invest 93:1940–1947, 1994.

656. Schreiner GF, Cotran RS, Pardo V, Unanue ER: A mononuclear cell component in experimental immunological glomerulonephritis. J Exp Med 147:369–384, 1978.

657. Hunsicker LG, Shearer TP, Plattner SB, and Weisenburger D: The role of monocytes in serum sickness nephritis. J Exp Med 150:413–425, 1979.

658. Holdsworth SR, Neale TJ, Wilson CB: The participation of macrophages and monocytes in experimental immune complex glomerulonephritis. Clin Immunol Immunopathol 15:510–524, 1980.

659. Parra G, Mosquera J, Rodriguez-Iturbe B: Migration inhibition factor in acute serum sickness nephritis. Kidney Int 38:1118–1124, 1990.

660. Becker GJ, Hancock WW, Stow JL, et al: Involvement of the macrophage in experimental chronic immune complex glomerulonephritis. Nephron 32:227–233, 1982.

661. Striker GE, Mannik M, Tung MY: Role of marrow-derived monocytes and mesangial cells in removal of immune complexes from renal glomeruli. J Exp Med 149:127–136, 1979.

662. Stad RK, Bogers WMJM, Muizert Y, et al: Deposition of IgA is associated with macrophage influx in the kidney of rats. Scand J Immunol 34:81–89, 1991.

663. Kanno H, Tachiwaki O, Nose M, Kyogoku M: Immune complex-degradation ability of macrophages in MRL/Mp-lpr/lpr lupus mice and its regulation by cytokines. Clin Exp Immunol 95:115–121, 1994.

664. Noble B, Ren K, Taverne J, et al: Mononuclear cells in glomeruli and cytokines in urine reflect the severity of experimental proliferative immune complex glomerulonephritis. Clin Exp Immunol 80:281–287, 1990.

665. Moxey-Mims MM, Noble B: Glomerular macrophage phagocytic activity in experimental immune complex nephritis. Kidney Int 45:1326–1332, 1994.

666. Garber SL, O'Morchoe PJ, O'Morchoe CCC: Effect of experimental glomerulonephritis on the cells in canine renal lymph with special reference to the veiled cell. Clin Exp Immunol 49:347–354, 1982.

667. Lan HY, Nikolic-Paterson DJ, Atkins RC: Trafficking of inflammatory macrophages from the kidney to draining lymph nodes during experimental glomerulonephritis. Clin Exp Immunol 92:336–341, 1993.

668. Postlethwaite AE, Kang AH: Collagen and collagen peptide–induced chemotaxis of human blood monocytes. J Exp Med 143:1299–1307, 1976.

669. Holdsworth SR, Neale TJ: Macrophage-induced glomerular injury. Cell transfer studies in passive autologous antiglomerular basement membrane antibody–initiated experimental glomerulonephritis. Lab Invest 51:172–180, 1984.

670. Holdsworth SR, Bellomo R: Differential effects of steroids on leukocyte-mediated glomerulonephritis in the rabbit. Kidney Int 26:162–169, 1984.

671. Tipping PG, Holdsworth SR: The mechanism of action of corticosteroids on glomerular injury in acute serum sickness in rabbits. Clin Exp Immunol 59:555–563, 1985.

672. Hara M, Batsford SR, Mihatsch MJ, et al: Complement and monocytes are essential for provoking glomerular injury in passive Heymann nephritis in rats. Terminal complement components are not the sole mediators of proteinuria. Lab Invest 65:168–179, 1991.

673. Magil AB, Frohlich JJ: Monocytes and macrophages in focal glomerulosclerosis in Zucker rats. Nephron 59:131–138, 1991.

674. van Goor H, van der Horst MLC, Fidler V, Grond J: Glomerular macrophage modulation affects mesangial expansion in the rat after renal ablation. Lab Invest 66:564–571, 1992.

675. Diamond JR, Pesek-Diamond I: Sublethal X-irradiation during acute puromycin nephrosis prevents late renal injury: Role of macrophages. Am J Physiol 260:F779–F786, 1991.

676. Holzman LB, Wiggins RC: Consequences of glomerular injury. Glomerular crescent formation. Semin Nephrol 11:346–353, 1991.

677. Holdsworth SR, Tipping PG: Macrophage-induced glomerular fibrin deposition in experimental glomerulonephritis in the rabbit. J Clin Invest 76:1367–1374, 1985.

678. Vissers MCM, Wiggins R, Fantone JC: Comparative ability of human monocytes and neutrophils to degrade glomerular basement membrane in vitro. Lab Invest 60:831–838, 1989.

679. Huard TK, Malinoff HL, Wicha MS: Macrophages express a plasma membrane receptor for basement membrane laminin. Am J Pathol 123:365–370, 1986.

680. Endemann G, Pronzcuk A, Friedman G, et al: Monocyte adherence to endothelial cells in vitro is increased by β-VLDL. Am J Pathol 126:1–6, 1987.

681. Kobayashi M, Koyama A, Narita M, Shigematsu H: Intraglomerular monocytes in human glomerulonephritis. Nephron 59:580–585, 1991.

682. Saito T, Ootaka T, Sato H, et al: Participation of macrophages in segmental endocapillary proliferation preceding focal glomerular sclerosis. J Pathol 170:179–185, 1993.

683. Schiffer MS, Michael AR: Renal cell turnover studied by Y chromosome (Y body) staining of the transplanted human kidney. J Lab Clin Med 92:841–848, 1978.

684. Magil AB, Wadsworth LD: Monocyte involvement in glomerular crescents. A histochemical and ultrastructural study. Lab Invest 47:160–166, 1982.

685. Sarno EN, Alvarenga FBF, Ruzany F, Gattass CR: Distribution of mononuclear phagocytes in glomerulonephritis with crescents. Nephron 32:265, 1982.

686. Hancock WW, Atkins RC: Cellular composition of crescents in human rapidly progressive glomerulonephritis identified using monoclonal antibodies. Am J Nephrol 4:177–181, 1984.

687. Magil AB: Histogenesis of glomerular crescents. Immunohistochemical demonstration of cytokeratin in crescent cells. Am J Pathol 120:222–229, 1985.

688. Jennette JC, Hipp CG: The epithelial antigen phenotype of glomerular crescent cells. Am J Clin Pathol 86:274–280, 1986.

689. Guettier C, Nochy D, Jacquot C, et al: Immunohistochemical demonstration of parietal epithelial cells and macrophages in human proliferative extra-capillary lesions. Virchows Arch A 409:739–748, 1986.

690. Harrison DJ, MacDonald MK: The origin of cells in the glomerular crescent investigated by the use of monoclonal antibodies. Histopathology 10:945–952, 1986.

691. Boucher A, Droz D, Adafer E, Noël L-H: Relationship between the integrity of Bowman's capsule and the composition of cellular crescents in human crescentic glomerulonephritis. Lab Invest 56:526–533, 1987.

692. Li HL, Hancock WW, Hooke DH, Dowling JP: Mononuclear cell activation and decreased renal function in IgA nephropathy with crescents. Kidney Int 37:1552–1556, 1990.

693. Li HL, Hancock WW, Dowling JP, Atkins RC: Activated (IL-2R⁺) intraglomerular mononuclear cells in crescentic glomerulonephritis. Kidney Int 39:793–798, 1991.

694. Arima S, Nakayama M, Naito M, et al: Significance of mononuclear phagocytes in IgA nephropathy. Kidney Int 39:684–692, 1991.

695. Schreiner GF, Kiely JM, Cotran RS, Unanue ER: Characterization of resident glomerular cells in the rat expressing Ia determinants and manifesting genetically restricted interactions with lymphocytes. J Clin Invest 68:920–931, 1981.

696. Schreiner GF, Cotran RS: Localization of an Ia-bearing glomerular cell in the mesangium. J Cell Biol 94:483–488, 1982.

697. Ren K, Brentjens J, Chen Y, et al: Glomerular macrophage proliferation in experimental immune complex nephritis. Clin Immunol Immunopathol 60:384–398, 1991.

698. Sterzel RB, Eisenbach GM, Seiler MW, Hoyer JR: Uptake of polyvinyl alcohol by macrophages in the glomerular mesangium of rats. Histologic and functional studies. Am J Pathol 111:247, 1983.

699. Sterzel RB, Perfetto M, Biemesderfer D, Kashgarian M: Disposal of ferritin in the glomerular mesangium of rats. Kidney Int 23:480–488, 1983.

700. Savill J: Apoptosis: A mechanism for regulation of the cell complement of inflamed glomeruli. Kidney Int 41:607–612, 1992.

701. Savill J: Apoptosis and the kidney. J Am Soc Nephrol 5:12–21, 1994.

702. Vaux DL: Toward an understanding of the molecular mechanisms of physiological cell death. Proc Natl Acad Sci USA 90:786–789, 1993.

703. Gold R, Schmied M, Giegerich G, et al: Differentiation between cellular apoptosis and necrosis by the combined use of in situ tailing and nick translation techniques. Lab Invest 71:219–225, 1994.

704. Boise LH, Gonzalez-Garcia M, Postema CE, et al: bcl-x, a bcl-2–related gene that functions as a dominant regulator of apoptotic cell death. Cell 74:597–608, 1993.

705. Reed JC: Bcl-2 and the regulation of programmed cell death. J Cell Biol 124:1–6, 1994.

706. Strasser A, Whittingham S, Vaux DL, et al: Enforced *BCL2* expression in B-lymphoid cells prolongs antibody responses and elicits autoimmune disease. Proc Natl Acad Sci USA 88:8661–8665, 1991.

707. Veis DJ, Sorenson CM, Shutter JR, Korsmeyer SJ: Bcl-2–deficient mice demonstrate fulminant lymphoid apoptosis, polycystic kidneys, and hypopigmented hair. Cell 75:229–240, 1993.

708. Schlegel PN, Matthews GJ, Cichon Z, et al: Clusterin production in the obstructed rabbit kidney: Correlations with loss of renal function. J Am Soc Nephrol 3:1163–1171, 1992.

709. Pearse MJ, O'Bryan M, Fisicaro N, et al: Differential expression of clusterin in inducible models of apoptosis. Int Immunol 4:1225–1231, 1992.

710. French LE, Wohlwend A, Sappino AP, et al: Human clusterin gene expression is confined to surviving cells during in vitro programmed cell death. J Clin Invest 93:877–884, 1994.

711. Wong P, Taillefer D, Lakins J, et al: Molecular characterization of human TRPM-2/clusterin, a gene associated with sperm maturation, apoptosis and neurodegeneration. Eur J Biochem 221:917–925, 1994.

712. Nath KA, Dvergsten J, Correa-Rotter R, et al: Induction of clusterin in acute and chronic oxidative renal disease in the rat and its dissociation from cell injury. Lab Invest 71:209–218, 1994.

713. Dvergsten J, Manivel JC, Correa-Rotter R, Rosenberg ME: Expression of clusterin in human renal diseases. Kidney Int 45:828–835, 1994.

714. Harrison DJ: Cell death in the diseased glomerulus. Histopathology 12:679–683, 1988.

715. Ledda-Columbano GM, Columbano A, Coni P, et al: Cell deletion by apoptosis during regression of renal hyperplasia. Am J Pathol 135:657–662, 1989.

716. Tsai CY, Wu TH, Sun KH, et al: Polyclonal IgG anti-dsDNA antibodies exert cytotoxic effect on cultured rat mesangial cells by binding to cell membrane and augmenting apoptosis. Scand J Rheumatol 22:162–171, 1993.

717. Watson ML, Rao JK, Gilkeson GS, et al: Genetic analysis of MRL-lpr mice: Relationship of the *Fas* apoptosis gene to disease manifestations and renal disease–modifying loci. J Exp Med 176:1645–1656, 1992.

718. Mysler E, Bini P, Drappa J, et al: The apoptosis-1/Fas protein in human systemic lupus erythematosus. J Clin Invest 93:1029–1034, 1994.

719. Savill J, Smith J, Sarraf C, et al: Glomerular mesangial cells and inflammatory macrophages ingest neutrophils undergoing apoptosis. Kidney Int 42:924–936, 1992.

720. Savill J, Dransfield I, Hogg N, Haslett C: Vitronectin receptor–mediated phagocytosis of cells undergoing apoptosis. Nature 343:170–173, 1990.

721. Arends MJ, Harrison DJ: Novel histopathologic findings in a surviving case of hemolytic uremic syndrome after bone marrow transplantation. Hum Pathol 20:89–91, 1989.

722. Johnson RJ, Klebanoff SJ, Couser WG: Oxidants in glomerular injury. *In* Wilson CB, Brenner BM, Stein JH (eds): Contemporary Issues in Nephrology, Vol 18. Churchill Livingstone, New York, 1988, pp 87–110.

723. Johnson KJ, Rehan A, Ward PA: The role of oxygen radicals in kidney disease. *In* Halliwell B (ed): Oxygen Radicals and Tissue Injury. Proceedings of an Upjohn Symposium. FASEB, Bethesda, MD, 1988, pp 115–121.

724. Shah SV: Role of reactive oxygen metabolites in experimental glomerular disease. Kidney Int 35:1093–1106, 1989.

725. Shah SV: Oxidant mechanisms in glomerulonephritis. Semin Nephrol 11:320–326, 1991.

726. Andreoli SP: Reactive oxygen molecules, oxidant injury and renal disease. Pediatr Nephrol 5:733–742, 1991.

727. Diamond JR: The role of reactive oxygen species in animal models of glomerular disease. Am J Kidney Dis 19:292–300, 1992.

728. Baud L, Fouqueray B, Philippe C, Ardaillou R: Reactive oxygen species as glomerular autacoids. J Am Soc Nephrol 2(suppl 2):S132–S138, 1992.

729. Kakuta S, Nakamura K, Shimomura M, et al: Role of reactive oxygen species in the development of glomerular injury. Contrib Nephrol 101:255–262, 1993.

730. Johnson RJ, Lovett D, Lehrer RI, et al: Role of oxidants and proteases in glomerular injury. Kidney Int 45:352–359, 1994.

731. Boyce NW, Tipping PG, Holdsworth SR: Glomerular macrophages produce reactive oxygen species in experimental glomerulonephritis. Kidney Int 35:778–782, 1989.

732. Cook HT, Smith J, Salmon JA, Cattell V: Functional characteristics of macrophages in glomerulonephritis in the rat. $O_2^-$ generation, MHC class II expression, and eicosanoid synthesis. Am J Pathol 134:431–437, 1989.

733. Oberle GP, Niemeyer J, Thaiss F, et al: Increased oxygen radical and eicosanoid formation in immune-mediated mesangial cell injury. Kidney Int 42:69–74, 1992.

734. Firnhaber C, Murphy ME: Nitric oxide and superoxide in cultured cells: Limited production and influence on DNA synthesis. Am J Physiol 265:R518–R523, 1993.

735. Feng L, Xia Y, Garcia GE, et al: IL-1, TNFα and LPS induce cyclooxygenase-2 (COX-2) expression in mesangial cells (MC) through an oxidant-dependent mechanism. J Am Soc Nephrol 5:679, 1994.

736. Feng L, Xia Y, Wilson CB: Expression of a novel oxidative stress–inducible protein tyrosine phosphatase (PTPase) in mesangial cells (MC) and the glomerulus in experimental glomerulonephritis (GN). J Am Soc Nephrol 5:746, 1994.

737. Babior BM: The respiratory burst of phagocytes. J Clin Invest 73:599–601, 1984.

738. Henson PM, Johnston RB Jr: Tissue injury in inflammation. Oxidants, proteinases, and cationic proteins. J Clin Invest 79:669–674, 1987.

739. Babior GL, Rosin RE, McMurrich BJ, et al: Arrangement of the respiratory burst oxidase in the plasma membrane of the neutrophil. J Clin Invest 67:1724–1728, 1981.

740. Gallin JI, Buescher ES, Seligmann BE, et al: Recent advances in chronic granulomatous disease. Ann Intern Med 99:657–674, 1983.

741. Johnston RB Jr, Keele BB Jr, Misra HP, et al: The role of superoxide anion generation in phagocytic bactericidal activity. Studies with normal and chronic granulomatous disease leukocytes. J Clin Invest 55:1357–1372, 1975.

742. Weiss SJ, King GW, LoBuglio AF: Evidence for hydroxyl radical generation by human monocytes. J Clin Invest 60:370–373, 1977.

743. Ichikawa I, Kiyama S, Yoshioka T: Renal antioxidant enzymes: Their regulation and function. Kidney Int 45:1–9, 1994.

744. Steinert BW, Anderson PJ, Oberley LW, Oberley TD: Kidney glomerular explants in serum-free media: Demonstration of intracellular antioxidant enzymes and active oxygen metabolites. In Vitro Cell Dev Biol 22:285–294, 1986.

745. Yoshioka T, Homma T, Meyrick B, et al: Oxidants induce transcriptional activation of manganese superoxide dismutase in glomerular cells. Kidney Int 46:405–413, 1994.

746. Yoshioka T, Kawamura T, Meyrick BO, et al: Induction of manganese superoxide dismutase by glucocorticoids in glomerular cells. Kidney Int 45:211–219, 1994.

747. Oberley TD, Coursin DB, Cihla HP, et al: Immunolocalization of manganese superoxide dismutase in normal and transgenic mice expressing the human enzyme. Histochem J 25:267–279, 1993.

748. Adler S, Baker PJ, Johnson RJ, et al: Complement membrane attack complex stimulates production of reactive oxygen metabolites by cultured rat mesangial cells. J Clin Invest 77:762–767, 1986.

749. Radeke HH, Meier B, Topley N, et al: Interleukin 1-α and tumor necrosis factor-α induce oxygen radical production in mesangial cells. Kidney Int 37:767–775, 1990.

750. Baud L, Hagege J, Sraer J, et al: Reactive oxygen production by cultured rat glomerular mesangial cells during phagocytosis is associated with stimulation of lipoxygenase activity. J Exp Med 158:1836–1852, 1983.

751. Sedor JR, Carey SW, Emancipator SN: Immune complexes bind to cultured rat glomerular mesangial cells to stimulate superoxide release. Evidence for an Fc receptor. J Immunol 138:3751–3757, 1987.

752. Radeke HH, Cross AR, Hancock JT, et al: Functional expression of NADPH oxidase components (α- and β-subunits of cytochrome $b_{558}$ and 45-kDa flavoprotein) by intrinsic human glomerular mesangial cells. J Biol Chem 266:21025–21029, 1991.

753. Satriano JA, Shuldiner M, Hora K, et al: Oxygen radicals as second messengers for expression of the monocyte chemoattractant protein, JE/MCP-1, and the monocyte colony-stimulating factor, CSF-1, in

754. Waddell TK, Fialkow L, Chan CK, et al: Potentiation of the oxidative burst of human neutrophils. A signaling role for L-selectin. J Biol Chem 269:18485–18491, 1994.

755. Varani J, Taylor CG, Riser B, et al: Mesangial cell killing by leukocytes: Role of leukocyte oxidants and proteolytic enzymes. Kidney Int 42:1169–1177, 1992.

756. Keane WF, O'Donnell MP, Kasiske BL, Kim Y: Oxidative modification of low-density lipoproteins by mesangial cells. J Am Soc Nephrol 4:187–194, 1993.

757. Rovin BH, Wurst E, Kohan DE: Production of reactive oxygen species by tubular epithelial cells in culture. Kidney Int 37:1509–1514, 1990.

758. Sellak H, Franzini E, Hakim J, Pasquier C: Reactive oxygen species rapidly increase endothelial ICAM-1 ability to bind neutrophils without detectable upregulation. Blood 83:2669–2677, 1994.

759. Poelstra K, Hardonk MJ, Koudstaal J, Bakker WW: Intraglomerular platelet aggregation and experimental glomerulonephritis. Kidney Int 37:1500–1508, 1990.

760. Mossmann H, Hoyer B, Walz W, et al: Antibody-dependent cellular cytotoxicity and chemiluminescence as a tool for studying the mechanism of anti–glomerular basement membrane nephritis. The role of the cytotoxic potential of polymorphonuclear granulocytes and monocytes. Immunology 53:545–552, 1984.

761. Shah SV, Baricos WH, Basci A: Degradation of human glomerular basement membrane by stimulated neutrophils. Activation of a metalloproteinase(s) by reactive oxygen metabolites. J Clin Invest 79:25–31, 1987.

762. Weiss SJ, Regiani S: Neutrophils degrade subendothelial matrices in the presence of alpha-1-proteinase inhibitor. Cooperative use of lysosomal proteinases and oxygen metabolites. J Clin Invest 73:1297–1303, 1984.

763. Kashihara N, Watanabe Y, Makino H, et al: Selective decreased de novo synthesis of glomerular proteoglycans under the influence of reactive oxygen species. Proc Natl Acad Sci USA 89:6309–6313, 1992.

764. Davies M, Coles GA, Harber MJ: Effect of glomerular basement membrane on the initiation of chemiluminescence and lysosomal enzyme release in human polymorphonuclear leucocytes: an in vitro model of glomerular disease. Immunology 52:151–159, 1984.

765. Vissers MCM, Winterbourn CC: The effect of oxidants on neutrophil-mediated degradation of glomerular basement membrane collagen. Biochim Biophys Acta 889:277–286, 1986.

766. Rehan A, Johnson KJ, Kunkel RG, Wiggins RC: Role of oxygen radicals in phorbol myristate acetate–induced glomerular injury. Kidney Int 27:503–511, 1985.

767. Ito S, Ueda Y, Sugisaki T, Iidaka K: Induction of glomerular injury by singlet oxygen. Nephron 60:204–209, 1992.

768. Stratta P, Canavese C, Mazzucco G, et al: Mesangiolysis and endothelial lesions due to peroxidative damage in rabbits. Nephron 51:250–256, 1989.

769. Yoshioka T, Ichikawa I, Fogo A: Reactive oxygen metabolites cause massive, reversible proteinuria and glomerular sieving defect without apparent ultrastructural abnormality. J Am Soc Nephrol 2:902–912, 1991.

770. Dileepan KN, Sharma R, Stechschulte DJ, Savin VJ: Effect of superoxide exposure on albumin permeability of isolated rat glomeruli. J Lab Clin Med 121:797–804, 1993.

771. Duque I, Garcia-Escribano C, Rodriguez-Puyol M, et al: Effects of reactive oxygen species on cultured rat mesangial cells and isolated rat glomeruli. Am J Physiol 263:F466–F473, 1992.

772. Rehan A, Johnson KJ, Wiggins RC, et al: Evidence for the role of oxygen radicals in acute nephrotoxic nephritis. Lab Invest 51:396–403, 1984.

773. Webb DB, Mackenzie R, Zoob SN, Rees AJ: Evidence against a role for superoxide ions in the injury of nephrotoxic nephritis in rats. Clin Sci 69:687–689, 1985.

774. Birtwistle RJ, Michael J, Howie AJ, Adu D: Reactive oxygen products in heterologous anti–glomerular basement membrane nephritis in rats. Br J Exp Pathol 70:207–213, 1989.

775. Boyce NW, Holdsworth SR: Hydroxyl radical mediation of immune renal injury by desferrioxamine. Kidney Int 30:813–817, 1986.

response to tumor necrosis factor-α and immunoglobulin G. Evidence for involvement of reduced nicotinamide adenine dinucleotide phosphate (NADPH)–dependent oxidase. J Clin Invest 92:1564–1571, 1993.

776. Adachi T, Fukuta M, Ito Y, et al: Effect of superoxide dismutase on glomerular nephritis. Biochem Pharmacol 35:341–345, 1986.

777. Lotan D, Kaplan BS, Fong JSC, et al: Reduction of protein excretion by dimethyl sulfoxide in rats with passive Heymann nephritis. Kidney Int 25:778–788, 1984.

778. Kaplan BS, Milner LS, Lotan D, et al: Interactions of dimethyl sulfoxide and nonsteroidal anti-inflammatory agents in passive Heymann's nephritis. J Lab Clin Med 107:425–430, 1986.

779. Shah SV: Evidence suggesting a role for hydroxyl radical in passive Heymann nephritis in rats. Am J Physiol 254:F337–F344, 1988.

780. Rahman MA, Emancipator SS, Sedor JR: Hydroxyl radical scavengers ameliorate proteinuria in rat immune complex glomerulonephritis. J Lab Clin Med 112:619–626, 1988.

781. Milner LS, de Chadarevian J-P, Goodyer PR, et al: Amelioration of murine lupus nephritis by dimethylsulfoxide. Clin Immunol Immunopathol 45:259–267, 1987.

782. Hayashi T, Noguchi Y, Kameyama Y: Suppression of development of anti-nuclear antibody and glomerulonephritis in NZB × NZWF₁ mice by persistent infection with lactic dehydrogenase virus: Possible involvement of superoxide anion as a progressive effector. Int J Exp Pathol 74:553–560, 1993.

783. Baliga R, Baliga M, Shah SV: Effect of selenium-deficient diet in experimental glomerular disease. Am J Physiol 263:F56–F61, 1992.

784. Yoshioka T, Bills T, Moore-Jarrett T, et al: Role of intrinsic antioxidant enzymes in renal oxidant injury. Kidney Int 38:282–288, 1990.

785. Kawamura T, Yoshioka T, Bills T, et al: Glucocorticoid activates glomerular antioxidant enzymes and protects glomeruli from oxidant injuries. Kidney Int 40:291–301, 1991.

786. Johnson RJ, Klebanoff SJ, Ochi RF, et al: Participation of the myeloperoxidase-H₂O₂-halide system in immune complex nephritis. Kidney Int 32:342–349, 1987.

787. Johnson RJ, Guggenheim SJ, Klebanoff SJ, et al: Morphologic correlates of glomerular oxidant injury induced by the myeloperoxidase-hydrogen peroxide-halide system of the neutrophil. Lab Invest 58:294–301, 1988.

788. Diamond JR, Bonventre JV, Karnovsky MJ: A role for oxygen free radicals in aminonucleoside nephrosis. Kidney Int 29:478–483, 1986.

789. Beaman M, Birtwistle R, Howie AJ, et al: The role of superoxide anion and hydrogen peroxide in glomerular injury induced by puromycin aminonucleoside in rats. Clin Sci 73:329–332, 1987.

790. Okasora T, Takikawa T, Utsunomiya Y, et al: Suppressive effect of superoxide dismutase on Adriamycin nephropathy. Nephron 60:199–203, 1992.

791. Paller MS, Hoidal JR, Ferris TF: Oxygen free radicals in ischemic acute renal failure in the rat. J Clin Invest 74:1156–1164, 1984.

792. Bird JE, Milhoan K, Wilson CB, et al: Ischemic acute renal failure and antioxidant therapy in the rat. The relation between glomerular and tubular dysfunction. J Clin Invest 81:1630–1638, 1988.

793. Rahman MA, Stork JE, Dunn MJ: The roles of eicosanoids in experimental glomerulonephritis. Kidney Int 32(suppl 22):S40–S48, 1987.

794. Lianos EA: Eicosanoid biosynthesis and role in renal immune injury. Prostaglandins Leukot Essent Fatty Acids 41:1–12, 1990.

795. Schreiner GF, Klahr S: Diet and kidney disease: The role of dietary fatty acids. Proc Soc Exp Biol Med 197:1–11, 1991.

796. Lianos EA: Biosynthesis and role of arachidonic acid metabolites in glomerulonephritis. Nephron 37:73–77, 1984.

797. Lewis RA, Austen KF: The biologically active leukotrienes. Biosynthesis, metabolism, receptors, functions, and pharmacology. J Clin Invest 73:889–897, 1984.

798. Schlondorff D: Prostaglandins and other arachidonate metabolites and the kidney. In Kinne RKH (ed): Renal Biochemistry. Elsevier Science, Amsterdam, 1985, pp 337–421.

799. Stahl RAK, Thaiss F: Eicosanoids: Biosynthesis and function in the glomerulus. Renal Physiol 10:1–13, 1987.

800. Ardaillou R, Baud L, Sraer J: Lipoxygenase products and their functions in glomeruli. Adv Exp Med Biol 259:49–74, 1989.

801. Lianos EA: Eicosanoids and the modulation of glomerular immune injury. Kidney Int 35:985–992, 1989.

802. Ardaillou R, Baud L, Sraer J: Leukotrienes and reactive oxygen species as mediators of glomerular injury. Am J Nephrol 9(suppl 1):17–22, 1989.

803. Zoja C, Benigni A, Remuzzi G: Role of eicosanoids as mediators

of glomerular injury in immune-mediated nephropathies. Contrib Nephrol 69:18–26, 1989.

804. Badr KF: Cell-cell interactions in the regulation of glomerular inflammation by arachidonate lipoxygenase products. In Wong PY-K, Serhan CN (eds): Cell-Cell Interactions in the Release of Inflammatory Mediators. Plenum Publishing, New York, 1991, pp 335–346.

805. Badr KF: Arachidonic acid metabolites in glomerular immune injury. Semin Nephrol 11:332–339, 1991.

806. Mené P, Simonson MS, Dunn MJ: Prostaglandins, thromboxane and leukotrienes in the control of mesangial function. Adv Exp Med Biol 259:167–197, 1989.

807. Homma T, Zhang JY, Shimizu T, et al: Cyclooxygenase-derived metabolites of 8,9-epoxyeicosatrienoic acid are potent mitogens for cultured rat glomerular mesangial cells. Biochem Biophys Res Commun 191:282–288, 1993.

808. Seilhamer JJ, Pruzanski W, Vadas P, et al: Cloning and recombinant expression of phospholipase A₂ present in rheumatoid arthritic synovial fluid. J Biol Chem 264:5335–5338, 1989.

809. Kramer RM, Hession B, Johansen B, et al: Structure and properties of a human non-pancreatic phospholipase A₂. J Biol Chem 264:5768–5775, 1989.

810. Ishizaki J, Ohara O, Nakamura E, et al: cDNA cloning and sequence determination of rat membrane–associated phospholipase A₂. Biochem Biophys Res Commun 162:1030–1036, 1989.

811. Komada M, Kudo I, Inoue K: Structure of gene coding for rat group II phospholipase A₂. Biochem Biophys Res Commun 168:1059–1065, 1990.

812. Clark JD, Lin L-L, Kriz R-W, et al: A novel arachidonic acid-selective cytosolic PLA₂ contains a Ca²⁺-dependent translocation domain with homology to PKC and GAP. Cell 65:1043–1051, 1991.

813. Sharp JD, White DL, Chiou XG, et al: Molecular cloning and expression of human Ca²⁺-sensitive cytosolic phospholipase A₂. J Biol Chem 266:14850–14853, 1991.

814. Lin L-L, Lin AY, DeWitt DL: Interleukin-1α induces the accumulation of cytosolic phospholipase A₂ and the release of prostaglandin E₂ in human fibroblasts. J Biol Chem 267:23451–23454, 1992.

815. Pruzanski W, Vadas P: Phospholipase A₂—a mediator between proximal and distal effectors of inflammation. Immunol Today 12:143–146, 1991.

816. Nakamura H, Nemenoff RA, Gronich JH, Bonventre JV: Subcellular characteristics of phospholipase A₂ activity in the rat kidney. Enhanced cytosolic, mitochondrial, and microsomal phospholipase A₂ enzymatic activity after renal ischemia and reperfusion. J Clin Invest 87:1810–1818, 1991.

817. Schalkwijk C, Pfeilschifter J, Marki F, van den Bosch H: Interleukin-1β– and forskolin-induced synthesis and secretion of group II phospholipase A₂ and prostaglandin E₂ in rat mesangial cells is prevented by transforming growth factor-β2. J Biol Chem 267:8846–8851, 1992.

818. Schalkwijk CG, de Vet E, Pfeilschifter J, van den Bosch H: Interleukin-1 beta and transforming growth factor-beta 2 enhance cytosolic high-molecular-mass phospholipase A₂ activity and induce prostaglandin E₂ formation in rat mesangial cells. Eur J Biochem 210:169–176, 1992.

819. Pfeilschifter J, Schalkwijk C, Briner VA, van den Bosch H: Cytokine-stimulated secretion of group II phospholipase A₂ by rat mesangial cells. Its contribution to arachidonic acid release and prostaglandin synthesis by cultured rat glomerular cells. J Clin Invest 92:2516–2523, 1993.

820. Konieczkowski M, Sedor JR: Cell-specific regulation of type II phospholipase A₂ expression in rat mesangial cells. J Clin Invest 92:2524–2532, 1993.

821. Schalkwijk CG, Vervoordeldonk M, Pfeilschifter J, van den Bosch H: Interleukin-1β–induced cytosolic phospholipase A₂ activity and protein synthesis is blocked by dexamethasone in rat mesangial cells. FEBS Lett 333:339–343, 1993.

822. Nakazato Y, Simonson MS, Herman WH, et al: Interleukin-1α stimulates prostaglandin biosynthesis in serum-activated mesangial cells by induction of a non-pancreatic (type II) phospholipase A₂. J Biol Chem 266:14119–14127, 1991.

823. Pfeilschifter J, Mühl H, Pignat W, et al: Cytokine regulation of group II phospholipase A₂ expression in glomerular mesangial cells. Eur J Clin Pharmacol 44(suppl 1):S7–S9, 1993.

824. Maxwell AP, Goldberg HJ, Tay AH, et al: Epidermal growth factor and phorbol myristate acetate increase expression of the mRNA for cytosolic phospholipase A$_2$ in glomerular mesangial cells. Biochem J 295:763–766, 1993.

825. Gronich J, Konieczkowski M, Gelb MH, et al: Interleukin 1α causes rapid activation of cytosolic phospholipase A$_2$ by phosphorylation in rat mesangial cells. J Clin Invest 93:1224–1233, 1994.

826. Nakazato Y, Okada H, Sato A, et al: Interleukin 4 downregulates cell growth and prostaglandin release of human mesangial cells. Biochem Biophys Res Commun 197:486–493, 1993.

827. Uchida K, Ballermann BJ: Sustained activation of PGE$_2$ synthesis in mesangial cells cocultured with glomerular endothelial cells. Am J Physiol 263:C200–C209, 1992.

828. DeRubertis FR, Craven PA: Eicosanoids in the pathogenesis of the functional and structural alterations of the kidney in diabetes. Am J Kidney Dis 22:727–735, 1993.

829. Simonson MS, Wolfe JA, Konieczkowski M, et al: Regulation of prostaglandin endoperoxide synthase gene expression in cultured rat mesangial cells: Induction by serum via a protein kinase-C–dependent mechanism. Mol Endocrinol 5:441–451, 1991.

830. Coyne DW, Nickols M, Bertrand W, Morrison AR: Regulation of mesangial cell cyclooxygenase synthesis by cytokines and glucocorticoids. Am J Physiol 263:F97–F102, 1992.

831. Feng L, Sun W, Xia Y, et al: Cloning two isoforms of rat cyclooxygenase: Differential regulation of their expression. Arch Biochem Biophys 307:361–368, 1993.

832. Rzymkiewicz D, Leingang K, Baird N, Morrison AR: Regulation of prostaglandin endoperoxide synthase gene expression in rat mesangial cells by interleukin-1β. Am J Physiol 266:F39–F45, 1994.

833. Martin M, Neumann D, Hoff T, et al: Interleukin-1–induced cyclooxygenase 2 expression is suppressed by cyclosporin A in rat mesangial cells. Kidney Int 45:150–158, 1994.

834. Nowak R: Cox II enzyme is new target for inflammation drugs. J NIH Res 5:54–57, 1993.

835. Schlondorff D: Renal complications of nonsteroidal anti-inflammatory drugs. Kidney Int 44:643–653, 1993.

836. Baird NR, Morrison AR: Amplification of the arachidonic acid cascade: Implications for pharmacologic intervention. Am J Kidney Dis 21:557–564, 1993.

837. Scharschmidt L, Simonson M, Dunn MJ: Glomerular prostaglandins, angiotensin II, and nonsteroidal anti-inflammatory drugs. Am J Med 81(suppl 2B):30–42, 1986.

838. Dunn MJ, Scharschmidt LA: Prostaglandins modulate the glomerular actions of angiotensin II. Kidney Int 31(suppl 20):S95–S101, 1987.

839. Mené P, Simonson MS, Dunn MJ: Eicosanoids, mesangial contraction, and intracellular signal transduction. Tohoku J Exp Med 166:57–73, 1992.

840. Wilson TW: Renal prostaglandin synthesis and angiotensin-converting enzyme inhibition. J Cardiovasc Pharmacol 19(suppl 6):S39–S44, 1992.

841. Radeke HH, Schwinzer B, Resch K: Activated T-lymphocytes induce growth inhibition and prostaglandin E$_2$ release from syngeneic glomerular mesangial cells. Clin Exp Immunol 90:483–490, 1992.

842. Albrightson CR, Nambi P, Zabko-Potapovich B, et al: Effect of thrombin on proliferation, contraction and prostaglandin production of rat glomerular mesangial cells in culture. J Pharmacol Exp Ther 263:404–412, 1992.

843. Schlondorff D, Aynedjian HS, Satriano JA, Bank N: In vivo demonstration of glomerular PGE$_2$ responses to physiological manipulations and experimental agents. Am J Physiol 252:F717–F723, 1987.

844. Farman N, Pardelles P, Bonvalet JP: PGE$_2$, PGF$_{2\alpha}$, 6-keto-PGF$_{1\alpha}$, and TxB$_2$ synthesis along the rabbit nephron. Am J Physiol 252:F53–F59, 1987.

845. Govindarajan S, Nast CC, Smith WL, et al: Immunohistochemical distribution of renal prostaglandin endoperoxide synthase and prostacyclin synthase: Diminished endoperoxide synthase in the hepatorenal syndrome. Hepatology 7:654–659, 1987.

846. Nagamatsu T, Saitoh N, Suzuki Y, et al: Studies on experimental immune complex nephritis (3) therapeutic effect of prostaglandin E$_1$ α-cyclodextrin host molecule (PGE • CD) on serum sickness nephritis in rats. Jpn J Pharmacol 35:407–414, 1984.

847. McLeish KR, Stelzer GT, Eades DS, Wallace JH: Alterations in serum antibody and peripheral T-lymphocyte subsets resulting from treatment of murine immune complex glomerulonephritis with PGE$_2$. Clin Immunol Immunopathol 34:100–108, 1985.

848. Lavelle KJ, Golichowski AM, Neff LC, Yum MN: Effect of prostaglandins on immune complex interaction with glomerular cells in vitro. Immunol Invest 14:57–71, 1985.

849. McLeish KR, Stelzer GT, Eades DS, et al: Serial changes in humoral and cellular immunity induced by prostaglandin E$_2$ treatment of murine immune complex glomerulonephritis. J Lab Clin Med 106:517–523, 1985.

850. Nagamatsu T, Kojima J, Ito M, et al: Antinephritic effects of PGE$_1$ and thiaprostaglandin E$_1$, TEI-5178 and TEI-6122, on crescentic-type anti-GBM nephritis in rats. Jpn J Pharmacol 51:521–530, 1989.

851. Cattell V, Smith J, Cook HT: Prostaglandin E1 suppresses macrophage infiltration and ameliorates injury in an experimental model of macrophage-dependent glomerulonephritis. Clin Exp Immunol 79:260–265, 1990.

852. Kher V, Barcelli U, Weiss M, Pollak VE: Effects of dietary linoleic acid enrichment on induction of immune complex nephritis in mice. Nephron 39:261–266, 1985.

853. Girard D, Aloisi RM, Bliven ML, et al: Cyclophosphamide and 15(S)-15 methyl PGE$_1$ correct the T/B lymphocyte ratios of NZB/NZW mice. Agents Actions 29:333–341, 1990.

854. Kiberd BA: The functional and structural changes of the glomerulus throughout the course of murine lupus nephritis. J Am Soc Nephrol 3:930–939, 1992.

855. Niwa T, Asada H, Yamada K: Prostaglandin E$_1$ infusion therapy in chronic glomerulonephritis—a double-blind, crossover trial. Prostaglandins Leukotrienes Med 19:227–233, 1985.

856. Lin C-Y: Improvement in steroid and immunosuppressive drug resistant lupus nephritis by intravenous prostaglandin E$_1$ therapy. Nephron 55:258–264, 1990.

857. Kreisberg JI, Patel PY: The effects of insulin, glucose and diabetes on prostaglandin production by rat kidney glomeruli and cultured glomerular mesangial cells. Prostaglandins Leukotrienes Med 11:431–442, 1983.

858. Schambelan M, Blake S, Sraer J, et al: Increased prostaglandin production by glomeruli isolated from rats with streptozotocin-induced diabetes mellitus. J Clin Invest 75:404–412, 1985.

859. Jensen PK, Steven K, Blaehr H, et al: Effects of indomethacin on glomerular hemodynamics in experimental diabetes. Kidney Int 29:490–495, 1986.

860. Stahl RAK, Thaiss F, Haberstroh U, et al: Cyclooxygenase inhibition enhances rat interleukin 1β–induced growth of rat mesangial cells in culture. Am J Physiol 259:F419–F424, 1990.

861. Yokoyama C, Miyata A, Ihara H, et al: Molecular cloning of human platelet thromboxane A synthase. Biochem Biophys Res Commun 178:1479–1484, 1991.

862. Ohashi K, Ruan K-H, Kulmacz RJ, et al: Primary structure of human thromboxane synthase determined from the cDNA sequence. J Biol Chem 267:789–793, 1992.

863. Zhang L, Chase MB, Shen R-F: Molecular cloning and expression of murine thromboxane synthase. Biochem Biophys Res Commun 194:741–748, 1993.

864. Spurney RF, Onorato JJ, Ruiz P, et al: Characterization of glomerular thromboxane receptors in murine lupus nephritis. J Pharmacol Exp Ther 264:584–590, 1993.

865. Spurney RF, Onorato JJ, Albers FJ, Coffman TM: Thromboxane binding and signal transduction in rat glomerular mesangial cells. Am J Physiol 264:F292–F299, 1993.

866. Wu X, Pippin J, Lefkowith JB: Platelets and neutrophils are critical to the enhanced glomerular arachidonate metabolism in acute nephrotoxic nephritis in rats. J Clin Invest 91:766–773, 1993.

867. Macconi D, Benigni A, Morigi M, et al: Enhanced glomerular thromboxane A$_2$ mediates some pathophysiologic effect of platelet-activating factor in rabbit nephrotoxic nephritis: Evidence from biochemical measurements and inhibitor trials. J Lab Clin Med 113:549–560, 1989.

868. Kaizu K, Marsh D, Zipser R, Glassock RJ: Role of prostaglandins and angiotensin II in experimental glomerulonephritis. Kidney Int 28:629–635, 1985.

869. Takahashi K, Schreiner GF, Yamashita K, et al: Predominant functional roles for thromboxane A$_2$ and prostaglandin E$_2$ during late nephrotoxic serum glomerulonephritis in the rat. J Clin Invest 85:1974–1982, 1990.

870. Saito H, Ideura T, Takeuchi J: Effects of a selective thromboxane $A_2$ synthetase inhibitor on immune complex glomerulonephritis. Nephron 36:38–45, 1984.

871. Shinkai Y, Cameron JS: Rabbit nephrotoxic nephritis: Effect of a thromboxane synthetase inhibitor on evolution and prostaglandin excretion. Nephron 47:211–219, 1987.

872. Longhofer SL, Frisbie DD, Johnson HC, et al: Effects of thromboxane synthetase inhibition on immune complex glomerulonephritis. Am J Vet Res 52:480–487, 1991.

873. Cook HT, Cattell V, Smith J, et al: Effect of a thromboxane synthetase inhibitor on eicosanoid synthesis and glomerular injury during acute unilateral glomerulonephritis in the rat. Clin Nephrol 26:195–202, 1986.

874. Rahman MA, Emancipator SN, Dunn MJ: Immune complex effects on glomerular eicosanoid production and renal hemodynamics. Kidney Int 31:1317–1326, 1987.

875. Stahl RAK, Adler S, Baker PJ, et al: Enhanced glomerular prostaglandin formation in experimental membranous nephropathy. Kidney Int 31:1126–1131, 1987.

876. Cybulsky AV, Lieberthal W, Quigg RJ, et al: A role for thromboxane in complement-mediated glomerular injury. Am J Pathol 128:45–51, 1987.

877. Bresnahan BA, Wu S, Fenoy FJ, et al: Mesangial cell immune injury. Hemodynamic role of leukocyte- and platelet-derived eicosanoids. J Clin Invest 90:2304–2312, 1992.

878. Rahman MA, Liu CN, Dunn MJ, Emancipator SN: Complement and leukocyte independent proteinuria and eicosanoid synthesis in rat membranous nephropathy. Lab Invest 59:477–483, 1988.

879. Stahl RAK, Thaiss F, Kahf S, et al: Immune-mediated mesangial cell injury—biosynthesis and function of prostanoids. Kidney Int 38:273–281, 1990.

880. Garcia-Estan J, Roman RJ, Lianos EA, Garancis J: Effects of complement depletion on glomerular eicosanoid production and renal hemodynamics in rat nephrotoxic serum nephritis. J Lab Clin Med 114:389–393, 1989.

881. Kelley VE, Sneve S, Musinski S: Increased renal thromboxane production in murine lupus nephritis. J Clin Invest 77:252–259, 1986.

882. Badr KF, Kelley VE, Rennke HG, Brenner BM: Roles for thromboxane $A_2$ and leukotrienes in endotoxin-induced acute renal failure. Kidney Int 30:474–480, 1986.

883. Remuzzi G, Imberti L, Rossini M, et al: Increased glomerular thromboxane synthesis as a possible cause of proteinuria in experimental nephrosis. J Clin Invest 75:94–101, 1985.

884. de Keijzer MH, Provoost AP, Zijlstra FJ: Enhanced urinary excretion of eicosanoids in fawn-hooded rats. Nephron 62:454–458, 1992.

885. Bruggeman LA, Horigan EA, Horikoshi S, et al: Thromboxane stimulates synthesis of extracellular matrix protein in vitro. Am J Physiol 261:F488–F494, 1991.

886. Cybulsky AV, Goodyer PR, Cyr M-D, McTavish AJ: Eicosanoids enhance epidermal growth factor receptor activation and proliferation in glomerular epithelial cells. Am J Physiol 262:F639–F646, 1992.

887. Stahl RAK, Thaiss F, Wenzel U, et al: A rat model of progressive chronic glomerular sclerosis: The role of thromboxane inhibition. J Am Soc Nephrol 2:1568–1577, 1992.

888. Kirschenbaum MA, Liebross BA, Serros ER: Effect of indomethacin on proteinuria in rats with autologous immune complex nephropathy. Prostaglandins 30:295–303, 1985.

889. Zoja C, Benigni A, Verroust P, et al: Indomethacin reduces proteinuria in passive Heymann nephritis in rats. Kidney Int 31:1335–1343, 1987.

890. Thaiss F, Mihatsch MJ, Schoeppe W, Stahl RAK: Thromboxane mediates glomerular haemodynamics in a model of chronic glomerular disease. Eur J Clin Invest 22:182–189, 1992.

891. Nagamatsu T, Pippin J, Schreiner GF, Lefkowith JB: Paradoxical exacerbation of leukocyte-mediated glomerulonephritis with cyclooxygenase inhibition. Am J Physiol 263:F228–F236, 1992.

892. Bertani T, Benigni A, Cutillo F, et al: Effect of aspirin and sulindac in rabbit nephrotoxic nephritis. J Lab Clin Med 107:261–268, 1986.

893. Ciabattoni G, Cinotti GA, Pierucci A, et al: Effects of sulindac and ibuprofen in patients with chronic glomerular disease. N Engl J Med 310:279–283, 1984.

894. Takahashi K, Badr KF: Functional significance of lipoxygenase metabolites of arachidonic acid in the glomerular microcirculation. Adv Prostaglandin Thromboxane Leukot Res 21:683–688, 1990.

895. Badr KF: Five-lipoxygenase products in glomerular immune injury. J Am Soc Nephrol 3:907–915, 1992.

896. Krump E, Borgeat P: Kinetics of 5-lipoxygenase activation, arachidonic acid release, and leukotriene synthesis in human neutrophils: Effects of granulocyte-macrophage colony-stimulating factor. Biochim Biophys Acta 1213:135–139, 1994.

897. Lianos EA, Rahman MA, Dunn MJ: Glomerular arachidonate lipoxygenation in rat nephrotoxic serum nephritis. J Clin Invest 76:1355–1359, 1985.

898. Rahman MA, Nakazawa M, Emancipator SN, Dunn MJ: Increased leukotriene $B_4$ synthesis in immune injured rat glomeruli. J Clin Invest 81:1945–1952, 1988.

899. Fauler J, Wiemeyer A, Marx K-H, et al: $LTB_4$ in nephrotoxic serum nephritis in rats. Kidney Int 36:46–50, 1989.

900. Lianos EA, Noble B: Glomerular leukotriene synthesis in Heymann nephritis. Kidney Int 36:998–1002, 1989.

901. Gimbrone MA, Jr, Brock AF, Schafer AI: Leukotriene $B_4$ stimulates polymorphonuclear leukocyte adhesion to cultured vascular endothelial cells. J Clin Invest 74:1552–1555, 1984.

902. Migliorisi G, Folkes E, Pawlowski N, Cramer EB: In vitro studies of human monocyte migration across endothelium in response to leukotriene $B_4$ and f-Met-Leu-Phe. Am J Pathol 127:157–167, 1987.

903. Lianos EA: Synthesis of hydroxyeicosatetraenoic acids and leukotrienes in rat nephrotoxic serum glomerulonephritis. Role of antiglomerular basement membrane antibody dose, complement, and neutrophiles. J Clin Invest 82:427–435, 1988.

904. Lefkowith JB, Nagamatsu T, Pippin J, Schreiner GF: Role of leukocytes in metabolic and functional derangements of experimental glomerulonephritis. Am J Physiol 261:F213–F220, 1991.

905. Yared A, Albrightson-Winslow C, Griswold D, et al: Functional significance of leukotriene $B_4$ in normal and glomerulonephritic kidneys. J Am Soc Nephrol 2:45–56, 1991.

906. Brady HR, Denton MD, Brenner BM, Serhan CN: Neutrophil adhesion to glomerular mesangial cells: Regulation by lipoxygenase-derived eicosanoids. Adv Exp Med Biol 314:347–359, 1991.

907. Ballermann BJ, Lewis RA, Corey EJ, et al: Identification and characterization of leukotriene $C_4$ receptors in isolated rat renal glomeruli. Circ Res 56:324–330, 1985.

908. Baud L, Sraer J, Perez J, et al: Leukotriene $C_4$ binds to human glomerular epithelial cells and promotes their proliferation in vitro. J Clin Invest 76:374–377, 1985.

909. Assem ESK, Abdullah NA: Release of thromboxane $B_2$ and leukotriene $C_4$ and reduction in renal perfusion in experimental anaphylactic reaction of isolated guinea pig kidney. Int Arch Allergy Appl Immunol 82:212–214, 1987.

910. Baud L, Sraer J, Delarue F, et al: Lipoxygenase products mediate the attachment of rat macrophages to glomeruli in vitro. Kidney Int 27:855–863, 1985.

911. Sraer J, Bens M, Oudinet J-P, Ardaillou R: Bioconversion of leukotriene $C_4$ by rat glomeruli and papilla. Prostaglandins 31:909–919, 1986.

912. Badr KF, Brenner, BM, Ichikawa I: Effects of leukotriene $D_4$ on glomerular dynamics in the rat. Am J Physiol 253:F239–F243, 1987.

913. Joris I, Majno G, Corey EJ, Lewis RA: The mechanism of vascular leakage induced by leukotriene $E_4$. Endothelial contraction. Am J Pathol 126:19–24, 1987.

914. Badr KF, Schreiner GF, Wasserman M, Ichikawa I: Preservation of the glomerular capillary ultrafiltration coefficient during rat nephrotoxic serum nephritis by a specific leukotriene $D_4$ receptor antagonist. J Clin Invest 81:1702–1709, 1988.

915. Katoh T, Lianos EA, Fukunaga M, et al: Leukotriene $D_4$ is a mediator of proteinuria and glomerular hemodynamic abnormalities in passive Heymann nephritis. J Clin Invest 91:1507–1515, 1993.

916. Wu S-H, Bresnahan BA, Lianos EA: Hemodynamic role of arachidonate 12- and 5-lipoxygenases in nephrotoxic serum nephritis. Kidney Int 43:1280–1285, 1993.

917. Albrightson CR, Short B, Dytko G, et al: Selective inhibition of 5-lipoxygenase attenuates glomerulonephritis in the rat. Kidney Int 45:1301–1310, 1994.

918. Wu S-H, Lianos EA: Modulatory effect of arachidonate 5-lipoxygenation on glomerular cell proliferation in nephrotoxic serum nephritis. J Lab Clin Med 122:703–710, 1993.

919. Badr KF: 15-Lipoxygenase products as leukotriene antagonists: Therapeutic potential in glomerulonephritis. Kidney Int 42(suppl 38):S-101–S-108, 1992.

920. Katoh T, Lakkis FG, Makita N, Badr KF: Co-regulated expression of glomerular 12/15-lipoxygenase and interleukin-4 mRNAs in rat nephrotoxic nephritis. Kidney Int 46:341–349, 1994.

921. Rifai A, Sakai H, Yagame M: Expression of 5-lipoxygenase and 5-lipoxygenase activation protein in glomerulonephritis. Kidney Int 43(suppl 39):S-95–S-99, 1993.

922. Hurd ER, Johnston JM, Okita JR, et al: Prevention of glomerulonephritis and prolonged survival in New Zealand Black/New Zealand White $F_1$ hybrid mice fed an essential fatty acid–deficient diet. J Clin Invest 67:476–485, 1981.

923. McLeish KR, Gohara AF, Johnson LJ, Sustarsic DL: Alteration in immune complex glomerulonephritis by arachidonic acid. Prostaglandins 23:383–389, 1982.

924. Dubois CH, Foidart JB, Dechenne CA, Mahieu PR: Effects of a diet deficient in essential fatty acids on the glomerular hypercellularity occurring in the course of nephrotoxic serum nephritis in rats. Kidney Int 21(suppl 11):S39–S45, 1982.

925. Prickett JD, Robinson DR, Steinberg AD: Dietary enrichment with the polyunsaturated fatty acid eicosapentaenoic acid prevents proteinuria and prolongs survival in NZB × NZW $F_1$ mice. J Clin Invest 68:556–559, 1981.

926. Robinson DR, Prickett JD, Polisson R, et al: The protective effect of dietary fish oil on murine lupus. Prostaglandins 30:51–75, 1985.

927. Kelley VE, Ferretti A, Izui S, Strom TB: A fish oil diet rich in eicosapentaenoic acid reduces cyclooxygenase metabolites, and suppresses lupus in MRL-*lpr* mice. J Immunol 134:1914–1919, 1985.

928. Yumura W, Hattori S, Morrow WJW, et al: Dietary fat and immune function. II. Effects on immune complex nephritis in (NZB × NZW)$F_1$ mice. J Immunol 135:3864–3868, 1985.

929. Rahman MA, Sauter DC, Young MR: Effects of dietary fish oil on the induction of experimental membranous nephropathy in the rat. Lab Invest 64:371–376, 1991.

930. Wheeler DC, Nair DR, Persaud JW, et al: Effects of dietary fatty acids in an animal model of focal glomerulosclerosis. Kidney Int 39:930–937, 1991.

931. Walton AJE, Snaith ML, Locniskar M, et al: Dietary fish oil and the severity of symptoms in patients with systemic lupus erythematosus. Ann Rheum Dis 50:463–466, 1991.

932. Kher V, Barcelli U, Weiss M, et al: Protective effect of polyunsaturated fatty acid supplementation in apoferritin induced murine glomerulonephritis. Prostaglandins Leukotrienes Med 22:323–334, 1986.

933. Papanikolaou N: Alteration of mercuric chloride–induced autoimmune glomerulonephritis in brown-Norway rats by herring oil, evening primrose oil and OKY-046, a selective TXA-synthetase inhibitor. Prostaglandins Leukotrienes Med 27:129–149, 1987.

934. Lefkowith JB, Schreiner G: Essential fatty acid deficiency depletes rat glomeruli of resident macrophages and inhibits angiotensin II–induced eicosanoid synthesis. J Clin Invest 80:947–956, 1987.

935. Schreiner GF, Rovin B, Lefkowith JB: The antiinflammatory effects of essential fatty acid deficiency in experimental glomerulonephritis. J Immunol 143:3192–3199, 1989.

936. Rovin BH, Lefkowith JB, Schreiner GF: Mechanisms underlying the anti-inflammatory effects of essential fatty acid deficiency in experimental glomerulonephritis. Inhibited release of a monocyte chemotactic by glomeruli. J Immunol 145:1238–1245, 1990.

937. Takahashi K, Kato T, Schreiner GF, et al: Essential fatty acid deficiency normalizes function and histology in rat nephrotoxic nephritis. Kidney Int 41:1245–1253, 1992.

938. Thomas ME, Schreiner GF: Contribution of proteinuria to progressive renal injury: Consequences of tubular uptake of fatty acid bearing albumin. Am J Nephrol 13:385–398, 1993.

939. Lefkowith JB, Morrison AR, Schreiner GF: Murine glomerular leukotriene $B_4$ synthesis. Manipulation by (n-6) fatty acid deprivation and cellular origin. J Clin Invest 82:1655–1660, 1988.

940. Fox PL, DiCorleto PE: Fish oils inhibit endothelial cell production of platelet-derived growth factor–like protein. Science 241:453–456, 1988.

941. Lefkowith JB, Pippin J, Nagamatsu T, Lee V: Urinary eicosanoids and the assessment of glomerular inflammation. J Am Soc Nephrol 2:1560–1567, 1992.

942. Pugliese F, Pierucci A, Simonetti BM, et al: Prostaglandins and other arachidonic acid metabolites in the pathogenesis of clinical and experimental glomerulonephritis. Int J Artif Organs 8:11–12, 1984.

943. Niwa T, Maeda K, Shibata M: Urinary prostaglandins and thromboxane in patients with chronic glomerulonephritis. Nephron 46:281–287, 1987.

944. Tönshoff B, Momper R, Kühl PG, et al: Increased thromboxane biosynthesis in childhood hemolytic uremic syndrome. Kidney Int 37:1134–1141, 1990.

945. Colina-Chourio JA, Rodriguez-Iturbe B, Baggio B, et al: Urinary excretion of prostaglandins ($PGE_2$ and $PGF_{2\alpha}$) and kallikrein in acute glomerulonephritis. Clin Nephrol 20:217–224, 1983.

946. Niwa T, Maeda K, Naotsuka Y, et al: Improvement of renal function with prostaglandin $E_1$ infusion in patients with chronic renal disease. Lancet 1:687, 1982.

947. Niwa T, Maeda K, Asada H, et al: Beneficial effects of prostaglandin $E_1$ in rapidly progressive glomerulonephritis. N Engl J Med 308:969, 1983.

948. Pierucci A, Simonetti BM, Pecci G, et al: Improvement of renal function with selective thromboxane antagonism in lupus nephritis. N Engl J Med 320:421–425, 1989.

949. Cinotti GA, Pierucci A, Mene P: Experimental and clinical action of thromboxane $A_2$ receptor antagonists. Contrib Nephrol 81:270–278, 1990.

950. Bearer EL, Friend DS: Lipids of the platelet membrane. Lab Invest 54:119–121, 1986.

951. Camussi G, Tetta C, Vercellone A: Platelets and platelet-derived cationic proteins in human and experimental glomerular pathology. Contrib Nephrol 69:27–36, 1989.

952. Johnson RJ: Platelets in inflammatory glomerular injury. Semin Nephrol 11:276–284, 1991.

953. Barnes JL: Platelets in renal disease. *In* Tetta C (ed): Immunopharmacology of the Renal System. Academic Press, San Diego, CA, 1993, pp 88–118.

954. Barnes JL, Venkatachalam MA: The role of platelets and polycationic mediators in glomerular vascular injury. Semin Nephrol 5:57–68, 1985.

955. Jorgensen L, Grothe AG, Larsen T, et al: Injury to cultured endothelial cells by thrombin-stimulated platelets. Lab Invest 54:408–415, 1986.

956. Tranqui I, Duperray A, Chenais F, et al: Influence of human platelet factors on the proliferation of rat mesangial glomerular cells. Thromb Res 38:245–251, 1985.

957. Wight TN, Raugi GJ, Mumby SM, Bornstein P: Light microscopic immunolocation of thrombospondin in human tissues. J Histochem Cytochem 33:295–302, 1985.

958. Silverstein RL, Nachman RL: Thrombospondin binds to monocytes-macrophages and mediates platelet-monocyte adhesion. J Clin Invest 79:867–874, 1987.

959. McGregor B, Colon S, Mutin M, et al: Thrombospondin in human glomerulopathies. A marker of inflammation and early fibrosis. Am J Pathol 144:1281–1287, 1994.

960. Kaplan C, Champeix P, Blanchard D, et al: Platelet antibodies in systemic lupus erythematosus. Br J Haematol 67:89–93, 1987.

961. Johnson RJ, Pritzl P, Iida H, Alpers CE: Platelet-complement interactions in mesangial proliferative nephritis in the rat. Am J Pathol 138:313–321, 1991.

962. Johnson RJ, Alpers CE, Pritzl P, et al: Platelets mediate neutrophil-dependent immune complex nephritis in the rat. J Clin Invest 82:1225–1235, 1988.

963. Johnson RJ, Garcia RL, Pritzl P, Alpers CE: Platelets mediate glomerular cell proliferation in immune complex nephritis induced by anti-mesangial cell antibodies in the rat. Am J Pathol 136:369–374, 1990.

964. Poelstra K, Heynen ER, Baller JFW, et al: Modulation of anti-Thy1 nephritis in the rat by adenine nucleotides. Evidence for an anti-inflammatory role for nucleotidases. Lab Invest 66:555–563, 1992.

965. Poelstra K, Brouwer E, Baller JFW, et al: Attenuation of anti-Thy1 glomerulonephritis in the rat by anti-inflammatory platelet-inhibiting agents. Am J Pathol 142:441–450, 1993.

966. Ideura T, Ogasawara M, Tomura S, et al: Effect of thrombocytopenia on the onset of immune complex glomerulonephritis. Nephron 60:49–55, 1992.

967. Barnes JL, Camussi G, Tetta C, Venkatachalam MA: Glomerular

localization of platelet cationic proteins after immune complex–induced platelet activation. Lab Invest 63:755–761, 1990.

968. Barnes JL: Glomerular localization of platelet secretory proteins in mesangial proliferative lesions induced by Habu snake venom. J Histochem Cytochem 37:1075–1082, 1989.

969. Bakker WW, Willink EJ, Donga J, et al: Antithrombotic activity of glomerular adenosine diphosphatase in the glomerular basement membrane of the rat kidney. J Lab Clin Med 109:171–177, 1987.

970. Deuel TF, Huang JS: Platelet-derived growth factor. Structure, function, and roles in normal and transformed cells. J Clin Invest 74:669–676, 1984.

971. Ross R, Bowen-Pope DF, Raines EW: Platelets, macrophages, endothelium, and growth factors. Their effects upon cells and their possible roles in atherogenesis. Ann N Y Acad Sci 454:254–260, 1985.

972. Deuel TF: Polypeptide growth factors: Roles in normal and abnormal cell growth. Annu Rev Cell Biol 3:443–492, 1987.

973. Hart CE, Forstrom JW, Kelly JD, et al: Two classes of PDGF receptor recognize different isoforms of PDGF. Science 240:1529–1534, 1988.

974. Johnson R, Iida H, Yoshimura A, et al: Platelet-derived growth factor: A potentially important cytokine in glomerular disease. Kidney Int 41:590–594, 1992.

975. Gesualdo L, Di Paolo S, Milani S, et al: Expression of platelet-derived growth factor receptors in normal and diseased human kidney. An immunohistochemistry and in situ hybridization study. J Clin Invest 94:50–58, 1994.

976. Deuel TF, Senior RM, Huang JS, Griffin GL: Chemotaxis of monocytes and neutrophils to platelet-derived growth factor. J Clin Invest 69:1046–1049, 1982.

977. Tzeng DY, Deuel TF, Huang JS, et al: Platelet-derived growth factor promotes polymorphonuclear leukocyte activation. Blood 64:1123–1128, 1984.

978. Tzeng DY, Deuel TF, Huang JS, Baehner RL: Platelet-derived growth factor promotes human peripheral monocyte activation. Blood 66:179–183, 1985.

979. Heldin CH, Wasteson A, Westermark B: Platelet-derived growth factor. Mol Cell Endocrinol 39:169–187, 1985.

980. Habenicht AJR, Goerig M, Grulich J, et al: Human platelet-derived growth factor stimulates prostaglandin synthesis by activation and by rapid de novo synthesis of cyclooxygenase. J Clin Invest 75:1381–1387, 1985.

981. Yahalom J, Eldor A, Fuks Z, Vlodavsky I: Degradation of sulfated proteoglycans in the subendothelial extracellular matrix by human platelet heparitinase. J Clin Invest 74:1842–1849, 1984.

982. Barnes JL, Hevey KA: Glomerular mesangial cell migration. Response to platelet secretory products. Am J Pathol 138:859–866, 1991.

983. Ogawa S, Naruse T: Effects of various antiplatelet drugs and a defibrinating agent on experimental glomerulonephritis in rats. J Lab Clin Med 99:428–441, 1982.

984. Koyama A, Inage H, Sano M, et al: Platelet involvement in the nephritis of acute serum sickness in rabbits: Protection by dipyridamole and FUT-175. Clin Exp Immunol 61:388–396, 1985.

985. Izumino K, Iida H, Asaka M, et al: Effect of the antiplatelet agents ticlopidine and dipyridamole on experimental immune complex glomerulonephritis in rats. Nephron 43:56–61, 1986.

986. Izumino K, Iida H, Asaka M, Sasayama S: Effect of the antiplatelet agents ticlopidine and dipyridamole on nephrotoxic serum nephritis in rats. Nephron 45:306–310, 1987.

987. Donadio JV Jr, Anderson CF, Mitchell JC III, et al: Membranoproliferative glomerulonephritis. A prospective clinical trial of platelet-inhibitor therapy. N Engl J Med 310:1421–1426, 1984.

988. Chan MK, Kwan SYL, Chan KW, Yeung CK: Controlled trial of antiplatelet agents in mesangial IgA glomerulonephritis. Am J Kidney Dis 9:417–421, 1987.

989. Barnes JL, Levine SP, Venkatachalam MA: Binding of platelet factor four (PF4) to glomerular polyanion. Kidney Int 25:759–765, 1984.

990. Wu V-Y, Cohen MP: Platelet factor 4 binding to glomerular microvascular matrix. Biochim Biophys Acta 797:76–82, 1984.

991. Prosdocimi M, Scattolo N, Mazzucato A, et al: Disappearance of human platelet factor 4 (PF4) in rabbits: Does an immediate component exist? Thromb Res 39:541–547, 1985.

992. Shirato I, Tomino Y, Koide H: Detection of 'activated platelets' in the urinary sediments using a scanning electron microscope in patients with IgA nephropathy. Am J Nephrol 10:186–190, 1990.

993. Taira K, Hewitson TD, Kincaid-Smith P: Urinary platelet factor four (Pf4) levels in mesangial IgA glomerulonephritis and thin basement membrane disease. Clin Nephrol 37:8–13, 1992.

994. Nakajima M, Hewitson TD, Mathews DC, Kincaid-Smith P: Platelet-derived growth factor mesangial deposits in mesangial IgA glomerulonephritis. Nephrol Dial Transplant 6:11–16, 1991.

995. Hanahan DJ: Platelet activating factor: A biologically active phosphoglyceride. Annu Rev Biochem 55:483–509, 1986.

996. Wardlaw AJ, Moqbel R, Cromwell O, Kay AB: Platelet-activating factor. A potent chemotactic and chemokinetic factor for human eosinophils. J Clin Invest 78:1701–1706, 1986.

997. Angle MJ, Pinckard RN, Showell HJ, McManus LM: Ontogeny of the responsiveness to intravenous platelet-activating factor. Lab Invest 57:321–328, 1987.

998. Snyder F (ed): Platelet Activating Factor and Related Lipid Mediators. Plenum Publishing, New York, 1987, pp 1–472.

999. Prescott SM, Zimmerman GA, McIntyre TM: Platelet-activating factor. J Biol Chem 265:17381–17384, 1990.

1000. Snyder F: Platelet-activating factor and related acetylated lipids as potent biologically active cellular mediators. Am J Physiol 259:C697–C708, 1990.

1001. Koltai M, Hosford D, Braquet P: Role of PAF and cytokines in microvascular tissue injury. J Lab Clin Med 119:461–466, 1992.

1002. Hwang SB: Specific receptors of platelet-activating factor, receptor heterogeneity, and signal transduction mechanisms. J Lipid Mediat 2:123–158, 1990.

1003. Hwang S-B: Function and regulation of extracellular and intracellular receptors of platelet activating factor. Ann N Y Acad Sci 629:217–226, 1991.

1004. Honda Z-I, Nakamura M, Miki I, et al: Cloning by functional expression of platelet-activating factor receptor from guinea-pig lung. Nature 349:342–346, 1991.

1005. Ye RD, Prossnitz ER, Zou A, Cochrane CG: Characterization of a human cDNA that encodes a functional receptor for platelet activating factor. Biochem Biophys Res Commun 180:105–111, 1991.

1006. Nakamura M, Honda Z-I, Izumi T, et al: Molecular cloning and expression of platelet-activating factor receptor from human leukocytes. J Biol Chem 266:20400–20405, 1991.

1007. Kunz D, Gerard NP, Gerard C: The human leukocyte platelet-activating factor receptor. cDNA cloning, cell surface expression, and construction of a novel epitope-bearing analog. J Biol Chem 267:9101–9106, 1992.

1008. Kester M, Thomas CP, Wang J, Dunn MJ: Platelet-activating factor stimulates multiple signaling pathways in cultured rat mesangial cells. J Cell Physiol 153:224–255, 1992.

1009. Chao W, Olson MS: Platelet-activating factor: Receptors and signal transduction. Biochem J 292:617–629, 1993.

1010. Perico N, Remuzzi G: Role of platelet-activating factor in renal immune injury and proteinuria. Am J Nephrol 10(suppl 1):98–104, 1990.

1011. Ortiz A, Gomez-Chiarri M, Lerma JL, et al: The role of platelet-activating factor (PAF) in experimental glomerular injury. Lipids 26:1310–1315, 1991.

1012. Schlondorff D, Satriano JA, Hagege J, et al: Effect of platelet-activating factor and serum-treated zymosan on prostaglandin $E_2$ synthesis, arachidonic acid release, and contraction of cultured rat mesangial cells. J Clin Invest 73:1227–1231, 1984.

1013. Bonventre JV, Weber PC, Gronich JH: PAF and PDGF increase cytosolic $[Ca^{2+}]$ and phospholipase activity in mesangial cells. Am J Physiol 254:F87–F94, 1988.

1014. Schlondorff D, Singhal P, Hassid A, et al: Relationship of GTP-binding proteins, phospholipase C, and $PGE_2$ synthesis in rat glomerular mesangial cells. Am J Physiol 254:F171–F178, 1989.

1015. Huang SJ, Monk PN, Downes CP, Whetton AD: Platelet-activating factor–induced hydrolysis of phosphatidylinositol 4,5-bisphosphate stimulates the production of reactive oxygen intermediates in macrophages. Biochem J 249:839–845, 1988.

1016. Prpic V, Uhing RJ, Weiel JE, et al: Biochemical and functional responses stimulated by platelet-activating factor in murine peritoneal macrophages. J Cell Biol 107:363–372, 1988.

1017. Hirafuji M, Maeyama K, Watanabe T, Ogura Y: Transient increase of cytosolic free calcium in cultured human vascular endothelial cells by platelet-activating factor. Biochem Biophys Res Commun 154:910–917, 1988.

1018. Dhar A, Paul AK, Shukla SD: Platelet-activating factor stimulation of tyrosine kinase and its relationship to phospholipase C in rabbit platelets: Studies with genistein and monoclonal antibody to phosphotyrosine. Mol Pharmacol 37:519–525, 1990.

1019. Dhar A, Shukla SD: Involvement of pp60$^{c\text{-}src}$ in platelet-activating factor–stimulated platelets. Evidence for translocation from cytosol to membrane. J Biol Chem 266:18797–18801, 1991.

1020. Gomez-Cambronero J, Wang E, Johnson G, et al: Platelet-activating factor induces tyrosine phosphorylation in human neutrophils. J Biol Chem 266:6240–6245, 1991.

1021. Chao W, Liu H, Hanahan DJ, Olson MS: Protein tyrosine phosphorylation and regulation of the receptor for platelet-activating factor in rat Kupffer cells. Effect of sodium vanadate. Biochem J 288:777–784, 1992.

1022. Chao W, Liu H, Hanahan DJ, Olson MS: Platelet-activating factor–stimulated protein tyrosine phosphorylation and eicosanoid synthesis in rat Kupffer cells. Evidence for calcium-dependent and protein kinase C–dependent and -independent pathways. J Biol Chem 267:6725–6735, 1992.

1023. Mazer B, Domenico J, Sawami H, Gelfand EW: Platelet-activating factor induces an increase in intracellular calcium and expression of regulatory genes in human B lymphoblastoid cells. J Immunol 146:1914–1920, 1991.

1024. Schulam PG, Kuruvilla A, Putcha G, et al: Platelet-activating factor induces phospholipid turnover, calcium flux, arachidonic acid liberation, eicosanoid generation, and oncogene expression in a human B cell line. J Immunol 146:1642–1648, 1991.

1025. Dell'Albani P, Condorelli DF, Mudo G, et al: Platelet-activating factor and its methoxy-analogue ET-18-OCH3 stimulate immediate early gene expression in rat astroglial cultures. Neurochem Int 22:567–574, 1993.

1026. Müller R, Bravo R, Burckhardt J, Curran T: Induction of c-*fos* gene and protein by growth factors precedes activation of c-*myc*. Nature 312:716–720, 1984.

1027. Bazan HEP, Tao Y, Bazan NG: Platelet-activating factor induces collagenase expression in corneal epithelial cells. Proc Natl Acad Sci USA 90:8678–8682, 1993.

1028. Arribas I, Martin Ambrosio R, Diez Marques ML, et al: Direct interactions between platelets and cultured rat mesangial cells. Prostaglandins Leukot Essent Fatty Acids 49:597–602, 1993.

1029. Tripathi YB, Lim RW, Fernandez-Gallardo S, et al: Involvement of tyrosine kinase and protein kinase C in platelet-activating-factor–induced c-*fos* gene expression in A-431 cells. Biochem J 286:527–533, 1992.

1030. Fu XY, Zhang JJ: Transcription factor p91 interacts with the epidermal growth factor receptor and mediates activation of the c-*fos* gene promoter. Cell 74:1135–1145, 1993.

1031. Pirotzky E, Bidault J, Burtin C, et al: Release of platelet-activating factor, slow-reacting substance, and vasoactive amines from isolated rat kidneys. Kidney Int 25:404–410, 1984.

1032. Pirotzky E, Pintos-Morell G, Burtin C, et al: Renal anaphylaxis. I. Antigen-initiated responses from isolated perfused rat kidney. Kidney Int 32:233–237, 1987.

1033. Pirotzky E, Page C, Morley J, et al: Vascular permeability induced by Paf-acether (platelet-activating factor) in the isolated perfused rat kidney. Agents Actions 16:17–18, 1985.

1034. Schwertschlag US, Dennis VW, Tucker JA, Camussi G: Nonimmunological alterations of glomerular filtration by s-PAF in the rat kidney. Kidney Int 34:779–785, 1988.

1035. Perico N, Delaini F, Tagliaferri M, et al: Effect of platelet-activating factor and its specific receptor antagonist on glomerular permeability to proteins in isolated perfused rat kidney. Lab Invest 58:163–171, 1988.

1036. Perico N, Remuzzi A, Dadan J, et al: Platelet-activating factor alters glomerular barrier size selectivity for macromolecules in rats. Am J Physiol 261:F85–F90, 1991.

1037. Goldstein BM, Gabel RA, Huggins FJ, et al: Effect of platelet activating factor (PAF) on blood flow distribution in the spontaneously hypertensive rat. Life Sci 35:1373–1378, 1984.

1038. Pirotzky E, Ninio E, Bidault J, et al: Biosynthesis of platelet-activating factor. VI. Precursor of platelet-activating factor and acetyltransferase activity in isolated rat kidney cells. Lab Invest 51:567–572, 1984.

1039. Schlondorff D, Goldwasser P, Neuwirth R, et al: Production of platelet-activating factor in glomeruli and cultured glomerular mesangial cells. Am J Physiol 250:F1123–F1127, 1986.

1040. Zanglis A, Lianos EA: Platelet activating factor biosynthesis and degradation in rat glomeruli. J Lab Clin Med 110:330–337, 1987.

1041. Morell GP, Pirotzky E, Erard D, et al: Paf-acether (platelet-activating factor) and interleukin-1–like cytokine production by lipopolysaccharide-stimulated glomeruli. Clin Immunol Immunopathol 46:396–405, 1988.

1042. Neuwirth R, Ardaillou N, Schlondorff D: Extra- and intracellular metabolism of platelet-activating factor by cultured mesangial cells. Am J Physiol 256:F735–741, 1989.

1043. Schlondorff D: Interactions of platelet activating factor and prostaglandins in the glomerulus and in mesangial cells. Adv Exp Med Biol 259:199–219, 1989.

1044. Weisman SM, Felsen D, Vaughan ED Jr: Platelet-activating factor is a potent stimulus for renal prostaglandin synthesis: Possible significance in unilateral ureteral obstruction. J Pharmacol Exp Ther 235:10–15, 1985.

1045. Camussi G: Potential role of platelet-activating factor in renal pathophysiology. Kidney Int 29:469–477, 1986.

1046. Badr KF, DeBoer DK, Takahashi K, et al: Glomerular responses to platelet-activating factor in the rat: Role of thromboxane A$_2$. Am J Physiol 256:F35–F43, 1989.

1047. Rodriguez-Puyol D, Lamas S, Olivera A, et al: Actions of cyclosporin A on cultured rat mesangial cells. Kidney Int 35:632–637, 1989.

1048. López-Farré A, Gómez-Garre D, Bernabeu F, et al: Renal effects and mesangial cell contraction induced by endothelin are mediated by PAF. Kidney Int 39:624–630, 1991.

1049. Neuwirth R, Satriano JA, DeCandido S, et al: Angiotensin II causes formation of platelet activating factor in cultured rat mesangial cells. Circ Res 64:1224–1229, 1989.

1050. Biancone L, Tetta C, Turello E, et al: Platelet-activating factor biosynthesis by cultured mesangial cells is modulated by proteinase inhibitors. J Am Soc Nephrol 2:1251–1261, 1992.

1051. Lianos EA, Zanglis A: Glomerular platelet-activating factor levels and origin in experimental glomerulonephritis. Kidney Int 37:736–740, 1990.

1052. Noris M, Perico N, Macconi D, et al: Renal metabolism and urinary excretion of platelet-activating factor in the rat. J Biol Chem 265:19414–19419, 1990.

1053. Macconi D, Noris M, Benfenati E, et al: Increased urinary excretion of platelet activating factor in mice with lupus nephritis. Life Sci 48:1429–1437, 1991.

1054. Noris M, Benigni A, Boccardo P, et al: Urinary excretion of platelet activating factor in patients with immune-mediated glomerulonephritis. Kidney Int 43:426–429, 1993.

1055. Benveniste J, Henson PM, Cochrane CG: Leukocyte-dependent histamine release from rabbit platelets. The role of IgE, basophils and a platelet-activating factor. J Exp Med 136:1356–1377, 1972.

1056. Camussi G, Tetta C, Deregibus MC, et al: Platelet-activating factor (PAF) in experimentally induced rabbit acute serum sickness: Role of basophil-derived PAF in immune complex deposition. J Immunol 128:86–94, 1982.

1057. Camussi G, Tetta C, Alberton M, et al: The role of platelet-activating factor in experimental immune complex pathology. Int J Tissue React 7:355–362, 1985.

1058. Camussi G, Tetta C, Meroni M, et al: Localization of cationic proteins derived from platelets and polymorphonuclear neutrophils and local loss of anionic sites in glomeruli of rabbits with experimentally induced acute serum sickness. Lab Invest 55:56–62, 1986.

1059. Camussi G, Tetta C, Coda R, et al: Platelet-activating factor–induced loss of glomerular anionic charges. Kidney Int 25: 73–81, 1984.

1060. Tetta C, Coda R, Camussi G: Human platelet cationic proteins bind to rat glomeruli, induce loss of anionic charges and increase glomerular permeability. Agents Actions 16:24–26, 1985.

1061. Carmussi G, Tetta C, Mazzucco G, et al: Platelet cationic proteins are present in glomeruli of lupus nephritis patients. Kidney Int 30:555–565, 1986.

1062. Bertani T, Livio M, Macconi D, et al: Platelet activating factor (PAF) as a mediator of injury in nephrotoxic nephritis. Kidney Int 31:1248–1256, 1987.

1063. Yoo J, Schlondorff D, Neugarten J: Protective effects of specific platelet-activating factor receptor antagonists in experimental glomerulonephritis. J Pharmacol Exp Ther 256: 841–844, 1991.

1064. Miyamoto M, Koike H, Sada T, et al: The effects of R-75,371 on antiglomerular basement membrane glomerulonephritis in rats. Lipids 26:1316–1319, 1991.

1065. Idia H, Fujita M, Izumino K, et al: Effects of the platelet-activating factor antagonists CV-6209 and CV-3988 on nephrotoxic serum nephritis in the rat. Nephron 60:471–476, 1992.

1066. Stahl RAK, Thaiss F, Oberle G, et al: The platelet activating factor receptor antagonist WEB 2170 improves glomerular hemodynamics and morphology in a proliferative model of mesangial cell injury. J Am Soc Nephrol 2:37–44, 1991.

1067. Baldi E, Emancipator SN, Hassan MO, Dunn MJ: Platelet activating factor receptor blockade ameliorates murine systemic lupus erythematosus. Kidney Int 38:1030–1038, 1990.

1068. Morigi M, Macconi D, Riccardi E, et al: Platelet-activating factor receptor blocking reduces proteinuria and improves survival in lupus autoimmune mice. J Pharmacol Exp Ther 258:601–606, 1991.

1069. Salvidio G, Brentjens J, Camussi G: Receptor antagonists of platelet-activating factor do not influence the development of passive Heymann nephritis. J Lipid Mediat 3:197–204, 1991.

1070. Camussi G, Pawlowski I, Saunders R, et al: Receptor antagonist of platelet activating factor inhibits inflammatory injury induced by in situ formation of immune complexes in renal glomeruli and in the skin. J Lab Clin Med 110:196–206, 1987.

1071. Ito S, Camussi G, Tetta C, et al: Hyperacute renal allograft rejection in the rabbit. The role of platelet-activating factor and of cationic proteins derived from polymorphonuclear leukocytes and from platelets. Lab Invest 51:148–161, 1984.

1072. Egido J, Robles A, Ortiz A, et al: Role of platelet-activating factor in Adriamycin-induced nephropathy in rats. Eur J Pharmacol 138:119–123, 1987.

1073. Egido J, Mampaso F, Gomez-Chiarri M, et al: Evidence suggesting a role for platelet-activating factor (PAF) in experimental nephrotic syndrome. Int J Tissue React 12:213–220, 1990.

1074. Yamada T, Tomioka K, Horie M, et al: Effects of YM264, a novel PAF antagonist, on puromycin aminonucleoside–induced nephropathy in the rat. Biochem Biophys Res Commun 176:781–785, 1991.

1075. Egido J, Ortiz A, Gomez-Chiarri M, et al: Involvement of lipid mediators in the pathogenesis of experimental nephrosis in rats: Its pharmacological modulation. Ren Fail 13:95–101, 1991.

1076. Ghiggeri GM, Cercignani G, Ginevri F, et al: Puromycin aminonucleoside metabolism by glomeruli and glomerular epithelial cells in vitro. Kidney Int 40:35–42, 1991.

1077. Wang Y, Bass PS, Evans B, et al: Glomerular epithelial cell endocytosis in puromycin-induced glomerulopathy. Nephron 62: 84–89, 1992.

1078. Gómez-Chiarri M, Ortíz A, Lerma JL, et al: Involvement of tumor necrosis factor and platelet-activating factor in the pathogenesis of experimental nephrosis in rats. Lab Invest 70:449–459, 1994.

1079. Eddy AA, Michael AF: Acute tubulointerstitial nephritis associated with aminonucleoside nephrosis. Kidney Int 33:14–23, 1988.

1080. Mampaso F, Egido J, Martinez-Montero JC, et al: Interstitial mononuclear cell infiltrates in experimental nephrosis: Effect of PAF antagonist. Nephrol Dial Transplant 4:1037–1044, 1988.

1081. Bergstein JM: Glomerular fibrin deposition and removal. Pediatr Nephrol 4:78–87, 1990.

1082. Edgington TS, Mackman N, Brand K, Ruf W: The structural biology of expression and function of tissue factor. Thromb Haemost 66: 67–79, 1991.

1083. DeLa Cadena RA, Wachtfogel YT, Colman RW: Contact activation pathway: Inflammation and coagulation. In Colman RW, Hirsh J, Marder VJ, Salzman EW (eds): Hemostasis and Thrombosis: Basic Principles and Clinical Practice, 3rd ed. JB Lippincott, Philadelphia, 1994, pp 219–240.

1084. Colman RW, Marder VJ, Salzman EW, Hirsh J: Overview of hemostasis. In Coleman RW, Hirsh J, Marder VJ, Salzman EW (eds): Hemostasis and Thrombosis: Basic Principles and Clinical Practice, 3rd ed. JB Lippincott, Philadelphia, 1994, pp 3–18.

1085. Cameron JS: Coagulation and thromboembolic complications in the nephrotic syndrome. Adv Nephrol 13:75–114, 1984.

1086. Kanfer A: Coagulation factors in nephrotic syndrome. Am J Nephrol 10(suppl 1):63–68, 1990.

1087. Bellomo R, Atkins RC: Membranous nephropathy and thromboembolism: Is prophylactic anticoagulation warranted? Nephron 63:249–254, 1993.

1088. Rabelink TJ, Zwaginga JJ, Koomans HA, Sixma JJ: Thrombosis and hemostasis in renal disease. Kidney Int 46:287–296, 1994.

1089. Takemura T, Yoshioka K, Akano N, et al: Glomerular deposition of cross-linked fibrin in human kidney diseases. Kidney Int 32:102–111, 1987.

1090. Yamabe H, Sugawara N, Ozawa K, et al: Glomerular deposition of Hageman factor in IgA nephropathy. Nephron 37:62–63, 1984.

1091. Terukina S, Aoki N: Fibronectin and deposits of fibrinolytic components in glomerular capillary walls. Am J Nephrol 5:248–254, 1985.

1092. Ikeya M, Nagase M, Honda N: Intraglomerular distribution of fibronectin in primary glomerular diseases. Clin Nephrol 24:53–59, 1985.

1093. Miura M, Tomino Y, Yagame M, et al: Immunofluorescent studies on alpha 2-plasmin inhibitor (α2-PI) in glomeruli from patients with IgA nephropathy. Clin Exp Immunol 62:380–386, 1985.

1094. Suzuki S, Sato H, Shimada H, et al: Significance of glomerular deposition of plasmin–alpha₂-plasmin inhibitor complexes in various glomerulopathies. Clin Nephrol 40:270–276, 1993.

1095. He C-J, Rondeau E, Medcalf RL, et al: Thrombin increases proliferation and decreases fibrinolytic activity of kidney glomerular epithelial cells. J Cell Physiol 146:131–140, 1991.

1096. Wiggins RC: Hageman factor in experimental nephrotoxic nephritis in the rabbit. Lab Invest 53:335–348, 1985.

1097. Yang AH, Chang HJ: Effects of fibrin matrix on growth of glomerular cells. Am J Pathol 140:569–579, 1992.

1098. Border WA, Wilson CB, Dixon FJ: Failure of heparin to affect two types of experimental glomerulonephritis in rabbits. Kidney Int 8:140–148, 1975.

1099. Hoyer JR, Michael AF, Hoyer LW: Immunofluorescent localization of antihemophilic factor antigen and fibrinogen in human renal disease. J Clin Invest 53:1375–1384, 1974.

1100. Colasanti G, Morel Maroger L, D'Amico G: Deposition of fibrin-stabilizing factor (F XIIIA and S), fibrinogen-related antigens, fibrinogen degradation products (FDPd and FDPe) and antihemolytic factor (F VIII) in renal disease: Analysis of 161 cases by immuno-fluorescence microscopy. Clin Nephrol 28:28–34, 1987.

1101. Mathieson PW, Thiru S, Peters DK, Oliveira DBG: Effects of ancrod and rtPA on fibrin accumulation, glomerular inflammation and renal function in nephrotoxic nephritis. Int J Exp Pathol 72: 679–693, 1991.

1102. Cole EH, Glynn MFX, Laskin CA, et al: Ancrod improves survival in murine systemic lupus erythematosus. Kidney Int 37:29–35, 1990.

1103. Tipping PG, Thomson NM, Holdsworth SR: A comparison of fibrinolytic and defibrinating agents in established experimental glomerulonephritis. Br J Exp Pathol 67:481–491, 1986.

1104. Tipping PG, Holdsworth SR: Fibrinolytic therapy with streptokinase for established experimental glomerulonephritis. Nephron 43:258–264, 1986.

1105. Pollak VE, Glueck HI, Weiss MA, et al: Defibrination with ancrod in glomerulonephritis: Effects on clinical and histologic findings and on blood coagulation. Am J Nephrol 2:195–207, 1982.

1106. Dosekun AK, Pollak VE, Glas-Greenwalt P, et al: Ancrod in systemic lupus erythematosus with thrombosis. Clinical and fibrinolysis effects. Arch Intern Med 144:37–42, 1984.

1107. Kant KS, Pollak VE, Dosekun A, et al: Lupus nephritis with thrombosis and abnormal fibrinolysis: Effect of ancrod. J Lab Clin Med 105:77–88, 1985.

1108. Glas-Greenwalt P, Kant KS, Dosekun A, et al: Ancrod: Normalization of fibrinolytic enzyme abnormalities in patients with systemic lupus erythematosus and lupus nephritis. J Lab Clin Med 105:99–107, 1985.

1109. Colaco CB, Elkon KB: The lupus anticoagulant. A disease marker in antinuclear antibody negative lupus that is cross-reactive with autoantibodies to double-stranded DNA. Arthritis Rheum 28:67–74, 1985.

1110. Glueck HI, Kant KS, Weiss MA, et al: Thrombosis in systemic lupus erythematosus. Relation to the presence of circulating anticoagulants. Arch Intern Med 145:1389–1395, 1985.

1111. Petri M, Rheinschmidt M, Whiting-O'Keefe Q, et al: The frequency of lupus anticoagulant in systemic lupus erythematosus. A study of sixty consecutive patients by activated partial thromboplastin time, Russell viper venom time, and anticardiolipin antibody level. Ann Intern Med 106: 524–531, 1987.

1112. Colucci M, Semeraro N, Montemurro P, et al: Urinary procoagulant and fibrinolytic activity in human glomerulonephritis. Relationship with renal function. Kidney Int 39:1213–1217, 1991.

1113. Angles-Cano E, Rondeau E, Delarue F, et al: Identification and cellular localization of plasminogen activators from human glomeruli. Thromb Haemost 54:688–692, 1985.

1114. Brown PAJ, Wilson HM, Reid FJ, et al: Urokinase-plasminogen activator is synthesized in vitro by human glomerular epithelial cells but not by mesangial cells. Kidney Int 45:43–47, 1994.

1115. Bergstein JM, Riley M, Bang NU: Analysis of the plasminogen activator activity of the human glomerulus. Kidney Int 33:868–874, 1988.

1116. Rondeau E, Angles-Cano E, Delarue F, et al: Polyunsaturated fatty acids increase fibrinolytic activity of human isolated glomeruli. Kidney Int 30:701–705, 1986.

1117. Sakakibara K, Urano T, Takada Y, Takada A: Urinary UK, t-PA and urinary trypsin inhibitor in health and glomerular diseases. Thromb Res 56:239–249, 1989.

1118. Colucci M, Zoja C, Remuzzi G, Semeraro N: Reduced fibrinolytic activity in glomeruli isolated from rabbits infused with tumor necrosis factor. Haemostasis 23:173–178, 1993.

1119. Rondeau E, Mougenot B, Lacave R, et al: Plasminogen activator inhibitor 1 in renal fibrin deposits of human nephropathies. Clin Nephrol 33:55–60, 1990.

1120. Becquemont L, Nguyen G, Peraldi MN, et al: Expression of plasminogen/plasmin receptors on human glomerular epithelial cells. Am J Physiol 267:F303–F310, 1994.

1121. Villamediana LM, Rondeau E, He C-J, et al: Thrombin regulates components of the fibrinolytic system in human mesangial cells. Kidney Int 38:956–961, 1990.

1122. Stark H, Miller K, Michael AF: Renal cortical fibrinolytic activity in rabbits with chronic immune complex nephritis. Isr J Med Sci 15:610–612, 1979.

1123. Feng L, Tang WW, Loskutoff DJ, Wilson CB: Dysfunction of glomerular fibrinolysis in experimental antiglomerular basement membrane antibody glomerulonephritis. J Am Soc Nephrol 3:1753–1764, 1993.

1124. Tomosugi N, Wada T, Naito T, et al: Role of plasminogen activator inhibitor on nephrotoxic nephritis and its modulation by tumor necrosis factor. Nephron 62:213–219, 1992.

1125. Malliaros J, Holdsworth SR, Wojta J, et al: Glomerular fibrinolytic activity in anti-GBM glomerulonephritis in rabbits. Kidney Int 44:557–564, 1993.

1126. Bevilacqua MP, Schleef RR, Gimbrone MA Jr, Loskutoff DJ: Regulation of the fibrinolytic system of cultured human vascular endothelium by interleukin 1. J Clin Invest 78:587–591, 1986.

1127. Schleef RR, Bevilacqua MP, Sawdey M, et al: Cytokine activation of vascular endothelium. Effects on tissue-type plasminogen activator and type 1 plasminogen activator inhibitor. J Biol Chem 263:5797–5803, 1988.

1128. Saksela O, Moscatelli D, Rifkin DB: The opposing effect of basic fibroblast growth factor and transforming growth factor beta on the regulation of plasminogen activator activity in capillary endothelial cells. J Cell Biol 105:957–963, 1987.

1129. Sawdey MS, Podor TJ, Loskutoff DJ: Regulation of type 1 plasminogen activator inhibitor gene expression in cultured bovine aortic endothelial cells. Induction by transforming growth factor-β, lipopolysaccharide, and tumor necrosis factor-α. J Biol Chem 264:10396–10401, 1989.

1130. Mawatari M, Okamura K, Matsuda T, et al: Tumor necrosis factor and epidermal growth factor modulate migration of human microvascular endothelial cells and production of tissue-type plasminogen activator and its inhibitor. Exp Cell Res 192:574–580, 1991.

1131. Hagège J, Peraldi MN, Rondeau E, et al: Plasminogen activator inhibitor-1 deposition in the extracellular matrix of cultured human mesangial cells. Am J Pathol 141:117–128, 1992.

1132. Sawdey MS, Loskutoff DJ: Regulation of murine type 1 plasminogen activator inhibitor gene expression in vivo. Tissue specificity and induction by lipopolysaccharide, tumor necrosis factor-α, and transforming growth factor-β. J Clin Invest 88:1346–1353, 1991.

1133. Tomooka S, Border WA, Marshall BC, Noble NA: Glomerular matrix accumulation is linked to inhibition of the plasmin protease system. Kidney Int 42:1462–1469, 1992.

1134. Kanalas JJ: Effect of the nephritogenic autoantibody of Heymann's nephritis on plasminogen-binding to Gp330 and activation by urokinase. Biochim Biophys Acta 1225:101–106, 1993.

1135. Briggs JD, Kwaan HC, Potter EV: The role of fibrinogen in renal disease. III. Fibrinolytic and anticoagulant treatment of nephrotoxic serum nephritis in mice. J Lab Clin Med 74:715–724, 1969.

1136. Akiba T, Tanaka K: Effects of fibrinolytic treatment on rabbit Masugi nephritis. Acta Pathol Jpn 33:773–787, 1983.

1137. Zoja C, Corna D, Macconi D, et al: Tissue plasminogen activator therapy of rabbit nephrotoxic nephritis. Lab Invest 62: 34–40, 1990.

1138. McCluskey RT, Andres GA: Does t-PA have a role in the treatment of crescentic glomerulonephritis? Lab Invest 62:1–4, 1990.

1139. Murakami T, Kawakami H: Urokinase, a scavenger of affected tubules in acute worsening during macroscopic hematuria of IgA nephropathy? Nephron 55:92–93, 1990. Letter.

1140. Tomura S, Oono Y, Kuriyama R, Takeuchi J: Plasma concentrations of fibrinopeptide A and fibrinopeptide B$_\beta$ 15-42 in glomerulonephritis and the nephrotic syndrome. Arch Intern Med 145:1033–1035, 1985.

1141. Belovezhdov N, Robeva R, Genova V: Blood coagulation in glomerulonephritis. Int Urol Nephrol 18:193–203, 1986.

1142. Kamitsuji H, Whitworth JA, Dowling JP, Kincaid-Smith P: Urinary crosslinked fibrin degradation products in glomerular disease. Am J Kidney Dis 7:452–455, 1986.

1143. Sakakibara K, Nagase M, Takada Y, Takada A: Relationship between urinary fibrinogen degradation products and various types of chronic nephritis. Thromb Res 45:403–411, 1987.

1144. Nagayama Y, Imura H, Muso R: Decrease in renal function following decreased fibrinogen and raised fibrin degradation products in lupus nephritis with nephrotic syndrome. Scand J Urol Nephrol 26:387–391, 1992.

1145. Nieuwenhuizen W: Soluble fibrin as a molecular marker for a pre-thrombotic state: A mini-review. Blood Coagul Fibrinolysis 4:93–96, 1993.

1146. Saldeen K, Christie N, Nelson WR, Movat HZ: Effect of a fibrin(ogen)-derived vasoactive peptide on polymorphonuclear leukocyte emigration. Thromb Res 37:85–89, 1985.

1147. Senior RM, Skogen WF, Griffin GL, Wilner GD: Effects of fibrinogen derivatives upon the inflammatory response. Studies with human fibrinopeptide B. J Clin Invest 77:1014–1019, 1986.

1148. Dang CV, Bell WR, Kaiser D, Wong A: Disorganization of cultured vascular endothelial cell monolayers by fibrinogen fragment D. Science 227:1487–1490, 1985.

1149. Rowland FN, Donovan MJ, Picciano PT, et al: Fibrin-mediated vascular injury. Identification of fibrin peptides that mediate endothelial cell retraction. Am J Pathol 117:418–428, 1984.

1150. Fair DS, Marlar RA, Levin EG: Human endothelial cells synthesize protein S. Blood 67:1168–1171, 1986.

1151. Tanabe S, Sugo T, Matsuda M: Synthesis of protein C in human umbilical vein endothelial cells. J Biochem (Tokyo) 109:924–928, 1991.

1152. Kisiel W, Canfield WM, Ericsson LH, Davie EW: Anticoagulant properties of bovine plasma protein C following activation by thrombin. Biochemistry 16:5824–5830, 1977.

1153. Kisiel W: Human plasma protein C. Isolation, characterization, and mechanism of activation by alpha-thrombin. J Clin Invest 64:761–769, 1979.

1154. Walker FJ, Chavin SI, Fay PJ: Inactivation of factor VIII by activated protein C and protein S. Arch Biochem Biophys 252: 322–328, 1987.

1155. Maruyama I, Majerus PW: Protein C inhibits endocytosis of thrombin-thrombomodulin complexes in A549 lung cancer cells and human umbilical vein endothelial cells. Blood 69:1481–1484, 1987.

1156. Suzuki K, Nishioka S, Hashimoto S: Protein C inhibitor. Purification from human plasma and characterization. J Biol Chem 258:163–168, 1983.

1157. Heeb MJ, Griffin J: Physiologic inhibition of human activated protein C by alpha$_1$-antitrypsin. J Biol Chem 263:11613–11616, 1988.

1158. Dahlback B: Purification of human vitamin-K dependent protein S and its limited proteolysis by thrombin. Biochem J 209:2007–2010, 1983.

1159. Mitchell CA, Jane SM, Salem HH: Inhibition of the anticoagulant activity of protein S by prothrombin. J Clin Invest 82:2142–2147, 1988.

1160. Greengard JS, Fernandez JA, Sun X, et al: Protein S: A natural substrate of the kidney and brain γ-carboxylases. International Congress on Thrombosis and Hemostasis, New York, July 1993. Abstract.

1161. Radtke K-P, Fernandez JA, Greengard JS, et al: Expression and localization of the serpin protein C inhibitor (PAI-3) in human and rhesus monkey kidney. International Congress on Thrombosis and Hemostasis, New York, July 1993. Abstract.

1162. Hancock WW, Tsuchida A, Kupiec-Weglinski JW, Sayegh MH: Pathogenetic role of cellular immunity in glomerulonephritis: Anti-IL2R monoclonal antibody prevents mononuclear and endothelial cell activation, cytokine production, and glomerular injury in nephrotoxic nephritis (NTN). J Am Soc Nephrol 3:592, 1992. Abstract.

1163. Tsuchida A, Salem H, Thomson N, Hancock WW: Tumor necrosis factor production during human renal allograft rejection is associated with depression of plasma protein C and free protein S levels and decreased intragraft thrombomodulin expression. J Exp Med 175:81–90, 1992.

1164. Debault LE, Emon NL, Olson JR, Esmon CT: Distribution of the thrombomodulin antigen in the rabbit vasculature. Lab Invest 54:172–178, 1986.

1165. Hancock WW: IL-1 and TNF depress glomerular endothelial thrombomodulin (TM) expression in vitro and in vivo. Kidney Int 38: 557, 1990. Abstract.

1166. He CJ, Kanfer A: Quantification and modulation of thrombomodulin activity in isolated rat and human glomeruli. Kidney Int 41:1170–1174, 1992.

1167. Mizutani M, Yuzawa Y, Maruyama I, et al: Glomerular localization of thrombomodulin in human glomerulonephritis. Lab Invest 69:193–202, 1993.

1168. Cosio FG, Harker C, Batard MA, et al: Plasma concentrations of the natural anticoagulants protein C and protein S in patients with proteinuria. J Lab Clin Med 106:218–222, 1985.

1169. Sorensen PJ, Knudsen F, Nielsen AH, Dyerberg J: Protein C activity in renal disease. Thromb Res 38:243–249, 1985.

1170. Mannucci PM, Valsecchi C, Bottasso B, et al: High plasma levels of protein C activity and antigen in the nephrotic syndrome. Thromb Haemost 55:31–33, 1986.

1171. Soff GA, Sica DA, Marlar RA, et al: Protein C levels in nephrotic syndrome: Use of a new enzyme-linked immunoadsorbent assay for protein C antigen. Am J Hematol 22:43–49, 1986.

1172. Vigano-D'Angelo S, D'Angelo A, Kaufman CE Jr, et al: Protein S deficiency occurs in the nephrotic syndrome. Ann Intern Med 107:42–47, 1987.

1173. Rostoker G, Goualt-Heilmann M, Levent M, et al: High level of protein C and protein S in nephrotic syndrome. Nephron 46:220–221, 1987. Letter.

1174. Allon M, Soffer O, Evatt BL, et al: Protein S and C antigen levels in proteinuric patients: Dependence on type of glomerular pathology. Am J Hematol 31:96–101, 1989.

1175. Perry GJ, Elston T, Khouri NA, et al: Antiendothelial cell antibodies in lupus: Correlations with renal injury and circulating markers of endothelial damage. Q J Med 86:727–734, 1993.

1176. Woo KT, Lee EJC, Lau YK, Lim CH: Antithrombin III in mesangial IgA nephritis. Thromb Res 40:483, 1985.

1177. Cochrane CG, Griffin JH: The biochemistry and pathophysiology of the contact system of plasma. Adv Immunol 33:241–306, 1982.

1178. MacDonald RJ, Margolius HS, Erdös EG: Molecular biology of tissue kallikrein. Biochem J 253:313–321, 1988.

1179. Brady JM, MacDonald RJ: The expression of two kallikrein gene family members in the rat kidney. Arch Biochem Biophys 278:342–349, 1990.

1180. Bascands J-L, Pecher C, Rouaud S, et al: Evidence for existence of two distinct bradykinin receptors on rat mesangial cells. Am J Physiol 264:F548–F556, 1993.

1181. Hutchison FN, Webster SK, Jaffa AA: Altered renal kallikrein and renin gene expression in nephrotic rats and modulation by converting enzyme inhibition. J Clin Invest 92:1073–1079, 1993.

1182. Proud D, Knepper MA, Pisano JJ: Distribution of immunoreactive kallikrein along the rat nephron. Am J Physiol 244:F510–F515, 1983.

1183. O'Connor DT, Barg AP, Amend W, Vincenti F: Urinary kallikrein excretion after renal transplantation. Relationship to hypertension, graft source, and renal function. Am J Med 73:475–481, 1982.

1184. Schwager I, Jungi TW: Effect of human recombinant cytokines on the induction of macrophage procoagulant activity. Blood 83:152–160, 1994.

1185. Bar-Shavit R, Kahn A, Wilner GD: Monocyte chemotaxis: Stimulation by specific exosite region in thrombin. Science 220:728–731, 1983.

1186. Edgington TS, Helin H, Gregory SA, et al: Cellular pathways and signals for the induction of biosynthesis of initiators of the coagulation protease cascade by cells of the monocyte lineage. *In* van

Furth R (ed): Mononuclear Phagocytes, Characteristics, Physiology and Function. Martinus Nijhoff, Boston, 1985, pp 687–696.

1187. Brentjens JR: Glomerular procoagulant activity and glomerulonephritis. Lab Invest 57:107–111, 1987.

1188. Carson SD, Johnson DR, Tracy SM: Tissue factor and the extrinsic pathway of coagulation during infection and vascular inflammation. Eur Heart J 14(suppl K):98–104, 1993.

1189. Wiggins RC, Glatfelter A, Brukman J: Procoagulant activity in glomeruli and urine of rabbits with nephrotoxic nephritis. Lab Invest 53:156–165, 1985.

1190. Tipping PG, Holdsworth SR: The participation of macrophages, glomerular procoagulant activity, and factor VIII in glomerular fibrin deposition. Studies on anti-GBM antibody–induced glomerulonephritis in rabbits. Am J Pathol 124:10–17, 1986.

1191. Tipping PG, Worthington LA, Holdsworth SR: Quantitation and characterization of glomerular procoagulant activity in experimental glomerulonephritis. Lab Invest 56:155–159, 1987.

1192. Silva FG, Hoyer JR, Pirani CL: Sequential studies of glomerular crescent formation in rats with anti–glomerular basement membrane–induced glomerulonephritis and the role of coagulation factors. Lab Invest 51:404–415, 1984.

1193. Tipping PG, Lowe MG, Holdsworth SR: Glomerular macrophages express augmented procoagulant activity in experimental fibrin-related glomerulonephritis in rabbits. J Clin Invest 82:1253–1259, 1988.

1194. Cole EH, Sweet J, Levy GA: Expression of macrophage procoagulant activity in murine systemic lupus erythematosus. J Clin Invest 78:887–893, 1986.

1195. Cole EH, Schulman J, Urowitz M, et al: Monocyte procoagulant activity in glomerulonephritis associated with systemic lupus erythematosus. J Clin Invest 75:861–868, 1985.

1196. de Prost D, Ollivier V, Ternisien C, Chollet-Martin S: Increased monocyte procoagulant activity independent of the lupus anticoagulant in patients with systemic lupus erythematosus. Thromb Haemost 64:216–221, 1990.

1197. Tipping PG, Dowling JP, Holdsworth SR: Glomerular procoagulant activity in human proliferative glomerulonephritis. J Clin Invest 81:119–125, 1988.

1198. Kanfer A, de Prost D, Guettier C, et al: Enhanced glomerular procoagulant activity and fibrin deposition in rats with mercuric chloride–induced autoimmune nephritis. Lab Invest 57:138–143, 1987.

1199. Brukman J, Wiggins RC: Procoagulant activity in kidneys of normal and bacterial lipopolysaccharide–treated rabbits. Kidney Int 32:31–38, 1987.

1200. Moldow CF, Bach RR, Staskus K, Rick PD: Induction of endothelial tissue factor by endotoxin and its presursors. Thromb Haemost 70:702–706, 1993.

1201. Bevilacqua MP, Pober JS, Wheeler ME, et al: Interleukin-1 activation of vascular endothelium. Effects on procoagulant activity and leukocyte adhesion. Am J Pathol 121:393–403, 1985.

1202. Bevilacqua MP, Pober JS, Majeau GR, et al: Interleukin 1 (IL-1) induces biosynthesis and cell surface expression of procoagulant activity in human vascular endothelial cells. J Exp Med 160:618–623, 1984.

1203. Stern DM, Bank I, Nawroth PP, et al: Self-regulation of procoagulant events on the endothelial cell surface. J Exp Med 162:1223–1235, 1985.

1204. Nawroth PP, Stern DM: Modulation of endothelial cell hemostatic properties by tumor necrosis factor. J Exp Med 163:740–745, 1986.

1205. Hancock W, Atkins R: Activation of coagulation pathways and fibrin deposition in human glomerulonephritis. Semin Nephrol 5:69–77, 1985.

1206. Neale TJ, Tipping PG, Carson SD, Holdsworth SR: Participation of cell-mediated immunity in deposition of fibrin in glomerulonephritis. Lancet 2:421–424, 1988.

1207. Morrissey JH, Fair DS, Edgington TS: Monoclonal antibody analysis of purified and cell-associated tissue factor. Thromb Res 52:247–261, 1988.

1208. Drake TA, Morrissey JH, Edgington TS: Selective cellular expression of tissue factor in human tissues: Implications for disorders of hemostasis and thrombosis. Am J Pathol 134:1087–1097, 1989.

1209. de Prost D, Kanfer A, Le Floch V: Quantitative assessment of procoagulant activity in isolated rat glomeruli. Kidney Int 28:566–568, 1985.

1210. Wiggins RC, Njoku N, Sedor JR: Tissue factor production by cultured rat mesangial cells. Stimulation by TNFα and lipopolysaccharide. Kidney Int 37:1281–1285, 1990.
1211. Yamabe H, Yoshikawa S, Ohsawa H, et al: Tissue factor production by cultured rat glomerular epithelial cells. Nephrol Dial Transplant 8:519–523, 1993.
1212. Ardaillou R, Bens M, Edgington TS: Glomerular tissue factor stimulates thromboxane synthesis in human platelets via thrombin generation. Kidney Int 41:361–368, 1992.
1213. Morrissey JH, Fakhrai H, Edgington TS: Molecular cloning of the cDNA for tissue factor, the cellular receptor for the initiation of the coagulation protease cascade. Cell 50:129–135, 1987.
1214. Scarpati EM, Wen D, Broze GJ Jr, et al: Human tissue factor: cDNA sequence and chromosome localization of the gene. Biochemistry 26:5234–5238, 1987.
1215. Spicer EK, Horton R, Bloem L, et al: Isolation of cDNA clones coding for human tissue factor: Primary structure of the protein and cDNA. Proc Natl Acad Sci USA 84:5148–5152, 1987.
1216. Kasinath BS: Resident glomerular cells in glomerular injury: Glomerular epithelial cells. Semin Nephrol 11:294–303, 1991.
1217. Delarue F, Virone A, Hagege J, et al: Stable cell line of T-SV40 immortalized human glomerular visceral epithelial cells. Kidney Int 40:906–912, 1991.
1218. Natori Y, O'Meara YM, Manning EC, et al: Production and polarized secretion of basement membrane components by glomerular epithelial cells. Am J Physiol 262:F131–F137, 1992.
1219. Weinstein T, Cameron R, Katz A, Silverman M: Rat glomerular epithelial cells in culture express characteristics of parietal, not visceral, epithelium. J Am Soc Nephrol 3:1279–1287, 1992.
1220. Schlondorff D: The glomerular mesangial cell: An expanding role for a specialized pericyte. FASEB J 1:272–281, 1987.
1221. Veis JH, Yamashita W, Liu YJ, Ooi BS: The biology of mesangial cells in glomerulonephritis. Proc Soc Exp Biol Med 195:160–167, 1990.
1222. Hawkins NJ, Wakefield D, Charlesworth JA: The role of mesangial cells in glomerular pathology. Pathology 22:24–32, 1990.
1223. Ardaillou R, Chansel D, Stefanovic V, Ardaillou N: Cell surface receptors and ectoenzymes in mesangial cells. J Am Soc Nephrol 2:S107–S115, 1992.
1224. Kashgarian M, Sterzel RB: The pathobiology of the mesangium. Kidney Int 41:524–529, 1992.
1225. Sterzel RB, Schulze-Lohoff E, Marx M: Cytokines and mesangial cells. Kidney Int 43(suppl 39):S-26–S-31, 1993.
1226. Floege J, Eng E, Young BA, Johnson RJ: Factors involved in the regulation of mesangial cell proliferation in vitro and in vivo. Kidney Int 43(suppl 39):S-47–S-54, 1993.
1227. Sraer JD, Adida C, Peraldi MN, et al: Species-specific properties of the glomerular mesangium. J Am Soc Nephrol 3:1342–1350, 1993.
1228. Sedor JR, Konieczkowski M, Huang S, et al: Cytokines, mesangial cell activation and glomerular injury. Kidney Int 43(suppl 39): S-65–S-70, 1993.
1229. Davies M: The mesangial cell: A tissue culture view. Kidney Int 45:320–327, 1994.
1230. Striker GE, Soderland C, Bowen-Pope DF, et al: Isolation, characterization, and propagation in vitro of human glomerular endothelial cells. J Exp Med 160:323–328, 1984.
1231. Castellot JJ, Hoover RL, Karnovsky MJ: Glomerular endothelial cells secrete a heparin-like inhibitor and a peptide stimulator of mesangial cell proliferation. Am J Pathol 125:493–500, 1986.
1232. MacKay K, Striker LJ, Elliot S, et al: Glomerular epithelial, mesangial, and endothelial cell lines from transgenic mice. Kidney Int 33:677–687, 1988.
1233. Ballermann BJ: Regulation of bovine glomerular endothelial cell growth in vitro. Am J Physiol 256:C182–C189, 1989.
1234. Savage COS, Bogle R: Resident glomerular cells in glomerular injury: Endothelial cells. Semin Nephrol 11:312–319, 1991.
1235. Marsden PA, Goligorsky MS, Brenner BM: Endothelial cell biology in relation to current concepts of vessel wall structure and function. J Am Soc Nephrol 1:931–948, 1991.
1236. Nitta K, Simonson MS, Dunn MJ: The regulation and role of prostaglandin biosynthesis in cultured bovine glomerular endothelial cells. J Am Soc Nephrol 2:156–163, 1991.
1237. Ballermann BJ, Marsden PA: Endothelium-derived vasoactive mediators and renal glomerular function. Clin Invest Med 14:508–517, 1991.

1238. Rabkin R, Tsao T, Elliot SJ, et al: Insulin uptake and processing by cultured mouse glomerular endothelial cells. Am J Physiol 265:C453–C459, 1993.
1239. Adler S, Eng B: Integrin receptors and function on cultured glomerular endothelial cells. Kidney Int 44:278–284, 1993.
1240. Laulajainen T, Julkunen I, Haltia A, et al: Establishment and characterization of a rat glomerular endothelial cell line. Lab Invest 69:183–192, 1993.
1241. Savage COS: The biology of the glomerulus: Endothelial cells. Kidney Int 45:314–319, 1994.
1242. Gardiner DS, Lindop GBM: The glomerular peripolar cell—an immunohistochemical study. APMIS 100:107–115, 1992.
1243. Kreisberg JI, Karnovsky MJ: Glomerular cells in culture. Kidney Int 23:439–447, 1983.
1244. Lovett DH, Sterzel RB: Cell culture approaches to the analysis of glomerular inflammation. Kidney Int 30:246–254, 1986.
1245. Striker GE, Lange MA, MacKay K, et al: Glomerular cells in vitro. Adv Nephrol 16:169–186, 1987.
1246. Floege J, Radeke HR, Johnson RJ: Glomerular cells in vitro versus the glomerulus in vivo. Kidney Int 45:360–368, 1994.
1247. Pabst R, Sterzel RB: Cell renewal of glomerular cell types in normal rats. An autoradiographic analysis. Kidney Int 24:626–631, 1983.
1248. Bertram JF, Soosaipillai MC, Ricardo SD, Ryan GB: Total numbers of glomeruli and individual glomerular cell types in the normal rat kidney. Cell Tissue Res 270:37–45, 1992.
1249. Nadasdy T, Laszik Z, Blick KE, et al: Proliferative activity of intrinsic cell populations in the normal human kidney. J Am Soc Nephrol 4:2032–2039, 1994.
1250. Troyer DA, Kreisberg JI: Isolation and study of glomerular cells. Methods Enzymol 191:141–152, 1990.
1251. Pfeilschifter J: Cross-talk between transmembrane signalling systems: a prerequisite for the delicate regulation of glomerular haemodynamics by mesangial cells. Eur J Clin Invest 19:347–361, 1989.
1252. Sterzel RB, Schulze-Lohoff E, Marx M: Cytokines and mesangial cells. Kidney Int 43(suppl 39):S-26–S-31, 1993.
1253. Sedor JR, Konieczkowski M, Huang S, et al: Cytokines, mesangial cell activation and glomerular injury. Kidney Int 43(suppl 39):S-65–S-70, 1993.
1254. Egido J, Gomez-Chiarri M, Ortiz A, et al: Role of tumor necrosis factor-α in the pathogenesis of glomerular diseases. Kidney Int 43(suppl 39):S-59–S-64, 1993.
1255. Knauss TC, Mené P, Ricanati SA, et al: Immune complex activation of rat glomerular mesangial cells: Dependence on the Fc region of antibody. Am J Physiol 257:F478–F485, 1989.
1256. Adler S, Stahl RAK, Baker PJ, et al: Biphasic effect of oxygen radicals on prostaglandin production by rat mesangial cells. Am J Physiol 252:F743–F749, 1987.
1257. Duff JL, Marrero MB, Paxton WG, et al: Angiotensin II induces 3CH134, a protein-tyrosine phosphatase, in vascular smooth muscle cells. J Biol Chem 268:26037–26040, 1993.
1258. Levin DE, Errede B: A multitude of MAP kinase activation pathways. J NIH Res 5:49–52, 1993.
1259. Huwiler A, Pfeilschifter J: Interleukin-1 stimulates de novo synthesis of mitogen-activated protein kinase in glomerular mesangial cells. FEBS Lett 350:135–138, 1994.
1260. Lovett DH, Martin M, Bursten S, et al: Interleukin 1 and the glomerular mesangium. III. IL-1–dependent stimulation of mesangial cell protein kinase activity. Kidney Int 34:26–35, 1988.
1261. Foster DA: Intracellular signalling mediated by protein-tyrosine kinases: Networking through phospholipid metabolism. Cell Signal 5:389–399, 1993.
1262. Kazlauskas A: Receptor tyrosine kinases and their targets. Curr Opin Genet Dev 4:5–14, 1994.
1263. Coyne DW, Morrison AR: Effect of the tyrosine kinase inhibitor, genistein, on interleukin-1 stimulated PGE₂ production in mesangial cells. Biochem Biophys Res Commun 173:718–724, 1990.
1264. Thomas PE, Wharram BL, Goyal M, et al: GLEPP1, a renal glomerular epithelial cell (podocyte) membrane protein-tyrosine phosphatase. Identification, molecular cloning, and characterization in rabbit. J Biol Chem 269:19953–19962, 1994.
1265. Perlmutter RM, Levin SD, Appleby MW, et al: Regulation of lymphocyte function by protein phosphorylation. Annu Rev Immunol 11:451–499, 1993.

1266. Trowbridge IS, Thomas ML: CD45: An emerging role as a protein tyrosine phosphatase required for lymphocyte activation and development. Annu Rev Immunol 12:85–116, 1994.

1267. Chan AC, Desai DM, Weiss A: The role of protein tyrosine kinases and protein tyrosine phosphatases in T cell antigen receptor signal transduction. Annu Rev Immunol 12:555–592, 1994.

1268. Pfeilschifter J, Leighton J, Pignat W, et al: Cyclic AMP mimics, but does not mediate, interleukin-1– and tumour-necrosis-factor–stimulated phospholipase A$_2$ secretion from rat renal mesangial cells. Biochem J 273:199–204, 1991.

1269. Huwiler A, Fabbro D, Pfeilschifter J: Possible regulatory functions of protein kinase C-α and -ε isoenzymes in rat renal mesangial cells. Stimulation of prostaglandin synthesis and feedback inhibition of angiotensin II–stimulated phosphoinositide hydrolysis. Biochem J 279:441–445, 1991.

1270. Mene P, Cinotti GA, Pugliese F: Signal transduction in mesangial cells. J Am Soc Nephrol 2(10 suppl):S100–S106, 1992.

1271. Hug H, Sarre TF: Protein kinase C isoenzymes: Divergence in signal transduction? Biochem J 291:329–343, 1993.

1272. Matsumoto K, Hatano M: Soluble immune complexes stimulate production of interleukin-1 by cultured rat glomerular mesangial cells. Am J Nephrol 11:138–143, 1991.

1273. Kasai S: Effects of glomerular macrophages on mesangial cells in rat serum sickness glomerulonephritis: A comparison of histological and co-culture studies. Pathol Int 44:107–114, 1994.

1274. Gomez-Guerrero C, Gonzalez E, Egido J: Evidence for a specific IgA receptor in rat and human mesangial cells. J Immunol 151:7172–7181, 1993.

1275. van den Dobbelsteen ME, van der Woude FJ, Schroeijers WE, et al: C1Q, a subunit of the first component of complement, enhances the binding of aggregated IgG to rat renal mesangial cells. J Immunol 151:4315–4324, 1993.

1276. Furness PN: Immune complex degradation by cultured rat mesangial cells. J Pathol 170:197–203, 1993.

1277. Amore A, Cavallo F, Bocchietto E, et al: Cytokine mRNA expression by cultured rat mesangial cells after contact with environmental lectins. Kidney Int 43(suppl 39):S-41–S-46, 1993.

1278. Lovett DH, Ryan JL, Sterzel RB: A thymocyte-activating factor derived from glomerular mesangial cells. J Immunol 130:1796–1801, 1983.

1279. Lovett DH, Sterzel RB, Ryan JL, Atkins E: Production of an endogenous pyrogen by glomerular mesangial cells. J Immunol 134:670–672, 1985.

1280. Lovett DH, Szamel M, Ryan JL, et al: Interleukin 1 and the glomerular mesangium. 1. Purification and characterization of a mesangial cell–derived autogrowth factor. J Immunol 136:3700–3705, 1986.

1281. Lovett DH, Larsen A: Cell cycle–dependent interleukin 1 gene expression by cultured glomerular mesangial cells. J Clin Invest 82:115–122, 1988.

1282. Sedor JR, Nakazato Y, Konieczkowski M: Interleukin-1 and the mesangial cell. Kidney Int 41:595–599, 1992.

1283. Ooi BS, MacCarthy EP, Hsu A: β-Endorphin amplifies the effect of interleukin-1 on mouse mesangial cell proliferation. J Lab Clin Med 110:159–163, 1987.

1284. Singhal PC, Gibbons N, Abramovici M: Long term effects of morphine on mesangial cell proliferation and matrix synthesis. Kidney Int 41:1560–1570, 1992.

1285. Singhal PC, Driesach AL, Abramovici M, et al: Specific receptors for beta-endorphin on mesangial cells. Nephron 62:66–70, 1992.

1286. Marti HP, McNeil L, Thomas G, et al: Molecular characterization of a low-molecular-mass matrix metalloproteinase secreted by glomerular mesangial cells as PUMP-1. Biochem J 285:899–905, 1992.

1287. Martin J, Lovett DH, Gemsa D, et al: Enhancement of glomerular mesangial cell neutral proteinase secretion by macrophages: Role of interleukin 1. J Immunol 137:525–529, 1986.

1288. Martin J, Davies M, Thomas G, Lovett DH: Human mesangial cells secrete a GBM-degrading neutral proteinase and a specific inhibitor. Kidney Int 36:790–801, 1989.

1289. Marti HP, Lee L, Kashgarian M, Lovett DH: Transforming growth factor-β1 stimulates glomerular mesangial cell synthesis of the 72-kd type IV collagenase. Am J Pathol 144:82–94, 1994.

1290. LaMarre J, Wollenberg GK, Gonias SL, Hayes MA: Cytokine binding and clearance properties of proteinase-activated α$_2$-macroglobulins. Lab Invest 65:3–14, 1991.

1291. Moestrup SK: The α$_2$-macroglobulin receptor and epithelial glycoprotein-330: Two giant receptors mediating endocytosis of multiple ligands. Biochim Biophys Acta 1197:197–213, 1994.

1292. Abbate M, Bachinsky D, Zheng G, et al: Location of gp330/α$_2$ m receptor–associated protein (α$_2$-MRAP) and its binding sites in kidney: Distribution of endogenous α$_2$-MRAP is modified by tissue processing. Eur J Cell Biol 61:139–149, 1993.

1293. Zheng G, Bachinsky DR, Stamenkovic I, et al: Organ distribution in rats of two members of the low-density lipoprotein receptor gene family, gp330 and LRP/alpha 2MR, and the receptor-associated protein (RAP). J Histochem Cytochem 42:531–542, 1994.

1294. Conz P, Bevilacqua PA, Ronco C, et al: Alpha-1-antichymotrypsin in renal biopsies. Nephron 56:387–390, 1990.

1295. Davis ID, Burke B, Freese D, et al: The pathologic spectrum of the nephropathy associated with alpha 1-antitrypsin deficiency. Hum Pathol 23:57–62, 1992.

1296. Asami T, Ohsawa S, Tomisawa S, et al: Glomerular deposition of alpha 2-macroglobulin in a child with steroid refractory nephrotic syndrome. Nephron 61:211–213, 1992.

1297. Khan TN, Sinniah R: Renal tubular antiproteinase (alpha-1-antitrypsin and alpha-1-antichymotrypsin) response in tubulo-interstitial damage. Nephron 65:232–239, 1993.

1298. Steinhoff J, Buhner U, Preuss R, Sack K: C-reactive protein and α$_2$ macroglobulin in urine as markers of renal transplant rejection. Transplant Proc 26:1768, 1994.

1299. Novick D, Engelmann H, Wallach D, Rubinstein M: Soluble cytokine receptors are present in normal human urine. J Exp Med 170:1409–1414, 1989.

1300. Kaczmarski RS, Mufti GJ: The cytokine receptor superfamily. Blood Rev 5:193–203, 1991.

1301. Aggarwal BB, Kohr WJ, Hass PE, et al: Human tumor necrosis factor. Production, purification, and characterization. J Biol Chem 260:2345–2354, 1985.

1302. Urban JL, Shepard HM, Rothstein JL, et al: Tumor necrosis factor: A potent effector molecule for tumor cell killing by activated macrophages. Proc Natl Acad Sci USA 83:5233–5237, 1986.

1303. Le J, Vilček J: Tumor necrosis factor and interleukin 1: Cytokines with multiple overlapping biological activities. Lab Invest 56:234–248, 1987.

1304. Remick DG, Kunkel RG, Larrick JW, Kunkel SL: Acute in vivo effects of human recombinant tumor necrosis factor. Lab Invest 56:583–590, 1987.

1305. Waldherr R, Cuzic S, Noronha IL: Pathology of the human mesangium in situ. Clin Investig 70:865–874, 1992.

1306. Baud L, Fouqueray B, Philippe C, Amrani A: Tumor necrosis factor alpha and mesangial cells. Kidney Int 41:600–603, 1992.

1307. Baud L, Ardaillou R: Tumor necrosis factor alpha in glomerular injury. Kidney Int 45(suppl 45):S-32–S-36, 1994.

1308. Baud L, Fouqueray B, Philippe C: Involvement of tumor necrosis factor-α in glomerular injury. Springer Semin Immunopathol 16:53–61, 1994.

1309. Bertani T, Abbate M, Zoja C, et al: Tumor necrosis factor induces glomerular damage in the rabbit. Am J Pathol 134:419–430, 1989.

1310. Hruby ZW, Cybulsky AV, Lowry RP: Effects of tumor necrosis factor on glomerular mesangial and epithelial cells in culture. Nephron 56:410–413, 1990.

1311. Talmadge JE, Bowersox O, Tribble H, et al: Toxicity of tumor necrosis factor is synergistic with γ-interferon and can be reduced with cyclooxygenase inhibitors. Am J Pathol 128:410–425, 1987.

1312. Meulders Q, He C-J, Adida C, et al: Tumor necrosis factor α increases antifibrinolytic activity of cultured human mesangial cells. Kidney Int 42:327–334, 1992.

1313. Jevnikar AM, Brennan DC, Singer GG, et al: Stimulated kidney tubular epithelial cells express membrane associated and secreted TNF alpha. Kidney Int 40:203–211, 1991.

1314. Yard BA, Daha MR, Kooymans-Couthino M, et al: IL-1α stimulated TNFα production by cultured human proximal tubular epithelial cells. Kidney Int 42:383–389, 1992.

1315. Dinarello CA: Biology of interleukin 1. FASEB J 2:108–115, 1988.

1316. Dinarello CA: Interleukin-1 and tumor necrosis factor: Effector cytokines in autoimmune diseases. Semin Immunol 4:133–145, 1992.

1317. Werber HI, Emancipator SN, Tykocinski ML, Sedor JR: The interleukin 1 gene is expressed by rat glomerular mesangial cells and is augmented in immune complex glomerulonephritis. J Immunol 138:3207–3212, 1987.

1318. Boswell JM, Yui MA, Endres S, et al: Novel and enhanced IL-1 gene expression in autoimmune mice with lupus. J Immunol 141:118–124, 1988.

1319. Matsumoto K: Production of interleukin-1 in macrophage cultures from rats with nephrotoxic serum nephritis. Int Arch Allergy Appl Immunol 87:435–438, 1988.

1320. Boswell JM, Yui MA, Burt DW, Kelley VE: Increased tumor necrosis factor and the IL-1β gene expression in the kidneys of mice with lupus nephritis. J Immunol 141:3050–3054, 1988.

1321. Matsumoto K, Hatano M: Production of interleukin 1 in glomerular cell cultures from rats with nephrotoxic nephritis. Clin Exp Immunol 75:123–128, 1989.

1322. Matsumoto K: Recombinant tumor necrosis factor stimulates interleukin-1 production in glomerular cultures from rats with nephrotoxic serum nephritis. Nephron 55:300–305, 1990.

1323. Nathan C, Sporn M: Cytokines in context. J Cell Biol 113:981–986, 1991.

1324. Bogdan C, Nathan C: Modulation of macrophage function by transforming growth factor beta, interleukin-4, and interleukin-10. Ann N Y Acad Sci 685:713–739, 1993.

1325. Dinarello CA: Interleukin-1. Adv Pharmacol 25:21–51, 1994.

1326. Arend WP: Interleukin-1 receptor antagonist. Adv Immunol 54:167–227, 1993.

1327. Lan HY, Nikolic-Paterson DJ, Zarama M, et al: Suppression of experimental crescentic glomerulonephritis by the interleukin-1 receptor antagonist. Kidney Int 43:479–485, 1993.

1328. Tomosugi NI, Cashman SJ, Hay H, et al: Modulation of antibody-mediated glomerular injury in vivo by bacterial lipopolysaccharide, tumor necrosis factor, and IL-1. J Immunol 142:3083–3090, 1989.

1329. Cavallo T, Granholm NA: Bacterial lipopolysaccharide transforms mesangial into proliferative lupus nephritis without interfering with processing of pathogenic immune complexes in NZB/W mice. Am J Pathol 137:971–978, 1990.

1330. Brennan DC, Yui MA, Wuthrich RP, Kelley VE: Tumor necrosis factor and IL-1 in New Zealand black/white mice. Enhanced gene expression and acceleration of renal injury. J Immunol 143:3470–3475, 1989.

1331. Gordon C, Ranges GE, Greenspan JS, Wofsy D: Chronic therapy with recombinant tumor necrosis factor-α in autoimmune NZB/NZW F₁ mice. Clin Immunol Immunopathol 52:421–434, 1989.

1332. Karkar AM, Koshino Y, Cashman SJ, et al: Passive immunization against tumour necrosis factor-alpha (TNF-alpha) and IL-1 beta protects from LPS enhancing glomerular injury in nephrotoxic nephritis in rats. Clin Exp Immunol 90:312–318, 1992.

1333. Hruby ZW, Shirota K, Jothy S, Lowry RP: Antiserum against tumor necrosis factor-alpha and a protease inhibitor reduce immune glomerular injury. Kidney Int 40:43–51, 1991.

1334. Wilson KP, Black JF, Thomson JA, et al: Structure and mechanism of interleukin-1β converting enzyme. Nature 370:270–275, 1994.

1335. Thornberry NA: Key mediator takes shape. Nature 370:251–252, 1994.

1336. Iwano M, Dohi K, Hirata E, et al: Induction of interleukin 6 synthesis in mouse glomeruli and cultured mesangial cells. Nephron 62:58–65, 1992.

1337. Brown Z, Fairbanks L, Strieter RM, et al: Human mesangial cell–derived interleukin 8 and interleukin 6: Modulation by an interleukin 1 receptor antagonist. Adv Exp Med Biol 305:137–145, 1991.

1338. Zoja C, Rambaldi A, Remuzzi G: Interleukin-1 and glomerular mesangial cells. Renal Physiol Biochem 16:89–92, 1993.

1339. Kakizaki Y, Kraft N, Atkins RC: Interferon-gamma stimulates the secretion of IL-1, but not IL-6, by glomerular mesangial cells. Clin Exp Immunol 91:521–525, 1993.

1340. Horii Y, Muraguchi A, Iwano M, et al: Involvement of IL-6 in mesangial proliferative glomerulonephritis. J Immunol 143:3949–3955, 1989.

1341. Ruef C, Budde K, Lacy J, et al: Interleukin 6 is an autocrine growth factor for mesangial cells. Kidney Int 38:249–257, 1990.

1342. Ikeda M, Ikeda U, Ohara T, et al: Recombinant interleukin-6 inhibits the growth of rat mesangial cells in culture. Am J Pathol 141:327–334, 1992.

1343. Coleman DL, Ruef C: Interleukin-6: An autocrine regulator of mesangial cell growth. Kidney Int 41:604–606, 1992.

1344. Brown Z, Fairbanks L, Strieter RM, et al: Human mesangial cell–derived interleukin 8 and interleukin 6: Modulation by an interleukin 1 receptor antagonist. Adv Exp Med Biol 305:137–145, 1991.

1345. Matsell DG, Gaber LW, Sehic E, Malik KU: Interleukin 1 and interleukin 6 inhibition of mesangial cell proliferation: Role of PGE₂. J Lipid Mediat 6:343–352, 1993.

1346. Matsell DG, Gaber LW, Malik KU: Cytokine stimulation of prostaglandin production inhibits the proliferation of serum-stimulated mesangial cells. Kidney Int 45:159–165, 1994.

1347. D'Souza RJ, Phillips HM, Jones PW, et al: Interactions of hydrogen peroxide with interleukin-6 and platelet-derived growth factor in determining mesangial cell growth: Effect of repeated oxidant stress. Clin Sci 85:747–751, 1993.

1348. Hartner A, Sterzel RB, Reindl N, et al: Cytokine-induced expression of leukemia inhibitory factor in renal mesangial cells. Kidney Int 45:1562–1571, 1994.

1349. Floege J, Topley N, Wessel K, et al: Monokines and platelet-derived growth factor modulate prostanoid production in growth arrested, human mesangial cells. Kidney Int 37:859–869, 1990.

1350. Jirik FR, Podor TJ, Hirano T, et al: Bacterial lipopolysaccharide and inflammatory mediators augment IL-6 secretion by human endothelial cells. J Immunol 142:144–147, 1989.

1351. van den Dobbelsteen ME, van der Woude FJ, Schroeijers WE, van Es LA: Soluble aggregates of IgG and immune complexes enhance IL-6 production by renal mesangial cells. Kidney Int 43:544–553, 1993.

1352. van den Dobbelsteen MEA, van der Woude FJ, Schroeijers WEM, et al: Binding of dimeric and polymeric IgA to rat renal mesangial cells enhances the release of interleukin 6. Kidney Int 46:512–519, 1994.

1353. Ryffel B, Car BD, Gunn H, et al: Interleukin-6 exacerbates glomerulonephritis (NZB × NZW)F₁ mice. Am J Pathol 144:927–937, 1994.

1354. Finck BK, Chan B, Wofsy D: Interleukin 6 promotes murine lupus in NZB/NZW F₁ mice. J Clin Invest 94:585–591, 1994.

1355. Kiberd BA: Interleukin-6 receptor blockage ameliorates murine lupus nephritis. J Am Soc Nephrol 4:58–61, 1993.

1356. Karkar AM, Tam FWK, Proudfoot AEI, et al: Modulation of antibody-mediated glomerular injury in vivo by interleukin-6. Kidney Int 44:967–973, 1993.

1357. Fukatsu A, Matsuo S, Tamai H, et al: Distribution of interleukin-6 in normal and diseased human kidney. Lab Invest 65:61–66, 1991.

1358. Tomino Y, Funabiki K, Ohmuro H, et al: Urinary levels of interleukin-6 and disease activity in patients with IgA nephropathy. Am J Nephrol 11:459–464, 1991.

1359. Dohi K, Iwano M, Muraguchi A, et al: The prognostic significance of urinary interleukin 6 in IgA nephropathy. Clin Nephrol 35:1–5, 1991.

1360. Lakkis FG, Cruet EN: Cloning of rat interleukin-13 (IL-13) cDNA and analysis of IL-13 gene expression in experimental glomerulonephritis. Biochem Biophys Res Commun 197:612–618, 1993.

1361. Mori T, Bartocci A, Satriano J, et al: Mouse mesangial cells produce colony-stimulating factor-1 (CSF-1) and express the CSF-1 receptor. J Immunol 144:4697–4702, 1990.

1362. Budde K, Coleman DL, Lacy J, Sterzel RB: Rat mesangial cells produce granulocyte-macrophage colony-stimulating factor. Am J Physiol 257:F1065–F1078, 1989.

1363. Waldherr R, Noronha IL, Niemir Z, et al: Expression of cytokines and growth factors in human glomerulonephritides. Pediatr Nephrol 7:471–478, 1993.

1364. Roy-Chaudhury P, Jones MC, MacLeod AM, et al: An immunohistological study of epidermal growth factor receptor and neu receptor and neu receptor expression in proliferative glomerulonephritis. Pathology 25:327–332, 1993.

1365. Takemura T, Yoshioka K, Murakami K, et al: Cellular localization of inflammatory cytokines in human glomerulonephritis. Virchows Arch 424:459–464, 1994.

1366. Simonson MS, Wang Y, Dunn MJ: Cellular signaling by endothelin peptides: Pathways to the nucleus. J Am Soc Nephrol 2(10 suppl):S116–S125, 1992.

1367. King AJ, Brenner BM: Endothelium-derived vasoactive factors and the renal vasculature. Am J Physiol 260:R653–662, 1991.

1368. Simonson MS, Dunn MJ: Endothelin peptides: A possible role in glomerular inflammation. Lab Invest 64:1–4, 1991.

1369. Schultz PJ: An emerging role for endothelin in renal disease. J Lab Clin Med 119:448–449, 1992.

1370. Perico N, Remuzzi G: Role of endothelin in glomerular injury. Kidney Int 43(suppl 39):S-76–S-80, 1993.

1371. Zoja C, Orisio S, Perico N, et al: Constitutive expression of endothelin gene in cultured human mesangial cells and its modulation by transforming growth factor-beta, thrombin, and a thromboxane $A_2$ analogue. Lab Invest 64:16–20, 1991.

1372. Kohan DE: Production of endothelin-1 by rat mesangial cells: Regulation by tumor necrosis factor. J Lab Clin Med 119:477–484, 1992. (Comment in J Lab Clin Med 119:448–449, 1992.)

1373. Marsden PA, Brenner BM: Transcriptional regulation of the endothelin-1 gene by TNF-alpha. Am J Physiol 262:C854–C861, 1992.

1374. Kasinath BS, Fried TA, Davalath S, Marsden PA: Glomerular epithelial cells synthesize endothelin peptides. Am J Pathol 141:279–283, 1992.

1375. Cybulsky AV, Stewart DJ, Cybulsky MI: Glomerular epithelial cells produce endothelin-1. J Am Soc Nephrol 3:1398–1404, 1993.

1376. Kohno M, Horio T, Yokokawa K, et al: Endothelin modulates the mitogenic effect of PDGF on glomerular mesangial cells. Am J Physiol 266:F894–F900, 1994.

1377. Simonson MS, Herman WH: Protein kinase C and protein tyrosine kinase activity contribute to mitogenic signaling by endothelin-1. Corss-talk between G protein–coupled receptors and pp60$^{c-src}$. J Biol Chem 268:9347–9357, 1993.

1378. Kohno M, Yokokawa K, Horio T, et al: Heparin inhibits endothelin-1 production in cultured rat mesangial cells. Kidney Int 45:137–142, 1994.

1379. Wang Y, Pouyssegur J, Dunn MJ: Endothelin stimulates mitogen-activated protein kinase p42 activity through the phosphorylation of the kinase in rat mesangial cells. J Cardiovasc Pharmacol 22(suppl 8):S164–S167, 1993.

1380. He CJ, Nguyen G, Li XM, et al: Transcriptional activation of the urokinase receptor gene by endothelin-1. Biochem Biophys Res Commun 186:1631–1638, 1992.

1381. Rebibou JM, He CJ, Delarue F, et al: Functional endothelin 1 receptors on human glomerular podocytes and mesangial cells. Nephrol Dial Transplant 7:288–292, 1992.

1382. Simonson MS, Rooney A: Characterization of endothelin receptors in mesangial cells: Evidence for two functionally distinct endothelin binding sites. Mol Pharmacol 46:41–50, 1994.

1383. Benigni A, Zoja C, Corna D, et al: A specific endothelin subtype A receptor antagonist protects against injury in renal disease progression. Kidney Int 44:440–444, 1993.

1384. Nakamura T, Ebihara I, Fukui M, et al: Renal expression of mRNAs for endothelin-1, endothelin-3 and endothelin receptors in NZB/W $F_1$ mice. Renal Physiol Biochem 16:233–243, 1993.

1385. Wolf G, Thaiss F, Schoeppe W, Stahl RA: Angiotensin II–induced proliferation of cultured murine mesangial cells: Inhibitory role of atrial natriuretic peptide. J Am Soc Nephrol 3:1270–1278, 1992.

1386. Yamamoto T, Feng L, Mizuno T, et al: Expression of mRNA for natriuretic peptide receptor subtypes in bovine kidney. Am J Physiol 267:F318–F324, 1994.

1387. Sugimoto T, Kikkawa R, Haneda M, Shigeta Y: Atrial natriuretic peptide inhibits endothelin-1–induced activation of mitogen-activated protein kinase in cultured rat mesangial cells. Biochem Biophys Res Commun 195:72–78, 1993.

1388. Hirata Y, Ishii M, Fukui K, et al: Differential effects of atrial natriuretic peptide and dopamine on urinary protein excretion in chronic glomerulonephritis. Clin Sci 80:131–136, 1991.

1389. Hirata Y, Ishii M, Fukui K, et al: Effects of atrial natriuretic peptide on urinary protein excretion in mesangial proliferative glomerulonephritis. Nephron 58:58–61, 1991.

1390. Ozdemir S, Saatci U, Besbas N, et al: Plasma atrial natriuretic peptide and endothelin levels in acute poststreptococcal glomerulonephritis. Pediatr Nephrol 6:519–522, 1992.

1391. Feng L, Tang WW, Ahn C, Wilson CB: Immediate early gene (IE) expression in anti–tubular basement membrane (TBM)-antibody associated tubulointerstitial nephritis (TIN). J Am Soc Nephrol 2:539, 1991. Abstract.

1392. Sawczuk IS, Hoke G, Olsson CA, et al: Gene expression in response to acute unilateral ureteral obstruction. Kidney Int 35:1315–1319, 1989.

1393. Sawczuk IS, Olsson CA, Hoke G, Buttyan R: Immediate induction of c-*fos* and c-*myc* transcripts following unilateral nephrectomy. Nephron 55:193–195, 1990.

1394. Safirstein R: Gene expression in nephrotoxic and ischemic acute renal failure. J Am Soc Nephrol 4:1387–1395, 1994.

1395. Schulze-Lohoff E, Fees H, Zanner S, et al: Inhibition of immediate-early-gene induction in renal mesangial cells by depletion of intracellular polyamines. Biochem J 298:647–653, 1994.

1396. Sakai T, Kriz W: The structural relationship between mesangial cells and basement membrane of the renal glomerulus. Anat Embryol 176:373–386, 1987.

1397. Drenckhahn D, Schnittler H, Nobiling R, Kriz W: Ultrastructural organization of contractile proteins in rat glomerular mesangial cells. Am J Pathol 137:1343–1351, 1990.

1398. Keane WF, Raij L: Relationship among altered glomerular barrier permselectivity, angiotensin II, and mesangial uptake of macromolecules. Lab Invest 52:599–604, 1985.

1399. Nouwen EJ, De Broe ME: EGF and TGF-α in the human kidney: Identification of octapal cells in the collecting duct. Kidney Int 45:1510–1521, 1994.

1400. Harris RC, Hoover RL, Jacobson HR, Badr KF: Evidence for glomerular actions of epidermal growth factor in the rat. J Clin Invest 82:1028–1029, 1988.

1401. Feng L, Pan Z, Xia Y, et al: Platelet-activating factor (PAF) induces expression of the growth factor, heparin-binding EGF (HB-EGF) in glomerular epithelial cells (GECs) which may contribute to immune glomerular injury. J Am Soc Nephrol 5:679, 1994. Abstract.

1402. Garcia GE, Feng L, Xia Y, et al: Expression of heparin-binding EGF (HB-EGF) in glomerulonephritis (GN). Recombinant (r) HB-EGHF decreased glomerular filtration rate (GFR). J Am Soc Nephrol 5:692, 1994. Abstract.

1403. Daniels BS: The role of the glomerular epithelial cell in the maintenance of the glomerular filtration barrier. Am J Nephrol 13:318–323, 1993.

1404. Kriz W, Hackenthal E, Nobiling R, et al: A role for podocytes to counteract capillary wall distention. Kidney Int 45:369–376, 1994.

1405. Harper PA, Robinson JM, Hoover RL, et al: Improved methods for culturing rat glomerular cells. Kidney Int 26:875–900, 1984.

1406. Oberley TD, Yang A-H, Gould-Kostka J: Selection of kidney cell types in primary glomerular explant outgrowths by in vitro culture conditions. J Cell Sci 84:69–92, 1986.

1407. Oberley TD, Steinert BW, Yang A-H, Anderson PJ: Kidney glomerular explants in serum-free media. Sequential morphologic and quantitative analysis of cell outgrowths. Virchows Arch B 50:209–235, 1986.

1408. Nøgaard JOR: Rat glomerular epithelial cells in culture. Parietal or visceral epithelial origin? Lab Invest 57:277–290, 1987.

1409. Adler S, Chen X, Eng B: Control of rat glomerular epithelial cell growth in vitro. Kidney Int 37:1048–1054, 1990.

1410. Yanagisawa M, Imai H, Fukushima Y, et al: Effects of tumour necrosis factor alpha and interleukin 1 beta on the proliferation of cultured glomerular epithelial cells. Virchows Arch 424:581–586, 1994.

1411. Floege J, Johnson RJ, Alpers CE, et al: Visceral glomerular epithelial cells can proliferate in vivo and synthesize platelet-derived growth factor B-chain. Am J Pathol 142:637–650, 1993.

1412. Moutabarrik A, Nakanishi I, Ishibashi M: Interleukin-6 and interleukin-6 receptor are expressed by cultured glomerular epithelial cells. Scand J Immunol 40:181–186, 1994.

1413. Klein DJ, Oegema TR Jr, Freeden TS, et al: Partial characterization of proteoglycans synthesized by human glomerular epithelial cells in culture. Arch Biochem Biophys 277:389–401, 1990.

1414. Thomas GJ, Jenner L, Mason RM, Davies M: Human glomerular epithelial cell proteoglycans. Arch Biochem Biophys 278:11–20, 1990.

1415. Kasinath BS: Glomerular endothelial cell proteoglycans—regulation by TGF-beta 1. Arch Biochem Biophys 305:370–377, 1993.

1416. Nakamura T, Miller D, Ruoslahti E, Border WA: Production of extracellular matrix by glomerular epithelial cells is regulated by transforming growth factor-beta 1. Kidney Int 41:1213–1221, 1992.

1417. Adler S: Heparin alters epidermal growth factor metabolism in cultured rat glomerular epithelial cells. Am J Pathol 139:169–175, 1991.

1418. Watanabe K, Kinoshita S, Nakagawa H: Gelatinase secretion by glomerular epithelial cells. Nephron 56:405–409, 1990.

1419. Johnson RJ, Yamabe H, Chen Y-P, et al: Glomerular epithelial cells secrete a glomerular basement membrane degrading metalloprotease. J Am Soc Nephrol 2:1388–1397, 1992.

1420. Cybulsky AV, Bonventre JV, Quigg RJ, et al: Extracellular matrix regulates proliferation and phospholipid turnover in glomerular epithelial cells. Am J Physiol 259:F326–F337, 1990.

1421. Cybulsky AV, Carbonetto S, Huang Q, et al: Adhesion of rat glomerular epithelial cells to extracellular matrices: Role of $\beta_1$ integrins. Kidney Int 42:1099–1106, 1992.

1422. Adler S: Characterization of glomerular epithelial cell matrix receptors. Am J Pathol 141:571–578, 1992.

1423. Cybulsky AV, McTavish AJ, Cyr MD: Extracellular matrix modulates epidermal growth factor receptor activation in rat glomerular epithelial cells. J Clin Invest 94:68–78, 1994.

1424. Castellot JJ Jr, Hoover RL, Harper PA, Karnovsky MJ: Heparin and glomerular epithelial cell–secreted heparinlike species inhibit mesangial-cell proliferation. Am J Pathol 120:427–435, 1985.

1425. Pugliese F, Singh AK, Kasinath BS, et al: Glomerular epithelial cell polyanion neutralization is associated with enhanced prostanoid production. Kidney Int 32:57–61, 1987.

1426. Singh AK, Rahman MA: Intracellular processing of immune complexes formed on the surface of glomerular epithelial cells. Am J Physiol 266:F246–F253, 1994.

1427. Stefanovic V, Ardaillou N, Vlahovic P, et al: Interferon-gamma induces dipeptidylpeptidase IV expression in human glomerular epithelial cells. Immunology 80:465–470, 1993.

1428. Green DF, Resnick L, Bourgoignie JJ: HIV infects glomerular endothelial and mesangial but not epithelial cells in vitro. Kidney Int 41:956–960, 1992.

1429. Green DF, Hwang KH, Ryan US, Bourgoignie JJ: Culture of endothelial cells from baboon and human glomeruli. Kidney Int 41:1506–1516, 1992.

1430. Mantovani A, Bussolino F, Dejana E: Cytokine regulation of endothelial cell function. FASEB J 6:2591–2599, 1992.

1431. Davies PF, Tripathi SC: Mechanical stress mechanisms and the cell. An endothelial paradigm. Circ Res 72:239–245, 1993.

1432. Brady HR, Serhan CN: Adhesion promotes transcellular leukotriene biosynthesis during neutrophil–glomerular endothelial cell interactions: Inhibition by antibodies against CD18 and L-selectin. Biochem Biophys Res Commun 186:1307–1314, 1992.

1433. Cosio FG, Sedmak DD, Nahman NS Jr: Cellular receptors for matrix proteins in normal human kidney and human mesangial cells. Kidney Int 38:886–895, 1990.

1434. Saeki T, Morioka T, Arakawa M, et al: Modulation of mesangial cell proliferation by endothelial cells in coculture. Am J Pathol 139:949–957, 1991.

1435. Hirschberg R, Kopple JD: Effects of growth hormone and IGF-1 on renal function. Kidney Int 36(suppl 27):S-20–S-26, 1989.

1436. Ohashi H, Rosen KM, Smith FE, et al: Characterization of type I IGF receptor and IGF-1 mRNA expression in cultured human and bovine glomerular cells. Regul Pept 48:9–20, 1993.

1437. Humes HD, Cieslinski DA, Coimbra TM, et al: Epidermal growth factor enhances renal tubule cell regeneration and repair and accelerates the recovery of renal function in postischemic acute renal failure. J Clin Invest 84:1757–1761, 1989.

1438. Hammerman MR, Miller SB: Therapeutic use of growth factors in renal failure. J Am Soc Nephrol 5:1–11, 1994.

1439. Doi T, Striker LJ, Elliot SJ, et al: Insulinlike growth factor-1 is a progression factor for human mesangial cells. Am J Pathol 134:395–404, 1989.

1440. Olson JL, Heptinstall RH: Nonimmunologic mechanisms of glomerular injury. Lab Invest 59:564–578, 1988.

1441. Diamond JR, Karnovsky MJ: Focal and segmental glomerulosclerosis: Analogies to atherosclerosis. Kidney Int 33:917–924, 1988.

1442. Rennke HG, Klein PS: Pathogenesis and significance of nonprimary focal and segmental glomerulosclerosis. Am J Kidney Dis 13:443–456, 1989.

1443. Walser M: Progression of chronic renal failure in man. Kidney Int 37:1195–1210, 1990.

1444. Striker GE, Peten EP, Yang CW, Striker LJ: Glomerulosclerosis: Studies of its pathogenesis in humans and animals. Contrib Nephrol 107:124–131, 1994.

1445. El Nahas AM: Renal scarring: A new look at an old problem. Springer Semin Immunopathol 16:63–69, 1994.

1446. Johnson RJ: The glomerular response to injury: Progression or resolution? Kidney Int 45:1769–1782, 1994.

1447. El Nahas AM: Growth factors and glomerular sclerosis. Kidney Int 41(suppl 36):S-15–S-20, 1992.

1448. Neuringer JR, Brenner BM: Glomerular hypertension: Cause and consequence of renal injury. J Hypertens Suppl 10:S91–S97, 1992.

1449. Neuringer JR, Brenner BM: Hemodynamic theory of progressive renal disease: A 10-year update in brief review. Am J Kidney Dis 22:98–104, 1993.

1450. Wolf G, Neilson EG: Molecular mechanisms of tubulointerstitial hypertrophy and hyperplasia. Kidney Int 39:401–420, 1991.

1451. Yee J, Kuncio GS, Neilson EG: Tubulointerstitial injury following glomerulonephritis. Semin Nephrol 11:361–366, 1991.

1452. Müller GA, Markovic-Lipkovski J, Rodemann HP: The progression of renal diseases: On the pathogenesis of renal interstitial fibrosis. Klin Wochenschr 69:576–586, 1991.

1453. Kuncio GS, Neilson EG, Haverty T: Mechanisms of tubulointerstitial fibrosis. Kidney Int 39:550–556, 1991.

1454. Jones CL, Buch S, Post M, et al: Pathogenesis of interstitial fibrosis in chronic purine aminonucleoside nephrosis. Kidney Int 40:1020–1031, 1991.

1455. Fine LG, Ong AC, Norman JT: Mechanisms of tubulo-interstitial injury in progressive renal diseases. Eur J Clin Invest 23:259–265, 1993.

1456. Agarwal A, Nath KA: Effect of proteinuria on renal interstitium: Effect of products of nitrogen metabolism. Am J Nephrol 13:376–384, 1993.

1457. Strutz F, Neilson EG: The role of lymphocytes in the progression of interstitial disease. Kidney Int 45(suppl 45):S-106–S-110, 1994.

1458. Alexopoulos E, Seron D, Harley RB, Cameron JS: Lupus nephritis: Correlation of interstitial cells with glomerular function. Kidney Int 37:100–109, 1990.

1459. Pichler R, Giachelli CM, Lombardi D, et al: Tubulointerstitial disease in glomerulonephritis. Potential role of osteopontin (uropontin). Am J Pathol 144:915–926, 1994.

1460. Giachelli CM, Pichler R, Lombardi D, et al: Osteopontin expression in angiotensin II–induced tubulointerstitial nephritis. Kidney Int 45:515–524, 1994.

1461. Tang WW, Feng L, Xia Y, Wilson CB: Extracellular matrix accumulation in immune-mediated tubulointerstitial injury. Kidney Int 45:1077–1084, 1994.

1462. Nath KA, Fischereder M, Hostetter TH: The role of oxidants in progressive renal injury. Kidney Int 45(suppl 45):S-111–S-115, 1994.

1463. Schwartz MM, Korbet SM: Primary focal segmental glomerulosclerosis: Pathology, histological variants, and pathogenesis. Am J Kidney Dis 22:874–883, 1993.

1464. Scheinman JI, Fish AJ, Matas AJ, Michael AF: The immunohistopathology of glomerular antigens. II. The glomerular basement membrane, actomyosin, and fibroblast surface antigens in normal, diseased, and transplanted human kidneys. Am J Pathol 90:71–88, 1978.

1465. Striker LM, Killen PD, Chi E, Striker GE: The composition of glomerulosclerosis. I. Studies in focal sclerosis, crescentic glomerulonephritis, and membranoproliferative glomerulonephritis. Lab Invest 51:181–192, 1984.

1466. Adler S, Striker LJ, Striker GE, et al: Studies of progressive glomerular sclerosis in the rat. Am J Pathol 123:553–562, 1986.

1467. Kemeny E, Fillit HM, Damle S, et al: Monoclonal antibodies to heparan sulfate proteoglycan: Development and application to the study of normal tissue and pathologic human kidney biopsies. Connect Tissue Res 18:9–25, 1988.

1468. Yoshioka K, Takemura T, Tohda M, et al: Glomerular localization of type III collagen in human kidney disease. Kidney Int 35:1203–1211, 1989.

1469. Oomura A, Nakamura T, Arakawa M, et al: Alterations in the extracellular matrix components in human glomerular diseases. Virchows Arch A 415:151–159, 1989.

1470. Leardkamolkarn V, Salant DJ, Abrahamson DR: Loss and rearrangement of glomerular basement membrane laminin during acute nephrotoxic nephritis in the rat. Am J Pathol 137:187–198, 1990.

1471. Dixey J, Moss J, Woodrow DF, et al: SLE nephritis: An ultrastructural immunogold study to evaluate the relationship between immune complexes and the basement membrane components type IV collagen, fibronectin and heparan sulphate proteoglycans. Clin Nephrol 34:95–102, 1990.

1472. Mohan PS, Carter WG, Spiro RG: Occurrence of type IV collagen in extracellular matrix of renal glomeruli and its increase in diabetes. Diabetes 39:31–37, 1990.

1473. Kim Y, Butkowski R, Burke B, et al: Differential expression of basement membrane collagen in membranous nephropathy. Am J Pathol 139:1381–1388, 1991.

1474. Fogel MA, Boyd CD, Leardkamolkarn V, et al: Glomerular basement membrane expansion in passive Heymann nephritis. Absence of increased synthesis of type IV collagen, laminin, or fibronectin. Am J Pathol 138:465–475, 1991.

1475. Nakamura T, Ebihara I, Shirato I, et al: Modulation of basement membrane component gene expression in glomeruli of aminonucleoside nephrosis. Lab Invest 64:640–647, 1991.

1476. Bergijk EC, Munaut C, Baelde JJ, et al: A histologic study of the extracellular matrix during the development of glomerulosclerosis in murine chronic graft-versus-host disease. Am J Pathol 140:1147–1156, 1992.

1477. Ebihara I, Suzuki S, Nakamura T, et al: Extracellular matrix component mRNA expression in glomeruli in experimental focal glomerulosclerosis. J Am Soc Nephrol 3:1387–1397, 1993.

1478. Truong LD, Pindur J, Barrios R, et al: Tenascin is an important component of the glomerular extracellular matrix in normal and pathologic conditions. Kidney Int 45:201–210, 1994.

1479. Schiffer MS, Michael AF, Kim Y, Fish AJ: Distribution of glomerular basement membrane antigens in diseased human kidneys. Lab Invest 44:234–240, 1981.

1480. Büyübabani N, Droz D: Distribution of the extracellular matrix components in human glomerular lesions. J Pathol 172:199–207, 1994.

1481. Mosquera JA: Increase production of fibronectin by glomerular cultures from rats with nephrotoxic nephritis. Macrophages induce fibronectin production in cultured mesangial cells. Lab Invest 68:406–412, 1993.

1482. French-Constant C, Van de Water L, Dvorak HF, Hynes RO: Reappearance of an embryonic pattern of fibronectin splicing during wound healing in the adult rat. J Cell Biol 109:903–914, 1989.

1483. Magnuson VL, Young M, Schattenberg DG, et al: The alternative splicing of fibronectin pre-mRNA is altered during aging and in response to growth factors. J Biol Chem 266:14654–14662, 1991.

1484. Tang WW, Feng L, Xia Y, et al: Expression of embryonic (E) fibronectins (FN) due to alternative splicing after immune renal injury. J Am Soc Nephrol 4:667, 1993. Abstract.

1485. Striker LJ, Peten EP, Elliot SJ, et al: Mesangial cell turnover: Effect of heparin and peptide growth factors. Lab Invest 64:446–456, 1991.

1486. Sterzel RB, Schulze-Lohoff E, Weber M, Goodman SL: Interactions between glomerular mesangial cells, cytokines, and extracellular matrix. J Am Soc Nephrol 2(10 suppl):S126–S131, 1992.

1487. Ruef C, Kashgarian M, Coleman DL: Mesangial cell-matrix interactions. Effects on mesangial cell growth and cytokine secretion. Am J Pathol 141:429–439, 1992.

1488. Takeuchi A, Yoshizawa N, Yamamoto M, et al: Basic fibroblast growth factor promotes proliferation of rat glomerular visceral epithelial cells in vitro. Am J Pathol 141:107–116, 1992.

1489. Haralson MA, Jacobson HR, Hoover RL: Collagen polymorphism in cultured rat kidney mesangial cells. Lab Invest 57:513–532, 1987.

1490. Jimenez SA, Freundlich B, Rosenbloom J: Selective inhibition of human diploid fibroblast collagen synthesis by interferons. J Clin Invest 74:1112–1116, 1984.

1491. Ishimura E, Sterzel RB, Budde K, Kashgarian M: Formation of extracellular matrix by cultured rat mesangial cells. Am J Pathol 134:843–855, 1989.

1492. Creely JJ, DiMari SJ, Howe AM, et al: Effects of epidermal growth factor on collagen synthesis by an epithelioid cell line derived from normal rat kidney. Am J Pathol 136:1247–1257, 1990.

1493. Person JM, Lovett DH, Raugi GJ: Modulation of mesangial cell migration by extracellular matrix components. Inhibition by heparinlike glycosaminoglycans. Am J Pathol 133:609–614, 1988.

1494. Kitamura M, Maruyama N, Mitarai T, et al: Extracellular matrix contraction by cultured mesangial cells: Modulation by transforming growth factor-β and matrix components. Exp Mol Pathol 56:132–143, 1992.

1495. Zahner G, Disser M, Thaiss F, et al: The effect of prostaglandin E2 on mRNA expression and secretion of collagens I, III, and IV and fibronectin in cultured rat mesangial cells. J Am Soc Nephrol 4:1778–1785, 1994.

1496. Shan Z, Tan D, Satriano J, et al: Intracellular glutathione influences collagen generation by mesangial cells. Kidney Int 46:388–395, 1994.

1497. Ziesche R, Roth M, Papakonstantinou E, et al: A granulocyte inhibitory protein overexpressed in chronic renal disease regulates expression of interleukin 6 and interleukin 8. Proc Natl Acad Sci USA 91:301–305, 1994.

1498. Hirano T: Interleukin-6 and its relation to inflammation and disease. Clin Immunol Immunopathol 62:S60–S65, 1992.

1499. Horii Y, Iwano M, Hirata E, et al: Role of interleukin-6 in the progression of mesangial proliferative glomerulonephritis. Kidney Int 43(suppl 39):S-71–S-75, 1993.

1500. Hynes RO: Integrins: Versatility, modulation, and signaling in cell adhesion. Cell 69:11–25, 1992.

1501. Cosio FG: Cell-matrix adhesion receptors: Relevance to glomerular pathology. Am J Kidney Dis 20:294–305, 1992.

1502. Adler S: Integrin receptors in the glomerulus: Potential role in glomerular injury. Am J Physiol 262:F697–F704, 1992.

1503. Ruoslahti E: Integrins. J Clin Invest 87:1–5, 1991.

1504. Petermann A, Fees H, Grenz H, et al: Polymerase chain reaction and focal contact formation indicate integrin expression in mesangial cells. Kidney Int 44:997–1005, 1993.

1505. Grenz H, Carbonetto, S, Goodman SL: Alpha 3 beta 1 integrin is moved into focal contacts in kidney mesangial cells. J Cell Sci 105:739–751, 1993.

1506. Mendrick DL, Kelly DM: Temporal expression of VLA-2 and modulation of its ligand specificity by rat glomerular epithelial cells in vitro. Lab Invest 69:690–702, 1993.

1507. Adler S, Chen X: Anti-Fx1A antibody recognizes a $\beta_1$-integrin on glomerular epithelial cells and inhibits adhesion and growth. Am J Physiol 262:F770–F776, 1992.

1508. O'Meara YM, Natori Y, Minto AWM, et al: Nephrotoxic antiserum identifies a $\beta_1$-integrin on rat glomerular epithelial cells. Am J Physiol 262:F1083–F1091, 1992.

1509. Kerjaschki D, Ojha PP, Susani M, et al: A $\beta_1$-integrin receptor for fibronectin in human kidney glomeruli. Am J Pathol 134:481–489, 1989.

1510. Rahilly MA, Fleming S: Differential expression of integrin alpha chains by renal epithelial cells. J Pathol 167:327–334, 1992.

1511. Racusen LC: Alterations in tubular epithelial cell adhesion and mechanisms of acute renal failure. Lab Invest 67:158–165, 1992.

1512. Leavesley DI, Schwartz MA, Rosenfeld M, Cheresh DA: Integrin $\beta_1$- and $\beta_3$-mediated endothelial cell migration is triggered through distinct signaling mechanisms. J Cell Biol 121:163–170, 1993.

1513. Weening JJ, Westenend PJ, Beukers JJB, Grond J: Experimental models of glomerulosclerosis. Contrib Nephrol 77:65–76, 1990.

1514. Simons JL, Provoost AP, Anderson S, et al: Pathogenesis of glomerular injury in the fawn-hooded rat: Early glomerular capillary hypertension predicts glomerular sclerosis. J Am Soc Nephrol 3:1775–1782, 1993.

1515. Simons JL, Provoost AP, De Keijzer MH, et al: Pathogenesis of glomerular injury in the fawn-hooded rat: Effect of unilateral nephrectomy. J Am Soc Nephrol 4:1362–1370, 1993.

1516. Provoost AP: Spontaneous glomerulosclerosis: Insights from the fawn-hooded rat. Kidney Int 45(suppl 45):S-2–S-5, 1994.

1517. Yoshida F, Matsuo S, Fujishima H, et al: Renal lesions of the FGS strain of mice: A spontaneous animal model of progressive glomerulosclerosis. Nephron 66:317–325, 1994.

1518. Perkinson DT, Baker PJ, Couser WG, et al: Membrane attack complex deposition in experimental glomerular injury. Am J Pathol 120:121–128, 1985.

1519. Rayner HC, Ross-Gilbertson VL, Walls J: The role of lipids in the pathogenesis of glomerulosclerosis in the rat following subtotal nephrectomy. Eur J Clin Invest 20:97–104, 1990.

1520. Floege J, Burns MW, Alpers CE, et al: Glomerular cell proliferation and PDGF expression precede glomerulosclerosis in the remnant kidney model. Kidney Int 41:297–309, 1992.

1521. Barnes JL, Hevey KA, Hastings RR, Bocanegra RA: Mesangial cell migration precedes proliferation in habu snake venom–induced glomerular injury. Lab Invest 70:460–467, 1994.

1522. Riser BL, Cortesm P, Zhao X, et al: Intraglomerular pressure and mesangial stretching stimulate extracellular matrix formation in the rat. J Clin Invest 90:1932–1943, 1992.

1523. Wardle EN: Cellular biology of glomerulosclerosis. Nephron 61:125–128, 1992.

1524. Cortes P, Riser BL, Zhao X, Narins RG: Glomerular volume expansion and mesangial cell mechanical strain: Mediators of glomerular pressure injury. Kidney Int 45(suppl 45):S-11–S-16, 1994.

1525. Harris RC, Akai Y, Yasuda T, Homma T: The role of physical forces in alterations of mesangial cell function. Kidney Int 45(suppl 45):S-17–S-21, 1994.

1526. Floege J, Johnson RJ, Gordon K, et al: Increased synthesis of extracellular matrix in mesangial proliferative nephritis. Kidney Int 40:477–488, 1991.

1527. Ishimura E, Sterzel RB, Morii H, Kashgarian M: Extracellular matrix protein: Gene expression and synthesis in cultured rat mesangial cells. Nippon Jinzo Gakkai Shi 34:9–17, 1992.

1528. Floege J, Alpers CE, Burns MW, et al: Glomerular cells, extracellular matrix accumulation, and the development of glomerulosclerosis in the remnant kidney model. Lab Invest 66:485–497, 1992.

1529. Creely JJ, DiMari SJ, Howe AM, Haralson MA: Effects of transforming growth factor-β on collagen synthesis by normal rat kidney epithelial cells. Am J Pathol 140:45–55, 1992.

1530. Sharma K, Ziyadeh FN: The emerging role of transforming growth factor-β in kidney diseases. Am J Physiol 266:F829–F842, 1994.

1531. Couchman JR, Beavan LA, McCarthy KJ: Glomerular matrix: Synthesis, turnover and role in mesangial expansion. Kidney Int 45:328–335, 1994.

1532. Truong LD, Majesky MW, Pindur J: Tenascin is synthesized and secreted by rat mesangial cells in culture and is present in extracellular matrix in human glomerular diseases. J Am Soc Nephrol 4:1771–1777, 1994.

1533. Coffey AK, Karnovsky MJ: Heparin inhibits mesangial cell proliferation in habu-venom-induced glomerular injury. Am J Pathol 120:248–255, 1985.

1534. Tang WW, Wilson CB: Heparin decreases mesangial matrix accumulation following selective antibody-induced mesangial cell injury. J Am Soc Nephrol 3:921–929, 1992.

1535. Floege J, Eng E, Young BA, et al: Heparin suppresses mesangial cell proliferation and matrix expansion in experimental mesangioproliferative glomerulonephritis. Kidney Int 43:369–380, 1993.

1536. Wolthuis A, Boes A, Berden JHM, Grond J: Heparins modulate extracellular matrix and protein synthesis of cultured rat mesangial cells. Virchows Arch B 63:181–189, 1993.

1537. Border WA, Okuda S, Languino LR, et al: Suppression of experimental glomerulonephritis by antiserum against transforming growth factor beta 1. Nature 346:371–374, 1990.

1538. Okuda S, Languino LR, Ruoslahti E, Border WA: Elevated expression of transforming growth factor-β and proteoglycan production in experimental glomerulonephritis. Possible role in expansion of the mesangial extracellular matrix. J Clin Invest 86:453–462, 1990.

1539. Border WA, Noble NA, Yamamoto T, et al: Antagonists of transforming growth factor-β: A novel approach to treatment of glomerulonephritis and prevention of glomerulosclerosis. Kidney Int 41:566–570, 1992.

1540. Border WA, Noble NA, Yamamoto T, et al: Natural inhibitor of transforming growth factor-β protects against scarring in experimental kidney disease. Nature 360:361–364, 1992.

1541. Border WA, Brees D, Noble NA: Transforming growth factor-beta and extracellular matrix deposition in the kidney. Contrib Nephrol 107:140–145, 1994.

1542. Bruijn JA, Roos A, de Geus B, de Heer E: Transforming growth factor-β and the glomerular extracellular matrix in renal pathology. J Lab Clin Med 123:34–47, 1994.

1543. Lianos EA, Orphanos V, Cattell V, et al: Glomerular expression and cell origin of transforming growth factor-beta 1 in anti–glomerular basement membrane disease. Am J Med Sci 307:1–5, 1994.

1544. Choi ME, Kim EG, Huang Q, Ballermann BJ: Rat mesangial cell hypertrophy in response to transforming growth factor-beta 1. Kidney Int 44:948–958, 1993.

1545. Kagami S, Border WA, Miller DE, Noble NA: Angiotensin II stimulates extracellular matrix protein synthesis through induction of transforming growth factor-β expression in rat glomerular mesangial cells. J Clin Invest 93:2431–2437, 1994.

1546. Jaffer F, Saunders C, Shultz P, et al: Regulation of mesangial cell growth by polypeptide mitogens. Inhibitory role of transforming growth factor beta. Am J Pathol 135:261–269, 1989.

1547. Yamamoto T, Noble NA, Miller DE, Border WA: Sustained expression of TGF-β1 underlies development of progressive kidney fibrosis. Kidney Int 45:916–927, 1994.

1548. Okuda S, Nakamura T, Yamamoto T, et al: Dietary protein restriction rapidly reduces transforming growth factor β1 expression in experimental glomerulonephritis. Proc Natl Acad Sci USA 88:9765–9769, 1991.

1549. Eddy AA: Protein restriction reduces transforming growth factor-β and interstitial fibrosis in nephrotic syndrome. Am J Physiol 266:F884–F893, 1994.

1550. Coimbra T, Wiggins R, Noh JW, et al: Transforming growth factor-β production in anti–glomerular basement membrane disease in the rabbit. Am J Pathol 138:223–234, 1991.

1551. Burmester JK, Qian SW, Roberts AB, et al: Characterization of distinct functional domains of transforming growth factor β. Proc Natl Acad Sci USA 90:8628–8632, 1993.

1552. Tamaki K, Okuda S, Ando T, et al: TGF-β1 in glomerulosclerosis and interstitial fibrosis of Adriamycin nephropathy. Kidney Int 45:525–536, 1994.

1553. Kanai H, Mitsuhashi H, Ono K, et al: Increased excretion of urinary transforming growth factor beta in patients with focal glomerular sclerosis. Nephron 66:391–395, 1994.

1554. Shull MM, Ormsby I, Kier AB, et al: Targeted disruption of the mouse transforming growth factors-β1 gene results in multifocal inflammatory disease. Nature 359:603–699, 1992.

1555. Kulkarni AB, Huh C-H, Becker D, et al: Transforming growth factors-β1 null mutation in mice causes excessive inflammatory response and early death. Proc Natl Acad Sci USA 90:770–774, 1993.

1556. Kulkarni AB, Karlsson S: Transforming growth factor-$\beta_1$ knockout mice. A mutation in one cytokine gene causes a dramatic inflammatory disease. Am J Pathol 143:3–9, 1993.

1557. Gresham HD, Ray CJ, O'Sullivan FX: Defective neutrophil function in the autoimmune mouse strain MRL/*lpr*. Potential role of transforming growth factor-β1. J Immunol 146:3911–3921, 1991.

1558. Keane WF, Mulcahy WS, Kasiske BL, et al: Hyperlipidemia and progressive renal disease. Kidney Int 39(suppl 31):S-41–S-48, 1991.

1559. Yoshimura A, Gordon K, Alpers CE, et al: Demonstration of PDGF B-chain mRNA in glomeruli in mesangial proliferative nephritis by in situ hybridization. Kidney Int 40:470–476, 1991.

1560. Floege J, Topley N, Resch K: Regulation of mesangial cell proliferation. Am J Kidney Dis 17:673–676, 1991.

1561. Johnson RJ, Raines EW, Floege J, et al: Inhibition of mesangial cell proliferation and matrix expansion in glomerulonephritis in the rat by antibody to platelet-derived growth factor. J Exp Med 175:1413–1416, 1992.

1562. Floege J, Johnson RJ, Couser WG: Mesangial cells in the pathogenesis of progressive glomerular disease in animal models. Clin Investig 70:857–864, 1992.

1563. Eng J, Floege J, Young BA, et al: Is mesangial cell proliferation required for extracellular matrix expansion in glomerular disease? Contrib Nephrol 107:156–162, 1994.

1564. Couser WG, Johnson RJ: Mechanisms of progressive renal disease in glomerulonephritis. Am J Kidney Dis 23:193–198, 1994.

1565. Feng L, Xia Y, Tang WW, Wilson CB: Cloning a novel form of rat PDGF A-chain with a unique 5'-UT: Regulation during development and in glomerulonephritis. Biochem Biophys Res Commun 194:1453–1459, 1993.

1566. Daniel TO, Kumjian DA: Platelet-derived growth factor in renal development and disease. Semin Nephrol 13:87–95, 1993.

1567. Elger M, Drenckhahn D, Nobiling R, et al: Cultured rat mesangial cells contain smooth muscle alpha-actin not found in vivo. Am J Pathol 142:497–509, 1993.

1568. Abboud HE, Grandaliano G, Pinzani M, et al: Actions of platelet-derived growth factor isoforms in mesangial cells. J Cell Physiol 158:140–150, 1994.

1569. Bhandari B, Grandaliano G, Abboud HE: Platelet-derived growth factor (PDGF) BB homodimer regulates PDGF A- and PDGF B-chain gene transcription in human mesangial cells. Biochem J 297:385–388, 1994.

1570. Choudhury GG, Biswas P, Grandaliano G, Abboud HE: Involvement of PKC-alpha in PDGF-mediated mitogenic signaling in human mesangial cells. Am J Physiol 265:F634–F642, 1993.

1571. Marx M, Daniel TO, Kashgarian M, Madri JA: Spatial organization of the extracellular matrix modulates the expression of PDGF-receptor subunits in mesangial cells. Kidney Int 43:1027–1041, 1993.

1572. Fukui M, Nakamura T, Ebihara I, et al: Low-protein diet attenuates increased gene expression of platelet-derived growth factor and transforming growth factor-β in experimental glomerular sclerosis. J Lab Clin Med 121:224–234, 1993.

1573. Akai Y, Iwano M, Kitamura Y, et al: Intraglomerular expression of IL-1 alpha and platelet-derived growth factor (PDGF-B) mRNA in experimental immune complex–mediated glomerulonephritis. Clin Exp Immunol 95:29–34, 1994.

1574. Nakamura T, Ebihara I, Nagaoka I, et al: Renal platelet-derived growth factor gene expression in NZB/W F$_1$ mice with lupus and ddY mice with lupus and ddy mice with IgA nephropathy. Clin Immunol Immunopathol 63:173–181, 1992.

1575. Alpers CE, Seifert RA, Hudkins KL, et al: Developmental patterns of PDGF B-chain, PDGF-receptor, and α-actin expression in human glomerulogenesis. Kidney Int 42:390–399, 1992.

1576. Alpers CE, Seifert RA, Hudkins KL, et al: PDGF-receptor localizes to mesangial, parietal epithelial, and interstitial cells in human and primate kidneys. Kidney Int 43:286–294, 1993.

1577. Fellström B, Klareskog L, Heldin CH, et al: Platelet-derived growth factor receptors in the kidney—upregulated expression in inflammation. Kidney Int 36:1099–1102, 1989.

1578. Ueno H, Colbert H, Escobedo JA, Williams LT: Inhibition of PDGF β receptor signal transduction by coexpression of a truncated receptor. Science 252:844–848, 1991.

1579. Duan D-SR, Pazin MJ, Fretto LJ, Williams LT: A functional soluble extracellular region of the platelet-derived growth factor (PDGF) β-receptor antagonizes PDGF-stimulated responses. J Biol Chem 266:413–418, 1991.

1580. Heidaran MA, Yu J-C, Jensen RA, et al: A deletion in the extracellular domain of the α platelet-derived growth factor (PDGF) receptor differentially impairs PDGF-AA and PDGF-BB binding affinities. J Biol Chem 267:2884–2887, 1992.

1581. Khachigian LM, Owensby DA, Chesterman CN: A tyrosinated peptide representing the alternatively spliced exon of the platelet-derived growth factor A-chain binds specifically to cultured cells and interferes with binding of several growth factors. J Biol Chem 267:1660–1666, 1992.

1582. Raines EW, Lane TF, Iruela-Arispe ML, et al: The extracellular glycoprotein SPARC interacts with platelet-derived growth factor (PDGF)-AB and -BB and inhibits the binding of PDGF to its receptors. Proc Natl Acad Sci USA 89:1281–1285, 1992.

1583. Mühl H, Geiger T, Pignat W, et al: PDGF suppresses the activation of group II phospholipase A$_2$ gene expression by interleukin 1 and forskolin in mesangial cells. FEBS Lett 291:249–252, 1991.

1584. Floege J, Topley N, Hoppe J, et al: Mitogenic effect of platelet-derived growth factor in human glomerular mesangial cells: Modulation and/or suppression by inflammatory cytokines. Clin Exp Immunol 86:334–341, 1991.

1585. Marinides GN, Suchard SJ, Mookerjee BK: Role of thrombospondin in mesangial cell growth: Possible existence of an autocrine feedback growth circuit. Kidney Int 46:350–357, 1994.

1586. Floege J, Eng E, Lindner V, et al: Rat glomerular mesangial cells synthesize basic fibroblast growth factor. Release, upregulated synthesis, and mitogenicity in mesangial proliferative glomerulonephritis. J Clin Invest 90:2362–2369, 1992.

1587. Floege J, Eng E, Young BA, et al: Infusion of platelet-derived growth factor or basic fibroblast growth factor induces selective glomerular mesangial cell proliferation and matrix accumulation in rats. J Clin Invest 92:2952–2962, 1993.

1588. Kim EG, Kwon HM, Burrow CR, Ballermann BJ: Expression of rat fibroblast growth factor receptor 1 as three splicing variants during kidney development. Am J Physiol 264:F66–F73, 1993.

1589. Diamond JR: Analogous pathobiologic mechanisms in glomerulosclerosis and atherosclerosis. Kidney Int 39(suppl 31):S-29–S-34, 1991.

1590. Grone EF, Abboud HE, Hohne M, et al: Actions of lipoproteins in cultured human mesangial cells: Modulation by mitogenic vasoconstrictors. Am J Physiol 263:F686–F696, 1992.

1591. Schreiner GF: The mesangial phagocyte and its regulation of contractile cell biology. J Am Soc Nephrol 2(10 suppl):S74–S82, 1992.

1592. Magil AB, Cohen AH: Monocytes and focal glomerulosclerosis. Lab Invest 61:404–409, 1989.

1593. Matsumoto K, Atkins RC: Glomerular cells and macrophages in the progression of experimental focal and segmental glomerulosclerosis. Am J Pathol 134:933–945, 1989.

1594. Diamond JR, Ding G, Frye J, Diamond I-P: Glomerular macrophages and the mesangial proliferative response in the experimental nephrotic syndrome. Am J Pathol 141:887–894, 1992.

1595. Ding G, Pesek-Diamond I, Diamond JR: Cholesterol, macrophages, and gene expression of TGF-β1 and fibronectin during nephrosis. Am J Physiol 264:F577–F584, 1993.

1596. Zoja C, Perico N, Corna D, et al: Thromboxane synthesis inhibition increases renal prostacyclin and prevents renal disease progression in rats with remnant kidney. J Am Soc Nephrol 1:799–807, 1990.

1597. Fries JWU, Sandstrom DJ, Meyer TW, Rennke HG: Glomerular hypertrophy and epithelial cell injury modulate progressive glomerulosclerosis in the rat. Lab Invest 60:205–218, 1989.

1598. Miller PL, Scholey JW, Rennke HG, Meyer TW: Glomerular hypertrophy aggravates epithelial cell injury in hephrotic rats. J Clin Invest 85:1119–1126, 1990.

1599. Nagata M, Kriz W: Glomerular damage after uninephrectomy in young rats. II. Mechanical stress on podocytes as a pathway to sclerosis. Kidney Int 42:148–160, 1992.

1600. Rennke HG: How does glomerular epithelial cell injury contribute to progressive glomerular damage? Kidney Int 45(suppl 45):S-58–S-63, 1994.

1601. Kriz W, Elger M, Nagata M, et al: The role of podocytes in the development of glomerular sclerosis. Kidney Int 45(suppl 42):S-64–S-72, 1994.

1602. Harris RC: Potential physiologic roles for epidermal growth factor in the kidney. Am J Kidney Dis 17:627–630, 1991.

1603. Yoshioka K, Takemura T, Murakami K, et al: Identification and localization of epidermal growth factor and its receptor in the human glomerulus. Lab Invest 63:189–196, 1990.

1604. Adler S, Eng B: Reversal of inhibition of rat glomerular epithelial cell growth by growth factors. Am J Pathol 136:557–563, 1990.

1605. Yoshida Y, Fogo A, Ichikawa I: Glomerular hemodynamic changes vs hypertrophy in experimental glomerular sclerosis. Kidney Int 35:654–660, 1989.

1606. Miller PL, Rennke HG, Meyer TW: Glomerular hypertrophy accelerates hypertensive glomerular injury in rats. Am J Physiol 261:F459–465, 1991.

1607. Schwartz MM, Bidani AK: Role of glomerular epithelial cell injury in the pathogenesis of glomerular scarring in the rat remnant kidney model. Am J Pathol 142:209–219, 1993.

1608. Muda AO, Feriozzi S, Cinotti GA, Faraggiana T: Glomerular hypertrophy and chronic renal failure in focal segmental glomerulosclerosis. Am J Kidney Dis 23:237–241, 1994.

1609. Davies M, Coles GA, Thomas GJ, et al: Proteinases and the glomerulus: Their role in glomerular diseases. Klin Wochenschr 68:1145–1149, 1990.

1610. Davies M, Martin J, Thomas GJ, Lovett DH: Proteinases and glomerular matrix turnover. Kidney Int 41:671–678, 1992.

1611. Laiho M, Keski-Oja J: Growth factors in the regulation of pericellular proteolysis: A review. Cancer Res 49:2533–2553, 1989.

1612. Mullins DE, Rifkin DB: Induction of proteases and protease inhibitors by growth factors. In Sporn MB, Roberts AB (eds): Handbook of Experimental Pharmacology, Vol 95, Peptide Growth Factors and Their Receptors II, Part 2. Springer-Verlag, Berlin, 1990, p 481.

1613. Bejarano PA, Langeveld JPM, Hudson BG, Noelken ME: Degradation of basement membranes by Pseudomonas aeruginosa elastase. Infect Immun 57:3783–3787, 1989.

1614. Dano K, Andreasen PA, Grondahl-Hansen J, et al: Plasminogen activators, tissue degradation, and cancer. Adv Cancer Res 44:139–266, 1985.

1615. Schleef RR, Loskutoff DJ: Fibrinolytic system of vascular endothelial cells. Role of plasminogen activator inhibitors. Haemostasis 18:328–341, 1988.

1616. Stack MS, Moser TL, Pizzo SV: Binding of human plasminogen to basement-membrane (type IV) collagen. Biochem J 284:103–108, 1992.

1617. Matrisian LM: Metalloproteinases and their inhibitors in matrix remodeling. Trends Genet 6:121–125, 1990.

1618. Matrisian LM, Hogan BLM: Growth factor–regulated proteases and extracellular matrix remodeling during mammalian development. Curr Top Dev Biol 24:219–259, 1990.

1619. Matrisian LM: The matrix-degrading metalloproteinases. Bioessays 14:455–463, 1992.

1620. Sorsa T, Konttinen YT, Lindy O, et al: Collagenase in synovitis of rheumatoid arthritis. Semin Arthritis Rheum 22:44–53, 1992.

1621. Marshall BC, Santana A, Xu Q-P, et al: Metalloproteinases and tissue inhibitor of metalloproteinases in mesothelial cells. Cellular differentiation influences expression. J Clin Invest 91:1792–1799, 1993.

1622. Carome MA, Striker LJ, Peten EP, et al: Human glomeruli express TIMP-1 mRNA and TIMP-2 protein and mRNA. Am J Physiol 264:F923–F929, 1993.

1623. Liotta LA, Steeg PS, Stetler-Stevenson WG: Cancer metastasis and angiogenesis: An imbalance of positive and negative regulation. Cell 64:327–336, 1991.

1624. Woessner JF Jr: Matrix metalloproteinases and their inhibitors in connective tissue remodeling. FASEB J 5:2145–2154, 1991.

1625. Marcotte PA, Kozan IM, Dorwin SA, Ryan JM: The matrix metalloproteinase pump-1 catalyzes formation of low molecular weight (pro)urokinase in cultures of normal human kidney cells. J Biol Chem 267:13803–13806, 1992.

1626. Kawanishi S, Imai E, Moriyama T, et al: Differential regulation of tissue inhibitor of metalloproteinases (TIMP)-1, TIMP-2 and stromelysin gene by interleukin 1 (IL-1) and TGF-beta in cultured rat mesangial cells. J Am Soc Nephrol 2:577, 1991.

1627. Tomosugi N, Okada Y, Wada T, et al: Production of metalloproteinase (MMP) and tissue inhibitor of metalloproteinase (TIMP) by human mesanagial cells (MC) and its regulation. J Am Soc Nephrol 2:584, 1991.

1628. Martin J, Knowlden J, Davies M, Williams JD: Characterization of neutral proteinase synthesis by cultured human glomerular cells. J Am Soc Nephrol 2:579, 1991.

1629. Lovett DH, Johnson RJ, Marti H-P, et al: Structural characterization of the mesangial cell type IV collagenase and enhanced expression in a model of immune complex–mediated glomerulonephritis. Am J Pathol 141:85–98, 1992.

1630. Marti H-P, McNeil L, Davies M, et al: Homology cloning of rat 72 kDa type IV collagenase: cytokine and second-messenger inducibility in glomerular mesangial cells. Biochem J 291:441–446, 1993.

1631. Lacave R, Rondeau E, Ochi S, et al: Characterization of a plasminogen activator and its inhibitor in human mesangial cells. Kidney Int 35:806–811, 1989.

1632. Iwamoto T, Nakashima Y, Sueishi K: Secretion of plasminogen activator and its inhibitor by glomerular epithelial cells. Kidney Int 37:1466–1476, 1990.

1633. Martin J, Knowlden J, Davies M, Williams JD: Identification and independent regulation of human mesangial cell metalloproteinases. Kidney Int 46:877–885, 1994.

1634. Wong AP, Cortez SL, Baricos WH: Role of plasmin and gelatinase in extracellular matrix degradation by cultured rat mesangial cells. Am J Physiol 263:F1112–1118, 1992.

1635. Allenberg M, Weinstein T, Silverman M:Activation of procollagenase IV by cytochalasin D and concanavalin A in cultured rat mesangial cells: Linkage to cytoskeletal reorganization. J Am Soc Nephrol 4:1760–1770, 1994.

1636. Walker PD, Kaushal GP, Shah SV: Presence of a distinct extracellular matrix–degrading metalloproteinase activity in renal tubules. J Am Soc Nephrol 5:55–61, 1994.

1637. Kitamura M, Shirasawa T, Maruyama N: Gene transfer of metalloproteinase transin induces aberrant behavior of cultured mesangial cells. Kidney Int 45:1580–1586, 1994.

1638. Vassalli J-D, Dayer J-M, Wohlwend A, Belin D: Concomitant secretion of prourokinase and of a plasminogen activator–specific inhibitor by cultured human monocytes-macrophages. J Exp Med 159:1653–1668, 1984.

1639. Shapiro SD, Campbell EJ, Kobayashi DK, Welgus HG: Immune modulation of metalloproteinase production in human macrophages. Selective pretranslational suppression of interstitial collagenase and stromelysin biosynthesis by interferon-gamma. J Clin Invest 86:1204–1210, 1990.

1640. Welgus HG, Campbell EJ, Bar-Shavit Z, et al: Human alveolar macrophages produce a fibroblast-like collagenase and collagenase inhibitor. J Clin Invest 76:219–224, 1985.

1641. Masure S, Proost P, Van Damme J, Opdenakker G: Purification and identification of 91-kDa neutrophil gelatinase. Release by the activating peptide interleukin-8. Eur J Biochem 198:391–398, 1991.

1642. Dinarello CA: Interleukin-1 and interleukin-1 antagonism. Blood 77:1627–1652, 1991.

1643. Kishimoto T: The biology of interleukin-6. Blood 74:1–10, 1989.

1644. MacNaul KL, Chartrain N, Lark M, et al: Discoordinate expression of stromelysin, collagenase, and tissue inhibitor of metalloproteinases-1 in rheumatoid human synovial fibroblasts. J Biol Chem 265:17238–17245, 1990.

1645. Lotz M, Guerne P-A: Interleukin-6 induces the synthesis of tissue inhibitor of metalloproteinases-1/erythroid potentiating activity (TIMP-1/EPA). J Biol Chem 266:2017–2020, 1991.

1646. Suematsu S, Matsuda T, Aozasa K, et al: IgG1 plasmacytosis in interleukin 6 transgenic mice. Proc Natl Acad Sci USA 86:7547–7551, 1989.

1647. Kerr LD, Miller DB, Matrisian LM: TGF-beta 1 inhibition of transin/stromelysin gene expression is mediated through a Fos binding sequence. Cell 61:267–278, 1990.

1648. Overall CM, Wrana JL, Sodek J: Independent regulation of collagenase, 72-kDa progelatinase, and metalloendoproteinase inhibitor expression in human fibroblasts by transforming growth factor-β. J Biol Chem 264:1860–1869, 1989.

1649. Laiho M, Saksela O, Andreasen PA, Keski-Oja J: Enhanced production and extracellular deposition of the endothelial-type plasminogen activator inhibitor in cultured human lung fibroblasts by transforming growth factor-beta. J Cell Biol 103:2403–2410, 1986.

1650. Kenagy RD, Nikkari ST, Welgus HG, Clowes AW: Heparin inhibits the induction of three matrix metalloproteinases (stromelysis, 92-kD gelatinase, and collagenase) in primate arterial smooth muscle cells. J Clin Invest 93:1987–1993, 1994.

1651. Lindeman RD, Tobin JD, Shock NW: Association between blood pressure and the rate of decline in renal function with age. Kidney Int 26:861–868, 1984.

1652. Neugarten J, Feiner HD, Schacht RG, et al: Aggravation of experimental glomerulonephritis by superimposed clip hypertension. Kidney Int 22:257–263, 1982

1653. Okuda S, Onoyama K, Fujimi S, et al: Influence of hypertension on the progression of experimental autologous immune complex nephritis. J Lab Clin Med 101:461–471, 1983.

1654. Tikkanen I, Miettinen A, Törnroth T, Fyhrquist F: Hypertension and progression of experimental nephritis. Interaction between immunological and hemodynamic factors. Scand J Urol Nephrol Suppl 90:45–50, 1985.

1655. Johnson RJ, Alpers CE, Yoshimura A, et al: Renal injury from angiotensin II-mediated hypertension. Hypertension 19:464–474, 1992.

1656. Springate JE, Feld LG, Ganten D: Renal function in hypertensive rats transgenic for mouse renin gene. Am J Physiol 266:F731–F737, 1993.

1657. Blantz RC, Gabbai F, Gushwa LC, Wilson CB: The influence of concomitant experimental hypertension and glomerulonephritis. Kidney Int 32:652–663, 1987.

1658. Neugarten J, Kaminetsky B, Feiner H, et al: Nephrotoxic serum nephritis with hypertension: amelioration by antihypertensive therapy. Kidney Int 28:135–139, 1985.

1659. Anderson S, Meyer TW, Rennke HG, Brenner BM: Control of glomerular hypertension limits glomerular injury in rats with reduced renal mass. J Clin Invest 76:612–619, 1985.

1660. Baldwin DS, Neugarten J: Role of hypertension in the evolution of renal diseases. Contrib Nephrol 54:63–76, 1987.

1661. Brunner HR: ACE inhibitors in renal disease. Kidney Int 42:463–479, 1992.

1662. Raij L, Azar S, Keane WF: Role of hypertension in progressive glomerular immune injury. Hypertension 7:398–404, 1985.

1663. Stein HD, Sterzel RB, Hunt JD, et al: No aggravation of the course of experimental glomerulonephritis in spontaneously hypertensive rats. Am J Pathol 122:520–530, 1986.

1664. Anderson S, Diamond JR, Karnovsky MJ, Brenner BM: Mechanisms underlying transition from acute glomerular injury to late glomerular sclerosis in a rat model of nephrotic syndrome. J Clin Invest 82:1757–1768, 1988.

1665. Anderson S, Brenner BM: Therapeutic benefit of converting-enzyme inhibition in progressive renal disease. Am J Hypertens 1:380S–383S, 1988.

1666. Lafayette RA, Mayer G, Park SK, Meyer TW: Angiotensin II receptor blockade limits glomerular injury in rats with reduced renal mass. J Clin Invest 90:766–771, 1992.

1667. Sorbi D, Fadly M, Hicks R, et al: Captopril inhibits the 72 kDa and 92 kDa matrix metalloproteinases. Kidney Int 44:1266–1272, 1993.

1668. Tanaka R, Kon V, Yoshioka T, et al: Angiotensin converting enzyme inhibitor modulates glomerular function and structure by distinct mechanisms. Kidney Int 45:537–543, 1994.

1669. Ritz E, Orth S, Weinreich T, Wagner J: Systemic hypertension versus intraglomerular hypertension in progression. Kidney Int 45:438–442, 1994.

1670. Dworkin LD, Benstein JA, Parker M, et al: Calcium antagonists and converting enzyme inhibitors reduce renal injury by different mechanisms. Kidney Int 43:808–814, 1993.

1671. Haller H: Calcium antagonists and cellular mechanisms of glomeruloscerosis and atherosclerosis. Am J Kidney Dis 21(suppl 3):26–31, 1993.

1672. Fogo A, Yoshida Y, Glick AD, et al: Serial micropuncture analysis of glomerular function in two rat models of glomerular sclerosis. J Clin Invest 82:322–330, 1988.

1673. Lax DS, Benstein JA, Tolbert E, Dworkin LD: Effects of salt restriction on renal growth and glomerular injury in rats with remnant kidneys. Kidney Int 41:1527–1534, 1992.

1674. Ardaillou R, Chansel D: Glomerular effects of angiotensin II: A reappraisal based on studies with non–peptide receptor antagonists. J Hypertens Suppl 11:S43–S47, 1993.

1675. Madhun ZT, Ernsberger P, Ke FC, et al: Signal transduction mediated by angiotensin II receptor subtypes expressed in rat renal mesangial cells. Regul Pept 44:149–157, 1993.

1676. Burns KD, Homma T, Harris RC: The intrarenal renin-angiotensin system. Semin Nephrol 13:13–30, 1993.

1677. Gabbai FB, De Nicola L, Thompson SC, et al: Effect of chronic converting enzyme inhibitor (CEI) in rats with chronic glomerulonephritis with (GC) and without hypertension (G). J Am Soc Nephrol 2:678, 1991. Abstract.

1678. Vanhoutte PM: Endothelium and control of vascular function. State of the art lecture. Hypertension 13:658–667, 1989.

1679. Wolf G, Neilson EG: Angiotensin II induces cellular hypertrophy in cultured murine proximal tubular cells. Am J Physiol 259:F768–F777, 1990.

1680. Wolf G, Neilson EG, Goldfarb S, Ziyadeh FN: The influence of glucose concentration on angiotensin II–induced hypertrophy of proximal tubular cells in culture. Biochem Biophys Res Commun 176:902–909, 1991.

1681. Bourcier T, Hassid A: Nitric oxide (NO) and atrial natriuretic peptides inhibit angiotensin II– and vasopressin-induced protein synthesis in cultured aortic smooth muscle cells by a cyclic GMP–independent mechanism. FASEB J 5:A780, 1991. Abstract.

1682. Wolf G, Haberstroh U, Neilson EG: Angiotensin II stimulates the proliferation and biosynthesis of type I collagen in cultured murine mesangial cells. Am J Pathol 140:95–107, 1992.

1683. Anderson PW, Do YS, Hsueh WA: Angiotensin II causes mesangial cell hypertrophy. Hypertension 21:29–35, 1993.

1684. Fogo A: Internephron heterogeneity of growth factors and sclerosis. Kidney Int 45(suppl 45):S-24–S-26, 1994.

1685. Rupprecht HD, Sukhatme VP, Rupprecht AP, et al: Serum response elements mediate protein kinase C dependent transcriptional induction of early growth response gene-1 by arginine vasopressin in rat mesangial cells. J Cell Physiol 159:311–323, 1994.

1686. De Nicola L, Blantz RC, Gabbai FB: Nitric oxide and angiotensin II. Glomerular and tubular interaction in the rat. J Clin Invest 89:1248–1256, 1992.

1687. Baylis C, Harton P, Engels K: Endothelial derived relaxing factor controls renal hemodynamics in the normal rat kidney. J Am Soc Nephrol 1:875–881, 1990.

1688. King AJ, Troy JL, Downes SJ, et al: Effects of N-monomethyl-L-arginine (L-NMMA) on basal renal hemodynamics and the response to amino acid (AA) infusion. Kidney Int 37:371, 1990. Abstract.

1689. Zatz R, de Nucci G: Effects of acute nitric oxide inhibition on rat glomerular microcirculation. Am J Physiol 261:F360–F363, 1991.

1690. Vane J: Control of the circulation by endothelial mediators. Int Arch Allergy Immunol 101:333–345, 1993.

1691. Lamas S, Michel T, Brenner BM, Marsden PA: Nitric oxide synthesis in endothelial cells: Evidence for a pathway inducible by TNF-alpha. Am J Physiol 261:C634–C641, 1991.

1692. Lamas S, Michel T, Collins T, et al: Effects of interferon-gamma on nitric oxide synthase activity and endothelin-1 production by vascular endothelial cells. J Clin Invest 90:879–887, 1992.

1693. Baylis C, Mitruka B, Deng A: Chronic blockade of nitric oxide synthesis in the rat produces systemic hypertension and glomerular damage. J Clin Invest 90:278–281, 1992.

1694. Ribeiro MO, Antunes E, de Nucci G, et al: Chronic inhibition of nitric oxide synthesis. A new model of arterial hypertension. Hypertension 20:298–303, 1992.

1695. Radner W, Hoger H, Lubec B, et al: L-Arginine reduces kidney collagen accumulation and N-epsilon-(carboxymethyl) lysine in the aging NMRI-mouse. J Gerontol 49:M44–M46, 1994.

1696. Fujihara CK, Michellazzo SM, De Nucci G, Zatz R: Sodium excess aggravates hypertension and renal parenchymal injury in rats with chronic NO inhibition. Am J Physiol 266:F697–F705, 1994.

1697. Mayhan WC, Faraci FM, Heistad DD: Impairment of endothelium-dependent responses of cerebral arterioles in chronic hypertension. Am J Physiol 253:H1435–H1440, 1987.

1698. Gabbai FB, Wilson CB, Blantz RC: Role of angiotensin II in experimental membranous nephropathy. Am J Physiol 254:F500–F506, 1988.

1699. Malinski T, Kapturczak M, Dayharsh J, Bohr D: Nitric oxide synthase activity in genetic hypertension. Biochem Biophys Res Commun 194:654–658, 1993.

1700. De Nicola L, Thomson SC, Wead LM, et al: Arginine feeding modifies cyclosporine nephrotoxicity in rats. J Clin Invest 92:1859–1865, 1993.

1701. Muhl H, Kunz D, Rob P, Pfeilschifter J: Cyclosporin derivatives inhibit interleukin 1 beta induction of nitric oxide synthase in renal mesangial cells. Eur J Pharmacol 249:95–100, 1993.

1702. Reyes AA, Karl IE, Kissane J, Klahr S.: L-Arginine administration prevents glomerular hyperfiltration and decreases proteinuria in diabetic rats. J Am Soc Nephrol 4:1039–1045, 1993.

1703. Ketteler M, Border WA, Noble NA: Cytokines and L-arginine in renal injury and repair. Am J Physiol 267:F197–F207, 1994.

1704. Shimamura T, Morrison AB: A progressive glomerulosclerosis occurring in partial five-sixths nephrectomized rats Am J Pathol 79:95–106, 1975.

1705. Hostetter TH, Olson JL, Rennke HG, et al: Hyperfiltration in remnant nephrons: a potentially adverse response to renal ablation. Am J Physiol 241:F85–F93, 1981.

1706. Grond J, Schilthuis MS, Koudstaal J, Elema JD: Mesangial function and glomerular sclerosis in rats after unilateral nephrectomy. Kidney Int 22:338–343, 1982.

1707. Brenner BM, Goldszer RC, Hostetter TH: Glomerular response to renal injury. Contrib Nephrol 33:48–66, 1982.

1708. Olson JL, Hostetter TH, Rennke HG, et al: Altered glomerular permselectivity and progressive sclerosis following extreme ablation of renal mass. Kidney Int 22:112–126, 1982.

1709. Brenner BM: Hemodynamically mediated glomerular injury and the progressive nature of kidney disease. Kidney Int 23:647–655, 1983.

1710. Hayslett JP: Functional adaptation to reduction in renal mass. Physiol Rev 59:137–164, 1979.

1711. Ichikawa I, Ikoma M, Fogo A: Glomerular growth promoters, the common key mediator for progressive glomerular sclerosis in chronic renal diseases. Adv Nephrol 20:127–148, 1991.

1712. Zatz R, Fujihara CK: Glomerular hypertrophy and progressive glomerulopathy. Is there a definite pathogenetic correlation? Kidney Int 45(suppl 45):S-27–S-29, 1994.

1713. Kiprov DD, Colvin RB, McCluskey RT: Focal and segmented glomerulosclerosis and proteinuria associated with unilateral renal agenesis. Lab Invest 46:275–281, 1982.

1714. Harris KPG, Baker F, Brown J, Walls J: Early increase in glomerular leucocyte number after a reduction in renal mass: Implications for the pathogenesis of glomerulosclerosis. Clin Sci 85:27–31, 1993.

1715. Diamond JR, Karnovsky MJ: Nonanticoagulant protective effect of heparin in chronic aminonucleoside nephrosis. Renal Physiol 9:366–374, 1986.

1716. Purkerson ML, Tollefsen, DM, Klahr S: N-desulfated/acetylated heparin ameliorates the progression of renal disease in rats with subtotal renal ablation. J Clin Invest 81:69–74, 1988.

1717. Brenner BM, Meyer TW, Hostetter TH: Dietary protein intake and the progressive nature of kidney disease: The role of hemodynamically mediated glomerular injury in the pathogenesis of progressive glomerular sclerosis in aging, renal ablation, and intrinsic renal disease. N Engl J Med 307:652–659, 1982.

1718. Meyer TW, Anderson S, Brenner BM: Dietary protein intake and progressive glomerular sclerosis: The role of capillary hypertension and hyperperfusion in the progression of renal disease. Ann Intern Med 98:832–838, 1983.

1719. Beukers JJB, Hoedemaeker PJ, Weening JJ: A comparison of the effects of converting-enzyme inhibition and protein restriction in experimental nephrosis. Lab Invest 59:631–640, 1988.

1720. Tapp DC, Wortham WG, Addison JF, et al: Food restriction retards body growth and prevents end-stage renal pathology in remnant kidneys of rats regardless of protein intake. Lab Invest 60:184–195, 1989.

1721. Masoro EJ, Yu BP: Diet and nephropathy. Lab Invest 60:165–167, 1989.

1722. Adams LG, Polzin DJ, Osborne CA, et al: Influence of dietary protein/calorie intake on renal morphology and function in cats with 5/6 nephrectomy. Lab Invest 70:347–357, 1994.

1723. Friend PS, Fernandes G, Good RA, et al: Dietary restrictions early and late. Effects on the nephropathy of the NBZ × NZW mouse. Lab Invest 38:629–632, 1978.

1724. Neugarten J, Feiner HD, Schacht RG, Baldwin DS: Amelioration of experimental glomerulonephritis by dietary protein restriction. Kidney Int 24:595–601, 1983.

1725. Petersen BH, Watson RD, Holmes DH: Protein malnutrition and complement activity in guinea pigs, germ free and conventional rats. J Nutr 110:2159–2165, 1980.

1726. Safai-Kutti S, Fernandes G, Wang Y, et al: Reduction of circulating immune complexes by calorie restriction in (NZB × NZW) F₁ mice. Clin Immunol Immunopathol 15:293–300, 1980.

1727. van Goor H, Fidler V, Weening JJ, Grond J: Determinants of focal and segmental glomerulosclerosis in the rat after renal ablation. Evidence for involvement of macrophages and lipids. Lab Investig 64:754–765, 1991.

1728. Gröne H-J, Walli AK, Gröne EF: Arterial hypertension and hyperlipidemia as determinants of glomerulosclerosis. Clin Investig 71:834–839, 1993.

1729. Kamanna VS, Roh DD, Kirschenbaum MA: Atherogenic lipoproteins: Mediators of glomerular injury. Am J Nephrol 13:1–5, 1993.

1730. Wheeler DC, Chana RS: Interactions between lipoproteins, glomerular cells and matrix. Miner Electrolyte Metab 19:149–164, 1993.

1731. Schlondorff D: Cellular mechanisms of lipid injury in the glomerulus. Am J Kidney Dis 22:72–82, 1993.

1732. Baba N, Shimokama T, Watanabe T: Effects of hypercholesterolemia on initial and chronic phases of rat nephrotoxic serum nephritis: Development of focal segmental glomerulosclerosis, analogous to atherosclerosis. Virchows Arch B 64:97–105, 1993.

1733. Avram MM: Low-density lipoprotein immunofluorescence at the site of renal injury in glomerulosclerosis: A potential pathogenetic role for lipids in renal disease. Am J Kidney Dis 22:69–71, 1993.

1734. Kamanna V, Kirschenbaum MA: Association between very-low-density lipoprotein and glomerular injury in obese Zucker rats. Am J Nephrol 13:53–58, 1993.

1735. Magil AB, Frohlich JJ, Innis SM, Steinbrecher UP: Oxidized low-density lipoprotein in experimental focal glomerulosclerosis. Kidney Int 43:1243–1250, 1993.

1736. van Goor H, van der Horst MLC, Atmosoerodjo J, et al: Renal apolipoproteins in nephrotic rats. Am J Pathol 142:1804–1812, 1993.

1737. Wheeler DC, Chana RS, Topley N, et al: Oxidation of low density lipoprotein by mesangial cells may promote glomerular injury. Kidney Int 45:1628–1636, 1994.

1738. Kramer A, Nauck M, Pavenstadt H, et al: Receptor-mediated uptake of IDL and LDL from nephrotic patients by glomerular epithelial cells. Kidney Int 44:1341–1351, 1993.

1739. Takemura T, Yoshioka K, Aya N, et al: Apolipoproteins and lipoprotein receptors in glomeruli in human kidney diseases. Kidney Int 43:918–927, 1993.

1740. Kasiske BL, O'Donnell MP, Kim Y, et al: Cholesterol synthesis inhibitors inhibit more than cholesterol synthesis. Kidney Int 45(suppl 45):S-51–S-53, 1994.

1741. Fine LG: How little kidney tissue is enough? N Engl J Med 325:1097–1099, 1991.

1742. Novick AC, Gephardt G, Guz B, et al: Long-term follow-up after partial removal of a solitary kidney. N Engl J Med 325:1058–1062, 1991.

1743. Doi T, Striker LJ, Quaife C, et al: Progressive glomerulosclerosis develops in transgenic mice chronically expressing growth hormone and growth hormone releasing factor but not in those expressing insulinlike growth factor-1. Am J Pathol 131:398–403, 1988.

1744. Quaife CJ, Mathews LS, Pinkert CA, et al: Histopathology associated with elevated levels of growth hormone and insulin-like growth factor 1 in transgenic mice. Endocrinology 124:40–48, 1989.

1745. MacKay K, Striker LJ, Pinkert CA, et al: Glomerulosclerosis and renal cysts in mice transgenic for the early region of SV40. Kidney Int 32:827–837, 1987.

1746. Weiher H, Noda T, Gray DA, et al: Transgenic mouse model of kidney disease: Insertional inactivation of ubiquitously expressed gene leads to nephrotic syndrome. Cell 62:425–434, 1990.

1747. Doi T, Striker LJ, Kimata K, et al: Glomerulosclerosis in mice transgenic for growth hormone. Increased mesangial extracellular matrix is correlated with kidney mRNA levels. J Exp Med 173:1287–1290, 1991.

1748. Yang C-W, Striker LJ, Kopchick JJ, et al: Glomerulosclerosis in mice transgenic for native or mutated bovine hormone gene. Kidney Int 43(suppl 39):S-90–S-94, 1993.

1749. Peten EP, Striker LJ, Garcia-Perez A, Striker GE: Studies by competitive PCR of glomerulosclerosis in growth hormone transgenic mice. Kidney Int 43(suppl 39):S-55–S-58, 1993.

1750. Yang C-W, Striker LJ, Pesce C, et al: Glomerulosclerosis and body growth are mediated by different portions of bovine growth hormone. Studies in transgenic mice. Lab Invest 68:62–70, 1993.

1751. Peten EP, Yang C-W, Striker GE, Striker LJ: Gene activation in glomerulosclerosis: A role for growth promoting hormones. Kidney Int 45(suppl 45):S-48–S-50, 1994.

1752. Fattori E, Rocca CD, Costa P, et al: Development of progressive kidney damage and myeloma kidney in interleukin-6 transgenic mice. Blood 83:2570–2579, 1994.

1753. Dickie P, Felser J, Eckhaus M, et al: HIV-associated nephropathy in transgenic mice expressing HIV-1 genes. Virology 185:109–119, 1991.

1754. Kopp JB, Klotman ME, Adler SH, et al: Progressive glomerulosclerosis and enhanced renal accumulation of basement membrane components in mice transgenic for human immunodeficiency virus type 1 genes. Proc Natl Acad Sci USA 89:1577–1581, 1992.

1755. Weiher H: Glomerular sclerosis in transgenic mice: The *Mpv-17* gene and its human homologue. Adv Nephrol 22:37–42, 1993.

1756. Dressler GR, Wilkinson JE, Rothenpieler UW, et al: Deregulation of *Pax-2* expression in transgenic mice generates severe kidney abnormalities. Nature 362:65–67, 1993.

1757. Kestilä M, Männikkö M, Holmberg C, et al: Congenital nephrotic syndrome of the Finnish type is not associated with the Pax-2 gene despite the promising transgenic animal model. Genomics 19:570–572, 1994.

1758. Isaka Y, Fujiwara Y, Ueda N, et al: Glomerulosclerosis induced by in vivo transfection of transforming growth factor-β or platelet-derived growth factor gene into the rat kidney. J Clin Invest 92:2597–2601, 1993.

1759. Kollias G, Evans DJ, Ritter M, et al: Ectopic expression of Thy-1 in the kidneys of transgenic mice induces functional and proliferative abnormalities. Cell 51:21–31, 1987.

1760. Giacomini P, Ciucci A, Nicotra MR, et al: Tissue-specific expression of the *HLA-DRA* gene in transgenic mice. Immunogenetics 34:385–391, 1991.

1761. Song YW, Tsao BP, Hahn BH: Contribution of major histocompatibility complex (MHC) to upregulation of anti-DNA antibody in transgenic mice. J Autoimmun 6:1–9, 1993.

1762. Lo D, Quill H, Burkly L, et al: A recessive defect in lymphocyte or granulocyte function caused by an integrated transgene. Am J Pathol 141:1237–1246, 1992.

1763. Breslow JL: Transgenic mouse models of lipoprotein metabolism and atherosclerosis. Proc Natl Acad Sci USA 90:8314–8318, 1993.

1764. Unanue ER, Dixon FJ: Experimental glomerulonephritis. V. Studies on the interaction of nephrotoxic antibodies with tissues of the rat. J Exp Med 121:697–714, 1965.

1765. Lerner RA, Dixon FJ: Transfer of ovine experimental allergic glomerulonephritis (EAG) with serum. J Exp Med 124:431, 1966.

1766. Unanue ER, Dixon FJ, Feldman JD: Experimental allergic glomerulonephritis induced in the rabbit with homologous renal antigens. J Exp Med 125:163–176, 1967.

1767. Weening JJ, Prins FA, Fransen JAM, et al: Methods in laboratory investigation. Ultrastructural localization and quantitation of nephritogenic antibodies in experimental glomerulonephritis. Lab Invest 55:372–376, 1986.

1768. Van Zyl Smit R, Rees AJ, Peters DK: Factors affecting severity of injury during nephrotoxic nephritis in rabbits. Clin Exp Immunol 54:366–372, 1983.

1769. Krakower CA, Greenspon SA: Localization of the nephrotoxic antigen within the isolated renal glomerulus. Arch Pathol 51:629–639, 1951.

1770. Krakower CA, Greenspon SA: The localization of the "nephrotoxic" antigen(s) in extraglomerular tissues. Observations including a measure of its concentration in certain locales. Arch Pathol 66:364–383, 1958.

1771. Yong LCJ, Rhodes GC: The clearance of heterologous antibodies in experimental antibasement membrane antibody mediated glomerulonephritis. Exp Pathol 39:79–87, 1990.

1772. Kefalides NA: Isolation of a collagen from basement membranes containing three identical α-chains. Biochem Biophys Res Commun 45:226–234, 1971.

1773. Wick G, Glanville RW, Timpl R: Characterization of antibodies to basement membrane (type IV) collagen in immunohistological studies. Immunobiology 156:372–381, 1979.

1774. Bender BL, Jaffe R, Carlin B, Chung, AE: Immunolocalization of entactin, a sulfated basement membrane component, in rodent tissues, and comparison with GP-2 (laminin). Am J Pathol 103:419–426, 1981.

1775. Michael AF, Yang J-Y, Falk RJ, et al: Monoclonal antibodies to human renal basement membranes: Heterogenic and ontogenic changes. Kidney Int 24:74–86, 1983.

1776. Jaffe R, Bender B, Santamaria M, Chung AE: Segmental staining of the murine nephron by monoclonal antibodies directed against the GP-2 subunit of laminin. Lab Invest 51:88–96, 1984.

1777. Scheinman JI, Tsai C: Monoclonal antibody to type IV collagen with selective basement membrane localization. Lab Invest 50:101–112, 1984.

1778. Sariola H, Timpl R, von der Mark K, et al: Dual origin of glomerular basement membrane. Dev Biol 101:86–96, 1984.

1779. Bonadio JF, Sage H, Cheng F, et al: Localization of collagen types IV and V, laminin, and heparan sulfate proteoglycan to the basal lamina of kidney epithelial cells in transfilter metanephric culture. Am J Pathol 116:289–296, 1984.

1780. Abrahamson DR: Origin of the glomerular basement membrane visualized after in vivo labeling of laminin in newborn rat kidneys. J Cell Biol 100:1988–2000, 1985.

1781. Abrahamson DR, Caulfield JP: Distribution of laminin within rat and mouse renal, splenic, intestinal, and hepatic basement membranes identified after the intravenous injection of heterologous antilaminin IgG. Lab Invest 52:169–181, 1985.

1782. Abrahamson DR, Perry EW: Evidence for splicing new basement membrane into old during glomerular development in newborn rat kidneys. J Cell Biol 103:2489–2498, 1986.

1783. Abrahamson DR: Structure and development of the glomerular capillary wall and basement membrane. Am J Physiol 253:F783–F794, 1987.

1784. Wick G, Müller PU, Timpl R: In vivo localization and pathological effects of passively transferred antibodies to type IV collagen and laminin in mice. Clin Immunol Immunopathol 23:656–665, 1982.

1785. Yaar M, Foidart JM, Brown KS, et al: The Goodpasture-like syndrome in mice induced by intravenous injections of anti–type IV collagen and anti-laminin antibody. Am J Pathol 107:79–91, 1982.

1786. Abrahamson DR, Caulfield JP: Proteinuria and structural alterations in rat glomerular basement membranes induced by intravenously injected anti-laminin immunoglobulin G. J Exp Med 156:128–145, 1982.

1787. Mackel AM, DeLustro F, LeRoy EC: Cell-mediated immunity to homologous basement membrane (type IV) collagen in C57BL/6 mice. Clin Immunol Immunopathol 21:204–216, 1981.

1788. Mackel AM, De Lustro F, LeRoy EC:Cross-reactivity of cell-mediated immunity between interstitial (type 1) and basement membrane (type IV) collagens. J Exp Med 156:1042–1056, 1982.

1789. Mackel AM, DeLustro F, LeRoy EC: Immune response to laminin, a noncollagenous glycoprotein of basement membrane, in a syngeneic murine system (41484). Proc Soc Exp Biol Med 171:98–108, 1982.

1790. Szarfman A, Terranova VP, Rennard SI, et al: Antibodies to laminin in Chagas' disease. J Exp Med 155:1161–1171, 1982.

1791. Bruijn JA, Oemar BS, Ehrich JHH, et al: Anti–basement membrane glomerulopathy in experimental trypanosomiasis. J Immunol 139:2482–2488, 1987.

1792. Feintzeig ID, Abrahamson DR, Cybulsky AV, et al: Nephritogenic potential of sheep antibodies against glomerular basement membrane laminin in the rat. Lab Invest 54:531–542, 1986.

1793. Makino H, Gibbons JT, Reddy MK, Kanwar YS: Nephritogenicity of antibodies to proteoglycans of the glomerular basement membrane-I. J Clin Invest 77:142–156, 1986.

1794. Miettinen A, Stow JL, Mentone S, Farquhar MG: Antibodies to basement membrane heparan sulfate proteoglycans bind to the laminae rarae of the glomerular basement membrane (GBM) and induce subepithelial GBM thickening. J Exp Med 163:1064–1084, 1986.

1795. Lelongt B, Kashihara N, Makino H, Kanwar YS: Influence of genetics on the nephritogenic potential of proteoglycans. Am J Pathol 141:561–569, 1992.

1796. Makino H, Lelongt B, Kanwar YS: Nephritogenicity of proteoglycans. II. A model of immune complex nephritis. Kidney Int 34:195–208, 1988.

1797. Makino H, Lelongt B, Kanwar YS: Nephritogenicity of proteoglycans. III. Mechanism of immune deposit formation. Kidney Int 34:209–219, 1988.

1798. van den Born J, van den Heuvel LPWJ, Bakker MAH, et al: A monoclonal antibody against GBM heparan sulfate induces an acute selective proteinuria in rats. Kidney Int 41:115–123, 1992.

1799. Hara M, Kihara I, Morita T, et al: Autoimmune antiglomerular basement membrane glomerulonephritis induced with isologous renal antigen in rats. Acta Pathol Jpn 31:367–377, 1981.

1800. Stuffers-Heiman M, Tjoeng-Mutsaerts N, Ferwerda W, Van Es LA: Immunological properties of glomerular basement membrane antigens solubilized by elastase digestion. J Immunol Methods 32:93–102, 1980.

1801. Unanue ER, Dixon FJ: Experimental glomerulonephritis. VI. The autologous phase of nephrotoxic serum nephritis. J Exp Med 121:715–725, 1965.

1802. de Almeida DB, Curi PR: Treatment of rat nephrotoxic nephritis. Use of 5-fluorouracil or methotrexate-5-fluorouracil association. Clin Exp Immunol 57:591–599, 1984.

1803. Hara S, Fukatsu A, Suzuki N, et al: The effects of a new immunosuppressive agent, FK506, on the glomerular injury in rats with accelerated nephrotoxic serum glomerulonephritis. Clin Immunol Immunopathol 57:351–362, 1990.

1804. Nagamatsu T, Kojima N, Kondo N, et al: Suppression by cyclosporin A of anti-GBM nephritis in rats. Jpn J Pharmacol 58:27–36, 1992.

1805. Sato T, Oite T, Nagase M, Shimizu F: Nephrotoxic serum nephritis in nude rats: The roles of host immune reactions. Clin Exp Immunol 84:139–144, 1991.

1806. Unanue ER, Lee S, Dixon FJ, Feldman JD: Experimental glomerulonephritis. VII. The absence of an autoimmune antikidney response in nephrotoxic serum nephritis. J Exp Med 122:565–578, 1965.

1807. Ito M, Yamada H, Okamoto K, Suzuki Y: Crescentic type nephritis induced by anti–glomerular basement membrane (GBM) serum in rats. Jpn J Pharmacol 33:1145–1154, 1983.

1808. Granados R, Mendrick DL, Rennke HG: Antibody-induced crescent formation in WKY rats: Potential role of antibody-dependent cell cytotoxicity (ADCC) in vivo. Kidney Int 37:414, 1990. Abstract.

1809. Hill PA, Lan HY, Nikolic-Paterson DJ, Atkins RC: The ICAM-1/LFA-1 interaction in glomerular leukocytic accumulation in anti-GBM glomerulonephritis. Kidney Int 45:700–708, 1994.

1810. Nishihara T, Kusuyama Y, Gen E, et al: Masugi nephritis produced by the antiserum to heterologous glomerular basement membrane. I. Results in mice. Acta Pathol Jpn 31:85–92, 1981.

1811. Kusuyama Y, Nishihara T, Gen E, Saito K: Effect of cyclophosphamide on murine nephrotoxic nephritis. Nephron 33:220–223, 1983.

1812. Wheeler J, Morley AR, Appleton DR: Anti–glomerular basement membrane (GBM) glomerulonephritis in the mouse: Development of disease and cell proliferation. J Exp Pathol 71:411–422, 1990.

1813. Kusuyama Y, Nishihara T, Saito K: Nephrotoxic nephritis in nude mice. Clin Exp Immunol 46:20–26, 1981.

1814. Okada K, Oite T, Kihara I, et al: Masugi nephritis in the nude mice and their normal littermates. Acta Pathol Jpn 32:1–11, 1982.

1815. Assmann KJM, Tangelder MM, Lange WPJ, et al: Anti-GBM nephritis in the mouse: Severe proteinuria in the heterologous phase. Virchows Arch A 406:285–300, 1985.

1816. Tipping PG, Boyce NW, Holdsworth SR: Relative contributions of chemo-attractant and terminal components of complement to anti–glomerular basement membrane (GBM) glomerulonephritis. Clin Exp Immunol 78:444–448, 1989.

1817. Schrijver G, Schalkwijk J, Robben JCM, et al: Antiglomerular basement membrane nephritis in beige mice. Deficiency of leukocyte neutral proteinases prevents the induction of albuminuria in the heterologous phase. J Exp Med 169:1435–1448, 1989.

1818. Makino H, Nishimura S, Takaoka M, Ota Z: Mechanism of hematuria. II. A scanning electron microscopic demonstration of the passage of blood cells through a glomerular capillary wall in rabbit Masugi nephritis. Nephron 50:142–150, 1988.

1819. Couser WG, Darby C, Salant DJ, et al: Anti–GBM antibody–induced proteinuria in isolated perfused rat kidney. Am J Physiol 249:F241–F250, 1985.

1820. Boyce NW, Holdsworth SR: Anti–glomerular basement membrane antibody–induced experimental glomerulonephritis: Evidence for dose-dependent, direct antibody and complement-induced, cell-independent injury. J Immunol 135:3918–3921, 1985.

1821. Boyce NW, Holdsworth SR: Direct antiGBM antibody induced alterations in glomerular permselectivity. Kidney Int 30:666–672, 1986.

1822. Allison ME, Wilson CB, Gottschalk CW: Pathophysiology of experimental glomerulonephritis in rats. J Clin Invest 53:1402, 1974.

1823. Eddy AA: Tubulointerstitial nephritis during the heterologous phase of nephrotoxic serum nephritis. Nephron 59:304–313, 1991.

1824. Wilson CB, Blantz RC: Nephroimmunopathology and pathophysiology. Am J Physiol 248:F319–F331, 1985.

1825. Savige JA, Dash AC, Rees AJ: Exaggerated glomerular albuminuria after cobra venom factor in anti–glomerular basement membrane disease. Nephron 52:29–35, 1989.

1826. Boyce NW, Holdsworth SR: Intrarenal hemodynamic alterations induced by anti-GBM antibody. Kidney Int 31:8–14, 1987.

1827. Timmermans V, Peake PW, Charlesworth JA, et al: Angiotensin II receptor regulation in anti–glomerular basement membrane nephritis. Kidney Int 38:518–524, 1990.

1828. Blantz RC, Tucker BJ, Gushwa LC, et al: Glomerular immune injury in the rat: The influence of angiotensin II and α-adrenergic inhibitors. Kidney Int 20:452–461, 1981.

1829. Wilson CB, Gushwa LC, Peterson OW, et al: Glomerular immune injury in the rat: Effect of antagonists of histamine activity. Kidney Int 20:628–635, 1981.

1830. Alfino PA, Neugarten J, Schacht RG, et al: Glomerular size-selective barrier dysfunction in nephrotoxic serum nephritis. Kidney Int 34:151–155, 1988.

1831. Sharma VK, Pratap VK, Mehrotra ML, Mishra SD: Goodpasture's syndrome-like lesions after intraperitoneal administration of rabbit antirat lung serum in rats. Indian J Chest Dis Allied Sci 25:101–107, 1983.

1832. Boyce NW, Fernando NS, Neale TJ, Holdsworth SR: Acute pulmonary and renal injury after administration of heterologous anti-lung antibodies in the rat. Characterization of ultrastructural binding sites, basement membrane epitopes, and inflammatory mediation systems. Lab Invest 64:272–278, 1991.

1833. Jennings L, Roholt OA, Pressman D, et al: Experimental anti–alveolar basement membrane antibody–mediated pneumonitis. I. The role of increased permeability of the alveolar capillary wall induced by oxygen. J Immunol 127:129–134, 1981.

1834. Downie GH, Roholt OA, Jennings L, et al: Experimental anti–alveolar basement membrane antibody–mediated pneumonitis. II. Role of endothelial damage and repair, induction of autologous phase, and kinetics of antibody deposition in Lewis rats. J Immunol 129:2647–2652, 1982.

1835. Yamamoto T, Wilson CB: Binding of anti–basement membrane antibody to alveolar basement membrane after intratracheal gasoline instillation in rabbits. Am J Pathol 126:497–505, 1987.

1836. O'Regan S, Turgeon C: Lack of antiglomerular basement membrane antibody binding to alveolar membranes after hydrocarbon exposure in rats. J Clin Lab Immunol 20:147–149, 1986.

1837. Steblay RW: Glomerulonephritis induced in sheep by injections of heterologous glomerular basement membrane and Freund's complete adjuvant. J Exp Med 116:253–272, 1962.

1838. Steblay RW, Rudofsky UH: Experimental autoimmune glomerulonephritis induced by anti–glomerular basement membrane antibody. II. Effects of injecting heterologous, homologous, or autologous glomerular basement membranes and complete Freund's adjuvant into sheep. Am J Pathol 113:125–133, 1983.

1839. James MP, Herdson PB, Gavin JB: Recurrence of antiglomerular basement membrane glomerulonephritis in sheep renal allografts. Pathology 13:335–344, 1981.

1840. Bygren P, Wieslander J, Heinegård D: Glomerulonephritis induced in sheep by immunization with human glomerular basement membrane. Kidney Int 31:25–31, 1987.

1841. Wilson CB, Dixon FJ: Renal injury from immune reactions involving antigens in or of the kidney. In Wilson CB, Brenner BM, Stein JH (eds): Contemporary Issues in Nephrology, Vol 3. Churchill Livingstone, New York, 1979, pp 35–66.

1842. Steblay RW, Rudofsky UH: Experimental autoimmune antiglomerular basement membrane antibody–induced glomerulonephritis. I. The effects of injecting sheep with human, homologous or autologous lung basement membranes and complete Freund's adjuvant. Clin Immunol Immunopathol 27:65–80, 1983.

1843. Lubec G: A new model for autoimmunity and the kidney. Nephron 57:129–130, 1991.

1844. Wick G, Von der Mark H, Dietrich H, Timpl R: Globular domain of basement membrane collagen induces autoimmune pulmonary lesions in mice resembling human Goodpasture disease. Lab Invest 55:308–317, 1986.

1845. Kazama T, Nakamura T, Morioka T, et al: A nephropathy induced by immunization of rats with EMS tumour. Clin Exp Immunol 62:104–111, 1985.

1846. Murphy-Ullrich JE, Oberley TD: Immune-mediated injury to basement membranes in mice immunized with murine laminin. Clin Immunol Immunopathol 31:33–43, 1984.

1847. Matsuo S, Brentjens JR, Andres G, et al: Distribution of basement membrane antigens in glomeruli of mice with autoimmune glomerulonephritis. Am J Pathol 122:36–49, 1986.

1848. Abrass CK, Cohen AH: Characterization of renal injury initiated by immunization of rats with heparan sulfate. Am J Pathol 130:103, 1988.

1849. Bannister KM, Ulich TR, Wilson CB: Induction, characterization, and cell transfer of autoimmune tubulointerstitial nephritis in the Lewis rat. Kidney Int 32:642–651, 1987.

1850. Reynolds J, Cashman SJ, Evans DJ, Pusey CD: Cyclosporin A in the prevention and treatment of experimental autoimmune glomerulonephritis in the brown Norway rat. Clin Exp Immunol 85:28–32, 1991.

1851. Sado Y, Watanabe K, Okigaki T, et al: Isolation and characterization of nephritogenic antigen from bovine glomerular basement membrane. Biochim Biophys Acta 798:96–102, 1984.

1852. Sado Y, Okigaki T, Takamiya H, Seno S: Experimental autoimmune glomerulonephritis with pulmonary hemorrhage in rats. The dose-effect relationship of the nephritogenic antigen from bovine glomerular basement membrane. J Clin Lab Immunol 15:199–204, 1984.

1853. Sado Y, Naito I, Akita M, Okigaki T: Strain specific responses of inbred rats on the severity of experimental autoimmune glomerulonephritis. J Clin Lab Immunol 19:193–199, 1986.

1854. Naito I, Sado Y: Early changes of rat experimental autoimmune glomerulonephritis induced with the nephritogenic antigen from bovine renal basement membranes. J Clin Lab Immunol 28:187–193, 1989.

1855. Sado Y, Kagawa M, Naito I, Okigaki T: Properties of bovine nephritogenic antigen that induces anti-GBM nephritis in rats and its similarity to the Goodpasture antigen. Virchows Arch B 60:345–351, 1991.

1856. Sado Y, Naito I, Okigaki T: Transfer of anti–glomerular basement membrane antibody–induced glomerulonephritis in inbred rats with isologous antibodies from the urine of nephritic rats. J Pathol 158:325–332, 1989.

1857. Sado Y, Kagawa M, Rauf S, et al: Isologous monoclonal antibodies can induce anti-GBM glomerulonephritis in rats. J Pathol 168:221–227, 1992.

1858. Nishikawa K, Andres G, Bhan AK, et al: Hyaluronate is a component of crescents in rat autoimmune glomerulonephritis. Lab Invest 68:146–153, 1993.

1859. Tsuji Y, Okuyama K, Kobayashi K, et al: Studies on cell-mediated immunity (CMI) in the glomeruli: Immunization with GBM antigen from Masugi nephritis in Wistar-Kyoto rats. Nippon Jinzo Gakkai Shi 36:95–102, 1994.

1860. Kalluri R, Gattone VH II, Noelken ME, Hudson BG: The α3 chain of type IV collagen induces autoimmune Goodpasture syndrome. Proc Natl Acad Sci USA 91:6201–6205, 1994.

1861. Goldman M, Baran D, Druet P: Polyclonal activation and experimental nephropathies. Kidney Int 34:141–150, 1988.

1862. Girolami JP, Orfila C, Cabos-Boutot G, et al: Early acute effects of mercuric chloride on synthesis and release of kallikrein and on distal tubular morphology of rat renal cortical slices. Renal Physiol Biochem 13:223–232, 1990.

1863. Lash LH, Zalups RK: Mercuric chloride–induced cytotoxicity and compensatory hypertrophy in rat kidney proximal tubular cells. J Pharmacol Exp Ther 261:819–829, 1992.

1864. Sapin C, Druet E, Druet P: Induction of anti–glomerular basement membrane antibodies in the Brown-Norway rat by mercuric chloride. Clin Exp Immunol 28:173–179, 1977.

1865. Sapin C, Mandet C, Druet E, et al: Immune complex type disease induced by HgCl₂: Genetic control of susceptibility. Transplant Proc 13:1404–1406, 1981.

1866. Michaelson JH, McCoy JP Jr, Bigazzi PE: Antibodies to glomerular basement membrane: Detection by an enzyme-linked immunosorbent assay in the sera of Brown Norway rats. Kidney Int 20:285–288, 1981.

1867. Bellon B, Capron M, Druet E, et al: Mercuric chloride induced autoimmune disease in Brown-Norway rats: Sequential search for anti–basement membrane antibodies and circulating immune complexes. Eur J Clin Invest 12:127–133, 1982.

1868. Druet E, Mahieu P, Foidart JM, Druet P: Magnetic solid-phase enzyme immunoassay for the detection of anti–glomerular basement membrane antibodies. J Immunol Methods 48:149–157, 1982.

1869. Pusey CD, Bowman C, Peters DK, Lockwood CM: Effects of cyclophosphamide on autoantibody synthesis in the Brown Norway rat. Clin Exp Immunol 54:697–704, 1983.

1870. Goter Robinson CJ, Abraham AA, Balazs T: Induction of anti-nuclear antibodies by mercuric chloride in mice. Clin Exp Immunol 58:300–306, 1984.

1871. Hoedemaeker PHJ: Glomerular antigens in experimental glomerulonephritis. Int Rev Exp Pathol 30:159–229, 1988.

1872. Aten J, Bosman CB, Rozing J, et al: Mercuric chloride–induced autoimmunity in the Brown Norway rat. Cellular kinetics and major histocompatibility complex antigen expression. Am J Pathol 133:127–138, 1988.

1873. Hue J, Pelletier L, Berlin M, Druet P: Autoimmune glomerulonephritis induced by mercury vapour exposure in the Brown Norway rat. Toxicology 79:119–129, 1993.

1874. Henry GA, Jarnot BM, Steinhoff MM, Bigazzi PE: Mercury-induced renal autoimmunity in the MAXX rat. Clin Immunol Immunopathol 49:187–203, 1988.

1875. Aten J, Veninga A, Bruijn JA, et al: Antigenic specificities of glomerular-bound autoantibodies in membranous glomerulopathy induced by mercuric chloride. Clin Immunol Immunopathol 63:89–102, 1992.

1876. Makker SP, Kanalas JJ: Renal antigens in mercuric chloride induced, anti-GBM autoantibody glomerular disease. Kidney Int 37:64–71, 1990.

1877. Guéry J-C, Druet E, Glotz D, et al: Specificity and crossreactive idiotypes of anti–glomerular basement membrane autoantibodies in HgCl₂-induced autoimmune glomerulonephritis. Eur J Immunol 20:93–100, 1990.

1878. Michaelson JH, McCoy JP Jr, Hirszel P, Bigazzi PE: Mercury-induced autoimmune glomerulonephritis in inbred rats. I. Kinetics and species specificity of autoimmune responses. Surv Synth Pathol Res 4:401–411, 1985.

1879. Druet E, Fournie G, Mandet C, et al: Genetic control of susceptibility to immune complex type nephritis induced by HgCl₂ in rats. Transplant Proc 11:1600–1603, 1979.

1880. Prouvost-Danon A, Abadie A, Sapin C, et al: Induction of IgE synthesis and potentiation of anti-ovalbumin IgE antibody response by HgCl₂ in the rat. J Immunol 126:699–702, 1981.

1881. Hirsch F, Couderc J, Sapin C, et al: Polyclonal effect of HgCl₂ in the rat, its possible role in an experimental autoimmune disease. Eur J Immunol 12:620–625, 1982.

1882. Pelletier L, Pasquier R, Guettier C, et al: HgCl₂ induces T and B cells to proliferate and differentiate in BN rats. Clin Exp Immunol 71:336–342, 1988.

1883. Sapin C, Druet P, Mandet C: Induction of susceptibility to HgCl₂ immune glomerulonephritis in the Lewis rat by immunocompetent cells from susceptible F₁ hybrids. Eur J Immunol 10:371–374, 1980.

1884. Hirsch F, Druet E, Vendeville B, et al: Production of monoclonal anti–glomerular basement membrane antibodies during autoimmune glomerulonephritis. Clin Immunol Immunopathol 33:425–430, 1984.

1885. Pelletier L, Pasquier R, Hirsch F, et al: Autoreactive T cells in mercury-induced autoimmune disease: In vitro demonstration. J Immunol 137:2548–2554, 1986.

1886. Aten J, Veninga A, De Heer E, et al: Susceptibility to the induction of either autoimmunity or immunosuppression by mercuric chloride is related to the major histocompatibility complex class II haplotype. Eur J Immunol 21:611–616, 1991.

1887. Kosuda LL, Greiner DL, Bigazzi PE: Mercury-induced renal autoimmunity in BN→LEW.1N chimeric rats. Cell Immunol 155:77–94, 1994.

1888. Bruijn JA, Van Elven EH, Corver WE, et al: Genetics of experimental lupus nephritis: Non–H-2 factors determine susceptibility for renal involvement in murine chronic graft-versus-host disease. Clin Exp Immunol 76:284–289, 1989.

1889. van Vliet E, Uhrberg M, Stein C, Gleichmann E: MHC control of IL-4–dependent enhancement of B cell Ia expression and Ig class switching in mice treated with mercuric chloride. Int Arch Allergy Immunol 101:392–401, 1993.

1890. Baran D, Vendeville B, Vial MC, et al: Effect of cyclosporine A on mercuric-induced glomerulonephritis in the Brown Norway rat. Clin Nephrol 25(suppl 1):S175–S180, 1986.

1891. Aten J, Bosman CB, De Heer E, et al: Cyclosporin A induces long-term unresponsiveness in mercuric chloride-induced autoimmune glomerulonephritis. Clin Exp Immunol 73:307–311, 1988.

1892. Madrenas J, Parfrey NA, Halloran PF: Interferon gamma–mediated renal MHC expression in mercuric chloride–induced glomerulonephritis. Kidney Int 39:273–281, 1991.

1893. Lillevang ST, Rosenkvist J, Andersen CB, et al: Single and combined effects of the vitamin D analogue KH1060 and cyclosporin A on mercuric-chloride–induced autoimmune disease in the BN rat. Clin Exp Immunol 88:301–306, 1992.

1894. Rossi F, Bellon B, Vial MC, et al: Beneficial effect of human therapeutic intravenous immunoglobulins (IVIg) in mercuric-chloride-induced autoimmune disease of Brown-Norway rats. Clin Exp Immunol 84:129–133, 1991.

1895. Bowman C, Mason DW, Pusey CD, Lockwood CM: Autoregulation of autoantibody synthesis in mercuric chloride nephritis in the Brown Norway rat. I. A role for T suppressor cells. Eur J Immunol 14:464–470, 1984.

1896. Chalopin JM, Lockwood CM: Autoregulation of autoantibody synthesis in mercuric chloride nephritis in the Brown Norway rat. II. Presence of antigen-augmentable plaque-forming cells in the spleen is associated with humoral factors behaving as auto-anti-idiotypic antibodies. Eur J Immunol 14:470–475, 1984.

1897. Lockwood CM: Regulation of autoantibody responses to glomerular basement membrane in man and experimental animals. Ciba Found Symp 108:227–242, 1984.

1898. Mathieson PW, Stapleton KJ, Oliveira DBG, Lockwood CM: Immunoregulation of mercuric chloride–induced autoimmunity in Brown Norway rats: A role for CD8⁺ T cells revealed by in vivo depletion studies. Eur J Immunol 21:2105–2109, 1991.

1899. Pelletier L, Rossert J, Pasquier R, et al: HgCl₂-induced perturbation of the T cell network in experimental allergic encephalomyelitis. Cell Immunol 137:379–388, 1991.

1900. Pelletier L, Galceran M, Pasquier R, et al: Down modulation of Heymann's nephritis by mercuric chloride. Kidney Int 32:227–232, 1987.

1901. Baran D, Lantz O, Dosquet P, et al: Interleukin-2 production in Brown-Norway rats with HgCl₂-induced autoimmune disease: paradoxical in vivo versus in vitro findings. Clin Exp Immunol 73:401–405, 1988.

1902. Eneström S, Hultman P: Immune-mediated glomerulonephritis induced by mercuric chloride in mice. Experientia 40:1234–1240, 1984.

1903. Hultman P, Eneström S: The induction of immune complex deposits in mice by peroral and parenteral administration of mercuric chloride: strain dependent susceptibility. Clin Exp Immunol 67:283–292, 1987.

1904. Hirszel P, Michaelson JH, Dodge K, et al: Mercury-induced autoimmune glomerulonephritis in inbred rats. II. Immunohistopathology, histopathology and effects of prostaglandin administration. Surv Synth Pathol Res 4:412–422, 1985.

1905. Hinglais N, Pelletier L, Vial MC, et al: Effect of prostaglandin E₁ in Brown Norway rats with mercury-induced autoimmune disease. Clin Immunol Immunopathol 40:401–409, 1986.

1906. Guéry J-C, Tournade H, Pelletier L, et al: Rat anti–glomerular basement membrane antibodies in toxin-induced autoimmunity and in chronic graft-vs.-host reaction share recurrent idiotypes. Eur J Immunol 20:101–105, 1990.

1907. Tournade H, Pelletier L, Pasquier R, et al: D-Penicillamine–induced autoimmunity in Brown-Norway rats. Similarities with HgCl₂-induced autoimmunity. J Immunol 144:2985–2991, 1990.

1908. Joshi BC, Dwivedi C, Powell A, Holscher M: Immune complex nephritis in rats induced by long-term oral exposure to cadmium. J Comp Pathol 91:11–15, 1981.

1909. Houssin D, Druet E, Hinglais N, et al: Glomerular and vascular IgG deposits in HgCl₂ nephritis: Role of circulating antibodies and of immune complexes. Clin Immunol Immunopathol 29:167–180, 1983.

1910. Fukatsu A, Brentjens JR, Killen PD, et al: Studies on the formation of glomerular immune deposits in Brown Norway rats injected with mercuric chloride. Clin Immunol Immunopathol 45:35, 1987.

1911. Michaud A, Sapin C, Leca G, et al: Involvement of hemostasis during an autoimmune glomerulonephritis induced by mercuric chloride in Brown Norway rats. Thromb Res 33:77–88, 1983.

1912. Roman-Franco AA, Turiello M, Albini B, et al: Anti–basement membrane antibodies and antigen-antibody complexes in rabbits injected with mercuric chloride. Clin Immunol Immunopathol 9:464–481, 1978.

1913. Bruijn JA, Hogendoorn PCW, Corver WE, et al: Pathogenesis of experimental lupus nephritis: A role for anti–basement membrane and anti–tubular brush border antibodies in murine chronic graft-versus-host disease. Clin Exp Immunol 79:115–122, 1990.

1914. Bruijn JA, van Leer EHG, Baelde HJJ, et al: Characterization and in vivo transfer of nephritogenic autoantibodies directed against dipeptidyl peptidase IV and laminin in experimental lupus nephritis. Lab Invest 63:350–359, 1990.

1915. Florquin S, Abramowicz D, De Heer E, et al: Renal immunopathology in murine host-versus-graft disease. Kidney Int 40:852–861, 1991.

1916. Wilson CB, Yamamoto T, Moullier PH, Blantz RC: Selective glomerular cell immune injury—anti–mesangial cell antibodies. *In* Davison AM, Briggs JD, Green R, et al (eds): Nephrology. Proceedings of the Xth International Congress of Nephrology, Vol 1. Baillière Tindall, London, 1988, pp 509–522.

1917. Matsuo S, Caldwell PRB, Brentjens JR, Andres G: In vivo interaction of antibodies with cell surface antigens. A mechanism responsible for in situ formation of immune deposits in the zona pellucida of rabbit oocytes. J Clin Invest 75:1369–1380, 1985.

1918. Brentjens JR, Andres G: Interaction of antibodies with renal cell surface antigens. Kidney Int 35:954–968, 1989.

1919. Vogt A, Batsford S: Local immune complex formation and pathogenesis of glomerulonephritis. Contrib Nephrol 43:51–63, 1984.

1920. Wilson CB: Immune reactions with antigens in or of the glomerulus. *In* Milgrom F, Albini B (eds): Immunopathology. S Karger, Basel, 1979, pp 127–131.

1921. Couser WG: In situ formation of immune complexes and the role of complement activation in glomerulonephritis. Clin Immunol Allergy 6:287–306, 1986.

1922. Kerjaschki D: Dysfunctions of cell biological mechanisms of visceral epithelial cell (podocytes) in glomerular diseases. Kidney Int 45:300–313, 1994.

1923. Heymann W, Hackel DB, Harwood S, et al: Production of nephrotic syndrome in rats by Freund's adjuvants and rat kidney suspensions. Proc Soc Exp Biol Med 100:660–664, 1959.

1924. Feenstra K, van den Lee R, Greben HA, et al: Experimental glomerulonephritis in the rat induced by antibodies directed against tubular antigens. The natural history: A histologic and immunohistologic study at the light microscopic and the ultrastructural level. Lab Invest 32:235–242, 1975.

1925. Sun X, Jones H Jr, Jones JA, et al: Apolipoprotein gene expression in analbuminemic rats and in rats with Heymann nephritis. Am J Physiol 262:F755–F761, 1992.

1926. Kaysen GA, Pan X-M, Couser WG, Staprans I: Defective lipolysis persists in hearts of rats with Heymann nephritis in the absence of nephrotic plasma. Am J Kidney Dis 22:128–134, 1993.

1927. Sun X, Martin V, Weiss RH, Kaysen GA: Selective transcriptional augmentation of hepatic gene expression in the rat with Heymann nephritis. Am J Physiol 264:F441–F447, 1993.

1928. Edgington TS, Glassock RJ, Dixon FJ: Autologous immune complex nephritis induced with renal tubular antigen. I. Identification and isolation of the pathogenetic antigen. J Exp Med 127:555–571, 1968.

1929. Naruse T, Fukasawa T, Miyakawa Y: Laboratory model of membranous glomerulonephritis in rats induced by pronase-digested homologous renal tubular epithelial antigen. Lab Invest 33:141–146, 1975.

1930. Chant S, Katz A, Silverman M: Pathogenicity of a highly purified brush border membrane preparation in Heymann nephritis. J Clin Lab Immunol 4:133–140, 1980.

1931. Barabas AZ, Cornish J, Lannigan R: Passive Heymann nephritis in the rat produced by a heterologous antibody to a heterologous kidney fraction 3 antigen. Br J Exp Pathol 63:667–670, 1982.

1932. Miettinen A: Nephritogenic antibodies against kidney brush border glycoproteins in rabbits injected with Freund's adjuvant. Lab Invest 47:67–75, 1982.

1933. Bakker WW, Bagchus WM, Vos JTWM, et al: The specificity of nephritogenic antibodies: I. Evidence on anti-T-cell specificity in nephritogenic antibodies detected by cytotoxicity and MIF assays. Immunobiology 159:235–243, 1981.

1934. Jeraj K, Vernier RL, Sisson SP, Michael AF: A new glomerular antigen in passive Heymann's nephritis. Br J Exp Pathol 65:485–498, 1984.

1935. Hogendoorn PCW, Bruijn JA, vd Broek LJCM, et al: Antibodies to purified renal tubular epithelial antigens contain activity against laminin, fibronectin, and type IV collagen. Lab Invest 58:278–286, 1988.

1936. Bagchus WM, Vos JTWM, Hoedemaeker PJ, Bakker WW: The specificity of nephritogenic antibodies. III. Binding of anti-F × 1A antibodies in glomeruli is dependent on dual specificity. Clin Exp Immunol 63:639–647, 1986.

1937. Cheng IKP, Dorsch SE, Hall BM: The regulation of autoantibody production in Heymann's nephritis by T lymphocyte subsets. Lab Invest 59:780–788, 1988.

1938. Edgington TS, Glassock RJ, Dixon FJ: Autologous immune complex pathogenesis of experimental allergic glomerulonephritis. Science 155:1432–1434, 1967.

1939. Glassock RJ, Edgington TS, Watson JI, Dixon FJ: Autologous immune complex nephritis induced with renal tubular antigen. II. The pathogenetic mechanism. J Exp Med 127:573–587, 1968.

1940. Abrass CK, Border WA, Glassock RJ: Circulating immune complexes in rats with autologous immune complex nephritis. Lab Invest 43:18–27, 1980.

1941. Zanetti M, Bellon B, Verroust P, Druet P: A search for circulating immune complex–like material during the course of autoimmune complex glomerulonephritis in Lewis and Brown Norway rats. Clin Exp Immunol 42:86–94, 1980.

1942. Cattran DC, Chodirker WB: Experimental membranous glomerulonephritis. The relationship between circulating free antibody and immune complexes to subsequent pathology. Nephron 31:260–265, 1982.

1943. Neale TJ, Wilson CB: Glomerular antigens in Heymann's nephritis: reactivity of eluted and circulating antibody. J Immunol 128:323–330, 1982.

1944. Hori MT, Abrass CK: Isolation and characterization of circulating immune complexes from rats with experimental membranous nephropathy. J Immunol 144:3849–3855, 1990.

1945. Abrass CK, Cohen AH: The role of circulating antigen in the formation of immune deposits in experimental membranous nephropathy. Proc Soc Exp Biol Med 183:348–357, 1986.

1946. Abrass CK: Autologous immune complex nephritis in rats. Influence of modification of mononuclear phagocyte system function. Lab Invest 51:162–171, 1984.

1947. Van Damme BJC, Fleuren GJ, Bakker WW, et al: Experimental glomerulonephritis in the rat induced by antibodies directed against tubular antigens. V. Fixed glomerular antigens in the pathogenesis of heterologous immune complex glomerulonephritis. Lab Invest 38:502–510, 1978.

1948. Couser WG, Steinmuller DF, Stilmant MM, et al: Experimental glomerulonephritis in the isolated perfused rat kidney. J Clin Invest 62:1275–1287, 1978.

1949. Fleuren GJ, Grond J, Hoedemaeker PHJ: The pathogenetic role of free-circulating antibody in autologous immune complex glomerulonephritis. Clin Exp Immunol 41:205–217, 1980.

1950. Neale TJ, Couser WG, Salant DJ, et al: Specific uptake of Heymann's nephritic kidney eluate by rat kidney: Studies in vivo and in isolated perfused kidneys. Lab Invest 46:450–453, 1982.

1951. Madaio MP, Salant DJ, Cohen AJ, et al: Comparative study of in situ immune deposit formation in active and passive Heymann nephritis. Kidney Int 23:498–505, 1983.

1952. Makker SP, Kirson IJ, Moorthy B: Enhancement of in situ immune complex formation in isolated perfused kidneys in Heymann's nephritis. Clin Exp Immunol 47:317–326, 1982.

1953. Madaio MP, Adler S, Groggel GC, et al: Charge selective properties of the glomerular capillary wall influence antibody binding in rat membranous nephropathy. Clin Immunol Immunopathol 39:131–138, 1986.

1954. Salant DJ, Darby C, Couser WG: Experimental membranous glomerulonephritis in rats. Quantitiative studies of glomerular immune deposit formation in isolated glomeruli and whole animals. J Clin Invest 66:71–81, 1980.

1955. Gabbai FB, Gushwa LC, Wilson CB, Blantz RC: An evaluation of the development of experimental membranous nephropathy. Kidney Int 31:1267–1278, 1987.

1956. Bertani T, Nolin L, Foidart J, et al: The effect of puromycin on subepithelial deposits induced by antibodies directed against tubular antigens: a quantitative study. Eur J Clin Invest 9:465–472, 1979.

1957. Couser WG, Salant DJ, Stilmant MM, et al: The effects of aminonucleoside of puromycin and nephrotoxic serum on subepithelial immune-deposit formation in passive Heymann nephritis. J Lab Clin Med 94:917–932, 1979.

1958. Bertani T, Remuzzi G, Poggi A, et al: Severe glomerular epithelial cell damage does not prevent passive Heymann nephritis in rats. Clin Exp Immunol 51:38–44, 1983.

1959. Laitinen L, Miettinen A, Tikkanen I, et al: Glomerular sialic acid in Heymann nephritis and diacetylbenzidine induced nephropathy in rats. Clin Sci 69:57–62, 1985.

1960. Couser WG, Jermanovich NB, Belok S, Stilmant MM: Effect of aminonucleoside nephrosis on immune complex localization in autologous immune complex nephropathy in rats. J Clin Invest 61:561–572, 1978.

1961. Salant DJ, Belok S, Stilmant MM, et al: Determinants of glomerular localization of subepithelial immune deposits. Effects of altered antigen to antibody ratio, steroids, vasoactive amine antagonists, and aminonucleoside of puromycin on passive Heymann nephritis in rats. Lab Invest 41:89–99, 1979.

1962. Challice J, Barabas AZ, Cornish J, et al: Passive Heymann nephritis in pre- and post-natal rats. Br J Exp Pathol 67:915–924, 1986.

1963. Rydel JJ, Schwartz MM, Singh AK: Sequential localization of antibody to multiple regions of the glomerular capillary wall in passive Heymann nephritis. Lab Invest 60:492–498, 1989.

1964. Zanetti M, Druet P: Passive Heymann's nephritis as a model of immune glomerulonephritis mediated by antibodies to immunoglobulins. Clin Exp Immunol 41:189–195, 1980.

1965. Abrass CK, McVay J, Glassock RJ: Evaluation of homologous and isologous passive Heymann nephritis: Influence on endogenous antibody production. J Immunol 130:195–202, 1983.

1966. Barabas AZ, Boyd N, Cornish J, Lannigan R: Progressive passive Heymann nephritis in the rat. Lab Invest 47:400–405, 1982.

1967. Barabas AZ, Cornish J, Lannigan R: Progressive passive Heymann nephritis: Induction of autologous antibodies to rat brush border by multiple injections of heterologous antiserum. Clin Exp Immunol 60:381–386, 1985.

1968. Barabas AZ, Cornish J, Lannigan R: Stimulation of circulating autoantibody levels in the rat with established progressive passive Heymann nephritis. Clin Exp Immunol 65:34–41, 1986.

1969. Abrass CK: Evaluation of sequential glomerular eluates from rats with Heymann nephritis. J Immunol 137:530–535, 1986.

1970. Behar M, Katz A, Silverman M: A rat hybridoma model of Heymann nephritis: Production of a monoclonal anti gp330 from a nephritis rat. Clin Invest Med 13:264–270, 1990.

1971. Specht Grijp-Glandorf RJ, De Heer E, Dekker-Nooren CC, et al: Specificity and cross-reactive idiotypes of anti-gp330 autoantibodies in active Heymann nephritis. Immunology 70:290–295, 1990.

1972. Miettinen A, Törnroth T, Tikkanen I, et al: Heymann nephritis induced by kidney brush border glycoproteins. Lab Invest 43:547–555, 1980.

1973. Kerjaschki D, Farquhar MG: The pathogenic antigen of Heymann nephritis is a membrane glycoprotein of the renal proximal tubule brush border. Proc Natl Acad Sci USA 79:5557–5561, 1982.

1974. Kerjaschki D, Farquhar MG: Immunocytochemical localization of the Heymann nephritis antigen (GP330) in glomerular epithelial cells of normal Lewis rats. J Exp Med 157:667–686, 1983.

1975. Brown D, McCluskey RT, Ausiello DA: The cell biology of Heymann nephritis: A model of human membranous glomerulonephritis. Am J Kidney Dis 10:74–76, 1987.

1976. Coudrier E, Kerjaschki D, Louvard D: Cytoskeleton organization and submembranous interactions in intestinal and renal brush borders. Kidney Int 34:309–320, 1988.

1977. Leung CCK, Cheewatrakoolpong B, O'Mara T, Black M: Passive Heymann nephritis induced by rabbit antiserum to membrane antigens isolated from rat visceral yolk-sac microvilli. Am J Anat 179:169–174, 1987.

1978. Sahali D, Mulliez N, Chatelet F, et al: Characterization of a 280-kD protein restricted to the coated pits of the renal brush border and the epithelial cells of the yolk sac. Teratogenic effect of the specific monoclonal antibodies. J Exp Med 167:213–218, 1988.

1979. Meads TJ, Wild AE: Apical expression of an antigen common to rabbit yolk sac endoderm and kidney proximal tubule epithelium. J Reprod Immunol 23:247–264, 1993.

1980. Sahali D, Mulliez N, Chatelet F, et al: Coexpression in humans by kidney and fetal envelopes of a 280 kDa-coated pit–restricted protein. Similarity with the murine target of teratogenic antibodies. Am J Pathol 140:33–44, 1992.

1981. Sahali D, Mulliez N, Chatelet F, et al: Comparative immunochemistry and ontogeny of two closely related coated pit proteins. The 280-kd target of teratogenic antibodies and the 330-kd target of nephritogenic antibodies. Am J Pathol 142:1654–1667, 1993.

1982. Ronco P, Neale TJ, Wilson CB, et al: An immunopathologic study of a 330-kD protein defined by monoclonal antibodies and reactive with anti–RTE-α5 antibodies and kidney eluates from active Heymann nephritis. J Immunol 136:125–130, 1986.

1983. Kerjaschki D: The pathogenesis of membranous glomerulonephritis from morphology to molecules. Virchows Arch B 58:253–271, 1990.

1984. Kerjaschki D: Molecular aspects of immune deposit formation in Heymann nephritis. Nephrol Dial Transplant 7(suppl 1):16–20, 1992.

1985. Kerjaschki D: Molecular pathogenesis of membranous nephropathy. Kidney Int 41:1090–1105, 1992.

1986. Cavallo T: Membranous nephropathy. Insights from Heymann nephritis. Am J Pathol 144:651–658, 1994.

1987. Kerjaschki D, Horvat R, Binder S, et al: Identification of a 400-kd protein in the brush borders of human kidney tubules that is similar to gp330, the nephritogenic antigen of rat Heymann nephritis. Am J Pathol 129:183–191, 1987.

1988. Natori Y, Hayakawa I, Shibata S: Heymann nephritis in rats induced by human renal tubular antigens: Characterization of antigen and antibody specificities. Clin Exp Immunol 69:33–40, 1987.

1989. Kanalas JJ, Makker SP: Isolation of a 330-kDa glycoprotein from human kidney similar to the Heymann nephritis autoantigen (gp330). J Am Soc Nephrol 1:792–798, 1990.

1990. Rantala I: Glomerular epithelial cell endocytosis of immune deposits in the nephrotic rat. An ultrastructural immunoperoxidase study. Nephron 29:239–244, 1981.

1991. Sharon Z, Schwartz MM, Pauli BU, Lewis EJ: Impairment of glomerular clearance of macroaggregates in immune complex glomerulonephritis. Kidney Int 22:8–12, 1982.

1992. Kamata K, Baird LG, Erikson ME, et al: Characterization of antigens and antibody specificities involved in Heymann nephritis. J Immunol 135:2400–2408, 1985.

1993. Bhan AK, Schneeberger EE, Baird LG, et al: Studies with monoclonal antibodies against brush border antigens in Heymann nephritis. Lab Invest 53:421–432, 1985.

1994. Chatelet F, Brianti E, Ronco P, et al: Ultrastructural localization by monoclonal antibodies of brush border antigens expressed by glomeruli. Am J Pathol 122:500–511, 1986.

1995. Chatelet F, Brianti E, Ronco P, et al: Ultrastructural localization by monoclonal antibodies of brush border antigens expressed by glomeruli. II. Extrarenal distribution. Am J Pathol 122:512–519, 1986.

1996. Assmann KJM, Lange WPH, Tangelder MM, Koene RAP: The organ distribution of gp-330 (Heymann antigen) and gp-90 in the mouse and the rat. Virchows Arch A 408:541–553, 1986.

1997. Ronco P, Allegri L, Melcion C, et al: A monoclonal antibody to brush border and passive Heymann nephritis. Clin Exp Immunol 55:319–332, 1984.

1998. Assmann KJM, Ronco P, Tangelder MM, et al: Comparison of antigenic targets involved in antibody-mediated membranous glomerulonephritis in the mouse and rat. Am J Pathol 121:112–122, 1985.

1999. Assmann KJM, Ronco P, Tangelder MM, et al: Involvement of an antigen distinct from the Heymann antigen in membranous glomerulonephritis in the mouse. Lab Invest 60:138–146, 1989.

2000. Van Leer EHG, Moullier Ph, Ronco P, Verroust P: Lymphocyte expression of a 90 kD brush border antigen. Clin Exp Immunol 67:572–580, 1987.

2001. Makker SP, Singh AK: Characterization of the antigen (gp600) of Heymann nephritis. Lab Invest 50:287–293, 1984.

2002. Singh AK, Makker SP: The distribution and molecular presentation of the brush border antigen of Heymann nephritis in various rat tissues. Clin Exp Immunol 60:579–585, 1985.

2003. Verroust PJ: Kinetics of immune deposits in membranous nephropathy. Kidney Int 35:1418–1428, 1989.

2004. van Leer EH, Ronco P, Verroust P, et al: Heymann nephritis: a model of human membranous glomerulopathy. A study of the role of additional antigens. Nephrol Dial Transplant 7(suppl 1):1–8, 1992.

2005. Singh AK, Makker SP: Circulatory antigens of Heymann nephritis. I. Identification and partial characterization. Immunology 57:467–472, 1986.

2006. Singh AK, Schwartz MM: Circulatory antigen of Heymann nephritis. II. Isolation of a 70,000 MW antigen from normal rat serum which cross-reacts with Heymann nephritis antigen. Immunology 59:451–458, 1986.

2007. Singh AK, Schwartz MM: Circulatory antigen of Heymann nephritis. III. Presence of the 70-kD circulatory protein in the immune deposits of Heymann nephritis. Clin Exp Immunol 85:469–475, 1991.

2008. Natori Y, Hayakawa I, Shibata S: Passive Heymann nephritis with acute and severe proteinuria induced by heterologous antibody against renal tubular brush border glycoprotein gp108. Lab Invest 55:63–70, 1986.

2009. Natori Y, Hayakawa I, Shibata S: Role of dipeptidyl peptidase IV (gp 108) in passive Heymann nephritis. Use of dipeptidyl peptidase IV–deficient rats. Am J Pathol 134:405–410, 1989.

2010. Behar M, Katz A, Silverman M: Biochemical investigation of the pathogenesis of Heymann nephritis. Kidney Int 30:9–15, 1986.

2011. Quigg RJ, Abrahamson DR, Cybulsky AV, et al: Studies with antibodies to cultured rat glomerular epithelial cells. Subepithelial immune deposit formation after in vivo injection. Am J Pathol 134:1125–1133, 1989.

2012. Raychowdhury R, Niles JL, McCluskey RT, Smith JA: Autoimmune target in Heymann nephritis is a glycoprotein with homology to the LDL receptor. Science 244:1163–1165, 1989.

2013. Pietromonaco S, Kerjaschki D, Binder S, et al: Molecular cloning of a cDNA encoding a major pathogenic domain of the Heymann nephritis antigen gp330. Proc Natl Acad Sci USA 87:1811–1815, 1990.

2014. Strickland DK, Ashcom JD, Williams S, et al: Primary structure of $\alpha_2$-macroglobulin receptor–associated protein. Human homologue of a Heymann nephritis antigen. J Biol Chem 266:13364–13369, 1991.

2015. Herz J, Goldstein JL, Strickland DK, et al: 39-kDa protein modulates binding of ligands to low density lipoprotein receptor–related protein/$\alpha_2$-macroglobulin receptor. J Biol Chem 266:21232–21238, 1991.

2016. Kounnas MZ, Argraves WS, Strickland DK: The 39-kDa receptor–associated protein interacts with two members of the low density lipoprotein receptor family, $\alpha_2$-macroglobulin receptor and glycoprotein 330. J Biol Chem 267:21162–21166, 1992.

2017. Orlando RA, Kerjaschki D, Kurihara H, et al: gp330 associates with a 44-kDa protein in the rat kidney to form the Heymann nephritis antigenic complex. Proc Natl Acad Sci USA 89:6698–6702, 1992.

2018. Kerjaschki D, Ullrich R, Diem K, et al: Identification of a pathogenic epitope involved in initiation of Heymann nephritis. Proc Natl Acad Sci USA 89:11179–11183, 1992.

2019. Kanalas JJ, Makker SP: Analysis of a 45-kDa protein that binds to the Heymann nephritis autoantigen gp330. J Biol Chem 268:8188–8192, 1993.

2020. Biemesderfer D, Dekan G, Aronson PS, Farquhar MG: Biosynthesis of the gp330/44-kDa Heymann nephritis antigenic complex: Assembly takes place in the ER. Am J Physiol 264:F1011–F1020, 1993.

2021. Orlando RA, Farquhar MG: Identification of a cell line that expresses a cell surface and a soluble form of the gp330/receptor-associated protein (RAP) Heymann nephritis antigenic complex. Proc Natl Acad Sci USA 90:4082–4086, 1993.

2022. Lundstrom M, Orlando RA, Saedi MS, et al: Immunocytochemical and biochemical characterization of the Heymann nephritis antigenic complex in rat L2 yolk sac cells. Am J Pathol 143:1423–1435, 1993.

2023. Kanalas JJ, Makker SP: Identification of the rat Heymann nephritis autoantigen (GP330) as a receptor site for plasminogen. J Biol Chem 266:10825–10829, 1991.

2024. Christensen EI, Gliemann J, Moestrup SK: Renal tubule gp330 is a calcium binding receptor for endocytic uptake of protein. J Histochem Cytochem 40:1481–1490, 1992.

2025. Kanalas JJ: Analysis of plasmin binding and urokinase activation of plasminogen bound to the Heymann nephritis autoantigen, gp330. Arch Biochem Biophys 299:255–260, 1992.

2026. Willnow TE, Goldstein JL, Orth K, et al: Low density lipoprotein receptor–related protein and gp330 bind similar ligands, including plasminogen activator-inhibitor complexes and lactoferrin, an inhibitor of chylomicron remnant clearance. J Biol Chem 267:26172–26180, 1992.

2027. Moestrup SK, Nielsen S, Andreasen P, et al: Epithelial glycoprotein-330 mediates endocytosis of plasminogen activator–plasminogen activator inhibitor type-1 complexes. J Biol Chem 268:16564–16570, 1993.

2028. Kounnas MZ, Chappell DA, Strickland DK, Argraves WS: Glycoprotein 330, a member of the low density lipoprotein receptor family, binds lipoprotein lipase in vitro. J Biol Chem 268:14176–14181, 1993.

2029. Mendrick DL, Chung DC, Rennke HG: Heymann antigen gp330 demonstrates affinity for fibronectin, laminin, and type I collagen and mediates rat proximal tubule epithelial cell adherence to such matrices in vitro. Exp Cell Res 188:23–35, 1990.

2030. Bachinsky DR, Zheng G, Niles JL, et al: Detection of two forms of gp330. Their role in Heymann nephritis. Am J Pathol 143:598–611, 1993.

2031. Van Leer EHG, Ronco P, Verroust P, et al: Epitope specificity of anti-gp330 autoantibodies determines the development of proteinuria in active Heymann nephritis. Am J Pathol 142:821–829, 1993.

2032. Camussi G, Brentjens JR, Noble B, et al: Antibody-induced redistribution of Heymann antigen on the surface of cultured glomerular visceral epithelial cells: Possible role in the pathogenesis of Heymann glomerulonephritis. J Immunol 135:2409–2416, 1985.

2033. Camussi G, Noble B, Van Liew J, et al: Pathogenesis of passive Heymann glomerulonephritis: Chlorpromazine inhibits antibody-mediated redistribution of cell surface antigens and prevents development of the disease. J Immunol 136:2127–2135, 1986.

2034. Allegri L, Brianti E, Chatelet F, et al: Polyvalent antigen-antibody interactions are required for the formation of electron-dense immune deposits in passive Heymann's nephritis. Am J Pathol 126:1–6, 1986.

2035. Brentjens JR, Andres GA: Interaction of antibodies with renal cell surface antigens. Kidney Int 35:954–968, 1989.

2036. Camussi G, Kerjaschki D, Gonda M, et al: Expression and modulation of surface antigens in cultured rat glomerular visceral epithelial cells. J Histochem Cytochem 37:1675–1687, 1989.

2037. Cybulsky AV, Quigg RJ, Badalamenti J, Salant DJ: Anti-F × 1A induces association of Heymann nephritis antigens with microfilaments of cultured glomerular visceral epithelial cells. Am J Pathol 129:373–384, 1987.

2038. Kerjaschki D, Miettinen A, Farquhar MG: Initial events in the formation of immune deposits in passive Heymann nephritis: gp330–anti-gp330 immune complexes form in epithelial coated pits and rapidly become attached to the glomerular basement membrane. J Exp Med 166:109–128, 1987.

2039. Fukatsu A, Yuzawa Y, Olson L, et al: Interaction of antibodies with human glomerular epithelial cells. Lab Invest 61:389–403, 1989.

2040. Salant DJ, Quigg RJ, Cybulsky AV: Heymann nephritis: Mechanisms of renal injury. Kidney Int 35:976–984, 1989.

2041. Susani M, Schulze M, Exner M, Kerjaschki D: Antibodies to glycolipids activate complement and promote proteinuria in passive Heymann nephritis. Am J Pathol 144:807–819, 1994.

2042. Fleuren GJ, Hoedemaeker PHJ: Triple-drug treatment of autologous immune complex glomerulonephritis. Clin Exp Immunol 41:218–224, 1980.

2043. Gronhagen-Riska C, von Willebrand E, Tikkanen T, et al: The effect of cyclosporin A on the interstitial mononuclear cell infiltration and the induction of Heymann's nephritis. Clin Exp Immunol 79:266–272, 1990.

2044. Matsukawa W, Hara S, Yoshida F, et al: Effects of a new immunosuppressive agent, FK506, in rats with active Heymann nephritis. J Lab Clin Med 119:116–123, 1992.

2045. Litwin A, Bash JA, Adams LE, et al: Immunoregulation of Heymann's nephritis. I. Induction of suppressor cells. J Immunol 122:1029–1038, 1979.

2046. Harmon WE, Grupe WE, Parkman R: Control of autologous immune complex nephritis. I. Suppression of the disease in the presence of T cell sensitization. J Immunol 124:1034–1038, 1980.

2047. Quiza CG, Leenaerts PL, Hall BM: Induction of unresponsiveness to Heymann's nephritis: Inhibited by monoclonal antibody to CD4 but not to CD8. Cell Immunol 133:456–467, 1991.

2048. de Heer E, Daha MR, Van Es LA: Lymph node cells from rats with Heymann's nephritis produce in vitro autoantibodies directed against purified renal tubular antigen. Immunology 52:743–752, 1984.

2049. de Heer E, Daha MR, Van Es LA: The autoimmune response in active Heymann's nephritis in Lewis rats is regulated by T-lymphocyte subsets. Cell Immunol 92:254–264, 1985.

2050. de Heer E, Daha MR, Burgers J, Van Es LA: Reestablishment of self tolerance by suppressor T-cells after active Heymann's nephritis. Cell Immunol 98:28–33, 1986.

2051. Noble B, Van Liew JB, Brentjens JR, Andres GA: Effect of reimmunization with F × 1A late in the course of Heymann nephritis. Lab Invest 47:427–436, 1982.

2052. Noble B, Van Liew JB, Andres GA, Brentjens JR: Factors influencing susceptibility of LEW rats to Heymann nephritis. Clin Immunol Immunopathol 30:241–254, 1984.

2053. Tikkanen I, Törnroth T, Miettinen A, Fyhrquist F: Heymann nephritis-DOCA-NaCl hypertension in the rat. Role of nephritis, DOCA, NaCl, and vascular lesions in the development of hypertension. Nephron 28:90–95, 1981.

2054. Okuda S, Oh Y, Onoyama K, et al: Autologous immune complex nephritis in streptozotocin-induced diabetic rats. Nephron 37:166–173, 1984.

2055. Okuda S, Oh Y, Tsuruda H, et al: Rapidly progressive renal deterioration in partially nephrectomized rats with experimental membranous nephropathy. Nephron 41:359–364, 1985.

2056. Milner LS, Lotan D, Mills M, et al: Colchicine reduces proteinuria in passive Heymann nephritis. Nephron 46:11–17, 1987.

2057. Nakazawa M, Emancipator SN, Lamm ME: Proteolytic enzyme treatment reduces glomerular immune deposits and proteinuria in passive Heymann nephritis. J Exp Med 164:1973–1987, 1986.

2058. Cybulsky AV, Salant DJ: Glomerular cell injury and proteinuria. Lab Invest 66:652–653, 1992.

2059. Yoneyama T, Nagase M, Ikeya M, et al: Intraglomerular fibronectin in rat experimental glomerulonephritis. Virchows Arch B 62:179–188, 1992.

2060. Ichikawa I, Hoyer JR, Seiler MW, Brenner BM: Mechanism of glomerulotubular balance in the setting of heterogeneous glomerular injury. Preservation of a close functional linkage between individual nephrons and surrounding microvasculature. J Clin Invest 69:185–198, 1982.

2061. Yoshioka T, Rennke HG, Salant DJ, et al: Role of abnormally high transmural pressure in the permselectivity defect of glomerular capillary wall: A study in early passive Heymann nephritis. Circ Res 61:531–538, 1987.

2062. Fetterman GH, Allison MEM, Wilson CB, Gottschalk CW: Structural changes of experimental glomerulonephritis in rats as revealed by microdissection. Pathol Annu 13:55, 1978.

2063. Mendrick DL, Noble B, Brentjens JR, Andres GA: Antibody-mediated injury to proximal tubules in Heymann nephritis. Kidney Int 18:328–343, 1980.

2064. Noble B, Andres GA, Brentjens JR: Passively transferred anti–brush border antibodies induce injury of proximal tubules in the absence of complement. Clin Exp Immunol 56:281–288, 1983.

2065. Zamlauski-Tucker MJ, Van Liew JB, Noble B: Pathophysiology of the kidney in rats with Heymann nephritis. Kidney Int 28:504–512, 1985.

2066. Sekse I, Iversen BM, Matre R, Ofstad J: Acute effect of passive Heymann nephritis on renal blood flow and glomerular filtration rate in rat: The effect of infusion of F (ab')₂ fraction of anti-F×1(A) antibody. Nephron 59:110–115, 1991.

2067. Hutchison FN, Webster SK: Effect of ANG II receptor antagonist on albuminuria and renal function in passive Heymann nephritis. Am J Physiol 263:F311–F318, 1992.

2068. Haddad A, Goldinger JM, Van Liew JB, Noble B: Kidney immunopathology and pathophysiology in rats immunized with proximal tubule cell brush border or basolateral membrane vesicles. Immunol Invest 16:213–225, 1987.

2069. Mutti A, Lucertini S, Valcavi P, et al: Urinary excretion of brush-border antigen revealed by monoclonal antibody: Early indicator of toxic nephropathy. Lancet 2:914–916, 1985.

2070. Klassen J, Sugisaki T, Milgrom F, McCluskey RT: Studies on multiple renal lesions in Heymann nephritis. Lab Invest 25:577–585, 1971.

2071. Noble B, Mendrick DL, Brentjens JR, Andres GA: Antibody-mediated injury to proximal tubules in the rat kidney induced by passive kidney transfer of homologous anti–brush border serum. Clin Immunol Immunopathol 19:289–301, 1981.

2072. Eddy AA, Ho GC, Thorner PS: The contribution of antibody-mediated cytotoxicity and immune-complex formation to tubulointerstitial disease in passive Heymann nephritis. Clin Immunol Immunopathol 62:42–55, 1992.

2073. Brodkin M, Noble B: Antibody-mediated proliferation of proximal tubule cells requires cross-linking of antigenic determinants. Clin Exp Immunol 72:315–320, 1988.

2074. Gutmann EJ, Niles JL, McCluskey RT, Brown D: Loss of antigens associated with the apical endocytotic pathway in proximal tubules from rats with Heymann nephritis. Am J Pathol 138:1243–1255, 1991.

2075. Gutmann EJ, Niles JL, McCluskey RT, Brown D: Colchicine-induced redistribution of an apical membrane glycoprotein (gp330) in proximal tubules. Am J Physiol 257:C397–C407, 1989.

2076. Barabas AZ, Lannigan R: Immune-complex nephritis in the rabbit produced by injections of rat renal tubular fraction 3 antigen. Br J Exp Pathol 62:94–102, 1981.

2077. Barabas AZ, Cornish J, Lannigan R: Passive Heymann–like nephritis in the rabbit. Br J Exp Pathol 66:357–364, 1985.

2078. Nicol MJ, Miller JH, Neale TJ: Tubular antigen–associated renal disease in New Zealand white rabbits. Clin Exp Immunol 63:629–638, 1986.

2079. Assmann KJM, Tangelder MM, Lange WPJ, et al: Membranous glomerulonephritis in the mouse. Kidney Int 24:303–312, 1983.

2080. Neale TJ, Wilson CB: Non-GBM glomerular antigen in spontaneous nephritis in rabbits. Kidney Int 14:715, 1978. Abstract.

2081. Neale TJ, Woodroffe AJ, Wilson CB: Spontaneous glomerulonephritis in rabbits: Role of a glomerular capillary antigen. Kidney Int 26:701–711, 1984.

2082. Caldwell PRB, Wigger HJ, Fernandez LT, et al: Lung injury induced by antibody fragments to angiotensin-converting enzyme. Am J Pathol 105:54–63, 1981.

2083. Barba LM, Caldwell PRB, Downie GH, et al: Lung injury mediated by antibodies to endothelium. I. In the rabbit a repeated interaction of heterologous anti–angiotensin-converting enzyme antibodies with alveolar endothelium results in resistance to immune injury through antigenic modulation. J Exp Med 158:2141–2158, 1983.

2084. Camussi G, Caldwell PRB, Andres G, Brentjens JR: Lung injury mediated by antibodies to endothelium. II. Study of the effect of repeated antigen-antibody interactions in rabbits tolerant to heterologous antibody. Am J Pathol 127:216–228, 1987.

2085. Matsuo S, Fukatsu A, Taub ML, et al: Glomerulonephritis induced in the rabbit by antiendothelial antibodies. J Clin Invest 79:1798–1811, 1987.

2086. Lynch JM, Lotner GZ, Betz SJ, Henson PM: The release of a platelet-activating factor by stimulated rabbit neutrophils. J Immunol 123:1219–1226, 1979.

2087. Camussi G, Aglietta M, Malavasi G, et al: The release of platelet-activating factor from human endothelial cells in culture. J Immunol 131:2397–2403, 1983.

2088. Camussi G, Pawlowski I, Bussolino F, et al: Release of platelet activating factor in rabbits with antibody-mediated injury of the lung: The role of leukocytes and of pulmonary endothelial cells. J Immunol 131:1802–1807, 1983.

2089. Ito S, Hirabayashi K, Nielsen N, et al: Von Willebrand factor in the rat kidney: Its localization and the effects of its in vivo interaction with specific antibodies. Nephron 66:200–207, 1994.

2090. Coffey AK, Karnovskey MJ: Heparin inhibits mesangial cell proliferation in Habu-venom-induced glomerular injury. Am J Pathol 120:248–255, 1985.

2091. Cattell V, Bradfield JWB: Focal mesangial proliferative glomerulonephritis in the rat caused by Habu snake venom: A morphologic study. Am J Pathol 87:511–524, 1977.

2092. Morita T, Kihara I, Oite T, et al: Mesangiolysis: Sequential ultrastructural study of Habu venom–induced glomerular lesions. Lab Invest 38:94–102, 1978.

2093. Mauer SM, Sutherland DER, Howard RJ, et al: The glomerular mesangium. III. Acute immune mesangial injury: A new model of glomerulonephritis. J Exp Med 137:553–570, 1973.

2094. Seelig HP, Seelig R, Roth E, Roth E: Antibodies reacting with the glomerular mesangium. Isolation and immunopathology. Virchows Arch A 366:313–330, 1975.

2095. Barbosa JE, Rossi MA, Mello de Oliveira JA, Sarti W: Nephropathy produced by Forssman antibody in guinea pigs: An experimental model of mesangial injury. Res Exp Med 185:283–290, 1985.

2096. Mendrick DL, Rennke HG: Immune deposits formed in situ by a monoclonal antibody recognizing a new intrinsic rat mesangial matrix antigen. J Immunol 137:1517–1526, 1986.

2097. Tsai CY, Wu TH, Sun KH, Yu CL: Effects of antibodies to double stranded DNA, purified from serum samples of patients with active systemic lupus erythematosus, on the glomerular mesangial cell. Ann Rheum Dis 51:162–167, 1992.

2098. Yamamoto T, Wilson CB: Antibody-induced mesangial cell damage: The model, functional alterations, and effects of complement. Kidney Int 29:296, 1986. Abstract.

2099. Yamamoto T, Wilson CB: Quantitative and qualitative studies of antibody-induced mesangial cell damage in the rat. Kidney Int 32:514–525, 1987.

2100. Ishizaki M, Masuda Y, Fukuda Y, et al: Experimental mesangioproliferative glomerulonephritis in rats induced by intravenous administration of anti-thymocyte serum. Acta Pathol Jpn 36:1191–1203, 1986.

2101. Bagchus WM, Hoedemaeker PJ, Rozing J, Bakker WW: Acute glomerulonephritis after intravenous injection of monoclonal anti-thymocyte antibodies in the rat. Immunol Lett 12:109–113, 1986.

2102. Bagchus WM, Hoedemaeker PJ, Rozing J, Bakker WW: Glomerulonephritis induced by monoclonal anti-Thy 1.1 antibodies. A sequential histological and ultrastructural study in the rat. Lab Invest 55:680–687, 1986.

2103. Seki T, Chang H-C, Moriuchi T, et al: A hydrophobic transmembrane segment at the carboxyl terminus of Thy-1. Science 227:649–651, 1985.

2104. Seki T, Moriuchi T, Chang H-C, et al: Structural organization of the rat Thy-1 gene. Nature 313:485–487, 1985.

2105. Crawford JM, Barton RW: Biology of disease. Thy-1 glycoprotein: structure, distribution, and ontogeny. Lab Invest 54:122–135, 1986.

2106. Ishizaki M, Sato S, Sano J, et al: The presence of Thy-1.1 antigen in rat glomerular mesangial cells. Biomed Res 1:438–442, 1980.

2107. Barclay AN: Different reticular elements in rat lymphoid tissue identified by localization of Ia, Thy-1 and MRC OX 2 antigens. Immunology 44:727–736, 1981.

2108. Harada K, Yamamoto T, Hara M, Kihara I: Antigenic association between kidney and thymocyte. Acta Pathol Jpn 32:483–489, 1982.

2109. Paul LC, Rennke HG, Milford EL, Carpenter CB: Thy-1.1 in glomeruli of rat kidneys. Kidney Int 25:771–777, 1984.

2110. Yamamoto T, Yamamoto K, Kawasaki K, et al: Immunoelectron microscopic demonstration of Thy-1 antigen on the surfaces of mesangial cells in the rat glomerulus. Nephron 43:293–298, 1986.

2111. Shires M, Goode NP, Crellin DM, Davison AM: Immunogold-silver staining of mesangial antigen in Lowicryl K4M- and LR gold-embedded renal tissue using epipolarization microscopy. J Histochem Cytochem 38:287–289, 1990.

2112. Miyata T, Isobe K, Dawson R, et al: Determination of the molecular nature and cellular localization of Thy-1 in human renal tissue. Immunology 69:391–395, 1990.

2113. Yamamoto T, Wilson CB: Complement dependence of antibody-induced mesangial cell injury in the rat. J Immunol 138:3758–3765, 1987.

2114. Blantz RC, Wilson CB: Acute effects of anti–glomerular basement membrane antibody on the process of glomerular filtration in the rat. J Clin Invest 58:899–911, 1976.

2115. Golbus SM, Wilson CB: Experimental glomerulonephritis induced by in situ formation of immune complexes in glomerular capillary wall. Kidney Int 16:148–157, 1979.

2116. Okada H, Suzuki H, Sakaguchi H, Saruta T: Dissociation of clinical manifestation and histopathology in the course of mesangial injury by anti-thymocyte antibody. Pathol Res Pract 189:437–442, 1993.

2117. Schreiber RD, Pangburn MK, Medicus RG, Muller-Eberhard HJ: Raji cell injury and subsequent lysis by the purified cytolytic alternative pathway of human complement. Clin Immunol Immunopathol 15:384–396, 1980.

2118. Koski CL, Ramm LE, Hammer CH, et al: Cytolysis of nucleated cells by complement: Cell death displays multihit characteristics. Proc Natl Acad Sci USA 80:3816–3820, 1983.

2119. Ramm LE, Whitlow MB, Mayer MM: Complement lysis of nucleated cells: Effect of temperature and puromycin on the number of channels required for cytolysis. Mol Immunol 21:1015–1021, 1984.

2120. Carney DF, Koski CL, Shin ML: Elimination of terminal complement intermediates from the plasma membrane of nucleated cells: The rate of disappearance differs for cells carrying C5b-7 or C5b-8 or a mixture of C5b-8 with a limited number of C5b-9. J Immunol 134:1804–1809, 1985.

2121. Bagchus WM, Jeunink MF, Elema JD: The mesangium in anti-Thy-1 nephritis. Influx of macrophages, mesangial cell hypercellularity, and macromolecular accumulation. Am J Pathol 137:215–223, 1990.

2122. van Diemen-Steenvoorde R, Lambers A, van der Wal A, et al: Macrophages are responsible for mesangial cell injury and extracellular matrix (ECM) expansion in anti–Thy-1 nephritis in rats. J Am Soc Nephrol 2:585, 1991. Abstract.

2123. Miyachi K, Fritzler MJ, Tan EM: Autoantibody to a nuclear antigen in proliferating cells. J Immunol 121:2228–2234, 1978.

2124. Ogata K, Ogata Y, Nakamura RM, Tan EM: Purification and N-terminal amino acid sequence of proliferating cell nuclear antigen (PCNA)/cyclin and development of ELISA for anti-PCNA antibodies. J Immunol 135:2623–2627, 1985.

2125. Johnson RJ, Iida H, Alpers CE, et al: Expression of smooth muscle phenotype by rat mesangial cells in immune complex nephritis. α-smooth muscle actin is a marker of mesangial cell proliferation. J Clin Invest 87:847–858, 1991.

2126. Alpers CE, Hudkins KL, Gown AM, Johnson RJ: Enhanced expression of "muscle-specific" actin in glomerulonephritis. Kidney Int 41:1134–1142, 1992.

2127. Stahl RA, Thaiss F, Wenzel U, Helmchen U: Morphologic and functional consequences of immune-mediated mesangiolysis: Development of chronic glomerular sclerosis. J Am Soc Nephrol 2(10 suppl):S144–S148, 1992.

2128. Yamamoto T, Mundy CA, Wilson CB, Blantz RC: Effect of mesangial cell lysis and proliferation on glomerular hemodynamics in the rat. Kidney Int 40:705–713, 1991.

2129. Aizawa C, Nosaka K, Imaki H, et al: Tubuloglomerular feedback response in rats with antithymocyte serum–induced glomerular lesions. Kidney Int 39(suppl 32):S-119–S-121, 1991.

2130. Bagchus WM, Donga J, Rozing J, et al: The specificity of nephritogenic antibodies. IV. Binding of monoclonal antithymocyte antibodies to rat kidney. Transplantation 41:739–745, 1986.

2131. Wilson CB, Dixon FJ, Fortner JG, Cerilli J: Glomerular basement membrane–reactive antibody in anti-lymphocyte globulin. J Clin Invest 50:1525–1535, 1971.

2132. Kawachi H, Orikasa M, Matsui K, et al: Epitope-specific induction of mesangial lesions with proteinuria by a MoAb against mesangial cell surface antigen. Clin Exp Immunol 88:399–404, 1992.

2133. Donker AJ, Venuto RC, Vladutiu AO, et al: Effects of prolonged administration of D-penicillamine or captopril in various strains of rats. Brown Norway rats treated with D-penicillamine develop autoantibodies, circulating immune complexes, and disseminated intravascular coagulation. Clin Immunol Immunopathol 30:142–155, 1984.

2134. Wilson CB: Nephritogenic antibody mechanisms involving antigens within the glomerulus. Immunol Rev 55:257–297, 1981.

2135. Neale TJ, Wilson CB: Glomerular antigens in glomerulonephritis. Springer Semin Immunopathol 5:221–249, 1982.

2136. Murphy-Ullrich JE, Oberley TD, Mosher DF: Glomerular and vascular injury in mice following immunization with heterologous and autologous fibronectin. Virchows Arch B 39:305–321, 1982.

2137. Zanetti M, Takami T: Mesangial immune deposits induced in rats by antibodies to fibronectin. Clin Immunol Immunopathol 31:353–363, 1984.

2138. Murphy-Ullrich JE, Oberley TD, Mosher DF: Detection of auto-antibodies and glomerular injury in rabbits immunized with denatured human fibronectin monomer. Am J Pathol 117:1–11, 1984.

2139. Shibata S, Miura K: A third glycopeptide (nephritogenoside) isolated from the glomerular basement membrane. J Biochem (Tokyo) 89:1737–1749, 1981.

2140. Natori Y, Shibata S: Enzyme linked immunosorbent assay for Heymann's antigen as a contaminating minor component in nephritogenic glycopeptide, nephritogenoside. Clin Exp Immunol 51:595–599, 1983.

2141. Shibata S, Takeda T, Natori Y: The structure of nephritogenoside. A nephritogenic glycopeptide with α-N-glycosidic linkage. J Biol Chem 263:12483–12485, 1988.

2142. Bariéty J, Oriol R, Hinglais N, et al: Distribution of blood group antigen A in normal and pathologic human kidneys. Kidney Int 17:820–826, 1980.

2143. Paul LC, van Es LA, Baldwin WM III: Antigens in human renal allografts. Clin Immunol Immunopathol 19:206–223, 1981.

2144. Hart DNJ, Fabre JW: Major histocompatibility complex antigens in rat kidney, ureter, and bladder. Localization with monoclonal antibodies and demonstration of Ia-positive dendritic cells. Transplantation 31:318–325, 1981.

2145. Hart DNJ, Fuggle SV, Williams KA, et al: Localization of HLA-ABC and DR antigens in human kidney. Transplantation 31:428–433, 1981.

2146. Fuggle SV, Errasti P, Daar AS, et al: Localization of major histocompatibility complex (HLA-ABC and DR) antigens in 46 kidneys. Differences in HLA-DR staining of tubules among kidneys. Transplantation 35:385–390, 1983.

2147. Trickett LP, Evans PR, MacIver AG, et al: Variable localization of blood group antigen in group A kidneys. Br J Exp Pathol 64:137–143, 1983.

2148. Leung CCK: Isolation, partial characterization, and localization of a rat renal tubular glycoprotein antigen. Antibody-induced birth defects. J Exp Med 156:372–384, 1982.

2149. Rosenmann E, Boss JH: Tissue antigens in normal and pathologic urine samples: A review. Kidney Int 16:337–344, 1979.

2150. Kerjaschki D, Sharkey DJ, Farquhar MG: Identification and characterization of podocalyxin—the major sialoprotein of the renal glomerular epithelial cell. J Cell Biol 98:1591–1596, 1984.

2151. Horvat R, Hovorka A, Dekan G, et al: Endothelial cell membranes contain podocalyxin—the major sialoprotein of visceral glomerular epithelial cells. J Cell Biol 102:484–491, 1986.

2152. Schnabel E, Dekan G, Miettinen A, Farquhar MG: Biogenesis of podocalyxin—the major glomerular sialoglycoprotein—in the newborn rat kidney. Eur J Cell Biol 48:313–326, 1989.

2153. Stamenkovic I, Skalli O, Gabbiani G: Distribution of intermediate filament proteins in normal and diseased human glomeruli. Am J Pathol 125:465–475, 1986.

2154. Gröne H-J, Weber K, Gröne E, et al: Coexpression of keratin and vimentin in damaged and regenerating tubular epithelia of the kidney. Am J Pathol 129:1–8, 1987.

2155. Miettinen A, Dekan G, Farquhar MG: Monoclonal antibodies against membrane proteins of the rat glomerulus. Immunochemical specificity and immunofluorescence distribution of the antigens. Am J Pathol 137:929–944, 1990.

2156. Dekan G, Miettinen A, Schnabel E, Farquhar MG: Binding of monoclonal antibodies to glomerular endothelium, slit membranes, and epithelium after in vivo injection. Localization of antigens and bound IgGs by immunoelectron microscopy. Am J Pathol 137:913–927, 1990.

2157. Fleming S, Lindop GBM, Gibson AAM: The distribution of epithelial membrane antigen in the kidney and its tumours. Histopathology 9:729–739, 1985.

2158. Gröne H-J, Weber K, Helmchen U, Osborn M: Villin—a marker of brush border differentiation and cellular origin in human renal cell carcinoma. Am J Pathol 124:294–302, 1986.

2159. Howie AJ: Epithelial membrane antigen in normal and proteinuric glomeruli and in damaged proximal tubules. J Pathol 148:55–60, 1986.

2160. Ozaki I, Ito Y, Fukatsu A, et al: A plasma membrane antigen of rat glomerular epithelial cells. Antigenic determinants involving N-linked sugar residues in a 140-kilodalton sialoglycoprotein of the podocytes. Lab Invest 63:707–716, 1990.

2161. Falkenberg FW, Müller E, Riffelmann HD, et al: The production of monoclonal antibodies against glomerular and other antigens of the human nephron. Renal Physiol 4:150–156, 1981.

2162. Sakai LY, Engvall E, Hollister DW, Burgeson RE: Production and characterization of a monoclonal antibody to human type IV collagen. Am J Pathol 108:310–318, 1982.

2163. Mendrick DL, Rennke HG, Cotran RS, et al: Monoclonal antibodies against rat glomerular antigens: Production and specificity. Lab Invest 49:107–117, 1983.

2164. Hancock WW, Atkins RC: Monoclonal antibodies to human glomerular cells: A marker for glomerular epithelial cells. Nephron 33:83–90, 1983.

2165. Foellmer HG, Madri JA, Furthmayr H: Monoclonal antibodies to type IV collagen: Probes for the study of structure and function of basement membranes. Lab Invest 48:639–649, 1983.

2166. Pressey A, Pusey CD, Dash A, et al: Production of a monoclonal antibody to autoantigenic components of human glomerular basement membrane. Clin Exp Immunol 54:178–184, 1983.

2167. Hancock WW, Kraft N, Clarke F, Atkins RC: Production of monoclonal antibodies to fibronectin, type IV collagen and other antigens of the human glomerulus. Pathology 16:197–206, 1984.

2168. Shimizu F, Orikasa M, Sato K, Oite T: Monoclonal antibodies to rat renal antigens. Immunology 52:319–323, 1984.

2169. Nakamura T: Monoclonal antibodies to human glomerular antigens. II. Using human adult kidney components as antigens. Clin Immunol Immunopathol 41:399–408, 1986.

2170. Nicol MJ, Miller JH, Neale TJ: Production of monoclonal antibody probes specific for nonbasement membrane glomerular capillary wall antigens in the rat. Hybridoma 6:337–347, 1987.

2171. Kawaguchi H, Yamaguchi Y, Itoh K: Monoclonal antibody (KI-13) against glomerular cytoskeletal protein, produced by immunization with cultured mesangial cells from rabbits. Jpn J Nephrol 28:1187–1195, 1986.

2172. Quackenbush EJ, Gougos A, Baumal R, Letarte M: Differential localization within human kidney of five membrane proteins expressed on acute lymphoblastic leukemia cells. J Immunol 136:118–124, 1986.

2173. Krawiec DR, Felsburg PJ, Gelberg HB, Dugan SJ: Development of monoclonal antibodies against canine glomerular antigens. Vet Immunol Immunopathol 24:199–209, 1990.

2174. Stewart KN, Roy-Chaudhury P, Lumsden L, et al: Monoclonal antibodies to cultured human glomerular mesangial cells. I. Reactivity with haematopoietic cells and normal kidney sections. J Pathol 163:265–272, 1991.

2175. Nishikawa K, Fukatsu A, Tamai H, et al: Formation of subepithelial dense deposits in rats induced by a monoclonal antibody against the glomerular cell surface antigen. Clin Exp Immunol 83:143–148, 1991.

2176. Verroust P, Ronco PM, Chatelet F: Monoclonal antibodies and identification of glomerular antigens. Kidney Int 30:649–655, 1986.

2177. Neale TJ, Callus MS, Donovan LC, Baird H: Definition of glomerular antigens by monoclonal antibodies produced against a human glomerular membrane fraction. Hybridoma 9:429–442, 1990.

2178. Kittelberger R, Neale TJ: Isolation and characterization of an unique kidney antigen of relevance in human renal disease. Biochem Biophys Res Commun 172:439–445, 1990.

2179. Bander NH: Study of the normal human kidney and kidney cancer with monoclonal antibodies. Uremia Invest 8:263–273, 1984-85.

2180. Luner SJ, Ghose T, Chatterjee S, et al: Monoclonal antibodies to kidney and tumor-associated surface antigens of human renal cell carcinoma. Cancer Res 46:5816–5820, 1986.

2181. Oosterwijk E, Ruiter DJ, Wakka JC, et al: Immunohistochemical analysis of monoclonal antibodies to renal antigens. Application in the diagnosis of renal cell carcinoma. Am J Pathol 123:301–309, 1986.

2182. Mendrick DL, Rennke HG: I. Induction of proteinuria in the rat by a monoclonal antibody against SGP-115/107. Kidney Int 33:818–830, 1988.

2183. Mendrick DL, Rennke HG: II. Epitope specific induction of proteinuria by monoclonal antibodies. Kidney Int 33:831–842, 1988.

2184. Kagami S, Okada K, Funai M, et al: A monoclonal antibody (1G10) recognizes a novel human mesangial antigen. Kidney Int 42:700–709, 1992.

2185. Orikasa M, Matsui K, Oite T, Shimizu F: Massive proteinuria induced in rats by a single intravenous injection of a monoclonal antibody. J Immunol 141:807–814, 1988.

2186. Huang TW, Langlois JC: Podoendin. A new cell surface protein of the podocyte and endothelium. J Exp Med 162:245–267, 1985.

2187. Kunz A, Brown D, Vassalli J-D, et al: Ultrastructural localization of glycocalyx domains in human kidney podocytes using the lectin-gold technique. Lab Invest 53:413–420, 1985.

2188. Sawada H, Stukenbrok H, Kerjaschki D, Farquhar MG: Epithelial polyanion (podocalyxin) is found on the sides but not the soles of the foot processes of the glomerular epithelium. Am J Pathol 125:309–318, 1986.

2189. Fries JWU, Rumpelt H-J, Thoenes W: Alterations of glomerular podocytic processes in immunologically mediated glomerular disorders. Kidney Int 32:742–748, 1987.

2190. Drenckhahn D, Franke R-P: Ultrastructural organization of contractile and cytoskeletal proteins in glomerular podocytes of chicken, rat, and man. Lab Invest 59:673–682, 1988.

2191. Blantz RC, Gabbai FB, Peterson O, et al: Water and protein permeability is regulated by the glomerular epithelial slit diaphragm. J Am Soc Nephrol 4:1957–1964, 1994.

2192. Takashima N, Kawachi H, Oite T, et al: Effect of chlorpromazine on kinetics of injected monoclonal antibody in MoAb-induced glomerular injury. Clin Exp Immunol 91:135–140, 1993.

2193. Assmann KJ, van Son JP, Dijkman HB, Koene RA: A nephritogenic rat monoclonal antibody to mouse aminopeptidase A. Induction of massive albuminuria after a single intravenous injection. J Exp Med 175:623–635, 1992.

2194. Izui S, Lambert PH, Miescher PA: In vitro demonstration of a particular affinity of glomerular basement membrane and collagen for DNA. A possible basis for a local formation of DNA–anti-DNA complexes in systemic lupus erythematosus. J Exp Med 144:428–443, 1976.

2195. Izui S, Lambert P-H, Fournié GJ, et al: Features of systemic lupus erythematosus in mice injected with bacterial lipopolysaccharides. Identification of circulating DNA and renal localization of DNA–anti-DNA complexes. J Exp Med 145:1115–1130, 1977.

2196. Lake RA, Morgan A, Henderson B, Staines NA: A key role for fibronectin in the sequential binding of native dsDNA and monoclonal anti-DNA antibodies to components of the extracellular matrix: its possible significance in glomerulonephritis. Immunology 54:389–395, 1985.

2197. Gupta RC, Simpson WA, Raghow R: Interaction of fibronectin with DNA/anti-DNA complexes from systemic lupus erythematosus: Role of activated complement C1 in modulation of the interactions. Clin Immunol Immunopathol 46:368–381, 1988.

2198. Yamamoto T, Nagase M, Honda N: Inhibitory effect of lysozyme on the intraglomerular immune complex formation in lupus mice. Clin Immunol Immunopathol 47:27–38, 1988.

2199. Jacob L, Viard JD, Allenet B, et al: A monoclonal anti–double-stranded DNA autoantibody binds to a 94-kDa cell-surface protein on various cell types via nucleosomes or a DNA-histone complex. Proc Natl Acad Sci USA 86:4669–4673, 1989.

2200. Schmiedeke TMJ, Stöckl FW, Weber R, et al: Histones have high affinity for the glomerular basement membrane. J Exp Med 169:1879–1894, 1989.

2201. Termaat RM, Brinkman K, Van Gompel F, et al: Cross-reactivity of monoclonal anti-DNA antibodies with heparan sulfate is mediated via bound DNA/histone complexes. J Autoimmun 3:531–545, 1990.

2202. Termaat R-M, Assmann KJM, Dijkman HBPM, et al: Anti-DNA antibodies can bind to the glomerulus via two distinct mechanisms. Kidney Int 42:1363–1371, 1992.

2203. Brinkman K, Termaat R, Berden JHM, Smeenk RJT: Anti-DNA antibodies and lupus nephritis: The complexity of crossreactivity. Immunol Today 11:232–234, 1990.

2204. Cukier R, Tron F: Monoclonal anti-DNA antibodies: An approach to studying SLE nephritis. Clin Exp Immunol 62:143–149, 1985.

2205. Jones FS, Pisetsky DS, Kurlander RJ: The clearance of a monoclonal anti-DNA antibody following administration of DNA in normal and autoimmune mice. Clin Immunol Immunopathol 39:49–60, 1986.

2206. O'Regan S, Turgeon C: Unilateral glomerular DNA–anti-DNA complex formation in situ. J Clin Lab Immunol 15:101–104, 1984.

2207. Cosio FG, Mahan JD, Sedmak DD: Experimental glomerulonephritis induced by antigen that binds to glomerular fibronectin. Am J Kidney Dis 15:160–168, 1990.

2208. Cosio FG, Bakaletz AP, Mahan JD: Role of precipitating and nonprecipitating antibodies in glomerular immune complex formation. Kidney Int 37:1429–1437, 1990.

2209. Stad RK, Bruijn JA, van Gijlswijk-Janssen DJ, et al: An acute model for IgA-mediated glomerular inflammation in rats induced by monoclonal polymeric rat IgA antibodies. Clin Exp Immunol 92:514–521, 1993.

2210. Nagasawa T: Interaction of concanavalin A and GBM glycoprotein in vivo. In Yoshitoshi Y, Ueda Y (eds): Glomerulonephritis. Proceedings of the International Symposium on Glomerulonephritis—Progression and Regression, December 6–8, 1977. University of Tokyo Press, Tokyo, 1979, pp 39–51.

2211. Davin J-C, Nagy J, Lombet J, et al: Experimental glomerulonephritis induced by the glomerular deposition of IgA–concanavalin A complexes. Contrib Nephrol 67:111–116, 1988.

2212. Davin J-C, Dechenne C, Lombet J, et al: Acute experimental glomerulonephritis induced by the glomerular deposition of circulating polymeric IgA–concanavalin A complexes. Virchows Arch A 415:7–20, 1989.

2213. Matsuo S, Yoshida F, Yuzawa Y, et al: Experimental glomerulonephritis induced in rats by a lectin and its antibodies. Kidney Int 36:1011–1021, 1989.

2214. Roth J, Brown D, Orci L: Regional distribution of N-acetyl-D-galactosamine residues in the glycocalyx of glomerular podocytes. J Cell Biol 96:1189–1196, 1983.

2215. Kizaki T, Takeda Z, Watanabe M, et al: Histochemical analysis of changes in lectin binding in murine glomerular lesions. Acta Pathol Jpn 39:31–41, 1989.

2216. Sekiyama S, Yoshida F, Yuzawa Y, et al: Mesangial proliferative glomerulonephritis induced in rats by a lentil lectin and its antibodies. J Lab Clin Med 121:71–82, 1993.

2217. Holthöfer H: Lectin binding sites in kidney. A comparative study of 14 animal species. J Histochem Cytochem 31:531–537, 1983.

2218. Wilson CB, Golbus SM, Neale TJ, Woodroffe AJ: Nephritogenic immune responses involving antigens in or of the glomerulus. In Read SE, Zabriskie JB (eds): Streptococcal Diseases and the Immune Response. Academic Press, New York, 1980, pp 463–475.

2219. Abramowsky CR, Powers KG, Aikawa M, Swinehart G: Dirofilaria immitis. 5. Immunopathology of filarial nephropathy in dogs. Am J Pathol 104:1–12, 1981.

2220. Grauer GF, Culham CA, Dubielzig RR, et al: Experimental Dirofilaria immitis–associated glomerulonephritis induced in part by in situ formation of immune complexes in the glomerular capillary wall. J Parasitol 75:585–593, 1989.

2221. Nakagaki K, Nogami S, Hayashi Y, et al: Dirofilaria immitis: Detection of parasite-specific antigen by monoclonal antibodies in glomerulonephritis in infected dogs. Parasitol Res 79:49–54, 1993.

2222. Nakagaki K, Hayasaki M, Ohishi I: Histopathological and immunopathological evaluation of filarial glomerulonephritis in Dirofilaria immitis infected dogs. Jpn J Exp Med 60:179–186, 1990.

2223. Houba V, Sturrock RF, Butterworth AE: Kidney lesions in baboons infected with Schistosoma mansoni. Clin Exp Immunol 30:439–449, 1977.

2224. Johnston WH, Latta H: Acute hematogenous pyelonephritis in the rabbit. Electron microscopic study of Escherichia coli localization and early acute inflammation. Lab Invest 38:439–446, 1978.

2225. Vogt A, Batsford S, Rodriguez-Iturbe B, Garcia R: Cationic antigens in poststreptococcal glomerulonephritis. Clin Nephrol 20:271–279, 1983.

2226. Lange K, Seligson G, Cronin W: Evidence for the in situ origin of poststreptococcal glomerulonephritis: Glomerular localization of endostreptosin and the clinical significance of the subsequent antibody response. Clin Nephrol 19:3–10, 1983.

2227. Cronin WJ, Lange K: Immunologic evidence for the in situ deposition of a cytoplasmic streptococcal antigen (endostreptosin) on the glomerular basement membrane in rats. Clin Nephrol 34:143–146, 1990.

2228. Yoshizawa N, Oshima S, Sagel I, et al: Role of a streptococcal antigen in the pathogenesis of acute poststreptococcal glomerulonephritis. Characterization of the antigen and a proposed mechanism for the disease. J Immunol 148:3110–3116, 1992.

2229. Gerfaux J, Chany-Fournier F, Bardos P, et al: Lectin-like activity of components extracted from human glomerular basement membrane. Proc Natl Acad Sci USA 76:5129–5133, 1979.

2230. Vogt A, Schmiedeke T, Stockl F, et al: The role of cationic proteins in the pathogenesis of immune complex glomerulonephritis. Nephrol Dial Transplant 5(suppl 1):6–9, 1990.

2231. Batsford SR: Cationic antigens as mediators of inflammation. Acta Pathol Microbiol Immunol Scand 99:1–9, 1991.

2232. Kaseda N, Uehara Y, Yamamoto Y, Tanaka K: Induction of in situ immune complexes in rat glomeruli using avidin, a native cation macromolecule. Br J Exp Pathol 66:729–736, 1985.

2233. Batsford SR, Takamiya H, Vogt A: A model of in situ immune complex glomerulonephritis in the rat employing cationized ferritin. Clin Nephrol 14:211–216, 1980.

2234. Batsford S, Oite T, Takamiya H, Vogt A: Anionic binding sites in the glomerular basement membrane: Possible role in the pathogenesis of immune complex glomerulonephritis. Renal Physiol 3:336–340, 1980.

2235. Oite T, Batsford SR, Mihatsch MJ, et al: Quantitative studies of in situ immune complex glomerulonephritis in the rat induced by planted cationized antigen. J Exp Med 155:460–474, 1982.

2236. Vogt A, Rohrbach R, Shimizu F, et al: Interaction of cationized antigen with rat glomerular basement membrane: In situ immune complex formation. Kidney Int 22:27–35, 1982.

2237. Oite T, Shimizu F, Kihara I, et al: An active model of immune complex glomerulonephritis in the rat employing cationized antigen. Am J Pathol 112:185–194, 1983.

2238. Ward HJ, Cohen AH, Border WA: In situ formation of subepithelial immune complexes in the rabbit glomerulus: Requirement of a cationic antigen. Nephron 36:257–264, 1984.

2239. Oite T, Shimizu F, Suzuki Y, Vogt A: Ultramicroscopic localization of cationized antigen in the glomerular basement membrane in the course of active, in situ immune complex glomerulonephritis. Virchows Arch B 48:107–118, 1985.

2240. Suzuki Y, Maruyama Y, Arakawa M, Oite T: Preservation of fixed anionic sites in the GBM in the acute proteinuric phase of cationic antigen mediated in-situ immune complex glomerulonephritis in the rat. Histochemistry 81:243–246, 1984.

2241. Boulton Jones JM, Chandrachud L, Mosely H: Inherited variations in glomerular handling of antigen between Lewis and DA rats. Clin Sci 71:565–572, 1986.

2242. Kagami S, Miyao M, Shimizu F, Oite T: Active in situ immune complex glomerulonephritis using the hapten-carrier system: Role of epitope density in cationic antigens. Clin Exp Immunol 74:121–125, 1988.

2243. Border WA, Ward HJ, Kamil ES, Cohen AH: Induction of membranous nephropathy in rabbits by administration of an exogenous cationic antigen. Demonstration of a pathogenic role for electrical charge. J Clin Invest 69:451–461, 1982.

2244. Kagami S, Kawakami K, Okada K, et al: Mechanism of formation of subepithelial electron-dense deposits in active in situ immune complex glomerulonephritis. Am J Pathol 136:631–639, 1990.

2245. Sawtell NM, Weiss MA, Pesce AJ, Michael JG: An immune complex glomerulopathy associated with glomerular capillary thrombosis in the laboratory mouse. A highly reproducible accelerated model utilizing cationized antigen. Lab Invest 56:256–263, 1987.

2246. Huang JT, Mannik M, Gleisner J: In situ formation of immune complexes in the choroid plexus of rats by sequential injection of a cationized antigen and unaltered antibodies. J Neuropathol Exp Neurol 43:489–499, 1984.

2247. Barnes JL, Reznicek MJ, Radnik RA, Venkatachalam MA: Anionization of an antigen promotes glomerular binding and immune complex formation. Kidney Int 34:156–163, 1988.

2248. Adler S, Baker P, Pritzl P, Couser WG: Effect of alterations in glomerular charge on deposition of cationic and anionic antibodies to fixed glomerular antigens in the rat. J Lab Clin Med 106:1–11, 1985.

2249. Feintzeig ID, Dittmer JE, Cybulsky AV, Salant DJ: Antibody, antigen, and glomerular capillary wall charge interactions: Influence of antigen location on in situ immune complex formation. Kidney Int 29:649–657, 1986.

2249a. Yang JJ, Jennett JC, Falk RJ: Immune complex glomerulonephritis is induced in rats immunized with heterologous myeloperoxidase. Clin Exp Immunol 97:466–473, 1994.

2250. Hunsicker LG, Shearer TP, Shaffer SJ: Acute reversible proteinuria induced by infusion of the polycation hexadimethrine. Kidney Int 20:7–17, 1981.

2251. Assel E, Neumann K-H, Schurek H-J, et al: Glomerular albumin leakage and morphology after neutralization of polyanions. 1. Albumin clearance and sieving coefficient in the isolated perfused rat kidney. Renal Physiol 7:357–364, 1984.

2252. Bertolatus JA, Foster SJ, Hunsicker LG: Stainable glomerular basement membrane polyanions and renal hemodynamics during hexadimethrine-induced proteinuria. J Lab Clin Med 103:632–642, 1984.

2253. Barnes JL, Radnik RA, Gilchrist EP, Venkatachalam MA: Size and charge selective permeability defects induced in glomerular basement membrane by a polycation. Kidney Int 25:11–19, 1984.

2254. Andrews PM, Bates SB: Dose-dependent movement of cationic molecules across the glomerular wall. Anat Rec 212:223–231, 1985.

2255. Bertolatus JA, Hunsicker LG: Glomerular sieving of anionic and neutral bovine albumins in proteinuric rats. Kidney Int 28:467–476, 1985.

2256. Pilia PA, Swain RP, Williams AV, et al: Glomerular anionic site distribution in nonproteinuric rats. A computer-assisted morphometric analysis. Am J Pathol 121:474–485, 1985.

2257. Barnes JL, Venkatachalam MA: Enhancement of glomerular immune complex deposition by a circulating polycation. J Exp Med 160:286–293, 1984.

2258. Furness PN, Drakeley S: Heparin causes partial removal of glomerular antigen deposits by a mechanism independent of its anticoagulant properties. J Pathol 168:217–220, 1992.

2259. Kanwar YS, Caulin-Glaser T, Gallo GR, Lamm ME: Interaction of immune complexes with glomerular heparan sulfate–proteoglycans. Kidney Int 30:842–851, 1986.

2260. Schaeverbeke J, Moreau Lalande H, Geloso-Meyer A, et al: Enhancement of glomerular permeability to anionic ferritin induced by kidney perfusion with collagenase. Biol Cell 53:179–186, 1985.

2261. Adler SG, Wang H, Ward HJ, et al: Electrical charge. Its role in the pathogenesis and prevention of experimental membranous nephropathy in the rabbit. J Clin Invest 71:487–499, 1983.

2262. Oite T, Shimizu F, Batsford SR, Vogt A: The effect of protamine sulfate on the course of immune complex glomerulonephritis in the rat. Clin Exp Immunol 64:318–322, 1986.

2263. Raj AS, Tuscan M, Shapiro B, et al: Amount of antibody is critical for immune complex displacement by charge competition from both rabbit glomeruli and anionic beads. Clin Exp Immunol 64:629–637, 1986.

2264. Fleuren G, Grond J, Hoedemaeker PJ: In situ formation of subepithelial glomerular immune complexes in passive serum sickness. Kidney Int 17:631–637, 1980.

2265. White RB, Lowrie L, Stork JE, et al: Targeted enzyme therapy of experimental glomerulonephritis in rats. J Clin Invest 87:1819–1827, 1991.

2266. Duan H-J, Nakazawa K, Ishigame H, et al: Masking of anionic sites by deposits in lamina rara externa in immune complex nephritis in rats. Virchows Arch B 60:165–171, 1991.

2267. Lambert PH, Goldman M, Rose LM, Morel PA: A possible role for idiotypic interactions in the pathogenesis of immune complex glomerulonephritis. Transplant Proc 14:543–546, 1982.

2268. Goldman M, Renversez JC, Lambert PH: Pathological expression of idiotypic interactions: Immune complexes and cryoglobulins. Springer Semin Immunopathol 6:33–49, 1983.

2269. Zanetti M, Wilson CB: A role for antiidiotypic antibodies in immunologically mediated nephritis. Am J Kidney Dis 7:445–451, 1986.

2270. Ford PM: Rheumatoid factor and experimental glomerular disease. Monogr Allergy 26:240–250, 1989.

2271. Zanetti M, Wilson CB: Participation of auto-anti-idiotypes in immune complex glomerulonephritis in rabbits. J Immunol 131:2781–2783, 1983.

2272. Goldman M, Rose LM, Hochmann A, Lambert PH: Deposition of idiotype–anti-idiotype immune complexes in renal glomeruli after polyclonal B cell activation. J Exp Med 155:1385–1399, 1982.

2273. Rose LM, Goldman M, Lambert P-H: The production of anti-idiotypic antibodies and of idiotype–anti-idiotype immune complexes after polyclonal activation induced by bacterial LPS. J Immunol 128:2126–2133, 1982.

2274. Goidl EA, Choy JW, Gibbons JJ, et al: Production of auto-antiidiotypic antibody during the normal immune response. VII. Analysis of the cellular basis for the increased auto-antiidiotype antibody production by aged mice. J Exp Med 157:1635–1645, 1983.

2275. Rose LM, Lambert PH: The natural occurrence of circulating idiotype–anti-idiotype complexes during a secondary immune response to phosphorylcholine. Clin Immunol Immunopathol 15:481–492, 1980.

2276. Rose LM, Goldman M, Lambert P-H: Simultaneous induction of an idiotype, corresponding anti-idiotypic antibodies, and immune complexes during African trypanosomiasis in mice. J Immunol 128:79–85, 1982.

2277. Schreiber RD, Müller-Eberhard HJ: Complement and renal disease. In Wilson CB, Brenner BM, Stein JH (eds): Contemporary Issues in Nephrology, Vol 3. Churchill Livingstone, New York, 1979, pp 67–105.

2278. Gyotoku Y, Abdelmoula M, Spertini F, et al: Cryoglobulinemia induced by monoclonal immunoglobulin G rheumatoid factors derived from autoimmune MRL/MpJ-lpr/lpr mice. J Immunol 138:3785–3792, 1987.

2279. Abdelmoula M, Spertini F, Shibata T, et al: IgG3 is the major source of cryoglobulins in mice. J Immunol 143:526–532, 1989.

2280. Berney T, Shibata T, Izui S: Murine cryoglobulinemia: Pathogenic and protective IgG3 self-associating antibodies. J Immunol 147:3331–3335, 1991.

2281. Lemoine R, Berney T, Shibata T, et al: Induction of "wire-loop" lesions by murine monoclonal IgG3 cryoglobulins. Kidney Int 41:65–72, 1992.

2282. Reininger L, Berney T, Shibata T, et al: Cryoglobulinemia induced by a murine IgG3 rheumatoid factor: Skin vasculitis and glomerulonephritis arise from distinct pathogenic mechanisms. Proc Natl Acad Sci USA 87:10038–10042, 1990.

2283. Spertini F, Donati Y, Welle I, et al: Prevention of murine cryoglobulinemia and associated pathology by monoclonal anti-idiotypic antibody. J Immunol 143:2508–2513, 1989.

2284. Izui S, Berney T, Shibata T, Fulpius T: IgG3 cryoglobulins in autoimmune MRL-lpr/lpr mice: Immunopathogenesis, therapeutic approaches and relevance to similar human diseases. Ann Rheum Dis 52(suppl 1):S48–S54, 1993.

2285. Fulpius T, Berney T, Lemoine R, et al: Glomerulopathy induced by IgG3 anti-trinitrophenyl monoclonal cryoglobulins derived from non-autoimmune mice. Kidney Int 45:962–971, 1994.

2286. Heieren MH, van der Woude FJ, Balfour HH Jr: Cytomegalovirus replicates efficiently in human kidney mesangial cells. Proc Natl Acad Sci USA 85:1642–1646, 1988.

2287. Madaio MP, Salant DJ, Adler S, et al: Effect of antibody charge and concentration on deposition of antibody to glomerular basement membrane. Kidney Int 26:397–403, 1984.

2288. Salant DJ, Adler S, Darby C, et al: Influence of antigen distribution on the mediation of immunological glomerular injury. Kidney Int 27:938–950, 1985.

2289. Salant DJ, Cybulsky AV, Feintzeig ID: Quantitation of exogenous and endogenous components of glomerular immune deposits. Kidney Int 30:255–263, 1986.

2290. Bannister KM, Wilson CB: Transfer of tubulointerstitial nephritis in the Brown Norway rat with anti–tubular basement membrane antibody: Quantitation and kinetics of binding and effect of decomplementation. J Immunol 135:3911–3917, 1985.

2291. Lerner RA, Glassock RJ, Dixon FJ: The role of anti–glomerular basement membrane antibody in the pathogenesis of human glomerulonephritis. J Exp Med 126:989–1004, 1967.

2292. Wilson CB, Dixon FJ: Anti–glomerular basement membrane antibody-induced glomerulonephritis. Kidney Int 3:74–89, 1973.

2293. Almkuist RD, Buckalew VM Jr, Hirszel P, et al: Recurrence of anti–glomerular basement membrane antibody mediated glomerulonephritis in an isograft. Clin Immunol Immunopathol 18:54–60, 1981.

2294. Wilson CB: Anti-GBM glomerulonephritis. In Rosen S (ed): Contemporary Issues in Surgical Pathology, Vol I, Pathology of Glomerular Disease. Churchill Livingstone, New York, 1983, pp 171–194.

2295. Johnson JP, Moore J Jr, Austin HA III, et al: Therapy of anti–glomerular basement membrane antibody disease: Analysis of prognostic significance of clinical, pathologic, and treatment factors. Medicine 64:219–227, 1985.

2296. Savage COS, Pusey CD, Bowman C, et al: Antiglomerular basement membrane antibody mediated disease in the British Isles 1980–1984. Br Med J 292:301–304, 1986

2297. Wilson CB: Immunologic diseases of the lung and kidney (Goodpasture's syndrome). In Fishman AP (ed): Pulmonary Diseases and Disorders, 2nd ed. McGraw-Hill, New York, 1988, pp 675–682.

2298. Pusey CD, Lockwood CM: Autoimmunity in rapidly progressive glomerulonephritis. Kidney Int 35:929–937, 1989.

2299. O'Donoghue DJ, Short CD, Brenchley PEC, et al: Sequential development of systemic vasculitis with anti-neutrophil cytoplasmic antibodies complicating anti–glomerular basement membrane disease. Clin Nephrol 32:251–255, 1989.

2300. Wilson CB: Goodpasture's syndrome. In Suki WN, Massry SG (eds): Therapy of Renal Diseases and Related Disorders, 2nd ed. Kluwer Academic Publishers, Boston, 1991, pp 333–342.

2301. Saxena R, Johansson C, Bygren P, Wieslander J: Autoimmunity and glomerulonephritis. Postgrad Med J 68:242–250, 1992.

2302. Wilson CB: Goodpasture's syndrome and other anti–basement membrane antibody disease. In Rich R (ed): Clinical Immunology: Principles and Practice. Mosby–Year Book, St. Louis (in press).

2303. Bell DD, Moffatt SL, Singer M, Munt PW: Antibasement membrane antibody disease without clinical evidence of renal disease. Am Rev Respir Dis 142:234–237, 1990.

2304. Tobler A, Schürch E, Altermatt HJ, Im Hof V: Anti–basement membrane antibody disease with severe pulmonary haemorrhage and normal renal function. Thorax 46:68–70, 1991.

2305. Churg A, Franklin W, Chan KL, et al: Pulmonary hemorrhage and immune-complex deposition in the lung. Complications in a patient with systemic lupus erythematosus. Arch Pathol Lab Med 104:388–391, 1980.

2306. Lam M, Krous HF, Llach F: Massive pulmonary hemorrhage and fulminant renal failure associated with immune complex glomerulonephritis. South Med J 74:1338–1342, 1981.

2307. Marino CT, Pertschuk LP: Pulmonary hemorrhage in systemic lupus erythematosus. Arch Intern Med 141:201–203, 1981.

2308. Haupt HM, Moore GW, Hutchins GM: The lung in systemic lupus erythematosus. Analysis of the pathologic changes in 120 patients. Am J Med 71:791–798, 1981.

2309. Chugh KS, Gupta VK, Singhal PC, Sehgal S: Case report: Poststreptococcal crescentic glomerulonephritis and pulmonary hemorrhage simulating Goodpasture's syndrome. Ann Allergy 47:104–106, 1981.

2310. Daniele RP, Henson PM, Fantone JC III, et al: Immune complex injury of the lung. Am Rev Respir Dis 124:738–755, 1981.

2311. Leatherman JW, Sibley RK, Davies SF: Diffuse intrapulmonary hemorrhage and glomerulonephritis unrelated to anti–glomerular basement membrane antibody. Am J Med 72:401–410, 1982.

2312. Verberckmoes R, Bobbaers H: Pulmonary problems in renal patients. Contrib Nephrol 33:67–85, 1982.

2313. Rankin JA, Matthay RA: Pulmonary renal syndromes. II. Etiology and pathogenesis. Yale J Biol Med 55:11–26, 1982.

2314. Fukuda Y, Yamanaka N, Ishizaki M, et al: Immune complex–mediated glomerulonephritis and interstitial pneumonia simulating Goodpasture's syndrome. Acta Pathol Jpn 32:361–370, 1982.

2315. Castañeda S, Herrero-Beaumont G, Valenzuela A, et al: Massive pulmonary hemorrhage: Fatal complication of systemic lupus erythematosus. J Rheumatol 12:186–187, 1985.

2316. Brasington RD, Furst DE: Pulmonary disease in systemic lupus erythematosus. Clin Exp Rheumatol 3:269–276, 1985.

2317. Boyce NW, Holdsworth SR: Pulmonary manifestations of the clinical syndrome of acute glomerulonephritis and lung hemorrhage. Am J Kidney Dis 8:31–36, 1986.

2318. Zell SC, Duxbury G, Shankel SW: Alveolar hemorrhage associated with a membranoproliferative glomerulonephritis and smooth muscle antibody. Am J Med 82:1073–1076, 1987.

2319. Wu M-J, Rajaram R, Shelp WD, et al: Vasculitis in Goodpasture's syndrome. Arch Pathol Lab Med 104:300–302, 1980.

2320. Stave GM, Croker BP: Thrombotic microangiopathy in anti–glomerular basement membrane glomerulonephritis. Arch Pathol Lab Med 108:747–751, 1984.

2321. Wahls TL, Bonsib SM, Schuster VL: Coexistent Wegener's granulomatosis and anti–glomerular basement membrane disease. Hum Pathol 18:202–205, 1987.

2322. Jayne DRW, Marshall PD, Jones SJ, Lockwood CM: Autoantibodies to GBM and neutrophil cytoplasm in rapidly progressive glomerulonephritis. Kidney Int 37:965–970, 1990.

2323. Nässberger L, Sjöholm AG, Thysell H: Antimyeloperoxidase antibodies in patients with extracapillary glomerulonephritis. Nephron 56:152–156, 1990.

2324. Bosch X, Mirapeix E, Font J, et al: Prognostic implication of anti–neutrophil cytoplasmic autoantibodies with myeloperoxidase specificity in anti–glomerular basement membrane disease. Clin Nephrol 36:107–113, 1991.

2325. Bygren P, Rasmussen N, Isaksson B, Wieslander J: Anti–neutrophil cytoplasm antibodies, anti-GBM antibodies and anti-dsDNA antibodies in glomerulonephritis. Eur J Clin Invest 22:783–792, 1992.

2326. Bosch X, Mirapeix E, Font J, et al: Anti-myeloperoxidase autoantibodies in patients with necrotizing glomerular and alveolar capillaritis. Am J Kidney Dis 20:231–239, 1992.

2327. McCance DR, Maxwell AP, Hill CM, Doherty CC: Glomerulonephritis associated with antibodies to neutrophil cytoplasm and glomerular basement membrane. Postgrad Med J 68:186–188, 1992.

2328. Bowman C, Ambrus K, Lockwood CM: Restriction of human IgG subclass expression in the population of auto-antibodies to glomerular basement membrane. Clin Exp Immunol 69:341–349, 1987.

2329. Noël LH, Aucouturier P, Monteiro RC, et al: Glomerular and serum immunoglobulin G subclasses in membranous nephropathy and anti–glomerular basement membrane nephritis. Clin Immunol Immunopathol 46:186–194, 1988.

2330. Weber M, Lohse AW, Manns M, et al: IgG subclass distribution of autoantibodies to glomerular basement membrane in Goodpasture's syndrome compared to other autoantibodies. Nephron 49:54–57, 1988.

2331. Segelmark M, Butkowski R, Wieslander J: Antigen restriction and IgG subclasses among anti-GBM autoantibodies. Nephrol Dial Transplant 5:991–996, 1990.

2332. Melvin T, Kim Y, Michael AF: Selective binding of IgG$_4$ and other negatively charged plasma proteins in normal and diabetic human kidneys. Am J Pathol 115:443–446, 1984.

2333. Gris P, Pirson Y, Hamels J, et al: Antiglomerular basement membrane nephritis induced by IgA1 antibodies. Nephron 58:418–424, 1991.

2334. Savige JA, Yeung SP, Bierre AR, Kincaid-Smith P: Lambda-light-chain–mediated anti-GBM disease. Nephron 52:144–148, 1989.

2335. Wilson CB, Marquardt H, Dixon FJ: Radioimmunoassay (RIA) for circulating antiglomerular basement membrane (GBM) antibodies. Kidney Int 6:114a, 1974. Abstract.

2336. Wilson CB: Radioimmunoassay for anti–glomerular basement membrane antibodies. *In* Rose NR, Friedman H (eds): Manual of Clinical Immunology, 2nd ed. American Society for Microbiology, Washington, DC, 1980, pp 376–379.

2337. Wieslander J, Bygren P, Heinegård D: Antiglomerular basement membrane antibody: Antibody specificity in different forms of glomerulonephritis. Kidney Int 23:855–861, 1983.

2338. Fish AJ, Kleppel M, Jeraj K, Michael AF: Enzyme immunoassay of anti–glomerular basement membrane antibodies. J Lab Clin Med 105:700–705, 1985.

2339. Weber M, Köhler H, Manns M, Meyer zum Büschenfelde K-H: Antiglomerular basement membrane antibodies in human sera: Detection by a modified micro-ELISA. Clin Immunol Immunopathol 35:285–294, 1985.

2340. Bowman C, Lockwood CM: Clinical application of a radio-immunoassay for auto-antibodies to glomerular basement membrane. J Clin Lab Immunol 17:197–202, 1985.

2341. Simon CA, Winkelmann RK: Bullous pemphigoid and glomerulonephritis. Report of four cases. J Am Acad Dermatol 14:456–463, 1986.

2342. van Joost T, Muntendam J, Heule F, et al: Subepidermal bullous autoimmune disease associated with immune nephritis. Immunomorphologic studies. J Am Acad Dermatol 14:214–220, 1986.

2343. Davenport A, Verbov JL, Goldsmith HJ: Circulating anti–skin basement membrane zone antibodies in a patient with Goodpasture's syndrome. Br J Dermatol 117:125–127, 1987.

2344. Sawamura D, Nomura K, Sugita Y, et al: Bullous pemphigoid antigen (BPAG1): cDNA cloning and mapping of the gene to the short arm of human chromosome 6. Genomics 8:722–726, 1990.

2345. Li K, Sawamura D, Giudice GJ, et al: Genomic organization of collagenous domains and chromosomal assignment of human 180-kDa bullous pemphigoid antigen-2, a novel collagen of stratified squamous epithelium. J Biol Chem 266:24064–24069, 1991.

2346. Uitto J, Christiano AM: Molecular genetics of the cutaneous basement membrane zone. Perspectives on epidermolysis bullosa and other blistering skin diseases. J Clin Invest 90:687–692, 1992.

2347. Lee LK, Pollock AS, Lovett DH: Asymmetric origins of the mature glomerular basement membrane. J Cell Physiol 157:169–177, 1993.

2348. Martinez-Hernandez A, Amenta PS: The basement membrane in pathology. Lab Invest 48:656–677, 1983.

2349. Timpl R: Structure and biological activity of basement membrane proteins. Eur J Biochem 180:487–502, 1989.

2350. Hudson BG, Wieslander J, Wisdom BJ Jr, Noelken ME: Goodpasture syndrome: Molecular architecture and function of basement membrane antigen. Lab Invest 61:256–269, 1989. (Erratum in Lab Invest 61:690, 1989.)

2351. Weber M: Basement membrane proteins. Kidney Int 41:620–628, 1992.

2352. al-Mutlaq H, Wheeler J, Robertson H, et al: Tissue distribution of amyloid P component as defined by a monoclonal antibody produced by immunization with human glomerular basement membranes. Histochem J 25:219–227, 1993.

2353. Fish AJ, Carmody KM, Michael AF: Spatial orientation and distribution of antigens within human glomerular basement membrane. J Lab Clin Med 94:447–457, 1979.

2354. Jeraj K, Michael AF, Fish AJ: Immunologic similarities between Goodpasture's and Steblay's antibodies. Clin Immunol Immunopathol 23:408–413, 1982.

2355. Wieslander J, Bygren P, Heinegård D: Different antibody response in experimental and spontaneous glomerulonephritis. Renal Physiol 3:341–346, 1980.

2356. Sisson S, Dysart NK Jr, Fish AJ, Vernier RL: Localization of the Goodpasture antigen by immunoelectron microscopy. Clin Immunol Immunopathol 23:414–422, 1982.

2357. Kefalides NA: Current status of chemistry and structure of basement membranes. *In* Kefalides NA (ed): Biology and Chemistry of Basement Membranes. Academic Press, New York, 1978, pp 215–228.

2358. Kefalides NA: Isolation of a collagen from basement membranes containing three identical α-chains. Biochem Biophys Res Commun 45:226–234, 1971.

2359. Hudson BG, Reeders ST, Tryggvason K: Type IV collagen: Structure, gene organization, and role in human diseases. J Biol Chem 268:26033–26036, 1993.

2360. Dixit SN, Mainardi CL, Beachey EH, Kang AH: 7S domain constitutes the amino-terminal end of type IV collagen: An immunochemical study. Coll Relat Res 3:263–270, 1983.

2361. Fessler LI, Fessler JH: Identification of the carboxyl peptides of mouse procollagen IV and its implications for the assembly and structure of basement membrane procollagen. J Biol Chem 257:9804–9810, 1982.

2362. Weber S, Engel J, Wiedemann H, et al: Subunit structure and assembly of the globular domain of basement-membrane collagen type IV. Eur J Biochem 139:401–410, 1984.

2363. Siebold B, Deutzmann R, Kühn K: The arrangement of intra- and intermolecular disulfide bonds in the carboxyterminal, non-collagenous aggregation and cross-linking domain of basement-membrane type IV collagen. Eur J Biochem 176:617–624, 1988.

2364. Timpl R: Recent advances in the biochemistry of glomerular basement membrane. Kidney Int 30:293–298, 1986.

2365. Spiro RG: Studies on the renal glomerular basement membrane. Nature of the carbohydrate units and their attachment to the peptide portion. J Biol Chem 242:1923–1932, 1967.

2366. Langeveld JPM, Noelken ME, Hård K, et al: Bovine glomerular basement membrane. Location and structure of the asparagine-linked oligosaccharide units and their potential role in the assembly of the 7 S collagen IV tetramer. J Biol Chem 266:2622–2631, 1991.

2367. Nayak BR, Spiro RG: Localization and structure of the asparagine-linked oligosaccharides of type IV collagen from glomerular basement membrane and lens capsule. J Biol Chem 266:13978–13987, 1991.

2368. Soininen R, Haka-Risku T, Prockop DJ, Tryggvason K: Complete primary structure of the α$_1$-chain of human basement membrane (type IV) collagen. FEBS Lett 225:188–194, 1987.

2369. Brazel D, Oberbäumer I, Dieringer H, et al: Completion of the amino acid sequence of the α1 chain of human basement membrane collagen (type IV) reveals 21 non-triplet interruptions located within the collagenous domain. Eur J Biochem 168:529–536, 1987.

2370. Hostikka SL, Tryggvason K: The complete primary structure of the α2 chain of human type IV collagen and comparison with the α1(IV) chain. J Biol Chem 263:19488–19493, 1988.

2371. Pöschl E, Pollner R, Kühn K: The genes for the α1(IV) and α2(IV) chains of human basement membrane collagen type IV are arranged head-to-head and separated by a bidirectional promoter of unique structure. EMBO J 7:2687–2695, 1988.

2372. Guo X, Kramer JM: The two *Caenorhabditis elegans* basement membrane (type IV) collagen genes are located on separate chromosomes. J Biol Chem 264:17574–17582, 1989.

2373. Morrison KE, Germino GG, Reeders ST: Use of the polymerase chain reaction to clone and sequence a cDNA encoding the bovine alpha 3 chain of type IV collagen. J Biol Chem 266:34–39, 1991.

2374. Morrison KE, Mariyama M, Yang-Feng TL, Reeders ST: Sequence and localization of a partial cDNA encoding the human α3 chain of type IV collagen. Am J Hum Genet 49:545–554, 1991.

2375. Turner N, Mason PJ, Brown R, et al: Molecular cloning of the human Goodpasture antigen demonstrates it to be the α3 chain of type IV collagen. J Clin Invest 89:592–601, 1992.

2376. Quinones S, Bernal D, Garcia-Sogo M, et al: Exon/intron structure of the human α3(IV) gene encompassing the Goodpasture antigen (α3(IV)NC1). Identification of a potentially antigenic region at the triple helix/NC1 domain junction. J Biol Chem 267:19780–19784, 1992.

2377. Mariyama M, Zheng K, Yang-Feng TL, Reeders ST: Colocalization of the genes for the α3(IV) and α4(IV) chains of type IV collagen to chromosome 2 bands q35-q37. Genomics 13:809–813, 1992.

2378. Zhou J, Mochizuki T, Smeets H, et al: Deletion of the paired α5(IV) and α6(IV) collagen genes in inherited smooth muscle tumors. Science 261:1167–1169, 1993.

2379. Pihlajaniemi T, Pohjolainen ER, Myers JC: Complete primary structure of the triple-helical region and the carboxyl-terminal domain of a new type IV collagen chain, alpha 5(IV). J Biol Chem 265:13758–13766, 1990.

2380. Hostikka SL, Eddy RL, Byers MG, et al: Identification of a distinct type IV collagen α chain with restricted kidney distribution and assignment of its gene to the locus of X chromosome–linked Alport syndrome. Proc Natl Acad Sci USA 87:1606–1610, 1990.

2381. Myers JC, Jones TA, Pohjolainen E-R, et al: Molecular cloning of α5(IV) collagen and assignment of the gene to the region of the X chromosome containing the Alport syndrome locus. Am J Hum Genet 46:1024–1033, 1990.

2382. Haralson MA, Federspiel SJ, Martinez-Hernandez A, et al: Synthesis of [Proα1(IV)]₃ collagen molecules by cultured embryo-derived parietal yolk sac cells. Biochemistry 24:5792–5797, 1985.

2383. Saus J, Wieslander J, Langeveld JPM, et al: Identification of the Goodpasture antigen as the α3(IV) chain of collagen IV. J Biol Chem 263:13374–13380, 1988.

2384. Johansson C, Butkowski R, Wieslander J: The structural organization of type IV collagen. Identification of three NC1 populations in the glomerular basement membrane. J Biol Chem 267:24533–24537, 1992.

2385. Butkowski RJ, Wieslander J, Kleppel M, et al: Basement membrane collagen in the kidney: Regional localization of novel chains related to collagen IV. Kidney Int 35:1195–1202, 1989.

2386. Marquardt H, Wilson CB, Dixon FJ: Isolation and immunological characterization of human glomerular basement membrane antigens. Kidney Int 3:57–65, 1973.

2387. Timpl R, Orkin RW, Robey PG, et al: Chemical and immunological studies on basement membrane collagen from a murine tumor. *In* Kefalides NA (ed): Biology and Chemistry of Basement Membranes. Academic Press, New York, 1978, pp 413–419.

2388. Wick G, Timpl R: Study on the nature of the Goodpasture antigen using a basement membrane–producing mouse tumour. Clin Exp Immunol 39:733–738, 1980.

2389. Wisdom BJ Jr, Gunwar S, Hudson MD, et al: Type IV collagen of Engelbreth-Holm-Swarm tumor matrix: Identification of constituent chains. Connect Tissue Res 27:225–234, 1992.

2390. Holdsworth SR, Golbus SM, Wilson CB: Characterization of collagenase solubilized human glomerular basement membrane antigens reacting with human antibodies. Kidney Int 16:797, 1979. Abstract.

2391. Wilson CB, Holdsworth SR, Neale TJ: Anti–basement membrane antibodies in immunologic renal disease. Aust N Z J Med 11(suppl 1):94–100, 1981.

2392. Wilson CB, Holdsworth SR: Anti–glomerular basement membrane (GBM) antibody-induced diseases. *In* Zurukzoglu W, Papadimitriou M, Pyrpasopoulos M, et al (eds): Proceedings of the 8th International Congress of Nephrology. S Karger, Basel, 1981, pp 910–916.

2393. Wieslander J: The Goodpasture antigen. Contrib Nephrol 80:56–67, 1990.

2394. Hudson BG, Kalluri R, Gunwar S, et al: Molecular characteristics of the Goodpasture autoantigen. Kidney Int 43:135–139, 1993.

2395. Hunt JS, Macdonald PR, McGiven AR: Isolation of human glomerular basement membrane antigens by affinity chromatography utilising Goodpasture's kidney antibody eluates. Renal Physiol 3:156–162, 1980.

2396. Hunt JS, Macdonald PR, McGiven AR: Characterisation of human glomerular basement membrane antigenic fractions isolated by affinity chromatography utilising anti–glomerular basement membrane autoantibodies. Biochem Biophys Res Commun 104:1025–1032, 1982.

2397. Wieslander J, Bygren P, Heinegård D: Isolation of the specific glomerular basement membrane antigen involved in Goodpasture syndrome. Proc Natl Acad Sci USA 81:1544–1548, 1984.

2398. Yoshioka K, Kleppel M, Fish AJ: Analysis of nephritogenic antigens in human glomerular basement membrane by two-dimensional gel electrophoresis. J Immunol 134:3831–3837, 1985.

2399. Pusey CD, Dash A, Kershaw MJ, et al: A single autoantigen in Goodpasture's syndrome identified by a monoclonal antibody to human glomerular basement membrane. Lab Invest 56:23–31, 1987.

2400. Gunwar S, Noelken ME, Hudson BG: Properties of the collagenous domain of the α3(IV) chain, the Goodpasture antigen, of lens basement membrane collagen. Selective cleavage of α(IV) chains with retention of their triple helical structure and noncollagenous domain. J Biol Chem 266:14088–14094, 1991.

2401. Gunwar S, Ballester F, Kalluri R, et al: Glomerular basement membrane. Identification of dimeric subunits of the noncollagenous domain (hexamer) of collagen IV and the Goodpasture antigen. J Biol Chem 266:15318–15324, 1991.

2402. Hellmark T, Johansson C, Wieslander J: Characterization of anti-GBM antibodies involved in Goodpasture's syndrome. Kidney Int 46:823–829, 1994.

2403. Kefalides NA, Ohno N, Wilson CB: Antigenic components of bovine lens capsule that cross-react serum from Goodpasture's syndrome. Fed Proc 43:779, 1984. Abstract.

2404. Wieslander J, Barr JF, Butkowski RJ, et al: Goodpasture antigen of the glomerular basement membrane: Localization to noncollagenous regions of type IV collagen. Proc Natl Acad Sci USA 81:3838–3842, 1984.

2405. Butkowski RJ, Langeveld JPM, Wieslander J, et al: Localization of the Goodpasture epitope to a novel chain of basement membrane collagen. J Biol Chem 262:7874–7877, 1987.

2406. Wieslander J, Langeveld J, Butkowski R, et al: Physical and immunochemical studies of the globular domain of type IV collagen. Cryptic properties of the Goodpasture antigen. J Biol Chem 260:8564–8570, 1985.

2407. Kleppel MM, Michael AF, Fish AJ: Comparison of non-collagenous type IV collagen components in the human glomerulus and ESH tumor. Biochim Biophys Acta 883:178–189, 1986.

2408. Wieslander J, Heinegård D: The involvement of type IV collagen in Goodpasture's syndrome. Ann N Y Acad Sci 460:363–374, 1985.

2409. Weber M, Köhler H, Manns M, et al: Identification of Goodpasture target antigens in basement membranes of human glomeruli, lung, and placenta. Clin Exp Immunol 67:262–269, 1987.

2410. Schuppan D, Besser M, Schwarting R, Hahn EG: Radioimmunoassay for the carboxy-terminal cross-linking domain of type IV (basement membrane) procollagen in body fluids. Characterization and application to collagen type IV metabolism in fibrotic liver disease. J Clin Invest 78:241–248, 1986.

2411. Saxena R, Isaksson B, Bygren P, Wieslander J: A rapid assay for circulating anti–glomerular basement membrane antibodies in Goodpasture syndrome. J Immunol Methods 118:73–78, 1989.

2412. Kleppel MM, Michael AF, Fish AJ: Antibody specificity of human glomerular basement membrane type IV collagen NC1 subunits. Species variation in subunit composition. J Biol Chem 261:16547–16552, 1986.

2413. Butkowski RJ, Wieslander J, Wisdom BJ, et al: Properties of the globular domain of type IV collagen and its relationship to the Goodpasture antigen. J Biol Chem 260:3739–3747, 1985.

2414. Butkowski RJ, Shen G-Q, Wieslander J, et al: Characterization of type IV collagen NC1 monomers and Goodpasture antigen in human renal basement membranes. J Lab Clin Med 115:365–373, 1990.

2415. Kalluri R, Gunwar S, Reeders ST, et al: Goodpasture syndrome. Localization of the epitope for the autoantibodies to the carboxyl-terminal region of the α3(IV) chain of basement membrane collagen. J Biol Chem 266:24018–24024, 1991.

2416. Neilson EG, Kalluri R, Sun MJ, et al: Specificity of Goodpasture autoantibodies for the recombinant noncollagenous domains of human type IV collagen. J Biol Chem 268:8402–8405, 1993.

2417. Turner N, Forstová J, Rees A, et al: Production and characterization of recombinant Goodpasture antigen in insect cells. J Biol Chem 269:17141–17145, 1994.

2418. Wieslander J, Kataja M, Hudson BG: Characterization of the human Goodpasture antigen. Clin Exp Immunol 69:332–340, 1987.

2419. Kefalides NA: The Goodpasture antigen and basement membranes: The search must go on. Lab Invest 56:1–3, 1987.

2420. Kefalides NA, Ohno N, Wilson CB: Heterogeneity of antibodies in Goodpasture syndrome reacting with type IV collagen. Kidney Int 43:85–93, 1993.

2421. Kefalides NA, Ohno N, Wilson CB, et al: Identification of antigenic epitopes in type IV collagen by use of synthetic peptides. Kidney Int 43:94–100, 1993.

2422. Johansson C, Butkowski R, Swedenborg P, et al: Characterization of a non-Goodpasture autoantibody to type IV collagen. Nephrol Dial Transplant 8:1205–1210, 1993.

2423. Gunwar S, Bejarano PA, Kalluri R, et al: Alveolar basement membrane: Molecular properties of the noncollagenous domain (hexamer) of collagen IV and its reactivity with Goodpasture autoantibodies. Am J Respir Cell Mol Biol 5:107–112, 1991.

2424. Weber M, Pullig O: Different immunologic properties of the globular NC1 domain of collagen type IV isolated from various human basement membranes. Eur J Clin Invest 22:138–146, 1992.

2425. Keller F, Lyreal Ser Y, Schuppan D: Raised concentrations of the carboxyl terminal propeptide of type IV (basement membrane) procollagen (NC1) in serum and urine of patients with glomerulonephritis. Eur J Clin Invest 22:175–181, 1992.

2426. Bernal D, Quinones S, Saus J: The human mRNA encoding the Goodpasture antigen is alternatively spliced. J Biol Chem 268:12090–12094, 1993.

2427. Feng L, Xia Y, Wilson CB: Alternative splicing of the NC1 domain of the human α3 (IV) collagen gene. Differential expression of mRNA transcripts that predict three protein variants with distinct carboxyl regions. J Biol Chem 269:2342–2348, 1994.

2428. Feng L, Xia Y, Tang WW, Wilson CB: Alternative splicing of the NC domain of the human alpha-3 type IV collagen (C4A3) gene generates multiple mRNA transcripts which predict three protein variants with distinct carboxyl termini. J Am Soc Nephrol 3:629, 1992. Abstract.

2429. Wilson CB: Individual and strain differences in renal basement membrane antigens. Transplant Proc 12(suppl 1):69–73, 1980.

2430. Wilson CB, Lehman DH, McCoy RC, et al: Antitubular basement membrane antibodies after renal transplantation. Transplantation 18:447–452, 1974.

2431. De Heer E, Davidoff A, van der Wal A, et al: Chronic renal allograft rejection in the rat. Transplantation-induced antibodies against basement membrane antigens. Lab Invest 70:494–502, 1994.

2432. Fish AJ, Yoshioka K, Kleppel M, et al: Heterogeneity of the autoimmune response in human antiglomerular basement membrane (antiGBM) nephritis. Fed Proc 43:1589, 1984. Abstract.

2433. Anand SK, Landing BH, Heuser ET, et al: Changes in glomerular basement membrane antigen(s) with age. J Pediatr 92:952–953, 1978.

2434. Langeveld JPM, Veerkamp JH, Duyf CMP, Monnens LH: Chemical characterization of glomerular and tubular basement membranes of men of different ages. Kidney Int 20:104–114, 1981.

2435. Evans DJ, Smith A: Goodpasture antigen in infant kidney. Clin Nephrol 19:215, 1983. Letter.

2436. Jeraj J, Fish AJ, Yoshioka K, Michael AF: Development and heterogeneity of antigens in the immature nephron. Reactivity with human antiglomerular basement membrane autoantibodies. Am J Pathol 117:180–183, 1984.

2437. Yoshioka K, Michael AF, Velosa J, Fish AJ: Detection of hidden nephritogenic antigen determinants in human renal and nonrenal basement membranes. Am J Pathol 121:156–165, 1985.

2438. Wingen A-M, Döhner H, Schärer K, Rauterberg EW: Evidence for developmental changes of type IV collagen in glomerular basement membrane. Nephron 45:302–305, 1987.

2439. Kashtan CE, Kleppel MM, Butkowski RJ, et al: Alport syndrome, basement membranes and collagen. Pediatr Nephrol 4:523–532, 1990.

2440. Gubler M, Levy M, Broyer M, et al: Alport's syndrome: A report of 58 cases and a review of the literature. Am J Med 70:493–505, 1981.

2441. DiBona GF: Alport's syndrome: A genetic defect of biochemical composition of basement membranes of glomerulus, lens, and inner ear? J Lab Clin Med 101:817–820, 1983.

2442. Spear GS: Hereditary nephritis (Alport's syndrome)—1983. Clin Nephrol 21:3–6, 1984.

2443. Bernstein J: The glomerular basement membrane abnormality in Alport's syndrome. Am J Kidney Dis 10:222–229, 1987.

2444. McCoy RC, Johnson HK, Stone WJ, Wilson CB: Variation in glomerular basement membrane antigens in hereditary nephritis. Lab Invest 34:325, 1976. Abstract.

2445. Olson DL, Anand SK, Landing BH, et al: Diagnosis of hereditary nephritis by failure of glomeruli to bind anti–glomerular basement membrane antibodies. J Pediatr 96:697–699, 1980.

2446. Jenis EH, Valeski JE, Calcagno PL: Variability of anti-GBM binding in hereditary nephritis. Clin Nephrol 15:111–114, 1981.

2447. McCoy RC, Johnson HK, Stone WJ, Wilson CB: Absence of nephritogenic GBM antigen(s) in some patients with hereditary nephritis, Kidney Int 21:642–652, 1982.

2448. Reznik VM, Griswold WR, Vazquez MD, et al: Glomerulonephritis with absent glomerular basement membrane antigens. Am J Nephrol 5:296–298, 1985.

2449. Gubler M-C, Antignac C, Deschênes G, et al: Genetic, clinical, and morphologic heterogeneity in Alport's syndrome. Adv Nephrol 22:15–35, 1993.

2450. Melvin T, Kim Y, Michael AF: Amyloid P component is not present in the glomerular basement membrane in Alport-type hereditary nephritis. Am J Pathol 125:460–464, 1986.

2451. Habib R, Gubler M-C, Hinglais N, et al: Alport's syndrome: Experience at Hôpital Necker. Kidney Int 21(suppl 11):S-20–S-28, 1982.

2452. Jeraj K, Kim Y, Vernier RL, et al: Absence of Goodpasture's antigen in male patients with familial nephritis. Am J Kidney Dis 2:626–269, 1983.

2453. Savage COS, Reed A, Kershaw M, et al: Use of a monoclonal antibody in differential diagnosis of children with haematuria and hereditary nephritis. Lancet 1:1459–1461, 1986.

2454. Savage COS, Pusey CD, Kershaw MJ, et al: The Goodpasture antigen in Alport's syndrome: Studies with a monoclonal antibody. Kidney Int 30:107–112, 1986.

2455. Ding J, Kashtan CE, Fan WW, et al: A monoclonal antibody marker for Alport syndrome identifies the Alport antigen as the α5 chain of type IV collagen. Kidney Int 46:1504–1506, 1994.

2456. Kashtan CE, Atkin CL, Gregory MC, Michael AF: Identification of variant Alport phenotypes using an Alport-specific antibody probe. Kidney Int 36:669–674, 1989.

2457. Kleppel MM, Kashtan C, Santi PA, et al: Distribution of familial nephritis antigen in normal tissue and renal basement membranes of patients with homozygous and heterozygous Alport familial nephritis. Relationship of familial nephritis and Goodpasture antigens to novel collagen chains and type IV collagen. Lab Invest 61:278–289, 1989.

2458. Kashtan CE, Rich SS, Michael AF, de Martinville B: Gene mapping in Alport families with different basement membrane antigenic phenotypes. Kidney Int 38:925–930, 1990.

2459. Kashtan C, Fish AJ, Kleppel M, et al: Nephritogenic antigen determinations in epidermal and renal basement membranes of kindreds with Alport-type familial nephritis. J Clin Invest 78:1035–1044, 1986.

2460. Kashtan CE, Kim Y: Distribution of the α1 and α2 chains of collagen IV and of collagens V and VI in Alport syndrome. Kidney Int 42:115–126, 1992.

2461. Kleppel MM, Kashtan CE, Butkowski RJ, et al: Alport familial nephritis. Absence of 28 kilodalton noncollagenous monomers of type IV collagen in glomerular basement membrane. J Clin Invest 80:263–266, 1987.

2462. Streeten BW, Robinson MR, Wallace R, Jones DB: Lens capsule abnormalities in Alport's syndrome. Arch Ophthalmol 105:1693–1697, 1987.

2463. Ding J, Zhou J, Tryggvason K, Kashtan CE: COL4A5 deletions in three patients with Alport syndrome and posttransplant antiglomerular basement membrane nephritis. J Am Soc Nephrol 5:161–168, 1994.

2464. Savage COS, Noel L-H, Crutcher E, et al: Hereditary nephritis: Immunoblotting studies of the glomerular basement membrane. Lab Invest 60:613–618, 1989.

2465. Kleppel MM, Fan WW, Cheong HI, et al: Immunochemical studies of the Alport antigen. Kidney Int 41:1629–1637, 1992.

2466. Hudson BG, Kalluri R, Gunwar S, et al: The pathogenesis of Alport syndrome involves type IV collagen molecules containing the α3(IV) chain: Evidence from anti-GBM nephritis after renal transplantation. Kidney Int 42:179–187, 1992.

2467. Kleppel MM, Fan WW, Cheong HI, Michael AF: Evidence for separate networks of classical and novel basement membrane collagen. Characterization of α3(IV)-Alport antigen heterodimer. J Biol Chem 267:4137–4142, 1992.

2468. Kalluri R, Weber M, Netzer K-O, et al: COL4A5 gene deletion and production of post-transplant anti-α3(IV) collagen alloantibodies in Alport syndrome. Kidney Int 45:721–726, 1994.

2469. Barker DF, Hostikka SL, Zhou J, et al: Identification of mutations in the COL4A5 collagen gene in Alport syndrome. Science 248:1224–1227, 1990.

2470. Zhou J, Barker DF, Hostikka SL, et al: Single base mutation in α5(IV) collagen chain gene converting a conserved cysteine to serine in Alport syndrome. Genomics 9:10–18, 1991.

2471. Boye E, Vetrie D, Flinter F, et al: Major rearrangements in the α5(IV) collagen gene in three patients with Alport syndrome. Genomics 11:1125–1132, 1991.

2472. Reeders ST: Molecular genetics of hereditary nephritis. Kidney Int 42:783–792, 1992.

2473. Flinter F, Bobrow M: The molecular genetics of Alport syndrome: Report of two workshops. J Med Genet 29:352–353, 1992.

2474. Weber M, Netzer KO, Pullig O: Molecular aspects of Alport's syndrome. Clin Invest 70:809–815, 1992.

2475. Zhou J, Hertz JM, Tryggvason K: Mutation in the α5(IV) collagen chain in juvenile-onset Alport syndrome without hearing loss or ocular lesions: Detection by denaturing gradient gel electrophoresis of a PCR product. Am J Hum Genet 50:1291–1300, 1992.

2476. Zhou J, Hertz JM, Leinonen A, Tryggvason K: Complete amino acid sequence of the human α5(IV) collagen chain and identification of a single-base mutation in exon 23 converting glycine 521 in the collagenous domain to cysteine in an Alport syndrome patient. J Biol Chem 267:12475–12481, 1992.

2477. Vetrie D, Boye E, Flinter F, et al: DNA rearrangements in the α5(IV) collagen gene (COL4A5) of individuals with Alport syndrome: Further refinement using pulsed-field gel electrophoresis. Genomics 14:624–633, 1992.

2478. Netzer K-O, Renders L, Zhou J, et al: Deletions of the COL4A5 gene in patients with Alport syndrome. Kidney Int 42:1336–1344, 1992.

2479. Renieri A, Seri M, Myers JC, et al: Alport syndrome caused by a 5′ deletion within the COL4A5 gene. Hum Genet 89:120–121, 1992.

2480. Knebelmann B, Deschenes G, Gros F, et al: Substitution of arginine for glycine 325 in the collagen α5(IV) chain associated with X-linked Alport syndrome: Characterization of the mutation by direct sequencing of PCR-amplified lymphoblas cDNA fragments. Am J Hum Genet 51:135–142, 1992.

2481. Antignac C, Zhou J, Sanak M, et al: Alport syndrome and diffuse leiomyomatosis: Deletions in the 5′ end of the COL4A5 collagen gene. Kidney Int 42:1178–1183, 1992.

2482. M'Rad R, Sanak M, Deschenes G, et al: Alport syndrome: A genetic study of 31 families. Hum Genet 90:420–426, 1992.

2483. Smeets HJM, Melenhorst JJ, Lemmink HH, et al: Different mutations in the COL4A5 collagen gene in two patients with different features of Alport syndrome. Kidney Int 42:83–88, 1992.

2484. Tryggvason K, Zhou J, Hostikka SL, Shows TB: Molecular genetics of Alport syndrome. Kidney Int 43:38–44, 1993.

2485. Netzer K-O, Pullig O, Frei U, et al: COL4A5 splice site mutation and α5(IV) collagen mRNA in Alport syndrome. Kidney Int 43:486–492, 1993.

2486. Zhou J, Gregory MC, Hertz JM, et al: Mutations in the codon for a conserved arginine-1563 in the COL4A5 collagen gene in Alport syndrome. Kidney Int 43:722–729, 1993.

2487. Saito A, Sakatsume M, Yamazaki H, et al: A deletion mutation in the 3′ end of the α5(IV) collagen gene in juvenile-onset Alport syndrome. J Am Soc Nephrol 4:1649–1653, 1994.

2488. Antignac C, Knebelmann B, Drouot L, et al: Deletions in the COL4A5 collagen gene in X-linked Alport syndrome. Characterization of the pathological transcripts in nonrenal cells and correlation with disease expression. J Clin Invest 93:1195–1207, 1994.

2489. Savige JA: The gene corresponding to the putative Goodpasture antigen is present in Alport's syndrome. Clin Exp Immunol 85:236–239, 1991.

2490. Thorner P, Jansen B, Baumal R, et al: Samoyed hereditary glomerulopathy. Immunohistochemical staining of basement membranes of kidney for laminin, collagen type IV, fibronectin, and Goodpasture antigen, and correlation with electron microscopy of glomerular capillary basement membranes. Lab Invest 56:435–443, 1987.

2491. Thorner P, Baumal R, Valli VEO, et al: Abnormalities in the NC1 domain of collagen type IV in GBM in canine hereditary nephritis. Kidney Int 35:843–850, 1989.

2492. Hood JC, Robinson WF, Huxtable CR, et al: Hereditary nephritis in the bull terrier: Evidence for inheritance by an autosomal dominant gene. Vet Rec 126:456–459, 1990.

2493. Cosio FG, Falkenhain ME, Sedmak DD: Association of thin glomerular basement membrane with other glomerulopathies. Kidney Int 46:471–474, 1994.

2494. Pettersson E, Törnroth T, Wieslander J: Abnormally thin glomerular basement membrane and the Goodpasture epitope. Clin Nephrol 33:105–109, 1990.

2495. Savige J: Hereditary abnormalities of renal basement membranes. Pathology 23:350–355, 1991.

2496. Kestilä M, Männikkö M, Holmberg C, et al: Exclusion of eight genes as mutated loci in congenital nephrotic syndrome of the Finnish type. Kidney Int 45:986–990, 1994.

2497. Tuttle SE, Sharma HM, Bay WH, Hebert LA: Glomerular basement membrane splitting and microaneurysm formation associated with nitrosourea therapy. Am J Nephrol 5:388–394, 1985.

2498. Carone FA, Makino H, Kanwar YS: Basement membrane antigens in renal polycystic disease. Am J Pathol 130:466–471, 1988.

2499. Milliner DS, Pierides AM, Holley KE: Renal transplantation in Alport's syndrome. Anti–glomerular basement membrane glomerulonephritis in the allograft. Mayo Clin Proc 57:35–43, 1982.

2500. Quérin S, Noël L-H, Grünfeld J-P, et al: Linear glomerular IgG fixation in renal allografts: incidence and significance in Alport's syndrome. Clin Nephrol 25:134–140, 1986.

2501. Teruel JL, Liaño F, Mampaso F, et al: Allograft antiglomerular basement membrane glomerulonephritis in a patient with Alport's syndrome. Nephron 46:43–44, 1987.

2502. Savige JA, Mavrova L, Kincaid-Smith P: Inhibitable anti-GBM antibody activity after renal transplantation in Alport's syndrome. Transplantation 48:704–705, 1989.

2503. Noël LH, Gubler MC, Bobrie G, et al: Inherited defects of renal basement membranes. Adv Nephrol 18:77–94, 1989.

2504. Berardinelli L, Pozzoli E, Raiteri M, et al: Renal transplantation in Alport's syndrome. Personal experience in twelve patients. Contrib Nephrol 80:131–134, 1990.

2505. Bobrie G, Noël L-H, Savage COS, et al: Kidney transplantation in Alport's syndrome and related diseases. Contrib Nephrol 80:76–80, 1990.

2506. Peten E, Pirson Y, Cosyns J-P, et al: Outcome of thirty patients with Alport's syndrome after renal transplantation. Transplantation 52:823–826, 1991.

2507. Göbel J, Olbricht CJ, Offner G, et al: Kidney transplantation in Alport's syndrome: Long-term outcome and allograft anti-GBM nephritis. Clin Nephrol 38:299–304, 1992.

2508. Heuvel LPWJvd, Schröder CH, Savage COS, et al: The development of anti–glomerular basement membrane nephritis in two children with Alport's syndrome after renal transplantation: Characterization of the antibody target. Pediatr Nephrol 3:406–413, 1989.

2509. Rassoul Z, Al-Khader AA, Al-Sulaiman M, et al: Recurrent allograft antiglomerular basement membrane glomerulonephritis in a patient with Alport's syndrome. Am J Nephrol 10:73–76, 1990.

2510. Kashtan CE, Butkowski RJ, Kleppel MM, et al: Posttransplant anti–glomerular basement membrane nephritis in related males with Alport syndrome. J Lab Clin Med 116:508–515, 1990.

2511. Cameron JS: Recurrent primary disease and de novo nephritis following renal transplantation. Pediatr Nephrol 5:412–421, 1991.

2512. Hind CRK, Bowman C, Winearls CG, Lockwood CM: Recurrence of circulating anti–glomerular basement membrane antibody three years after immunosuppressive treatment and plasma exchange. Clin Nephrol 21:244–246, 1984.

2513. Mehler PS, Brunvand MW, Hutt MP, Anderson RJ: Chronic recurrent Goodpasture's syndrome. Am J Med 82:833–835, 1987.

2514. Klasa RJ, Abboud RT, Ballon HS, Grossman L: Goodpasture's syndrome: Recurrence after a five-year remission. Case report and review of the literature. Am J Med 84:751–755, 1988.

2515. Lim EC, Terasaki PI: Outsome of kidney transplantation in different diseases. In Terasaki P (ed): Clinical Transplants. UCLA Tissue Typing Laboratory, Los Angeles, 1990, pp 461–469.

2516. Rees AJ, Peters DK, Compston DAS, Batchelor JR: Strong association between HLA-DRW2 and antibody-mediated Goodpasture's syndrome. Lancet 1:966–968, 1978.

2517. Perl SI, Pussell BA, Charlesworth JA, et al: Goodpasture's (anti-GBM) disease and HLA-DRw2. N Engl J Med 305:463–464, 1981.

2518. Rees AJ, Peters DK, Amos N, et al: The influence of HLA-linked genes on the severity of anti-GBM antibody–mediated nephritis. Kidney Int 26:444–450, 1984.

2519. Burns A, So A, Pusey C, Rees A: HLA restrictions in Goodpasture's syndrome. In Hatano M, Honda N, et al (eds): Nephrology. Proceedings of the XIth International Congress of Nephrology. Springer-Verlag, Tokyo, 1991, Abstract 375A.

2520. Mercier B, Bourbigot B, Raguenes O, et al: HLA class II typing of Goodpasture's syndrome affected patients. J Am Soc Nephrol 3:658, 1992. Abstract.

2521. Rees AJ, Demaine AG, Welsh KI: Association of immunoglobulin Gm allotypes with antiglomerular basement membrane antibodies and their titer. Hum Immunol 10:213–220, 1984.

2522. Huey B, McCormick K, Capper J, et al: Associations of HLA-DR and HLA-DQ types with anti-GBM nephritis by sequence-specific oligonucleotide probe hybridization. Kidney Int 44:307–312, 1993.

2523. Fujinami RS: Virus-induced autoimmunity through molecular mimicry. Ann N Y Acad Sci 540:210–217, 1988.

2524. Horsfall AC: Molecular mimicry and autoantigens in connective tissue diseases. Mol Biol Rep 16:139–147, 1992.

2525. Okuhara K, Yoshimoto M, Fujisawa S, et al: Anti-streptococcal cell membrane and anti-human glomerular basement membrane titers in sera of patients with poststreptococcal acute glomerulonephritis and anaphylactoid purpura. Jpn Circ J 47:1293–1297, 1983.

2526. Bengtsson U: Glomerulonephritis and organic solvents. Lancet 2:566, 1985.

2527. Roy AT, Brautbar N, Lee DBN: Hydrocarbons and renal failure. Nephron 58:385–392, 1991.

2528. Bombassei GJ, Kaplan AA: The association between hydrocarbon exposure and anti–glomerular basement membrane antibody–mediated disease (Goodpasture's syndrome). Am J Ind Med 21:141–153, 1992.

2529. Mutti A, Alinovi R, Bergamaschi E, et al: Nephropathies and exposure to perchloroethylene in dry-cleaners. Lancet 340:189–193, 1992.

2530. Carlier B, Schroeder E, Mahieu P: A rapidly and spontaneously reversible Goodpasture's syndrome after carbon tetrachloride inhalation. Acta Clin Belg 35:193–198, 1980.

2531. Bernis P, Hamels J, Quoidbach A, et al: Remission of Goodpasture's syndrome after withdrawal of an unusual toxic. Clin Nephrol 23:312–317, 1985.

2532. Bonzel K-E, Müller-Wiefel DE, Ruder H, et al: Anti–glomerular basement membrane antibody-mediated glomerulonephritis due to glue sniffing. Eur J Pediatr 146:296–300, 1987.

2533. Lechleitner P, Defregger M, Lhotta K, et al: Goodpasture's syndrome. Unusual presentation after exposure to hard metal dust. Chest 103:956–957, 1993.

2534. Wilson CB: Drug and toxin-induced nephritides: Antikidney antibody and immune complex mediation. In Porter G (ed): Nephrotoxic Mechanisms of Drugs and Environmental Toxins. Plenum Publishing, New York, 1982, pp 383–392.

2535. Williams PS, Davenport A, McDicken I, et al: Increased incidence of anti–glomerular basement membrane antibody (anti-GBM) nephritis in the Mersey Region, September 1984–October 1985. Q J Med 68:727–733, 1988.

2536. Peces R, Riera JR, Arboleya LR, et al: Goodpasture's syndrome in a patient receiving penicillamine and carbimazole. Nephron 45:316–320, 1987.

2537. Pusey CD, Bowman C, Morgan A, et al: Kinetics and pathogenicity of autoantibodies induced by mercuric chloride in the brown Norway rat. Clin Exp Immunol 81:76–82, 1990.

2538. Kurki P, Helve T, von Bonsdorff M, et al: Transformation of

membranous glomerulonephritis into crescentic glomerulonephritis with glomerular basement membrane antibodies. Serial determinations of anti-GBM before the transformation. Nephron 38:134–137, 1984.

2539. Rajaraman S, Pinto JA, Cavallo T: Glomerulonephritis with coexistent immune deposits and antibasement membrane activity. J Clin Pathol 37:176–181, 1984.

2540. Pettersson E, Törnroth T, Miettinen A: Simultaneous anti–glomerular basement membrane and membranous glomerulonephritis: Case report and literature review. Clin Immunol Immunopathol 31:171–180, 1984.

2541. Zevin D, Ben-Bassat M, Weinstein T, et al: Rejection-related nephrotic syndrome associated with massive antiglomerular and antitubular basement membrane deposits. Isr J Med Sci 21:915–918, 1985.

2542. Lubec G: Anti–glomerular basement membrane disease after lithotripsy. Lancet 335:1405, 1990.

2543. Weber M, Pullig O, Boesken WH: Anti–glomerular basement membrane disease after renal obstruction. Lancet 336:512–513, 1990.

2544. Guerin V, Rabian C, Droz D, et al: Anti–glomerular-basement-membrane disease after lithotripsy. Lancet 335:856–857, 1990.

2545. Torffvit O, Agardh C-D, Cederholm B, Wieslander J: A new enzyme-linked immunosorbent assay for urine and serum concentrations of the carboxyterminal domain (NC1) of collagen IV: Application in type I (insulin-dependent) diabetes. Scand J Clin Lab Invest 49:431–439, 1989.

2546. Lerner RA, Dixon FJ: The induction of acute glomerulonephritis in rabbits with soluble antigens isolated from normal homologous and autologous urine. J Immunol 100:1277–1287, 1968.

2547. Lombard CM, Colby TV, Elliott CG: Surgical pathology of the lung in anti–basement membrane antibody–associated Goodpasture's syndrome. Hum Pathol 20:445–451, 1989.

2548. Yoshioka K, Iseki T, Okada M, et al: Identification of Goodpasture antigens in human alveolar basement membrane. Clin Exp Immunol 74:419–426, 1988.

2549. Rees AJ, Lockwood CM, Peters DK: Enhanced allergic tissue injury in Goodpasture's syndrome by intercurrent bacterial infection. Br Med J 2:723–726, 1977.

2550. Donaghy M, Rees AJ: Cigarette smoking and lung haemorrhage in glomerulonephritis caused by autoantibodies to glomerular basement membrane. Lancet 2:1390–1393, 1983.

2551. Leaker B, Walker RG, Becker GJ, Kincaid-Smith P: Cigarette smoking and lung haemorrhage in anti–glomerular-basement-membrane nephritis. Lancet 2:1039, 1984.

2552. Keogh AM, Ibels LS, Allen DH, et al: Exacerbation of Goodpasture's syndrome after inadvertent exposure to hydrocarbon fumes. Br Med J 288:188, 1984.

2553. Queluz TH, Pawlowski I, Brunda MJ, et al: Pathogenesis of an experimental model of Goodpasture's hemorrhagic pneumonitis. J Clin Invest 85:1507–1515, 1990.

2554. Escolar Castellón J de D, Roche Roche PA, Escolar Castellón A, Miñana Amada C: The modifications produced in allergic alveolitis and in Goodpasture's syndrome due to exposure to cigarette smoke. Histol Histopathol 6:535–547, 1991.

2555. Batsford SR, Rohrbach R, Takamiya H, et al: Autoantibody specific for the glomerular mesangium and Bowman's capsule in man. Clin Nephrol 12:163–167, 1979.

2556. Lowance DC, Mullins JD, McPhaul JJ Jr: Immunoglobulin A (IgA)–associated glomerulonephritis. Kidney Int 3:167–176, 1973.

2557. Tomino Y, Sakai H, Endoh M, et al: Cross-reactivity of eluted antibodies from renal tissues of patients with Henoch-Schönlein purpura nephritis and IgA nephropathy. Am J Nephrol 3:315–318, 1983.

2558. O'Donoghue DJ, Darvill A, Ballardie FW: Mesangial cell autoantigens in immunoglobulin A nephropathy and Henoch-Schönlein purpura. J Clin Invest 88:1522–1530, 1991.

2559. McPhaul JJ Jr, Stastny P, Freeman RB: Specificities of antibodies eluted from human cadaveric renal allografts. Multiple mechanisms of renal allograft injury. J Clin Invest 67:1405–1414, 1981.

2560. Dolcher MP, Marchini B, Sabbatini A, et al: Autoantibodies from mixed cryoglobulinaemia patients bind glomerular antigens. Clin Exp Immunol 96:317–322, 1994.

2561. Cines DB, Lyss AP, Reeber M, et al: Presence of complement-fixing anti–endothelial cell antibodies in systemic lupus erythematosus. J Clin Invest 73:611–625, 1984.

2562. Rosenbaum J, Pottinger BE, Woo P, et al: Measurement and characterisation of circulating anti–endothelial cell IgG in connective tissue diseases. Clin Exp Immunol 72:450–456, 1988.

2563. Fukatsu A, Tamai H, Nishikawa K, et al: The kidney disease of Crow-Fukase (POEMS) syndrome: A clinico-pathological study of four cases. Clin Nephrol 36:76–82, 1991.

2564. Leung DYM, Moake JL, Havens PL, et al: Lytic anti–endothelial cell antibodies in haemolytic-uraemic syndrome. Lancet 2:183–186, 1988.

2565. Heurkens AHM, Hiemstra PS, Lafeber GJM, et al: Anti–endothelial cell antibodies in patients with rheumatoid arthritis complicated by vasculitis. Clin Exp Immunol 78:7–12, 1989.

2566. Bodolay E, Bojan F, Szegedi G, et al: Cytotoxic endothelial cell antibodies in mixed connective tissue disease. Immunol Lett 20:163–168, 1989.

2567. van der Zee JM, Siegert CEH, De Vreede TA, et al: Characterization of anti–endothelial cell antibodies in systemic lupus erythematosus (SLE). Clin Exp Immunol 84:238–244, 1991.

2568. D'Cruz DP, Houssiau FA, Ramirez G, et al: Antibodies to endothelial cells in systemic lupus erythematosus: A potential marker for nephritis and vasculitis. Clin Exp Immunol 85:254–261, 1991.

2569. McCrae KR, DeMichele A, Samuels P, et al: Detection of endothelial cell–reactive immunoglobulin in patients with anti-phospholipid antibodies. Br J Haematol 79:595–605, 1991.

2570. Wangel AG, Kontiainen S, Scheinin T: Anti–endothelial cell antibodies in insulin-dependent diabetes mellitus. Clin Exp Immunol 88:410–413, 1992.

2571. Paul LC, Busch GJ, Paradysz JM, Carpenter CB: Definition, genetics, and possible significance of a newly defined endothelial antigen in the rat. Transplantation 36:533–539, 1983.

2572. Pescovitz MD, Sachs DH, Lunney JK, Hsu S-M: Localization of class II MHC antigens on porcine renal vascular endothelium. Transplantation 37:627–630, 1984.

2573. Baldwin WM III, Claas FHJ, van Rood JJ, van Es LA: Antigenic composition of human renal vascular endothelium assessed by kidney perfusion. Tissue Antigens 23:256–262, 1984.

2574. Gibbs VC, Wood DM, Garovoy MR: The response of cultured human kidney capillary endothelium to immunologic stimuli. Hum Immunol 14:259–269, 1985.

2575. Sedmak DD, Orosz CG: The role of vascular endothelial cells in transplantation. Arch Pathol Lab Med 115:260–265, 1991.

2576. Yap HK, Sakai RS, Bahn L, et al: Anti–vascular endothelial cell antibodies in patients with IgA nephropathy: Frequency and clinical significance. Clin Immunol Immunopathol 49:450–462, 1988.

2577. Wang M-X, Walker RG, Kincaid-Smith P: Clinicopathologic associations of anti–endothelial cell antibodies in immunoglobulin A nephropathy and lupus nephritis. Am J Kidney Dis 22:378–386, 1993.

2578. Abbott F, Jones S, Lockwood CM, Rees AJ: Autoantibodies to glomerular antigens in patients with Wegener's granulomatosis. Nephrol Dial Transplant 4:1–8, 1989.

2579. Paul LC, Stuffers-Heiman M, Van Es LA, DeGraeff J: Antibodies directed against brush border antigens of proximal tubules in renal allograft recipients. Clin Immunol Immunopathol 14:238–243, 1979.

2580. Douglas MFS, Rabideau DP, Schwartz MM, Lewis EJ: Evidence of autologous immune-complex nephritis. N Engl J Med 305:1326–1329, 1981.

2581. Zanetti M, Mandet C, Duboust A, et al: Demonstration of a passive Heymann nephritis–like mechanism in a human kidney transplant. Clin Nephrol 15:272–277, 1981.

2582. Thorpe LW, Cavallo T: Renal tubule brush border antigens: Failure to confirm a pathogenetic role in human membranous glomerulonephritis. J Clin Lab Immunol 3:125–127, 1980.

2583. Collins AB, Andres GA, McCluskey RT: Lack of evidence for a role of renal tubular antigen in human membranous glomerulonephritis. Nephron 27:297–301, 1981.

2584. Nagai T, Tamura T: Urinary excretion of thermostable kidney antigen (BE antigen) in patients with various renal diseases. Nephron 33:216–219, 1983.

2585. Deal JE, Groves RW, Harmer AW, et al: Renal disease, epidermal necrosis, and epithelial cell antibodies. Br Med J 303:161–163, 1991.

2586. Martin S, Brenchley PE, Postlethwaite RJ, et al: Detection of anti–epithelial cell antibodies in association with pediatric renal trans-

2587. Colletti RB, Guillot AP, Rosen S, et al: Autoimmune enteropathy and nephropathy with circulating anti–epithelial cell antibodies. J Pediatr 118:858–864, 1991.

2588. Matsumoto K: Renal tubular epithelial antigen-containing immune complexes stimulate interleukin-1 production by monocytes from patients with glomerulonephritis. Int Urol Nephrol 24:319–326, 1992.

2589. Cederholm B, Wieslander J, Bygren P, Heinegård D: Patients with IgA nephropathy have circulating anti–basement membrane antibodies reacting with structures common to collagen I, II, and IV. Proc Natl Acad Sci USA 83:6151–6155, 1986.

2590. Cederholm B, Wieslander J, Bygren P, Heinegård D: Circulating complexes containing IgA and fibronectin in patients with primary IgA nephropathy. Proc Natl Acad Sci USA 85:4865–4868, 1988.

2591. Shinkai Y, Karai M, Osawa G, et al: Antimouse laminin antibodies in IgA nephropathy and various glomerular diseases. Nephron 56:285–296, 1990.

2592. Saxena R, Bygren P, Butkowski R, Wieslander J: Entactin: A possible auto-antigen in the pathogenesis of non-Goodpasture anti-GBM nephritis. Kidney Int 38:263–272, 1990.

2593. Saxena R, Bygren P, Cederholm B, Wieslander J: Circulating anti-entactin antibodies in patients with glomerulonephritis. Kidney Int 39:996–1004, 1991.

2594. Foidart J-M, Hunt J, Lapiere C-M, et al: Antibodies to laminin in preeclampsia. Kidney Int 29:1050–1057, 1986.

2595. Gabrielli A, Candela M, Ricciatti AM, et al: Antibodies to mouse laminin in patients with systemic sclerosis (scleroderma) recognize galactosyl ($\alpha$1-3)-galactose epitopes. Clin Exp Immunol 86:367–373, 1991.

2596. Goroncy-Bermes P, Dale JB, Beachey EH, Opferkuch W: Monoclonal antibody to human renal glomeruli cross-reacts with streptococcal M protein. Infect Immun 55:2416–2419, 1987.

2597. Fillit H, Damle SP, Gregory JD, et al: Sera from patients with poststreptococcal glomerulonephritis contain antibodies to glomerular heparan sulfate proteoglycan. J Exp Med 161:277–289, 1985.

2598. Kefalides NA, Pegg MT, Ohno N, et al: Antibodies to basement membrane collagen and to laminin are present in sera from patients with poststreptococcal glomerulonephritis. J Exp Med 163:588–602, 1986.

2599. Kraus W, Beachey EH: Renal autoimmune epitope of group A streptococci specified by M protein tetrapeptide Ile-Arg-Leu-Arg. Proc Natl Acad Sci USA 85:4516–4520, 1988.

2600. Kraus W, Dale JB, Beachey EH: Identification of an epitope of type 1 streptococcal M protein that is shared with a 43-kDa protein of human myocardium and renal glomeruli. J Immunol 145:4089–4093, 1990.

2601. Fitzsimons EJ Jr, Weber M, Lange CF: The isolation of cross-reactive monoclonal antibodies: Hydridomas to streptococcal antigens cross-reactive with mammalian basement membrane. Hybridoma 6:61–69, 1987.

2602. Kraus W, Ohyama K, Snyder DS, Beachey EH: Autoimmune sequence of streptococcal M protein shared with the intermediate filament protein, vimentin. J Exp Med 169:481–492, 1989.

2603. Kraus W, Seyer JM, Beachey EH: Vimentin–cross-reactive epitope of type 12 streptococcal M protein. Infect Immun 57:2457–2461, 1989.

2604. Froude J, Gibofsky A, Buskirk DR, et al: Cross-reactivity between streptococcus and human tissue: A model of molecular mimicry and autoimmunity. Curr Top Microbiol Immunol 145:5–26, 1989.

2605. Stollerman GH: Rheumatogenic streptococci and autoimmunity. Clin Immunol Immunopathol 61:131–142, 1991.

2606. Oldstone MBA, Schwimmbeck P, Dyrberg T, Fujinami R: Mimicry by virus of host molecules: Implications for autoimmune disease. Prog Immunol 6:787–795, 1986.

2607. Oldstone MBA: Molecular mimicry and autoimmune disease. Cell 50:819–820, 1987.

2608. Oldstone MBA: Molecular mimicry as a mechanism for the cause and as a probe uncovering etiologic agent(s) of autoimmune disease. Curr Top Microbiol Immunol 145:127–135, 1989.

2609. Cohen IR: A heat shock protein, molecular mimicry and autoimmunity. Isr J Med Sci 26:673–676, 1990.

2610. Gustafson KS, Vercellotti GM, Bendel CM, Hostetter MK: Molecular mimicry in *Candida albicans*. Role of an integrin analogue in adhesion of the yeast to human endothelium. J Clin Invest 87:1896–1902, 1991.

2611. Williams RC Jr: A second look at rheumatoid factor and other "autoantibodies." Am J Med 67:179–181, 1979.

2612. Linder E, Hormia M, Lehto VP, Törnroth T: Identification of cytoskeletal intermediate filaments of vascular endothelial cells as targets for autoantibodies in patient sera. Clin Immunol Immunopathol 21:217–227, 1981.

2613. Guilbert B, Dighiero G, Avrameas S: Naturally occurring antibodies against nine common antigens in human sera. I. Detection, isolation, and characterization. J Immunol 128:2779–2787, 1982.

2614. Dighiero G, Guilbert B, Avrameas S: Naturally occurring antibodies against nine common antigens in humans sera. II. High incidence of monoclonal Ig exhibiting antibody activity against actin and tubulin and sharing antibody specificities with natural antibodies. J Immunol 128:2788–2792, 1982.

2615. Haspel MV, Onodera T, Prabhakar BS, et al: Virus-induced autoimmunity: Monoclonal antibodies that react with endocrine tissues. Science 220:304–306, 1983.

2616. Satoh J, Prabhakar BS, Haspel MV, et al: Human monoclonal autoantibodies that react with multiple endocrine organs. N Engl J Med 309:217–220, 1983.

2617. Essani K, Satoh J, Prabhakar BS, et al: Anti-idiotypic antibodies against a human multiple organ-reactive autoantibody. Detection of idiotypes in normal individuals and patients with autoimmune diseases. J Clin Invest 76:1649–1656, 1985.

2618. Schwartz RS, Stollar BD: Origins of anti-DNA antibodies. J Clin Invest 75:321–327, 1985.

2619. Madaio MP, Carlson J, Cataldo J, et al: Murine monoclonal anti-DNA antibodies bind directly to glomerular antigens and form immune deposits. J Immunol 138:2883–2889, 1987.

2620. Foster MH, Cizman B, Madaio MP: Nephritogenic autoantibodies in systemic lupus erythematosus: Immunochemical properties, mechanisms of immune deposition, and genetic origins. Lab Invest 69:494–507, 1993.

2621. Sabbaga J, Peres Line SR, Potocnjak P, Madaio MP: A murine nephritogenic monoclonal anti-DNA autoantibody binds directly to mouse laminin, the major non-collagenous protein component of the glomerular basement membrane. Eur J Immunol 19:137–143, 1989.

2622. Lafer EM, Rauch J, Andrzejewski C Jr, et al: Polyspecific monoclonal lupus autoantibodies reactive with both polynucleotides and phospholipids. J Exp Med 153:897–909, 1981.

2623. Rauch J, Tannenbaum H, Stollar BD, Schwartz RS: Monoclonal anti-cardiolipin antibodies bind to DNA. Eur J Immunol 14:529–534, 1984.

2624. Faaber P, Capel PJA, Rijke GPM, et al: Cross-reactivity of anti-DNA antibodies with proteoglycans. Clin Exp Immunol 55:502–508, 1984.

2625. André-Schwartz J, Datta SK, Shoenfeld Y, et al: Binding of cytoskeletal proteins by monoclonal anti-DNA lupus autoantibodies. Clin Immunol Immunopathol 31:261–271, 1984.

2626. Tron F, Jacob L, Bach J-F: Binding of a murine monoclonal anti-DNA antibody to Raji cells. Implications for the interpretation of the Raji cell assay for immune complexes. Eur J Immunol 14:283–286, 1984.

2627. Jacob L, Lety M-A, Louvard D, Bach J-F: Binding of a monoclonal anti-DNA autoantibody to identical protein(s) present at the surface of several human cell types involved in lupus pathogenesis. J Clin Invest 75:315–317, 1985.

2628. Faaber P, Rijke TPM, van de Putte LBA, et al: Cross-reactivity of human and murine anti-DNA antibodies with heparan sulfate. The major glycosaminoglycan in glomerular basement membranes. J Clin Invest 77:1824–1830, 1986.

2629. Raz E, Brezis M, Rosenmann E, Eilat D: Anti-DNA antibodies bind directly to renal antigens and induce kidney dysfunction in the isolated perfused rat kidney. J Immunol 142:3076–3082, 1989.

2630. Vlahakos DV, Forster MH, Adams S, et al: Anti-DNA antibodies form immune deposits at distinct glomerular and vascular sites. Kidney Int 41:1690–1700, 1992.

2631. Termaat R-M, Assmann KJM, van Son JPHF, et al: Antigen-specificity of antibodies bound to glomeruli of mice with systemic lupus erythematosus–like syndromes. Lab Invest 68:164–173, 1993.

2632. Frampton G, Hobby P, Morgan A, et al: A role for DNA in anti-DNA antibodies binding to endothelial cells. J Autoimmun 4:463–478, 1991.

2633. Chan TM, Frampton G, Staines NA, et al: Different mechanisms by which anti-DNA MoAbs bind to human endothelial cells and glomerular mesangial cells. Clin Exp Immunol 88:68–74, 1992.

2634. Kramers C, Hylkema MN, van Bruggen MCJ, et al: Anti-nucleosome antibodies complexed to nucleosomal antigens show anti-DNA reactivity and bind to rat glomerular basement membrane in vivo. J Clin Invest 94:568–577, 1994.

2635. Morioka T, Woitas R, Fujigaki Y, et al: Histone mediates glomerular deposition of small size DNA anti-DNA complex. Kidney Int 45:991–997, 1994.

2636. Uwatoko S, Gauthier VJ, Mannik M: Autoantibodies to the collagen-like region of C1Q deposit in glomeruli via C1Q in immune deposits. Clin Immunol Immunopathol 61:268–273, 1991.

2637. Takaya M, Ichikawa Y, Kobayashi N, et al: Serum thrombomodulin and anticardiolipin antibodies in patients with systemic lupus erythematosus. Clin Exp Rheumatol 9:495–499, 1991.

2638. Moreland LW, Gay RE, Gay S: Collagen autoantibodies in patients with vasculitis and systemic lupus erythematosus. Clin Immunol Immunopathol 60:412–418, 1991.

2639. Barbara JA, Thomas AC, Smith PS, et al: Membranous nephropathy with graft-versus-host disease in a bone marrow transplant recipient. Clin Nephrol 37:115–118, 1992.

2640. Brownlee M, Pongor S, Cerami A: Covalent attachment of soluble proteins by nonenzymatically glycosylated collagen. Role in the in situ formation of immune complexes. J Exp Med 158:1739–1744, 1983.

2641. Gonzalez-Cabrero J, Egido J, Mampaso F, et al: Characterization of circulating idiotypes containing immune complexes and their presence in the glomerular mesangium in patients with IgA nephropathy. Clin Exp Immunol 76:204–209, 1989.

2642. Pollet S, Depner T, Moore P, et al: Mesangial glomerulopathy and IgM rheumatoid factor in rheumatoid arthritis. Nephron 51:107–111, 1989.

2643. Miyazaki M, Endoh M, Suga T, et al: Rheumatoid factors and glomerulonephritis. Clin Exp Immunol 81:250–255, 1990.

2644. Germuth FG, Rodriguez E: Experimental circulating immune complex glomerulonephritis. Uremia Invest 8:183–187, 1984-85.

2645. Brentjens JR, Andres G: Immunopathogenesis of renal vasculitis. Semin Nephrol 5:3–14, 1985.

2646. Salvidio G, Andres G: Immune deposits and immune complex disease. Clin Exp Rheumatol 4:281–288, 1986.

2647. Mannik M: Experimental models for immune complex–mediated vascular inflammation. Acta Med Scand [Suppl] 715:145–155, 1987.

2648. Mannik M: Mechanisms of tissue deposition of immune complexes. J Rheumatol 14(suppl 13):35–42, 1987.

2649. Gauthier VJ, Abrass CK: Circulating immune complexes in renal injury. Semin Nephrol 12:379–394, 1992.

2650. Furness PN: The formation and fate of glomerular immune complex deposits. J Pathol 164:195–202, 1991.

2651. Wilson CB, Neale TJ, Holdsworth SR: Nephritogenic immune reactions involving immune complex formation in the circulation and in situ within the kidney. Aust N Z J Med 11(suppl 1):88–93, 1981.

2652. Lowe MG, Holdsworth SR, Tipping PG: T lymphocyte participation in acute serum sickness glomerulonephritis in rabbits. Immunol Cell Biol 69:81–87, 1991.

2653. Wilson CB, Dixon FJ: Antigen quantitation in experimental immune complex glomerulonephritis. I. Acute serum sickness. J Immunol 105:279–290, 1970.

2654. Fujita M, Iida H, Asaka M, et al: Effect of the immunosuppressive agent, ciclosporin, on experimental immune complex glomerulonephritis in rats. Nephron 57:201–205, 1991.

2655. Wilson CB, Dixon FJ: Quantitation of acute and chronic serum sickness in the rabbit. J Exp Med 134:7S–18S, 1971.

2656. Noble B, Van Liew JB, Brentjens JR: A transition from proliferative to membranous glomerulonephritis in chronic serum sickness. Kidney Int 29:841–848, 1986.

2657. Nakazawa K, Ohno S, Naramoto A, et al: Immune deposits in the glomerular extracellular matrix detected by the quick-freezing and deep-etching method. Nephron 62:203–212, 1992.

2658. Wang YM, al-Nawab MD, Evans B, et al: Glomerular epithelial-cell endocytosis of horseradish peroxidase–polylysine conjugate in immune-complex glomerulonephritis. Nephrol Dial Transplant 5:771–776, 1990.

2659. al-Nawab MD, Jones NF, Davies DR: Glomerular epithelial cell endocytosis of immune deposits in human lupus nephritis. Nephrol Dial Transplant 6:316–323, 1991.

2660. al-Nawab MD, Bass PS, Das AK, Davies DR: Immunoelectron microscopy of cationized bovine serum albumin–induced glomerulonephritis in the rabbit. J Pathol 167:33–40, 1992.

2661. Neuland C, Albini B, Brentjens J, et al: Antigen concentration in tissues of rabbits with systemic chronic serum sickness. Int Arch Allergy Appl Immunol 64:385–394, 1981.

2662. Alpers CE, Hudkins KL, Pritzl P, Johnson RJ: Mechanisms of clearance of immune complexes from peritubular capillaries in the rat. Am J Pathol 139:855–867, 1991.

2663. Ishidate T, Ward HJ, Hoyer, J R: Quantitative studies of tubular immune complex formation and clearance in rats. Kidney Int 38:1075–1084, 1990.

2664. Peress NS, Tompkins DC: Rat CNS in experimental chronic serum sickness: Integrity of the zonulae occludentes of the choroid plexus epithelium and brain endothelium in experimental chronic serum sickness. Neuropathol Appl Neurobiol 5:279–288, 1979.

2665. Noble B, Olson KA, Milgrom M, Albini B: Tissue deposition of immune complexes in mice receiving daily injections of bovine serum albumin. Clin Exp Immunol 42:255–262, 1980.

2666. Noble B, Milgrom M, Van Liew JB, Brentjens JR: Chronic serum sickness in the rat: Influence of antigen dose, route of antigen administration and strain of rat on the development of disease. Clin Exp Immunol 46:499–507, 1981.

2667. Yamamoto T, Kihara I, Hara M, et al: Bovine serum albumin (BSA) nephritis in rats. II. Histological findings and complement activation by immune complex in SHR rats. Br J Exp Pathol 64:660–669, 1983.

2668. Yamamoto K, Oite T, Kihara I, Shimizu F: Experimental glomerulonephritis induced by human IgG in rats. Clin Exp Immunol 57:575–582, 1984.

2669. McLeish KR, Stelzer GT, Gohara AF, Wallace JH: Variable susceptibility to immune complex glomerulonephritis among mice sharing the same major histocompatibility complex. Immunol Invest 15:541–547, 1986.

2670. Noble B, Brentjens JR: Experimental serum sickness. Methods Enzymol 162:484–501, 1988.

2671. Albini B, Brentjens J, Olson K, et al: Studies on the immune response of rabbits and chickens with chronic serum sickness. *In* Milgram F, Albini B (eds): Immunopathology. Sixth International Convocation on Immunology. S Karger, Basel, 1979, pp 207–211.

2672. Bishop SA, Stokes CR, Lucke VM: Experimental proliferative glomerulonephritis in the cat. J Comp Pathol 106:49–60, 1992.

2673. Bishop SA, Bailey M, Lucke VM, Stokes CR: Antibody response and antibody affinity maturation in cats with experimental proliferative immune complex glomerulonephritis. J Comp Pathol 107:91–102, 1992.

2674. Stills HF Jr, Bullock BC, Clarkson TB: Increased atherosclerosis and glomerulonephritis in cynomolgus monkeys (*Macaca fascicularis*) given injections of BSA over an extended period of time. Am J Pathol 113:222–234, 1983.

2675. Hebert LA, Cosio FG, Birmingham DJ, et al: Experimental immune complex-mediated glomerulonephritis in the nonhuman primate. Kidney Int 39:44–56, 1991.

2676. Hogendoorn PC, Bruijn JA, Gelok EW, et al: Development of progressive glomerulosclerosis in experimental chronic serum sickness. Nephrol Dial Transplant 5:100–109, 1990.

2677. Miyazaki S, Kawasaki K, Yaoita E, et al: Bovine serum albumin (BSA) nephritis in rats. III. Antigen distribution in various organs. Clin Exp Immunol 59:293–299, 1985.

2678. Miyazaki S, Kawasaki K, Yaoita E, et al: Bovine serum albumin nephritis in rats. V. Kinetic studies of antigen localization in various organs and the phagocytic role of polymorphonuclear leukocytes. Am J Pathol 119:412–419, 1985.

2679. Kawasaki K, Miyazaki S, Yaoita E, et al: Bovine serum albumin (BSA) nephritis in rats. IV. A sequential evaluation of mononuclear phagocyte system (MPS) function. Acta Pathol Jpn 36:429–437, 1986.

2680. Kawasaki K, Miyazaki S, Yamamoto T, Kihara I: Identification and quantitation of cells that process immune complexes in nephritic rats induced with bovine serum albumin. J Leukoc Biol 40:355–365, 1986.

2681. Noble B, Steward MW, Vladutiu A, Brentjens JR: Relationship of the quality and quantity of circulating anti-BSA antibodies to the severity of glomerulonephritis in rats with chronic serum sickness. Clin Exp Immunol 67:277–282, 1987.

2682. Park EK, Hong SK, Andres G, Noble B: Proximal tubule function in chronic serum sickness glomerulonephritis of rats. Proc Soc Exp Biol Med 178:105–113, 1985.

2683. Lawler W: Experimental mesangial proliferative glomerulopathy. J Pathol 133:107–122, 1981.

2684. Natali PG, Tan EM: Experimental renal disease induced by DNA-antiDNA immune complexes. J Clin Invest 51:345–355, 1972.

2685. Sweny P: Ultraviolet light-denatured DNA/anti-ultraviolet light-denatured DNA immune-complex nephritis in rabbits. J Lab Clin Med 95:791–800, 1980.

2686. Hagstrom GL, Bloom PM, Yum MN, et al: Ferritin- and apoferritin-induced immune complex glomerulonephritis in mice. Nephron 24:127–133, 1979.

2687. McLeish KR, Gohara AF, Gunning WT III: Chronic serum sickness in the mouse. Relationship of antigen dose to glomerular pathology. Nephron 31:82–88, 1982.

2688. Iskandar SS, Jennette JC, Wilkman AS, Becker RL: Interstrain variations in nephritogenicity of heterologous protein in mice. Lab Invest 46:344–351, 1982.

2689. Iskandar SS, Jennette JC: Interaction of antigen load and antibody response in determining heterologous protein nephritogenicity in inbred mice. Lab Invest 48:726–734, 1983.

2690. Iskandar SS, Gifford DR, Emancipator SN: Immune complex acute necrotizing glomerulonephritis with progression to diffuse glomerulosclerosis. A murine model. Lab Invest 59:772–779, 1988.

2691. Kelley VE, Winkelstein A: Effect of prostaglandin $E_1$ treatment on murine acute immune complex glomerulonephritis. Clin Immunol Immunopathol 16:316–323, 1980.

2692. McLeish KR, Gohara AF, Gunning WT III: Suppression of antibody synthesis by prostaglandin E as a mechanism for preventing murine immune complex glomerulonephritis. Lab Invest 47:147–152, 1982.

2693. McLeish KR, Gohara AF, Stelzer GT, Wallace JH: Treatment of murine immune complex glomerulonephritis with prostaglandin $E_2$: Dose-response of immune complex deposition, antibody synthesis, and glomerular damage. Clin Immunol Immunopathol 26:18–23, 1983.

2694. Koyama A, Niwa Y, Shigematsu H, et al: Studies on passive serum sickness. II. Factors determining the localization of antigen-antibody complexes in the murine renal glomerulus. Lab Invest 38:253–262, 1978.

2695. Germuth FC Jr, Rodriguez E, Lorelle CA, et al: Passive immune complex glomerulonephritis in mice: Models for various lesions found in human disease. I. High avidity complexes and mesangiopathic glomerulonephritis. Lab Invest 41:360–365, 1979.

2696. Germuth FG Jr, Rodriguez E, Lorelle CA, et al: Passive immune complex glomerulonephritis in mice: Models for various lesions found in human disease. II. Low avidity complexes and diffuse proliferative glomerulonephritis with subepithelial deposits. Lab Invest 41:366–371, 1979.

2697. Emancipator SN, Lamm ME: IgA nephropathy: Pathogenesis of the most common form of glomerulonephritis. Lab Invest 60:168–183, 1989.

2698. Emancipator SN: Immunoregulatory factors in the pathogenesis of IgA nephropathy. Kidney Int 38:1216–1229, 1990.

2699. Waldo FB: Role of IgA in IgA nephropathy. J Pediatr 116:S78–S85, 1990.

2700. Schena FP, Gesualdo L, Montinaro V: Immunopathological aspects of immunoglobulin A nephropathy and other mesangial proliferative glomerulonephritides. J Am Soc Nephrol 2:S167–S172, 1992.

2701. van Es LA: Pathogenesis of IgA nephropathy. Kidney Int 41:1720–1729, 1992.

2702. International Symposium on IgA Nephropathy: The 25th year. Proceedings. Nancy, France, August 31–September 2, 1992. Contrib Nephrol 104:1–219, 1993.

2703. Harper SJ, Feehally J: The pathogenic role of immunoglobulin A polymers in immunoglobulin A nephropathy. Nephron 65:337–345, 1993.

2704. Williams DG: Pathogenesis of idiopathic IgA nephropathy. Pediatr Nephrol 7:303–311, 1993.

2705. Yoshikawa N, Nakamura H, Ito H: IgA nephropathy in children and adults. Springer Semin Immunopathol 16:105–120, 1994.

2706. Endo Y, Kanbayashi H: Etiology of IgA nephropathy syndrome. Pathol Int 44:1–13, 1994.

2707. Emancipator SN: IgA nephropathy: Morphologic expression and pathogenesis. Am J Kidney Dis 23:451–462, 1994.
2708. Ibels LS, Györy AZ: IgA nephropathy: Analysis of the natural history, important factors in the progression of renal disease, and a review of the literature. Medicine (Baltimore) 73:79–102, 1994.
2709. Rifai A: Experimental models for IgA-associated nephritis. Kidney Int 31:1–7, 1987.
2710. Hebert LA: Disposition of IgA-containing circulating immune complexes. Am J Kidney Dis 12:388–392, 1988.
2711. Emancipator SN, Rao CS, Amore A, et al: Macromolecular properties that promote mesangial binding and mesangiopathic nephritis. J Am Soc Nephrol 2:S149–S158, 1992.
2712. Montinaro V, Gesualdo L, Schena FP: Primary IgA nephropathy: The relevance of experimental models in the understanding of human disease. Nephron 62:373–381, 1992.
2713. Rifai A: Immunopathogenesis of experimental IgA nephropathy. Springer Semin Immunopathol 16:81–95, 1994.
2714. Chen A, Wei C-H, Lee W-H, Lin C-Y: Experimental IgA nephropathy: Factors influencing IgA–immune complex deposition in the glomerulus. Springer Semin Immunopathol 16:97–103, 1994.
2715. Rifai A, Small PA Jr, Teague PO, Ayoub EM: Experimental IgA nephropathy. J Exp Med 150:1161–1173, 1979.
2716. Rifai A, Small P Jr, Ayoub EM: Experimental IgA nephropathy. Factors governing the persistence of IgA-antigen complexes in the circulation of mice. Contrib Nephrol 40:37–44, 1984.
2717. Rifai A, Millard K: Glomerular deposition of immune complexes prepared with monomeric or polymeric IgA. Clin Exp Immunol 60:363–368, 1985.
2718. Rafai A, Mannik M: Clearance kinetics and fate of mouse IgA immune complexes prepared with monomeric or dimeric IgA. J Immunol 130:1826–1832, 1983.
2719. Chen A, Wong SS, Rifai A: Glomerular immune deposits in experimental IgA nephropathy. A continuum of circulating and in situ formed immune complexes. Am J Pathol 130:216–222, 1988.
2720. Rifai A, Chen A, Imai H: Complement activation in experimental IgA nephropathy: An antigen-mediated process. Kidney Int 32:838–844, 1987.
2721. Montinaro V, Esparza AR, Cavallo T, Rifai A: Antigen as mediator of glomerular injury in experimental IgA nephropathy. Lab Invest 64:508–519, 1991.
2722. Chen A, Ding S-L, Sheu L-F, et al: Experimental IgA nephropathy. Enhanced deposition of glomerular IgA immune complex in proteinuric states. Lab Invest 70:639–647, 1994.
2723. Emancipator SN, Ovary Z, Lamm ME: The role of mesangial complement in the hematuria of experimental IgA nephropathy. Lab Invest 57:269–276, 1987.
2724. Isaacs K, Miller F, Lane B: Experimental model for IgA nephropathy. Clin Immunol Immunopathol 20:419–426, 1981.
2725. Isaacs K, Miller F: Dextran-induced IgA nephropathy. Contrib Nephrol 40:45–50, 1984.
2726. Hirabayashi A, Hamaguchi N, Shigemoto K, et al: Experimental IgA nephropathy induced by oral administration of dextran. Hiroshima J Med Sci 35:53–58, 1986.
2727. Isaacs KL, Miller F: Antigen size and charge in immune complex glomerulonephritis. II. Passive induction of immune deposits with dextran–anti-dextran immune complexes. Am J Pathol 111:298–306, 1983.
2728. Gesualdo L, Ricanati S, Hassan MO, et al: Enzymolysis of glomerular immune deposits in vivo with dextranase/protease ameliorates proteinuria, hematuria, and mesangial proliferation in murine experimental IgA nephropathy. J Clin Invest 86:715–722, 1990.
2729. Emancipator SN, Gallo GR, Lamm ME: Experimental IgA nephropathy induced by oral immunization. J Exp Med 157:572–582, 1983.
2730. Genin C, Laurent B, Sabatier JC, et al: IgA mesangial deposits in C3H/HeJ mice after oral immunization with ferritin or bovine serum albumin. Clin Exp Immunol 63:385–394, 1986.
2731. Coppo R, Mazzucco G, Martina G, et al: Gluten-induced experimental IgA glomerulopathy. Lab Invest 60:499–506, 1989.
2732. Sato M, Ideura T, Koshikawa S: Experimental IgA nephropathy in mice. Lab Invest 54:377–384, 1986.
2733. Ward DM, Spiegelberg HL, Wilson CB: Persistence of IgA aggregates in the glomerular mesangium in mice. Kidney Int 16:801, 1979. Abstract.
2734. Stad RK, Bogers WMJM, Muizert Y, et al: Deposition of IgA is

associated with macrophage influx in the kidney of rats. Scand J Immunol 34:81–89, 1991.
2735. Dong W, Sell JE, Pestka JJ: Quantitative assessment of mesangial immunoglobulin A (IgA) accumulation, elevated circulating IgA immune complexes, and hematuria during vomitoxin-induced IgA nephropathy. Fundam Appl Toxicol 17:197–207, 1991.
2736. Rasooly L, Pestka JJ: Vomitoxin-induced dysregulation of serum IgA, IgM and IgG reactive with gut bacterial and self antigens. Food Chem Toxicol 30:499–504, 1992.
2737. Greene DM, Bondy GS, Azcona-Olivera JI, Pestke JJ: Role of gender and strain in vomitoxin-induced dysregulation of IgA production and IgA nephropathy in the mouse. J Toxicol Environ Health 43:37–50, 1994.
2738. Rasooly L, Abouzied MM, Brooks KH, Pestka JJ: Polyspecific and autoreactive IgA secreted by hybridomas derived from Peyer's patches of vomitoxin-fed mice: Characterization and possible pathogenic role in IgA nephropathy. Food Chem Toxicol 32:337–348, 1994.
2739. Rasooly L, Pestka JJ: Polyclonal autoreactive IgA increase and mesangial deposition during vomitoxin-induced IgA nephropathy in the BALB/c mouse. Food Chem Toxicol 32:329–336, 1994.
2740. Imai H, Nakamoto Y, Asakura K, et al: Spontaneous glomerular IgA deposition in ddY mice: An animal model of IgA nephritis. Kidney Int 27:756–761, 1985.
2741. Muso E, Yoshida H, Takeuchi E, et al: Pathogenic role of polyclonal and polymeric IgA in a murine model of mesangial proliferative glomerulonephritis with IgA deposition. Clin Exp Immunol 84:459–465, 1991.
2742. Takeuchi E, Doi T, Shimada T, et al: Retroviral gp70 antigen in spontaneous mesangial glomerulonephritis of ddY mice. Kidney Int 35:638–646, 1989.
2743. Wakui H, Imai H, Nakamoto Y, et al: Anti-histone autoantibodies in ddY mice, an animal model for spontaneous IgA nephritis. Clin Immunol Immunopathol 52:248–256, 1989.
2744. Shimizu M, Tomino Y, Abe M, et al: Retroviral envelope glycoprotein (gp 70) is not a prerequisite for pathogenesis of primary immunoglobulin A nephropathy in ddY mice. Nephron 62:328–331, 1992.
2745. Masuda Y, Ishizaki M, Yamanaka N, et al: Evidence of delayed mesangial transport of human IgA in glomeruli of ddY mice pretreated with sheep anti–type IV collagen serum. Acta Pathol Jpn 39:289–295, 1989.
2746. Duan HJ, Nagata T: Glomerular extracellular matrices and anionic sites in aging ddY mice: A morphometric study. Histochemistry 99:241–249, 1993.
2747. Tomino Y, Nakamura T, Ebihara I, et al: Altered steady-state levels of mRNA coding for extracellular matrices in renal tissues of ddY mice, an animal model of IgA nephropathy. J Clin Lab Anal 5:106–113, 1991.
2748. Tomino Y, Shimizu M, Koide H, et al: Effect of monoclonal antibody CD4 on glomerulonephritis of ddY mice, a spontaneous animal model of IgA nephropathy. Am J Kidney Dis 21:427–432, 1993.
2749. Tsushima Y, Tomino Y, Shimizu M, et al: IgA deposits might not influence the production of extracellular matrix in glomeruli of ddY mice, a spontaneous animal model for IgA nephropathy. Nephron 66:81–86, 1994.
2750. Harris CH, Krawiec DR, Gelberg HB, Shapiro SZ: Canine IgA glomerulonephropathy. Vet Immunol Immunopathol 36:1–16, 1993.
2751. Jessen RH, Nedrud JG, Emancipator SN: A mouse model of IgA nephropathy induced by Sendai virus. Adv Exp Med Biol 216B:1609–1618, 1987.
2752. Jessen RH, Emancipator SN, Jacobs GH, Nedrud JG: Experimental IgA-IgG nephropathy induced by a viral respiratory pathogen. Dependence on antigen form and immune status. Lab Invest 67:379–386, 1992.
2753. Russell MW, Brown TA, Mestecky J: Role of serum IgA. Hepatobiliary transport of circulating antigen. J Exp Med 153:968–976, 1981.
2754. Brown TA, Russell MW, Mestecky J: Hepatobiliary transport of IgA immune complexes: Molecular and cellular aspects. J Immunol 128:2183–2186, 1982.
2755. Gromly AA, Smith PS, Seymour AE, et al: IgA glomerular deposits in experimental cirrhosis. Am J Pathol 104:50–54, 1981.

2756. Woodroffe AJ, Gormly AA, Clarkson AR, et al: Experimental cirrhosis and deposition of glomerular IgA immune complexes. Contrib Nephrol 40:51–54, 1984.
2757. Iida H, Izumino K, Matsumoto M, et al: Glomerular deposition of IgA in experimental hepatic cirrhosis. Acta Pathol Jpn 35:561–567, 1985.
2758. Melvin T, Burke B, Michael AF, Kim Y: Experimental IgA nephropathy in bile duct ligated rats. Clin Immunol Immunopathol 27:369–377, 1983.
2759. Amore A, Coppo R, Roccatello D, et al: Experimental IgA nephropathy secondary to hepatocellular injury induced by dietary deficiencies and heavy alcohol intake. Lab Invest 70:68–77, 1994.
2760. Emancipator SN, Gallo GR, Razaboni R, Lamm ME: Experimental cholestasis promotes the deposition of glomerular IgA immune complexes. Am J Pathol 113:19–26, 1983.
2761. Gallo GR, Emancipator SN, Lamm ME: Experimental cholestasis and deposition of glomerular IgA immune complexes. Contrib Nephrol 40:55–61, 1984.
2762. Abramowsky CR, Christiansen DM: Secretory immunoglobulin deposits in renal glomeruli of children with extrahepatic biliary atresia: Studies in a human counterpart of experimental ligation of the bile ducts. Hum Pathol 18:1126–1131, 1987.
2763. Ward DM, Lee S, Wilson CB: Direct antigen binding to glomerular immune complex deposits. Kidney Int 30:706–711, 1986.
2764. Fornasieri A, Moullier PM, Wilson CB: Dynamic interchange and factors influencing disappearance of antigen (Ag) and/or antibody (Ab) within glomerular (G) immune deposits (ID). Kidney Int 37:413, 1990. Abstract.
2765. Mannik M, Striker GE: Removal of glomerular deposits of immune complexes in mice by administration of excess antigen. Lab Invest 42:483–489, 1980.
2766. Haakenstad AO, Striker GE, Mannik M: Removal of glomerular immune complex deposits by excess antigen in chronic mouse model of immune complex disease. Lab Invest 48:323–331, 1983.
2767. Ford PM, Kosatka I: In situ formation of antigen-antibody complexes in the mouse glomerulus. Immunology 38:473–479, 1979.
2768. Ford PM, Kosatka I: The effect of in situ formation of antigen-antibody complexes in the glomerulus on subsequent glomerular localization of passively administered immune complexes. Immunology 39:337–344, 1980.
2769. Ford PM, Kosatka I: A mechanism of enhancement of immune complex deposition following in situ immune complex formation in the mouse glomerulus. Immunology 43:433–439, 1981.
2770. Haakenstad AO: Removal of glomerular deposits induced by either preformed immune complexes or by a chronic immune complex model in NZB/W mice. J Immunol 138:4192–4199, 1987.
2771. Raz E, Michaeli J, Brezis M, et al: Improvement of immune-complex nephritis associated with hepatitis B surface antigen excess. Am J Nephrol 9:162–166, 1989.
2772. Mannik M, Agodoa LYC, David KA: Rearrangement of immune complexes in glomeruli leads to persistence and development of electron-dense deposits. J Exp Med 157:1516–1527, 1983.
2773. Lew AM, Tovey DG, Steward MW: Localization of covalent immune complexes on the epithelial side of the glomerular basement membrane in mice. Int Arch Allergy Appl Immunol 75:242–249, 1984.
2774. Gauthier VJ, Mannik M: Only the initial binding of cationic immune complexes to glomerular anionic sites is mediated by charge-charge interactions. J Immunol 136:3266–3271, 1986.
2775. Agodoa LYC, Gauthier VJ, Mannik M: Precipitating antigen-antibody systems are required for the formation of subepithelial electron-dense immune deposits in rat glomeruli. J Exp Med 158:1259–1271, 1983.
2776. Geltner D, Franklin EC, Frangione B: Antiidiotypic activity in the IgM fractions of mixed cryoglobulins. J Immunol 125:1530–1535, 1980.
2777. Sindrey M, Barratt J, Hewitt J, Naish P: Infective endocarditis-associated glomerulonephritis in rabbits: Evidence of a pathogenetic role for antiglobulins. Clin Exp Immunol 45:253–260, 1981.
2778. Ford PM, Kosatka I: The effect of human IgM rheumatoid factor on renal glomerular immune complex deposition in passive serum sickness in the mouse. Immunology 46:761–768, 1982.
2779. Ford PM, Kosatka I: In situ immune complex formation in the mouse glomerulus: Reactivity with human IgM rheumatoid factor and the effect on subsequent immune complex deposition. Clin Exp Immunol 51:285–291, 1983.
2780. Ford PM: Interaction of rheumatoid factor with immune complexes in experimental glomerulonephritis—possible role of antiglobulins in chronicity. J Rheumatol 10(suppl 11):81–84, 1983.
2781. Germuth FG, Rodriguez E: Effect of human IgM rheumatoid factor on the glomerular site of localization of passively administered immune complexes in mice. Immunology 53:395–398, 1984.
2782. Devey ME, Hogben DN: The effect of rheumatoid factor on the clearance of endogenous immune complexes formed in low-affinity mice during the induction of immune complex disease. Int Arch Allergy Appl Immunol 83:206–209, 1987.
2783. Siegert CEH, Daha MR, Halma C, et al: IgG and IgA autoantibodies to C1q in systemic and renal diseases. Clin Exp Rheumatol 10:19–23, 1992.
2784. Penner E, Albini B, Glurich I, et al: Dissociation of immune complexes in tissue sections by excess of antigen. Int Arch Allergy Appl Immunol 67:245–253, 1982.
2785. Suzuki Y, Oite T, Shimizu F, et al: Solubilization of immune complex deposits by native 7S IgG molecules in lupus glomerulonephritis—a possible antigen excess effect on rheumatoid factor–IgG complexes. Clin Exp Immunol 58:663–671, 1984.
2786. Tomino Y, Sakai H, Takaya M, et al: Solubilization of intraglomerular deposits of IgG immune complexes by human sera or gamma-globulin in patients with lupus nephritis. Clin Exp Immunol 58:42–48, 1984.
2787. Cavalot F, Miyata M, Vladutiu A, et al: Glomerular lesions induced in the rabbit by physicochemically altered homologous IgG. Am J Pathol 140:581–600, 1992.
2788. Chen A, Chou W-Y, Ding S-L, Shaio M-F: Glomerular localization of nephritogenic protein complexes on a nonimmunologic basis. Lab Invest 67:175–185, 1992.
2789. Nakazawa M, Emancipator SN, Lamm ME: Removal of glomerular immune complexes in passive serum sickness nephritis by treatment in vivo with proteolytic enzymes. Lab Invest 55:551–556, 1986.
2790. Döring G, Goldstein W, Botzenhart K, et al: Elastase from polymorphonuclear leucocytes: A regulatory enzyme in immune complex disease. Clin Exp Immunol 64:597–605, 1986.
2791. Batsford SR: Cationic antigens as mediators of inflammation. APMIS 99:1–9, 1991.
2792. Koyama A, Inage H, Kobayashi M, et al: Role of antigenic charge and antibody avidity on the glomerular immune complex localization in serum sickness of mice. Clin Exp Immunol 64:606–614, 1986.
2793. Koyama A, Inage H, Kobayashi M, et al: Effect of chemical modification of antigen on characteristics of immune complexes and their glomerular localization in the murine renal tissues. Immunology 58:535–540, 1986.
2794. Koyama A, Inage H, Kobayashi M, et al: Effect of chemical cationization of antigen on glomerular localization of immune complexes in active models of serum sickness nephritis in rabbits. Immunology 58:529–534, 1986.
2795. Yamamoto T, Miyazaki S, Kawasaki K, et al: Rat bovine serum albumin (BSA) nephritis. VI. The influence of chemically altered antigen. Clin Exp Immunol 65:51–56, 1986.
2796. Bass PS, Drake AF, Wang Y, et al: Cationization of bovine serum albumin alters its conformation as well as its charge. Lab Invest 62:185–188, 1990.
2797. Batsford SR, Mihatsch MJ, Rawiel M, et al: Surface charge distribution is a determinant of antigen deposition in the renal glomerulus: Studies employing 'charge-hybrid' molecules. Clin Exp Immunol 86:471–477, 1991.
2798. Gallo GR, Caulin-Glaser T, Lamm ME: Charge of circulating immune complexes as a factor in glomerular basement membrane localization in mice. J Clin Invest 67:1305–1313, 1981.
2799. Gallo GR, Caulin-Glaser T, Lamm ME: Role of electrostatic charge interactions in glomerular deposition of immune complexes. Pathobiol Annu 12:203–211, 1982.
2800. Mannik M, Stapleton SA, Burns MW, et al: Glomerular subendothelial and subepithelial immune complexes, containing the same antigen, are removed at different rates. Clin Exp Immunol 84:367–372, 1991.
2801. Mannik M, Kobayashi M, Alpers CE, Gauthier VJ: Antigens of varying size persist longer in subepithelial than in subendothelial immune deposits in murine glomeruli. J Immunol 150:2062–2071, 1993.

2802. Furness PN, Turner DR: Chronic serum sickness glomerulonephritis: Passive immunisation inhibits the removal of glomerular antigen and electron dense deposits. Virchows Arch A 413:551–553, 1988.

2803. Furness PN, Turner DR: Chronic serum sickness glomerulonephritis: Modification of the immune response influences the rate of removal of mesangial electron-dense deposits. J Pathol 156:137–145, 1988.

2804. Fries JWU, Mendrick DL, Rennke HG: Determinants of immune complex–mediated glomerulonephritis. Kidney Int 34:333–345, 1988.

2805. Fujigaki Y, Nagase M, Honda N: Intraglomerular basement membrane translocation of immune complex (IC) in the development of passive in situ IC nephritis of rats. Am J Pathol 142:831–843, 1993.

2806. Caulin-Glaser T, Gallo GR, Lamm ME: Nondissociating cationic immune complexes can deposit in glomerular basement membrane. J Exp Med 158:1561–1572, 1983.

2807. Gauthier VJ, Mannik M, Striker GE: Effect of cationized antibodies in preformed immune complexes on deposition and persistence in renal glomeruli. J Exp Med 156:766–777, 1982.

2808. Gauthier VJ, Mannik M: A small proportion of cationic antibodies in immune complexes is sufficient to mediate their deposition in glomeruli. J Immunol 145:3348–3352, 1990.

2809. Caulin-Glaser T, Emancipator SN, Gallo GR, Lamm ME: Charge-related deposition of immune complexes in the glomerular basement membrane is independent of Fc effector function. Am J Pathol 119:288–293, 1985.

2810. Gauthier VJ, Striker GE, Mannik M: Glomerular localization of preformed immune complexes prepared with anionic antibodies or with cationic antigens. Lab Invest 50:636–644, 1984.

2811. Mannik M, Gauthier VJ, Stapleton SA, Agodoa LYC: Immune complexes with cationic antibodies deposit in glomeruli more effectively than cationic antibodies alone. J Immunol 38:4209–4217, 1987.

2812. Iskandar SS, Zhang J, Rodriguez E: Nephropathy induced in a nephritis-resistant inbred mouse strain with the use of a cationized antigen. Am J Pathol 123:67–72, 1986.

2813. Ebling F, Hahn BH: Restricted subpopulations of DNA antibodies in kidneys of mice with systemic lupus. Comparison of antibodies in serum and renal eluates. Arthritis Rheum 23:392–403, 1980.

2814. Dang H, Harbeck RJ: A comparison of anti-DNA antibodies from serum and kidney eluates of NZB × NZW F₁ mice. J Clin Lab Immunol 9:139–145, 1982.

2815. Gavalchin J, Nicklas JA, Eastcott JW, et al: Lupus prone (SWR × NZB)F₁ mice produce potentially nephritogenic autoantibodies inherited from the normal SWR parent. J Immunol 134:885–894, 1985.

2816. Gavalchin J, Seder RA, Datta SK: The NZB × SWR model of lupus nephritis. I. Cross-reactive idiotypes of monoclonal anti-DNA antibodies in relation to antigenic specificity, charge, and allotype. Identification of interconnected idiotype families inherited from the normal SWR and the autoimmune NZB parents. J Immunol 138:128–137, 1987.

2817. Gavalchin J, Datta SK: The NZB × SWR model of lupus nephritis. II. Autoantibodies deposited in renal lesions show a distinctive and restricted idiotypic diversity. J Immunol 138:138–148, 1987.

2818. Dang H, Harbeck RJ: The in vivo and in vitro glomerular deposition of isolated anti–double-stranded-DNA antibodies in NZB/W mice. Clin Immunol Immunopathol 30:265–278, 1984.

2819. Datta SK, Patel H, Berry D: Induction of a cationic shift in IgG anti-DNA autoantibodies. Role of T helper cells with classical and novel phenotypes in three murine models of lupus nephritis. J Exp Med 165:1252–1268, 1987.

2820. Furness PN: Chronic serum sickness glomerulonephritis: Heparin enhances the removal of glomerular antigen. J Pathol 161:233–237, 1990.

2821. Melnick GF, Ladoulis CT, Cavallo T: Decreased anionic groups and increased permeability precedes deposition of immune complexes in the glomerular capillary wall. Am J Pathol 105:114–120, 1981.

2822. Duan HJ, Nakazawa K, Ishigame H, et al: Masking of anionic sites by deposits in lamina rara externa in immune complex nephritis in rats. Virchows Arch B 60:165–171, 1991.

2823. Chan EKL, Boyd ND, Alexander F, et al: Effect of cationic proteins on the glomerular deposition of anionic proteins and immune complexes. Nephron 43:93–104, 1986.

2824. Agodoa LYC, Gauthier VJ, Mannik M: Antibody localization in the glomerular basement membrane may precede in situ immune deposit formation in rat glomeruli. J Immunol 134:880–884, 1985.

2825. Ford PM, Kosatka I: Cationised IgM rheumatoid factor: In-vivo glomerular localization and immunoabsorptive capacity in the mouse. Clin Exp Immunol 62:150–158, 1985.

2826. Agodoa LYC, Mannik M: Removal of subepithelial immune complexes with excess unaltered or cationic antigen. Kidney Int 32:13–18, 1987.

2827. Cohen S, Vernier RL, Michael AF: The effect of charge on the renal distribution of ferritin. Am J Pathol 110:170–181, 1983.

2828. Gallo GR, Caulin-Glaser T, Emancipator SN, Lamm ME: Nephritogenicity and differential distribution of glomerular immune complexes related to immunogen charge. Lab Invest 48:353–362, 1983.

2829. Border WA, Kamil ES, Ward HJ, Cohen AH: Antigenic charge as a determinant of immune complex localization in the rat glomerulus. Lab Invest 40:442–449, 1981.

2830. Isaacs KL, Miller F: Role of antigen size and charge in immune complex glomerulonephritis. I. Active induction of disease with dextran and its derivatives. Lab Invest 47:198–205, 1982.

2831. Wright NG, Mohammed NA, Eckersall PD, Nash AS: Experimental immune complex glomerulonephritis in dogs receiving cationised bovine serum albumin. Res Vet Sci 38:322–328, 1985.

2832. Nash AS, Mohammed NA, Wright NG: Experimental immune complex glomerulonephritis and the nephrotic syndrome in cats immunised with cationised bovine serum albumin. Res Vet Sci 49:370–372, 1990.

2833. Springate JE, Van Liew JB, Noble B, Feld LG: Progressive glomerular injury after recovery from acute glomerulonephritis in rats. Clin Immunol Immunopathol 61:309–319, 1991.

2834. Lachmann PJ: Complement genetics and host defence. Int J Med Microbiol 274:316–324, 1990.

2835. Davies KA, Schifferli JA, Walport MJ: Complement deficiency and immune complex disease. Springer Semin Immunopathol 15:397–416, 1994.

2836. Noble BK: Immunologically complex kidneys. Lancet 342:1250–1251, 1993.

2837. Miller GW, Nussenzweig V: A new complement function: Solubilization of antigen-antibody aggregates. Proc Natl Acad Sci USA 72:418–422, 1975.

2838. Takahashi M, Takahashi S, Hirose S: Solubilization of antigen-antibody complexes: A new function of complement as a regulator of immune reactions. Prog Allergy 27:134–166, 1980.

2839. Fujita T, Takata Y, Tamura N: Solubilization of immune precipitates by six isolated alternative pathway proteins. J Exp Med 154:1743–1751, 1981.

2840. Schifferli JA, Bartolotti SR, Peters DK: Inhibition of immune precipitation by complement. Clin Exp Immunol 42:387–394, 1980.

2841. Schifferli JA, Woo P, Peters DK: Complement-mediated inhibition of immune precipitation. I. Role of the classical and alternative pathways. Clin Exp Immunol 47:555–562, 1982.

2842. Naama JK, Mitchell WS, Zoma A, et al: Complement-mediated inhibition of immune precipitation in patients with immune complex diseases. Clin Exp Immunol 51:292–298, 1983.

2843. Bartolotti SR, Peters DK: Delayed removal of renal-bound antigen in decomplemented rabbits with acute serum sickness. Clin Exp Immunol 32:199–206, 1978.

2844. Bartolotti SR, Peters DK: Complement fixation in acute serum sickness: Assembly of glomerular-bound C3-convertase. Clin Exp Immunol 37:391–398, 1979.

2845. Aguado MT, Mannik M: Clearance kinetics and organ uptake of complement-solubilized immune complexes in mice. Immunology 60:255–260, 1987.

2846. Furness PN, Turner DR: Chronic serum sickness glomerulonephritis: Removal of glomerular antigen and electron-dense deposits is largely dependent on plasma complement. Clin Exp Immunol 74:126–130, 1988.

2847. Schifferli JA, Morris SM, Dash A, Peters DK: Complement-mediated solubilization in patients with systemic lupus erythematosus, nephritis or vasculitis. Clin Exp Immunol 46:557–564, 1981.

2848. Medof ME, Scarborough D, Miller G: Ability of complement to release systemic lupus erythematosus immune complexes from cell receptors. Clin Exp Immunol 44:416–425, 1981.

2849. Aguado MT, Perrin LH, Miescher PA, Lambert PH: Decreased capacity to solubilize immune complexes in sera from patients with systemic lupus erythematosus. Arthritis Rheum 24:1225–1229, 1981.

2850. Sakurai T, Fujita T, Kono I, et al: Complement-mediated solubilization of immune complexes in systemic lupus erythematosus. Clin Exp Immunol 48:37–42, 1982.

2851. Medof ME, Prince GM, Oger JJ-F: Kinetics of interaction of immune complexes with complement receptors on human blood cells: Modification of complexes during interaction with red cells. Clin Exp Immunol 48:715–725, 1982.

2852. Schreiber RD, Pangburn MK, Bjornson AB, et al: The role of C3 fragments in endocytosis and extracellular cytotoxic reactions by polymorphonuclear leukocytes. Clin Immunol Immunopathol 23:335–357, 1982.

2853. Medof ME, Iida K, Mold C, Nussenzweig V: Unique role of the complement receptor $CR_1$ in the degradation of C3b associated with immune complexes. J Exp Med 156:1739–1754, 1982.

2854. Taylor RP, Burge J, Horgan C, Shasby DM: The complement-mediated binding of soluble antibody/dsDNA immune complexes to human neutrophils. J Immunol 130:2656–2662, 1983.

2855. Medof ME, Lam T, Prince GM, Mold C: Requirement for human red blood cells in inactivation of C3b in immune complexes and enhancement of binding to spleen cells. J Immunol 130:1336–1340, 1983.

2856. Nielsen CH, Svehag SE, Marquart HV, Leslie RG: Interactions of opsonized immune complexes with whole blood cells: Binding to erythrocytes restricts complex uptake by leucocyte populations. Scand J Immunol 40:228–236, 1994.

2857. Taylor RP, Pocanic F, Reist C, Wright EL: Complement-opsonized IgG antibody/dsDNA immune complexes bind to CR1 clusters on isolated human erythrocytes. Clin Immunol Immunopathol 61:143–160, 1991.

2858. Madi N, Paccaud J-P, Steiger G, Schifferli JA: Immune complex binding efficiency of erythrocyte complement receptor 1 (CR1). Clin Exp Immunol 84:9–15, 1991.

2859. Iida K, Nussenzweig V: Functional properties of membrane-associated complement receptor CR1. J Immunol 130:1876–1880, 1983.

2860. Schifferli JA, Ng YC, Peters DK: The role of complement and its receptor in the elimination of immune complexes. N Engl J Med 315:488–494, 1986.

2861. Weiss L, Fischer E, Haeffner-Cavaillon N, et al: The human C3b receptor (CR1). Adv Nephrol 18:249–269, 1989.

2862. Shifferli JA, Taylor RP: Physiological and pathological aspects of circulating immune complexes. Kidney Int 35:993–1003, 1989.

2863. Hebert LA, Cosio FG, Birmingham DJ, Mahan JD: Biologic significance of the erythrocyte complement receptor: A primate perquisite. J Lab Clin Med 118:301–308, 1991.

2864. Pascual M, Schifferli JA: The binding of immune complexes by the erythrocyte complement receptor 1 (CR1). Immunopharmacology 24:101–106, 1992.

2865. Iida K, Mornaghi R, Nussenzweig V: Complement receptor ($CR_1$) deficiency in erythrocytes from patients with systemic lupus erythematosus. J Exp Med 155:1427–1438, 1982.

2866. Wilson JG, Wong WW, Schur PH, Fearon DT: Mode of inheritance of decreased C3b receptors on erythrocytes of patients with systemic lupus erythematosus. N Engl J Med 307:981–986, 1982.

2867. Inada Y, Kamiyama M, Kanemitsu T, et al: Studies on immune adherence (C3b) receptor activity of human erythrocytes: Relationship between receptor activity and presence of immune complexes in serum. Clin Exp Immunol 50:189–197, 1982.

2868. Taylor RP, Horgan C, Buschbacher R, et al: Decreased complement mediated binding of antibody/³H-dsDNA immune complexes to the red blood cells of patients with systemic lupus erythematosus, rheumatoid arthritis, and hematologic malignancies. Arthritis Rheum 26:736–744, 1983.

2869. Ross GD, Yount WJ, Walport MJ, et al: Disease-associated loss of erythrocyte complement receptors ($Cr_1$, C3b receptors) in patients with systemic lupus erythematosus and other diseases involving autoantibodies and/or complement activation. J Immunol 135:2005–2014, 1985.

2870. Wilson JG, Jack RM, Wong WW, et al: Autoantibody to the C3b/C4b receptor and absence of this receptor from erythrocytes of a patient with systemic lupus erythematosus. J Clin Invest 76:182–190, 1985.

2871. Cook JM, Kazatchkine MD, Bourgeois P, et al: Anti–C3b-receptor (CR1) antibodies in patients with systemic lupus erythematosus. Clin Immunol Immunopathol 38:135–138, 1986.

2872. Kazatchkine MD, Fearon DT, Appay MD, et al: Immunohistochemical study of the human glomerular C3b receptor in normal kidney and in seventy-five cases of renal diseases. Loss of C3b receptor antigen in focal hyalinosis and in proliferative nephritis of systemic lupus erythematosus. J Clin Invest 69:900–912, 1982.

2873. Emancipator SN, Iida K, Nussenzweig V, Gallo GR: Monoclonal antibodies to human complement receptor (CR1) detect defects in glomerular diseases. Clin Immunol Immunopathol 27:170–175, 1983.

2874. Matre R, Tönder O: C4 receptors in the human glomeruli. Int Arch Allergy Appl Immunol 63:312–316, 1980.

2875. Matre R, Nilsen R, Thunold S, Tønder O: The localization of glomerular C3b receptor by immunoelectron microscopy. Scand J Immunol 16:351–354, 1982.

2876. Cornacoff JB, Herbert LA, Smead WL, et al: Primate erythrocyte–immune complex–clearing mechanism. J Clin Invest 71:236–247, 1983.

2877. Hebert LA, Cosio FG: The erythrocyte–immune complex–glomerulonephritis connection in man. Kidney Int 31:877–885, 1987.

2878. Cosio FG, Hebert LA, Birmingham DJ, et al: Clearance of human antibody/DNA immune complexes and free DNA from the circulation of the nonhuman primate. Clin Immunol Immunopathol 42:1–9, 1987.

2879. Hebert LA, Birmingham DJ, Shen X-P, Cosio FG: Stimulating erythropoiesis increases complement receptor expression on primate erythrocytes. Clin Immunol Immunopathol 62:301–306, 1992.

2880. Birmingham DJ, Hebert LA, Cosio FG, Van Aman ME: Immune complex erythrocyte complement receptor interactions in vivo during induction of glomerulonephritis in nonhuman primates. J Lab Clin Med 116:242–252, 1990.

2881. Cosio FG, Xiao-Ping S, Birmingham DJ, et al: Evaluation of the mechanisms responsible for the reduction in erythrocyte complement receptors when immune complexes form in vivo in primates. J Immunol 145:4198–4206, 1990.

2882. Hebert LA, Birmingham DJ, Mahan JD, et al: Effect of chronically increased erythrocyte complement receptors on immune complex nephritis. Kidney Int 45:493–499, 1994.

2883. Colasanti G, Moran J, Bellini A, D'Amico G: Significance of glomerular C3b receptors in human renal diseases. Renal Physiol 3:387–394, 1980.

2884. Bolton WK, Schrock JH, Davis JS, IV: Rheumatoid factor inhibition of in vitro binding of IgG complexes in the human glomerulus. Arthritis Rheum 25:297–303, 1982.

2885. Kasinath BS, Maaba MR, Schwartz MM, Lewis EJ: Demonstration and characterization of C3 receptors on rat glomerular epithelial cells. Kidney Int 30:852–861, 1986.

2886. Lavelle KJ: Interaction of immune complexes with cultured rabbit glomerular cells. Nephron 32:351–358, 1982.

2887. Sánchez-Crespo M, Alonso F, Barat A, Egido J: Rat serum sickness: Possible role of inflammatory mediators allowing deposition of immune complexes in the glomerular basement membrane. Clin Exp Immunol 49:631–638, 1982.

2888. Chia YC, Cattell V: The role of platelets in mesangial localization: carbon uptake in thrombocytopenic rats. Br J Exp Pathol 66:465–474, 1985.

2889. Lightfoot RW Jr, Drusin RE, Christian CL: Properties of soluble immune complexes. J Immunol 105:1493–1500, 1970.

2890. Haakenstad AO, Striker GE, Mannik M: The disappearance kinetics and glomerular deposition of small-latticed soluble immune complexes. Immunology 47:407–414, 1982.

2891. Mannik M: Physicochemical and functional relationships of immune complexes. J Invest Dermatol 74:333–338, 1980.

2892. Mannik M, David KA: Covalently cross-linked immune complexes prepared with multivalent cross-linking antigens. J Immunol 127:1999–2006, 1981.

2893. Cochrane CG, Hawkins DJ: Studies on circulating immune complexes. III. Factors governing the ability of circulating complexes to localize in blood vessels. J Exp Med 127:137–154, 1968.

2894. Shigematsu H, Takizawa J, Akikusa B, Niwa Y: Arthus-type nephritis. II. Glomerular clearing system against poorly soluble and insoluble immune complexes. Acta Pathol Jpn 31:379–389, 1981.

2895. Clark WF, Turnbull DI, Driedger AA, et al: Intrarenal insoluble immune complex formation. J Clin Lab Immunol 4:21–25, 1980.

2896. Kim YW, Halsey JF: Metabolism and clearance of antibody-excess immune complexes in lactating mice. J Immunol 129:619–622, 1982.

2897. Cameron JS, Clark WF: A role for insoluble antibody-antigen complexes in glomerulonephritis? Clin Nephrol 18:55–61, 1982.
2898. Hogendoorn PC, van Dorst EB, van der Burg SH, et al: Antigen size influences the type of glomerular pathology in chronic serum sickness. Nephrol Dial Transplant 8:703–710, 1993.
2899. Hosoi S, Shinomiya K, Mikawa H: The use of monoclonal antibodies in demonstrating the effect of antibody heterogeneity on immune complex size. Clin Immunol Immunopathol 32:378–386, 1984.
2900. Griswold WR, Brams M: Antibody affinity and acute immune complex disease. J Clin Lab Immunol 14:181–183, 1984.
2901. Pincus T, Haberkern R, Christian CL: Experimental chronic glomerulitis. J Exp Med 127:819–831, 1968.
2902. Steward MW, Collins MJ, Stanley C, Devey ME: Chronic antigen-antibody-complex glomerulonephritis in mice. Br J Exp Pathol 62:614–622, 1981.
2903. Devey ME, Bleasdale K, Collins M, Steward MW: Experimental antigen-antibody complex disease in mice. The role of antibody levels, antibody affinity and circulating antigen-antibody complexes. Int Arch Allergy Appl Immunol 68:47–53, 1982.
2904. Devey ME, Bleasdale K, Stanley C, Steward MW: Failure of affinity maturation leads to increased susceptibility to immune complex glomerulonephritis. Immunology 52:377–383, 1984.
2905. Devey ME, Bleasdale K: Antigen feeding modifies the course of antigen-induced immune complex disease. Clin Exp Immunol 56:637–644, 1984.
2906. Moulder K, Steward MW: Capillary-localized low-affinity antibody-antigen complexes act as a focus for the deposition of high-affinity complexes. Clin Exp Immunol 77:275–280, 1989.
2907. Quinn DG, Fennell JS, Sheils O, et al: Effect of cyclosporin on immune complex deposition in murine glomerulonephritis. Immunology 72:550–554, 1991.
2908. Lew AM, Steward MW: Glomerulonephritis: The use of grafted hybridomas to investigate the role of epitope density, antibody affinity and antibody isotype in active serum sickness. Immunology 52:367–376, 1984.
2909. Lew AM, Staines NA, Steward MW: Glomerulonephritis induced by pre-formed immune complexes containing monoclonal antibodies of defined affinity and isotype. Clin Exp Immunol 57:413–422, 1984.
2910. Chen X-M, Tanaka T, Kobayashi Y, et al: Experimental glomerulonephritis induced by immune complexes of monoclonal antibodies produced by immunoglobulin class-switch variants. Lab Invest 57:665–672, 1987.
2911. Reinhardt MC, Devey M, Collins M, et al: The effect of protein deficiency on the development of chronic antigen-antibody complex disease in mice. Clin Exp Immunol 44:528–537, 1981.
2912. Iskandar SS, Jennette JC: Influence of antibody avidity on glomerular immune complex localization. Am J Pathol 112:155–159, 1983.
2913. Germuth FG Jr, Rodriguez E, Wise O: Passive immune complex glomerulonephritis in mice. III. Clearance kinetics and properties of circulating complexes. Lab Invest 46:515–519, 1982.
2914. Mannik M: Pathophysiology of circulating immune complexes. Arthritis Rheum 25:783–787, 1982.
2915. Griffin FM Jr: Effects of soluble immune complexes on Fc receptor– and C3b receptor–mediated phagocytosis by macrophages. J Exp Med 152:905–919, 1980.
2916. Ezekowitz RAB, Bampton M, Gordon S: Macrophage activation selectively enhances expression of Fc receptors for IgG2a. J Exp Med 157:807–812, 1983.
2917. Halma C, Daha MR, Van Es LA: In vivo clearance by the mononuclear phagocyte system in humans: An overview of methods and their interpretation. Clin Exp Immunol 89:1–7, 1992.
2918. Frank MM: The reticuloendothelial system and bloodstream clearance. J Lab Clin Med 122:487–488, 1993.
2919. Ravetch JV, Kinet JP: Fc receptors. Annu Rev Immunol 9:457–492, 1991.
2920. Fridman WH: Fc receptors and immunoglobulin binding factors. FASEB J 5:2684–2690, 1991.
2921. Unkeless JC, Boros P, Fein M: Structure, signalling and function of FcγR. In Gallin JI, Goldstein IM, Snyderman R (eds): Inflammation: Basic Principles and Clinical Correlates, 2nd ed. Raven Press, New York, 1992, pp 497–510.
2922. Tuijnman WB, Van Wichen DF, Schuurman H-J: Tissue distribution of human IgG Fc receptors CD16, CD32 and CD64: An immunohistochemical study. APMIS 101:319–329, 1993.
2923. van de Winkel JGJ, Capel PJA: Human IgG Fc receptor heterogeneity: Molecular aspects and clinical implications. Immunol Today 14:215–221, 1993.
2924. Boros P, Muryoi T, Spiera H, et al: Autoantibodies directed against different classes of FcγR are found in sera of autoimmune patients. J Immunol 150:2019–2024, 1993.
2925. Fridman WH, Teillaud JL, Bouchard C, et al: Soluble Fc γ receptors. J Leukoc Biol 54:504–512, 1993.
2926. Clarkson SB, Kimberly RP, Valinsky JE, et al: Blockade of clearance of immune complexes by an anti–Fc-γ receptor monoclonal antibody. J Exp Med 164:474–489, 1986.
2927. Mahan JD, Hebert LA, McAllister C, et al: Platelet involvement in experimental immune complex–mediated glomerulonephritis in the nonhuman primate. Kidney Int 44:716–725, 1993.
2928. Morgan EL, Weigle WO: Regulation of the immune response: III. The role of macrophages in the potentiation of the immune response by Fc fragments. J Immunol 126:1302–1306, 1981.
2929. Neville ME, Lischner HW: Activation of FC receptor–bearing lymphocytes by immune complexes. I. Stimulation of lymphokine production by nonadherent human peripheral blood lymphocytes. J Immunol 128:1063–1069, 1982.
2930. Miyama-Inaba M, Suzuki T, Paku YH, Masuda T: Feedback regulation of immune responses by immune complexes; possible involvement of a suppressive lymphokine by FcRγ-bearing B cell. J Immunol 128:882–887, 1982.
2931. Segal DM, Titus JA, Dower SK: The FcR-mediated enodocytosis of model immune complexes by cells from the P388D₁ mouse macrophage line. II. The role of ligand-induced self-aggregation in promoting internalization. J Immunol 130:138–144, 1983.
2932. Segal DM, Dower SK, Titus JA: The FcR-mediated endocytosis of model immune complexes by cells from the P388D₁ mouse macrophage line. I. Internalization of small, nonaggregating oligomers of IgG. J Immunol 130:130–137, 1983.
2933. Michl J, Unkeless JC, Pieczonka MM, Silverstein SC: Modulation of Fc receptors of mononuclear phagocytes by immobilized antigen-antibody complexes. Quantitative analysis of the relationship between ligand number and Fc receptor response. J Exp Med 157:1746–1757, 1983.
2934. Parren PWHI, Warmerdam PAM, Boeije LCM, et al: On the interaction of IgG subclasses with the low affinity FcγRIIa (CD32) on human monocytes, neutrophils, and platelets. Analysis of a functional polymorphism to human IgG2. J Clin Invest 90:1537–1546, 1992.
2935. Brunkhorst BA, Strohmeier G, Lazzari K, et al: Differential roles of FcγRII and FcγRIII in immune complex stimulation of human neutrophils. J Biol Chem 267:20659–20666, 1992.
2936. Dransfield I, Buckle AM, Savill JS, et al: Neutrophil apoptosis is associated with a reduction in CD16 (Fc gamma RIII) expression. J Immunol 153:1254–1263, 1994.
2937. Looney RJ: Structure and function of human and mouse Fc gamma RII. Blood Cells 19:353–359, 1993.
2938. Dusi S, Donini M, Della Bianca V, et al: In human neutrophils the binding to immunocomplexes induces the tyrosine phosphorylation of Fc gamma RII but this phosphorylation is not an essential signal for Fc-mediated phagocytosis. Biochem Biophys Res Commun 201:30–37, 1994.
2939. Lin CT, Shen Z, Boros P, Unkeless JC: Fc receptor–mediated signal transduction. J Clin Immunol 14:1–13, 1994.
2940. Fanger MW, Graziano RF, Guyre PM: Production and use of anti-FcR dispecific antibodies. Immunomethods 4:72–81, 1994.
2941. Finbloom DS, Plotz PH: Studies of reticuloendothelial function in the mouse with model immune complexes. I. Serum clearance and tissue uptake in normal C3H mice. J Immunol 123:1594–1599, 1979.
2942. Finbloom DS, Plotz PH: Studies of reticuloendothelial function in the mouse with model immune complexes. II. Serum clearance, tissue uptake, and reticuloendothelial saturation in NZB/W mice. J Immunol 123:1600–1603, 1979.
2943. Jimenez RAH, Mannik M: Evaluation of aggregated IgG in mice as an Fc receptor specific probe of the hepatic mononuclear phagocyte system. Clin Exp Immunol 49:200–208, 1982.
2944. Russell PJ, Steinberg AD: Studies of peritoneal macrophage function in mice with systemic lupus erythematosus: Depressed phago-

cytosis of opsonized sheep erythrocytes in vitro. Clin Immunol Immunopathol 27:387–402, 1983.

2945. Meryhew NL, Shaver C, Messner RP, Runquist OA: Mononuclear phagocyte system dysfunction in murine SLE: Abnormal clearance kinetics precede clinical disease. J Lab Clin Med 117:181–193, 1991.

2946. Kimberly RP: Of mice and men: Insights into the complexity of mononuclear phagocyte system blockade provided by autoimmune mouse strains. J Lab Clin Med 117:173–174, 1991.

2947. Abrass CK, Hori M: Alterations in Fc receptor function of macrophages from streptozotocin-induced diabetic rats. J Immunol 133:1307–1312, 1984.

2948. Finbloom DS, Abeles D, Rifai A, Plotz PH: The specificity of uptake of model immune complexes and other protein aggregates by the murine reticuloendothelial system. J Immunol 125:1060–1065, 1980.

2949. Finbloom DS, Magilavy DB, Harford JB, et al: Influence of antigen on immune complex behavior in mice. J Clin Invest 68:214–224, 1981.

2950. Rifai A, Finbloom DS, Magilavy DB, Plotz PH: Modulation of the circulation and hepatic uptake of immune complexes by carbohydrate recognition systems. J Immunol 128:2269–2275, 1982.

2951. Day JF, Thornburg RW, Thorpe SR, Baynes JW: Carbohydrate-mediated clearance of antibody-antigen complexes from the circulation. The role of high mannose oligosaccharides in the hepatic uptake of IgM antigen complexes. J Biol Chem 255:2360–2365, 1980.

2952. Emlen W, Mannik M: Effect of preformed immune complexes on the clearance and tissue localization of single-stranded DNA in mice. Clin Exp Immunol 40:264–272, 1980.

2953. Emlen W, Mannik M: Clearance of circulating DNA–anti-DNA immune complexes in mice. J Exp Med 155:1210–1215, 1982.

2954. Bogers WMJM, Stad R-K, Janssen DJ, et al: Kupffer cell depletion in vivo results in preferential elimination of IgG aggregates and immune complexes via specific Fc receptors on rat liver endothelial cells. Clin Exp Immunol 86:328–333, 1991.

2955. Lawrence S, Lockwood CM, Peters DK: Studies on NEM-treated erythrocyte clearance in the rabbit, with special reference to the effects of circulating immune complexes. Clin Exp Immunol 44:433–439, 1981.

2956. Raij L, Sibley RK, Keane WF: Mononuclear phagocytic system stimulation. Protective role from glomerular immune complex deposition. J Lab Clin Med 98:558–567, 1981.

2957. Barcelli U, Rademacher R, Ooi YM, Ooi BS: Modification of glomerular immune complex deposition in mice by activation of the reticuloendothelial system. J Clin Invest 67:20–27, 1981.

2958. Nagamatsu T, Suzuki Y: Antinephritic effect of prostaglandin $E_1$ on serum sickness nephritis in rats (4). Enhanced clearance of macromolecules by the reticuloendothelial system with prostaglandin $E_1$. Jpn J Pharmacol 44:369–372, 1987.

2959. Xu JJ, Qian TS, Xin CY, et al: Protective role of BCG in the rabbit model of mesangial proliferative glomerulonephritis. Nephrol Dial Transplant 6:554–556, 1991.

2960. Siag WM, Jones JM: Effects of staphylococcal protein A on distribution of immune complexes in rats and uptake by phagocytic cells. Clin Immunol Immunopathol 31:102–108, 1984.

2961. Quirós J, Gonzalez-Cabrero J, Egido J, et al: Beneficial effect of fibronectin administration on chronic nephritis in rats. Arthritis Rheum 33:685–692, 1990.

2962. Cederholm B, Linne T, Wieslander J, et al: Fibronectin-immunoglobulin complexes in the early course of IgA and Henoch-Schönlein nephritis. Pediatr Nephrol 5:200–204, 1991.

2963. Kabbash L, Brandwein S, Esdaile J, et al: Reticuloendothelial system Fc receptor function in systemic lupus erythematosus. J Rheumatol 9:374–379, 1982.

2964. Parris TM, Kimberly RP, Inman RD, et al: Defective Fc receptor–mediated function of the mononuclear phagocyte system in lupus nephritis. Ann Intern Med 97:526–532, 1982.

2965. Kimberly RP, Parris TM, Inman RD, McDougal JS: Dynamics of mononuclear phagocyte system Fc receptor function in systemic lupus erythematosus. Relation to disease activity and circulating immune complexes. Clin Exp Immunol 51:261–268, 1983.

2966. Frank MM, Lawley TJ, Hamburger MI, Brown EJ: Immunoglobulin G Fc receptor–mediated clearance in autoimmune diseases. Ann Intern Med 98:206–218, 1983.

2967. van der Woude FJ, Piers DA, van der Giessen M, et al: Abnormal reticuloendothelial function in patients with active vasculitis and idiopathic membranous glomerulopathy. A study with $^{99m}$Tc-labeled heat-damaged autologous red blood cells. Eur Nucl Med 8:60–64, 1983.

2968. Lawrence S, Pussell BA, Charlesworth JA: Mesangial IgA nephropathy: Detection of defective reticulophagocytic function in vivo. Clin Nephrol 19:280–283, 1983.

2969. Smiley JD, Moore SE Jr: Immune-complex vasculitis: Role of complement and IgG-Fc receptor functions. Am J Med Sci 298:267–277, 1989.

2970. Lawley TJ, Hall RP, Fauci AS, et al: Defective Fc-receptor functions associated with the HLA-B8/DRw3 haplotype. Studies in patients with dermatitis herpetiformis and normal subjects. N Engl J Med 304:185–192, 1981.

2971. Kimberly RP, Gibofsky A, Salmon JE, Fotino M: Impaired Fc-mediated mononuclear phagocyte system clearance in HLA-DR2 and MT1-positive healthy young adults. J Exp Med 157:1698–1703, 1983.

2972. Katayama S, Chia D, Nasu H, Knutson DW: Increased Fc receptor activity in monocytes from patients with rheumatoid arthritis: A study of monocyte binding and catabolism of soluble aggregates of IgG in vitro. J Immunol 127:643–647, 1981.

2973. Kávai M, Zsindely A, Sonkoly I, et al: Monocyte activation by immune complexes of patients with SLE. Adv Exp Med Biol 141:575–582, 1982.

2974. Sato M, Kinugasa E, Ideura T, Koshikawa S: Phagocytic activity of polymorphonuclear leucocytes in patients with IgA nephropathy. Clin Nephrol 19:166–171, 1983.

2975. Ooi YM, Ooi BS: Identification of a monocyte phagocytic defect in a subpopulation of patients with nephritis. Kidney Int 23:851–854, 1983.

2976. Gelfand MC, Frank MM, Green I, Shin ML: Binding sites for immune complexes containing IgG in the renal interstitium. Clin Immunol Immunopathol 13:19–29, 1979.

2977. Matre R, Tönder O, Wesenberg F: Human renal glomeruli possess no Fcγ receptors. Clin Immunol Immunopathol 17:157–162, 1980.

2978. Schrieber L, Penny R: Tissue distribution of IgG Fc receptors. Clin Exp Immunol 47:535–540, 1982.

2979. Aarli A, Matre R, Thunold S: IgG Fc receptors on epithelial cells of distal tubuli and on endothelial cells in human kidney. Int Arch Allergy Appl Immunol 95:64–69, 1991.

2980. Santiago A, Mori T, Satriano J, Schlondorff D: Regulation of Fc receptors for IgG on cultured rat mesangial cells. Kidney Int 39:87–94, 1991.

2981. Radeke HH, Gessner JE, Uciechowski P, et al: Intrinsic human glomerular mesangial cells can express receptors for IgG complexes (hFc gamma RIII-A) and the associated Fc epsilon RI gamma-chain. J Immunol 153:1281–1292, 1994.

2982. Ren K, Van Liew JB, Noble B: The effect of cyclosporin A on disease progression in proliferative immune complex glomerulonephritis. Clin Immunol Immunopathol 66:107–113, 1993.

2983. Wada T, Tomosugi N, Naito T, et al: Prevention of proteinuria by the administration of anti–interleukin 8 antibody in experimental acute immune complex-induced glomerulonephritis. J Exp Med 180:1135–1140, 1994.

2984. Michael AF, Kean WF, Raij L, et al: The glomerular mesangium. Kidney Int 17:141–154, 1980.

2985. Michael AF: The glomerular mesangium. Contrib Nephrol 40:7–16, 1984.

2986. Latta H, Fligiel S: Mesangial fenestrations, sieving, filtration, and flow. Lab Invest 52:591–598, 1985.

2987. Lee S, Vernier RL: Immunoelectron microscopy of the glomerular mesangial uptake and transport of aggregated human albumin in the mouse. Lab Invest 42:44–58, 1980.

2988. Keane WF, Raij L: Determinants of glomerular mesangial localization of immune complexes. Role of endothelial fenestrae. Lab Invest 45:366–371, 1981.

2989. Mancilla-Jimenez R, Bellon B, Kuhn J, et al: Phagocytosis of heat-aggregated immunoglobulins by mesangial cells. An immunoperoxidase and acid phosphatase study. Lab Invest 46:243–253, 1982.

2990. Cattell V, Gaskin De Urdaneta A, Arlidge S, et al: Uptake and clearance of ferritin by the glomerular mesangium. I. Phagocytosis by mesangial cells and blood monocytes. Lab Invest 47:296–303, 1982.

2991. Seiler MW, Hoyer JR, Sterzel RB: Role of macrophages in the glomerular mesangial uptake of polyvinyl alcohol in rats. Lab Invest 49:26–37, 1983.

2992. Boyce NW, Holdsworth SR: Quantitation of the intrarenal uptake of immunoglobulin aggregates by macrophages in diffuse proliferative glomerulonephritis. Clin Exp Immunol 64:638–645, 1986.

2993. Sterzel RB, Ehrich JHH, Lucia H, et al: Mesangial disposal of glomerular immune deposits in acute malarial glomerulonephritis of rats. Lab Invest 46:209–214, 1982.

2994. Burkholder PM: Functions and pathophysiology of the glomerular mesangium. Lab Invest 46:239–241, 1982.

2995. Shinkai Y: Experimental glomerulonephritis induced in rabbits by horseradish peroxidase. Mesangial uptake and processing of immune complexes. Lab Invest 46:577–583, 1982.

2996. Furness PN: Degradation of insoluble immune complexes by glomerular mesangial cells and macrophages in culture. Exp Nephrol 1:372–375, 1993.

2997. Gomez-Guerrero C, Gonzalez E, Hernando P, et al: Interaction of mesangial cells with IgA and IgG immune complexes: A possible mechanism of glomerular injury in IgA nephropathy. Contrib Nephrol 104:127–137, 1993.

2998. Chen A, Chen WP, Sheu LF, Lin CY: Pathogenesis of IgA nephropathy: In vitro activation of human mesangial cells by IgA immune complex leads to cytokine secretion. J Pathol 173:119–126, 1994.

2999. Keane WF, Raij L: Impaired mesangial clearance of macromolecules in rats with chronic mesangial ferritin-antiferritin immune complex deposition. Lab Invest 43:500–508, 1980.

3000. Border WA, Cohen AH: Role of immunoglobulin class in mediation of experimental mesangial glomerulonephritis. Clin Immunol Immunopathol 27:187–199, 1983.

3001. Kimura M, Nakamura M, Nagase M, et al: Reticuloendothelial system and glomerular deposition of heat-aggregated human IgG. Jpn J Exp Med 55:89–98, 1985.

3002. Borges HF, Goldstein C, Kim M, Michael AF: The glomerular mesangium: Kinetics using radiolabeled ferritin and the effects of aggregated IgG. Clin Immunol Immunopathol 33:80–86, 1984.

3003. Seiler MW, Terrell CH, Finnegan A, et al: Studies of glomerular mesangial uptake and processing of macromolecules. I. Effect of polyvinyl alcohol–induced macrophages on uptake of iron dextran. Lab Invest 54:616–623, 1986.

3004. Furness PN: Stimulation of mesangial phagocytes does not influence the removal of established glomerular immune complex deposits. Int J Exp Pathol 71:529–536, 1990.

3005. Grond J, Elema JD: Glomerular mesangium. Analysis of the increased activity observed in experimental acute aminonucleoside nephrosis in the rat. Lab Invest 45:400–409, 1981.

3006. Goode NP, Davison AM, Gowland G, et al: Persistence of inert macromolecules (Imposil) in the rat mesangium and glomerular functional disturbance. J Pathol 144:179–187, 1984.

3007. Batsford SR, Weghaupt R, Takamiya H, Vogt A: Studies on the mesangial handling of protein antigens: Influence of size, charge and biologic activity. Nephron 41:146–151, 1985.

3008. Schneeberger EE, Collins AB, Stavrakis G, McCluskey RT: Diminished mesangial accumulation of intravenously injected soluble immune complexes in rats with autologous immune complex nephritis. Lab Invest 42:440–449, 1980.

3009. Suzuki Y, Kihara I, Morita T, et al: Accelerated immune complex nephritis due to mesangial overloading in spontaneous hypertensive (SHR) rats. Jpn J Exp Med 49:373–382, 1979.

3010. Raij L, Azar S, Keane W: Mesangial immune injury, hypertension, and progressive glomerular damage in Dahl rats. Kidney Int 26:137–143, 1984.

3011. Cosio FG, Bakaletz AP: Role of fibronectin on the clearance and tissue uptake of antigen and immune complexes in rats. J Clin Invest 80:1270–1279, 1987.

3012. Simpson LO: Role of glomerular basement membrane thixotropy and influence of glomerular vascular pressure in the pathogenesis of immune complex–induced glomerulonephritis. A new hypothesis. Nephron 27:105–112, 1981.

3013. Ooi BS, Weiss MA, Hamoui T: Effect of renal vein constriction on the localization of immune complexes in the kidney. Kidney Int 16:681–687, 1979.

3014. Glassock RJ: Immune complex–induced glomerular injury in viral diseases: An overview. Kidney Int 40(suppl 35):S-5–S-7, 1991.

3015. Oldstone MBA, Buchmeier MJ, Doyle MV, Tishon A: Virus-induced immune complex disease: Specific anti-viral antibody and Clq binding material in the circulation during persistent lymphocytic choriomeningitis virus infection. J Immunol 124:831–838, 1980.

3016. Oldstone MBA, Tishon A, Buchmeier MJ: Virus-induced immune complex disease: Genetic control of C1q binding complexes in the circulation of mice persistently infected with lymphocytic choriomeningitis virus. J Immunol 130:912–918, 1983.

3017. Snyder HW Jr, Jones FR, Day NK, Hardy WD Jr: Isolation and characterization of circulating feline leukemia virus-immune complexes from plasma of persistently infected pet cats removed by ex vivo immunosorption. J Immunol 128:2726–2730, 1982.

3018. Dong Z-W, Witkin SS, Fernandes G, et al: Circulating immune complexes, antigens, and antibodies related to the murine mammary tumor virus in C3H mice. J Immunol 129:872–876, 1982.

3019. Portis JL, Coe JE: Deposition of IgA in renal glomeruli of mink affected with Aleutian disease. Am J Pathol 96:227–236, 1979.

3020. Yoshiki T, Hayasaka T, Fukatsu R, et al: The structural proteins of murine leukemia virus and the pathogenesis of necrotizing arteritis and glomerulonephritis in SL/Ni mice. J Immunol 122:1812–1820, 1979.

3021. Sanfilippo F, Genovesi EV, Collins JJ: Immunotherapy of murine leukemia. V. Protection against friend leukemia virus-induced immune complex glomerulonephritis by passive serum therapy. J Natl Cancer Inst 67:703–717, 1981.

3022. Bergholm A-M, Holm SE: Experimental poststreptococcal glomerulonephritis in rabbits. Acta Pathol Microbiol Immunol Scand [C] 91:263–270, 1983.

3023. Bergholm A-M, Holm SE: Effect of early penicillin treatment on the development of experimental poststreptococcal glomerulonephritis. Acta Pathol Microbiol Immunol Scand [C] 91:271–281, 1983.

3024. Stinson MW, Nisengard RJ, Neiders ME, Albini B: Serology and tissue lesions in rabbits immunized with *Streptococcus mutans*. J Immunol 131:3021–3027, 1983.

3025. Albini B, Nisengard RJ, Glurich I, et al: *Streptococcus mutans*–induced nephritis in rabbits. Am J Pathol 118:408–418, 1985.

3026. Thörig L, Daha MR, Eulderink F, et al: Experimental *Streptococcus sanguis* endocarditis: Immune complexes and renal involvement. Clin Exp Immunol 40:469–477, 1980.

3027. Yasuda PH, Hoshino-Shimizu S, Yamashiro EH, De Brito T: Experimental leptospirosis (*L. interrogans* serovar *icterohaemorrhagiae*) of the guinea pig: Leptospiral antigen, gamma globulin and complement C3 detection in the kidney). Exp Pathol 29:35–43, 1986.

3028. Haines H, Farmer JN: Glomerular filtration rate and plasma solutes in BALB/c mice infected with *Plasmodium berghei*. Parasitol Res 77:411–414, 1991.

3029. Delvinquier B, Goumard P, Dubarry M, et al: Renal deposits of lipoprotein-immunoglobulin complexes in *Plasmodium chabaudi*–infected mice. J Immunol 133:2243–2249, 1984.

3030. Boonpucknavig S, Boonpucknavig V, Tanvanich S, et al: Development of immune-complex glomerulonephritis and amyloidosis in Syrian golden hamsters infected with *Opisthorchis viverrini*. J Med Assoc Thai 75(suppl 1):7–19, 1992.

3031. Van Marck EAE, Deelder AM, Gigase PLJ: *Schistosoma mansoni*: Anodic polysaccharide antigen in glomerular immune deposits of mice with unisexual infection. Exp Parasitol 52:62–68, 1981.

3032. El-Dosoky I, Van Marck EAE, Deelder AM: Presence of *Schistosoma mansoni* antigens in liver, spleen and kidney of infected mice: A sequential study. Z Parasitenkd 70:491–497, 1984.

3033. El-Sherif AK, Befus D: Predominance of IgA deposits in glomeruli of *Schistosoma mansoni* infected mice. Clin Exp Immunol 71:39–44, 1988.

3034. Sobh M, Moustafa F, Ramzy R, et al: *Schistosoma mansoni* nephropathy in Syrian golden hamsters: Effect of dose and duration of infection. Nephron 59:121–130, 1991.

3035. Costa RS, Monteiro RC, Lehuen A, et al: Immune complex–mediated glomerulopathy in experimental Chagas' disease. Clin Immunol Immunopathol 58:102–114, 1991.

3036. Oliveira AV, Rossi MA, Roque-Barreira MC, et al: The potential role of *Leishmania* antigens and immunoglobulins in the pathogenesis of glomerular lesions of hamsters infected with *Leishmania donovani*. Ann Trop Med Parasitol 79:539–543, 1985.

3037. Oliveira AV, Roque-Barreira MC, Sartori A, et al: Mesangial pro-liferative glomerulonephritis associated with progressive amyloid deposition in hamsters experimentally infected with *Leishmania donovani*. Am J Pathol 120:256–262, 1985.

3038. Sartori A, de Oliveira AV, Roque-Barreira MC, et al: Immune complex glomerulonephritis in experimental kala-azar. Parasite Immunol 9:93–103, 1987

3039. Nieto CG, Navarrete I, Habela MA, et al: Pathological changes in kidneys of dogs with natural *Leishmania* infection. Vet Parasitol 45:33–47, 1992.

3040. Sartori A, Roque-Barreira MC, Coe J, Campos-Neto A: Immune complex glomerulonephritis in experimental kala-azar. II. Detection and characterization of parasite antigens and antibodies eluted from kidneys of *Leishmania donovani*–infected hamsters. Clin Exp Immunol 87:386–392, 1992.

3041. Albano Edelweiss MI, Lizardo-Daudt HM: Naturally existing model of glomerulonephritis mediated by immune complexes associated with hydatidosis in sheep. Nephron 57:253–254, 1991.

3042. Codner EC, Caceci T, Saunders GK, et al: Investigation of glomer-ular lesions in dogs with acute experimentally induced *Ehrlichia canis* infection. Am J Vet Res 53:2286–2291, 1992.

3043. Sami S, Fischer-Scherl T, Hoffmann RW, Pfeil-Putzien C: Immune complex–mediated glomerulonephritis associated with bacterial kidney disease in the rainbow trout (*Oncorhynchus mykiss*). Vet Pathol 29:169–174, 1992.

3044. Dixon FJ: Murine lupus—an overview. Arthritis Rheum 25:721–725, 1982.

3045. Theofilopoulos AN, Dixon FJ: Experimental murine systemic lupus erythematosus. *In* Lahita RG (ed): Systemic Lupus Erythematosus. John Wiley & Sons, New York, 1987, pp 121–202.

3046. Theofilopoulos AN, Dixon FJ: Murine models of systemic lupus erythematosus. Adv Immunol 37:269–390, 1985.

3047. Stollar BD: The biochemistry and genetics of DNA and anti-DNA antibodies. Chin Rheumatol 9(suppl 1):30–38, 1990.

3048. Jacob L, Viard J-P, Louvard D, Bach J-F: Recent advances in the pathogenesis of systemic lupus erythematosus. Adv Nephrol 19:237–256, 1990.

3049. Harley JB, Scofield RH: Systemic lupus erythematosus: RNA-pro-tein autoantigens, models of disease heterogeneity, and theories of etiology. J Clin Immunol 11:297–316, 1991.

3050. Jacob L, Viard J-P: Anti-DNA antibodies and their relationships with anti-histone and anti-nucleosome specificities. Eur J Med 1:425–431, 1992.

3051. Frampton G, Perry GJ, Chan TM, Cameron JS: Significance of anticardiolipin and antiendothelial cell antibodies in the nephritis of lupus. Contrib Nephrol 99:7–16, 1992.

3052. Datta SK, Rajagopalan S, O'Keefe TL, et al: Pathogenic anti-DNA autoantibodies and pathogenic autoantibody-inducing T cells. Immunol Ser 55:133–153, 1992.

3053. Asherson RA, Cervera R: Antiphospholipid syndrome. J Invest Dermatol 100:21S–27S, 1993.

3054. Steinberg AD: Systemic lupus erythematosus: theories of pathogen-esis and approach to therapy. Clin Immunol Immunopathol 72:171–176, 1994.

3055. Reichlin M: Systemic lupus erythematosus. Antibodies to ribonu-clear proteins. Rheum Dis Clin North Am 20:29–43, 1994.

3056. Osman C, Swaak AJ: Lymphocytotoxic antibodies in SLE: A re-view of the literature. Clin Rheumatol 13:21–27, 1994.

3057. Tan EM: Autoantibodies in pathology and cell biology. Cell 67:841–842, 1991.

3058. Tan EM: Molecular biology of nuclear autoantigens. Adv Nephrol 22:213–236, 1993.

3059. Steinberg AD, Raveche ES, Laskin CA, et al: Genetic, environmen-tal, and cellular factors in the pathogenesis of systemic lupus ery-thematosus. Arthritis Rheum 25:734–743, 1982.

3060. Theofilopoulos AN, Balderas RS, Gozes Y, et al: Surface and functional characteristics of B cells from lupus-prone murine strains. Clin Immunol Immunopathol 23:224–244, 1982.

3061. Prud'homme GJ, Balderas RS, Dixon FJ, Theofilopoulos AN: B cell dependence on and response to accessory signals in murine lupus strains. J Exp Med 157:1815–1827, 1983.

3062. Hang L, Slack JH, Amundson C, et al: Induction of murine autoim-mune disease by chronic polyclonal B cell activation. J Exp Med 157:874–883, 1983.

3063. Prud'homme GJ, Park CL, Fieser TM, et al: Identification of a B cell differentiation factor(s) spontaneously produced by proliferat-ing T cells in murine lupus strains of the *lpr/lpr* genotype. J Exp Med 157:730–742, 1983.

3064. Klinman DM: Polyclonal B cell activation in lupus-prone mice precedes and predicts the development of autoimmune disease. J Clin Invest 86:1249–1254, 1990.

3065. Merino R, Iwamoto M, Fossati L, Izui S: Polyclonal B cell activa-tion arises from different mechanisms in lupus-prone (NZB × NZW)F₁ and MRL/MpJ-*lpr/lpr* mice. J Immunol 151:6509–6516, 1993.

3066. Granholm NA, Cavallo T: Autoimmunity, polyclonal B-cell acti-vation and infection. Lupus 1:63–74, 1992.

3067. Andrews BS, Eisenberg RA, Theofilopoulos AN, et al: Spontaneous murine lupus-like syndromes. Clinical and immunopathological manifestations in several strains. J Exp Med 148:1198–1215, 1978.

3068. Kiberd BA: Murine lupus nephritis. A structure-function study. Lab Invest 65:51–60, 1991.

3069. Accinni L, Dixon FJ: Degenerative vascular disease and myocardial infarction in mice with lupus-like syndrome. Am J Pathol 96:477–492, 1979.

3070. Tarkowski A, Jonsson R, Sanchez R, et al: Features of renal vas-culitis in autoimmune MRL *lpr/lpr* mice: Phenotypes and functional properties of infiltrating cells. Clin Exp Immunol 72:91–97, 1988.

3071. Nose M, Nishimura M, Kyogoku M: Analysis of granulomatous arteritis in MRL/Mp autoimmune disease mice bearing lymphopro-liferative genes. The use of mouse genetics to dissociate the devel-opment of arteritis and glomerulonephritis. Am J Pathol 135:271–280, 1989.

3072. Itoh J, Nose M, Kyogoku M: Pathogenic significance of serum components in the development of autoimmune polyarthritis in MRL/Mp mice bearing the lymphoproliferation gene. Am J Pathol 139:511–521, 1991.

3073. Mathieson PW, Qasim FJ, Esnault VLM, Oliveira DBG: Animal models of systemic vasculitis. J Autoimmun 6:251–264, 1993.

3074. Theofilopoulos AN, Dixon FJ: Etiopathogenesis of murine SLE. Immunol Rev 55:179–216, 1981.

3075. Izui S, Elder JH, McConahey PJ, Dixon FJ: Identification of retro-viral gp70 and anti-gp70 antibodies involved in circulating immune complexes in NZB × NZW mice. J Exp Med 153:1151–1160, 1981.

3076. Izui S, Hara I, Hang LM, et al: Association of elevated serum glycoprotein gp70 with increased gp70 immune complex formation and accelerated lupus nephritis in autoimmune male BXSB mice. Clin Exp Immunol 56:272–280, 1984.

3077. Cavallo T, Graves K, Granholm NA, Izui S: Association of glyco-protein gp70 with progression or attenuation of murine lupus ne-phritis. J Clin Lab Immunol 18:63–67, 1985.

3078. Stetler DA, Sipes DE, Jacob ST: Anti-RNA polymerase I antibodies in sera of MRL *lpr/lpr* and MRL +/+ autoimmune mice. Corre-lation of antibody production with delayed onset of lupus-like dis-ease in MRL +/+ mice. J Exp Med 162:1760–1770, 1985.

3079. Stetler DA, Cavallo T: Anti–RNA polymerase I antibodies: Poten-tial role in the induction and progression of murine lupus nephritis. J Immunol 138:2119–2123, 1987.

3080. Fisher CL, Eisenberg RA, Cohen PL: Quantitation and IgG subclass distribution of antichromatin autoantibodies in SLE mice. Clin Im-munol Immunopathol 46:205–213, 1988.

3081. Andrews J, Hang L, Theofilopoulos AN, Dixon FJ: Lack of rela-tionship between serum gp70 levels and the severity of systemic lupus erythematosus in MRL/*l* mice. J Exp Med 163:458–462, 1986.

3082. Krieg AM, Steinberg AD: Retroviruses and autoimmunity. J Au-toimmun 3:137–166, 1990.

3083. Krieg AM, Gourley MF, Steinberg AD: Association of murine lupus and thymic full-length endogenous retroviral expression maps to a bone marrow stem cell. J Immunol 146:3002–3005, 1991.

3084. Gourley MF, Kisch WJ, Mojcik CF, et al: Molecular aspects of systemic lupus erythematosus: Murine endogenous retroviral expression. DNA Cell Biol 11:253–257, 1992.

3085. Fronek Z, Timmerman LA, Alper CA, et al: Major histocompatibil-ity complex genes and susceptibility to systemic lupus erythemato-sus. Arthritis Rheum 33:1542–1553, 1990.

3086. Schur PH, Marcus-Bagley D, Awdeh Z, et al: The effect of ethnic-ity on major histocompatibility complex complement allotypes and extended haplotypes in patients with systemic lupus erythematosus. Arthritis Rheum 33:985–992, 1990.

3087. Drake CG, Kotzin BL: Genetic and immunological mechanisms in the pathogenesis of systemic lupus erythematosus. Curr Opin Immunol 4:733–740, 1992.

3088. Arnett FC, Reveille JD: Genetics of systemic lupus erythematosus. Rheum Dis Clin North Am 18:865–892, 1992.

3089. Jevnikar AM, Grusby MJ, Glimcher LH: Prevention of nephritis in major histocompatibility complex class II–deficient MRL-*lpr* mice. J Exp Med 179:1137–1143, 1994.

3090. Singer PA, Theofilopoulos AN: Novel origen of *lpr* and *gld* cells and possible implications in autoimmunity. J Autoimmun 3:123–135, 1990.

3091. Cohen PL, Eisenberg RA: *Lpr* and *gld*: Single gene models of systemic autoimmunity and lymphoproliferative disease. Annu Rev Immunol 9:243–269, 1991.

3092. Kimura M, Ogata Y, Shimada K, et al: Nephritogenicity of the *lpr^cg* gene on the MRL background. Immunology 76:498–504, 1992.

3093. Rosenblatt N, Hartmann K-U, Loor F: The *Yaa* mutation induces the development of autoimmunity in mice heterozygous for the *gld* (generalized lymphadenopathy disease) mutation. Cell Immunol 156:519–528, 1994.

3094. Merino R, Iwamoto M, Gershwin ME, Izui S: The *Yaa* gene abrogates the major histocompatibility complex association of murine lupus in (NZB × BXSB)F$_1$ hybrid mice. J Clin Invest 94:521–525, 1994.

3095. Gillette-Ferguson I, Sidman CL: A specific intercellular pathway of apoptotic cell death is defective in the mature peripheral T cells of autoimmune *lpr* and *gld* mice. Eur J Immunol 24:1181–1185, 1994.

3096. Wu J, Zhou T, He J, Mountz JD: Autoimmune disease in mice due to integration of an endogenous retrovirus in an apoptosis gene. J Exp Med 178:461–468, 1993.

3097. Chu J-L, Drappa J, Parnassa A, Elkon KB: The defect in *Fas* mRNA expression in MRL/*lpr* mice is associated with insertion of the retrotransposon, *ETn*. J Exp Med 178:723–730, 1993.

3098. Adachi M, Watanabe-Fukunaga R, Nagata S: Aberrant transcription caused by the insertion of an early transposable element in an intron of the Fas antigen gene of *lpr* mice. Proc Natl Acad Sci USA 90:1756–1760, 1993.

3099. Nagata S: Mutations in the Fas antigen gene in *lpr* mice. Semin Immunol 6:3–8, 1994.

3100. Wu J, Zhou T, Zhang J, et al: Correction of accelerated autoimmune disease by early replacement of the mutated *lpr* gene with the normal *Fas* apoptosis gene in the T cells of transgenic MRL-*lpr/lpr* mice. Proc Natl Acad Sci USA 91:2344–2348, 1994.

3101. Sobel ES, Kakkanaiah VN, Cohen PL, Eisenberg RA: Correction of *gld* autoimmunity by co-infusion of normal bone marrow suggests that *gld* is a mutation of the Fas ligand gene. Int Immunol 5:1275–1278, 1993.

3102. Takahashi T, Tanaka M, Brannan CI, et al: Generalized lymphoproliferative disease in mice, caused by a point mutation in the Fas ligand. Cell 76:969–976, 1994.

3103. Ramsdell F, Seaman MS, Miller RE, et al: *gld/gld* mice are unable to express a functional ligand for Fas. Eur J Immunol 24:928–933, 1994.

3104. Cohen PL, Eisenberg RA: The *lpr* and *gld* genes in systemic autoimmunity: Life and death in the *Fas* lane. Immunol Today 13:427–428, 1992.

3105. Steinberg AD: MRL-*lpr-lpr* disease: Theories meet Fas. Semin Immunol 6:55–69, 1994.

3106. Eisenberg RA, Sobel ES, Reap EA, et al: The role of B cell abnormalities in the systemic autoimmune syndromes of *lpr* and *gld* mice. Semin Immunol 6:49–54, 1994.

3107. Hanabuchi S, Koyanagi M, Kawasaki A, et al: Fas and its ligand in a general mechanism of T-cell-mediated cytotoxicity. Proc Natl Acad Sci USA 91:4930–4934, 1994.

3108. Rozzo SJ, Eisenberg RA, Cohen PL, Kotzin BL: Development of the T cell receptor repertoire in *lpr* mice. Semin Immunol 6:19–26, 1994.

3109. Carson DA, Ribeiro JM: Apoptosis and disease. Lancet 341:1251–1254, 1993.

3110. Tan EM: Autoimmunity and apoptosis. J Exp Med 179:1083–1086, 1994.

3111. Kofler R, Noonan DJ, Levy DE, et al: Genetic elements used for a murine lupus anti-DNA autoantibody are closely related to those for antibodies to exogenous antigens. J Exp Med 161:805–815, 1985.

3112. Kofler R, Perlmutter RM, Noonan DJ, et al: Ig heavy chain variable region gene complex of lupus mice exhibits normal restriction fragment length polymorphism. J Exp Med 162:346–351, 1985.

3113. Theofilopoulos AN: Molecular genetics of murine lupus. Agents Actions 19:282–294, 1986.

3114. Kofler R, Noonan DJ, Strohal R, et al: Molecular analysis of the murine lupus-associated anti-self response: Involvement of a large number of heavy and light chain variable region genes. Eur J Immunol 17:91–95, 1987.

3115. Theofilopoulos AN, Kofler R, Singer PA, Dixon FJ: Molecular genetics of murine lupus models. Adv Immunol 46:61–109, 1989.

3116. Eilat D: The role of germline gene expression and somatic mutation in the generation of autoantibodies to DNA. Mol Immunol 27:203–210, 1990.

3117. Diamond B, Katz JB, Paul E, et al: The role of somatic mutation in the pathogenic anti-DNA response. Annu Rev Immunol 10:731–757, 1992.

3118. Marion TN, Tillman DM, Jou N-T, Hill RJ: Selection of immunoglobulin variable regions in autoimmunity to DNA. Immunol Rev 128:123–149, 1992.

3119. Stewart AK, Huang C, Long AA, et al: VH-gene representation in autoantibodies reflects the normal human B-cell repertoire. Immunol Rev 128:101–122, 1992.

3120. Stollar BD: Molecular analysis of anti-DNA antibodies. FASEB J 8:337–342, 1994.

3121. Burlingame RW, Rubin RL, Balderas RS, Theofilopoulos AN: Genesis and evolution of antichromatin autoantibodies in murine lupus implicates T-dependent immunization with self antigen. J Clin Invest 91:1687–1696, 1993.

3122. Tsao BP, Ebling FM, Roman C, et al: Structural characteristics of the variable regions of immunoglobulin genes encoding a pathogenic autoantibody in murine lupus. J Clin Invest 85:530–540, 1990.

3123. Young F, Tucker L, Rubinstein D, et al: Molecular analysis of a germ line–encoded idiotypic marker of pathogenic human lupus autoantibodies. J Immunol 145:2545–2553, 1990.

3124. Foster MH, Sabbaga J, Line SRP, et al: Molecular analysis of spontaneous nephrotropic anti-laminin antibodies in an autoimmune MRL-*lpr/lpr* mouse. J Immunol 151:814–824, 1993.

3125. Katz MS, Foster MH, Madaio MP: Independently derived murine glomerular immune deposit–forming anti-DNA antibodies are encoded by near-identical V$_H$ gene sequences. J Clin Invest 91:402–408, 1993.

3126. Ohnishi K, Ebling FM, Mitchell B, et al: Comparison of pathogenic and non-pathogenic murine antibodies to DNA: Antigen binding and structural characteristics. Int Immunol 6:817–830, 1994.

3127. Demaison C, Chastagner P, Thèze J, Zouali M: Somatic diversification in the heavy chain variable region genes expressed by human autoantibodies bearing a lupus-associated nephritogenic anti-DNA idiotype. Proc Natl Acad Sci USA 91:514–518, 1994.

3128. Theofilopoulos AN, Singer PA, Kofler R, et al: B and T cell antigen receptor repertoires in lupus/arthritis murine models. Springer Semin Immunopathol 11:335–368, 1989.

3129. Singer PA, Theofilopoulos AN: T-cell receptor Vβ repertoire expression in murine models of SLE. Immunol Rev 118:103–127, 1990.

3130. Adams S, Zordan T, Sainis K, Datta SK: T cell receptor V$_β$ genes expressed by IgG anti-DNA autoantibody–inducing T cells in lupus nephritis: Forbidden receptors and double-negative T cells. Eur J Immunol 20:1435–1443, 1990.

3131. Tsokos GC: Lymphocyte abnormalities in human lupus. Clin Immunol Immunopathol 63:7–9, 1992.

3132. Theofilopoulos AN, Balderas RS, Baccala R, Kono DH: T-cell receptor genes in autoimmunity. Ann N Y Acad Sci 681:33–46, 1993.

3133. Seaman WE, Wofsy D, Greenspan JS, Ledbetter JA: Treatment of autoimmune MRL/*lpr* mice with monoclonal antibody to Thy-1.2: A single injection has sustained effects on lymphoproliferation and renal disease. J Immunol 130:1713–1718, 1983.

3134. Wofsy D, Seaman WE: Reversal of advanced murine lupus in NZB/NZW F$_1$ mice by treatment with monoclonal antibody to L3T4$^+$. J Immunol 138:3247–3253, 1987.

3135. Jacob CO, van der Meide PH, McDevitt HO: In vivo treatment of (NZB × NZW)F$_1$ lupus-like nephritis with monoclonal antibody to γ interferon. J Exp Med 166:798–803, 1987.

3136. Carteron NL, Schimenti CL, Wofsy D: Treatment of murine lupus with F(ab')₂ fragments of monoclonal antibody to L3T4. Suppression of autoimmunity does not depend on T helper cell depletion. J Immunol 142:1470–1475, 1989.

3137. Gutierrez-Ramos JC, Andreu JL, Revilla Y, et al: Recovery from autoimmunity of MRL/*lpr* mice after infection with an interleukin-2/vaccinia recombinant virus. Nature 346:271–274, 1990.

3138. Baccalà R, González-Quintial R, Theofilopoulos AN: Lack of evidence for central T-cell tolerance defects in lupus mice and for Vβ-deleting endogenous superantigens in rats and humans. Res Immunol 143:288–290, 1992.

3139. Jabs DA, Burek CL, Hu Q, et al: Anti-CD4 monoclonal antibody therapy suppresses autoimmune disease in MRL/Mp-*lpr/lpr* mice. Cell Immunol 141:496–507, 1992.

3140. Fossati L, Merino R, Iwamoto M, et al: Lack of association of Vβ8⁺ T cells with lupus-like syndrome in MRL-*lpr/lpr* mice. Eur J Immunol 24:1717–1720, 1994.

3141. de Alborán I, Gonzalo JA, Kroemer G, et al: Attenuation of autoimmune disease and lymphocyte accumulation in MRL/*lpr* mice by treatment with anti-V_β8 antibodies. Eur J Immunol 22:2153–2158, 1992.

3142. Poljak RJ: An idiotype–anti-idiotype complex and the structural basis of molecular mimicking. Proc Natl Acad Sci USA 91:1599–1600, 1994.

3143. Irigoyen M, Manheimer-Lory A, Gaynor B, Diamond B: Molecular analysis of the human immunoglobulin VλII gene family. J Clin Invest 94:532–538, 1994.

3144. Isenberg DA, Staines NA: DNA antibody idiotypes. An analysis of their role in health and disease. J Autoimmun 3:339–356, 1990.

3145. Shefner R, Manheimer-Lory A, Davidson A, et al: Idiotypes in systemic lupus erythematosus. Clues for understanding etiology and pathogenicity. Chem Immunol 48:82–108, 1990.

3146. Watts R, Isenberg DA: DNA antibody idiotypes: An analysis of their clinical connections and origins. Int Rev Immunol 5:279–293, 1990.

3147. Diamond B, Rauch J: An idiotype systems update. Lupus 1:323–324, 1992.

3148. Shoenfeld Y: Idiotypic induction of autoimmunity: A new classification of autoimmune diseases. Isr J Med Sci 30:11–14, 1994.

3149. Koizumi T, Puccetti A, Migliorini P, et al: Molecular heterogeneity of auto-anti-idiotypic antibodies in MLR-*lpr/lpr* mice. Eur J Immunol 21:2185–2193, 1991.

3150. Isenberg DA, Collins C: Detection of cross-reactive anti-DNA antibody idiotypes on renal tissue-bound immunoglobulins from lupus patients. J Clin Invest 76:287–294, 1985.

3151. Kalunian KC, Panosian-Sahakian N, Ebling FM, et al: Idiotypic characteristics of immunoglobulins associated with systemic lupus erythematosus. Studies of antibodies deposited in glomeruli of humans. Arthritis Rheum 32:513–522, 1989.

3152. Muryoi T, Sasaki T, Hatakeyama A, et al: Clonotypes of anti-DNA antibodies expressing specific idiotypes in immune complexes of patients with active lupus nephritis. J Immunol 144:3856–3861, 1990.

3153. Suzuki M, Hatakeyama A, Kameoka J, et al: Anti-DNA idiotypes deposited in renal glomeruli of patients with lupus nephritis. Am J Kidney Dis 18:232–239, 1991.

3154. Knupp CJ, Uner AH, Tatum AH, Gavalchin J: The onset of nephritis in the (NZB × SWR)F₁ murine model for systemic lupus erythematosus correlates with an increase in the ratio of CD4 to CD8 T lymphocytes specific for the nephritogenic idiotype (IdLNF1). Clin Immunol Immunopathol 65:167–175, 1992.

3155. Shoenfeld Y, Mozes E: Pathogenic idiotypes of autoantibodies in autoimmunity: Lessons from new experimental models of SLE. FASEB J 4:2646–2651, 1990.

3156. Mozes E, Mendlovic S: The role of anti–DNA idiotype antibodies in systemic lupus erythematosus. Crit Rev Immunol 10:329–345, 1990.

3157. Isenberg DA, Katz D, Le Page S, et al: Independent analysis of the 16/6 idiotype lupus model. A role for an environmental factor? J Immunol 147:4172–4177, 1991.

3158. Waisman A, Mendlovic S, Ruiz PJ, et al: The role of the 16/6 idiotype network in the induction and manifestations of systemic lupus erythematosus. Int Immunol 5:1293–1300, 1993.

3159. Tincani A, Balestrieri G, Allegri F, et al: Induction of experimental SLE in naive mice by immunization with human polyclonal anti-

DNA antibody carrying the 16/6 idiotype. Clin Exp Rheumatol 11:129–134, 1993.

3160. Shoenfeld Y: The significance of experimental models of systemic lupus erythematosus and antiphospholipid syndrome induced by idiotypic manipulation. Isr J Med Sci 30:10–18, 1994.

3161. Segal R, Globerson A, Zinger H, Mozes E: Induction of experimental systemic lupus erythematosus (SLE) in mice with severe combined immunodeficiency (SCID). Clin Exp Immunol 89:239–243, 1992.

3162. Segal R, Globerson A, Zinger H, Mozes E: Inhibition of autoantibody production in experimental SLE by pre-immunization with DNA. Autoimmunity 17:149–156, 1994.

3163. Isenberg DA, Shoenfeld Y, Madaio MP, et al: Anti-DNA antibody idiotypes in systemic lupus erythematosus. Lancet 2:417–422, 1984.

3164. Puccetti A, Migliorini P, Sabbaga J, Madaio MP: Human and murine anti-DNA antibodies induce the production of anti-idiotypic antibodies with autoantigen-binding properties (epibodies) through immune-network interactions. J Immunol 145:4229–4237, 1990.

3165. Rombach E, Stetler DA, Brown JC: Induction of an anti-Fab, anti-DNA and anti–RNA polymerase I autoantibody response network in rabbits immunized with SLE anti-DNA antibody. Clin Exp Immunol 94:466–472, 1993.

3166. Zouali M, Diamond B: Idiotype-mediated intervention in systemic lupus erythematosus. J Autoimmun 3:381–388, 1990.

3167. Pisetsky DS: Autoantibodies and their idiotypes. Curr Opin Rheumatol 3:731–737, 1991.

3168. Mackworth-Young CG, Madaio MP: Anti-DNA idiotype network: Therapeutic considerations. Lupus 1:339–340, 1992.

3169. Hahn BH, Ebling FM: Suppression of NZB/NZW murine nephritis by administration of a syngeneic monoclonal antibody to DNA. Possible role of anti-idiotypic antibodies. J Clin Invest 71:1728–1736, 1983.

3170. Jacob L, Tron F: Induction of anti-DNA autoanti-idiotypic antibodies in (NZB × NZW)F₁ mice: Possible role for specific immune suppression. Clin Exp Immunol 58:293–299, 1984.

3171. Hahn BH, Ebling FM: Suppression of murine lupus nephritis by administration of an anti-idiotypic antibody to anti-DNA. J Immunol 132:187–190, 1984.

3172. Hahn BH: Suppression of autoimmune diseases with anti-idiotypic antibodies: Murine lupus nephritis as a model. Springer Semin Immunopathol 7:25–34, 1984.

3173. Hahn BH, Ebling FM: Idiotype restriction in murine lupus: High frequency of three public idiotypes on serum IgG in nephritic NZB/NZW F₁ mice. J Immunol 138:2110–2118, 1987.

3174. Lebrun P, Burny W, Cosyns JP, Saint-Remy JM: Injections of complexes made of dsDNA and specific polyclonal antibodies extend MRL *lpr* mouse survival: A pilot study. Lupus 3:47–53, 1994.

3175. Ravirajan CT, Staines NA: Involvement in lupus disease of idiotypes Id.F-423 and Id.IV-228 defined, respectively, upon foetal and adult MRL/Mp-*lpr/lpr* DNA-binding monoclonal autoantibodies. Immunology 74:342–347, 1991.

3176. Uner AH, Knupp CJ, Tatum AH, Gavalchin J: Treatment with antibody reactive with the nephritogenic idiotype, IdᴸᴺF₁, suppresses its production and leads to prolonged survival of (NZB × SWR)F₁ mice. J Autoimmun 7:27–44, 1994.

3177. Harata N, Sasaki T, Osaki H, et al: Therapeutic treatment of New Zealand mouse disease by a limited number of anti-idiotypic antibodies conjugated with neocarzinostatin. J Clin Invest 86:769–776, 1990.

3178. Abdou NI, Wall H, Lindsley HB, et al: Network theory in autoimmunity. In vitro suppression of serum anti-DNA antibody binding to DNA by anti-idiotypic antibody in systemic lupus erythematosus. J Clin Invest 67:1297–1304, 1981.

3179. Ballow M: Mechanisms of action of intravenous immunoglobulin therapy and potential use in autoimmune connective tissue diseases. Cancer 68(6 suppl)1430–1436, 1991.

3180. Jordan SC, Toyoda M: Treatment of autoimmune diseases and systemic vasculitis with pooled human intravenous immune globulin. Clin Exp Immunol 97(suppl 1):31–38, 1994.

3181. Silvestris F, Cafforio P, Dammacco F: Pathogenic anti–DNA idiotype–reactive IgG in intravenous immunoglobulin preparations. Clin Exp Immunol 97:19–25, 1994.

3182. Koffler D, Agnello V, Thoburn R, Kunkel HG: Systemic lupus erythematosus: Prototype of immune complex nephritis in man. J Exp Med 134:169S–179S, 1971.

3183. Sasaki T, Muryoi T, Hatakeyama A, et al: Circulating anti-DNA immune complexes in active lupus nephritis. Am J Med 91:355–362, 1991.

3184. Sasaki T, Hatakeyama A, Shibata S, et al: Heterogeneity of immune complex–derived anti-DNA antibodies associated with lupus nephritis. Kidney Int 39:746–753, 1991.

3185. Seegal BC, Accinni L, Andres GA, et al: Immunologic studies of autoimmune disease in NZB/NZW F₁ mice. Binding of fluorescein-labeled antinucleoside antibodies in lesions of lupus-like nephritis. J Exp Med 130:203–216, 1969.

3186. Andres GA, Accinni L, Beister SM, et al: Localization of fluorescein-labeled antinucleoside antibodies in glomeruli of patients with active systemic lupus erythematosus nephritis. J Clin Invest 49:2106–2118, 1970.

3187. Malide D, Londoño I, Russo P, Bendayan M: Ultrastructural localization of DNA in immune deposits of human lupus nephritis. Am J Pathol 143:304–311, 1993.

3188. Pisetsky DS, Grudier JP, Gilkeson GS: A role for immunogenic DNA in the pathogenesis of systemic lupus erythematosus. Arthritis Rheum 33:153–159, 1990.

3189. Terada K, Okuhara E, Kawarada Y, Hirose S: Demonstration of extrinsic DNA from immune complexes in plasma of a patient with systemic lupus erythematosus. Biochem Biophys Res Commun 174:323–330, 1991.

3190. Terada K, Okuhara E, Kawarada Y: Antigen DNA isolated from immune complexes in plasma of patients with systemic lupus erythematosus hydridizes with the *Escherichia coli* lac Z gene. Clin Exp Immunol 85:66–69, 1991.

3191. Terada K, Hirose S, Okuhara E: Production of antibodies specific for double stranded antigen DNA cloned from immune complexes in plasma of a SLE patient. Biochem Biophys Res Commun 183:797–802, 1992.

3192. Bernstein K, Bolshoun D, Gilkeson G, et al: Detection of glomerular-binding immune elements in murine lupus using a tissue-based ELISA. Clin Exp Immunol 91:449–455, 1993.

3193. Bernstein KA, Bolshoun D, Lefkowith JB: Serum glomerular binding activity is highly correlated with renal disease in MRL/lpr mice. Clin Exp Immunol 93:418–423, 1993.

3194. Field M, Brennan FM, Melson RD, et al: MRL mice show an age-related impairment of IgG aggregate removal from the circulation. Clin Exp Immunol 61:195–202, 1985.

3195. Field M, Brennan FM, McCarthy D, et al: MRL-lpr/lpr mice show an impairment of IgG aggregate removal which relates to parameters of disease activity. Immunology 61:463–467, 1987.

3196. Mullins WW Jr, Plotz PH, Schrieber L: Soluble immune complexes in lupus mice: Clearance from blood and estimation of formation rates. Clin Immunol Immunopathol 42:375–385, 1987.

3197. Magilavy DB, Hundley TR, Steinberg AD, Katona IM: Hepatic reticuloendothelial system activation in autoimmune mice: Differences between (NZB × NZW)F₁ and MRL-lpr/lpr strains. Clin Immunol Immunopathol 42:386–398, 1987.

3198. Dang-Vu AP, Pisetsky DS, Weinberg JB: Functional alterations of macrophages in autoimmune MRL-lpr/lpr mice. J Immunol 138:1757–1761, 1987.

3199. Russell PJ, Cameron FH: Studies of macrophage function in murine systemic lupus erythematosus. 4. Failure to reverse the defect in Fc-mediated phagocytosis and binding by in vitro stimulants or prostaglandins. Pathology 18:59–63, 1986.

3200. Halma C, Breedveld FC, Daha MR, et al: Elimination of soluble ¹²³I-labeled aggregates of IgG in patients with systemic lupus erythematosus. Arthritis Rheum 34:442–452, 1991.

3201. Davies KA, Peters AM, Beynon HLC, Walport MJ: Immune complex processing in patients with systemic lupus erythematosus. In vivo imaging and clearance studies. J Clin Invest 90:2075–2083, 1992.

3202. Mohan C, Adams S, Stanik V, Datta SK: Nucleosome: A major immunogen for pathogenic autoantibody-inducing T cells of lupus. J Exp Med 177:1367–1381, 1993.

3203. Rumore PM, Steinman CR: Endogenous circulating DNA in systemic lupus erythematosus. Occurrence as multimeric complexes bound to histone. J Clin Invest 86:69–74, 1990.

3204. Losman JA, Fasy TM, Novick KE, et al: Nucleosome-specific antibody from an autoimmune MRL/Mp-lpr/lpr mouse. Arthritis Rheum 36:552–560, 1993.

3205. Schmiedeke T, Stoeckl F, Muller S, et al: Glomerular immune deposits in murine lupus models may contain histones. Clin Exp Immunol 90:453–458, 1992.

3206. Sainis K, Datta SK: CD4⁻ T cell lines with selective patterns of autoreactivity as well as CD4⁺ CD8⁻ T helper cell lines augment the production of idiotypes shared by pathogenic anti-DNA autoantibodies in the NZB × SWR model of lupus nephritis. J Immunol 140:2215–2224, 1988.

3207. Silvestris F, Yancey WB Jr, Malone C, et al: Parallelism of serum anti-F(ab′)₂ and anti-cationic IgG reactivities in patients with systemic lupus erythematosus. Clin Immunol Immunopathol 59:256–270, 1991.

3208. Suenaga R, Abdou NI: Cationic and high affinity serum IgG anti-dsDNA antibodies in active lupus nephritis. Clin Exp Immunol 94:418–422, 1993.

3209. Suzuki N, Harada T, Mizushima Y, Sakane T: Possible pathogenic role of cationic anti-DNA autoantibodies in the development of nephritis in patients with systemic lupus erythematosus. J Immunol 151:1128–1136, 1993.

3210. Gompertz NR, Isenberg DA, Turner BM: Correlation between clinical features of systemic lupus erythematosus and levels of antihistone antibodies of the IgG, IgA, and IgM isotypes. Ann Rheum Dis 49:524–527, 1990.

3211. Termaat RM, Brinkman K, Nossent JC, et al: Anti–heparan sulphate reactivity in sera from patients with systemic lupus erythematosus with renal or non-renal manifestations. Clin Exp Immunol 82:268–274, 1990.

3212. Wesierska-Gadek J, Penner E, Lindner H, et al: Autoantibodies against different histone H1 subtypes in systemic lupus erythematosus sera. Arthritis Rheum 33:1273–1278, 1990.

3213. Subiza JL, Caturla A, Pascual-Salcedo D, et al: DNA–anti-DNA complexes account for part of the antihistone activity found in patients with systemic lupus erythematosus. Arthritis Rheum 32:406–412, 1989.

3214. Viard J-P, Choquette D, Chabre H, et al: Anti-histone reactivity in systemic lupus erythematosus sera: A disease activity index linked to the presence of DNA:anti-DNA immune complexes. Autoimmunity 12:61–68, 1992.

3215. Stöckl F, Schmiedeke T, Muller S, et al: Glomerular histone and ubiquitin deposits in biopsies of SLE patients. J Am Soc Nephrol 1:541, 1990.

3216. Stöckl F, Muller S, Batsford S, et al: A role for histones and ubiquitin in lupus nephritis? Clin Nephrol 41:10–17, 1994.

3217. Termaat R-M, Brinkman K, van Gompel F, et al: Cross-reactivity of monoclonal anti-DNA antibodies with heparan sulfate is mediated via bound DNA/histone complexes. J Autoimmun 3:531–545, 1990.

3218. Kramers C, Termaat RM, ter Borg EJ, et al: Higher anti–heparan sulphate reactivity during systemic lupus erythematosus (SLE) disease exacerbations with renal manifestations; a long term prospective analysis. Clin Exp Immunol 93:34–38, 1993.

3219. Kashihara N, Makino H, Szekanecz Z, et al: Nephritogenicity of anti-proteoglycan antibodies in experimental murine lupus nephritis. Lab Invest 67:752–760, 1992.

3220. Sabbaga J, Pankewycz OG, Lufft V, et al: Cross-reactivity distinguishes serum and nephritogenic anti-DNA antibodies in human lupus from their natural counterparts in normal serum. J Autoimmun 3:215–235, 1990.

3221. Viard J-P, Bach J-F, Jacob L: Splenocytes from MRL/Mp-lpr/lpr mice spontaneously produce antibodies against a cell-surface protein cross-reacting with DNA. Clin Immunol Immunopathol 45:516–521, 1987.

3222. Jacob L, Lety M-A, Monteiro RC, et al: Altered cell-surface protein(s), crossreactive with DNA, on spleen cells of autoimmune lupic mice. Proc Natl Acad Sci USA 84:1361–1363, 1987.

3223. Savage COS: Endothelial cell antibodies: Pathogenetic or epiphenomenon? Nephrol Dial Transplant 9:1362, 1994.

3224. Love PE, Santoro SA: Antiphospholipid antibodies: Anticardiolipin and the lupus anticoagulant in systemic lupus erythematosus (SLE) and in non-SLE disorders. Ann Intern Med 112:682–698, 1990.

3225. Frampton G, Hicks J, Cameron JS: Significance of anti-phospholipid antibodies in patients with lupus nephritis. Kidney Int 39:1225–1231, 1991.

3226. Hashimoto Y, Kawamura M, Ichikawa K, et al: Anticardiolipin antibodies in NZW × BXSB F₁ mice. A model of antiphospholipid syndrome. J Immunol 149:1063–1068, 1992.

3227. Pérez-Vázquez ME, Cabiedes J, Cabral AR, Alarcón-Segovia D: Decrease in serum antiphospholipid antibody levels upon development of nephrotic syndrome in patients with systemic lupus erythematosus: Relationship to urinary loss of IgG and other factors. Am J Med 92:357–362, 1992.

3228. Spronk PE, Bootsma H, Nikkels PGJ, Kallenberg CGM: A new class of lupus nephropathy associated with antiphospholipid antibodies. Br J Rheumatol 33:686–693, 1994.

3229. Pereira LF, Marco FM, Boimorto R, et al: Histones interact with anionic phospholipids with high avidity; its relevance for the binding of histone-antihistone immune complexes. Clin Exp Immunol 97:175–180, 1994.

3230. Jones DRE, Hopkinson ND, Powell RJ: Autoantibodies in pet dogs owned by patients with systemic lupus erythematosus. Lancet 339:1378–1380, 1992.

3231. Gilkeson GS, Pritchard AJ, Pisetsky DS: Specificity of anti-DNA antibodies induced in normal mice by immunization with bacterial DNA. Clin Immunol Immunopathol 59:288–300, 1991.

3232. Gilkeson GS, Ruiz P, Howell D, et al: Induction of immune-mediated glomerulonephritis in normal mice immunized with bacterial DNA. Clin Immunol Immunopathol 68:283–292, 1993.

3233. Tsao BP, Cheroutre H, Ohnishi K, et al: Nephritis in normal mice expressing transgenes encoding an antibody to DNA. Arthritis Rheum 33:S19, 1990.

3234. Duchosal MA, McConahey PJ, Robinson CA, Dixon FJ: Transfer of human systemic lupus erythematosus in severe combined immunodeficient (SCID) mice. J Exp Med 172:985–988, 1990.

3235. Duchosal MA, Eming SA, McConahey PJ, Dixon FJ: The hu-PBL-SCID mouse model. Long-term human serologic evolution associated with the xenogeneic transfer of human peripheral blood leukocytes into SCID mice. Cell Immunol 139:468–477, 1992.

3236. Ashany D, Hines J, Gharavi A, et al: Analysis of autoantibody production in SCID-systemic lupus erythematosus (SLE) chimeras. Clin Exp Immunol 88:84–90, 1992.

3237. Portanova JP, Claman HN, Kotzin BL: Autoimmunization in murine graft-vs-host disease. 1. Selective production of antibodies to histones and DNA. J Immunol 135:3850–3856, 1985.

3238. Bruijn JA, Van Elven EH, Hogendoorn PCW, et al: Murine chronic graft-versus-host disease as a model for lupus nephritis. Am J Pathol 130:639–641, 1988.

3239. Portanova JP, Ebling FM, Hammond WS, et al: Allogeneic MHC antigen requirements for lupus-like autoantibody production and nephritis in murine graft-vs-host disease. J Immunol 141:3370–3376, 1988.

3240. Morris SC, Cohen PL, Eisenberg RA: Experimental induction of systemic lupus erythematosus by recognition of foreign Ia. Clin Immunol Immunopathol 57:263–273, 1990.

3241. van Leer EHG, Bruijn JA, Prins FA, et al: Redistribution of glomerular dipeptidyl peptidase type IV in experimental lupus nephritis. Demonstration of decreased enzyme activity at the ultrastructural level. Lab Invest 68:550–556, 1993.

3242. Bruijn JA, Bergijk EC, de Heer E, et al: Induction and progression of experimental lupus nephritis: Exploration of a pathogenetic pathway. Kidney Int 41:5–13, 1992.

3243. Kubota T, Iizuka H, Bachovchin WW, Stollar BD: Dipeptidyl peptidase IV (DP IV) activity in serum and on lymphocytes of MRL/Mp-lpr/lpr mice correlates with disease onset. Clin Exp Immunol 96:292–296, 1994.

3244. Hultman P, Enestrom S: Mercury induced antinuclear antibodies in mice: Characterization and correlation with renal immune complex deposits. Clin Exp Immunol 71:269–274, 1988.

3245. Hultman P, Skogh T, Enestrom S: Circulating and tissue immune complexes in mercury-treated mice. J Clin Lab Immunol 29:175–183, 1989.

3246. Clagett JA, Wilson CB, Weigle WO: Interstitial immune complex thyroiditis in mice. The role of autoantibody to thyroglobulin. J Exp Med 140:1439–1456, 1974.

3247. Meade CJ, Brandon DR, Smith W, et al: The relationship between hyperglycaemia and renal immune complex deposition in mice with inherited diabetes. Clin Exp Immunol 43:109–120, 1981.

3248. Abrass CK: Evaluation of the presence of circulating immune complexes and their relationship to glomerular IgG deposits in streptozotocin-induced diabetic rats. Clin Exp Immunol 57:17–24, 1984.

3249. Fornasieri A, Li M, Armelloni S, et al: Glomerulonephritis induced by human IgMK-IgG cryoglobulins in mice. Lab Invest 69:531–540, 1993.

3250. Takahashi S, Nose M, Sasaki J, et al: IgG3 production in MRL/lpr mice is responsible for development of lupus nephritis. J Immunol 147:515–519, 1991.

3251. Denman AM: Cryoglobulins and the immunopathological manifestations of autoimmune disease. Clin Exp Immunol 87:169–171, 1992.

3252. Shibata T, Berney T, Spertini F, Izui S: Rheumatoid factors in mice bearing the lpr or gld mutation. Selective production of rheumatoid factor cryoglobulins in MRL/MPJ-lpr/lpr mice. Clin Exp Immunol 87:190–195, 1992.

3253. Itoh J, Nose M, Takahashi S, et al: Induction of different types of glomerulonephritis by monoclonal antibodies derived from an MRL/lpr lupus mouse. Am J Pathol 143:1436–1443, 1993.

3254. Sugisaki T, Takase S: Composition of immune deposits present in glomeruli of NZB/W F₁ mice. Clin Immunol Immunopathol 61:296–308, 1991.

3255. Howard TW, Iannini MJ, Burge JJ, Davis JS IV: Rheumatoid factor, cryoglobulinemia, anti-DNA, and renal disease in patients with systemic lupus erythematosus. J Rheumatol 18:826–830, 1991.

3256. Burkholder PM: Glomerular disease in captive galagos. Vet Pathol 18(suppl 6):6–22, 1981.

3257. Chalifoux LV, Bronson RT, Sehgal P, et al: Nephritis and hemolytic anemia in owl monkeys (Aotus trivirgatus). Vet Pathol 18(suppl 6):23–37, 1981.

3258. Boyce JT, Giddens WE Jr, Seifert R: Spontaneous mesangioproliferative glomerulonephritis in pigtailed macaques (Macaca nemestrina). Vet Pathol 18(suppl 6):82–88, 1981.

3259. Abramowsky CR, Aikawa M, Swinehart GL, Snajdar RM: Spontaneous nephrotic syndrome in a genetic rat model. Am J Pathol 117:400–408, 1984.

3260. Arthur JE, Lucke VM, Newby TJ, Bourne FJ: An immunohistological study of feline glomerulonephritis using the peroxidase-antiperoxidase method. Res Vet Sci 37:12–17, 1984.

3261. MacDougall DF, Cook T, Steward AP, Cattell V: Canine chronic renal disease: Prevalence and types of glomerulonephritis in the dog. Kidney Int 29:1144–1151, 1986.

3262. Jeraj KP, Vernier RL, Polzin D, et al: Idiopathic immune complex glomerulonephritis in dogs with multisystem involvement. Am J Vet Res 45:1699–1705, 1984.

3263. Wright NG, Nash AS: Experimental ampicillin glomerulonephropathy. J Comp Pathol 94:357–361, 1984.

3264. Jeraj KP, Hardy R, O'Leary TP, et al: Immune complex glomerulonephritis in a cat with renal lymphosarcoma. Vet Pathol 22:287–290, 1984.

3265. Sabnis SG, Gunson DE, Antonovych TT: Some unusual features of mesangioproliferative glomerulonephritis in horses. Vet Pathol 21:574–581, 1984.

3266. Frelier PF, Pritchard J, Armstrong DL, et al: Spontaneous mesangiocapillary glomerulonephritis in Finn cross lambs from Alberta. Can J Comp Med 48:215–218, 1984.

3267. Stark H, Alkalay A, Ben-Bassat M, et al: Levan-induced glomerulitis in rabbits: A possible role for direct complement activation in situ. Br J Exp Pathol 66:165–171, 1985.

3268. Blum JR, Cork LC, Morris JM, et al: The clinical manifestations of a genetically determined deficiency of the third component of complement in the dog. Clin Immunol Immunopathol 34:304–315, 1985.

3269. Cork LC, Morris JM, Olson JL, et al: Membranoproliferative glomerulonephritis in dogs with a genetically determined deficiency of the third component of complement. Clin Immunol Immunopathol 60:455–470, 1991.

3270. Jansen JH, Hogasen K, Mollnes TE: Extensive complement activation in hereditary porcine membranoproliferative glomerulonephritis type II (porcine dense deposit disease). Am J Pathol 143:1356–1365, 1993.

3271. Foltz CJ, Cork LC, Winkelstein JA: Absence of glomerulonephritis in guinea pigs deficient in the fourth component of complement. Vet Pathol 31:201–206, 1994.

# Primary Glomerular Diseases

*Richard J. Glassock*
*Arthur H. Cohen*
*Sharon G. Adler*

Disorders of glomerular structure and function constitute one of the major problems encountered in the practice of nephrology. Beginning with Richard Bright, the study of glomerular diseases has focused on the relationship of clinical findings to morbid anatomy. Until comparatively recently, these studies were based largely on information from patients with fatal disease.[1]* Thus, only a portion of the spectrum of glomerulopathic processes was uncovered, and a vast area of natural history remained uncharted. The introduction and wide application of percutaneous renal biopsy permitted exploration of these hitherto hidden facets of glomerular disease.[2, 3] Disorders originally thought to be homogeneous have been increasingly subdivided and reclassified, and new entities have emerged. Much knowledge is now available regarding the relationship of clinical findings to underlying pathology, natural history, and response to treatment.[1] As is evident from Chapter 29, the discipline of immunopathology has provided substantial evidence for the important role of immunologic mechanisms in many glomerular diseases.[1] Environmental agents (e.g., bacteria, viruses, drugs) have increasingly been incriminated in the genesis of many glomerular lesions. Remarkable progress has been made in unraveling the complicated biochemistry and function of the glomerular capillary wall.[4–8] The pathophysiologic alterations that attend glomerular injury are now better understood, and the potential role of nonimmunologic factors, independent of the initiation of disease, in the progression of glomerular disease to end-stage renal failure is now well appreciated (see also Chapters 43 and 44). Thus, the clinical nephrologist dealing with glomerular

disease must at once be a consummate bedside observer, an accomplished morphologist and pathologic physiologist, and at least an amateur immunopathologist.

The nomenclature of glomerular disease has undergone periodic and often confusing revisions.[1, 9–12] New clinicopathologic entities previously believed to be homogeneous become subdivided when they are restudied with more sophisticated techniques. Lesions believed to represent individual disease entities may be recognized as secondary complications of diverse pathogenic processes. Thus, the classification of glomerular disease is constantly evolving.

One must approach the glomerular disorders at several levels simultaneously: first, by clinical features (the major clinical syndromes); second, by morphology (the integrated light, electron, and immunofluorescence microscopic patterns); third, according to the responsible pathogenic mechanisms (discussed in Chapter 29); and finally, according to known etiologic factors or agents. Clinical syndromes, morphologic appearances, and presumed pathogenic mechanisms do not demonstrate a precise relationship except in a few circumstances.[1] Further, etiologic factors are at present unknown for the majority of the disorders to be described.

## THE MAJOR CLINICAL SYNDROMES

The major clinical manifestations of the glomerular diseases may be grouped by patterns (Table 30–1) representing various combinations of the cardinal expressions of glomerular injury, namely, proteinuria; hematuria; reduced glomerular filtration rate (GFR); and alterations in $Na^+$ excretion leading to edema, circulatory congestion, and hy-

---

*For a more extensive bibliography of literature appearing before 1989, the interested reader is referred to the third or fourth edition of this book.[1]

**TABLE 30–1. The Major Clinical Syndromes of Glomerular Disease**

Acute glomerulonephritis
Rapidly progressive glomerulonephritis
Chronic glomerulonephritis
Persistent urinary abnormalities with few or no symptoms
Nephrotic syndrome

pertension. The pathophysiologic alterations responsible for these manifestations of glomerular injury are discussed in detail in Chapter 43.

Acute glomerulonephritis or the acute nephritic syndrome is a clinical pattern characterized by a relatively abrupt onset of variable degrees of hematuria, proteinuria, diminished GFR, $Na^+$ and fluid retention, circulatory congestion, hypertension, and occasionally oliguria. This syndrome is also typified by a tendency to spontaneous recovery and a frequent association with preceding microbial infection.

Rapidly progressive glomerulonephritis (RPGN), on the other hand, is a clinical syndrome characterized by a more insidious onset and a picture dominated by progressive loss of renal function and, frequently, oliguria. There is little tendency for spontaneous recovery, and the temporal association with microbial infection is inconstant.

Chronic glomerulonephritis or the chronic nephritic syndrome is a vague, all-inclusive term referring to progressive renal functional impairment of insidious onset accompanied by varying degrees of proteinuria, hematuria, and hypertension. The course is usually relentlessly progressive, but it may be protracted, extending over decades. In its end stages, it may be difficult or impossible clinically to distinguish whether a glomerular, tubulointerstitial, or vascular disease was primarily responsible for the loss of renal function.

Persistent urinary abnormalities with few or no symptoms (asymptomatic proteinuria or hematuria) is a clinical pattern manifested chiefly by mild to moderate proteinuria, usually much less than 3 g/d, occurring with or without hematuria but accompanied by few or no systemic abnormalities such as hypertension, reduced renal function, hypoproteinemia, or edema. Hematuria, either gross or microscopic, may occur in a recurrent or persistent fashion and often is not accompanied by abnormal proteinuria.

The nephrotic syndrome is a term employed to characterize the insidious onset of heavy proteinuria, usually more than 3.5 g/d in an adult, accompanied by a distinct lowering of the plasma albumin concentration, usually below 3 g/dL.[13] A variable tendency toward edema, hypertension, lipidemia, and lipiduria is also seen in this group of patients.

These clinical syndromes may appear in the context of a primary glomerular disease or in association with infectious, drug-induced, multisystem, or hereditary diseases (see Chapter 31). It should also be readily apparent that the division of clinical manifestations into separate clinical syndromes is arbitrary and that much overlap exists; however, the classification of the expression of glomerular injury into common themes serves a useful purpose for the clinician in that identification of the major clinical features directs at-

tention to the consideration of specific clinicopathologic entities. It also provides a framework on which may be added information regarding pathology, pathogenesis, and etiology, with the final aim of constructing a complete picture of the disease process, assessing prognosis, and designing rational therapy.

## DEFINITION OF PRIMARY GLOMERULAR DISEASES

The primary glomerular diseases constitute a heterogeneous collection of disorders in which the glomeruli are the sole or predominant tissue involved. Extrarenal manifestations are the result of the functional abnormalities that accompany the glomerular injury itself. For the most part, the primary glomerular diseases are also idiopathic (i.e., of unknown cause), although predominant glomerular injury in some circumstances is consequent to a well-defined event, such as bacterial infection or drug exposure. Thus, the terms primary and idiopathic are not necessarily synonymous. On the other hand, glomerular injury may be a feature of diseases in which multiple extrarenal organs or systems are involved. As primary glomerular diseases are subjected to closer scrutiny, it is apparent that clinically covert involvement of organs other than the kidney (skin, lung) may occur frequently, and diseases classically regarded in the multisystem category may present initially with manifestations solely confined to the kidney.

The distinction between diseases in which the glomeruli are solely or predominantly involved and those in which glomerular injury is but a part of a multisystem, hereditary, or biochemical disturbance is unquestionably arbitrary. Undoubtedly, as intensive investigation yields further insight into the mechanisms underlying the so-called primary glomerular diseases, multisystem or hereditary features will be uncovered. Many primary glomerular diseases have already been found to have an underlying genetic basis, and it is likely that the mechanisms underlying the linkage between susceptibility genes and injurious pathologic processes will be elucidated in the future.[14, 15]

## ACUTE GLOMERULONEPHRITIS

Patients presenting with features of the acute nephritic syndrome often have some evidence of a recent infection of the pharynx or the skin or both with a group A β-hemolytic streptococcus.[1, 16–18] However, an acute nephritic syndrome clinically resembling that related to streptococcal infection may occur after many other bacterial, viral, and parasitic infections,[1, 18–20] such as pneumococcal[20, 21] or *Klebsiella* pneumonia,[22] staphylococcal or gram-negative sepsis,[23] meningococcemia,[24] gonococcemia,[25] secondary syphilis,[26] brucellosis,[27] leptospirosis,[28] typhoid fever,[29] *Mycoplasma* pneumonia,[30] varicella,[31] mumps,[32] measles,[33] infectious mononucleosis,[34, 35] hepatitis B[36] (see Chapter 31), Hantaan virus (Puumala virus) infection,[37] cytomegalovirus infection,[38] coxsackievirus infection,[39, 40] *Chlamydia psittaci* infection,[41] typhus,[42] Rocky Mountain spotted fever,[43–45] histoplasmosis,[46] trichinosis,[47] schistosomiasis,[48] falciparum malaria,[49] and toxoplasmosis[50, 51] (see also Chapter 31). Many of these infectious diseases can also evoke other clinical syndromes, such as nephrotic syndrome and RPGN. Furthermore, many other primary glomerular diseases not known to be related to preceding infectious disease may produce a picture of acute nephritis. Predominant among these diseases are idiopathic mesangiocapillary glomerulonephritis (MCGN) and mesangial proliferative glomerulonephritis, with or without immunoglobulin (Ig) M or C3 mesangial deposits, and Berger disease (IgA nephropathy; see later). An acute nephritic syndrome has also been observed in association with Guillain-Barré-Strohl syndrome,[52] with Charcot-Marie-Tooth disease,[53] and after irradiation and chemotherapy of renal tumors in children.[54]

The multisystem diseases that may provoke the acute nephritic syndrome, such as systemic lupus erythematosus (SLE), Schönlein-Henoch purpura, essential mixed cryoimmunoglobulinemia, and infective endocarditis, are described more fully in Chapter 31. An acute hypersensitivity interstitial nephritis arising as a complication of drug therapy and described more completely in Chapter 31 may also be associated with clinical findings closely resembling those of acute glomerulonephritis. The passage of time, careful serologic studies, and examination of renal biopsy material nearly always distinguish these entities from classic streptococcus-related, postinfectious glomerulonephritis (poststreptococcal glomerulonephritis, PSGN). Because the manifestations of acute PSGN may be regarded as a prototype for the acute nephritic syndrome, it is discussed in detail. The other infection-associated forms of glomerulonephritis are discussed in Chapter 31.

## Poststreptococcal Glomerulonephritis

### EPIDEMIOLOGY

The association of acute glomerulonephritis with certain infections has been suspected since the time of Richard Bright. Studies in the early part of the 20th century clearly established the relationship of acute nephritis to infection with group A (β-hemolytic) streptococci.[1] The classic studies of Rammelkamp and co-workers[55–57] clearly showed that only certain strains of the group A streptococcus, in particular type 12, were capable of evoking nephritis. In contradistinction, all strains of group A streptococci are capable of evoking acute rheumatic fever, although some evidence favors the existence of "rheumatogenic" strains of streptococci.[1] These observations explain in part the variable attack rate of nephritis in outbreaks of streptococcal disease and the relative constancy of attack rate for acute rheumatic fever.[55–58] It is now recognized that in addition to type 12, many other types, including 1, 2, 3, 4, 18, 25, 49, 55, 57, and 60, are potentially nephritogenic.[18, 55–58] In addition, types 31, 52, 56, 59, and 61 are suspected of being nephritogenic. Acute glomerulonephritis may also on occasion be associated with non–group A streptococcal infection, particularly group C (*Streptococcus zooepidemicus*).[59] Even among outbreaks of infection with potentially nephritogenic strains, the attack rate of glomerulonephritis is variable, indicating either that intrastrain variation in nephritogenic-

ity exists or that there is an unidentified host factor relating to susceptibility to nephritis.[1, 18, 60] Subclinical episodes occur about four times more frequently than easily recognized clinical disease, which makes attack rates difficult to determine without careful prospective studies.[58] Asymptomatic family contacts of patients with PSGN can frequently be shown to have abnormal urinalyses (hematuria).[1, 20] Rheumatic fever and acute PSGN coexist only rarely.[1]

Although rheumatic fever follows only pharyngeal infection with group A streptococci, nephritis may follow either skin or pharyngeal infection. In fact, outbreaks of streptococcal impetigo are more commonly associated with nephritis than are upper respiratory infections in certain geographic zones.[61–64] For example, the well-studied epidemics in Minnesota and in Trinidad were predominantly associated with streptococcal impetigo,[62, 63, 65, 66] the latter in association with an outbreak of scabies.[62] Certain strains, most notably types 2, 49, 55, 57, and 60, are chiefly associated with impetigo and nephritis.[61, 64] Type 49 is especially common and has a worldwide distribution. Some potentially nephritogenic strains cannot be typed by M protein content and are identified by agglutination methods (T strains).[1, 18, 56]

Among epidemics of infection with streptococci of proven nephritogenicity (i.e., all affected individuals infected with an identical strain), the apparent "clinical attack rate" is in the vicinity of 10% to 12%[1, 57, 66, 67]; however, there is much variation in the prevalence of nephritis among sporadic infections with group A streptococci of potentially nephritogenic types.[55–57] The reason for this variability is not known. True attack rates are difficult to define without thorough investigation, including serial urinalyses and measurement of complement components (see later).[58, 60] Even such detailed studies may underestimate the true attack rate, because glomerulonephritis may ensue without any detectable clinical or laboratory abnormalities.[68] Studies of outbreaks of streptococcal infection among families have indicated that susceptibility to PSGN may be genetically determined, but as yet no phenotypic markers consistently related to such susceptibility have been described.[58, 68] Finally, the nephritogenic factor in group A streptococci may be only loosely linked to M protein type. A considerable body of evidence has accumulated that suggests that other antigens, independent of M protein, may be the factors that confer nephritogenicity on group A streptococci.[1, 18, 69–73] One such antigen derived from cell membranes, and called endostreptosin by Lange and co-workers,[72–74] may well be the responsible nephritogenic antigen. It is present in nephritogenic strains of both group A and C streptococci. Asymptomatic family contacts of patients with PSGN who demonstrate abnormal urinalyses may also have raised antiendostreptosin antibody levels.[1, 72, 73] Other non–cell membrane antigens of streptococci, as well as autologous antigens, have also been implicated in the pathogenesis of this disorder.[75–80]

### CLINICAL FEATURES

PSGN is principally a disease of children, although it may occur at nearly any age.[1, 18, 81–83] It is rarely seen in children younger than 2 years. For unknown reasons, it shows a predilection for males. A broad range of severity of disease exists, from entirely asymptomatic cases detected only by the incidental finding of microscopic hematuria to oliguric acute renal failure.[84] In its classic form, the clinical onset of PSGN is abrupt. A latent period between the onset of recognizable streptococcal infection and the first manifestations of nephritis is usually present, averaging about 10 days, but occasionally latent periods in excess of 3 weeks have been seen.[1, 82] Short latent periods of a few days generally indicate an exacerbation of pre-existing disease, sometimes referred to as "synpharyngitic nephritis." This is most frequently due to an underlying IgA nephropathy (see later). In pharyngeal-associated PSGN, the latent period ranges from 6 to 21 days and averages about 10 days.[61] Latent periods are difficult to determine in impetigo-associated PSGN. Oliguria and gross hematuria with a smoky or rusty appearance to the urine are commonly reported by the patient. Anuria is relatively infrequent and, when present for more than a few days, may indicate the development of crescentic glomerulonephritis (see later). Dysuria may be present in cases with severe hematuria, giving rise to confusion with urinary tract infection, especially when leukocytes are also present in the urinary sediment (see later). Hematuria is microscopic in as many as two thirds of cases. Some degree of edema and hypertension is found in more than 75% of cases. This may lead to the erroneous diagnosis of congestive heart failure or essential hypertension unless the urine sediment is examined carefully. The edema typically involves the face, eyelids, and hands initially and is notably worse on first rising. Ascites may appear in children. Hypertension is usually mild to moderate and not accompanied by the retinal alterations of malignant hypertension or end-stage renal disease.[1, 16] Hypertension is usually most evident at or near the onset of clinical manifestations of renal disease and subsides promptly with the onset of diuresis. A rise in diastolic pressure from 70 to 85 mm Hg may be the sole manifestation of the hypertensive process in children. Evidence of circulatory congestion, such as dyspnea, cough, engorged neck veins, cardiomegaly, gallop rhythms, or even frank pulmonary edema, may at times dominate the clinical picture,[1, 16] especially in elderly patients.[81, 83] The circulatory congestion is the result of primary renal Na$^+$ and fluid retention rather than intrinsic myocardial disease. Although echocardiograms may show left ventricular dysfunction, this abnormality is not well correlated with hypertension or fluid retention.[85] In such instances, an incorrect diagnosis of primary cardiovascular disease may be made if examination of the urinary sediment is initially omitted or performed carelessly.

Atypical manifestations seem to be especially common in older patients.[81–83] Encephalopathy is occasionally a complication of acute PSGN, especially in children. Confusion, headache, somnolence, or even convulsions may occur. At times, the encephalopathic manifestations dominate the clinical picture and suggest a primary neurologic disorder, especially in children.[86] Although hypertension is present in most patients exhibiting abnormalities of central nervous system function, the role of elevated blood pressure in the genesis of these clinical features is not certain. Systemic symptoms such as mild fever, nausea, and loin or abdominal pain may develop but, when severe, should increase the

suspicion of a systemic disease such as SLE or vasculitis. Occasionally, acute PSGN mimics Schönlein-Henoch purpura (see Chapter 31). Infective endocarditis should always be suspected in patients presenting with fever, anemia, heart murmurs, and nephritis.[1]

Although many or all of these symptoms and signs may be present, it is important to re-emphasize the variability of presenting features. One should always consider the diagnosis of acute PSGN in patients with unexplained acute onset of edema, oliguria, hypertension, circulatory congestion, or encephalopathy. In addition, many subclinical cases may be discovered only on examination of the urine sediment in the course of investigating family members of individuals with clear-cut disease.[1, 58, 68, 86]

## LABORATORY FINDINGS

Hematuria is nearly always present and may be either gross (macroscopic) or microscopic. Several cases have been reported in which the clinical features of acute glomerulonephritis have been present and confirmed by renal biopsy but in which urinalyses were nearly or completely normal and hypertension was absent.[1, 58, 86] Therefore, even a relatively benign urine sediment should not distract the physician from the possibility of an underlying acute PSGN.[1] When gross hematuria is present, a characteristic rusty or smoky hue may be present if urine pH is acid. On microscopic examination of the urine sediment, red blood cell casts are commonly found but may be difficult to identify unless a generous sample of urine is centrifuged lightly, the sediment is gently resuspended, and the specimen is freshly examined and is of acid pH. Dysmorphic erythrocytes dominate the urinary sediment.[87, 88] Renal tubule epithelial cells, leukocytes, and occasionally leukocyte casts may also be seen, as well as large numbers of hyaline and granular casts. Waxy casts and broad casts are more suggestive of either an exacerbation of pre-existing nephritis or an underlying systemic disease such as SLE or systemic vasculitis. Proteinuria is nearly always present but is less than 3 g/d in more than 75% of cases and less than 500 mg/d in more than half the cases.[89, 90] Severe cases may be associated with massive proteinuria. The proteinuria is typically "nonselective" (see later) and often contains greatly increased amounts of fibrin degradation products and fibrinopeptides.[86, 91]

The GFR is often but not invariably depressed during the acute stages of the disease. Elderly patients may have pronounced decline in GFR.[83] However, mild decreases in GFR (less than 50%) may be accompanied by profound degrees of fluid retention and circulatory congestion. Thus, serum creatinine levels may not increase above the upper range of normal even in patients with overt signs of serious Na$^+$ and fluid retention. Early in its course, serum levels of endothelin and atrial natriuretic peptide are increased, accompanied by Na$^+$ retention and volume expansion.[91a] Renal plasma flow is typically less reduced or even increased relative to GFR; thus, the filtration fraction is nearly always decreased.[92] Maximal tubule reabsorption of glucose and tubule secretion of p-aminohippurate are usually well preserved relative to GFR.[92] Urinary concentrating ability is also well preserved, and blood urea nitrogen may be

**TABLE 30–2. Selected Serologic Findings in Primary Glomerular Disease***

| Disease | Complement Components | | | ASO, ADNase B | Cryo Ig | aGBM | ANCA | CIC | C3 NeF |
|---|---|---|---|---|---|---|---|---|---|
| | *C1q* | *C4* | *C3* | | | | | | |
| Acute poststreptococcal GN | N or sl ↓ | N or sl ↓ | ↓↓ | + + + | + + | − | − | + + + | ± |
| Idiopathic crescentic GN | | | | | | | | | |
|   Type I | N | N | N | − | − | + + + | − | − | − |
|   Type II | ↓ | ↓ | ↓↓ | − | + + | − | ± | + + | − |
|   Type III | N | N | N | − | − | ± | + + + | ± | − |
|   Type IV | N | N | N | − | − | + + | + + + | ± | − |
|   Type V | N | N | N | − | − | − | − | ± | − |
| Primary IgA nephropathy (Berger disease) | N | N | N | − | ± | − | − | + + (IgA) | − |
| Minimal-change disease | N or sl ↓ | N | N | − | − | − | − | ±−+ + | − |
| Mesangial proliferative GN | N | N | N | − ± | − | − | − | ±−+ | − |
| Focal glomerular sclerosis | N or sl ↓ | N | N | − | − | − | − | ±−+ + | − |
| Membranous GN | N | N | N | − | − | − | − | ±−+ + | − |
| Mesangiocapillary GN | | | | | | | | | |
|   Type I | ↓ | ↓ | ↓↓↓ | + | + + | − | − | + + | ± |
|   Type II | N | N | ↓↓↓ | + | − | − | − | + | + + + |
| Focal and segmental proliferative GN | N | N | N | − | − | ± | − | ± | − |
| Fibrillary GN | N | N | N | − | − | − | − | ± | − |

*− = most often normal; ± = occasionally slightly abnormal; + = occasionally modestly abnormal; + + = often abnormal; + + + = regularly abnormal; N = normal levels; sl ↓ = slightly reduced; ↓ to ↓↓↓ = definitely to severely reduced; ASO = antistreptolysin O titer; ADNase B = anti–deoxyribonuclease B titer; Cryo Ig = cryoimmunoglobulins; aGBM = anti–glomerular basement membrane antibody; ANCA = anti–neutrophil cytoplasmic antibody; CIC = circulatory immune complexes by any *one* of several assays (e.g., Raji cell, C1q binding); C3 NeF = C3 nephritic factor (see also Chapter 29); GN = glomerulonephritis.

increased disproportionately to serum creatinine. Urinary $Na^+$ excretion and $Ca^{2+}$ excretion are greatly reduced.[93] Fractional excretion of $Na^+$ ($FE_{Na}$) is typically less than 0.5% during the acute phases of the disease. Among patients having free access to hypotonic fluids, a mild dilutional hyponatremia may be found. Hyperchloremic acidosis with mild hyperkalemia (type IV renal tubular acidosis) is often present even in patients without oliguria. The impairment of $H^+$ and $K^+$ excretion may be due to extracellular volume expansion with concomitant suppression of plasma renin activity and aldosterone secretion coupled with reduced distal delivery of solute.[94] Oliguric acute renal failure is relatively uncommon but when present may be attended by life-threatening hyperkalemia or fluid overload.[1, 84, 90, 95–97]

Throat or skin cultures frequently but not invariably reveal group A streptococci.[1, 68] Members of the immediate family of an affected person may also have positive throat or skin cultures even in the absence of symptoms or signs of nephritis. Immunity to the streptococcal M protein is type specific, long lasting, and protective.[1, 61] This phenomenon and the relatively limited number of serotypes associated with nephritogenicity offer one explanation for the rarity of proven second episodes of acute PSGN after initial healing of the renal lesion.[1, 89, 98] Most second episodes of presumed PSGN represent exacerbations of underlying disease that may be evoked by both streptococcal and nonstreptococcal infections.[98] The antibody response to the extracellular products of streptococci has little importance in

protective immunity but provides useful markers of the presence or absence of recent infection[1] (Table 30–2). These antibodies include antistreptolysin O (ASO), antistreptokinase, antihyaluronidase, anti–deoxyribonuclease B, and anti–nicotyladenine dinucleotidase.[1] In 90% or more of patients with pharyngeal infection, ASO titers above 200 U are attained within 3 to 5 weeks after infection and then decline slowly to normal in several months.[98] However, early treatment of pharyngitis with antimicrobials may blunt or eliminate the expected rise in ASO titer, and certain strains of type 12 group A streptococci neither display β-hemolysis in blood agar nor produce streptolysin S or O.[56] Contrariwise, many non-nephritogenic group B streptococci reveal β-hemolysis in blood agar culture plates.[1, 56] The magnitude of the rise in ASO titer bears little relationship to the risk for development of nephritis or its severity.[1] ASO titers rise little or not at all in acute glomerulonephritis associated with streptococcal impetigo.[99] In these circumstances, anti–deoxyribonuclease B and antihyaluronidase titers are of special value in diagnosis; elevated values are found in well above 90% of cases.[1, 99] Serial measurements with a twofold or greater rise in titer are highly indicative of recent infection but do not define the potential nephritogenicity of the infection. Single measurements are of less value, especially because "normal" values vary according to season, age of the patient, and socioeconomic population group from which the patient is drawn.[1, 99] False-positive test results for ASO may be found in patients with severe hypercholesterolemia; cholesterol inhibits the interaction of streptolysin O with erythrocytes. Rarely, paraproteins with ASO activity have been described.[100]

Thus, among patients with typical historical and clinical features of acute glomerulonephritis, the serial determination of antibody responses to extracellular production of streptococci by use of several serologic tests, such as ASO and anti–deoxyribonuclease B, considerably enhances the likelihood of obtaining definitive evidence of recent streptococcal infection. The Streptozyme test, which combines several antistreptococcal antibody assays, is a useful screening test.[101] The antibody level to endostreptosin also increases, and this immune response may be prolonged in patients with PSGN.[72–74] On occasion, autoantibody to collagen or laminin may be detected.[102] Antibodies to other streptococcal cell wall glycoproteins may also be noted.[1, 74, 80] Throat or skin cultures are less satisfactory than serologic studies but, if obtained early from appropriate sites, may be positive for group A β-hemolytic streptococci in one fourth or more of patients not previously treated with antimicrobial agents.

One of the most important laboratory parameters used in the investigation of patients with acute glomerulonephritis is the serial estimation of complement components[82, 103, 104] (see Table 30–2). With occasional exceptions,[105] the serum levels of hemolytic complement activity ($CH_{50}$) and C3 protein are abnormally reduced in specimens obtained early in the course of disease, and the values return to normal in less than 8 weeks.[1, 82, 103–108] Serum C3 levels usually fall to less than 50% of normal. The degree and duration of depression of the other early complement components (C1q, C2, and C4) are usually much less than those of C3.[103, 104, 109] The levels of C3 are usually lower in those patients in whom factors capable of cleaving native C3 can be demonstrated in the serum (e.g., C3 nephritic factor; see later).[110–112] The level of complement factor B is usually not depressed.[110] Mild depression of C5 levels is common, but C6 and C7 are most often normal.[109, 110] Plasma levels of fluid-phase terminal complement components (soluble C5b–C9) rise acutely and then fall to normal.[104] Properdin levels are decreased in about 60% of cases, usually in association with reduced C3 levels.[110] These findings suggest prominent involvement of the alternative pathway of complement activation.[103] Profound and persisting depressed C3 levels should alert the physician to suspect an underlying idiopathic MCGN, atheromatous emboli, endocarditis, occult sepsis, SLE (see later), hemolytic-uremic syndrome, or a congenital deficiency state.[103] The degree of depression of C3 levels has no relationship to severity of disease or ultimate prognosis.

Anemia and modest hypoalbuminemia are largely the result of the retention of fluid and circulatory congestion. Red blood cell mass is usually normal in patients without oliguric renal failure.[113] A full-blown nephrotic syndrome may be found in as many as 20% of hospitalized patients.[89, 90] Transient hyperlipemia may often be present in the acute stages of PSGN.[1]

Circulating cryoglobulins (type III) may be found in most patients during the acute illness[114, 115] (see Table 30–2 and Chapter 31). They contain polyclonal IgG, alone or in combination with IgM or C3. Antibody activity to altered autologous IgG may be found in the cryoglobulins (see

later).[116] Circulating immune complexes are also frequently detectable by any of several currently available methods,[117–120] but these may be epiphenomena unrelated to the occurrence of nephritis[70, 119, 120] (see later and Chapter 29). Fibrinogen, factor VIII, and plasmin activity are often elevated during acute stages and correlate with severity, and thrombocytopenia may be seen.[121–125] Circulating high-molecular-weight fibrinogen complexes are frequently present, particularly in severe cases.[123] Persistence of these complexes may have unfavorable prognostic implications. Increased levels of bioactive plasma circulating platelet-activating factor are seen during the acute phase of glomerulonephritis.[126] Defective phagocyte function in vitro has been observed.[127] Patients with PSGN have altered responsiveness to streptococcal cell membrane antigens in vitro.[128] Some patients may have altered cellular responses to glomerular basement membrane (GBM) antigens in vitro, but a humoral response to native GBM antigens is not a usual feature of classic acute PSGN.[129] As noted before, circulating antibodies to basement membrane constituents (e.g., type IV collagen) may be found, but these may also be epiphenomena unrelated to the occurrence of nephritis.[102] A variety of streptococcal antigens have been implicated in the pathogenesis of the glomerular lesion, including an extracellular 46-kd plasma binding protein, a 43-kd protein capable of activating the alternative complement pathway, and a cytoplasmic streptococcal antigen (endostreptosin).[74, 130, 130a]

## PATHOLOGY

**Light Microscopy.** Much of the early information accumulated on PSGN was derived from severe or fatal cases, and a much more comprehensive picture has emerged in the last several decades from the widespread use of percutaneous renal biopsy. Renal biopsy specimens taken early in the course of disease reveal a more or less typical but not pathognomonic lesion.[1, 16, 63, 86, 90] The glomeruli are bloodless, hypercellular, and enlarged, and they fill Bowman space. The capillary lumens are occluded by proliferating mesangial and endothelial cells accompanied by a variable degree of infiltration with polymorphonuclear leukocytes, monocytes, and eosinophils within capillary lumens and the mesangium.[1, 131] All glomeruli are affected, and the involvement is more or less uniform among glomeruli. The capillary walls are usually thin and delicate except for occasional irregularities that, after thin sectioning and the use of Masson trichrome or toluidine blue stains, can be seen to be due to the presence of discrete "gumdrop" or "domed" deposits on the epithelial side of the basement membrane.[1, 63] Red blood cells may be seen within Bowman space or in tubule lumens. The term "generalized and diffuse endocapillary proliferative glomerulonephritis" has been used to describe these findings (Fig. 30–1). When infiltration by polymorphonuclear leukocytes is prominent, the qualifying term "exudative" may be added.

Extensive accumulation of cells (monocytes or epithelial cells) in Bowman space leading to the formation of crescents is uncommon and, if present, may be associated with oliguria or progressive renal failure (see later). A few focal

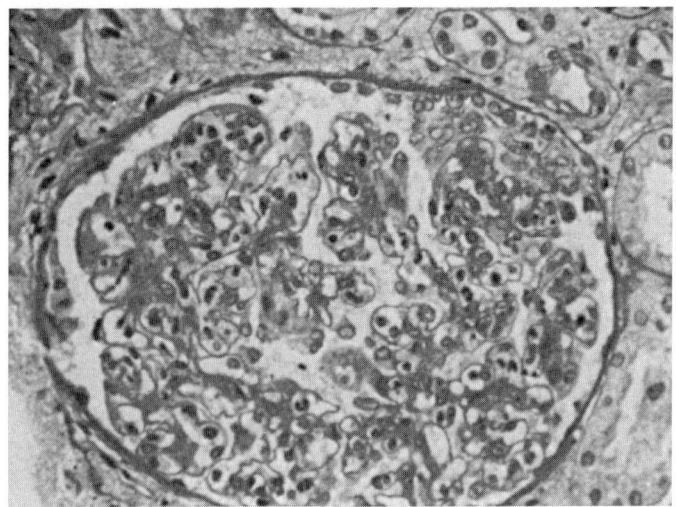

**Figure 30–1.** Light microscopic appearance of poststreptococcal glomerulonephritis. The glomerulus is diffusely hypercellular as a result of the accumulation of numerous neutrophils and monocytes and an increase in intrinsic glomerular cells. A small cellular crescent is present at 1 o'clock. (Periodic acid–Schiff; magnification × 1100.)

and segmental crescents may be seen in biopsy specimens from patients with apparently mild and reversible disease[131]; but when such lesions involve 30% or more of glomeruli, the prognosis is more guarded (see later). At times, the increased cellularity is primarily axial or mesangial, resulting in lobular accentuation of the glomerular tufts.[132] Interstitial edema, focal tubule cell degeneration, and scattered mononuclear cell infiltrates may be seen. The blood vessels are usually normal, although examples of arteriolitis and necrotizing arteritis have been reported.[133] In cases examined by biopsy after clinical resolution, the extreme degree of hypercellularity subsides, and the capillary lumens again become patent. Prominence of the axial zones persists, and at times some diffuse or segmental mesangial proliferation remains.[1, 9] Moreover, nearly every glomerulus retains some abnormal morphologic features at this stage. Progression of pure endocapillary lesions to extensive crescentic disease in a few weeks has been documented.[96, 97, 134–136] On the other hand, resolution of crescents with clinical healing is not

unusual, in contrast to other glomerulopathies with crescents. Rarely, a lesion of membranous glomerulonephritis (MGN) may evolve.[137] The evolution of PSGN in the succeeding months to years is described in the section on course and therapy.

**Electron Microscopy.** The most characteristic and constant finding is the presence of discrete electron-dense, dome-shaped deposits projecting outward from the epithelial side of the basement membrane[1, 16, 63, 138] (Fig. 30–2). These "humps" are the ultrastructural counterpart of the red deposits seen in thin sections stained with Masson trichrome technique. Characteristically, the humps are separated from the basement membrane by a clear zone continuous with the lamina rara externa. The overlying epithelial cell cytoplasm is condensed adjacent to the hump, and the deposits are most often located at the site of the epithelial cell slit pore. These humps are especially frequent in biopsy specimens obtained early in the clinical course but diminish in number after 4 to 8 weeks, when they may still be

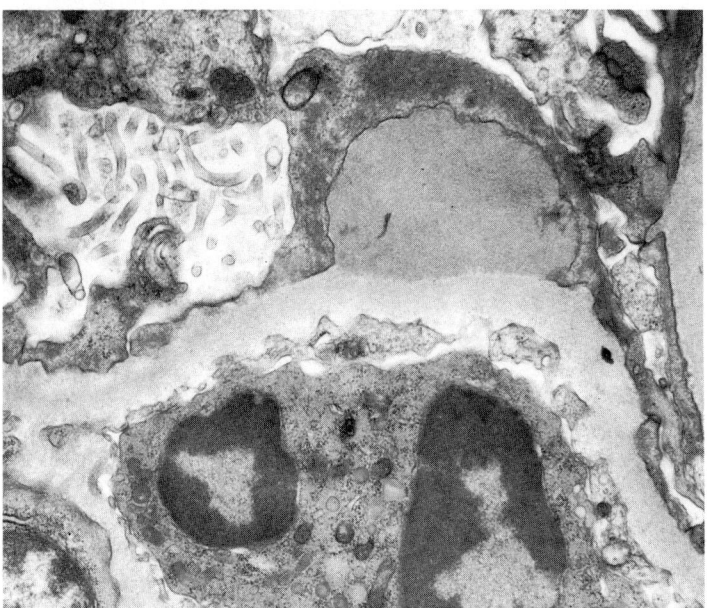

**Figure 30–2.** Electron microscopic appearance of poststreptococcal glomerulonephritis demonstrating a large, hump-shaped subepithelial deposit in the glomerular capillary. The epithelial cell cytoplasm is condensed over the deposit, and the foot processes are effaced. A polymorphonuclear leukocyte is in the capillary lumen. (Magnification × 27,000.)

recognized as lucent rather than dense structures.[139] They may disappear completely or may be incorporated into the basement membranes in a small number of capillaries and persist for several years.[139] Occasionally, the humps are more numerous and involve contiguous areas. These "atypical humps" are more likely to persist and be associated with incomplete clinical resolution.[90] Humps may also be found in other forms of postinfectious glomerulonephritis, infective endocarditis, Schönlein-Henoch purpura, and idiopathic MCGN (types I and II).[1, 140, 141] Subendothelial deposits of varying sizes may also be present in capillary walls with or without subepithelial humps, especially in renal biopsy specimens taken early in the course of disease. There may also be mesangial deposits. Furthermore, short (or, less commonly, long) intramembranous dense deposits may be observed and may bear morphologic similarity with dense deposit disease (see later).

Polymorphonuclear leukocytes may be seen impinging on basement membrane denuded of endothelial cell cytoplasm, particularly adjacent to the aggregated humps on the epithelial side. Epithelial cell foot processes may be focally juxtaposed with obliteration of the slit pore complex, especially in the areas of extensive humps.[1] Mesangial cells are notably increased in number, with an associated increase in matrix.[1] Monocytes may also be identified in the glomerulus, not only in the capillaries but also infiltrating the mesangium, where their presence has been associated with a good prognosis and complete resolution of the abnormalities in a small number of patients.[131]

**Immunofluorescence.** Considering the uniform degree of alterations observed by light microscopy and the presence of electron-dense deposits, the immunofluorescence findings are surprisingly variable (Fig. 30–3). Three patterns are observed, designated starry-sky, mesangial, and garland by Sorger and colleagues.[142–145]

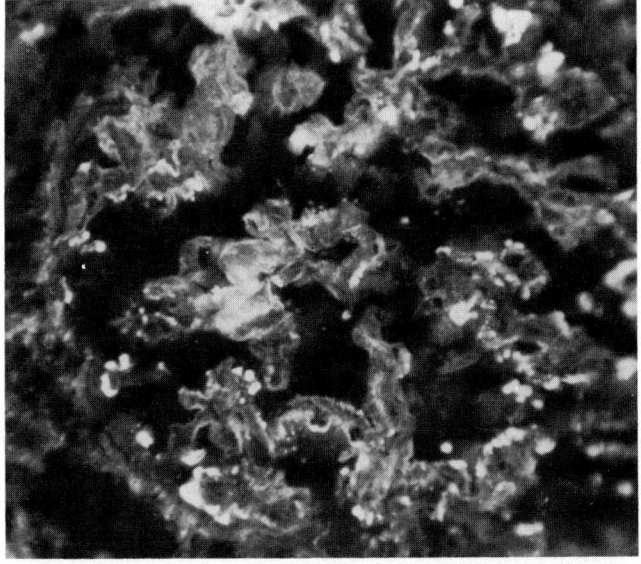

**Figure 30–3.** Immunofluorescence view of poststreptococcal glomerulonephritis. Large, granular, rounded deposits on the capillary wall and minor mesangial deposits are present. This is similar to the starry-sky pattern (see text), although the peripheral deposits are somewhat larger here. (Antihuman IgG; magnification × 1000.)

The starry-sky pattern is observed in about 30% of renal biopsy samples and is characterized by diffuse and irregular, finely granular glomerular capillary wall and mesangial deposits of immunoglobulin or C3. Few or rare large capillary wall deposits are seen. This pattern is observed during the first 2 weeks of the illness and is often associated with marked glomerular endothelial and mesangial hypercellularity and leukocyte infiltration.

The mesangial pattern is seen in about 45% of renal biopsy specimens and is characterized by the predominant deposition of immunoglobulin or C3 in the axial or stalk regions of the glomerulus. Hypercellularity is confined to the mesangium. This pattern is more frequently seen in younger persons and is associated with a favorable long-term prognosis.[143, 144] It is also noted during the subsiding phase of the illness.[144]

The garland pattern is seen in about 25% of renal biopsy specimens and is characterized by decoration of the peripheral glomerular capillary walls with densely packed and contiguous immunoglobulin or C3 deposits and by relatively few mesangial deposits. This pattern often confers a lobular appearance to the glomerular tufts but is occasionally also associated with a membranous lesion.[145] The garland pattern is more frequently seen in males and in patients presenting with heavy proteinuria, and it may be indicative of a poor long-term prognosis.[143, 144] Repeated renal biopsies have disclosed segmental glomerulosclerosis in this group of patients.[146] The peripheral capillary wall deposits may correspond to atypical humps seen on electron microscopy.

IgG is the predominant immunoglobulin deposited, although small amounts of IgM and IgA may be found. C3 is the predominant complement protein deposited, and C1q and C4 are seldom found except in small amounts. C3 deposits may often be more intense than immunoglobulin deposits. Properdin is frequently present. Sometimes the immunofluorescence findings are negative even though electron microscopy demonstrates deposits. A discrepancy between IgG and C3 deposition, a prominent tendency for properdin deposition, and a relative deficiency of C1q in the deposits suggest involvement of the alternative pathway of complement activation.[103–106] Fibrin may be found in a segmental fashion within the mesangium or in association with focal and segmental crescents. Tubule cells may contain intracytoplasmic droplets rich in albumin, fibrin, and other proteins. Granular deposits of immunoglobulins or C3 in mesangial zones have been noted to persist for months or even years despite clinical healing. Deposits of IgG, C3, and fibrin have been observed in the arteries in a biopsy specimen from a patient with necrotizing arteritis and typical PSGN.[133] Electron-dense deposits composed of IgG and C3 have been seen in splenic vessels in a patient with acute PSGN who underwent splenectomy for traumatic rupture.[147] Rarely, a linear pattern of glomerular immunoglobulin deposition may be seen in later biopsies, but there is no convincing evidence that this constitutes the development of anti-GBM antibody.[1] On rare occasions, linear deposits of IgG and C3 on the tubule basement membranes and circulating anti–tubule basement membrane antibodies have developed after typical severe PSGN.[89, 148] The pathogenic mechanisms that led to this peculiar immunologic abnormality are not clear.

## PATHOGENESIS

Although many morphologic, clinical, and serologic features suggest that acute PSGN is an immune complex disease, the precise nature of the antigen-antibody system remains undefined.[1, 70, 73–75, 79, 116, 130, 149–151] Many attempts have been made to localize soluble streptococcal antigenic products in the glomeruli of acute glomerulonephritis, but the results have been negative, inconclusive, or difficult to repeat.[1, 74, 130, 149, 152] Lange, Treser, and co-workers[1, 74, 151–152] have identified an antigen derived from nephritogenic streptococci (endostreptosin) in the mesangium of early but not late biopsy material of patients with typical PSGN. It is noteworthy that this antigen has not yet been identified in the humps so characteristic of this lesion.[74, 151, 152] Immune complexes containing IgG and C3 are often present in the circulation.[1, 117–120] Similar amounts of immune complexes are also found in acute rheumatic fever without nephritis or in streptococcal impetigo without nephritis.[70] Streptococcal extracellular antigens have been detected in circulating immune complexes of patients with PSGN and acute rheumatic fever.[70, 79] Unique streptococcal antigens associated with nephritogenic strains of streptococci were found in the immune complexes associated with PSGN but not acute rheumatic fever. McIntosh, Rodriguez-Iturbe, and co-workers[1, 150, 153] have suggested that the complexes are composed of an altered form of autologous IgG and an IgG to these altered or neoantigenic determinants. They further suggest that a streptococcal exoenzyme (? sialidase) is responsible for the alteration in autologous IgG. Circulating antibodies to native constituents of the glomerular capillary wall may occasionally occur in PSGN. The possibility exists that an antigen derived from the streptococcus (endostreptosin or other cationic cytoplasmic antigens)[74, 130] may bind to glomerular structures in vivo and serve as a "planted antigen" for development in situ of immune complexes.[77, 130] Streptococcal streptokinase does not appear to be involved.[75] Using lectin binding, Mosquera and Rodriguez-Iturbe[154] found that there is sialic acid–depleted material in glomeruli early in the course of PSGN, suggesting loss of anionic sites in capillaries and mesangium. The role of cell-mediated immunity in the glomerular injury remains uncertain; however, monocytes are frequently found infiltrating the mesangium in acute cases, and cell-mediated immunity to altered GBM antigens may be demonstrable in vitro.[129]

## COURSE AND PROGNOSIS

The immediate prognosis for acute PSGN is favorable, especially in children. Elderly patients also appear to have a favorable short-term evolution.[83] With modern management, less than 1% of pediatric patients die in the acute stages of the illness.[1, 18, 89, 131, 155] The long-term evolution and prognosis of acute PSGN, however, remain controversial.[1, 17, 18, 155–165] Unfortunately, in many studies, the documentation of streptococcal etiology has not been pursued with the thoroughness necessary to achieve a homogeneous population for study.[68] Studies of the prognosis of acute PSGN have been undertaken in connection with epidemics such as those occurring on the Red Lake Indian Reservation in Minnesota in 1953[56] and again in 1966[66] or in geographic areas with a high prevalence of epidemic and endemic PSGN such as Trinidad[1, 65, 158] or Maracaibo, Venezuela.[165] Many of these studies involved PSGN predominantly due to skin infections with type 49 group A streptococci and were associated with glomerulonephritis, usually of a mild nature, in susceptible children and young adults.[66] Long-term follow-up of pediatric patients with epidemic or endemic PSGN has revealed a paucity of chronic sequelae.[68, 155, 158, 159, 166] Apparent failure to recover from acute glomerulonephritis is also uncommon in sporadic cases of PSGN studied in some children, although complete disappearance of urinary abnormalities may not occur for 2 years or more.[1, 17, 159, 166] The prognosis for full recovery is less certain when severe nephrotic syndrome is present at initial discovery.[156] Persistence of albuminuria is a marker of underlying renal disease.[167]

It would appear that in the majority of pediatric patients with well-documented sporadic or epidemic acute PSGN in whom there is no evidence of pre-existing renal disease, persistent heavy proteinuria, or extensive crescentic glomerular lesions at the onset, the prognosis is excellent, at least for the intermediate term of up to 10 to 20 years.[68, 155, 158, 159, 165–167] An initial biopsy revealing extensive crescents by light microscopy, atypical humps by electron microscopy, or a garland lesion by immunofluorescence may indicate a less favorable prognosis especially in the face of persisting or worsening proteinuria or hypertension.[143–145] Although the complete disappearance of urinary abnormalities may be delayed for several years, ultimate recovery can usually be expected.[167] Serial or sequential biopsies may display mild segmental glomerular abnormalities and mild persistent mesangial prominence with immunoglobulin or C3 deposition. Whether the outcome in children observed for two or three decades or more will remain essentially benign remains to be seen. The studies cited earlier would seem to indicate that at least for children with disease severe enough to require hospitalization, the outcome may not always be benign.[89, 156]

The situation in adults appears to be different from that in children. Jennings and Earle,[132] in a classic study published in 1961, described 36 adults with sporadic acute glomerulonephritis presumed to be streptococcal. After short-term follow-up, nonhealing occurred in 12, predominantly among men. In many of these patients, the documentation of recent streptococcal infection was incomplete, and C3 levels were not determined. Biopsies that revealed prominent mesangial thickening and hypercellularity, often with lobular expansion, were associated with nonhealing. Some of these cases could possibly have been what is now recognized as MCGN, mesangial proliferative glomerulonephritis, or IgA nephropathy (Berger disease, see later). The long-term prognosis of PSGN in elderly persons may be poor.[83] Melby and colleagues[168] found a higher mortality rate in elderly patients, especially if they were dialysis dependent. Such patients may be predisposed to more extensive crescent formation and experience more problems with circulatory congestion. Patients without crescents have a favorable short-term outlook despite markedly abnormal initial GFR values.[83]

Many other studies have also demonstrated the development of histologic and clinical "chronicity" after acute glomerulonephritis in adults, although the extent has varied from survey to survey, and in many reports a poststreptococcal cause was not unequivocally documented.[1, 160] Baldwin and co-workers[89, 163, 164] have reported the results of a long-term study of patients with acute glomerulonephritis of presumed poststreptococcal etiology, 70% of whom were adults. Many were black or of Puerto Rican extraction. Nephrotic syndrome was present initially in 20%, and the serum creatinine concentration exceeded 2 mg/dL in more than half the patients. Thus, these patients were in general afflicted with a more severe form of acute glomerulonephritis. After the initial episode, proteinuria declined such that at the end of 2 years, only about 20% of patients observed had abnormal protein excretion. However, by the end of the ninth year of follow-up, the frequency of abnormal proteinuria had nearly doubled. There was a suggestion of a similar pattern for the evolution of hypertension. Serial renal biopsies revealed a slow resolution of endocapillary (mesangial) proliferation, but a significant increase in the number of sclerotic glomeruli developed with time. This was due largely to an increase in the number of obsolescent glomeruli, but in addition, some glomeruli were affected by a segmental sclerosing process. Thirty percent to 40% of the patients observed for 5 years or more had some clinical evidence of persisting renal disease, and a mildly abnormal blood urea nitrogen concentration or creatinine level was observed in 20% to 30%. Progression to end-stage renal failure was documented in several instances.[163, 164] The development of renal failure or nephrotic syndrome subsequent to complete clinical recovery from the initial episode was rare. Many normotensive patients had exaggerated natriuresis in response to an acute saline load, similar to that seen in benign essential hypertension. Volume depletion with salt restriction did not correct the exaggerated natriuresis observed.[169] However, this phenomenon has not been confirmed by other investigators.[170] The late progression of disease observed by Baldwin and co-workers[163, 164] could have been a manifestation of nonimmunologic factors initiated early in the course of the severe disease (e.g., glomerular capillary hypertension) and persisting throughout the later course (see Chapter 44). As noted before, the garland pattern of immunofluorescence in renal biopsy specimens from patients with PSGN is associated with a more chronic course and persistent proteinuria.[143–145] The mesangial and starry-sky patterns demonstrate a more favorable course in the long term.[143–145]

In contradistinction, in long-term follow-up of cases of acute PSGN in Trinidad (up to 20 years), predominantly in adults, a low frequency of clinical features of chronicity (i.e., abnormal urinalysis, hypertension, or decreased renal function) has been noted.[1, 158, 161, 162] Furthermore, a study from South Australia, with a high percentage of adult patients observed for an extended period, indicated that recovery from PSGN in adults is the rule even though complete histologic and clinical healing may take as long as 9 years. Only 4 of 57 cases demonstrated progressive disease in this well-studied group. Patients with severe lesions on initial biopsies, especially crescents, may not fare as well.[17]

In summary, it would appear that ultimate recovery from sporadic acute PSGN in adults is less predictable than that in children, especially when associated with initially severe impairment of renal function, persistent proteinuria, or nephrotic syndrome. Initial renal biopsy in severe cases may provide information of prognostic significance. The development of crescentic glomerulonephritis does seem to be more common in adults, but this may be a matter of selection. Elderly patients with acute PSGN appear to have a poor long-term prognosis.[1, 168] The long-term prognosis in acute PSGN occurring in association with epidemics appears to be more favorable than for cases occurring in a sporadic fashion. For some patients carrying the diagnosis of chronic (nonspecific) sclerosing glomerulonephritis who present in end-stage renal failure, the disease may have been initiated by a remote episode of acute PSGN. Perhaps such patients might be recognized by a persistent high level of antibody to endostreptosin or other streptococcal cell membrane antigens.[74] Because many cases of PSGN go unrecognized owing to their mild nature, it is easy to understand why a history of a distinct episode of acute nephritis may be infrequently obtained from such patients. Finally, even with the information provided by renal biopsy available, it may still be difficult to be certain whether serologic or bacteriologic evidence of recent streptococcal infection was causally related to disease or simply a coincidental finding. Recurrence of true PSGN is uncommon.[171, 172]

## PREVENTION AND TREATMENT

The prevention of acute PSGN depends on development of means to reliably induce long-term protective immunity to the group A streptococcus or alternatively on the eradication of the organism in the population. Neither seems feasible at present. However, with increased knowledge of the biochemistry and immunology of the group A streptococcus, the development of a protective vaccine having few or no side effects or hazards should be possible. For the moment, antimicrobial therapy (penicillin, erythromycin, or azithromycin) of affected persons and their immediate families and personal contacts is all that is available to limit the spread of infection. Personal hygiene, of course, is an additional important factor in preventing the spread of cutaneous streptococcal infection. Whether early antimicrobial therapy of streptococcal pharyngitis will reduce the risk of development of PSGN, as it does for acute rheumatic fever, is not yet clearly known. On the basis of the limited data available, it does not appear likely that early antimicrobial therapy of streptococcal pharyngitis will have a significant impact on the subsequent likelihood of developing PSGN, but it may attenuate its severity.[1] Widespread use of antibiotics and better hygiene have greatly reduced the occurrence of PSGN, at least in developed countries.

The treatment of acute PSGN is largely symptomatic.[18] Prolonged bed rest is of no value and does not seem to improve or alter the long-term prognosis.[1] Fluid and sodium restriction and loop diuretics (e.g., furosemide) are valuable in the treatment of patients with circulatory congestion, hypertension, and edema. $K^+$-sparing diuretics (e.g., amiloride, spironolactone, triamterene) are contraindicated. Antihypertensive agents are occasionally required. Hydralazine, $Ca^{2+}$ channel blockers, and nitroprusside are the most useful agents. Because plasma renin activity levels are reduced, β-blocking agents (e.g., propranolol, metoprolol) or angiotensin-converting enzyme (ACE) inhibition would not be expected to be of great value alone but may be useful combined with vasodilators and diuretics in cases with severe hypertension. Nonetheless, captopril has been shown to improve GFR and lower blood pressure in patients with PSGN.[173] Digitalis glycosides should not be given unless organic heart disease is unequivocally present or there is pulmonary venous congestion refractory both to lowering the systemic arterial blood pressure and to adequate diuresis. In patients unresponsive to diuretics, hemodialysis, hemofiltration, or peritoneal dialysis should be considered. Protein intake may be temporarily restricted in azotemic patients. Hyperkalemia may be treated with ion exchange resins or dialysis.[1]

Most patients with typical disease uncomplicated by crescentic involvement (see later) can be expected to undergo a diuresis within a week or so of the onset of illness, although longer periods of impaired function with ultimate complete recovery have been observed.[1] Prolonged severe oliguria or anuria and persisting massive proteinuria are ominous signs; under these conditions, a renal biopsy may be indicated to assess prognosis or the presence of unsuspected underlying primary (not poststreptococcal) or systemic glomerular disease, such as SLE, MCGN, or vasculitis. Steroids and cytotoxic agents have no proven role in the management of acute PSGN and may be harmful. Whether early treatment of the uncommon poststreptococcal crescentic glomerulonephritis with combined steroid, cytotoxic, anticoagulant, or intensive plasma exchange is of any benefit remains to be tested in a definitive fashion; however, anecdotal cases treated with these regimens have shown promising results (see later).[174]

## Noninfectious Diseases That Evoke Acute Glomerulonephritis

Multisystem and hereditary diseases that may evoke a clinical picture resembling PSGN are discussed in Chapter 31. These diseases include SLE, Schönlein-Henoch pur-

pura, various forms of systemic vasculitis, and Goodpasture disease. Idiopathic diseases with primary glomerular involvement that may be associated at times with the clinical features of acute glomerulonephritis are discussed in later sections of this chapter. These diseases include MCGN, IgA nephropathy (Berger disease), focal and segmental proliferative glomerulonephritis, and mesangial proliferative glomerulonephritis. Nonglomerular diseases evoking a syndrome resembling acute glomerulonephritis are discussed in the relevant chapters. These include acute hypersensitivity interstitial nephritis, hemolytic-uremic syndrome, thrombotic thrombocytopenic purpura, atheroembolic renal disease, and occasionally malignant hypertension. Cases of acute glomerulonephritis secondary to irradiation of solid tumors,[54] Guillain-Barré-Strohl syndrome,[52] and self-administered diphtheria-pertussis-tetanus vaccine have been reported.[175]

## RAPIDLY PROGRESSIVE GLOMERULONEPHRITIS

Much confusion exists regarding classification and terminology of the group of disorders having in common features of glomerulonephritis with a fulminant, progressively downhill course, often accompanied by oliguria or anuria. Subacute glomerulonephritis was the term used at one time to emphasize the protracted course and to contrast it with the ordinarily self-limited course of acute glomerulonephritis. Ellis introduced the term "rapidly progressive nephritis" as a variant of type I (acute) nephritis. Because patients who manifest this clinical behavior often but not invariably display extensive accumulation of cells within Bowman space (crescents), the pathologic terms "crescentic" or "extracapillary proliferative glomerulonephritis" have often been used to identify this clinical syndrome (Fig. 30–4). Conversely, the clinical term "rapidly progressive glomerulonephritis" has been used to describe the biopsy picture of crescentic glomerulonephritis.[1, 176–180] Because some patients with the clinical picture of RPGN may be found on biopsy to have diffuse endocapillary proliferative

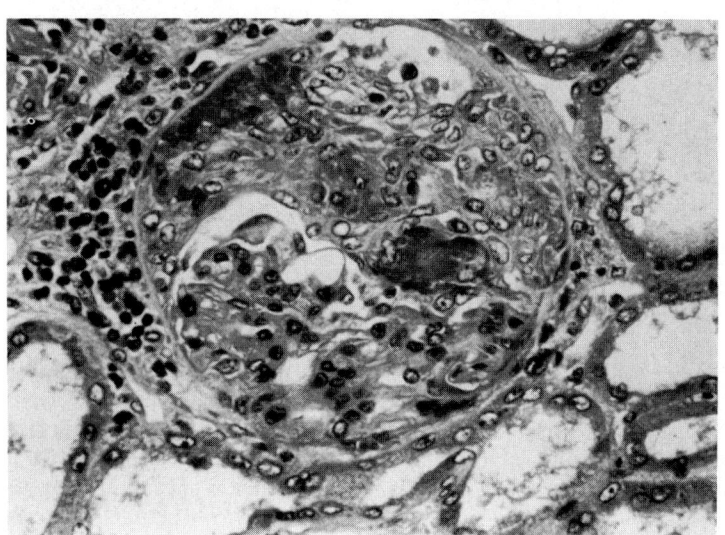

**Figure 30–4.** Light microscopic appearance of crescentic glomerulonephritis. A large crescent, composed of mononuclear cells and darkly stained, admixed fibrin, compresses the glomerular tuft (below). This form of injury is commonly observed in anti-GBM nephritis and in necrotizing vasculitis. (Hematoxylin-eosin; magnification × 500.)

or necrotizing glomerulonephritis with scanty crescentic lesions, it would seem preferable to avoid the use of a clinical term to describe pathologic appearances. Further difficulties arise when some disease entities not primarily involving the glomeruli masquerade clinically as an RPGN syndrome (e.g., thrombotic microangiopathies, atheroembolic renal disease, acute tubule necrosis, acute interstitial nephritis). Finally, some patients with extensive glomerular involvement with crescents may have a prolonged course (up to 10 years) before end-stage renal failure ensues.[176, 180]

In this section, RPGN is used to refer to the clinical syndrome of rapid and progressive decline in renal function occurring in association with features of glomerulonephritis (dysmorphic hematuria and glomerular proteinuria), which without treatment usually results in end-stage renal failure in a matter of weeks or months. However, with aggressive treatment, the prognosis for patients with RPGN has greatly improved.[181]

Overall, RPGN is an uncommon clinical syndrome. The estimated incidence is 7 cases/1,000,000 population per year.[179] Nevertheless, there are wide geographic differences in apparent incidence, and outbreaks of ''miniepidemics'' have occurred on a limited basis.

The glomerular disease is characterized principally, but not exclusively, by extensive crescent formation (see Fig. 30–4). The cells of the crescents are now believed to be derived from blood-borne monocytes (macrophages) that have migrated into Bowman space through areas of localized capillary damage,[177, 182] from surrounding renal interstitium, and from parietal epithelial cells lining Bowman space.[177, 183, 184] Epithelial cells predominate early in the course of events and when Bowman capsule is intact; monocytes, macrophages, and T cells may predominate later and when Bowman capsule is disrupted. Initial events involved in crescent formation occur at the capillary wall, where antibody deposition or formation/deposition of immune complexes activates intercellular adhesion molecules (e.g., intercellular adhesion molecule-1). Subsequently, activated monocytes and leukocytes express ligands, localize in the capillary wall, and elaborate enzymes and reactive oxygen species that lead to capillary wall disruption.[186] Fibrinogen escapes into the urinary space through large defects (gaps) in the capillary wall.[178, 183, 185] Synthesis of hyaluronate locally may activate T cells through a hyaluronate receptor (CD44) on their surface.[187] Activated cells elaborate interleukin-1, interleukin-2, tumor necrosis factor-α, and transforming growth factor-β. Transforming growth factor-β may stimulate collagen production and inhibit plasminogen activators, thus retarding local fibrinolysis.[186, 187] Activated monocytes may express a membrane-bound procoagulant factor (e.g., prothrombinase), promoting fibrin polymerization.[188–192] Fibrin polymers can be demonstrated between the cells and are free in the urinary space[192, 193] (Fig. 30–5); later, collagen and fibroblastic cells can be seen. The fibroblasts may originate from the periglomerular interstitium and gain access to Bowman space through defects in Bowman capsule. The leakage of fibrinogen and its polymerization into fibrin by thrombin-dependent and thrombin-independent mechanisms may be crucial to the development of extracapillary proliferation and transformation of monocytes. The organization of the crescent

into a fibrous scar may be dependent on migration of fibroblasts from interstitium into Bowman space. Monocytes may participate in this process by secretion of monokines influencing fibroblastic behavior.[194]

A classification of RPGN with extensive crescentic glomerular involvement is given in Table 30–3. As shown, four broad categories of disease are included, namely, infectious disease, multisystem disease, drug-induced disease, and primary renal disease. The infectious, multisystem, and drug-induced diseases are discussed in Chapter 31. Primary forms of RPGN are of two general types: in one, crescentic disease occurs de novo; in the other, crescents are superimposed on another chronic primary glomerular disease process. The former is discussed here, and the latter is discussed in other sections related to the primary underlying disorder. With the discovery of the importance of certain autoantibodies (e.g., anti-GBM antibodies and antineutrophil cytoplasmic autoantibodies [ANCAs]) in various forms of crescentic glomerulonephritis, many cases previously regarded as idiopathic could now be classified according to a presumed pathogenetic mechanism or associated serologic finding (see later). In addition, the underlying immunopathologic appearances provided further clues to the heterogeneity of RPGN. Thus, anti-GBM antibodies with linear deposits of IgG (and no extrarenal manifestations, such as pulmonary hemorrhage) formed one group (type I). Granular deposits of IgG without anti-GBM antibody or ANCA production formed another group (type II). Scanty deposits of IgG with concomitant ANCA formed another group (type III). Linear deposits of IgG with both anti-GBM antibodies and ANCA formed another group (type IV). Scanty deposits of IgG with neither anti-GBM antibodies nor ANCA formed a final group (type V). Because nearly all primary crescentic glomerulonephritis can be categorized into one of the foregoing subsets, idiopathic crescentic glomerulonephritis may not be a truly relevant or appropriate term. In fact, some doubt the existence of a true idiopathic category.[195, 196] Although the subsets have many clinical similarities, they are discussed separately. Patients with

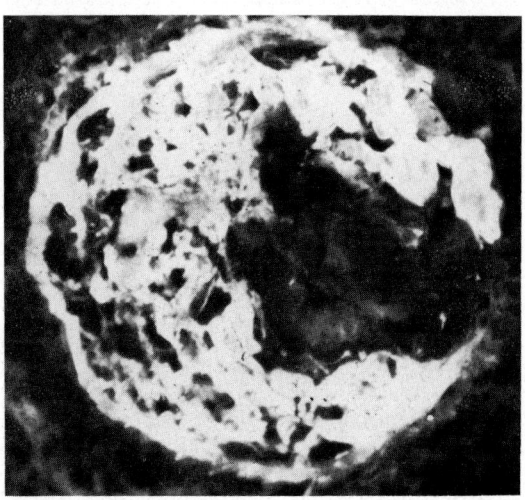

**Figure 30–5.** Immunofluorescence microscopic view of crescentic glomerulonephritis revealing extensive deposits of fibrinogen and fibrin polymers in Bowman space. (Antihuman fibrinogen; magnification × 500.)

**TABLE 30–3. Classification of Disorders Associated with Extensive Glomerular Crescents and Rapidly Progressive Glomerulonephritis**

**Primary Glomerular Diseases**
Primary diffuse crescentic glomerulonephritis
   Type I: anti-GBM–mediated disease, *without* pulmonary
      hemorrhage (with anti-GBM)
   Type II: immune complex–associated disease (without anti-GBM
      or ANCA)*
   Type III: pauci-immune (with ANCA)†
   Type IV: mixed pattern (with anti-GBM and ANCA)
   Type V: pauci-immune (without ANCA or anti-GBM)
Superimposed on another primary glomerular disease
   Mesangiocapillary glomerulonephritis (especially type II)
   Membranous glomerulonephritis (with or without anti-GBM)
   IgA nephropathy
   Fibrillary and immunotactoid glomerulonephritis
   Focal sclerosis (rare)

**Associated with Infectious Disease‡**
Poststreptococcal glomerulonephritis
Infective endocarditis
Visceral abscesses
Hepatitis B and C
*Mycoplasma* infection
Histoplasmosis
Influenza (?)

**Associated with Multisystem Disease‡**
Systemic lupus erythematosus
Goodpasture disease (anti-GBM *with* pulmonary hemorrhage)
Schönlein-Henoch purpura
Systemic polyangiitis
   Microscopic polyangiitis (with ANCA)
   Wegener granulomatosis (with ANCA)
   Churg-Strauss syndrome
   Other variants
Mixed (IgG/IgM) cryoimmunoglobulinemia (hepatitis C)
Relapsing polychondritis
Carcinoma (lung, bladder, prostate)
Lymphoma

**Associated with Medications‡**
Allopurinol
Rifampin
D-Penicillamine
Bucillamine
Hydralazine

*ANCA = antineutrophil cytoplasmic antibody.
†May be a forme fruste of microscopic polyangiitis. Most patients have ANCA.
‡See also Chapter 31 for details on associations with infections, multisystem diseases, and medication.

multisystem involvement, including pulmonary hemorrhage, are discussed in more detail in Chapter 31.

## Primary Diffuse Crescentic Glomerulonephritis

Primary diffuse crescentic glomerulonephritis refers to a condition that reveals extensive (more than 50%, most often more than 70%) involvement of glomeruli with crescents, with or without accompanying glomerular tuft hypercellularity, and that manifests progressive deterioration of renal function in days, weeks, or a few months rather than years or decades.[178, 185, 197–199] Clear-cut evidence of a multisystem,

drug-induced, or infectious disease is lacking. Without therapy, less than 10% to 20% of such patients will escape the necessity of regular dialysis therapy within 6 months of onset of disease. The diagnosis can be established only by excluding known causes of this disorder. The exclusion of these known causes may be difficult, because infectious origins may be covert and the manifestations of multisystem disease may be subtle or develop only well after the initial manifestation of renal disease.[199] Whereas the term primary crescentic glomerulonephritis has been applied to this group of disorders, it should be recognized that the pathogenetic mechanisms that underlie the clinicopathologic group known as primary crescentic glomerulonephritis are heterogeneous.[178, 185, 195–206] A tentative classification, based on pathogenesis or associated disease states, is given in Table 30–3. Overall, primary crescentic glomerulonephritis is an uncommon disorder. Hydrocarbon exposure may be a risk factor in the development of the disorder.[207]

## PRIMARY CRESCENTIC GLOMERULONEPHRITIS, TYPE I (Anti–Glomerular Basement Membrane Antibody–Mediated Crescentic Glomerulonephritis Without Pulmonary Hemorrhage)

This subset is identified on the basis of evidence of antibodies reacting with GBM—either free in the circulation, as detected by immunoserologic assays, or bound to glomeruli.[1, 178, 185, 195–205] The latter can be suspected on the basis of an "ultralinear" deposition of IgG (or rarely IgA)[206] on GBM, sometimes accompanied by IgG (or rarely IgA) deposited in a similar pattern on tubule basement membrane.[1, 204] The anti-GBM nature of the immunoglobulin deposits may be proved by elution of specific antibody from tissue samples, although this is rarely necessary in clinical practice.[1, 200, 204] Depending on the series examined, this subset constitutes 10% to 20% of the overall group of cases defined as primary diffuse crescentic glomerulonephritis. Patients with anti-GBM antibody–mediated disease accompanied by overt pulmonary hemorrhage are categorized separately as having Goodpasture disease (discussed in Chapter 31).

**Clinical Findings.** The patients tend to be young or middle aged and male, although with the introduction and wide use of immunoserologic tests for anti-GBM antibody, more older persons and females are being recognized and the male/female ratio approaches 1.3:1 (see Chapters 29 and 31).[1, 177, 178, 185, 195–205] Two peaks of prevalence relative to age are seen: ages 21 to 30 and ages 51 to 70 years. Males are usually younger than females at onset.[214] The primary form of anti-GBM antibody–associated glomerulonephritis without pulmonary hemorrhage is seen more often in older women (see also Goodpasture disease, Chapter 31). The disorder appears to be rare in Asian and in Afro-Caribbean persons. A preceding upper respiratory or influenza-like illness and recent exposure to hydrocarbon fumes have commonly been noted,[207] but the etiologic significance of such findings is poorly understood at present; they may be found in many patients with other forms of renal disease.[1, 209] The onset may occasionally be abrupt and in many respects resembles acute glomerulonephritis except that severe oliguria or even anuria is more common. In most instances, the onset is insidious, with presenting complaints mainly referable to the development of uremia or fluid retention.[1, 204, 205, 208, 210] Arthralgias may occasionally be observed. Fever, myalgias, and abdominal pain are other less commonly observed features.[1, 204, 205, 208, 210] When present, vasculitis should be suspected (see Chapter 31). Gastrointestinal complaints or neurologic disturbances are noted in rare instances.[204] Hypertension is typically mild. The absence of overt pulmonary hemorrhage serves to distinguish this group from Goodpasture disease (see Chapter 31); however, because pulmonary bleeding in Goodpasture disease may be mild and evanescent and easily overlooked, many cases initially categorized as primary crescentic glomerulonephritis (type I) may ultimately behave more like Goodpasture disease. Careful inspection of high-quality chest radiographs, examination of sputum for hemosiderin-laden macrophages, serial measurement of the alveolar-arterial oxygen gradient, and scanning of pulmonary parenchyma after parenteral administration of $^{59}$Fe-loaded erythrocytes may be of value in detecting covert pulmonary hemorrhage[1, 201] (see also Chapter 31). Ewan and co-workers[211] also described the ratio of pulmonary uptake of carbon monoxide to the pulmonary clearance of $C^{15}O$ as being of particular value for the detection and serial evaluation of intra-alveolar hemorrhage. Smoking cigarettes may provoke pulmonary hemorrhage,[212] as may intercurrent infection,[213] cocaine use, and hydrocarbon inhalation.[209]

**Laboratory Findings.** The urine usually reveals dysmorphic red blood cells and red blood cell casts but on occasion may appear more benign than would be predicted from the clinical course. Although massive proteinuria may be seen, the features of overt nephrotic syndrome are not common.[204, 205, 208, 210] GFR is initially decreased and progressively declines, often with appalling rapidity. The serum levels of $CH_{50}$, C3, and C1q are usually normal (see Table 30–2), although there may be a modest decline in C3 with the onset of renal failure and treatment with dialysis, and C1q or $CH_{50}$ may occasionally be elevated.[1, 106]

Circulating anti-GBM antibody can be demonstrated early in the course of the majority of patients (more than 95%) when radioimmunoassay is used.[1, 204, 205, 208, 210, 214, 215] The anti-GBM antibody is most often the IgG class, but rarely it may be IgA. IgG1 subclass is found more commonly in males; IgG4 subclass is found more often in females.[216] The antibody reacts with a 25- to 27-kd antigen sequestered within the globular, noncollagenous (NC1) domain of the α3-chain of type IV collagen. Ninety percent of the anti-GBM antibody is directed to this epitope, but small amounts of antibody to other portions of the type IV collagen molecule or to other extracellular matrix antigens may be detected. The dominant epitope is a 36–amino acid segment of the COOH-terminal portion of the noncollagenous domain of the α3-chain of type IV collagen.[204, 217, 218] This epitope is present in highest concentrations in the GBM but is also found on tubule basement membrane, alveolar basement membrane, and choroid plexus[4, 215–219] (see Chapter 29). Antibodies to entactin (nidogen) may be seen in patients who do not have the classic anti-α3, type

IV collagen antibodies.[219] Mildly increased ASO titers may be found in about 30% of cases without other evidence of a streptococcal cause.[208] Human leukocyte antigen (HLA) DR2 is found in more than 85% of patients.[14, 220] The *DRB1\*1501* and *DRB1\*0602* alleles are also frequently associated with this disease.[221] Circulating immune complexes, cryoimmunoglobulins, and antinuclear antibodies are absent. ANCAs are found to coexist in some patients (less than 30%).[215, 222] These patients are discussed with primary crescentic glomerulonephritis type IV and also in Chapter 31. Thrombocytopenia, thrombocytosis, or microangiopathic hemolytic anemia may be seen occasionally. Fibrin degradation products are frequently elevated in the urine and serum, the latter as much a consequence of decreased elimination as of increased production.

**Pathology**

*Light Microscopy.* The most striking feature is the accumulation of cells within Bowman space (i.e., crescents), usually affecting 50% or more of the glomeruli[1, 177, 178, 185, 201–205, 208] (see Fig. 30–4). In severe cases, virtually every glomerulus may be affected. The glomerular tufts may be compressed by the circumferential collection of cells filling Bowman space. The cellular composition of the crescent depends on the stage of evolution of disease and whether Bowman capsule is intact.[223] When the capsule has been disrupted, monocytes and macrophages may predominate, and interstitial fibroblasts may migrate into the proliferating cells and participate in the organization of the crescent into a fibrous scar. When the capsule is intact, epithelial cells (perhaps of parietal origin) are the predominant cell type.[223] T lymphocytes may also be found in the crescents.[224] Mitoses, monocytes, giant cells, and polymorphonuclear leukocytes may be seen in the crescent.[225–228] Silver stains may reveal segmental and extensive destruction of the glomerular and Bowman capsule basement membranes.[229] Material having the tinctorial properties of fibrin may occasionally be seen in Bowman space, but this is usually not striking. There may be variable amounts of periglomerular inflammation. Organization with fibroblasts and collagen deposition occurs, and the crescent becomes increasingly less cellular. With time, there is usually progressive global glomerular sclerosis and fibrosis. This process of organization of the crescent and glomerular obsolescence can occur in as brief a period as a few weeks.[225] However, in an unpredictable fashion, the crescents may resolve without cellular residue.[90, 96] The glomerular tuft may not show any striking degree of proliferation of the endocapillary cells.[1, 95] Such proliferation is much more a characteristic feature of postinfectious nephritis, SLE, Schönlein-Henoch purpura, vasculitis, IgA nephropathy, and infective endocarditis (see Chapter 31). The glomerular tuft may show some areas of fibrinoid necrosis, polymorphonuclear leukocyte infiltration, and collapse of capillary loops. Arteritis is not usually seen but may be found associated with SLE, necrotizing vasculitis, cryoglobulinemia, Schönlein-Henoch purpura, and rarely anti-GBM disease.[230] Red blood cell casts may be seen in tubules that show a variable degree of alteration, including proliferation of proximal tubule cells. There may be an associated extensive tubulointerstitial nephritis, particularly, but not exclusively, when immunofluorescence studies reveal extensive linear immunoglobulin or complement deposits along tubule basement membranes.[231, 232]

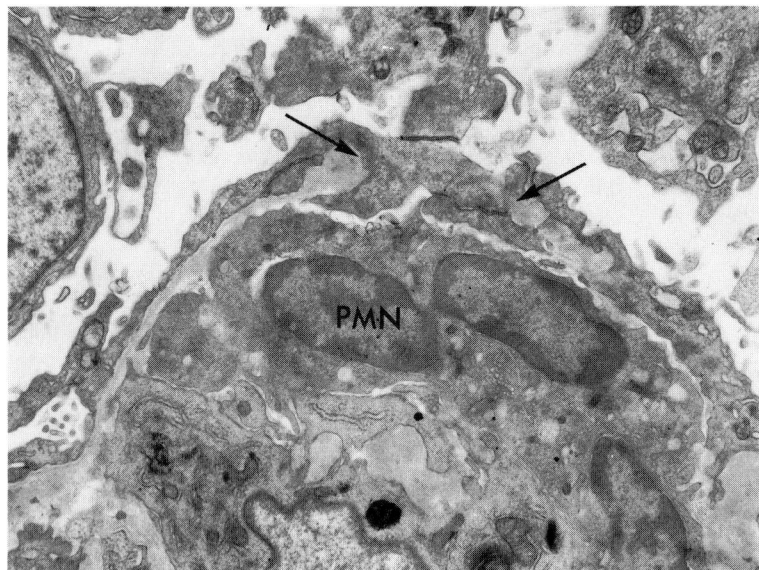

**Figure 30–6.** Electron microscopic appearance of crescentic glomerulonephritis. The capillary wall shows large discontinuities in basement membrane *(between arrows).* A polymorphonuclear leukocyte (PMN) fills the lumen and is directly apposed to the remaining basement membrane. It is through such "gaps" that fibrin is thought to gain access to the urinary space and initiate crescent formation. (Magnification × 13,600.)

***Electron Microscopy.*** The major ultrastructural alterations include widened and subendothelial zones of capillary walls, segmental detachment of endothelial cells, and fibrin in capillary lumens and directly apposed to basement membranes and in the urinary space intermixed with the cells, but in the crescent, capillary collapse involving a portion or all of the tuft may be observed. Gaps or focal discontinuities are often found along the GBM (Fig. 30–6) or Bowman capsule membrane.[229] Bonsib[233] has elegantly demonstrated the widespread nature of discontinuities using scanning electron microscopy. It is these gaps that allow migration of circulating monocytes and interstitial fibroblasts into Bowman space.[1, 185, 204–209, 228, 229] A few cases with widely spaced electron-dense deposits have been seen.[219, 234]

***Immunofluorescence.*** Immunofluorescence findings are valuable in distinguishing the underlying pathogenetic mechanisms involved.[1, 185, 204–209, 231, 232] In the type I lesion under discussion, the glomerular capillaries reveal a smooth, linear deposit of IgG (or rarely IgA), often but not invariably accompanied by C3 deposition in a similar pattern[1, 185, 231, 232, 235] (Fig. 30–7). In severely damaged glomeruli, it may be difficult to recognize the linear pattern, and C3 deposits may become irregular or even granular. There are some patients whose biopsies reveal both linear IgG and clear-cut granular C3, the latter associated with discrete electron-dense deposits. In addition, the linear IgG deposits may evolve into a granular pattern, giving rise to confusion with other types of primary RPGN.[234] Granular deposits may also be associated with antientactin autoantibodies.[219]

This ultralinear pattern of IgG deposition is identical to that seen in patients with Goodpasture disease (see also Chapters 29 and 31). Linear deposits of IgG with or without C3 may also be found along tubule basement membrane.[232] Regardless of the pattern of IgG or C3 deposition, fibrin-related antigens are found frequently in the crescent and in Bowman space or in tubule lumens[1, 193] (see Fig. 30–5). The relative paucity of factor VIII in the crescents (at least in biopsy specimens taken late in the course of the disease)

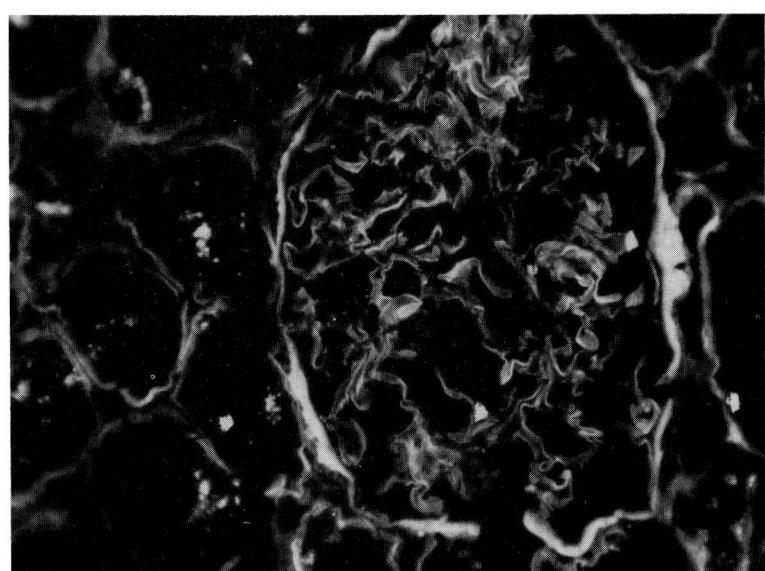

**Figure 30–7.** Immunofluorescence view of anti-GBM nephritis. Linear fixation of IgG along the glomerular basement membrane, as well as many tubule and Bowman capsule basement membranes, can be observed. (Antihuman IgG; magnification × 1000.)

despite marked deposition of fibrin-related antigens suggests that fibrinogen polymerization may not always be the consequence of the intrinsic pathway of coagulation or, alternatively, that fibrinolysis is impaired in Bowman space with early resolution of factor VIII deposits and persistence of fibrin.[193]

**Pathogenesis.** The diffuse linear IgG pattern is indicative of an anti-GBM pathogenesis[177, 185, 204–209, 236] (see Chapters 29 and 31). This may also occur in association with pulmonary hemorrhage (Goodpasture disease). The reason for the failure of development of overt pulmonary hemorrhage in this subgroup is not at all clear. The circulating and tissue-bound anti-GBM antibody reacts in vitro with alveolar basement membrane as it does in patients with fully developed Goodpasture disease. The autoantibody reacts with epitopes on the α3-chain of type IV collagen[4, 217, 218, 237] but may also react with other epitopes on the collagen molecule (see earlier). The antigen in the lung may be sequestered in a form making it less available for reaction with circulating antibody. Lung biopsies have not been performed in patients with otherwise normal lungs to see whether antibody to alveolar basement membrane antigen is deposited in vivo. Other permeability factors may be involved in enhancing the antibody-induced pulmonary injury. Cigarette smoking or other environmental hazards (e.g., hydrocarbons, cocaine, viral pneumonitis)[207–209] injurious to the lung greatly enhance the likelihood of pulmonary hemorrhage.[212] Perhaps type I primary crescentic glomerulonephritis represents instances of Goodpasture disease in which pulmonary involvement is so mild as to be clinically unrecognizable. Cell-mediated immunity may also be involved in the pathogenesis of the glomerular lesions.[224]

**Course and Therapy.** In general, the outlook for recovery in this group is poor unless treatment is instituted early in the course of disease.[238–242] One may assess prognosis on the basis of several findings in renal biopsies. A poor prognosis is indicated when any of the following are present: 1) universal glomerular involvement with circumferential crescents; 2) severe tubule atrophy and interstitial fibrosis with or without arterionephrosclerosis; and 3) extensive glomerular fibrosis and organization of crescents.[241] Profound loss of renal function (i.e., GFR less than 5 mL/min) and oliguria are ominous prognostic features but not universally indicative of an irreversible stage of disease (see later). The initial titer of anti-GBM antibody does not seem to have any consistent bearing on ultimate outcome.[201, 202, 243]

In the absence of therapy, the majority of patients with primary crescentic glomerulonephritis type I progress to irreversible end-stage renal failure requiring dialysis support or transplantation. Spontaneous recovery is rare.[201, 202, 204–209, 239–245] Possession of the HLA-B7, -DR2 phenotype may be related to a worse prognosis and more severe crescentic involvement.[220] The risk of recurrent disease in transplanted kidneys is not precisely known but might be in the vicinity of 10% to 30%.[1, 201, 208] The risk of recurrent disease may be higher in nonimmunosuppressed identical twin transplants or when grafting is performed soon after onset of disease when high levels of anti-GBM antibody may be present. If transplantation is delayed for several months when anti-GBM antibody titers are low or undetectable and immunosuppression is employed, clinical recurrence rates should be low (possibly less than 10%).[204–209, 246, 247] Anti-GBM disease may rarely appear de novo after transplantation,[246–247] especially in patients with Alport syndrome (see Chapter 31). Relapses may occur months or years later even in the absence of rising titers of anti-GBM antibody.[248, 249] Contrariwise, relapse of serologic findings may not necessarily be accompanied by recurrence of clinical abnormalities.[249, 250]

Because this clinicopathologic entity is rare, only a few limited controlled studies of treatment have yet been conducted. As discussed in more detail in the section on Goodpasture disease (Chapter 31), limited controlled trials and anecdotal experience with intensive plasma exchange (plasmapheresis) (i.e., removal of 2 to 4 L daily or every other day using 5% albumin as replacement fluid)[204, 240] combined with oral steroids and cytotoxic agents (cyclophosphamide or azathioprine) have suggested that the progressive nature of the disease can be abrogated provided that therapy is initiated early in the course of disease before the development of oliguria or the need for dialysis support.[197, 198, 204–209, 244, 250–257] Intensive plasma exchange with immunosuppression is usually continued on a daily basis until circulating antibody levels fall to low or undetectable levels (usually within 14 days). Subsequently, immunosuppression is gradually discontinued in several weeks to months later. Glucocorticoids, even in high doses such as "pulses" of intravenous methylprednisolone, have not yet been shown to be of great value in this subcategory of crescentic glomerulonephritis.[258–262] Because fibrin-related antigens are frequently demonstrated in the lesions, the use of anticoagulants in conjunction with steroids and cytotoxic agents has theoretic merit.[263, 264] However, studies have been unable to demonstrate any effect of conventional doses of heparin on renal function or histologic appearance in anti-GBM nephritis in rabbits. Warfarin has been effective in experimental crescentic glomerulonephritis only in doses associated with a high mortality from hemorrhage.[265] The beneficial effect of defibrination with use of ancrod on the course of anti-GBM antibody nephritis in the rabbit has not yet been tested in a controlled fashion in humans.[266] It remains possible that tissue plasminogen activator therapy could be beneficial.[267] Because of the coagulation disorders present in uremia, the use of anticoagulants is particularly risky.[1] Patients with anti-GBM antibody disease may be at special risk because of the possible presence of covert pulmonary hemorrhage. The need to perform a renal biopsy may pose an additional problem. When renal biopsies are performed in patients undergoing plasma exchange, the replacement fluid should include fresh frozen plasma to avoid bleeding problems.

When intensive plasma exchange and immunosuppression are begun *before* serum creatinine concentration has risen above 8 mg/dL, approximately 90% of patients can be expected to retain native renal function 1 year later; when therapy is started *after* the serum creatinine concentration rises above 8 mg/dL, only about 10% will improve sufficiently to recover native renal function. Those who show improvement often remain in remission for years, and relapses of anti-GBM antibody production are uncommon.[204–209] Circulating anti-GBM antibody levels quickly decrease with intensive plasma exchange, although a few patients may have persisting low levels for many months or even years.[204–209]

# PRIMARY CRESCENTIC GLOMERULONEPHRITIS, TYPE II (Immune Complex–Mediated Crescentic Glomerulonephritis)

The lesion is identified by virtue of extensive glomerular deposits of immunoglobulin and complement in a "granular" pattern suggestive of localization of circulating immune complexes or formation in situ of immune complexes in the glomerular capillary circulation or mesangium, often accompanied by serologic findings consistent with circulating immune complexes (e.g., reduced serum levels of complement components, cryoimmunoglobulins, positive circulating immune complex assay responses). Depending on the series examined, this subset accounts for 10% to 20% of all patients with primary diffuse crescentic glomerulonephritis.[1, 177, 185, 197, 198] If IgA is the predominant immunoglobulin deposited, then the patients are classified as having IgA nephropathy or Schönlein-Henoch purpura. Many patients having these clinical characteristics will eventually be proved to have a multisystem rather than a primary glomerular disease (e.g., SLE, cryoimmunoglobulinemia) or crescentic disease superimposed on another primary glomerular disease (e.g., MGN, MCGN) (see Chapter 31).

**Clinical Features.** The patients tend to be middle aged or older, and no striking sex predominance is consistently observed. Constitutional symptoms such as fever and malaise are common. Hypertension, if present, is usually mild. In other respects, these cases resemble type I crescentic glomerulonephritis. Some patients may have occult visceral sepsis[268] or an inapparent PSGN. Some patients may have atypical forms of a multisystem disease, such as SLE, presenting with exclusive renal involvement (see Chapter 31).

**Laboratory Findings.** Urinary findings indicate glomerular injury, namely, hematuria and proteinuria. GFR is initially decreased and declines thereafter at variable rates. Serum levels of C3 and other complement components are frequently decreased. Cryoimmunoglobulins and circulating immune complexes are often detectable. The prevalence of HLA-DR2 and complement factor BfF is increased.[269] Anti-GBM and ANCA antibody assay responses are consistently negative (see later). Other laboratory features resemble type I crescentic glomerulonephritis.

**Pathology**

*Light Microscopy.* The glomerular lesions are similar to those of type I crescentic glomerulonephritis with variable extent of crescent formation. Proliferative endocapillary lesions or fibrinoid necrosis of the tufts is more common, particularly in infection-related disease. Special stains (e.g., Masson trichrome) can often demonstrate proteinaceous deposits in mesangium or subendothelial space. If the deposits are principally located in the subepithelial space and extensive endocapillary proliferation with monocyte or polymorphonuclear leukocyte infiltration is present, one should suspect an underlying and unrecognized infectious etiology (such as PSGN, infective endocarditis, or occult visceral sepsis). If the deposits are extensive and predominantly subendothelial and associated with extensive mesangial interposition, one should suspect an unrecognized SLE, cryoimmunoglobulinemia, or MCGN (type I). Other light microscopic features resemble those of type I crescentic glomerulonephritis; however, giant cells in the crescents seem to be less common.[1, 177, 185, 197]

*Electron Microscopy.* The major distinguishing feature is the presence of electron-dense deposits scattered throughout the mesangium and irregularly in the subendothelial space. The extent and orientation of the observed deposits may be helpful in differentiating the primary disorder from other secondary forms of RPGN. However, in the former instance, deposits tend to be relatively scant. If the deposits are principally subepithelial and have a hump-like configuration, a postinfectious cause should be sought. Subepithelial deposits with spike-like projections of basement membrane material are indicative of an underlying MGN. An organized substructure ("fingerprinting") of massive subendothelial deposits suggests mixed IgG/IgM cryoimmunoglobulinemia or SLE (see also Chapter 31). Electron-dense transformation of GBM may indicate an underlying MCGN (type II, dense deposit disease). As mentioned earlier, the presence of electron-dense deposits, usually small and subepithelial in location, does not completely exclude anti-GBM antibody–mediated disease.[234] Hence, the need for immunofluorescence as an important component of the evaluation of crescentic glomerulonephritis is again emphasized. Other features by electron microscopy resemble type I crescentic glomerulonephritis. The ultrastructure of the crescent itself is not greatly different among the various categories of idiopathic RPGN.[1]

*Immunofluorescence.* The principal distinguishing feature is scattered mesangial and peripheral capillary wall deposits of IgG or IgM, often, but not always, accompanied by C3.[1, 177, 185, 197] Extensive IgG, IgM, and IgA deposits, especially if accompanied by C1q, C4, and C3, should give rise to suspicion of SLE. Predominant IgA deposits should permit classification as a case of IgA nephropathy or Schönlein-Henoch purpura (see Chapter 31). Isolated C3 deposits in mesangium or peripheral capillaries should make one suspect an underlying MCGN. Deposits of fibrin-related antigens are similar to type I except that with necrosis, more extensive glomerular capillary staining may be seen.[1]

**Pathogenesis.** The pathogenesis of this subset is unknown, but its morphologic resemblance to models of immune complex–mediated disease has led to the conclusion that it is the result of glomerular deposition or in situ formation of immune complexes composed of unknown environmental or autologous antigens and their respective antibodies. Many of the cases are probably due to occult infections (? viruses) or unusual responses to other environmental agents.

**Course and Therapy.** Although without therapy most patients will progress to end-stage renal disease, in contradistinction to type I crescentic glomerulonephritis, there is a tendency for spontaneous improvement, particularly among cases with less severe crescentic involvement, prominent endocapillary proliferation, and a prodrome suggesting an infectious cause.[1] At present, it is not possible to provide any reasonable estimate of the frequency of such spontaneous resolution. Many of the same caveats mentioned in connection with type I crescentic glomerulonephritis apply here. For example, persistent oliguria, extensive glomerular obsolescence, and tubulointerstitial lesions augur an unfavorable evolution. Unfortunately, few controlled studies of treatment have been conducted in this uncommon clinicopathologic entity. Therefore, recommendations are largely based on anecdotal observations and personal experience.

There are few data available that would permit the physician to make a rational choice among the forms of therapy mentioned in the context of type I crescentic glomerulonephritis, namely, intensive plasma exchange, pulse methylprednisolone, or glucocorticoid-immunosuppressive therapy.[1, 252, 270–273] At present, a trial of pulse methylprednisolone would seem to be the safest and possibly the most effective approach.[270–273] Three or four pulses (200 to 1000 mg intravenous methylprednisolone given slowly for several hours) on a daily or every-other-day basis followed by daily or every-other-day oral prednisone (1 mg/kg) for several weeks, followed by gradual tapering, would seem to constitute an adequate trial. Limited data would suggest that 75% to 80% of patients treated in this fashion experience improvement in renal function and avoid, at least in the short term, the necessity of dialysis support.[270] Patients receiving this form of therapy should be carefully monitored; sudden death has occurred after administration of very large doses of glucocorticoids in an intravenous bolus.[272]

Intensive plasma exchange combined with lower doses of oral prednisone and a cytotoxic drug *may* also be effective, particularly in patients who have already had advanced renal failure in dialysis, but proof based on randomized prospective trials is lacking. There does not appear to be any advantage gained by introducing intensive plasma exchange for patients with impaired renal function not requiring dialysis.[274] The addition of cyclophosphamide (oral or intravenous) to a regimen of glucocorticoids (oral or intravenous) *may* be more effective in cases of crescentic glomerulonephritis in which prominent vasculitic manifestations are present and in which ANCAs are absent (see later). The long-term prognosis for such patients is uncertain. As in all cases of crescentic glomerulonephritis, treatment, if undertaken at all, should be instituted *early,* before advanced and irreversible features ensue.[274] Renal biopsies should be performed on an urgent basis in suspected cases to assess the potential for therapeutic response or spontaneous recovery. The risks of therapy (e.g., infection, bleeding) versus potential benefits must be taken into account in therapeutic decisions in individual cases. For patients with clinical and pathologic features indicative of advanced irreversible disease, dialysis and transplantation (if feasible) should be offered. The risk of recurrence of disease in the renal allograft is not known but is probably low if a reasonable time (e.g., 6 months) elapses between onset of disease and transplantation.

## PRIMARY CRESCENTIC GLOMERULONEPHRITIS, TYPE III

The existence of a third category of primary diffuse crescentic glomerulonephritis is no longer in dispute. This cat-

egory is a distinct clinicopathologic entity categorized by the absence of immunoglobulin deposits (either linear or granular) or electron-dense deposits.[177, 178, 185, 197, 274–279] Because of the lack of clear-cut immunoglobulin deposition and the tendency for necrotizing features, the term ''pauci-immune necrotizing crescentic glomerulonephritis'' has been used to describe this entity.[275, 280, 281] It has been shown that 75% to 90% of patients in this category have circulating ANCA, similar to the findings in systemic necrotizing vasculitis and Wegener granulomatosis[274–281] (see Chapter 31). Thus, many of these patients may in fact be suffering from a form of vasculitis in which the kidney is the sole or predominant organ involved (e.g., renal limited microscopic polyangiitis). Indeed, it is probably correct to regard a patient with type III crescentic glomerulonephritis and a positive test response for ANCA as having a forme fruste of vasculitis (see Chapter 31). Depending on the series examined, this subset constitutes 50% to 70% of the overall group of cases defined as primary crescentic glomerulonephritis.[177, 178, 185, 197, 274–279]

**Clinical Features.** This disorder tends to involve middle-aged and older patients, with a slight predilection for males.[275, 281] Constitutional symptoms are common (e.g., fever, weight loss), and many cases may have manifestations suggestive of a systemic vasculitis (i.e., fever, arthralgias, abdominal pain). Indeed, there is overlap between this group and those that are more readily classified as vasculitis on the basis of clinically evident extrarenal organ involvement (e.g., skin, muscle, lung). The coexistence of pulmonary infiltrates and ANCA in the absence of anti-GBM antibody may be sufficient to categorize patients under the heading of a vasculitis (e.g., Wegener syndrome)[1] (see Chapter 31), but pulmonary hemorrhage can occur without necrotizing granulomas.[281a]

**Laboratory Findings.** The urinalysis and renal function parameters resemble those of any form of crescentic glomerulonephritis. Anti-GBM antibody, circulating immune complexes, and cryoimmunoglobulins are not usually found in the circulation, and serum complement component concentrations are most often normal or elevated. The erythrocyte sedimentation rate and C-reactive protein levels are often greatly elevated. As stated before, ANCAs, usually of the IgG class, are found in 75% to 90% of patients.[281–283] A perinuclear ANCA pattern on alcohol-fixed slides is most commonly observed.[281–283] This pattern is frequently associated with antimyeloperoxidase autoantibodies.[281] A smaller number of patients have a diffuse cytoplasmic ANCA pattern, commonly associated with autoantibodies to proteinase-3.[281–283] Approximately two thirds or more of patients with circulating ANCA have antimyeloperoxidase autoantibodies.[281] Therefore, patients with type III primary crescentic glomerulonephritis who demonstrate high-titer autoantibodies to proteinase-3 should be carefully examined for other manifestations of Wegener granulomatosis, a disorder much more frequently associated with anti–proteinase-3 autoantibodies (see Chapter 31). Similarly, perinuclear ANCA patterns may be observed in patients with ulcerative colitis, cystic fibrosis, Crohn disease, primary biliary cirrhosis, Felty syndrome, sclerosing cholangitis, and autoimmune hepatitis.[278] The specific antigens reacting with these autoantibodies are not well understood; however, many are unrelated to myeloperoxidase. Therefore, in patients positive for perinuclear ANCA patterns, confirmation with specific leukocyte antigen immunoassays is preferred.[278, 281, 283] These antibodies quickly decline with effective therapy. Immunoglobulin levels (IgG, IgM, IgA) may be increased. Rheumatoid factors are usually absent. Occasionally, ANCA and anti-GBM antibodies may coexist (see later).[284–286]

### Pathology

*Light Microscopy.* The only distinctive feature is the absence of proteinaceous deposits on examination with special stains. Segmental or diffuse necrotizing glomerular lesions are frequently present,[281–283] which may be indicative of an underlying vasculitis. Leukocytoclastic vasculitis may be noted in the medulla.[276]

*Electron Microscopy.* Electron-dense deposits are not seen in the mesangium or capillary walls. Extensive destruction of GBM may be found. The ultrastructure of the crescent is similar to other varieties described.[1]

*Immunofluorescence.* By definition, immunoglobulin deposits are absent. Unfortunately, the distinction between absent, scanty, trace, and positive is subjective, and it could be argued that some traces of immunoglobulin deposits are present in every case.[280, 281] Because renal biopsy is a static record of a dynamic process, it is also possible that immunoglobulin deposits were present at an earlier time but have decreased consequent to phagocytosis and digestion by infiltrating monocytes and polymorphonuclear leukocytes. Fibrin-related antigen deposition in the crescent and glomerular capillaries resembles other forms of RPGN.[1, 280, 281]

**Course and Therapy.** Anecdotal data indicate that this category may at times be associated with a favorable outcome, even in the absence of specific therapy, so long as occult multisystem disease and irreversible glomerular or tubulointerstitial lesions are absent. Nevertheless, because of the likelihood of progression to end-stage renal disease, most patients undergo some form of therapy. Because of the strong suspicion of underlying vasculitis in the presence of positive test results for ANCA, many patients are treated with combinations of glucocorticoids and alkylating agents (cyclophosphamide). Initiation of therapy with pulse intravenous methylprednisolone may be preferred when renal function is deteriorating rapidly,[270] but data regarding the necessity for initiating therapy with high-dose intravenous glucocorticoids (e.g., greater than 500 mg per dose) are unconvincing. On the other hand, glucocorticoid therapy alone seems inadequate in most cases. Daily oral or intermittent intravenous cyclophosphamide has been used, with approximately equal efficacy and safety. With early and aggressive therapy, approximately 70% to 85% of patients respond initially,[270] although later relapses may occur,[287] especially with too rapid tapering of immunosuppression in the face of persisting positive ANCA test responses.[288] Conversion from cyclophosphamide to azathioprine therapy may also be associated with relapse, especially with persistent positive ANCA test responses. Late occurrence of progressive renal failure and heavy proteinuria may be seen if patients are treated after severe glomerular disease has already developed. The use of ACE inhibitors may slow the rate of progression in this group of patients. The safety and efficacy of intensive plasma exchange have not been well

defined in this group. Such therapy, when combined with immunosuppression, *may* have value in patients who have already advanced to dialysis-dependent renal failure.[274, 289] No convincing evidence is available to support the use of intensive plasma exchange therapy as an adjunct to immunosuppression when patients have not advanced to a stage of disease that requires dialysis therapy.[274, 288–290] Renal biopsies revealing extensive irreversible glomerular or tubulointerstitial lesions and prolonged severe reduction in GFR with oliguria are probable reasons to avoid the risks of vigorous regimens of treatment. These patients should be reasonable candidates for dialysis or transplantation. The risk of recurrence in renal allografts is unknown but is probably low.[1]

## PRIMARY CRESCENTIC GLOMERULONEPHRITIS, TYPE IV

Primary crescentic glomerulonephritis type IV represents a combination of type I (anti-GBM) and type III (ANCA associated)[284–286] (see also Chapter 31). It is a relatively uncommon condition accounting for less than 5% of all cases of primary crescentic glomerulonephritis. The ANCA pattern is typically perinuclear and of the antimyeloperoxidase variety. However, on occasion, the ANCA pattern may be of the cytoplasmic variety and may be directed to proteinase-3. This category seems to be observed more commonly in older women.[284] Lung hemorrhage may be seen as in Goodpasture disease (see Chapter 31). Sometimes the autoantibodies occur contemporaneously and at other times sequentially, with anti-GBM antibody production often preceding ANCA production.[284–286] The clinical and morphologic findings are similar to those described in type I and type III primary crescentic glomerulonephritis. The prognosis appears to be poor in that many patients will have end-stage renal disease despite aggressive therapy.[284]

## PRIMARY CRESCENTIC GLOMERULONEPHRITIS, TYPE V

The existence of this category of primary crescentic glomerulonephritis, characterized by the lesions of pauci-immune crescentic glomerulonephritis (see type III) but in which no ANCA or anti-GBM antibodies can be detected, remains in dispute. Most series identify this uncommon group as true *idiopathic* crescentic glomerulonephritis. The clinical features, course, and therapy are similar to those described for type III primary crescentic glomerulonephritis.

## Superimposition of Diffuse Glomerular Crescents on Other Primary Glomerular Diseases

Extensive glomerular crescentic involvement may be superimposed on other primary glomerular lesions.[1] Such a process is most likely to occur in idiopathic MCGN (see later).

The dense deposit disease variant (type II MCGN) of this

disorder seems most susceptible to this complication. Other disorders with such superimposition include long-standing idiopathic membranous glomerulonephritis, focal and segmental glomerular sclerosis, fibrillary or immunotactoid glomerulonephritis, and IgA nephropathy. These are discussed elsewhere in this chapter or in Chapter 31.

# CHRONIC GLOMERULONEPHRITIS

Chronic glomerulonephritis should properly be viewed as the clinical expression of a wide variety of glomerular diseases having a protracted course, often asymptomatic for lengthy periods, and associated with a relentless obliteration of nephron mass.[1] The mechanisms responsible for this progressive course vary widely but include continued activity of the basic disease process, superimposed hypertensive arterionephrosclerosis, hyperlipidemia, chronic tubulointerstitial injury, and hemodynamically mediated glomerular sclerosis (see Chapter 44). In early stages, the sole manifestations may be minor abnormalities in urine sediment, increased protein excretion, and mildly reduced renal function. In its final stages, this syndrome is accompanied by a complex series of biochemical and metabolic disturbances, the uremic state, which is dealt with in detail in Chapter 49. The evolution from earliest detectable changes to terminal uremia may encompass several decades. Many of the entities described under the heading of other glomerulopathic syndromes may gradually merge with the syndrome of chronic nephritis. For example, symptomless proteinuria may be regarded in some patients as an early stage in the evolution of the chronic nephritic syndrome. Furthermore, nephrotic syndrome may be a prominent manifestation in the evolution of lesions falling under the general rubric of chronic glomerulonephritis. In addition, this syndrome may develop de novo as an idiopathic process not clearly related to an underlying definable disease or clinicopathologic entity.

In some patients, hypertension may be the dominant feature, although it will nearly always be accompanied by some sign of renal disease (e.g., proteinuria, abnormal urine sediment, or reduced GFR). As many as 20% or more of white patients believed on clinical grounds to have essential hypertension will be shown to have a primary glomerular disease on biopsy (particularly IgA nephropathy). Most of these patients will be younger than 30 years and will often manifest microhematuria and proteinuria. On the other hand, black patients with presumed essential hypertension nearly always have arteriolonephrosclerosis on renal biopsy.[290a]

The clinical differentiation of chronic nephritis from other nonglomerular disorders such as essential hypertension and chronic tubulointerstitial nephritis is difficult in advanced stages, but some useful clues are often present. For example, the presence of heavy proteinuria or the finding of dysmorphic red blood cells or red blood cell casts in the urine sediment is usually indicative of an underlying glomerular disease.[87, 88] However, patients whose clinical features suggest glomerulonephritis may reveal only vascular and nonspecific glomerular alterations on renal biopsy.[291] Marked ophthalmoscopic abnormalities and renal cortical scarring as seen on pyelograms may be indicative of arteriolonephrosclerosis and hypertensive vascular disease. Radiographic evidence of calyceal distortion or scarring and asymmetric renal atrophy may be seen in chronic bacterial interstitial nephritis. In individual cases, however, the clinical diagnosis of the nature of the underlying renal disease in patients presenting with end-stage renal failure and atrophic kidneys is as often wrong as right.[292] In some instances, the evolution of chronic nephritis is clearly initiated by a definable process or clinicopathologic entity, such as PSGN, MGN, or IgA nephropathy. These glomerular diseases may exist in a covert, subclinical form for years before giving rise to detectable clinical abnormalities.

## Pathology and Immunopathology

Because renal biopsies are not often performed in patients with advanced renal atrophy and approaching end-stage renal failure, it is difficult to reconstruct a complete picture of the histologic evolution of the heterogeneous disorders encompassed by the general term "chronic glomerulonephritis." Complicating vascular disease resulting from severe hypertension, intercurrent parenchymal bacterial infection, and metabolic and hemodynamic disturbances related to the loss of nephron mass all contribute in an important way to the parenchymal changes that are observed. In gross appearance, the kidneys are usually but not invariably much reduced in size. The symmetric atrophy is due to cortical thinning, and the pelvocalyceal systems are not distorted. Cysts and neoplasms may be present, even before the institution of dialysis (see Chapter 38). At the level of the light microscope, there is a great variation in findings. In advanced instances, particularly when the renal mass is markedly contracted or when tissue is removed after a period of hemodialysis treatments, the glomeruli may all be nearly totally sclerotic in association with severe tubule loss, interstitial fibrosis, and marked vascular disease. Fibrinoid necrosis may be present in the afferent arteriole in cases complicated by malignant hypertension. Lymphocytic infiltration of the interstitium may be seen, but the pleomorphic cellular infiltrate (principally T cells) so common in chronic bacterial tubulointerstitial nephritis is usually inconspicuous. Crystals of urates and oxalate may be found in localized areas, and microscopic nephrocalcinosis may also be observed. By immunofluorescence or electron microscopy, residual mesangial IgA deposits, linear IgG deposits, or diffuse subepithelial electron-dense deposits permit recognition of a distinctive underlying disease process. Frequently, however, only nonspecific IgM or C3 deposits are seen.[293]

In some cases, often described as idiopathic (nonspecific) sclerosing chronic glomerulonephritis, there is a mixed picture of totally sclerotic glomeruli coexisting with reasonably normal or even hypertrophied glomeruli. Segmental sclerosis may be noted in some. Less involved glomeruli may reveal nonspecific IgM or C3 deposits. This picture is reminiscent of that seen in cases of focal glomerular sclerosis with nephrotic syndrome and in biopsy specimens from patients with persisting proteinuria and mildly reduced renal function years after an episode of PSGN. Thus, some of the patients present de novo in later life with an apparent idiopathic (nonspecific) sclerosing chronic glomerulonephritis or the insidious progression of focal glomerular sclerosis. The resolution of this problem is an important aspect of the prevention of chronic renal failure. Other cases may be described simply as chronic or "persistent" proliferative glomerulonephritis if some degree of glomerular hypercellularity is present.[1]

## Course and Therapy

The evolution of "chronic nephritis" and end-stage renal failure is discussed in some detail in relation to specific clinical and clinicopathologic entities in other sections of this chapter, and little more needs to be said here. Patients who present with few or no symptoms and only urine sediment abnormalities, proteinuria, and little impairment of renal function are often regarded as having "latent" chronic glomerulonephritis.[1] The duration of this latent stage may be extremely long and varied. Exacerbations may be related to any type of infection, usually without the latent period preceding the initial episode of acute PSGN,[98] often called synpharyngitic nephritis. Many of these patients have an underlying IgA nephropathy (see later). These exacerbations are characterized by a transient decline in renal function, worsening of the proteinuria, and abnormalities of urine sediment. They resolve spontaneously, usually without any serious further impairment in renal function.

Once a definite and unequivocal abnormality in renal function is noted, the course to end-stage renal failure is reasonably rapid and predictable although influenced by the severity of hypertension, dietary protein intake, dietary phosphorus intake, antihypertensive therapy, intercurrent infection, use of nephrotoxic drugs, congestive heart failure, salt depletion, hyperparathyroidism, and other metabolic disturbances. The course of an individual patient depends on the nature of the underlying glomerular lesions.[1] The mechanisms responsible for the progressive loss of renal function in chronic glomerulonephritis are largely unknown; however, it is not necessary for the basic initiating process to persist for later progression to occur. Adaptive hemodynamic events, intrinsic to the glomerular circulation and arising as a consequence of loss of filtering surface area, are set into motion early in the course of glomerular disease[294] (see Chapter 44). These events, which include increase in glomerular capillary pressure and flow, may inexorably damage residual capillaries and lead to a vicious circle of relentless obliteration of the capillary network.[294] Vigorous antihypertensive therapy, especially with agents that reduce intracapillary pressure (e.g., ACE inhibitors), nonsteroidal anti-inflammatory drugs (NSAIDs), and protein or phosphate restriction may all act to slow progression of disease by modifying these hemodynamic events that serve to perpetuate and promote progression of disease (see Chapter 44). The data bearing on the efficacy of therapy directed at the basic disease process, rather than complicating events, are reviewed in the context of the individual lesions discussed elsewhere in this chapter.

## PERSISTING URINARY ABNORMALITIES WITH FEW OR NO SYMPTOMS

### Recurrent or Persistent Hematuria with or Without Abnormal Proteinuria

The finding of hematuria with or without mild proteinuria and in the absence of any readily identifiable systemic disease or anatomic lesion in the upper or lower urinary tract is a familiar and vexing clinical problem. The list of conditions of a nonglomerular nature that may produce hematuria is extensive.[1, 87, 88, 295–297] Hematuria of glomerular origin may be microscopic or macroscopic (gross), persistent or recurrent, and the pattern occurring in individual patients is not indicative of the nature or severity of the underlying glomerular lesions.[1, 297] Determination of the morphologic features of erythrocytes in freshly voided urine may be a helpful clue to the separation of glomerular from nonglomerular (extrarenal parenchymal) disease. Fragmented, distorted, poorly hemoglobinized (dysmorphic) erythrocytes are predictive of underlying renal parenchymal or glomerular disease.[87, 88, 297–307] Acanthocytes (distorted erythrocytes with blebs) in the urine have the highest diagnostic utility for identifying a glomerular source of hematuria.[305, 307] Other dysmorphic erythrocytes (echinocytes, anulocytes, schistocytes, stomatocytes, codocytes, knizocytes) are less specific.[306] Thus, dysmorphism of erythrocytes in the urine is not necessarily equivalent to glomerular disease. Nevertheless, distorted and misshapen erythrocytes are far more commonly found in the urine of patients suffering from renal parenchymal as opposed to lower urinary tract disorders. Urinary erythrocyte mean corpuscular volume of less than 72 fL may be highly predictive of glomerular erythrocyturia.[308–310] Flow cytometry using fluorescein-labeled anti–human hemoglobin antibodies may also be useful in detecting glomerular hematuria.[311] Dipstick methods of detecting hematuria (glomerular or nonglomerular) have low false-negative but high false-positive rates.[312] Heavy proteinuria (>1 to 2 g/d), presence of erythrocyte casts, and granular casts containing immunoglobulins are also indicative of glomerular disease.

The terminology used to describe this clinical syndrome is varied and includes primary or idiopathic hematuria, symptomless hematuria, primary benign hematuria, "benign and curable form of hemorrhagic acute nephritis," and persistent or recurrent renal hematuria.[1, 313–316] The term "isolated hematuria" is used when abnormal erythrocyte excretion is not accompanied by abnormal proteinuria.[317]

The clinical syndrome of recurrent or persistent hematuria due to an underlying glomerular disorder constitutes a heterogeneous group of primary renal disorders and in addition may be the mode of presentation of a variety of heredofamilial, multisystem, and infectious diseases (such as SLE, Schönlein-Henoch purpura, Alport syndrome, Fabry disease, and sickle-cell disease), as discussed in Chapter 31. In addition, hematuria may be the presenting feature in children with underlying idiopathic hypercalciuria.[318]

In general, persons in nearly any age group may be affected by the primary glomerular diseases that evoke this

**TABLE 30–4. Light, Electron, and Immunofluorescence Microscopic Patterns Observed in "Asymptomatic" Hematuria with or Without Proteinuria Due to Primary Glomerular Disease**

**Light Microscopy**
Basic lesions
  Normal glomeruli
  Minimal glomerular changes
  Mesangial proliferative glomerulonephritis
  Diffuse endocapillary proliferative glomerulonephritis
  Focal and segmental proliferative glomerulonephritis
  MCGN
Superimposed lesions
  Focal and segmental glomerular sclerosis
  Focal or diffuse crescents

**Electron Microscopy**
Basement membrane abnormalities: thin–basement membrane
  nephropathy, reduplication, basket-weave abnormalities, splitting
Electron-dense deposits (subendothelial, intramembranous,
  subepithelial, mesangial)
Nonamyloid fibrillar deposits
No deposits

**Immunofluorescence Microscopy**
Predominant mesangial IgA and C3 deposits (IgA nephropathy or
  Berger disease)
Predominant mesangial IgM and C3 deposits (IgM nephropathy)
Predominant C3 deposits with scanty immunoglobulin
Other patterns of immunoglobulin and C3 deposits (including
  "linear" immunoglobulin)
No immunoglobulin or C3 deposits

syndrome; however, most reported cases are children and young adults.[1, 313–317] Patients may present with persistent microscopic hematuria discovered on routine urinalysis or with bouts of gross hematuria, frequently brought on by excessive exercise, febrile illnesses, and immunizations.[301, 302] Constitutional symptoms, hypertension, edema, and abnormal GFRs are typically absent at the time of discovery. However, the finding of hematuria in patients with hypertension may indicate the presence of an underlying glomerular lesion, particularly IgA nephropathy (see later).[1, 315] Bilateral loin pain is a common symptom, particularly in some categories of disease (e.g., IgA nephropathy and loin pain–hematuria syndrome; see later). Proteinuria, when present, is mild (i.e., <1 g/d); more severe proteinuria suggests forms of glomerular disease discussed later under the topic of nephrotic syndrome.[1, 316] Normal values for complement components, rheumatoid factor, cryoglobulins, antinuclear antibodies, and ASO and anti–deoxyribonuclease B titers are found.[1, 319] A diligent search for the nonrenal symptoms and signs of heredofamilial and multisystem diseases must be conducted before the patient is diagnosed as having idiopathic or primary renal hematuria.[1] Examining the urine sediment of first-degree relatives and family contacts may be useful; both heredofamilial disease (such as Alport syndrome, Fabry disease, thin–basement membrane nephropathy) and postinfectious glomerulonephritis may occur in an asymptomatic form in these persons.[320–323] A familial occurrence of idiopathic hematuria without clinical hearing loss and the incidental discovery of hematuria in siblings (benign familial hematuria) have been described[322] (see thin–basement membrane nephropathy). Because there was no tendency for the development of progressive renal failure, it is uncertain whether these cases represent variants of Alport syndrome, mild PSGN occurring in families, or a distinct heredofamilial disorder such as thin–basement membrane nephropathy[313] (see also Chapter 31).

Considered as a group, patients with primary glomerular disease and hematuria display a wide variety of morphologic abnormalities.[1, 315–319] By light microscopy (Table 30–4), 5% to 15% reveal optically normal or only minimally altered glomeruli, 30% to 50% of cases reveal a focal and segmental proliferative glomerular lesion ("focal glomerulonephritis")[1, 316, 319] (Fig. 30–8) with or without segmental glomerular sclerosis, and about 20% to 50% reveal a more diffuse mesangial proliferative glomerular lesion sometimes resembling resolving acute PSGN. The remainder reveal more advanced lesions with sclerosis, adhesions, or severe and diffuse proliferative glomerulonephritis with variable crescentic involvement, an unsuspected primary interstitial nephritis, arterionephrosclerosis, or other primary glomerular diseases.[314, 315] Renal biopsies in patients with isolated hematuria are more likely to reveal normal or minimally

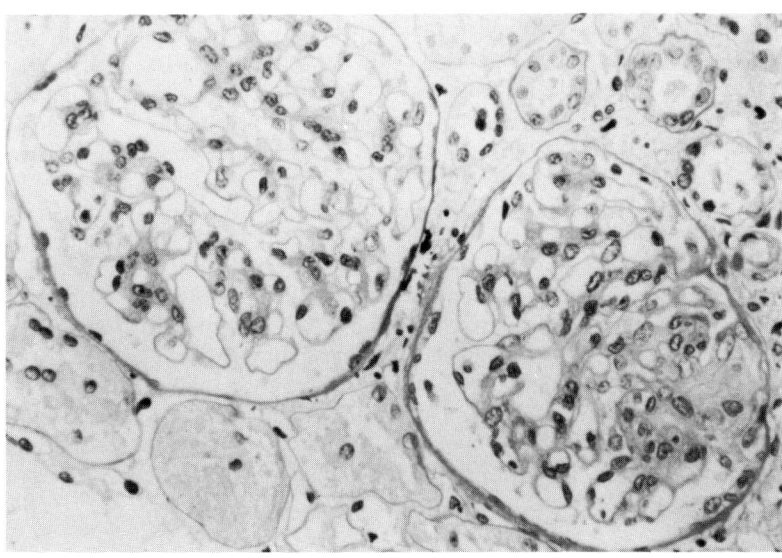

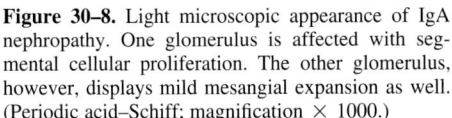

**Figure 30–8.** Light microscopic appearance of IgA nephropathy. One glomerulus is affected with segmental cellular proliferation. The other glomerulus, however, displays mild mesangial expansion as well. (Periodic acid–Schiff; magnification × 1000.)

altered glomeruli by light microscopy.[317, 323] Focal glomerulonephritis is a lesion and not a clinical diagnosis and occurs frequently in association with systemic diseases such as Schönlein-Henoch purpura, SLE, Wegener granulomatosis, polyarteritis, Goodpasture disease, Alport syndrome, and infective endocarditis and in association with other infectious illnesses.[1]

Electron microscopic findings have varied, but subepithelial, subendothelial, and paramesangial electron-dense deposits have all been reported.[314, 315] Humps, when found, suggest an association with recent streptococcal or other bacterial infection. A variable proportion (as high as 25%) demonstrate thin, attenuated GBMs (less than 265 nm, or less than 5% of normal).[323] Such a finding delineates a specific subgroup known as thin–basement membrane nephropathy (see later). These patients frequently have normal-appearing glomeruli by light microscopy and have persistent microscopic—rather than recurrent macroscopic—erythrocyturia. The long-term prognosis for this group appears benign, but occasional progression to renal failure has been reported. Such patients do not have hearing abnormalities and do not have a clear-cut X-linked inheritance pattern, so they may be distinguished from Alport syndrome[323] (see Chapter 31). This lesion may occur in association with familial hematuria or in patients with isolated hematuria[317] (see also Chapter 31).

Immunofluorescence studies have revealed a variable picture with respect to the extent, pattern, and type of immunoglobulin deposition.[1, 316, 319, 324–327] In many patients, extensive mesangial deposits of IgA and, to a lesser extent, IgG are found (Berger disease, see later and Fig. 30–10).[1, 328, 329] In some series, 50% or more of patients with primary glomerular hematuria have IgA nephropathy.[1] Predominant segmental or generalized mesangial deposits of IgM or IgG with C3 or isolated C3 deposits[1, 316, 319, 324–327, 330–332] have been found frequently, and in a variable percentage, the immunofluorescence findings are entirely negative.[314, 321–323, 330, 331] Some patients have C3 deposits confined to arterioles or arteries.[317, 330, 332] In most cases, regardless of the type of immunoglobulin deposited, the pattern has been one of diffuse mesangial and irregular granular deposition, sometimes with extension into the peripheral capillaries in a focal and segmental fashion. Rarely, linear IgG deposits may be found and circulating anti-GBM autoantibodies detected, even with normal pulmonary or renal function.[326] Such cases represent the mildest form of clinically recognized anti-GBM antibody associated with glomerulonephritis (see also Goodpasture disease, Chapter 31).

In general, the prognosis is good for both adults and children. Of all cases of idiopathic hematuria due to glomerular disease, within 5 years of discovery 50% or more will have experienced spontaneous remission and few will have developed a decline in GFR or increase in blood pressure.[1] However, in those patients demonstrating extensive mesangial IgA deposits, the long-term prognosis may be unfavorable (see later). If hematuria is accompanied by proteinuria of more than 1 g/d, the prognosis is more guarded and a renal biopsy is more likely to uncover proliferative or chronic sclerosing glomerular changes.[1, 316]

# IgA NEPHROPATHY
## (Berger Disease, IgA/IgG Mesangial Nephropathy)

In an immunofluorescence study of a group of patients with apparently idiopathic hematuria, Berger and Hinglais noted IgA and, to a lesser extent, IgG or IgM deposits in a granular pattern chiefly involving the mesangium.[1, 328, 329, 333–342] The immunoglobulin was accompanied by a deposition of C3 and fibrin-related antigens in a similar pattern, but not by C1q or C4. These findings have been amply confirmed in succeeding years, and this pathologic entity has come to be known as Berger disease, glomerulonephritis with mesangial IgA/IgG deposits, IgA mesangial nephropathy, or simply IgA nephropathy. The typical immunofluorescence findings are associated with a wide spectrum of histologic glomerular changes ranging from normal to extensive crescentic glomerulonephritis.[1, 343–347] Electron-dense deposits are found in mesangial and paramesangial areas. IgA nephropathy is distributed widely and is believed to be the most common form of primary glomerular disease throughout the world.[348] The apparent prevalence of IgA nephropathy varies widely in different geographic areas.[348] It is seen in about 10% of all renal biopsies performed for primary glomerular disease in North America, 20% in Europe, and as high as 30% to 40% in the Asian-Pacific area.[348] These differences could be explained by regional differences in the performance of routine urinalysis in children and young adults or the indications for renal biopsy rather than a true difference in geographic incidence.[349] The fact that lesions of IgA nephropathy tend to be milder in series reported from Asia would be consistent with this explanation; routine urinalyses are performed on school-aged children, and many Asian nephrologists consider renal biopsies to be strongly indicated in patients with abnormal urinalyses, even without proteinuria. Genetic factors and environmental influences could also contribute to geographic differences in prevalence. It is common in Native Americans (Zuni and Navajo)[350] but uncommon in African-Americans).[351] Extensive mesangial IgA deposits may also be seen in a variety of multisystem, neoplastic, and infectious diseases (Table 30–5). Clinically inapparent glomerular IgA deposits may be seen in approximately 5% of individuals at autopsy,[352] whereas the prevalence of clinically apparent IgA nephropathy in the general population is about 25 to 50 cases/100,000.[348, 349]

**Clinical Features.** Although the clinical spectrum of presenting features is varied, the most common feature leading to the diagnosis by renal biopsy is recurring episodes of gross (macroscopic) hematuria.[1, 335, 336, 338–344] Macroscopic hematuria is a more common initial feature among cases described in Europe. The disorder may be found at any age, but it is uncommon before the age of 10 or after the age of 50 years. More than 80% of patients are between the ages of 16 and 35 years at time of discovery of the lesion.[1, 335, 336, 338–344] It is uncommon in African-Americans.[351, 353] When IgA nephropathy does appear in black persons, the usual predilection for males is not observed.[353] The male/female ratio may be as high as 6:1 but averages about 2:1.[1, 335, 336, 338–344] Lower ratios may be observed in Asian patients.

**TABLE 30–5. Classification of Predominant Mesangial Immunoglobulin A Deposition in Glomerular Disease***

**Primary**
IgA nephropathy (Berger disease)

**Secondary**
Multisystem disease
  *Schönlein-Henoch purpura*
  Celiac disease
  Dermatitis herpetiformis
  Crohn disease
  Seronegative arthropathy (ankylosing spondylitis, Reiter syndrome, psoriasis)
  Sicca syndrome
Neoplasia
  IgA monoclonal gammopathy
  Mucin-secreting carcinoma
  *Carcinoma of lung, larynx, pharynx, pancreas*
  Mycosis fungoides
  Sézary syndrome
Infection
  Leprosy
  Toxoplasmosis
  Human immunodeficiency virus infection
Other
  *Chronic liver disease* (including alcoholic liver disease)
  Portosystemic shunts
  Familial immunothrombocytopenia
  Episcleritis
  Pulmonary hemosiderosis
  Recurrent mastitis
  Various pulmonary diseases
  Buerger disease

*Most common causes are in italics. See Chapter 31 for details regarding secondary causes.

Episodes of hematuria (gross or microscopic) frequently follow quickly on some nonspecific virus-like syndrome or intercurrent infection, such as acute tonsillitis (e.g., synpharyngitic nephritis). Thus, such cases are often initially confused with PSGN.[354] Bouts of severe hematuria and renal insufficiency may also occur after tonsillectomy.[1] Frequently, with the onset of hematuria, mild constitutional symptoms such as malaise, myalgia, vague back or loin discomfort, and low-grade fever are present. Thus, it is not surprising that many patients are initially diagnosed as having a urinary tract infection and are treated with antibiotics or inappropriately subjected to urologic investigations, such as cystoscopy.[355] Gross hematuria is more prevalent among patients with polymeric IgA immune complexes.[356] Dysuria may be a prominent complaint, leading to an erroneous diagnosis of bacterial hemorrhagic cystitis. Blood pressure is usually normal, although mild to severe hypertension may be present in patients with more advanced disease. Malignant hypertension may be the presenting feature.[357] Edema and nephrotic syndrome are reported at frequencies ranging from 0% to 30%, usually approximately 10%.[1, 339, 344] Renal vein thrombosis is unusual. Reversible acute renal failure associated with episodes of macroscopic hematuria may occur, sometimes in a recurrent fashion.[1, 358–361] Such patients often present after acute upper respiratory infection. Renal biopsies may show acute tubule necrosis, extensive erythrocyte casts, and segmental crescents

involving less than 50% of the glomeruli. Spontaneous recovery is the rule, even though temporary dialysis may be required.[361] Rapidly progressive renal failure (with extensive crescents) is distinctly uncommon.[1, 358] Cyclic neutropenia,[362] episcleritis,[363] sicca syndrome,[364] recurrent mastitis,[365] and various pulmonary disorders[365a] including pulmonary hemosiderosis[366] and IgA immune complex–mediated pneumonitis[367] have been reported to occur in association with Berger disease. Gut permeability may be transiently abnormal.[368] Crohn disease may be associated with IgA nephropathy and acute renal failure.[369] Buerger disease can also be associated with IgA nephropathy.[369a] Recurrent bloody peritoneal dialysate has been reported in a male patient with Berger disease during respiratory tract infections.[370] IgA nephropathy may be a relatively common lesion among white (but not black) patients believed to have essential hypertension who also manifest hematuria.[371]

As discussed later, the distinction between Berger disease and Schönlein-Henoch purpura, both conditions revealing extensive glomerular mesangial IgA deposits, is based entirely on clinical features (see also Chapter 31). In fact, these diseases are most likely related pathogenetically, if not etiologically, and form parts of a spectrum of a single disease. Schönlein-Henoch purpura may be diagnosed when a nonthrombopenic leukocytoclastic vasculitic purpura, often occurring in association with arthralgias and abdominal pain, is present concomitant with glomerulonephritis and mesangial IgA deposits (see also Chapter 31). On the other hand, Berger disease is distinguished by the lack of purpura, abdominal pain, or arthralgias. Thus, Berger disease can be viewed as a monosymptomatic form of Schönlein-Henoch purpura. Otherwise typical cases of IgA nephropathy have evolved into Schönlein-Henoch purpura, and both IgA nephropathy and Schönlein-Henoch purpura have occurred in siblings.

Glomerular mesangial IgA deposition may also be seen in otherwise normal healthy subjects. It may also be seen in association with chronic alcoholic liver disease or with ankylosing spondylitis, Reiter syndrome, psoriasis, mycosis fungoides, Sézary syndrome, nontropical sprue (celiac disease, gluten-sensitive enteropathy), sicca syndrome, recurrent mastitis, various pulmonary diseases, Buerger disease, familial immunothrombocytopenia, dermatitis herpetiformis, various carcinomas, leprosy, toxoplasmosis, and human immunodeficiency virus infection (see Table 30–5 and Chapter 31), and in association with IgG and IgM in SLE nephritis.[364–381] Berger disease may also occur in siblings and identical twins, sometimes in association with deafness (thus resembling Alport syndrome; see also Chapter 31).[382–385] Immune abnormalities may also be found in otherwise healthy family members. Multiple cases have been found among families. Large pedigrees have been described in eastern Kentucky, France, and Australia.[1, 386] A variety of genetic markers have been shown to be associated with IgA nephropathy, but none consistently across geographic areas. These associations include *HLA-BW35, DR1, DR4, C4* allotypes, *C3* alleles, and factor B and IgA switch region polymorphisms[386] (see later). IgA deposits may be present in the glomerular mesangium of some persons who are outwardly normal in all other respects.[352, 387]

**Laboratory Findings.** The urinalysis is almost always

abnormal, with microscopic hematuria occasionally persisting between episodes of macroscopic hematuria. A glomerular source of hematuria is suggested by dysmorphic erythrocytes in urine,[295] but a mixed pattern of normal and dysmorphic urinary erythrocytes is common.[1] Abnormal proteinuria is characteristically mild and may be absent at times.[1, 338–340] Protein excretion is less than 1.0 g/d in more than 60% of cases.[1] Nephrotic range proteinuria occurs in about 10% of patients.[1, 388] Increased urinary IgG excretion may be associated with a poor prognosis.[389] On occasion, a steroid-sensitive relapsing form of nephrotic syndrome may be observed, often associated with minimal glomerular changes on renal biopsy.[390–392] Renal function is usually normal at time of discovery; however, as discussed later, slowly progressive decline in GFR occurs in many cases, although some patients exhibit a stable course for many years of observation.[1, 393–395] Episodes of acute deterioration of GFR and macroscopic hematuria may occur in association with intercurrent respiratory infections. Most of these episodes are spontaneously reversible.[361] Sometimes patients exhibit a prolonged stable course despite impaired renal function.[396–398] Renal biopsies are of value in estimating prognosis in individual patients (see later).

Serum IgA levels are increased in about 50% of cases.[399, 400] Most investigators have found evidence of an increased serum concentration of polymeric (20–21S) IgA.[400–405] The polymeric IgA seems to chiefly consist of the IgA1 subclass.[400–405] Complement component protein levels (e.g., C3, C4) are typically normal or elevated[406]; however, C3 fragments may be increased in 50% to 75% of patients, suggesting C3 activation in vivo, perhaps by the alternative pathway.[407, 408] Cold-induced complement activation has been described.[409] IgA-fibronectin aggregates are increased in the serum in 50% to 95% of patients, whereas elevated levels of IgA-fibronectin aggregates are found in less than 10% of non–IgA-associated glomerulonephritis.[410, 411] A positive value for IgA-fibronectin aggregates may be helpful in distinguishing IgA nephropathy from other glomerular diseases. Platelet-derived growth factor and interleukin-6 may be present in the urine, but elevated urinary levels of interleukin-6 may also be found in association with urinary tract infections.[465–467] Patients with IgA nephropathy also have decreased plasma ω-3 fatty acid concentrations.[468]

Some investigators have found increased levels of an IgM, cold-reactive antibody to saline-extractable, organ-specific nuclear antigen in a high percentage of patients.[412] Other studies have suggested the frequent presence of circulating IgA-containing immune complexes.[403, 405, 413–420] These immune complexes do not usually bind C1q and are best detected by non–complement-dependent assays. The levels of circulating immune complexes increase after an oral challenge with cow's milk in about 10% to 15% of patients.[420] Similar immune complexes are found in liver disease and Schönlein-Henoch purpura.[413] They contain polymeric IgA.[403] IgG-containing immune complexes are less common.[343] It has been suggested that the codeposition of mesangial IgG or IgM may be responsible for complement deposition, thereby contributing to the development of glomerular injury.[421]

In sporadic or familial cases, the *DQw7, DQA1b,* and *DRw12* alleles are increased.[422–431] The association of IgA nephropathy with diabetes mellitus may be more than coincidental.[425] Rare cases with congenital C9 deficiency have also been described.[432] HLA antigens, most notably B12, B27, Bw35, DR1, DR4, DQw7, and DR12, are increased in frequency in patients with Berger disease compared with control subjects, although this is not true for all geographic areas.[384, 422–431] Homozygosity at the *C4* null allele occurs more frequently in patients with IgA nephropathy and Schönlein-Henoch purpura.[433] C4A deficiency due to inheritance of the *C4A* null allele may be associated with a particularly poor prognosis.[434]

Cryoglobulins and rheumatoid factor are most often absent, as are the usual IgG antinuclear factors associated with SLE.[344] However, IgA rheumatoid factor has been identified by a number of investigators and may have pathogenic significance.[435, 436] A wide variety of autoantibodies, including IgG anti–mesangial cell, antineutrophil cytoplasmic, antiendothelial, and anti–extracellular matrix antibodies, have been described.[437–442] The exact role of these antibodies in the pathogenesis of disease is uncertain. In patients with crescentic disease or vasculitis, IgA ANCAs have been observed.[440, 441] Some workers have found an increased prevalence of antibody to bovine plasma proteins, soy protein, respiratory pathogens, gliadin, herpesvirus, *Haemophilus parainfluenzae,* and common gut flora.[443–452] The role of these antigen-antibody systems in the pathogenesis of IgA nephropathy remains uncertain (see later). A defect in IgA-specific suppressor T cell activity has been described.[453] In general, T and B cell subsets are not different from normal subjects or other patients with glomerular disease.[454] Some but not all studies have shown an increase in peripheral IgA-bearing lymphocytes. Lectin-treated lymphocytes from patients with IgA nephropathy (as well as other glomerular diseases) produce permeability factors in vitro.[455] Peripheral blood monocytes contain increased messenger RNA for endothelin-1 during acute exacerbations. The levels correlate with severity of glomerular lesions and urinary protein excretion.[456] Pharyngeal washings contain increased amounts of IgA.[457] IgA-specific helper T cells may be increased.[458] Tonsillar cells spontaneously secrete more IgA than normal.[459] The clearance of IgG-coated autologous erythrocytes may be prolonged, indicating a defect in the mononuclear phagocyte system.[460, 461] Erythrocyte receptors for the C3b component of complement (CR1) are more numerous in azotemic patients with Berger disease than in other azotemic persons or nonazotemic patients with Berger disease.[462, 463] Soluble IgA aggregates are less readily phagocytosed by macrophages in vitro.[463] Some investigators have found increased whole blood and plasma viscosity and altered red blood cell deformability.[464] Urinary excretion of interleukin-6 and platelet factor 4 are increased, particularly during acute exacerbations.[465–467] The levels remain normal in thin–basement membrane nephropathy[465–467] (see later). Linolenic acid may be decreased in serum, and the abnormality is corrected by supplementation of the diet with ω-3 fatty acids.[468]

Skin biopsies from the volar surface of the forearm reveal dermal capillary deposits of IgA, C3, properdin, and fibrin but not C1q, C4, or IgA secretory piece in 20% to 50% of cases.[469–472] This pattern is also found in renal biopsies (see later). Similar cutaneous deposits are also found in involved and uninvolved skin in Schönlein-Henoch purpura and infrequently in the absence of prominent glomerular mesangial IgA in other disease states (e.g., vasculitis, SLE).[470–473] Thus, demonstration of dermal vasculature deposits of IgA may be a useful adjunct in the evaluation of recurrent hematuric syndromes. Indeed, a patient with recurrent hematuria with elevated IgA levels who has IgA and C3 but not IgG or IgM deposits in the dermal vasculature almost certainly will be found to have IgA mesangial deposits on renal biopsy. The role of renal biopsy in such circumstances is primarily prognostic rather than diagnostic (see later). The overall value of skin biopsy in IgA nephropathy is limited because of variations in sensitivity and specificity.[471] Hene and co-workers,[472] in a prospective study, estimated the sensitivity and specificity of skin biopsy in dermal capillary IgA deposits in IgA nephropathy to be 75% and 88%, respectively.

### Pathology

***Light Microscopy.*** Almost any glomerular lesion seen in primary glomerular disease, with the possible exception of MGN, may be observed by routine light microscopy.[1, 472–476] The major abnormality, involving virtually all glomeruli, is expansion of the mesangium, usually affecting all lobules. When Masson trichrome or a related stain is used, fuchsinophilic deposits are often identified in the mesangium; the deposits are usually globular and large and are limited by the paramesangial matrix. Mesangial enlargement is often accompanied by an increase in mesangial cellularity, most commonly affecting lobules to an unequal degree, and is the factor responsible for inclusion of Berger disease in the group of focal glomerulonephritides, as emphasized in early studies that first defined this as a clinicopathologic entity (see Fig. 30–8). There is also a constant increase in mesangial matrix. Increased cellularity is considered an early "lesion," whereas predominance of matrix implies a late lesion with glomerular scarring.

Superimposed on this basic pattern of glomerular injury is a spectrum of other changes, including focal and segmental or global sclerosis, crescent formation affecting a variable percentage of glomeruli, and adhesions.[473, 477] The extent of crescentic involvement may be difficult to measure, especially when only a few glomeruli are present in the biopsy specimen.[478, 479] Acute renal failure in association with macroscopic hematuria and less than 50% glomerular involvement with crescents may resolve spontaneously.[361] When more than 50% of the glomeruli are involved with circumferential crescents, RPGN is frequently noted.[361] When acute renal failure develops, the decline in renal function is more related to tubule swelling, necrosis, obstruction with erythrocyte casts, and interstitial changes than to the glomerular disease.[361, 480] Virtually all of biopsies performed during episodes of gross hematuria have disclosed crescents.[358, 361] This lesion may be associated with a better prognosis, as opposed to a chronic sclerosing lesion.

It is the presence of segmental sclerosis, often with "hyalinosis," that might allow confusion of IgA nephropathy with focal and segmental glomerulosclerosis if only light microscopy is used for studying renal biopsy specimens.[473] Some investigators believe that the finding of segmental sclerosis is more commonly associated with significant pro-

teinuria and a more serious prognosis.[1, 348, 474] Others have described increasing mesangial sclerosis or crescentic involvement on repeated biopsies as an indicator of a worse outcome.[481] Tubule atrophy and interstitial fibrosis usually reflect the degree of glomerular obsolescence, and small quantities of interstitial lymphocytes and plasma cells may be observed in some biopsy samples.[482–485] Cellular infiltration of the interstitium consists of macrophages, T cells, and B cells. Increased numbers of interstitial B cells may be indicative of a poor prognosis.[486, 487] Acute tubule necrosis resulting in transient acute renal failure has been documented during gross hematuria and may be related to the tubulotoxic effects of released hemoglobin.[358, 361] "Hyalinization" of arterioles is evident in many specimens[488] and may correlate with progressive disease. Patients with malignant hypertension have the typical arterial and arteriolar lesions of malignant nephrosclerosis.[489] A subgroup of patients with nephrotic syndrome has been described whose glomeruli are nearly normal by light microscopy; IgA mesangial deposits are present. Most of these patients respond to glucocorticoid therapy (see later).[390–392, 490]

***Electron Microscopy.*** In almost all instances, finely granular to homogeneous electron-dense deposits are identified in the mesangium of all lobules of all glomeruli (Fig. 30–9). However, in a small number of biopsies, despite prominent IgA and other proteins demonstrated by immunofluorescence, ultrastructural studies have failed to disclose typical deposits or have shown only ill-defined densities. This has been noted especially in biopsy specimens in which only IgA is present.[1, 491] Deposits have also been identified in subendothelial locations, usually near the mes-

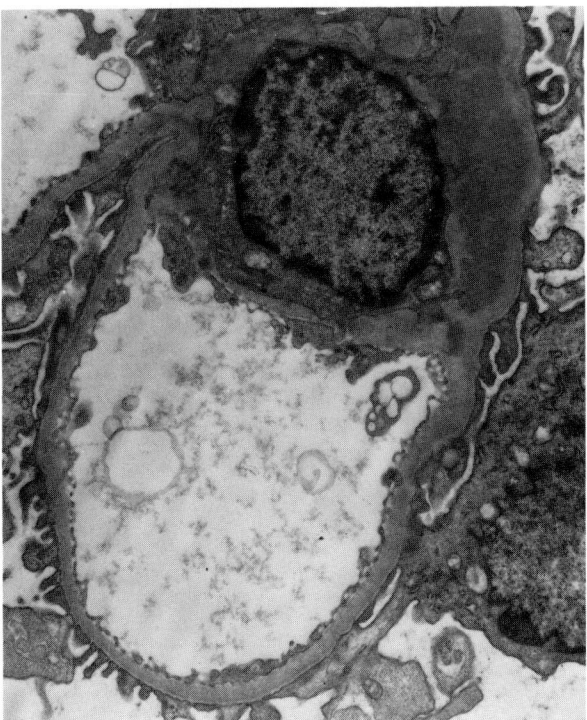

**Figure 30–9.** Electron microscopic appearance of IgA nephropathy. Several confluent deposits, limited to the mesangium, are evident. (Magnification × 12,000.)

angium, and with less frequency in epimembranous sites, occasionally as humps similar to those seen in PSGN. Epithelial foot processes are generally well preserved, and mesangial cell interposition is infrequent.[1] There is increased mesangial matrix in advanced cases.[492] Diffuse foot process effacement may be seen in patients with nephrotic syndrome, either associated with segmental glomerulosclerosis or in patients with what appears to be minimal-change nephrotic syndrome with IgA mesangial deposits.[490] Electron-dense deposits of uncertain nature are often noted in the basement membrane of Bowman capsule of many glomeruli.[1, 493] In advanced lesions, considerable distortion, layering, and splitting of the basement membranes may be noted.[493, 494] There may also be "lysis" of the basement membrane, in which thinning, rarefaction, and replacement of lamina densa occur in association with subepithelial deposits and polymorphonuclear leukocytes in lumens in direct contact with basement membrane. These changes have been correlated with advanced light microscopic lesions and heavy proteinuria, but not hematuria.[495]

*Immunofluorescence.* By definition, IgA as the sole or predominant immunoglobulin and almost always localized to the mesangium is found in all biopsy specimens[1] (Fig. 30–10). However, the frequency with which IgG is found, often in the same intensity as IgA, had previously suggested to some that this entity should be termed IgA/IgG mesangial nephropathy. Indeed, in several series, IgG was detected in more than 90% of the biopsies[329, 345] in the same pattern as IgA. C3, likewise, is usually observed in about the same proportion of specimens as IgG. Although not emphasized in the original description, IgM has been detected to a much lesser intensity in 3% to 72% of biopsies in several reports.[346, 403] The λ light chain predominates in the IgA deposits, unlike that of serum.[496] C1q and C4 are almost never found.[346] These findings suggest prominent involvement of the alternative pathway of complement activation. Other immunoreactants, including fibrinogen and

properdin, have been detected when sought. IgD and IgE, infrequently looked for, have also not been noted.[346] In almost all instances, IgA, IgG, and C3 have been limited to the mesangium; on occasion, however, capillary wall localization has been noted, but usually with less intensity. Capillary wall deposits, whether documented by immunofluorescence or electron microscopy, have been associated with more severe manifestations and a worse prognosis.[497] Secretory piece is usually not present in the deposits. However, J chain may be found in conjunction with IgA or IgM deposits, particularly after acid urea treatment of the specimen.[498] Secretory piece will bind to deposits in vitro.[499] These findings support the polymeric nature of the IgA deposit.

Cytomegalovirus antigen has been found by immunofluorescence in the mesangial deposits in 100% of a group of subjects studied in one report, but this has not been confirmed.[500, 501] Antigens of the outer membrane of *H. parainfluenzae* have been detected in the glomerular deposits of 44 of 44 patients with IgA nephropathy and only 2 of 39 patients with other non–IgA-associated glomerular diseases.[450] Patients with IgA nephropathy also have increased levels of circulating antibody to *H. parainfluenzae*.[450] This finding has not yet been confirmed, but if it is true, it may have special significance for the underlying pathogenic mechanism in IgA nephropathy. In situ hybridization studies have failed to reveal specific deposition of antigens of Epstein-Barr or herpes simplex viruses.[502] Hepatitis B surface antigenemia is commonly associated with IgA nephropathy in Asia.[503] Eluates of IgA react with glomeruli of some but not all patients with IgA.[504–506] Eluted antibodies react with tonsillar cells of the same patient.[507] Some of the IgA may react with single-stranded DNA.[439] Both IgA1, and IgA2 are found in the deposits,[403, 508, 509] but most investigators have found predominant IgA1.[509] Shared idiotypes in the deposited IgA are not disease specific, suggesting a polyclonal nature of the deposits.[510] The IgA in the circulation may be galactose deficient and may have an abnormal metabolism because of defective hepatic transport.[511]

Sera from patients with IgA nephropathy reveal impaired ability to solubilize immune deposits in vitro.[512] The membrane attack complex of complement has been demonstrated in mesangial regions at sites corresponding to IgA deposits, especially in advanced or severe glomerular lesions.[513] S protein, a regulatory component of the membrane attack complex, has also been identified in glomeruli, especially if adhesions or crescents are present, suggesting that the presence of S protein reflects certain types of injury.[514] Furthermore, activation of the terminal components of complement may exacerbate glomerular damage.[421, 514] Platelet-derived growth factor and a heterogeneous charge glycoprotein have been found in the IgA deposits.[515, 516] Fibronectin and vitronectin are also increased in the mesangium.[517]

In a report describing findings on repeated biopsy 45 days after the documentation of IgA deposits, Bergstein[518] observed the absence of immunoglobulin and complement deposits in glomeruli, despite continuation of hematuria. This interesting observation raises the possibility that some patients with IgA nephropathy may, at some time during the course of the disease, have no immunoglobulin deposits

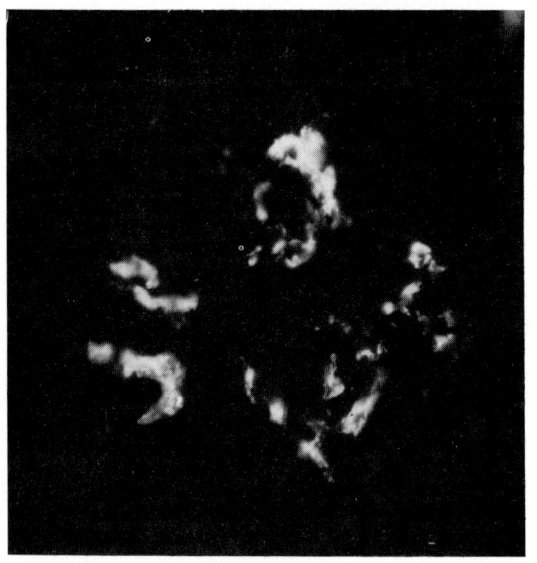

**Figure 30–10.** Immunofluorescence view of IgA nephropathy. Heavy IgA deposits are localized to the mesangial areas of this glomerulus. Note the lack of capillary wall staining. (Antihuman IgG; magnification × 1000.)

and may explain immunofluorescence-negative focal glomerulonephritides associated with hematuria (see later).[1] However, this observation has not been confirmed by numerous reports of repeated biopsies in many other patients with IgA nephropathy. IgA deposits may also be found in glomeruli in otherwise normal persons. A few patients have been described with coexisting IgA nephropathy and MGN; granular capillary wall deposits of IgG are present along with mesangial IgA deposits.[519–522]

**Pathogenesis.** The pathogenesis of Berger disease is unknown.[1, 343, 344, 446, 523] The presence of granular deposits of IgA and C3 but not early-acting complement components in both glomerular mesangium and dermal capillaries and the similarity to Schönlein-Henoch purpura with its attendant systemic features suggest that it is a circulating immune complex–mediated disease involving prominent activation of the alternative complement pathway. The deposition of IgA with J chain but not with secretory component suggests that polymeric IgA1 is involved.[403] Strong evidence exists that the deposited IgA is chiefly polymeric IgA1 capable of activating the alternative pathway of complement.[509, 518] Frequent reports of IgA nephropathy in patients with syndromes affecting IgA secretory epithelium in the gut, respiratory tract, or rarely the breast suggest that in at least some patients, the antibody is produced as a part of a specific host immune response to a variety of offending antigens in these areas. IgA, produced in the bone marrow, may also be involved.[524, 525] IgA antibody to dietary components (e.g., gluten, bovine albumin)[443–446] and to infectious agents, such as cytomegalovirus, herpesvirus, *H. parainfluenzae,* and adenovirus, may be found in some patients with IgA nephropathy.[438–450, 526] This strengthens the potential relationship between mucosal immunity and IgA nephropathy; however, not all studies support the concept that the increases in IgA in some patients with IgA nephropathy and the IgA-containing immune complexes are directed to antigens related to mucosal epithelium. IgA rheumatoid factors seen in some patients with IgA nephropathy suggest a nonmucosal origin of the immunoglobulin.[435, 436] In addition, an increase in IgA-secreting lymphocytes has been observed in the peripheral blood of patients with Berger disease,[527] as have enhanced IgA-specific helper T cells and diminished numbers of IgA-specific suppressor T cells.[528] Still other patients with Berger disease manifest abnormalities in the clearance of IgA immune complexes rather than in the synthesis of IgA or IgA immune complexes. Impaired clearance of IgA immune complexes and IgA aggregates and diminished numbers of phagocytes with receptors for the Fc portion of IgA have been reported.[529, 530] Also, impairment of immune complex solubilization by C3b has been reported in patients with Berger disease.[530] Some evidence has accumulated that the IgA molecule itself is abnormal (e.g., galactose deficient) in IgA nephropathy.[511]

In addition, some investigators have demonstrated that circulating IgA or IgG antibodies will react with mesangium of some but not all patients with IgA nephropathy, with fibroblasts cocultured with pharyngeal cells from patients with IgA nephropathy,[531] or with a cytoplasmic antigen in cultured human mesangial cells.[442, 532] These studies raise the possibility of an autoimmune reaction to a normal or ''planted'' mesangial antigen.[533]

A genetic predisposition to IgA nephropathy has been commented on before; in some instances, it is linked to HLA, but in others, no association with HLA can be found.[386] Immunologic abnormalities in the IgA system can be found in many apparently healthy relatives of patients with IgA nephropathy.[386, 534] Demaine and co-workers[535] noted an intriguing association of IgA nephropathy with restriction of fragment length polymorphisms in the IgA heavy chain switch region. Experimental models of IgA nephropathy have been produced by oral immunization[421, 536] (see also Chapter 29), by dextran injections,[537] and by induction of chronic hepatic injury.[538, 539] Because the liver is involved in processing gut-derived IgA complexed with antigen and IgA deposits are found in glomeruli in alcoholic liver disease, a defect in hepatic processing of IgA complexed with gut-derived antigens has been postulated to account for IgA nephropathy.[538–541]

**Course and Therapy.** Most patients continue to have episodes of gross or microscopic hematuria, but long symptom-free intervals may occasionally occur. Spontaneous complete remissions occur in less than 4% of adult patients, usually more than 4 years from the onset of disease or its discovery.[542] Pediatric patients may have a higher frequency of spontaneous complete remissions. The development of progressive chronic renal failure is poorly predictable, at least on clinical grounds. In extensive long-term follow-up of patients in France, Italy, and Spain, 20% to 30% have progressive renal insufficiency 20 years or more after initial discovery of disease.[1, 334, 340, 482–485] Actuarial renal survival in 11 series involving more than 1900 patients was 78% to 87% at 10 years after initial diagnosis.[483] It can be estimated that about 1% to 2% of patients will enter end-stage renal failure each year from time of diagnosis. Individualized prognosis is more difficult, but attempts have been made by use of multivariate analysis.[543] Not all series have demonstrated such a tendency to a progressive course.[398] Some patients may have a transient and reversible decline in renal function associated with synpharyngitic episodes of gross hematuria. Some patients' disease is rapidly progressive to end-stage renal failure in less than 4 years from the time of diagnosis.[544]

Clinical features that indicate a poor prognosis include male sex, older age at onset, decreased GFR at discovery, persistent nephrotic range proteinuria, and moderate hypertension.[482–485, 545, 546] Some studies have also shown an influence of HLA specificities on prognosis.[386, 427, 546] The influence on prognosis of the macroscopic or microscopic character of hematuria is debated; however, most studies have suggested that persistent microscopic hematuria combined with proteinuria is associated with the worst prognosis.[483] The presence of HLA-Bw35 or -DR4 has conferred a worse prognosis in some series.[546] The serum IgA level, severity and frequency of episodes of hematuria, and cutaneous deposits of IgA have no consistent bearing on prognosis, but many authors have noted that glomerular crescent involvement is more common in patients with recurrent macroscopic hematuria.[348, 358]

The effects of pregnancy on IgA nephropathy have been assessed in retrospective studies.[547–550] Whereas an unexpected rapid downhill course to end-stage renal failure was observed in a small number of patients in certain series, in general, pregnancy was safe and successful in the absence of preconception hypertension or azotemia (serum creatinine concentration ≤ 2.3 mg/dL).[547–550] In one study, 63% of the gestations were associated with hypertension, one quarter of which were severe, 22% with diminished renal function, and a significant number with worse renal histologic changes than of patients who had never been pregnant.[547, 549] Other studies have shown increased perinatal mortality if the initial GFR is less than 70 mL/min.[550]

Renal pathologic findings that indicate a poor prognosis include diffuse proliferative glomerular lesions, especially if accompanied by segmental or diffuse crescents, focal and segmental glomerular sclerosis or tubule atrophy, arteriolar sclerosis, and interstitial fibrosis.[1, 482–485, 545, 546, 551, 552] Peripheral capillary IgA and C3 deposits may confer a worse prognosis.[483]

For the majority of patients, no specific therapy is required. However, for patients with features indicative of a poor prognosis (e.g., proteinuria greater than 1 g/d, impaired GFR, persistent hypertension, sclerosing or crescentic glomerular lesions, or tubulointerstitial fibrosis), a more aggressive approach may be indicated. Unfortunately, few therapies have been proved to be effective when studied in appropriately designed prospective randomized trials.[553–555] The effect of glucocorticoids on long-term outcome is controversial, but meta-analyses and limited trials have suggested a potential beneficial effect, particularly if glucocorticoid therapy is begun relatively early in the course of disease in patients with modest proteinuria (greater than 1 g/d) and well-preserved renal function (GFR greater than 70 mL/min).[556–564] Steroids are clearly beneficial in the uncommon patient with nephrotic syndrome and mild glomerular lesions.[391, 392] An argument has been made that these patients actually represent a subset of minimal-change nephropathy.[392] The use of cytotoxic agents has not been rigorously examined in controlled trials but does not seem indicated in any case because of the unpredictable and indolent course.[553–555] In patients with a demonstrably progressive course, cytotoxic drugs combined with glucocorticoids or cytotoxic agents combined with anticoagulant and antithrombotic drugs[565] may be of benefit, but the paucity of long-term controlled trials clearly places these therapeutic approaches in the realm of experimental treatment.[565] Whereas cyclosporine may transiently decrease proteinuria, such therapy is usually associated with a further decline in GFR.[566] Prophylactic penicillin, sulfonamide, and broad-spectrum antibiotics have been tried, although the frequency of bouts of gross hematuria may decrease.[553–555] A single case report described benefit from plasmapheresis.[567] Because phenytoin lowers IgA levels, Clarkson and colleagues[568] embarked on a trial of this agent in Berger disease several years ago. Although early results were encouraging and elevated IgA levels returned to normal, no consistent effect on the progression of disease or of modification of IgA-containing immune complexes has yet been consistently observed.[569–571] In an attempt to improve complement-mediated solubilization of immune complexes, long-term therapy with danazol has been tried, but no clear-cut beneficial effects have yet been reported.[572] Tonsillectomy may reduce frequency of hematuric episodes in patients with recurrent tonsillitis,[553–555] but episodes of acute

renal failure may occur in proximity to tonsillectomy.[1] Aspirin and dipyridamole were not any more effective than placebo in preserving renal function in a prospective trial that observed patients for a mean of 33 months.[573] Combinations of dipyridamole and low-dose warfarin in small controlled trials have been claimed to slow the rate of progression of renal disease in high-risk groups.[565] In addition, dipyridamole alone, and perhaps other agents having similar effects on platelet aggregation, will decrease the magnitude of proteinuria in many patients with IgA nephropathy as well as in patients with other glomerular diseases (e.g., MGN, focal and segmental glomerular sclerosis).[574] Eicosapentaenoic acid (ω-3 fatty acid) therapy and low dosage or short duration of treatment in small trials[575–577] were of no benefit. More recently, a large prospective randomized placebo-controlled trial in patients with IgA nephropathy and more than 1 g of protein excretion per day using 12 g of ω-3 fatty acids has been reported.[578] Treated patients received 1.87 g of eicosapentaenoic acid and 1.36 g of docosahexaenoic acid. Striking benefits were seen in the treated patients. Only 3 of 55 patients receiving ω-3 fatty acids had an increase in serum creatinine concentration exceeding 50% above the baseline values compared with 14 of 56 receiving the placebo (olive oil). End-stage renal disease developed in 5 patients receiving ω-3 fatty acids and in 14 receiving placebo. No differences were seen in urinary protein excretion. Blood pressure was treated to the same extent in both groups.[578] Low-antigen (elimination) diets and gluten-free diets have also decreased IgA levels and improved protein excretion rates in some patients with IgA nephropathy.[579, 580] These therapeutic approaches need further confirmation. Plasma exchange plus immunosuppressive therapy may be of value in the rare patient with rapidly progressive glomerulonephritis associated with extensive (75%) crescentic involvement, but full recovery even with such treatment is unlikely.[567, 581] ACE inhibitors lower protein excretion and are associated with better preservation of renal function, perhaps because of intrarenal effects.[582–584] NSAIDs may also retard the progression of IgA nephropathy.[1, 553, 555] High-dose intravenous immunoglobulin (1.0 g/kg/d for two doses repeated three times in the succeeding months) followed by intramuscular injections of lower doses on an intermittent basis may be associated with partial recovery of renal function in patients with severe and rapidly progressive disease.[585] Many patients with an acute reduction in renal function associated with macroscopic hematuria and moderate (<50%) crescentic glomerular involvement recover spontaneously, even if dialysis is required.[361, 586] Because of occurrence of IgA deposits in dermatitis herpetiformis, dapsone has been tried, but without success.[553–555]

The disease may commonly recur in renal allografts, although short-term follow-up has only rarely indicated any serious clinical consequences.[587–589] Indeed, long-term observations suggest that recurrence rates are greater than 50% with follow-up of 5 years or longer.[588, 589] Overall, however, kidney graft survival is increased rather than decreased in IgA nephropathy, perhaps because of the presence of IgA-blocking antibody.[589a] Inapparent IgA nephropathy in a sibling donor has led to the inadvertent transmission of disease with an allograft. Occasionally, IgA deposits in an allograft may spontaneously resolve.[1]

In summary, IgA nephropathy (Berger disease) is one of the most common primary renal diseases and can be readily diagnosed by correlative light and immunofluorescence microscopy. A reasonably accurate prognosis can be made with use of selected clinical and morphologic features. Although the etiology and pathogenesis of IgA nephropathy are still unknown, they are likely to be multifactorial. The IgA nephropathy lesion may be a *phenotypic* expression of a heterogeneous collection of disorders of diverse pathogenesis. At present, patients with an intrinsically unfavorable prognosis should receive therapy with ACE inhibitors or oral high-dose ω-3 fatty acids. Some patients, including those with nephrotic syndrome with minimal-change disease, may also benefit from oral glucocorticoids or a combination of dipyridamole and low-dose warfarin. Antigen-elimination or gluten-free diets may be useful, but both require further confirmation before they can be widely applied. Patients with severe disease, including crescentic glomerulonephritis, could be treated either with plasma exchange and immunosuppression or with high-dose immunoglobulins. Patients with acute renal failure associated with intercurrent upper respiratory illnesses and who show relatively few crescents but mainly tubulointerstitial disease on biopsy can be treated conservatively, including dialysis as necessary, while awaiting spontaneous recovery. Patients with normal renal function, less than 1 g/d protein excretion in urine, and mild pathologic findings should be treated conservatively and receive ACE inhibitors if blood pressure is elevated. The overall prognosis of IgA nephropathy is favorable; 10-year renal survival exceeds 80% in most cases.

## OTHER PRIMARY GLOMERULAR DISEASES THAT EVOKE HEMATURIA WITH OR WITHOUT PROTEINURIA

Among patients with this syndrome who do not fall into the category of IgA nephropathy, a variety of histopathologic lesions and immunopathologic lesions have been found (see Table 30–4). The clinical features of this group are similar to those of Berger disease, although increased IgA levels and other serologic findings are not usually encountered. Loin pain may be seen frequently, and males and females may be involved with equal frequency. Proteinuria, if present, is typically mild, and as in the case of Berger disease, one should suspect other underlying diseases if massive proteinuria is present (see Chapter 31 and later discussion of nephrotic syndrome). Renal function is typically normal, and hypertension is absent. A strong family history may be seen occasionally. Hearing abnormalities of Alport syndrome, the typical angiokeratoma of Fabry disease, and other clinical and biochemical clues of heredofamilial disease should be sought in all cases (see also Chapter 31). Light microscopic studies of renal biopsy specimens reveal a spectrum ranging from normal histologic appearance to minimal glomerular abnormalities to diffuse proliferative glomerulonephritis (mesangial or endocapillary proliferative glomerulonephritis) and focal and segmental proliferative glomerulonephritis.[1] Some patients may represent instances of resolving postinfectious glomerulonephritis or the early manifestations of a systemic disease process, such as SLE, Goodpasture disease, or vasculitis. Still others represent instances of primary glomerular disease more frequently associated with massive proteinuria (see nephrotic syndrome) but not yet advanced to a nephrotic stage or have undergone a partial spontaneous or therapy-induced remission (e.g., MCGN, focal glomerular sclerosis, MGN). When these cases have been excluded, either by appropriate serologic studies or biopsy of kidney or other tissue, and Berger disease is excluded by absence of IgA deposits, the remaining patients still display a diversity of glomerular lesions and immunopathologic findings. The light microscopic findings have been alluded to before. The electron microscopic findings are helpful. Excessive thinning or attenuation of peripheral GBM may identify a thin–basement membrane nephropathy or an underlying familial disease related to Alport syndrome[1, 323, 590–593] (see later). Occasionally, thinning, reduplication, and fragmentation of the GBM identical to that found in otherwise typical examples of Alport syndrome may be found in patients who have no clear-cut hereditary occurrence of hematuria or deafness (see also Chapter 31).

Several patterns of immunoglobulin or C3 deposition may be seen: 1) diffuse granular mesangial IgM and C3; 2) diffuse granular mesangial IgG and C3; 3) diffuse linear IgG and C3; or 4) isolated mesangial C3 deposits. A variable percentage of patients reveal no immunoglobulin or C3 deposits. The immunopathogenetic significance of these immunoglobulin or C3 deposits is unknown, although occasionally linear IgG deposits may represent anti-GBM antibody deposition.[324–334]

The long-term course of this group of patients is not well defined. If glomerular abnormalities are minimal or mild and if persistent heavy proteinuria is absent, the outlook appears good. The majority of patients can be expected to undergo spontaneous remission of hematuria, and progressive renal failure is exceptional. Because of the benign nature of this group of disorders, no therapy is recommended.

### Thin–Basement Membrane Nephropathy

This entity, also frequently called benign recurrent hematuria, has been separated from other causes of renal hematuria by its characteristic electron microscopic findings.[1, 323, 589–594] The thickness of the peripheral capillary GBM is decreased to 265 nm or less (normal 375 ± 75 nm for males, 325 ± 40 nm for females). Light microscopic findings are normal; however, immunofluorescence may reveal diffuse mesangial C3 deposition in some patients.[323] IgA nephropathy and thin–basement membrane nephropathy may coexist, sometimes in a familial distribution.[593]

The typical presentation of patients with thin–basement membrane nephropathy is similar to that of IgA nephropathy. Young to middle-aged adults predominate. Males and females are affected about equally. However, macroscopic hematuria is uncommon, unlike in IgA nephropathy.[323, 591] The degree of proteinuria is variable and of little diagnostic significance, but approximately 70% of patients do not have any detectable abnormal protein excretion at the time of presentation. Persistence of microscopic hematuria is the rule. Occasionally, family members may also have microscopic hematuria, but no clear pattern of inheritance has been observed.[323, 591-594] Hearing is normal. If audiograms demonstrate high-tone neural deafness, it is likely that the patient has Alport syndrome (see also Chapter 31). Many patients are O-positive, Rh-positive.[594] No serologic tests are available to identify this disease without recourse to renal biopsy.

Among patients with apparently idiopathic renal hematuria with normal blood pressure and renal function, thin–basement membrane nephropathy was encountered in 23% in a prospective study.[323] In the same study, IgA nephropathy was found in 34% of patients; the remaining 43% had either entirely normal renal tissue or other glomerular or tubulointerstitial diseases.[323] Among patients with idiopathic renal hematuria with normal renal tissue by light microscopy, thin–basement membrane nephropathy was seen in approximately 43%. Thin–basement membrane nephropathy was uncommonly found if *macroscopic* hematuria was the mode of presentation, but among those with *persisting microscopic* hematuria and proteinuria of less than 200 mg/d and normal glomeruli by light microscopy, 65% had thin–basement membrane nephropathy.[323] Although precise diagnosis of this entity requires a renal biopsy with electron microscopy, thin–basement membrane nephropathy should be suspected when an adult man or woman younger than 40 years presents with persisting microscopic hematuria, normal renal function, and normal blood pressure with or without non-nephrotic range proteinuria, especially if urinalyses in family members reveal microscopic hematuria and hearing is normal. Urinary interleukin-6 and platelet factor 4 levels should also be normal.[465-467]

The prognosis is regarded as good, although a few patients with progressive renal failure have been described.[323, 590-595] No therapy for this disorder is available. Because patients with thin–basement membrane nephropathy may resemble those with classic X-linked Alport syndrome (except for deafness), one should be cautious about prognostication. A monoclonal antibody reactive with the Goodpasture epitope on the noncollagenous domains of type IV collagen binds to the basement membrane in thin–basement membrane nephropathy but not to the basement membrane in classic X-linked Alport syndrome[595] (see also Chapter 31). Thus, it appears that thin–basement membrane nephropathy and Alport syndrome are two distinct disorders. The biochemical defect responsible for thin–basement membrane nephropathy remains unknown.

### Loin Pain–Hematuria Syndrome

Although not a glomerular disease in the strictest sense, this syndrome is nonetheless an important cause of recurrent hematuria and should be differentiated from the primary glomerular lesions mentioned. This syndrome, delineated in 1967,[596-598] typically occurs in young women; however, males have also been affected. Use of oral contraceptive agents has been implicated in its pathogenesis.[596-599] Presenting features include recurrent bouts of gross hematuria, bilateral or unilateral dull and aching loin pain, and low-grade fever giving rise to confusion with IgA nephropathy, renal infections, tumors, and urolithiasis. A search for dysmorphic erythrocytes is often helpful in the differential

diagnosis. Proteinuria, if present, is usually mild. Blood pressure and GFR are usually normal. There are no distinctive laboratory findings, but increased fibrinopeptide A levels, enhanced platelet aggregation, and decreased prostaglandin $I_2$ (prostacyclin)–stimulating factor activity have been noted.[600, 603] Arteriograms sometimes reveal abnormal narrowing of the terminal branches of the intrarenal vessels.[598] Segmental areas of renal ischemia may be found with radionuclide scans (personal observation). Renal biopsies reveal normal glomeruli, mural thickening of interlobular arteries, often associated with C3, but no immunoglobulin deposits.[599-601] Occasionally, IgM deposits will be found.[602] The origin of the loin pain is uncertain. It may be due to microvascular thrombosis and infarction of the kidney from neural-driven vasospasm. There is a strong psychologic overlay in many patients. Addiction to narcotics is common.[599] It may be associated with IgA or IgM nephropathy.[602] The long-term prognosis is uncertain, but some patients may benefit symptomatically from discontinuance of oral contraceptives or treatment with antithrombotic or anticoagulant agents.[596-600] The role of vasodilators, such as $Ca^{2+}$ channel antagonists, is unclear. Complete renal denervation by autotransplantation of the kidney has been tried as a desperate measure in a few patients.[603] Most patients experience immediate relief of loin pain, but later recurrences are common (at least 30%, probably higher). Because of the strong psychologic background, nephrectomy is not advised even though it has been resorted to in a few cases.[603]

### Isolated Non-nephrotic Glomerular Proteinuria (Asymptomatic Proteinuria Without Hematuria; Isolated Proteinuria)

This group is defined by the presence of mild glomerular proteinuria (principally albumin), usually less than 2 g/d, with a normal urine sediment in the absence of systemic disease.[1, 604-606] The proteinuria in these cases may be persistent ("fixed and reproducible") or transient. It may (orthostatic) or may not (constant) be related to posture. This abnormality is nearly always discovered incidentally and is distressing to patients and physicians alike. Such patients typically have normal renal function, normal blood pressure, and none of the biochemical abnormalities of the nephrotic state (e.g., hypoalbuminemia). In some cases, particularly those with constant proteinuria, such an abnormality will be the initial feature of an illness of serious import. For example, idiopathic MGN, focal glomerular sclerosis, IgA nephropathy, and amyloidosis may all initially present with isolated mild to moderate proteinuria. Isolated proteinuria may also be present in patients with asymptomatic essential hypertension and mild or latent diabetic nephropathy. The excretion of small quantities of albumin (15 to 200 $\mu$g/min), well below the limit of detection of usual assays (microalbuminuria), may be an early sign of developing overt diabetic glomerulopathy (see also Chapters 31 and 39). Mild transient proteinuria may accompany febrile states, congestive heart failure, vigorous exercise, and self-limited infectious illnesses.[1, 607-609]

It is important to exclude overflow proteinuria (e.g., excessive filtration) of low-molecular-weight plasma proteins (e.g., light chains) and tubule proteinuria in patients with modest degrees of isolated constant proteinuria. This can best be accomplished by immunochemical determination of light chain ($\kappa$ and $\lambda$) excretion, by cellulose acetate electrophoresis of urinary protein, and by comparison of $\beta_2$-microglobulin and albumin excretion rates.

## POSTURAL PROTEINURIA

Orthostatic or postural proteinuria has been defined as a clinical syndrome requiring the absence of qualitative proteinuria during recumbency and its appearance during quiet upright ambulation or on standing.[1, 604–606] The total daily protein excretion usually is less than 1.5 g but may be much higher, the majority being excreted during upright ambulation. Similar patterns of protein excretion may be observed in patients with documented primary glomerular disease. Patients with orthostatic proteinuria tend to have more selective proteinuria on recumbency, whereas those with definite glomerulonephritis do not.

Renal biopsy studies in patients with fixed and reproducible orthostatic proteinuria have revealed that approximately 8% had unequivocal evidence of readily classifiable primary glomerular disease; 45% had minimal to moderate glomerular changes of a nonspecific nature; and in 47%, the glomeruli could not be distinguished from normal by light microscopy.[1, 605] Sinniah and co-workers[610] found that 30% of patients with orthostatic proteinuria had normal or minimally altered glomeruli, whereas 70% had mild mesangial prominence. No immunoglobulin or C3 deposits were found in any case.

Constant proteinuria, present in both upright and recumbent positions, is, in general, related to well-defined underlying glomerular disease and thus is associated with a less benign prognosis. As previously mentioned, the combination of non-nephrotic persistent proteinuria and abnormal findings in the urine sediment is commonly but not invariably indicative of underlying glomerular disease and is often associated with a progressive decline in GFR or the appearance of hypertension.[606, 611]

In the study of Sinniah's group,[610] about 0.95% of otherwise healthy young adult men in Singapore were discovered to have isolated proteinuria. In 40% of this group, the proteinuria was constant, regardless of position, and persisted for several periods of study. In 60%, the proteinuria was orthostatic only. Renal biopsies in the group with constant and persistent isolated proteinuria revealed normal or minimally altered glomeruli in 13%, mild mesangial prominence with or without focal sclerosis in 67%, and definite diffuse or focal proliferative glomerulonephritis in only about 15% of cases. Interestingly, predominant IgA deposits were found in 34% and prominent C3 deposits in 60%. IgM deposits were uncommon, accounting for only 7% of biopsies. In the group with orthostatic proteinuria only, glomerular lesions were mild, consisting of minor changes in 30% and mild mesangial prominence in 70%. Immunofluorescence findings in renal biopsy were uniformly negative in this group. Occasionally, primary vascular or interstitial lesions predominated.

Long-term follow-up studies of patients presenting with orthostatic proteinuria in general have confirmed its benign nature.[1, 604–606, 612] These studies have noted a steadily declining frequency of proteinuria in such patients. The prognosis of constant proteinuria that persists for several periods of observation is less benign and depends on the nature of the underlying lesion.[1, 604–606, 612] Hypertension and reduced GFR may appear after many years. For patients with idiopathic, constant, non-nephrotic proteinuria or orthostatic proteinuria, no treatment is indicated. Apart from providing the patient with a means of reassurance or as an additional measure of prognosis, renal biopsies do not contribute in an important way to the management of persistent non-nephrotic proteinuria, although specific disease entities, such as amyloidosis, may on occasion be encountered in the absence of other clinical findings. Many experienced clinicians limit renal biopsy to those patients demonstrating constant proteinuria in excess of 1 to 2 g/d, consistently demonstrable in a period of several months' observation, that is not readily explained by some systemic disease process (e.g., diabetes mellitus, multiple myeloma). Patients with "benign" essential hypertension and arteriolonephrosclerosis with impaired renal function not infrequently excrete abnormal quantities of protein, which on occasion can reach levels of 1 to 2 g/d. Separation of these patients from those with underlying glomerular disease (e.g., IgA nephropathy, fibrillary glomerulonephritis) is difficult or impossible without resorting to renal biopsy.[613] African-Americans with presumed essential hypertension accompanied by non-nephrotic proteinuria (<2.0 g/d) nearly always have underlying arteriolonephrosclerosis rather than primary glomerular disease.[290a, 613]

## THE NEPHROTIC SYNDROME

Schreiner[614] originally defined the nephrotic syndrome as a "clinical entity having multiple causes and characterized by increased glomerular permeability manifested by massive proteinuria and lipiduria. There is a variable tendency toward edema, hypoalbuminemia, and hyperlipidemia. Protein excretion rates are usually in excess of 3.5 g/day/1.73 m² body surface area in the absence of a depressed GFR." In the modern era of ready availability of percutaneous biopsy and sophisticated serologic and immunopathologic technology, the great variability of underlying lesions and etiologic agents that can evoke the nephrotic syndrome is now apparent.[615] The nephrotic syndrome is the predictable consequence of continued heavy proteinuria, modified by various homeostatic responses. However, the clinician should resist the temptation to ascribe some special significance to the arbitrary value of 3.5 g/d/1.73 m², dividing nephrotic from non-nephrotic proteinuria. It is true, however, that such heavy proteinuria more often than not indicates a glomerulopathy of some sort rather than one of the tubulointerstitial or vascular disorders of the kidney. Virtually all of the glomerulopathies that can provoke the biochemical features of the nephrotic syndrome can instead be associated with mild to moderate proteinuria, not infrequently asymptomatic, and it must be stressed that profound hypoalbuminemia often leads to a reduction of protein excretion well below the values mentioned yet is associated with a glomerular lesion causing enhanced permeability to plasma proteins (see also Chapter 43). The absolute rate of protein excretion above 3.5 g/d (or 2.5 mg/min) has little diagnostic significance, although protein excretion rates above 10 g/d (7 mg/min) are more commonly seen in focal and segmental glomerular sclerosis, MGN, MCGN, and amyloidosis (see later).

The multiplicity of etiologic factors, associated conditions, underlying disease, and pathogenesis make it difficult to review nephrotic syndrome without encompassing all of the diseases that constitute the general group of glomerular diseases[1, 615] (Table 30–6). Indeed, except for those processes that rapidly destroy the entire nephron population, virtually any glomerular lesion may be associated, at least temporarily, with proteinuria of sufficient magnitude to result in hypoalbuminemia and thus set into motion the pathophysiologic processes responsible for the constellation of findings we call the nephrotic syndrome.

Therefore, this discussion is organized as follows. First, the clinical parameters common to most patients displaying massive proteinuria are enumerated. Second, the complications and general management of the nephrotic state are discussed. Third, the clinical and pathologic entities most closely associated with nephrotic syndrome are reviewed. Multisystem, neoplastic, and heredofamilial disorders, which may commonly present in a variety of ways in addition to the nephrotic syndrome, are discussed in Chapter 31. Diabetic glomerulopathy, an extremely important cause of the nephrotic syndrome, is discussed in detail in Chapter 39. Nephrotic syndrome arising secondarily to defined events such as microbial infection, neoplasia, drugs, and specific disease entities is also discussed in Chapter 31. The nephrotic syndrome due to primary glomerular disease (also known as idiopathic nephrotic syndrome) is dealt with here. The pathophysiology of edema formation and the mechanisms of abnormal transglomerular passage of plasma proteins are discussed in Chapter 43.

This discussion emphasizes that nephrotic syndrome is a systemic biochemical disturbance with many important consequences. The development of nephrotic syndrome may be accompanied by progressive loss of renal function, depending on underlying disease. Continued activity of the injurious process (e.g., immune complex deposition or formation in the glomeruli), hemodynamic adaptations, concomitant systemic arterial hypertension, hyperlipidemia, nephrotoxic drugs, and the noxious potential of abnormal filtration of macromolecules into Bowman space and into the tubule lumen all may play pivotal roles in the progressive nature of the disease. The disappearance of abnormal proteinuria is a favorable sign, and few patients with nephrotic syndrome who enter into complete remissions progress to end-stage renal disease. Even a partial remission of the nephrotic syndrome confers significant protection from progressive renal disease.[616]

## Clinical and Laboratory Abnormalities

### PROTEINURIA

Although it was initially believed that abnormal protein excretion in ''nephrosis'' was the result of some abnormality in tubule function, it is now clear that an abnormality in

glomerular permeability is fundamental to those conditions producing heavy proteinuria.[1, 615, 617–619] The basic structure of the glomerular capillary wall and the mechanisms whereby the capillary prevents the passage of serum proteins into Bowman space have been discussed in Chapters 1, 7, and 43.[1, 615, 617–619]

In brief, proteinuria arising from defects in glomerular permeability can result from abnormalities in the charge-selective or size-selective barrier.[6, 617–619] Predominantly charge-selective barrier defects arise from diffuse biochemical changes in glomerular structure (visceral epithelial cells or GBM) often unassociated with recognizable abnormalities at the level of the light microscope; however, special staining techniques may reveal a marked decrease in anionic constituents of the capillary wall. On the other hand, size-selective barrier defects are usually associated with recognizable abnormalities of glomerular structure, including deposition of proteins, alterations in basement membrane structure, and mesangial abnormalities.[620] Heavy proteinuria can and does arise when only a small percentage of the total filtering surface area develops a size-selective barrier defect characterized by abnormally large effective pore radius (heteroporosity of capillary wall). Protein excretion rates in the nephrotic syndrome vary widely and are influenced considerably by the GFR, the prevailing glomerular plasma flow rate and transglomerular hydraulic pressure gradient, the activity of the renin-angiotensin system, the production and plasma concentration of albumin, and the dietary protein intake.[1, 6, 618, 621–627] The permeability characteristics of glomeruli can be measured in vitro, and this technique may be useful in identifying circulating factors that alter glomerular permselectivity.[628–630] The simple expression of abnormal proteinuria in quantitative terms (grams per day) in the arbitrary definition of nephrotic range proteinuria does not take into account the important influence of the factors that influence proteinuria. A dramatic fall in plasma albumin concentration might lead to a reduction in the rate of urinary excretion of albumin even though the fundamental defect in glomerular capillary wall function remains unaltered. Contrariwise, an infusion of albumin to raise the serum albumin concentration can be accompanied by a dramatic rise in urinary protein excretion. For this reason, it has been suggested that protein excretion rates should be presented as clearance rates for specific proteins (e.g., albumin clearance) or as clearance ratios (e.g., clearance of albumin/clearance of creatinine).[1, 631] The advantage of the latter measurement is that urine collections need not be timed, because the volume term cancels in the clearance ratio.

Expression of protein concentration relative to creatinine concentration in untimed urine specimens is a convenient way to avoid vagaries and uncertainties of a 24-hour urine collection.[1, 631] Urinary protein/creatinine concentration ratios in excess of 3.0 usually indicate nephrotic range proteinuria. Increases in albumin excretion follow expansion of plasma volume with isoncotic dextran, despite a decrease in serum albumin concentration.

Overall, there is a significant inverse correlation between protein excretion rates and serum albumin concentrations, but some patients maintain normal serum albumin concentrations for extended periods despite heavy proteinuria. This

**TABLE 30–6. Classification of the Disease States Associated with the Development of Nephrotic Syndrome**

**Idiopathic Nephrotic Syndrome due to Primary Glomerular Disease (see Table 30–8)**

**Nephrotic Syndrome Associated with Specific Etiologic Events or in Which Glomerular Disease Arises as a Complication of Other Diseases**

1. Medications
   *Organic, inorganic, elemental mercury**
   *Organic gold*
   *Penicillamine*, bucillamine
   *"Street" heroin*
   *Probenecid*
   *Captopril*
   *NSAIDs*
   *Lithium*
   *Interferon alfa*
   Chlorpropamide
   Rifampin
   Paramethadione (Paradione), trimethadione (Tridione)
   Mephenytoin (Mesantoin)
   Tolbutamide†
   Phenindione†
   Warfarin
   Clonidine†
   Perchlorate†
   Bismuth†
   Trichloroethylene†
   Silver†
   Insect repellent†
   Contrast media
2. Allergens, venoms, immunizations
   *Bee sting*
   *Pollens*
   Poison ivy and poison oak
   Antitoxins (serum sickness)
   Snake venom
   Diphtheria, pertussis, tetanus toxoid
   Vaccines
3. Infections
   a. *Bacterial–PSGN, infective endocarditis, "shunt nephritis,"* leprosy, syphilis (congenital and secondary), *Mycoplasma* infection, tuberculosis,† chronic bacterial pyelonephritis with vesicoureteral reflux
   b. *Viral*—hepatitis B, hepatitis C, cytomegalovirus, infectious mononucleosis (Epstein-Barr virus), herpes zoster, vaccinia, human immunodeficiency virus type I
   c. *Protozoal*— *malaria* (especially quartan malaria), toxoplasmosis
   d. *Helminthic—schistosomiasis*, trypanosomiasis, filariasis
4. Neoplastic‡
   a. *Solid tumors* (carcinoma and sarcoma): *lung, colon, stomach, breast,* cervix, kidney, thyroid, ovary, melanoma, pheochromocytoma, adrenal, oropharynx, carotid body,† Wilms tumor, prostate, mesothelioma, oncocytoma
   b. *Leukemia and lymphoma: Hodgkin disease,* chronic lymphatic leukemia, multiple myeloma (amyloidosis), Waldenström macroglobulinemia, lymphoma

5. Multisystem disease‡
   *Systemic lupus erythematosus*
   Mixed connective tissue disease
   Dermatomyositis
   Rheumatoid arthritis
   Goodpasture disease
   *Schönlein-Henoch purpura* (see also IgA nephropathy, Berger disease)
   Systemic vasculitis (including Wegener granulomatosis)
   Takayasu arteritis
   Mixed cryoglobulinemia
   Light and heavy chain disease (Randall-type)
   Partial lipodystrophy
   Sjögren syndrome
   Toxic epidermolysis
   Dermatitis herpetiformis
   Sarcoidosis
   Ulcerative colitis
   *Amyloidosis* (primary and secondary)
6. Heredofamilial and metabolic disease‡
   *Diabetes mellitus*
   Hypothyroidism (myxedema)
   Graves disease
   Amyloidosis (familial Mediterranean fever and other hereditary forms, Muckle-Wells syndrome)
   Alport syndrome
   Fabry disease
   Nail-patella syndrome
   Lipoprotein glomerulopathy
   Sickle-cell disease
   $\alpha_1$-Antitrypsin deficiency
   Asphyxiating thoracic dystrophy (Juene syndrome)
   von Gierke disease
   Charcot-Marie-Tooth disease
   Weber-Christian syndrome
   Congenital nephrotic syndrome (Finnish-type)
   Drash syndrome
   Cystinosis (adult)
   Galloway-Mowat syndrome
   Hurler syndrome
   Familial dysautonomia
   Familial nephrotic syndrome
7. Miscellaneous‡
   *Pregnancy-associated* (preeclampsia, recurrent, transient)
   *Chronic renal allograft failure*
   Accelerated or malignant nephrosclerosis
   Unilateral renal arterial hypertension
   Intestinal lymphangiectasia
   Chronic jejunoileitis†
   Spherocytosis†
   Renal artery stenosis
   Congenital heart disease† (cyanotic)
   Severe congestive heart failure†
   Constrictive pericarditis†
   Tricuspid insufficiency†
   Massive obesity
   Vesicoureteric reflux nephropathy
   Papillary necrosis
   Gardner-Diamond syndrome
   Castleman disease
   Kartagener syndrome
   Buckley syndrome
   Kimura disease
   Silica exposure

*Diseases and other agents in italics are the more commonly encountered causes of nephrotic syndrome.
†Single case reports or small series in which cause-and-effect relationship cannot be established. Other factors (e.g., mercurial diuretics in heart failure) may have been true inciting event.
‡See Chapter 31 for detailed discussion of the secondary forms of nephrotic syndrome.

is particularly likely to occur in athletic, well-nourished subjects who are consuming high-protein diets. On the other hand, profound hypoalbuminemia may occur with modest urinary protein excretion rates.[1] This occurrence could be the consequence of alterations in systemic capillary permeability such that a greater fraction of the total albumin pool resides in the extravascular compartment (interstitial space), a more profound disturbance in hepatic albumin synthesis than is usually seen, or loss of albumin into the small intestine (protein-losing enteropathy). The dietary protein intake greatly influences both urinary protein excretion rate and hepatic albumin synthesis.[621, 632] High protein intake by patients with nephrotic syndrome results in an increase in both urinary albumin excretion and hepatic albumin synthesis; thus, plasma albumin concentration and plasma and total albumin mass change little. The augmented protein excretion associated with high protein intake can be prevented by concomitant therapy with ACE inhibitors,[621, 632] thus resulting in a rise in plasma albumin concentration and albumin mass. Low-protein diets are associated with reduced urinary protein excretion rates, probably because of changes in glomerular hemodynamics, and no change in plasma albumin concentration because of a reduction in hepatic albumin synthesis.[632]

As indicated before, certain drugs, perhaps because of their effects on preglomerular and postglomerular capillary vascular resistance, have significant effects on the magnitude of proteinuria. Both NSAIDs and ACE inhibitors reduce proteinuria by 30% to 60%, especially if given to patients who have been "salt depleted."[622, 623, 625–627] The effects are reversible and cannot be fully explained by a concomitant decline in GFR.[622, 623] They are most likely the result of intraglomerular hemodynamic changes, but other effects on capillary wall function cannot be excluded. Similar antiproteinuric effects may also be observed with other antihypertensive agents that are not believed to have major effects on intraglomerular hemodynamics (e.g., β-adrenergic antagonists).[622] On the other hand, prednisolone can increase glomerular permeability of plasma proteins, independent of an effect on GFR.[624]

In proteinuria of glomerular origin, a number of plasma proteins are found in the urine, and several authors have suggested that determination of the fractional clearance of excreted proteins as a function of their molecular size is an indirect estimate of the extent of damage to the glomerular capillary wall.[1, 606, 633, 634] The clearance ratios of most proteins found in the urine of nephrotic subjects may be readily determined by immunochemical methods. In general, although many important exceptions occur, there is an inverse linear relationship between the log of the molecular weight (as an estimate of the molecular dimensions) and the log of the ratio of the clearance of individual proteins to that of albumin or transferrin. The angle subtended by such a linear regression (θ) may be used as a semiquantitative index of the selectivity of proteinuria.[1, 606, 633, 634] The lower the numeric value for this angle, the less the selectivity of proteinuria. If the theory is correct, lower selectivity indicates greater damage to the structural integrity of the glomerular capillary wall and impairment of its function as a size-selective barrier. Such an analysis fails to take into account the well-recognized importance of the molecular

charge of a protein in addition to its molecular dimensions as a determinant of movement across the glomerular capillary wall.[635] One of the principal assumptions underlying this technique is that, once filtered, the reabsorption of these proteins is not selective (i.e., it is in proportion only to their concentrations in the tubule fluid). Thus, the urine concentrations of these proteins are assumed to be related to their concentrations in the glomerular filtrate. As pointed out by several authors, this simple assumption may not always be correct.[633, 635]

A much simpler although intrinsically less reliable technique is to select two individual proteins of different molecular dimensions and to express selectivity as a ratio of the observed clearances. Cameron and Blandford[634] selected IgG and transferrin for these purposes, whereas other authors have used a variety of other combinations. The use of such clearance ratios has been demonstrated to bear a relationship, albeit an imperfect one, to underlying renal histology or response to treatment.[636] Measurement of fractional IgG clearance has been of particular value in the assessment of the severity of the size-selective barrier defect of glomerular permeability.[635] As discussed in Chapter 43, an isolated increase in fractional albumin clearance would be indicative of a defect in the charge-selective permeability barrier because at physiologic pH, albumin behaves like a polyanion.[6, 635] The urinary excretion of retinol-binding protein and $\beta_2$-microglobulin may also be used to detect the presence of glomerular morphologic abnormalities and thereby a poorer prognosis.[637] Another method, although clinically more difficult, for assessing glomerular permeability according to molecular size and charge is the use of dextran or polyvinylpyrrolidone (neutral), dextran sulfate (anionic), or diethylaminoethyl-dextran (cationic). The theory underlying their usefulness is discussed in more detail in Chapter 43. Modestly increased fractional clearance of larger neutral polymers (>4.2 nm) and reduced fractional clearance of smaller polymers (2 to 3.5 nm) may be observed in many nephrotic patients with structural glomerular lesions. This may represent a defect in the size-selective barrier in a small population of glomeruli and reduced "pore density" in the remainder.[618, 635] These abnormalities correspond to increased values for fractional IgG clearances.[635]

Finally, one should remember that severe (gross) hematuria with hypotonic urine produces an artifactual increase in proteinuria. This can be readily distinguished from glomerular proteinuria by urinary protein electrophoreses; most of the released protein from erythrocyte lysis migrates as hemoglobin in the beta globulin region.[638]

## ALTERED PLASMA PROTEIN CONCENTRATION

**Hypoalbuminemia.** Serum albumin levels are depressed below normal in many but not all patients with massive proteinuria.[1, 606, 626, 639] There is an approximate correlation between the degree of proteinuria and the extent of hypoalbuminemia, but as previously mentioned, many exceptions occur.[1, 626] Albumin levels measured immunochemically or electrophoretically are usually less than those measured by salt fractionation techniques. Fractional albumin catabolism is increased in most but not all patients.[1, 632] However, because of hypoalbuminemia and reduced albumin pool size, the absolute albumin catabolic rate is either normal or reduced.[1, 632, 640] Absolute hepatic albumin synthesis is most often increased. On the average, absolute hepatic albumin synthesis rates increase from $145 \pm 9$ mg/kg/d (normal) to $213 \pm 17$ mg/kg/d (nephrotic).[640] The rise in hepatic synthetic rate of albumin is highly correlated with urinary albumin excretion but not with plasma oncotic pressure or serum albumin concentration. The increase in hepatic albumin synthesis is transcriptionally regulated, but the exact promoter is poorly understood.[644] A fall in plasma oncotic pressure alone may not be the stimulus to increase albumin synthesis.[632]

A substantial fraction of overall albumin catabolism occurs in the kidney in proteinuric states. Total extrarenal catabolism is decreased in proportion to the declining serum albumin concentration. Total and plasma albumin mass is decreased,[621, 632] and the ratio of intravascular to extravascular (interstitial) albumin mass rises from normal values of about 0.8 to values in excess of 1.1 in nephrotic patients.[1, 606, 615] The interstitial albumin concentration falls to a greater extent than do plasma albumin concentrations. Thus, the transcapillary oncotic pressure gradient may decline to a much lesser extent than would have been predicted by the magnitude of hypoalbuminemia.[641] This may be a major protective factor for plasma volume in edematous patients with nephrotic syndrome, at least when plasma oncotic pressure is above 8 mm Hg. The transcapillary escape rate of albumin may be variably increased. In some cases, excessive gastrointestinal loss of protein has been documented.[642] Nitrogen balance is generally negative, but positive balance may be achieved by high protein intake. Increased dietary intake of protein in nephrotic states leads to an increase in urinary protein excretion and no or rather modest increase in plasma albumin concentration, except when severe malnutrition is present or when ACE inhibitors are administered concomitantly.[1, 621, 632] Restriction of protein intake in nephrotic states is followed by a reduction in urinary protein excretion and little or no change in plasma albumin levels.[643] Infusion of hyperoncotic dextran diminishes albumin degradation rates and albumin synthesis, suggesting that plasma oncotic pressure may be an important regulator of albumin synthesis.[1, 632] The availability of drug binding sites may be restricted by hypoalbuminemia and lead to high levels of free drug, enhancing the potential for toxic reactions (see later). Parallel transverse bands in the fingernails (Muehrcke lines) may appear in association with severe hypoalbuminemia.[1]

**Other Plasma Proteins.** In addition to the well-recognized deficiency of albumin, other plasma proteins may have altered serum or plasma concentrations.[645-650] Depressed levels may signify enhanced urinary loss or decreased synthesis, but few metabolic turnover studies have been conducted to be certain of the precise mechanism for altered plasma protein composition in nephrotic states. Serum levels of alpha$_2$ and beta globulins are increased as determined by cellulose acetate electrophoresis. Alpha$_1$-globulin levels may be normal or decreased.[1, 647] Studied by immunochemical methods, IgG levels may be significantly decreased, whereas IgA, IgM, or IgE levels are usually normal or even elevated. The changes in immunoglobulin levels seem to depend on the nature of the underlying lesions. IgG levels may be decreased in minimal-change disease despite the lack of urinary losses of IgG, whereas similar declines in IgG levels in other nephrotic states may reflect urinary losses (see later). Deficiencies in factor B of the alternative pathway of complement activation may impair the opsonization of bacteria and thus contribute to enhanced susceptibility to infection.[1, 646, 647] C1q, C2, C8, and C9 levels may be decreased, independent of the underlying disease. C3 may be lost in the urine in some glomerular lesions but usually not in sufficient amounts to result in a lowering of serum level.[1, 646] C1s, C4, and C1 inhibitor levels are normal. C3 and C4bp levels may be increased.

There may be an increase in fibrinogen levels and an elevation of the levels of factors V, VII, VIII–von Willebrand, and X, with a mildly increased platelet count.[647, 651-656] Antithrombin III (heparin cofactor) levels may be normal or greatly reduced, especially with severe hypoalbuminemia (less than 2.0 g/dL), probably because of excessive urinary losses.[1, 647, 651, 654] Protein C and protein S levels are usually normal or increased in nephrotic syndrome, but the functional activity of these proteins may be reduced, contributing to the "hypercoagulable" state.[1, 647, 657] Increased platelet aggregation has been noted. Elevated β-thromboglobulin levels may be a sign of underlying spontaneous thrombosis.[658, 659] Fibrin degradation products in urine are more a reflection of altered permeability than of glomerular coagulation.[660] Decreased levels of factors XI and XII, prekallikrein, and kallikrein inhibitor suggest in vivo Hageman factor activation.[647, 654, 655] Factors IX and XII may be depressed in nephrotic syndrome, in part owing to excessive urinary losses.[661] Antiplasmin, α$_1$-antitrypsin levels, plasminogen activator, and endothelial prostacyclin-stimulating factors may also be decreased.[1, 647, 655] An increase in the catabolic rate of fibrinogen and increased fibrinogen synthesis have been noted. Plasma viscosity may be increased because of the combined effects of hypercholesterolemia and hyperfibrinogenemia.[1, 647, 655]

Overall, the proaggregatory and procoagulant factors are enhanced; antiaggregatory, anticoagulant, and fibrinolytic mechanisms are impaired.[655] When superimposed on endothelial injury or stasis of flow and hyperlipidemia, these findings may contribute to the well-recognized tendency to spontaneous thrombosis observed in patients with nephrotic syndrome (see later).

Urinary loss of proteins having important metal-binding (e.g., iron, copper, zinc) or hormone-binding functions[1, 639, 648, 649, 662-666] may contribute to associated clinical findings. Urinary loss of erythropoietin may contribute to the anemia commonly observed in patients with heavy proteinuria.[650] In addition, abnormal filtration of trace elements into the tubule urine may predispose to tubule injury (see later). Zinc deficiency may contribute to dysgeusia, poor wound healing, impotence, and impaired cell-mediated immunity.[663, 664] Profound depression of serum transferrin concentration may lead to a microcytic, hypochromic anemia resistant to iron therapy.[660] Serum ferritin levels are increased in this circumstance. Transcortin deficiency may lead to an alteration in ratio of free to bound cortisol in patients receiving pharmacologic doses of glucocorticoids, thus altering the metabolism of and tissue response to these agents.[647, 667, 668] Thyroxine-binding globulin deficiency may affect thyroid function tests. Although total serum thyroxine and triiodothyronine levels may fall and triiodothyronine resin uptake rise because of thyroxine-binding globulin deficiency, free thyroxine and triiodothyronine levels, thyroidal radioactive iodine uptake, and thyroid-stimulating hormone levels remain normal.[647, 669]

Loss of cholecalciferol-binding globulin may result in an acquired vitamin D deficiency state with low plasma levels of 25-hydroxycholecalciferol, reduction in plasma $Ca^{2+}$, impaired gastrointestinal absorption of $Ca^{2+}$, elevated plasma parathyroid hormone, secondary hyperparathyroidism, osteomalacia, and osteitis fibrosa.[1, 670–672] Total 1,25-dihydroxycholecalciferol levels are normal or modestly decreased, but the free levels are normal or increased. These findings may develop before any decrease in GFR and aggravate the metabolic disturbances that occur as GFR decreases. Only a portion of the low total serum $Ca^{2+}$ levels seen in hypoalbuminemic nephrotic patients is due to decreased plasma protein-bound $Ca^{2+}$. A reduction in plasma renin substrate may impair generation of angiotensin II, even with increased levels of plasma renin concentration.[673] However, plasma renin substrate is often elevated in nephrotic syndrome.[674] Urinary losses of lecithin–cholesterol acyltransferase may contribute to the disordered lipoprotein metabolism in nephrotic syndrome (see later). Severe hypoproteinemia may lead to a persistent metabolic alkalosis.[675] For each gram per deciliter reduction in plasma albumin, the steady-state plasma $HCO_3^-$ concentration rises by 3.7 mEq/L, and the anion gap falls by 3.0 mEq/L. Orosomucoid deficiency may impair activation of lipoprotein lipase.

## HYPERLIPIDEMIA AND LIPIDURIA

In many but not all cases, there is an increase in serum total cholesterol, phospholipid, and triglyceride levels.[1, 647, 676–683] For poorly understood reasons, occasional patients with severe nephrotic syndrome do not have hyperlipidemia (e.g., SLE, amyloidosis). The low-density lipoproteins (LDLs) and very low density lipoproteins (VLDLs) are usually increased.[647, 676–683] Triglycerides and VLDLs are regularly increased only when the serum albumin concentration is less than 1 to 2 g/dL[683] (Table 30–7). Thus, lactescent serum in a nephrotic patient is usually indicative of severe hypoproteinemia. High-density lipoprotein (HDL)

levels may be normal, increased, or reduced, depending on severity of proteinuria and the nature of the underlying lesion and permeability defect.[683, 684] $HDL_2$ decreases more than $HDL_3$, and urinary excretion of apolipoprotein A increases.[685] Plasma concentrations of apolipoproteins B, C-II, and E are increased, and the ratio of apolipoprotein C-III to apolipoprotein C-II is elevated.[680] The plasma concentration of Lp(a) is greatly increased in parallel with increased total cholesterol, LDL and VLDL, and apolipoprotein B levels, but this elevation is not well correlated with urinary albumin excretion or serum albumin concentration.[686–689] Lp(a) may act as a potent inhibitor of plasminogen and thus contribute to the hypercoagulable state commonly observed in nephrotic syndrome (see later). A highly significant inverse correlation between cholesterol and triglycerides and serum albumin, oncotic pressure, or plasma viscosity can be demonstrated,[676–678, 689a, 690] and the level of cholesterol is directly related to the magnitude of urinary albumin excretion.[691] Interestingly, hyperlipidemia may precede the development of diminished albumin concentration in some experimental models of massive proteinuria and may persist well after serum albumin levels have returned to normal in some patients after spontaneous or therapy-induced partial or complete remission of proteinuria. Age, nutritional state, obesity, coexistent diabetes mellitus, and other factors may influence the level and patterns observed. Lipoprotein electrophoresis patterns vary, but about 60% of patients reveal type II a or b, 30% type V, and 10% or less type III or IV.[1, 639, 645, 682] There is little effect of heparin on the hyperlipemia.[682] The binding of serum cholesterol to plasma proteins is diminished.[692]

The mechanisms that underlie the disturbances in lipid metabolism in nephrotic syndrome are at least partly understood.[1, 647, 676–684] Currently available data suggest that reduced plasma oncotic pressure from hypoalbuminemia or enhanced loss of a regulatory factor in urine results in enhanced hepatic lipoprotein ($VLDL_2$, apolipoprotein B) production and interferes with the peripheral use or catabolism of lipoproteins.[676–684] Apolipoprotein B is the principal apolipoprotein demonstrating enhanced production.[684] The basic mechanism underlying increased hepatic lipoprotein synthesis is not well understood and may be multifactorial. Mevalonate availability is increased, and cholesterol ester transfer protein activity is greatly increased.[680] The enhancement of hepatic lipoprotein synthesis is not directly linked to hepatic albumin synthesis and may be stimulated by a loss of a regulatory substance in the urine.[680, 681]

The peripheral conversion of VLDLs to intermediate-density lipoproteins and LDLs may be impaired at low plasma oncotic pressure, explaining the tendency for precipitous rises in triglyceride-rich VLDLs and declining values for cholesterol-rich LDLs when severe hypoalbuminemia develops.[680–683, 693] The mechanism of impaired receptor-mediated conversion of VLDLs to LDLs is uncertain but may be due to defects in lipoprotein lipase activity, lecithin–cholesterol acyltransferase activity, deficient apolipoprotein C-II content of VLDL, deficiencies of cofactors (?orosomucoid), or accumulation of free fatty acids or lysolecithin due to lack of albumin-dependent binding sites.[1, 676–684, 693] HDLs may be lost in urine in severely proteinuric states and lead to low plasma HDL levels.[680, 685] In some

**TABLE 30–7. Lipoprotein Abnormalities in the Nephrotic Syndrome***

| Serum Albumin Concentration (g/dL) | Plasma Levels of Lipoproteins | | | | |
|---|---|---|---|---|---|
| | VLDL | $LDL_1$ | $LDL_2$ | $HDL_2$ | $HDL_3$ |
| 2–3.5 | nl or ↑ | ↑ | ↑ | ↑ nl or ↓ | ↑ or nl |
| 1.0–2.0 | ↑↑ | ↑↑ | ↑ | ↓ | nl |
| <1.0 | ↑↑↑ | ↑ | ↓ | ↓↓ | ↓ |

*VLDL = very low density lipoprotein; LDL = low-density lipoprotein; HDL = high-density lipoprotein; nl = normal level.

disorders, HDL levels actually rise. Thus, although total cholesterol levels rise in most nephrotic patients, the ratio of LDL- to HDL-cholesterol may vary from normal to extremely high values. Because this ratio may be more predictive of the risk of atherosclerosis, not all hypercholesterolemic nephrotic patients may be at equivalent risk of vascular complications related to enhanced atherogenesis[694–700] (see later).

A pronounced lowering of plasma lipids on infusion of hyperoncotic albumin or dextran suggests that colloid osmotic pressure of plasma is an important determinant of the defect causing hyperlipidemia in the nephrotic syndrome.[676–681] A part of the effect may also be due to changes in plasma viscosity.[690] The dissociation of plasma albumin concentration and lipidemia suggests that other factors may be operative, including an effect of the abnormal filtration of protein into the proximal tubule or possibly the loss of some critical factor in the urine of nephrotic patients.[1, 676–681] Kaysen and co-workers[701] have provided data that support the conclusion that the renal loss of albumin (or other regulatory proteins) is the primary cause of deranged cholesterol metabolism rather than enhanced hepatic albumin synthesis. Lipiduria is chiefly manifested by the presence in the urine of doubly refractile lipid bodies (probably epithelial cells) containing cholesterol esters or fat-filled casts (oval fat bodies). These are signs of the disordered lipid metabolism and possibly the excessive filtration of lower molecular weight HDL.[685, 702] Several apolipoproteins are deposited (or accumulate) in the mesangium in experimental nephrotic syndrome.[703]

## SODIUM HOMEOSTASIS AND EDEMA FORMATION

The mechanisms of edema formation are also discussed in Chapters 20 and 43.[704–706] The presence and severity of edema are related in a general way to the extent of depression of albumin concentration; however, notable exceptions may occur.[606] As noted before, initially a drop in interstitial oncotic pressure concomitant with the decline in plasma oncotic pressure tends to preserve the transcapillary oncotic pressure gradient and retard the development of edema.[641, 704–706] The limited ability of the interstitial oncotic pressure to fall further despite worsening of plasma albumin concentration and plasma oncotic pressure (below about 8 mm Hg) ultimately leads to enhanced flow of fluid into the interstitial space at rates that cannot be accommodated by a further increase in lymphatic flow, so edema fluid accumulates.[707]

It seems likely that the Na$^+$ retention in nephrotic states is related to intrarenal events[704–706, 708–711] and is not dependent on a change in activity of the renin-angiotensin-aldosterone system.[712–714] Indeed, values for plasma volume, plasma renin, and plasma aldosterone are highly variable in nephrotic subjects with edema.[715] In general, expanded plasma volume and suppressed plasma renin are more often observed in patients with proliferative glomerular lesions, especially with reduced GFR. Lowered plasma volume and enhanced plasma renin are more often observed in patients with minimal glomerular lesions and the acute onset of severe proteinuria.[713, 715] Water immersion of nephrotic sub-

jects with edema will result in a diuresis, natriuresis (albeit blunted compared with normal subjects), phosphaturia, and calciuria. These effects can occur without major change in plasma aldosterone concentration, and the intensity of the augmented excretion of Na$^+$ is related directly to the preimmersion plasma volume.[716–719]

Alterations in Na$^+$ excretion in nephrotic syndrome are largely the consequence of intrarenal defects and not the result of reductions in effective arterial volume.[704–706, 709–712] Indeed, as mentioned, most patients with nephrotic syndrome are normovolemic or hypervolemic, although they may have a more pronounced fall in plasma volume during orthostasis because of ineffective regulation of transcapillary fluid exchange.[705–707] Resistance to the natriuretic action of atrial natriuretic peptide is commonly seen, which is most likely due to postreceptor abnormalities such as enhanced cyclic guanine monophosphate phosphodiesterase activity.[704–706, 720, 721] The plasma levels of atrial natriuretic peptide are variable but may be increased.[704–706, 710, 711]

## Complications and General Management

### EDEMA

The edema of nephrotic syndrome is in many instances a bothersome but not debilitating clinical feature, but it can occasionally be severe and associated with accumulation of peritoneal or pleural fluid. Pericardial effusions are rare in uncomplicated nephrotic syndrome. In the periphery, edema is characteristically soft and easily pitting and accumulates in areas of low interstitial tissue pressure and high compliance, such as the periorbital areas. It is usually worse about the face on arising and increases in dependent areas with activity and upright posture.

Treatment of edema consists of mild sodium restriction and, in selected cases, the judicious use of diuretics. Many patients experience spontaneous diuresis during recumbency. Potent loop diuretics such as furosemide, bumetanide, or ethacrynic acid have become popular, although thiazide diuretics (hydrochlorothiazide or chlorthalidone) may suffice in many cases. Metolazone may be effective when used alone or in combination with furosemide in severe or refractory nephrotic edema. Because marked kaliuresis may occur with the use of these diuretics, a K$^+$-sparing diuretic such as spironolactone, amiloride, or triamterene may be employed concomitantly to prevent hypokalemia. However, these agents should not be used when GFR is substantially decreased because of the danger of precipitating hyperkalemia. Diuretics should be used cautiously in patients with profound hypoalbuminemia. Hyperoncotic salt-poor albumin infusions should be reserved for patients for whom orthostatic hypotension and hypovolemia are a significant problem or in cases of severe and refractory edema. Albumin infusions transiently increase plasma volume and oncotic pressure and may restore diuretic responsiveness, but most of the infused albumin is excreted in the urine 24 to 48 hours after completion of the infusion.[722] When plasma oncotic pressure is profoundly depressed (less than 8 mm Hg),[707] as in the case of severe hypoalbuminemia, there may be a tendency for accumulation of interstitial fluid even in the low-pressure pulmonary circuit. Even minor increases in left atrial filling pressure may induce florid pulmonary edema in such patients. Treatment for this complication is similar to that for the pulmonary edema of left ventricular failure, with the addition of measures to increase plasma oncotic pressure, while at the same time ensuring that left atrial (pulmonary wedge) pressure is not further increased. The combination of intravenous furosemide and hyperoncotic albumin infusion would seem to be a reasonable therapeutic approach to this uncommon problem. Extracorporeal ultrafiltration is rarely, if ever, required unless GFR is markedly reduced.

## HYPOVOLEMIA AND ACUTE RENAL FAILURE

The plasma volume of nephrotic patients may be increased, normal, or occasionally decreased.[704–706, 715, 723, 724] Patients with decreased plasma volume constitute the minority. Elevated plasma renin activity, increased plasma aldosterone concentration, and enhanced transcapillary escape of albumin may be seen in the hypovolemic subset, which is generally associated with the acute onset of nephrotic syndrome, severe hypoalbuminemia, or overly vigorous diuresis.[724] Patients with hypertension, reduced GFR, and structural glomerular lesions (especially proliferative glomerulonephritis) often have expanded plasma volume and reduced plasma renin activity.[723] Patients with massive proteinuria and extremely low plasma albumin levels or those with minimal glomerular lesions may have low plasma volume and, depending on concentration of renin substrate, increased plasma renin. However, plasma volume may even be increased in patients with minimal glomerular lesions. The extent of the edema does not necessarily correspond to the degree of change in plasma volume. Hypovolemic subjects with severe hypoalbuminemia may have cardiovascular instability with further diuretic-induced contraction of plasma volume; volume-expanded patients are often symptomatically benefited by a diuresis.[704–706, 723] A sudden fall in GFR and blood pressure after the use of ACE inhibitors may be a feature indicative of volume depletion in nephrotic syndrome.

When proteinuria is massive and albumin levels are profoundly depressed, the circulating plasma volume may be so diminished as to produce marked orthostatic hypotension or circulatory collapse even in the absence of diuretics. Reversible acute renal failure has been reported to develop in a few patients in such circumstances.[725, 726] Treatment with infusions of hyperoncotic albumin or other plasma volume expanders is indicated in this situation. However, acute renal failure may also be observed in certain forms of nephrotic syndrome with massive proteinuria, in the absence of features of volume depletion.[1, 727–730] This could be due to severe disturbance in visceral epithelial cells so as to result in nearly total obliteration of the slit pores and severe reduction in hydraulic conductivity.[731] Alternatively, severe proteinuria conceivably could result in occlusion of distal nephron lumens from cast formation or extratubule compression from interstitial edema.[732] Some patients with acute impairment of GFR may respond dramatically to vigorous treatment with loop diuretics, which suggests a role for

interstitial edema or intratubular obstruction in producing a form of intranephron obstructive uropathy.[732] The form of acute renal failure seen in patients with minimal-change lesions in relapse without signs of hypovolemia may also respond to corticosteroids[730]; but irreversible forms of acute renal failure have also been described, usually in patients with structural glomerular lesions, such as focal glomerular sclerosis[729] (see later). Acute renal failure may also be seen in association with nephrotic syndrome due to NSAIDs (see Chapter 28), or it may accompany a diuretic-induced hypersensitivity acute interstitial nephritis or bilateral acute renal vein thrombosis (see later and Chapters 33 and 35).

## PROTEIN MALNUTRITION

Prolonged, massive proteinuria may lead to severe negative nitrogen balance and protein-calorie malnutrition.[643–645] Urinary protein excretion varies directly with protein intake. Hepatic synthesis of protein can be augmented by high-protein diets; in the presence of adequate calorie intake, this is usually accompanied by increased albumin catabolism, the consequence of increased urinary protein excretion. Plasma albumin levels, therefore, do not change to any great extent when dietary protein is either increased or decreased,[643] unless ACE inhibitors or NSAIDs are administered concomitantly.[621–623, 643, 733, 734] Nonetheless, for patients with normal GFR, dietary management should include a generous intake of protein of high biologic value, about 1.0 g/kg/d plus urinary losses, and adequate calorie intake (more than 35 kcal/kg/d).[1] When higher protein diets are used, small doses of ACE inhibitors should be used simultaneously to prevent the expected augmentation of urinary protein excretion and to foster hepatic albumin synthesis.[621, 733] For patients with nephrotic syndrome and slowly progressive renal failure, modest protein restriction (e.g., 0.65 g/kg/d plus urinary losses) supplemented with amino acids may be indicated, provided that severe protein-calorie malnutrition is absent. Supplementation with intravenous hyperoncotic albumin or plasma protein preparations is usually unsatisfactory because of the excessive cost and the rapid urinary losses.

The urinary losses or increased fractional catabolism of plasma proteins having an important transport or binding function may lead to specific deficiency states, as discussed previously. Cholecalciferol deficiency may be amenable to vitamin D supplementation, but the optimal type of vitamin D preparation and dosage have not yet been fully evaluated.[671] 25-Hydroxycholecalciferol would be the most desirable preparation for treatment. Losses of copper, zinc, and iron may be replaced by oral supplements.

From time to time, persistent extremely heavy proteinuria may produce profound nutritional problems, striking hyperlipidemia, and refractory, incapacitating edema. Often, the lesion responsible for this disastrous state of affairs is unresponsive to therapy (e.g., focal glomerular sclerosis, advanced MGN, amyloidosis, diabetic glomerulosclerosis). For such patients, maneuvers to temporarily or permanently ablate renal function may be in order, especially if advanced renal failure is also present. Toxic doses of mercurial diuretics, percutaneous transfemoral embolization, balloon occlusion of renal arteries, and surgical nephrectomy have been employed in these circumstances.[735–737] Toxic doses of mercurial diuretics are ineffective unless GFR is already markedly decreased.

Indomethacin,[738, 739] meclofenamate,[740] or other NSAIDs as well as ACE inhibitors in carefully titrated doses may also be used in an attempt to nonspecifically decrease proteinuria.[622, 623, 733, 734, 739] These agents are more effective after diuresis and when taken with low-sodium diets.[619, 622, 623, 734] Doses of indomethacin of 150 to 300 mg/d may be required and may be associated with further reduction of GFR (usually modest in degree), aggravation of $Na^+$ retention, hyponatremia, hyperkalemia, hypertension, and peptic ulcer disease; on occasion, acute renal failure accompanied by an acute interstitial nephritis may ensue. The occurrence of hypotension or hyperkalemia may limit the use of ACE inhibitors, particularly when these agents are used concomitantly with NSAIDs. If not effective after a few weeks of high dosage, these agents should be discontinued.

## HYPERLIPIDEMIA AND ACCELERATED CARDIOVASCULAR DISEASE

Prolonged hyperlipidemia, especially with elevated LDL, elevated Lp(a), and decreased HDL, has the potential of accelerating the development of coronary artery atherosclerosis and increasing the risk of acute myocardial infarction in patients with nephrotic syndrome.[694–700, 741–744] The attendant hypercoagulable state may participate in enhancing the risk of acute coronary artery thrombosis.[1, 745] However, there is a lack of agreement regarding the magnitude of this risk.[694–700, 741–744] The majority view holds that the persistence of hyperlipidemia in nephrotic syndrome constitutes a significant risk factor for the subsequent development of atherosclerosis and coronary artery disease. Indeed, there appears to be an excess of cardiovascular deaths and major cardiac events in patients with the nephrotic syndrome, even after adjustment of concomitant risk factors (e.g., smoking, hypertension).[697, 698] The overall risk of accelerated atherogenesis with nephrotic hyperlipidemia is probably related to the nature of the underlying disease, the presence and severity of concomitant hypertension, smoking and other risk factors, the duration of the hyperlipidemic state, Lp(a) concentration, and the ratio of LDL- to HDL-cholesterol. Thus, management of hyperlipidemia is a controversial aspect in the overall care of patients with the nephrotic syndrome.

Despite the lack of prospective data proving benefit in terms of reduction in cardiovascular morbidity or mortality, the prevailing view is that treatment of hyperlipidemia is indicated in patients in whom the disturbance of lipid metabolism is expected to persist for long periods.[746, 747] Obviously, attention must first be placed on the reduction of other risk factors, such as hypertension, obesity, and smoking. Dietary treatment of the hyperlipidemia of nephrotic syndrome is generally unsuccessful, but a vegetarian diet rich in polyunsaturated fat and low in cholesterol may be helpful in some cases.[748] High–soluble fiber diets (oat or rice bran, psyllium colloid) or supplementation with ω-3 fatty acids may be of added benefit, but these approaches have not been rigorously studied. Moderate exercise and

the avoidance of heavy alcohol intake should be encouraged. Pharmacologic therapy of hyperlipidemia is needed in most cases, but such therapy may result in some patients in undesirable side effects (e.g., myonecrosis, hepatic injury).[746, 747] Although clofibrate and other fibric acid derivatives, such as gemfibrozil, may reduce triglyceride and to a lesser extent total cholesterol levels, free drug concentrations are increased because of hypoalbuminemia, and toxic muscle effects may be observed when usual doses of this agent are employed.[749, 750] Dosage of clofibrate must be reduced by one half to two thirds to avoid this complication. The prevention of accelerated atherosclerosis by such therapy is unproved. Other agents that sequester bile acids in the gut, such as colestipol and cholestyramine, reduce plasma cholesterol levels modestly[751] but may also impair intestinal absorption of vitamin D, thereby aggravating vitamin D deficiency (see earlier),[752] which could have disastrous effects on children. Probucol lowers cholesterol by 25% to 30%, but HDL-cholesterol levels may also fall so that the LDL/HDL ratio is unaffected.[753] However, probucol may reduce atherogenic oxidized cholesterol and in experimental animals with certain forms of glomerular disease may have dramatic antiproteinuric effects (e.g., experimental MGN).[754] Hydroxymethylglutaryl–coenzyme A reductase inhibitors, such as lovastatin, pravastatin, and simvastatin, cause a substantial decline in total cholesterol and LDL-cholesterol and a modest increase in HDL-cholesterol. Thus, these agents exert a favorable effect on the LDL/HDL ratio.[746, 747, 755, 756] However, the long-term efficacy and safety in patients with nephrotic syndrome, as is the case with all other hypercholesterolemic agents, are unknown, and side effects may ensue. Nevertheless, because of desirable effects on hypercholesterolemia and an acceptable profile of side effects, these agents have become the treatment of choice for nephrotic hyperlipidemia. Even though hydroxymethylglutaryl–coenzyme A inhibitors can reduce LDL-cholesterol by 30% to 50% in nephrotic syndrome and thus favorably affect the atherogenic profile, these agents may not be nearly so effective in decreasing Lp(a) levels,[757, 758] and the underlying factors that promote atherogenesis may thus be only partially remedied. In patients at high risk of cardiovascular disease (e.g., strong family history, smoking, hypertension, prior or current coronary artery disease), it would seem reasonable to attempt to lower the cholesterol level, particularly with an agent that favorably affects HDL-cholesterol levels, but the clinician should recognize that so long as the patient has heavy proteinuria and hypoalbuminemia, it may be impossible to normalize the plasma cholesterol level. Furthermore, any modest decrease in the cholesterol level will have uncertain effects in terms of reducing the risk of coronary artery or atherosclerotic disease. As a potential added benefit of reducing total cholesterol level, some experimental studies in animals have implicated cholesterol and perhaps other lipids in the progression of renal disease[679] (reviewed in Chapter 44).

## INCREASED SUSCEPTIBILITY TO BACTERIAL INFECTIONS

Before the introduction of antibiotics and steroid therapy, a major cause of death in children with nephrotic syndrome was pulmonary, meningeal, or peritoneal infection due to *Streptococcus, Haemophilus,* or *Klebsiella* species.[1, 759, 760] This unusual susceptibility to encapsulated bacterial infection may have been due to acquired IgG deficiency, a frequent complication in patients with massive proteinuria, regardless of the underlying histologic lesions (see later).[760] Deficiency of factor B with defective opsonization or nonspecific depression of immunologic responses in protein-calorie malnutrition or in association with underlying disease may also be contributory.[761] Prophylactic antibiotics, pneumococcal vaccination, or parenteral hyperimmune serum globulin may occasionally be indicated in high-risk patients (infants and elderly adults). Vaccination may be best administered during remission, because immunization may not be effective if given during relapse.[762] Viral infections are ordinarily tolerated well unless immunosuppressive agents are being given.

## RENAL TUBULE ABNORMALITIES

Proximal tubule dysfunction with renal glycosuria, hyperphosphaturia, generalized aminoaciduria, hypouricemia, and $K^+$ and proximal $HCO_3^-$ wasting (Fanconi syndrome) have been observed in some patients with massive proteinuria, particularly those with prominent histologic features of focal and segmental glomerular sclerosis and with tubule atrophy and interstitial fibrosis.[1, 763] In a few cases, this has led to a distinctive syndrome of rickets or osteomalacia and renal tubular acidosis.[764] These abnormalities imply an unfavorable prognosis.[763] Impaired water excretion due to persistent antidiuretic hormone secretion may lead to hyponatremia,[765] but this is unusual except in patients receiving diuretics. Increased tubule secretion of creatinine may well result in overestimation of GFR by creatinine clearances in patients with heavy proteinuria.[766] Finally, altered glomerular permeability to macromolecules may contribute to progressive tubulointerstitial and glomerular injury.[767]

## INCREASED THROMBOEMBOLIC TENDENCY

The frequency of renal vein thrombosis, pulmonary arterial or venous thrombosis in situ, pulmonary emboli, and peripheral venous or arterial thrombosis is increased in patients with nephrotic syndrome.[1, 654, 655, 768–777] The precise mechanism is not clear, although some abnormalities of clotting tests performed in vitro suggest a hypercoagulable state. Deficiency in antithrombin III,[776] abnormalities in the activity of protein S or C,[656] deficient fibrinolysis, increased platelet aggregability, enhanced erythrocyte aggregation,[1, 775] and increased plasma levels of procoagulant factors (e.g., fibrinogen, Lp(a),[686, 687] factor VIII) may all participate in the thrombotic tendency.[1, 654, 655, 768–777] Stasis, hyperlipidemia, hyperviscosity, steroid therapy, and endothelial cell injury may be other important factors. Platelet activation or aggregation may be a common underlying abnormality. The renal venous circulation is particularly vulnerable to thrombosis.[1, 769, 777] Renal vein thrombosis is currently regarded as a complication of nephrotic syndrome and is therefore discussed here.

## RENAL VEIN THROMBOSIS

**Clinical Findings.** The association of renal vein thrombosis and proteinuria was first described by the French nephrologist Rayer in 1840.[1] Since then, several hundred cases have been recorded in the literature.[1, 769, 770] Thrombosis or occlusion of one or both renal veins may arise from extrinsic compression by a tumor or retroperitoneal mass; from invasion of the renal veins or inferior vena cava by tumor (most commonly a renal cell carcinoma); or as a result of trauma, hemoconcentration, or an underlying hypercoagulable state. Renal vein thrombosis may also be a superimposed feature of a number of glomerulopathies, chiefly MGN, MCGN, lupus nephritis, and amyloidosis accompanied by the nephrotic syndrome.[1, 769, 770] For poorly understood reasons, nephrotic syndrome due to diabetes mellitus, focal sclerosis, and minimal-change disease does not carry a high risk of renal vein thrombosis. Overall, the prevalence of renal vein thrombosis is higher in primary than in secondary glomerular disease. For poorly understood reasons, the reported prevalence of renal vein thrombosis in MGN and MCGN varies widely (5% to 54%),[1, 654, 655, 769, 770] averaging about 20% to 30%. The risk of renal vein thrombosis is increased when the serum albumin level falls below 2.0 g/dL, in the presence of increased levels of $\alpha_2$-antiplasmin,[771] or with decreased levels of antithrombin III.[1, 776]

Acute bilateral renal vein thrombosis in the absence of pre-existing renal disease may occur in children with dehydration or in association with neoplastic invasion of renal veins or inferior vena cava and need not always be associated with heavy proteinuria. Flank pain, acute decline in GFR, hematuria, and changes in urinary protein excretion are features of acute renal vein thrombosis superimposed on nephrotic syndrome.[769] Chronic renal vein thrombosis, on the other hand, may frequently be clinically covert. Unilateral chronic renal vein thrombosis may arise in patients with heavy proteinuria demonstrable in urine emanating from both ureters.[1, 768–779] Pulmonary emboli and hemoptysis, back pain, thrombophlebitis in the lower extremity, asymmetric edema, glycosuria, hyperchloremic acidosis, greatly elevated urinary fibrin degradation products,[780] left varicocele, and dilated abdominal veins are additional clinical clues to the presence of renal vein thrombosis.[1, 777] An intravenous pyelogram may demonstrate enlarged kidneys, with differences in renal size and function, particularly when thrombosis has occurred relatively rapidly without opportunity for collateral circulation to develop.[1, 769] The calyces may appear elongated in cases in which renal edema is prominent. In chronic renal vein thrombosis, the collateral circulation may produce notching in the proximal ureter. Chest films and lung scans may reveal defects typical of pulmonary arterial embolization[769]; however, such abnormalities are also found in nephrotic subjects without demonstrable renal vein thrombosis. They may represent in situ thrombosis or embolization from other venous beds.

Abdominal ultrasonography, Doppler ultrasound venography, or magnetic resonance imaging may be useful techniques for screening patients suspected of having renal vein thrombosis, but the sensitivity and specificity of these techniques are variable. False-positive rather than false-negative studies are the rule, so a negative study may allow further investigation to be avoided.[780] Confirmation of renal vein thrombosis may be obtained by arteriography with delayed films during the venous phase, by inferior venacavograms, or, preferably, by retrograde selective renal vein angiograms.[1, 768, 769] The last procedure should be preceded by gentle manual injection of contrast material into the low inferior vena cava to demonstrate the absence of an inferior vena caval thrombosis. Blind passage of a retrograde catheter into the cava may dislodge loose clots and is hazardous. If the inferior vena cava is free of clots, the catheters may be advanced to the level of the renal veins and selective injections made to outline the proximal renal veins and their intrarenal division. When renal function is normal, the high rate of renal blood flow may render this procedure difficult; the contrast material is rapidly washed out, and artifacts resembling thrombi may be produced by turbulent mixing of contrast material in renal venous blood.

Renal biopsies in patients with documented renal vein thrombosis and nephrotic syndrome not unexpectedly reveal a variety of changes but most frequently demonstrate the typical light and electron microscopic and immunofluorescence features of MGN or MCGN.[1, 769] Several authors have drawn attention to the tendency for peripheral margination of polymorphonuclear leukocytes, the presence of interstitial edema, fibrosis, and tubule atrophy out of proportion to the degree of glomerular alterations as morphologic clues to the presence of a complicating acute renal vein thrombosis.[1, 769] In instances of unilateral renal vein thrombosis, the uninvolved kidney has usually shown the typical glomerular alterations of MGN or MCGN.[1, 774, 779]

**Association with Nephrotic Syndrome.** Several explanations can be offered for the association of renal vein thrombosis and the nephrotic syndrome. First, renal vein thrombosis may always be a secondary complicating event and therefore may occur in association with any of a variety of lesions that cause the nephrotic syndrome. The presence of bilateral glomerular disease in cases showing only unilateral renal vein obstruction and the repeated failure to reproduce the syndrome and characteristic renal lesions by experimental techniques may be cited in favor of this explanation.[1, 769] The frequent occurrence of renal vein thrombosis as a complication of the experimental model of MGN in rats is further evidence in support of this viewpoint.[1, 769] Second, it has been suggested that an increase in renal vein pressure from thrombosis of the renal vein, extrinsic occlusion of the inferior vena cava above the renal veins, constrictive pericarditis, extreme obesity, and tricuspid valve disease may all lead to a disturbance of glomerular capillary wall function and massive proteinuria.[1] Congestive heart failure has also been reported in the older literature to be associated with nephrotic syndrome[1, 781]; however, apparently all of these patients received mercurial diuretics, a well-recognized cause of nephrotic syndrome.[1, 781] Apart from renal vein thrombosis, the occurrence of nephrotic syndrome in states of increased renal vein pressure in which mercurial diuretics were not administered is rare.[1] The few cases of nephrotic syndrome associated with constrictive pericarditis, with remission after pericardiectomy, did not include study of renal tissue

or mention the diuretic therapy that was employed. Remissions of proteinuria after relief of elevated renal vein pressure do not always occur.[1] Experimental increases in renal vein pressure by ligature in dogs do not produce massive proteinuria unless contralateral nephrectomy is performed.[1, 782] The immunofluorescence and electron microscopic findings usually observed in the human disorder are not found in the experimental animal.[1, 783]

In view of all the available evidence, then, it appears likely that nearly every case of renal vein thrombosis can be explained as a complicating event in a patient with occult or overt primary or secondary glomerulopathy. It is possible that the increase in renal vein pressure may exacerbate proteinuria or cause an asymptomatic mild proteinuria to become massive. It seems highly unlikely that an increase in renal vein pressure ever produces a glomerulopathy and the nephrotic syndrome.

**Effect on Prognosis.** The prognosis of any glomerular disease may be made worse by superimposition of acute renal vein thrombosis, but it is not certain yet whether the slow development of chronic renal vein thrombosis accelerates the rate of progression of disease to end-stage renal failure.[1, 769] Several anecdotal reports suggest that on occasion, the occurrence of bilateral renal vein thrombosis is associated with a more rapid decline in GFR than would have occurred otherwise. For example, in amyloidosis, the development of acute renal vein thrombosis is usually associated with a sudden decline in renal function and marked worsening of proteinuria.[784]

Renal vein thrombosis certainly does expose the patient to an increased risk of pulmonary emboli, although venous thromboses in other sites clearly also contribute to increased risk of pulmonary emboli in nephrotic patients. Once renal vein thrombosis is documented by radiographic or other techniques, the clinician is faced with a serious dilemma. Clearly, if pulmonary embolism or thrombosis has occurred, long-term anticoagulation is indicated. Nevertheless, the real dangers of anticoagulation in nephrotic or azotemic patients must be stressed. Even in the absence of demonstrated pulmonary emboli, anticoagulation of patients with documented renal vein thrombosis may be of prophylactic value for the occurrence of pulmonary emboli, and in cases of acute renal vein thrombosis, massive proteinuria has partially or totally remitted and renal function improved in association with demonstrable recanalization of renal veins during anticoagulation therapy.[1, 785–787] In most chronic renal vein thrombosis cases, however, anticoagulation has little effect on renal function, and thrombosis may recur in the recanalized vessels when anticoagulants are discontinued. Whether the reduction in proteinuria is in fact the direct result of such therapy has not been established, because spontaneous recovery has been seen in other patients with nephrotic syndrome–associated glomerulopathy. The value of elective surgical thrombectomy in acute renal vein thrombosis has not been determined. In most cases in which this procedure has been undertaken, GFR has either improved or been maintained and proteinuria has diminished somewhat, but complete remissions of proteinuria have generally not occurred.[1, 788, 789]

Because of the reported high prevalence of covert chronic renal vein thrombosis in adults with nephrotic syndrome (particularly due to MGN), one may be justified in performing renal vein angiograms in patients with biopsy-proven MGN, particularly if any clues of a possible renal vein thrombosis are present and if the patient is at high risk of thromboembolic disease owing to the severity of the nephrotic state. The dilemma arises again, because it has not yet been shown in a well-controlled study that oral anticoagulant therapy or parenteral heparin reduces the prevalence of pulmonary emboli or retards the progression of an already indolent disease process. Furthermore, the risks of prolonged anticoagulant therapy are not inconsiderable. More prospective data bearing on the benefit-risk ratio of long-term anticoagulants in nephrotic syndrome, with and without renal vein thrombosis, are needed. Nevertheless, a carefully performed Markov decision analysis, using reasonable estimates of the risk of thrombosis and life-threatening embolism and the likelihood of serious bleeding from oral warfarin, has concluded that more fatal embolic events will be *prevented* than serious bleeding events *induced* by a prophylactic anticoagulation approach to patients at high risk (e.g., patients with MGN and the nephrotic syndrome).[790] Therefore, unless contraindicated, it may be prudent to recommend long-term oral anticoagulation to patients with certain forms of glomerular disease producing the nephrotic syndrome, particularly MGN, when the nephrotic syndrome is anticipated to persist for extended periods. Because the greatest risk for thromboembolic events is seen in patients with a serum albumin concentration less than 2.0 to 2.5 g/dL, a prophylactic anticoagulation approach may be most strongly indicated in the subgroup with more profound hypoalbuminemia. Patients with nephrotic syndrome who are immobilized for any reason should probably receive short-term low-dose parenteral heparin. Patients with a documented thrombotic or embolic event should receive long-term oral anticoagulation for as long as they are nephrotic.

## IMMUNOLOGIC ABNORMALITIES

A number of disturbances of humoral and cell-mediated immunity occur in patients with the nephrotic syndrome. Some of these are related to specific underlying disease and are discussed elsewhere. Features common to many patients with nephrotic syndrome, regardless of cause or underlying disease, include decrease in IgG levels and decreased serum levels of factor B (see earlier). Most patients not receiving concomitant immunosuppressive therapy will have normal or suboptimal responses to active immunization and are at increased risk for bacterial infection (see earlier).

In vitro tests of cell-mediated immunity are frequently abnormal. Altered ratios of $CD4^+$ to $CD8^+$ lymphocyte subsets have also been described[791, 792] (see specific diseases later). Lymphocytes from nephrotic patients also produce factors capable of altering vascular permeability.[793-795] A soluble immune response suppressor factor produced by T lymphocytes can be found in urine of patients with nephrotic syndrome, especially minimal-change disease.[796, 797] The mechanisms responsible for these changes are unknown but could be due to the altered milieu of the nephrotic patient (e.g., increased immunoregulatory intermediate-density lipoproteins; hypoalbuminemia; hypo-

transferrinemia; zinc deficiency; augmented prostaglandin synthesis; prior therapy with immunosuppressive agents, especially cyclophosphamide) or to an underlying abnormality of the immune system causally related in some way to the disease process evoking nephrotic syndrome (see later).[1, 796, 797] Whatever the case, nephrotic patients do not appear to be at great risk for the unusual opportunistic infections or malignant neoplasms associated with the acquired immunodeficiency syndrome, unless they have received frequent or prolonged therapy with immunosuppressive agents such as glucocorticoids or cytotoxic drugs.

## Primary Glomerular Diseases That Evoke the Nephrotic Syndrome (Idiopathic Nephrotic Syndrome)

In this section are discussed those clinicopathologic entities in which the nephrotic syndrome develops in the absence of any underlying heredofamilial or multisystem disease (including neoplasia) or drug or microbial exposure. Before the introduction of percutaneous renal biopsy, this group of disorders was usually regarded as a single disease entity having a common cause and pathogenesis. Although some progress has been made in understanding etiology, much knowledge has been accumulated regarding morphology and pathogenesis. It is now possible to classify idiopathic nephrotic syndrome into several reasonably well defined groups of clinicopathologic entities.[1, 13, 606] Furthermore, a plethora of data is now available relating the clinical appearance to the morphologic lesion, natural history, and response to treatment. The classification presented here represents commonly held views and is based predominantly on light microscopic appearance of renal biopsy specimens, supplemented by immunofluorescence and electron microscopic examination. Even so, it is likely that some of the groups presented here as discrete entities in fact represent heterogeneous disorders of various causes and pathogeneses. Thus, the classification of the glomerular lesions responsible for idiopathic nephrotic syndrome must be viewed as being in a constant state of development.

A working classification of the most common morphologic varieties of the primary glomerular lesions observed in idiopathic nephrotic syndrome and their relative frequencies in adults and children are presented in Tables 30–8 and 30–9, respectively.[1, 16, 606] The relative frequency of these different entities differs widely according to the age of the patient, whether the population is unselected or referred, indications for renal biopsy, geography, socioeconomic status, and criteria used by pathologists to assign patients to one or another category.[798-800] An examination of more narrowly defined age groups reveals distinctive age-related glomerular disease. For example, among patients between the ages of 2 and 6 years, the prevalence of minimal-change disease may be as high as 95%[1, 16, 606]; among adults older than 60 years, MGN is seen in 40% of cases and amyloidosis in 9% to 13%.[1, 16, 798-800]

Prospective epidemiologic studies in children with the nephrotic syndrome, conducted by the International Study of Kidney Disease in Children (ISKDC), have permitted

**TABLE 30–8. Classification of Histologic Lesions Observed in Idiopathic Nephrotic Syndrome Due to Primary Glomerular Disease**

**Minimal Glomerular Abnormalities (Minimal-Change Lesion, "Lipoid Nephrosis")**

**Mesangial Proliferative Glomerulonephritis***

**Focal and Segmental Glomerular Sclerosis†** (Focal Sclerosis)
With segmental sclerosis and hyalinosis superimposed on minimal-change lesion *or* mesangial proliferative glomerulonephritis
With global sclerosis superimposed on minimal-change lesion *or* mesangial proliferative glomerulonephritis

**Diffuse Mesangial Sclerosis**

**Membranous Glomerulonephritis (Membranous Nephropathy)**

**Mesangiocapillary Glomerulonephritis (Membranoproliferative Glomerulonephritis)**
With subendothelial deposits (type I)
With intramembranous dense deposits (dense deposit disease, type II)
With other structural variations or superimposed features (type III and others)

**Endocapillary Proliferative Glomerulonephritis‡**
Diffuse lesions with or without superimposed crescents or adhesions
Focal and segmental lesions‡ with or without superimposed crescents or adhesions (focal and segmental proliferative glomerulonephritis)

**Fibrillary or Immunotactoid Glomerulonephritis**

**Other Chronic, Sclerosing Lesions**

**Other Lesions§**

---

*The immunopathology of this lesion varies, but a proportion will reveal mesangial IgM or IgA deposits.
†Whether focal sclerosis is a discrete entity or merely a nonspecific lesion superimposed on a more basic and fundamental lesion is controversial.
‡The immunopathology of these lesions varies, but many will reveal extensive IgA deposits and be categorized as Berger disease.
§Including collagen III glomerulopathy and lipoprotein glomerulopathy.

development of predictive formulas that make possible "a more accurate prebiopsy identification of the underlying primary glomerular lesions."[1] These formulas are based on a multivariate analysis of clinical characteristics of well-defined, unselected populations of nephrotic children, including age, sex, blood pressure, urinalysis findings, C3 level, serum creatinine concentration, serum albumin level, and selectivity of proteinuria. Such multivariate analyses have been less successful in adults in the development of prebiopsy predictions, probably as the result of a greater diversity of glomerular lesions in this population.[1] In children, these predictive criteria are of greater use in enhancing the diagnostic suspicions of a lesion other than minimal-change disease, so as to lead to an early renal biopsy and delay in glucocorticoid therapy until the true nature of the lesion is documented.[1] Although considerable emphasis has been placed on renal biopsy findings here, the precise role of renal biopsy as a diagnostic tool in adults and children with idiopathic nephrotic syndrome is widely debated.[1, 801–807] Some believe that a renal biopsy is not required for appropriate management; a brief course (8 to 16 weeks) of oral glucocorticoids in sufficient dosage will adequately separate the steroid-responsive patients, having a favorable long-term evolution, from the steroid-unresponsive patients, who are more likely to have underlying structural glomerular alterations and a progressive course.[802, 803]

Whereas this may be true in children younger than 8 years, the increased frequency of a variety of structural glomerular lesions having different evolutionary patterns and potential responsiveness to therapy other than glucocorticoids has led many to conclude that (in the absence of contraindications and in experienced hands) a renal biopsy provides additional useful information permitting a more accurate prognosis and perhaps a more rational approach to design of a therapeutic regimen, with minimal additional risk. Nonetheless, by use of decision analysis techniques and estimated prevalence of treatment-responsive and nonresponsive lesions, it has been suggested that a policy of an initial trial of therapy without renal biopsy will yield satisfactory results in adults.[801, 807] On the other hand, many studies have shown that renal biopsy contributes to management decisions in adults in an important way. One often overlooked advantage of renal biopsy is the finding of a superimposed glomerular lesion in patients with underlying primary or secondary renal disease (e.g., acute PSGN superimposed on diabetic glomerulosclerosis).[808]

## MINIMAL-CHANGE DISEASE

In 1913, Munk[809] coined the term "lipoid nephrosis" to describe a group of patients with heavy proteinuria unaccompanied by abnormalities of the glomeruli examined by light microscopy. Prominent lesions consisting of lipid droplets in the cells of the proximal tubules were noted. This suggested that proteinuria might be the result of defective reabsorption of normally filtered protein. However, more careful scrutiny of biopsy material revealed a lesion of the glomerular epithelial cells consisting of juxtaposition

**TABLE 30–9. Prevalence* of Most Common Histopathologic Lesions in Idiopathic Nephrotic Syndrome Due to Primary Glomerular Disease**

| Lesion | Age-Associated Prevalence (%) | | | |
|---|---|---|---|---|
| | <15 y | 15–29 y | 30–49 y | >50 y |
| Minimal-change disease | 83 | 31 | 30 | 23 |
| | | | 28 | |
| Focal glomerular sclerosis | 8 | 22 | 9 | 12 |
| | | | 15 | |
| MGN | 1 | 5 | 32 | 34 |
| | | | 25 | |
| MCGN | 5 | 21 | 8 | 8 |
| | | | 12 | |
| Other proliferative lesions, including mesangial, endocapillary, and crescentic glomerulonephritis | 3 | 21 | 21 | 23 |
| | | | 20 | |
| | 100% | | 100% | |

---

*Data derived from biopsy series at Guys Hospital, London, England. These prevalences may not be representative of other geographic areas or selected racial populations.
From Cameron JS, Glassock RJ (eds): The Nephrotic Syndrome. Marcel Dekker, New York, 1988.

of the normal club-shaped foot processes and obliteration of the slit pore membrane complex.[810] This process has also been described as swelling, obliteration, fusion, retraction, or effacement of the epithelial cell foot processes.[811] The GBM remained essentially unaltered, at least by standard morphologic examination.

The etiology and pathogenesis of this disorder await definition, but the clinical and morphologic features are sufficiently distinct to consider this a clinicopathologic entity.[1, 811, 812] The term lipoid nephrosis has now fallen into disuse. The terms minimal-change lesion, minimal-change disease, and minimal-change nephropathy have become more widely used to emphasize the relative paucity of glomerular changes visible by light microscopy. Many nephrologists believe that the minimal-change lesion is a part of a spectrum of morphologic responses to a single underlying disease process.[813–815] Incorporated into this spectrum are the lesions of focal and segmental glomerular sclerosis superimposed on the minimal-change lesion and the milder forms of diffuse mesangial proliferative glomerulonephritis (see later). Whereas this triad of glomerular lesions (minimal-change lesions, focal and segmental glomerular sclerosis, and mesangial proliferative glomerulonephritis) share certain clinical, immunohistologic, and ultrastructural features and have been observed to evolve one to another with time in individual patients, it is hazardous to conclude on these clinical and morphologic criteria that they in fact represent a single disease entity rather than an expression of heterogeneity of etiology and pathogenesis. Nevertheless, observations demonstrating circulating nonimmunoglobulin permeability factors in patients with this group of diseases may provide a unifying pathogenetic theme for minimal-change disease, focal and segmental glomerular sclerosis, and pure mesangial proliferative glomerulonephritis.[619, 816–820]

**Clinical Features.** One of the characteristic features of the minimal-change lesion is its predilection to affect young children, with a peak occurrence between the ages of 2 and 6 years. The incidence among children younger than 10 years is approximately 1.8 to 5 cases/1,000,000 per year.[1, 821, 822] For reasons that are poorly understood, minimal-change disease is more common in Asian populations.[823] Minimal-change lesions account for about 80% and 20% of the cases of idiopathic nephrotic syndrome due to primary glomerular disease in children and adults, respectively,[1, 16, 795, 820, 824] and may be seen in elderly patients.[798, 820] Minimal-change lesions are found in more than 85% of cases of nephrotic syndrome due to primary glomerular disease in children between the ages of 2 and 6 years.[1, 16, 821] The reported variation in the prevalence of this lesion is probably accounted for by differences in selection, referral bias, geography, and histologic interpretation. Males predominate by about 2:1 to 2.5:1 in children, whereas the sex ratio is closer to unity in adults.[1, 16, 825] The lesion has been reported to occur in siblings.[1, 826] Viral upper respiratory infection is a common antecedent feature, and the interval between the infection and the onset of proteinuria is usually short.[1, 827] There is no evidence to implicate streptococci.[827] A background of allergy, atopy, or recent immunizations may be found frequently.[827–831] The abrupt onset of a full-blown nephrotic syndrome with heavy proteinuria, hypoal-

buminemia, and hyperlipidemia is the rule. The tendency for a relapsing course and responsiveness to therapy are discussed later. Gross hematuria is unusual. Hypertension is relatively uncommon. Elevated diastolic pressure was found in only 13% of the ISKDC series,[1, 16] but systolic hypertension may occur more commonly than is generally believed. Acute renal failure may occur, most likely as a result of ischemic tubule necrosis,[832] but this is uncommon.[1] Thromboembolic events and serious bacterial infections (peritonitis, meningitis) may occur during relapse.[1, 833] Glucocorticoids may also play a prothrombogenic role.[833]

**Laboratory Findings** (see Table 30–2). Urinalyses reveal heavy proteinuria that, when measured, is usually in the nephrotic range when adjusted for surface area or serum albumin. In children, protein excretion rates exceed 40 mg/h/m$^2$. Microscopic hematuria is seen in 15% to 20% of cases, but macroscopic hematuria is rare.[821] Serum creatinine concentration may be mildly increased in as many as one third of cases at the time of initial presentation.[1, 821, 835] Severe depression of renal function may be seen if hypovolemia is marked. Cases of reversible oliguric renal failure have been described (see later).[1, 832, 834, 835] Inulin clearances may be depressed during periods of relapse, and the ratio of endogenous creatinine clearance to inulin clearance may be elevated.[766] The reduction in GFR is predominantly due to a reduction in epithelial slit pore density and an increase in the length of the pathway fluid must traverse between the capillary lumen and Bowman space.[731, 836] Filtration fraction is almost always greatly reduced.[836–838] Serum Na$^+$ concentration may be decreased, in part owing to extreme hyperlipidemia. Hematocrit and hemoglobin may be increased if plasma volume is seriously reduced. Platelet counts are modestly increased. Erythrocyte sedimentation rate is increased because of hypoalbuminemia and hyperfibrinogenemia, but seldom to more than 50 mm/h (Westergren method). Plasma viscosity and red blood cell aggregation are increased, thus promoting thrombosis.[833, 833a] Fractional clearances of neutral polyvinylpyrrolidone (effective molecular radius 2.0 to 4.6 nm) or dextran are reduced in relapse and return to normal in remission. Fractional albumin clearance is increased disproportionately compared with fractional IgG clearance, which strongly suggests a defect in the charge-selective permselectivity barrier (see later).[839–842]

Serum albumin concentration is often greatly depressed. Total cholesterol, triglyceride, VLDL, and LDL levels are regularly increased. HDL levels may also be elevated. Plasminogen and antithrombin III levels may be low and participate in a thrombotic tendency.[833, 843] A circulating anticoagulant to factor XII has been described.[844] C3, C4, and properdin levels are usually elevated or within normal limits. C1q levels may occasionally be decreased.[1] IgG levels may be profoundly depressed during relapse.[1, 16, 760] This may account for the notorious susceptibility of such children to infection with pneumococci. IgE or IgM levels may be increased,[1, 845] the former in the presence of associated atopy. Elevated IgE levels may be associated with a requirement for higher steroid dosage to induce a remission. Elevated IgM levels may persist after remission.[1, 760] IgA levels are usually normal or modestly decreased.[760] IgM rheumatoid factors are increased in relapse and early

**TABLE 30–10. Classification of Diseases Associated with Minimal-Change Lesions**

**Primary (Idiopathic)**
With atopy and HLA-B12
Without atopy

**Secondary**
Hodgkin disease
Non-Hodgkin lymphoma
Solid tumors (renal cell carcinoma, lung, oncocytoma, pancreatic
    carcinoma, mesothelioma, colon, prostate)
Angiolymphoblastic lymphadenopathy
IgA nephropathy
Diabetes mellitus
Syphilis
Human immunodeficiency virus
Drugs (nonsteroidal anti-inflammatory agents, interferon, lithium
    carbonate, gold, rifampin, trimethadione, methimazole)

Modified from Nadasky T, Selin F, Hogg R: Minimal change nephrotic syndrome. *In* Tisher CC, Brenner BM (eds): Renal Pathology, 2nd ed. JB Lippincott, Philadelphia, 1994, p 330.

remission.[1, 846] Antibody levels to endostreptosin may be greatly reduced, even during remission.[1] Plasma renin activity and plasma aldosterone levels are frequently, but not always, increased.[1, 847] Plasma volume and blood volume may be normal, reduced, or elevated (see earlier).[1, 723, 724] HLA-B12 antigen is associated with those patients who display associated atopic manifestations and a frequently relapsing steroid-dependent course.[848] Atopic children with the HLA-B12 antigen have greatly increased risk for development of minimal-change lesions and the nephrotic syndrome.[849] Additional series describing increased prevalence of HLA-DR7, -DQw3, -DRw8, -B8, and -B13 have been reported.[849–853] Steroid-sensitive children with minimal-change disease may display certain HLA specificities, particularly DQw2 and the extended haplotype *AI, B8, DR3, DRw52* and *SCOI* and *B44, DR7, DRw35, FC31*.[852] The latter extended haplotype is also associated with gluten-sensitive enteropathy. A soluble immune response suppressor (13 to 18 kd), produced by $CD8^+$ lymphocytes may be found during relapse.[797] Interleukin-2 receptor–positive cells are increased in relapse, but this is not specific for minimal-change disease.[854, 855] The numbers of circulating $CD4^+$ and $CD8^+$ lymphocytes are more variable.[855] Substances having characteristics of circulating immune complexes have been described that appear during relapse and may or may not disappear during remission.[856–859]

Certain neoplastic diseases, primarily Hodgkin disease, have been associated with nephrotic syndrome due to underlying minimal-change lesion.[1, 860–863] Solid tumors that have also been associated with minimal-change disease with the nephrotic syndrome include undifferentiated, uroepithelial, pancreatic, prostatic, colon, lung, and renal cell carcinomas; oncocytoma; mesothelioma; and chordomas[1, 863] (Table 30–10; see Chapter 31). Syphilis and human immunodeficiency virus infection have been associated with minimal-change disease[864] (see Chapter 31). Nephrotic syndrome appearing secondarily to use of NSAIDs (indomethacin, fenoprofen, ibuprofen) has often revealed minimal glomerular changes associated with lymphocytic interstitial nephritis (see Chapter 31).

In children, the proteinuria is most often highly selective (e.g., IgG/transferrin clearance less than 0.10).[1, 636] The combination of highly selective proteinuria, normal or nearly normal GFR, normal serum C3 concentration, unremarkable urine sediment, and normal blood pressure is highly predictive of a minimal-change, steroid-responsive lesion in children with nephrotic syndrome[1, 636]; however, in adults, poorly selective proteinuria may be seen in a small number of cases.[812] As with many other varieties of the nephrotic syndrome, there is a tendency for thromboembolic events to occur, but renal vein thrombosis is unusual. On radiographic examination, the kidneys may be of normal size or enlarged.

**Pathology**

*Light Microscopy.* The distinguishing feature is the paucity of glomerular alterations as seen by light microscopy[1, 812–822] (Fig. 30–11). Increase in the overall cellularity of the mesangium is usually minor; but when it is

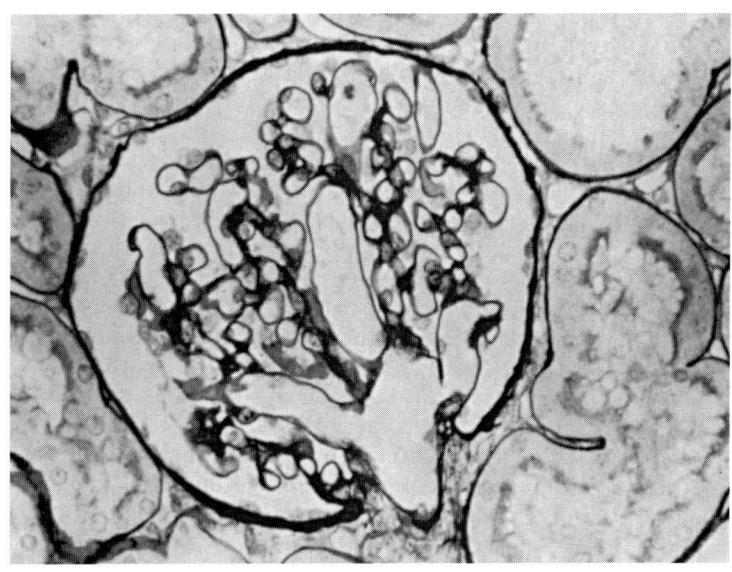

**Figure 30–11.** Light microscopic appearance of minimal-change lesion. This glomerulus has no abnormalities; note the lack of increased cellularity and the normal capillary walls. (Periodic acid–methenamine silver; magnification × 1000.)

more prominent, it may make a clear-cut distinction with mesangial proliferative glomerulonephritis difficult[1, 865–867] (see later). The epithelial cells may be enlarged with a more basophilic cytoplasm. In older patients, there may be an increase in mesangial matrix or an occasional obsolescent glomerulus, which is probably the consequence of aging or coexisting vascular disease. The capillary walls are thin and delicate. The parietal epithelial cells are normal, and proteinaceous material may be found in Bowman space. The glomerular volume is normal in minimal-change disease.[868] Large glomeruli may be a harbinger of the later development of focal and segmental glomerular sclerosis and steroid unresponsiveness (see later). If the glomerular volume is normal in a patient with otherwise typical minimal-change disease, the risk of subsequent progression to focal and segmental glomerular sclerosis is less than 5%.[868] Focal and segmental or global sclerosing lesions may be superimposed on this fundamental lesion, and this finding has potential prognostic and therapeutic significance,[1, 869, 870] as discussed later. Serial renal biopsies sometimes reveal transition into focal and segmental glomerular sclerosis or IgM nephropathy (see later). The exact frequency of this transition is debated but may be as high as 50% to 60%,[871] especially in patients with enlarged glomeruli on initial biopsy.[868] The proximal tubules may contain fine lipid droplets that are doubly refractile and similar to the material found in degenerating epithelial cells in the urine (oval fat bodies).[1] Focal areas of tubule atrophy, tubule basement membrane thickening, and interstitial fibrosis are usually absent or inconspicuous, especially in children.[1] If such tubule and interstitial lesions are well developed, it should heighten suspicion that a superimposed focal glomerular lesion is present but not represented in the available sections of the renal biopsy tissue sample. This is an indication for serial sectioning of the remaining biopsy material. Adequate numbers of glomeruli from both the outer cortical zones and the inner juxtamedullary zones are essential for accurate interpretation, because focal and segmental glomerular sclerosis in its earlier stages affects inner juxtamed-

ullary glomeruli preferentially (see later).[1, 870] Vascular changes, when present, are usually related to the age of the patient or to associated but unrelated hypertensive disease and are common features in elderly adults.[1, 872] Biopsies from patients with early MGN may likewise show minimal alterations by light microscopy, indistinguishable from those of minimal-change lesions.[1, 811] Therefore, a definitive assessment often cannot be made if material is examined by light microscopy alone, because these two entities may be clinically indistinguishable.

***Electron Microscopy.*** The electron microscope regularly detects abnormalities of the epithelial cells of the glomerular capillaries that are typical but not specific.[1, 811–821] Juxtaposition of the foot processes of the visceral epithelial cells and obliteration of the slit pore membrane complex are noted in most glomeruli and glomerular capillaries (Fig. 30–12). The extent of this lesion correlates with the severity of reduction in GFR.[837, 838] Epithelial cell vacuolization and detachment from the underlying basement membrane may be present, although more commonly they occur in evolving or well-developed focal and segmental glomerulosclerosis.[873, 874] Microvillous transformation of the free surfaces of the epithelial cells is common. The GBM is usually of normal thickness, with minor and inconstant changes in fine structure. Platelet aggregates and fibrin polymers may be recognized in the capillary lumens[1] but may be more indicative of evolving focal and segmental glomerular sclerosis. Small electron-dense deposits are infrequently found in the paramesangial location in otherwise typical cases, even in the apparent absence of immunoglobulin deposits.[875] The similarity of clinical findings, with the exception of steroid responsiveness, in patients with underlying minimal-change glomerular lesions with superimposed focal glomerular sclerosis has been repeatedly emphasized.[1, 876] Thus, an initial biopsy diagnosis of uncomplicated minimal-change disease on the basis of light microscopy alone in a patient with idiopathic nephrotic syndrome should be viewed with some skepticism. The possibility always exists that this diagnosis may be incorrect, particularly if the patient subsequently

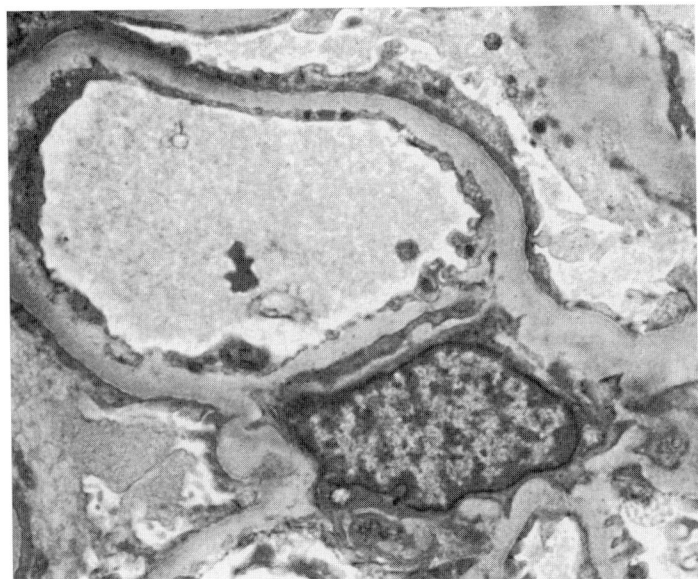

**Figure 30–12.** Electron microscopic view of minimal-change lesion showing complete effacement of foot processes of epithelial cells. No electron-dense deposits can be seen along capillary walls. Note occasional subendothelial nodularities of the basement membrane. (Magnification × 12,250.)

proves to be resistant to steroid therapy. Glomerular enlargement and separation of epithelial cells from underlying basement membrane, development of a lucent zone filled with amorphous or fibrillary material between the epithelial cells and the basement membrane, and extensive visceral epithelial cell vacuolization may be early ultrastructural features of superimposed focal and segmental glomerular sclerosis.[818, 873, 874, 877]

***Immunofluorescence.*** Immunofluorescence findings are noteworthy for the lack of deposition of immunoglobulin and complement in glomeruli in most uncomplicated cases.[1, 878] Some investigators have described the occasional presence of small flecks or comma-shaped deposits of IgM in the mesangium, especially at the vascular pole, or similar deposits of IgG or IgM diffusely throughout the mesangium.[1, 865, 879, 880] The significance of these deposits remains controversial.[1, 879, 880–884] The preponderance of studies have shown that such deposits, so long as the light microscopic and ultrastructural features are consistent with minimal-change disease, do not seem to indicate any predilection for steroid unresponsiveness or tendency for evolution to progressive disease.[1] Nonetheless, some studies have shown that heavy and diffuse mesangial IgG or IgM deposits, especially in conjunction with mild to moderate mesangial hypercellularity, portend a greater likelihood of unresponsiveness to steroids (as high as 50%) and a greater propensity for evolution to progressive disease,[1, 865, 882, 883] especially to focal and segmental glomerular sclerosis. In some of these cases, the degree of mesangial hypercellularity was so mild as to permit categorization on the basis of light microscopy into the minimal-change lesion. Whether well-marked mesangial IgM deposition delineates a separate entity (IgM nephropathy) or is simply a part of the spectrum of minimal-change disease–focal sclerosis–mesangial proliferative glomerulonephritis alluded to before will require further study.[1, 865, 882, 883] Whatever the cause, diffuse, heavy mesangial IgM deposits in minimal-change disease may simply be a marker of more disturbed mesangial function with subsequent trapping of circulating macromolecules in an altered microenvironment.[1, 880]

On occasion, mesangial IgE deposits have been observed,[885] but not consistently.[886] Fibrin polymers may be found in a fibrillar pattern within the glomerular capillary lumen, particularly during relapses. Albumin may be found as fine droplets in many proximal tubule cells, but other proteins, such as IgG, IgM, and fibrin-related antigens, are usually not seen in a similar distribution.[1] Rarely, linear deposits of IgG may be found in patients with concomitant acute renal failure. There is no evidence that these deposits represent anti-GBM antibody.[834] CD4+ and CD8+ T cells may also be found within glomeruli in the minimal-change disease lesion, with or without concomitant IgM deposition.[887]

**Pathogenesis.** The pathogenesis of the minimal-change lesion is unknown. Histologic and ultrastructural changes similar to this lesion may be induced by infusion of hyperoncotic albumin, by aminonucleoside of puromycin or doxorubicin (Adriamycin), or by the injection of polycations into the renal artery.[1, 888, 889] Glomerular net negative charge is reduced in relapse, but the mechanism responsible for this change is unknown.[890a] The anionic constituents of the glomerular capillary wall are reduced or blocked from reaction with polycationic marker molecules.[836, 839] Mononuclear cells from patients with minimal-change disease may induce a reduction in glomerular polyanion, but this effect is not specific for minimal-change disease.[889, 890] The negative charge on erythrocytes is reduced in minimal-change disease (and MGN) in remission.[891]

The basic abnormality may reside in the GBM or in the epithelial cells. Studies using neutral dextran and comparison of fractional clearances of albumin and IgG have strongly supported the notion that minimal-change disease is the prototypical example of a charge-selective barrier defect, but the precise reason for loss of this barrier is unknown.[839, 840, 891–895] The urinary albumin excreted during relapse is less anionic than normal serum albumin[896]; this change could contribute to the hypoalbuminemia characteristic of this condition.

As previously mentioned, an identical histologic lesion may commonly be found to underlie the nephrotic syndrome in Hodgkin disease[1, 860, 897] as well as rarely in other malignant neoplasms (see Tables 30–6 and 30–10 and Chapter 31). Remissions may occur in association with viral infections (e.g., measles) that transiently depress cell-mediated hypersensitivity.[1] As discussed later, the lesion responds dramatically to corticosteroids and alkylating cytotoxic drugs. These findings and others have led some to postulate that minimal-change lesions are the result of a disorder of T cell function.[796, 898, 899] In support of this view, it has been noted that lymphocytes or mononuclear cells from patients with minimal-change disease may display depressed cellular reactivity in vitro to mitogens such as concanavalin A or phytohemagglutinin and when activated may induce changes in glomerular polyanion or permeability in vitro.[1, 619, 795, 819, 890, 900–904] These alterations can be partially corrected by indomethacin, which suggests a role for prostaglandins in vivo.[905] Altered cell reactivity to renal antigens may be present.[906] Suppressor T cell function may be enhanced[907] or depressed. The latter effect may be a long-lasting effect of prior cyclophosphamide therapy.[908–910] Graft-versus-host reactions induced by lymphocytes may be decreased.[911] Such patients also frequently possess circulating lymphocytotoxins[912, 913] and may release permeability-enhancing factors from lymphocytes, some of which reduce glomerular polyanion content.[795, 900–904] Circulating factors capable of suppressing mitogenic response of lymphocytes and the mixed leukocyte culture reaction have been described, but the specificity of this finding is also open to question.[914–921] The recurrence of typical steroid-responsive minimal glomerular lesions in a renal allograft clearly implicates some systemic permeability factor in the pathogenesis of this disorder.[922] Preliminary findings suggest that the permeability factor is a nonimmunoglobulin protein of molecular mass less than 100 kd. It is similar to that found in patients with focal and segmental glomerular sclerosis.[816, 820] No consistent abnormalities in T or B cell subpopulations have been described in patients with minimal-change disease, during either relapse or remission.[854, 855, 923, 924] Cyclophosphamide therapy may temporarily decrease the CD4+ to CD8+ T cell ratios.[925] Defective suppressor T cell function is more likely to occur in patients who have received cyclophosphamide therapy.[908] Monocyte suppressor activity may be responsible for some of the abnormalities described in minimal-change disease, including reduced IgG levels, which are profoundly depressed in relapse (see earlier).[760] However, immunoglobulin synthesis by blood mononuclear cells is increased in relapse.[926] IgM levels are elevated and persist during remission.[760] Likewise, the coexistence of atopy and other allergic manifestations with minimal-change lesions, as well as occasional precipitation of the latter by immunization, has led some to suggest an anaphylactic or reaginic antibody response as being important.[1] Such patients often possess the HLA-B12 antigen.[1, 848] HLA-DR7 may also be increased in patients with minimal-change disease without atopy.[849] Elevated levels of immunoconglutinin suggest complement activation in vivo, yet complement component levels are most often normal.[927]

To confound the issue of pathogenesis further, several investigators have found circulating material having characteristics of immune complexes in a high percentage of children with presumed minimal-change disease during relapse.[857, 858] Levels fell slowly during steroid-induced or spontaneous remission.[857] These immune complexes did not bind C1q.[859] Other investigators using assays dependent on C1q fixation and other methods have also reported occasional positive results, especially in adults with the disease.[1, 857] These immune complexes are likely epiphenomena unrelated to underlying pathogenesis. As noted previously, IgM rheumatoid factor may be present during a relapse, which suggests the formation of immune complexes.[846] Fc receptor function of the spleen may be impaired during relapse, but this finding does not correlate with circulating immune complex levels and may persist after remission.[928]

In summary, many clues strongly suggest involvement of immune-mediated processes in this disorder particularly related to T cell dysregulation.[898, 929] The diversity of findings might suggest a degree of pathogenetic heterogeneity in this lesion. Abnormalities in T cell function, particularly suppressor T cell function and the generation of lymphokines capable of reversibly altering glomerular polyanion content and enhancing permeability to albumin, seem likely to be involved.

**Course and Therapy.** This disorder is characterized chiefly by a remitting and relapsing course and its striking susceptibility to corticosteroid therapy.[1, 930–944] It also has a favorable long-term course. Less than 5% of children with minimal-change disease will have end-stage renal disease after 25 years of follow-up.[944] Spontaneous remissions apparently occur frequently, although the true frequency is difficult to judge because steroid therapy is intentionally withheld from few patients, and information regarding histology is lacking from the presteroid era.[945, 946] Spontaneous remissions may occur in as many as 50% of patients, but they may not occur for several years after initial presentation.[1, 13, 947–949] Children are often noted to have fewer relapses after puberty and after 10 to 15 years of follow-up; few patients continue to exhibit a remitting and relapsing course.[16, 944] Several broad patterns of clinical evolution are found, and these are best described in the context of steroid treatment: 1) lasting complete remission of abnormal proteinuria and manifestations of the nephrotic state with a single course of glucocorticoid treatment (primary re-

sponder, nonrelapser); 2) steroid-induced remission but with relapses occurring less than twice in the first 6 months of the initial response (primary responder, infrequent relapser); 3) steroid-induced remission but with two or more relapses within 6 months of the initial response (primary responder, frequent relapser); 4) steroid-induced remission but with relapses occurring during steroid withdrawal or shortly thereafter (steroid-dependent responder); 5) no response after an initial response (secondary nonresponder); 6) no response to initial therapy, but remission occurring after completion of therapy (primary nonresponder, late responder); 7) no remission at any time with therapy (continuing nonresponder); and 8) spontaneous remission without treatment (spontaneous responder).[931, 932, 947–949]

The optimal dose, schedule of administration, and total duration of steroid therapy have not yet been fully standardized and probably differ for children and adults with this disorder.[937–943] The newly diagnosed child may be *initially* treated with oral prednisone or prednisolone, 60 mg/m²/d (equivalent to about 1.5 mg/kg/d in adults) but usually not more than 80 mg/d, given as a single daily dose. Such therapy results in the complete disappearance of abnormal proteinuria in more than 90% of patients within 4 weeks. At 4 to 6 weeks (or earlier, if remission occurs), therapy can be changed to 35 to 40 mg/m² (about 0.9 mg/kg in adults) in a single dose every other morning (alternate-day schedule).[1, 940–942, 948–950] This therapy may be continued for an additional 4 to 6 weeks, unless a remission occurs during the alternate-day therapy. Treatment is often continued for a full 6 weeks after a complete remission of proteinuria occurs. Too early or too abrupt withdrawal of steroids may result in a relapse, perhaps because of partial pituitary-adrenal suppression and relative adrenal insufficiency.[950–953] Altered prednisone or prednisolone pharmacokinetics could play a role in responsiveness of patients to standard oral dosage regimens.[954] Children who have persistent nephrotic syndrome after a full 8- to 12-week course of glucocorticoid therapy are commonly regarded as nonresponders or steroid-resistant patients. Renal biopsies in this group of patients frequently, although not invariably, demonstrate lesions other than those of minimal-change disease. Steroid resistance may also be acquired late in the course of disease.[1, 955] Patients receiving intravenous albumin in an attempt to promote diuresis require longer periods of therapy to induce remissions and have a higher rate of relapse.[956] Thus, albumin infusions should be avoided during initial treatment.

Adults respond more slowly than children do, and therapy for more than 8 weeks is often required to clearly delineate the steroid responsiveness of the lesion.[937–939, 941, 942] Japanese adults may be an exception to this rule; they appear to be more steroid responsive.[939] Adults older than 40 years at the time of diagnosis may require as much as 16 to 20 weeks of glucocorticoid therapy before a complete remission occurs.[937, 938] Because of the variability of the duration (and intensity) of therapy required to obtain a response, it is difficult to clearly define the population of steroid-resistant adults with minimal-change disease. An alternate-day regimen (2 mg/kg every other day, 125 mg maximal dose) may be as effective as the daily (followed by alternate-day) regimen described before.[957] High-dose intravenous methylprednisone may also be effective in inducing remissions but is seldom needed,[958–960] and relapses are more frequent.

Using a daily followed by alternate-day oral steroid regimen, 93% of children with minimal-change lesions fell into the category of primary responders in the ISKDC study mentioned before.[1, 932] Subsequent follow-up for 10 months indicated that 38% of the primary responders were nonrelapsers, 19% were infrequent relapsers, and 42% were frequent relapsers,[1, 961] including the steroid-dependent category. Of the last group, 5% were secondary responders, according to the previous definitions. Primary nonresponders constituted 7% of the entire group; 70% of these were late responders and 30% continuing nonresponders. The data for adults are similar, but with advancing age, the prevalence of complete remissions at 8 weeks rapidly declines.[937, 938] More protracted therapy seems to be associated with a lower frequency of relapses but, of course, a greater prevalence of steroid-related side effects. Patients who have their first relapse within 6 months of the initial response tend to be frequent relapsers and usually require more intensive therapy. For this group, continuation of prednisone for an additional 6 months on an alternate-day basis (35 mg/m² in children or 0.8 to 1.0 mg/kg in adults every other day) may be associated with a lower prevalence of later relapse.[1] One must balance the hazards of continuation of moderate doses of steroids for prolonged periods against the potential complications of sustaining the nephrotic state. Patients requiring high doses of glucocorticoids to maintain a remission (greater than 0.4 mg/kg/d; ''high-dose'' steroid dependency) should be strongly considered for alternative therapeutic regimens (see later). The processes responsible for steroid unresponsiveness, either to initial therapy or after a series of relapses, is not known, but such patients could represent those acquiring superimposed focal and segmental sclerosing lesions (see later).

Patients with unquestioned minimal-change lesions on an adequate biopsy examination who do not respond to the steroid regimens outlined may subsequently respond to higher doses; more prolonged therapy; or the addition of cyclophosphamide, chlorambucil, azathioprine, levamisole, or cyclosporine (see later) to the treatment program.[1, 934, 963] Areas of focal tubule changes, focal and global glomerular obsolescence, mild mesangial thickening, or hypercellularity do not greatly alter the initial response to therapy or the subsequent course.[931, 932] Although the data from ISKDC are the most representative of an unselected population of pediatric patients with minimal-change lesions, it should be noted that, in children, the frequency of a primary lasting response to initial steroid therapy varies considerably, from 7% to 40% in published series.[1, 825, 947–964] On the average, 60% or more of children having an initial response to steroid subsequently display a relapsing course.[941, 942, 964] Adults appear to behave in a similar fashion. Patients with HLA-B12 appear to be at higher risk for a relapsing course.[848] Relapses may continue to occur after many years, although the frequency tends to decline 10 years or more after the diagnosis is established.[944, 965, 966] Occasionally, relapses may occur after long disease-free intervals, often precipitated by an allergic reaction or a viral illness.[966–968] A small number of patients (<10%) may acquire steroid

unresponsiveness after repeated episodes of relapse and remission.[955] Some of these will display features of focal glomerular sclerosis on late renal biopsies or reveal glomerulomegaly on initial biopsy.[868] However, such lesions are also observed in patients who continue to respond to steroids.

Because of the tendency for relapses and the risk of pneumococcal infection during full-blown nephrotic syndrome, many pediatricians recommend pneumococcal vaccination during steroid-induced remissions. This might also apply to elderly adults. Prophylactic subcutaneous minidose heparin, 5000 U every 12 hours, is also used by some physicians during relapse to decrease risk of thromboembolism.

Patients who continue to exhibit frequent relapses despite prolonged or repeated cycles of steroid therapy or who acquire high-dose steroid dependency constitute a difficult problem. Such patients may experience growth retardation,[934] adverse social and psychologic effects from acne, moon facies, emotional irritability, and menstrual irregularity. Peptic ulceration, cataracts, osteoporosis, aseptic necrosis of the femoral head, and psychiatric disturbances may also occur, and the advisability of continued steroid therapy in the presence of these complications is questionable.

For such patients, the physician has several alternatives. First, discontinue steroids altogether and manage the patient symptomatically with diuretics, sodium restriction, and dietary manipulation in the hope of an ultimate spontaneous remission. If proteinuria and hypoalbuminemia are not severe, this approach may be satisfactory, although the patient will still have an enhanced susceptibility to infection and hyperlipidemia, and the nutritional consequences of protein depletion may be unacceptable. The possible but yet unproven relationship of prolonged elevation of cholesterol and triglycerides to the accelerated development of cardiovascular disease cannot be discounted. There is also an increased tendency to thromboembolic events in the untreated nephrotic state. Second, attempt adjunctive therapy with the cytotoxic alkylating agents cyclophosphamide,[1, 934, 941, 942, 962, 963, 969] chlorambucil,[970] nitrogen mustard,[971] or other agents (such as azathioprine, cyclosporine, or levamisole). Many reports have documented that cyclophosphamide given in conjunction with steroids will induce longer lasting remissions in the frequently relapsing group or on occasion convert an initially steroid-unresponsive patient to a steroid-responsive state.[1, 963, 969–976] Similar well-designed long-term controlled studies have also demonstrated the efficacy of chlorambucil, but there is no clear evidence to indicate the superiority of chlorambucil to cyclophosphamide.[970, 975–981]

The subset of patients who are clearly steroid dependent (who experience relapses during or shortly after glucocorticoid withdrawal) are a special problem. Short-term (8- to 10-week) courses of cyclophosphamide in conjunction with a steroid-induced remission are associated with a poor long-term outcome. Only 20% to 30% of these patients experience a long-term relapse-free interval. Longer periods of therapy, about 12 weeks, are associated with improved long-term results.[963, 976]

These agents may be given without any loss of effectiveness in dosages not generally associated with significant leukopenia[1]; 2 mg/kg/d of cyclophosphamide for 8 to 12 weeks or 0.15 to 0.2 mg/kg/d of chlorambucil for 8 to 10 weeks is considered effective,[1, 941, 942, 963, 977–982] depending on whether the patient being treated is steroid dependent. Treatment duration longer than 12 weeks or use of cyclophosphamide doses greater than 2.5 to 3 mg/d is unnecessary and may increase the hazards or long-term complications of therapy. Cyclophosphamide may be the preferred agent, but either agent should be used only in cases in which continued steroid therapy is associated with unacceptable side effects. Cyclophosphamide appears to be more effective when given in conjunction with steroids but may also induce remissions when given alone.[979] Intravenous nitrogen mustard is also effective but is accompanied by more side effects and possesses no particular advantages over short-term therapy with cyclophosphamide or chlorambucil.[971] However, among the small group of patients who continue to relapse after a course of cyclophosphamide or chlorambucil, intravenous nitrogen mustard may induce a more prolonged remission.[971] In the context of the beneficial effects of cyclophosphamide, one should recall the association of Hodgkin disease and the minimal-change lesions and the impressive remissions that occur in connection with treatment of Hodgkin disease with alkylating agents and radiotherapy and the relative resistance of this lesion to glucocorticoids.[1, 983, 984]

In an assessment of the long-term benefits of cyclophosphamide, several authors have noted that 75% of frequently relapsing patients treated with cyclophosphamide in connection with a steroid-induced remission remained free of proteinuria for 1 year and about 40% were still in remission 5 years later.[963, 977, 985] The effects of cyclophosphamide were similar in adults and children with minimal-change lesions. Uncontrolled studies have suggested that steroid-resistant patients with minimal changes on initial biopsy may respond to cyclophosphamide or become steroid responsive after having received a course of cyclophosphamide[942, 963, 975, 986]; but a prospective, controlled study of steroid-unresponsive children (with minimal glomerular changes or focal and segmental sclerosis on renal biopsy) failed to show any significant advantage of therapy with cyclophosphamide over continued intermittent or alternate-day steroids.[975, 987] The number of patients with delayed responses was about equal in both treatment groups.[975] Second courses of cyclophosphamide in patients who relapse after the initial course of cyclophosphamide therapy are associated with an outcome similar to that found with the initial course of treatment. However, more than two courses of cyclophosphamide is not recommended owing to the cumulative risks.[1, 941]

The use of cytotoxic alkylating agents in this condition is, of course, not without hazards that limit their applicability.[1] Reversible alopecia is common. Chlorambucil therapy may produce seizures in children. Increased susceptibility to cholinesterase-inhibiting muscle relaxants, hyponatremia, pulmonary toxic effects, and hemorrhagic cystitis may occur. With the use of cyclophosphamide, hemorrhagic cystitis is uncommon if fluid intake is encouraged and administration of the drug in the evening is avoided. Long-term use may be associated with the late development of bladder contractures and fibrosis or atypical (premalignant) cell changes in bladder epithelium.[1] Both cyclophosphamide and chlorambucil also enhance susceptibility to certain viral and fungal diseases, and fatal or nearly fatal episodes of measles and disseminated varicella have been reported.[1] In the young susceptible child, varicella is a particularly worrisome threat, and these agents should be used with great caution in children who have not yet had measles or chickenpox and who have no demonstrable immunity. Attenuated viral vaccines are contraindicated during treatment.

One of the most serious side effects of therapy with alkylating agents is the high frequency of gonadal failure. This appears to be a dose-dependent phenomenon and may be reversible if the therapeutic trial is kept brief (i.e., less than 8 weeks) and the total cumulative amount administered is less than about 200 mg/kg of cyclophosphamide or less than 10 mg/kg of chlorambucil.[942, 988] This problem is of less concern in older patients. Females may be less susceptible to irreversible gonadal failure than are males. The coadministration of oral contraceptives to menstruating females may reduce gonadal toxicity of alkylating agents. The oncogenic or mutagenic potential of cyclophosphamide or chlorambucil employed on a short-term basis is not yet fully known but should be considered a potential hazard.[942, 989, 990] A number of cases of malignant neoplasms, particularly acute leukemia, cancer of bladder, renal carcinoma, and squamous cell carcinoma of the skin, have now been reported in patients receiving prolonged therapy (usually longer than 1 year) with cyclophosphamide or chlorambucil for non-neoplastic conditions.[1, 990] The acquisition of the −5/−7 karyotype after cyclophosphamide therapy places the patient at a high risk for development of acute nonlymphocytic leukemia.[991]

Although cyclophosphamide or chlorambucil appears to exert a beneficial effect on minimal-change lesions, azathioprine and other purine analogues have long been thought to have no substantial effect on the course of disease.[992] Cade and co-workers[993] have demonstrated a possible beneficial effect of azathioprine given without glucocorticoids for patients with minimal-change disease who are resistant to steroid therapy or who are steroid dependent. After 12 to 24 months of continuous azathioprine therapy, all patients became proteinuria free. Those with more selective proteinuria entered into a complete remission in shorter periods than did those with nonselective proteinuria. Limited experience has suggested that azathioprine may also be useful in maintaining remission in difficult to treat patients.[994] A controlled clinical trial would seem to be warranted; in the meantime, azathioprine could be used as an alternative to cyclophosphamide or chlorambucil in selected instances.[995]

Levamisole, a nonspecific T cell–stimulating factor, has been used to treat minimal-change disease with some success in preliminary trials.[996, 997] The British Association for Pediatric Nephrology carried out a controlled trial of levamisole in frequently relapsing and steroid-dependent minimal-change disease.[998] Levamisole was given in doses of 2.5 mg/kg every other day. Relapses were decreased from 85% in control subjects to 45% in levamisole-treated subjects at 3 months. Neutropenia was uncommon. Lower doses of levamisole (approximately 2.5 mg/kg twice weekly) *may* be useful in maintaining remission in steroid-dependent patients with high-dose steroid dependency,[999] but this has not been unequivocally demonstrated. A preliminary report of a randomized trial failed to show any benefit of biweekly levamisole in frequently relapsing steroid-dependent disease.[999a] In addition, Chinese workers have claimed that bacille Calmette-Guérin vaccination in gradually decreasing doses combined with levamisole greatly increases the likelihood of persistent remissions.[1000] This has not been confirmed in a prospective randomized trial. Doxantrazole and disodium cromoglycate are ineffective.[1] Hypoallergenic diets and desensitization to specific allergens have been successful in a limited number of instances.

Cyclosporine is emerging as a potentially promising agent in the management of minimal-change disease, particularly in steroid-resistant patients and in patients who have severe side effects from prolonged or recurrent glucocorticoid therapy and who fail to satisfactorily respond to cyclophosphamide or for some other reason cannot be treated with alkylating agents.[1001–1008] Cyclosporine in doses of 4 to 6 mg/kg/d, usually in conjunction with low-dose, alternate-day prednisone (0.5 to 0.6 mg/kg every other day), induces a complete remission in a high percentage of steroid-responsive adult and pediatric patients, perhaps as high as 85% to 90%.[962, 964, 1002–1004] Unfortunately, lasting remissions after discontinuation of therapy are uncommon (probably around 20% to 30%), and prolonged therapy may be associated with side effects, including nephrotoxic injury. Nephrotoxic effects of cyclosporine are largely seen in patients who receive a dosage greater than 5.5 mg/kg/d.[1004] Furthermore, nephrotoxic injury is not regularly associated with an increase in serum creatinine concentration.[1008] Older patients appear to be at greater risk for significant cyclosporine-associated nephrotoxic effects.[1004, 1008] The response of steroid-unresponsive patients is less predictable. About 50% to 65% of steroid-resistant adults and children with minimal-change disease respond with complete remission to a course of cyclosporine.[941, 942, 1002–1004] Responses, if they are to occur at all, are usually noted within the first 4 months of treatment.[1004] Unfortunately, relapses are particularly likely to occur after discontinuance of cyclosporine.[1002–1004] Alkylating agents are the preferred therapy for frequently relapsing steroid-dependent patients with minimal-change disease, because of the ability to achieve more prolonged remissions.[963, 1005] Alkylating agents or cyclosporine could be used for steroid-resistant patients.[1006] Patients with steroid-dependent frequently relapsing disease who receive cyclosporine and who have remissions may be continued on therapy at the lowest dose possible (e.g., 2 to 4 mg/kg/d) for prolonged periods (up to 1 to 2 years) to sustain remissions. Such patients may then be withdrawn from cyclosporine therapy with a high probability that relapse will not occur.[1008]

Blood level monitoring of cyclosporine is desirable but not mandatory. Whole blood cyclosporine levels (monoclonal antibody assay) should be maintained at less than 100 to 200 ng/mL, and dosage should not exceed 5.5 mg/kg/d.[1004, 1009] Children with severe hypercholesterolemia may require higher doses (as high as 10 to 14 mg/kg/d) to achieve therapeutic levels.[1010]

The long-term use of ACE inhibitors may decrease urinary protein excretion to 60% of baseline values but seldom induces complete remissions. Nevertheless, in steroid-resistant nephrotic syndrome or in patients with difficult to manage frequently relapsing disease, real benefit may accrue from concomitant administration of ACE inhibitors.[1011, 1012]

Very low protein diets are not recommended, but a vegetarian soy diet decreases urinary protein excretion and improves hyperlipidemia.[1013] A fluoroquinolone antimicrobial, pefloxacin, was serendipitously found to be associated with remission of nephrotic syndrome in adults with steroid-dependent or frequently relapsing disease.[1014] Remission occurred in 60% of patients treated with 400 mg of pefloxacin twice daily for 1 month, with few relapses when therapy was withdrawn. This new approach to therapy is deserving of a prospective trial. Use of this agent in focal and segmental glomerulosclerosis has been disappointing[1014a] (see later).

Long-term follow-up of children and adults with clear-cut, biopsy-proven minimal-change lesions indicates an overall favorable prognosis.[1, 16, 934, 944, 1015, 1016] In children with idiopathic nephrotic syndrome (of whom 75% or more can be assumed to have minimal-change lesions), the mortality rate was high in presteroid, preantibiotic years.[1, 13] Since then, short-term mortality and morbidity have declined rapidly. Cameron and co-workers[977] estimated the 20- to 25-year survival of steroid-responsive patients with minimal-change disease to be in excess of 95%, with most of the mortality observed in adults treated with steroids. Late onset of chronic renal failure is uncommon,[1, 944, 1015] and the major reasons for mortality are cardiovascular disease and infection, the latter often attributable to steroid and alkylating agent therapy. Because of the intrinsically favorable prognosis, some experienced clinicians prefer not to treat adults with minimal-change disease who are minimally symptomatic with steroids but rather to await a spontaneous remission and manage conservatively with diet and diuretics.

In summary, the long-term prognosis of patients with idiopathic nephrotic syndrome with minimal-change lesions is excellent if one restricts the diagnosis to patients of any age having 1) minimal glomerular changes by light microscopy, 2) diffuse epithelial cell lesion only by electron microscopy, 3) absence or minimal deposition of immunoglobulin by immunofluorescence microscopy, and 4) complete remission after an appropriate course of steroid therapy. Even so, it is likely that multiple relapses will occur. Steroid therapy should be regarded chiefly as palliative rather than curative; more prolonged therapy is required in adults. Given sufficient time, a high percentage of untreated patients will undergo spontaneous remission, although such patients will be exposed to the risks of the underlying pathophysiologic disturbances of continued massive proteinuria during the nephrotic period. Adjunctive therapy of patients with minimal-change disease with cytotoxic drugs or other immunosuppressants does not greatly affect the occurrence of renal failure and probably does not significantly affect long-term survival. However, these agents do decrease the exposure of the patient to the undesirable effects of the nephrotic milieu and the potentially toxic exposure to glucocorticoids. The cost of these potentially beneficial effects is the risk of infection, gonadal or bladder toxicity (for cyclophosphamide and chlorambucil), hepatitis, and the potential emergence of neoplasia. If treatment with an alkylating agent is of short duration, the risks are small, and for many patients with disabling steroid toxic effects or severe nephrotic syndrome, such treatment can be justified. Cyclosporine therapy is of value in selected patients and may induce prolonged remissions after extended therapy. Doses of cyclosporine above 5.5 mg/kg/d should be avoided because of the possibility of cumulative nephrotoxic effects. Levamisole, azathioprine, and ACE inhibitors may be of benefit in some circumstances. Chronic renal failure is an uncommon outcome usually associated with acquisition of steroid resistance and a glomerular lesion of focal and segmental glomerulosclerosis (see later).

## MESANGIAL PROLIFERATIVE GLOMERULONEPHRITIS

Among patients with the nephrotic syndrome, "pure" mesangial proliferative glomerulonephritis is a relatively uncommon glomerular lesion and is usually defined by its light microscopic features.[1, 13, 1017–1020] It is found as an uncomplicated lesion in less than 10% of biopsies in patients with idiopathic nephrotic syndrome, although some series have demonstrated an overall prevalence of proliferative glomerulonephritis (other than MCGN) as high as 20%. Some of the "other proliferative" group may fall into the category of mesangial proliferative glomerulonephritis; others will have focal and segmental proliferative, extracapillary proliferative, or endocapillary proliferative glomerulonephritis (see later). Because the differentiation between the mild prominence of mesangial cells as observed in minimal-change lesions and definite mesangial proliferation is so subjective and highly susceptible to artifacts of sectioning and specimen preparation, it is easy to understand how patients in this category of lesions may sometimes be classified with minimal-change disease and vice versa.[1, 1020–1030] Furthermore, because of the nonspecificity of the character and distribution of the proliferative lesions by light microscopy alone, patients with resolving postinfectious glomerulonephritis and systemic diseases (e.g., SLE, Schönlein-Henoch purpura) may fit into this category (Table 30–11). By convention, patients with mesangial proliferative glomerulonephritis with extensive mesangial IgA deposits are categorized as having Berger disease (see earlier). Nonamyloid fibrillar deposits would lead to categorization as fibrillary or immunotactoid glomerulonephritis (see later). Here we discuss the clinical features of patients with idiopathic nephrotic syndrome due to primary glomerular disease in which well-developed mesangial proliferative lesions are present, without features (such as IgA deposits) that would permit categorization as a separate entity.[1020, 1021] "Asymptomatic" hematuria with or without proteinuria is another common clinical expression of this underlying primary glomerular lesion.

**Clinical Features.** The dominant feature is the insidious onset of heavy proteinuria with or without the other biochemical features of the nephrotic state.[1, 13, 1017–1021] GFR is usually normal.[1021] Any age can be affected, but patients are usually older children and young adults. Males predominate slightly over females. Familial cases have been described. Hematuria is present in the majority of cases and is occasionally macroscopic or recurrent. A precipitating event or evidence of an infectious event is most often lacking. Mild hypertension is present in about 30% of cases. On clinical grounds alone, it is difficult to separate this group of patients from those with minimal-change disease or other histopathologic variants of the idiopathic nephrotic syndrome.[1, 1017–1021] Pregnancy is generally well tolerated.[1023]

**Laboratory Findings** (see Table 30–2). The laboratory features are not distinctive. The typical biochemical features of nephrotic syndrome are usually present. Hematuria is frequently present. Renal function is decreased at discovery in about 25% of patients. IgG levels may be modestly reduced. Complement component levels are most often normal, but a rare patient has decreased C4 levels associated with a null allele at *C4* locus.[1024] Circulating IgM- or IgG-containing immune complexes may be found in some patients. ASO titers are usually normal. Proteinuria is usually nonselective. There is no known association with HLA antigens, except in unusual familial cases.[1030]

### Pathology

*Light Microscopy.* The glomeruli are characterized by definite but variable degrees of increase in cellularity of the mesangium, usually affecting all lobules of all glomeruli to an equal degree (Fig. 30–13). Four or five nuclei may be seen per mesangial zone in mild forms and more than five nuclei in more severe forms.[1, 1017–1021, 1025, 1026] The capillary walls are thin and delicate and usually free of deposits. The capillary lumens are patent. In the uncomplicated variety, adhesions and segmental sclerosis are lacking. With the use of Masson trichrome stain, fuchsinophilic deposits in the mesangium have been identified in almost half of the biopsy samples. Similar staining deposits of uncertain nature may be noted in the basement membranes of Bowman capsules. Aside from "hyalinization" of the walls of arterioles, significant tubule, interstitial, or other vascular lesions are not evident. However, as the disease progresses, segmentally or totally sclerotic glomeruli and their tubule and interstitial consequences superimpose on the basic lesion described[1, 813, 865, 866, 1029] (see focal sclerosis).

*Electron Microscopy.* Ultrastructural studies have indicated that in up to 50% of the biopsy specimens, finely granular or homogeneous electron-dense deposits are iden-

---

**TABLE 30–11. Classification of Diseases Associated with Mesangial Proliferative Glomerulonephritis**

**Primary (Idiopathic)**
With predominant IgA mesangial deposits (Berger disease)
With predominant mesangial IgM and C3 deposits
With other patterns of immunoglobulin and C3 deposits
No immunoglobulin or C3 deposits

**Secondary to Underlying Disease**
Resolving postinfectious glomerulonephritis
Systemic lupus erythematosus
Schönlein-Henoch purpura
Rheumatoid arthritis
Alport syndrome
Goodpasture syndrome
Kimura disease
D-Penicillamine

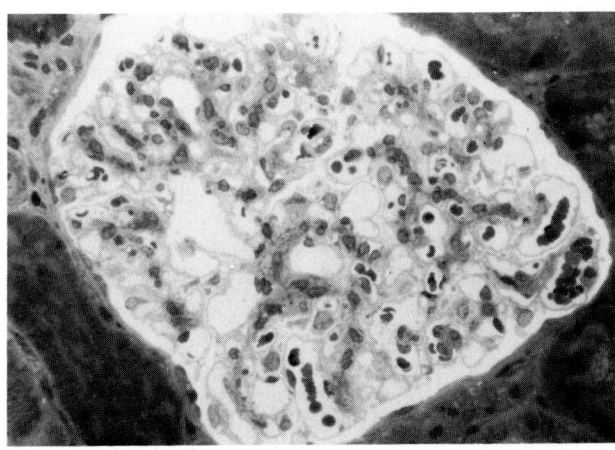

**Figure 30–13.** Light microscopic appearance of mesangial proliferative glomerulonephritis. There is a mild, diffuse increase in mesangial cellularity and an absence of capillary wall changes. (Toluidine blue; magnification × 1000.)

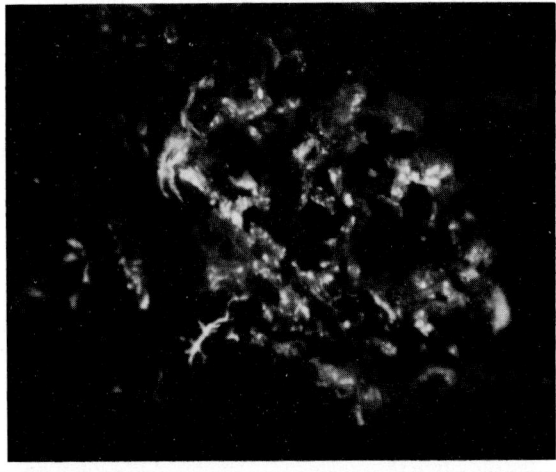

**Figure 30–15.** Immunofluorescence view of mesangial proliferative glomerulonephritis revealing extensive mesangial IgM deposits. (Antihuman IgM; magnification × 1000.)

tified in the mesangium (Fig. 30–14). As noted previously, similar deposits may be seen in biopsies categorized as minimal-change lesions, even when immunofluorescence findings are negative.

The precise relationship between mesangial electron-dense deposits has not yet been settled, but some investigators believe such deposits contain IgM and are the hallmark of a discrete clinicopathologic entity (IgM mesangial nephropathy, see later). Ill-defined densities, lucent zones, vacuoles, and striated membranous structures have been observed in the mesangium of glomeruli of some biopsy specimens, whereas aside from increased cellularity, no other mesangial changes have been noted in others. Epithelial foot processes are diffusely swollen and effaced and occasionally have disruption of the cytoplasm, with denudation of the urinary aspect of the basement membranes. Minor basement membrane changes, usually in the form of thickening or irregularities, are often evident. Capillary wall deposits are seldom found.[1, 1025]

*Immunofluorescence.* A frequent although not invariable finding in this disorder is the presence of IgM deposits, primarily in the mesangium but also occasionally as small granularities, in the capillary walls[1] (Fig. 30–15). This feature has led some to use the more descriptive term "IgM mesangial nephropathy."* The true pathogenetic role of such deposits is disputed.[880, 881, 1027–1029, 1031, 1032] Some investigators believe the IgM deposits to be a nonspecific manifestation of altered mesangial function,[1, 1033] whereas others believe that these deposits are involved in some way in the initiation of the disease process.[1, 1031, 1032, 1034–1037] In many instances, C3 has been observed in a similar distribution, although not in all cases.[1, 865] IgG and IgA are variably present and usually with a lesser intensity than IgM and C3.[1, 865, 1038] By definition, predominant IgA deposits result in categorization as Berger disease (see earlier). In several series, the immunofluorescence findings have been reported

*References 1, 865, 866, 883, 1021, 1022, 1028–1030.

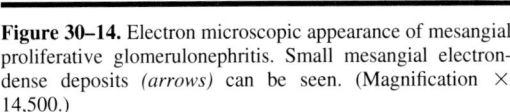

**Figure 30–14.** Electron microscopic appearance of mesangial proliferative glomerulonephritis. Small mesangial electron-dense deposits *(arrows)* can be seen. (Magnification × 14,500.)

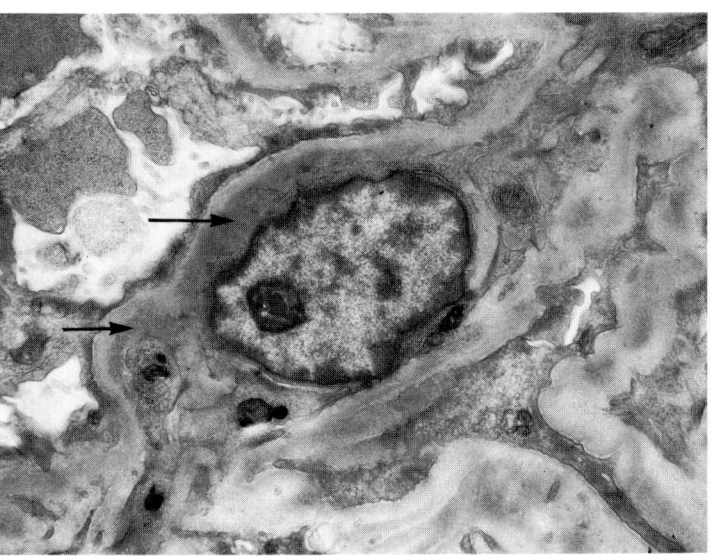

as negative for immunoglobulin deposits in most cases.[1, 1017] One view of this group would be to assume that they represent instances of minimal-change disease with more prominent mesangial cell hypercellularity, but this is controversial.[1038, 1039] IgM deposits in mesangium may also be seen in steroid-responsive minimal-change disease (see earlier), calling into question the clinical significance of IgM mesangial deposits.[1, 881] Familial cases with prominent IgM deposits with a common HLA haplotype have been described.[1030] On occasion, only diffuse mesangial C1q, C3, or C4 deposits may be found[1040] (see also C1q nephropathy later). Isolated C3 deposition is suggestive of resolving acute postinfectious glomerulonephritis; C4 deposition may be associated with decreased C4 levels and the presence of a null allele at the *C4B* locus.[1024] C1q deposits are more often found in conjunction with IgG or IgM deposition. This lesion, often designated C1q nephropathy, may present with recurrent hematuria, abnormal proteinuria, and the nephrotic syndrome.[1041, 1042] These patients lack the usual features of SLE, but renal lesions have similarities to mesangial proliferative glomerulonephritis observed in SLE[1041] (see C1q nephropathy later). Spontaneous remissions can occur.

**Pathogenesis.** The pathogenesis of this lesion is unknown. In view of the variable immunofluorescence findings, the lesion may be the consequence of a number of underlying mechanisms. Diffuse granular IgM and C3 deposits in mesangium and circulating immune complexes suggest an immune complex disease in some cases, but the antigen is unknown.[1, 813]

**Course and Therapy.** The long-term evolution of this lesion is not well understood. Because of the relative infrequency of the lesion, no randomized, controlled trials of therapy have been conducted. It seems clear that progression to renal failure does occur in some patients, usually in association with failure to respond to glucocorticoids and the development of superimposed focal and segmental sclerosis.[1, 1037] A variable percentage (50% or more) of patients will have a complete remission of proteinuria after glucocorticoid therapy. The finding of hematuria may predict a poorer response to steroids. Steroid responders usually represent those with only mild mesangial proliferation uncomplicated by focal and segmental lesions.[1, 882, 1027, 1035] Whether the steroid responder represents a variant of minimal-change lesions with more prominent mesangial hypercellularity or a different entity is a matter of dispute. Nonetheless, patients who do respond to steroids with complete or partial remission have a more favorable prognosis.[1, 882, 883, 1017] Spontaneous remissions and multiple relapses have also been described.[1, 1033]

The role of adjunctive cytotoxic drug therapy (e.g., cyclophosphamide, chlorambucil, or azathioprine) is also not well understood.[1] Several uncontrolled studies have noted beneficial effects in steroid-unresponsive or partially responsive patients.[1, 1017, 1019, 1043] Tejani and co-workers[933, 1028] found a 58% response rate in patients with steroid-sensitive, frequently relapsing IgM nephropathy. The response rate of steroid-unresponsive patients is much less. Controlled clinical trials of patients with lesions believed to be mesangial proliferative have come to different conclusions.[1] Some studies have suggested a beneficial effect of long-term indomethacin therapy.[1043]

In summary, a therapeutic trial of steroids similar to that employed in the treatment of minimal-change lesions might be tried in patients with mesangial proliferative glomerulonephritis, especially if extensive IgM or C3 deposits are absent and proliferation is mild. In the absence of a steroid response, the optimal therapy is uncertain at best, but some have used cytotoxic agents or indomethacin with some success.

The clinical and pathologic similarities of mesangial proliferative glomerulonephritis and minimal-change disease and the observations by serial biopsy that one may evolve from the other have led Habib and colleagues to propose that the two are part of the same disease process, both of which may be complicated by superimposition of focal and segmental sclerosing lesions as the disease progresses.[1, 813] This unifying hypothesis has virtue but cannot, of course, be proved by morphologic studies alone. In the experience of Waldherr and colleagues,[1, 1017] more than 50% of patients with definite mesangial proliferative glomerulonephritis have a protracted, steroid-unresponsive course, and as many as 70% have superimposed focal and segmental glomerular sclerosis on initial or follow-up biopsies,[1017] which portends a poor prognosis (see next section and Table 30–6). Such patients also seem to have a higher frequency of recurrent disease in renal allografts,[1044] which may be as high as 40% to 60% (see also Chapter 31).

## FOCAL GLOMERULAR SCLEROSIS

Arnold Rich[870] in 1957 described what appeared to be at that time a new pathologic finding in an autopsy study of 20 patients presumed on clinical grounds to have idiopathic nephrotic syndrome due to minimal-change lesions. Focal and segmental sclerosing lesions of glomeruli, particularly involving the deeper juxtamedullary zones of the cortex, were found. Nine of the 20 patients died of uremia, and hypertension was present in more than 50%. Later, McGovern,[1045] Habib and Gubler,[1046] and other authors pointed out the frequency of this lesion in idiopathic nephrotic syndrome of children and adults.[1] The poor response to therapy and the progressive loss of renal function found in association with this lesion have been repeatedly emphasized.[1, 1047–1052] Some investigators have regarded this lesion as a nonspecific feature superimposed on other fundamental lesions, such as minimal-change lesion or mesangial proliferative glomerulonephritis[1, 813, 1053, 1054]; others have regarded it as a discrete clinicopathologic entity, especially when it is found fully developed in initial renal biopsy specimens taken from patients with otherwise idiopathic nephrotic syndrome.[1] In the absence of knowledge regarding etiology and pathogenesis, it is impossible to be certain which view is the correct one.

Idiopathic focal glomerular sclerosing lesions may be viewed as consisting of three distinct subcategories based on the histopathologic characteristics of glomeruli and the distribution of the sclerosing lesions: 1) focal and segmental glomerular sclerosis and hyalinosis superimposed on minimal-change lesions (FSSH/MCL); this category may be further subdivided into a group based on the site or sites of sclerosis within affected glomeruli and another group characterized by concomitant presence of glomerular enlargement[868, 1056, 1057]; 2) focal and segmental sclerosis and hyalinosis superimposed on mesangial proliferative glomerulonephritis (FSSH/MesPGN); and 3) focal and global glomerular sclerosis representing a further progression of 1 or 2 or secondary to underlying vascular disease in the presence of minimal-change lesions.[1, 1055–1058] Focal and segmental glomerular sclerosis may also arise secondary to a wide variety of other glomerular and multisystem disorders (Table 30–12). These other lesions are associated with infections, drugs and medications, reduced renal mass, or processes that directly damage epithelial cells or induce hemodynamic alterations favoring glomerular sclerosis.[1058] In some patients, the glomerular sclerosis is the consequence of a previous proliferative or necrotizing lesion.

**Clinical Features.** Overall, focal glomerular sclerosis is found in about 7% to 15% of children and 15% to 20% of adults with idiopathic nephrotic syndrome. With few exceptions, most series have noted a male preponderance.[1, 1047–1054] Black patients are at increased risk for development of this lesion and may have a worse prognosis. In Cameron's clinic, where patients of all ages are seen, the mean age at onset was 21 years, and 60% of the patients older than 15 years presented with nephrotic syndrome before age 40 years.[1] In Habib's experience with children, about 60% of the cases were found in children younger than 5 years.[1] The nephrotic syndrome is the principal clinical manifestation, although in 10% to 30% of patients, only isolated mild proteinuria or proteinuria accompanied by hematuria and hypertension was found.[1] Gross hematuria is more likely to be seen in cases with prominent mesangial proliferation. Hypertension is relatively common, particularly if GFR is reduced.

On clinical grounds alone, it is difficult to separate this group of patients from those with uncomplicated minimal-change disease or mesangial proliferative glomerulonephritis.[1] There is no particular association with infection, although symptoms may be exacerbated by upper respiratory infections and immunizations. Some patients may present with what appears to be idiopathic disease and demonstrate chronic human immunodeficiency virus infection; the pathologic process in these cases is usually distinctive (see Chapter 31). Asymptomatic persistent proteinuria may be present for long periods before overt nephrotic syndrome develops.[1] Among cases with focal and segmental sclerosing lesions found on initial biopsy, the nephrotic syndrome tends to persist and is regarded as being steroid resistant in the majority of cases (see later). Similar lesions may also be encountered late in the course of an otherwise steroid-responsive, frequently relapsing category of nephrotic syndrome in which early biopsies revealed only minimal-change lesions. Thus, in Habib's experience with children in whom biopsies were performed at various intervals, 34 of 98 cases revealing focal glomerular sclerosing lesions followed a clinical course characterized by exacerbations and remissions.[1, 813] Focal glomerular sclerosing lesions are found frequently in nephrotic syndrome that occurs with familial aggregation, although minimal-change lesions may show familial occurrence as well.[1, 1059–1064] Friedman, Rao, and others[1065–1068] have emphasized the frequency of this lesion in heroin addicts with nephrotic syndrome, particularly among black persons (see later), although a wide variety of glomerular lesions may be encountered in this group of patients (see Chapter 31). The lesion seems to be relatively common among patients with atopic manifestations and renal disease.[1069]

**Laboratory Findings** (see Table 30–2). Urinary excretion rate of protein is nearly always abnormal. Proteinuria is typically nonselective, although some exceptions have been noted,[1] especially early in the course.[1070] Hematuria is common, especially if lesions are superimposed on mesangial proliferative glomerulonephritis.[1] C3 levels are nearly always normal, whereas IgG levels may be significantly depressed.[1] C1q levels may vary but are usually normal. Sterile pyuria, lymphocyturia, glycosuria, aminoaciduria, and phosphaturia may be found, and the occurrence of abnormalities of these tubule functions is more common than in other varieties of the nephrotic syndrome.[1, 1071] Circulating immune complexes may be found in 10% to 30% of cases.[859] Erythrocytosis may be present. As noted previously, a circulating vascular permeability factor may be present, particularly in patients who progress rapidly to end-stage renal disease.[816, 820, 900, 1072] Some groups have noted increased prevalence of HLA-DR4 and -DR8.[869, 1062, 1063]

**Pathology**

*Light Microscopy.* The light microscopic features that permit categorization as focal and segmental sclerosis are lesions affecting a variable minority of the glomeruli, often those in the deeper, juxtamedullary cortex.[1, 867–870, 1055–1058] The unaffected glomeruli may appear normal by light microscopy (FSSH/MCL) or reveal diffuse mesangial proliferation (FSSH/MesPGN).[1017] The individual glomerular lesion consists of a segmental sclerosis due to increased mesangial matrix and basement membrane[1, 869, 870, 1074] (Fig. 30–16). Evaluation of transplanted kidneys removed shortly after engraftment in instances of recurrent focal sclerosis has indicated that the majority of the affected glomeruli are

---

**TABLE 30–12. Classification of Focal and Segmental Glomerular Sclerosis**

**Primary (Idiopathic)**
Focal and segmental glomerular sclerosis with hyalinosis
 Superimposed on minimal-change lesion
 Superimposed on mesangial proliferative glomerulonephritis
 Glomerular tip lesion
 Collapsing glomerulopathy
 Superimposed on another primary glomerular lesion (e.g., IgA, nephropathy, MGN)

**Secondary**
Infectious: human immunodeficiency virus infection
Medication/drugs: heroin abuse, NSAID, analgesic abuse
Reduced renal mass: oligonephronia, unilateral renal agenesis, renal dysplasia, vesicoureteral reflux, cortical necrosis, surgical ablation, renal allograft
Normal renal mass: diabetes mellitus, hypertensive arteriolosclerosis, Alport syndrome, obesity, sickle-cell disease, von Gierke disease, cystinosis, sarcoidosis, cyanotic congenital heart disease, Galloway-Mowat syndrome malignant neoplasms, light and heavy chain disease, familial dysautonomia, radiation nephritis, Guillain-Barré syndrome
Consequent to postinflammatory/postnecrotic scarring: IgA nephropathy, SLE, vasculitis

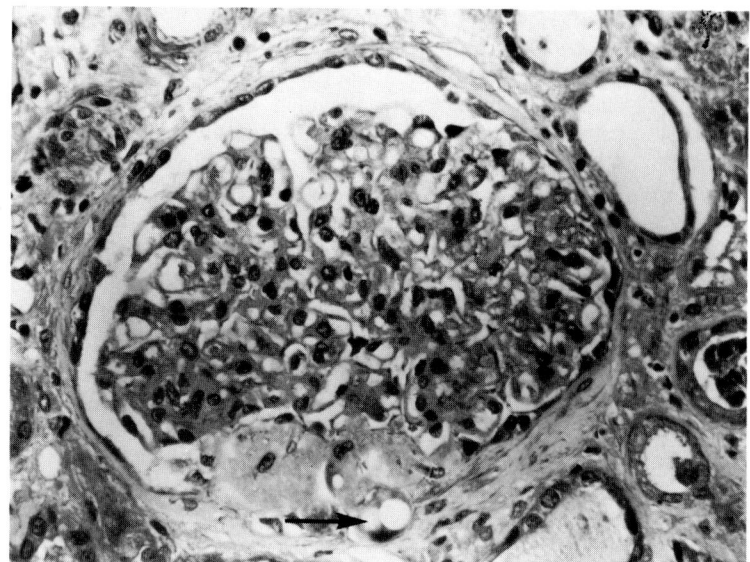

**Figure 30–16.** Light microscopic view of focal and segmental glomerular sclerosis. A localized segment of sclerosis, adherent to Bowman capsule, is evident at the 6 o'clock position. At its periphery is a large protein deposit (hyalinosis), within which are several large lipid vacuoles *(arrow)*. There is mild mesangial hypercellularity in the remainder of the tuft. (Masson trichrome; magnification × 900.)

in juxtamedullary locations.[1075] Hyaline material ("insudative lesion") is characteristically deposited in the subendothelial areas of affected loops and may occasionally contain lipid inclusions.[1] Occasional synechia and foamy (lipid-laden) histiocytes may be encountered in the sclerotic segment.[1]

Localized epithelial cell hypertrophy and hyperplasia frequently occur. The epithelial cells are often coarsely vacuolated and contain protein reabsorption droplets.[1, 874, 1076] On the other hand, early lesions may consist only of localized detachment of visceral epithelial cells from underlying basement membrane. A reasonably characteristic finding is the presence of a clear zone, or halo, overlying the sclerotic segment and between the basement membrane and the visceral epithelial cell.[1, 1076] The segmental lesions may begin either at the vascular pole (hilum) or at the tubule pole, which can eventually extend to any portion of the glomerular tuft.[1073] The extent of segmental lesions may vary from glomerulus to glomerulus; as the disorder progresses, a picture of global sclerosis may result.[1] Thus, advanced cases may often be regarded as "nonspecific" chronic sclerosing glomerulonephritis. Segmental crescentic lesions may also be seen.[1077] Immunofluorescence findings may be helpful in differentiating focal glomerular sclerosis from the capillary tuft collapse and fibrosis that accompany the later stages of a focal and segmental proliferative or necrotizing glomerulonephritis (see later).[1, 1078] Tubule changes are common, consisting of focal thickening of basement membrane and atrophy.[1, 1071] The finding of focal tubule changes in a biopsy specimen that otherwise demonstrates minimal glomerular changes should heighten the suspicion of the presence of an underlying superimposed focal glomerular sclerosis.[1, 869] Similar focal and segmental glomerular sclerosing lesions may also be seen in the late stages of a focal and segmental proliferative glomerulonephritis[1078] (e.g., IgA nephropathy) and in association with heroin abuse,[1066–1068] analgesic abuse, chronic allograft failure,[1079] vesicoureteral reflux,[1080] sarcoidosis,[1081] Alport syndrome, essential hypertension, sickle-cell disease,[1082] massive obesity,[1083] glycogen storage disease, cystinosis, Guillain-Barré syndrome,[1084]

x-irradiation or gamma irradiation,[1085] neoplasia, and human immunodeficiency virus infection (see Chapter 31).[1058, 1086] They can be superimposed on many other primary glomerular diseases, such as IgA or membranous glomerulopathy (see Table 30–12), and can occur consequent to a severe reduction in nephron mass[1058, 1087–1089] and as a part of "chronic allograft rejection."

The occurrence of focal and global glomerular sclerosis (i.e., the focal distribution of complete glomerular obsolescence) is regarded as a variant of the minimal-change lesion or a late stage of focal glomerular sclerosis.[1, 1046] This lesion is usually accompanied by significant degrees of interstitial and tubule damage and, in Habib's experience, accounts for about 30% of pediatric cases categorized as focal glomerular sclerosis.[1, 1046] Focal and global glomerular sclerosis may also be seen in Drash syndrome (Wilms tumor and pseudohermaphroditism) (see Chapter 31). A few globally sclerotic glomeruli may be seen in adults with otherwise typical steroid-responsive minimal-change lesions.

Weiss and colleagues[1090] described a group of patients with nephrotic syndrome and progressive renal failure whose glomeruli exhibited what appeared to be an aggressive form of segmental glomerular sclerosis. Most glomeruli were involved with an exaggerated early lesion with extensive capillary collapse and extensive visceral epithelial cell hypertrophy and hyperplasia.[1090, 1091] This variant is known as "collapsing glomerulopathy" and is seen most often in black persons and in males. This disorder is commonly associated with heavy proteinuria (more than 70% of patients have more than 10 g/d protein excretion) and a progressive course (more than 50% of patients have end-stage renal disease by 2 years after diagnosis).[1091]

Howie and colleagues[1092–1095] have described what they termed the glomerular tip lesion, an evolving form of segmental glomerular sclerosis in which the tubule pole of the capillary tufts (tip) is involved.[1055–1057] This form of injury can affect virtually all glomeruli. Some but not all studies have found that the proteinuria in these patients is steroid responsive.[1057, 1095] They have also described the lesion in other glomerulopathies.[1092, 1095] Others have found that a better prognosis correlates with segmental sclerosis of the tubule pole rather than the vascular pole.[1096, 1097]

***Electron Microscopy.*** By electron microscopy, most or all glomeruli show diffuse or segmental foot process alterations, especially if heavy proteinuria is present. Extensive foot process effacement is more likely to be seen in the idiopathic lesion. Diffuse mesangial cell hyperplasia may also be observed.[1, 1017] Extensive mesangiolysis may be found to underlie the sclerotic lesion. Ballooning of the capillary wall and microaneurysms are commonly observed in this circumstance.[1055, 1057] Extensive capillary microaneurysms are also seen in diabetic glomerulosclerosis and in light and heavy chain glomerulopathies (Randall type) (see also Chapter 31). Those glomeruli that are abnormal by light microscopy reflect the genesis of the lesions. In the early stages, intracapillary or mesangial foam cells are observed, usually concomitant with or followed by increase in mesangial matrix and segmental capillary collapse. The foam cells, often located in these abnormal segments, undergo degeneration and disintegrate; their cytoplasmic debris becomes incorporated, along with gradually increasing electron-dense deposits, within concavities of occluded capillaries, surrounded by peripheral basement membranes that are adherent to Bowman capsule (Fig. 30–17). These large deposits are the ultrastructural counterpart of the "hyalinosis" of light microscopy and of the IgM and C3 deposits demonstrated by immunofluorescence microscopy.[1] Paramesangial and subendothelial finely granular electron-dense deposits are also seen. The epithelial cells of capillaries of either involved or noninvolved glomeruli undergo degeneration, with subsequent denudation of the basement membranes, and reparative changes.[1, 877] Vacuolization is often a prominent finding.[873, 874] These abnormalities include the incorporation of cellular debris and newly formed thin basement membranes between the overlying epithelial cell, which had presumably migrated to the damaged area, and the original capillary basement membrane. This finding is most likely the explanation for the halo over the sclerotic segment frequently observed in light microscopic prepara-

tions[1] (see Figs. 30–16 and 30–17). However, the degenerative changes of the podocytes are not limited to focal glomerular sclerosis but are common to many glomerulopathies associated with heavy proteinuria.[1] Extensive hyperplasia of the visceral epithelial cell is seen in the collapsing variant.[1091]

***Immunofluorescence.*** IgM, C1q, and C3 deposition may be seen in an irregular, granular, or nodular distribution in association with the focal sclerotic lesions seen by light microscopy[1, 813] (Fig. 30–18). Unaffected glomeruli are usually negative but on occasion may contain variable amounts of IgM and C3 in a mesangial distribution[1, 813, 1098] or rarely in a segmental capillary wall distribution.[1098] In vitro complement fixation is positive.[1] IgG and IgA deposition is less common. Reabsorption droplets of albumin may be seen in a few but not all tubules and also in some but not all glomerular visceral epithelial cells. Linear IgG deposits with C3 have been found in a small group of patients, most of whom were heroin addicts.[1] Circulating anti-GBM antibodies were not found, and the pathogenetic importance of the linear deposits of IgG is unknown but probably related to nonimmunologic factors. Diffuse mesangial IgA deposits suggest that the focal and segmental sclerosing lesions in fact represent the scarred residue of IgA nephropathy. HLA-DR and intercellular adhesion molecule-1 expression is increased in tubule cells. CD8+ lymphocytes may be seen in the glomeruli, and CD4+ lymphocytes may be seen in the tubulointerstitial areas.[1099]

***Pathogenesis.*** The pathogenesis of this disorder is unknown. The mesangial deposition of IgM and C3 in a granular pattern suggests an immune complex disease. It is also possible that a primary disorder of the capillary tuft leads to nonspecific trapping of IgM with subsequent binding of C1q and C3. It has been suggested that the occurrence of segmental areas of platelet deposition and fibrin polymers in certain patients with minimal-change lesions provides an explanation of how focal glomerular sclerosis could develop on a substrate of minimal-change lesions.[1] Lesions resembling focal glomerular sclerosis may be

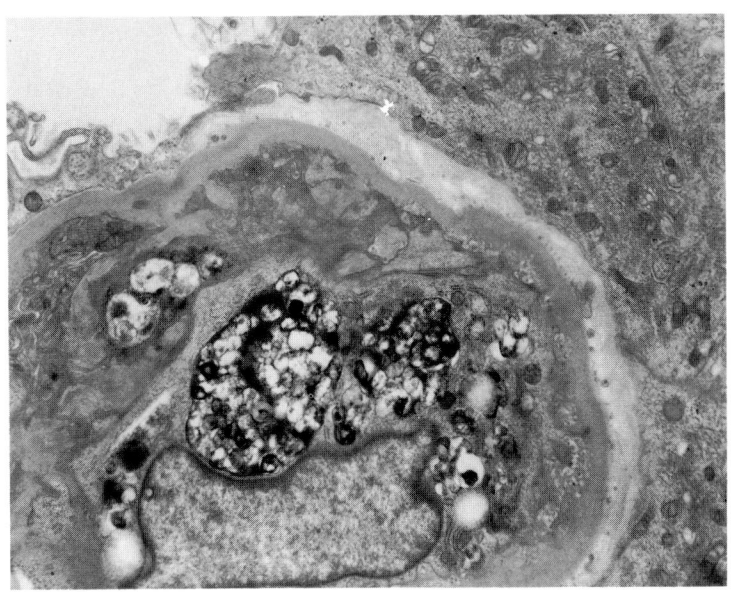

**Figure 30–17.** Electron microscopic appearance of focal and segmental glomerular sclerosis. A portion of glomerulus with segmental sclerosis is shown. The lumen is obliterated by a cell with large, lipid-containing lysosomes; the visceral epithelial cell is separated from the basement membrane by a lucent zone that includes cytoplasmic debris and thin layers of basement membrane material. (Magnification × 12,250.)

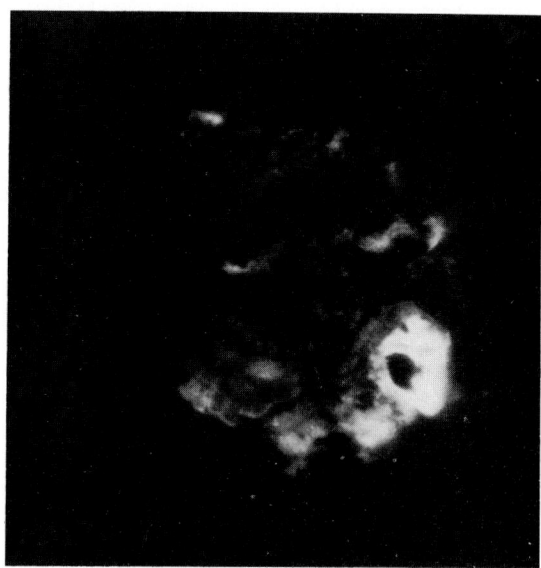

**Figure 30–18.** Immunofluorescence view of focal and segmental glomerular sclerosis showing segmental and peripheral localization of IgM, corresponding to hyalinosis. There is a small amount of mesangial staining as well. (Antihuman IgM; magnification × 950.)

found in aging rats and humans and after persistent proteinuria induced by aminonucleoside of puromycin or doxorubicin.[1100–1103] The occurrence of similar lesions in animals subjected to continuous "overload" proteinuria by infusion of heterologous albumin[1104] indicates that focal glomerular sclerosis may be the consequence and not the cause of proteinuria.[1103, 1105–1107, 1107a] The mesangium may also be affected as shown by reduction in the net negative charge of mesangial matrix.[1108] The extent of the epithelial lesions, including localized necrosis and detachment of cells and foot processes, also suggests that focal glomerular sclerosis is a manifestation of a reparative process indicative of severe epithelial cell injury.[1, 1103] Rapid recurrence of lesions in renal allografts clearly implicates a systemic factor in the pathogenesis of this lesion.[1109–1116] Preliminary studies have suggested the presence of a nonimmunoglobulin factor that induces altered glomerular permselectivity.[816, 820, 1058, 1072]

The development of similar lesions in the remnant kidney after subtotal nephrectomy has suggested that focal glomerular sclerosis may be the result of a hemodynamic alteration in residual nephrons (see Chapter 44). Compensatory capillary hypertension resulting from loss of nephron mass may induce epithelial and endothelial cell injury and mesangial dysfunction and may lead to progressive focal and segmental sclerotic lesions.[1086–1089, 1117–1120] Protein feeding aggravates and protein restriction and antihypertensive therapy impede the development of these lesions (see also Chapter 44). Disordered lipid metabolism due to urinary loss of enzymes (lecithin–cholesterol acyltransferase) has also been suggested to play a role in epithelial cell injury and glomerular sclerosis.[679, 1121–1123] Altered T cell function may also play a role.[1124] Enhanced intraglomerular coagulation could participate in the evolution of the segmental sclerotic lesions.[1125, 1126] Mesangial injury with mesangiolysis may play a role in the evolution of the lesion in some circumstances. Growth factors (such as transforming

growth factor-β and platelet-derived growth factor) and other cytokines undoubtedly participate in the evolution of the lesions.[1020, 1119, 1127, 1128]

It is difficult to imagine how light microscopic and clinical studies alone will answer this challenging question, because the focal nature of the process introduces a serious problem of sampling error, especially in the case of superficial needle or open renal biopsies.

**Course and Therapy.** A proportion of patients with nephrotic syndrome in whom renal biopsies performed early in the course of disease reveal focal and segmental glomerular sclerosis superimposed on either minimal-change disease or mesangial proliferative glomerulonephritis demonstrate a progressive decline in GFR, the development of hypertension, and persistent proteinuria unresponsive to treatment.[1, 1047, 1048, 1129–1131] In an extensive retrospective review of 75 children with nephrotic syndrome and focal and segmental glomerular sclerosis, after an average follow-up of 57 months, end-stage renal failure had developed in 21%, reduced GFR was noted in 23%, and persisting nephrotic syndrome with normal renal function was observed in 31%. Only 11% of the patients had a complete remission. None of the morphologic or immunohistologic features in this series was predictive of outcome.[1130] Others have noted adverse outcome with severe mesangial proliferation, arteriosclerosis, hilar glomerulosclerosis, and interstitial fibrosis.[1017, 1049, 1052, 1131, 1132] Korbet and co-workers,[1052] in another retrospective review of mostly adults, found a cumulative 10-year renal survival of 25% to 55% when nephrotic syndrome was present, compared with an 85% to 90% 10-year renal survival when nephrotic syndrome was absent. If protein excretion consistently exceeded 14 g/d, all patients had entered end-stage renal failure by 6 years of follow-up. Black patients fared much worse than whites. Most instances of end-stage renal disease developed within the first 15 years of follow-up. Persisting hypertension, older age at onset, male sex, and initially abnormal GFR also portended a progressive course. In patients with onset in the pediatric age group, the 20-year renal survival approximated 60%, whereas in the adult-onset disorder, the 20-year renal survival was usually less than 40%.[1052] Patients who are initially discovered with asymptomatic proteinuria may ultimately have frank nephrotic syndrome. Spontaneous remissions and exacerbations of both isolated proteinuria and the nephrotic syndrome may occur, although this is relatively uncommon except in children.[1, 1052]

Three general patterns of evolution are observed with respect to glucocorticoid therapy. A lasting remission of proteinuria and freedom from later progressive renal failure are seen in 20% to 35%, a relapsing and remitting course with late-onset renal failure is seen in 10% to 15%, and a glucocorticoid-unresponsive pattern with progressive renal failure is seen in 50% to 70%.[1049, 1052, 1130] The prognosis may be better when lesions are found late in the course of disease, especially in children with steroid-responsive, frequently relapsing nephrotic syndrome,[1129] although this has not been universally observed.[1130]

The prognosis is also greatly influenced by the severity of proteinuria. Persisting nephrotic proteinuria was associated with a 10-year survival of only 45%, whereas persisting non-nephrotic proteinuria had a 10-year survival of more than 90%.[1047, 1133] Certain patients may exhibit profuse proteinuria (>10 g/d) and severe hyperlipidemia and have a rapidly progressive decline in renal function,[1048, 1134] especially in association with collapsing lesions.[1091] Brown and co-workers[1048] have referred to this condition as malignant focal sclerosis. Thus, failure to respond to steroids and to have a clinical remission spontaneously is associated with a poor prognosis.[813, 1050–1052] Among the pediatric patients described by Habib and co-workers[813] with global sclerosis of glomeruli, there was a tendency for longer survival and for the occurrence of only transient episodes of nephrotic syndrome. The recurrence of nephrotic syndrome and a focal glomerular sclerosis in the transplanted kidney has been documented and may be as high as 40%. Patients with profuse proteinuria, a rapid course to renal failure, and mesangial proliferative lesions appear to be at the greatest risk for recurrence.[1113, 1115] Pregnant patients with FSSH and impaired renal function do poorly, with a high prevalence of toxemia and renal functional deterioration.[1135]

Relatively few controlled studies of treatment are available in patients displaying fully developed FSSH/MCL or FSSH/MesPGN in early biopsies. In an extensive review, Korbet and co-workers[1052] found that glucocorticoid therapy alone (in varying doses and duration) was associated with a complete remission in 25% and a partial remission in 3% of children. In adults, glucocorticoids alone were associated with a 52% complete remission and a 10% partial remission rate. Banfi and colleagues[1136] found a 60% complete remission rate in adults treated with more prolonged courses of glucocorticoids (averaging about 9 months).[942] Somewhat higher remission rates have been achieved in children by Mendoza and associates[940] with use of an aggressive therapeutic regimen involving prolonged treatment with intravenous methylprednisolone commonly accompanied by oral cyclophosphamide. Preliminary results of a controlled study conducted by the Cooperative Study of Adult Glomerular Disease have shown a tendency for a greater frequency of complete or partial remissions and protection from progressive renal failure in a group treated with alternate-day prednisone compared with placebo (Coggins CH, personal communication, 1976). Patients with the late development of these lesions on a background of minimal-change lesions may remain steroid responsive, but those who have focal glomerular sclerosis superimposed on mesangial proliferative glomerulonephritis usually do poorly.[1017, 1018] These and other studies suggest that focal sclerosis is a partially steroid-responsive lesion but requires more prolonged treatment or higher doses or both in comparison to minimal-change disease for maximal beneficial effects to be achieved.[941, 942, 1137] As many as 60% to 75% of patients can be induced into a complete or partial remission, if one is willing to accept the hazards of more prolonged, high-dose glucocorticoid therapy. Although no minimally effective duration of therapy has been established, and it probably varies widely from patient to patient, 4 to 6 months of glucocorticoid therapy has been recommended.[942] Therapy is usually initiated with daily glucocorticoids followed by conversion to an alternate-day regimen.

The results of treatment with cytotoxic drugs in both controlled and uncontrolled studies have also been inconsis-

tent and difficult to evaluate.[942, 987, 1138] However, the development of a partial remission after combined glucocorticoid and cyclophosphamide therapy (2.0 to 2.5 mg/kg/d for 10 to 12 weeks) may afford significant protection from end-stage renal disease.[942] About 50% of patients with apparent steroid-unresponsive FSSH who receive cyclophosphamide experience some reduction in proteinuria.[942, 1138] Cyclophosphamide therapy appears to be of value in the frequently relapsing steroid-dependent varieties of FSSH, although this has not been tested in a rigorously designed prospective trial. Intensive therapy with intravenous methylprednisolone and oral cyclophosphamide may result in lasting remissions in a portion of patients with steroid-resistant nephrotic syndrome secondary to FSSH.[940, 1139]

Cyclosporine in doses of 4 to 5.5 mg/kg/d may be of value in the treatment of FSSH, especially in steroid-responsive or steroid-dependent forms.* Approximately 90% of children and 50% to 60% of adults with steroid-dependent or frequently relapsing forms of FSSH respond initially to a course of cyclosporine with a complete remission.[1002] Unfortunately, steroid-resistant patients do not do as well; only 40% of children and only 15% to 20% of adults manifest a complete remission after treatment with cyclosporine.[1002] However, many patients (approximately 40%) do experience a modest decrease in proteinuria to subnephrotic levels.[1002–1006] If lowered protein excretion places the patient at a lower risk for subsequent renal failure, then therapy with cyclosporine may be worthwhile even in the absence of complete remission. Patients with FSSH and impaired GFR or extensive chronic tubulointerstitial lesions before initiation of therapy do poorly with cyclosporine treatment, manifest a low response rate, and are at high risk for nephrotoxic effects. Therefore, if cyclosporine is to be used in the treatment of FSSH, it should be limited to patients with steroid-dependent or frequently relapsing steroid-responsive disease who also have normal or nearly normal values of renal function and whose biopsy samples do not display significant chronic tubulointerstitial lesions.[1002–1006] The dose of cyclosporine should not exceed 5.5 mg/kg/d, and patients who fail to respond within 4 months should not be treated for longer periods.[1004] More prolonged treatment of cyclosporine-responsive patients with low maintenance doses may be beneficial, but repeated biopsies may be required to assess ongoing nephrotoxic effects of cyclosporine.[1009] Not infrequently, such biopsies may reveal progression of glomerular sclerosis despite improved urinary protein excretion rates.[1008]

The addition of anticoagulants and inhibitors of platelet aggregation to a regimen of steroids and cytotoxic agents has shown promising results in preliminary trials, but further long-term observations in larger numbers of patients are required before this therapeutic approach can be widely recommended. Dipyridamole treatment alone has been noted to reduce the magnitude of proteinuria.[1141] A preliminary trial using carefully titrated doses of meclofenamate (an NSAID) has been encouraging.[1142, 1143] Such therapy seems to reduce protein excretion and result in stabilization of renal function. Carefully monitored controlled trials of this drug or other NSAIDs seem warranted.[1143, 1144] Quino-

_____

*References 941, 942, 1002, 1004–1006, 1008, 1140.

lone antibiotics are ineffective and may have adverse side effects.[1014a] ACE inhibitors reduce protein excretion rates by 40% to 60% in the majority of patients with FSSH.[941, 942, 1011, 1012] A similar reduction in protein excretion rate is seen in patients with other glomerular diseases, especially if combined with modest sodium chloride dietary restriction.[584, 626, 1011, 1012] The mechanism of this effect is not fully understood but is probably in part related to changes in renal hemodynamics, including a decrease in transglomerular hydraulic pressure gradients. Because glomerular capillary hypertension and proteinuria may both contribute to progressive glomerular disease, it is reasonable to hope that therapy with ACE inhibitors will offer significant benefits in terms of reducing the rate of progression. Because systemic arterial blood pressure also declines, the effect may not necessarily be an ACE inhibitor–specific event; rather, it may be related to the overall reduction in arterial blood pressure.[622] In addition, ACE inhibitors may affect other angiotensin-dependent events, such as transforming growth factor-β–driven increases in extracellular matrix accumulation. Furthermore, the improvement in glomerular permselectivity could also translate into a reduction of tubulointerstitial or visceral epithelial injury.[1107, 1107a] Therefore, there is good reason to believe that long-term administration of ACE inhibitors will be of benefit to patients with FSSH who manifest continued heavy proteinuria, hypertension, or progressive renal failure. Prospective controlled randomized trials are under way to test this hypothesis. Modest dietary protein restriction combined with ACE inhibitor therapy could also be of value, especially if malnutrition can be avoided and the magnitude of proteinuria is decreased (see also Chapter 44).

As mentioned before, patients with FSSH are at high risk for recurrent disease in renal allografts.[1113, 1115] Approximately 30% to 40% of patients with FSSH will have a recurrence of disease in the renal allograft.[1113] This risk rises to approximately 80% in secondary grafts if the first graft was lost to recurrent disease.[1113, 1115] Plasma exchange or protein A absorption reduces proteinuria, perhaps by removal of a putative nonimmunoglobulin permeability factor.[816, 820, 1112, 1115, 1116] Responses to these forms of therapy are often short lived.[1115, 1116] NSAIDs and ACE inhibitors may prolong the antiproteinuric effect of plasma exchange.[1142, 1143] Patients with recurrent disease also have a greater risk of rejection and transplant loss.[1114] This could be due to the effect of hyperlipidemia on cyclosporine metabolism.[1010] LDL apheresis or plasma exchange may also have beneficial effects on proteinuria in the native kidney disease, which suggests that lipids may contribute additionally to altered permselectivity.[1145] Significant questions remain to be answered concerning the possible role of prophylactic plasma exchange or immunoabsorption in patients with FSSH undergoing renal transplantation. Whether much higher doses of oral cyclosporine will lower the risk of recurrent disease is presently unknown. The risk of recurrent disease does not seem to be substantially different in the cyclosporine era than it was in the azathioprine era.[1114–1116]

In summary, an initial renal biopsy in a patient with nephrotic syndrome that reveals well-developed FSSH is a relatively ominous prognostic finding. However, despite the likelihood of steroid unresponsiveness, a trial of glucocorticoids, with more prolonged versions of regimens used for minimal-change disease, is probably indicated because a pronounced reduction of proteinuria or a complete remission improves the prognosis. The therapy of the steroid-unresponsive or partially steroid-responsive patient is a problem. Cyclophosphamide or cyclosporine could be tried, but the data presently available make it difficult to determine whether such approaches are of great value in the long term. Nevertheless, if no contraindication exists (such as impaired renal function or significant tubulointerstitial lesions on renal biopsy), a trial of cyclosporine therapy, not longer than 4 months, is probably worthwhile. Some completely steroid-unresponsive patients progress relentlessly despite vigorous attempts at therapy. The partially steroid-responsive or steroid-dependent patient would appear to be a better candidate for adjunctive therapy with cyclophosphamide or cyclosporine. ACE inhibitor therapy is probably indicated in most patients with persistent proteinuria, especially in the presence of systemic arterial hypertension.

## MEMBRANOUS GLOMERULONEPHRITIS (Membranous Nephropathy)

The term idiopathic MGN refers to a distinctive clinicopathologic entity commonly associated with the nephrotic syndrome, appearing in the absence of systemic disease or known precipitating factors.[1, 1146, 1147] The membranous designation refers to the characteristic diffuse thickening of the capillary wall, originally thought to be the consequence of increased basement membrane material. The synonyms for this disorder (epimembranous, perimembranous, or extramembranous glomerulonephritis) emphasize the occurrence of immune complex deposits in a subepithelial location adjacent to the GBM proper.[1, 1146] Although this disorder is operationally defined by the exclusion of known infections, neoplasia, drug exposure, or multisystem disease processes, in practice this may prove to be extraordinarily difficult to accomplish. It is abundantly clear that some cases of so-called idiopathic MGN in fact represent cases due to some underlying disease (especially hepatitis B virus infection, neoplasia, or SLE) that has not yet expressed itself in a readily identifiable form.[1, 1148–1164] A listing of the diseases that can evoke a lesion similar or identical to idiopathic MGN is given in Table 30–13.[1, 13, 615, 1086–1164]

**Clinical Features.** Although idiopathic MGN may occur at any age, it is unusual in children and adolescents, and about 80% to 95% of patients are older than 30 years at the time of diagnosis.[1, 1146, 1147] The peak occurrence is in the fifth decade.[1] In most series in adults, there has been a male preponderance.[1, 1146, 1147] Among adults with the idiopathic nephrotic syndrome, MGN is a commonly encountered lesion, accounting for 25% to 30% of all cases.[1, 16, 1146] Among patients older than 50 years with idiopathic nephrotic syndrome, 35% to 40% have an underlying MGN.[1, 16, 1146]

The clinical presentation is less varied than in many of the glomerulopathies in that the majority (in excess of 80%) have heavy proteinuria and other features of the nephrotic syndrome and the remainder present with symptomless proteinuria with or without hematuria.[1, 16, 1146] The onset is

**TABLE 30–13. Membranous Glomerulonephritis: Classification of Possible Etiologic Factors**

**Primary (Idiopathic)**

**Secondary to an Underlying Disease**
Infectious: hepatitis B,* hepatitis C, malaria, syphilis (congenital and secondary), leprosy, schistosomiasis, filariasis, PSGN (rare), hydatid disease
Multisystem: SLE,* mixed connective tissue disease, rheumatoid arthritis, Sjögren syndrome, dermatomyositis, sarcoidosis, graft-versus-host disease, Crohn disease, ankylosing spondylitis
Neoplastic: carcinoma* (lung, colon, stomach, breast, other), lymphoma, leukemia (rare)
Medications: organic gold,* mercury* (organic, inorganic, elemental),* D-penicillamine,* trimethadione, probenecid, captopril, ketoprofen, fenoprofen
Heredofamilial and metabolic: sickle-cell disease, thyroiditis, diabetes (?)
Miscellaneous: de novo in renal allografts,* Gardner-Diamond syndrome, bullous pemphigoid, Fanconi syndrome, Kimura disease, Weber-Christian syndrome, urticarial vasculitis, Castleman disease

*These diseases account for about 75% of the secondary forms of membranous glomerulonephritis. See Chapter 31 for detailed discussion of secondary forms.

usually insidious and without antecedent upper respiratory infection. Hypertension and azotemia occur late in the course of the disease. Chemical or overt diabetes mellitus appears to be more common than might be expected by chance alone in such patients.[1160, 1161] This may be related to a common underlying HLA phenotype related to susceptibility to both diabetes mellitus and MGN (see later). A neoplastic process, usually a carcinoma, may be found in 4% to 11% of patients with MGN and in as many as 20% of patients older than 60 years with MGN.[1086, 1148, 1164] Most often, the neoplasia is overt or is readily diagnosed at the time of onset of the nephrotic syndrome, but in one third to three quarters of cases, it is occult at the time of discovery of the nephrotic syndrome.[1086, 1148, 1163, 1164] Most patients with MGN secondary to a malignant neoplasm are older than 50 years at the time of diagnosis.[1148] Thus, on occasion, MGN is regarded erroneously as idiopathic when initially diagnosed. Similarly, chronic hepatitis B infection may be present in occult form[1153] and MGN appearing as otherwise idiopathic nephrotic syndrome may be the initial manifestation of SLE[1150, 1151] (see Table 30–13 and Chapter 31). Rheumatoid arthritis may also be seen in patients with MGN or on exposure to a variety of drugs,[1146, 1148] particularly gold (see also Chapter 31). Pregnancy is generally tolerated well, although there is some increase in fetal wastage and nephrotic syndrome and renal function may worsen.[1166] As stated previously, renal vein thrombosis is commonly observed in patients with MGN.[790] The true prevalence is disputed, related to difficulties in securing a firm diagnosis, but is believed to be between 5% and 50%. The overall average prevalence is approximately 20%. The risk for development of renal vein thrombosis appears to be increased if the serum albumin concentration falls below 2 to 2.5 g/dL.[776, 1165]

**Laboratory Findings** (see Table 30–2). Proteinuria is nearly always present and is above 3.5 g/d in more than

80% of cases. At times, the proteinuria may be severe (>20 g/d). Most commonly, it is nonselective, but highly selective proteinuria may occur in as many as 20% of cases.[1, 1146] Increased excretion of the membrane attack complex neoantigen (C5b-C9) or C3dg may be indicative of MGN in an "active" stage. High levels of C5b-C9 in the urine are seen in patients with MGN who are presumably actively depositing or forming immune complexes in situ.[1167–1176] Activation of complement at the subepithelial site may play a role in altered glomerular permselectivity in MGN.[1168, 1171, 1175] Microscopic hematuria is common, whereas gross hematuria is rare.[1146] A heavy proteinuria may also nonspecifically increase C5b-C9 urinary excretion.[1176] Urinary excretion of platelet-activating factor can also be increased.[1177] The levels of C3 and other complement components are nearly always normal; reduced levels suggest a multisystem infectious or topical form of the disease, such as SLE[1146] (see later and Chapter 31). HLA-DR3 is found in 65% to 75% of white patients compared with 20% to 25% of control subjects.[1, 1178, 1180] The frequency of HLA-B8 is also increased.[1179–1182] The HLA haplotype *DR3, Bf\*F, B18,* or *DR3, BF\*S, B8* may be associated with a more progressive course.[1, 1180] Japanese patients show a strong association with HLA-DR2[1179, 1183, 1184] and -Dqw1.[1179] *C4A* null alleles are also found more frequently in MGN in whites.[1185] Circulating immune complex–like material has been described by some but not all investigators.[1, 859, 1186] Such material seems more likely to be present in cases with underlying renal vein thrombosis or in cases secondary to SLE, viral infection, or neoplasia.[1186] These immune complexes may be enriched with IgG4 low-avidity antibodies.[1187] Antinuclear antibody, rheumatoid factor, and anti-GBM antibody should not be present in uncomplicated, truly idiopathic cases. Cryoglobulinemia should suggest the presence of an underlying disorder, especially SLE or occult hepatitis B or hepatitis C[1188, 1189] (see also Chapter 31). Erythrocytosis may be present.[1190] Although acute or chronic, unilateral or bilateral renal vein thrombosis is frequently associated with a histologic picture of MGN, overwhelming evidence exists that renal vein thrombosis is a consequence of the glomerulopathy rather than its cause (see earlier).

**Pathology**

*Light Microscopy.* The typical and characteristic light microscopic feature of well-developed MGN is a diffuse and uniform thickening of the capillary wall, usually without any significant proliferation of endothelial, mesangial, or epithelial cells[1, 1146, 1147] (Fig. 30–19). Mild to moderate mesangial cell proliferation, especially when accompanied by parietal epithelial cell abnormalities[1191] and coexistent FSSH,[1192, 1192a] may indicate a worse prognosis. The capillary lumens are widely patent in early stages. Silver impregnation techniques may reveal the presence of "spikes" of argyrophilic material projecting outward toward the urinary space[1, 1146, 1147] (see Fig. 30–19). These have been shown to consist of laminin and the α3- and α4-chains of type IV collagen but not the α1- or α2-chains of type IV collagen.[1193–1195] Such spike-like transformation may also occasionally be seen in glomerular amyloidosis (see Chapter 31). The space between the spikes has a negative periodic acid–Schiff (PAS) reaction, is weakly eosinophilic, and stains orange-red with trichrome stains and red with azocar-

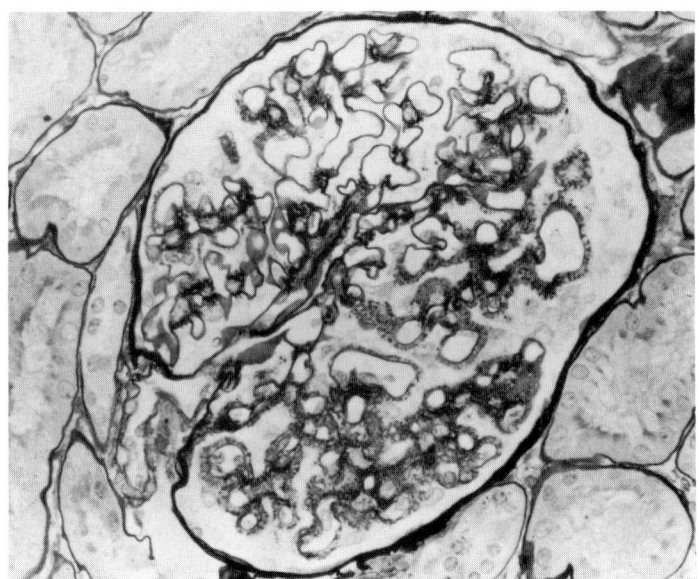

**Figure 30–19.** Light microscopic appearance of membranous glomerulonephritis. Numerous epimembranous projections of basement membrane material are present in most but not all capillary walls. (Periodic acid–methenamine silver; magnification × 1000.)

mine or chromotrope-R.[1146, 1147] In early or mild cases, the capillary wall may appear normal by light microscopy or may display numerous small round basement membrane vacuoles (best seen with silver impregnation stains) when sectioned tangentially.[1, 1146, 1147] With progression of the lesions, the capillary wall becomes increasingly thickened and encroaches on the capillary lumen. The glomerulus therefore may acquire a "rigid" appearance. At this stage, silver stains reveal large numbers of elongated spikes, some of which have joined together to form silver-positive circles enclosing an eosinophilic, PAS-negative deposit. The outer aspects of the circles are composed of α3- and α4-chains of type IV collagen,[1193, 1194] with lesser amounts of laminin; the thickened basement membrane on the endothelial aspect contains α1- and α2-chains of type IV collagen.[1193, 1194] In advanced states, the capillary wall is thickened, appearing reduplicated or moth-eaten with PAS and silver stains, and significant superimposed focal and segmental glomerular sclerosis may be found. Extensive interstitial fibrosis and tubule atrophy may be found at this stage. Interstitial infiltration with CD4+ and CD8+ T cells also occurs.[1196] A "segmental" form has also been described in which only a portion of the capillary loops is involved with deposits and basement membrane alterations. This may be an early or resolving form of the more diffuse and global disease or may represent a discrete entity. It may indicate a more favorable prognosis.

The occurrence of acute or chronic renal vein thrombosis has occasionally been associated with significant edema and fibrotic changes in the interstitium, and there may be margination of polymorphonuclear leukocytes in the peripheral glomerular capillaries.[1, 768, 769] However, these changes are inconstant. With the development of glomerular obsolescence, tubule atrophy becomes pronounced, and in the end stages, the pathologic picture may be difficult to distinguish from nonspecific chronic glomerulonephritis. Vascular changes are common in advanced disease but usually are lacking in the early stages. Focal and segmental crescents are uncommon manifestations, but rarely fulminant diffuse

crescentic glomerulonephritis may develop late in the course owing to superimposition of anti-GBM or anti–tubule basement membrane disease or other mechanisms[1, 1197–1202] (see Chapter 31). The evolution of diffuse endocapillary proliferative glomerulonephritis into typical MGN is distinctly unusual,[137] except during therapy of proliferative glomerulonephritis in SLE (see Chapter 31). Focal and segmental epimembranous deposits may be superimposed on a variety of other primary or secondary glomerular lesions.[1203, 1204]

***Electron Microscopy.*** The electron microscopic findings serve to clarify and amplify the changes seen by light microscopy and have important diagnostic and prognostic significance.[1, 1146, 1147] Some workers have found a series of changes by electron microscopy that correspond to the stages of disease; others have not.[1] In early cases (stage I), the GBM is normal in thickness and appearance, but small, discrete, subepithelial deposits of slightly greater electron density than the lamina densa appear at the level of the slit pore membrane.[1] These deposits produce some distortion of the structure of the foot processes. In more advanced cases (stage II), projections of basement membrane–like material corresponding to the silver-positive spikes seen by light microscopy are seen to develop between the enlarging deposits[1] (Fig. 30–20). This gives an irregular contour to the epithelial side of the GBM, which, however, remains of normal thickness. In time, the deposits become larger and more heterogeneous in size and distribution, and they may also vary in their degree of electron density. Spikes of GBM-like material may nearly encircle a deposit, giving a dome-like appearance (stage III). The foot processes are greatly distorted. Finally, the basement membrane–like material encloses the deposit, which now has become less electron-dense, giving the capillary wall a thickened or "Swiss cheese" appearance (stage IV). These abnormalities have been well demonstrated by scanning electron microscopy of glomerular capillaries devoid of cells.[1205] With remission of proteinuria, the deposits become more lucent but usually do not disappear unless basement membrane

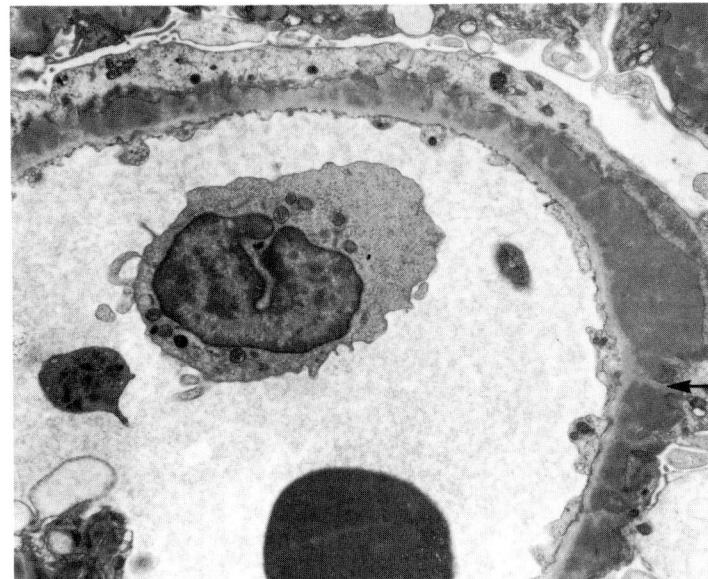

**Figure 30–20.** Electron microscopic view of membranous glomerulonephritis. Numerous epimembranous electron-dense deposits, often separated by projection of basement membrane material *(arrow),* can be seen. (Magnification × 8300.)

alterations are initially minimal.[1] Superimposition of electron-dense or electron-lucent deposits suggests renewed disease activity. The size and extent of the deposits are roughly correlated with the magnitude of proteinuria; the thickness of GBM and extent of effacement of foot processes correlate with the decline in GFR.[731, 1209] Electron-dense deposits in mesangium are scanty; pronounced deposits should increase suspicion of an underlying SLE, cancer, drug reaction,[1206, 1206a] or infectious disease. Peritubular or tubule basement membrane deposits may be seen, particularly when underlying SLE is responsible (see Chapter 31).

In general, the stage of the lesion, as determined by light and electron microscopy, correlates with the duration of the illness. However, in some cases, the lesions may remain stable for long periods and show little tendency for progression; in others, the lesions may progress with little change in the clinical course.[1] A remission of proteinuria, either spontaneous or therapeutically related, may at times be accompanied by some resolution of findings, including decreasing density of the deposits. In relapsing nephrotic syndrome, the appearance of deposits correlates with clinical features; the deposits are lucent during remission and dense during relapse.[1207] Decreasing GFR is generally associated only with advanced lesions unless acute renal vein thrombosis, crescentic glomerulonephritis, or acute hypersensitivity interstitial nephritis has supervened. Chronic interstitial fibrosis and tubule atrophy correlate better with reduced GFR than do glomerular lesions,[1208] but thickness of GBM may correlate with the extent of reduction of GFR.[1209]

***Immunofluorescence.*** The immunofluorescence findings are typical and highly reproducible from case to case.[1] IgG is nearly always present in a uniform granular distribution outlining all of the capillary loops but usually sparing the mesangium (Fig. 30–21). Extensive mesangial deposits of immunoglobulins usually indicate an underlying disease, particularly SLE.[1206a] The capillary wall deposits are usually IgG4. IgG3 is most often absent or minimal.[1210] In early cases, the capillary wall deposits are small and may have a

"linear" or continuous appearance at lower power magnification. In advanced cases, the deposits are larger and still uniform in size but focally may show coalescence. In advanced cases, or after prolonged remission of proteinuria, the IgG deposits may be weak and irregular or even absent, corresponding to the decreasing electron density seen by electron microscopy. IgM and IgA deposits are scanty. C3 is usually present in a pattern and intensity similar to IgG.[1] Deposition of C1q and C4 are seen much less often and with less intensity than C3. Heavy C1q deposits are indicative of underlying SLE rather than of idiopathic MGN.[1210] The membrane attack complex of complement (C5b-C9) and C3dg are found in the deposits.[1167, 1171, 1173] Fibrin-related antigens may be found along the capillary wall or in the mesangium, but usually this is not a striking finding. Hageman factor is frequently deposited in the glomerular

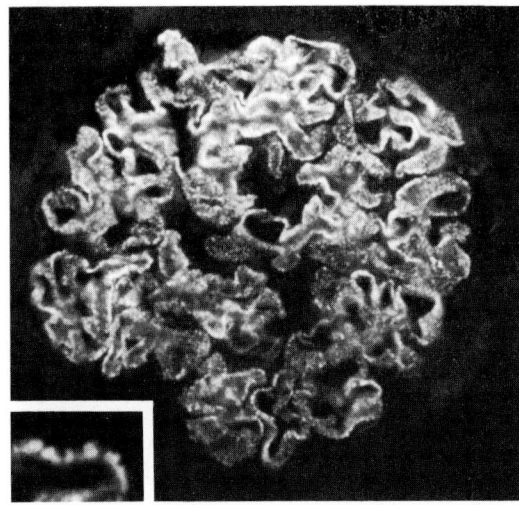

**Figure 30–21.** Immunofluorescence view of membranous glomerulonephritis. The capillary walls reveal diffuse granular deposits of IgG, which are present in a subepithelial location *(inset).* (Antihuman IgG; magnification × 500.)

capillary wall, particularly in those cases complicated by renal vein thrombosis.[1211] A few authors have found deposits of renal tubule epithelial antigens in a distribution similar to IgG in idiopathic cases and in association with urate nephropathy or obstructive disease with tubule damage, but this has not been regularly confirmed.[1213–1215] These patients may also have circulating autoantibody to renal tubule epithelial antigens.[1, 1212] Deposits of other endogenous antigens (e.g., DNA, thyroglobulin, tumor-associated antigens) or exogenous antigens (e.g., hepatitis B e antigen, treponemal proteins) may be found in cases secondary to underlying disease (see also Chapters 29 and 31). In an unconfirmed report, porcine insulin antigens have been found in the deposits of immunoglobulin in patients with insulin-dependent diabetes mellitus (treated with porcine insulin) associated with MGN.[1216] When IgG, IgA, and IgM are all deposited with equal intensity, especially with concomitant mesangial deposits of immunoglobulin and intense deposits of C1q, a diagnosis of SLE should be entertained.

**Pathogenesis.** The pathogenesis of MGN in humans is controversial[1147, 1217] (see Chapter 29). HLA studies cited before strongly suggest that a genetic basis of susceptibility exists. Three possible mechanisms have been suggested. First, the lesion may be due to glomerular localization of preformed, circulating immune complexes composed of a low-molecular-weight oligovalent antigen and low-affinity IgG antibody.[1218] The source of the antigen in this postulated mechanism is unknown but could be endogenous (e.g., normal tissue antigen) or environmental (e.g., virus) or related to occupational or environmental heavy metal or organic solvent exposure. Attempts to identify nonglomerular autologous antigens in the deposits of idiopathic MGN have, with few exceptions, been negative, as have attempts to elute antibody with reactivity to nonrenal autologous tissue antigens.[1212–1215] A number of cases initially presumed to be idiopathic have been documented to have deposits of environmental antigens such as hepatitis B virus (see Chapter 31). Circulating immune complexes are inconsistently found, and no one has yet proved that the circulating immune complex material is the same as that which is deposited in glomeruli.[1186]

Second, the lesions may arise consequent to a reaction of circulating antibody with an intrinsic glomerular antigen discontinuously distributed along the lamina rara externa or in association with the clathrin-coated endocytotic pits at the base of visceral epithelial cells,[1217, 1219] resulting in the formation of immune complexes in situ (see Chapter 29). Whereas this mechanism certainly accounts for the development of subepithelial glomerular deposits in some laboratory models[1217, 1219, 1220] (e.g., passive Heymann nephritis, Chapter 29), antibody reactive in vitro with a normal glomerular capillary wall antigen (other than classic anti-GBM antibody) has only rarely been described in MGN of humans,[1221–1223] and elution studies have seldom been carried out with the sophistication necessary to identify such an antibody were it present. The relative difficulty with which circulating immune complexes are identified in this disorder would support this mechanism.

Third, the lesions could develop as a result of a reaction of circulating antibody with an antigen normally extrinsic to the glomerulus but planted there by virtue of some bio-

chemical or electrostatic affinity for GBM (see also Chapter 29). Although it is theoretically possible, little evidence has yet been accumulated to support (or deny) a potential role for this mechanism in humans.

The mechanism of proteinuria in MGN involves the appearance of a population of large-radius pores leading to increased heteroporosity of the capillary wall and increased fractional IgG clearance relative to the fractional albumin clearance.[1224] Local deposition and activation of the C5b-C9 membrane attack complex and local complement-mediated injury may in part explain the proteinuria,[1167, 1171, 1173] although complement-independent mechanisms are also almost certainly involved.[1225, 1226] An increase in the local production of reactive oxygen species (hydroxyl radical, superoxide anion, and hydrogen peroxide) leading to lipid peroxidation of cell membranes and alterations in collagen cross-linking may be involved in the proteinuria of MGN.[754] Antioxidant agents, such as probucol, have significant antiproteinuric effects in animal models but have not yet been tested in human subjects.[754] The alterations in extracellular matrix seen in MGN do not necessarily depend on activation of complement and formation of the C5b-C9 complex.[1227] Circulating permeability-promoting factors do not appear to be involved in the proteinuria of MGN.[1227a] The extent of deposits does not correlate with the magnitude of proteinuria; however, as stated before, the electron lucency or density of the deposits does correlate with proteinuria.

**Course and Therapy.** The course of untreated idiopathic MGN is indolent and slowly progressive, at times punctuated by clinical remissions and exacerbations of the nephrotic syndrome.[1, 1228–1240] The overall prognosis in children is excellent; less than 5% progress to renal failure within 5 years, and 10-year survival is above 90%.[1, 1228] The majority of children experience a complete remission of proteinuria (frequently spontaneous) within 5 years of diagnosis.[1] The frequency of spontaneous complete remissions of proteinuria in adults varies among series but averages about 25%.[1, 1229–1240] An additional 20% to 35% of cases sustain a spontaneous partial remission (i.e., protein excretion less than 2 g but more than 200 mg/d) and maintain a stable GFR for extended periods.[1, 1146]

An extensive retrospective survey conducted by the Mayo Clinic group demonstrated a 10-year survival of patients of about 75%, regardless of whether the patients were treated with steroids or immunosuppressive drugs or remained untreated; 20% had end-stage renal failure, of which 60% occurred within 2.5 years of diagnosis (so-called rapidly progressive MGN).[1232] Similar findings have been reported from France, also involving untreated patients,[1] and from Japan,[1233] Finland,[1234] and Scotland.[1235] A group from Italy described 100 untreated patients with MGN observed for up to 10 years, 63% of whom presented with nephrotic range proteinuria.[1236] Of the group with nephrotic syndrome at presentation, approximately 50% underwent spontaneous remissions within 5 years, and approximately 30% had progressive renal impairment after 8 years of follow-up. Proteinuria of greater than 4 g/d that persists for more than 8 months is highly predictive of future progressive renal failure.[1237, 1238] Patients with at least one spontaneous or treatment-associated remission have a favorable prognosis, even though relapses are common.[1239]

Patients who have a progressive course (20% to 30% of the total population) in the first 10 years usually manifest impairment of GFR within the first 2 to 3 years of initial diagnosis.[1240] A relapsing and remitting course similar to that observed with minimal-change disease may be seen in 10% to 15% of cases.[1230, 1241] Male sex, older age at onset, severe proteinuria (>10 g/d), poorly controlled hypertension, severe hypercholesterolemia, reduced GFR at onset, and renal biopsy findings of advanced glomerular disease (stage III or IV), tubule atrophy, and interstitial fibrosis have all been associated with a poor prognosis and a high risk for subsequent development of progressive renal failure.[1232, 1236–1238, 1240] These clinical parameters may be used to predict long-term course and guide therapy.[1237–1240, 1242, 1243] Adults who present initially with non-nephrotic proteinuria have a much more favorable prognosis, with a 10-year survival rate of 85% to 90%.[1236] As indicated before, some patients may experience an aggressive course.[1232] Patients who still have normal renal function 5 years or more from the time of diagnosis are relatively unlikely to subsequently have end-stage renal failure, provided that massive proteinuria (>10 g/d) does not develop.[1233] In the untreated patients observed by Davison and co-workers,[1231] doubling of the serum creatinine concentration was noted in a mean of 30 months in 44% of patients. In a similar group of untreated patients, a doubling of the serum creatinine concentration within the first 2 years after discovery was found in about 30%.[1, 1244] Progressive renal failure occurring within a few months of diagnosis should suggest a complicating hypersensitivity interstitial nephritis[1245] (due to diuretics, NSAIDs, or antimicrobials); the development of superimposed crescentic glomerulonephritis (see earlier); the development of severe, acute bilateral renal vein thrombosis; or profound hypovolemia from massive proteinuria.

Because of the indolent nature of this disorder and the tendency for spontaneous remission, the evaluation of the beneficial effect of therapy from short-term, uncontrolled observations is difficult or impossible.[1246–1250] Much of the existing literature, primarily describing uncontrolled studies, does not indicate a substantial beneficial effect of steroid therapy on either proteinuria or ultimate prognosis.[1248–1251] In a small controlled trial in adults, Black and colleagues[1252] found no effect of prednisone on proteinuria, but the dosage employed was usually 40 mg/d or less. However, too few patients were included for the beneficial effect to have been detected if one were present. A prospective, randomized, controlled double-blind study of idiopathic MGN presenting with nephrotic syndrome and well-preserved GFR in the United States,[1244, 1253] using higher doses than those employed in the Medical Research Council trial (i.e., 120 to 150 mg of prednisone every other day for 8 weeks or more), demonstrated a significant reduction in average proteinuria and the prevalence of complete or partial remissions of proteinuria in the treated group compared with the placebo group.[1244] However, at the end of the follow-up period, no difference in the prevalence of patients remaining in complete remission was noted. The most striking effect of steroids noted in this study was a significant reduction of the occurrence of progressive renal failure in the steroid-treated group. Almost 30% of the placebo-treated group had an estimated 50% or greater reduction in

GFR, often within 2 years of discovery of disease, whereas a similar decline occurred in less than 10% of the steroid-treated group. According to clinical and morphologic data, the treated and placebo groups were comparable at the time of randomization. Renal vein thrombosis was not routinely sought in this study, but pulmonary emboli did not occur in either placebo or steroid group. Thus, it did not seem likely that the differences could be accounted for by nonrandom allocation of more patients with occult renal vein thrombosis to the placebo group. The rate of progression of disease in the placebo group did appear to be more rapid than that described previously in untreated cases from some geographic areas.[1232, 1236] The number of patients experiencing undesired side effects of steroid therapy was small, and no mortality attributable to such therapy was observed, at least in the first several years of observation. Long-term follow-up is required to determine whether the effect of steroids on progressive renal disease will be sustained. It is surprising that such a short course of steroids had such long-term effects. This study has been criticized because the prognosis of the placebo group was much worse than that observed in other studies of untreated patients.[1232, 1236] In addition, other controlled trials of glucocorticoids in different dosages have not confirmed these observations,[1254] including another Medical Research Council trial that employed a prednisone regimen identical to that employed in the U.S. Collaborative Study mentioned before.[1255] Whether higher doses or longer periods of glucocorticoid therapy would be more beneficial is unknown. Hopper[1256] and Bolton and colleagues[1257] in uncontrolled studies have suggested that higher dosage or more prolonged therapy (i.e., 6 months to several years) with daily or alternate-day steroids is associated with an improved outcome; however, such therapy is associated with a higher prevalence of undesirable side effects. Steroid therapy may be more effective in patients with stage I disease.[1258] If progression to impaired GFR has already occurred before discovery of disease, it is uncertain whether steroid therapy will be beneficial, although Hopper[1256] has suggested that high-dose, alternate-day steroid therapy will often stabilize or improve renal function in such patients.[1256] Short and colleagues[1259] have also suggested that short courses of high-dose intravenous methylprednisolone may also be beneficial in the short term in patients with deteriorating GFR, but such responses may be short lived, and no clear-cut benefit on protein excretion rates has been noted. The other causes of declining GFR occurring as a complication of the underlying disease must always be carefully evaluated when GFR declines rapidly in the first few months or years after diagnosis. On balance, studies conducted to date indicate that oral glucocorticoids *do not* have a major impact on the natural history of MGN, except for the uncommon steroid-responsive/relapsing subgroup.[941, 942, 1230]

The precise role of cytotoxic agents in therapy is also uncertain,[941, 942, 1260–1281] but a role for these agents in the management of MGN has been suggested by several controlled and uncontrolled studies[1260–1281] and by meta-analyses of controlled trials.[1281] The addition of cyclophosphamide to alternate-day or daily steroids has been associated with stable or improving renal function or decrease in proteinuria.[1273, 1274, 1281] Ponticelli and colleagues[1266, 1269, 1273] have shown in a controlled study that sequential therapy with high-dose intravenous methylprednisolone, oral methylprednisolone, and oral chlorambucil for 6 months can result in increased likelihood of complete or partial remission and better maintenance of renal function, with follow-up now averaging 10 years. Similar benefits for oral cyclophosphamide combined with prednisone have also been described in both controlled and uncontrolled studies, but the beneficial effects are not consistent.[1265, 1276] Prolonged therapy (6 to 12 months) may be required. Delayed treatment also seems to be effective despite presence of impaired renal function. If therapy is delayed until renal function is significantly impaired, however, the beneficial effects of treatment may be reduced.[1273] Early stages of the disease may be more responsive to treatment.[1258, 1273] The improvement in outcome, at least for the first 3 years after treatment, can be attributed to the addition of an alkylating agent to the regimen,[1273] but the question of whether long-term outcome is greatly improved is still in doubt. Because the long-term outcome in the treated group in some trials is approximately the same as that of untreated patients in other studies, questions have been raised regarding the significance of the shorter term observations that are indicative of an improved outcome.[1250] Nevertheless, it seems clear that the short-term course of MGN can be improved, at least in most patients, by the addition of an alkylating agent, either chlorambucil or cyclophosphamide, to the regimen.[1273, 1279, 1281] Patients who present with already developed or progressive abnormalities in renal function with continued heavy proteinuria may also be "rescued" by aggressive regimens consisting of glucocorticoids and alkylating agents.[1268, 1270, 1275, 1278] Prolonged therapy is required, and side effects may be more frequent,[1275] especially in elderly patients.[1275a] Oral cyclophosphamide or chlorambucil appears to be more effective than intravenous pulses of cyclophosphamide.[1277, 1278] Complete or partial remissions of proteinuria can be obtained in 30% to 50% of patients, frequently accompanied by stability of renal function. Combinations of azathioprine and prednisone may also promote stable renal function, but this has not been tested in a controlled fashion.[1271] Indomethacin, meclofenamate, and other NSAIDs in patients with profuse proteinuria and declining renal function may be beneficial but require further evaluation. Cyclosporine in doses of 4 to 5.5 mg/kg/d has slowed the rate of progression and decreased protein excretion in a limited number of trials.[1282–1285] Further controlled and randomized trials are required before this agent can be added to the therapeutic armamentarium.[1286] Low-protein diets generally have little effect, except to modestly decrease proteinuria.[1287] The ω-3 fatty acids decrease protein excretion in animal models, but the effect on progressive renal functional abnormalities in humans is unknown.[1288] ACE inhibitors decrease proteinuria by 30% to 50% without a significant change in GFR or renal hemodynamics.[1289, 1290] Whether these agents exhibit renoprotective effects in the long term is presently unknown. Intravenous administration of immunoglobulins (0.4 g/kg/d) in repeated doses for extended periods has been associated with an increased prevalence of complete and partial remissions in patients with normal renal function.[1291] This approach to therapy, although expensive, is deserving of further evalu-

ation in a controlled fashion. The role of prophylactic anticoagulants has been discussed in the preceding section on renal vein thrombosis. Evidence favoring their routine use in MGN has been reported.[790] MGN has developed de novo in renal allografts,[1292, 1293] but for poorly understood reasons, it has a low recurrence rate in renal transplants,[1294, 1295] except when superimposed crescentic disease is present[1296] (see also Chapter 59).

In summary, idiopathic MGN is an indolent disease in most circumstances, and spontaneous complete remissions eventually occur in about 25% of patients. The overall prognosis can be estimated at the time of diagnosis by application of clinical and pathologic criteria, particularly by analyzing protein excretion rates, GFR, and biopsy findings of chronic interstitial lesions. Patients with a favorable long-term prognosis (e.g., children, adults with non-nephrotic proteinuria) need not receive specific treatment. Adult patients (particularly women younger than 40 years) with nephrotic syndrome but with normal renal function and only modest proteinuria (<10 g/d) could be managed conservatively without steroids or cytotoxic agents and observed for either spontaneous remission or progression. Patients with persisting severe proteinuria (particularly men older than 40 years), symptomatic nephrotic syndrome, or progressive renal failure may be treated best by combinations of cytotoxic drugs (oral cyclophosphamide) and glucocorticoids or sequential chlorambucil and glucocorticoids (see earlier). Patients with advanced chronic renal failure (not due to interstitial nephritis or crescentic nephritis), as estimated by serum creatinine levels above 3 to 4 mg/dL, are probably best managed by conservative means and optimal control of blood pressure with ACE inhibitors while awaiting dialysis or renal transplantation. The role of cyclosporine, NSAIDs, intravenous immunoglobulins, and long-term ACE inhibition deserves further exploration.

## MESANGIOCAPILLARY GLOMERULONEPHRITIS (Membranoproliferative Glomerulonephritis, Hypocomplementemic Persistent Glomerulonephritis, Lobular Glomerulonephritis)

The glomerulopathies characterized by proliferation of cells within the glomerular tufts have been subdivided into several more or less well defined clinicopathologic groups. One such group is MCGN, so called because of the presence of both a prominent increase in mesangial cellularity and the circumferential extension of mesangial cells and cytoplasm into the peripheral capillary wall.[1, 1297–1300] These changes lead to the appearance of a thickened and reduplicated ("tram track" or "double-contoured") capillary wall by light microscopy. As pointed out later, some forms of glomerulopathy with subepithelial deposits may take on the added feature of endocapillary (mesangial) proliferation with circumferential mesangial interposition (mixed membranous and proliferative glomerulonephritis). These lesions may also be classified as MCGN.[1301] Because prolonged depression of serum complement levels is a common but not invariable feature, hypocomplementemic persistent glomerulonephritis is a term also used to describe this condition[1297–1299, 1302] and to contrast it with acute PSGN, in which the depression of serum complement levels is transitory. Furthermore, biopsy specimens in certain cases of MCGN demonstrate a marked increase in mesangial matrix and a tendency to form centrilobular nodules, in addition to the increase in mesangial cells.[1, 1297–1299, 1303] Because of this appearance, such cases have been termed lobular glomerulonephritis.[1303] The lesions of MCGN may also be complicated at times by superimposed focal or diffuse crescents[1, 1297–1299] and the lesions of focal and segmental glomerulosclerosis.

MCGN may be a primary glomerular disease or secondary to a variety of infectious, hereditary, or multisystem diseases (such as SLE)[1, 1297–1299] (Table 30–14). The primary (idiopathic) forms are heterogeneous and have been further categorized on the basis of light ultrastructural and immunofluorescence patterns.[1297] By light microscopy, several patterns may be seen in MCGN[1299]: 1) diffuse mesangial interposition with capillary wall thickening and reduplication (classic form); 2) nodular expansion of the mesangium; 3) exudative lesions; 4) focal and segmental mesangial interposition with or without sclerosis; 5) massive capillary wall deposits; and 6) crescentic lesions. The classic and

## TABLE 30–14. Classification of Mesangiocapillary Glomerulonephritis (Membranoproliferative Glomerulonephritis)

**Primary (Idiopathic)**
Type I (subendothelial deposits)
Type II (dense deposit disease)
Other variants (type III, type IV, others)

**Secondary***
Systemic lupus erythematosus
Mixed (IgG/IgM) essential cryoglobulinemia
Chronic active hepatitis (hepatitis B, hepatitis C)
Light or heavy chain nephropathy
Sickle-cell disease
Scleroderma
Sjögren syndrome
Celiac disease
Sarcoidosis
Cyanotic congenital heart disease
Infective endocarditis
Visceral abscesses
"Shunt" nephritis
Quartan malaria
Schistosomal nephropathy
Mycoplasma infection
Malignant neoplasm (lymphoma, leukemia, carcinoma)
Antitrypsin deficiency
Complement deficiency (C2, C3) with or without partial
  lipodystrophy
De novo in renal allografts
Hemolytic-uremic syndrome
After bone marrow transplantation
Kartagener syndrome
Renal artery dysplasia
Chronic allograft failure
Radiation nephritis
Angiofollicular lymph node hyperplasia (Castleman disease)
Buckley syndrome
Familial

*See Chapter 31 for details on secondary causes.

nodular patterns are most frequent, accounting for approximately 60% of cases. By electron and immunofluorescence microscopy, a variety of deposits are observed. The pattern of deposits gives rise to the classification by ultrastructural type. With light microscopy, the nodular form of MCGN may be confused with intercapillary diabetic glomerular sclerosis, light and heavy chain nephropathy (Randall-type), fibrillary glomerulonephritis, and amyloidosis (see Chapter 31), but electron microscopic and immunofluorescence findings can usually resolve the classification. Ultrastructural analysis gives rise to three or more patterns.[1297, 1300] Type I MCGN is characterized by subendothelial electron-dense deposits, and type II MCGN by the presence of extremely electron-dense deposits within the GBM. Other variants (e.g., type III MCGN) have also been described[1, 1301–1312] (see later). Because of the similarity of clinical features, MCGN is used in this section as a generic term to encompass all of the variants currently recognized.

**Clinical Features.** The disorders considered together as MCGN seem to affect all age groups.[1, 1299, 1300] The majority of patients, however, have the onset of disease after the age of 5 years and before the age of 30 years. In the extensive pediatric population described by Levy, Gubler, and Habib,[1313] 90% of the cases of type I MCGN and 70% of type II MCGN were discovered between 8 and 16 years of age. There is a slight predominance of females in type I and a nearly equal sex ratio in type II disease.[1297–1300, 1307–1317] The lesion is found in 6% to 12% of renal biopsies performed in the course of evaluating glomerular disease (averaging about 10%) and accounts for 7% of idiopathic nephrotic syndrome in children and about 12% in adults.[1, 1299, 1300] In more recent years, the prevalence of MCGN has been decreasing; in many centers, it has become an uncommon lesion.[1318] This decrease has been mainly confined to type I lesions.[1318]

The clinical presentation is varied.[1, 1297–1300, 1319] As many as 50% of patients present initially with a well-developed nephrotic syndrome; about 30% present with asymptomatic proteinuria, usually accompanied by recurrent gross or microscopic hematuria; and another 20% to 30% present with features of the acute nephritic syndrome.[1, 1297–1300, 1319] An acute nephritic onset seems more common in type II disease.[1297–1300, 1307, 1313] An upper respiratory infection precedes the onset of renal disease in as many as half of the cases. Increased ASO titers and other evidence of streptococcal infection may antedate the onset of disease in up to 40% of cases.[1, 1313] Hypertension, usually mild, occurs in about one third of cases.[1, 1297–1299] A severe hypertensive crisis, however, may be induced by high-dose steroid therapy. Partial lipodystrophy (Barraquer-Simons disease) may be seen, especially in type II MCGN, even in the absence of clinical manifestations of renal disease.[1320–1324] Some patients may show X-linked transmission.[1325] Congenital complement protein or regulatory protein deficiency state may also predispose to MCGN type I.[1, 1326, 1327] Decreased GFR occurs in approximately 50% of the cases and, if present at onset of disease, usually indicates a poor prognosis.[1297–1300] The reduction in GFR is associated with a reduction in filtration surface area and an increase in renal interstitial volume.[1327] Regardless of the mode of presentation, hematuria and proteinuria are nearly always found together.

**Laboratory Features** (see Table 30–2). Proteinuria and hematuria are almost invariably present. Nephrotic range proteinuria is seen in more than half of the cases.[1, 1297–1300] Milder degrees of proteinuria, nearly always accompanied by hematuria, are seen in the remainder. Urinary protein selectivity, as measured by differential protein clearances, is moderate or poor in more than 90% of the cases.[1] An important diagnostic marker for this group of disorders is the frequent depression of hemolytic complement activity of serum accompanied by lowering of the serum level of the C3 component as measured immunochemically or functionally.[1, 110, 1326] Indeed, the first recognition as a distinct entity arose from serial studies of serum hemolytic complement activity and C3 component analysis in children with persistent or progressive glomerulonephritis.[1] As discussed previously, serum total hemolytic complement activity and C3 levels are also usually depressed in acute postinfectious glomerulonephritis but characteristically return to normal values within 3 to 8 weeks.[110–112] The failure of complement levels to return to normal within 2 months of the onset of an acute nephritic syndrome is highly suggestive of underlying MCGN.

Overall depression of the C3 component of complement is found at initial study in about 75% of cases.[1, 1297–1300, 1326] A marked decrease to less than 30 mg/dL is seen in about 30% to 40% of patients,[1326] particularly among patients with type II disease. In type I MCGN, the C3 levels are often decreased with or without a concomitant decrease in other complement components (C1q, C4, C5b-C9).[1326] This pattern is seen in approximately one third of cases of type I MCGN and suggests activation of the alternative rather than of the classic pathway. In type II MCGN, there is isolated C3 depression, and factor B depression is seen in 80% of patients. In type III MCGN, C3 depression is accompanied by reduction in the terminal components in more than 80% of patients.[1326] The average C3 concentration at discovery is 68% of normal in type I disease and 47% of normal in type II disease.[1328] Low levels persist longer in type II disease.[1297] Serum levels of C3 may fluctuate without any change in the clinical course or therapy.[1, 1297–1300] The serum levels of early-acting components, such as C1q and C4, are usually normal in type II disease[1326] but may be variably decreased in type I disease.[1326] Serum levels of properdin may be normal, or if C3 is decreased, they may be modestly depressed.[1, 1326] The serum level of factor B is usually within normal limits or slightly decreased, and it may be greatly decreased in type II disease.[1326] The metabolic turnover of C3 is usually increased at a time when C3 serum levels are depressed.[1, 1329] In addition to elevated fractional catabolic rates for C3, depressed synthesis of C3 may be found, which likewise contributes to the lowering of the C3 levels.[1, 1326, 1329] A heat-stable factor, present in the serum of many but not all patients, is capable of cleaving C3 in fresh normal plasma in the presence of magnesium egtazic acid (this chelating agent selectively inhibits the classic pathway).[1, 1326, 1329–1331] This factor, commonly referred to as C3 nephritic factor (C3 NeF) is an IgG autoantibody to the C3 convertase of the alternative complement pathway (C3b,Bb)[1, 1332–1335] (see also Chapter 29). It apparently stabilizes this converting enzyme by protecting it from inhibitor proteins, resulting in continuous degradation of native

C3.[1, 1326] With low synthetic levels of C3, the serum level thereby falls. C3 NeF is found in more than 60% of patients with type II MPGN, and substances with similar activity may be found in 10% to 20% of patients with type I disease as well as in other acute proliferative glomerulonephritides.[1, 1326, 1328] Occasionally, the C3 lytic activity found in sera of patients with MCGN will not be related to an IgG autoantibody to C3b,Bb.[1336, 1337] The levels of C3 NeF and of depressed C3 component are unaffected by bilateral nephrectomy or the clinical state of disease but do have a tendency to return to normal with time[1, 1338, 1339] and show little relationship to clinical activity.[1339] In some patients, cleavage products of C3 or factor B may be detected in fresh plasma by immunoelectrophoretic or radioimmunoassay analysis.[1] C3 cleaving activity may also be found in sera from patients with SLE and acute glomerulonephritis, but this activity is often heat labile and inhibited by ethylenediaminetetraacetic acid.[1, 110] This activity appears, therefore, to be dependent on the classic complement pathway and probably represents circulating immune complexes. Low levels of C3 are uncommon in other varieties of idiopathic nephrotic syndrome[1, 106, 107] (see Table 30–2) but may be depressed in advanced liver disease, monoclonal gammopathies, leukemia, and metastatic carcinoma, presumably because of defective synthesis rather than increased catabolism.[1] IgG levels may be elevated in MCGN.[1340] Cryoimmunoglobulins and immune complexes may be detected in the circulation by a variety of techniques, particularly in type I disease.[1341, 1342] High levels of IgG/IgM cryoimmunoglobulins, normal or slightly reduced levels of C3, and low levels of C4 should suggest an underlying chronic hepatitis C virus infection (see also Chapter 31). More than 75% of cases of type I disease may have a particular B cell alloantigen, suggesting a genetic basis of susceptibility.[1, 1343] HLA-B7 is associated with type II disease.[1344] Familial β1H deficiency associated with dense deposit disease has been observed.[1345]

GFR is frequently decreased but may be normal even when severe glomerular lesions are found in the biopsy sample. Normocytic, normochromic, Coombs-negative anemia is found in more than half the cases and may be severe and out of proportion to the degree of azotemia.[1] Red blood cell survival is shortened, and there may be a microangiopathic component to the anemia. Another possible explanation for the anemia is that activated terminal complement components may act on the nonsensitized red blood cell to initiate "innocent bystander lysis."[1346] Platelet survival may also be curtailed and fibrinogen turnover increased.[1347] The erythrocyte sedimentation rate may be normal or low.[1, 1297, 1300]

**Pathology.** The hallmarks of this group of glomerular lesions are pronounced abnormalities of mesangial areas and the peripheral capillary walls, hence the descriptive term mesangiocapillary. Mesangiolysis may be a common lesion underlying the morphologic pattern of MCGN. A variety of subgroups have been based on light microscopic, electron microscopic, and immunofluorescent appearance (see earlier).[1299, 1348a] The classification that is based on the ultrastructural appearance and location of deposits is used here. Two types that occur more frequently and are much better defined than the others are considered in detail; the remainder are described briefly.[1, 1297–1300, 1348–1351] The current terminology for the two major variants is MCGN, type I and type II. Type I is often known as the classic form; type II is commonly referred to as dense deposit disease. In most large series, type I MCGN accounts for 65% to 75% of cases, type II MCGN for about 20% to 30%, and other variants for the remainder. Some include the other variants under the category of type I disease.

### Type I Mesangiocapillary Glomerulonephritis

LIGHT MICROSCOPY. The major alteration is variable expansion, with increase in cellularity and matrix, of the mesangium. This usually affects almost all lobules to an equal degree. When especially pronounced, this results in mild or marked accentuation of the lobular architecture of the tufts[1, 1297–1300, 1348–1351] (Fig. 30–22). Because of an excessive increase in mesangial matrix that leads to the formation of prominent nodules, this variant is sometimes referred to as lobular glomerulonephritis or the nodular form of MCGN; however, most authors agree that the lobular pattern merely represents variants of the same morphologic entity and that a subdivision into lobular and nonlobular forms is not warranted.[1297–1300] In any event, in addition to the increased cells and matrix of the mesangium, leukocytes, predominantly neutrophils, may be found infiltrating into the mesangium,[1, 1297–1300, 1314] giving rise to the term exudative MCGN.[1299] The capillary walls are almost always thickened; with appropriate stains, a double-contoured or tram track appearance, due to the extension and interposition of mesangial cells and matrix, is easily appreciated.[1, 1348a] Mesangiolysis may be a prominent finding.[1348a] Because of the staining properties of basement membrane and mesangial matrix, the double-contoured capillary wall (incorrectly referred to as split basement membrane) can best be appreciated with silver impregnation stains or with PAS reagent. Fuchsinophilic deposits, as observed with the trichrome stain, may occasionally be seen in subendothelial sites.[1351] The occurrence of focal and global sclerosis has been associated with progressive disease.[1298] Focal and segmental forms of glomerular involvement have also been described.[1352, 1353]

Crescents, either focal and segmental or diffuse and circumferential, may be a feature of up to 10% of biopsies;

they may be present at initial examination or may occur during progression of the disease and may also be noted in recurrence of this form of glomerulonephritis in a transplanted kidney.[1, 1354] When extensive crescents are present, they are usually indicative of a poor prognosis (see later). As a general rule, however, the extent of glomerular alterations is not a useful prognostic factor.[1355] Tubule and interstitial changes early in the course of the disease are often inconspicuous or absent, whereas interstitial fibrosis, tubule atrophy, and interstitial mononuclear inflammatory cells are often observed in patients with a progressive decline in GFR or later in the course of the disease.[1356] Some investigators have found that impairment of GFR is dependent on the severity of the tubule and interstitial changes, rather than the severity of the glomerular involvement, especially in patients with normal serum creatinine concentrations.[1356]

ELECTRON MICROSCOPY. The ultrastructural abnormalities are distinctive but not diagnostic. The major feature is the extension and interposition of cells and matrix between the glomerular capillary basement membranes and endothelial cells.[1, 1297–1300, 1303, 1357] The cells are presumed to be of mesangial origin, but they may also be derived from infiltrating cells (e.g., monocytes). Monocytes or neutrophils may also infiltrate into the space between mesangial matrix and basement membrane. There is increase in matrix and cells in the mesangium. Electron-dense deposits are often identified in subendothelial locations or within the internal lamina of GBM (endomembranous deposits) (Fig. 30–23), usually associated with mesangial cell interposition, and in the mesangium. Despite the universal presence of deposits in the peripheral capillary walls seen by immunofluorescence microscopy, not all specimens have readily identifiable subendothelial dense deposits by electron microscopy.[1316] Small to moderate numbers of epimembranous deposits, either as humps or often with adjacent basement membrane projections, may be present in some biopsy samples.[1, 1297–1300, 1357] When this is a prominent feature and associated with segmental spike-like projections of GBM, it is sometimes recognized as a distinct subgroup of MCGN (type III of Burkholder).[1, 1358, 1359] All the deposits are usually homogeneous to finely granular in appearance, similar

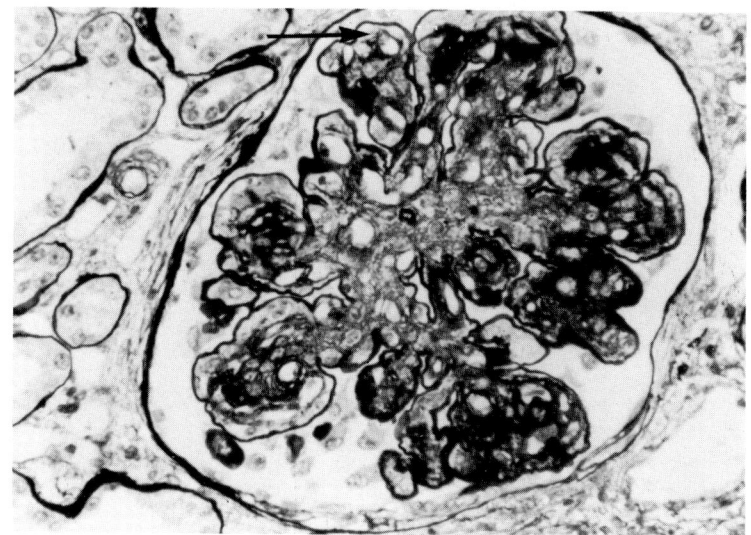

**Figure 30–22.** Light microscopic appearance of MCGN, type I. The tuft is lobulated; the mesangial regions have increased cells; and double-contoured capillary walls *(arrow)* are evident. (Periodic acid–methenamine silver; magnification × 1200.)

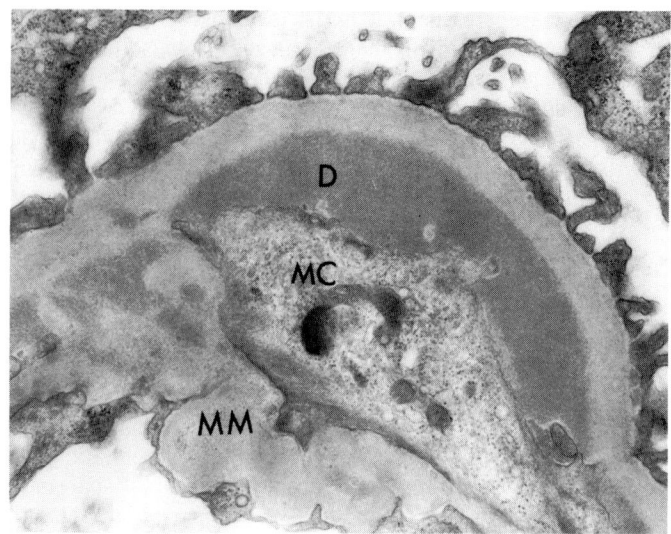

**Figure 30–23.** Electron microscopic appearance of MCGN, type I. A portion of capillary wall, showing mesangial interposition in association with subendothelial deposits, is seen. MC = mesangial cell; MM = mesangial matrix; D = deposits. (Magnification × 27,000.)

to those observed in most other glomerulopathies with deposits. However, a single case has been described with a fingerprint organizational pattern of the deposits similar to those frequently noted in SLE.[1316] A nonamyloid fibrillar structure should suggest the group of disorders discussed later and in Chapter 31 as fibrillary or immunotactoid glomerulonephritis. Organized deposits are also seen in IgG/IgM cryoglobulinemia and in light and heavy chain nephropathy (Randall type). Epithelial foot process loss or effacement almost always occurs. A variable increase in mesangial matrix, as described before (light microscopy) is also observed.[1, 1297–1300] Extensive electron-dense deposits in both subendothelial and subepithelial locations should suggest SLE (Chapter 31).

IMMUNOFLUORESCENCE MICROSCOPY. The findings in both the lobular and the nonlobular forms are similar[1, 1297–1300, 1348, 1357, 1360] (Fig. 30–24). Prominent C3 deposits are found in an irregular and granular distribution, tending to outline the periphery of the lobule, with variable localiza-

tion in the mesangium. Properdin and, to a lesser degree, factor B are found in a similar distribution.[1317] Immunoglobulins, especially IgM and IgG, are found in an inconsistent and segmental granular capillary wall and, less often, mesangial distribution and are not demonstrated in as many as one third to one half of the cases.[1, 1316, 1348] IgA deposits may be present in a third of the specimens[1] and may be an indication of coexisting liver disease[1] (see Chapter 31). The early-acting complement components, such as C1q and C4, are found only slightly less often than C3, usually in association with prominent immunoglobulin deposits.[1, 1297–1300] Although no clear-cut difference in clinical course has been demonstrated, some authors have divided type I MCGN into subcategories, depending on the types of immunofluorescence patterns: type A, C3 only; type B, C3 predominant with some IgG or IgM; type C, C3 and immunoglobulin in equal intensity. Each may have different degrees of mesangial or peripheral capillary wall involvement.[1348, 1360] Extensive IgG, IgM, IgA, C1q, C4, and C3 deposition should

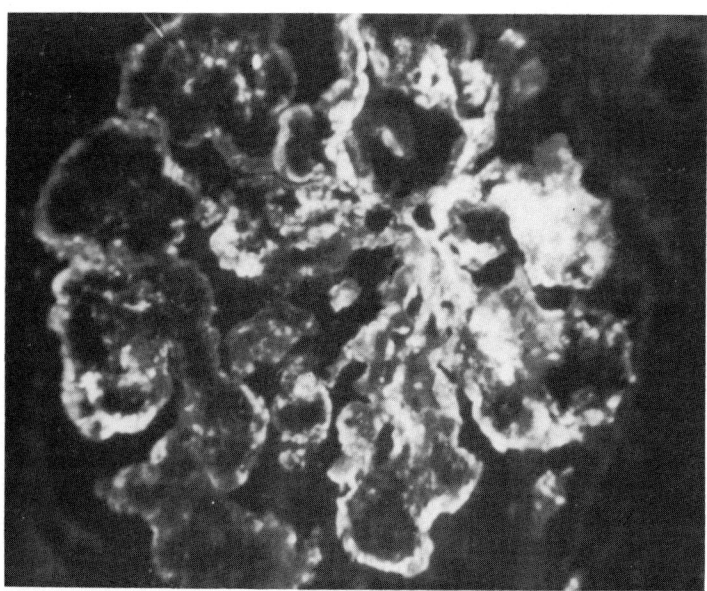

**Figure 30–24.** Immunofluorescence microscopic view of MCGN, type I, showing lobular accentuation with granular peripheral capillary and mesangial C3 deposits. (Antihuman C3; magnification × 1000.)

suggest occult SLE (see Chapter 31). Monoclonal light or heavy chains may be seen in MCGN associated with plasma cell dyscrasias. The IgM component of mixed (IgG/IgM) cryoglobulinemia is also monoclonal, usually containing a κ light chain (see Chapter 31).

### Type II Mesangiocapillary Glomerulonephritis

LIGHT MICROSCOPY. The morphologic findings in this variant are distinctive and unique.[1, 1297–1300, 1304–1309, 1360–1366] The structural hallmark is a peculiar transformation of the normal staining qualities of the glomerular capillary basement membranes, best appreciated by electron microscopy, but usually readily detectable with the light microscope. The glomeruli, all of which are usually abnormal, have increased mesangial cellularity and matrix, sometimes to a degree sufficient to result in a prominent lobular pattern and thickened capillary walls. The basement membranes have a ribbon-like refractile appearance and are colored intensely with many histochemical stains (Fig. 30–25). This change often affects all or most of the capillary walls and can be so distinctive as to be diagnostic with this method of examination.[1364] Occasionally, they are not readily detectable, so that ultrastructural studies may be required for diagnosis.[1365] Rarely, the dense deposits have been documented to evolve from proliferative glomerulonephritis.[1366] Depending on the staining method used, the basement membranes usually stain more intensely than normal basement membranes do. Thioflavine T staining is a sensitive but nonspecific method for the identification of this glomerulopathy.[1367, 1368] Although the altered basement membrane accounts for the major capillary wall changes, circumferential mesangial interposition, resulting in a double-contoured appearance to the capillary wall, is usually present in a variable number of capillaries.[1362] The mesangial changes, as mentioned before, are highly variable. With Masson trichrome stain, rounded fuchsinophilic deposits are often observed in the mesangium.[1351] In addition, in approximately one third of the biopsy specimens, large subepithelial hump-like deposits can be detected in some capillary walls.[1363] Increased numbers of leukocytes, especially neutrophils, are often present in capillary lumens. The combination of basement membrane thickening with mesangial interposition and the presence of intraluminal leukocytes results in narrowing or loss of patency of the capillaries. Crescents, either cellular or fibrocellular, occur in a variable number of cases. Their presence, even when affecting a large percentage of the glomerular population, is not always associated with rapidly progressive loss of renal function.[1] The light microscopic lesions of focal and segmental glomerulosclerosis may be prominent, particularly in patients with mild proteinuria, normal C3 levels, and a stable course.[1369]

The same basement membrane changes affecting the capillaries are also noted in the basement membranes of Bowman capsules and the tubules, although not always with the same degree of involvement as in the tuft.[1361] The medullary collecting tubules are said to be unaffected. Interstitial changes in the form of leukocyte infiltration and fibrosis, although present early, increase with duration of the disorder.

ELECTRON MICROSCOPY. The ultrastructural appearance is diagnostic and gives rise to separate classification of this disorder. It was because of the characteristic alterations of the glomerular capillary walls that this disease received its common name, dense deposit disease.[1, 1370] The GBMs are greatly widened (500 to 1500 nm, usual range) and appear as extremely electron-dense structures[1364] (Fig. 30–26). This density affects variable portions of the basement membranes. In each glomerulus, some capillary walls are normal; others may be completely or partially involved. In such instances, the densities are fusiform, globular, or sausage shaped. The transition between normal and abnormal is often abrupt and clear-cut. The dense material is homogeneous, having no distinct substructure even at extremely high magnifications. Peripheral migration and interposition of mesangial cells and matrix are often evident, but not to the same degree as in type I disease. Subepithelial electron-dense humps, similar to the deposits observed in PSGN, are occasionally present. As under light microscopy, there is variable increase in cells and matrix of the mesangium. Mesangial electron-dense deposits, usually rounded, are present in many instances.[1, 1363, 1364] The foot processes of visceral epithelial cells are almost always completely effaced. The electron-dense transformation also affects the

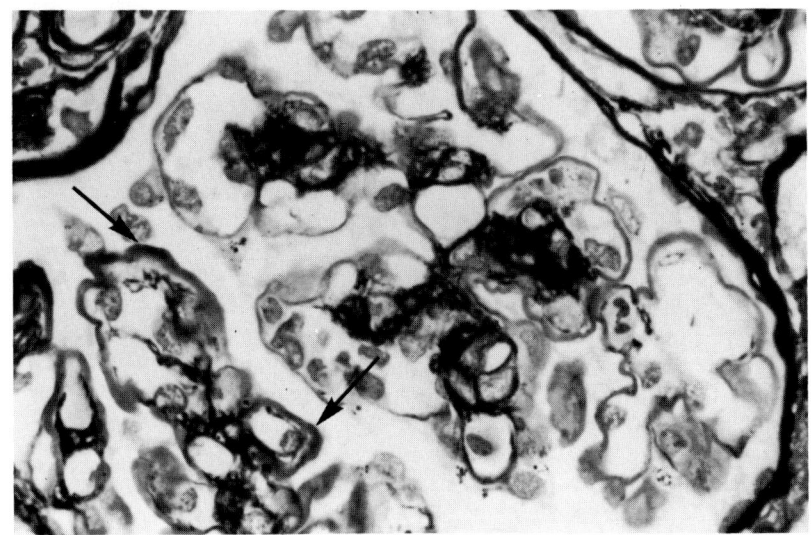

**Figure 30–25.** Light microscopic appearance of MCGN, type II (dense deposit disease). The capillary basement membranes are thickened *(arrows)* but stain less intensely than usual with silver impregnation methods, compared with the black mesangial matrix. (Periodic acid–methenamine silver; magnification × 2500.)

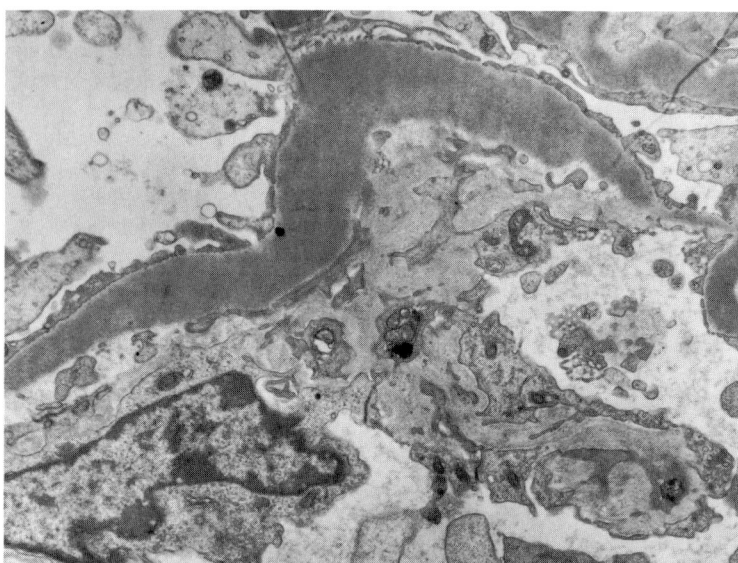

**Figure 30–26.** Electron microscopic view of MCGN, type II. The peripheral capillary basement membranes are thickened and deeply stained; note the more normal density of the mesangial matrix. (Magnification × 10,000.)

basement membranes of Bowman capsules, proximal tubules, and occasionally interstitial capillaries and arterioles.[1, 1364, 1371] Similar lesions have also been observed in splenic tissue.[1372] In these locations, it is more common for the "deposits" to be segmental rather than to involve the entire length of the structure. The tubule basement membrane deposits may be so characteristic as to be highly suggestive of an ultrastructural diagnosis of MCGN type II, even in the absence of glomeruli for examination.[1361]

IMMUNOFLUORESCENCE MICROSCOPY. The immunofluorescence findings in type II MCGN are less variable than in type I. There is virtually uniform agreement that C3 is heavily deposited in the glomeruli.[1, 1348, 1363] Several different but usually simultaneous patterns are evident. Most commonly, C3 is observed in a discontinuous linear ("railroad track") pattern outlining the capillary walls, Bowman capsules, tubules, and occasionally arterioles in a distribution identical to the basement membrane abnormalities. In addition, there may be granular C3 deposits in many capillary walls and large globular masses of C3 in many mesangial areas[1363] (Fig. 30–27). Linear capillary wall staining is due to the presence of two closely approximated parallel lines (railroad tracks) of C3, which, when compared with the same preparations stained with PAS reagent, is present on both sides of the basement membrane, rather than within it, as might be suggested by conventional light or electron microscopy. "Mesangial rings" corresponding to the granular deposits in the mesangium observed by light and electron microscopy are also found.[1363] Other complement components are found in less than 50% of the biopsies.[1362–1364] Some investigators have reported C3 as the sole complement component deposit, whereas others have noted C4 and C1q with lesser intensity and a more sparse distribution.[1, 1363] Properdin, when sought, has been identified in more cases than C4 and C1q.[1362, 1363] Immunoglobulins (especially IgG and IgA) are usually absent; IgM is noted in approximately 50% of the biopsies.[1297–1300] The membrane attack complex (C5b-C9) of complement has been localized to the capillary walls containing dense deposits; the membrane attack complex is along the periphery of the deposits

but not within them as demonstrated by immunoelectron microscopy.[1373]

***Other Morphologic Variants of Mesangiocapillary Glomerulonephritis.*** Several investigators have described additional variants of MCGN.[1352, 1353, 1358, 1359] In general, not enough experience has been accumulated to ascertain whether they represent variations of type I MCGN or, perhaps, are distinct entities. These variants are distinguished almost exclusively on the basis of electron microscopic study.

Burkholder[1359] described a type that is characterized by capillary walls with isolated epimembranous deposits, separated by projections of basement membrane material (sim-

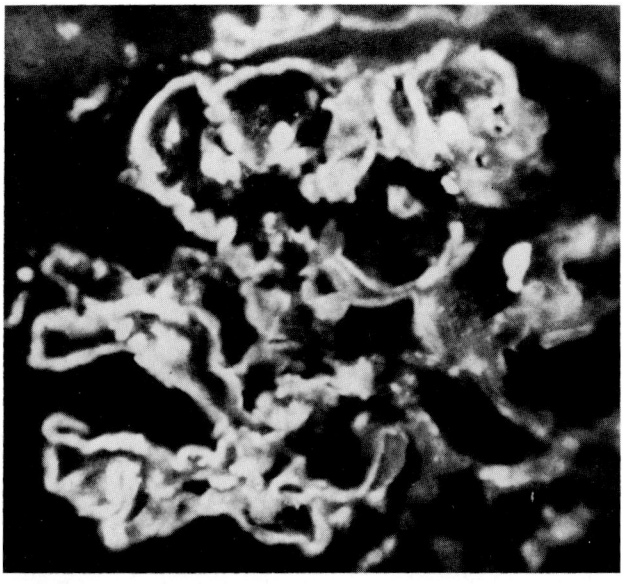

**Figure 30–27.** Immunofluorescence microscopic appearance of MCGN, type II. The capillary walls are heavily stained with C3; note also partial staining of the basement membrane of Bowman capsule *(top)* and the nodular deposits in the mesangium. (Antihuman C3; magnification × 1000.)

ilar to MGN) in addition to the presence of the changes characteristically evident in type I MCGN. This type has also been referred to as mixed membranous and proliferative glomerulonephritis (see earlier).[1301, 1358] Davis and co-workers[1308] described two patients with reduced serum C3 levels, proteinuria and hematuria, and a protracted but mild clinical course. Their biopsy specimens had mesangial proliferative changes and the presence of numerous small and irregular electron-dense deposits within short segments of capillary basement membranes and within Bowman capsule and tubule basement membranes. In addition, intramembranous and subendothelial lucent zones containing vesicles were identified in the capillary walls. Mesangial migration and interposition were not features. C3 was noted in capillary walls and mesangium in a granular pattern; IgM was also present. Strife and colleagues[1374] and Anders and co-workers[1352] described unusual ultrastructural changes in patients with clinical features similar to those of other forms of MCGN and nondistinguishing light and immunofluorescence microscopy. Jackson and co-workers[1319] have described this type III lesion to be detected in clinically asymptomatic patients and to be associated with less glomerular hypercellularity than type I MCGN. With the use of silver impregnation staining of material for electron microscopy, they described a complex alteration of the capillary wall that was characterized by disruption and layering of and elaboration of new basement membrane material. This was associated with the presence of subendothelial and epimembranous deposits that were in proximity. Finally, Morel-Maroger and colleagues[1375, 1376] have described a form of MGN with modest endocapillary proliferation with reduced C3 concentrations in children from tropical Africa with the nephrotic syndrome (also called tropical extramembranous nephropathy; see Chapter 31). MCGN has also been described in SLE; cryoglobulinemia; hepatitis B and C virus infection; schistosomal nephropathy; "shunt nephritis"; polyarteritis; cirrhosis with antitrypsin deficiency[1377]; hereditary C3, C2, and C1 deficiency[1378]; C3 convertase deficiency; renal artery dysplasia; Buckley syndrome[1379]; celiac disease[1380]; sarcoidosis[1381]; Sjögren syndrome; a Goodpasture-like syndrome with autoantibodies to smooth muscle antigens[1382]; malignant neoplasms; light and heavy chain nephropathy (Randall type); post–bone marrow transplantation; chronic renal allograft rejection; hemolytic-uremic syndrome; radiation nephritis; Kartagener syndrome; and Castleman disease (see Chapter 31) and as a familial disorder (see Table 30–14 and Chapter 31).

**Pathogenesis.** The pathogenesis of the various lesions in this category is largely unknown.[1, 1382] The morphologic and immunopathologic diversity most certainly indicates a high degree of heterogeneity of underlying mechanisms. Glomerular deposition of circulating immune complexes, probably involving some as yet unidentified environmental or autologous antigen, probably accounts for the majority of cases of type I lesions, especially those with heavy granular deposits of immunoglobulin. The pathogenesis of the subgroup with isolated C3 deposits is less certain. The association of alterations in C3 metabolism, suggesting pronounced activation of the alternative pathway of complement, indicates some pathogenetic link between glomerular disease and complement activation, but as yet no experi-

mental model of MCGN has been produced by prolonged complement activation.[1383] C3 NeF may be a marker or epiphenomenon rather than involved in causation of disease, but this is far from proved. Low complement levels may be primarily involved in enhancing susceptibility to occult and opportunistic infection and favoring development and persistence of circulating immune complexes[1378, 1383–1385] (Chapter 29).

Type II MPGN seems to be fundamentally a structural alteration of renal basement membranes, perhaps by incorporation of a sialic acid–rich glycoprotein.[1] Because the ultrastructural lesions recur frequently in renal allografts before C3 is deposited and regardless of the nature and severity of the complement abnormalities in the circulation,[1338] it is believed that the activation of the alternative pathway and formation of C3 NeF is secondary to some more fundamental biochemical disturbance in renal basement membrane biosynthesis or degradation.[1313]

**Course and Therapy.** The various disorders included under the generic heading MCGN display a relentless but slowly progressive course, albeit at highly variable rates. A reduced GFR and severe hypertension at discovery of disease indicate a poor prognosis, as does the presence of persistent nephrotic syndrome, extensive interstitial fibrosis and tubule atrophy,[1349, 1355, 1356] and the histologic identification of superimposed diffuse crescentic disease.[1354] The 10-year survival in patients studied by Cameron[1, 1386] with type I MCGN and persistent nephrotic syndrome was only 40%, whereas 85% of those with only non-nephrotic proteinuria survived for 10 years. D'Amico and Ferrario,[1299] in a later review, found a 10-year renal survival of 60% to 65%. Schmitt and co-workers[1355] found a worse prognosis of only 49% 5-year renal survival. The reason for the differences in renal survival rates between these analyses is not clear. The prognosis of the lobular and nonlobular varieties is similar, at least in children.[1, 1298] Although there may be occasional spontaneous clinical remissions of nephrotic proteinuria,[1386] serial biopsies have demonstrated stable or progressive findings.[1] The prognosis for type II disease has generally been worse than for type I, especially if superimposed crescentic disease, obliteration of capillary loops, or chronic tubulointerstitial lesions are present.[1355, 1369, 1387] The prognosis in children is not greatly different from that in adults.

A variety of therapeutic regimens have been employed, most often in an uncontrolled fashion.[1, 1297–1300, 1307, 1308] Therefore, it is difficult to draw any firm conclusions regarding the beneficial effects of treatment. McAdams, McEnery, and West[1388–1392] noted an apparent benefit on renal survival of continuous low-dose prednisone, although experience with this form of treatment is limited. Other uncontrolled studies have supported the notion that prolonged steroid therapy may be beneficial, at least in children. Low-dose, alternate-day oral prednisone administered for several years is often associated with improvement in GFR, reduction in protein excretion, and improvement in glomerular disease.[1393, 1394] The results of the ISKDC controlled trial of alternate-day steroids did not confirm these results.[1]

The value of combined steroid–cytotoxic drug regimens or therapy with anticoagulants and inhibitors of platelet aggregation remains uncertain. An uncontrolled trial using combinations of intravenous methylprednisolone, oral glucocorticoids, and cyclophosphamide observed a 79% remission rate, but relapses were common when the treatment was discontinued.[1395] In a small group of adult patients treated in an uncontrolled fashion with cyclophosphamide, oral anticoagulants, and dipyridamole, Kincaid-Smith[1396] found a 3-year survival rate of 82%, whereas in a retrospective survey of untreated patients, all of whom were observed before the introduction of the regimen mentioned before, there were no survivors at 3 years. This is an unusually high mortality for the untreated disease. Other anecdotal reports have supported a beneficial effect of combined anticoagulation and immunosuppression.[1397, 1398] Controlled trials using this approach in Australia and Canada have not demonstrated a consistently beneficial effect.[1, 1399] Michielsen and co-workers[1400] have noted temporary decline in proteinuria and have claimed decreased mortality rate in an uncontrolled trial of indomethacin in MCGN. Encouraging results have also been reported with use of anticoagulants and inhibitors of platelet aggregation without cytotoxic drugs, but serious bleeding complications may occur.[1401] Donadio and colleagues[1297, 1402] have shown in a controlled trial that long-term treatment with dipyridamole (375 mg/d) and aspirin (950 mg/d) slows the rate of decline in GFR in type I MCGN. These findings have been extended in another controlled trial in small numbers of patients with MCGN, primarily of the type I category. Acetylsalicylic acid at 500 mg/d combined with dipyridamole at 75 mg/d resulted in a decrease in urinary protein excretion but no difference in renal functional impairment in 36 months.[1402a] Diet and blood pressure control were optimized in both arms of this trial. The dosage of the drugs and the duration of the trial may not have been adequate to detect the difference in progressive loss of GFR. Plasma exchange therapy has been tried with some success in patients with MCGN and extensive crescents.[1403–1405] ACE inhibitors reduce proteinuria, but it is not yet known whether they will retard the rate of progression of renal disease.[622, 941, 942] Cyclosporine seems to have little effect on the disease except in MCGN associated with Buckley syndrome.[941, 942, 1002] Interferon alfa, glucocorticoids, cyclophosphamide, and perhaps plasma exchange may be useful in the treatment of MCGN associated with chronic hepatitis C virus infection and mixed essential (IgG/IgM) cryoglobulinemia (see Chapter 31).

In summary, MCGN is an increasingly uncommon disorder. It can be suspected in a patient with idiopathic nephrotic syndrome on the basis of hematuria and persistently low serum C3 levels. Several morphologic variants have been described on the basis of light, immunofluorescence, and electron microscopy. The prognosis is poor for many patients. However, because of the variable course and the tendency for slow progression, long-range and suitably controlled trials of therapy are required to definitively establish the efficacy of new approaches to therapy. At present, either long-term, low-dose, alternate-day prednisone therapy or combinations of dipyridamole and aspirin appear to be reasonable candidates for therapy. Plasma exchange and immunosuppression could be used for patients who exhibit extensive crescent formation or who have underlying disease, such as mixed (IgG/IgM) cryoglubinemia. Other

proposed forms of treatment are likely to entail substantial risks; therefore, the clinician should take a cautious and conservative stance regarding treatment and await the results of ongoing trials before embarking on any long-range program, particularly those involving prolonged use of cytotoxic agents, cyclosporine, or high-dose steroids. Interferon alfa may be of use when chronic hepatitis C virus infection can be documented to underlie the lesion. Long-term therapy with ACE inhibitors would be the preferred approach for management of hypertension. Recurrent disease in the transplanted kidney is common, perhaps universal, in type II MCGN and also occurs commonly in type I MCGN.[1297–1300, 1338, 1385, 1406, 1407]

# Other Primary Glomerular Lesions Associated with the Idiopathic Nephrotic Syndrome

A variety of other glomerular lesions have been found to underlie the occurrence of nephrotic syndrome, with or without hematuria, in which there is no obvious extrarenal involvement. Some of these lesions may also be seen in patients with non-nephrotic proteinuria or asymptomatic hematuria. They are covered here because of the not infrequent progression to typical nephrotic syndrome. Some of these clinical pathologic entities may indeed be secondary to some systemic disturbance, but this is usually not obvious when the patients initially present (see also Chapter 31 for additional description of those with multisystem involvement).

## FIBRILLARY AND IMMUNOTACTOID GLOMERULONEPHRITIS

The lesions of fibrillary and immunotactoid glomerulonephritis comprise a group of disorders called the nonamyloid fibrillary glomerulopathies (Table 30–15) because of the presence of fibrillar or microtubular structures within glomeruli that do not stain with Congo red or thioflavine T and that contain immunoglobulins[1408–1417] (see also Chapter 31). They were first delineated by Roseman and Eliakim[1418] and Avasthi and associates[1419] in 1977 and more extensively by Duffy and co-workers[1420] in 1983. Immunotactoid glomerulonephritis was separated from fibrillary glomerulonephritis by Schwartz and Lewis[1421] in 1985.

Since the original descriptions, numerous case reports have appeared, and the entities are now well established but still account for only a minority of cases of nephrotic syndrome due to primary glomerular lesions. They are seen in about 1% of all nontransplant renal biopsies, similar in frequency to that observed for amyloidosis.[1409] The typical clinical presentation is with hematuria and variable degrees of proteinuria often accompanied by hypertension and impaired renal function.[1408–1417] The average age at discovery is between 40 and 50 years, but typical cases have been described in patients between the ages of 10 and 80 years.[1409] The overall male/female ratio is 1.6. African-Americans appear to be rarely affected.[1409] In most cases, there are no clinical manifestations of extrarenal involvement, but rare cases of cutaneous vasculitis resembling

**TABLE 30–15. Classification of Fibrillary Glomerulopathies**

**Amyloid (Congo red–positive)**
Primary amyloidosis (AL)
Multiple myeloma associated (AL)
Secondary and heredofamilial (AA and other)

**Nonamyloid (Congo red–negative)**
*Immunoglobulin containing*
Fibrillary glomerulonephritis
Immunotactoid glomerulonephritis
Mixed (IgG/IgM) cryoglobulinemia
Monoclonal immunoglobulin deposition disease (lymphomas)
Light or heavy chain nephropathy (Randall type) (usually nonfibrillar)
Lupus nephritis
Collagen III glomerulopathy (rare)

*Immunoglobulins absent*
Diabetes mellitus (nodular glomerulosclerosis)
Fibronectin mesangiopathy
Nail-patella syndrome and collagen III glomerulopathy
Diffuse mesangial sclerosis (Drash syndrome)
Advanced chronic sclerosing glomerular disease (nonspecific)
Fibrillary glomerulonephritis (rare cases)

Schönlein-Henoch purpura and pulmonary hemorrhage have been observed.[1422, 1423]

Laboratory findings are those of nephrotic syndrome with normal serum complement values.[1408–1417] Cryoglobulins are absent.[1409] Occasionally, fluorescent antinuclear antibody test results are positive. The erythrocyte sedimentation rate is greatly elevated. Some patients have evidence of underlying lymphoproliferative disease with the production of monoclonal immunoglobulins (see later). At the light microscopic level, a variety of lesions are observed, including MGN, proliferative glomerulonephritis, MCGN, crescentic glomerulonephritis, or nodular glomerulosclerosis.[1408–1417b] The capillary walls are usually greatly thickened with an increase in mesangial matrix. The deposits in the capillary wall are Congo red–negative, thioflavine T–negative, PAS-positive, and PAS–silver methenamine–positive. Amyloid P component may be present.[1409–1417] Electron microscopy is the definitive study because it reveals the fibrillar/microtubular nature of the deposits (see Table 30–15).

Two categories are recognized on the basis of their ultrastructural appearance; however, it is debated whether they represent two diseases or simply different phenotypes of the same fundamental lesion.[1408–1413] Fibrillary glomerulonephritis is often diagnosed when the deposits are composed of randomly oriented fibrils 10 to 30 nm in diameter (averaging 20 nm) located extracellularly within the glomerulus, usually in the mesangium and capillary walls.[1410–1413] The deposits are found in both subepithelial and subendothelial locations. By immunofluorescence, the deposits contain IgG and to a lesser extent IgM, IgA, and C3. The deposits commonly contain IgG4 and in less than 15% are monoclonal IgG κ.[1411] Rarely, the fibrillar deposits are negative for immunoglobulins.[1424] A familiar case with fibronectin deposits and mesangial abnormalities has been described.[1426] In comparison, primary amyloid (AL) fibrils are typically oriented randomly, are less than 10 nm in

diameter, and are monoclonal, either κ or λ (see Chapter 31). In fibrillary glomerulonephritis, it is uncommon for patients to have concomitant lymphoproliferative disease, such as a B cell lymphoma.[1411]

On the other hand, immunotactoid glomerulopathy, as originally described by Schwartz and Lewis,[1408, 1421] was named because of the deposits of microtubular structures often in a parallel array. The microtubules have diameters ranging between 18 and 90 nm (averaging 25 to 45 nm).[1408, 1409, 1414, 1421] The deposits always contain IgG and lesser amounts of C3. The variation in size of the fibrillar structures is greater than that observed for fibrillary glomerulonephritis. Nevertheless, there is some overlap in the size of fibrils between fibrillary and immunotactoid glomerulonephritis.[1411, 1412] Not uncommonly, monoclonality of the deposits can be detected, and several patients have had lymphoproliferative disorders leading to classification as a secondary glomerulopathy[1411, 1415, 1425] (see Chapter 31). Circulating and urinary monoclonal proteins have also been detected.[1411, 1415] On occasion, cryoimmunoglobulins of the mixed IgG/IgM variety have given rise to similar ultrastructural and immunopathologic appearances (see Chapter 31). The clinical manifestations of immunotactoid glomerulopathy are similar to those observed in fibrillary glomerulonephritis. Slow progression to end-stage renal disease is frequently seen, especially in patients with superimposed crescents and severe proliferation.[1412] Progression to end-stage renal disease may be seen somewhat more frequently in immunotactoid than in fibrillary glomerulonephritis.[1412] Treatment of fibrillary and immunotactoid glomerulopathies is generally unsatisfactory, although chemotherapy of an associated lymphoproliferative disorder may occasionally result in clinical resolution.[1408–1417, 1425] Both fibrillary and immunotactoid glomerulopathy have been noted to recur in renal allografts.[1409, 1411, 1417]

## COLLAGEN III GLOMERULOPATHY
### (Collagenofibrotic Glomerulopathy)

This lesion is also categorized as one of the nonamyloid fibrillary glomerular lesions because of the occurrence of Congo red–negative, thioflavine T–negative fibrillar deposits in glomeruli.[1427–1431] However, these deposits are known to be composed of collagen type III not normally present in glomeruli. These findings resemble those in nail-patella syndrome (see Chapter 31), but no bone or cutaneous abnormalities are found. This lesion was first described by Arakawa and co-workers[1427] in 1979, and several cases of this rare disorder have now been described from Japan, Italy, and the United States.[1428, 1431] Typically, patients with this disorder present with nephrotic or subnephrotic proteinuria occasionally complicated by hematuria, hypertension, and anemia.[1427–1431] Renal function is initially normal and then progressively declines. There is no family history of disease, and no osseous, nail, or cutaneous abnormalities are found.[1428] The erythrocyte sedimentation rate is greatly increased; otherwise, all laboratory findings are nonspecific.[1428, 1431] By light microscopy, the glomeruli are enlarged and lobulated, and the capillary wall shows double contours similar to those seen in MCGN.[1428–1431] The capillary walls are thickened with eosinophilic, PAS-negative,

PAS–silver methenamine–negative, Congo red–negative, and aniline blue–positive fibrillar deposits that are strongly reactive with trichrome stains.[1428] Acellular nodules, resembling those of intercapillary diabetic glomerulosclerosis, may also be seen.[1428] Chronic tubulointerstitial lesions may be encountered with accumulation of collagenous material around tubules. Electron microscopy reveals that the deposits are composed of randomly oriented collagen fibrils with typical periodicity having average diameters greater than 30 nm.[1428–1431] Immunofluorescence reveals scattered and nonspecific IgG, IgM, and C3 deposits. Monoclonal antibody studies have identified the collagen deposits as type III collagen.[1428] The pathogenesis of this disorder is unknown, but it may be related to nail-patella syndrome and be a molecular disorder of extracellular matrix formation (see Chapter 31). The course of disease is usually slowly progressive, and there is no known effective therapy.[1428–1431]

## LIPOPROTEIN GLOMERULOPATHY

This is a rare glomerular disease first described in Japan by Watanabe and co-workers[1432] in 1980 and Saito and colleagues[1433] in 1989. Patients usually present with nephrotic syndrome without extrarenal features to suggest a secondary disease.[1434] The plasma lipid profile is usually abnormal with a type III lipoprotein phenotype.[1434] However, unlike in familial lipoproteinemia, apolipoprotein E levels are greatly increased and the apolipoprotein E polymorphism is present. Lecithin–cholesterol acyltransferase levels are normal. Apolipoprotein E isoforms have usually been of the 2/3 or 4/4 type.[1434, 1435] Total cholesterol and lipid levels are rarely normal, but the apolipoprotein E levels are always increased.[1435] No familial tendency has yet been described.

The glomerular lesions consist of extensive deposition of lipoproteins, principally consisting of apolipoprotein E.[1434, 1435] Glomerular ''thrombi,'' mesangiolysis, and capillary ballooning (microaneurysms) are particularly common.[1432–1435] IgG deposition is variable, but IgA deposition has been observed.[1436] Persistence of nephrotic syndrome and slow progression are the rule. Probucol therapy may be effective and is likely to be the treatment of choice.[1436]

## C1q NEPHROPATHY

C1q nephropathy is an uncommon cause of the nephrotic syndrome. It was first delineated by Jennette and Hipp[1041, 1437] in 1985 and accounts for less than 3% of patients undergoing renal biopsy for heavy proteinuria.[1041, 1437, 1438] It is characterized by heavy mesangial deposition of C1q usually accompanied by IgG, IgM, or both. C3 deposition is also common. Electron-dense deposits are found in mesangial areas.[1438] By light microscopy, a variety of patterns are observed, including minimal changes, mesangial proliferative glomerulonephritis, or focal and segmental proliferative glomerulonephritis.[1437–1439] Typically, a nephrotic syndrome is present without any evidence of a multisystem disorder, including SLE.[1437] Males predominate and black persons are commonly affected.[1438] Laboratory findings are nonspecific, and low complement levels and anti-DNA antibodies are not seen. Most patients fail to respond to steroid treatment, and the renal survival is about 85% at 3 years.[1439] Initial elevated serum creatinine concentration is a poor prognostic sign. The pathogenesis is unknown but could be due to C1q binding to polyanionic antigens within mesangial deposits of immune complexes.[1041, 1440]

## FOCAL AND SEGMENTAL PROLIFERATIVE GLOMERULONEPHRITIS

A focal and segmental proliferative glomerular lesion has been described occasionally in patients who present clinically with the idiopathic nephrotic syndrome. However, with the passage of time and with more sophisticated diagnostic techniques, most of these cases in fact have been proved to be cases of initially unsuspected systemic or heredofamilial diseases, such as SLE, Schönlein-Henoch purpura, systemic angiitis, or Alport syndrome. IgA nephropathy is a common cause of focal and segmental proliferative glomerulonephritis and may also occasionally present initially as nephrotic syndrome. The distinguishing features of this lesion are that only segments of the glomerular tuft are affected and that normal glomeruli are also present. The proliferating cells are both endocapillary (mesangial) and extracapillary (i.e., focal and segmental crescents). In the extensive survey of idiopathic nephrotic syndrome in children carefully studied by Habib and co-workers,[814] no examples of this histologic variety were encountered. Similarly, few cases in adults were encountered in the United States Cooperative Study of the Adult Idiopathic Nephrotic Syndrome.[1244] Hematuria is commonly observed in this group. Most authors have indicated a generally favorable outcome in this group and a lack of response to steroids, although data on natural history in those cases presenting with nephrotic syndrome are scanty.[1]

## DIFFUSE CRESCENTIC GLOMERULONEPHRITIS

This lesion is distinctly uncommon in patients who present with the insidious onset of idiopathic nephrotic syndrome. Habib's group[814] described only 20 cases among 512 children, and the disorder is similarly uncommon in adults. Patients with this lesion usually have only a minority of the glomeruli affected with crescents. This lesion frequently progresses to more advanced disease (RPGN, see earlier), and the overall prognosis is poor. The response to therapy among those patients presenting with nephrotic syndrome is unknown. Spontaneous remissions may occur in those with prominent endocapillary proliferation and a background of infectious illness.

## DIFFUSE ENDOCAPILLARY PROLIFERATIVE GLOMERULONEPHRITIS

This lesion is usually the result of a prior infectious illness (see PSGN) and consists of extensive endocapillary proliferation with or without crescents. The capillary loops are frequently abnormal and may contain deposits. Exudative lesions may also be present. The findings in the peripheral capillary wall serve to distinguish this lesion from mesangial proliferative glomerulonephritis discussed earlier. This is an uncommon lesion among patients presenting with insidious onset of nephrotic syndrome. The natural history and response to therapy of this lesion are not well understood.

## DIFFUSE MESANGIAL SCLEROSIS

The appearance of heavy proteinuria at birth or shortly thereafter can often be traced to a heredofamilial disorder (Finnish-type congenital nephrotic syndrome, Chapter 31), to an underlying infectious disease (i.e., congenital syphilis or toxoplasmosis),[1441, 1442] or to an idiopathic primary glomerular disease. In the last category, several types of lesions have been observed. Diffuse mesangial sclerosis,[1, 1443] focal and segmental glomerular sclerosis, and mesangial proliferative glomerulonephritis have all been described, sometimes with a familial pattern of development. Diffuse mesangial sclerosis is a congenital glomerulopathy causing nephrotic syndrome in infants.[1443] It is often familial and demonstrates a progressive and treatment-resistant course. The female/male ratio is 1.6. It occurs in two forms, isolated diffuse mesangial sclerosis as a primary renal lesion, and in association with Drash syndrome of male pseudohermaphroditism and Wilms tumor (see Chapter 31). It appears to be a heterogeneous phenotype genetically related to abnormalities of the *WT1* gene locus on chromosome 11p13.[1443] Because of the high frequency of Wilms tumor in Drash syndrome, prophylactic bilateral nephrectomy may be advisable.[1443] The lesion of diffuse mesangial sclerosis consists of widespread glomerular involvement, resulting in global sclerosis in the absence of hypercellularity. Collagen fibrils may be observed. These cases generally begin within a few weeks of birth to as late as the first year and progress inexorably to renal failure and death before the age of 3 years. Severe nephrotic syndrome is the rule. No effective form of therapy is known. Transplantation may occasionally be possible. No recurrence in the allograft has yet been noted.

### *Acknowledgments*

The authors wish to thank Nancy Stinnett, Charlotte Townsend, and Carol Mitchell for their expert secretarial assistance and Jo-Anne Glassock for her invaluable library research.

## REFERENCES

1. Glassock RJ, Adler SG, Ward HJ, Cohen AH: Primary glomerular diseases. *In* Brenner BM, Rector FC Jr (eds): The Kidney, 4th ed. WB Saunders, Philadelphia, 1991, p 1182.
2. Iverson P, Brun C: Aspiration biopsy of the kidney. Am J Med 11:324, 1951.
3. Brun C, Raaschou F: Kidney biopsies. Am J Med 24:676, 1958.
4. Hudson BG, Wieslander J, Wisodom BJ, Noelken ME: Biology of disease. Goodpasture's syndrome: Molecular architecture and function of basement membrane antigen. Lab Invest 61:256, 1989.
5. Timpl R, Wiedmann H, Van Delden V, et al: A network model in the organization of type IV collagen molecules in basement membranes. Eur J Biochem 120:203, 1981.
6. Deen WM, Myers BD, Brenner BM: The glomerular barrier to macromolecules: Theoretical and experimental consideration in nephrotic syndrome. *In* Brenner BM, Stein JH (eds): Contemporary Issues in Nephrology. Churchill Livingstone, New York, 1982, p 1.
7. Schnabel E, Kriz W: Structure of the kidney. *In* Massry S, Glassock R (eds): Textbook of Nephrology, 3rd ed. Williams & Wilkins, Baltimore, 1995, pp 10–33.
8. Kashtan C, Fish A: Basement membrane and cellular components of the nephron. *In* Massry S, Glassock R (eds): Textbook of Nephrology, 3rd ed. Williams & Wilkins, Baltimore, 1995, pp 34–40.
9. Rosen S, Galvanek E, Levy M, Habib R: Glomerular disease. Hum Pathol 12:964, 1981.
10. Rosen S: Classification of glomerular disease. *In* Rosen S (ed): Pathology of Glomerular Disease. Churchill Livingstone, New York, 1983, p 1.
11. Cameron JS: A clinician's view of the classification of glomerulonephritis. *In* Kincaid-Smith P, Mathew TH, Becker EL (eds): Glomerulonephritis, Morphology, Natural History and Treatment. John Wiley & Sons, New York, 1973, p 63.
12. Churg J, Bernstein J, Glassock R: Renal Disease: Classification and Atlas of Glomerular Disease, 2nd ed. Igaku-Shoin Medical Publishers, New York, 1994.
13. Cameron JS, Glassock RJ: The Nephrotic Syndrome. Marcel Dekker, New York, 1988.
14. Rees A: The immunogenetics of glomerulonephritis. Kidney Int 45:377–383, 1994.
15. Rambausek MH, Waldherr R, Ritz E: Immunogenetic findings in glomerulonephritis. Kidney Int 43:S-3–S-8, 1993.
16. Lewy JE, Salinas-Madrigal L, Herdson PB, et al: Clinicopathologic correlations in acute poststreptococcal glomerulonephritis. Medicine (Baltimore) 50:453, 1971.
17. Lien JWK, Mathew TH, Meadows R: Acute post-streptococcal glomerulonephritis in adults: A long-term study. Q J Med 48:99, 1979.
18. Tejani A, Ingiulli A: Post-streptococcal glomerulonephritis: Current clinical and pathologic concepts. Nephron 55:1–5, 1990.
19. Glassock RJ: Immune complex–induced glomerular injury in viral diseases: An overview. Kidney Int 40:S-5–S-7, 1991.
20. Smith MC, Cooke JH, Zimmerman DM, et al: Asymptomatic glomerulonephritis after nonstreptococcal upper respiratory infections. Ann Intern Med 91:697, 1979.
21. Kaehny WD, Ozawa T, Schwartz MI, et al: Acute nephritis and pulmonary alveolitis following pneumococcal pneumonia. Arch Intern Med 138:806, 1978.
22. Forrest JW Jr, John F, Milk LR, et al: Immune complex glomerulonephritis associated with *Klebsiella pneumoniae* infection. Clin Nephrol 7:76, 1977.
23. Beaufils M: Glomerular disease complicating abdominal sepsis. Kidney Int 19:609, 1981.
24. Rainford DJ, Woodrow DF, Sloper JC, et al: Postmeningococcal acute glomerular nephritis. Clin Nephrol 9:249, 1978.
25. Ebright JR, Komorowski R: Gonococcal endocarditis associated with immune complex glomerulonephritis. Am J Med 68:793, 1980.
26. Sterzel RB, Krause PH, Zobl H, Kuhn K: Acute syphilitic nephrosis. A transient glomerular immunopathy. Clin Nephrol 2:164, 1974.
27. Dunea G, Kark RM, Lannigan R, et al: *Brucella* nephritis. Ann Intern Med 70:783, 1969.
28. Griffin RJ, Iseri LT, Boyle AJ, Myers BB: Studies of renal function in Weil's disease. Am J Med 10:514, 1951.
29. Sitprija V, Pipatanagul V, Boonpucknavig V, Boonpucknavig S: Glomerulitis in typhoid fever. Ann Intern Med 81:210, 1974.
30. Vitullo BB, O'Regan S, de Chadarevian J-P, Kaplan BS: *Mycoplasma* pneumonia associated with acute glomerulonephritis. Nephron 21:284, 1978.
31. Lin C-Y, Hsu H-C: Nephrotic syndrome associated with varicella infection. Pediatrics 75:1127, 1985.
32. Monteiro GE, Lillicrap CA: Case of mumps nephritis. Br Med J 4:721, 1967.
33. Lin C-Y, Hsu H-C: Measles and acute glomerulonephritis. Pediatrics 71:398–401, 1983.
34. Woodroffe AJ, Row PG, Meadows R, Lawrence JR: Nephritis in infectious mononucleosis. Q J Med 43:451, 1974.

35. Lee S, Kjellstrand CM: Renal disease in infectious mononucleosis. Clin Nephrol 9:236, 1978.
36. Ronco P, Verroust P, Morel-Maroger L: Viruses and glomerulonephritis. Nephron 31:97–102, 1982.
37. Mustonen J, Helin H, Pietila K, et al: Renal biopsy findings and clinicopathologic correlations in nephropathia epidemica. Clin Nephrol 41:121–126, 1994.
38. Ozawa T, Stewart JA: Immune-complex glomerulonephritis associated with cytomegalovirus infection. Am J Clin Pathol 72:103, 1979.
39. Bayatpour M, Zbitnew A, Dempster G, Miller KP: Role of coxsackie virus B in the pathogenesis of acute glomerulonephritis. Can Med Assoc J 109:873, 1973.
40. Fraser JRE, Cunningham AL, Muller HK, et al: Glomerulonephritis in the acute phase of Ross River virus disease (epidemic polyarthritis). Clin Nephrol 29:149, 1988.
41. Jeffrey RF, More IAR, Carrington D, et al: Acute glomerulonephritis following infection with *Chlamydia psittaci*. Am J Kidney Dis 20:94–96, 1992.
42. Allen AC, Spitz SA: A comparative study of pathology of scrub typhus (tsutsugamushi disease) and other rickettsial diseases. Am J Pathol 21:603, 1945.
43. Bradford WD, Croker BP, Tisher CC: Kidney lesions in Rocky Mountain spotted fever. Am J Pathol 97:381, 1979.
44. Perez-Fontan M, Huarte E, Tellez A, et al: Glomerular nephropathy associated with chronic Q fever. Am J Kidney Dis 11:298, 1988.
45. Quigg RJ, Gaines R, Wakely PE, Schoolwerth AC: Acute glomerulonephritis in a patient with Rocky Mountain spotted fever. Am J Kidney Dis 17:339–342, 1991.
46. Bullock WE, Artz RP, Bhathena D, Tung KSK: Histoplasmosis. Association with circulating immune complexes, eosinophilia, and mesangiopathic glomerulonephritis. Arch Intern Med 139:700, 1979.
47. Quattery JM, Milne J, House RK: Observations on hepatic and renal dysfunction in trichinosis. Anatomic changes in these organs occurring in a case of trichinosis. Am J Med 21:567, 1956.
48. Barsoum RS: Schistosomal glomerulopathies. Kidney Int 44:1–12, 1993.
49. Houba V: Immunopathology of nephropathies associated with malaria. Kidney Int 16:3, 1979.
50. Wickbom B, Winberg J: Coincidence of congenital toxoplasmosis and acute nephritis with nephrotic syndrome. Acta Paediatr Scand 61:470, 1972.
51. Ginsburg BE, Wasserman J, Huldt G, et al: Case of glomerulonephritis associated with acute toxoplasmosis. Br Med J 3:664, 1974.
52. Rodriguez-Iturbe B, Garcia R, Rubio L, et al: Acute glomerulonephritis in the Guillain-Barré-Strohl syndrome: A report of nine cases. Ann Intern Med 78:391, 1973.
53. Lemieux G: Charcot-Marie-Tooth disease and nephritis. Can Med Assoc J 96:1193, 1967.
54. Hopper J: Nephritis after irradiation and chemotherapy for nephroblastoma. Lancet 1:1281, 1974.
55. Rammelkamp CH Jr, Weaver RS: Acute glomerulonephritis. The significance of variations in the incidence of disease. J Clin Invest 32:345, 1953.
56. Rammelkamp CH Jr: Acute hemorrhagic glomerulonephritis. *In* McCarty M (ed): Streptococcal Infections. Columbia University Press, New York, 1954.
57. Stetson CA, Rammelkamp CH, Krause RM, et al: Epidemic acute nephritis: Studies on etiology, natural history and prevention. Medicine (Baltimore) 34:431, 1955.
58. Rodriguez-Iturbe B, Rubio L, Garcia R: Attack rate of poststreptococcal nephritis in families. A prospective study. Lancet 1:401, 1981.
59. Barnham M, Thornton TJ, Lange K: Nephritis caused by *Streptococcus zooepidemicus* (Lancefield group C). Lancet 1:945, 1983.
60. Read SE, Reid H, Poon-King T, et al: HLA and predisposition to the nonsuppurative sequelae of group A streptococcal infections. Transplant Proc 9:543, 1977.
61. Dillon HC: Streptococcal infections of the skin and their complications: Impetigo and nephritis. *In* Wannamaker IW, Matsen JM (eds): Streptococci and Streptococcal Diseases. Academic Press, New York, 1972, p 571.
62. Svartman M, Porter EV, Finklea JF, et al: Epidemic scabies and acute glomerulonephritis in Trinidad. Lancet 1:249, 1972.
63. Fish AJ, Herdman RC, Michael AF, et al: Epidemic acute glomerulonephritis associated with type 49 streptococcal pyoderma. II. Correlative study of light, immunofluorescent and electron microscopic findings. Am J Med 48:28, 1970.
64. Dillon HC Jr, Reeves MSA: Streptococcal immune responses and nephritis after skin infection. Am J Med 56:333, 1974.
65. Porter EV, Siegel AC, Simon NM, et al: Streptococcal infections and epidemic acute glomerulonephritis in South Trinidad. J Pediatr 72:871, 1968.
66. Kaplan EL, Anthony BF, Chapman SS, Wannamaker IW: Epidemic acute glomerulonephritis associated with type 49 streptococcal pyoderma. I. Clinical and laboratory findings. Am J Med 48:9, 1970.
67. Anthony BF, Kaplan EL, Wannamaker IW, et al: Attack rates of acute nephritis after type 49 streptococcal infections of the skin and respiratory tract. J Clin Invest 48:1697, 1969.
68. Rodriguez-Iturbe B: Epidemic post-streptococcal glomerulonephritis. Kidney Int 25:129, 1984.
69. Treser G, Semar M, Sagel I, et al: Independence of nephritogenicity of group A streptococci from their M types. Clin Exp Immunol 9:57, 1971.
70. Villarreal H, Fischetti VA, Van de Rijn I, Zabriskie JB: The occurrence of a protein in the extracellular products of streptococci isolated from patient with acute glomerulonephritis. J Exp Med 149:459, 1979.
71. Treser G, Ahmed V, Rodriguez I: Studies on the probable antigen of acute post-streptococcal glomerulonephritis. Proc Am Soc Nephrol 18:94, 1974.
72. Lange K, Seligson G, Cronin W: Evidence for the in-situ origin of post-streptococcal glomerulonephritis: Glomerular localization of endostreptosin and clinical significance of subsequent antibody response. Clin Nephrol 19:3, 1983.
73. Lange K, Ahmed V, Kleinberger H, Treser G: A hitherto unknown streptococcal antigen and its probable relation to acute post-streptococcal glomerulonephritis. Clin Nephrol 5:207, 1976.
74. Cronin WJ, Lange K: Immunologic evidence for the in situ deposition of a cytoplasmic streptococcal antigen (endostreptosin) on the glomerular basement membrane in rats. Clin Nephrol 34:143–146, 1990.
75. Mezzano S, Burgos E, Mahabir R, et al: Failure to detect unique reactivity to streptococcal streptokinase in either the sera or renal biopsy specimens of patients with acute poststreptococcal glomerulonephritis. Clin Nephrol 38:305–310, 1992.
76. Rodriguez-Iturbe B, Katujar VN, Coello J: Neuraminidase activity and free sialic acid levels in the serum of patients with acute poststreptococcal glomerulonephritis. N Engl J Med 304:1506, 1981.
77. Vogt A, Batsford S, Rodriguez-Iturbe B, Garcia R: Cationic antigens in poststreptococcal glomerulonephritis. Clin Nephrol 20:271, 1983.
78. Vilches AR, Williams DG: Persistent anti-DNA antibodies and DNA–anti-DNA complexes in poststreptococcal glomerulonephritis. Clin Nephrol 21:97, 1984.
79. Friedman J, van de Rijn I, Ohkuni H, et al: Immunological studies of post-streptococcal sequelae. Evidence for presence of streptococcal antigens in circulating immune complexes. J Clin Invest 74:1027, 1984.
80. Yoshimoto M, Hosoi S, Fujisawa S, et al: High levels of antibodies to streptococcal cell membrane antigens specifically bound to monoclonal antibodies in acute poststreptococcal glomerulonephritis. J Clin Microbiol 25:680, 1987.
81. Lee HA, Stirling G, Sharpstone P: Acute glomerulonephritis in middle-aged and elderly patients. Br Med J 2:1361, 1966.
82. Madaio MP, Harrington JT: The diagnosis of acute glomerulonephritis. N Engl J Med 309:1299, 1983.
83. Washio M, Oh Y, Okuda S, et al: Clinicopathological study of poststreptococcal glomerulonephritis in the elderly. Clin Nephrol 41:265–270, 1994.
84. Ferrario F, Kourilsky O, Morel-Maroger L: Acute endocapillary glomerulonephritis in adults: A histologic and clinical comparison between patients with and without initial acute renal failure. Clin Nephrol 19:17, 1983.
85. Balat A, Baysal K, Kocak H: Myocardial functions of children with acute poststreptococcal glomerulonephritis. Clin Nephrol 39:151–155, 1993.
86. Dodge WF, Spargo BH, Travis LB, et al: Poststreptococcal glomer-

ulonephritis, a prospective study in children. N Engl J Med 286:273, 1972.

87. Fairley KF, Birch DF: Hematuria: A simple method for identifying glomerular bleeding. Kidney Int 21:105, 1982.

88. Fassett RG, Horgan BA, Mathew TH: Detection of glomerular bleeding by phase-contrast microscopy. Lancet 1:1432, 1982.

89. Baldwin DS, Gluck MC, Schacht RG, Gallo G: The long-term course of poststreptococcal glomerulonephritis. Ann Intern Med 80:342, 1974.

90. Hinglais N, Garcia-Torres R, Kleinknecht D: Long-term prognosis in acute glomerulonephritis. The predictive value of early clinical and pathologic features observed in 65 patients. Am J Med 56:52, 1974.

91. Cortes P, Potter EV, Kwaan HC: Characterization and significance of urinary fibrin degradation products. J Lab Clin Med 82:377, 1973.

91a. Ozdemir S, Saatchi U, Besbas N, et al: Plasma atrial natriuretic peptide and endothelin levels in acute poststreptococcal glomerulonephritis. Pediatr Nephrol 6:519, 1992.

92. Parrish AE, Kramer NC, Hatch FE, et al: The relation between glomerular function and histology in acute glomerulonephritis. J Lab Clin Med 58:197, 1961.

93. Wilson RJ: Renal excretion of calcium and sodium in acute nephritis. Br Med J 4:713, 1969.

94. Don BR, Schambelan M: Hyperkalemia in acute glomerulonephritis due to transient hyporeninemic hypoaldosteronism. Kidney Int 38:1159–1163, 1990.

95. Leonard CD, Nagle RB, Striker GE, et al: Acute glomerulonephritis with prolonged oliguria. Ann Intern Med 73:703, 1970.

96. Anand SK, Trygstad CW, Sharma HM, Northway JD: Extracapillary proliferative glomerulonephritis in children. Pediatrics 56:434, 1975.

97. Ferrario F, Kourlisky O, Morel-Maroger L: Acute endocapillary glomerulonephritis in adults: A histological and clinical comparison between patients with and without initial acute renal failure. Clin Nephrol 19:17–23, 1983.

98. Seegal D, Lyttle JD, Loch EN, et al: On the exacerbation in chronic glomerulonephritis. J Clin Invest 19:569, 1940.

99. Dillon HC: Pyoderma and nephritis. Annu Rev Med 18:207, 1967.

100. Seligmann M, Danon F, Basch A, Bernard J: IgG myeloma cryoglobulin with antistreptolysin activity. Nature 220:711, 1968.

101. Bergner-Rabinowitz S, Fleiderman S, Ferne M, et al: The new streptozyme test for streptococcal antibodies. Clin Pediatr 14:804, 1975.

102. Kefalides WA, Pegg M, Ohno N, et al: Antibodies to basement membrane collagen and to laminin are present in sera from patient with poststreptococcal glomerulonephritis. J Exp Med 163:588, 1986.

103. Hebert LA, Cosio FG, Neff JC: Diagnostic significance of hypocomplementemia. Kidney Int 39:811–821, 1991.

104. Matsell DG, Roy S III, Tamerius JD, et al: Plasma terminal complement complexes in acute poststreptococcal glomerulonephritis. Am J Kidney Dis 17:311–316, 1991.

105. McLean RH, Schrager MA, Rothfield NF, Berman MM: Normal complement in early poststreptococcal glomerulonephritis. Br Med J 2:1326, 1977.

106. Lewis EJ, Carpenter CB, Schur PH: Serum complement levels in human glomerulonephritis. Ann Intern Med 75:55, 1971.

107. Cameron JS, Vick RM, Ogg CS, et al: Plasma C3 and C4 concentrations in the management of glomerulonephritis. Br Med J 3:668, 1973.

108. Sjoholm AG: Complement components and complement activation in acute poststreptococcal glomerulonephritis. Int Arch Allergy Appl Immunol 58:3, 1979.

109. Schreiber RD, Muller-Eberhard JJ: Complement and renal disease. In Wilson CB, Brenner BM, Stein JH (eds): Contemporary Issues in Nephrology, Vol 3. Churchill Livingstone, New York, 1979, p 67.

110. Williams DG, Pteres DK, Fallows J, et al: Studies of serum complement in the hypocomplementemic nephritides. Clin Exp Immunol 18:391, 1974.

111. Pickering RJ, Gewurz H, Good RA: Complement inactivation by serum from patients with acute and hypocomplementemic chronic glomerulonephritis. J Lab Clin Med 72:298, 1968.

112. Halbwachs L, Leveille M, Lesavre P, et al: Nephritic factor of the classical pathway of complement. Immunoglobulin G autoantibody directed against the classical pathway C3 convertase enzyme. J Clin Invest 65:1249, 1980.

113. Dodge WF, Travis LB, Haggard ME, et al: Studies of physiology during the early stage of acute glomerulonephritis in children. In Metcoff J (ed): Acute Glomerulonephritis. Little, Brown, Boston, 1967, p 319.

114. McIntosh RM, Kulvinskas C, Kaufman DB: Cryoglobulins II. The biological and chemical properties of cryoproteins in acute poststreptococcal glomerulonephritis. Int Arch Allergy Appl Immunol 41:700, 1971.

115. McIntosh RM, Griswold WR, Chernack WB, et al: Cryoglobulins. III. Further studies on the nature, incidence, clinical, diagnostic, prognostic and immunopathologic significance of cryoproteins in renal disease. Q J Med 44:285, 1975.

116. McIntosh RM, Garcia R, Rubio L, et al: Evidence of an autologous immune complex pathogenic mechanism in acute poststreptococcal glomerulonephritis. Kidney Int 14:501, 1978.

117. Rodriguez-Iturbe B, Carr RI, Garcia R, et al: Circulating immune complexes and serum immunoglobulins in acute poststreptococcal glomerulonephritis. Clin Nephrol 13:1, 1980.

118. Yoshizawa N, Treser G, McClung JA, et al: Circulating immune complexes in patients with uncomplicated group A streptococcal pharyngitis and patients with acute poststreptococcal glomerulonephritis. Am J Nephrol 3:23, 1983.

119. Mezzano S, Olavarria F, Ardiles L, et al: Incidence of circulating immune complexes in patients with acute poststreptococcal glomerulonephritis and in patients with streptococcal impetigo. Clin Nephrol 26:61, 1987.

120. Sesso RC, Ramos OL, Periera AB: Detection of IgG-rheumatoid factor in sera of patients with acute poststreptococcal glomerulonephritis and its relationship with circulating immune complexes. Clin Nephrol 26:55, 1986.

121. Ekert H, Powell H, Muntz R: Hypercoagulability in acute glomerulonephritis. Lancet 1:965, 1972.

122. Ekberg M, Nilsson IM: Factor VIII and glomerulonephritis. Lancet 1:1111, 1975.

123. Alkjaersig NK, Fletcher AP, Lewis ML, et al: Pathophysiological response of blood coagulation systems in acute glomerulonephritis. Kidney Int 10:319, 1976.

124. Adhikari M, Coovadia HM, Greig DBW, Christensen S: Factor VIII procoagulant activity in children with nephrotic syndrome and poststreptococcal glomerulonephritis. Nephron 22:301, 1978.

125. Kaplan BS, Esseltine D: Thrombocytopenia in patients with acute poststreptococcal glomerulonephritis. J Pediatr 93:974, 1978.

126. Mezzano S, Kunick M, Olavarria F, et al: Detection of platelet activating-factor in plasma of patients with streptococcal nephritis. J Am Soc Nephrol 4:235, 1993.

127. Ruley EJ, Huang SW, Plant J, Morris N: Defective phagocyte adherence in acute poststreptococcal glomerulonephritis—clinical and laboratory observations. J Pediatr 89:748, 1976.

128. Bhat JG, Gombos EA, Baldwin DS: Depressed cellular immune response to streptococcal antigens in poststreptococcal glomerulonephritis. Clin Immunol Immunopathol 7:2130, 1977.

129. Fillit HM, Read SE, Sherman RL, et al: Cellular reactivity to altered glomerular basement membrane in glomerulonephritis. N Engl J Med 298:861, 1978.

130. Yoshizawa N, Oshima S, Sagel I, et al: Role of a streptococcal antigen in the pathogenesis of acute poststreptococcal glomerulonephritis. Characterization of the antigen and a proposed mechanism for the disease. J Immunol 148:3110, 1992.

130a. Poon-King R, Bannan J, Viteri A, et al: Identification of an extracellular plasmin binding protein from nephritogenic streptococci. J Exp Med 178:759, 1993.

131. Baldwin DS, Gluck MC, Schacht RG, Gallo G: The long-term prognosis of post-streptococcal glomerulonephritis. Ann Intern Med 80:342, 1974.

132. Jennings RB, Earle DP: Poststreptococcal glomerulonephritis: Histopathologic and clinical studies of the acute, subsiding acute and early chronic latent phases. J Clin Invest 40:1525, 1961.

133. Inglefinger JR, McCluskey RT, Scheenberger EE, Grupe WE: Necrotizing arteritis in acute poststreptococcal glomerulonephritis. J Pediatr 91:228, 1977.

134. Gill DG, Turner DR, Chantler C, Cameron JS: The progression of acute proliferative poststreptococcal glomerulonephritis to severe epithelial crescent formation. Clin Nephrol 8:445, 1977.

135. Fairley K, Matthews DC, Becker GJ: Rapid development of diffuse crescents in poststreptococcal glomerulonephritis. Clin Nephrol 26:256, 1987.

136. Modai D, Pik A, Behar M, et al: Biopsy proven evolution of poststreptococcal glomerulonephritis to a rapidly progressive glomerulonephritis. Clin Nephrol 23:198, 1985.

137. Richet G, Fillastre JP, Morel-Maroger L, Bariety J: Change from diffuse proliferative to membranous glomerulonephritis. Serial biopsies in four cases. Kidney Int 5:57, 1974.

138. Andres GL, Accinni L, Hsu KC, et al: Electron microscopic studies of human glomerulonephritis with ferritin conjugated antibody. J Exp Med 123:399, 1966.

139. Tornroth T: The fate of subepithelial deposits in acute poststreptococcal glomerulonephritis. Lab Invest 35:461, 1976.

140. Urizar RE, Singh JK, Muhammad J: Henoch-Schönlein anaphylactoid purpura nephropathy. Electron microscopic lesions mimicking acute poststreptococcal nephritis. Hum Pathol 9:223, 1978.

141. Habib R, Levy M: Membranoproliferative glomerulonephritis. *In* Hamburger J, Crosnier J, Grünfeld J-P (eds): Nephrology. Wiley-Flammarion, Paris, 1979.

142. Sorger K, Gessler U, Hübner FK, et al: Subtypes of post-infectious glomerulonephritis. Synopsis of clinical and pathological features. Clin Nephrol 17:114, 1982.

143. Sorger K, Balun J, Hübner FK, et al: The garland type of acute post-infectious glomerulonephritis: Morphological characteristics and follow-up studies. Clin Nephrol 20:17, 1983.

144. Edelstein CL, Bates WD: Subtypes of acute postinfectious glomerulonephritis: A clinico-pathological correlation. Clin Nephrol 38:311–317, 1992.

145. Nand N, Argent NB, Morley AR, Ward MK: Garland pattern poststreptococcal glomerulonephritis. Nephrol Dial Transplant 7:155–157, 1992.

146. Sorger S, Gessler MN, Hübner FK, et al: Follow-up studies of three subtypes of acute postinfectious glomerulonephritis ascertained by renal biopsy. Clin Nephrol 27:111, 1987.

147. Ossi E, Prezyna A, Sepulveda M, et al: Immune deposits in the spleen of a patient with acute poststreptococcal glomerulonephritis. Clin Immunol Immunopathol 6:306, 1976.

148. Morel-Maroger L, Kourilsky D, Mignon F, Richet G: Antitubular basement membrane antibodies in rapidly progressive poststreptococcal glomerulonephritis: Report of a case. Clin Immunol Immunopathol 2:185, 1974.

149. Lange K, Treser G: Acute poststreptococcal glomerulonephritis: Mechanisms and sequelae—attempts at a unifying concept. Clin Nephrol 1:55, 1973.

150. McIntosh RM, Rabideau D, Allen JE, et al: Acute poststreptococcal glomerulonephritis in Maracaibo. II. Studies of the incidence, nature, and significance of circulating anti-immunoglobulins. Ann Rheum Dis 38:257, 1979.

151. Yoshizawa N, Treser G, Sagel I, et al: Demonstration of antigenic sites in glomeruli of patients with acute poststreptococcal glomerulonephritis by immunofluorescence and immunoferritin technique. Am J Pathol 70:131, 1973.

152. Treser G, Ahmed U, Rodriguez-Iturbe B: Studies on the probable antigen of acute poststreptococcal glomerulonephritis. Kidney Int 6:107A, 1974.

153. Rodriguez-Iturbe B, Silva-Beauperthny Y, Piarra G, et al: Similar immune response to normal human IgG in patients with rheumatoid arthritis and acute poststreptococcal glomerulonephritis. Am J Clin Pathol 76:270, 1981.

154. Mosquera JA, Rodriguez-Iturbe B: Granular binding sites for peanut agglutinin in acute postinfectious glomerulonephritis. Clin Nephrol 26:227, 1986.

155. Drachman R, Aladjem M, Vardy PA: Natural history of an acute glomerulonephritis epidemic in children: An 11- to 12-year follow-up. Isr J Med Sci 18:603, 1982.

156. Vogl W, Renke M, Mayer-Eichberger D, et al: Long-term prognosis in endocapillary glomerulonephritis of poststreptococcal type in children and adults. Nephron 74:58, 1986.

157. Mota-Hernandez F, Briseno-Mondragon E, Gordillo-Paniagun G: Glomerular lesions and final outcome in children with glomerulonephritis of acute onset. Nephron 16:272, 1976.

158. Nissenson AR, Mayon-White R, Potter EV, et al: Continued absence of clinical renal disease seven to twelve years after poststreptococcal acute glomerulonephritis in Trinidad. Am J Med 67:255, 1979.

159. Travis LB, Dodge WF, Beathard GA, et al: Acute glomerulonephritis in children: A review of the natural history with emphasis on prognosis. Clin Nephrol 1:169, 1973.

160. Kaplan EL, Vernier RL: Progressive nephritis after strep infection questioned. Am J Med 64:910, 1978.

161. Potter EV, Abidh S, Sharrett AR, et al: Clinical healing two to six years after poststreptococcal glomerulonephritis in Trinidad. N Engl J Med 298:767, 1978.

162. Potter EV, Lipschultz SA, Abidh S, et al: Twelve to seventeen-year follow-up of patients with poststreptococcal acute glomerulonephritis in Trinidad. N Engl J Med 307:725, 1982.

163. Baldwin DS: Poststreptococcal glomerulonephritis. A progressive disease? Am J Med 62:1, 1977.

164. Baldwin DS, Schacht RG: Late sequelae of poststreptococcal glomerulonephritis. Annu Rev Med 27:49, 1976.

165. Garcia R, Rubio L, Rodriguez-Iturbe B: Long-term prognosis of epidemic poststreptococcal glomerulonephritis in Maracaibo: Follow-up studies 11–12 years after the acute episode. Clin Nephrol 15:291, 1981.

166. Popovic-Ralovic M, Kostic M, Antic-Pew A, et al: Medium and long-term prognosis of patients with acute post-streptococcal glomerulonephritis. Nephron 58:393–399, 1991.

167. Buzio C, Allegri L, Mutti A, et al: Significance of albuminuria in the follow-up of acute poststreptococcal glomerulonephritis. Clin Nephrol 41:259–264, 1994.

168. Melby PC, Musick WD, Luger AM, Khana R: Poststreptococcal glomerulonephritis in the elderly. Report of a case and review of the literature. Am J Nephrol 7:235, 1987.

169. Schacht RG, Steele JM Jr, Lowenstein J, Baldwin DS: Failure of sodium restriction to abolish exaggerated natriuresis in poststreptococcal glomerulonephritis. Nephron 18:333, 1977.

170. Nissenson AR, Mayon-White R, Potter EV, et al: Effect of sodium loading on sodium excretion in patients recovered from poststreptococcal acute glomerulonephritis. Cardiovasc Med 6:779, 1977.

171. Velhote V, Saldanha LB, Malheirops P, et al: Acute glomerulonephritis: Three episodes documented by light and electron microscopy and immunofluorescence studies—a case report. Clin Nephrol 26:307, 1986.

172. Glotz D, Jouvin MH, Nochy D, et al: Recurrent acute glomerulonephritis. Am J Kidney Dis 17:228–230, 1991.

173. Parra G, Rodriguez-Iturbe B, Colina-Chourio J, Garcia R: Short-term treatment with captopril in hypertension due to acute glomerulonephritis. Clin Nephrol 29:58, 1988.

174. Robson AM, Cole BR, Kienstra RA, et al: Severe glomerulonephritis complicated by coagulopathy. Treatment with anticoagulant and immunosuppressive drugs. J Pediatr 90:881, 1977.

175. Boulton-Jones JM, Sissons JG, Naish PF, et al: Self-induced glomerulonephritis. Br Med J 3:387, 1974.

176. Baldwin DS, Neugarten J, Feiner HD, et al: The existence of a protracted course in crescentic glomerulonephritis. Kidney Int 31:790, 1987.

177. Couser WG: Rapidly progressive glomerulonephritis: Classification, pathogenetic mechanisms and therapy. Am J Kidney Dis 11:449, 1988.

178. Salant DJ: Immunopathogenesis of crescentic glomerulonephritis and lung purpura. Kidney Int 32:408, 1987.

179. Andrassy K, Kuster S, Waldherr R, Ritz E: Rapidly progressive glomerulonephritis: Analysis of prevalence and clinical course. Nephron 59:206–212, 1991.

180. Takeda S, Kida H, Yokoyama H, et al: Two distinct types of crescentic glomerulonephritis. Clin Nephrol 37:285–293, 1992.

181. Rondeau E: Current treatment of crescentic glomerulonephritis. J Nephrol 6:14–21, 1993.

182. Yoshioka K, Takemura T, Akano N, et al: Cellular and non-cellular compositions of crescents in human glomerulonephritis. Kidney Int 32:284, 1987.

183. Jennette JC, Hipp CG: The epithelial antigen phenotype of glomerular crescent cells. Am J Clin Pathol 86:274, 1986.

184. Atkins RC, Holdsworth SR, Glasgow EF, Matthews F: The macrophage in human rapidly progressive glomerulonephritis. Lancet 1:830, 1976.

185. Glassock R: A clinical and immunopathologic dissection of rapidly progressive glomerulonephritis. Nephron 22:253, 1978.

186. Nishikawa K, Guo YJ, Miyasaka M, et al: Antibodies to intercellular adhesion molecule 1/lymphocyte function–associated antigen

1 prevent crescent formation in rat autoimmune glomerulonephritis. J Exp Med 177:667–677, 1993.

187. Nishikawa K, Andres G, Bhan A, et al: Hyaluronate is a component of crescents in rat autoimmune glomerulonephritis. Lab Invest 68:146–153, 1993.

188. Cattell V, Jamieson SW: The origin of glomerular crescents in experimental nephrotoxic serum nephritis in the rabbit. Lab Invest 39:584, 1978.

189. Thomson NM, Holdsworth SR, Glasgow EF, et al: Mechanisms of injury in experimental glomerulonephritis. *In* Kincaid-Smith P, d'Apice AJF, Atkins RC (eds): Progress in Glomerulonephritis. John Wiley & Sons, New York, 1979, p 1851.

190. Atkins RC, Glasgow EF, Holdsworth SR, et al: Tissue culture of isolated glomeruli from patients with glomerulonephritis. Kidney Int 17:515, 1980.

191. Schwartz BS, Levy GA, Edington TS: Immune complex induced human monocyte procoagulant activity: Cellular kinetics and metabolic requirements. J Immunol 128:1037, 1982.

192. Holdsworth SR, Tipping DG: Macrophage-induced glomerular fibrin deposits in experimental glomerulonephritis in the rabbit. J Clin Invest 76:1367, 1985.

193. Hoyer J, Michael AF, Hoyer L: Immunofluorescent localization of antihemophilic factor antigen and fibrinogen in human renal disease. J Clin Invest 53:1375, 1974.

194. Korn JH, Pickles FR, Ewan VA, et al: Mononuclear cell modulation of fibroblast procoagulant activity. J Lab Clin Med 99:657, 1982.

195. Angangco R, Thiru S, Esnault VLM, et al: Does truly 'idiopathic' crescentic glomerulonephritis exist? Nephrol Dial Transplant 9:630–636, 1994.

196. Ferrario F, Tadros MT, Napodano P, et al: Critical re-evaluation of 41 cases of "idiopathic" crescentic glomerulonephritis. Clin Nephrol 41:1–9, 1994.

197. Couser WG: Idiopathic rapidly progressive glomerulonephritis. Am J Nephrol 2:57, 1982.

198. Lewis EJ, Schwartz MM: Idiopathic crescentic glomerulonephritis. Semin Nephrol 2:193, 1982.

199. Neild GH, Cameron JS, Ogg CS, et al: Rapidly progressive glomerulonephritis with extensive crescent formation. Q J Med 52:395, 1983.

200. Lerner RA, Glassock RJ, Dixon FJ: The role of antiglomerular basement membrane antibody in the pathogenesis of human glomerulonephritis. J Exp Med 126:989, 1967.

201. Briggs WA, Johnson JP, Tiechman S, et al: Antiglomerular basement membrane antibody–mediated glomerulonephritis and Goodpasture's syndrome. Medicine (Baltimore) 58:348, 1979.

202. Savage COS, Pusey CD, Bowman C, et al: Anti–glomerular basement membrane antibody–mediated disease in the British Isles 1980–1984. Br Med J 292:301, 1986.

203. Senekjian HO, Knight HO, Weinman EJ: The spectrum of renal diseases associated with anti–basement membrane antibodies. Arch Intern Med 140:79, 1980.

204. Turner N, Rees AJ: Antiglomerular basement membrane disease. *In* Cameron J, Davison A, Grünfeld JP, Ritz E (eds): Oxford Textbook of Clinical Nephrology. Oxford Medical Publishers, London, 1992.

205. Kelly PT, Haponik EF: Goodpasture's syndrome: Molecular and clinical advances. Medicine (Baltimore) 73:171–185, 1994.

206. Border WA, Bachler RW, Bhathena D, Glassock RJ: IgA antibasement membrane nephritis with pulmonary hemorrhage. Ann Intern Med 91:21, 1979.

207. Ravnskov U: Possible mechanisms of hydrocarbon-associated glomerulonephritis. Clin Nephrol 23:294, 1985.

208. Wilson CB, Dixon FJ: Antiglomerular basement membrane antibody–induced glomerulonephritis. Kidney Int 3:74, 1973.

209. Zimmerman SW, Groehler K, Beirne GJ: Hydrocarbon exposure and chronic glomerulonephritis. Lancet 2:199, 1975.

210. Walker RG, Scheinkestel C, Becker GJ, et al: Clinical and morphological aspects of the management of crescentic anti–glomerular basement membrane antibody (anti-GBM) nephritis/Goodpasture's syndrome. Q J Med 54:75, 1985.

211. Ewan PW, Jones HA, Rhodes CG, Hughes J: Detection of intrapulmonary hemorrhage with carbon monoxide uptake. Application in Goodpasture's syndrome. N Engl J Med 295:1391, 1976.

212. Donaghy M, Rees AJ: Cigarette smoking and lung haemorrhage in glomerulonephritis caused by autoantibodies to glomerular basement membrane. Lancet 2:1390, 1983.

213. Rees AJ, Lockwood CM, Peters DK: Enhanced allergic tissue injury in Goodpasture's syndrome by intercurrent bacterial infection. Br Med J 2:723, 1977.

214. McPhaul JJ Jr, Dixon FJ: The presence of anti–glomerular basement membrane antibodies in peripheral blood. J Immunol 103:1168, 1969.

215. Lockwood CM, Bowman C, Bakes D, et al: Autoimmunity in glomerulonephritis. Adv Nephrol 16:291, 1987.

216. Segelmark M, Butkowski R, Wieslander J: Antigen restriction and IgG subclasses among anti-GBM autoantibodies. Nephrol Dial Transplant 5:991–996, 1990.

217. Hellmark T, Johansson C, Wieslander J: Characterization of anti-GBM antibodies involved in Goodpasture's syndrome. Kidney Int 46:823–829, 1994.

218. Hudson BG, Kalluri R, Gunwar S, et al: Molecular characteristics of the Goodpasture autoantigen. Kidney Int 43:135–139, 1993.

219. Saxena R, Bygren P, Butkowski R, Wieslander J: Entactin: A possible autoantigen in the pathogenesis of non-Goodpasture anti-GBM nephritis. Kidney Int 38:263–272, 1990.

220. Rees AJ, Peters DK, Compston DAS, Batchelor JR: Strong association between HLA DRW2 and antibody-mediated Goodpasture's syndrome. Lancet 1:966, 1978.

221. Huey B, McCormick K, Capper J, et al: Associations of HLA-DQ types with anti-GBM nephritis by sequence-specific oligonucleotide probe hybridization. Kidney Int 44:307–312, 1993.

222. Savage COS, Lockwood CM: Antineutrophil antibodies in vasculitis. Adv Nephrol 19:225, 1990.

223. Boucher A, Droz D, Adafer E, Noel L-H: Relationship between the integrity of Bowman's capsule and the composition of cellular crescents in human crescentic glomerulonephritis. Lab Invest 56:526, 1987.

224. Bolton WK, Innes DJ, Sturgill BC, Kaiser DL: T cells and macrophages in rapidly progressive glomerulonephritis: Clinicopathologic correlations. Kidney Int 32:869, 1987.

225. Morita T, Suzuki Y, Churg J: Structure and development of the glomerular crescent. Am J Pathol 72:349, 1973.

226. Burkholder PM: Ultrastructural demonstration of injury and perforation of glomerular capillary basement membrane in acute proliferative glomerulonephritis. Kidney Int 5:47, 1974.

227. Min KW, Gyorkey F, Gyorkey P, et al: The morphogenesis of glomerular crescents in rapidly progressive glomerulonephritis. Kidney Int 5:47, 1974.

228. Bohman S-O, Olsen S, Petersen VP: Glomerular ultrastructure in extracapillary glomerulonephritis. Acta Pathol Microbiol Scand Suppl 249:29, 1974.

229. Stejskal J, Pirani CL, Okada M, et al: Discontinuities (gaps) of the glomerular capillary wall and basement membrane in renal disease. Lab Invest 28:149, 1973.

230. Wu M-J, Rajaram R, Shelp WD, et al: Vasculitis in Goodpasture's syndrome. Arch Pathol Lab Med 104:300, 1980.

231. Olsen S, Petersen VP, Hansen ES: Immunofluorescent studies of extracapillary glomerulonephritis. Acta Pathol Microbiol Scand Suppl 249:20, 1974.

232. Andres G, Brentjens J, Kohli R, et al: Histology of human tubulo-interstitial nephritis associated with antibodies in renal basement membranes. Kidney Int 13:480, 1978.

233. Bonsib SM: Glomerular basement membrane discontinuities: Scanning electron microscopic study of acellular glomeruli. Am J Pathol 119:357, 1985.

234. Savige J, Dowling J, Kincaid-Smith P: Superimposed glomerular immune complexes in anti–glomerular basement membrane disease. Am J Kidney Dis 14:145, 1989.

235. McPhaul JJ Jr, Mullins JD: Glomerulonephritis mediated by antibody to glomerular basement membrane. Immunological, clinical and histopathological characteristics. J Clin Invest 57:351, 1976.

236. Glassock RJ: The pathogenesis of crescentic glomerulonephritis. *In* Remuzzi G (ed): Glomerulonephritis. Wichtig Editore, Milan, 1984.

237. Saus J, Wieslander J, Langeveld JPM, et al: Identification of the Goodpasture's antigen in the $\alpha_3$ (IV) strain of collagen IV. J Biol Chem 263:1337, 1988.

238. Johnson JP, Moore J Jr, Austin HA III, et al: Therapy of antiglomerular basement membrane antibody disease: Analysis of prognostic significance of clinical, pathologic and treatment factors. Medicine (Baltimore) 64:219, 1985.

239. Merkel F, Pullig O, Marx M, et al: Course and prognosis of anti–

basement membrane antibody mediated disease: Report of 35 cases. Nephrol Dial Transplant 9:372–376, 1994.

240. O'Meara Y, Salant D: Management of glomerular disease of primary and secondary origin. Curr Opin Nephrol Hypertens 1:124–132, 1992.

241. Herody M, Bobrie G, Gouarin C, et al: Anti-GBM disease: Predictive value of clinical, histological and serological data. Clin Nephrol 40:249–255, 1993.

242. Heilman RL, Offord KP, Holley KE, Velosa JA: Analysis of risk factors for patient and renal survival in crescentic glomerulonephritis. Am J Kidney Dis 9:98, 1987.

243. Flores JC, Taube D, Savage COS, et al: Clinical and immunological evolution of oligoanuric anti-GBM nephritis treated by haemodialysis. Lancet 1:5, 1986.

244. Hind CRK, Paraskevakou H, Lockwood CM, et al: Prognosis after immunosuppression of patients with crescentic nephritis requiring dialysis. Lancet 1:263, 1983.

245. Peters DK, Rees AJ, Lockwood CM, Pusey CD: Treatment and prognosis in anti–basement membrane antibody–mediated nephritis. Transplant Proc 14:513, 1982.

246. Boyce N, Holdsworth S, Atkins R, Dowling J: De novo anti-GBM antibody induced glomerulonephritis in a renal transplant. Clin Nephrol 23:148, 1985.

247. Almquist RD, Buckalew VM Jr, Hirszel P, et al: Recurrence of anti–glomerular basement membrane antibody mediated glomerulonephritis in an isograft. Clin Immunol Immunopathol 18:54, 1981.

248. Ulu MJ, Moorthy AV, Beisne GJ: Relapse in anti–glomerular basement membrane antibody mediated crescentic glomerulonephritis. Clin Nephrol 13:97, 1980.

249. Hind CRK, Bowman C, Winearls CG, Lockwood CM: Recurrence of circulating anti–glomerular basement membrane antibody three years after immunosuppressive treatment and plasma exchange. Clin Nephrol 21:244, 1984.

250. Strauch BS, Charney A, Doctorouff S, Kashgarian M: Goodpasture's syndrome with recovery after renal failure. JAMA 229:444, 1974.

251. Pusey CD, Lockwood CM: Plasma exchange for glomerular disease. *In* Robinson RR (ed): Nephrology. Springer-Verlag, New York, 1984, p 1474.

252. Lockwood CM, Rees AJ, Pearson TA, et al: Immunosuppression and plasma exchange in the treatment of Goodpasture's syndrome. Lancet 1:711, 1976.

253. Lang CH, Brown DC, Staley N, et al: Goodpasture's syndrome treated with immuno-suppression and plasma exchange. Arch Intern Med 137:1076, 1977.

254. Johnson JP, Whitman W, Briggs WA, Wilson CB: Plasmapheresis and immunosuppressive agents in anti–basement membrane antibody–induced Goodpasture's syndrome. Am J Med 64:354, 1978.

255. Kincaid-Smith P, d'Apice AJF: Plasmapheresis in rapidly progressive glomerulonephritis. Am J Med 65:564, 1978.

256. Lockwood CM, Pussell B, Wilson CB, Peters DK: Plasma exchange in nephritis. Adv Nephrol 8:383, 1979.

257. McKenzie PE, Taylor AE, Woodroffe AJ, et al: Plasmapheresis in glomerulonephritis. Clin Nephrol 12:97, 1979.

258. Bolton WK: Pulse methylprednisolone therapy of rapidly progressive glomerulonephritis. Contrib Nephrol 3:213, 1981.

259. Thysell H, Bygren P, Bengtsson U, et al: Immunosuppression and the additive effect of plasma exchange in treatment of rapidly progressive glomerulonephritis. Acta Med Scand 212:107, 1982.

260. Glassock RJ: The role of high-dose steroids in nephritic syndromes: The case for a conservative approach. *In* Narins R (ed): Controversies in Nephrology and Hypertension. Churchill Livingstone, New York, 1984, p 409.

261. Bolton WK: The role of high dose steroids in nephritic syndromes: The case for aggressive use. *In* Narins R (ed): Controversies in Nephrology and Hypertension. Churchill Livingstone, New York, 1984, p 421.

262. Bruns FJ, Fraley DS, Adler S, Segel DP: Megadose methylprednisolone versus plasmapheresis in treatment of rapidly progressive glomerulonephritis (RPGN). Kidney Int 19:121, 1981.

263. Kincaid-Smith P: Anticoagulants are of value in the treatment of renal disease. Am J Kidney Dis 3:299, 1984.

264. Border WA, Glassock RJ: Coagulation in renal disease. *In* Suki W, Eknoyan G (eds): The Kidney in Systemic Disease. John Wiley & Sons, New York, 1980.

265. Vassalli P, McCluskey RT: The pathogenetic role of the coagulation process in rabbit Masugi nephritis. Am J Pathol 45:653, 1964.

266. Thomson N, Moran J, Simpson I, Peters DK: Defibrination with ancrod in nephrotoxic serum nephritis. Kidney Int 10:343, 1976.

267. Zoya C, Corna D, Macconi D, et al: Tissue plasminogen activator therapy of rabbit nephrotoxic nephritis. Lab Invest 62:34, 1990.

268. Beaufils M, Morel-Maroger L, Sraer JD, et al: Acute renal failure of glomerular origin during visceral abscesses. N Engl J Med 295:185, 1976.

269. Muller G, Gebhardt M, Kompf J, et al: Association between rapidly progressive glomerulonephritis and properdin factor BfF and different HLA-D region products. Kidney Int 25:115, 1984.

270. Bolton WK: Use of pulse methylprednisolone in primary and multisystem glomerular diseases. *In* Robinson RR (ed): Nephrology. Springer-Verlag, New York, 1984, p 1464.

271. Rose GM, Cole BR, Robson AM: The treatment of severe glomerulopathies in children using high-dose intravenous methylprednisolone pulses. Am J Kidney Dis 1:148, 1981.

272. McDougal BA, Whittier FC, Dross DE: Sudden death after bolus steroid therapy for acute rejection. Transplant Proc 8:493, 1976.

273. O'Neill WM, Etheridge WB, Bloomer HA: High-dose corticosteroids. Their use in treating idiopathic rapidly progressive glomerulonephritis. Arch Intern Med 139:514, 1979.

274. Glassock RJ: Intensive plasma exchange in crescentic glomerulonephritis: Help or no help? Am J Kidney Dis 20:270–275, 1992.

275. Jennette JC, Falk RJ: Antineutrophil cytoplasmic autoantibodies and associated diseases: A review. Am J Kidney Dis 15:517–529, 1990.

276. Falk RJ, Hogan S, Carey TS, Jennette JC, and the Glomerular Disease Collaborative Network: Clinical course of anti-neutrophil cytoplasmic autoantibody–associated glomerulonephritis and systemic vasculitis. Ann Intern Med 1131:656–663, 1990.

277. Geffriaud-Ricourard C, Noel LH, Chauveau D, et al: Clinical spectrum associated with ANCA of defined antigen specificities in 98 selected patients. Clin Nephrol 39:125–136, 1993.

278. Kallenberg CGM, Mulder AHL, Tervaert JW: Antineutrophil cytoplasmic antibodies: A still-growing class of autoantibodies in inflammatory disorders. Am J Med 93:675–682, 1992.

279. Robinson AJ: Antineutrophil cytoplasmic antibodies (ANCA) and the systemic necrotizing vasculitides. Nephrol Dial Transplant 9:119–126, 1994.

280. Cohen AH, Border WA, Shankel E, Glassock RJ: Crescentic glomerulonephritis: Immune or nonimmune pathogenesis. Am J Nephrol 1:78, 1981.

281. Falk RJ, Jennette JC: Antineutrophil cytoplasmic autoantibodies with specificity and/or myeloperoxidase in patients with systemic vasculitis and idiopathic necrotizing and crescentic glomerulonephritis. N Engl J Med 318:1651, 1988.

281a. Jones CL, Shields M, Eddy AA, et al: Pulmonary hemorrhage and necrotizing glomerulonephritis without glomerular immune deposits: Report of two cases. Am J Kidney Dis 18:257–263, 1991.

282. Jennette JC, Falk RJ: Diagnostic classification of antineutrophil cytoplasmic autoantibody–associated vasculitides. Am J Kidney Dis 18:184–187, 1991.

283. Kallenberg CGM, Brouwer E, Weening JJ, et al: Anti-neutrophil cytoplasmic antibodies: Current diagnostic and pathophysiological potential. Kidney Int 46:1–15, 1994.

284. Bonsib SM, Goeken JA, Kemp JD, et al: Coexistent anti-neutrophil cytoplasmic antibody and antiglomerular basement membrane antibody associated disease: Report of six cases. Mod Pathol 6:526–530, 1993.

285. Weber MFA, Andrassy K, Pullig O, et al: Antineutrophil-cytoplasmic antibodies and antiglomerular basement membrane antibodies in Goodpasture's syndrome and in Wegener's granulomatosis. J Am Soc Nephrol 2:1227–1234, 1992.

286. Jayne DRW, Marshall PD, Jones SJ, Lockwood CM: Autoantibodies to GBM and neutrophil cytoplasm in rapidly progressive glomerulonephritis. Kidney Int 37:965–970, 1990.

287. Belghiti D, Levy Y, Rifle G, et al: Relapses of idiopathic diffuse crescentic glomerulonephritis, without immune deposits: Report of 6 cases. Am J Nephrol 7:22, 1983.

288. Gaskin G, Savage COS, Ryan JJ, et al: Anti-neutrophil cytoplasmic antibodies and disease activity during long-term follow-up of 70 patients with systemic vasculitis. Nephrol Dial Transplant 6:689–694, 1991.

289. Pusey CD, Rees AJ, Evans DJ, et al: Plasma exchange in focal necrotizing glomerulonephritis without anti-GBM antibodies. Kidney Int 40:757–763, 1991.
290. Glockner WM, Sieberth HG, Wickmann HE, et al: Plasma exchange and immunosuppression in rapidly progressive glomerulonephritis: A controlled multi-center study. Clin Nephrol 29:1, 1988.
290a. Fogo A, Smith M, Cleveland W, et al: Renal biopsy findings in the African-American Study of Kidney Disease (AASK). J Am Soc Nephrol 5:560, 1995. Abstract.
291. Katz SM, Lavin L, Swartz C: Glomerular lesions in benign essential hypertension. A study of eight biopsy specimens with laboratory evidence suggestive of glomerular abnormalities. Arch Pathol Lab Med 102:199, 1979.
292. Rakowski TA, Argy WP, Curtis JJ, Schreiner GF: Percutaneous renal biopsy in end-stage renal failure. Clin Res 23:37A, 1975.
293. Velosa J, Miller K, Michael AF: Immunopathology of the end-stage kidney. Immunoglobulin and complement component deposition in nonimmune disease. Am J Pathol 84:149, 1976.
294. Brenner BM: Hemodynamically mediated glomerular injury and the progressive nature of kidney disease. Kidney Int 23:647, 1983.
295. Birch DF, Fairley KF, Whitworth JA, et al: Urinary erythrocyte morphology in the diagnosis of glomerular hematuria. Clin Nephrol 20:78, 1983.
296. Mohr DN, Offord KP, Owen RA, Melton LJ: Asymptomatic hematuria and urologic disease. JAMA 256:224, 1986.
297. Glassock RJ: Hematuria and pigmenturia. In Massry S, Glassock R (eds): Textbook of Nephrology, 3rd ed. Williams & Wilkins, Baltimore, 1995, pp 557–566.
298. Fassett RG, Horgan B, Gove D, Mathew TH: Scanning electron microscopy of glomerular and non-glomerular red blood cells. Clin Nephrol 20:11, 1983.
299. DeSanto MG, Nuzzi F, Capodicasa G, et al: Phase contrast microscopy of the urine sediment in the diagnosis of glomerular and nonglomerular bleeding. Nephron 45:35, 1987.
300. Hauglustaine D, Bollens W, Michielsen D: Detection of glomerular bleeding using a simple staining method for light microscopy. Lancet 2:761, 1982.
301. Fassett RG, Owen JE, Fairley J, et al: Urinary red cell morphology during exercise. Br Med J 285:1455, 1982.
302. Kincaid-Smith P: Haematuria and exercise-related haematuria. Br Med J Clin Res 285:1595, 1982. Editorial.
303. Fairley KF, Birch DF: Microscopic urinalysis in glomerulonephritis. Kidney Int 44:S-9–S-12, 1993.
304. Fogazzi GB, Passerini P: Urinary sediment—its use in recognizing complications of the nephrotic syndrome. Nephrol Dial Transplant 9:70–71, 1994.
305. Kohler H, Wandel E, Brunck B: Acanthocyturia—a characteristic marker for glomerular bleeding. Kidney Int 40:115–120, 1991.
306. Tomita M, Kitamoto Y, Nakayama M, Sato T: A new morphological classification of urinary erythrocytes for differential diagnosis of glomerular hematuria. Clin Nephrol 37:84–89, 1992.
307. Kohler H, Wandel E: Acanthocyturia detects glomerular bleeding. Nephrol Dial Transplant 8:879, 1993.
308. Goldwasser P, Antignani S, Norbergs A, et al: Urinary red blood cell volume differentiates glomerular and non-glomerular hematuria. Kidney Int 33:191, 1988.
309. Docci D, Maldini M, Delvecchio C, et al: Urinary red blood cell volume analysis in the investigation of haematuria. Nephrol Dial Transplant 5:S-69–S-70, 1990.
310. Shichiri M, Hosoda K, Nishio Y, et al: Red-cell-volume distribution curves in diagnosis of glomerular and non-glomerular haematuria. Lancet 1:908, 1988.
311. Tanaka M, Kitamoto Y, Sato T, Ishii T: Flow cytometric analysis of hematuria using fluorescent antihemoglobin antibody. Nephron 65:354–358, 1993.
312. Bonnardeaux A, Somerville P, Kaye M: A study on the reliability of dipstick urinalysis. Clin Nephrol 41:167–172, 1994.
313. West CD: Asymptomatic hematuria and proteinuria in children: Causes and appropriate diagnostic studies. J Pediatr 89:173, 1976.
314. Sinniah R, Pwee HS, Lim CH: Glomerular lesions in asymptomatic microscopic hematuria discovered on routine medical examination. Clin Nephrol 5:216, 1976.
315. Pardo V, Berian MG, Levi DF, Strauss J: Primary benign hematuria. Clinicopathologic study of 65 patients. Am J Med 67:817, 1979.
316. Hendler ED, Kashgarian M, Hayslett JP: Clinicopathological correlations of primary haematuria. Lancet 1:458, 1972.
317. Trachtman H, Weiss R, Bennett B, Griefer I: Isolated hematuria in children: Indication for renal biopsy. Kidney Int 25:94, 1984.
318. Roy S, Stapelton F, Noe H, Jenkins F: Hematuria preceding renal calculus formation in children with hypercalciuria. J Pediatr 99:712, 1981.
319. van de Putte LBA, de la Riviere GG, van Breda Vriesman PJC: Recurrent or persisting hematuria and mesangial immune complex deposition. N Engl J Med 290:1165, 1974.
320. Copley JB, Hasbargen J: Idiopathic hematuria. A prospective evaluation. Arch Intern Med 147:434, 1987.
321. Blumenthal SS, Fritsche C, Lemann J: Establishing the diagnosis of benign familial hematuria. The importance of examining the urinary sediment of family members. JAMA 259:2263, 1988.
322. Rogers PW, Kurtzman NA, Bunn SM, White MG: Familial benign essential hematuria. Arch Intern Med 131:257, 1976.
323. Tiebosch ATMG, Frederik PM, van Breda Vriesman PJC, et al: Thin basement membrane nephropathy in adults with persistent hematuria. N Engl J Med 320:14, 1989.
324. Yoshikawa N, Ilkuma K, Shinomura M, et al: IgG associated primary glomerulonephritis in children. Clin Nephrol 42:281–287, 1994.
325. Sato M, Kojima H, Nakeshima K, et al: Primary glomerulonephritis with predominant mesangial deposits of IgG, a distinct entity. Nephron 64:122–128, 1993.
326. Knoll G, Rabin E, Burus B: Antiglomerular antibody induced nephritis with normal pulmonary and renal function. Am J Nephrol 13:494–496, 1993.
327. Roy LP, Fish AJ, Vernier RL, Michael AF: Recurrent macroscopic hematuria, focal nephritis and mesangial deposition of immunoglobulin and complement. J Pediatr 82:767, 1973.
328. Berger J, Hinglais N: Les depots intercapillaires d'IgA-IgG. J Urol Nephrol (Paris) 74:694, 1968.
329. Berger J: IgA glomerular deposits in renal disease. Transplant Proc 1:939, 1969.
330. Osfila C, Pieraggi MT, Suc J-M: Mesangial isolated C3 deposition in patients with recurrent or persistent hematuria. Lab Invest 43:1, 1980.
331. Grekas D, Morley AR, Wilkinson R, Kerr DNS: Isolated C3 deposition in patients without systemic disease. Clin Nephrol 21:270, 1984.
332. Pollock CA, Ibels LS, Eckstein RP, et al: Afferent arteriolar C3 disease. A distinct pathological entity. Am J Kidney Dis 14:31, 1989.
333. Berger J: Idiopathic mesangial deposition of IgA. In Hamburger J, Crosnier J, Grünfeld JP (eds): Nephrology. John Wiley & Sons, New York, 1979, p 535.
334. Noel LH, Gascon M, Berger J: Primary IgA nephropathy: From the first described cases to the present. Semin Nephrol 7:351, 1987.
335. Niaudet P, Murcia I, Beaufils H, et al: Primary IgA nephropathy in children: Prognosis and treatment. Adv Nephrol 22:121–140, 1993.
336. Schena FP: A retrospective analysis of the natural history of primary IgA nephropathy worldwide. Am J Med 89:209–215, 1990.
337. Southwest Pediatric Nephrology Study Group: A multicenter study of IgA nephropathy in children. Kidney Int 22:643, 1982.
338. Clarkson AR, Seymour AE, Thompson AJ, et al: IgA nephropathy: A syndrome of uniform morphology, diverse clinical features and uncertain prognosis. Clin Nephrol 8:459, 1977.
339. Colasanti G, Banfi G, Barbiano di Belgiorioso G, et al: Idiopathic IgA mesangial nephropathy: Clinical features. Contrib Nephrol 40:147, 1984.
340. Clarkson AR, Woodroffe AJ, Bannister KM, et al: The syndrome of IgA nephropathy. Clin Nephrol 21:7, 1984.
341. Glassock RJ: IgA nephropathy: 25 years of progress. Contrib Nephrol 104:212–219, 1993.
342. Glassock RJ: Highlights and trends: IgA symposium. Contrib Nephrol 111:201–208, 1995.
343. Emancipator S, Schena FP (eds): Immunoglobulin A nephropathy. Semin Nephrol 7:275, 1987.
344. Clarkson AR: IgA nephropathy. In Andreucci VE (ed): Topics in Renal Medicine. Martinus Nijhoff, Boston, 1987.
345. Waldherr R, Rambausek M, Rauterberg W, et al: Immunohistochemical features of mesangial IgA glomerulonephritis. Contrib Nephrol 40:99, 1984.

346. Jennette JC: Immunohistology of IgA nephropathy. Am J Kidney Dis 12:348, 1988.

347. Sinniah R: Idiopathic IgA mesangial nephropathy: Histological features. Contrib Nephrol 40:156, 1984.

348. D'Amico G: The commonest glomerulonephritis in the world: IgA nephropathy. Q J Med 64:709, 1987.

349. Power D, Murhead N, Simpson J, et al: IgA nephropathy is not a rare disease in the United Kingdom. Nephron 27:180, 1985.

350. Hoy WE, Hughson MO, Smith SM, Megill DM: Mesangial proliferative glomerulonephritis in southwestern American Indians. Am J Kidney Dis 21:486–496, 1993.

351. Crowley-Nowick PA, Julian BA, Wyatt RJ, et al: IgA nephropathy in blacks: Studies of IgA2 allotypes and clinical course. Kidney Int 39:1218–1224, 1991.

352. Waldherr R, Rambausek M, Ducker WD, Ritz E: Frequency of mesangial IgA deposits in a non-selected autopsy series. Nephrol Dial Transplant 4:943–946, 1989.

353. Jennette JC, Wall SD, Wilkman AS: Low incidence of IgA nephropathy in blacks. Kidney Int 28:944, 1985.

354. Rekola S, Bergstrand A, Lindberg A: Are β-hemolytic streptococci involved in the pathogenesis of mesangial IgA nephropathy? Proc Eur Dial Transplant Assoc Eur Renal Assoc 21:698, 1984.

355. Michael J, Jones NF, Davies DR, Tighe JR: Recurrent haematuria: Role of renal biopsy and investigative morbidity. Br Med J 1:686, 1976.

356. Hernando P, Egido J, deNicholas R, Sancho J: Clinical significance of polymeric and monomeric IgA complexes in patients with IgA nephropathy. Am J Kidney Dis 8:410, 1986.

357. Perez-Fontan M, Miguel J, Picazo ML, et al: Idiopathic IgA nephropathy presenting as malignant hypertension. Am J Nephrol 6:182, 1986.

358. Kincaid-Smith P, Bennett WM, Dowling JP, Ryan GB: Acute renal failure and tubular necrosis associated with hematuria due to glomerulonephritis. Clin Nephrol 19:206, 1983.

359. Praga M, Costa JR, Shandas GJ, et al: Acute renal failure in cirrhosis associated with macroscopic hematuria of glomerular origin. Arch Intern Med 147:173, 1987.

360. Praga M, Gutierrez-Millet V, Navas JJ, et al: Acute worsening of renal function during episodes of macroscopic hematuria in IgA nephropathy. Kidney Int 28:69, 1985.

361. Delclaux C, Jacquot C, Callard P, Kleinknecht D: Acute reversible renal failure with macroscopic haematuria in IgA nephropathy. Nephrol Dial Transplant 8:195–199, 1993.

362. Nash H, Binns GF, Clarkson AR, Beare TH: Concomitant IgA nephropathy and cyclical neutropaenia. Aust N Z J Med 8:184, 1978.

363. Nomoto Y, Sakai H, Endoh M, Tomino Y: Scleritis and IgA nephropathy. Arch Intern Med 140:783, 1980.

364. Andrassy K, Lichtenberg G, Rambausek M: Sicca syndrome in mesangial IgA glomerulonephritis. Clin Nephrol 24:60, 1985.

365. Thomas M, Ibels LS, Abbot N: IgA nephropathy associated with mastitis and haematuria. Br Med J 291:867, 1985.

365a. Endo Y, Hara M: Glomerular IgA deposits in pulmonary disease. Kidney Int 29:557, 1986.

366. Yum MN, Lampton LM, Bloom PM, Edwards JL: Asymptomatic IgA nephropathy associated with pulmonary hemosiderosis. Am J Med 64:1056, 1978.

367. Harland RW, Becker CG, Brandes JC, et al: Immunoglobulin A (IgA) immune complex pneumonitis in a patient with IgA nephropathy. Ann Intern Med 116:220–222, 1992.

368. Layward L, Hattersley JM, Patel HR, et al: Gut permeability in IgA nephropathy. Nephrol Dial Transplant 5:569–571, 1990.

369. Hirsch DJ, Jindal KK, Trillo A, Cohen AO: Acute renal failure in Crohn's disease due to IgA nephropathy. Am J Kidney Dis 20:189–190, 1992.

369a. Remy P, Jacquot C, Nocky D, et al: Buerger's disease associated with IgA nephropathy. Report of two cases. Br Med J 296:683, 1988.

370. Ritz E: Recurrent bloody dialysate during upper respiratory tract infection in mesangial IgA glomerulonephritis. Nephron 46:213, 1987.

371. Kapoor A, Mowbray J, Porter K, Peart S: Significance of haematuria in hypertensive patients. Lancet 1:231, 1980.

372. Katz A, Dyck F, Beard A: Celiac disease associated with immune complex glomerulonephritis. Clin Nephrol 11:39, 1979.

373. Jennette JC, Ferguson AL, Moore MA, Freeman DG: IgA nephropathy associated with seronegative spondylarthropathies. Arthritis Rheum 25:144, 1982.

374. Helin H, Mustanen J, Rennala T, Pasternack A: IgA nephropathy associated with celiac disease and dermatitis herpetiformis. Arch Pathol Lab Med 107:324, 1983.

375. Woodroffe AJ: IgA glomerulonephritis and liver disease. Aust N Z J Med 11:109, 1981.

376. Kalsi J, Delacroix DC, Hodgson HJF: IgA in alcoholic cirrhosis. Clin Exp Immunol 52:499, 1983.

377. Sinniah R: Mucin secreting cancer with mesangial IgA deposits. Pathology 14:303, 1982.

378. Ramirez G, Stinson JB, Zawada ET, Moatomed F: IgA nephritis associated with mycosis fungoides. Report of two cases. Arch Intern Med 141:1287, 1981.

379. Spichtin HP, Truniger B, Mikatsch MJ, et al: Immunothrombocytopenia and IgA nephritis. Clin Nephrol 14:304, 1980.

380. Woodrow G, Innes A, Boyd SM, Burden RP: A case of IgA nephropathy with coeliac disease responding to a gluten-free diet. Nephrol Dial Transplant 8:1382–1383, 1993.

381. Pasternack A, Collin P, Mustonen J, et al: Glomerular IgA deposits in patients with celiac disease. Clin Nephrol 34:56–60, 1990.

382. Tolkoff-Rubin NE, Cosimi AB, Fuller J, et al: IgA nephropathy in HLA-identical siblings. Transplantation 26:430, 1978.

383. Sabatier JC, Genin C, Cessenat H, et al: Mesangial IgA glomerulonephritis in HLA-identical brothers. Clin Nephrol 11:35, 1979.

384. Julian B, Quiggins P, Thompson J, et al: Familial IgA nephropathy: Evidence of an inherited mechanism of disease. N Engl J Med 312:202, 1985.

385. Chahin J, Ortiz A, Mendez L, et al: Familial IgA nephropathy associated with bilateral sensorineural deafness. Am J Kidney Dis 19:592–596, 1992.

386. Levy M, Lesasavre I: Genetic factors in IgA nephropathy (Berger's disease). Adv Nephrol 21:23–51, 1992.

387. Silva FG, Chander P, Pirani CL, Hardy MA: Disappearance of glomerular mesangial IgA deposits after renal allograft transplantation. Transplantation 33:214, 1982.

388. Neelakertappa K, Gallo GR, Baldwin DS: Proteinuria in IgA nephropathy. Kidney Int 33:716, 1988.

389. Widstam-Attorps U, Berg U, Bohman SO, Lefvert AK: Proteinuria and renal function in relation to renal morphology. A clinicopathological study of IgA nephropathy at the time of kidney biopsy. Clin Nephrol 38:245–253, 1992.

390. Furuse A, Himatsu M, Adachi N, et al: Dramatic response to corticosteroid therapy of nephrotic syndrome associated with IgA nephropathy. Int J Pediatr Nephrol 6:205, 1985.

391. Sinnassamy P, O'Regan S: Mesangial IgA deposits with steroid-responsive nephrotic syndrome. Probable minimal lesion nephrosis. Am J Kidney Dis 5:267, 1985.

392. Southwest Pediatric Nephrology Study Group: Association of IgA nephropathy with steroid-responsive nephrotic syndrome. Am J Kidney Dis 5:157, 1985.

393. Joshua H, Sharon Z, Gutglas E, et al: IgA-IgG nephropathy. A clinicopathologic entity with slow evolution and favorable prognosis. Am J Clin Pathol 67:289, 1977.

394. Hood SA, Velosa JA, Holley KE, Donadio JV Jr: IgA-IgG nephropathy: Predictive indices of progressive disease. Clin Nephrol 16:55, 1981.

395. D'Amico G, Fessario F, Colasanti G, et al: IgA mesangial nephropathy (Berger's disease) with rapid decline in renal function. Clin Nephrol 16:251, 1981.

396. D'Amico G, Barbiano di Belgioroso G, Imbasciati E, et al: Idiopathic IgA mesangial nephropathy: Natural history. Contrib Nephrol 40:208, 1984.

397. Droz D, Kramar A, Nawar T, Noel LH: Primary IgA nephropathy: Prognostic factors. Contrib Nephrol 40:202, 1984.

398. D'Amico G, Colasanti G, Barbiano di Belgioroso G, et al: Long-term follow-up of IgA mesangial nephropathy: Clinicohistological study in 374 patients. Semin Nephrol 7:355, 1987.

399. D'Amico G, Imbasciati E, Barbiano di Belgioroso G, et al: Idiopathic IgA mesangial nephropathy: Clinical and histological study of 374 patients. Medicine (Baltimore) 64:49, 1985.

400. Jones CL, Powell HR, Kincaid-Smith P, Roberton DM: Polymeric IgA and immune complex concentrations in IgA-related renal disease. Kidney Int 38:323–331, 1990.

401. Cosio PG, Lam S, Folami AO, et al: Immune regulation of immunoglobulin production in IgA nephropathy. Clin Immunol Immunopathol 23:430, 1982.
402. Trascasa ML, Egido J, Sancho J, Hernando L: Evidence of high polymeric IgA levels in serum of patients with Berger's disease and its modification with phenytoin treatment. Eur Dial Transplant Assoc 16:513, 1979.
403. Egido J, Sancho J, Blasco R, et al: Immunologic aspects of IgA nephropathy in humans. In Robinson RR (ed): Nephrology. Springer-Verlag, New York, 1984, p 652.
404. Newkirk MM, Klein MH, Katz A, et al: Estimation of polymeric IgA in human serum: An assay based on binding of radiolabeled human secretory component with applications in the study of IgA nephropathy. IgA monoclonal gammopathy, and liver disease. J Immunol 130:1176, 1983.
405. Sancho J, Egido J, Sanchez-Crespo M, Blasco R: Detection of monomeric and polymeric IgA containing immune complexes in serum and kidney from patients with alcoholic liver disease. Clin Exp Immunol 47:327, 1981.
406. Julian BA, Wyatt RJ, McMorrow RG, Galla JH: Serum complement proteins in IgA nephropathy. Clin Nephrol 20:251, 1983.
407. Geiger H: A study of complement components C3, C5, C6, C7, C8, C9 in chronic membranoproliferative glomerulonephritis, systemic lupus erythematosus, poststreptococcal nephritis, idiopathic nephrotic syndrome and anaphylactoid purpura. Z Kinderheilkd 119:269, 1975.
408. Wyatt RJ, Kanayama Y, Julian B, et al: Complement activation in IgA nephropathy. Kidney Int 31:1019, 1987.
409. Day NK, Geiger H, McLean R, et al: The association of respiratory infection, recurrent hematuria, and focal glomerulonephritis with activation of the complement system in the cold. J Clin Invest 52:1698, 1973.
410. Baldree LA, Wyatt RJ, Julian BA, et al: Immunoglobulin A–fibronectin aggregate levels in children and adults with immunoglobulin A nephropathy. Am J Kidney Dis 22:1–4, 1993.
411. Jennette JC, Wieslander J, Tuttle R, Falk RJ, and the Glomerular Disease Collaborative Network: Serum IgA-fibronectin aggregates in patients with IgA nephropathy and Henoch-Schönlein purpura: Diagnostic value and pathogenic implications. Am J Kidney Dis 18:466–471, 1991.
412. Nomoto Y, Suga T, Miura M, et al: Characterization of an acidic nuclear protein recognized by autoantibodies in sera from patients with IgA nephropathy. Clin Exp Immunol 65:513, 1986.
413. Woodroffe AJ, Gormly AA, McKenzie PE, et al: Immunologic studies in IgA nephropathy. Kidney Int 18:366, 1980.
414. Stachura I, Singh G, Whiteside TL: Immune abnormalities in IgA nephropathy (Berger's disease). Clin Immunol Immunopathol 20:373, 1981.
415. Coppo R, Basolo B, Martina G, et al: Circulating immune complexes containing IgA, IgG, IgM in patients with primary IgA nephropathy and with Henoch-Schönlein nephritis. Correlation with clinical and histologic signs of activity. Clin Nephrol 18:230, 1982.
416. Lesavre P, Digeon M, Bach JF: Analysis of circulating IgA and detection of immune complexes in primary IgA nephropathy. Clin Exp Immunol 48:61, 1982.
417. Hall RP, Stachura I, Cason J, et al: IgA containing circulating immune complexes in patients with IgA nephropathy. Am J Med 74:56, 1983.
418. Valentijn RM, Kauffmann RH, de la Riviere GB, et al: Presence of circulating macromolecular IgA in patients with hematuria due to primary IgA nephropathy. Am J Med 74:375, 1983.
419. Tomino Y, Sakai H, Endoh M, et al: Detection of immune complexes in polymorphonuclear leukocytes by double immunofluorescence in patients with IgA nephropathy. Clin Immunol Immunopathol 24:61, 1982.
420. Sato M, Takayama K, Wakasa M, Koshikawa S: Estimation of circulating immune complexes following oral challenge with cow's milk in patients with IgA nephropathy. Nephron 47:43, 1987.
421. Emancipator SN, Ovary Z, Lamm ME: The role of mesangial complement in the hematuria of experimental IgA nephropathy. Lab Invest 57:269, 1987.
422. Moore R: MHC gene polymorphism in primary IgA nephropathy. Kidney Int 43:S-9–S-12, 1993.
423. Freedman BI, Spray BJ, Heise ER: HLA associations in IgA nephropathy and focal and segmental glomerulosclerosis. Am J Kidney Dis 23:352–357, 1994.
424. Li PKT, Burns AP, So AKL, et al: The DQw7 allele at the HLA-DQB locus is associated with susceptibility to IgA nephropathy in Caucasians. Kidney Int 39:961–965, 1991.
425. Gans ROB, Ueda Y, Ito S, et al: The occurrence of IgA-nephropathy in patients with diabetes mellitus may not be coincidental: A report of five cases. Am J Kidney Dis 20:255–260, 1992.
426. Mustonen J, Pasternack A, Helin H, et al: Circulating immune complexes, the concentration of serum IgA and the distribution of HLA antigens in IgA nephropathy. Nephron 29:170, 1981.
427. Berthoux FC, Genin C, le Petit J-C, Laurent B: Immunogenetics of mesangial IgA nephritis. Contrib Nephrol 40:118, 1984.
428. Richman AV, Mahoney JJ, Fuller TJ: Higher prevalence of HLA-B12 in patients with IgA nephropathy. Ann Intern Med 90:201, 1979.
429. Hiki Y, Kobayashi Y, Tateno S, et al: Strong association of HLA-DR4 with benign IgA nephropathy. Nephron 32:222, 1982.
430. Fauchet B, Gueguen M, Genetet B, et al: HLA-DR antigen and IgA nephropathy (Berger's disease). N Engl J Med 302:1033, 1980.
431. Kashiwabara H, Shishido H, Tomura S, et al: Strong association between IgA nephropathy and HLA-DR4 antigen. Kidney Int 22:377, 1982.
432. Yoshioka K, Takemura T, Akano N, et al: IgA nephropathy in patients with congenital C9 deficiency. Kidney Int 42:1253–1258, 1992.
433. McLean RH, Wyatt RJ, Julian BA: Complement phenotypes in glomerulonephritis: Increased frequency of homozygous null C4 phenotypes in IgA nephropathy and Henoch-Schönlein purpura. Kidney Int 26:855, 1985.
434. Wyatt RJ, Julian BA, Woodford SY, et al: C4A deficiency and poor prognosis in patients with IgA nephropathy. Clin Nephrol 36:1–5, 1991.
435. Sinico RA, Fornasieri A, Oreni N, et al: Polymeric IgA rheumatoid factor in idiopathic IgA mesangial nephropathy (Berger's disease). J Immunol 137:536, 1986.
436. Czerkinsky C, Koopman WJ, Jackson S, et al: Circulating immune complexes and IgA rheumatoid factor in patients with mesangial immunoglobulin A nephropathies. J Clin Invest 77:1931, 1986.
437. Cederholm B, Wieslander J, Bygren P, Heinegard D: Patients with IgA nephropathy have circulating anti–basement membrane antibodies reacting with structures common to collagen I, II and IV. Proc Natl Acad Sci USA 83:6151, 1986.
438. Wang MX, Walker RG, Kincaid-Smith P: Endothelial cell antigens recognized by IgA autoantibodies in patients with IgA nephropathy: Partial characterization. Nephrol Dial Transplant 7:805–810, 1992.
439. Frampton G, Walker RG, Perry GJ, et al: IgA affinity to ssDNA or endothelial cells and its deposition in glomerular capillary walls in IgA nephropathy. Nephrol Dial Transplant 5:841–846, 1990.
440. Saulsbury FT, Kirkpatrick PR, Bolton WK: IgA antineutrophil cytoplasmic antibody in Henoch-Schönlein purpura. Am J Nephrol 11:295–300, 1991.
441. Savige JA, Gallicchio M: IgA antimyeloperoxidase antibodies associated with crescentic IgA glomerulonephritis. Nephrol Dial Transplant 7:952–955, 1992.
442. O'Donoghue D, Fehally J: Auto-antibodies in IgA nephropathy. Contrib Nephrol 111:93–103, 1995.
443. Fornasieri A, Sinico RA, Malidfassi P, et al: IgA-antigliadin antibodies in IgA mesangial nephropathy (Berger's disease). Br Med J 295:78, 1987.
444. Laurent J, Branellec A, Heslan J-M, et al: An increase in circulating IgA antibodies to gliadin in IgA mesangial glomerulonephritis. Am J Nephrol 7:178, 1987.
445. Yagami M, Tomino Y, Eguchi K, et al: Levels of circulating IgA immune complexes after gluten-rich diets in patients with IgA nephropathy. Nephron 49:104, 1988.
446. Nagy J, Scott H, Brandtzaeg P: Antibodies to dietary antigens in IgA nephropathy. Clin Nephrol 29:275, 1988.
447. Rostoker G, Andre C, Branellec A, et al: Lack of antireticulin and IgA antiendomysium antibodies in sera of patients with primary IgA nephropathy associated with circulating IgA antibodies to gliadin. Nephron 48:81, 1988. Letter.
448. Darvin J-C, Malaise M, Foidart J, Mahieu P: Anti-α galactosyl antibodies and immune complexes in children with Henoch-Schönlein purpura or IgA nephropathy. Kidney Int 31:1132, 1984.
449. Yap HK, Sakai RS, Woo T, et al: Detection of bovine serum albumin in the circulating IgA immune complexes of patients with IgA nephropathy. Clin Immunol Immunopathol 43:395, 1987.

450. Suzuki S, Nakatomi Y, Sato H, et al: *Haemophilus parainfluenzae* antigen and antibody in renal biopsy samples and serum of patients with IgA nephropathy. Lancet 343:12–16, 1994.

451. Nagy J, Uj M, Szucs G, et al: Herpes virus antigens and antibodies in kidney biopsies and sera of IgA glomerulonephritic patients. Clin Nephrol 21:259, 1984.

452. Tomino Y, Yagame M, Omata F, et al: A case of IgA nephropathy associated with adeno- and herpes simplex viruses. Nephron 47:258, 1987.

453. Sakai H, Nomoto Y, Armori S: Decrease of IgA-specific suppressor T cell activity in patients with IgA nephropathy. Clin Exp Immunol 38:243, 1979.

454. Fiorini G, Fornasieri A, Sinico R, et al: Lymphocyte populations in the peripheral blood from patients with IgA nephropathy. Nephron 31:354, 1982.

455. Bakker WW, Beukhof JR, Van Luijk WHJ, Van der Hem GK: Vascular permeability increasing factor (VPF) in IgA nephropathy. Clin Nephrol 18:165, 1982.

456. Nakamura T, Ebihara I, Shirato I, et al: Endothelin 1 mRNA expression by peripheral blood monocytes in IgA nephropathy. Lancet 342:1147–1148, 1993.

457. Tomino Y, Endoh M, Kaneshige H, et al: Increase of IgA in pharyngeal washings from patients with IgA nephropathy. Am J Med Sci 286:15, 1983.

458. Sakai H, Endoh M, Tomino Y, Nomoto Y: Increase of IgA specific helper T cells in patients with IgA nephropathy. Clin Exp Immunol 50:77, 1982.

459. Bene MC, Faure G, Hurault de Ligny B, et al: Immunoglobulin A nephropathy. Quantitative immunohistomorphometry of the tonsillar plasma cells evidences an inversion of the immunoglobulin A versus immunoglobulin G secreting cell balance. J Clin Invest 71:1342, 1983.

460. Lawrence S, Pussell BA, Charlesworth JA: Mesangial IgA nephropathy: Detection of defective reticulophagocytic function in vivo. Clin Nephrol 16:280, 1983.

461. Sato M, Kinugasa E, Ideura T, Koshikawa S: Phagocytic activity of polymorphonuclear leucocytes in patients with IgA nephropathy. Clin Nephrol 19:166, 1983.

462. Ida K, Koyama Y, Nakamura H, et al: Abnormal expression of complement receptor (CRI) in IgA nephritis: Increase in erythrocytes and loss of glomeruli in patient with impaired renal function. Clin Immunol Immunopathol 40:393, 1986.

463. Egido J, Sancho J, Rivera F, Sanchez-Crespo M: Handling of soluble IgA aggregates by the mononuclear phagocytic system in mice. A comparison with IgG aggregates. Immunology 46:1, 1982.

464. Shand B, Bailey R, Simpson L: Blood rheology in IgA nephropathy. Clin Nephrol 29:288, 1988.

465. Ohta K, Takano N, Seno A, et al: Detection and clinical usefulness of urinary interleukin-6 in the diseases of the kidney and the urinary tract. Clin Nephrol 38:185–189, 1992.

466. Tomino Y, Funabiki K, Ohmuro H, et al: Urinary levels of interleukin-6 and disease activity in patients with IgA nephropathy. Am J Nephrol 11:459–464, 1991.

467. Taira K, Hewitson TD, Kincaid-Smith P: Urinary platelet factor four (Pf4) levels in mesangial IgA glomerulonephritis and thin basement membrane disease. Clin Nephrol 37:8–13, 1992.

468. Holman RT, Johnson SB, Bibus D, et al: Essential fatty acid deficiency profiles in idiopathic immunoglobulin A nephropathy. Am J Kidney Dis 23:648–654, 1994.

469. Baart de la Faille-Kuyper EH, Kater L, Dorhout-Mees EJ, Kooiker CJ: Immunohistochemical studies comparing clinically normal skin and kidney tissues in 46 patients with nephropathy. Neth J Med 16:60, 1973.

470. Baart de la Faille-Kuyper EH, Kater L, Kuijten RH, et al: Occurrence of vascular IgA deposits in clinically normal skin of patients with renal disease. Kidney Int 9:424, 1976.

471. Hasbargen J, Copley J: Utility of skin biopsy in the diagnosis of IgA nephropathy. Am J Kidney Dis 6:100, 1985.

472. Hene R, Valthius P, van den Wiel A, et al: The relevance of IgA deposits in vessel walls of clinical normal skin. A prospective study. Arch Intern Med 146:745, 1986.

473. Whitworth JA, Turner DA, Leibowitz S, Cameron JS: Focal segmental sclerosis or scarred focal proliferative glomerulonephritis. Clin Nephrol 9:229, 1978.

474. Alamartine E, Sabatier JC, Berthoux FC: Comparison of patholog-ical lesions on repeated renal biopsies in 73 patients with primary IgA glomerulonephritis: Value of quantitative scoring and approach to final prognosis. Clin Nephrol 34:45–51, 1990.

475. Emancipator SN: IgA nephropathy: Morphologic expression and pathogenesis. Am J Kidney Dis 23:451–462, 1994.

476. Schena FP, Gesualdo L, Montinaro V: Immunopathological aspects of immunoglobulin A nephropathy and other mesangial proliferative glomerulonephritides. J Am Soc Nephrol 2:5167–5172, 1992.

477. Magil AB, Ballon HS: IgA nephropathy: Evaluation of prognostic factors in patients with moderate disease. Nephron 47:246, 1987.

478. Hotta O, Taguma Y, Kurosawa K, et al: Predictive value of small crescents in IgA nephropathy: Analysis of four patients showing a deteriorated renal function during a long follow up period. Clin Nephrol 40:125–130, 1993.

479. Hotta O, Taguma Y, Sudo K, Kurosawa K: Limitation of kidney biopsy in detecting crescentic lesions in IgA nephropathy. Nephron 65:472–473, 1993.

480. MacKensen-Haen S, Eissele R, Bohle A: Contribution on the correlation between morphometric parameters gained from the renal cortex and renal function in IgA nephritis. Lab Invest 59:239, 1988.

481. Tateno S, Kobayashi Y: Quantitative analysis of mesangial areas in serial biopsied patients with IgA nephropathy. Nephron 46:28, 1987.

482. Bogenschutz O, Bohle A, Batz C, et al: IgA nephritis: On the importance of morphological and clinical parameters in the long-term prognosis of 239 patients. Am J Nephrol 10:137–147, 1990.

483. D'Amico G: Influence of clinical and histological features on actuarial renal survival in adult patients with idiopathic IgA nephropathy, membranous nephropathy, and membranoproliferative glomerulonephritis: Survey of the recent literature. Am J Kidney Dis 20:315–323, 1992.

484. Donadio JV, Bergstralh EJ, Offord KP, et al, and the Mayo Collaborative Group: Clinical and histopathologic associations with impaired renal function in IgA nephropathy. Clin Nephrol 41:65–71, 1994.

485. Katafuchi R, Oh Y, Hori K, et al: An important role of glomerular segmental lesions on progression of IgA nephropathy: A multivariate analysis. Clin Nephrol 41:191–198, 1994.

486. Frasca GM, Vangelista A, Biagini G, Bonomini V: Immunological tubulointerstitial deposits in IgA nephropathy. Kidney Int 22:184, 1982.

487. Alexopoulos E, Seron D, Hartley RB, et al: The role of interstitial infiltrates in IgA nephropathy: A study with monoclonal antibodies. Nephrol Dial Transplant 4:187–195, 1989.

488. Feiner HD, Cabilis C, Baldwin DS, et al: Intrarenal vascular sclerosis in IgA nephropathy. Clin Nephrol 18:183, 1982.

489. Sabais R, Botey A, Darnell A, et al: Malignant or accelerated hypertension in IgA nephropathy. Clin Nephrol 27:1, 1987.

490. Lai KN, Lai FMM, Chan KW, et al: An overlapping syndrome of IgA nephropathy and lipoid nephrosis. Am J Clin Pathol 86:716, 1986.

491. Katz A, Underdown BJ, Minta JO, Lepow IH: Glomerulonephritis with mesangial deposits of IgA unassociated with systemic disease. Can Med Assoc J 114:209, 1976.

492. Sinniah R, Churg J: Effect of IgA deposits on the glomerular mesangium in Berger's disease. Ultrastruct Pathol 4:9, 1983.

493. Navas-Palacios JJ, Gutierrez-Miller V, Usera-Sarraga G: IgA nephropathy: An ultrastructural study. Ultrastruct Pathol 2:151, 1981.

494. Shigematsu H, Kobayashi Y, Tateno S, et al: Ultrastructural glomerular loop abnormalities in IgA nephritis. Nephron 30:1, 1982.

495. Yoshikawa N, Yoshiara S, Yoshiya K, et al: Lysis of the glomerular basement membrane in children with IgA nephropathy and Henoch-Schönlein nephritis. J Pathol 150:119, 1986.

496. Lai KN, Lai FMM, Lo S, Lam CWK: Light chain composition of IgA in IgA nephropathy. Am J Kidney Dis 11:425, 1988.

497. Yoshimuira M, Kida H, Abe T, et al: Significance of IgA deposits on the glomerular capillary walls in IgA nephropathy. Am J Kidney Dis 9:404, 1987.

498. Komatsu N, Nagura H, Watanabe K: Mesangial deposition of J chain linked polymeric IgA in IgA nephropathy. Nephron 33:61, 1983.

499. Bene M-C, Faure G, Duheille J: IgA nephropathy: Characterization of the polymeric nature of mesangial deposits by in vitro binding of free secretory component. Clin Exp Immunol 47:527, 1982.

500. Gregory MC, Hammond ME, Brewer ED: Renal deposition of

cytomegalovirus antigen in immunoglobulin-A nephropathy. Lancet 2:11, 1988.

501. Park JS, Song JH, Yang WS, et al: Cytomegalovirus is not specifically associated with immunoglobulin A nephropathy. J Am Soc Nephrol 4:1623–1626, 1994.

502. Sinniah R, Khan TN, Dodd S: An in situ hybridization study of herpes simplex and Epstein-Barr viruses in IgA nephropathy and non-immune glomerulonephritis. Clin Nephrol 40:137–141, 1993.

503. Lai KN, Lai FMM, Tam JS, Vallance-Owen F: Strong association between IgA nephropathy and hepatitis B surface antigenemia in endemic areas. Clin Nephrol 29:229, 1988.

504. Tomino Y, Sakai H, Endoh M, et al: Cross-reactivity of eluted antibodies from renal tissues of patients with Henoch-Schönlein purpura nephritis and IgA nephropathy. Am J Nephrol 3:315, 1983.

505. Tomino Y, Endoh M, Nomoto Y, Sakai H: Specificity of eluted antibody from renal tissues of patients with IgA nephropathy. Am J Kidney Dis 1:276, 1982.

506. Tomino Y, Endoh M, Nomoto Y, Sakai H: Specificity of IgA antibody in IgA nephropathy. Nephron 29:103, 1981.

507. Tomino Y, Sakai H, Endoh M, et al: Cross-reactivity of IgA antibodies between renal mesangial areas and nuclei of tonsillar cells in patients with IgA nephropathy. Clin Exp Immunol 51:605, 1983.

508. Andre C, Berthoux F, Andre F, et al: Prevalence of IgA$_2$ deposits in IgA nephropathies. N Engl J Med 303:1343, 1980.

509. Conley ME, Cooper MD, Michael AF: Selective deposition of immunoglobulin A1 in immunoglobulin A nephropathy, anaphylactoid purpura nephritis and systemic lupus erythematosus. J Clin Invest 66:1432, 1980.

510. van den Wall Bake AW, Bruijn JA, Accavitti MA, et al: Shared idiotypes in mesangial deposits in IgA nephropathy are not disease-specific. Kidney Int 44:65–74, 1993.

511. Mestecky J, Haskim O, Tomana M: Alterations in the IgA carbohydrate chains influence the cellular distribution of IgA1. Contrib Nephrol 111:66–72, 1995.

512. Tomino Y, Sakai H, Suga T, et al: Impaired solubilization of glomerular immune deposits by sera from patients with IgA nephropathy. Am J Kidney Dis 3:48, 1983.

513. Rantenberg EW, Lieberknecht H-M, Wingen AM, Ritz E: Complement membrane attack (MAC) idiopathic IgA glomerulonephritis. Kidney Int 31:830, 1987.

514. Tomino Y, Yagami M, Eguchi K, et al: Immunofluorescent studies on S protein in glomeruli from patients with IgA nephropathy. Am J Pathol 129:402, 1987.

515. Imai H, Wakui M, Ishino T, et al: Glomerular deposition of complex-forming glycoprotein heterogenous in charge (protein HC) in IgA nephropathy. Clin Nephrol 37:169–176, 1992.

516. Nakajima M, Hewitson JD, Mathews DC, Kincaid-Smith P: Platelet-derived growth factor mesangial deposits in mesangial IgA glomerulonephritis. Nephrol Dial Transplant 6:11–16, 1991.

517. Kanahara K, Yorioka N, Arita M, et al: Immunohistochemical studies of extracellular matrix components and integrins in IgA nephropathy. Nephron 66:29–37, 1994.

518. Bergstein J: IgA nephropathy. Clin Nephrol 9:258, 1978. Letter.

519. Doi T, Kanatsu K, Nagai H, et al: An overlapping syndrome of IgA nephropathy and membranous nephropathy? Nephron 35:24, 1983.

520. Jennette JC, Newman WJ, Diaz-Buxo JA: Overlapping IgA and membranous nephropathy. Am J Clin Pathol 88:74, 1987.

521. Magil A, Webber D, Chan V: Glomerulonephritis associated with hepatitis B surface antigenemia: Report of a case with features of both membranous and IgA nephropathy. Nephron 42:335, 1986.

522. Kobayashi Y, Fujii K, Hiki Y, Chen XM: Coexistence of IgA nephropathy and membranous nephropathy. Acta Pathol Jpn 35:1293, 1985.

523. van Es LA: Pathogenesis of IgA nephropathy. Kidney Int 41:1720–1729, 1992.

524. van den Wall Bake AW, Daha MR, Valentijn RM, van Es LA: The bone marrow as a possible origin of the IgA1 deposited in the mesangium in IgA nephropathy. Semin Nephrol 7:329, 1987.

525. Mestecky J, Tomana M, Czerkinsky C, et al: IgA-associated renal diseases: Immunochemical studies of IgA$_1$ proteins, circulating immune complexes, and cellular interactions. Semin Nephrol 7:332, 1987.

526. Drew PA, Nieuwhof WN, Clarkson AR, Woodroffe AJ: Increased concentration of serum IgA antibody to pneumococcal polysaccharides in patients with IgA nephropathy. Clin Exp Immunol 67:124, 1987.

527. Schena FP, Mastrolitti G, Fracasso AR, et al: Increased immunoglobulin secreting cells in the blood of patients with active idiopathic IgA nephropathy. Clin Nephrol 26:163, 1986.

528. Cagnoli L, Beltrandi E, Pasquali S, et al: B and T cell abnormalities in patients with primary IgA nephropathy. Kidney Int 28:646, 1985.

529. Sancho J, Egido J, Rivera F, Hernando L: Immune complexes in IgA nephropathy: Presence of antibodies against diet antigens and delayed clearance of specific polymeric IgA immune complexes. Clin Exp Immunol 54:194, 1983.

530. Schena FP, Pastore A, Sinico RA, et al: Studies on the mechanisms producing solubilization of immune precipitates in the serum of patients with primary IgA nephropathy. Semin Nephrol 7:336, 1987.

531. Tomino Y, Sakai H, Miura M, et al: Specific binding of circulating IgA antibodies in patients with IgA nephropathy. Am J Kidney Dis 6:149, 1985.

532. Ballardie FW, Brenchley PEC, Williams S, O'Donoghue D: Autoimmunity in IgA nephropathy. Lancet 2:588, 1988.

533. Bene M-C, Favre G: Berger's disease: Recent advances in immunology and genetics. Adv Nephrol 16:281, 1987.

534. Egido J, Blasco R, Sancho J, Hernando L: Immunological abnormalities in healthy relatives of patients with IgA nephropathy. Am J Nephrol 5:14, 1985.

535. Demaine A, Rambausek M, Knight J, et al: Relation of mesangial IgA glomerulonephritis to polymorphism of immunoglobulin heavy chain switch region. J Clin Invest 81:611, 1988.

536. Emancipator SN, Gallo GR, Lamm ME: Experimental IgA nephropathy induced by oral immunization. J Exp Med 157:572, 1983.

537. Isaacs K, Miller F, Lane B: Experimental model for IgA nephropathy. Clin Immunol Immunopathol 20:419, 1981.

538. Gormly AA, Smith PS, Seymour AE, et al: IgA glomerular deposits in experimental cirrhosis. Am J Pathol 104:50, 1981.

539. Woodroffe AJ, Lomax-Smith JD: Pathogenetic mechanisms of IgA nephropathy from studies of experimental models. *In* Robinson RR (ed): Nephrology. Springer-Verlag, New York, 1984, p 645.

540. Delacroix DL, Elkon KB, Geubel AP, et al: Changes in size, subclass, and metabolic properties of serum immunoglobulin A in liver diseases and in other diseases with high serum immunoglobulin. Am J Clin Invest 71:358, 1983.

541. Bene MC, De Korwin JD, de Ligny BH, et al: IgA nephropathy and alcoholic liver cirrhosis. A prospective necropsy study. Am J Clin Pathol 89:769, 1988.

542. Costa RS, Droz D, Noël LH: Longstanding spontaneous clinical remission and glomerular involvement in primary IgA nephropathy (Berger's disease). Am J Nephrol 7:440, 1987.

543. Beukhof JR, Karduan P, Schaafsma W, et al: Toward individual prognosis in IgA nephropathy. Kidney Int 29:549, 1986.

544. Nichols K, Walker R, Dowling J, Kincaid-Smith P: "Malignant" IgA nephropathy. Am J Kidney Dis 5:42, 1985.

545. Ibels LS, Gyory AZ: IgA nephropathy: Analysis of the natural history. Important factors in the progression of renal disease, and a review of the literature. Medicine (Baltimore) 73:79–102, 1994.

546. Alamartine E, Sabatier JC, Guerin C, et al: Prognostic factors in mesangial IgA glomerulonephritis: An extensive study with univariate and multivariate analyses. Am J Kidney Dis 18:12–19, 1991.

547. Kincaid-Smith P, Fairley KF: Renal disease in pregnancy. Three controversial areas: Mesangial IgA nephropathy, focal glomerular sclerosis (focal and segmental hyalinosis and sclerosis), and reflux nephropathy. Am J Kidney Dis 9:328, 1987.

547a. Jungers P, Forget D, Houiller P, et al: Pregnancy in IgA nephropathy, reflux nephropathy and focal glomerular sclerosis. Am J Kidney Dis 9:334, 1987.

548. Packham DK, North RA, Fairley KF, et al: IgA glomerulonephritis and pregnancy. Clin Nephrol 30:15, 1988.

549. Packham D, Whitworth JA, Fairley KF, Kincaid-Smith P: Histological features of IgA glomerulonephritis as predictors of pregnancy outcome. Clin Nephrol 30:22, 1988.

550. Abe S: Pregnancy in IgA nephropathy. Kidney Int 40:1098–1102, 1991.

551. Croker BP, Dawson DV, Sanfilippo F: IgA nephropathy: Correlation of clinical and histologic features. Lab Invest 48:19, 1983.

552. Lec S-M, Rao VM, Franklin WA, Spargo B: IgA nephropathy: Morphologic predictors of progressive renal disease. Hum Pathol 13:314, 1982.

553. Clarkson AR, Woodroffe AJ, Bannister KM, et al: Therapy in IgA nephropathy. Contrib Nephrol 104:189–197, 1993.
554. Clarkson AR, Woodroffe AJ: Therapeutic perspectives in mesangial IgA nephropathy. Contrib Nephrol 40:187, 1984.
555. Clarkson AR, Woodroffe AJ, Aarons IA, et al: Therapeutic options in IgA nephropathy. Am J Kidney Dis 12:443, 1988.
556. Lai KN, Lai FM, Ho CP, Chan KW: Corticosteroid therapy in IgA nephropathy with nephrotic syndrome: A long-term controlled trial. Clin Nephrol 26:174, 1986.
557. Kobayashi Y, Fujii K, Hiki Y, Tateno S: Steroid therapy in IgA nephropathy: A prospective pilot study in moderate proteinuric cases. Q J Med 61:935, 1986.
558. Kobayashi Y, Fujii K, Hiki Y, et al: Steroid therapy in IgA nephropathy. A retrospective study in heavy proteinuric cases. Nephron 48:12, 1988.
559. Andreoli SP, Bergstein JM: Treatment of severe IgA nephropathy in children. Pediatr Nephrol 3:248–252, 1989.
560. Schena FP, Montenegro M, Scivittaro V: Meta-analysis of randomized controlled trials in patients with primary IgA nephropathy (Berger's disease). Nephrol Dial Transplant 5:S-47–S-52, 1990.
561. Kobayashi Y, Hiki Y, Fujii K, et al: Moderately proteinuric IgA nephropathy: Prognostic prediction of individual clinical courses and steroid therapy in progressive cases. Nephron 53:250–256, 1989.
562. Waldo FB, Alexander R, Wyatt RJ, Kohaut EC: Alternate-day prednisone therapy in children with IgA-associated nephritis. Am J Kidney Dis 13:55–60, 1989.
563. Woo KT, Edmondson R, Yap HP, et al: Effects of triple therapy on the progression of mesangial proliferative glomerulonephritis. Clin Nephrol 27:56, 1987.
564. Julian BA, Barker C: Alternate-day prednisone therapy in IgA nephropathy. Contrib Nephrol 104:198–206, 1993.
565. Woo KT, Lee GSL, Lau YK, et al: Effects of triple therapy in IgA nephritis: A follow-up study of 5 years later. Clin Nephrol 36:60–66, 1991.
566. Lai KN, Lai M-M, Vallance-Owen J: A short-term controlled trial of cyclosporine A in IgA nephropathy. Transplant Proc 20(suppl 4):297, 1988.
567. Giachino O, Roccatelli D, Lajdo D, et al: Plasmapheresis in a patient with rapidly progressive idiopathic IgA nephropathy: Removal of IgA containing circulating immune complexes and clinical recovery. Nephron 40:488, 1985.
568. Clarkson AR, Seymour AE, Woodroffe AJ, et al: Controlled trial of phenytoin therapy in IgA nephropathy. Clin Nephrol 13:215, 1980.
569. Egido J, Sanchez Crespo M, Sancho J, Hernando L: Phenytoin in the treatment of IgA mesangial glomerulonephritis (Berger's disease). Clin Nephrol 15:164, 1981.
570. Egido J, Rivera F, Sancho J, et al: Phenytoin in IgA nephropathy: A long-term controlled trial. Nephrology 38:30, 1984.
571. Coppo R, Basolo B, Bulzomi MR, Piccoli G: Ineffectiveness of phenytoin treatment on IgA-containing circulating immune complexes in IgA nephropathy. Nephron 36:275, 1984.
572. Tomino Y, Sakai H, Hanzawa S, et al: Clinical effect of danazol in patients with IgA nephropathy. Jpn J Med 26:162, 1987.
573. Chan MK, Kwan SYL, Chan KW, Yeung CK: Controlled trial of antiplatelet agents in mesangial IgA glomerulonephritis. Am J Kidney Dis 9:417, 1987.
574. Camara S, de la Cruz JP, Frutos M, et al: Effects of dipyridamole on the short-term evolution of glomerulonephritis. Nephron 58:13–16, 1991.
575. Bennett WM, Walker RG, Kincaid-Smith P: Treatment of IgA nephropathy with eicosopentanoic acid (EPA): A 2-year prospective trial. Clin Nephrol 31:128, 1989.
576. Pettersson EE, Rekola S, Berglund L, et al: Treatment of IgA nephropathy with omega-3-polyunsaturated fatty acids: A prospective, double-blind, randomized study. Clin Nephrol 41:183–190, 1994.
577. Cheng IKP, Chan PCK, Chan MK: The effect of fish-oil dietary supplement on the progression of mesangial IgA glomerulonephritis. Nephrol Dial Transplant 5:241–246, 1990.
578. Donadio JV Jr, Bergstralh EJ, Offord KP, et al, for the Mayo Nephrology Collaborative Group: A controlled trial of fish oil in IgA nephropathy. N Engl J Med 331:1194–1199, 1994.
579. Ferri C, Puccini R, Longombardo G, et al: Low-antigen-content diet in the treatment of patients with IgA nephropathy. Nephrol Dial Transplant 8:1193–1198, 1993.
580. Coppo R, Roccatello D, Amore D, et al: Effects of a gluten-free diet in primary IgA nephropathy. Clin Nephrol 33:72–86, 1990.
581. Lai KN, Lai FM-M, Leung A, et al: Plasma exchange in patients with rapidly progressive IgA nephropathy: A report of two cases and review of the literature. Am J Kidney Dis 10:66, 1987.
582. Cattran DC, Greenwood C, Ritchie S: Long-term benefits of angiotensin-converting enzyme inhibitor therapy in patients with severe immunoglobulin A nephropathy: A comparison to patients receiving treatment with other antihypertensive agents and to patients receiving no therapy. Am J Kidney Dis 23:247–254, 1994.
583. Maschio G, Cagnoli L, Claroni F, et al: ACE inhibition reduces proteinuria in normotensive patients with IgA nephropathy: A multicentre, randomized, placebo-controlled study. Nephrol Dial Transplant 9:265–269, 1994.
584. Coppo R, Amore A, Gianoglio B, et al: Angiotensin II local hyperreactivity in the progression of IgA nephropathy. Am J Kidney Dis 21:593–602, 1993.
585. Rostoker G, Desvaux-Belghiti D, Pilatte Y, et al: High-dose immunoglobulin therapy for severe IgA nephropathy and Henoch-Schönlein purpura. Ann Intern Med 120:476–484, 1994.
586. Lupo A, Rugin G, Cagnoli L, et al: Acute changes in renal function in IgA nephropathy. Semin Nephrol 7:359, 1987.
587. Berger J, Yaneva H, Nabarra B, Barbanel C: Recurrence of mesangial deposition of IgA after renal transplantation. Kidney Int 7:232, 1975.
588. Pettersson E, Honkanen E, Tornroth T: Recurrence of IgA nephropathy with nephrotic syndrome in renal allograft. Nephron 41:114, 1985.
589. Odum J, Peh CA, Clarkson AR, et al: Recurrent mesangial IgA nephritis following renal transplantation. Nephrol Dial Transplant 9:309–312, 1994.
589a. Lim E, Chia D, Terasaki P: Studies of sera from IgA nephropathy patients to explain high kidney graft survival. Hum Immunol 32:81–86, 1991.
590. Abe S, Amagasaki Y, Iyori S: Thin–basement membrane syndrome in adults. J Clin Pathol 40:318, 1987.
591. Dische FE, Weston MJ, Parsons N: Abnormally thin basement membranes associated with hematuria, proteinuria, or renal failure in adults. Am J Nephrol 5:103, 1985.
592. Coleman M, Haynes WD, Oumopoulos P, et al: Glomerular basement membrane abnormalities associated with apparently idiopathic hematuria: Ultrastructural morphometric studies. Hum Pathol 17:1022, 1986.
593. Cosio FG, Falkenhain ME, Sedmak DD: Association of thin glomerular basement membrane with other glomerulopathies. Kidney Int 46:471–474, 1994.
594. McLay ALC, Jackson R, Meyboom F, Boulton Jones JM: Glomerular basement membrane thinning in adults: Clinicopathological correlations of a new diagnostic approach. Nephrol Dial Transplant 7:191–199, 1992.
595. Dische FE, Brooke IP, Cashman SJ, et al: Reactivity of monoclonal antibody PI with glomerular basement membrane in thin-membrane nephropathy. Nephrol Dial Transplant 4:611–617, 1989.
596. Little PJ, Sloper JS, de Wardener HE: A syndrome of loin pain and hematuria associated with diseases of peripheral renal arteries. Q J Med 36:253, 1967.
597. Burden RP, Etherington MD, Dathan JK, et al: The loin-pain haematuria syndrome. Lancet 1:897, 1979.
598. Weisberg L, Bloom P, Simmons R, Ulner E: Loin-pain hematuria syndrome. Am J Nephrol 13:229–237, 1993.
599. Boyd W, Burden RP, Aber GM: Intra-renal vascular changes in patients receiving oestrogen containing compounds—a clinical histological and angiographic study. Q J Med 44:115, 1975.
600. Siegler R, Brewer E, Hammond E: Platelet activation and prostaglandin supporting capacity in the loin pain–hematuria syndrome. Am J Kidney Dis 12:156, 1988.
601. Fletcher P, Al-Khader AA, Parsons V, Aber GM: The pathology of intrarenal vascular lesions associated with the loin-pain–haematuria syndrome. Nephron 24:150, 1979.
602. Nortman DF, Rever BL, Stanley TM, Kurokawa K: The loin pain–hematuria syndrome in two cases of IgA and IgM nephropathy. Arch Intern Med 141:1782, 1981.
603. Dimski DS, Herbert LA, Sedmak D, et al: Renal auto-transplanta-

tion in the loin pain–hematuria syndrome: A cautionary note. Am J Kidney Dis 20:180–184, 1992.

604. Robinson RR, Krueger RP: Postural proteinuria. *In* Edelmann CM Jr (ed): Pediatric Kidney Diseases. Little, Brown, Boston, 1979, p 597.

605. Robinson RR: Isolated proteinuria in asymptomatic patients. Kidney Int 18:395, 1980.

606. Glassock R: Proteinuria. *In* Massry S, Glassock R (eds): Textbook of Nephrology, 3rd ed. Williams & Wilkins, Baltimore, 1995, pp 600–604.

607. Carrie BJ, Hilberman M, Schroeder JS, Myers BD: Albuminuria and the permselective properties of the glomerular wall in cardiac failure. Kidney Int 17:507, 1980.

608. Reuben DB, Wachter TJ, Brown PC, Driscoll JL: Transient proteinuria in emergency medical admissions. N Engl J Med 306:1031, 1982.

609. Albright R, Brensilver J, Cortell S: Proteinuria in congestive heart failure. Am J Nephrol 3:272, 1983.

610. Sinniah R, Law CH, Pwee HS: Glomerular lesions in patients with asymptomatic persistent and orthostatic proteinuria discovered on routine medical examination. Clin Nephrol 7:1, 1977.

611. Morrin PAF: Urinary sediment in the interpretation of proteinuria. Ann Intern Med 98:254, 1983.

612. Springberg PD, Garrett LE Jr, Thompson AL, et al: Fixed and reproducible orthostatic proteinuria: Results of a 20 year follow-up study. Ann Intern Med 97:516, 1982.

613. Harvey JM, Howie AJ, Lee SJ, et al: Renal biopsy findings in hypertensive patients with proteinuria. Lancet 340:1435–1436, 1992.

614. Schreiner GE: The nephrotic syndrome. *In* Strauss MB, Welt LG (eds): Diseases of the Kidney, 2nd ed. Little, Brown, Boston, 1971, p 503.

615. Cameron JS, Glassock R (eds): The Nephrotic Syndrome. Marcel Dekker, New York, 1988.

616. Mallick NP: Epidemiology and natural course of idiopathic nephrotic syndrome. Clin Nephrol 35:S-3–S-7, 1991.

617. Kaysen GA, Myers BD, Couser WG, et al: Biology of disease. Mechanisms and consequences of proteinuria. Lab Invest 54:479, 1986.

618. Brenner BM, Hostetter TH, Humes HD: Molecular basis of proteinuria of glomerular origin. N Engl J Med 298:826, 1978.

619. Savin VJ: Mechanisms of proteinuria in noninflammatory glomerular diseases. Am J Kidney Dis 31:347–362, 1993.

620. Ota Z, Shikata K, Ota K: Nephrotic tunnels in glomerular basement membrane as revealed by a new electron microscopic method. J Am Soc Nephrol 4:1965–1973, 1994.

621. Kaysen GA, Jones H, Martin V, Hutchison F: A low-protein diet restricts albumin synthesis in nephrotic rats. J Clin Invest 83:1623, 1989.

622. Vriesendorp R, de Zeeuw D, de Jong PE, et al: Reduction of urinary protein and prostaglandin $E_2$ excretion in the nephrotic syndrome by non-steroidal anti-inflammatory drugs. Clin Nephrol 25:105, 1986.

623. Heeg JE, de Jong P, van der Hern G, de Zeeuw D: Reduction of proteinuria by angiotensin-converting enzyme inhibition. Kidney Int 32:78, 1987.

624. Wetzels J, Sluiter H, Hortsma A, et al: Prednisolone can increase glomerular permeability to proteins in nephrotic syndrome. Kidney Int 33:1169, 1988.

625. Sharma R, Lovell HB, Wiegmann TB, Savin VJ: Vasoactive substance induces cytoskeletal changes in cultured rat glomerular epithelial cells. J Am Soc Nephrol 3:1131–1138, 1992.

626. Praga M, Borstein B, Andres A, et al: Nephrotic proteinuria without hypoalbuminemia: Clinical characteristics and response to angiotensin-converting enzyme inhibitor. Am J Kidney Dis 17:330–338, 1991.

627. Kloke HJ, Wetzels JFM, van Hamersvelt HW, et al: Angiotensin-converting enzyme inhibition and the combination of a beta blocker and a diuretic are equally effective in lowering proteinuria in patients with glomerulonephritis. Nephrol Dial Transplant 8:808–813, 1993.

628. Richardson WP, Hassanein R, Pinnick RV, Savin VJ: Ultrafiltration coefficients of glomeruli from human biopsies. Kidney Int 34:845–852, 1988.

629. Savin VJ, Lindskey HB, Nagle RB, Cachia R: Ultrafiltration coef-

630. ficient and glomerular capillary resistance in a model of immune complex glomerulonephritis. Kidney Int 21:28–35, 1982.

630. Savin VJ, Sharma R, Lovell HB, Welling DJ: Measurement of albumin reflection coefficient with isolated rat glomeruli. J Am Soc Nephrol 3:1260–1269, 1992.

631. Shaw AB, Pisdon P, Lewis-Jackson J: Protein-creatinine index and Albustix in assessment of proteinuria. Br Med J 287:929, 1983.

632. Kaysen GA: Plasma composition in the nephrotic syndrome. Am J Nephrol 13:347–359, 1993.

633. Pollak VE, First MR, Pesce AJ: Value of the sieving coefficient in the interpretation of renal protein clearances in kidney disease. Nephron 13:82, 1974.

634. Cameron JS, Blandford G: The simple assessment of selectivity of heavy proteinuria. Lancet 2:242, 1966.

635. Myers BD, Okarma TB, Friedman S, et al: Mechanisms of proteinuria in human glomerulonephritis. J Clin Invest 70:732, 1982.

636. Laurent J, Philippon C, Lagrue G, et al: Proteinuria selectivity index—prognostic value in lipoid nephrosis and related diseases. Nephron 65:185–189, 1993.

637. Sesso R, Santos AP, Nishida SK, et al: Prediction of steroid responsiveness in the idiopathic nephrotic syndrome using urinary retinol-binding protein and beta-2-microglobulin. Ann Intern Med 116:905–909, 1992.

638. Tapp DC, Copley J: Effect of red blood cell lysis on protein quantitation in hematuric states. Am J Nephrol 8:190, 1988.

639. Bernard DB: Metabolic abnormalities in nephrotic syndrome. *In* Brenner BM, Stein JH (eds): Pathophysiology and Complications in Nephrotic Syndrome. Contemporary Issues in Nephrology. Churchill Livingstone, New York, 1982, p 86.

640. Ballmer PE, Weber BK, Roy-Chaudhury P, et al: Elevation of albumin synthesis rates in nephrotic patients, measured with [1-$^{13}$C]leucine. Kidney Int 41:132–138, 1992.

641. Koomans HA, Kortland W, Geers AB, et al: Lowered protein content of tissue fluid in patients with the nephrotic syndrome: Observations during pressure and recovery. Nephron 40:391, 1985.

642. Schultze G, Ahuja S, Faber U, Molzahn M: Gastrointestinal protein loss in the nephrotic syndrome. Studies with $^{51}$Cr–albumin. Nephron 25:227, 1980.

643. Hutchison F, Gambertoglio J, Jiminez I, et al: Effect of reduced dietary protein intake on albumin homeostasis and albuminuria in man. Kidney Int 27:141, 1985.

644. Pedraza-Chaverri J, Huberman A: Actinomycin D blocks the hepatic functional albumin mRNA increase in aminonucleoside-nephrotic rats. Nephron 59:648–650, 1991.

645. Bernard DB: Extrarenal complications of the nephrotic syndrome. Kidney Int 33:1184, 1988.

646. Strife CF, Jackson E, Forrestal J, West CD: Effect of the nephrotic syndrome on the concentration of serum complement components. Am J Kidney Dis 86:37, 1986.

647. Harris RC, Ismail N: Extrarenal complications of the nephrotic syndrome. Am J Kidney Dis 23:477–497, 1994.

648. Howard RL, Buddington B, Alfrey AC: Urinary albumin, transferrin and iron excretion in diabetic patients. Kidney Int 40:923–926, 1991.

649. Pedraza-Chaverri J, Torres-Rodriguez GA, Cruz C, et al: Copper and zinc metabolism in aminonucleoside-induced nephrotic syndrome. Nephron 66:87–92, 1994.

650. Vaziri ND, Kaupke CJ, Barton CH, Gonzales E: Plasma concentration and urinary excretion of erythropoietin in adult nephrotic syndrome. Am J Med 92:35–40, 1992.

651. Panicucci F, Sagripanti A, Vispi M, et al: Comprehensive study of haemostasis in nephrotic syndrome. Nephron 33:9–13, 1983.

652. Previato G, Loschiano C, Lupo A, et al: Clinical significance of plasma factor VIII levels in renal disease. Clin Nephrol 16:200, 1981.

653. Coppola R, Guerra L, Ruggeri ZM, et al: Factor VIII/von Willebrand factor in glomerular nephropathies. Clin Nephrol 16:217, 1981.

654. Llach F: Nephrotic syndrome: Hypercoagulability, renal vein thrombosis and other thromboembolic complications in nephrotic syndrome. *In* Brenner BM, Stein JH (eds): Contemporary Issues in Nephrology, Vol 9. Churchill Livingstone, New York, 1982, p 121.

655. Cameron JS: Coagulation and thromboembolic complications in the nephrotic syndrome. Adv Nephrol 13:75, 1984.

656. Vaziri N, Ali Khani S, Patel B, et al: Increased levels of protein C

concentrations, total and free protein S in nephrotic syndrome. Nephron 49:20, 1988.

657. Vigano-d'Angelo S, d'Angelo A, Kaufman CE, et al: Protein S deficiency occurs in the nephrotic syndrome. Ann Intern Med 107:42, 1987.

658. Adler AJ, Lundin AP, Feinroth MV, et al: β-Thromboglobulin levels in the nephrotic syndrome. Am J Med 69:551–554, 1980.

659. Kuhlmann U, Steuser J, Rhyner K, et al: Platelet aggregation and β-thromboglobulin levels in nephrotic patients with and without thrombosis. Clin Nephrol 15:229, 1981.

660. Loschiavo C, Previato G, Valvo E, et al: Clinical significance of urinary fibrinogen degradation products in renal disease. Study of two methods and correlation with histological findings of intraglomerular coagulation. Nephron 28:200, 1981.

661. Vaziri ND, Tuyetngo J-L, Ibsen KH, et al: Deficiency and urinary losses of factor XII in adult nephrotic syndrome. Nephron 32:342, 1982.

662. Cartwright GE, Gubler CJ, Wintrobe MM: Studies on copper metabolism. XI. Copper and iron metabolism in the nephrotic syndrome. J Clin Invest 33:685, 1954.

663. Freeman RM, Richards CJ, Rames LK: Zinc metabolism in aminonucleoside induced nephrosis. Am J Clin Nutr 28:699, 1975.

664. Reimold EW: Changes in zinc metabolism during the course of the nephrotic syndrome. Am J Dis Child 134:46, 1980.

665. Ellis D: Anemia in the course of nephrotic syndrome secondary to transferrin depletion. J Pediatr 90:953, 1977.

666. Hancock FE, Onstad JW, Wolf PL: Transferrin loss into the urine with hypochromic, microcytic anemia. Am J Clin Pathol 65:73, 1976.

667. Bergrem H: Pharmacokinetics and protein binding of prednisolone in patients with nephrotic syndrome and patients undergoing hemodialysis. Kidney Int 23:876, 1983.

668. Frey FJ, Frey BM: Altered prednisolone kinetics in patients with the nephrotic syndrome. Nephron 32:45, 1982.

669. Feinstein EI, Kaptien EM, Nicoloff JT, Massry SG: Thyroid function in patients with nephrotic syndrome and normal renal function. Am J Nephrol 2:70, 1982.

670. Schmidt-Gayk H, Schmitt W, Grawunder C, et al: 25-Hydroxy-vitamin D levels in nephrotic syndrome. Lancet 2:105, 1977.

671. Goldstein DA, Oda Y, Kurokawa K, Massry SG: Blood levels of 25-hydroxy vitamin D in nephrotic syndrome. Ann Intern Med 87:664, 1977.

672. Chan Y-L, Mason RS, Parmentier M, et al: Vitamin D metabolism in nephrotic rats. Kidney Int 24:336, 1985.

673. Medina A, Davies DL, Brown JJ, et al: A study of the renin-angiotensin system in the nephrotic syndrome. Nephron 12:233, 1974.

674. Boer P, Roos JC, Geyskes GG, Dorhout Mees EJ: Observations on plasma renin substrate in the nephrotic syndrome. Nephron 26:121, 1980.

675. McAuliffe J, Lind LJ, Leith D, Fencl V: Hypoproteinemic alkalosis. Am J Med 81:86, 1986.

676. Warwick GL, Parkard CJ: Lipoprotein metabolism in the nephrotic syndrome. Nephrol Dial Transplant 8:385–396, 1993.

677. Joles J, Kaysen G: Lipid metabolism in the nephrotic syndrome. Contemp Issues Nephrol 24:63–84, 1991.

678. Kaysen GA: Hyperlipidemia of the nephrotic syndrome. Kidney Int 39:S-8–S-15, 1991.

679. Keane WF: Lipids and the kidney. Kidney Int 46:910–920, 1994.

680. Wheeler DC, Bernard DB: Lipid abnormalities in the nephrotic syndrome: Causes, consequences and treatment. Am J Kidney Dis 23:331–346, 1994.

681. Kaysen GA, Don B, Schambelan M: Proteinuria, albumin synthesis and hyperlipidemia in the nephrotic syndrome. Nephrol Dial Transplant 6:141–149, 1991.

682. Newmark SR, Anderson CF, Donadio JV Jr, Ellefson RD: Lipoprotein profiles in adult nephrotics. Mayo Clin Proc 50:359, 1975.

683. Baxter JH, Goodman HC, Havel RJ: Serum lipid and lipoprotein alterations in nephrosis. J Clin Invest 39:455, 1960.

684. Joven J, Villabona C, Vilella E, et al: Abnormalities of lipoprotein metabolism for patients with the nephrotic syndrome. N Engl J Med 323:579–584, 1990.

685. Short CD, Durrington PN, Mallick NP, et al: Serum and urinary high-density lipoproteins in glomerular disease with proteinuria. Kidney Int 29:1224, 1986.

686. Thomas ME, Freestone A, Varghese Z, et al: Lipoprotein(a) in patients with proteinuria. Nephrol Dial Transplant 7:597–601, 1992.

687. Wanner C, Rader D, Bartens W, et al: Elevated plasma lipoprotein(a) in patients with the nephrotic syndrome. Ann Intern Med 119:263–269, 1993.

688. Stenvinkel P, Berglund L, Heimburger O, et al: Lipoprotein(a) in nephrotic syndrome. Kidney Int 44:1116–1123, 1993.

689. Faucher C, Doucet C, Baumelou A, et al: Elevated lipoprotein(a) levels in primary nephrotic syndrome. Am J Kidney Dis 22:808–813, 1993.

689a. Conwill DE, Granger DN, Cook BH, et al: The effect of serum oncotic pressure on serum cholesterol levels: A study in ''normal'' and nephrotic subjects. South Med J 70:456, 1977.

690. Yedgar S, Eilam O, Shafrir E: Regulation of plasma lipid levels by plasma viscosity in nephrotic rats. Am J Physiol 248:E10, 1985.

691. Warwick GL, Fox JG, Boulton-Jones JM: The relationship between urinary albumin excretion rate and serum cholesterol in primary glomerular disease. Clin Nephrol 41:135–137, 1994.

692. Perez GO, Levine S, Gomez E, Hsia SL: Serum-cholesterol–binding reserve in patients with the nephrotic syndrome. Nephron 24:146, 1979.

693. Garber DW, Gottlieb B, Marsh JB, Sparks C: Catabolism of very low density lipoproteins in experimental nephrosis. J Clin Invest 74:1375, 1984.

694. Wass V, Cameron JS: Cardiovascular disease and the nephrotic syndrome: The other side of the coin. Nephron 27:58, 1981.

695. Mallick NP, Short CD: The nephrotic syndrome and ischaemic heart disease. Nephron 27:54, 1981.

696. Stampfer MJ, Sacks FM, Salvini S, et al: A prospective study of cholesterol, apolipoproteins, and the risk of myocardial infarction. N Engl J Med 325:373–381, 1991.

697. Ordonez JD, Hiatt RA, Killebrew EJ, Fireman BH: The increased risk of coronary heart disease associated with nephrotic syndrome. Kidney Int 44:638–642, 1993.

698. Radhakrishnan J, Appel AS, Valeri A, Appel GB: The nephrotic syndrome, lipids, and risk factors for cardiovascular disease. Am J Kidney Dis 22:135–142, 1993.

699. Ravnskov U: Hypercholesterolemia does not cause coronary heart disease—evidence from the nephrotic syndrome. Nephron 66:356–357, 1994.

700. Olbricht CJ, Koch KM: Persistent nephrotic syndrome, high cholesterol and mortality. Nephron 66:358–359, 1994.

701. Kaysen GA, Gambertoglio J, Felts J, Hutchison F: Albumin synthesis and hyperlipemia in nephrotic patients. Kidney Int 31:1368, 1987.

702. de Mendoza SG, Kashyap ML, Chen CY, Lutmer RF: High-density lipoproteinemia in nephrotic syndrome. Metabolism 25:1143, 1976.

703. van Goor H, van der Horst MLC, Atmosoerodjo J, et al: Renal apolipoproteins in nephrotic rats. Am J Pathol 142:1804–1812, 1993.

704. Humphreys MH: Mechanisms and management of nephrotic edema. Kidney Int 45:266–281, 1994.

705. Perico N, Remuzzi G: Renal handling of sodium in the nephrotic syndrome. Am J Nephrol 13:413–421, 1993.

706. Perico N, Remuzzi G: Edema of the nephrotic syndrome: The role of the atrial peptide system. Am J Kidney Dis 22:355–366, 1993.

707. Joles JA, Rabelink TJ, Braam B, Koomans HA: Plasma volume regulation: Defences against edema formation (with special emphasis on hypoproteinemia). Am J Nephrol 13:399–412, 1993.

708. Ichikawa I, Rennke HG, Hoyer JR, et al: Role for intrarenal mechanisms in the impaired salt excretion of experimental nephrotic syndrome. J Clin Invest 71:91, 1983.

709. Kaysen GP, Paukert TT, Menke DJ, et al: Plasma volume expansion is necessary for edema formation in the rat with Heymann nephritis. Am J Physiol 248:F247, 1985.

710. Perico N, Delaini F, Lupini C, Remuzzi G: Renal response to atrial peptides is reduced in experimental nephrons. Am J Physiol 252:F654, 1987.

711. Tulassay T, Rascher W, Lang RE, Seyberth S: Atrial natriuretic peptide and other vasoactive peptides in nephrotic syndrome. Kidney Int 31:1391, 1987.

712. Brown EA, Markandu ND, Sagnella GA, et al: Lack of effect of captopril on the sodium retention of the nephrotic syndrome. Nephron 37:43, 1984.

713. Brown EA, Markandu ND, Rouston JE, et al: Is the renin-angiotensin-aldosterone system involved in the sodium retention in the nephrotic syndrome? Nephron 32:102, 1982.
714. Brown EA, Markandu ND, Sagnella GA, et al: Evidence that some mechanism other than the renin system causes sodium retention in nephrotic syndrome. Lancet 2:1237, 1982.
715. Geers A, Koomans H, Roos J, et al: Functional relationships in the nephrotic syndrome. Kidney Int 26:324, 1984.
716. Berlyne GM, Brown C, Adler A, et al: Water immersion in nephrotic syndrome. Arch Intern Med 141:1275, 1981.
717. Sutton JV, Brown C, Adler AJ, et al: Renal phosphate handling in nephrotic syndrome during water immersion. Nephron 32:108, 1982.
718. Brown C, Sutton JV, Adler A, et al: Renal calcium and magnesium handling in water immersion in nephrotic patients. Nephron 33:17, 1983.
719. Krishna GG, Danovitch GM: Effects of water immersion on renal function in the nephrotic syndrome. Kidney Int 21:395, 1982.
720. Valentin JP, Qiu C, Muldowney WP, et al: Cellular basis for blunted volume expansion natriuresis in experimental nephrotic syndrome. J Clin Invest 90:1302–1312, 1992.
721. Orisio S, Perico N, Benatti L, et al: Renal cyclophilin-like protein gene expression parallels changes in sodium excretion in experimental nephrosis and is positively modulated by atrial natriuretic peptide. J Am Soc Nephrol 3:1710–1716, 1993.
722. Davison AM, Lambie AT, Verth AH, Cash JD: Salt-poor albumin in the management of nephrotic syndrome. Br Med J 1:481, 1974.
723. Meltzer JI, Keinn HJ, Laragh JH, et al: Nephrotic syndrome: Vasoconstrictor and hypervolemia types indicated by renin sodium profiling. Ann Intern Med 91:688, 1979.
724. Dorhout Mees EJ, Roos JC, Boer P, et al: Observations on edema formation in the nephrotic syndrome in adults with minimal lesions. Am J Med 67:378, 1979.
725. Yamamuchi H, Hopper J Jr: Hypovolemic shock and hypotension as a complication in the nephrotic syndrome. Ann Intern Med 60:242, 1964.
726. Reimold EW, Marks JF: Hypovolaemic shock complicating nephrotic syndrome in children. J Pediatr 69:658, 1966.
727. Chamberlain MJ, Pringle A, Wrong OM: Oliguric renal failure in nephrotic syndrome. Q J Med 35:215, 1966.
728. Conolly ME, Wrong OM, Jones NF: Reversible acute renal failure in idiopathic nephrotic syndrome with minimal glomerular change. Lancet 1:665, 1968.
729. Raij L, Keane WF, Leonard A, Shapiro F: Irreversible acute renal failure in idiopathic nephrotic syndrome. Am J Med 61:207, 1976.
730. Holdsworth DR, Stephens P, Dowling JP, Atkins RC: Reversible acute renal failure in the nephrotic syndrome with minimal glomerular pathology. Med J Aust 2:532, 1977.
731. Drumond MC, Kristal B, Myers BD, Deen WM: Structural basis for reduced glomerular filtration capacity in nephrotic humans. J Clin Invest 94:1187–1195, 1994.
732. Lowenstein J, Schacht RG, Baldwin DS: Renal failure in minimal change nephrotic syndrome. Am J Med 70:227, 1981.
733. Hutchison FM, Schambelan M, Kaysen G: Modulation of albuminuria by dietary protein and converting enzyme inhibition. Am J Physiol 253:F719, 1987.
734. Zoja C, Benigni A, Verroust P, et al: Indomethacin reduces proteinuria in passive Heymann nephritis in rats. Kidney Int 31:1335, 1987.
735. Avram MM, Lepner HI, Gan AC: Medical nephrectomy. The use of metallic salts for the control of massive proteinuria in the nephrotic syndrome. Proc Am Soc Artif Intern Organs 22:431, 1976.
736. Henrich WL, Goldman M, Dotter CT, et al: Therapeutic renal arterial occlusion for elimination of proteinuria—medical nephrectomy. Arch Intern Med 136:840, 1976.
737. McCarron DA, Rubin RJ, Barnes BA, et al: Therapeutic bilateral renal infarction in end-stage renal disease. N Engl J Med 294:652, 1976.
738. Donker AJM, Brentjens JRH, van der Hem GK, Arisz L: Treatment of the nephrotic syndrome with indomethacin. Nephron 22:374, 1978.
739. Baumelou A, Legrain M: Medical nephrectomy with antiinflammatory non-steroidal drugs. Br Med J 284:234, 1982.
740. Torres VE, Velosa JA, Holley KE, et al: Meclofenamate treatment of recurrent idiopathic nephrotic syndrome with focal segmental glomerulosclerosis after renal transplantation. Mayo Clin Proc 59:146, 1984.
741. Curry RC Jr, Roberts WC: Status of the coronary arteries in the nephrotic syndrome (analysis of 20 necropsy patients aged 15 to 35 years to determine if coronary atherosclerosis is accelerated). Am J Med 63:183, 1977.
742. Mukherjee AP, Toh BH, Chan GEL, et al: Vascular complications in the nephrotic syndrome. Br Med J 4:273, 1970.
743. Alexander JH, Schapel GJ, Edwards KDG: Increased incidence of coronary heart disease associated with combined elevation of serum triglyceride and cholesterol concentrations in the nephrotic syndrome in man. Med J Aust 2:119, 1974.
744. Cameron JS, Wass V, Jarrett RJ, Chilvers C: Nephrotic syndrome and cardiovascular disease. Lancet 2:1017, 1979.
745. Kallen R, Brynes R, Aronson B, et al: Premature coronary atherosclerosis in a 5-year-old with corticosteroid-refractory nephrotic syndrome. Am J Kidney Dis 131:976, 1977.
746. D'Amico G, Gentile MG: Pharmacological and dietary treatment of lipid abnormalities in nephrotic patients. Kidney Int 39:S-65–S-69, 1991.
747. Grundy SM: Management of hyperlipidemia of kidney disease. Kidney Int 37:847–853, 1990.
748. D'Amico G, Gentile MG, Manna G, et al: Effect of vegetarian soy diet on hyperlipidaemia in nephrotic syndrome. Lancet 339:1131–1134, 1992.
749. Hoak JC, Conner WE, Armstrong ML, Warner ED: Effect of clofibrate on serum and hepatic lipids in nephrotic rats. Lab Invest 19:370, 1968.
750. Bridgman JF, Rosen SM, Thorp JM: Complications during clofibrate treatment of nephrotic-syndrome hyperlipoproteinaemia. Lancet 2:506, 1972.
751. Rabelink AJ, Hene RJ, Erkelens DW, et al: Effects of simvastatin and cholestyramine on lipoprotein profile in hyperlipidaemia of nephrotic syndrome. Lancet 2:1335, 1988.
752. Freundlich M, Bourgoignie J, Zilleruelo G, et al: Calcium and vitamin D metabolism in children with nephrotic syndrome. J Pediatr 108:383, 1986.
753. Iida H, Izumino K, Asaka M, et al: Effect of probucol on hyperlipidemia in patients with nephrotic syndrome. Nephron 47:280, 1987.
754. Neale TJ, Ojha PP, Exner M, et al: Proteinuria in passive Heymann nephritis is associated with lipid peroxidation and formation of adducts on type IV collagen. J Clin Invest 94:1577–1584, 1994.
755. Vega GL, Grundy SM: Lovastatin therapy in nephrotic hyperlipidemia. Kidney Int 33:1160, 1988.
756. Martins Prata M, Nogueira AC, Reimao Pinto J, et al: Long-term effect of lovastatin on lipoprotein profile in patients with primary nephrotic syndrome. Clin Nephrol 41:277–283, 1994.
757. Jacob BG, Richter WO, Schwandt P: Lovastatin, pravastatin, and serum lipoprotein(a). Ann Intern Med 112:713–714, 1990.
758. Wanner C, Bohler J, Eckardt HG, et al: Effects of simvastatin on lipoprotein(a) and lipoprotein composition in patients with nephrotic syndrome. Clin Nephrol 41:138–143, 1994.
759. Rubin HM, Blau EB, Michaels RH: Hemophilus and pneumococcal peritonitis in children with nephrotic syndrome. Pediatrics 56:598, 1975.
760. Giangiacomo J, Cleary TG, Cole BR, et al: Serum immunoglobulins in the nephrotic syndrome. N Engl J Med 293:8, 1975.
761. McLean RH, Forsgren A, Bjorstein B, et al: Decreased serum factor-B concentration associated with decreased opsonization of Escherichia coli in idiopathic nephrotic syndrome. Pediatr Res 11:910, 1977.
762. Garin EH, Sausville PJ, Richard GA: Impaired primary antibody response in experimental nephrotic syndrome. Clin Exp Immunol 52:595, 1983.
763. Praga M, Anders A, Hernandez E, et al: Tubular dysfunction in nephrotic syndrome: Incidence and prognostic implications. Nephrol Dial Transplant 6:683–688, 1991.
764. Stanbury SW, Macaulay D: Defects of renal tubular function in the nephrotic syndrome. Q J Med 26:7, 1957.
765. Gur A, Adefuin PY, Siegel NJ, Hayslett JP: A study of the renal handling of water in lipoid nephrosis. Pediatr Res 10:197, 1976.
766. Carrie BJ, Golbetz HV, Michaels AS, Myers BD: Creatinine: An inadequate filtration marker in glomerular disease. Am J Med 69:177, 1980.
767. Remuzzi G, Bertani T: Is glomerulosclerosis a consequence of

altered glomerular permeability to monomolecules? Kidney Int 38:384–394, 1990.

768. Llach F, Arieff AI, Massry SG: Renal vein thrombosis and nephrotic syndrome: A prospective study of 36 adult patients. Ann Intern Med 83:8, 1975.

769. Llach F: Renal Vein Thrombosis. Futura Publishing, Mount Kisco, NY, 1983.

770. Llach F: Hypercoagulability, renal vein thrombosis and other thrombotic complications of nephrotic syndrome. Kidney Int 28:429, 1985.

771. Du XH, Glas-Greenwalt P, Kant KS, et al: Nephrotic syndrome and renal vein thrombosis: Pathogenetic importance of a plasmin inhibitor ($\alpha_2$-antiplasmin). Clin Nephrol 24:186, 1985.

772. Trew PA, Biava CG, Jacobs RP, Hopper J: Renal vein thromboses in membranous glomerulopathy. Incidence and association. Medicine (Baltimore) 57:69, 1978.

773. Harrington JT, Kassirer JP: Renal vein thrombosis. Ann Rev Med 33:255, 1982.

774. Wagoner RD, Stanson AW, Holley KE, Winter CS: Renal vein thrombosis in idiopathic membranous glomerulopathy and nephrotic syndrome: Incidence and significance. Kidney Int 23:368, 1983.

775. Thomson C, Forbes CD, Prentice CRM, Kennedy AC: Changes in blood coagulation and fibrinolysis in the nephrotic syndrome. Q J Med 43:399, 1974.

776. Kauffman RH, Veltkamp JJ, van Tilburg NH, van Es LA: Acquired antithrombin-III deficiency and thrombosis in the nephrotic syndrome. Am J Med 65:607, 1978.

777. Cade R, Spooner G, Juncos L: Chronic renal vein thrombosis. Am J Med 63:387, 1977.

778. Avasthi PS, Greene ER, Scholler C, Fowler CR: Noninvasive diagnosis of renal vein thrombosis by ultrasonic echo-Doppler flowmetry. Kidney Int 23:882, 1983.

779. Morris JF, Ginn HE, Thompson DD: Unilateral renal vein thrombosis associated with the nephrotic syndrome. Am J Med 34:867, 1963.

780. Rostoker G, Texier JP, Jeandel B, et al: Asymptomatic renal-vein thrombosis in adult nephrotic syndrome ultrasonography and urinary fibrin-fibrinogen products: A prospective study. Eur J Med 1:19–22, 1992.

781. Burston J, Darmady EM, Stranack F: Nephrosis due to mercurial diuretics. Br Med J 1:1277, 1958.

782. Omae T, Masson GM, Corcoran AC: Experimental production of nephrotic syndrome following renal vein constriction in rats. Proc Soc Exp Biol Med 97:821, 1958.

783. Fisher ER, Sharkey D, Pardo V, Vuzevski V: Experimental renal vein constriction: Its relation to renal lesions observed in human renal vein thrombosis and the nephrotic syndrome. Lab Invest 18:689, 1968.

784. Barclay GPT, Cameron H, Mae D, Loughridge L: Amyloid disease of the kidney and renal vein thrombosis. Q J Med 29:137, 1960.

785. Balabamian MB, Schnetzler DE, Kaloyanides GJ: Nephrotic syndrome, renal vein thrombosis and renal failure. Report of a case with recovery of renal function, loss of proteinuria and dissolution of thrombus after anticoagulant therapy. Am J Med 54:768, 1973.

786. Pollak VE, Pirani CL, Sesking C, Griffel B: Bilateral renal vein thrombosis. Clinical and electron microscopic studies of a case with complete recovery after anticoagulant therapy. Ann Intern Med 65:1056, 1966.

787. Duffy JL, Letteri J, Cinque T, et al: Renal vein thrombosis and the nephrotic syndrome. Report of two cases with successful treatment of one. Am J Med 54:663, 1973.

788. Fein RL, Chart A, Leviton A: Renal vein thrombectomy for treatment of renal vein thrombosis associated with the nephrotic syndrome. J Urol 99:1, 1968.

789. Cohn LH, Lee J, Hopper J: The treatment of bilateral renal vein thrombosis and nephrotic syndrome. Surgery 64:387, 1968.

790. Sarasin FP, Schifferli JA: Prophylactic oral anticoagulation in nephrotic patients with idiopathic membranous nephropathy. Kidney Int 45:578–585, 1994.

791. Sasdelli M, Cagnoli L, Candi P, et al: Cell-mediated immunity in idiopathic glomerulonephritis. Clin Exp Immunol 46:27, 1981.

792. Cagnoli L, Tabacchi P, Pasquali S, Cecci M: T-cell subset alterations in idiopathic glomerulonephritis. Clin Exp Immunol 50:70, 1982.

793. Tanaka R, Yoshikawa N, Nakamura H, Ito H: Infusion of blood mononuclear products from nephrotic children increases albuminuria in rats. Nephron 60:35–41, 1992.

794. Sobel A, Heslan J-M, Branellec A, Lagrue G: Vascular permeability factor produced by lymphocytes of patients with nephrotic syndrome. Adv Nephrol 10:315, 1981.

795. Boulton Jones JM, Tulloch I, Dore B, McLay A: Changes in the glomerular capillary wall induced by lymphocyte products and serum of nephrotic patients. Clin Nephrol 20:72, 1983.

796. Schnaper HW, Avne TM: Identification of the lymphokine-soluble immune response suppressor in urine of nephrotic children. J Clin Invest 76:341, 1985.

797. Schnaper HW: A regulatory system for soluble immune response suppressor production in steroid-responsive nephrotic syndrome. Kidney Int 38:151–159, 1990.

798. Abrass CK: Glomerulonephritis in the elderly. Am J Med 5:409, 1985.

799. Mattoo TK, Al-Sowailem AM: Spectrum of renal pathology in 100 selected children with nephrotic syndrome. Ann Saudi Med 13:420–422, 1993.

800. Donadio JV: Treatment of glomerulonephritis in the elderly. Am J Kidney Dis 16:307–311, 1990.

801. Danovitch GM, Nissenson AR: The role of renal biopsy in determining therapy and prognosis in renal disease. Am J Nephrol 2:179, 1982.

802. Levey A, Lau J, Pauker S, Kassirer J: Idiopathic nephrotic syndrome. Puncturing the biopsy myth. Ann Intern Med 107:697, 1987.

803. Hlatky MA: Is renal biopsy necessary in adults with nephrotic syndrome? Lancet 2:1264, 1982.

804. Donadio JV Jr: The limitations of renal biopsy. Am J Kidney Dis 1:249, 1982.

805. Morel-Maroger L: The value of renal biopsy. Am J Kidney Dis 1:244, 1982.

806. Striker GE: Controversy: The role of renal biopsy in modern medicine. Am J Kidney Dis 1:241, 1982.

807. Kassirer J: Nephrology forum: Is renal biopsy necessary for optimal management of the idiopathic nephrotic syndrome? Kidney Int 24:561, 1983.

808. Bertani T, Mecca G, Sacchi G, Remuzzi G: Superimposed nephritis: A separate entity among glomerular disease. Am J Kidney Dis 7:205, 1986.

809. Munk F: Die Nephrosen. Med Klin 12:1019, 1047, 1073, 1946.

810. Farquhar MG, Vernier RL, Good RA: An electron microscopic study of the glomerulus in nephrosis, glomerulonephritis and lupus erythematosus. J Exp Med 106:649, 1957.

811. Jao W, Pollak VE, Norris VE, et al: Lipoid nephrosis: An approach to the clinicopathologic analysis and dismemberment of idiopathic nephrotic syndrome with minimal glomerular changes. Medicine (Baltimore) 52:445, 1973.

812. Cameron JS, Turner DR, Ogg CS, et al: The nephrotic syndrome in adults with "minimal change" glomerular lesions. Q J Med 43:461, 1974.

813. Habib R, Churg J, Bernstein J, et al: Minimal change disease, mesangial proliferative glomerulonephritis and focal sclerosis: Individual entities or a spectrum of disease? *In* Robinson RR (ed): Nephrology. Springer-Verlag, New York, 1984, p 634.

814. Habib R, Levy M, Gubler MC: Clinicopathologic correlations in the nephrotic syndrome. Paediatrician 8:325, 1979.

815. Lichtig C, Ben-Izhak O, On A, et al: Childhood minimal change disease and focal segmental glomerulosclerosis: A continuous spectrum of disease? Am J Nephrol 11:325–331, 1991.

816. Savin VJ, Chonko AM, Sharma R, et al: Factor present in serum of patients with minimal change nephrotic syndrome or focal sclerosing glomerulopathy causes an immediate increase in glomerular protein permeability in vitro. J Am Soc Nephrol 1:567, 1990.

817. Koyama A, Fujisaki M, Kobayashi M, et al: A glomerular permeability factor produced by human T cell hybridomas. Kidney Int 40:453–460, 1991.

818. Iijima K, Yoshikawa N, Connolly DT, Nakamura H: Human mesangial cells and peripheral blood mononuclear cells produce vascular permeability factor. Kidney Int 44:959–966, 1993.

819. Sewell RF, Short CD: Minimal-change nephropathy: How does the immune system affect the glomerulus? Nephrol Dial Transplant 8:108–112, 1993.

820. Dantal J, Bigot E, Bogers W, et al: Effect of plasma protein adsorption on protein excretion in kidney-transplant recipients with recurrent nephrotic syndrome. N Engl J Med 330:7–14, 1994.
821. Grupe WE: Minimal change disease. Semin Nephrol 2:241, 1982.
822. Wyatt RJ, Marx MB, Kuzee M, Holland NH: Current estimates of the incidence of steroid responsive idiopathic nephrosis in Kentucky children 1–9 years of age. Int J Pediatr Nephrol 3:63, 1982.
823. Sharples P, Poulton J, White RHR: Steroid-responsive nephrotic syndrome is more common in Asians. Arch Dis Child 60:1014, 1985.
824. Sharpstone P, Ogg CS, Cameron JS: Nephrotic syndrome due to primary renal disease in adults. I. Survey of incidence in southeast England. Br Med J 2:533, 1969.
825. White RHR, Glasgow IEF, Mills RJ: Clinicopathological analysis of nephrotic syndrome in childhood. Lancet 1:1353, 1970.
826. Bader PI, Grove J, Trygstad CW: Familial nephrotic syndrome. Am J Med 56:34, 1974.
827. Reeves WG, Cameron JS, Ogg CS: Seasonal nephrotic syndrome. Kidney Int 3:412, 1973.
828. Sandberg DH, Bernstein CW, McIntosh RM, et al: Severe steroid-responsive nephrosis associated with hypersensitivity. Lancet 1:338, 1977.
829. Lagrue G, Laurent J: Allergy and lipoid nephrosis. Adv Nephrol 12:151, 1983.
830. Lagrue G, Laurent J: Is lipoid nephrosis an ''allergic'' disease? Transplant Proc 14:485, 1982.
831. Meadow SR, Sarsfield JK: Steroid-responsive nephrotic syndrome and allergy: Clinical studies. Arch Dis Child 56:509, 1981.
832. Sakarcan A, Timmons C, Seikaly M: Reversible idiopathic acute renal failure in children with primary nephrotic syndrome. J Pediatr 126:723–728, 1994.
833. Ueda N: Effect of corticosteroids on some homeostatic parameters in children with minimal change nephrotic syndrome. Nephron 56:374–378, 1990.
833a. Bohler T, Linderkamp O, Leo A, et al: Increased aggregation with normal surface charge and deformability of red blood cells in children with nephrotic syndrome. Clin Nephrol 38:119–124, 1992.
834. Jacquot C, Radeau E, Nochy D, et al: Nephrotic syndrome, linear glomerular IgG deposits, and minimal glomerular changes. Report of a case. Arch Intern Med 141:670, 1981.
835. Esparza AR, Hahn SI, Garella S, Abuelo JG: Spectrum of acute renal failure in nephrotic syndrome with minimal (or minor) glomerular lesions: Role of hemodynamic factors. Lab Invest 45:510, 1981.
836. Robson AM, Giangiacomo J, Kienstra RA, et al: Normal glomerular permeability and its modification by minimal-change nephrotic syndrome. J Clin Invest 54:1190, 1974.
837. Berg U, Bohlin A-B: Renal hemodynamics in minimal-change nephrotic syndrome. Int J Pediatr Nephrol 3:187, 1982.
838. Bohman S-O, Jaremko G, Bohlin A-B, Berg U: Foot process fusion and glomerular filtration rate in minimal-change nephrotic syndrome. Kidney Int 25:696, 1984.
839. Winetz JA, Robertson CR, Golbetz HV, et al: The nature of the glomerular injury in minimal-change and focal sclerosing glomerulopathies. Am J Kidney Dis 1:91, 1981.
840. Carrie BJ, Salyer WR, Myers BD: Minimal-change nephropathy: An electrochemical disorder of the glomerular membrane. Am J Med 70:262, 1981.
841. Bridges CR, Myers BD, Brenner BM, Deen WM: Glomerular charge alterations in human minimal-change nephropathy. Kidney Int 22:677, 1982.
842. Ghiggeri GM, Candiano G, Ginerri F, et al: Renal selectivity properties towards endogenous albumin in minimal-change nephropathy. Kidney Int 32:69, 1987.
843. Lau SO, Tkachuck JY, Hasegawa DK, Edson JR: Plasminogen and antithrombin III deficiencies in the childhood nephrotic syndrome associated with plasminogenuria and antithrombinuria. J Pediatr 96:390, 1980.
844. Batemen D, Gokal R, Prescott R, et al: Minimal-change glomerulonephritis associated with circulating anticoagulant to factor XII. Br Med J 281:358, 1980.
845. Schulte-Wisserman H, Gertz W, Straub E: IgE in patients with glomerulonephritis and minimal-change nephrotic syndrome. Eur J Pediatr 131:105, 1979.
846. Endoh M, Miyazaki M, Suga T, et al: Rheumatoid factors in patients with minimal change nephrotic syndrome. Clin Nephrol 35:93–97, 1991.
847. Chonko AM, Bay WH, Stein JH, Ferris TF: The role of renin and aldosterone in the salt retention of edema. Am J Med 63:881, 1977.
848. Trompeter RS, Barratt TM, Kay R, et al: HLA, atopy, and cyclophosphamide in steroid-responsive childhood nephrotic syndrome. Kidney Int 17:113, 1980.
849. Alfiler CA, Roy LP, Doran T, et al: HLA-DRw7 and steroid-responsive nephrotic syndrome of childhood. Clin Nephrol 14:71, 1980.
850. Noss G, Bachmann HJ, Olbing H: Association of minimal-change nephrotic syndrome (MCNS) with HLA-B8 and B13. Clin Nephrol 15:172, 1981.
851. Thomson PD, Barratt TM, Stokes CR: HLA antigens and atopic features in steroid-responsive nephrotic syndrome of childhood. Lancet 2:765, 1976.
852. Laugueruela CC, Buettner TL, Cole BR, et al: HLA extended haplotypes in steroid-sensitive nephrotic syndrome of childhood. Kidney Int 38:145–150, 1990.
853. Kobayashi Y, Chen X-M, Hiki Y, et al: Association of HLA DRW8 and DQW3 with minimal-change nephrotic syndrome in Japanese adults. Kidney Int 28:193, 1985.
854. Kobayashi K, Yoshikawa N, Nakamura H: T-cell subpopulations in childhood nephrotic syndrome. Clin Nephrol 41:253–258, 1994.
855. Fiser RT, Arnold WC, Charlton RK, et al: T-lymphocyte subsets in nephrotic syndrome. Kidney Int 40:913–916, 1991.
856. Poston RN, Cerio R, Cameron JS: Circulating immune complexes in minimal-change nephritis. N Engl J Med 298:1089, 1979.
857. Levinsky RJ, Malleson PN, Barratt TM: Circulating immune complexes in steroid responsive nephrotic syndrome. N Engl J Med 298:127, 1978.
858. Cairns SA, London A, Mallick NP: Immune complexes in minimal-change glomerulopathy. N Engl J Med 302:1033, 1980.
859. Abrass C, Hall C, Border WA, et al, and the Collaborative Study of Idiopathic Nephrotic Syndrome: Circulating immune complexes in adults with idiopathic nephrotic syndrome. Kidney Int 17:545, 1980.
860. Sherman RL, Susin M, Weksler ME, Becker EL: Lipoid nephrosis in Hodgkin's disease. Am J Med 52:699, 1972.
861. Schroeter NJ, Rushing D, Parker JP, Beltaos E: Minimal-change disease nephrotic syndrome associated with malignant mesothelioma. Arch Intern Med 146:1834, 1986.
862. Whelan JV, Hirzel D: Minimal-change nephropathy associated with pancreatic carcinoma. Arch Intern Med 148:975, 1988.
863. Martinez-Vea A, Panisello J, Garcia C, et al: Minimal change glomerulopathy and carcinoma. Report of 2 cases and a review of the literature. Am J Nephrol 13:69–72, 1993.
864. Krane N, Espenau P, Walker PD, et al: Renal disease and syphilis: A report of nephrotic syndrome with minimal-change disease. Am J Kidney Dis 9:176, 1987.
865. Cohen AH, Border WA, Glassock RJ: Nephrotic syndrome with glomerular mesangial IgM deposits. Lab Invest 38:610, 1978.
866. Bhasin HK, Abuelo JG, Nayak R, Esparza A: Mesangial proliferative glomerulonephritis. Lab Invest 39:21, 1978.
867. Bohle A, Fischback H, Wehner H, et al: Minimal-change lesion with nephrotic syndrome and focal glomerular sclerosis (variations of minimal proliferative glomerulonephritis with the nephrotic syndrome). Clin Nephrol 2:52, 1974.
868. Fogo A, Hawkins EP, Berry PL, et al: Glomerular hypertrophy in minimal change disease predicts subsequent progression to focal glomerular sclerosis. Kidney Int 38:115–123, 1990.
869. Hoyer JR: Focal segmental glomerulosclerosis. Semin Nephrol 2:253, 1982.
870. Rich AR: A hitherto unrecognized vulnerability of the juxtamedullary glomeruli in lipoid nephrosis. Bull Johns Hopkins Hosp 100:173, 1957.
871. Tejani A: Morphologic transitions in minimal-change nephrotic syndrome. Nephron 39:157, 1985.
872. Allen MJ, Thomas AC, Eastwood JB: Minimal change glomerulonephritis in the elderly: The role of renal biopsy. Clin Nephrol 28:99, 1987.
873. Chiang ML, Hawkins EP, Berry PL, et al: Diagnostic and prognostic significance of glomerular epithelial cell vacuolization and podocyte effacement in children with minimal lesion nephrotic syndrome and focal and segmental glomerulosclerosis: An ultrastructural study. Clin Nephrol 30:8, 1988.

874. Yoshikawa N, Ito H, Akamatsu R, et al: Glomerular podocyte vacuolization in focal segmental glomerulosclerosis. Arch Pathol Lab Med 100:394, 1986.

875. Kleinknecht G, Gubler MD: Nephrosis. *In* Hamburger J, Crosnier J, Grünefeld JP (eds): Nephrology. John Wiley & Sons, New York, 1979, p 433.

876. Lim VS, Sibley R, Spargo B: Adult lipoid nephrosis: Clinicopathological correlations. Ann Intern Med 81:314, 1974.

877. Cohen AH, Mampaso F, Zamboni L: Glomerular podocyte degeneration in human renal disease: An ultrastructural study. Lab Invest 37:30, 1977.

878. Abu-Farsakh H, Berry PL, Hill LL, et al: Mesangial IgG in childhood minimal change disease: Clinical relevance. Clin Nephrol 39:245–248, 1993.

879. Drummond KN, Michael AF, Good RA, Vernier RL: The nephrotic syndrome of childhood: Immunologic, clinical and pathologic correlation. J Clin Invest 45:620, 1966.

880. Vilches AR, Cameron JS, Turner DR: Minimal change-disease with mesangial IgM deposits. N Engl J Med 303:1480, 1980.

881. Ji-Yun Y, Melvin T, Sibley R, Michael AF: No evidence for a specific role of IgM in mesangial proliferation in idiopathic nephrotic syndrome. Kidney Int 25:100, 1984.

882. Saha H, Mustoneu J, Pasternak A, Halin H: Clinical follow-up of 54 patients with IgM nephropathy. Am J Nephrol 9:124, 1989.

883. Gonzalo A, Mampaso F, Gallego N, et al: Clinical significance of IgM mesangial deposits in nephrotic syndrome. Nephron 41:246, 1985.

884. Prasad DR, Zimmerman SW, Burkholder PM: Immunohistologic features of minimal-change nephrotic syndrome. Arch Pathol Lab Med 101:315, 1977.

885. Gerber MA, Paronetto F: IgE in glomeruli of patients with nephrotic syndrome. Lancet 1:1097, 1971.

886. Roy LP, Westberg NG, Michael AF: Nephrotic syndrome—no evidence for a role of IgE. Clin Exp Immunol 3:553, 1973.

887. Garcia del Moral R, Gomez-Morales M, Cortes V, et al: Mononuclear cell subsets in IgM mesangial proliferative glomerulonephritis. Nephron 65:215–221, 1993.

888. Vehaskari VM, Root ER, Germuth FG Jr, Robson AM: Glomerular charge and urinary protein excretion: Effects of systemic and intrarenal polycation infusion in the rat. Kidney Int 22:127, 1982.

889. Cotran R, Rennke HG: Anionic sites and the mechanisms of proteinuria. N Engl J Med 309:1050, 1983.

890. Bakker W, van Luijk W, Hene R, et al: Loss of glomerular polyanion in vitro induced by mononuclear blood cells from patients with minimal-change nephrotic syndrome. Am J Nephrol 6:107, 1986.

890a. Kitano Y, Yoshikawa N, Nakamura H: Glomerular anionic sites in minimal change nephrotic syndrome and focal segmental glomerulosclerosis. Clin Nephrol 40:199–204, 1993.

891. Boulton-Jones J, McWilliams G, Chandrachud L: Variation in the charge of red cells in patients with different glomerulopathies. Lancet 2:186, 1986.

892. Bennett CM, Glassock RJ, Chang RLS, et al: Permselectivity of the glomerular capillary wall: Studies of experimental glomerular nephritis in the rat using dextran sulfate. J Clin Invest 57:1287, 1976.

893. Davies DJ, Brewer DB, Hardwicke J: Urinary proteins and glomerular morphometry in protein overload proteinuria. Lab Invest 30:232, 1978.

894. Michael AF, Blau E, Vernier RL: Glomerular polyanion alteration in aminonucleoside nephrosis. Lab Invest 23:649, 1970.

895. Bridges CR, Myers BD, Brenner BM, Deen WM: Glomerular charge alterations in human minimal-change nephropathy. Kidney Int 22:677, 1982.

896. Ghizzeri GM, Candiano G, Ginevri F, et al: Renal selectivity properties towards endogenous albumin in minimal-change nephropathy. Kidney Int 32:69, 1977.

897. Walker F, O'Neill S, Carmody M, O'Dwyer WF: Nephrotic syndrome in Hodgkin's disease. Int J Pediatr Nephrol 4:35, 1983.

898. Shalhoub RJ: Pathogenesis of lipoid nephrosis: A disorder of T-cell function. Lancet 2:556, 1974.

899. Mallick NP: The pathogenesis of minimal change nephropathy. Clin Nephrol 7:87, 1977.

900. Maruyama K, Tomizawa S, Seki Y, et al: Inhibition of vascular permeability factor production in minimal change nephrotic syndrome. Nephron 62:27–30, 1992.

901. Tomizawa S, Maruyama K, Nagasawa N, et al: Studies of vascular permeability factor derived from T lymphocytes and inhibitory effect of plasma on its production in minimal-disease nephrotic syndrome. Nephron 41:157, 1985.

902. Lagrue G, Branellec LA, Blanc C, et al: A vascular permeability factor in lymphocyte culture supernatants from patients with nephrotic syndrome. II. Pharmacological and physiochemical properties. Biomedicine 23:73, 1975.

903. Trompeter RS, Barratt TM, Layward L: Vascular permeability and the nephrotic syndrome. Lancet 2:900, 1978.

904. Lagrue G, Xheneumont LS, Branellec A, et al: A vascular permeability factor elaborated from lymphocytes. I. Demonstration in patients with nephrotic syndrome. Biomedicine 23:37, 1975.

905. Chapman SJ, Brown Z, Williams DG, et al: Abnormalities of lymphocyte function in minimal-change nephrotic syndrome and focal glomerular sclerosis and the in vitro effect of indomethacin. Arch Dis Child 55:491, 1980.

906. Eyres K, Mallick NP, Taylor G: Evidence for cell-mediated immunity to renal antigens in minimal-change nephrotic syndrome. Lancet 1:118, 1976.

907. Wu MJ, Moorthy AV: Suppressor cell function in patients with primary glomerular disease. Clin Immunol Immunopathol 22:442, 1982.

908. Taube D, Brown Z, Williams DG: Long term impairment of suppressor cell function by cyclophosphamide in minimal-change nephropathy and its association with therapeutic response. Lancet 1:235, 1981.

909. Taube D, Brown Z, Williams DG: Cyclophosphamide and suppressor cell function. Lancet 1:720, 1981.

910. Chapman S, Taube D, Brown Z, Williams DG: Impaired lymphocyte transformation in minimal-change nephropathy in remission. Clin Nephrol 18:34, 1982.

911. Matsumoto K: Impaired local graft-versus-host reaction in lipoid nephrosis. Nephron 31:281, 1982. Letter.

912. Ooi BS, Orlina AR, Masaitis L: Lymphocytotoxins in primary renal disease. Lancet 2:1348, 1974.

913. Thomson NM, Kraft N: Normal human serum also contains the lymphotoxin found in minimal-change nephropathy. Kidney Int 31:1186, 1987.

914. Martini A, Vitiello MA, Siena S, et al: Multiple serum inhibitors of lectin-induced lymphocyte proliferation in nephrotic syndrome. Clin Exp Immunol 45:178, 1981.

915. Beale MG, Hoffsten PE, Robson AM, MacDermott RP: Inhibitory factors of lymphocyte transformation in sera from patients with minimal-change nephrotic syndrome. Clin Nephrol 13:271, 1980.

916. Menchaca JA, Lefkowitz S: Hyperlipoproteinaemia, cellular immunity, and nephrotic syndrome. Lancet 1:1084, 1980.

917. Taube D, Chapman S, Brown Z, Williams DG: Depression of normal lymphocyte transformation by sera of patients with minimal-change nephropathy and other forms of nephrotic syndrome. Clin Nephrol 15:286, 1981.

918. Fodor P, Saitua M, Rodriquez E, et al: T-cell dysfunction in minimal change nephrotic syndrome of childhood. Am J Dis Child 136:713–717, 1982.

919. Szewezyk Z, Klinger M, Maiga K: Lymphocytic transformation in minimal-change nephrotic syndrome. Lancet 1:433, 1977.

920. Iitaka K, West DD: A serum inhibitor of blastogenesis in idiopathic nephrotic syndrome transferred by lymphocytes. Clin Immunol Immunopathol 12:62, 1979.

921. Tomizawa S, Suzuki S, Oguri M, Kuroume T: Studies of T lymphocyte function and inhibitory factors in minimal-change nephrotic syndrome. Nephron 24:179, 1979.

922. Mauer SM, Hellerstein S, Cohn LRA, et al: Recurrence of steroid-responsive nephrotic syndrome after renal transplantation. J Pediatr 95:261, 1979.

923. Sasdelli M, Rovinetti C, Cagnoli L, et al: Lymphocyte subpopulations in minimal-change nephropathy. Nephron 25:72, 1980.

924. Kerpen HL, Bhat JG, Kantor LR, et al: Lymphocyte subpopulations in minimal-change nephrotic syndrome. Clin Immunol Immunopathol 14:130, 1979.

925. Feehally J, Beattie JJ, Brenchley PFC, et al: Modulation of cellular immune function by cyclophosphamide in children with minimal-change nephropathy. N Engl J Med 310:415, 1984.

926. Beale MG, Nash GS, Bertovich MJ, MacDermott RP: Immunoglobulin synthesis by peripheral blood mononuclear cells in minimal-change nephrotic syndrome. Kidney Int 23:380, 1983.

927. Ngu JL, Barratt JM, Soothill JF: Immunoconglutinin and complement changes in steroid-sensitive relapsing nephrotic syndrome of children. Clin Exp Immunol 6:109, 1970.
928. Davin JC, Fordart JB, Mahieu PR: Fc-receptor function in minimal-change nephrotic syndrome of childhood. Clin Nephrol 20:280, 1983.
929. Schnaper HW: Immune dysfunction and the pathogenesis of steroid-responsive nephrotic syndrome. Kidney 21:25, 1989.
930. Kida H, Iida H, Doki K: Period of freedom from relapses as an indication of cure in minimal-change nephrotic syndrome in adults. Nephron 19:153, 1977.
931. Report of the International Study of Kidney Disease in Children: Primary nephrotic syndrome in children: Clinical significance of histopathologic variants of minimal change and of diffuse mesangial hypercellularity. Kidney Int 20:765, 1981.
932. Report of the International Study of Kidney Disease in Children: The primary nephrotic syndrome in children. Identification of patients and minimal-change nephrotic syndrome from initial response to prednisone. J Pediatr 98:561, 1981.
933. Tejani A: Relapsing nephrotic syndrome. Nephron 45:81, 1987.
934. Berns JS, Gaudio KM, Krassner LS, et al: Steroid-responsive nephrotic syndrome of childhood: A long-term study of clinical course, histopathology, efficacy of cyclophosphamide therapy and effects on growth. Am J Kidney Dis 9:108, 1987.
935. Trachtman H, Carroll F, Phadke K, et al: Paucity of minimal-change lesion in children with early frequently relapsing steroid-responsive nephrotic syndrome. Am J Nephrol 7:13, 1987.
936. Nair RB, Date A, Kirubakaran MG, Shastry JCM: Minimal-change nephrotic syndrome in adults treated with alternate-day steroids. Nephron 47:209, 1987.
937. Nolasco F, Cameron JS, Heywood EF, et al: Adult-onset minimal-change nephrotic syndrome: A long-term follow-up. Kidney Int 29:1215, 1986.
938. Korbet SM, Schwartz MM, Lewis EJ: Minimal-change glomerulopathy of adulthood. Am J Nephrol 8:29, 1988.
939. Fujimoto S, Yamamoto Y, Hisanaga S, et al: Minimal change nephrotic syndrome in adults: Response to corticosteroid therapy and frequency of relapse. J Kidney Dis 17:687–692, 1991.
940. Mendoza SA, Tune BM: Treatment of childhood nephrotic syndrome. J Am Soc Nephrol 3:889–894, 1992.
941. Glassock RJ: Therapy of idiopathic nephrotic syndrome in adults. Am J Nephrol 13:422–428, 1993.
942. Ponticelli C, Passerini P: Treatment of the nephrotic syndrome associated with primary glomerulonephritis. Kidney Int 46:595–604, 1994.
943. Primack WA, Schulman SL, Kaplan BS: An analysis of the approach to management of childhood nephrotic syndrome by pediatric nephrologists. Am J Kidney Dis 23:524–527, 1994.
944. Tarshish P, Bernstein J, Tobin J, Edelmann C: Course of minimal change nephrotic syndrome. A report of the International Study of Kidney Disease in Children. J Am Soc Nephrol 4:208, 1993. Abstract.
945. Arneil GC, Lam C: Long-term assessment of steroid therapy in childhood nephrosis. Lancet 2:819, 1966.
946. Arneil GC: 164 children with nephrosis. Lancet 2:1103, 1961.
947. Wingen A, Muller-Wiefel D, Scharer K: Spontaneous remissions in frequently relapsing and steroid-dependent idiopathic nephrotic syndrome. Clin Nephrol 23:35, 1985.
948. Report of the International Study of Kidney Disease in Children: Nephrotic syndrome in children: A randomized trial comparing two prednisone regimens in steroid-responsive patients who relapse early. J Pediatr 95:239, 1979.
949. Arbeitsgemeinschaft für Pädiatrische Nephrologie: Alternate-day versus intermittent prednisone in frequently relapsing nephrotic syndrome. Lancet 1:401, 1979.
950. Leisti S, Hallman N, Koskimies O, et al: Association of post-medication hypocortisolism with first relapse of idiopathic nephrotic syndrome. Lancet 2:795, 1977.
951. Leisti S, Koskimies O, Perheentupa J, et al: Idiopathic nephrotic syndrome. Prevention of early relapse. Br Med J 1:892, 1978.
952. Leisti S, Koskimies O: Risk of relapse in steroid-sensitive nephrotic syndrome: Effect of stage of post-prednisone adrenocortical suppression. J Pediatr 103:553, 1983.
953. Arbeitsgemeinschaft für Pädiatrische Nephrologie: Short versus standard prednisone therapy for initial treatment of idiopathic nephrotic syndrome in children. Lancet 1:380, 1988.
954. Green DC, Winter RJ, Kawahara FS, et al: Pharmacokinetic studies of prednisolone in children. J Pediatr 93:299, 1978.
955. Srivastava RN, Agarwal RK, Moudgil A, Bhuyan U: Late resistance to corticosteroids in nephrotic syndrome. J Pediatr 108:70, 1986.
956. Yoshimura A, Idenra T, Iwasaki S, et al: Aggravation of minimal change nephrotic syndrome by administration of human albumin. Clin Nephrol 37:109–114, 1992.
957. Wang F, Looi LM, Chua CT: Minimal-change glomerular disease in Malaysian adults and use of alternate-day steroid therapy. Q J Med 51:312, 1982.
958. Imbasciati E, Gusmano R, Edefonti A, et al: Controlled trial of methylprednisolone pulses and low dose oral prednisone for the minimal change nephrotic syndrome. Br Med J 291:1305, 1985.
959. Yeung CK, Wang KL, Ng WL: Intravenous methylprednisolone pulse therapy in minimal-change nephrotic syndrome. Aust N Z J Med 13:349, 1983.
960. Ponticelli C, Imbasciati E, Case N, et al: Intravenous methylprednisolone in minimal-change nephrotic syndrome. Br Med J 280:685, 1980.
961. Bernstein J, Edelmann CM: Minimal-change nephrotic syndrome. Histopathology and steroid responsiveness. Arch Dis Child 57:816, 1982.
962. Meyrier A, Simon P: Treatment of corticoresistant idiopathic nephrotic syndrome in the adult: Minimal-change disease and focal and segmental glomerulosclerosis. Adv Nephrol 17:127, 1988.
963. Ponticelli C, Passerini P: Alkylating agents and purine analogues in primary glomerulonephritis with nephrotic syndrome. Nephrol Dial Transplant 6:381–388, 1991.
964. Niaudet D, Habib R, Gagnodoux MF, et al: Treatment of severe childhood nephrosis. Adv Nephrol 17:151, 1988.
965. Ooi BS, Chen BTM, Tan K, Khoo OT: Longitudinal studies of lipoid nephrosis. Arch Intern Med 130:883, 1972.
966. Pru C, Kjellstrand CM, Cohn RA, Vernier RL: Late recurrence of minimal-lesion nephrotic syndrome. Ann Intern Med 100:69, 1984.
967. Cuoghi D, Vangelista A, Baraldi A, Cheli E: Relapse of nephrotic syndrome following remission for 20 years. Int J Pediatr Nephrol 4:211, 1983.
968. Engle JE, Schoolwerth AC: Late recurrence of corticosteroid-responsive nephrotic syndrome of childhood. JAMA 243:1840, 1980.
969. Barratt TM, Soothill JF: Controlled trial of cyclophosphamide in steroid-sensitive relapsing nephrotic syndrome of childhood. Lancet 2:479, 1970.
970. Grupe W, Makker SP, Ingelfinger JR: Chlorambucil treatment of frequently relapsing nephrotic syndrome. N Engl J Med 295:746, 1976.
971. Schoeneman MJ, Spitzer A, Greifer I: Nitrogen mustard therapy in children with frequent relapsing nephrotic syndrome and steroid toxicity. Am J Kidney Dis 2:526, 1983.
972. Barratt TM, Cameron JS, Chantler C, et al: Comparative trial of 2 weeks and 8 weeks cyclophosphamide in steroid-sensitive relapsing nephrotic syndrome of childhood. Arch Dis Child 48:286, 1973.
973. McCrory WW, Shibuya M, Lu W-H, Lewy JE: Therapeutic and toxic effects observed with different dosage programs of cyclophosphamide in treatment of steroid-responsive but frequently relapsing nephrotic syndrome. J Pediatr 82:614, 1973.
974. Chin J, Drummond KN: Long-term follow-up of cyclophosphamide therapy in frequently relapsing minimal-lesion nephrotic syndrome. J Pediatr 84:825, 1974.
975. Report of the International Study of Kidney Disease in Children: Prospective, controlled trial of cyclophosphamide therapy in children with the nephrotic syndrome. Lancet 2:423, 1974.
976. Arbeitsgemeinshaft für Pädiatrische Nephrologie: Cyclophosphamide treatment of steroid-dependent nephrotic syndrome: Comparison of 8-week with 12-week course. Arch Dis Child 62:1102, 1987.
977. Cameron JS, Chantler C, Ogg CS, White RHR: Long-term stability of remission in nephrotic syndrome after treatment with cyclophosphamide. Br Med J 4:7, 1974.
978. Pennisi AJ, Grushkin CM, Lieberman E: Cyclophosphamide in the treatment of idiopathic nephrotic syndrome. Pediatrics 57:948, 1976.
979. Al-Khader AA, Lien JWK, Aber GM: Cyclophosphamide alone in the treatment of adult patients with minimal-change glomerulonephritis. Clin Nephrol 11:26, 1979.

980. Siegel NJ, Gaudio KM, Krassner LS, et al: Steroid-dependent nephrotic syndrome in children: Histopathology and relapses after cyclophosphamide treatment. Kidney Int 19:454, 1981.

981. Williams SA, Makker SP, Ingelfinger JR, Grupe WE: Long-term evaluation of chlorambucil including effects of dose in frequently relapsing nephrotic syndrome. Pediatr Res 2:560, 1977.

982. Arbeitsgemeinschaft für Pädiatrische Nephrologie: Effect of cytotoxic drugs on frequently relapsing nephrotic syndrome with and without steroid dependence. N Engl J Med 306:457, 1982.

983. Ghosh L, Muehreke RC: The nephrotic syndrome. A prodrome to lymphoma. Ann Intern Med 72:379, 1970.

984. Plager J, Stutzman L: Acute nephrotic syndrome as a manifestation of active Hodgkin's disease. Am J Med 50:56, 1971.

985. Kashtan C, Melvin T, Kim Y: Long-term follow-up of patients with steroid-dependent, minimal-change nephrotic syndrome. Clin Nephrol 29:79, 1988.

986. Bergstrand A, Bollgren I, et al: Idiopathic nephrotic syndrome of childhood: Cyclophosphamide induced conversion from steroid refractory to highly sensitive disease. Clin Nephrol 1:302, 1973.

987. Report of the International Study of Kidney Disease in Children: Cyclophosphamide therapy in focal and segmental glomerulosclerosis. Pediatr Res 16:320A, 1982.

988. Callis L, Nieto J, Vila A, Rende J: Chlorambucil treatment in minimal lesion nephrotic syndrome: A reappraisal of its gonadal toxicity. J Pediatr 97:653, 1980.

989. Lewis EJ: Chlorambucil for childhood nephrosis. A word of caution. N Engl J Med 302:963, 1980.

990. Puri HC, Campbell RA: Cyclophosphamide and malignancy. Lancet 1:1306, 1977.

991. Brusamolino E, Pagnucco G, Bernasconi C: Acute leukemia occurring in a primary neoplasia (secondary leukemia). A review of biological, epidemiological and clinical aspects. Haematologica 71:60, 1986.

992. Barratt TM, Cameron JS, Chantler C: Controlled trial of azathioprine in treatment of steroid-responsive nephrotic syndrome of childhood. Arch Dis Child 52:462, 1977.

993. Cade R, Mars D, Privette M, et al: Effect of long-term azathioprine administration in adults with minimal-change glomerulonephritic and nephrotic syndrome resistant to corticosteroids. Arch Intern Med 146:737, 1986.

994. Kamil E, Kayyana R, Moudgil X, et al: Use of azathioprine in difficult childhood nephrotic syndrome. J Am Soc Nephrol 4:278, 1993. Abstract.

995. Adams DA, Gordon A, Maxwell M: Azathioprine treatment of immunologic renal disease. JAMA 199:459–463, 1967.

996. Tanphaichitr P, Tanphaichitr D, Sueeratanan J, Chatasingh S: Treatment of nephrotic syndrome with levamisole. J Pediatr 96:490, 1980.

997. Mehta KP, Ali V, Kutty M, Kolhatkar U: Immunoregulatory treatment for minimal-change nephrotic syndrome. Arch Dis Child 61:153, 1988.

998. British Association for Pediatric Nephrology: Levamisole for corticosteroid-dependent nephrotic syndrome in childhood. Lancet 337:1555–1557, 1991.

999. Dayal U, Dayal AK, Shastry JCM, Raghupathy P: Use of levamisole in maintaining remission in steroid-sensitive nephrotic syndrome in children. Nephron 66:408–412, 1994.

999a. Weiss R: Randomized, double blind placebo controlled trial of levamisole in children with frequently relapsing/steroid dependent nephrotic syndrome. J Am Soc Nephrol 4:289, 1993. Abstract.

1000. Xu J, Qian T, Jiang J, et al: Clinical studies in the use of BCG and levamisole in the treatment of glomerulonephritis. Nephrol Dial Transplant 6:548–553, 1991.

1001. Meyrier A: Treatment with cyclosporin of patients with idiopathic nephrotic syndrome. Semin Immunopathol 9:441, 1987.

1002. Glassock RJ: Role of cyclosporine in glomerular diseases. Cleve Clin J Med 61:363–369, 1994.

1003. Meyrier A: Treatment of glomerular disease with cyclosporin A. Nephrol Dial Transplant 4:923–931, 1989.

1004. Meyrier A: Treatment of nephrotic syndrome with cyclosporin A. What remains in 1994? Nephrol Dial Transplant 9:596–598, 1994.

1005. Ponticelli C, Edefonti A, Ghio L, et al: Cyclosporin versus cyclophosphamide for patients with steroid-dependent and frequently relapsing idiopathic nephrotic syndrome: A multicentre randomized controlled trial. Nephrol Dial Transplant 8:1326–1332, 1993.

1006. Ponticelli C, Rizzoni G, Edefonti A, et al: A randomized trial of cyclosporine in steroid-resistant idiopathic nephrotic syndrome. Kidney Int 43:1377–1384, 1993.

1007. Melocoton TL, Kamil ES, Cohen AH, Fine RN: Long-term cyclosporine A treatment of steroid-resistant and steroid-dependent nephrotic syndrome. Am J Kidney Dis 18:583–588, 1991.

1008. Meyrier A, Noel L-H, Auriche P, Callard P: Long-term renal tolerance of cyclosporin A treatment in adult idiopathic nephrotic syndrome. Kidney Int 45:1446–1456, 1994.

1009. Feutren G, Mihatsch MJ, for the International Kidney Biopsy Registry of Cyclosporin in Autoimmune Diseases: Risk factors for cyclosporine-induced nephropathy in patients with autoimmune diseases. N Engl J Med 326:1654–1660, 1992.

1010. Ingulli E, Tejani A: Severe hypercholesterolemia inhibits cyclosporin A efficacy in a dose-dependent manner in children with nephrotic syndrome. J Am Soc Nephrol 3:254–259, 1992.

1011. Gansevoort RT, de Zeeuw D, de Jong PE: Long-term benefits of the antiproteinuric effect of angiotensin converting enzyme inhibitors in non-diabetic renal disease. Am J Kidney Dis 22:202–206, 1993.

1012. Praga M, Hernandez E, Montoyo C, et al: Long-term beneficial effects of angiotensin-converting enzyme inhibition in patients with nephrotic proteinuria. Am J Kidney Dis 20:240–248, 1992.

1013. Gentile MG, Fellin G, Cofano F, et al: Treatment of proteinuric patients with a vegetarian soy diet and fish oil. Clin Nephrol 40:315–320, 1993.

1014. Pruna A, Metivier F, Akposso K, et al: Pefloxacin as first-line treatment in nephrotic syndrome. Lancet 340:728–729, 1992.

1014a. Geffriaud-Ricouard C, Jungers P, Chauveau D, Grunfeld, JP: Inefficacy and toxicity of pefloxacin in focal and segmental glomerulosclerosis with steroid-resistant nephrotic syndrome. Lancet 341:1475, 1993. Letter.

1015. Trainin EB, Gomez-Leon G: Development of renal insufficiency after long-standing steroid-responsive nephrotic syndrome. Int J Pediatr Nephrol 2:55, 1982.

1016. Koskimies O, Vilska J, Rapola J, Hallman N: Long-term outcome of primary nephrotic syndrome. Arch Dis Child 57:544, 1982.

1017. Waldherr R, Gubler MC, Levy M, et al: The significance of pure diffuse mesangial proliferation in idiopathic nephrotic syndrome. Clin Nephrol 10:171, 1978.

1018. Schoeneman MJ, Bennett B, Griefer I: The natural history of focal segmental glomerulosclerosis with and without mesangial hypercellularity in children. Clin Nephrol 9:45, 1978.

1019. Brown EA, Upadhyaya K, Hayslett JP, et al: The clinical course of mesangial proliferative glomerulonephritis. Medicine (Baltimore) 58:295, 1979.

1020. Murphy WM, Jukkola AF, Roy S: Nephrotic syndrome with mesangial-cell proliferation in children—a distinct entity. Am J Clin Pathol 72:27, 1979.

1021. Saha H, Mustonen J, Pasternak A, Helm H: Clinical follow-up of 54 patients with IgM nephropathy. Am J Nephrol 9:124, 1989.

1022. Cohen AH, Border WA: Mesangial proliferative glomerulonephritis. Semin Nephrol 2:228, 1982.

1023. Packham DK, North RA, Fairley KF, et al: Pregnancy in women with diffuse mesangial proliferative glomerulonephritis. Clin Nephrol 29:193, 1988.

1024. Bryan JA, Campbell WG, Wells JO, Bourke E: Mesangial glomerulonephropathy with decreased circulating C4 and predominant mesangial C4 deposition in association with one null gene at C4B locus. Nephron 43:128, 1986.

1025. Mampaso F, Leyva-Cobian F, Martinez-Montero JG, et al: Mesangial proliferative glomerulonephritis with unusual intramembranous granular dense deposits. Clin Nephrol 19:92, 1983.

1026. Churg J, Habib R, White RHR: Pathology of the nephrotic syndrome in children. A report for the International Study of Kidney Disease in Children. Lancet 1:1299, 1970.

1027. Cavallo T, Johnson MP: Immunopathologic study of minimal-change glomerular disease with mesangial IgM deposits. Nephron 27:281, 1981.

1028. Tejani A, Nicastri AD: Mesangial IgM nephropathy. Nephron 35:1, 1983.

1029. Jennette JC: Evolution of mesangial IgM nephropathy into focal segmental glomerulosclerosis. Am J Nephrol 1:222, 1981.

1030. Scolari F, Scaini P, Savoldi S, et al: Familial IgM mesangial nephropathy: A morphologic and immunogenetic study of three pedigrees. Am J Nephrol 10:261–268, 1990.

1031. Murphy MJ, Bailey RR, McGiven AR: Is there an IgM nephropathy? Aust N Z J Med 13:35, 1983.

1032. Helin H, Munstonen J, Pasternack A, Antonen J: IgM-associated glomerulonephritis. Nephron 31:11, 1982.

1033. Vilches AR, Turner DR, Cameron JS, et al: Significance of mesangial IgM deposition in ''minimal-change'' nephrotic syndrome. Lab Invest 46:10, 1982.

1034. Mampaso F, Gonzalo A, Teruel J, et al: Mesangial deposits of IgM in patients with the nephrotic syndrome. Clin Nephrol 16:230, 1981.

1035. Pardo V, Riesgo L, Zillernelo G, Strauss J: The clinical significance of mesangial IgM deposits and mesangial hypercellularity in minimal-change nephrotic syndrome. Am J Kidney Dis 3:264, 1984.

1036. Gonzalo A, Mampaso F, Gallego N, et al: Clinical significance of IgM mesangial deposits in the nephrotic syndrome. Nephron 41:246, 1985.

1037. Aubert J, Humain L, Chatelaut F, de Torrente A: IgM-associated mesangial proliferative glomerulonephritis and focal and segmental hyalinosis with nephrotic syndrome. Am J Nephrol 5:449, 1985.

1038. Larsen S: Immunofluorescent microscopy findings in minimal- or no-change disease and slight generalized mesangio-proliferative glomerulonephritis. Fluorescency microscopy results correlated to symptoms and clinical course. Acta Pathol Microbiol Scand 86:534, 1978.

1039. Larsen S: Immune deposits in generalized mesangioproliferative glomerulonephritis. Fluorescency microscopy findings correlated to symptoms, clinical course and immunosuppressive therapy. Acta Pathol Microbiol Scand 86:543, 1978.

1040. Manno C, Proscia AR, Laraia E, et al: Clinicopathological features in patients with isolated C3 mesangial proliferative glomerulonephritis. Nephrol Dial Transplant 5(suppl 1):78–80, 1990.

1041. Jennette JC, Falk RJ: C1q nephropathy. In Massry S, Glassock R (eds): Textbook of Nephrology, 3rd ed. Williams & Wilkins, Baltimore 1995, pp 749–752.

1042. Davenport A, Maciver AG, Mackenzie JC: C1q nephropathy: Do C1q deposits have any prognostic significance in the nephrotic syndrome? Nephrol Dial Transplant 7:391–396, 1992.

1043. German Glomerulonephritis Research Group: A controlled multicenter trial of cyclophosphamide and indomethacin in chronic glomerulonephritis. In Kluthe R, Vogt A, Batsford SR (eds): Glomerulonephritis. John Wiley & Sons, New York, 1977, p 196.

1044. Zimmerman CE: Renal transplantation for focal segmental glomerulosclerosis. Transplantation 29:172, 1979.

1045. McGovern VJ: Persistent nephrotic syndrome: A renal biopsy study. Australas Ann Med 13:306, 1964.

1046. Habib R, Gubler MD: Les lesions glomerulaires focales des syndromes nephrotiques idiopathiques de l'enfant. Apropos de 49 observations. Nephron 8:382, 1971.

1047. Beaufils H, Alphonse JC, Guedon J, Legrain M: Focal glomerulosclerosis: Natural history and treatment: A report of 70 cases. Nephron 21:75, 1978.

1048. Brown CB, Cameron JS, Turner DR, et al: Focal segmental glomerulosclerosis with rapid decline in renal function (''malignant FSGS''). Clin Nephrol 10:51, 1978.

1049. Arbus GS, Poncell S, Bacheyie GS, Baumal R: Focal segmental glomerulosclerosis with idiopathic nephrotic syndrome: Three types of clinical response. J Pediatr 101:41, 1982.

1050. Wehrmann M, Bohle A, Held H, et al: Long-term prognosis of focal sclerosing glomerulonephritis. An analysis of 250 cases with particular regard to tubulointerstitial changes. Clin Nephrol 33:115–122, 1990.

1051. Mongeau JG, Robitaille PO, Clermont MJ, et al: Focal segmental glomerulosclerosis (FSG) 20 years later. From toddler to grown up. Clin Nephrol 40:106, 1993.

1052. Korbet SM, Schwartz MM, Lewis EJ: Primary focal segmental glomerulosclerosis: Clinical course and response to therapy. Am J Kidney Dis 23:773–783, 1994.

1053. Kashgarian M, Hayslett JP, Siegel NJ: Lipoid nephrosis and focal sclerosis. Distinct entities or spectrum of disease. Nephron 13:105, 1974. Editorial.

1054. Siegel NJ, Kashgarian M, Spargo BH, Hayslett J: Minimal-change and focal sclerotic lesions in lipoid nephrosis. Nephron 13:130, 1974.

1055. Howie AJ, Lee SJ, Green NJ, et al: Different clinicopathological types of segmental sclerosing glomerular lesions in adults. Nephrol Dial Transplant 8:590–599, 1993.

1056. Schwartz MM, Korbet SM: Primary focal segmental glomerulosclerosis: Pathology, histological variants and pathogenesis. Am J Kidney Dis 22:874–883, 1993.

1057. Morita M, White RHR, Coad NAG, Raafat F: The clinical significance of the glomerular location of segmental lesions in focal segmental glomerulosclerosis. Clin Nephrol 33:211–219, 1990.

1058. D'Agati V: The many masks of focal segmental glomerulosclerosis. Kidney Int 46:1223–1241, 1994.

1059. Burke EC, Holley KE, Stickler GB: Familial nephrotic syndrome with nephrocalcinosis and tubular dysfunction. J Pediatr 82:202, 1973.

1060. Weening JJ, Beukers JJB, Grond J, Elema JD: Genetic factors in focal segmental glomerulosclerosis. Kidney Int 29:789, 1986. Editorial review.

1061. McCurdy FA, Butera PJ, Wilson R: The familial occurrence of focal segmental glomerulosclerosis. Am J Kidney Dis 10:467, 1987.

1062. Glicklich D, Haskell L, Senitzer D, Weiss RA: Possible genetic predisposition to idiopathic focal segmental glomerulosclerosis. Am J Kidney Dis 12:30, 1988.

1063. Trainin EB, Gomez-Leon G: HLA identity in siblings with focal glomerulosclerosis. Int J Pediatr Nephrol 4:55, 1983.

1064. Tejani A, Nicastri A, Phadke K, et al: Familial focal segmental glomerulosclerosis. Int J Pediatr Nephrol 4:231, 1983.

1065. Friedman EA, Rao TK, Nicastri AD: Heroin-associated nephropathy. Nephron 13:421, 1974.

1066. Rao TK, Nicastri AD, Friedman EA: Natural history of heroin-associated nephropathy. N Engl J Med 290:19, 1974.

1067. Treser G, Cherubin C, Lonegan ET, et al: Renal lesions in narcotic addicts. Am J Med 57:687, 1974.

1068. Grishman E, Chung J, Porush JG: Glomerular morphology in nephrotic heroin addicts. Lab Invest 35:415, 1976.

1069. Falleroni AE, Earle DP, Patterson R: Atopy in adults with glomerular diseases: A preliminary report. J Chronic Dis 29:599, 1976.

1070. White RHR, Mills RJ, Beetham R, Paine RN: The significance of variation in the selectivity of proteinuria. Clin Nephrol 3:42, 1975.

1071. McVicar M, Exeni R, Susin M: Nephrotic syndrome and multiple tubular defects in children, an early sign of focal segmental sclerosis. J Pediatr 97:918, 1980.

1072. Artero M, Sharma R, Savin V, Vincenti F: Association of recurrent focal glomerulosclerosis (FGS) with increased albumin permeability of glomeruli incubated with patient sera. J Am Soc Nephrol 2:791, 1991.

1073. Remuzzi A, Pergolizzi R, Mauer MS, Bertani T: Three-dimensional morphometric analysis of segmental glomerulosclerosis in the rat. Kidney Int 38:851–856, 1990.

1074. Miyata J, Takebayashi S, Taguchi T, et al: Evaluation and correlation of clinical and histological features of focal segmental glomerulosclerosis. Nephron 44:115, 1986.

1075. Verani RR, Hawkins EP: Recurrent focal segmental glomerulosclerosis: A pathologic study of the early lesion. Am J Nephrol 6:263, 1986.

1076. Schwartz MM, Lewis EJ: Focal and segmental glomerulosclerosis: The cellular lesion. Kidney Int 28:968, 1985.

1077. Gottlieb RP, Caputo C, Damjanov I: Glomerular crescents in focal glomerulosclerosis with hyalinosis. Am J Kidney Dis 18:720–722, 1991.

1078. Whitworth JA, Turner DR, Leibowitz S, Cameron JS: Focal segmental sclerosis or scarred focal proliferative glomerulonephritis. Clin Nephrol 9:229, 1978.

1079. Malekzadeh M, Heuser EJ, Ettenger RB, et al: Focal glomerulosclerosis and renal transplantation. J Pediatr 95:249, 1979.

1080. Kincaid-Smith P: Glomerular and vascular lesions in chronic atrophic pyelonephritis and reflex nephropathy. Adv Nephrol Necker Hosp 5:3–17, 1975.

1081. Lee SM, Michael AF: Focal glomerular sclerosis and sarcoidosis. Arch Pathol Lab Med 102:572, 1978.

1082. McCoy RC: Ultrastructural alterations in the kidney of patients with sickle cell disease and the nephrotic syndrome. Lab Invest 21:85, 1969.

1083. Weisinger JR, Kempson RL, Eldridge FL, Swenson RS: The nephrotic syndrome: A complication of massive obesity. Ann Intern Med 81:440, 1974.

1084. Carless D, Rigby R, Axelsen R, Boyle R: A case of Guillain-Barré syndrome with focal segmental glomerulosclerosis. Am J Nephrol 13:160–163, 1993.

1085. Jaenke RS, Phemister RD, Norrdin RW: Progressive glomerulosclerosis and renal failure following perinatal gamma radiation in the beagle. Lab Invest 42:643, 1980.
1086. Eagen J, Lewis EJ: Glomerulopathies of neoplasia. Kidney Int 11:297, 1977.
1087. Olson JL, Hostetter TH, Rennke HG, et al: Altered glomerular permselectivity and progressive sclerosis following extreme ablation of renal mass. Kidney Int 22:112, 1982.
1088. Brenner BM, Meyer TW, Hostetter TH: Dietary protein intake and the progressive nature of kidney disease: The role of hemodynamically mediated glomerular injury in the pathogenesis of progressive glomerular sclerosis in aging, renal ablation, and intrinsic renal disease. N Engl J Med 307:652, 1982.
1089. Brenner BM: Hemodynamically mediated glomerular injury and the progressive nature of kidney disease. Kidney Int 23:647, 1983.
1090. Weiss MA, Daquioag E, Margolin G, Pollak VE: Nephrotic syndrome, progressive irreversible renal failure, and glomerular "collapse": A new clinicopathologic entity? Am J Kidney Dis 8:20, 1986.
1091. Detwiler RK, Falk RJ, Hogan SL, Jennette JC: Collapsing glomerulopathy: A clinically and pathologically distinct variant of focal segmental glomerulosclerosis. Kidney Int 45:1416–1424, 1994.
1092. Howie AJ, Brewer DB: The glomerular tip lesion: A previously undescribed type of segmental glomerular abnormality. J Pathol 142:205, 1984.
1093. Howie AJ, Brewer DB: Further studies in the glomerular tip lesion: Early and late stages and life table analysis. J Pathol 147:245, 1985.
1094. Howie AJ: Changes at the glomerular tip: A feature of membranous nephropathy and other diseases associated with proteinuria. J Pathol 150:13, 1986.
1095. Beaman M, Howie AJ, Hardwicke J, et al: The glomerular tip lesions: A steroid-responsive nephrotic syndrome. Clin Nephrol 27:217, 1987.
1096. Thomsen OF, Ladefoged J: Glomerular tip lesions in renal biopsies with focal segmental IgM. Acta Pathol Microbiol Immunol Scand 99:836–843, 1991.
1097. Yoshikawa N, Ito H, Akamatsu R, et al: Focal and segmental glomerulosclerosis with and without nephrotic syndrome in children. J Pediatr 109:65, 1986.
1098. Gephardt GN, Tubbs RR, Popowniak KL, McMahon JT: Focal and segmental glomerulosclerosis: Immunohistologic study of 20 renal biopsy specimens. Arch Pathol Lab Med 110:902, 1986.
1099. Markovic-Lypkovski J, Muller C, Risler T, et al: Mononuclear leukocytes, expression of HLA class II antigens and intercellular adhesion molecule 1 in focal segmental glomerulosclerosis. Nephron 59:286–293, 1991.
1100. Glasser RJ, Velosa JA, Michael AF: Experimental model of focal sclerosis. I. Relationship to protein excretion in aminonucleoside nephrosis. Lab Invest 36:519, 1977.
1101. Velosa JA, Glasser RJ, Nevins TE, Michael AF: Experimental model of focal sclerosis. II. Correlation with immunopathologic changes, macromolecular kinetics, and polyanion loss. Lab Invest 36:527, 1977.
1102. Bolton WK, Benton FR, MacKay JG, Sturgill BC: Spontaneous glomerular sclerosis in aging man. Nephron 20:307, 1978.
1103. Bolton WK, Westervelt FB, Sturgill BC: Nephrotic syndrome and focal glomerular sclerosis in aging man. Nephron 20:307, 1978.
1104. Marks MI, Drummond KN: Nephropathy and persistent proteinuria after albumin administration in the rat. Lab Invest 23:416, 1970.
1105. Kreisberg JI, Karnovsky MJ: Focal glomerular sclerosis in the fawn-hooded rat. Am J Pathol 92:637, 1978.
1106. Remuzzi G, Bertani T: Is glomerulosclerosis a consequence of altered glomerular permeability to macromolecules? Kidney Int 38:384–394, 1990.
1107. Thomas ME, Schreiner GF: Contribution of proteinuria to progressive renal injury: Consequences of tubular uptake of fatty acid bearing albumin. Am J Nephrol 13:385–398, 1993.
1107a. Agarwal A, Nath KA: Effect of proteinuria on renal interstitium: Effect of products of nitrogen metabolism. Am J Nephrol 13:376–384, 1993.
1108. Ueda Y, Ono Y, Sagiya A, et al: Mesangial anionic sites are decreased in human focal glomerular sclerosis. Clin Nephrol 37:280–284, 1992.
1109. Hoyer JR, Vernier RL, Najarian JS, et al: Recurrence of idiopathic nephrotic syndrome after renal transplantation. Lancet 2:343, 1972.
1110. Leumann EP, Briner J, Donckerwolcke RAM, et al: Recurrence of focal segmental glomerulosclerosis in the transplanted kidney. Nephron 25:65, 1980.
1111. Axelsen RA, Seymour AE, Mathew TH, et al: Recurrent focal glomerulosclerosis in renal transplants. Clin Nephrol 21:110, 1984.
1112. Artero ML, Sharma R, Savin VJ, Vincenti F: Plasmapheresis reduces proteinuria and serum capacity to injure glomeruli in patients with recurrent focal glomerulosclerosis. Am J Kidney Dis 23:574–581, 1994.
1113. Artero M, Biava C, Amend W, et al: Recurrent focal glomerulosclerosis: Natural history and response to therapy. Am J Med 92:375–384, 1992.
1114. Kim E-M, Striegel J, Kim Y, et al: Recurrence of steroid-resistant nephrotic syndrome in kidney transplants is associated with increased acute renal failure and acute rejection. Kidney Int 45:1440–1445, 1994.
1115. Dantal J, Baatard R, Hourmant M, et al: Recurrent nephrotic syndrome following renal transplantation in patients with focal glomerulosclerosis. Transplantation 52:827–831, 1991.
1116. Li PK, Lai M-MF, Leung CB, et al: Plasma exchange in the treatment of early recurrent focal glomerulosclerosis after renal transplantation. Report and review. Am J Nephrol 13:289–292, 1993.
1117. El Nahas AM: Glomerulosclerosis: Insights into pathogenesis and treatment. Nephrol Dial Transplant 4:843–853, 1989.
1118. Simons JL, Provoost AP, Anderson S, et al: Modulation of glomerular hypertension defines susceptibility to progressive glomerular injury. Kidney Int 46:396–404, 1994.
1119. Johnson RJ: The glomerular response to injury: Progression or resolution? Kidney Int 45:1769–1782, 1994.
1120. Couser WG, Johnson RJ: Mechanisms of progressive renal disease in glomerulonephritis. Am J Kidney Dis 23:193–198, 1994.
1121. Moorhead JF, El-Nahas M, Harry D, et al: Focal glomerular sclerosis and nephrotic syndrome with partial lecithin:cholesterol acyl transferase deficiency and discoidal high density lipoprotein in plasma and urine. Lancet 1:936, 1983.
1122. Moorhead JF, Chan MK, El-Nahas M, Varghese Z: Lipid nephrotoxicity in chronic progressive glomerular and tubulointerstitial disease. Lancet 2:1309, 1982.
1123. Diamond JR, Karnovsky M: Focal and segmental glomerulosclerosis: Analogies to atherosclerosis. Kidney Int 33:917, 1988.
1124. Matsumoto K, Osakabe K, Katayama H, Hatano M: Concanavalin A–induced suppressor cell activity in focal glomerular sclerosis. Nephron 31:27, 1982.
1125. Futrakul P, Poshyachinda M, Mitrakul C: Focal sclerosing glomerulonephritis: A kinetic evaluation of hemostasis and the effect of anticoagulant therapy: A controlled study. Clin Nephrol 10:180, 1978.
1126. Purkerson ML, Valdes A, Yates J, et al: Inhibition of thromboxane synthesis ameliorates the progressive kidney disease of rats with subtotal renal ablation. Proc Natl Acad Sci USA 82:193, 1985.
1127. Border WA, Okuda S, Languino LR, Ruoslahti E: Transforming growth factor-β regulates production of proteoglycans by mesangial cells. Kidney Int 37:689–695, 1990.
1128. Yamamoto T, Noble NA, Miller DE, Border WA: Sustained expression of TGF-β1 underlies development of progressive kidney fibrosis. Kidney Int 45:916–927, 1994.
1129. Mongeau J-G, Corneille L, Pobitaille P, et al: Primary nephrosis in childhood associated with focal glomerular sclerosis: Is long-term prognosis that severe? Kidney Int 20:743, 1981.
1130. Southwest Pediatric Nephrology Study Group: Focal and segmental glomerulosclerosis in children with idiopathic nephrotic syndrome. Kidney Int 27:442, 1985.
1131. Korbet SM, Schwartz MM, Lewis EJ: The prognosis of focal segmental glomerular sclerosis of adulthood. Medicine (Baltimore) 65:304, 1986.
1132. Ito H, Yoshikawa N, Aozai F, et al: Twenty-seven children with focal segmental glomerulosclerosis: Correlation between the segmental location of the glomerular lesions and prognosis. Clin Nephrol 22:9, 1984.
1133. Velosa JA, Holley KE, Torres VE, Offord KP: Significance of proteinuria in the outcome of renal function in patients with focal segmental glomerulosclerosis. Mayo Clin Proc 58:568, 1983.
1134. Ramirez F, Travis LB, Cunningham RJ, et al: Focal segmental glomerulosclerosis, crescent and rapidly progressive renal failure. Int J Pediatr Nephrol 3:175, 1982.

1135. Packham DK, North RA, Fairley KF, et al: Pregnancy in women with primary focal and segmental hyalinosis and sclerosis. Clin Nephrol 29:185, 1988.

1136. Banfi G, Moriggi M, Sabadini E, et al: The impact of prolonged immunosuppression on the outcome of idiopathic focal-segmental glomerulosclerosis with nephrotic syndrome in adults. A collaborative retrospective study. Clin Nephrol 36:53–59, 1991.

1137. Pei Y, Cattran D, Delmore T, et al: Evidence suggesting undertreatment in adults with idiopathic focal segmental glomerulosclerosis. Am J Med 82:938, 1987.

1138. Geary DF, Farine M, Thorner P, Baumal R: Response to cyclophosphamide in steroid-resistant focal segmental glomerulosclerosis: A reappraisal. Clin Nephrol 21:109, 1984.

1139. Griswold WR, Tune BM, Reznik VM, et al: Treatment of childhood prednisone-resistant nephrotic syndrome and focal segmental glomerulosclerosis with intravenous methylprednisolone and oral alkylating agents. Nephron 46:73, 1987.

1140. Tejani A, Butt K, Trachtman H, et al: Cyclosporine A–induced remission of relapsing nephrotic syndrome in children. Kidney Int 33:729, 1988.

1141. Okada S, Kurata N, Ota Z, Ofuji T: Effect of dipyridamole on proteinuria of nephrotic syndrome. Lancet 1:719, 1981.

1142. Velosa JA, Torres V, Donadio JV, et al: Treatment of severe nephrotic syndrome with meclofenamate: An uncontrolled study. Mayo Clin Proc 60:586, 1985.

1143. Kooijmans-Coutinho MF, Tegzess AM, Bruijn JA, et al: Indomethacin treatment of recurrent nephrotic syndrome and focal segmental glomerulosclerosis after renal transplantation. Nephrol Dial Transplant 8:469–473, 1993.

1144. Velosa JA, Torres VE: Benefits and risks of nonsteroidal anti-inflammatory drugs in steroid-resistant nephrotic syndrome. Am J Kidney Dis 8:345, 1986.

1145. Muso E, Yashiro M, Matsuhima M, et al: Does LDL-apheresis in steroid-resistant nephrotic syndrome affect prognosis? Nephrol Dial Transplant 9:257–264, 1994.

1146. Coggins CH, Frommer JP, Glassock RJ: Membranous nephropathy. Semin Nephrol 2:264, 1982.

1147. Remuzzi G, Bertani T, Schieppati A: Idiopathic membranous nephropathy. Lancet 342:1277–1280, 1993.

1148. Glassock RJ: Secondary membranous glomerulonephritis. Nephrol Dial Transplant 7:S-64–S-71, 1992.

1149. Cahen R, Francois B, Trolliet P, et al: Aetiology of membranous glomerulonephritis: A prospective study of 82 adult patients. Nephrol Dial Transplant 4:172–180, 1989.

1149a. Warms PC, Rosenbaum B, Michelis MF: Idiopathic membranous glomerulonephritis occurring with diabetes mellitus. Arch Intern Med 132:735, 1973.

1150. Shearn MA, Hopper J, Biava CG: Membranous lupus nephropathy initially seen as idiopathic membranous nephropathy. Arch Intern Med 140:1521, 1980.

1151. Adu D, Williams DG, Taube D, et al: Late-onset systemic lupus erythematosus and lupus-like disease in patients with apparent idiopathic glomerulonephritis. Q J Med 52:471, 1983.

1152. Kleinknecht C, Levy M, Gagnadoux M-F, Habib R: Membranous glomerulonephritis with extra-renal disorders in children. Medicine (Baltimore) 58:219, 1979.

1153. Takekoshi Y, Shida N, Saheki Y, et al: Strong association between membranous nephropathy and hepatitis-B surface antigenaemia in Japanese children. Lancet 2:1065, 1978.

1154. Samuels B, Lee JC, Engleman EP, Hopper J: Membranous nephropathy in patients with rheumatoid arthritis: Relationship to gold therapy. Medicine (Baltimore) 57:319, 1978.

1155. Schwartzberg M, Burnstein SL, Calabro JJ, Jacobs JB: The development of membranous glomerulonephritis in a patient with rheumatoid arthritis and Sjögren's syndrome. J Rheum 6:65, 1979.

1156. Yamada A, Mitsuhashi K, Miyakawa Y, et al: Membranous glomerulonephritis associated with eosinophilic lymph-folliculosis of the skin (Kimura's disease): Report of a case and review of the literature. Clin Nephrol 18:211, 1982.

1157. Dupont AG, Verbeelen DL, Six RO: Weber-Christian panniculitis with membranous glomerulonephritis. Am J Med 75:527, 1983.

1158. Taylor RG, Fisher C, Hoffbrand BI: Sarcoidosis and membranous glomerulonephritis: A significant association. Br Med J 284:1297, 1982.

1159. Weetman AP, Pinching AJ, Pussel BA, et al: Membranous glomer-

ulonephritis and autoimmune thyroid disease. Clin Nephrol 15:50, 1981.

1160. Kobayashi K, Harada A, Onoyama K, et al: Idiopathic membranous glomerulonephritis associated with diabetes mellitus. Light, immunofluorescence and electron microscopic study. Nephron 28:163, 1981.

1161. Rao KV, Crosson JT: Idiopathic membranous glomerulonephritis in diabetic patients. Arch Intern Med 140:624, 1980.

1162. Ibarrola AS, Sobrini B, Guisantes J, et al: Membranous glomerulonephritis secondary to hydatid disease. Am J Med 70:311, 1981.

1163. Brueggemeyer CD, Ramirez G: Membranous nephropathy: A concern for malignancy. Am J Kidney Dis 9:23, 1987.

1164. Burstein DM, Korbet SM, Schwartz MM: Membranous glomerulonephritis and malignancy. Am J Kidney Dis 22:5–10, 1993.

1165. Bellomo R, Wood C, Wagner I, et al: Idiopathic membranous nephropathy in an Australian population: The incidence of thrombo-embolism and its impact on the natural history. Nephron 63:240–241, 1993.

1166. Packham DK, North RA, Fairley KF, et al: Membranous glomerulonephritis and pregnancy. Clin Nephrol 28:56, 1987.

1167. Cybulsky AV, Rennke HG, Feintzeig ID, Salant DJ: Complement-induced glomerular epithelial cell injury. Role of the membrane attack complex in rat membranous nephropathy. J Clin Invest 77:1096, 1986.

1168. DeHeer E, Daha MR, Bhakdi S, et al: Possible involvement of terminal complement complex in active Heymann nephritis. Kidney Int 27:388, 1985.

1169. Schulze M, Donadio JV, Pruchno CJ, et al: Elevated urinary excretion of the $C_{5b-9}$ complex in membranous nephropathy. Kidney Int 40:533–538, 1991.

1170. Ogrodowski JL, Hebert LA, Sedmak D, et al: Measurement of $C_{5b-9}$ in urine in patients with the nephrotic syndrome. Kidney Int 40:1141–1147, 1991.

1171. Couser WG, Schulze M, Pruchno CJ: Role of $C_{5b-9}$ in experimental membranous nephropathy. Nephrol Dial Transplant 7:S-25–S-31, 1992.

1172. Brenchley PE, Coupes B, Short CD, et al: Urinary $C_{3dg}$ and $C_{5b-9}$ indicate active immune disease in human membranous nephropathy. Kidney Int 41:933–937, 1992.

1173. Coupes B, Brenchley PEC, Short CD, Mallick NP: Clinical aspects of $C_{3dg}$ and $C_{5b-9}$ in human membranous nephropathy. Nephrol Dial Transplant 7:S-32–S-34, 1992.

1174. Coupes BM, Kon SP, Brenchley PEC, et al: The temporal relationship between urinary $C_{3dg}$ and $C_{5b-9}$ and clinical parameters in human membranous nephropathy. Nephrol Dial Transplant 8:399–401, 1993.

1175. Savin VJ, Johnson RJ, Couser WG: $C_{5b-9}$ increases albumin permeability of isolated glomeruli in vitro. Kidney Int 46:382–387, 1994.

1176. Kusanoki Y, Akutsuo Y, Itami N, et al: Urinary excretion of terminal complement components complexes in glomerular disease. Nephron 59:27–32, 1991.

1177. Noris M, Benigni A, Boccardo P, et al: Urinary excretion of platelet activating factor in patients with immune-mediated glomerulonephritis. Kidney Int 43:426–429, 1993.

1178. Klouda PT, Manos J, Acheson EJ, et al: Strong association between idiopathic membranous nephropathy and HLA-DRW3. Lancet 2:770, 1979.

1179. Ogahara S, Naito S, Abe K, et al: Analysis of HLA class II genes in Japanese patients with idiopathic membranous glomerulonephritis. Kidney Int 41:175–182, 1992.

1180. Freedman BI, Spray BJ, Dunston GM, Heise ER: HLA associations in end-stage renal disease due to membranous glomerulonephritis: HLA-DR3 associations with progressive renal injury. Am J Kidney Dis 23:797–802, 1994.

1181. Chevrier D, Giral M, Braud V, et al: Membranous nephropathy and $TAP_1$ gene polymorphism. N Engl J Med 331:133–134, 1994.

1182. Sacks SH, Warner C, Campbell RD, Dunham I: Molecular mapping of the HLA class II region in HLA-DR3 associated idiopathic membranous nephropathy. Kidney Int Suppl 43:S-13–S19, 1993.

1183. Tomura S, Kashiwabara H, Tuchida H, et al: Strong association of idiopathic membranous nephropathy with HLA-DR2 and MT1 in Japanese. Nephron 36:242, 1984.

1184. Hiki Y, Kobayashi Y, Itoh I, Kashiwagi N: Strong association of HLA DR2 and MT1 with idiopathic membranous nephropathy in Japan. Kidney Int 25:953, 1984.

1185. Sacks SH, Nomura S, Warner C, et al: Analysis of complement C4 loci in Caucasoids and Japanese with idiopathic membranous nephropathy. Kidney Int 42:882–887, 1992.

1186. Ooi YM, Ooi BS, Pollak VE: Relationship of levels of circulating immune complexes to histologic patterns of nephritis: A comparative study of membranous glomerulonephritis. J Lab Clin Med 90:891, 1977.

1187. Doi T, Kanatsu K, Mayumi M, et al: Analysis of IgG immune complexes in sera from patients with membranous nephropathy: Role of IgG4 subclass and low-avidity antibodies. Nephron 57:131–136, 1991.

1188. Yoshikawa N, Ito H, Yamada Y, et al: Membranous glomerulonephritis associated with hepatitis B antigen in children: A comparison with idiopathic membranous glomerulonephritis. Clin Nephrol 23:28, 1985.

1189. Milner LS, Dusheiko GM, Jacobs D, et al: Biochemical and serological characteristics of children with membranous nephropathy (South African children) secondary to hepatitis B infection: Correlation with hepatitis e antigen, hepatitis B DNA and hepatitis D. Nephron 49:184, 1988.

1190. Stack JI, Zabetakis PM: Erythrocytosis associated with idiopathic membranous glomerulopathy. Clin Nephrol 12:87, 1979.

1191. Gaffney EF, Panner BJ: Membranous glomerulonephritis: Clinical significance of glomerular hypercellularity and parietal epithelial abnormalities. Nephron 29:209, 1981.

1192. Wakai S, Magil AB: Focal glomerulosclerosis in idiopathic membranous glomerulonephritis. Kidney Int 41:428–434, 1992.

1192a. Lee HS, Koh HI: Nature of progressive glomerulosclerosis in human membranous nephropathy. Clin Nephrol 39:7–16, 1993.

1193. Haramoto T, Makino H, Ikeda S, et al: Ultrastructural localization of the three major basement membrane components—type IV collagen, heparan sulfate proteoglycan and laminin—in human membranous glomerulonephritis. Am J Nephrol 14:30–36, 1994.

1194. Kim Y, Butkowski R, Burke B, et al: Differential expression of basement membrane collagen in membranous nephropathy. Am J Pathol 139:1382–1388, 1991.

1195. Fukatsu A, Matsuo S, Killen PD, et al: The glomerular distribution of type IV collagen and laminin in human membranous glomerulonephritis. Hum Pathol 19:64, 1988.

1196. Alexopoulos E, Leontsini M, Papadimitriou M: Relationship between interstitial infiltrates and steroid responsiveness of proteinuria in membranous nephropathy. Nephrol Dial Transplant 9:623–629, 1994.

1197. Klassen J, Elwood C, Grossberg AL, et al: Evolution of membranous nephropathy into antiglomerular-basement membrane glomerulonephritis. N Engl J Med 290:1340, 1974.

1198. Nicholson GP, Amin UF, Alleyne GAO: Membranous nephropathy with crescents. Clin Nephrol 4:198, 1975.

1199. Moorthy AV, Zimmerman SW, Burkholder PM, Harrington AR: Association of crescentic glomerulonephritis with membranous glomerulonephropathy: A report of three cases. Clin Nephrol 6:319, 1976.

1200. Levy M, Gagnadoux M-F, Beziau A, Habib R: Membranous glomerulonephritis associated with anti-tubular and anti-alveolar basement membrane antibodies. Clin Nephrol 10:158, 1978.

1201. Abreo K, Abreo F, Mitchell B, Schloemer G: Idiopathic crescentic membranous glomerulonephritis. Am J Kidney Dis 8:257, 1986.

1202. Koethe J, Gerig J, Glickman J, et al: Progression of membranous nephropathy to acute crescentic rapidly progressive glomerulonephritis and response to pulse methyl prednisolone. Am J Nephrol 6:224, 1986.

1203. Bertani T, Appel GB, D'Agati V, et al: Focal segmental membranous glomerulonephropathy associated with other diseases. Am J Kidney Dis 2:439, 1983.

1204. Gaffney EO, Alexander RW, Donnelly WH: Segmental membranous glomerulonephritis. Arch Pathol Lab Med 106:409, 1982.

1205. Weidner N, Lorentz WBJ: Scanning electron microscopy of the acellular glomerular basement membranes in idiopathic membranous glomerulopathy. Lab Invest 54:84, 1986.

1206. Honig C, Mouradian JA, Montoliu J, et al: Mesangial electron-dense deposits in membranous nephropathy. Lab Invest 42:427, 1980.

1206a. Davenport A, Maciver AG, Hall CL, Mackenzie JC: Do mesangial immune complex deposits affect the renal prognosis in membranous glomerulonephritis? Clin Nephrol 41:271–276, 1994.

1207. Tornroth T, Honkanen E, Pettersson E: The evolution of membranous glomerulonephritis reconsidered: New insights from a study on relapsing disease. Clin Nephrol 28:107–117, 1987.

1208. Riemenschneider T, Mackensen-Haen S, Christ H, Bohle A: Correlation between endogenous creatinine clearance and relative interstitial volume of the renal cortex in patients with diffuse membranous glomerulonephritis having a normal serum creatinine concentration. Lab Invest 43:145, 1980.

1209. Toth T, Takebayashi S: Idiopathic membranous glomerulonephritis: A clinicopathologic and quantitative morphometric study. Clin Nephrol 38:14–19, 1992.

1210. Haas M: IgG subclass deposits in glomeruli of lupus and nonlupus membranous nephropathies. Am J Kidney Dis 23:358–364, 1994.

1211. Berger J, Yaneva H: Hageman factor deposition in membranous glomerulopathy. Transplant Proc 14:472, 1982.

1212. Gonzalez-Cabrero J, de Nicolas R, Ortiz A, et al: Presence of circulating antibodies against brush border antigens (Fx1A) in a patient with membranous nephropathy and bilateral pyeloureteral stenosis. Comparison with idiopathic membranous nephropathy. Nephrol Dial Transplant 7:293–299, 1992.

1213. Naruse T, Miyakawa Y, Kitamura K, Shibata S: Membranous glomerulonephritis mediated by renal tubular epithelial antigen-antibody complex. J Allergy Clin Immunol 54:311, 1974.

1214. Whitworth JA, Leibowitz S, Kennedy MC, et al: Absence of glomerular renal tubular epithelial antigen in membranous glomerulonephritis. Clin Nephrol 5:159, 1976.

1215. Thorpe LW, Cavallo T: Renal tubule brush border antigens: Failure to confirm a pathogenetic role in human membranous glomerulonephritis. J Clin Lab Immunol 3:2, 125, 1980.

1216. Faruta T, Seino J, Saito T, et al: Insulin deposits in membranous nephropathy associated with diabetes mellitus. Clin Nephrol 37:65–69, 1992.

1217. Kerjaschki D: Molecular pathogenesis of membranous nephropathy. Kidney Int 41:1090–1105, 1992.

1218. Friend PS, Michael AF: Hypothesis: Immunologic rationale for the therapy of membranous lupus nephropathy. Clin Immunol Immunopathol 10:35, 1978.

1219. Eddy AA, Fritz IB: Localization of clusterin in the epimembranous deposits of passive Heymann nephritis. Kidney Int 39:247–252, 1991.

1220. Fleuren GJ, Lee RVD, Greben HA, et al: Experimental glomerulonephritis in the rat induced by antibodies directed against tubular antigen. IV. Investigations into the pathogenesis of the model. Lab Invest 38:198, 1978.

1221. Zager RA, Couser WG, Andrews BS, et al: Membranous nephropathy: A radioimmunological search for anti-renal tubular epithelial antibodies and circulating immune complexes. Nephron 24:10, 1979.

1222. Douglas BFS, Rabideau DP, Schwartz BB, Lewis EJ: Evidence of autologous immune complex nephritis. N Engl J Med 305:1326, 1981.

1223. Zanetti M, Mandet C, Duboust A, et al: Demonstration of a passive Heymann nephritis–like mechanism in a human kidney transplant. Clin Nephrol 15:272, 1981.

1224. Shemesh O, Ross JC, Deen WM, et al: Nature of the glomerular capillary injury in human membranous glomerulopathy. J Clin Invest 77:868, 1986.

1225. Groggel GC, Stevenson J, Hovingh P, et al: Changes in heparan sulfate correlate with increased glomerular permeability. Kidney Int 33:517, 1988.

1226. Couser WG, Baker PJ, Adler S: Complement and the direct mediation of immune glomerular injury: A new perspective. Kidney Int 28:879, 1985. Editorial review.

1227. Floege J, Johnson RJ, Gordon K, et al: Altered glomerular extracellular matrix synthesis in experimental membranous nephropathy. Kidney Int 42:573–585, 1992.

1227a. Swan S, Sharma R, Sharma M, et al: Proteinuria of membranous nephropathy does not depend on the circulating factor of focal sclerosing glomerulopathy. J Am Soc Nephrol 3:883, 1992.

1228. Ramirez F, Brouhard BH, Travis LB, Ellis EN: Idiopathic membranous nephropathy in children. J Pediatr 101:677, 1982.

1229. Hopper J Jr, Trew PA, Biava CG: Membranous nephropathy: Its relative benignity in women. Nephron 29:18, 1981.

1230. Manos J, Short CD, Acheson EJ, et al: Relapsing idiopathic membranous nephropathy. Clin Nephrol 18:286, 1982.

1231. Davison AM, Cameron JS, Kerr DNS, et al: The natural history of renal function in untreated idiopathic membranous glomerulonephritis in adults. Clin Nephrol 21:61, 1984.

1232. Donadio JV, Torres VE, Velosa J, et al: Idiopathic membranous nephropathy: The natural history of untreated patients. Kidney Int 33:708, 1988.

1233. Kida H, Asamoto T, Yokoyama H, et al: Long-term prognosis of membranous glomerulonephritis. Clin Nephrol 25:64, 1986.

1234. Honkanen E: Survival in idiopathic membranous glomerulonephritis. Clin Nephrol 25:122, 1986.

1235. MacTier R, Boulton-Jones J, Payton CD, McLay A: The natural history of membranous nephropathy in the west of Scotland. Q J Med 60:793, 1986.

1236. Schieppati A, Mosconi L, Perna A, et al: Prognosis of untreated patients with idiopathic membranous nephropathy. N Engl J Med 329:85–89, 1993.

1237. Cattran DC, Pei Y, Greenwood C: Predicting progression in membranous glomerulonephritis. Nephrol Dial Transplant 7:S-48–S-52, 1992.

1238. Pei Y, Cattran D, Greenwood C: Predicting chronic renal insufficiency in idiopathic membranous glomerulonephritis. Kidney Int 42:960–966, 1992.

1239. Passerini P, Pasquali P, Cesana B, et al: Long-term outcome of patients with membranous nephropathy after complete remission of proteinuria. Nephrol Dial Transplant 4:525–529, 1989.

1240. Honkanen E, Tornroth T, Gronhagen-Riska C, Sankila R: Long-term survival in idiopathic membranous glomerulonephritis: Can the course be clinically predicted? Clin Nephrol 41:127–134, 1994.

1241. Rosen S, Tornroth T, Bernard P: Membranous glomerulonephritis. *In* Tisher CC, Brenner BM, (eds): Renal Pathology: With Clinical and Functional Correlations, 2nd ed. JB Lippincott, Philadelphia, 1994, p 280.

1242. Ponticelli C: Prognosis and treatment of membranous nephropathy. Kidney Int 29:927, 1986.

1243. Tu W-H, Petitti DB, Biava CG, et al: Membranous nephropathy: Predictors of terminal renal failure. Nephron 36:118, 1984.

1244. Collaborative Study of the Adult Idiopathic Nephrotic Syndrome: A controlled study of short-term prednisone treatment in adults with membranous nephropathy. N Engl J Med 301:1301, 1979.

1245. Fuller TJ, Barcenas CG, White MG: Diuretic-induced interstitial nephritis. Occurrence in a patient with membranous glomerulonephritis. Arch Intern Med 235:1998, 1976.

1246. Cameron JS: Membranous nephropathy: The treatment dilemma. Am J Kidney Dis 1:371, 1982.

1247. Garattini S, Bertani T, Remuzzi G: What is the basis for the use of steroids in the treatment of idiopathic membranous nephropathy? Nephron 45:1, 1987.

1248. Cameron JS: Membranous nephropathy and its treatment. Nephrol Dial Transplant 7:S-72–S-79, 1992.

1249. Pollak VE: Treatment of membranous glomerulonephropathy. Am J Kidney Dis 19:68–71, 1992.

1250. Lewis EJ: Idiopathic membranous nephropathy—to treat or not to treat. N Engl J Med 329:127–129, 1993.

1251. D'Achiardi-Rey R, Pollak VE: Membranous glomerulonephropathy: There is no significant effect of treatment with corticosteroids. Am J Kidney Dis 1:386, 1982.

1252. Black DAK, Rose G, Brewer BB: Controlled trial of prednisone in adult patients with the nephrotic syndrome. Br Med J 3:421, 1970.

1253. Coggins CH: Is membranous nephropathy treatable? Am J Nephrol 1:219, 1981.

1254. Cattran DC, Delmore J, Roscoe J, et al: A randomized controlled trial of prednisone in patients with idiopathic membranous glomerulonephritis. N Engl J Med 320:210, 1989.

1255. Cameron JS, Healy MJR, Adu D: The Medical Research Council trial of short-term, high-dose, alternate-day prednisolone in idiopathic membranous nephropathy with a nephrotic syndrome in adults. Q J Med 74:133, 1990.

1256. Hopper J Jr: Membranous glomerulonephritis. Ann Intern Med 79:285, 1973.

1257. Bolton WK, Atuk NO, Sturgill BC, Westervelt FB: Therapy of the idiopathic nephrotic syndrome with alternate-day steroids. Am J Med 62:60, 1977.

1258. Fuiano G, Stanziale P, Balletta M, et al: Effectiveness of steroid therapy in different stages of membranous nephropathy. Nephrol Dial Transplant 4:1022–1029, 1989.

1259. Short CD, Solomon LR, Gokal R, Mallick NP: Methylprednisolone in patients with membranous nephropathy and declining renal function. Q J Med 65:929, 1987.

1260. Medical Research Council Working Party: Controlled trial of azathioprine and prednisone in chronic renal disease. Br Med J 2:239, 1971.

1261. Warwick G, Boulton-Jones JM: Immunosuppression for membranous nephropathy. Lancet 2:1361, 1988.

1262. Western Canadian Glomerulonephritis Study Group: Controlled trial of azathioprine in the nephrotic syndrome secondary to idiopathic membranous nephropathy. Can Med Assoc J 115:1209, 1976.

1263. Donadio JV, Holley KE, Anderson CF, Taylor WF: Controlled trial of cyclophosphamide in idiopathic membranous nephropathy. Kidney Int 6:431, 1974.

1264. Lagrue G, Bernard D, Bariety J: Traitement par le chlorambucil et l'azathioprine dans les glomérulonéphrites primitives. Résultats d'une étude controllée. J Urol Nephrol 9:655, 1975.

1265. Suki WN, Chavez A: Membranous nephropathy: Response to steroids and immunosuppression. Am J Nephrol 1:11, 1981.

1266. Ponticelli C, Zucchelli P, Imbasciati E, et al: Controlled trial of methylprednisolone and chlorambucil in idiopathic membranous nephropathy. N Engl J Med 310:946, 1984.

1267. Ponticelli C, Zucchelli P, Passerini P, et al: Treatment of idiopathic membranous nephropathy. Adv Nephrol 16:195, 1987.

1268. West ML, Jindal KK, Bear RA, Goldstein MB: A controlled trial of cyclophosphamide in patients with membranous glomerulonephritis. Kidney Int 32:579, 1987.

1269. Ponticelli C, Zucchelli P, Passerini P, et al: A randomized trial of methylprednisolone and chlorambucil in idiopathic membranous nephropathy. N Engl J Med 320:8, 1989.

1270. Mathieson PW, Turner AN, Maidment CGH, et al: Prednisolone and chlorambucil treatment in idiopathic membranous nephropathy with deteriorating renal function. Lancet 2:869, 1988.

1271. Williams PS, Bone JM: Immunosuppression can arrest renal failure due to idiopathic membranous glomerulonephritis. Nephrol Dial Transplant 4:181–186, 1989.

1272. Bruns FJ, Adler S, Fraley DS, Segel DP: Sustained remission of membranous glomerulonephritis after cyclophosphamide and prednisone. Ann Intern Med 114:725–730, 1991.

1273. Ponticelli C, Zucchelli P, Passerini P, Cesana B: Methylprednisolone plus chlorambucil as compared with methylprednisolone alone for the treatment of idiopathic membranous nephropathy. The Italian Idiopathic Membranous Nephropathy Treatment Study Group. N Engl J Med 327:599–603, 1992.

1274. Murphy BF, McDonald I, Fairley KF, Kincaid-Smith P: Randomized controlled trial of cyclophosphamide, warfarin and dipyridamole in idiopathic membranous glomerulonephritis. Clin Nephrol 37:229–234, 1992.

1275. Jindal K, West M, Bear R, Goldstein M: Long-term benefits of therapy with cyclophosphamide and prednisone in patients with membranous glomerulonephritis and impaired renal function. Am J Kidney Dis 19:61–67, 1992.

1275a. Passerini P, Como G, Vigano E, et al: Idiopathic membranous nephropathy in the elderly. Nephrol Dial Transplant 8:1321–1325, 1993.

1276. Alexopoulos E, Sakellariou G, Memmos D, et al: Cyclophosphamide provides no additional benefit to steroid therapy in the treatment of idiopathic membranous nephropathy. Am J Kidney Dis 21:497–503, 1993.

1277. Falk RJ, Hogan SL, Muller KE, Jennette JC, and the Glomerular Disease Collaborative Network: Treatment of progressive membranous glomerulopathy. A randomized trial comparing cyclophosphamide and corticosteroids with corticosteroids alone. Ann Intern Med 116:438–445, 1992.

1278. Reichert LJM, Huysmans FTM, Assmann K, et al: Preserving renal function in patients with membranous nephropathy: Daily oral chlorambucil compared with intermittent monthly pulses of cyclophosphamide. Ann Intern Med 121:328–333, 1994.

1279. Piccoli A, Pillon L, Passerini P, Ponticelli C: Therapy for idiopathic membranous nephropathy: Tailoring the choice by decision analysis. Kidney Int 45:1193–1202, 1994.

1280. Kibriya MG, Tishkov I, Nikolov D: Immunosuppressive therapy with cyclophosphamide and prednisolone in severe idiopathic membranous nephropathy. Nephrol Dial Transplant 9:138–143, 1994.

1281. Imperiale T, Goldfarb S, Berns J: Are cytotoxic agents beneficial in idiopathic membranous nephropathy? A meta-analysis of the controlled trials. J Am Soc Nephrol 5:1553–1558, 1995.

1282. De Santo N, Capodicasa G, Giordano C: Treatment of idiopathic membranous nephropathy unresponsive to methylprednisolone and chlorambucil with cyclosporin. Am J Nephrol 7:74, 1987.

1283. Rostoker G, Belghiti D, Maadi AB, et al: Long-term cyclosporin A therapy for severe idiopathic membranous nephropathy. Nephron 63:335–341, 1993.

1284. Guasch A, Suranyi M, Newton L, et al: Short-term responsiveness of membranous glomerulopathy to cyclosporine. Am J Kidney Dis 20:472–481, 1992.

1285. Cattran D, Greenwood C, Ritchie S, et al, and Canadian Glomerulonephritis Study Group: A controlled trial of cyclosporine in patients with progressive membranous nephropathy. Kidney Int 47:1130–1135, 1988.

1286. Laurens W, Ruggeneti P, Perna A, et al: A randomized and controlled study to assess the effect of cyclosporin in nephrotic patients with membranous nephropathy and reduced renal function (cyclomen). J Nephrol 7:237–247, 1994.

1287. Remuzzi A, Perticucci E, Battaglia C, et al: Low protein diet and glomerular size-selective function in membranous glomerulopathy. Am J Kidney Dis 17:317–322, 1991.

1288. Weisse WJ, Natori Y, Levine JS, et al: Fish oil has protective and therapeutic effects on proteinuria in passive Heymann nephritis. Kidney Int 43:359–368, 1993.

1289. Gansevoort RT, Heeg J, Vuesendorp R, et al: Acute proteinuria drugs in patients with idiopathic membranous glomerulopathy. Nephrol Dial Transplant 6(suppl 1):91–96, 1991.

1290. Thomas DM, Hillis AN, Coles GA, et al: Enalapril can treat the proteinuria of membranous glomerulonephritis without detriment to systemic or renal hemodynamics. Am J Kidney Dis 18:38–43, 1991.

1291. Palla R, Cirami C, Panichi V, et al: Intravenous immunoglobulin therapy of membranous nephropathy: Efficacy and safety. Clin Nephrol 35:98–104, 1991.

1292. Briner J, Binswanger U, Largiader F: Recurrent and de novo membranous glomerulonephritis in renal cadaver allotransplants. Clin Nephrol 13:189, 1980.

1293. Dische FE, Herbertson BM, Melcher DH, Morley AR: Membranous glomerulonephritis in transplant kidneys: Recurrent or de novo disease in four patients. Clin Nephrol 15:154, 1981.

1294. Lieberthal W, Bernard DB, Donohoe JF, et al: Rapid recurrence of membranous nephropathy in a related renal allograft. Clin Nephrol 12:222, 1979.

1295. Iskandar SS, Jennette JC: Recurrence of membranous glomerulopathy in an allograft. Case report and review of the literature. Nephron 29:270, 1981.

1296. Hill GS, Robertson J, Grossman R, et al: An unusual variant of membranous nephropathy with abundant crescent formation and recurrence in the transplanted kidney. Clin Nephrol 10:114, 1978.

1297. Donadio JV Jr, Holley KE: Membranoproliferative glomerulonephritis. Semin Nephrol 2:214, 1982.

1298. Cameron JS, Turner DR, Heaton J, et al: Idiopathic mesangiocapillary glomerulonephritis. Comparison of types I and II in children and adults and long-term prognosis. Am J Med 74:175, 1983.

1299. D'Amico G, Ferrario F: Mesangiocapillary glomerulonephritis. J Am Soc Nephrol 2:S159–S166, 1993.

1300. Holley KE, Donadio J: Membranoproliferative glomerulonephritis. In Tisher CC, Brenner BM (eds): Renal Pathology: With Clinical and Functional Correlations, 2nd ed. JB Lippincott, Philadelphia, 1994, pp 294–329.

1301. Burkholder PM, Marchand A, Krueger RP: Mixed membranous and proliferative glomerulonephritis. A correlative light, immunofluorescence and electron microscopic study. Lab Invest 23:459, 1970.

1302. West GD, McAdams AJ, McConville JM, et al: Hypocomplementemic and normocomplementemic persistent (chronic) glomerulonephritis: Clinical and pathologic characteristics. J Pediatr 67:1089, 1965.

1303. Mandalenakis N, Mendoza N, Pirani CL, Pollak VD: Lobular glomerulonephritis and membranoproliferative glomerulonephritis. Medicine (Baltimore) 50:319, 1971.

1304. Barbiano di Belgiojoso G, Ferrario F: Membranoproliferative glomerulonephritis. In Massry S, Glassock R (eds): Textbook of Nephrology, 3rd ed. Williams & Wilkins, Baltimore, 1995, pp 734–738.

1305. Berger J, Galle P: Depots denses au sein des membranes basales du rein. Etude en microscopes optique et electronique. Presse Med 49:2351, 1963.

1306. Gallé P, Mahieu P: Electron dense alteration of kidney basement membranes. A renal lesion specific of a systemic disease. Am J Med 58:749, 1975.

1307. Habib R, Gubler M-C, Loirat C, et al: Dense deposit disease: A variant of membranoproliferative glomerulonephritis. Kidney Int 7:204, 1975.

1308. Davis AE, Schneeberger FE, McCluskey RT, Grupe WE: Mesangial proliferative glomerulonephritis with irregular intramembranous deposits. Another variant of hypocomplementemic nephritis. Am J Med 63:481, 1977.

1309. King JT, Valenzuela R, McCormack JL, Osborne DG: Granular dense deposit disease. Lab Invest 39:591, 1978.

1310. Strife CF, McEnery P, McAdams AJ, et al: A third ultrastructural variant of membranoproliferative glomerulonephritis. Kidney Int 8:454, 1975.

1311. Strife CF, Jackson EC, McAdams AJ: Type III membranoproliferative glomerulonephritis: Long-term clinical and morphologic evaluation. Clin Nephrol 21:323, 1984.

1312. Klein M, Poucell S, Arbus GS, et al: Characteristics of a benign subtype of dense deposit disease: Comparison with the progressive form of this disease. Clin Nephrol 20:163, 1983.

1313. Levy M, Gubler M-C, Habib R: New concepts in membranoproliferative glomerulonephritis. In Kincaid-Smith P, d'Apice AJF, Atkins RC (eds): Progress in Glomerulonephritis. John Wiley & Sons, New York, 1979, p 177.

1314. Zucchelli P, Sasdelli M, Cagnoli L, et al: Membranoproliferative glomerulonephritis: Correlations between immunological and histological findings. Nephron 17:449, 1976.

1315. Vargas R, Thomson KJ, Wilson D, et al: Mesangiocapillary glomerulonephritis with dense "deposits" in the basement membrane of the kidney. Clin Nephrol 5:73, 1976.

1316. Davis BK, Cavallo T: Membranoproliferative glomerulonephritis. Am J Pathol 84:283, 1976.

1317. Donadio JV Jr, Slack TK, Holley KE, Ilstrup DM: Idiopathic membranoproliferative (mesangiocapillary) glomerulonephritis: A clinicopathologic study. Mayo Clin Proc 54:141, 1979.

1318. Barbiano de Belgioroso G, Baroni M, Pagliari B, et al: Is membranoproliferative glomerulonephritis really decreasing? Nephron 40:380, 1985.

1319. Jackson EC, McAdams J, Strife F, et al: Differences between membranoproliferative glomerulonephritis types I and III in clinical presentation, glomerular morphology, and complement perturbation. Am J Kidney Dis 9:115, 1987.

1320. Eisenger AJ, Shortland JR, Moorhead PJ: Renal disease in partial lipodystrophy. Q J Med 41:343, 1972.

1321. Peters DK, Charlesworth JA, Sissons JG, et al: Mesangiocapillary nephritis, partial lipodystrophy, and hypocomplementemia. Lancet 2:535, 1973.

1322. Sissons JGP, West RJ, Fallows J, et al: The complement abnormalities of lipodystrophy. N Engl J Med 294:461, 1976.

1323. Bennett WM, Bardana EJ, Wuepper K, et al: Partial lipodystrophy. C3 nephritic factor and clinically inapparent mesangiocapillary glomerulonephritis. Am J Med 62:757, 1977.

1324. Ipp MM, Minta JO, Gelfand EW: Disorders of the complement system in lipodystrophy. Clin Immunol Immunopathol 7:281, 1977.

1325. Stutchfield PR, White RHR, Cameron AH, et al: X-linked mesangiocapillary glomerulonephritis. Clin Nephrol 26:150, 1986.

1326. Varade WS, Forristal J, West CD: Patterns of complement activation in idiopathic membranoproliferative glomerulonephritis, types I, II and III. Am J Kidney Dis 16:196–206, 1990.

1327. Hattori M, Kim Y, Steffes MW, Maver SM: Structural-functional relationships in type I mesangiocapillary glomerulonephritis. Kidney Int 43:381–386, 1993.

1328. Ooi YM, Vallota EH, West CD: Classical component pathway activation in membranoproliferative glomerulonephritis. Kidney Int 9:246, 1976.

1329. Colten HR, Levey RH, Rosen FS, Alper CA: Decreased synthesis of C3 in membranoproliferative glomerulonephritis. J Clin Invest 52:20a, 1973.

1330. Vallota EH, Gotze O, Spiegelberg H, et al: A serum factor in chronic hypocomplementemic nephritis distinct from immunoglobulins and activating the alternate pathway of complement. J Exp Med 139:1249, 1974.

1331. Gotze O, Müller-Eberhard HJ: The C3 activator system: An alternate pathway of complement activation. J Exp Med 134:90, 1971.

1332. Spitzer RE, Vallota EH, Forristal J, et al: Serum C3 lytic system in patients with glomerulonephritis. Science 164:436, 1969.

1333. Schreiber RD, Gotze O, Müller-Eberhard HJ: Nephritic factor: Its structure and function and its relationship to initiating factor of the alternative pathway. Scand J Immunol 5:705, 1976.

1334. Williams DG, Bartlett A, Duffers P: Identification of nephritic factor as an immunoglobulin. Clin Exp Immunol 33:425, 1978.

1335. Daha MR, Austen KF, Fearon DT: Heterogeneity, polypeptide chain composition and antigenic reactivity of C3 nephritic factor. J Immunol 120:1389, 1978.

1336. Bartlow BG, Roberts JL, Lewis EL: Nonimmunoglobulin C3 activating factor in membranoproliferative glomerulonephritis. Kidney Int 15:294, 1979.

1337. Roberts JL, Levy M, Chioros PG, et al: A serum C3-activating factor: Its characterization and its presence in glomerular deposits. J Immunol 127:1131, 1981.

1338. Droz D, Nabarra B, Noel L-H, et al: Recurrence of dense deposits in transplanted kidneys. I. Sequential survey of the lesions. Kidney Int 15:386, 1979.

1339. Ohi H, Tanuma NY: Does nephrotic factor relate to disease activity in hypocomplementemic membranoproliferative glomerulonephritis? Nephron 62:116–117, 1991.

1340. Thompson RA: IgG levels in patients with chronic membranoproliferative glomerulonephritis. Br Med J 1:282, 1972.

1341. Ooi YM, Vallota EH, West CD: Serum immune complexes in membranoproliferative and other glomerulonephritides. Kidney Int 11:275, 1977.

1342. Davis CA, Marder H, West CP: Circulating immune complexes in membranoproliferative glomerulonephritis. Kidney Int 20:728, 1981.

1343. Friend PS, Yunis EJ, Noreen HJ, Michael AF: B-cell alloantigen associated with chronic mesangiocapillary glomerulonephritis. Lancet 1:562, 1977.

1344. Welch TR, Beischel L, Balakrishnan K, et al: Major histocompatibility complex–extended haplotypes in membranoproliferative glomerulonephritis. N Engl J Med 314:1476, 1988.

1345. Levy M, Halbwachs-Mecarelli L, Gubler M-C, et al: H deficiency in two brothers with atypical dense intramembranous deposit disease. Kidney Int 30:949, 1986.

1346. Arroyave CM, Vallota E, Müller-Eberhard HJ: Lysis of human erythrocytes due to activation of the alternate complement pathway by nephritic factor (C3NF). J Immunol 113:764, 1974.

1347. George CRP: A kinetic evaluation of hemostasis in renal disease. N Engl J Med 291:1111, 1974.

1348. Barbiano di Belgioroso G, Tarantino A, Bazzi C, et al: Immunofluorescence patterns in chronic membranoproliferative glomerulonephritis (MPGN). Clin Nephrol 6:303, 1976.

1348a. Nakamoto Y, Yasuda T, Imai H, Miura AB: Circumferential mesangial interposition: A form of mesangiolysis. Nephrol Dial Transplant 7:373–378, 1992.

1349. Bohle A, Gartner HV, Fischbach H, et al: The morphological and clinical features of membranoproliferative glomerulonephritis in adults. Virchows Arch A 363:213, 1974.

1350. Anders D, Thoenes W: Basement membrane–change in membranoproliferative glomerulonephritis. Virchows Arch A 369:87, 1975.

1351. Cohen AH: Masson's trichrome stain in the evaluation of renal biopsies: An appraisal. Am J Clin Pathol 65:631, 1976.

1352. Anders D, Agricola B, Sippel M, Thoenes W: Basement membrane changes in membranoproliferative glomerulonephritis. II. Characterization of a third type by silver impregnation of ultra thin sections. Virchows Arch A 376:1, 1977.

1353. Strife CF, McAdams AJ, West CD: Membranoproliferative glomerulonephritis characterized by focal, segmental proliferative lesions. Clin Nephrol 18:9, 1982.

1354. McCoy RC, Clapp J, Seigler HF: Membranoproliferative glomerulonephritis. Progression from the pure form to the crescentic form with recurrence after transplantation. Am J Med 59:288, 1975.

1355. Schmitt H, Bohle H, Reinke T, et al: Long-term prognosis of membranoproliferative glomerulonephritis type I. Significance of clinical and morphological parameters. Nephron 55:242–250, 1990.

1356. Mackensen-Haen S, Grund KE, Schinmeister J, Bohle A: Impairment of the glomerular filtration rate by glomerular and interstitial factors in membranoproliferative glomerulonephritis with normal serum creatinine concentration. Virchows Arch A 382:11, 1979.

1357. Davis AE, Schneeberger EE, Grupe WE, McCluskey RT: Membranoproliferative glomerulonephritis (MPGN type I) and dense deposit disease (DDD) in children. Clin Nephrol 9:184, 1978.

1358. Abreo K, Moorthy AV: Type III membranoproliferative glomerulonephritis. Arch Pathol Lab Med 106:413, 1982.

1359. Burkholder PM: Atlas of Human Glomerular Pathology. Harper & Row, Hagerstown, MD, 1974, p 189.

1360. Levy M, Gubler M-C, Sich M, et al: Immunopathology of membranoproliferative glomerulonephritis with subendothelial deposits (type I MPGN). Clin Immunol Immunopathol 10:477, 1978.

1361. Campbell-Boswell MV, Linder D, Naylor BR, Brooks RE: Kidney tubule basement membrane alterations in type II membranoproliferative glomerulonephritis. Virchows Arch A 382:49, 1979.

1362. Lamb V, Tisher CC, McCoy RC, Robinson RR: Membranoproliferative glomerulonephritis with dense intramembranous alterations. A clinicopathologic study. Lab Invest 36:607, 1977.

1363. Kim Y, Vernier RL, Fish AJ, Michael AF: Immunofluorescence studies of dense deposit disease. The presence of railroad track and mesangial rings. Lab Invest 40:474, 1979.

1364. Habib R, Gubler M-C, Loirat C, et al: Dense deposit disease. A variant of membranoproliferative glomerulonephritis. Kidney Int 7:204, 1975.

1365. Sibley R, Kim Y: Dense intramembranous deposit disease. New pathologic features. Kidney Int 25:660, 1984.

1366. Sato H, Saito T, Seino J, et al: Dense deposit disease: Its possible pathogenesis suggested by an observation of a patient. Clin Nephrol 27:41, 1987.

1367. Date A, Neela P, Shastry JCM: Thioflavin T fluorescence in membranoproliferative glomerulonephritis. Nephron 32:90, 1982.

1368. Churg J, Duffy JL, Bernstein J: Identification of dense deposits disease. Arch Pathol Lab Med 103:67, 1979.

1369. Kashtan CE, Burke B, Burch G, et al: Dense intramembranous deposit disease: A clinical comparison of histological subtype. Clin Nephrol 33:1–6, 1990.

1370. Droz D, Zanetti M, Nöel LH, Leibowitch J: Dense deposits disease. Nephron 19:1, 1977.

1371. Jenis EH, Sander R, Hill GS, et al: Glomerulonephritis with basement membrane dense deposits. Arch Pathol 97:84, 1974.

1372. Thorner P, Baumal R: Extraglomerular dense deposits in dense deposit disease. Arch Pathol Lab Med 106:628, 1982.

1373. Falk RJ, Sisson SP, Dalmasso AP, et al: Ultrastructural localization of the membrane attack complex complement in human renal tissues. Am J Kidney Dis 9:121, 1987.

1374. Strife CF, McEnery PT, McAdams AJ, West CD: Membranoproliferative glomerulonephritis with disruption of the glomerular basement membrane. Clin Nephrol 7:65, 1977.

1375. Morel-Maroger L, Saimot AG, Sloper JC, et al: "Tropical nephropathy" and "tropical intramembranous glomerulonephritis." Br Med J 1:541, 1975.

1376. Coovida HM, Adhikari M, Morel-Maroger L: Clinicopathologic features of the nephrotic syndrome in South African children. Q J Med 48:77, 1979.

1377. Strife CF, Mug G, Chuck G, et al: Membranoproliferative glomerulonephritis and antitrypsin deficiency in children. Pediatrics 71:88, 1983.

1378. Pussel BA, Nayef M, Bourke E, et al: Complement deficiency and nephritis. A report of a family. Lancet 1:675, 1980.

1379. Lagrue G, Laurent J, Dubertret L, Branellec A: Buckley's syndrome and membranoproliferative glomerulonephritis. Nephron 31:279, 1982.

1380. Swarbrick ET, Fairclough PD, Campbell PJ, et al: Coeliac disease, chronic active hepatitis and mesangiocapillary glomerulonephritis in the same patient. Lancet 2:1084, 1980.

1381. Molle D, Baumelou A, Beaufils H, et al: Membranoproliferative glomerulonephritis associated with pulmonary sarcoidosis. Am J Nephrol 6:386, 1986.

1382. Zell SC, Duxbury G, Shankel SW: Alveolar hemorrhage associated with a membranoproliferative glomerulonephritis and smooth muscle antibody. Am J Med 82:1073, 1987.

1383. Simpson IJ, Moran J, Evans DJ, Peters DK: Prolonged complement activation in mice. Kidney Int 13:467, 1978.

1384. Schifferli J, Ng YC, Peters DK: The role of complement and its receptor in the elimination of immune complexes. N Engl J Med 315:488, 1986.

1385. Liebowitch J, Halbwachs L, Wattel S, et al: Recurrence of dense deposits in transplanted kidneys: II. Serum complement and nephritic factor profiles. Kidney Int 15:396, 1979.

1386. Cameron JS, Turner DR, Heaton J, et al: Idiopathic mesangiocapillary glomerulonephritis: Comparison of types I and II in children and adults and long-term prognosis. Am J Med 74:175, 1983.

1387. The Southwest Pediatric Nephrology Study Group: Dense deposit disease in children. Prognostic value of clinical and pathologic observations. Am J Kidney Dis 6:161, 1985.

1388. McAdams AJ, McEnery PT, West CD: Mesangiocapillary glomerulonephritis: Changes in glomerular morphology with long-term alternate-day prednisone therapy. J Pediatr 86:23, 1975.

1389. McEnery PT, McAdams AJ, West CD: Membranoproliferative glomerulonephritis: Improved survival with alternate-day prednisone therapy. Clin Nephrol 13:117, 1980.

1390. West CD: Childhood membranoproliferative glomerulonephritis: An approach to management. Kidney Int 29:1077, 1986.

1391. McEnery PT, McAdams AJ, West CD: The effect of prednisone in a high-dose alternate-day regimen on the natural history of idiopathic membranoproliferative glomerulonephritis. Medicine (Baltimore) 64:401, 1985.

1392. McEnery PT, McAdams AJ: Regression of membranoproliferative glomerulonephritis type II (dense deposit disease): Observation in six children. Am J Kidney Dis 12:138, 1988.

1393. Ford DM, Briscoe DM, Shanely PF, Lum GM: Childhood membranoproliferative glomerulonephritis type I: Limited steroid therapy. Kidney Int 41:1606–1612, 1992.

1394. Warady B, Guggenheim S, Sedman A, Lum G: Prednisone therapy of membranoproliferative glomerulonephritis in children. J Pediatr 107:703, 1985.

1395. Faedda R, Satta A, Tanda F, et al: Immunosuppressive treatment of membranoproliferative glomerulonephritis. Nephron 67:59–65, 1994.

1396. Kincaid-Smith P: The natural history and treatment of mesangiocapillary glomerulonephritis. In Kincaid-Smith P, Mathew T, Becker E (eds): Glomerulonephritis. Morphology, Natural History and Treatment. John Wiley & Sons, New York, 1973, p 591.

1397. Kher KK, Makker SP, Aikawa M, Kirson IJ: Regression of dense deposits in type II membranoproliferative glomerulonephritis: Case report of clinical course in a child. Clin Nephrol 17:100, 1982.

1398. Chapman SJ, Cameron JS, Chantler C, Turner D: Treatment of mesangiocapillary glomerulonephritis in children with combined immunosuppression and anticoagulation. Arch Dis Child 55:446, 1980.

1399. Cattran DC, Cardella CJ, Roscoe JM, et al: Results of a controlled drug trial in membranoproliferative glomerulonephritis. Kidney Int 27:436, 1985.

1400. Michielsen P, Van Damme B, Dotremont G, et al: Indomethacin treatment of membranoproliferative and lobular glomerulonephritis. In Kincaid-Smith P, Mathew TH, Becker EL (eds): Glomerulonephritis. Morphology, Natural History, and Treatment. John Wiley & Sons, New York, 1973, p 611.

1401. Zimmerman SW, Moorthy AV, Dreher WH, et al: Prospective trial of warfarin and dipyridamole in patients with membranoproliferative glomerulonephritis. Am J Med 75:920, 1983.

1402. Donadio JV, Anderson CF, Mitchell JC, et al: Membranoproliferative glomerulonephritis: A prospective trial of platelet inhibitor therapy. N Engl J Med 310:1421, 1984.

1402a. Zauner I, Bohler J, Braun N, et al, for the Collaborative Glomerulonephritis Therapy Study Group: Effect of aspirin and dipyridamole on proteinuria in idiopathic membranoproliferative glomerulonephritis: A multicentre prospective clinic trial. Nephrol Dial Transplant 9:619–622, 1994.

1403. Montoliu J, Bergada E, Arrizabalaga P, Revert L: Acute renal failure in dense deposit disease: Recovery after plasmapheresis. Br Med J 284:940, 1982.

1404. McGinley E, Watkins R, McLay A, Boulton-Jones JM: Plasma exchange in treatment of mesangiocapillary glomerulonephritis. Nephron 40:385, 1985.

1405. Morton MR, Bannister KM: Renal failure due to mesangiocapillary glomerulonephritis in pregnancy: Use of plasma exchange therapy. Clin Nephrol 40:74–78, 1993.

1406. Curtis JJ, Wyatt RJ, Bhathena D, et al: Renal transplantation for patients with type I and type II membranoproliferative glomerulonephritis: Serial complement and nephritic factor measurements and the problem of recurrence of disease. Am J Med 66:216, 1979.

1407. Glicklich D, Matas A, Sublay L, et al: Recurrent membranoproliferative glomerulonephritis type I in successive renal transplants. Am J Nephrol 7:143, 1987.

1408. Korbet SM, Schwartz M, Rosenberg B, et al: Immunotactoid glomerulopathy. Medicine (Baltimore) 64:228–243, 1995.

1409. Korbet SM, Schwartz M, Lewis EJ: Immunotactoid glomerulopathy. Am J Kidney Dis 17:247–257, 1991.

1410. Iskander SS, Falk RJ, Jennette JC: Clinical and pathologic features of fibrillary glomerulonephritis. Kidney Int 42:1401–1407, 1992.

1411. Alpers CE: Immunotactoid (microtubular) glomerulopathy: An entity distinct from fibrillary glomerulonephritis? Am J Kidney Dis 19:185–191, 1992.

1411a. Schwartz M: Renal amyloidosis and other fibrillar glomerular diseases. Curr Opin Nephrol Hypertens 2:238–245, 1993.

1412. Fogo A, Qureshi N, Horn RG: Morphologic and clinical features of fibrillary glomerulonephritis versus immunotactoid glomerulopathy. Am J Kidney Dis 22:367–377, 1993.

1413. Alpers CE: Fibrillary glomerulonephritis and immunotactoid glomerulopathy: Two entities, not one. Am J Kidney Dis 22:448–451, 1993.

1414. Schwartz MM: Immunotactoid glomerulopathy: The case for Occam's razor. Am J Kidney Dis 22:446–447, 1993. Editorial.

1415. Touchard G, Bauwens M, Goujon JM, et al: Glomerulonephritis with organized microtubular monoclonal immunoglobulin deposits. Adv Nephrol Necker Hosp 23:149–175, 1994.

1416. Korbet SM, Schwartz MM, Lewis EJ: The fibrillary glomerulopathies. Am J Kidney Dis 23:751–765, 1994.

1417. Jennette JC, Iskandar SS, Falk RJ: Fibrillary glomerulonephritis. In Tisher CC, Brenner BM (eds): Renal Pathology: With Clinical and Functional Correlations, 2nd ed. JB Lippincott, Philadelphia, 1994, pp 553–563.

1417a. Nakajima M, Hewitson TD, Mathews DC, et al: Atypical structured glomerular deposits: An immunohistochemical study. Am J Nephrol 11:151–156, 1991.

1417b. Okada H, Konishi K, Suzuki H, et al: Idiopathic progressive glomerulopathy with extensive subendothelial and mesangial immune deposit formation. Clin Nephrol 41:338–341, 1994.

1418. Rosemann E, Eliakim M: Nephrotic syndrome with amyloid-like deposits. Nephron 18:301–308, 1977.

1419. Avasthi PS, Erickson DG, Williams RC, Tung KSK: Benign monoclonal gammaglobulinemia and glomerulonephritis. Am J Med 62:324–329, 1977.

1420. Duffy JL, Khurana E, Susin M, et al: Fibrillary renal deposits and nephritis. Am J Pathol 113:279–280, 1983.

1421. Schwartz M, Lewis ET: The quarterly case. Nephrotic syndrome in a middle aged man. Ultrastruct Pathol 1:575, 1985.

1422. Orfila C, Meeus F, Bernadet P, et al: Immunotactoid glomerulopathy and cutaneous vasculitis. Am J Nephrol 11:67–72, 1991.

1423. Rovin BH, Bou-Khalil P, Sedmak D: Pulmonary-renal syndrome in a patient with fibrillary glomerulonephritis. Am J Kidney Dis 22:713–716, 1993.

1424. Churg J, Venkataseshan VS: Fibrillary glomerulonephritis without immunoglobulin deposits in the kidney. Kidney Int 44:837–842, 1993.

1425. Kohan DE, Perkins SL, Terreros DA: Immune complex glomerulonephritis with unusual microfibrillar deposits associated with primary bone marrow lymphoma. Am J Kidney Dis 21:47–51, 1993.

1426. Mazzucco G, Maran E, Rollino C, Monga G: Glomerulonephritis with organized deposits: A mesangiopathic not immune-complex mediated disease? A pathologic study of two cases in the same family. Hum Pathol 23:63–68, 1992.

1427. Arakawa M, Hueki H, Hirana H, et al: Idiopathic mesangio-degenerated glomerulopathy, a new group entity of glomerular disease. Jpn J Nephrol 21:914–915, 1979.

1428. Imbasciati E, Gheradi G, Morozumi K, et al: Collagen type III glomerulopathy: A new idiopathic glomerular disease. Am J Nephrol 11:422–429, 1991.

1429. Ikeda K, Yokoyama H, Tomosugi N, et al: Primary glomerular fibrosis: A new nephropathy caused by diffuse intra-glomerular increase in atypical type III collagen fibers. Clin Nephrol 33:155–159, 1990.

1430. Mizuiri S, Hasegawa A, Kikuchi A, et al: A case of collagen or fibrotic glomerulopathy associated with hepatic perisinusoidal fibrosis. Nephron 63:183–187, 1993.

1431. Dowling JP, Forbes IK, Chou ST: Collagen type III glomerulopathy: Extension beyond the glomerulus. Kidney Int 46:937–938, 1994.

1432. Watanabe Y, Ozaki I, Yoshida F, et al: A case of nephrotic syndrome with glomerular lipoprotein deposition with capillary ballooning and mesangiolysis. Nephron 51:265–270, 1980.

1433. Saito T, Sato H, Kudo K, et al: Lipoprotein glomerulopathy: Glomerular lipoprotein thrombi in a patient with hyperlipoproteinuria. Am J Kidney Dis 13:148–153, 1989.

1434. Oikawa S, Suzuki N, Sakuma E, et al: Abnormal lipoprotein and apolipoprotein pattern in lipoprotein glomerulopathy. Am J Kidney Dis 18:553–558, 1991.

1435. Saito T, Sato H, Oikawa S, et al: Lipoprotein glomerulopathy. Report of normolipidemic case and review of the literature. Am J Nephrol 13:64–68, 1993.

1436. Amenomori M, Haneda M, Morikawa J, et al: A case of lipoprotein glomerulopathy successfully treated with probucol. Nephron 67:109–113, 1994.

1437. Jennette JC, Hipp CG: C1q nephropathy: A distinct pathologic entity usually causing nephrotic syndrome. Am J Kidney Dis 6:103–110, 1985.

1438. Iskandar SS, Browning MC, Lorentz WB: C1q nephropathy: A pediatric clinicopathologic study. Am J Kidney Dis 18:459–465, 1991.

1439. Jennette JC, Wilkman AS, Hogan SL, Falk RJ: Clinical and pathologic features of C1q nephropathy (C1qN). J Am Soc Nephrol 4:681, 1993.

1440. Jennette JC, Hipp CG: Immunohistopathologic evaluation of C1q in 800 renal biopsy specimens. Am J Clin Pathol 83:415–420, 1985.

1441. Huttunen N-P: Congenital nephrotic syndrome of Finnish type. Arch Dis Child 51:344, 1976.

1442. Hoyer JR, Michael AF, Good RA, Vernier RL: The nephrotic syndrome of infancy: Clinical, morphologic, and immunologic studies of four infants. Pediatrics 40:233, 1967.

1443. Habib R, Gubler M-C, Antignac C, Gagnadoux MF: Diffuse mesangial sclerosis: A congenital glomerulopathy with the nephrotic syndrome. Adv Nephrol 22:43–66, 1993.

# Secondary Glomerular Diseases

*Sharon G. Adler*
*Arthur H. Cohen*
*Richard J. Glassock*

The previous chapter (Chapter 30) dealt with diseases in which the structure or function of the glomerular capillary network was disturbed as a result of processes that were largely limited to the kidney and in which extrarenal perturbations were primarily the result of abnormalities of renal function. This chapter deals with clinicopathologic entities in which glomerular involvement is but a part, often a minor part, of the overall disease-induced disturbances in single or multiple nonrenal organs or tissues, or disorders in which glomerular involvement arises consequent to a readily identifiable event—such as an infection, drug exposure, or neoplasm—even though the kidney may be the sole or major organ involved. These diseases encompass many of the so-called collagen-vascular diseases, glomerular disturbances in neoplasia, infectious diseases with prominent organ involvement (e.g., infective endocarditis, chronic viral hepatitis), and the heredofamilial disorders that may affect the integrity of the glomerular capillary circulation. Although the division of glomerular diseases along these broad lines may seem arbitrary, it offers the virtue of a clinical categorization more useful for practicing nephrologists than a strictly morphologic or pathogenetic compartmentalization, which is more useful for pathologists. The clinical manifestations of extrarenal organ involvement in many of the diseases discussed here may be subtle or may not evolve contemporaneously with the clinical manifestations of renal involvement. Thus, the clinician should be cautious in assigning a given patient a diagnosis of primary glomerular disease until a thorough search for possible inciting events or underlying multisystem diseases has been conducted and has proved unrevealing.

## GLOMERULAR INVOLVEMENT IN MULTISYSTEM DISEASES

### Systemic Lupus Erythematosus

Renal involvement as one of the manifestations of systemic lupus erythematosus (SLE) has been recognized for more than half a century.[1-4] A more complete picture of the genesis and behavior of the renal complications has been constructed in the past two decades.[5-10] The extrarenal symptoms and signs of SLE are extensive, and the reader is referred to several comprehensive treatises[2, 3, 5-7] for coverage of these subjects. Criteria for the classification of patients with SLE based on clinical and laboratory findings, first established in 1971 by the American Rheumatism Association, were revised in 1982.[10] According to the latter criteria, if 4 of the following 11 manifestations are present, the patient may be classified as having SLE: 1) malar rash, 2) discoid rash, 3) photosensitivity, 4) oral ulcers, 5) arthritis, 6) serositis (pleuritis/pericarditis), 7) renal disorder (proteinuria > 500 mg/d or cellular casts), 8) neurologic disorder (seizures or psychosis), 9) hematologic disorder (hemolytic anemia, leukopenia, lymphocytopenia, or thrombocytopenia), 10) immunologic disorder (positive lupus erythematosus cell test result, anti-DNA antibody, anti-Sm antibody, or false-positive serologic test result for syphilis), and 11) positive antinuclear antibody test result. Although these criteria have reasonable sensitivity (96%) and specificity (96%), they were designed principally for classification and not for diagnostic purposes. Clearly, SLE remains a clinical diagnosis, and some patients fail to meet the requisite number of criteria for classification as bona fide cases.[11, 12]

The prevalence of renal involvement in well-documented cases of SLE varies according to the criteria used to define renal disease. It also depends on the fundamental interests of the groups reporting collected series. On the basis of a clinical definition—such as abnormal proteinuria, urine sediment, and renal function—the reported frequency of renal involvement varies between about 35% and 90% of cases.[3–10] Various claims have been made, however, that nephritis is more uncommon or benign in certain subsets of patients with SLE, such as those with specific antibody patterns,[13, 14] with nonscarring cutaneous lesions and negative test results for antinuclear antibody,[15, 16] and with high[17] or low[18] helper/suppressor T cell ratios. Some overt clinical evidence of renal involvement at the time of diagnosis is expected in about two thirds of patients with well-documented SLE. If light microscopic evaluation of renal biopsy or autopsy material is performed, the incidence of renal involvement approaches 90%.[3–10, 19–21] Nearly all patients with SLE, regardless of the presence of clinical evidence of renal involvement, have some abnormality found when the more sophisticated techniques of immunofluorescence and electron microscopy are included in the examination of biopsy material.[22–25]

As with the extrarenal manifestations, the diversity of modes of presentation and clinical courses in SLE renal disease is great. Some patients may present with predominantly extrarenal manifestations and only subtle or no clinical signs of renal involvement, showing little tendency for the later development of renal failure. Other patients may present predominantly with signs of renal disease, such as nephrotic syndrome, accompanied by vague or transient extrarenal manifestations. Unless a diligent laboratory search is made for evidence of SLE, particularly serologic study for antinuclear factors, the latter group of patients may be diagnosed erroneously as having idiopathic glomerular disease[16, 26] (see also Chapter 30). A few patients may present with florid, life-threatening extrarenal complications or explosively severe renal disease. Modification of these various modes of presentation and clinical expression by prior treatment can further increase the complexity of the diagnostic problem. Although patients tend to retain a particular pattern of clinical expression (e.g., dominance of extrarenal symptoms and signs with minimal renal disease), many exceptions to this generalization can be cited.

## CLINICAL FINDINGS

SLE is predominantly a disease of young women, but it may affect persons of almost any age or either sex.[3–10, 27] The clinical manifestations of SLE are similar in males and females but the clinical features may differ between black and white patients. About 90% of patients are female, and the peak age of onset is in the third decade.[1–10] It is a relatively common disease—in the United States about 1 in 500 adult women is afflicted. Familial cases are common.[27] Male-to-male transmission of disease may occur.[1–4] Multiple organ systems are involved, including the serous membranes of the pleura and pericardium, joints, skin, heart and heart valves, lungs, gastrointestinal tract, blood and blood-forming organs, liver, and central nervous system (CNS). This broad spectrum of organ system involvement is responsible for the plethora of symptoms and signs.[1–6] Exacerbation of disease may occur after sun exposure, drug use (especially estrogens, penicillin, and hydralazine), or dietary modification (e.g., alfalfa ingestion).[5, 28] Cigarette smoking is associated with an adverse renal outcome.[28a]

Pulmonary hemorrhage may be a prominent manifestation of SLE,[29, 30] occasionally resembling Goodpasture syndrome (see later discussion). Ascites and pleural effusions may be manifestations of severe vasculitis.[31] Viral diseases (such as herpes zoster or herpes simplex) may complicate the clinical picture.[32] Sjögren syndrome and SLE may coexist.[33] Acute renal failure may ensue secondary to severe glomerular or predominantly acute tubulointerstitial nephritis.[34–37] Distal tubule defects, including renal tubular acidoses, have been reported,[38] and reversible tubule functional defects have been noted in association with flares in activity of glomerulonephritis.[39] Lymphoma may develop.[40] Raynaud phenomenon is present in about 40% of cases and often occurs in association with mild nonprogressive renal disease.[41] SLE in the elderly usually presents with atypical manifestations (serositis, pneumonia) and only mild renal disease.[42] Avascular polyarticular osteonecrosis may develop.[43] A syndrome closely resembling thrombotic thrombocytopenic purpura may evolve,[44] especially in patients with antiphospholipid antibodies (see later discussion).[45–48] Drug-induced SLE (from hydralazine or procainamide) may be associated with decreased complement levels or renal disease, but such patients usually do not display these features.[49, 50] The presence of antibodies to guanosine may be useful in identifying patients with lupus-like symptoms associated with procainamide ingestion.[50]

Overt renal disease appears to be equally common among children and adults with SLE and tends to be present at the outset rather than to develop later in the course of the disease.[6, 51–55] Two reviews summarize the course of pediatric patients with lupus nephritis,[6, 55] which, overall, is similar to the experience in adults. Persistent hypertension, anemia, an elevated serum creatinine level, and renal biopsy findings of either increased activity or chronicity correlated with the development of progressive renal insufficiency.[55] A small, uncontrolled study has suggested that SLE-related renal death may occur more frequently in black and Hispanic children who are younger than 10 years of age at the onset of illness.[56] Infants are rarely affected with renal disease,[53] but infants of mothers carrying anti-Ro antibodies with or without overt SLE may express a transient lupus-like syndrome characterized by rash and cardiac conduction defects.[54]

All the recognized clinical syndromes associated with glomerular disease can occur in patients with SLE (see Chapter 30). The nephrotic syndrome occurs commonly, often with associated renal insufficiency, and is the predominant clinical manifestation in about two thirds of patients with renal involvement.[1–10] The reported occurrence of nephrotic syndrome in SLE varies widely, however, according to the selection bias present. It has been estimated that SLE accounts for about 6% to 10% of all cases of nephrotic syndrome, whereas the incidence of SLE is nearly 16%[57] among female patients with nephrotic syndrome. About one in every six patients with SLE and renal involvement has a reduced glomerular filtration rate (GFR) at the time of recognition of disease. Hypertension tends to occur but may be independent of other signs of renal involvement[58] and may be of great prognostic importance.[59] Atherosclerotic coronary artery disease occurs with greater frequency in patients with SLE.[60, 61] The clinical activity of SLE may decline with the development of renal failure, and features of active disease are somewhat uncommon in patients with SLE receiving regular maintenance dialysis,[62–65] but exceptional cases continue to have severe extrarenal manifestations despite advanced uremia requiring hemodialysis. This subset has a poor prognosis.[66]

Patients with SLE have been reported to suffer arterial and venous thrombotic complications, often associated with the presence of a circulating anticoagulant.[44–48, 67–69] The presence of a lupus anticoagulant can be suspected on the basis of a prolonged partial thromboplastin time that does not correct with a 1:1 dilution with normal plasma.[67] It may also be discerned by the presence of a false-positive Venereal Disease Research Laboratory (VDRL) or serologic test for syphilis, anticardiolipin or antiphospholipid antibodies, or a prolonged kaolin clotting time or Russell viper venom test. Not all test results are positive in all patients.[67, 68] Some of these patients may present with or develop features of thrombotic thrombocytopenic purpura, including neurologic abnormalities.[44] Livedo reticularis is common, as is recurrent fetal wastage.[67, 68] Leg ulcers, hemolytic anemia, thrombocytopenia, transverse myelitis, and pulmonary hypertension may also occur more frequently in SLE patients with the antiphospholipid syndrome.[67] One group found a correlation between glomerular thrombi and the immunoglobulin G (IgG) isotype anticardiolipin antibody.[68] Another group correlated the IgM isotype to increased risk of leg ulcers and arterial thromboses and the IgG isotype to thrombocytopenia, recurrent fetal loss, and recurrent venous thromboses.[67] Although some suggested that patients with SLE and the lupus anticoagulant have milder renal disease, others have found that for the most part, renal function and histologic findings do not differ from those for patients without the lupus anticoagulant.[69] The presence of a thrombotic microangiopathy with glomerular fibrin deposits, however, portended a worse prognosis.[46–48, 70] Renal infarcts and loin pain may occur.[47] Most studies report that antiphospholipid and anticardiolipin antibodies are resistant to treatment with steroids and cytotoxic drugs,[68] although a minority view suggests that the IgM isotype may respond.[67] Long-term anticoagulant therapy is indicated for patients experiencing venous or arterial thrombosis.

In addition to the patients in whom glomerular fibrin thrombi may occur, patients with glomerular hyaline thrombi caused by large immune complexes have been described.[1, 10] Speculations regarding the cause of the

thrombosis have included endothelial cell injury in SLE from circulating immune complexes and complement activation[70]; specific antibodies directed against phospholipid coagulation factors[71]; impaired generation of prostaglandin $I_2$ (prostacyclin)[72]; deficiency or abnormalities of antithrombin III[73, 74]; and platelet activation.[72] Kant and co-workers[75] described a subset of lupus patients, most of whom had proliferative glomerulonephritis, who were predisposed to the development of glomerular capillary thrombosis without necrosis. These patients were characterized by the presence of circulating anticoagulant, normal serum complement levels, and undetectable anti–double-stranded DNA (anti-dsDNA) antibody. Renal biopsy specimens from these patients tended to show less glomerular complement deposition and more segmental sclerosis and crescents. A significant correlation was noted between the presence of glomerular thrombosis on a renal biopsy specimen and the subsequent development of glomerular scarring.[75] A small number of lupus patients with glomerular hyaline thrombi have been treated with ancrod, a defibrinating agent, occasionally with favorable responses.[72] As mentioned, some patients with SLE may present with or develop features of thrombotic thrombocytopenic purpura, including neurologic abnormalities.[42–48]

## LABORATORY EVALUATION

**Antibody Production.** Autoantibody production (Fig. 31–1) is a major characteristic of the SLE syndrome, with antibody-producing cells increased in both the bone marrow[76] and the peripheral circulation.[77] The presence of antibodies to nuclear antigens, most notably DNA but others as well, has been included in the American Rheumatism Association classification of SLE.[10] The circulating antibodies in patients with SLE, however, often have wide cross-reactivity.[78–80] The common cross-recognized sites on antigens appear to be phosphodiester-linked phosphate groups that may be present on glycosoaminoglycans, cardiolipin, other phospholipids, cytoskeleton, Raji cells, B and T cells, erythrocytes, platelets, endothelial cells, and DNA. However, the role of cross-reactivity of antibodies as a mechanism for antibody deposition in SLE nephritis is uncertain.[81] Autoantibodies that are bound to the kidneys of unrelated patients with SLE share idiotypes, suggesting a derivation from a common germ cell gene.[82]

*Antinuclear Antibodies.* The presence of antinuclear antibodies (as tested by indirect immunofluorescence and substrate-containing nuclei of mammalian source [e.g., mouse liver, chicken erythrocyte, human leukocytes]) in a patient's serum is greater than 90% sensitive but only about 70% specific for SLE. Antinuclear antibodies are also found frequently in patients with rheumatoid arthritis, Sjögren syndrome, scleroderma, and polymyositis and in chronic active hepatitis, infectious mononucleosis, infective endocarditis, normal aging, malaria, and lepromatous leprosy.[83] It is, therefore, not the presence of antinuclear antibody that makes the diagnosis of SLE but rather its presence as one of a constellation of laboratory and clinical signs and symptoms.[10] Antinuclear antibody, as detected by indirect immunofluorescence techniques (fluorescent antinuclear antibody [FANA]), is found in most patients with active

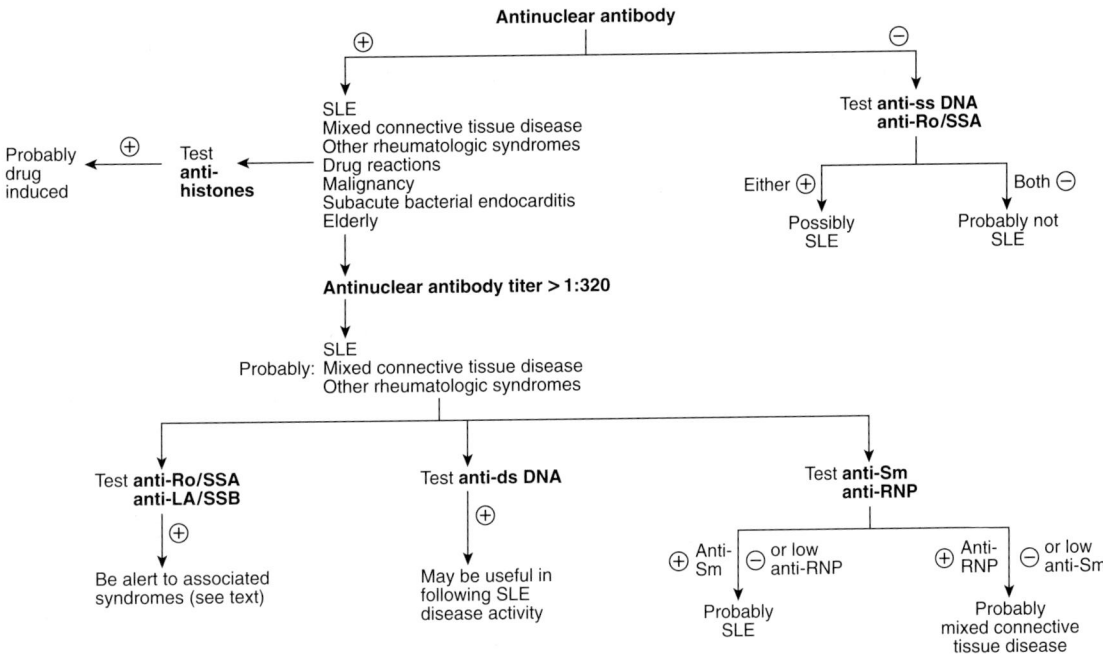

**Figure 31–1.** Suggested pathway for the use of some available antibody tests in patients suspected of having SLE.

disease, provided they have not been treated with steroids or immunosuppressive agents,[84] but about 5% to 10% of patients fulfilling the diagnostic criteria established for the classification of SLE (see earlier list) have negative FANA results[16, 85, 86] when the test is performed using mouse liver or kidney cryostat sections as the nuclear substrate.[83, 85–87] The sensitivity of the FANA test can be improved by careful attention to the choice of substrate and by the use of well-standardized reagents.[88] Of these FANA-negative patients, more than half can be shown to have positive FANA results if tissue culture cell line KB or HEp-2 is substituted for mouse epithelial cells as the nuclear substrate.[88] It has been suggested that the FANA negativity of these patients is due to a relative deficiency of single-stranded DNA (ssDNA) antigens in mouse tissue and not to a true absence of antinuclear antibodies in the patients.[88] In the remaining FANA-negative patients, antibody to ssDNA can occasionally be detected by radioimmunoassay.[83] FANA titer bears no relation to presence or severity of renal disease.[89] Some patients with active disease have antinuclear antibody detectable only after in vitro dissociation of circulating antigen-antibody complexes.[90] Antinuclear antibody is usually of the IgG class, but IgM, IgA, and IgE antinuclear antibodies have also been described.[91–93] Particular patterns of nuclear fluorescence (nucleolar, homogeneous, speckled, or rim) were once thought to be indicative of specific disease processes[94] or useful as correlates of active renal disease.[95] With the observation that a single serum sample can cause different patterns depending on serum dilution, the usefulness of pattern recognition has been questioned.[83]

*Antibodies to DNA.* The presence of antibodies to native, undenatured dsDNA in sera from patients is more specific but less sensitive than FANA in helping to make a diagnosis of SLE.[96] Estimates of the incidence of anti-dsDNA antibody in SLE patients range from 40% to 92%[98]; such antibody is present in about 70% of untreated SLE patients with active disease.[83] These antibodies were identified using the Farr radioimmunoassay, often with the use of dsDNA antigen that did not always meet high standards for specificity (i.e., ssDNA was often present as well).

An immunofluorescence test based on the circular native DNA in the kinetoplast of *Crithidia luciliae* (a single-celled hemoflagellate) is useful in detecting anti-dsDNA antibody in patients with SLE,[99–102] especially of the complement-fixing variety.[101] Anti-dsDNA antibodies of IgG class that fix complement and are of high avidity are said to correlate best with renal disease,[95, 101–107] but not all studies are in agreement.[105, 106, 108–113] Anti-DNA antibodies bearing particular idiotypes may be deposited in the glomeruli of both mice and patients with SLE nephritis.[114, 115] The prevalence of antibodies to denatured ssDNA in patients with SLE is high but the specificity is low. Anti-ssDNA antibodies are commonly found in patients with Sjögren syndrome, rheumatoid arthritis, drug-induced lupus erythematosus, scleroderma, discoid lupus, and chronic active hepatitis.[83] Occasional patients with SLE develop predominantly anti-ssDNA antibodies and thus may have negative results in assays based on binding to native or dsDNA.[86] Circulating free DNA may rarely be found in patients with active SLE.[116] Such DNA may be released from apoptotic or necrotic cells and provide antigen for the formation of immune complexes (see later discussion).

*Antibodies to Non-DNA Nuclear and Cytosolic Antigens.* Antibodies to four ribonuclear antigens (Sm, nRNP, Ro/SSA, La/SSB) are frequently found in patients with SLE and other autoimmune diseases. Two of these antigens, Sm and nRNP, are derived from a ribonuclease-sensitive, saline-extractable nuclear antigen (ENA) of calf thymus.[117]

The major component of ENA is native ribonucleoprotein (nRNP), which is ribonuclease sensitive. The Sm antigen is a ribonuclease-insensitive, minor antigen of ENA. Antibodies to Sm (anti-Sm) are highly specific for SLE, but not highly prevalent, and are found in about 25% of patients with SLE.[83, 97] Anti-Sm precipitates five small nuclear RNAs, U1, U2, U4, U5, and U6,[118] and their associated nuclear proteins (snRNPs). The function of these snRNPs is unclear, but some evidence suggests that U1 may be involved in RNA splicing.[118, 119] Some clinical studies have suggested that, in anti-ENA–positive patients, the presence of anti-Sm (i.e., in the absence of anti-nRNPs) may be associated with greater risk for the development of renal and CNS disease[120] compared with patients who are anti-Sm–negative and anti-RNP–positive (i.e., in comparison with patients who may have mixed connective tissue disease; see later discussion). On the other hand, one retrospective study[121] suggested that, in patients with definite SLE, the presence of anti-Sm antibodies was associated with an increased risk of cutaneous vasculitis, cardiopulmonary manifestations, and fatal outcome.[121]

Anti-nRNP is found in 30% to 46% of patients with SLE[83, 97] and with variable frequencies in patients with other collagen-vascular diseases.[122] It has been suggested that the presence of anti-RNP defines a subset of patients (mixed connective tissue disease) with symptoms of scleroderma, SLE, and polymyositis, including Raynaud phenomenon, pulmonary hypertension, myositis, abnormal esophageal motility, sclerodactyly, arthralgias, nondeforming arthritis, and calcinosis with skin tightening (see later discussion).[123] Glomerulonephritis has been said to occur in about 20% of these patients, in contrast to its higher prevalence in patients with classic SLE. In addition, it is usually associated with membranous glomerulonephritis when renal involvement does occur, and end-stage renal disease is uncommon.[124] Other groups have suggested that the frequency of renal involvement may be higher than 20%,[125] and more severe histologic forms have been described.[126–128] Whether this syndrome represents a distinct clinical entity or should be considered a part of the spectrum of SLE is still controversial.[129, 130]

Anti-Ro/SSA and anti-La/SSB are antibodies occasionally found in the sera of patients with SLE (frequency of 25% to 30% and 5% to 15%, respectively),[97] Sjögren syndrome (frequency of about 70%),[131, 132] and, rarely, polymyositis, scleroderma, rheumatoid arthritis, and primary biliary cirrhosis. Anti-Ro/SSA interacts with a cytoplasmic RNA molecule and its complexed proteins (small cytoplasmic RNPs).[133] Anti-La/SSB, originally thought to interact also with a cytoplasmic antigen, actually recognizes a nuclear antigen, snRNP, distinct from ENA.[134] These antibodies are occasionally present in SLE patients who are FANA-negative (see earlier discussion). Their clinical importance relates to the SLE syndromes associated with them. Maternal anti-Ro/SSA has been linked to neonatal lupus, a transient illness of newborns associated with cardiac conduction abnormalities, a characteristic rash, and a high neonatal mortality. Ten percent to 20% of the mothers of these children are known to have SLE; an additional 20% later develop it.[54] Other serologic abnormalities for SLE are often absent in these patients. Another syndrome,

subacute cutaneous lupus erythematosus, has been associated with anti-Ro/SSA in 63% of patients. Illness in these patients is characterized by presentation with a psoriasis-like rash, differing from discoid lupus in that it does not scar or develop follicular plugging. Photosensitivity appears to be even more common than in classic SLE.[3, 4, 16] Although these patients generally present initially with dermatologic manifestations, many develop systemic illness,[135] including glomerulonephritis.[16] Patients with homozygous C2 deficiency and SLE almost always have anti-Ro/SSA antibodies.[136] Finally, an FANA-negative SLE-like syndrome characterized by large and small vessel vasculitis, CNS involvement, and cutaneous ulcers has also been associated with anti-Ro/SSA antibodies.[136] The presence of anti-Ro/SSA is correlated with human leukocyte antigen (HLA) DRw3.[133]

Anti-La/SSB antibodies rarely occur in the absence of anti-Ro/SSA. The combination of the two antibodies was associated with a decreased frequency of glomerulonephritis to 9% in one study. In contrast, patients with anti-Ro/SSA alone (who are FANA-positive) have a 53% frequency of glomerular involvement.[133] Black female SLE patients who have antibodies to Ro/SSA, Sm, and nRNP but not to La/SSB appear to develop severe nephritis.[137]

**Other Antibodies.** The spectrum of lupus-associated antibodies has been reviewed.[115] Antibodies to histones may develop in patients with SLE, but they are more common in patients with drug-induced lupus.[138–141] Antibodies to endothelial cells are occasionally seen, perhaps explaining some of the vasculitic lesions.[140] As previously noted, antibodies to phospholipids may be seen in patients with "lupus anticoagulant."[45–48] Small numbers of patients with SLE have been noted to have antibodies to heparan sulfate that cross-react with DNA[80] and antibodies to the ribosomal P protein.[142] Autoantibodies to the C1q component of complement are also found, particularly with active renal disease.[143] In addition, some patients with SLE demonstrate circulating antineutrophil cytoplasmic antibody (see also the section on vasculitis).[144] In the presence of a positive FANA, however, antineutrophil cytoplasmic antibodies (ANCAs) demonstrable solely by immunofluorescence microscopy or by fluorescence-activated cell sorting are of uncertain significance. However, FANA-positive patients with specific anti–proteinase 3 or antimyeloperoxidase antibodies may have simultaneous underlying necrotizing vasculitis (see later). Antibodies to extracellular matrix have also been observed in SLE, including those to laminin,[145] heparan sulfate proteoglycan,[146] and entactin (nidogen).[147]

***Complement.*** $CH_{50}$ and serum complement components (C1q, C4, C2, C3, and C5) are frequently depressed during active renal disease.[148–153] Hypercatabolism of C3 may be present even with normal serum levels.[150] Increased serum concentration of C3 fragments is often present.[149] Hyposynthesis of C3 may contribute to low C3 levels in advanced renal disease and in association with severe hypercatabolism.[150] The serum C4 levels are often particularly low in active SLE, and levels may decline in advance of a clinical flare of disease,[154] but this is not always the case. This may be due to conversion of C4 to C4d and measurement of both active and degraded proteins in the assay.[155] C4 levels may be less sensitive as an indicator of disease activity because of a broader range of normal values and because of the existence of *C4A* null alleles in SLE. Therefore, some groups believe that monitoring C3 levels is a better way to assess patients for disease activity.[156] The serum level of properdin is less often depressed than in acute poststreptococcal glomerulonephritis and is not well correlated with the depression in C3 levels. During active stages of the disease, serum may contain a C3-cleaving activity similar to that observed in acute poststreptococcal glomerulonephritis, and its presence may be used as a rough indication of activity.[154] Serum concentration of factor B may be modestly depressed, especially if C3 is markedly decreased. This may be an indication of activation of the alternative complement pathway by means of the amplification loop involving C3b (see Chapter 30). Factor B may also be depressed in massive proteinuria because of excessive urinary losses. C3 is occasionally markedly depressed without significant evidence of active renal disease, especially in patients with active and widespread skin lesions.[151, 157] The correlations of complement component concentrations (e.g., C3, C4) and clinical activity of disease are poor,[158] but serial measurements may show reasonable predictive value with relapses, in about a third of patients. Normalization of serum complement is associated with an improved renal outcome. Thus, some have stressed the importance of directing therapy toward the goal of normalization of serum complement levels.[159] However, no scientifically rigorous studies show that normalization of serum complement as a primary goal of therapy improves outcome. In pregnant women, C3 and C4 concentrations may be used to differentiate exacerbations of SLE from preeclampsia.[160]

Lupus-like syndromes have been observed in association with several isolated complement deficiency states, particularly of C1r, C1s, C2, C4, C5, and C8. Such patients may have depressed total hemolytic activity of serum $CH_{50}$ despite normal levels of C3.[161] Hereditary angioedema patients, with absence of C1 inhibitor protein, have a 2% incidence of a lupus-like syndrome.[162] Patients with active SLE have depressed complement-mediated immune complex–solubilizing activity in vitro. This defect may account, in part, for the deposition and resistance of immune complexes in tissue. Many patients with SLE also have decreased density of C3b receptors (CR1) on erythrocytes and phagocytic cells.[163–166, 166a] Diminished C3b receptor density in these patients is probably an acquired rather than a congenital abnormality[166] and may also be found on the visceral epithelial cells of the glomerulus.[165, 166] A correlation between the number of C3b receptor sites on erythrocytes and in the glomerulus has been reported.[167] This defect may also contribute to the prolonged circulation of immune complexes.

***Circulating Immune Complexes.*** Circulating immune complexes (CICs) are often found, but the prevalence depends on the type of assay employed.[158] Some assays show a good correlation with the presence and severity of renal disease.[168–177] Solid-phase C1q assay seems to correlate best with clinical manifestations,[172] but this may be due to autoantibodies to C1q rather than to CICs.[143] Raji cell test results may be falsely positive because of IgM antilymphocyte cell membrane autoantibodies in serum. Circulating DNA and DNA–anti-DNA immune complexes have also

been found[177] but not by all investigators.[178] The complexes that do contain DNA and anti-DNA have been found to contain low-molecular-weight dsDNA (about 30 to 35 base pairs) and a particular anti-DNA antibody that protects DNA from endogenous DNase.[179] For clinical purposes, the measurement of CICs in patients with SLE is of dubious value.

**Genetic Studies.** The prevalence of HLA-B7 and -B8 is increased in SLE, and the HLA-B8 antigen may be associated with a more severe form of renal involvement.[180] SLE patients with anti-Ro/SSA activity have a high incidence of HLA-DR3.[136] HLA-A10, -B18, and -DR2 tend to be associated with SLE-like syndromes in C2-deficient patients.[181] Familial cases have been described,[182, 183] especially in association with complement deficiencies[183, 184] and IgA deficiency.[185] Null alleles at C2 and C4 loci in the major histocompatibility complex are frequently found in patients with SLE.[183, 186, 187] The most common extended haplotype associated with SLE in whites is HLA-DR3, C4AQ0, C4B1, C2′, Bf5, HLA-B8, HLA-CW⁻, HLA-A1. In a study of 90 Hungarian patients, homozygosity at the GM3;5,13 allele for the IgG heavy chain was associated with an increased risk of symptomatic renal disease in individuals with SLE.[188] Taken together, these findings suggest that an underlying inherited deficiency of complement or complement receptors may be pathogenetically involved in many patients with SLE.

***Lupus Band Test.*** Granular deposits of IgG and complement components are frequently found in the dermal-epidermal junction of involved and clinically normal skin of patients with SLE but only in the involved skin in patients with discoid lupus erythematosus.[189–193] Such deposits rarely correlate with active renal disease and depressed C3 levels.

***Urinalysis.*** A carefully done urinalysis frequently but not invariably reveals some abnormality in patients with histologically evident renal involvement.[1, 21–25] In severe cases, especially with vasculitis, the urine sediment may contain dysmorphic erythrocytes, white blood cells, and hyaline and broad casts; this is referred to as telescoped urine.[194]

Urinary protein clearance determinations in patients with nephrotic syndrome are usually poorly selective. Fractional IgG clearances increase relative to that of albumin, indicating a major role for disturbances in the size-selective barrier.[195] During active disease, the concentration of free light chains in the urine usually exceeds 20 µg/mL.[196] Serum and urinary fibrin degradation products may also be increased, the latter particularly during active disease,[197, 198] but clinically helpful correlations have not always been found.

***Miscellaneous.*** Rheumatoid factor and mixed polyclonal IgG-IgM cryoimmunoglobulins (cryoIgs) may be present in patients with active renal disease. High levels of cryoIg may be a clue to underlying SLE in patients presenting with otherwise idiopathic (primary) glomerular disease. Rheumatoid factor and cryoIgs are inversely correlated in patients with renal disease.[148] cryoIg correlates best with severe proliferative glomerular disease. cryoIg may contain DNA and anti-DNA antibody and fibronectin. Leukopenia, biologically false-positive VDRL, positive Coombs test, lymphocytotoxins, and other autoantibodies may also be detected.[199–201] The false-positive VDRL is due to an autoantibody to a phosphate ester containing an epitope common to DNA, cardiolipin, and a circulating procoagulant protein.[202]

Defects in suppressor cell activity and abnormalities in T cell subsets have been described.[17] The patterns of T lymphocyte subset functional defects have been related to the specificities of circulating anti–T cell autoantibodies. Many different patterns of abnormal T cell expression have been observed in patients with SLE. One group of patients has low CD4+/CD8+ subset ratios (<1.0) and circulating autoantibodies that impair the suppressor-inducer function of CD4+ (helper-inducer cells) and thereby reduce the generation of CD8+ suppressor-cytotoxic cells. Another group of patients has high CD4+/CD8+ subset ratios (>2.0) and circulating autoantibodies that interfere directly with CD8+ suppressor cell function (probably a cytolytic effect). Another group with moderately low (1.0 to 1.2) CD4+/CD8+ subset ratios has circulating autoantibody to the CD4+ suppressor-inducer cell but has no effect on CD8+ suppressor cell function. A final group has slightly decreased CD4+/CD8+ subset ratios (>1.2, <2.0), but its anti–T cell autoantibodies have no effect on either CD4+ or CD8+ cells. Thus, the dysregulation of T cell subsets in SLE often involves the CD8+ suppressor-cytotoxic and the CD4+ helper-inducer cells.[18, 203] CD4+ helper cell function is relatively intact, even though the CD4+/CD8+ subset ratio may be decreased in some patients. An unusual T helper population, found in the peripheral blood of normal individuals at a frequency of approximately 0.3%, was found to be markedly expanded in patients with active lupus nephritis. These cells, which are CD4−/CD8− and α,β T cell receptor–positive, appear to contribute to the production of cationic IgG class pathogenic anti-DNA autoantibodies.[204]

Monocyte-dependent suppression of immunoglobulin (Ig) synthesis has been observed, and monocyte procoagulant activity appears to correlate with endocapillary proliferation.[205] Antilymphocytic antibodies may cross-react with antigens of the CNS and be involved in CNS manifestations.[206] Antineuronal antibodies are prevalent in patients with CNS lupus but are nonspecific.[207] Circulating anti-Sm antibody and free DNA also correlate with CNS disease.[208, 209] Defective reticuloendothelial Fc receptor function of the spleen has been described in patients with active SLE.[210] The C3-dependent rosette phenomenon is suppressed during active disease.[211] C-reactive protein levels are usually normal or mildly increased during exacerbations of SLE, but the erythrocyte sedimentation rate is frequently greatly elevated in association with superimposed infection.[212] A rising erythrocyte sedimentation rate with stable normal C-reactive protein levels in a febrile patient with SLE strongly supports a diagnosis of an exacerbation of disease rather than infection.

Cholesterol levels in patients with SLE[213] and nephrotic syndrome sometimes do not correlate well with the level of serum albumin.[213] However, this probably does not occur more frequently than in patients with primary glomerular disorders.[6, 213, 214] Testosterone levels are lower and estrogen levels higher than normal in many men with SLE.

Researchers continue to search for noninvasive methods of assessing renal prognosis. One study of 22 patients suggested that the presence of a low filtration fraction was 61% sensitive and 88% specific in predicting a fall in GFR in a 1-year follow-up period.[215] Radioimmunoassay of urinary albumin has been reported useful in detecting subclinical lupus nephritis by some[216] but not all[217] workers. Contradictory evidence surrounds the widely held belief that low C3 or C4 levels and a high or rising titer of autoantibody to native DNA may augur a poor prognosis or an impending exacerbation of lupus nephritis.[153, 156, 218, 219] As mentioned, a high fractional urinary clearance of IgG may indicate severe renal disease.[195]

## PATHOLOGY

Since the 1960s, several classifications have been proposed for the various forms of glomerular injury encountered in SLE. With widespread use of renal biopsies, it has become apparent that distinct patterns of involvement may occur, either in different forms at different times in the same patient or with the same features during the entire course of the disease. The first classification was initially proposed by Muehrcke and co-workers[220] and was subsequently modified by many investigators.[1, 6, 9, 220–222] The schema proposed by Baldwin and associates and used by the World Health Organization (WHO)[1, 222–224] is used in this discussion (Table 31–1).

It is commonly believed that most, if not all, patients with SLE, regardless of clinical manifestations, have glomerular Ig and complement component deposits.[1] Although many studies have found evidence of near-universal immunopathologic glomerular involvement, a few reports indicate that some patients with SLE may have no detectable renal lesions by light or immunofluorescence microscopy.[225] From a practical and conceptual point of view, it is convenient to consider that the basic immunologic abnormality in the kidney is the accumulation or deposition of Ig and complement components in the mesangium.[1] Such deposition depends on a variety of factors, including mesangial and mononuclear phagocyte function, size, composition, and, perhaps, charge of the immune complexes or antigen, as well as other poorly defined considerations (see Chapter 29). This pattern of immune deposition represents the background on which the more severe glomerular lesions are imposed.[1] Depending on the composition and circulatory load of immune complexes, capillary wall localization may also occur. The local glomerular reaction and cellular constituents from the circulating blood may result in varying patterns of glomerular injury seen by light microscopy. Alternatively, immune complexes may form in situ as a consequence of circulating antibody reacting with a planted nonglomerular antigen such as ssDNA or an intrinsic glomerular antigen[226, 227] (see also Chapter 29). It is with this information in mind that a reasonable understanding of the subdivisions of lupus glomerulonephritis (LGN) may be achieved. In addition to classification of the glomerular lesions according to general appearance by light, electron, and immunofluorescence microscopy, it is essential to recognize that certain lesions are associated with active disease (e.g., glomerular hypercellularity including leukocytic infiltration, nuclear karyorrhexis, fibrinoid necrosis, cellular crescents, subendothelial deposits, hematoxylin bodies, hyaline thrombi, vasculitis, interstitial mononuclear infiltrates, and edema), whereas others indicate chronic changes

**TABLE 31–1. Summary of the Light Microscopic, Electron Microscopic, and Immunofluorescence Microscopic Features of Renal Lesions in Systemic Lupus Erythematosus***

| Category (WHO Class) | Light Microscopic Features | Electron Microscopic Features (Electron-Dense Deposits) | Immunofluorescence Microscopic Features (Deposits of Ig/C) |
|---|---|---|---|
| Normal (I) | Normal | — | — |
| Mesangial proliferative glomerulonephritis (II) | Normal or diffuse mesangial widening and hypercellularity | Mes: + +<br>SE: ±<br>Epi:0 | Mes: + +<br>CW: ±<br>SE: ±<br>Epi: 0 |
| Focal and segmental proliferative glomerulonephritis (III) | Diffuse mesangial hypercellularity with focal and segmental accentuation, segmental necrosis, hyaline thrombi | Mes: + + +<br>SE: +<br>Epi: 0 | Mes: + +<br>CW: +<br>SE: +<br>Epi: 0 |
| Diffuse proliferative glomerulonephritis (IV) | Pronounced diffuse hypercellularity, mesangial interposition, subendothelial deposits (wire loops), segmental necrosis, hyaline thrombi, hematoxylin bodies, cellular infiltration, crescents | Mes: + + +<br>SE: + + +<br>Epi: + + + + | Mes: + + +<br>CW: + +<br>SE: + + +<br>Epi: + + + + extraglomerular tubulointerstitial deposits |
| Membranous lupus glomerulonephritis (V) | Mild mesangial hypercellularity, epimembranous deposits, spikes | Mes: + + +<br>SE: ±<br>Epi: + + | Mes: + + + +<br>CW: ±<br>SE: ±<br>Epi: + + |
| Advanced sclerosing glomerulonephritis | Superimposed focal and segmental or global sclerosis on category IV or V | Mes: +<br>CW ± | Mes: +<br>CW: ± |
| Interstitial nephritis | Marked acute and chronic tubulointerstitial inflammation with minor glomerular lesions | Tubule basement membrane + + Variable glomerular deposits | Tubule basement membrane + + Variable glomerular deposits |

*WHO = World Health Organization; Mes = mesangial; CW = capillary wall; SE = subendothelial deposits; Epi = epimembranous deposits; 0 to + + + + = semiquantitative assessment of intensity of deposition.

in the form of scarring or reparative processes (e.g., tubule atrophy, interstitial fibrosis, glomerular sclerosis, fibrous crescents, adhesions, arteriolosclerosis).[1, 228, 229] These active or chronic lesions have been claimed to have importance in determining prognosis and therapy.[1, 218, 224, 229–237] The scheme for determining activity and chronicity indices is depicted in Table 31–2.

This classification of the glomerular lesions can be expanded to include the simultaneous occurrence of more than one type of glomerular injury (e.g., membranous and focal proliferative glomerulonephritis).[224, 232] Renal biopsy is therefore a potentially useful tool in the overall management of patients with lupus nephritis.[237] Indeed, some believe that renal biopsy is an indispensable part of the evaluation of patients with SLE. However, as discussed later, renal biopsies are seldom used *diagnostically* in SLE, because the diagnosis is usually established on the basis of clinical and laboratory findings. Thus, the principal role of renal biopsy in SLE is to help in more accurate prognostication, to supplement clinical information for the selection of the most appropriate therapeutic approach, and to exclude other lesions that may complicate the course of SLE (such as acute tubule necrosis or acute hypersensitivity interstitial nephritis). Although a rough correlation exists between renal pathology and the clinical and laboratory features, exceptions are not uncommon. Transformation of one morphologic pattern to another limits the utility of renal biopsy in predicting outcome, and with the modern approach to management, the contributions of renal pathology to overall prognosis are only marginal compared with the information provided from clinical assessment. Nonethe-

less, renal biopsy may be quite useful in determining the *initial* approach to management. Unfortunately, the true role of renal biopsy in SLE has never been tested in a randomized prospective manner.[233–237]

**Normal Glomeruli (WHO Class I).** This extremely infrequent pattern is characterized by complete absence of any structural alterations or immune deposits.[1]

**Mesangial (Mesangiopathic) Glomerulonephritis (WHO Class II).** In this form of glomerular damage, immune deposits are found in mesangial regions almost exclusively; there may be no structural abnormalities or increased cellularity by light microscopy (class IIa), or there

**TABLE 31–2. Systemic Lupus Erythematosus Nephritis: Index of Activity and Chronicity***

| Active Lesions | Chronic Lesions |
|---|---|
| Glomeruli<br>  Hypercellularity<br>  Fibrinoid necrosis<br>  Karyorrhexis†<br>  Crescents (cellular*)<br>  Wire loops<br>  Hyaline thrombi<br>  Leukocyte infiltration<br>Tubules/interstitium<br>  Mononuclear infiltration | Glomerulosclerosis<br>Fibrous crescents<br>Interstitial fibrosis<br>Tubule atrophy |

*Score 0 to 3 for each item.
†Multiply score by 2.
Modified from Austin HA 3d, Muenz LR, Joyce KM, et al.: Prognostic factors in lupus nephritis: Contribution of renal histologic data. Am J Med 75:382, 1983.

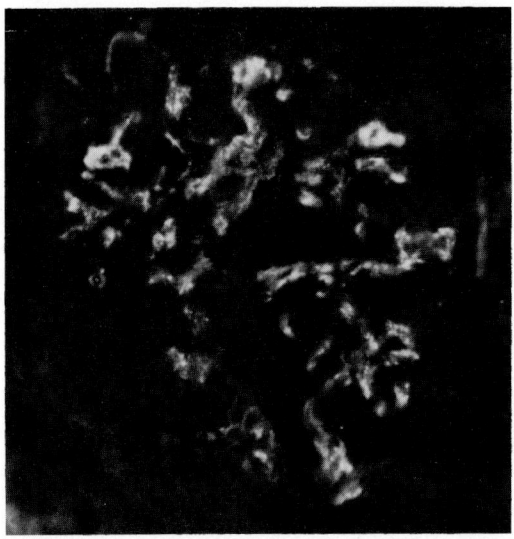

**Figure 31–2.** Immunofluorescence microscopic appearance of mesangial LGN. Deposits are present in the mesangium and occasionally in the capillary walls. (Antihuman C3; magnification × 400.)

may be a uniform increase of cells (mesangial cells or monocytes) in the mesangium (class IIb). By immunofluorescence microscopy, granular Ig (IgG, less commonly IgM and IgA) and complement (C3, C4, C1q) are observed (Fig. 31–2), but rare instances of linear IgG have been noted.[23] Ultrastructural examination usually reveals relatively small electron-dense deposits in the mesangium, most prominent in the regions beneath the paramesangial basement membranes (Fig. 31–3). When significantly large, the deposits may be detected by light microscopy with the use of Masson trichrome or related stains. The capillary walls are largely unaffected, the only significant lesions being segmental effacement of the epithelial cell foot processes.

Some reports have described small and widely scattered subendothelial deposits in a few capillaries. Tubule, interstitial, and vascular alterations are usually lacking.[1, 237]

**Focal and Segmental Proliferative Lupus Glomerulonephritis (WHO Class III).** This form of glomerular injury is characterized by the presence of IgG, IgM, IgA, C1q, C4, C3, and properdin in the capillary walls of virtually all glomeruli, usually in small quantities, in addition to the earlier mentioned uniform mesangial deposits.[1] Dense, coarser accumulations are often observed, however, and correspond to portions of the glomeruli with segmental hypercellular lesions noted by light microscopy. In general, IgG is the main Ig identified, but IgM and, less often, intense IgA are also present in the glomeruli. Superimposed on the mesangial changes described earlier are segmental areas of increased cellularity seen by light microscopy (Fig. 31–4). The increased cellularity is due to the accumulation of polymorphonuclear leukocytes and monocytes in capillary lumina, a modest increase in the number of endothelial cells, a greater increase in mesangial cells, and occasionally segmental cellular crescents (admixed with fibrin) overlying the affected areas. Cell death, with nuclear karyorrhexis and pyknosis, may be a common accompaniment of these abnormalities. Relatively small subendothelial deposits may be identified in affected capillary walls. By definition, less than half of the glomerular population displays these segmental alterations, whereas the remainder are involved with only the mesangial changes described earlier. With the electron microscope, deposits are observed in subendothelial sites, in addition to the omnipresent mesangial deposits (Fig. 31–5). The capillary deposits are frequently small or medium sized, but they may also be large. Intramembranous and epimembranous deposits are also noted but with less frequency. The various proliferative and cellular abnormalities are obvious at the ultrastructural level; in addition, epithelial foot processes are effaced in most capillary walls.[1, 148, 225, 230–239]

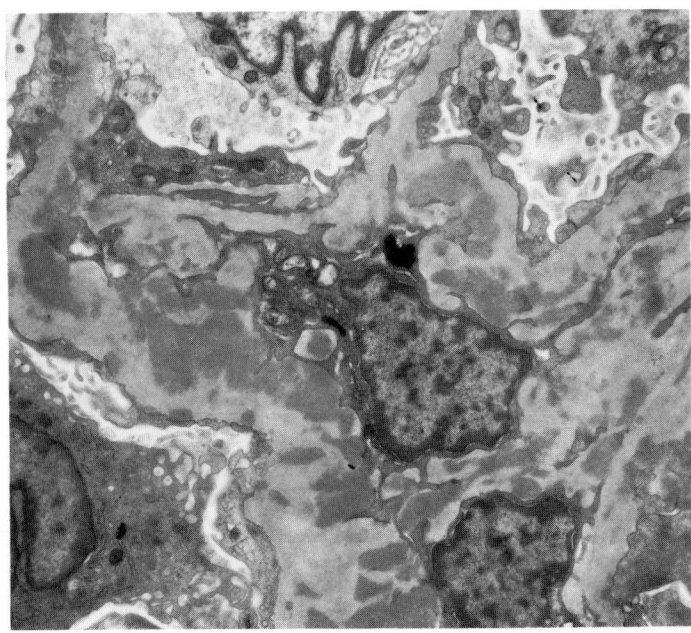

**Figure 31–3.** Electron microscopic appearance of mesangial LGN. Note prominent dense deposits in the mesangium. (Magnification × 12,000.)

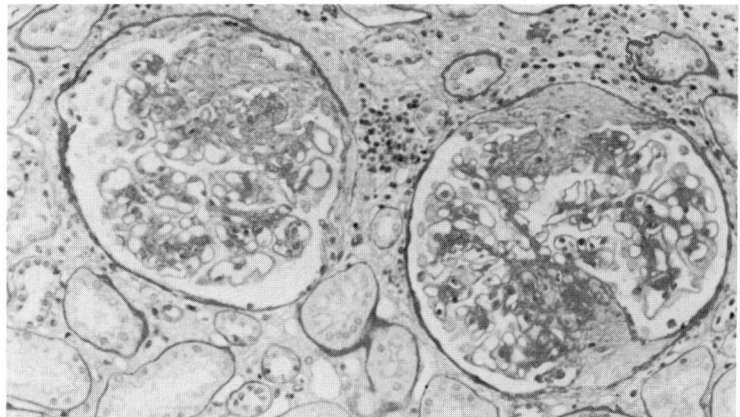

**Figure 31–4.** Light microscopic appearance of focal and segmental proliferative LGN. Two glomeruli demonstrate segmental cellular proliferation: the mesangial regions of less-affected lobules have mild expansion. (Periodic acid–Schiff; magnification × 375.)

**Diffuse Proliferative Lupus Glomerulonephritis (WHO Class IV).** This form of injury is basically the same as the focal and segmental proliferative variety, except that the changes are more pronounced and more widespread, involving more than half of the glomerular population. Hence, the immunofluorescence microscopic findings are indicative of heavy granular Ig (IgG, IgM, IgA, and sometimes IgE) and complement (C1q, C4, C3, C5–9) deposits in all sites, especially in the subendothelial aspect of capillary walls, where they are large, globular, and more numerous than elsewhere (Fig. 31–6). Fibrin deposition is more frequently observed, especially in the urinary space, where it may be associated with crescent formation. Light microscopy is characterized by severe changes in all or almost all glomeruli; all tufts are equally involved (Fig. 31–7). Extensive hypercellularity occurs, because of an increase in mesangial and endothelial cells and the presence of numerous and varied leukocytes in both luminal and extraluminal sites. Many cells show evidence of degeneration, and there are more pyknotic nuclei in contrast to cells in the focal proliferative variant of glomerulonephritis. Although considered the sole feature pathognomonic for SLE by light

microscopy, hematoxylin bodies are observed, albeit infrequently, in this form of glomerular injury. They are amorphous, ill-defined, lilac-stained structures that vary in size but are generally slightly smaller than nuclei. They are usually clustered together and are observed in areas of necrosis, in the mesangium, or occasionally free in capillary lumens.[240, 241] Capillary walls are greatly thickened and may have a "wire loop" appearance, which is due to the presence of large, circumferential subendothelial deposits. Sometimes these deposits achieve such a large size that they protrude into the lumen of the capillaries, where they take the form of hyaline thrombi. Epimembranous deposits, much smaller in size and often associated with basement membrane projections, are also noted in many capillary walls.

Small or large segmental or circumferential crescents may be noted in some or all glomeruli. When most glomeruli are affected, these structures appear similar to those seen in crescentic glomerulonephritis (see Chapter 30). It is often easy to distinguish crescentic LGN from other glomerulopathies with crescents, because the capillary tuft is still characterized by the changes basic to the diffuse prolifera-

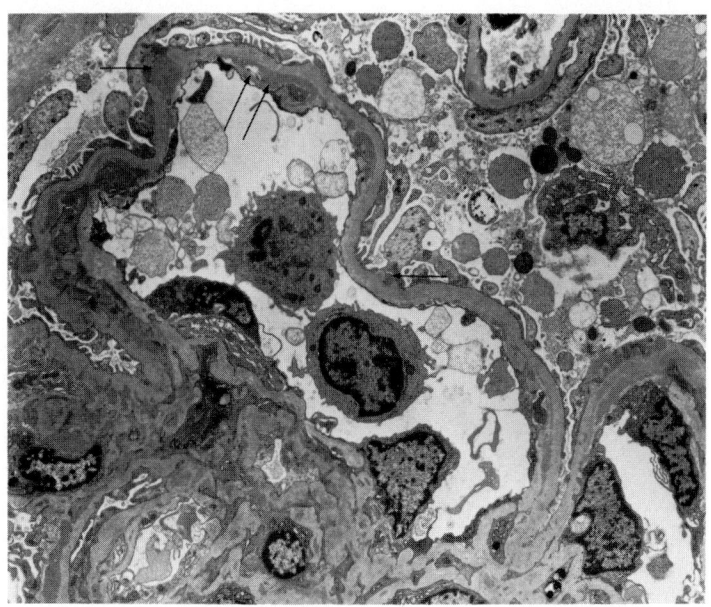

**Figure 31–5.** Electron microscopic appearance of focal and segmental proliferative LGN. The deposits are in the mesangium and in the capillary wall, where they are both epimembranous *(single arrow)* and subendothelial *(double arrow)* in location. (Magnification × 4900.)

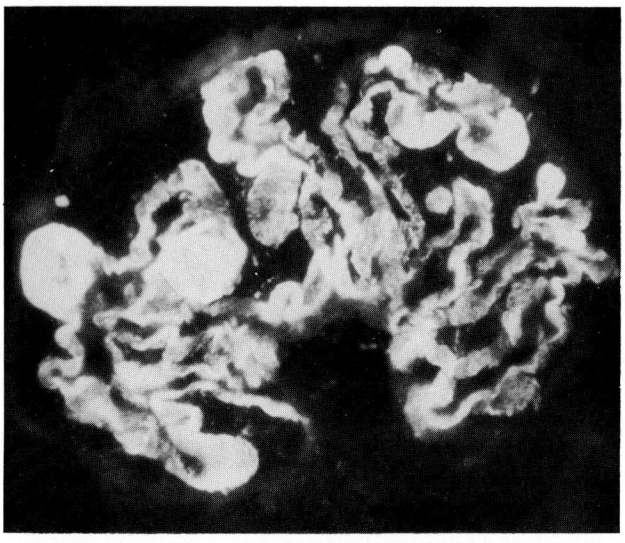

**Figure 31–6.** Immunofluorescence microscopic appearance of diffuse proliferative LGN. Note heavy deposits in mesangium and peripheral capillary walls. (Antihuman IgG; magnification × 600.)

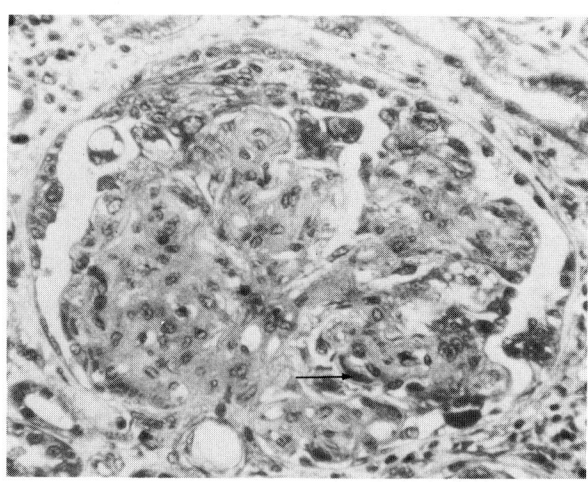

**Figure 31–7.** Light microscopic appearance of diffuse proliferative LGN. The glomerulus is hypercellular and has a small segmental cellular crescent at 12 o'clock position. Note the thickened capillary walls and the large subendothelial fuchsinophilic deposit *(arrow)*. (Masson trichrome; magnification × 500.)

tive lesions. Biopsy specimens from patients with diffuse proliferative glomerulonephritis occasionally have glomeruli that in many respects resemble those seen in type I idiopathic mesangiocapillary glomerulonephritis (see Chapter 30).

The ultrastructural findings mimic those seen by light microscopy (Fig. 31–8); specifically, large electron-dense deposits are observed in all glomerular locations, being especially prominent in subendothelial sites, where they may become extremely large and completely encase the capillary lumina. Epimembranous and intramembranous deposits are also common, but they occur in fewer numbers

and distribution than the subendothelial deposits. Mesangial cell migration and interposition are common findings, whether or not the glomeruli are lobular in appearance. The aforementioned hematoxylin bodies have been morphogenetically traced to degenerating leukocytes, which (presumably after their nuclei have combined with any of the antinuclear antibodies) are ingested by mesangial cells and undergo further degradation, ultimately appearing as a structure with a dense, sometimes lobulated center of nuclear origin, surrounded by a variable amount of cytoplasmic remnants.[1, 223] Glomerular capillary thrombosis, composed primarily of fibrin and distinct from the earlier mentioned hyaline thrombi, has been emphasized by Kant

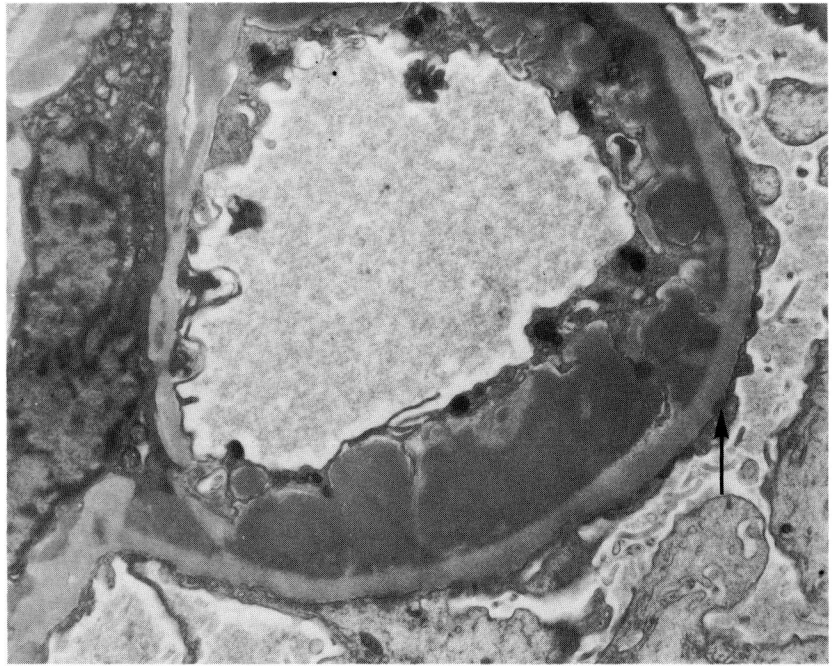

**Figure 31–8.** Electron microscopic appearance of diffuse proliferative LGN. Note the large confluent subendothelial deposits; a few small epimembranous deposits are also present *(arrow)*. (Magnification × 12,000.)

and co-workers[75] and is predictive of ultimate glomerular sclerosis.

**Membranous Lupus Glomerulonephritis (WHO Class V).** This form of injury is characterized primarily by the granular deposition of Ig (IgG, IgM, IgA) and complement (C1q, C4, C3, C5–9) along all capillary walls in a pattern similar to that observed in idiopathic membranous glomerulonephritis (Fig. 31–9; see Chapter 30 and Fig. 30–21). All Ig classes and complement components may be evident, however; IgG and C1q deposits are usually more prominent. Mesangial deposits may also be present and almost always are detected by electron microscopy. Four variants of membranous glomerulonephritis in SLE are recognized. In one variant, the findings are virtually identical to those in idiopathic membranous glomerulonephritis (class Va).[242-244] In another, diffuse mesangial alterations are concomitantly present (class Vb). In another, segmental hypercellularity or sclerosis is present (class Vc). Finally, the features of membranous glomerulonephritis may coexist with the lesions of diffuse proliferative glomerulonephritis (class Vd). This latter category resembles diffuse proliferative glomerulonephritis both clinically and serologically.[218, 242, 244] Severe crescentic glomerulonephritis may be superimposed.[245] Although mesangial deposits detected ultrastructurally[244, 246] and mesangial hypercellularity have been reported in some patients with non-LGN, these findings should raise the suspicion of the pathologist that the patient may have SLE, even in the absence of serologic and clinical confirmation at the time of the biopsy.[244] Other features, such as subendothelial dense deposits and tubuloreticular

structures and extraglomerular deposits (see later discussion), may also be clues to the diagnosis of lupus.[244]

**Glomerular Sclerosis (WHO Class VI).** Some investigators categorize separately renal biopsy specimens that have as their most apparent abnormality the presence of completely or segmentally sclerotic glomeruli. Although completely sclerotic glomeruli may be observed in focal or diffuse proliferative LGN, on occasion glomerular sclerosis may be the predominant alteration. Because of the lack of other changes, Baldwin and co-workers differentiated glomerular sclerosis into its own category.[1, 6] They speculated that, in some individuals with lupus, the primary glomerular response to injury may be sclerosing rather than proliferative changes. Most other investigators, however, do not categorize such renal lesions separately but consider them to be either end-stage abnormalities of diffuse proliferative glomerulonephritis (when most glomeruli are involved) or arrested or healed focal proliferative lesions (when only isolated glomeruli are affected).[1, 230]

**Vascular Abnormalities.** Various types of vascular abnormalities may be encountered in the kidneys. Perhaps the most common are the typical arterial and arteriolar changes of hypertension.[1, 59, 224, 247, 248] A vasculopathy similar to that of malignant hypertension has been observed, however. Small arteries and afferent arterioles are preferentially affected. There is intramural (usually intimal) plasma protein accumulation, with endothelial cell swelling or destruction and luminal narrowing. This may be associated with occlusive luminal precipitates, either in the form of true fibrin thrombi or as aggregated Ig, complement, and fibrin. In this

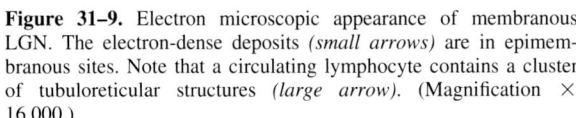

**Figure 31–9.** Electron microscopic appearance of membranous LGN. The electron-dense deposits *(small arrows)* are in epimembranous sites. Note that a circulating lymphocyte contains a cluster of tubuloreticular structures *(large arrow).* (Magnification × 16,000.)

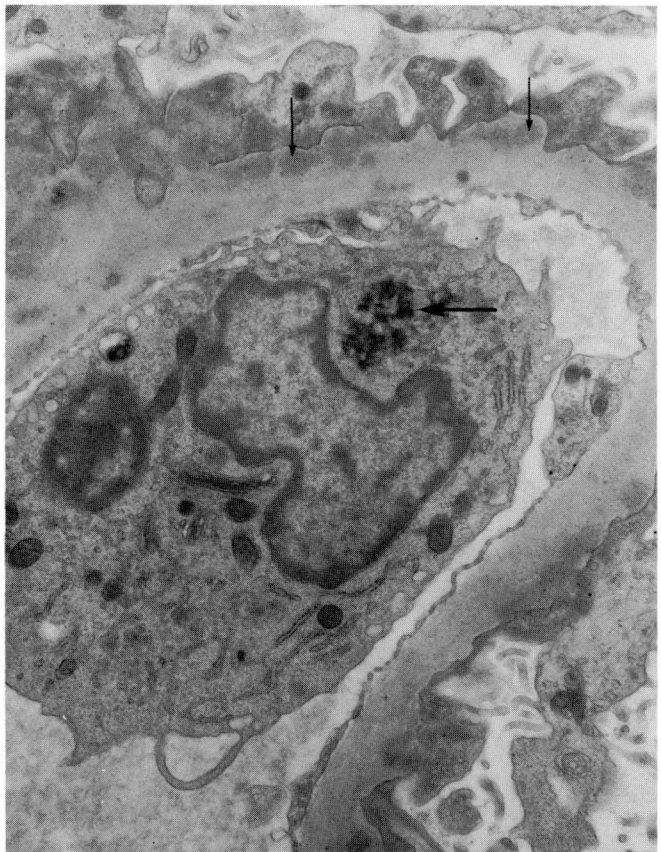

form of vascular injury, there is usually no accompanying inflammation.[1, 6, 249] The patients described by Baldwin and colleagues[1] were all suffering from severe hypertension, whereas the group reported by Bhathena and co-workers[249] were normotensive at the time of renal biopsy, but most ultimately developed hypertension. A true necrotizing arteritis, with leukocytic infiltration and destruction of the vessel wall, is distinctly unusual. When present, it is usually associated with diffuse proliferative glomerulonephritis, although only mild glomerular involvement may occur.[1, 245, 250] Such patients may also have circulating antineutrophil cytoplasmic antibodies (see later section on vasculitis). The presence of renal vascular lesions reportedly augurs for poorer renal survival than occurs in patients without them, but similar overall survival is observed in patients with and without vascular lesions.[59, 247, 248]

**Interstitial Inflammation.** Interstitial cellular infiltration is a frequent biopsy finding, especially in diffuse proliferative glomerulonephritis, but also in the focal proliferative, less often in the membranous, and rarely in the mesangial variant.[1] With careful study of trichrome-stained sections, fuchsinophilic deposits may be noted in tubule basement membranes and occasionally in the interstitium. When severe, the inflammation may be associated with tubule atrophy or necrosis,[251] tubule basement membrane thickening, and interstitial fibrosis. Immunofluorescence may reveal deposits of Ig and complement along basement membrane, and dense deposits may be seen by electron microscopy. Monocytes may be identified by cell markers.[252] Deposits are more readily detected by immunofluorescence than by electron microscopy; they may be found in the interstitium, tubule basement membranes, peritubular capillaries, arteries, and Bowman capsule basement membrane. The prevalence of extraglomerular deposits generally correlates with the activity of glomerular lesions and the severity of glomerular hypercellularity. Several groups[253–255] have noted little correlation between tubulointerstitial deposits and interstitial inflammation, but good correlation has been reported between inflammation and the degree of renal impairment. Scanning electron microscopic studies have allowed a better understanding of the structural alterations in tubule basement membrane.[255]

**Tubuloreticular Structures.** Certain peculiarities noted with considerable frequency in glomeruli from patients with SLE deserve special comment. Tubuloreticular structures (i.e., clustered microtubules measuring about 250 nm in diameter) have been described in the cytoplasm of endothelial cells in nearly all biopsies.[1] Although they may also be noted in other diseases and even in nondiseased individuals, their presence, especially in large numbers, is most consistent with LGN.[1, 256, 257] Tubuloreticular structures have also been noted as an integral feature of human immunodeficiency virus (HIV) infection, especially in renal endothelial cells (see later discussion).[258, 259] As indicated earlier, in several studies, the finding of such tubuloreticular structures was the only clue to a diagnosis of LGN in children who, at the time of renal biopsy for nephrotic syndrome, had no other clinical or laboratory manifestations of the disease.[260, 261] These structures have also been described in lymphocytes, and, on rare occasions, they can be noted in these cells found in glomerular capillaries (see Fig. 31–9).

**Organized Deposits.** Although electron-dense deposits are usually composed of homogeneous or finely granular electron-dense material, some have an unusual organization pattern. Most prominent is a crystalline acrilinear, parallel-arranged substructure, having the appearance of a fingerprint; other patterns are also noted but less frequently.[1, 262, 263] The fingerprint organization has been observed by the authors in about 20% of biopsy specimens from patients with lupus; this organization has been seen in non-LGN, especially in association with cryoIg. Deposits with a similar substructure have also been described in extrarenal sites. Fingerprint deposits may be the only diagnostic clue to the ultimate development of lupus.[263]

**Tubule Abnormalities.** Another feature that is common to many biopsy specimens, especially those involved with diffuse proliferative glomerulonephritis, is the presence of electron-dense deposits in tubule basement membranes, the interstitium, the walls of peritubular capillaries, and occasionally in the basement membranes of the Bowman capsule. Acute tubule cell necrosis may also be seen, especially in patients with acute renal failure associated with use of nonsteroidal anti-inflammatory drugs (NSAIDs).[251, 264] These deposits correspond to the extraglomerular renal Ig and complement components described earlier. Such deposits are often associated with interstitial nephritis.[1, 251]

**Transformations.** Many reports have documented the transformation of one form of glomerular injury to another.[1, 265–270] In general, the more common progression is from mesangial to focal or diffuse proliferative lesions or from focal to diffuse proliferative lesions, but transformation to a less severe lesion has been shown to be common. Diffuse proliferative lesions can transform to membranous lesions, almost always under the influence of therapy. Less common transitions include membranous to diffuse proliferative lesions and diffuse proliferative to focal proliferative lesions. Patients with mild focal or diffuse proliferative lesions who have heavy proteinuria or evidence of serologic activity (e.g., elevated anti-DNA antibody, depressed C4 or C3 levels) seem more likely to progress to diffuse proliferative LGN. One study, however, has shown that transformations are not readily predictable on the basis of clinical, laboratory, or pathologic features at the time of the initial renal biopsy, but younger patients tend to have more stable glomerular disease.[269]

Amyloidosis (AA type) is a rare complication of long-standing lupus nephritis.[271]

## CLINICOPATHOLOGIC CORRELATIONS

Only an approximate correlation exists between the clinical findings and the patterns of glomerular and interstitial involvement as seen by light, electron, or immunofluorescence microscopy (Table 31–3). The extent and distribution of electron-dense deposits and Ig and complement deposits, especially in a subendothelial distribution, seem to correlate better with clinical and serologic findings than does a light microscopy–based categorization. Many studies, however, have found that detailed light microscopic analysis of renal biopsies of patients with lupus can contribute significantly toward accurate prognostic predictions. Specifically, the

**TABLE 31–3. Clinicopathologic Correlations in Lupus Glomerulonephritis: Clinical Features and Histologic Patterns**

| | Pathologic Findings (%) | | | |
|---|---|---|---|---|
| Clinical Findings | *Minimal Change or Mild Mesangial Proliferation* | *Focal and Segmental Proliferative Glomerulonephritis* | *Diffuse Proliferative Glomerulonephritis* | *Membranous Glomerulonephritis* |
| No clinical findings of renal involvement | 40 | 30 | 25 | <5 |
| Renal abnormalities present | 7 | 16 | 65 | 12 |
| Nephrotic syndrome with or without renal failure | <1 | 8 | 70 | 22 |
| Hematuria or non-nephrotic proteinuria | 10 | 21 | 63 | 6 |

presence of lesions indicative of chronicity has been cited as a poor prognostic factor.[229, 236, 272, 273] A light microscopic scoring system, emphasizing chronic changes (chronicity index) rather than morphologic classification, has been suggested to be valuable in predicting renal outcome and as a guide to therapy. Specific findings suggesting a poor prognosis include extensive glomerular sclerosis, fibrous crescents, tubule atrophy, and interstitial fibrosis.[229, 236, 272] Not all investigators agree, however, that renal biopsies and activity and chronicity scoring are valuable in estimating prognosis.[273–275] Furthermore, some have suggested that scoring is not reproducible, in either clinical or research settings.[276, 277]

Lesions indicative of activity of the underlying disease process may also indicate the potential for reversibility with aggressive treatment. A light microscopic scoring system emphasizing active lesions (activity index) may be valuable in assessing potential responsiveness to therapy and prognosis.[276] Specific lesions indicative of activity include endocapillary proliferation, nuclear karyorrhexis, cellular crescents, fibrinoid necrosis, subendothelial deposits (and wire loops), interstitial mononuclear cell infiltration, and vasculitis.[200, 202, 231, 234, 235]

According to the WHO scheme, morphologic classification may show some correspondence with clinical features. Many investigators now view focal proliferative glomerulonephritis (class III) as an early, more limited form of diffuse proliferative glomerulonephritis (class IV). Only a minority of such patients, however, are actually documented to experience a transformation from class III to class IV disease. On presentation, few patients have nephrotic syndrome and renal failure at the outset is distinctly uncommon. Whereas some investigators have found end-stage renal disease (ESRD) to be uncommon in patients with focal proliferative glomerulonephritis,[238] others found no difference in clinical course between those with focal and those with diffuse proliferative glomerulonephritis, especially when more than half of glomeruli are involved with segmental lesions.[274, 275] Membranous LGN, on the other hand, is commonly associated with the nephrotic syndrome, and the subsequent gradual development of renal failure is similar to that seen in the idiopathic variety.[278, 279] Rapid progression to renal failure may occur when membranous changes are complicated by crescent formation.[245] The diffuse proliferative glomerular lesions are also associated with nephrotic syndrome, and in at least half of cases, GFR is reduced.[6] Renal failure often occurs, and in the presence of extensive crescentic disease, severe hypertension or vasculitis may be rapidly progressive.[6, 245] It should be noted, however, that clinically "silent" diffuse proliferative glomerulonephritis occurs.[250]

Nonetheless, as has been mentioned, the clinical features of renal involvement have an imperfect relationship to the extent and severity of underlying glomerular lesions. Severe diffuse proliferative lesions have been encountered in patients with no or only mild clinical evidence of renal involvement (see Table 31–3). Such patients are more likely, however, to reveal some serologic evidence of active disease, such as high levels of anti-DNA antibody, low C3 and C4 levels, CIC, or cryoIg. The dissociation between clinical findings and histologic severity in SLE has suggested to some that an initial staging renal biopsy be performed in all patients with SLE, regardless of the presence or absence of clinical features of renal involvement, to provide a better guide to therapy. Unfortunately, no study has yet demonstrated that such an approach contributes in a favorable way to the survival of patients or decreases the morbidity in SLE. Retrospective studies have supported the notion that careful follow-up of clinical and laboratory data provides adequate information concerning prognosis and therapy.[234, 235, 280, 281] Renal biopsy can provide data only on the extent of severity of disease at a single point in time, and its value as a prognostic tool and therapeutic guide is greatly diminished by the tendency for exacerbations and transformations of diseases from one category to another.[268, 269] To further compound the difficulties inherent in using renal biopsy as a prognostic and therapeutic guide, the glomerular lesions do not always fit nicely into the discrete categories used here for discussion purposes. This is especially true for the proliferative lesions. Nonetheless, careful analysis of a renal biopsy, especially with attention given to features of activity and chronicity, sometimes provides useful guides to prognosis and treatment.[269–274, 276] For example, finding membranous glomerulopathy in a patient with SLE and nephrotic syndrome and a normal GFR, or detecting advanced glomerulosclerosis and interstitial fibrosis in a patient with SLE and a moderately reduced GFR, would provide helpful information before deciding on a therapeutic regimen. It is also helpful to distinguish the rapid deterioration of renal function that may be associated with diffuse proliferative glomerulonephritis from that of acute tubule cell necrosis or acute interstitial nephritis, such as might occur secondary to an adverse reaction to a drug (especially antimicrobials or NSAIDs).[264]

Baldwin and co-workers[6] did not find any relationship between the histologic classification and the initial antinuclear antibody titer, Ig class of antinuclear factor, or presence or absence of rheumatoid factor. This lack of parallelism between serology and histology has also been found by many others.[1, 9, 158, 282–285] Some workers have found correlations, albeit imperfect, with levels of anti-DNA antibody, C3 or C4 levels, CIC measurements, or cryoIgs.[148, 222, 286–288] In practice, however, such significant overlap exists in these measurements in individual patients with varying histologic findings that it is often difficult, if not impossible, to be consistently correct in predicting renal histologic type on the basis of serologic data alone. In individual cases, a high degree of correlation may exist between serologic parameters (e.g., anti-DNA antibody, C3 or C4 levels) and evidence of activity of renal disease.[158] Falling C4 or C3 levels and rising CIC levels may have the best predictive value.[156, 289, 290] Anti-DNA antibody levels and antibody avidity correlate poorly with features of activity.[113–116]

## PATHOGENESIS

The pathogenetic mechanisms operative in lupus glomerulopathy are dealt with extensively in Chapter 29. In brief, lupus nephritis is a classic example of immune complex glomerulonephritis.[1, 291] Deposits may be found in all three glomerular regions (subendothelial, subepithelial, and mesangial). The mechanism of deposition probably differs among WHO classes. Early evidence suggested that deposition of CICs was the principal mechanism by which the glomeruli were damaged. This is most likely to be true for immune complexes in the mesangium, whereas those in the capillary wall may also reflect in situ complex formation. The underlying cause of autoantibody production in lupus remains undetermined. Both polyclonal B cell activation and antigen-driven mechanisms have been suggested.[292] The relative roles of B and T cells in autoantibody production have been reviewed.[293] The result, however, is a synthesis of autoantibodies interacting with a wide array of self-antigens, including nuclear (DNA, histone, Sm, RNP), cytoplasmic (Ro, La), cellular (lymphocyte, platelet, endothelial), and basement membrane (heparan sulfate, laminin, collagen IV) components.[294] Several studies have suggested that binding of DNA to glomerular basement membrane (GBM) followed by in situ reaction with anti-DNA antibody may participate in the genesis of the glomerular lesions of SLE in experimental models.[295] In vitro, binding of CICs to GBM also occurs.[296] In humans, glomerular anti-DNA antibodies have frequently been identified in lupus nephritis,[297, 298] but direct evidence of DNA in these immune deposits is rare.[298] Although circulating anti-DNA immune complexes have occasionally been identified,[299] their participation in the deposition of glomerular DNA–anti-DNA immune complexes has been further questioned because free DNA is uncommon in the serum of lupus patients[300] and DNA immune complexes represent only a small proportion of the total CICs.[178] The recognition that anti-DNA

antibodies may cross-react with other antigens having exposed phosphodiester phosphate groups[78–80] raises the possibility that in some cases the antigens in glomerular immune complexes may not necessarily be DNA.[301–303] Instead, they may be intrinsic renal antigens.[304] Some investigators suggest that histones may facilitate DNA–anti-DNA binding in the glomerulus.[81, 138, 139] Cationic charge and specific idiotypes of anti-DNA antibodies[305–308] appear to predispose to nephritis. Other antibodies such as antilaminin have also been implicated in nephritis.[115, 140, 141] Nephritis has also been associated with the presence of CD4$^-$/CD8$^-$ and α/β T cell receptor–positive T helper cells.[204]

Susceptibility to SLE is an inherited trait.[309] The gene or genes that determine this susceptibility are located on chromosome 6 in proximity to the major histocompatibility complex.[309] SLE is commonly associated with an extended HLA-complement haplotype. Over three quarters of patients with SLE and many of their first-degree relatives have null genes at C4a, C4b, or C2, and the prevalence of a partial or complete deficiency of a component of the complement cascade is greatly increased.[186] Partial complement deficiency is in strong linkage disequilibrium with DR3. These findings, coupled with the well-recognized deficiency of Fc or C3b receptor density on erythrocytes and phagocytic cells[310] and the fact that an intact complement system is required for solubilization of immune complexes,[311] could indicate that processing of immune complexes is abnormal in SLE. This could be a major factor in promoting immune complex tissue deposition and injury.

## COURSE AND PROGNOSIS

The prognosis for patients with SLE has been improving decade by decade. This improvement has variably been ascribed to the early recognition of milder forms of the illness, therapeutic benefits of steroids and cytotoxic agents, and the possibility that the disease is evolving into a more benign form.[273, 312] Patients presenting initially with SLE and only mild clinical evidence of renal disease, in whom biopsies show minimal or mild diffuse mesangial alterations, scant mesangial electron-dense deposits, and diffuse exclusively mesangial IgG deposits, uncommonly progress to renal failure,[6, 9, 312] unless renal histologic transformation occurs.[268] In general, mortality occurs either as a result of the extrarenal manifestations of the disease (primarily CNS)[1, 313] or as a consequence of overaggressive treatment and infection. Some of these patients, however, have been observed to develop subsequent progressive renal disease and more diffuse glomerular involvement.[314]

It is difficult to predict which patients in this category will remain stable and which patients will have progressive disease. Black patients and patients in lower socioeconomic strata have a worse prognosis.[315] Heavy proteinuria, evidence of serologic activity, and more extensive capillary wall involvement, especially extensive crescents and fibrinoid necrosis, seem to indicate a greater likelihood of progression.[273, 276] The presence of well-developed lesions of chronicity may be predictive of later development of renal failure,[229–231, 271, 316] particularly when results for groups of patients, rather than for individuals, are assessed. Tubule atrophy, interstitial fibrosis, and segmental glomerulosclerosis indicate a poor prognosis for maintenance of renal function.[229–231, 272, 316] However, some have argued that no precise numerical cutoff point on the chronicity index scale can be discerned that is sufficiently sensitive and specific in predicting outcomes for individual patients.[275] The renal outcome for patients with focal proliferative glomerulonephritis is relatively good,[6] unless transformation to a diffuse lesion ensues, an eventuality in up to one third of patients.[231, 276, 314]

The clinical course of membranous glomerulonephritis in patients with SLE is often reported to be similar to that of the idiopathic variety.[278, 279] More recently, it has been reported that the renal prognosis is poor for patients with membranous LGN whose histologic findings are characterized by superimposed focal or diffuse proliferative glomerulonephritis.[279, 317, 318, 318a] Among patients with pure membranous glomerulonephritis related to SLE, the average 5-year survival is about 90%. However, Radhakrishnan and colleagues[318] examined the long-term course of 50 patients with lupus membranous nephropathy (WHO class Va, Vb) seen at Columbia-Presbyterian Hospital. Ninety-three percent of the patients had proteinuria greater than 1 g/d and 64% were frankly nephrotic. Eighty percent had received various therapies directed to the renal lesion, and 41% of these responded with a decrease in proteinuria to less than 1 g/d. After 6 years of follow-up, 22% had progressed to renal failure and 8% had died. Approximately 18% of the patients transformed to proliferative glomerulonephritis and 48% had persistent abnormal proteinuria. No clinical or pathologic parameter was predictive of a progressive course except for thickening of the GBM.[318] Transformation of membranous glomerulonephritis to diffuse proliferative glomerulonephritis is associated with a worsening prognosis, as is the presence of lesions of chronicity such as glomerular sclerosis or tubule atrophy. Patients with pure membranous lupus nephritis or with accompanying mild mesangial alterations (WHO class Va, Vb) generally do well, even without specific therapy, except for an increased prevalence of thrombosis, often with associated antiphospholipid autoantibodies.[279] As indicated previously, treatment with various glucocorticoid or immunosuppressive regimens induces complete or partial remissions in 35% to 50% of patients. Progression to renal insufficiency may occur in those patients with persisting heavy proteinuria.[279] The prognosis for patients with superimposed diffuse or focal proliferative lesions (WHO class Vc, Vd) is more guarded, and remissions occur less frequently with therapy.[279, 317, 318, 318a]

The prognosis for diffuse proliferative LGN with extensive subendothelial deposits, especially if the disorder is associated with azotemia at the onset, is considerably worse than for all other groups.[1, 6] Severe hypertension coexisting with renal failure appears to be an especially ominous sign.[59] Earlier studies by Baldwin and associates[1] and Pollak and colleagues[319] found a 5-year survival of about 25% in this group of patients, most of whom were given large doses of corticosteroids.[6] Compilations of survival statistics among patients with diffuse proliferative glomerulonephritis have indicated a greatly improved survival[232, 272, 320] compared with the earlier reports. The precise reason for the steady improvement in long-term prognosis of this variant is uncertain, but it is likely to be due in part to earlier recognition and more widespread use of aggressive therapeutic regimens.[312] Many centers now report 5-year survival in excess of 80% and 10-year survival in excess of 60%.[1, 272] Mortality in these patients seems to be related to cerebritis, infection, and atherosclerotic disease.[1] Notwithstanding the overall improvement in survival as a group, individual patients continue to be observed with progressive disease despite all forms of therapy. The factors that are responsible for this heterogeneity of behavior among patients with similar initial degrees of severity, as assessed by function or morphologic findings, continue to be elusive. Patients who present with well-advanced renal failure and evidence of extensive chronic changes on biopsy generally do not respond to therapy with improved renal function.[229]

## PREGNANCY

In the presence of heavy proteinuria or amenorrhea secondary to cytotoxic drugs, false-positive urinary gonadotropin test (pregnancy test) results may be seen in patients with SLE. Measurements of serum gonadotropin by radioimmunoassay, however, are elevated only in premenopausal patients with true pregnancies.[321] It is commonly reported that SLE is exacerbated by pregnancy, usually in the third trimester or in the early puerperium. Early reports of increased disease activity varied from 10% to 75% of pregnant SLE patients.[1] More recently, lower exacerbation rates have been reported, probably related to the liberal use of steroids and cytotoxic agents during pregnancy.[322–325] Clinical flares and fetal wastage occur less frequently when conception occurs during periods of remission.[322–325] In a series of 64 pregnancies in 41 patients, 37% of pregnancies resulted in full-term infants, 30% of infants were premature, and 33% of pregnancies were spontaneously (29%) or medically (4%) aborted.[326] Patients with a circulating anticoagulant were more likely to experience recurrent fetal loss but were not more likely to experience maternal complications than patients without a lupus anticoagulant.[326] Azotemia (with serum creatinine levels greater than 1.5 mg/dL) and hypertension during pregnancy are both associated with increased fetal wastage, whereas nephrotic syndrome alone is not. During pregnancy, 44% of patients in one series developed hypertension. Renal function declined in 19% but recovered post partum in 17%.[326] Persistently low serum complement levels are said to be useful in distinguishing a lupus flare from an uncomplicated or preeclamptic pregnancy in patients with lupus.[160, 327]

## THERAPY

The effects of glucocorticoids on the extrarenal manifestations are dramatic and well described.[1, 3, 4, 9] There is no reason to question seriously their value in the management of the disabling and sometimes life-threatening complications that affect organ systems other than the kidney. The long-term effect of steroid therapy on survival and renal disease in SLE is still debated, however.[328] With mild extrarenal disease, distressing problems such as fever, skin lesions, and arthralgias may be controlled satisfactorily with antimalarials,[329] acetylsalicylic acid, or NSAIDs. The use of the last may be associated with transient functional reductions in GFR,[330, 331] the development of an acute interstitial nephritis, or acute tubule cell necrosis.[264] In the absence of clinical evidence of renal disease (or if a biopsy specimen shows only normal or mild changes), symptomatic therapy with or without low-dose daily or alternate-day steroids is generally satisfactory.[1] For patients who require large doses of steroids to control the extrarenal manifestations, the addition of a cytotoxic drug as a steroid-sparing agent may obviate some of the unfortunate consequences of long-term high-dose steroid therapy. The long-term hazards of such cytotoxic drug therapy must be kept in mind, however.[332, 333]

In patients with definite but mild or moderate renal disease accompanied by focal glomerular lesions by light microscopy, a prudent course is to manage the disease with the lowest dose of steroids possible and to observe the patient carefully for signs of exacerbation or development of more diffuse renal disease. Serologic monitoring (i.e., anti-DNA, $CH_{50}$, C3, C4) may be of value in such cases. Some investigators have suggested that therapy directed at normalization of these parameters (especially $CH_{50}$) may be associated with greatly improved protein excretion rates and a trend toward improved histologic findings.[159, 290] The value of long-term cytotoxic drug therapy has not been established in long-term controlled clinical trials[333–335] in this group of patients, but such adjunctive cytotoxic drug therapy may have a steroid-sparing effect in selected cases. More data are required to evaluate the long-term beneficial effects of a prophylactic approach using a combination of steroids and cytotoxic drugs in these patients; a conservative regimen involving the lowest dosage of medications consistent with relative freedom from symptoms and careful follow-up of urinalysis and serologic findings seems most reasonable.

Membranous glomerulonephritis may be treated in a fashion similar to that described for focal glomerular lesions.[278, 279, 318, 336] Complete remission of the nephrotic syndrome usually does not occur, but there may be a partial remission and disappearance of symptoms and signs.[6] A complete remission, including the disappearance of subepithelial electron-dense deposits, has been observed in some patients treated in an uncontrolled fashion with a combination of high-dose steroids (i.e., prednisone at 40 mg/d for 6 months or more) and a cytotoxic drug (azathioprine or cyclophosphamide at 1.0 to 2.5 mg/kg/d).[337] Overall, however, there is no convincing evidence that an aggressive therapeutic program including prolonged high-dose steroids or combinations of lower-dose daily or alternate-day steroids and cytotoxic agents greatly alters the natural history of the relatively benign forms of nonproliferative or mildly proliferative membranous lupus nephritis (WHO class Va, Vb). In fact, overly aggressive therapy of patients with membranous LGN is not uncommonly associated with serious side effects such as opportunistic infection, aseptic necrosis of the hips, and psychosis. Given the emerging sense that the more proliferative forms of membranous LGN (WHO class Vc, Vd) may have a poorer prognosis, however, more aggressive therapy may be indicated in these subgroups.[317, 318, 318a] Transformation to diffuse proliferative glomerulonephritis also requires more aggressive management. Renal vein thrombosis may require the addition of long-term anticoagulants to the regimen.

The serious prognosis of diffuse proliferative LGN merits an aggressive therapeutic approach. Many years ago, Pollak and associates[338] demonstrated in an uncontrolled study that low-dose steroids are ineffective but that a high-dose regimen (i.e., 40 mg of prednisone per day for at least 6 months) improved prognosis. Baldwin and co-workers[1] reported similar results in diffuse proliferative glomerulonephritis treated with daily oral steroids in high doses. The patients with advanced disease, significant azotemia, extensive crescent formation, and numerous obsolescent glomeruli did poorly despite therapy. Conversely, MacKay and co-workers[339] and Cade and colleagues[340] did not find steroids alone to be effective in patients with severe disease. Other studies have also called into question the wisdom of using long-term, daily, oral glucocorticoids in the management of the renal complications of SLE, especially if a renal biopsy demonstrates substantial changes of chronicity and manifests few features of activity.[270, 272, 316] Studies from the National Institutes of Health (NIH) have shown statistically significant benefits for patients with severe forms of LGN treated with steroids and pulse cyclophosphamide (500 to 1000 mg/m² intravenously every 1 to 3 months) compared with similar patients treated with steroids alone.[341] Patients treated with steroids alone were shown to develop progressive alterations on repeated renal biopsy, indicative of chronicity.[271] Although controversy regarding the validity and interpretation of the NIH data remains,[333, 342] it seems reasonable to conclude that daily oral steroids alone, even if given chronically in high dosages, may not be altogether satisfactory for the management of the diffuse proliferative variety of SLE nephritis, particularly in the presence of reduced GFR and changes of chronicity on renal biopsy. Improvement in renal and systemic manifestations may occur, but complications of chronic steroid therapy generally limit its long-term usefulness. It is not surprising, therefore, that alternative forms of treatment have been diligently sought.[1, 3, 4, 6, 333, 335–370] Large and repeated boluses of parenteral methylprednisolone (pulse therapy) have been claimed in uncontrolled and small controlled studies to be beneficial in treating severe diffuse proliferative lesions, particularly when renal deterioration has been of short duration.[357–359, 366] Whether the short-term effects can be sustained by intermittent intravenous bolus therapy has not been tested in a definitive fashion. Dosage is usually 500 to 1000 mg of methylprednisolone daily for 3 to 5 days, followed by oral prednisone, 60 mg daily or every other day, for 1 to 2 months with gradual tapering. Repeated pulses given at regular intervals with a lower dosage of oral prednisone in between the pulses have also been advocated as a useful regimen.[317]

Various cytotoxic drugs—usually oral azathioprine or cyclophosphamide in doses of 1.5 to 3 mg/kg/d or cyclophosphamide, 500 to 1000 mg/m² intravenously every 1 to 3 months, in combination with low-dose steroids (usually daily oral prednisone, 5 to 30 mg/d, or equivalent doses of prednisone on an alternate-day regimen)—have been employed in a number of therapeutic trials.[1, 333, 342, 371, 372] Uncontrolled studies in the first half of the 1970s reported that the combined use of steroids and cytotoxic agents was steroid sparing, at the same time that it induced improvements in proteinuria and creatinine clearance.[1] The second half of the 1970s was characterized by prospective randomized controlled trials assessing the efficacy of these regimens in lupus nephritis.[344] These studies tended to be of relatively short duration and included small numbers of patients. The results of these randomized, controlled studies have not always supported the findings of uncontrolled observations.[340–342, 352, 366] However, a meta-analysis of eight randomized trials conducted between 1972 and 1982[344] demonstrated evidence of superiority of immunosuppressive drugs (azathioprine or cyclophosphamide) combined with prednisone over prednisone therapy alone in terms of slowing the rate of decline in GFR or preventing end-stage renal failure but not in preventing death. No clear evidence was found in this analysis favoring cyclophosphamide over azathioprine. A randomized study conducted by Cade and associates[340] demonstrated that the addition of azathioprine or azathioprine plus heparin to prednisone therapy was superior to prednisone alone, the 5-year survival in treated patients approaching 70%. Similar findings were reported by Sztejnbok and colleagues.[352] On the other hand, reports of two randomized studies conducted by Hahn and coworkers[354] and Donadio and colleagues[360] showed no differences in outcome between groups of patients treated with azathioprine or cyclophosphamide plus prednisone and those treated with steroids alone over an 18-month period. Thus, during the early 1980s, the relative merit of cytotoxic therapy for the treatment of lupus nephritis was a highly charged issue. The infectious and other extrarenal complications of cytotoxic therapy seemed to offset to some degree the protection from flares of SLE or progressive renal function impairment provided by these drugs.[332, 333, 360]

In the mid-1980s, investigators from the NIH were able to demonstrate a trend toward a beneficial effect using prednisone combined with oral cyclophosphamide and azathioprine and a definite benefit over steroids alone using prednisone combined with intravenous cyclophosphamide administered every 3 months, but only after a minimum of 5 years of follow-up.[341, 371] In addition, data also suggested that long-term therapy with cytotoxic agents combined with prednisone may be more beneficial than prednisone alone in protecting against the development of chronic irreversible fibrotic changes in the kidney.[229, 270, 316, 341, 371] Combinations of prednisone with azathioprine plus cyclophosphamide or prednisone with intermittent intravenous cyclophosphamide achieved the best results. Critics of the NIH study have cautioned against dogmatic interpretations of these data, however, given the relatively small number of patients randomized to each of the five study arms; the inclusion of a significant minority of patients with renal biopsies of WHO classes II, III, and V; and the noncontemporaneous nature of some of the study arms.[333, 342] Others have argued that the long-term intensive steroid and cytotoxic therapy advocated by the NIH group may be excessive for a subgroup of patients with class IV nephritis with normal serum creatinine values, who may have an excellent long-term prognosis.[372] Despite these shortcomings, the use of oral steroids and intravenous cyclophosphamide has become commonplace for patients with class IV nephritis as evidenced by numerous small uncontrolled trials[345–347] and the overwhelming choice of this therapy by nephrologists polled at a 1993 computer-interactive session of the Amer-

ican Society of Nephrology. Infection, hemorrhagic cystitis, neoplasm, and suppression of ovarian function remain concerns when prescribing long-term cyclophosphamide.[333, 342] Indeed, patients receiving prolonged intravenous courses of cyclophosphamide, particularly older women, frequently developed sustained amenorrhea.[348]

More recently, the NIH group has conducted a prospective trial for patients with severe diffuse proliferative lupus nephritis to examine the effects of monthly pulses of intravenous methylprednisolone, or monthly pulses of intravenous cyclophosphamide for 6 months (short course), or monthly pulses of intravenous cyclophosphamide for 6 months followed by dosage every 3 months for 2 years (long course).[349] Each group also received roughly equivalent maintenance doses of oral glucocorticoids. The majority of patients entered into this trial had heavy proteinuria, reduced renal function, and active renal disease on biopsy. After a minimum of 5 years of follow-up, doubling of the serum creatinine level occurred in 50% of the pulse methylprednisolone group and 25% developed ESRD. Short courses of intravenous cyclophosphamide were associated with doubling of the serum creatinine value in 33% and 25% developed ESRD, not greatly different from those receiving only intravenous methylprednisolone. More prolonged intravenous cyclophosphamide therapy reduced the frequency of doubling of the serum creatinine level to 15% and the occurrence of ESRD to 10%. Fewer exacerbations of lupus nephritis were seen in patients receiving cyclophosphamide. The total number of infections, including herpes zoster, did not occur at different rates in the three groups. Only one malignancy (cervical carcinoma in situ) was seen in the patients receiving long-term intravenous cyclophosphamide. Ovarian failure was particularly common in patients receiving intravenous cyclophosphamide for the long course. Osteonecrosis and cataract formation occurred equally in all three groups. Hemorrhagic cystitis did not occur. Because these patients had ''severe'' diffuse proliferative lupus nephritis, it would not be appropriate to conclude that intravenous cyclophosphamide is more efficacious than pulse intravenous methylprednisolone for all cases of lupus nephritis, as milder forms of the disease might respond quite well to less intensive therapy.[349] Water intoxication has been reported in patients given cyclophosphamide, 30 to 50 mg/kg intravenously, and hyponatremia should be considered and avoided when administering intravenous bolus doses of cyclophosphamide to patients with SLE.[373] Although hemorrhagic cystitis and bladder carcinomas are known complications in patients taking cyclophosphamide,[373a] 2-mercaptoethane sulfonate (mesna), which is used to prevent bladder toxicity during cancer chemotherapy,[374] may also be used for this purpose in patients with SLE.

In numerous small, usually uncontrolled series, intensive plasma exchange combined with low-dose steroids and cytotoxic agents had been claimed to produce a beneficial effect, particularly in patients with severe diffuse proliferative nephritis and renal failure,[356, 361–364] but some studies were unable to show clinical improvement.[364] The results of a national cooperative prospective study including patients randomly assigned to receive prednisone and cyclophosphamide either with or without plasma exchange failed to find benefit in the plasma exchange group with regard to renal survival or overall survival of the patient.[370] Although it is still possible that a subset of patients who benefit from intensive plasma exchange may yet be identified,[368] on the basis of current knowledge, there are few convincing data to support the use of plasma exchange as it was performed by the Lupus Nephritis Study Group[370] for the treatment of patients with LGN. Some have proposed that maximization of benefit might occur if plasmapheresis is followed sequentially by cytotoxic therapy[375, 376] rather than administered simultaneously as it was by the Lupus Nephritis Study Group. A controlled trial is under way to test this hypothesis.[377] A limited number of patients with LGN have been treated with total lymphoid irradiation with improvements in serologic and systemic manifestations of lupus but only transient improvement in proteinuria and GFR.[378, 379] Lack of long-term efficacy and substantial infectious complications reported by others[367] limit the value of this form of therapy for lupus nephritis. The relative merits of this form of therapy remain to be established. Finally, the usefulness of cyclosporine for the treatment of LGN is under investigation. The preliminary data are encouraging.[350, 380–382] Interestingly, patients with SLE who are treated with cyclosporine improve clinically despite unchanged levels of anti-DNA and complement.[382] Further controlled trials are warranted before this experimental form of therapy can be broadly recommended for the treatment of LGN. Fish oil, ω-3 fatty acids, and eicosapentaenoic acid therapy failed to benefit patients with lupus nephritis studied under controlled conditions.[383–385] A thromboxane receptor antagonist[386] induced modest acute improvements in GFR, but its long-term usefulness is untested. Long-term benefit has been claimed for the use of the antithrombotic agent ancrod along with steroids and nitrogen mustard,[387] but confirmatory controlled trials are lacking. Intravenous Ig appeared efficacious in a small number of children with lupus nephritis who were unresponsive to 2 months of therapy with steroids and oral cyclophosphamide.[388] Novel therapies targeted to eliminate autoreactive T and B cell clones are being developed and may ultimately prove efficacious for some patients with lupus nephritis.[389] Extracorporeal immunoadsorption, using DNA or anti-DNA immunoadsorbents, is another interesting experimental form of therapy deserving further exploration.[365]

In summary, well-designed, long-range studies of patients with diffuse proliferative glomerulonephritis and SLE have suggested that the addition of cytotoxic drugs to a regimen of low- or intermittent-dose prednisone may offer benefit in this subset of patients with SLE. Patients most likely to benefit include those in whom steroid side effects have been disabling, advanced chronic renal failure is not present, and renal biopsy specimens do not show extensive fibrosis but do show features of active glomerular disease. It is hoped that such treatment will lead to long-term stabilization of renal function. Because of the risks involved in the use of these toxic agents, however, the patient should be advised of the morbidity and mortality that may result from their administration.

Some patients may do quite well with initial therapy consisting of high doses of oral or intravenous glucocorticoids, and several experienced clinicians have suggested that a trial of intensive glucocorticoid therapy should be

given before resorting to potent cytotoxic agents. On the other hand, others have recommended institution of combined glucocorticoid-cytotoxic regimens when severe lupus nephritis (WHO class III, IV, or Vc, Vd) is diagnosed, especially if renal function is impaired. Whether intravenous pulses of cyclophosphamide[347, 371] are preferred to oral cyclophosphamide cannot be definitively answered, but the intravenous route of administration may have a lower profile of side effects (perhaps because of the lower cumulative dosage delivered). If cyclophosphamide is used initially, the duration of therapy required for optimal effect is unclear. Short courses, for example, 2 to 6 months in duration,[372] which avoid many of the risks of cumulative toxicity, may be associated with subsequent exacerbations and some prefer to convert patients to maintenance oral azathioprine (1 to 2 mg/kg/d) and low-dose glucocorticoids to avoid the cumulative toxicity of cyclophosphamide. More prolonged therapy with intravenous cyclophosphamide may be preferred for patients with aggressive disease and features suggestive of a poor prognosis, but the cost of side effects, particularly amenorrhea and/or the later development of alkylating agent–associated myelodysplastic syndromes, must be taken into account.

## DIALYSIS AND TRANSPLANTATION

Despite the improving rates of renal survival and survival of patients in SLE, some patients develop renal insufficiency that advances to ESRD. In the past, most of these patients died. With the more ready availability of dialysis and transplantation, lupus patients with ESRD survive longer.[63, 390] Early death of lupus patients who have started dialysis is often related to infection and occurs more frequently in patients taking high-dose steroids as a consequence of exacerbations of disease with rapid loss of renal function. The mortality of SLE patients receiving chronic dialysis who develop end-stage renal failure after a protracted course is not greatly different from that found in non-SLE patients receiving dialysis.[63, 391, 392] Late deaths are often caused by severe coronary atherosclerotic disease.[392] Survival rates of patients having dialysis have been reported to compare favorably with survival in other ESRD patients.[63, 391–393]

Clinical and serologic remission of SLE is common as azotemia develops, suggesting that nonimmunologic factors are involved in the development of ESRD.[63, 392] Spontaneous remissions of renal failure have been reported in end-stage LGN.[63, 392, 394, 395] Some of these, however, may actually represent healed hypertensive lesions, acute interstitial nephritis or tubule cell necrosis, or other nonimmunologic factors.[263] Renal transplantation is usually well tolerated, and recurrence in the transplanted kidney is uncommon.[396–399] In most series, overall allograft outcome and outcome of SLE patients compare favorably to those observed in patients with primary glomerular disease.[397–399] As mentioned,[59, 234] hypertension may be an important factor determining the long-term course for patients with SLE, including the period of dialysis and transplantation for those who progress to end-stage renal failure.

# Schönlein-Henoch Purpura

Heberden[400] is credited with the first description of this disorder, subsequently characterized as anaphylactoid purpura. Schönlein[401] provided the first description of the purpuric and articular manifestations, and Henoch[402] later described the gastrointestinal and renal manifestations. Osler[2] also recognized the importance of renal manifestations in this syndrome. Because of the finding of prominent cutaneous leukocytoclastic vasculitis[403] and the systemic manifestations, Schönlein-Henoch purpura is often classified with the other systemic vasculitides (see later discussion). Synonyms for this disorder include Schönlein-Henoch syndrome, anaphylactoid purpura, and rheumatoid purpura.

## CLINICAL AND LABORATORY FINDINGS

This syndrome consists of dermal, abdominal, articular, and renal manifestations.[403–408] The dermal lesions are the most characteristic and chiefly involve the lower extremities and buttocks. They consist of an initial urticarial lesion evolving into dusky red-purple purpuric macules that do not blanch on pressure.[409] The purpura may become generalized and result in palpable lesions, occasionally with small bullae, and desquamation may ensue. Morphologically, these lesions consist of a leukocytoclastic vasculitis.[403, 409] They may be associated with mild edema of the lower extremities, unrelated to either hypoalbuminemia or vascular congestion.[409] The purpuric rash is often accompanied by constitutional symptoms such as fever and malaise.[404, 409] The abdominal manifestations, including colic, vomiting, melena, or hematochezia, occur in about a fourth of patients.[409] The patients may present with nonmigratory transient arthralgias, occasionally with effusions, particularly of the ankle and knee joints.[409] Joint deformities and articular erosions do not occur. Epistaxis or hemoptysis may occasionally develop. A tendency for frequent relapses after exposure to cold and to potential allergens may exist,[409, 410] suggesting to some authors a possible etiologic role for these agents. Acute toxoplasmosis, mycoplasmal infection, gonococcemia, meningococcemia, and *Yersinia* enterocolitis have been associated with findings strikingly similar to those of Schönlein-Henoch purpura.[411–415]

Similar symptoms have also been associated with the use of medications[416, 417] and vaccinations.[418–420] The disorder may easily be confused with poststreptococcal glomerulonephritis when systemic manifestations are prominent in the latter.[421, 422] One patient with staphylococcal endocarditis and a clinical syndrome consistent with anaphylactoid purpura had a renal biopsy showing crescentic glomerulonephritis and mesangial IgA deposits, confirming a relationship between infection and the development of this clinical syndrome.[423] Familial cases may occur.[424] The severity of the dermal, gastrointestinal, and articular manifestations bears no constant relationship to the severity of the renal lesion.[403–410]

The incidence of clinical renal manifestations varies considerably.[403–410] The findings include gross or microscopic hematuria, proteinuria, and, uncommonly, progressive renal failure.[403–410, 425–429] Nephrotic syndrome, usually accompanied by hematuria, develops in as many as half of patients referred for renal evaluation.[427] This is probably an overestimate of the true prevalence of nephrotic syndrome, as many mild cases are never diagnosed. The subsequent development of progressive renal disease is said to be uncommon if it does not occur within the first 3 or 4 years after the onset of clinical symptoms; however, late-onset progressive renal failure may be seen.[427] In one pediatric study, 39% of children with either nephrotic syndrome or nephritis within 90 days of initial presentation progressed to ESRD. In the same period, no patient with a normal urinalysis or with hematuria and non-nephrotic proteinuria progressed to end-stage renal failure.[430] Males are most often affected, and the median age at onset is about 4 years, but typical cases have been recorded in adults.[425–426]

Manifestations are similar in adults and children, but renal disease tends to be more severe in the adult population.[404] The condition is often misdiagnosed initially, particularly in adults. For example, the abdominal pain has led to exploratory laparotomy in many instances. Punctate hemorrhages have been found in the intestine, sometimes associated with perforation or intussusception. There is a strong background of allergy in one fourth of patients.[407, 411] Several patients have been described with recurrent bouts of acute nephritic syndrome seemingly related to food allergy, but usually there is no clear association with any particular allergen.[411] Although an upper respiratory tract infection frequently precedes the onset and the antistreptolysin titers are occasionally moderately elevated, there is no convincing evidence linking this syndrome with group A streptococcal infection.[412] Rarely, pulmonary hemorrhage occurs.[431] Hematuria is rarely the result of ureteritis rather than glomerulonephritis.[432] One patient with transient circulating inhibitors to coagulation factors VIII and IX has been described.[433]

Occasional cases of Schönlein-Henoch purpura may mimic poststreptococcal glomerulonephritis and vice versa.[421, 422] Serum complement component values are usually within normal limits,[406, 409, 421] but modestly reduced $CH_{50}$ and properdin levels with normal C3 levels are found in about a third of patients.[434] Evidence of alternative pathway complement activation may be present.[435] Serum IgA concentration is increased in about half of patients.[436, 437] IgA rheumatoid factor was found in 54% of 24 children with anaphylactoid purpura compared with 4% of healthy control adults and children.[438] Cryoglobulins may occasionally be found.[439, 440] CICs containing IgA and IgG are frequently found in serum during active disease, remission, or relapse.[441–445] IgA ANCAs may be found in patients with active disease.[446] Antibodies to α-galactose are increased in Schönlein-Henoch purpura and also in patients with poststreptococcal glomerulonephritis. IgA anti–α-galactosyl antibodies may be more specific for anaphylactoid purpura and are most likely observed with exacerbations of hematuria.[447] The concentration of both IgA and IgG complexes has been said to correlate with the development of renal manifestations.[441, 444] The frequency of HLA-Bw35 is increased in some series.[448] Biopsy specimens of affected or unaffected skin nearly always reveal dermal capillary deposits of IgA, IgG, C3, properdin, and fibrin but not C4, C1q, or IgA secretory piece (see later discussion). IgA deposits have also been identified in intestinal vessels.[449, 450] Proteinuria is most often poorly selective.[406]

## PATHOLOGY

**Light Microscopy.** The basic pattern of glomerular involvement is that of a mesangial injury or mesangial proliferative glomerulonephritis with varying degrees of hypercellularity, similar to lesions in IgA nephropathy. Segmental capillary thrombosis, possibly related to the development of necrosis and crescents, is often present.[223] To classify the degree of involvement and to correlate it with clinical manifestations and prognostic indices, the following categories have been established: I) minimal alterations, II) pure mesangial proliferation, III) a) focal and b) diffuse mesangial proliferation with less than 50% crescents, IV) a) focal and b) diffuse mesangial proliferation with 50% to 75% crescents, V) a) focal and b) diffuse mesangial proliferation with greater than 75% crescents, and VI) "pseudo" mesangiocapillary glomerulonephritis.[1, 406, 451] In general, nephrotic syndrome is present in only about 25% of groups I, II, and III, and hematuria is present in all groups. Patients with groups II and IIIa histologic findings tend to have better outcomes, with either return of normal renal function or persistent microscopic hematuria and proteinuria, whereas patients in groups IIIb, IV, and V have persistent proteinuria and hematuria or progress to terminal renal failure.[451] Occasional patients develop rapidly progressive renal failure accompanied by exuberant crescent formation (see Chapter 30). Large fuchsinophilic deposits may be seen in the mesangium with Masson trichrome stain. Less commonly, typical humps may be observed. Renal arteritis is unusual. The cutaneous lesion is one of leukocytoclastic vasculitis, characterized by the presence of fragmented nuclei of leukocytes in and around the walls of small dermal vessels and with surrounding dermal hemorrhages.[403]

**Electron Microscopy.** By electron microscopy, the principal abnormalities are found in the mesangium. Focal proliferation, increase in mesangial matrix, and electron-dense deposits may be seen.[1, 452, 453] Similar electron-dense deposits may be found scattered in the subendothelial areas adjacent to the mesangium. The deposits have been shown to contain IgA by immunoelectron microscopy.[454] The findings are similar to those of Berger disease (see Chapter 30, Figs. 30–8 through 30–10). The deposits are not as extensive as in SLE. The capillary lumen may contain platelets and fibrin. Although not described in earlier reports, subepithelial deposits were noted by Heaton and co-workers[451] in 6 of 25 biopsy specimens studied; in 3 specimens, these deposits were virtually identical to the humps classically described in acute poststreptococcal glomerulonephritis. Similar deposits have been described in several other reports.[422, 455, 456] In any location, the deposits are easier to identify in thick sections embedded in plastic and stained with toluidine blue than in the material prepared for electron microscopic study.[451] Basement membrane lysis or dissolution, especially in association with subepithelial deposits and neutrophils in capillary lumens, is found in more than half of biopsies. These changes correlate well with the more severe glomerular damage as assessed by light microscopy and by heavy proteinuria.[457]

## IMMUNOFLUORESCENCE

In contrast to the frequently focal and segmental nature of the glomerular lesions by light microscopy, one of the striking features observed is the widespread involvement of glomeruli seen by immunofluorescence study. These abnormalities are granular deposits of IgA and, to a lesser extent, IgG or IgM (see also Chapter 30, Fig. 30–10).[1, 407, 453, 455, 458, 459] Secretory piece is absent but J chain may be detected, indicating the polymeric nature of the IgA deposits. The later-acting components of the complement sequence, C3 and properdin, are more frequently found than C1q or C4.[1, 458, 459] The deposits are largely mesangial in distribution, with an occasional segmental paramesangial capillary deposit. Fibrin-related antigens are frequently deposited in the mesangial areas.[453, 455]

Both clinically involved and uninvolved skin may reveal IgA, C3, and C5 deposits but not C1q, C4, or IgA secretory piece.[460, 461] These deposits are located in the walls of superficial capillaries. Fibrin-related antigens may be seen in and around vascular structures. Similar findings in the glomeruli and skin have been noted in Berger disease (see Chapter 30), suggesting a relationship between these two disorders.[460, 461] Dermatitis herpetiformis is another disorder in which IgA and late-acting complement components may be found in skin lesions, but the distribution of the deposits is at the tips of the dermal papillae in this disorder rather than in the blood vessels.[462] These findings should be contrasted with those in SLE, in which both involved and uninvolved skin show deposits of IgG, IgM, IgA, C1q, C3, and C4 in the dermal-epidermal junction (lupus band test; see earlier discussion). In a small number of patients studied, IgA and complement deposits have been described in vasculitic lesions in affected gastrointestinal tract.[449, 450]

## PATHOGENESIS

The pathogenesis of Schönlein-Henoch purpura is unknown, but the mesangial location and the granular nature of the immune deposits suggest an immune complex disease.[1, 440–444] Demonstrations of circulating IgA and IgG immune complexes support this view.[441] Elevated serum levels of polymeric IgA have been reported. In the setting of mucosal infection, these levels increase further and remain higher for a longer duration than in control subjects with mucosal infection, suggesting abnormal regulation of IgA-associated immunity.[463] Similarly, deposits of IgA in dermal and intestinal vessels and recurrence of disease in renal allografts (see later discussion) suggest a systemic pathogenetic process.[449, 450, 463a] One group has reported decreased Fc receptor function of circulating monocytes and splenic macrophages in children with Schönlein-Henoch purpura, suggesting an abnormality in the immune complex clearance process.[463b] The development of the syndrome in a patient with an IgA monoclonal gammopathy offers an additional clue to pathogenesis.[470] The presence of IgA with the late-acting complement components, including properdin, suggests the activation of the alternative complement pathway.[435] The plasma of children with anaphylactoid purpura shows diminished ability to generate prostaglandin $I_2$ in vitro when cultured with human umbilical arterial rings.[463c] Serum levels of prostaglandin $I_2$, thromboxane $A_2$, and prostaglandin $E_2$ are elevated in children during the acute phase of illness.[464] Anti–mesangial cell antibodies with IgG isotype have been identified in the serum of patients with Schönlein-Henoch purpura, correlating with the degree of hematuria.[465] Their presence in patients with IgA nephropathy as well suggests a common pathogenesis.[465] The frequent presence of circulating IgA-fibronectin aggregates in the serum of patients with IgA nephropathy and Schönlein-Henoch purpura further substantiates a commonality between these entities.[466] The role of bacterial, viral, fungal, protozoan, or other agents in this order is not well established.[415, 416]

## COURSE AND THERAPY

In general, Schönlein-Henoch purpura is a benign, self-limited disorder, but there may be episodic and recurrent bouts of rash, arthralgias, gastrointestinal symptoms, and hematuria for several months or even years after the initial onset.[404–409]

In patients with focal and segmental proliferative glomerular lesions, the overall mortality is less than 10% at 5 and 10 years after onset.[406, 409, 428, 467, 468] In a large series of patients seen by Meadow and co-workers,[406] 2 years or more after diagnosis, 55% were entirely normal, 22% had residual urinary abnormalities but normal GFR, 10% had both abnormal urine sediment and reduced GFR, and 8% had a severe reduction in GFR, were receiving dialysis, or had died of renal failure. The occurrence of the acute nephritic syndrome at the onset, a persistent nephrotic syndrome, and older age were indicators of a poor prognosis. All renal deaths occurred in patients with clinical and histologic pictures of crescentic glomerulonephritis. In a group of patients who recovered or improved clinically, repeated biopsies also showed lessening of severe glomerular alterations. Hypercellularity diminished or disappeared, and focal lesions decreased in number and extent of glomerular involvement. Furthermore, IgA deposits diminished considerably or even disappeared in a few patients. Capillary wall deposits (and accompanying diffuse hypercellularity) also disappeared with clinical improvement.[468]

In a long-term follow-up of 78 patients, averaging 23 years, Goldstein and co-workers[467] noted that 44% of patients who presented with nephrotic syndrome or acute nephritis had persisting hypertension or progressive decline in GFR, and 82% of those who presented with hematuria only were normal. More than one third of pregnancies were complicated. Later deterioration in clinical status after initial apparent full recovery was found in approximately 20% to 25% of patients, indicating the necessity for long-term follow-up of patients with Schönlein-Henoch purpura.

Treatment is generally considered to be ineffective in altering the course of the renal disease. However, in one study, prednisone therapy given to patients without renal signs or symptoms at presentation seemed to prevent subsequent renal involvement.[468] In view of the frequency of spontaneous remissions, the intrinsically favorable course, and the lack of a tendency for the focal lesion to progress, an aggressive management program is generally not indicated. Patients with the more ominous crescentic lesions[469]

accompanied by nephrotic syndrome or progressive renal failure have been treated with steroids, cytotoxic drugs, anticoagulants, or intensive plasma exchange, but not in a controlled and randomized fashion.[470, 471] The few cases reported do not allow any firm conclusions, but improvement in renal function has been noted in some patients, especially after plasma exchange and immunosuppressive therapy.[469] Steroids may provide temporary relief from severe extrarenal complications such as abdominal pain but have little effect on the renal lesion. This disorder may recur in patients with renal allografts, and although the exact risk of such an event is not clearly understood, it appears to be uncommon.[472–475] Recurrent disease in allografts may be more frequent in those with continued active skin or gastrointestinal manifestations.[472, 473]

## Goodpasture Syndrome

Ernest Goodpasture, in 1919, described an unusual case of an 18-year-old man who died of an influenzal illness characterized by hemoptysis, alveolar hemorrhage and necrosis, and proliferative glomerulonephritis.[476] In the succeeding years, many hundreds of cases characterized by a similar association of glomerulonephritis and pulmonary hemorrhage have been reported in the literature.[1, 477–489] (See also sections on anti-GBM antibody–mediated nephritis in Chapters 29 and 30.) Synonyms for Goodpasture syndrome are lung purpura with nephritis, pulmonary hemorrhage and glomerulonephritis, hemorrhagic pneumonia and nephritis, hemorrhagic pulmonary–renal syndrome, pulmonary hemosiderosis with glomerulonephritis, and anti-GBM antibody–mediated nephritis with pulmonary hemorrhage. Stanton and Tange,[477] in 1958, were the first to use the eponym to describe cases of pulmonary hemorrhage and necrotizing glomerulonephritis. Because of the essentially clinical character of the findings that distinguished Goodpasture syndrome from other varieties of progressive nephritis, the underlying pathologic features of early reported cases varied. Indeed, in the original case described by Goodpasture himself, and in many others described subsequently, there was evidence of arteritis, suggesting that these disorders might be more properly classified as some variant of systemic vasculitis,[1] but rare examples of well-documented Goodpasture syndrome with systemic vasculitis have been reported.[479] In any case, with the discovery of the role of anti-GBM antibodies in the pathogenesis of Goodpasture syndrome in 1967, the diagnostic criteria that permitted differentiation of this syndrome from other causes of lung hemorrhage and glomerulonephritis were firmly established.[1, 480] In this section, Goodpasture syndrome is defined as a disorder consisting of the triad of 1) glomerulonephritis, commonly of the rapidly progressive or crescentic variety; 2) lung hemorrhage; and 3) anti-GBM antibody formation (Fig. 31–10; see also Chapter 29). It should be emphasized that lung hemorrhage and renal disease may also coexist in conditions such as SLE, hypersensitivity angiitis, Wegener granulomatosis, Schönlein-Henoch purpura, mixed IgG-IgM cryoglobulinemia, renal vein thrombosis with pulmonary embolism, congestive heart failure with uremia, rheumatoid arthritis (RA) with sys-

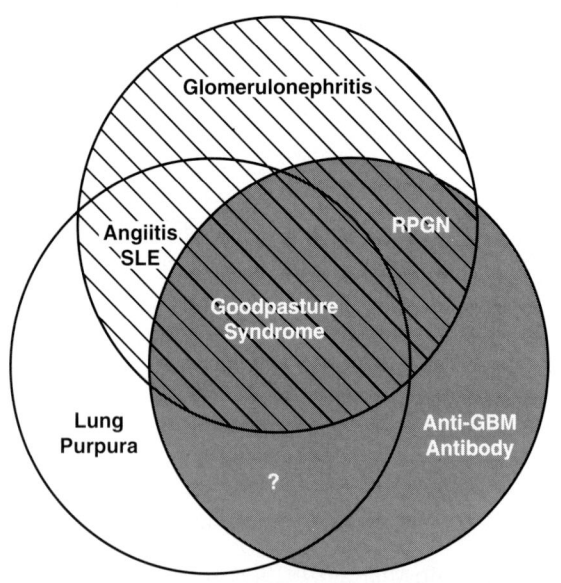

**Figure 31–10.** Venn diagram illustrating the triad of features characteristic of Goodpasture syndrome and the interrelations of lung purpura (lung hemorrhage), glomerulonephritis, and anti-GBM antibody in other diseases. RPGN = idiopathic (type I) crescentic glomerulonephritis.

temic vasculitis, mixed connective tissue disease, and legionnaire disease.[1, 478, 480–483]

ANCA-associated vasculitis (see later) is a particularly common cause of pulmonary hemorrhage and glomerulonephritis, in which anti-GBM antibodies may or may not be found concomitantly. ANCA of the IgM class may be particularly prone to be associated with lung hemorrhage.[490] Sometimes both anti-GBM and ANCAs coexist (see later).

It should also be emphasized that the pulmonary hemorrhage may be clinically silent, may follow the glomerulonephritic presentation in 30% of cases rather than precede it, or may occur coincidentally with it, and, in some cases, the lung may not be involved.[491] In the last case, the term anti-GBM nephritis has been used. However, because most current evidence suggests that both Goodpasture syndrome and anti-GBM nephritis involve the same antigen-antibody system (see later), the differentiation between these two entities is becoming more of a technicality than a useful distinction. Some have suggested that the eponym Goodpasture syndrome should be defined as encompassing all disorders in which glomerulonephritis and pulmonary hemorrhage coexist.[484, 485] We prefer to restrict the term to patients who satisfy evidence of anti-GBM antibody production.

As pointed out in Chapters 29 and 30, evidence of anti-GBM antibody formation may be obtained in several ways; first by the demonstration of linear, ribbon-like deposits of IgG along the glomerular capillary walls by immunofluorescence study of renal biopsy material[1, 482, 483, 486–489] (see also Chapter 30, Fig. 30–7). These deposits are frequently accompanied by C3, usually in an irregular or interrupted linear fashion.[1, 489] By themselves, such linear deposits are not diagnostic of anti-GBM antibody formation, because a similar pattern has been found in a variety of other glomer-

ular diseases (e.g., diabetic nephropathy, SLE, necrotizing vasculitis, chronic poststreptococcal nephritis, and focal glomerular sclerosis).[1, 482, 489] When such deposits are observed in association with crescentic glomerulonephritis, however, they can confidently be assumed to represent in vivo fixation of anti-GBM antibody. As pointed out in Chapter 30, linear deposits of IgG in crescentic glomerulonephritis can also occur in the absence of overt or covert pulmonary hemorrhage (primary crescentic glomerulonephritis, type I). Deposits of albumin in a similar pattern and a lack of C3 deposits should also make one suspect a non–anti-GBM mechanism for the linear IgG deposits, such as underlying diabetic nephropathy.

Second, circulating anti-GBM antibody may be demonstrated by indirect immunofluorescence, passive hemagglutination, and immunoenzymatic or radioimmunoassay procedures.[1, 489, 492–494] Although not extremely sensitive, the indirect immunofluorescence assay is specific; if it is performed early in the course of disease, it is positive in more than three fourths of patients with Goodpasture syndrome, whereas control subjects have uniformly negative results.[494] Radioimmunoassay for anti-GBM antibody using a semi-purified or purified antigenic preparation extracted from particulate GBM by enzymes or protein-dissociating agents is highly specific (false-positive results in less than 2%) and highly sensitive (false-negative results in less than 10%) in cases of proven anti-GBM antibody nephritis.[489, 494] The circulating anti-GBM antibody is typically of the IgG class, but a rare case of IgA-mediated disease has been reported.[495]

The autoantibodies react chiefly with well-defined epitopes on the noncollagenous domain (NC1) of type IV collagen,[496–498] encoded on chromosome 2, region q35-q37. A few patients also demonstrate autoantibody to other domains on the type IV collagen molecule.[498] The most common epitope is on a 26-kd peptide that is derived from an α chain (α3) specific for basement membrane collagen.[499–501] Data suggest that the primary antigenic site comprises amino acid residues 198 to 233 on the COOH-terminal region of α3NC1.[502] This epitope has been found not only in the GBM but also in the basement membranes of alveoli, the anterior lens, and neuromuscular junctions.[503] The structure on which the epitope is identified (α3NC1 hexamer) is identical in the alveolus and the glomerulus. However, the degree of cross-linking of subunits is greater in the alveolar basement membrane, and the amount is about one third of that found in the GBM.[504] This epitope may be normally sequestered in the NC1 domain and requires partial denaturation for full exposure to antibody[496] (see also Chapter 29). The anti-GBM antibody frequently also reacts with non-GBM antigens of the Bowman capsule, renal tubules, and pulmonary alveoli. Not all IgG anti-GBM antibody fixes complement in vitro.[505] The renally deposited IgG is often of IgG1 subclass.[506, 507]

Third, if sufficient renal or lung tissue is available, elution studies may be carried out to demonstrate directly the antibody nature and specificity of deposited IgG.[505, 506] Such studies are rarely necessary, because the combination of light microscopy, direct immunofluorescence of renal biopsy material, and assay of circulating antibody usually establishes the presence or absence of pathogenetic anti-GBM antibody.

In summary, it is appropriate to consider Goodpasture syndrome or disease as having three essential elements, pulmonary hemorrhage, nephritis, and anti-GBM antibody (see Fig. 31–10). However, some patients with idiopathic crescentic glomerulonephritis (type I) display only two of these features (anti-GBM antibody and nephritis). Pulmonary hemorrhage may be mild and evanescent or recurrent in Goodpasture syndrome. Cigarette smoking or exposure to inhaled volatile compounds may provoke episodes of pulmonary hemorrhage.[508-510] Pulmonary hemorrhage without anti-GBM antibodies can be provoked by cocaine inhalation. Finally, it should be pointed out that pulmonary hemorrhage may exist in conjunction with anti-GBM antibody, minor glomerular abnormalities, and few, if any, findings on urinalysis.[491, 511, 512] Thus, Goodpasture syndrome is now recognized to include a broad spectrum of clinical features, ranging from massive pulmonary hemorrhage with little overt evidence of renal disease to fulminant crescentic glomerulonephritis and little overt evidence of pulmonary bleeding. Some cases designated as idiopathic pulmonary hemosiderosis may represent the former, and type I primary rapidly progressive glomerulonephritis may represent the latter (see Chapters 29 and 30).

## CLINICAL FINDINGS

Before wide application of assays for circulating anti-GBM antibody, most reported patients were young adult men, the usual age at onset being between 20 and 30 years,[1, 482, 484, 485, 489, 494] but nearly any age or either sex may be affected. Patients from 4 to older than 80 years of age have been observed, and older women are affected only somewhat less frequently than are men. Hemoptysis is the most common extrarenal symptom and occurs to some degree in most patients.[1, 494] The degree of hemoptysis may vary from a few flecks of blood in the sputum to massive exsanguinating or suffocating intra-alveolar hemorrhage. Pulmonary symptoms precede or are discovered coincident with the renal lesion in more than 70% of cases.[494] The latent period between the first episode of hemoptysis and the discovery of renal disease (usually in the form of abnormal urinalysis) may vary from a few weeks to several years, but it averages about 3 months. Recurrent episodes of mild hemoptysis may antedate the renal lesion by several years. Azotemia may be present at or near the time of discovery of hemoptysis or renal disease in 50% to 70% of cases.[494] In the extensive survey of Wilson and Dixon,[494] 26 of 32 patients developed end-stage renal failure within 1 year of diagnosis (average 3.5 months), whereas only 3 patients had mild nonprogressive glomerular disease.[1] Since then, there have been a few well-documented instances of mild renal involvement associated with a stable course or recovery, with or without treatment.[511, 512] Patients with predominantly pulmonary symptoms and subtle renal abnormalities, such as microscopic hematuria, may do well for long periods without aggressive immunosuppressive therapy.[511, 512] Although antibody production usually subsides with time, symptomatic recurrences have been reported in association with the recrudesence of circulating antibody.[513, 514] One study of 20 patients reported an overall improved prognosis in Goodpasture syndrome, partly because of identification of more mildly affected patients and partly because of improved supportive management.[515] Familial occurrence has been reported, and miniepidemics have also been observed.[516-518] Occasionally, exacerbations have appeared to be associated with exposure to environmental agents including products used in hair permanents, hydrocarbon fumes, cigarette smoking, hard metal dust (inert tungsten carbide and cobalt) exposure,[519] or cocaine inhalation.

Pallor and anemia out of proportion to the degree of hemoptysis and renal failure are common.[518, 520] Cough, dyspnea, and basilar rales are common. These findings may wax and wane even without overt hemoptysis. An upper respiratory tract infection may precede the onset in 10% to 30% of patients, but fever, rash, and chest pain are relatively uncommon. Arthritic complaints, however, may be noted and may be related to concomitant or complicating vasculitis. Mild to moderate elevation of diastolic blood pressure is found in less than 20% of patients.[518, 520] Rarely, the disorder may occur as a complication of other diseases such as membranous glomerulonephritis (see Chapter 30), the nail-patella syndrome,[521] or an underlying malignant lymphoma or lymphocytic malignancy.[522] D-Penicillamine has been associated with pulmonary hemorrhage and extracapillary glomerulonephritis, but the typical immunopathologic features of Goodpasture syndrome are usually lacking.[523] Anti-GBM antibody disease may also appear de novo after renal allotransplantation in patients with Alport syndrome (see later discussion). Occasionally, cases may be encountered in clusters, suggesting an infectious etiology.[524] Influenza A2 viral infection has been associated with typical Goodpasture syndrome and anti-GBM antibody formation, but a cause-and-effect relationship remains unproved.[525] Occasionally, relapses may occur after the initial episode[526, 527]; on rare occasions multiple relapses may occur,[513] often in association with superimposed infection.[528] Cigarette smoking increases the risk of hemoptysis.

## LABORATORY FINDINGS

Urinalyses are nearly always abnormal, with both hematuria and proteinuria being present. Red blood cell casts are often evident. Massive proteinuria and the nephrotic syndrome are unusual, probably because of the early and rapid deterioration of GFR. Anti–streptolysin O levels are not usually increased, and antinuclear antibodies are rarely found.[489, 520] Hemolytic complement and C3 levels are nearly always normal. CICs, rheumatoid factor, and cryoIgs are almost always absent.[489, 520] Circulating anti-GBM antibodies are found in more than 90% of patients at the onset of disease (see earlier discussion). The titer of antibody does not correlate closely with the severity of renal or pulmonary findings.[494, 520] Antibody levels peak at the time of clinical presentation and usually decline thereafter, with or without treatment. Treatment may accelerate the rate of decline of circulating antibody levels, however. Persistence of detectable antibody in the circulation for more than 6 months is uncommon; however, rare patients with relapsing courses have been reported.[513, 514] The prevalence of HLA-DR2 in patients with anti-GBM antibody nephritis is greatly increased compared with control subjects (88% versus 32%).[529-531] Simultaneous presence of HLA-B8 and HLA-

DR2 is associated with a more serious prognosis primarily because of more exuberant crescent formation.[531] ANCAs may coexist in some patients or develop subsequent to the disappearance of anti-GBM antibodies[532] (see section on vasculitis). Antibodies to proteinase 3 or myeloperoxidase have been reported concomitant or in tandem with anti-GBM antibodies, suggesting, in some patients, an associated vasculitis[520, 533] (see also Chapter 29). It is unclear whether anti-GBM antibodies are the cause or the result of the associated vasculitis in the patients in whom both antibodies are found.

Anemia is of a microcytic, hypochromic type.[518] Serum iron levels may be low despite relatively scant hemoptysis, perhaps caused in part by extensive intrapulmonary iron sequestration. The iron sequestration may be demonstrable by [59]Fe scanning of lungs.[534] Hemosiderin-laden macrophages may be detected in the sputum, but this is a nonspecific finding. Pulmonary bleeding can be detected by fluffy hilar and basilar infiltrates and may result in an increase in the arterial-alveolar $PO_2$ gradient. Ewan and colleagues[535] described a sensitive method for detection of pulmonary bleeding based on the affinity of carbon monoxide (CO) for hemoglobin. Thus, the uptake of inhaled CO is increased and the excretion of $C^{15}O$ is delayed in pulmonary hemorrhage. Single-breath CO uptake is compared with pulmonary clearance, the latter using $C^{15}O$; decreased clearance is strongly suggestive of bleeding. This test is of value in following the progress of Goodpasture syndrome, but the ratio measurement requires access to a cyclotron. Perhaps serial CO uptake measurements alone are of value. These can be performed in most pulmonary function laboratories.

## PATHOLOGY

**Light Microscopy.** Patients with mild renal failure or those with only urinary abnormalities and normal GFR may demonstrate only focal and segmental glomerular hypercellularity, often with segmental necrosis of glomerular tufts and small crescents.[1, 494, 520, 536, 537] Normal glomerular architecture has also been observed by light microscopy.[1, 494, 537] The focal and segmental proliferative lesion may persist or resolve, but it more often progresses to the ominous picture of crescentic glomerulonephritis. One feature frequently noted is the lack of endocapillary proliferation and the extreme and circumferential nature of crescent formation. The degree and extent of crescent formation may have prognostic significance. Tubulointerstitial changes, including edema and leukocytic infiltration, are prominent and may be linked to the concomitant deposition of anti–tubule basement membrane antibody.[1, 538] Multinucleate giant cells may be common in some patients in both interstitium and crescents. Severe tubulointerstitial lesions can be related to the degree and duration of renal failure.[1, 537, 538] By light microscopy, these morphologic features are indistinguishable from many of the other forms of crescentic glomerulonephritis and rapidly progressive renal failure (especially type I idiopathic crescentic glomerulonephritis). The lungs reveal extensive intra-alveolar hemorrhage with disruption of the alveolar septa and intra-alveolar hemosiderin-laden

macrophages.[1, 484, 485, 518] Renal vasculitis may be seen on rare occasions.[518, 537]

**Electron Microscopy.** Electron microscopic observations of the kidney are virtually identical to the findings in the idiopathic variety of anti-GBM antibody–mediated rapidly progressive crescentic glomerulonephritis (see Chapter 30). The major change is lucent widening of the subendothelial space of the capillaries, which corresponds to the site of binding of anti–basement membrane antibody as documented by immunoelectron microscopy.[539] As mentioned, gaps and discontinuities of the GBM are frequently observed. Similar gaps, which may also be seen in the Bowman capsule, may permit interstitial fibroblasts to gain access to the Bowman space, thus facilitating organization of the crescent into a fibrous scar.[528, 530, 540, 541] Electron-dense deposits are usually not found; several reports, however, have documented electron-dense capillary wall deposits that evolved over time.[542–544] Subendothelial fibrin deposits may mimic electron-dense deposits of immune complex disease, but they more commonly manifest as subendothelial lucent zones. Membranous glomerulonephritis may coexist with anti-GBM antibody–mediated nephritis.[543]

**Immunofluorescence.** Immunofluorescence findings are typical. Linear deposits of IgG and, less frequently, IgM outlining the capillary loops are found (see also Chapter 30, Fig. 30–7). Rarely, IgA may be the predominant Ig, being deposited in a linear pattern.[1, 495] IgG1 and IgG4 subclasses have been found in the deposits and in circulating anti-GBM antibodies.[507] Deposits of C3 are often found in a segmental or interrupted linear fashion but may be absent in as many as 20% to 30% of patients.[1, 505, 537] C3 may also be in a distinctly granular pattern in capillary walls and may be associated with a coexisting membranous glomerulonephritis.[543] C1q is absent in many patients.[537] Fibrin-related antigens are also found, chiefly in the crescents or in areas of tuft necrosis. Lung tissue reveals similar linear or segmental linear deposits of IgG (or rarely IgA) along the alveolar capillary membranes,[1, 495, 537] but the deposits may be focal. Lung biopsies, even from patients with overt pulmonary hemorrhage, may not always reveal linear deposits of IgG, even when circulating antibody levels are elevated. Eluates of lung react with GBM and vice versa.[506] Circulating antibody reacts with normal lung alveolar basement membrane and also tends to react with epithelial basement membranes of the Bowman capsule and renal tubules.

## PATHOGENESIS

The pathogenesis of anti-GBM antibody–induced disease has been discussed in Chapters 29 and 30. Glomerular injury is mediated by interaction of circulating autoantibody with intrinsic GBM glycoproteins, almost always an epitope on the NC1 domain of collagen α3(IV).[499–501] This causes activation of the complement cascade, and glomerular infiltration by polymorphonuclear leukocytes and monocytes. The antigen is located principally on the inner aspect of the lamina densa.[520, 539] Patients with Goodpasture syndrome may also develop antibody to a variety of other basement membrane constituents, including antibody to an alternative epitope on the 7S portion of the type IV collagen molecule.[497, 520] In experimental animals, antibody to heparan sulfate proteoglycan resulted in linear immunofluorescence along the glomerular capillary wall but no nephritogenic response.[498] Coagulation mechanisms and monocytes participate actively in generation of crescents.[545-548] Fibrinogen leaking into the Bowman space through gaps in GBM is polymerized to fibrin through action of procoagulant factors, primarily membrane-bound prothrombinase associated with activated monocytes. Interleukin-1 generated by activated blood-borne monocytes may attract fibroblasts from renal interstitium and lead to organization and scar. Lung injury may be induced in a similar fashion. In fact, it is clear that the target peptide subunits of collagen IV in the lung and in the kidney are identical in structure but differ in quantity and cross-linkage.[504] However, the relative lack of correlation between levels of anti-GBM antibody (presumably cross-reactive with alveolar basement membrane) and pulmonary manifestations is difficult to account for and has led a few to question the pathogenetic significance of the antibody. Furthermore, pulmonary hemorrhage may occur in non–anti-GBM antibody–mediated renal diseases. It is possible that nonantibody factors also participate in pulmonary injury. Alternatively, anti-GBM antibody–GBM antigen complexes may participate in pulmonary capillary damage.[549, 550] The etiology of production of anti-GBM autoantibodies is unknown. Genetic predisposition coupled to exposure to an environmental agent that damages alveolar walls and releases autoantigen (e.g., inhaled hydrocarbons, cigarette smoke, cocaine, viruses) may be involved.

## COURSE AND THERAPY

In most untreated patients with crescentic glomerulonephritis, progressive renal failure eventually requires dialysis support.[1, 485, 494, 520] Severe bouts of hemoptysis, some life threatening, are typical. Long remissions of pulmonary hemorrhage may occur inexplicably, despite progressive renal disease.[520, 551-555] Spontaneous recovery from renal disease is uncommon, but it appears that some patients, particularly those with mild renal involvement, may remain stable or even improve under certain circumstances, at times coincident with treatment by steroids or cytotoxic drugs.[520, 551-555] Some patients treated with steroids and cytotoxic drugs, however, did not fulfill the diagnostic criteria used here for Goodpasture syndrome.

Uncontrolled observations suggest that high-dose parenteral (pulse therapy) or oral glucocorticoid treatment produces a prompt improvement in the pulmonary hemorrhagic manifestations and may induce a lasting remission from troublesome bouts of hemoptysis.[518, 520, 556] Unfortunately, steroids alone seem to have little demonstrable beneficial effect on the rapidly progressive glomerular disease.[557] The role of anticoagulation in treatment is unclear, but it can be expected to be exceptionally hazardous in these patients because of the unpredictable appearance of pulmonary hemorrhage. With recovery after lung hemorrhage, there are no long-term sequelae except for a mild increase in pulmonary diffusing capacity; other pulmonary function test results return to normal.[558]

Although only limited controlled studies have been reported, the dramatic results using intensive plasma exchange (plasmapheresis) initially reported by the group at Hammersmith Hospital in England, and subsequently confirmed by many additional investigators in the United States, New Zealand, and Australia, cannot be overlooked.[515, 520, 559-566] Indeed, the prompt disappearance of pulmonary bleeding and the reversal of renal function deterioration by prompt and aggressive therapy with plasma exchange combined with steroids and cytotoxic drugs in many patients with Goodpasture syndrome make it difficult to justify a controlled clinical trial. Some patients, however, have shown no improvement even with aggressive plasma exchange therapy.[567] Because IgM ANCAs may be found in some patients with lung hemorrhage and such antibodies are removed poorly or not at all by membrane plasma cell separators, it is best to employ centrifugal methods when plasma exchange is used to treat lung hemorrhage and the underlying relationship to immunopathogenetic mechanism is unknown.[490] As with other forms of rapidly progressive renal failure, early and aggressive therapy is required. Poor results can be expected in oliguric patients or in those with renal failure severe enough to require dialysis support (e.g., >8 mg/dL creatinine), although occasionally patients respond to plasma exchange therapy with severe dialysis-dependent renal failure. Initial therapy with daily 3- to 4-L plasma exchanges combined with cyclophosphamide at 2 to 3 mg/kg/d plus prednisone at 1 mg/kg/d has been recommended, while following the levels of renal function, anti-GBM antibody, and pulmonary function.[520, 568] When renal function or pulmonary hemorrhage is stabilized, the frequency and volume of plasma exchange can be cautiously reduced in accordance with the foregoing parameters. With more specific knowledge of the inciting antigen in most patients, specific immunoadsorption eventually may supplant the use of plasmapheresis. Exacerbations related to intercurrent infections may occur.[509, 527, 528] Cyclophosphamide may be especially hazardous in older people, and the total duration of cytotoxic drug therapy should be kept to a minimum. Maintenance steroids may be required, especially for patients with recurrent hemoptysis. Many patients treated with early and aggressive plasma exchange and immunosuppression recover normal or nearly normal renal function, and all evidence of anti-GBM antibody production ceases.[575] The mechanism of termination of autoantibody production in this circumstance remains unknown.

Before the introduction of plasma exchange therapy, bilateral nephrectomy was occasionally performed in cases of life-threatening pulmonary hemorrhage; it now appears that bilateral nephrectomy is rarely, if ever, indicated. Some patients with partial recovery of renal function with aggressive therapy have later developed slowly progressive renal failure associated with heavy proteinuria. The mechanism underlying this evolution remains unknown, but nonimmunologic factors (e.g., glomerular hypertension) may be involved. Patients with persisting proteinuria and/or declining renal function should probably receive long-term therapy with angiotensin-converting enzyme (ACE) inhibitors, especially in the presence of systemic arterial hypertension (see Chapter 30).

Recurrent disease has occurred in renal allografts.[515, 520, 569-574] The precise risk of recurrence is difficult to establish, but if recurrence is defined as development of linear IgG deposits in the graft, its prevalence may be as high as

30%. Fortunately, graft loss caused by recurrent disease is uncommon as long as patients did not undergo transplantation during the active stages of disease, when high circulating anti-GBM antibody levels are present.[574] Grafts may also survive even if low levels of circulating antibody are present at the time of transplantation.[574] Patients receiving grafts from an identical twin should receive post-transplantation immunosuppression as a prophylactic measure. Allografts have also developed linear IgG glomerular deposits when the original disease was not known to be an anti-GBM antibody–mediated disorder.[575] Cyclosporine has not proved to be an effective immunosuppressive agent for patients with Goodpasture syndrome, except in an occasional anecdotal case report.[576]

## Systemic Necrotizing Vasculitis

The term systemic necrotizing vasculitis refers to a heterogeneous group of disorders in which polymorphous manifestations occur as a result of involvement of blood vessels in many different organ systems with an inflammatory and necrotizing lesion.[1, 577–581] Synonyms are polyarteritis, systemic angiitis, and systemic necrotizing vasculitis. Weight loss, anemia, fever, palpable purpura, arthritis, abdominal pain, mononeuritis multiplex, myocardial failure and infarction, pulmonary infiltrates, asthma, hemoptysis, splenic infarction, myopathy, pancreatitis, testicular pain, and CNS dysfunction are a few of the more common manifestations.[1, 578–581] These manifestations and the underlying pathologic findings may be grouped into more or less distinctive syndromes, but much clinical and morphologic overlap exists. Depending on the criteria used (clinical or morphologic), some degree of renal involvement occurs in 70% to 90% of patients.[582] However, the severity of the renal disease with respect to clinical manifestations and structural changes varies widely according to the size of the blood vessels involved. Numerous in-depth reviews have stressed the broad spectrum of disease that can be associated with vasculitis.[583–589] Classification of the systemic vasculitides has historically been a problem, because pathogenetic understanding has been lacking for most of the clinically recognized entities. Zeek's classification, published in 1953[579] and updated by Fauci et al in 1978,[580] was based on clinical and histologic features. These classifications comprised disorders grouped by symptom complexes, such as hypersensitivity angiitis, rheumatic arteritis, polyarteritis nodosa, giant cell arteritis, and then later Wegener granulomatosis, lymphomatoid granulomatosis, and thromboangiitis obliterans. Other classifications have evolved based on the size of the involved vessels (e.g., large, medium, small arteries versus venules), the presence of underlying causes (such as infection, malignancy, drugs, connective tissue disorders, rejection), and the presence or absence of ANCAs. The classification of the systemic vasculitides has been reviewed.[590] However, the importance of ANCA in the classification, diagnosis, and treatment of systemic vasculitis has so altered the nephrologist's approach to these disorders that a brief overview is warranted. More extensive reviews on ANCA have been published.[591–595a]

ANCAs (antibodies to neutrophil cytoplasmic antigens) were first noted in the serum of patients with segmental necrotizing glomerulonephritis in 1982.[596] Their usefulness as serologic markers in patients with Wegener granulomatosis and other systemic vasculitides was appreciated by the mid-1980s.[596–598] ANCAs interact with lysosomal enzymes present in the azurophilic granules of neutrophils.

The earliest method utilized to detect these antibodies was indirect immunofluorescence. With this technique, neutrophils isolated from heparinized peripheral blood were plated onto glass slides, fixed with ethanol, incubated with patients' sera, and secondarily incubated with labeled anti-human Ig. In the positive sera, two patterns of immunofluorescence were noted. The cytoplasmic pattern (cANCA) showed positive staining distributed throughout the neutrophil cytoplasm, whereas the perinuclear pattern (pANCA) showed positive staining predominantly surrounding the nucleus.[595, 597–599] Despite the differences noted in pattern distribution by immunofluorescence microscopy, the antigens to which the antibodies are directed are both located in lysosomes. The differences in localization are actually due to fixation artifact. After ethanol fixation, the positively charged lysosomal granules, which are the target antigen for the pANCA pattern, are released from the lysosomes and move toward and surround the negatively charged nucleus, facilitating the perinuclear pattern. The usefulness of the indirect immunofluorescence method is limited by its lack of standardization and by the presence of false-positives, particularly in patients who have antinuclear antibodies, which may be confused with a pANCA pattern (pANCA may be differentiated from a positive antinuclear antibody by fixing the cells with formalin instead of ethanol). Furthermore, the indirect immunofluorescence result may be positive if the patient has antibodies to cytoplasmic antigens other than proteinase 3 and myeloperoxidase, the predominant target antigens for cANCA and pANCA, respectively (see later).[591–599] The clinical significance of a positive ANCA directed at other antigens is not clear.

Better standardization and improved specificity are now achieved by performing assays for ANCA with specific test antigens. The majority of patients with a cANCA indirect immunofluorescence pattern have Wegener granulomatosis and have antibodies directed against conformational epitopes on proteinase 3.[600] Proteinase 3 is a 29-kd lysosomal neutral serine protease identical to p29 (a naturally occurring neutrophil peptide with antibiotic properties), AG7 (azurophilic granule 7), and myeloblastin (a growth factor derived from myeloid cells).[593, 601] Apart from its antibiotic properties, its functions include degradation of basement membrane proteins such as elastin, fibronectin, laminin, vitronectin, and type IV collagen.[593] The majority of patients with a pANCA indirect immunofluorescence pattern have non-Wegener vasculitis (e.g., microscopic polyangiitis, Churg-Strauss syndrome, idiopathic crescentic glomerulonephritis) and have antibodies directed against myeloperoxidase.[595, 595a, 601] Less commonly, ANCAs may be directed against other antigens, including elastase, lactoferrin, CAP57, cathepsin G, α-enolase, and histone eosinophil peroxidase.[599–606] Using these as target antigens (particularly proteinase 3 and myeloperoxidase), the specificity of a positive ANCA indirect immunofluorescence can be ascertained and the degree of positivity can be quantitated. This is achieved by radioimmunoassay, enzyme-linked immunosorbent assay, Western blotting, dot blotting, or immunoprecipitation.

The presence of cANCA identified by either indirect immunofluorescence or the more specific methodologies outlined earlier is 90% to 98% sensitive and specific for active Wegener granulomatosis.[593, 597, 607, 608] The sensitivity and specificity are higher in patients with active disease than in those in the initial phase of presentation or in remission. However, the sensitivity and specificity are dependent on the definition one uses to diagnose Wegener granulomatosis. If a narrow diagnostic set of criteria is utilized (such as a requirement for the presence of granulomatous respiratory tract inflammation), then cANCA testing is highly sensitive but less specific. If a less restrictive set of criteria is utilized for establishing the diagnosis, the specificity is high but the sensitivity decreases.[609] Furthermore, the probability that a positive cANCA test result will correctly predict the diagnosis depends not entirely on the sensitivity and specificity of the assay but also on the prevalence of the disease in the population studied. Thus, the predictive value of the test would be greatest when utilized for patients with classic signs and symptoms of Wegener granulomatosis (close to 99%); less for patients with nonspecific pulmonary-renal symptoms, systemic vasculitis, or rapidly progressive glomerulonephritis; and least for asymptomatic patients undergoing screening.[607, 608] In the last population, even if the sensitivity and specificity of the test are as high as 95%, because the prevalence of the disease is low (<1% of the populace), the number of false-positives would outnumber the true-positives. Thus, a positive cANCA result cannot be taken to be synonymous with Wegener granulomatosis in the absence of clinical correlation.[610] Furthermore, a significant minority of patients with Wegener granulomatosis have pANCA rather than cANCA reactivity. The predictive value for a specific diagnosis is lower for pANCA than for cANCA, because the former is less closely linked to a specific disease entity. Positive ANCA (cytoplasmic or perinuclear) has been observed in hydralazine-associated nephritis[611]; in interstitial nephritis[612]; in patients with malignancy and monoclonal gammopathy,[613, 614] HIV infection,[615] tuberculosis,[610] and cystic fibrosis[616]; and concomitant with Goodpasture disease with anti-GBM autoantibodies[617, 618] (see also Chapter 30). In some of these instances, the presence of ANCA may not be a false-positive, as vasculitis may indeed be present. Positive pANCA results are frequently reported in ulcerative colitis (60% to 75%), Crohn disease (10% to 20%), autoimmune chronic active hepatitis (60% to 70%), primary biliary cirrhosis (30% to 40%), primary sclerosing cholangitis (60% to 85%), RA with (90% to 100%) or without (20% to 75%) Felty syndrome,[593] and malignancy,[613] and in some chronic dialysis patients without vasculitis.[619] In the setting of vasculitis, no difference in prognosis is discernible among patients with cytoplasmic versus perinuclear ANCA.[608, 620]

Apart from its usefulness as an important adjunct to the history, physical findings, and histology in the diagnosis of vasculitic syndromes, the cANCA titer appears to be helpful in guiding the long-term management of patients with Wegener granulomatosis. The clinical utility of following ANCA titers in patients with vasculitis is discussed later in the section on Wegener granulomatosis.

Finally, some evidence suggests that ANCA may participate in the pathogenesis of the vasculitic syndromes. An initiating step in the development of vasculitis may be the secretion of cytokines as a result of infection or other inflammatory stimulus. In patients with Wegener granulomatosis and microscopic polyarteritis, serum levels of tumor necrosis factor-α and interleukin-2 receptor are elevated.[621, 622] In addition, these cytokines, as well as interleukin-1β, are present in the kidney predominantly in infiltrating cells at periglomerular, interstitial, and perivascular sites, as well as in crescents and in the walls of necrotic arterioles and arteries.[622] In vitro, cytokines such as tumor necrosis factor-α and interleukin-8 have been shown to facilitate the movement of neutrophil lysosomal ANCA antigens to the cell surface, where they are capable of interacting with the serum ANCA.[623, 624] The usually intracytoplasmic lysosomal enzyme proteinase 3 has been identified on the surface of neutrophils from patients with Wegener granulomatosis and sepsis.[625] In addition, neutrophils (particularly when primed by cytokines) degranulate and secrete toxic oxygen radicals in vitro,[626] a process that may contribute to endothelial cell damage.[627] Neutrophils actively secreting hydrogen peroxide have been identified in renal biopsy specimens from patients with Wegener granulomatosis.[628] Capillary wall damage may also be mediated by the binding of ANCA to proteinase 3, thereby impeding the activity of natural inhibitors of proteinase 3. Theoretically, this may facilitate potentially injurious proteolytic actions of proteinase 3 at the level of the basement membrane.[594, 629] Additional in vitro data suggest that ANCA may interact with proteinase 3 on the surface of activated endothelial cells,[629, 630] although proteinase 3 has not been found on the surface of endothelial cells ex vivo.[631] Antiendothelial antibodies have been found in patients with vasculitis by some investigators[632–634] but not by others.[635]

The etiology of systemic vasculitis is unknown. Some cases can be traced to a reaction to a drug (allopurinol, rifampin, penicillamine, bucillamine, hydralazine, sulfonamides), whereas others may be triggered by an infection (e.g., hepatitis B or bacterial infection).[635a] Chronic parvovirus B19 infection has also been implicated in some cases (see later).[636] Such an infection could explain rapid clearing of clinical signs and symptoms after treatment with intravenous Igs, which presumably contain parvovirus-neutralizing antibodies.

A genetic predisposition may exist in some cases of vasculitis. For example, the ANCA-associated vasculitides in which anti–proteinase 3 autoantibodies are formed are seen in patients with hereditary α1-antitrypsin deficiency.[637] In addition, the HLA-DQw7 specificity is associated with ANCA-positive vasculitis.[637a] To provide a framework for this discussion, the classification initially proposed by Zeek[579] and later modified by Fauci and associates[580, 581, 638] is employed.

## WEGENER GRANULOMATOSIS

In 1939, Wegener[639] described a series of patients with necrotizing granulomatous arteritis of the upper and lower respiratory tracts, including the sinuses, middle ear, and nasopharynx. Many subsequent reports have amply confirmed the existence of this disorder as a discrete clinicopathologic entity.[580, 581, 638, 639] The disease affects patients of any age but is more common in older males. It is often associated with a localized, cavitary necrotic pneumonitis and evidence of glomerular injury. Purulent rhinorrhea, painful sinusitis, otitis, keratoconjunctivitis, cough, hemoptysis, necrotizing skin lesions, arthralgias, arthritis, coronary artery disease, neuritis, fever, and abdominal pain are common findings.[580, 581, 638–646] Saddle-nose deformity may also occur. More uncommon findings include oral ulcers, proptosis caused by retro-orbital mass lesions, visual abnormalities, hearing loss, pleuritis, pleural effusions, headache, temporal bone granulomas, and cholesteatoma. Palatal ulcers have not been seen.[580, 581] Rarely, auricular chondritis occurs. Histoplasmosis and tuberculosis can mimic Wegener granulomatosis but the ANCA is usually negative in those diseases.[645] Renal involvement is characterized by hematuria, varying degrees of proteinuria, and progressive decline in GFR. Ureteric obstruction and perirenal hematomas may develop.[638] Hypertension is uncommon. IgA serum levels may be increased.[1, 638, 646] HLA-B8 has been found in higher frequency than in control subjects, as have HLA-B2 and -DR2.[647] Eighty-five percent of patients have some sign of renal involvement, but only 11% present with renal impairment initially.[646] Finally, pulmonary hemorrhage may develop, sometimes with concomitant anti-GBM autoantibodies and ANCA.[617, 618]

Reliable serologic markers for Wegener granulomatosis (and other types of vasculitis) had been elusive until the identification of ANCA. Intensive investigation into the relevance of ANCA in various forms of vasculitis has provided not only a diagnostic aid (see earlier) but also a useful adjunct to clinical criteria in the assessment of specific disease activity. Van der Woude and co-workers[597] were among the first to draw attention to the specificity and sensitivity of these autoantibodies in the various forms of vasculitis including Wegener granulomatosis.

Some caution is advised, however, in the use of ANCA titers as estimates of clinical activity. Although most investigators find relationships between ANCA titers and disease activity,[597, 646–649] this association has not been found universally.[650, 651] In most studies, disappearance of ANCA is associated with clinical remission.[620, 649] However, autoantibodies may persist in some patients despite clinical quiescence,[620, 650, 651] and serologic relapse may precede clinical relapse by many months, making a cause-and-effect relationship uncertain.[651–653] Titers appear to be more predictive of activity in the longitudinal follow-up of an individual patient than in cross-sectional comparisons of groups of patients. One prospective, randomized clinical trial assessed the value of using ANCA titers as a guide to treatment for the prevention of relapse in patients with Wegener granulomatosis.[653] In the experimental group, a fourfold increment in the titer of the immunofluorescence test for ANCA triggered either institution of or an increment in prednisone and cyclophosphamide therapy. In the control group, the same treatment was instituted when a clinically apparent relapse occurred. During a 2-year follow-up period, the patients in the experimental group had no relapses, compared with nine relapses in the 11 control patients. A cumulatively lower immunosuppressive dose was used in the patients treated prophylactically than in those treated when symptoms were evident.[653]

The renal lesions include diffuse or segmental necrotizing glomerulonephritis accompanied by a granulomatous reaction associated with blood vessel walls. In a report of 85 patients with Wegener granulomatosis, however, granulomata and arteritis were rarely found on percutaneous renal biopsy,[581, 646] thus emphasizing the lack of diagnostic usefulness of renal biopsy. Conversely, lung biopsy commonly reveals the typical granulomatous vasculitis. Extensive crescents may be seen in patients with rapidly progressive renal failure. A possible forme fruste in which renal involvement is lacking or mild has been described.[581, 646] Immunofluorescence findings may vary, but scattered Ig and C3 granular deposits may be seen. Electron-dense deposits in capillary walls may be detected by electron microscopy.[1, 581, 646] The pathogenesis is presumed to be immune complex deposition, but the antigen is unknown.

The dismal outlook for patients with Wegener granulomatosis has been dramatically altered by combined treatment with steroids and cytotoxic drugs.[1, 581, 638, 647] Although no controlled trials have been conducted, the results are sufficiently dramatic and the progressively downhill course without therapy so predictable that it is doubtful that a controlled study will ever be done. The average life expectancy without treatment is only about 5 months, and 1-year survival is less than 20%.[580, 581, 638, 646] With steroids alone, life expectancy is about doubled, and with the addition of cytotoxic drugs, 1-year survival is in excess of 80%. Ninety-three percent of 85 patients treated at NIH with cytotoxic agents (primarily cyclophosphamide) achieved long-term remissions of 7 months to 13.2 years, with a mean of 48 months.[638, 646] Intravenous pulse cyclophosphamide has been applied to patients with Wegener granulomatosis with or without plasma exchange.[620, 642–644, 654, 655] A prospective nonrandomized trial included 70 patients with ANCA-positive pauci-immune crescentic glomerulonephritis (the majority of whom had Wegener granulomatosis) observed for a mean period of 2 years. Oral and intravenous cyclophosphamide appeared to be equally efficacious when used in conjunction with corticosteroids.[620] Relapses may occur more frequently with the intravenous route.[620, 654, 655] Trimethoprim-sulfamethoxazole is of benefit only in patients with limited disease.[644] Methotrexate may be useful but has a high complication rate.[644] Monoclonal antibody and intravenous Ig therapies are promising approaches to treatment.[656, 658, 659] Azathioprine may be used but is less effective than alkylating agents and is not recommended as ''first-line'' therapy.[660, 661] Intravenous Ig and protein A immunoadsorption[369] have been utilized in a small number of patients with some success.[656–658] A few reports have documented the ability of cytotoxic agents with or without plasma exchange (see also Chapter 30)[662–664] to achieve remission even in patients with apparent ESRD, resulting in the discontinuation of hemodialysis in some of these patients, albeit with impaired creatinine clearances.[665–673] In some of these patients, subsequent slow development of chronic renal failure was observed despite adequate immunosuppression, suggesting perhaps a nonimmunologic mechanism.[673] Whereas some have reported that the activity of Wegener granulomatosis diminishes with the advent of ESRD, others have reported instances in which apparently idiopathic glomerulonephritis leading to ESRD was rapidly followed by the pulmonary manifestations of Wegener granulomatosis, making the diagnosis apparent only after hemodialysis was initiated.[673–675] Relapses of disease have occurred when patients' therapy was converted from cyclophosphamide to azathioprine, especially when ANCAs were still present. Neoplasms (particularly lymphocytic leukemia) have been observed in patients with Wegener granulomatosis who were treated with cytotoxic agents for long periods.[676–679] Patients who recover but later develop proteinuria and progressive renal insufficiency and who are serologically "inactive" may benefit from treatment with ACE inhibitors.[679a] Occasional reports have indicated long-term remissions after broad-spectrum antibiotic (trimethoprim-sulfamethoxazole) therapy[680] but usually only in pulmonary or upper airway–limited disease.[644]

**Miscellaneous Forms of Vasculitis.** Glomeruli are not commonly involved in the other varieties of vasculitis, including temporal arteritis,[681] mucocutaneous lymph node syndrome (Kawasaki disease),[682] hypocomplementemic cutaneous vasculitis (McDuffie syndrome), Cogan syndrome, Eales disease, Behçet disease,[683–686] and rheumatic arteritis.[687] There are several descriptions of glomerular lesions in Takayasu arteritis.[686] The kidney is occasionally involved in the syndrome of immunoblastic lymphadenopathy.[687] Patients with widespread vasculitis secondary to RA (malignant rheumatoid disease) may develop renal complications.[688, 688a, 689] Rheumatoid vasculitis is an uncommon complication of long-standing RA. It may present with subcutaneous nodules, cutaneous ulcers, palpable purpura, pleuritis with effusion, pericarditis, coronary artery disease, distal gangrene, nail fold infarcts, or mononeuritis multiplex. Rheumatoid factor levels are greatly elevated, as are the erythrocyte sedimentation rate and C-reactive protein level. The C3 and C4 complement components are greatly depressed. CICs and cryoIgs (type III) may be present (see later). Most patients are HLA-DR4–positive, and there is a strong association with homozygosity at the HLA-DRB1-*0401 allele at the HLA-DR4 locus.[689] The vasculitis that accompanies essential mixed IgG-IgM cryoimmunoglobulinemia is discussed in the section on paraproteinemias.

## PERIARTERITIS NODOSA

Periarteritis nodosa is also called polyarteritis nodosa, classic polyarteritis, macroscopic form of polyarteritis, and Kussmaul-Maier disease. In this form of systemic vasculitis, systemic symptoms such as polyarthralgias, weight loss, abdominal pain, ischemic skin lesions (ulcers, necrosis), and fever are frequently present. Mononeuritis multiplex is the typical clinical feature of peripheral nerve involvement. Males are affected twice as often as females, and peak incidence is in the sixth decade of life.[1, 582] Hypertension is common, is usually related to increased levels of plasma renin, and may be severe or malignant.[579] Testicular pain is a common feature. Infarction of various organs, including the myocardium, small intestine, and portions of the kidney,

is common and is due to occlusion of major vessels.[579] Cutaneous involvement is relatively uncommon but may manifest as urticaria, morbilliform rash, subcutaneous nodules, ischemic infarction and ulceration, gangrene, and livedo reticularis. Palpable purpura is not usually seen. Renal involvement occurs in 80% to 90% of patients, who typically present initially with hematuria.[578, 580, 582] Amphetamine abuse and chronic viral hepatitis may also be associated with similar lesions.[690] The urine sediment may contain broad renal failure casts together with signs of active disease, the so-called telescoped urine. Nephrotic syndrome is uncommon, and progressive renal failure is usually a late manifestation.[582] $Na^+$ wasting and vasopressin (Pitressin)-resistant hyposthenuria are atypical presentations.[691] Eosinophilia is usually absent. Serum C3 concentration may be reduced, normal, or increased. CICs are frequently present and contain IgG, IgA, IgM, and complement components. cryoIg is occasionally present. A significant number of patients (10% to 30%) may be found to be carriers of hepatitis B virus (see later discussion). The erythrocyte sedimentation rate is often greatly elevated (over 100 mm/h, Westergren method). C-reactive protein is also greatly elevated.[692] Perinuclear ANCAs or antimyeloperoxidose antibodies, or both, are present in 25% to 50% of patients.[592, 593, 620]

Pathologically, the kidney in early stages reveals acute inflammation of the medium-sized blood vessels, particularly the interlobar and arcuate arteries[582, 690] (Fig. 31–11). All or part of the wall may be involved. The elastic lamina is disrupted and fragmented and the vessel wall undergoes fibrinoid necrosis with later formation of aneurysms.[1, 580, 693] Ischemic infarction of irregular zones of kidney may be observed in severe cases. Glomerular lesions are predominantly those of ischemia with hyperplasia of the juxtaglomerular apparatus, occasional segmental or diffuse proliferation, and accompanying fibrinoid necrosis. In the healing stages, there is gradual resolution of inflammation, with increasing luminal obliteration and fibrosis in the aneurysms, which may be detected by selective renal angiograms.[1, 694] Characteristically, lesions of various ages are observed. The disruption of the elastic lamina is an important differential diagnostic point, because it distinguishes healed arteritis from the lesions secondary to essential hypertension, in which reduplication rather than disruption is seen.[582, 689] The glomerular lesions often consist of ischemic collapse, but extensive crescents may be seen occasionally.[582, 689, 693] Percutaneous needle biopsy specimens are not likely to reveal a lesion of vasculitis unless a major vessel is included in the specimen. Many patients have only scant deposits of IgG or complement components distributed throughout the abnormal capillary walls and mesangium.[588, 589]

## HYPERSENSITIVITY ANGIITIS OR MICROSCOPIC POLYANGIITIS

The terms hypersensitivity angiitis and microscopic polyangiitis are used to describe this group of patients to emphasize the frequent association with drug or infectious exposure and the involvement of small vessels (venules and capillaries).[586] Constitutional symptoms similar to those observed in periarteritis nodosa are seen in this disorder as

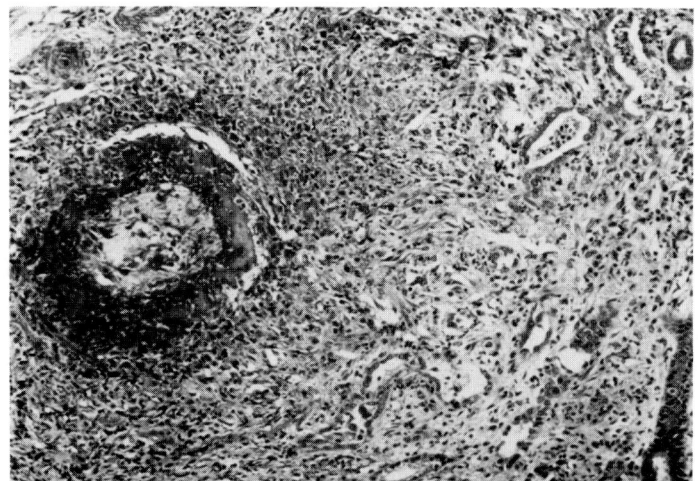

**Figure 31–11.** Light microscopic appearance of necrotizing vasculitis. An arcuate artery has extensive fibrinoid necrosis of the wall and occlusion of the lumen. Pronounced inflammation is seen surrounding the artery and in the adjacent interstitium. (Masson trichrome; magnification × 250.)

well, but hypertension is frequently absent or mild.[1, 582, 586, 589] In general, the patients who develop microscopic polyangiitis are older, averaging about 45 years. Pulmonary involvement may be manifested by asthmatic symptoms and is frequently associated with eosinophilia,[1, 582, 586] although in some classifications, the presence of pulmonary vasculitis precludes a diagnosis of periarteritis nodosa.[620] Cutaneous involvement is common, leading to palpable purpura. Urinalysis reveals hematuria, telescoped sediment, and proteinuria. The last may sometimes be massive. Microangiopathic hemolytic anemia may be observed in this form of systemic vasculitis. Many patients have detectable ANCAs[595a, 597] typically reactive with myeloperoxidase.[695] A history of upper respiratory tract infection or allergic reactions to drugs such as antimicrobial agents is common.[578, 579, 696] Uremia is a frequent occurrence and may develop early in the course of the disease.[578, 579, 696, 697] Many such patients outwardly resemble those with rapidly progressive glomerulonephritis,[697, 698] and may be classified as having type III primary crescentic glomerulonephritis (pauci-immune crescentic glomerulonephritis; see also Chapter 30).[588, 621] Pulmonary hemorrhage also may occur, giving rise to confusion with Goodpasture syndrome.[484, 485, 582, 699] Scattered inflammation and necrotizing lesions involving both small arteries and arterioles may be found in patients with SLE, Schönlein-Henoch purpura, and, rarely, acute poststreptococcal glomerulonephritis and bacterial endocarditis. In such cases, the vessel involvement is not as widespread as that observed in hypersensitivity angiitis. In some cases, the evidence for vasculitis in sites other than the glomerular capillaries or kidney may be scant or nonexistent.

Microscopically, the lesions of hypersensitivity angiitis involve blood vessels of small caliber, including the glomerular capillaries. The lesions are described as a leukocytoclastic vasculitis and often involve postcapillary venules with infiltration of polymorphonuclear leukocytes and monocytes, fibrinoid necrosis, extravasation of erythrocytes, and nuclear debris. The vascular lesions often appear to be at about the same stage of evolution at any point in time. The predominant changes are frequently in the glomeruli; there are segments of necrosis, often with prolifer-

ation of endocapillary cells and segmental or circumferential crescents. Other glomeruli may show localized fibrous scars or collapse of portions of tufts.[1, 484, 485, 583–589, 695]

Electron microscopy does not reveal any characteristic alterations, and electron-dense deposits are seen infrequently. Immunofluorescence studies have usually revealed scant and irregular mesangial and capillary wall deposits of IgG and IgM and complement components[1, 693, 695] (pauci-immune crescentic glomerulonephritis). There is usually a striking deposition of fibrin-related antigens in the Bowman space and in the areas of segmental tuft necrosis. Albumin and other nonimmunologic proteins may also be found in areas of necrosis. Similar findings are seen in some of the affected blood vessels in the kidney or elsewhere.

Immune complex deposition in the walls of vessels has been suggested as a pathogenetic mechanism to explain both microscopic and macroscopic polyarteritis. The inability to find Ig and complement consistently has led many to doubt this hypothesis and to suggest other mechanisms such as cell-mediated immunity or leukocytic activation. However, even in experimental serum sickness arteritis, a disease that is unquestionably of immune complex pathogenesis, the deposits of immune reactants are scant and evanescent. A pathogenetic role for ANCAs has been suggested. As in periarteritis nodosa, some cases may be traced to occult hepatitis B virus infection or other chronic, persistent infectious diseases. α-Antitrypsin deficiency, congenital complement deficiency states, renal cholesterol embolization, Takayasu arteritis, temporal arteritis, T cell lymphoma, and Kawasaki disease have been described as associations.[681, 686, 699, 700]

In an early study of the effect of steroids in this group of disorders conducted by the Medical Research Council, no clear-cut improvements in survival were demonstrated, but many patients showed rapid symptomatic improvement.[701] Hypertension clearly had a deleterious effect on survival. In a retrospective survey, Frohnert and Sheps[702] found a 5-year survival of 48% in steroid-treated cases versus 13% in untreated cases. Prompt recognition and early aggressive treatment were said to decrease the incidence of renal disease, but prolonged treatment was necessary to maintain remission. To what extent this can be attributed to steroids, rather than appropriate concomitant therapy such as antihypertensives, is not known. Large doses of parenteral methylprednisolone have been claimed to be associated with dramatic improvement of clinical findings and renal function.[703] The addition of cytotoxic drugs, including azathioprine, cyclophosphamide, or methotrexate, has been noted to decrease mortality even more,* although in elderly patients such therapy may actually increase mortality.[689] Ninety-three percent of patients so treated survived an average of 26 months, and complete remission was obtained in as many as 20%. In a study from the NIH involving the treatment of 27 patients with diverse forms of systemic vasculitis with steroids and oral cyclophosphamide, complete remission was induced in 26. One patient subsequently died with active vasculitis.[647] Intravenous pulse cyclophosphamide has also been used with beneficial effects, although the relapse rate may be higher than with oral therapy.[654, 655, 705]

Preliminary data of Falk and colleagues,[620] examining patients during a 2-year follow-up period, suggest that oral and intravenous routes of cyclophosphamide administration are equally efficacious. Similar findings were noted by Pall and associates.[706] However, further confirmation and longer follow-up are needed before making definitive recommendations regarding the relative efficacy of these treatment modalities.[620] Combinations of intensive plasma exchange, steroids, and cytotoxic drugs have also been used in patients with vasculitis and rapidly progressive renal failure.[568, 661–663, 709–720] Prospective trials involving patients with polyangiitis or Churg-Strauss syndrome failed to show that plasmapheresis, when added to prednisone, was more efficacious therapy than immunosuppression alone, especially when patients were not dependent on dialysis.[707, 708] Furthermore, complications associated with plasmapheresis occurred in a substantial number of the treatments, including technical difficulties, hypotension, and allergy to the infused replacement fluid.[708] Whether the addition of plasma exchange to a regimen of immunosuppression is beneficial to dialysis-dependent patients remains uncertain.[663] A search for an inciting agent (drug, infection), followed by its removal or treatment, is indicated in all cases, but in general this is not rewarding. A review by Furlong and colleagues[583] described a mortality of nearly 30% after 25 months of follow-up of patients with a variety of types of necrotizing vasculitis demonstrating renal involvement. About 20% of these patients developed end-stage renal failure and were treated by maintenance dialysis. These investigators emphasized the variable course that patients demonstrated regarding progressive versus indolent disease. Few patients with vasculitis who have undergone transplantation have been reported in the literature.[709]

## LYMPHOMATOID GRANULOMATOSIS

This rare disorder is distinguished from other forms of systemic vasculitis by the invasion of the small vessels of various organs by atypical lymphocytoid and plasmacytoid cells.[580, 581, 721] The lesions often have the characteristics of a lymphoproliferative disease. Granulomas are not as copi-

ous as in Wegener granulomatosis, and the vasculitis is neither necrotizing nor leukocytoclastic. Infarction and necrosis of tissue occur by means of compromised blood flow caused by extensive infiltration of the vascular wall.

Lung involvement is common, taking the form of nodular cavitary lesions. The skin and the CNS may also be involved, but the upper respiratory tract is usually spared. Renal involvement is present in about half of patients and is usually mild; it consists of infiltrates of the abnormal cells. Death is often the consequence of the pulmonary or CNS lesions in untreated patients or patients who do not respond to therapy.[580, 581] Malignant lymphoma develops in up to half of these patients.[721] Steroids and cyclophosphamide may be effective in achieving remissions and prolonging survival, but the mortality rate still exceeds 50%.[721] No prospective, randomized controlled study has been done to evaluate the efficacy of therapy.

## ALLERGIC GRANULOMATOUS ANGIITIS

Churg and Strauss[722] in 1951 described 13 cases of a syndrome distinct from both periarteritis nodosa and hypersensitivity angiitis.[580, 581, 723, 724] The patients, of various ages, presented chiefly with severe intractable asthma, fever, and eosinophilia. In some cases, the asthma abated with onset of systemic symptoms referable to vasculitis. Hypertension was uncommon. Mortality was high; heart failure, cerebral hemorrhage, pulmonary disease, and, less commonly, uremia were the causes of death. A characteristic pathologic feature was the presence of necrotizing granulomas containing epithelioid giant cells and the occurrence of eosinophils in many tissues, associated with an arteritis (often granulomatous) involving medium-sized blood vessels similar to that seen in periarteritis nodosa. Both an acute interstitial nephritis with large numbers of eosinophils and a necrotizing lesion of the glomerulus, similar to that seen in hypersensitivity angiitis, were found. Steroids appear to be effective in the management of this condition; the addition of a cytotoxic agent may provide additional benefit as in other examples of vasculitis.

# Renal Involvement in Other Multisystem Diseases

## MIXED CONNECTIVE TISSUE DISEASE

Mixed connective tissue disease is characterized by an admixture of features resembling SLE, polymyositis, and scleroderma.[725] Prominent clinical manifestations are Raynaud phenomenon, dysphagia, sclerodactyly, myalgia and weakness, and nondeforming arthritis. Renal disease is relatively uncommon, affecting only about 10% to 15% of patients, and it is usually mild and nonprogressive.[725–728] Progressive forms of proliferative glomerulonephritis have been described,[729] however, and ESRD with crescentic glomerulonephritis is rare but has been observed. Very high titers of antibody to a saline-extractable, ribonuclease-sensitive nuclear antigen (RNP) are found in most patients.[726] Other autoantibodies to nuclear antigens (e.g., anti-ssDNA

---

*References 584, 589, 620, 644, 664, 703, 704.

or anti-dsDNA) may be found in low titers. Anti-Sm antibodies are usually absent but may be found in low titers. Serum complement component levels are usually normal.[726, 728] When present, renal lesions are usually of the membranous or diffuse proliferative variety.[727, 728] The response to glucocorticoid therapy is generally favorable, but severe renal disease may occasionally require more aggressive management.

## RHEUMATOID ARTHRITIS

Typically, glomerular disease is uncommon in patients with RA.[730, 731] Glomerular amyloidosis may complicate severe and long-standing RA.[730–732] Patients treated with penicillamine or gold (chrysotherapy) may develop membranous glomerulonephritis (see later discussion). HLA-DR specificities may be linked to the susceptibility to membranous glomerulonephritis in gold- or penicillamine-induced disease.[733, 734] Patients with RA have a high incidence of HLA-DR4.[734]

Several reports have suggested that, in addition to the described glomerular lesions, immune complex–mediated glomerulonephritis unrelated to gold or penicillamine therapy may be an integral part of the spectrum of multisystem involvement in RA.[1] Samuels and co-workers[735] described eight patients with RA and membranous glomerulonephritis. Only three patients were receiving gold at the onset of proteinuria; three others had been treated previously with this agent. The authors suggested that RA can be associated de novo with membranous glomerulonephritis and that chrysotherapy does not necessarily play a role in the genesis of the abnormality. Additional small series of cases have been published confirming this postulate.[735–739] A few other patients have been described who have various proliferative immune complex–mediated glomerulonephritides.[740–742] These include necrotizing glomerulonephritis either alone or as a part of rheumatoid vasculitis[743–745] and mesangial proliferative glomerulonephritis with predominant IgA or IgM mesangial deposits.[746–748] This latter group of patients often presents with hematuria, proteinuria, or both. In a series involving 74 patients with RA who had renal biopsies, 31% had mesangial proliferative glomerulonephritis (four of which were IgA nephropathy), 27% had amyloidosis, and only 18% had membranous nephropathy. The remainder had miscellaneous glomerular and tubulointerstitial disorders or nondiagnostic biopsies.[724] A similar spectrum of lesions has been documented in children.[747] Because RA is characterized by persistently high levels of CICs, it is surprising that glomerular disease does not develop more frequently.

## SERONEGATIVE ARTHROPATHIES

In 1970, Linder and Pasternak[749] described glomerulonephritis in one patient with ankylosing spondylitis. IgG and C3 deposits were found in glomeruli. Since then, IgA nephropathy,[750–753] membranous glomerulonephritis,[754] and other immune complex glomerulopathies[755] have been reported in association with HLA-B27–positive ankylosing spondylitis and Reiter syndrome.[751] In addition, mesangial proliferative glomerulonephritis with IgM or with C3 de-

posits alone has been documented.[750] Similar associations between Behçet disease and various forms of glomerulonephritis, particularly with mesangial IgA deposits,[756–759] have also been reported, including focal proliferative glomerulonephritis,[759–763] diffuse proliferative and crescentic glomerulonephritis,[756] segmental necrotizing glomerulonephritis, and secondary amyloidosis.[764] Whether the association with glomerulonephritis in these syndromes is etiologically significant or just fortuitous is not clear. The usefulness of glucocorticoids[761] or plasmapheresis[762] for the renal disease seen in such patients is difficult to assess because of the small numbers of patients treated.

## ACUTE RHEUMATIC FEVER

A mild to moderate glomerulitis, frequently accompanied by mild hematuria and proteinuria, occurs transiently in an appreciable number of patients with acute rheumatic fever.[765] Histologically, a focal proliferative or mild diffuse endocapillary proliferative glomerular lesion is seen, and arteritis is uncommon.[765] An interstitial nephritis may also be seen.[1] Electron microscopy reveals electron-dense deposits in the mesangium, but the humps typical of acute poststreptococcal glomerulonephritis are usually not seen.[765] Rare case reports document the coexistence of acute rheumatic fever with acute poststreptococcal glomeruloncphritis characterized by subepithelial humps.[766–768] CICs develop as commonly in patients with acute rheumatic fever as they do in those with acute poststreptococcal glomerulonephritis.[769] This glomerulopathy is nonprogressive and is usually not accompanied by the nephrotic syndrome.

## RELAPSING POLYCHONDRITIS

Renal involvement has been reported in 22% of patients presenting with relapsing polychondritis.[770] More common systemic manifestations include auricular chondritis (85%), nasal cartilage changes (54%) including saddle-nose deformity (29%), arthritis (52%), scleritis or episcleritis (47%), laryngotracheal-bronchial symptoms (48%), hearing loss (30%), and less commonly costochondritis, cutaneous symptoms, and cardiac valvular dysfunction.[771, 772] Non-nephrotic proteinuria and microhematuria, occasionally with erythrocyte casts, characterized the renal presentation.[770] In patients undergoing renal biopsy for these manifestations, hypertension and azotemia were common.[770] Mesangial cell proliferation, segmental necrotizing glomerulonephritis, crescentic glomerulonephritis, and tubule interstitial changes were the dominant histologic features. Membranous glomerulonephritis may occasionally be observed. Arteritis was absent in the kidney. Antibodies to major and minor collagen components, most commonly to type II[772] but also to types IX, X,[772] and IV (Adler S, personal observation), have been noted. Their contribution to the pathogenesis of the renal disease is uncertain. Renal involvement is associated with shorter survival time.[770] Steroids, cytotoxic agents, and plasmapheresis have been used with some improvement.[770] Cyclosporine has been used to treat the systemic disease, but its effects on the glomerular process are not known.[773]

## SJÖGREN SYNDROME

Sjögren syndrome may be associated in rare instances with a glomerular lesion manifested as heavy proteinuria and consisting either of an otherwise typical membranous glomerulopathy, or less frequently, a focal proliferative mesangiocapillary or cryoglobulin-associated glomerulonephritis.[774–776] Immunofluorescence deposits of IgG, IgM, and C3 in a granular distribution suggest an immune complex–mediated disease.[1] More frequently, acute or chronic interstitial nephritis is seen. Occasionally, granular peritubular deposits of IgG and C3 are seen without significant glomerular deposits.[1] Such patients seem to respond impressively to combinations of steroids and cytotoxic agents. Severe cryoimmunoglobulinemia may also be present[1] (see later discussion). Plasmapheresis has also been used in individual patients in whom severe cryoglobulinemia is present.[776]

## SARCOIDOSIS

Several patients have been described in whom glomerulonephritis coexisted with sarcoidosis. The various glomerular lesions included membranous nephropathy most commonly but also endocapillary proliferative, crescentic, focal, and segmental sclerosing glomerulonephritis. Ig and complement deposits in a granular pattern and electron-dense deposits have been observed. The lesions may be produced by CICs. Nephrotic syndrome has been a common clinical manifestation, occasionally with concurrent renal vein thrombosis.[777–779]

More common renal manifestations of sarcoidosis include interstitial nephritis, interstitial fibrosis, nephrolithiasis, obstructive uropathy, and abnormalities of tubule function including nephrogenic (and occasionally central) diabetes insipidus and renal tubular acidosis. Dramatic responses to glucocorticoids may occur.

## ERYTHEMA MULTIFORME AND TOXIC EPIDERMAL NECROLYSIS

Sporadic case reports have appeared in which evidence of clinical renal involvement has accompanied these disorders.[780] The findings are chiefly those of microscopic he-

maturia and mild proteinuria, but a few cases of more severe renal disease have been reported. Krumlovsky and associates[780] recorded the development of acute renal failure and nephrotic syndrome associated with a membranous and proliferative glomerulonephritis in a patient with toxic epidermal necrolysis. In this review, 22 of 128 patients with toxic epidermal necrolysis were found to have some clinical evidence of renal disease.[780] Because of the similarity of these skin diseases to SLE, a diligent search for serologic evidence of lupus should be made in every case.

Reports of psoriasis, Sézary syndrome, mycosis fungoides, dermatitis herpetiformis, and celiac disease associated with IgA nephropathy have been described (see Chapter 30). The exact relation of these disorders to the glomerulopathy is uncertain.

## DYSPROTEINEMIAS AND PARAPROTEINEMIAS

### Cryoimmunoglobulinemia

Abnormal circulating Igs that precipitate in the cold may occur in a variety of disease states, including SLE, acute poststreptococcal glomerulonephritis, systemic vasculitis, leukemia, hepatitis C and other acute and chronic infections, Sjögren syndrome, Waldenström macroglobulinemia, and multiple myeloma.[781–799] They may also be found in the absence of an identifiable systemic illness (essential cryoglobulinemia). The ability of these proteins to precipitate at 4°C may be related to their content of fibronectin (cold-insoluble globulin). Frequently, cryoglobulins are composed of Igs with rheumatoid factor activity.[790, 797, 800, 801] Data suggest that the development of glomerulonephritis is dependent on the cryoglobulin activity of the Ig, whereas skin vasculitis requires both cryoglobulin and rheumatoid factor activity.[800] This suggests that there are basic pathogenetic differences between skin and renal vasculitis. The subject of cryoglobulinemia has been dealt with by extensive monographs.[797, 798, 800]

Any of the major Ig classes can be found, but IgG and IgM are the most frequent. Three basic types of cryoimmunoglobulinemia are recognized[787, 790, 797] (Table 31–4):

**TABLE 31–4. Cryoimmunoglobulinemia: Classification and Clinical Correlations**

| Type | Ig Class/Concentration | Associated Diseases |
|---|---|---|
| I. Monoclonal cryoIg | IgM > IgG > IgA > BJP* >500 mg/dL in 60% | Multiple myeloma Waldenström macroglobulinemia |
| II. Mixed cryoIg with monoclonal component | IgM/IgG > > IgG/IgG Rheumatoid factor + + >500 mg/dL in 40% | Sjögren syndrome Waldenström macroglobulinemia Lymphoma Hepatitis C |
| III. Mixed polyclonal cryoIg | IgM/IgG < 100 mg/dL in 80% | Chronic infections SLE Systemic vasculitis Neoplasia |

*BJP = Bence Jones protein.
After Brouet JC, Claurel JP, Danon F, et al: Biologic and clinical significance of cryoglobulins: A review of 86 cases. Am J Med 57:775, 1974.

Type I) A single monoclonal Ig class having no recognizable antibody activity is present. This type is most frequently associated with hematopoietic malignancy. Type II) A mixture of two or more Ig classes, one of which is a monoclonal antibody directed to epitopes on IgG (aIgA) (mixed type). This variety is also called mixed (IgG-IgM) cryoimmunoglobulinemia because of the frequent presence of IgM and IgG in the cryoprecipitates; the monoclonal IgM possesses rheumatoid factor activity and is commonly associated with glomerular disease. The frequent association of this disorder with infection suggests that many cases may be due to occult infections with viruses or bacteria (particularly hepatitis C virus; see later). Type III) One or more different Ig classes are present, none of which are homogeneous (polyclonal type), but anti-IgG activity is present. This type is most frequently associated with inflammatory or autoimmune disorders, such as poststreptococcal glomerulonephritis and SLE. cryoIg-containing antibodies to native DNA can appear in the serum in response to infectious stimuli (e.g., parasitic infestation), even if features of SLE are lacking.[802, 803]

## MIXED (IgG-IgM) CRYOIMMUNOGLOBULINEMIA (TYPE II)

The development of cold-precipitable mixed IgG-IgM with rheumatoid factor activity may be associated with findings such as purpuric and necrotizing skin lesions in exposed areas, acroparesthesia, Raynaud phenomenon, urticaria, neuritis, arthralgia, fever, and hepatosplenomegaly.[1, 784, 797, 804] The proteins may circulate as separate or perhaps loosely associated entities, but in some fashion they aggregate or precipitate in peripheral blood vessels or glomeruli.[1, 784, 797] Glomerular involvement may develop acutely, particularly after dehydration or transient exposure to the cold and may be associated with oliguric acute renal failure.[1, 782, 788, 790–799, 805] Perhaps the increased protein concentration in the glomerular capillaries is a factor that enhances their vulnerability in these disorders. Immune complexes from patients with essential mixed cryoglobulinemia stimulate the synthesis of interleukin-1 by monocytes, perhaps thereby contributing to local inflammatory processes.[806] Fragments of laminin are present in the serum in high concentrations in patients with essential mixed cryoglobulinemia with visceral involvement, and this increase appears to correlate with disease activity.[807] The latter may result from local tissue injury, rather than cause it. The development of cryoIg-associated glomerulonephritis may also be related to defective reticuloendothelial system Fc receptor function.[808]

Strong evidence exists that links chronic infection with hepatitis C virus and type II mixed cryoglobulinemia (see later).[809–814] Hepatitis B virus infection, although sometimes concomitantly present, does not often seem to be involved in the cause of cryoglobulinemia.[814] Anti–hepatitis C viral antibody, hepatitis C viral core antigens, and hepatitis C RNA can be found in cryoglobulins and in the renal deposits of patients with hepatitis C virus infection associated with mixed (IgG-IgM) cryoglobulinemia.[809–814] Interferon alfa therapy may transiently improve the clinical features.[810]

It has been estimated that 50% to 75% of patients with "essential" mixed IgG-IgM cryoglobulinemia have underlying chronic hepatitis C virus infection.[811]

Type I cryoIgs appear to precipitate in the cold more rapidly than do those of the type II variety, and plasma viscosity may increase in both varieties, causing symptoms of retinal or renal dysfunction. Leukocyte counts may also be falsely elevated in cryoimmunoglobulinemia when automated counter methodologies are employed because of formation of macroaggregates. The erythrocyte sedimentation rate is higher at 37°C than at room temperature. The C4 concentration is often depressed to a greater extent than is C3 concentration.[813]

Other clinical syndromes may occur, including nephrotic syndrome and asymptomatic proteinuria and hematuria, with or without functional renal impairment.[782, 797] Pulmonary involvement with hemorrhage may also occur.[804, 815] Mixed type II cryoIg may be found in association with typical renal and systemic clinical manifestations in heroin addicts without concomitant evidence of infectious endocarditis, probably because of concomitant hepatitis C virus infection (see later), but hepatitis B virus infection could also be a contributing factor.[816, 817] In one series, 3 of 13 patients with type II essential mixed cryoglobulinemia eventually developed a lymphoproliferative disease years after their initial presentation.[798] Renal disease is especially common if the concentration of circulating cryoIg exceeds 1 g/dL.

In patients with acute renal failure, light microscopy usually reveals a diffuse endocapillary proliferative or mesangiocapillary lesion with crescents in a few glomeruli and numerous subendothelial deposits (Fig. 31–12) and large, rounded intraluminal thrombi. The thrombi may represent large subendothelial deposits, or they may be actual intraluminal precipitates of cryoglobulins, sometimes within monocytes. These cells are particularly prevalent in these lesions as revealed by nonspecific esterase stains.[1, 791–798] Frank vasculitis is seen in one third of renal biopsy speci-

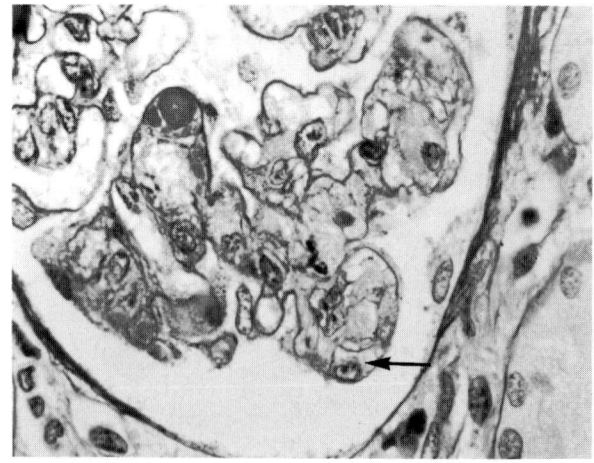

**Figure 31–12.** Light microscopic appearance of essential mixed (IgG-IgM) cryoimmunoglobulinemia. A hyaline thrombus fills a capillary lumen; there are segmental changes of mesangial interposition *(arrow).* (Periodic acid–Schiff; magnification × 1000.)

mens. Immunofluorescence microscopy reveals granular capillary wall and mesangial deposits and intraluminal masses of C3, IgM, and IgG that are immunologically similar to the circulating cryoglobulins[817, 818] (Fig. 31–13). Typically, only trace amounts of Clq are present.[817] IgM may also be found in the interstitium.[817] Electron microscopy may reveal large intracapillary deposits (Fig. 31–14) and may show electron-dense deposits with a crystalline substructure.[1, 817, 819, 820]

Reduction in the level of cryoglobulins by intensive plasma exchange may be associated with a reversal of the lesion and a clinical remission.[791, 801, 802] Combinations of prednisone and cyclophosphamide may be helpful in controlling the manifestations of the disease. The use of pulse methylprednisolone therapy often followed by long-term oral prednisolone and cytotoxic therapy has been shown to be efficacious in treating renal and systemic manifestations of cryoglobulinemia.[801, 820, 821] Treatment with high-dose interferon alfa (2 million to 10 million U three times per week for 2 to 12 months) has been helpful in cases associated with hepatitis C virus infection, but relapses are not uncommon.[810, 813]

## Waldenström Macroglobulinemia

Waldenström macroglobulinemia, a syndrome of a homogeneous increase in monoclonal IgM associated with lymphoid cell proliferation, may occasionally be associated with glomerular lesions.[1, 789, 822–824a] Proteinuria is common but usually mild, and it may at times be related to excessive excretion of low-molecular-weight Bence Jones protein.[822–824] Hematuria may also be present, and giant kidneys have been observed. Fifty percent to 60% of patients with macroglobulinemia may exhibit neoplastic involvement of the kidney.[825] Plasmacytoid cells and IgM in the urine usually confirm the diagnosis. Massive proteinuria and the nephrotic syndrome may develop and are frequently associ-

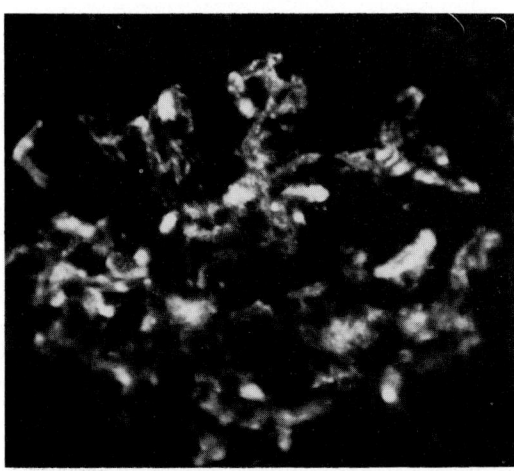

**Figure 31–13.** Immunofluorescence microscopic appearance of essential mixed (IgG-IgM) cryoimmunoglobulinemia. Diffuse mesangial staining and large rounded (probably intracapillary) masses, the latter corresponding to thrombi, are evident. (Antihuman IgM; magnification × 225.)

ated with azotemia. Renal amyloidosis is uncommon but may be found, especially in patients presenting with nephrotic syndrome. Monoclonal (type I) cryoimmunoglobulinemia may develop.[789, 824] Rarely, anti-GBM antibody disease may appear. A unique but uncommon feature is the development of acute renal failure, associated with intraglomerular occlusive thrombi or coagula consisting of the IgM protein but unassociated with hypercellularity or capillary wall changes.[822] By light microscopy, these masses are eosinophilic, periodic acid–Schiff–positive, and red or green with trichrome stains, indicating their glycopeptide nature. They show no reaction to fibrin and lipid stains.[822] Intratubular cast formation such as that found in multiple myeloma is rarely seen. Immunofluorescence microscopy demonstrates massive intracapillary deposits of the paraprotein, usually not accompanied by C3. Treatment by intensive plasma exchange and alkylating agents is indicated.[1, 822]

## Benign Monoclonal Gammopathy

Benign monoclonal gammopathy is characterized by a monoclonal elevation of IgG, IgA, IgM, or other Ig classes in the absence of known inciting disease, such as parasitic infestations, lymphomas, visceral malignancies, chronic infections, hypersensitivity disorders, multiple myeloma, or Waldenström macroglobulinemia.[826] Patients with this disorder usually have less than 2.0 g/dL of the monoclonal protein in the serum. Such patients may display mild proteinuria (other than Bence Jones proteinuria), hematuria, and, rarely, the nephrotic syndrome.[1, 782] Renal biopsy specimens have revealed various glomerular alterations that usually are mild. These include periodic acid–Schiff–negative intraglomerular deposits that may be accompanied by endocapillary proliferation.[789] Deposits of the circulating Ig not accompanied by complement components may be found by immunofluorescence microscopy. This renal disease is usually nonprogressive; however, more than 20% of these patients go on to manifest an overt plasma cell neoplasm.[826] Amyloidosis was found in two of seven patients described by Verroust and associates,[826a] and these authors have also described a case of membranous glomerulopathy developing in a patient with benign monoclonal IgM gammopathy.[1] Additional cases of proliferative glomerulonephritis have been described.[827–830] Crescentic glomerulonephritis has been reported in a variety of paraproteinemias, some of which developed into frank malignancies.[831, 832]

## Multiple Myeloma

Hypercalcemia, hyperuricosuria, renal tubular acidosis, "myeloma kidney," and rarely plasma cell infiltration of the renal parenchyma dominate the renal manifestations of multiple myeloma. In patients with myeloma kidney, heavy Bence Jones proteinuria may be observed.[833] The clinical presentation is characterized by acute or chronic progressive renal insufficiency. In contrast, less commonly, when the glomerulus is affected, renal disease takes the form of either AL amyloid deposition, monoclonal Ig deposit dis-

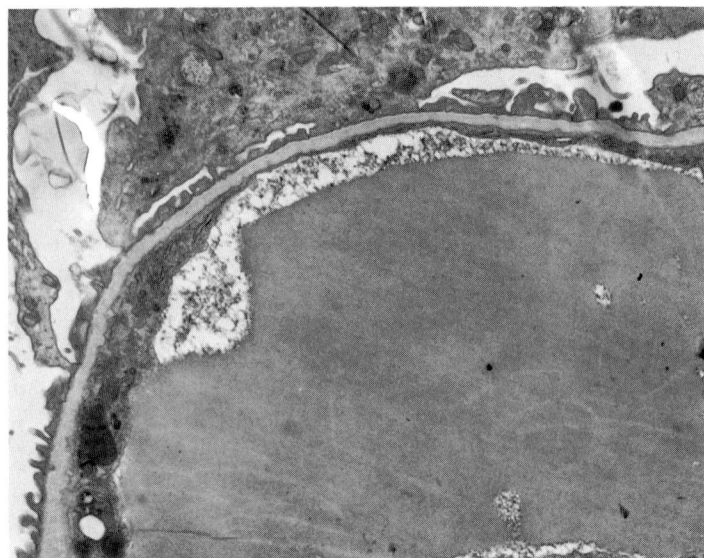

**Figure 31–14.** Electron microscopic appearance of essential mixed (IgG-IgM) cryoimmunoglobulinemia. This material often has a fibrillar substructure. (Magnification × 11,400.)

ease, or immune complex glomerulopathy.[834, 835] Patients present with heavy proteinuria reflecting both overflow of the abnormal monoclonal Ig and nonselective glomerular proteinuria, consisting largely but not exclusively of albumin. Hematuria and elevated serum creatinine levels are common.[836]

The pathogenetic causes for glomerular paraprotein deposition in myeloma are unknown. Specific physicochemical properties of the paraprotein, such as size, charge, aggregability, and glycosylation, have been implicated, but none of these factors explains all cases observed and numerous exceptions are reported.[837] However, data clearly demonstrate that intrinsic physicochemical properties of the paraprotein, rather than features of the host, define the disorder. When injected into mice, myeloma proteins from patients reproduce in the mouse kidneys the renal lesions observed in the patients.[838]

Renal insufficiency was once thought to independently confer a poor prognosis for survival in patients with multiple myeloma. However, tumor burden and responsiveness to therapy now seem to be more important prognostic factors, with severe and irreversible renal failure often a surrogate marker for more extensive disease.[836, 839] Treatment strategies for patients with myeloma kidney and/or monoclonal Ig deposit disease are somewhat controversial. Noncontroversial elements include treatment of hypercalcemia and hyperuricemia and hydration to prevent intrarenal precipitation of Ig molecules.[836] Although also frequently recommended, the additive effect of urinary alkalinization in preventing Ig precipitation is probably minimal if adequate hydration is achieved.[837] Plasmapheresis in combination with chemotherapy has been advocated as beneficial in improving renal function by some but not all. The majority of patients so treated had myeloma kidney rather than glomerular involvement.[840, 841] Renal transplantation has been performed in patients with ESRD.[842] However, susceptibility to infection, overall short survival of patients, and the potential for recurrence in the transplanted kidney limit the appropriateness of this intervention in this setting to rare individuals.[842]

## Monoclonal Immunoglobulin Deposition Diseases (Light and/or Heavy Chain Nephropathies)

Light and heavy chain nephropathies, also called monoclonal Ig deposit diseases (Randall type),[843–845] are uncommon disorders in which deposits of monoclonal Ig light and/or heavy chains and electron-dense material are found within the glomerular and tubule basement membranes. These disorders are often, but not always, seen in association with multiple myeloma or other plasma cell dyscrasia.[843–845] In these disorders, there is typically deposition of the abnormal light chain in renal basement membranes: tubule, glomerular, and vascular. In addition, there is often concomitant deposition in the glomerular mesangium (Fig. 31–15). This last feature results in varying degrees of glomerular damage, most commonly in the form of nodular glomerulosclerosis[844–855] (Fig. 31–16), but glomeruli may be structurally normal or hypercellular, sometimes with crescents.[844–855] Immunohistochemical studies have disclosed, in almost all instances, basement membrane fixation of a monoclonal light and/or heavy chain, and deposits of complement have been observed.[844, 845, 855, 856] In about 80% of reported cases, κ light chain has been described; the reason for this predominance is unclear.[854] The GBM deposits have been localized by immunoelectron microscopy to the lamina rara interna.[854] In this location in the mesangium, they usually appear as finely granular material of varying electron density, which, in the capillary walls, occurs in a continuous pattern[844, 845, 847–855] (Fig. 31–17). Some reports have emphasized the presence of fine fibrils (11 to 14 nm) within the deposits,[847] whereas a single unconfirmed study indicated long-spacing collagen within the mesangium.[1]

The histologic appearance of nodular glomerular lesions is similar to diabetic nodular glomerulosclerosis of Kimmelstiel-Wilson, and, as a result, the differentiation between these two entities may be difficult at the light microscopic level of examination.[1, 844–845, 847–855] The nodules are usually hypocellular in diabetes and may also have a reduced cell

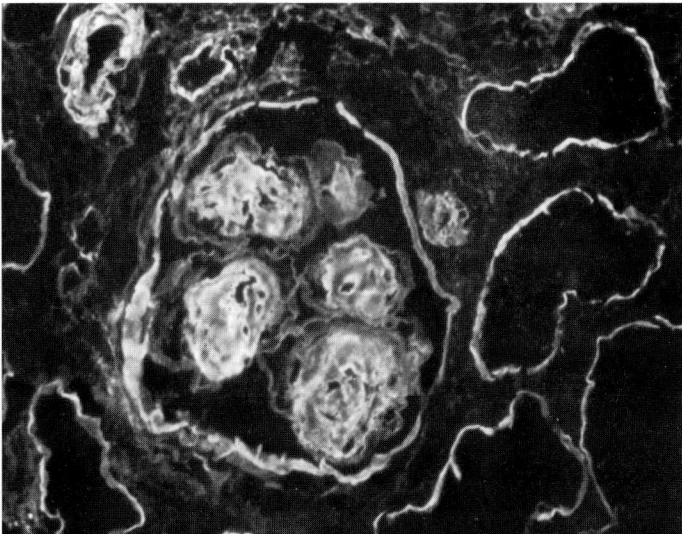

**Figure 31–15.** Immunofluorescence microscopic appearance of light chain nephropathy. There is linear staining for κ light chain along tubule basement membranes and GBM and mesangial nodules. (Magnification × 300.)

population in light chain disease. Capillary microaneurysms, traditionally considered an integral feature of diabetes, have also been shown to occur with considerable frequency in light chain disease.[855] The staining characteristic of the nodules may be helpful: they are strongly periodic acid–Schiff–positive but irregularly argyrophilic in light and/or heavy chain disease and less periodic acid–Schiff–positive and more likely to be argyrophilic in diabetes, the latter in well-developed but not far-advanced lesions. Perhaps the most important distinguishing feature is in the arterioles: the demonstration of hyalinization of both afferent and efferent vessels is virtually limited to diabetes. The ultrastructural findings are reasonably distinctive. In diabetes, the basement membranes are thickened and the lamina densa is homogeneous in staining; in light and/or heavy chain disease, the lamina densa may be thickened, but frequently a continuous layer of finely granular dense material is present in the lamina densa. This substance may also be found in the mesangium, impregnating increased matrix, and is almost always observed along the outer aspects of tubule basement membranes. The most characteristic distinguishing feature is, of course, determined by immunofluorescence microscopy. In light and/or heavy chain disease,

there is linear staining for the abnormal Ig chain along tubule basement membranes, GBMs, and mesangial nodules, but glomerular staining may sometimes be scant or even absent. In diabetes, the linear staining is for albumin and IgG. Amyloid P component is lacking.[1]

Monoclonal Ig deposition diseases may occur in the absence of overt multiple myeloma,[844, 845, 847, 850, 854] with somewhat more than 60% of reported cases having well-documented myeloma or another lymphoplasmacytic disorder at the time of or after discovery of the nephropathy.[854] The remainder of the patients do not have a significant increase in plasma cells. Some studies have documented the production of abnormal monoclonal protein by numerically and morphologically normal plasma cells.[847]

The usual renal manifestations consist of heavy proteinuria and renal insufficiency.[844, 845, 847] Proteinuria may be of glomerular origin with nephrotic syndrome or may be exclusively of the abnormal chain. Abnormal monoclonal light chain excretion may also be seen in patients with diabetes.[852–855] Hematuria is rarely observed. Renal insufficiency may progress to end-stage renal failure necessitating dialysis or transplantation; recurrence of renal damage was well documented in a single case.[849] In a study by Alpers

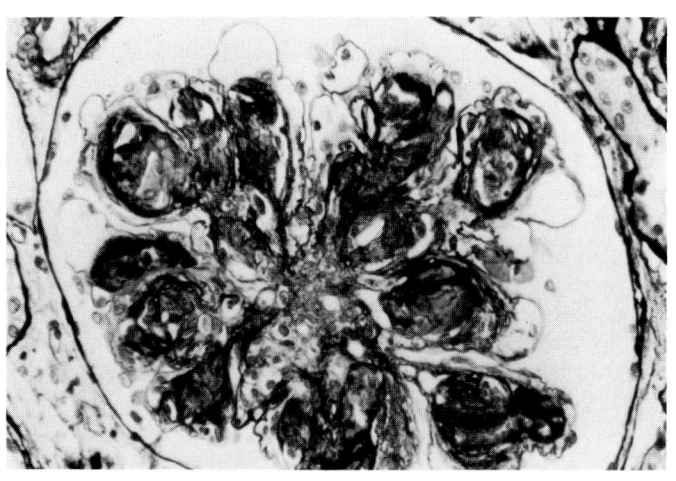

**Figure 31–16.** Light microscopic appearance of glomerulus in light chain nephropathy. Nodular transformation of the tuft, with an increased mesangial matrix, is evident. Aneurysmal dilation of the capillaries is also present. (Periodic acid–methenamine silver; magnification × 400.)

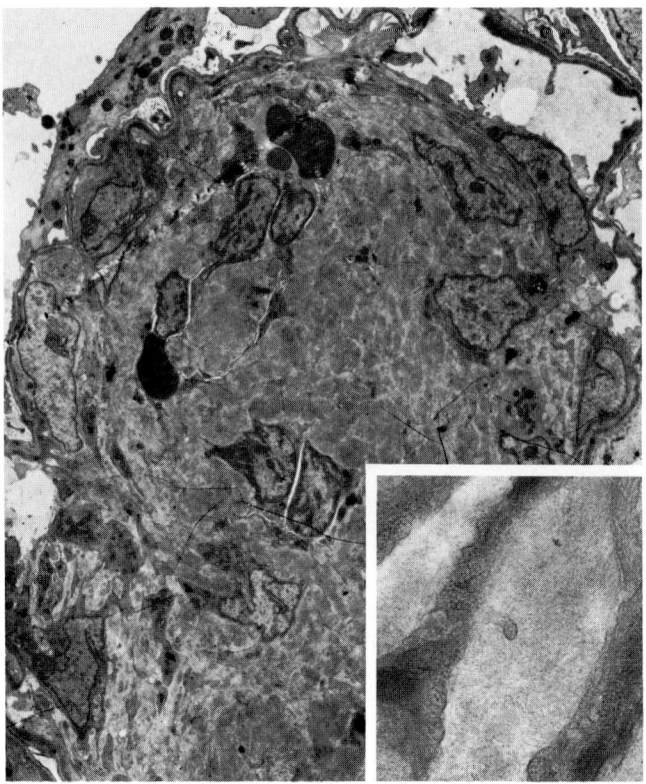

**Figure 31–17.** Electron microscopic appearance of light chain nodular glomerulosclerosis in multiple myeloma. The mesangial nodule consists of numerous confluent deposits. The overlying capillaries are dilated, and the basement membranes are more electron dense. (Magnification × 3500.) *Inset.* High magnification of mesangial deposits showing finely fibrillar substructure. (Magnification × 35,700.)

and co-workers,[856] all 11 patients with κ light chain disease showing glomerulosclerosis were alive after 6 months to 17 years of follow-up. Four developed ESRD, and two received renal transplants without recurrence.

The renal deposition is but a part of a systemic disease process.[844, 845, 853–855, 856a] Although the major clinical manifestations are of renal damage, monoclonal Ig deposits have been noted in liver, heart, skin, nerve and choroid plexus, spleen, thyroid, adrenal glands, gastrointestinal tract, and large vessels.[844, 845, 847] Disordered function of liver and heart are relatively common.[854] Treatment with cytotoxic drugs (melphalan and prednisone) may diminish proteinuria and improve renal function.[854] The 5-year renal survival is about 40%.[853]

## Amyloidosis

Amyloidosis represents a diverse family of chronic infiltrative disorders characterized by the presence of extracellular deposits of insoluble fibrillar proteins. There are several varieties of amyloidosis, each of which is identified by the immunochemical nature of the amyloid protein fibrils[858, 859] (Table 31–5). The common features of all the amyloid proteins are their β-pleated sheet configuration on x-ray diffraction examination, their fine fibrillar nonbranching appearance by electron microscopy, and their apple-green birefringence when tissue is examined under polarized light after staining with Congo red. Amyloid proteins codeposit with glycosaminoglycans, usually in association with amyloid P component.[860, 861]

The diagnosis of amyloidosis is suspected on the basis of clinical features (see later) and is established by biopsy,

although the best approach to tissue selection is controversial. In AL or AA amyloidosis, subcutaneous fat pad aspiration is positive as often as 70% to 80% of the time[862] and bone marrow biopsy approximately 50% of the time.[863] Rectal biopsy has been estimated to be up to 73% positive if sufficient submucosal tissue is obtained at biopsy,[864] and the sensitivity of an adequate kidney biopsy in proteinuric patients approaches 100%. The increased concern regarding hemostasis after liver biopsy does not seem to apply to renal biopsies. Other potential sites for tissue examination include the gingiva and skin (low sensitivity), gastric mucosa, and small intestine. Gastric examination may be positive by endoscopic brush cytology as well as by biopsy.[865] Synovial tissue removed after carpal tunnel release is invariably positive, but often such tissue is not sent for diagnostic evaluation.

A number of noninvasive studies may suggest the presence of amyloidosis. Serum protein electrophoresis or immunoelectrophoresis discloses a monoclonal paraprotein in almost two thirds of patients, and when urine is also examined, the yield increases to 86%.[866] Immunoelectropheresis and immunofixation are occasionally required to detect small quantities of protein that may be obscured on a screening serum or urine electrophoresis.[866] Two-dimensional echocardiography is highly sensitive in detecting cardiac amyloid.[867] The presence of Howell-Jolly bodies on the peripheral blood smear may connote splenic involvement.[866] Radionuclide scanning has been utilized to detect amyloid deposits. Original enthusiasm for $^{99m}$Tc has dissipated because of lack of sensitivity of this assay.[866, 868] Scintigraphy with $^{123}$I-labeled serum amyloid P component appears promising for AA and AL amyloid.[869] Imaging of β$_2$-microglobulin (β$_2$-M)–containing amyloid has been re-

**TABLE 31–5. Classification of Amyloidosis**

| Historical Classification | Major Molecular Component | Glomerular Involvement |
|---|---|---|
| Primary (AL) | | |
|   Associated with multiple myeloma | Ig light chains | + |
|   No identifiable plasma cell dyscrasia | | + |
| Secondary (AA) | | |
|   Associated with chronic infectious, immune, inflammatory, and neoplastic disorders | Serum amyloid A apolipoprotein (AA) | + |
| $\beta_2$-Microglobulin ($\beta_2$-M) | | |
|   Long-term hemodialysis | $\beta_2$-Microglobulin | − |
| Heredofamilial (AF) | | |
|   Nephropathic varieties | | |
|     Familial Mediterranean fever | AA | + |
|     Muckle-Wells | ? | + |
|     Ostertag | ? | + |
|     Zalin | Apolipoprotein A-1 | + |
|   Neuropathic varieties | | |
|     Type I, Japanese, Portuguese, Swedish | $Met^{30}$ prealbumin | − |
|     Type II, German, Swiss, Indiana, Maryland | $Gly^{49}/Ile^{33}$ prealbumin | − |
|     Type III, English, Irish, Scottish, Iowa | Apolipoprotein A-1 ($Gly^{26} \rightarrow Arg^{26}$) | − |
|     Type IV, Finnish | Gelsolin | + |
|      | | + |
|     Danish | $Met^{110}$ prealbumin | − |
|     Appalachian | $Ala^{60}$ prealbumin | − |
|     Icelandic | Cystatin C | − |
|     Trisomy 21, Dutch cerebral amyloid angiopathy, Alzheimer disease | Alzheimer $\beta$-protein | − |
| Endocrine associated (EA) | | |
|   Type II diabetes, pancreas (IAPP) | Islet polypeptide | − |
|   Medullary thyroid carcinoma | Calcitonin | − |
| Senile (AS) | | |
|   Cardiac (ASC) | Prealbumin | − |
|   Isolated atrial (IAA) | Atrial natriuretic peptide | − |
|   Brain (ASB) | A4 or B | − |
| Localized (AL) | Ig light chains | − |

ported after intravenous injection with radiolabeled $\beta_2$-M.[870] Renal involvement may occur in the absence of a recognized underlying disease (primary amyloidosis), in which the AL type of protein fibril predominates, or may be the result of secondary involvement, wherein protein AA occurs in association with a variety of inflammatory, immune, infectious, hereditary, or neoplastic states. Some manifestations of renal disease are found in three fourths or more of patients with amyloidosis. In addition to the primary and secondary syndromes, amyloidosis may be associated with a wide variety of other disorders (see Table 31–5).

## PRIMARY AMYLOIDOSIS

**Clinical Features, Course, and Therapy.** Primary amyloidosis is due to tissue infiltration of organs by the $NH_2$-terminal portion of the variable region of Ig light chains (AL). It is presumed that this protein product is derived from a monoclonal population of plasma cells, thus placing primary amyloidosis in the spectrum of plasma cell dyscrasias. Bone marrow examination most often shows increased numbers of plasma cells, making the distinction from multiple myeloma difficult at times. Primary amyloidosis is more likely to be present than multiple myeloma if the number of bone marrow plasma cells is less than 25%, the monoclonal protein in serum or urine is present in small amounts, and there is no associated anemia, hypercalcemia, or lytic bone lesions.[866] The amyloid protein of both primary amyloidosis and multiple myeloma is of the AL type.

Primary amyloidosis should be suspected clinically when the function of the heart, kidney, liver, synovium, skin, tongue, and/or gastrointestinal tract is compromised by the presence of an infiltrative substance. Men are affected more often than women, with the median age at presentation 63 years for the former and 59 for the latter.[866] Few cases have been reported before the age of 40.[866] Most often, multiple organ involvement is present, with the kidney most frequently affected (50%), followed by heart (40%), carpal tunnel (26%), peripheral or autonomic nervous system (19%), liver (16%), and purpuric skin lesions (5% to 15%).[866, 871]

Nonspecific symptoms such as weight loss, weakness, and fatigue are common. Renal involvement is manifested predominantly by edema. Thirty percent to 40% of patients with primary amyloidosis develop nephrotic syndrome,[866, 871] and some present with lesser amounts of proteinuria. More than half have some degree of azotemia at presentation. The degree of glomerular amyloid deposition correlates poorly with renal function.[872] Most but not all patients have poorly selective proteinuria, and the urinary proteins may include a broad range of plasma proteins and monoclonal protein (the latter in 76% of patients).[873] Elevated serum cholesterol levels are observed somewhat less frequently than in other forms of nephrotic syndrome.[874] The urinalysis is characteristically benign, but microhematuria and cellular casts are rarely observed.[875] Hypertension is uncommon, occurring in 20% to 50% of patients, a figure lower than one might expect given the prevalence of renal insufficiency in this population.[876] In contrast, orthostatic hypotension as a feature of the autonomic neuropathy is characteristic. Adrenal insufficiency may occur.[866] Renal enlargement has been reported but is neither specific nor sensitive as an aid in diagnosis. Renal tubule functional compromise occasionally occurs, including renal tubular acidosis and impairment in urinary concentrating capacity.

The median survival of patients with primary amyloidosis is 20.4 months, with a 5-year survival rate of 19.6%.[866] The presence of congestive heart failure,[866] elevated serum creatinine level,[873, 877] and interstitial fibrosis on renal biopsy specimens[872] affect overall prognosis unfavorably. Patients with urinary λ monoclonal proteins have shorter survival times (12 months) than patients with κ monoclonal protein (30 months) and are more likely to have nephrotic-range proteinuria.[873]

Treatment strategies remain controversial, as the response rate to alkylating therapy is low (approximately 18%) and the risk of inducing a dysmyelopoietic syndrome or frank leukemia is high (approximately 4%), especially when the course of treatment exceeds a year.[877] However, in one retrospective study, patients who responded to therapy with prednisone and alkylating agents survived a mean of 89.4 months, compared with 14.7 months for patients who failed to respond.[877]

Occasionally, dramatic responses to treatment with melphalan, prednisone, and colchicine are seen.[878] The presence of renal insufficiency marginally decreases the likelihood of a positive response to treatment.[877] The efficacy of colchicine and dimethyl sulfoxide in the treatment of primary amyloidosis is uncertain, but anecdotal reports suggest some benefit, particularly for the former.[879]

Approximately 18% of patients with primary amyloidosis are dialyzed, and the median survival time for these patients is 8.2 months after the start of dialytic therapy.[880] Two thirds died of complications of cardiac amyloid.[880] No survival advantage was noted for peritoneal dialysis over hemodialysis.[880] Few patients with amyloidosis have received transplants. Most transplant recipients have AA rather than AL amyloid. Recurrent amyloidosis has been reported in allografts, and cadaveric graft survival during a 3-year follow-up is less in some series and approximately equal in others compared with that of patients undergoing transplantation for primary glomerular disorders.[866, 881] Transplant patients with amyloidosis have shorter survival times than transplant recipients who do not have amyloidosis.[881] Colchicine is utilized to minimize the risk of recurrence in the allograft in secondary forms of amyloidosis[882, 883] and by extension is often recommended in the setting of AL amyloid, although its efficacy in this setting requires additional study.

## SECONDARY AMYLOIDOSIS

The major infiltrative protein in AA amyloidosis is a proteolytic cleavage product of serum amyloid A (AA)

protein, an apolipoprotein acute-phase reactant whose synthesis by the liver increases under the influence of interleukin-1.[884, 885] It exists as multiple isoforms, consists of 76 to 83 amino acids, and has a mass of approximately 86 kd. Its accumulation in serum and subsequent deposition in tissues occur in a wide variety of chronic infectious, inflammatory, immune, genetic, and neoplastic disorders (Table 31–6).

**Clinical Features, Course, and Therapy.** In the preantibiotic era, infectious causes of secondary amyloidosis were most common, with tuberculosis, syphilis, and osteomyelitis predominating. Before the emergence of drug-resistant tuberculosis, the latter had virtually disappeared as a cause of amyloidosis, and syphilis and osteomyelitis had become minor contributors.[863] Although the overall incidence of amyloidosis from infectious causes has declined, our ability to maintain longer term survival in patients suffering traumatic paraplegia or quadriplegia has resulted in an increase in amyloidosis in this group,[886] probably as a result of chronic urinary tract infections and/or decubitus ulcers. In these individuals with amyloidosis, glomerular involvement approaches 25%. Initial nephrotic syndrome followed by progressive renal insufficiency is the rule. Chronic skin infections associated with subcutaneous her-

**TABLE 31–6. Conditions Complicated by Secondary Amyloidosis (AA)**

**Chronic Inflammatory Disorders**
Rheumatoid arthritis
Ankylosing spondylitis
Psoriatic arthritis
Sjögren syndrome
Reiter syndrome
Behçet syndrome
Juvenile rheumatoid arthritis
Whipple disease
Inflammatory bowel disease
SLE (rare)
Polymyositis
Scleroderma
Third-degree burns
Takayasu arteritis

**Chronic Infectious Diseases**
Tuberculosis
Osteomyelitis
Paraplegia
Heroin abuse (skin popping associated with chronic suppuration)
Bronchiectasis
Leprosy
Syphilis
Cystic fibrosis
HIV infection
Xanthogranulomatous pyelonephritis

**Neoplastic Disorders**
Multiple myeloma
Hodgkin disease
Renal cell carcinoma
Medullary carcinoma of the thyroid
Waldenström macroglobulinemia
Uterine cervical cancer

**Familial Disorders**
Familial Mediterranean fever
Glycogen storage disease, type Ib
Astrocytoma

oin injection (''skin popping'') have also been associated with AA amyloidosis and progressive renal insufficiency.[887] Almost half of the 64 patients in a series had RA as an underlying cause, and an additional 17 patients had other rheumatologic and/or immunologic disorders,[863] making immune and inflammatory causes the most important predisposing factors currently. The underlying disease was present for a mean of 18.3 years (range 0.2 to 42.7 years) at the time of diagnosis of amyloidosis, with 73% of patients chronically ill for more than a decade at diagnosis.[863]

Familial Mediterranean fever (FMF) involves a unique subset of patients with secondary amyloidosis. Unlike most other hereditary forms of amyloidosis, in which a variety of different deposited proteins have been identified (see Table 31–5), in FMF the deposited protein is AA amyloid. The disorder is inherited in an autosomal recessive pattern and most commonly affects Sephardic Jews, Turks, Armenians, and Arabs,[1, 888–890] but the disease has also been reported in patients from Iran, France, Italy, Greece, Holland, Spain, and Sweden.[891] Glomerular amyloidosis with proteinuria (often nephrotic syndrome) and progressive renal insufficiency occurs frequently. (Occasionally, other forms of glomerular involvement have been reported, including mesangial proliferative glomerulonephritis with either IgA or IgM predominating.[888, 891]) Two phenotypic presentations of FMF occur with amyloidosis. In one, multiple febrile episodes of serositis and synovitis beginning in childhood precede the development of amyloidosis by many years. In the second, the patient presents predominantly with the renal findings of glomerular amyloid deposition, characterized by nephrotic syndrome and progressive renal insufficiency. The prevalence of amyloidosis among reported patients with FMF varies substantially (range 0% to 60%). This broad range probably reflects genetic variation, small sample size in some of the reports, and differences among the investigators regarding criteria for performing biopsies to diagnose amyloidosis. In Israel, 6% of the ESRD population has FMF,[892] and renal failure contributes to mortality in more than half the cases.[889]

Overall survival is similar for patients with AA (24 months) and AL amyloid (20.4 months). Azotemia at presentation is strongly associated with shorter survival time.[863] With AA amyloid (as with AL), interstitial fibrosis on biopsy predicts a poor renal outcome and the degree of glomerular amyloid deposition correlates poorly with renal function.[872]

Therapy should be directed at treating the underlying disorder. Rarely, remissions have been reported after antibiotic therapy for underlying infection, chemotherapy for rheumatic disease, or resection of inflammatory bowel disease or neoplasms.[863, 893–896] Colchicine is useful in preventing attacks of serositis and synovitis in FMF[882, 896, 897] and in slowing the accumulation of amyloid in native kidneys or preventing its deposition in renal allografts after transplantation.[883, 892] In one study in which colchicine therapy was utilized for FMF, amyloid deposits recurred in 10 of 19 allografts, but actuarial graft survival was 84%, 73%, and 57% at 12, 60, and 120 months, respectively.[892] A colchicine dose of at least 1.5 mg/d appears to be necessary to accrue benefit after renal transplantation.[883] Dimethyl sulfoxide may be useful in limited circumstances.[898, 899]

**β₂-Microglobulin Amyloidosis (Dialysis Associated).** This form of amyloidosis has been described in patients during long-term hemodialysis. It commonly involves deposits in synovium and long bones, causing carpal tunnel syndrome and destructive arthropathy, and rarely deposits in viscera.[900–903] This entity is described more fully in Chapter 56. Two patients have been described who were not dialysis dependent but in whom glomerular amyloid deposits of β₂-M have been found.[904]

**Heredofamilial Amyloidosis.** The most common heredofamilial amyloidosis syndrome is the autosomal recessive disorder FMF. It was discussed in the section on secondary amyloidosis because of its association with AA amyloid. The remaining familial amyloidosis syndromes are, for the most part, rare diseases that are inherited in an autosomal dominant pattern. The deposited amyloid in most, but not all, of these syndromes consists of thyroxine-binding prealbumin molecules (also called transthyretins). They differ, often, by a single amino acid substitution.[905] Traditionally, these syndromes have been subclassified into nephropathic and neuropathic varieties (see Table 31–5). The latter classification is not intended to be mutually exclusive, because renal involvement occurs in some of the neuropathic types.[891] Although neurologic symptoms predominate, glomerular involvement has been reported in patients with neuropathic type III (apolipoprotein A-I, Gly²⁶ → Arg²⁶ substitution) and type IV (gelsolin, Asp¹⁸⁷ → Asn) amyloid protein deposition. In the latter form of amyloidosis, also known as Finnish amyloidosis, two patients who were homozygous for the mutant gelsolin gene on chromosome 9 reached ESRD.[906–908] More often, the renal manifestations in the neuropathic form of Finnish amyloidosis are more subtle, consisting of non-nephrotic proteinuria and mild, if any, azotemia.[909] In the type III neuropathic form of amyloidosis, the deposited amyloid protein was identified in one Iowa kindred as apolipoprotein A-I altered by a single amino acid substitution of arginine for glycine at position 26. An identical substitution has also been noted in another kindred, whose manifestations have been predominantly renal and hepatic.[910] Thus, it has been noted that the clinical presentations of amyloidosis may vary, even if the accumulating protein is identical, and conversely, that chemically different amyloid proteins may induce clinical presentations that are quite similar.[905] No glomerular involvement has been reported to date in type I or II neuropathic amyloidosis; in the Danish, Appalachian, or Icelandic forms; or in the forms associated with Alzheimer β-protein.

In contrast, glomerular involvement causing proteinuria, and ultimately progressive renal insufficiency, is characteristic of the familial nephropathic amyloidoses. In the most common familial form of nephropathic amyloidosis, FMF, the accumulating protein is AA amyloid. In another form, a kindred is described in whom the accumulating protein is apolipoprotein A-I. In this kindred, the amyloid protein is not characterized by the single amino acid substitution seen in the type III neuropathic patients.[905] In the remaining heredofamilial nephropathic amyloidoses, the nature of the infiltrating protein is unknown. Therapy for the non-FMF heredofamilial forms of amyloid is uncertain.

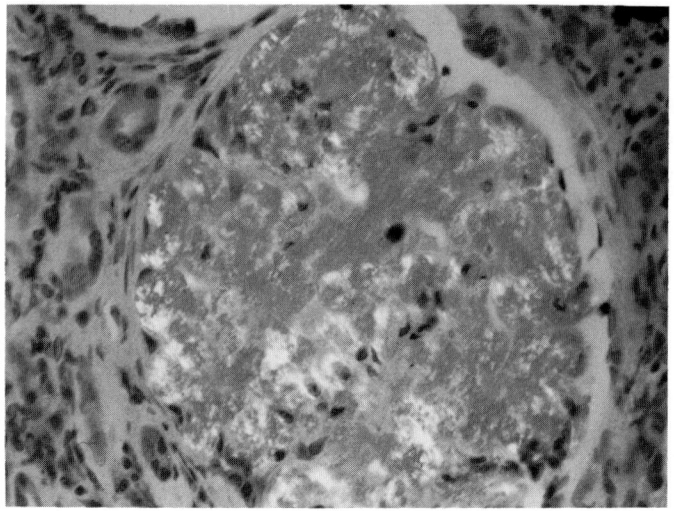

**Figure 31–18.** Light microscopic appearance of glomerular amyloidosis. Congo red–stained glomerulus, which is completely infiltrated by amyloid, demonstrates the characteristic birefringence. (Magnification × 450.)

## PATHOLOGY

**Light Microscopy.** The histopathologic features of the kidney are similar in primary and secondary forms of amyloidosis.[911] In mild early stages, the glomerular changes may be inconsequential, and the correct diagnosis can be made only by use of special stains. With Congo red stain, there are reddish pink deposits in the mesangium, peripheral capillary walls, and blood vessels that demonstrate apple-green birefringence when examined in polarized light (Fig. 31–18). Metachromasia is observed with methyl violet staining, and fluorescence is observed with thioflavin-T stains viewed under ultraviolet light. Thick sections (6 to 10 μm) should be used when these stains are applied. Similar amyloid deposits may be seen in the vasa recta, interlobular vessels, arterioles, collecting ducts, and interstitium. These interstitial deposits may be associated with defects in tubule function such as nephrogenic diabetes insipidus or impaired tubule reabsorption of $HCO_3^-$.[1, 911]

In standard hematoxylin-eosin–stained sections, the mesangium may appear solidified with an eosinophilic material. With increasing severity, the glomeruli become hypocellular and replaced with deposits of amyloid. In this stage, standard light microscopy may suggest diabetic glomerulosclerosis, light chain deposit disease, or nonspecific chronic glomerulonephritis. In some instances, marked thickening of the capillary walls with silver-positive spikes may occur, simulating idiopathic membranous glomerulopathy (Fig. 31–19). Giant cells may surround the deposits of amyloid in the familial variety of Ostertaag.[912] Amyloid casts in the tubules may be seen.

**Electron Microscopy.** Ultrastructural findings are diagnostic and of great value in confirming the presence of amyloid, if this is still doubtful after examination by light microscopy.[1, 911] A characteristic and pathognomonic lesion is the presence of fine, 8- to 10-nm fibrils arranged randomly or sometimes in bundles[1, 911, 912] (Fig. 31–20). They are readily differentiated from collagen fibrils because of their lack of periodicity. These fibrils are found in the mesangium and within the GBMs on either subepithelial or subendothelial aspects.[1, 911] In mild involvement, the mesangium alone is involved; with more severe disease capillary walls of the site of amyloid fibril deposition are involved.[913–916] The deposits may occasionally be found in the subepithelial space in a spicular arrangement.[917] One group has suggested that fibrillar amyloid deposits are more likely

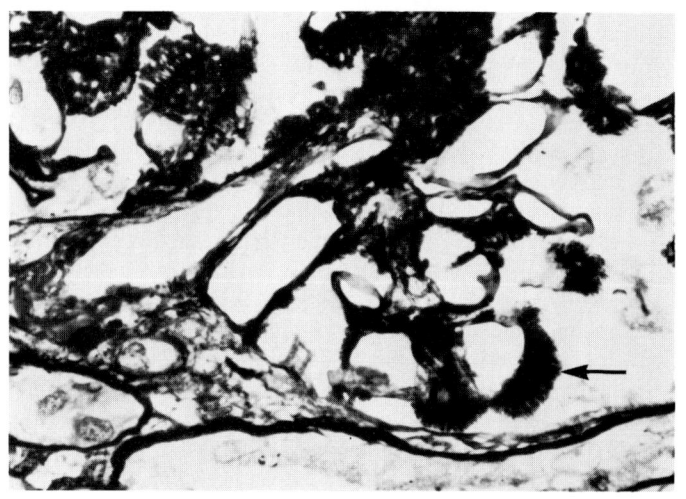

**Figure 31–19.** Light microscopic appearance of glomerular amyloidosis. Periodic acid–methenamine silver stain of glomerulus reveals closely packed long ''spikes'' in some capillary walls *(arrow)*. (Magnification × 1000.)

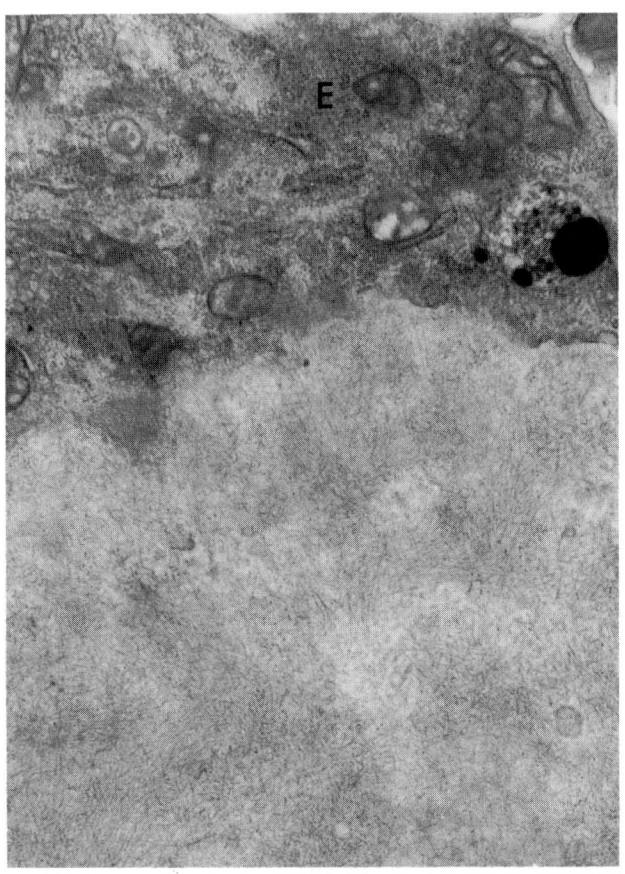

**Figure 31–20.** Electron microscopic appearance of glomerular amyloidosis. Note the fine, haphazardly arranged fibrils replacing the basement membrane. E = epithelial cell. (Magnification × 35,000.)

to be composed of AA amyloid and that granular amyloid deposits, when they occur, are more likely to be AL.[918]

**Immunofluorescence.** The findings are variable, but the most frequent finding is the presence of amorphous intracapillary and mesangial masses staining weakly for Ig, light chains, and C3.[904, 911] Gallo and colleagues[913] reported the distinction between AA and AL types in 88% of the patients studied; they used immunofluorescence and antisera to Igs, light chains, and AA protein. Other serum proteins, including albumin and fibrinogen, are also found in the deposits. These immunofluorescence findings are not sufficiently characteristic to have diagnostic value; in primary amyloidosis, however, the corresponding light chains (κ or λ) may be found in the deposits.

## PATHOGENESIS

The amyloidoses are now recognized to result from the deposition of a family of different proteins, all of which share the properties of apple-green birefringence after staining with Congo red and the β-pleated sheet conformation observed by x-ray crystallography. The wide variety of different proteins in this "family" is catalogued in Table 31–5. Overproduction of these proteins contributes to their deposition in some cases, particularly in AL amyloidosis complicating multiple myeloma. Furthermore, in secondary

amyloidosis and FMF, the acute-phase reactant serum AA apolipoprotein may deposit as AA amyloid, in part as a result of increased synthesis. In $\beta_2$-M–induced amyloidosis, serum levels of $\beta_2$-M are increased, yet deposition correlates poorly with serum levels.[903a] The latter suggests that an increased serum level, resulting from either overproduction or diminished excretion or degradation, is insufficient cause for the accumulation of amyloid in tissues. Thus, other characteristics have been sought. In some amyloid proteins, particularly involving prealbumin or the transthyretins, single amino acid substitutions distinguish the deposited protein from its normal counterpart (see Table 31–5). This suggests the possibility that deposition in these cases is directly related to a physicochemical change in molecular character caused by an alteration in the peptide sequence. In AL amyloid, the deposited light chain is usually a proteolytic cleavage fragment of the original light chain.[919] Occasionally, unaltered light chains appear to be involved.[920] Other characteristics, apart from mutation and cleavage, have been described as potential mediators of amyloid deposition. In $\beta_2$-M deposition, the involved protein appears to be more acidic than normal $\beta_2$-M and to have characteristics of advanced glycosylation.[921] Glycosylated $\beta_2$-M induced transient increments in macrophage tumor necrosis factor-$\alpha$ and interleukin-1 secretion and chemotaxis for mononuclear cells.[922] Finally, virtually all amyloid proteins codeposit with amyloid P protein and glycosaminoglycans. The role of these associated molecules in the deposition of amyloid is under investigation.[923]

## Immunotactoid Glomerulopathy and Fibrillary Glomerulonephritis
### (See also Chapter 30)

Several reports describe filamentous glomerular deposits containing Igs that do not stain with Congo red in patients undergoing renal biopsy for proteinuria or hematuria.[924] Most of these patients do not have any systemic involvement and the disease appears as a primary glomerular disease; therefore, they are discussed more extensively in Chapter 30.[924, 925] However, some patients have an underlying lymphoproliferative disease and monoclonal Ig deposits in serum and/or urine.[843] Patients are most often (but not always) adult. All have proteinuria (70% in the nephrotic range), and the majority are hypertensive and have microhematuria. Chronic renal insufficiency is common on presentation, and acute renal failure has been reported. Most often, the history, physical examination, and serologic evaluation fail to distinguish these patients from others with the idiopathic nephrotic syndrome. However, a minority of patients, usually those with large fibrils (>30 nm in diameter) or microtubule structures, appear to have an underlying lymphoplasmacytic disorder as evidenced by monoclonal paraproteins in either serum, urine, or the glomerular deposits.[926] Thus, it has been suggested, but remains to be confirmed, that the larger microtubule structures (immunotactoids) are clinically as well as pathologically distinct from the smaller (12 to 20 nm) and less crystalline deposits (fibrillary glomerulonephritis).[925, 926]

By light microscopy, the glomeruli have mild hypercellularity of the mesangium with concomitant increased mesangial volume (Fig. 31–21). Capillary walls are thickened. In both the mesangium and capillary walls, there is infiltration of the matrix and basement membranes, respectively, by amorphous periodic acid–Schiff–positive material. In the latter locations, the basement membranes may appear irregularly thickened with a reticulated pattern similar to that in advanced membranous glomerulonephritis. Hyaline thrombi may occasionally be observed, and crescents may also be present. Congo red and thioflavin-T stains are uniformly negative.[927, 928] Immunofluorescence microscopy has disclosed Ig and C3 deposits in mesangial regions and capillary walls in a granular pattern. There are some differences among series as to the composition of the deposits. Korbet and co-workers[924, 929] found IgG in most biopsy specimens. However, some contained IgG κ and IgG λ, and others were monoclonal. Furthermore, there were a few biopsy specimens that had more than one IgG subclass and one contained only IgG3. Alpers and colleagues[930] also found IgG κ in six of seven cases. IgM and IgA are variably present in low intensity. Immunofluorescence findings, combined with the ultrastructural abnormalities, have led to the designation of immunotactoid glomerulopathy as a synonym for this disorder.[924, 929]

Ultrastructurally, the deposits are nonbranching fibrils that are distributed throughout the mesangial matrix and basement membranes, most commonly in the lamina densa and in subepithelial locations (Fig. 31–22). The fibrils are randomly arranged and are of medium to slightly deep electron density. They have been found to range in diameter from 10 to 45 nm. In each specimen, all fibrils tended to be of the same size, but they differed from specimen to specimen. In glomerular capillary walls, the fibrils occasionally coexist with granular electron-dense deposits. The fibrils are noted only infrequently in tubule basement membranes and in the interstitium.

Progression to end-stage renal failure has been described in at least half of the reported patients. No effective therapy has been found. Few patients have received renal transplants. One patient with a short-term follow-up did not have any evidence of clinical recurrence of the glomerulopathy,[924, 929] whereas another had a massive recurrence of fibrillary deposits at 5.5 years.[930]

## POEMS Syndrome (Crow-Fukase Syndrome)

First described in 1956,[931] POEMS syndrome, also called Crow-Fukase syndrome,[932] is a disorder characterized by polyneuropathy, organomegaly, endocrinopathy, a monoclonal paraprotein, and skin changes. This disorder is often considered in the initial differential diagnosis of patients with multiple myeloma because of the presence of a monoclonal paraprotein. Some but not the majority of patients have this clinical syndrome as a complicating feature of

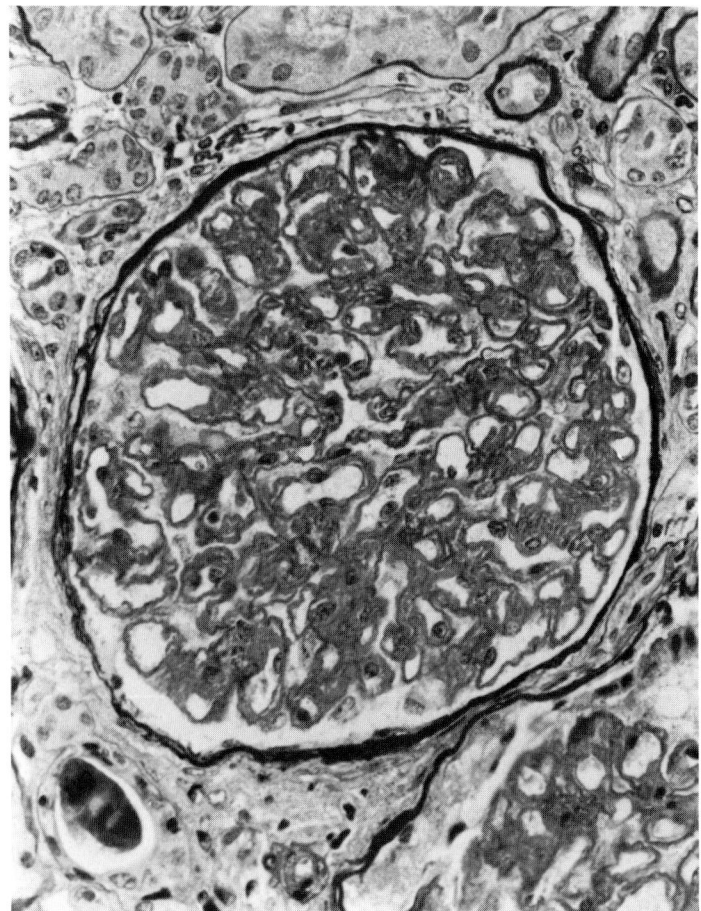

**Figure 31–21.** Light microscopic appearance of fibrillary glomerulonephritis. The mesangium is mildly widened and the capillary basement membranes are thickened, sometimes with a double contour. (Periodic acid–Schiff; magnification × 300.)

myeloma. An association with Castleman disease has been reported.[932, 933] The neuropathy may be central (62% have papilledema) or peripheral. Organomegaly is usually manifested by hepatosplenomegaly; the endocrinopathy by glucose intolerance, amenorrhea, or impotence; and the skin changes by edema, thickened skin, and angiomas. In the largest series of patients,[932] renal involvement was not commented on. However, numerous case reports have documented renal involvement, albeit with varying histologic appearances.[934–936] Microangiopathic changes are common,[935–936] but other histologic pictures have also been observed, including mesangial proliferation, mesangiolysis, and mesangiocapillary changes.[935–938] Immunofluorescence microscopy is usually negative. Presenting manifestations of renal involvement include proteinuria and hematuria with mild renal insufficiency, but progression to renal failure may occur.[935, 936] Initiated early, steroid therapy improved renal function in a small number of patients.[935] Increased amounts of interleukin-6 have been found in the serum and ascites, as well as in mesangial and subendothelial regions of the glomerulus, in peritubular capillaries, and in occasional tubule cells.[938, 939] Its pathogenetic significance is uncertain.

# LIVER DISEASES

## Viral Hepatitis

### HEPATITIS B

The spectrum of hepatitis B–associated glomerular disease has been reviewed.[940–942] Several major renal syndromes may occur in patients with hepatitis B: a serum sickness–like syndrome, membranous nephropathy, mesangiocapillary glomerulonephritis, and systemic necrotizing vasculitis, and most commonly polyarteritis nodosa and crescentic glomerulonephritis.[940–943]

Serum sickness–like symptoms accompany hepatitis B in 10% to 25% of infected patients, including fever, rash, arthralgias, arthritis, and rarely transient proteinuria with or without hematuria.[944, 945] The renal histology that accompanies the proteinuria and hematuria is unknown, because patients with these mild and self-limited renal manifestations rarely have biopsies. Spontaneous resolution of both renal and extrarenal manifestations is the rule.

Membranous nephropathy associated with hepatitis B was first described in 1969,[946] and in 1971 the Australia antigen (hepatitis B surface antigen) was identified in glomerular capillary walls along with Ig and C3.[947] Since then, all three hepatitis B antigens—hepatitis B surface, core, and e antigens (HBs, HBc, and HBe antigens)—have been identified in the subepithelial immune complexes of patients with membranous nephropathy and hepatitis B,[941, 948] as has specific anti-HBe antibody.[949] The majority of patients reported with hepatitis B–associated membranous nephropathy are children from Asia,[950, 951] although the disorder has been seen globally.[950] In the Pacific, transmission is hypothesized to occur either horizontally from infected mothers or, at an early age, vertically from infected household contacts.[951] Thus, serologically, patients tend to express a pattern consistent with the chronic carrier state. The most

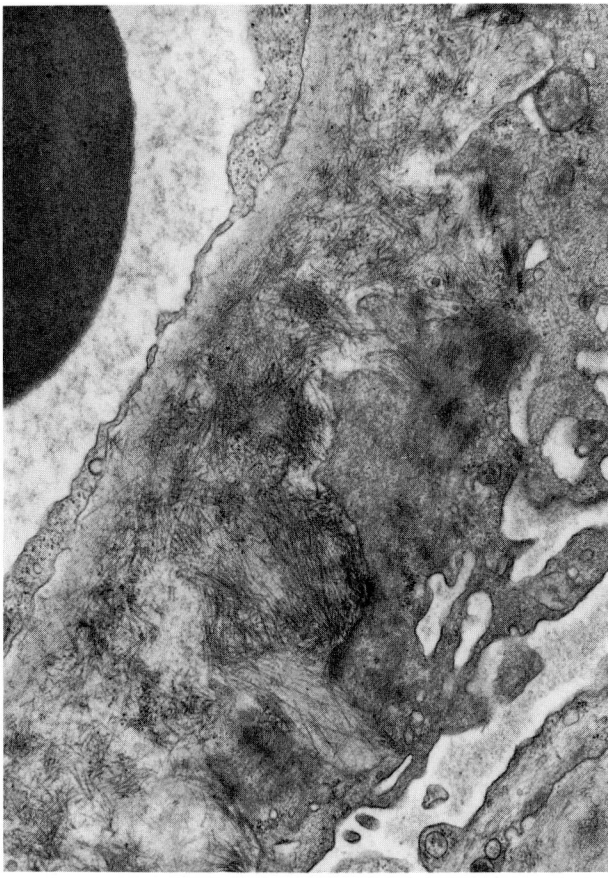

**Figure 31–22.** Ultrastructure of fibrillary glomerulonephritis. The fibrils are mainly electron-dense and randomly arranged along the subepithelial aspect of the basement membrane. (Magnification × 17,400.)

common serologic pattern is positivity for HBs and HBe antigen, as well as anti-HBc antibody, in the absence of HBs and HBe antibodies.[942] In Taiwan, 95% of the membranous nephropathy in children that is not ascribable to systemic lupus is in children with chronic hepatitis B.[951] There is a striking male preponderance. Peak incidence occurs at a mean of 6 to 7 years of age,[951, 952] usually without a clinically apparent preceding history of acute hepatitis,[952] but serum transaminase levels are often mildly elevated.[951] Proteinuria (nephrotic or non-nephrotic) and hematuria (usually microscopic, occasionally gross) are the presenting manifestations. Hypertension is uncommon. Most patients present with normal or only mildly elevated serum creatinine levels.[940–942] There is a variable incidence of hypocomplementemia. In children, spontaneous remission is the rule and is estimated to occur in 65% of patients 1 year after presentation, 85% after 2 years, and 95% after 5 to 7 years.[942] Remission is often but not always associated with disappearance of HBe antigenemia and conversion to positive HBe antibody state.[942, 948, 951] Treatment with steroids is inadvisable, as it may stimulate viral replication[951, 953] and its withdrawal has been associated with worsening hepatitis.[954] Interferon therapy has been particularly ineffective in children[955] but may be transiently beneficial in adults (see later), and other antiviral protocols are under investigation.[956, 957]

Adults from nonendemic areas who have hepatitis B and membranous nephropathy often acquire the infection in association with homosexuality, intravenous drug abuse, multiple sexual partners, or institutionalized living quarters. Other individuals at risk include people with occupational exposure to blood and patients with acquired immunodeficiency syndrome (AIDS).[950] Adults are more likely than children to have clinically apparent acute hepatitis in the 2 to 6 months preceding the onset of nephrotic proteinuria. Coexistent chronic active hepatitis is common[957] but not invariable. The spontaneous remission rate in adults is *substantially* less than in children,[958] approximately 30% to 60%.[941] Spontaneous remission has been reported in a patient with AIDS.[959] In one series, progressive renal insufficiency was observed in 29% of affected adults and ESRD occurred in 10%.[958] Therapy with interferon alfa only occasionally provides long-lasting complete remission.[957, 958]

Other histologic forms of glomerular disease have occasionally been reported in association with hepatitis B, including mesangiocapillary glomerulonephritis, mesangial proliferative glomerulonephritis (often with mesangial IgA deposits), and crescentic glomerulonephritis.[941–943, 960, 961] The relationship to hepatitis is less clear for these entities, particularly for IgA nephropathy.[961] Concurrent IgA nephropathy and chronic hepatitis B occur commonly in Asia.[961]

Polyarteritis nodosa associated with hepatitis B is more common in Western nations than in Asia. In a hyperendemic region of Alaska, its annual incidence is 7.7 cases/100,000 population.[962] Its clinical presentation is similar to that of patients with idiopathic polyarteritis nodosa,[963] including fever, weight loss, cutaneous leukocytoclastic vasculitis, livedo reticularis, myalgias, mono- or polyneuropathy, serous otitis, and arthritis. Orchitis and pulmonary manifestations may be less frequent in patients with hepatitis B as the underlying etiology.[964] Symptomatic acute hepatitis in the preceding 6 months is common, and serum transaminase levels are elevated in slightly less than half of patients at presentation.[964] Liver biopsy most often discloses chronic active or chronic persistent hepatitis. Typical serologic characteristics include the presence of HBs antigen and anti-HBc.[965] ANCAs may be positive in up to 9% of patients.[964] Saccular or fusiform aneurysms are most common in the renal and celiac circulations.[966] Vasculitic changes in medium-sized renal vessels such as those discoverable by angiography (see Chapter 30) may be the only abnormalities involving the kidney. However, a variety of histomorphologic changes have been described including ischemic changes; infarcts[967]; and in glomeruli, membranous, mesangial proliferative, membranoproliferative, diffuse proliferative, and, rarely, crescentic glomerulonephritis.[941, 943, 967] The spectrum of presenting renal manifestations includes hypertension (frequently malignant[967, 968]), microscopic or gross hematuria, proteinuria, and azotemia.[963, 968, 969] Rare spontaneous resolution has been reported.[965] However, if the patient with hepatitis B and polyarteritis nodosa is untreated, mortality and morbidity are high because of progressive systemic vasculitis.[962, 963, 970] In uncontrolled experiences, overall prognosis appears to be improved by steroids and cyclophosphamide[962, 963, 967, 970, 971] despite the concern that these agents may enhance viral

replication and exacerbate hepatitis.[951, 953] Plasmapheresis and dapsone have been employed anecdotally[972–975] with some success. Combination therapy including plasmapheresis and corticosteroids directed at the immune-mediated vasculitis and vidarabine antiviral therapy has been employed for 33 patients in a prospective nonrandomized trial[975] and appears promising. Within 18 months, 72.7% of treated patients had no clinical or serologic evidence of vasculitis. Seroconversion from HBe antigen to antibody positivity occurred after a single treatment cycle in 36.3% of patients and after a second treatment of either vidarabine or interferon alfa in 45.4%. Viral replication was no longer present in 51.1% of patients at the last follow-up. There were eight deaths, three of which were attributable to continued vasculitic activity early in the course of treatment despite therapy.[975]

A cryoglobulinemia-associated vasculitis has also been reported in patients with chronic hepatitis B.[976]

## HEPATITIS C

Approximately 80% of all transfusion-associated hepatitis (formerly non-A, non-B hepatitis) is thought to be due to the RNA virus now called hepatitis C virus. Fully 25% of acute hepatitis in the United States is ascribable to infection with this agent. The sequelae of this infection include prolonged antibody carriage, persistent or intermittent elevation of transaminase values in the majority of patients (although "silent" cases are not uncommon), chronic active or chronic persistent hepatitis in as many as 60% of infected individuals, and cirrhosis in 10% to 20%.[977] Extrahepatic involvement has also been reported, including patients with polyarteritis nodosa[978] and glomerulonephritis with[979–981] and without[981–983] cryoglobulinemia.

Although individual case reports document hepatitis C associated with mesangial proliferative glomerulonephritis[982] and membranous nephropathy,[983] the majority of patients reported to date have had type I mesangiocapillary glomerulonephritis.[979, 981] Hepatitis C virus was acquired by the majority of these patients by parenteral means, through either transfusion (38%) or intravenous drug abuse (50%). All patients had both antibody to hepatitis C and hepatitis C RNA demonstrable in blood. Clinical characteristics included hypertension (62%), edema (75%), hepatomegaly (50%), and palpable purpura (25%). Abnormal serum transaminase levels were present for longer than 6 months in 75% of patients. Rheumatoid factor and hypocomplementemia were present in all patients, and mixed IgG-IgM cryoglobulins were demonstrable in almost two thirds (see section on cryoglobulinemia). Viral RNA was identified in the cryoprecipitate of 60% of patients in whom cryoglobulins were present. The urinalysis demonstrated nearly universal microscopic hematuria and proteinuria, the latter being in the nephrotic range for more than half of the patients. Creatinine clearance was diminished in all of the patients.[981] Virtually all of the affected patients had chronic active or persistent hepatitis or frank cirrhosis.

Therapy for the glomerulonephritis associated with hepatitis C viral infection is currently controversial. Steroids and cytotoxic agents are relatively contraindicated as they may enhance viral replication, as has been seen for hepatitis

B.[951, 952, 954] Interferon alfa has been used most extensively for patients with chronic active hepatitis[984, 985] but also for patients with mixed (IgG-IgM) cryoglobulinemia[986] and glomerulonephritis.[981] Benefits accruing during therapy with interferon alfa include eradication of detectable virus in blood, improvements in liver histology, and decrements in serum cryoglobulins, transaminases, and creatinine, as well as in proteinuria. However, in 25% to 40% of patients who experience improvement during therapy, relapse occurs with discontinuation of therapy.[981, 984–986] Controlled trials are required to determine the optimal dose and duration of therapy, as well as risk-benefit analyses, for patients with hepatitis C–associated glomerulonephritis with mixed IgG-IgM cryoglobulinemia.

## Cirrhosis of the Liver

Severe chronic liver disease of almost any type may occasionally be associated with a diffuse glomerular sclerotic process, often referred to as cirrhotic glomerular sclerosis.[987–989] This lesion usually is not associated with any clinical manifestations other than mild proteinuria or hematuria. Morphologically, two basic patterns of glomerular involvement may be distinguished.[989] The more common one is characterized by mild increase in mesangial matrix with little or no increase in cellularity and thin capillary walls.[989] Immunofluorescence microscopy has often revealed the presence of IgA, most commonly in the mesangium but also occasionally extending into the capillary walls. In about 66% of the kidneys studied, IgG or IgM was also present but in lesser quantities.[990, 991] Some investigators have found that IgM is the dominant or sole Ig deposit and is present in as many as 70% of patients with cirrhosis.[987] In addition, in the mesangium and subendothelial portions of the capillary walls, numerous small (500 to 1000 nm) lucent zones containing small clusters of dense, granular structures are noted[989, 990] (Fig. 31–23). These are morphologically similar to structures present in lecithin–cholesterol acyltransferase deficiency (see later discussion). The second pattern is similar to mesangiocapillary glomerulonephritis with dominant IgA deposits and often the ultrastructural peculiarities previously mentioned.[990] IgA depos-

its are found in a significant proportion of patients with alcoholic cirrhosis without associated seropositivity for HBs antigen. Monomeric and polymeric IgA may be contained within immune complex material from the serum and kidney in these patients.[992] Mallory body (alcoholic hyaline) antigen has also been found within immune complexes and in glomeruli of cirrhosis-associated IgA nephropathy.[993] The mechanism of IgA deposition in alcoholic liver disease is probably multifactorial. Serum IgA levels are elevated in the majority of patients.[994] Defective elimination of IgA-containing immune complexes has been demonstrated. An IgA-IgG aggregate utilized to simulate IgA immune complexes is cleared slowly by the liver in patients with cirrhosis compared with normal persons and individuals with IgA nephropathy. Although splenic clearance is disproportionately increased, this increment fails to normalize the overall clearance rate.[995] Clearance time via specific asialoglycoprotein receptors is also prolonged in patients with cirrhosis, suggesting defective processing of IgA or IgA immune complexes.[995] Thus, IgA deposition in the liver of cirrhotic patients may reflect abnormalities in both the synthesis and the clearance of IgA and its associated immune complexes. A review of cirrhotic liver disease demonstrated that half of patients coming to necropsy had involvement of glomeruli, predominantly in the form of mesangial IgA deposits with lesser prevalence of proliferative glomerulonephritis, membranous glomerulonephritis, crescentic glomerulonephritis, and mesangiocapillary glomerulonephritis.[996, 997] An additional necropsy study showed similar mesangial proliferative changes with IgA and IgM deposits even in patients with noncirrhotic alcoholic liver disease at a prevalence exceeding that observed in control subjects.[998] Glomerular changes associated with noncirrhotic alcoholic liver disease were more common in Native Americans than in whites or Hispanics.[998] When IgA nephropathy occurs, it is usually clinically silent but may be associated with proteinuria, sediment changes, or, rarely, a syndrome simulating Schönlein-Henoch purpura.[998, 999] Resolution of proteinuria and hematuria has been reported after liver transplantation. Whether remission is ascribable to the concomitant immunosuppression or to the normalization of hepatic function is unclear.[1000]

The association of primary biliary cirrhosis, cutaneous vasculitis, and membranous nephropathy has been re-

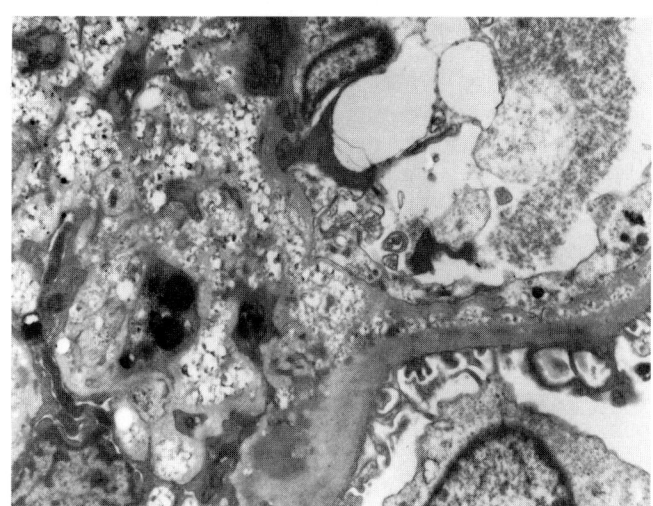

**Figure 31–23.** Electron microscopic appearance of glomerular alterations in hepatic cirrhosis. A mesangial electron-dense deposit, corresponding to IgA, is present. In addition, irregular lucencies containing dense granular and rounded membranous structures are in the mesangium and subendothelial space. (Magnification × 13,500.)

ported.[1001] It is also of interest that there appears to be an increased incidence of poststreptococcal glomerulonephritis in patients with cirrhosis.[1002] In addition, Moroz and co-workers[1003] observed three children with $\alpha_1$-antitrypsin deficiency and cirrhosis who had mesangiocapillary glomerulonephritis noted at postmortem examination. In one well-studied case, IgG, IgA, IgM, C3, and $\alpha_1$-antitrypsin were documented in glomerular capillary wall (subendothelial) deposits. Other forms of familial liver disease associated with nephritis have also been described.[1004] Two additional cirrhotic children with $\alpha_1$-antitrypsin deficiency and mesangiocapillary glomerulonephritis type I have since been reported[1005]; however, it appears that complement deficiency unrelated to mesangiocapillary glomerulonephritis is a common occurrence in antitrypsin deficiency of the ZZ phenotype.

## NEOPLASIA

The occurrence of massive proteinuria in association with malignant neoplasia is an uncommon but highly instructive event.[1006, 1006a] Lee and co-workers[1007] collected 11 cases from their personal experience of 101 patients with nephrotic syndrome in a 10-year period. The renal lesions antedated the discovery of tumor in two thirds of the patients, and all patients were over 40 years old. This subject has been reviewed extensively by Eagen and Lewis[1006] and again by Cotran and Alpers,[1008] Dabbs and colleagues,[1009] Brueggemeyer and Ramirez,[1010] and Davidson and Thomson.[1011] Some form of glomerular disease, principally manifested as heavy proteinuria or progressive renal failure, has been observed to occur in association with carcinomas of the lung, breast, stomach, colon, ovary, carotid body, oropharynx, cervix, skin (malignant melanoma and basal cell carcinoma), thymoma, kidney, penis, bladder, and prostate and also with pheochromocytoma, Wilms tumor, Hodgkin disease, lymphosarcoma, Burkitt lymphoma, chronic lymphatic leukemia, malignant mesothelioma, atrial myxoma, and eosinophilic lymphofolliculosis of the skin (Kimura disease).[1, 1010–1036] Although both renal amyloidosis and renal vein thrombosis may complicate many of these disorders, they were excluded in most cases. Carcinomas of the lung, stomach, breast, and colon appear to be the most frequent. In most cases involving a carcinoma in which biopsy material was studied adequately, typical membranous glomerulonephritis was present.* Minimal-change disease may also be associated with a variety of malignancies including Hodgkin disease, pancreatic carcinoma, malignant mesothelioma, carcinoma of the colon, retroperitoneal sarcoma, renal cell carcinoma, renal oncocytoma, and prostatic carcinoma.† Zech and colleagues[1019] studied the etiologies of nephrotic syndrome in adults older than 60 years and determined that nearly one fourth of the cases of membranous glomerulonephritis were associated with malignant disease. An eluate of renal tissue has been shown to react with autochthonous tumor or a soluble extract in a case of bronchogenic carcinoma.[1037] A melanoma antigen has been detected in the glomerular Ig deposits in a case of malignant melanoma,[1018] and a circulating antibody absorbable by tumor antigens reacted with the glomerular deposits in a case of colon carcinoma.[1016] Carcinoembryonic antigen was detected in the glomerular deposits.[1015] Renal tubule antigen-antibody complexes were found in glomeruli of three patients with renal cell carcinoma,[1038] but this has not been confirmed.[1039] Removal of the bulk of tumor may be associated with the remission of nephrotic syndrome, which may recur with development of metastases.[1006–1010] It is likely that tumor-associated antigens in the presence of an antibody response can form CICs that may deposit in the kidney and evoke glomerular damage. Furthermore, some cancer patients in whom glomerulopathies develop may be unable to produce adequate amounts of antibody to promote immune elimination of excess antigen and immune complex load.

Patients older than 50 years with nephrotic syndrome in whom membranous glomerulonephritis is demonstrated by renal biopsy should be scrutinized carefully for underlying carcinoma, especially of lung, stomach, and colon. Brueggemeyer and Ramirez[1010] found a yearly incidence rate of 0.8% for carcinoma in patients presenting with membranous glomerulonephritis after age 40 years. The associated carcinoma usually presented within 18 months of when nephrotic syndrome appeared. Several investigators have called attention to the development of vasculitis or crescentic glomerulonephritis in patients with malignancies.[1040] Immunofluorescence findings have varied and have included granular IgG deposits[1041, 1042] and one case in which the glomeruli were devoid of Ig deposits. In a selected group of patients with cancer but without clinical renal disease, Pascal and colleagues[1041] observed that 55% had Ig, complement, or electron-dense deposits in glomeruli. They concluded that cancer patients may have a high incidence of subclinical immune complex disease, possibly related to the presence of tumor-associated antigens and corresponding antibodies. The high prevalence of CICs or cryoIg among patients with various forms of cancer supports this suggestion.

The situation is somewhat different in Hodgkin disease and lymphomas, but here, too, nephrotic syndrome may precede the discovery of neoplasia sometimes by several years.[1009, 1031–1033, 1042, 1043] Remissions of nephrotic syndrome occur after chemotherapy or even locally applied radiation in the case of Hodgkin disease, and the reappearance of proteinuria may herald the relapse of the malignancy. Spontaneous remissions of nephrotic syndrome have also been noted to precede relapses of Hodgkin disease.[1033] In Hodgkin disease, malignant lymphoma, and thymoma, most cases have minimal changes revealed by light and electron microscopy, but membranous glomerulonephritis and other varieties of glomerulopathies have also been observed.[1, 1042] These include cryoglobulinemic glomerulonephritis and various proliferative glomerulonephritides. The association of T cell–derived Hodgkin disease or lymphoma and nephrotic syndrome with minimal-change lesion supports a pathogenetic link between T cell abnormalities and glomerular diseases with minimal histologic injury.[1043] The well-known sensitivity of minimal-change lesions to cytotoxic agents such as cyclophosphamide, and a similar beneficial effect on Hodgkin disease, are unexplained.

*References 1006, 1007, 1009, 1014, 1016, 1026.
†References 1, 1006, 1007, 1009, 1027, 1029, 1033, 1036.

Glomerular lesions may also occur in chronic lymphocytic leukemia and related B cell lymphomas. The observed lesions include mesangiocapillary glomerulonephritis (with type I or type II cryoimmunoglobulinemia), fibrillary glomerulonephritis, membranous glomerulonephritis, and focal and segmental glomerulosclerosis.[1034] Therapy with alkylating agents sometimes improves the patient's condition.[1032] Cutaneous T cell lymphomas can be associated with IgA nephropathy, membranous glomerulonephritis, and minimal-change disease, sometimes with marked visceral epithelial cell hypertrophy.[1035] Interferon alfa therapy is effective in these disorders.[1035]

## INFECTIOUS DISEASES

Glomerular diseases that arise as a consequence of infection are discussed here. The reader should also consult the relevant sections in Chapter 30 concerning poststreptococcal glomerulonephritis. Hepatitis B and C virus infections have been reviewed in the preceding section.

### Nonstreptococcal Postinfectious Acute Glomerulonephritis

A variety of nonstreptococcal infections may be associated with features of acute glomerulonephritis. Rather than the fully developed syndrome with edema, hypertension, and circulatory congestion, this nephritis is usually mild, often manifested only by hematuria and proteinuria. The organisms and diseases responsible for such nephritis include staphylococcal, pneumococcal, *Legionella, Mycoplasma,* and *Klebsiella* pneumonitis; cat-scratch disease; meningococcal infections; typhoid fever; syphilis; leptospirosis; histoplasmosis; varicella; mumps; cytomegalovirus, herpesvirus, echovirus, coxsackievirus, and Epstein-Barr virus (infectious mononucleosis) infections; hepatitis B; rubella; vaccinia; Q fever; trichinosis; toxoplasmosis; and falciparum malaria.[1, 1044–1059] The finding of rash, hepatic disturbances, or thrombocytopenia should increase the suspicion that meningococcus infection, syphilis, typhoid fever, Rocky Mountain spotted fever, cat-scratch disease, infectious mononucleosis, toxoplasmosis, or other virus infections (e.g., hepatitis B, cytomegalovirus infection) are etiologically involved.[1, 1048–1053] Severe eosinophilia may suggest trichinosis, histoplasmosis,[1054] or an acute hypersensitivity interstitial nephritis (see Chapter 33). Although detailed pathologic descriptions are available in relatively few cases, a histologic picture of mild diffuse proliferative or focal and segmental proliferative glomerulonephritis has usually been observed. In staphylococcal sepsis, humps similar to those in acute poststreptococcal glomerulonephritis have been found by electron microscopy. A case of proliferative glomerulonephritis secondary to pneumococcal pneumonia with alternative pathway C activation was described by Hyman and colleagues.[1055] Infection with other organisms possessing polysaccharide or lipopolysaccharide components to their structure presumably would have a similar propensity to activate the alternative pathway. Acute diffuse interstitial nephritis, more completely described in

Chapter 33, may also occur after many infectious diseases—most notably pneumococcal or streptococcal bacteremia, typhoid fever, infectious mononucleosis, brucellosis, and leptospirosis—and may complicate antimicrobial drug therapy for a variety of infections. In most cases, the glomerulonephritis attending these conditions is nonprogressive, and spontaneous recovery is the rule. On occasion, however, a rapidly progressive form of glomerulonephritis with extensive crescents develops. This is more likely when the infection is protracted, as might occur in infective endocarditis or in occult visceral abscess (as exemplified by pulmonary or abdominal abscesses or osteomyelitis). Because it is believed that glomerular injury is mediated by phlogogenic CICs composed of soluble products of the infecting organism and antibody to these products, it is easy to conceptualize that chronicity and heavy body burden of infection combine with brisk antibody response to facilitate the development of large quantities of immune complexes and magnified glomerular injury.

### Infective Endocarditis

The development of glomerulonephritis in patients with persistent bacteremia associated with endocarditis has been recognized since the early part of the century.[1, 1060–1063] Renal failure secondary to glomerulonephritis was a common cause of death in the preantimicrobial era. Despite the more widespread use of blood cultures in the evaluation of obscure cases of fever and despite better antimicrobial management, cases of glomerulonephritis resulting from infective endocarditis still occur sporadically. In general, glomerulonephritis appears among patients who present late for treatment, in whom the site of valvular involvement diminishes the likelihood of a prompt diagnosis, or who develop disease with fastidious or antimicrobial-resistant organisms. More frequently, this disorder is being observed among heroin addicts with right-sided endocarditis and negative blood culture results. Although early investigators believed that endocarditis-associated glomerulonephritis was caused by emboli, the presence of glomerulonephritis in patients with right-sided endocarditis in the absence of right-to-left shunting effectively challenges this hypothesis. The immune-mediated basis of this glomerulonephritis is supported by the findings of CICs,[1064] glomerular Ig and complement,[1065–1067] and detection of bacterial antigen in glomerular immune complexes.[1068] A wide variety of organisms may be responsible, but staphylococci and streptococci predominate.[1, 1063, 1065, 1069–1071] A report from the Glomerulonephritis Registry of the United Kingdom revealed that 1.7% of all patients had persisting infection as a cause of their glomerular disease and that infective endocarditis was the predominant disorder.[1047] Approximately 22% of patients with endocarditis develop either focal or diffuse glomerulonephritis.[1072]

The clinical manifestations of renal involvement are variable and include microscopic or gross hematuria and proteinuria, which are often discovered incidentally. Nephrotic syndrome occurs in up to 25% of patients. Hypertension is uncommon. In one series, the serum creatinine value exceeded 2 mg/dL only when other contributing factors such as hypotension, radiocontrast medium administration, or antibiotic nephrotoxicity were present.[1072] Renal dysfunction did not contribute to patients' mortality.[1072] Rapidly progressive renal failure with extensive crescentic involvement has been reported.[1072, 1073] The serum levels of C3 and C4 are often reduced.[1066, 1072] Normalization of serum complement is associated with bacteriologic cure.[1066] A non-Ig C3 lytic factor may be present.[1074] Rheumatoid factor is often present, sometimes in high titer.[1066] cryoIg is often found.[1069] CICs are almost always present in untreated or inadequately treated patients.[1064]

The most typical abnormality detected by light microscopy is a focal and segmental proliferative glomerular lesion, sometimes with focal fibrinoid necrosis or capillary thrombi.[1065–1067, 1076] This lesion was at one time referred to as a focal embolic nonsuppurative glomerulonephritis,[1062] but there is no evidence to implicate emboli of bacterial vegetations in the pathogenesis.[1076] This focal glomerulonephritic lesion is usually associated with mild proteinuria or hematuria. A more diffuse proliferative glomerulonephritis, with or without crescents, may occasionally be seen.[1065]

Electron microscopy reveals dense subepithelial and subendothelial deposits, along with varying degrees of mesangial proliferation. Immunofluorescence microscopy almost always shows granular capillary and mesangial deposits of IgG, IgM, and C3.[1065–1067, 1076] Antibody to or soluble antigens of the infecting organism have been demonstrated in the glomeruli, leading to the conclusion that the renal lesion is the result of immune complex deposition.[1065, 1068, 1075] At times no Ig is demonstrable within the glomeruli, suggesting that a staphylococcal toxin may directly damage the glomerular capillary or that cell-mediated immune responses are involved. In addition, in one reported case and in another seen by the authors, anti-GBM antibody has been eluted from diseased glomeruli.[1075] The significance of this observation is completely unknown. The manifestations of glomerulonephritis commonly subside with control of infection within days to weeks of initiation of antibiotic treatment. Rarely, microscopic hematuria or low-grade proteinuria persists for months to years[1072]; progressive disease rarely may ensue, however (most commonly resulting from crescentic glomerulonephritis). Vigorous therapy with plasma exchange and immunosuppression may be beneficial in these circumstances.[1073, 1074] Use of such therapy should be tempered by the possible risk of exacerbation of the underlying infectious process, as well as by the other side effects common to use of immunosuppressive strategies.

## Shunt Nephritis

Ventriculovascular shunts, once commonly placed for the treatment of hydrocephalus, become colonized with microorganisms in up to 27% of cases.[1, 1076–1083] The majority of infections are with *Staphylococcus albus* (75%), but diphtheroids (8%), *Staphylococcus aureus* (3%), and other less common organisms (*Listeria monocytogenes, Bacillus subtilis, Peptococcus, Serratia, Corynebacterium bovis,* numerous fungi) have been reported.[1077] Ventriculoperitoneal shunts are more resistant to infection than are ventriculo-

atrial shunts. Up to 4% of patients with infected shunts develop glomerulonephritis,[1084] and more than 80 cases have appeared in the literature. Fever occurs in 84% of patients and is the most common presenting manifestation. Blood and even cerebrospinal fluid cultures may be negative, and bacterial identification may be possible on occasion only after culture of the removed shunt.[1085] Glomerulonephritis appears a mean of 4.4 years after shunt placement but has occurred as early as a few weeks or as delayed as 14 years later.[1082] Microscopic or gross hematuria is frequent, associated with moderate proteinuria, azotemia, anemia, hepatosplenomegaly,[1082] purpura, arthralgias, and adenopathy. Nephrotic syndrome occurs in about 30%, and hypertension, leukopenia, and thrombocytopenia are rather uncommon.[1082] Rheumatoid factor, cryoIg, and CICs may be present, and C-reactive protein levels may be elevated.[1078–1083] Hypocomplementemia occurs with glomerulonephritis but not with uncomplicated shunt colonization or infection.[1083] Serial measurements of serum complement may be useful in aiding in the evaluation of resolution of glomerulonephritis[1081] with treatment.

By light microscopy, the glomeruli have either a mesangial proliferative or mesangiocapillary glomerulonephritis type I appearance. Diffuse granular and capillary deposits of IgG, IgM, and C3 have been found.[1081] Furthermore, the infecting bacterial antigen has been identified in the glomerular deposits.[1079] Like infective endocarditis, therefore, this entity can be regarded as an immune complex disease.

In both infective endocarditis and shunt nephritis, early recognition and prompt antimicrobial therapy, including removal of the ventriculoatrial shunt, lead to clinical healing of the glomerular lesions.[1, 1078, 1081] In some instances, glomerulonephritis does not resolve for several years after elimination of the infective stimulus.[1083] Persistence of renal insufficiency, marked by azotemia, proteinuria, microhematuria, and rarely hypertension, occurs in one third of cases. Progression to ESRD has been reported.[1082] Steroids and cytotoxic agents have not been beneficial in anecdotal reports.[1087] In rare cases, a form of rapidly progressive glomerulonephritis may develop, associated with extensive crescentic disease.[1077]

## Visceral Sepsis

The development of glomerular lesions in association with severe visceral infection (pulmonary, retroperitoneal, hepatic abscess) is well appreciated.[1080] Such patients resemble those with infective endocarditis. Progressive renal failure, at times accompanied by oliguria, is not uncommon. Extrarenal manifestations of purpura and arthralgias occur in about a third of cases and are usually related to circulating cryoglobulins. Serum C3 levels are often low, and cryoIg and CICs are often present. Glomerular lesions consist of focal and segmental proliferative mesangiocapillary or crescentic glomerulonephritis. The lesions may resolve with effective antimicrobial therapy and drainage. When treatment of the infectious etiology is ineffective or incomplete, the nephritis may progress to end-stage renal failure.

## Other Bacterial and Fungal Infections

As discussed in other sections (see also Chapter 30), proteinuria, hematuria, and even nephrotic syndrome may occur during the course of acute poststreptococcal glomerulonephritis, infective endocarditis, and infected ventriculoatrial shunts. In this section, glomerular disease, often evoking heavy proteinuria as a specific complication of other infectious diseases, is described. In the nephrotic syndrome associated with congenital and secondary syphilis, renal biopsy specimens usually demonstrate a picture of membranous glomerulonephritis with variable degrees of proliferation.[1088, 1089] Granular deposits of IgG and C3 and subepithelial electron-dense deposits are found. Both treponemal antigen[1089] and antibody[1090] have been demonstrated in or eluted from the glomerular deposits. An immune complex disease is thus established by the pattern and nature of Ig deposits.[1090] The response to penicillin treatment is usually favorable, but spontaneous improvement in the proteinuria of secondary syphilis may occur. The acute nephritic syndrome with pathologic findings similar to those of acute poststreptococcal glomerulonephritis may rarely occur in secondary syphilis. Tuberculosis, aspergillosis,[1091] leprosy,[1092] and other chronic granulomatous bacterial or fungal infections may also be associated with nephrotic syndrome. At times, this is the result of development of amyloidosis. Types I and II mesangiocapillary glomerulonephritis have been reported in hypocomplementemic patients with single or recurrent episodes of meningococcal meningitis.[1093, 1094] It is unclear, however, if the infection is causally related to the glomerulonephritis or if the defect in the complement system underlies both the propensity to glomerular disease and infection.[1093, 1094] *Mycoplasma* infection has also been associated with acute nephrotic syndrome caused by minimal-change disease or crescentic glomerulonephritis.[1056] Chronic bacterial pyelonephritis is not usually associated with massive proteinuria; in a few cases, however, a typical nephrotic syndrome has occurred, perhaps because of the chance occurrence of an unrelated glomerular disease.[1095] Chronic vesicoureteric reflux[1096–1098] with or without infection has been associated with lesions of focal glomerular sclerosis, membranous glomerulonephritis, or minimal-change nephrotic syndrome.

## Protozoal and Other Parasitic Infections

Malaria is an important cause of nephrotic syndrome, especially in Uganda and Nigeria, where as many as one third of nephrotic children have quartan malaria.[1099] Its most serious consequences are experienced with infection by *Plasmodium malariae* (quartan malaria), although transient mesangiocapillary or mesangial proliferative glomerulonephritis occasionally accompanies falciparum malaria.[1099] The incidence of nephrotic syndrome as a cause for hospital admission in the malarial endemic areas of Uganda is 20 to 60 times that observed in the United States.[1, 1099–1101] The peak age at onset of nephrotic syndrome is between 5 and 8 years. Hypertension is uncommon at presentation but develops as renal insufficiency progresses. Proteinuria is poorly selective in up to 80% of patients.[1102] Some patients have diminished C3 levels and circulating rheumatoid factor. Malarial parasitemia and CICs containing C3 and antimalarial antibody can frequently be found. Histologically, the glomerular changes are varied. In the studies in Ugandan children, diffuse proliferative glomerulonephritis was found in 35%, focal glomerulonephritis in 14%, minimal glomerular changes in 22%, and membranous nephropathy in 12%.[1100] Some form of proliferative glomerulonephritis occurred in most of the cases with proven quartan malaria. In contrast, in an extensive survey of Nigerian children, a characteristic lesion was found and designated quartan malarial nephropathy.[1101] This lesion consists of a thickening of the capillary wall with a focal or generalized double contour or plexiform appearance of the basement membrane on silver impregnation technique. Segmental mesangial sclerosis progressing to global sclerosis was also a feature. Similar lesions have also been described in Senegalese children with nephrotic syndrome not clearly related to malarial infection.[1, 1099] Electron microscopy revealed thick basement membranes with subendothelial deposits and lacunae within the basement membrane. Immunofluorescence has generally revealed granular deposits of IgG and IgM, often with C3 distributed along the glomerular capillary wall. *P. malariae* antigen was detected in a similar distribution in several cases, and eluted IgG contained antibody activity to the malarial parasite.[1, 1099] It is therefore suggested that the pathogenesis of malarial nephropathy involves deposition of immune complexes consisting of soluble malarial parasite antigen plus antibody. It is also possible, however, that autologous nonglomerular antigens participate in this immune complex disease. Neither spontaneous remission nor remission after antimalarial therapy is common, and the usual course involves slow progressive renal functional loss during a period of 3 to 5 years.[1103] The response to steroids or cytotoxic drugs is generally poor. Some cases discovered early that display highly selective proteinuria or mild proliferative changes on biopsy may improve with steroid treatment.

Nephrotic syndrome has also occurred after lepromatous and nonlepromatous leprosy,[1099] filariasis,[1099] toxoplasmosis,[1104] and schistosomiasis.[1105] The last has been extensively reviewed.[1099, 1105] Glomerular disease is most commonly associated with *Schistosoma mansoni*, but geographic differences have been reported. The presence of hepatic fibrosis markedly increases the incidence of glomerular disease, presumably as a function of diminished immune complex clearance. *Schistosoma haematobium* causes histopathologic glomerular changes, most often without overt clinical signs or symptoms.[1105] In overt nephropathy, numerous histopathologic changes may be found. The most common change is mesangial proliferative glomerulonephritis, of which cases approximately two thirds remit with antiparasitic treatment combined with immunosuppression.[1100] A more inflammatory glomerular lesion with infiltration by neutrophils, monocytes, platelets, fibrin, and crescentic changes has been described in patients with hepatosplenic schistosomiasis and superimposed salmonellosis.[1105] Prognosis is good when therapy eradicates both infestations.[1105] Other forms of schistosomal glomerulonephritis, including mesangiocapillary glomerulonephritis, focal sclerosis, and AA amyloidosis, respond poorly to therapy, and progressive renal failure occurs.[1099, 1105]

# Viral Infections

Hepatitis B has also been associated with glomerular disease, on occasion manifested as nephrotic syndrome (see earlier discussion). Hepatitis B is particularly associated with the development of membranous or mesangiocapillary glomerulonephritis, or vasculitis (see earlier). At times, the infection is occult and not accompanied by the usual features of acute or chronic hepatic parenchymal disease. Depressed serum C3, circulating cryoIg, CICs, hypergammaglobulinemia, and positive results for HBs antigen would be expected to occur. The hepatitis C virus could also be implicated in glomerular disease associated with chronic active hepatitis and mixed (IgG-IgM) cryoglobulinemia (see earlier).

## HUMAN IMMUNODEFICIENCY VIRUS–ASSOCIATED NEPHROPATHY

Initially described in 1984 as a proteinuric syndrome occurring predominantly in black male intravenous drug abusers with AIDS, HIV-associated nephropathy is now recognized frequently to antedate signs and symptoms of full-blown AIDS.[1106-1119] It occurs even in otherwise asymptomatic carriers of HIV and affects individuals without a history of drug abuse.[1106, 1120] Thus, HIV nephropathy has been described in patients with any of the risk factors for AIDS, including homosexual or heterosexual intercourse, maternal-fetal transmission, transfusion with contaminated blood or blood products, and intravenous drug abuse.[1121] Clinically, patients with HIV-associated nephropathy present with nonselective proteinuria, often in the nephrotic range. Edema, hypercholesterolemia, and hypertension are uncommon. Although hypoalbuminemia is the rule, it is as likely to be reflective of a hypercatabolic and/or undernourished state as of a concomitant nephrotic syndrome.[1122] Microscopic hematuria or pyuria occurs in a minority of patients. The precise incidence of clinically significant HIV nephropathy among HIV-positive individuals is unknown, but it appears to be relatively uncommon. Some have challenged whether a specific lesion exists, because a variety of renal lesions, nonspecific for HIV infections, have been observed in some series.[1116, 1118, 1123] In one study, 30% of HIV-infected outpatients without demonstrable dipstick proteinuria had microalbuminuria, a prevalence higher than that noted in normal subjects but not significantly different from that of febrile hospitalized control subjects.[1124] Similar results were observed for urinary $\beta_2$-M measurements.[1124] Renal ultrasonography demonstrates hyperechoic kidneys of generous size.[1125] Rapid progression to ESRD occurs in adults[1106, 1122]; however, more protracted courses have been reported in adults[1106, 1122, 1125] and are the rule in children.[1126]

The majority of patients reported have a variant of focal and segmental glomerulosclerosis with characteristic tubulointerstitial changes (see later). However, a growing number of HIV-infected patients are reported to have IgA mesangial immune deposits.[1126-1128a] In these patients, microscopic hematuria was universal, and circulating IgA immune complexes, IgA rheumatoid factor, and IgA antibodies to HIV antigens were detected in serum.[1127] Although these patients did not have significant liver disease, it is

likely that chronic pulmonary infection or diarrhea was present, potentially implicating the respiratory and/or gastrointestinal mucosal immune system in the pathogenesis of this disorder. Unlike the case of focal and segmental glomerulosclerosis, loss of renal function in these patients is not fulminant.[1127]

The pathologic aspects are distinctive and may even be unique. The kidneys are nearly always grossly enlarged. Even in the presence of advanced uremia, there is no reduction in renal size,[1111, 1112, 1125] unlike the situation observed in heroin-associated nephropathy (see later discussion). Microscopically, there are alterations in glomeruli, tubules, and interstitium.[1121] Changes of focal and segmental glomerulosclerosis that are frequently in the early stage of morphogenesis are common. By light microscopy, clusters of visceral epithelial cells are enlarged, coarsely vacuolated, and contain protein reabsorption droplets (Fig. 31–24). The affected capillary lumina are occluded by large foam cells. As the lesion progresses, plasma protein precipitates occlude many capillaries (hyalinosis), some capillary walls collapse, and mesangial matrix increases (collapsing glomerulopathy). In most instances, there is concomitant degeneration or necrosis of tubule cells, usually in the absence of precipitating factors such as nephrotoxic medications or hypotension. Protein reabsorption droplets are found in tubule epithelium. A peculiar and regularly observed feature is microcystic dilatation of tubules that are filled with pale-staining casts (Fig. 31–25); all segments of the nephron may be affected. The casts are a precipitate of filtered plasma protein, often with Tamm-Horsfall protein. There is an accompanying diffuse interstitial edema, sometimes associated with a leukocytic infiltrate.

Immunofluorescence microscopy typically discloses segmental IgM, C3, and C1q in glomeruli, but diffuse mesangial IgM or IgA may be detected. There are no regular granular capillary wall deposits.

The ultrastructure of the glomerular lesions does not differ appreciably for many of the basic findings in idiopathic focal and segmental glomerulosclerosis and hyalinosis (see Chapter 30). There are, however, additional cellular changes of note and importance.[1110, 1120, 1121, 1126] Perhaps the most consistent change involves the endothelium. There are numerous and large tubuloreticular structures in the cytoplasm of the endothelial cells of glomeruli as well as in all other renal vascular structures.[1116, 1120, 1121] The tubuloreticular structures are morphologically identical to those seen in SLE (see earlier discussion). Their presence in a biopsy specimen from a patient with focal and segmental glomerulosclerosis may indicate HIV infection before its clinical or laboratory recognition.[1120, 1121, 1128, 1129] Other ultrastructural cellular abnormalities may be present in renal tissue in HIV-associated nephropathy. These include a variety of nuclear bodies and confronting cisterna in cytoplasm. These abnormalities may be found in tubule and interstitial cells.

The pathogenesis of HIV-associated nephropathy is unknown. The pronounced cellular abnormalities, however, especially of glomerular and tubule epithelium, have suggested to several investigators the concept of a viral etiology.[1110, 1121] Indeed, HIV genome was documented in glomerular and tubule epithelium in biopsy specimens from patients with this lesion.[1130] Furthermore, HIV has been

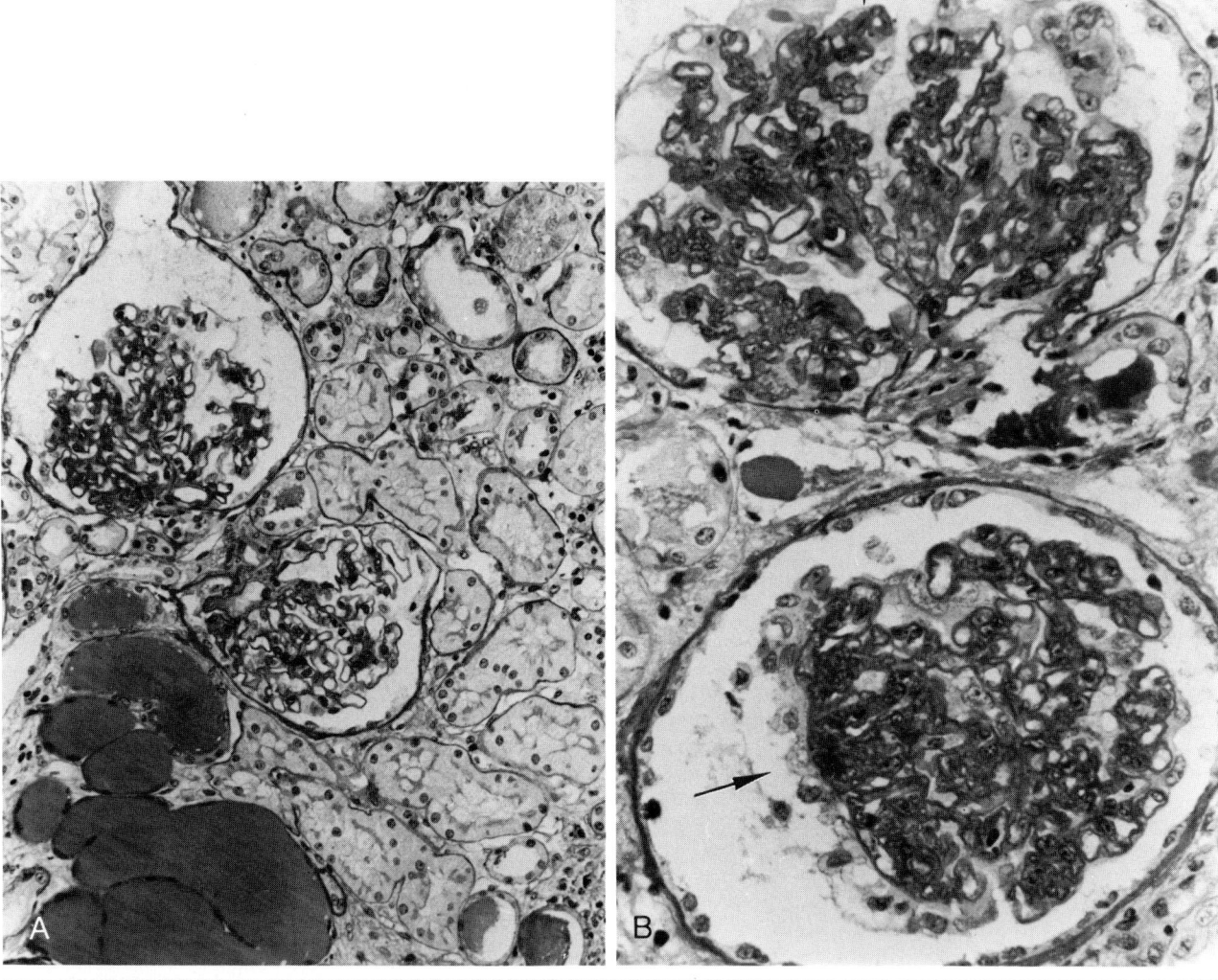

**Figure 31–24.** Light microscopic appearance of HIV-associated nephropathy. *A.* Low-magnification view demonstrates clusters of dilated tubules filled with relatively pale-staining cast matrix and two glomeruli, the larger of which has segmental capillary collapse. (Periodic acid–Schiff; magnification × 350.) *B.* Glomeruli with segmental sclerosis *(arrow)* and capillary collapse *(arrowhead).* Many visceral epithelial cells are enlarged and coarsely vacuolated. These lesions are often referred to as collapsing glomerulopathy. (Periodic acid–Schiff; magnification × 315.)

shown to be capable of infecting cultured glomerular endothelial and mesangial cells by some[1131] but not all investigators.[1132] It is uncertain whether HIV alone is responsible or whether other viruses, hereditary or environmental factors, or concomitant drugs or toxins are also necessary for the fully developed lesions. HIV nephropathy has been demonstrated in mice transgenic for a noninfectious HIV-1 DNA construct lacking the *gag* and *pol* genes. Glomerular and tubule histopathologic changes similar to those seen in patients have been described. Sclerotic glomeruli in mice expressed the viral protein Rev. These findings directly implicate HIV-1 genes in the pathogenesis of HIV nephropathy.[1133]

In addition to HIV-associated nephropathy, other glomerular lesions have been described in HIV-infected patients. In some of the early reports,[1106–1109] mesangioproliferative glomerulonephritis with immune deposits was documented, usually at autopsy, in patients with mild proteinuria. Mesangial IgA deposits have been reported, both with and without crescents.[1128, 1128a] Several cases of minimal-change disease have also been described.[1134, 1135] Furthermore, membranous, mesangiocapillary, and acute postinfectious forms of glomerulonephritis have been described.[1108, 1118, 1123, 1136–1138] Thrombotic microangiopathy has also been observed.[1113, 1114, 1118, 1123] Some of the patients with membranous glomerulonephritis had concomitant hepatitis B infection and localization of hepatitis B viral antigens to the glomerular deposits.[1136]

Although exceptions exist, the fully developed lesion of HIV-associated nephropathy still appears to carry a poor prognosis, both for renal survival and for overall survival of the patient, especially for patients who have overt AIDS. Often, rapid progression to renal failure occurs.[1139] Therapy for the nephropathy is controversial. Anecdotal reports suggest that azidothymidine may induce remissions and slow or reverse the course of progressive renal insufficiency and diminish proteinuria.[1140, 1141] Experience with steroids and cytotoxic agents, now common for *Pneumocystis carinii*

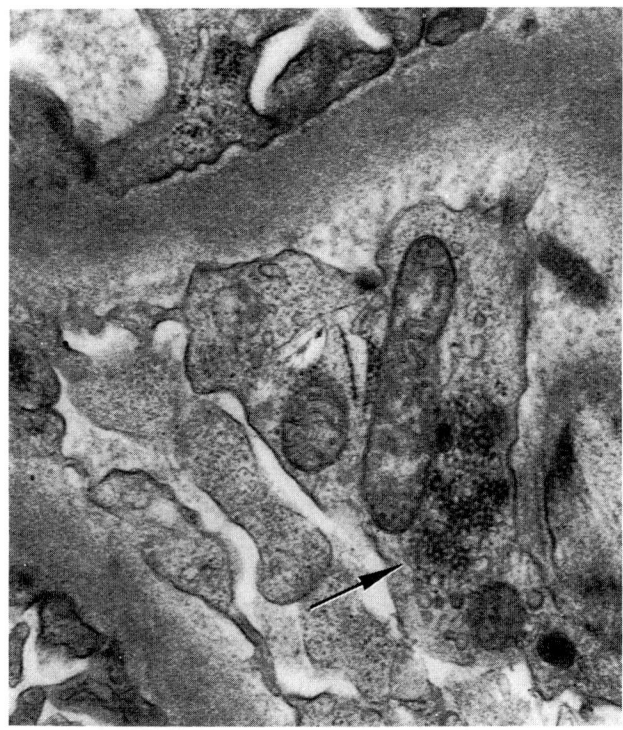

**Figure 31–25.** Electron photomicrograph of HIV-associated nephropathy. A glomerular endothelial cell contains a cluster of tubuloreticular structures *(arrow)*. (Magnification × 28,150.)

infections, thrombocytopenia, and lymphoma in AIDS patients, is limited when applied to the nephropathy. However, anecdotal reports document beneficial responses in proteinuria and serum creatinine when oral prednisone is administered for 2 to 6 weeks.[1141, 1142] Clearly, this therapy, if chosen, should be used in a highly selective fashion, given the potential for exacerbations or susceptibility to secondary infections.

Most patients with HIV-associated nephropathy evolve to ESRD within a year of presentation with nephropathy[1111, 1139] and succumb to the complications of AIDS regardless of whether they are maintained with dialysis. Renal transplantation has been performed in dozens of HIV-positive patients. Some were known to be HIV-positive before surgery, and others were either discovered to be positive after the surgery or contracted the disease at or after transplantation. In the majority, opportunistic infections were associated with significant morbidity and mortality,[1143, 1144] effectively contraindicating renal transplantation for the vast majority of HIV-infected patients. Cyclosporine therapy is poorly tolerated by patients with AIDS. Side effects include hyperkalemia, rising serum creatinine level, and falls in hemoglobin, platelets, leukocytes, total T cells, and CD4+ and CD8+ T cells.[1145] Rarely, a syndrome similar to hemolytic-uremic syndrome may be seen in HIV-infected patients.[1113]

Other examples of nephrotic syndrome appearing in association with viral infections include herpes zoster, infectious mononucleosis, and cytomegalovirus, although the relationship between cytomegalovirus and glomerular disease is controversial.[1046a] Glomerulonephritis has also been reported in association with mumps virus,[1046b] adenovirus, echovirus, coxsackievirus, and influenza virus A and B.[1]

# HEREDOFAMILIAL DISEASES
(Table 31–7)

## Diabetic Glomerulopathy

The renal and genitourinary disorders that accompany diabetes mellitus are more completely described in Chapter 39, and only a brief analysis is provided here. The glomerular lesions of diabetes mellitus consist of diffuse or nodular glomerulosclerosis.[1, 1146, 1147] The hallmark of the diabetic glomerulosclerotic lesion is a generalized increase in mesangial matrix, usually accompanied by a diffuse thickening of the glomerular capillary wall. The nodular glomerulosclerotic lesion (Kimmelstiel-Wilson lesion) is considered pathognomonic of diabetic glomerulopathy, but it may at times be confused with light chain glomerulopathy, the lobular form of type I mesangiocapillary glomerulonephritis, or amyloid, and it may rarely occur in the absence of diabetes as an idiopathic lesion.[1148–1152] The excretion of κ light chains in urine of some patients with typical newly diagnosed diabetes mellitus may give rise to confusion with light chain nephropathy.[1153] Special stains for immunofluorescence microscopy ordinarily alleviate any diagnostic difficulty.[1] Typically, patients with diabetic glomerulopathy have been recognized to have glucose intolerance for 10 years or more and have demonstrated microalbuminuria or isolated, non-nephrotic proteinuria for several years before the onset of heavy proteinuria and an overt nephrotic state.[1] The risk for developing abnormal proteinuria increases from 5 to 15 years after the onset of insulin-dependent diabetes mellitus and then declines, suggesting that nephropathy affects only a subset of diabetic patients. Progression to ESRD is more rapid in patients diagnosed during or after puberty than in those initially affected in childhood.[1] When nephrotic syndrome supervenes, the edema may be more severe than would be expected on the basis of the extent of lowering of serum albumin levels alone. This is perhaps a reflection of the diffuse capillary lesion in diabetic patients or subclinical congestive heart failure caused by atherosclerotic myocardial disease. In type I (insulin-dependent) diabetes, microalbuminuria appears to be valuable in predicting clinical proteinuria.[1] Although early studies suggested that this may also be of predictive value in patients with type II (maturity-onset; non–insulin-dependent) diabetes mellitus,[1, 1154] later work has refuted the earlier contention. The optic fundi represent an important clinical signpost in the evaluation of a patient with possible diabetic glomerulosclerosis. Gellman and colleagues,[1155] in a comprehensive study of diabetes mellitus, found that more than 90% of patients who had some evidence of diabetic retinopathy (i.e., microaneurysms) revealed some histologic glomerular abnormality consistent with diabetic glomerulopathy. Therefore, a nephrotic patient with retinal microaneurysms and overt diabetes mellitus almost always has a lesion consistent with or pathognomonic of diabetic glomerulopathy. In rare instances,

**TABLE 31–7. Heredofamilial Diseases with Prominent Glomerular Involvement**

| Disease | Mode of Inheritance |
| --- | --- |
| Classic hereditary chronic nephritis with deafness (Alport syndrome) | a. Autosomal dominant with preferential segregation with X chromosome<br>b. Autosomal dominant, partially lethal for male fetus<br>c. Autosomal dominant, sex influenced<br>d. X linked |
| Variant hereditary chronic nephritis (with or without deafness)<br>With hyperprolinemia<br>With ichthyosis<br>With macrothrombocytopenia<br>With Charcot-Marie-Tooth disease<br>With ocular abnormalities<br>With leiomyomatosis | a. Same as above or unknown |
| Familial benign hematuria with thin GBM | Autosomal dominant or autosomal recessive |
| Angiokeratoma corporis diffusum universale (Fabry disease) | X linked |
| Osteo-onychodysplasia (nail-patella syndrome) | Autosomal recessive (ABO linked) |
| Congenital (Finnish-type) nephrotic syndrome | Autosomal recessive |
| Diabetic nephropathy | a. Insulin dependent, HLA linked<br>b. Non–insulin dependent, non–HLA linked |
| Sickle-cell disease | Autosomal intermediate dominant |
| SLE (particularly with C2, C1r, C1s, C5, and C8 deficiency) | HLA linked (A10, B8, DR2), polygenic |
| Partial lipodystrophy and membranoproliferative glomerulonephritis | Autosomal dominant |
| $\alpha_1$-Antitrypsin deficiency with glomerulonephritis or vasculitis | Autosomal dominant |
| Membranoproliferative glomerulonephritis with hepatic fibrosis and subepidermal immunoprotein deposits | Autosomal recessive |
| Urticaria-deafness-amyloidosis (Muckle-Wells syndrome) | Autosomal dominant |
| FMF with amyloidosis | Autosomal recessive |
| Hereditary amyloidosis with polyneuropathy | Autosomal dominant |
| Intestinal malabsorption of vitamin $B_{12}$ (Imerslund syndrome) | Autosomal recessive |
| Hereditary osteolysis with glomerulonephritis | Autosomal dominant |
| Asphyxiating thoracic dystrophy (Jeune syndrome) | Autosomal recessive |
| Lecithin acyltransferase deficiency | Autosomal recessive |

however, nephrotic syndrome with the specific lesion of nodular glomerulosclerosis has occurred in the absence of retinopathy or overt glucose intolerance, but light and/or heavy chain nephropathy was not excluded.[1149–1152]

Whereas the development of overt proteinuria (greater than 500 mg/d) in a patient with insulin-dependent diabetes with overt retinopathy is highly indicative of an underlying diabetic intercapillary glomerulosclerosis, this is not always the case in patients with non–insulin-dependent diabetes. Some but not all studies have shown a greatly increased frequency of nondiabetic glomerular disease in patients with non–insulin-dependent diabetes presenting with abnormal proteinuria and/or reduced renal function.[1156, 1157] Gambara and co-workers[1156] found that 33 of 52 patients with non–insulin-dependent diabetes and overt renal disease had nondiabetic glomerular lesions, including several specific lesions such as acute endocapillary proliferative glomerulonephritis, minimal-change disease, crescentic glomerulonephritis, membranous glomerulonephritis, amyloidosis, and ischemic nephropathy. For some reason, IgA nephropathy is rare in non–insulin-dependent diabetes. For these reasons, one should suspect nondiabetic glomerular lesions when a patient with this type of diabetes mellitus presents with abnormal urinalyses or impaired renal function, especially in the absence of overt retinopathy or concomitant hypertension.

As discussed, most patients with diabetic nephropathy display a typical clinical course and do not require renal biopsy for diagnostic or prognostic purposes. A steep in-crease in the slope of the decline in GFR (reciprocal of the serum creatinine) over time, however, may indicate superimposed renal disease or urologic complications.[1] One should suspect associated immune-mediated glomerulonephritis in patients with diabetic nephropathy who display hematuria, red blood cell casts, and unusually rapid progression to renal failure.[1158, 1159] Screening urinalysis in patients with diabetic nephropathy has revealed hematuria in as many as 30% and red blood cell casts in 13% of cases.[1160] This indicates that significant hematuria with red blood cell casts may be a clinical feature of isolated diabetic nephropathy. Furthermore, primary immune complex glomerulonephritides may occur at a higher frequency in patients with diabetic nephropathy than in the nondiabetic population. IgA nephropathy and membranous glomerulopathy are examples of immunologic forms of glomerular injury occurring more frequently in diabetics.[1160]

A number of abnormalities have been noted in patients with diabetes mellitus that may ultimately be related to the development of diabetic nephropathy.[1, 1161] Platelets in patients with diabetes have been shown to express increased growth-promoting activity of cultured smooth muscle cells and fibroblasts.[1162] Increased plasma inactive renin levels are associated with abnormal proteinuria and other microvascular complications.[1163] Increased levels of sorbitol and diminished intracellular myoinositol concentration have been noted in cells from diabetic patients where glucose uptake is insulin independent (e.g., lens, renal tissue, peripheral nerves). Sorbinil inhibition of aldose reductase (the enzyme responsible for converting glucose to sorbitol) diminished proteinuria in experimental animals.[1164] Nonenzymatic glycosylation of structural and functional proteins has been proposed as a mechanism for the development of many diabetic complications, including nephropathy.[1165] Glycosylation of ferritin and albumin appears to increase the clearance of these molecules across the glomerular capillaries.[1166, 1167] Atrial natriuretic peptide is increased in experimental diabetes in association with an increased GFR, reduced afferent glomerular resistance, and an increase in glomerular capillary pressures and flows.[1168] Blockade of this peptide with specific antisera or receptor antagonist modulates the diabetes-associated rise in GFR.[1168, 1168a] Finally, the diabetic renal glomerulus contracts less well in response to angiotensin II than do nondiabetic glomeruli.[1169]

Systemic hypertension accelerates the progression of diabetic nephropathy. Long-term studies (6 to 10 years of mean follow-up) have clearly shown that the reduction of mean arterial pressure achieved by using diuretics, β-blockers, and hydralazine slows the progressive loss of renal function in patients with overt diabetic nephropathy.[1170, 1171] However, according to the hypothesis of Brenner and associates,[1172] hyperglycemia and its attendant volume expansion or perhaps metabolic perturbations may set the stage for sustained glomerular damage by inducing intraglomerular hypertension. Various mechanisms have been proposed to account for intraglomerular hypertension. A hormonal agent or changes in sympathetic nervous system function may be capable of inducing reductions in afferent arteriolar resistance, which would in turn allow greater intraglomerular pressures and flows as a maladaptation to reductions in functional nephron mass.[1172] Intraglomerular hypertension can be lowered by administering ACE inhibitors, thus providing a unique renoprotective effect from the damage associated with intraglomerular hypertension. ACE inhibitors maintain elevated renal blood flow in the diabetic but diminish intraglomerular hypertension by efferent arteriolar dilatation. In experimental diabetic animals, ACE inhibitors protected against proteinuria and progressive structural diabetic glomerular disease.[1173] In humans, ACE inhibitors diminished proteinuria in diabetics with microalbuminuria,[1174] moderate proteinuria, and established nephrotic syndrome.[1175-1177] Furthermore, in patients with overt nephropathy, two studies have demonstrated either a decline in the rate of loss of GFR[1178] or a decline in the rate of doubling of the serum creatinine value,[1179] plus a decline in proteinuria, in patients receiving ACE inhibitors compared with control subjects not receiving these drugs. The frequency of death, dialysis, and transplantation was also found to be lower in the patients treated with ACE inhibitors.[1179] These beneficial effects were noted despite similar control of systemic hypertension in the patients receiving ACE inhibitors and those receiving conventional antihypertensive agents.[1178-1180] Furthermore, these benefits also appeared to occur even in patients with overt nephropathy who were not hypertensive.[1179] Thus, ACE inhibitors can currently be recommended for the treatment of diabetic renal disease in all patients with overt nephropathy lacking contraindications (e.g., hyperkalemia, pregnancy). For patients with incipient nephropathy, ACE inhibitors diminished microalbuminuria[1174, 1181-1183] and, in one study, decreased the rate

of loss of GFR.[1174] ACE inhibitors also decreased the incidence of progression from incipient to overt proteinuria in nonhypertensive patients with microalbuminuria.[1181] However, definitive proof that this ultimately results in the maintenance of renal function will require long-term clinical trials.

$Ca^{2+}$ channel blockers have not been systematically studied for long periods in large numbers of patients with diabetic nephropathy. The few studies available are inconsistent in outcome. A number of short-term studies showed no effect on proteinuria[1183a] or worsening of proteinuria[1184, 1185] with the dihydropyridine class of $Ca^{2+}$ channel blockers, especially in patients with non–insulin-dependent diabetes. Other studies showed decrements in proteinuria with either dihydropyridine[1186] or nondihydropyridine $Ca^{2+}$ channel blockers.[1184] The long-term effects of $Ca^{2+}$ channel blockers on GFR in patients with diabetic nephropathy have not been studied for follow-up periods of sufficient duration to make recommendations regarding their efficacy. Studies of young diabetic patients without renal disease reveal that GFR varies with increasing and decreasing dietary protein intake as it does in nondiabetics.[1187] A 3-week crossover study demonstrated that low-protein diets diminished GFR and microalbuminuria in diabetic patients.[1188] A randomized prospective trial was performed in which patients with insulin-dependent diabetes and overt nephropathy were observed for a mean of 34.7 months and randomized to a diet with a protein content of either 0.6 g/kg or more than 1 g/kg.[1189] The rate of change of GFR was less in the group prescribed a low-protein diet than in the high dietary protein group. Thus, dietary protein restriction may be of some benefit in slowing the progression of overt diabetic nephropathy. The effect of low-protein diets on the long-term progression of diabetic nephropathy remains to be firmly established. Rasch[1190] demonstrated that diabetic nephropathy could be prevented in diabetic rats with tight glycemic control. Mauer and co-workers[1191] made the same point by transplanting diabetic kidneys into normal rats. Once normoglycemia was established by this method, a marked regression in prior mesangial thickening was noted. Urinary albumin excretion was abolished, despite the persistence of GBM thickening. Most studies now suggest that tight glycemic control prevents or slows the transition from no nephropathy to incipient nephropathy, as well as the progression from incipient to overt nephropathy. Numerous studies demonstrate decreased microalbuminuria and/or improved GFR in patients treated with an insulin pump or multiple insulin injections to achieve tight glycemic control.[1192-1195] The largest of these studies involved 1400 patients, with a mean follow-up period of 6.5 years.[1195] In the tight glycemic control group, a glycosylated hemoglobin value of approximately 7% was achieved. A substantial lowering of risk for the development and progression of nephropathy was observed,[1195] albeit at the cost of a two- to threefold increased rate of significant hypoglycemia. There is little direct evidence that strict glycemic control substantially retards the progression of established diabetic nephropathy; when combined with optimal control of systemic arterial hypertension, however, some additive benefit may be obtained. Furthermore, tight glycemic control should be achieved in patients with overt nephropathy in order to minimize progressive retinopathy and neuropathy.

When far advanced, however, diabetic glomerulopathy is a progressive disorder that is not amenable to any known form of treatment. Therapy is further complicated by associated extrarenal vascular disease and progressive debilitation. Fortunately, the earlier inferior results of uremia therapy in the diabetic population are showing steady improvement.[1196] Better overall survival with hemodialysis and continuous ambulatory peritoneal dialysis represents significant advances. Optimal rehabilitation is now achieved by renal transplantation in carefully selected patients.[1197] Although the best survival of patients has been offered by living-related donation, the advent of cyclosporine has significantly improved the outlook for the diabetic patient receiving a cadaveric renal allograft by sparing steroid dosage.

## Hereditary Nephritis (Alport Syndrome)

### CLINICAL AND LABORATORY FINDINGS

Dickinson,[1198] in 1875, reported on the familial association of hematuria in three generations of a single family. Guthrie,[1199] Kendall and Hertz,[1200] and finally Alport,[1201] in 1927, studied various members of the same family and described the additional features of albuminuria and azotemia. Alport is credited with drawing attention to the important clinical feature of deafness, and his name is regularly attached to this syndrome. Since then, a number of additional family pedigrees have been described.[1202–1206]

The disorder is frequently discovered in children or young adults.[1204–1206] Males are affected more commonly than females.[1207] Recurrent gross or microscopic hematuria is the most common presenting feature and is often exacerbated by exercise or nonspecific respiratory tract infections.[1204–1207] There is no special relation to streptococcal infections. The hematuria may be accompanied by flank pain or vague abdominal discomfort. Massive proteinuria is uncommon, but typical full-blown nephrotic syndrome has been reported.[1205–1209] Bacteriuria and urinary tract infection may be found but probably not more so than in any chronic renal disease; the radiographic features of chronic bacterial pyelonephritis or reflux nephropathy are not found, however. Slowly progressive renal failure is common, especially in males, and mild hypertension is usually a late complication.[1, 1208, 1209] A number of cases of renal failure have been described in females.[1, 1210]

Sensorineural deafness, particularly to high-frequency sound, is common, occurring in 30% to 50% of patients, but may be detected in some patients only by formal audiometry.[1, 1205, 1206, 1210] There is no clear-cut relation between the severity of the hearing abnormality and renal disease. Other associated findings include various ocular abnormalities (spherophakia, lenticonus, myopia, retinal flecks, cataracts, retinitis pigmentosa, and amaurosis), thrombocytopathia (megathrombocytopenia),[1, 1205, 1207, 1210–1213] and leukocyte inclusions.[1214] These abnormalities may occur without clinically detectable deafness. Perimacular retinal lesions have received attention as specific markers for the disease in a significant proportion of patients.[1215] Other abnormalities have been reported sporadically, including hyperprolinemia and cerebral dysfunction, hypoparathyroidism, aminoaciduria,[1215] thyroiditis,[1216] and leiomyomas.[1216a, 1217] Serum complement levels and Ig levels are typically normal. Antithyroid antibodies may sometimes be present.[1216, 1218]

Detailed family studies have indicated variable modes of inheritance. In the majority of families (at least 50%), transmission occurs via X-linked inheritance. However, autosomal dominance with variable penetrance and expressivity and autosomal recessive transmission have been reported.[1205, 1206, 1219, 1220] Sporadic cases have also been observed.[1205, 1206] In families with clear-cut X-linked transmission, the gene has been mapped to the middle of the long arm of the X chromosome (Xq21.3).[1205, 1206, 1220] In these families renal failure is common in males. In an extensive study of Utah kindreds with this disease, O'Neill and co-workers[1207] found strong support for X-linked inheritance. Thus, male offspring of affected men did not inherit the disease. Women with Alport syndrome transmitted the disease equally to about a third to a half of their sons or daughters. The disease is usually mild and only partially expressed in females but is fully expressed and severe in males. This difference could be accounted for by the Lyon hypothesis, which states that only one X chromosome is active in each cell in females. Thus, a heterozygous female has two cell types, one with the active mutant gene and the other without it. Some have suggested that affected males may have a deficiency of male offspring.[1221] It is of interest to note that in the family originally described by Alport and others, the disease appears to have disappeared spontaneously. More recently, no new cases of nephritis have been discovered in the original family tree.[1202]

It should be pointed out that other hereditary conditions may also be associated with various combinations of proteinuria, hematuria, and azotemia, including Fabry disease, the nail-patella syndrome, sickle-cell disease, urticaria-deafness-amyloidosis syndrome, FMF and amyloidosis, polycystic kidney disease, medullary cystic kidney disease, and partial or total progressive lipodystrophy. The syndrome of benign familial hematuria with thin or attenuated glomerular basement membranes (see also Chapter 30), which is usually not a progressive disorder, may be related to Alport syndrome, because many of the former patients were not formally tested by audiometry.[1222–1224]

### PATHOLOGY

**Light Microscopy.** The findings by light microscopy are varied and nonspecific; the tissue diagnosis rests primarily on electron microscopy and indirect immunofluorescence.[1224, 1225] On the basis of studies of autopsy tissues, the later stages of this disorder had been described diversely as glomerulonephritis, interstitial nephritis, or pyelonephritis. Because of the more frequent use of renal biopsies, earlier lesions have now been well characterized. Although Alport syndrome is considered to be a glomerular disease, early in the course of the disease some patients may have no abnormalities detected by light microscopy.[1, 1226] Other patients have mild focal and segmental increase in cellularity and matrix of the mesangium, usually affecting less than 50%

of the glomeruli, and variable thickening of the GBM.[1227] Persistent fetal glomeruli are observed in about a quarter of patients, especially those younger than 10 years.[1225] As the disease progresses, the glomeruli undergo segmental and then complete sclerosis and often have capsular adhesions.[1225, 1226] Although two siblings with Alport syndrome presenting with acute renal failure and extensive crescentic glomerulonephritis have been described,[1228] crescents are distinctly unusual. The tubule and interstitial changes generally parallel those in the glomeruli. As more glomeruli undergo sclerosis, greater degrees of tubule atrophy and interstitial fibrosis are observed. There is often a mixed interstitial inflammatory infiltrate in advanced cases. Once believed to be the hallmark of the disease, large numbers of interstitial foam cells, most likely of macrophage origin, are present in about 40% of the cases.[1, 1225, 1226] These large cells have pale, foamy cytoplasm and contain neutral fat, mucopolysaccharides, cholesterol, and phospholipids.[1229] Because these cells are found in a large variety of glomerular diseases, their presence should not be considered in any way diagnostic of Alport syndrome (Fig. 31–26).

**Immunofluorescence.** Immunofluorescence has generally been negative in most patients studied. C3 may occasionally be observed in a focal and irregular pattern, however, and IgM, sometimes with C3, has been localized in peripheral capillaries of glomeruli from a small number of patients.[1225, 1226] A significant finding was described by McCoy and co-workers,[1230] who noted that glomeruli of patients with Alport syndrome do not react with anti-GBM antibodies. These investigators suggested that this was evidence that basement membranes of patients with Alport syndrome lack a nephritogenic antigen. They also described a patient with this syndrome who developed anti-GBM antibodies after allotransplantation. This observation has since been confirmed, and anti-GBM antibody disease can develop in allografts in patients with Alport syndrome.[1231] Presumably, this is due to the presence of immunogenic GBM antigens in the allograft and the fact that patients with Alport syndrome lack native tolerance to certain GBM antigens. As a diagnostic aid, therefore, it seems that performing indirect immunofluorescence using an anti-GBM serum (e.g., derived from a patient with Goodpasture syndrome) on tissue from patients with suspected Alport syndrome would be helpful. If the tissue does not bind anti-GBM antibodies, a diagnosis of Alport syndrome is appropriate.[1232] Melvin and co-workers[1233] have also noted the lack of amyloid P component normally found in GBM in these structures in biopsy specimens from patients with Alport syndrome. Amyloid P component and Goodpasture antigen are both absent in some patients.[1206, 1233] Skin biopsy specimens (after acid urea denaturation) may also show deficient expression of an epitope that reacts with anti-GBM antibodies derived from patients with Goodpasture syndrome (see earlier discussion).[1234] Thus, with appropriate reagents, it is possible that Alport syndrome might be diagnosed without resorting to renal biopsy.

**Electron Microscopy.** Ultrastructural studies of glomeruli in Alport syndrome are mandatory, and the changes are often diagnostic. The characteristic alterations affect the basement membranes, which are thickened with longitudinal splitting or layering, reticulation, and fragmentation (basket weave pattern).[1206, 1226, 1235–1237] Thickening and splitting of the glomerular basement membrane are seen more often in males with heavy proteinuria.[1238] There is wide variation in basement membrane appearance, including a normal structure in a small number of patients (Fig. 31–27). The basement membranes are split into layers about 30 to 100 nm in width; the intervening lucent zones often contain small, dense or vacuolated, rounded particles 30 × 90 nm. Extremely thin and attenuated basement membranes are found either adjacent to or between segments of basement membranes involved with these changes or affecting the entire length of a peripheral capillary. This is especially true in children. These structures sometimes reach a thickness of less than 1.5 nm, which is roughly 25% or less of the normal thickness.[1236, 1237] The subepithelial aspects of the basement membrane are typically scalloped.[1239] The earliest changes may be an abnormal thinning and attenuation of the GBM. Not all kindreds with otherwise typical features of hereditary nephritis have these ultrastructural changes. Similar, if not identical, alterations of GBM have been noted in glomeruli from patients affected by other diseases, including IgA nephropathy, postinfectious glomerulonephritis, focal and segmental sclerosis, and other glomerulopathies. For this reason, the specificity of the changes for Alport syndrome has been questioned.[1240] Although Hill and co-workers[1240] observed that in some instances the basement membrane changes were widespread, there were often features of the other diseases (such as the presence of characteristic electron-dense deposits) to permit differentiation from Alport syndrome. Kohaut and associates[1241] and others,[1226] on the other hand, noted that the basement membrane changes in a variety of glomerular diseases were most likely to affect small segments of the capillary walls, whereas they were widespread in Alport syndrome. It is concluded that ultrastructural evaluation of basement membranes is a useful way to diagnose hereditary nephritis.

Other changes that are noted in glomeruli include varia-

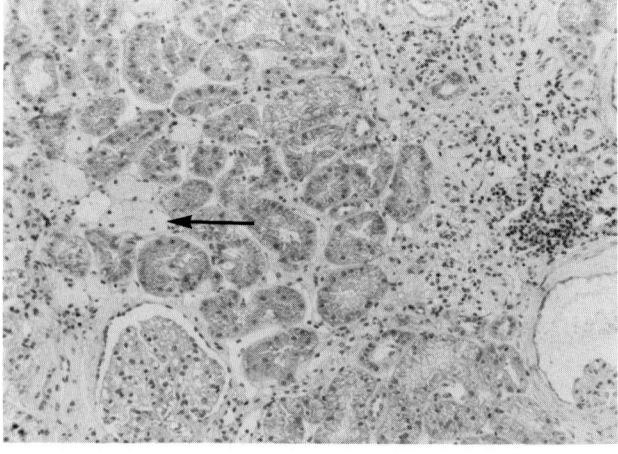

**Figure 31–26.** Light microscopic appearance of hereditary nephritis (Alport syndrome). Nonspecific glomerular changes are present; there are clusters of atrophic tubules and interstitial lymphocytes. Note the commonly found but nondiagnostic interstitial foam cells *(arrow)*. (Hematoxylin-eosin; magnification × 250.)

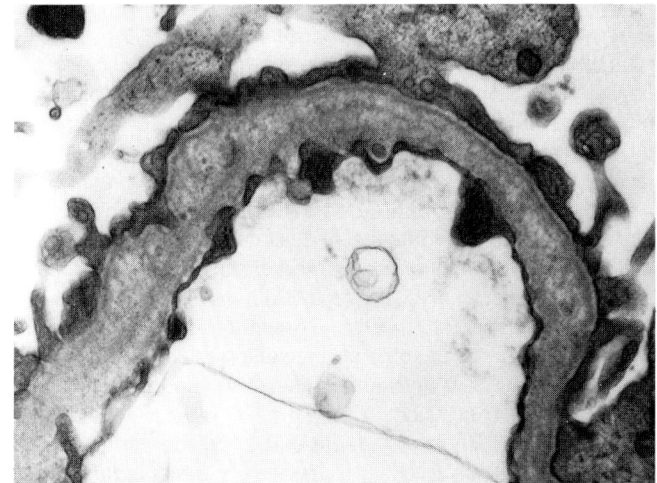

**Figure 31–27.** Ultrastructural appearance of GBM in hereditary nephritis (Alport syndrome). The basement membrane is thickened, layered, and irregular in contour. (Magnification × 9000.)

ble obliteration of epithelial foot processes, variable increase in mesangial matrix, and variable increase in mesangial cellularity, as described earlier for light microscopy.[1, 1226] Similar alterations (layering, reticulation, dense inclusions) have also been described in the basement membranes of Bowman capsules and renal tubules, but usually to a lesser degree.[1226, 1235, 1242] Because they may be commonly observed in many other diseases, their significance is unknown and their diagnostic value is limited.

As mentioned, the typical basement membrane lesions are not present in all cases.[1239] Grünfeld and co-workers have suggested that the absence of the lesion is generally associated with a less severe clinical course.[1222] Serial biopsy specimens from many patients have shown a progression of the characteristic changes, so that greater proportions of the capillary walls are involved.[1222, 1227] On the other hand, Beathard and Granholm[1242] reported a kindred with hereditary nephritis who on initial biopsy had normal findings, whereas a second biopsy in two patients 8 years later disclosed the usual basement membrane lesions. This suggests that, in certain affected individuals, the anatomic abnormalities may not develop for many years and that a normal biopsy specimen does not exclude the disease. In one study, capillary loop size is similar in Alport patients and age-matched control subjects younger than 10 years but is significantly smaller in patients older than 10 years.[1243]

## PATHOGENESIS

The primary defect in Alport syndrome associated with X-linked inheritance is the result of mutations (including single base pair substitutions, deletions, insertions, and duplications) in the COL4A5 gene encoding a novel α5 peptide chain of type IV collagen.[1206, 1219, 1244–1249] However, the structural abnormalities observed in the Alport GBM probably involve more than the peptide chain encoded by the mutated gene. Serum amyloid P component is absent in some kindreds.[1233] Type IV collagen peptide chains α1(IV) and α2(IV), determined by genes on chromosome 2[1206, 1250] normally restricted to the mesangial and subendothelial glomerular regions, are present diffusely in the GBM of patients with Alport syndrome who have biopsies at a time

when glomeruli appear normal by light microscopy.[1250] With progressive renal insufficiency and glomerular obsolescence, these classic type IV collagen peptide chains disappear, in association with an increase in collagen V and VI.[1250] Furthermore, it has been known for some time that the basement membranes of patients with Alport syndrome often do not react with anti-GBM antibodies,[1231–1233] suggesting absence, alteration, or unavailability of the COL4A3-determined α3 NC1 domain.[1249, 1251] In affected males and mosaic females, urea-denatured skin biopsy specimens reveal a similar lack of an epitope on the globular (NC1) domain of type IV collagen, introducing the possibility that the diagnosis of Alport syndrome may be achievable by skin biopsy in some patients.[1234] The precise mechanism by which these diffuse structural basement membrane defects occur is currently unknown. However, the data indicate that mutations in the COL4A5 gene alter the local expression and incorporation of other collagens into the basement membrane. Cationic components of GBM are also deficient.[1252] Genetic screening is difficult because of the large number of mutations and the lack of "hot spots" on the genomic sequence involved.[1206] In the related condition of hereditary nephritis with deafness and diffuse leiomyomatosis, the deletion of the 5' end of the COL4A5 gene extends into the adjacent COL4A6 gene.[1216, 1217]

## COURSE AND THERAPY

Recurrent hematuria may be present for many years before the onset of renal failure, which subsequently is only slowly progressive.[1, 1204, 1210, 1238, 1253] Affected males usually enter terminal renal failure before the fifth decade of life, whereas females rarely develop renal failure.[1253] Some investigators have noted that progressive renal failure is most often correlated with more complex splitting and layering of the GBMs.[1254] No satisfactory form of treatment is available.[1, 1204–1208] The disease does not usually recur in renal allografts.[1231] As noted, however, a more fascinating immunopathologic observation has been made in allografted kidneys. This observation entails the appearance of circulating antibody directed against the Goodpasture epitope on *COL4A3* in a minority of patients with Alport syndrome who undergo renal transplantation.[1233, 1234, 1255-1257] Graft loss from this complication has been reported.[1257] However, in many of these patients, linear IgG was present in glomeruli, but renal function was unaffected.[1257] This more benign course appears to be more prevalent in patients in whom linear GBM staining is accompanied by the absence of measurable anti-GBM antibody in the serum.[1257] In other patients, the binding of this antibody to the GBM in allografts has led to crescentic nephritis reminiscent of that seen in other anti-GBM nephritides.[1258, 1259]

A perhaps related disorder, benign familial hematuria with thin basement membranes (see Chapter 30), is characterized by persistent or recurrent hematuria and little or no tendency for progression to impairment of renal function. Renal tissue is almost always normal by light microscopy. The GBMs, as observed ultrastructurally, are nearly uniformly extremely thin and attenuated, without, however, the layering or splitting of Alport syndrome. Many patients with abnormally thin basement membranes apparently do not have a familial history. The typical presentation is hematuria with or without proteinuria and, rarely, renal failure. A favorable prognosis is usually noted. This entity is discussed in greater detail in Chapter 30.[1260-1262]

## Angiokeratoma Corporis Diffusum Universale (Fabry Disease)

Fabry disease is an X-linked inborn error of glycosphingolipid metabolism with deficient tissue activity of a specific lysosomal enzyme, α-galactosidase A.[1263-1267] The disorder is transmitted by the presence of a defective gene on the long arm of the X chromosome, Xq22 > q24.[1267, 1268] In the hemizygote, the gene is highly penetrant, and intrafamilial as well as interfamilial variations in the clinical expression of the enzyme defect have been observed. The entire sequence of the human gene has been encoded, and a full-length complementary DNA is available.[1269, 1270] Specific molecular derangements differ from family to family. Gene rearrangements,[1271, 1272] exonic point mutations,[1271, 1273] and base pair deletions[1274] have all been reported. The enzyme deficiency leads to the accumulation of neutral glycosphingolipids (globotriaosylceramide) in many tissues, including the kidney. The clinical manifestations are protean. The most common skin lesions are reddish purple macules ranging in size from micrometers to several millimeters, most often in the distribution of the abdomen, buttocks, hips, genitalia, and upper thighs. Other less characteristic findings include palmar erythema, splinter hemorrhages, and conjunctival and buccal mucous membrane telangiectasias. Autonomic neuropathy is manifested by acral paresthesias, hypohidrosis, impaired pupillary constriction, diminished saliva and tear formation, and disordered intestinal motility.[1275, 1276] Premature coronary and cerebrovascular arterial disease with cardiac dysrhythmias is common.[1275, 1276] Strokes and myocardial ischemia may be found. Other reported cardiac features include valvular lesions and hypertrophic nonobstructive cardiomyopathy.[1276, 1277] Corneal opacities (verticillata) are seen in virtually all hemizygotes and most heterozygotes. Other ocular

findings include edema of the retina and eyelids, posterior capsular cataracts, and tortuous retinal and conjunctival vessels.[1275] Anemia, lymphadenopathy, hepatosplenomegaly, aseptic necrosis of the bone, myopathy, hypogammaglobulinemia, and hypoalbuminemia have been reported.[1278] Renal disease, manifested by hematuria and mild proteinuria, is common in male hemizygotes and is reported occasionally in female heterozygotes. Females typically lack the cutaneous features. The diagnosis can be made easily, however, on the basis of characteristic morphologic findings, especially the ultrastructural abnormalities.[1279, 1280]

In men, ESRD frequently develops by the fifth decade of life.[1275, 1278] Patients with blood groups B and AB have an earlier onset of disease and a more severe symptomatic course, perhaps related to accumulation of a terminal α-galactose substance occurring during the synthesis of the B antigen on the red blood cell membrane.[1281] In individuals whose clinical presentation suggests α-galactosidase A deficiency, measuring the enzyme in peripheral blood leukocytes is helpful in confirming the diagnosis. Although hemizygotes usually have almost no measurable enzymatic activity, as little as 6% to 20% activity may mask the clinical syndrome.[1275, 1278] Because female heterozygotes may have enzyme activity levels in the low normal range, leukocyte α-galactosidase A determinations are insensitive in identifying carriers.[1276-1278] The carrier state is better identified by measuring urinary ceramide digalactoside and trihexoside.[1276] Prenatal diagnosis can be made by measuring amniocyte enzyme levels.[1278]

Renal morphologic features have been studied in both symptomatic and asymptomatic individuals. As demonstrated by Gubler and co-workers,[1264] the accumulation of glycosphingolipid may be observed in hemizygous patients early in life; the major site of this lipid is in the glomerular epithelial cells, most prominently the visceral epithelial cells, and, to a lesser degree, the parietal cells lining the Bowman capsule (Fig. 31–28). By light microscopy, the cells are enlarged, with abundant cytoplasm filled with numerous clear, small, uniform vacuoles, imparting a foamy appearance. In paraffin-embedded sections, the vacuoles do

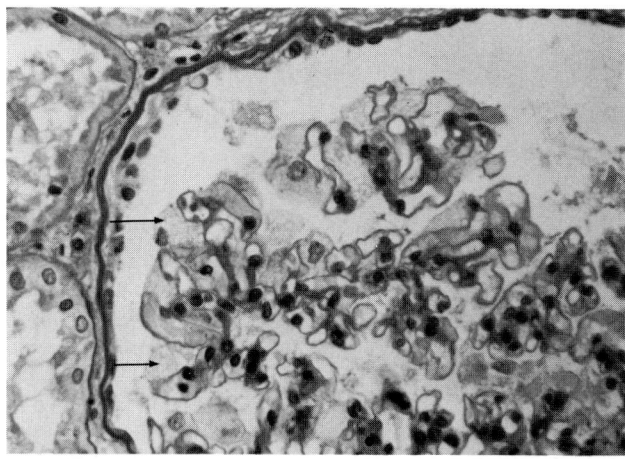

**Figure 31–28.** Light microscopic appearance of Fabry disease. The visceral epithelial cells are enlarged and finely vacuolated *(arrows)*. (Periodic acid–Schiff; magnification × 500.)

not stain with periodic acid–Schiff or other reagents; if, however, the tissue is examined before being placed in lipid-soluble solutions, the vacuoles can be shown to contain double refractile lipid with the use of cross-polarized filters, Sudan black staining, or oil red O. This material may also be observed in glomerular endothelial and mesangial cells. Tubule epithelial cells are often involved, the distal convoluted tubules and loops of Henle more severely than the proximal tubules. Endothelial and muscle cells of arteries can also be sites of lipid storage. In heterozygous individuals, the same changes are present but to a considerably lesser degree.[1, 1264, 1282]

The ultrastructural features are characteristic. The vacuoles are noted to be single membrane-bound dense bodies of variable size; these structures are most often lamellated and round, with a concentric onionskin appearance, or ovoid, with a parallel arrangement of layers (myelin figures or zebra bodies) (Fig. 31–29). The dense bodies are rarely amorphous. In either event, high resolution and magnification indicate that the material has similar features (i.e., regularly arranged light and dark layers of 4- to 5-nm periodicity). Electron microscopy has shown that every type of renal cell is involved—glomerular visceral and parietal epithelium; mesangial and endothelial cells; arterial, arteriolar, and peritubule capillary endothelial cells; arterial smooth muscle; and interstitial cells—even when apparently normal by light microscopy (see Fig. 31–28). Although the distal tubules and loops of Henle are involved, the proximal tubule cells are not always affected. In addition to these changes of lipid storage, glomerular podocytes usually have some degree of foot process effacement. Initially, the GBMs are normal; as the disease progresses, including presumably the vascular changes, however, the effects of ischemia are noted, including thickening and collapse of the basement membranes, focal segmental and global glomerular sclerosis, and tubule atrophy and interstitial fibrosis. As a possible diagnostic aid, ultrastructural examination of the urine sediment for the characteristic cellular structures, both free and intracellular, has been performed. Immunofluorescence microscopy has rarely been reported; the findings have been negative, except when segmental sclerosis is present, at which time segmental IgM and complement are demonstrated.[1, 1282, 1283]

Apart from providing the patient with a source of the deficient or ineffective enzyme, no treatment is available. Neither phlebotomy to remove senescent erythrocytes (a source of plasma ceramide trihexoside) nor infusion of the enzyme, leukocytes, platelets, and fetal liver cells nor plasma exchange has been successful in improving the biochemical defect for significant periods. Initial enthusiasm for renal transplantation[1284, 1285] as a source of the enzyme has been countered with less optimistic findings.[1286, 1287] Tubule secretion of the enzyme by the transplant is enhanced by acute alkalinization of the blood and is diminished by acute acidification. However, chronic acidification fails to maintain diminished urinary excretion of the enzyme. Thus, manipulation of acid-base balance on a long-term basis fails to increase serum enzyme levels after transplantation.[1288] Although significant enzyme repletion is an unlikely prospect after renal transplantation, long-term kidney function in patients with Fabry disease has been reported.[1289] One group urged caution in transplanting organs in patients with Fabry disease because of an unexpectedly high 1- to 5-year mortality from sepsis.[1290] Patients with ESRD resulting from α-galactosidase A deficiency, however, appear to have cellular and humoral immune responses no different from those seen in other uremic patients.[1291] Glycosphingolipid deposits recur in transplanted kidneys but have not been reported to cause functional graft loss. Enzyme replacement is currently impractical and expensive; recombinant DNA technology, however, offers a potential method of producing pharmacologic quantities of the deficient enzyme.

## Hereditary Osteo-onychodysplasia (Nail-Patella Syndrome)

The nail-patella syndrome, an autosomal dominant disease, occurs at a frequency of approximately 22 per million.[1292, 1293] It is genetically linked to the loci for ABO blood groups and for adenylate cyclase on chromosome 9[1294–1299] and is manifested in children or young adults by the presence of dystrophic nails, absence of one or both patellas, deformity of the elbow joints, iliac horns, and an

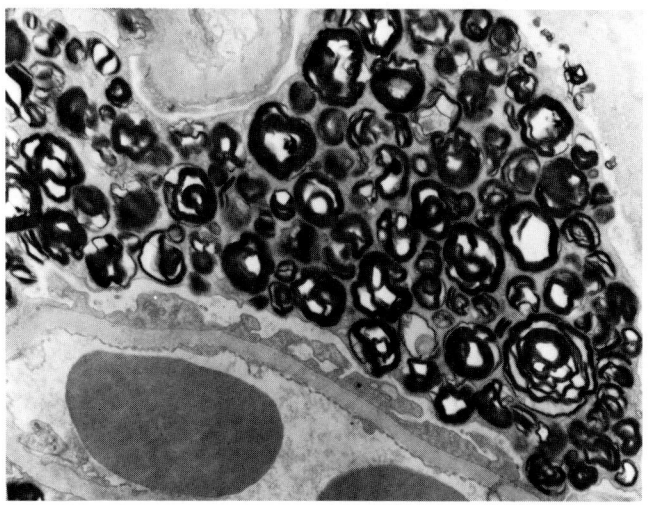

**Figure 31–29.** Electron microscopic appearance of Fabry disease. Numerous zebra bodies are present in visceral epithelial cells. Note similar structures also in an endothelial cell of the glomerular capillary in the lower left corner. (Magnification × 5500.)

assortment of other skeletal abnormalities.[1293-1297] More than half of the patients with skeletal abnormalities have an abnormal urine sediment, impaired urinary concentrating ability, or abnormalities in urine acidification or protein excretion.[1296] The most frequent presenting signs and symptoms include proteinuria, microhematuria, hypertension, and edema.[1294] The nephrotic syndrome and progressive renal failure occur occasionally.[1293-1301] Membranous glomerulonephritis and anti-GBM antibody–mediated nephritis[1300, 1301] have been reported superimposed on the congenital defect. Congenital malformations of the urinary tract and renal stones occur in a disproportionate number of patients. Although direct proof is lacking, it has been suggested that nail-patella syndrome may be a true collagen disease, reflecting an abnormality in the synthesis, structure, or degradation of collagen. In support of this conjecture is the finding that in two of three patients tested, the GBM failed to bind a monoclonal antibody directed against the Goodpasture epitope.[1302] This suggests, first, that there may be heterogeneity in basement membrane composition in this disorder. Furthermore, it suggests that in some patients the novel collagen peptide α3(IV), which carries the Goodpasture epitope, may be absent, altered, or unavailable for binding. It is unclear whether this abnormality is a primary or a secondary event. The glomerular changes by light microscopy are nonspecific, generally showing variable degrees of focal and segmental sclerosis, segmental thickening of the capillary wall, and hypercellularity. Electron microscopy reveals a unique and characteristic lesion consisting of a mottled and moth-eaten appearance of the GBM caused by localized areas of rarefaction. The presence of intramembranous fibrils having the periodicity of collagen is considered to be specific for this lesion (Fig. 31–30) and is best demonstrated with the use of phosphotungstic acid stain.[1296, 1297] Because of the collagen deposition, nail-patella syndrome is believed to be related to collagen III glomerulopathy (see Chapter 30), a primary renal disease without associated nail or osseous abnormalities characterized by extensive glomerular deposition of type III collagen. IgM and C3 immunofluorescent deposits have been observed in sclerotic segments, but the disease is considered to be a generalized disorder of the mesenchyme. Genetic counseling may be useful to patients as they consider family planning. Looij and colleagues,[1303] using their own as well as published data, concluded that for patients in families with clinically apparent renal disease, the risk of having a child with congenital nephropathy is 1 in 4 and the risk of having a child who progresses to ESRD is 1 in 10. Characteristically, the course is rather benign, with renal failure a late feature.[1295-1297] No treatment is known to be effective; occasional patients have received transplants.[1304]

## Congenital Nephrotic Syndrome (Finnish Type)

Congenital nephrotic syndrome is a rare disease characterized by the development of massive proteinuria at or within 3 months of birth. It occurs with a high incidence in Finland and in families of Finnish extraction but may also be seen in patients of non-Finnish extraction. The placenta is usually large (more than 25% of birth weight), and the affected individuals have low birth weight relative to gestational age. Massive proteinuria, ascites, anasarca, and polycythemia but normal or nearly normal GFR are present initially. Failure to thrive and superimposed infectious complications are common.[1309] Sometimes IgM levels are elevated. IgG levels tend to be low. Infusions of gamma globulin change the character of the proteinuria from highly selective to nonselective.[1310] The diagnosis may be established in utero with a characteristic family history and elevated α-fetoprotein levels in the amniotic fluid and maternal sera.[1311-1314] Associated abnormalities include pyloric stenosis and severe gastroesophageal reflux, resulting in aspiration pneumonia and thrombotic complications.[1, 1309]

This disorder is inherited as an autosomal recessive trait, and heterozygotes are clinically normal, but renal biopsies have not been performed on heterozygotes. The gene frequency may be as high as 0.2 in some areas of Finland. The disorder has occurred in only one of a pair of dizygotic twins, which seems to negate any possible intrauterine influence on the development of the disease.[1304-1308]

Renal biopsy or autopsy material reveals a microcystic

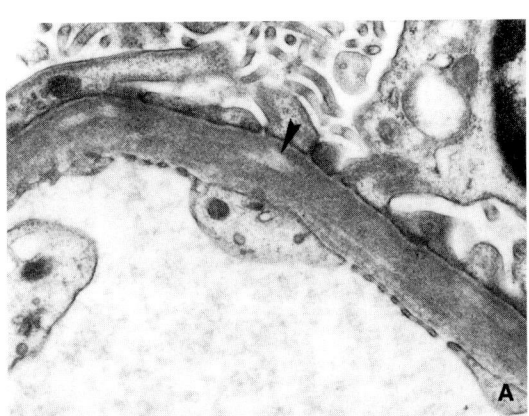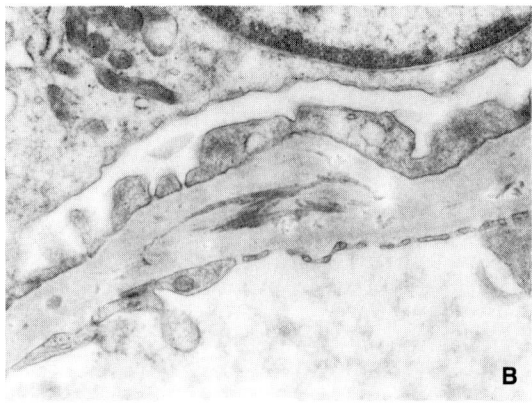

**Figure 31–30.** *A.* Electron photomicrograph of portion of GBM in nail-patella syndrome. The basement membrane is thickened, containing irregular lucencies *(arrowhead).* (Magnification × 15,000.) *B.* Similar segment stained with phosphotungstic acid and demonstrating dense fibrils representing collagen. (Magnification × 15,000.)

appearance to the cortex with a sclerosing process affecting glomeruli (Fig. 31–31). The cystic appearance is the result of dilatation of proximal convoluted tubules. Some glomeruli appear normal. Electron microscopy reveals diffuse abnormalities of the foot processes in addition to collapse and sclerosis of glomerular tufts. Immunofluorescence is generally negative, but there are occasional reports of irregular IgG and C3 deposits in glomeruli. The precise pathogenesis is unknown, but a study demonstrated the absence of heparan sulfate anionic sites in the GBM of patients with this disease.[1315] Thus, it has been proposed that there is an underlying defect in the rate of GBM proteoglycan synthesis. None of the patients in this study were of Finnish extraction.[1315] The course is a progressive one in that most patients die of complications of nephrotic syndrome or renal failure in the first year of life. Few survive long enough to be considered candidates for dialysis and transplantation.[1305–1308] Treatment with steroids and cytotoxic drugs has been entirely ineffective.[1307] Patients who have received transplants exhibit dramatic improvement in psychomotor retardation. Although post-transplantation nephrotic syndrome has been observed, it is not clear that this is due to recurrence of the original disease.[1316]

Another form of congenital glomerulopathy, diffuse mesangial sclerosis, has been reported[1317] (see also Chapter 30). More frequently seen in children between the ages of 3 months and 3 years, it is occasionally diagnosed at birth or within the first 3 months of life. Histopathologically, it is characterized by sclerotic glomeruli surrounded by hypertrophied and vacuolated glomerular visceral epithelial cells. Cystically dilated tubules are present, most prominently in the deep cortex. Clinically, these patients present with proteinuria, most often with the nephrotic syndrome, and relatively rapid progression to ESRD. Occasional patients have had features of the Drash syndrome—either Wilms tumor or male pseudohermaphrodism or both.[1317, 1318] Other associated features have also been reported, including cataracts, corneal clouding, microcephaly, strabismus, nystagmus, and hypertelorism. The syndrome has occurred in siblings. It is unresponsive to therapy and may recur in renal allografts.[1317] The development of nephrotic syndrome in these patients after transplantation could be due to complicating cytomegalovirus infection or rejection.[1316]

Other examples of familial aggregation of nephrotic syndrome usually appearing several months after birth have been reported.[1308, 1309, 1315] These patients, in all likelihood, are afflicted by distinctly different disorders, and the prognosis is usually good in comparison with the congenital nephrotic syndrome. It should be pointed out that congenital syphilis, HIV infection (especially in the offspring of narcotic addicts), malaria, cytomegalovirus infection, and toxoplasmosis in the neonate have been associated with massive proteinuria. Although male pseudohermaphrodism (46,XY) and ocular abnormalities are common accompaniments of Drash syndrome, this syndrome has also been reported in a 46,XX female.[1318] The lesion in the kidney is diffuse mesangial sclerosis (see also Chapter 30). Prophylactic bilateral nephrectomy has been recommended because of the extremely high prevalence of bilateral Wilms tumor. The Galloway-Mowat syndrome, consisting of microcephaly, hypotonia, developmental abnormalities, and ear anomalies, is also associated with congenital nephrotic syndrome.[1319] The typical renal pathologic picture consists of flocculent material and narrow fibrils (6 to 8 nm in length) deposited in a structurally distorted GBM. Roos syndrome, consisting of microcephaly, infantile spasms, and psychomotor retardation, is also a familial disorder appearing in infancy commonly accompanied by nephrotic syndrome.[1320] The renal pathology in Roos syndrome is focal and segmental glomerulosclerosis with extensive mesangiolysis. Spondyloepithelial dysplasia, mental retardation, conductive hearing loss, and retinitis pigmentosa may be another syndrome associated with focal and segmental glomerulosclerosis and nephrotic syndrome in infancy.[1321] Renal vein thrombosis may also be a complication of the nephrotic syndrome developing in neonatal life and may be associated with the rapid development of renal failure.

## Sickle-Cell Disease

The vast majority of patients with sickle-cell anemia or sickle-cell trait have no clinically apparent renal disease, although virtually all of the former and many of the latter experience papillary necrosis and associated urinary concentrating defects.[1322, 1323] Microscopic or gross hematuria is often observed, presumably the result of microinfarcts in the medulla and papillae.[1322]

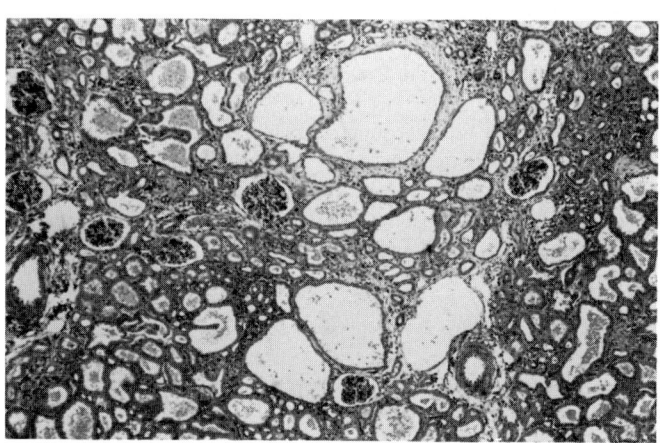

**Figure 31–31.** Light microscopic appearance of congenital nephrotic syndrome. Cystically dilated cortical tubules can be seen; glomerular abnormalities are inconspicuous. (Hematoxylin-eosin; magnification × 150.)

Glomerular disease is less common than tubulointerstitial disease. In a prospective study, the prevalence of proteinuria (>1+ on dipstick) was 31% in patients with hemoglobin SS disease and 16% in patients with hemoglobin SC or sickle cell–thalassemia.[1324] The majority of patients with proteinuria had less than 3 g/d. An elevated serum creatinine level was present in 7% of patients.[1324]

ESRD may occur in as many as 18% of patients with sickle-cell anemia.[1325] Immunosuppressive therapy has generally been disappointing. ACE inhibitors acutely decrease proteinuria even without altering systemic blood pressure, inulin clearance, or effective renal plasma flow.[1323, 1324] The effectiveness of ACE inhibitors in diminishing proteinuria and the observations of glomerular hypertrophy in patients with sickle-cell anemia implicate hemodynamic factors in the initiation and/or progression of the glomerulopathy.[1326] However, the effectiveness of ACE inhibitors in diminishing proteinuria and preventing loss of renal function over the long term remains to be demonstrated. Both dialysis and transplantation are feasible in these patients, and graft survival is comparable to that observed in the general transplant population.[1327, 1328] However, long-term survival is poor, largely because of complications of the systemic disease.[1327, 1328]

Renal biopsy specimens in patients with sickle-cell disease have revealed enlarged and congested glomeruli displaying sickled erythrocytes within the capillary lumen.[1323, 1325, 1329] Various degrees of mild proliferation involving the mesangial cells are commonly seen. There is mild to moderate capillary wall thickening because of a reduplication of the GBM, which resembles mesangiocapillary glomerulonephritis.[1, 1329, 1330] Iron can be seen in the endothelial and epithelial cells and hemosiderin in the tubule epithelial cells.[1330] In particular, patients with nephrotic syndrome develop lesions resembling mesangiocapillary glomerulonephritis with an increased lobulation; however, focal and segmental glomerulosclerosis and membranous glomerulonephritis have also been described.[1323, 1329, 1331, 1332] Similar lesions have been seen in sickle cell–thalassemia.

Electron microscopy has revealed the accumulation of granular deposits measuring about 25 nm in the mesangium and subepithelial areas. There is also frequently a mild mesangial proliferation and peripheral mesangial interposition.[1330] Electron-dense deposits are usually not seen. Immunofluorescence findings may be negative; irregular granular deposits of IgG and C3 in the peripheral capillary location have been observed in several patients, however.[1331] These have generally been associated with cases of nephrotic syndrome and a picture of membranous or mesangiocapillary glomerulonephritis.[1, 1331] One group of investigators reported finding deposits of a renal tubule antigen in a distribution similar to the granular IgG and C3 deposits, raising the possibility that sickle-cell disease may be associated with renal tubule injury, release of immunogenic tubule antigens, and the production of renal tubule antigen-antibody complexes that provoke glomerular injury.[1321, 1332]

The course of renal disease is generally that of persistent and massive proteinuria, with slowly progressive glomerulosclerosis and the ultimate development of renal failure.[1, 1322, 1323] Treatment of the renal disease is generally unsatisfactory, and although only a few cases have been studied,

no beneficial effects of steroids or cytotoxic agents have been noted. It is possible that long-term ACE inhibitor therapy may delay the progression of the disease because the underlying glomerular lesions may be hemodynamically mediated.[1323] Renal transplantation should no longer be considered contraindicated in these patients.[1327, 1328] Graft survival and survival of patients are comparable to those of the general transplant population. Appreciable morbidity and mortality temper enthusiasm for transplantation in these patients, however.[1327, 1328] Sickle-cell crisis is still common in patients who have received transplants.[1333]

## Partial or Total Lipodystrophy (Barraquer-Simons Disease)

Lipodystrophy occurs in a partial form, in which lipoatrophy usually involves the neck, arms, cheeks, and abdomen.[1334] This entity is associated with increased fat deposits in the hips and legs.[1334] It has also been described in a more diffuse form, total lipodystrophy, in which diminished adipose tissue is generalized, or in a patchy distribution associated with a variety of metabolic disturbances including euthyroid hypermetabolism, hyperproteinemia, hyperlipidemia, hyperinsulinism, insulin resistance, and nonketotic hyperglycemia.[1335, 1336] Occasional patients have signs and symptoms that overlap between partial and total lipodystrophy. Because the pathogenesis and pathophysiology of these disturbances are poorly understood, a convenient classification has been suggested based on the time of onset of the syndrome.[1336] Total lipodystrophy is subdivided into congenital and acquired forms. Partial lipodystrophy appears to be uniformly acquired and is often preceded by a viral syndrome.[1335, 1336] Renal disease is common in patients with lipodystrophic disorders, but lipoatrophy may precede the onset of overt renal disease by as much as 20 years. The most consistent renal syndrome observed is mesangiocapillary glomerulonephritis, type II (dense deposit disease; see also Chapter 30), which is seen most commonly in patients with partial lipodystrophy. These patients are usually found to have asymptomatic proteinuria and microscopic hematuria on routine screening examination; however, the nephrotic syndrome is occasionally present. A diminished serum concentration of the third component of complement in association with C3 nephritic factor is also frequently present, but neither is a requirement or a sufficient element for the presence of renal disease.[1337] Pyelonephritis and chronic and acute glomerulonephritis have all been reported in patients with partial or total lipodystrophy based on the clinical findings of albuminuria, macroscopic and microscopic hematuria, pyuria, acute flank pain, fever, edema, hyperlipidemia, hypertension, and azotemia.[1336] Because many of these patients did not undergo renal biopsy, the relation of the signs and symptoms to mesangiocapillary glomerulonephritis is not known. Hydronephrosis and collecting system dilatation have also been reported.[1336]

Apart from its renal manifestations, generalized lipodystrophy may also manifest itself in tall stature, muscular hypertrophy, hirsutism, macroglossia, abdominal distention, acanthosis nigricans, subcutaneous nodules, hepatomegaly, genital enlargement, febrile adenopathy, cerebral atrophy, cerebral ventricular dilatation, mental retardation, hemiplegia, and cardiomegaly.[1336–1338] Occasional patients with partial lipodystrophy share these signs and symptoms. When present, the mesangiocapillary proliferative lesion often progresses rapidly to ESRD. Dense deposits have recurred in both cadaveric and living related donor transplants.[1339] The pathogenesis of this syndrome and the relation among the complement abnormalities, the disturbances in fat and glucose metabolism, and renal disease remain obscure.

## Other Heredofamilial Diseases

The hereditary amyloidoses (FMF, Muckle-Wells syndrome, and familial amyloidosis with polyneuropathy) have been commented on in earlier sections of this chapter. Glomerulonephritis and vasculitis associated with $\alpha_1$-antitrypsin deficiency have also been discussed earlier. The association of Charcot-Marie-Tooth disease with nephritis was discussed earlier. Hurler syndrome (type I mucopolysaccharidosis) may be associated with the nephrotic syndrome.[1340] Renal biopsy specimens reveal extensive vacuolization of visceral epithelial cells and numerous intracellular inclusions. After many years, patients with type I glycogen storage disease (von Gierke disease) may develop proteinuria, progressive renal failure, and hypertension. Renal biopsy specimens reveal focal and segmental glomerulosclerosis and hyalinosis. Many of these patients had greatly elevated GFRs preceding or coincident with onset of proteinuria, implying a hemodynamic basis for glomerular injury.[1341, 1342]

Juvenile intestinal malabsorption of vitamin $B_{12}$ with megaloblastic anemia (Imerslund syndrome) is an autosomal recessive disorder associated with isolated proteinuria and glomerular lesions.[1343] Asphyxiating thoracic dystrophy (Jeune syndrome) is another lethal autosomal recessive disorder sometimes associated with glomerular lesions in addition to tubule defects and interstitial nephritis.[1344] Hereditary osteolysis, an autosomal dominant disorder, may at times be associated with chronic glomerulonephritis.[1345] This disease is characterized by recurring bouts of acute arthralgia and progressive deformity of wrists and ankles.

Hereditary lecithin-cholesterol acyltransferase (LCAT) deficiency is an autosomal recessive condition resulting in low levels or dysfunction of the enzyme LCAT that is responsible for cholesterol esterification.[1346–1354] Therefore, when this syndrome is considered in a differential diagnosis, studies of LCAT mass by radioimmunoassay[1353a] or studies of LCAT biologic activity[1353b] should be performed. Complementary DNA clones for human LCAT have been isolated and utilized to analyze the genetic defect in affected families.[1349] Initial reports failed to identify gene rearrangements or abnormal gene fragments.[1349] Instead, missense mutations,[1349, 1350] single base pair substitutions,[1353] and short base pair insertions[1352] have been identified. LCAT deficiency is characterized by hematuria, nonselective proteinuria, bone marrow foam cells, normal C3 levels, anemia (normochromic, normocytic with target cells), corneal opacities, increased triglyceride and cholesterol levels, premature atherosclerosis, and hyperuricemia. Urinalysis may be completely normal or may disclose the presence of erythrocytes or hyaline or granular casts. Mild proteinuria

is usually present early in life, progressing to frank nephrotic syndrome in the fourth to fifth decade. The development of nephrotic syndrome usually heralds a rapid loss of renal function and accompanying hypertension. The major lesions are in the glomeruli. By light microscopy, the basement membranes are irregular and thickened, often with small, clear, rounded, lucent bubbles, some of which may also be found in the mesangial matrix. Foam cells are found in scattered glomerular capillaries, in the interstitium, and in the walls of arteries and arterioles. The ultrastructural changes are distinctive and unique; mesangial matrix and basement membranes are permeated by small and large lucent zones in which are found small rounded dense structures (Fig. 31–32). These lesions may also be found in basement membranes of tubules and Bowman capsule and in arteries and arterioles. They represent tissue lipid deposits.[1346–1348] Dietary therapy to lower serum lipid levels and plasma infusion to restore enzyme levels have not been effective in altering outcome in patients with LCAT deficiency.[1354] Renal transplantation does not increase plasma LCAT activity. Histologic recurrence has been reported in transplanted kidneys.[1346]

As noted previously, atypical SLE may be associated with congenital partial or complete deficiency of various complement components, including C1r, C1s, C2, C4, C5, and C8. C2 deficiency is particularly common and is associated with the HLA-A10, -B8, -DR2 haplotypes. Cystinosis[1355, 1356] (Fig. 31–33) and hereditary spherocytosis may also be associated with glomerular lesions, particularly focal glomerulosclerosis. Nephrotic syndrome may complicate cystinosis, particularly in the adult-onset variety. These patients have blonde hair, photophobia, hypothyroidism, crystalline corneal deposits, rickets, and Fanconi syndrome. The glomerular lesions are focal and segmental glomerulosclerosis with cystine crystals found in the glomerular epithelial cells and tubule epithelial cells. Bone marrow aspirates may also contain cystine crystals. End-stage renal failure is common. Although the glomerular lesions do not specifically recur in the transplanted kidney, cystine crystals may be found in the host cells infiltrating the glomeruli and tubules.[1355, 1356]

Scattered reports of the occurrence of various forms of glomerulonephritis in a familial pattern have been observed. These have most commonly been IgA nephropathy, but mesangiocapillary glomerulonephritis, IgM nephropathy, and thin–basement membrane disease have also been described in multiple members of the same family[1357] (see also Chapter 30).

## MEDICATIONS, IMMUNIZATIONS, AND ALLERGENS

A large variety of medications has been reported to be associated with glomerular lesions, frequently presenting with a nephrotic syndrome.[1, 1358–1401] In some patients, the association is so close or has occurred so frequently as to suggest a cause-and-effect relationship.[1, 1359–1368] In others, however, the relationship is more tenuous, and the nephrotic syndrome may have occurred by chance alone in these patients. In a few examples (probenicid, trimethadi-

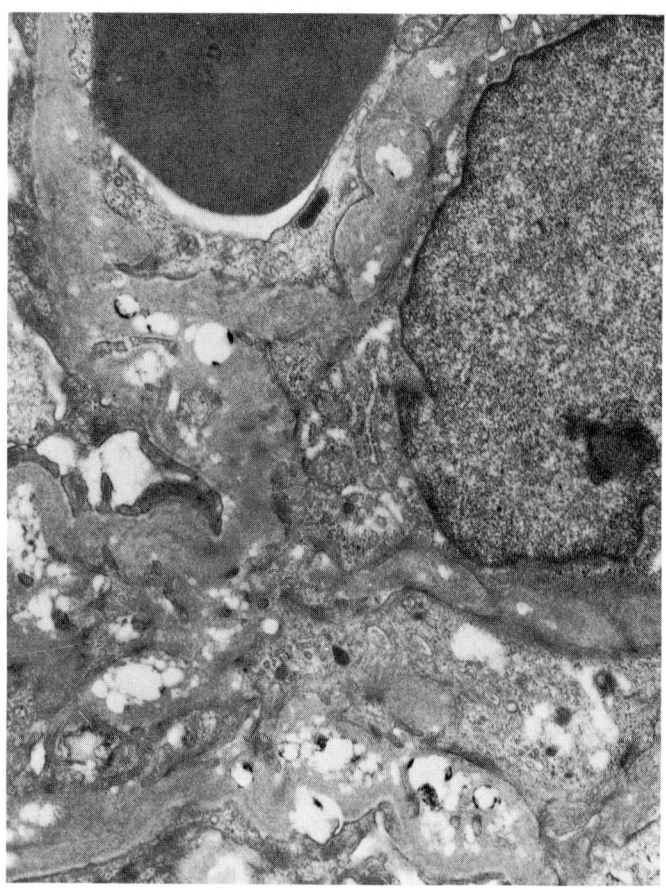

**Figure 31–32.** Electron photomicrograph from a patient with LCAT deficiency depicting multiple clear lacunae, with dense, rounded membranous structures, throughout mesangial matrix and in basement membranes. (Magnification × 14,500.) (Courtesy of A Magil.)

one), repeated exposure has led to the recurrence of a similar syndrome. Manifestations of hypersensitivity reactions, such as urticaria, occur not uncommonly, particularly after exposure to gold, penicillamine, probenicid, and the anticonvulsant group of medications. Susceptibility to drug-induced nephrotic syndrome may be genetically determined and linked to HLA, particularly to HLA-DR3 and -DR4 (see Chapter 30).

The nephrotic syndrome in intravenous heroin abuse is associated with a variety of glomerular lesions but chiefly

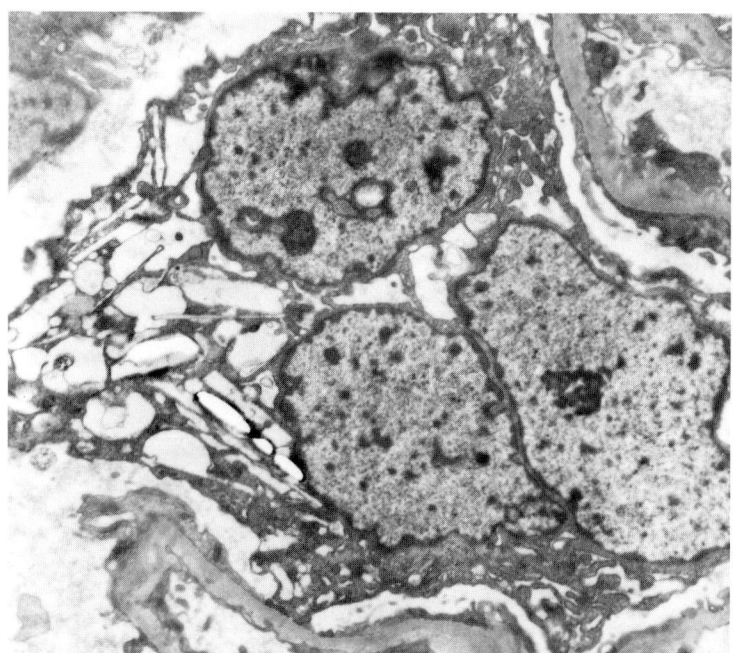

**Figure 31–33.** Electron photomicrograph of portion of glomerulus in cystinosis. The visceral epithelial cell is enlarged and multinucleate and contains numerous elongated spaces representing dissolved crystals. (Magnification × 5800.)

those of focal glomerular sclerosis and mesangiocapillary glomerulonephritis.[1, 1374–1376] Segmental granular deposits containing IgM, C1q, and C3 in a subendothelial location are seen frequently.[1] Focal glomerular sclerosis and nephrotic syndrome in heroin addicts appear to have a poor prognosis in that more than three fourths of such patients develop end-stage renal failure within 4 years of the onset of proteinuria.[1375] All forms of treatment appear to be ineffective, and the lesion may progress despite discontinuance of heroin.[1375] Some of these patients have reduced complement levels, circulating C3NF-like activity, and C1q precipitins,[1] suggesting CICs. In most cases, assay for HBs antigen or anti–hepatitis C antibodies has been negative, but a relation to hepatitis virus cannot be excluded. Concomitant cryoglobulinemia, decreased serum levels of C4, hepatosplenomegaly, and vasculitis are strongly suggestive of chronic hepatitis C virus–associated mixed (IgG-IgM) cryoimmunoglobulinemia (see earlier). An immune response to contaminants in the street or brown heroin or to other infectious agents to which addicts are unduly susceptible could also be important in the pathogenesis. Some studies have cast doubt on the specificity of the association between heroin abuse and nephrotic syndrome.[1] As mentioned, some heroin addicts develop amyloidosis. Many intravenous drug abusers, including heroin users, may develop HIV-associated nephropathy (see earlier discussion). The main distinguishing point between heroin nephropathy and HIV-associated nephropathy is the finding of large kidneys in HIV-associated nephropathy and normal to small kidneys in heroin-associated nephropathy. Renal biopsy findings are also distinctive, but focal and segmental glomerulosclerosis is common to both entities.

Preparations containing organic mercurials given orally, parenterally, or topically have been associated with proteinuria and nephrotic syndrome.[1369, 1377] Elemental mercury and inorganic mercurial salts taken accidentally or intentionally also have produced massive proteinuria.[1, 1369, 1377] The pathologic findings in these cases have often been available, but either minimal glomerular changes or membranous glomerulopathy has usually been observed by light microscopy.[1369] Most of the biopsy material showing only minimal glomerular changes was not studied by electron microscopy or immunofluorescence and therefore might represent early examples of membranous glomerulopathy. Partial or complete remissions may occur spontaneously on withdrawal of the offending agent. With the introduction and wide usage of potent nonmercurial diuretics, reports of the nephrotic syndrome with heart failure and constrictive pericarditis have virtually ceased.[1]

Gold, given parenterally or orally in the therapy of RA, may cause hematuria, proteinuria, or the nephrotic syndrome. Frequently, there is an associated dermatitis.[1] Renal biopsy specimens usually have demonstrated mild membranous glomerulonephritis and infrequently minimal-change disease; the syndrome is usually reversible with discontinuance of the drug.[1] HLA-DR2 and -DR3 may be linked to susceptibility to development of nephrotic syndrome on exposure to gold therapy.[1371, 1372] The pathogenesis of the nephrotic syndrome secondary to exposure to heavy metals such as mercury and gold is unknown. The release of antigens through a toxic effect on the renal tubule followed by

the formation of autologous renal tubule antigen-antibody complexes is one possible explanation (see Chapter 29). It is also possible that the heavy metal forms a complex with a nonrenal autologous tissue protein, rendering it immunogenic and thus capable of forming antigen-antibody complexes. Nephrotic syndrome may occur with oral gold therapy in about 1% of patients so treated. Lower serum and renal gold concentrations, however, may explain the lower risk than with parenteral therapy.[1371] D-Penicillamine usage appears to be clearly related to the occasional occurrence of nephrotic syndrome[1, 1382]; usually membranous glomerulonephritis with granular subepithelial deposits of IgG and C3 has been found. However, on occasion, crescentic glomerulonephritis,[1384] rarely involving anti-GBM antibodies,[1382] has been reported. Bucillamine has also been associated with rapidly progressive (crescentic) glomerulonephritis.[1378] Individuals with RA not receiving penicillamine or gold therapy may also develop membranous glomerulonephritis de novo. Nephrotic syndrome secondary to bismuth tartrate therapy has been reported, but no pathologic reports are available to assess a possible cause-and-effect relationship.[1360] Lithium therapy for depression has occasionally been implicated in the development of nephrotic syndrome, often with minimal-change disease on renal biopsy.[1361] Nephrotic syndrome and focal and segmental glomerulosclerosis complicating lithium therapy have also been reported.[1386]

Treatment with certain anticonvulsant agents including mesantoin, trimethadione, and paradione may be associated with the nephrotic syndrome.[1359, 1360] Massive proteinuria generally abates with discontinuance of the drug and may recur with reinstitution; some patients display persistent proteinuria, however. Little information is available on pathology, but minimal glomerular change and membranous glomerulonephritis have been observed. The pathogenesis is unknown, but some investigators have reported production of massive proteinuria in rats treated with trimethadione.[1359] Single case reports have appeared describing the nephrotic syndrome as a complication of perchlorate treatment[1367] of thyrotoxicosis. Tolbutamide and chlorpropamide therapy of mild diabetes mellitus, interferon therapy for mycosis fungoides, and phenindione have all been associated with nephrotic syndrome.[1366] Probenicid has been associated with massive proteinuria on a number of occasions, and re-exposure to the drug has produced a recrudescence of massive proteinuria.[1368] Allopurinol, penicillin, sulfonamides, and thiazides have occasionally been linked to the development of proliferative glomerulonephritis, sometimes in association with systemic vasculitis.[1386] Clonidine antihypertensive therapy has been implicated in nephrotic-range proteinuria and hyperglycemia.[1387] Captopril therapy for severe hypertension has occasionally produced heavy proteinuria caused by membranous glomerulonephritis.[1388] Cross-sensitivity does not occur with enalapril, and the substitution of enalapril for captopril has been associated with resolution of proteinuria.[1389] In addition, the new appearance of proteinuria in patients receiving captopril has generally been associated with large doses, and, in some patients, improvement in proteinuria has been noted even with continuation of therapy.[1390] The use of rifampin, warfarin, amoxicillin, and penicillamine has been associated with rapidly progressive glomerulone-phritis.[1362, 1391, 1392]

With the widespread use of the NSAIDs came the de-scription of a relatively infrequent syndrome of acute renal failure accompanied by the nephrotic syndrome. Implicated NSAIDs have included fenoprofen, sulindac, naproxen, zomepirac, ibuprofen, ketoprofen, and salicylate,[1393–1394] but it is likely that all NSAIDs share a common propensity to cause nephrotic syndrome infrequently. Membranous glomerulonephritis may also occasionally be seen in associa-tion with NSAIDs. Spontaneous relapse of naproxen-asso-ciated nephrotic syndrome has been reported. The interval between the beginning of therapy and the onset of docu-mented renal injury ranged from a few months to more than a year. The typical clinical picture includes edema, ne-phrotic-range proteinuria, hypoalbuminemia, mild to severe azotemia, and often hypertension. Oliguria and the need for dialysis have been common. Eosinophilia, eosinophiluria, rash, and fever are often absent. Renal biopsy most often discloses minimal-change glomerulopathy in association with acute tubulointerstitial nephritis. Immunofluorescence microscopy has usually been negative, but trace amounts of amorphous IgG deposits have occasionally been identi-fied.[1396] Studies of the infiltrating interstitial cells show them to be predominantly T lymphocytes. Studies suggest a cell-mediated immunopathogenesis for this disorder.[1399] Although discontinuation of the drug usually results in complete recovery, some authors[1396] have suggested the early use of corticosteroids in these patients to prevent renal scarring.[1396] Recombinant interferon-α has produced similar lesions, and immune complex glomerulonephritis has some-times been observed. On occasion, an unusual lesion con-sisting of widening of the capillary wall caused by thick-ening of the lamina rara interna may be associated with nephrotic syndrome and renal insufficiency in patients re-ceiving interferon alfa treatment for leukemia.[1380]

A number of cases of multiple recurrences of nephrotic syndrome associated with milk or pollen allergy have been reported. Most of these have been children who presumably have had minimal-change lesions. Some of these latter cases were associated with the eventual onset of renal fail-ure and may have had focal glomerular sclerosis. It is dif-ficult to be sure if milk or pollen hypersensitivity is the cause of nephrotic syndrome or merely a precipitating fac-tor, but elimination diets have reduced frequency of re-lapses. Poison oak, polio vaccination, smallpox vaccination, bee stings, snake bite, wool, insect repellants, antilympho-cyte globulin, and radiographic contrast materials have on rare occasions been reported to be associated with the ne-phrotic syndrome.[1] Nephrotic syndrome has been observed in patients after bone marrow transplantation.[1381, 1383] This could be attributed to graft-versus-host reactions or to the effect of high-dose chemotherapy included as part of the conditioning regimen.[1381] Membranous glomerulonephritis and prominent mesangiolysis with glomerulosclerosis have been found in renal biopsies.[1381, 1383] A peculiar form of glomerular disease has been reported to occur in 1% to 2% of patients who have received renal allografts and been treated with cyclosporine. Glomerular involvement and other smaller vessels display evidence of thrombotic micro-angiopathy that usually results in graft loss.[1400, 1401] Occa-

sional case reports, however, indicate resolution after cyclo-sporine is reduced or discontinued. Depletion of endothelial prostaglandin $I_2$ induced by the drug may be part of the underlying pathogenetic mechanism, similar to that which occurs in the microangiopathic lesions seen in thrombotic thrombocytopenic purpura and hemolytic-uremic syndrome (see also Chapter 30).

## RECURRENT GLOMERULONEPHRITIS

Recurrence of glomerulonephritis in renal allografts and isografts, in both primary and secondary glomerular dis-ease, is dealt with in greater detail in Chapter 59. It is also discussed in connection with specific diseases in this and other chapters. This subject has been extensively re-viewed.[1402–1406] The overall recurrence rate in renal allo-grafts for all forms of glomerulonephritis averages about 20%, but the specific disease-related recurrence varies widely from zero or quite rare (Alport syndrome and SLE) to near certainty if the graft enjoys long-term survival (in-sulin-dependent diabetes mellitus, IgA nephropathy, mes-angiocapillary glomerulonephritis type II).[1402–1406]

Many recurrences are not associated with clinical find-ings and are diagnosed only as a consequence of transplant renal biopsy. The clinical manifestations of recurrence in-clude proteinuria, hematuria nephrotic syndrome, and rap-idly progressive glomerulonephritis. Many recurrent dis-eases have limited impact on overall graft survival (e.g., IgA nephropathy), whereas others contribute significantly to graft failure (e.g., focal and segmental glomerulosclero-sis, mesangiocapillary glomerulonephritis). In some, recur-rence may not strictly affect donor tissue, but rather the influx of host cells afflicted with a metabolic disorder in-vading the transplanted kidney gives rise to the appearance of recurrence (Fabry disease, cystinosis). Diseases that progress rapidly in the recipient may have a greater ten-dency to recur in the allograft. Living related donor kidneys may be at somewhat greater risk for recurrence than cadav-eric kidneys, but this is controversial. Multiple recurrences may develop in repeated allografts, especially in focal and segmental glomerulosclerosis. Cyclosporine therapy may be associated with a somewhat lower rate of recurrence com-pared with that in patients receiving azathioprine immuno-suppression maintenance, but this difference is not strik-ing.[1402–1406]

The management of recurrent disease is similar to that of the original disease, although in some cases aggressive management, including plasma exchange for recurrent focal and segmental glomerulosclerosis, may be quite successful, at least temporarily. More specific details regarding therapy of recurrent disease is given in the sections dealing with the individual disease entities. De novo glomerular disease oc-curring in renal allografts that is distinctly different from the original disease is described elsewhere (Chapter 59) but may include membranous glomerulonephritis, focal and segmental glomerulosclerosis, mesangiocapillary glomeru-lonephritis, glomerular thrombotic microangiopathy, dia-betic glomerulosclerosis, and crescentic glomerulonephri-tis.[1406] The last is especially likely to occur in Alport syndrome and is due to the development of anti-GBM auto-antibodies[1258, 1259] (see earlier). A specific transplant (allo-graft) glomerulopathy may accompany chronic rejection. This lesion may evoke significant proteinuria and thus resemble recurrent glomerulonephritis.

## MISCELLANEOUS DISORDERS

Glomerular abnormalities, as both morphologic curiosities and clinically significant lesions, have been described in massively obese individuals.[1407–1413] Asymptomatic glomerular enlargement has been reported by Suzuki and Cohen.[1407, 1408] The patients described had either no urinary abnormalities or mild proteinuria. On the other hand, Weisinger and co-workers[1411] and Warnke and Kempson[1412] reported a total of five massively obese individuals with nephrotic syndrome; the major morphologic findings in all who had renal biopsies consisted of focal and segmental glomerular sclerosis.[1411, 1412] Rare patients have normal renal biopsy specimens[1409]; most have focal sclerosing lesions,[1410, 1413] but a variety of renal lesions may be found.[1410] In all patients, the proteinuria diminished significantly with considerable reduction in weight. In a review of 22 massively obese subjects with proteinuria, Verani and co-workers[1413] noted the frequent occurrence of focal and segmental glomerulosclerosis. No association was found between the extent of the obesity and the glomerular lesions, but a relationship was found between left ventricular enlargement and hypercholesterolemia and the presence of glomerular lesions, supporting the notion that the association between obesity and glomerular lesions may be mediated by hemodynamic factors and perhaps fostered by lipid disturbances.

Glomerular enlargement and prominence of the axial portion of the glomerulus are frequently observed in cyanotic congenital heart disease and in conditions in which chronic hypoxia and polycythemia are present,[1414–1416] such as chronic cor pulmonale accompanying emphysema and cystic fibrosis. There appears to be a relation between the hematocrit level and the glomerular diameter in these states. Progressive renal insufficiency with prominent glomerulomegaly and focal and segmental glomerulosclerosis are observed.[1416] The increase in glomerular size is not reflected in an increase in renal weight, tubule maximum for *p*-aminohippuric acid, or GFR. The urinary findings are mild or nonexistent, and the precise mechanism of the glomerular changes involved is unknown, but it could involve hemodynamic changes.[1414, 1415]

Glomerulonephritis has been reported in patients without SLE or with seronegative lupus who nevertheless have circulating antibodies to cardiolipin or who demonstrate the lupus anticoagulant (primary antiphospholipid syndrome).[1417, 1418] Hypertension occurs in more than half and nephrotic syndrome in somewhat less than half. Although the majority of patients reported have a thrombotic microangiopathy, the authors have also seen membranous nephropathy as well as typical IgA nephropathy in a patient with an IgA anticardiolipin antibody.

Patients with unilateral renal agenesis,[1419, 1420] hypoplasia of the kidney, or subtotal nephrectomy may later develop progressive proteinuria and even nephrotic syndrome and progressive renal failure. Glomerular lesions have most commonly been focal and segmental glomerulosclerosis. It has been postulated that long-standing adaptive hemodynamic changes in glomerular pressure and plasma flow are responsible for this association.

Renal arterial stenosis, either unilateral or bilateral, is a rare cause of heavy proteinuria and nephrotic syndrome. Surgical correction of the lesion may result in the prompt disappearance of proteinuria. This phenomenon is presumably related to renin proteinuria and thus may be due to an alteration in glomerular function secondary to the increased production of angiotensin II by the ischemic juxtaglomerular apparatus.[1421] Dermatitis herpetiformis, a chronic pruritic skin disease characterized by crops of herpetic vesicles and malabsorption, may be associated with nephrotic syndrome. CICs have been detected in some of these cases. Glomerular IgA deposits are found.[1422] Severe preeclampsia of pregnancy may be associated with massive proteinuria and the biochemical features of nephrotic syndrome.[1423] Interestingly, such patients often develop nephrotic syndrome in later pregnancies rather than in their first. Such proteinuria abates rapidly on termination of pregnancy. Glomerular lesions consist chiefly of endothelial cell swelling and mesangial cell prominence. Electron-dense deposits are not observed; fibrin-related antigens, increased amounts of fibronectin, Ig, and complement components are frequently detected in the mesangium and along the capillary walls by immunofluorescence, however. Localized intrarenal vascular coagulation may be responsible for some of the observed disturbances.

As already noted, the nephrotic syndrome may develop as a complication of chronic rejection of renal allografts or as a manifestation of recurrence of the original disease in the graft (see specific clinicopathologic entities).[1402, 1405, 1424] De novo nephrotic syndrome in renal allografts is usually membranous glomerulonephritis. De novo membranous glomerulonephritis in renal allografts is associated with cationic IgG spectrotypes in the serum and with increased amounts of small (9S) IgG-containing immune complexes.[1425] Mesangiocapillary or focal glomerular sclerosis may also be seen, but it is uncertain whether these patterns are independent of chronic rejection. Takayasu arteritis, myxedema, thyroiditis, osteomyelitis without amyloidosis, ulcerative colitis, and retroperitoneal fibrosis have been associated with nephrotic syndrome on rare occasions. McDuffie syndrome, consisting of hypocomplementemia with cutaneous vasculitis, ulcerative colitis, and type A immune-mediated gastritis, has also been associated with glomerular lesions.[1426–1428] Renal vein thrombosis, constrictive pericarditis, congestive heart failure, and tricuspid insufficiency have been discussed previously.[1] Silicoproteinosis nephropathy may occasionally produce the nephrotic syndrome[1429–1431] and crescentic glomerulonephritis resulting from IgA nephropathy.[1431] The glomerular lesions in this condition can resemble Fabry disease.[1429]

The glomerular lesions encountered in dysproteinemias, neoplasias, infections, drug reactions, and heredofamilial disorders have been commented on earlier in this chapter. Sarcoidosis and Sjögren syndrome have been associated with membranous glomerulonephritis or focal and segmental glomerulosclerosis.[1432] Steroid therapy of these diseases may result in complete remissions. Kimura disease, consisting of pruritus, eosinophilia, greatly elevated IgE levels, retroauricular masses, subcutaneous granulomas, lymphoid and vascular proliferation, and extensive tissue eosinophil infiltration, is frequently associated with the nephrotic syndrome.[1433] A variety of glomerular lesions have been observed, including membranous glomerulonephritis, proliferative glomerulonephritis, and minimal-change disease. Long-term glucocorticoid therapy often leads to a favorable outcome. Castleman disease, consisting of fever, night sweats, lymphadenopathy, hepatosplenomegaly, polyclonal hyperimmunoglobulinemia, circulating factor VIII inhibitors, greatly elevated interleukin-6 serum levels, and angiofollicular lymph node hyperplasia, is occasionally associated with nephrotic syndrome and/or hematuria.[1434] A wide variety of glomerular lesions may be observed, including minimal-change disease, membranous glomerulonephritis, mesangial proliferative glomerulonephritis, mesangiocapillary glomerulonephritis, crescentic glomerulonephritis, and amyloidosis. Aggressive immunosuppressive regimens may have beneficial effects on the renal disease.

### Acknowledgments

The authors thank Carlos A. Ayala, Susan Darett, Charlotte Townsend, and Carol Mitchell for excellent secretarial assistance. Jo-Anne Glassock provided very valuable library assistance.

## REFERENCES

1. Glassock RJ, Cohen AH, Adler SG, Ward HJ: Secondary glomerular diseases. In Brenner BM, Rector FC Jr (eds): The Kidney, 4th ed. WB Saunders, Philadelphia, 1991, p 1280.
2. Osler W: The visceral lesions of purpura and allied conditions. Br Med J 1:517, 1914.
3. Wallace D, Dubois E: Dubois' Lupus Erythematosus. Lea & Febiger, Philadelphia, 1987.
4. Lahita R: Systemic Lupus Erythematosus. John Wiley & Sons, New York, 1987.
5. Balow JE, Austin HA III: Lupus nephritis. In Massy SG, Glassock RJ (eds): Textbook of Nephrology, 2nd ed. Williams & Wilkins, Baltimore, 1991–1992, pp 787–796.
6. Cameron JS: Lupus and nephritis in children. Adv Nephrol 22:59–117, 1993.
7. Hayslett JP, Kashgarian M: Nephropathy of septic lupus erythematosus. Clinical manifestations of systemic lupus erythematosus (SLE). In Schrier RW, Gottschalk CW (eds): Diseases of the Kidney, 4th ed. Little, Brown, Boston, 1988, pp 2253–2271.
8. Cameron JS, Turner DR, Ogg CS, et al: Systemic lupus with nephritis: A long-term study. Q J Med 48:1, 1979.
9. Balow J: Lupus nephritis (NIH conference). Ann Intern Med 106:79, 1987.
10. Tan EM, Cohen AS, Fries JF, et al: The 1982 revised criteria for the classification of systemic lupus erythematous. Arthritis Rheum 25:1271, 1982.
11. Canoso JJ, Cohen AS: A review of the use, evaluations, and criticisms of the preliminary criteria for the classification of systemic lupus erythematosus. Arthritis Rheum 22:917, 1979.
12. Manu P: Serial probability analysis of the 1982 revised criteria for the classification of systemic lupus erythematosus. N Engl J Med 309:1460, 1983. Letter.
13. Wasicek CA, Reichlin M: Clinical and serologic differences between systemic lupus erythematosus patients with antibodies to Ro and La. J Clin Invest 69:835, 1982.
14. Sharp GC: Subsets of SLE and mixed connective tissue disease. Am J Kidney Dis 2(suppl 1):201, 1982.
15. Sontheimer RD, Thomas JR, Gilliam JN: Subacute cutaneous lupus erythematosus: A cutaneous marker for a distinct lupus erythematosus subset. Arch Dermatol 115:1409, 1979.
16. Maddison PJ, Provost TT, Reichlin M: Serologic findings in patients with "ANA-negative" systemic lupus erythematosus. Medicine (Baltimore) 60:87, 1981.
17. Hamilton MD, Infield JB: T cells in systemic lupus erythematosus. Arthritis Rheum 22:1, 1979.
18. Smolen JS, Chused TM, Leiserson WM, et al: Heterogeneity of immunoregulatory T-cell subsets in systemic lupus erythematosus. Am J Med 72:783, 1982.
19. Leehey DJ, Katz AI, Azaran AH, et al: Silent diffuse lupus nephritis: Long-term follow-up. Am J Kidney Dis 2(suppl 1):188, 1982.
20. Cavallo T, Cameron WR, Lapenas D: Immunopathology of early and clinically silent lupus nephropathy. Am J Pathol 87:1, 1977.
21. Bennett W, Houghton D, Bardana E, Striker G: Staging of renal involvement in systemic lupus erythematosus when clinical involvement is absent. Clin Res 24:161A, 1976.
22. Woolf A, Croker B, Osofsky SG, Kredich DW: Nephritis in children and young adults with systemic lupus erythematosus and normal urinary sediment. Pediatrics 64:678, 1979.
23. Koffler D, Agnello V, Carr I, Kunkel HG: Variable patterns of immunoglobulin and complement deposition in the kidneys of patients with systemic lupus erythematosus. Am J Pathol 56:305, 1969.
24. Dujovne I, Pollak VE, Pirani CL, Dillard MG: The distribution and character of glomerular deposits in systemic lupus erythematosus. Kidney Int 2:33, 1972.
25. Dillard MG, Tilman RL, Sampson CC: Lupus nephritis: Correlations between clinical course and presence of electrondense deposits. Lab Invest 32:261, 1975.
26. Ascer J, Walker JA, Lief PD, et al: Triad of glomerulonephritis, antinuclear antibodies, and positive skin immunofluorescence. Am J Med 74:83, 1983.
27. Lahita RG, Chiorazzi N, Gibofsky A, et al: Familial systemic lupus erythematosus in males. Arthritis Rheum 26:39, 1983.
28. Roberts JL, Hayashi JA: Exacerbation of SLE associated with alfalfa ingestion. N Engl J Med 308:1361, 1983.
28a. Ward MM, Studenski S: Clinical prognostic factors in lupus nephritis. The importance of hypertension and smoking. Arch Intern Med 152:2082, 1992.
29. Eagen JW, Memoli VA, Roberts JL, et al: Pulmonary hemorrhage in systemic lupus erythematosus. Medicine (Baltimore) 57:545, 1978.
30. Mintz G, Galindo IF, Fernandez-Diaz J, et al: Acute massive pulmonary hemorrhage in systemic lupus erythematosus. J Rheumatol 5:39, 1978.
31. Schocket AL, Lain D, Kohler PF, Steigerwald J: Immune complex vasculitis as a cause of ascites and pleural effusions in systemic lupus erythematosus. J Rheumatol 5:33, 1978.
32. Moutsopoulos HM, Gallagher JD, Decker JL, Steinberg AD: Herpes zoster in patients with systemic lupus erythematosus. Arthritis Rheum 21:798, 1978.
33. Sobel JD, Alroy G, Falor Z, et al: Systemic lupus erythematosus, Sjögren's syndrome and glomerular nephritis. Postgrad Med J 53:97, 1977.
34. Cunningham E, Provost T, Brentjens J, et al: Acute renal failure secondary to interstitial lupus nephritis. Arch Intern Med 138:1560, 1978.
35. Tron F, Ganeval D, Droz D: Immunologically mediated acute renal failure of nonglomerular origin in the course of systemic lupus erythematosus (SLE): Report of two cases. Am J Med 67:529, 1979.
36. Park M, D'Agati V, Appel GB, Pirani CL: Tubulointerstitial disease in lupus nephritis: Relationship to immune deposits, interstitial inflammation, glomerular changes, renal function, and prognosis. Nephron 44:309, 1986.
37. Henry R, Williams AV, McFadden NR, Pilea PA: Histopathologic evaluation of lupus patients with transient renal failure. Am J Kidney Dis 6:417, 1986.
38. Carvana RJ, Barish CF, Buckalew VM: Complete distal renal tubular acidosis in systemic lupus: Clinical and laboratory findings. Am J Kidney Dis 6:59, 1985.

39. ter Borg EJ, de Jong PE, Meijer SS, Kallenberg CGM: Tubular dysfunction in proliferative lupus nephritis. Am J Nephrol 11:16, 1991.

40. Green JA, Dawson AA, Walker W: Systemic lupus erythematosus and lymphoma. Lancet 2:753, 1978.

41. Dimant J, Ginzler E, Schlesinger M, et al: The clinical significance of Raynaud's phenomenon in systemic lupus erythematosus. Arthritis Rheum 22:815, 1979.

42. Baker SB, Rovira JR, Campion EW, Mills JA: Late onset systemic lupus erythematosus. Am J Med 66:727, 1979.

43. Klippel JH, Gerber LH, Pollak L, Decker JL: Avascular necrosis in systemic lupus erythematosus: Silent symmetric osteonecroses. Am J Med 67:83, 1979.

44. Gelfand J, Truong L, Stern L, et al: Thrombotic thrombocytopenic purpura syndrome in systemic lupus erythematosus: Treatment with plasma infusion. Am J Kidney Dis 6:154, 1985.

45. Hughson MD, Nadasdy T, McCarty GA, et al: Renal thrombotic microangiopathy in patients with systemic lupus erythematosus and the antiphospholipid syndrome. Am J Kidney Dis 20:150–158, 1992.

46. Scolari F, Savoldi S, Costantino E, et al: Antiphospholipid syndrome and glomerular thrombosis in the absence of overt lupus nephritis. Nephrol Dial Transplant 8:1274–1276, 1993.

47. Mandreoli M, Zucchelli P: Renal vascular disease in patients with primary antiphospholipid antibodies. Nephrol Dial Transplant 8:1277–1280, 1993.

48. Frampton G, Hicks J, Cameron JS: Significance of anti-phospholipid antibodies in patients with lupus nephritis. Kidney Int 39:1225–1231, 1991.

49. Whittle TS, Ainsworth SK: Procainamide-induced systemic lupus erythematosus: Renal involvement with deposition of immune complexes. Arch Pathol Lab Med 100:469, 1976.

50. Weisbart RH, Yee WS, Colburn KK, et al: Anti-guanosine antibodies: A new marker for procainamide-induced systemic lupus erythematosus. Ann Intern Med 104:310, 1986.

51. Garin EH, Donnelly WH, Fennel RS, Richard GA: Nephritis in systemic lupus erythematosus in children. J Pediatr 89:366, 1979.

52. Fish AJ, Blau EB, Westberg NG, et al: Systemic lupus erythematosus within the first two decades of life. Am J Med 62:99, 1977.

53. Ty A, Fine B: Membranous nephritis in infantile systemic lupus erythematosus associated with chromosomal abnormalities. Clin Nephrol 12:137, 1979.

54. Franco HL, Weston WL, Peebles C, et al: Autoantibodies directed against sicca syndrome antigens in the neonatal lupus syndrome. J Acad Dermatol 4:67, 1981.

55. McCurdy DK, Lehman TJA, Bernstein B, et al: Lupus nephritis: Prognostic factors in children. Pediatrics 89:240, 1992.

56. Tejani A, Nicastri AD, Chen C-K, et al: Lupus nephritis in black and Hispanic children. Am J Dis Child 137:481, 1983.

57. Hamburger J, Richet G, Crosnier J, Antoine B, et al: Nephrology, Vol II. WB Saunders, Philadelphia, 1968, Chap. 24.

58. Budman DR, Steinberg AD: Hypertension and renal disease in systemic lupus erythematosus. Arch Intern Med 136:1003, 1976.

59. Gruppo Italiano per lo Studio della Nefrite Lupica (GISNEL): Frequency and prognostic value of renal vascular lesions (RVL) in patients with systemic lupus erythematosus. Kidney Int 37:437, 1990. Abstract.

60. Haider YS, Roberts WC: Coronary arterial disease in systemic lupus erythematosus: Quantification of degrees of narrowing in 22 necropsy patients (21 women) aged 16 to 37 years. Am J Med 70:755, 1981.

61. Homcy CJ, Liberthson RR, Fallon JT, et al: Ischemic heart disease in systemic lupus erythematosus in the young patient: Report of six cases. Am J Cardiol 49:478, 1982.

62. Rao TKS: Hemodialysis and transplantation in systemic diseases: the facts. In Friedman EA (ed): Strategy in Renal Failure. John Wiley & Sons, New York, 1978, p 321.

63. Nossent HC, Swaak TJG, Berden JHM: Systemic lupus erythematosus: Analysis of disease activity in 55 patients with end-stage renal failure treated with hemodialysis or continuous ambulatory peritoneal dialysis. Am J Med 89:169–174, 1990.

64. Cheigh TS, Stenzel KH: End-stage renal disease in systemic lupus erythematosus. Am J Kidney Dis 21:2–8, 1993.

65. Cheigh TS, Kim H, Stenzel KH, et al: Systemic lupus erythematosus in patients with end-stage renal disease: Long-term follow-up

66. Sires RL, Adler SG, Louie JS, Cohen AH: Poor prognosis in end-stage lupus nephritis due to nonautologous vascular access site associated septicemia and lupus flares. Am J Nephrol 9:279, 1989.

67. Alarcón-Segovia D, Delezé M, Oria CV, et al: Antiphospholipid antibodies and the antiphospholipid syndrome in systemic lupus erythematosus. A prospective analysis of 500 consecutive patients. Medicine (Baltimore) 68:353, 1989.

68. Cameron JS, Frampton G: The "antiphospholipid syndrome" and the "lupus anticoagulant." Pediatr Nephrol 4:663, 1990.

69. Farrugia E, Torres VE, Gastineau D, et al: Lupus anticoagulant in systemic lupus erythematosus: A clinical and renal pathological study. Am J Kidney Dis 20:463, 1992.

70. Angles-Cano E, Sultan Y, Clauvel JP: Predisposing factors to thrombosis in systemic lupus erythematosus: Possible relation to endothelial cell damage. J Lab Clin Med 94:312, 1979.

71. Aberg H, Nilsson IM: Recurrent thrombosis in a young woman with a circulating anticoagulant directed against factors XI and XII. Acta Med Scand 192:419, 1972.

72. Kant KS, Dosekun AK, Chandran KGP, et al: Deficiency of a plasma factor stimulating vascular prostacyclin generation in patients with lupus nephritis and glomerular thrombi and its correction by ancrod: In-vivo and in-vitro observations. Thromb Res 27:651, 1982.

73. Cosgriff TM, Martin BA: Low functional and high antigenic antithrombin III level in a patient with the lupus anticoagulant and recurrent thrombosis. Arthritis Rheum 24:94, 1981.

74. Jarrett MP, Green D, Chung-Hsin T: Relation between antithrombin III and clinical and serological parameters in systemic lupus erythematosus. J Clin Pathol 36:357, 1983.

75. Kant KS, Pollak VE, Weiss MA, et al: Glomerular thrombosis in systemic lupus erythematosus: Prevalence and significance. Medicine (Baltimore) 60:71, 1981.

76. Fauci AS, Moutsopoulos HM: Polyclonal triggered B cells in the peripheral blood and bone marrow of normal individuals and in patients with systemic lupus erythematosus and primary Sjögren's syndrome. Arthritis Rheum 24:577, 1981.

77. Tsokos GC, Balow JE: Spontaneous pokeweed mitogen–induced plaque forming cells in systemic lupus erythematosus. Clin Immunol Immunopathol 21:172, 1981.

78. Koike T, Tomioka H, Kumagi A: Antibodies cross-reactive with DNA and cardiolipin in patients with systemic lupus erythematosus. Clin Exp Immunol 50:298, 1982.

79. Shoenfeld Y, Rauch H, Massicotte H, et al: Polyspecificity of monoclonal lupus autoantibodies produced by human hybridomas. N Engl J Med 308:414, 1983.

80. Faaber P, Rijke TPM, Van de Putte LBA, et al: Cross-reactivity of human and murine anti-DNA antibodies with heparan sulfate: The major glycosaminoglycan in glomerular basement membranes. J Clin Invest 77:1824, 1986.

81. Brinkman K, Termaat R, Berden JHM, Smeenk RJT: Anti-DNA antibodies and lupus nephritis: The complexity of crossreactivity. Immunol Today 11:232, 1990.

82. Isenberg DA, Collins C: Detection of cross-reactive anti-DNA antibody idiotypes on renal tissue-bound immunoglobulins from lupus patients. J Clin Invest 76:287, 1985.

83. Reichlin M: Diagnosis, criteria and serology. In Schur P (ed): Clinical Management of Systemic Lupus Erythematosus. Grune & Stratton, New York, 1983, Chap. 5.

84. Kunkel HG, Tan EM: Autoantibodies and disease. Adv Immunol 4:351, 1964.

85. Bohan A: Seronegative systemic lupus erythematosus. J Rheumatol 6:534, 1979.

86. Wasicek CA, Maddison PJ, Reichlin M: Occurrence of antibodies to single-stranded DNA in ANA-negative patients. Clin Exp Immunol 37:190, 1979.

87. Moses S, Berland P: Laboratory criteria for a diagnosis of systemic lupus erythematosus. JAMA 242:1039, 1979.

88. Maddison PJ, Provost TT, Reichlin M: Serological findings in patients with "ANA-negative" systemic lupus erythematosus. Medicine (Baltimore) 60:87, 1981.

89. Weitzman RI, Walker SE: Relation to titered peripheral pattern ANA to anti-DNA and disease activity in systemic lupus erythematosus. Ann Rheum Dis 34:44, 1977.

90. Harbeck RJ, Barbana EJ, Kohler PF, Carr RL: DNA–anti-DNA complexes: Their detection in systemic lupus erythematosus sera. J Clin Invest 52:789, 1973.

91. Rothfield NF, Stollar DB: The relation of immunoglobulin class, pattern of antinuclear antibody, and complement fixing antibodies to DNA in sera from patients with systemic lupus erythematosus. J Clin Invest 46:1785, 1967.

92. Puritz EM, Yount WJ, Newell M, Utsinger PD: Immunoglobulin classes and IgG subclasses of human antinuclear antibodies. Clin Immunol Immunopathol 2:98, 1973.

93. Barone C, Bartoloni C, Gentiloni N, et al: Systemic lupus erythematosus with only IgE-class antinuclear antibodies. Arthritis Rheum 24:1441, 1981.

94. Otman DD, Kurata N, Tan EM: Profiles of antinuclear antibodies in systemic rheumatic diseases. Ann Intern Med 83:464, 1975.

95. Schur PH, Sandson J: Immunologic factors and clinical activity in systemic lupus erythematosus. N Engl J Med 278:533, 1968.

96. Emlen W, Pisetsky D, Taylor R: Antibodies to DNA: A perspective. Arthritis Rheum 29:1417, 1986.

97. Synkowski DR, Reichlin M, Provost TT: Serum autoantibodies in SLE and correlation with cutaneous features. J Rheumatol 9:380, 1982.

98. Weinstein A, Bordwell B, Stone B, et al: Antibodies to native DNA and serum complement (C3) level: Application to diagnosis with classification of systemic lupus erythematosus. Am J Med 74:206, 1983.

99. Clough JD, Valenzuela R: Relationship of renal histopathology in SLE nephritis to immunoglobulin class of anti-DNA. Am J Med 66:80–85, 1980.

100. Aarden LA, deGroot ER, Feltkamp TE: Immunology of DNA. III: *Crithidia luciliae,* a simple substrate for the determination of anti-dsDNA with the immunofluorescent technique. Ann N Y Acad Sci 254:505, 1975.

101. Huber O, Greenberg ML, Huber J: Complement fixing anti–double-stranded DNA with the *Crithidia* method: Better indicator of active SLE than anti-DNA with the Farr method. J Lab Clin Med 93:32, 1979.

102. Ballou SP, Kushner I: Anti–native DNA detection by the *Crithidia luciliae* method: An improved guide to the diagnosis and clinical management of systemic lupus erythematosus. Arthritis Rheum 22:321, 1979.

103. Feldman MD, Huston DP, Karsh J, et al: Correlation of serum IgG, IgM, and anti–native-DNA antibodies with renal and clinical indexes of activity in systemic lupus erythematosus. J Rheumatol 9:52, 1982.

104. Leon SA, Green A, Ehrlich GE, et al: Avidity of antibodies in SLE: Relation to severity of renal involvement. Arthritis Rheum 20:23, 1977.

105. Sontheimer RD, Gilliam JN: DNA antibody class, subclass, and complement fixation in systemic lupus erythematosus with and without nephritis. Clin Immunol Immunopathol 10:459, 1978.

106. Asano Y, Nakamoto Y: Avidity of anti–native DNA antibody and glomerular immune complex localization in lupus nephritis. Clin Nephrol 10:134, 1978.

107. Chubick A, Sontheimer RD, Gilliam JN, Ziff M: An appraisal of tests for native DNA antibodies in connective tissue diseases: Clinical usefulness of *Crithidia luciliae* assay. Ann Intern Med 89:186, 1978.

108. Winfield JB, Faiferman I, Koffler D: Avidity of anti-DNA antibodies in serum and IgG glomerular eluates from patients with systemic lupus erythematosus: Association of high avidity antinative DNA antibody with glomerulonephritis. J Clin Invest 59:90, 1977.

109. Tron F, Bach JF: Relationships between antibodies to native DNA and glomerulonephritis in systemic lupus erythematosus. Clin Exp Immunol 28:426, 1977.

110. Davis P, Percy JS, Russell AS: Correlation between levels of DNA antibodies and clinical disease activity in SLE. Ann Rheum Dis 36:157, 1977.

111. Manak RC, Voss EW Jr: Anti-DNA antibody purified from sera of human patients with systemic lupus erythematosus: II. Ligand binding properties of purified antibodies. Immunochemistry 15:653, 1978.

112. Devens B, Chia D, Barnett EV: Anti-DNA antibody: Avidity and valence measurements, studies using sera from immunized rabbits and from two systemic lupus erythematosus patients. J Immunol Methods 19:187, 1978.

113. Beaulien A, Quisnorio FP, Friou GJ, et al: IgG antibodies to double-stranded DNA in systemic lupus erythematosus sera: Independent variation and complement fixing activity and total antibody content. Arthritis Rheum 22:565, 1979.

114. Sasaki T, Hatakeyama A, Shibata S, et al: Heterogeneity of immune complex–derived anti-DNA antibodies associated with lupus nephritis. Kidney Int 39:746, 1991.

115. Foster MH, Cizman B, Madaio MP: Nephritogenic autoantibodies in systemic lupus erythematosus: Immunochemical properties, mechanisms of immune deposition, and genetic origins. Lab Invest 69:494, 1993.

116. Fournie G: Circulating DNA and lupus nephritis. Kidney Int 33:487, 1988.

117. Mattioli M, Reichlin M: Physical association of two nuclear antigens and mutual occurrence of their antibodies: The relationship of Sm and RNA protein (Mo) systems in SLE sera. J Immunol 110:1318, 1973.

118. Lerner EA, Lerner MR, Hardin JA, et al: Deciphering the mysteries of RNA-containing lupus antigens. Arthritis Rheum 25:761, 1982.

119. Rogers J, Wall R: A mechanism for RNA splicing. Proc Natl Acad Sci USA 77:1877, 1980.

120. Sharp GC: Anti-nRNP and anti-Sm antibodies. Arthritis Rheum 25:757, 1982.

121. Beaufils M, Kouki F, Mignon F, et al: Clinical significance of anti-Sm antibodies in systemic lupus erythematosus. Am J Med 74:201, 1983.

122. Maddison PJ, Mogavero H, Reichlin M: Patterns of clinical disease associated with antibodies to nuclear ribonucleoprotein. J Rheumatol 5:407, 1978.

123. Sharp GC, Irvin WS, Tan EJ, et al: Mixed connective tissue disease: An apparently distinct rheumatic disease syndrome associated with a specific antibody to an extractable nuclear antigen (ENA). Am J Med 52:148, 1972.

124. Nimelstein SH, Brody S, McShane D, Holman HR: Mixed connective tissue disease: A subsequent evaluation of the original 25 patients. Medicine (Baltimore) 59:239, 1980.

125. Bennett RM, Spargo BJ: Immune complex nephropathy in mixed connective tissue disease. Am J Med 63:534, 1977.

126. Cohen IM, Swerdlin HR, Steinberg SM, Stone RA: Mesangial proliferative glomerulonephritis with mixed connective tissue disease (MCTD). Clin Nephrol 13:93, 1980.

127. Palferman TG, McIntosh CS, Kershaw M: Mixed connective tissue disease with associated glomerulonephritis and hypocomplementaemia. Br Med J 56:177, 1980.

128. Bennett RM, O'Connell DJ: Mixed connective tissue disease: A clinicopathologic study of 20 cases. Semin Arthritis Rheum 10:25, 1980.

129. Sharp GC: Subsets of SLE and mixed connective tissue disease. Am J Kidney Dis 2(suppl 1):201, 1982.

130. LeRoy EC: Overlap features of connective tissue disease. Arthritis Rheum 25:889, 1982.

131. Alspaugh MA, Tan EM: Antibodies to cellular antigens in Sjögren's syndrome. J Clin Invest 55:1067, 1975.

132. Alspaugh MA, Maddison PJ: Resolution of the identity of certain antigen-antibody systems in systemic lupus erythematosus and Sjögren's syndrome: An interlaboratory collaboration. Arthritis Rheum 22:796, 1979.

133. Wasicek CA, Reichlin M: Clinical and serologic differences between systemic lupus erythematosus patients with antibodies to Ro versus patients with antibodies to Ro and La. J Clin Invest 69:835, 1982.

134. Lerner MR, Boyle JA, Hardin JA, Steitz JA: Two novel classes of small ribonucleoproteins detected by antibodies associated with lupus erythematosus. Science 211:400, 1981.

135. Gilliam JN, Sontheimer RD: Distinctive cutaneous subsets in the spectrum of lupus erythematosus. J Am Acad Dermatol 4:471, 1981.

136. Reichlin M: Clinical and immunologic significance of antibodies to Ro and La in systemic lupus erythematosus. Arthritis Rheum 25:767, 1982.

137. McCarty GA, Harley JB, Reichlin M: A distinctive autoantibody profile in black female patients with lupus nephritis. Arthritis Rheum 11:1560, 1993.

138. Termaat RM, Assmann KJM, Dijkman HBPM, et al: Anti-DNA antibodies can bind to the glomerulus via two distinct mechanisms. Kidney Int 43:1363–1371, 1992.

139. Morioka T, Woitas R, Fujigaki Y, et al: Histone mediates glomerular deposition of small size DNA anti-DNA complex. Kidney Int 45:991–997, 1994.

140. D'Cruz DP, Houssiau FA, Ramirez G, et al: Antibodies to endothelial cells in systemic lupus erythematosus: A potential marker for nephritis and vasculitis. Clin Exp Immunol 85:254, 1991.

141. Termaat RM, Assmann KJM, Van Son JPHF, et al: Antigen-specificity of antibodies bound to glomeruli of mice with systemic lupus erythematosus–like syndromes. Lab Invest 68:164–172, 1993.

142. Bonfa E, Golombek SJ, Kaufman LD, et al: Association between lupus psychosis and anti-ribosomal P protein antibodies. N Engl J Med 317:265, 1987.

143. Siegert CEH, Daha MR, Westedt ML: IgG autoantibodies to C1q are correlated with nephritis, hypocomplementemia, and dsDNA antibodies in systemic lupus erythematosus. J Rheumatol 18:230–234, 1991.

144. Rustagi PK, Currie M, Logue GL: Complement-activating and neutrophil cytoplasmic antibody in systemic lupus erythematosus. Am J Med 78:971, 1985.

145. Bruijn J, van Leer E, Baelde H, et al: Characterization and in vivo transfer of nephritogenic autoantibodies directed against dipeptidyl peptidase IV and laminin in experimental lupus nephritis. Lab Invest 63:350, 1990.

146. Kramers C, Termaat RM, ter Borg EJ, et al: Higher anti–heparan sulphate reactivity during systemic lupus erythematosus (SLE) disease exacerbations with renal manifestations; a long term prospective analysis. Clin Exp Immunol 93:34–38, 1993.

147. Saxena R, Bygren P, Cederholm B, Wieslander J: Circulating anti-entactin antibodies in patients with glomerulonephritis. Kidney Int 39:996–1004, 1991.

148. Hill GS, Hinglais N, Iron F, Bach JF: Systemic lupus erythematosus: Morphologic correlations and clinical data at the time of biopsy. Am J Med 64:61, 1978.

149. Perrin LH, Lambert PH, Miescher PA: Complement breakdown products in the plasma from patients with systemic lupus erythematosus and patients with membranoproliferative or other glomerulonephritis. J Clin Invest 56:165, 1975.

150. Petz LD, Powers R, Fries JR, et al: The in vitro metabolism of the third component of complement in systemic lupus erythematosus. Arthritis Rheum 20:1304, 1977.

151. Singsen BH, Bernstein BH, King KK, Hanson V: Systemic lupus erythematosus in childhood: Correlation between change in disease activity and serum complement levels. J Pediatr 89:358, 1976.

152. Schreiber RD, Muller-Eberhard HJ: Complement and renal disease. In Wilson CB (ed): Immunologic Mechanisms of Renal Disease. Churchill Livingstone, New York, 1979, p 67.

153. Garin EH, Donnelly WH, Shulman ST, et al: The significance of serial measurements of serum complement C3 and C4 components and DNA binding capacity in patients with lupus nephritis. Clin Nephrol 12:148, 1979.

154. Williams PG, Peters DK, Fallows J, et al: Studies of serum complement in the hypocomplementemic nephritides. Clin Exp Immunol 18:391, 1974.

155. West CD: Relative value of serum C3 and C4 levels in predicting relapse in systemic lupus erythematosus. Am J Kidney Dis 18:686–688, 1991.

156. Ricker DM, Hebert LA, Rohde R, et al: Serum C3 levels are diagnostically more sensitive and specific for systemic lupus erythematosus activity than are serum C4 levels. Am J Kidney Dis 18:678–685, 1991.

157. Marshall DA, Nesbitt LT Jr, Biundo JJ: Serum complement related to skin lesions of systemic lupus erythematosus. South Med J 67:1275, 1974.

158. Valentijn R, van Overhagen H, Hazevoet HM, et al: The value of complement and immune complex determinations in monitoring disease activity in patients with systemic lupus erythematosus. Arthritis Rheum 28:904, 1985.

159. Laitman RS, Glicklich D, Sablay L, et al: Effect of long-term normalization of serum complement levels on the course of lupus nephritis. Am J Med 87:132, 1989.

160. Buyon JP, Cronstein BN, Morris M, et al: Serum complement values (C3 and C4) to differentiate between systemic lupus activity and pre-eclampsia. Am J Med 81:194, 1986.

161. Sissons JG, Peters DK, Williams DG, et al: Skin lesions, angioedema, and hypocomplementaemia. Lancet 2:1350, 1974.

162. Donaldson VH, Hess EV, McAdams AJ: Lupus-erythematosus–like disease in three unrelated women with hereditary angioneurotic edema. Ann Intern Med 86:312, 1977.

163. Miyakawa Y, Yamada A, Kosaka K, et al: Defective immune adherence (C3b) receptor on erythrocytes from patients with systemic lupus erythematosus. Lancet 1:493, 1981.

164. Wilson JG, Wong WW, Shur PH, Fearon DT: Mode of inheritance of decreased C3b receptors on erythrocytes of patients with systemic lupus erythematosus. N Engl J Med 307:981, 1982.

165. Kazatchkine MD, Fearon DT, Appay MD, et al: Immunohistochemical study of the human glomerular C3b receptor in normal kidney and in seventy-five cases of renal disease: Loss of C3b receptor antigen in focal hyalinosis and in proliferative nephritis of systemic lupus erythematosus. J Clin Invest 69:900, 1982.

166. Moldenhauer F, David J, Fielder AHK, et al: Inherited deficiency of erythrocyte complement receptor type 1 does not cause susceptibility to systemic lupus erythematosus. Arthritis Rheum 30:961, 1987.

166a. Walport M, Ng YC, Lachmann PJ: Erythrocytes transfused into patients with SLE and hemolytic anaemia lose complement receptor type 1 from their cell surface. Clin Exp Immunol 69:501, 1987.

167. Minota S, Terai C, Nojima Y, et al: Correlative expression of C3b receptors in the glomerulus and on erythrocytes. Clin Immunol Immunopathol 38:85, 1986.

168. Agnello V, Koffler D, Eisenberg JW, et al: C1q precipitins in the sera of patients with systemic lupus erythematosus and other hypocomplementemic states: Characterization of high and low molecular weight types. J Exp Med 134:2285, 1971.

169. Levinsky RJ, Cameron JS, Soothill JF: Serum immune complexes and disease activity in lupus nephritis. Lancet 1:564, 1977.

170. Davis P, Cumming RH, Verrierjoine J: Relationship between anti-DNA antibodies, complement consumption and circulating immune complexes in systemic lupus erythematosus. Clin Exp Immunol 28:226, 1977.

171. Caro PO, Jeny LM, Sladowski JP, Osterland CK: Circulating immune complexes in systemic lupus erythematosus. Clin Exp Immunol 29:197, 1977.

172. Abrass CK, Nies KM, Louie JS, et al: Correlations of circulating immune complexes and disease activity in patients with systemic lupus erythematosus. Arthritis Rheum 21:539, 1978.

173. Volanakis JE, Halla JJ, Fallahi S, Schrohenloker RE: Detection of immune complexes in connective tissue diseases: a comparison of three radioassays. In Peters H (ed): Protides of the Biological Fluids, 26th Colloquium. Pergamon Press, New York, 1979, p 251.

174. Tung SK, Woodroffe AJ, Ahlin JD, et al: Application of the solid phase C1q and Raji cell radioimmune assays for the detection of circulating immune complexes in glomerulonephritis. J Clin Invest 62:61, 1978.

175. Donadio JV, McDuffie FC, Ilstrup DM: Circulating immune complexes in SLE. J Rheumatol 5:423, 1978.

176. Greisman SG, Redecha PB, Kimberly RP, Christian CL: Differences among immune complexes: Association of C1q in SLE immune complexes with renal disease. J Immunol 138:739, 1987.

177. Bruneau C, Benveniste J: Circulating DNA–anti-DNA complexes in systemic lupus erythematosus: Detection and characterization by ultracentrifugation. J Clin Invest 64:191, 1979.

178. Izui S, Lambert PH, Miescher PA: Failure to detect circulating DNA–anti-DNA complexes by four radioimmunological methods in patients with systemic lupus erythematosus. Clin Exp Immunol 30:354, 1977.

179. Emlen W, Ansari R, Burdick G: DNA–anti-DNA immune complexes: Antibody protection of a discrete DNA fragment from DNase digestion in vitro. J Clin Invest 74:185, 1984.

180. Rigby RJ, Dawkins RL, Wetherall JD, Hawkins BR: HLA in systemic lupus erythematosus: Influence on severity. Tissue Antigens 12:25, 1978.

181. Schur PH: Genetics of complement deficiencies associated with lupus-like syndromes. Arthritis Rheum 21:51, 1978.

182. Lippman SM, Arnett FC, Conley CL, et al: Genetic factors predisposing to autoimmune diseases: Autoimmune hemolytic anemia, chronic thrombocytopenic purpura, and systemic lupus erythematosus. Am J Med 73:827, 1982.

183. Roberts JL, Schwartz MM, Lewis EJ: Hereditary C2 deficiency and systemic lupus erythematosus associated with severe glomerulonephritis. Clin Exp Immunol 31:328, 1978.

184. Lehman TJA, Hanson V, Singsen BH, et al: Serum complement abnormalities in the antinuclear antibody–positive relatives of children with systemic lupus erythematosus. Arthritis Rheum 22:954, 1979.

185. Cleland LG, Bell DA: The occurrence of systemic lupus erythematosus in two kindreds in association with selective IgA deficiency. J Rheumatol 5:288, 1978.

186. Howard PF, Hochberg MC, Bias WB, et al: Relationship between C4 null genes, HLA-D region antigens, and genetic susceptibility to systemic lupus erythematosus in Caucasian and black Americans. Am J Med 81:187, 1986.

187. Fielder HL, Walport MJ, Batchelor JR, et al: Family study of the major histo-compatibility complex in patients with systemic lupus erythematosus: Importance of null alleles of C4A and C4B in determining disease susceptibility. Br Med J 286:425, 1983.

188. Stenszky V, Kozma L, Szegedi G, Farid NR: Interplay of immunoglobulin G heavy chain markers (Gm) and HLA in predisposing to systemic lupus nephritis. J Immunogenet 13:11, 1986.

189. Landry M, Sanis WM Jr: Systemic lupus erythematosus: Studies of the antibodies bound to skin. J Clin Invest 53:1871, 1973.

190. Gilliam HN, Cheatum DE, Hurd ER, et al: Immunoglobulin in clinically uninvolved skin in systemic lupus erythematosus in association with renal disease. J Clin Invest 53:1434, 1974.

191. Pennebaker JB, Gilliam JN, Ziff B: Immunoglobulin classes of DNA binding activity in serum and skin in systemic lupus erythematosus. J Clin Invest 60:1331, 1977.

192. Lief PD, Barland P, Bank N: Diagnosis of lupus nephritis by skin immunofluorescence in the absence of extrarenal manifestations of systemic lupus erythematosus. Am J Med 63:441, 1977.

193. Noel L-H, Droz D, Rothfield NF: Clinical and serologic significance of cutaneous deposits of immunoglobulins, C3 and C1q, in SLE patients with nephritis. Clin Immunol Immunopathol 10:318, 1978.

194. Krupp MA: Urinary sediment in visceral angiitis: Quantitative studies. Arch Intern Med 71:54, 1943.

195. Chagnac A, Kiberd B, Farinas C, et al: Outcome of the acute glomerular injury in lupus nephritis. J Clin Invest 84:922, 1989.

196. Spriggs B, Epstein EN: Clinical and laboratory correlates of L-chain proteinuria in systemic lupus erythematosus. J Rheumatol 1:287, 1974.

197. Bond RE, Donadio JV Jr, Holley JE, Bowie EJ: Fibrinolytic split products: A clinicopathological correlative study in adults with lupus glomerulonephritis and various renal diseases. Arch Intern Med 132:182, 1973.

198. Hardin JA, Cronlung M, Haber E, Block KJ: Activation of blood clotting in patients with systemic lupus erythematosus. Am J Med 65:420, 1978.

199. Zvaifler NJ: Lymphocytotoxic antibody activity in cryoprecipitates from serum of patients with SLE. Arthritis Rheum 19:844, 1976.

200. Sakane T, Steinberg AD, Reeves JP, Green I: Studies of immune functions of patients with systemic lupus erythematosus: T-cell subsets and antibodies to T-cell subsets. J Clin Invest 64:1260, 1979.

201. Searles RP, Messner RP, Bankhurst AD: Cross-reactivity of anti-lymphocyte and antinuclear antibodies in systemic lupus erythematosus. Clin Immunol Immunopathol 14:292, 1979.

202. Espinoza LR, Hartmann RC: Significance of lupus anticoagulant. Am J Hematol 22:331, 1986.

203. Steinberg AD, Smith HR, Laskin CA, et al: Studies of immune abnormalities in systemic lupus erythematosus. Am J Kidney Dis 2(suppl 1):101, 1982.

204. Shivakumar S, Tsokos GC, Datta SK: T cell receptor α/β expressing double-negative (CD4−/CD8−) and CD4+ T helper cells in humans augment the production of pathogenic anti-DNA autoantibodies associated with lupus nephritis. J Immunol 143:103–112, 1989.

205. Cole EH, Schulman J, Urowitz M, et al: Monocyte procoagulant activity in glomerulonephritis associated with systemic lupus erythematosus. J Clin Invest 75:861, 1985.

206. Bresnihan B, Olwen M, Grigor R, Hughes GRV: Brain reactivity of lymphocytotoxic antibodies in systemic lupus erythematosus with and without cerebral involvement. Clin Exp Immunol 30:333, 1977.

207. van Dam AP: Diagnosis and pathogenesis of CNS lupus. Rheumatol Int 11:1, 1991.

208. Winfield JB, Brunner CM, Koffler D: Serologic studies in patients with systemic lupus erythematosus and central nervous system dysfunction. Arthritis Rheum 21:289, 1978.

209. Steinman CR: Circulating DNA in systemic lupus erythematosus: Association with central nervous system involvement with systemic vasculitis. Am J Med 67:429, 1979.

210. Frank MM, Hamburger ML, Lawley TJ, et al: Defective reticuloendothelial system Fc-receptor function in systemic lupus erythematosus. N Engl J Med 300:518, 1979.

211. Scheinberg MA, Filho GI, Mendes NF, Vertzman P: Suppression of C3 rosette formation by serum from patients with systemic lupus erythematosus: A corollary of disease activity. J Rheumatol 5:19, 1978.

212. Honig S, Gorevic P, Weissmann R: C-reactive protein in systemic lupus erythematosus. Arthritis Rheum 20:1065, 1977.

213. Shearn MA: Normocholesterolemic nephrotic syndrome of systemic lupus erythematosus. Am J Med 36:250, 1954.

214. Groggel GC, Cheung AK, Ellis-Benigni K, et al: Treatment of nephrotic hyperlipoproteinemia with gemfibrozil. Kidney Int 36:266–271, 1989.

215. Favre H, Miescher PA: Filtration fraction in index of renal disease activity in patients with systemic lupus erythematosus. Proc Eur Dial Transplant Assoc Eur Ren Assoc 21:717, 1984.

216. Terai C, Nojima Y, Takano K, et al: Determination of urinary albumin excretion by radioimmunoassay in patients with subclinical lupus nephritis. Clin Nephrol 27:79, 1987.

217. Parving HH, Sorensen SF, Mogensen CE, Helin P: Urinary albumin and B$_2$-microglobulin excretion rates in patients with systemic lupus erythematosus. Scand J Rheumatol 9:49, 1988.

218. Schwartz MM, Lan S, Bonsib SM, et al: Clinical outcome of three discrete histologic patterns of injury in severe lupus glomerulonephritis. Am J Kidney Dis 13:273–283, 1989.

219. Klein MH, Thorner PS, Yoon SJ, et al: Determination of circulating immune complexes, C3 and C4 complement components and anti-DNA antibody in different classes of lupus nephritis. Int J Pediatr Nephrol 5:75–82, 1984.

220. Muehrcke R, Kark R, Pirani C, Pollak V: Lupus nephritis: A clinical and pathologic study based on renal biopsies. Medicine (Baltimore) 46:1, 1967.

221. Comerford FR, Cohen AS: The nephropathy of systemic lupus erythematosus. Medicine (Baltimore) 46:425, 1967.

222. Appel BG, Silva FG, Pirani CL, et al: Renal involvement in systemic lupus erythematosus (SLE): A study of 56 patients emphasizing histologic classification. Medicine (Baltimore) 57:371, 1978.

223. Churg J: Renal Disease: Classification and Atlas of Glomerular Diseases. Igaku-Shoin, Tokyo, 1982.

224. Kashgarian M: Lupus nephritis: Lessons from the path lab. Kidney Int 45:928–938, 1994.

225. Morel-Maroger L, Mery JP, Droz D, et al: The course of lupus nephritis: Contribution of serial renal biopsies. Adv Nephrol 6:79, 1976.

226. Izui S, Lambert P-H, Miescher PA: In vitro demonstration of a particular affinity of glomerular basement membrane and collagen for DNA: A possible basis for a local formation of DNA–anti-DNA complexes in systemic lupus erythematosus. J Exp Med 144:428, 1976.

227. Izui S, Lambert P-H, Fournie GJ, et al: Features of systemic lupus erythematosus in mice injected with bacterial lipopolysaccharides: Identification of circulating DNA and renal localization of DNA–anti-DNA complexes. J Exp Med 115:1115, 1977.

228. Couser WG, Salant DJ, Madaio MP, et al: Factors influencing glomerular and tubulointerstitial patterns of injury in SLE. Am J Kidney Dis 2:126, 1982.

229. Austin HA III, Mueng LR, Joyce KM, et al: Prognostic factors in lupus nephritis: Contribution of renal histologic data. Am J Med 75:382, 1983.

230. Leaker B, Fairley K, Dowling J, Kincaid-Smith P: Lupus nephritis: Clinical and pathological correlations. Q J Med 62:163, 1987.

231. Nossent HC, Henzen-Logmans SC, Vroom TM, et al: Contribution of renal biopsy data in predicting outcome in lupus nephritis. Arthritis Rheum 33:970, 1990.

232. Lewis EJ, Kawala K, Schwartz M: Histologic features that correlate with prognosis of patients with lupus nephritis. Am J Kidney Dis 10:192, 1987.

233. Austin HA III, Boumpas DT, Vaughn EM, Balow JE: Predicting

renal outcomes in severe lupus nephritis: Contributions of clinical and histologic data. Kidney Int 45:544–550, 1994.

234. Gruppo Italiano per lo Studio della Nefrite Lupica (GISNEL): Lupus nephritis: Prognostic factors and probability of maintaining life-supporting renal function 10 years after the diagnosis. Am J Kidney Dis 19:473–479, 1992.

235. Esdaile JM, Federgreen W, Quintal H, et al: Predictors of one year outcome in lupus nephritis: The importance of renal biopsy. Q J Med 81:907–918, 1991.

236. Esdaile JM, Levinton C, Federgreen W, et al: The clinical and renal biopsy predictors of long-term outcome in lupus nephritis: A study of 87 patients and review of the literature. Q J Med 72:779, 1989.

237. Schwartz MM: The role of renal biopsy in the management of lupus nephritis. Semin Nephrol 5:255, 1985.

238. Grishman E, Churg J: Focal segmental lupus nephritis. Clin Nephrol 17:5, 1982.

239. Magil AB, Ballon HS, Rae A: Focal proliferative lupus nephritis: A clinicopathologic study using the WHO classification. Am J Med 72:620, 1982.

240. Schurch W: Morphologie und Lokalisation der Hämatoxylinkörperchen bei Lupus Nephritis. Virchows Arch A 359:331, 1973.

241. Cohen AH, Zamboni L: Ultrastructural appearance and morphogenesis of renal glomerular hematoxylin bodies. Am J Pathol 89:105, 1977.

242. Schwartz MM, Kawala K, Roberts JL, et al: Clinical and pathological features of membranous glomerulonephritis of systemic lupus erythematosus. Am J Nephrol 4:301, 1984.

243. Gonzales-Dettoni H, Tron F: Membranous glomerulopathy in systemic lupus erythematosus. Adv Nephrol 14:347, 1985.

244. The Southwest Pediatric Nephrology Study Group: Comparison of idiopathic and systemic lupus erythematosus associated membranous glomerulonephropathy in children. Am J Med Dis 7:115, 1986.

245. Williams WW, Shah D, Morgan AG, Alleyne GAO: Membranous glomerulonephropathy with crescents in systemic lupus erythematosus. Am J Nephrol 5:168, 1985.

246. Honig C, Mouradian JA, Montolin J, et al: Mesangial electron-deposits in membranous nephropathy. Lab Invest 42:4279, 1980.

247. Katz SM, Korn S, Umlas SL, DeHoratius RJ: Renal vascular lesions in systemic lupus erythematosus. Ann Clin Lab Sci 20:147, 1990.

248. Banfi G, Bertani T, Boeri V, et al: Renal vascular lesions as a marker of poor prognosis in patients with lupus nephritis. Am J Kidney Dis 18:240, 1991.

249. Bhathena DB, Sobel BJ, Midgal SD: Noninflammatory renal microangiopathy of systemic lupus erythematous ("lupus vasculitis"). Am J Nephrol 1:144, 1981.

250. Stamenkovic I, Favre H, Donath A, et al: Renal biopsy in SLE irrespective of clinical findings: Long-term follow-up. Clin Nephrol 26:109, 1986.

251. Schwartz MM, Fennell JS, Lewis EJ: Pathologic changes in the renal tubule in systemic lupus erythematosus. Hum Pathol 13:534, 1982.

252. Alexopoulos E, Seron D, Hartley RB, Cameron JS: Lupus nephritis: Correlation of interstitial cells with glomerular function. Kidney Int 37:100–109, 1990.

253. Park M, D'Agati A, Appel G, Pirani CL: Tubulointerstitial disease in lupus-nephritis: Relationship to immune deposits, interstitial inflammation, glomerular changes, renal function, and prognosis. Nephron 44:309, 1986.

254. Banfi G, Mazzucco G, Barbiano de Belgiojoso G, et al: Morphologic parameters in lupus nephritis: Their relevance for classification and relationships with clinical and histological findings and outcome. Q J Med 55:153, 1986.

255. Weidner N, Lorentz WB: Scanning electron microscopy of acellular glomerular and tubular basement membrane in lupus nephritis. Am J Clin Pathol 85:135, 1986.

256. Gyorkey F, Min KW, Sincovics JG, et al: Systemic lupus erythematosus and myxovirus. N Engl J Med 280:333, 1969.

257. Grausz H, Earlye L, Stephens BG, et al: Diagnostic import of virus-like particles in the glomerular endothelium of patients with systemic lupus erythematosus. N Engl J Med 283:506, 1970.

258. Chander P, Soni A, Suri A, et al: Renal ultrastructural markers in AIDS-associated nephropathy. Am J Pathol 126:513, 1987.

259. Cohen AH, Nast CC: HIV-associated nephropathy: A unique combined glomerular tubular and interstitial lesion. Mod Pathol 1:87, 1988.

260. Kallen RJ, Lee S-K, Aronson AJ, Spargo BH: Idiopathic membranous glomerulopathy preceding the emergence of systemic lupus erythematosus in two children. J Pediatr 90:72, 1977.

261. Libit SA, Burke B, Michael AF, Vernier RL: Extramembranous glomerulonephritis in childhood: Relationship to systemic lupus erythematosus. J Pediatr 88:394, 1976.

262. Grishman E, Porush JC, Rosen SM, Churg J: Lupus nephritis with organized deposits in the kidneys. Lab Invest 16:717, 1967.

263. Algers CE, Hopper J Jr, Bernstein MJ, Biava CG: Late development of systemic lupus erythematosus in patients with glomerular "fingerprint" deposits. Ann Intern Med 100:66, 1984.

264. Cohen AH, Wang HY, Border WA, Glassock RJ: Acute renal failure due to acute tubular necrosis in lupus nephritis. Kidney Int 23:119, 1983. Abstract.

265. Niaudet P, Berterottiere D, Lacoste M, et al: Évolution des lésions rénales du lupus erythemateux disséminé. Ann Pediatr (Paris) 38:427, 1991.

266. Zimmerman SW, Jenkins PG, Shelp WD, et al: Progression from minimal to focal to diffuse proliferative lupus nephritis. Lab Invest 32:665, 1975.

267. Hall-Craggs M, Ramos E: Transformation of diffuse proliferative glomerulonephritis to membranous nephritis in a patient with systemic lupus erythematosus. Nephron 28:42, 1981.

268. Mahajan SK, Ordonez NG, Spargo BH, Katz AI: Changing histopathology patterns in lupus nephropathy. Clin Nephrol 10:1, 1978.

269. Lee HS, Mujais SK, Kasinath BS, et al: Course of renal pathology in patient with systemic lupus erythematosus. Am J Med 77:612, 1984.

270. Hecht B, Siegel N, Adler M, et al: Prognostic indices in lupus nephritis. Medicine (Baltimore) 55:163, 1976.

271. Ellington KT, Truong L, Olivero JJ: Renal amyloidosis in systemic lupus erythematosus. Am J Kidney Dis 21:676–678, 1993.

272. Balow JE, Austin HA, Muenz LR, et al: Effect of treatment on the evolution of renal abnormalities in lupus nephritis. N Engl J Med 311:491, 1984.

273. Appel GB, Cohen DJ, Pirani CL, et al: Long-term follow-up of patients with lupus nephritis: A study based on the classification of the World Health Organization. Am J Med 83:877, 1987.

274. Schwartz MM, Lan S-P, Bernstein J, et al: Role of pathology indices in the management of severe lupus glomerulonephritis. Kidney Int 42:743, 1992.

275. Schwartz MM, Lan S-P, Bernstein J, et al: Irreproducibility of the activity and chronicity indices limits their utility in the management of lupus nephritis. Am J Kidney Dis 21:374, 1993.

276. Schwartz MM, Kawala K, Corwin H, Lewis E: The prognosis of segmental glomerulonephritis in systemic lupus erythematosus. Kidney Int 32:274, 1987.

277. Wernick RM, Smith DL, Houghton DC, et al: Reliability of histologic scoring for lupus nephritis: A community-based evaluation. Ann Intern Med 19:805, 1993.

278. Donadio JV, Burgess JH, Holley KE: Membranous lupus nephropathy: A clinicopathologic study. Medicine (Baltimore) 56:527, 1977.

279. Pasquali S, Banfi G, Zucchelli P: Lupus membranous nephropathy: Long-term outcome. Clin Nephrol 39:175–182, 1993.

279a. Gonzalez-Detroni H, Tron F: Membranous glomerulopathy in systemic lupus erythematosus. Adv Nephrol 14:347, 1985.

280. Whiting O'Keefe Q, Henke JE, Shearn MA, et al: The information content from renal biopsy in systemic lupus erythematosus. Ann Intern Med 96:718, 1982.

281. Fries JF, Porta J, Liang MH: Marginal benefit of renal biopsy in systemic lupus erythematosus. Arch Intern Med 138:1386, 1978.

282. Kalmin ND, Bartholomew WR, Wicher K: Relative values of laboratory assays in systemic lupus erythematosus. Am J Clin Pathol 75:846, 1981.

283. Bardana EJ, Harbeck RJ, Pirofsky B, Carr RL: The prognostic and therapeutic implications of DNA–anti-DNA immune complexes in systemic lupus erythematosus. Am J Med 59:515, 1975.

284. Huston KA, Gupta RC, Donadio JV, et al: Circulating immune complexes in systemic lupus erythematosus. J Rheumatol 5:423, 1978.

285. Balow JE: Clinicopathologic correlation in lupus nephritis. Ann Intern Med 91:587, 1979.

286. Gladman DD, Urowitz MB, Keystone EC: Serologically active clinically quiescent systemic lupus erythematosus: A discordance between clinical and serologic features. Am J Med 66:210, 1979.

287. Lough JD, Valenzuela R: Relationship of renal histopathology in SLE nephritis to immunoglobulin class of anti-DNA. Am J Med 68:80, 1980.

288. Friend PS, Kim Y, Michael AF, Donadio JV: Pathogenesis of membranous nephropathy in systemic lupus erythematosus: Possible role of nonprecipitating DNA antibody. Br Med J 1:25, 1977.

289. Kohler PF, Ten-Bensel R: Serial complement component alteration in acute glomerulonephritis and systemic lupus erythematosus. Clin Exp Immunol 4:191, 1969.

290. Rothfield N: Lupus nephritis. In Schur P (ed): Clinical Management of Systemic Lupus Erythematosus. Grune & Stratton, New York, 1983.

291. Bruijn JA, Bergijk EC, DeHeer E, et al: Induction and progression of experimental lupus nephritis: Exploration of a pathogenetic pathway. Kidney Int 41:5–13, 1992.

292. Mills JA: Systemic lupus erythematosus. N Engl J Med 330:1871, 1994.

293. Datta SK, Rajagopalan S, O'Keefe TL, et al: Pathogenic anti-DNA autoantibodies and pathogenic autoantibody-inducing T cells. Immunol Ser 55:133, 1991.

294. Atta MS, Powell RJ, Hopkinson ND, Todd I: Human anti-fibronectin antibodies in systemic lupus erythematosus: Occurrence and antigenic specificity. Clin Exp Immunol 96:20, 1994.

295. Raz E, Brezis M, Rosenmann E, et al: Anti-DNA antibodies bind directly to renal antigens and induce kidney dysfunction in the isolated perfused rat kidney. J Immunol 142:3076, 1989.

296. Kramers C, Hylkema MN, van Bruggen MC, et al: Anti-nucleosome antibodies complexed to nucleosomal antigens show anti-DNA reactivity and bind to rat glomerular basement membrane in vivo. J Clin Invest 94:568, 1994.

297. Malide D, Londoño I, Russo P, et al: Ultrastructural localization of DNA in immune deposits of lupus nephritis. Am J Pathol 143:304, 1993.

298. Morioka T, Woitas R, Fujigaki Y, et al: Histone mediates glomerular deposition of small size DNA anti-DNA complex. Kidney Int 45:991, 1994.

299. Sasaki T, Muryoi T, Hatakeyama A, et al: Circulating anti-DNA immune complexes in active lupus nephritis. Am J Med 91:355, 1991.

300. Steinman CR: Circulating DNA in systemic lupus erythematosus, isolation and characterization. J Clin Invest 73:834, 1984.

301. Reichlin M, Martin A, Taylor-Albert E, et al: Lupus autoantibodies to native DNA cross-react with the A and D SnRNP polypeptides. J Clin Invest 93:443, 1994.

302. Sabbaga J, Pankewycz OG, Lufft V, et al: Cross-reactivity distinguishes serum and nephritogenic anti-DNA antibodies in human lupus from their natural counterparts in normal serum. J Autoimmun 3:215, 1990.

303. Waer M: The role of anti-DNA antibodies in lupus nephritis. Clin Rheumatol 1:111, 1990.

304. Termat RM, Brinkman K, Nossent JC, et al: Anti–heparan sulphate reactivity in sera from patients with systemic lupus erythematosus with renal or non-renal manifestations. Clin Exp Immunol 82:268, 1990.

305. Suzuki N, Harada T, Mizushima Y, et al: Possible pathogenic role of cationic anti-DNA autoantibodies in the development of nephritis in patients with systemic lupus erythematosus. J Immunol 151:1128, 1993.

306. Suzuki M, Hatakeyama A, Kameoka J, et al: Anti-DNA idiotypes deposited in renal glomeruli of patients with lupus nephritis. Am J Kidney Dis 18:232, 1991.

307. Vlahakos DV, Foster MH, Adams S, et al: Anti-DNA antibodies form immune deposits at distinct glomerular and vascular sites. Kidney Int 41:1690, 1992.

308. Tsao BP, Ebling FM, Roman C, et al: Structural characteristics of the variable regions of immunoglobulin genes encoding a pathogenic autoantibody in murine lupus. J Clin Invest 85:530, 1990.

309. Arnett FC, Reveille JD: Genetics of systemic lupus erythematosus. Rheum Dis Clin North Am 18:865, 1992.

310. Wilson JG, Wong WW, Schur PH, Fearon DT: Mode of inheritance of decreased C3b receptors on erythrocytes of patients with systemic lupus erythematosus. N Engl J Med 307:981, 1982.

311. Miller GW, Nussenzeig V: A new complement function: Solubilization of antigen-antibody aggregates. Proc Natl Acad Sci USA 72:418, 1975.

312. Coggins CH: Overview of treatment of lupus nephropathy. Am J Kidney Dis 2(suppl 1):197, 1982.

313. Cheatum DE, Hurd ER, Strunk SW, Ziff M: Renal histology and clinical course of systemic lupus erythematosus: A prospective study. Arthritis Rheum 16:670, 1973.

314. Ginzler EM, Nicastri AD, Chen CK, et al: Progression of mesangial and focal to diffuse lupus nephritis. N Engl J Med 291:693, 1974.

315. Petri M, Perez-Gutthann S, Longenecker JC, Hochberg M: Morbidity of systemic lupus erythematosis: Role of race and socioeconomic status. Am J Med 91:345–353, 1991.

316. Austin HA III, Muenz LR, Joyce KM, et al: Diffuse proliferative lupus nephritis: Identification of specific pathologic features affecting renal outcome. Kidney Int 25:689, 1984.

317. Schwartz MM, Lau SS (The Lupus Nephritis Collaborative Study Group): Clinical outcome of three discrete lesions in severe lupus glomerulonephritis. Kidney Int 31:217, 1988. Abstract.

318. Radhakrishnan J, Szabolcs S, d'Agati V, et al: Lupus membranous nephropathy: Course and prognosis in 50 patients. J Am Soc Nephrol 4:284, 1993. Abstract.

318a. Adler SG, Johnson K, Louie JS, et al: Lupus membranous glomerulonephritis: Different prognostic subgroups obscured by imprecise histologic classifications. Mod Pathol 3:186, 1990.

319. Pollak VE, Pirani CL, Kark RM: Effect of large doses of prednisone on the renal lesions and lifespan of patients with lupus erythematosus. J Lab Clin Med 57:495, 1961.

320. Dinant HJ, Decker JL, Klippel JH, et al: Alternative modes of cyclophosphamide and azathioprine therapy in lupus nephritis. Ann Intern Med 96:728, 1982.

321. Wei N, Wu T, Klippel JH: False positive pregnancy tests in systemic lupus erythematosus. J Rheumatol 9:303, 1982.

322. Fraga A, Mintz G, Orozco J, et al: Sterility and fertility rates, fetal wastage and maternal mortality in systemic lupus erythematosus. J Rheumatol 1:293, 1974.

323. Zulman JI, Talal N, Hoffman GS, Epstein WV: Problems associated with the management of pregnancies in patients with systemic lupus erythematosus. J Rheumatol 7:37, 1980.

324. Hayslett JP, Lynn RI: Effect of pregnancy in patients with lupus nephropathy. Kidney Int 18:207, 1980.

325. Bobrie G, Liote F, Houiller P, et al: Pregnancy in lupus nephritis and related disorders. Am J Kidney Dis 9:339, 1987.

326. Packham DK, Lam SS, Nicholls K, et al: Lupus nephritis and pregnancy. Q J Med 83:315–324, 1992.

327. Porcel JM: Complement in pregnant women with systemic lupus erythematosus. Med Clin (Barc) 102:594, 1994.

328. Albert DA, Hadler NM, Ropes MW: Does corticosteroid therapy affect the survival of patients with systemic lupus erythematosus? Arthritis Rheum 22:945, 1979.

329. The Canadian Hydroxychloroquine Study Group: A randomized study of the effect of withdrawing hydroxychloroquine sulfate in systemic lupus erythematosus. N Engl J Med 324:150, 1991.

330. Kimberly RP: Renal prostaglandins in systemic lupus erythematosus. Lancet 2:553, 1978.

331. Kimberly RP, Gill J, Bowden RE, et al: Elevated urinary prostaglandins and the effects of aspirin on renal function in lupus erythematosus. Ann Intern Med 89:336, 1978.

332. Elliott HW, Essenhigh DM, Morley HR: Cyclophosphamide treatment of systemic lupus erythematosus: Risk of bladder cancer exceeds benefit. Br Med J 284:1160, 1982.

333. Donadio JV, Glassock RJ: Immunosuppressive drug therapy in lupus nephritis. Am J Kidney Dis 21:239, 1993.

334. Donadio JV, Holley KE, Wagoner RD, et al: Further observations on the treatment of lupus nephritis with prednisone and combined prednisone and azathioprine. Arthritis Rheum 17:573, 1974.

335. Snaith ML, Holt JM, Oliver DO, et al: Treatment of patients with systemic lupus erythematosus, including nephritis, with chlorambucil. Br Med J 2:197, 1973.

336. Donadio JV Jr: Treatment of membranous nephropathy in systemic lupus erythematosus. Nephrol Dial Transplant 7(suppl 1):97, 1992.

337. Nanra RS, Kincaid-Smith P: Lupus nephritis: Clinical course in relation to treatment. In Kincaid-Smith P, Mathew TH, Becker EL (eds): Glomerulonephritis: Morphology, Natural History, and Treatment, Part II. John Wiley & Sons, New York, 1973, p 1193.

338. Pollak VE, Pirani CL, Kark RM: Effect of large doses of prednisone on the renal lesions and life span of patients with lupus glomerulonephritis. J Lab Clin Med 57:495, 1961.

339. MacKay IR, Chan D, Robson G: Prednisolone treatment of lupus nephritis. Aust Ann Med 2:123, 1970.

340. Cade R, Spooner G, Schlein E, et al: Comparison of azathioprine, prednisone and heparin alone or combined in treating lupus nephritis. Nephron 10:37, 1973.

341. Austin HA, Klippel JH, Balow JE, et al: Therapy of lupus nephritis: Controlled trial of prednisone and cytotoxic drugs. N Engl J Med 314:614, 1986.

342. Ponticelli C: Current treatment recommendations for lupus nephritis. Drugs 40:19, 1990.

343. Pollak VE, Kant KS, Hariharan S: Diffuse and focal proliferative lupus nephritis: Treatment approaches and results. Nephron 59:177–193, 1991.

344. Felson DT, Anderson J: Evidence for superiority of immunosuppressive drugs and prednisone over prednisone alone in lupus nephritis. Results of a pooled analysis. N Engl J Med 331:1528–1533, 1984.

345. Lehman TJA, Sherry DD, Wagner-Weiner L, et al: Intermittent intravenous cyclophosphamide therapy for lupus nephritis. J Pediatr 114:1055–1060, 1989.

346. Eiser AR, Grishman E, Dreznin S: Intravenous pulse cyclophosphamide in the treatment of type IV lupus nephritis. Clin Nephrol 40:155–159, 1993.

347. Valeri A, Radhakrishnan J, Estes D, et al: Intravenous pulse cyclophosphamide treatment of severe lupus nephritis: A prospective five-year study. Clin Nephrol 42:71–78, 1994.

348. Boumpas DT, Austin HA III, Vaughan EM, et al: Risk for sustained amenorrhea in patients with systemic lupus erythematosus reclining intermittent pulse cyclophosphamide therapy. Ann Intern Med 119:366–369, 1993.

349. Boumpas DT, Austin HA III, Vaughn EM, et al: Controlled trial of pulse methylprednisolone versus two regimens of pulse cyclophosphamide in severe lupus nephritis. Lancet 340:741–745, 1992.

350. Favre H, Miescher PA, Huang YP, et al: Ciclosporin in the treatment of lupus nephritis. Am J Nephrol 9(suppl 1):57–60, 1989.

351. McCune W, Golbus J, Zeldes W, et al: Clinical and immunologic effects of monthly administration of intravenous cyclophosphamide in severe systemic lupus erythematosus. N Engl J Med 318:1423, 1988.

352. Sztejnbok M, Stewart A, Diamond H, Kaplan D: Azathioprine in the treatment of systemic lupus erythematosus. Arthritis Rheum 14:639, 1971.

353. Dillard MG, Dujoune I, Pollack VE, Pirani CL: The effect of treatment with prednisone and nitrogen mustard on the renal lesions and life span of patients with lupus glomerulonephritis. Nephron 10:273, 1973.

354. Hahn BH, Kantor OS, Osterland K: A controlled trial of prednisone and azathioprine plus prednisone in the treatment of systemic lupus erythematosus. Clin Res 22:642A, 1974.

355. Ginzler E, Diamond H, Guttadauria M, Kaplan D: Prednisone and azathioprine compared to prednisone plus low-dose azathioprine and cyclophosphamide in the treatment of diffuse lupus nephritis. Arthritis Rheum 19:639, 1976.

356. Jones JV, Bucknall RC, Cumming RH, et al: Plasmapheresis in the management of acute systemic lupus erythematosus? Lancet 1:709, 1976.

357. Cathcart E, Idelson BA, Scheinberg MA, Couser WG: Beneficial effects of methyl prednisolone "pulse" therapy in diffuse proliferative lupus nephritis. Lancet 1:163, 1976.

358. Kimberly RP, Lockshin MD, Sherman RL, et al: High dose intravenous methylprednisolone pulse therapy in systemic lupus erythematosus. Am J Med 70:817, 1981.

359. Liebling MR, McLaughlin K, Boonsue S, et al: Monthly pulses of methylprednisolone in SLE nephritis. J Rheumatol 9:543, 1982.

360. Donadio JV, Holley KE, Ferguson RH, Ilstrup DM: Treatment of lupus nephritis with prednisone and combined prednisone and cyclophosphamide. N Engl J Med 299:1151, 1978.

361. Jones J, Vernier RL, Cumming RH, et al: Evidence for a therapeutic effect of plasmapheresis in patients with systemic lupus erythematosus. Q J Med 48:555, 1979.

362. Jones JV, Fraser ID, Bothamley J, et al: A therapeutic role for plasmapheresis in the management of acute systemic lupus erythematosus. Plasma Ther 1:33, 1979.

363. Clark WF, Lindsay RM, Cattran DC, et al: Monthly plasmapheresis for systemic lupus erythematosus with diffuse proliferative glomerulonephritis: A pilot study. Can Med Assoc J 125:171, 1981.

364. Wei N, Klippel JH, Huston DP, et al: Randomised trial of plasma exchange in mild systemic lupus erythematosus. Lancet 1:17–22, 1983.

365. Terman DS, Buffaloe G, Mattioli C, et al: Extracorporeal immunoadsorption: Initial experience in human systemic lupus erythematosus. Lancet 2:824, 1979.

366. Ponticelli C, Zucchelli P, Banfi G, et al: Treatment of diffuse proliferative lupus nephritis by intravenous high dose methylprednisolone. Q J Med 201:16, 1982.

367. Ben-Chetrit E, Gross DJ, Braverman A, et al: Total lymphoid irradiation in refractory systemic lupus erythematosus. Ann Intern Med 105:58, 1986.

368. Leaker BR, Becker GJ, Dowling JP, Kincaid-Smith PS: Rapid improvement in severe lupus glomerular lesions following intensive plasma exchange associated with immunosuppression. Clin Nephrol 25:236, 1986.

369. Palmer A, Cairns T, Dische F, et al: Treatment of rapidly progressive glomerulonephritis by extracorporeal immunoadsorption, prednisone and cyclophosphamide. Nephrol Dial Transplant 6:536, 1991.

370. Lewis EJ, Hunsicker LG, Lan S-P, et al: A controlled trial of plasmapheresis therapy in severe lupus nephritis. N Engl J Med 326:1373, 1992.

371. Steinberg AD, Steinberg SC: Long-term preservation of renal function in patients with lupus nephritis receiving treatment that includes cyclophosphamide versus those treated with prednisone only. Arthritis Rheum 34:945, 1991.

372. Levey AS, Lan S-P, Corwin HL, et al: Progression and remission of renal disease in the Lupus Nephritis Collaborative Study. Results of treatment with prednisone and short-term oral cyclophosphamide. Ann Intern Med 116:114–123, 1992.

373. Bressler RB, Huston DP: Water intoxication following moderate dose intravenous cyclophosphamide. Arch Intern Med 145:548, 1985.

373a. Thrasher JB, Miller GJ, Wettlaufer JN: Bladder leiomyosarcoma following cyclophosphamide therapy for lupus nephritis. J Urol 143:119, 1990.

374. Hows JM, Mehta A, Ward L, et al: Comparison of mesna with forced diuresis to prevent cyclophosphamide induced haemorrhagic cystitis in marrow transplantation: A prospective randomised study. Br J Cancer 50:753–756, 1984.

375. Dau PC, Callahan J, Parker R, Golbus J: Immunologic effects of plasmapheresis synchronized with pulse cyclophosphamide in systemic lupus erythematosus. J Rheumatol 18:270, 1991.

376. Schroeder JD, Evler HH, Loffler H: Synchronization of plasmapheresis and pulse cyclophosphamide in severe systemic lupus erythematosus. Ann Intern Med 107:344, 1987.

377. Clark WF, Dau PC, Euler HH, et al: Plasmapheresis and subsequent pulse cyclophosphamide versus pulse cyclophosphamide alone in severe lupus: Design of the LPSG trial. J Clin Apheresis 6:40, 1991.

378. Chagnac A, Kiberd BA, Farinas MC, et al: Outcome of the acute glomerular injury in proliferative lupus nephritis. J Clin Invest 84:922, 1989.

379. Myers BD, Chagnac A, Golbetz H, et al: Extent of glomerular injury in active and resolving lupus nephritis: A theoretical analysis. Am J Physiol 260:F717, 1991.

380. Miescher PA, Miescher A: Combined cyclosporine-steroid treatment of systemic-lupus erythematosus. *In* Schindler R (ed): Cyclosporin in Autoimmune Diseases. Springer-Verlag, Berlin, 1985, p 334.

381. Radhakrishnan J, Kunis CL, D'Agati V, et al: Cyclosporine treatment of lupus membranous nephropathy. Clin Nephrol 42:147, 1994.

382. Feutren G, Querin S, Chatenoud L, et al: The effects of cyclosporine in twelve patients with severe systemic lupus. *In* Schindler R (ed): Cyclosporin in Autoimmune Diseases. Springer-Verlag, Berlin, 1985, p 366.

383. Clark WF, Parbtani A, Naylor CD, et al: Fish oil in lupus nephritis: Clinical findings and methodological implications. Kidney Int 44:75, 1993.

384. Clark WF, Parbtani A, Huff MW, et al: Omega-3 fatty acid dietary

supplementation in systemic lupus erythematosus. Kidney Int 36:653, 1989.

385. Westberg G, Tarkowski A: Effect of MaxEPA in patients with SLE. A double-blind, crossover study. Scand J Rheumatol 19:137, 1990.

386. Pierucci A, Simonetti BM, Pecci G, et al: Improvement of renal function with selective thromboxane antagonism in lupus nephritis. N Engl J Med 320:421, 1989.

387. Hariharan S, Pollak VE, Kant KS, et al: Diffuse proliferative lupus nephritis: Long-term observations in patients treated with ancrod. Clin Nephrol 34:61, 1990.

388. Lin C-Y, Hsu H-C, Chiang H: Improvement of histological and immunological change in steroid and immunosuppressive drug–resistant lupus nephritis by high-dose intravenous gamma globulin. Nephron 53:303, 1989.

389. Wacholtz MC, Lipsky PE: Treatment of lupus nephritis with CD5 PLUS, an immunoconjugate of an anti-CD5 monoclonal antibody and ricin A chain. Arthritis Rheum 35:837–839, 1992.

390. Coplon NN, Deskin CJ, Petersen J, et al: The long-term clinical course of systemic lupus erythematosus in end-stage renal disease. N Engl J Med 308:186, 1983.

391. Correia P, Cameron JS, Ogg GS, et al: End stage renal failure in systemic lupus nephritis. Clin Nephrol 22:293, 1985.

392. Cheigh JS, Stenzel KH, Rubin AL, et al: Systemic lupus erythematosus in patients with chronic renal failure. Am J Med 75:602, 1983.

393. Zebb M, Helderman JH: Dialysis and transplantation in end-stage lupus nephritis. N Engl J Med 308:218, 1983.

394. Ng ROK, Craddock PR: End-stage renal disease in systemic lupus erythematosus. N Engl J Med 308:1357, 1983.

395. Wallace DJ, Dubois EL: Prognostic subsets, natural course and causes of death in systemic lupus erythematosus. In Wallace DJ, Dubois E (eds): Dubois' Lupus Erythematosus, 3rd ed. Lea & Febiger, Philadelphia, 1987, p 580.

396. Amend WJC, Vincenti F, Feduska NJ, et al: Recurrent systemic lupus erythematosus involving renal allografts. Ann Intern Med 94:444, 1981.

397. Nossent HC, Swaak TJG, Berden JHM: Systemic lupus erythematosus after renal transplantation: Patient and graft survival and disease activity. Ann Intern Med 114:183–188, 1991.

398. Goss JA, Cole BR, Jendrisak MD, et al: Renal transplantation for systemic lupus erythematosus and recurrent lupus nephritis. A single-center experience and a review of the literature. Transplantation 52:805, 1991.

399. Cattran DC, Aprile M: Renal transplantation in lupus erythematosus. Ann Intern Med 114:991, 1991.

400. Jones JV: Schönlein versus Henoch. Br Med J 4:677, 1973.

401. Schönlein JL: Allgemeine und specielle Pathologie and Therapie, 3rd ed, Vol 2. Literatur-Comptoir, Freiburg, Germany, 1837, p 48.

402. Henoch E: Über eine eigentümliche Form von Purpura. Berl Klin Wochenschr 11:641, 1874.

403. Pinkus H, Mehregan AH: A Guide to Dermatohistopathology, 2nd ed. Appleton-Century-Crofts, New York, 1976, p 222.

404. Cream JH, Gumpel JM, Peachey RDG: Schönlein-Henoch purpura in the adult: A study of 77 adults with anaphylactoid or Schönlein-Henoch purpura. Q J Med 39:461, 1970.

405. Ballard HS, Eisinger RP, Gallo G: Renal manifestations of the Henoch-Schönlein syndrome in adults. Am J Med 49:328, 1970.

406. Meadow SR, Glasgow EF, White RHR, et al: Schönlein-Henoch nephritis. Q J Med 41:241, 1972.

407. Habib R, Levy M: Anaphylactoid purpura nephritis: observations with sixty childhood cases. Clin Pediatr 12:445, 1973.

408. Cameron JS: The nephritis of Schönlein-Henoch purpura: Current problems. In Kincaid-Smith P, d'Apice AJF, Atkins RL (eds): Progress in Glomerulonephritis. John Wiley & Sons, New York, 1979, p 283.

409. Allen DM, Diamond LK, Howell PA: Anaphylactoid purpura in children (Schönlein-Henoch syndrome). Am J Dis Child 99:147, 1960.

410. Rogers PW, Bunn SM Jr, Kurtzman NA, White MG: Schönlein-Henoch syndrome associated with exposure to cold. Arch Intern Med 128:782, 1971.

411. Ackroyd JF: Allergic purpura including purpura due to foods, drugs, and infections. Am J Med 14:605, 1953.

412. Vernier RL, Worthen HG, Peterson RD, et al: Anaphylactoid purpura: I. Pathology of the skin and kidney and frequency of streptococcal infection. Pediatrics 27:181, 1961.

413. Ginsburg BE, Wasserman J, Huldt G, Bergstrand A: Case of glomerulonephritis associated with acute toxoplasmosis. Br Med J 3:664, 1974.

414. Sussman M, Jones JH, Almeida JD, Lachmann PJ: Deficiency of the second component of complement associated with presence of mycoplasma in the serum. Clin Exp Immunol 14:531, 1973.

415. Rasmussen NH: Henoch-Schönlein purpura after *Yersinia*. Arch Dis Child 57:322, 1982.

416. Fagan JE: Henoch-Schönlein purpura and γ-benzene hexachloride. Pediatrics 67:310–311, 1980. Letter.

417. Goebel KM, Mueller-Brodman W: Reversible overt nephropathy with Henoch-Schönlein purpura due to puroxicam. Br Med J 284:311, 1982.

418. Robertson PW, Leonard BJ: Some delayed complications of inoculation. Br Med J 2:1029, 1956.

419. Lane JM: Vaccination and Henoch-Schönlein purpura (concluded). N Engl J Med 280:781, 1969.

420. Blumberg S, Bierfang D, Kantrowitz FG: A possible association between influenza vaccination and small-vessel vasculitis. Arch Intern Med 140:847, 1980.

421. Ayoub EM, Hoyer J: Anaphylactoid purpura: Streptococcal antibody titers and B₁C globulin levels. J Pediatr 75:193, 1969.

422. Urizar EE, Singh JK, Muhammad T, Hines O: Henoch-Schönlein anaphylactoid purpura nephropathy: Electron microscopic lesions mimicking acute poststreptococcal nephritis. Hum Pathol 9:223, 1978.

423. Montoliu J, Miro JM, Campistol JM, et al: Henoch-Schönlein purpura complicating staphylococcal endocarditis in a heroin addict. Am J Nephrol 7:137, 1987.

424. Lofters WS, Penco GF, Luke KH, Yaworsky RG: Henoch-Schönlein purpura occurring in three members of a family. Can Med Assoc J 109:46, 1973.

425. Oliver TK Jr, Barnett HL: The incidence and prognosis of nephritis associated with anaphylactoid purpura in children. Am J Dis Child 90:544, 1955.

426. Wedgewood RJP, Klaus MH: Anaphylactoid purpura (Schönlein-Henoch syndrome): A long-term follow-up study with special reference to renal involvement. Pediatrics 16:196, 1955.

427. Meadow SR: The prognosis of Henoch-Schönlein nephritis. Clin Nephrol 9:87, 1978.

428. Linne T, Aperia A, Broberger O, et al: Renal function and biopsy changes during the course of Henoch-Schönlein glomerulonephritis. Acta Paediatr Scand 72:97, 1983.

429. Koskimies O, Mir S, Rapola J, Wilska S: Henoch-Schönlein nephritis: Long-term prognosis of unselected patients. Arch Dis Child 56:482, 1981.

430. Farine M, Poucell S, Geary DL, Baumal R: Prognostic significance of urinary findings and renal biopsy in children with Henoch-Schönlein nephritis. Clin Pediatr 25:257, 1986.

431. Payton CD, Allison MEM, Boulton-Jones JM: Henoch-Schönlein purpura presenting with pulmonary hemorrhage. Scott Med J 32:26, 1987.

432. Martini A, Ravelli A, Beluffi G: Urinary microscopy in the diagnosis of hematuria in Henoch-Schönlein purpura. Eur J Pediatr 144:591, 1986.

433. Guyon JB, Seiller F, Deries X, et al: Inhibitors of factors VIII and IX in a child with Henoch-Schönlein syndrome. Am J Pediatr Hematol Oncol 7:376, 1985.

434. Garcia-Fuentes M, Martin A, Chantler C, Williams DG: Serum complement components in Henoch-Schönlein purpura. Arch Dis Child 53:417, 1978.

435. Spitzer RE, Vromson JR, Farnett ML, et al: Alteration of the complement system in children with Henoch-Schönlein purpura. Clin Immunol Immunopathol 11:52, 1978.

436. Trygstad CW, Stiehm ER: Elevated serum IgA globulin in anaphylactoid purpura. Pediatrics 47:1023, 1971.

437. Smila S, Kouvalainen K, Lanning M: Serum immunoglobulin levels in the course of anaphylactoid purpura in children. Acta Paediatr Scand 66:537, 1977.

438. Saulsbury FT: IgA rheumatoid factor in Henoch-Schönlein purpura. J Pediatr 108:71, 1986.

439. Williams DG, Garcia-Fuentes M, Chantler C: Cryoglobulins and the complement system in Henoch-Schönlein nephritis. Kidney Int 12:151, 1977.

440. Mookerjee BK, Maddison PJ, Reichlin M: Mesangial IgA-IgG deposition in mixed cryoglobulinemia. Am J Med Sci 276:224, 1978.

441. Levinsky RJ, Barratt TM: IgA immune complexes in Henoch-Schönlein purpura. Lancet 2:1100, 1979.
442. Woodroffe AJ, Gormly AA, McKenzie PE, et al: Immunologic studies in IgA nephropathy. Kidney Int 18:366, 1980.
443. Coppo R, Basolo B, Martina G, et al: Circulating immune complexes containing IgA, IgM, and IgG in patients with primary IgA nephropathy and with Henoch-Schönlein nephritis: Correlation with clinical and histologic signs of activity. Clin Nephrol 18:230, 1982.
444. Egido J, Sancho J, Mampaso F, et al: A possible common pathogenesis of the mesangial IgA glomerulonephritis in patients with Berger's disease and Schönlein-Henoch syndrome. Proc Eur Dial Transplant Assoc 17:660, 1980.
445. Coppo R, Basolo B, Mazzucco G, et al: IgA$_1$ and IgA$_2$ in circulating immune complexes and in renal deposits of Berger's and Schönlein-Henoch glomerulonephritis. Proc Eur Dial Transplant Assoc 19:648, 1982.
446. Shaw G, Ronda N, Bevan JS, et al: Antineutrophil cytoplasmic antibodies (ANCA) of IgA class correlate with disease activity in adult Henoch-Schönlein purpura. Nephrol Dial Transplant 7:1238–1241, 1992.
447. Darvin J-C, Malaise M, Foidart J, Mahieu P: Anti–α-galactosyl antibodies and immune complexes in children with Henoch-Schönlein purpura or IgA nephropathy. Kidney Int 31:1132, 1987.
448. Nyulassy S, Bue M, Sasinba M, et al: The HLA system in glomerulonephritis. Clin Immunol Immunopathol 7:319, 1977.
449. Stevenson JA, Leong LA, Cohen AH, Border WA: Henoch-Schönlein purpura. Simultaneous demonstration of IgA deposits in involved skin, intestines and kidneys. Arch Pathol Lab Med 106:192, 1982.
450. Toucharo G, Marie P, Beanchant M, et al: Vascular IgA and C3 deposition in gastrointestinal tract of patients with Henoch-Schönlein purpura. Lancet 1:771, 1983.
451. Heaton JM, Turner DR, Cameron JS: Localization of glomerular ''deposits'' in Henoch-Schönlein nephritis. Histopathology 1:93, 1977.
452. Brun C, Bryld C, Fenger L, Jorgensen F: Glomerular lesions in adults with the Schönlein-Henoch syndrome: A light and electron microscopic study. Acta Pathol Microbiol Scand [A] 79:569–583, 1971.
453. Urizar RE, Michael A, Sisson S, Vernier RL: Anaphylactoid purpura: II. Immunofluorescent and electron microscopic studies of the glomerular lesions. Lab Invest 19:437, 1968.
454. Yoshiara S, Yoshikawa N, Matsuo T: Immunoelectron microscopic study of childhood IgA nephropathy and Henoch-Schönlein nephritis. Virchows Arch A 412:95, 1987.
455. Sinniah R, Feng PH, Chen BJM: Henoch-Schönlein syndrome: A clinical and morphological study of renal biopsies. Clin Nephrol 9:219, 1978.
456. Kim CK, Aikawa M, Makker SP: Electron-dense subepithelial glomerular deposits in Henoch-Schönlein purpura syndrome. Arch Pathol Lab Med 103:595, 1979.
457. Yoshikawa N, Yoshiara S, Yoshiya K, et al: Lysis of the glomerular basement membrane in children with IgA nephropathy and Henoch-Schönlein purpura. J Pathol 150:119, 1986.
458. Levy M, Broyer M, Habib R: Pathology and immunopathology of Schönlein-Henoch glomerulonephritis. *In* Kincaid-Smith P, d'Apice AJF, Atkins RL (eds): Progress in Glomerulonephritis. John Wiley & Sons, New York, 1979, p 261.
459. Evans DJ, Williams D, Peters DK, et al: Glomerular deposition of properdin in Henoch-Schönlein syndrome and idiopathic focal nephritis. Br Med J 3:326, 1973.
460. Baart de la Faille-Kuyper EH, Van der Meer JB, Kater L, Mul N: Alternate pathway complement activation by IgA in Schönlein-Henoch syndrome. Neth J Med 17:5, 1974.
461. Baart de la Faille-Kuyper EH, Kater L, Kuipten RH, et al: Occurrence of vascular IgA deposits in clinically normal skin of patients with renal disease. Kidney Int 9:424, 1976.
462. Provost TT, Tomasi B: Evidence for complement activation by the alternate pathway in skin diseases: II. Dermatitis herpetiformis. Clin Immunol Immunopathol 3:178, 1974.
463. Jones CL, Powell HR, Kincaid-Smith P, Robertson DM: Polymeric IgA and immune complex concentrations in IgA-related renal disease. Kidney Int 38:323, 1990.
463a. Nast CC, Ward HJ, Koyle MA, Cohen AH: Recurrent Henoch-Schönlein purpura following renal transplantation. Am J Kidney Dis 9:39, 1987.

463b. Davin JC, Foidart JB, Mahieu PR: Fc-receptor function in Henoch-Schönlein disease of childhood. Proc Eur Dial Trans Assoc 19:590, 1982.
463c. Turi S, Belch JJF, Beattie TJ, Forbes CD: Abnormalities of vascular prostaglandins in Henoch-Schönlein purpura. Arch Dis Child 6:173, 1986.
464. Tönshoff B, Momper R, Schweer H, et al: Increased biosynthesis of vasoactive prostanoids in Schönlein-Henoch purpura. Pediatr Res 32:137, 1992.
465. O'Donoghue DJ, Darvill A, Ballardie FW: Mesangial cell autoantigens in immunoglobulin A nephropathy and Henoch-Schönlein purpura. J Clin Invest 88:1522, 1991.
466. Jennette JC, Wieslander J, Tuttle R, et al: Serum IgA-fibronectin aggregates in patients with IgA nephropathy and Henoch-Schönlein purpura: Diagnostic value and pathogenic implications. Am J Kidney Dis 18:466, 1991.
467. Goldstein AR, White RHR, Akuse R, Chantler C: Long-term follow-up of childhood Henoch-Schönlein nephritis. Lancet 339:280, 1992.
468. Mollica F, LiVolti S, Garozzo R, Russo G: Effectiveness of early prednisone treatment in preventing the development of nephropathy in anaphylactoid purpura. Eur J Pediatr 151:40, 1992.
469. Austin HA III, Balow JE: Henoch-Schönlein nephritis: Prognostic features and the challenge of therapy. Am J Kidney Dis 2:512, 1983.
470. Dosa S, Cairns SA, Mallick NP, et al: Relapsing Henoch-Schönlein syndrome with renal involvement in a patient with an IgA monoclonal gammopathy: A study of the result of immunosuppressant and cytotoxic therapy. Nephron 26:145, 1980.
471. Kauffmann RH, Houwert DA: Plasmapheresis in rapidly progressive Henoch-Schönlein glomerulonephritis and the effect on circulating IgA immune complexes. Clin Nephrol 16:155, 1981.
472. Baliah T, Kim KH, Anthone S, et al: Recurrence of Henoch-Schönlein purpura (HSP) glomerulonephritis in transplanted kidney. Transplantation 18:343, 1974.
473. Weiss JH, Bhathena DB, Curtis JJ, et al: A possible relationship between Henoch-Schönlein syndrome and IgA nephropathy (Berger's disease). Nephron 22:582, 1978.
474. Nast CC, Ward HJ, Koyle MA, Cohen AH: Recurrent Henoch-Schönlein purpura following renal transplantation. Am J Kidney Dis 9:39, 1987.
475. Bachman V, Biava C, Amend W, et al: The clinical course of IgA nephropathy and Henoch-Schönlein purpura following renal transplantation. Transplantation 42:511, 1986.
476. Goodpasture EW: The significance of certain pulmonary lesions in relation to the etiology of influenza. Am J Med Sci 158:863, 1919.
477. Stanton MC, Tange JD: Goodpasture's syndrome (pulmonary haemorrhage associated with glomerulonephritis). Aust Ann Med 7:132, 1958.
478. Heptinstall RH, Salmon MV: Pulmonary hemorrhage with extensive glomerular disease of the kidney. J Clin Pathol 12:272, 1959.
479. Wu M-J, Rajarm R, Shelp D, et al: Vasculitis in Goodpasture's syndrome. Acta Pathol Lab Med 104:300, 1980.
480. Lerner RA, Glassock RJ, Dixon FJ: The role of antiglomerular basement membrane antibody in the pathogenesis of human glomerulonephritis. J Exp Med 126:989, 1967.
481. Martinez JS, Kohler PF: Variant ''Goodpasture's syndrome''? Ann Intern Med 75:67, 1971.
482. Glassock RJ: A clinical and immunopathologic dissection of rapidly progressive glomerulonephritis. Nephron 22:253, 1978.
483. Leatherman JW, Sibley RK, Davies SF: Diffuse intrapulmonary hemorrhage and glomerulonephritis unrelated to antiglomerular basement membrane antibody. Am J Med 72:401, 1982.
484. Boyce N, Holdsworth SR: Pulmonary manifestations of the clinical syndrome of acute glomerulonephritis and lung hemorrhage. Am J Kidney Dis 8:31, 1986.
485. Holdsworth S, Boyce N, Thomson N, Atkins R: The clinical spectrum of acute glomerulonephritis and lung hemorrhage (Goodpasture's syndrome). Q J Med 55:75, 1985.
486. Duncan DA, Drummond KN, Michael AF, Vernier RL: Pulmonary hemorrhage and glomerulonephritis: Report of six cases and study of the renal lesion by fluorescent antibody technique and electron microscopy. Ann Intern Med 62:920, 1965.
487. McPhaul JJ, Mullins JD: Glomerulonephritis mediated by antibody to glomerular basement membrane: Immunological, clinical and histopathological characteristics. J Clin Invest 57:351, 1976.

488. Teague C, Doak P, Simpson I, et al: Goodpasture's syndrome: Analysis of 29 cases. Kidney Int 13:492, 1978.
489. Wilson CB, Dixon FJ: Renal injury from immune reactions involving antigens in or of the kidney. *In* Brenner BM, Stein J (eds): Contemporary Issues in Nephrology, Vol 3. Churchill Livingstone, New York, 1979, p 35.
490. Esnault VLM, Soleimani B, Keogan MT, et al: Association of IgM with IgG anti-neutrophil cytoplasmic antibodies in patients presenting with pulmonary hemorrhage. Kidney Int 41:1304–1310, 1992.
491. Lamriben L, Kourilsky O, Mougenot B, et al: Goodpasture's syndrome with asymptomatic renal involvement. Disappearance of antiglomerular basement membrane antibodies and deposits after treatment. Nephrol Dial Transplant 8:1267–1269, 1993.
492. Graindorge PP, Mahieu PR: Radioimmunologic method for detection of antitubular basement membrane antibodies. Kidney Int 14:594, 1978.
493. Buffaloe GW, Evans JE, McIntosh RW, et al: Antibodies in human glomerular basement membrane: New methodology for detection in serum. Clin Exp Immunol 39:316, 1979.
494. Wilson CB, Dixon FJ: Anti–glomerular basement membrane antibody–induced glomerulonephritis. Kidney Int 3:74, 1973.
495. Border WA, Baehler RW, Bhathena D, Glassock RJ: IgA anti–basement membrane nephritis with pulmonary hemorrhage. Ann Intern Med 91:21, 1979.
496. Butkowski RJ, Langewild JPM, Wieslander J, et al: Localization of the Goodpasture syndrome to a novel chain of basement membrane collagen. J Biol Chem 262:7874, 1977.
497. Wieslander J, Kataja M, Hudson BG: Characterization of the human Goodpasture antigen. Clin Exp Immunol 69:332, 1987.
498. Makino H, Gibbons JT, Reddy MK, Kanwar YS: Nephrogenicity of antibodies to proteoglycans of the glomerular basement membrane. J Clin Invest 77:142, 1986.
499. Turner N, Mason PJ, Brown R, et al: Molecular cloning of the human Goodpasture antigen demonstrates it to be the α3 chain of type IV collagen. J Clin Invest 89:592–601, 1992.
500. Morrison KE, Mariyama M, Yang-Feng TL, et al: Sequence and localization of a partial cDNA encoding the human α3 chain of type IV collagen. Am J Hum Genet 49:545, 1991.
501. Kefalides NA, Ohno N, Wilson CB: Heterogeneity of antibodies in Goodpasture syndrome reacting with type IV collagen. Kidney Int 43:85, 1993.
502. Kalluri R, Gunwar S, Reeders ST, et al: Goodpasture syndrome: Localization of the epitope for the autoantibodies to the carboxyl-terminal region of the α3(IV) chain of basement membrane collagen. J Biol Chem 266:24018–24024, 1991.
503. Hudson BG, Kalluri R, Gunwar S, et al: Molecular characteristics of the Goodpasture autoantigen. Kidney Int 43:135–139, 1993.
504. Gunwar S, Bejarano PA, Kalluri R, et al: Alveolar basement membrane: Molecular properties of the noncollagenous domain (hexamer) of collagen IV and its reactivity with Goodpasture autoantibodies. Am J Respir Cell Mol Biol 5:107, 1991.
505. McPhaul JJ, Dixon FJ: Characterization of immunoglobulin G anti–glomerular basement membrane antibodies eluted from kidneys of patients with glomerulonephritis: II. IgG subtypes and in vitro complement fixation. J Immunol 107:678, 1971.
506. Koffler D, Sandson J, Carr R, Kinkel HG: Immunologic studies concerning the pulmonary lesions in Goodpasture's syndrome. Am J Pathol 54:293, 1969.
507. Weber M, Lohse A, Manus M, et al: IgG subclass distribution of autoantibodies to glomerular basement membrane in Goodpasture's syndrome compared to other autoantibodies. Nephron 49:54, 1988.
508. Bernis P, Hamels J, Quoidbach A, et al: Remission of Goodpasture's syndrome after withdrawal of an unusual toxin. Clin Nephrol 23:312, 1985.
509. Keogh A, Ibels LS, Allen DH, Isbister JP: Exacerbation of Goodpasture's syndrome after inadvertent exposure to hydrocarbon fumes. Br Med J 288:188, 1983.
510. Ravnskov V: Possible mechanisms of hydrocarbon-associated glomerulonephritis. Clin Nephrol 23:294, 1985.
511. Zimmerman SW, Varanasi UR, Hoff B: Goodpasture's syndrome with normal renal function. Am J Med 66:163, 1979.
512. Bell DD, Moffatt SL, Singer M, Munt PW: Antibasement membrane antibody disease without clinical evidence of renal disease. Am Rev Respir Dis 142:234–237, 1990.
513. Mehler PS, Brunvand MW, Hutt MP, Anderson RJ: Chronic recurrent Goodpasture's syndrome. Am J Med 82:833, 1987.
514. Hind CRK, Bowman G, Winearls CG, Lockwood CM: Recurrence of circulating anti–glomerular basement membrane antibody three years after immunosuppressive treatment and plasma exchange. Clin Nephrol 21:244, 1984.
515. Simpson IJ, Doak PB, Williams LC, et al: Plasma exchange in Goodpasture's syndrome. Am J Nephrol 2:301, 1982.
516. Gossain VV, Gerstein AR, James AW: Goodpasture's syndrome: A familial occurrence. Am Rev Respir Dis 105:621, 1972.
517. d'Apice AJF, Kincaid-Smith P, Becker GJ, et al: Goodpasture's syndrome in identical twins. Ann Intern Med 88:61, 1978.
518. Benoit FL, Rulon DB, Theil GB, et al: Goodpasture's syndrome: A clinicopathologic entity. Am J Med 37:424, 1964.
519. Lechleitner P, Defregger M, Lhotta K, et al: Goodpasture's syndrome. Unusual presentation after exposure to hard metal dust. Chest 103:956, 1993.
520. Turner N, Lockwood CM, Rees AJ: Antiglomerular basement membrane antibody-mediated nephritis. *In* Schrier RW, Gottschalk CW (eds): Diseases of the Kidney, 5th ed. Little, Brown, Boston, 1993, pp 1865–1894.
521. Curtis JJ, Bhathena D, Leach RP, et al: Goodpasture's syndrome in a patient with the nail-patella syndrome. Am J Med 61:401, 1976.
522. Wilson CB: Nephritogenic immune responses involving basement membranes and other antigens in or of the glomerulus. *In* Cummings NB, Michael AF, Wilson CB (eds): Immune Mechanisms of Renal Disease. Plenum Medical Book, New York, 1983, p 240.
523. Sternlieb I, Bennett B, Scheinberg IH: D-Penicillamine-induced Goodpasture's syndrome in Wilson's disease. Ann Intern Med 82:673, 1975.
524. Perez GO, Bjornsson S, Ross AH, et al: A mini-epidemic of Goodpasture's syndrome: Clinical and immunological studies. Nephron 13:161, 1974.
525. Wilson CB, Smith RC: Goodpasture's syndrome associated with influenza A₂ virus infection. Ann Intern Med 76:91, 1972.
526. Dahlberg PJ, Kurtz SB, Donadio JV, et al: Recurrent Goodpasture's syndrome. Mayo Clin Proc 53:533, 1978.
527. Wu MJ, Moorthy AV, Beirne GJ: Relapse in anti–glomerular basement membrane antibody–mediated crescentic glomerulonephritis. Clin Nephrol 13:9, 1980.
528. Rees AJ, Lockwood CM, Peters DK: Enhanced allergic tissue injury in Goodpasture's syndrome by concurrent bacterial infection. Br Med J 2:723, 1977.
529. Rees AJ, Peters DK, Compston DAS, Batchelor JR: Strong association between HLA-DRw2 and antibody-mediated Goodpasture's syndrome. Lancet 1:966, 1978.
530. Perl SI, Pussell BA, Charlesworth JA, et al: Goodpasture's (anti-GBM) disease and HLA-DRw2. N Engl J Med 305:463, 1981.
531. Rees AJ, Peters DK, Amos N, et al: The influence of HLA-linked genes on the severity of anti-GBM antibody mediated nephritis. Kidney Int 26:444, 1984.
532. Jayne DRW, Marshall PD, Jones SJ, Lockwood CM: Autoantibodies to GBM and neutrophil cytoplasm in rapidly progressive glomerular nephritis. Kidney Int 37:965, 1990.
533. Weber MF, Andrassy K, Pullig O, et al: Anti–neutrophil-cytoplasmic antibodies and antiglomerular basement membrane antibodies in Goodpasture's syndrome and in Wegener's granulomatosis. J Am Soc Nephrol 2:1227, 1992.
534. Azen EA, Clatanoff DV: Prolonged survival in Goodpasture's syndrome. Arch Intern Med 114:453, 1964.
535. Ewan PW, Jones HA, Rhodes CG, Hughes JMB: Detection of intrapulmonary hemorrhage with carbon monoxide uptake: Application in Goodpasture's syndrome. N Engl J Med 295:1391, 1976.
536. Senekjian HO, Knight HO, Weinman EJ: The spectrum of renal diseases associated with antibasement membrane antibodies. Arch Intern Med 140:79, 1980.
537. Wilson CB: Anti-GBM glomerulonephritis. *In* Rosen S (ed): Pathology of Glomerular Disease. Churchill Livingstone, New York, 1983, p 171.
538. Andres G, Brentjens J, Kohli R, et al: Histology of human tubulo-interstitial nephritis associated with antibodies to renal basement membranes. Kidney Int 13:480, 1978.
539. Sisson S, Sysart NK Jr, Fish AJ, Fernier RL: Localization of the Goodpasture antigen by immunoelectron microscopy. Clin Immunol Immunopathol 23:414, 1982.
540. Stejskal J, Pirani CL, Okada M, et al: Discontinuities (gaps) of the

glomerular capillary wall and basement membrane in renal disease. Lab Invest 28:149, 1973.

541. Min KW, Gyorkey F, Gyorkey P, et al: The morphogenesis of glomerular crescents in rapidly progressive glomerulonephritis. Kidney Int 5:47, 1974.

542. Savage JA, Dowling J, Kincaid-Smith P: Superimposed glomerular immune complexes in anti–glomerular basement membrane disease. Am J Kidney Dis 14:145, 1989.

543. Pettersson E, Tornroth T, Miettinen A: Simultaneous antiglomerular basement membrane and membranous glomerulonephritis: Case report and literature review. Clin Immunol Immunopathol 31:171, 1984.

544. Agodoa LCY, Striker GE, George CRP, et al: The appearance of nonlinear deposits of immunoglobulin in Goodpasture's syndrome. Am J Med 61:407, 1976.

545. Atkins RC: The macrophage in human rapidly progressive glomerulonephritis. Lancet 1:830, 1976.

546. Schreiner GF, Cotran RS, Pardo V: A mononuclear cell component in experimental crescentic glomerulonephritis. J Exp Med 147:369, 1978.

547. Cattell V, Jamieson SW: The origin of glomerular crescents in experimental nephrotoxic serum nephritis in the rabbit. Lab Invest 39:584, 1978.

548. Thomson NM, Holdsworth SR, Glasgow EG, et al: Mechanisms of injury in experimental glomerulonephritis. In Kincaid-Smith P, D'Apice AJF, Atkins RC (eds): Progress in Glomerulonephritis. John Wiley & Sons, New York, 1979, p 1851.

549. Pasternack A, Tornroth T, Linder E: Evidence of both anti-GBM and immune complex mediated pathogenesis in the initial phase of Goodpasture's syndrome. Clin Nephrol 9:77, 1978.

550. Siegel RR: Basis of pulmonary disease resolution after nephrectomy in Goodpasture's syndrome: A report of five cases and a review of the literature. Am J Med 48:162, 1970.

551. Freeman RM, Vertel RM, Easterling RE: Goodpasture's syndrome: Prolonged survival with chronic hemodialysis. Arch Intern Med 117:643, 1966.

552. Couser WG: Goodpasture's syndrome: A response to nitrogen mustard. Am J Med Sci 268:175, 1974.

553. Strauch BS, Charney A, Doctorouff S, Kashgarian M: Goodpasture's syndrome with recovery after renal failure. JAMA 229:444, 1974.

554. Maxwell DR, Ozawa T, Nielsen RL, Luft FC: Spontaneous recovery from rapidly progressive glomerulonephritis. Br Med J 2:643, 1979.

555. Munro JF, Geddes AM, Lamb WL: Goodpasture's syndrome: Survival after acute renal failure. Br Med J 4:95, 1967.

556. De Torrente A, Popovtzer M, Guggenheim SE, Schrier R: Serious pulmonary hemorrhage, glomerulonephritis and massive steroid therapy. Ann Intern Med 83:218, 1975.

557. Bolton WK: Crescentic glomerulonephritis. In Glassock RJ (ed): Current Therapy in Nephrology and Hypertension. BC Decker, Philadelphia, 1984, p 213.

558. Conlon PJ Jr, Walshe JJ, Daly C, et al: Antiglomerular basement membrane disease: The long-term pulmonary outcome. Am J Kidney Dis 23:794–796, 1994.

559. Lockwood CM, Boutoln-Jones JM, Lowenthal RM, et al: Recovery from Goodpasture's syndrome after immunosuppressive treatment and plasmapheresis. Br Med J 2:252–254, 1975.

560. Cove-Smith JR, McLeod AA, Blamey RW, et al: Transplantation, immunosuppression and plasmapheresis in Goodpasture's syndrome. Clin Nephrol 9:126, 1978.

561. Rossen RD, Hersh EM, Sharp JJ, et al: Effect of plasma exchange on circulating immune complexes and antibody formation in patients treated with cyclophosphamide and prednisone. Am J Med 63:674, 1977.

562. Johnson JP, Whitman W, Briggs WA, Wilson CB: Plasmapheresis and immunosuppressive agents in anti–basement membrane antibody–induced Goodpasture's syndrome. Am J Med 64:354, 1978.

563. McKenzie PE, Taylor AE, Woodroffe AJ, et al: Plasmapheresis in glomerulonephritis. Clin Nephrol 12:97, 1979.

564. Rosenblatt SG, Knight W, Bannayan GA, et al: Treatment of Goodpasture's syndrome with plasmapheresis: A case report and review of the literature. Am J Med 66:689, 1979.

565. Thysell H, Bygren P, Bengtsson V, et al: Immunosuppression and the additive effect of plasma exchange in treatment of rapidly progressive glomerulonephritis. Acta Med Scand 212:107, 1982.

566. Levin M, Rigden SPA, Pincott JR, et al: Goodpasture's syndrome: Treatment with plasmapheresis, immunosuppression with anticoagulation. Arch Dis Child 58:697, 1983.

567. McLeish KR, Maxwell DR, Luft FC: Failure of plasma exchange and immunosuppression to improve renal function in Goodpasture's syndrome. Clin Nephrol 10:71, 1978.

568. Lockwood CM, Pussell B, Wilson CB, Peters DK: Plasma exchange in nephritis. Adv Nephrol 8:383, 1979.

569. McPhaul JJ, Thompson AL, Lordan RE, et al: Evidence suggesting persistence of nephritogenic immunopathogic mechanisms in patients receiving renal allografts. J Clin Invest 52:1059, 1973.

570. Beliel OM, Coburn JW, Shinaberger JHJ, Glassock RJ: Recurrent glomerulonephritis due to anti-glomerular basement membrane antibodies in two successive allografts. Clin Nephrol 1:377, 1973.

571. Cameron JS, Turner DR: Recurrent glomerulonephritis in allografted kidneys. Clin Nephrol 7:47, 1977.

572. Gluckman JC, Beaufils H, Berger J, et al: Rapidly progressive glomerulonephritis with linear fluorescence in a kidney transplant. Clin Nephrol 1:40, 1973.

573. Almkvist RD, Buckalew VM, Hirszel P: Recurrence of anti-glomerular basement membrane antibody mediated glomerulonephritis in an isograft. Clin Immunol Immunopathol 18:54, 1981.

574. Couser WG, Wallace H, Monaco AP, Lewis EJ: Successful renal transplantation in patients with circulating antibody to glomerular basement membrane: Report of two cases. Clin Nephrol 1:381, 1973.

575. Bergrem H, Jervell J, Brodwall EK, et al: Goodpasture's syndrome: A report of seven patients including long-term follow-up of three who received a kidney transplant. Am J Med 68:54, 1980.

576. Querin S, Schurch W, Beaulieu R: Ciclosporin in Goodpasture's syndrome. Nephron 60:355, 1992.

577. Fahr T: Maligne Nephrosklerose und Periateritis nodosa. Dtsch Med Wochenschr 67:1223, 1941.

578. Nuzum JW Jr, Nuzum JW: Polyarteritis nodosa: A statistical review of 175 cases from the literature and report of a "typical" case. Arch Intern Med 94:942, 1954.

579. Zeek PM: Periarteritis nodosa and other forms of necrotizing angiitis. N Engl J Med 248:764, 1953.

580. Fauci AS, Haynes BF, Katz P: The spectrum of vasculitis: Clinical, pathologic, immunologic, and therapeutic considerations. Ann Intern Med 89:660, 1978.

581. Cupps TR, Fauci T: The Vasculitides. WB Saunders, Philadelphia, 1981.

582. Davson J, Ball J, Platt R: The kidney in periarteritis nodosa. Q J Med 17:175, 1948.

583. Furlong TJ, Ibels LS, Eckstein RP: The clinical spectrum of necrotizing glomerulonephritis. Medicine (Baltimore) 66:192, 1987.

584. Parfrey P, Hutcheson T, Jothy S, et al: The spectrum of diseases associated with necrotizing glomerulonephritis and its prognosis. Am J Kidney Dis 6:387, 1985.

585. Serra A, Cameron JS: Clinical and pathologic aspects of renal vasculitis. Semin Nephrol 5:55, 1985.

586. Savage CO, Winearls C, Evans D, et al: Microscopic polyarteritis: Presentation, pathology and prognosis. Q J Med 56:467, 1985.

587. Leavitt R, Fauci A: Polyangiitis overlap syndrome: Classification and prospective clinical experience. Am J Med 81:79, 1986.

588. Velosa JA: Idiopathic crescentic glomerulonephritis or systemic vasculitis. Mayo Clin Proc 62:145, 1987.

589. Balow JE: Renal vasculitis [clinical conference]. Kidney Int 27:954–964, 1985.

590. Churg J: Nomenclature of vasculitic syndromes: A historical perspective. Am J Kidney Dis 18:148, 1991.

591. Falk RJ: ANCA-associated renal disease. Kidney Int 38:998, 1990.

592. Gross WL, Schmitt WH, Csernok E: ANCA and associated diseases: Immunodiagnostic and pathogenetic aspects. Clin Exp Immunol 91:1, 1993.

593. Kallenberg CGM, Mulder L, Cohen Taervert JW: Antineutrophil cytoplasmic antibodies: A still-growing class of autoantibodies in inflammatory disorders. Am J Med 93:675, 1992.

594. Robinson AJ: Antineutrophil cytoplasmic antibodies (ANCA) and the systemic necrotizing vasculitides. Nephrol Dial Transplant 9:119, 1994.

595. Falk RJ, Hogan S, Carey TS, et al: Clinical course of anti-neutrophil cytoplasmic autoantibody–associated glomerulonephritis and systemic vasculitis. Ann Intern Med 113:656–663, 1990.

595a. Falk RJ, Jennette JC: Anti-neutrophil cytoplasmic autoantibodies with specificity for myeloperoxidase in patients with systemic vasculitis and idiopathic necrotizing and crescentic glomerulonephritis. N Engl J Med 318:1651, 1988.

596. Davies DJ, Moran JE, Niall JF, Ryan GB: Segmental necrotising glomerulonephritis with antineutrophil antibody: Possible arbovirus aetiology? Br Med J 285:606, 1982.

597. Van der Woude FJ, Rasmussen N, Lobatto S: Autoantibodies against neutrophils and monocytes: Tool/N diagnosis and marker of disease activity in Wegener's granulomatosis. Lancet 1:425, 1985.

598. Lockwood CM, Bakes D, Jones S, et al: Association of alkaline phosphatase with an autoantigen recognised by circulating antineutrophil antibodies in systemic vasculitis. Lancet 1:716–720, 1987.

599. Wieslander J: How are antineutrophil cytoplasmic autoantibodies detected? Am J Kidney Dis 18:154–158, 1991.

600. Bini P, Gabay JE, Teitel A, et al: Antineutrophil cytoplasmic autoantibodies in Wegener's granulomatosis recognize conformational epitopes on proteinase 3. J Immunol 149:1409, 1992.

601. Rao NV, Wehner NG, Marshall BC, et al: Characterization of proteinase 3, a neutral serine proteinase. J Biol Chem 266:9540, 1991.

602. Lockwood CM, Ronda N: Spectrum of autoimmune responses in systemic vasculitis. Ann Ital Med Intern 7:203–208, 1992. Editorial.

603. Moodie FDL, Leaker B, Cambridge G, et al: Alpha-enolase: A novel cytosolic autoantigen in ANCA positive vasculitis. Kidney Int 43:675–681, 1993.

604. Esnault VLM, Short AK, Audrain MAP, et al: Autoantibodies to lactoferrin and histone in systemic vasculitis identified by antimyeloperoxidase solid phase assays. Kidney Int 46:153–160, 1994.

605. Ulmer M, Rautmann A, Cross WL: Immunodiagnostic aspects of autoantibodies against myeloperoxidase. Clin Nephrol 37:161–168, 1992.

605a. Sinico RA, Pozzi C, Radice A, et al: Clinical significance of antineutrophil cytoplasmic autoantibodies with specificity for lactoferrin in renal diseases. Am J Kidney Dis 22:253–260, 1993.

606. Lesavre P: Antineutrophil cytoplasmic autoantibodies antigen specificity. Am J Kidney Dis 18:159, 1991.

607. Jennette JC: Antineutrophil cytoplasmic autoantibody–associated diseases: A pathologist's perspective. Am J Kidney Dis 18:164, 1991.

608. Niles JL, Pan GL, Collins AB, et al: Antigen-specific radioimmunoassays for anti-neutrophil cytoplasmic antibodies in the diagnosis of rapidly progressive glomerulonephritis. J Am Soc Nephrol 2:27, 1991.

609. Jennette JC, Falk RJ: Antineutrophil cytoplasmic autoantibodies and associated diseases: A review. Am J Kidney Dis 15:517, 1990.

610. Davenport A: "False positive" perinuclear and cytoplasmic antineutrophil cytoplasmic antibody results leading to misdiagnosis of Wegener's granulomatosis and/or microscopic polyarteritis. Clin Nephrol 37:124–130, 1992.

611. Almroth G, Eneström S, Hed J, et al: Autoantibodies to leucocyte antigens in hydralazine-associated nephritis. J Intern Med 231:37, 1992.

612. Lockwood CM: Antineutrophil cytoplasmic autoantibodies: The nephrologist's perspective. Am J Kidney Dis 18:171, 1991.

613. Edgar JDM, Rooney DP, McNamee P, McNeill TA: An association between ANCA positive renal disease and malignancy. Clin Nephrol 40:22, 1993.

614. Esnault VLM, Jayne DRW, Keogan MT, et al: Antineutrophil cytoplasm antibodies in patients with monoclonal gammopathies. J Clin Lab Immunol 32:153, 1990.

615. Klaasen RJL, Goldschmeding R, Dolman K, et al: Anti-neutrophil cytoplasmic autoantibodies in patients with symptomatic HIV infection. Clin Exp Immunol 87:24, 1992.

616. Efthimiou J, Spickett G, Lane D, et al: Antineutrophil cytoplasmic antibodies, cystic fibrosis and infection. Lancet 337:1037, 1991.

617. Jayne DRW, Marshall PD, Jones SJ, Lockwood CM: Autoantibodies to GBM and neutrophil cytoplasm in rapidly progressive glomerulonephritis. Kidney Int 37:965, 1990.

618. Weber MFA, Andrassy K, Pullig O, et al: Antineutrophil-cytoplasmic antibodies and antiglomerular basement membrane antibodies in Goodpasture's syndrome and in Wegener's granulomatosis. J Am Soc Nephrol 2:1227, 1992.

619. Weidemann S, Andrassy K, Ritz E: ANCA in haemodialysis patients. Nephrol Dial Transplant 8:839–845, 1993.

620. Falk RJ, Hogan S, Carey TS, et al: Clinical course of anti-neutrophil cytoplasmic autoantibody–associated glomerulonephritis and systemic vasculitis. Ann Intern Med 113:656, 1990.

621. Arimura Y, Minoshima S, Kamiya Y, et al: Serum myeloperoxidase and serum cytokines in anti-myeloperoxidase antibody–associated glomerulonephritis. Clin Nephrol 40:256–264, 1993.

622. Noronha IL, Kruger C, Andrassy K, et al: In situ production of TNF-α, IL-1b, IL-2R in ANCA-positive glomerulonephritis. Kidney Int 43:682, 1993.

623. Csernok E, Schmitt WH, Martin E, et al: Membrane surface proteinase 3 expression and intracytoplasmic immunoglobulin on neutrophils from patients with ANCA-associated vasculitides. In Gross WL (ed): ANCA Associated Vasculitides: Immunodiagnostic and Pathogenetic Value of Anti-Neutrophil Cytoplasmic Antibodies. Plenum Publishing, London, 1994.

624. Evert BH, Jennette JC, Falk RJ: The pathogenic role of antineutrophil cytoplasmic autoantibodies. Am J Kidney Dis 18:188–195, 1991.

625. Csernok E, Ernst M, Schmitt WH, et al: Translocation of PR-3 on the cell surface of neutrophils: Association with disease activity in Wegener's granulomatosis. Arthritis Rheum 34:79, 1991.

626. Falk RJ, Terrell RS, Charles LA, Jennette JC: Anti-neutrophil cytoplasmic autoantibodies induce neutrophils to degranulate and produce oxygen radicals in vitro. Proc Natl Acad Sci USA 87:4115, 1990.

627. Ewert B, Falk RJ, Jennette JC: Anti-neutrophil cytoplasmic antibodies stimulate neutrophils to injure endothelial monolayers in vitro. Am J Kidney Dis 18:203, 1991.

628. Brouwer E, Huitema MG, Mulder AH, et al: Neutrophil activation in vitro and in vivo in Wegener's granulomatosis. Kidney Int 45:1120, 1994.

629. Mayet WJ, Hermann EW, Csernok E, et al: In vitro interactions of c-ANCA (antibodies to proteinase 3) with human endothelial cells. Adv Exp Med Biol 336:109–113, 1993.

630. Mayet WJ, Meyer zum Buschenfelde KH: Antibodies to proteinase 3 increase adhesion of neutrophils to human endothelial cells. Clin Exp Immunol 94:440, 1993.

631. Braun MG, Csernok E, Gross WL, et al: Proteinase 3, the target antigen of anticytoplasmic antibodies circulating in Wegener's granulomatosis. Am J Pathol 139:831, 1991.

632. Savage COS, Pottinger BE, Gaskin G, et al: Vascular damage in Wegener's granulomatosis and microscopic polyarteritis: Presence of anti–endothelial cell antibodies and their relation to anti–neutrophil cytoplasm antibodies. Clin Exp Immunol 85:14, 1991.

633. Wang M-X, Walker RG, Kincaid-Smith P: Clinicopathologic associations of anti–endothelial cell antibodies in immunoglobulin A nephropathy and lupus nephritis. Am J Kidney Dis 22:378–386, 1993.

634. Chan TM, Frampton G, Jayne DRW, et al: Clinical significance of anti–endothelial cell antibodies in systemic vasculitis: A longitudinal study comparing anti–endothelial cell antibodies and anti–neutrophil cytoplasm antibodies. Am J Kidney Dis 22:387–392, 1993.

635. Varagunam M, Nwosu Z, Adu D, et al: Little evidence for anti–endothelial cell antibodies in microscopic polyarteritis and Wegener's granulomatosis. Nephrol Dial Transplant 8:113, 1992.

635a. Angangco R, Thiru S, Oliveira DBG: Pauci-immune glomerulonephritis associated with bacterial infection. Nephrol Dial Transplant 8:754–756, 1993.

636. Funkel T, Torok T, Ferguson P, et al: Chronic parvovirus B-19 infection and systemic necrotizing vasculitis: Opportunistic infection or aetiological agent. Lancet 343:1255–1258, 1994.

637. Esnault VLM, Testa A, Audrain M, et al: Alpha 1-antitrypsin genetic polymorphism in ANCA-positive systemic vasculitis. Kidney Int 43:1329–1332, 1993.

637a. Spencer SJW, Burns A, Gaskin G, et al: HLA class III specificities in vasculitis with antibodies to neutrophil cytoplasmic antigens. Kidney Int 41:1059–1063, 1992.

638. Hoffman GS, Kerr GS, Leavitt RY, et al: Wegener's granulomatosis: An analysis of 158 patients. Ann Intern Med 116:488–498, 1992.

639. Wegener F: Über eine eigenartige rhinogene Granulomatose mit besonderer Beteiligung des Arteriensystems und der Nieren. Beitr Pathol Anat 102:36, 1939.

640. Fahey JL, Leonard E, Churg J, Godman G: Wegener's granulomatosis. Am J Med 17:168, 1954.
641. Godman GG, Churg J: Wegener's granulomatosis: Pathology and review of the literature. Arch Pathol 58:533, 1954.
642. Grotz W, Wanner C, Keller E, et al: Crescentic glomerulonephritis in Wegener's granulomatosis: Morphology, therapy, outcome. Clin Nephrol 35:243–251, 1991.
643. Haubitz M, Frei U, Rother U, et al: Cyclophosphamide pulse therapy in Wegener's granulomatosis. Nephrol Dial Transplant 6:531–535, 1991.
644. Gross WL, Rasmussen N: Treatment of Wegener's granulomatosis: The view from two non-nephrologists. Nephrol Dial Transplant 9:1219–1225, 1994.
645. Papo T, Boisnic S, Piette JC, et al: Disseminated histoplasmosis with glomerulonephritis mimicking Wegener's granulomatosis. Am J Kidney Dis 21:542–544, 1993.
646. Fauci AS, Haynes BF, Kat P, Wolff SM: Wegener's granulomatosis: Prospective clinical and therapeutic experience with 85 patients for 21 years. Ann Intern Med 98:76, 1983.
647. Elkon KB, Sutherland DC, Rees AJ, et al: HLA antigen frequencies in systemic vasculitis: Increase in HLA-DR2 in Wegener's granulomatosis. Arthritis Rheum 26:102, 1983.
648. Cohen Tervaert JW, van der Woude FJ, Fauci AS, et al: Association between active Wegener's granulomatosis and anticytoplasmic antibodies. Arch Intern Med 149:2461, 1989.
649. Specks U, Wheatley CL, McDonald TJ, et al: Anticytoplasmic autoantibodies in the diagnosis and follow-up of Wegener's granulomatosis. Mayo Clin Proc 64:28, 1989.
650. Geffriaud-Ricouard C, Noel LH, Chauveau D, et al: Clinical spectrum associated with ANCA of defined antigen specificities in 98 selected patients. Clin Nephrol 39:125, 1993.
651. Keri GS, Fleisher TA, Hallahan CW, et al: Limited prognostic value of changes in antineutrophil cytoplasmic antibody titer in patients with Wegener's granulomatosis. Arthritis Rheum 36:365, 1993.
652. Pettersson E, Heigl Z: Antineutrophil cytoplasmic antibody titers in relation to disease activity in patients with necrotizing vasculitis: A longitudinal study. Clin Nephrol 37:219, 1992.
653. Cohen Tervaert JW, Huitema MG, Hene RJ, et al: Prevention of relapses in Wegener's granulomatosis by treatment based on antineutrophil cytoplasmic antibody titre. Lancet 336:1990, 1990.
654. Hoffman GS, Leavitt RY, Fleisher TA, et al: Treatment of Wegener's granulomatosis with intermittent high-dose intravenous cyclophosphamide. Am J Med 89:403–410, 1990.
655. Cupps TR: Cyclophosphamide: To pulse or not to pulse? Am J Med 89:399–402, 1990.
656. Jayne DRW, Davies MJ, Fox CJV, et al: Treatment of systemic vasculitis with pooled intravenous immunoglobulin. Lancet 337:1137–1139, 1991.
657. Tuso P, Moudgil A, Hay J, et al: Treatment of antineutrophil cytoplasmic autoantibody positive systemic vasculitis and glomerulonephritis with pooled intravenous gammaglobulin. Am J Kidney Dis 20:504, 1992.
658. Rossi F, Jayne DRW, Lockwood CM, Kazatchkine MD: Anti-idiotypes against anti-neutrophil cytoplasmic antigen autoantibodies in normal human polyspecific IgG for therapeutic use and in the remission sera of patients with systemic vasculitis. Clin Exp Immunol 83:298–303, 1991.
659. Lockwood CM, Thiru S, Isaacs JO, et al: Long-term remission of intractable systemic vasculitis with monoclonal antibody therapy. Lancet 341:1620–1622, 1993.
660. Baker SB, Robinson DR: Unusual renal manifestations of Wegener's granulomatosis: Report of two cases. Am J Med 64:883, 1978.
661. Bonroncle BA, Smith EJ, Cuppage FE: Treatment of Wegener's granulomatosis with Imuran. Am J Med 42:314, 1967.
662. Rondeau E, Levy M, Dosquet P, et al: Plasma exchange and immunosuppression for rapidly progressive glomerulonephritis: Prognosis and complications. Nephrol Dial Transplant 4:196–200, 1989.
663. Cole E, Cattran D, Magil A, et al: A prospective randomized trial of plasma exchange as additive therapy in idiopathic crescentic glomerulonephritis. Am J Kidney Dis 20:261–269, 1992.
664. Glassock RJ: Intensive plasma exchange in crescentic glomerulonephritis: Help or no help? Am J Kidney Dis 20:270–275, 1992.
665. Raitt JW: Wegener's granulomatosis: Treatment with cytotoxic agents and adrenocorticoids. Ann Intern Med 74:344, 1967.
666. Aldo MA, Benson MD, Comerford AS: Treatment of Wegener's granulomatosis with immunosuppressive agents: Description of renal ultrastructure. Arch Intern Med 127:298, 1970.
667. Moorthy AV, Chesney RW, Segar WE, Groshong T: Wegener's granulomatosis in childhood: Prolonged survival following cytotoxic therapy. J Pediatr 91:616, 1977.
668. van der Woude FJ, Hoorntje SJ, Weening JJ, et al: Renal involvement in Wegener's granulomatosis: Report of three unusual cases. Nephron 32:185, 1982.
669. Minta JO, Winkler CJ, Bissar WD, Greenberg M: A selective and complete absence of C1q in a patient with vasculitis and nephritis. Clin Immunol Immunopathol 22:225, 1982.
670. Dabbagh S, Chevalier RL, Sturgill BC: Prolonged anuria and aortic insufficiency in a child with Wegener's granulomatosis. Clin Nephrol 17:155, 1982.
671. Hannedouche T, Godin M, Courtois H, et al: Necrotizing glomerulonephritis and renal cholesterol embolization. Nephron 42:271, 1986.
672. Berry S, Greene J III, Park HS, et al: Return of renal function after renal insufficiency with cyclophosphamide therapy in Wegener's granulomatosis. Arch Intern Med 141:544, 1981. Letter.
673. Kuross S, Davin T, Kjellstrand CM: Wegener's granulomatosis with severe renal failure: Clinical course and results of dialysis and treatment. Clin Nephrol 16:172, 1981.
674. Cuevas J, Pelegre A, Morlans M, et al: Wegener's granulomatosis and hemodialysis. Clin Nephrol 18:109, 1982.
675. Thasia G, Woodworth J, Abullo J, et al: Severe glomerulonephritis with late emergence of classic Wegener's granulomatosis. Medicine (Baltimore) 66:181, 1987.
676. Wheeler GE: Cytoxan-associated leukemia in Wegener's granulomatosis. Ann Intern Med 94:361, 1981.
677. Westberg NS, Swolin B: Acute myelogenous leukemia appearing in two patients after prolonged continuous chlorambucil therapy for Wegener's granulomatosis. Acta Med Scand 199:373, 1976.
678. Chang J, Geary CB: Therapy-linked leukemia. Lancet 1:97, 1977. Letter.
679. Sant GR, Ucci AA, Meares EM: Renal immunoblastic sarcoma complicating immunosuppressive therapy for Wegener's granulomatosis. Urology 21:632, 1983.
679a. Leaker B, Neild GH: Effect of enalapril on proteinuria and renal function in patients with healed severe crescentic glomerlonephritis. Nephrol Dial Transplant 6:936–938, 1991.
680. West BC, Todd JR, King JW: Wegener's granulomatosis and trimethoprim-sulfamethoxazole. Ann Intern Med 106:840, 1987.
681. Truong L, Kopelman RG, Williams GS, Pirani CL: Temporal arteritis and renal disease. Am J Med 78:171, 1985.
682. Salcedo JR, Greenberg L, Kapur S: Renal histology of mucocutaneous lymph node syndrome (Kawasaki disease). Clin Nephrol 29:47, 1988.
683. Alcalay M, Reboux J-F, Touchard G, et al: Vasculasite leucocytoclasique hypocomplémentemique (syndrome de MacDuffie). Nouv Presse Med 7:3125, 1978.
684. Gamble CN, Weisner KB, Shapiro RF, Boyer WJ: The immune complex pathogenesis of glomerulonephritis and pulmonary vasculitis in Behçet's disease. Am J Med 66:103, 1979.
684a. Yang CW, Park IS, Kim SY, et al: Antineutrophil cytoplasmic autoantibody associated vasculitis and renal failure in Behçet disease. Nephrol Dial Transplant 8:871–873, 1993.
685. Ludivico CL, Myers AR, Maurer K: Hypocomplementemic urticarial vasculitis with glomerulonephritis and pseudotumor cerebri. Arthritis Rheum 22:1024, 1979.
686. Lai KN, Chan KW, Ho CP: Glomerulonephritis associated with Takayasu's arteritis: Report of three cases and review of the literature. Am J Kidney Dis 7:197, 1986.
687. Weisenburger D, Armitage J, Dick F: Immunoblastic lymphadenopathy and pulmonary infiltrates, hypocomplementemia and vasculitis. Am J Med 63:849, 1977.
688. Sinclair RJG, Bruickshank B: A clinical and pathological study of sixteen causes of rheumatoid arthritis with extensive visceral involvement (rheumatoid disease). Q J Med 25:313, 1956.
688a. Korpela M, Mustonen J, Helin H, Pasternak A: Immunological comparison of patients with rheumatoid arthritis with and without nephropathy. Ann Rheum Dis 49:214, 1990.
689. Weyland C, Hicok K, Conn D, Gorongy T: The influence of HLA-DRB1 genes on disease severity in rheumatoid arthritis. Ann Intern Med 117:801–806, 1992.

690. Citron BP, Halpern M, McCarron M, et al: Necrotizing angiitis associated with drug abuse. N Engl J Med 283:1003, 1970.

691. Darmady EM, Griffiths WJ, Spencer H, et al: Renal tubular failure associated with polyarteritis nodosa. Lancet 1:378, 1955.

692. Hind CR, Savage COS, Winerals CG, Pepip M: Objective monitoring of disease activity in polyarteritis by measurement of C-reactive protein concentration. Clin Nephrol 21:341, 1984.

693. Droz D, Noel LH, Leibowitch M, Barbanel C: Glomerulonephritis and necrotizing angiitis. Adv Nephrol 8:343–363, 1979.

694. Dornfeld I, Lecky JW, Peter JB: Polyarteritis and intrarenal renal artery aneurysms. JAMA 215:1950, 1971.

695. Falk RJ: ANCA-associated renal disease. Kidney Int 38:998, 1990.

696. Brentjens JR, Andres GE: Immunopathogenesis of vasculitis. Semin Nephrol 5:3, 1985.

697. Harrison CV, Loughridge LW, Milne MD: Acute oliguric renal failure in acute glomerulonephritis and polyarteritis nodosa. Q J Med 33:39, 1964.

698. Kaufer A, Sraer J-D, Feintuch J-J, et al: Acute renal insufficiency in association with periarteritis nodosa. Nouv Presse Med 5:1883, 1976.

699. Fortin PR, Fraser RS, Watts CS, Esdaile JM: Alpha-1 antitrypsin deficiency and systemic necrotizing vasculitis. J Rheumatol 18:1613, 1991.

700. Foley JF, Linder J, Koh J, et al: Cutaneous necrotizing granulomatous vasculitis with evolution to T cell lymphoma. Am J Med 82:839, 1987.

701. Report to the Medical Research Council by the Collagen Diseases and Hypersensitivity Panel: Treatment of polyarteritis nodosa with cortisone: Results after three years. Br Med J 1:1399, 1960.

702. Frohnert PP, Sheps SG: Long-term follow-up study of periarteritis nodosa. Am J Med 43:8, 1967.

703. Bolton WK: The role of high dose steroids in nephrotic syndromes: The case for an aggressive approach. In Narins RG (ed): Controversies in Nephrology and Hypertension. Churchill Livingstone, New York, 1984, p 421.

704. Leib ES, Restivo C, Paulus HE: Immunosuppressive and corticosteroid therapy of polyarteritis nodosa. Am J Med 67:941, 1979.

705. Kunis CL, Kiss B, Williams G, et al: Intravenous "pulse" cyclophosphamide therapy of crescentic glomerulonephritis. Clin Nephrol 37:1–7, 1992.

706. Pall AA, Luqmani RA, Adu D, et al: Controlled trial of pulse cyclophosphamide (PCY) and prednisolone (PP) versus continuous cyclophosphamide (CCY) and prednisolone (CP) in the treatment of systemic vasculitis. Nephrol Dial Transplant 9:204, 1994.

707. Guillevin L, Fain O, Lhote F, et al: Lack of superiority of steroids plus plasma exchange to steroids alone in the treatment of polyarteritis nodosa and Churg-Strauss syndrome. A prospective, randomized trial in 78 patients. Arthritis Rheum 35:208, 1992.

708. Lhote F, Guillevin L, Leon A, et al: Complications of plasma exchange in the treatment of polyarteritis nodosa and Churg-Strauss angiitis and the contribution of adjuvant immunosuppressive therapy: A randomized trial in 72 patients. Artif Organs 12:27, 1988.

709. Montalbert C, Carvallo A, Broumand B, et al: Successful renal transplantation in polyarteritis nodosa. Clin Nephrol 14:206, 1980.

710. D'Apice AJF: Plasmapheresis for the management of renal disease. In Massry S, Glassock R (eds): Textbook of Nephrology, 2nd ed. Williams & Wilkins, Baltimore, 1989, p 1571.

711. Shumak KH, Rock GA: Therapeutic plasma exchange. N Engl J Med 310:762, 1984.

712. Pusey CD, Lockwood CM: Physiological response to removal of macromolecules by apheresis. In Tindall RSA (ed). Therapeutic Apheresis and Plasma Perfusion. Alan R Liss, New York, 1982, p 91.

713. Stevens ME, McConnell M, Bone JM: Aggressive treatment with pulse methylprednisolone or plasma exchange is justified in rapidly progressive glomerulonephritis. Proc Eur Dial Transplant Assoc 19:724, 1982.

714. Balow JE, Austin HA III, Tsokos GC: Plasmapheresis therapy in immunologically mediated rheumatic and renal disease. Clin Immunol Rev 3:235, 1984.

715. Lockwood C, Peters DK: Plasma exchange in glomerulonephritis. Annu Rev Med 31:167, 1980.

716. Heaf G, Jorgensen F, Melsen LP: Treatment and prognosis of extracapillary glomerulonephritis. Nephron 35:217, 1986.

717. Glockner WM, Sieberta HG, Wichmann HE, et al: Plasma ex-

change and immunosuppression in rapidly progressive nephritis. Clin Nephrol 29:1, 1988.

718. Coward RA, Hamdy NAT, Shortland JS, Brown CB: Renal micropolyarteritis: A treatable condition. Nephrol Dial Transplant 1:31, 1986.

719. Houwert DA, Kater L, Hene RJ, Struyvenberg A: Plasma exchange in immune complex diseases. Proc Eur Dial Transplant Assoc 6:520, 1979.

720. Hind CRK, Pareskevakou H, Lockwood CM, et al: Prognosis after immunosuppression of patients with crescentic nephritis requiring dialysis. Lancet 1:263, 1983.

721. Fauci AS, Haynes BF, Costa J, et al: Lymphomatoid granulomatosis: Prospective clinical and therapeutic experience over 10 years. N Engl J Med 306:68, 1982.

722. Churg J, Strauss L: Allergic granulomatosis, allergic angiitis and periarteritis nodosa. Am J Pathol 27:277, 1951.

723. Chumbley LC, Harrison EC Jr, DeRemee RA: Allergic granulomatosis and angiitis (Churg-Strauss syndrome): Report and analysis of 30 cases. Mayo Clin Proc 52:477, 1977.

724. Clutterbuck EJ, Evans DJ, Pusey CD: Renal involvement in Churg-Strauss syndrome. Nephrol Dial Transplant 5:161–167, 1990.

725. Sharp GC, Irvin WG, Tan EM, et al: Mixed connective tissue disease: An apparently distinct rheumatic disease syndrome associated with a specific antibody to an extractable nuclear antigen (ENA). Am J Med 52:148, 1972.

726. Sharp GC: Subsets of SLE and mixed connective tissue disease. Am J Kidney Dis 2(suppl 1):201, 1982.

727. Fuller TJ, Richman AV, Auerbach D, et al: Immune-complex glomerulonephritis in a patient with mixed connective tissue disease. Am J Med 62:761, 1977.

728. Bennett RM, Spargo BH: Immune complex nephropathy in mixed connective tissue disease. Am J Med 63:5344, 1977.

729. Cohen IM, Swerdlin AHR, Steenberg SM, Stone RA: Mesangial proliferative glomerulonephritis in mixed connective tissue disease. Clin Nephrol 13:93, 1980.

730. Missen GAK, Taylor JD: Amyloidosis in rheumatoid arthritis. J Pathol Bacteriol 71:179, 1956.

731. Bourke BE, Woodrow DF, Scott JT: Proteinuria in rheumatoid arthritis: Drug induced or amyloid? Ann Rheum Dis 40:240, 1981.

732. Falck HM, Tornroth T, Skrifvars B, Wegelius O: Resolution of renal amyloidosis secondary to rheumatoid arthritis. Acta Med Scand 205:651, 1979.

733. Wooley PH, Griffin J, Panayi GS, et al: HLA-DR antigens and toxic reactions to sodium aurothiomalate and D-penicillamine in patients with rheumatoid arthritis. N Engl J Med 303:300, 1980.

734. Stastny P: Association of the B-cell alloantigen DRw4 with rheumatoid arthritis. N Engl J Med 298:869, 1978.

735. Samuels B, Lee JC, Engleman EP, Hopper J Jr: Membranous nephropathy in patients with rheumatoid arthritis: Relationship to gold therapy. Medicine (Baltimore) 57:319, 1978.

736. Honkanen E, Tornroth T, Pettersson E, Skrifvars B: Membranous glomerulonephritis in rheumatoid arthritis not related to gold or D-penicillamine therapy: A report of four cases and review of the literature. Clin Nephrol 27:87, 1987.

737. Short CD, Soloman LR, Mallick NP, Mackay JD: Rheumatoid disease presenting as a nephrotic syndrome. Ann Rheum Dis 47:256, 1988.

738. Higuchi A, Suzuki Y, Okada T: Membranous glomerulonephritis in rheumatoid arthritis unassociated with gold or penicillamine treatment. Ann Rheum Dis 46:488, 1987.

739. Figueroa JE, Waxman J: Membranous nephropathy in rheumatoid arthritis. South Med J 75:480, 1982.

740. Davis JA, Cohen AH, Weisbart R, Paulus HE: Glomerulonephritis in rheumatoid arthritis. Arthritis Rheum 22:1018, 1979.

741. Banfi G, Imbasciati E, Guerra L, et al: Extracapillary glomerulonephritis with necrotizing vasculitis in D-penicillamine–treated rheumatoid arthritis. Nephron 33:56, 1983.

742. Farhangi M, Luger AM, Morris AD: Pathogenic role of a monoclonal IgA (kappa) anti-IgG-paraprotein associated with hemorrhagic diathesis, rheumatoid arthritis, vascular purpura, and acute membranoproliferative glomerulonephritis. J Clin Immunol 2:75, 1982.

743. Kuznetsky KA, Schwartz MM, Lohmann LA, Lewis EJ: Necrotizing glomerulonephritis in rheumatoid arthritis. Clin Nephrol 26:257, 1986.

744. Akikusa B, Irabu N, Kamei K, et al: Glomerulonephritis in patients

with rheumatoid arthritis (RA): Report of five cases and review of the literature. Acta Pathol Jpn 36:235, 1986.

745. Boers M, Croonen AM, Dijkmans BAC, et al: Renal findings in rheumatoid arthritis: Clinical aspects of 132 necropsies. Ann Rheum Dis 46:658, 1987.

746. Helin H, Korpela M, Mustonen J, Pasternak A: Mild mesangial glomerulopathy: A frequent finding in rheumatoid arthritis patients with hematuria or proteinuria. Nephron 42:224, 1986.

747. Levy M, Prieur A-M, Gubler M-C, et al: Renal involvement in juvenile chronic arthritis: Clinical and pathologic features. Am J Kidney Dis 9:138, 1987.

748. Mahallaway MN, Sabour MS: Renal lesions in rheumatoid arthritis. Lancet 2:852, 1959.

749. Linder E, Pasternak A: Immunofluorescence studies on kidney biopsies in ankylosing spondylitis. Acta Pathol Microbiol Scand [B] 78:517–525, 1970.

750. Shu K-H, Lian J-D, Yang Y-F, et al: Glomerulonephritis in ankylosing spondylitis. Clin Nephrol 25:169, 1986.

751. Jennette JC, Ferguson AL, Moore MA, Freeman DG: IgA nephropathy associated with seronegative spondyloarthropathies. Arthritis Rheum 25:144, 1982.

752. Burry AF, McGiven AR, Kirk JA, et al: A renal lesion in ankylosing spondylitis. Nephron 26:171, 1980.

753. Sissons JGP, Woodrow DF, Curtis JR, et al: Isolated glomerulonephritis with mesangial IgA deposits. Br Med J 3:611, 1975.

754. Botey A, Torres A, Revert L: Membranous nephropathy in ankylosing spondylitis. Nephron 29:203, 1981.

755. Malavuja AN, Rain V, Mittal V, et al: Glomerulonephritis in seronegative spondylarthritis syndrome. Arthritis Rheum 24:751, 1981.

756. Olsson PJ, Gafney E, Alexander RW, et al: Proliferative glomerulonephritis with crescent formation in Behçet's syndrome. Arch Intern Med 140:713, 1980.

757. Akutsu Y, Itami N, Tanaka M, et al: IgA nephritis in Behçet's disease: Case report and review of the literature. Clin Nephrol 34:52, 1990.

758. Furukawa T, Hisau O, Furuta S, Shigematsu H: Henoch-Schönlein purpura with nephritis in a patient with Behçet's disease. Am J Kidney Dis 13:497, 1989.

759. Wilkey D, Yocum DE, Oberley TD, et al: Budd-Chiari syndrome and renal failure in Behçet disease: Report of a case and review of the literature. Am J Med 75:541, 1983.

760. Yokayama Y, Kuno T, Aoki M: Focal proliferative glomerulonephritis with Behçet's syndrome. Ryu Machi 13:281, 1978.

761. Gamble CN, Weigner IB, Shapiro RF, Boyer WJ: The immune complex pathogenesis of glomerulonephritis and pulmonary vasculitis in Behçet's disease. Am J Med 66:1031, 1979.

762. Landwehr DM, Cooke CL, Rodriguez GE: Rapidly progressive glomerulonephritis in Behçet's syndrome. JAMA 244:1709, 1980.

763. Donnelly S, Jothy S, Barre P: Crescentic glomerulonephritis in Behçet's syndrome—results of therapy and review of the literature. Clin Nephrol 31:213, 1989.

764. Rosenthal T, Bauk H, Aladjem M, et al: Systemic amyloidosis in Behçet's disease. Ann Intern Med 83:220, 1975.

765. Grishman E, Cohen S, Salomon ME, Churg J: Renal lesions in acute rheumatic fever. Am J Pathol 51:1045, 1967.

766. Escudero J, Stanislawsky E, Escudero X: Fulminant acute rheumatic fever with multisystem involvement. Am Heart J 105:161, 1983.

767. Matsell DG, Baldree LA, DiSessa TG, et al: Acute poststreptococcal glomerulonephritis and acute rheumatic fever: Occurrence in the same patient. Child Nephrol Urol 10:112–114, 1990.

768. Gibney R, Reineck HJ, Bannayan GA, Stein JH: Renal lesions in acute rheumatic fever. Ann Intern Med 94:322, 1981.

769. Van de Rijn I, Fillet H, Brandeis W, et al: Serial studies on circulating immune complexes in post-streptococcal sequelae. Clin Exp Immunol 34:318, 1978.

770. Chang-Miller A, Okamura M, Torres VE, et al: Renal involvement in relapsing polychondritis. Medicine (Baltimore) 66:202, 1987.

771. Isaak BL, Liesegang TJ, Michet CJ Jr, et al: Ocular and systemic findings in relapsing polychondritis. Ophthalmology 93:681, 1986.

772. Yang CL, Brinckmann J, Rui HF, et al: Autoantibodies to cartilage collagens in relapsing polychondritis. Arch Dermatol 285:245, 1993.

773. Anstey A, Mayou S, Morgan K, et al: Relapsing polychondritis: Autoimmunity to type II collagen and treatment with cyclosporin A. Br J Dermatol 125:588, 1991.

774. Khan MA, Akhtar M, Taher SM: Membranoproliferative glomerulonephritis in a patient with primary Sjögren's syndrome. Report of a case with review of the literature. Am J Nephrol 8:235, 1988.

775. Schlesinger I, Carlson TS, Nelson D: Type III membranoproliferative glomerulonephritis in primary Sjögren's syndrome. Community Med 53:629, 1989.

776. Van Eer MY, Netten PM, Schrijver G, et al: Sjögren's syndrome complicated by cryoglobulinaemia and acute renal failure. Neth J Med 39:23, 1991.

777. Martl HP, Laissue J, Mihatsch M, et al: Renal manifestations of sarcoidosis. Schweiz Med Wochenschr 118:413, 1988.

778. Salomon MI, Poon TP, Hsu KC, et al: Membranous glomerulopathy in a patient with sarcoidosis. Arch Pathol 100:479, 1975.

779. Goldszer RC, Galvarek EG, Lazarus M: Glomerulonephritis in a patient with sarcoidosis: Report of a case and review of the literature. Arch Pathol Lab Med 105:478, 1981.

780. Krumlovsky FA, Delgreco F, Herdson PB, Lazar P: Renal disease associated with toxic epidermal necrolysis (Lyell's disease). Am J Med 57:817, 1974.

781. McIntosh RM, Griswold WR, Chernack WB, et al: Cryoglobulins: III. Further studies on the nature, incidence, clinical, diagnostic, prognostic and immunopathologic significance of cryoproteins in renal disease. Q J Med 44:285, 1975.

782. Adam C, Morel-Maroger L, Richet G: Cryoglobulins in glomerulonephritis not related to systemic disease. Kidney Int 3:334, 1973.

783. McIntosh RW, Kulvinskas C, Kaufman DB: Cryoglobulins: II. The biological and chemical properties of cryoproteins in acute poststreptococcal glomerulonephritis. Int Arch Allergy Appl Immunol 41:700, 1971.

784. Tarantino A, de Vecchi A, Montaguino G, et al: Renal disease in essential mixed cryoglobulinemia: long-term follow-up of 44 patients. Q J Med 50:1, 1981.

785. Vilches AR, Williams DG: Persistent anti-DNA antibodies and DNA anti-DNA complexes in post-streptococcal glomerulonephritis. Clin Nephrol 22:97, 1984.

786. Houewert DA, Hene RJ, Struyvenberg A, Kater L: Effect of plasmapheresis, corticosteroids and cyclophosphamide in essential mixed cryoglobulinemia associated with glomerulonephritis. Proc Eur Dial Transpl 17:650, 1980.

787. Grey H, Kohler PF: Cryoimmunoglobulins. Semin Hematol 10:87, 1973.

788. Adam C, Morel-Maroger L, Richet G: Cryoglobulins in glomerulonephritis not related to systemic disease. Kidney Int 3:334, 1973.

789. Morel-Maroger L, Verroust P: Glomerular lesions in dysproteinemias. Kidney Int 5:249, 1974.

790. Brouet JC, Clauvel JP, Danon F, et al: Biologic and clinical significance of cryoglobulins: A report of 86 cases. Am J Med 57:775, 1974.

791. Zago-Novaretti M, Khuri F, Miller KB, et al: Waldenstrom's macroglobulinemia with an IgM paraprotein that is both a cold agglutinin and a cryoglobulin and has a suppressive effect on progenitor cell growth. Transfusion 34:910, 1994.

792. Zimmerman SW, Dreher WH, Burkholder PM, et al: Nephropathy and mixed cryoglobulinemia: Evidence for an immune complex pathogenesis. Nephron 16:103, 1976.

793. Ponticelli C, Imbasciati E, Tarantino A, Pietrogrande M: Acute anuric glomerulonephritis in monoclonal cryoglobulinaemia. Br Med J 2:948, 1977.

794. Beaufils M, Morel-Maroger L: Pathogenesis of renal disease in monoclonal gammopathies. Nephron 20:125, 1978.

795. McPhaul JJ Jr: Cryoimmunoglobulinemia in patients with primary renal disease and systemic lupus erythematosus. Clin Exp Immunol 31:131, 1978.

796. Gamble CN, Ruggles SW: The immunopathogenesis of glomerulonephritis associated with mixed cryoglobulinemia. N Engl J Med 299:81, 1978.

797. D'Amico G, Colasanti G, Farrario F, et al: Renal involvement in essential mixed cryoglobulinemia: A peculiar type of immune complex mediated disease. Adv Nephrol 17:219, 1988.

798. Frankel AH, Singer DR, Winearls CG, et al: Type II essential mixed cryoglobulinaemia: Presentation, treatment and outcome in 13 patients. Q J Med 82:101–124, 1992.

799. Agnello V, Chung RT, Kaplan LM: A role for hepatitis C virus infection in type II cryoglobulinemia. N Engl J Med 327:1490, 1992.

800. Reininger L, Berney T, Shibata T, et al: Cryoglobulinemia induced by a murine IgG3 rheumatoid factor: Skin vasculitis and glomerulonephritis arise from distinct pathogenic mechanisms. Proc Natl Acad Sci USA 87:10038, 1990.

801. Ponticelli C, Minetti G, D'Amico G (eds): Antiglobulins, Cryoglobulins and Glomerulonephritis. Martinus Nijhoff, Dordrecht, Netherlands, 1986, p 1.

802. Roberts JL, Lewis EJ: Identification of antinative DNA antibodies in cryoglobulinemia states. Am J Med 65:437, 1978.

803. Roberts JL, Lewis EJ: Immunochemical demonstration of cryoprecipitable anti–native DNA antibody and DNA in the serum of patients with glomerulonephritis. J Immunol 124:127, 1980.

804. Cordonnier D, Vialfel P, Renversy J, et al: Renal disease in 18 patients with mixed type II IgM-IgG cryoglobulinemia: Monoclonal lymphoid infiltration (2 cases) and membrano-proliferative glomerulonephritis (14 cases). Adv Nephrol 12:177, 1983.

805. Gilboa N, Durante D, Guggenheim S, et al: Immune deposit nephritis and single-component cryoglobulinemia associated with chronic lymphocytic leukemia. Nephron 24:223, 1979.

806. Chantry D, Winearls CG, Maini RN, Feldmann M: Mechanism of immune complex–mediated damage: Induction of interleukin 1 by immune complexes and synergy with inferior-gamma and tumor necrosis factor-alpha. Eur J Immunol 19:189, 1989.

807. Gabrielli A, Marchegiani G, Rupoli S, et al: Assessment of disease activity in essential cryoglobulinemia by serum levels of a basement membrane antigen, laminin. Arthritis Rheum 31:1558, 1988.

808. Hamburger MI, Gorevic PD, Lawley TJ, et al: Mixed cryoglobulinemia: Association of glomerulonephritis with defective reticuloendothelial system Fc receptor function. Trans Am Assoc Physicians 92:104, 1979.

809. Misiani R, Bellavita P, Fenili D: Hepatitis C virus infection in patients with essential mixed cryoglobulinemia. Ann Intern Med 117:573–577, 1992.

810. Johnson RJ, Gretch DR, Yamabe H, et al: Membranoproliferative glomerulonephritis associated with hepatitis C virus infection. N Engl J Med 328:465–470, 1993.

811. Cacoub P, Fabiani FL, Musset L, et al: Mixed cryoglobulinemia and hepatitis C virus. Am J Med 96:124–132, 1994.

812. D'Amico G: Hepatitis C virus and essential mixed cryoglobulinemia. Nephrol Dial Transplant 8.579–581, 1993.

813. Levey JM, Bjornsson B, Banner B, et al: Mixed cryoglobulinemia in chronic hepatitis C infection: A clinicopathologic analysis of 10 cases and review of recent literature. Medicine (Baltimore) 73:53–67, 1994.

814. Galli M, Monti G, Invernizzi F, et al: Hepatitis B virus–related markers in secondary and in essential mixed cryoglobulinemias: A multicentric study of 596 cases. Ann Ital Med Intern 7:209–214, 1992.

815. Bombardieri S, Paoletti PK, Ferri C, et al: Lung involvement in essential mixed cryoglobulinemia. Am J Med 66:748, 1979.

816. Levo Y: Hepatitis B virus and essential mixed cryoglobulinemia. Ann Intern Med 94:282, 1981.

817. Agnello V: Case records of the Massachusetts General Hospital. N Engl J Med 323:1756, 1990.

818. Seneco R, Winearls C, Sabadini E, et al: Identification of the glomerular immune deposits in cryoglobulinemic glomerulonephritis. Kidney Int 34:109, 1988.

819. Feiner H, Gallo G: Ultrastructure in glomerulonephritis associated with cryoglobulinemia. Am J Pathol 88:145, 1977.

820. Roberts J: Cryoglobulinemia. In Glassock RJ (ed): Current Therapy in Nephrology and Hypertension. BC Decker, Philadelphia, 1984, p 162.

821. De Vecchi A, Montaguino G, Pozzi C, et al: Intravenous methylprednisolone in cryoglobulinemia. Clin Nephrol 19:221, 1983.

822. Morel-Maroger L, Basch A, Danon F, et al: Pathology of the kidney in Waldenström's macroglobulinemia. N Engl J Med 283:123, 1970.

823. Argani I, Kopkie GF: Macroglobulinemia nephropathy. Acute renal failure in macroglobulinemia of Waldenström. Am J Med 36:151, 1964.

824. Beaufils M, Morel-Maroger L: Pathogenesis of renal disease in monoclonal gammopathies: Current concepts. Nephron 20:125, 1978.

824a. Tsuji M, Ochiai S, Taka T, et al: Non-amyloidogenic nephrotic syndrome in Waldenström's macroglobulinemia. Nephron 54:176–178, 1990.

825. Grossman ME, Bia MJM, Goldwein MI, et al: Giant kidneys in Waldenström's macroglobulinemia. Arch Intern Med 137:1613, 1977.

826. Kyle RA: Monoclonal gammopathy of undetermined significance: Natural history in 241 cases. Am J Med 64:814, 1978.

826a. Verroust P, Mery JP, Morel-Maroger L, et al: Glomerular lesions in monoclonal gammopathies and mixed essential cryoglobulinemias. IgG-IgM. Adv Nephrol 1:161, 1971.

827. Avasthi PS, Erickson DG, Williams RC Jr, Tung KSK: Benign monoclonal gammaglobulinemia and glomerulonephritis. Am J Med 62:324, 1977.

828. Zlotnick A, Rosenmann E: Renal pathologic findings associated with monoclonal gammopathies. Arch Intern Med 135:40, 1975.

829. Sobel AT, Antonucci M, Intrator L, et al: Association of a monoclonal gammopathy, a chronic glomerulopathy, and an auto-immune hyperlipidaemia: Course under treatment. Nouv Presse Med 5:2375, 1976.

830. Dhar SK, Smith EC, Fresco R: Proliferative glomerulonephritis in monoclonal gammopathy. Nephron 19:288, 1977.

831. Meyrier A, Simon P, Migan F, et al: Rapidly progressive glomerulonephritis and monoclonal gammopathies. Nephron 38:156, 1984.

832. Kebler R, Kithier K, McDonald FD, Cadnapaphouchai P: Rapidly progressive glomerulonephritis and monoclonal gammopathy. Am J Med 78:133, 1985.

833. Hayes JS, Jankey N, Cuthberg AL, Das PM: Massive proteinuria in light chain disease. Arch Intern Med 138:785, 1978.

834. Hill GS, Morel-Maroger L, Méry JP, et al: Renal lesions in multiple myeloma: Their relationship to associated protein abnormalities. Am J Kidney Dis 2:423, 1983.

835. Silva FG, Meyrier A, Morel-Maroger L, Pirani CL: Proliferative glomerulonephropathy in multiple myeloma. J Pathol 130:229, 1980.

836. Iggo N, Parsons V: Renal disease in multiple myeloma: Current perspectives. Nephron 56:229–233, 1990.

837. Cohen AH, Adler SG: Nephrotoxicity of myeloma proteins. Plasma Ther Transfus Technol 5:531–541, 1984.

838. Solomon AS, Weiss DT, Kattine AA: Nephrotoxic potential of Bence Jones proteins. N Engl J Med 324:1845–1851, 1991.

839. Alexanian R, Barlogie B, Dixon D: Renal failure in multiple myeloma. Pathogenesis and prognostic implications. Arch Intern Med 150:1693–1695, 1990.

840. Johnson WJ, Kyle RA, Pineda AA, et al: Treatment of renal failure associated with multiple myeloma. Arch Intern Med 150:863–869, 1990.

841. Zucchelli P, Pasquali S, Cagnoli L, Ferrari G: Controlled plasma exchange trial in acute renal failure due to multiple myeloma. Kidney Int 33:1175–1180, 1988.

842. Walker F, Bear RA: Renal transplantation in light-chain multiple myeloma. Case report and review of the literature. Am J Nephrol 3:31–37, 1983.

843. Alpers CE: Glomerulopathies of dysproteinurias, abnormal immunoglobulin deposition and lymphoproliferative disorders. Curr Opin Nephrol Hypertens 3:349–355, 1994.

844. Preud'Homme JL, Aucouturier P, Touchard G, et al: Monoclonal immunoglobulin deposition disease (Randall type). Relationship with structural abnormalities of immunoglobulin chains. Kidney Int 46:965–972, 1994.

845. Buxbaum JN, Chuba JV, Hellman GC, et al: Monoclonal immunoglobulin deposition disease: Light chain and light and heavy chain deposition diseases and their relation to light chain amyloidosis. Ann Intern Med 112:455–464, 1990.

846. Tubbs RR, Gephart GN, McMahon J, et al: Light chain nephropathy. Am J Med 71:263, 1981.

847. Cohen AH: Pathology of light chain nephropathies. In Robinson RR (ed): Nephrology. Springer-Verlag, New York, 1984, p 895.

848. Gallo G, Feiner HD, Katz LA, et al: Nodular glomerulopathy associated with nonamyloidotic kappa light chain deposits and excess immunoglobulin light chain synthesis. Am J Pathol 99:621, 1980.

849. Colvin R: Case records of the Massachusetts General Hospital (case 1–1981). N Engl J Med 304:33, 1981.

850. Gipstein RM, Cohen AH, Adams DA, et al: Kappa light chain nephropathy without evidence of myeloma cells. Am J Nephrol 2:276, 1982.

851. Seymour AE, Thompson AJ, Smith PS, et al: Kappa light chain glomerulosclerosis in multiple myeloma. Am J Pathol 101:557, 1980.

852. Morel-Maroger L, Verroust P, Preud'Homme J-L: Glomerular lesions in plasma cell dyscrasias. *In* Rosen S (ed): Pathology of Glomerular Disease. Churchill Livingstone, New York, 1983, p 207.

853. Ganeval D, Mignon F, Preud'Homme JL, et al: Visceral deposition of monoclonal light chains and immunoglobulins: A study of renal and immunopathologic abnormalities. Adv Nephrol 11:25, 1982.

854. Ganeval D, Noel LH, Preud'Homme J-L, et al: Light chain deposition disease: Its relation with AL-type amyloidosis. Kidney Int 26:1, 1984.

855. Sinniah R, Cohen AH: Glomerular capillary aneurysms in light chain nephropathy: An ultrastructural proposal of morphogenesis. Am J Pathol 118:298, 1985.

856. Alpers CE, Tu WH, Hopper J, Biava CG: Single light chain subclass (kappa chain) immunoglobulin deposition in glomerulonephritis. Hum Pathol 16:294, 1985.

856a. Aucouturier P, Khamlichi AA, Touchard G, et al: Brief report: Heavy-chain deposition disease. N Engl J Med 329:1389–1393, 1993.

857. Heilman RL, Velosa JA, Holley KE, et al: Long-term follow-up and response to chemotherapy in patients with light-chain deposition disease. Am J Kidney Dis 20:34–41, 1992.

858. Cohen AS, Cathcart ES, Skinner M: Amyloidosis: Current trends in its investigation. Arthritis Rheum 21:153, 1978.

859. Scheinberg MA, Wohlgeth JR, Cathcart ES: Humoral and cellular aspects of amyloid disease: Present status. Prog Allergy 27:250, 1980.

860. Baltz ML, Caspi D, Evans DJ, et al: Circulating serum amyloid P component is the precursor of amyloid P component in tissue amyloid deposits. Clin Exp Immunol 66:691, 1986.

861. Kisilevsky R: Heparan sulfate proteoglycans in amyloidogenesis: An epiphenomenon, a unique factor, or the tip of a more fundamental process? Lab Invest 63:589, 1990.

862. Westermark P, Stenvist B, Natvig J: Demonstration of protein AA in subcutaneous fat tissue obtained by fine needle biopsy. Ann Rheum Dis 38:68, 1979.

863. Gertz AG, Kyle RA: Secondary systemic amyloidosis. Response and survival in 64 patients. Medicine (Baltimore) 70:246, 1991.

864. Gipstein RM, Cohen AH, Gordon EM: Kappa light chain glomerulopathy: Early diagnosis and treatment. *In* Nose Y, Malchesky PS, Smith JW (eds): Plasmapheresis. ISAO Press, Cleveland, OH, 1983, pp 263–267.

865. Korat O, Yachnis AT, Ernst CS: Cytologic detection of amyloid in duodenal and ureteral brushings. Diagn Cytopathol 4:133, 1988.

866. Gertz AG, Kyle RA: Primary systemic amyloidosis—a diagnostic primer. Mayo Clin Proc 64:1505, 1989.

867. Hamer JP, Janssen S, van Rijswijk MH, Lie KI: Amyloid cardiomyopathy in systemic nonhereditary amyloidosis. Clinical, echocardiographic and electrocardiographic findings in 30 patients with AA and 24 patients with AL amyloidosis. Eur Heart J 13:623, 1992.

868. Lomena F, Rosello R, Pons F, et al: Abnormal scintigraphic evolution in AA hepatic amyloidosis. Clin Nucl Med 13:194, 1988.

869. Hawkins PN, Lavender JP, Pepys MB: Evaluation of systemic amyloidosis by scintigraphy with $^{123}$I-labeled serum amyloid P component. N Engl J Med 323:508, 1990.

870. Floege J, Burchert W, Brandis A, et al: Imaging of dialysis-related amyloid (AM-amyloid) deposits with $^{131}$I-$\beta_2$-microglobulin. Kidney Int 38:1169–1176, 1990.

871. Brandt K, Cathcart ES, Cohen AS: A clinical analysis of the course and prognosis of forty-two patients with amyloidosis. Am J Med 44:955, 1968.

872. Bohle A, Wehrmann M, Eissele R, et al: The long-term prognosis of AA and AL renal amyloidosis and the pathogenesis of chronic renal failure in renal amyloidosis. Pathol Res Pract 189:316, 1993.

873. Gertz MA, Kyle RA: Prognostic value of urinary protein in primary systemic amyloidosis. Am J Clin Pathol 94:313, 1990.

874. Isobe T, Osserman EF: Patterns of amyloidosis and their association with plasma cell dyscrasia, monoclonal immunologlobulins and Bence Jones proteins. N Engl J Med 290:473, 1974.

875. Cohen AS: Amyloidosis. N Engl J Med 277:522, 574, 628, 1967. Review.

876. Danby P, Harri KPG, Williams B, et al: Adrenal dysfunction in patients with renal amyloid. Q J Med 76:915, 1990.

877. Gertz MA, Kyle RA, Greipp PR: Response rates and survival in primary systemic amyloidosis. Blood 77:257, 1991.

878. Goddard IR, Jackson R, Jones JM: AL amyloidosis: Therapeutic response in two patients with renal involvement. Nephrol Dial Transplant 6:592–594, 1991.

879. Cohen AS, Rubinow A, Anderson JJ, et al: Survival of patients with primary (AL) amyloidosis. Colchicine-treated cases from 1976 to 1983 compared with cases in previous years (1961 to 1973). Am J Med 82:1182, 1987.

880. Gertz MA, Kyle RA, O'Fallon WM: Dialysis support of patients with primary systemic amyloidosis. A study of 211 patients. Arch Intern Med 152:2245, 1992.

881. Pasternack A, Ahonen J, Kuhlback B: Renal transplantation in 45 patients with amyloidosis. Transplantation 42:598, 1986.

882. Zemer D, Pras M, Sohar E, et al: Colchicine in the prevention and treatment of the amyloidosis of familial Mediterranean fever. N Engl J Med 314:1011, 1986.

883. Livneh A, Zemer D, Siegal B, et al: Colchicine prevents kidney transplant amyloidosis in familial Mediterranean fever. Nephron 60:418, 1992.

884. Benditt EP, Ericksen N: Amyloid protein SAA is associated with high density lipoprotein from human serum. Proc Natl Acad Sci USA 74:4025–4028, 1977.

885. Ramadori G, Sipe JD, Dinarello CA: Pretranslational modulation of acute phase hepatic protein synthesis by murine recombinant interleukin-1 (IL-1) and purified human IL-1. J Exp Med 162:930, 1985.

886. Barton CH, Vaziri ND, Gordon S, Tilles S: Renal pathology in end-stage renal disease associated with paraplegia. Paraplegia 22:31–41, 1984.

887. Gross E, Frangione B, Gallo G: AA protein-related renal amyloidosis in drug addicts. Am J Pathol 112:195, 1983.

888. Said R, Hamzeh Y, Said S, et al: Spectrum of renal involvement in familial Mediterranean fever. Kidney Int 41:414, 1992.

889. Sohar E, Gafni J, Pras M, Heller H: Familial Mediterranean fever: A survey of 470 cases and review of the literature. Am J Med 43:227, 1967.

890. Gafni J, Sohar E, Zeiner D: Amyloid nephropathy. *In* Hamburger J, Crosnier J, Grünfeld J (eds): Nephrology. John Wiley & Sons, New York, 1979, p 689.

891. Alexander R, Atkins EL: Familial renal amyloidosis: Case reports, literature review and classification. Am J Med 59:121, 1975.

892. Shmueli D, Lustig S, Nakache R, et al: Renal transplantation in patients with amyloidosis due to familial Mediterranean fever. Transplant Proc 24:1783, 1992.

893. Dikman SH, Kahn T, Gribetz D, Churg J: Resolution of renal amyloidosis. Am J Med 63:430, 1977.

894. Tang AL, Davies DR, Wing AJ: Remission of nephrotic syndrome in amyloidosis associated with a hypernephroma. Clin Nephrol 32:225, 1989.

895. Lauzurica R, Felip A, Serra A, et al: Xanthogranulomatous pyelonephritis and systemic amyloidosis: Report of 2 new cases and the natural history of this association. J Urol 146:1603–1606, 1991.

896. Reimann HA: Recovery from amyloidosis. JAMA 104:1070, 1935.

897. Zemer D, Revach M, Pras M, et al: A controlled trial of colchicine in preventing attacks of familial Mediterranean fever. N Engl J Med 291:932, 1974.

898. Nurmi MJ, Ekfors TO, Rajala PO, Puntala PV: Intravesical dimethyl sulfoxide instillations in the treatment of secondary amyloidosis of the bladder. J Urol 143:808, 1990.

899. Okuma Y, Kuroda M, Hashimoto C, et al: Improvement of severe diarrhea by dimethylsulfoxide in a case of AA type secondary amyloidosis. Nippon Naika Gakkai Zasshi 78:698, 1989.

900. Gejyo F, Odani S, Yamada T, et al: Beta-2 microglobulin: A new form of amyloid protein associated with chronic hemodialysis. Kidney Int 30:385, 1986.

901. Ishikawa I, Horiguchi T, Kitoda H, et al: Beta-2 microglobulin–derived amyloid deposition in acquired cystic disease of kidneys with renal cell carcinoma. Nephron 46:101, 1987.

902. Campistal JM, Torres A, Lopez-Cases A, et al: Visceral involvement of dialysis amyloidosis. Am J Nephrol 7:390, 1987.

903. Noel LH, Zingreff J, Bardin T, et al: Tissue distribution of dialysis amyloidosis. Clin Nephrol 27:175, 1987.

904. Fitzmaurice RJ, Bartley C, McClure J, Ackrill P: Immunohistological characterization of amyloid deposits in renal biopsy specimens. J Clin Pathol 44:200, 1991.

905. Zalin AM, Jones S, Fitch NJS, Ramsden DB: Familial nephropathic non-neuropathic amyloidosis: Clinical features, immunohistochemistry and chemistry. Q J Med 81:945, 1991.

906. Maury CPJ: Homozygous familial amyloidosis, Finnish type: Demonstration of glomerular gelsolin-derived amyloid and non-amyloid tubular gelsolin. Clin Nephrol 40:53, 1993.

907. Levy E, Haltia M, Fernandez-Madrid I, et al: Mutation in gelsolin gene in Finnish hereditary amyloidosis. J Exp Med 172:1865, 1990.

908. Kwiatkowski DJ, Mehl R, Yin HL: Genomic organization and biosynthesis of secreted and cytoplasmic forms of gelsolin. J Cell Biol 106:375, 1988.

909. Meretoja J, Jokinen EJ, Collan Y, Lähdevirta J: Renal biopsy findings in familial amyloidosis with corneal lattice dystrophy. Acta Pathol Microbiol Scand [A] 80(suppl 233):228, 1972.

910. Libby CA, Talbert ML: Case records of the Massachusetts General Hospital, case 50–1987. N Engl J Med 317:1520, 1987.

911. Hill GS: Multiple myeloma, amyloidosis, and macroglobulinemia. *In* Heptinstall RH (ed): Pathology of the Kidney. Little, Brown, Boston, 1983, p 1014.

912. Weiss JW, Page DL: Amyloid nephropathy of Ostertag with special reference to renal glomerular giant cells. Am J Pathol 72:447, 1973.

913. Gallo GR, Feiner HD, Chuba JV, et al: Characterization of tissue amyloid by immunofluorescence microscopy. Clin Immunol Immunopathol 39:479, 1988.

914. Picken MM, Gallo G, Buxbaum J, Frangione B: Characterization of renal amyloid derived from the variable region of the lambda light chain subgroup II. Am J Pathol 124:82, 1986.

915. Picken MM, Pelton K, Frangione B, Gallo G: Primary amyloidosis A: Immunohistochemical and biochemical characterization. Am J Pathol 129:536, 1987.

916. Shirahama T, Cohen AS: Fine structure of the glomerulus in human and experimental renal amyloidosis. Am J Pathol 51:869, 1967.

917. Ansell ID, Joekes AM: Spicular arrangement of amyloid in renal biopsy. J Clin Pathol 25:1056, 1972.

918. Yang GCH, Gallo GR: Protein A–gold immunoelectron microscopic study of amyloid fibrils, granular deposits, and fibrillar luminal aggregates in renal amyloidosis. Am J Pathol 137:1223, 1990.

919. Eulitz M: Amyloid formation from immunoglobulin chains. Biol Chem Hoppe Seyler 373:629, 1992.

920. Eulitz M, Linke RP: The precursor molecule of a V lambda II-immunoglobulin light chain–derived amyloid fibril protein circulates precleaved. Biochem Biophys Res Commun 194:1427–1434, 1993.

921. Miyata T, Oda O, Inagi R, et al: $\beta_2$-Microglobulin modified with advanced glycosylation end product is a major component of hemodialysis-associated amyloidosis. J Clin Invest 92:1243, 1993.

922. Miyata T, Inagi R, Iida Y, et al: Involvement of $\beta_2$-microglobulin modified with advanced glycosylation end products in the pathogenesis of hemodialysis-associated amyloidosis. Induction of human monocyte chemotaxis and macrophage secretion of tumor necrosis factor-$\alpha$ and interleukin-1. J Clin Invest 93:521, 1994.

923. Linker A, Carney HD: Presence and role of glycosaminoglycans in amyloidosis. Lab Invest 57:297, 1987.

924. Korbet SM, Schwartz MM, Lewis EJ: Immunotactoid glomerulopathy. Am J Kidney Dis 17:247–257, 1991.

925. Iskandar SS, Falk RJ, Jennette JC: Clinical and pathologic features of fibrillary glomerulonephritis. Kidney Int 42:1401–1407, 1992.

926. Alpers CE: Immunotactoid (microtubular) glomerulopathy: An entity distinct from fibrillary glomerulonephritis? Am J Kidney Dis 19:185–191, 1992.

927. Sadjadi SA, Sobel HJ: Congo red–negative amyloidosis-like glomerulopathy: Report of a case. Am J Kidney Dis 9:231, 1987.

928. Schifferli JA, Merot Y, Cruchaud A, Chatelanat F: Immunotactoid glomerulopathy with leukocytoclastic skin vasculitis and hypocomplementemia: A case report. Clin Nephrol 27:1512, 1987.

929. Korbet SM, Schwartz MM, Rosenberg BF, et al: Immunotactoid glomerulopathy. Medicine (Baltimore) 64:228, 1985.

930. Alpers CE, Rennke HG, Hopper J Jr, Biava CG: Fibrillary glomerulonephritis: An entity with unusual immunofluorescence features. Kidney Int 31:781, 1987.

931. Crow RS: Peripheral neuritis in myelomatosis. Br Med J 2:802, 1956.

932. Nakanishi T, Sobue T, Toyokura Y, et al: The Crow-Fukase syndrome: A study of 102 cases in Japan. Neurology 34:712, 1984.

933. Frizzera G: Castleman's disease and related disorders. Semin Diagn Pathol 5:346, 1988.

934. Miralles GD, O'Fallon JR, Talley NJ: Plasma cell dyscrasia with

polyneuropathy. The spectrum of POEMS syndrome. N Engl J Med 327:1919, 1992.

935. Fukatsu A, Tamai H, Nishikawa K, et al: The kidney disease of Crow-Fukase (POEMS) syndrome: A clinicopathological study of four cases. Clin Nephrol 36:76, 1991.

936. Chazot C, Dijoud F, Trolliet P, et al: Crow-Fukase disease/POEMS syndrome presenting with severe microangiopathic involvement of the kidney. Nephrol Dial Transplant (in press).

937. Mizuiri S, Mitsuo K, Sakai K, et al: Renal involvement in POEMS syndrome. Nephron 59:153, 1991.

938. Nakazawa K, Itoh N, Shigematsu H, Koh C-S: An autopsy case of Crow-Fukase syndrome with a high level of IL-6 in the ascites. Special reference to glomerular lesions. Acta Pathol Jpn 42:651, 1992.

939. Fukatsu A, Ito Y, Yuzawa Y, et al: A case of POEMS syndrome showing elevated serum interleukin 6 and abnormal expression of interleukin 6 in the kidney. Nephron 62:47, 1992.

940. Pucello LP, Agnello V: Membranoproliferative glomerulonephritis associated with hepatitis B and C viral infections: From virus-like particles in the cryoprecipitate to viral like particles in para-mesangial deposits, problematic investigations prone to artifacts. Curr Opin Nephrol Hypertens 3:465–470, 1994.

941. Johnson RJ, Couser WG: Hepatitis B infection and renal disease: Clinical, immunopathogenic and therapeutic considerations. Kidney Int 37:663, 1990.

942. Venkataseshan VS, Lieberman K, Kim DV, et al: Hepatitis B–associated glomerulonephritis: Pathology, pathogenesis, and clinical courses. Medicine (Baltimore) 69:200, 1990.

943. Li PKT, Lai FM-M, Ho SS, et al: Acute renal failure in hepatitus B virus–related membranous nephropathy with mesangiocapillary transition and crescentic transformation. Am J Kidney Dis 19:76–80, 1992.

944. Onion DK, Crumpacker CS, Gilliland BC: Arthritis of hepatitis associated with Australia antigen. Ann Intern Med 75:291, 1971.

945. Duffy J, Lidsky MD, Sharp JT, et al: Polyarthritis, polyarteritis and hepatitis B. Medicine (Baltimore) 55:19, 1976.

946. Feizi T, Gitlin N: Immune complex disease of the kidney associated with chronic hepatitis and cryoglobulinaemia. Lancet 2:873, 1969.

947. Combes B, Stastny PN, Shorey J, et al: Glomerulonephritis with deposition of Australia antigen-antibody complexes in glomerular basement membrane. Lancet 2:234, 1971.

948. Takekoshi Y, Tanaka M, Miyakawa Y, et al: Free "small" and IgG associated "large" hepatitis Be antigen in the serum and glomerular capillary walls of two patients with membranous glomerulonephritis. N Engl J Med 300:814, 1979.

949. Hattori S, Furuse A, Matsuda I: Presence of HBe antibody in glomerular deposits in membranous glomerulonephritis is associated with hepatitis B virus infection. Am J Nephrol 8:384, 1988.

950. Levy M, Chan N: Worldwide perspective of hepatitis B–associated glomerulonephritis in the 80s. Kidney Int 40(suppl 35):S-24, 1991.

951. Lin C-Y: Clinical features and natural course of HBV-related glomerulopathy in children. Kidney Int 40(suppl 35):S46, 1991.

952. Southwest Pediatric Nephrology Study Group: Hepatitis B surface antigenemia in North American children with membranous glomerulonephropathy. J Pediatr 106:571, 1985.

953. Schullard GH, Smith CI, Merigan TC, et al: Effects of immunosuppressive therapy on viral markers in chronic active hepatitis B. Gastroenterology 81:987, 1981.

954. Hoofnagle JH, Davis MD, Pappas C, et al: A short course of prednisone in chronic type B hepatitis. Ann Intern Med 104:12, 1986.

955. Lai CL, Lok AS, Lin HJ, et al: Placebo-controlled trial of recombinant alpha 2-interferon in Chinese HBsAg-carrier children. Lancet 2:877–880, 1987.

956. Lin C-Y, Lo S: Treatment of hepatitis B virus–associated membranous nephropathy with adenine arabinoside and thymic extract. Kidney Int 39:301, 1991.

957. Lisker-Melman M, Webb D, DiBisceglie AM, et al: Glomerulonephritis caused by chronic hepatitis B virus infection: Treatment with recombinant human alpha-interferon. Ann Intern Med 111:479, 1989.

958. Lai KN, Li PKT, Lui SF, et al: Membranous nephropathy related to hepatitis B virus in adults. N Engl J Med 324:1457, 1991.

959. Schectman JM, Kimmel PL: Remission of hepatitis B–associated membranous glomerulonephritis in human immunodeficiency virus infection. Am J Kidney Dis 17:716, 1991.

960. Lai FM-M, Li PKT, Suen MWM, et al: Crescentic glomerulonephritis related to hepatitis B virus. Mod Pathol 5:262, 1992.
961. Iida H, Izumino K, Asaka M, et al: IgA nephropathy and hepatitis B virus. IgA nephropathy unrelated to hepatitis B surface antigenemia. Nephron 54:18–20, 1990.
962. McMahon BJ, Heyward WL, Templin DW, et al: Hepatitis B–associated polyarteritis nodosa in Alaskan Eskimos: Clinical and epidemiological features and long-term follow-up. Hepatology 9:97–101, 1989.
963. Lightfoot RW Jr, Michel BA, Block DA, et al: The American College of Rheumatology 1990 criteria for the classification of polyarteritis nodosa. Arthritis Rheum 33:1088, 1990.
964. Guillevin L, Lhote F, Jarrousse B, et al: Polyarteritis nodosa related to hepatitis B virus. A retrospective study of 66 patients. Ann Med Interne 143(suppl 1P):63, 1992.
965. Trepo CG, Zuckerman AJ, Bird RC, Prince AM: The role of circulating hepatitis B antigen/antibody immune complexes in the pathogenesis of vascular and hepatic manifestations in polyarteritis nodosa. J Clin Pathol 27:863, 1974.
966. Ewald EA, Griffin D, McCune WJ: Correlation of angiographic abnormalities with disease manifestations and disease severity in polyarteritis nodosa. J Rheumatol 14:952, 1987.
967. Azar N, Guillevin L, Huong Du LT, et al: Symptomatic urogenital manifestations of polyarteritis nodosa and Churg-Strauss angiitis: Analysis of 8 of 165 patients. J Urol 142:136, 1989.
968. Razzak IA, Bauer FW, Itzel W: Hepatitis-B-antigenemia with panarteritis, diffuse proliferative glomerulitis and malignant hypertension. Am J Gastroenterol 68:476, 1974.
969. Guillevin J, Lhote F, Sauvage F, et al: Treatment of polyarteritis nodosa related to hepatitis B virus with interferon-alpha and plasma exchanges. Ann Rheum Dis 53:334, 1994.
970. Frohnert PP, Sheps SG: Long-term follow-up study of periarteritis nodosa. Am J Med 43:8, 1967.
971. Oriente P, Riccio A, Farinaro C, et al: Cyclosphosphamide treatment in polyarteritis nodosa. Clin Rheumatol 5:193, 1986.
972. Lockwood CM, Worlledge S, Nicholas A, et al: Reversal of impaired splenic functions in patients with nephritis or vasculitis (or both) by plasma exchange. N Engl J Med 300:524–530, 1979.
973. Guillevin L: Treatment of polyarteritis nodosa with dapsone. Scand J Rheumatol 15:95–96, 1986.
974. Chalopin JM, Rifle G, Turc JM, et al: Immunological findings during successful treatment of HBsAg-associated polyarteritis nodosa by plasmapheresis alone. Br Med J 1:368, 1980.
975. Guillevin L, Lhote F, Leon A, et al: Treatment of polyarteritis nodosa related to hepatitis B virus with short term steroid therapy associated with antiviral agents and plasma exchanges. A prospective trial in 33 patients. J Rheumatol 20:289, 1993.
976. Levo Y, Gorevic PD, Kassab HJ, et al: Association between hepatitis B virus and essential mixed cryoglobulinemia. N Engl J Med 296:1501, 1977.
977. Alter MJ, Margolis HS, Krawczynski K, et al: The nature history of community-acquired hepatitis C in the United States. N Engl J Med 327:1899–1905, 1992.
978. Cacoub P, Lunel-Fabiani F: Polyarteritis nodosa and hepatitis C virus infection. Ann Intern Med 116:605, 1992.
979. Pascual M, Perrin L, Giostra E, Schifferli JA: Hepatitis C virus in patients with cryoglobulinemia type II. J Infect Dis 162:569–570, 1990.
980. De Bandt M, Ribard P, Meyer O, et al: Type II IgM monoclonal cryoglobulinemia and hepatitis C virus infection. Clin Exp Rheumatol 9:659–660, 1991.
981. Johnson RJ, Gretch DR, Yamabe H, et al: Membranoproliferative glomerulonephritis associated with hepatitis C virus infection. N Engl J Med 328:465–70, 1993.
982. Horikoshi S, Okada T, Shirato I, et al: Diffuse proliferative glomerulonephritis with hepatitis C virus–like particles in paramesangial dense deposits in a patient with chronic hepatitis C virus hepatitis. Nephron 64:462–464, 1993.
983. Rollino C, Roccatello D, Giachino O, et al: Hepatitis C virus infection and membranous glomerulonephritis. Nephron 59:319–320, 1991.
984. DiBisceglie AM, Martin P, Kassianides CK, et al: Recombinant interferon alfa therapy for chronic hepatitis C. A randomized double-blind placebo-controlled trial. N Engl J Med 321:1506–1510, 1989.

985. Davis GL, Balart LA, Schiff ER, et al: Treatment of chronic hepatitis C with recombinant interferon alfa. A multicenter randomized, controlled trial. N Engl J Med 321:1501–1506, 1989.
986. Casato M, Lagana B, Antonelli G, et al: Long-term results of therapy with interferon-α for type II essential mixed cryoglobulinemia. Blood 78:3142–3147, 1991.
987. Kawaguchi K, Koike M: Glomerular lesions associated with liver cirrhosis: An immunohistochemical and clinicopathologic analysis. Hum Pathol 17:1137, 1986.
988. Bloodworth JMB Jr, Sommers SC: "Cirrhotic glomerulosclerosis," a renal lesion associated with hepatic cirrhosis. Lab Invest 8:962, 1959.
989. Berger J, Yaneva M, Nabarra B: Glomerular changes in patients with cirrhosis of the liver. Adv Nephrol 7:3, 1978.
990. Callard P, Feldmann G, Prandi D, et al: Immune complex type of glomerulonephritis in cirrhosis of the liver. Am J Pathol 80:329, 1975.
991. Nochy D, Callard P, Bellon B, et al: Association of overt glomerulonephritis and liver disease: A study of 34 patients. Clin Nephrol 6:422, 1976.
992. Sancho J, Egido J, Sanchez R, et al: Detection of monomeric and polymeric IgA containing immune complexes in serum and kidney from patients with alcoholic liver disease. Clin Exp Immunol 47:327, 1981.
993. Burns J, D'Ardenne AJ, Morton JA, McGae J: Immune complex nephritis in alcoholic cirrhosis: Mallory body antigen in complexes by means of monoclonal antibodies to Mallory bodies. J Clin Pathol 36:751, 1983.
994. Bene MC, Dekorwin JD, deLigny BH, et al: IgA nephropathy and alcoholic liver cirrhosis. A prospective necropsy study. Am J Clin Pathol 89:767, 1988.
995. Roccatello D, Picciotto G, Torchio M, et al: Removal systems of immunoglobulin A and immunoglobulin A containing complexes in IgA nephropathy and cirrhosis patients. The role of asialoglycoprotein receptors. Lab Invest 69:714, 1993.
996. Newell GC: Cirrhotic glomerulonephritis: Incidence, morphology, clinical features and pathogenesis. Am J Kidney Dis 9:183, 1987.
997. Glassock RJ, Nast CC, Cohen AH: The renal response to infection. Adv Exp Med Biol 252:163, 1989.
998. Smith SM, Hoy WE: Frequent association of mesangial glomerulonephritis and alcohol abuse: A study of 3 ethnic groups. Mod Pathol 2:138, 1989.
999. Aggarwal M, Manske CL, Lynch PJ, Paller MS: Henoch-Schönlein vasculitis as a manifestation of IgA associated disease in cirrhosis. Am J Kidney Dis 20:400, 1992.
1000. Ghabra M, Piraino B, Greenberg A, Banner B: Resolution of cirrhotic glomerulonephritis following successful liver transplantation. Clin Nephrol 35:6, 1991.
1001. Rai GS, Hamlyn AN, Dahl MGC, et al: Primary biliary cirrhosis, cutaneous capillaritis, and IgM-associated membranous glomerulonephritis. Br Med J 1:817, 1977.
1002. Patek AJ Jr, Seegal D, Bevans M: The coexistence of cirrhosis of the liver and glomerulonephritis: Report of 14 cases. Am J Med Sci 221:77, 1951.
1003. Moroz SP, Cutz E, Bulte JW, Sass-Kortsak A: Membranoproliferative glomerulonephritis in childhood cirrhosis associated with alpha$_1$-antitrypsin deficiency. Pediatrics 57:232, 1976.
1004. Dobrin RS, Hoyer JR, Nevins TE, et al: Association of familial liver disease, subepidermal immunoproteins, and membranoproliferative glomerulonephritis. J Pediatr 90:901, 1977.
1005. Strife CF, Hug G, Chuck G, et al: Membranoproliferative glomerulonephritis and alpha$_1$-antitrypsin deficiency in children. Pediatrics 71:88, 1983.
1006. Eagen JW, Lewis EJ: Glomerulopathies of neoplasia. Kidney Int 11:297, 1977.
1006a. Norris SH: Paraneoplastic glomerulopathies. Semin Nephrol 13:258, 1993.
1007. Lee JC, Yamauchi H, Hopper J Jr: The association of cancer and the nephrotic syndrome. Ann Intern Med 64:41, 1966.
1008. Cotran RS, Alpers CE: Neoplasia and glomerular injury. Kidney Int 30:465, 1986.
1009. Dabbs D, Striker LM-M, Mignon F, Striker G: Glomerular lesions in lymphoma and leukemia. Am J Med 80:63, 1986.
1010. Brueggemeyer CD, Ramirez G: Membranous nephropathy: A concern for malignancy. Am J Kidney Dis 9:23, 1987.

1011. Davidson AM, Thomson D: Malignancy-associated glomerular disease. *In* Cameron S, Davison J, Greenfield JP, Ritz E (eds): Oxford Textbook of Clinical Nephrology. Oxford Medical Publishers, London, 1992.
1012. Loughridge LW, Lewis MG: Nephrotic syndrome in malignant disease of non-renal origin. Lancet 1:256, 1971.
1013. Richard-Mendes da Costa C, Dupont E, Hamers R, et al: Nephrotic syndrome in bronchogenic carcinoma: Report of two cases with immunochemical studies. Clin Nephrol 2:245, 1974.
1014. Weintroub S, Stavorovsky M, Griffel B: Membranous glomerulonephritis: An initial symptom of gastric carcinoma? Arch Surg 110:833, 1978.
1015. Costanza ME, Pinn VE, Schwartz RS, Nathanson L: Carcinoembryonic antigen-antibody complexes in a patient with colonic carcinoma and nephrotic syndrome. N Engl J Med 289:520, 1973.
1016. Couser WG, Wagonfeld JB, Spargo BH, Lewis EJ: Glomerular deposition of tumor antigen in membranous nephropathy associated with colonic carcinoma. Am J Med 57:962, 1974.
1017. Lumeng J, Moran J: Carotid body tumor associated with mild membranous glomerulonephritis. Ann Intern Med 65:1266, 1966.
1018. Olson JL, Philips T, Lewis MG, Solez K: Malignant melanoma with renal dense deposits containing tumor antigens. Clin Nephrol 12:74, 1979.
1019. Zech P, Colon S, Pointer P, et al: The nephrotic syndrome in adults aged over 60: Etiology, evolution and treatment of 76 cases. Clin Nephrol 18:232, 1982.
1020. Stuart K, Fallon B, Cardi M: Development of the nephrotic syndrome in a patient with prostatic carcinoma. Am J Med 80:295, 1986.
1021. Schroeter NJ, Rushing DA, Parker JP, Beltaos E: Minimal-change nephrotic syndrome associated with malignant mesothelioma. Arch Intern Med 146:1834, 1986.
1022. Qunibi W, Al-Sibai M, Akhtar M: Mesangioproliferative glomerulonephritis associated with Kimura's disease. Clin Nephrol 30:111–114, 1988.
1023. Whelan T, Maker J, Kragel P, et al: Nephrotic syndrome associated with Kimura's disease. Am J Kidney Dis 11:353, 1988.
1024. Dussol B, Berland Y, Casanova P: Crescentic glomerulonephritis associated with gastric adenocarcinoma. Nephrologie 13:163, 1992.
1025. Haskell LP, Fusco MJ, Wadler S, et al: Crescentic glomerulonephritis associated with prostatic carcinoma: Evidence of immune-mediated glomerular injury. Am J Med 88:189–192, 1990.
1026. Cudkowicz ME, Sayegh MH, Rennke H: Membranous nephropathy in a patient with renal cell carcinoma. Am J Kidney Dis 17:349–351, 1991.
1027. McDonald P, Kalra PA, Coward RA: Thymoma and minimal-change glomerulonephritis. Nephrol Dial Transplant 7:357–359, 1992.
1028. Kalra PA, Raghavan C, Hasson R, et al: Nephrotic-range proteinuria associated with right atrial myxoma. Clin Nephrol 37:294–296, 1992.
1029. Peces R, Sanchez L, Gorostidi M, Alvarez J: Minimal change nephrotic syndrome associated with Hodgkin's lymphoma. Nephrol Dial Transplant 6:155–158, 1991.
1030. Poch E, Almirall J, Torras A, et al: Rapidly progressive glomerulonephritis and systemic vasculitis in non-Hodgkin lymphoma. Nephrol Dial Transplant 6:51–54, 1991.
1031. Rault R, Holley JL, Banner BF, El-Shahawy M: Glomerulonephritis and non-Hodgkin's lymphoma: A report of two cases and review of the literature. Am J Kidney Dis 20:84–89, 1992.
1032. Delmez JA, Safdar SH, Kissane JM: The successful treatment of recurrent nephrotic syndrome with the MOPP regimen in a patient with a remote history of Hodgkin's disease. Am J Kidney Dis 23:743–746, 1994.
1033. Korzets Z, Golan E, Manor Y, et al: Spontaneously remitting minimal change nephropathy preceding a relapse of Hodgkin's disease by 19 months. Clin Nephrol 38:125–127, 1992.
1034. Moulin B, Ronco PM, Mougenot B, et al: Glomerulonephritis in chronic lymphocytic leukemia and related B-cell lymphomas. Kidney Int 42:127–135, 1992.
1035. Moe SM, Baron JM, Coventry S, et al: Glomerular disease and urinary Sézary cells in cutaneous T-cell lymphomas. Am J Kidney Dis 21:545–547, 1993.
1036. Traynor A, Kuzel T, Samuelson E, Kanwar Y: Miminal-change glomerulopathy and glomerular visceral epithelial hyperplasia associated with alpha-interferon therapy for cutaneous T-cell lymphoma. Nephron 67:94–100, 1994.
1037. Lewis MG, Loughridge LW, Phillips TM: Immunological studies in nephrotic syndrome associated with extrarenal malignant disease. Lancet 2:134, 1971.
1038. Ozawa T, Pluss R, Lacher J, et al: Endogenous immune complex nephropathy associated with malignancy: I. Studies on the nature and significance of glomerular bound antigen antibody, isolation and characterization of tumor antigen and antibody and circulating immune complexes. Q J Med 44:563, 1975.
1039. McCanse LR, Moore JD, Markel L, Mebust WK: Renal cell carcinoma presenting with nephrotic syndrome: A case report and review of the literature. J Urol 114:938, 1975.
1040. Biava CG, Gonwa TA, Naughton JL, Hopper J Jr: Crescentic glomerulonephritis associated with non-renal malignancies. Am J Nephrol 4:208, 1984.
1041. Pascal RR, Tannaccone PM, Rollwagon FM, et al: Electron microscopy and immunofluorescence of glomerular immune complex deposits in cancer patients. Cancer Res 36:43, 1976.
1042. Beaufils H, Jouanneau C, Chomette L: Kidney and cancer: Results of immunofluorescence. Microscopy 40:303, 1985.
1042. Striker LM-M, Mignon F, Dabbs D, Striker GE: Glomerular lesions in lymphomas and leukemias. *In* Robinson R (ed): Nephrology. Springer-Verlag, New York, 1984, p 905.
1043. Belghiti D, Vernant JP, Hirbec G, et al: Nephrotic syndrome associated with T-cell lymphoma. Cancer 47:1878, 1981.
1044. Eknoyan G, Dillman RO: Renal complications of infectious diseases. Med Clin North Am 52:979, 1978.
1045. Kaehny WD, Ozawa T, Schwartz MI, et al: Acute nephritis and pulmonary alveolitis following pneumococcal pneumonia. Arch Intern Med 138:806, 1978.
1046. Forrest JW Jr, John F, Milk LR, et al: Immune complex glomerulonephritis associated with *Klebsiella pneumoniae* infection. Clin Nephrol 7:76, 1977.
1046a. Sissons JG, Sinclair JH, Borysiewicz LK: Pathogenesis of human cytomegalovirus disease and the kidney. Kidney Int 35(suppl):S8, 1991.
1046b. Lin CY, Chen WP, Chiang H: Mumps associated with nephritis. Child Nephrol Urol 10:68, 1990.
1047. Boulton-Jones J, Davison A: Persisting infection as a cause of renal disease in patients submitted to renal biopsy: A report of the glomerulonephritis registry of the United Kingdom MRC. Q J Med 58:123, 1986.
1048. Rainford DJ, Woodrow DF, Sloper JC, et al: Postmeningococcal acute glomerular nephritis. Clin Nephrol 9:249, 1978.
1049. Sterzel RB, Krause PH, Zobl H, Kuhn K: Acute syphilitic nephrosis: A transient glomerular immunopathy. Clin Nephrol 2:164, 1974.
1050. Sitprija V, Pipatanagul V, Boonpucknavig V, Boonpucknavig S: Glomerulitis in typhoid fever. Ann Intern Med 81:210, 1974.
1051. Woodroffe AJ, Row PG, Meadows R, Lawrence JR: Nephritis in infectious mononucleosis. Q J Med 43:451, 1974.
1052. Lee S, Kjellstrand CM: Renal disease in infectious mononucleosis. Clin Nephrol 9:326, 1978.
1053. Ozawa T, Stewart JA: Immune-complex glomerulonephritis associated with cytomegalovirus infection. Am J Clin Pathol 72:103, 1979.
1054. Bullock WE, Artz RP, Bhathena D, Tung KSK: Histoplasmosis: Association with circulating immune complexes, eosinophilia, and mesangiopathic glomerulonephritis. Arch Intern Med 139:700, 1979.
1055. Hyman LR, Jenia EH, Hill GS, et al: Alternate C3 pathway activation in pneumococcal glomerulonephritis. Am J Med 58:810, 1975.
1056. Akano N, Yoshioka K, Matsui K, et al: Transient massive proteinuria associated with *Mycoplasma pneumoniae* infection. Am J Kidney Dis 18:123–125, 1991.
1057. Campbell JH, Warwick G, Boulton-Jones M, et al: Rapidly progressive glomerulonephritis and nephrotic syndrome associated with *Mycoplasma pneumoniae* pneumonia. Nephrol Dial Transplant 6:518, 1991.
1058. D'Agati V, McEachrane S, Dicker R, Nielsen E: Cat scratch disease and glomerulonephritis. Nephron 56:431, 1990.
1059. Quigg RJ, Gaines R, Wakely PE Jr, Schoolwerth AC: Acute glomerulonephritis in a patient with Rocky Mountain spotted fever. Am J Kidney Dis 17:339, 1991.

1060. Löhlein M: Über hämmorrhagische Nierenaffektionen bei chronischer ulzeröser Endokarditis (Embolische, nichteitrige Herd Nephritis). Med Klin 10:375, 1910.

1061. Baehr G: Glomerular lesions of subacute bacterial endocarditis. J Exp Med 15:330, 1912.

1062. Baehr G, Laude H: Glomerulonephritis as a complication of subacute streptococcus endocarditis. JAMA 75:789, 1920.

1063. Craddock C, Richards N, Powell R, Morgan A: Novel C3 nephrotic factor activity in the glomerulonephritis of staphylococcal endocarditis. Q J Med 65:895, 1987.

1064. Bayer AS, Theophilopoulous AN, Eisenberg R, et al: Circulating immune complexes in infective endocarditis. N Engl N Med 295:1500, 1976.

1065. Morel-Maroger L, Sraer JD, Herreman G, Godeau P: Kidney in subacute endocarditis: Pathological and immunofluorescent findings. Arch Pathol 94:205, 1972.

1066. Williams RC, Kunkel HG: Rheumatoid factor complement and conglutinin aberrations in patients with subacute bacterial endocarditis. J Clin Invest 41:666, 1962.

1067. Boulton-Jones JM, Sissons JG, Evans DJ, Peters DK: Renal lesions of subacute infective endocarditis. Br Med J 2:11, 1974.

1068. Yum M, Wheat LJ, Maxwell D, et al: Immunofluorescent localization of *Staphylococcus aureus* antigen in acute bacterial endocarditis nephritis. Am J Clin Pathol 70:832, 1978.

1069. Hurwitz D, Quismorio FP, Friow GJ: Cryoglobulinemia in patients with infectious endocarditis. Clin Exp Immunol 19:131, 1975.

1070. Hall GH, Hart RJC, Davies SW, et al: Glomerulonephritis associated with *Coxiella burnetii* endocarditis. Br Med J 2:275, 1975.

1071. Perez-Fontan M, Huarte E, Tellez A, et al: Glomerular nephropathy associated with chronic Q fever. Am J Kidney Dis 11:298, 1988.

1072. Neugarten J, Baldwin DS: Glomerulonephritis in bacterial endocarditis. Am J Med 77:297, 1984.

1073. Rovzar MA, Logan J, Ogden D, Graham A: Immunosuppressive therapy and plasmapheresis in rapidly progressive glomerulonephritis associated with bacterial endocarditis. Am J Kidney Dis 7:428, 1986.

1074. Montseny JJ, Kleinknecht D, Meyrier A: Rapidly progressive glomerulonephritis of infectious origin. Ann Med Interne 144:308, 1993.

1075. Levy RL, Hong R: The immune nature of subacute bacterial endocarditis (SBE) nephritis. Am J Med 54:645, 1973.

1076. Gutman RA, Striker GE, Gilliland BC, Cutler RE: The immune complex glomerulonephritis of bacterial endocarditis. Medicine (Baltimore) 51:1, 1972.

1077. Adler SG, Cohen AH: Glomerulonephritis with bacterial endocarditis, ventriculo-vascular shunts and visceral infections. *In* Schrier RS, Gottschalk CW (eds): Diseases of the Kidney. Little, Brown, Boston, 1992, pp 1681–1688.

1078. Kaufman DB, McIntosh R: The pathogenesis of the renal lesion in a patient with streptococcal disease, infected ventriculoatrial shunt, cryoglobulinemia and nephritis. Am J Med 50:262, 1971.

1079. McKenzie SA, Hayden SK: Two cases of "shunt nephritis." Pediatrics 54:806, 1974.

1080. Beaufils M, Morel-Maroger L, Sraer JD, et al: Acute renal failure of glomerular origin during visceral abscesses. N Engl J Med 295:185, 1976.

1081. Black JA, Challacombe DN, Ockenden BG: Nephrotic syndrome associated with bacteremia after shunt operations for hydrocephalus. Lancet 2:921, 1965.

1082. Arze RS, Rashid H, Morley R, et al: Shunt nephritis: Report of two cases and review of the literature. Clin Nephrol 19:48, 1983.

1083. Levy M, Gubler MC, Habib R: Pathology and immunopathology of shunt nephritis in children: Report of 10 cases. *In* Proceedings of the 8th International Congress of Nephrology. S Karger, Basel, 1981, p 290.

1084. Schoenbaum SC, Gardner P, Shillito J: Infections of cerebrospinal fluid shunts: Epidemiology, clinical manifestations, and therapy. Infect Dis 131:543, 1975.

1085. Fukuda Y, Ohtomo Y, Kaneko K, Yabuta K: Pathologic and laboratory dynamics following the removal of the shunt in shunt nephritis. Am J Nephrol 13:78, 1993.

1086. Wyatt RJ, Walsh JW, Holland NH: Shunt nephritis. Role of complement system in its pathogenesis and management. J Neurosurg 55:99, 1981.

1087. Stickler GB, Shin MH, Burke EC, et al: Diffuse glomerulonephritis associated with ventriculoatrial shunt. N Engl J Med 279:1077, 1968.

1088. Sanchez-Bayle M, Ecija JL, Estepa R, et al: Incidence of glomerulonephritis in congenital syphilis. Clin Nephrol 20:27, 1983.

1089. Hruby Z, Kuniar J, Rabczyski J, et al: The variety of clinical and histopathologic presentations of glomerulonephritis associated with latent syphilis. Int Urol Nephrol 24:541, 1992.

1090. Gamble C, Reardan J: Immunopathogenesis of syphilitic glomerulonephritis: Elution of anti-treponemal antibody from glomerular immune-complex deposits. N Engl J Med 292:449, 1975.

1091. Slater DN, Brown CB, Ward AM, et al: Immune complex crescentic glomerulonephritis associated with pulmonary aspergillosis. Histopathology 7:957, 1983.

1092. Cologlu AS: Immune complex glomerulonephritis in leprosy. Lepr Rev 50:213, 1979.

1093. Fernandez-Sola J, Monforte R, Ponz E, et al: Persistent low C3 levels associated with meningococcal meningitis and membranoproliferative glomerulonephritis. Am J Nephrol 10:426, 1990.

1094. Hulton S-A, Risdon RA, Dillon JJ: Mesangiocapillary glomerulonephritis associated with meningococcal meningitis, C3 nephritic factor and persistently low complement C3 and C5. Pediatr Nephrol 6:239, 1992.

1095. Kincaid-Smith PS: Natural history and treatment of reflux nephropathy. *In* Robinson R (ed): Nephrology. Springer-Verlag, New York, 1984, p 959.

1096. Torres VE, Verlosa JA, Holley KE, et al: The progression of vesicoureteral reflux nephropathy. Ann Intern Med 92:776, 1980.

1097. Bhathena DB, Weiss JH, Holland NH, et al: Focal and segmental glomerular sclerosis in reflux nephropathy. Am J Med 68:886, 1980.

1098. Cotran RS: Glomerulosclerosis in reflux nephropathy. Kidney Int 21:528, 1982.

1099. Chugh KS, Sakhuja V: Glomerular diseases in the tropics. Am J Nephrol 10:437–450, 1990. Editorial.

1100. Kibukamusoke JW, Hutt MSR, Wilks NE: The nephrotic syndrome in Uganda and its association with quartan malaria. Q J Med 36:393, 1967.

1101. Hendrickse RG: The quartan malarial nephrotic syndrome. Adv Nephrol 6:229, 1976.

1102. Adeniyi A, Hendrickse RG, Houba V: Selectivity of proteinuria and response to prednisolone or immunosuppressive drugs in children with malarial nephrosis. Lancet 1:644, 1970.

1103. Hendrickse RG, Adeniyi A: Quartan malarial nephrotic syndrome in children. Kidney Int 16:64, 1979.

1104. Shanin B, Popadopanton ZL, Jenis EH: Congenital nephrotic syndrome associated with congenital toxoplasmosis. J Pediatr 85:366, 1974.

1105. Barsoum RS: Schistosomal glomerulopathies. Kidney Int 44:1, 1993.

1106. Rao TK, Filipone EJ, Nicastri AD, et al: Associated focal and segmental glomerulosclerosis in the acquired immunodeficiency syndrome. N Engl J Med 310:669, 1984.

1107. Pardo V, Aldana M, Colton RM, et al: Glomerular lesions in the acquired immunodeficiency syndrome. Ann Intern Med 101:429, 1984.

1108. Gardenswartz MH, Lerner CW, Seligson GR, et al: Renal disease in patients with AIDS: A clinicopathologic study. Clin Nephrol 21:197, 1984.

1109. Patrick AL, Roberts LA, Burton EN, et al: Focal and segmental glomerulosclerosis in the acquired immunodeficiency syndrome. West Indian Med J 35:200, 1986.

1110. Chander P, Soni A, Suri A, et al: Renal ultrastructure markers in AIDS associated nephropathy. Am J Pathol 126:513, 1987.

1111. Rao TKS, Friedman EA, Nicastri AD: The types of renal disease in the acquired immunodeficiency syndrome. N Engl J Med 316:1062, 1987.

1112. Bourgoignie JJ, Meneses R, Pardo V: The nephropathy related to acquired immunodeficiency syndrome. Adv Nephrol 17:113, 1988.

1113. D'Agati V, Suh JI, Carbone L, et al: Pathology of HIV associated nephropathy. A detailed morphologic and comparative study. Kidney Int 35:1358–1370, 1989.

1114. Bourgoignie JJ: Renal complications of human immunodeficiency virus type 1. Kidney Int 37:1571–1584, 1990.

1115. Seney FD, Burns DK, Silva FG: Acquired immunodeficiency syndrome and the kidney. Am J Kidney Dis 16:1–13, 1990.

1116. Mazbar SA, Schoenfeld PY, Humphreys MH: Renal involvement in patients infected with HIV: Experience at San Francisco General Hospital. Kidney Int 37:1325–1332, 1990.

1117. Korbet SM, Schwartz MM: Human immunodeficiency virus infection and nephrotic syndrome. Am J Kidney Dis 20:97–103, 1992.

1118. Nochy D, Glotz D, Dosquet P, et al: Renal disease associated with HIV infection: A multicentric study of 60 patients from Paris hospitals. Nephrol Dial Transplant 8:11–19, 1993.

1119. Artiz-Butcher C: The spectrum of kidney diseases in patients with human immunodeficiency virus infection. Curr Opin Nephrol Hypertens 2:355–364, 1995.

1120. Chander D, Agarwal A, Soni A, et al: Renal cytomembranous inclusions in idiopathic renal disease as predictive markers for the acquired immunodeficiency syndrome. Hum Pathol 19:1060, 1988.

1121. Cohen AH, Nast CC: HIV-associated nephropathy: A unique combined glomerular, tubular and interstitial lesion. Mod Pathol 1:87, 1988.

1122. Langs C, Gallo GR, Schacht RG, et al: Rapid renal failure in AIDS-associated focal glomerulosclerosis. Arch Intern Med 150:287–292, 1990.

1123. Brunkhorst R, Brunkhorst U, Eisenbach GM, et al: Lack of clinical evidence for a specific HIV associated glomerulopathy in 203 patients with HIV infection. Nephrol Dial Transplant 7:87–92, 1992.

1124. Kimmel PL, Umana WD, Bosch JP: Abnormal urinary protein excretion in HIV-infected patients. Clin Nephrol 39:17–21, 1993.

1125. Carbone L, D'Agati V, Cheng JT, et al: Course and prognosis of human immunodeficiency virus–associated nephropathy. Am J Med 87:389–395, 1989.

1126. Strauss J, Zilleruelo G, Abitbol C, et al: Human immunodeficiency nephropathy. Pediatr Nephrol 7:220–225, 1993.

1127. Katz A, Bargman JM, Miller DC, et al: IgA nephritis in HIV-positive patients: A new HIV-associated nephropathy? Clin Nephrol 38:61–68, 1992.

1128. Kimmel PL, Phillips TM, Ferreira-Centeno A, et al: Brief report: Idiotypic IgA nephropathy in patients with human immunodeficiency virus infection. N Engl J Med 327:702–706, 1992.

1128a. Jinda KK, Trillo A, Bishop G, et al: Crescentic IgA nephropathy as a manifestation of human immune deficiency virus infection. Am J Nephrol 11:147–150, 1991.

1129. Alpers CE, Harawi S, Rennke HG: Focal glomerulosclerosis with tubulo reticular inclusions: Possible predictive value for acquired immunodeficiency syndrome (AIDS). Am J Kidney Dis 12:240, 1988.

1130. Cohen AH, Sun CJ, Shapshak P, Imagawa DT: Demonstration of human immunodeficiency virus in renal epithelium in HIV associated nephropathy. Mod Pathol 2:125, 1989.

1131. Green DF, Resnick L, Bourgoignie JJ: HIV infects glomerular endothelial and mesangial but not epithelial cells in vitro. Kidney Int 41:956–960, 1992.

1132. Alpers CE, McClure J, Burstein SL: Human mesangial cells are resistant to productive infection by multiple strains of human immunodeficiency virus types 1 and 2. Am J Kidney Dis 19:126–130, 1992.

1133. Kopp JB, Klotman ME, Adler SH, et al: Progressive glomerulosclerosis and enhanced renal accumulation of basement membrane components in mice transgenic for human immunodeficiency virus type 1 genes. Proc Natl Acad Sci USA 89:1577–1581, 1992.

1134. Singer DR, Jenkins AP, Gupton S, Evans DJ: Minimal change nephropathy in the acquired immunodeficiency syndrome. Br Med J 291:868, 1985.

1135. Cases A, Montoliu J, Baradad M, et al: Nefropatia por canibios minimos asociada a un sindrome de immunodeficiencia adquirida. Med Clin (Barc) 86:604, 1986.

1136. Collins AB, Bhan AK, Dienstag JL, et al: Hepatitis B immune complex glomerulonephritis: Simultaneous glomerular deposition of hepatitis B surface and E antigens. Clin J Immunopathol 26:137, 1983.

1137. Guerra IL, Abraham AA, Kimmel PL, et al: Nephrotic syndrome associated with chronic persistent hepatitis B in an HIV antibody positive patient. Am J Kidney Dis 10:385, 1988.

1138. Kim KK, Factor SM: Membranoproliferative glomerulonephritis and plexogenic pulmonary arteriopathy in a homosexual man with acquired immunodeficiency syndrome. Hum Pathol 18:1293, 1987.

1139. Langs C, Gallo GR, Schacht RG, et al: Rapid renal failure in AIDS-associated focal glomerulosclerosis. Arch Intern Med 150:287, 1990.

1140. Lam M, Park MC: HIV-associated nephropathy—beneficial effect of zidovudine therapy. N Engl J Med 323:1775–1776, 1990.

1141. Cook PP, Appel RG: Prolonged clinical improvement in HIV-associated nephropathy with zidovudine therapy. J Am Soc Nephrol 1:842, 1990. Letter.

1142. Smith MC, Pawar R, Carey JT, et al: Effect of corticosteroid therapy on human immunodeficiency virus–associated nephropathy. Am J Med 97:145, 1994.

1143. Lang P, Niaudet P: Update and outcome of renal transplant patients with human immunodeficiency virus. Transplant Proc 23:1352–1353, 1991.

1144. Rubin RH, Tolkoff-Rubin NE: The problem of human immunodeficiency virus infection and transplantation. Transpl Int 1:36, 1988.

1145. Phillips A, Wainberg MA, Coates R, et al: Cyclosporine-induced deterioration in patients with AIDS. Can Med Assoc J 140:1456–1460, 1989.

1146. Watkins PJ, Blamey JD, Brewer DB, et al: The natural history of diabetic renal disease. Q J Med 41:437, 1972.

1147. Schreiner GE: The nephrotic syndrome. In Strauss MB, Welt LG (eds): Diseases of the Kidney, 2nd ed. Little, Brown, Boston, 1971, p 503.

1148. Gonzalo A, Navarro J, Mampaso F, Ortuno J: Nodular glomerulosclerosis without glucose intolerance: Long-term follow up. Nephron 66:481–482, 1994.

1149. Suzuki S, Maruyama Y, Nakamura T, et al: Nodular glomerulosclerosis of unknown origin associated with the nephrotic syndrome. Nephron 66:462–469, 1994.

1150. Innes A, Furness PN, Cotton RE, et al: Diabetic glomerulosclerosis without diabetes mellitus: Two case reports and a review of the literature. Nephrol Dial Transplant 7:642–646, 1993.

1151. Harrington AR, Hare HG, Chambers WN, Valtin H: Nodular glomerulosclerosis suspected during life in a patient without demonstrable diabetes mellitus. N Engl J Med 275:206, 1972.

1152. Strauss FG, Argy WP Jr, Schreiner GF: Diabetic glomerulosclerosis in the absence of glucose intolerance. Ann Intern Med 75:239, 1971.

1153. Groop L, Makipernaa A, Stenman S, et al: Urinary excretion of kappa light chains in patients with diabetes mellitus. Kidney Int 37:1120–1125, 1990.

1154. Mogensen CE: Microalbuminuria predicts clinical proteinuria and early mortality in maturity-onset diabetes. N Engl J Med 310:356, 1984.

1155. Gellman DD, Pirani CL, Soothill JF, et al: Diabetic nephropathy: A clinical and pathologic study based on renal biopsies. Medicine (Baltimore) 38:321, 1959.

1156. Gambara V, Mecca G, Remuzzi G, Bertani T: Heterogeneous nature of renal lesions in type II diabetes. J Am Soc Nephrol 3:1458–1466, 1993.

1157. Waldherr R, Ilkenhans C, Ritz E: How frequent is glomerulonephritis in diabetes mellitus type II? Clin Nephrol 37:271–273, 1992.

1158. Appel GB, D'Agati V, Bergman M, Pirani CL: Nephrotic syndrome and immune complex glomerulonephritis associated with chlorpropamide therapy. Am J Med 74:337, 1983.

1159. Cavallo T, Pinto JA, Rajaraman S: Immune complex disease complicating diabetic glomerulosclerosis. Am J Nephrol 4:347, 1984.

1160. O'Neill WM, Wallin JD, Walker PD: Hematuria and red cell casts in typical diabetic nephrology. Am J Med 74:389, 1983.

1161. The KROC Collaborative Study Group: Blood glucose control and the evolution of diabetic retinopathy and albuminuria: A preliminary multicenter trial. N Engl J Med 311:365, 1984.

1162. Hamet P, Sugimoto H, Umeda F, et al: Abnormalities of platelet-derived growth factors in insulin-dependent diabetes. Metabolism 34:25, 1985.

1163. Luetscher JA, Kraemer FB, Wilson DM, et al: Increased plasma inactive renin in diabetes mellitus. N Engl J Med 312:1412, 1985.

1164. Beyer-Mears A: The polyol pathway, sorbinil, and renal dysfunction. Metabolism 35:46, 1986.

1165. Brownlee M, Vlassara H, Cerami A: Non-enzymatic glycosylation and the pathogenesis of diabetic complications. Ann Intern Med 101:527, 1984.

1166. Ghiggeri GM, Candiano G, Delfino G, Queirolo C: Electrical charge of serum and urinary albumin in normal and diabetic humans. Kidney Int 28:168, 1985.

1167. Williams SK, Siegal RK: Preferential transport of nonenzymatically glucosylated ferritin across the kidney glomerulus. Kidney Int 28:146, 1985.

1168. Ortola FV, Ballermann BJ, Anderson S, et al: Elevated plasma atrial natriuretic peptide levels in diabetic rats: Potential mechanisms of hyperfiltration. J Clin Invest 80:670, 1987.

1168a. Zhang PL, Mackenzie HS, Troy JL, et al: Effects of an atrial natriuretic peptide receptor antagonist on glomerular hyperfiltration in diabetic rats. J Am Soc Nephrol 4:1564, 1994.

1169. Kikkawa R, Kitamura E, Fujiwara Y, et al: Impaired contractile responsiveness of diabetic glomeruli to angiotensin II: A possible indication of mesangial dysfunction in diabetes mellitus. Biochem Biophys Res Commun 136:1185, 1986.

1170. Mogensen CE: Long-term antihypertensive treatment inhibiting progression of diabetic nephropathy. Br Med J 285:685, 1982.

1171. Parving H-H, Smidt UM, Hommel E, et al: Effective antihypertensive treatment postpones renal insufficiency in diabetic nephropathy. Am J Kidney Dis 22:188, 1993.

1172. Zatz R, Brenner BM: Diabetic microangiopathy: The hemodynamic view. Am J Med 80:443, 1986.

1173. Zatz R, Dunn BR, Meyer TW, et al: Prevention of diabetic glomerulopathy by pharmacological amelioration of glomerular capillary hypertension. J Clin Invest 77:1925, 1986.

1174. Marre M, Leblanc H, Suarez L, et al: Converting enzyme inhibition and kidney function in normotensive diabetic patients with persistent microalbuminuria. Br Med J 294:1448, 1987.

1175. Hommel E, Parving H-H, Mathiesen E, et al: Effect of captopril on kidney function in insulin-dependent diabetic patients with nephropathy. Br Med J 293:467, 1986.

1176. Taguma Y, Kitamoto Y, Futaki G, et al: Effect of captopril on heavy proteinuria in azotemic diabetics. N Engl J Med 26:1617, 1985.

1177. Björck S, Nyberg G, Mulec CH, et al: Beneficial effects of angiotensin converting enzyme inhibition on renal function in patients with diabetic nephropathy. Br Med J 293:471, 1986.

1178. Björck S, Mulec H, Johnsen SA, et al: Renal protective effect of enalapril in diabetic nephropathy. Br Med J 304:339, 1992.

1179. Lewis EJ, Hunsicker LG, Bain RP, et al: The effect of angiotensin converting enzyme inhibition on diabetic nephropathy. N Engl J Med 329:1456, 1993.

1180. Ravid M, Savin H, Jutrin I, et al: Long-term stabilizing effect of angiotensin-converting enzyme inhibition on plasma creatinine and on proteinuria in normotensive type II diabetic patients. Ann Intern Med 118:577, 1993.

1181. Mathiesen ER, Hommel E, Giese J, Parving H-H: Efficacy of captopril in postponing nephropathy in normotensive insulin dependent diabetic patients with microalbuminuria. Br Med J 303:81, 1991.

1182. Mogensen CE, and the European Microalbuminuria Captopril Study Group: Captopril delays progression to overt renal disease in insulin-dependent diabetes mellitus. J Am Soc Nephrol 3:336, 1992.

1183. Brichard SM, Santoni JP, Thomas JR, et al: Long-term reduction of microalbuminuria after 1 year of angiotensin converting enzyme inhibition by perindopril in hypertensive insulin-treated diabetic patients. Diabete Metab 16:30, 1989.

1183a. Holdaas H, Hartmann A, Lien MG, et al: Contrasting effects of lisinopril and nifedipine on albuminuria and tubular transport functions in insulin dependent diabetes with nephropathy. J Intern Med 229:163, 1991.

1184. Demarie BK, Bakris GL: Effects of different calcium antagonists on proteinuria associated with diabetes mellitus. Ann Intern Med 113:987, 1990.

1185. Mimran A, Insua A, Ribstein J, et al: Comparative effect of captopril and nifedipine in normotensive patients with incipient diabetic nephropathy. Diabetes Care 11:850, 1988.

1186. Melbourne Diabetic Nephropathy Study Group: Comparison between perindopril and nifedipine in hypertensive and normotensive diabetic patients with microalbuminuria. Br Med J 302:210, 1991.

1187. Kupin WL, Cortes P, Dumler F, et al: Effect on renal function of change from high to moderate protein intake in type I diabetic patients. Diabetes 36:73, 1986.

1188. Cohen D, Dodds R, Viberti G: Effect of protein restriction in insulin-dependent diabetics at risk of nephropathy. Br Med J 294:795, 1982.

1189. Zeller K, Whittaker E, Sullivan L, et al: Effect of restricting dietary protein on the progression of renal failure in patients with insulin-dependent diabetes mellitus. N Engl J Med 324:78, 1991.

1190. Rasch R: Prevention of diabetic glomerulopathy in streptozotocin diabetic rats by insulin treatment: The mesangial region. Diabetologia 17:243, 1979.

1191. Mauer SM, Brown DM, Steffes MW: Studies on the reversibility of kidney changes in experimental diabetes in the rat. Acta Endocrinol 97(suppl 242):29, 1981.

1192. Feldt-Rasmussen B, Mathiesen ER, Jensen T, et al: Effect of improved metabolic control on loss of kidney function in type 1 (insulin-dependent) diabetic patients: An update of the Steno studies. Diabetologia 34:164, 1991.

1193. Dahl-Jorgensen K, Hansen KF, Kierulf P, et al: Reduction of urinary albumin excretion after 4 years of continuous subcutaneous insulin infusion in insulin-dependent diabetes mellitus: The Oslo study. Acta Endocrinol (Copenh) 117:19, 1988.

1194. Reichard P, Nilsson B-Y, Rosenqvist U: The effect of long-term intensified insulin treatment on the development of microvascular complications of diabetes mellitus. N Engl J Med 329:304, 1993.

1195. The Diabetes Control and Complication Trial Research Group: The effect of intensive treatment of diabetes on the development and progression of long-term complications in insulin-dependent diabetes mellitus. N Engl J Med 329:977, 1993.

1196. Friedman EA: Clinical imperatives in diabetic nephropathy. Kidney Int 23(suppl 14):S16, 1983.

1197. Najarian JS, Sutherland DER, Morrow CE, et al: Kidney transplant for high-risk patients. Kidney Int 23(suppl 14):S10, 1983.

1198. Dickinson WH: Diseases of the Kidney and Urinary Derangements, Part 2. Longmans, Green, London, 1875, p 379.

1199. Guthrie LB: "Idiopathic" or congenital hereditary and family haematuria. Lancet 1:1243, 1902.

1200. Kendall G, Hertz AF: Hereditary familial congenital hemorrhagic nephritis. Guys Hosp Rep 66:137, 1912.

1201. Alport AC: Hereditary familial congenital hemorrhagic nephritis. Br Med J 1:504, 1927.

1202. Crawfurd MD'A, Toghill PJ: Alport's syndrome of hereditary chronic nephritis and deafness. Q J Med 37:563, 1968.

1203. Spear GS, Whitworth JM, Konigsmark BW: Hereditary nephritis with nerve deafness: Immunofluorescent studies on the kidney with a consideration of discordant immunoglobulin complement immunofluorescent patterns. Am J Med 49:52, 1970.

1204. Gubler M, Levy M, Broyer M, et al: Alport's syndrome: A report of 58 cases and a review of the literature. Am J Med 70:493, 1981.

1205. Chugh KS, Sakhuja V, Agarwal A, et al: Hereditary nephritis (Alport's syndrome)—clinical profile and inheritance in 28 kindreds. Nephrol Dial Transplant 8:690–695, 1993.

1206. Kashtan CE, Michael AF: Alport syndrome: From bedside to genome to bedside. Am J Kidney Dis 22:627–640, 1993.

1207. O'Neill WM, Atkin CL, Bloomer HA: Hereditary nephritis: A reexamination of its clinical and genetic features. Ann Intern Med 88:176, 1978.

1208. Chazan JA, Zacks J, Cohen JJ, Garella S: Hereditary nephritis: Clinical spectrum and mode of inheritance in five new kindreds. Am J Med 50:764, 1971.

1209. Knepshield JH, Roberts PL, Davis CJ, Moser RH: Hereditary chronic nephritis complicated by nephrotic syndrome. Arch Intern Med 122:156, 1968.

1210. Grünfeld J-P, Noel L-H, Hafex S, Droz D: Renal prognosis in women with hereditary nephritis. Clin Nephrol 23:267, 1985.

1211. Epstein CJ, Sahud M, Piel CF, et al: Hereditary macrothrombocytopathia, nephritis and deafness. Am J Med 52:299, 1972.

1212. Sarles HE, Rodin PE, Poduska PR, et al: Hereditary nephritis, retinitis pigmentosa and chromosomal abnormalities. Am J Med 45:312, 1968.

1213. Parsa KP, Lee DBN, Zamboni L, Glassock RJ: Hereditary nephritis, deafness and abnormal thrombopoiesis: Study of a new kindred. Am J Med 60:665, 1976.

1214. Peterson LC, Rao KV, Crosson JT, White JG: Fechtner syndrome-Q variant of Alport's syndrome with leukocyte inclusions and macrothrombocytopenia. Blood 65:397, 1985.

1215. Spear GS: Hereditary nephritis (Alport's syndrome)—1983. Clin Nephrol 21:3, 1984.

1216. De Marchi S, Cecchin E: Asymptomatic autoimmune thyroiditis and thyroid dysfunction in Alport's syndrome. A report of three families. Nephrol Dial Transplant 6:79–85, 1991.

1216a. Antignac C, Zhou J, Sanak M, et al: Alport syndrome and diffuse leiomyomatosis: Deletions in the 5′ end of the COL4A5 collagen gene. Kidney Int 42:1178–1183, 1992.

1217. Garcia-Torres R, Orozco L: Alport-leiomyomatosis syndrome: An update. Am J Kidney Dis 22:641–648, 1993.

1218. Lambert M, Pirson Y, De Nayer P, van Ypersele de Strihou C: No association between Alport's syndrome and antithyroid antibodies. Nephrol Dial Transplant 7:1082–1084, 1992.

1219. Trygvasson K, Zhou J, Hostikka SL, Shows TB: Molecular genetics of Alport syndrome. Kidney Int 43:38, 1993.

1220. Gubler M-C, Antignac C, Deschenes G, et al: Genetic, clinical, and morphologic heterogeneity in Alport's syndrome. Adv Nephrol Necker Hosp 22:15–35, 1993.

1221. Tishler PV: Hereditary nephritis. Ann Intern Med 89:285, 1978.

1222. Grünfeld J-P, Bois EP, Hinglais N: Progressive and non-progressive hereditary chronic nephritis. Kidney Int 4:216, 1973.

1223. Rogers PW, Kurtzman NA, Bunn SM, White MG: Familial benign essential hematuria. Arch Intern Med 131:257, 1976.

1224. Grünfeld J-P: The clinical spectrum of hereditary nephritis. Kidney Int 27:83, 1985.

1225. Zollinger HU, Mihatsch MJ: Renal Pathology in Biopsy: Light Electron and Immunofluorescent Microscopy and Clinical Aspects. Springer-Verlag, Berlin, 1978, p 466.

1226. Rumpelt HJ: Hereditary nephropathy (Alport's syndrome): Spectrum and development of glomerular lesions. In Rosen S (ed): Pathology of Glomerular Disease. Churchill Livingstone, New York, 1983, p 225.

1227. Gaboardi F, Edefonti A, Imbusciati E, et al: Alport's syndrome (progressive hereditary nephritis). Clin Nephrol 2:143, 1974.

1228. Harris JP, Ralcowski TA, Argy WP Jr, Schreiner GE: Alport's syndrome presenting as crescentic glomerulonephritis: A report of two siblings. Clin Nephrol 10:245, 1978.

1229. Neustein HB, O'Brien JS, Rosser RJ, Fillerup DL: Chronic nephritis and renal foam cells: Cholesterol ester storage. Arch Pathol 93:503, 1972.

1230. McCoy RC, Johnson HK, Stone WJ, Wilson CB: Absence of nephritogenic GBM antigen(s) in some patients with hereditary nephritis. Kidney Int 21:642, 1982.

1231. Milliner DS, Pierides AM, Holley KE: Renal transplantation in Alport's syndrome: Anti-glomerular basement membrane glomerulonephritis in the allograft. Mayo Clin Proc 57:35, 1982.

1232. Olson DL, Anand SK, Landing BH, et al: Diagnosis of hereditary nephritis by failure of glomeruli to bind anti–glomerular basement membrane antibodies. J Pediatr 96:697, 1980.

1233. Melvin T, Kim Y, Michael AF: Amyloid P component is not present in the glomerular basement membrane in Alport-type hereditary nephritis. Am J Pathol 125:460, 1986.

1234. Kashtan C, Fish AJ, Kleppel M, et al: Nephritogenic antigen determinants in epidermal and renal basement membranes of kindreds hereditary nephritis. Am J Pathol 125:460, 1986.

1235. Churg J, Sherman RL: Pathologic characteristics of hereditary nephritis. Arch Pathol 95:374, 1973.

1236. Spear GS, Slusser RJ: Alport's syndrome, emphasizing electron microscopic studies of the glomerulus. Am J Pathol 69:213, 1972.

1237. Rumpelt HJ, Langer KH, Scharer K, et al: Split and extremely thin glomerular basement membranes in hereditary nephropathy (Alport's syndrome). Virchows Arch [A] 364:225, 1974.

1238. Basta-Jovanovic G, Venkataseshan VS, Churg J: Correlation of glomerular basement membrane alterations with clinical data in progressive hereditary nephritis (Alport's syndrome). Am J Kidney Dis 16:51–56, 1990.

1239. Bernstein J: The glomerular basement membrane abnormality in Alport's syndrome. Am J Kidney Dis 10:222, 1987.

1240. Hill GS, Jenis EH, Goodloe S Jr: The nonspecificity of the ultrastructural alterations in hereditary nephritis with additional observation on benign familial hematuria. Lab Invest 31:516, 1974.

1241. Kohaut EC, Singer DB, Nevels BK, Hill LL: The specificity of split renal membranes in hereditary nephritis. Arch Pathol Lab Med 100:475, 1976.

1242. Beathard GA, Granholm NA: Development of the characteristic ultrastructural lesion of hereditary nephritis during the course of the disease. Am J Med 62:751, 1977.

1243. Rumpelt HJ, Steinke A, Thoenes W: Alport-type glomerulopathy: Evidence for diminished capillary loop size. Clin Nephrol 37:57, 1992.

1244. Hostikka SL, Eddy RL, Byers MG, et al: Identification of a distinct type IV collagen a chain with restricted kidney distribution and assignment of its gene to the locus of X-chromosome–linked Alport syndrome. Proc Natl Acad Sci USA 87:1606, 1990.

1245. Barker DF, Hostikka SL, Zhou J, et al: Identification of mutations in the COL4A5 collagen gene in Alport syndrome. Science 248:1224, 1990.

1246. Kleppel MM, Kashtan C, Santi PA, et al: Distribution of familial nephritis antigen in normal tissue and renal basement membranes of patients with homozygous and heterozygous Alport familial nephritis: Relationships of familial nephritis and Goodpasture antigens to novel collagen chains and type IV collagen. Lab Invest 61:278–289, 1989.

1247. Knebelmann B, Antignac C, Gubler MC, Grünfeld JP: Molecular genetics of Alport syndrome: The clinical consequences. Nephrol Dial Transplant 8:677–679, 1993.

1248. Netzer KO, Renders L, Zhou J, et al: Deletions of the COL4A5 gene in patients with Alport syndrome. Kidney Int 42:1336–1344, 1992.

1249. Kalluri R, Weber M, Netzer K, et al: COL4A5 gene deletion and production of post-transplant anti-α3(IV) collagen alloantibodies in Alport syndrome. Kidney Int 45:721–726, 1994.

1250. Kashtan CE, Kim Y: Distribution of the α1 and α2 chains of collagen IV and of collagens V and VI in Alport syndrome. Kidney Int 42:115–126, 1992.

1251. Hudson BG, Kalluri R, Gunwar S, et al: The pathogenesis of Alport syndrome involves type IV collagen molecules containing the α3(IV) chain: Evidence from anti-GBM nephritis after renal transplantation. Kidney Int 42:179, 1992.

1252. Van den Heuvel LPWJ, Savage COS, Wong M, et al: The glomerular basement membrane defect in Alport-type hereditary nephritis: Absence of cationic antigenic components. Nephrol Dial Transplant 4:770–775, 1989.

1253. Pochet JM, Bobrie G, Landais P, et al: Renal prognosis in Alport's and related syndromes: Influence of the mode of inheritance. Nephrol Dial Transplant 4:1016–1021, 1989.

1254. Yoshikawa N, White RHR, Cameron AH: Familial hematuria: Clinicopathological correlations. Clin Nephrol 17:172, 1982.

1255. Kashtan CE, Butkowski RJ, Kleppel M, et al: Posttransplant anti–glomerular basement membrane nephritis in related males with Alport syndrome. J Lab Clin Med 116:508, 1990.

1256. Göbel J, Olbricht CJ, Offner G, et al: Kidney transplantation in Alport's syndrome: Long-term outcome and allograft anti-GBM nephritis. Clin Nephrol 38:299, 1992.

1257. Peter E, Pirson Y, Cosyns J-P, et al: Outcome of thirty patients with Alport's syndrome after renal transplantation. Transplantation 52:832, 1991.

1258. Goldman M, Depierreux M, De Pauw L, et al: Failure of two subsequent renal grafts by anti-GBM glomerulonephritis in Alport's syndrome: Case report and review of the literature. Transpl Int 3:82, 1990.

1259. Oliver TB, Gouldesbrough DR, Swainson CP: Acute crescentic glomerulonephritis associated with antiglomerular basement membrane antibody in Alport's syndrome after second transplantation. Nephrol Dial Transplant 6:893–895, 1991.

1260. Rogers PW, Kurtzman NA, Bunn SM Jr, White MG: Familial benign essential hematuria. Arch Intern Med 131:257, 1973.

1261. Tina LU, Jenis E, Jose P, et al: The glomerular basement membrane in benign familial hematuria. Clin Nephrol 17:1, 1982.

1262. Piel CF, Biava CG, Goodman JR: Glomerular basement membrane alteration in familial nephritis and "benign" hematuria. J Pediatr 101:359, 1982.

1263. Fabry J: Ein Beitrag zur Kenntnis der Purpura Hemorrhagica nodularis (Purpura papulosa Hemorrhagica Hebrae). Arch Dermatol 43:187, 1898.

1264. Gubler MC, Lenoir G, Grünfeld J-P, et al: Early renal changes in homozygous and heterozygous patients with Fabry's disease. Kidney Int 13:223, 1978.

1265. Desnick RJ, Allen KY, Desnick SJ, et al: Fabry's disease: Enzymatic diagnosis of hemizygotes and heterozygotes. J Lab Clin Med 81:157, 1973.

1266. Desnick RJ, Astrin KH, Bishop DF: Fabry disease: Molecular genetics of the inherited nephropathy. Adv Nephrol 18:113–128, 1989.

1267. Morgan SH: Anderson-Fabry disease and other inherited metabolic storage disorders with significant renal involvement. In Cameron S, Davison J, Grünfeld JP, Ritz E (eds): Oxford Textbook of Clinical Nephrology. Oxford Medical Publishers, London, 1992.

1268. Shows TB, Brown JA, Halley LL, et al: Assignment of alpha galactosidase gene to the q22qter region of the X-chromosome in man. Cytogenet Cell Genet 22:541, 1978.

1269. Bishop DF, Kornreich R, Eng CE, et al: Human alpha-galactosidase: Characterization and eukaryotic expression of the full-length cDNA and structural organization of the gene. *In* Salvayre R, Douste-Blazy L, Gatt S (eds): Lipid Storage Disorders: Biological and Medical Aspects. New York, Plenum Publishing, 1988, pp 809–822.

1270. Kornreich R, Desnic RJ, Bishop DF: Nucleotide sequences of the human alpha-galactosidase A gene. Nucleic Acids Res 17:3301, 1989.

1271. Bernstein HS, Bishop DF, Astrin KH, et al: Fabry disease: Six gene rearrangements and an exonic point mutation in the alpha galacto-sidase gene. J Clin Invest 83:1390, 1989.

1272. Kornreich R, Bishop DF, Desnick RJ: Alpha galactosidase A gene rearrangements causing Fabry disease. J Biol Chem 265:9319, 1990.

1273. Sakuraba H, Oshima A, Fujuhara Y, et al: Identification of point mutations in the alpha galactosidase A gene in classical and atypi-cal hemizygotes with Fabry disease. Am J Hum Genet 47:784, 1990.

1274. Ishii S, Sakuraba H, Shimmoto M, et al: Fabry disease: Detection of 13-bp deletion in alpha-galactosidase A gene and its application to gene diagnosis of heterozygotes. Ann Neurol 29:560, 1991.

1275. Abreo K, Oberley TD, Gilbert EF, et al: A 29-year-old man with recurrent episodes of fever, abdominal pain and vomiting. Am J Med Genet 18:249, 1984.

1276. Davison DM: Case reports of the Massachusetts General Hospital. N Engl J Med 310:106, 1984.

1277. Kramer W, Thormann J, Mueller K, Frenzel H: Progressive cardiac involvement by Fabry's disease despite successful renal allotrans-plantation. Int J Cardiol 7:72, 1985.

1278. Desnick RJ, Sweeley CC: Fabry's disease: Alpha-galactosidase A deficiency. *In* Stanbury JB, Wyngaarden JB, Fredrickson DS, et al (eds): The Metabolic Basis of Inherited Disease, 5th ed. McGraw-Hill, New York, 1983, p 906.

1279. Farge D, Nadler S, Wolfe LS, et al: Diagnostic value of kidney biopsy in heterozygous Fabry's disease. Arch Pathol Lab Med 109:85, 1985.

1280. Rodriguez F, Hoffman ED, Ordinario AT, Baliga M: Fabry's dis-ease in a heterozygous woman. Arch Pathol Lab Med 109:89, 1985.

1281. Wherret JR, Hakomori S: Characterization of blood group B gly-colipid, accumulating in the pancreas of a patient with Fabry's disease. J Biol Chem 218:3046, 1973.

1282. Ferraggiana T, Churg J, Grishman E, et al: Light- and electron-microscopic histochemistry of Fabry's disease. Am J Pathol 103:247, 1981.

1283. Burkholder PM, Updike SJ, Ware RA, Reese DG: Clinicopatho-logic, enzymatic, and genetic features in a case of Fabry's disease. Arch Pathol Lab Med 104:17, 1980.

1284. Philippart M, Franklin SS, Gordon A: Reversal of an inborn sphin-golipoidosis (Fabry's disease) by kidney transplantation. Ann Intern Med 77:195, 1972.

1285. Clarke JTR, Guttman RD, Wolfe LS, et al: Enzyme replacement therapy by renal allotransplantation in Fabry's disease. N Engl J Med 287:1215, 1972.

1286. Wilson RE: Transplantation in patients with unusual causes of renal failure. Clin Nephrol 5:51, 1976.

1287. Vanden Berg FA, Rietra PJ, Kolk-Vegter AJ, et al: Therapeutic implications of renal transplantation in a patient with Fabry's dis-ease. Acta Med Scand 200:249, 1976.

1288. Berty RM, Adler S, Basu A, Glew RH: Effect of acid-base changes on urinary hydrolases in Fabry's disease after renal transplantation. J Lab Clin Med 115:696–703, 1990.

1289. Helin I: Fabry's disease: A brief review in connection with a Scan-dinavian survey. Scand J Urol Nephrol 13:335, 1979.

1290. Maizel SE, Simmons RL, Kjellstrand C, Fryd DS: Ten-year expe-rience in renal transplantation for Fabry's disease. Transplant Proc 13:57, 1981.

1291. Donati D, Sabbadini MG, Capsoni F, et al: Immune function and renal transplantation in Fabry's disease. Proc Eur Dial Transplant Assoc 21:686, 1984.

1292. Muth RG: The nephropathy of hereditary osteo-onychodysplasia. Ann Intern Med 62:1270, 1965.

1293. Barratt TM: Congenital nephrotic syndrome. *In* Cameron S, Davi-son J, Grünfeld JP, Ritz E (eds): Oxford Textbook of Clinical Nephrology. Oxford Medical Publishers, London, 1992, pp 2218–2220.

1294. Ben-Bassat M, Cohen L, Rosenfeld J: The glomerular basement membrane in nail-patella syndrome. Arch Pathol 72:350, 1971.

1295. Hoyer JR, Michael AF, Vernier RL, Sisson S: Renal disease in nail-patella syndrome: Clinical and morphologic studies. Kidney Int 2:231, 1972.

1296. Bennett WM, Musgrave JE, Campbell RA, et al: The nephropathy of the nail-patella syndrome: Clinicopathologic analysis of 11 kindreds. Am J Med 54:304, 1973.

1297. Morita T, Laughlin LO, Kawano K, et al: Nail-patella syndrome: Light and electron microscopic studies of the kidney. Arch Intern Med 131:217, 1973.

1298. Schleutermann DA, Bias WB, et al: Linkage of the loci for the nail patella syndrome and adenylate kinase. Am J Hum Genet 21:606, 1969.

1299. Renwick JH, Lawler SD: Genetical linkage between the ABO and the nail patella loci. Ann Hum Genet 19:312, 1955.

1300. Mackay IG, Doig A, Thomson D: Membranous nephropathy in a patient with nail-patella syndrome nephropathy. Scott Med J 30:47, 1985.

1301. Curtis JJ, Bhathena D, Leack RP, et al: Goodpasture's syndrome in a patient with the nail-patella syndrome. Am J Med 61:401, 1976.

1302. Sutcliffe NP, Cashman SJ, Savage COS, et al: Variability of the antigenicity of the glomerular basement membrane in nail-patella syndrome. Nephrol Dial Transplant 4:262, 1989.

1303. Looij BJ Jr, Slaa RL, Hogewind BL, et al: Genetic counselling in hereditary osteo-onychodysplasia with nephropathy. J Med Genet 25:682, 1988.

1304. Verdich J: Nail-patella syndrome associated with renal failure re-quiring transplantation. Acta Derm Venereol (Stockh) 60:440, 1980.

1305. Hoyer JR, Anderson CE: Congenital nephrotic syndrome. Clin Per-inatol 8:333, 1981.

1306. Norio R: Heredity in the congenital nephrotic syndrome: A genetic study of 57 Finnish families with a review of reported cases. Ann Pediatr Finn 9(suppl 27):94, 1966.

1307. Hallman N, Norio R, Kouvalainen K: Main features of the congen-ital nephrotic syndrome. Acta Paediatr Scand Suppl 172:75, 1967.

1308. Sibley R, Mahan J, Mauer S, Vernier R: A clinicopathologic study of forty-eight infants with nephrotic syndrome. Kidney Int 27:544, 1985.

1309. Mahan JD, Mauer SM, Sibley RK: Congenital nephrotic syndrome: Evolution of medical management and results of renal transplanta-tion. J Pediatr 105:549, 1984.

1310. Harris HW Jr, Umetsu D, Geha R, Harmon WE: Altered immuno-globulin status in congenital nephrotic syndrome. Clin Nephrol 25:308, 1986.

1311. Rouslatti E: Congenital nephrotic syndrome: Prenatal diagnosis and genetic counselling by estimation of amniotic fluid and maternal serum alpha-fetoprotein. Lancet 2:123, 1976.

1312. Milunsky A, Alpert E, Frigoletto FD, et al: Prenatal diagnosis of congenital nephrotic syndrome. Pediatrics 59:770, 1977.

1313. Wiggelinkjiuzen J, Nelson MM, Berger GMB, Kaschula ROC: Alpha-fetoprotein in the antenatal diagnosis of the congenital ne-phrotic syndrome. J Pediatr 89:452, 1976.

1314. Thom H, Johnstone ED, Gibson JI, et al: Fetal proteinuria in diag-nosis of congenital nephrosis detected by raised alpha-fetoprotein in maternal serum. Br Med J 1:16, 1977.

1315. Vernier RL, Klein DJ, Sisson SP, et al: Heparan sulfate–rich an-ionic sites in the human glomerular basement membrane: decreased concentration in congenital nephrotic syndrome. N Engl J Med 309:1001, 1983.

1316. Laine J, Jalanko H, Holthofer H, et al: Post-transplantation nephro-sis in congenital nephrotic syndrome of the Finnish type. Kidney Int 44:867–874, 1993.

1317. Habib R, Gubler M-C, Antignac C, Gagnadoux M-F: Diffuse mes-angial sclerosis: A congenital glomerulopathy with nephrotic syn-drome. Adv Nephrol Necker Hosp 22:43–57, 1993.

1318. Melocoton TL, Salusky IB, Hall TR, et al: A case report of Drash syndrome in a 46,XX female. Am J Kidney Dis 18:503–508, 1991.

1319. Cohen AH, Turner MC: Kidney in Galloway-Mowat syndrome: Clinical spectrum with description of pathology. Kidney Int 45:1407–1415, 1994.

1320. Joh K, Usui N, Aizawa S, et al: Focal segmental glomerulosclerosis associated with infantile spasms in five mentally retarded children: A morphological analysis of mesangiolysis. Am J Kidney Dis 17:569–577, 1991.

1321. Boganovic R, Komar P, Cvoric A, et al: Focal glomerular sclerosis and nephrotic syndrome in spondyloepiphyseal dysplasia. Nephron 66:219–224, 1994.

1322. Buckalew VM Jr: Sickle cell nephropathy. *In* Robinson RR (ed): Nephrology. Springer-Verlag, New York, 1984, p 916.

1323. Falk R, Jennette JC: Sickle cell nephropathy. Adv Nephrol Necker Hosp 23:133–146, 1994.

1324. Falk RJ, Scheinman J, Phillips G, et al: Prevalence and pathologic features of sickle cell nephropathy and response to inhibition of angiotensin-converting enzyme. N Engl J Med 326:910–915, 1992.

1325. Thomas AN, Pattison C, Serjeant GR: Causes of death in sickle-cell disease in Jamaica. Br Med J 285:633–635, 1982.

1326. Bhathena DB, Sondheimer JH: The glomerulopathy of homozygous sickle hemoglobin disease: Morphology and pathogenesis. J Am Soc Nephrol 1:1241–1252, 1991.

1327. Chatterjee SN: National study on natural history of renal allografts in sickle cell disease or trait. Transplant Proc 21(suppl):33, 1987.

1328. Gonzales-Carillo M, Rudge CJ, Parsons V, et al: Renal transplantation in sickle cell disease. Clin Nephrol 18:209, 1982.

1329. Effenbeing IB, Patchefsky A, Schwartz W, Weinstein AG: Pathology of the glomerulus in sickle cell anemia with and without nephrotic syndrome. Am J Pathol 77:357, 1974.

1330. McCoy RC: Ultrastructural alterations in the kidney of patients with sickle cell disease and the nephrotic syndrome. Lab Invest 21:85, 1969.

1331. Pardo V, Strauss J, Kramer H, et al: Nephropathy associated with sickle cell anemia: Autologous immune complex nephritis: II. Clinicopathologic study of seven patients. Am J Med 59:650, 1975.

1332. Ozawa T, Mass M, Guggenheim S, et al: Autologous immune complex nephritis associated with sickle cell trait: Diagnosis of the haemoglobinopathy after renal structural and immunological studies. Br Med J 1:369, 1976.

1333. Spector D, Zachary JB, Sterioff S, Millan J: Painful crises following renal transplantation in sickle cell anemia. Am J Med 64:835, 1978.

1334. Mitchel SW: Singular case of absence of adipose matter in upper half of the body. Am J Med Sci 90:105, 1985.

1335. Lawrence RD: Lipodystrophy and hepatomegaly with diabetes, lipemia, and other metabolic disturbances. Lancet 1:724, 773, 1946.

1336. Senior B, Gellis SS: The syndromes of total lipodystrophy and partial lipodystrophy. Pediatrics 33:593, 1964.

1337. McLean RH, Hoenage ID: Partial lipodystrophy and familial C3 deficiency. Hum Pathol 30:149, 1980.

1338. Schwartz R, Schafer IA, Renold AE: Generalized lipoatrophy, hepatic cirrhosis, disturbed carbohydrate metabolism and accelerated growth (lipotrophic diabetes). Am J Med 28:973, 1960.

1339. Cahill J, Waldron S, O'Neill G, Duffy BS: Partial lipodystrophy and renal disease. Ir J Med Sci 152:451, 1983.

1340. Taylor J, Thornes P, Geary D, et al: Nephrotic syndrome and hypertension. Two children with Hurler's syndrome. J Pediatr 108:726, 1986.

1341. Chen YT, Coleman R, Scheinman JI, et al: Renal disease in type I glycogen storage disease. N Engl J Med 318:7, 1988.

1342. Obara K, Saito T, Sato H, et al: Renal histology in two adult patients with type I glycogen storage disease. Clin Nephrol 39:59–64, 1993.

1343. Collan Y, Lahdevirta J, Jokinen EJ: Selective vitamin $B_{12}$ malabsorption with proteinuria. Nephron 23:297, 1979.

1344. Herdman RC, Langer LO: The thoracic asphyxiant dystrophy and renal disease. Am J Dis Child 116:192, 1968.

1345. Marie J, Levéque B, Lyon G, et al: Acro-ostéolyse essential compliqué d'insuffance rénale d'évolution finale. Presse Med 71:249, 1963.

1346. Gjone E: Familial lecithin–cholesterol acyltransferase deficiency: A new metabolic disease with renal involvement. Adv Nephrol 10:167, 1981.

1347. Magil A, Chase W, Frohlich J: Unusual renal biopsy findings in a patient with familial lecithin–cholesterol acyltransferase deficiency. Hum Pathol 13:283, 1982.

1348. Weber P, Owen JS, Desai K, Clemens MR: Hereditary lecithin–cholesterol acyltransferase deficiency. Am J Clin Pathol 88:510, 1987.

1349. Rogne S, Skretting G, Larsen F, et al: The isolation and characterization of a cDNA clone for human lecithin:cholesterol acyltransferase and its use to analyse the genes in patients with LCAT deficiency and fish eye disease. Biochem Biophys Res Commun 148:161–169, 1987.

1350. Humphries SE, Chaves ME, Tata F, et al: A study of the structure of the gene for lecithin: cholesterol acyltransferase in four unrelated individuals with familial lecithin:cholesterol acyltransferase deficiency. Clin Sci 74:91, 1988.

1351. Maeda E, Naka Y, Matozaki T, et al: Lecithin:cholesterol acyltransferase (LCAT) deficiency with a missense mutation in exon 6 of the LCAT gene. Biochem Biophys Res Commun 178:460, 1991.

1352. Gotoda T, Yamada N, Murase T, et al: Differential phenotypic expression by three mutant alleles in familial lecithin:cholesterol acyltransferase deficiency. Lancet 338:778, 1991.

1353. Taramelli R, Pontoglio M, Candiani G, et al: Lecithin:cholesterol acyltransferase deficiency: Molecular analysis of a mutated allele. Hum Genet 85:195, 1990.

1353a. Albers JJ, Adolphson JL, Chen C-H: Radioimmunoassay of human plasma lecithin–cholesterol acyltransferase. J Clin Invest 67:141, 1981.

1353b. Chen C-H, Albers JJ: Characterization of proteolysomes containing apoprotein A-I: A new substitute for the measurement of lecithin–cholesterol acyltransferase activity. J Lipid Res 23:680, 1982.

1354. Murayama N, Asano Y, Hosoda S, et al: Decreased sodium influx and abnormal red cell membrane lipids in a patient with familial lecithins: Cholesterol acyltransferase deficiency. Am J Hematol 16:129, 1984.

1355. Hauglustaine D, Corbeel L, Van Damme B, et al: Glomerulonephritis in late-onset cystinosis: Report of two cases and review of the literature. Clin Nephrol 6:529, 1976.

1356. Scharer K, Manz F: Nephropathic cystinosis. J Nephrol 7:165–174, 1994.

1357. Scolari F, Amoroso A, Savoldi S, et al: Familial occurrence of primary glomerulonephritis: Evidence for a role of genetic factors. Nephrol Dial Transplant 7:587–596, 1992.

1358. Hoehn D: Nephrosis probably due to excessive use of "Sta-Way" insect repellent. JAMA 128:513, 1945.

1359. Heymann W: Nephrotic syndrome after use of trimethadione and paramethadione in petit mal. JAMA 202:893, 1967.

1360. Beattie JW: Nephrotic syndrome following sodium bismuth tartrate therapy in rheumatoid arthritis. Ann Rheum Dis 12:144, 1953.

1361. Richman AV, Masco HL, Rifkin SI, Acharya MK: Minimal change disease and the nephrotic syndrome associated with lithium therapy. Ann Intern Med 92:70, 1980.

1362. Schnall C, Wiener JS: Nephrosis during tolbutamide administration. JAMA 167:214, 1958.

1363. Lange K: Nephropathy induced by D-penicillamine. Clin Nephrol 10:63, 1978.

1364. Hofle KH, Schoop W: Acute nephrotic syndrome caused by Mesantoin treatment. Dtsch Med Wochenschr 84:837, 1959.

1365. Steinbeck AW: Nephrotic syndrome developing after snakebite. Med J Aust 1:543, 1960.

1366. Tait GB: Nephropathy during phenindione therapy. Lancet 2:1198, 1960.

1367. Lee RE, Ulstrom RA, Vernier RL: Nephrotic syndrome as a complication of perchlorate treatment of thyrotoxicosis. N Engl J Med 264:1121, 1961.

1368. Ferris TF, Morgan WS, Levitin H: Nephrotic syndrome caused by probenicid. N Engl J Med 265:381, 1961.

1369. Becker CG, Becker EL, Maher JF, Schreiner GE: Nephrotic syndrome after contact with mercury: A report of five cases, three after use of ammoniated mercury ointment. Arch Intern Med 110:178, 1962.

1370. Hall C, Fothergill N, Blackwell M, et al: The natural course of gold nephropathy: A long-term study in 21 patients. Br Med J 295:745, 1987.

1371. Atero F, Rodriguez-France R, Parano MJ, et al: Nephrotic syndrome after oral gold. Br J Rheum 25:315, 1986. Letter.

1372. Nagi A, Alexander F, Barabas AZ: Gold nephropathy in rats: Light and electron microscopy studies. Exp Mol Pathol 15:354, 1971.

1373. Borra S, Hawkins D, Duquid W, Kaye M: Acute renal failure and nephrotic syndrome after angiocardiography with meglumine diatrizoate. N Engl J Med 284:592, 1971.

1374. Cunningham EE, Brentjens JR, Zielezny MA, et al: Heroin nephropathy: A clinicopathologic and epidemiologic study. Am J Med 68:47, 1980.

1375. Rao TK, Nicastri AD, Friedman EA: Natural history of heroin-associated nephropathy. N Engl J Med 290:19, 1974.

1376. Dubrow A, Mittman N, Ghali V, Flamenbaum W: The changing spectrum of heroin associated nephropathy. Am J Kidney Dis 5:36, 1985.

1377. Kazantzis G, Schiller KFR, Asscher AW, Drew RG: Albuminuria and the nephrotic syndrome following exposure to mercury and its compounds. Q J Med 31:403, 1962.

1378. Yoshida A, Morozumi K, Takeda A, et al: A case of rapidly progressive glomerulonephritis associated with bucillamine-treated rheumatoid arthritis. Am J Kidney Dis 20:411–413, 1992.

1379. Wooley PH, Griffin J, Panayi GS, et al: HLA-DR antigens and toxic reaction to sodium aurothiomalate and D-penicillamine with rheumatoid arthritis. N Engl J Med 303:300, 1980.

1380. Lederer E, Truong L: Unusual glomerular lesion in a patient receiving long-term interferon alpha. Am J Kidney Dis 20:516–518, 1992.

1381. Hebert MJ, Fish D, Madore F, et al: Mesangiolysis associated with bone marrow transplantation: New insights on possible etiologic factors. Am J Kidney Dis 23:882–883, 1994.

1382. Peces R, Riera JR, Arboleya LR: Goodpasture's syndrome in a patient receiving penicillamine and carbimazole. Nephron 45:316, 1987.

1383. Barbara JAJ, Thomas AC, Smith PS, et al: Membranous nephropathy with graft-versus-host disease in a bone marrow transplant recipient. Clin Nephrol 37:115–118, 1992.

1384. Ntoso KA, Tomaszewski JE, Jimenez SA: Penicillamine-induced rapidly progressive glomerulonephritis in patients with progressive systemic sclerosis: Successful treatment of two patients and a review of the literature. Am J Kidney Dis 8:159, 1986.

1385. Santella RN, Rimmer JM, MacPherson BR: Focal segmental glomerulosclerosis in patients receiving lithium carbonate. Am J Med 84:951–954, 1988.

1386. Young JL, Boswell RB, Nies AS: Severe allopurinol hypersensitivity: Association with thiazides and prior renal compromise. Arch Intern Med 134:553, 1979.

1387. Josselson J, Sadler JH: Nephrotic-range proteinuria and hyperglycemia associated with clonidine therapy. Am J Med 80:545–546, 1986.

1388. Prins EJL, Hoorntje SJ, Weening JJ, Donker AJM: Nephrotic syndrome in patients on captopril. Lancet 2:306, 1979.

1389. Webb DJ, Atkinson AB: Enalapril following captopril-induced nephrotic syndrome. Scott Med J 31:30, 1986.

1390. Jackson B, Maher D, Matthews PG, et al: Lack of cross sensitivity between captopril and enalapril. Aust N Z J Med 18:21, 1988.

1391. Murray AN, Cassidy MJ, Templecamp C: Rapidly progressive glomerulonephritis associated with rifampicin therapy for pulmonary tuberculosis. Nephron 46:373, 1987.

1392. Turney JH, Michael J, Adu D: Acute crescentic glomerulonephritis developing during warfarin therapy. Postgrad Med J 62:1159, 1986.

1393. Brezin JH, Katz SM, Schwartz AB, Chinitz JL: Reversible renal failure and nephrotic syndrome associated with non-steroidal anti-inflammatory drugs. N Engl J Med 301:1271, 1979.

1394. Curt GA, Kaldany A, Whitley LG, et al: Reversible rapidly progressive renal failure with nephrotic syndrome due to fenoprofen calcium. Ann Intern Med 92:72, 1980.

1395. Heller M: Nephrotic syndrome associated with sulindac. N Engl J Med 304:424, 1981.

1396. Bender WL, Whelton A, Darwish MO, et al: Interstitial nephritis, proteinuria, and renal failure caused by nonsteroidal anti-inflammatory drugs: Immunologic characterization of the inflammatory infiltrate. Am J Med 76:1006, 1984.

1397. Valles M, Tova JL: Salicylate and minimal-change nephrotic syndrome. Ann Intern Med 107:116, 1987. Letter.

1398. Schwartzman M, D'Agati V: Spontaneous relapse of naproxen-related nephrotic syndrome. Am J Med 82:329, 1987.

1399. Stachura I, Jayakumar S, Bourke E: T and B lymphocyte subsets in fenoprofen nephropathy. Am J Med 75:9, 1983.

1400. Van Buren D, Van Buren CT, Flecher SM, et al: De novo hemolytic uremic syndrome in renal transplant recipient immunosuppressed with cyclosporine. Surgery 98:54, 1985.

1401. Gibson J, Bleasel A, Duggin G, et al: Cyclosporine A–associated proteinuria. Med J Aust 146:325, 1987.

1402. Cameron JS: Recurrent renal disease after renal transplantation. Curr Sci 3:602–607, 1994.

1403. O'Meara Y, Green A, Carmody M, et al: Recurrent glomerulonephritis in renal transplants: Fourteen years' experience. Nephrol Dial Transplant 4:730–734, 1989.

1404. Neumayer HH, Kienbaum M, Graf S, et al: Prevalence and long-term outcome of glomerulonephritis in renal allografts. Am J Kidney Dis 22:320–325, 1993.

1405. Ramos EL, Tisher CC: Recurrent diseases in the kidney transplant. Am J Kidney Dis 24:142–154, 1994.

1406. Heidet L, Gagnadoux MF, Beziau A, et al: Recurrence of de novo membranous glomerulonephritis on renal grafts. Clin Nephrol 41:314–318, 1994.

1407. Suzuki M: Pickwickian syndrome and endocardial fibroclastosis: A possible pathogenetic correlation. Am J Med 53:123, 1972.

1408. Cohen AH: Massive obesity and the kidney: A morphologic and statistical study. Am J Pathol 81:117, 1975.

1409. Wesson DE, Kurtzman N, Frommer J: Massive obesity and nephrotic syndrome with a normal renal biopsy. Nephron 40:235, 1985.

1410. Kisiske B, Crosson JT: Renal disease in patients with massive obesity. Arch Intern Med 146:1105, 1986.

1411. Weisinger JR, Kempson RL, Eldridge FL, Swenson RS: The nephrotic syndrome: A complication by massive obesity. Ann Intern Med 81:440, 1974.

1412. Warnke RA, Kempson RL: The nephrotic syndrome in massive obesity: A study by light, immunofluorescence, and electron microscopy. Arch Pathol Lab Med 102:431, 1978.

1413. Verani RR: Obesity-associated focal segmental glomerulosclerosis: Pathological features of the lesion and relationship with cardiomegaly and hyperlipidemia. Am J Kidney Dis 20:629–634, 1992.

1414. Spear GS: The glomerulus in cyanotic congenital heart disease and primary pulmonary hypertension: A review. Nephron 1:238, 1964.

1415. Ingelfinger JR, Kissane JM, Robson AM: Glomerulomegaly in a patient with cyanotic congenital heart disease. Am J Dis Child 120:69, 1970.

1416. Hagley MT, Murphy DP, Mullins D, Zarconi J: Decline in creatinine clearance in a patient with glomerulomegaly associated with a congenital cyanotic heart disease. Am J Kidney Dis 20:177–179, 1992.

1417. Amigo M-C, Garcia-Torres R, Robles M, et al: Renal involvement in primary antiphospholipid syndrome. J Rheumatol 19:1181–1185, 1992.

1418. Simon LS: Case records of the Massachusetts General Hospital. N Engl J Med 322:754, 1990.

1419. Kiprov DD, Colvin RB, McClusky RT: Focal and segmental glomerulosclerosis and proteinuria associated with unilateral renal agenesis. Lab Invest 46:275, 1982.

1420. Gutierrez-Millet V, Nieto J, Praga M, et al: Focal glomerulosclerosis and proteinuria in patients with solitary kidneys. Arch Intern Med 146:705, 1986.

1421. Eiser AR, Katz SM, Swartz C: Reversible nephrotic range proteinuria with renal artery stenosis: A clinical example of renin-associated proteinuria. Nephron 30:374, 1982.

1422. Helin H, Mustonen J, Reunala T, Pasternack A: IgA nephropathy associated with celiac disease and dermatitis herpetiformis. Arch Pathol Lab Med 107:324, 1983.

1423. Heptinstall RH: Pathology of the Kidney. Little, Brown, Boston, 1983, p 963.

1424. Cameron JS: Glomerulonephritis in renal transplants. Transplantation 34:237, 1982.

1425. Ward HJ, Koyle MA: Immunopathologic features of denovo membranous nephropathy in renal allograft. Transplantation 45:524, 1988.

1426. Blumberg A, Stamm B, Wegmann W, Schaub N: Immune-mediated type A gastritis and glomerulonephritis. Am J Kidney Dis 21:210–212, 1993.

1427. Thomas DM, Nicholls AJ, Feest TG: Ulcerative colitis and glomerulonephritis: Is there an association? Nephrol Dial Transplant 5:628–629, 1990.

1428. Kobayashi S, Nagase M, Hidaka S, et al: Membranous nephropathy associated with hypocomplementemic urticarial vasculitis: Report of two cases and a review of the literature. Nephron 66:1–7, 1994.

1429. Banks DE, Milutinovic J, Desnick RJ, et al: Silicon nephropathy mimicking Fabry's disease. Am J Nephrol 3:279, 1983.

1430. Osorio A, Thun M, Novak RF, et al: Silica and glomerulonephritis: Case report and review of the literature. Am J Kidney Dis 9:224, 1987.

1431. Bonnin A, Mousson C, Justrabo E, et al: Silicosis associated with crescentic glomerulonephritis and IgA mesangial nephropathy. Nephron 47:229, 1987.
1432. Khan IH, Simpson JG, Catto GRD, MacLead AM: Membranous nephropathy and granulomatous interstitial nephritis in sarcoidosis. Nephron 66:459–461, 1994.
1433. Matsuda O, Makiguchi K, Ishibashi K, et al: Long-term effects of steroid treatment on nephrotic syndrome associated with Kimura's disease and a review of the literature. Clin Nephrol 37:119–123, 1992.
1434. Chan TM, Cheng IKP, Wong KL, Chan KW: Resolution of membranoproliferative glomerulonephritis complicating angiofollicular lymph node hyperplasia (Castleman's disease). Nephron 65:628–632, 1993.

# 32

# Urinary Tract Infection, Pyelonephritis, and Reflux Nephropathy

*Robert H. Rubin*
*Ramzi S. Cotran*
*Nina E. Tolkoff-Rubin*

Urinary tract infection (UTI), the most common of all bacterial infections, affects humans throughout their life span. Twenty percent to 35% of all women experience at least one episode of UTI sometime in their lives. UTI occurs in all populations, from the neonate to the geriatric patient, but has a particular impact on females of all ages, males at the two extremes of life, kidney transplant patients, and anyone with functional or structural abnormalities of the urinary excretory system. Because of the wide range of individuals affected and because UTI is frequently superimposed on other medical problems, physicians in virtually all specialties are called on to deal with this clinical problem.[1]

Not only is UTI common, but the range of clinical effects it can produce is exceptionally broad, from acute pyelonephritis with gram-negative sepsis to asymptomatic bacteriuria and even so-called symptomatic abacteriuria. Because the clinical syndromes may vary so much, and the population affected and the physicians who provide care may be equally diverse, a coherent approach to the problem of UTI is essential—an approach that addresses the following questions:

1. What is the pathogenesis of UTI, and how can such pathogenetic events be interrupted?
2. What is the frequency of UTI in different population groups, and what impact does it have on them?

3. How does one best diagnose, prevent, and treat the infectious disease aspects of UTI?
4. Does UTI have any long-term effects on the human host other than direct infectious disease morbidity and mortality? The particular areas of concern are the contributions of UTI to the development of chronic renal disease, hypertension, or both; its effects on longevity and survival; and, finally, its effects on the outcome of pregnancy.

It is the purpose of this chapter to answer these questions and to provide a coherent approach for physicians caring for this most common of genitourinary tract diseases.

## PROBLEMS IN DEFINITION

Generically, pyelonephritis means inflammation of the kidney and its pelvis, but from a historical point of view and through common usage, the term has come to designate a disorder of the kidney resulting from bacterial invasion. This is certainly true in the case of acute pyelonephritis, with its relatively simple histopathologic features—acute interstitial inflammation and tubule cell necrosis. The role of active bacterial infection in chronic pyelonephritis is more complex. Heptinstall,[2] on the basis of Hodson's radiologic studies[3] and their morphologic confirmation by Smith,[4] urged that the term "chronic pyelonephritis" be restricted to cases that show unequivocal evidence of pelvocalyceal inflammation, fibrosis, and deformity. If these criteria are adhered to, it will be found that in the majority of patients with chronic pyelonephritis, the bacterial urinary infection is superimposed on an anatomic urinary tract anomaly, urinary obstruction, or, most commonly, vesicoureteral reflux (VUR).

The point to emphasize, therefore, is that a great variety of etiologic agents can cause chronic tubulointerstitial disease, but it is only when the pyelocalyceal system is involved that bacterial infection seems to play a major role. Further, urinary infection in the absence of an underlying urinary tract abnormality or of VUR infrequently causes serious chronic renal disease.

A few other terms need to be defined. Cystitis refers to infection limited to the bladder. Significant bacteriuria occurs when more than $10^5$ pathogenic bacteria are present per milliliter of urine, with or without symptoms. Asymptomatic bacteriuria is significant bacteriuria without the presence of symptoms requiring medical consultation; a preferable term is covert bacteriuria, defined as significant bacteriuria detected by means of screening or revealed on examination of healthy populations.[5] Reflux nephropathy refers to the renal scarring associated with VUR[6]; although this is frequently caused or accompanied by bacterial infection, some patients are free of bacteriuria when the condition is discovered.

# BACTERIOLOGY OF URINARY TRACT INFECTION

## General Considerations: The Urine Culture

The cornerstone of the approach to patients with possible UTI is the evaluation of the results of a quantitative urine culture. This is due to two factors: on the one hand, there is an incomplete correlation between the clinical symptoms of urinary tract inflammation and the presence of true UTI, so objective evidence of the presence and type of infection is of great importance; on the other hand, there is frequently great difficulty in obtaining a spontaneously voided urine specimen uncontaminated by the normal flora of the distal urethra, vagina, or skin. Therefore, certain guidelines are necessary for evaluating the results of urine cultures.

The first clue to the importance of a positive urine culture report comes from the nature of the organism or organisms isolated on culture. In more than 95% of UTIs, the infecting organism is a gram-negative bacillus, *Enterococcus faecalis,* or, in the case of sexually active women, *Staphylococcus saprophyticus*[7] (Table 32–1). In contrast, the organisms that commonly colonize the distal urethra and skin of both men and women and the vagina of women—*Staphylococcus epidermidis,* diphtheroids, lactobacilli, *Gardnerella vaginalis,* and a variety of anaerobes (Table 32–2)—rarely cause UTI.[8] The problem in interpretation comes from the vaginal contamination in some women, approximately 20% of whom may harbor Enterobacteriaceae in the vagina at any one point in time.[9, 10] In these situations, further information can be gained from the number of different bacterial species identified in the single culture. In

**TABLE 32–1. Bacteriologic Findings Among 250 Outpatients and 150 Inpatients with Urinary Tract Infection**

| Bacterial Species | Outpatients (%) | Inpatients (%) |
|---|---|---|
| *Escherichia coli* | 89.2 | 52.7 |
| *Proteus mirabilis* | 3.2 | 12.7 |
| *Klebsiella pneumoniae* | 2.4 | 9.3 |
| Enterococci | 2.0 | 7.3 |
| *Enterobacter aerogenes* | 0.8 | 4.0 |
| *Pseudomonas aeruginosa* | 0.4 | 6.0 |
| *Proteus* species (excluding P. mirabilis) | 0.4 | 3.3 |
| *Serretia marcescens* | 0.0 | 3.3 |
| *Staphylococcus epidermidis** | 1.6 | 0.7 |
| *Staphylococcus aureus* | 0.0 | 0.7 |

*It is likely that most of the outpatient *S. epidermidis* strains in healthy, sexually active young women were *S. saprophyticus.*
Modified from Rubin RH: Infections of the urinary tract. Scientific American Medicine, Dale DC, Federman DD, Eds. Section 7, Subsection XXIII. © 1995 Scientific American, Inc. All rights reserved.

more than 95% of true UTIs, a single bacterial species is responsible for the infection. Polymicrobial infection can be present in a few clinical situations: when a long-term urinary catheter or other foreign body (e.g., necrotic tumors, stones) is in place, when the patient has a neurogenic bladder, or when there is a fistulous communication between the urinary tract and the gastrointestinal or genital tracts. Otherwise, the isolation of two or more bacterial species on urine culture usually signifies a contaminated specimen.[6]

Microscopic examination of the urine at the time of clinical presentation can yield important information that can be helpful in the interpretation of urine cultures. Examination of a drop of urine that has been stained with Gram stain is particularly helpful. The finding of at least one organism per oil immersion field has a 95% sensitivity for detecting bacteriuria at a level of $10^5$ colony-forming units (CFUs) per milliliter or greater; a finding of more than five organisms has a 95% specificity.[11] On urinalysis, the presence of squamous epithelial cells strongly suggests contamination and the need for a repeated specimen. The finding of pyuria on urinalysis can also be helpful if the appropriate technique for demonstrating pyuria is employed. The usual method for measuring the number of leukocytes in the urine is to count the number of white blood cells present per high-power field in the resuspended sediment of a centrifuged aliquot of urine. With use of this method, as many as 50% of patients with significant bacteriuria will not have

**TABLE 32–2. Common Bacterial Contaminants of Urine Cultures That Are Unlikely Causes of True Urinary Tract Infections**

*Staphylococcus epidermidis*
Corynebacteria (diphtheroids)
*Lactobacillus*
*Gardnerella vaginalis*
Anaerobic bacteria

pyuria (>five leukocytes per high-power field),[12] with a coefficient of variation of approximately 40%.[13] In contrast, Mabeck[14] has used leukocyte excretion rates for a period of 3 hours and has found a high correlation between a leukocyte excretion rate of more than 400,000 cells/h and the presence of significant bacteriuria.

The leukocyte excretion rate is too cumbersome for routine clinical use, but several studies have shown that a positive leukocyte excretion test result correlates well with the finding of more than 10 leukocytes/mm³ when a randomly collected urine specimen is examined in a counting chamber (such as a hemocytometer) and the number of leukocytes is determined.[15, 16] Using this simple method for enumerating leukocytes in the urine of individuals suspected of harboring UTI (which has a coefficient of variation of approximately 4%[13]), Stamm[17] has noted the following: 1) More than 96% of symptomatic men and women with significant bacteriuria have more than 10 leukocytes/mm³ in their urine; less than 1% of asymptomatic, nonbacteriuric individuals have such evidence of pyuria. 2) Most symptomatic women with pyuria but without significant bacteriuria have urinary infection with either bacterial uropathogens present in colony counts of less than 10⁵/mL of urine or *Chlamydia trachomatis*. 3) Individuals, particularly women, with asymptomatic bacteriuria probably should be divided into two subgroups: those with true asymptomatic infection (associated with pyuria) and those with transient, self-limited bladder colonization. 4) Catheterized patients with bacteriuria and pyuria have true infection. Thus, the presence or absence of pyuria in an aliquot of the same urine submitted to culture can be an extremely useful parameter, provided that the appropriate technique is employed to test for it.

The other major criterion for determining the validity of culture results is the number of CFUs found per milliliter of urine cultured. Kass[18, 19] and Savage and associates[20] made a major contribution to this field by demonstrating that quantitative culturing of the urine allowed the separation of individuals into two populations: those who consistently had large numbers of bacteria in their urine (>10⁵ CFU/mL) and experienced morbidity on that basis; and those with few bacteria in their urine ("insignificant bacteriuria"), which were contaminants. For example, in patients with clinically manifested pyelonephritis, more than 10⁵ CFU/mL are found in more than 80%.[6, 18, 21] When patients with bacteremic pyelonephritis were considered, it was found that 82% had more than 10⁵ CFU/mL; 12% had between 10⁴ and 10⁵ CFU/mL; and the remainder had fewer bacteria in the urine.[22] When a single species of gram-negative bacillus is isolated in numbers greater than 10⁵ CFU/mL, true infection is confirmed in 92% of instances; in contrast, such confirmation is made in only 70% of instances of gram-positive isolates. Isolation of 10³ to 10⁵ organisms/mL represents true infection in 74% of patients with gram-negative isolates but in only 30% of those with gram-positive isolates.[23] Overall, as many as 20% to 30% of individuals with true bacterial UTIs will have 10³ to 10⁵ CFU/mL, the great majority of these with lower UTI (as opposed to pyelonephritis).[24–26]

The circumstances associated with lower densities of bacteria being found in the urine when the patient has true infection include the acute urethral syndrome, antibacterial chemotherapy, rapid diuresis, extreme acidification of the urine, obstruction of the urinary tract, extraluminal infection, and infection caused by fastidious organisms.[19, 24–28] Clinically, the acute urethral syndrome and rapid diuresis account for the majority of such cases.

## Etiologic Agents

### BACTERIAL PATHOGENS

As discussed subsequently, the usual mechanism by which bacteria invade the urinary tract is by the ascending route, with the gastrointestinal tract being the reservoir from which the bacteria emerge. Not surprisingly, then, the Enterobacteriaceae and *E. faecalis* are the most important causes of UTI in all population groups, accounting for more than 95% of all UTIs. Of the Enterobacteriaceae, *Escherichia coli* is by far the most common invader, causing some 90% of UTIs in outpatients and approximately 50% in hospitalized patients (see Table 32–1). The likelihood of a non–*E. coli* UTI or the possibility that the bacterial isolate will be antibiotic resistant is influenced by three major factors: whether the flora of the gastrointestinal tract reservoir has been modified, whether the urinary tract has been instrumented, and whether structural or functional obstruction of the urinary tract is present. Thus, in Table 32–1, there is a shift to the non–*E. coli* and more antibiotic resistant organisms as one moves from outpatient to hospitalized patients. Hospitalized patients usually have their gastrointestinal flora modified by their environmental exposure to such organisms as *Serratia marcescens* and *Pseudomonas aeruginosa* and by frequent treatment with broad-spectrum antimicrobial agents, and they may have been subjected to urinary tract instrumentation (as with Foley catheters) at a relatively high rate. Obviously, these adverse prognostic factors are much more common in hospitalized patients than in outpatients.[6, 29]

In addition, certain bacterial pathogens are especially associated with UTI in a particular population group. One notable example is the recognition that *S. saprophyticus* is an important cause of symptomatic UTI in young, sexually active women.[30–33] *S. saprophyticus* is an uncommon cause of infection in men.[34] Other associations that have been reported include an increased frequency of *Proteus* infections in boys aged 1 to 12 years, and *E. faecalis* infection in elderly men with prostatism.[35] Because of the urea-splitting properties of *Proteus,* chronic infection with these organisms leads to an alkaline urine and promotes the occurrence of struvite stones.[35, 36]

Although the aerobic fecal flora are the important pathogens for the urinary tract, it is less clear what role, if any, anaerobic bacteria play in UTI.[37] It is clear that anaerobes, particularly gram-positive ones, are present in the distal urethra of both sexes,[7, 38, 39] so associations with clinical disease must be made with great care. One association that does appear convincing is that between the presence of true anaerobic UTI and anatomic obstruction,[34, 40, 41] especially obstruction due to malignant disease. Thus, *Bacteroides* sepsis has been found to be frequent in malignant disease of the genitourinary tract.[42] Presumably, colonizing anaerobes from the gastrointestinal tract and distal urethra are frequently introduced into the bladder but fail to establish sustained infection unless the normal host defenses (see later) of the urinary tract have been significantly altered.[43] The local anaerobic environment associated with malignant disease would presumably provide an especially favorable condition for invasive infection with anaerobic bacterial species.

In more than 95% of instances, UTI develops through the ascending route, from urethra to bladder to kidney. However, if bacteremia occurs from some other site, seeding of the urinary tract, particularly the kidney, can occur, with the most common manifestation being a positive urine culture. Renal abscesses (usually with *Staphylococcus aureus*) can also be initiated in this fashion. Hematogenous seeding of the urinary tract is particularly characteristic of such virulent organisms as *S. aureus, P. aeruginosa,* and *Salmonella* species; indeed, a positive urine culture may be the first laboratory evidence of disseminated infection due to these organisms.[6, 29] Hematogenously derived infection of the urinary tract is particularly common in instances of *Salmonella* sepsis. Thus, approximately 25% of patients with *Salmonella typhi* infection have positive urine cultures.[44] An unusual example of this phenomenon occurs in areas of the world where urinary tract schistosomiasis due to *Schistosoma haematobium* is common. In such patients, bacteremic seeding of the urinary tract with *Salmonella* species results in infection of the schistosomes and chronic *Salmonella* bacteriuria. Re-entry to the bloodstream by the salmonella from the seeded urinary tract can then occur on a regular basis. Interestingly, such infections can be controlled only by eradicating the schistosomal infection first.[44, 45]

Other bacteria that have been unusual causes of hematogenous UTI include *Brucella,*[46] *Nocardia,*[47] and *Actinomyces* species.[48] Far more important are cases of urinary tract tuberculosis. The kidney is the most common extrapulmonary site of tuberculosis; the tubercle bacilli reach the kidney from the lung by the hematogenous route, usually with later spread down the urinary tract to the ureter, bladder, and, in the male patient, prostate, seminal vesicle, and epididymis.[49]

## FUNGAL PATHOGENS

By far the most frequent form of fungal infection of the urinary tract is that caused by *Candida species.* Most such infection occurs in patients with indwelling Foley catheters who have been receiving broad-spectrum antibacterial therapy, particularly when diabetes mellitus is also present or corticosteroids are being administered. Although the great majority of these infections remain limited to the bladder and clear with removal of the catheter, cessation of the antibacterial therapy, and control of the diabetes, the urinary tract is the source of approximately 10% of episodes of candidemia—usually in association with urinary tract manipulation or obstruction.[50, 51] Spontaneously occurring lower UTI due to *Candida* species is far less common, although papillary necrosis, calyceal invasion, and fungal ball obstruction have all been described as resulting from ascending candidal UTI not related to catheterization. Candidal obstructive uropathy is particularly important in children with congenital anatomic abnormalities of the urinary tract and in kidney transplant recipients.[51–54] In the transplant patient, obstructive uropathy due to candiduria is a particularly dangerous situation, being associated with a high risk of systemic dissemination from the urinary tract.[55]

The urinary tract is more commonly the site of metastatic spread in cases of disseminated candidiasis than the portal of entry from which dissemination spreads. Indeed, as with hematogenously spread bacterial infection, the appearance of *Candida* species, particularly *C. albicans* or *C. tropicalis,* in the urine of a nonpregnant, nondiabetic, noncatheterized individual can be an early warning of disseminated candidiasis.[56] Other *Candida* species and the closely related yeast *Torulopsis glabrata* are less invasive for the urinary tract but can on occasion cause catheter-related UTI and, less commonly, focal pyelonephritis or disseminated infection.[57]

Similarly, hematogenous spread to the kidney and other sites within the genitourinary tract may be seen in any systemic fungal infection, but particularly coccidioidomycosis[58] and blastomycosis.[59, 60] In coccidioidomycosis, renal seeding is more common; in blastomycosis, lower genitourinary tract involvement is the rule. Among immunosuppressed patients, a common hallmark of disseminated cryptococcal infection is the appearance of this organism in the urine. In addition, *Cryptococcus neoformans* may cause a syndrome of papillary necrosis, pyelonephritis, and pyuria akin to that seen in tuberculosis.[61] Thus, in the appropriate clinical and epidemiologic settings, the possibility of hematogenous seeding with a variety of fungal organisms should be considered in addition to tuberculosis and chlamydial infection (see later) in patients with bacteriologically sterile pyuria.

## OTHER PATHOGENS

Several other classes of microorganisms can invade the urinary tract, most notably *C. trachomatis,* the genital mycoplasmas, and certain viruses. *C. trachomatis* has been clearly shown to be an important cause of the acute urethral syndrome (see later).[25, 27] Whether this organism could have an impact on the upper urinary tract remains to be demonstrated.

The two genital mycoplasmas are *Ureaplasma urealyticum* (formerly called T-strain mycoplasma) and *Mycoplasma hominis.* Both have been associated more with genital infection than with UTI, but *U. urealyticum* does cause a significant number of cases of urethritis (albeit fewer than *C. trachomatis*)[62] and both have been implicated as causes of chronic pyelonephritis,[63] although this remains controversial.[64] Perhaps the best argument that these organisms may play a role in upper UTI is the report of the association of *U. urealyticum* with renal stones.[65]

A variety of viruses can have an impact on the urinary tract, either in association with glomerular disease or, most commonly, associated with asymptomatic viral excretion. For the purposes of this chapter, two groups of viruses are of importance because they can mimic some of the effects of bacterial and fungal infection. Adenovirus types 11 and 21, particularly type 11, have been shown to cause between one fourth and one half of cases of hemorrhagic cystitis in schoolchildren.[66] They appear to have less of an impact on adults. Rosen and associates[67] have described a 6-year-old boy with hyperimmunoglobulin M immunodeficiency who had chronic renal failure secondary to tubulointerstitial nephritis associated with the presence of BK polyomavirus in the renal parenchyma and the urine. This finding and previous observations[55, 68] demonstrating a high frequency of BK viruria, possibly associated with the development of ureteral stenosis, in kidney transplant patients suggest that this virus could cause a variety of effects on the kidney and uroepithelium in immunosuppressed patients. In addition, there is a report associating childhood acute hemorrhagic cystitis with polyomavirus excretion.[69] Because studies of this class of virus have, until recently, been handicapped by insensitive diagnostic techniques, further studies are needed to determine the frequency with which they cause urinary tract disease.

## PATHOGENESIS

The first consideration in discussing the pathogenesis of UTI is the route by which microorganisms, especially bacteria, reach the urinary tract in general and the kidney in particular. Two potential routes have been proposed: the hematogenous route, with seeding of the kidney during the course of bacteremia; and the ascending route, from the urethra to the bladder, then by the ureters to the kidneys.[70, 71]

### Hematogenous Infection

In humans, blood-borne infection of the kidneys and urinary tract accounts for less than 3% of the cases of UTI and pyelonephritis. When one considers the organisms that are capable of causing pyelonephritis by the hematogenous route, a list different from that outlined in Table 32–1 is compiled. Whereas E. coli, the other Enterobacteriaceae, S. saprophyticus, and E. faecalis account for approximately 95% of UTIs, the major causes of hematogenous infection are S. aureus, Salmonella species, P. aeruginosa, and Candida species.[6] Studies in animals, reviewed in detail elsewhere,[72] shed considerable light on the pathogenetic mechanisms responsible for this dichotomy.

Because the kidneys receive 20% to 25% of the cardiac output, any microorganism that reaches the bloodstream can be delivered to the kidneys. However, only certain organisms are effective pathogens in this circumstance. Detailed studies with E. coli in animal models of hematogenous pyelonephritis have shown that of large numbers of organisms injected into the circulation, only a fraction of this inoculum is actually trapped within the kidney. Thus, in rats, when $5 \times 10^8$ E. coli organisms are injected intravenously, only $10^3$ to $10^4$ can be found within the kidney. Even then the kidney is resistant to these organisms. The number of organisms remains relatively constant, but no inflammation or tissue destruction occurs, bacteriuria does not develop, and the kidneys eventually become sterile (usually within 10 days). There appears to be a difference

in virulence among different E. coli strains (see later); a few strains can establish sustained infection.[73]

In mice, infections can be produced by intravenous injection of E. coli and other gram-negative bacilli, provided that a minimal number of intrarenal bacteria are deposited.[74] However, to achieve this critical, intrarenal infecting inoculum, a bloodstream level of bacteria is required that is extremely close to the lethal dose in these animals, and thus only a 15% frequency of renal infection is obtained.[75] It appears, then, that the inability of most strains of E. coli to cause infection is related not only to their intrinsic nonpathogenicity by this route of infection but also to the small proportion of the injected dose that is actually deposited in the kidney. Presumably, intrinsic bacterial clearing mechanisms within the renal tissue are able to clear the kidneys of these small numbers of organisms without sequelae.

This is not to say that the kidney is immune to blood-borne infection with other bacterial species. Both Proteus and Pseudomonas species can readily cause hematogenous pyelonephritis in mice[75] and occasionally in rats.[72, 76–78] Acute and chronic infection can be produced in intact rat kidneys by the intravenous injection of E. faecalis.[79, 80] Perhaps most germane to the human experience is the observation that the intravenous injection of S. aureus regularly results in acute suppurative infections of the kidneys.[81] Virulence of staphylococcal strains can be correlated with coagulase positivity and the production of hemolysins by the organism.[82, 83] Thus, a variety of virulent species are capable of establishing infection in the kidney in the face of sublethal numbers of organisms in the bloodstream— exactly opposite to the situation with E. coli.

Although the intact kidney is resistant to hematogenous E. coli infection, a variety of interventions affecting renal structure and function can increase the susceptibility of the kidney and favor the initiation of pyelonephritis by the hematogenous route. Of such interventions, the one that has been most commonly exploited, and the simplest to induce experimentally, is complete obstruction to urine flow. With E. coli as the infecting organism, it is usually possible to induce renal infection in 100% of animals by the intravenous injection of $5 \times 10^8$ organisms after ligation of one of the ureters.[72, 84] In a classic early study, Lepper[85] found that temporary ligation of the ureters for periods as short as an hour increased renal susceptibility to infection. Other interventions include intrarenal obstruction due either to scarring[86, 87] or to intratubular precipitation of drugs, such as sulfonamides[88]; vascular factors, such as renal vein constriction,[89] arterial constriction,[90] hemorrhagic hypotension,[91] or acute or chronic hypertension[92, 93]; $K^+$ depletion[94]; analgesics[95]; renal massage[96]; polycystic kidney disease[97]; experimentally induced diabetes mellitus[98–100]; and the administration of estrogens.[101]

The mechanism by which obstruction increases the susceptibility of the kidney to infection is unclear. Freedman and co-workers[102] showed that neither increased trapping of circulating bacteria nor simple stagnation of urine can account for the initiation of infection. Experimental evidence suggests that the main cause may be increased tissue pressure in the kidney, possibly interfering with the renal microcirculation during the obstructive phase.[103, 104]

These experimental observations offer several important insights that are relevant to human infection:

1. In patients with normal urinary tract anatomy, the simultaneous demonstration of *E. coli* in the urine and the blood strongly suggests the kidney as a portal of entry for the bacteremia. In contrast, the simultaneous demonstration of *S. aureus* or *Salmonella* infection (or candidal infection in noncatheterized patients) in the blood and urine suggests a portal of entry outside the urinary tract with spread to the kidney and underscores the need for a careful search for the primary source of the infection. *P. aeruginosa* and possibly *Proteus* infection can manifest either pattern.

2. Patients with increased intrarenal pressures due to urinary tract obstruction may be at risk for metastatic infection with a variety of organisms, including those like *E. coli*, that are usually not pathogenic for the kidney when bacteremia is present.

3. A kidney subjected to trauma, such as after renal massage in the experimental model, may be at particular risk for the development of pyelonephritis. This observation may be especially relevant to kidney transplantation and patients undergoing physical trauma.

## Ascending Infection

There is considerable clinical evidence that most infections of the kidney result from ascension of fecally derived organisms from the urethra and periurethral tissues into the bladder and then by the ureter to the renal pelvis, with subsequent invasion of the renal medullae at this site.[6, 10, 70, 71, 105–107] Ascending infection was first documented experimentally by Vivaldi and associates[108] after inoculation of *Proteus mirabilis* into the urinary bladder of rats and was subsequently confirmed in a variety of experimental models.[72, 109]

In discussing the pathogenesis of ascending infection, it is useful to examine the various steps necessary for the spread of organisms from the periurethral region to the kidney.

### URETHRAL AND INTROITAL COLONIZATION

The crucial first step in the pathogenesis of UTI is the colonization of the distal urethra, the periurethral tissue, and, in the female patient, the vaginal vestibule with potential urinary tract pathogens. Studies of this phenomenon have been almost entirely restricted to women. It is clear that the reservoir from which urinary tract pathogens emerge is the gastrointestinal tract and that, in women, the proximity of the anus and the urethra potentiates colonization with fecal flora.[6, 10, 13] Although an effort has been made to correlate the occurrence of this initial step with personal hygiene habits, methods of menstrual protection, and types of intimate clothing, no clear-cut relationship has emerged.[13, 16]

Whether sustained bacteriuria results from the colonization of the vaginal vestibule and distal urethra depends on the interaction of two factors: whether the colonizing species possesses surface adhesins that promote the attachment of the organisms to the epithelial surface (see later) and whether the mucosal cells of a particular woman have a

particularly high affinity for these bacterial adhesins. Periurethral and vaginal mucosal cells derived from women subjected to recurrent UTI adhere to pathogenic *E. coli* strains to a much greater extent than do cells derived from women who are free of this problem.[110–119] It now appears that women who do not secrete blood group antigens in their body fluids (nonsecretors) are particularly susceptible to recurrent UTI and that their uroepithelial cells bind significantly greater numbers of uropathogenic *E. coli* than do the cells of women who are secretors. This binding is accomplished through specific bacterial ligand–epithelial cell receptor interaction. Thus, in predicting whether a UTI will develop in a woman who is colonized with *E. coli,* key variables are the woman's own genetic constitution (which determines the ''stickiness'' of her uroepithelium for uropathogens, such stickiness being correlated with secretor status) and the genetic constitution of the bacterial strain that is colonizing (i.e., whether it possesses adhesins that mediate attachment).[120, 121]

Vaginal colonization and bacteriuria can be promoted as well by contraceptive practices. In particular, the use of a diaphragm with a spermicide (which inhibits the normal vaginal flora) promotes vaginal colonization with potential uropathogens.[122] In practical terms, this can be extremely important in managing women susceptible to recurrent UTI—substituting a different form of contraception can lead to effective prevention of UTI recurrence. Whether such other factors as the hormonal changes of the menstrual cycle, personal hygiene practices, or alterations in vaginal pH also promote vaginal colonization is at present unclear.

Men are normally protected against the initiation of UTI because of the anatomic separation of the urethral meatus and the anus, the length of the male urethra, and the bactericidal activity of prostatic secretions. Lack of circumcision has been linked to an increased risk of UTI, as have homosexual activity that involves anal intercourse and, rarely, heterosexual vaginal intercourse (with a partner colonized with a uropathogen). However, because sustained colonization of the distal urethra in the man is difficult to accomplish, even in these circumstances, bacteriuria is unusual in the absence of prostatic dysfunction or other urogenital abnormalities.[123–128]

### ENTRY OF PATHOGENS INTO THE BLADDER

The processes by which bacteria ascend from the urethra into the bladder are at present incompletely understood. O'Grady and colleagues[129] have suggested that bacteria ascend not uncommonly during micturition, possibly related to a turbulent stream or reflux into the bladder after the completion of voiding. Presumably, whether infection is established will then depend on the nature of the organisms that reach the bladder and their interaction with uroepithelial cells. Although such hypotheses are reasonable, the only clearly demonstrated mechanism by which bacteria are introduced into the bladder is by instrumentation of the urethra and bladder—cystoscopy, urologic surgery, and the placement of a Foley catheter.

Several investigators have attempted to define other pathogenetic mechanisms. Bran and associates[130] have shown that even gentle manual manipulation of the urethra results in the introduction of bacteria into the bladder. If such minor trauma can have these effects, the question arises whether urethral trauma occurring during normal sexual intercourse is responsible for the increased frequency of UTI in adult women. This has been an area of great controversy. Kunin and McCormack[131] reported that the frequency of bacteriuria in the general female population was 12.8 times greater than among nuns of a similar age. Kelsey and colleagues[132] reported that the frequency of bacteriuria was inversely related to the interval since last intercourse in a population of women attending a clinic for sexually transmitted diseases. Nicolle and associates[133] reported a high association between the development of significant bacteriuria in women and intercourse in the previous 24 hours and noted that the frequency of intercourse was higher in infected women than in uninfected women. In this study, 75% of the episodes of UTI in women with a history of recurrent UTIs occurred within 24 hours of intercourse.

If intercourse is an important pathogenetic event in the development of UTI, then therapy directed at the immediate postintercourse period should be effective. Indeed, Vosti,[134] in a retrospective study, noted that a single dose of antibiotic taken after intercourse is effective in preventing UTI in a group of women susceptible to recurrent UTI. Buckley and colleagues[43] have shown that bacteria are introduced during intercourse but that for the most part these bacteria are components of the normal flora of the vagina and distal urethra (*S. epidermidis,* diphtheroids, and lactobacilli), which rarely cause UTI. The implications of this study were that bacteria are regularly introduced into the bladder during intercourse but that unless virulent organisms colonize the distal urethra and vagina, sustained bacteriuria will not result.

On balance, it appears that sexual intercourse alone will not establish bacteriuria and that bacteriuria can occur in the absence of intercourse, but when intercourse is coupled with the presence of virulent bacteria and other factors, it will lead to an increased frequency of infection. Kunin[135] has suggested that among such other factors are urodynamic considerations (the frequency and timing of voiding, the volume of residual urine left in the bladder), hormonal changes, variations in the toxicity and antibacterial properties of the urine, personal hygiene habits, patterns of masturbation, and virulence properties of the resident bacterial flora. Menstruation has been suggested as another factor, perhaps in altering the resident flora.[133, 136]

## BACTERIAL MULTIPLICATION IN THE BLADDER AND BLADDER DEFENSE MECHANISMS

Whatever the mode of entry of bacteria into the bladder, it has long been known that the normal bladder is capable of clearing itself of organisms within 2 to 3 days of their introduction either accidentally, as by urethral catheterization, or experimentally in human volunteers and laboratory animals. This property of the normal bladder represents an important defense mechanism against urinary infection and appears to depend on interactions among at least three factors: 1) the eradication of bacteria by voiding, 2) the presence of bacteriostatic substances in the urine, and 3) the intrinsic mucosal bladder defense mechanisms.

Dilution resulting from the constant inflow of urine from the kidneys followed by periodic voiding undoubtedly plays a role in the clearing of bacteria from the bladder. Using human urine, Cox and Hinman[137] showed that periodic dilution and emptying of a simulated bladder in vitro resulted in maintenance of the original number of bacteria inoculated ($10^6$), whereas in the absence of periodic emptying, the number increased up to $10^9$ within 12 hours. On the other hand, when *E. coli* at $10^6$ to $10^7$ organisms/mL was introduced into the urinary bladder of four human volunteers, the numbers decreased to $10^3$ organisms/mL after 9 hours, and the urine samples were sterile for all four subjects at 72 hours. It was concluded that two defense mechanisms operated to keep the normal bladder sterile: periodic voiding (the hydrokinetic defense mechanism); and an intrinsic property probably of the vesical mucosa, which accounts for killing of bacteria in the small volume of residual urine that coats the bladder mucosa after normal voiding, calculated to be between 0.09 and 2.43 mL by Hinman and Cox.[138]

The theoretic calculations and experiments of Cox and Hinman are predicated on two assumptions: 1) the multiplication rate of bacteria in urine in the bladder is the same as that in vitro, and 2) the effect of dilution by inflow of fresh urine and voiding is simply volume dependent. Although urine is thought to serve as a good culture medium in vitro, O'Grady and Cattell[139] and O'Grady and Pennington[140] suggested that these two assumptions may not always be correct. They showed that the growth of *E. coli* in urine in the bladder could be significantly lower than growth in vitro in the same aliquot of urine. Lower multiplication rates in vitro could occur owing to incomplete mixing and aeration; they found that whereas the maximal rate of multiplication in vivo results in doubling of the number of bacteria every 20 minutes, the doubling time is lengthened to 50 minutes if the urine is not artificially aerated. Furthermore, periodic differences in the composition of urine may enhance the action of a variety of bacteriostatic factors known to exist in urine: undissociated organic acids that are particularly active in the presence of low pH,[141] high urea and $NH_4^+$ concentrations, lysozyme,[142] and immunoglobulins G and A.[143] Urine of high osmolality destroyed some 90% of *E. coli* organisms and markedly prolonged the time for log phase growth, compared with more dilute urine, although high osmolality does inhibit bacterial phagocytosis.[144, 145] Thus, it is possible that the inhibitory effect of urine on bacterial growth, which is maximal under suitable conditions of pH and osmolality in vivo, may be one of the factors that serves to reduce bacterial multiplication in the bladder.

Because neither dilution of the bacteria by voiding nor inhibition of bacterial growth in urine is sufficient to cause total eradication of bacteria from the bladder under usual circumstances, antibacterial mechanisms residing in or close to the bladder mucosa have been postulated. This "mucosal factor" was demonstrated experimentally by Vivaldi and colleagues,[91] who applied radioactively labeled *E. coli* directly to the exposed bladder mucosa of rabbits. By the end of 1 hour, only 0.3% of the inoculum had survived,

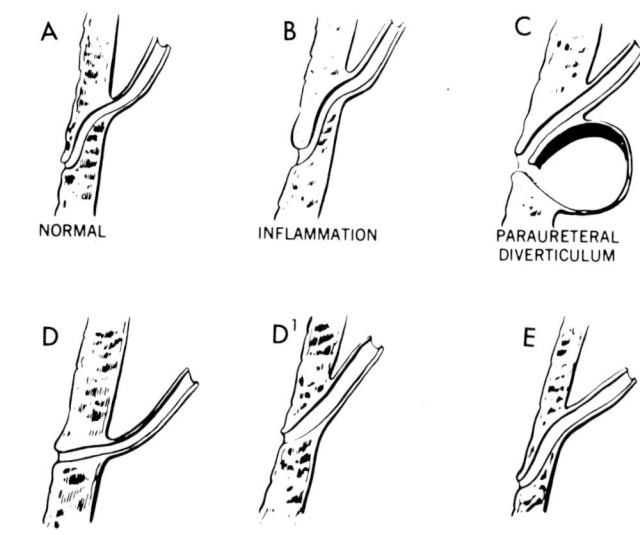

A NORMAL

B INFLAMMATION

C PARAURETERAL DIVERTICULUM

D ABSENCE OF INTRAVESICAL URETER

D¹ PARTIAL ABSENCE OF INTRAVESICAL URETER

E FLACCID NEUROGENIC BLADDER WALL

**Figure 32–1.** Intravesical position of the ureter in the normal person *(A)* and in patients with vesicoureteral reflux. Types *D* and *D¹* are by far the most common in children and infants. (*A* to *E* from King LR, Surian MA, Wendel RM, Burden JJ: Vesicoureteral reflux. A classification based on cause and the results of treatment. JAMA 203:169–174, 1968. Copyright 1968, American Medical Association.)

even though radioactivity in the mucosa persisted. The nature of this mucosal factor is unknown. Phagocytosis by neutrophils or mucosal epithelial cells and the local excretion of bacteriostatic organic acids, immunoglobulin G, immunoglobulin A, peroxidase, and lysozyme have been implicated but not documented convincingly.[146, 147]

Whatever the mechanism, some property of the intact bladder mucosa probably limits the multiplication of invading bacteria, thus accelerating their clearance by dilution and voiding. Whether infection becomes established depends on the balance between bacterial proliferation and the effectiveness of bladder defenses. Clinically, clearing does not occur in the presence of frank residual urine, inadequate micturition, foreign bodies or stones in the bladder, increased vesical pressure, or previous inflammation of the bladder mucosa. The role of residual urine, foreign bodies, and pre-existing inflammatory lesions is readily recognized. Residual urine not only increases the number of bacteria remaining in the bladder but also lowers the ratio between the surface area of the bladder mucosa and the volume of urine exposed to it, thus reducing the effectiveness of potential antibacterial mucosal factors. Lapides[148] also stressed the role of distention and increased hydrostatic pressure in inhibiting clearance. In a careful study, Fiveash and colleagues[149] found significant increases in the degree and duration of bacteriuria in rabbits with bladder neck obstruction compared with those having nonobstructed bladders.

The efficacy of bladder bacterial clearance mechanisms is demonstrated not only by the experimental studies but also by the clinical observations of Mabeck.[150] These observations of a group of Swedish women with acute, uncomplicated UTI showed that more than 70% of women with lower UTI who are treated with a placebo will clear their infections within 1 month.

## Vesicoureteral Reflux

From clinical and experimental studies, it is now well established that VUR allows infected urine to ascend to the kidney and, furthermore, that it is the most common factor predisposing to chronic pyelonephritic scarring, particularly in infants and children.[151]

In humans, the normal vesicoureteral valve is extremely competent. A number of studies have documented that VUR does not occur or occurs rarely under normal conditions in adults, children,[152–155] neonates (whether premature or full term),[156–158] or even the fetus.[159] In the normal urinary tract, VUR is prevented by virtue of the length of the intramural segment of the ureter; the ureter is obliquely inserted into a tunnel in the bladder wall (Fig. 32–1), so the intravesical portion of the ureter is compressed by the bladder musculature during micturition.[160, 161] Failure of this valve mechanism is most commonly due to shortening of the intravesical portion of the ureter (primary VUR).[162, 163] This shortening is thought to be caused by abnormal embryologic development of an ectopically located ureteric bud, so the ureteric orifices are displaced laterally. The intravesical portion of the ureter lengthens with growth, increasing the competence of the valve mechanisms and rendering it less susceptible to reflux.[163] Thus, VUR is much more likely to occur in younger children and, indeed, may disappear completely with age.[164] Although primary maldevelopment of the ureteric bud is a logical explanation for congenital VUR, proof for such a sequence is lacking.

In children, VUR may also be secondary, occurring in association with other anomalies usually manifested by obstruction.[151] Neonates with neurogenic bladder disorders such as myelodysplasia, in which high-pressure obstruction occurs, have no demonstrable VUR but eventually develop secondary VUR with typical ureteric "golf-hole" orifices as well as ureteric dilatation and tortuosity. Forty-five percent of patients with meningomyeloceles develop VUR by age 5 years, some with renal scarring.[165]

Bladder-sphincter dysfunctional disturbances in toddlers and children are associated with high-pressure VUR.[165–168] The elevated pressures apparently result from uninhibited bladder contractions followed by voluntary constriction of perineal musculature. In a study of 458 children with bladder dysfunction, Griffiths and Scholtmeiger[169] identified two different types of reflux and dysfunction complexes with contrasting urodynamic characteristics. In one, the bladder contracted poorly during voiding, and overactivity of the urethral closure mechanism was present. In this group, VUR was bilateral and was associated with upper urinary tract anomalies and renal scarring. In the second type, there was bladder instability and powerful voiding contractions of the bladder; this type was associated with unilateral reflux and rare renal scarring.

Of the congenital anatomic anomalies, VUR occurs commonly in the presence of paraurethral diverticulum[170]; in 25% to 50% of boys with posterior urethral valves[170, 171]; in 10% of those with ureteropelvic junction obstruction[172]; and in association with ureteral duplications, hypospadias, and ureteroceles. With the increasing application of ultrasound techniques to examine the fetus during pregnancy, a number of studies have now addressed the etiology and long-term implications of a dilated urinary tract, specifically hydronephrosis, identified antenatally. Although obstructive uropathy is assumed to be the cause of fetal hydronephrosis, VUR is found to be present in 10% to 40% of these infants studied postnatally, often with advanced grades of reflux. The hope would be that the aggressive treatment of these neonates, 75% to 80% of whom are boys, would help preserve renal function and facilitate kidney growth.[173–176]

Congenital VUR is five times more common in boys than in girls and tends to occur in families. When asymptomatic siblings of children with VUR are studied with sensitive radiologic procedures, approximately 40% have been shown to also have reflux, some with evidence of clinically silent scarring. Approximately two thirds of the offspring of parents with known VUR have evidence of reflux as well when they are studied by voiding cystourethrogram.[177–179] On the basis of segregation analysis of 88 affected families, Chapman and colleagues[180] concluded that the best model was that of a single dominant gene acting together with a random environmental effect. Computer modeling indicated that the gene frequency was 1 in 600 and that mutation was uncommon.

VUR is seen in 18% of adults who have spinal cord injuries and in a variable percentage of adults with bladder tumors, prostatic hypertrophy, and urinary tract stones.[181] It can also follow fulguration of lesions in the area of the orifice or simple trauma, such as extraction of a ureteral calculus by means of a ''basket.''[151]

Still unresolved is the question of whether bladder infection can precede and, in a way, cause VUR. Bladder infection can cause reflux in some experimental animals, but studies in adult primates with chronic cystitis demonstrate no reflux.[181] A series of studies on renal infection and reflux in monkeys by Roberts[181] and by others suggest, however, that bladder infection increases the duration of reflux and renders a partially competent ureterovesical junction overtly refluxing. The clinical evidence suggests that infection is not a necessary cause of reflux but that it can precipitate reflux in a ureterovesical junction that is congenitally defective or, indeed, can increase the grade of reflux.[182]

VUR, which can be unilateral or bilateral, may vary considerably in severity. Severity of reflux is graded by means of voiding cystourethrography in a number of ways.[183] The grading system adopted by the International Reflux Study Committee is as follows[184] (Fig. 32–2):

Grade I: Reflux partly up the ureter
Grade II: Reflux up to the pelvis and calyces without dilatation; normal calyceal fornices
Grade III: Same as grade II, but with mild or moderate dilatation and tortuosity of the ureter and no blunting of the fornices
Grade IV: Moderate dilatation and tortuosity of the ureters, pelvis, and calyces; complete blunting of fornices
Grade V: Gross dilatation and tortuosity of the ureter, pelvis, and calyces; absent papillary impressions in the calyces

A variety of technical and clinical factors can influence the grade of the reflux as seen on voiding cystogram, however, and few attempts have been made to standardize this procedure.[183, 185]

Radionuclide cystography is emerging as an alternative and, in many ways, superior technique for evaluating VUR.[186] Indirect radionuclide cystography, in which the radionuclide is injected intravenously, is noninvasive but detects only high-pressure gross VUR and requires good renal function. On the other hand, cystography after direct instillation of radionuclide (technetium Tc 99m pertechnetate) has proved to be a sensitive, quantitative, and safe procedure that also serves as a test for evaluating functional bladder disorders.[186]

Although the significance of VUR was appreciated as early as 1903 by Sampson, it was Hodson and Edwards[187] who demonstrated renal pyelonephritic scarring by radiographic means. Since then, a great deal of evidence linking VUR, renal infection, and renal scarring has accumulated,[151, 188–191] and the findings can be summarized as follows.

1. In various series, VUR can be demonstrated by voiding cystourethrography in 30% to 50% of children with recurrent infection and in 85% to 100% of children and 50% of adults with chronic pyelonephritic scarring.[170, 189] Furthermore, even in children and adults with renal scars who do not exhibit reflux, anatomic abnormalities of the

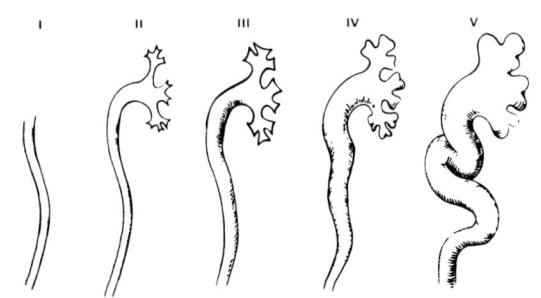

**Figure 32–2.** Grades of reflux. International Reflux Study classification. I. Ureter only. II. Ureter, pelvis, and calyces. No dilatation, normal calyceal fornices. III. Mild or moderate dilatation and/or tortuosity of ureter and mild or moderate dilatation of renal pelvis but no or slight blunting of fornices. IV. Moderate dilatation and/or tortuosity of ureter and moderate dilatation of renal pelvis and calyces. Complete obliteration of sharp angle of fornices but maintenance of papillary impressions in majority of calyces. V. Gross dilatation and tortuosity of ureter. Gross dilatation of renal pelvis and calyces. Papillary impressions are no longer visible in majority of calyces.

ureteral orifices (lateral ectopia and abnormal configuration) are seen cystoscopically, which suggests that reflux had been present in the past.[162]

2. Alternatively, between 30% and 60% of children with VUR exhibit pyelonephritic scarring, the higher figure being derived from surgical clinics and the lower from medical studies.[192]

3. Renal scarring of the pyelonephritic type is found in up to 25% of children with UTI,[193–204] and as mentioned, about 30% to 50% of these have VUR.

4. Several studies have documented the progressive development of clubbing of the calyces and renal scarring after discovery of VUR in previously normal kidneys.[205–211] Progressive scarring appears in the severer forms of reflux and, as discussed later, almost always in the presence of infected urine. It must be stressed, however, that in many infants and children with VUR, pyelonephritic scarring never develops, and VUR may disappear either spontaneously or with antibacterial therapy in up to 80% of ureters after long follow-up.[193] Even severe reflux associated with scarring may disappear, although reflux is more likely to cease when it is mild or moderate and when the kidneys are unscarred. Among adults, about 90% with severe VUR have renal scars.[211, 212]

5. All stages of pyelonephritis—from acute suppurative inflammation to typical chronic pyelonephritic scarring—can be produced in experimental animals by inducing VUR and concomitant lower UTI.[213, 214]

## INTRARENAL REFLUX

Whereas VUR is responsible for the ascent of bacteria into the renal pelvis, considerable evidence now suggests that the spread of infection from the pelvis into the cortex occurs by virtue of a phenomenon known as intrarenal reflux. Brodeur and associates,[215] Amat,[216] and Rolleston and colleagues[217] found that in some children with urinary infection, contrast medium instilled into the bladder during voiding cystourethrography permeated the renal parenchyma as far as the renal capsule. Intrarenal reflux occurred with the severer grades of VUR (Fig. 32–3). Curiously, intrarenal reflux was focal in distribution and affected predominantly the two polar regions of the kidney, areas that are frequently the site of chronic scars. It was suggested that such intrarenal reflux could form the basis for the spread and distribution of infection. Intrarenal reflux has since been reported by others,[218–221] although, for a number of reasons, conventional techniques may often fail to demonstrate it.

The importance of intrarenal reflux in the pathogenesis of pyelonephritic scarring has been confirmed by two series of elegant experimental studies. Hodson and associates[188, 213] induced VUR in piglets by incising the anterior wall of the intramural ureter. When bladder pressures were raised in these animals by placement of a silver ring around the proximal urethra, intrarenal reflux could be readily demonstrated (Fig. 32–4). Particularly in the presence of infected urine, the precise foci that exhibited intrarenal reflux developed acute inflammation and subsequent scarring (Figs. 32–5 and 32–6), and the distribution of intrarenal scars was remarkably similar to that occurring in

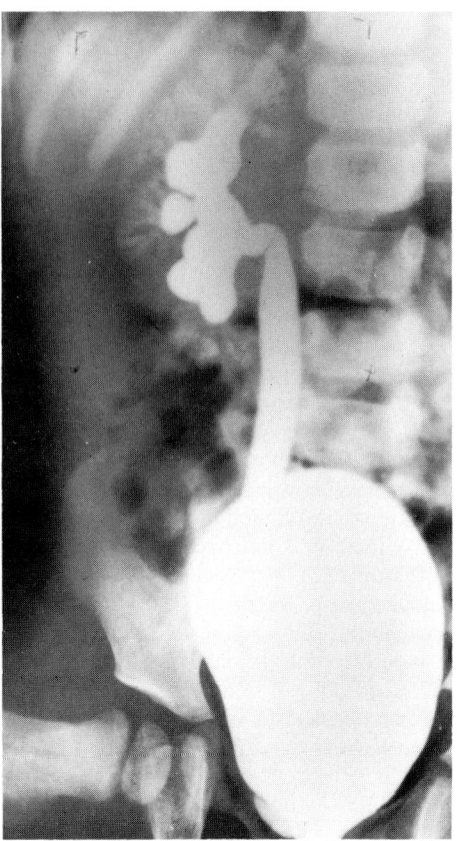

**Figure 32–3.** Cystogram showing severe grade of VUR (grade IV) with scattered intrarenal reflux into all zones of the kidney. (From Hodson CJ: Reflux nephropathy. Med Clin North Am 62:1201, 1978.)

human kidneys in that it affected mainly the lower and upper poles.

Ransley and Risdon[214] confirmed and extended these studies and made the observation that intrarenal reflux in the multipapillary kidneys of both human infants and young pigs occurred only in renal papillae with particular morphologic characteristics.[222–224] They found two basic forms of renal papillae. 1) Nonrefluxing papillae are conic, and their papillary ducts open obliquely near the tip of the papilla onto a convex surface through slit-like orifices (Fig. 32–7A). These papillae may be simple, representing a single renal reniculus, or compound, in which two or more reniculi have fused. Such papillae are never associated with intrarenal reflux, because even in the presence of VUR, their orifices are closed by the rise of pressure within the calyx. 2) Refluxing papillae are larger as a result of fusion of several adjacent reniculi (Fig. 32–7B). They have concave rather than convex tips, and the papillary ducts open with gaping orifices that cannot be closed by an increase in intracalyceal pressure. Of great significance is that both in infants and in young pigs, refluxing papillae are present predominantly in the upper and lower poles (which are more susceptible to renal scarring); the simple and compound types are present mostly in the midzones (Table 32–3). In addition, although the number of refluxing papillae is less in the human than in the pig, approximately two thirds of human kidneys contained at least one poten-

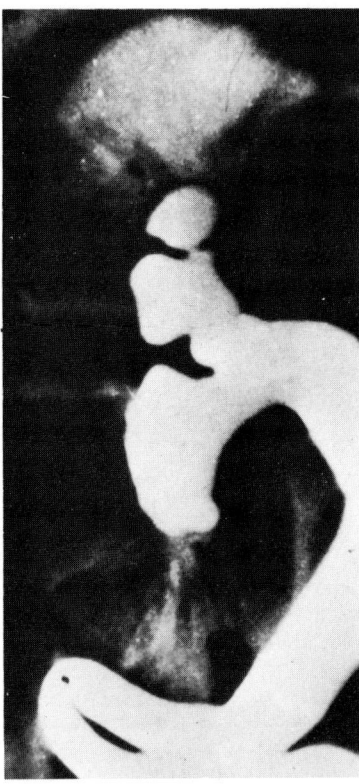

**Figure 32–4.** Intrarenal reflux in the pig. Note that there is major involvement of the upper pole but somewhat less involvement of the lower pole. Compare the distribution of polar intrarenal reflux with that of acute inflammation (Fig. 32–5) and scarring (Fig. 32–6). (From Hodson CJ, Maling RM, McManamon PJ, Lewis MJ: The pathogenesis of reflux nephropathy [chronic atrophic pyelonephritis]. Br J Radiol 13[suppl]:1, 1975.)

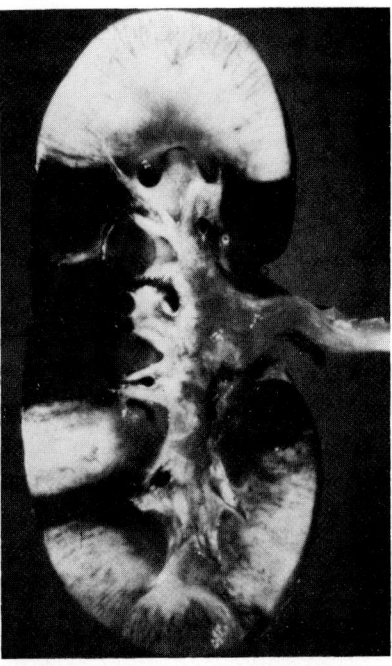

**Figure 32–5.** Large acute lesions of acute bacterial inflammation from infected intrarenal reflux in the pig. The subsequent contraction of these lesions gives rise to focal scars (see Fig. 32–6). (From Hodson CJ: Reflux nephropathy. Med Clin North Am 62:1201, 1978.)

tially refluxing papilla, and in one fifth of the kidneys, the percentage of nonconvex papillae was 30% or more. Tamminen and Kaprio[225] reported similar findings in the kidneys of infants and children dying of nonrenal causes.

In summary, there are two main determinants for the progression of ascending infection from the bladder into the renal parenchyma:

1. VUR most commonly is apparently due to a congenital anatomic abnormality of the insertion of the ureter into the bladder.

2. Intrarenal reflux is determined by the presence of morphologically distinct papillae with open ducts, which allows spread of organisms into the renal parenchyma in the presence of high intracalyceal pressure. VUR and intrarenal reflux, in combination, are almost certainly the major mechanisms responsible for the renal inflammation and scarring characteristic of chronic pyelonephritis.

These findings of VUR, intrarenal reflux, and papillary morphologic characteristics can also explain some perplexing clinical observations in children. It has been amply shown that in the majority of children with VUR who develop renal scars, scarring is already evident at the initial radiologic investigation, which is usually performed because of recurrent UTI. Scarring thus appears to occur early in life, possibly even in utero. For example, Rolleston and

associates[185] found that 147 (42%) of 350 infants (age range, 3 days to 12 months; mean age, 3 months) had VUR, 49 with gross reflux. Twenty-nine of the 49 infants with gross VUR (60%) had kidneys that were already damaged by 12 months of age. No damage was found associated

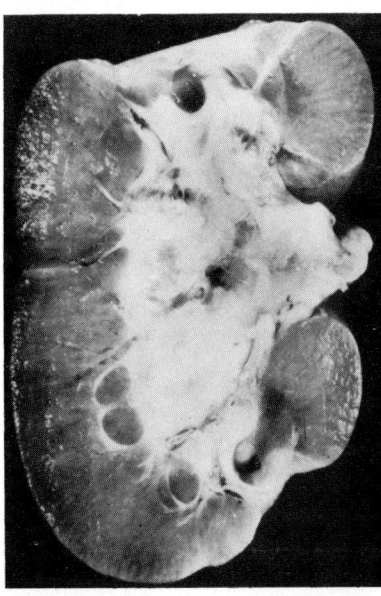

**Figure 32–6.** Typical polar scars 3 months after infected intrarenal reflux in the pig. Note dilatation of the calyx underlying the scars. (From Hodson CJ, Maling RM, McManamon PJ, Lewis MJ: The pathogenesis of reflux nephropathy [chronic atrophic pyelonephritis]. Br J Radiol 13[suppl]:1, 1975.)

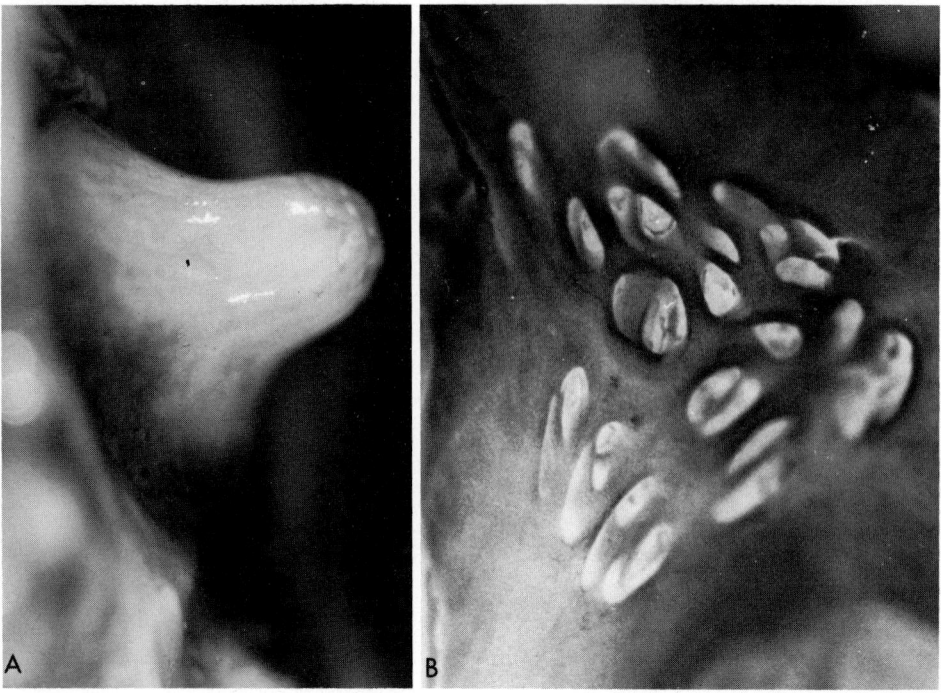

**Figure 32–7.** *A.* A simple, nonrefluxing papilla from pig kidney. Note the conic form, with papillary ducts opening near the tip onto a convex surface. *B.* A compound refluxing papilla with a concave surface and wide-open papillary duct orifices. (*A* and *B* from Ransley PG, Risdon RA: The pathogenesis of reflux nephropathy. Br J Radiol 14[suppl]:1, 1978.)

with the lesser degrees of VUR. Bailey[189] noted that 10 infants presenting with UTI and VUR from 9 days to 7 weeks of life already had evidence of renal scarring. Indeed, the development of new scars in children is unusual beyond the age of 5 years (and possibly the age of 2 years), regardless of proven episodes of UTI.[226] Ransley and Risdon[224] proposed the "big bang" theory of scar formation to account for such findings: In the presence of gross VUR, the first few episodes of clinical or subclinical UTI in infants and children will affect potentially refluxing papillae, leaving nonrefluxing papillae intact. The nonrefluxing papillae are immune to damage by further episodes of UTI. Normal kidney parenchyma drained by nonrefluxing papillae will continue to resist the challenge of UTI and VUR. These findings also point to the importance of early detection of UTI and the gross forms of VUR if renal scarring is to be prevented.

### STERILE REFLUX

Although the association between VUR in the infected child and renal scarring is unequivocal, the question of whether reflux results in renal damage in the absence of bacterial infection (sterile reflux) deserves consideration. This is a particularly attractive notion, because VUR can disappear from one or both involved ureters; sterile reflux would then account for those cases of pyelonephritic scarring not associated with infection and not exhibiting obvious signs of reflux when they are discovered (see later). It has been shown that renal inflammation and scarring can result from high-pressure VUR[213, 227–229] in the total absence of infection, particularly if there is sustained bladder decompensation (i.e., when bladder pressure does not return to normal between micturitions in the presence of outflow obstruction). However, there is still considerable controversy as to the frequency with which such damage occurs clinically.

Several authors have reported progressive renal dysfunction or end-stage kidney disease apparently associated with sterile reflux.[185, 230–235] Others have found no consistent correlation between the frequency of UTI and the occurrence of progressive damage in patients with VUR. Unfortunately, it is difficult to acquire clinical evidence on both

**TABLE 32–3. Distribution of Compound Types II and III (Refluxing) Papillae in Normal Young Human and Porcine Kidneys**

| Species | Both Upper and Lower Poles | Upper Pole Only | Lower Pole Only | None |
|---|---|---|---|---|
| Human* (n = 33) | 6 (18%) | 14 (42%) | 4 (12%) | 9 (27%) |
| Pig (n = 25) | 24 (96%) | 1 (4%) | 0 (0%) | 0 (0%) |

*Only one kidney showed a refluxing papilla in the midzone.
From Ransley PG, Risdon RA: Renal papillary morphology in infants and young children. Urol Res 3:111, 1977.

these points. Most patients with reflux nephropathy already have renal scars when they are first seen, and the finding of sterile urine at this time does not mean that infection has never occurred. Progression of an established scar may simply reflect contraction of the scar with hypertrophy of the surrounding parenchyma from a previous infection rather than progression in the presence of sterile urine.[236] Furthermore, a large group of children with reflux who were observed for up to 15 years developed no new renal scars when a sterile urine was maintained by prophylactic antibacterial therapy.[237, 238] On the basis of their review of the clinical literature, Ransley and Risdon[223] contended that the occurrence of a completely new scar in a previously normal kidney with continuously sterile urine has not been reported. However, infected reflux may so modify the morphologic features of some apparently nonrefluxing papillae as to allow intrarenal reflux and progressive scarring but only in the presence of reinfection. In addition, the development of hypertension or glomerular injury in some patients with reflux nephropathy may be responsible for functional deterioration unrelated to the direct effects of VUR.

Hodson[151] and others believed that high-pressure obstructed situations, which occur in children with reflux associated with congenital obstruction (i.e., posterior urethral valves), may lead to sterile renal damage akin to the experimental models described earlier. Ransley and colleagues,[227] however, argued that the renal scarring in these patients is more probably due to coexistent renal dysplasia or unrecognized UTI.

The balance of evidence on this issue suggests that renal involvement in reflux nephropathy occurs early in childhood, before age 5 years, largely as a result of superimposition of bacterial infection on VUR and intrarenal reflux.[239] Because most potentially refluxing papillae will thus be affected early on, additional progressive scarring occurs rarely owing to the transformation of papillae from nonrefluxing to refluxing types. This accounts for the occurrence of new segmental scars or sequential scarring of an already scarred kidney, but such progression is rare. If sterile intrarenal reflux induces renal damage, it does so in the presence of severe obstructive uropathy with high intrapelvic pressures. Such may be the case in children with posterior urethral valves or other obstructive congenital anomalies.

Before this discussion of the significance of VUR in the pathogenesis of renal pyelonephritic scarring is concluded, a few points regarding VUR and renal disease should be emphasized. First, most patients with VUR are detected during investigations for UTI, the most common marker for this disorder. The actual frequency of VUR in the general population, and in particular in patients with other renal manifestations such as proteinuria or hypertension, is unknown. Second, there is evidence that VUR, when sought, may be detected in patients with nonpyelonephritic forms of chronic renal disease, including chronic glomerulonephritis and nephrosclerosis.[240–243] Bishop and colleagues,[242] for example, found VUR in 12 of 40 patients with chronic glomerulonephritis who were maintained on long-term hemodialysis. In all but one ureter, reflux was mild or moderate. In four of these patients, reflux occurred after long-term dialysis, which suggests that hemodialysis may in some way provoke VUR. In 85 consecutive adult patients with end-stage renal disease, Huland and associates[243] found 11 patients with chronic glomerulonephritis or nephrosclerosis who had VUR (grades I and II). Third, in addition to renal scarring, VUR in children is associated with reduced renal growth, and there is some question as to whether VUR or UTI or both play a role in such growth retardation.[244–246] Finally, in patients with VUR, renal function may deteriorate for reasons other than UTI, particularly hypertension, an associated glomerulopathy, urinary obstruction, or analgesic abuse. All these points emphasize the complexity of assessing the interrelationships among VUR, UTI, and chronic renal disease.

## Bacterial Virulence Factors Influencing Infection

### ESCHERICHIA COLI

One of the most striking characteristics of UTI is that a single species of bacteria, *E. coli*, not only accounts for the great majority of UTIs but also can cause a wide range of clinical disease, from asymptomatic bacteriuria to cystitis to full-blown pyelonephritis. This observation by itself raises a series of important questions: Are there differences between the *E. coli* strains that cause these different clinical forms of UTI? In particular, are there ''nephritogenic'' strains of *E. coli*, that is, strains that possess the ability to adhere, ascend, and invade the anatomically normal urinary tract? Conversely, are nonvirulent strains able to adhere, ascend, and invade the anatomically abnormal urinary tract? Is there a difference between the characteristics of the *E. coli* strains causing the acute inflammatory condition that we recognize as acute pyelonephritis and those causing chronic renal scarring and progressive loss of renal function?

On the basis of a series of landmark studies done in the past two decades that have combined clinical epidemiology with molecular biology and well-designed animal models, it is now possible to say that the answer to all of these questions is clearly yes; that is, strains of *E. coli* that invade the urinary tract are not merely the most prevalent components of the fecal flora. Rather, they are specific clones that possess a variety of virulence characteristics that facilitate intestinal carriage, persistence in the vagina, and then ascension and invasion of the anatomically normal urinary tract. In the presence of foreign bodies, VUR, or obstruction, these events can occur in the absence of such characteristics, which emphasizes that host characteristics are as important as the nature of the invading organism in determining the outcome of the infection.[247–250]

The first evidence that *E. coli* strains causing pyelonephritis were different from other isolates came from serotyping studies, in which the O (somatic or surface cell wall) antigen, H (flagellar) antigen, and K (capsular) antigen of isolates from well-defined clinical populations were determined. Whereas the serotypes associated with asymptomatic bacteriuria do not differ from those present in the fecal reservoir,[251] strains from symptomatic patients are significantly different both when serotyping is carried out and when molecular genetic analyses are performed.[248] Thus, *E.*

*coli* strains bearing eight of the approximately 170 different O antigens (O1, O2, O4, O6, O7, O16, O18, and O75) account for approximately 80% of the cases of pyelonephritis caused by this species, with a small number of K antigens (K1, K2, K5, K12, and K13 or K51) being identifiable on more than 70% of the pyelonephritis isolates. In contrast, the H antigens appear not to be independently associated with virulence.[251–257]

It is likely that these O antigens are not themselves responsible for the uropathogenicity of these strains of *E. coli;* rather, the genes that determine the O antigen structure are closely linked to other genes that are responsible for the pathogenicity of these isolates.[258, 259] In contrast, the acidic polysaccharide capsular K antigens do appear to be directly pathogenic by inhibiting both phagocytosis and complement-mediated bactericidal activity.[260, 261] This appears to increase the resistance of *E. coli* to the inflammatory response and to foster persistence of the bacteria within the kidney.[262] The amount of K antigen expressed appears to be especially important, because strains of *E. coli* particularly rich in K antigen appear to be more successful both in reaching the bladder and in ascending to and invading the kidney than are strains with low amounts of K antigen.[255, 260–264]

Not only do strains of *E. coli* isolated from patients with asymptomatic bacteriuria have a serotype distribution indistinguishable from that of fecal isolates, but the surface characteristics of these isolates are different. The morphologic features of many of these strains have undergone apparent mutation from "smooth" to "rough" bacterial colony, reflecting the loss of carbohydrate components of the O antigen.[253, 265] These strains exhibit the following characteristics: loss of reactivity to O-typing sera, lesser adherence to uroepithelial cells, increased ability to activate the alternative complement pathway, and sensitivity to normal human serum.[252, 253, 265–268] The frequency of these less virulent strains appears to increase with the duration of time over which asymptomatic bacteriuria is present. New infections that follow successful efforts to eradicate asymptomatic bacteriuria in schoolgirls are more often associated with symptoms than are the continuing or relapsing infections in untreated or unsuccessfully treated patients.[265, 269]

Thus, minimal requirements in defining uropathogenic *E. coli* include an intact O antigen (smooth colony morphologic appearance on a culture plate) and the negatively charged K antigen, which together render bacteria resistant to phagocytosis. Strains of *E. coli* from patients with acute pyelonephritis are homogeneous in terms of surface physicochemical properties: smooth-type bacterial envelope, elevated negative charge, and the ability to undergo hydrophobic interactions.[270–273] Strains from patients with cystitis or asymptomatic bacteriuria are much more heterogeneous in terms of these characteristics. Thus, one might postulate that these surface characteristics are not important in the pathogenesis of lower UTI or asymptomatic bacteriuria but are essential for renal infection, that is, these are nephritogenic characteristics.

The reservoir from which bacteria causing UTI are derived is the large intestine. Sustained colonization of the large intestine with later spread to the urinary tract is one of the requirements that must be fulfilled for a strain to be pathogenic for the urinary tract. Sustained intestinal colonization appears to be associated with the same factors that mediate attachment to the uroepithelium after initial colonization of the introital and periurethral area in women.[250, 274]

Adherence to the uroepithelium is accomplished by the interaction of specific adhesins on the surfaces of the uropathogenic strains with specific receptors on the uroepithelium. The adhesins are lectins, frequently expressed on the tips of pili or fimbriae extending out from the bacterial surface; the receptors are specific carbohydrate components that are part of surface glycolipids or glycoproteins expressed on the uroepithelial surface. Early in the study of the pili, it became apparent that two different classes of pili, which appeared to be identical under the electron microscope, could be distinguished on the basis of whether their binding to uroepithelial cells could be blocked by the presence of mannose. Initially, these were termed type 1 (mannose-sensitive) and type 2 (mannose-resistant) pili.[275–279]

Type 1 or common pili mediate mannose-sensitive adherence and are commonly present on gram-negative bacteria, including non–*E. coli* species isolated from patients with UTI.[252, 280] These adhesins mediate binding to mannose residues on the Tamm-Horsfall protein in the urine,[281] to the carbohydrate portion of secretory immunoglobulin A,[252] and to phagocytic cells.[282] They also bind much less avidly to uroepithelial cells than do the other adhesins.[250, 252] Given these characteristics, it is not surprising that the presence of type 1 pili does not appear to be particularly associated with the development of the clinical manifestations of acute pyelonephritis. On the other hand, the increased binding to phagocytic cells mediated by these type 1 pili may enhance tissue destruction and lead to scarring as a result of the release of free oxygen radicals and other tissue-destroying enzymes that are products of an enhanced inflammatory response.[283–285]

Type 2 pili, in contrast, are intimately involved in all the steps leading to acute pyelonephritis. These are not only the most important of the adhesin-receptor systems but also the most important uropathogenic virulence factors that have been defined. These adhesins, whose binding is resistant to the effects of mannose, have been given a variety of names reflecting their association with pyelonephritis and a particular receptor: P pili, P fimbriae, Pap (pyelonephritis-associated) pili, and Gal-Gal pili. Their binding specificity is to the globoseries of glycolipid receptors that have a common disaccharide $\alpha$Gal(1–4)-$\beta$Gal. These receptors are identical to the glycosphingolipids of the P blood group system and are found on the uroepithelial tissues of the urinary tract, kidneys, and large intestine but not on phagocytic cells. Thus, these uropathogenic strains are able to attach to the host mucosal surface while avoiding binding to host polymorphonuclear cells, a significant survival advantage for these organisms. The presence of P pili on uropathogenic *E. coli* strains is maintained stably, presumably related to the chromosomal as opposed to the extrachromosomal localization of the genes coding for these pili.[250, 252, 280, 286–289]

Expression of these pili is under a phase-variation control mechanism in which individual bacterial cells alternate between being phenotypically pilus-positive and pilus-negative through a process involving DNA methylation by deoxyadenosine methylase.[290] As previously stated, only the tips of the pili express the adhesin that interacts with the specific receptor; a number of other polypeptides form the remainder of the pilus. Thus, a family of these P pili with variability of both the tip peptide and the structural polypeptides is created. The more copies of the genes encoding these pili that are present in a given isolate, the more uropathogenic the isolate. Experimental vaccines made of isolated P pili appear to be promising in protecting against pyelonephritis after challenge with either the original strain from which the vaccine was derived or heterologous strains. These observations re-emphasize the importance of adhesin-receptor interaction in the pathogenesis of pyelonephritis, the conservation of polypeptides within the family of P pili, and the possibility of an effective vaccine for human use in the future.[291–295]

The fact that P pili do not bind to human polymorphonuclear leukocytes (because the globoseries of glycolipids is not found on these cells) has an influence on whether bacteremia occurs in the setting of pyelonephritis. Essentially all *E. coli* blood isolates from normal individuals with pyelonephritis express P pili; non–P-piliated isolates are only isolated from the blood of individuals with pyelonephritis and compromised host defenses, particularly defects in leukocyte function.[296–298]

The receptor glycolipids are present in all three glycosphingolipids associated with the P blood group (Table 32–4). The three antigens P, P1, and P$^K$ are found on erythrocytes from people with blood group P1 (approximately 75% of the population), whereas P2 cells (approximately 25% of the population) lack the P1 antigen and may have less of the P$^K$ antigen. It has been suggested that a similar difference in the amount of globoseries glycolipids on urogenital epithelium and renal cells may affect their affinity for bacterial attachments and, hence, explain the difference in susceptibilities to infection of different individuals; that is, the density or the availability (or both) of such receptors is a major determinant of host susceptibility and explains the increased frequency of pyelonephritis among children of blood group P1.[288, 299–301]

Other less well characterized adhesins have been reported to be present on uropathogenic strains of *E. coli:* S fimbriae, which bind to terminal sialic acid residues on both epithelial cells and phagocytes[302]; adhesins that bind to the blood group M antigen[303]; and an afimbrial adhesin.[304, 305] A reasonable hypothesis at present is that a major (if not the

major) determinant of uropathogenicity is the sum of the adhesive interactions between the invading strain of bacteria and the uroepithelium, although that mediated by the family of P pili appears quantitatively most important.

In addition to surface adhesins, which are clearly associated with uropathogenicity, a variety of other characteristics have been linked with virulence. These include the production of hemolysin, the presence of the iron-binding protein aerobactin, the ability of the bacteria to resist the bactericidal effect of normal human serum, the production of colicin V, the ability to ferment salicin and perhaps other substrate, and the ability to induce an inflammatory response. This last is induced by endotoxin, particularly when it is presented to the mucosal surface in the context of P pili. Indeed, it has been suggested that the acute symptoms of UTI are due to the inflammatory response to endotoxin presented by bacteria attaching to the mucosal surface.[249, 252]

Perhaps the most completely studied of these additional virulence factors is hemolysin production and the presence of aerobactin. Hemolysin does not appear to play a role in the causation of inflammation but is present in the majority of P pili–positive isolates. It has been shown to kill cultured human renal proximal tubule epithelial cells, which could be important in the pathogenesis of renal injury; indeed, an α-hemolysin vaccine protects against renal injury in a murine model of pyelonephritis.[306–309] In addition to the injurious effects of hemolysin on tubule cells, it is possible that bacterial growth is promoted by the induction of hemolysis, thus freeing erythrocyte iron, an important growth factor for bacteria. Not surprisingly, then, aerobactin, which would facilitate the uptake of iron by bacteria, is also associated with virulence.[275, 310]

Although it is clear that multiple virulence factors are probably operative, what is not clear are how many or which of these are independent variables or are just closely linked to more important factors. Invasive UTI is caused by a few clones of *E. coli* with a number of characteristics in common (see earlier) that are closely linked on the bacterial chromosome. Whether one or more of the other listed factors is an independent virulence factor remains to be determined.[311]

The virulence characteristics of uropathogenic *E. coli* described thus far have been defined in terms of their ability to invade the normal urinary tract, enter the bloodstream, and elicit a variety of acute inflammatory responses. These include an elevated temperature; an increased erythrocyte

**TABLE 32–4.** P$^K$, P, and P1 Blood Group Antigens and Corresponding Glycosphingolipids Isolated from Human Erythrocyte Membranes (the Receptor for P Pili Is Outlined)

| Blood Group Antigen | Structure of Glycosphingolipid |
|---|---|
| P$^K$ | [α-D-Gal*p*-(1–4)-β-D-Gal*p*-] (1–4)-β-D-Glc*p*-Cer (trihexosyl ceramide) |
| P | β-D-GalNac*p*-(1–3)- [α-D-Gal*p*-(1–4)-β-D-Gal*p*-] (1–4)-β-D-Glc*p*-Cer (globoside) |
| P1 | [α-D-Gal*p*-(1–4)-β-D-Gal*p*-] (1–4)-β-D-GlcNac*p*-(1–3)-β-D-Gal*p*-(1–4)-D-Glc*p*-Cer |

Modified from Winberg J: P-fimbriae, bacterial adhesion, and pyelonephritis. Arch Dis Child 59:180, 1984.

sedimentation rate; an acute cytokine response involving interleukin-1, interleukin-6, and tumor necrosis factor; and an increased level of C-reactive protein (an acute-phase reactant that is particularly responsive to acute infection in children). Studies of interleukin-6 release suggest that much of the acute inflammatory response is generated in the kidney in response to invasion by these uropathogens, with the secondary systemic response as a consequence of bloodstream invasion or the systemic release of these locally produced cytokines.[275, 312–315] Consistent with these observations is the report that individuals who are nonsecretors are particularly likely to engender such an acute inflammatory response.[315] Of all the uropathogenic clones, it has been suggested that *E. coli* O1:K1:H7 is the one that is associated with the greatest proinflammatory activity.[316]

Surprisingly, however, infections associated with an acute inflammatory response are not associated with chronic or progressive scarring. Studies performed with both boys and girls have demonstrated that strains of *E. coli* that fail to induce the acute inflammatory response and that do not exhibit the uropathogenic phenotype are the ones responsible for virtually all renal scarring in association with VUR.[312, 317–320] Once again, nonsecretor status carried an increased risk of injury, in this instance for chronic scarring.[321, 322] The mechanisms responsible for this are currently unclear. However, the finding that a peptide isolated from the broth filtrate of such strains induces a far stronger specific T lymphocyte response than does any component of the filtrate from the proinflammatory strains is clearly of interest and raises the possibility of an immune mechanism being at work.[323, 324]

## OTHER BACTERIAL SPECIES

Information is beginning to accumulate as to the pathogenetic mechanisms involved when non–*E. coli* strains invade the urinary tract. Reflecting its position as the most common non–*E. coli* cause of UTI, *P. mirabilis* is the other bacterial species that has received the most attention. So-called mannose-resistant/*Proteus*-like (MR/P) fimbriae and flagellae have been identified on strains isolated from patients with UTI. These are expressed preferentially on isolates from patients with pyelonephritis and appear to be responsible for binding to the uroepithelium. Of great interest, there is considerable structural homology between these fimbriae and the P pili of *E. coli*.[325, 326] Again, as with *E. coli*, other fimbriae have been found that appear not to mediate attachment to the uroepithelium.[327] The possibility that other surface structures of *P. mirabilis* are important is suggested by the observation that an outer membrane protein vaccine prepared from a uropathogenic strain offered considerable protection in a murine model of pyelonephritis.[328]

After attachment to the uroepithelium, three *P. mirabilis* enzymes have been linked to virulence: urease, hemolysin, and a protease. Elegant studies in a mouse model of ascending infection, using isogenic mutant strains as well as the wild-type UTI isolate, have shown that the presence of urease greatly lowered the infecting inoculum necessary to produce sustained infection, was associated with a far more virulent form of pyelonephritis, and resulted in the formation of urinary tract calculi.[329–331] Both urease and, even more, hemolysin are cytotoxic for renal proximal tubule cells.[330, 331] Finally, an immunoglobulin A protease elaborated by this organism, which destroys immunoglobulin A normally present in the urine, may play a role in promoting the occurrence of ascending infection.[332]

*Klebsiella* isolates from patients with pyelonephritis were serum resistant and were more likely to be aerobactin-positive and to possess type 1 fimbriae than were isolates from patients with asymptomatic bacteriuria or cystitis.[333] However, it is clear that our understanding of the mechanisms of molecular pathogenesis involved in *Klebsiella*-induced pyelonephritis are at present incomplete.

Studies of *E. faecalis* strains have suggested that urinary tract isolates are notable for their ability to adhere to the uroepithelium. If they enter the bloodstream from this site, they undergo a change that can be reproduced by the presence of human serum that renders them better able to adhere to the endocardium, thus producing endocarditis.[334]

## Host Factors Influencing Infection

### FACTORS PREDISPOSING TO PYELONEPHRITIS

Several factors are important clinically in predisposing the kidney to infection.

**Urinary Tract Obstruction.** Reference has already been made to the role of obstruction in hematogenous and ascending pyelonephritis. Clinically, renal infections are associated with a variety of obstructive lesions (see Chapter 41). Experimentally, even temporary obstruction markedly increases susceptibility to infection; indeed, almost 100% of rats become infected after ligation of the ureter followed by intravenous injection of *E. coli*. Obstruction at the level of the urinary bladder interferes with the mechanisms by which the normal bladder eradicates bacteria in at least three ways: first, the increase in residual urine volume raises the number of bacteria remaining in the bladder after voiding; second, bladder distention decreases the surface area of the mucosa relative to the total volume of the bladder and thus decreases the effect of the postulated mucosal bactericidal factors; and finally, there is some experimental evidence that bladder wall distention diminishes flow of blood to the bladder mucosa and hence the delivery of leukocytes and antibacterial factors. The net result is that even "nonuropathogenic" strains can cause ascending infection and bacteremic pyelonephritis.[335]

Whereas complete ureteral obstruction markedly increases the susceptibility of the kidney to infection and also results in reactivation of healing lesions, gradual or partial ureteral obstruction induced either surgically or by irradiation of ureters[72] affects renal susceptibility to hematogenous infection to only a slight degree. It is probable, therefore, that the association between partial obstruction and pyelonephritis in humans is due to an effect on the ascending mechanism of infection, either by interfering with ureteral urodynamics or by accentuating the effect of VUR.

**Vesicoureteral Reflux.** The role of vesicoureteral and intrarenal reflux in predisposing to ascending infection is discussed earlier.

**Instrumentation of the Urinary Tract.** Any instrumentation of the urinary tract increases the possibility of infection. The following risk factors have been shown to play a role in the pathogenesis of catheter-associated infection: duration of catheterization, absence of use of a urinometer, microbial colonization of the drainage bag, diabetes mellitus, absence of antibiotic use, female patient, complex urologic problem (i.e., a requirement for a catheter other than to passively drain the urine perioperatively or to monitor urine output), abnormal renal function, and errors in catheter care.[336] Once a urethral catheter is in place, even with closed drainage systems, the daily frequency of bacteriuria is 3% to 10%, with the great majority of patients becoming bacteriuric by the end of 1 month.[337]

**Pregnancy.** The interrelationships among pregnancy, bacteriuria, and pyelonephritis are described later.

**Diabetes Mellitus.** Patients with diabetes mellitus have an increased risk for development of symptomatic UTI, including pyelonephritis.[338-340] The postulated causative factors for this increased frequency of upper UTI are that the metabolic derangements in diabetes lead to increased urinary glucose concentrations; a defect in leukocyte function; and the propensity for obesity, vulvovaginitis, neuropathy, and angiopathy.

There is, however, no epidemiologic evidence that diabetic patients are more likely to acquire bacteriuria than are nondiabetic persons except possibly for women older than 50 years. In no studies do diabetic men appear at increased risk for UTI. A number of studies have analyzed a selected diabetic population but have failed to analyze concurrently a nondiabetic group matched for sex, age, and underlying illnesses. O'Sullivan and associates[341] were unable to detect increased numbers of UTI in a diabetic group when it was compared directly with a nondiabetic population. In a separate study, pregnant women with diabetes did not have significantly increased rates of UTI.[342]

It must be concluded that an increased risk for bacteriuria in diabetic patients, after they were subjected to careful analysis, has not been established. However, there is substantial evidence that diabetic patients are at greater risk for the development of serious complications once infection has occurred. The complications include septicemia, papillary necrosis, renal abscesses, and emphysematous pyelonephritis.

## NONINFECTIOUS RENAL DISORDERS

Various forms of glomerular, tubule, and vascular renal diseases have been reported to show an increased frequency of secondary pyelonephritis. Most reports are based on pathologic studies, without bacteriologic confirmation. It seems probable that in some cases the high frequency represents noninfectious interstitial nephritis rather than infection. In the case of analgesic nephropathy, however, it is well recognized that many patients have bouts of proven urinary infection.

**Differential Susceptibility of Renal Cortex Versus Medulla.** Experimental studies of hematogenous pyelonephritis have revealed a distinct difference in susceptibility to bacterial infection between the renal medulla and cortex. Gorrill[343] first demonstrated that after intravenous inocula-

tion of *E. coli* in animals with ligated ureters, the number of organisms rose logarithmically with time in the medulla, but there was a lag before the increase began in the cortex. Rocha and Fekety[344] then induced localized foci of injury by electrocautery in the cortex and medulla of rabbits; subsequent intravenous injection of bacteria resulted in infection in more than 85% of instances after injury to the medulla, whereas no infection occurred after cortical injury. The most critical experiments were those of Freedman and Beeson,[345] which showed that as few as 10 bacteria injected into the medulla could produce infection, whereas $10^5$ organisms were required in the cortex. Immunofluorescence studies confirmed that in some models of pyelonephritis, bacterial multiplication occurred first in the interstitium of the medulla and then spread to the cortex.[346, 347] However, this vulnerability of the medulla is not a universal finding in all models of pyelonephritis: in some species, both cortical and medullary lesions can be found at the same time; in others, the first lesions are clearly in the cortex.

Although older evidence implicated the anticomplementary action of ammonia as the cause of the exquisite susceptibility of the medulla,[348] more probable explanations are the reduced blood flow to the medulla, delayed mobilization of leukocytes, and medullary hypertonicity.[348-350] In addition to affecting granulocyte mobilization and bacterial multiplication, medullary hypertonicity also interferes with antigen-antibody reactions, serum bactericidal effect,[351] and phagocytosis by leukocytes.[352]

## IMMUNOLOGIC REACTIONS

Interest in the immunologic reactions occurring in the course of pyelonephritis has focused on two events:

1. The possible role of acquired immunity directed against bacterial antigens in determining the outcome of infection. Theoretically, these reactions could be protective, serving to eliminate bacteria from renal tissue; conversely, they could enhance establishment of the infection or cause progression of the tissue damage.

2. The possibility that bacterial infection may somehow stimulate an autoimmune reaction against renal tissue, thus accounting for the progression of renal lesions after infection has been eradicated.[353]

**Antibody Production in Pyelonephritis.** There is ample clinical and experimental evidence that pyelonephritis induces both systemic and local antibody response against the infecting bacteria, principally against the O antigen.[354, 355] Local antibody production by pyelonephritic kidneys has been demonstrated by immunofluorescence techniques[356] and by sensitive methods that detect in vitro synthesis of immunoglobulin and specific antibody by renal tissue.[357] Immunoglobulin G, M, and A synthesis can be localized to areas of lymphocyte infiltration by use of a modification of the Jerne-plaque procedure.[358] K antigens (which have more significant virulence than do O antigens in *E. coli* infection) induce serum and local antibody much less frequently and in lower titers.[359] In humans, K antibodies appear rather irregularly in the urine during acute pyelonephritis, and indeed, the *E. coli* K1 strain seems to induce tolerance to the K1 antigen. Antibodies to both type 1 and P fimbriae have also been reported.[360, 361]

Despite some conflicting results, the antibody response seems to serve a protective role against both hematogenous and ascending infection.[354, 355, 360] Immunization with antibodies to O antigen reduces the frequency of infection and abscesses in both hematogenous and ascending *E. coli* pyelonephritis in rats, and K antibodies are even more efficiently protective. Transfer of urine from animals immunized intravesically with killed *E. coli* protects against ascending pyelonephritis, and this immunity is diminished by absorption of the urine with K antigen.[354] Antibodies against bacterial pili also afford protection from experimental ascending pyelonephritis.[291–295] However, it is clear that antibody synthesis is only one of the factors that protect against further bacterial growth and tissue damage. In some experimental models, passively administered antibodies do not afford protection, or infection may disappear despite a lack of antibody response.

**Cell-Mediated Immunity in Pyelonephritis.** A role for cell-mediated immunity against bacterial antigens in either the pathogenesis of pyelonephritis or protection against bacterial invasion has not been clearly defined. The finding that a specific T cell response against bacterial peptides can be demonstrated suggests that this issue should be reopened.[323, 324]

**Possible Autoimmune Mechanisms in Pyelonephritis.** There has been considerable interest in the possibility that renal infection can stimulate an autoimmune reaction against renal antigens, which could contribute to the perpetuation of renal damage in the absence of continued bacterial proliferation.[353] It is theoretically possible, for example, that the tubule injury in acute pyelonephritis may release tubule antigens into the circulation and initiate an antibody-mediated tubulointerstitial disease. However, several studies failed to demonstrate antikidney antibodies in the serum of patients or animals with bacterial pyelonephritis or locally synthesized immunoglobulin G and immunoglobulin M in experimental pyelonephritis. Further, neither granular staining for immunoglobulin G and complement (suggesting immune complex tubule disease) nor linear deposition (suggesting anti–tubule basement membrane disease) has been demonstrated by immunofluorescence microscopy in experimental or human pyelonephritis.[362–364] However, Losse and colleagues[365] did find antibodies directed against an antigenic determinant of *E. coli* in rabbit experimental pyelonephritis that also reacted against antigens derived from kidney and liver tissue. A telling argument against an antibody-mediated autoimmune reaction to pyelonephritis is that pyelonephritis can remain localized to one kidney, often leading to its complete destruction, while the contralateral kidney remains normal. This occurs in patients with unilateral obstruction and has been repeatedly demonstrated in experimental animals.

The profound mononuclear cell infiltrate characteristic of chronic pyelonephritis has also raised the question of whether cell-mediated immune reactions to renal antigens may be involved in the progression of the renal lesions. Indeed, Kalmanson and associates[366] reported a number of experiments supporting such a possibility. Histologic lesions resembling chronic pyelonephritis were found to de-

velop in normal rats joined by parabiosis to rats with chronic enterococcal pyelonephritis after bacteria had been eliminated from the infected rats by means of antibiotic therapy. In addition, peritoneal lymphocytes from animals with chronic enterococcal pyelonephritis produced inhibition of macrophage migration when they were incubated with homologous renal antigen. However, using the same experimental model, Cotran and Galvanek[363] found that whereas significant stimulation of pyelonephritic lymphocytes occurred after exposure to the bacterial antigen (*E. faecalis* cell wall), there was little stimulation after incubation with renal antigen. Although this discrepancy with regard to cell-mediated immunity to renal antigen cannot be resolved, the presence of cell-mediated immunity to bacterial antigen is interesting in light of experiments by van Zwieten and colleagues.[367] These workers induced mononuclear cell infiltrates in sensitized guinea pigs and rats by intracortical injections of aggregated but not soluble bovine gamma globulin. The reactivity could be transferred with lymph node cells but not with serum, which suggests that delayed hypersensitivity reactions occur in the kidney if the antigen is in a particulate form. It is possible, therefore, that the mononuclear infiltrate in chronic pyelonephritis may in part reflect a delayed hypersensitivity reaction to particulate bacterial antigen.

On balance, however, it is doubtful that T cell–mediated immune reactions have an important bearing on the establishment or the course of pyelonephritis. Miller's group[368] showed that ablation of 99% of T lymphocytes by thymectomy and serial sublethal irradiation did not perceptibly alter the bacteriologic or pathologic course of experimental pyelonephritis. In these experiments, the response to both O and K antigens appeared to be T cell independent. Asscher and associates[369] also concluded that delayed hypersensitivity reactions do not play a role in the pathogenesis of kidney scarring associated with *E. coli* infection of rat kidney.

There has been interest in the possibility that immune reactions to Tamm-Horsfall protein may play a role in renal damage. Tamm-Horsfall protein is a urinary mucoprotein formed by the cells of the ascending thick limb and distal convoluted tubule and is normally restricted largely to renal tubule cells, urine itself beyond the distal convoluted tubule, and renal casts.[370] It has been shown to leak into the interstitium in human and experimental reflux nephropathy, obstructive uropathy, and some other tubulointerstitial disorders.[371, 372] The first evidence was of a humoral reaction to Tamm-Horsfall protein developing within 3 weeks of the onset of either VUR or ureteric obstruction in pigs[373]; this has since been corroborated.[374] A further protocol involved rabbits "immunized" by rabbit urine. A focal interstitial nephritis developed in 19 of 23 animals killed between 16 and 48 weeks after the commencement of the study. A similar response followed challenge by isolated rabbit Tamm-Horsfall protein, whereas there was no response to a challenge by Tamm-Horsfall protein–depleted urine. However, no relationship was demonstrable between cellular Tamm-Horsfall protein extravasation and interstitial fibrosis in another study of rats subjected to unilateral ureteral obstruction for periods varying from 6 hours to 3 weeks,[375, 376] which can be regarded as a short-term study of this problem. Serum autoantibodies to Tamm-Horsfall protein have been detected in patients with acute pyelonephritis and VUR,[377, 378] but their relationship to renal damage is unclear. Thus, the pathogenetic role of Tamm-Horsfall protein in immunologic renal injury must be judged uncertain.[379]

**Evolution of the Renal Lesion.** The usual course of uncomplicated *E. coli* acute pyelonephritis in both experimental animals and humans is one of healing rather than of progressive damage. In most experimental models of *E. coli* pyelonephritis, the phase of acute suppurative inflammation in the kidney lasts 1 to 3 weeks. The tissue destruction is largely the result of bacterial multiplication and inflammation. With healing, there are an increase in the number of mononuclear cells, a decrease in neutrophils in the interstitium, and replacement of necrotic tubules by fibrous tissue and foci of tubule atrophy. These changes are accompanied by a decrease in the number of bacteria cultured from the kidneys; by the 6th to the 10th week, the kidneys are sterile and the resultant renal lesion is a triangular, depressed scar extending from the cortex, with its apex in the medulla and pelvis. However, a variety of bacterial and host factors can modify this sequence of events and lead to progressive damage. Whereas *Staphylococcus* infections may eventually heal, they tend to remain active for longer periods and to result in considerable tissue destruction. In *Klebsiella* infection, the original infecting strain persists in the kidney for at least 24 weeks, probably owing to the lack of production of circulating antibodies to these organisms.[380] *Proteus* infections, although associated with a vigorous antibody response, do not heal as a consequence of the urinary obstruction resulting from the deposition of magnesium ammonium phosphate calculi.

In human pyelonephritis, persistence of the original infecting organism is more likely to occur with unusual organisms, such as *Proteus* and *Klebsiella,* and is frequently associated with obstructive uropathy, renal calculi, renal carbuncle, or bacterial prostatitis. However, bacterial persistence within the renal parenchyma as a cause of progressive damage has been difficult to demonstrate convincingly in humans. It is probable that most instances of recurrences of UTI with the same pathogen (defined as ''relapse'') are due to its persistence in the lower urinary tract (bladder, periurethral tissues, and prostate) rather than in the kidney. Indeed, serologic studies of UTI suggest that the majority of recurrences are actually reinfections with a different strain of the same bacterial species or with a pathogen of a different species. This is particularly true in young women with uncomplicated recurrent cystitis. As we shall see later, the large majority of these infections do not lead to renal damage except in the presence of obstruction or VUR.

Because a variable but small number of patients with the typical morphologic lesion of chronic pyelonephritis give no evidence of bacterial infection, the question has arisen whether progression of renal lesions can still occur after the bacteria have been totally eradicated. Several mechanisms have been postulated to explain such events.[353, 381]

1. The role of autoimmune mechanisms is discussed in detail earlier. Suffice it to say here that there is no conclusive evidence that either antibody- or cell-mediated autoimmune reactions play a major role in progressive renal damage in chronic pyelonephritis.[362]

2. Vascular changes caused by the initial inflammation with consequent ischemia may conceivably produce progressive tissue destruction even when bacteria disappear. This explanation derives credence from the frequency with which vascular thickening and angiographic abnormalities are seen in human chronic pyelonephritis and the similarity between lesions induced by ischemia and infection.[382, 383] However, interpretation of human data is hampered by the frequent occurrence of hypertensive vascular changes, which contribute to renal parenchymal atrophy, and by our inability to determine whether the vascular changes precede the parenchymal damage or are merely an expression of it. Kincaid-Smith and Hodson[384] have reported remarkable myointimal as well as perivascular thickening in a study in which VUR and urinary infection were maintained in four pigs for more than 2 years. They suggest that these lesions may contribute to both the hypertension and the parenchymal atrophy that developed in these pigs. (Vascular lesions, however, were not present in noninfected animals with VUR.) Both clinical and experimental evidence suggests that superimposition of secondary hypertension in the course of chronic pyelonephritis measurably hastens deterioration of renal function and reduction of renal mass.[385-387] It is possible, therefore, that progressive renal insufficiency in some cases of chronic pyelonephritis may be due to vascular disease rather than pyelonephritic scarring.

3. The possibility that sterile reflux may induce progressive renal damage is discussed earlier. Granted that sterile reflux may be harmful, how is the damage induced? Urodynamic factors (water-hammer effect),[384] vascular narrowing and ischemia, and leakage of urinary constituents (e.g., Tamm-Horsfall protein) into the interstitium[372, 374, 375] have all been implicated as possible mechanisms but, to date, without conclusive proof.

4. It has been suggested that the ability of bacteria to survive in the kidney as bacterial variants that lack part or all of their cell wall (spheroplasts, protoplasts, or L-forms) may account for persistent or progressive renal infection. Such variants may remain viable in the hypertonic environment of the renal medulla and induce pathologic changes either as variants or after reversion to bacterial forms. However, despite scattered clinical studies reporting the presence of such forms in the urine after UTI[388] and in renal biopsy specimens of patients with sterile pyuria,[389] other studies have failed to detect such forms. Experimentally, protoplasts can indeed produce renal lesions but only after they have reverted to the parent bacterial form.[390, 391] More than two decades after the suggestion was first made, the role of bacterial variants is still unclear.

In concluding this discussion of factors affecting the evolution of renal lesions in pyelonephritis, the work of Glauser and associates[392] should be noted. These authors evaluated the importance of suppuration, persistent infection, and scar formation in the evolution of *E. coli* chronic pyelonephritis by treating rats with different antibiotic regimens at different stages of the disease. They found that the magnitude of the suppuration in the acute phase of pyelonephritis was the most significant factor in predicting the eventual development of small, chronically scarred kidneys. Persistent low-grade infection did not lead to chronic pyelonephritis if the acute suppuration was suppressed; antigen load and antibody- or cell-dependent autoimmune processes did not appear to play a significant role in the progression of infection. Essentially similar conclusions were reached by Ransley and Risdon,[393] based on experiments in pigs. The clinical evidence summarized is for the most part consistent with these conclusions and further emphasizes the need for prompt and effective antibiotic treatment of the earliest pyelonephritic lesions, particularly in infants with VUR.

## PATHOLOGY

### Acute Pyelonephritis

Typical descriptions of the pathologic changes in acute pyelonephritis in humans are based on severely affected kidneys from patients dying with sepsis. Changes in uncomplicated acute pyelonephritis, such as occurs in pregnancy or after single attacks of obstructive acute pyelonephritis, are less well known. However, from studies on experimental animals with ascending pyelonephritis, it is clear that the acute lesions can vary considerably in severity from some that affect only the pelvic mucosa (pyelitis) to others that involve entire lobules of the medulla and cortex.

On macroscopic examination, kidneys from patients with severe acute pyelonephritis are enlarged and contain a variable number of abscesses on the capsular surface and on cut sections of the cortex and medulla. Tissue between infected areas appears normal. Occasionally, areas of inflammation extend from the cortex into the medulla in the shape of a wedge. In the presence of obstruction, the calyces are enlarged, the papillae are blunted, and the pelvic mucosa is sometimes congested and thickened. The papillae may be completely normal in some cases or may show outright papillary necrosis in others.

Histologic changes are characterized by involvement of the tubules and interstitium. The interstitium is edematous and infiltrated by a variety of inflammatory cells, predominantly neutrophils. Within abscesses, the tubules show necrosis, and many tubules contain polymorphonuclear leukocytes. The patchiness of the inflammation is particularly striking. Thus, completely normal tubules and interstitium may lie adjacent to a large necrotizing renal abscess. Even in areas of the most severe inflammation, normal glomeruli can be seen, and indeed, intraglomerular inflammation is rare except in some forms of monilial glomerulonephritis. In the presence of total ureteral obstruction, the inflammatory reaction sometimes affects the entire kidney.

The morphologic appearance of acute renal infections associated with reflux in children has, to our knowledge, rarely been described. In experimental acute reflux nephropathy in the pig, large acute inflammatory lesions corresponding to zones of intrarenal reflux have been referred to as "acute lobar nephronia" by Hodson[151] (see Fig. 32–5).

The sequence of events in the healing of acute pyelonephritis has been deduced from experimental studies. The neutrophilic exudate is rapidly replaced by one that is predominantly mononuclear, with macrophages and plasma cells and, later, lymphocytes. There are formation of granulation tissue, deposition of collagen, and eventual replacement of abscesses by scars that can be seen on the cortical surface as fibrous depressions. Such scars are characterized microscopically by atrophy of tubules, interstitial fibrosis, and lymphocyte infiltration. Progressive scarring has also been documented radiologically in children with reflux nephropathy and in reflux nephropathy in the pig. Such scars have a characteristically depressed cortical surface associated with a blunt and often deformed calyx (see Fig. 32–6).

## Chronic Pyelonephritis and Reflux Nephropathy

### TERMINOLOGY AND FREQUENCY

Despite the long-standing controversy over the use of the term chronic pyelonephritis, there is now reasonable agreement as to the morphologic changes sufficient to distinguish this condition from the many other tubulointerstitial diseases (see earlier).

Radiologic studies demonstrated the relatively specific anatomic features used in the diagnosis of chronic pyelonephritis. Hodson[3] drew attention to the association between cortical scarring and a corresponding deformity of the underlying calyx as a diagnostic feature that differentiated pyelonephritic from other types of renal scarring. This suggestion was confirmed in a morphologic study by Smith.[4] The requirement for calyceal deformity for the diagnosis of chronic pyelonephritis, subsequently expounded by Heptinstall,[2] measurably limits the differential diagnosis and the possible causes for the renal scarring. Only a limited number of conditions can lead to a morphologic picture of chronic corticomedullary tubulointerstitial damage coupled with calyceal abnormality, and they are as follows.

1. VUR. As detailed earlier, renal damage in VUR is associated with intrarenal reflux and is most frequently due to infected reflux. This is the most common cause of entities referred to as "chronic atrophic" or chronic nonobstructive pyelonephritis. The term "reflux nephropathy" is slowly replacing chronic pyelonephritis to describe this condition. Besides emphasizing the role of VUR, the term has the virtue of including two types of changes associated with VUR: the more common and widely recognizable focal scarring, which is attributed to scarring at the site of compound papillae with intrarenal reflux; and the diffuse renal damage affecting all papillae and usually associated with high-pressure obstructive reflux. It must be stressed that whereas the majority of children with chronic pyelonephritic scars demonstrate VUR, only about half of adults do.[394, 395] However, up to 89% of adults will have abnormal ureteral orifices, which suggests (but by no means proves) that ureteral reflux may have occurred in the past.[395]

2. Urinary obstruction. It is frequently difficult to differentiate uninfected obstruction from a combination of obstruction and infection, but discrete parenchymal scars usually indicate the coexistence of infection.

3. Analgesic nephropathy, with or without bacterial infection. This is usually readily distinguished by the widespread papillary necrosis (see Chapter 34).

4. Unusual forms of noninfectious acute papillary necro-

sis due to such conditions as sickle cell disease and dehydration in infants. Chrispin and associates[396, 397] described infants with severe acute gastroenteritis who had papillary necrosis and subsequent corticopapillary scarring that resembled chronic pyelonephritis.

5. Segmental hypoplasia (the Ask-Upmark kidney). This condition, previously considered a developmental anomaly, is now also thought to be caused by VUR in the majority of cases.[398, 399]

A small number of patients will exhibit corticomedullary scarring and calyceal deformity in the apparent absence of the aforementioned conditions or of bacterial infection. The more diligently one looks for a recognized cause, the fewer of these cases are reported. Such cases were described more frequently before the widespread use of voiding cystourethrography to exclude reflux and before calyceal deformity was appreciated as the diagnostic criterion for chronic pyelonephritis.[400] In children with urinary tract anomalies, some scars show histologic evidence of renal dysplasia (e.g., dysplastic tubules, embryonic cartilage) and are almost certainly coexistent developmental abnormalities of the renal parenchyma. Nonetheless, a few cases with no apparent cause still appear in most series.[401–403]

For these reasons, chronic pyelonephritis can be subdivided into three types: 1) chronic pyelonephritis with reflux (reflux nephropathy), 2) chronic pyelonephritis with obstruction (chronic obstructive pyelonephritis), and 3) idiopathic chronic pyelonephritis.

If the morphologic criteria are adhered to, we have found the incidence of chronic pyelonephritic scarring at autopsy to be 1.85% in two series of patients examined at the Boston City Hospital between 1965 and 1972. This figure is remarkably close to that of Farmer and Heptinstall.[402] Admittedly, the numbers may be somewhat larger or smaller in hospitals serving other population groups. For example, the higher figure of Kleeman and colleagues[71] was derived from a Veterans Administration Hospital with a population of patients that showed a high frequency of urologic abnormalities.

The frequency of chronic pyelonephritis as a cause of end-stage kidney disease is also variable. The Human Renal Transplant Registry reports a frequency of about 13%, and data from the European Dialysis and Transplant Association show that 22% of adults with end-stage kidney disease suffer from chronic pyelonephritis. Unfortunately, the criteria for diagnosis of chronic pyelonephritis in these series are not certain. Chronic pyelonephritis was found in 11% of 95 consecutive pretransplant nephrectomy specimens examined grossly, microscopically, and bacteriologically by Schwartz and Cotran.[401] A series from New South Wales lists the diagnoses etiologically.[403] Of 317 histologically studied cases of adult end-stage renal disease, 8% had reflux nephropathy; 1%, idiopathic chronic pyelonephritis; and 6%, obstruction, congenital malformations, or renal calculi. In Kincaid-Smith's series[394] of 147 pretransplant nephrectomy specimens, 30 (20%) of the patients had chronic pyelonephritis; of these, about half had demonstrable reflux. In a later account of her series, 15.3% of patients with end-stage renal failure had clinical and radiologic features of reflux nephropathy.[404] In Christchurch Hospital, 12% of patients who entered dialysis and transplant pro-

grams had reflux nephropathy.[405] In children younger than 16 years, reflux nephropathy accounts for 19% to 34% of patients entering renal replacement programs.[406]

## GROSS PATHOLOGY

The most characteristic changes are seen on gross rather than microscopic examination. The most common morphologic appearance of chronic pyelonephritis and reflux nephropathy is that referred to as coarse renal scarring or focal scarring, consisting of corticopapillary scars overlying dilated, blunted, or deformed calyces (Fig. 32–8). The remarkable pelvocalyceal deformity is not easy to visualize grossly on pathologic examination but is particularly obvious in tracings of the calyces made on excretory urograms (Fig. 32–9). The kidneys are usually smaller than normal, and extreme reductions in size of one of the two kidneys are not unusual. Involvement can be bilateral or unilateral, depending on whether reflux or obstruction has occurred on one or both sides; with bilateral involvement, the kidneys are usually asymmetrically scarred. The scars vary in size but are usually broad, involve a whole lobe, are rather shallow, and have a flatter surface than do healed infarcts (see Fig. 32–8B). The areas between scars may be smooth but are usually finely granular, reflecting hypertrophic changes. Although any part of the kidney may be involved, the large majority of scars are in the upper and lower poles, consistent with the frequency of intrarenal reflux in these areas. The medulla is distorted, and affected papillae are flattened. In cases with obstruction, the pelvis and calyces are distinctly dilated, but they may be of normal caliber in the absence of obstruction (in late cases) or after obstruction has been relieved. The pelvic and calyceal mucosa can be thickened and granular, particularly in cases of chronic reflux. Kincaid-Smith[404] emphasized the importance of examining the ureters, because thickening of the ureteral wall with or without dilatation is a reliable sign of the pre-existence of VUR (Fig. 32–10).

A second morphologic variety, referred to as diffuse or generalized reflux nephropathy by radiologists, occurs in patients with severe VUR together with obstruction (e.g., children with posterior urethral valves).[407] The scarring is so generalized that the cortical surface appears to be relatively smooth or finely granular. In these cases, the pelvis and calyces are diffusely dilated, and the renal parenchyma shows widespread atrophy resembling postobstructive atrophy (see Fig. 32–10). In these kidneys, the presence of a thickened pelvic and ureteral wall (or the cystoscopic appearance of ureteral orifices) suggests previous VUR. Lying somewhere between those with coarse scars and those with generalized damage are kidneys in which two or more areas of coarse scarring are associated with generalized dilatation of calyces and overall reduction in kidney size, labeled mixed damage by Hodson.[407]

## MICROSCOPIC FINDINGS

The histologic appearance is one of tubule damage and interstitial inflammation and scarring, and it varies according to the evolutionary stage of the lesion. Old, extensive scars can be composed almost entirely of atrophic or dilated

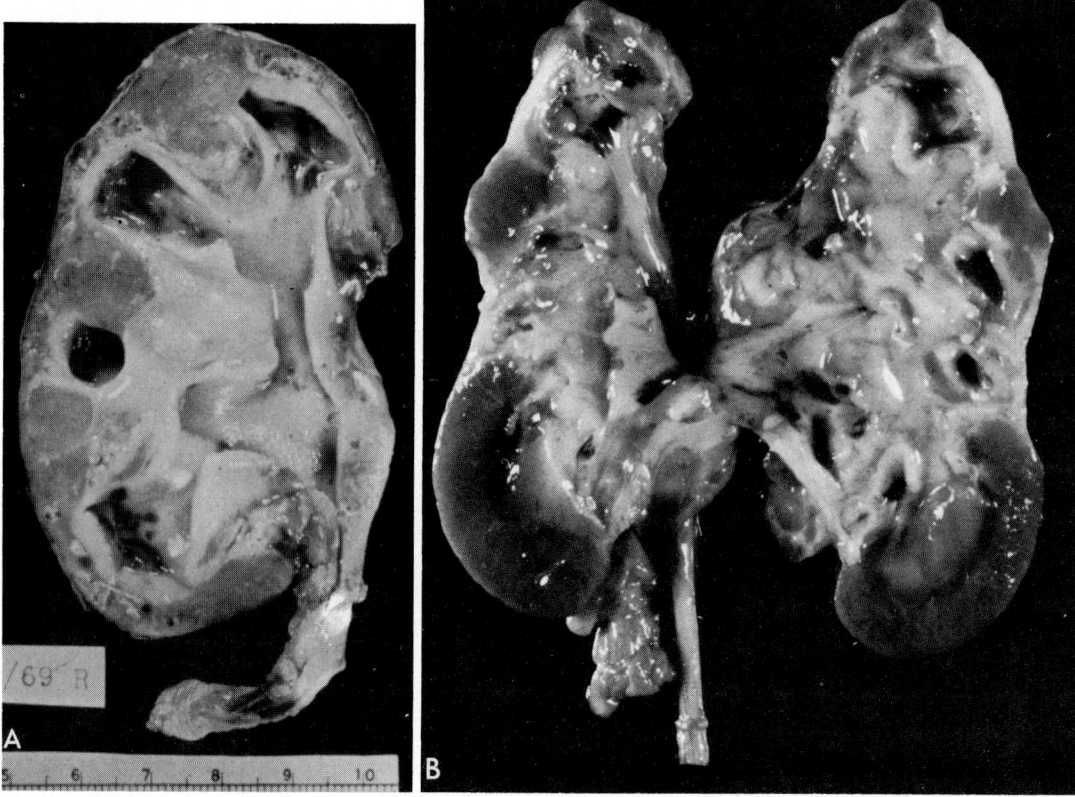

**Figure 32–8.** *A.* Chronic pyelonephritis. Note irregularly scarred kidney, dilated and blunted calyces, and a thickened ureter that suggests chronic VUR. *B.* Typical pyelonephritic broad scars in a patient with reflux nephropathy. The scars involve entire lobes. Note prominent underlying calyceal dilatation. (*B* from Bhathena DB, Holland NH, Weiss JH, et al: Morphology of coarse renal scars in reflux-associated nephropathy in man. *In* Hodson CJ, Kincaid-Smith P [eds]: Reflux Nephropathy. Masson Publishing USA, New York, 1979, p 243.)

tubules, separated by fibrous tissue, with remaining large blood vessels (Fig. 32–11). More recent scars show variable amounts of interstitial mononuclear inflammation, tubule atrophy and necrosis, increase in interstitial fibrous tissue, and periglomerular fibrosis. Many tubules are dilated, lined by flattened epithelium, and filled with colloid casts (thyroidization). The inflammatory infiltrate is variable. Lymphocytes and monocytes predominate, but occasionally one can see large foci of plasma cells; in the presence of active inflammation, neutrophils can be plentiful. Pus casts are also frequently present, particularly when there is active infection. However, pus casts can also be present in the absence of bacteriuria, presumably owing to ischemic damage.

Vascular changes within the scars can be either mild or more severe. Both arteries and arterioles may show medial and intimal thickening; the intimal thickening is of the fine, concentric cellular type. In some cases, there is clear-cut elastic reduplication. Vascular changes within the scarred areas are present even in patients who are not hypertensive, although they become more severe in the presence of hypertension. In the nonscarred areas, hyaline arteriolar changes are limited to those patients with secondary hypertension.

The pelvis and calyces are universally affected. Usually there is infiltration of the subendothelial connective tissue by inflammatory cells, which often form large masses or lymphoid follicles (see Fig. 32–11). Neutrophils, eosino-

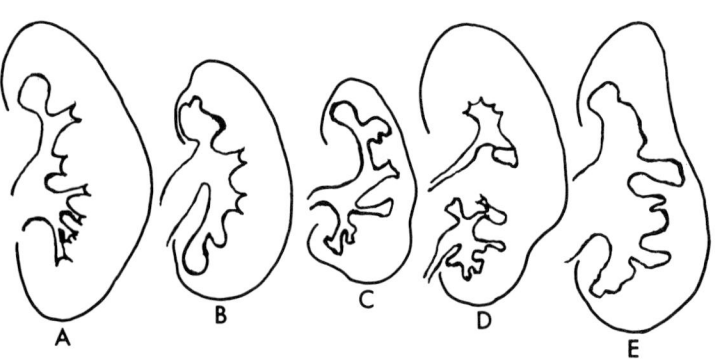

**Figure 32–9.** Tracings of urograms showing common patterns of scarring and calyceal deformities in reflux nephropathy. *A.* Upper pole. *B.* Severe bipolar. *C.* Generalized, with one lower pole lobe spared. *D.* Duplex kidney, with severe deformities in the lower pole. *E.* Generalized diffuse calyceal involvement. (*A* to *E* from Hodson CJ: Reflux nephropathy. Med Clin North Am 62:1201, 1978.)

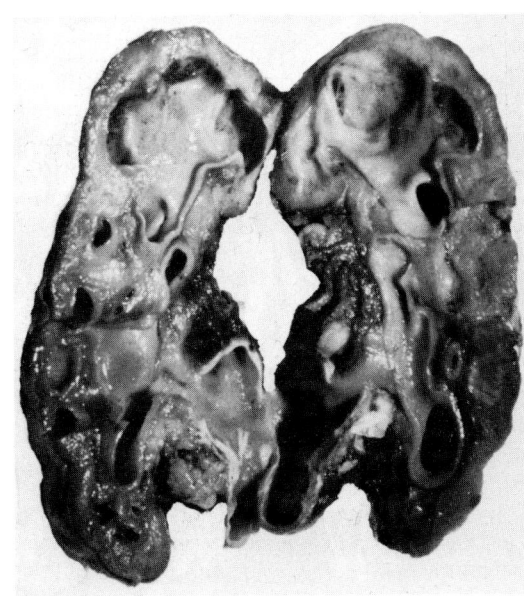

**Figure 32–10.** Kidney showing the "generalized" or diffuse form of reflux nephropathy. There is more or less uniform dilatation of calyces and thinning of renal parenchyma. Note thickening of the pelvis and base of the ureter. (From Hodson CJ: Formation of renal scars with special reference to reflux nephropathy. Contrib Nephrol 16:83, 1979, S Karger AG, Basel.)

phils, and occasionally giant cells may also be present. The mucosal epithelium may be severely thickened and infiltrated with inflammatory cells. The amount of collagen in the underlying connective tissue is usually also increased.

Of interest is the presence of interstitial deposits of Tamm-Horsfall protein precipitates in the kidneys with chronic pyelonephritis associated with reflux or obstruction. Tamm-Horsfall protein can be localized specifically by immunofluorescence microscopy, but its presence in casts and in interstitial tissue can be suspected by histologic examination as a strongly periodic acid–Schiff (PAS) reaction–positive amorphous or fibrillar material. Interstitial deposits of Tamm-Horsfall protein have been detected in kidneys from patients with chronic pyelonephritis, reflux nephropathy, urinary tract obstruction, and other interstitial diseases.[371, 408] These deposits are sometimes surrounded by

an intense inflammatory infiltrate consisting of mononuclear cells, occasional neutrophils, and even giant cells. Deposits probably result from tubule disruption, with discharge of urinary contents into the interstitium. Tamm-Horsfall protein has also been seen in thin-walled renal veins and lymphatics, possibly from pyelovenous or pyelolymphatic ruptures.[409, 410] Interstitial Tamm-Horsfall protein deposits have also been demonstrated in experimental reflux nephropathy,[372] and the question has been raised whether they may play a role in inducing tissue damage and fibrosis either by direct toxic effects or by inducing an immunologic reaction in the interstitium. This issue is discussed earlier.

In a careful morphologic study of 23 cases of coarse renal scarring associated with VUR, Bhathena and associates[411] detected histologic evidence of renal dysplasia, including immature medullary segments and islands of cartilage, in nine scars. Whether this type of scar represents an intrinsic embryologic anomaly of the ureteric bud or whether intrauterine VUR plays a role in its genesis is unknown.

Although glomeruli may be entirely normal or show only periglomerular fibrosis, a variety of glomerular changes may be present. These have been well described and illustrated by Heptinstall.[412] Ischemic changes, consisting of solidification of glomerular tufts and deposition of collagen within Bowman space, are frequent, as are small shrunken glomeruli. Focal or diffuse proliferation and necrosis can also be present; these have been considered secondary to hypertension. Kincaid-Smith[413, 414] has drawn attention to the association of chronic pyelonephritis and reflux nephropathy with a glomerular lesion best described as focal segmental sclerosis and hyalinosis, similar to that seen in some patients with focal sclerosis and the nephrotic syndrome. She noted in patients with reflux nephropathy that those with proteinuria were more likely to progress to renal failure, even in the absence of hypertension, overt infection, or persistent VUR. Renal biopsy specimens showed focal and segmental hyalinosis and sclerosis in most of these patients. Similar findings have since been described by numerous other investigators. The pathogenesis and clinical significance of these glomerular lesions are discussed in detail later.

**Figure 32–11.** Pyelonephritic scar composed of atrophic or dilated tubules, a few sclerosed or sclerosing glomeruli, and thickened vessels. Note the dilated calyx with prominent lymphoid infiltrate beneath the mucosa.

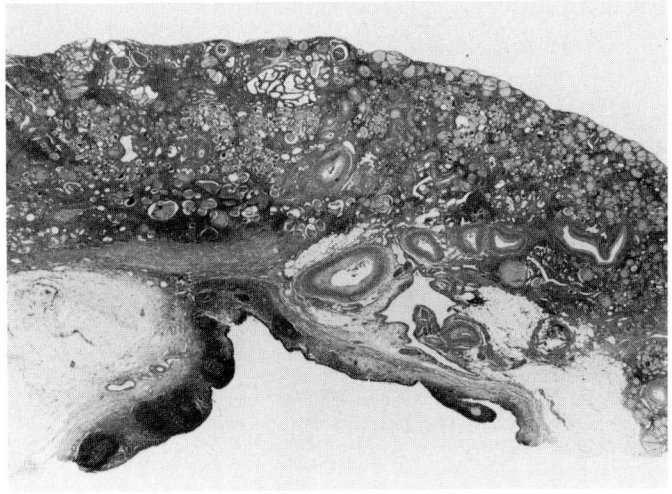

## NATURAL HISTORY OF BACTERIURIA AND PYELONEPHRITIS

### Frequency and Epidemiology of Urinary Tract Infection

The frequency of UTI and its clinical impact are different for the two sexes at different stages of life (Fig. 32–12). Approximately 1% of neonates are bacteriuric, with a two-fold to fourfold higher frequency among boys presumably due to an increased occurrence of urogenital congenital anomalies.[415, 416] Equally striking is a fourfold increase in bacteriuria among premature infants (2.9% versus 0.7% among full-term infants)[417]; approximately half of these premature infants will demonstrate VUR.[416]

Once the neonatal period is past, the lack of circumcision has been shown to potentiate the development of febrile UTI and pyelonephritis in boys without urogenital abnormalities,[418] an observation that continues into young adulthood.[419]

After infancy and until age 55 years, when prostatic hypertrophy starts becoming apparent in men, UTI is predominantly a female disease. From infancy until age 10 years, the frequency of UTI in girls is about 1.2%, with approximately one third of these infections being symptomatic. After an initial episode of bacteriuria, approximately 80% of schoolgirls will have one or more recurrences; 80% of these recurrences are due to reinfections rather than relapses of sequestered deep tissue infection. It has been estimated that a minimum of 5% to 6% of schoolgirls will have at least one episode of UTI between the ages of 5 and 18 years. Approximately 20% of schoolgirls with bacteriuria have demonstrable VUR.[416, 420, 421]

When cohorts of schoolgirls with and without bacteriuria are observed for periods as long as 18 years, some important observations emerge.[422, 423] Although the urine may

have remained sterile for long periods in many of these bacteriuric schoolgirls, bacteriuria usually redeveloped shortly after marriage or during the first pregnancy.[422] There is an increase in the number of episodes of bacteriuria and the number of hospitalizations for UTI over the one to two decades of follow-up among the initially bacteriuric schoolgirls. This increase is most marked during pregnancy, with a 63.8% frequency of pregnancy-associated bacteriuria in women who were bacteriuric as schoolgirls, as opposed to a 26.7% frequency for those who were not. Of potentially great clinical and pathogenetic importance is the observation that 10.8% of the children of the bacteriuric schoolgirls who were studied became bacteriuric themselves, as opposed to none of the children of the nonbacteriuric control patients.[423] Persistence of bacteriuria appears to be more common in children with VUR than in those with normal urinary tracts.[424]

Among adult women, the incidence and prevalence of bacteriuria are related to age, degree of sexual activity, and form of contraception employed. Approximately 1% to 3% of women between the ages of 15 and 24 years have bacteriuria; the incidence increases by 1% to 2% for each decade thereafter up to a level of about 10% to 15% by the sixth or seventh decades. Approximately 40% to 50% of women will have at least one UTI in their lifetimes.[37, 416] There is an incomplete correlation between the findings of bacteriuria and the occurrence of clinical symptoms. Dysuria occurs each year in approximately 20% of women between the ages of 24 and 64 years, half of whom come to medical attention. Of the group seeking medical care, one third has the acute urethral syndrome (see later), and two thirds (approximately 6% of the adult female population) has significant bacteriuria in association with clinical symptoms referable to the urinary tract.[425–427]

Bacteriuria, whether asymptomatic or clinically overt, is unusual in males before they reach their 50s in the absence of urinary tract instrumentation.[416] The frequency of bacteriuria among schoolboys is between 0.04% and 0.14%.[418, 419, 428] Although the frequency of structural and neurologic defects of the urinary tract is much higher in schoolboys than in schoolgirls with UTI, such abnormalities are not invariable. Indeed, if the first episode of bacteriuria in boys is delayed until after the age of 10 years, the frequency of structural abnormalities is low, the prognosis is excellent, and recurrence is infrequent after an adequate course of antimicrobial therapy.[429] One male population that appears to be at an increased risk for UTI is sexually active male homosexuals, who become infected with the same nephritogenic strains of *E. coli* that infect women.[430] Several investigators have noted a high frequency of *Proteus* infection, as opposed to *E. coli* infection, among boys with UTI, perhaps related to a high rate of colonization of the preputial sac with *Proteus* species.[431, 432]

As the aging process progresses and prostatic disease becomes more common, the frequency of UTI in men rises dramatically. By age 70 years, the frequency of bacteriuria reaches a level of 3.5% in otherwise healthy men and a level of greater than 15% in hospitalized men.[13] With the onset of chronic debilitating illness and long-term institutionalization, bacteriuria rates in both sexes reach levels of 25% to 50%,[433, 434] with the frequency in women now only slightly greater than that in men.[435, 436]

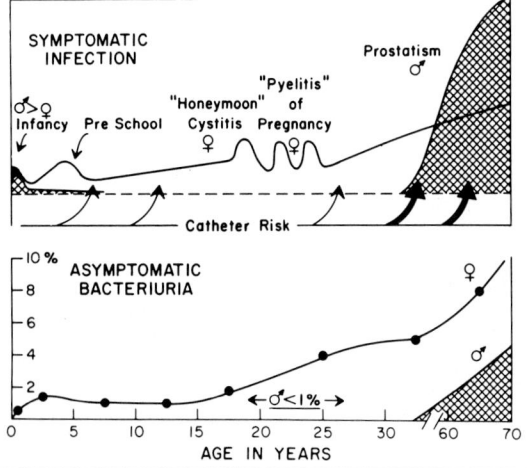

**Figure 32–12.** Overview of the frequency of symptomatic UTI and of asymptomatic bacteriuria according to age and sex. (Modified from the original concept of Jawetz; from Kunin CM: Detection, Prevention and Management of Urinary Tract Infections, 3rd ed. Lea & Febiger, Philadelphia, 1979.)

Certain populations of patients are at increased risk for UTI. This risk is most marked in pregnant women, who have a 4% to 10% frequency of bacteriuria—a rate at least twice that for similarly aged nonpregnant women.[437–442] As many as 60% of pregnant women with asymptomatic bacteriuria early in pregnancy will develop symptomatic infection if untreated, with approximately one fourth to one third developing symptomatic pyelonephritis.[416, 442, 443] About 25% to 33% of women with pregnancy-associated bacteriuria have infection at postpartum follow-up, even if this is done as many as 10 to 14 years post partum, as opposed to 5% of similarly aged women who never had pregnancy-associated bacteriuria. Approximately 30% of women with a history of bacteriuria of pregnancy have changes on the excretory urogram that suggest chronic pyelonephritis. This is not to say, however, that bacteriuria of pregnancy is responsible for these changes. Current data would suggest that the kidneys of the women with postpartum infection after pregnancy-associated infection were probably damaged during childhood, with recurrent infection being exacerbated by the hormonal and mechanical changes induced by pregnancy. There is little evidence that infection developing for the first time during pregnancy is responsible for long-term effects.[6, 442, 444, 445] Indeed, the frequency of bacteriuria during pregnancy is significantly higher in women with a history of past childhood UTI.[445] As in other populations, the occurrence of pyelonephritis among pregnant women is particularly associated with infection with uropathogenic strains possessing P pili to mediate adherence to the uroepithelium.[446]

Epidemics of pyelonephritis have been reported in newborn infants being provided care on neonatal wards. These have been shown to be due to the patient-to-patient spread of P-fimbriated *E. coli* strains on the ward, resulting in intestinal colonization of these children. Once such intestinal colonization with uropathogenic strains occurs, invasion of the urinary tract can then develop.[447–449]

In sexually active women, coitus is an important factor in the pathogenesis of symptomatic UTI,[450, 451] with prompt urination after intercourse offering some protection.[451] In addition, diaphragm use, probably by inducing changes in vaginal flora, is significantly associated with an increased risk of symptomatic UTI.[122, 451–453] In contrast, tampon use, oral contraceptives, and direction of wiping after a bowel movement are not.[451]

Patients with anatomic or neurologic disorders of the urinary tract of any type that result in obstruction or incomplete voiding have an increased frequency of UTI and pyelonephritis.[6, 29] A particularly important group of such patients are those rendered paraplegic or quadriplegic as a result of spinal cord injury. Bacteriuria, urosepsis, and the eventual development of VUR and progressive renal scarring are common in these individuals. It is of great interest that the organisms causing UTI in these patients are the same nonuropathogenic strains of bacteria associated with scarring in children with VUR.[454] Risk factors associated with the development of UTI in these patients include overdistention of the bladder, VUR, high-pressure voiding, large postvoid residuals, the presence of stones in the urinary tract, bladder outlet obstruction, indwelling catheterization, and urinary diversion.[455]

Recipients of kidney transplants are another population at particular risk for UTI, with a reported frequency of 35% to 79% of such infections if no antimicrobial prophylaxis is administered. The major factors associated with the occurrence of UTI in this population include the technical complications associated with the ureteral anastomosis, a UTI present before transplantation that has not been eradicated (by antibiotics or native nephrectomy before or at the time of transplantation), the postoperative urinary catheter, the physical and immunologic trauma that the kidney suffers, and the immunosuppressive therapy that is administered. The first two of these have been largely eliminated because of advances in the preparation of the patient for transplantation and in the technical aspects of the operation. However, the requirement for bladder catheters for 1 to 7 days after transplantation provides a reservoir from which infection is derived. In animal models, the combination of bacteria inoculated into the bladder and trauma to the kidney results in pyelonephritis, whereas bladder infection without renal trauma results only in a transient cystitis. It is reasonable to postulate that the kidney is rendered susceptible to invasive infection as a result of the physical trauma of the transplant procedure as well as the immunologic trauma. Once infection develops, its impact can be greatly amplified by the effects of immunosuppressive therapy.[456–458]

UTI occurring in the first 3 months after transplantation is frequently associated with invasion of the allograft, bacteremia, and a high rate of relapse when it is treated with a conventional course of antibiotics. In contrast, UTI occurring at a later time is usually benign, can be managed with a conventional 10- to 14-day course of antibiotics, is rarely associated with bacteremia or requires hospitalization, and has an excellent prognosis. Exceptions to this general pattern should be evaluated for functional or anatomic abnormalities of the urinary tract, such as a stone, obstructive uropathy, or a poorly functioning bladder.[456, 458]

## Clinical Impact of Urinary Tract Infection

The most important issues regarding UTI have to do with whether there are long-term consequences of bacteriuria over and above the direct infectious disease morbidity and mortality these infections cause. The particular questions that have received the most attention are the following:

1. Does UTI, particularly when it is chronic or recurrent, lead to significant loss of renal function, to hypertension, or to both? If it does, is there a particular subset of patients at special risk for these complications?

2. Does UTI have an adverse effect on the outcome of pregnancy—on the mother, the fetus, or both?

3. Is UTI associated with an increased mortality? If it is, is it a causative factor or just a marker for poor health, and will effective therapy decrease the mortality rate?

### URINARY TRACT INFECTION, RENAL FAILURE, AND HYPERTENSION

As previously discussed, it is now clear that in the past the diagnosis of pyelonephritis was loosely applied to a wide variety of tubulointerstitial inflammatory conditions. With more stringent criteria for pathologic diagnosis, several workers in the 1960s began to question the hypothesis that uncomplicated UTI could lead to progressive renal injury.[459, 460] Murray and Goldberg[461] reported the results of a retrospective review of all the cases of chronic renal disease seen at the Hospital of the University of Pennsylvania between 1969 and 1972. They identified 101 individuals with chronic interstitial nephritis, approximately one third of the patients with chronic renal disease—a figure similar to that attributed previously to chronic pyelonephritis.[462, 463] However, in none of these 101 cases of chronic interstitial nephritis was infection the primary cause of the renal disease; instead, analgesic abuse and anatomic abnormalities of the urinary tract accounted for the majority of cases. It was suggested, however, that in approximately one third of these patients, infection played an important secondary role—but only when it was superimposed on such primary problems as anatomic abnormalities, calculous disease, or analgesic abuse.[461]

These notions have since been confirmed in several prospective, long-term studies of bacteriuria in adults. Freedman and Andriole[462] observed 250 women with UTI for periods up to 12 years and found no evidence for deterioration in renal function or blood pressure elevation. Similarly, Asscher and associates[463] studied 107 women with bacteriuria and 88 matched control subjects for a period of 5 years and found that untreated bacteriuria, in the absence of hypertension or obstructive uropathy, was not associated with progressive renal dysfunction. Freeman and colleagues[464] prospectively studied 249 men with bacteriuria for periods up to 10 years and again found no deterioration in renal function in the absence of severe urologic disease or concomitant noninfectious renal disease. Even in a particularly high-risk group of adult patients—the 25% of adult patients with asymptomatic bacteriuria who had renal scars demonstrable by urography at the time of entry into the study—renal damage did not seem to progress, and no new scars developed unless such complicating factors as obstruction, hypertension, analgesic abuse, or diabetes mellitus were present concurrently.[462–464]

Thus, in adults, there is little evidence that UTI beginning in adult life, by itself, leads to progressive chronic renal injury. It is still possible that bacteriuria, when superimposed on other urinary tract lesions, could accelerate the development of renal damage. There is no justification at this time, then, to advocate mass screening of adults for asymptomatic bacteriuria; bacteriuria screening in the adult population should be restricted to patients with urinary tract or renal disease of other primary causes or to patients with a history of recurrent symptomatic infection (see later).

In contrast to the experience in adults, bacteriuria may have a significant impact on children. As discussed in detail earlier, current information suggests that most renal damage caused by UTI develops in childhood, usually in association with an anatomic or functional abnormality, particularly VUR. Studies of children between the ages of 5 and 15 years have demonstrated that if scarring has not occurred by the age of 5 years, the kidneys, sometimes in the face of continued bacteriuria and VUR, remained unscarred and renal growth remained unimpaired. It is primarily the children who have pyelonephritis before age 5 years who manifest not only renal scarring but also a decreased glomerular filtration rate and a failure of compensatory renal growth.[465–467] Experimental studies in young rats have confirmed that ascending pyelonephritis inhibits renal growth.[468]

Edwards and associates[469] have reported extremely encouraging results with long-term continuous low-dose antimicrobial prophylaxis in children who initially presented with symptomatic UTI and were found to have VUR. Whereas Lenaghan and colleagues[470] noted a 20% frequency of fresh scarring and a 66% frequency of increased scarring in children treated with intermittent antimicrobial therapy, Edwards and associates,[469] in an apparently similar population of children, found only one new scar and only one extension among 75 children treated continuously for a 7- to 15-year period.

Thus, there is little question that the combination of VUR and UTI can have potentially disastrous consequences, which might be amenable to early recognition and prolonged therapy. Long-term studies of these children have shown that once scarring has occurred, the prognosis depends on the severity of initial damage and the presence of proteinuria, which is a measure of the degree of secondary glomerulosclerosis. As discussed elsewhere in this book, secondary glomerulosclerosis is thought to be due to glomerular hyperfiltration and hypertension in remnant nephrons, causing changes in permselectivity to macromolecules that are delivered to the kidney. Progressive damage to the remaining glomeruli then ensues, with progression of the degree of proteinuria from microalbuminuria to frank nephrotic syndrome and progressive azotemia.[471–473]

Chronic pyelonephritis appears to be the most common cause of hypertension in children, accounting for some 30% of childhood hypertension, and is also a frequent cause of secondary hypertension in adults.[473] Hypertension as a complication of chronic pyelonephritis is discussed in detail later.

## URINARY TRACT INFECTION AND THE OUTCOME OF PREGNANCY

The clearest demonstration that untreated, asymptomatic bacteriuria has an adverse effect on the human host comes from studies carried out in the pregnant woman. As previously discussed, approximately half of such untreated women subsequently have symptomatic UTI, and 25% to 30% have acute pyelonephritis.[13, 437–443] Such pyelonephritis may be associated with the development of the adult respiratory distress syndrome and disseminated intravascular coagulation.[474] An association of pregnancy bacteriuria with anemia, hypertension, decreased glomerular filtration rate, and decreased urinary concentrating ability, which is alleviated by therapy, has also been noted.[475]

More controversial has been the question of an increased risk of maternal toxemia and neonatal prematurity, low birth weight, and perinatal mortality in pregnancies complicated by bacteriuria. Kincaid-Smith[476] and McFadyen[475] both have reported an increased rate of spontaneous abortion in pregnancies complicated by bacteriuria. In addition, there appears to be a higher frequency of low-birth-weight-for-date infants born to bacteriuric mothers, particularly those with hypertension or in whom treatment programs have failed to eradicate the bacteria.[475–478] In addition to the increase in low-birth-weight infants, acute UTI is associated with an increased fetal mortality rate.[478]

Perhaps the definitive word on this subject has come from two reports derived from data generated in a multicenter study of more than 55,000 pregnant women.[479, 480] Sever and colleagues[479] noted a higher frequency of low birth weights and stillbirths resulting from the pregnancies of the 3.5% of women with symptomatic UTI. From the same database, Naeye[480] reported a frequency of perinatal death of 42 per 1000 when the mothers were bacteriuric as opposed to 21 per 1000 when they were not. In this study, virtually all the excess mortality occurred when the UTI was present within 15 days of delivery, with the highest death rates occurring when UTI coexisted with maternal hypertension and acetonuria. Women who had pyuria and bacteriuria close to the time of delivery had a 24% greater frequency of amniotic fluid infection than did women without pyuria. Hypertension was 88% more frequent in mothers who had pyuria and bacteriuria than in those who did not have pyuria. In addition, bacteriuria was associated with growth-retarded placentas. The mechanisms by which bacteriuria exerts its effects on the outcome of pregnancy are unclear, although it has been suggested that an adverse effect of bacterial endotoxin on the placental circulation plays an important role.[481]

Thus, routine screening for and treatment of bacteriuria of pregnancy are indicated for both the mother's and the child's health. Although complete evidence that treatment will prevent all of the complications of pregnancy-associated bacteriuria will probably never become available, the withholding of therapy for such bacteriuria, whether symptomatic or asymptomatic, must be regarded as both ethically wrong and medically unsupportable.[482, 483]

Long-term studies of schoolgirls with previously diagnosed bacteriuria and renal scarring have shown that when they reach adulthood and become pregnant, they have a greater than threefold increased risk of hypertension and a greater than sevenfold risk of preeclampsia. Despite these findings, with skilled obstetric management, the outcome of the pregnancy in terms of the health of both the mother and the child should be satisfactory.[484]

### URINARY TRACT INFECTION AND SURVIVAL OF THE PATIENT

The final question regarding the biologic impact of UTI has to do with the patient's survival. Although it is absolutely clear that gram-negative sepsis originating in the urinary tract can have lethal consequences, occasionally even with the best of treatment, the question has been raised whether survival of the patient can be adversely influenced outside of the direct infectious disease effects of UTI. Several reports have suggested that bacteriuria, particularly in the elderly, is associated with an increased risk of subsequent mortality.[485–488] Although a cause-and-effect relationship between bacteriuria and death was usually postulated, more recent data have questioned this relationship. It would now appear that the occurrence of bacteriuria is related to the degree of functional impairment present and is a marker

for how seriously ill the individual is. Bacteriuria is not an independent variable that evolves with mortality. It is not surprising, then, that antimicrobial therapy aimed at bacteriuria has no effect on subsequent mortality rates. Indeed, in the elderly patient, antimicrobial therapy has little long-term benefit in terms of the occurrence of the bacteriuria itself. Therefore, there appears to be little justification for either screening adult patients, particularly elderly patients, for asymptomatic bacteriuria or treating them with antimicrobial agents.[433, 489–492]

## CLINICAL PRESENTATIONS

The clinical evaluation of the patient with UTI can be surprisingly difficult because the range of clinical illness is remarkably broad: from the dysuria-frequency syndrome to full-blown pyelonephritis, from symptomatic to asymptomatic bacteriuria (the acute urethral syndrome). It is also clear that the ability of the clinician to accurately define the cause of the urinary tract symptoms or the anatomic site of involvement is limited. On the one hand, the patient who presents with frank rigors, a temperature of 104°F, exquisite loin pain, and signs suggesting gram-negative sepsis clearly has acute pyelonephritis. On the other hand, the absence of such findings does not rule out the presence of renal involvement, that is, covert pyelonephritis. In dealing with the patient who presents with possible UTI, the tasks of the clinician are the following:

1. To define the microbial etiologic agent of the symptoms and the ideal form of antimicrobial management.
2. To make a judgment as to the anatomic site within the urinary tract that is the site of infection. That is, does infection involve the kidney as well as the lower urinary tract, or is it restricted to the lower urinary tract? In the male patient, does it involve the prostate as well as the bladder?
3. To ascertain the risk of complicating structural or functional disease of the urinary tract that might alter clinical management and, when indicated, carry out such diagnostic tests as cystoscopy, voiding cystourethrography, ultrasonography, or excretory urography.

These next sections are devoted to an approach designed to allow fulfillment of these tasks in each category of patients who present with possible UTI.

### Acute Urinary Tract Infection

#### ACUTE UNCOMPLICATED CYSTITIS

By far the most common clinical symptoms associated with UTI that brings patients to medical attention are those referable to the lower urinary tract: dysuria (burning or discomfort on urination), frequency, nocturia, and suprapubic discomfort. Approximately 10% of women of reproductive age come to medical attention each year with these symptoms.[425–427] Of these, two thirds have significant bacteriuria, whereas one third (those with the acute urethral syndrome) do not. Of the patients with significant bacteriuria, 50% to 70% have infection restricted to the bladder, but fully 30% to 50% will have covert infection of the upper urinary tract as well.[6, 10, 25–27, 125, 427, 493] As demonstrated in Table 32–5, the differentiation between patients with and without covert renal involvement cannot be done on clinical grounds alone. This lack of sensitivity of clinical evaluation in delineating the anatomic site of UTI has led to two practices: the treatment of most forms of UTI with identical therapeutic regimens, and an intensive effort by many investigators to develop noninvasive techniques for localizing the anatomic site of infection. However, as described subsequently, such techniques have proved to be too insensitive to be useful in the clinical management of the individual patient. Therefore, management of the patient with the dysuria-frequency syndrome has to be based on the recognition of the possibility that infection more serious than simple cystitis may be present (see later).[6, 125, 493, 494]

The greatest advances in this area have come from the partial unraveling of the causes of the acute urethral syndrome. Stamm and colleagues[24, 25, 495] and Roberts and associates[27] have convincingly shown that women with the acute urethral syndrome can be divided essentially into two groups. Approximately 70% have pyuria on urinalysis and have true infection. An occasional patient in this category has tuberculosis, fungal disease of the urinary tract, or, rarely, an intra-abdominal or pelvic abscess adjoining the urinary tract causing "sympathetic inflammation."[27] For the most part, however, these patients have infection with *C. trachomatis* or with the usual bacterial uropathogens (e.g., *E. coli, S. saprophyticus*) but in "less than significant" numbers ($10^2$ to $10^4$/mL). The remaining 30% of patients with the acute urethral syndrome, but no pyuria, have no known microbial etiologic agent for their symptoms. Presumably, these symptoms result from trauma related to intercourse, local irritation or allergy, or some other as yet undefined process.

Confirmation of these microbiologic results comes from treatment data. Stamm and colleagues[495] have reported a double-blind, randomized study of doxycycline (100 mg given twice daily by mouth for 10 days) versus placebo in the management of patients with the acute urethral syn-

drome. The results were striking: 11 of 12 women with the acute urethral syndrome due to "true but less than significant bacteriuria" with coliform organisms or *S. saprophyticus* became asymptomatic with therapy, whereas only 4 of 10 women given placebo responded; all 5 women with documented *C. trachomatis* infection responded to doxycycline, whereas only 2 of 6 responded to placebo. In contrast, doxycycline failed to have any discernible clinical effect on patients with the acute urethral syndrome without pyuria. Although less well documented bacteriologically, a similar experience was reported by Tolkoff-Rubin and associates[496] with trimethoprim-sulfamethoxazole; this drug and doxycycline are active against both bacterial uropathogens and *C. trachomatis.*

## RECURRENT CYSTITIS

Recurrent symptoms of lower urinary tract inflammation may be due to either relapsing infection or reinfection. Relapse in either sex is caused by reappearance of the same organism from a sequestered focus, usually within the kidney or prostate, shortly after completion of therapy. In reinfection, the course of therapy has successfully eradicated the infection, and there is no sequestered focus, but organisms are reintroduced from the fecal reservoir. More than 80% of all recurrences are due to reinfection.[125]

Among schoolgirls with symptomatic UTI, about 20% will remain infection free after each course of treatment, with 25% having repeated bouts of infection.[416] Among the group of adult women susceptible to recurrent UTIs (defined as three or more infections in a calendar year), the attack rate over several years is approximately 0.15 infections per month, with virtually all such infections being symptomatic. Approximately one third of such infections are followed by an infection-free interval of at least 6 months, the average infection-free interval being approximately 1 year. Unfortunately, even prolonged remission in these individuals does not mean cure because infections tend to recur even after an infection-free interval of a year or longer.[497]

The most important cause of recurrent symptoms of

**TABLE 32–5. Relationship Among Clinical Syndromes, Presence of Significant Bacteriuria, and Anatomic Site of Urinary Tract Infection in a General Practice Population**

| Manifestation | % of Population with Symptom | | |
|---|---|---|---|
| | Insignificant or Absent Bacteriuria (Acute Urethral Syndrome) | Renal Bacteriuria | Bladder Bacteriuria |
| Symptoms suggesting lower UTI | | | |
| Frequency | 95 | 98 | 70 |
| Burning | 70 | 68 | 70 |
| Suprapubic pain | 70 | 68 | 51 |
| Symptoms suggesting upper UTI | | | |
| Loin pain | 50 | 48 | 19 |
| Fever | 35 | 44 | 4 |
| Rigors | 15 | 32 | 15 |
| Nausea and vomiting | 25 | 24 | 8 |
| Macroscopic hematuria | 25 | 20 | 12 |

Modified from Fairley F, Carson NE, Gutch RC, et al: Site of infection in acute urinary tract infection in general practice. Lancet 2:615, 1971.

lower urinary tract inflammation in adult men is prostatitis due to either *E. coli* or the other bacterial uropathogens seen in women or *C. trachomatis.* Acute bacterial prostatitis is a febrile illness associated with chills; perineal, back, or pelvic pain; dysuria; and urinary frequency and urgency. There may be bladder outlet obstruction; on physical examination, the prostate is enlarged, tender, and indurated. Chronic prostatitis, in contrast, may be more occult; asymptomatic infection is manifested as recurrent bacteriuria or variable low-grade fever with back or pelvic discomfort. Urinary symptoms are usually due to reintroduction of infection into the bladder from a chronic prostatic focus that has been inadequately treated and only temporarily suppressed by a previous course of antimicrobial therapy.[6, 29, 416]

## ACUTE PYELONEPHRITIS

The clinical findings associated with full-blown acute pyelonephritis are familiar: recurrent rigors and fever, back and loin pain (with exquisite tenderness on percussion of the costovertebral angle), often with colicky abdominal pain, nausea and vomiting, dysuria, frequency, and nocturia. Although bacteremia may complicate the course of symptomatic pyelonephritis in any patient, such bacteremias are seldom associated with the more serious sequelae of gram-negative sepsis, that is, the triggering of the complement, clotting, and kinin systems, which may lead to septic shock, disseminated intravascular coagulation, or both. When shock or disseminated intravascular coagulation occurs in the setting of pyelonephritis, the possibility of complicating obstruction must be ruled out. In one particularly important form of obstructive uropathy, which is associated with acute papillary necrosis, the sloughed papilla may obstruct the ureter. This form should be particularly suspected in diabetic patients with severe pyelonephritis and high-grade bacteremia, especially if the response to therapy is delayed.

In children younger than 2 years, fever, vomiting, non-specific abdominal complaints, or failure to thrive may be the only manifestations of significant acute pyelonephritis. Indeed, UTI accounts for approximately 10% of these febrile episodes. In older children, clinical manifestations resemble more closely those seen in the adult, although the reappearance of enuresis may be a marker of the decreased urinary concentrating ability sometimes associated with renal infection (see later).[498, 499]

## COMPLICATED URINARY TRACT INFECTION

This term encompasses a wide range of clinical syndromes that include asymptomatic bacteriuria, cystitis, pyelonephritis, and frank urosepsis. The common element is the presence of bacterial infection of the urinary tract in patients with structurally abnormal (e.g., ureteral or bladder neck obstruction, polycystic kidney disease, obstructing stones, or the presence of a catheter or some other foreign body) or functionally abnormal (e.g., a neurogenic bladder from spinal cord injury, diabetes mellitus, or multiple sclerosis) urinary tracts, intrinsic renal disease, or a systemic process that renders the patient particularly susceptible to

bacterial invasion. The range of organisms causing such infections is far broader than that noted in patients with uncomplicated infection, and the level of antibiotic resistance of these bacteria is also greater than that seen in isolates from the general population. Because the therapeutic requirements and management strategies for complicated UTI are different from those for uncomplicated infection (see later), this differentiation is clinically important.[126, 494]

Two unusual forms of renal infection are macroscopic renal and perinephric abscesses. In the past, most such abscesses were secondary to hematogenous infection with *S. aureus* or, less commonly, group A streptococci. These were primarily located in the renal cortex. Today, most are secondary to UTI with the usual Enterobacteriaceae, complicated by renal calculi and obstruction of urine flow from either the kidney or the ureter. Such abscesses are typically located at the corticomedullary junction. Less commonly, pre-existing renal cysts may become infected and develop into abscesses; rarely, there may be contiguous spread from neighboring sites of suppuration, such as the colon or overlying rib. Renal abscesses may extend into the perinephric space. The usual presentation of renal and perinephric abscesses is insidious, with chronic symptoms of fever, weight loss, night sweats, and anorexia, often associated with flank or back pain. At times, when infection is under pressure, usually because of obstruction, a more acute presentation occurs with associated bacteremia. Symptoms specific to the urinary tract, such as dysuria, hematuria, and urinary retention, are sometimes noted. On physical examination, costovertebral angle tenderness or even a palpable mass may be found, but in 30% to 50% of patients, the examination results are normal. Routine laboratory tests are of variable value: leukocytosis may be present; anemia is not unusual; and urinalysis may reflect signs of inflammation, such as pyuria, proteinuria, or both. In more than half of patients, the same organism may be isolated on urine culture as that present in the abscess. Definitive diagnosis, however, is dependent on the demonstration of a mass lesion, as by excretory urography with nephrotomograms. Gallium and ultrasonic scans and computed tomography may also yield evidence of an inflammatory mass lesion in and around the kidney. If prompt drainage and therapy with antibiotics is not carried out, such abscesses may be complicated by extension to the peritoneal cavity, the chest, or the skin.[29, 500, 501]

# Chronic Pyelonephritis and Reflux Nephropathy

Unlike the dramatic clinical presentation of many patients with acute pyelonephritis, chronic disease typically has a more insidious course. Clinical signs and symptoms may be divided into two categories: those related directly to infection and those related to the degree and location of injury within the kidney. Surprisingly, the infectious aspects of the disease may be minor. Although intermittent episodes of full-blown pyelonephritis may occur, these are the exception. More common is asymptomatic bacteriuria, symptoms referable to the lower urinary tract (dysuria and frequency), vague complaints of flank or abdominal discomfort, and intermittent low-grade fevers.

Much more striking than the infectious or inflammatory symptoms are the physiologic derangements that result from the long-standing tubulointerstitial injury. These derangements include hypertension, inability to conserve $Na^+$, a decreased concentrating ability, and a tendency to the development of hyperkalemia and acidosis. Although all of these are seen to a greater or lesser extent in all forms of renal disease, in patients with tubulointerstitial nephropathy such as this, the degree of physiologic derangement is out of proportion to the degree of renal failure (or serum creatinine elevation). Thus, in other forms of renal disease, physiologic derangements are minimal at serum creatinine levels of 2 to 3 mg/dL; in the patient with chronic pyelonephritis and reflux nephropathy with serum creatinine at this level, polyuria, nocturia, hyperkalemia, and acidosis may all be observed. Clinically, it is particularly important to recognize that such patients are especially susceptible to dehydration because of their inability to excrete a concentrated urine.

The diagnosis of chronic pyelonephritis is either a pathologic one or one based on specific radiologic findings of excretory urography. As defined by Hodson,[3, 407] these consist of focal, coarse cortical scarring with underlying retraction of the papillae and blunting and dilatation of the calyces. Scars are most frequently observed in the upper and lower poles. In patients with diffuse injury related to the presence of significant VUR, there are usually more marked cortical thinning and generalized calyceal dilatation (see Fig. 32–10). In more recent years, renal cortical scintigraphy with use of $^{99m}Tc$-labeled dimercaptosuccinic acid has emerged as the most sensitive means for detecting renal changes due to acute pyelonephritis as well as the most sensitive way of detecting renal scarring. This is particularly true when tomographic imaging (so-called single-photon emission tomography) is employed as part of the scan. What is less clear, however, is the clinical importance of detecting small areas of renal abnormality by radioscintigraphy (which can be confirmed pathologically and thus are not artifacts) that are not demonstrable by excretory urography. Our practice at present is to regard such findings as "an early warning of potential danger" and to observe such individuals closely with intensive medical therapy (see later).[502–511]

The laboratory findings are as nonspecific as the clinical findings. Although pyuria is usually present, it may be absent, particularly if no active infection is present. Less common is the presence of white blood cell casts on urinalysis. Bacteriuria may or may not be demonstrable.

The determination of 24-hour protein excretion may be an important prognostic indicator in patients with chronic pyelonephritis and reflux nephropathy. The majority of patients with this condition excrete less than 1 g of protein per day. Alt and associates[512] reported an average 24-hour protein excretion of 1.12 g in patients with creatinine clearances of less than 40 mL/min, with minimal proteinuria in those when creatinine clearances exceeded 65 mL/min. However, heavy proteinuria, including the nephrotic syndrome, may develop in a subset of patients. Renal biopsies in such patients reveal the superimposition of focal and segmental glomerulosclerosis on the basic tubulointerstitial injury. These patients have a particularly poor prognosis and progress to end-stage renal disease (see later).

## Natural History of Vesicoureteral Reflux and Reflux Nephropathy

The natural history of VUR and reflux nephropathy is variable, depending on the severity of the VUR, the concurrence of other congenital anomalies or obstruction, the age at presentation, the surgical or antibacterial intervention, and the development of such complications as hypertension and glomerulosclerosis.

It is useful in discussing the natural history to separate the issue of coarse scar formation in the kidney from the progressive deterioration of renal function not related to new scar formation; although coarse scar formation is closely linked to VUR and infection, the progressive deterioration of renal function can result from a variety of secondary mechanisms.

### FORMATION OF SCARS

The two main conclusions of the studies summarized earlier are that 1) scar development usually represents the combined effects of infection, VUR, and intrarenal reflux and 2) the severity of VUR is the single most important determinant of whether renal damage will occur. The importance of infection in the development of new scars was shown by Smellie and associates,[237, 238] who found only two fresh scars developing among 75 compliant children observed for 15 years and given low-dose prophylactic antibacterial therapy. It has been suggested that infection and high pressure may alter some borderline papillae to the refluxing state. These factors explain the few instances reported of new scars developing in already scarred kidneys; however, this occurrence is distinctly rare.[513]

### PROGRESSIVE RENAL FAILURE

The progressive renal failure seen in patients with reflux nephropathy is frequently caused not by infection nor continued VUR but by other complicating or related conditions. These include 1) retardation of renal growth, 2) obstruction or other congenital anomalies, 3) hypertension, and 4) progressive glomerulosclerosis.

**Retardation of Renal Growth.** The effect of VUR on renal growth is important, because normal renal growth is an indication of a healthy kidney and has a linear relationship with the child's height.[514] Earlier studies had reported retardation or arrest of renal growth in children with UTI with or without VUR.[244] Several studies have examined this issue in some detail. Winberg and colleagues[515] observed 22 infants with acute pyelonephritis who had no visible scarring at first presentation. No scars developed after 9 years of follow-up, but there was a significant reduction in the parenchymal thickness of the patients' kidneys compared with that of control subjects, regardless of the presence of VUR. Claesson and associates[516] studied renal growth profiles in 26 patients with unilateral scarring and found that renal tissue loss was compensated for almost completely by hypertrophy of the contralateral kidney, which took place even in the presence of VUR. The glomerular filtration rate was normal in these patients after 10 to 15 years of follow-up. A renal growth spurt eventually follows growth impairment, but this may be postponed until puberty in both scarred and unscarred kidneys for unknown reasons. Winberg's conclusion was that focal scarring and growth impairment are two different consequences of renal infection.

Smellie and colleagues[237] reported the effects of VUR on renal growth in 70 children with initial UTI and VUR managed with continuous antibacterial prophylaxis. Renal growth was abnormal in 11 of 11 kidneys drained by refluxing ureters, and 10 of these 11 kidneys were exposed to recurrence of urinary infection. In pairs of kidneys with unilateral VUR, there was a significant difference in growth only if the refluxing ureter drained a scarred kidney. Seven kidneys that grew least well had established severe scarring associated with persisting gross VUR, and each had a period of infection during observation. It was concluded that the prognosis for renal growth is generally excellent with VUR, particularly if the kidneys are unscarred and there is no recurrence of infection. The prognosis for growth is poorest for patients with gross, persistent VUR, severe generalized scarring, and an increased tendency toward recurrent infection.

In the report of the Newcastle Covert Bacteriuria Research Group,[517] schoolgirls 4 to 18 years of age with covert bacteriuria, observed for 5 years, had below-average renal growth only when the kidneys were scarred, regardless of whether they had received antibacterial therapy. However, none of the girls in this group became hypertensive or had abnormal blood chemistry profiles during the follow-up.

The balance of the evidence suggests that renal growth may be transiently impaired in children with VUR, but mainly in those with renal scarring and usually in the presence of infection. However, this reduction in renal growth does not seem to be a major determinant of the later progressive deterioration of renal function in patients with reflux nephropathy.[467, 468, 513–517]

**Obstruction and Other Congenital Anomalies.** Children with UTI with or without VUR may have a variety of renal and lower urinary tract anomalies that contribute to renal damage. These include[238] duplex kidneys, cysts, hydronephrosis due to ureteropelvic obstruction, renal calculi, vesicoureteral or urethral obstruction, and bladder diverticula. These anomalies predispose to repeated renal infection. The coexistence of VUR and an obstructive anomaly such as posterior urethral valves is particularly harmful, and it is under these conditions that sterile reflux may cause renal damage.

**Hypertension.** The association between chronic pyelonephritis or reflux nephropathy and hypertension is well documented; the frequency of the hypertension varies with both age and severity of the disease.[473] In Bengtsson's series,[518] more than 90% of the patients observed to terminal uremia became hypertensive, but Gower[519] found hypertension in only 12% of patients with unilateral pyelonephritis and in 28% of those with bilateral pyelonephritis whose renal function was normal. Kincaid-Smith and associates[404]

found hypertension in 27% of 145 adults with reflux nephropathy. The degree of hypertension was related to the severity of the reflux nephropathy.

Reflux nephropathy is one of the most common causes of hypertension in children. Gill and colleagues[520] found that 83% of 100 severely hypertensive children had associated renal disease and that 14% of these had reflux nephropathy. Most of Holland's[521, 522] 177 children with malignant hypertension and scarred atrophic kidneys had reflux nephropathy, and Rance and associates[523] found that 30% of 96 children with persistent hypertension had chronic pyelonephritis, making it the most common etiologic factor in the group. About 10% of children with renal scarring become hypertensive,[524] and 15% of patients with reflux nephropathy who reach adulthood have hypertension.

The pathogenesis of hypertension in reflux nephropathy is unclear. In humans, there is some evidence both for and against a role for hyperreninemia.[525–528] Although it has been difficult to produce hypertension in rats and rabbits that have been made pyelonephritic, studies in pigs show that hypertension develops in some animals 1 to 2 years after the induction of VUR with scarring and that such hypertension is associated with pronounced arterial lesions and activation of the renin-angiotensin system (Hodson CJ, unpublished data). Hypertension also occurs in unilateral reflux nephropathy, but there is uncertainty whether such hypertension can be prevented or ameliorated by unilateral nephrectomy.[527]

**Proteinuria and Progressive Glomerulosclerosis.** There is a prognostically important association among the development of proteinuria, focal segmental glomerulosclerosis, and progressive renal insufficiency in patients with reflux nephropathy.[471–473, 529] Although several authors had reported occasional severe proteinuria or overt nephrotic syndrome in patients diagnosed as having chronic pyelonephritis,[530, 531] it was Kincaid-Smith[404, 413, 414, 532] who first stressed the occurrence of proteinuria and glomerulosclerosis in patients with chronic pyelonephritis and reflux nephropathy. In 55 adult patients with reflux nephropathy, she found that 19 had proteinuria. All but 1 of 11 patients whose renal function subsequently declined had significant proteinuria, with the mean being 2.36 g in 24 hours, whereas all patients whose serum creatinine level remained stable had either no proteinuria (7 patients) or proteinuria of less than 1 g in 24 hours (2 patients). The degree of proteinuria correlated well with the presence and extent of glomerular lesions, most of which consisted of focal and segmental glomerulosclerosis and hyalinosis.

A number of other studies have confirmed the association among proteinuria, glomerulosclerosis, and reflux nephropathy.[533–537] In the study of Bhathena and colleagues[537] of 23 patients with end-stage reflux nephropathy, all had focal glomerulosclerosis, and their average protein excretion ranged from 1.2 to 5.8 g/24 h. In 29 of the 54 patients described by Torres and associates,[535] the 24-hour urinary protein excretion ranged from 0.5 to 10.4 g. There was a significant positive correlation between the 24-hour protein excretion and the simultaneous determination of creatinine clearance. The clinical course to end-stage renal disease was not appreciably altered by the late surgical correction of the VUR, by the occurrence of infection, or by hypertension. In our series[379, 538] of patients with chronic pyelone-phritis or reflux nephropathy, half of those with focal glo-merulosclerosis had radiologic or morphologic evidence of bilateral renal disease and a serum creatinine level of more than 2.5 mg/dL, and 63% had a 24-hour urinary protein excretion of greater than 1 g. In contrast, patients without focal sclerosis had normal serum creatinine levels, minimal proteinuria, and unilateral disease.

The precise mechanism responsible for the development of proteinuria and glomerulosclerosis in patients with reflux nephropathy is still unclear. Immunologic injury by circu-lating immune complexes was suggested by the presence of immunoglobulin M and C3 in the mesangium and in scle-rotic areas in more than half of the patients reported.[535, 539] However, the search for bacterial products as antigens within the glomeruli has proved negative.[538] Autologous antigens, such as brush border antigen or Tamm-Horsfall protein, have also been incriminated as antigens causing autoimmune glomerular injury, but we and others[537] have failed to localize this protein in the mesangium of patients with focal sclerosis and reflux nephropathy. The presence of the membrane attack complex of complement in sclerotic areas[540] and evidence of alternative complement pathway activation suggest a role for complement in the glomerular injury, but it is improbable that this is the primary event. A second possible explanation for the development of focal sclerosis is mesangial dysfunction occurring as a result of the hydrodynamic changes consequent to VUR and resem-bling the changes shown with ureteral obstruction in exper-imental animals.[540, 541]

Vascular changes consisting of intimal hyperplasia and medial hypertrophy are found in most patients with focal sclerosis and reflux nephropathy and may well play a role in the development of focal sclerosis. However, these vas-cular changes occur in the absence of hypertension or be-fore the development of hypertension in patients with reflux nephropathy and proteinuria.

The most attractive explanation for glomerulosclerosis in reflux nephropathy is that it results from the adaptive changes occurring in glomeruli because of reductions in renal mass[542, 543] (see also Chapter 44). With certain excep-tions, the clinical data are consistent with this hypothesis. In most series, proteinuria and glomerulosclerosis are most prominent in patients with bilateral disease and impaired renal function, although they have occasionally been re-ported in patients with unilateral disease and those with normal renal function. In patients with normal renal func-tion, it is probable that the adapted glomeruli have main-tained normal function and that this continues until pro-gressive sclerosis of the remaining glomeruli leads to a reduction of glomerular filtration rate. Occasionally, pro-teinuria occurs in patients with unilateral reflux neph-ropathy,[212, 544] and the glomerulosclerosis is present in the normal hypertrophied kidney. Although this has been cited as evidence against the hemodynamic mechanism, it is con-sistent with it because hemodynamic changes have been well documented in uninvolved kidneys of patients with unilateral scars.[545] Finally, morphometric studies confirm the hypertrophy of glomeruli in biopsy specimens of pa-tients with reflux nephropathy and show a relationship among renal size, glomerular size, and renal function in these patients.[546]

Whatever the mechanisms, it is now clear that progres-sive glomerulosclerosis is a major determinant of the devel-opment of chronic renal failure in reflux nephropathy.

# DIAGNOSTIC EVALUATION

## History and Physical Examination

Despite the incomplete relationship between clinical symptoms and the presence of infection at various sites in the urinary tract, useful information can be gained from a skillfully obtained history. When a patient with a single acute episode of symptomatic UTI is examined, the first consideration is whether there are signs or symptoms sug-gesting the presence or imminent development of systemic sepsis: spiking fevers, rigors, tachypnea, colicky abdominal pain, and exquisite loin pain. Such patients require imme-diate attention and probably parenteral therapy within a hospital setting. If the patient is not acutely septic, attention turns to such concerns as previous history of UTIs, renal disease, or such conditions as diabetes mellitus, multiple sclerosis, other neurologic conditions, history of renal stones, or previous genitourinary tract manipulation—con-ditions that could predispose to UTI and affect the efficacy of therapy. A careful neurologic examination can be partic-ularly important in suggesting the possibility of a neuro-genic bladder.

The patient with a history of recurrent UTIs merits spe-cial attention in terms of obtaining a clear history of sexual activity, response to therapy, and temporal relationships of recurrences to the cessation of therapy. Thus, women with recurrent bacterial UTIs temporally related to intercourse could benefit from the administration of antibiotics after each sexual exposure (see later).[134] The woman with the acute urethral syndrome due to *C. trachomatis* infection may respond only temporarily to antichlamydial therapy because of reinfection from the untreated sexual partner (so-called ping-ponging infection); cure occurs when both individuals are treated simultaneously. Women with recur-rent UTIs who have relapsing infection as opposed to rein-fection often give a different history of the temporal rela-tionship between the end of therapy and the onset of new symptoms. The majority of women with relapsing infection relapse within 4 to 7 days of completing a course of therapy of 14 days or less, whereas those with recurrent reinfection usually have a longer interval between episodes unless bladder dysfunction or some other disturbance of urinary tract function is present. Similarly, men with persistent prostatic foci of infection often relapse promptly after a similar conventional course of therapy.[21, 29] In addition, a history of prostatic obstruction to urine flow should be sought (e.g., narrowing of the urine stream, hesitancy, noc-turia, or dribbling).

When the patient with possible chronic pyelonephritis and reflux nephropathy is examined, two types of informa-tion should be sought: the history of UTI in childhood and during pregnancy; and the possible presence of such patho-physiologic consequences as hypertension, proteinuria, polyuria, nocturia, and frequency.

## Urinary Findings

The criteria used to evaluate the presence of infection by culture and the presence of pyuria on microscopic examination have been described previously. Because of the ubiquity of UTIs in all age groups, the expense of culturing urine by conventional techniques, and the emphasis on attempting to diagnose UTI in the home or in the physician's office (as opposed to the hospital setting), a great deal of attention has been paid to the development of simple tests for bacteriuria that require a minimum of expertise and equipment. These may be summarized as follows.

### CHEMICAL TESTS FOR THE PRESENCE OF BACTERIURIA

Four major chemical tests have been evaluated as rapid diagnostic tools. By far the most commonly used is the Griess nitrate reduction test, which is dependent on the bacterial reduction of nitrate in the urine to nitrite, with a variety of commercially available tapes or dipsticks employed to measure the presence of nitrites. This test is most accurate on first-morning urine specimens and is reasonably accurate in identifying infection due to Enterobacteriaceae but fails to detect infection due to gram-positive organisms and *Pseudomonas*. False-negative results may also be caused by lack of dietary nitrate or during diuresis, because bladder incubation time is necessary for bacteria to reduce the nitrates. Because of its simplicity, this test is best used as part of a home or epidemiologic screening program, particularly if multiple specimens can be evaluated from a single individual.[7, 8, 416, 547] The combination of the nitrate test with a test for leukocyte esterase on a single, inexpensive dipstick that can be read in less than 2 minutes has greatly increased the utility of this approach. This system provides a useful assessment for the presence of more than $10^5$ Enterobacteriaceae per milliliter of urine and of pyuria. A negative test result has a predictive value of 97%. False-negative test results can be caused by proteinuria and the presence of gentamicin or cephalexin in the urine. Overall, this test has an 87% sensitivity and 67% specificity (false-positive results usually result from vaginal contamination). This approach is far more effective in screening urine specimens from patients with symptoms as opposed to screening asymptomatic patients, such as occurs in obstetric practice.[11, 548–552]

The other commonly employed chemical test is the reduction of triphenyltetrazolium chloride to triphenylformazan (which has a red color) by bacteria. False-positive test results are caused by the ingestion of large amounts of vitamin C or a urine pH less than 6.5. False-negative test results are due to deterioration of the reagent (common) and infection with staphylococci, some enterococci, and *Pseudomonas* species. Other tests that have been employed are a glucose oxidase test (bacteria consume the small amount of glucose present in the nondiabetic urine) and an assay for urinary catalase (which most uropathogens possess, but so do inflammatory cells of any cause). Unfortunately, these are even less accurate than the first two methods.[8, 416]

### DIP-SLIDE METHODS

Far more useful are a variety of dip-slide methods in which plastic paddles with agar on their surfaces are immersed into the urine, drained, and incubated. An agar medium selective for gram-negative organisms (such as MacConkey agar) is usually present on one side of the paddle or slide, and a nonselective medium that supports the growth of most bacterial species, including gram-positive organisms, is present on the other side. After overnight incubation, the number of colonies on both agar surfaces is then compared with standardized pictures of inoculated dip slides to achieve a semiquantitative estimation of the number of organisms present. Positive slides can then be sent to a reference laboratory for species identification and antibiotic susceptibility testing. The technique is useful for office or home screening.[8, 416, 553, 554]

### SEMIAUTOMATED METHODS

There are three semiautomated techniques available for the noncultural diagnosis of UTI designed for the laboratory that processes many urine cultures per day (i.e., not for home or single-practitioner office settings). The first of these is the Bac-T-Screen, in which the specimen is passed through a filter paper disk that is then stained and rinsed before being read on a colorimeter. This technique has a threshold of more than $10^4$ bacteria/mL, with a sensitivity of approximately 88% but a specificity as low as 66%. Clogging of the instrument remains a problem, as does pigment deposition on the filter, which results in uninterpretable results.[11, 555]

The second semiautomated method uses bioluminescence to detect bacteriuria. Bacterial ATP is measured as an index of bacterial numbers by use of the firefly luciferin/luciferase bioluminescent reaction. This system has a sensitivity of about 97% at a threshold of $10^4$ bacteria/mL and a specificity of 70% to 80%. It is most useful in detecting urine negative for bacteria; this test has a negative predictive value of greater than 99%.[11, 556]

Finally, particle counting by electrical impedance is a growth-independent method that can also measure leukocytes separately. At present, there is a significant false-positive rate (20% to 25%), but this is promising technology.[11, 556]

## Infection-Localizing Tests

Although there may be great similarity in the clinical presentation of patients with upper and lower UTIs, there can be vast differences in the response to therapy and type of pathologic process. Bladder infection is a superficial mucosal infection at an anatomic site to which high concentrations of antibiotics can be easily delivered, whereas renal infection (and prostatic infection in men) is a deep parenchymal infection at a tissue site where natural host defenses are rendered less effective by a hostile physicochemical environment and to which antimicrobial delivery may be limited. One would predict that the type of antimicrobial therapy necessary to eradicate infection from the urinary tract would be different for these two anatomic sites, with renal infection (and prostatic infection) requiring a more intensive or prolonged course of therapy, or both, than bladder infection.[6, 24]

The problem has been to develop a means of assessing the anatomic site of infection, given the 30% to 50% frequency of covert renal infection in patients with symptoms referable only to the lower urinary tract.[6, 10, 24, 557, 558] The only direct method of localizing the infection site is bilateral ureteral catheterization.[10, 24] Although too invasive for general use, it remains the standard with which all other methods of localization are compared. A less invasive procedure is the bladder washout procedure introduced by Fairley and colleagues.[558] In this procedure, a Foley catheter is introduced into the bladder, the bladder is irrigated with an antibiotic solution (usually neomycin or neomycin and polymyxin), and several urine samples are collected. Patients with lower UTI have sterile urine during the collection period after the washout, whereas patients with renal infection have bacteria in all of the samples after washout. The major drawback with this technique is its inability to distinguish between unilateral and bilateral renal infection. However, because it is easy to perform, safe, and inexpensive and does not require an expert cystoscopist, it has replaced the ureteral catheterization studies as the method with which all noninvasive techniques are compared.

Three types of noninvasive techniques have been employed in an attempt to differentiate between renal and bladder infection: assay of renal medullary function by measurement of maximal urinary concentrating capacity; measurement of urinary enzymes as an index of tissue injury and inflammation; and measurements of the immunologic response to infection. The basis for each of these tests is the pathologic differences between upper and lower tract infections: renal medullary infection occurs at a site where critical aspects of urine formation are taking place, and where inflammatory and immunologic responses are brisk and extensive; bladder infection occurs in the superficial mucosa, where little is occurring functionally and where both inflammatory and immunologic responses are limited.[557]

## URINARY CONCENTRATING ABILITY

As previously observed, acute or chronic tubulointerstitial inflammation of the kidney is commonly associated with a defect in concentrating ability, best measured by a maximal urinary concentrating test.[559–561] The defect in urinary concentrating ability in pyelonephritis appears to be due to the elaboration of prostaglandins in the renal medulla associated with inflammation, because it can be blocked by the administration of the prostaglandin synthetase inhibitor indomethacin.[562, 563] A typical result was reported by Ronald and associates[561] in a group of 38 patients whose site of infection was directly localized by ureteral catheterization. They demonstrated that renal but not bladder bacteriuria was associated with a decreased concentrating ability and that bilateral renal infection was associated with a greater defect than unilateral infection. In patients with unilateral infection, they were able to show a defect in the involved kidney and normal concentrating ability in the uninfected

kidney. Eradication of infection was associated with return of concentrating ability. This approach to infection localization is flawed by frequent overlap in values in patients with bladder, unilateral renal, and bilateral renal infection. Thus, in addition to being inconvenient to perform, such tests are too insensitive to be useful in routine management of patients.[557]

## MEASUREMENT OF URINARY ENZYMES

Wacker and Dorfman[564] found that urinary lactate dehydrogenase activity was elevated in 25% of patients with pyelonephritis. However, in addition to false-negative results, the presence of blood and heavy proteinuria will cause false-positive results. Urinary β-glucuronidase activity has been found to be higher in patients with pyelonephritis than in patients with lower tract infection.[565] Ronald and colleagues,[566] using ureteral catheterization for localization, found slightly higher β-glucuronidase activity in patients with renal infection than in control subjects or patients with bladder infection. However, considerable overlap was seen in these three groups, and the test was not useful in the individual patient. Turck[567] reported a similar experience. Viganò and associates[568] reported promising results with the measurement of the renal tubule cell enzyme N-acetyl-β-D-glucosaminidase. In a study of children with UTI, they reported urinary levels of 906 ± 236 mol/h/mg of urinary creatinine in those with pyelonephritis as opposed to levels of 145 ± 23 mol/h/mg in those with lower UTI and 151.6 ± 10 mol/h/mg in normal children. Excretion of this enzyme fell in children with pyelonephritis in association with clinical response to antimicrobial therapy. Unfortunately, there is considerable overlap between patients with pyelonephritis and cystitis in other studies.[569]

Thus, measurement of tubule cell enzymes or antigens in the urine is a promising approach to the problem of UTI anatomic localization, but the best test system for accomplishing this remains to be defined.

## MEASUREMENT OF C-REACTIVE PROTEIN

Jodal and colleagues[570, 571] reported that consistently elevated levels of C-reactive protein in serum, as detected by an immunodiffusion technique, were seen in children with pyelonephritis. Children with acute cystitis, on the other hand, did not have elevated C-reactive protein levels. Sequential determination of C-reactive protein values in children with pyelonephritis showed that effective therapy led to a progressive decrease in these levels. However, localization of infection in these studies was made primarily on clinical grounds, and the assigned diagnosis did not correlate with bladder washout studies in 5 of 25 patients studied. The C-reactive protein level may also be elevated in a variety of other inflammatory conditions, and false-positive values may be observed.[572] Hellerstein and associates,[573] in a study of children in whom infection was localized by the bladder washout technique, failed to show any correlation with the C-reactive protein determination. In our experience, this test is even less sensitive in evaluating adult UTI.

## MEASUREMENT OF ANTIBODY RESPONSES TO BACTERIA

Renal infection is associated with the net synthesis of specific antibody directed against antigens of the infecting organism.[574] A variety of investigators have attempted to apply immunologic techniques to the problems of UTI anatomic localization. Percival and colleagues,[575] using a bacterial agglutination test, found elevated serum antibody levels in patients with symptoms of acute pyelonephritis, with these titers falling in response to antimicrobial therapy. Patients with clinically inapparent pyelonephritis also had high antibody levels, whereas patients with bladder infections had normal titers. Clark and associates[576] localized the site of infection by ureteral catheterization, examined the hemagglutinating antibody response, and confirmed that some patients with renal infection had higher hemagglutinating antibody titers than those of patients with bladder bacteriuria. However, a wide range of titers and a considerable overlap between the two groups of patients was once again observed, so that such serum studies are of limited use in the individual patient.[11]

The most widely used infection-localizing technique employed in more recent years has been the assay for antibody-coated bacteria (ACB assay) in the urine. Thomas,[577] Jones,[578] and their colleagues, using an immunofluorescence assay, showed that bacteria originating from the kidney were coated with antibody, whereas bacteria associated with lower UTIs were antibody-negative. Their work was confirmed by several investigators,[579–581] although some problems have emerged as the assay has been used more widely. The following appears to be a fair summary[6, 29] of the current status of this assay.

1. False-positive test results occur when vaginal or rectal flora contaminate a urine specimen; when heavy proteinuria appears, as in patients with the nephrotic syndrome; and when infection invades the uroepithelium outside the kidney (prostatitis, hemorrhagic cystitis, or bladder infections in the presence of bladder tumors or catheters).[581–583]

2. False-negative ACB test results have been noted in 16% to 38% of adult patients with acute pyelonephritis[584] and in most children.[585] In contrast, the ACB assay appears to have an accuracy of 95% or better in patients with chronic pyelonephritis.[578] This is presumably related to the 10- to 15-day lag with first infections between initiation of renal bacterial invasion and the ACB test result's turning positive[586]; lesser amounts of time are required with repeated infection because of an anamnestic antibody response.[29]

3. The frequency of positive ACB test results in women with acute uncomplicated UTI appears to vary among different populations of patients. These differences may be related to the ease of access to medical care and the amount of time that elapses between the onset of symptoms and initiation of medical care.[29]

4. The ACB-positive population is heterogeneous in its response to single-dose antimicrobial therapy; 50% to 60% of women with acute uncomplicated UTI who are ACB-positive respond to such therapy, as opposed to approximately 95% of those with ACB-negative infection.[6, 587]

Because of these observations, the ACB test is not recommended for routine management of patients. Clearly, continuing efforts to develop better noninvasive tests for UTI localization are indicated.

## Radiologic and Urologic Evaluations

The primary objective of radiologic and urologic evaluations in UTI is to delineate abnormalities that would lead to changes in the medical or surgical management of the patient. Such studies are particularly useful in the evaluation of children and adult men. In women, there is more controversy regarding their appropriate deployment. The following guidelines[6] would appear to be reasonable.

1. Either an excretory urogram or an ultrasound study is indicated to rule out obstruction in patients requiring hospital admission for bacteremic pyelonephritis, particularly if the infection is slow to respond to appropriate therapy. Patients with septic shock in this setting require such procedures on an emergency basis, because such patients often cannot be effectively resuscitated unless their "pus under pressure" is relieved by some form of drainage procedure that bypasses the obstruction.

2. Children with first or second UTIs, particularly those younger than 5 years, merit both excretory urography and voiding cystourethrography for detection of obstruction, VUR, and renal scarring. Dimercaptosuccinic acid scanning may be used in lieu of intravenous pyelography to detect scars but will not delineate anomalies in the pyelocalyceal system or the ureters. This effort is aimed at identifying not only those who might benefit from surgical correction but also those with lesser degrees of scarring and VUR who would benefit from prolonged antimicrobial prophylaxis. Because active infection by itself can produce VUR, it is usually recommended that the radiologic procedures be delayed until 4 to 8 weeks after the eradication of infection.

This approach is not ideal in that 60% to 90% of the studies that are undertaken will be negative, the cost is relatively high, and the exposure of young children to both radiation and bladder catheterization is undesirable. However, there have been few other parameters available for delineating the pediatric population at highest risk for anatomic abnormalities of the urinary tract. In particular, the noninvasive infection-localizing techniques have been of little diagnostic value in this population of patients.

3. Most men with bacterial UTI have some anatomic abnormality of the urinary tract, most commonly bladder neck obstruction secondary to prostatic enlargement. Therefore, anatomic investigation, starting with a good prostatic examination and then proceeding to excretory urography or urinary tract ultrasound studies with postvoiding views, should be seriously considered in all male patients with UTI.

4. Although there is general agreement that first UTIs in women do not merit radiologic or urologic study, the management of recurrent infection is more controversial. In such women, the once routine cystoscopic study with urethral dilatation has fallen out of fashion, largely because of the careful work of Stamey.[10] In addition, several studies

have demonstrated the lack of cost-effectiveness of radiologic and urologic studies in the evaluation of women with recurrent UTIs. Fair and co-workers[588] have reviewed the results of urograms in 164 women with histories of UTI, finding a 5.5% frequency of abnormalities but with none of these having an impact on clinical management. Engel and colleagues[589] reviewed the records of 153 women who had undergone urography and cystoscopy for the evaluation of infection. Abnormalities were observed in 11%; only one abnormality, a colovesical fistula, influenced clinical management. Fowler and Pulaski[590] studied 126 women with recurrent UTIs using urography, cystography, and cystoscopy and found only three instances (all patients with urethral diverticula) in which the results of the studies influenced clinical management of the patients' UTIs. Similar findings have been reported by others.[591]

Therefore, it would appear that the routine anatomic evaluation of women with recurrent UTI cannot be recommended. This is not to say that a few patients might not benefit from such studies. Characteristics that select a population of women who might benefit from such anatomic studies include patients who fail to respond to appropriate antimicrobial therapy or who rapidly relapse after such therapy; patients with continuing hematuria; patients with infection with urea-splitting bacteria; patients with symptoms of continuing inflammation, such as night sweats; and patients with symptoms of possible obstruction, such as persistent back or pelvic pain despite adequate antimicrobial therapy.[592, 593] In our experience, a disappointing response to antimicrobial therapy has been the most useful indicator for the need for radiologic and urologic evaluation.

# TREATMENT

## General Principles of Antimicrobial Therapy

The rational deployment of antimicrobial agents in the management of UTI is based on certain important clinical pharmacologic principles. Superficial mucosal infection, such as bladder infection, can be easily cured by the delivery of effective concentrations of antibiotic into the urine, with serum levels being of less importance. Thus, penicillin, which would not be used to treat *E. coli* or *Proteus* infection outside the urinary tract, is effective in treating bladder infections due to these organisms.[24] Similarly, tetracycline in the concentrations achieved in the urine, but not in serum or tissue, can be effective in treating UTIs due to "resistant" gram-negative bacilli including *P. aeruginosa.*[594, 595]

Therapy of deep tissue infection, such as that involving the kidney or the prostate, likewise requires delivery of effective concentrations of drug to the site of involvement. In addition, effective serum concentrations would seem to be advantageous. Whether bactericidal as opposed to bacteriostatic therapy, or synergistic two-drug therapy as opposed to single-drug therapy, is better suited for this purpose remains to be determined. These considerations are given particular emphasis by studies demonstrating in an experimental pyelonephritis model that the prompt reduction of intrarenal suppuration, as is achieved with effective antimicrobial therapy, was important in the prevention of chronic pyelonephritic scars.[392, 393, 596]

The goals in treating UTI are to prevent or treat systemic sepsis, to relieve symptoms, to eradicate sequestered infection, to eliminate uropathogenic bacterial strains from fecal and vaginal reservoirs, and to prevent long-term sequelae—all at minimal cost, with the lowest rate of side effects, and with the least selection of an antibiotic-resistant bacterial flora. These goals can be best achieved by prescribing different forms of therapy for different types of UTI.

## Specific Recommendations

### ACUTE UNCOMPLICATED CYSTITIS IN YOUNG WOMEN

Therapy of healthy women of reproductive age who present with symptoms of lower urinary tract inflammation (dysuria, frequency, urgency, nocturia, or suprapubic discomfort) in the absence of signs and symptoms of vaginitis (vaginal discharge or odor, pruritus, dyspareunia, external dysuria without frequency, and vulvovaginitis on examination) should be approached with two objectives in mind: eradication of superficial mucosal infection of the lower urinary tract, and eradication of uropathogenic clones from the vagina and lower gastrointestinal tract. To accomplish these tasks, short-course therapy with trimethoprim-sulfamethoxazole or a fluoroquinolone appears to be the treatment of choice; both of these are superior to β-lactam therapy.[126, 494] Both fluoroquinolones and trimethoprim achieve high concentrations in vaginal secretions, more than sufficient to eradicate the usual *E. coli* and other major uropathogens (with the notable exception of enterococci). At the same time, the antibacterial spectrum of activity of these drugs is such that the normal anaerobic and microaerophilic vaginal flora, which provides colonization resistance against the major uropathogens, is left intact.[126, 494] In contrast, β-lactam drugs, such as amoxicillin, appear to promote vaginal colonization with uropathogenic *E. coli.*[597]

There are two forms of short-course therapy: single-dose therapy[598–610] and a 3-day course of therapy.[126, 494, 610–615] There is now compelling evidence that 3 days of therapy is superior to a single dose. Both regimens, when trimethoprim-sulfamethoxazole or a fluoroquinolone (e.g., ciprofloxacin, ofloxacin, lomefloxacin, or enoxacin) is employed, are probably equally efficacious in eradicating bladder infection in women. However, single-dose therapy is not as effective in eradicating the uropathogenic clones from the vaginal or intestinal reservoir. As a result, early recurrence, predominantly due to reinfection from these reservoirs, is significantly more common with single-dose therapy. Longer courses of therapy (i.e., >5 days) for healthy women of reproductive age who present with symptoms suggesting cystitis are not only more expensive but are associated with a higher frequency of side effects (drug-induced rashes and fevers, particularly with trimethoprim-sulfamethoxazole; gastrointestinal upset; and candidal vaginitis) without evidence of higher rates of cure for this particular form of UTI.[126, 494, 610–615]

It should be emphasized, however, that short-course therapy is specifically designed for the treatment of superficial mucosal infection and to serve as a guide for those with unsuspected deep tissue infection who would benefit from a more extended course of therapy (e.g., women with occult pyelonephritis). Short-course therapy should therefore never be given to individuals who fall into the following categories of patients with a high probability of deep tissue infection: any man with UTI (in whom tissue invasion of at least the prostate should be assumed), anyone with overt pyelonephritis, patients with symptoms of longer than 7 days' duration, patients with underlying structural or functional defects of the urinary system, immunosuppressed individuals, patients with indwelling catheters, or patients with a high probability of infection with antibiotic-resistant organisms.[494, 601, 610]

Acute uncomplicated UTI in otherwise healthy women is so common, the range of organisms causing the infection is so well defined, the susceptibility of these organisms to the antimicrobial agents recommended is so uniform, and the efficacy and lack of side effects of short-course therapy are now so well established that all have combined to lead to a cost-effective approach that minimizes both laboratory studies and the need for visits to the physician (Fig. 32–13). The first step is to initiate short-course therapy in response to the complaint of dysuria and frequency without evidence of vaginitis. If a urine specimen is readily available, a leukocyte esterase dipstick test can be carried out (which has a reported sensitivity of 75% to 96% in this situation)[616]; urine culture and microscopic examination of the urine are reserved for the patient with atypical presentations. Alternatively, a reliable patient who reports a typical clinical presentation by telephone could have short-course therapy prescribed without initial examination of the urine. Because short-course therapy is both safe and inexpensive, and because most practitioners begin therapy on the basis of symptoms before culture data are available, this approach appears to be cost-effective.[126, 601, 610, 617]

The critical practitioner-patient interaction comes after the completion of therapy: if the patient is asymptomatic, nothing further needs to be done. If the patient is still symptomatic, both urinalysis and urine culture are necessary. If the symptomatic patient has a negative urinalysis and bacterial culture, no clear microbial etiologic agent is present and the physician's attention should be directed toward analgesia and concerns about trauma, personal hygiene, allergy to clothing dyes, or primary gynecologic conditions. If the patient is pyuric but not bacteriuric, the possibility of *C. trachomatis* urethritis should be considered, particularly if the woman is sexually active with multiple partners. Optimal therapy for *C. trachomatis* infection consists of a 7- to 14-day regimen of a tetracycline or sulfonamide for the patient and her sexual partner. Finally, patients with symptomatic bacteriuria due to an organism susceptible to the antibiotic that had been prescribed in a short-course regimen should be regarded as having covert renal infection. A more prolonged course of therapy should be administered, initially 14 days, with the potential for a more extended course if needed. Again, either a fluoroquinolone or trimethoprim-sulfamethoxazole (assuming the isolate is sensitive) would be the most effective drug in this circumstance.[126, 601, 610, 617]

## RECURRENT URINARY TRACT INFECTION IN YOUNG WOMEN

Recurrent bacterial UTI is common in women, accounting for more than 5 million visits to physicians in the United States each year.[607] Approximately 20% of young women suffering a first episode of UTI will have recurrent infection.[126] A variety of regimens have been designed to prevent repeated reinfections, which account for more than 90% of UTI recurrences. Before the physician embarks on these antimicrobial approaches, however, such simple interventions as voiding immediately after sexual intercourse and switching from a diaphragm and spermicide–based contraceptive strategy to some other approach should be implemented. If these measures are not effective, it is then time to consider which of a variety of preventive strategies is most appropriate for a particular patient. For such preventive regimens to be acceptable, they should be effective at low doses and have minimal side effects and should have minimal impact on the make-up and antibiotic susceptibility of the bowel flora, the reservoir from which UTIs are derived.

One strategy that is moderately efficacious in treating recurrent bacterial UTI is to acidify the urine with either methenamine mandelate or methenamine hippurate plus ascorbic acid, which results in the release of formaldehyde when the urine pH is maintained at 5.5 or lower. An extremely high rate of compliance by the patient and frequent checks of the urine pH are necessary for such a regimen to succeed. In the one direct comparison of this regimen with a placebo or low-dose trimethoprim-sulfamethoxazole regimen, the frequency of UTI per patient-year in a population of women susceptible to recurrent reinfections was 3.4 for placebo treatment, 1.6 for the methenamine mandelate plus

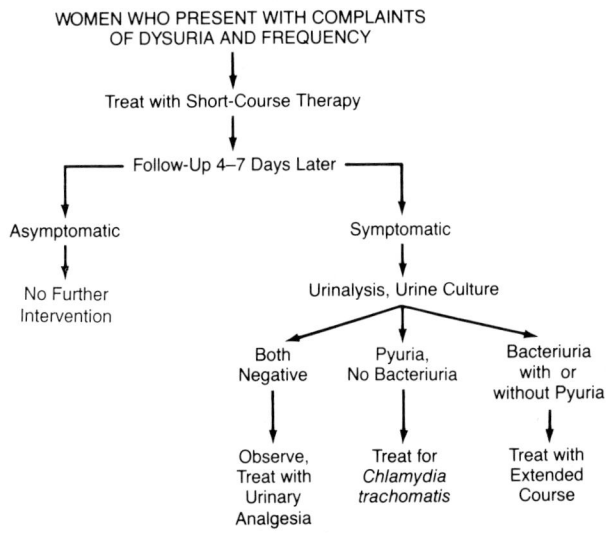

**Figure 32–13.** Clinical approach to the woman with dysuria and frequency. (Modified from Tolkoff-Rubin NE, Wilson ME, Zuromskis P, et al: Single-dose amoxicillin therapy of acute uncomplicated urinary tract infections in women. Antimicrob Agents Chemother 25:626, 1984.)

ascorbic acid regimen, and 0.15 for the trimethoprim-sulfamethoxazole program.[618]

Several prospective studies have now demonstrated the efficacy of either nitrofurantoin, 50 mg, or nitrofurantoin macrocrystals, 100 mg, at bedtime for prophylaxis against recurrent reinfection of the urinary tract. Such a regimen has little if any effect on the fecal flora and presumably acts by providing intermittent urinary antibacterial activity.[619] Although this regimen is effective, a report from Sweden[620] has suggested that long-term nitrofurantoin prophylaxis against UTI is associated with an alarming rate of adverse side effects. These adverse effects include chronic interstitial pneumonitis, acute pulmonary hypersensitivity reactions, liver damage, blood dyscrasias, skin reactions, and neuropathy. In addition, nitrofurantoin should not be used in patients with renal impairment.

Perhaps the most popular prophylactic regimen currently used in women susceptible to recurrent UTI is low-dose trimethoprim-sulfamethoxazole; as little as half a tablet (trimethoprim 40 mg, sulfamethoxazole 200 mg) three times weekly at bedtime is associated with an infection frequency of less than 0.2 per patient-year. The efficacy of this prophylactic regimen appears to remain unimpaired even after several years.[619, 621] This regimen would be cost-effective in most practice settings for women suffering more than two UTIs per year. Like trimethoprim-sulfamethoxazole, the fluoroquinolones may be used in a low-dose prophylactic regimen.[622] The efficacy of these prophylactic regimens is further delineated by their potency in preventing UTI in the far more challenging population of kidney transplant recipients.[456] A variation on these efficacious continuous prophylaxis programs is to use a fluoroquinolone or trimethoprim-sulfamethoxazole as postcoital prophylaxis.[623]

An important unanswered question is the duration of prophylactic therapy against recurrent UTI. Our practice has been to continue such therapy for 6 months and then to discontinue it. If infection then recurs, prophylaxis is reinstituted for periods of 1 to 2 years or longer. Although obvious side effects of such a program have not been apparent, more subtle long-term adverse effects on otherwise healthy women remain a concern. In particular, Freeman and co-workers,[464] in a study of men with chronic UTI treated with a sulfonamide for 25 months, observed a significantly increased rate of cardiovascular mortality compared with that seen in patients treated with placebo, nitrofurantoin, or methenamine mandelate. Because of concerns regarding long-term adverse effects, compliance, and cost in the long-term prophylaxis of recurrent UTI, one final approach has been taken to this problem: to provide women having histories of recurrent infections with a supply of trimethoprim-sulfamethoxazole, a fluoroquinolone, or another effective single-dose regimen drug. The patient is then instructed to initiate single-dose therapy with the onset of symptoms; further medical attention is sought only when the symptoms do not abate or the number of treated episodes exceeds four in a 6-month period.[126, 624]

The approach to the minority of patients with relapsing infection is different. Two factors may contribute to the pathogenesis of relapsing infection in women: deep tissue infection of the kidney that is suppressed but not eradicated by a 14-day course of antibiotics, and structural abnormal-ity of the urinary tract (e.g., calculi). At least some of these patients will respond to a 6-week course of therapy.[625, 626] Because the strategy in dealing with relapsing infection and repeated reinfection is so different, the critical decision to be made by the clinician concerns the form of recurrent infection present in the individual patient. Certain clues to this are available from the past history and bacteriologic information. Most relapses occur within 1 week of the cessation of antimicrobial therapy, and virtually all within 1 month, so information concerning the timing of the recurrences can be helpful. Knowledge of the bacterial species isolated and the antibiotic susceptibility pattern of the species can help in deciding whether it is the same organism or different from the original pathogen. However, this kind of information is too often either unavailable or inadequate for making this assessment. We have found that the response to short-course therapy in such women is helpful in making the management decision: if the patient responds to short-course therapy, it is likely that she has been having recurrent reinfection and is thus a candidate for long-term prophylaxis; if the patient fails short-course therapy, it is probable that she has been having relapsing infection and is thus a candidate for an intensive course of prolonged therapy. Thus, one can more exactly delineate those patients in whom the greatest clinical benefit would compensate for the increased costs and side effects of prolonged treatment (Fig. 32–14).

## ACUTE UNCOMPLICATED CYSTITIS IN OLDER WOMEN

Several aspects of UTI in postmenopausal women merit special attention. The frequency of both symptomatic and asymptomatic bacteriuria is considerably higher than in younger age groups, probably as a result of at least two factors: many postmenopausal women have significant amounts of residual urine in their bladders after voiding as a consequence of childbirth and loss of pelvic tone; and the lack of estrogens causes a marked change in the susceptibility of the uroepithelium and vagina to pathogens. This is at least partly due to such changes in the vaginal microflora as the loss of lactobacilli, which causes a rise in vaginal pH.[126, 627–630] Whereas symptoms referable to the lower urinary tract in younger women are almost invariably due to uropathogens and C. trachomatis (see earlier), other possibilities exist in older women. In particular, in symptomatic women with pyuria and negative cultures, the possibility of genitourinary tuberculosis, systemic fungal infection, and diverticulitis or a diverticular abscess impinging on the bladder or ureters merits consideration, rather than the chlamydial infection that represents a major cause of such infections in younger women.

The antimicrobial strategies discussed before for the management of acute cystitis in younger women are applicable in postmenopausal women as well. In addition, however, other interventions have an important role in this population. Several studies have now shown that estrogen replacement therapy, either locally by use of a vaginal cream or systemically with oral therapy, restores the atrophic genitourinary tract mucosa of the postmenopausal woman, is associated with a reappearance of lactobacilli in

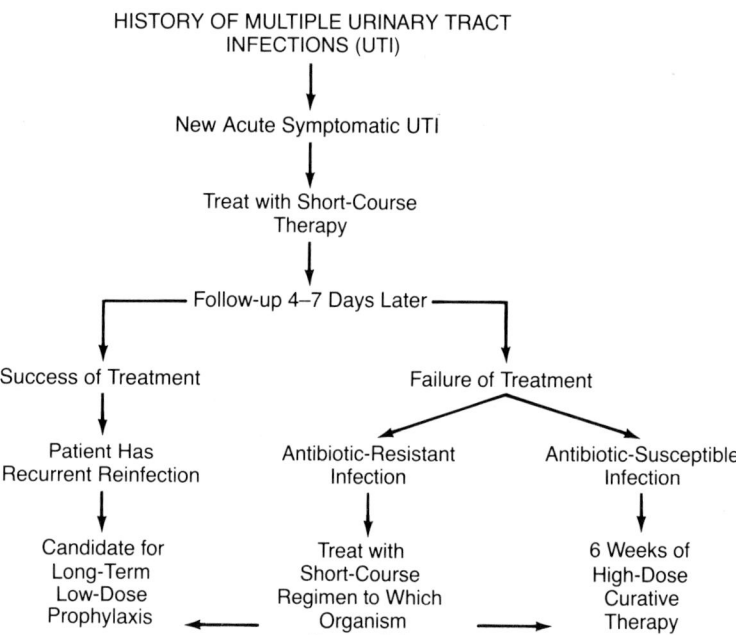

**Figure 32–14.** Clinical approach to the woman with recurrent UTIs.

the vaginal flora and a resultant fall in vaginal pH, and decreases vaginal colonization by Enterobacteriaceae.[630–632] Raz and Stamm,[630] in a carefully controlled study, demonstrated unequivocally that these physiologic effects were translated into significant protection against recurrent UTI in postmenopausal women.

In a study that may be translatable to other populations, Avorn and co-workers[633] have reported that the regular intake of cranberry juice significantly reduced the frequency of both bacteriuria and pyuria in a population of elderly women. Although the possibility of this effect has been postulated for many years, it has in the past been linked to urinary acidification. Because consistent acidification with oral intake of cranberry juice requires the consistent ingestion of prodigious volumes, this approach had fallen out of favor. What is noteworthy in this study is that the therapeutic effect was clearly independent of any changes in urine pH. Rather than an acidification effect, it has been postulated that cranberry juice contains materials that inhibit the attachment of bacterial adhesins to the uroepithelium.[633–635]

## ACUTE UNCOMPLICATED PYELONEPHRITIS IN WOMEN

Patients with clear-cut symptomatic pyelonephritis have deep tissue infection, have or are at risk for bacteremia, and merit intensive antimicrobial therapy. The key principle in the management of these patients is the immediate delivery of effective concentrations of an antimicrobial agent to which the invading organism is susceptible both to the bloodstream and to the urinary tract. A variety of strategies are available to accomplish this; the following general principles are a useful guide.[126, 494]

1. There are three goals in the antimicrobial therapy of symptomatic pyelonephritis: control or prevention of the development of urosepsis (i.e., the consequences of blood-

stream invasion), eradication of the invading organism, and prevention of recurrences.

2. It is useful to divide the therapeutic program to accomplish these aims into two parts: the immediate control of systemic sepsis, which usually requires parenteral therapy; and the eradication of the infecting organism (and prevention of early recurrence) with an oral agent, after initial control of the systemic sepsis and acute inflammatory consequences of pyelonephritis.

3. Initial antimicrobial programs to obtain control of systemic sepsis are prescribed to fulfill two objectives: the infecting organism has a greater than 99% probability of being sensitive to the regimen chosen; and adequate blood levels of the drugs can be reliably achieved promptly in the particular patient. At present, there is no evidence to suggest that one antibiotic or program is inherently superior to another for control of systemic sepsis provided that these two requirements are fulfilled. Thus, the objection to ampicillin, amoxicillin, or first-generation cephalosporins as initial therapy for pyelonephritis when the nature and susceptibility of the infecting organism are unknown (as is usually the case) is due to the fact that 20% to 30% of isolates are now resistant to these drugs. Similarly, the merits of intravenous therapy have to do with the reliability of drug delivery, rather than something inherently more desirable about intravenous drugs (indeed, as is well recognized, vascular access devices have their own infectious disease complications). In patients with milder disease, who are free of nausea and vomiting, advantage can be taken of the excellent antimicrobial spectrum and bioavailability with oral administration (with the easy achievement of high blood levels with oral administration *provided that the gastrointestinal tract is functioning adequately*) of such drugs as trimethoprim-sulfamethoxazole and the fluoroquinolones to prescribe oral therapy for the entire therapeutic course.

4. Once the patient has been afebrile for 24 hours (usually within 72 hours of initiation of therapy), there is no

inherent benefit to maintaining parenteral therapy. At this point, prescription of trimethoprim-sulfamethoxazole or a fluoroquinolone to complete a 14-day course of therapy appears to be the most effective means of eradicating both tissue infection and residual clones of uropathogen present in the gastrointestinal tract that could cause early recurrence if left in place. One important point that bears emphasis in this regard: parenteral trimethoprim-sulfamethoxazole and fluoroquinolones are effective drugs for initial control of systemic sepsis, but there is no special benefit of initiating therapy with one of these to be able to continue the same drug orally. Initial control with any effective parenteral regimen, followed by oral trimethoprim-sulfamethoxazole or fluoroquinolone for eradication, is the cornerstone of the therapeutic strategy.

With these principles in mind, what, then, should be used as initial parenteral therapy? If possible, a Gram stain of the urine should be done to establish whether enterococcal infection could be present. If gram-positive cocci are present, or that information is not available, initial therapy should include intravenous ampicillin (or vancomycin) plus gentamicin to provide adequate coverage of both enterococci and the more common gram-negative uropathogens. If only gram-negative bacilli are present, there is a large number of choices ranging from parenteral trimethoprim-sulfamethoxazole and fluoroquinolones to gentamicin, such broad-spectrum cephalosporins as ceftriaxone, aztreonam, the β-lactam/β-lactamase inhibitor combinations (ampicillin-sulbactam, ticarcillin-clavulanate, and piperacillin-tazobactam), and imipenem-cilastatin. In general, these last agents on the list (beginning with aztreonam) are reserved for patients with more complicated histories, previous episodes of pyelonephritis, and recent urinary tract manipulations.[126, 494]

## URINARY TRACT INFECTION IN PREGNANCY

As previously discussed, pregnant women are the one population in whom screening for asymptomatic bacteriuria is not only cost-effective but obligatory to prevent consequences for the developing fetus and the mother. Treatment of pregnant women with asymptomatic bacteriuria or symptoms of lower urinary tract inflammation (dysuria and frequency, akin to acute uncomplicated cystitis in the nonpregnant woman of reproductive age) is similar to that in nonpregnant women: short-course therapy.[126, 636] Although studies comparing single-dose with 3-day regimens are not available, and both have been effective in pregnant women, our preference is for a 3-day regimen. There are two major differences, however, in the approach to pregnant women with UTI: the drugs that can be safely used are far more limited, and intensive follow-up with the institution of prophylaxis for the duration of the pregnancy is an important management consideration.

Sulfonamides, nitrofurantoin, ampicillin, and cephalexin have been considered relatively safe for use in early pregnancy; sulfonamides are avoided near term because of a possible role in the development of kernicterus. Trimethoprim is usually avoided because of evidence of toxic effects

in the fetus at high doses in experimental animals, although it has been used successfully in humans during pregnancy without evidence of toxicity or teratogenicity. Fluoroquinolones are avoided because of possible adverse effects on fetal cartilage development. Our preference is the use of nitrofurantoin, ampicillin, or cephalexin—the drugs that have been used most extensively in pregnancy—in pregnant women with asymptomatic or minimally symptomatic UTI whenever possible. In pregnant women with overt pyelonephritis, admission to the hospital for parenteral therapy should be the standard of care; β-lactam drugs, aminoglycosides, or both are the cornerstone of therapy.[126, 636–638]

Effective prevention of UTI, including pyelonephritis, can be accomplished during pregnancy with postcoital prophylaxis with nitrofurantoin, cephalexin, or ampicillin; or these drugs may be given at bedtime without relation to coitus. Patients who should be considered for such prophylaxis during pregnancy include patients with histories of acute pyelonephritis during pregnancy, patients with bacteriuria during pregnancy who have had a recurrence after a treatment course, and patients with a history of recurrent UTI before pregnancy that has required a prophylaxis program outside the added stresses of pregnancy.[639, 640]

## URINARY TRACT INFECTIONS IN MEN

UTI is uncommon in men younger than 50 years, although UTI without associated urologic abnormalities can occur under the following circumstances: in homosexual men, in men having intercourse with women colonized with uropathogens, and in the face of the acquired immunodeficiency syndrome with a CD4$^+$ lymphocyte count of less than 200/mm$^3$. Such individuals should never be treated with short-course therapy; rather, 10- to 14-day regimens of trimethoprim-sulfamethoxazole or a fluoroquinolone should be regarded as standard therapy unless antimicrobial intolerance or an unusual pathogen requires an alternative approach.[125, 126, 641, 642]

In men older than 50 years with UTI, tissue invasion of the prostate, the kidneys, or both should be assumed, even in the absence of overt signs of infection at these sites. Acute bacterial prostatitis, because of the inflammation usually present, initially responds well to the same array of antimicrobial agents used to treat UTIs in other populations. However, after a conventional course of therapy of 10 to 14 days, relapse is common. Recurrent infection in men usually connotes a sustained focus within the prostate that has not been eradicated by previous courses of therapy. Several factors at work here make eradication of prostatic foci so difficult: many antimicrobial agents do not diffuse well across the prostatic epithelium into the prostatic fluid, where the infection lies; the prostate may harbor calculi, which can serve to block drainage of portions of the prostate gland or act as foreign bodies around which persistent infection can be hidden; and an enlarged (and inflamed) prostate gland can cause bladder outlet obstruction, resulting in pools of stagnant urine in the bladder that are difficult to sterilize.[125, 126, 643–645]

As a result of these factors, it is now recognized that intensive therapy for at least 4 to 6 weeks and as many as

12 weeks is required to sterilize the urinary tract in many of these men. The drugs of choice for this purpose, assuming the invading organisms are susceptible, are trimethoprim-sulfamethoxazole, trimethoprim (in the individual allergic to sulfonamide), and the fluoroquinolones. Prolonged treatment with each of these has a greater than 60% chance of eradicating infection. Most of the failures are due to one of two factors: the anatomic factors listed before are too abnormal to permit cure; the infection that is present is due to *E. faecalis* or *P. aeruginosa*, two organisms with a particularly high rate of relapse after treatment with the antimicrobial agents currently available. When relapse occurs, a choice then has to be made among three therapeutic approaches: long-term antimicrobial suppression, repeated treatment courses for each relapse, and surgical removal of the infected prostate gland under coverage of systemic antimicrobial therapy. The choice from among these approaches depends on the age, sexual activity, and general condition of the patient; the degree of bladder outlet obstruction present; and the level of suspicion that prostate cancer could be present.[125, 126, 643–645]

In addition to the usual uropathogens causing a UTI in men, one additional entity merits attention. After instrumentation of the urinary tract, most commonly after repeated insertion of a Foley catheter, infection with *S. aureus* may occur; the use of antistaphylococcal therapy and the removal of the foreign body are required for cure.

## TREATMENT OF CHILDHOOD URINARY TRACT INFECTION

The treatment of full-blown pyelonephritis in the child is similar to that in the adult: broad-spectrum parenteral therapy until the antimicrobial susceptibility pattern of the infecting organism is known, followed by narrow-spectrum least toxic therapy parenterally until the patient is afebrile for 24 to 48 hours. A prolonged 1- to 3-month course of oral therapy is then instituted. Follow-up urine cultures within a week of completion of therapy and at frequent intervals for the next year are indicated. In children with acute, uncomplicated UTI, although many will respond to short-course therapy, conventional 7- to 14-day regimens appear to be preferable. One potential exception to this observation is adolescent girls, for whom the increased compliance associated with short-course therapy can be a significant advantage. The one major difference in the approach to children as opposed to adults is that fluoroquinolones cannot be used in children because of possible adverse effects on developing cartilage.[646–651]

Recurrent UTI in children, particularly in those with renal scarring or demonstrable VUR, is dealt with by long-term prophylaxis with such agents as trimethoprim-sulfamethoxazole (2 mg/kg/dose once or twice per day of the trimethoprim component, which gives 10 mg/kg/dose of the sulfamethoxazole component), nitrofurantoin (2 mg/kg/d as single dose), or methenamine mandelate (50 mg/kg/d in three divided doses). Sulfonamides are less effective because of the emergence of resistance. Trimethoprim-sulfamethoxazole and nitrofurantoin macrocrystals have been particularly effective in this regard.[650–654] Results of trials comparing medical therapy with surgical correction of

VUR in children have failed to show significant benefit from the surgical approach in terms of renal function, progressive scarring, or renal growth despite the fact that the technical aspects of the surgical repair could be accomplished satisfactorily. As a result, current views are to attempt to prevent scarring aggressively with prolonged antimicrobial therapy and close monitoring, with surgical correction reserved for the child who, in a 2- to 4-year period, appears to be failing medical therapy.[655–664]

## COMPLICATED URINARY TRACT INFECTION

The term complicated UTI, by its nature, encompasses a heterogeneous group of patients with a wide variety of structural and functional abnormalities of the urinary tract and kidney. In addition, the range of organisms causing infection in these patients is particularly broad, with a high percentage of these organisms being resistant to one or more of the antimicrobial agents frequently used in other populations of patients with UTI. Having said this, the following general principles appear to be reasonable in approaching patients with complicated UTI.[125, 126, 492, 494]

1. Therapy should be aimed primarily at symptomatic UTI, because there is little evidence that treatment of asymptomatic bacteriuria in this population of patients either alters the clinical condition of the patient or is likely to be successful. The one exception to this rule is if the asymptomatic patient is scheduled for instrumentation of the urinary tract. In this instance, sterilization of the urine before manipulation and continuation of antimicrobial therapy for 3 to 7 days after manipulation can prevent serious morbidity and even mortality from urosepsis.

2. Because of the broad range of infecting pathogens and their varying sensitivity patterns, culture data are essential in prescribing therapy for symptomatic patients. If therapy should be needed before such information is available, initial therapy must be far broader spectrum than in other groups of patients. Thus, in a patient with apparent pyelonephritis or urosepsis in a complicated setting, initial therapy with such regimens as ampicillin plus gentamicin, imipenem-cilastatin, or piperacillin-tazobactam is indicated. In the patient who is more subacutely ill, trimethoprim-sulfamethoxazole or a fluoroquinolone appears to be a reasonable first choice.

3. Every effort should be made to correct the underlying complicating factor, whenever possible, in conjunction with the antimicrobial therapy. If this is possible, a prolonged 4- to 6-week "curative" course of therapy in conjunction with the surgical manipulation is appropriate. If such correction is not possible, shorter courses of therapy (7 to 14 days), aimed at controlling symptoms, appear to be more appropriate. Frequent symptomatic relapses are worth an attempt at long-term suppressive therapy.

A particular subgroup of patients susceptible to complicated UTI are patients with neurogenic bladders secondary to spinal cord injury. In these, intermittent self-catheterization with clean catheters and methenamine prophylaxis have been shown to decrease the morbidity associated with UTI.[455, 665]

## CATHETER-ASSOCIATED URINARY TRACT INFECTION

Infections of the urinary tract are by far the most common cause of hospital-acquired infection. Most such nosocomial UTIs are due to the use of bladder catheters. More than 900,000 episodes of catheter-associated bacteriuria occur in acute care hospitals in the United States each year. Approximately 2% to 4% of these patients develop gram-negative sepsis, and such events can contribute to the mortality of patients.[126, 666]

Important in determining the effectiveness of antibiotic treatment of catheter-associated UTI is the development of a biofilm on the surface of the catheter. Bacteria adhering to the surface of the catheter initiate the formation of a complex biologic structure containing the bacteria, bacterial glycocalyces, Tamm-Horsfall protein, apatite, struvite, and other constituents. This structure protects bacteria from antimicrobial therapy, which leads to prompt relapse once therapy is stopped. Thus, replacement of the bladder catheter should be part of the treatment of catheter-associated UTI, when treatment is thought to be indicated.[126, 667, 668]

Although bacteriuria is inevitable with chronic catheterization, certain guidelines can be employed to delay the onset of such infections and to minimize the rate of acquisition of antibiotic-resistant pathogens (Table 32–6). Critically important in this regard are sterile insertion and care of the catheter, use of a closed drainage system, and prompt removal. Whether such additions as silver ion–coated catheters, the use of disinfectants in collecting bags, and other local strategies offer additional benefit is still unclear. Systemic antimicrobial therapy can delay the onset of bacteriuria and can be useful in those clinical situations in which the time of catheterization is clearly limited (e.g., in association with gynecologic or vascular surgery and kidney transplantation).[126, 669–671]

Treatment of catheter-associated UTI requires good clinical judgment. In any patient symptomatic from the infection (e.g., exhibiting fever, chills, dyspnea, and hypotension), immediate therapy with effective antibiotics is indicated, with use of the same antimicrobial strategies described before for other forms of complicated UTI. In an asymptomatic patient, no therapy is indicated. Patients with long-term indwelling catheters rarely become symptomatic unless the catheter is obstructed or is eroding through the bladder mucosa. In those patients who do become symptomatic, antibiotics should be given and close attention should be directed to changing the catheter or changing the type of urinary drainage.

## CANDIDAL INFECTION OF THE URINARY TRACT

Clear-cut guidelines for the treatment of candidal infection of the urinary tract are currently not available, particularly because there are currently no criteria that are generally accepted to distinguish between colonization and infection.[672] Until more information is available, the following approach is the one that we currently employ.

1. In patients with catheter-associated candidal UTI, re-

**TABLE 32–6. Guidelines for Bladder Catheter Care to Prevent Infection**

1. Use catheter only when absolutely necessary; remove as soon as possible.
2. Insert catheters aseptically and maintain by trained personnel only; the use of "catheter teams" is preferable.
3. A sterile closed drainage system is mandatory. The catheter and drainage tube must never be disconnected except when irrigation is necessary to relieve obstruction. Strict aseptic technique is employed under these circumstances.
4. Urine for culture should be obtained by aspirating the catheter with a 21-gauge needle after the catheter is prepared with povidone-iodine.
5. Maintain downhill, unobstructed flow, with the collection bag always below the level of the bladder and emptied at frequent intervals.
6. Replace indwelling catheters when obstruction or concretions are demonstrated.
7. Separate catheterized patients whenever possible; in particular, a patient with a sterile bladder catheter system should always be kept separate from patients with infected urine, and strict hand-washing procedures should be observed by staff caring for these patients.

Modified from Kaye D, Santoro J: Urinary tract infection. *In* Mandell GL, Douglas RG Jr, Bennett JE (eds): Principles and Practice of Infectious Diseases. Copyright © 1979 John Wiley & Sons. Reprinted by permission of John Wiley & Sons, Inc.

moval of the preceding catheter, insertion of a three-way catheter, and infusion of an amphotericin rinse for a period of 3 to 5 days appear to have a greater than 75% success rate in eradicating this infection. Success is increased if such contributing factors as hyperglycemia, corticosteroid use, and antibacterial therapy can be eliminated.[673]

2. In patients with candiduria without an indwelling catheter, insertion of a catheter for an amphotericin rinse appears to introduce another hazard, the risk of bacteriuria. Our preference is to treat such individuals with fluconazole, 200 to 400 mg/d for 10 to 14 days. In a population of organ transplant patients, such an approach has been successful in more than 75% of patients with candiduria.[674]

3. Any patient with candiduria who is to undergo instrumentation of the urinary tract requires systemic therapy with amphotericin or fluconazole to prevent the consequences of transient candidemia.[51]

## SPECIAL FORMS OF PYELONEPHRITIS

### Renal Tuberculosis

Approximately 10% of the new cases of tuberculosis reported annually are extrapulmonary, and among these cases, the genitourinary tract is the leading site.[49, 675–678] Unfortunately, many cases of renal tuberculosis remain clinically silent for years while irreversible renal destruction takes place. Thus, unexplained "sterile" pyuria or hematuria should prompt the clinician to undertake an evaluation for renal tuberculosis.[49]

Genitourinary tuberculosis usually results from "silent" bacillemia accompanying pulmonary tuberculosis. However, active lesions in the kidney may not become manifest clinically for many years, often at a time when little evidence of active pulmonary disease exists. If routine screening of urine specimens for tubercle bacilli is undertaken in a group of patients hospitalized specifically for active pulmonary infection, a number of silent urinary infections will be detected.[49] In the general population, symptoms referable to the urinary tract rather than the lung are those most likely to lead the patient with renal tuberculosis to the physician. In one series describing 41 cases of genitourinary tuberculosis observed from 1962 through 1974, concomitant pulmonary findings were present in only 66% of newly diagnosed cases of genitourinary tuberculosis.[675] In the same series, dysuria (34%), hematuria (27%), flank pain (10%), and pyuria (5%) were the most frequent presenting symptoms for active urinary tuberculosis. Constitutional symptoms occurred in only 14% of cases, and no symptoms attributable to tuberculosis could be elicited in 20% of patients. An abnormal urinalysis was found in well over half these cases. A positive skin test result (purified protein derivative) was present in 95% of cases, and urine cultures grew *Mycobacterium tuberculosis* in 90%. Excretory urograms were abnormal in 93% of patients examined. Thus, genitourinary tuberculosis should not be a difficult diagnosis to make if patients with localizing urinary symptoms plus abnormal urinalyses are screened for tuberculosis after routine urine cultures have been found to be negative. The pathologic changes—granulomatous inflammation and caseous necrosis—often (but not always) begin in the medulla and papilla, causing papillary necrosis, but soon involve the cortex and occasionally the perirenal tissues. Coalescence of the lesions sometimes leads to large caseous cavities.

Radiographic examinations are rarely pathognomonic for renal tuberculosis, but the intravenous urogram and computed tomographic scan may be helpful in the differential diagnosis of tuberculosis from other infectious and granulomatous entities.[679] The gross strictures, cavities, and calcifications of advanced renal tuberculosis are distinctive.[49]

Current recommendations for the treatment of genitourinary tuberculosis are as follows.[49]

1. Uncomplicated urinary tract tuberculosis, likely to be due to drug-sensitive organisms, is well treated with an initial 2 months of daily rifampin, isoniazid, and pyrazinamide followed by 4 months of daily rifampin and isoniazid. Such a regimen is particularly useful in women. In men, in whom concern regarding sequestered foci within the prostate is an issue, we prefer to continue such a program for an additional 3 to 6 months. If pyrazinamide is not tolerated, rifampin and isonizad therapy for 9 months is recommended for women, with a preference for an additional 3 to 6 months in men.

2. At present, there is little published experience with these relatively short regimens in patients with caseating destruction of the kidneys or in men with overt genital disease. In such instances, we would prefer to prolong the isoniazid and rifampin components so that a minimum of 12 to 18 months of therapy with at least two bactericidal agents is delivered.

3. Anyone with possible drug-resistant tuberculosis should have therapy instituted with isoniazid, rifampin, and pyrazinamide, to ensure the use of at least two bactericidal agents, plus one of the following: ethambutol, ofloxacin, or streptomycin. Once drug sensitivity results are available, the regimen can be modified accordingly. If two bactericidal agents can be employed, we prefer a minimum of 12 months of therapy in patients with drug-resistant disease. If only one bactericidal agent plus ethambutol is possible, a minimum of 24 months of therapy is recommended.

4. Preliminary experience with the treatment of tuberculosis in the setting of acquired immunodeficiency syndrome suggests that 9 to 12 months of therapy may be adequate, particularly with the initial 2 months of isoniazid, rifampin, and pyrazinamide being part of this regimen. However, the possibility of relapse in this population of immunocompromised patients must be considered. In selected patients with progressive acquired immunodeficiency syndrome, longer courses of therapy or reinstitution of therapy should be considered.

5. In patients who cannot tolerate at least two of the three primary bactericidal agents because of side effects, one bactericidal agent plus a second agent such as ethambutol should be used for a period of 24 months.

Additional issues that should be addressed include the following: antimicrobial sensitivity testing should be carried out on all primary isolates (owing to the increase in drug-resistant tuberculosis in more recent years); proof of cure must be documented by culture; and follow-up urograms or ultrasound examinations must be performed to rule out the development of obstructive uropathy as a consequence of the healing process. Such a development would obligate surgical correction to salvage renal function.[49]

## Xanthogranulomatous Pyelonephritis

This is a form of chronic bacterial pyelonephritis characterized by destruction of renal parenchyma and the presence of granulomas, abscesses, and collections of lipid-filled macrophages (foam cells).[680–685]

Although the disease remains uncommon, accounting for 6 per 1000 surgically proven cases of chronic pyelonephritis,[680] it has apparently increased in frequency in more recent years.[681] It occurs at any age, from 11 months to 89 years, but is most frequent in adults in the fifth through seventh decades. Women are affected more often than men (2:1), and except in a rare patient with bilateral disease,[686] the lesions affect only one kidney. Most patients present with renal pain, recurrent UTI, fever (of undetermined nature), malaise, anorexia, weight loss, and constipation. Duration of treatment before diagnosis is between 3 months and 9 years. Seventy-three percent of patients give a history of previous calculous disease, obstructive uropathy, or diabetes mellitus, and 38% have undergone urologic procedures. A renal mass is present in 60% of cases and hypertension in about 40%.

In gross appearance, the kidney is usually enlarged, and the capsule and perirenal tissue are often thickened and adherent. The process may be localized to one tumor mass involving one pole of the kidney or may be diffuse and multifocal. On section, the pelvis and calyces are dilated and contain either purulent fluid or calculi (often staghorn calculi) or both. The renal parenchyma, particularly surrounding the dilated calyces, is replaced by orange-yellow, soft inflammatory tissue, often with surrounding small abscesses. The tumor can be mistaken grossly for renal cell carcinoma, but the presence of calculi, obstruction, abscesses, and purulent material and the localization of yellow tissue adjacent to the pelvis and calyces point to an inflammatory disorder (Fig. 32–15). However, there have been reports of coexistent renal cell carcinoma in the same[687–689] or contralateral kidneys.

On microscopic examination, the orange-yellow areas are made up of inflammatory tissue consisting of an admixture of large foamy macrophages, smaller macrophages with granular cytoplasm, neutrophils, lymphocytes, plasma cells, and fibroblasts. Neutrophils and necrotic debris are particularly abundant surrounding the pelvic mucosa. An occasional foreign body giant cell may be present. The cytoplasm of the foamy macrophages and particularly of the small granular monocytes stains strongly with PAS.

The radiographic picture is varied.[690, 691] The heterogeneous pattern is due to diverse combinations of localized or diffuse lesions; the radiologic appearance depends on the presence of obstruction, calculi, or other anomalies. On excretory urograms, a stone-bearing, nonfunctioning kidney is present in about 80% of cases. Calyceal deformity and irregularity are also common, particularly in the diffuse type. The localized lesions appear as cystic or cavitary masses that show no ''puddling'' of contrast medium. On angiograms, most xanthogranulomatous renal masses are hypovascular or avascular. There is spreading of intrarenal arteries without peripheral arborization, but usually there are no pathologic vessels; however, some cases have shown increased vascularity. Furthermore, the avascular solitary mass of xanthogranulomatous pyelonephritis cannot be definitively distinguished from necrotic avascular adenocarcinoma by angiography alone. Computed tomography is helpful in the diagnosis and particularly in identifying extension of the inflammation to the perirenal fat.[692–694] Magnetic resonance imaging may also aid in the diagnosis.[695]

The diagnosis of xanthogranulomatous pyelonephritis should be considered in patients with a history of chronic infection and certain radiologic features.[691] The radiologic findings include unilateral renal enlargement; a nonfunctioning kidney on intravenous urograms; the presence of renal calculi, ureteral calculi, or both; angiographic demonstration of an avascular mass or masses with stretched attenuated intrarenal vessels, prominent capsular periureteric vessels, and an irregular impaired nephrogram with prominent avascular areas; and suggestive changes by computed tomography or magnetic resonance imaging. With these features, some 40% of cases can be diagnosed or suspected preoperatively.[694, 695]

Bacterial cultures of the urine are almost invariably positive. *P. mirabilis* and *E. coli* are the most frequent organisms cultured.[696] Series reporting a high frequency of *E. coli* also showed a low frequency of staghorn calculi. Methicillin-resistant *S. aureus* can also cause the condition.[697]

The pathogenesis of xanthogranulomatous pyelonephritis is unclear, although it seems certain that the condition is caused by bacterial infection and accentuated by urinary obstruction. Similar cells with PAS reaction–positive granules have been produced by *Proteus, E. coli,* and staphylococcal infection in rats. Electron microscopy shows that the foamy macrophages initially contain bacteria and subsequently contain numerous phagolysosomes filled with myelin figures and amorphous material.[698] The presence of these phagolysosomes has suggested that there may be a lysosomal defect of macrophages that interferes with the digestion of bacterial products.[698]

Most kidneys with xanthogranulomatous pyelonephritis are removed surgically, largely because a correct preoperative diagnosis is made infrequently, but studies suggest that diagnosis by a combination of clinical and radiologic features is possible in 40% of cases.[694] In the focal disease, unnecessary radical surgery may be prevented in the poor-risk patient. Recurrences in the other kidney have not been reported after surgery. The disease has also been reported in transplant recipients.[699]

## Malakoplakia

Malakoplakia is a rare, histologically distinct inflammatory reaction usually caused by enteric bacteria and affecting many organs but most commonly the urinary tract. In most cases, the condition is confined to the urinary bladder mucosa, where it appears as soft, yellow, slightly raised, often confluent plaques 3 to 4 cm in diameter. It is most common in middle-aged women with chronic UTI. The microscopic picture is typical. Plaques are composed of closely packed, large macrophages with occasional lymphocytes and multinucleate giant cells. The macrophages have abundant, foamy, PAS reaction–positive cytoplasm; in addition, laminated mineralized concretions, known as Michaelis-Gutmann bodies, are typically present within macrophages and in the interstitial tissue. The Michaelis-Gutmann bodies measure 4 to 10 μm in diameter, stain strongly with PAS, and contain calcium (Fig. 32–16). On

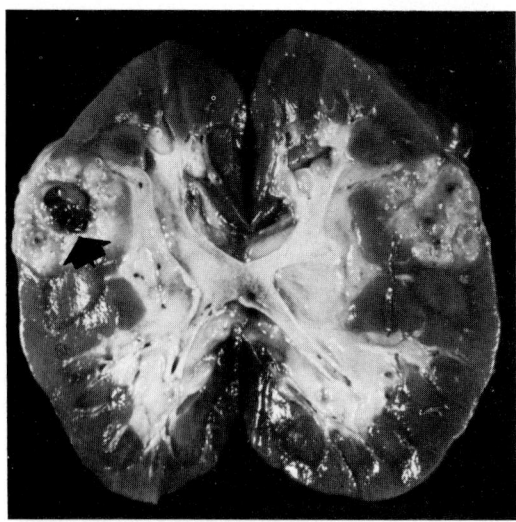

**Figure 32–15.** Xanthogranulomatous pyelonephritis, localized form. The orange-yellow granulomatous mass surrounds a black calculus *(arrow)* in a calyceal diverticulum. Note resemblance to renal cell carcinoma.

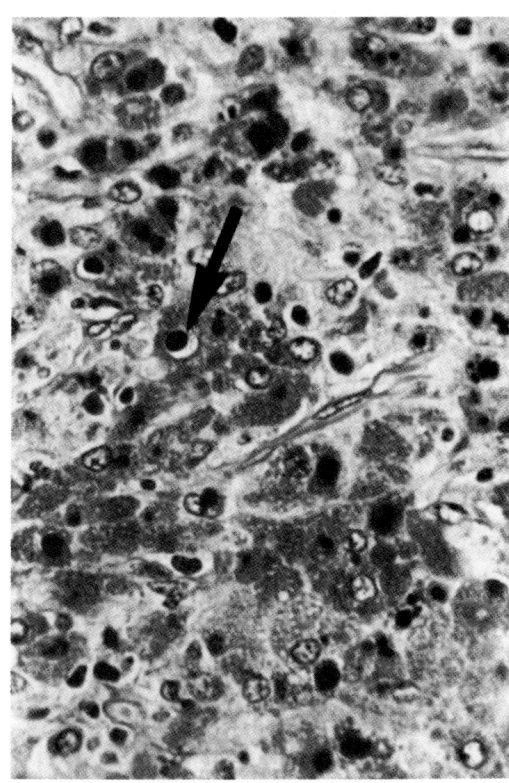

**Figure 32–16.** Michaelis-Gutmann bodies of malakoplakia *(arrow).*

electron microscopic studies, they show a typical crystalline structure with a central dense core, an intermediate halo, and a peripheral lamellated ring.[700] Intracellular bacteria and giant phagolysosomes can be demonstrated within macrophages.[700–702]

Identical lesions have been discovered in the prostate, ureteral and pelvic mucosa, bones, lungs, testes, gastrointestinal tract, skin, and kidneys. Renal malakoplakia occurs in the same clinical setting as xanthogranulomatous pyelonephritis[703]—chronic infection and obstruction—and indeed, except for the presence of Michaelis-Gutmann bodies, there is considerable overlap in the gross histologic features of both conditions. *E. coli* is the most common organism cultured from urine. Clinical findings usually include flank pain and signs of active renal infection. Bilateral involvement has been reported, as has a clinical presentation simulating acute renal failure.[704, 705]

The pathogenesis of malakoplakia is unclear, but about half of the cases are associated with immunodeficiency or autoimmune disorders, including hypogammaglobulinemia, therapeutic immunosuppression, malignant neoplasms, chronic debilitating disorder, rheumatoid arthritis, and the acquired immunodeficiency syndrome.[701] A current scenario is that the lesions result from a defect in macrophage function blocking the lysosomal enzymatic degradation of engulfed bacteria and overloading the cytoplasm with undigested bacterial debris. Microtubule defects impairing the movement of lysosomes to phagocytic vacuoles and decreased lysosomal enzyme release within phagocytes have been postulated.[706–708] The Michaelis-Gutmann bodies are

thought to result from the deposition of calcium phosphate and other minerals on these overloaded phagosomes.

Another histologic entity that overlaps with both malakoplakia and xanthogranulomatous pyelonephritis is so-called megalocytic interstitial nephritis; in this variant, the interstitial infiltrate is polymorphous with predominance of histiocytes containing crystalloid material.[708]

## REFERENCES

1. Kunin CM: Detection, Prevention and Management of Urinary Tract Infections, 4th ed. Lea & Febiger, Philadelphia, 1987.
2. Heptinstall RH: The enigma of chronic pyelonephritis. J Infect Dis 120:104, 1969.
3. Hodson CJ: Radiological diagnosis of pyelonephritis. Proc R Soc Med 52:669, 1959.
4. Smith JF: The diagnosis of the scars of chronic pyelonephritis. J Clin Pathol 15:522, 1962.
5. Report by the Medical Research Council Bacteriuria Committee: Recommended terminology of urinary tract infection. Br Med J 2:717, 1979.
6. Risdon RA: Pyelonephritis and reflux nephropathy. *In* Tisher C, Brenner B (eds): Renal Pathology. JB Lippincott, Philadelphia, 1989, pp 775–808.
7. Tolkoff-Rubin NE, Rubin RH: Urinary tract infection. *In* Cotran RS (ed): Tubulo-interstitial Nephropathies. Churchill Livingstone, New York, 1983, pp 49–82.
8. Pollack HM: Laboratory techniques for detection of urinary tract infection and assessment of value. Am J Med 75:79, 1983.
9. Kunin CM, Polyak F, Postel E: Periurethral bacterial flora in women: Prolonged intermittent colonization with *Escherichia coli.* JAMA 243:134, 1980.
10. Stamey TA: Urinary tract infections in the female: A perspective. *In* Remington JS, Swartz MN (eds): Current Clinical Topics in Infectious Disease, Vol 2. McGraw-Hill, New York, 1981, p 31.
11. Morgan MG, McKenzie H: Controversies in the laboratory diagnosis of community-acquired urinary tract infection. Eur J Clin Microbiol Infect Dis 12:491, 1993.
12. Mcguckin M, Cohen L, McGregor RR: Significance of pyuria in urinary sediment. J Urol 120:452, 1978.
13. Standfeld JM: The measurement and meaning of pyuria. Arch Dis Child 37:257, 1982.
14. Mabeck CE: Studies in urinary tract infections. IV. Urinary leukocyte excretion in bacteriuria. Acta Med Scand 186:193, 1969.
15. Gadeholt H: Quantitative estimation of cells in urine. Acta Med Scand 183:369, 1968.
16. Brumfitt W: Urinary cell counts and their value. J Clin Pathol 18:550, 1965.
17. Stamm WE: Measurement of pyuria and its relation in bacteriuria. Am J Med 75:53, 1983.
18. Kass EH: Asymptomatic infections of the urinary tract. Trans Assoc Am Physicians 69:56, 1956.
19. Kass EH: Bacteriuria and the diagnosis of infections of the urinary tract, with observations on the use of methenamine as a urinary antiseptic. Arch Intern Med 100:709, 1957.
20. Savage WE, Hajj SN, Kass EH: Demographic and prognostic characterizations of bacteriuria in pregnancy. Medicine (Baltimore) 46:385, 1967.
21. Jackson GG, Grieble HG, Knudsen KB: Urinary findings diagnostic of pyelonephritis. JAMA 166:14, 1958.
22. Roberts FJ: Quantitative urine culture in patients with urinary tract infection and bacteriuria. Am J Clin Pathol 85:616, 1986.
23. Little PJ, Paddie BA, Sincock AR: Significance of bacterial and white cell counts in midstream urines. J Clin Pathol 33:58, 1980.
24. Stamm WE, Wagner KF, Amsel R, et al: Causes of the acute urethral syndrome. N Engl J Med 303:409, 1980.
25. Stamm WE, Counts GW, Running KR, et al: Diagnosis of coliform infection in acutely dysuric women. N Engl J Med 307:463, 1982.
26. Kunin CM, White LV, Hua TH: A reassessment of the importance of ''low-count'' bacteriuria in young women with acute urinary symptoms. Ann Intern Med 119:454, 1993.

27. Roberts AP, Robinson RE, Beard RW: Some factors affecting bacterial colony counts in urinary infection. Br Med J 1:400, 1967.
28. Platt R: Quantitative definition of bacteriuria. Am J Med 75:44, 1983.
29. Rubin RH: Infection of the urinary tract. In Rubenstein E, Federman DD (eds): Scientific American Textbook of Medicine, Sect 7. Scientific American, New York, 1994, pp 1–13.
30. Latham RH, Running K, Stamm WE: Urinary tract infections in young women caused by Staphylococcus saprophyticus. JAMA 250:3063, 1983.
31. Pead L, Marshall R, Morris J: Staphylococcus saprophyticus as a urinary pathogen: A six-year perspective survey. Br Med J 291:1157, 1985.
32. Marrie TJ, Kwan C, Noble MA, et al: Staphylococcus saprophyticus as a cause of urinary tract infections. J Clin Microbiol 16:427, 1982.
33. Pollack HM: Laboratory techniques for detection of urinary tract infection and assessment of value. Am J Med 75:79, 1983.
34. Kaufman CA, Hertz CS, Sheaepen JN: Staphylococcus saprophyticus: Role in urinary infections in men. J Urol 130:493, 1983.
35. Maskell R, Pead L, Hollett RJ: Urinary pathogens in the male. Br J Urol 47:691, 1975.
36. Vermeulen CW, Goetz RL: Experimental urolithiasis. VIII. Furadantin in treatment of experimental Proteus infection with stone formation. J Urol 72:99, 1954.
37. Kunin CM: Urinary tract infections in females. Clin Infect Dis 18:1, 1994.
38. Marrie TJ, Swantee CA, Harlen M: Aerobic and anaerobic urethral flora of healthy females in various physiological age groups and of females with urinary tract infections. J Clin Microbiol 11:654, 1980.
39. Bowie WR, Potlock HM, Forsyth PS, et al: Bacteriology of the urethra in normal men and men with nongonococcal urethritis. J Clin Microbiol 6:482, 1977.
40. Finegold SM, Miller LG, Merrill SL, Posnick DJ: Significance of anaerobic and capnophilic bacteria isolated from the urinary tract. In Kass FH (ed): Progress in Pyelonephritis. FA Davis, Philadelphia, 1965.
41. Alling B, Brandberg A, Seeberg S, Svanborg H: Aerobic and anaerobic microbial flora in the urinary tract of geriatric patients during long-term care. J Infect Dis 127:34, 1973.
42. Singer C, Kaplan MH, Armstrong D: Bacteremia and fungemia complicating neoplastic disease. Am J Med 62:731, 1977.
43. Buckley RM. Jr, Mcguckin M, MacGregor RR: Urine bacterial counts after sexual intercourse. N Engl J Med 298:321, 1978.
44. Rubin RH, Weinstein L: Salmonellosis: Microbiologic, Pathologic and Clinical Features. Stratton Intercontinental Medical Book Corp, New York, 1977.
45. Farid Z, Bassily S, Kent DC, et al: Chronic urinary Salmonella carriers with intermittent bacteremia. J Trop Med Hyg 73:153, 1970.
46. Abernathy RS, Price WE, Spink WW: Chronic brucellar pyelonephritis simulating tuberculosis. JAMA 159:1534, 1955.
47. Cruz PT, Clancy CF: Nocardiosis. Nocardial osteomyelitis and septicemia. Am J Pathol 28:607, 1952.
48. Rosenblum PS: Renal actinomycosis: A case report. Urol Cutan Rev 53:329, 1949.
49. Pasternack MS, Rubin RH: Urinary tract tuberculosis. In Schrier RW, Gottschalk CW (eds): Diseases of the Kidney, 5th ed. Little, Brown, Boston, 1993, p 909.
50. Goldberg PK, Kozinn PJ, Wise GJ, et al: Incidence and significance of candiduria. JAMA 241:582, 1979.
51. Ang BSP, Telenti A, King B, et al: Candidemia from a urinary tract source: Microbiological aspects and clinical significance. Clin Infect Dis 17:662, 1993.
52. Scerpella EG, Alhalel R: An unusual cause of acute renal failure: Bilateral ureteral obstruction due to Candida tropicalis fungus balls. Clin Infect Dis 18:440, 1994.
53. Guze LB, Haley LD: Fungus infections of the urinary tract. Yale J Biol Med 30:292, 1958.
54. Guziel LP, Stone WJ, Schaffner W, et al: Case report. Primary renal candidiasis with renal granulomata and salt-losing nephropathy. Am J Med Sci 269:123, 1975.
55. Rubin RH: Infection in the organ transplant patient. In Rubin RH, Young LS (eds): Clinical Approach to Infection in the Compromised Host, 3rd ed. Plenum Publishing, New York, 1994, p 629.
56. Edwards JE. Jr, Lehrer RI, Stiehm ER, et al: Severe candidal infections: Clinical perspective, immune defense mechanisms, and current concepts of therapy. Ann Intern Med 89:91, 1978.
57. Kauffman CA, Tan JS: Torulopsis glabrata renal infection. Am J Med 57:217, 1974.
58. Petersen EA, Friedman BA, Crowder ED, et al: Coccidioidouria: Clinical significance. Ann Intern Med 85:34, 1976.
59. Eickenberg H-U, Amin M, Lich R. Jr: Blastomycosis of the genitourinary tract. J Urol 113:650, 1975.
60. Bissada NK, Finkbeiner AE, Redman JF: Prostatic mycosis; nonsurgical diagnosis and management. Urology 9:427, 1977.
61. Randall RE. Jr, Story WK, Toone EC, et al: Cryptococcal pyelonephritis. N Engl J Med 279:60, 1968.
62. Bowie WR, Wang SP, Alexander ER, et al: Etiology of nongonococcal urethritis. J Clin Invest 59:735, 1977.
63. McCormack WM: Role of the genital mycoplasmas in extragenital disease. In Hobson D, Holmes KK (eds): Nongonococcal Urethritis and Related Infections. American Society for Microbiology, Washington, DC, 1977, p 98.
64. Thosen AC: Occurrence of mycoplasmas in urinary tracts of patients with acute pyelonephritis. J Clin Microbiol 8:84, 1978.
65. Pettersson S, Brorson JE, Grenabo L, Hedelin H: Ureaplasma urealyticum in infectious urinary tract stones. Lancet 1:526, 1983.
66. Nufson MA, Belske RB: A review of adenovirus in the etiology of acute hemorrhagic cystitis. J Urol 115:191, 1976.
67. Rosen S, Harmon W, Krensky AM, et al: Tubulo-interstitial nephritis associated with polyomavirus (BK type) infection. N Engl J Med 308:1192, 1983.
68. Coleman DV, MacKenzie EFD, Gardner SD, et al: Human polyomavirus (BK) infection and ureteric stenosis in renal allograft recipients. J Clin Pathol 31:338, 1978.
69. Hashida Y, Gaffney PC, Yunis EJ: Acute hemorrhagic cystitis of childhood and papovavirus-like particles. J Pediatr 89:85, 1976.
70. Beeson PB: Factors in the pathogenesis of pyelonephritis. Yale J Biol Med 28:81, 1955.
71. Kleeman CR, Hewitt WL, Guze LB: Pyelonephritis. Medicine (Baltimore) 39:3, 1960.
72. Cotran RS: Experimental pyelonephritis. In Rouiller C, Miller AF (eds): The Kidney, Vol II. Academic Press, New York, 1969, pp 269–345.
73. Woods JW: Non-obstructive Escherichia coli pyelonephritis in the rat. Proc Soc Exp Biol Med 104:116, 1960.
74. Gorrill RH, Klyhn LM, McNeil EM: The initiation of infection in the mouse kidney after intravenous injection of bacteria. J Pathol Bacteriol 91:157, 1966.
75. Gorrill RH: The fate of Pseudomonas aeruginosa, Proteus mirabilis and Escherichia coli in the mouse kidney. J Pathol Bacteriol 89:81, 1975.
76. Teplitz C, Raultson GL, Walker HL, et al: Spontaneous hematogenous Pseudomonas pyelonephritis in rats. J Infect Dis 114:75, 1964.
77. Shapiro AP, Kobernick JL: Effects of unilateral nephrectomy and mixed infection on blood pressure of rats with experimental chronic pyelonephritis. Circ Res 7:936, 1959.
78. Braude AI, Shapiro AP, Siemienski J: Hematogenous pyelonephritis in rats. III. Relationship of bacterial species for the pathogenesis of acute pyelonephritis. J Bacteriol 77:270, 1959.
79. Guze LB: Experimental pyelonephritis: Observations on the course of enterococcal infection in the kidney of the rat. In Quinn EL, Kass EH (eds): The Biology of Pyelonephritis. Little, Brown, Boston, 1960, pp 11–26.
80. Guze LB, Goldner BH, Kalmanson GM: Pyelonephritis. I. Observations on the course of chronic nonobstructed enterococcal infection in the kidney of the rat. Yale J Biol Med 33:372, 1961.
81. Freedman LR: Experimental pyelonephritis. VI. Observations on susceptibility of the rabbit kidney to infection by a virulent strain of Staphylococcus aureus. Yale J Biol Med 32:272, 1960.
82. Foster EA: Hemolysin production in the development of staphylococcal lesions. Science 149:1395, 1965.
83. Foster EA: Tissue injury by toxins in experimental staphylococcal infections. Am J Pathol 51:913, 1969.
84. Guze LB, Beeson PB: Experimental pyelonephritis. I. Effect of urethral ligation on the course of bacterial infection in the kidney of the rat. J Exp Med 104:83, 1956.
85. Lepper MH: The production of coliform infection in the urinary tract of rabbits. J Pathol Bacteriol 24:192, 1921.
86. DeNavasquez S: Further studies in experimental pyelonephritis produced by various bacteria, with special reference for renal scarring as a factor in pathogenesis. J Pathol Bacteriol 71:27, 1956.

87. Rocha H, Guze LB, Freedman LR, Beeson PB: Experimental pyelonephritis. III. The influence of localized injury in different parts of the kidney on susceptibility to bacillary infection. Yale J Biol Med 30:341, 1958.
88. Rocha H, Guze LB, Beeson PB: Experimental pyelonephritis. V. Susceptibility of rats for hematogenous pyelonephritis following chemical injury to the kidneys. Yale J Biol Med 32:120, 1959.
89. Brumfitt W, Heptinstall RH: Experimental pyelonephritis: The effects of renal vein constriction on bacterial localization and multiplication in the rat kidney. Br J Exp Pathol 40:145, 1959.
90. Godley JA, Freedman LR: Experimental pyelonephritis. XI. A comparison of temporary occlusion of renal artery and vein on susceptibility of rat kidney for infection. Yale J Biol Med 36:268, 1964.
91. Vivaldi E, Munoz J, Cotran RS, Kass EH: Factors affecting the clearance of bacteria within the urinary tract. *In* Kass EH (ed): Progress in Pyelonephritis. FA Davis, Philadelphia, 1965, pp 531–535.
92. Jones RK, Shapiro AP: Increased susceptibility to pyelonephritis during acute hypertension by angiotensin II and norepinephrine. J Clin Invest 42:179, 1963.
93. Shapiro AP, Kobernick JL: Susceptibility of rats with renal hypertension for pyelonephritis and predisposition of rats with chronic pyelonephritis to hormonal hypertension. Circ Res 9:869, 1961.
94. Woods JW, Welt LG, Hollander WJ: Susceptibility of rats for experimental pyelonephritis during potassium depletion. J Clin Invest 40:599, 1961.
95. Miescher P, Schnyder V, Kresh V: Zur Pathogenese den "interstitiellen Nephritis" bei Abusus phenacetin-hatigen Analgetica. Tierexperimentelle Untersuchungen. Schweiz Med Wschr 88:432, 1958.
96. Braude AI, Shapiro AP, Siemienski J: Hematogenous pyelonephritis in rats. I. Its pathogenesis when produced by a simple new method. J Clin Invest 34:1489, 1955.
97. Kime SW. Jr, McNamara JJ, Lu Se S, et al: Experimental polypeptic renal disease in rats: Electron microscopy, function, and susceptibility to pyelonephritis. J Lab Clin Med 60:64, 1962.
98. Boschell BR, Hunter EO Jr, Warren TL, Lipton CH. Jr: Experimental pyelonephritis in the alloxan diabetic animal. Diabetes 12:56, 1963.
99. Browder AA, Petersdorf RG: Experimental pyelonephritis in rats with alloxan diabetes. Proc Soc Exp Biol Med 115:332, 1961.
100. Cod JA, Davis JH: Altered host response to experimental pyelonephritis in alloxan diabetic rats. J Surg Res 7:1, 1967.
101. Andriole VT, Cohn GL: The effect of diethylstilbestrol on the susceptibility of rats to hematogenous pyelonephritis. J Clin Invest 43:1136, 1964.
102. Freedman LR, Kaminskas R, Beeson PB: Experimental pyelonephritis. VII. Evidence on the mechanisms by which obstruction of urine flow enhances susceptibility to pyelonephritis. Yale J Biol Med 33:65, 1960.
103. Andriole VT, Lytton B: The effect and critical duration of increased tissue pressure on susceptibility to bacterial infection. Br J Exp Pathol 46:308, 1965.
104. Schwartz MM, Venkatachalam MA, Cotran RS: Reversible inner medullary vascular obstruction in acute unilateral hydronephrosis in the rat. Am J Pathol 86:425, 1977.
105. Asscher AW: Urinary tract infection in women. *In* Jones F (ed): Recent Advances in Renal Disease. Churchill Livingstone, Edinburgh, 1975.
106. Kass EH: Pathogenesis of pyelonephritis. *In* Mostofi FK, Smith DE (eds): The Kidney. Williams & Wilkins, Baltimore, 1965, pp 204–212.
107. Heptinstall RH: Pathology of the Kidney, 2nd ed. Little, Brown, Boston, 1974.
108. Vivaldi E, Cotran RS, Zangwill DP, Kass EH: Ascending infection as a mechanism in the pathogenesis of experimental non-obstructive pyelonephritis. Proc Soc Exp Biol Med 102:242, 1959.
109. Sommer JL: Experimental pyelonephritis in the rat with observations on ureteral reflux. J Urol 86:375, 1961.
110. Cox CE, Lacy SS, Hinman F, Jr: The urethra and its relationship to urinary tract infections. II. The urethral flora of the female with recurrent urinary infection. J Urol 99:632, 1968.
111. Stamey TA, Sexton CC: The role of vaginal colonization with Enterobacteriaceae in recurrent urinary infections. J Urol 113:214, 1975.
112. Schaeffer AJ, Stamey TA: Pathogenesis of Enterobacteriaceae isolated from the vaginal vestibule. *In* Kass EH, Brumfitt W (eds):

Infections of the Urinary Tract. University of Chicago Press, Chicago, 1979.
113. Fowler JE, Stamey TA: Studies of introital colonization in women with recurrent urinary infections. VIII. The role of bacterial adherence. J Urol 117:472, 1977.
114. Bollgren I, Winberg J: The periurethral aerobic flora in girls highly susceptible for urinary infections. Acta Pediatr Scand 65:81, 1976.
115. Harding GKM, Buckwold FJ, Marrie TJ, et al: Prophylaxis of recurrent urinary tract infection in female patients: Efficacy of low-dose thrice-weekly therapy with trimethoprim-sulfamethoxazole. JAMA 242:1975, 1979.
116. Ronald AR, Harding GKM: Urinary infection prophylaxis in women. Ann Intern Med 9:268, 1981.
117. Fowler JE, Stamey TA: Studies of introital colonization in women with recurrent urinary infections. VII. The role of bacterial adherence. J Urol 117:472, 1977.
118. Kallenius G, Winberg J: Bacterial adherence to periurethral cells in girls prone to urinary tract infections. Lancet 2:540, 1978.
119. Schaeffer AJ, Jones JM, Dunn JK: Association of in vitro *Escherichia coli* adherence to vaginal and buccal epithelial cells with susceptibility of women to recurrent urinary tract infections. N Engl J Med 304:1062, 1981.
120. Sheinfeld J, Schaeffer AJ, Cordon-Cardo C, et al: Association of the Lewis blood-group phenotype with recurrent urinary tract infections in women. N Engl J Med 320:773, 1989.
121. Stapleton A, Nudelman E, Clausen H, et al: Binding of uropathogenic *Escherichia coli* R45 to glycolipids extracted from vaginal epithelial cells is dependent on histo–blood group secretor status. J Clin Invest 90:965, 1992.
122. Hooton TM, Hillier S, Johnson C, et al: *Escherichia coli* bacteriuria and contraceptive method. JAMA 265:64, 1991.
123. Barnes RC, Daifuku R, Roddy RE, Stamm WE: Urinary tract infection in sexually active homosexual men. Lancet 1:171, 1986.
124. Spach DH, Stapleton AE, Stamm WE: Lack of circumcision increases the risk of urinary tract infection in young men. JAMA 267:679, 1992.
125. Lipsky BA: Urinary tract infections in men: Epidemiology, pathophysiology, diagnosis, and treatment. Ann Intern Med 110:138, 1989.
126. Stamm WE, Hooton TM: Management of urinary tract infections in adults. N Engl J Med 329:1328, 1993.
127. Ulleryd P, Lincoln K, Scheutz F, Sandberg T: Virulence characteristics of *Escherichia coli* in relation to host response in men with symptomatic urinary tract infection. Clin Infect Dis 18:579, 1994.
128. Fair WR, Timothy MM, Churg HD: Antibacterial nature of prostatic fluid. Nature 218:444, 1968.
129. O'Grady FW, Richards B, McSherry MA, et al: Introital enterobacteria, urinary infection, and the urethral syndrome. Lancet 2:1208, 1970.
130. Bran JL, Levinson ME, Kaye D: Entrance of bacteria in the female urinary bladder. N Engl J Med 286:626, 1972.
131. Kunin CM, McCormack RC: An epidemiologic study of bacteriuria and blood pressure among nuns and working women. N Engl J Med 278:635, 1968.
132. Kelsey MC, Mead MG, Gruneberg RN, Oriel JD: Relationship between sexual intercourse and urinary tract infection in women attending a clinic for sexually transmitted diseases. J Med Microbiol 12:511, 1979.
133. Nicolle LE, Harding GKM, Preiksaitis J, Ronald AR: The association of urinary tract infection with sexual intercourse. J Infect Dis 146:579, 1982.
134. Vosti KL: Recurrent urinary tract infections: Prevention by prophylactic antibodies after sexual intercourse. JAMA 231:934, 1975.
135. Kunin CM: Sexual intercourse and urinary infections. N Engl J Med 298:336, 1978.
136. Evans DA, Hennekens CH, Miao L, et al: Oral contraceptive use and bacteriuria in a community-based study. N Engl J Med 299:536, 1978.
137. Cox CE, Hinman F: Experiments with induced bacteriuria, vesical emptying and bacterial growth on the mechanisms of bladder defense to infection. J Urol 86:739, 1961.
138. Hinman FJ, Cox CE: Residual urine volume in normal male subjects. J Urol 97:641, 1967.
139. O'Grady F, Cattell WR: Kinetics of urinary tract infection. II. The bladder. Br J Urol 38:156, 1966.

140. O'Grady F, Pennington JH: Bacterial growth in in vitro system-stimulating conditions in the urinary bladder. Br J Exp Pathol 47:152, 1966.

141. Bodel P, Cotran RS, Kass EH: Cranberry juice and the antibacterial action of hippuric acid. J Lab Clin Med 54:881, 1959.

142. Wilson AT: Urinary lysozyme. I. Identification and management. J Pediatr 36:39, 1950.

143. Burden DW: Immunoglobulins in the urinary tract. Discussion on a possible role of urinary tract infection. In Brumfitt W, Asscher AW (eds): Urinary Tract Infection. Oxford University Press, London, 1973, p 148.

144. Cicmanec JF, Shank RA, Evans T: Overnight concentration of urine: Natural defense mechanism against urinary tract infection. Urology 26:157, 1985.

145. Gargan RA, Hamilton-Miller JMT, Brumfitt W: Effect of alkalinisation and increased fluid intake on bacterial phagocytosis and killing in urine. Eur J Clin Microbiol Infect Dis 12:534, 1993.

146. Norden CW, Green GM, Kass EH: Antibacterial mechanisms of the urinary bladder. J Clin Invest 47:2689, 1968.

147. Hand WL, Smith JW, Sanford JP: The antibacterial effect of normal and infected urinary bladder. J Lab Clin Med 77:605, 1971.

148. Lapides J: Role of hydrostatic pressure and distention in urinary tract infection. In Kass EH (ed): Progress in Pyelonephritis. FA Davis, Philadelphia, 1965, pp 578–580.

149. Fiveash JG, Foster EA, Paquin AJ: Experimental Escherichia coli bacteriuria in the rabbit. In Kass EH (ed): Progress in Pyelonephritis. FA Davis, Philadelphia, 1965, pp 581–590.

150. Mabeck CE: Treatment of uncomplicated urinary tract infection in nonpregnant women. Postgrad Med 48:69, 1972.

151. Hodson CJ, Cotran RS: Vesicoureteral reflux, reflux nephropathy, and chronic pyelonephritis. In Cotran RS (ed): Contemporary Issues in Nephrology, Vol 10, Tubulointerstitial Nephropathies. Churchill Livingstone, New York, 1983, pp 83–120.

152. Kjellberg SR, Ericsson NO, Rudheu U: The Lower Urinary Tract in Childhood. Year Book Medical Publishers, Chicago, 1957.

153. Politano VA: Ureterovesical junction. J Urol 107:239, 1972.

154. Jones BW, Hestem DW: Vesicoureteric reflux in children. J Urol 81:114, 1968.

155. Bailey R: Vesicoureteral reflux in healthy infants and children. In Hodson CJ, Kincaid-Smith P (eds): Reflux Nephropathy. Masson Publishing USA, New York, 1979, p 59.

156. Peters JP, Johnson DE, Jackson JP: The incidence of vesicoureteral reflux in the premature child. J Urol 97:259, 1967.

157. Levitt SB, Sandler HJ: Absence of vesicoureteral reflux in the neonate with myelodysplasia. J Urol 114:118, 1975.

158. Lich R, Homerton LW, Goode LS, Davis LA: The ureterovesical junction of the newborn. J Urol 92:436, 1964.

159. Booth EJ, Bell TE, McLaine C, Evans APT: Fetal vesicoureteric reflux. J Urol 113:258, 1975.

160. Castro JE, Fine H: Passive antireflux mechanisms in the human and cadaver. Br J Urol 41:559, 1969.

161. Retik AB: Vesicoureteral reflux. In Edelmann CM Jr (ed): Pediatric Kidney Disease. Little, Brown, Boston, 1978.

162. Stephens FD: Cytoscopic appearance of the ureteric orifices associated with reflux nephropathy. In Hodson CJ, Kincaid-Smith P (eds): Reflux Nephropathy. Masson Publishing USA, New York, 1979, p 119.

163. Risdon RA: Reflux nephropathy. Diagn Histopathol 4:61, 1981.

164. Baker R, Maxted W, Maybath J, Shuman I: Relation of age, sex, and infection to reflux. Data indicating high spontaneous cure in the pediatric population. J Urol 95:271, 1966.

165. Koff SA, Lapides J, Piazza DH: Association of urinary tract infection and reflux with uninhibited bladder contractions and voluntary sphincteric obstruction. J Urol 122:373, 1979.

166. van Gool JD, Kuitjen RH, Donckerwolcke RA, et al: Bladder-sphincter dysfunction, urinary infection and vesico-ureteral reflux with special reference to cognitive bladder training. Contrib Nephrol 39:190, 1984.

167. Koff SA, Muttagh D: The uninhibited bladder in children: Effect of treatment on vesicoureteral reflux resolution. Contrib Nephrol 39:211, 1984.

168. Noe HN: The role of dysfunctional voiding in failure or complication of ureteral implantation for primary reflux. J Urol 134:1172, 1985.

169. Griffiths JD, Scholtmeiger RJ: Vesicoureteral reflux and lower urinary tract dysfunction: Evidence for 2 different reflux/dysfunction complexes. J Urol 137:240, 1987.

170. Fowler R: The many faces of vesicoureteral reflux. Factors contributing to renal damage. Aust N Z J Surg 54:417, 1984.

171. Parkhouse HF, Barratt TM, Dillon MJ, et al: Long-term outcome of boys with posterior urethral valves. Br J Urol 62:59, 1988.

172. Lebowitz RL, Blickman JG: The coexistence of ureteropelvic function, obstruction and reflux. Am J Radiol 140:231, 1983.

173. Dejter SW Jr, Gibbons MD: The fate of infant kidneys with fetal hydronephrosis but initially normal postnatal sonography. J Urol 142:661, 1989.

174. Elder JS: Commentary: Importance of antenatal diagnosis of vesicoureteral reflux. J Urol 148:1750, 1992.

175. Ring E, Petritsch P, Riccabona M, et al: Primary vesicoureteral reflux in infants with a dilated fetal urinary tract. Eur J Pediatr 152:523, 1993.

176. Zerin JM, Ritchey ML, Chang AC: Incidental vesicoureteral reflux in neonates with antenatally detected hydronephrosis and other renal abnormalities. Radiology 187:157, 1993.

177. Kenda RB, Kenig T, Budihna N: Detecting vesico-ureteral reflux in asymptomatic siblings of children with reflux by direct radionuclide cystography. Eur J Pediatr 150:735, 1991.

178. Noe HN, Wyatt RJ, Peeden JN Jr, Rivas ML: The transmission of vesicoureteral reflux from parent to child. J Urol 148:1869, 1992.

179. Buonomo C, Treves ST, Jones B, et al: Silent renal damage in symptom-free siblings of children with vesicoureteral reflux: Assessment with technetium Tc 99m dimercaptosuccinic acid scintigraphy. J Pediatr 122:721, 1993.

180. Chapman CJ, Bailey RR, Janus ED: Vesicoureteral reflux: Segregation analysis. Am J Med Genet 20:577, 1985.

181. Roberts JA: The monkey as a model of urinary tract infection and reflux nephropathy in man. In Davison AM (ed): Nephrology, Vol II. WB Saunders, Philadelphia, 1988, pp 844–853.

182. King LR, Levitt SB: Vesicoureteral reflux. In Walsh PC, Perlmutter AD, Gittes RF, Stamey TA (eds): Campbell's Urology, 5th ed. WB Saunders, Philadelphia, 1986.

183. Friedland GW: The voiding cystourethrogram: An unreliable examination. In Hodson CJ, Kincaid-Smith P (eds): Reflux Nephropathy. Masson Publishing USA, New York, 1979, p 91.

184. International Reflux Study Committee: Medical versus surgical treatment of primary vesicoureteral reflux. Prospective International Reflux Study in Children. J Urol 125:277, 1981.

185. Rolleston GL, Shannon FT, Utley WL: Follow-up of vesicoureteral reflux in the newborn. Kidney Int 8:S59, 1975.

186. Chapman SG, Chantler G, Haycock GB, et al: Radionuclide cystography in vesicoureteric reflux. Arch Dis Child 63:650, 1988.

187. Hodson CJ, Edwards D: Chronic pyelonephritis and vesicoureteral reflux. Clin Radiol 2:19, 1960.

188. Hodson CJ: Reflux Nephropathy. Med Clin North Am 62:1201, 1978.

189. Bailey RR: An overview of reflux nephropathy. In Hodson CJ, Kincaid-Smith P (eds): Reflux Nephropathy. Masson Publishing USA, New York, 1979, p 3.

190. Lerner GR, Fleischman LE, Perlmutter AD: Reflux nephropathy. Pediatr Clin North Am 34:747, 1987.

191. Williams DI: Vesicoureteral reflux. In Williams DI (ed): Urology in Childhood. Springer-Verlag, Basel, 1974.

192. Smellie JM, Normand ICS: Bacteriuria, reflux and renal scarring. Arch Dis Child 50:581, 1975.

193. Smellie JM, Normand ICS: Reflux nephropathy in childhood. In Hodson CJ, Kincaid-Smith P (eds): Reflux Nephropathy. Masson Publishing USA, New York, 1978, p 14.

194. Smellie JM, Hodson CJ, Edwards D, Normand ICS: Clinical and urological features of urinary infection in childhood. Br Med J 2:1222, 1964.

195. Savage DCL, Wilson MI, McHardy ML, et al: Covert bacteriuria of childhood. Arch Dis Child 48:8, 1973.

196. Asscher AW, McLachlan MSF, Jones RV, et al: Screening for asymptomatic urinary tract infection in schoolgirls. Lancet 2:1, 1973.

197. Newcastle Asymptomatic Bacteriuria Group: Asymptomatic bacteriuria in schoolchildren in Newcastle-upon-Tyne. Arch Dis Child 50:902, 1975.

198. Lindberg U, Claesson I, Hanson LA, Jodal U: Asymptomatic bacteriuria in school girls. Acta Pediatr Scand 64:425, 1975.

199. Edwards B, White RHR, Maxted H, et al: Screening methods for covert bacteriuria in school girls. Br Med J 1:463, 1975.

200. Smellie JM, Normand ICS: Experience of follow-up of children with

urinary tract infections. *In* O'Grady F, Brumfitt W (eds): Urinary Tract Infection. Oxford University Press, London, 1968.

201. Wein J, Schoenberg HW: A review of 402 girls with recurrent urinary tract infection. J Urol 107:329, 1972.

202. Winberg J, Andersen HJ, Bergstrom TB, et al: Epidemiology of symptomatic urinary tract infection in childhood. Acta Pediatr Scand Suppl 252:1, 1974.

203. Shannon FT: Urinary tract infection in infancy. N Z Med J 75:282, 1972.

204. Drew JH, Acton CM: Radiological findings in newborn infants with urinary infection. Arch Dis Child 51:628, 1976.

205. Penn IA, Briedahl PD: Ureteric reflux and renal damage. Aust N Z J Surg 37:163, 1967.

206. Bergstrom T, Larson H, Lincoln K, Winberg J: Studies of urinary tract infection in infancy and childhood. 1280 patients with neonatal infection. J Pediatr 80:858, 1972.

207. Rolleston GL, Maling TMJ, Hodson CJ: Intrarenal reflux and the scarred kidney. Arch Dis Child 49:531, 1974.

208. Filly R, Friedland GW, Govan DE, Fair WR: Development and progression of clubbing and scarring in children with recurrent urinary tract infection. Radiology 113:145, 1974.

209. Lenaghan D, Whitaker JG, Hensen F, Stephens FD: The natural history of reflux and long-term effects of reflux on the kidney. J Urol 115:728, 1976.

210. Shah KJ, Robins DG, White RHR: Renal scarring and vesico-ureteric reflux. Arch Dis Child 53:210, 1978.

211. Kincaid-Smith P, Becker GJ: Reflux nephropathy in the adult. *In* Hodson CJ, Kincaid-Smith P (eds): Reflux Nephropathy. Masson Publishing USA, New York, 1979, p 21.

212. Zuchelli P, Gaggi R: Vesicoureteral reflux and reflux nephropathy in adults. Contrib Nephrol 61:220, 1987.

213. Hodson CJ, Maling RM, McManamon PJ, Lewis MJ: The pathogenesis of reflux nephropathy (chronic atrophic pyelonephritis). Br J Radiol Suppl 13:1, 1975.

214. Ransley PG, Risdon RA: The pathogenesis of reflux nephropathy. Br J Radiol Suppl 14:1, 1978.

215. Brodeur AE, Goyer RA, Melick W: A potential hazard of barium cystography. Radiology 85:1080, 1965.

216. Amat AD: Calicotubular backflow with vesico-ureteral reflux. JAMA 213:293, 1970.

217. Rolleston GL, Shannon FT, Utley WLF: Relationship of infantile vesico-ureteric reflux to renal damage. Br Med J 1:460, 1970.

218. Bourne HH, Condon NR, Hoyt TS, Nixon GW: Intrarenal reflux and renal damage. J Urol 110:255, 1976.

219. Rose JS, Glassberg KI, Waterhouse K: Intrarenal reflux and its relationship to renal scarring. J Urol 113:400, 1975.

220. Ransley PF: Intrarenal reflux: Anatomical, dynamic and radiological studies—part I. Urol Res 5:61, 1977.

221. Maling RMJ, Rolleston GL: Intrarenal reflux in children demonstrated by micturating angiography. Clin Radiol 25:81, 1974.

222. Ransley PG, Risdon RA: Renal papillary morphology in infants and young children. Urol Res 3:111, 1977.

223. Ransley PG, Risdon RA: The pathogenesis of reflux nephropathy. Contrib Nephrol 16:90, 1979.

224. Ransley PG, Risdon RA: The renal papilla, intrarenal reflux, and chronic pyelonephritis. *In* Hodson CJ, Kincaid-Smith P (eds): Reflux Nephropathy. Masson Publishing USA, New York, 1979, p 126.

225. Tamminen TE, Kaprio EA: The relation of the shape of the renal papilla and of collecting duct openings to intrarenal reflux. Br J Urol 49:345, 1977.

226. Bailey RR: Long-term follow-up of infants with gross vesicoureteric reflux. Contrib Nephrol 39:146, 1984.

227. Ransley PG, Risdon RA, Godley ML: High-pressure sterile vesico-ureteral reflux and renal scarring: An experimental study in the pig and minipig. Contrib Nephrol 39:320, 1984.

228. Heptinstall RH, Hodson CJ: Pathology of sterile reflux in the pig. Contrib Nephrol 39:344, 1984.

229. Jorgensen TM, Olsen S, Djurhuus JC, Norgaard JP: Renal morphology in experimental vesicoureteric reflux in pigs. Scand J Urol Nephrol 18:49, 1984.

230. Hutch JA, Smith DR: Sterile reflux. Report of 24 cases. Urol Int 24:460, 1969.

231. Stephens FD: Urologic aspects of recurrent urinary tract infection in children. J Pediatr 80:725, 1972.

232. Bakshandeh K, Lynne C, Carrion H: Vesicoureteral reflux and end-stage renal disease. J Urol 116:557, 1976.

233. Bailey RR: Sterile reflux—is it harmless? *In* Hodson CJ, Kincaid-Smith P (eds): Reflux Nephropathy. Masson Publishing USA, New York, 1979, p 334.

234. Stickler BG, Kelalis PP, Burke EC, Segar WE: Primary interstitial nephritis with reflux: A cause of hypertension. Am J Dis Child 122:144, 1971.

235. Salvatierra O Jr, Tanagho EA: Reflux as a cause of end-stage kidney disease: Report of 32 cases. J Urol 117:441, 1977.

236. (VUR + IRR) + UTI = CPN. Lancet 2:301, 1978. Editorial.

237. Smellie JM, Edwards D, Normand ICS, Prescod N: Effect of VUR on renal growth in children with urinary tract infection. Arch Dis Child 56:593, 1981.

238. Smellie JM, Normand ICM, Katz G: Children with urinary infection: A comparison of those with and without VUR. Kidney Int 20:717, 1981.

239. Holland NH, Jackson EC, Kazee M, et al: Relation of urinary tract infection and vesicoureteral reflux to scars: Follow-up of thirty eight patients. J Pediatr 116:S65, 1990.

240. Mosconi CEV, Ianhez LE, Borrelli M, et al: Vesicoureteral reflux in patients in end-stage chronic renal failure. Urol Int 4:357, 1975.

241. Mosconi CEV, Ianhez LE, Borrelli M, Campos Friere JG: Bladder dysfunction in uremic patients. Acta Urol Belg 42:418, 1974.

242. Bishop MC, Moss SW, Oliver O, et al: The significance of vesico-ureteral reflux in non-pyelonephritic patients supported by long-term hemodialysis. Clin Nephrol 8:354, 1977.

243. Huland H, Buchard P, Kollerman M, Augustin I: Vesicoureteral reflux in end-stage renal disease. J Urol 121:10, 1979.

244. McCrae CV, Shannon FT, Utley WLF: Effect on renal growth or reimplantation of refluxing ureters. Lancet 1:1310, 1974.

245. Willscher MK, Bauer SB, Zammuto PJ, Retik AB: Renal growth and urinary infection following anti-reflux surgery in infants and children. J Urol 115:722, 1976.

246. Ransley PG, Risdon RA, Godley ML: Effects of vesicoureteric reflux on renal growth and function. Br J Urol 60:193, 1987.

247. Mabeck CE, Orskov R, Orskov I: *Escherichia coli* serotypes and renal involvement. Lancet 1:1312, 1971.

248. Cougant DA, Levin BR, Lidin-Javson G, et al: Genetic diversity and relationship among strains of *Escherichia coli* in the intestine and these causing urinary tract infections. Prog Allergy 33:203, 1983.

249. Schoolnik GK, O'Hanley P, Lark D, et al: Uropathogenic *Escherichia coli:* Molecular mechanisms of adherence. Adv Exp Med Biol 224:53, 1987.

250. Svanborg-Eden C, Hausson S, Jodal Y, et al: Host-parasite interaction in the urinary tract. J Infect Dis 157:421, 1988.

251. Liden-Jenson F, Hanson LA, Kaijsen B, et al: Comparison of *Escherichia coli* from bacteriuric patients with those from feces of healthy school children. J Infect Dis 136:346, 1977.

252. Svanborg-Eden C, de Man P: Bacterial virulence in urinary tract infection. Infect Dis Clin North Am 1:731, 1987.

253. Hanson LA: Host-parasite relationships in urinary tract infections. J Infect Dis 127:726, 1973.

254. Olling S, Hanson LA, Holmgren J, et al: The bactericidal effect of normal human serum on E. coli strains from normals and from patients with urinary tract infection. Infection 1:24, 1973.

255. Kaijser B, Hanson LA, Jodal U, et al: Frequency of E. coli K antigens in urinary tract infections in children. Lancet 1:663, 1977.

256. Achtman M, Mercer A, Kusecek B, et al: Six widespread bacterial clones among *Escherichia coli* K1 isolates. Infect Immun 39:315, 1983.

257. Sandberg T, Stenquist K, Svanborg-Eden C, et al: Host-parasite relationship in urinary tract infections during pregnancy. Prog Allergy 33:228, 1983.

258. Vosti KL, Goldberg LN, Monto AS, Pantz LA: Host-parasite interactions in patients with infections due to *Escherichia coli*. I. The serogrouping of E. coli from intestinal and extraintestinal sources. J Clin Invest 43:2377, 1964.

259. Van den Bosch JF, Postima P, Koopman PAR, et al: Virulence of urinary and fecal *Escherichia coli* in relation to serotype, haemolysis and hemagglutination. J Hyg 88:567, 1982.

260. Guze LB, Montgomerie JZ, Potter CS, Kalmanson GM: Pyelonephritis. XVI. Correlates of parasite virulence in acute ascending *Escherichia coli* pyelonephritis in mice undergoing diuresis. Yale J Biol Med 46:203, 1973.

261. Howard CJ, Glynn AA: The virulence for mice of strains of *Escherichia coli* related to the effects of K antigens on their resistance for phagocytosis and killing by complement. Immunology 20:767, 1971.

262. Svanborg-Eden C, Hagberg L, Hull R, et al: Bacterial virulence versus host resistance in the urinary tracts of mice. Infect Immun 55:1224, 1987.

263. Kaijser B, Vatilne G: *Escherichia coli* K antigen. Bakt Hyg 243:271, 1979.

264. Hanson LA, Fasth A, Jodal Y, et al: Biology and pathology of urinary tract infections. J Clin Pathol 34:695, 1981.

265. Lindberg U, Hanson LA, Lidin-Janson G, et al: Studies of *Escherichia coli* shown in asymptomatic bacteriuria of school girls. *In* Kass EH, Brumfitt W (eds): Infections of the Urinary Tract. University of Chicago Press, Chicago, 1978, p 44.

266. Lidin-Janson G, Lindberg U: Asymptomatic bacteriuria in school girls. VI. The correlations between urinary and fecal *Escherichia coli*. Relations to the duration of the bacteriuria and the sampling technique. Acta Paediatr Scand 66:349, 1977.

267. Bjorksten B, Knigsen B: Interaction of human serum and neutrophils with *Escherichia coli* chains: Differences between strains isolated from urine of patients with pyelonephritis or asymptomatic bacteriuria. Infect Immun 22:308, 1978.

268. Svanborg-Eden C, Eriksson B, Hanson LA, et al: Adhesion to normal human non-epithelial cells of *Escherichia coli* from children with various forms of urinary tract infections. J Pediatr 93:398, 1978.

269. Hanson LA, Phlstedt S, Fasth A, et al: Antigens of *Escherichia coli*, human immune response, and the pathogenesis of urinary tract infections. J Infect Dis Suppl 136:5144, 1977.

270. Stendahl O, Normann B, Edebo L: Influence of O and K antigens on the surface properties of *Escherichia coli* in relation to phagocytosis. Acta Pathol Microbiol Scand B 87:85, 1977.

271. Ohmann L, Normann B, Stendahl O: Physicochemical surface properties of *Escherichia coli* strains isolated from different types of urinary tract infections. Infect Immun 32:951, 1981.

272. Jacobson SH, Tullus K, Brauncr A: Hydrophobic properties of *Escherichia coli* causing acute pyelonephritis. J Infect 19:17, 1989.

273. Brauner A, Katouli M, Tullus K, Jacobson SH: Cell surface hydrophobicity, adherence to HeLa cell cultures and haemagglutination pattern of pyelonephritogenic *Escherichia coli* strains. Epidemiol Infect 105:255, 1990.

274. Leffler H, Svanborg-Eden C, Schoolnick G, Wastrom T: Glycosphingolipids as receptors for bacterial adhesion, host glycolipid diversity. *In* Boedekke ED (ed): Adherence of Organisms in the Gut Mucosa, Vol 2. CRC Press, Boca Raton, FL, 1984, p 177.

275. Svanborg-Eden C, Hanson LA, Jodal U, et al: Variable adherence to normal human urinary tract epithelial cells of *Escherichia coli* strains associated with various forms of urinary tract infection. Lancet 2:490, 1976.

276. Svanborg-Eden C, Hanson HA: *E. coli* pili as mediators of attachment for human urinary tract epithelial cells. Infect Immun 21:229, 1978.

277. Svanborg-Eden C, Gotschlich EC, Korhonen TK, et al: Aspects of structure and function of pili on *Escherichia coli*. Prog Allergy 33:189, 1983.

278. Orskov I, Orskov F, Birch-Anderasen A: A fimbria *E. coli* antigen, F7, determining uroepithelial adherence. Comparison with type I fimbriae which attach to urinary slime. Infect Immun 27:657, 1980.

279. Hagberg L, Jodal U, Karhonen TK, et al: Adhesion, hemagglutination and virulence of *E. coli* causing urinary tract infections. Infect Immun 31:564, 1981.

280. Dyguid JP, Old DC: Adhesive properties of Enterobacteriaceae. *In* Brachay EH (ed): Bacterial Adherence. Chapman & Hall, London, 1988, p 187.

281. Orskov O, Ferencz A, Orskov F: Tamm-Horsfall protein or uromucoid is the normal urinary slime that binds type I fimbriated *E. coli*. Lancet 1:887, 1980.

282. Bar-Shavit Z, Ofek I, Goldman R, et al: Mannose residues on phagocytes as receptors for the attachment of *Escherichia coli* and *Salmonella typhi*. Biochem Biophys Res Commun 78:455, 1977.

283. Svanborg C, de Man P, Sandberg T: Renal involvement in urinary tract infection. Kidney Int 39:541, 1991.

284. Topley N, Steadman R, Mackenzie R, et al: Type 1 fimbriate strains of *Escherichia coli* initiate renal parenchymal scarring. Kidney Int 36:609, 1989.

285. Mundi H, Bjorkseten B, Svanborg C, et al: Extracellular release of reactive oxygen species from human neutrophils upon interaction with *Escherichia coli* strains causing renal scarring. Infect Immun 59:4168, 1991.

286. Kallenius G, Mollby R: Adhesion of *Escherichia coli* attaching to human urinary tract epithelial cells correlated to mannose-resistant agglutination of human erythrocytes. FEMS Microbiol Lett 5:295, 1979.

287. Leffler H, Svanborg-Eden C: Chemical definition of a glycosphingolipid receptor for *Escherichia coli* attaching to human urinary tract epithelial cells and agglutinating erythrocytes. FEMS Microbiol Lett 8:127, 1980.

288. Svanborg-Eden C, Hagberg L, Hanson LA, et al: Bacterial adherence: A pathogenetic mechanism in urinary tract infections caused by *Escherichia coli* Prog Allergy 33:175, 1983.

289. Lindberg FP, Lund B, Normark S: Genes of pyelonephritogenic *E. coli* required for digalactoside-specific agglutination of human cells. EMBO J 3:1167, 1984.

290. Nou X, Skinner B, Braaten B, et al: Regulation of pyelonephritis-associated pili phase-variation in *Escherichia coli*: Binding of the PapI and the Lrp regulatory proteins is controlled by DNA methylation. Mol Microbiol 7:545, 1993.

291. Denich K, Blyn LB, Craiu A, et al: DNA sequences of three papA genes from uropathogenic *Escherichia coli* strains: Evidence of structural and serological conservation. Infect Immun 59:3849, 1991.

292. Plos K, Carter T, Hull S, et al: Frequency and organization of pap homologous DNA in relation to clinical origin of uropathogenic *Escherichia coli*. J Infect Dis 161:518, 1990.

293. Johanson IM, Plos K, Marklund BI, Svanborg C: Pap, papG and prsG DNA sequences in *Escherichia coli* from the fecal flora and the urinary tract. Microb Pathog 15:121, 1993.

294. Pecha B, Low D, O'Hanley P: Gal-Gal pili vaccines prevent pyelonephritis by piliated *Escherichia coli* in a murine model. Single component Gal-Gal pili vaccines prevent pyelonephritis by homologous and heterologous piliated *E. coli* strains. J Clin Invest 83:2101, 1989.

295. Roberts JA, Kaack MB, Baskin G, et al: P-fimbriae vaccines. II. Cross reactive protection against pyelonephritis. Pediatr Nephrol 3:391, 1989.

296. Svanborg-Eden C, Bjursten LM, Hull R, et al: Influence of adhesion in the interaction of *Escherichia coli* with human phagocytes. Infect Immun 44:407, 1984.

297. Johnson JR, Roberts PL, Stamm WE: P fimbriae and other virulence factors in *Escherichia coli* urosepsis: Association with patients' characteristics. J Infect Dis 156:225, 1987.

298. Otto G, Sandberg T, Marklund BI, et al: Virulence factors and pap genotype in *Escherichia coli* isolates from women with acute pyelonephritis, with or without bacteremia. Clin Infect Dis 17:448, 1993.

299. Winberg J: P-fimbriae, bacterial adhesion and pyelonephritis. Arch Dis Child 59:180, 1984.

300. Tomisawa S, Kogure T, Kuroume T, et al: P blood group and proneness to urinary tract infection in Japanese children. Scand J Infect Dis 21:403, 1989.

301. Lomberg H, Eden CS: Influence of P blood group phenotype on susceptibility to urinary tract infection. FEMS Microbiol Immunol 1:363, 1989.

302. Korhonen TK, Vaisanen-Rhen V, Rhen M, et al: *Escherichia coli* fimbriae recognize sialyl galactosides. J Bacteriol 159:762, 1984.

303. Vaisanen-Rhen V, Korhonen T, Jokinen M, et al: Blood group M specific haemagglutination in pyelonephritogenic *Escherichia coli*. Lancet 1:1192, 1982.

304. Labigne-Roussel A, Falkow S: Distribution and degree of heterogeneity of the afimbrial adhesion encoding operon (afa) among uropathogenic *Escherichia coli* isolates. Infect Immun 56:640, 1988.

305. Le Bouguenec C, Garcia MI, Ouin V, et al: Characterization of plasmid-borne afa-3 gene clusters encoding afimbrial adhesins expressed by *Escherichia coli* strains associated with intestinal or urinary tract infections. Infect Immun 61:5106, 1993.

306. Connell H, de Man P, Jodal U, et al: Lack of association between hemolysin production and acute inflammation in human urinary tract infection. Microb Pathog 14:463, 1993.

307. Arthur M, Johnson CE, Rubin RH, et al: Molecular epidemiology of adhesin and hemolysin virulence factors among uropathogenic *Escherichia coli*. Infect Immun 57:303, 1989.

308. Mobley HL, Green DM, Trifillis AL, et al: Pyelonephritogenic *Escherichia coli* and killing of cultured human renal proximal tubular epithelial cells: Role of hemolysin in some strains. Infect Immun 58:1281, 1990.

309. O'Hanley P, Lalonde G, Ji G: Alpha hemolysin contributes to the

pathogenicity of piliated digalactoside-binding *Escherichia coli* in the kidney: Efficacy of an alpha hemolysin vaccine in preventing renal injury in the BALB/c mouse model of pyelonephritis. Infect Immun 59:1153, 1991.

310. Orskov I, Williams PH, Svanborg-Eden C, Orskov F: Assessment of biological and colony hybridization assays for detection of the aerobactin system in *Escherichia coli* from urinary tract infections. Med Microbiol Immunol 178:143, 1989.

311. O'Hanley P, Low D, Romero I, et al: Gal-Gal binding and hemolysin phenotypes and genotype associated with uropathogenic *E. coli*. N Engl J Med 313:414, 1985.

312. Hedges S, Stenqvist K, Lidin-Janson G, et al: Comparison of urine and serum concentrations of interleukin-6 in women with acute pyelonephritis or asymptomatic bacteriuria. J Infect Dis 166:653, 1992.

313. de Man P, Jodal U, Svanborg C: Dependence among host response parameters used to diagnose urinary tract infection. J Infect Dis 163:331, 1991.

314. Rugo HS, O'Hanley P, Bishop AG, et al: Local cytokine production in a murine model of *Escherichia coli* pyelonephritis. J Clin Invest 89:1032, 1992.

315. Lomberg H, Jodal U, Leffler H, et al: Blood group non-secretors have an increased inflammatory response to urinary tract infection. Scand J Infect Dis 24:77, 1992.

316. Marild S, Jodal U, Orskov I, et al: Special virulence of the *Escherichia coli* O1:K1:H7 clone in acute pyelonephritis. J Pediatr 115:40, 1989.

317. Lomberg H, de Man P, Svanborg-Eden C: Bacterial and host determinants of renal scarring. APMIS 97:193, 1989.

318. de Man P, Jodal U, van Kooten C, Svanborg C: Bacterial adherence as a virulence factor in urinary tract infection. APMIS 98:1053, 1990.

319. Plos K, Lomberg H, Hull S, et al: *Escherichia coli* in patients with renal scarring: Genotype and phenotype of Galα1→4Galβ, Forssman- and mannose-specific adhesins. Pediatr Infect Dis J 10:15, 1991.

320. de Man P, Claeson I, Hohanson IM, et al: Bacterial attachment as a predictor of renal abnormalities in boys with urinary tract infection. J Pediatr 115:915, 1989.

321. Lomberg H, Hellstrom M, Jodal U, Svanborg-Eden C: Secretor state and renal scarring in girls with recurrent pyelonephritis. FEMS Microbiol Immunol 1:371, 1989.

322. Jacobson SH, Lomberg H: Overrepresentation of blood group non-secretors in adults with renal scarring. Scand J Urol Nephrol 24:145, 1990.

323. Kurnick JT, McCluskey RT, Bhan AK, et al: *E. coli*–specific T-lymphocytes in experimental pyelonephritis. J Immunol 141:3220, 1988.

324. Wilz SW, Kurnick JT, Pandolfi F, et al: T lymphocyte responses to antigens of gram negative bacteria in pyelonephritis. Clin Immunol Immunopathol 69:36, 1993.

325. Bahrani FK, Johnson DE, Robbins D, Mobley HL: *Proteus mirabilis* flagella and MR/P fimbriae: Isolation, purification, N-terminal analysis, and serum antibody response following experimental urinary tract infection. Infect Immun 59:3574, 1991.

326. Bahrani FK, Mobley HL: *Proteus mirabilis* MR/P fimbriae: Molecular cloning, expression, and nucleotide sequence of the major fimbrial subunit gene. J Bacteriol 175:457, 1993.

327. Massad G, Lockatell CV, Johnson DE, Mobley HL: *Proteus mirabilis* fimbriae: Construction of an isogenic pmfA mutant and analysis of virulence in a CBA mouse model of ascending urinary tract infection. Infect Immun 62:536, 1994.

328. Moayeri N, Collins CM, O'Hanley P: Efficacy of a *Proteus mirabilis* outer membrane protein vaccine in preventing experimental *Proteus* pyelonephritis in a BALB/c mouse model. Infect Immun 59:3778, 1991.

329. Johnson DE, Russell RG, Lockatell CV, et al: Contribution of *Proteus mirabilis* urease to persistence, urolithiasis, and acute pyelonephritis in a mouse model of ascending urinary tract infection. Infect Immun 61:2748, 1993.

330. Mobley HL, Chippendale GR: Hemagglutinin, urease, and hemolysin production by *Proteus mirabilis* from clinical sources. J Infect Dis 161:525, 1990.

331. Mobley HL, Chippendale GR, Swihart KG, Welch RA: Cytotoxicity of the HpmA hemolysin and urease of *Proteus mirabilis* and *Proteus vulgaris* against cultured human renal proximal tubular epithelial cells. Infect Immun 59:2036, 1991.

332. Senior BW, Loomes LM, Kerr MA: The production and activity in vivo of *Proteus mirabilis* IgA protease in infections of the urinary tract. J Med Microbiol 35:203, 1991.

333. Podschun R, Sievers D, Fischer A, Ullmann U: Serotypes, hemagglutinins, siderophore synthesis, and serum resistance of *Klebsiella* isolates causing human urinary tract infections. J Infect Dis 168:1415, 1993.

334. Guzman CA, Pruzzo C, LiPira G, Calegari L: Role of adherence in pathogenesis of *Enterococcus faecalis* urinary tract infection and endocarditis. Infect Immun 57:1834, 1989.

335. Johnson DE, Russell RG, Lockatell CV, et al: Urethral obstruction of 6 hours or less causes bacteriuria, bacteremia, and pyelonephritis in mice challenged with "nonuropathogenic" *Escherichia coli*. Infect Immun 61:3422, 1993.

336. Platt R, Polk BF, Murdock B, et al: Risk factors for nosocomial urinary tract infection. Am J Epidemiol 124:977, 1986.

337. Garibaldi RA, Mooney BR, Epstein BJ, et al: An evaluation of daily bacteriologic monitoring to identify preventable episodes of catheter-associated urinary tract infection. Infect Control 3:466, 1982.

338. Ooi BS, Chen B, Yu M: Prevalence and site of bacteriuria in diabetes mellitus. Postgrad Med J 50:497, 1974.

339. Young KR, Clancy CF: Urinary tract infections complicating diabetes mellitus. Med Clin North Am 39:1665, 1955.

340. Baldimos MC: Diabetic nephropathy. *In* Marble A, White P, Bradley RF, Kroll LP (eds): Joslin's Diabetes Mellitus, 11th ed. Lea & Febiger, Philadelphia, 1971.

341. O'Sullivan DJ, Fitzgerald MG, Meynell MJ, Malins JM: Urinary tract infection: A comparative study in the diabetic and general populations. Br Med J 1:786, 1961.

342. Pometta D, Rees SB, Younger D, Kass EH: Asymptomatic bacteriuria in diabetes mellitus. N Engl J Med 276:1118, 1967.

343. Gorrill RH: The effect of obstruction of the ureter on the renal localization of bacteria. J Pathol Bacteriol 72:59, 1956.

344. Rocha H, Fekety FR Jr: Delayed granulocyte mobilization in the renal medulla. *In* Kass EH (ed): Progress in Pyelonephritis. FA Davis, Philadelphia, 1964, p 211.

345. Freedman LR, Beeson PB: Experimental pyelonephritis. IV. Observations on infections resulting from direct inoculation of bacteria in different zones of the kidney. Yale J Biol Med 30:406, 1958.

346. Cotran RS, Vivaldi E, Zangwill DP, Kass EH: Retrograde *Proteus* pyelonephritis in rats. Bacteriologic, pathologic, and fluorescent antibody studies. Am J Pathol 43:1, 1963.

347. Sanford JP, Hunter BW, Donaldson P: Localization and fate of *Escherichia coli* in hematogenous pyelonephritis. J Exp Med 116:285, 1962.

348. Beeson PB, Rowley D: The anticomplementary effect of renal tissue. Its association with ammonia formation. J Exp Med 110:685, 1959.

349. Rocha H, Fekety FR: Acute inflammation in the renal cortex and medulla following thermal injury. J Exp Med 119:131, 1964.

350. Andriole VT: Acceleration of the inflammatory response of the renal medulla by water diuresis. J Clin Invest 45:847, 1966.

351. Hubert EG, Montgomerie JZ, Kalmanson GM, Guze LB: Effect of renal physicochemical milieu on serum bactericidal activity. Am J Med Sci 253:225, 1967.

352. Takahashi K, Matsumoto T, Ogata N, et al: Direct inactivation of human polymorphonuclear leukocytes by hyperosmotic urea comparable to the renal medulla. J Urol 149:386, 1993.

353. Mayrer AR, Miniter P, Andriole VT: Immunopathogenesis of chronic pyelonephritis. Am J Med 75:59, 1983.

354. Hanson LA, Ahlstedt S, Fasth HA, et al: Antigens of E. coli in human immunoresponse and the pathogenesis of urinary tract infections. J Infect Dis 136:S144, 1977.

355. Kaijser B, Larrson P, Olling S: Protection against ascending E. coli pyelonephritis in rats and significance of local immunity. Infect Immunol 20:78, 1978.

356. Cotran RS: Retrograde *Proteus* pyelonephritis in rats. Localization of antigen and antibody in treated sterile pyelonephritic kidneys. J Exp Med 117:813, 1963.

357. Lehmann JD, Smith JW, Miller TE, et al: Local immune response in experimental pyelonephritis. J Clin Invest 427:2541, 1968.

358. Smith JA, Holmgren J, Ahlstedt S, Hanson LA: Local antibody production in experimental pyelonephritis. Amount, ability and immunoglobulin class. Infect Immunol 10:411, 1974.

359. Smith JW, Kaijser B: The local immune response to E. coli O- and K-antigen in experimental pyelonephritis. J Clin Invest 58:276, 1976.

360. Hanson LA, Fasth A, Jodal U, et al: Biology and pathology of urinary tract infections. J Clin Pathol 34:695, 1981.
361. DeRee JM, Van den Bosch JF: Serological response to the P fimbriae of uropathogenic *Escherichia coli* in pyelonephritis. Infect Immun 55:2204, 1987.
362. Cotran RS, Piessens WF: Pathogenesis of chronic pyelonephritis. The role of humoral and cell-mediated reactions to bacterial and renal antigen. *In* Giovannetti S, Bonomini V, D'Amico G (eds): Proceedings of the 6th International Congress on Nephrology (Florence). S Karger, Basel, 1976.
363. Cotran RS, Galvanek EG: Immunopathology of human tubular interstitial diseases: Localization of immunoglobulins and Tamm-Horsfall protein. Contrib Nephrol 16:126, 1979.
364. McCluskey RT, Colvin RG: Immunologic aspects of renal, tubular and interstitial disease. Annu Rev Med 29:191, 1978.
365. Losse H, Intorp HW, Lison AE, Funke C: Evidence of an autoimmune mechanism in pyelonephritis. Kidney Int 8(suppl 4):S44, 1975.
366. Kalmanson GM, Glassock RJ, Harwick HJ, Guze MB: Cellular immunity in experimental pyelonephritis. Kidney Int 8(suppl 4):S35, 1975.
367. van Zwieten MJ, Leber PD, Bhan AK, McCluskey RT: Experimental and cell-mediated interstitial nephritis induced with exogenous antigens. J Immunol 118:589, 1977.
368. Miller TE, Burnham S, Simpson G: Selective deficiency of thymus-derived lymphocytes in experimental pyelonephritis. Kidney Int 8:88, 1975.
369. Asscher AW, Jones BM, MacKenzie R: Delayed hypersensitivity to *E. coli* in the rat: A study of its possible relevance to the pathogenesis of kidney scars. Br J Exp Pathol 58:549, 1977.
370. Hoyer JR, Seiler MW: Tamm-Horsfall protein. Kidney Int 16:279, 1979.
371. Zager RA, Cotran RS, Hoyer JR: Histological localization of Tamm-Horsfall protein in interstitial deposits in renal disease. Lab Invest 38:52, 1978.
372. Cotran RS, Hodson CJ: Extratubular localization of Tamm-Horsfall protein in experimental reflux nephropathy in the pig. *In* Hodson CJ, Kincaid-Smith P (eds): Reflux Nephropathy. Masson Publishing USA, New York, 1979, p 213.
373. Hodson CJ, Davies A, Prescod A: Renal parenchymal radiographic measurement in infants and children. Pediatr Radiol 3:16, 1975.
374. Mayrer AR, Dziukas LJ, Hodson CJ, Andriole VT: Antibody to Tamm-Horsfall protein in porcine reflux nephropathy. Kidney Int 19:187, 1981.
375. Mayrer AR, Kashgarian M, Ruddle NH, et al: Tubulointerstitial nephritis and immunologic responses to Tamm-Horsfall protein in rabbits' challenged homologous urine or Tamm-Horsfall protein. J Immunol 128:2634, 1982.
376. Dziukas LJ, Sterzel RB, Hoyer JR, Hodson CJ: Unilateral ureteric obstruction in rats. J Lab Invest 47:185, 1982.
377. Fasth A, Bjure J, Hjalmas K, et al: Serum autoantibodies to Tamm-Horsfall protein and their relation to renal damage and glomerular filtration rate in children with urinary tract malformations. Contrib Nephrol 39:285, 1984.
378. Lynn KI, Bailey RR, Groufsky A, et al: Antibodies to Tamm-Horsfall urinary glycoprotein in patients with urinary tract infection, reflux nephropathy, urinary obstruction and paraplegia. Contrib Nephrol 39:296, 1984.
379. Cotran RS: Pathogenetic mechanisms in the progress of reflux nephropathy: The roles of glomerulosclerosis and extravasation of Tamm-Horsfall protein. *In* Zurukzoglu W, et al (eds): Advances in Basic and Clinical Nephrology. S Karger, Basel, 1981, p 368.
380. Sanford JP, Hunter BW, Atkins LL, Barnett JA: Immunity and obstructive uropathy as determinants in the pathogenesis of experimental pyelonephritis with observations in the distribution of antibody in highly nephrotic kidneys. *In* Kass EH (ed): Progress in Pyelonephritis. FA Davis, Philadelphia, 1965.
381. Cotran RS: Interstitial nephritis. *In* Churg J, Spargo BH, Mostofi FK, Abell MR (eds): Kidney Disease: Present Status. Williams & Wilkins, Baltimore, 1979, p 254.
382. Gill M, Pudvan WR: The angiographic diagnosis of renal parenchymal diseases. Radiology 96:81, 1970.
383. Hodson CJ: Radiology and the kidney. Contrib Nephrol 5:41, 1977.
384. Kincaid-Smith P, Hodson CJ: Lesions in the pig kidney with chronic reflux nephropathy. *In* Hodson CJ, Kincaid-Smith P (eds): Reflux Nephropathy. Masson Publishing USA, New York, 1979.
385. Gill DG, Mendes da Costa B, Cameron JS, et al: Analysis of 100 children with severe and persistent hypertension. Arch Dis Child 51:951, 1976.
386. Holland NH, Kotchen T, Bhathena D: Hypertension in children with chronic pyelonephritis. Kidney Int 8:S243, 1975.
387. Holland NH: Reflux nephropathy and hypertension. *In* Hodson CJ, Kincaid-Smith P (eds): Reflux Nephropathy. Masson Publishing USA, New York, 1970, p 257.
388. Gutman LT, Turck M, Petersdorf RG, Wedgwood RJ: Significance of bacterial variants in urine of patients with chronic bacteriuria. J Clin Invest 44:1945, 1965.
389. Fairley KF, Becker JF, Butler HM, et al: Diagnosis in the difficult case. Kidney Int 8:S12, 1975.
390. Guze LB, Kalmanson GM: Observations on the host parasite relationship in "protoplast" infection of the kidney. *In* Kass EH (ed): Progress in Pyelonephritis. FA Davis, Philadelphia, 1965.
391. Alderman MH, Freedman RL: Experimental pyelonephritis. X. Direct injection of E. coli protoplasts into the medulla of the rabbit kidney. Yale J Biol Med 36:157, 1963.
392. Glauser MP, Lyons JM, Braude AI: Prevention of chronic experimental pyelonephritis by suppression of acute suppuration. J Clin Invest 61:403, 1978.
393. Ransley PG, Risdon RA: Reflux nephropathy: Effects of antimicrobial therapy on the evolution of early pyelonephritic scar. Kidney Int 20:733, 1981.
394. Kincaid-Smith P: The Kidney. A Clinicopathologic Study. Blackwell Scientific Publications, Oxford, 1975.
395. Vermillion CD, Heale CD: Ureteral reflux in infancy. Relation to pyelonephritic scarring in adults. Rocky Mt Med J 72:200, 1975.
396. Chrispin AR, Hull D, Lillie JG, Risdon RA: Renal tubular necrosis and papillary necrosis after gastroenteritis in infants. Br Med J 1:410, 1970.
397. Chrispin AR: Medullary necrosis in infancy. Br Med Bull 28:233, 1972.
398. Benz G, Willich E, Scharer K: Segmental renal hypoplasia in childhood. Pediatr Radiol 5:86, 1976.
399. Arant BS Jr, Sotelo-Avila C, Bernstein J: Segmental hypoplasia of the kidney (Ask-Upmark). J Pediatr 95:931, 1979.
400. Angell ME, Relman AS, Robbins SL: "Active" chronic pyelonephritis without evidence of bacterial infection. N Engl J Med 278:1303, 1968.
401. Schwartz MM, Cotran RS: Primary renal disease in transplant recipients. Hum Pathol 7:455, 1976.
402. Farmer EF, Heptinstall RH: Chronic non-obstructive pyelonephritis—a reappraisal. *In* Kincaid-Smith P, Fairley KF (eds): Renal Infection and Renal Scarring. Mercedes, Melbourne, 1970.
403. Stewart JF, McCarthy SW, Storey BG, et al: Diseases causing end-stage renal failure in New South Wales. Br Med J 1:440, 1975.
404. Kincaid-Smith PS, Bastos MG, Becker GJ: Reflux nephropathy in the adult. Contrib Nephrol 39:94, 1984.
405. Bailey RR: Clinical presentations and diagnosis of vesicoureteric reflux and reflux nephropathy. *In* Davison A (ed): Nephropathy II. WB Saunders, Philadelphia, 1988, pp 835–843.
406. Bailey RR, Lynn KL: End-stage reflux nephropathy. Contrib Nephrol 39:102, 1984.
407. Hodson CJ: Reflux nephropathy. Scoring the damage. *In* Hodson CJ, Kincaid-Smith P (eds): Reflux Nephropathy. Masson Publishing USA, New York, 1979, p 29.
408. Resnick JS, Sisson S, Vernier RL: Tamm-Horsfall protein: Abnormal localization in renal disease. Lab Invest 38:550, 1978.
409. Solez K, Heptinstall RH: Intra-renal urinary extravasation with formation of venous polyps containing Tamm-Horsfall protein. J Urol 119:180, 1977.
410. Heptinstall RH, Bhagavan BS, Solez K: Urinary deposits in veins and interstitium of the kidney: Their possible role in causing renal damage. Contrib Nephrol 16:70, 1979.
411. Bhathena DB, Holland NH, Weiss JH, et al: Morphology of coarse renal scars in reflux-associated nephropathy in man. *In* Hodson CJ, Kincaid-Smith P (eds): Reflux Nephropathy. Masson Publishing USA, New York, 1979, p 240.
412. Heptinstall RH: Pathology of the Kidney. Little, Brown, Boston, 1983.
413. Kincaid-Smith P: Glomerular lesions—atrophic PN and reflux nephropathy. Kidney Int 8:S81, 1975.
414. Kincaid-Smith P: Glomerular and vascular lesions in chronic atrophic PN and reflux nephropathy. Adv Nephrol 5:3, 1975.

415. Abbott GD: Neonatal bacteriuria: A prospective study in 1,460 infants. Br Med J 1:267, 1972.

416. Kunin CM: Detection, Prevention and Management of Urinary Tract Infections, 3rd ed. Lea & Febiger, Philadelphia, 1979.

417. Edelman CM Jr, Ogwo JE, Fine BP, Martinez AB: The prevalence of bacteriuria in full-term and premature newborn infants. J Pediatr 82:125, 1973.

418. Rushton HG, Majd M: Pyelonephritis in male infants: How important is the foreskin? J Urol 148:733, 1992.

419. Spach DH, Stapleton AE, Stamm WE: Lack of circumcision increases the risk of urinary tract infection in young men. JAMA 267:679, 1992.

420. Kunin CM: The natural history of recurrent bacteriuria in school girls. N Engl J Med 282:1443, 1970.

421. Kunin CM: Epidemiology and natural history of urinary tract infection in school age children. Pediatr Clin North Am 18:50, 1971.

422. Kunin CM: Emergence of bacteriuria, proteinuria and symptomatic urinary tract infections among a population of school girls followed for 7 years. Pediatrics 41:968, 1968.

423. Gillenwater JW, Harrison RB, Kunin CM: Natural history of bacteriuria in school girls: A long-term case control study. N Engl J Med 301:396, 1979.

424. Jones ERV, Miller ST, McLachlan MSF, et al: Treatment of bacteriuria in school girls. Kidney Int Suppl 8:585, 1975.

425. Waters WE, Elwood PC, Asscher AW, et al: Clinical significance of dysuria. Br Med J 2:754, 1970.

426. Freedman LR, Phair JP, Saki M, et al: The epidemiology of urinary tract infections in Hiroshima. Yale J Biol Med 37:262, 1975.

427. Sanford JP: Urinary tract symptoms and infections. Annu Rev Med 26:485, 1976.

428. Silverberg DS: City-wide screening for urinary abnormalities in school boys. Can Med Assoc J 111:410, 1974.

429. Cohen M: The first urinary tract infection in male children. Am J Dis Child 130:810, 1976.

430. Baines RC, Daifuku R, Roddy RE, Stamm WE: Urinary tract infection in sexually active homosexual men. Lancet 1:171, 1986.

431. Saxena DR, Bassett DCJ: Sex-related incidence in *Proteus* infection of the urinary tract in childhood. Arch Dis Child 50:899, 1975.

432. Hallet RJ, Pead L, Maskell R: Urinary infection in boys. Lancet 2:1107, 1976.

433. Nicolle LE, Bjornson J, Harding GKM, Mac-Donell JA: Bacteriuria in elderly institutionalized men. N Engl J Med 309:1420, 1983.

434. Freedman LR: Urinary tract infections in the elderly. N Engl J Med 309:1451, 1983.

435. Bentzen A, Vejlsgaard R: Asymptomatic bacteriuria in elderly subjects. Dan Med Bull 27:101, 1980.

436. Dontas AS, Kasviki-Charvati P, Papanayiotou PC, Marketos SG: Bacteriuria and survival in old age. N Engl J Med 304:939, 1981.

437. Kass EH: The role of asymptomatic bacteriuria in the pathogenesis of pyelonephritis. *In* Quinn EL, Kass EH (eds): Biology of Pyelonephritis. Little, Brown, Boston, 1960.

438. Andriole VT: Urinary tract infections in pregnancy. Urol Clin North Am 2:485, 1975.

439. Kincaid-Smith P: Bacteriuria in pregnancy. *In* Kass EH (ed): Progress in Pyelonephritis. FA Davis, Philadelphia, 1965, p 11.

440. Whalley P: Bacteriuria of pregnancy. Am J Obstet Gynecol 7:723, 1967.

441. Gower PE, Haswell B, Sidaway ME, de Wardener HE: Follow-up of 164 patients with bacteriuria of pregnancy. Lancet 1:990, 1968.

442. Polk BF: Urinary tract infection in pregnancy. Clin Obstet Gynecol 22:285, 1979.

443. Brumfitt W: The effects of bacteriuria in pregnancy on maternal and fetal death. Kidney Int Suppl 8:S113, 1975.

444. Zinner SH, Kass EH: Long-term (10 to 14 years) follow-up of bacteriuria of pregnancy. N Engl J Med 285:820, 1971.

445. Martinell J, Jodal U, Lidin-Janson G: Pregnancies in women with and without renal scarring after urinary infections in childhood. BMJ 300:840, 1990.

446. Stenqvist K, Lidin-Janson G, Sandberg T, Eden CS: Bacterial adhesion as an indicator of renal involvement in bacteriuria of pregnancy. Scand J Infect Dis 21:193, 1989.

447. Tullus K, Horlin K, Svenson SB, Kallenius G: Epidemic outbreaks of acute pyelonephritis caused by nosocomial spread of P fimbriated E. coli in children. J Infect Dis 150:728, 1984.

448. Tullus K, Kuhn I, Kallenius G, et al: Fecal colonization with pyelo-

nephrogenic E. coli in neonates as a major factor for pyelonephritis. Eur J Clin Microbiol 5:643, 1986.

449. Tullus K, Kallenius G: Epidemiological aspects of p-fimbriated E. coli. IV. Extraintestinal E. coli infections before the age of one year and their relation to fecal colonization with p-fimbriated E. coli. Acta Paediatr Scand 76:463, 1987.

450. Nicolle LE, Harding GK, Preiksaitis J, Ronald AR: The association of urinary tract infection with sexual intercourse. J Infect Dis 146:579, 1982.

451. Strom BL, Collins M, West SL, et al: Sexual activity, contraceptive use, and other risk factors for systematic and asymptomatic bacteriuria: A case-control study. Ann Intern Med 107:816, 1987.

452. Fihn SD, Latham RH, Roberts P, et al: Association between diaphragm use and urinary tract infection. JAMA 254:240, 1985.

453. Fihn SD, Johnson C, Pinkstaff C, Stamm WE: Diaphragm use and urinary tract infections: Analysis of urodynamic and microbiological factors. J Urol 136:853, 1986.

454. Benton J, Chawla J, Parry S, Stickler D: Virulence factors in *Escherichia coli* from urinary tract infections in patients with spinal injuries. J Hosp Infect 22:117, 1992.

455. The prevention and management of urinary tract infections among people with spinal cord injuries. National Institute on Disability and Rehabilitation Research Consensus Statement. J Am Paraplegia Soc 15:194, 1992.

456. Rubin RH: Infection in the organ transplant recipient. *In* Rubin RH, Young LS (eds): Clinical Approach to Infection in the Compromised Host, 3rd ed. Plenum Publishing, New York, 1994, p 629.

457. Korzeniowski OM: Urinary tract infection in the impaired host. Med Clin North Am 75:391, 1991.

458. Rubin RH, Fang LST, Cosimi AB, et al: Usefulness of the antibody-coated bacteria assay in the management of urinary tract infection in the renal transplant patient. Transplantation 27:18, 1979.

459. Pawlowski J, Blosdoric J, Kimmelstiel P: Chronic pyelonephritis: A morphologic and bacteriologic study. N Engl J Med 286:965, 1960.

460. Freedman L: Chronic pyelonephritis at autopsy. Ann Intern Med 66:697, 1967.

461. Murray T, Goldberg MJ: Chronic interstitial nephritis: Etiologic factors. Ann Intern Med 82:453, 1975.

462. Freedman LR, Andriole V: The long-term follow-up of women with urinary tract infections. *In* Villarreal H (ed): Proceedings of the 5th International Congress of Nephrology. S Karger, Basel, 1972, p 230.

463. Asscher AW, Chick S, Radfors N, et al: Natural history of asymptomatic bacteriuria in non-pregnant women. *In* Brumfitt W, Asscher AW (eds): Urinary Tract Infection. Oxford University Press, London, 1973, p 51.

464. Freeman RB, Smith WM, Richardson JA, et al: Long-term therapy for chronic bacteriuria in men: U.S. Public Health Service Cooperative Study. Ann Intern Med 83:133, 1975.

465. Lindberg U, Claesson I, Hanson LA, Jodal U: Asymptomatic bacteriuria in school girls. VIII. Clinical course during a 3-year follow-up. J Pediatr 92:194, 1978.

466. Cardiff-Oxford Bacteriuria Study Group: Sequelae of covert bacteriuria in school girls: A four-year follow-up survey. Lancet 1:889, 1978.

467. Berg UB: Long-term followup of renal morphology and function in children with recurrent pyelonephritis. J Urol 148:1715, 1992.

468. Hannerz L, Celsi G, Eklof AC, et al: Ascending pyelonephritis in young rats retards kidney growth. Kidney Int 35:1133, 1989.

469. Edwards D, Normand ICS, Prescott N, Smellie JM: Disappearance of reflux during long-term prophylaxis of urinary tract infection in children. Br Med J 2:285, 1977.

470. Lenaghan D, Whitaber JG, Jemsen F, Stephens FD: The natural history of reflux and long-term effects of reflux on the kidney. J Urol 115:728, 1976.

471. Becker GJ, Kincaid-Smith P: Reflux nephropathy: The glomerular lesion and progression of renal failure. Pediatr Nephrol 7:365, 1993.

472. Coppo R, Porcellini MG, Gianoglio B, et al: Glomerular permselectivity to macromolecules in reflux nephropathy: Microalbuminuria during acute hyperfiltration due to amino acid infusion. Clin Nephrol 40:299, 1993.

473. Jacobson SH, Eklof O, Eriksson CG, et al: Development of hypertension and uraemia after pyelonephritis in childhood: 27 year follow up. BMJ 299:703, 1989.

474. Cunningham FG, Luca MJ, Hankins GD: Pulmonary injury complicating antepartum pyelonephritis. Am J Obstet Gynecol 156:797, 1987.

475. McFadyen IR: Pregnancy bacteriuria and *Escherichia coli*. J R Soc Med 73:227, 1980.
476. Kincaid-Smith P: Bacteriuria and urinary infection in pregnancy. Clin Obstet Gynecol 11:533, 1968.
477. Harris RE, Thomas VL, Shelokov A: Asymptomatic bacteriuria in pregnancy: Antibody-coated bacteria, renal function, and intrauterine growth retardation. Am J Obstet Gynecol 126:20, 1976.
478. McGrady GA, Daling JR, Peterson DR: Maternal urinary tract infection and adverse fetal outcomes. Am J Epidemiol 121:377, 1985.
479. Sever JL, Ellenberg JH, Edmonds D: Urinary tract infection during pregnancy: Maternal and pediatric findings. *In* Kass EH, Brumfitt W (eds): Infections of the Urinary Tract. University of Chicago Press, Chicago, 1979, p 12.
480. Naeye RL: Cause of the excessive rates of perinatal mortality and prematurity in pregnancies complicated by maternal urinary tract infections. N Engl J Med 300:819, 1979.
481. Coid CR, Landsoun ABG, McFadyen IR: Urinary tract infection in pregnancy. *In* Coid CR (ed): Infections in Pregnancy. Academic Press, London, 1977, p 289.
482. Zinner SH: Bacteriuria and babies revisited. N Engl J Med 300:853, 1979.
483. Gilstrap LC, Leveno KJ, Cunningham FG, et al: Renal infection and pregnancy outcome. Am J Obstet Gynecol 141:709, 1981.
484. McGladdery SL, Aparicio S, Verrier-Jones K, et al: Outcome of pregnancy in an Oxford-Cardiff cohort of women with previous bacteriuria. Q J Med 83:533, 1992.
485. Dontas AS, Kasviki-Charvati P, Chem L, et al: Bacteriuria and survival in old age. N Engl J Med 304:939, 1981.
486. Evans DA, Kass EH, Hennekens CH, et al: Bacteriuria and subsequent mortality in women. Lancet 1:156, 1982.
487. Sourander LB, Kasnanen A: A 5 year follow-up of bacteriuria in the aged. Gerontol Clin 14:274, 1972.
488. Platt R, Polk BF, Murdock B, Rosner B: Mortality associated nosocomial urinary tract infection. N Engl J Med 307:637, 1982.
489. Nordenstam GR, Brandberg CA, Oden AS, et al: Bacteriuria and mortality in an elderly population. N Engl J Med 314:1152, 1986.
490. Nicolle LE, Mayhew WJ, Bryan L: Prospective randomized comparison of therapy and no therapy for asymptomatic bacteriuria in institutionalized elderly women. Am J Med 83:27, 1987.
491. Nicolle LE, Henderson E, Bjornsen J, et al: The association of bacteriuria with resident characteristics and survival in elderly institutionalized men. Ann Intern Med 106:682, 1987.
492. Abrutyn E, Mossey J, Berlin JA, et al: Does asymptomatic bacteriuria predict mortality and does antimicrobial treatment reduce mortality in elderly ambulatory women? Ann Intern Med 120:827, 1994.
493. Johnson JR, Stamm WE: Diagnosis and treatment of acute urinary tract infections. Infect Dis Clin North Am 1:773, 1987.
494. Rubin RH, Shapiro ED, Andriole VT, et al: Evaluation of new antiinfective drugs for the treatment of urinary tract infection. Clin Infect Dis 15(suppl 1):S216, 1992.
495. Stamm WE, Running K, McKevitt M, et al: Treatment of acute urethral syndrome. N Engl J Med 304:956, 1981.
496. Tolkoff-Rubin NE, Weber D, Fang LST, et al: Single-dose therapy with trimethoprim-sulfamethoxazole for urinary tract infection in women. Rev Infect Dis 4:444, 1982.
497. Kraft JA, Stamey TA: The natural history of symptomatic recurrent bacteriuria in women. Medicine (Baltimore) 56:55, 1977.
498. Smellie JM, Hodson CJ, Edwards D, et al: Clinical and radiological features of urinary infection in childhood. Br Med J 2:1222, 1964.
499. Hoberman A, Chao HP, Keller DM, et al: Prevalence of urinary tract infection in febrile infants. J Pediatr 123:17, 1993.
500. Thorley JD, Jones SR, Sanford JP: Perinephric abscesses. Medicine (Baltimore) 53:441, 1974.
501. Patterson JE, Andriole VT: Renal and perirenal abscesses. Infect Dis Clin North Am 1:907, 1987.
502. Bjorgvinsson E, Majd M, Eggli KD: Diagnosis of acute pyelonephritis in children: Comparison of sonography and $^{99m}$Tc-DMSA scintigraphy. AJR 157:539, 1991.
503. Itoh K, Asano Y, Tsukamoto E, et al: Single photon emission computed tomography with Tc-99m–dimercaptosuccinic acid in patients with upper urinary tract infection and/or vesicoureteral reflux. Ann Nucl Med 5:29, 1991.
504. Rushton HG, Majd M, Jantausch B, et al: Renal scarring following reflux and nonreflux pyelonephritis in children: Evaluation with $^{99m}$technetium-dimercaptosuccinic acid scintigraphy. J Urol 147:1327, 1992.
505. Rushton HG, Majd M: Dimercaptosuccinic acid renal scintigraphy for the evaluation of pyelonephritis and scarring: A review of experimental and clinical studies. J Urol 148:1726, 1992.
506. Majd M, Rushton HG: Renal cortical scintigraphy in the diagnosis of acute pyelonephritis. Semin Nucl Med 22:98, 1992.
507. Kass EJ, Fink-Bennett D, Cacciarelli AA, et al: The sensitivity of renal scintigraphy and sonography in detecting nonobstructive acute pyelonephritis. J Urol 148:606, 1992.
508. Jakobsson B, Nolstedt L, Svensson L, et al: $^{99m}$Technetium-dimercaptosuccinic acid scan in the diagnosis of acute pyelonephritis in children: Relation to clinical and radiological findings. Pediatr Nephrol 6:328, 1992.
509. Shanon A, Feldman W, McDonald P, et al: Evaluation of renal scars by technetium-labeled dimercaptosuccinic acid scan, intravenous urography, and ultrasonography: A comparative study. J Pediatr 120:399, 1992.
510. Eggli DF, Tulchinsky M: Scintigraphic evaluation of pediatric urinary tract infection. Semin Nucl Med 23:199, 1993.
511. Benador D, Benador N, Slosman DO, et al: Cortical scintigraphy in the evaluation of renal parenchymal changes in children with pyelonephritis. J Pediatr 124:17, 1994.
512. Alt JM, Janig H, Schrurek HJ, Stollet H: Study of renal protein excretion in chronic pyelonephritis. Contrib Nephrol 16:37, 1939.
513. Torres VE, Neves JR, Svensson J: Vesicoureteral reflux in the adult. II. Pathogenesis. J Urol 130:10, 1983.
514. Hodson CJ: The 1980 Neuhauser Lecture. Am J Radiol 137:451, 1981.
515. Winberg J, Claesson I, Jacobsson B, et al: Renal growth after acute pyelonephritis in childhood: An epidemiological approach. *In* Hodson CJ, Kincaid-Smith P (eds): Reflux Nephropathy. Masson Publishing USA, New York, 1979, p 309.
516. Claesson I, Jacobsson B, Jodal V, Winberg J: Compensatory kidney growth in children with urinary tract infection and unilateral renal scarring: An epidemiological study. Kidney Int 20:759, 1981.
517. Newcastle Covert Bacteriuria Research Group: Covert bacteria in schoolgirls in Newcastle-upon-Tyne: A 5-year follow-up study. Arch Dis Child 56:585, 1981.
518. Bengtsson U: Long-term pattern in chronic pyelonephritis. Contrib Nephrol 16:31, 1979.
519. Gower PE: A prospective study of patients with radiological pyelonephritis, papillary necrosis and obstructive atrophy. Q J Med 45:315, 1976.
520. Gill DG, Mendes da Costa B, Cameron JS, et al: Analysis of 100 children with severe and persistent hypertension. Arch Dis Child 51:951, 1976.
521. Holland NH, Kotchen T, Bhathena D: Hypertension in children with chronic pyelonephritis. Kidney Int 8:S243, 1975.
522. Holland NH: Reflux nephropathy and hypertension. *In* Hodson CJ, Kincaid-Smith P (eds): Reflux Nephropathy. Masson Publishing USA, New York, 1979, p 257.
523. Rance CP, Arbus GS, Balfe JW, Kooh SW: Persistent systematic hypertension in infants and children. Pediatr Clin North Am 21:735, 1976.
524. Wallace DMA, Rothwell DL, Williams DI: The long-term followup of surgically-treated vesicoureteral reflux. Br J Urol 50:479, 1978.
525. Bailey RR, McRae CU, Mailing TMJ, et al: Renal vein renin concentration in the hypertension of unilateral reflux nephropathy. J Urol 120:21, 1978.
526. Savage JM, Shah V, Dillon MJ, et al: Renin and blood pressure in children with renal scarring and vesicoureteral reflux. Lancet 2:441, 1978.
527. Bailey RR, Lynn KL, McRae CU: Unilateral reflux nephropathy and hypertension. Contrib Nephrol 39:116, 1984.
528. Savage JM, Koh CT, Shah V, et al: Five-year prospective study of plasma renin activity and blood pressure in patients with corresponding reflux nephropathy. Arch Dis Child 62:678, 1987.
529. Cotran RS: Glomerulosclerosis in reflux nephropathy. Kidney Int 21:528, 1982.
530. Delano BG, Goodwin NJ, Thomson GE, et al: Chronic pyelonephritis as a cause of massive proteinuria of nephrotic syndrome. Arch Intern Med 129:73, 1972.
531. Woods HF, Walls J: Nephrotic syndrome in vesicoureteral reflux. Br Med J 2:917, 1976.
532. Kincaid-Smith P: Clinical implications of reflux in the adult. *In* Zurukzoglu W, et al (eds): Advances in Basic and Clinical Nephrology. S Karger, Basel, 1981, p 359.

533. Senekjian HO, Stinebaugh BJ, Mattioli CA, Suki WN: Irreversible renal failure following vesicoureteral reflux. JAMA 241:160, 1979.

534. Aladjem M, Schoeneman JJ, Bennett B, et al: Focal segmental glomerulosclerosis with proteinuria and chronic interstitial nephritis. N Y State J Med 78:579, 1978.

535. Torres VE, Velosa JA, Holley KE, et al: The progression of vesicoureteral reflux nephropathy. Ann Intern Med 92:776, 1980.

536. Zimmerman SW, Uehling DT, Burkholder PM: Vesicoureteral reflux nephropathy: Evidence for immunologically mediated glomerular injury. Urology 2:531, 1973.

537. Bhathena DB, Weiss JH, Holland NH, et al: Focal and segmental glomerular sclerosis in reflux nephropathy (chronic pyelonephritis). Am J Med 68:886, 1980.

538. Schwartz MM, Cotran RS: Primary renal disease in transplant recipients. Hum Pathol 7:455, 1976.

539. Velosa J, Miller K, Michael AF: Immunopathology of end-stage kidney. Immunoglobulin and complement deposition in nonimmune disease. Am J Pathol 84:149, 1976.

540. Yoshioka K, Takemura T, Matsubara K, et al: Immunohistochemical studies of reflux nephropathy. The role of extracellular matrix, membrane, attack complex, and immune cells in glomerulosclerosis. Am J Pathol 129:223, 1987.

541. Raij L, Keane WF, Osswald H, Michael AF: Mesangial function in ureteral obstruction in the rat. Blockade of the efferent limb. J Clin Invest 64:1204, 1979.

542. Hostetter RH, Olson JL, Rennke HG, et al: Hyperfiltration in remnant nephrons: A potentially adverse response to renal ablation. Am J Physiol 241:F85, 1981.

543. Olson JL, Hostetter TH, Rennke HG, et al: Altered charge and size-selective properties of the glomerular wall: A response to reduced renal mass. Kidney Int 22:112, 1982.

544. Bailey RR, Swainson CP, Lynn KL, Burry AF: Glomerular lesions in the "normal" kidney in patients with unilateral reflux nephropathy. Contrib Nephrol 39:126, 1984.

545. Verrier Jones K, Asscher W, Verrier Jones R, et al: Renal functional changes in schoolgirls with covert asymptomatic bacteriuria. Contrib Nephrol 39:152, 1984.

546. Khatib ML, Becker GJ, Kincaid-Smith P: Morphometric aspects of reflux nephropathy. Kidney Int 32:261, 1987.

547. Bartlett RC, O'Neill D, McLaughlin JC: Detection of bacteriuria by leukocyte esterase, nitrate, and the automicrobic system. Am J Clin Pathol 82:683, 1984.

548. Guignard JP, Torrado N: Nitrite indicator strip test for bacteriuria. Lancet 1:47, 1978.

549. Lejeune B, Baron R, Guillois B, Mayeux D: Evaluation of a screening test for detecting urinary tract infection in newborns and infants. J Clin Pathol 44:1029, 1991.

550. Evans PJ, Leaker BR, McNabb WR, Lewis RR: Accuracy of reagent strip testing for urinary tract infection in the elderly. J R Soc Med 84:598, 1991.

551. Lachs MS, Nachamkin I, Edelstein PH, et al: Spectrum bias in the evaluation of diagnostic tests: Lessons from the rapid dipstick test for urinary tract infection. Ann Intern Med 117:135, 1992.

552. Bachman JW, Heise RH, Naessens JM, Timmerman MG: A study of various tests to detect asymptomatic urinary tract infections in an obstetric population. JAMA 270:1971, 1993.

553. Kunin CM: New methods in detecting urinary tract infections. Urol Clin North Am 2:423, 1975.

554. Martin MJ, McGuckin MB: Evaluation of a dip-slide in a university outpatient service. J Urol 120:193, 1978.

555. Hoyt SM, Ellner PD: Evaluation of the bacteriuria detection device. J Clin Microbiol 18:882, 1983.

556. Smith TK, Hudson AJ, Spencer RC: Evaluation of six screening methods for detecting significant bacteriuria. J Clin Pathol 41:904, 1988.

557. Fang LST, Tolkoff-Rubin NE, Rubin RH: Efficacy of single-dose and conventional amoxicillin therapy in urinary tract infection localized by the antibody-coated bacteria technique. N Engl J Med 298:413, 1979.

558. Fairley KF, Carson NE, Gutch RC, et al: Site of infection in acute urinary tract infection in general practice. Lancet 2:615, 1971.

559. Norden CW, Levy PS, Kass EH: Predictive effect of urinary concentrating ability and hemagglutinizing antibody taken upon response to antimicrobial therapy in bacteriuria of pregnancy. J Infect Dis 121:588, 1970.

560. Clark H, Ronald AR, Cutler RE, Turck M: The correlation between site of infection and maximal concentrating ability in bacteriuria. J Infect Dis 120:47, 1969.

561. Ronald AR, Cutler RE, Turck M: Effect of bacteriuria on the renal concentrating mechanism. Ann Intern Med 70:723, 1969.

562. Levison SP, Levison ME: Effect of indomethacin and sodium meclofenamate on the renal concentrating defect in experimental enterococcal pyelonephritis in rats. J Lab Clin Med 88:958, 1976.

563. Levison SP, Levison ME: Papillary plasma flow in experimental pyelonephritis in rats: Effect of antibiotic therapy and indomethacin. J Lab Clin Med 92:570, 1978.

564. Wacker W, Dorfman L: Urinary lactic dehydrogenase activity. JAMA 181:148, 1962.

565. Bank N, Baline SH: Urinary beta-glucuronidase activity in patients with urinary tract infection. N Engl J Med 272:70, 1965.

566. Ronald AR, Silverblatt F, Clark H, et al: Failure of urinary beta-glucuronidase activity to localize the site of urinary tract infection. Appl Microbiol 21:990, 1971.

567. Turck M: Importance of localization of urinary tract infection in women. *In* Kass EH, Brumfitt W (eds): Infections of the Urinary Tract. University of Chicago Press, Chicago, 1978, p 114.

568. Viganò A, Assael BM, Dalla Villa A, et al: *N*-Acetyl-β-D-glucosaminidase (NAG) and NAG isoenzymes in children with upper and lower urinary tract infections. Clin Chim Acta 130:297, 1983.

569. Johnson CE, Vacca CV, Fattlar D, et al: Urinary *N*-acetyl-beta-glucosaminidase and the selection of children for radiologic evaluation after urinary tract infection. Pediatrics 86:211, 1990.

570. Jodal U, Lindberg U, Lincoln K: Level diagnosis of symptomatic urinary tract infections in childhood. Acta Paediatr Scand 64:201, 1975.

571. Jodal U, Hanson LA: Sequential determination of C-reactive protein in acute childhood pyelonephritis. Acta Paediatr Scand 65:319, 1976.

572. Sabel KG, Hanson LA: The clinical usefulness of C-reactive protein (CRP) determinations in bacterial meningitis and septicemia in infancy. Acta Paediatr Scand 63:381, 1974.

573. Hellerstein S, Duggan E, Welchert E, Mansour F: Serum C-reactive protein and the site of urinary tract infections. J Pediatr 100:21, 1982.

574. Rubin RH, Cotran RS: Immunological aspects of pyelonephritis with a critical survey of antibody-coated bacteria test. *In* Losse H, Asscher AW (eds): Pyelonephritis, Vol IV, Urinary Tract Infections. Georg Thieme Verlag, Stuttgart, 1980, p 124.

575. Percival A, Brumfitt W, DeLouvois J: Serum antibody levels as an indication of clinically apparent pyelonephritis. Lancet 2:1027, 1964.

576. Clark H, Ronald AR, Turck M: Serum antibody response in renal versus bladder bacteria. J Infect Dis 123:539, 1971.

577. Thomas V, Shelokov A, Forland M: Antibody-coated bacteria in the urine and the site of urinary tract infection. N Engl J Med 290:588, 1974.

578. Jones SR, Smith JW, Sanford JP: Localization of urinary tract infections by detection of antibody-coated bacteria in urine sediment. N Engl J Med 290:591, 1974.

579. Montplaisir S, Cote PA, Martineau B, et al: Localisation du site de l'infection urinaire chez l'enfant par la recherche de bactéries vecouvertes d'anticorps. Can Med Assoc J 115:1096, 1976.

580. Thomas VL, Harris RE, Gilstrap LC III: antibody-coated bacteria in the urine of hospitalized patients with acute pyelonephritis. J Infect Dis Suppl 131:S57, 1975.

581. Montplaisir S, Courteau C, Roche AJ: Antibody-coated bacteria in contaminated urine specimens. N Engl J Med 296:758, 1977.

582. Braude R, Block C: Proteinuria and antibody-coated bacteria in the urine. N Engl J Med 297:617, 1977.

583. Riedasch F, Ritz E, Mohring K, Bommer J: Antibody coating of urinary bacteria: Relation to site of infection and invasion of uroepithelium. Clin Nephrol 10:239, 1978.

584. Rumans LW, Vosti KL: The relationship of antibody-coated bacteria to clinical syndromes; as found in unselected populations with bacteriuria. Arch Intern Med 138:1077, 1978.

585. Hellerstein S, Kennedy E, Nussbaum L, Rice K: Localization of the site of urinary tract infections by means of antibody-coated bacteria in the urinary sediments. J Pediatr 92:188, 1978.

586. Smith JW, Jones SR, Kaijser B: Significance of antibody-coated bacteria in urinary sediment in experimental pyelonephritis. J Infect Dis 135:577, 1977.

587. Savard-Fenton M, Fenton BW, Roller LB, et al: Single-dose amoxi-

cillin therapy with follow-up urine culture: Effective initial management for acute uncomplicated urinary tract infections. Am J Med 73:808, 1982.

588. Fair WR, McClennan BL, Jost RG: Are excretory urograms necessary in evaluating women with urinary tract infection? J Urol 121:313, 1979.

589. Engel G, Schaeffer AJ, Grayback JT, Wendel EF: The role of excretory urography and cystoscopy in the evaluation and management of women with recurrent urinary tract infection. J Urol 123:190, 1980.

590. Fowler JE Jr, Pulaski ET: Excretory urography, cystography and cystoscopy in the evaluation of women with urinary tract infection: A prospective study. N Engl J Med 304:462, 1981.

591. Delange EE, Jones B: Unnecessary intravenous urography in young women with recurrent urinary tract infections. Clin Radiol 34:551, 1983.

592. Sandberg T, Stokland E, Brolin I, et al: Selective use of excretory urography in women with acute pyelonephritis. J Urol 141:1290, 1989.

593. Nickel JC, Wilson J, Morales A, Heaton J: Value of urologic investigation in a targeted group of women with recurrent urinary tract infections. Can J Surg 34:591, 1991.

594. Stamey TA, Fair WR, Timothy MM, et al: Serum versus urinary antimicrobial concentrations in cure of urinary tract infections. N Engl J Med 291:1159, 1974.

595. Muscher DM, Minuth JN, Thorsteinsson SB, Holmes T: Effectiveness of achievable urinary concentrations of tetracyclines against "tetracycline-resistant" pathogenic bacteria. J Infect Dis 131(suppl P):S40, 1975.

596. Glauser MP, Lyons JM, Brande A: Synergism of ampicillin and gentamicin against obstructive pyelonephritis due to *Escherichia coli* in rats. J Infect Dis 139:133, 1979.

597. Herthelius M, Mollby R, Nord CE, Winberg J: Amoxicillin promotes vaginal colonization with adhering *Escherichia coli* present in faeces. Pediatr Nephrol 3:443, 1989.

598. Ronald AR, Boutros P, Mourtoda H: Bacteriuria localization and response to single-dose therapy in women. JAMA 235:1854, 1976.

599. Nicolle LE, Ronald AR: Recurrent urinary tract infections in adult women: Diagnosis and treatment. Infect Dis Clin North Am 1:793, 1987.

600. Bailey RR: Single-Dose Therapy of Urinary Tract Infection. ADIS Health Science Press, Sydney, 1983.

601. Tolkoff-Rubin NE, Wilson ME, Zuromskis P, et al: Single-dose amoxicillin therapy of acute uncomplicated urinary tract infection in women. Antimicrob Agents Chemother 25:626, 1984.

602. Harbord RB, Gruneborg RN: Treatment of urinary tract infection with a single dose of amoxicillin, co-trimoxazole, or trimethoprim. Br J Med 303:409, 1981.

603. Ludwig P, Buckwold F, Harding G, et al: Single-dose therapy of acute cystitis in adult females: Prospective randomized comparison of four regimes. *In* Nelson JD, Grass C (eds): Current Chemotherapy and Infectious Disease—1980. American Society for Microbiology, Washington, DC, 1980, p 1297.

604. Counts GW, Stamm WE, McKevitt M, et al: Treatment of cystitis in women with a single-dose of trimethoprim-sulfamethoxazole. Rev Infect Dis 4:484, 1982.

605. Fairley KF, Whitworth JA, Kincaid-Smith P, Durman O: Single-dose therapy in management of urinary tract infection. Med J Aust 2:75, 1978.

606. Kallenius F, Winberg J: Urinary tract infections treated with a single dose of short-acting sulfonamide. Br Med J 1:1175, 1979.

607. Johnson JR, Stamm WE: Diagnosis and treatment of acute urinary tract infections. Infect Dis Clin North Am 1:773, 1987.

608. Greenberg RN, Reilly PM, Luppen KL, et al: Randomized study of single-dose three-day, and seven-day treatment of cystitis in women. J Infect Dis 153:277, 1986.

609. Fihn SD, Johnson C, Roberts PL, et al: Trimethoprim-sulfamethoxazole for acute dysuria in women: A single-dose or 10-day course. A double-blind, randomized trial. Ann Intern Med 108:350, 1988.

610. Tolkoff-Rubin NE, Rubin RH: New approaches to the treatment of urinary tract infection. Am J Med 82(suppl 4A):270, 1987.

611. Johnson JR, Stamm WE: Urinary tract infections in women: Diagnosis and treatment. Ann Intern Med 111:906, 1989.

612. Inter-Nordic Urinary Tract Infection Study Group: Double-blind comparison of 3-day versus 7-day treatment with norfloxacin in symptomatic urinary tract infections. Scand J Infect Dis 20:619, 1988.

613. Hooton TM, Johnson C, Winter C, et al: Single dose and three day regimens of ofloxacin versus trimethoprim-sulfamethoxazole for acute cystitis in women. Antimicrob Agents Chemother 35:1479, 1991.

614. Norrby SR: Short term treatment of uncomplicated lower urinary tract infections in women. Rev Infect Dis 12:458, 1990.

615. Hooton TM, Stamm WE: Management of acute uncomplicated urinary tract infection in adults. Med Clin North Am 75:339, 1991.

616. Pappas PG: Laboratory in the diagnosis and management of urinary tract infections. Med Clin North Am 75:313, 1991.

617. Carlson KJ, Mulley AG: Management of acute dysuria: A decision-analysis model of alternative strategies. Ann Intern Med 102:244, 1985.

618. Harding GKM, Ronald AR: A controlled study of antimicrobial prophylaxis of recurrent urinary infection in women. N Engl J Med 291:597, 1974.

619. Ronald AR, Harding GKM: Urinary infection prophylaxis in women. Ann Intern Med 9:268, 1981.

620. Holmber L, Boman G, Bottinger LE, et al: Adverse reactions to nitrofurantoin. Analysis of 921 reports. Am J Med 69:733, 1980.

621. Harding GKM, Buckwald FJ, Marrie TJ, et al: Prophylaxis of recurrent urinary tract infection in female patients: Efficacy of low dose, thrice weekly therapy with trimethoprim-sulfamethoxazole. JAMA 242:1975, 1979.

622. Tolkoff-Rubin NE, Rubin RH: Ciprofloxacin in the management of urinary tract infection. Urology 31:359, 1988.

623. Stapleton A, Latham RH, Johnson C, Stamm WE: Postcoital antimicrobial prophylaxis for recurrent urinary tract infection: A randomized, double-blind, placebo-controlled trial. JAMA 264:703, 1990.

624. Wong ES, McKevitt M, Running K, et al: Management of recurrent urinary tract infections with patient-administered single dose therapy. Ann Intern Med 102:302, 1985.

625. Turck M, Anderson KN, Petersdorf RG: Relapse and reinfection in chronic bacteriuria. N Engl J Med 275:70, 1966.

626. Turck M, Ronald AR, Petersdorf RG: Relapse and reinfection in chronic bacteriuria. II. The correlation between site of infection and pattern of recurrence in chronic bacteriuria. N Engl J Med 278:422, 1968.

627. Sobel JD, Muller G: Pathogenesis of bacteriuria in elderly women—the role of *Escherichia coli* adherence to vaginal epithelial cells. J Gerontol 39:682, 1984.

628. Romano JM, Kaye D: UTI in the elderly: Common yet atypical. Geriatrics 36:113, 1981.

629. Molander U, Milson I, Ekelund P, et al: Effect of oral oestriol on vaginal flora and cytology and urogenital symptoms in the postmenopause. Maturitas 12:113, 1990.

630. Raz R, Stamm WE: A controlled trial of intravaginal estriol in postmenopausal women with recurrent urinary tract infections. N Engl J Med 329:753, 1993.

631. Parsons CL, Schmidt JD: Control of recurrent lower urinary tract infection in postmenopausal women. J Urol 12:1224, 1982.

632. Brandberg A, Mellstrom D, Samside G: Low dose oral estriol treatment in elderly women with urogenital infections. Acta Obstet Gynecol Scand Suppl 140:33, 1987.

633. Avorn J, Monane M, Gurwitz JH, et al: Reduction of bacteriuria and pyuria after ingestion of cranberry juice. JAMA 271:751, 1994.

634. Zafriri D, Ofek I, Adar R, et al: Inhibitory activity of cranberry juice on adherence of type 1 and P fimbriated *Escherichia coli* to eukaryotic cells. Antimicrob Agents Chemother 33:92, 1989.

635. Ofek I, Goldhar J, Zafriri D, et al: Anti-*Escherichia* adhesin activity of cranberry and blueberry juices. N Engl J Med 324:1599, 1991.

636. Zinner SH: Management of urinary tract infections in pregnancy: A review with comments on single dose therapy. Infection 20(suppl 4):S280, 1992.

637. Little PJ: The treatment of bacteriuria of pregnancy with low dosage nitrofurantoin. *In* Kass EH (ed): Symposium on Pyelonephritis. Churchill Livingstone, Edinburgh, 1967, p 17.

638. Harris RE, Gilstrap LC, Pretty A: Single dose antimicrobial therapy for asymptomatic bacteriuria during pregnancy. Obstet Gynecol 59:546, 1982.

639. Pfau A, Sacks TG: Effective prophylaxis for recurrent urinary tract infections during pregnancy. Clin Infect Dis 14:810, 1992.

640. Sandberg T, Brorson JE: Efficacy of long term antimicrobial prophylaxis after acute pyelonephritis in pregnancy. Scand J Infect Dis 23:221, 1991.

641. Wong ES, Stamm WE: Sexual acquisition of urinary tract infection in a man. JAMA 250:3087, 1983.

642. Hoepelman AI, van Buren M, van den Broek J, Borleffs JC: Bacteriuria in men infected with HIV-1 is related to their immune status (CD4+ cell count). AIDS 6:179, 1992.

643. Meares EM Jr: Acute and chronic prostatitis: Diagnosis and treatment. Infect Dis Clin North Am 1:855, 1987.

644. Gleckman R, Crowley M, Natsios GA: Therapy of recurrent invasive urinary tract infections of men. N Engl J Med 301:878, 1979.

645. Smith JW, Jones SR, Reed WP, et al: Recurrent urinary tract infection in men: Characteristics and response to therapy. Ann Intern Med 91:544, 1979.

646. Avner ED, Ingelfinger JR, Herrin JT, et al: Single-dose amoxicillin therapy of uncomplicated pediatric urinary tract infections. J Pediatr 102:623, 1983.

647. Mofatt M, Embrec J, Grimm P, Law B: Short-course antibiotic therapy for urinary tract infections in children. A methodological review of the literature. Am J Dis Child 142:57, 1988.

648. Madrigal G, Odio CM, Mohs E, et al: Single-dose antibiotic therapy is not as effective as conventional regimens for management of acute urinary tract infections in children. Pediatr Infect Dis J 7:316, 1988.

649. Fine JS, Jacobsen MS: Single-dose versus conventional therapy of urinary tract infections in female adolescents. Pediatrics 75:916, 1985.

650. Durbin WA Jr, Peter G: Management of urinary tract infections in infants and children. Pediatr Infect Dis 3:564, 1984.

651. McCracken GH Jr: Options in antimicrobial management of urinary tract infections in infants and children. Pediatr Infect Dis J 8:552, 1989.

652. Smellie JM, Gruneberg RN, Leahey A, et al: Long-term low-dose cotrimoxazole in prophylaxis of childhood urinary tract infection: Clinical aspects. Br Med J 2:203, 1976.

653. Marks MI: Cystitis. In Feigin RD, Cherry JD (eds): Textbook of Pediatric Infectious Diseases. WB Saunders, Philadelphia, 1981, p 352.

654. Belman AB, Skoog SJ: Nonsurgical approach to the management of vesicoureteral reflux in children. Pediatr Infect Dis J 8:556, 1989.

655. Birmingham Reflux Study Group: Prospective trial of operative versus non-operative treatment of severe vesicoureteric reflux in children: Five years' observation. Br Med J 295:237, 1987.

656. Duckett JW, Walker RD, Weiss R: Surgical results: International Reflux Study in Children—United States branch. J Urol 148:1674, 1992.

657. Weiss R, Duckett J, Spitzer A: Results of a randomized clinical trial of medical versus surgical management of infants and children with grades III and IV primary vesicoureteral reflux (United States). The International Reflux Study in Children. J Urol 148:1667, 1992.

658. Tamminen-Mobius T, Brunier E, Ebel KD, et al: Cessation of vesicoureteral reflux for 5 years in infants and children allocated to medical treatment. The International Reflux Study in Children. J Urol 148:1662, 1992.

659. Hjalmas K, Lohr G, Tamminen-Mobius T, et al: Surgical results in the International Reflux Study in Children (Europe). J Urol 148:1657, 1992.

660. Olbing H, Claesson I, Ebel KD, et al: Renal scars and parenchymal thinning in children with vesicoureteral reflux: A 5-year report of the International Reflux Study in Children (European branch). J Urol 148:1653, 1992.

661. Jodal U, Koskimies O, Hanson E, et al: Infection pattern in children with vesicoureteral reflux randomly allocated to operation or long term antibacterial prophylaxis. The International Reflux Study in Children. J Urol 148:1650, 1992.

662. Arant BS Jr: Medical management of mild and moderate vesicoureteral reflux: Followup studies of infants and young children. A preliminary report of the Southwest Pediatric Nephrology Study Group. J Urol 148:1683, 1992.

663. McLorie GA, McKenna PH, Jumper BM, et al: High grade vesicoureteral reflux: Analysis of observational therapy. J Urol 144:537, 1990.

664. Smellie JM: Commentary: Management of children with severe vesicoureteral reflux. J Urol 148:1676, 1992.

665. Banovac K, Wade N, Gonzalez F, et al: Decreased incidence of urinary tract infections in patients with spinal cord injury: Effect of methenamine. J Am Paraplegia Soc 14:52, 1991.

666. Kreger BE, Craven DE, Carling PC, McCabe WR: Gram negative bacteremia. III. Reassessment of etiology, epidemiology and ecology in 612 patients. Am J Med 68:332, 1980.

667. Nickel JC, Gristina AG, Costerton JW: Electron microscopic study of an infected Foley catheter. Can J Surg 28:50, 1985.

668. Nickel JC, Ruseka I, Wright JB, Costerton JW: Tobramycin resistance of Pseudomonas aeruginosa cells growing as a biofilm on urinary catheter material. Antimicrob Agents Chemother 27:619, 1985.

669. Warren JW: Catheter-associated urinary tract infections. Infect Dis Clin North Am 1:823, 1987.

670. Platt R, Polk BF, Murdock B, Rosner B: Risk factors for nosocomial urinary tract infection. Am J Epidemiol 124:977, 1986.

671. Johnson JR, Roberts PL, Olsen RJ, et al: Prevention of catheter-associated urinary tract infection with a silver oxide–coated urinary catheter: Clinical and microbiologic correlates. J Infect Dis 162:1145, 1990.

672. Wong-Beringer A, Jacobs RA, Guglielmo BJ: Treatment of funguria. JAMA 267:2780, 1992.

673. Jacobs LG, Skidmore EA, Cardoso LA, Ziv F: Bladder irrigation with amphotericin B for treatment of fungal urinary tract infections. Clin Infect Dis 18:313, 1994.

674. Hibberd PH, Rubin RH: Clinical aspects of fungal infection in organ transplant recipients. Clin Infect Dis 19(suppl 1):533, 1994.

675. Simon HB, Weinstein AJ, Pasternak MS, et al: Genitourinary tuberculosis. Clinical features in a general hospital population. Am J Med 63:410, 1977.

676. Garcia-Rodriguez JA, Garcia Sanchez JE, Munoz Bellido JL, et al: Genitourinary tuberculosis in Spain: Review of 81 cases. Clin Infect Dis 18:557, 1994.

677. Christiansen WJ: Genitourinary tuberculosis: Review of 102 cases. Medicine (Baltimore) 53:377, 1974.

678. Narayana AS: Overview of renal tuberculosis. Urology 19:231, 1982.

679. Hartman DS: Radiologic-pathologic correlation of the infectious granulomatous diseases of the kidney. Monogr Urol 6:3, 1985.

680. Malek RS, Eza S, Elder JS: Xanthogranulomatous pyelonephritis: A critical analysis of 26 cases and of the literature. J Urol 119:589, 1978.

681. Parson MA, Harris SC, Longstaff AJ, Grainger RG: Xanthogranulomatous pyelonephritis: A pathological, clinical and etiological analysis of 87 cases. Diagn Histopathol 6:203, 1983.

682. Goodman M, Curry T, Russell T: Xanthogranulomatous pyelonephritis: A local disease with systemic manifestations. Report of 23 cases and review of the literature. Medicine (Baltimore) 58:171, 1979.

683. Braun G, Moussali L, Balamzar JL: Xanthogranulomatous pyelonephritis in children. J Urol 133:326, 1985.

684. Clapton WK, Boucat HA, Dewan PA, et al: Clinicopathological features of xanthogranulomatous pyelonephritis in infancy. Pathology 25:110, 1993.

685. Hammadeh MY, Nicholls G, Calder CJ, et al: Xanthogranulomatous pyelonephritis in childhood: Preoperative diagnosis is possible. Br J Urol 73:83, 1994.

686. Rossi P, Myers DH, Furey R, Bonfils-Roberts EA: Angiography in bilateral xanthogranulomatous pyelonephritis. Radiology 93:20, 1968.

687. Cowley JP, Connolly CE, Hehir M, O'Brien SF: Renal carcinoma with staghorn calculus, perinephritic abscess, and xanthogranulomatous pyelonephritis in same kidney. Urology 21:635, 1983.

688. Piscioli F, Luciani L: Association of xanthogranulomatous pyelonephritis with small renal cell carcinoma. Case report and review of the literature. Eur Urol 10:62, 1984.

689. List AR, Johansson SL, Nilson AE, Pettersson S: Xanthogranulomatous pyelonephritis and renocolic fistula and coexistent contralateral renal carcinoma. Scand J Urol Nephrol 17:139, 1983.

690. Crane LM, McClellan L: Xanthogranulomatous pyelonephritis. J Can Assoc Radiol 27:45, 1976.

691. Gammill S, Rabinowitz JG, Peace R, et al: New thoughts concerning xanthogranulomatous pyelonephritis. Am J Roentgenol 125:154, 1975.

692. Subramanyam BR, Megibow AJ, Rashavendra BN, Bosniak MA: Diffuse xanthogranulomatous pyelonephritis: Analysis by computed tomography and sonography. Urol Radiol 4:5, 1982.

693. Solomon A, Braf Z, Papo J, Merimsky E: Computerized tomography in xanthogranulomatous pyelonephritis. J Urol 130:323, 1983.

694. Goldman SM, Hartman DS, Fishman EK: Computerized tomography of xanthogranulomatous PN: Radiological-pathological correlations. Am J Radiol 141:963, 1984.

695. Mulapulos GP, Patel SK, Pessis D: MR imaging of xanthogranulomatous PN. J Comput Assist Tomogr 10:154, 1986.

696. Oosterhof G, Delacre K: Xanthogranulomatous pyelonephritis. Urol Int 41:180, 1986.

697. Treadwall TL, Craven DC, Delfin H, et al: Xanthogranulomatous pyelonephritis caused by methicillin-resistant *Staphylococcus aureus.* Am J Med 76:533, 1984.

698. Khalyl-Mawad J, Greco MA, Schinella RA: Ultrastructural demonstration of intracellular bacteria in xanthogranulomatous pyelonephritis. Hum Pathol 13:41, 1982.

699. Carson CC, Weinerth JL: Xanthogranulomatous pyelonephritis in renal transplant recipient. Urology 23:50, 1984.

700. Lambrid PA, Yardley JH: Urinary tract malakoplakia. Report of a fatal case with ultrastructural observations of Michaelis-Gutmann bodies. Johns Hopkins Med J 126:1, 1970.

701. Stanton MJ, Maxted W: Malakoplakia: A study of the literature and current concepts of pathogenesis, diagnosis, and treatment. J Urol 125:139, 1981.

702. McClurg FR, D'Agostino AN, Martin JH, Race GJ: Ultrastructural demonstration of intracellular bacteria in three cases of malakoplakia of the bladder. Am J Clin Pathol 60:780, 1973.

703. Schwartz DT, Mascatello VJ, David Nelson MA: Malakoplakia of the kidney. South Med J 76:11427, 1983.

704. Bowers JH, Cathey WJ: Malakoplakia of the kidney with renal failure. Am J Clin Pathol 55:765, 1971.

705. Cadnapaphornchai P, Rosenberg BF, Taber S, et al: Renal parenchymal malakoplakia: An unusual cause of renal failure. N Engl J Med 299:1110, 1978.

706. Lou TY, Teplitz C: Malakoplakia: Pathogenesis and ultrastructural morphogenesis. A problem of altered macrophage (phagolysosomal) response. Hum Pathol 5:191, 1974.

707. Malfunctioning microtubules. Lancet 1:697, 1978. Editorial.

708. Abdou NI, NaPombejara C, Sagawa A, et al: Malakoplakia: Evidence for monocyte lysosomal abnormality correctable by cholinergic agonist in vitro and in vivo. N Engl J Med 297:1413, 1977.

# Tubulointerstitial Diseases

*Carolyn J. Kelly*
*Eric G. Neilson*

## HISTORICAL PERSPECTIVE

The tubulointerstitial compartment comprises everything that is not glomerular.[1] It is formed first during embryogenesis, and its structures quickly become the principal mass of mature kidney.[2] The understanding of its function is deeply rooted in the study of its structure. That the kidney is composed of tubules has been known since the 16th century.[3] Bowman's[4] report in 1842 that malpighian bodies were connected to tubules forged the basis of the filtration theory of urine formation. By 1852, the interstitium had received anatomic recognition as a separate compartment of its own.[5] Biermer, in 1860, first observed interstitial infiltrates in the absence of infection[6]; at the same time, Taylor and Pavy[7] introduced a model of experimental interstitial injury after exposure to mercury bichloride. This was soon followed by an early description of lead nephropathy.[8] By 1868, Dickinson[9] had devoted an entire chapter of his book on albuminuria to diseases of tubule nephritis. Ponfick's[10] description in 1869 of stiletto fibroblast-like cells in the interstitium of the kidney led to the suggestion that interstitial alterations in Bright disease may be responsible for the contracted kidneys of end-stage renal failure.[11] In 1898, Councilman[12] provided the first comprehensive report on the cause and effect of acute interstitial nephritis. This work led to Pearce's[13] critical discussion of different models of tubulointerstitial injury in 1910 and set the stage for Vollhard and Fahr[14] to assign interstitial nephritis a place in their 1914 classification of renal diseases.

Longcope,[15] in 1913, began injecting rabbits with heterologous proteins to produce lymphocyte infiltration and fibrosis in the renal interstitium, which led to a century of study of immune-mediated interstitial nephritis. In 1943, Melnick[16] reported that antibiotics would produce interstitial nephritis in humans, and Spühler and Zollinger[17] later suggested the same for analgesics, starting an expansive catalogue of drugs that could inflict injury on the interstitial compartment. In 1966, Unanue[18] described interstitial nephritis in rabbits developing glomerulonephritis. This observation refocused attention on the immunologic basis of interstitial injury with the suggestion that glomerular and interstitial processes may be related. In 1971, Steblay and Rudofsky[19] produced anti–tubule basement membrane (anti-TBM) disease in guinea pigs, and in 1974, Lehman and Wilson[20] demonstrated that such diseases could be transferred with immune lymphocytes in rats. In 1984, an inheritable model of spontaneous interstitial nephritis was described in mice.[21] This work, through to the present era, has stimulated an intense study of immunologic and cell-mediated mechanisms of interstitial nephritis with use of the tools of cellular and molecular biology.[22]

Progressive inflammation or injury to the renal interstitium typically destroys extensive amounts of kidney tissue and, as a result, usually produces a considerable decrement in renal function. Interstitial inflammation can begin either from within the interstitial compartment or as a secondary event after glomerular or vascular injury. The clinical distinction between acute and chronic interstitial inflammation can be confirmed at a pathologic or tissue level, but these distinctions are not useful in biochemical or immunologic terms because these processes are largely a continuum of protracted effects. It is also difficult to make useful comparisons of the pathogenesis of interstitial lesions between experimental animals and humans, because nearly all we know about this process in humans comes from work in experimental systems.

Whereas some forms of injury to the tubulointerstitial compartment are the result of toxic insult or exposure to infection and drugs, much of the inflammatory process is immunologic in nature; the mononuclear infiltrates that appear as part of tubulointerstitial disease lead to the release of paracrine cytokines, which collectively create a microenvironment impaired in function and appearance.[22, 23] Knowledge of such events has also led to an examination of immune effects on somatic epithelium expressing renal target antigens. That the immune system is capable of signaling somatic cells directly, as well as of just destroying them in phenotypically distinct ways, is one of the more interesting outgrowths of current research.[24]

# STRUCTURE-FUNCTION RELATIONSHIPS

Simple correlations between disturbances in glomerular structure and functional impairment of the kidney are surprisingly imperfect.[25, 26] Glomerular disease is only one aspect of the anatomic representation in renal dysfunction. Damage to the tubulointerstitial compartment is another and, perhaps, more accurate gauge of renal performance (Fig. 33–1).

The concept of tubulointerstitial damage mediating impaired renal function is not new.[17] Many studies have pointed to the guarded prognostic significance of severe interstitial disease in lupus nephritis,[27, 28] membranous nephropathy,[29] and chronic glomerulonephritis.[30] Functional comparative parameters, such as inulin clearance, maximal concentrating ability, and $NH_4^+$ excretion, are often best correlated with a semiquantitative scoring of tubulointerstitial disease and inflammation.[26]

The analyses on this topic by Bohle and co-workers[31, 32] have employed quantitative morphometric comparisons between tubulointerstitial damage and renal function. Tubulointerstitial changes were studied in a wide variety of glomerulopathies arising from disparate pathogenetic mechanisms, and decreasing maximal urine osmolality was correlated best with increasing interstitial volume, decreasing cross-sectional area of proximal tubule epithelium, and decreasing cross-sectional area of epithelium from the thick segment of the loop of Henle. T lymphocytes near or among epithelial cells were also evident in these cases. Other key morphologic components of tubulointerstitial nephritis include the presence of edema, activated fibroblasts, collagen, proteoglycans, lymphocytes, monocytes, antibody, and complement as imaged by light microscopy, immunofluorescence, or histochemistry. Some of these reports suggest that such interstitial changes may also predict the long-term prognosis in chronic glomerulonephritis.[31, 32]

The structure-function relationship between tubulointerstitial disease and renal function can be understood at a hypothetic level by several mechanisms that are not mutually exclusive. The first and simplest explanation for this relationship is that urine flow is impeded by tubule obstruction on an anatomic basis as a result of inflammation.[23, 31] Interstitial inflammation and fibrosis may also occlude the tubules and cause increased intratubular pressure. In the absence of direct measurements, an analogy may be found in rats that, after unilateral ureteral ligation, develop retrograde Tamm-Horsfall casts in the proximal nephron.[33] Tubule atrophy or debris within tubules would, therefore, essentially represent a clogged drain.

A second hypothetic mechanism implicates an increase

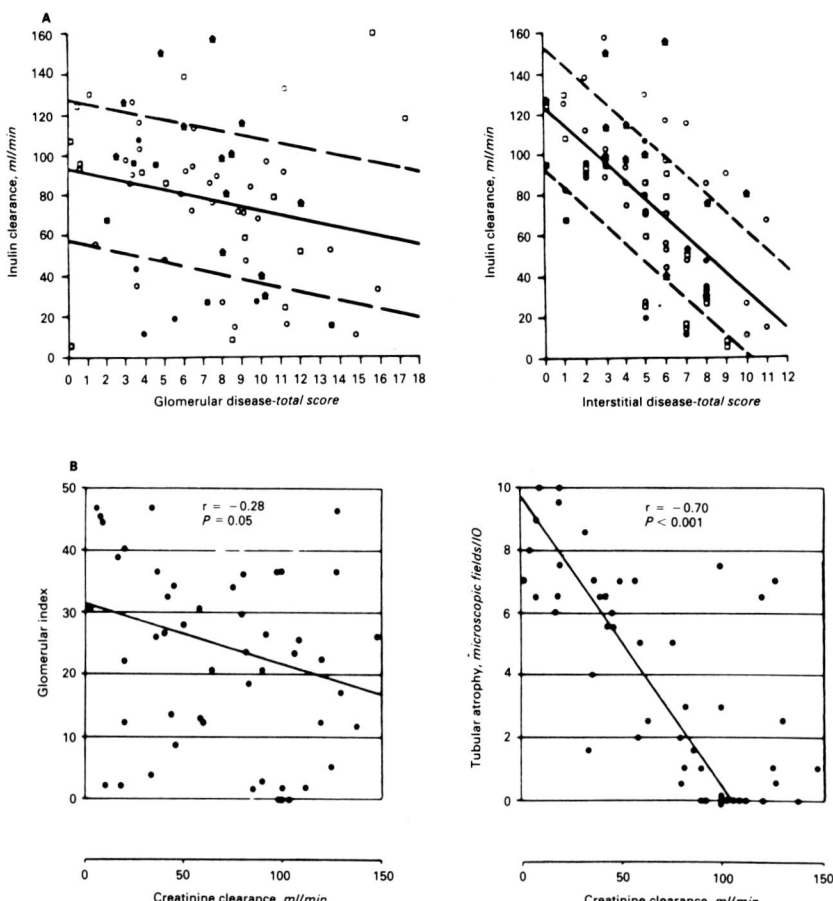

**Figure 33–1.** Structure-function relationships. *A* and *B* are from two publications[26, 30] that address structural and morphometric changes in renal biopsy specimens of patients with glomerular or interstitial disease. In *A,* grading scale evaluations of biopsies are correlated with inulin clearance (acute glomerulonephritis; chronic glomerulonephritis; interstitial nephritis; nephrosclerosis; miscellaneous); $y = 92 - 0.02x$ for glomerular disease, and $y = 122 - 8.8x$ for interstitial disease. In *B,* comparisons are also made between biopsies graded for degrees of normal architecture (glomerular index and tubule atrophy scores) plotted against creatinine clearance. The findings in these two studies indicate that falling glomerular filtration correlates better with progressive interstitial changes than with changes in the glomerular tuft. (*A* from Schainuck LI, Striker GE, Cutler RE, Benditt EP: Structural-functional correlations in renal disease. II. The correlations. Hum Pathol 1:631–641, 1970. *B* from Risdon RA, Sloper JC, De Wardener HE: Relationship between renal function and histological changes found in renal-biopsy specimens from patients with persistent glomerular nephritis. Lancet 2[564]:363–366, © by The Lancet Ltd, 1968.)

in vascular resistance with progressive tubule injury and fibrosis.[31] The volume of peritubular capillaries is decreased in areas of interstitial inflammation, edema, or fibrosis.[34] The number and cross-sectional area of the postglomerular capillaries diminish with increasing interstitial width.[35] These studies demonstrate that tubulointerstitial processes may render this compartment relatively avascular and therefore somewhat ischemic. Impairment of glomerular arteriolar outflow may also lead to increased intraglomerular hypertension. An increased cross-sectional area of the glomerular capillary tuft has been observed in cases of membranous and membranoproliferative glomerulonephritis with chronic sclerosing interstitial nephritis.[36] Increased intracapillary pressures within the glomerulus may be reflected in this change. Intraglomerular hypertension may also lead to mesangial sclerosis and glomerular damage.[37] These mechanisms are most applicable when injury is still relatively mild. For this second mechanism to achieve a credible level of effect, however, the net reduction in cross-sectional area of peritubular vessels must increase postglomerular resistance sufficiently such that the compensatory increase in glomerular hydraulic pressure cannot fully restore filtration to normal levels. Tubuloglomerular feedback can also assume increasing importance in the transition from acute to chronic glomerulonephritis when autoregulation of renal blood flow is disrupted by permanent structural change,[38] such as after tubulointerstitial fibrosis. Loss of autoregulation here, as a third hypothesis, could indicate insensitivity of the afferent arteriole to a tubuloglomerular feedback signal or, alternatively, loss of the signal. Perhaps more significant is the effect of interstitial pressure on the sensitivity of the feedback mechanism.[39] Such modulation may be transmitted through the local renin-angiotensin system or by alterations in local prostaglandin production.

In slightly damaged tubules, as a fourth explanation, there can be atrophy of interstitial regions and attenuation of epithelium along the proximal tubules and thick ascending limbs of the loops of Henle. The normal renal osmotic gradient is diminished consequently by a decrease in $Na^+$ transport in the thick ascending limb. This leads to a diminution in the abstraction of water from the filtrate and results in hyposthenuria and polyuria. Such an increase in solute content and water within the tubule fluid decreases glomerular filtration by adaptively regulating the filtering process in the face of tubule insufficiency.[40–43] Such adaptations include reductions in glomerular capillary pressure ($P_{GC}$) and filtration coefficient ($K_f$).[43, 44] Feedback also occurs in cortical and juxtamedullary nephrons and results in a reduction of renin output from the juxtaglomerular apparatus.[43, 45] Consequently, the vasoconstrictive influence of angiotensin II on the vas efferens decreases, and filtration drops from the decrease in arteriolar tone.[23]

In summary, these collective effects probably contribute to the structure-function interactions relating interstitial damage to progressive deterioration in renal function. Whereas active and acute elements of tubulointerstitial disease correspond to potentially recoverable renal function, tubule atrophy and fibrosis probably represent function lost permanently.

# MECHANISMS OF TUBULOINTERSTITIAL INJURY

## Tubulointerstitial Antigens

Nephritogenic antigens are derived from surrounding interstitial cells and their extracellular structures, or they are added to this microenvironment by extraction and implantation from the circulation.[23, 46] Some renal structures may also mimic other nonrenal moieties and become antigenic on the basis of sequence or conformational similarity. The extent of known renal antigens can be arbitrarily divided into several categories.[46]

**Antigens from Renal Cells and Tubule Basement Membranes.** Antibodies that react to cellular brush border have been observed in Heymann nephritis,[47–50] and although the membranous lesion stands out as an early feature of this disease, interstitial infiltrates and injury are also seen with time.[51–53] The antigen complex goes by several names, including Fx1A, gp330, and Heymann nephritis antigen complex.[54–57] The antigen system seems multimeric and involves more than one gene. Tamm-Horsfall protein is also on the tubule cell surface and can be secreted into tubule fluid by cells of the ascending limb of Henle. Tamm-Horsfall protein, or uromodulin, is a glycoprotein that has been sequenced and studied biochemically.[58–60] The protein can also form immune deposits along the base of the tubule cells and to some extent in the lymphatic drainage of the ascending limb.[61, 62] These deposits are associated with mild interstitial inflammation[62–64] and are most noticeable after lower tract obstruction.[65, 66] In another system, *kd/kd* mice spontaneously develop interstitial nephritis.[21, 67, 68] The antigen has been partially identified by use of functional properties of the T cell repertoire. A 56,000-dalton protein produces a delayed-type hypersensitivity response in the $CD8^+$ cell population from *kd/kd* spleen cells[68] (C. Kelly, work in progress). Finally, the antigen of anti-TBM disease is called 3M-1.[69, 70] It has an observed molecular mass of 48,000 to 54,000 daltons in humans down to 30,000 daltons in mice.[46, 70–73] There is polymorphism of expression in rats and humans, and allotypic differences in its expression among humans may occasionally result in anti-TBM disease after renal transplantation.[74–78] The gene in rats is inherited as a dominant trait and maps to linkage groups I and IV.[79, 80] The antibody binding site has some protein sequence homology with intermediate filament-associated proteins.[81]

**Drug/Hapten Conjugates as Nephritogenic Antigens.** Extrarenal antigens that form interstitial immune deposits producing inflammation either develop locally in situ or precipitate as a circulating complex.[82–84] The antigen in that deposit, however, does not have to be chemically linked to the tubule basement membrane as a conjugate for interstitial nephritis to ensue. This has been observed with members of the penicillin family,[84] with cephalosporins,[82] after treatment with phenytoin,[83] and after prolonged exposure to aurothiomalate or mercuric chloride.[85, 86] Antibodies and inflammatory cells then find these new antigens, and interstitial disease ensues in the susceptible host.

**Antigens Based on Molecular Mimicry.** Mimicry has

always held a special place in the beliefs regarding the origins of autoimmunity and inflammation.[87] The universe of epitopes, although theoretically limitless, nevertheless presents some shared redundancies among self-proteins and the external environment.[88–90] Some antibodies to nephritogenic streptococci cross-react with type IV collagen,[88] for example, and some antibodies to *Escherichia coli* cross-react with Tamm-Horsfall protein.[89] The role of virus-infected tubulointerstitial cells presenting new or modified antigen is not yet fully explored, although interstitial nephritis can appear after viral exposure.[91–94] Whereas most examples of shared epitope expression are derived from infectious agents,[87] work in the autoimmunity of DNA has also provided examples in which anti-DNA antibodies also equally recognize extracellular matrix components such as laminin[95] or heparan sulfate.[96]

**Extrarenal Antigens in Preformed or In Situ Immune Deposits.** Immune deposit formation in the tubulointerstitium can result in interstitial nephritis. Rabbits with chronic serum sickness provide a good example of this process,[97] as do systemic lupus with DNA deposits, immunoglobulin A nephropathy, Sjögren nephropathy, cryoglobulinemia, and occasionally chronic idiopathic interstitial nephritis in humans.[46, 98] The localization of such deposits depends on the charge and structure of the antigen and antibody, renal flow mechanics, the presence of Fc receptors, the effectiveness of clearance from the circulation, the receptivity of the vasculature, and many other unknown factors.[46, 99]

## Immune Response Genes

Currently, it is fair to state that most forms of tubulointerstitial disease are mediated by an immunologic process. Target antigens are incapable of inciting an immune response by themselves. Rather, antigen must be processed by antigen-presenting cells (most commonly a macrophage or dendritic cell) and presented on the surface of that cell in association with class I or class II major histocompatibility complex (MHC) antigens.[100] As a general rule, helper T cells, which induce antibody-producing B cells and effector T cells, recognize processed antigen in the context of class II MHC determinants (in humans, these are human leukocyte antigen [HLA] D region antigens; in mice, they are H-2 AαAβ/EαEβ); cytotoxic T cells respond to antigen in the context of class I MHC molecules (in humans, HLA-A, HLA-B, and HLA-C antigens; in mice, H-2 K/D).

The ability to mount an immune response to antigen is furthermore known to be a genetic trait, which often maps to the major histocompatibility locus. These immune response genes are associated with susceptibility to disease. Two decades of intensive investigation have resulted in the suggestion that the ability to respond to antigen may depend on any of four distinct processes. These processes are illustrated by various experimental models. The first model requires the proper association of antigen and MHC molecules. In this determinant selection theory,[101] tolerance or unresponsiveness is explained by evidence that some self-antigens and the available major histocompatibility determinants of a host do not constitute an effective stimulatory event. Hence, the appropriate activation of T cells is impos-

sible. This is illustrated in mice with interstitial nephritis in which antigen associated with MHC genes of one haplotype leads to autoimmune interstitial injury, but not in others.[102] The second model predicts that the presence of T cells with receptors complementary to self-antigen plus MHC product might lead to autoimmunity. Some cases of nonresponsiveness may be explained, therefore, by a lack of T cells that react to antigen in the context of MHC determinants. Such findings form the basis of the clonal deletion theory[103] and probably reflect the failure of some strains of rats to develop acute interstitial nephritis.[104] Third, in certain individuals, the lack of interference by suppressor T cells that act to specifically repress an immune response to self-antigen might facilitate the expression of disease. Suppressor T cell function is restricted by genes in the MHC. Susceptibility to interstitial injury may depend on the selective absence of these regulatory programs in some individuals.[105] Finally, T cell contact with antigen expressed on epithelium lacking appropriate costimulators may produce anergy.[106, 107] The immune basis for tubulointerstitial disease, in its simplest terms, probably represents the abrogation of tolerance to self-determinants in the kidney.[108] In other words, it is implicit that an autoimmune process must ignore or bypass the protective mechanisms that exist to preclude a response to autologous tissues.

## Antibody-Mediated Immunity

Most forms of interstitial nephritis in humans are not associated with antibody deposition. In lesions in which immunofluorescence demonstrates deposited antibody, it is seen in association with tubulointerstitial cells, along the tubule basement membranes, or as immune complexes. Anti-TBM antibodies are observed in several different clinical settings. Seventy percent of patients with anti–glomerular basement membrane (anti-GBM) disease, for example, also display a linear deposition of anti-TBM antibodies.[109] It is not known whether these antibodies recognize the NC1 domain of type α3(IV) collagen as do the anti-GBM antibodies.[110] Some cases of drug-associated interstitial nephritis show linear anti-TBM antibody staining, but the majority do not.[23, 84] Tubule basement membrane staining occasionally occurs as a primary renal disease in the absence of anti-GBM antibodies, and in this case, the antigen recognition appears to be the same as in experimental anti-TBM disease (see earlier).[69, 70] Anti-TBM antibodies also appear commonly in the setting of renal transplantation.[78, 111, 112] Most of these antibodies probably result from antigenic polymorphisms when an antigen-expressing kidney is transplanted into a nonexpressing recipient.[78, 111, 112] Anti-TBM antibodies do not predictably modify the length of successful engraftment.

Primary immune deposit–mediated interstitial nephritis is uncommon.[23] Such deposits are probably formed in situ because circulating immune complexes would be more likely to be deposited in the glomeruli. Indeed, interstitial immune deposits are observed more regularly after glomerular inflammation.[113, 114] The best example of spontaneous immune deposit interstitial nephritis is in the setting of lupus in mice and humans.[47, 115] Other renal lesions, such as cryoglobulinemia, immunoglobulin A nephropathy, Sjögren syndrome, and membranous disease, can also produce similar lesions on occasion.[46] In such cases, pre-existent proteinuria probably facilitates delivery of immune reactants to the tubulointerstitial compartment.[51, 52, 116–118] Even though hypersensitivity reactions can be part of the clinical picture of interstitial nephritis, immunoglobulin E has only rarely been seen among tubulointerstitial immune deposits.

Because mononuclear interstitial infiltration often occurs in the absence of any antibodies, the pathologic role of antibody can be uncertain. This role can be directly assessed only in experimental models after passive transfer into a naive host.[119–122] In a few but not all species or strains of experimental animal, this is sufficient to engage an inflammatory process. This selective expression of disease after antibody transfer suggests the additional need for cellular immune response genes for the full measure of injury to be seen.

The nephritogenic antibody response has been most extensively studied in experimental anti-TBM disease. The role of these anti-TBM antibodies (anti–3M-1 antibodies) varies, depending on the species under study.[120, 123–126] The antibody responses in rats and mice have provided a great deal of insight into the requirements for immune response genes in this disease.[79, 104] All mice are 3M-1[+], and all strains tested make anti–3M-1 antibodies, but only selected strains like SJL, SWR, and BALB/c develop disease after immunization, which suggests, as in guinea pigs, that other immune response or susceptibility genes are required for the expression of cellular lesions.[102, 127] Anti–3M-1 antibodies eluted from the tubules of susceptible and nonsusceptible mice have a similar epitope binding pattern, express a similar spectrum of idiotypes, have broad class representation, and are of similar titer.[122] Anti–3M-1 antibodies may even subserve a protective function in immunized mice because they decrease MHC class II expression by tubule epithelium expressing 3M-1.[128]

The 3M-1–reactive B cell repertoire has been quantitatively assessed in BN rats.[69] These studies indicated the presence of approximately 58 distinct B cell clones involved in the anti–3M-1 antibody response and also demonstrated some biased $V_H$ gene use among these autoantibodies. Epitopic recognition of 3M-1 by these antibodies was strikingly similar despite their considerable variability in affinity. Many of these antibodies also expressed a disease-protective cross-reactive idiotype. This cross-reactive idiotype localizes to the CDR3 region of the heavy chain. Computer modeling of the idiotype suggests a conformational structure largely dependent on hydroxyl groups within the CDR3 region of $V_H$.[129]

The idiotypes on the T and B cell repertoires in anti-TBM disease can also be recognized by the immune system. This recognition induces anti-idiotypic antibodies that often have immunoregulatory properties.[130–133] The B and T cell repertoires in anti-TBM disease broadly express a cross-reactive idiotype.[134] A heterologous antiserum to this cross-reactive determinant was effective both as a prophylactic regimen to abrogate disease and as a therapeutic modality to arrest the progression of disease.

Other antibody responses that have been experimentally studied and shown to produce immune deposits and exper-

imental interstitial lesions include those to the Heymann nephritis antigen complex in brush border[47, 49, 50, 55, 115] and to Tamm-Horsfall protein.[61, 64]

## Cell-Mediated Immunity

Cell-mediated immune responses were historically implicated in the pathogenesis of interstitial nephritis because of both in vivo (delayed-type hypersensitivity) and in vitro (lymphoblast transformation) evidence of hypersensitivity to specific inciting antigens.[135] Phenotypic analysis of infiltrating mononuclear cells in human interstitial nephritis of different causes has demonstrated that in most cases, the majority (>50%) of infiltrating mononuclear cells are T lymphocytes.[136–140] The remaining cells are predominantly monocytes. Significant numbers of B cells, plasma cells, or natural killer cells are only occasionally seen. In most cases, the CD4/CD8 ratio of the interstitial infiltrate is at least 1 and usually greater than 1. Several studies have observed lower CD4/CD8 ratios in nonsteroidal anti-inflammatory drug–associated interstitial nephritis than in interstitial nephritis related to metabolic derangements, granulomatous diseases, or autoimmune diseases.[139, 141] Such observations do not have direct functional implications; experimental work has shown that T cell phenotype correlates poorly with classically assigned functions in interstitial disease.[142, 143] The predominant T cell population may also be altered by immunosuppressive therapy before biopsy or the stage of disease at the time of biopsy. Corticosteroids can markedly deplete the number of lymphocytes seen in interstitial nephritis. Other phenotypic characteristics of interstitial nephritis include augmented expression of class II MHC antigens on T cells and tubule epithelial cells[140, 141] and augmented tubule cell expression of adhesion molecules, such as intercellular adhesion molecule-1. Expression of class II MHC is seen in less than 5% of tubule cells from normal kidneys. Augmented class II MHC and adhesion molecule expression on tubule cells may facilitate their ability to serve as antigen-presenting cells (see later).

It is difficult in human interstitial nephritis to define the antigenic specificity, antigen recognition requirements, or cytokine expression profiles of infiltrating cells. Insight into such issues has been facilitated by work in experimental models. CD4[+] T helper cells become activated by antigen-presenting cells expressing class II MHC antigens and other costimulatory molecules.[144, 145] This process may occur in the peripheral lymphoid system or locally within the kidney by tissue-associated macrophages or other antigen-presenting cells. When priming occurs in the periphery, the processed antigenic peptides expressed by antigen-presenting cells, in conjunction with class II MHC molecules, may either be additionally expressed in the kidney or be cross-reactive with renal antigens. Experimental work supports the notion that renal parenchymal cells (including proximal tubule epithelial cells, glomerular epithelial cells, and mesangial cells) can be antigen-presenting cells.[107, 146–149] Antigen-presenting function by renal parenchymal cells extends to both endogenous and exogenous antigens. For a tubule-specific antigen (the target antigen of anti-TBM disease), presentation by tubule epithelial cells can be inhibited by antibodies to the target antigen,[147] an effect probably mediated through transcriptional inhibition of class II MHC antigen expression by such antibodies.[107, 146–150]

The histologic appearance of human interstitial disease can vary from granulomatous interstitial nephritis with an intense cellular infiltrate to sparse infiltrates with striking microcystic change. Whereas this kind of variable appearance may reflect different stages of an immune-mediated lesion or different target antigens, it may also reflect the biologic activity of discrete populations of stimulated T cells. Some experimental interstitial lesions are histologically analogous to a cutaneous delayed-type hypersensitivity reaction. This type of lesion is frequently seen in experimental anti-TBM disease. The kidneys of these immunized animals display focal aggregates of mononuclear cells, including T cells, B cells, natural killer cells, and macrophages.[120] More intensive infiltration is sometimes associated with granuloma formation. Impressive granuloma formation in the interstitium is consistently seen when Lewis rats are immunized with a renal tubule antigen preparation derived from BN rats, emulsified with tuberculin and pertussis.[151] In murine anti-TBM disease, the aforementioned histologic appearance can be largely reproduced after adoptive transfer of a T cell clone that mediates both delayed-type hypersensitivity to the target antigen and cytotoxic injury to renal tubule cells.[152] Whereas injury induced by a T cell clone confirms that a single cell can initiate a lesion, it does not imply that other cells are not involved. The resultant damage to interstitial and tubule cells and the architecture is the end result of interactions between many cell types. A number of cytokines and enzymes elaborated by activated macrophages and T cells have the potential to alter renal parenchymal cell biology. These biologically active products include matrix-degrading enzymes, such as collagenases and elastases,[153] as well as cytokines (such as transforming growth factor-β [TGF-β], tumor necrosis factor-α, and interleukin [IL]–1), which may lead to the pathologic overexpression of extracellular matrix.[154–158]

The cytotoxic activity of renal antigen-reactive T cell clones may well account for tubule cell destruction and resultant tubule atrophy. Cultured cytotoxic T cells synthesize proteins with serine esterase activity[159, 160] as well as pore-forming proteins, which can effect membrane damage much like the activated membrane attack complex of the complement cascade.[161–163] Such enzymatic activity provides a cogent structural explanation for target cell lysis. Whereas cytotoxicity provides a direct explanation for tubule cell dropout, cytotoxic T lymphocytes may also injure renal parenchymal cells by noncytotoxic mechanisms, largely through cytokine release, leading to changes in basement membrane synthesis, altered tubule cell function, or proliferation of interstitial fibroblasts. Whether the relative expression of functionally distinct types of T cell clones varies within the course of a spontaneous interstitial lesion or whether certain antigens predominantly activate clones of discrete function remains to be determined.

## Cytokine and Amplification Processes

The term "amplification process" refers to events resulting from the deposition of specific antibody, deposition of immune complexes, or infiltration of T cells, which augment inflammation and injury. These processes include the activation of the complement cascade; the release of a wide array of cytokines and proteinases from T cells; and the attraction and activation of a number of nonspecific immune effector cells including macrophages and eosinophils,[153] both of which have a wide array of secretory products. Although these events have traditionally been viewed as amplifying damage, secondary events may also serve to quench further tissue injury.

Complement is only variably present in both human and experimental interstitial nephritis. When complement components are demonstrable by immunofluorescence, they are seen in association with deposition of immunoglobulin G and immune complexes[97, 114, 164] or immunoglobulin E and eosinophils.[97, 114, 164, 165] Complement can also be activated through the alternative pathway by ammonia, in the absence of antibody.[166] This reaction, triggered by amidated C3, may be an important one for progressive localized injury because it occurs as a secondary event in several nonimmune models of renal injury.[167, 168] Complement activation can be proinflammatory, through the release of chemotactic components, but may also contribute to the clearance of immune complexes and thereby to tissue healing.[99] Parenchymal cells and infiltrating cells can also express proinflammatory molecules, called intercrines, which act in an attractive capacity.[169]

T cell–related amplification mechanisms influence renal parenchymal cell biology through the release of cytokines. Among CD4+ T cells, discrete subsets express different profiles of cytokines (Th1 cells express IL-2 and interferon-γ [IFN-γ]; Th2 cells express IL-4 and IL-10).[170] This distinction has been widely studied in mice but also has relevance to humans. The relative expression of one subset versus another in situ may have profound effects on the expression of an immune response. Infiltration of T cells expressing IL-2, IFN-γ, and tumor necrosis factor-α, for example, might be expected to clonally expand (the IL-2 effect) and induce the expression of adhesion molecules and class II MHC molecules on organ parenchymal cells. IFN-γ and tumor necrosis factor-α will activate macrophages and lead to the release of cytotoxic mediators, including oxygen radicals and nitric oxide.[171]

## Fibrogenesis and Atrophy

The process of fibrogenesis can be viewed as an aberrant extension of normal regulatory events operating in the turnover of cellular components and extracellular matrix. Although many details of this complex process remain to be elucidated in kidney, several general features are probably shared with paradigms in other organ systems, such as liver, lung, and skin.[172, 173] In the kidney, there are several interstitial cell types that may act as targets for inflammatory mediators and whose activation is directly responsible for new or modified synthesis of extracellular matrix. Among these are tubule interstitial fibroblasts, epithelial cells, and vascular endothelium.[174] Some of these cells probably change phenotype once they are activated by inflammation.[175–177]

It appears that fibrogenic cells can migrate to an inflammatory lesion. Platelet-derived growth factor and TGF-β, as cytokines, can also act as powerful, local fibroblast chemoattractants, as does a cleavage fragment of complement C5.[178–180] Cleavage of fibronectin and collagen types I and II can also enhance cell motility.[174, 181] Movement of fibroblasts through the extracellular matrix is further facilitated by the secretion of metalloproteinases released by macrophages or by fibroblasts themselves.[182] Countering these attractants are the inhibitory fibroblastic growth effects of IL-1 and tumor necrosis factor-α.[183, 184] Finally, fibroblasts themselves can secrete TGF-β, thereby amplifying the process.[185]

Fibroblasts are a heterogeneous population of cells that are particularly sensitive to factors elaborated by mononuclear cells.[173, 174] Many of these lymphoid cells initiate a cytokine bath in the microenvironment that is either proinflammatory or counterinflammatory.[173] The phenotype of the fibroblast response seems to depend on the microenvironment from which they were harvested originally.[173, 175] Tubulointerstitial fibroblasts, for example, are less repressed in their secretion of collagen types I, III, IV, and V in response to TGF-β, epidermal growth factor, and IL-2 than are dermal fibroblasts.[175] Cytokine-induced responses for collagen types I and III in tubulointerstitial fibroblasts tend to be discordant; for collagen types I and IV, IFN-γ and epidermal growth factor inhibit whereas TGF-β stimulates the secretory process. T cells from guinea pigs with anti-TBM disease recognizing the 3M-1 antigen, for example, secrete cytokines that will activate fibroblast growth and collagen expression in renal cells.[186, 187]

Murine proximal tubule cells[150] as well as rat renal epithelial cells[188] are also capable of synthesizing type I and type III collagens and are modulated by a variety of growth factors.[175] These epithelial cells represent, perhaps, the most common cell in the kidney; in addition to fibroblasts, the tubule epithelium may be a significant contributor to the process of fibrogenesis. Epithelium also provides a basement membrane containing type IV collagen that forms the outer boundary of the tubule casement. This basement membrane structure attenuates with progressive inflammation, presumably because of a change in the biosynthesis of the tubule epithelium that maintains it. Cytokines like IFN-γ may play an attenuating role in this remodeling,[175] but antigen-binding cytokines secreted by helper T lymphocytes in the kidney can also specifically repress the cellular transcription and secretion of basement membrane type IV collagen.[158] This immune-mediated repression of transcription of type IV collagen may modulate the remodeling of the interstitial infrastructure and contribute to the process of tubule atrophy attendant to prolonged renal inflammation.

After fibroblasts acquire a synthetic phenotype, expand their population, and migrate into residential areas of active inflammation, they begin to deposit a fibronectin matrix that provides a scaffold for the association of interstitial collagens.[189, 190] In the initial stages of collagen deposition and fibril formation, type III collagen appears in greater amounts than type I. As fibrogenesis progresses, however, there is a proportional decrease in type III collagen.[191] The regulators of collagen and fibronectin synthesis are not really known, but both moieties are stimulated by the action of TGF-β and IL-1, whereas IFN-γ tends to inhibit the transcription of type I collagen.[189, 190, 192, 193] The synthesis of collagenase and stromelysin is also inhibited by TGF-β, whereas the synthesis of a metalloproteinase inhibitor is stimulated.[193] This reciprocal effect produces a net increase in the amount of interstitial collagen. The specific mechanisms that reduce or block the fibrogenic response in the tubulointerstitium remain speculative.

## ACUTE INTERSTITIAL NEPHRITIS

In walking healthy populations who have a renal biopsy during a workup of hematuria or proteinuria, about 1% will have primary interstitial nephritis.[194] Significant interstitial nephritis was also observed in a series of 8000 autopsies in up to 1% of unselected cases.[195] It has been further reported in series from single centers that 1% to 15% of all renal biopsies in patients with apparent renal disease will have acute interstitial nephritis.[196, 197] This figure is somewhat consistent with chart review data indicating that chronic interstitial nephritis accounts for approximately 25% of cases leading to permanent renal failure.[198] Primary acute interstitial nephritis is now recognized as a common renal ailment.

## Pathology

The hallmark of acute primary interstitial nephritis is the infiltration of inflammatory cells into the interstitial compartment with sparing of glomeruli. Lesions that reduce renal function are usually diffuse, but it is said that drug-induced interstitial injury is often patchy, beginning deep in the cortex.[199] Glomerular involvement producing a nil lesion in association with interstitial nephritis is frequently observed with use of nonsteroidal anti-inflammatory drugs.[200] The infiltrating cell population in acute interstitial nephritis is composed mainly of T cells and monocytes, but plasma cells and eosinophils may be seen.[22, 201–203] The T cells are of a mixed phenotype with a distinct preference for CD4+ lymphocytes.[120, 140, 204–206] Together with interstitial edema, this infiltrate causes the tubules to be pushed away from each other rather than to lie in close apposition. The tubule basement membrane may be disrupted in more severe cases.[202] Staining of the tubule basement membrane for immunoglobulin G, immunoglobulin M, or complement may occasionally be seen by immunofluorescence, with both linear and granular patterns having been reported. Most forms of acute interstitial nephritis do not have immune deposits present.[22, 23] In nearly all cases, the tubule epithelium involved in the inflammatory process will aberrantly express MHC class II antigens and adhesion molecules like intercellular adhesion molecule-1.[149, 203] Both of these determinants are important for the engagement of T cells. In some instances, this engagement enhances inflammation; in others, it attenuates the process.[107]

In the chronic lesion, the cellular infiltrate is largely replaced by interstitial fibrosis, which accounts for the irregular and contracted gross appearance of the kidney. The tubule epithelial cells are atrophied, and the tubule lumens are dilated. Chronic is a relative term, because fibrotic changes can be seen within 7 to 10 days of initiation of an inflammatory process. Chronic vascular and glomerular changes, consisting of nephrosclerosis and glomerulosclerosis, are often present at later stages of the disease, so that pathologic determination of the primary cause may be impossible.

A third pathologic category can be seen in either the acute or chronic setting, namely, that of granuloma formation.[207] In acute granulomatous interstitial nephritis, the granulomas are sparse and non-necrotic, giant cells are rare, and an accompanying interstitial infiltrate is common. The granulomas of the chronic lesion contain more giant cells and, if due to tuberculosis, may become necrotic.[208] Drugs are a common cause of this lesion in the acute setting, and most of the drugs associated with acute interstitial nephritis have been reported to cause granuloma formation.[209] Sarcoidosis[210, 211] or tuberculosis[212] should be considered when granulomas are seen in chronic disease. When renal granulomas are seen in Wegener granulomatosis, they are almost always accompanied by glomerular and vascular disease.[213]

## Clinical Features

The characteristic features of acute interstitial nephritis are both clinical and pathologic. The typical presentation of acute tubulointerstitial disease is that of a sudden decrement in renal function, most commonly in an asymptomatic patient who has experienced an intervening illness or who has begun a new medication. Occasionally, the nephritis is severe enough to result in total renal failure. It is important, consequently, to consider this diagnosis in any patient with an unexplained precipitous diminution in renal function. Several features of acute interstitial nephritis may help in distinguishing it from acute tubule necrosis or glomerulonephritis. Some predisposing factors are usually identifiable in both acute tubule necrosis and acute interstitial nephritis. Furthermore, in the case of infection, there will often be fever and localizing signs, and with drug-induced acute tubulointerstitial disease, the patient commonly exhibits an allergic process, such as a maculopapular rash, fever, or eosinophilia. The frequency of such signs has been evaluated in patients with acute interstitial nephritis taking penicillin-like drugs. In these patients, rash was present in less than 50%, whereas fever occurred in 75% and eosinophilia in 80%. The entire triad, however, was present in less than 33%.[214, 215] Immunoglobulin E levels are occasionally increased in these patients.[216] Such signs, however, seem to be uncommon when acute interstitial nephritis is caused by the nonsteroidal anti-inflammatory drugs.[200] Lumbar pain, and occasionally unilateral lumbar pain, can be seen in either acute interstitial nephritis or acute tubule necrosis.[197, 217] This is possibly due to distention of the renal capsule from diffuse swelling of the kidney.

The time course of renal failure in acute interstitial nephritis is most commonly several days to weeks. Interestingly, this appears to parallel, in the majority of cases, the kinetics of a primary immune response, with immune reactivity peaking at approximately 2 weeks. However, on occasion, renal failure can be precipitous, especially in those patients re-exposed to a nephropathic agent[218]; conversely, it can be protracted, with a steadily declining glomerular filtration rate noted over months. The protracted course is more common with diuretic-induced interstitial nephritis.[219] The onset of drug-induced nephritis ranges from days to weeks after initiation of drug therapy. A previous allergic history is only rarely obtained. A classic setting for a drug reaction is a febrile patient with an infectious process who defervesces on appropriate antibiotic therapy and in whom recrudescent fever occurs several days later.

Valuable information can also be obtained from the urinalysis because several features may strongly speak for or against the diagnosis of acute interstitial nephritis. The cumulative experience from several different studies suggests that a chemical (dipstick) evaluation will reveal mild to moderate proteinuria and hematuria in more than 75% of cases of tubulointerstitial disease.[199, 220, 221] Gross hematuria has been reported in 44% of cases, but that seems high to us. The sediment, also in approximately 75% of patients, will show red and white blood cells. White blood cell casts are occasionally observed. Red blood cell casts have been reported in primary acute interstitial nephritis[222] but are so infrequent that they should suggest an alternative glomerular diagnosis. The finding of eosinophils in the urine is suggestive of allergic interstitial nephritis. This is optimally observed by using a Hansel stain on the sediment from a urine specimen.[223, 224] Although two reports[199, 220] indicate that eosinophiluria is a common concomitant of acute tubulointerstitial disease due to drug allergy, this has not been a uniform experience.[225] The absence of eosinophiluria should never discourage the diagnostic pursuit of acute interstitial nephritis.

Serum creatinine values are usually elevated and often first draw attention to the renal failure. The magnitude of proteinuria in acute tubulointerstitial disease is usually modest and nearly always less than 3 g/24 h.[218] Nephrotic range proteinuria is not usually seen in acute interstitial nephritis unless there is a coexisting glomerular lesion after exposure to nonsteroidal anti-inflammatory drugs.[200] Many patients with acute interstitial nephritis also have a fractional excretion of $Na^+$ greater than 1.[226] They are often oliguric, but nonoliguric renal failure also occurs.[199, 220, 227] Oliguria may be related to interstitial inflammation severe enough to cause tubule obstruction and impede urine flow. Actual compromise of the ureteral lumen has also been documented in severe acute interstitial nephritis with marked edema and cellular infiltration of the ureteral submucosa and muscularis.[228] Tubule defects and tubule syndromes, such as Fanconi syndrome and renal tubular acidosis, are rarely observed in acute interstitial nephritis and are more common with chronic tubulointerstitial diseases.

Some imaging procedures may provide helpful diagnostic information. The kidney in acute interstitial nephritis is usually normal or slightly increased in size by echographic or pyelographic criteria.[218] This finding can have practical implications; for example, the patient who presents with presumed end-stage renal disease but normal-sized kidneys may have acute interstitial nephritis or another acute process. Interestingly, some reports have correlated markedly increased cortical echogenicity with diffuse interstitial infiltrates on renal biopsy,[229] although no correlation exists between echogenicity and specific lesions.[230] Acute interstitial nephritis may be suggested by such a finding in a patient with acute renal failure. Gallium scanning has also been suggested as a useful diagnostic tool.[199, 231, 232] Unfortunately, because a variety of other renal processes can similarly result in gallium uptake (including minimal-change glomerulonephritis, cortical necrosis, and acute tubule necrosis[233, 234]), and because biopsy-proven acute tubulointerstitial disease can be associated with a negative finding on gallium scan,[232] the predictive value of this test may be limited.

Many features of the patient's history, presentation, urinalysis, and laboratory evaluation may suggest the diagnosis of acute interstitial nephritis. Unfortunately, none of these findings is pathognomonic, and ultimately the diagnosis can be established with certainty only by renal biopsy. A biopsy should be performed in patients with acute renal failure who present with suggestive signs or symptoms of an interstitial process or who, alternatively, lack a typical clinical picture for glomerulonephritis and acute tubule necrosis and in whom obstructive nephropathy and prerenal azotemia have been excluded. Algorithms for this decision process are available.[235]

## Etiology

The causative factors leading to acute interstitial nephritis are usually limited to a few broad categories. In our experience, drugs are the predominant etiologic agents today, followed by infection, particularly in children, and then the autoimmune idiopathic lesions.

### DRUGS

A list of potentially offending pharmacologic agents is presented in Table 33–1. Although a multitude of agents have been reported to cause acute interstitial nephritis, far fewer are implicated commonly.[236–238] The β-lactam antibiotics (including the cephalosporins[239]) are the best-studied group because of the past frequency of use of methicillin, a drug no longer in common use.[199, 214] Autopsy studies reveal that penicillin moieties can bind to the tubule basement membrane in patients treated with penicillin-related antibiotics who do not have associated interstitial disease,[84, 240] which suggests that immune response genes are also necessary for pathogenesis. After methicillin, generic penicillin and ampicillin have been commonly implicated in acute tubulointerstitial disease.[241] Nafcillin has only rarely been observed to produce such disease.[242] It should be remembered that recurrent acute interstitial nephritis, after an initial insult with one penicillin derivative, has occurred with the use of a different penicillin, or even with a cephalosporin.[218]

In addition to the penicillin-like antibiotics, many other antimicrobials have been associated with acute interstitial nephritis. Prominent among these are the sulfonamides[220] and rifampin.[243–245] The sulfonamides have also been reported to cause a vasculitis, and rifampin appears to be

**TABLE 33–1. Acute Interstitial Nephritis**

| Drugs[236] | Infection |
|---|---|
| **Antibiotics** | **Bacteria** |
| Penicillins[241, 242] | *Legionella*[260] |
| Rifampin[243–245] | *Brucella*[261] |
| Sulfa[220, 409, 410] | *Corynebacterium* |
| Vancomycin[411] | *diphtheriae*[225] |
| Ciprofloxacin[412] | *Streptococcus*[262] |
| Cephalosporins[239] | *Staphylococcus*[263] |
| Erythromycin[413] | *Yersinia*[264] |
| Minocycline[414, 415] | *Salmonella*[265] |
| Trimethoprim- | *Escherichia coli*[266] |
| sulfamethoxazole[246] | *Campylobacter*[267] |
| Acyclovir[416] | **Viruses** |
| Ethambutol[417] | Epstein-Barr virus[268] |
| **Nonsteroidal anti-inflammatory** | Cytomegalovirus[93] |
| drugs[200, 256] | Hantaan virus[94] |
| **Diuretics**[418] | Human immunodeficiency |
| Thiazides[251] | virus[91] |
| Furosemide[252] | Herpes simplex virus[269] |
| Triamterene[419] | Polyomavirus[270] |
| **Miscellaneous** | Hepatitis B virus[271] |
| Captopril[420] | **Other** |
| Cimetidine[254] | *Mycoplasma*[272] |
| Ranitidine[253] | *Rickettsia*[273, 274] |
| Phenobarbital[421] | *Leptospira*[276] |
| Phenindione[247] | *Mycobacterium tuberculosis*[275] |
| Phenytoin[248] | *Schistosoma mekongi*[277] |
| Allopurinol[249, 250] | *Toxoplasma*[278] |
| Interferon[422] | |
| Interleukin-2[423, 424] | **Idiopathic** |
| Anti-CD4 antibody[425] | Anti–tubule basement membrane |
| Hairy vetch poisoning[426] | disease[23, 109] |
| | Tubulointerstitial nephritis and |
| | uveitis syndrome[427, 428] |
| | Kawasaki disease[429] |

most often associated with acute tubulointerstitial disease in conjunction with intermittent or discontinuous dosing. Drugs other than antibiotics have also been reported to cause acute interstitial nephritis. These include trimethoprim-sulfamethoxazole,[246] phenindione,[247] phenytoin,[248] allopurinol,[249, 250] thiazides,[251] furosemide,[252] ranitidine,[253] and cimetidine.[254]

In the past decade, the nonsteroidal anti-inflammatory drugs have also been observed to produce serious nephrologic injury.[200] It has become evident with more experience that at least four types of renal injury are associated with nonsteroidal anti-inflammatory drugs: acute renal ischemic renal insufficiency, analgesic-associated nephropathy, a flank pain–renal failure syndrome, and acute interstitial nephritis. Acute interstitial nephritis appears in two forms. The first is an occasional pure lesion, with or without papillary necrosis but without any glomerular disease. Its counterpart in 86% of cases, however, is a combined lesion of minimal-change glomerulonephritis and interstitial infiltrates.[255] Patients with the combined lesion can present with nephrotic range proteinuria, nephrotic syndrome, and renal failure. Thus, the nonsteroidal anti-inflammatory drugs, particularly fenoprofen,[256] must be added to diabetes mellitus and amyloidosis as considerations in the differential diagnosis of advanced renal failure with massive proteinuria. A further basis of distinction in regard to nonsteroidal anti-inflammatory drug–induced acute tubulointerstitial disease is the observation that signs of a hypersensitivity reaction are frequently missing.[200] The interstitial lesion can appear as early as 1 week after medication is begun but more commonly is seen after several months to a year of use.[256] Most patients respond to removal of the offending nonsteroidal anti-inflammatory drug after a few months without steroid therapy.[256, 257]

## INFECTION

Acute pyelonephritis is frequently associated with transient interstitial infiltrates containing polymorphonuclear leukocytes. In the patient who presents with acute pyelonephritis and renal compromise, serious consideration should be given to the presence of reflux, obstruction, papillary necrosis, volume depletion, or urosepsis with acute tubule necrosis as an explanation for diminished glomerular filtration rate. It has also become clear that invasive pyelonephritis is closely associated with bacterial virulence.[258]

Acute interstitial nephritis and renal failure, however, can frequently be seen in the setting of systemic infection.[22, 23] Whereas drugs are clearly the most common etiologic agent for acute interstitial nephritis in adults, studies from the pediatric literature suggest that infections, particularly streptococcal, are pre-eminent.[225, 259] The interstitial lesion as indicated by Councilman[12] seems to be a response to disseminated infection and not simply a matter of hematogenous seeding of the kidney with bacteria. This view is supported by the mononuclear character of the interstitial infiltrate and by the observation of a low rate of bacterial isolation from the involved kidney. The possibility of an idiosyncratic (or genetically restricted) response to a microbial antigen that is cross-reactive with renal parenchymal tissue is a provocative one.[88, 89] In addition to streptococcal infection, acute interstitial nephritis has been associated with the infectious diseases of *Legionella*,[260] *Brucella*,[261] *Corynebacterium diphtheriae*,[225] *Streptococcus*,[262] *Staphylococcus*,[263] *Yersinia*,[264] *Salmonella*,[265] *E. coli*,[266] *Campylobacter*,[267] Epstein-Barr virus,[268] cytomegalovirus,[93] Hantaan virus,[94] human immunodeficiency virus,[91] herpes simplex virus,[269] polyomavirus,[270] hepatitis B virus,[271] *Mycoplasma*,[272] *Rickettsia*,[273, 274] *Mycobacterium tuberculosis*,[275] *Leptospira*,[276] *Schistosoma mekongi*,[277] and *Toxoplasma*.[278] The definitive distinction between these entities is ultimately made by culture or, in some cases, by serology or biopsy.

The human immunodeficiency virus has not been shown to directly cause an isolated interstitial nephritis; however, it has been emphasized that tubulointerstitial lesions are common in this disease because of a variety of factors.[91] These include opportunistic infections with cytomegalovirus, cryptococcosis or histoplasmosis, nephrocalcinosis, and sulfa derivatives. Similarly, renal allograft recipients may be susceptible to such etiologic agents as Epstein-Barr virus and cytomegalovirus.[279] The various forms of Hantaan virus infection, particularly through airborne transmission from dispursing rodent dander, have also been growing in frequency in Western Europe and North America.[94] Renal failure from infection-related acute interstitial nephritis generally resolves with treatment of the underlying infection, and steroid therapy is usually not recommended or needed.

## IDIOPATHIC ACUTE INTERSTITIAL NEPHRITIS

Idiopathic interstitial nephritis is said to be an uncommon lesion. Interestingly, however, in one series of 30 patients with acute interstitial nephritis, no etiologic factor could be demonstrated in 30% of the group.[197] The predominance of mononuclear cells in the interstitial infiltrate, the presence of constitutional symptoms, and the spontaneous nature of the lesion all suggest a possible immunologic basis. In humans, anti–3M-1 antibodies have been observed in several different clinical settings. As discussed before, linear deposition of anti-TBM antibodies has been observed in 70% of patients with anti-GBM disease,[109] and they probably include several specificities. For example, although it is now clear that anti-GBM antibodies principally recognize the NC1 domain of type $\alpha3(IV)$ collagen as the Goodpasture antigen,[110, 280] it is not known for sure whether this is the same specificity for the anti-TBM antibodies in that serum. Several cases of drug-associated interstitial nephritis have been reported to show linear anti-TBM antibody staining, but the majority of patients with drug-associated interstitial nephritis do not have these deposits.[23] Anti-TBM staining occurs without anti-GBM antibodies occasionally as a primary renal disease, and in this case the antigen recognition appears to be 3M-1.[81] Most commonly, however, anti-TBM antibodies appear in the setting of renal transplantation.[78, 111, 112] Most of these antibodies probably result from 3M-1 polymorphisms when a 3M-1$^+$ transplanted kidney is placed in a 3M-1$^-$ recipient.[72, 104] Anti-TBM antibodies do not appear to cause predictable changes in the length of successful engraftment.[281] Unlike drug-induced lesions, the idiopathic forms of interstitial nephritis are infrequently associated with rash or eosinophilia, although fever is common.[197] The absence of obvious predisposing factors for acute interstitial nephritis should not bias one against consideration of this diagnosis in an otherwise appropriate clinical setting. Its potentially subtle nature forms the basis for many diagnostic renal biopsies.

One particular category of idiopathic patient has received special attention: patients with tubulointerstitial nephritis and uveitis (the so-called TINU syndrome).[282–285] These patients are usually adolescent girls, or occasionally adults, who present with constitutional symptoms, reduced renal function and tubule dysfunction, bone marrow or lymphoid granulomas, and uveitis during some point in the course of disease. On renal biopsy, there is interstitial nephritis, sometimes fibrosis (particularly in adults), and no evidence of sarcoidosis, tuberculosis, toxoplasmosis, Wegener granulomatosis, or Sjögren syndrome. The etiology is unknown, but a report has suggested an association with *Chlamydia* infection.[284] The prognosis in children seems to be excellent with or without treatment with steroids, whereas the course is more guarded in adults. The adult group is generally treated with corticosteroids, and partial recovery of renal function may occur over several weeks.

## Course and Treatment

As a general rule, many cases of acute interstitial nephritis resolve with removal of the offending agent. The likelihood of complete recovery, however, appears to be inversely proportional to the duration of renal failure; in one study, serum creatinine levels averaged approximately 1 mg/dL in patients with acute renal failure of less than 2 weeks' duration, compared with an average value of 3 mg/dL in those who were diagnosed and treated after 3 weeks of acute renal failure.[197, 286] Prolonged and active tubulointerstitial injury and a subsequent lack of total resolution have their pathologic correlate in irreversible interstitial fibrosis. An additional prognostic factor appears to be the extent to which the interstitium is involved with mononuclear cell infiltrates. Scattered infiltrates are associated with return of impairment.[197] Unless an offending agent can be identified and removed, progression to end-stage renal disease is more likely. In the case of idiopathic acute interstitial nephritis, although spontaneous resolution occurs, more than 50% of patients are left with residual renal dysfunction. The presence of anti-TBM antibodies in spontaneous disease may occasionally portend especially severe injury.

The primary therapeutic principle in acute interstitial nephritis is to identify the likely inciting factor and remove or treat it. An algorithm for offering therapy for this family of lesions has been devised.[235] Withdrawal of a drug or offending agent often results in improvement in renal function within several days in many patients. In the absence of a prompt response, early institution of chemotherapy may be appropriate. For example, we believe a time frame exists for the use of steroids in acute interstitial disease. This trial of corticosteroids consists of a dose equivalent to 1 mg/kg/d of prednisone in patients with absent infection. Improvement in renal function should begin within 1 to 2 weeks of initiation of treatment, in which case the course can be discontinued after 4 to 6 weeks. If no improvement is seen within the first 2 weeks, the addition of a second agent, such as cyclophosphamide (2 mg/kg/d), may be considered; if successful, this treatment should be continued up to 1 year with appropriate monitoring of the white blood cell count. Lack of any evidence of improvement after 6 weeks of combined therapy constitutes grounds for discontinuation of both agents. In the authors' experience, this program has been particularly effective in the setting of sarcoidosis. Three points are worth mentioning, however. First, no prospective, randomized, well-controlled trials assessing the value of chemotherapy in this setting in humans are available. Anecdotal case reports provide provocative temporal relationships between the institution of steroid therapy and improvement in renal function. Two reports[199, 287] looking at such treatment in a series of patients with acute interstitial nephritis similarly indicate its likely value. Second, although there are rare reports of improvement in renal function after prolonged renal failure due to acute tubulointerstitial disease, the presence of marked interstitial fibrosis on renal biopsy specimens suggests a more appropriate diagnosis of chronic interstitial nephritis and militates against the use of chemotherapy.[174, 203] Finally, the case report of rifampin-related acute interstitial nephritis in a patient receiving 40 mg of prednisone daily suggests that this drug may not always prove completely efficacious.[288] Anecdotal reports have supported the use of cytotoxic therapy in some patients; such effect has been demonstrated in the experimental literature.[289, 290] Up to one third of patients

with drug-induced acute interstitial nephritis (and more in the case of rifampin) also require dialytic therapy before resolution of the disease. Plasmapheresis, specifically, may be a reasonable consideration in patients with anti-TBM antibodies or in unusual cases of acute lupus interstitial nephritis.[235]

# CHRONIC INTERSTITIAL NEPHRITIS

## Pathology

The pathologic features of chronic tubulointerstitial nephritis are remarkably conserved among a wide variety of presumed causes. These include tubule cell atrophy with flattened epithelial cells and tubule dilatation, interstitial fibrosis, and areas of mononuclear cell infiltration within the interstitial compartment and between tubules. Tubule basement membranes are frequently thickened. Neutrophils or lymphocytes may also be seen within tubule epithelium (so-called tubulitis), with resulting cellular luminal casts; these findings are typically seen with acute interstitial disease but are not inconsistent with pathologic or clinical chronic interstitial nephritis.[291] The cellular infiltrate in chronic interstitial disease is composed of lymphocytes with only occasional neutrophils, plasma cells, or eosinophils. Rare cases may demonstrate interstitial edema, hemorrhage, and a cellular infiltrate with predominant neutrophils. Immunofluorescent evaluation of biopsy specimens from chronic interstitial disease occasionally reveals the presence of C3 or immunoglobulin along the tubule basement membrane, typically in a linear distribution.

In chronic interstitial disease, the glomeruli can remain remarkably normal by light microscopy, even when a lowered glomerular filtration demonstrates marked functional impairment. As chronic interstitial injury progresses, glomerular abnormalities are more evident and consist of periglomerular fibrosis, segmental sclerosis, and ultimately global sclerosis. Progressive glomerular sclerosis also occurs with aging, and this must be considered in interpretation of a biopsy specimen. By immunofluorescence studies, the response of glomeruli to staining is usually negative, with only occasional faint segmental mesangial staining for C3 and immunoglobulin M.[291] Small arteries and arterioles typically show fibrointimal thickening of variable severity, but vasculitis is not a feature of chronic interstitial disease.

## Clinical Features

Unless a patient is found to have an abnormal urinalysis or elevated serum creatinine level from a screening test, patients with chronic interstitial disease present either because of systemic symptoms of a primary disease (see later) or because of nonspecific symptoms of renal failure. These nonspecific symptoms depend on the severity of the renal failure but may include lassitude, weakness, nausea, nocturia, and sleep disturbances. In a series of patients with biopsy-documented chronic interstitial disease, the creatinine clearance at presentation was below 50 mL/min in

75% of the cases and below 15 mL/min in roughly 33% of them. Typical laboratory findings in these patients included non-nephrotic range proteinuria, microscopic hematuria and pyuria, glycosuria (25% of cases), and, surprisingly, positive urine cultures in 28% of patients.[291] Acidifying and concentrating defects are common. Some causes of chronic interstitial disease display characteristic patterns of tubule dysfunction (proximal or distal renal tubule acidosis) or marked early concentrating defects (primary medullary dysfunction).[292] More often, the pattern of tubule dysfunction is not highly restricted. Serum uric acid levels are usually lower than expected for the degree of renal failure, presumably because of tubule defects in the reabsorption of uric acid. Anemia occurs relatively early in the course of certain forms of chronic interstitial disease, presumably because of early destruction of erythropoietin-producing interstitial cells. Approximately 50% of patients presenting with chronic interstitial disease have hypertension (>140/90 mm Hg). This figure is unrelated to the degree of renal failure and persists at glomerular filtration rates lower than 15 mL/min.[291]

## Etiology

The pathologic and clinical scenario described in the preceding can occur in association with a number of diseases of diverse etiology. Distinguishing features of many of these causes are discussed individually in the following. For many of these entities, biopsies are infrequently performed, which limits clinicopathologic correlations. Table 33–2 provides a more exhaustive list of common and rare causes of chronic interstitial disease. Some causes that are discussed fully in other chapters are additionally listed here. A number of drugs are also associated with chronic interstitial nephritis.

### ENDEMIC NEPHROPATHY

Balkan nephropathy is a form of chronic interstitial disease endemic to areas of Bulgaria, Yugoslavia, and Rumania. Its cause remains unknown, although it has been attributed over the years to long-term lead exposure, infection, environmental agents (including fungus-contaminated foodstuffs), and genetic factors, alone or in combination. The disease typically manifests clinically in the fourth or fifth decade of life and is only rarely seen in individuals younger than 20 years.[293] Initial pathologic abnormalities may occur decades before the development of end-stage renal disease: the consensus is that this is a slowly progressive disease. There is no specific diagnostic test for Balkan nephropathy, which makes early diagnosis difficult. Asymptomatic patients typically have elevated excretion of "tubule" proteins (lysozyme, light chains, $\beta_2$-microglobulin, retinol-binding protein), increased enzymuria (N-acetyl-$\beta$-D-glucosaminidase), and submaximal urine concentrating ability.[293] Excretion of $\beta_2$-microglobulin is a sensitive indicator of early damage.[294] Serum complement values are typically normal, as is the serum protein electrophoresis, and there are no detectable anti-GBM or anti-TBM antibodies. The kidneys are normal in size in the latent stages of

the disease and become small with progressive disease. Various series have reported that anywhere from 2% to 47% of patients with Balkan nephropathy have uroepithelial tumors.[293]

### SARCOIDOSIS

Sarcoidosis most commonly affects the kidney through disordered $Ca^{2+}$ metabolism.[295] Approximately 10% to 15% of patients with sarcoidosis have hypercalcemia (even more have normocalcemic hypercalciuria), which can lead to

**TABLE 33–2. Chronic Interstitial Nephritis**

**Hereditary Diseases**
Autosomal dominant polycystic kidney disease[430]
Medullary cystic disease–juvenile nephronophthisis[431]

**Metabolic Disturbances**
Hypercalcemia/nephrocalcinosis[432]
Hyperoxaluria[433]
Hypokalemia[370]
Hyperuricemia[198, 367]
Cystinosis[434]
Methylmalonic acidemia[435]

**Drugs and Toxins**
Analgesics[436]
Cadmium[403]
Lead[403]
Lithium[437]
Cyclosporine[438]
Cisplatin[439]
Nitrosoureas[440]
Slimming regimens with Chinese herbs[441]
Germanium lactate citrate[442]

**Immune Mediated**
Renal allograft rejection[443, 444]
Systemic lupus erythematosus[445]
Wegener granulomatosis[446]
Vasculitis[447]
Sjögren syndrome[448]
Sarcoidosis[449]

**Hematologic Disturbances**
Multiple myeloma[308]
Light chain deposition disease[313]
Paroxysmal nocturnal hemoglobinuria[450]
Lymphoma[451]
Sickle cell disease[452]

**Infection**
Direct infection[453]
Malacoplakia[454]
Xanthogranulomatous pyelonephritis[455]

**Obstructive and Mechanical Disorders**
Tumors[456]
Stones[198]
Outlet obstruction[379, 385]
Vesicoureteral reflux[457]

**Miscellaneous**
Endemic nephropathy[293]
Radiation nephritis[330]
Progressive glomerular disease[389]
Aging[458]
Hypertension[459]
Ischemia[460]
Extracorporeal shock wave lithotripsy[461]

concentrating defects, depress glomerular filtration, or result in nephrocalcinosis or nephrolithiasis.

Although autopsy series have demonstrated that noncaseating granulomas are present within the renal interstitium in 15% to 30% of patients with sarcoidosis,[296] it is unusual for these pathologic abnormalities to result in clinically apparent renal dysfunction. Granulomatous interstitial nephritis can also coexist with hypercalcemia, and in some cases renal insufficiency is improved or corrected simply by volume expansion and treatment of hypercalcemia. Despite these qualifications, there clearly is a small subset of patients with sarcoidosis who develop granulomatous interstitial nephritis that leads to renal insufficiency. Some reports have also emphasized the tubule defects present in such patients, including glycosuria, concentrating defects, and renal tubular acidosis.[297] It is unusual to see renal sarcoidosis without other apparent organ involvement.[295] The population at risk for granulomatous interstitial nephritis appears to be a distinct subset of all patients with sarcoidosis. Reported cases are predominantly in men,[297, 298] whereas at least 50% (and in the African-American population >50%) of patients with sarcoidosis are women.[299] One series has emphasized that patients with sarcoidosis and granulomatous interstitial nephritis may also present atypically, lacking skin, eye, and pulmonary involvement.[298] In this series, patients presented with systemic symptoms and hypercalcemia, which suggests malignant neoplasm or infection.

The pathologic findings in renal sarcoidosis consist of interstitial noncaseating granulomas composed of giant cells, histiocytes, and lymphocytes. The extent of such granulomas is variable, but in some cases, they may virtually replace the majority of the cortical volume, severely distorting the tubule architecture.[297] Focal areas of lymphocytic infiltrate and periglomerular fibrosis are commonly seen in addition to granulomas. Immunofluorescence and electron microscopic studies typically show no immune deposits.[297, 300]

These patients often have an impressive therapeutic response to corticosteroid therapy, with improvement in glomerular filtration[298] and, on repeated biopsy, loss of granulomas and lymphocytic infiltrate. The often concomitant hypercalcemia is also corticosteroid responsive.[301] Healing of this lesion may result in interstitial fibrosis. Cyclophosphamide is occasionally used in patients refractory to or intolerant of corticosteroids.

Rarely, patients with sarcoidosis have primary glomerular disease, including focal glomerulosclerosis and membranous nephropathy. Arteritis has also been described.[302] Other diseases characterized by granuloma formation, including tuberculosis, silicosis, and histoplasmosis, can cause hypercalcemia and renal insufficiency on that basis. They do not appear to frequently cause granulomatous interstitial nephritis, although case reports exist.[212]

## MULTIPLE MYELOMA

Acute and chronic renal failure is common in patients with multiple myeloma and can be attributable to multiple interacting mechanisms, including cast nephropathy (''myeloma kidney'') and coexistent volume depletion, hypercalcemia, nephrocalcinosis, and uric acid nephropathy.

The classic pathologic changes in myeloma kidney include the presence of proteinaceous casts in dilated, atrophic distal nephron segments with surrounding multinucleate giant cells, probably of monocyte-macrophage origin.[303] The casts typically contain both Tamm-Horsfall protein and the pathologic light chain.[304, 305] Coexisting abnormalities may include plasma cell and mononuclear cell infiltration of the interstitium, calcifications in the interstitium, and amyloid deposits in the vessels and glomeruli. Immunofluorescence staining may reveal light chain deposition along both the glomerular and tubule basement membranes.[306]

The pathogenesis of cast nephropathy has been an area of investigative interest for many years. Attention has focused on the role of filtered light chains for the following reasons: 1) the majority of myeloma patients with renal failure have Bence Jones proteinuria[307]; 2) patients with plasma cell dyscrasias without Bence Jones proteinuria do not typically develop renal failure[308]; and 3) light chains are an integral part of the intraluminal proteinaceous casts.[304, 305] The current consensus is that light chains are nephrotoxic both through their ability to directly injure tubule epithelial cells and through intrarenal obstruction from cast formation.[309] Light chains are normally synthesized by plasma cells in excess of heavy chains, and as low-molecular-weight (approximately 22,000) proteins they are filtered at the glomerulus. Light chains are normally reabsorbed by the proximal tubule, probably by receptor-mediated endocytosis through low-affinity, high-capacity binding sites on the apical membrane of proximal tubule cells.[310] This process is saturable, so that in the setting of excess light chain production, the proximal tubule reabsorptive capacity is overwhelmed, which leads to eventual urinary excretion of light chains as ''Bence Jones'' proteins.[309, 311–313] Hemodynamic studies have suggested that elevated intratubular pressures account for the decline in glomerular filtration in experimental cast nephropathy.[314]

The observation that there is no consistent relationship between quantitative excretion of pathologic light chains and glomerular filtration[315, 316] has led to extensive physicochemical analysis of light chain properties that correlate with tubule toxic effects or the propensity to precipitate intraluminally. The physicochemical factors important for light chain precipitation include light chain concentration,[317] perhaps isoelectric point,[314, 318–320] acidic intraluminal pH of the distal nephron,[321] tubule flow rate,[317] and presence of Tamm-Horsfall protein.[322] In addition, elevated intratubular concentrations of $Na^+$ and $Ca^{2+}$ augment light chain aggregation with Tamm-Horsfall protein.[322] Experimental work has demonstrated that colchicine can prevent obstruction from cast-forming light chains. The mechanism underlying this effect may be due to an alteration in Tamm-Horsfall glycoprotein, because Tamm-Horsfall protein purified from colchicine-treated rats does not aggregate with potentially toxic light chains and possesses less carbohydrate than does Tamm-Horsfall glycoprotein from control rats.[317]

On the basis of these findings, appropriate therapy for presumed cast nephropathy in multiple myeloma includes chemotherapy to ameliorate excess light chain production;

treatment of hypercalcemia; alkalinization of the urine in conjunction with induction of polyuria by hypotonic fluids (if tolerated); and avoidance of radiocontrast agents, which may enhance the nephrotoxicity of light chains.[308, 321] Because furosemide can increase distal tubule $Na^+$ and $Ca^{2+}$ concentrations, loop diuretics should be used with caution, particularly in the setting of volume depletion.[317] Colchicine is effective in familial Mediterranean fever in preventing amyloidosis[323] and, based on experimental studies, may be effective in ameliorating cast nephropathy as well.

## RADIATION NEPHRITIS

It is uncommon to see patients with radiation nephritis any longer because recognition of radiation-induced renal damage has altered protocols for the administration of therapeutic radiation. Radiation nephritis can present in several forms.[324] An acute form is usually seen within a year after radiation and presents with hypertension, anemia, and edema. A more insidious chronic form presents primarily with diminished glomerular filtration, hypertension, and occasionally proteinuria.[325] There is another subset of patients who may develop hypertension within several years after radiation but have no significant azotemia.[324] A fraction of this group can develop malignant hypertension with accelerated loss of renal function. A final pattern of less severe renal injury after radiation is that of isolated proteinuria. This can first occur more than a decade after radiation and may be persistent or intermittent.[325] The common pathologic finding in those patients with chronic radiation nephritis is interstitial fibrosis.[325, 326] Because hypertension so commonly accompanies radiation nephritis, it is difficult to separate the effects of the radiation and hypertension on the fibrotic process.

Experimental models of radiation nephritis have helped elucidate the pathogenesis of radiation injury. The initial injury is to endothelial cells and results in endothelial cell swelling. Subsequent vascular occlusion develops with resultant tubule atrophy.[327] Irradiated renal parenchymal cells display impaired proliferation and are highly susceptible to multiple forms of injury.[328] At the organ level, the irradiated kidney initially undergoes a period of augmented blood flow, which is followed by a fall in renal blood flow and glomerular filtration rate.[329–331] It is possible that the fall in renal blood flow is accompanied by augmented renin release and, secondarily, angiotensin II–dependent hypertension.[332] Hypertension in some patients with radiation nephritis has been reversible with removal of a unilaterally irradiated kidney.[333, 334]

Radiation nephritis is dose dependent, affecting the majority of those exposed to more than 2300 rad.[325, 335] It can be prevented by kidney shielding or, alternatively, by fractionating doses, which increases renal tolerance to the damaging effects of radiation.[336] Even with fractionated schedules, patients exposed to other nephrotoxins (chemotherapeutic agents, antibiotics, radiocontrast agents) are at an increased risk for toxic effects.

## ANALGESIC NEPHROPATHY

Long-term ingestion of large quantities of analgesics has been associated in epidemiologic studies with chronic interstitial nephritis and papillary necrosis.[337] Because discontinuation of heavy analgesic use can slow or arrest progression of the renal disease,[338] this is an important diagnosis to make. The incidence of analgesic nephropathy varies in different countries and between different geographic areas of the United States.[339] It is a relatively common cause of chronic renal failure in Scotland, Belgium, and Australia, accounting for 10% to 20% of patients with end-stage renal disease in those countries.[340–342] In the United States, case-control studies from the Philadelphia area did not detect an excess risk of renal disease in daily users of analgesics,[343] whereas this was apparent in North Carolina.[344] These two populations differed markedly by the degree of regular analgesic use, consistent with previous suggestions that variation in the frequency of analgesic nephropathy tracks closely with patterns of analgesic use.

Analgesic nephropathy is recognized more frequently (five to seven times) in women than in men. Patients typically take analgesics for chronic headaches, abdominal discomfort, or nonspecific joint pain. The caffeine component of certain over-the-counter analgesics may encourage dependence. Because over-the-counter analgesics are widely available, the typical patient may not come to medical attention until renal failure is advanced. On presentation, patients frequently have nocturia (decreased urine concentrating ability), sterile pyuria, and hypertension. The hypertension may be exacerbated by volume depletion, which suggests that it is renin dependent.[345] Anemia is frequently seen, attributable to both the renal failure and chronic blood loss from peptic ulcer disease. Uroepithelial malignant neoplasms occur with increased frequency in these patients.[346, 347] Current clinical practice is to screen patients annually with urine cytology. A new onset of hematuria in such a patient warrants an aggressive workup.

Several generalities have emerged from the epidemiologic study of analgesic nephropathy. One is that its development requires prolonged regular ingestion of combination analgesics (six tablets daily for more than 3 years).[348] It has frequently been stated that analgesic nephropathy requires ingestion of combinations of analgesics, including aspirin, acetaminophen, phenacetin, caffeine, or codeine. A case-control study of analgesic use in North Carolina, however, demonstrated an increased odds risk for those patients with excessive ingestion of only acetaminophen.[344] Several case reports of chronic interstitial disease and end-stage renal disease after long-term heavy ingestion of nonsteroidal anti-inflammatory agents increase this concern over the toxicity of single agents.[349, 350] Whether chronic interstitial disease related to nonsteroidal anti-inflammatory drugs is an immune-mediated extension of the well-defined acute lesion or a toxic nephropathy is unclear.

The pathologic abnormalities in analgesic nephropathy are nonspecific and typical of chronic interstitial disease with papillary necrosis. At the time of clinical presentation, the kidneys are typically small. Papillary necrosis is usually present but not required for the diagnosis. At a light microscopic level, the interstitium is fibrotic with tubule atrophy and occasional mononuclear cell infiltration.[351] There may be concomitant focal glomerular sclerosis and interstitial calcifications as well.

Acetaminophen (a hepatic metabolite of phenacetin) is

highly concentrated in the papillary tip, especially during antidiuresis. It is further metabolized in the kidney to a number of reactive metabolites.[352, 353] The toxicity of these metabolites may be exacerbated by the actions of other analgesics, such as aspirin or other nonsteroidal anti-inflammatory agents, which inhibit the activity of the hexose monophosphate shunt, thereby diminishing the intracellular supply of glutathione and reducing potential.[198, 354] In addition, the inhibition of prostaglandin synthesis can exacerbate medullary damage from ischemia.[355]

## URIC ACID NEPHROPATHY

Although it is widely accepted that overproduction of uric acid and hyperuricemia (especially in acutely treated myeloproliferative disease) can cause acute renal failure,[356, 357] it is less clear that chronic hyperuricemia independently results in chronic interstitial nephritis and progressive renal failure. Historically, chronic hyperuricemia associated with chronic interstitial disease was called "gouty nephropathy." In a review of the causes of chronic interstitial nephritis in the late 1970s, Murray and Goldberg[198] attributed 11% of chronic interstitial disease primarily to disorders of uric acid metabolism and cited uric acid as a contributing factor in an additional 7% of cases. This association was challenged in the early 1980s by Berger and Yu,[358] who could not demonstrate an association of hyperuricemia with chronic interstitial disease that could not be attributed to hypertension, vascular disease, stones, or aging. The existence of gouty nephropathy received another challenge by the finding that infusion of ethylenediaminetetraacetic acid (EDTA) into patients with gout and interstitial disease elicited an abnormal increase in lead excretion, which suggests that heavy metal intoxication may be the primary event resulting in hypertension, interstitial disease, and hyperuricemia.[359]

Despite the clear associations between lead intoxication and hyperuricemia, it is still controversial whether chronic hyperuricemia alone can lead to interstitial disease. It is an important question, especially because many patients with chronic renal failure have serum uric acid levels above 10 mg/dL attributable to diminished glomerular filtration and the effects of diuretics.[360] Although underexcretion of uric acid is often clinically assumed not to be harmful to the kidney, this assumption may not be true. If hyperuricemia in chronic renal failure can accelerate progression, then it is an important metabolic abnormality to treat specifically. Lowering of the serum uric acid level in chronic renal failure can be most safely accomplished through protein and purine restriction.[360]

## HYPERCALCEMIA

Disorders of $Ca^{2+}$ metabolism leading to hypercalcemia or increased $Ca^{2+}$ turnover have a multiplicity of effects on the kidney. Hypercalcemia can decrease glomerular filtration through renal vasoconstriction,[361] a decrease in the glomerular ultrafiltration coefficient,[362] and volume contraction due to the vasopressin-resistant concentrating defect.[363] Disorders of $Ca^{2+}$ metabolism may also lead to nephrocalcinosis, with deposition of $Ca^{2+}$ in the kidney, around the

tubule basement membranes, and especially around distal tubules and collecting ducts. Such deposition secondarily leads to mononuclear cell infiltration and tubule necrosis.

$Ca^{2+}$ deposition begins in the medullary tubules, followed by deposition in the cortical proximal and distal tubules and within the interstitial space.[364, 365] In addition to frank hypercalcemia, nephrocalcinosis can occur in normocalcemic disorders of augmented gut absorption of $Ca^{2+}$ (sarcoidosis, vitamin D intoxication), skeletal breakdown (neoplasms or multiple myeloma), or classic distal renal tubular acidosis. Therapy is directed toward the primary disease, in addition to measures aimed at reducing the serum $Ca^{2+}$ level and correcting acid-base disturbances.

## HYPOKALEMIC NEPHROPATHY

It is rare for sustained hypokalemia to cause chronic interstitial nephritis. There are both inherited and acquired forms of hypokalemic nephropathy.[366–368] The inherited form is HLA linked and characterized by primary renal wasting of $K^+$, normal blood pressure, but elevated renin, aldosterone, and urinary prostaglandin E excretion. These patients have an interstitial nephritis with progressive renal failure. A pathologic characteristic of both acquired and inherited forms is the finding of vacuoles in the proximal convoluted tubules,[369, 370] the composition of which is unknown.

An insight into the possible pathogenesis of hypokalemic nephropathy comes from studies of experimental hypokalemia in the rat.[167] In this setting, hypokalemia stimulates ammoniagenesis (because of the associated intracellular acidosis), which then elicits complement activation, initiating the influx of immune cells into the interstitium.

## OXALOSES

Hyperoxaluria occurs in the setting of inborn errors of metabolism,[371] increased bowel absorption of oxalate,[372] or acute massive oxalate loads.[373] In all three settings, renal dysfunction can occur. Primary hyperoxaluria is due to a defect in either the 2-oxoglutarate:glyoxylate carboligase (type 1) or the 2-glyceric dehydrogenase (type 2). These patients develop chronic renal failure typically before reaching adulthood.[371] Patients with inflammatory bowel disease or ileal-jejunal bypass surgery have increased bowel absorption of oxalate and can develop chronic renal insufficiency, which can be progressive. Ethylene glycol ingestion or ascorbic acid overdoses result in acute massive oxalate loads and acute renal failure associated with intrarenal obstruction by intratubular precipitation of oxalic acid crystals.[373] In each setting, the pathogenesis appears to be intraluminal obstruction by oxalate crystals, followed by progressive tubule atrophy and fibrosis.

## OBSTRUCTIVE NEPHROPATHY

The etiology and pathophysiology of urinary tract obstruction are discussed in detail elsewhere. Complete or partial urinary tract obstruction is accompanied by a decline in glomerular filtration and a plethora of tubule abnormalities, including diminished reabsorption of solutes,[374–376] impaired excretion of $H^+$ and $K^+$,[377] and a vasopressin-resistant concentrating defect (nephrogenic diabetes insipidus).[378] These functional alterations are accompanied by pathologic changes in both the tubulointerstitium and glomeruli consisting of interstitial fibrosis, tubule atrophy, and occasionally focal glomerular sclerosis.

The pathophysiologic mechanism of urinary tract obstruction has been studied extensively. In models of both unilateral and bilateral ureteral obstruction, there is a fall in glomerular filtration attributable to both a fall in single-nephron glomerular filtration and a decrease in the number of filtering nephrons. The fall in single-nephron glomerular filtration occurs because of diminished plasma flow, diminished net hydraulic pressure, and a depressed ultrafiltration coefficient.[379] Mediators that have been identified as relevant to the diminished single-nephron glomerular filtration include angiotensin II,[380, 381] thromboxane $A_2$,[380] antidiuretic hormone,[382] and leukotrienes.[383] Diminished production of nitric oxide may also play a role, because dietary arginine can augment glomerular filtration in postobstructed kidneys.

In both chronic and acute ureteral obstruction, there are mononuclear cells in the interstitium.[384, 385] They are most evident surrounding distal tubule cells but are present throughout the cortex and medulla. In experimental models of obstruction, the majority of these cells are macrophages or $CD8^+$ lymphocytes.[385] The cells disappear after release of obstruction. Whereas the relationship of these cells to renal functional abnormalities has not been fully elucidated, manipulations that diminish the cellular infiltrate (such as irradiation) are associated with a less marked decrement in glomerular filtration after obstruction.[386] Because angiotensin II[387] and thromboxane $A_2$ can be expressed by such infiltrating cells,[386] the infiltrate may be of functional significance. Insight into why leukocytes migrate into a kidney experiencing elevated intratubular pressures comes from the observation that a lipid chemoattractant is released by the obstructed kidney.[388] Growth factors, such as TGF-β1, released by infiltrating cells may in addition contribute to the interstitial fibrosis[389] and glomerular sclerosis[390] accompanying chronic urinary tract obstruction.

## LEAD NEPHROPATHY

Occupational exposure to lead in the United States is currently restricted by governmental regulations. Continuing sources of exposure occur, however, from old water pipes, pottery, crystal, and lead-based paint in older dwellings. Several epidemiologic analyses support the association of excess lead burden with chronic renal failure.[391] Lead nephropathy is underdiagnosed because no simple blood test is diagnostic. The diagnosis is suggested by an augmented (>0.6 mg) 24-hour urinary excretion of lead after two 1-g doses of disodium EDTA.[392] EDTA is not nephrotoxic at these doses. Because the lead content in bones of patients with chronic renal failure unrelated to lead intoxication is not elevated, this test can also be used in patients with chronic renal insufficiency.[393] The correlation between chelatable lead and bone lead concentration determined by atomic absorption spectroscopy is excellent.[393] For those patients with low urine output, the collec-

tion times after EDTA administration can be prolonged up to several days. Blood lead levels reflect only recent, not chronic, exposure and can be normal in patients with multisystem damage from lead.[392] Despite this, epidemiologic studies have also documented a correlation between blood lead concentrations and diastolic blood pressure[394] as well as blood lead concentrations, zinc protoporphyrin, and creatinine clearance.[391]

Lead is preferentially deposited in the $S_3$ portion of the proximal tubule.[395] Nuclear inclusions within proximal tubule cells are characteristic of lead nephropathy.[396] The pathophysiologic correlate of this is that lead exposure can result in proximal tubule dysfunction (especially in children), with either isolated tubule defects or a full Fanconi syndrome.[397] These defects are potentially reversible. It is unusual to see chronic renal failure from lead in children.

In adults, lead nephropathy is pathologically a chronic interstitial nephritis, with interstitial fibrosis, atrophy, and nephrosclerosis.[398] Patients frequently have recurrent gout,[399] and the majority of the patients have hyperuricemia and hypertension. Ingestion of moonshine liquor, with its high lead content, is an important historical clue to the diagnosis.[400, 401] EDTA has been advocated as therapy in addition to its use as a diagnostic test.[392] The goal of chelation therapy is to normalize the EDTA mobilization test. In some patients, this may arrest or reverse progression of renal failure.

## CADMIUM NEPHROPATHY

Cadmium nephropathy can develop in individuals with prolonged low-level exposure to excess cadmium. Such individuals are likely to be employed in smelters. In vivo, cadmium is bound to metallothionein, and these complexes are pinocytosed by proximal tubule cells.[402] The liver and kidney are the two major organs in which cadmium accumulates. Its half-life in the body is more than 10 years.

Like blood levels of lead, the blood levels of cadmium fall after an acute exposure because of extensive tissue deposition.[403] Once a threshold of renal deposition is exceeded, excess cadmium is excreted in the urine.[404] Cadmium intoxication also produces proximal tubule dysfunction, hypercalciuria, and a high frequency of metabolic bone disease and nephrolithiasis. The major clinical manifestation of an unfortunate massive environmental exposure to cadmium (through contaminated water and rice in Japan) was bone pain (called *itai itai,* or ''ouch-ouch'' disease).[405] The tubule dysfunction seen with cadmium is not reversible. Epidemiologic studies have documented an excess mortality from chronic renal failure in areas contaminated by cadmium.[406]

The mechanism by which cadmium and lead elicit chronic inflammation and fibrosis is relatively unstudied. Some work has suggested that exogenous agents such as these, which markedly augment expression of inducible heat shock proteins, can lead to interstitial renal damage initiated by T cells reactive to an immunodominant peptide of such inducible heat shock proteins.[407]

## Course and Therapy

Most forms of chronic interstitial nephritis display slowly progressive renal functional deterioration. General therapeutic principles include treating primary diseases and identifying and eliminating any exogenous agents (drugs, heavy metals) or conditions (obstruction, infection) associated with the chronic interstitial lesion. Other prudent maneuvers include good control of blood pressure[408] (particularly angiotensin-converting enzyme inhibition) and treatment of electrolyte disturbances (particularly metabolic acidosis, hyperuricemia, and hyperphosphatemia). More specific therapies, such as chelation in lead nephropathy and corticosteroids in sarcoidosis, have been discussed before. Many of the entities discussed present with moderate to advanced renal failure and have no specific therapy. For these reasons, it is often not indicated to perform a renal biopsy when chronic interstitial nephritis is suspected, because the pathologic diagnosis will not affect therapy. With the exception of sarcoidosis, there are as yet no strong indications for immunosuppressive therapies in chronic interstitial nephritis.

### *Acknowledgments*

This work was supported, in part, by grants from the National Institutes of Health (DK-07006, DK-46282, DK-30280, DK-41110, DK-45191, and DK-42155). The authors would like to thank Dr. Gunter Wolf for identifying some of the early non-English literature.

## REFERENCES

1. Lemley KV, Kriz W: Anatomy of the renal interstitium. Kidney Int 39:370, 1991.
2. Ekblom P: Developmentally regulated conversion of mesenchyme to epithelium. FASEB J 3:2141, 1989.
3. Eustachio E (ed): Opuscula Anatomica. Luchinus, Vincent, 1564.
4. Bowman W: On the structure and use of malpighian bodies of the kidney, with observations on the circulation through the gland. Philos Trans Soc Lond 4:57, 1842.
5. Kolliker A: Mikroskopische Anatomie oder Gewebelehre des Menschen. Wilhelm Engelmann, Berlin, 1852.
6. Biermer A: Ein ungewohnlicher Fall von Scharlach. Virchows Arch Pathol Anat 19:537, 1860.
7. Pavy FW, Taylor AS: Poisoning by white precipitate: Physiological effects of this substance on animals. Guys Hosp Rep 6:504, 1860.
8. Lanceraux E: Note relative à un cas de paralysie saturnine avec alteration des cordons nerveux et des muscles paralyses. Gaz Med Paris 17:709, 1862.
9. Dickinson WH (ed): On the Pathology and Treatment of Albuminuria. William Wood & Co, New York, 1868.
10. Ponfick E: Studien über die Schicksale Korniger Farbstoffe im Organismus. Virchows Arch 48:1, 1869.
11. Traube L: Zur Pathologie der Nierenkrankheiten. Ges Beitrage 2:966, 1870.
12. Councilman WT: Acute interstitial nephritis. J Exp Med 3:393, 1898.
13. Pearce RM: The problems of experimental nephritis. Arch Intern Med 5:133, 1910.
14. Vollhard F, Fahr TH (eds): Die Bright'sche Nierenkrankheiten. Springer, Berlin, 1914.
15. Longcope WT: The production of experimental nephritis by repeated protein intoxication. J Exp Med 18:678, 1913.
16. Melnick PJ: Acute interstitial nephritis with uremia. Arch Pathol 36:499, 1943.
17. Spühler O, Zollinger HU: Die chronische interstitielle Nephritis. Z Klin Med 131:1, 1953.
18. Unanue ER, Dixon FJ, Feldman JD: Experimental allergic glomerulonephritis induced in the rabbit with homologous renal antigens. J Exp Med 125:163, 1966.
19. Steblay RW, Rudofsky U: Renal tubular disease and autoantibodies against basement membrane induced in guinea pigs. J Immunol 107:589, 1971.
20. Lehman DH, Wilson CB: Role of sensitized cells in antitubular basement membrane interstitial nephritis. Int Arch Allergy Appl Immunol 51:168, 1976.
21. Neilson EG, McCafferty E, Feldman A, et al: Spontaneous interstitial nephritis in kdkd mice. I. An experimental model of autoimmune renal disease. J Immunol 133:2560, 1984.
22. Kelly CJ, Tomaszewski J, Neilson EG: Immunopathogeneic mechanisms of tubulointerstitial injury. In Tisher CC, Brenner BM (eds): Renal Pathology. JB Lippincott, 1994, p 699.
23. Neilson EG: Pathogenesis and therapy of interstitial nephritis [clincial conference]. Kidney Int 35:1257, 1989.
24. Yee J, Neilson EG: The immune modulation of biologic systems in renal cells. Kidney Int 43:128, 1993.
25. Brenner BM: Nephron adaptation to renal injury or ablation. Am J Physiol 249:F334, 1985.
26. Schainuck LI, Striker GE, Cutler RE, Benditt EP: Structural-functional correlations in renal disease. II. The correlations. Hum Pathol 1:631, 1970.
27. Muehrcke RC, Kark RM, Pirani CL, Pollak VE: Lupus nephritis: A clinical and pathologic study based on renal biopsies. Medicine 36:1, 1957.
28. Schwartz MM, Fennell JS, Lewis EJ: Pathologic changes in the renal tubule in systemic lupus erythematosus. Hum Pathol 13:534, 1982.
29. Andropoulos E, Seron D, Hartley RB, et al: Immune mechanisms in idiopathic membranous nephropathy: The role of the interstitial infiltrates. Am J Kidney Dis 13:404, 1989.
30. Risdon RA, Sloper JC, De Wardener HE: Relationship between renal function and histological changes found in renal-biopsy specimens from patients with persistent glomerular nephritis. Lancet 2:363, 1968.
31. Bohle A, Mackensen-Haen S, von Gise H: Significance of tubulointerstitial changes in the renal cortex for the excretory function and concentration ability of the kidney: A morphometric contribution. Am J Nephrol 7:421, 1987.
32. Bohle A, Mackensen-Haen S, von Gise H, et al: The consequences of tubulointerstitial changes for renal function in glomerulopathies. Pathol Res Pract 186:135, 1990.
33. Dziukas LJ, Sterzel RB, Hodson CJ, Hoyer JR: Renal localization of Tamm-Horsfall protein in unilateral obstructive uropathy in rats. Lab Invest 47:185, 1982.
34. Ljungquist A: The intrarenal arterial pattern in the normal and diseased human kidney. Acta Med Scand Suppl 5:401, 1963.
35. Bohle A, von Gise H, Mackensen-Haen S, Stark-Jakob B: The obliteration of the postglomerular capillaries and its influence upon the function of both glomeruli and tubuli. Functional interpretation of morphologic findings. Klin Wochenschr 59:1043, 1981.
36. Mackensen S, Grund KE, Sindjic M, Bohle A: Influence of the renal cortical interstitium on the serum creatinine concentration and creatinine clearance in different chronic sclerosing interstitial nephritides. Nephron 24:30, 1979.
37. Brod J, Benesova D: A comparative study of functional and morphological renal changes in glomerulonephritis. Acta Med Scand 157:23, 1957.
38. Iversen BM, Ofstad J: Loss of renal blood flow autoregulation in chronic glomerulonephritic rats. Am J Physiol 23:F284, 1990.
39. Persson AEG, Boberg U, Hahne B, et al: Interstitial pressure as a modulator of tubuloglomerular feedback control. Kidney Int 22:S-122, 1982.
40. Peterson OW, Gushwa LC, Wilson CB, et al: Tubuloglomerular feedback activity after glomerular injury. Am J Physiol 26:F67, 1989.
41. Thurau K, Boylan JW: Acute renal success: The unexpected logic of oliguria in acute renal failure. Am J Med 61:308, 1976.
42. Wright FS, Okusa MD: Functional role of tubuloglomerular feedback control of glomerular filtration. Adv Nephrol 19:119, 1990.
43. Persson AEG, Gushwa LC, Blantz RC: Feedback pressure-flow responses in normal and angiotensin-prostaglandin–blocked rats. Kidney Int 247:F925, 1984.
44. Ichikawa I: Hemodynamic influence of altered distal salt delivery on glomerular microcirculation. Kidney Int 22:S-109, 1982.
45. Muller-Suur R, Persson AEG, Ulfendahl HR: Tubuloglomerular feedback in juxtamedullary nephrons. Kidney Int 22:S-104, 1982.
46. Wilson CB: Nephritogenic tubulointerstitial antigens. Kidney Int 39:501, 1991.

47. Salant D, Cybulsky A: Experimental glomerulonephritis. Methods Enzymol 162:421, 1988.

48. Klassen J, Sugisaki T, Milgrom F, McCluskey RT: Studies on multiple renal lesions in Heymann nephritis. Lab Invest 25:577, 1971.

49. Couser W: Mediation of immune glomerular injury. J Am Soc Nephrol 1:13, 1990.

50. Brown D, McCluskey RT, Ausiello DA: The cell biology of Heymann nephritis: A model of human membranous glomerulonephritis. Am J Kidney Dis 10:74, 1987.

51. Noble B, Andres GA, Brentjens JR: Passively transferred anti–brush border antibodies induce injury of proximal tubules in the absence of complement. Clin Exp Immunol 56:281, 1983.

52. Noble B, Mendrick DL, Brentjens JR, Andres GA: Antibody-mediated injury to proximal tubules in the rat kidney induced by passive transfer of homologous anti–brush border serum. Clin Immunol Immunopathol 19:289, 1981.

53. Gronhagen-Riska C, von Willebrand E, Honkanen E, et al: Interstitial cellular infiltration detected by fine-needle aspiration biopsy in nephritis. Clin Nephrol 34:189, 1990.

54. Kerjaschki D, Farquhar MG: The pathogenic antigen of Heymann nephritis is a membrane glycoprotein of the renal proximal tubule brush border. Proc Natl Acad Sci USA 79:5557, 1982.

55. Kerjaschki D, Farquhar MG: Immunocytochemical localization of the Heymann nephritis antigen (GP330) in glomerular epithelial cells of normal Lewis rats. J Exp Med 157:667, 1983.

56. Pietromonaco S, Kerjaschki D, Binder S, et al: Molecular cloning of a cDNA encoding a major pathogenic domain of the Heymann nephritis antigen gp330. Proc Natl Acad Sci USA 87:1811, 1990.

57. Raychowdhury R, Niles JL, McCluskey RT, Smith JA: Autoimmune target in Heymann nephritis is a glycoprotein with homology to the LDL receptor. Science 244:1163, 1989.

58. Ronco P, Brunisholz M, Geniteau-Legendre M, et al: Physiopathologic aspects of Tamm Horsfall protein: A phylogenetically conserved marker of the thick ascending limb of Henle's loop. Adv Nephrol 16:231, 1987.

59. Hoyer JR, Seiler MW: Pathophysiology of Tamm-Horsfall protein. Kidney Int 16:279, 1979.

60. Hession C, Decker JM, Sherblom AP, et al: Uromodulin (Tamm-Horsfall glycoprotein): A renal ligand for lymphokines. Science 237:1479, 1987.

61. Seiler MW, Hoyer JR: Ultrastructural studies of tubulointerstitial immune complex nephritis in rats immunized with Tamm-Horsfall protein. Lab Invest 45:321, 1981.

62. Fasth A, Hoyer JR, Seiler MW: Renal tubular immune complex formation in mice immunized with Tamm-Horsfall protein. Am J Pathol 125:555, 1986.

63. Mayrer AR, Kashgarian M, Ruddle NH, et al: Tubulointerstitial nephritis and immunologic responses to Tamm-Horsfall protein in rabbits challenged with homologous urine or Tamm-Horsfall protein. J Immunol 128:2634, 1982.

64. Hoyer JR: Tubulointerstitial immune complex nephritis in rats immunized with Tamm-Horsfall protein. Kidney Int 17:284, 1980.

65. Fasth AL, Hoyer JR, Seiler MW: Extratubular Tamm-Horsfall protein deposits induced by ureteral obstruction in mice. Clin Immunol Immunopathol 47:47, 1988.

66. Thomas DBL, Davies M, Williams JD: Tamm-Horsfall protein: An aetiological agent in tubulointerstitial disease? Exp Nephrol 1:281, 1993.

67. Kelly CJ, Korngold R, Mann R, et al: Spontaneous interstitial nephritis in kdkd mice. II. Characterization of a tubular antigen-specific, H-2K–restricted Lyt-2$^+$ effector T cell that mediates destructive tubulointerstitial injury. J Immunol 136:526, 1986.

68. Kelly CJ, Neilson EG: Contrasuppression in autoimmunity. Abnormal contrasuppression facilitates expression of nephritogenic effector T cells and interstitial nephritis in kdkd mice. J Exp Med 165:107, 1987.

69. Clayman MD, Martinez-Hernandez A, Michaud L, et al: Isolation and characterization of the nephritogenic antigen producing anti–tubular basement membrane disease. J Exp Med 161:290, 1985.

70. Clayman MD, Michaud L, Brentjens J, et al: Isolation of the target antigen of human anti–tubular basement membrane antibody-associated interstitial nephritis. J Clin Invest 77:1143, 1986.

71. Butkowski RJ, Langwald JPM, Wieslander J, et al: Characterization of a tubular basement membrane component reactive with autoantibodies associated with tubulointerstitial nephritis. J Biol Chem 265:21091, 1990.

72. Butkowski RJ, Kleppel MM, Katz A, et al: Distribution of tubulointerstitial nephritis antigen and evidence for multiple forms. Kidney Int 40:838, 1991.

73. Yoshioka K, Morimoto Y, Iseki T, Maki S: Characterization of tubular basement membrane antigens in human kidney. J Immunol 136:1654, 1986.

74. Hart DNJ, Fabre JW: Kidney-specific alloantigen system in the rat. Characterization and role in transplantation. J Exp Med 151:651, 1980.

75. Paul LC, Carpenter CB: Antigenic determinants of tubular basement membranes and Bowman's capsule in rats. Kidney Int 21:800, 1982.

76. Sugisaki T, Kano K, Andres G, Milgrom F: Antibodies to tubular basement membrane elicited by stimulation with allogeneic kidney. Kidney Int 21:557, 1982.

77. Wilson CB: Individual and strain differences in renal basement membrane antigens. Transplant Proc 12(suppl 1):69, 1980.

78. Lehman DH, Lee S, Wilson CB, Dixon FJ: Induction of antitubular basement membrane antibodies in rats by renal transplantation. Transplantation 17:429, 1974.

79. Matsumoto AK, McCafferty E, Neilson EG, Gasser DL: Mapping of the genes for tubular basement membrane antigen and a submaxillary gland protease in the rat. Immunogenetics 20:117, 1984.

80. Guery C-J, Hedrick HJ, Mercier P, et al: Mapping of a gene for the M 48000 tubular basement membrane antigen in the rat. Immunogenetics 29:350, 1989.

81. Neilson EG, Sun MJ, Kelly CJ, et al: Molecular characterization of a major nephritogenic domain in the autoantigen of anti–tubular basement membrane disease. Proc Natl Acad Sci USA 88:2006, 1991.

82. Joh K, Shibasaki T, Azuma T, et al: Experimental drug-induced allergic nephritis mediated by antihapten antibody. Int Arch Allergy Appl Immunol 88:337, 1989.

83. Hyman LR, Ballow M, Knieser MR: Diphenylhydantoin interstitial nephritis. Roles of cellular and humoral immunologic injury. J Pediatr 92:915, 1978.

84. Border WA, Lehman DH, Egan JD, et al: Antitubular basement-membrane antibodies in methicillin-associated interstitial nephritis. N Engl J Med 291:381, 1974.

85. Druet E, Sapin C, Gunther E, et al: Mercuric chloride–induced anti–glomerular basement membrane antibodies in the rat. Genetic control. Eur J Immunol 7:348, 1977.

86. Ueda S, Wakashin M, Wakashin Y, et al: Experimental gold nephropathy in guinea pigs: Detection of autoantibodies to renal tubular antigens. Kidney Int 29:539, 1986.

87. Oldstone MBA: Molecular mimicry and autoimmune disease. Cell 80:819, 1987.

88. Fitzsimons EJJ, Weber M, Lange CF: The isolation of cross-reactive monoclonal antibodies: Hybridomas to streptococcal antigens cross-reactive with mammalian basement membrane. Hybridoma 6:61, 1987.

89. Fasth A, Ahlstedt S, Hanson LA, et al: Cross-reactions between the Tamm-Horsfall glycoprotein and *Escherichia coli*. Int Arch Allergy Appl Immunol 63:303, 1980.

90. Kraus W, Beachey EH: Renal autoimmune epitope of a group A streptococci specified by M protein tetrapeptide Ile-Arg-Leu-Arg. Proc Natl Acad Sci 85:4516, 1988.

91. Bourgoignie JJ, Pardo V: The nephropathology in human immunodeficiency virus (HIV-1) infection. Kidney Int 35:S19, 1991.

92. Woodroffe AJ, Row PA, Meadows R, Lawrence JR: Nephritis in infectious mononucleosis. Q J Med 43:451, 1974.

93. Platt JL, Sibley RK, Michael AF: Interstitial nephritis associated with cytomegalovirus infection. Kidney Int 28:550, 1985.

94. van Ypersele de Strihou C, Mery JP: Hantavirus-related acute interstitial nephritis in western Europe. Expansion of a world-wide zoonosis. Q J Med 73:941, 1989.

95. Madaio MP, Carlson J, Cataldo J, et al: Murine monoclonal anti-DNA antibodies bind directly to glomerular antigens and form immune deposits. J Immunol 138:2883, 1987.

96. Faaber P, Rijke TPM, Van de Putte LBA, et al: Cross-reactivity of human and murine anti-DNA antibodies with heparan sulfate. J Clin Invest 77:1824, 1986.

97. Brentjens JR, O'Connell DW, Pawlowski IB, Andres GA: Extraglomerular lesions associated with deposition of circulating antigen-antibody complexes in kidneys of rabbits with chronic serum sickness. Clin Immunol Immunopathol 3:112, 1974.

98. Makker SP: Tubular basement membrane antibody-induced interstitial nephritis in systemic lupus erythematosus. Am J Med 69:949, 1980.

99. Neilson EG, Phillips SM: The immunobiology of nephritis. Prog Allergy 27:167, 1980.

100. Germain RN, Margulies DH: The biochemistry and cell biology of antigen processing and presentation. Annu Rev Immunol 11:403, 1993.

101. Schwartz RH: T-lymphocyte recognition of antigen in association with gene products of the major histocompatibility complex. Annu Rev Immunol 3:237, 1985.

102. Neilson EG, Phillips SM: Murine interstitial nephritis. I. Analysis of disease susceptibility and its relationship of pleiomorphic gene products defining both immune-response genes and a restrictive requirement for cytotoxic T cells at H-2K. J Exp Med 155:1075, 1982.

103. Kappler JW, Roehm N, Marrack N: T cell tolerance by clonal elimination in the thymus. Cell 49:273, 1987.

104. Neilson EG, Gasser DL, McCafferty E, et al: Polymorphism of genes involved in anti–tubular basement membrane disease in rats. Immunogenetics 17:55, 1983.

105. Kelly CJ, Silvers WK, Neilson EG: Tolerance to parenchymal self. Regulatory role of major histocompatibility complex–restricted, OX8$^+$ suppressor T cells specific for autologous renal tubular antigen in experimental interstitial nephritis. J Exp Med 162:1892, 1985.

106. Singer GG, Yokoyama H, Bloom RD, et al: Stimulated renal tubular epithelial cells induce anergy in CD4$^+$ T cells. Kidney Int 44:1030, 1993.

107. Neilson EG: Is immunologic tolerance of self modulated through antigen presentation by parenchymal epithelium. Kidney Int 44:927, 1993.

108. Heeger PS, Neilson EG: Overcoming tolerance in autoimmune renal disease. Curr Opin Nephrol Hyp 3:123–132, 1994.

109. Andres G, Brentjens J, Kohli R, et al: Histology of human tubulointerstitial nephritis associated with antibodies to renal basement membranes. Kidney Int 13:480, 1978.

110. Kalluri IR, Gunwar S, Reeders S, et al: Goodpasture syndrome. Localization of the epitope for the autoantibodies to the carboxyl-terminal region of the alpha 3(IV) chain of basement membrane collagen. J Biol Chem 266:24018, 1991.

111. Klassen J, Kano K, Milgrom F, et al: Tubular lesions produced by autoantibodies to tubular basement membrane in human renal allografts. Arch Allergy Appl Immunol 45:675, 1973.

112. Wilson CB, Lehman DH, McCoy RC, et al: Antitubular basement membrane antibodies after renal transplantation. Transplantation 18:447, 1974.

113. Andrews BS, Eisenberg RA, Theofilopoulos AN, et al: Spontaneous murine lupus-like syndromes. Clinical and immunopathological manifestations in several strains. J Exp Med 148:1198, 1978.

114. Lehman DH, Wilson CB, Dixon FJ: Extraglomerular immunoglobulin deposits in human nephritis. Am J Med 58:765, 1975.

115. Salant DJ, Quigg RJ, Cybulsky AV: Heymann nephritis: Mechanisms of renal injury. Kidney Int 35:976, 1989.

116. Mendrick DL, Noble B, Brentjens JR, et al: Antibody-mediated injury to proximal tubules in Heymann's nephritis. Kidney Int 18:328, 1980.

117. Brentjens JR, Matsuo S, Fukatsu A, et al: Immunologic studies in two patients with antitubular basement membrane nephritis. Am J Med 86:603, 1989.

118. Brentjens JR, Andres G: Lesions of the kidney caused by the interaction of antibodies with antigens on the surface of renal cells. Kidney Int 35:954, 1989.

119. Steblay RW, Rudofsky U: Transfer of experimental autoimmune renal cortical tubular and interstitial disease in guinea pigs by serum. Science 180:966, 1973.

120. Zakheim B, McCafferty E, Phillips SM, et al: Murine interstitial nephritis. II. The adoptive transfer of disease with immune T lymphocytes produces a phenotypically complex interstitial lesion. J Immunol 133:234, 1984.

121. Hall CL, Colvin RB, Carey K, McCluskey R: Passive transfer of autoimmune disease with isologous IgG1 and IgG2 antibodies to the tubular basement membrane in strain XIII guinea pigs. J Exp Med 146:1246, 1977.

122. Clayman MD, Michaud L, Neilson EG: Murine interstitial nephritis. VI. Characterization of the B cell response in anti–tubular basement membrane disease. J Immunol 139:2242, 1987.

123. Zanetti M, Wilson CB: Characterization of anti–tubular basement membrane antibodies in rats. J Immunol 130:2173, 1983.

124. Ulich TR, Bannister KM, Wilson CB: Tubulointerstitial nephritis induced in the Brown Norway rat with chaotropically solubilized bovine tubular basement membrane: The model and the humoral and cellular responses. Clin Immunol Immunopathol 36:187, 1985.

125. Hyman LR, Colvin RB, Steinberg AD: Immunopathogenesis of autoimmune tubulointerstitial nephritis. I. Demonstration of differential susceptibility in strain II and strain XIII guinea pigs. J Immunol 116:327, 1976.

126. Bannister KM, Wilson CB: Transfer of tubulointerstitial nephritis in the Brown Norway rat with anti–tubular basement membrane antibody: Quantitation and kinetics of binding and effect of decomplementation. J Immunol 135:3911, 1985.

127. Rudofsky UH, Dilwith RL, Tung TSK: Susceptibility differences of inbred mice to induction of autoimmune renal tubulointerstitial lesions. Lab Invest 43:463, 1980.

128. Haverty TP, Watanabe M, Neilson EG, Kelly CJ: Protective modulation of class II MHC gene expression in tubular epithelium by target antigen–specific antibodies. Cell-surface directed down-regulation of transcription can influence susceptibility to murine tubulointerstitial nephritis. J Immunol 143:1133, 1989.

129. Karp SL, Kieber-Emmons T, Sun MJ, et al: The molecular structure of a cross-reacting idiotype on autoantibodies recognizing parenchymal self. J Immunol 150:1993.

130. Brown CA, Carey K, Colvin RB: Inhibition of autoimmune tubulointerstitial nephritis in guinea pigs by heterologous antisera containing anti-idiotype antibodies. J Immunol 123:2102, 1979.

131. Neilson EG, Phillips M: Suppression of interstitial nephritis by auto-anti-idiotypic immunity. J Exp Med 155:179, 1982.

132. Neilson EG, McCafferty E, Phillips SM, et al: Antiidiotypic immunity in interstitial nephritis. II. Rats developing anti–tubular basement membrane disease fail to make an antiidiotypic regulatory response: The modulatory role of an RT7.1$^+$, OX8$^-$ suppressor T cell mechanism. J Exp Med 159:1009, 1984.

133. Zanetti M, Mampaso F, Wilson CB: Anti-idiotype as a probe in the analysis of autoimmune tubulointerstitial nephritis in the Brown-Norway rats. J Immunol 131:1268, 1983.

134. Clayman MD, Sun MJ, Michaud L, et al: Clonotypic heterogeneity in experimental interstitial nephritis. Restricted specificity of the anti–tubular basement membrane B cell repertoire is associated with a disease-modifying crossreactive idiotype. J Exp Med 167:1296, 1988.

135. McLeish KR, Senitzer D, Gohara AF: Acute interstitial nephritis in a patient with aspirin hypersensitivity. Clin Immunol Immunopathol 14:64, 1979.

136. Rosenberg ME, Schendel PB, McCurdy FA, Platt JL: Characterization of immune cells in kidneys from patients with Sjögren's syndrome. Am J Kidney Dis 11:20, 1988.

137. Stachura I, Si L, Madan E, Whiteside T: Mononuclear cell subsets in human renal disease. Enumeration in tissue sections with monoclonal antibodies. Clin Immunol Immunopathol 30:362, 1984.

138. Husby G, Tung KS, Williams RC Jr: Characterization of renal tissue lymphocytes in patients with interstitial nephritis. Am J Med 70:31, 1981.

139. Bender WL, Whelton A, Beschorner WE, et al: Interstitial nephritis, proteinuria, and renal failure caused by nonsteroidal anti-inflammatory drugs. Immunologic characterization of the inflammatory infiltrate. Am J Med 76:1006, 1984.

140. Boucher A Droz D, Adafer E, Noel LH: Characterization of mononuclear cell subsets in renal cellular interstitial infiltrates. Kidney Int 29:1043, 1986.

141. Cheng HF, Nolasco F, Cameron JS, et al: HLA-DR display by renal tubular epithelium and phenotype of infiltrate in interstitial nephritis (Erratum in Nephrol Dial Transplant 4:580, 1989). Nephrol Dial Transplant 4:205, 1989.

142. Kelly CJ, Clayman MD, Neilson EG: Immunoregulation in experimental interstitial nephritis: Immunization with renal tubular antigen in incomplete Freund's adjuvant induces major histocompatibility complex–restricted, OX8$^+$ suppressor T cells which are antigen-specific and inhibit the expression of disease. J Immunol 136:903, 1986.

143. Neilson EG, McCafferty E, Mann R, et al: Murine interstitial nephritis. III. The selection of phenotypic (Lyt and L3T4) and idiotypic (RE-ld) T cell preferences by genes in Igh-1 and H-2K characterizes

the cell-mediated potential for disease expression: Susceptible mice provide a unique effector T cell repertoire in response to tubular antigen. J Immunol 134:2375, 1985.

144. Babbitt BP, Allen PM, Matsueda G, et al: Binding of immunogenic peptides to Ia histocompatibility molecules. Nature 317:359, 1985.

145. Unanue ER, Allen PM: The basis for the immunoregulatory role of macrophages and other accessory cells. Science 236:551, 1987.

146. Hagerty DT, Allen PM: Processing and presentation of self and foreign antigens by the renal proximal tubule. J Immunol 148:2324, 1992.

147. Hines WH, Haverty TP, Elias JA, et al: T cell recognition of epithelial self. Autoimmunity 5:37, 1989.

148. Mendrick DL, Kelly DM, Rennke HG: Antigen processing and presentation by glomerular visceral epithelium in vitro. Kidney Int 39:71, 1991.

149. Rubin Kelley VR, Singer GG: The antigen presentation function of renal tubular epithelial cells. Exp Nephrol 1:102, 1993.

150. Haverty TP, Kelly CJ, Hines WH, et al: Characterization of a renal tubular epithelial cell line which secretes the autologous target antigen of autoimmune experimental interstitial nephritis. J Cell Biol 107:1359, 1988.

151. Bannister KM, Ulich TR, Wilson CB: Induction, characterization, and cell transfer of autoimmune tubulointerstitial nephritis in the Lewis rat. Kidney Int 32:642, 1987.

152. Meyers CM, Kelly CJ: Effector mechanisms in organ-specific autoimmunity. I. Characterization of a CD8$^+$ T cell line that mediates murine interstitial nephritis. J Clin Invest 88:408, 1991.

153. Nathan C: Secretory products of macrophages. J Clin Invest 79:319, 1987.

154. Mizel SB, Dayer J-M, Krane SM, Mergenhagen SE: Stimulation of rheumatoid synovial cell collagenase and prostaglandin production by partially purified lymphocyte activating factor (interleukin 1). Proc Natl Acad Sci USA 78:2474, 1981.

155. Roberts AB, Sporn MB, Assoian RK, et al: Transforming growth factor type β: Rapid induction of fibrosis and angiogenesis in vivo and stimulation of collagen formation in vitro. Proc Natl Acad Sci USA 83:4167, 1986.

156. Sporn MB, Roberts AB: Peptide growth factors are multifunctional. Nature 332:217, 1988.

157. Beutler B, Cerami A: Cachectin and tumour necrosis factor as two sides of the same biological coin. Nature 320:584, 1986.

158. Haverty TP, Kelly CJ, Hoyer JR, et al: Tubular antigen-binding proteins repress transcription of type IV collagen in the autoimmune target epithelium of experimental interstitial nephritis. J Clin Invest 89:517, 1992.

159. Masson D, Tschopp J: A family of serine esterases in lytic granules of cytolytic T lymphocytes. Cell 49:679, 1987.

160. Gershenfeld HK, Weissman IL: Cloning of a cDNA for a T cell–specific serine protease from a cytotoxic T lymphocyte. Science 232:854, 1986.

161. Lowrey DM, Aebischer T, Olsen K, et al: Cloning, analysis, and expression of murine perforin 1 cDNA, a component of cytolytic T cell granules with homology to complement component C9. Proc Natl Acad Sci USA 86:247, 1989.

162. Podack ER, Young J. D-E, Cohn ZA: Isolation and biochemical and functional characterization of perforin 1 from cytolytic T cell granules. Proc Natl Acad Sci USA 82:8629, 1985.

163. Zalman LS, Martin DE, Jung G, Muller-Eberhard HJ: The cytolytic protein of human lymphocytes related to the ninth component (C9) of human complement: Isolation from anti-CD3 activated peripheral blood mononuclear cells. Proc Natl Acad Sci USA 84:2426, 1987.

164. Couser WG: Mechanisms of glomerular injury: An overview. Semin Nephrol 11:254, 1991.

165. Hyun J, Galen MA: Acute interstitial nephritis. A case characterized by increase in serum IgG, IgM, and IgE concentrations. Eosinophilia, and IgE deposition in renal tubules. Arch Intern Med 141:679, 1981.

166. Nath KA, Hostetter MK, Hostetter TH: Pathophysiology of chronic tubulo-interstitial disease in rats. Interactions of dietary acid load, ammonia, and complement C3. J Clin Invest 76:667, 1985.

167. Tolins JP, Hostetter MK, Hostetter TH: Hypokalemic nephropathy in the rat: Role of ammonia in chronic tubular injury. J Clin Invest 79:1447, 1987.

168. Clark EC, Nath KA, Hostetter MK, Hostetter TH: Role of ammonia in tubulointerstitial injury. Miner Electrolyte Metab 16:315, 1990.

169. Heeger PGW, Sun MJ, Meyers C, et al: Isolation and characteriza-

tion of cDNA from renal tubular cells encoding Murine Rantes, a small cytokine from the Scy superfamily. Kidney Int 41:220, 1992.

170. Mossman TR, Coffman RL: TH1 and TH2 cells: Different patterns of lymphokine secretion lead to different functional properties. Annu Rev Immunol 7:145, 1989.

171. Nathan C: Nitric oxide as a secretory product of mammalian cells. FASEB J 6:3051, 1992.

172. Libby P, Friedman GB, Saloman RN: Cytokines as modulators of cell proliferation in fibrotic diseases. Am Rev Respir Dis 140:1114, 1989.

173. Freundlich B, Bomalaski JS, Neilson EG, Jimenez SA: Immune regulation of fibroblast proliferation and collagen synthesis by soluble factors from mononuclear cells. Immunol Today 7:303, 1986.

174. Kuncio GS, Neilson EG, Haverty TP: Mechanisms of tubulointerstitial fibrosis. Kidney Int 41:550, 1992.

175. Alvarez RJ, Haverty TP, Watanabe M, et al: Biosynthetic and proliferative heterogeneity of anatomically distinct fibroblasts probed with paracrine cytokines. Kidney Int 41:14, 1992.

176. Muller GA, Rodemann HP: Characterization of human renal fibroblasts in health and disease: I. Immunophenotyping of cultured tubular epithelial cells and fibroblasts derived from kidneys with histologically proven interstitial fibrosis. Am J Kidney Dis 17:680, 1991.

177. Rodemann HP, Muller GA: Characterization of human renal fibroblasts in health and disease: II. In vitro growth, differentiation, and collagen synthesis of fibroblasts from kidneys with interstitial fibrosis. Am J Kidney Dis 17:684, 1991.

178. Postlethwaite AE, Snyderman R, Kang AH: Generation of a fibroblast chemotactic factor in serum by activation of complement. J Clin Invest 64:1379, 1979.

179. Shimokado K, Raines EW, Madtes DK, et al: A significant part of macrophage-derived growth factor consists of at least two forms of PDGF. Cell 43:277, 1985.

180. Wahl S, Hunt D, Wakefield L, et al: Transforming growth factor beta (TGF-β) induces monocyte chemotaxis and growth factor production. Proc Natl Acad Sci USA 84:5788, 1987.

181. Postlethwaite AE, Seyer JM, Kang AH: Chemotactic attraction of human fibroblasts to type I, II, III collagens and collagen-derived peptides. Proc Natl Acad Sci USA 75:871, 1978.

182. Wahl LM, Winter CC: Regulation of guinea pig macrophage collagenase production by dexamethasone and colchicine. Arch Biochem Biophys 230:661, 1984.

183. Schidt JA, Mizel SB, Cohen D, Green I: Interleukin-1, a potential regulator of fibroblast proliferation. J Immunol 128:2177, 1982.

184. Vilcek J, Palombell VJ, Hinriksen-DeStefano D, et al: Fibroblast growth enhancing activity of tumor necrosis factor and its relationship to other polypeptide growth factors. J Exp Med 163:632, 1986.

185. Roberts A, Flanders KC, Kondaiah P, et al: Transforming growth factor β: Biochemistry and roles in embryogenesis, tissue repair and remodeling, and carcinogenesis. Recent Prog Horm Res 44:57, 1988.

186. Neilson EG, Jimenez SA, Phillips SM: Cell-mediated immunity in interstitial nephritis. III. T lymphocyte–mediated fibroblast proliferation and collagen synthesis: An immune mechanism for renal fibrogenesis. J Immunol 125:1708, 1980.

187. Neilson EG, Phillips SM, Jimenez S: Lymphokine modulation of fibroblast proliferation. J Immunol 128:1484, 1982.

188. Creely JJ, Commers PA, Haralson MA: Synthesis of type III collagen by cultured kidney epithelial cells. Connect Tissue Res 18:107, 1988.

189. Bornstein P, Sage H: Regulation of collagen gene expression. Prog Nucleic Acid Res Mol Biol 37:67, 1989.

190. Vaheri A, Salonen E-M, Varito T: Fibronectin in formation and degradation of the pericellular matrix. Ciba Found Symp 114:111, 1985.

191. Wahl SM: Fibrosis: Bacterial-cell-wall–induced hepatic granulomas. *In* Gallin JI, Goldstein IM, Snyderman R, et al (eds): Inflammation: Basic Principles and Clinical Correlates. Raven Press, New York, 1988, p 841.

192. Dean DC, Newby RF, Bourgeois J: Regulation of fibronectin biosynthesis by dexamethasone, transforming growth factor β, cAMP in human cell lines. J Cell Biol 106:2159, 1988.

193. Kerr LD, Miller DB: TGFβ-1 inhibition of transin/stromelysin gene expression is mediated through a fos binding sequence. Cell 61:267, 1990.

194. Pettersson E, von Bonsdorff M, Tornroth T, Lindholm H: Nephritis among young Finnish men. Clin Nephrol 22:217, 1984.

195. Zollinger HU, Mihatsch MJ: Morphology of acute interstitial nephropathies. Contrib Nephrol 16:118, 1979.

196. Wilson DB: Value of renal biopsy in acute intrinsic renal failure. Br Med J 2:447, 1978.

197. Laberke HG, Bohle A: Acute interstitial nephritis: Correlations between clinical and morphological findings. Clin Nephrol 14:263, 1980.

198. Murray T, Goldberg M: Chronic interstitial nephritis: Etiologic factors. Ann Intern Med 82:453, 1975.

199. Galpin JE, Shinaberger JH, Stanley TM, et al: Acute interstitial nephritis due to methicillin. Am J Med 65:756, 1978.

200. Murray MD, Brater DC: Renal toxicity of the nonsteroidal anti-inflammatory drugs. Annu Rev Pharmacol Toxicol 33:435, 1993.

201. Cameron JS: Tubular and interstitial factors in the progression of glomerulonephritis. Pediatr Nephrol 6:292, 1992.

202. Olsen TS, Wassef NF, Olsen HS, Hansen HE: Ultrastructure of the kidney in acute interstitial nephritis. Ultrastruct Pathol 10:1, 1986.

203. Muller GA, Markovic-Lipkovski J, Rodemann HP: The progression of renal diseases: On the pathogenesis of renal interstitial fibrosis. Klin Wochenschr 69:576, 1991.

204. Muller GA, Muller CA, Markovic LJ, et al: Renal, major histocompatibility complex antigens and cellular components in rapidly progressive glomerulonephritis identified by monoclonal antibodies. Nephron 49:132, 1988.

205. Patel R, Connor G, Patel DR, et al: T cell subsets in idiopathic glomerulonephritis. Int Arch Allergy Appl Immunol 79:182, 1986.

206. Saito T, Atkins RC: Contribution of mononuclear leucocytes to the progression of experimental focal glomerular sclerosis. Kidney Int 37:1076, 1990.

207. Langer KH, Thoenes W: Characterization of cells involved in the formation of granuloma. An ultrastructural study on macrophages, epitheloid cells, and giant cells in experimental tubulo-interstitial nephritis. Virchows Arch [B] 36:177, 1981.

208. Mignon F, Mery JP, Mougenot B, et al: Granulomatous interstitial nephritis. Adv Nephrol 13:219, 1984.

209. Singer DR, Simpson JG, Catto GR, Johnston AW: Drug hypersensitivity causing granulomatous interstitial nephritis. Am J Kidney Dis 11:357, 1988.

210. van Dorp WT, Jie K, Lobatto S, et al: Renal failure due to granulomatous interstitial nephritis after pulmonary sarcoidosis. Nephrol Dial Transplant 2:573, 1987.

211. Hannedouche T, Grateau G, Noel LH, et al: Renal granulomatous sarcoidosis: Report of six cases. Nephrol Dial Transplant 5:18, 1990.

212. Somvanshi PP, Patni PD, Khan MA: Renal involvement in chronic pulmonary tuberculosis. Indian J Med Sci 43:55, 1989.

213. Fannin SW, Hagley MT, Seibert JD, Koenig TJ: Bronchocentric granulomatosis, acute renal failure, and high titer antineutrophil cytoplasmic antibodies: Possible variants of Wegener's granulomatosis. J Rheumatol 20:507, 1993.

214. Ditlove J, Werdmann P, Bernstein M, Massry SG: Methicillin nephritis. Medicine (Baltimore) 56:483, 1977.

215. Appel GB, Garvey G, Silva F, et al: Acute intestinal nephritis due to amoxicillin therapy. Nephron 27:313, 1981.

216. Ooi BS, Pesce AJ, First MR, et al: IgE levels in interstitial nephritis. Lancet 1:1254, 1974.

217. van Ypersele de Strihou C: Acute oliguric interstitial nephritis. Kidney Int 16:751, 1979.

218. Appel GB, Kunis CL: Acute tubulointerstitial nephritis. Contemp Issues Nephrol 10:151, 1983.

219. Lyons H, Pinn VW, Cortell S, et al: Allergic interstitial nephritis causing reversible renal failure in four patients with idiopathic nephrotic syndrome. N Engl J Med 288:124, 1973.

220. Linton AL, Clark WF, Driedger AA, et al: Acute interstitial nephritis due to drugs: Review of the literature with a report of nine cases. Ann Intern Med 93:735, 1980.

221. Ooi BS, Jao W, First MR, et al: Acute interstitial nephritis. A clinical and pathologic study based on renal biopsies. Am J Med 59:614, 1975.

222. Sigala JF, Biava CG, Hulter HN: Red blood cell casts in acute interstitial nephritis. Arch Intern Med 138:1419, 1978.

223. Corwin HL, Bray RA, Haber MH: The detection and interpretation of urinary eosinophils. Arch Pathol Lab Med 113:1256, 1989.

224. Nolan CR 3, Anger MS, Kelleher SP: Eosinophiluria—a new method of detection and definition of the clinical spectrum. N Engl J Med 315:1516, 1986.

225. Ellis D, Fried WA, Yunis EJ, Blau EB: Acute interstitial nephritis in children: A report of 13 cases and review of the literature. Pediatrics 67:862, 1981.

226. Lins RL, Verpooten GA, De Clerck DS, De Broe ME: Urinary indices in acute interstitial nephritis. Clin Nephrol 26:131, 1986.

227. van Ypersele de Strihou C, Vandenbroucke JM, Levy M, et al: Diagnosis of epidemic and sporadic interstitial nephritis due to Hantaan-like virus in Belgium. Lancet 2:1493, 1983. Letter.

228. Simenhoff ML, Guild WR, Dammin GJ: Acute diffuse interstitial nephritis. Review of the literature and case report. Am J Med 44:618, 1968.

229. Rosenfield AT, Siegel NJ: Renal parenchymal disease: Histopathologic-sonographic correlation. Am J Radiol 137:793, 1981.

230. Patel PJ: Renal parenchymal disease: Histopathologic-sonographic correlation. Urol Int 41:289, 1986.

231. Wood BC, Sharma JN, Germann DR, et al: Gallium citrate Ga 67 imaging in noninfectious interstitial nephritis. Arch Intern Med 138:1665, 1978.

232. Graham GD, Lundy MM, Moreno AJ: Failure of gallium-67 scintigraphy to identify reliably noninfectious interstitial nephritis: Concise communication. J Nucl Med 24:568, 1983.

233. Kumar B: Significance of delayed 67-gallium localization in the kidneys. J Nucl Med 17:872, 1976.

234. Linton AL, Richmond JM, Clark WF, et al: Gallium67 scintigraphy in the diagnosis of acute renal disease. Clin Nephrol 24:84, 1985.

235. Heeger P, Neilson EG: 1992. Treatment of interstitial nephritis. In Glassock R (ed): Current Therapy in Nephrology and Hypertension, Vol 3. BC Decker, Philadelphia, 1992, p 108.

236. Murray KM, Keane WR: Review of drug-induced acute interstitial nephritis. Pharmacotherapy 12:462, 1992.

237. Paller MS: Drug-induced nephropathies. Med Clin North Am 74:909, 1990.

238. Jorkasky DK, Singer I: Drug-induced tubulo-interstitial nephritis: Special cases. Semin Nephrol 8:62, 1988.

239. Quin JD: The nephrotoxicity of cephalosporins. Adverse Drug React Acute Poisoning Rev 8:63, 1989.

240. Colvin RB, Burton JR, Hyslop NE Jr, et al: Penicillin-associated interstitial nephritis. Ann Intern Med 81:404, 1974. Letter.

241. Appel GB: A decade of penicillin related acute interstitial nephritis—more questions than answers. Clin Nephrol 13:151, 1980.

242. Guharoy SR, Kar S, McGalliard J: Suspected nafcillin-induced interstitial nephritis. Ann Pharmacother 27:170, 1993.

243. Gabow PA, Lacher JW, Neff TA: Tubulointerstitial and glomerular nephritis associated with rifampin. Report of a case. JAMA 235:2517, 1976.

244. Katz MD, Lor E: Acute interstitial nephritis associated with intermittent rifampin use. Drug Intell Clin Pharm 20:789, 1986.

245. Neugarten J, Gallo GR, Baldwin DS: Rifampin-induced nephrotic syndrome and acute interstitial nephritis. Am J Nephrol 3:38, 1983.

246. Smith EJ, Light JA, Filo RS, Yum MN: Interstitial nephritis caused by trimethoprim-sulfamethoxazole in renal transplant recipients. JAMA 244:360, 1980.

247. Storch D, Christmann D, Vetter JM, et al: Acute nephritis and allergic vasculitis due to pheninindione [author's translation]. Sem Hop Paris 55:1330, 1979.

248. Hoffman EW: Phenytoin-induced interstitial nephritis. South Med J 74:1160, 1981.

249. Arellano F, Sacristan JA: Allopurinol hypersensitivity syndrome: A review. Ann Pharmacother 27:337, 1993.

250. Magner P, Sweet J, Bear RA: Granulomatous interstitial nephritis associated with allopurinol therapy. Can Med Assoc J 135:496, 1986.

251. Magil AB, Ballon HS, Cameron EC, Rae A: Acute interstitial nephritis associated with thiazide diuretics. Clinical and pathologic observations in three cases. Am J Med 69:939, 1980.

252. Jennings M, Shortland JR, Maddocks JL: Interstitial nephritis associated with furosemide. J R Soc Med 79:239, 1986.

253. Gaughan WJ, Sheth VR, Francos GC, et al: Ranitidine-induced acute interstitial nephritis with epithelial cell foot process fusion. Am J Kidney Dis 22:337, 1993.

254. Ozawa TT, Smith P Jr, Vance D, et al: Acute interstitial nephritis induced by cimetidine. J Tenn Med Assoc 80:411, 1987.

255. Pirani CL, Valeri A, D'Agati V, Appel GB: Renal toxicity of nonsteroidal anti-inflammatory drugs. Contrib Nephrol 55:159, 1987.

256. Porile JL, Bakris GL, Garella S: Acute interstitial nephritis with

glomerulopathy due to nonsteroidal anti-inflammatory agents: A review of its clinical spectrum and effects of steroid therapy. J Clin Pharmacol 30:468, 1990.

257. Brezin JH, Katz SM, Schwartz AB, Chinitz JL: Reversible renal failure and nephrotic syndrome associated with non-steroidal anti-inflammatory drugs. N Engl J Med 310:1271, 1979.

258. Svanborg C, de Man P, Sandberg T: Renal involvement in urinary tract infection. Kidney Int 39:541, 1991.

259. Burghard R, Brandis M, Hoyer PF, et al: Acute interstitial nephritis in childhood. Eur J Pediatr 142:103, 1984.

260. Haines JD Jr, Calhoon H: Interstitial nephritis in a patient with Legionnaires' disease. Postgrad Med 81:77, 1987.

261. Patino R, Blanco J, Yubero B: Interstitial nephritis caused by *Brucella*. Rev Clin Esp 129:93, 1973.

262. Haddow JE, Robotham JL: Acute interstitial nephritis in children—a process produced by streptococcal infection and by chemotherapeutic agents. A review. J Maine Med Assoc 69:1, 1978.

263. Martinez-Costa X, Ribera E, Segarra A, et al: Acute interstitial nephritis secondary to tricuspid endocarditis caused by *Staphylococcus aureus*. Ann Med Interne 6:595, 1989.

264. Sato T: Acute renal failure due to interstitial nephritis associated with *Yersinia pseudotuberculosis* infection. Pediatr Nephrol 7:327, 1993. Letter.

265. Laing RB, Nathwani D, Adamson DJ: *Salmonella typhimurium* infection leading to acute interstitial nephritis. Infection 19:254, 1991. Letter.

266. Singhal PC, Horowitz B, Molho L: Acute interstitial nephritis following Enterobacteriaceae sepsis. Ann Allergy 61:205, 1988.

267. Rautelin HI, Outinen AV, Kosunen TW: Tubulointerstitial nephritis as a complication of *Campylobacter jejuni* enteritis. Scand J Nephrol 21:151, 1987.

268. Kopolovic J, Pinkus G, Rosen S: Interstitial nephritis in infectious mononucleosis. Am J Kidney Dis 12:76, 1988.

269. Silbert PL, Matz LR, Christiansen K, et al: Herpes simplex virus interstitial nephritis in a renal allograft [see comments]. Clin Nephrol 33:264, 1990.

270. Rosen S, Harmon W, Krensky AM, et al: Tubulo-interstitial nephritis associated with polyomavirus (BK type) infection. N Engl J Med 308:1192, 1983.

271. Jones JM, Davison AM: Persistent infection as a cause of renal disease in patients submitted to renal biopsy: A report from the Glomerulonephritis Registry of the United Kingdom MRC. Q J Med 58:123, 1986.

272. Pasternack A, Helin H, Vanttinen T: Acute tubulointerstitial nephritis in a patient with *Mycoplasma pneumoniae* infection. Scand J Infect Dis 11:85, 1979.

273. Walker DH, Mattern WD: Acute renal failure in Rocky Mountain spotted fever. Arch Intern Med 139:443, 1979.

274. Schumann V, Fritschka E, Helmchen U, et al: Interstitial nephritis in typhus. Dtsch Med Wochenschr 118:893, 1993.

275. al-Sulaiman MH, Dhar JM, al-Hasani MK, et al: Tuberculous interstitial nephritis after kidney transplantation. Transplantation 50:162, 1990.

276. Lai KN, Aarons I, Woodroffe AJ, Clarkson AR: Renal lesions in leptospirosis. Aust N Z J Med 12:276, 1982.

277. Byram JE, von Lichtenberg F: Experimental infection with *Schistosoma mekongi* in laboratory animals: Parasitological and pathological findings. Malacological Rev 2:125, 1980.

278. Guignard JP, Torrado A: Interstitial nephritis with toxoplasmosis. J Pediatr 85:381, 1974.

279. Rubin RH, Wolfson JS, Cosimi AB, Tolkoff-Rubin NE: Infection in the renal transplant recipient. Am J Med 70:405, 1981.

280. Neilson EG, Kalluri R, Sun MJ, et al: Specificity of Goodpasture antibodies for the recombinant noncollagenous (NC1) domains of type IV collagen. J Biol Chem 268:8402, 1993.

281. Kelly CJ, Roth DA, Meyers CM: Immune recognition and response to the renal interstitium. Kidney Int 39:518, 1991.

282. Burnier M, Jaeger P, Campiche M, Wauters JP: Idiopathic acute interstitial nephritis and uveitis in the adult. Report of 1 case and review of the literature. Am J Nephrol 6:312, 1986.

283. Riminton S, O'Donnell J: Tubulo-interstitial nephritis and uveitis (TINU) syndrome in an adult. Aust N Z J Med 23:57, 1993. Letter.

284. Stupp R, Mihatsch MJ, Matter L, Streuli RA: Acute tubulo-interstitial nephritis with uveitis (TINU syndrome) in a patient with serologic evidence for *Chlamydia* infection. Klin Wochenschr 68:971, 1990.

285. van Leusen R, Assmann KJ: Acute tubulo-interstitial nephritis with uveitis and favourable outcome after five months of continuous ambulatory peritoneal dialysis (CAPD). Neth J Med 33:133, 1988.

286. Muller GA, Markovic-Lipkovski J, Frank J, Rodemann HP: The role of interstitial cells in the progression of renal diseases. J Am Soc Nephrol 2:S198, 1992.

287. Laberke HG: Treatment of acute interstitial nephritis. Klin Wochenschr 58:531, 1980.

288. Qunibi WY, Godwin J, Eknoyan G: Toxic nephropathy during continuous rifampin therapy. South Med J 73:791, 1980.

289. Agus D, Mann R, Clayman M, et al: The effects of daily cyclophosphamide administration on the development and extent of primary experimental interstitial nephritis in rats. Kidney Int 29:635, 1986.

290. Shih W, Hines WH, Neilson EG: Effects of cyclosporin A on the development of immune-mediated interstitial nephritis. Kidney Int 33:1113, 1988.

291. Eknoyan G, McDonald MA, Appel D, Truong LD: Chronic tubulo-interstitial nephritis: Correlation between structural and functional findings. Kidney Int 38:736, 1990.

292. Cogan MG: Tubulo-interstitial nephropathies: A pathophysiological approach. West J Med 132:134, 1980.

293. Radonic M, Radosevic Z: Clinical features of Balkan endemic nephropathy. Food Chem Toxicol 3:189, 1992.

294. Karlsson FA, Lenkei R: Urinary excretion of albumin and beta-2-microglobulin in a population from an area where Balkan nephrology is endemic. Scand J Clin Lab Invest 37:169, 1977.

295. Muther RS, McCarron DA, Bennett WM: Renal manifestations of sarcoidosis. Arch Intern Med 141:643, 1981.

296. Lebacq E, Verhaegen H, Desmet V: Renal involvement in sarcoidosis. Postgrad Med J 46:526, 1970.

297. Muther RS, McCarron DA, Bennett WM: Granulomatous sarcoid nephritis: A cause of multiple renal tubular abnormalities. Clin Nephrol 14:190, 1980.

298. McCurley T, Salter J, Glick A: Renal insufficiency in sarcoidosis. Arch Pathol Lab Med 114:488, 1990.

299. Mayock AL, Bertrand P, Morrison CE, Scott JH: Manifestations of sarcoidosis: Analysis of 145 patients with a review of nine series selected from the literature. Am J Med 35:67, 1963.

300. Simonsen O, Thysell H: Sarcoidosis with normocalcemic granulomatous nephritis. Nephron 40:411, 1985.

301. Korzets Z, Schneider M, Taragan R, et al: Acute renal failure due to sarcoid granulomatous infiltration of the renal parenchyma. Am J Kidney Dis 6:250, 1986.

302. Coburn PW, Hobbs C, Johnston GS, et al: Granulomatous sarcoid nephritis. Am J Med 42:273, 1967.

303. Sedmak DD, Tubbs RR: The macrophagic origin of multinucleated giant cells in myeloma kidney: An immunohistologic study. Hum Pathol 18:304, 1987.

304. Rota S, Mougenot B, Baudouin B, et al: Multiple myeloma and severe renal failure: A clinicopathologic study of outcome and prognosis in 34 patients. Medicine (Baltimore) 66:126, 1987.

305. Cohen AH, Border WA: An immunomorphogenetic study of renal biopsies. Lab Invest 42:248, 1980.

306. Koss MN, Pirani CL, Osserman EF: Experimental Bence-Jones cast nephropathy. Lab Invest 35:579, 1976.

307. DeFronzo RA, Cooke CR, Wright JR, et al: Renal function in patients with multiple myeloma. Medicine (Baltimore) 57:151, 1978.

308. Smolens P: The kidney in dysproteinemic states. Am Kidney Found Nephrol Lett 4:27, 1987.

309. Sanders PW, Herrera GA, Lott RL, Galla JH: Morphologic alterations of the proximal tubules in light chain–related renal disease. Kidney Int 33:881, 1988.

310. Batuman V, Dreisbach AW, Cyran J: Light chain binding sites on renal brush border membranes. Am J Physiol 258:F1259, 1990.

311. Sanders PW, Herrera GA, Galla JH: Human Bence Jones protein toxicity in rat proximal tubule epithelium in vivo. Kidney Int 32:851, 1987.

312. Sanders PW, Herrera GA, Lott RL, Galla JH: Morphologic alterations of the proximal tubules in light chain–related renal disease. Kidney Int 33:881, 1988.

313. Sanders PW, Herrera GA, Kirk KA, et al: Spectrum of glomerular and tubulointerstitial renal lesions associated with monotypical immunoglobulin light chain deposition. Lab Invest 64:527, 1991.

314. Weiss JH, Williams RH, Galla JH, et al: Pathophysiology of acute Bence-Jones protein nephrotoxicity in the rat. Kidney Int 20:198, 1981.

315. Kapadis SB: Multiple myeloma: A clinicopathologic study of 62 consecutively autopsied cases. Medicine (Baltimore) 59:380, 1980.

316. Kyle RA: Multiple myeloma: Review of 869 cases. Mayo Clin Proc 50:29, 1975.

317. Sanders PW, Booker BB: Pathobiology of cast nephropathy from human Bence Jones proteins. J Clin Invest 89:630, 1992.

318. Smolens P, Venkatachalam M, Stein JH: Myeloma kidney cast nephropathy in a rat model of multiple myeloma. Kidney Int 24:192, 1983.

319. Cline DH, Pesce AJ, Thomson RE: Nephrotoxicity of Bence-Jones protein in the rat: Importance of protein isoelectric point. Kidney Int 16:345, 1979.

320. Coward RA, Delamore IW, Mallick NP, et al: The importance of urinary immunoglobulin light chain isoelectric point (pI) in nephrotoxicity in multiple myeloma. Clin Sci 66:229, 1984.

321. Holland MD, Galla JH, Sanders PW, Luke RG: Effect of urinary pH and diatrizoate on Bence Jones protein nephrotoxicity in the rat. Kidney Int 27:46, 1985.

322. Sanders PW, Booker BB, Bishop JB, Cheung HC: Mechanisms of intranephronal proteinaceous cast formation by low molecular weight proteins. J Clin Invest 85:570, 1990.

323. Zemer D, Pras M, Sohar E, et al: Colchicine in the prevention and treatment of the amyloidosis of familial Mediterranean fever. N Engl J Med 314:1001, 1986.

324. Luxton RW: Radiation nephritis: A long-term study of 54 patients. Lancet 2:1221, 1961.

325. Redd BL Jr: Radiation nephritis: Review, case report and animal study. Am J Roentgenol 83:88, 1960.

326. Grossman BJ: Radiation nephritis. J Paediatr 47:424, 1955.

327. Scanlon GT: Vascular alteration in the irradiated rabbit kidney: A microangiographic study. Radiology 94:401, 1970.

328. Withers HR, Mason KA, Thomas HD Jr: Late radiation response of kidney assayed by tubule-cell survival. Br J Radiol 59:587, 1986.

329. Robbins MEC, Hopewell JW, Gunn Y: Effects of single doses of x-rays on renal function in unilaterally irradiated pigs. Radiother Oncol 4:143, 1985.

330. Gup AK, Schlegel JV, Caldwell T, Schlosser J: Effect of irradiation on renal function. J Urol 97:36, 1967.

331. Concannon JP, Summers RE, Brewer R, et al: High oxygen tension and radiation effect on the kidney. Radiology 82:508, 1964.

332. Bloomfield DK, Schneider DH, Vertes V: Renin and angiotensin II: Studies in malignant hypertension after X-irradiation for seminoma. Ann Intern Med 68:146, 1968.

333. Ljungquist A, Unge G, Lagergren C, Notter G: The intrarenal vascular alterations in radiation nephritis and their relationship to the development of hypertension. Acta Pathol Microbiol Scand 79:629, 1971.

334. Wacholz BW, Casarett GW: Radiation hypertension and nephrosclerosis. Radiat Res 41:39, 1970.

335. Kunkler PB, Farr RF, Luxton RW: Limits of renal tolerance to x-rays. Br J Radiol 25:190, 1952.

336. Thames HD, Withers HR, Peters LJ, Fletcher GH: Changes in early and late radiation responses with altered dose fractionation: Implications for dose-survival relationships. Int J Radiat Oncol 8:219, 1982.

337. Dubach UC, Rosner B, Pfister E: Epidemiologic study of abuse of analgesics containing phenacetin: Renal morbidity and mortality (1968–1979). N Engl J Med 308:357, 1983.

338. Gonwa TA, Hamilton RW, Buckalew VM Jr: Chronic renal failure and end-stage renal disease in northwest North Carolina: Importance of analgesic-associated nephropathy. Arch Intern Med 141:462, 1981.

339. McAnally JF, Winchester JF, Schreiner GE: Analgesic nephropathy: An uncommon cause of end-stage renal disease. Arch Intern Med 143:1897, 1983.

340. Kincaid-Smith P: Analgesic nephropathy. Ann Intern Med 68:949, 1968.

341. Pommer W, Glaeske G, Molzahn M: The analgesic problem in the Federal Republic of Germany: Analgesic consumption, frequency of analgesic nephropathy and regional differences. Clin Nephrol 26:273, 1986.

342. Prescott LF: Analgesic nephropathy: A reassessment of the role of phenacetin and other analgesics. Drugs 23:75, 1982.

343. Murray T, Stolley PD, Anthony JC, et al: Epidemiologic study of regular analgesic use and end-stage renal disease. Arch Intern Med 143:1687, 1983.

344. Sandler PD, Smith JC, Weinberg CR, et al: Analgesic use and chronic renal disease. N Engl J Med 320:1238, 1989.

345. Nanra RS, Taylor JS, Deleon AH, White KH: Analgesic nephropathy: Etiology, clinical syndrome and clinicopathologic correlations in Australia. Kidney Int 13:79, 1978.

346. Lornoy W, Becaus I, De Vleeschouwer M, et al: Renal cell carcinoma, a new complication of analgesic nephropathy. Lancet 1:1271, 1986.

347. Bach PH, Bridges JW: Chemically induced renal papillary necrosis and upper urothelial carcinoma. Part 1. Crit Rev Toxicol 15:217, 1986.

348. Murray TG: Analgesic use and kidney disease. Arch Intern Med 141:423, 1981.

349. Griffiths ML: End-stage renal failure caused by regular use of anti-inflammatory analgesic medication for minor sports injuries. S Afr Med J 81:377, 1992.

350. Boletis J, Williams AJ, Shortland JR, Brown CB: Irreversible renal failure following mefenamic acid. Nephron 51:575, 1989.

351. Gault MH, Blennerhassett J, Muehrcke RC: Analgesic nephropathy: A clinicopathologic study using electron microscopy. Am J Med 51:740, 1971.

352. Mudge GH, Gemborys MW, Duggins GG: Covalent binding of metabolics of acetaminophen to kidney protein and depletion of renal glutathione. J Pharmacol Exp Ther 206:218, 1978.

353. McMurtry RJ, Snodgrass WR, Mitchell JR: Renal necrosis, glutathione depletion and covalent binding after acetaminophen. J Toxicol Appl Pharmacol 46:87, 1978.

354. Walker RJ, Duggin GG: Drug nephrotoxicity. Annu Rev Pharmacol Toxicol 28:331, 1988.

355. Brezis M, Rosen S, Epstein FH: The pathophysiological implications of medullary hypoxia. Am J Kidney Dis 13:253, 1989.

356. Kjellstrand CM, Campbell DD, von Hartitzsch B, et al: Hyperuricemic acute renal failure. Arch Intern Med 133:349, 1974.

357. Passwell J, Boichis H, Cohen BE: Hyperuricemic nephropathy. Am J Dis Child 120:154, 1970.

358. Yu TA-F, Berger L: Impaired renal function in gout: Its association in hypertensive vascular disease and intrinsic renal disease. Am J Med 72:95, 1982.

359. Batuman V, Maesaka JK, Haddad B, et al: The role of lead in gout nephropathy. N Engl J Med 304:520, 1981.

360. Porter GA: Uric acid nephropathy. In Bennett WM (ed): Drugs and Renal Disease. Churchill Livingstone, New York, 1986, p 142.

361. Edvall CA: Renal function in hyperparathyroidism: A clinical study of 30 cases with special reference to selective renal clearance and renal vein catheterization. Acta Chir Scand 229(suppl):1, 1958.

362. Humes HD, Ichikawa I, Troy JL, Brenner BM: Evidence for a parathyroid hormone–dependent influence of calcium on the glomerular filtration. J Clin Invest 61:32, 1978.

363. Beck N, Singh H, Reed SW: Pathogenic role of cyclic AMP in the impairment of urinary concentrating ability in acute hypercalcemia. J Clin Invest 54:1049, 1974.

364. Ganote CE, Philipshorn DS, Chen E: Acute calcium nephrotoxicity: An electron microscopic and semiquantitative light microscopic study. Arch Pathol Lab Med 99:650, 1975.

365. Nguyen HT, Wodward JD: Intranephronic calculosis in rats. Am J Pathol 100:39, 1980.

366. Wallace MR, Bruton D, North A, et al: End-stage renal failure due to familial hypokalemic interstitial nephritis with identical HLA tissue types. N Z J 98:5, 1985.

367. Kraikitpanitch S, Lindeman RD, Mandal AK: Severe hyperuricemia, hypokalemic alkalosis and tubulointerstitial nephritis. Am J Med Sci 271:77, 1976.

368. Gullner HG, Bartter FC, Gill JR Jr, et al: A sibship with hypokalemic alkalosis and renal proximal tubulopathy. Arch Intern Med 143:1534, 1983.

369. Biava GG, Dyrda I, Genest J, et al: Kaliopenic nephropathy: A correlated light and electron microscopy study. Lab Invest 12:443, 1963.

370. Cremer W, Bock KD: Symptoms and causes of chronic hypokalemia nephropathy in man. Clin Nephrol 7:112, 1977.

371. Williams HE: Oxalic acid and the hyperoxaluric syndromes. Kidney Int 13:410, 1978.

372. Cryer PE, Garber AJ, Hoffsten P, et al: Renal failure after small intestinal bypass for obesity. Arch Intern Med 135:1610, 1975.

373. Collins JM, Hennes DM, Halzgaug CR, et al: Recovery after pro-

longed oliguria due to ethylene glycol intoxication: The prognostic value of several percutaneous renal biopsies. Arch Intern Med 125:1059, 1970.

374. Buerkert J, Head M, Klahr S: Effects of acute bilateral ureteral obstruction on deep nephron and terminal collecting duct function in the young rat. J Clin Invest 59:1055, 1977.

375. Buerkert J, Martin D, Head M, et al: Deep nephron function after release of acute unilateral ureteral obstruction in the young rat. J Clin Invest 62:1228, 1978.

376. Hanley MJ, Davidson K: Isolated nephron segments from rabbit models of obstructive nephropathy. J Clin Invest 69:165, 1982.

377. Batlle DC, Arruda JAL, Kurtzman NA: Hyperkalemic distal renal tubular acidosis associated with obstructive uropathy. N Engl J Med 304:373, 1981.

378. Campbell HT, Bello-Reuss E, Klahr S: Hydraulic water permeability and transepithelial voltage in the isolated perfused rabbit cortical collecting tubule following unilateral ureteral obstruction. J Clin Invest 75:219, 1985.

379. Klahr S, Harris KPG, Purkerson ML: Effects of obstruction on renal function. Pediatr Nephrol 2:34, 1988.

380. Purkerson ML, Klahr S: Prior inhibition of vasoconstriction normalizes GFR in postobstructed kidneys. Kidney Int 35:1305, 1989.

381. Yarger WE, Schocken DD, Harris RH: Obstructive nephropathy in the rat: Possible roles for the renin-angiotensin system, prostaglandins, and thromboxanes in postobstructive renal function. J Clin Invest 65:400, 1980.

382. Reyes AA, Robertson G, Klahr S: Role of vasopressin in rats with bilateral ureteral obstruction. Proc Soc Exp Biol Med 197:49, 1991.

383. Klahr S: New insights into the consequences and mechanisms of renal impairment in obstructive nephropathy. Am J Kidney Dis 18:689, 1991.

384. Nagle RB, Johnson ME, Jervis HR: Proliferation of renal interstitial cells following injury induced by ureteral obstruction. Lab Invest 35:18, 1976.

385. Schreiner G, Harris KPG, Purkerson ML, et al: The immunological aspects of acute ureteral obstruction: Immune cell infiltrate in the kidney. Kidney Int 34:487, 1988.

386. Harris KP, Schreiner GF, Klahr S: Effect of leukocyte depletion on the function of the postobstructed kidney in the rat. Kidney Int 36:210, 1989.

387. Costerousse O, Allegrini J, Lopez M, Alhenc-Gelas F: Angiotensin I–converting enzyme in human circulating mononuclear cells: Genetic polymorphism of expression in T-lymphocytes. Biochem J 290:33, 1993.

388. Rovin BH, Harris KP, Morrison A, et al: Renal cortical release of a specific macrophage chemoattractant in response to ureteral obstruction. Lab Invest 63:213, 1990.

389. Yee J, Kuncio GS, Neilson EG: Tubulointerstitial nephritis following glomerulonephritis. Semin Nephrol 11:361, 1991.

390. Border WA, Noble NA, Yamamoto T, et al: Natural inhibitor of transforming growth factor-β protects against scarring in experimental kidney disease. Nature 360:361, 1992.

391. Staessen JA, Lauwerys RR, Buchet J-P, et al: Impairment of renal function with increasing blood lead concentrations in the general population. N Engl J Med 327:151, 1992.

392. Wedeen RP, Malik DK, Batuman V: Detection and treatment of occupational lead nephropathy. Arch Intern Med 139:53, 1979.

393. Van de Vyver FL, D'Hease PC, Visser WJ, et al: Bone lead in dialysis patients. Kidney Int 33:601, 1988.

394. Harlan WR, Landis JR, Schmouder RL: Relationship of blood lead and blood pressure in the adolescent and adult U.S. population. JAMA 253:530, 1985.

395. Cramer K, Goyer RA, Jagenburg R, Wilson MH: Renal ultrastructure, renal function, and parameters of lead toxicity in workers with different periods of lead exposure. Br J Ind Med 31:113, 1974.

396. Mistry P, Lucier GW, Fowler BA: High-affinity lead-binding proteins in rat kidney cytosol mediate cell-free nuclear translocation of lead. J Pharmacol Exp Ther 232:462, 1985.

397. Chisolm JJ, Baltrop D: Recognition and management of children with increased lead absorption. Arch Dis Child 54:249, 1979.

398. Emmerson BT: Chronic lead nephropathy. Kidney Int 4:1, 1973.

399. Craswell PW, Price J, Boyle PD, et al: Chronic renal failure with gout: A marker of chronic lead poisoning. Kidney Int 26:319, 1984.

400. Crutcher JC: Clinical manifestations and therapy of acute lead intoxication due to the ingestion of illicitly distilled alcohol. Ann Intern Med 59:707, 1963.

401. Wedeen RP: The role of lead in renal failure. Clin Exp Dial Apheresis 6:113, 1982.

402. Suzuki CA, Cherian G: Renal toxicity of cadmium metallothionein and enzymuria in rats. J Pharmacol Exp Ther 240:314, 1987.

403. Wedeen RP: Environmental renal disease: Lead, cadmium, and Balkan endemic nephropathy. Kidney Int 40(suppl 34):S4, 1991.

404. Roels HA, Lauwerys R, Buchet JP: In vivo measurement of liver and kidney cadmium in workers exposed to this metal: Its significance with respect to cadmium in blood and urine. Environ Res 26:217, 1981.

405. Nogawa K: Biologic indicators of cadmium nephrotoxicity in persons with low-level cadmium exposure. Environ Health Perspect 54:163, 1984.

406. Lauwerys R, DeWals P: Environmental pollution by cadmium and mortality from renal diseases. Lancet 1:383, 1981.

407. Weiss RA, Kelly CJ, Madaio MP: Heat shock protein–reactive T cells eluted from the kidneys of nephritis mice are nephritogenic and cytotoxic to stressed renal tubular cells. J Am Soc Nephrol 4:641, 1993.

408. Hannedouche T, Albouze G, Chauveau P, et al: Effects of blood pressure and antihypertensive treatment on progression of advanced chronic renal failure. Am J Kidney Dis 21:131, 1993.

409. Robson M, Levi J, Dolberg L, Rosenfeld JB: Acute tubulo-interstitial nephritis following sulfadiazine therapy. Isr J Med Sci 6:561, 1970.

410. Segasothy M, Pang KS: Acute interstitial nephritis due to endosulfan. Nephron 62:118, 1992. Letter.

411. Codding CE, Ramseyer L, Allon M, et al: Tubulointerstitial nephritis due to vancomycin. Am J Kidney Dis 14:512, 1989.

412. Gaut PL, Carron WC, Ching WT, Meyer RD: Intravenous/oral ciprofloxacin therapy versus intravenous ceftazidime therapy for selected bacterial infections. Am J Med 87:169, 1989.

413. Rosenfeld J, Gura V, Boner G, et al: Interstitial nephritis with acute renal failure after erythromycin. Br Med J 286:938, 1983.

414. Wilkinson SP, Stewart WK, Spiers EM, Pears J: Protracted systemic illness and interstitial nephritis due to minocycline. Postgrad Med J 65:53, 1989.

415. Walker RG, Thomson NM, Dowling JP, Ogg CS: Minocycline-induced acute interstitial nephritis. Br Med J 1:524, 1979.

416. Rashed A, Azadeh B, Abu-Romeh SH: Acyclovir-induced acute tubulo-interstitial nephritis. Nephron 56:436, 1990.

417. Garcia-Martin F, Mampaso F, de Arriba G, et al: Acute interstitial nephritis induced by ethambutol. Nephron 59:679, 1991. Letter.

418. Prichard BN, Owens CW, Woolf AS: Adverse reactions to diuretics. Eur Heart J 13:96, 1992.

419. Sica DA, Gehr TW: Trimterene and the kidney. Nephron 51:454, 1989.

420. Smith WR, Neill J, Cushman WC, Butkus DE: Captopril-associated acute interstitial nephritis. Am J Nephrol 9:230, 1989.

421. Sawaishi Y, Komatsu K, Takeda O, et al: A case of tubulo-interstitial nephritis with exfoliative dermatitis and hepatitis due to phenobarbital hypersensitivity. Eur J Pediatr 151:69, 1992.

422. Averbuch SD, Austin HA 3, Sherwin SA, et al: Acute interstitial nephritis with the nephrotic syndrome following recombinant leukocyte α interferon therapy for mycosis fungoides. N Engl J Med 310:32, 1984.

423. Diekman MJ, Vlasveld LT, Krediet RT, et al: Acute interstitial nephritis during continuous intravenous administration of low-dose interleukin-2. Nephron 60:122, 1992. Letter.

424. Vlasveld LT, van de Wiel–van Kemenade E, de Boer AJ, et al: Possible role for cytotoxic lymphocytes in the pathogenesis of acute interstitial nephritis after recombinant interleukin-2 treatment for renal cell cancer. Cancer Immunol Immunother 36:210, 1993.

425. Choy EH, Kingsley GH, Panayi GS: Treatment with anti-CD4 monoclonal antibody and acute interstitial nephritis. Arthritis Rheum 36:723, 1993.

426. Panciera RJ, Mosier DA, Ritchey JW: Hairy vetch (Vicia villosa Roth) poisoning in cattle: Update and experimental induction of disease. J Vet Diagn Invest 4:318, 1992.

427. Yoshioka K, Takemura T, Kanasaki M, et al: Acute interstitial nephritis and uveitis syndrome: Activated immune cell infiltration in the kidney. Pediatr Nephrol 5:232, 1991.

428. Rosenbaum JT: Bilateral anterior uveitis and interstitial nephritis. Am J Ophthalmol 105:534, 1988.

429. Veiga PA, Pieroni D, Baier W, Feld LG: Association of Kawasaki disease and interstitial nephritis. Pediatr Nephrol 6:421, 1992.

430. Kelly CJ, Neilson EG: The interstitium in cystic kidney disease. *In* Gardner KD, Bernstein J (eds): The Cystic Kidney. Kluwer Academic Publishers, Amsterdam, 1989, p 43.

431. Kelly CJ, Neilson EG: Medullary cystic disease: An inherited form of autoimmune interstitial nephritis? Am J Kidney Dis 10:389, 1987.

432. Adams ND, Rowe JC: Nephrocalcinosis. Clin Perinatol 19:179, 1992.

433. Wandzilak TR, Williams HE: The hyperoxaluric syndromes. Endocrinol Metab Clin North Am 19:851, 1990.

434. Broyer M, Guillot M, Gubler MC, Habib R: Infantile cystinosis: A reappraisal of early and late symptoms. Adv Nephrol 10:137, 1981.

435. Rutledge SL, Geraghty M, Mroczek E, et al: Tubulointerstitial nephritis in methylmalonic acidemia. Pediatr Nephrol 7:81, 1993.

436. Fillastre JP, Moulin B, Josse S: Aetiology of nephrotoxic damage to the renal interstitium and tubuli. Toxicol Lett 46:45, 1989.

437. Walker RG, Bennet WM, Davies BM, Kincaid-Smith P: Structural and functional effects of long-term lithium therapy. Kidney Int 11:S13, 1982.

438. Myers BD, Ross J, Newton L, et al: Cyclosporine-associated chronic nephropathy. N Engl J Med 311:699, 1984.

439. Gonzalez-Vitale JC, Hayes DM, Cvitkovic E, et al: The renal pathology in clinical trials for *cis*-platinum (II) diaminedichloride. Cancer 39:1362, 1977.

440. Schacht RG, Baldwin DS: Chronic interstitial nephritis and renal failure due to nitrosourea therapy. Kidney Int 14:661, 1978.

441. Vanherweghem JL, Depierreux M, Tielemans C, et al: Rapidly progressive interstitial renal fibrosis in young women: Association with slimming regimen including Chinese herbs. Lancet 341:387, 1993.

442. Hess B, Raisin J, Zimmermann A, et al: Tubulointerstitial nephropathy persisting 20 months after discontinuation of chronic intake of germanium lactate citrate. Am J Kidney Dis 21:548, 1993.

443. Faull RJ, Russ GR: Tubular expression of intercellular adhesion molecule-1 during renal allograft rejection. Transplantation 48:226, 1989.

444. Cosimi AB, Conti D, Delmonico FL, et al: In vivo effects of monoclonal antibody to ICAM-1 (CD54) in nonhuman primates with renal allografts. J Immunol 144:4604, 1990.

445. Schwartz MM: Lupus vasculitis. Contrib Nephrol 99:35, 1992.

446. Jennette JC, Falk RJ: Antineutrophil cytoplasmic autoantibodies and associated diseases: A review. Am J Kidney Dis 15:517, 1990.

447. Matsutani H, Mizusawa J, Shimoda M, et al: Severe glomerulonephritis and tubulo-interstitial nephritis accompanied with urticaria and vasculitis. Child Nephrol Urol 10:214, 1990.

448. Siamopoulos KC, Mavridis AK, Elisaf M, et al: Kidney involvement in primary Sjögren's syndrome. Scand J Rheumatol Suppl 61:156, 1986.

449. Casella FJ, Allon M: The kidney in sarcoidosis. J Am Soc Nephrol 3:1555, 1993.

450. Zachee P, Henckens M, Van Damme B, et al: Chronic renal failure due to renal hemosiderosis in a patient with paroxysmal nocturnal hemoglobinuria. Clin Nephrol 39:28, 1993.

451. Srinivasa NS, McGovern CH, Solez K, et al: Progressive renal failure due to renal invasion and parenchymal destruction by adult T-cell lymphoma. Am J Kidney Dis 16:70, 1990.

452. Falk RJ, Scheinman J, Phillips G, et al: Prevalence and pathologic features of sickle cell nephropathy and response to inhibition of angiotensin-converting enzyme. N Engl J Med 326:910, 1992.

453. Meyrier A, Condamin MC, Fernet M, et al: Frequency of development of early cortical scarring in acute primary pyelonephritis. Kidney Int 35:696, 1989.

454. Dobyan DC, Truong LD, Eknoyan G: Renal malacoplakia reappraised. Am J Kidney Dis 22:243, 1993.

455. Goodman M, Curry T, Russell T: Xanthogranulomatous pyelonephritis: A local disease with systemic manifestations. Report of 23 cases and review of the literature. Medicine (Baltimore) 58:171, 1979.

456. Petkovic SD: Treatment of bilateral renal pelvic and ureteral tumors. A review of 45 cases. Eur Urol 4:397, 1978.

457. Stickler GB, Kelalis PP, Burke EC, Segar WE: Primary interstitial nephritis with reflux. Am J Dis Child 122:144, 1971.

458. Preston RA, Stemmer CL, Materson BJ, et al: Renal biopsy in patients 65 years of age or older. An analysis of the results of 334 biopsies. J Am Geriatr Soc 38:669, 1990.

459. Farrington K, Levison DA, Greenwood RN, et al: Renal biopsy in patients with unexplained renal impairment and normal kidney size. Q J Med 70:221, 1989.

460. Truong LD, Farhood A, Tasby J, Gillum D: Experimental chronic renal ischemia: Morphologic and immunologic studies. Kidney Int 41:1676, 1992.

461. Karalezli G, Gogus O, Beduk Y, et al: Histopathologic effects of extracorporeal shock wave lithotripsy on rabbit kidney. Urol Res 21:67, 1993.

# Toxic Nephropathy

*Robert E. Cronin*
*William L. Henrich*

As the kidney concentrates and excretes metabolic waste, chemicals, and many drugs, it is often exposed to toxic concentrations of these substances. The term "toxic nephropathy" encompasses renal disorders produced by a broad range of drugs, diagnostic agents, and chemicals. Nephrotoxic substances may cause injury at a number of sites along the nephron and produce characteristic clinical syndromes (Table 34–1). The mechanisms responsible for these abnormalities are several and are described in general terms here and again more specifically as individual nephrotoxic agents are discussed.

**Proximal Tubule Injury.** Although proximal tubule necrosis is a common manifestation of nephrotoxic agents like aminoglycosides, cisplatin, and heavy metals, proximal tubule dysfunction without tubule necrosis may also be an important aspect of nephrotoxicity. Histopathologic studies in several experimental models of acute renal failure demonstrate early nonlethal dysfunction, such as mitochondrial swelling, blebbing of the endoplasmic reticulum, and sloughing of portions of the plasma membrane.[1] With more severe injury, tubule cell death, intratubule plugging with cellular debris, and interstitial edema develop, leading to a reduction in renal blood flow and a marked fall in glomerular filtration rate (GFR).

**Renal Medullary Injury.** Nephrotoxic injury may be present without histologic evidence of proximal tubule necrosis. Thus, other nephron segments can be the focus of injury for some toxins. With a mild nephrotoxic insult to the kidney, impaired urinary concentration, a medullary event, is often the first and sometimes the only apparent injury. Under the best of circumstances, portions of the nephron traveling through the renal medulla are borderline hypoxic as a result of the normally low oxygen tension in this area of the kidney. In addition to their susceptibility to hypoxia, cells of the medullary thick ascending limb are at risk for nephrotoxic injury from polyene antibiotics,[2, 3] cyclosporine,[4] and radiocontrast agents.[5] Drugs that block $Na^+$ reabsorption in the medullary thick ascending limb (e.g., furosemide, ouabain) diminish cell damage, which suggests that if metabolic demand is reduced during periods of ischemia or nephrotoxic insult, cell necrosis may be avoidable.[5, 6]

**Intratubule Obstruction.** Agents that have a low solubility in tubule urine when given in high doses may precipitate within the nephron and obstruct the flow of urine, leading to a reduction in GFR. Such agents should be considered only relative nephrotoxins, because they may be given safely and precipitation is avoided by maintaining high tubule flow rates and optimizing urine pH.

**Distal Tubule Dysfunction.** Hyperkalemia is produced by several agents that interfere with the renin-angiotensin-aldosterone axis. These abnormalities include impaired production of renin, reduced production of aldosterone, and tubule insensitivity to the action of aldosterone. Renal tubular acidosis is caused by agents that interfere with $H^+$ secretion by distal tubule cells. Hypokalemia can result from enhanced excretion of $K^+$ by agents that cause renal tubular acidosis. Nephrogenic diabetes insipidus results from blockade of the effects of antidiuretic hormone on collecting tubule cells.

**Unknown Site.** Isolated hypokalemia and isolated hypomagnesemia can occur after administration of several therapeutic agents. The mechanisms responsible are not clear;

**TABLE 34–1. Mechanisms of Nephrotoxic Injury**

| Site | Example |
|---|---|
| Proximal tubule necrosis | Aminoglycoside antibiotics, cisplatin, radiocontrast agents, heavy metals, foscarnet |
| Proximal tubule dysfunction (e.g., glucosuria, aminoaciduria, proteinuria) | Aminoglycoside antibiotics |
| Medullary thick ascending limb injury | Amphotericin, radiocontrast agents, cyclosporine |
| Intratubule obstruction | Acyclovir, sulfadiazine |
| Distal tubule dysfunction | |
| Hyperkalemia | Nonsteroidal anti-inflammatory drugs, converting enzyme inhibitors, cyclosporine, pentamidine, trimethoprim-sulfamethoxazole |
| Renal tubular acidosis | Amphotericin |
| Hypokalemia | Amphotericin |
| Nephrogenic diabetes insipidus | Amphotericin, aminoglycosides, lithium, demeclocycline |
| Unknown | |
| Hypokalemia | Aminoglycosides |
| Hypomagnesemia | Cisplatin, cyclosporine, pentamidine, aminoglycosides |

injury to specific cell types involved in the transport of these ions seems most likely.

**Oxygen Free Radical Production.** Oxygen is primarily used by mitochondria to generate ATP. A small fraction, 1% to 2%, is converted to reactive oxygen species, which are capable of lipid peroxidation of cell and organelle membranes. Antioxidants (superoxide dismutase, catalase, glutathione, vitamin E, ascorbic acid) are protective tissue chemicals that react with and remove these reactive species, but the supply of these antioxidants can be depleted under severe hypoxic or nephrotoxic stress. Evidence for the participation of free radicals in nephrotoxic injury has been presented for aminoglycoside antibiotics and radiocontrast agents.[7–9]

## NEPHROTOXICITY OF AMINOGLYCOSIDE ANTIBIOTICS

The aminoglycoside antibiotics (neomycin, gentamicin, tobramycin, amikacin, netilmicin) are bactericidal agents that have nephrotoxic injury as their major adverse effect. The incidence of nephrotoxic effects from these aminoglycosides has increased since their introduction in 1969, when the reported incidence was 2% to 3%. In 1993, the incidence was reported to be 20%,[10] a figure that has changed little in the past two decades despite the proliferation of nomograms and pharmacokinetic programs devised to prevent renal injury. The percentage of patients who will have a nephrotoxic effect rises with the duration of therapy, reaching almost 50% with 14 days or more of therapy (Fig. 34–1).

Aminoglycosides penetrate the cytoplasmic membrane of bacteria and act on ribosomes, causing misreading of the genetic code and, ultimately, death of the microorganism. Aminoglycosides are polycationic, a property that is responsible for their poor oral absorption, poor penetration of the cerebrospinal fluid, and rapid renal excretion. The poly-

cationic charge also appears to be important in causing nephrotoxicity (see later).

## Clinical Features

The most common clinical presentation of aminoglycoside nephrotoxic injury is nonoliguric acute renal failure with a clinical course that is often milder than that of oliguric acute renal failure (Table 34–2). The onset of renal failure is usually slower and the daily rise in serum creatinine tends to be lower than that observed in acute renal failure from other causes. In more than 50% of patients with nephrotoxic injury, the decline in renal function occurs

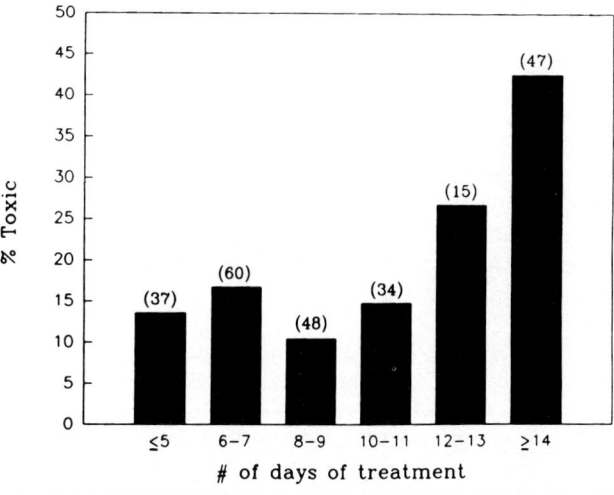

**Figure 34–1.** Relationship between duration of aminoglycoside administration and percentage of patients with a nephrotoxic effect. Numbers in parentheses are patients in the group. (From Leehy DJ, Braun BI, Tholl DA, et al: Can pharmacokinetic dosing decrease nephrotoxicity associated with aminoglycoside therapy? J Am Soc Nephrol 4[1]:81–90, 1993.)

only after therapy has been completed.[10] Recovery from the nephrotoxic effects of aminoglycoside therapy is usually slow, often requiring 4 to 6 weeks. In some patients, particularly those with previous renal insufficiency, recovery to baseline renal function may be incomplete.[11] The explanation for incomplete recovery to baseline function is probably permanent loss of nephrons. Supporting evidence for this explanation comes from animal studies that show residual areas of interstitial fibrosis in the renal cortex.[12, 13] In addition to reducing the GFR, aminoglycoside administration can cause enzymuria, proteinuria, aminoaciduria,[14] glucosuria,[14, 15] and a variety of electrolyte disorders including hypomagnesemia,[16, 17] hypocalcemia,[16, 17] and hypokalemia.[18]

## Pathophysiology

The mechanisms involved in aminoglycoside nephrotoxicity have been well studied. Because of their highly basic charge, aminoglycosides penetrate cell membranes poorly. However, to impair bacterial growth, and presumably to damage kidney cells, at least a small fraction of the administered aminoglycoside must gain access to the cell interior. Serum protein binding of aminoglycosides is minimal,[19, 20] and the renal clearance of gentamicin is close to that of inulin, which indicates little secretion or reabsorption. A small fraction of filtered gentamicin is known to gain access to proximal tubule cells. Of all the tissues in the body, the renal cortex stands alone in its ability to concentrate aminoglycosides severalfold more than plasma. The relatively non-nephrotoxic streptomycin is the only exception to this rule. The proximal, but not distal, tubule cells concentrate aminoglycosides and are the cells that demonstrate significant damage in experimental nephrotoxic injury in the rat.[21] Morphologic changes in proximal tubule cells can be detected within hours of drug administration.[22] Gentamicin gains access to proximal tubule cells through pinocytosis occurring at the brush border membrane on the luminal surface of the cell. Studies of renal cortical tissue slices (in which gentamicin presumably cannot gain access to the tubule from the luminal side) also demonstrate tissue uptake of gentamicin, which indicates uptake at the basolateral (contraluminal) surface as well.[23] Whereas transtubule secretion of gentamicin and netilmicin can be demonstrated by micropuncture techniques,[24] glomerular filtration is quantitatively the most important route of aminoglycoside elimination.

Once inside the cell, gentamicin binds to subcellular or-

ganelles or is taken up into lysosomes. The typical electron microscopic findings after the administration of gentamicin are an increase in the number of secondary lysosomes and the presence within them of myeloid bodies.[25] Aminoglycosides induce a lysosomal phospholipidosis.[26, 27] This probably occurs because the electrostatic attachment of aminoglycosides to anionic membrane phospholipids interferes with the normal action of phospholipases.[28, 29] How aminoglycoside-induced lysosomal dysfunction might lead to cell injury and death is unclear, but release of aminoglycosides into the cytoplasm through permeabilized lysosomes could interfere with the phosphatidylinositol cascade and stimulation by agonists, as has been shown in a cell culture model.[30] The findings of this study are consistent with the possibility that aminoglycosides bind to phosphatidylinositol 4,5-bisphosphate and prevent the hydrolysis of phospholipase C on stimulation by agonists.

The role of free radicals in the pathogenesis of aminoglycoside nephrotoxicity is unsettled. In vivo[31] and in vitro[7, 8] models of gentamicin nephrotoxicity show evidence supporting the production of free radicals, but studies designed to assess whether free radical scavengers protect against gentamicin nephrotoxicity have given conflicting results.[8, 32]

Tissue accumulation of aminoglycoside is an important factor in the generation of nephrotoxic injury. In the rat, gentamicin, tobramycin, or kanamycin given as a subcutaneous injection accumulates in high concentrations in the renal cortex, but streptomycin, an aminoglycoside with no nephrotoxicity, disappears rapidly. The half-life of gentamicin in renal tissue is 109 hours; once concentrated in renal tissues, gentamicin may take several months to be excreted.[33] The transport and accumulation of aminoglycosides in the renal cortex are mediated by a low-affinity, high-capacity system that is not easily saturable.[34, 35] The tissue accumulation of gentamicin is different from that of netilmicin, with a lower renal cortical accumulation noted for netilmicin. These findings are consistent with the observation that netilmicin has a lower absorptive flux and a higher secretory flux in the proximal tubule compared with gentamicin.[34, 35] Thus, whereas both the apical and basolateral membranes of proximal tubule cells participate in aminoglycoside uptake, the apical membrane is quantitatively far more important.[36, 37] Other aminoglycosides and organic polycations appear to compete for the same transport system with a relative affinity that is directly related to the net cationic charge of the molecule.[34]

The membrane binding sites for aminoglycosides appear to be anionic phospholipids, phosphatidylinositol 4,5-bisphosphate being one of the most important.[38, 39] Ischemia enhances apical membrane binding and internalization of gentamicin, an effect that is paralleled by a marked increase in the membrane content of phosphatidylinositol[40] (Fig. 34–2).

The risk for development of aminoglycoside nephrotoxic injury is affected by a number of factors (Table 34–3). The method of administration of aminoglycosides has a marked effect on renal cortical uptake. Multiple injections cause greater tissue accumulation and nephrotoxic injury than does the same total dose on a weight basis given as a single bolus.[41] Other risk factors associated with increased tissue accumulation of aminoglycosides are male sex,[42] Na+ de-

### TABLE 34–2. Clinical Features of Aminoglycoside Nephrotoxicity

Nonoliguric acute renal failure
Slow (4–6 wk) recovery of renal function
Proximal tubule dysfunction (enzymuria, proteinuria, aminoaciduria, glucosuria)
Hypomagnesemia
Hypocalcemia
Hypokalemia

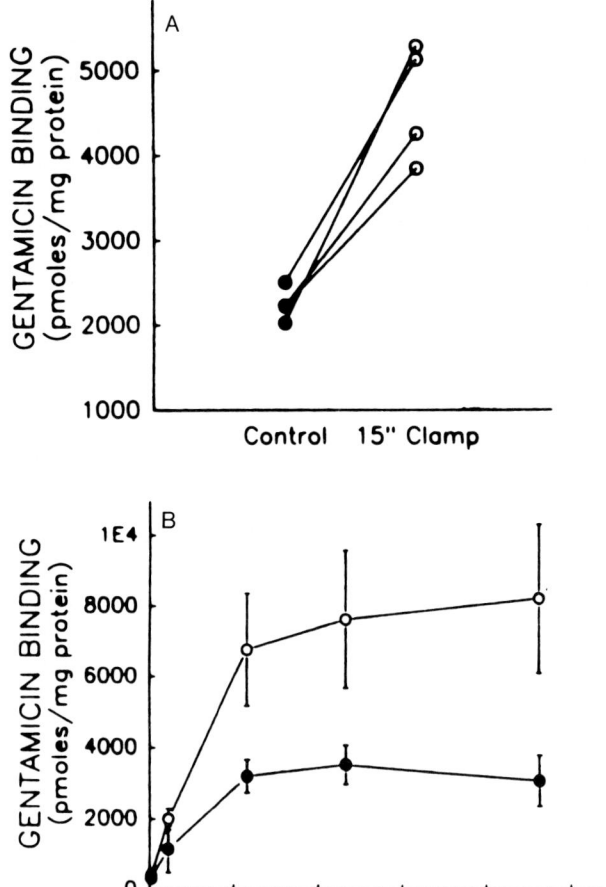

**Figure 34–2.** Effect of ischemia on gentamicin binding to brush border membrane vesicles. *A.* Equilibration gentamicin binding to brush border membrane vesicles was determined in control vesicles *(solid circles)* and in vesicles after 15 minutes of total renal ischemia *(open circles)*. *B.* Effect of gentamicin concentration on gentamicin binding to control and ischemic brush border membrane vesicles. *(A and B from Molitoris BA, Meyer C, Dahl R, et al: Mechanism of ischemia-enhanced aminoglycoside binding and uptake by proximal tubule cells. Am J Physiol 264:F907–F916, 1993.)*

tors are also involved. Administration of gentamicin to rats for 6 weeks leads to renal failure followed by recovery in spite of continued administration of the drug.[55] Although recovery of renal function occurs, the renal cortical concentration of gentamicin remains high. This study suggests that the regenerating or immature proximal tubule cells are resistant to the nephrotoxic effect of these antibiotics; however, the mechanism of this protective effect remains to be clarified.

How the aminoglycosides cause cell injury and cell death is unknown, but interactions with the cell membrane as well as with intracellular structures such as lysosomes, mitochondria,[56, 57] and microsomes[58–60] are likely to be involved. Bennett and co-workers[61] demonstrated in the rat that transport of organic acid (*p*-aminohippuric acid) is stimulated before development of overt renal failure, an effect possibly reflecting an early change in membrane permeability. The reported effects of gentamicin on membrane fluidity conflict, with two studies indicating a decrease[62, 63] but another reporting an increase.[64] The timing of the measurement may be important, because the report showing increased fluidity examined the brush border vesicles before a reduction in GFR.[64] Also, this study detected a gentamicin-induced decrease in the maximal velocity ($V_{max}$) of $Na^+$-$P_i$ cotransport and $Na^+/H^+$ exchange activity without an effect on $Na^+$-glucose or $Na^+$-proline cotransport activity, which suggests that the gentamicin effects within the apical membrane are highly selective. In addition to tubule changes induced by gentamicin, at least one glomerular defect has been reported. Baylis and colleagues,[65] using micropuncture techniques, demonstrated in the rat that gentamicin caused a marked decline in the glomerular capillary ultrafiltration coefficient ($K_f$) at a time when both whole kidney GFR and single-nephron GFR had fallen by 30% to 50%. Neither tubule obstruction nor renal ischemia appeared to be involved in the reduction of GFR.

Combining an aminoglycoside with a known nephrotoxin, such as amphotericin, cisplatin, and possibly x-ray contrast material, can enhance nephrotoxicity.[66–68] The combined use of aminoglycosides with cephalosporin or penicillin antibiotics does not seem to lead to enhanced nephrotoxicity. The combined use of aminoglycosides with vancomycin may be associated with a slightly greater fre-

pletion,[43] $K^+$ depletion,[17] endotoxemia,[44] obesity,[45] and ischemia.[40, 46] In contrast, a number of factors and interventions are associated with reduced renal tissue accumulation of aminoglycosides and a reduced nephrotoxic effect, including administration of organic polycations,[34] alkalinization of the urine,[47] thyroid hormone administration,[48] potassium chloride loading,[49] and experimental diabetes mellitus.[35] Polyaspartic acid protects the rat against gentamicin nephrotoxicity through an effect that does not depend on decreased renal cortical uptake of the drug.[50–52] The protective effect appears to depend on polyaspartic acid's preventing gentamicin from interacting with anionic phospholipids[53] and is present even when gentamicin is administered in a dose three times higher than what is normally a nephrotoxic dose.[54]

Whereas the intracellular concentration of aminoglycosides correlates roughly with nephrotoxic effect, other fac-

**TABLE 34–3. Factors Affecting the Development of Aminoglycoside Nephrotoxicity**

| Enhancing | Reducing |
|---|---|
| Male sex | Organic polycations |
| $Na^+$ depletion | Urinary alkalinization |
| $K^+$ depletion | Thyroid hormone |
| Endotoxemia | $K^+$ loading |
| Obesity | Experimental diabetes |
| Renal ischemia | |
| Liver disease | |
| Advanced age | |
| Diuretic use | |
| Shock | |
| Volume depletion | |
| Previous renal insufficiency | |

quency of nephrotoxic injury (see later). Advanced age, shock, use of furosemide, liver disease, volume depletion, and previous renal insufficiency enhance aminoglycoside nephrotoxicity.[10, 69]

The specific aminoglycoside preparation used might also be an important factor in the frequency of nephrotoxic injury. Laboratory and clinical studies demonstrate a direct relationship between the number of free amino groups on the aminoglycoside molecule and the risk of a nephrotoxic effect. In a prospective clinical study, nephrotoxic injury developed in 26% of 72 patients given gentamicin and 12% of 74 patients given tobramycin.[70] However, an ototoxic effect was seen in 10% of patients receiving both drugs.

Aminoglycosides will continue to be valuable agents for the treatment of serious gram-negative infections. The nomograms and formulas designed to estimate the aminoglycoside dosage in patients with renal failure may be helpful in planning the initial dose of drug. For accurate determination of subsequent doses, peak levels (blood sample drawn 1 hour after injection) and trough levels (blood sample drawn immediately before the next calculated dose) are useful to ensure that adequate bactericidal serum levels are achieved. Individualized pharmacokinetic dosing programs for aminoglycosides are available in many hospitals, often in cooperation with the pharmacy service. Whereas these dosing programs appear to decrease the number of treatment failures, there is little indication that their use reduces the nephrotoxic effects.[10, 71, 72] Leehey and co-workers[10] compared the frequency of aminoglycoside nephrotoxic injury in a group of patients given drug doses based on an estimate of creatinine clearance with that in two groups given doses based on a bayesian pharmacokinetic computer program. The frequency of nephrotoxic injury was not different among the groups and averaged 20%. Peak[69, 73] and trough[74] aminoglycoside blood levels have been proposed as indicators of aminoglycoside nephrotoxicity. However, there is little evidence to support the belief that the blood level of these agents is an important risk factor for or indicator of nephrotoxic injury. When observed prospectively, mean peak and trough levels were not associated with nephrotoxic effects.[10] Bennett and colleagues[75] have shown in the rat that a single large dose of gentamicin producing a high peak blood level was less nephrotoxic than the same amount given in divided doses in which the resulting peak blood levels were much lower. A rising trough level, rather than indicating an impending nephrotoxic effect, represents drug retention because of an already reduced GFR.

## Prevention

In attempting to minimize clinical nephrotoxic effects, several points should be emphasized. Aminoglycoside nephrotoxicity is directly dependent on the dose and duration of drug administration.[10] Thus, the nephrotoxic effect is more likely to be apparent when large doses of aminoglycosides are given for prolonged periods, or when usual doses are given to individuals with renal impairment who have diminished capacity to excrete the drugs. The goal of treatment should be the lowest dose and shortest course of therapy compatible with a clinical cure. The clinical success of once-daily aminoglycoside dosing schedules indicates

that the efficacy of these valuable agents can be retained while toxicity is reduced.[76–79] Empirically started aminoglycoside therapy for an infection subsequently proved to be due to an aerobic gram-negative bacillus should be changed to a less toxic agent, even if the patient is responding satisfactorily during the initial aminoglycoside therapy. Empirical aminoglycoside therapy in a patient with presumed sepsis or other serious infection must be re-evaluated when culture results are available. A clinical response in the absence of positive cultures is not usually sufficient justification for prolonged treatment with an empirically started aminoglycoside. It is appropriate to think of aminoglycosides as nephrotoxins for all patients who receive them. In most patients, the nephrotoxic effect is subclinical and beyond detection with the usual tests (e.g., serum creatinine concentration, creatinine clearance). Nevertheless, serial monitoring of renal function (e.g., serum creatinine level every other day) should be carried out in patients receiving these aminoglycosides. Concomitant administration of other potential nephrotoxins (radiographic contrast material, amphotericin, cisplatin, diuretics) should be avoided. Extracellular fluid volume and renal perfusion should be optimized during aminoglycoside therapy, because renal tissue accumulation of aminoglycosides is enhanced during states of volume depletion. The dosage and frequency should be based on the best index of GFR available. A steady-state serum creatinine concentration will often suffice. In elderly patients or patients with diminished renal function, however, creatinine clearance is preferable. When the clinical response to aminoglycoside treatment is inadequate, assessment of plasma drug levels is often helpful, particularly when impaired renal function is present.

## NEPHROTOXICITY OF PENICILLINS AND CEPHALOSPORINS

True nephrotoxic reactions with these classes of drugs are rare. The only agent with a clear potential to cause nephrotoxic injury is cephaloridine, an antibiotic that has not been used for more than 10 years. More often, acute interstitial nephritis is the cause of altered renal function with these agents. The topic of acute interstitial nephritis is covered in Chapter 33.

## NEPHROTOXICITY OF OTHER ANTI-INFECTIOUS AGENTS

### Vancomycin

This drug is valuable for the treatment of gram-positive infections, particularly for methicillin-resistant staphylococcal infections, *Staphylococcus epidermidis* infections, and *Clostridium difficile* diarrhea. It is particularly useful for patients undergoing hemodialysis, when weekly or twice weekly intravenous injections may be all the drug that is required. The early formulations of this drug carried a substantial nephrotoxic potential, but current preparations are largely free of this adverse effect. When vancomycin is used alone, the frequency of nephrotoxic injury is reported to be 5%, defined as a rise in the serum creatinine level of 0.5 mg/dL.[80] Whether aminoglycoside administration with vancomycin has a synergistic nephrotoxic effect is unclear. Retrospective and prospective studies report that 5% to 35% of patients given this combination experience a nephrotoxic reaction.[80–84] Because the frequency of aminoglycoside nephrotoxic injury in a separate control group given aminoglycosides alone from these same institutions is not known, it is impossible to determine whether these figures represent synergy or simply the nephrotoxic effects of aminoglycosides alone.

## Sulfonamides

Most cases of sulfonamide-induced renal disease represent acute interstitial nephritis. However, in the presence of an acid urine (pH less than 5.5), several of these agents are capable of precipitating in tubule urine and causing an acute intratubule obstructive nephropathy. The use of high doses of sulfadiazine and sulfamethoxazole for acquired immunodeficiency syndrome–related diseases has led to a resurgence of this form of acute renal failure.[85–88] The crystals caused by sulfadiazine resemble shocks of wheat and are formed by its primary metabolite, acetylsulfadiazine.[86] Renal failure can be prevented by increasing fluid intake during therapy and by maintaining an alkaline urine, which increases solubility of these drugs in the urine.

## Amphotericin

Amphotericin B is a polyene antibiotic containing a hydrophilic backbone as well as a lipophilic region. These characteristics allow the drug to form complexes with sterol moieties in cell membranes, disrupt them, and increase their permeability.[89] Amphotericin also causes renal vasoconstriction leading to renal ischemia.[90, 91] Amphotericin B use has increased with the rise in the number of fungal infections in patients with acquired immunodeficiency syndrome and the increasing number of immunosuppressed organ transplant recipients.

The nephrotoxic effect of amphotericin B is initially a distal tubule phenomenon characterized by a loss of urine concentration, distal renal tubular acidosis, and wasting of $K^+$ and $Mg^{2+}$.[92] However, long-term administration of amphotericin in the rat also leads to medullary injury, an effect that appears to be due to hypoxia. Chronic amphotericin nephrotoxic injury may be mediated in part by elevated endothelin levels.[93] Nearly all patients receiving amphotericin will experience a rise in the serum creatinine level. Fortunately, azotemia is rarely severe, and a small dosage reduction or short-term interruption of therapy is usually sufficient to reverse the azotemia such that drug administration can be restarted. The most important risk factor for nephrotoxic injury is salt depletion.[94–96] This has led to the common practice of saline loading before and during drug administration.[97, 98] Newer preparations, including liposome-encapsulated amphotericin B and lipid complex formulations of the drug, hold a promise that nephrotoxic potential may be less in future years.[99, 100]

## Acyclovir and Ganciclovir

Acyclovir is an antiviral agent used in the treatment of herpes infections. When given by the intravenous route in doses of 500 $mg/m^2$, it can be both nephrotoxic and neurotoxic.[101, 102] Acyclovir, which is excreted by the kidney through the processes of glomerular filtration and tubule secretion, has a low solubility in urine. Nephrotoxic injury results from intratubule precipitation leading to tubule obstruction. Clinical signs of nephrotoxicity include nausea, flank pain, and hematuria.[103] Urinalysis may show needle-shaped crystals under polarizing light. Interstitial inflammation may be seen adjacent to areas of intratubule obstruction.[103] Although an occasional patient may require hemodialysis,[102] most experience nonoliguric acute renal failure. Withdrawal of therapy usually leads to recovery of near-normal renal function within several days.[104] Patients who experience nephrotoxic effects may be rechallenged with a lower dose, usually less than 250 $mg/m^2$.[103] Volume depletion predisposes to nephrotoxic effects, and most cases can probably be prevented by vigorous hydration before and during infusion.

Ganciclovir, an antiviral agent related structurally to acyclovir and used in the treatment of chorioretinitis, does not seem to be nephrotoxic.

## Pentamidine

Intravenous pentamidine is commonly used to treat *Pneumocystis carinii* pneumonia, but a nephrotoxic effect occurs in 25% to 65% of patients.[105, 106] Nephrotoxic injury after nebulized pentamidine is a rarity.[107] Pharmacokinetic studies indicate that the intravenous half-life of pentamidine is approximately 6.5 hours.[108] The apparent volume of distribution of pentamidine is large, averaging 205 L in five adults with normal renal function (creatinine clearance > 80 mL/min). The kidney accounts for less than 5% of plasma clearance of pentamidine, and, not unexpectedly, dialysis removes little drug.[108]

Like aminoglycoside antibiotics, accumulation of pentamidine in renal tissue occurs after multiple doses,[109] and the drug can be detected in plasma and urine weeks after completion of therapy.[110] Whereas the mechanism of nephrotoxicity is incompletely understood, pentamidine is clearly a tubule toxin. Hypocalcemia,[110] hypomagnesemia with an inappropriately high fractional excretion of $Mg^{2+}$,[110] and hyperkalemia[109, 110a] occur with prolonged therapy. The simultaneous use of amphotericin with pentamidine appears to be synergistic in causing nephrotoxic effects.[111]

## Foscarnet

Foscarnet is a pyrophosphate analogue that acts by inhibiting DNA polymerase, RNA polymerase, and reverse transcriptase, depending on the virus species.[112, 113] Intravenous foscarnet is used in the management of cytomegalovirus infection in transplant recipients and, more recently, in patients with human immunodeficiency virus infection and clinical acquired immunodeficiency syndrome. It is used topically for herpes genitalis. The kidney is the only apparent organ of excretion, and the drug is not biotransformed. A nephrotoxic effect occurs in up to 66% of patients.[114, 115] Histopathologic postmortem examination showed proximal tubule necrosis in one patient dying of acute renal failure after foscarnet treatment.[114] In a group of 27 patients, intravenous saline administration before and during drug administration (2.5 L/24 h) virtually eliminated nephrotoxic effects.[114] Hypocalcemia, hyperphosphatemia, and increased serum parathyroid hormone level developed in some patients during foscarnet treatment.[114–116] The etiology of hyperphosphatemia is not certain, but suggested possibilities include foscarnet deposition in bone with release of stored phosphorus or inhibition of $Na^+$-$P_i$ cotransport in the proximal tubule by foscarnet.[115] Hypocalcemia and elevated serum parathyroid hormone levels suggest resistance of bone to the effect of parathyroid hormone. Foscarnet can be successfully administered to patients undergoing hemodialysis, with an initial dose of 60 mg/kg after each dialysis session and maintaining peak plasma levels between 500 and 800 $\mu$M.[117]

# NEPHROTOXICITY OF RADIOCONTRAST AGENTS

Acute renal failure due to radiocontrast agents is more likely to occur in the presence of advanced age, renal insufficiency, diabetes mellitus, severe congestive heart failure, multiple myeloma, volume depletion, low cardiac output states, and high-dose contrast studies (>125 mL)[118, 119] (Table 34–4). The frequency of nephrotoxic injury varies, depending on the underlying risk factors and the sensitivity of the measure used to determine nephrotoxic effects. In a study using a sensitive index of renal dysfunction (an increase in the level of serum creatinine of greater than 0.3 mg/dL and greater than 20% on day 1, 2, or 3 and day 5, 6, or 7), the frequency of nephrotoxic injury was 2% in nondiabetic, nonazotemic patients and 16% in diabetic, nonazotemic patients.[120] Diabetic patients with azotemia had a 38% frequency of nephrotoxic reactions. In another study of 59 diabetic patients with advanced azotemia (mean serum creatinine level of 5.9 mg/dL) undergoing coronary angiography, nephrotoxic reactions to the contrast agent developed in 50%, as defined by a serum creatinine level that was 25% above baseline levels 48 hours after angiography. Nine patients (15%) required hemodialysis.[121]

The warning against use of radiocontrast agents in the presence of multiple myeloma appears to be relative rather than absolute. In a retrospective review of 476 patients with multiple myeloma undergoing radiocontrast studies, the frequency of acute renal failure was 0.6% to 1.25%, substantially higher than the reported frequency of 0.15% in the general population as reported by Byrd and Sherman[122] yet not so prohibitive that contrast agents could not be used if the clinical indications were compelling.[123]

Renal failure may be oliguric or nonoliguric; nonoliguric renal failure is more common in patients with more nearly normal previous renal function. Most episodes of contrast agent nephrotoxicity are mild and sometimes not clinically apparent, characterized by a reversible rise in serum creatinine level of 1 to 3 mg/dL; dialysis therapy is rarely needed and usually only in those patients whose baseline serum creatinine level is high (e.g., >3 mg/dL).[121, 124–128] Unlike ischemia-induced acute renal failure, in which the urinary $Na^+$ concentration is characteristically high, radiocontrast nephrotoxicity may be associated with a low urinary $Na^+$ concentration (<10 mEq/L).[129, 130] The effect of radiocontrast material on urinalysis is variable. Renal tubule epithelial cell casts or coarsely granular casts may or may not be present in the presence or absence of functional deterioration.[125, 131] A persistent nephrogram during the 24 to 48 hours after the administration of the radiocontrast agent is a characteristic and sensitive indicator of contrast agent nephropathy, but there are many false-positive results, which gives it a low predictive value of 19%.[126]

Pathologic findings are restricted to the proximal tubule. The characteristic finding is an intense vacuolization of the proximal tubule called osmotic nephrosis,[132, 133] but the origin of the vacuoles is uncertain, and they have not been shown to contain iodine.[5, 133] Heyman and co-workers[5] have suggested that endocytosis is not the cause; rather, the vacuoles represent invaginations of the lateral cell membrane of the proximal tubules.

The pathogenesis of radiocontrast agent nephrotoxicity has been elusive. A healthy kidney is resistant to injury by radiocontrast agents. Most animal models require that renal function be compromised in some way before exposure to contrast material will impair function.[5, 134] One study correlated renal functional injury with damage to the more distal and highly oxygen dependent medullary thick ascending limb, an effect that may result from damage to $Na^+,K^+$-ATPase in the basolateral membrane.[5] Renal vasoconstriction develops transiently after administration of radiocontrast agents and could play a role in the pathogenesis of contrast agent nephrotoxicity. This vasoconstriction appears to be a $Ca^{2+}$-dependent effect because it can be blocked with $Ca^{2+}$ channel blockers but not $\alpha$-blockers.[135, 136] In vitro and in vivo studies show that both ionic and nonionic contrast agents induce release of the potent vasoconstrictor endothelin, which suggests a possible local mediator of contrast agent–induced vasoconstriction.[137] However, ioversol, a nonionic, low-molecular-weight contrast medium, is less nephrotoxic than iothalamate and has a reduced tendency to stimulate release of endothelin both in vivo and in vitro. This finding lends support to the idea that radiocontrast agent toxicity is linked to endothelin release.[138] Evidence against the role of renal vasoconstriction as an important element of radiocontrast agent nephrotoxicity comes from the observations that intracardiac injection of radiocontrast material is not associated with a fall in total renal blood flow in most patients with chronic renal fail-

**TABLE 34–4. Clinical Risk Factors in Radiocontrast Agent Nephrotoxicity**

| | |
|---|---|
| Advanced age | Multiple myeloma |
| Renal insufficiency | Volume depletion |
| Diabetes mellitus | Low cardiac output states |
| Congestive heart failure | High-dose contrast studies |

ure[139] and that the clinical use of dopamine, a renal vasodilator, in high-risk patients with chronic renal failure before and during angiography does not reduce the frequency of nephrotoxic injury.[140]

Prevention of the nephrotoxic effects of radiocontrast agents includes cautious volume expansion with saline before the procedure, a mannitol- or furosemide-induced diuresis during the procedure, and the use of the lowest possible dose of contrast agent. Whereas the nonionic contrast agents cause fewer allergic, cardiovascular, and endothelial reactions than do the ionic agents,[141] there is still uncertainty about whether their use leads to reduced nephrotoxic effects. In vitro studies suggest that cellular injury is less likely from nonionic agents.[142] However, clinical studies are in disagreement on this point; some show no benefit of nonionic agents in lowering the frequency of nephrotoxic injury in high-risk patients,[143-146] and others show less nephrotoxic effect.[147] A meta-analysis of 45 trials dealing with this question indicates that low-osmolality contrast material is associated with reduced nephrotoxic effects.[148]

# NEPHROTOXICITY OF MEDICATION USED IN TRANSPLANTATION

## Cyclosporine

Cyclosporine causes acute reversible as well as chronic, largely irreversible nephrotoxic effects (Table 34–5). During the early phase of cyclosporine treatment in humans, vasoconstriction develops in the systemic circulation and leads to arterial hypertension.[149, 150] At the level of the kidney, cyclosporine causes vasoconstriction of both the afferent and efferent glomerular arterioles.[151] This leads to a reduction in glomerular plasma flow and GFR and the rapidly reversible prerenal azotemia seen with large doses. However, tubule reabsorption and secretion remain largely intact.[152] Cyclosporine appears to enhance the renal vascular reactivity to certain vasoconstrictors[153] while also diminishing the responsivity to certain vasodilators, possibly mediated by a reduced endothelial capacity to produce nitric oxide.[151] Activation of the renin-angiotensin and sympathetic nervous systems, although present, seems not to play an important role in this vasoconstriction. However, increased intracellular $Ca^{2+}$ concentration, endothelial injury with release of endothelin,[154-156] and reduced vasodilator prostaglandin production appear to be prominently involved. In vitro studies show that the afferent and efferent glomerular arterioles vasoconstrict in a concentration-dependent way after exposure to cyclosporine, with the afferent arteriole being more sensitive.[157] A receptor antagonist for endothelin was able to block cyclosporine-induced vasoconstriction in the afferent arteriole, but not that in the efferent arteriole. In another study, afferent arteriole vasoconstriction, but not efferent arteriole vasoconstriction, was blocked by a cyclooxygenase inhibitor, which indicates that locally released cyclooxygenase products mediate sustained cyclosporine vasoconstriction.[158] Within hours of each oral dose of cyclosporine in kidney transplant recipients, there is a reduction in renal plasma flow and GFR. $Ca^{2+}$ channel blockers can provide some protection against early cyclosporine nephrotoxic effects in laboratory animals and humans.[159-163] In addition, several reports of long-term transplant recipients receiving cyclosporine suggest that $Ca^{2+}$ channel blockers improve graft survival and diminish long-term cyclosporine nephrotoxic injury,[164-166] but other studies have not found a beneficial effect.[167] Cyclosporine influences the production of several prostaglandins in vitro and in vivo.[168-172] Misoprostol, a prostaglandin E (PGE) analogue, can largely reverse the acute vasoconstrictive effects of cyclosporine in experimental animals[172] and can reduce the frequency of acute rejection in kidney transplant recipients treated with cyclosporine.[173] However, another PGE analogue, enisoprost, failed to improve renal function when it was given to human renal allograft recipients acutely[174] or to those chronically exposed to cyclosporine.[175] Also, blockade of thromboxane $A_2$ in experimental animals affords some protection against the vasoconstriction.[176]

Chronic cyclosporine nephrotoxic injury, as described in heart transplant recipients and patients with autoimmune disease with initially normal renal function, is characterized by a 35% to 45% reduction in GFR compared with that in patients not treated with cyclosporine. Also, the ability of cyclosporine to reduce short-term renal allograft loss but not to improve long-term allograft survival suggests that a similar nephrotoxic effect is occurring in kidney transplant recipients as well. Long-term cyclosporine administration causes an obliterative arteriolopathy that results in a form of interstitial nephritis and a progressive, largely irreversible decline in renal function. A peculiar form of tubulointerstitial damage called striped interstitial fibrosis is probably due to tubule collapse induced by constriction of the afferent arteriole. An analogue of cyclosporine, cyclosporin G, appears to be less nephrotoxic in the rat model.[177]

Cyclosporine is also a direct cellular toxin, causing hyperkalemia, hypophosphatemia, impaired urine concentration, and hyperchloremic metabolic acidosis.

## FK 506

FK 506 is a potent immunosuppressive agent that is similar to cyclosporine in its effect on T cell function; it binds to an immunophilin, FK 506–binding protein, and prevents signal transduction pathways in the lymphocyte.[178] It has been used primarily in liver transplant recipients, but it has also found a use in kidney and heart transplant recipients. Early use of this drug was confined initially to one center, and although nephrotoxic injury was reported as an adverse consequence, details about its effect on kidney

**TABLE 34–5. Etiologic Factors in Cyclosporine Nephrotoxicity**

Enhanced renal vascular reactivity to certain vasoconstrictors
Decreased responsivity to certain vasodilators
Activation of the renin–angiotensin II system
Increased intracellular $Ca^{2+}$ concentration
Endothelial injury with endothelin release
Reduced vasodilator prostaglandin production

function and comparisons with other immunosuppressive agents were scant.

In two groups of liver transplant recipients 4 weeks after transplantation,[179] FK 506 caused less systemic hypertension compared with cyclosporine but had similar effects on the kidney (i.e., a significant reduction in renal blood flow and GFR). FK 506 and cyclosporine have similar depressing effects on the level of urinary thromboxane $B_2$, plasma renin activity, and plasma aldosterone; FK 506 had a significantly greater effect in reducing the urinary excretion of 6-keto-PGF$_{1\alpha}$, the stable metabolite of prostacyclin (PGI$_2$), the renal vasodilator. A subsequent study from these same investigators in liver transplant recipients demonstrated a significantly lower GFR at 12 months in the FK 506 group compared with the cyclosporine group (45 $\pm$ 4 versus 64 $\pm$ 6 mL/min per body surface area, $P < .05$) (Fig. 34–3). Severe early nephrotoxic reactions were seen in some patients who received only FK 506.[180] Renal tubule damage from FK 506 results in a 50% frequency of hyperkalemia.[181] Like that of cyclosporine, long-term administration of FK 506 produces striped interstitial fibrosis in the renal cortex, which suggests that despite their chemical dissimilarity, they probably share a common pathway in producing nephrotoxic effects.[182]

# NEPHROTOXICITY OF ANTINEOPLASTIC DRUGS

## Alkylating Agents

### CISPLATIN

Cisplatin (*cis*-diamminedichloroplatinum II) is a highly effective antineoplastic agent with a broad spectrum of antitumor activity.[183–188] The drug has been shown to be effective in several different types of cancer, particularly small-cell cancer of the lung and testicular, ovarian, head and neck, and bladder cancers.[183–188] In addition to being useful against primary solid tumors, cisplatin has been helpful in improving the outlook for patients who suffer from metastatic testicular and ovarian carcinomas.[189] The major toxic effect of cisplatin therapy has been the nephrotoxic injury that occurs with successive treatments of the drug. The toxic effect observed in patients was predicted by early studies that showed renal injury as a major problem.[190] An unusual feature of cisplatin nephrotoxicity is that the renal damage is irreversible in many cases.

The usual pattern of cisplatin nephrotoxicity is that of a dose-related and progressive form of renal failure noted after one or more doses of the drug. This toxic effect may be gradual and subtle or, on occasion, abrupt. The hallmark of the nephrotoxic reaction is a tubulointerstitial pattern of injury without heavy proteinuria. Tubule proteinuria and prominent tubule casts may be a particularly impressive feature of the clinical presentation.[191] $\beta_2$-Microglobulin excretion has also been demonstrated to antedate renal failure, which suggests that renal tubule damage may occur on a subclinical level before an increase in the serum creatinine concentration.[192] The pathologic process of the lesion is one of tubule damage with impressive light and electron microscopic changes that show hyaline droplets in the proximal tubule cells, degeneration of the tubule basement membrane, and areas of focal tubule necrosis.[193] The glomeruli and blood vessels are largely spared from these processes. As might be expected, a variety of clinically apparent tubule defects occur in the presence of cisplatin nephrotoxicity: renal $Mg^{2+}$ wasting, hyperphosphaturia, and disorders of renal $Ca^{2+}$ and amino acid handling have all been reported.[194–196] The renal $Mg^{2+}$ wasting associated with cisplatin is particularly notable,[197] mainly because the hypomagnesemia that results may be severe and may be accompanied by hypocalcemia and tetany. In particularly large series of patients who received 70 mg/m$^2$ cisplatin every 3 weeks, 52% of patients were hypomagnesemic. The peak frequency of hypomagnesemia occurred 3 weeks after therapy. The hypomagnesemia associated with cisplatin has been observed to be exacerbated by the concomitant use of

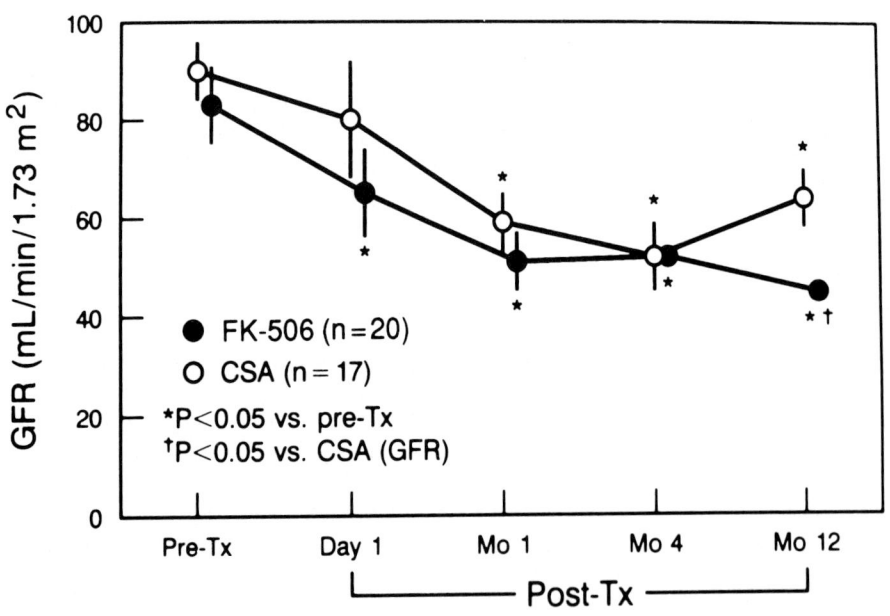

**Figure 34–3.** Changes in glomerular filtration rate (GFR) in patients treated with FK 506 and cyclosporine (CSA) before and after liver transplantation.

other drugs, particularly the aminoglycoside antibiotics.[198–200] This defect in renal $Mg^{2+}$ handling usually abates after a period of weeks and is easily treated with oral magnesium supplementation. There are exceptions to this pattern, however; some patients have had persistent hypomagnesemia lasting for years.

The exact mechanism of cisplatin nephrotoxicity is unclear. Experimental studies have shown that there is an abrupt fall in the effective renal plasma flow within 3 hours of the first dose of cisplatin.[201] Cisplatin is known to be filtered by the glomeruli and concentrated in the glomerular filtrate from which it gains entrance into proximal tubule cells. It is activated in the presence of a low intracellular $Cl^-$ concentration, and the aquated or activated agent forms intrastrand and interstrand cross-links between DNA molecules.[202] Renal damage is seen in both the proximal tubule $S_3$ portion and the distal tubule and collecting duct.[202, 203] Glomeruli are relatively well preserved despite the extensive damage to tubule elements.[204] More research is needed to clarify the effects of cisplatin on potent oxidative (cytochrome P-450 oxidase) and reducing substances (glutathione transferase) that are well known to be so abundant in renal tubule cells. As mentioned before, renal tubule dysfunction may persist well after cisplatin therapy has been completed; if this occurs, hypocalcemia may be a common feature of the clinical presentation.[205] A worrisome feature of cisplatin is that despite measures to avoid toxicity, silently progressive renal tubulointerstitial damage leading to a gradual decline in GFR can occur both experimentally and clinically.[206, 207]

The first step in avoiding nephrotoxic effects of cisplatin is to avoid the concomitant use of other agents that are known to induce nephrotoxic injury, such as aminoglycoside antibiotics. In addition, given the relationship of the toxicity to the dose administered, careful attention to the necessary dose is of key importance. Doses of cisplatin exceeding 25 to 33 $mg/m^2/wk$ predispose to nephrotoxic injury and other toxic effects, including ototoxic effects and myelosuppression.[208]

It is clear that a significant reduction in the frequency of cisplatin nephrotoxic effects can be obtained by the induction of a brisk diuresis. A urine output of at least 100 mL/h for several hours before and after a dose of cisplatin reduces the nephrotoxic effect.[196] Several studies have shown that the use of mannitol or furosemide to produce a natriuresis allows therapy with cisplatin up to 100 to 120 $mg/m^2$ without toxicity.[209] The administration of cisplatin is also better tolerated if the dose is administered in hypertonic saline, which does not alter the pharmacokinetics of cisplatin.[210–212] Some authors now suggest that the saline infusion precede the dose of cisplatin by 12 hours and be extended for another 12 hours after the completion of the cisplatin dose.[212] Additional renal protective measures that may be undertaken to prevent cisplatin nephrotoxic injury include the simultaneous administration of sodium thiosulfate, which is recommended for patients who are to receive in excess of 200 $mg/m^2$ of cisplatin. Sodium thiosulfate alters the pharmacokinetics of cisplatin, which results in a reduction in the fall in the white blood cell count and platelet count and also less neurotoxic reaction and vomiting. In one study, the concomitant use of sodium thiosulfate al-

lowed a significant dose intensification of cisplatin chemotherapy in individuals receiving biweekly administration of the antineoplastic drug.[208] In this particular study, whereas sodium thiosulfate was effective in reducing nephrotoxic injury, other types of toxic effect, including myelosuppression, were not reduced. The therapeutic goal of this therapy is to shorten the cycle intervals of the cisplatin therapy and thereby increase dosage intensity.

In addition to sodium thiosulfate as a drug to reduce the toxicity of cisplatin, other protective agents have undergone testing, including ethiofos (WR-2721), diethyldithiocarbamate, and ORG 2766.[213] Each of these drugs requires further testing to determine whether it reduces the nephrotoxic effect. Strategies to reduce the accumulation of cisplatin in the kidney include the use of probenecid, but this approach has not been tested extensively.[214] Finally, new platinum compounds are expected to reduce the dependence of the oncologist on cisplatin, including carboplatin (cis-diammine(1,1-cyclobutanedicarboxylato)platinum). A list of several antineoplastic agents and the type of toxic effect caused is provided in Table 34–6.

## CARBOPLATIN

Carboplatin was approved for clinical use in 1989 and has less nephrotoxicity than cisplatin; however, myelosuppression and thrombocytopenia remain as features of carboplatin toxicity.[215–217]

This drug was synthesized to be a non-nephrotoxic platinum analogue.[218] Carboplatin is available for use as chemotherapy for small-cell cancer of the lung and ovarian and head and neck cancers. The usual dose of carboplatin is 400 to 500 $mg/m^2$ every 4 weeks when it is used as a single agent.[219] In combination with other chemotherapy, carboplatin doses of 250 $mg/m^2$ have been well tolerated.[217] Several dose escalation studies have shown that nephrotoxic effect is detectable in increasing frequency at doses greater than 900 $mg/m^2$.[220, 221] However, most of the nephrotoxic effects occurred in patients who had received cisplatin previously or who were receiving other nephrotoxic drugs during preparation for autologous bone marrow transplantation. As for specific nephrotoxic injury with carboplatin, hypomagnesemia appears to be the most common manifestation.[222]

## CYCLOPHOSPHAMIDE

Cyclophosphamide is a highly useful antineoplastic agent with significant antitumor activity against lymphomas and hematologic malignant neoplasms. Primary side effects of the drug include a myelosuppressive effect, gastrointestinal symptoms, and hemorrhagic cystitis. The primary renal effect of cyclophosphamide has been that of hyponatremia, which has been observed with doses of 50 mg/kg.[223] This hyponatremia involves impaired water excretion because urine osmolality is high in the face of a decreased plasma osmolality. This effect is dissipated by approximately 24 hours after the drug has been discontinued and is caused by a direct antidiuretic effect in the distal nephron and not by increased levels of vasopressin.[224]

**TABLE 34–6. Types of Antineoplastic Agents That Cause Nephrotoxic Injury**

| Drug | Type of Toxic Effect |
|---|---|
| *Alkylating Agents* | |
| Cisplatin | TIN,* occasionally irreversible; often acute renal failure |
| Carboplatin | Less nephrotoxic than cisplatin; can cause acute renal failure secondary to TIN |
| Cyclophosphamide | Associated with hyponatremia due to distal tubule effect; also causes hemorrhagic cystitis |
| Streptozocin | Nitrosourea compound; renal dysfunction in 65% of patients; causes acute renal failure secondary to TIN |
| Semustine and carmustine | Nitrosourea compounds that can lead to chronic deterioration in renal function 3 y after therapy; semustine is more nephrotoxic than carmustine |
| Ifosfamide | Associated with nephrogenic diabetes insipidus and direct toxic injury to proximal and distal tubule |
| *Antibiotics* | |
| Mitomycin C | Associated with hemolytic-uremic syndrome |
| Mithramycin | Nephrotoxic injury in as many as 40% of patients with long-term treatment; causes proximal and distal tubule damage |
| *Antimetabolites* | |
| Methotrexate | Volume expansion reduces nephrotoxic risk; intratubule deposition of 7-hydroxymethotrexate a factor in toxicity; also causes direct tubule damage; associated with nonoliguric acute renal failure |
| Cytosine arabinoside | Associated with TIN |
| 6-Thioguanine | Parenteral administration and high doses associated with azotemia and acute renal failure syndrome |
| 5-Fluorouracil | Associated with acute renal failure, often in combination with other drugs; less nephrotoxic than methotrexate |
| *Other Agents* | |
| Interleukin-2 | High doses cause acute renal failure in ~90%; avoid use with nonsteroidal anti-inflammatory drugs |

*TIN = tubulointerstitial nephritis.

## STREPTOZOCIN

Streptozocin is a nonmyelosuppressive nitrosourea that is used in the treatment of patients with metastatic carcinoma of the pancreas and carcinoid tumors.[225] Some kidney dysfunction occurs in approximately 65% of the patients who are exposed to this drug.[226–228] In most cases, proteinuria antedates the development of azotemia. It appears that the rate of streptozocin administration plays a larger role in the development of nephrotoxic injury than does the total cumulative dose. A total weekly dose of 1 to 1.5 g/m$^2$ is safe and effective. However, a cumulative dose of greater than 4 g/m$^2$ has been associated with a higher frequency of toxic effects.

Tubule atrophy and interstitial fibrosis are the lesions most often described in association with streptozocin administration. The proximal tubule cells are more commonly affected, and there is often an exuberant interstitial infiltrate.

The avoidance of nephrotoxic injury with streptozocin involves using the drug in a dosage schedule in which less than 1.5 g/m$^2$/wk (0.5 g/m$^2$ daily for 5 days) is employed. Repeated courses may be given every 3 to 4 weeks. Patients who receive the drug should be monitored for the appearance of proteinuria or other renal tubule defects. A general rule is that if these abnormalities are detected early, the discontinuation of the drug will result in resolution of the toxic effect.

## SEMUSTINE AND CARMUSTINE

Semustine is a nitrosourea useful in the therapy of malignant melanoma and some lymphomas. This drug is lipid soluble and therefore has also been used as a chemotherapeutic agent in the treatment of malignant brain tumors because it crosses the blood-brain barrier easily. High-dose therapy (1500 mg/m$^2$) in children with brain tumors resulted in a pattern of insidious renal failure leading to renal insufficiency some 3 to 5 years after the onset of therapy.[229] The pathologic renal change in these patients included a modest lymphocytic infiltrate accompanied by interstitial fibrosis. The use of more than 1400 mg/m$^2$ for therapy of malignant melanoma in adults has resulted in a similar interstitial nephritis in these patients.[230] However, doses less than 1400 mg/m$^2$ are not typically associated with nephrotoxic effects in adults.

Carmustine is another nitrosourea compound that has been associated with a mild interstitial infiltrate and tubule changes. The main side effect appears to be a proclivity of this drug to cause an interstitial pneumonitis.

## IFOSFAMIDE

Ifosfamide is an alkylating agent that has the major side effect of hemorrhagic cystitis but has also been associated with renal tubule injury. The frequency of clinical nephrotoxic effects is believed to be less than 10%, but some cases of irreversible renal failure have been noted. Patients with pre-existing renal dysfunction may be more vulnerable to the nephrotoxic effects of ifosfamide.[231, 232] Doses of ifosfamide at 6 g/m² (given during a 5-day period) result in detectable increases in both proximal and distal tubule enzymes in the urine.[233] Clinically, the occurrence of nephrogenic diabetes insipidus has been linked to therapy with ifosfamide.[231–235] In addition, Elias and colleagues[236] have reported that 72% of patients administered doses of ifosfamide of 8 to 18 g/m² (given over 4 days) had renal tubular acidosis, and 24% of the patients went on to develop a serum creatinine concentration greater than 2.0 mg/dL. The pathogenesis of these lesions is not clear and is difficult to determine because of the frequent combination of ifosfamide with other chemotherapeutic agents such as cisplatin.

## Antibiotics

### MITOMYCIN C

Nephrotoxic injury from mitomycin C is unusual with cumulative doses less than 30 mL/m². This drug is useful in the therapy of gastrointestinal carcinomas when it is used in combination with 5-fluorouracil. A cancer-associated hemolytic-uremic syndrome has been reported in the majority of patients who were treated with mitomycin C in excess of 60 mL/m².[237–240] In one large study in which the frequency of mitomycin C nephrotoxic injury was assessed, a dose-related renal dysfunction developed in less than 1% of patients.

There appear to be no predictive laboratory tests to prospectively identify those patients at risk for mitomycin C–induced hemolysis and uremia. Renal biopsy changes that have been reported with mitomycin C toxicity include glomerular sclerosis and marked interstitial scarring. Fibrin deposits have been noted within glomeruli and small blood vessels. These findings coupled with the clinical observations of a hemolytic process suggest that mitomycin C may precipitate a microangiopathic hemolytic anemia in certain circumstances. In one case,[241] plasma exchange therapy resulted in improvement of thrombocythemia and the microangiopathic hemolytic anemia but not in renal function.

### MITHRAMYCIN (PLICAMYCIN)

Mithramycin is an antibiotic with antitumor activity against testicular cancers and glioblastomas.[242] The drug is usually administered daily for several consecutive days or on a schedule of three times per week in a dose between 15 and 50 g/kg. Toxic renal effects from the drug may approach a frequency of 40% of patients when it is given on a daily schedule.[243] Mithramycin-induced inhibition of RNA in neoplastic cells persisted for 48 hours, whereas inhibition of RNA in normal cells was reversed within this period.[244] This study also demonstrated that the nephrotoxic

effect was reduced by the use of alternate-day dosing. However, nephrotoxic injury was not eliminated; 6 of 54 patients died of azotemia while following the alternate-day dosing schedule.[245] In the further evaluation of patients on the alternate-day schedule, Kennedy[248] reported trace to 1+ proteinuria in 78% of patients and some evidence of chronic renal dysfunction in all of the patients tested. However, there are no correlations available between the type of kidney damage incurred and the clinical syndrome of mithramycin toxicity. Several other types of toxic effect have been observed with mithramycin, including liver dysfunction,[246] thrombocytopenia,[247] and hypocalcemia.[248]

The mechanism for the nephrotoxic injury observed with mithramycin is unknown. This drug forms a complex with DNA and inhibits DNA-dependent RNA synthesis.[249] Moreover, the proximal tubule concentration of mithramycin is believed to be high.[244] The drug has a short half-life because it is not extensively metabolized and has a relatively rapid appearance in urine, which presumably favors a high concentration of mithramycin in proximal tubule cells. Both proximal and distal tubule necrosis and tubule atrophy have been observed after mithramycin administration; as with cisplatin, glomeruli are usually not involved.

Mithramycin is widely used as an agent to treat the hypercalcemia of malignancy. In this setting, a single infusion of 25 μg/kg has been shown to decrease bone resorption and to improve serum Ca²⁺ concentration in about 90% of patients. When used in the setting of hypercalcemia, mithramycin is not usually nephrotoxic, although exceptions exist.[250] It is therefore recommended that renal function be monitored whenever mithramycin is used.

## Antimetabolites

### METHOTREXATE

Methotrexate is an antimetabolite that has been proved to be an effective chemotherapeutic agent in combination regimens for choriocarcinoma, acute lymphocytic leukemia, bladder cancers, squamous cell cancers of the head and neck, osteogenic sarcoma, breast carcinoma, and non-Hodgkin lymphoma. Standard doses of methotrexate are not associated with nephrotoxic injury unless the patient has some elements of underlying renal dysfunction.[251] However, high-dose therapy given without concomitant volume expansion or urine alkalinization is associated with nephrotoxic effects in at least 10% of treated patients.[252, 253] The intratubule deposition of 7-hydroxymethotrexate is believed to be at least partly responsible for the nephrotoxic effect.[253, 254]

Evidence for the importance of intratubule hydroxymethotrexate deposition is provided by the fact that the prophylactic use of volume expansion and an adequate urine output (>3 L/d) and of urine alkalinization appears to have reduced the nephrotoxicity of methotrexate.[255] Another possibility for methotrexate toxicity is direct tubule injury; hence, proximal tubule necrosis has been documented without the presence of intratubule deposits.[256] Finally, it is not clear whether methotrexate has a consistent effect of causing vasoconstriction of the afferent arteriole, although this has been suspected in some instances in which methotrexate has been administered to children for osteogenic sarcoma.

The clinical course of methotrexate toxicity is usually that of a nonoliguric renal failure. It is important to recognize this early because any reduction in GFR may result in high levels of methotrexate, thereby incurring risk for other toxic effects of the drug. There are also reports of methotrexate causing nephrotoxic injury when it is combined with other agents; this has been true for the use of methotrexate with nonsteroidal anti-inflammatory drugs (NSAIDs)[257] and procarbazine.[258]

## CYTOSINE ARABINOSIDE

Cytosine arabinoside is an antimetabolite with antitumor activity against non-Hodgkin lymphoma and acute leukemia. Interstitial nephritis has been reported with the use of this drug in combination with other drugs.[259] However, the precise contribution of cytosine arabinoside to the interstitial nephritis observed is unclear.

## 6-THIOGUANINE

Intravenous doses of 6-thioguanine exceeding 800 mg/m$^2$ have been associated with an increase in blood urea nitrogen and creatinine levels in treated individuals. The use of oral 6-thioguanine has not been shown to be nephrotoxic. The development of acute renal failure after intravenous administration of 6-thioguanine is usually reversible within several weeks of discontinuation of therapy.[260]

## 5-FLUOROURACIL

5-Fluorouracil is a mainstay of tumor therapy for cancers of the gastrointestinal tract. Nephrotoxic injury has been reported in approximately 10% of patients who receive 5-fluorouracil in combination with other agents, including mitomycin C.[261] Some of these patients with acute renal failure appear to have a microangiopathic hemolytic anemia, whereas others follow a more insidious course to renal failure. A high percentage of fatalities have occurred with either type of renal failure, however. Necropsy studies revealed evidence for fibrin deposition in the smaller arterioles of the kidneys.

## Other Agents

### INTERLEUKIN-2

This drug is a glycoprotein that possesses killer cell function. The drug is now commercially available because of the large production made possible through recombinant DNA technology. High-dose parenteral interleukin-2 infusions result in acute renal failure in approximately 90% of the patients subjected to such therapy.[262] This hemodynamic effect on the GFR is rapidly reversible, however. Patients with pre-existent renal failure subjected to such therapy were observed to have a prolonged course of acute renal failure. Because the effect of interleukin-2 given as an acute

bolus appears to be mediated through a vasoconstrictor mechanism in the kidney, it is recommended that the drug not be given with NSAID use. Constant infusions of interleukin-2 are presently being used to avoid the high frequency of toxic effects.[263, 264]

# NEPHROTOXICITY OF TUMOR CELL LYSIS

The rapid lysis of tumor cells can lead to several discrete forms of acute renal failure. First, acute uric acid nephropathy is an acute renal failure syndrome characterized by acute oliguria due to uric acid precipitation within the tubules.[265, 266] This syndrome is usually due to the overproduction and overexcretion of uric acid in patients with lymphoma or a myeloproliferative disease and follows the initiation of chemotherapy or radiation therapy. Less frequent causes of uric acid nephropathy are tissue catabolism due to seizure activity or due to the treatment of solid tumors, overproduction of uric acid due to the rare syndrome of hypoxanthine guanine phosphoribosyltransferase deficiency, or hyperuricosuria due to decreased uric acid reabsorption of the proximal tubule.[265-267] Although flank pain may occur in the syndrome, more often there are no symptoms referable to the urinary tract. The uric acid concentration is typically above 15 mg/dL; urinalysis may or may not show uric acid crystals. Overexcretion of uric acid is proved by determining the uric acid/creatinine ratio on a spot urine specimen; a ratio of greater than 1 suggests overexcretion of uric acid, whereas a value below 0.6 to 0.75 is more typical of other forms of acute renal failure.[268] The therapy of acute uric acid nephropathy begins with prophylaxis with allopurinol in higher than normal doses (500 to 600 mg/d). Fluid loading to maintain a urine output of 2.5 to 3 L/d is also suggested; sodium bicarbonate may also be administered to yield a more alkaline urine (urine pH of approximately 6.5). Once renal failure occurs in this syndrome, therapy consists of allopurinol and administration of fluids and loop diuretics. Hemodialysis has been used in those patients in whom a diuresis cannot be induced.

The second common clinical syndrome resulting from tumor lysis is characterized by hyperphosphatemia, hyperkalemia, hypocalcemia, and hyperuricemia.[269, 270] In this syndrome, the release of cellular contents from tumor cells leads to several metabolic derangements and acute renal failure (Fig. 34–4). This illness is most often associated with treatment of Burkitt lymphoma[271] but has also been described after therapy for ductal carcinoma of the breast and metastatic seminoma.[272] This disease may be particularly devastating in patients with pre-existent renal dysfunction. If the patient has been hypercalcemic as a consequence of the tumor before treatment, then the sudden increase in serum PO$_4$$^{3-}$ levels may result in marked metastatic calcification. In fact, the intrarenal precipitation of calcium phosphate has been suggested as the cause of acute renal failure in this setting.[273] Therapy is directed at vigorous diuresis, allopurinol administration, and dialysis if necessary to reduce the serum PO$_4$$^{3-}$ level.[274]

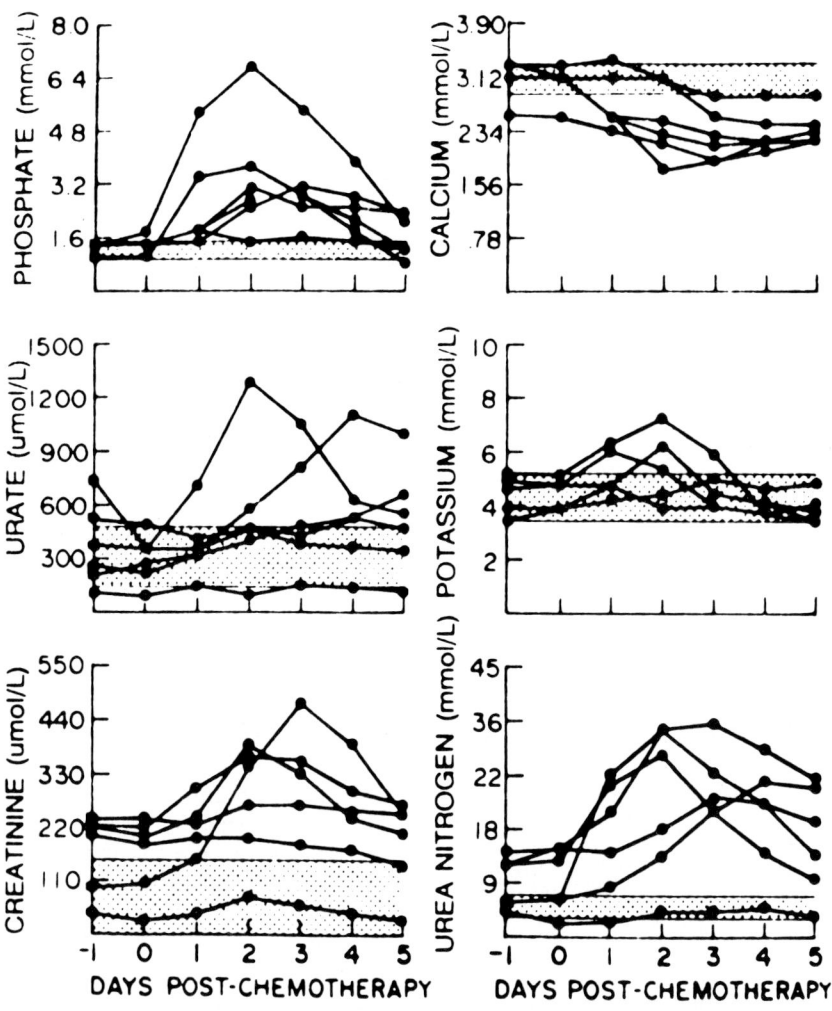

**Figure 34–4.** Changes in several parameters in patients with the acute tumor lysis syndrome. (From Hande KR, Garrow GC: Acute tumor lysis syndrome in patients with high-grade non-Hodgkin's lymphoma. Reprinted from American Journal of Medicine: Vol 94; 1993 [pgs 133–138].)

# NEPHROTOXICITY OF HEAVY METALS

## Lead

Lead intoxication is an ancient disease with a fascinating history. The Greek poet and physician Nikander was the first to note the clinical syndrome in 200 BC.[275] The first reports of clinical nephrotoxic effects associated with exposure to lead were provided by Lancerceaux in 1862. Other early descriptions of lead poisoning were provided by Ramazzini,[276] who described classic lead poisoning in potters and portrait painters in 1713, and by Thackrah,[277] who associated long-term exposure to lead in plumbers and lead manufacturers with clinical disease. Finally, Legge[278] proposed in 1934 that absorption of lead occurred through several routes, most notably by inhalation of lead particles and from the skin. The clinical syndrome associated with acute and sometimes chronic lead intoxication includes gastrointestinal colic, paralysis, visual disturbances, and encephalopathy.

As far as the kidney is concerned, acute lead nephropathy has most often been observed in children with resultant damage to the proximal tubule and aminoaciduria, phosphaturia, and glycosuria.[279, 280] This constellation of findings is consistent with the Fanconi syndrome and appears to be rapidly reversible by chelation therapy. The pathologic renal process in this case typically shows intranuclear inclusions in proximal tubule cells[281] as well as several mitochondrial defects. Perhaps the largest study performed on the effects of exposure of children to lead was performed by Nye[282] in 1929. This study was performed in Australia and consisted of a series of observations made on children who had been exposed to household lead-based paint. This series of observations made the association of previous lead intoxication with renal failure, hypertension, and gout.[282–284] At issue in these investigations was whether long-term sequelae of exposure of children to lead could result in chronic renal failure later. A prospective analysis of 62 subjects with significant lead poisoning (plasma lead level >100 mg/dL) was undertaken with a control group consisting of 8 siblings (plasma lead level <40 mg/dL).[285] Multiple regression analysis failed to demonstrate a significant influence of the presence of plumbism on blood pressure.

Moreover, only 4 of the 62 study subjects had an elevated serum creatinine value. There were no significant differences in renal function or blood pressure between the study subjects and the control groups. Another review of this subject[286] concluded that definitive proof that chronic renal failure may be a consequence of lead exposure was lacking. However, long-term exposure to lead has been associated with a high prevalence of renal dysfunction in previous studies.[287–291] In addition, Hu[292] studied 192 subjects with well-documented lead poisoning who had a follow-up of 50 years. These patients were carefully matched to a control group. The result showed that the patients with previous lead exposure had a sevenfold greater chance of having hypertension; in addition, these subjects had a lower hematocrit than control subjects did. Interestingly, creatinine clearances were similar in the patients with lead exposure and the control subjects. Thus, the exact relationship between early lead exposure and chronic renal failure remains unresolved in the setting of childhood exposure. A number of studies have provided evidence for excess mortality from renal disease in adults who have had lead exposure.[293–296] Most of these are industrial exposures in lead smelters or in battery assembly plants. Another common route of exposure is in the preparation of moonshine whiskey.

The classic clinical presentation for lead nephropathy is that of a benign urine sediment, less than 2 g/d of urinary protein excretion, hyperuricemia, and hypertension. Gouty arthritis affects about half of the patients with lead nephropathy.[297] The association between gout and chronic renal failure is strong enough to merit a lead chelation screening test with ethylenediaminetetraacetic acid (EDTA) in patients with chronic renal failure who have gout. The combination of hypertension with previous lead exposure limits the ability of clinicians to determine which disorder is responsible for renal dysfunction. The pathologic renal process with lead exposure includes a nonspecific tubule atrophy and an element of interstitial fibrosis with minimal inflammatory infiltrates; lysosomal dense bodies may also be evident in the proximal tubule.[298, 299] Inclusion bodies may be less prominent in far-advanced interstitial damage from lead. The kidneys are usually small and contracted and have irregular cortical surfaces. The initial primary insult to the kidney appears to occur through damage to the proximal tubule, a finding that has been confirmed in animal models of this disease.[300]

The diagnosis of lead nephropathy may be difficult. In one study of workers exposed to lead pollutant in a battery factory,[301] there were no noninvasive simple tests that distinguished the exposed workers from unexposed control subjects. The main finding of this study was that the renal excretion of 6-keto-PGF$_{1\alpha}$ was reduced in patients who had been exposed to lead. In addition, these workers also had an enhanced excretion of thromboxane. The significance of these observations in unclear, but it does suggest that the kidney may be more vulnerable to the effects of drugs that reduce the synthesis of locally produced vasodilators, such as NSAIDs. The blood lead concentration is relatively insensitive in assessing cumulative body stores that have been acquired over many years of exposure. This is the case because blood lead levels tend to fall rapidly after short-term exposure is completed. The main repository of lead in the body is bone; however, if blood levels are high (>80 μg/dL), this would suggest an increased body burden of lead. Levels above 40 μg/dL are considered high in children. Of note is that sustained blood lead levels greater than 10 μg/dL may be associated with lead-induced disease.[302, 303] The best available method of screening for lead intoxication is the use of two 1-g doses of the agent EDTA calcium disodium.[304] Subsequent to the injections, a 24-hour urine sample is collected. Adults excrete up to 650 μg of lead chelate in the urine; patients with a serum creatinine level greater than 1.5 mg/dL should have a 48-hour or 72-hour urine specimen collected because the excretion of lead may be delayed in these individuals. In all samples, creatinine must also be measured to verify an accurate collection. The chelatable lead found in the urine correlates well with bone lead stores.[305, 306] Other methods that may be used in the future to measure the amount of lead in the body include photofluorography.[307]

The therapy of lead nephropathy consists of three weekly 1-g treatments of EDTA calcium disodium administered intramuscularly. The end point of therapy is a lead chelate product that is normal. Studies that have tested the utility of 2,3-dimercaptosuccinic acid and iron as a chelator have produced promising results, although no major improvement in renal function has been documented.[308] The chelation therapy is effective in reversing acute lead nephropathy, but there is no evidence that this therapy reverses the established interstitial disease. The failure to demonstrate an improvement in renal function in these patients does not mean that the therapy has not been effective; on the contrary, Koster and co-workers[309] documented a high mobilization of lead in patients with high renal failure. Finally, it is important for the physician to realize that the repeated exposure of the patient to the EDTA chelator may create a separate toxic effect.[310] However, this is believed to be an unusual occurrence and does not warrant discontinuing the practice of lead chelation as the mainstay of therapy.

## Cadmium

Cadmium is a metal with a wide variety of industrial uses, including the manufacturing of glass, metal alloys, and electrical equipment. The first cases of acute poisoning by cadmium were reported as early as 1958, but the first recognition of cadmium as a definite industrial toxin was made in 1948.[311] Chronic exposure to cadmium reaches a plateau in the blood after about 4 months.[312] Urinary excretion of cadmium for creatinine in the urine is a reliable indicator of total body cadmium burden.[312] A progressive increase in cadmium excretion is observed in both humans and experimental animals with increasing dosage of cadmium. In one study of exposed workers, the average concentration of cadmium in blood was 5.5 μg/dL and 5.4 μg per gram of creatinine.[313] On the basis of sampling of a number of workers exposed to cadmium in Belgium, Roels and co-workers[313] have estimated a threshold for cadmium toxicity as follows: individuals with 2 μg of cadmium per gram of creatinine were noted to have mainly biochemical alterations; individuals excreting 4 μg of cadmium per gram of creatinine were noted to have the excretion of some high-molecular-weight proteins and some antigens or enzymes; and individuals who excreted 10 μg of cadmium per gram of creatinine were also noted to excrete low-molecular-weight proteins in the urine. The recommendation of the American Conference of Governmental Industrial Hygienists was that a value of 5 μg of cadmium per gram of creatinine in the urine is the occupational exposure limit to cadmium. In the study of Nogawa and colleagues,[314] the appearance of metallothionine in the urine was used as an index of renal toxic injury. These investigators found that the prevalence rate for metallothionineuria was calculated to be 4.2 μg per gram of creatinine for men and 4.8 μg per gram of creatinine for women. If the appearance of $\beta_2$-microglobulin in the urine is used as an index of tubule damage from cadmium, a value of 3.8 μg of cadmium per gram of creatinine for men and 4.1 μg of cadmium per gram of creatinine for women could be used as the urinary levels that would predict toxic effects.[314] The reason that cadmium toxicity has been linked to metallothionine is that cadmium accumulation in proximal tubule cells is linked to binding to metallothionine; metallothionine is synthesized in the liver and transfers bound cadmium to the kidney through the blood.[315] This cadmium-metallothionine complex is nephrotoxic because it is stored in lysosomes of proximal tubule cells. The concentration of cadmium in renal biopsy specimens has been estimated at approximately 8.7 μg per gram of protein; in this study, the highest concentrations of cadmium were associated with the most pronounced tubule interstitial changes.[316] Other methods of diagnosing cadmium toxic injury in the kidney have been used; in this regard, Jung and associates[317] have suggested that the combination of $\alpha_1$-microglobulin and N-acetyl-β-D-glucosaminidase be used to determine the amount of nephrotoxic injury from cadmium.

The long-term effects of exposure to cadmium are often subtle. Toffoletto and co-workers[318] found that urinary cadmium excretion greater than 10 μg per gram of creatinine was associated with evidence of renal tubule damage at a prevalence rate of about 8.4% in 105 workers exposed to cadmium for more than 10 years. In 16 workers previously exposed to cadmium, Jarup and colleagues[319] noted that all individuals who had cadmium exposure had evidence of persistent tubule damage as documented by increased excretion of $\beta_2$-microglobulin in the urine. Moreover, the GFR was reduced from about 77 to 72 mL/min in a 5-year period. This reduction in GFR exceeds the usual rate of reduction in the GFR that could be accounted for by age alone. Other studies[320–322] have documented similar changes in renal function over time. Nephrotoxic injury is manifested clinically by aminoaciduria, glycosuria, renal tubular acidosis, and, as mentioned before, the excretion of methallothionine and $\beta_2$-microglobulin. Given the deposition of cadmium in bone as well as in kidney, it is not surprising that many patients have a combination of renal failure and severe osteopenia[323] that may lead to fractures. Tsuchiya and associates[324] have described an outbreak of cadmium intoxication in Japan; there the disease is known as *itai itai* (''ouch ouch'') because of the painful fractures that are associated with the renal dysfunction. Renal involvement in the disease is characterized by a prominent tubule interstitial infiltrate with little involvement of glomeruli.

If cadmium exposure is eliminated, the usual trend is for renal function to stabilize, but continued deterioration is not usual. The consensus is that in most instances, cadmium-induced tubule interstitial disease is not reversible. In this regard, the treatment of cadmium intoxication with EDTA calcium disodium has not improved renal function dramatically. This is believed to be so because the binding of cadmium with metallothionine in the proximal tubule is the event that produces damage. New therapies with other chelating agents have been reported,[325, 326] but the efficacy of these treatments is uncertain at present. Nephrolithiasis may be a limiting factor in treating a bone disorder that is associated with cadmium. The presence of hypercalciuria is the main factor that leads to the development of osteopenia. It is interesting to note that the presence of overt chronic renal failure is relatively unusual given the fact that the disorder causes so much in the way of proximal tubule dysfunction.

## Mercury

Mercury intoxication usually occurs as a result of accidental exposure to mercury vapor; mercury is present in alloy plants, in mirror plants, and in some batteries.[327] If ingested in the elemental form, mercury is harmless. However, transformation to the organic salt produces injury. The major site of mercury damage in the kidney is the proximal tubule; short-term mercury exposure leads to frank tubule necrosis, which is reversible in most cases.[328] In patients with short-term mercury intoxication, the administration of 2,3-dimercaprol leads to some improvement in the natural history of the disease.[315] Intracellular mercury has an affinity for sulfhydryl groups in lysosomes and may produce toxic effects in this location.[315, 329] A blood mercury level greater than 3 μg/dL or a urine level above 50 μg per gram of creatinine is considered abnormal, but the relationship of these values to overt disease is not always clear.[330] The consequences of endemic methyl mercury poisoning were reported from Japan and revealed that neurologic sequelae of mercury ingestion dominated the clinical picture.[331] This outbreak of mercury intoxication occurred as a result of industrial pollution in a bay that was heavily fished. In this group of patients with severe neurologic effects from mercury ingestion, the renal disease was surprisingly benign, consisting only of tubule proteinuria and no changes in serum creatinine concentration or significant albuminuria. The histologic postmortem evaluation of these individuals revealed few overt renal changes. Thus, the nephrotoxic effect of mercury appears to be an acute poisoning syndrome in which proximal tubule necrosis occurs. Marked changes in renal function with long-term ingestion are not impressive.

## Uranium

Uranium is used as an investigational agent to produce experimental acute renal failure in laboratory animals. Human exposure is limited to low-level industrial sources. In one study, the evaluation of uranium workers revealed modest tubule dysfunction as characterized by an increased excretion of amino acids and $\beta_2$-microglobulin in uranium workers versus control subjects. In addition, acute tubule necrosis was reported in atomic bomb workers during the Manhattan Project in the 1940s,[332] but chronic renal failure due to uranium exposure has not been reported. If suspicion of uranium exposure exists, screening of the urine for $\beta_2$-microglobulin as well as testing for renal function abnormalities should be undertaken. In general, uranium levels in excess of 30 $\mu$g/L in the urine suggest an overabundance of uranium.

## Other Heavy Metals

Arsenic and arsine gas have been shown to cause acute renal failure, but this may be a result of the hemolysis or rhabdomyolysis that may accompany the ingestion of these substances, as well as severe hypotension.[333] Other metals that have been associated with renal injury include thallium, copper, nickel, antimony, and silver; however, reports of these substances causing nephrotoxic effects are unusual. Chromium has also been associated with proximal renal tubule damage in acute renal failure, but this is also unusual.[334]

## NEPHROTOXICITY OF ANTIRHEUMATIC AGENTS

### Penicillamine

Penicillamine has been used to treat rheumatoid arthritis, scleroderma, and cystinuria. If therapy is prolonged, as it commonly is in rheumatoid arthritis, renal complications from the drug are not uncommon.[335] In one large series of patients receiving penicillamine, a nephrotic syndrome developed in 7% secondary to membranous nephropathy.[336] Proteinuria usually develops within the first 6 to 8 months of therapy, but the onset of proteinuria may be delayed up to 6 years. Proteinuria disappeared in these patients when the drug was stopped; in four of seven patients who were administered the drug again, proteinuria returned.[337] The usual pathologic finding in patients treated with penicillamine who had nephrotic syndrome is that of membranous nephropathy.[337, 338] Deposits of immunoglobulins have been identified in the glomerular basement membrane, and circulating antibodies to penicillamine have been demonstrated.[335] A genetic predisposition of patients with human leukocyte antigens B8 and DR3 histocompatibility antigens to gold-induced proteinuria is also true of penicillamine.[339] A more serious but less common complication of penicillamine is the development of acute renal failure due to a crescentic, rapidly progressive glomerulonephritis.[340, 341] Pulse prednisone, cyclophosphamide, and plasmapheresis have all been used to treat this disorder with some success.[341] In one study, the effect of continuing penicillamine or gold treatment was examined in 53 patients with biopsy-proven penicillamine (32 patients) or gold (21 patients) nephropathy.[342] Thirty-two of the patients stopped penicillamine or gold therapy as soon as proteinuria was detected,

whereas 21 patients continued therapy for 2 to 11 months. There were no significant differences observed in the initial or maximal proteinuria, the duration of the proteinuria, or in the initial or latest creatinine clearances between the groups of patients. The results suggest that penicillamine and gold may be continued for short periods without causing permanent renal damage. However, despite the fact that there appears to be little impact of continued therapy on the filtration rate, it is not recommended that this strategy be undertaken except in cases in which the gold or penicillamine is absolutely essential for therapeutic control.

## Gold

The prevalence of proteinuria in therapeutic gold administration is approximately 30%. The magnitude of proteinuria in patients treated with gold is usually less than 3.5 g/d. Renal biopsy findings in patients who have been treated with gold for a long period typically reveal membranous glomerulopathy. However, other lesions have been described; minimal change disease and biopsy-demonstrated mesangial and subendothelial electron-dense deposits have also been described.[343] A decline in the GFR is unusual in gold-treated patients, but both severe renal failure and nephrotic syndrome have been reported.[344] Of interest is that parenteral gold administration is more likely to be associated with proteinuria than is oral administration of gold.[345] The cause of gold nephropathy is unknown; particles of gold have been detected in proximal tubule endothelium, and tubule proteinuria and $\beta_2$-microglobulinuria have also been reported. There does not seem to be a close relationship between the dose of gold and the renal lesion that develops. An autoimmune tubulointerstitial nephritis and an immune complex glomerulopathy develop in animals receiving gold therapy. As mentioned before, gold- and penicillamine-induced toxic effects are associated with the human leukocyte antigens DR3 and B8. Idiopathic membranous nephropathy is also associated with the same human leukocyte antigen haplotype.[339]

## Nonsteroidal Anti-inflammatory Drugs

The frequency of nephrotoxic effects due to NSAIDs is low, and generally the drugs are regarded as safe and well tolerated. The most common overall side effect from the use of the drugs involves injury of the gastrointestinal tract, where ulcer disease and gastrointestinal bleeding result from the use of the drugs. However, the growing use of these agents (between 30 and 40 million people consume NSAIDs daily in the United States) means that even with a relatively low frequency rate, nephrotoxic effects will be seen commonly. There are several forms of nephrotoxic injury due to the use of NSAIDs, including a syndrome with acute renal failure related to hemodynamic changes in the kidney, a direct nephrotoxic effect that is usually manifested as a tubulointerstitial nephritis, and syndromes of proteinuria and hypertension.

Several of the effects of NSAIDs on the kidney are linked to the inhibition of renal prostaglandin synthesis.

Prostaglandins are derivatives of arachidonic acid, a 20-carbon tetraenoic acid, which is acetylated to membrane phospholipids. Classes of prostaglandins produced in the kidney are varied; the main categories include $PGI_2$, thromboxane $A_2$, and $PGE_2$ (Fig. 34–5). Prostaglandins exert physiologic actions at the location where they are synthesized; thus, they are really autacoids rather than hormones because they are made to act locally rather than at distant loci. $PGE_2$ and $PGF_2$ are synthesized primarily by interstitial cells, whereas $PGI_2$ is synthesized by cortical arterioles and glomeruli. $PGE_2$ and thromboxane $A_2$ are also produced in the renal cortex by glomeruli[346, 347] (Table 34–7).

The basic concept regarding the hemodynamic role of prostaglandins in the kidney has evolved to the following scheme: 1) Under euvolemic conditions, there is typically a low rate of prostaglandin synthesis, thereby making it difficult to demonstrate that prostaglandins exert any maintenance role on renal function. 2) When prostaglandin synthesis is stimulated, it is usually in circumstances in which the systemic circulation has become destabilized. Under these conditions, prostaglandins have been shown to exert a moderating influence on renal function by opposing the stimulus to prostaglandin synthesis. For example, vasopressin stimulates prostaglandin synthesis and release, but prostaglandins antagonize the hydro-osmotic effects of vasopressin on collecting tubule epithelium. Similarly, angiotensin II and norepinephrine (both renal vasoconstrictors) are potent stimulators of $PGI_2$ and $PGE_2$ formation. $PGI_2$ and $PGE_2$ are renal vasodilators that then attenuate any vasoconstrictor response to angiotensin II.[351] Hence, prostaglandins have a number of important roles to play in the renal circulation, including renal vasodilatation, renin secretion, and $Na^+$ and water excretion. The consequences of inhibiting prostaglandin synthesis with powerful nonsteroidal drugs include an increase in vascular tone, an antinatriuretic effect, an antirenin effect, and an antidiuretic effect. This intraplay between vasoconstrictor and vasodilator forces in the kidney is dynamic and has been shown to exist in vivo in several models.[348–351] In addition to opposing the vasoconstrictive effects of circulating hormones, prostaglandins oppose the vasoconstrictive influence in the renal sympathetic nervous system.[352–354] Thus, there is a balance between vasodilators and vasoconstrictor forces that influence renal circulation. In the presence of NSAIDs, compensatory vasodilatation is inhibited and the vasoconstrictive forces dominate, which leads to a decline in renal blood flow and to renal insufficiency. The clinical settings in which this construct becomes relevant include conditions in which blood volume or effective arterial blood volume is compromised. Enhanced vasoconstrictor activity is commonly seen in congestive heart failure, cirrhosis, nephrotic syndrome, some forms of hypertension, sepsis, anesthesia, diabetes, and volume depletion due to blood loss, diuretics, or extrarenal fluid losses.[355–362]

Prostaglandins also affect $Na^+$ excretion both indirectly and directly. Acting as renal vasodilators, prostaglandins may cause an increase in the filtered load of $Na^+$.[363, 364] In addition, prostaglandins augment medullary blood flow to the kidney, thereby reducing hypertonicity of the medullary interstitium and leading to a decrease in water reabsorption in the descending limb of the loop of Henle. Because of this effect, the $Na^+$ concentration at the loop is reduced, which leads to a reduction in passive $Na^+$ reabsorption along the water-impermeable thin ascending limb.[365–367] In addition, prostaglandins exert a vasodilatory effect at the efferent arteriolar site of the glomerular capillary, and this leads to a reduction in the filtration fraction and peritubular oncotic pressure. Peritubular hydraulic pressure increased by the sum of the changes in Starling forces causes a decrease in tubule $Na^+$ reabsorption.[368, 369] In addition to these effects on Starling forces, there is some evidence that prostaglandins act directly to inhibit $Na^+$ reabsorption. A number of in vivo and in vitro studies have shown that prostaglandins have a natriuretic effect by the inhibition of

## Metabolism of Arachidonic Acid

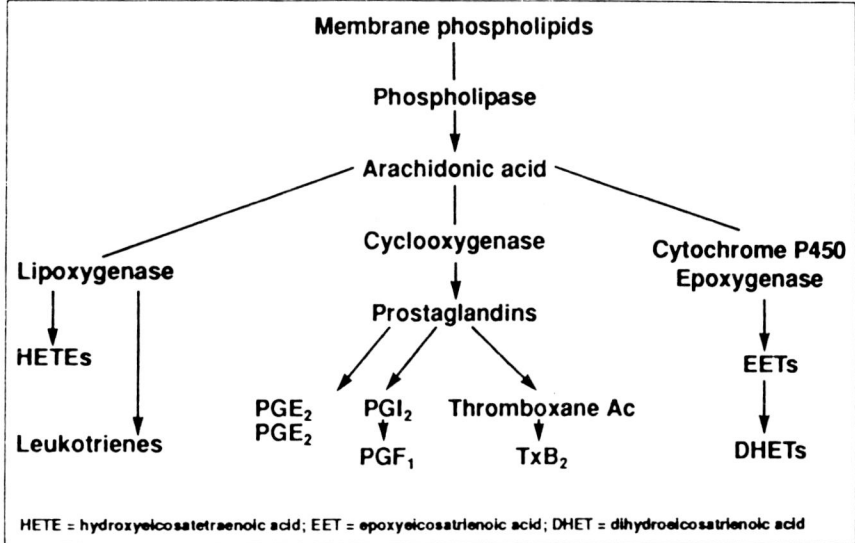

Figure 34–5. Metabolism of arachidonic acid. (From Houston MC: Nonsteroidal anti-inflammatory drugs and antihypertensives. Reprinted from American Journal of Medicine Supplement: Vol 90:5A; 1991 [pgs 42S–47S].)

**TABLE 34–7. Effects of Prostaglandins on Renal Function**

| Location of Synthesis and Action | Prostaglandin | Action | Physiologic Effects |
|---|---|---|---|
| Arterioles | $PGI_2$, $PGE_2$ | Vasodilatation | Maintain renal blood flow, direct more flow to intact cortical region and medulla |
| Glomeruli | $PGI_2$, $PGE_2$ | Vasodilatation | Modulate glomerular filtration rate |
| | Thromboxane $A_2$ | Vasoconstriction | |
| Distal tubules | $PGE_2$, $PGI_2$ | Inhibition of cyclic AMP | Interfere with vasopressin action |
| | $PGE_2$ | Decreased $Na^+$ transport | Natriuresis |
| Juxtaglomerular apparatus | $PGE_2$, $PGI_2$ | Possibly cyclic AMP stimulation | Increase renin release |

$Na^+$ transport in the loop of Henle, distal nephron, and collecting tubule.[370–374] Other studies show that prostaglandins may play a key permissive role in the $Na^+$ excretion that follows volume expansion and an increase in renal perfusion pressure.[375–377] NSAIDs are also able to partially blunt the natriuretic effect of some diuretics, mainly working through an effect on renal vasomotor tone.[377] This resistance to the natriuretic effects of diuretics has been seen in several circumstances[378–382] and has been confirmed in a study using the model of head-out water immersion after indomethacin administration in salt-depleted subjects.[383]

Prostaglandins also impair the ability of the kidney to concentrate the urine maximally, and NSAIDs impair urinary dilution. Both in vivo and in vitro experiments have shown that prostaglandins oppose the hydro-osmotic effects of vasopressin-induced prostaglandin synthesis.[384, 385] This serves to limit free water reabsorption by the collecting duct. Vasopressin also stimulates $PGE_2$ synthesis in the epithelial cells, thereby inducing its own antagonist. Thus, the antidiuretic effect is modulated by having vasopressin and $PGE_2$ play opposing roles in collecting duct epithelium. The clinical importance of this effect is that NSAIDs would be expected to impair renal water excretion and, in so doing, lead to a tendency toward water retention and hyponatremia.

$PGE_2$ and $PGI_2$ are known to be renin agonists, probably working through an increase in cyclic AMP in the juxtaglomerular cell.[386, 387] In addition, prostaglandins appear to be important in the normal functioning of the arterial baroreceptor that governs renin release and in the macula densa renin release as well.[388–390] By contrast, the β-adrenergic pathway to renin release appears to operate normally despite prostaglandin synthesis inhibition.[391–395] The practical clinical point made by these experiments in renin release is that in the presence of NSAID administration, positive $K^+$ balance may occur through an effect of the NSAID to cause hyporeninemia and hypoaldosteronism. This endogenous hyporenin-hypoaldosterone state could thereby favor the retention of $K^+$ and lead to hyperkalemia. There may also be an effect of the NSAIDs to reduce $Na^+$ delivery to distal exchange sites in the nephron, and this would also favor positive $K^+$ balance.

A number of clinical syndromes that follow the administration of NSAIDs are listed in Table 34–8. In terms of the frequency of occurrence of these syndromes, the renal insufficiency due to enhanced vasoconstriction is the leading consequence of NSAID use. As might be expected from the preceding discussion, there is a population of patients

who are at greater risk for this form of renal insufficiency from NSAIDs. This includes patients with congestive heart failure, cirrhosis (particularly with ascites), underlying renal disease, advanced age (older than 65 years), volume depletion or shock, septicemia, hypertension, concomitant diuretic therapy, and postoperative "third-space" fluid sequestration.[395–400] Urinalysis is usually unremarkable in the majority of patients during the acute deterioration of function. In addition, the fractional excretion of $Na^+$ may be low (<1%) in some of these patients who experience this form of renal failure.[401] If recognized early, the renal failure is reversible with discontinuation of the NSAIDs. In one survey of 27 patients with NSAID-induced vasoconstrictive renal failure,[402] only 3 patients required dialysis, and only 1 patient required permanent dialysis.[400] Hyperkalemia may be a pronounced feature of this disorder, occurring in about 25% of the cases. The unifying antecedent state for these patients who develop this form of NSAID-related disease

**TABLE 34–8. Syndromes of Nonsteroidal Anti-inflammatory Drug Nephrotoxicity**

| Syndrome | Characteristics |
|---|---|
| Acute renal failure | Prostaglandin inhibition leads to enhanced renal vasoconstriction; occurs in settings in which vasoconstrictors are stimulated, such as congestive heart failure, nephrotic syndrome, cirrhosis, volume depletion, and perhaps some pre-existent renal disease. |
| Interstitial nephritis | Usually results in heavy proteinuria, but it also can present with renal failure without proteinuria. Takes weeks to months to resolve. |
| Hyperkalemia | Occurs secondary to a decrease in renin release and therefore results in a hyporenin-hypoaldosterone syndrome; a decline in GFR may also contribute. |
| $Na^+$ and water retention | Usually a mild retention of $Na^+$ occurs because of the antinatriuretic effects of inhibiting prostaglandin synthesis; water retention is possible through an enhanced effect of vasopressin. |
| Hypertension | Usually a mild to modest increment in blood pressure ensues, but this can be more pronounced in patients with underlying hypertension. |

is that of a high-renin, high-angiotensin state[403–410] (Table 34–9).

Of particular note are two groups of patients who are susceptible to this form of renal failure. Patients with underlying renal disease have been shown to be particularly susceptible, given the fact that up to 30% of the patients may have worsening of renal function when they are exposed to an NSAID.[411–413] Renal disease may lead to an increased prostaglandin production and therefore make renal function dependent in part on prostaglandins to maintain renal blood flow and glomerular filtration.[414–416] Another group that may be more vulnerable is the elderly, for several reasons: 1) they often have lower albumin levels, which reduces protein binding of the NSAID and results in higher free drug levels; 2) they have reduced total body water, which leads to an increased concentration of the NSAID; and 3) they have decreased hepatic metabolism of the NSAID, an effect that would lead to increased drug levels. The sum of all these factors may cause an increased toxic effect from NSAIDs. Many of these points are summarized in an excellent paper by Blackshear and colleagues.[417]

Two additional points should be made regarding this form of NSAID-induced acute renal failure. First, the question has arisen whether some NSAIDs are "renal protective." This issue has been discussed in the context of sulindac, a drug that requires hepatic conversion from the inactive sulindac sulfoxide to an active sulfide.[418] Whereas there appears to be some reduced risk for vasoconstriction-induced renal insufficiency in patients who take sulindac versus other nonsteroidal drugs,[413, 419–423] the kidney can activate the prodrug[424, 425] and lead to vasoconstrictive renal failure or hyperkalemia.[426–429] In addition, Schlondorff[410] has pointed out that sulindac has a long half-life; because of this, the active sulindac sulfide can accumulate in the plasma for several days to weeks, eventually reaching levels that are two to four times higher than those observed in patients with normal hepatic and renal function.

A remaining unanswered question is that of the long-term toxic effect of NSAIDs. These drugs have been shown to cause papillary necrosis either alone or in combination with aspirin.[430–434] At present, the long-term sequelae of NSAIDs and the abuse potential of these agents are not known. This is a particularly pertinent question given the abuse potential of powerful NSAIDs and that ibuprofen is

### TABLE 34–10. Clinical Features of Nonsteroidal Anti-inflammatory Drug–Associated Tubulointerstitial Nephritis

Heavy proteinuria (>3.0 g/d)
Tubulointerstitial infiltrate on biopsy specimen; glomeruli well preserved
Nonoliguric course typical
Eosinophilia/eosinophiluria not common
Variable time (weeks to months) to development
Role of steroids in resolution unclear

available as an over-the-counter drug and naproxen has been released as an over-the-counter drug. A brief communication pointed out that long-term consumption of NSAIDs (alone or in combination with other drugs) could lead to papillary necrosis.[435] Of interest is that this disorder, in contrast to classic analgesic nephropathy, was more common in male patients (1.9:1) and was not typical of the usual psychologic profile associated with chronic drug use. Another study using epidemiologic analysis concluded that regular use of NSAIDs may increase the risk for chronic kidney disease in some patients.[436]

Another form of NSAID-induced kidney disease is that of interstitial nephritis (Table 34–10). The NSAID that is most often associated with this lesion is fenoprofen, but all NSAIDs have been linked to at least one case of this syndrome.[433, 437, 438] The key features are that the time for the syndrome to develop is variable, with a mean of 5.4 months; only 19% of patients have a fever, rash, or eosinophilia; and 83% of patients with this disorder have the nephrotic syndrome. The renal biopsy findings in this disorder typically include a focal interstitial infiltrate with some fibrosis. Immunofluorescence studies are usually not remarkable, but in some cases, weak and variable staining for immunoglobulins G, A, and M and C3 is seen in interstitial membranes. Electron-dense deposits have been noted in the mesangium in three patients.[437] The pathogenesis of this disorder is not known. A delayed hypersensitivity response to the NSAID appears to be a tenable hypothesis, but the involvement of the glomeruli in causing nephrotic syndrome without a lesion is really unclear. Another intriguing possibility is that inhibition of cyclooxygenase will shunt arachidonic acid metabolites to the lipoxygenase pathway and produce leukotrienes.[439, 440] Leukotrienes mediate inflammation, increase vascular permeability, and are chemotactic for white blood cells, including T lymphocytes and eosinophils.[441, 442] Torres[443] has summarized this scheme in detail.

In addition to causing nephrotic syndrome due to tubulointerstitial disease, NSAIDs have also been associated with minimal-change (or "nil lesion") disease and the nephrotic syndrome.[444, 445] The value of using corticosteroids to resolve this form of nephrotic syndrome is at present unknown; anecdotal reports of success with use of prednisone therapy are available.[446]

Na$^+$ retention is a common consequence of NSAID use and occurs in as many as 25% of patients who use the drugs. This positive Na$^+$ balance is usually transient and of no major clinical importance. However, spectacular accu-

### TABLE 34–9. Nonsteroidal Anti-inflammatory Drug–Induced Hemodynamic Deterioration of Renal Function

Usually a higher dose involved
Course may be oliguric or nonoliguric
Predisposing conditions
    Extracellular fluid volume depletion
    Congestive heart failure
    Cirrhosis (particularly with ascites)
    Nephrotic syndrome
    Underlying renal disease
    Third-space fluid sequestration
    Diuretic therapy
Usually reversible; usually does not require dialysis

**TABLE 34–11. Nonsteroidal Anti-inflammatory Drugs and Hypertension**

Increase in blood pressure usually modest
Patients receiving diuretics or β-blockers most vulnerable
$Ca^{2+}$ channel blockers less susceptible
Elderly and African-American persons perhaps at greater risk

mulations of $Na^+$ have been observed in patients taking NSAIDs,[447] and therefore close observation is advised in patients who are more apt to develop pulmonary edema. Diuretic resistance due to NSAIDs is discussed earlier and should be kept in mind, particularly in patients in intensive care units where large doses of parenteral diuretics may be partially blunted by the concomitant use of NSAIDs.

As mentioned before, the ability of prostaglandins to oppose the hydro-osmotic effects of vasopressin may set up a condition in which urine dilution is impaired when NSAIDs are used. Were this to occur, positive water balance would ensue, and hyponatremia could result. Such a case has been described previously.[448]

Hyperkalemia may also occur with the use of NSAIDs; monitoring should be performed in patients who require an NSAID and who have borderline high $K^+$ concentrations ($\geq 5.0$ mEq/L). Hyperkalemia has been observed to follow NSAID administration in patients with normal and abnormal renal function.[449–452] The mechanism of this effect is believed to be through the hyporenin-hypoaldosterone state that is created by the use of the NSAID. The physiologic opposite of this clinical state of NSAID-induced hyporeninemic hypoaldosteronism is that of Bartter syndrome, which is characterized by hyperreninemic hyperaldosteronism, hypokalemia, and an exaggerated renal prostaglandin synthesis and release. Of note is that several of the manifestations of Bartter syndrome have been ablated by NSAID administration.[453–456]

The last complication of NSAID use to be discussed is the ability of NSAIDs to cause hypertension (Table 34–11). From a theoretic point of view, the ability of NSAIDs to lower renin and aldosterone levels might be considered an effect that would lower blood pressure; however, NSAIDs also have the effect of reducing $Na^+$ and water excretion, and this could lead to an expansion of extracellular fluid volume and hypertension. When the effects of NSAIDs have been examined in a large population of patients, the following points emerge. First, in controlled studies, an average increase of between 6 and 8 mm Hg of mean blood pressure is seen in patients who are treated with NSAIDs. This increase in blood pressure appears to be most pronounced in patients who are already hypertensive and less pronounced in patients who are normotensive when they begin therapy. Second, patients who take diuretics or β-blockers seem to be more vulnerable to the hypertensive effect of NSAIDs than of other agents (Fig. 34–6). In this regard, it is particularly interesting to note that propranolol has been shown to increase $PGI_2$ formation,[457] which thus makes the drug more susceptible to the antihypertensive effects of NSAIDs. Third, $Ca^{2+}$ channel blockers, direct vasodilators, and clonidine appear to be less vulnerable to the effects of NSAIDs on blood pressure. Angiotensin-converting enzyme inhibitors (ACEIs) are also relatively unaffected by the use of NSAIDs, but there have been a few case reports of the deterioration of renal function that can follow the concomitant use of an ACEI and an NSAID.[458] Fourth, the patients most at risk for an NSAID-related increase in blood pressure appear to be those with low-renin hypertension (i.e., the elderly and African-Americans). Physicians should be cognizant of this interaction and be particularly mindful of the effects of NSAIDs on blood pressure in patients who are already taking antihypertensive medicines and who require an NSAID temporarily. The pathogenesis of NSAID-induced hypertension is not known with certainty; however, the elimination of the vasodilator $PGI_2$ from the resistance of blood vessels is believed

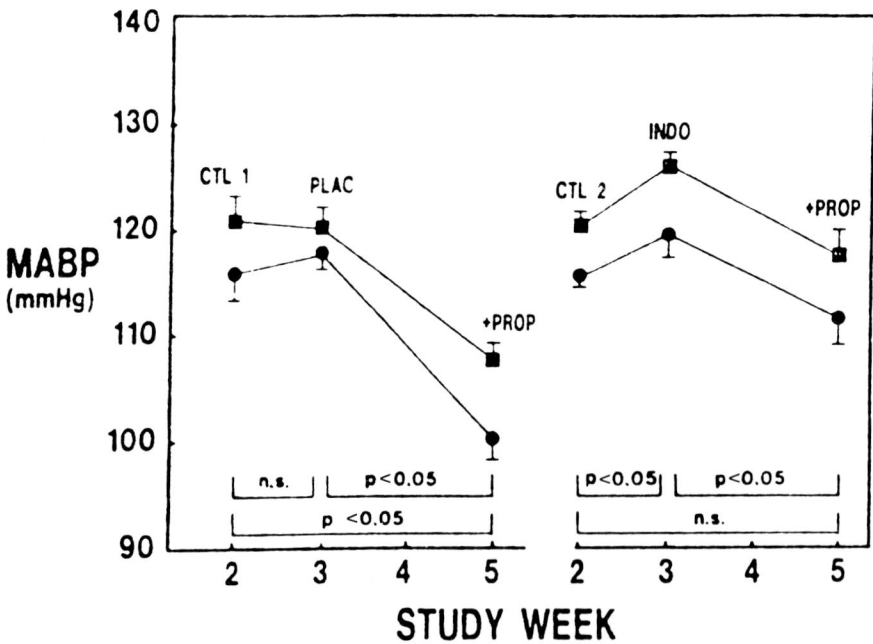

**Figure 34–6.** Effects of indomethacin on blood pressure in the upright position (■) and supine position (●). MAPB = mean arterial blood pressure. (From Beckmann ML, Gerber JG, Byyny RL, et al: Propranolol increases prostacyclin synthesis in patients with hypertension. Hypertension 12:582–588, 1988. Reproduced with permission. Hypertension. Copyright 1988 American Heart Association.)

to play some role in the development of hypertension in these individuals.[459–466] The large reviews that have examined this subject have shown only a modest but usually significant effect of NSAID on blood pressure.[467–469] In summary, it is important for the physician to be aware of this interaction and to be particularly mindful of this potential problem in patients who have antecedent hypertension and who require NSAIDs.

# ANGIOTENSIN-CONVERTING ENZYME INHIBITORS AND THE KIDNEY

ACEIs have been observed to cause reversible acute renal failure in the setting of hypertension and congestive heart failure. The reason for this phenomenon appears to be related to the role angiotensin II plays in sustaining the renal circulation under conditions of hypoperfusion.[470] GFR is largely governed by the relative tone of the afferent and efferent arterioles. When renal perfusion pressure declines, the afferent arteriole vasodilates, and total renal vascular resistance declines. This vasorelaxation is a compensatory myogenic reflex to the decline in renal perfusion pressure. In addition, depending on the level to which renal perfusion declines, an increase in efferent arteriolar resistance may be required to maintain the intracapillary glomerular pressure at a level sufficiently high to sustain glomerular filtration. The net effect of this increase in efferent resistance is to sustain GFR in the context of some increase in renal vascular resistance, thereby increasing the filtration fraction.[470, 471] The increase in efferent vascular tone that occurs under renal hypoperfusion conditions is in large part due to the vasoconstrictive effect of angiotensin II. What emerges from the number of studies that have been performed to examine this question is that the renal autoregulatory adjustments required to maintain GFR in prerenal conditions are highly dependent on a sustained efferent resistance, which is in turn dependent on angiotensin II. It is under these conditions that the administration of an ACEI could lead to a fall in GFR. What appears to occur is that the ACEI blunts the vasoconstrictive effect of angiotensin II at the efferent arteriole and therefore leads to a decline in efferent arteriolar resistance. This decline in efferent arteriolar resistance leads to a fall in the glomerular capillary pressure and then to a fall in GFR.[470]

The clinical settings in which this physiologic mechanism becomes important are as follows. First, in a setting of significant (usually more than 70%) stenosis of both renal arteries, efferent tone is increased to maximize the GFR. Second, in a setting of unilateral obstruction to a solitary functioning kidney, efferent tone again sustains the GFR necessary to maintain homeostasis. In both of these examples, there is ischemia to the whole renal mass, thereby making the kidney and GFR dependent on efferent resistance to sustain blood flow. Third, when cardiac output is low or there is an intense prerenal vasoconstriction, perfusion pressure may be low enough to mimic the conditions in which there is actual physical stenosis of the renal arteries. Such an occurrence would be in a setting of mod-

erate to severe congestive heart failure. Under these circumstances, efferent arteriolar tone again sustains GFR, and the use of an ACEI would result in a loss of efferent tone and a consequent decline in the GFR. A fourth circumstance in which this physiologic construct holds is severe small vessel disease of the kidney, as might be seen in severe nephrosclerosis. Even though the main renal arteries are patent, the obstruction to renal perfusion occurs more distally in arcuate and interlobular vessels, leading to another type of functional renal ischemia. These complex interrelationships between angiotensin II and efferent tone have made the use of ACEIs more complicated than that of other antihypertensive or unloading agents. Furthermore, the proliferation of ACEIs on the market and the widespread use of these drugs have brought the problem of silent ischemic disease of the kidney to greater attention.[472] It is estimated that approximately 10% to 15% of patients with end-stage renal disease may have occlusive renal artery obstruction or partial obstruction as a cofactor in the cause of the renal failure.[473] Similarly, it is common to observe a decline in renal function in the setting of ACEI therapy and heart failure.[474] This is more pronounced if cardiac filling pressures decline during the course of therapy with the ACEI.

The sum of all these interrelationships is that if renal insufficiency or a decline in renal function follows the use of an ACEI, underlying renal artery disease should be suspected. In fact, it has been proposed that ACEI challenge be used to screen for renal artery stenosis and other types of renin-mediated hypertension in kidney transplant patients.[472, 475] It is also clear that in severely hypertensive patients who come to medical attention when renal pressure declines too far, renal insufficiency may ensue. This was pointed out in studies by Ying and co-workers[476] and by Textor and colleagues,[477] who showed that acute renal insufficiency could develop in patients with bilateral renal artery stenosis or unilateral stenosis to a solitary functioning kidney if renal perfusion pressure was lowered below the autoregulatory threshold by drugs other than ACEIs. In both of the studies, successful revascularization or angioplasty of the renal artery reversed the effect.

When a decline in renal function follows the use of an ACEI, consideration for stenotic renal artery disease should be undertaken. If decline in renal function occurs on exposure to an ACEI in the context of congestive heart failure, a reduction in the dose of the ACEI, a liberalization of the salt diet of the patient, or a decrease in diuretic therapy may improve renal function without obviating the effect of the

---

**TABLE 34–12. Renal Complications of Angiotensin-Converting Enzyme Inhibitor Therapy**

Hemodynamic deterioration occurs in the setting of bilateral renal artery stenosis or unilateral stenosis in a solitary functioning kidney; may also occur in congestive heart failure, volume depletion, polycystic kidney disease
Membranous nephropathy
Interstitial nephritis
Acute tubule necrosis

ACEI on afterload. Screening tests for renal artery stenosis include captopril scintigraphy using *o*-iodohippurate or EDTA.[478–483] Some investigators have advocated the use of the peripheral plasma renin activity test to screen for this lesion,[484] but the test may lose its value in patients with bilateral artery stenosis, renal parenchymal disease, and essential hypertension. These patients may have high values that are affected by ACEI therapy.[485] The use of duplex scanning for diagnosis of renal artery disease is promising but remains impractical for many patients with obesity or previous abdominal surgery.[486] The best diagnostic test for diagnosis of this disorder is renal arteriography. Other renal complications of ACEI therapy are provided in Table 34–12. A few cases of membranous nephropathy have been reported after the drug has been used,[487, 488] but the overall frequency of this complication and that of tubulointerstitial nephritis are believed to be low.

# TOXIC NEPHROPATHY DUE TO HYDROCARBON EXPOSURE

A large literature suggests that long-term hydrocarbon exposure may predispose individuals to the development of several different types of renal disease.[489] Acute tubule necrosis, chronic interstitial nephritis, and glomerulonephritis have all been described.[488–497] In a study of this question, three groups of healthy men working in separate areas of a manufacturing plant were evaluated.[489] Group 1 was exposed to paint-based hydrocarbons; group 2 (101 volunteers) worked in the transmission assembly area of the plant and was exposed to petroleum-based mineral oils; and group 3 was composed of 92 automated press operators with minimal exposure to lubricants or solvents. The group 1 workers had a significantly higher prevalence of elevated serum creatinine concentration and a higher prevalence of abnormal urinary total protein, *N*-acetylglucosaminidase, γ-glutamyltransferase, and leucine aminopeptidase than group 2 or group 3 did. Group 2 had a normal serum creatinine concentration but a significantly higher prevalence of abnormal urinary total protein, transferrin-binding protein, *N*-acetylglucosaminidase, and leucine aminopeptidase than group 3 did. Blood pressures were similar in all three groups. The elevation in the serum creatinine concentration seen in group 1 was mild, and the elevation of urinary proteins observed in group 2 was also modest.

The pathogenesis of hydrocarbon-induced renal disease is not known with certainty; however, the possibility that solvents cause renal damage and thereby release a tubule antigen that results in an autoimmune reaction is a theory that is still held in some regard. Some animal studies that suggest the tubulointerstitial nephritis that follows chronic hydrocarbon exposure can be ameliorated by pretreatment of the animal with radiation support an autoimmune mechanism for this disease.[498] Another hypothesis is that potentially toxic immune factors arise independently of hydrocarbon exposure and that hydrocarbons facilitate the deposit of these mediators in renal tissue.[499] Alternatively, the immune system could be damaged by hydrocarbons, thereby leading to impaired clearance of antigenic material that then lodges in glomerular capillary loops and incites an inflammatory response.[500]

## REFERENCES

1. Molitoris BA: New insights into the cell biology of ischemic acute renal failure. J Am Soc Nephrol 1:1263–1270, 1991.
2. Brezis M, Rosen S, Silva P, et al: Polyene toxicity in renal medulla: Injury mediated by transport activity. Science 224:66–68, 1984.
3. Shanley PF, Brezis M, Spokes K, et al: Transport-dependent cell injury in the S₃ segment of the proximal tubule. Kidney Int 29:1033–1037, 1986.
4. Stillman IE, Brezis M, Greenfeld Z, et al: Cyclosporine nephropathy: Morphometric analysis of the medullary thick ascending limb. Am J Kidney Dis 20:162–167, 1992.
5. Heyman SN, Brezis M, Reubinoff CA, et al: Acute renal failure with selective medullary injury in the rat. J Clin Invest 82:401–412, 1988.
6. Heyman SN, Brezis M, Greenfeld Z, et al: Protective role of furosemide and saline in radiocontrast-induced acute renal failure in the rat. Am J Kidney Dis 14:377–385, 1989.
7. Walker PD, Shah SV: Gentamicin enhanced production of hydrogen peroxide by renal cortical mitochondria. Am J Physiol 253:C495–C499, 1987.
8. Walker PD, Shah SV: Evidence suggesting a role for hydroxyl radical in gentamicin-induced acute renal failure in rats. J Clin Invest 81:334–341, 1988.
9. Yoshioka T, Fogo A, Beckman JK: Reduced activity of antioxidant enzymes underlies contrast media–induced renal injury in volume depletion. Kidney Int 41:1008–1015, 1992.
10. Leehey DJ, Braun BI, Tholl DA, et al: Can pharmacokinetic dosing decrease nephrotoxicity associated with aminoglycoside therapy? J Am Soc Nephrol 4:81–90, 1993.
11. Luft FC: Clinical significance of renal changes engendered by aminoglycosides in man. J Antimicrob Chemother 13(suppl A):23–30, 1984.
12. Houghton DC, English J, Bennett WM: Chronic tubulointerstitial nephritis and renal insufficiency associated with long-term "subtherapeutic" gentamicin. J Lab Clin Med 112:694–703, 1988.
13. Cronin RE, Bulger RE, Southern P, et al: Natural history of aminoglycoside nephrotoxicity in the dog. J Lab Clin Med 95:463–474, 1980.
14. Schwartz JH, Schein P: Fanconi syndrome associated with cephalothin and gentamicin therapy. Cancer 41:769–772, 1978.
15. Melnick JZ, Baum M, Thompson JR: Aminoglycoside-induced Fanconi's syndrome. Am J Kidney Dis 23:118–122, 1994.
16. Bar RJ, Wilson HE, Mazzaferri EL: Hypomagnesemic hypocalcemia secondary to renal magnesium wasting: A possible consequence of high dose gentamicin therapy. Ann Intern Med 82:646–649, 1975.
17. Patel R, Savage A: Symptomatic hypomagnesemia associated with gentamicin therapy. Nephron 23:50–52, 1979.
18. Brinker KR, Bulger RE, Dobyan DC, et al: Effect of potassium depletion on gentamicin nephrotoxicity. J Lab Clin Med 98:292–301, 1981.
19. Pastoriza-Munoz E, Timmerman D, Feldman S, et al: Ultrafiltration of gentamicin and netilmicin in vivo. J Pharmacol Exp Ther 220:604–608, 1982.
20. Senekjian HO, Knight TF, Weinman EJ: Micropuncture study of the handling of gentamicin by the rat kidney. Kidney Int 19:416–423, 1981.
21. Pastoriza-Munoz E, Bowman RL, Kaloyanides GJ: Renal tubular transport of gentamicin in the rat. Kidney Int 15:440–450, 1979.
22. Silverblatt FJ, Kuehn C: Autoradiography of gentamicin uptake by the rat proximal tubule cell. Kidney Int 15:335–345, 1979.
23. Kluwe WM, Hook JB: Analysis of gentamicin uptake by rat renal cortical slices. Toxicol Appl Pharmacol 45:531–539, 1978.
24. Sheth AU, Senekjian HO, Babino H, et al: Renal handling of gentamicin by the Munich-Wistar rat. Am J Physiol 241:F645–F648, 1981.
25. Kosek JC, Mazze RI, Cousins MJ: Nephrotoxicity of gentamicin. Lab Invest 30:48–57, 1974.
26. Feldman S, Wang M, Kaloyanides GJ: Aminoglycosides induce a phospholipidosis in the renal cortex of the rat: An early manifestation of nephrotoxicity. J Pharmacol Exp Ther 220:514–520, 1982.

27. Josepovitz C, Farruggella T, Levine R, et al: Effect of netilmicin on the phospholipid composition of subcellular fractions of rat renal cortex. J Pharmacol Exp Ther 235:810–819, 1985.

28. Carlier MD, Laurent G, Claes PJ, et al: Inhibition of lysosomal phospholipases by aminoglycoside antibiotics: In vitro comparative studies. Antimicrob Agents Chemother 23:440–449, 1983.

29. Hostetler KY, Hall LB: Inhibition of kidney lysosomal phospholipases A and C by aminoglycoside antibiotics: Possible mechanism of aminoglycoside toxicity. Proc Natl Acad Sci USA 79:1663–1667, 1982.

30. Ramsammy LS, Josepovitz C, Kaloyanides GJ: Gentamicin inhibits agonist stimulation of the phosphatidylinositol cascade in primary cultures of rabbit proximal tubular cells and in rat renal cortex. J Pharmacol Exp Ther 247:989–996, 1988.

31. Ramsammy L, Ling KY, Josepovitz C, et al: Effect of gentamicin on lipid peroxidation in rat renal cortex. Biochem Pharmacol 34:3895–3900, 1985.

32. Kaloyanides GJ, Ramsammy L, Josepovitz C: Assessment of three therapeutic interventions for modifying gentamicin nephrotoxicity in the rat. *In* Bach PH, Delacruz L, Gregg NJ, Wilks MF (eds): Proceedings of the Fourth International Symposium of Nephrotoxicity. Marcel Dekker, New York, 1990, p 103.

33. Luft FC, Kleit SA: Renal parenchymal accumulation of aminoglycoside antibiotics in rats. J Infect Dis 130:656–659, 1974.

34. Josepovitz C, Pastoriza-Munoz E, Timmerman D, et al: Inhibition of gentamicin uptake in rat renal cortex in vivo by aminoglycosides and organic polycations. J Pharmacol Exp Ther 223:314–321, 1982.

35. Pastoriza-Munoz E, Josepovitz C, Ramsammy L, et al: Renal handling of netilmicin in the rat with streptozotocin-induced diabetes mellitus. J Pharmacol Exp Ther 241:166–173, 1987.

36. Collier VU, Lietman PS, Mitch WE: Evidence for luminal uptake of gentamicin in the perfused rat kidney. J Pharmacol Exp Ther 210:247–251, 1979.

37. Chiu PJS, Long JF: Urinary excretion and tissue accumulation of gentamicin and para-aminohippurate in post-ischemic kidneys. Kidney Int 15:618–623, 1979.

38. Ramsammy LS, Kaloyanides GJ: Effect of gentamicin on the transition temperature and permeability to glycerol of phosphatidylinositol-containing liposomes. Biochem Pharmacol 36:1179–1181, 1987.

39. Sastrasinh M, Knauss TC, Weinberg JM, et al: Identification of the aminoglycoside binding site in rat renal brush border membranes. J Pharmacol Exp Ther 222:350–358, 1982.

40. Molitoris BA, Meyer C, Dahl R, et al: Mechanism of ischemia-enhanced aminoglycoside binding and uptake by proximal tubule cells. Am J Physiol 264:F907–F916, 1993.

41. Bennett WM, Plamp C, Gilbert DN, et al: The effects of dosage regimen on experimental gentamicin nephrotoxicity: Dissociation of peak serum levels from renal failure. J Infect Dis 140:576–580, 1979.

42. Bennett WM, Parker RA, Elliot WC, et al: Sex-related differences in the susceptibility of rats to gentamicin nephrotoxicity. J Infect Dis 145:370–373, 1982.

43. Bennett WM, Hartnett MN, Gilbert D, et al: Effect of sodium intake on gentamicin nephrotoxicity in the rat. Proc Soc Exp Biol Med 151:736–738, 1976.

44. Tardif D, Beauchamp D, Bergeron MG: Influence of endotoxin on the intracortical accumulation kinetics of gentamicin in rats. Antimicrob Agents Chemother 34:576–580, 1990.

45. Corcoran GB, Salazar DE, Schentag JJ: Excessive aminoglycoside nephrotoxicity in obese patients. Am J Med 85:279, 1988.

46. Spiegel DM, Shanley PF, Molitoris BA: Mild ischemia predisposes the S3 segment to gentamicin toxicity. Kidney Int 38:459–464, 1990.

47. Chiu PJS, Miller GH, Long JF, et al: Renal uptake and nephrotoxicity of gentamicin during urinary alkalinization in rats. Clin Exp Pharmacol Physiol 6:317–326, 1979.

48. Cronin R, Inman L, Eche T, et al: Effect of thyroid hormone on gentamicin accumulation in rat proximal tubule lysosomes. Am J Physiol 257:F86–F91, 1989.

49. Thompson JR, Simonsen R, Spindler MA, et al: Protective effect of KCl loading in gentamicin nephrotoxicity. Am J Kidney Dis 15:583–591, 1990.

50. Williams PD, Hottendorf GH: Inhibition of renal membrane binding and nephrotoxicity of gentamicin by polyasparagine and polyaspartic acid in the rat. Res Commun Chem Pathol Pharmacol 47:317–320, 1985.

51. Gilbert DN, Wood CA, Kohlhepper SJ, et al: Polyaspartic acid prevents experimental aminoglycoside nephrotoxicity. J Infect Dis 159:945–953, 1989.

52. Ramsammy LS, Josepovitz C, Lane BP, et al: Polyaspartic acid protects against gentamicin nephrotoxicity in the rat. J Pharmacol Exp Ther 250:149–153, 1989.

53. Ramsammy L, Josepovitz C, Lane B, et al: Polyaspartic acid inhibits gentamicin-induced perturbations of phospholipid metabolism. Am J Physiol 258:C1141–C1149, 1990.

54. Swan SK, Gilbert DN, Kohlhepp SJ, et al: Pharmacologic limits of the protective effect of polyaspartic acid on experimental gentamicin nephrotoxicity. Antimicrob Agents Chemother 37:347–348, 1993.

55. Gilbert DN, Houghton DC, Bennett WL, et al: Reversibility of gentamicin nephrotoxicity in rats: Recovery during continuous drug administration. Proc Soc Exp Biol Med 160:99–103, 1979.

56. Simmons CF, Bogusky RT, Humes HD: Inhibitory effects of gentamicin on renal mitochondrial oxidative phosphorylation. J Pharmacol Exp Ther 214:709–715, 1980.

57. Mela-Riker LM, Widener LL, Houghton DC, et al: Renal mitochondrial integrity during continuous gentamicin treatment. Biochem Pharmacol 35:979–984, 1986.

58. Buss WC, Piatt MK, Kauten R: Inhibition of mammalian microsomal protein synthesis by aminoglycoside antibiotics. J Antimicrob Chemother 14:231–241, 1984.

59. Buss WC, Piatt MK: Gentamicin administered in vivo reduces protein synthesis in microsomes subsequently isolated from rat kidneys but not from rat brains. J Antimicrob Chemother 15:715–721, 1985.

60. Bennett WM, Mela-Riker LM, Houghton DC, et al: Microsomal protein synthesis inhibition: An early manifestation of gentamicin nephrotoxicity. Am J Physiol 255:F265–F269, 1988.

61. Bennett WM, Plamp CE, Parker RA, et al: Alterations in organic ion transport induced by gentamicin nephrotoxicity in the rat. J Lab Clin Med 95:32–39, 1980.

62. Kirschbaum BB: Interactions between renal brush border membranes and polyamines. J Pharmacol Exp Ther 229:409–416, 1984.

63. Morigama T, Nakahama H, Fukahara Y, et al: Decrease in the fluidity of brush-border membrane vesicles induced by gentamicin. A spin-labelling study. Biochem Pharmacol 48:1169–1174, 1989.

64. Levi M, Cronin RE: Early selective effects of gentamicin on renal brush-border membrane Na-P$_i$ cotransport and Na-H exchange. Am J Physiol 258:F1379–F1387, 1990.

65. Baylis C, Rennke HR, Brenner BM: Mechanisms of the defect in glomerular ultrafiltration associated with gentamicin administration. Kidney Int 12:344–353, 1977.

66. Barshay ME, Kaye JH, Goldman R, et al: Acute renal failure in diabetic patients after intravenous infusion pyelography. Clin Nephrol 1:35–39, 1973.

67. Churchill DN, Seely J: Nephrotoxicity associated with combined gentamicin–amphotericin B therapy. Nephron 19:176–181, 1977.

68. Dentino ME, Luft FC, Yum MN, et al: Long term effect of *cis*-diamminedichloride platinum (CDDP) on renal function and structure in man. Cancer 41:1274–1281, 1978.

69. Moore RD, Smith CR, Lipsky JJ, et al: Risk factors for nephrotoxicity in patients treated with aminoglycosides. Ann Intern Med 100:352–357, 1984.

70. Smith CR, Lipsky JJ, Laskin OL, et al: Double-blind comparison of the nephrotoxicity and auditory toxicity of gentamicin and tobramycin. N Engl J Med 302:1106–1109, 1980.

71. Dillon KR, Dougherty SH, Casner P, et al: Individualized pharmacokinetic versus standard dosing of amikacin: Comparison of therapeutic outcomes. J Antimicrob Chemother 24:581–589, 1989.

72. Burton ME, Ash CL, Hill DP Jr, et al: A controlled trial of the cost benefit of computerized bayesian aminoglycoside administration. Clin Pharmacol Ther 49:685–694, 1991.

73. Sawyers CL, Moore RD, Lerner SA, et al: A model for predicting nephrotoxicity in patients treated with aminoglycosides. J Infect Dis 153:1062–1068, 1986.

74. Dahlgren JG, Anderson ET, Hewitt WL: Gentamicin blood levels: A guide to nephrotoxicity. Antimicrob Agents Chemother 8:58–62, 1975.

75. Bennett WM, Plamp CE, Gilbert DN, et al: The influence of dosage regimen on experimental nephrotoxicity: Dissociation of peak serum levels from renal failure. J Infect Dis 140:576–579, 1979.

76. Gilbert DN: Once-daily aminoglycoside therapy. Antimicrob Agents Chemother 35:399–405, 1991.

77. Levison ME: New dosing regimens for aminoglycoside antibiotics. Ann Intern Med 117:693–694, 1992.

78. Prins JM, Buller HR, Kuijper EJ, et al: Once versus thrice daily gentamicin in patients with serious infections. Lancet 341:335–339, 1993.

79. Maller R, Ahrne H, Holmen C, et al: Once- versus twice-daily amikacin regimen: Efficacy and safety in systemic gram-negative infections. Scandinavian Amikacin Once Daily Study Group. J Antimicrob Chemother 31:939–948, 1993.

80. Farber BF, Moellering RC: Retrospective study of the toxicity of preparations of vancomycin from 1974 to 1981. Antimicrob Agents Chemother 23:138–141, 1983.

81. Sorrell TC, Collignon PJ: A prospective study of adverse reactions associated with vancomycin therapy. J Antimicrob Chemother 16:235–241, 1985.

82. Mellor JA, Kindgom J, Cafferkey M, et al: Vancomycin toxicity: A prospective study. J Antimicrob Chemother 15:773–780, 1985.

83. Downs NJ, Neihart RE, Dolezal JM, et al: Mild nephrotoxicity associated with vancomycin use. Arch Intern Med 149:1777–1781, 1989.

84. Rybak MJ, Albrecht LM, Burke SC, et al: Nephrotoxicity of vancomycin, alone and with an aminoglycoside. J Antimicrob Chemother 25:679–687, 1990.

85. Carbone LG, Bendixen B, Appel GB: Sulfadiazine-associated obstructive nephropathy occurring in a patient with the acquired immune deficiency syndrome. Am J Kidney Dis 12:72–75, 1988.

86. Simon DI, Brosius FC III, Rothstein DM: Sulfadiazine-induced crystalluria revisited. The treatment of *Toxoplasma* encephalitis in patients with acquired immune deficiency syndrome. Arch Intern Med 150:2379–2384, 1990.

87. Sasson JP, Dratch PL, Shortsleeve MJ: Renal US findings in sulfadiazine-induced crystalluria. Radiology 185:739–740, 1992.

88. Hein R, Brunkhorst R, Thon WF, et al: Symptomatic sulfadiazine crystalluria in AIDS patients: A report of two cases. Clin Nephrol 39:254–256, 1993.

89. Andreoli TE, Monahan M: The interaction of polyene antibiotics with thin lipid membranes. J Gen Physiol 52:300–325, 1968.

90. Cheng JT, Witty RT, Robinson RR, et al: Amphotericin B nephrotoxicity: Increased renal resistance and tubule permeability. Kidney Int 22:626–633, 1982.

91. Sawaya BP, Weihprecht H, Campbell WR, et al: Direct vasoconstriction as a possible cause for amphotericin B–induced nephrotoxicity in rats. J Clin Invest 87:2097–2107, 1991.

92. Douglas JB, Healy JK: Nephrotoxicity effect of amphotericin B, including renal tubular acidosis. Am J Med 46:154–162, 1969.

93. Heyman SN, Clark BA, Kaiser N, et al: In-vivo and in-vitro studies on the effect of amphotericin B on endothelin release. J Antimicrob Chemother 29:69–77, 1992.

94. Heyman SN, Stillman IE, Brezis M, et al: Chronic amphotericin nephropathy: Morphometric, electron microscopic, and functional studies. J Am Soc Nephrol 4:69–80, 1993.

95. Gerkens JF, Branch RA: The influence of sodium status and furosemide on canine acute amphotericin nephrotoxicity. J Pharmacol Exp Ther 214:306–311, 1980.

96. Tolins JP, Raij L: Chronic amphotericin B nephrotoxicity in the rat, protective effects of prophylactic salt loading. Am J Kidney Dis 11:313–317, 1988.

97. Heidemann HTH, Gerkens JF, Spickard WA, et al: Amphotericin B nephrotoxicity in humans decreased by salt repletion. Am J Med 75:476–481, 1983.

98. Fisher MA, Talbot GH, Maislin G, et al: Risk factors for amphotericin B–associated nephrotoxicity. Am J Med 87:547–552, 1989.

99. Kan VL, Bennett JE, Amantea MA, et al: Comparative safety, tolerance, and pharmacokinetics of amphotericin B lipid complex and amphotericin B desoxycholate in healthy male volunteers. J Infect Dis 164:418–421, 1991.

100. Moreau P, Milpied N, Fayette N, et al: Reduced renal toxicity and improved clinical tolerance of amphotericin B mixed with intralipid compared with conventional amphotericin B in neutropenic patients. J Antimicrob Chemother 30:535–541, 1992.

101. Berns JS, Cohen RM, Stumacher RJ, et al: Renal aspects of therapy for human immunodeficiency virus and associated opportunistic infections. J Am Soc Nephrol 1:1061–1080, 1991.

102. Krieble BF, Rudy DW, Glick MR, et al: Case report: Acyclovir neurotoxicity and nephrotoxicity—a role for hemodialysis. Am J Med Sci 305:36–39, 1993.

103. Sawyer MH, Webb DE, Balow JE, et al: Acyclovir-induced renal failure. Clinical course and histology. Am J Med 84:1067–1071, 1988.

104. Bianchetti MG, Roduit C, Oetliker OH: Acyclovir-induced renal failure: Course and risk factors. Pediatr Nephrol 5:238–239, 1991.

105. Wharton JM, Coleman DL, Wofsy CB, et al: Trimethoprim-sulfamethoxazole or pentamidine for *Pneumocystis carinii* pneumonia in the acquired immunodeficiency syndrome. Ann Intern Med 105:47–44, 1986.

106. Sattler FR, Cowan R, Nielsen DM, et al: Trimethoprim-sulfamethoxazole compared with pentamidine for treatment of *Pneumocystis carinii* pneumonia in the acquired immunodeficiency syndrome. Ann Intern Med 109:280–287, 1988.

107. Miller RF, Delany S, Semple SJG: Acute renal failure after nebulised pentamidine. Lancet 1:1271–1272, 1989.

108. Conte JE, Upton RA, Lin ET: Pentamidine pharmacokinetics in patients with AIDS with impaired renal function. J Infect Dis 156:885–890, 1987.

109. Lachaal M, Venuto RC: Nephrotoxicity and hyperkalemia in patients with acquired immunodeficiency syndrome treated with pentamidine. Am J Med 87:260–263, 1989.

110. Shah GM, Alvarado P, Kirschenbaum MA: Symptomatic hypocalcemia and hypomagnesemia with renal magnesium wasting associated with pentamidine therapy in a patient with AIDS. Am J Med 89:380–382, 1990.

110a. Kleymah TR, Roberts C, Ling BN: A mechanism for pentamidine-induced hyperkalemia: Inhibition of distal nephron sodium transport. Ann Intern Med 122:103–106, 1995.

111. Antoniskis D, Larsen RA: Acute, rapidly progressive renal failure with simultaneous use of amphotericin B and pentamidine. Antimicrob Agents Chemother 34:470–472, 1990.

112. Oberg B: Antiviral effects of phosphonoformate (PFA, foscarnet sodium). Pharmacol Ther 19:387–415, 1983.

113. Sundquist B, Oberg B: Phosphonoformate inhibits reverse transcriptase. J Gen Virol 45:273–281, 1979.

114. Deray G, Martinez F, Katlama C, et al: Foscarnet nephrotoxicity: Mechanism, incidence and prevention. Am J Nephrol 9:316–321, 1989.

115. Jacobson MA, O'Donnell JJ, Mills J: Foscarnet treatment of cytomegalovirus retinitis in patients with AIDS. Antimicrob Agents Chemother. 33:736–741, 1989.

116. Cacoub P, Deray G, Baumelou A, et al: Acute renal failure induced by foscarnet: 4 cases. Clin Nephrol 29:315–318, 1988.

117. MacGregor RR, Graziani AL, Weiss R, et al: Successful foscarnet therapy for cytomegalovirus retinitis in an AIDS patient undergoing hemodialysis: Rationale for empiric dosing and plasma level monitoring. J Infect Dis 164:785–787, 1991.

118. Cronin RE: Renal failure following radiologic procedures. Am J Med Sci 296:342–356, 1989.

119. Rich MW, Crecelius CA: Incidence, risk factors, and clinical course of acute renal insufficiency after cardiac catheterization in patients 70 years of age or older. A prospective study. Arch Intern Med 150:1237–1242, 1990.

120. Lautin EM, Freeman NJ, Schoenfeld AH, et al: Radiocontrast-associated renal dysfunction: Incidence and risk factors. AJR 157:49–58, 1991.

121. Manske CL, Sprafka JM, Strony JT, et al: Contrast nephropathy in azotemic diabetic patients undergoing coronary angiography. Am J Med 89:615–620, 1990.

122. Byrd L, Sherman RL: Radiocontrast-induced acute renal failure: A clinical and pathophysiologic review. Medicine (Baltimore) 58:270–279, 1979.

123. McCarthy CS, Becker JA: Multiple myeloma and contrast media. Radiology 183:519–521, 1992.

124. Harkonen S, Kjellstrand CM: Exacerbation of diabetic renal failure following intravenous pyelography. Am J Med 63:939–946, 1977.

125. Weinrauch LA, Healy RW, Leland OS, et al: Coronary angiography and acute renal failure in diabetic azotemic nephropathy. Ann Intern Med 86:56–59, 1977.

126. D'Elia JA, Gleason RE, Alday M, et al: Nephrotoxicity from angiographic contrast material. A prospective study. Am J Med 72:719–725, 1982.

127. Martin-Paredero V, Dixon SM, Baker JD, et al: Risk of renal failure after major angiography. Arch Surg 118:1417–1420, 1983.

128. Taliercio CP, Vlietstra RE, Fisher LD, et al: Risks for renal dysfunction with cardiac angiography. Ann Intern Med 104:501–504, 1986.

129. Fang LS, Sirota RA, Ebert TH, et al: Low fractional excretion of sodium with contrast media–induced acute renal failure. Arch Intern Med 140:531–533, 1980.
130. D'Elia JA, Kaldany A, Weinbrauch LA, et al: Inadequacy of fractional excretion of sodium test. Arch Intern Med 141:818, 1981. Letter.
131. Gelman ML, Rowe JW, Coggins CH, et al: Effects of an angiographic contrast agent on renal function. Cardiovasc Med 4:313–320, 1979.
132. Moreau JF, Droz D, Sabto J, et al: Osmotic nephrosis induced by water-soluble tri-iodinated contrast media in man. Radiology 115:329–336, 1975.
133. Moreau JF, Droz D, Noel LH, et al: Tubular nephrotoxicity of water-soluble iodinated contrast media. Invest Radiol 15:S54–S60, 1980.
134. Vari RC, Natarajan LA, Whitescarver SA, et al: Induction, prevention and mechanisms of contrast media-induced acute renal failure. Kidney Int 33:699–707, 1988.
135. Bakris GL, Burnett JC Jr: A role for calcium in radiocontrast-induced reductions in renal hemodynamics. Kidney Int 27:465–468, 1985.
136. Caldicott WJH, Hollenberg NK, Abrams HL: Characteristics of response of renal vascular bed to contrast media. Evidence of vasoconstriction induced by renin-angiotensin system. Invest Radiol 5:539–547, 1970.
137. Heyman SN, Clark BA, Kaiser N, et al: Radiocontrast agents induce endothelin release in vivo and in vitro. J Am Soc Nephrol 3:58–65, 1992.
138. Heyman SN, Clark BA, Cantley L, et al: Effects of ioversol versus iothalamate on endothelin release and radiocontrast nephropathy. Invest Radiol 28:313–318, 1993.
139. Weisberg LS, Kurnik PB, Kurnik BR: Radiocontrast-induced nephropathy in humans: Role of renal vasoconstriction. Kidney Int 41:1408–1415, 1992.
140. Weisberg LS, Kurnik PB, Kurnik BR: Dopamine and renal blood flow in radiocontrast-induced nephropathy in humans. Ren Fail 15:61–68, 1993.
141. Bettmann MA: Angiographic contrast agents: Conventional and new media compared. AJR 139:787–794, 1982.
142. Messana JM, Cieslinski DA, Nguyen VD, et al: Comparison of the toxicity of the radiocontrast agents, iopamidol and diatrizoate, to rabbit renal proximal tubule cells in vitro. J Pharmacol Exp Ther 244:1139–1144, 1988.
143. Schwab SJ, Hlatky MA, Pieper KS: Contrast nephrotoxicity: A randomized controlled trial of a nonionic and an ionic radiographic contrast agent. N Engl J Med 320:149–153, 1989.
144. Parfrey PS, Griffiths SM, Barrett BJ, et al: Contrast material–induced renal failure in patients with diabetes mellitus, renal insufficiency, or both. N Engl J Med 320:143–149, 1989.
145. Barrett BJ, Parfrey PS, Vavasour HM, et al: Contrast nephropathy in patients with impaired renal function: High versus low osmolar media. Kidney Int 41:1274–1279, 1992.
146. Moore RD, Steinberg EP, Powe NR, et al: Nephrotoxicity of high-osmolality versus low-osmolality contrast media: Randomized clinical trial. Radiology 182:649–655, 1992.
147. Lautin EM, Freeman NJ, Schoenfeld AH, et al: Radiocontrast-associated renal dysfunction: A comparison of lower-osmolality and conventional high-osmolality contrast media. AJR 157:59–65, 1991.
148. Barrett BJ, Carlisle EJ: Metaanalysis of the relative nephrotoxicity of high- and low-osmolality iodinated contrast media. Radiology 188:171–178, 1993.
149. Kopp JB, Klotman PE: Cellular and molecular mechanisms of cyclosporin nephrotoxicity. J Am Soc Nephrol 1:162–179, 1990.
150. Curtis JJ: Hypertension after renal transplantation: Cyclosporine increases the diagnostic and therapeutic considerations. Am J Kidney Dis 13(suppl 1):28–32, 1989.
151. Takenaka T, Hashimoto Y, Epstein M: Diminished acetylcholine-induced vasodilation in renal microvessels of cyclosporine-treated rats. J Am Soc Nephrol 4:42–50, 1992.
152. English J, Evan A, Houghton DC, et al: Cyclosporine-induced acute renal dysfunction in the rat: Evidence of arteriolar vasoconstriction with preservation of tubular function. Transplantation 44:135–141, 1987.
153. Garr MD, Paller MS: Cyclosporine augments renal but not systemic vascular reactivity. Am J Physiol 258:F211–F217, 1990.
154. Zoja C, Furci L, Ghilardi F, et al: Cyclosporin-induced endothelial cell injury. Lab Invest 55:455–462, 1986.
155. Lau DCW, Wong K, Hwang WS: Cyclosporine toxicity on cultured rat microvascular endothelial cells. Kidney Int 35:604–613, 1989.
156. Kon V, Sugiura M, Inagami T, et al: Role of endothelin in cyclosporine-induced glomerular dysfunction. Kidney Int 37:1487–1491, 1990.
157. Lanese DM, Conger JD: Effects of endothelin receptor antagonist on cyclosporine-induced vasoconstriction in isolated rat renal arterioles. J Clin Invest 91:2144–2149, 1993.
158. Munger KA, Takahashi K, Awazu M, et al: Maintenance of endothelin-induced renal arteriolar constriction in rats is cyclooxygenase dependent. Am J Physiol 264:F637–F644, 1993.
159. Rooth P, Dawidson I, Diller K, et al: Protection against cyclosporine-induced impairment of renal microcirculation by verapamil in mice. Transplantation 45:433–437, 1988.
160. Wagner K, Henkel M, Heinemeyer G, et al: Interaction of calcium blockers and cyclosporine. Transplant Proc 20(suppl 2):561–568, 1988.
161. Dawidson I, Rooth P, Fry WR, et al: Prevention of acute cyclosporine-induced renal blood flow inhibition and improved immunosuppression with verapamil. Transplantation 48:575–580, 1989.
162. Dawidson I, Rooth P, Alway C, et al: Verapamil prevents post-transplant delayed function and cyclosporine A nephrotoxicity. Transplant Proc 22:1379–1380, 1990.
163. Weir MR, Klassen DK, Shen SY, et al: Acute effects of intravenous cyclosporine on blood pressure, renal hemodynamics, and urine prostaglandin production of healthy humans. Transplantation 49:41–47, 1990.
164. Feehally J, Walls J, Mistry N, et al: Does nifedipine ameliorate cyclosporin A nephrotoxicity? Br Med J 295:310, 1987.
165. Hauser AC, Derfler K, Stockenhuber F, et al: Effect of calcium-channel blockers on renal function in renal-graft recipients treated with cyclosporine. N Engl J Med 324:1517, 1991. Letter.
166. Palmer BF, Dawidson I, Sagalowsky A, et al: Improved outcome of cadaveric renal transplantation due to calcium channel blockers. Transplantation 52:640–645, 1991.
167. Pirsch JD, D'Alessandro AM, Roecker EB, et al: A controlled, double-blind, randomized trial of verapamil and cyclosporine in cadaver renal transplant patients. Am J Kidney Dis 21:189–195, 1993.
168. Kawaguchi A, Goldman MH, Shapiro R, et al: Increase in urinary thromboxane $B_2$ in rats caused by cyclosporine. Transplantation 40:214–216, 1985.
169. Perico N, Benigni A, Zoja C, et al: Functional significance of exaggerated renal thromboxane $A_2$ synthesis induced by cyclosporine A. Am J Physiol 251:F581–F587, 1986.
170. Coffman TM, Carr DR, Yarger WE, et al: Evidence that renal prostaglandin and thromboxane production is stimulated in chronic cyclosporine nephrotoxicity. Transplantation 43:282–285, 1987.
171. Voss BL, Hamilton KK, Samara S, et al: Cyclosporine suppression of endothelial prostacyclin generation. Transplantation 45:793–796, 1988.
172. Paller MS: Effects of the prostaglandin $E_1$ analog misoprostol on cyclosporine nephrotoxicity. Transplantation 45:1126–1131, 1988.
173. Moran M, Mozes MF, Maddux MS, et al: Prevention of acute graft rejection by the prostaglandin $E_1$ analogue misoprostol in renal-transplant recipients treated with cyclosporine and prednisone. N Engl J Med 322:1183–1188, 1990.
174. Adams MB: Enisoprost in renal transplantation. Transplantation 53:338–345, 1992.
175. Pollak R, Knight R, Mozes MF, et al: A trial of the prostaglandin $E_1$ analogue, enisoprost, to reverse chronic cyclosporine-associated renal dysfunction. Am J Kidney Dis 20:336–341, 1992.
176. Perico N, Rossini M, Imberti O, et al: Thromboxane receptor blockade attenuates chronic cyclosporine nephrotoxicity and improves survival in rats with renal isograft. J Am Soc Nephrol 2:1398–1404, 1992.
177. Burdmann EA, Rosen S, Lindsley J, et al: Production of less chronic nephrotoxicity by cyclosporine G than cyclosporine A in a low-salt rat model. Transplantation 55:963–966, 1993.
178. Van Duyne GD, Standaert RF, Karplus PA, et al: Atomic structure of FKBP-FK506, an immunophilin-immunosuppressant complex. Science 252:839–842, 1991.
179. Textor SC, Wiesner R, Wilson DJ, et al: Systemic and renal hemodynamic differences between FK 506 and cyclosporine in liver transplant recipients. Transplantation. 55:1332–1339, 1993.
180. Porayko MK, Textor SC, Krom RAF, et al: Nephrotoxic effects of primary immunosuppression with FK-506 and cyclosporine regimens after liver transplantation. Mayo Clin Proc 69:105–111, 1994.

181. Fung JJ, Alessiani M, Abu-Elmagd M, et al: Adverse effects associated with the use of FK 506. Transplant Proc 23:3105–3108, 1991.
182. Randhawa PS, Shapiro R, Jordan ML, et al: The histopathological changes associated with allograft rejection and drug toxicity in renal transplant recipients maintained on FK506. Am J Surg Pathol 17:60–68, 1993.
183. Levin L, Hryniuk W: The application of dose intensity to problems in chemotherapy of ovarian and endometrial cancer. Semin Oncol 14(4):12–19, 1987.
184. Samson MK, Rivkin SE, Jones SE, et al: Dose-response and dose-survival advantage for high versus low dose cisplatin combined with vinblastine and bleomycin in disseminated testicular cancer. Cancer 53:1029–1035, 1984.
185. Nichols CR, Williams SD, Loehrer PJ, et al: Randomized study of cisplatin dose intensity in poor-risk germ cell tumors: A Southeastern Cancer Study Group and Southwest Oncology Group Protocol. J Clin Oncol 9:1163–1172, 1991.
186. Wiernik PH, Yeap B, Vogl SE, et al: Hexamethylmelamine and low or moderate dose cisplatin with or without pyridoxine for treatment of advanced ovarian carcinoma: A Study of the Eastern Cooperative Oncology Group. Cancer Invest 10:1–9, 1992.
187. McGuire WP, Hoskins WJ, Brady MF, et al: A phase III trial of dose intense versus standard dose cisplatin and cytoxan in advanced ovarian cancer. Proc Am Soc Clin Oncol 11:718–722, 1992.
188. Kaye SB, Lewis CR, Paul J, et al: Randomised study of two doses of cisplatin with cyclophosphamide in epithelial ovarian cancer. Lancet 340:329–333, 1992.
189. Einhorn LH, Williams SD: The role of cis-platinum in solid tumor therapy. N Engl J Med 300:289–293, 1979.
190. Schaeppi U, Heyman IA, Fleischman RW, et al: cis-Diamminedichloroplatinum(II) (NSC-119 875): Preclinical toxicologic evaluation of intravenous injection in dogs, monkeys and mice. Toxicol Appl Pharmacol 25:230–241, 1973.
191. Hardaker WT, Stone RA, McCoy R: Platinum nephrotoxicity. Cancer 34:1030–1034, 1974.
192. Fleming J, Collis C, Peckham MJ: Renal damage after cis-platinum. Lancet 2:960–963, 1979.
193. Weiner MW, Jacobs C: Mechanism of cisplatin nephrotoxicity. Fed Proc 42:2974–2977, 1983.
194. Schilsky RL, Barlock A, Ozols RF: Persistent hypomagnesemia following cisplatin chemotherapy for testicular cancer. Cancer Treat Rep 66:1767–1769, 1982.
195. Bitran JD, Desser RK, Billings M, et al: Acute nephrotoxicity following cis-dichlorodiammine-platinum. Cancer 49:1874–1888, 1982.
196. Vogelzang NJ, Torkelson JL, Kennedy BJ: Hypomagnesemia, renal dysfunction and Raynaud's phenomenon in patients treated with cisplatin, vinblastine and bleomycin. Cancer 56:2765–2770, 1985.
197. Buckley JE, Clark VL, Meyer TJ, Pearlman NW: Hypomagnesemia after cisplatin combination chemotherapy. Arch Intern Med 144:2347–2348, 1984.
198. Lerner SA, Seligsohn R, Matz GJ: Comparative clinical studies of ototoxicity and nephrotoxicity of amikacin and gentamicin. Am J Med 62:919–923, 1977.
199. Aso Y, Ohtawara YU, Suzuki K, et al: The effect of gentamicin and mercuric chloride on cyclic AMP and lipoperoxide in rat kidneys. Nippon Jinzo Gakkai Shi 6:583–590, 1982.
200. Kaloyanides GJ, Ramasammy LS: Alterations of biophysical properties of liposomes predict aminoglycoside toxicity: Inhibitory effect of polyaspartic acid. In Bach PH, Delacrey L, Gregg NJ, Wilks MF, (eds): Proceedings of the Fourth International Symposium on Nephrotoxicity. Marcel Dekker, New York, 1990, p 109.
201. Offerman JJG, Meijer S, Sleijfer DTh, et al: Acute effects on cis-diamminedichloroplatinum (CDDP) on renal function. Cancer Chemother Pharmacol 12:36, 1984.
202. Walker EM, Fazekas-May MA, Bowen WR: Nephrotoxic and ototoxic agents. Clin Toxicol 10:323, 1990.
203. Wolf W, Manaka RC: Synthesis and distribution of $^{195m}$Pt cis-dichlorodiammine platinum (II). J Clin Hematol Oncol 7:79, 1976.
204. Marcussen N: Atubular glomeruli in cisplatin-induced chronic interstitial nephropathy: An experimental stereological investigation. APMIS 98:1087–1097, 1990.
205. Bianchetti MG, Kanaka C, Ridolfi-Luthy A, et al: Persisting renotubular sequelae after cisplatin in children and adolescents. Am J Nephrol 11:127–130, 1991.
206. Guinee DG, Van Zee B, Houghton DC: Clinically silent progressive renal tubulointerstitial disease during cisplatin chemotherapy. Cancer 71:4050–4054, 1993.
207. Brillet G, Deray G, Dubois M, et al: Chronic cisplatin nephropathy in rats. Nephrol Dial Transplant 8:206–212, 1993.
208. Kim S, Howell SB, McClay E, et al: Dose intensification of cisplatin chemotherapy through biweekly administration. Ann Oncol 4:221–227, 1993.
209. Hayes DM: High-dose cis-platinum diammine dichloride: Amelioration of renal toxicity by mannitol diuresis. Cancer 39:1372–1376, 1977.
210. Ozols RF, Corden BJ, Jacob J, et al: High dose cisplatin in hypertonic saline. Ann Intern Med 100:19–24, 1984.
211. Bajorin DF, Bosl GJ, Jacob et al: Pharmacokinetics of cis-diamminedichloroplatinum (II) after administration in hypertonic saline. Cancer Res 46:5969–5972, 1986.
212. Ozols RF, Corden BJ, Jacob J, et al: High-dose cisplatin in hypertonic saline. Ann Intern Med 100:19–24, 1984.
213. Gandara DR, Perez EA, Wiebe V, De Gregorio MW: Cisplatin chemoprotection and rescue: Pharmacologic modulation of toxicity. Semin Oncol 18(suppl 3):49–55, 1991.
214. Ross RD, Gale CR: Reduction of the renal toxicity of cis-dichlorodiammineplatinum (II) by probenecid. Cancer Treat Rep 63:781, 1979.
215. Edmonson JH, McCormack GW, Krook JE, et al: Pilot study of cyclophosphamide plus carboplatin in advanced ovarian carcinoma. Cancer Treat Rep 71:199–200, 1987.
216. Van Echo DA, Egorin MJ, Whitacre MY, et al: A phase I clinical and pharmacologic trial of carboplatin daily for 5 days. Cancer Treat Rep 65:1103–1107, 1984.
217. Egorin MJ, Van Echo DA, Tipping SJ, et al: Pharmacokinetics and dosage reduction of cis-diammine (1,1-cyclobutanedicarboxylate) platinum in patients with impaired renal function. Cancer Res 44:5432–5436, 1984.
218. Christian MC: Carboplatin. In De Vita VT Jr, Hellman S, Rosenberg SA (eds): Principles and Practice of Oncology, 3rd ed. JB Lippincott, Philadelphia, 1989, pp 1–16.
219. Edmonson JH, McCormack GW, Krook JE, et al: Pilot study of cyclophosphamide plus carboplatin in advanced ovarian carcinoma. Cancer Treat Rep 71:199–200, 1987.
220. Gore ME, Calvert AH, Smith LE: High dose carboplatin in the treatment of lung cancer and mesothelioma: A phase I dose escalation study. Eur J Cancer Clin Oncol 23:1391–1397, 1987.
221. Shea TC, Flaherty M, Elias A, et al: A phase I clinical and pharmacokinetic study of carboplatin and autologous bone marrow support. J Clin Oncol 7:651–661, 1989.
222. Vogelzang NJ: Nephrotoxicity from chemotherapy: Prevention and management. Oncology 5:97–102, 1991.
223. DeFronzo RA, Colvin OM, Braine H, et al: Cyclophosphamide and the kidney. Cancer 33:483–491, 1974.
224. Bode U, Seif SM, Levine AS: Studies on the antidiuretic effect on cyclophosphamide: Vasopressin release and sodium excretion. Med Pediatr Oncol 8:295–303, 1980.
225. Weiss RB: Streptozocin: A review of its pharmacology, efficacy, and toxicity. Cancer Treat Rep 66:427–438, 1982.
226. Sadoff L: Nephrotoxicity of streptozocin (NSC 85988). Cancer Chemother Rep 54:457–459, 1970.
227. Meyerowik RL, Sartiano GP, Cavallo T: Nephrotoxic and cytoproliferative effects of streptozocin. Cancer 38:1550–1555, 1976.
228. Hricik DE, Goldsmith GH: Uric acid nephrolithiasis and acute renal failure secondary to streptozocin nephrotoxicity. Am J Med 84:153–156, 1988.
229. Schact RG, Feiner HD, Gallo GR, et al: Nephrotoxicity of nitrosoureas. Cancer 48:1328–1334, 1981.
230. Micetich KC, Jensen-Akula M, Mandard JC, Fisher RI: Nephrotoxicity of semustine (methyl-CCNU) in patients with malignant melanoma receiving adjuvant chemotherapy. Am J Med 71:967–972, 1981.
231. Goren MP, Wright RK, Pratt CB, et al: Potentiation of ifosfamide neurotoxicity, hematotoxicity, and tubular nephrotoxicity by prior cis-diamminedichloroplatinum (II) therapy. Cancer Res 47:1457–1460, 1987.
232. Goren MP, Wright RK, Horowitz ME, et al: Ifosfamide-induced subclinical tubular nephrotoxicity. Cancer Treat Rep 71:127–130, 1987.
233. Zalupski M, Baker LH: Ifosfamide. J Natl Cancer Inst 80:556–566, 1988.

234. Skinner R, Pearson AD, Price L, et al: Nephrotoxicity after ifosfamide. Arch Dis Child 65:732–738, 1990.
235. Burk CD, Restaino I, Kaplan BS, et al: Ifosfamide induced renal tubular dysfunction and rickets in children with Wilms tumor. J Pediatr 117:331–335, 1990.
236. Elias AD, Eder JP, Shea T, et al: High dose ifosfamide with mesna uroprotection: A phase I study. J Clin Oncol 8:170–178, 1990.
237. Lesesne JB, Rothschild N, Erickson B, et al: Cancer associated hemolytic-uremic syndrome: Analysis of 85 cases from a national registry. J Clin Oncol 7:781–789, 1989.
238. Valavaara R, Nordman E: Renal complications of mitomycin C therapy with special reference to the total dose. Cancer 55:47–50, 1985.
239. Cattell V: Mitomycin-induced hemolytic uremic kidney: An experimental model in the rat. Am J Pathol 121:88–95, 1985.
240. Verwey J, de Vries J, Pinedo HM: Mitomycin C–induced renal toxicity, a dose-dependent side effect? Eur J Clin Oncol 23:195–199, 1987.
241. Price TM, Murgo AJ, Keveney JJ, et al: Renal failure and hemolytic anemia associated with mitomycin C. A case report. Cancer 55:51–56, 1985.
242. Kennedy BJ, Brown JH, Yarbro JW: Mithramycin (NSC-24559) therapy for primary glioblastomas. Cancer Chemother Rep 48:59–63, 1965.
243. Kennedy BJ: Metabolic and toxic effects of mithramycin during tumor therapy. Am J Med 49:494–503, 1970.
244. Kennedy BJ, Sandberg-Wolheim M, Loken M, et al: Studies with tritiated mithramycin in C3H mice. Cancer Res 27:1534–1538, 1967.
245. Kennedy BJ: Metabolic and toxic effects during mithramycin therapy. Am J Med 49:494–503, 1970.
246. Green L, Donehower RC: Hepatic toxicity of low doses of mithramycin in hypocalcemia. Cancer Treat Rep 68:1379–1381, 1984.
247. Perlia CP, Gubish NJ, Wolter J, et al: Mithramycin treatment of hypercalcemia. Cancer 25:389–394, 1970.
248. Kiag DT, Lokien MK, Kennedy BJ: Mechanism of the hypocalcemic effect of mithramycin. J Clin Endocrinol Metab 48:341–344, 1979.
249. Chabner BA, Meyers CD: Clinical pharmacology of cancer chemotherapy. *In* De Vita VT Jr, Hellman S, Rosenberg SA (eds): Principles and Practice of Oncology, 3rd ed. JB Lippincott, Philadelphia, 1989, pp 349–388.
250. Singer FR, Neer RM, Murray TM, et al: Mithramycin treatment of intractable hypercalcemia due to parathyroid carcinoma. N Engl J Med 283:634, 1970.
251. Bleyer WA: The clinical pharmacology of methotrexate. Cancer 41:36–51, 1978.
252. Ackland SP, Schilsky RL: High-dose methotrexate: A critical reappraisal. J Clin Oncol 5:2017–2031, 1987.
253. Jacobs SA, Stoller RG, Chabner BA, et al: 7-Hydroxymethotrexate as a urinary metabolite in human subjects and rhesus monkeys receiving high-dose methotrexate. J Clin Invest 57:534–538, 1976.
254. Glode LM, Pitman SW, Ensminger WD, et al: A phase I study of high-dose aminopterin with leucovorin rescue in patients with advance metastatic tumor. Cancer Res 39:3707–3714, 1979.
255. Pitman SW, Frei E III: Weekly methotrexate-calcium leukovorin rescue: Effect of alkalinization on nephrotoxicity; pharmacokinetics in the CNS; and use in CNS non-Hodgkin's lymphoma. Cancer Treat Rep 61:695–701, 1977.
256. Abelson HT, Garnick MB: Renal failure induced by cancer chemotherapy. *In* Rieselbach RE, Garnick MB (eds): Cancer and the Kidney. Lea & Febiger, Philadelphia, 1982, pp 769–813.
257. Thyss A, Milano G, Kubar J, et al: Clinical and pharmacokinetic evidence of a life-threatening interaction between methotrexate and ketoprofen. Lancet 1:256–258, 1988.
258. Price P, Thompson H, Bessell EM, et al: Renal impairment following the combined use of high dose methotrexate and procarbazine. Cancer Chemother Pharmacol 21:265–267, 1988.
259. Slavin RE, Dias MA, Saral R: Cytosine arabinoside induced gastrointestinal toxic alteration in sequential chemotherapeutic protocols. A clinical pathological study of 33 patients. Cancer 42:1747–1759, 1978.
260. Presant CA, Denes AE, Klein L, et al: Phase I and preliminary phase II observations of high-dose intermittent 6-thioguanine. Cancer Treat Rep 64:1109–1113, 1980.
261. Hanna WT, Krauss S, Regester RF, Murphy WM: Renal disease after mitomycin C therapy. Cancer 48:2583–2588, 1981.
262. Belldegrun A, Webb DE, Austin HA 3d, et al: Effects of interleukin-2 on renal function in patients receiving immunotherapy for advanced cancer. Ann Intern Med 106:817–822, 1987.
263. Sosman JA, Kohler PC, Hank J, et al: Repetitive weekly cycles of recombinant human interleukin-2: Responses of renal carcinoma with acceptable toxicity. J Natl Cancer Inst 80:60–63, 1988.
264. West WH, Tauer KW, Yannelli JR, et al: Constant-infusion recombinant interleukin-2 in adoptive immunotherapy of advanced cancer. N Engl J Med 316:898–905, 1987.
265. Rose BD: Pathophysiology of Renal Disease, 2d ed. McGraw-Hill, New York, 1987, pp 418–425.
266. Kjellstrand CM, Campbell DC, von Hartikch B, Buselmeier TJ: Hyperuricemic acute renal failure. Arch Intern Med 133:349–359, 1974.
267. Hricik DE, Goldsmith GH: Uric acid nephrolithiasis and acute renal failure secondary to streptozotocin nephrotoxicity. Am J Med 84:153–156, 1988.
268. Kelton J, Kelley WN, Holmes EW: A rapid method for the detection of acute uric acid nephropathy. Arch Intern Med 138:612–615, 1978.
269. Zusman J, Brown DM, Nesbit ME: Hyperphosphataemia, hyperphosphaturia and hypocalcaemia in acute lymphoblastic leukemia. N Engl J Med 289:1335–1340, 1973.
270. Chastyl RC, Liu-Yin JA: Acute tumor lysis syndrome. Br J Hosp Med 49:488–492, 1993.
271. Hande KR, Garrow GC: Acute tumor lysis syndrome in patients with high grade non-Hodgkin's lymphoma. Am J Med 94:133–138, 1993.
272. Barton JC: Tumor lysis syndrome in nonhematopoietic neoplasms. Cancer 64:738–740, 1989.
273. Cadman E, Lundberg W, Bertino J: Hyperphosphatemia and hypocalcemia accompanying rapid cell lysis in a patient with Burkitt's cell leukemia. Am J Med 62:283–290, 1977.
274. Ettinger DS, Harker WG, Gerry HW, et al: Hyperphosphatemia, hypocalcemia, and transient renal failure. Results of cytotoxic treatment of acute lymphoblastic leukemia. JAMA 239:2472–2474, 1978.
275. Major RH: Classic Descriptions of Disease with Biographical Sketches of the Authors, 2nd ed. Charles C Thomas, Springfield, IL, 1939.
276. Ramazzini B; Wright WC, trans: De Morbis Artificium Diatriba. University of Chicago Press, Chicago, 1913.
277. Thackrah CT: The Effects of Arts, Trades and Professions and Civic Sates, and Habits of Living on Health and Longevity with Suggestions for the Removal of Many of the Agents Which Produce Disease and Shorten the Duration of Life, 2nd ed. Longman, Rees, Orme, Brown, Green & Longman, London, 1832.
278. Legge Sir T: Industrial Maladies. Oxford University Press, London, 1934.
279. Bariety J, Druet P, Laliberte F: Glomerulonephritis with α and β 1C-globulin deposits induced in rats by mercuric chloride. Am J Pathol 65:293–302, 1971.
280. Barry PSI: A comparison of concentrations of lead in human tissues. Br J Med 32:119–139, 1975.
281. Goyer RA, Wilson MH: Lead-induced inclusion bodies. Results of ethylenediaminetetraacetic acid treatment. Lab Invest 32:149–156, 1975.
282. Nye LJJ: An investigation of the extraordinary incidence of chronic nephritis in young people in Queensland. Med J Aust 2:145–159, 1929.
283. Lilis R, Gavirlescu N, Nestorescu B, et al: Nephropathy in chronic renal lead poisoning. Br J Ind Med 25:196–202, 1968.
284. Inglis JA, Henderson DA, Emmerson BT: The pathology and pathogenesis of chronic nephropathy occurring in Queensland. J Pathol 124:65–76, 1978.
285. Moel DI, Sachs HK: Renal function 17 to 23 years after chelation therapy for childhood plumbism. Kidney Int 42:1226–1231, 1992.
286. Nuyts GD, Daelemans RA, Jorens G, et al: Does lead play a role in the development of chronic renal disease? Nephrol Dial Transplant 6:307–315, 1991.
287. Pinto de Almeida AR, Carvalho FM, Spinola AG, et al: Renal dysfunction in Brazilian lead workers. Am J Nephrol 7:455–458, 1987.
288. Behringer D, Craswell P, Mohl C, et al: Urinary lead excretion in uremic patients. Nephron 42:323–329, 1986.
289. Cramer K, Goyer RA, Jagenburg R, Wilson MH: Renal ultrastructure, renal function, and parameters of lead toxicity in workers with different periods of lead exposure. Br J Ind Med 31:113–127, 1974.
290. Cooper WC, Wong O, Kheifets L: Mortality among employees of lead battery plants and lead producing plants, 1947–1980. Scand J Work Environ Health 11:331–345, 1985.

291. Searle J, Craswell P, Boyle P, et al: The current status of chronic lead nephropathy in Queensland. Aust N Z J Med 11:600–601, 1981.
292. Hu H: A 50-year follow-up of childhood plumbism. Am J Dis Child 145:681–687, 1991.
293. Cooper WC, Gaffey WR: Mortality of lead workers. J Occup Med 17:100–107, 1975.
294. Malcolm D, Barnett HAR: A mortality study of lead workers, 1925–76. Br J Ind Med 39:402–404, 1982.
295. McMichael AJ, Johnson HM: Long-term mortality profile of heavily-exposed lead smelter workers. J Occup Med 24:375–378, 1982.
296. Selevan SG, Landrigan PJ, Stern FB, et al: Mortality of lead smelter workers. Am J Epidemiol 122:673–683, 1985.
297. Craswell PW, Price J, Boyle PD, et al: Chronic renal failure with gout: A marker of chronic lead poisoning. Kidney Int 26:169–173, 1979.
298. Coffman TM, Yarger WE, Klotman PE: Functional role of thromboxane production by acutely rejecting renal allografts in rats. J Clin Invest 75:1242–1248, 1985.
299. Warren GV, Korbet SM, Schwartz MM, et al: Minimal change glomerulopathy associated with nonsteroidal antiinflammatory drugs. Am J Kidney Dis 13:127–130, 1989.
300. Vyskocil A, Pancl J, Tusl M, et al: Dose-related proximal tubular dysfunction in male rats chronically exposed to lead. J Appl Toxicol 9:395–399, 1989.
301. Cardenas A, Roels H, Bernard AM, et al: Markers of early renal changes induced by industrial pollutants. II. Application to workers exposed to lead. Br J Ind Med 50:28–36, 1993.
302. Piomelli A, Seaman C, Zullow D, et al: Threshold for lead damage to heme synthesis in urban children. Proc Natl Acad Sci USA 79:3335–3339, 1982.
303. Wedeen RP: Blood lead levels, dietary calcium, and hypertension. Ann Intern Med 102:403–404, 1985. Editorial.
304. Wedeen RP, Mallik DK, Batumen V: Detection and treatment of occupational lead nephropathy. Arch Intern Med 139:53–57, 1979.
305. Inglis JA, Henderson DA, Emmerson BT: The pathology and pathogenesis of chronic lead nephropathy occurring in Queensland. J Pathol 124:65–76, 1978.
306. Van de Vyver FL, D'Haese PC, Visser WJ: Bone lead in dialysis patients. Kidney Int 33:601–607, 1988.
307. Craswell P: Chronic lead nephropathy. Annu Rev Med 38:319–323, 1987.
308. Haust H, Inwood M, Spence JD, et al: Intramuscular administration of iron during long-term chelation therapy with 2,3-dimercaptosuccinic acid in a man with severe lead poisoning. Clin Biochem 22:189–196, 1989.
309. Koster J, Erhardt A, Stoeppler M, et al: Mobilizable lead in patients with chronic renal failure. Eur J Clin Invest 19:228–233, 1989.
310. Yver L, Marechaud R, Picaud D, et al: Insuffisance rénale aigue au cours d'un saturnisme professionel. Nouv Presse Med 7:1541–1543, 1978.
311. Bernard A, Lauwerys R: Cadmium in the human population. Experientia 40:143–151, 1984.
312. Bernard A, Roels A, Buchet JP, et al: Cadmium and health: The Belgian experience. IARC Sci Publ (118):15–33, 1992.
313. Roels H, Bernard AM, Cardenas A, et al: Markers of early renal changes induced by industrial pollutants. III. Application to workers exposed to cadmium. Br J Ind Med 50:37–48, 1993.
314. Nogawa K, Kido T, Shaikh ZA: Dose-response relationship for renal dysfunction in a population environmentally exposed to cadmium. IARC Sci Publ (118):311–318, 1992.
315. Wedeen RP: Occupational renal disease. Am J Kidney Dis 3:241–257, 1984.
316. Lindqvist K, Nystrom K, Stegmayr B, et al: Cadmium concentration in human kidney biopsies. Scand J Urol Nephrol 23:213–217, 1989.
317. Jung E, Pergande M, Graubaum HJ, et al: Urinary proteins and enzymes as early indicators of renal dysfunction in chronic exposure in cadmium. Clin Chem 39:757–765, 1993.
318. Toffoletto F, Apostoli P, Ghezzi I, et al: Ten-year follow-up of biological monitoring of cadmium-exposed workers. IARC Sci Publ (118):107–111, 1992.
319. Jarup L, Persson B, Edling C, Elinder CG: Renal function impairment in workers previously exposed to cadmium. Nephron 64:75–81, 1993.
320. Kahan E, Derazne E, Rosenboim J, Ashkenazi R: Adverse health effects in workers exposed to cadmium. Am J Ind Med 21:527–537, 1992.

321. Mueller P, Paschal DC, Hammel RR, et al: Chronic renal effects in three studies of men and women occupationally exposed to cadmium. Arch Environ Contam Toxicol 23:125–136, 1992.
322. Shibuya Y: A long-term surveillance of occupational health hazards faced by cadmium workers. Kitasato Arch Exp Med 63:37–48, 1990.
323. Kido R, Nogawa K, Hochi Y, et al: The renal handling of calcium and phosphorus in environmental cadmium-exposed subjects with renal dysfunction. J Appl Toxicol 13:43–47, 1993.
324. Tsuchiya K: Health effects of cadmium with special references to studies in Japan. IARC Sci Publ (118):35–49, 1992.
325. Shimada H, Kamenosono T, Kawagoe M, et al: Mobilization of renal and hepatic cadmium by dithiocarbamates in rats. J Pharmacobiodyn 14:555–560, 1991.
326. Jones MM, Gale GR, Singh PK, et al: The rate of the in vivo dithiocarbamate-induced mobilization of hepatic and renal cadmium deposits. Toxicology 48:313–323, 1989.
327. Landrigan PJ: Occupational and community exposures to toxic metals: Lead, cadmium, mercury and arsenic. West J Med 137:531–539, 1982.
328. Gerstner HB, Huff JE: Selected case histories and epidemiologic examples and human mercury poisoning. Clin Toxicol 11:131–150, 1977.
329. Wedeen RP: Occupational and environmental renal diseases. Curr Nephrol 11:65, 1988.
330. Kazantzis G: Mercury. In Waldron HA (ed): Metals in the Environment. Academic Press, New York, 1980, pp 221–261.
331. Nomiyama K: Recent progress and perspectives in cadmium health effects studies. Sci Total Environ 14:199–232, 1980.
332. Dounce AL: The mechanism of action of uranium compounds in the animal body. In Voegtlin C, Hodge HC (eds): Pharmacology and Toxicology of Uranium Compounds, Div VI, Vol 1. McGraw-Hill, New York, 1949.
333. Fowler BA, Weissberg JB: Arsine poisoning. N Engl Med 291:1171–1174, 1972.
334. Kaufman DB, DiNickola W, McIntosh R: Acute potassium dichromate poisoning. Am J Dis Child 119:374, 1970.
335. Lachmann PJ: Nephrotic syndrome from penicillamine. Postgrad Med J Suppl 23:23–27, 1968.
336. Stein HB, Patterson AC, Offer RC, et al: Adverse effects of D-penicillamine in rheumatoid arthritis. Ann Intern Med 92:24–29, 1980.
337. Bacon PA, Tribe CR, Mackenzie JC, et al: Penicillamine nephropathy in rheumatoid arthritis—a clinical pathological and immunological study. Q J Med 55:661–684, 1976.
338. Chisolm JJ, Baltrop D: Recognition and management of children with increased lead absorption. Arch Dis Child 54:249–262, 1979.
339. Wooley PH, Griffin JK, Panayi GS, et al: HLA-DR antigens and toxic reaction to sodium aurothiomalate and D-penicillamine in patients with rheumatoid arthritis. N Engl J Med 303:300–302, 1980.
340. Verroust PJ: Kinetics of immune deposits in membranous nephropathy. Kidney Int 35:1418–1428, 1989.
341. Ntoso KA, Tomaszewski JE, Jimenez SA, Neilson EG: Penicillamine-induced rapidly progressive glomerulonephritis in patients with primary systemic sclerosis: Successful treatment of two patients and a review of the literature. Am J Kidney Dis 8:159–163, 1986.
342. Hall OL: The natural course of gold and penicillamine nephropathy: A longterm study of 54 patients. Adv Exp Biol 252:247–256, 1989.
343. Francis KL, Jenis EH, Hensen GE, et al: Gold-associated nephropathy. Arch Pathol Lab Med 108:234–238, 1984.
344. Blum M, Liron M, Aviram A: Nephrotic syndrome with reversible severe renal failure after gold therapy. Int J Clin Pharmacol Ther Toxicol 22:562–564, 1984.
345. Katz WA, Blodgett RC, Pietrusko RG: Proteinuria in gold-treated rheumatoid arthritis. Ann Intern Med 101:176–179, 1984.
346. Dunn MJ, Howe D: Prostaglandins lack a direct inhibitory action on electrolyte and water transport in the kidney and the erythrocyte. Prostaglandins 13:417–429, 1977.
347. Henrich WL: Nephrotoxicity of non-steroidal anti-inflammatory agents. In Schrier R, Gottschalk C (eds): Diseases of the Kidney, 5th ed. Little, Brown, Boston, 1992, pp 1201–1218.
348. Aiken JW, Vane JR: Intrarenal prostaglandin release attenuates the renal vasoconstrictor activity of angiotensin. J Pharmacol Exp Ther 184:678–687, 1973.
349. Finn W, Arendshorst WJ: Effect of prostaglandin synthetase inhibitors on renal blood flow in the rat. Am J Physiol 231:1541–1545, 1976.

350. Satoh S, Zimmerman BG: Influence of the renin-angiotensin system on the effect of prostaglandin synthesis inhibitors in the renal vasculature. Circ Res 36 (suppl I):89–96, 1975.

351. Swain JA, Heyndricks GR, Boettcher DR, Vatner SF: Prostaglandin control of renal circulation in the unanesthetized dog and baboon. Am J Physiol 229:826–830, 1975.

352. Lonigro AJ, Itsokovitz HD, Crowshaw K, McGiff JC: Dependency of renal blood flow on prostaglandin synthesis in the dog. Circ Res 32:712–717, 1973.

353. Needleman P, Marshall GR, Johnson EM Jr: Determinants and modification of adrenergic and vascular resistance in the kidney. Am J Physiol 227:665–669, 1974.

354. Susic H, Malik KU: Prostacyclin and prostaglandin E$_2$ effects on adrenergic transmission in the kidney of the anesthetized dog. J Pharmacol Exp Ther 218:588–592, 1981.

355. Clive DM, Stoff JS: Renal syndromes associated with nonsteroidal antiinflammatory drugs. N Engl J Med 310:563–572, 1984.

356. Stillman MT, Schleisinger PA: Nonsteroidal anti-inflammatory drug nephrotoxicity. Arch Intern Med 150:268–270, 1990.

357. Unsworth J, Sturman S, Lunec J, et al: Renal impairment associated with non-steroidal anti-inflammatory drugs. J Rheum Dis 46:233–236, 1987.

358. Patrono C, Dunn MJ: The clinical significance of inhibition of renal prostaglandin synthesis. Kidney Int 32:1–12, 1987.

359. Carmichael J, Shankel SW: Effects of nonsteroidal anti-inflammatory drugs on prostaglandins and renal function. Am J Med 78:992–1000, 1985.

360. Adams DH, Michael J, Bacon PA, et al: Non-steroidal anti-inflammatory drugs and renal failure. Lancet 1:57–59, 1986.

361. Murray MD, Brater DC: Adverse effects of nonsteroidal anti-inflammatory drugs on renal function. Ann Intern Med 112:559–560, 1990.

362. Leehey DJ, Uckerman MT, Rahman MA: Role of prostaglandins and thromboxane in the control of renal hemodynamics in experimental liver cirrhosis. J Lab Clin Med 113:309–315, 1989.

363. Dunn MJ, Zambrask E: Renal effects of drugs that inhibit prostaglandin synthesis. Kidney Int 18:609–617, 1980.

364. Levenson DJ, Simmons CE Jr, Brenner BM: Arachidonic acid metabolism, prostaglandins and the kidney. Am J Med 72:354–374, 1979.

365. Fulgraff G, Meiforth A: Effects of prostaglandin E$_2$ on excretion and reabsorption of sodium and fluid in rat kidneys (micropuncture studies). Pflugers Arch 330:243–256, 1971.

366. Ganguli M, Tobian L, Azar S, et al: Evidence that prostaglandin synthesis inhibitors increase the concentration of sodium and chloride in rat renal medulla. Circ Res 40:135–139, 1977.

367. Shimizu K, Kurosawa T, Maeda T, et al: Free water excretion and washout of renal medullary urea by prostaglandin E. Jpn Heart J 10:437–455, 1969.

368. Ichicawa I, Brenner BM: Mechanism of inhibition of proximal tubule fluid reabsorption after exposure of the rat kidney to the physical effects of expansion of extracellular fluid volume. J Clin Invest 64:1466–1474, 1979.

369. Ichicawa I, Brenner BM: Importance of efferent arteriolar vascular tone in regulation of proximal tubular fluid reabsorption and glomerulotubular balance in the rat. J Clin Invest 65:1192–1201, 1980.

370. Higashihara E, Stokes JB, Kokko JP, et al: Cortical and papillary micropuncture examination of chloride transport in segments in the rat kidney during inhibition of prostaglandin production. J Clin Invest 64:1277–1287, 1979.

371. Iino Y, Imai M: Effects of prostaglandins on Na transport in isolated collecting tubules. Pflugers Arch 373:125–133, 1978.

372. Roman RJ, Kauker ML: Renal effect of prostaglandin synthetase inhibition in rats: Micropuncture studies. Am J Physiol 235:F111–F118, 1978.

373. Stokes JB, Kokko JP: Inhibition of sodium transport by prostaglandin E$_2$ across the isolated, perfused rabbit collecting tubule. J Clin Invest 49:1099–1104, 1977.

374. Work J, Baehler TR, Kotchen A, et al: Effect of prostaglandin inhibition on sodium chloride reabsorption in the diluting segment of the conscious dog. Kidney Int 17:24–30, 1980.

375. Carmines PK, Bell DP, Roman RJ, et al: Prostaglandins in the sodium excretory response to altered renal arterial pressure in dogs. Am J Physiol 248:F8–F14, 1985.

376. Wilson DR, Honrath U, Sonnenberg H: Prostaglandin synthesis inhibition during volume expansion: Collecting duct function. Kidney Int 22:1–7, 1982.

377. Nies AS, Gal J, Fadul S, et al: Indomethacin-furosemide interaction: The importance of renal blood flow. J Pharmacol Exp Ther 226:27–32, 1983.

378. Berg XJ: Acute effects of acetylsalicylate acid in patients with chronic renal insufficiency. Eur J Clin Pharmacol 11:111–116, 1977.

379. Mirouze D, Zisper RD, Reynolds TB: Effect of inhibitors of prostaglandin synthesis on induced cirrhosis. Hepatology 3:50–55, 1983.

380. Patak RV, Moorkejeree BK, Bentzel CJ, et al: Antagonism of the effects of furosemide by indomethacin in normal and hypertensive man. Prostaglandins 10:649–659, 1975.

381. Tiggeler RG, Koene RA, Wijdeveld PG: Inhibition of furosemide-induced natriuresis by indomethacin in patients with nephrotic syndrome. Clin Sci Mol Med 2:149–151, 1977.

382. Williamson HE, Bourland UA, Marchand GR: Inhibition of furosemide-induced increase in renal blood flow by indomethacin. Proc Soc Exp Biol Med 148:297–301, 1975.

383. Epstein M, Lifschitz MD, Hoffman DS, et al: Relationship between renal prostaglandin E and renal sodium handling during water immersion in normal man. Circ Res 45:71–80, 1979.

384. Dunn MJ, Hood VL: Prostaglandins and the kidney. Am J Physiol 233:F169–F184, 1977.

385. Dunn MJ, Zambraski E: Renal effects of drugs that inhibit prostaglandin synthesis. Kidney Int 18:609–617, 1980.

386. Henrich WL, Campbell WB: Importance of intracellular calcium in tissue renin release. Clin Res 32:242A, 1984. Abstract.

387. Berl T, Henrich W, Erickson AL, et al: Prostaglandins in the beta adrenergic and baroreceptor-mediated secretion of renin. Am J Physiol 236:F472–F477, 1979.

388. Blackshear JL, Spielman WS, Knox FG, Romero JC: Dissociation of renin release and renal vasodilation by prostaglandin synthesis inhibitors. Am J Physiol 237:F20–F24, 1979.

389. Gerber JG, Olson RD, Nies AS: Control of canine renin release: Macula densa requires prostaglandin synthesis. J Physiol (Lond) 319:419–429, 1981.

390. Henrich WL: Prostaglandins in renin secretion. Kidney Int 19:822–830, 1981.

391. Henrich WL, Campbell WB: Relationship between prostaglandins and the β-adrenergic pathway to renin secretion. An in vitro study. Am J Physiol 247:E343–E348, 1984.

392. Henrich WL, Berl T, McDonald KM, et al: Angiotensin II, renal nerves, and prostaglandins in renal hemodynamics during hemorrhage. Am J Physiol 235:F46–F51, 1978.

393. Henrich WL, Anderson RJ, Berns AS, et al: Role of renal nerves and prostaglandins in control of renal hemodynamics and plasma renin activity during hypotensive hemorrhage in the dog. J Clin Invest 61:744–750, 1978.

394. Henrich WL, Campbell WB: The β-adrenergic pathway to renin release: Relations with the prostaglandin system. Endocrinology 113:2247–2254, 1983.

395. Antillon M, Cominelli F, Lo S, et al: Effects of oral prostaglandins on indomethacin-induced renal failure in patients with cirrhosis and ascites. J Rheumatol 20:46–49, 1990.

396. Bernheim JL, Korzets Z: Indomethacin-induced renal failure. Ann Intern Med 91:792, 1979. Letter.

397. Blum M, Bauminger S, Algueti A, et al: Urinary prostaglandin E$_2$ in chronic renal disease. Clin Nephrol 15:87–89, 1981.

398. Brandstetter RD, Marr DD: Reversible oliguric renal failure associated with ibuprofen treatment. Br Med J 1194–1195, 1978.

399. Favre L, Glasson PH, Riondel A, et al: Interaction of diuretics and non-steroidal anti-inflammatory drugs in man. Clin Sci 64:407, 1983.

400. Fong HJ, Cohen AH: Ibuprofen-induced acute renal failure with acute tubular necrosis. Am J Nephrol 2:28–31, 1982.

401. Galler M, Folkert VW, Schlondorf D: Reversible acute renal insufficiency and hyperkalemia following indomethacin therapy. JAMA 246:154–155, 1981.

402. Garella S, Matarese RA: Renal effects of prostaglandins and clinical adverse effects of nonsteroidal anti-inflammatory agents. Medicine (Baltimore) 63:165–181, 1984.

403. Kimberly RP, Bowden RE, Keiser HR, et al: Reduction of renal function by newer nonsteroidal anti-inflammatory drugs. Am J Med 64:804–807, 1978.

404. Kimberly RP, Plotz PH: Aspirin-induced depression of renal function. N Engl J Med 296:418–428, 1977.

405. Lipsett MB, Goldman R: Phenylbutazone toxicity: Report of a case of acute renal failure. Ann Intern Med 41:1075–1079, 1954.

406. McCarthy JT, Torres VE, Romero JC, et al: Acute intrinsic renal failure induced by indomethacin. Role of prostaglandin synthetase inhibition. Mayo Clin Proc 57:289–296, 1982.

407. Fawaz-Estrup F, Ho G Jr: Reversible acute renal failure induced by indomethacin. Arch Intern Med 141:1670–1671, 1981.

408. Tan SY, Franco R, Stockard H, et al: Indomethacin-induced prostaglandin inhibition with hyperkalemia. A reversible cause of hyporeninemic hypoaldosteronism. Ann Intern Med 90:783–785, 1979.

409. Zipser RD, Hoefs JC, Speckart PF, et al: Prostaglandins: Modulators of renal function and pressor resistance in chronic liver disease. J Clin Endocrinol Metab 48:895–900, 1979.

410. Schlondorff D: Renal complications of nonsteroidal anti-inflammatory drugs. Kidney Int 44:643–653, 1993.

411. Gurwitz JH, Avorn J, Ross-Deghan D, et al: Nonsteroidal anti-inflammatory drug-associated azotemia in the very old. JAMA 264:471–475, 1990.

412. Simon LS, Basch CM, Young DY, Robinson DR: Effects of naproxen on renal function in older patients with mild to moderate renal dysfunction. Br J Rheumatol 31:163–168, 1992.

413. Whelton A, Stout RL, Spilman PS, Klassen DK: Renal effects of ibuprofen, piroxicam, and sulindac in patients with asymptomatic renal failure. Ann Intern Med 112:568–576, 1990.

414. Marasco WA, Gikas PW, Aziz-Baumgartner R, et al: Ibuprofen-associated renal dysfunction. Pathophysiologic mechanisms of acute renal failure hyperkalemia, tubular necrosis, and proteinuria. Arch Intern Med 147:2107–2116, 1987.

415. Patrono C, Pierucci A: A renal effect of nonsteroidal anti-inflammatory drugs in chronic glomerular disease. Am J Med 82(suppl 2B):71–83, 1986.

416. Laxer RM, Silverman E, Balfe D, et al: Indomethacin and ibuprofen-induced reversible acute renal failure in a patient with systemic lupus erythematosus. Neth J Med 30:181–186, 1987.

417. Blackshear JL, Davidman M, Stillman MT: Identification of risk for renal insufficiency from non-steroidal anti-inflammatory drugs. Arch Intern Med 43:1130–1134, 1983.

418. Bunning RD, Barth WF: Sulindac. A potentially renal-sparing non-steroidal anti-inflammatory drug. JAMA 248:2864–2867, 1982.

419. Daskalopoulos G, Kronborg I, Katkov W, et al: Sulindac and indomethacin suppress the diuretic action of furosemide in patients with cirrhosis and ascites: Evidence that sulindac affects renal prostaglandins. Am J Kidney Dis 6:217–222, 1985.

420. Dixey JJ, Noormohamed FH, Lant AF: The effects of naproxen and sulindac on renal function and their interaction with hydrochlorothiazide and piretanide in man. Br J Clin Pharmacol 23:55–63, 1987.

421. Swainson CP, Griffiths P: Acute and chronic effects of sulindac on renal function in chronic renal disease. Clin Pharmacol Ther 37:298–300, 1985.

422. Klassen DK, Stout RL, Spilman PS, et al: Sulindac kinetics and effects on renal function and prostaglandin excretion in renal insufficiency. J Clin Pharmacol 29:1037–1042, 1989.

423. Eriksson L-O, Sturfelt G, Thysell H, et al: Effects of sulindac and naproxen on prostaglandin excretion in patients with impaired renal function and rheumatoid arthritis. Am J Med 89:313–321, 1990.

424. Brater MJS, Bednar MM, McGiff JC: Renal metabolism of ibuprofen, naproxen and sulindac on prostaglandins in men. Kidney Int 27:66–72, 1985.

425. Miller MJS, Bednar MM, McGiff JC: Renal metabolism of sulindac: Functional implications. J Pharmacol Exp Ther 231:449–456, 1984.

426. Cibattoni G, Cinotti GA, Pierucci A: Effects of sulindac and ibuprofen in patients with chronic glomerular disease: Evidence for the dependence of renal function on prostacyclin. N Engl J Med 310:279–288, 1984.

427. Laffi G, Daskalopoulos G, Kronborg I, et al: Effects of sulindac and ibuprofen in patients with cirrhosis and ascites. An explanation for the renal-sparing effect of sulindac. Gastroenterology 90:182–187, 1986.

428. Quintero E, Gines P, Arroyo V: Sulindac reduces the urinary excretion of prostaglandins and impairs renal function in cirrhosis with ascites. Nephron 42:298–303, 1986.

429. Husserl FE, Lange RK, Kantrow CM Jr: Renal papillary necrosis and pyelonephritis accompanying fenoprofen therapy. JAMA 242:1896–1898, 1979.

430. Lourie SH, Denman SJ, Schroeder ET: Association of renal papillary necrosis and ankylosing spondylitis. Arthritis Rheum 20:917–921, 1977.

431. Morales A, Steyn J: Papillary necrosis following phenylbutazone ingestion. Arch Surg 103:420–421, 1971.

432. Gokal R, Matthews DR: Renal papillary necrosis after aspirin and alclofenac. Br Med J 2:1517–1518, 1977.

433. Abraham PA, Keane WF: Glomerular and interstitial disease induced by non-steroidal anti-inflammatory drugs. Am J Nephrol 4:1–6, 1984.

434. Brezin J, Ratz S, Schwartz A, et al: Reversible renal failure and nephrotic syndrome associated with non-steroidal anti-inflammatory drugs. N Engl J Med 301:1271–1273, 1979.

435. Segasothy M, Samad SA, Zulfiquar A, Bennett WM: Renal dysfunction and renal papillary necrosis with long term use of NSAIDs as a sole or predominant analgesic: A new form of analgesic nephropathy. J Am Soc Nephrol 4:759, 1993.

436. Sandler DP, Burr FR, Weinberg C: Non-steroidal anti-inflammatory drugs and the risk for chronic renal disease. Ann Intern Med 115:165–172, 1991.

437. Finkelstein A, Fraley DS, Stachura I, et al: Fenoprofen nephropathy: Lipoid nephrosis and interstitial nephritis. A possible T-lymphocyte disorder. Am J Med 72:81–87, 1982.

438. Katz S, Capaldo R, Everts E, et al: Association with reversible renal failure and acute interstitial nephritis. JAMA 246:243–245, 1981.

439. Goetzl E: Selective feed-back inhibition of the 5 lipoxygenation of the arachidonic acid in human T-lymphocytes. Biochem Biophys Res Commun 101:344–350, 1981.

440. Siegel MI, McConnell RT, Porter NA, Cuatrecasas P: Arachidonate metabolism via lipoxygenase and 12L-hydroperoxy-5,8,10,14-eicosatetraenoic acid perioxidase sensitive to anti-inflammatory drugs. Proc Natl Acad Sci USA 77:308–312, 1980.

441. Payan DG, Goetzl EJ: The dependence of human T-lymphocyte migration on the 5-lipoxygenation of endogenous arachidonic acid. J Clin Immunol 1:266, 1981.

442. Goetzl E: Mediators of immediate hypersensitivity derived from arachidonic acid. N Engl J Med 303:822–825, 1980.

443. Torres VE: Present and future of the nonsteroidal anti-inflammatory drugs in nephrology. Mayo Clin Proc 57:389–393, 1982.

444. Morgenstern SJ, Burns FJ, Fraley DS, et al: Ibuprofen-associated lipid nephrosis without interstitial nephritis. Am J Kidney Dis 16:50–52, 1989.

445. Schwartzman M, Dagati V: Spontaneous relapse of naproxen-related nephrotic syndrome. Am J Med 82:329–332, 1987.

446. Crespigny PJ, Becker GJ, Ihle U: Renal failure and nephrotic syndrome associated with sulindac. Clin Nephrol 30:52–55, 1988.

447. Sohooley RT, Wagley PF, Lietman PS: Edema associated with ibuprofen therapy. JAMA 237:1716–1717, 1977.

448. Walshe JJ, Venuto RC: Acute oliguric renal failure induced by indomethacin: Possible mechanism. Ann Intern Med 91:47–49, 1979.

449. Findling JW, Beckstrom D, Rawsthorne L: Indomethacin-induced hyperkalemia in three patients with gouty arthritis. JAMA 244:1127–1128, 1980.

450. Goldszer RC, Coodley EL, Rosner MJ, et al: Hyperkalemia associated with indomethacin. Arch Intern Med 141:802–804, 1980.

451. Kutyrina JM, Andosova SO, Tareyeva IE: Indomethacin-induced hyporeninaemic hypoaldosteronism. Lancet 1:785, 1979.

452. Tan SY, Franco R, Stockard H, Mulrow PJ: Indomethacin-induced prostaglandin inhibition with hyperkalemia. A reversible cause of hyporeninemic hypoaldosteronism. Ann Intern Med 90:783, 1979.

453. Donker AJM: The effect of indomethacin on renal function and glomerular protein loss. *In* Dunn MJ, Patrons C, Cinotti GA (eds): Prostaglandins and the Kidney: Biochemistry, Physiology, Pharmacology and Clinical Applications. Plenum Publishing, New York, 1990, pp 251–262.

454. Gill JR Jr, Frolich JC, Bowden RE, et al: Bartter's syndrome: A disorder characterized by high urinary prostaglandins and a dependence of hyperreninemia on prostaglandin synthesis. Am J Med 61:43–51, 1976.

455. Halushka PV, Privatera PJ, Hurwitz G, et al: Bartter's syndrome: Urinary prostaglandin E-like material and kallikrein: Indomethacin effects. Ann Intern Med 87:281–286, 1977.

456. Veroerckmoes R, Van Damme B, Clement J, et al: Bartter's syndrome with hyperplasia of renomedullary cells: Successful treatment with indomethacin. Kidney Int 9:302–307, 1976.

457. Beckmann ML, Gerber JG, Byyny RL, et al: Propranolol increases prostacyclin synthesis in patients with hypertension. Hypertension 12:582–588, 1988.

458. Seelig CB, Maloley PA, Campbell JR: Nephrotoxicity associated with concomitant ACE inhibitor and NSAID therapy. South Med J 83:1144–1148, 1990.

459. Diederich D, Yang Z, Buhler FR, et al: Impaired endothelium-dependent relaxations in hypertensive resistance arteries involve cyclooxygenase pathway. Am J Physiol 258:H445–H448, 1990.

460. Panza JA, Quyyumi AA, Brush JE Jr, Epstein SE: Abnormal endothelium-dependent vascular relaxation in patients with essential hypertension. N Engl J Med 323:22–27, 1990.

461. Vane JR, Anggard EE, Botting RM: Regulatory functions of the vascular endothelium. N Engl J Med 323:27–35, 1990.

462. Linder L, Wolfgang K, Buhler FR, et al: Indirect evidence for release of endothelium-derived relaxing factor in human forearm circulation in vivo. Circulation 81:1762–1767, 1990.

463. Kato T, Iwama Y, Okumura K, et al: Prostaglandin $H_2$ may be the endothelium-derived contracting factor released by acetylcholine in the aorta of the rat. Hypertension 15:475–481, 1990.

464. Minuz P, Barrow SE, Crockcroft JR, et al: Prostacyclin and thromboxane biosynthesis in mild essential hypertension. Hypertension 15:469–474, 1990.

465. Luscher TF: Imbalance of endothelium-derived relaxing and contracting factors. Am J Hypertens 3:317–330, 1990.

466. Houston MC: Nonsteroidal anti-inflammatory drugs and antihypertensives. Am J Med 90(5A):42S–47S, 1991.

467. Minuz P, Barrow SE, Crockcroft JR, et al: Effects of non-steroidal anti-inflammatory drugs on prostacyclin and thromboxane biosynthesis in patients with mild essential hypertension. Br J Clin Pharmacol 30:519–526, 1990.

468. Abe K, Sato M, Takeuchi K, et al: The roles of renal prostaglandin in the regulatory mechanism of renal excretory function and blood pressure in hypertension. Adv Prostaglandin Thromboxane Leukotriene Res 19:216–220, 1989.

469. Pope JE, Anderson JJ, Felson DT: A meta-analysis of the effects of nonsteroidal anti-inflammatory drugs on blood pressure. Arch Intern Med 153:477–484, 1993.

470. Henrich WL: Functional and organic ischemic renal disease. *In* Seldin DW, Giebisch GH (eds): The Kidney: Physiology and Pathophysiology, 2nd ed. Raven Press, New York, 1992, pp 3289–3304.

471. Badr KF, Ichikawa K: Prerenal failure: A deleterious shift from renal compensation to decompensation. N Engl J Med 319:623–629, 1988.

472. Curtis JJ, Luke RG, Whelchel JD, et al: Inhibition of angiotensin-converting enzyme in renal transplant recipients with hypertension. N Engl J Med 308:377–381, 1983.

473. Jacobson HR: Ischemic renal disease: An overlooked clinical entity? Kidney Int 34:729–743, 1988.

474. Packer M, Lee WH, Medina N, et al: Influence of diabetes mellitus on changes in left ventricular performance and renal function produced by converting enzyme inhibition in patients with severe chronic renal failure. Am J Med 823:1119–1126, 1987.

475. Nath KA, Crumbley AJ, Murray BM, Sibley RK: N Engl J Med 309:666–667, 1983. Letter.

476. Ying CY, Tifft CP, Gavras H, et al: Renal revascularization in the azotemic hypertensive patient resistant to therapy. N Engl J Med 311:1070–1075, 1984.

477. Textor SC, Novick AC, Tarazi RC, et al: Critical perfusion pressure for renal function in patients with bilateral atherosclerotic renal vascular disease. Ann Intern Med 102:308–314, 1985.

478. Bender W, LaFrance N, Walter WG: Mechanism of deterioration in renal function in patients with renovascular hypertension treated with enalapril. Hypertension 6:I193–I197, 1984.

479. Fommei E, Ghione S, Palla L: Renal scintigraphic captopril test in the diagnosis of renovascular hypertension. Hypertension 10:212–220, 1987.

480. Gruenewald SM, Collins LT: Renovascular hypertension: Quantitative renography as a screening test. Radiology 149:287–291, 1983.

481. Jackson B, McGrath BP, Matthews G, et al: Differential renal function during angiotensin converting enzyme inhibition in renovascular hypertension. Hypertension 8:650–654, 1986.

482. Miyanmori I, Yasuhara S, Takeda Y, et al: Effects of converting inhibition on split renal function in renovascular hypertension. Hypertension 8:415–421, 1986.

483. Nally JV Jr: Renal scintigraphy in the evaluation of renovascular hypertension: A note of optimism yet caution. J Nucl Med 28:1501–1505, 1987.

484. Schohn DC, Jahn HA, Schmitt RL: Predictability of a standardization captopril-test in hypertension in end-stage renal failure. Kidney Int 34:S145–S148, 1988.

485. Thibonnier M, Joseph A, Sassano P: Diagnostic value of a single dose of captopril in renin and aldosterone-dependent surgically curable hypertension. Cardiovasc Rev Rep 3:1659–1668, 1982.

486. Kohler TR, Zierler RE, Martin RL: Non-invasive diagnosis of renal artery stenosis by ultrasonic duplex scanning. J Vasc Surg 4:450–456, 1986.

487. Donker AJM: Nephrotoxicity of angiotensin converting enzyme inhibition. Kidney Int 31:S132–S137, 1987.

488. Cleland JGF, Dargie HJ, Gillen G, et al: Captopril in heart failure: A double-blind study of the effects on renal function. J Cardiovasc Pharmacol 8:700–706, 1986.

489. Yaqoob M, Bell GM, Stevenson A, et al: Renal impairment with chronic hydrocarbon exposure. Q J Med 86:165–174, 1993.

490. Barrientos A, Ortuno MT, Morales JM, et al: Acute renal failure after use of diesel fuel as shampoo. Arch Intern Med 137:1217, 1977.

491. Crisp AJ, Balla AK, Hoffbrand BI: Acute tubular necrosis after exposure to diesel oil. Br Med J 2:177, 1979.

492. Narvarte J, Saba SR, Ramirez G: Occupational exposure to organic solvents causing chronic tubulointerstitial nephritis. Arch Intern Med 149:154–159, 1989.

493. Anderson K: Acute nephritis due to turpentine absorbed by the skin. Br Med J 3:881, 1912.

494. Cagnoli I, Cassanova S, Pasquali S, Zuccheli P: Relationship between hydrocarbon exposure and the nephrotic syndrome. Br Med J 280:1068–1069, 1980.

495. Beirne GJ, Brennan JT: Glomerulonephritis associated with hydrocarbon solvents. Arch Environ Health 25:365–369, 1972.

496. Daniell WE, Couser WG, Rosenstock L: Occupational solvent exposure and glomerulonephritis. A case report and review of the literature. JAMA 259:2280–2283, 1988.

497. Klavis G, Drommer W: Goodpasture's syndrome and the effects of benzene. Arch Toxicol 26:40–55, 1970.

498. Ogawa M, Moti T, Mori Y, et al: Study on chronic renal injuries induced by carbon tetrachloride: Selective inhibition of the nephrotoxicity by irradiation. Nephron 60:68–73, 1992.

499. Yamamoto T, Wilson CB: Binding of anti–basement membrane after intratracheal gasoline instillation in rabbits. Am J Pathol 126:497–505, 1987.

500. Ravnskov U: Possible mechanisms of hydrocarbon-associated glomerulonephritis. Clin Nephrol 23:294–298, 1985.

# Microvascular Diseases
# of the Kidney

*Fadi G. Lakkis*
*Orville C. Campbell*
*Kamal F. Badr*

## THE HEMOLYTIC-UREMIC SYNDROME AND THROMBOTIC THROMBOCYTOPENIC PURPURA

The hemolytic-uremic syndrome (HUS) and thrombotic thrombocytopenic purpura (TTP) are closely related diseases characterized by microangiopathic hemolytic anemia and variable organ impairment.[1] Traditionally, the diagnosis of HUS is made when renal failure is a predominant feature of the syndrome, as is common in children.[2] In adults, neurologic impairment frequently predominates, and the syndrome is then referred to as TTP.[3, 4] Thrombotic microangiopathy is the underlying pathologic lesion in both syndromes,[5] and the clinical and laboratory findings in patients with either HUS or TTP overlap to a large extent.[1] This has prompted several investigators to regard the two syndromes as a continuum of a single disease entity.[1, 6]

### Clinical Features

A report by Moschowitz[7] in 1925 described a 16-year-old girl who had fever, anemia, petechiae, renal failure, and neurologic impairment. In 1936, Baehr and colleagues[8] described the presence of thrombocytopenia and reticulocytosis in a similar case. In both reports, TTP was the term used to describe the syndrome. More than 500 cases and several large series of patients have been reported since.[9-13] TTP is usually a sporadic disease with a frequency of approximately one case per million population.[12] It is more common in women (female/male ratio of 3:2 to 5:2) and in whites (white/black ratio of 3:1).[9, 13] Although peak occurrence is in the third and fourth decades of life, TTP can

affect any age group.[11, 14] TTP is an acute illness that is often accompanied by nonspecific constitutional symptoms, such as malaise, nausea, and vomiting.[9] The classic triad of microangiopathic hemolytic anemia, thrombocytopenia, and neurologic symptoms occurs in approximately 75% of the patients.[9] Hemorrhagic manifestations (83% to 96% of the cases) occur anywhere on the body and manifest as petechiae, purpura, ecchymoses, or bleeding from other sites.[13] Neurologic symptoms (84% to 92% of cases) are common at presentation and include headache, altered mental status, paresis, aphasia, dysphasia, paresthesias, visual problems, seizures, and coma.[13-15] Fever occurs in 98% of patients during the course of illness and is the most common symptom in TTP.[9] Renal involvement in TTP (80% to 90% of patients) is usually mild but can range from abnormal urinalysis to severe renal insufficiency requiring dialysis therapy[16] (see later). Severe acute renal failure or anuria occurs in less than 10% of the cases.[9]

The term HUS was introduced in 1955 by Gasser and co-workers[17] in their description of an acute fatal syndrome in children characterized by hemolytic anemia, thrombocytopenia, and severe renal failure. Gastrointestinal prodromes (vomiting, diarrhea, and abdominal pain) commonly occur a few days to a few weeks before the onset of HUS.[2, 17-19] Hemolytic anemia and renal involvement are uniformly present in HUS.[2] Acute renal failure is detected in 90% of patients, and anuria occurs in one third of the cases[20] (see later). Neurologic symptoms and signs are similar to those seen with TTP but occur less often (40% of patients).[21, 22] As with TTP, purpura and fever are frequently present.[2] The source of bleeding is most commonly the gastrointestinal tract. HUS is characteristically a disease of young children. The average annual incidence is 2.65

cases/100,000 for ages 5 years and younger and 0.97 cases/100,000 for ages 18 years and younger.[23] Both sporadic HUS and epidemic HUS occur in children.[2] The epidemic form is the typical presentation and is characteristically preceded by diarrhea.[24]

Additional clinical findings in either TTP or HUS result from microvascular thromboses in the intestines, pancreas, skeletal muscle, and heart. Gastrointestinal involvement may lead to symptoms of acute abdomen with occasional perforation.[12, 25, 26] Microinfarcts in the pancreas may cause pancreatitis[27] and rarely insulin-dependent diabetes mellitus.[28, 29] Acute rhabdomyolysis has been reported in association with HUS.[30] Cardiac manifestations include congestive heart failure and arrhythmias.[31] Ocular involvement presenting as retinal, choroidal, or vitreous hemorrhage is also observed in HUS and TTP patients.[32, 33]

Despite the historical distinction between HUS and TTP,[3] the two syndromes overlap to a large extent and may indeed represent a spectrum of a single disease.[1, 6] Occurrence of HUS is not restricted to children,[34, 35] nor is TTP limited to adults.[11, 14] An epidemic form of HUS, similar to the one seen in children, has been described in adult nursing home patients.[36] The underlying pathologic process, thrombotic microangiopathy, is identical in both syndromes and can affect multiple organs.[5] Renal damage does not reliably differentiate HUS from TTP because 80% to 90% of TTP patients have some evidence of renal involvement[16] and 40% to 80% have depressed renal function.[12, 37] Similarly, neurologic involvement is not characteristic of TTP because it is frequently observed in patients with the clinical diagnosis of HUS.[21, 22] These observations suggest that the two syndromes are variable presentations of the same disease and have prompted the use of the term HUS/TTP to describe patients with thrombotic microangiopathy.[1]

## Laboratory Findings

The hallmark laboratory finding, essential for the diagnosis of HUS/TTP, is microangiopathic hemolytic anemia. The peripheral smear reveals increased schistocyte number (burr cells, helmet cells, and other erythrocyte fragments).[38] In adults, hemoglobin levels are less than 10 g/dL in 99% of the cases and less than 6.5 g/dL in 40%.[39] Reticulocyte counts are uniformly elevated. Other indicators of intravascular hemolysis include elevated lactate dehydrogenase, increased indirect bilirubin, and low haptoglobin levels.[15] The Coombs test result is negative, indicating that the anemia is not immunologically mediated. Moderate leukocytosis may accompany the hemolytic anemia, but white blood cell counts of 20,000/mm³ are rarely exceeded.[9] Thrombocytopenia is uniformly present in HUS/TTP, and platelet counts below 60,000/mm³ are usual.[10–12] The presence of giant platelets in the peripheral smear and reduced platelet survival time are consistent with peripheral consumption or destruction of platelets.[40] In children, the duration of thrombocytopenia is variable and does not correlate with the course of renal disease.[41]

Biopsy samples of bone marrow usually show erythroid hyperplasia and increased number of megakaryocytes. Prothrombin time, partial thromboplastin time, fibrinogen level, and coagulation factors are normal, thus differentiating HUS/TTP from disseminated intravascular coagulopathy.[15, 42] Mild fibrinolysis with minimal elevation in fibrin degradation products may be observed, however. Complement levels are decreased in some patients.[43] Diagnostic central nervous system studies in HUS/TTP have not been extensively evaluated. Punctate lesions in the white matter were detected by magnetic resonance imaging, but not by computed tomography, in two patients with classic TTP presentation.[44, 45]

## Renal Involvement

Evidence of renal involvement is present in the majority of patients with HUS/TTP.[2, 12, 16, 20] Microscopic hematuria and subnephrotic proteinuria are the most consistent findings. In a retrospective study of 216 patients with a clinical picture of TTP, hematuria was detected in 78% and proteinuria in 75% of the cases.[16] Sterile pyuria and casts were present in 31% and 24% of the patients, respectively.[16] Gross hematuria is rare.[16] More than 90% of patients with an HUS presentation have significant renal failure, one third of whom are anuric.[20] Dialysis is required in a large percentage of these patients.[46] The mean duration of renal failure is 2 weeks.[20] Severe acute renal failure or anuria occurs in less than 10% of classic TTP cases.[9] The degree of elevation of blood urea nitrogen on presentation may be a prognostic indicator in patients with HUS/TTP.[16]

**Pathology.** The characteristic lesion in HUS/TTP is thrombotic microangiopathy.[5, 47] Microthrombi have been demonstrated in arterioles and capillaries of the kidney, brain, skin, pancreas, heart, spleen, and adrenal glands.[15] The microthrombi are composed predominantly of platelet aggregates and thin layers of fibrin.[15, 48] The platelet thrombi stain strongly for von Willebrand factor (vWF),[49] which has been implicated in the pathogenesis of HUS/TTP (see later). Subendothelial hyaline deposits and endothelial cell swelling also contribute to the occlusion of the arteriolar and capillary lumens.[15, 49] Venules are rarely affected, and vasculitis is usually absent.[15]

Three patterns of renal lesions have been described in HUS/TTP: glomerular, arterial, or both.[50] In younger children, the pathologic process is mainly confined to the glomeruli. On light microscopic examination, it is characterized by thickening of capillary walls, endothelial cell swelling, and narrowing or obliteration of capillary lumens. Widening of the subendothelial space may result in a double-contour or double-tracks appearance of the glomerular capillary walls. Clumps of red blood cells, platelets, or thrombi may be seen in the glomerular capillaries. Widening of the mesangium may be present without evidence of mesangial cell proliferation.[51] Arterial involvement in children with HUS is usually minimal. In older children and in adults, significant arterial changes coexist with glomerular lesions.[50, 52] Thrombi are present in the interlobular arteries, which also demonstrate intimal edema and myointimal cell proliferation.[52] This process may result in arterial fibroplasia. The glomerular lesions in these patients are ischemic in origin.[50] The glomerular capillary walls are wrinkled, the glomerular tuft may be atrophied, and Bowman capsule is thickened. In some patients, the glomerular changes described in younger children coexist with the pattern of arterial injury.[53] Acute cortical or tubule necrosis may occur in HUS/TTP patients.[50]

Immunofluorescence studies performed on renal biopsy specimens of patients with HUS/TTP invariably demonstrate fibrinogen along the glomerular capillary walls and in the arterial thrombi.[54] Granular deposits of C3 and immunoglobulin M may be observed in the vessel walls and in glomeruli.[55] Electron microscopic studies demonstrate swelling of the glomerular endothelial cells and detachment from the glomerular basement membrane.[1] Electron-lucent "fluffy" material fills the space between the glomerular basement membrane and the detached endothelium. The glomerular basement membrane itself remains intact. Similar findings are present in arteries and arterioles.[56]

## Etiology

Epidemiologic and laboratory data suggest that bacterial cytotoxins may be causative agents in HUS/TTP.[57] Outbreaks of hemorrhagic colitis in children have led to the isolation of a new *Escherichia coli* strain (serotype O157:H7) that produces Shiga-like cytotoxins.[58, 59] Because of the cytotoxic activity of these toxins on Vero cells, they are referred to as verotoxins.[58, 60] Strong epidemiologic evidence links cytotoxin-producing *E. coli*, serotype O157:H7 in particular, to sporadic cases and outbreaks of HUS[24, 36, 61, 62] and TTP.[63, 64] In an epidemic of diarrhea due to cytotoxin-producing *E. coli* O157:H7, HUS developed in 4 of 37 patients (ages 1 to 78 years) and TTP developed in 4 others.[65] In HUS outbreaks, 75% of patients show greater than fourfold increases in verotoxin-neutralizing antibodies.[36, 62] Less commonly, HUS/TTP is associated with gastrointestinal and respiratory infections caused by other cytotoxin-producing bacteria, such as *Shigella dysenteriae* type 1,[66] *Salmonella typhi*,[67] *Campylobacter jejuni*,[68] *Streptococcus pneumoniae*,[69] and *Yersinia pseudotuberculosis*[70] (Table 35–1). HUS/TTP accompanying viral infections has also been described.[71–74] The TTP syndrome has been associated with the acquired immunodeficiency syndrome.[75, 76]

Drug-induced HUS/TTP is well recognized.[15] It is most commonly diagnosed in patients receiving chemotherapeutic agents,[77, 78] the majority of whom were treated with mitomycin C.[79] HUS occurs in 5% to 15% of patients who have received a cumulative dose of 20 to 30 mg/m$^2$ or more. The onset of hemolytic anemia and renal failure is usually sudden, and mortality is high despite supportive therapy.[79] Treatment with plasma exchange, however, may be successful in some cases.[80] HUS/TTP has also been reported after chemotherapy with other agents (see Table 35–1). Thrombotic microangiopathy, unrelated to chemotherapy, has been described in conjunction with vascular tumors; acute promyelocytic leukemia; and prostatic, gastric, and pancreatic carcinomas.[81] Sporadic cases of HUS/TTP have been reported in bone marrow and solid organ transplant patients receiving immunosuppressive treatment with either cyclosporine[82–86] or FK 506.[87, 88] In renal allograft recipients, cyclosporine-induced HUS occurs in the first week after transplantation, and renal failure

**TABLE 35–1. Hemolytic-Uremic Syndrome and Thrombotic Thrombocytopenic Purpura: Causes and Associations**

**Infectious Agents**
*Bacteria*
*Escherichia coli* O157:H7 (verotoxin producing)[24, 36, 57, 61–64]
*Shigella dysenteriae* type 1[57, 66]
*Salmonella typhi* [67]
*Campylobacter jejuni* [68]
*Streptococcus pneumoniae* [69]
*Yersinia pseudotuberculosis*[70]
*Pseudomonas* species[111]
*Bacteroides*[111]

*Viruses*
Togavirus (rubella)[73]
Coxsackievirus[111]
Echoviruses[71, 72]
Influenza virus[111]
Epstein-Barr virus[74]
Rotaviruses[111]
Human immunodeficiency virus[75, 76]

**Drugs**
*Immunosuppressants*
Cyclosporine[82–86]
FK 506[87, 88]

*Chemotherapeutics*
Mitomycin C[79]
Cisplatin[78]
Daunorubicin[77]
Cytosine arabinoside[77]
Methyl CCNU[77]
Chlorozotocin[77]
Neocarcinostatin[77]

*Others*
Oral contraceptives[92]
Quinine[93]
Penicillin[94]
Penicillamine[95]
Metronidazole[96]

**Toxins**
Carbon monoxide[97]
Bee sting[98]
Arsenic[99]
Iodine[100]

**Pregnancy**[101–105]
Pre partum
Post partum

**Disorders**
Malignant neoplasm[123]
Transplantation[185, 186]
Systemic lupus erythematosus[111]
Polyarteritis nodosa[111]
Primary glomerulopathies[111]

reverses with the cessation of cyclosporine.[89, 90] HUS/TTP may occur after bone marrow transplantation independent of previous radiation or cyclosporine therapy.[91] Other drugs[92–96] and toxins[97–100] less commonly associated with HUS/TTP are listed in Table 35–1.

Association between HUS/TTP and pregnancy is also well recognized.[101] Neurologic involvement predominates in the prepartum form, whereas severe renal failure is more typical in postpartum HUS/TTP.[102] Fetal mortality from pregnancy-associated TTP approaches 80%, but successful plasma exchange treatment permitting near-term delivery has been reported.[103, 104] Like preeclampsia, pregnancy-associated TTP usually resolves with delivery.[101] It is possible that these two syndromes are a continuum of the microvascular abnormalities that occur during gestation. They differ, however, in that consumptive coagulopathy is present in severe preeclampsia but is characteristically absent in HUS/TTP.[105, 106] The etiologic agents in pregnancy-associated HUS/TTP are not established. The absence of thrombocytopenia or other manifestations of HUS/TTP in surviving infants excludes the possibility of an etiologic agent that crosses the placenta.[101] Several case reports have suggested a genetic predisposition for pregnancy-associated HUS/TTP.[107–109] A hereditary form of recurrent HUS/TTP has also been described in children and adults.[19, 110] Other diseases associated with HUS/TTP, such as primary glomerular and autoimmune disorders, are listed in Table 35–1.

Although the etiologic mechanisms in HUS/TTP are not well defined, the available data suggest that environmental factors (infection, drugs, toxins) combined with genetic predisposition in some patients are responsible for initiation of thrombotic microangiopathy. To date, the link between bacterial toxins and HUS offers the strongest etiologic evidence.[57]

## Pathogenesis

Experimental data strongly suggest that endothelial cell injury is the primary event in the pathogenesis of HUS/TTP.[1, 4, 111] Endothelial damage triggers a cascade of events that includes local intravascular coagulation, fibrin deposition, and platelet activation and aggregation. The end result is the histopathologic finding of thrombotic microangiopathy common to the different forms of the HUS/TTP syndrome. The following describes the different mediators and events involved in the pathogenesis of HUS/TTP.

**Endothelial Injury.** Many of the infectious agents and drugs implicated in the etiology of HUS/TTP are toxic to the vascular endothelium. The Shiga-like toxins, which include the verotoxins produced by *E. coli* O157:H7, inhibit eukaryotic protein synthesis and directly damage human vascular endothelial cells.[112, 113] The glycolipid receptor for verotoxins is present on the membranes of endothelial cells[112] and has been shown to be more prevalent in the renal cortex than in the medulla.[114] Although measurement of circulating Shiga-like toxins in humans after intestinal infection has not been reported, it is plausible that small amounts may enter the bloodstream.[111] The extreme potency of these toxins in inhibiting protein synthesis (IC$_{50}$ in the picomolar range)[112] supports the concept that even minute amounts of toxin entering the circulation could initiate endothelial cell injury in HUS/TTP. Injection of purified verotoxin-1 (Shiga-like toxin-1) in rabbits showed specific binding of the toxin to endothelial cells as well as histopathologic findings of thrombotic microangiopathy.[115]

Bacterial and viral neuraminidases have indirect toxic effects on endothelial cells.[4, 111] *S. pneumoniae*–derived neuraminidase removes sialic acid from the membranes of erythrocytes, platelets, and glomerular capillary endothelial cells, thus exposing a cryptic antigen known as Thomsen-Friedenreich antigen. It is postulated that exposure of this antigen leads to formation of immunoglobulin M antibodies, which in turn could cause platelet aggregation and possibly endothelial damage.[116–118] Complement-fixing antibodies to endothelial antigens have been detected in the plasma of HUS/TTP patients but not in normal subjects, which further suggests a role for immunologic mechanisms in endothelial injury.[119, 120] Antiendothelial antibodies are also present in patients with various autoimmune diseases, which could explain the occurrence of HUS/TTP in patients with systemic lupus erythematosus and polyarteritis nodosa.[120]

Drugs associated with HUS/TTP have also been demonstrated to cause endothelial damage. These include mitomycin[121] and cyclosporine.[122] Cancer- or chemotherapy-induced endothelial lesions in the kidney could result from generation of small soluble circulating immune complexes and autoantibodies that damage endothelial cells directly and trigger aggregation and deposition of platelets around the lesions.[123]

**Local Thrombosis and Fibrin Deposition.** Microthrombi and fibrin deposits are characteristically found in the glomerular capillaries of patients with HUS/TTP.[15, 50] Fibrinolytic mechanisms in the glomerulus mediated by tissue-type plasminogen activator and urokinase may play a role in the removal of such deposits.[124] Bergstein and coworkers[125] have demonstrated the presence of an inhibitor of glomerular fibrinolysis (plasminogen activator inhibitor-1) in plasma from 17 children with HUS. These investigators demonstrated that increased circulating levels of plasminogen activator inhibitor-1 correlate with poor outcome in HUS.[126] Moreover, removal of plasminogen activator inhibitor-1 by peritoneal dialysis correlated with improvement in renal function.[126] Increased plasma levels of tissue-type plasminogen activator inhibitors have also been measured in patients with TTP.[127] The sources of inhibitors of fibrinolysis are the platelets and the endothelial cells.[128] Primary endothelial injury could also cause decreased production of physiologic anticoagulants, such as thrombomodulin, and lead to thrombosis at the site of injury.[129]

**von Willebrand Factor, Prostacyclin, and Platelet Aggregation.** Platelet aggregates are a major constituent of microthrombi found in HUS/TTP.[15] Controversy exists as to whether platelet aggregation is a consequence of endothelial damage or a primary platelet abnormality.[130] Because higher molecular weight polymers of vWF support platelet adhesion to the subendothelium and promote platelet aggregation, vWF is suspected of playing a pathogenetic role in HUS/TTP.[131, 132] Patients with relapsing TTP have large circulating polymers of vWF during remissions but not during relapses.[133] It is postulated, therefore, that inefficient clearance of the vWF polymers secreted by the endothelial cells leads to microvascular thrombosis. The polymers are consumed during TTP relapse, and their levels thus decrease. In HUS patients, vWF antigens are elevated and the largest polymers are decreased during acute illness.[134] This pattern returns to normal with clinical improvement but persists in patients with progressive renal disease.[135] A platelet-aggregating factor (p37) has been detected in the plasma of HUS[136] and TTP[137] patients, but its pathogenetic role is not clear. Circulating antibodies to the Thomsen-Friedenreich antigen[116-118] or cancer- and chemotherapy-related immune complexes[123] could also enhance platelet aggregation in HUS/TTP.

The discovery that endothelial cells produce a potent inhibitor of platelet aggregation, prostacyclin (prostaglandin $I_2$ [$PGI_2$]), led to the investigation of its role in HUS/TTP.[1, 4] Several investigators have demonstrated decreased endothelial production of $PGI_2$ in HUS and TTP patients.[138, 139] The presence of a circulating inhibitor of endothelial cell production of $PGI_2$ has been reported in patients with HUS.[140] Interestingly, patients with preeclampsia do not have the increase in $PGI_2$ observed in normal pregnancies, which suggests that this could contribute to the thrombocytopenia and microangiopathic hemolytic anemia of severe preeclampsia.[141, 142] It is not clear, however, whether reduced $PGI_2$ production is a primary pathogenetic event in HUS/TTP or an epiphenomenon of microangiopathic hemolysis. Moreover, clinical trials of $PGI_2$ infusion in HUS/TTP patients gave equivocal results[143] (see later).

**Cytokines.** Because interleukin (IL)-1 and tumor necrosis factor (TNF) mediate endothelial injury in septic shock,[144] their role in HUS/TTP has been examined. Kaplan and associates[111] demonstrated that IL-1 and TNF synergize with the cytotoxic action of Shiga-like toxin-1 on umbilical vein endothelial cells. Furthermore, IL-1, TNF, and lipopolysaccharide up-regulate the receptors for verotoxin on the surface of endothelial cells by approximately 100-fold.[145] Elevated plasma levels of IL-1β and TNF were demonstrated in 13 patients with acute TTP and were found to decrease as the patients went into remission.[146] Increased levels of soluble IL-2 receptor and of IL-6 correlated with poorer prognosis in these patients. The data suggest that monocyte-derived cytokines (IL-1, IL-6, and TNF) may contribute to the pathogenesis of HUS/TTP. Fitzpatrick and co-workers[147] demonstrated increased levels of IL-8, a chemokine that attracts and activates neutrophils, in children with HUS. IL-8 was not detected in the 17 normal children but was significantly elevated in 20 of 25 diarrhea-associated HUS cases and in 3 of 9 children with non-diarrhea-associated HUS. IL-8 levels correlated with polymorphonuclear cell counts and with circulating α₁-antitrypsin–complexed elastase, a marker of neutrophil degranulation. The highest values of IL-8 were seen in children who died in the acute phase of the disease. Antineutrophil cytoplasmic antibody was not detected in any of the patients, and TNF-α was increased in only one patient. Direct evidence for the role of these cytokines in the pathogenesis of HUS/TTP remains to be determined.

## Prognosis and Treatment

If HUS/TTP is left untreated, mortality approaches 90%.[9] A study of the outcome of 678 patients with HUS by Gianantonio and co-workers[20] showed a trend toward better survival between the late 1950s and 1972. Mortality in children dropped from approximately 47% to 6.25%. A later analysis of 108 HUS/TTP patients (ages 16 to 77 years) treated between 1979 and 1990 revealed a 9% mortality rate.[148] Survival has significantly increased because of

improved management of HUS/TTP complications and because of treatment modalities used (see later).

Several prognostic factors have been postulated to predict the outcome in patients with HUS/TTP. Younger children presenting in the summer with the "typical" diarrheal prodrome have a better prognosis than do older children, in whom HUS occurs in the colder months of the year and is not heralded by diarrhea.[149] A high blood polymorphonuclear count at time of onset of disease in children is associated with higher probability of poor outcome.[150, 151] A retrospective 10-year follow-up of 73 children with HUS demonstrated that severe renal involvement, determined by duration of oliguria or anuria, is associated with a higher frequency of long-term complications, such as hypertension, reduced renal function, and proteinuria.[152] Adults presenting with HUS tend to have poorer prognosis than that of children. In a study of 43 adults with HUS, the overall mortality was 14%, and approximately 70% required hemodialysis.[153] The same study suggested that HUS secondary to an underlying disease, such as scleroderma or cancer, carries a poorer prognosis. The degree of renal dysfunction and severity of vascular lesions in renal biopsy specimens are also indicators of poor outcome in HUS/TTP.[16, 154]

Supportive therapy including dialysis, antihypertensive medications, blood transfusions, and management of neurologic complications contributes to the improved survival of HUS/TTP patients.[4, 148] Platelet transfusions are avoided because of the risk of precipitous worsening of clinical status.[13, 148, 155, 156] It is postulated that transfused platelets in combination with high circulating levels of vWF multimers induce further organ damage.[148]

Among the different therapeutic modalities used to treat patients with HUS/TTP, plasma exchange (plasmapheresis combined with fresh frozen plasma replacement) is currently the treatment of choice. Significant benefit from plasma exchange was observed in 1977 in adults with acute TTP.[157] Several reports have since confirmed the efficacy of this treatment modality in both children[158, 159] and adults[160-162] with HUS/TTP. Response rates vary between 60% and 80%.[162] Although significant benefit has also been observed with plasma infusion alone,[163-165] one randomized prospective trial has demonstrated that plasma exchange is more effective than is plasma infusion for the treatment of TTP.[162] After a 6-month follow-up period, patients treated with plasma exchange had a 78% response rate and 22% mortality compared with 49% response rate and 37% mortality among patients receiving plasma infusions only. No unanimous protocol has been established regarding the frequency and duration of plasma exchange. It is generally agreed that plasma exchange should be performed daily until remission is achieved, remission being normalization of platelet count or resolution of neurologic symptoms.[165] Hemoglobin level, percentage of schistocytosis, reticulocyte count, and renal indices do not appear to be determinants of initial response to therapy because they may be abnormal for an undefined period after remission.[161] Continuation of plasma exchange for several sessions after remission has been advocated to prevent relapses.[148, 161] TTP relapses occur between 1 and 140 months (median, 20 months) after the initial episode in up to 40% of the patients.[166] Because 85% of children with HUS recover after supportive therapy alone, plasma exchange is generally reserved for patients with poor prognostic indicators.[2, 167]

When administered alone, corticosteroids induce remission in less than 30% of patients with TTP.[148] Inconclusive data suggest that corticosteroids used in combination with plasma therapy decrease relapse rates and may improve survival in some patients.[13, 148] Other immunosuppressive agents have been used to treat TTP either alone or in combination with plasma therapy. These include vincristine,[168, 169] azathioprine,[170] and cyclophosphamide.[171] The rationale for their use is the demonstration of vWF autoantibodies in a subset of TTP patients.[170] Their effectiveness has not been proved.

Although platelet thrombi are invariably present in the thrombotic angiopathies, therapy with aspirin and dipyridamole has proved ineffective.[148, 172] Antiplatelet agents, however, may induce a more rapid recovery of the platelet count.[4, 173] Some investigators recommend their use in combination with plasma exchange on the basis of inconclusive evidence that relapse rate is lower in patients receiving antiplatelet agents.[162, 166, 173] Increased frequency of bleeding complications should be kept in mind, however.[162] Fibrinolytic therapy with either streptokinase or urokinase is ineffective and increases the risk of bleeding.[174, 175] Prospective studies of heparin treatment in HUS/TTP patients also failed to demonstrate any benefit.[176] Intravenous administration of immunoglobulins as a means of neutralizing platelet aggregation factors has been tried in TTP patients.[177–179] Controlled studies, however, are required to establish whether benefits from this treatment outweigh its disadvantages (anaphylaxis and infections).[180] Splenectomy performed on TTP patients to reduce platelet consumption can be associated with fatal complications.[148] In the absence of solid evidence that splenectomy is beneficial, its use is not recommended for the treatment of HUS/TTP.[39, 148] Experimental evidence indicating reduced bioavailability of PGI$_2$ in thrombotic microangiopathies suggested the use of PGI$_2$ infusions. Data on outcome for patients are contradictory, however.[4] Reports of dramatic remission in intractable TTP are available,[181, 182] but PGI$_2$ infusions have proved ineffective in other patients.[183] Moreover, the hypotensive effects of PGI$_2$ limit its usefulness.[4] On the basis of findings of decreased serum levels of vitamin E and reduced antioxidant potential of erythrocytes, oral vitamin E supplements have been administered to children with HUS. In a series of 16 patients treated with vitamin E, 100% survival and complete recovery of renal function were attained despite the presence of poor prognostic features.[184] A controlled trial is needed to confirm this observation, however.

Cancer- or chemotherapy-induced HUS/TTP carries a poor prognosis despite treatment. Snyder and co-workers[123] demonstrated improved survival in this group of patients using extracorporeal immunoadsorption with protein A columns to remove circulating immune complexes. Patients whose malignant neoplasms were in complete or partial remission at the time of development of HUS/TTP had a significantly higher estimated 1-year survival rate (74%) compared with a historical control group of patients receiving other treatments (22%).

In summary, plasma exchange is currently the treatment of choice for patients with thrombotic microangiopathies. High relapse rates present a therapeutic challenge in TTP patients. Whether concomitant use of corticosteroids or antiplatelet agents reduces the risk of relapse remains to be determined. Immunoadsorption with use of protein A columns may be of benefit in cancer-associated HUS/TTP.

**Treatment of Renal Failure in HUS/TTP.** Severe renal insufficiency resulting from HUS/TTP often requires dialysis. Kidney transplantation has also been performed. Regardless of the etiologic agent, HUS/TTP may recur in the renal allograft independent of cyclosporine use.[185, 186] The risk of recurrence, however, does not preclude transplantation. Similarly, the risk of cyclosporine-induced HUS is not a deterrent to use of this essential immunosuppressive agent because the syndrome is usually reversible after cyclosporine is discontinued.[4]

# SYSTEMIC SCLEROSIS

Systemic sclerosis is a generalized connective tissue disorder. It is characterized by fibrosis, degenerative changes, and vascular lesions affecting the skin, joints, skeletal muscles, and multiple internal organs.[187, 188] Involvement of the kidneys, the "most dangerous" complication of systemic sclerosis, commonly presents as a renal crisis characterized by malignant hypertension and rapidly progressive renal failure.[189] This discussion focuses on the renal complications of systemic sclerosis after a brief clinical overview of the disease.

## Clinical Features

Systemic sclerosis is a rare disease with an incidence of approximately 20 new cases per million population per year in the United States.[190] It characteristically affects women between the ages of 30 and 50 years.[191] The overall frequency in women is three times that in men, and the female/male ratio increases to 15:1 during the childbearing years.[6] Children and younger men are rarely affected.[192] Although there is no overall racial predilection, young black women have a 10-fold higher frequency of systemic sclerosis than that of young white women.[192]

The etiology of systemic sclerosis is unknown. Epidemiologic studies, however, have demonstrated association with several environmental factors.[193] An epidemic of chemically induced systemic sclerosis–like syndrome occurred in Spain in 1981 among people who ingested aniline-denatured rapeseed oil.[194] Silicone breast implants,[195, 196] drugs (bleomycin),[197] and silica exposure from gold and coal mining[198] are associated with systemic sclerosis–like illnesses. L-Tryptophan ingestion leads to cutaneous scleroderma changes that usually accompany the other manifestations of the eosinophilia-myalgia syndrome.[199–201] Systemic sclerosis has also been described in association with chronic graft-versus-host disease.[202] A genetic predisposition in systemic sclerosis is only weakly discernible. Association with human leukocyte antigens DR3 and DR5[203, 204] and an increased prevalence of antinuclear antibodies[17] in asymptomatic family members have been reported.

Involvement of the skin and subcutaneous tissue is the predominant feature of systemic sclerosis.[187] This explains the use of the traditional term scleroderma to describe the disease.[190] Systemic sclerosis is classified clinically on the basis of the extent of cutaneous involvement and the presence of features that overlap with other connective tissue diseases.[187–189] In the diffuse cutaneous or classic form of the disease, thickening of the skin is observed on the face, trunk, and distal and proximal extremities. Hardening of the skin usually starts in the hands and manifests initially as swelling and decreased range of motion of the fingers.[190] This phase is followed by sclerosis that leads to a taut, shiny appearance of the skin and tapering of the fingertips (sclerodactyly). The skin changes later involve the face (pinched nose and pursed lips), trunk, and lower extremities. Rapid progression of the cutaneous induration with extension into the underlying tendon sheaths and joints is a harbinger of visceral involvement.[205] The limited cutaneous form, on the other hand, is more indolent. The cutaneous thickening is usually confined to the face and fingers, and progression to visceral involvement is delayed. This variant of the disease is also referred to as the CREST syndrome, an acronym identifying the following features: calcinosis, Raynaud phenomenon, esophageal hypomotility, sclerodactyly, and telangiectasias. Renal and cardiac involvement is rare.[206] Localized scleroderma exclusively involving the skin includes two dermatologic conditions known as morphea (plaque-like) and linear scleroderma.[187–189] They generally carry a good prognosis, and visceral involvement is extremely rare.[207] Overlap syndrome or mixed connective tissue disease occurs in patients who have diffuse or limited cutaneous sclerosis combined with features of other autoimmune disorders. These include systemic lupus erythematosus, dermatomyositis/polymyositis, Sjögren syndrome, and primary biliary cirrhosis.[208] Some investigators have suggested use of the term undifferentiated autoimmune connective tissue disorder because many of these patients later "differentiate" into either systemic sclerosis or systemic lupus erythematosus.[208, 209]

Among the extrarenal manifestations of systemic sclerosis,[187–189] Raynaud phenomenon is the most prevalent (93% to 97% of the patients) and is usually the first symptom in patients with limited cutaneous disease. It results from increased vasomotor tone and could lead to infarctions of the fingertips. A bedside test, nail fold capillaroscopy, has been suggested for differentiation of systemic sclerosis–associated Raynaud phenomenon from benign Raynaud phenomenon and that associated with autoimmune disorders.[210] Patients with systemic sclerosis have significant capillary dropout in the nail beds. Telangiectasias on the skin of the face and upper torso are commonly present in patients with either diffuse or limited cutaneous sclerosis. Arthralgias or arthritis occurs in the majority of the patients. Tendon involvement and joint contractures are significantly more common in the diffuse cutaneous form of the disease (90% of cases).[187] Myopathy presenting as muscle atrophy and fibrosis occurs in approximately 20% of these patients and usually involves the shoulder and pelvic girdle muscles.[211] Esophageal hypomotility and diminished tone of the lower

esophageal sphincter are present in 75% of systemic sclerosis cases.[187] The symptoms include dysphagia and gastroesophageal reflux. Ulcerations and strictures of the distal esophagus have been described.[187] Gastrointestinal involvement can extend to the small and large bowels, resulting in hypomotility, dilatation, malabsorption from bacterial overgrowth, and occasionally volvulus or perforation. Diffuse pulmonary fibrosis occurs in 45% of the patients, causing restrictive lung disease. Intimal proliferation in the small pulmonary arteries can lead to pulmonary hypertension, particularly in the CREST syndrome.[212] Myocardial fibrosis in systemic sclerosis manifests as conduction disturbances and occasionally refractory congestive heart failure.[213, 214] Pericarditis and pericardial effusions have been described.[215] An infrequent finding in systemic sclerosis is fibrosis of the thyroid gland leading to clinical hypothyroidism.[216]

## Laboratory Findings

The most common serologic abnormality in systemic sclerosis is a positive antinuclear antibody response ($\geq$1:16), which occurs in 70% of the patients.[187, 188] The specificity of the antinuclear antibody test is increased if the immunofluorescence pattern is speckled or nucleolar. Although more specific, antibodies to DNA topoisomerase I (anti–Scl-70)[217] are found in only 30% of the patients with diffuse cutaneous involvement and 15% of those with the limited form. Anticentromere antibodies[217] are present in half of the patients, most of whom have limited systemic sclerosis. Anticentromere antibodies are particularly specific for the CREST syndrome.[217, 218] Approximately 30% of the patients have positive test results for rheumatoid factor.[1] Antibodies to double-stranded DNA are rarely noted.[187] Mild lymphopenia and anemia are often present in patients with visceral involvement.

Pulmonary function tests reveal a mixture of restrictive and obstructive changes.[187] The chest radiograph shows a reticular pattern most prominent in the lower two thirds of the lung fields that can progress to diffuse honeycombing.[187] Hand radiographs may show soft tissue calcifications and occasionally resorption of the terminal phalanges.[189] Pseudodiverticula due to atrophy of the colonic muscularis mucosae can be detected on barium enema examination.[187]

## Renal Involvement

The association between systemic sclerosis and renal failure was first reported by Auspitz[219] in 1863 and later noted by Osler.[220] A causal relationship between the two was generally accepted after several studies detailed the clinical and renal histologic abnormalities in patients with systemic sclerosis who died of uremia.[221, 222]

Involvement of the kidney in systemic sclerosis manifests as a slowly progressing chronic renal disease or as scleroderma renal crisis (SRC) characterized by malignant hypertension and acute azotemia.[189] The two presentations are not mutually exclusive. On the basis of autopsy studies, the frequency of renal disease in systemic sclerosis approaches 80%.[223] Clinical indicators of chronic renal involvement in systemic sclerosis include proteinuria, hypertension, and decreased glomerular filtration rate. The proteinuria is usually subnephrotic and occurs in 15% to 36% of the patients.[191, 224] Hypertension is present in 24% and elevated blood urea nitrogen in 19%.[224] Estimates of the frequency of chronic renal disease in systemic sclerosis vary, depending on which markers of disease are employed.[189] Renal manifestations rarely antedate the other features of systemic sclerosis.

SRC is defined by sudden onset of accelerated or malignant arterial hypertension followed by rapidly progressive oliguric renal failure.[189, 225] The reported frequency of SRC varies between 5% and 15%.[206, 226, 227] It occurs most commonly during the first 5 years after diagnosis, but in 5% to 10% of cases, there is no previous history of systemic sclerosis.[205] Patients with the diffuse cutaneous form are at much higher risk for development of SRC than are those with limited cutaneous systemic sclerosis. The symptoms are predominantly those of accelerated or malignant hypertension.[189, 225] Presenting complaints include severe headaches, blurring of vision, encephalopathy, convulsions, and acute left ventricular failure. Grade III or grade IV retinopathy is present in the majority of the cases. Oliguria and rapidly rising serum creatinine level follow shortly after.[189, 225] Proteinuria is universal but is rarely nephrotic. The urinalysis reveals microscopic hematuria and granular casts. Plasma renin activity is markedly elevated during SRC, but it is unclear whether this is a primary phenomenon or a result of renal ischemia.[224, 225] SRC progresses rapidly to severe renal failure requiring dialysis. Before the advent of angiotensin-converting enzyme (ACE) inhibitors, the majority of patients died of hypertensive complications within 1 to 3 months.[224-226] Other clinical manifestations of SRC include microangiopathic hemolytic anemia with thrombocytopenia,[228] which also occurs in association with other forms of malignant hypertension.[229] HUS has been reported in a patient with mixed connective tissue disease who had combined features of systemic sclerosis and systemic lupus erythematosus.[230]

No reliable predictors of the advent of SRC exist. The previous presence of proteinuria, renal insufficiency, or hypertension in a patient with diffuse systemic sclerosis does not necessarily portend progression to SRC.[205] A rise in plasma renin activity does not seem to herald the onset of SRC either.[205, 225] A higher frequency of SRC and hypertension has been noted among African-Americans with systemic sclerosis.[225] It is not clear, however, whether this observation is simply a reflection of the overall increased frequency of essential and malignant hypertension in the African-American population.

In summary, SRC is a form of malignant arteriolar nephrosclerosis associated with more dramatic worsening of renal function and poorer prognosis than in other forms of malignant hypertension.

**Pathology.** Autopsy studies demonstrate renal histopathologic changes in the majority of systemic sclerosis patients in whom SRC has not developed.[231] Subintimal proliferation with luminal narrowing of small and medium-sized arteries in the kidney is the most prominent finding.

The arterial changes coexist with varying degrees of tubule atrophy, interstitial fibrosis, and glomerular obsolescence. These histopathologic findings have been described in patients with systemic sclerosis even before the onset of hypertension.[224]

Arterial changes also characterize the SRC kidney.[223, 224] On microscopic examination, small and medium-sized arteries (interlobular and arcuate arteries in the renal cortex) show intimal edema and intimal cell proliferation. Accumulation of mucoid substance, composed of glycoproteins and mucopolysaccharides, may separate the endothelium from the internal elastic lamina. Myointimal cells, absent from normal arteries, possibly participate in the intimal thickening seen in systemic sclerosis. The common end point of these vascular changes is luminal narrowing and subsequent tissue ischemia (Fig. 35–1). The presence of adventitial and periadventitial fibrosis differentiates the renovascular lesions of systemic sclerosis from those of other forms of malignant hypertension.[223, 232] The typical lesion in smaller renal arteries and afferent arterioles in systemic sclerosis is fibrinoid necrosis.[233] Interestingly, these changes can be seen in patients who do not have hypertension or SRC.[223, 232] Lymphocytes and inflammatory cells are typically absent from the vascular lesions.

Glomerular disease in SRC is probably ischemic in origin and consists of basement membrane thickening, obliteration of the capillary loops, and glomerulosclerosis.[231, 233] Hyperplasia of the juxtaglomerular apparatus has been observed but is not specific for SRC.[234] Tubule epithelial degeneration and scattered interstitial fibrosis are also present. Immunofluorescence findings are generally nonspecific and may reveal immunoglobulin M, complement, and fibrin deposits in small renal arteries.[235] In a few cases, antinuclear antibodies have been eluted from renal biopsy tissue.[235, 236]

## Pathogenesis

A reductionist approach to the pathogenesis of systemic sclerosis is to regard the disease as primarily an abnormality of small and medium-sized arteries. A combination of vasospasm, subintimal cellular proliferation, and increased production of collagen in and around the vessel wall leads to luminal narrowing and subsequent tissue ischemia and sclerosis. This hypothesis, however, does not rule out the possibility that autoimmune-mediated events could contribute to the cutaneous and visceral fibrosis that characterizes systemic sclerosis.

**Vasospasm.** Abnormal vasomotor control is a dominant feature of systemic sclerosis as evidenced by the presence of Raynaud phenomenon in the vast majority of patients.[191] In addition to vasospasm of the digital arteries, a cold stimulus has been shown to decrease renal,[224, 232] coronary,[237, 238] and pulmonary perfusion.[239] The cause of abnormal vasomotor control is not known. Increased circulating levels of catecholamines do not seem to be a significant mediator of Raynaud phenomenon.[240] Renin and angiotensin II levels in systemic sclerosis increase after cold exposure and could possibly contribute to arterial vasospasm.[232] In addition to the juxtaglomerular apparatus, vascular smooth muscle cells produce renin.[241] In a vessel "primed"

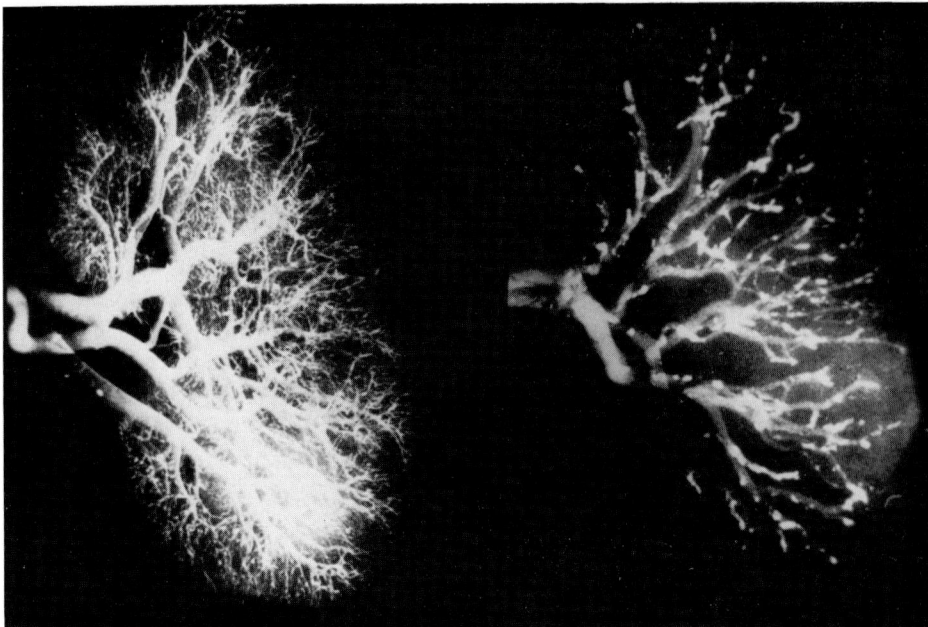

**Figure 35–1.** Latex injection of post-mortem normal kidney *(left)* and kidney from a patient with scleroderma renal crisis *(right)*. Note obstruction to flow at the level of the medium-sized interlobular arteries.

by renin-angiotensin, severe vasospasm can be precipitated by cold exposure, physical stress, caffeine, or nicotine.[189] More recently, the role of endothelin has been examined.[242] Knock and colleagues[242] demonstrated significantly increased endothelin-binding density in microvessels of skin from patients with systemic sclerosis and primary Raynaud phenomenon compared with that of normal control subjects. The potent vasoconstrictive effects of endothelin suggest that it may play a role in the arterial vasospasm observed in systemic sclerosis.

**Increased Collagen Production.** Fibroblast secretion of collagen, the main extracellular matrix component of connective tissue, is markedly increased in systemic sclerosis.[243] Several investigators have provided evidence that transforming growth factor-β could mediate increased collagen production in systemic sclerosis.[244–246] Gabrielli and co-workers[245] demonstrated increased immunostaining for transforming growth factor-β in the vascular endothelium and dermal fibroblasts of systemic sclerosis patients. Impaired production of interferon-γ by T lymphocytes isolated from patients with systemic sclerosis and fibrosing alveolitis has been observed.[247] This defect can contribute to fibrosis because interferon-γ is known to suppress collagen synthesis by fibroblasts.[248] Other investigators have provided evidence for production of abnormal collagen in patients with systemic sclerosis.[249, 250] Douvas[250] demonstrated that Scl-70 (DNA topoisomerase I) binds to collagen genes from scleroderma tissue but not to genes from normal tissue. The pathogenetic significance of this observation is unclear.

**Endothelial Cell Abnormalities.** Damage to the endothelial cell has been postulated as a primary event in the pathogenesis of systemic sclerosis.[65] Cytotoxicity of the patient's serum to cultured endothelial cells has been demonstrated.[251, 252] It is possible that platelet aggregation at the site of endothelial denudement could lead to the release of platelet-derived growth factor and transforming growth factor-β. Both cytokines are mitogenic to smooth muscle

cells and fibroblasts in addition to stimulating collagen production. Theoretically, this would account for the subintimal cell proliferation and the fibrosis seen in systemic sclerosis. Increased platelet-derived growth factor levels and circulating platelet aggregates have been demonstrated in patients with systemic sclerosis.[253, 254] Antiplatelet therapy, however, failed to provide any clinical benefit.[189]

**Immunologic Mediators.** Although several antinuclear autoantibodies have been detected in patients with systemic sclerosis, their contribution to the disease process is not established. Indirect evidence of immunologic mechanisms in systemic sclerosis has come to light.[255] Increased γδ T lymphocytes, activated helper T cells, intercellular adhesion molecules, and soluble IL-2 receptor have been demonstrated in patients.[255–259] Fibroblasts cultured from the skin of patients with systemic sclerosis produce much higher levels of IL-6 than do normal fibroblasts and may contribute to T cell activation.[260] It is unclear whether these immunologic changes constitute primary events in systemic sclerosis or are epiphenomena.

**Pathogenesis of Scleroderma Renal Crisis.** The different mechanisms discussed could contribute to the underlying renal vascular disease of systemic sclerosis. It is postulated that SRC is caused by a Raynaud-like phenomenon in the kidney.[225] Severe vasospasm leads to cortical ischemia and enhanced renin and angiotensin II production, which in turn perpetuate renal vasoconstriction. Hormonal changes (pregnancy),[261] physical and emotional stress, or cold temperature[224] may trigger the Raynaud-like arterial vasospasm. The role of the renin-angiotensin system in perpetuating renal ischemia is underscored by the significant benefit of ACE inhibitors in the treatment of SRC (see later).

## Management of Renal Complications

The one form of therapy that appears to have made a major difference in the prognosis of SRC is aggressive treatment of hypertension with ACE inhibitors.[225, 227, 262] In one study, 1-year survival was only 18% for patients treated before the availability of an ACE inhibitor, compared with 76% for those treated with the drug.[227] Progression to severe renal failure requiring dialysis was observed in only half of the patients treated with ACE inhibitors. This suggests that ACE inhibition can forestall progression of SRC in some but not all of the patients.[263] The management of SRC with ACE inhibitors does not exclude the concomitant use of other antihypertensive agents. Diuretics are best avoided, however, because of their ability to stimulate more renin release.[189]

In those patients with SRC who progress to severe renal insufficiency despite antihypertensive treatment, dialysis becomes a necessity. Both peritoneal dialysis and hemodialysis have been employed.[264, 265] The End-Stage Renal Disease Network report on 311 patients with systemic sclerosis–induced end-stage renal disease who underwent dialysis between 1983 and 1985[264] revealed a 33% survival rate at 3 years. On the bright side, recovery of renal function sufficient to render the patient dialysis independent occurred in 6.8% of the cases in this series. Other reports have documented reversal of SRC-induced renal failure with ACE inhibitors even after dialysis had been initiated.[227, 266] Interestingly, Raynaud phenomenon of the hands and Raynaud-type vasospasm of peritoneal blood vessels (manifesting as decreased peritoneal clearance) were observed in systemic sclerosis patients using unheated peritoneal dialysate fluid.[265]

Kidney transplantation for systemic SRC-induced end-stage renal disease has been performed successfully,[264, 267, 268] and recurrence of systemic sclerosis in the transplanted kidney was documented in one case.[236]

The different agents used for treatment of the nonrenal complications of systemic sclerosis are reviewed elsewhere.[269, 270] Of note is that the use of D-penicillamine may help prevent renal involvement.[271] Because D-penicillamine contains sulfhydryl groups, it can potentiate the toxicity of a sulfhydryl-containing ACE inhibitor such as captopril.

## RADIATION NEPHRITIS

Renal injury from irradiation was first described in 1904 by Baerman and Linser.[272] Failure to recognize the sensitivity of the renal capillary endothelium to irradiation led to a significant number of radiation nephritis cases reported in the literature between 1940 and 1960.[273] A landmark clinical study published in 1961 by Luxton[274, 275] established the clinical features of this entity and defined the tolerance limit of the kidney to irradiation. This led to preventive shielding of the kidneys in patients receiving radiation therapy and to a marked decline in the frequency of radiation nephritis.[276] Total body irradiation preceding bone marrow transplantation, however, has resulted in increased awareness of radiation nephritis in the last several years.[277, 278] Understanding the pathogenesis of this disease may provide insight into the prevention and treatment of renal complications that follow the use of radiation necessary for the management of otherwise fatal malignant neoplasms.

## Clinical Features

The long-term consequences of renal irradiation in excess of 2500 rad can be divided into five clinical syndromes.[274, 275] Acute radiation nephritis occurs in approximately 40% of patients after a latency period of 6 to 13 months. It is characterized clinically by abrupt onset of hypertension, proteinuria, edema, and progressive renal failure. The proteinuria is generally mild but can occasionally result in nephrotic syndrome.[279] The urinalysis may also demonstrate microscopic hematuria.[274] In most cases, the progressive renal failure results in end-stage kidneys.[274] Acute radiation nephritis can be accompanied by intravascular hemolysis.[280] Chronic radiation nephritis, on the other hand, has a latency period that varies between 18 months and 14 years after the initial insult. It is insidious in onset and is characterized by hypertension, proteinuria, and gradual loss of renal function.[274] The third syndrome manifests as benign proteinuria with normal renal function 5 to 19 years after exposure to radiation.[274] A fourth group of patients exhibits only benign hypertension 2 to 5 years later and may have variable proteinuria.[274] Late malignant hypertension arises 18 months to 11 years after irradiation in patients with either chronic radiation nephritis or benign hypertension.[274] High-renin hypertension resulting from irradiation of one kidney has been described.[281] Removal of the affected kidney reverses the hypertension. Radiation-induced damage to the renal arteries with subsequent renovascular hypertension has been reported.[282]

A syndrome of renal insufficiency analogous to acute radiation nephritis has been observed in bone marrow transplant patients who had received total body irradiation.[277, 278, 283, 284] In a long-term study of 103 adult survivors of bone marrow transplantation, Lawton and co-workers[278] reported late renal dysfunction in 14 patients. The syndrome developed at a median of 9 months (range, 4.5 to 26 months) after transplantation and was characterized by progressive decline in glomerular filtration rate, hypertension, and anemia. Eight of the 14 patients had non-nephrotic range proteinuria and microscopic hematuria. Renal biopsies performed on seven of these patients revealed changes consistent with those of acute radiation nephritis (see later). All of the affected patients had received 1400 rad of total body irradiation before bone marrow transplantation, whereas none of the patients receiving lower doses of irradiation had late hypertension or decreased glomerular filtration rate. Chemotherapy administered as part of the preparative regimen could potentiate the effects of irradiation on the kidneys.[285, 286] Increased sensitivity of the kidney to radiation injury has been observed with the use of actinomycin D,[286] bleomycin-vinblastine,[287] and cyclophosphamide.[283] The frequency of radiation nephritis after total body irradiation and bone marrow transplantation in children is higher than that observed in adults and is associated with severe hemolytic anemia.[277] Clinically, the presentation may be indistinguishable from that of HUS.

Radiographic studies may help in the diagnosis of acute radiation nephritis. Computed tomography with contrast enhancement demonstrates sharply demarcated, dense, persistent nephrograms corresponding to the irradiated areas.[288, 289] Increased uptake of technetium Tc 99 in the damaged areas of the kidneys is also observed after renal irradiation.[290]

## Pathology

The pathologic hallmark of acute radiation nephritis is glomerular capillary endothelial injury.[276] Because inflammatory cells are not observed in the renal parenchyma, the term nephritis is actually a misnomer. Keane and colleagues[276] analyzed renal biopsy specimens obtained from two patients in whom renal insufficiency developed within a year after abdominal irradiation. On light microscopic examination, mild endothelial cell swelling and basement membrane splitting were consistently observed in the glomerular capillaries. Electron microscopic examination revealed marked subendothelial expansion with deposition of basement membrane–like material adjacent to the endothelial cells. The endothelial cell lining was absent in some capillary loops. Results of immunofluorescence studies were negative. Similar pathologic findings were also noted in a biopsy specimen taken 3 months after the patient received 4500 rad to the kidney.[279] Similar glomerular endothelial injury has been observed in the renal biopsy specimens of patients who had renal insufficiency and hypertension after total body irradiation and bone marrow transplantation.[277, 278] Some of these biopsy samples also revealed arteriolar intimal thickening and tubule atrophy.

## Pathogenesis

Sequential morphologic studies performed on rat kidneys after exposure to irradiation suggest that injury begins in the glomerular endothelium and the tubule epithelium.[291–293] Radiation could directly damage DNA, leading to decreased regeneration of these cells and denudement of the basement membrane in the glomerular capillaries and the tubules. How this initial insult eventually leads to glomerulosclerosis, tubule atrophy, and interstitial fibrosis is unclear. It is postulated that degeneration of the endothelial cell layer may result in intravascular thrombosis in capillaries and smaller arterioles.[280, 294] This intrarenal angiopathy would then explain the progressive renal fibrosis and the hypertension that characterize radiation nephritis.

## Treatment

Aggressive treatment of hypertension in patients with radiation nephritis may slow the progression of disease. Evidence in experimental animals suggests that ACE inhibitors may have a renoprotective effect on radiation nephritis independent of their antihypertensive action.[295] Hypertension due to unilateral disease may respond to nephrectomy.[281] Radiation-induced renovascular hypertension may require angioplasty or surgical repair.[282] Uncontrolled hypertension in patients with radiation nephritis who progress to end-stage renal disease warrants bilateral nephrectomy.[296] Because radiation nephritis is generally an irreversible process, preventive measures should be observed during the administration of radiation therapy. These include selective shielding of the kidneys and use of the minimal effective dose of fractionated radiation when possible.[297] The use of

radioprotectors such as glutathione or cysteine concomitant with irradiation is still in the experimental phase.[298]

## ATHEROEMBOLIC RENAL DISEASE

Atheroembolic disease typically results from multiple showers of cholesterol-containing microemboli that are dislodged from atheromatous plaques in large arteries[299, 300] and occlude small vessels (150 to 200 $\mu$m in diameter) in the kidney as well as in other organs (retina, brain, pancreas, muscles, and skin).[301] It usually occurs in an elderly individual who has evidence of atherosclerotic disease elsewhere and, in the majority of cases, follows aortic surgery or renal or coronary arteriography.[301, 302] Spontaneous atheroembolic disease has also been reported. Renal manifestations include deterioration of function (sudden or gradual),[303] mild proteinuria,[303] microscopic hematuria,[303] and leukocyturia.[302] Urine volume may remain normal or fall to oliguric levels, depending on severity. The resultant renal ischemia may induce or exacerbate pre-existing hypertension.

Antemortem diagnosis of atherosclerotic renal emboli is difficult.[302] The demonstration of cholesterol emboli in the retina is helpful, but a firm diagnosis is established only by demonstration of pathognomonic cholesterol crystals in the smaller arteries and arterioles in renal biopsy or autopsy specimens[301] (Fig. 35–2). These may also be seen in asymptomatic skeletal muscle or skin.[301] No specific treatment is available.

## SICKLE CELL NEPHROPATHY

Sickle cell anemia can lead to profound multisystem complications, one of which stems from a single amino acid substitution of valine for glutamic acid at the sixth position in the hemoglobin B chain. Transmitted autosomally, it can be expressed heterozygously and cause modest findings or homozygously and lead to profound consequences. Herrick's[304] 1910 description of clinical findings associated with sickle-shaped red blood cells in a black medical student stimulated inquiry, which led to the description and demonstration by Pauling and co-workers[305] of altered electrophoretic motility of hemoglobin in patients with this disorder. Sickle cell anemia is present in 1 in 400 African-Americans; the trait is present in more than 10% of the African-American population.[306] The most significant clinical manifestation of sickling is the pain crisis. The pathophysiologic mechanism of the sickling is still unclear. However, certain changes in red blood cell properties are present when sickling occurs. These include the increase of dense cells during the beginning of the pain crisis followed by a decrease during resolution; red blood cell distribution width and hemoglobin distribution width also increase during the initial phase of the pain crisis and decrease during the resolution phase.[307]

### Morphologic Changes

**Light Microscopy.** The most obvious morphologic change is the glomerular enlargement, especially of the

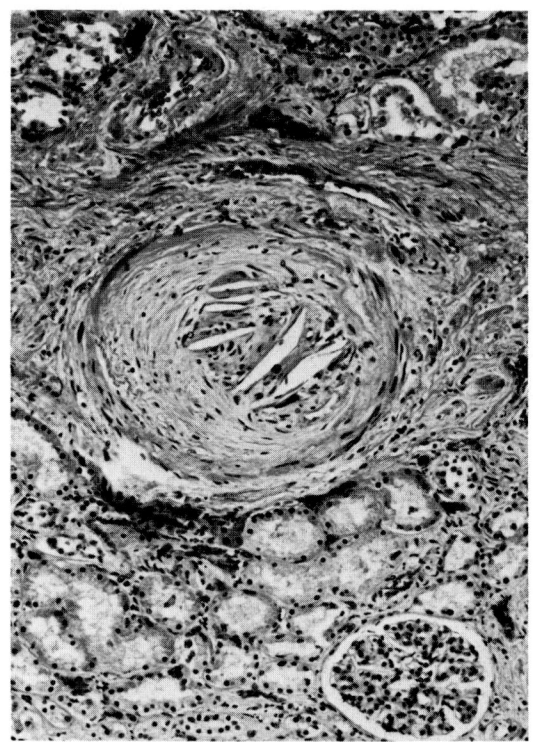

**Figure 35–2.** Atheroemboli lodged in an interlobular artery of a kidney obtained post mortem. The elongated clefts are actually voids where cholesterol crystals were located before fixation and staining. Note the exuberant intimal thickening and the cellular proliferation, which completely occlude the lumen. (Material courtesy of W Margaretten.)

juxtamedullary glomeruli.[308, 309] The mechanism for this glomerular enlargement has not been elucidated; however, it may be related to increased blood viscosity due to sickling. Other microscopic findings include iron deposits and sclerosis. Also, medullary interstitial fibrosis is found in a majority of patients.[309–311] Morphologic changes in patients with sickle cell trait consist of a reduction in the number of vasa recta and loss of the normal papillary bundle architecture.

**Microradioangiographic Studies.** These studies show almost total obliteration of vasa recta. The remaining medullary capillaries are dilated and spiral and many times end blindly.[312]

**Stereomicroscopic Studies.** The examinations show papillae to possess markedly dilated vasculature and show the presence of small tumors. Also, more than 50% of patients display calcium deposits on the papillary surface.[313]

**Magnetic Resonance Imaging.** Magnetic resonance imaging studies have borne out a pattern characteristic of sickle cell nephropathy: a decreased T2-weighted renal cortical signal. This is attributable to renal cortical iron deposition from intravascular hemolysis.[314]

## Renal Functional Changes

One of the most prominent renal functional changes and abnormalities caused by sickle cell anemia is the defect in concentrating ability. Sickle cell anemia can cause obliter-

ation of the vasa recta, which can lead to profound consequences in terms of generation of the medullary gradient needed for maximal urine concentration.[315] Transfusion therapy will reverse this concentrating defect in patients up to 15 years old. This not only suggests but shows that sickling is a major contributor to this concentrating defect.[316] After age 15 years, maximal urine osmolarity (400 to 450 mOsm) is attained under conditions of water deprivation.[315, 317, 318] The cause of this concentrating defect is largely due to impaired sodium chloride transport in the medullary ascending limb of Henle. This in turn affects the inner medullary function. Patients with sickle cell disease can still excrete technetium-labeled water under solute-loading conditions, which is accomplished by the thick ascending limb in the outer medulla.[315] Therefore, the achieved urine concentration reflects the tonicity of the outer medullary segment.[316]

Another prominent renal defect seen in patients with sickle cell disease is an incomplete form of distal tubule acidosis. It has been shown that there is impairment of titratable acid excretion after ammonium chloride loading, and $NH_4^+$ excretion is either normal or decreased.[311, 319–322] Patients with sickle cell trait show no evidence of this acidification abnormality.[316] There is an increase in glomerular filtration rate and renal blood flow that correlates with glomerular enlargement. Furthermore, it has been suggested that prostaglandins may participate in the mediation of the increase in glomerular filtration and decreased $Na^+$ reabsorption in the medullary thick ascending limb of Henle.[323] It has also been shown that when patients with sickle cell disease are loaded with $K^+$, there is an impaired capacity to excrete $K^+$ despite normal renin and aldosterone responses.[319, 321, 322] Proximal tubule function is increased in sickle cell disease; this can lead to hyperphosphatemia because of increased $PO_4^{3-}$ reabsorption and overestimation of glomerular filtration rate due to the increase in creatinine secretion.[322]

## Clinical Features

**Gross Hematuria.** The occurrence of gross hematuria is not an uncommon clinical feature in patients with sickle cell disease, sickle cell trait, and hemoglobin SC disease. However, the frequency has not been well established. One study showed that among African-Americans presenting with gross hematuria, one third had sickle cell disease.[324] Hemizygous individuals do have hematuria at some point.[325] It is unclear as to what events precipitate hematuria. However, it is thought that sickling in the medullary capillary bed is induced or influenced by relative hypoxia; hypertonicity, which may extract water from erythrocytes and concentrate hemoglobin S; and local acidemia. Therapeutic approaches that antagonize these precipitants of sickling have been shown to decrease the quantity of hematuria. These approaches include the administration of distilled water; sodium bicarbonate; and diuretics, including furosemide, ethacrynic acid, and mannitol.[326] There has been a report that oral urea leads to the abatement of hematuria in patients with sickle cell trait.[327] When all else fails to control hematuria, nephrectomy is at times performed; how-

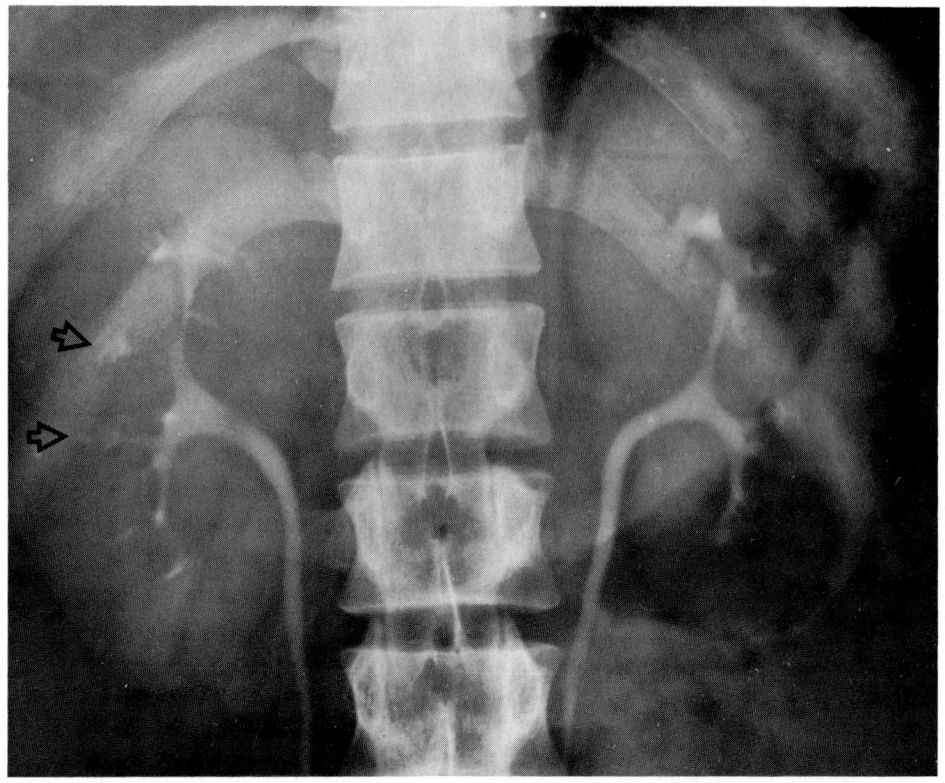

**Figure 35–3.** Renal papillary necrosis with various forms of cavitation in a 33-year-old man with sickle cell hemoglobinopathy and hematuria. Kidneys are normal size and smooth in contour. Central cavitation is present in many papillae, particularly in right interpolar areas *(arrows)*. (From Davidson AJ, Hartman DS: Radiology of the Kidney and Urinary Tract, 2nd ed. WB Saunders, Philadelphia, 1994, p 184.)

ever, recurrent bleeding can occur from the contralateral kidney.[324, 328]

**Papillary Necrosis and Renal Infarction.** Papillary infarction and subsequent necrosis develop in an indolent fashion secondary to chronic and recurrent sickling.[313] It is unusual to have renal failure associated with papillary necrosis. The characteristic findings of papillary necrosis on intravenous pyelography include a central cavitation of the papillae, papillary effacement, linear streaks from the angles of the fornices, and cavitation at the angle of the fornices (Fig. 35–3). Cortical infarction has been reported in patients with sickle cell disease and sickle cell trait.[329, 330] There are also case reports of perirenal hematoma due to extravasation after infarction.[331–333]

**Glomerulopathy.** A glomerulopathy may develop in patients with sickle cell disease but not in patients with sickle cell trait. Histopathologic lesions include mesangial expansion, basement membrane duplication consistent with membranoproliferative glomerulopathy, and glomerular sclerosis. About 26% of patients with sickle cell disease will have 1+ or greater proteinuria.[334] Treatment of these patients with enalapril may reduce proteinuria up to 79%; this suggests the presence of glomerular capillary hypertension.[334] Also, 40% of patients with sickle cell disease may have microalbuminuria; this may become the key in diagnosing early glomerular damage, as is the case in diabetes.[334] The nephrotic syndrome will develop in about 4% of sickle cell disease patients; renal failure will develop in more than 60%; and about half of these patients with renal failure will die in 2 years.[335] The ultimate cause of the nephropathy

associated with sickle cell disease is uncertain, but a hemodynamic basis is considered highly likely. Some investigators have reported immunoglobulin G, immunoglobulin M, and complement deposits in the glomeruli of affected kidneys.[336, 337]

## Kidney Transplantation and Sickle Cell Disease

When the patient with sickle cell nephropathy reaches end-stage renal disease, the issue of therapeutic options arises (i.e., dialysis versus kidney transplantation). Most patients are currently receiving dialysis. It remains controversial whether kidney transplantation should be a therapeutic intervention because transplantation fails to alter the patient's underlying disease. Even further, kidney transplantation in these patients may be associated with increased episodes of pain crises.[338, 339] Miner and co-workers[338] presented evidence in a case report for recurrence of sickle cell nephropathy as the cause for deterioration of renal function in an allograft recipient.

## REFERENCES

1. Remuzzi G: HUS and TTP: Variable expression of a single entity. Kidney Int 32:292, 1987.
2. Stewart CL, Tina LU: Hemolytic uremic syndrome. Pediatr Rev 14:218, 1993.
3. Nalabandian RM, Henry RL, Bick RL: Thrombotic thrombocytopenic purpura: An extended editorial. Semin Thromb Hemost 5:216, 1979.

4. Ruggenenti P, Remuzzi G: Thrombotic thrombocytopenic purpura and related disorders. Hematol Oncol Clin North Am 4:219, 1990.
5. Symmers W: Thrombotic microangiopathic haemolytic anaemia (thrombotic microangiopathy). Br Med J 2:897, 1952.
6. Kaplan BS, Drummond KN: The hemolytic-uremic syndrome is a syndrome. N Engl J Med 298:964, 1978.
7. Moschowitz E: Acute febrile pleiochromic anemia with hyaline thrombosis of the terminal arterioles and capillaries: An undescribed disease. Arch Intern Med 36:89, 1925.
8. Baehr G, Klemperer P, Schifrin A: An acute febrile anemia and thrombocytopenic purpura with diffuse platelet thrombosis of capillaries and arterioles. Trans Assoc Am Physicians 51:43, 1936.
9. Amorosi EL, Ultmann JE: Thrombotic thrombocytopenic purpura: Report of 16 cases and review of the literature. Medicine (Baltimore) 45:139, 1966.
10. Cuttner J: Thrombotic thrombocytopenic purpura: A ten year experience. Blood 56:302, 1980.
11. Kennedy SS, Zacharski LR, Beck JR: Thrombotic thrombocytopenic purpura: Analysis of 48 unselected cases. Semin Thromb Hemost 6:341, 1980.
12. Petitt RM: Thrombotic thrombocytopenic purpura: A thirty year review. Semin Thromb Hemost 6:350, 1980.
13. Ridolfi RL, Bell WR: Thrombotic thrombocytopenic purpura: Report of 25 cases and review of the literature. Medicine (Baltimore) 60:413, 1981.
14. Monnens LAH, Retera RJM: Thrombotic thrombocytopenic purpura in a neonatal infant. J Pediatr 71:118, 1967.
15. Kwaan HC: Clinicopathologic features of thrombotic thrombocytopenic purpura. Semin Hematol 24:71, 1987.
16. Eknoyan G, Riggs SA: Renal involvement in patients with thrombotic thrombocytopenic purpura. Am J Nephrol 6:117, 1986.
17. Gasser C, Gautier E, Steck A, et al: Hamolytisch-uramische Syndromes bilaterale Nierenrindennekrosen bei akuten erworbenchenschr hamolytischen Anamien. Schweiz Med Wochenschr 85:905, 1955.
18. Kibel M, Barnard PJ: The haemolytic-uremic syndrome. A survey in South Africa. S Afr Med J 42:692, 1966.
19. Drummond KN: Hemolytic uremic syndrome—then and now. N Engl J Med 312:116, 1985.
20. Gianantonio CA, Vitacco M, Mendilaharzu F, et al: The hemolytic uremic syndrome. Nephron 11:174, 1973.
21. Rooney JC, Anderson RM, Hopkins IJ: Clinical and pathological aspects of central nervous system involvement in the haemolytic uraemic syndrome. Aust Paediatr J 7:28, 1971.
22. Sheth KJ, Swick HM, Haworth N: Neurological involvement in hemolytic-uremic syndrome. Ann Neurol 19:90, 1986.
23. Rogers MF, Rutherford GW, Alexander SR, et al: A population-based study of hemolytic uremic syndrome in Oregon, 1979–1982. Am J Epidemiol 123:137, 1986.
24. Spika JS, Parsons JE, Nordenberg D, Gunn RA: Hemolytic uremic syndrome and diarrhea associated with *Escherichia coli* 0157:H7 in a day care center. J Pediatr 109:287, 1986.
25. Whitington PF, Friedman AL, Chesney RW: Gastrointestinal disease in the hemolytic uremic syndrome. Gastroenterology 76:278, 1979.
26. Hellstrom HR, Nash EC, Fischer ER: Thrombotic thrombocytopenic purpura as a cause of massive gastrointestinal hemorrhage, report of a case. Gastroenterology 36:132, 1959.
27. Jackson B, Files JC, Morrison FS, Scott-Conner CEH: Thrombotic thrombocytopenic purpura and pancreatitis. Am J Gastroenterol 84:667, 1989.
28. Andreoli SP, Bergstein JM: Development of insulin-dependent diabetes mellitus during the hemolytic-uremic syndrome. J Pediatr 100:541, 1982.
29. Andreoli S, Bergstein J: Exocrine and endocrine pancreatic insufficiency and calcinosis after hemolytic uremic syndrome. J Pediatr 110:816, 1987.
30. Andreoli SP, Bergstein JM: Acute rhabdomyolysis associated with hemolytic-uremic syndrome. J Pediatr 103:78, 1983.
31. Ridolfi RL, Hutchins GM, Bell WR: The heart and conduction system in thrombotic thrombocytopenic purpura. Ann Intern Med 91:357, 1979.
32. Siegler RL, Brewer ED, Swartz M: Ocular involvement in hemolytic-uremic syndrome. J Pediatr 112:594, 1988.
33. Percival SPB: Ocular findings in thrombotic thrombocytopenic purpura (Moschowitz's disease). Br J Ophthalmol 54:73, 1970.
34. Karlsberg RP, Lacher JW, Bartecchi C: Adult hemolytic-uremic syndrome: Familial variant. Arch Intern Med 137:1155, 1977.
35. Shapiro CM, Kanter A, Lopas H, et al: Hemolytic-uremic syndrome in adults. JAMA 213:567, 1970.
36. Carter AO, Borczyk AA, Carlson JA, et al: A severe outbreak of *Escherichia coli* O157:H7-associated hemorrhagic colitis in a nursing home. N Engl J Med 317:1496, 1987.
37. Dunea G, Muehrcke RC, Nakamato S, Schwartz FD: Thrombotic thrombocytopenic purpura with acute anuric renal failure. Am J Med 41:1000, 1966.
38. Symmers WC: Thrombotic microangiopathy: Histological diagnosis during life. Lancet 1:592, 1956.
39. Bukowski RM: Thrombotic thrombocytopenic purpura: A review. *In* Spaet TH (ed): Progress in Hemostasis and Thrombosis. Grune & Stratton, New York, 1982, p 287.
40. Berberich FR, Cuene SA, Chard RL, et al: Thrombotic thrombocytopenic purpura. Three cases with platelet and fibrinogen survival studies. J Pediatr 84:503, 1974.
41. Kaplan BS, Proesmans W: The hemolytic uremic syndrome of childhood and its variants. Semin Hematol 24:148, 1987.
42. Harker LA, Slichter SJ: Platelet and fibrinogen consumption in man. N Engl J Med 287:999, 1972.
43. Kaplan BS, Thomson PC, MacNab GM: Serum complement levels in haemolytic-uraemic syndrome. Lancet 2:1505, 1973.
44. Tardy B, Page Y, Convers P, et al: Thrombotic thrombocytopenic purpura: MR findings. Am J Neuroradiol 14:489, 1993.
45. De la Sayette V, Gallet E, Le Doze F, et al: Thrombotic thrombocytopenic purpura: A case diagnosed by MRI. Rev Neurol (Paris) 147:314, 1991.
46. Ekberg M, Holmberg L, Denneberg T: Hemolytic uremic syndrome: Results of treatment with hemodialysis. Acta Paediatr Scand 66:693, 1977.
47. Habib R, Mathieu H, Royer P: Le syndrome hémolytique et urémique de l'enfant. Nephron 4:139, 1967.
48. Nishioka GJ, Chilcoat CC, Aufdemorte TB, Clare N: The gingival biopsy in the diagnosis of thrombotic thrombocytopenic purpura. Oral Surg Oral Med Oral Pathol 65:580, 1988.
49. Asada Y, Sumiyoshi A, Hayashi T, et al: Immunohistochemistry of vascular lesion in thrombotic thrombocytopenic purpura, with special reference to factor VIII–related antigen. Thromb Res 38:469, 1985.
50. Levy M, Gagnadoux MF, Habib R: Pathology of hemolytic uremic syndrome in children. *In* Remuzzi G, Mecca G, De Gaetano G (eds): Hemostasis, Prostaglandins and Renal Disease. Raven Press, New York, 1980, pp 383–397.
51. Shigematsu H, Dikman SH, Churg J, et al: Mesangial involvement in hemolytic uremic syndrome. Am J Pathol 85:349, 1976.
52. Kanfer A, Morel-Maroger L, Solez K, et al: The value of renal biopsy in hemolytic-uremic syndrome in adults. *In* Remuzzi G, Mecca G, De Gaetano G (eds): Hemostasis, Prostaglandins, and Renal Disease. Raven Press, New York, 1980, pp 399–406.
53. Morel-Maroger L, Kanfer A, Solez K, et al: Prognostic importance of vascular lesions in acute renal failure with microangiopathic hemolytic anemia (hemolytic-uremic syndrome): Clinicopathologic study in 20 adults. Kidney Int 15:548, 1979.
54. Koffler D, Paronetto F: Fibrinogen deposition in acute renal failure. Am J Pathol 49:383, 1966.
55. Gonzalo A, Mampaso F, Gallego N, et al: Hemolytic-uremic syndrome with hypocomplementemia and deposits of IgM and C3 in the involved renal tissue. Clin Nephrol 16:193, 1981.
56. Feldman JD, Mardiney MR, Unanue ER, et al: The vascular pathology of thrombotic thrombocytopenic purpura: An immunohistochemical and ultrastructural study. Lab Invest 15:927, 1966.
57. Ashkenazi S: Role of bacterial cytotoxins in hemolytic uremic syndrome and thrombotic thrombocytopenic purpura. Annu Rev Med 44:11, 1993.
58. Konowalchuk J, Speirs JI, Stavric S: Vero response to a cytotoxin of *Escherichia coli*. Infect Immun 18:775, 1977.
59. Riley LW, Remis RS, Helgerson SD, et al: Hemorrhagic colitis associated with a rare *Escherichia coli* serotype. N Engl J Med 308:681, 1983.
60. Karmali MA: Infections by verocytotoxin-producing *Escherichia coli*. Clin Microbiol Rev 2:15, 1989.
61. Karmali MA, Steele BT, Petric M, Lim C: Sporadic cases of haemolytic-uraemic syndrome associated with faecal cytotoxin and cytotoxin-producing *Escherichia coli* in stools. Lancet 1:619, 1983.

62. Karmali MA, Petric M, Lim C, et al: The association between hemolytic uremic syndrome and infection by verotoxin-producing *Escherichia coli*. J Infect Dis 151:775, 1985.

63. Morrison DM, Tyrell DLJ, Jewell LD: Colonic biopsy in verotoxin-induced hemorrhagic colitis and thrombotic thrombocytopenic purpura (TTP). Am J Clin Pathol 86:108, 1985.

64. Kovacs MJ, Roddy J, Gregoire S, et al: Thrombotic thrombocytopenic purpura following hemorrhagic colitis due to *Escherichia coli* 0157:H7. Am J Med 88:177, 1990.

65. Griffin PM, Ostroff SM, Tauxe RV, et al: Illnesses associated with *Escherichia coli* 0157:H7 infections. A broad clinical spectrum. Ann Intern Med 109:705, 1988.

66. Raghupathy P, Date A, Shastry JCM, et al: Haemolytic-uraemic syndrome complicating *Shigella* dysentery in South Indian children. Br Med J 1:1518, 1978.

67. Baker NM, Mills AE, Rachman I, Thomas JEP: Haemolytic-uraemic syndrome in typhoid fever. Br Med J 2:84, 1974.

68. Denneberg TM, Friedberg M, Homberg L, et al: Combined plasmapheresis and hemodialysis treatment for severe hemolytic uremic syndrome following *Campylobacter* colitis. Acta Paediatr Scand 71:243, 1982.

69. Morel-Maroger L: Adult hemolytic-uremic syndrome. Kidney Int 18:125, 1983.

70. Prober CG, Tune B, Hoder L: *Yersinia pseudotuberculosis* septicemia. Am J Dis Child 133:623, 1979.

71. Ray CH, Tucker VL, Harris DJ, et al: Enteroviruses associated with hemolytic-uremic syndrome. Pediatrics 46:378, 1970.

72. O'Regan S, Robitaille P, Mongeau JB, McLaughlin B: The hemolytic uremic syndrome associated with ECHO 22 infection. Clin Pediatr 19:125, 1980.

73. Ueda K, Shingaki Y, Sato T, et al: Hemolytic anemia following postnatally acquired rubella during the 1975–1977 rubella epidemic in Japan. Clin Pediatr 24:155, 1985.

74. Shashaty GC, Atamaer MA: Hemolytic uremic syndrome associated with infectious mononucleosis. Am J Dis Child 127:720, 1974.

75. Segal GH, Tubbs RR, Ratliff NB, et al: Thrombotic thrombocytopenic purpura in a patient with AIDS. Cleve Clin J Med 57:360, 1990.

76. Nair JM, Bellevue R, Bertoni M, Dosik H: Thrombotic thrombocytopenic purpura in patients with the acquired immunodeficiency syndrome (AIDS)–related complex. A report of two cases. Ann Intern Med 109:209, 1988.

77. Murgo AJ: Thrombotic microangiopathy in the cancer patient including those induced by chemotherapeutic agents. Semin Hematol 24:161, 1987.

78. Weinblatt ME, Kahn E, Scimeca PG, Kochen JA: Hemolytic uremic syndrome associated with cisplatin therapy. Am J Pediatr Hematol Oncol 9:295, 1987.

79. Verweij J, van der Burg ME, Pinedo HM: Mitomycin C–induced hemolytic uremic syndrome. Six case reports and review of the literature on renal, pulmonary and cardiac side effects of the drug. Radiother Oncol 8:33, 1987.

80. Garibotto G, Acquarone N, Saffioti S, et al: Successful treatment of mitomycin C–associated hemolytic uremic syndrome by plasmapheresis. Nephron 51:409, 1989.

81. Lesesne JB, Rothschild N, Erickson B, et al: Cancer-associated hemolytic-uremic syndrome: Analysis of 85 cases from a national registry. J Clin Oncol 7:781, 1989.

82. Galli FC, Damon LE, Tomlanovich SJ, et al: Cyclosporine-induced hemolytic uremic syndrome in a heart transplant recipient. Heart Lung Transplant 12:440, 1993.

83. Noel C, Saunier P, Hazzan M, et al: Incidence and clinical profile of microvascular complications in renal allografted patients treated with cyclosporine. Ann Med Interne (Paris) 143(suppl 1):33, 1992.

84. Butkus DE, Herrera GA, Raju SS: Successful renal transplantation after cyclosporine-associated hemolytic-uremic syndrome following bilateral lung transplantation. Transplantation 54:159, 1992.

85. Atkinson K, Biggs JC, Hayes J, et al: Cyclosporin A associated nephrotoxicity in the first 100 days after allogeneic bone marrow transplantation: Three distinct syndromes. Br J Haematol 54:59, 1983.

86. Bonser RS, Adu D, Franklin I, et al: Cyclosporin-induced haemolytic uraemic syndrome in liver allograft recipient. Lancet 2:1337, 1984.

87. Randhawa PS, Shapiro R, Jordan ML, et al: The histopathological changes associated with allograft rejection and drug toxicity in renal transplant recipients maintained on FK506. Clinical significance and comparison with cyclosporine. Am J Surg Pathol 17:60, 1993.

88. Holman MJ, Gonwa TA, Cooper B, et al: FK506-associated thrombotic thrombocytopenic purpura. Transplantation 55:205, 1993.

89. Giroux L, Smeesters C, Corman J, et al: Hemolytic uremic syndrome in renal allografted patients treated with cyclosporin. Can J Physiol Pharmacol 65:1125, 1987.

90. Wolfe JA, McCann RL, San Filippo F: Cyclosporin associated microangiopathy in renal transplantation: A severe but potentially reversible form of early graft injury. Transplantation 41:541, 1986.

91. Oursler DP, Holley KE, Wagoner RD: Hemolytic uremic syndrome after bone marrow transplantation without total body irradiation. Am J Nephrol 13:167, 1993.

92. Schoolwerth AC, Sandler RS, Klahr S, et al: Nephrosclerosis postpartum in women taking oral contraceptives. Arch Intern Med 136:178, 1976.

93. Gottschall JL, Elliot W, Liano E, et al: Quinine-induced immune thrombocytopenia associated with hemolytic uremic syndrome: A new clinical entity. Blood 77:306, 1991.

94. Parker JC, Barrett DA 2nd: Microangiopathic hemolysis and thrombocytopenia related to penicillin drugs. Arch Intern Med 127:474, 1971.

95. Ahmed R, Sumalnop V, Spain DM, et al: Thrombohemolytic thrombocytopenic purpura during penicillamine therapy. Arch Intern Med 138:1292, 1983.

96. Powell HR, Davidson PM, McCredie DA, et al: Haemolytic-uremic syndrome after treatment with metronidazole. Med J Aust 149:222, 1988.

97. Stonesifer LD, Bone RC, Hiller FC: Thrombotic thrombocytopenic purpura in carbon monoxide poisoning. Arch Intern Med 140:104, 1980.

98. Jones AM, Armitage JO, Stone DV: Self-limited TTP-like syndrome after bee sting. JAMA 242:2212, 1979.

99. Symmers WC: Thrombotic microangiopathy (TTP) associated with acute haemorrhagic leukoencephalitis and sensitivity to oxophenarsine. Brain 79:511, 1956.

100. Ehrich WE, Seifter J: Thrombotic thrombocytopenic purpura caused by iodine. Arch Pathol 47:446, 1949.

101. Miller JM Jr, Pastorek JG: Thrombotic thrombocytopenic purpura and hemolytic uremic syndrome in pregnancy. Clin Obstet Gynecol 34:64, 1991.

102. Hayslett JP: Current concepts. Postpartum renal failure. N Engl J Med 312:1556, 1985.

103. Rozdzinski E, Hertenstein B, Schmeiser T, et al: Thrombotic thrombocytopenic purpura in early pregnancy with maternal and fetal survival. Ann Hematol 64:245, 1992.

104. Maina A, Donvito V, Giachino O, et al: Thrombotic thrombocytopenic purpura in pregnancy with maternal and fetal survival. Case report. Br J Obstet Gynaecol 97:443, 1992.

105. Krane NK: Acute renal failure in pregnancy. Arch Intern Med 148:2347, 1988.

106. Inglis TCM, Steward J, George JJ: Haemostatic and rheological changes in normal pregnancy and preeclampsia. Br J Haematol 50:461, 1982.

107. Wiznitzer A, Mazor M, Leiberman JR, et al: Familial occurrence of thrombotic thrombocytopenic purpura in two sisters during pregnancy. Am J Obstet Gynecol 166:20, 1992.

108. Wallace DC, Loveric A, Clubb JS, et al: Thrombotic thrombocytopenic purpura in four siblings. Am J Med 58:724, 1975.

109. Fuchs WE, George JN, Dotin LN, Sears DA: Thrombotic thrombocytopenic purpura occurrence two years apart during late pregnancy in two sisters. JAMA 19:235, 1976.

110. Berns JS, Kaplan BS, Mackow RC, Hefter LG: Inherited hemolytic uremic syndrome in adults. Am J Kidney Dis 19:331, 1992.

111. Kaplan BS, Cleary TG, Obrig TG: Recent advances in understanding the pathogenesis of the hemolytic uremic syndromes. Pediatr Nephrol 4:276, 1990.

112. Obrig TG, Vecchio PHD, Brown EJ, et al: Direct cytotoxic action of Shigatoxin action on human vascular endothelial cells. Infect Immun 56:2372, 1988.

113. Tesh VL, Samuel JE, Perera L, et al: Evaluation of the role of Shiga and Shiga-like toxins in remediating direct damage to human vascular endothelial cells. J Infect Dis 164:344, 1991.

114. Boyd B, Lingwood C: Verotoxin receptor glycolipid in human renal tissue. Nephron 51:207, 1989.

115. Richardson SE, Rotman TA, Jay V, et al: Experimental verocytotoxemia in rabbits. Infect Immun 60:4154, 1992.
116. Klein PJ, Bulla M, Newman RA, et al: Thomsen-Friedenreich antigen in haemolytic-uraemic syndrome. Lancet 2:1024, 1977. Letter.
117. Novak RW, Martin CR, Orsini EN: Hemolytic-uremic syndrome and T-cryptantigen exposure by neuraminidase-producing pneumococci: An emerging problem? Pediatr Pathol 1:409, 1983.
118. McGraw ME, Lendon M, Stevens RF, et al: Haemolytic uremic syndrome and the Thomsen-Friedenreich antigen. Pediatr Nephrol 3:135, 1989.
119. Leung DYM, Moake JL, Havens PL, et al: Lytic anti–endothelial cell antibodies in haemolytic-uraemic syndrome. Lancet 2:183, 1988.
120. Dillon MJ, Tizard EJ: Anti-neutrophil cytoplasmic antibodies and anti-endothelial cell antibodies. Pediatr Nephrol 5:256, 1991.
121. Cattell V: Mitomycin-induced hemolytic uremic kidney. An experimental model in the rat. Am J Pathol 121:88, 1985.
122. Zoja C, Furci L, Ghilardi F, et al: Cyclosporin induced endothelial cell injury. Lab Invest 55:455, 1986.
123. Snyder HW Jr, Mittelman A, Oral A, et al: Treatment of cancer chemotherapy–associated thrombotic thrombocytopenic purpura/hemolytic uremic syndrome by protein A immunoadsorption of plasma. Cancer 71:1882, 1993.
124. Bergstein JM, Riley M, Bang NU: Analysis of the plasminogen activator activity of the human glomerulus. Kidney Int 33:868, 1988.
125. Bergstein JM, Kuederli U, Bang NU: Plasma inhibitor of glomerular fibrinolysis in the hemolytic-uremic syndrome. Am J Med 73:322, 1982.
126. Bergstein JM, Riley M, Bang NU: Role of plasminogen-activator inhibitor type 1 in the pathogenesis and outcome of the hemolytic uremic syndrome. N Engl J Med 327:755, 1992.
127. Glas-Greenwalt P, Hall JM, Panke TW, et al: Fibrinolysis in health and disease: Abnormal levels of plasminogen activator, plasminogen activator inhibitor, and protein C in thrombotic thrombocytopenic purpura. J Lab Clin Med 108:415, 1986.
128. Hekman CM, Loskutoff DJ: Fibrinolytic pathways and the endothelium. Semin Thromb Hemost 13:514, 1987.
129. Esmon CT: Protein C: Biochemistry, physiology and clinical implications. Blood 62:1155, 1983.
130. Lian EC-Y: Pathogenesis of thrombotic thrombocytopenic purpura. Semin Hematol 24:82, 1987.
131. Bloom AL: von Willebrand factor: Clinical features of inherited and acquired disorders. Mayo Clin Proc 66:743, 1991.
132. Moake JL, McPherson PD: von Willebrand factor in thrombotic thrombocytopenic purpura and the hemolytic-uremic syndrome. Transfus Med Rev 4:163, 1990.
133. Moake JL, Rudy CK, Troll JH, et al: Unusually large plasma factor VIII: von Willebrand factor multimers in chronic relapsing thrombotic thrombocytopenic purpura. N Engl J Med 307:1432, 1982.
134. Moake JL, Byrnes JJ, Troll JH, et al: Abnormal factor VIII: von Willebrand factor patterns in plasma of patients with the hemolytic-uremic syndrome. Blood 64:592, 1984.
135. Rose PE, Enayat SM, Sunderland R, et al: Abnormalities of factor VIII related protein multimers in the haemolytic uraemic syndrome. Arch Dis Child 59:1135, 1984.
136. Monnens L, Van De Meer W, Langenhuysen C, et al: Platelet aggregating factor in the epidemic form of hemolytic uremic syndrome in childhood. Clin Nephrol 24:135, 1985.
137. Siddiqui FA, Lian ECY: Novel platelet-agglutinating protein from a thrombotic thrombocytopenic purpura patient. J Clin Invest 76:1330, 1985.
138. Remuzzi G, Misiani R, Mecca G, et al: Thrombotic thrombocytopenic purpura—a deficiency of plasma factor regulating platelet–vessel wall interaction. N Engl J Med 299:311, 1978.
139. Walters S, Levin M, Smith C, et al: Intravascular platelet activation in the hemolytic uremic syndrome. Kidney Int 33:107, 1988.
140. Levin M, Elkon KB, Nokes TJC, et al: Inhibitor of prostacyclin production in sporadic haemolytic uremic syndrome. Arch Dis Child 58:703, 1983.
141. Goodman RP, Killam AP, Brash AR, et al: Prostacyclin production during pregnancy: Comparison of production during normal pregnancy and pregnancy complicated by hypertension. Am J Obstet Gynecol 142:817, 1982.
142. Ylikorkala O, Makila UM, Viinikka L: Amniotic fluid prostacyclin and thromboxane in normal, preeclamptic, and some other complicated pregnancies. Am J Obstet Gynecol 141:487, 1981.
143. Defreyn G, Prosemans W, Machin SJ, et al: Abnormal prostacyclin metabolism in the hemolytic uremic syndrome: Equivocal effects of prostacyclin infusions. Clin Nephrol 18:43, 1982.
144. Abbas AK, Lichtman AH, Pober JS: Cellular and Molecular Immunology. WB Saunders, Philadelphia, 1991, p 225.
145. van de Kar NC, Monnens LA, Karmali MA, van Hinsbergh VW: Tumor necrosis factor and interleukin-1 induce expression of the verocytotoxin receptor globotriaosylceramide on human endothelial cells: Implications for the pathogenesis of the hemolytic uremic syndrome. Blood 80:2755, 1992.
146. Wada H, Kaneko T, Ohiwa M, et al: Plasma cytokine levels in thrombotic thrombocytopenic purpura. Am J Hematol 40:167, 1992.
147. Fitzpatrick MM, Shah V, Trompeter RS, et al: Interleukin-8 and polymorphoneutrophil leucocyte activation in hemolytic uremic syndrome of childhood. Kidney Int 42:951, 1992.
148. Bell WR, Braine HG, Ness PL, Kickler TS: Improved survival in thrombotic thrombocytopenic purpura–hemolytic uremic syndrome. Clinical experience in 108 patients. N Engl J Med 325:398, 1991.
149. Trompeter RS, Schwartz R, Chantler C, et al: Haemolytic-uraemic syndrome: An analysis of prognostic features. Arch Dis Child 58:101, 1983.
150. Walters MDS, Matthei IU, Kay R, et al: The polymorphonuclear leukocyte count in childhood haemolytic uraemic syndrome. Pediatr Nephrol 3:130, 1989.
151. Martin DL, MacDonald KL, White KE, et al: The epidemiology and clinical aspects of the hemolytic uremic syndrome in Minnesota. N Engl J Med 323:1161, 1990.
152. DeJong M, Monnens L: Haemolytic-uraemic syndrome: A 10-year follow-up study of 73 patients. Nephrol Dial Transplant 3:379, 1988.
153. Schieppati A, Ruggenenti P, Plata R, et al: Renal function at hospital admission as prognostic factor in adult haemolytic uraemic syndrome. J Am Soc Nephrol 2:1640, 1992.
154. Morel-Maroger L, Kanfer A, Solez K, et al: Prognostic importance of vascular lesions in acute renal failure with microangiopathic hemolytic anemia (hemolytic uremic syndrome): Clinicopathologic study in 20 adults. Kidney Int 15:548, 1979.
155. Harkness DR, Byrnes JJ, Lian ECY, et al: Hazard of platelet transfusion in thrombotic thrombocytopenic purpura. JAMA 246:1931, 1981.
156. Gordon LI, Kwaan HC, Rossi EC: Deleterious effects of platelet transfusions and recovery thrombocytosis in patients with thrombotic microangiopathy. Semin Hematol 24:194, 1987.
157. Bukowski RM, King JW, Hewlett JS: Plasmapheresis in the treatment of thrombotic thrombocytopenic purpura. Blood 50:413, 1977.
158. Beattie TJ, Murphy AV, Willoughby MLN, et al: Plasmapheresis in the haemolytic-uraemic syndrome in children. Br Med J 282:1667, 1981.
159. Gillor A, Bulla M, Roth B, et al: Plasmapheresis as a therapeutic measure in hemolytic-uremic syndrome in children. Klin Wochenschr 61:363, 1983.
160. Hakim RM, Schulman G, Churchill WH, et al: Successful management of thrombocytopenia, microangiopathic anemia, and acute renal failure by plasmapheresis. Am J Kidney Dis 5:170, 1985.
161. Blitzer JB, Granfortuna JM, Gottlieb AJ, et al: Thrombotic thrombocytopenic purpura: Treatment with plasmapheresis. Am J Hematol 24:329, 1987.
162. Rock GA, Shumak KH, Buskard NA, et al: Comparison of plasma exchange with plasma infusion in the treatment of thrombotic thrombocytopenic purpura. N Engl J Med 325:393, 1991.
163. Byrnes JJ, Khurana M: Treatment of thrombotic thrombocytopenic purpura with plasma. N Engl J Med 297:1386, 1977.
164. Misiani R, Appiani AC, Edefonti A, et al: Haemolytic uraemic syndrome: Therapeutic effect of plasma infusion. Br Med J 285:1304, 1982.
165. Shepard KV, Bukowski RM: The treatment of thrombotic thrombocytopenic purpura with exchange transfusions, plasma infusions and plasma exchange. Semin Hematol 24:178, 1987.
166. Rose M, Eldor A: High incidence of relapses in thrombotic thrombocytopenic purpura. Am J Med 83:437, 1987.
167. Siegler RL: Management of hemolytic-uremic syndrome. J Pediatr 112:1019, 1988.
168. Gutterman LA, Stevenson TD: Treatment of thrombotic thrombocytopenic purpura with vincristine. JAMA 247:1433, 1982.
169. Schreeder MT, Prchal JT: Successful treatment of thrombotic thrombocytopenic purpura by vincristine. Am J Hematol 14:75, 1983.

170. Moake LJ, Rudy CK, Troll JH, et al: Therapy of chronic relapsing thrombotic thrombocytopenic purpura with prednisone and azathioprine. Am J Hematol 20:73, 1985.

171. Wallach HW, Oren ME, Herskowitz A: Treatment of thrombotic thrombocytopenic purpura with plasma infusion and cyclophosphamide. South Med J 72:1346, 1979.

172. Rosove MH, Ho WG, Goldfinger D: Ineffectiveness of aspirin and dipyridamole in the treatment of thrombotic thrombocytopenic purpura. Ann Intern Med 96:27, 1981.

173. del-Zoppo GJ: Antiplatelet therapy in thrombotic thrombocytopenic purpura. Semin Hematol 24:130, 1987.

174. Diekmann L: Treatment of the hemolytic-uremic syndrome with streptokinase and heparin. Klin Padiatr 192:430, 1980.

175. Loirat C, Beaufils F, Sonsino E, et al: Urokinase treatment for hemolytic uremic syndrome in childhood: A multicenter controlled trial from the French Society of Pediatric Nephrology. Int J Pediatr Nephrol 3:46, 1982. Abstract.

176. Proesmans W, ki Muaka B, Van Damme B, et al: The use of heparin in childhood hemolytic uremic syndrome. In Remuzzi G, Mecca G, De Gaetano G (eds): Hemostasis, Prostaglandins, and Renal Disease. Raven Press, New York, 1980, p 407.

177. Wong P, Itoh K, Yoshida S: Treatment of thrombotic thrombocytopenic purpura with intravenous gamma globulin. N Engl J Med 314:385, 1986. Letter.

178. Chin D, Chyczij H, Etches W, et al: Treatment of thrombotic thrombocytopenic purpura with intravenous gamma globulin. Transfusion 27:115, 1987.

179. Gilcher RO, Goldman SN: Refractory TTP responding to IV gamma globulin. Blood 64:237, 1987.

180. Berkman SA, Lee ME, Gale RP: Clinical uses of intravenous immunoglobulins. Ann Intern Med 112:278, 1990.

181. Guelpa G, Trono D, Audetat F, Hochstrasser D: Purpura thrombotique thrombocytopénique traité par la prostacycline. Schweiz Med Wochenschr 116:647, 1986.

182. Payton CD, Belch JJF, Boulton Jones JM: Successful treatment of thrombotic thrombocytopenic purpura by epoprostenol infusion. Lancet 1:927, 1985. Letter.

183. Johnson JE, Mills GM, Batson AG, et al: Ineffective epoprostenol therapy for thrombotic thrombocytopenic purpura. JAMA 250:3089, 1983.

184. Powell HR, McCredie DA, Taylor CM, et al: Vitamin E treatment of haemolytic uraemic syndrome. Arch Dis Child 59:401, 1984.

185. Grino JM, Caralps A, Carreras L, et al: Apparent recurrence of hemolytic uremic syndrome in azathioprine-treated allograft recipients. Nephron 49:301, 1988.

186. Hebert D, Sibley RK, Mauer SM: Recurrence of hemolytic uremic syndrome in renal transplant recipients. Kidney Int 19:S51, 1986.

187. Medsger TA: Systemic sclerosis and localized scleroderma. In Schumacher HR (ed): Primer on the Rheumatic Diseases. Arthritis Foundation, Atlanta, 1988, pp 111–117.

188. Steen VD: Systemic sclerosis. Rheum Dis Clin North Am 16:641, 1990.

189. Donohoe JF: Scleroderma and the kidney. Kidney Int 41:462, 1992.

190. Steen VD, Conte C, Santora D, et al: Twenty-year incidence survey of systemic sclerosis. Arthritis Rheum 31:S21, 1988. Abstract.

191. Tuffanelli DL, Winkelmann RK: Systemic scleroderma: A clinical study of 727 cases. Arch Dermatol 84:359, 1961.

192. Steen VD, Medsger TA Jr: Epidemiology and natural history of systemic sclerosis. Rheum Dis Clin North Am 16:1, 1990.

193. Silman AJ: Epidemiology of scleroderma. Curr Opin Rheumatol 3:967, 1991.

194. Toxic Epidemic Syndrome Study Group: Toxic epidemic syndrome, Spain, 1981. Lancet 2:697, 1982.

195. Spiera H, Kerr LD: Scleroderma following silicone implantation: A cumulative experience of 11 cases. J Rheumatol 20:958, 1993.

196. Gutierrez V, Espinoza LR: Progressive systemic sclerosis complicated by severe hypertension: Reversal after silicone implant removal. Am J Med 89:390, 1990.

197. Finch WR, Rodnan GP, Buckingham RB, et al: Bleomycin-induced scleroderma. J Rheumatol 7:651, 1980.

198. Rodnan GP, Benedek TG, Medsger TA, Cammarata RJ: The association of progressive systemic sclerosis (scleroderma) with coal miners' pneumoconiosis and other forms of silicosis. Ann Intern Med 66:323, 1967.

199. Morgan JM, Adams SJ: Scleroderma and autoimmune thrombocytopenia associated with ingestion of L-tryptophan. Br J Dermatol 128:581, 1993.

200. Oursler JR, Farmer ER, Roubenoff R, et al: Cutaneous manifestations of the eosinophilia-myalgia syndrome. Br J Dermatol 127:138, 1992.

201. Kaufman LD: The eosinophilia-myalgia syndrome: Current concepts and future directions. Clin Exp Rheumatol 10:87, 1992.

202. Furst DE, Clements PJ, Graze P, et al: A syndrome resembling progressive systemic sclerosis after bone marrow transplantation. A model for scleroderma? Arthritis Rheum 22:904, 1979.

203. Whiteside T, Medsger TA, Rodnan GP: HLA-DR antigens in progressive systemic sclerosis (scleroderma). J Rheumatol 10:128, 1983.

204. Briggs DC, Laurent R, Black CM, Welsh KI: A strong association between null alleles at the C4A locus in the major histocompatibility complex and systemic sclerosis. Arthritis Rheum 29:1274, 1986.

205. Steen VD, Medsger TA Jr, Osial TA Jr, et al: Factors predicting development of renal involvement in progressive systemic sclerosis. Am J Med 76:779, 1984.

206. Eason RJ, Tan PL, Gow PJ: Progressive systemic sclerosis in Auckland: A ten year review with emphasis on prognostic features. Aust N Z J Med 11:657, 1981.

207. Birdi N, Laxer RM, Thorner P, et al: Localized scleroderma progressing to systemic disease. Case report and review of the literature. Arthritis Rheum 36:410, 1993.

208. Kallenberg CG: Overlapping syndromes, undifferentiated connective tissue disease, and other fibrosing conditions. Curr Opin Rheumatol 4:837, 1992.

209. Black C, Isenberg DA: Mixed connective tissue disease—goodbye to all that. Br J Rheumatol 31:695, 1992.

210. Maricq HR, LeRoy EC, D'Angelo WA, et al: Diagnostic potential of in vivo capillary microscopy in scleroderma and related disorders. Arthritis Rheum 23:183, 1980.

211. Clements PJ, Furst DE, Campion DS, et al: Muscle disease in progressive systemic sclerosis: Diagnostic and therapeutic considerations. Arthritis Rheum 21:62, 1978.

212. Salerni R, Rodnan GP, Leon DF, Shaver JA: Pulmonary hypertension in the CREST syndrome variant of progressive systemic sclerosis (scleroderma). Ann Intern Med 86:394, 1977.

213. Ridolfi RL, Bulkley BH, Hutchins GM: The cardiac conduction system in progressive systemic sclerosis: Clinical and pathologic features of 35 patients. Am J Med 61:361, 1976.

214. Follansbee WP, Curtiss EI, Medsger TA, et al: Physiologic abnormalities of cardiac function in progressive systemic sclerosis with diffuse scleroderma. N Engl J Med 310:142, 1984.

215. McWhorter JE, LeRoy EC: Pericardial disease in scleroderma (systemic sclerosis). Am J Med 57:566, 1974.

216. Gordon MB, Klein I, Dekker A, et al: Thyroid disease in progressive systemic sclerosis: Increased frequency of glandular fibrosis and hypothyroidism. Ann Intern Med 95:431, 1981.

217. Sturgess A: Recently characterised autoantibodies and their clinical significance. Aust N Z J Med 22:279, 1992.

218. Kallenberg CG: Early detection of connective tissue disease in patients with Raynaud's phenomenon. Rheum Dis Clin North Am 16:11, 1990.

219. Auspitz H: Ein Beitrag zur Lehre vom Haut-Sklerem der Erwachsenen. Wien Med Wochenschr 13:739, 1863.

220. Osler W: The Principles and Practice of Medicine. Appleton-Century-Crofts, New York, 1892, p 993.

221. Moore HC, Sheehan HL: The kidney of scleroderma. Lancet 1:68, 1952.

222. Rodnan GP, Schreiner G, Black R: Renal involvement in progressive systemic sclerosis (scleroderma). Am J Med 23:445, 1957.

223. D'Angelo WA, Fries JF, Masi AT, Shulman LE: Pathologic observations in systemic sclerosis. Am J Med 46:428, 1969.

224. Cannon PJ, Hassar M, Case DB, et al: The relationship of hypertension and renal failure in scleroderma (progressive systemic sclerosis) to structural and functional abnormalities of the renal cortical circulation. Medicine (Baltimore) 54:1, 1974.

225. Traub YM, Shapiro AP, Rodnan GP, et al: Hypertension and renal failure (scleroderma renal crisis) in progressive systemic sclerosis: Review of a 25 year experience with 68 cases. Medicine (Baltimore) 62:335, 1983.

226. Medsger TA Jr, Masi AT, Rodnan GP, et al: Survival with systemic sclerosis (scleroderma). Ann Intern Med 75:396, 1971.

227. Steen VD, Constantino JP, Shapiro AP, et al: Outcome of renal crisis in systemic sclerosis: Relation to availability of angiotensin converting enzyme (ACE) inhibitors. Ann Intern Med 113:352, 1990.

228. Salyer WR, Salyer DC, Heptinstall RH: Scleroderma and microangiopathic hemolytic anemia. Ann Intern Med 78:895, 1973.

229. Kincaid-Smith P: Participation of intravascular coagulation in the pathogenesis of glomerular and vascular lesions. Kidney Int 7:242, 1975.

230. Braun J, Sieper J, Schwarz A, et al: Widespread vasculopathy with hemolytic uremic syndrome, perimyocarditis and cystic pancreatitis in a young woman with mixed connective tissue disease. Case report and review of the literature. Rheumatol Int 13:31, 1993.

231. Trostle DC, Bedetti CD, Steen VD, et al: Renal vascular histology and morphometry in systemic sclerosis: A case control autopsy study. Arthritis Rheum 31:393, 1988.

232. Kovalchik MT, Guggenheim SJ, Silverman MH, et al: The kidney in progressive systemic sclerosis: A prospective study. Ann Intern Med 89:881, 1978.

233. McCoy RC, Tisher CC, Pepe PF, Cleveland LA: The kidney in progressive systemic sclerosis. Lab Invest 35:124, 1976.

234. Stone RA, Tisher CC, Hawkins HK, et al: Juxtaglomerular hyperplasia and hyperreninemia in progressive systemic sclerosis complicated by acute renal failure. Am J Med 36:119, 1974.

235. Lapenas D, Rodnan GP, Cavallo T: Immunopathology of the renal vascular lesion of progressive systemic sclerosis (scleroderma). Am J Pathol 91:243, 1978.

236. Woodhall PB, McCoy RC, Gunnells JC, Seigler HF: Apparent recurrence of progressive systemic sclerosis in a renal allograft. JAMA 236:1032, 1976.

237. Miller D, Waters DD, Warmca W, et al: Is variant angina the coronary manifestation of a generalized vasospastic disorder? N Engl J Med 304:763, 1981.

238. Kahan A, Deveaux JY, Amor B, et al: Nifedipine and thallium-201 myocardial perfusion in progressive systemic sclerosis. N Engl J Med 314:1397, 1986.

239. Fahey PJ, Utell MJ, Condemi JJ, et al: Raynaud's phenomenon of the lung. Am J Med 76:263, 1984.

240. Sapira JD, Rodnan GP, Scheib ET, et al: Studies of endogenous catecholamines in patients with Raynaud's phenomenon secondary to progressive systemic sclerosis (scleroderma). Am J Med 52:330, 1972.

241. Dzau VJ: Significance of the vascular renin-angiotensin pathway. Hypertension 8:553, 1986.

242. Knock GA, Terenghi G, Bunker CB, et al: Characterization of endothelin-binding sites in human skin and their regulation in primary Raynaud's phenomenon and systemic sclerosis. J Invest Dermatol 101:73, 1993.

243. LeRoy EC: Increased collagen synthesis by scleroderma skin fibroblasts in vitro. J Clin Invest 54:880, 1974.

244. Smith EA, LeRoy EC: A possible role for transforming growth factor-beta in systemic sclerosis. J Invest Dermatol 95:125S, 1990.

245. Gabrielli A, Di-Loreto C, Taborro R, et al: Immunohistochemical localization of intracellular and extracellular associated TGF beta in the skin of patients with systemic sclerosis (scleroderma) and primary Raynaud's phenomenon. Clin Immunol Immunopathol 68:340, 1993.

246. Falanga V, Gerhardt CO, Dasch JR, et al: Skin distribution and differential expression of transforming growth factor beta 1 and beta 2. J Dermatol Sci 3:131, 1992.

247. Prior C, Haslam PL: In vivo levels and in vitro production of interferon-gamma in fibrosing interstitial lung diseases. Clin Exp Immunol 88:280, 1992.

248. Rosenbloom J, Feldman G, Freundlich B, Jimenez SA: Inhibition of excessive scleroderma fibroblast collagen production by recombinant gamma-interferon. Arthritis Rheum 29:851, 1986.

249. Bashey RI, Jimenez SA, Perlish JS: Characterization of secreted collagen from normal and scleroderma fibroblasts in culture. J Mol Med 2:153, 1977.

250. Douvas A: Does Scl-70 modulate collagen production in systemic sclerosis? Lancet 2:475, 1988.

251. Kahaleh MB, Sherer GK, LeRoy EC: Endothelial injury in scleroderma. J Exp Med 149:1326, 1979.

252. Meyer O, Haim T, Dryll A, et al: Vascular endothelial cell injury in progressive systemic sclerosis and other connective tissue diseases. Clin Exp Rheumatol 1:29, 1983.

253. Pandolfi A, Florita M, Altomare G, et al: Increased plasma levels of platelet-derived growth factor activity in patients with progressive systemic sclerosis. Proc Soc Exp Biol Med 191:1, 1989.

254. Kahaleh MB, Osborn I, LeRoy EC: Elevated levels of circulating platelet aggregates and beta-thromboglobulin in scleroderma. Ann Intern Med 96:610, 1982.

255. Needleman BW: Immunologic aspects of scleroderma. Curr Opin Rheumatol 4:862, 1992.

256. Sfikakis PP, Tesar J, Baraf H, et al: Circulating intercellular adhesion molecule-1 in patients with systemic sclerosis. Clin Immunol Immunopathol 68:88, 1993.

257. LeRoy EC: A brief overview of the pathogenesis of scleroderma (systemic sclerosis). Ann Rheum Dis 51:286, 1992.

258. Sollberg S, Peltonen J, Uitto J, Jimenez SA: Elevated expression of beta 1 and beta 2 integrins, intercellular adhesion molecule 1, and endothelial leukocyte adhesion molecule 1 in the skin of patients with systemic sclerosis of recent onset. Arthritis Rheum 35:290, 1992.

259. Kahaleh MB, Yin TG: Enhanced expression of high-affinity interleukin-2 receptors in scleroderma: Possible role for IL-6. Clin Immunol Immunopathol 62:97, 1992.

260. Feghali CA, Bost KL, Boulware DW, Levy LS: Mechanisms of pathogenesis in scleroderma. I. Overproduction of interleukin 6 by fibroblasts cultured from affected skin sites of patients with scleroderma. J Rheumatol 19:1207, 1992.

261. Silman AJ: Pregnancy and scleroderma. Am J Reprod Immunol 28:238, 1992.

262. Lopez-Ovejero JA, Saal SD, D'Angelo WA, et al: Reversal of vascular and renal crises of scleroderma by oral angiotensin-converting enzyme blockade. N Engl J Med 300:1417, 1979.

263. Whitman HH III, Case DB, Laragh JH, et al: Variable response to oral angiotensin-converting-enzyme blockade in hypertensive scleroderma patients. Arthritis Rheum 25:241, 1982.

264. Nissenson AR, Port FK: Outcome of end-stage renal disease in patients with rare causes of renal failure. III. Systemic/vascular disorders. Q J Med 273:63, 1990.

265. Copley JB, Smith BJ: Continuous ambulatory peritoneal dialysis and scleroderma. Nephron 40:353, 1985.

266. London RD, Dikman SH, Spiera H: Recovery of renal function in undifferentiated connective tissue disease after treatment with angiotensin-converting enzyme inhibitors. Am J Kidney Dis 18:716, 1991.

267. Richardson JA: Hemodialysis and kidney transplantation for renal failure from scleroderma. Arthritis Rheum 16:265, 1973.

268. Merino GE, Sutherland DER, Kjellstrand CM, et al: Renal transplantation for progressive systemic sclerosis with renal failure. Am J Surg 133:745, 1977.

269. Steen V: Treatment of systemic sclerosis. Curr Opin Rheumatol 3:979, 1991.

270. Medsger TA Jr: Treatment of systemic sclerosis. Ann Rheum Dis 50(suppl 4):877, 1991.

271. Steen VD, Medsger TA Jr, Rodnan GP: D-Penicillamine therapy in progressive systemic sclerosis (scleroderma). Ann Intern Med 97:652, 1982.

272. Baerman G, Linser P: Über die lokale und allgemeine Wirkung der Röntgenstrahlen. Munch Med Wochenschr 51:1996, 1904.

273. Asscher AW, Wilson C, Anson SG: Sensitization of blood vessels to hypertensive damage by X-irradiation. Lancet 1:580, 1961.

274. Luxton RW: Radiation nephritis: A long-term study of fifty-four patients. Lancet 2:1221, 1961.

275. Luxton RW, Kunkler RB: Radiation nephritis. Acta Radiol 2:169, 1964.

276. Keane WF, Crosson JT, Staley NA, et al: Radiation-induced renal disease: A clinicopathologic study. Am J Med 60:127, 1976.

277. Guinan EC, Tarbell NJ, Niemeyer CM, et al: Intravascular hemolysis and renal insufficiency after bone marrow transplantation. Blood 72:451, 1988.

278. Lawton CA, Cohen EP, Barber-Derus SW, et al: Late renal dysfunction in adult survivors of bone marrow transplantation. Cancer 67:2795, 1991.

279. Jennette JC, Ordonez NG: Radiation nephritis causing nephrotic syndrome. Urology 22:631, 1983.

280. Steele BT, Lirenman DS: Acute radiation nephritis and the hemolytic uremic syndrome. Clin Nephrol 11:272, 1979.

281. Shapiro A, Cavallo T, Cooper W, et al: Hypertension in radiation nephritis. Report of a patient with unilateral disease, elevated renin

activity levels, and reversal after unilateral nephrectomy. Arch Intern Med 137:848, 1977.

282. Staab GE, Tegtmeyer J, Constable WC: Radiation-induced renovascular hypertension. Am J Roentgenol 126:634, 1976.

283. Bergstein J, Andreoli SP, Provisor AJ, Yum M: Radiation nephritis following total-body irradiation and cyclophosphamide in preparation for bone marrow transplantation. Transplantation 41:63, 1984.

284. Tarbell NJ, Guinan EC, Niemeyer C, et al: Late onset of renal dysfunction in survivors of bone marrow transplantation. Int J Radiat Oncol Biol Phys 15:99, 1988.

285. Arneil GC, Emmanuel IG, Flatman GE, et al: Nephritis in two children after irradiation and chemotherapy for nephroblastoma. Lancet 1:960, 1974.

286. Phillips TL, Fu KK: Quantification of combined radiation therapy and chemotherapy effects on critical normal tissues. Cancer 37:1186, 1976.

287. Churchill DN, Hong K, Gault MH: Radiation nephritis following combined abdominal radiation and chemotherapy (bleomycin-vinblastine). Cancer 41:2162, 1978.

288. Anderson BL, Lauver JW, Ross P, Fitzgerald RH: Demonstration of radiation nephritis by computed tomography. Comput Radiol 6:187, 1982.

289. Moore L, Curry NS, Jenrette JM: Computed tomography of acute radiation nephritis. Urol Radiol 8:89, 1986.

290. Desai A: Renal imaging after partial renal irradiation. Clin Nucl Med 7:113, 1982.

291. Madrazo A, Suzuki Y, Churg J: Radiation nephritis: Acute changes following high dose of radiation. Am J Pathol 54:507, 1969.

292. Madrazo A, Suzuki Y, Churg J: Radiation nephritis: Chronic changes after high doses of radiation. Am J Pathol 61:37, 1970.

293. Madrazo A, Churg J: Radiation nephritis: Chronic changes following moderate doses of radiation. Lab Invest 34:283, 1976.

294. Cogan MG, Arieff AI: Radiation nephritis and intravascular coagulation. Clin Nephrol 10:74, 1978.

295. Juncos LI, Carrasco-Duenas S, Cornejo JC, et al: Longterm enalapril and hydrochlorothiazide in radiation nephritis. Nephron 64:249, 1993.

296. Luscher TF, Wanner C, Hauri D, et al: Curable renal parenchymatous hypertension: Current diagnosis and management. Cardiology 72(suppl):33, 1985.

297. Maisin JR: Chemical protection against long-term effects in mice exposed to supralethal doses of X rays. C R Seances Soc Biol Paris 176:68, 1982.

298. Coia LR, Hanks GE: Complications from large field intermediate dose infradiaphragmatic radiation: An analysis of the patterns of care outcome studies for Hodgkin's disease and seminoma. Int J Radiat Oncol Biol Phys 15:29, 1988.

299. Bucher A, Roald B: Cholesterol embolization after intravenous streptokinase therapy in acute myocardial infarction. Tidsskr Nor Laegeforen 113:1844, 1993.

300. Cross SS: How common is cholesterol embolism? J Clin Pathol 44:859, 1991.

301. Smith MC, Ghose MK, Henry AR: The clinical spectrum of renal cholesterol embolization. Am J Med 71:174, 1981.

302. Wilson DM, Salazer TL, Farkouh ME: Eosinophiluria in atheroembolic renal disease. Am J Med 91:186, 1991.

303. Preston RA, Stemmer CL, Materson BJ, et al: Renal biopsy in patients 65 years of age or older: An analysis of the results in 334 biopsies. J Am Geriatr Soc 38:669, 1990.

304. Herrick JB: Peculiar elongated and sickle-shaped red blood corpuscles in a case of severe anemia. Arch Intern Med 6:517, 1910.

305. Pauling R, Itano HA, Singer SJ, Wells IC: Sickle cell anemia: A molecular disease. Science 110:543, 1949.

306. Vichinsky E, Hurst D, Earles A, et al: Newborn screening for sickle cell disease: Effect on mortality. Pediatrics 81:749, 1988.

307. Ballas S, Smith E: Red blood cell changes during the evolution of the sickle cell painful crisis. Blood 79:2154, 1992.

308. Pitcock JA, Muirhead EE, Hatch FE, et al: Early renal changes in sickle cell anemia. Arch Pathol 90:403, 1970.

309. Bernstein JN, Whitten CF: A histological appraisal of the kidney and sickle cell anemia. Arch Pathol 70:407, 1960.

310. Elfenbein I, Patchefsky A, Schwartz AW, Weinstein AG: Pathology of the glomerulus and sickle cell anemia with and without the nephrotic syndrome. Am J Pathol 77:357, 1974.

311. Alleyene GAO, Statius van Eps LW, Addae SK, et al: The kidney in sickle cell anemia. Kidney Int 7:371, 1975.

312. Statius van Eps LW, Pinedo-Veels C, de Vries GH, de Koning J: Nature of the concentrating defect in sickle cell nephropathy. Lancet 1:450, 1970.

313. Abrahams C: Stereopathy of the renal papilla: A stereo microscopic autopsy. Hum Pathol 16:488, 1985.

314. Siegelman ES, Outwater E, Hanau CA, et al: Abdominal iron distribution in sickle cell disease: MR findings in transfusion and nontransfusion dependent patients. J Comput Assist Tomogr 18:63, 1994.

315. Hatch FE, Culbertson JW, Diggs LW: Nature of renal concentrating defect in sickle cell disease. J Clin Invest 46:336, 1967.

316. de Jong PE, Statius van Eps LW: Sickle cell nephropathy: New insights into its pathophysiology. Kidney Int 27:711, 1985.

317. Keitel HG, Thompson D, Itano HA: Hyposthenuria in sickle cell anemia: A reversible defect. J Clin Invest 35:998, 1956.

318. Levitt MF, Hauser AD, Levy MS, Polimeros D: The renal concentrating defect in sickle cell disease. Am J Med 29:611, 1960.

319. DeFronzo RA, Taufield PA, Black H, et al: Impaired renal tubular potassium secretion in sickle cell disease. Ann Intern Med 90:310, 1979.

320. Ho Ping Kong H, Alleyne GAO: Studies on acid excretion in adults with sickle-cell anemia. Clin Sci 45:505, 1971.

321. Bourke E: The kidney in sickle cell anemia. J Assoc Acad Minor Phys 3:41, 1992.

322. Allon M: Renal abnormalities in sickle cell disease. Arch Intern Med 150:501, 1990.

323. Allon M, Lawson L, Eckman JR, et al: Effects of nonsteroidal inflammatory drugs on renal function in sickle cell anemia. Kidney Int 34:500, 1988.

324. Chapman ZA, Reeder PS, Friedman IA, Baker LA: Gross hematuria in sickle cell trait and sickle cell hemoglobin C disease. Am J Med 19:773, 1955.

325. Lucas WM, Bullock WH: Hematuria in sickle cell disease. J Urol 83:733, 1960.

326. Harrow BR, Sloane JA, Liebman N: Roentgenologic demonstration of renal papillary necrosis in sickle-cell trait. N Engl J Med 268:969, 1963.

327. Pariser S, Katz A: Treatment of sickle cell trait hematuria with oral urea. J Urol 151:401, 1994.

328. Lund HG, Cordonnier JJ, Forbes KA: Gross hematuria in sickle cell disease. J Urol 71:151, 1954.

329. Kimmelstil P: Vascular occlusion and ischemic infarction in sickle cell disease. Am J Med Sci 216:11, 1948.

330. Femi-Pearse D, Odunjo EO: Renal cortical infarcts in sickle cell trait. Br Med J 3:34, 1968.

331. Miller WA, Peck D, Lowman RM: Perirenal hematoma in association with renal infarction in sickle cell trait. Radiology 92:351, 1969.

332. Miller RE, Hartley EC, Clark EC, Lupton CH: Sickle cell nephropathy. Ala J Med Sci 1:233, 1964.

333. Sickles EA, Korobkin M: Perirenal hematoma as a complication of renal infarction in sickle-cell trait. Am J Roentgenol 122:800, 1974.

334. Falk RJ, Scheinman J, Phillips G, et al: Prevalence and pathologic features of sickle cell nephropathy and response to inhibition of angiotensin-converting enzyme. N Engl J Med 326:910, 1992.

335. Bakir AA, Hathiwala SC, Ainis H, et al: Prognosis of the nephrotic syndrome in sickle cell glomerulopathy. A retrospective study. Am J Nephrol 7:110, 1987.

336. Pardo V, Kramer H, Levi D, Strauss J: Glomerular changes in patients with sickle cell disease and the nephrotic syndrome. Am J Pathol 70:4A, 1973.

337. Strauss J, Pardo V, Koss MM, et al: Nephropathy associated with sickle cell anemia: An autologous immune complex nephritis. Am J Med 58:382, 1975.

338. Miner DJ, Jorkasky DK, Perloff LJ, et al: Recurrent sickle cell nephropathy in a transplanted kidney. Am J Kidney Dis 10:306, 1987.

339. Barber WH, Deierhoi MH, Julian BA, et al: Renal transplantation in sickle cell anemia and sickle cell disease. Clin Transplant 1:169, 1987.

# 36

# The Kidney and Hypertension in Pregnancy

*Mark S. Paller*
*Thomas F. Ferris*

Nephrologists have long been interested in the care of pregnant women because preeclampsia, the most common cause of hypertension in pregnancy, causes renal disease. In addition, the extraordinary changes in cardiovascular and renal function that occur during pregnancy have fascinated clinical investigators. An appreciation of these dramatic changes in renal function and hemodynamics is needed in the care of the pregnant woman, and understanding changes in pregnancy gives insight into physiologic mechanisms in the nonpregnant state. This chapter covers the changes in cardiovascular and renal function during pregnancy with particular attention to the changes that occur with the development of hypertension and preeclampsia. Also, improvements in the care of women with underlying renal disease have resulted in more of these women becoming pregnant. The effect of pregnancy on the mother and fetus when underlying renal disease is present is examined.

## RENAL ANATOMY AND FUNCTION DURING PREGNANCY
### Anatomic Changes

The kidney increases 1 cm in length during pregnancy. This increase in renal size is due to an increase in renal vascular volume and capacity of the collecting system as well as to hypertrophy of the kidney. In experimental animals, the length of the proximal tubules of the kidney increased by 20% in the first trimester.[1] Kidney volume (excluding the renal pelvis) increased by up to 30% when it was assessed by ultrasonography in 24 pregnant women.[2] Kidney volume decreased to normal values within 1 week post partum.

A more remarkable change is the increased capacity of the dilated renal collecting system, also known as physiologic hydronephrosis of pregnancy. Hormonal influence is one likely cause of the dilatation of the urinary collecting system because it can be reproduced in animals by the administration of estrogen and progesterone and may be seen in women taking oral contraceptives.[3] Pregnancy also induces increased synthesis of prostaglandin $E_2$ ($PGE_2$), which inhibits ureteral peristalsis in dogs and may be responsible for ureteral hypomotility and distention in pregnant women as well.[4] In addition, mechanical obstruction can at times contribute to ureteral distention, particularly on the right side where intraureteral pressures are higher above than below the pelvic brim. Smooth muscle relaxation also contributes to an increased occurrence of vesicoureteral reflux during pregnancy.[5] Although dilatation of the renal pelvis and ureters begins in the first trimester, it may persist for as long as 12 weeks post partum.

## CARDIOVASCULAR AND RENAL PHYSIOLOGY IN PREGNANCY

### Blood Pressure

One of the most striking features of pregnancy is that blood pressure and peripheral vascular resistance fall soon after conception. Peripheral vasodilatation is evident in the palmar erythema and spider telangiectases that frequently develop during pregnancy. The fall in vascular resistance is thought to be due to increased synthesis of vasodilating prostaglandins, particularly prostacyclin (prostaglandin $I_2$, $PGI_2$), which causes resistance to circulating vasoconstrictors like angiotensin II and norepinephrine.

MacGillivray and co-workers[6] found in 226 primigravid women on their first visit to an obstetric clinic that blood pressure was 103 ± 11 mm Hg systolic and 56 ± 10 mm Hg diastolic sitting and 113 ± 10 mm Hg systolic and 57 ± 10 mm Hg diastolic supine. Although a rise in both systolic and diastolic pressures occurs after the 28th week of gestation, blood pressure at term remained 109 ± 12 mm Hg systolic and 69 ± 9 mm Hg diastolic sitting and 116 ± 10 mm Hg systolic and 71 ± 12 mm Hg diastolic supine.

### Cardiac Output

Cardiac output increases in the first trimester of pregnancy, reaching a maximum of 30% to 40% above the nonpregnant level by the 24th week of gestation.[7] In spite of the rise in cardiac output, blood pressure falls because of the decrease in vascular resistance. When hypertension occurs in pregnancy, cardiac output tends to fall in response to reflex activation of the parasympathetic nervous system but usually remains higher than in the nonpregnant state.[8]

### Blood Volume

Blood volume increases approximately 50% in pregnancy beginning in the first trimester with a rise in both plasma volume and red blood cell volume. A greater increase in plasma than in red blood cell volume causes the "physiologic anemia" of pregnancy. Expansion of maternal extracellular volume continues throughout pregnancy with a cumulative $Na^+$ retention of between 500 and 900 mEq.[9] $Na^+$ retention proceeds at the rate of approximately 20 to 30 mEq/wk, which results in a mean weight gain of 12.5 kg. The major stimulus for the kidney to retain $Na^+$ is the decrease in peripheral vascular resistance, a recognized stimulus for $Na^+$ retention. When pregnant baboons were studied serially with Swan-Ganz catheters from the onset of pregnancy, decreases in right atrial, systemic, and pulmonary vascular resistance were found by the fourth week of gestation.[10] Plasma volume was not observed to be expanded until 8 weeks later.

The expanded extracellular volume may cause edema, which is present in 35% to 83% of healthy pregnant women, the frequency depending on the effort made to detect it.[11] Edema is benign because pregnant women with edema have fewer infants of low birth weight, and there is no association of edema with increased perinatal mortality or poor fetal development.[12] In contrast, inadequate maternal weight gain is associated with increased frequency of low birth weight and stillbirth. The edema in pregnancy is usually localized to the legs, whereas involvement of the face and hands with an angioneurotic appearance is more characteristic of preeclampsia. In late pregnancy, other factors contributing to leg edema may be compression of the inferior vena cava by the enlarged uterus and a reduction in colloid osmotic pressure. Limiting the time a pregnant woman spends standing and sleeping in a lateral recumbent position usually minimizes the edema.

### Renal Blood Flow and Glomerular Filtration Rate

Early in pregnancy, substantial increases in renal blood flow occur (Fig. 36–1). In one case studied prospectively, renal plasma flow had increased 45% by the ninth week of pregnancy.[13] When renal plasma flow has been estimated from $p$-aminohippuric acid clearance studies, the mean renal plasma flow was 809 mL/min in the first trimester, 695 mL/min in the last 10 weeks of pregnancy, and 482 mL/min after delivery.[13–17] The increase in renal blood flow is caused by an increase in cardiac output and a decrease in renal vascular resistance. The increase in cardiac output is probably less important than renal vasodilatation because cardiac output, which increases approximately 40%, does not increase blood flow uniformly to all regional beds. In contrast to the large increase in renal blood flow, there is no increase in cerebral or hepatic blood flow during pregnancy.

Studies in pregnant rats, in which precise micropuncture determinations of glomerular filtration rate (GFR) and renal

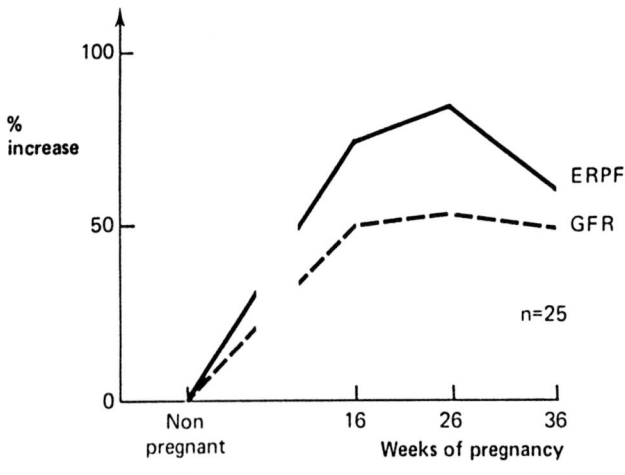

**Figure 36–1.** Effect of pregnancy on glomerular filtration rate (GFR) and effective renal plasma flow (ERPF). (From Davison JM: Overview: Kidney function in pregnant women. Am J Kidney Dis 9:248, 1987.)

blood flow can be performed, have demonstrated proportional reductions in afferent and efferent arteriolar resistance causing the decrease in renal vascular resistance and the increase in renal blood flow.[18] Conscious, chronically instrumented rats demonstrate similar changes in GFR and renal plasma flow in midpregnancy, averaging 26% and 20%, respectively.[19] Estimates of renal vascular resistance have suggested a 50% decrease in renal vascular resistance by the end of the first trimester of pregnancy.

Despite significant renal vasodilatation, the renal response to both volume expansion and hemorrhage is maintained in pregnant rats and rabbits.[20–22] Tubuloglomerular feedback activity is also as vigorous in pregnant rats as in nonpregnant rats.[23] These renal responses suggest that the kidneys react to and sense the expanded plasma volume normally. In addition, pregnant rats retain the ability to respond to an amino acid infusion with a further increase in renal blood flow and GFR proportionately as great as that in nonpregnant rats.[24]

The cause of pregnancy-induced renal vasodilatation is not known. Pregnancy results in large increases in the urinary excretion of $PGE_2$ and $PGI_2$.[25–28] Exogenous administration of $PGE_2$ and $PGI_2$ results in renal vasodilatation and an increase in renal blood flow. However, several investigators demonstrated that the increase in renal blood flow in pregnant rats was not reversed by the administration of cyclooxygenase inhibitors, which prevents synthesis of all prostaglandins, both vasodilators and vasoconstrictors.[29, 30] Mechanisms other than the production of prostaglandins may contribute to renal vasodilatation during pregnancy. Prolactin may be a hormonal mediator of renal vasodilatation because the pattern of prolactin excretion during pregnancy parallels that of renal blood flow. When rats were made pseudopregnant by prolactin injection, they developed an increase in GFR and renal blood flow similar to that seen in early pregnancy.[31, 32] Hyperprolactinemia can also induce renal vasodilatation and an increase in renal blood flow in male rats.[33] However, the ability of prolactin to stimulate renal blood flow and GFR has not been universally observed.[34] Pseudopregnancy, like prolactin administration, stimulates renal $PGE_2$ production similar to that observed during true pregnancy.[35] Thus, the renal vasodilatory effects of prolactin could be mediated through increased renal prostaglandin synthesis.

The most important consequence of the increase in renal blood flow during pregnancy is an increase in glomerular filtration. The pattern of the change in GFR is similar to that observed for renal blood flow, with an early increase in GFR by approximately 45%. GFR determinations by inulin clearance revealed a mean GFR of 96 mL/min in nonpregnant women that increased to 143 mL/min in the first trimester of pregnancy.[17] Bucht and Werko[36] reported that inulin clearance increased from 122 ± 24 to 170 ± 23 mL/min from the 8th to the 32nd week of pregnancy. Unlike renal plasma flow, which tends to decrease toward nonpregnant levels in the last few weeks of pregnancy, GFR remains elevated until term (see Fig. 36–1). The level of dietary protein correlates positively with GFR in pregnancy, as it does in the nonpregnant state.[37]

Micropuncture studies of pregnant rats suggest that the increase in GFR is solely a consequence of the increase in renal blood flow.[38] Comparison of superficial nephron single-nephron GFR and glomerular plasma flow rate ($Q_A$) with whole kidney values revealed proportional increases, which suggests that the renal vasodilatation was uniformly distributed throughout the kidney.[38] When Baylis[38] studied euvolemic Munich-Wistar rats on day 12 of a 21-day gestation, she found these rats to be in filtration pressure equilibrium. Values for mean glomerular hydraulic pressure gradient ($\Delta P$) and afferent and efferent arteriolar oncotic pressure were no different from those measured in nonpregnant rats. There were also no major changes in the glomerular capillary ultrafiltration coefficient $K_f$ because the estimated minimal value was similar in gravid and virgin rats.[38] At some disagreement with these findings are those of Dal Canton and colleagues,[39] who studied hydropenic, 15-day-pregnant Munich-Wistar rats. In their studies, the increase in GFR was dependent on a small increase in glomerular capillary hydraulic pressure as well as an increase in glomerular plasma flow. These rats were in filtration pressure disequilibrium and had a decrease in mean $K_f$ of 14%. A possible explanation for these discrepant results is that the former study was performed in euvolemic rats whereas the latter was performed in hydropenic rats and that there were substantial differences in volume status of these animals. In either case, however, the major determinant of the pregnancy-induced increase in GFR is an increase in renal blood flow.

The practical consequences of these changes in renal blood flow and GFR are that normal laboratory values change in the healthy pregnant woman. For example, blood urea nitrogen values in normal pregnancy average 8.7 ± 1.5 mg/dL, and serum creatinine levels average 0.46 ± 0.13 mg/dL.[13]

## The Renin-Angiotensin-Aldosterone System in Pregnancy

The level of plasma angiotensin II is dependent on several factors: the renin concentration in plasma, the concentration of its substrate angiotensinogen, the activity of the converting enzyme, and tissue angiotensinase activity. Under most circumstances, the concentration of renin in plasma is the most important determinant of plasma angiotensin II concentration, but in pregnancy, there is an increase in both plasma renin and angiotensinogen. There is a threefold to fourfold increase in angiotensinogen concentration, and plasma renin concentration is approximately eight times higher than in nonpregnant women.[40–43] With the combined rise in renin and substrate concentration, plasma renin activity, which measures the amount of angiotensin generated with incubation of plasma, is approximately 15 times higher than in nonpregnant women.

The paradox of pregnancy is that high renin secretion occurs during expansion of the extracellular volume and increased delivery of filtered $Na^+$ to the distal tubule, both of which should cause renin secretion to fall by baroreceptor and macula densa mechanisms. The increased renin secretion is probably largely due to the increase in $PGI_2$ synthesis, which directly increases renal renin secretion and causes resistance to angiotensin II in the peripheral vasculature. The suggestion that the elevated renin secretion in pregnancy is due to a salt-losing tendency of pregnancy caused by increased GFR and elevated progesterone secretion, which acts as an antagonist to aldosterone at the renal tubule, has not proved to be the case; a 300 mEq sodium intake for 7 days, intravenous saline, or prolonged mineralocorticoid administration does not suppress renin or aldosterone secretion to the levels seen in nonpregnant subjects.[26] The elevation in plasma angiotensin II in pregnancy maintains arterial blood pressure, because angiotensin blockade with saralasin or an angiotensin I–converting enzyme inhibitor causes a reduction in arterial pressure.[26]

The molecular precursor of renin, prorenin, circulates in plasma and constitutes 80% to 90% of potential human plasma renin activity and is elevated throughout pregnancy.[40, 41] Prorenin is converted to active renin by acid, storage in the cold, and incubation with proteolytic enzymes. The role of prorenin except as a precursor of renin is unknown because there is no evidence of conversion of plasma prorenin to renin under physiologic conditions.[40, 44, 45] The uterus, placenta, and ovaries synthesize prorenin in high concentration, and release of prorenin from the uterus occurs with reduction in uterine blood flow.[46, 47]

Uterine prorenin may function as a local hormone controlling blood flow to the uterus and placenta by maintaining a high uterine angiotensin II concentration. Unlike its vasoconstrictor effect on most vascular beds, angiotensin II increases uterine blood flow in the pregnant dog, rabbit, and monkey.[48, 49] Because angiotensin II increases uterine $PGE_2$ synthesis, the increase in blood flow with angiotensin may be due to concomitant increase in prostaglandin synthesis. Sealey and co-workers[50] suggested that the presence of prorenin in the afferent arteriole of the kidney and in the uterus might result in tachyphylaxis to angiotensin II because a high local concentration of angiotensin II would cause resistance to circulating angiotensin II. It is interesting that the sheep uterus does not contain prorenin, and angiotensin II does not increase uterine blood flow in that species.[51, 52]

Angiotensin II is also an angiogenesis factor, inducing new blood vessel growth in experimental circumstances.[53] Uterine prorenin may be involved in the extensive neovascularization that occurs in the uterus and placenta during pregnancy. Inhibitors of both prostaglandin and angiotensin II synthesis decrease uterine blood flow in pregnant rabbits.[48, 54, 55] Thus, uterine prostaglandin synthesis is dependent not only on the cyclooxygenase enzyme necessary for prostaglandin synthesis but also on the angiotensin-coverting enzyme.

## Prostaglandin Synthesis in Pregnancy

Pregnancy is associated with increase in both $PGI_2$ and thromboxane synthesis. Placental tissues are capable of generating $PGI_2$, and the umbilical artery has a 10- to 100-fold greater capacity to synthesize $PGI_2$ than other arteries do.[56–60] A reduction in $PGI_2$ synthesis has been demonstrated in umbilical artery specimens from women with preeclampsia.[57–60] The major urinary metabolite of $PGI_2$, 2,3-dinor-6-keto-$PGF_{1\alpha}$, was found by Fitzgerald and co-

workers[61] to be 1321 ± 160 ng/g creatinine in pregnant women compared with 254 ± 31 ng/g creatinine in nonpregnant women. Thromboxane synthesis was also elevated with increased urinary excretion of 2,3-dinor-thromboxane $B_2$ and 11-dehydro-thromboxane $B_2$ in the last trimester.[62]

The stimulus for the increase in prostaglandin synthesis during pregnancy is not known. In pregnant animals, resistance to angiotensin II, norepinephrine, and arginine vasopressin occurs early in pregnancy and has been found to be due to increased synthesis of prostaglandins.[35, 63] Pseudopregnancy, induced by mating female rats with sterile males, increases urinary $PGE_2$ excretion for up to 10 days with a fall in peripheral vascular resistance and resistance to angiotensin II and norepinephrine.[35] The findings in pseudopregnancy indicate that conception is not needed to increase prostaglandin synthesis and suggest that a hormonal change triggered by the central nervous system occurs. It is curious that pregnancy has many similarities to Bartter syndrome, a disorder characterized by insensitivity to angiotensin II, high plasma renin and angiotensin II concentrations, low to normal blood pressure, and increased prostaglandin synthesis.[64] In both conditions, prostaglandin synthesis inhibitors increase angiotensin II sensitivity and reduce renin secretion.[64, 65]

## Renal Tubule Function

Pregnancy is the most striking example in humans of the need for glomerular tubule balance to prevent extraordinary losses of $Na^+$. A 50% increase in GFR during pregnancy necessitates an equal increase in $Na^+$ reabsorption by the renal tubules. For an $Na^+$ concentration of 140 mEq/L in glomerular filtrate and a GFR of 100 mL/min, the daily filtered $Na^+$ equals 140 mEq/L × 0.1 L/min × 1440 min/d, or 20,160 mEq. An increase of 50% in GFR increases daily $Na^+$ filtration to 30,240 mEq, which necessitates that the renal tubules absorb 10,080 mEq more $Na^+$ than in the nonpregnant state to avoid $Na^+$ wasting. Most of the increase in $Na^+$ reabsorption occurs in the proximal tubule, but all segments of the nephron are involved. Physical factors such as capillary hydraulic pressure and oncotic pressure in the renal interstitial space alter proximal $Na^+$ reabsorption, whereas many hormonal factors are involved in distal portions of the nephron.

Most evidence suggests that pregnant women maintain $Na^+$ balance normally when sodium intake is either increased or decreased. With a sodium intake of 10 mEq, pregnant women reduced urinary $Na^+$ excretion as readily as nonpregnant women did without excessive weight loss.[25] Conversely, when pregnant women had a sodium intake of 300 mEq, they came into balance after 4 days, and the excretion of a short-term intravenous $Na^+$ load was as rapid in pregnant as in nonpregnant women.[25, 66] Thus, despite changes in extracellular fluid volume and the renal demands of increased $Na^+$ reabsorption, $Na^+$ balance is maintained in a normal manner.

Pregnant women also maintain normal water balance and retain the ability to produce a maximally concentrated and maximally dilute urine. In a study of 75 normotensive pregnant women, the maximal urine osmolality after water deprivation was 900 mOsm/kg $H_2O$, a value not different from that in nonpregnant women.[67] The ability to concentrate the urine is surprising because pregnant women have two features that would limit urine concentrating ability—an increase in renal blood flow and increased renal production of $PGE_2$, an antagonist of arginine vasopressin in the collecting tubule. Renal diluting ability is also normal during pregnancy. After a water load, urine osmolalities in pregnant women range between 25 and 88 mOsm/kg $H_2O$, values similar to those observed in nonpregnant women.[68] Twenty-four–hour urine volumes tend to be similar in nonpregnant and pregnant women early and late in pregnancy, although some studies have found an increase in urine volume of up to 25% in midpregnancy.[69, 70] Because there is no abnormality in renal water handling, an increase in urine volume would suggest an increase in water intake mediated by increased thirst.

Despite unaltered renal water handling, pregnant women have a decrease in serum $Na^+$ of approximately 5 mEq/L and a decrease in plasma osmolality of approximately 10 mOsm/kg $H_2O$.[71] Pregnant women have a decrease in the osmotic threshold for vasopressin secretion, although the sensitivity for vasopressin release is not altered[72] (Fig. 36–2). Nonpregnant women secrete vasopressin when plasma osmolality exceeds 285 mOsm/kg $H_2O$, whereas pregnant women secrete vasopressin when plasma osmolality exceeds 276 to 278 mOsm/kg $H_2O$.[69, 70] They respond in a

quantitatively normal manner to increases or limitations in water availability except that their set-point is reduced by approximately 10 mOsm/kg $H_2O$. Nonosmotic release of vasopressin is not altered by pregnancy in either rats or women.[73, 74]

Although a change in the osmotic threshold for vasopressin release is one factor that contributes to the hypo-osmolality in pregnancy, other factors also exist because pregnant Brattleboro rats, which have congenital lack of vasopressin, also develop hypo-osmolality.[75] To maintain hypo-osmolality, thirst would also have to be altered. Whereas nonpregnant women have an osmotic thirst threshold (derived from analogue scales relating the desire to drink water to plasma osmolality) of 290 mOsm/kg $H_2O$ and perceive thirst (the conscious desire to drink) at 298 mOsm/kg $H_2O$, pregnant women have an osmotic thirst threshold of 280 mOsm/kg $H_2O$ and perceive thirst at 288 mOsm/kg $H_2O$.[70] The decrease in thirst threshold may actually precede the change in threshold for vasopressin release. Thirst threshold reaches its minimal value within 5 to 8 weeks of pregnancy, whereas the decreased threshold for vasopressin release reaches its minimum at 10 to 12 weeks of gestation.

The mechanism of the resetting of thirst and of vasopressin osmoreceptors is not entirely clear, but changes in the concentration of chorionic gonadotropin may be involved. Infusion of human chorionic gonadotropin into nonpregnant

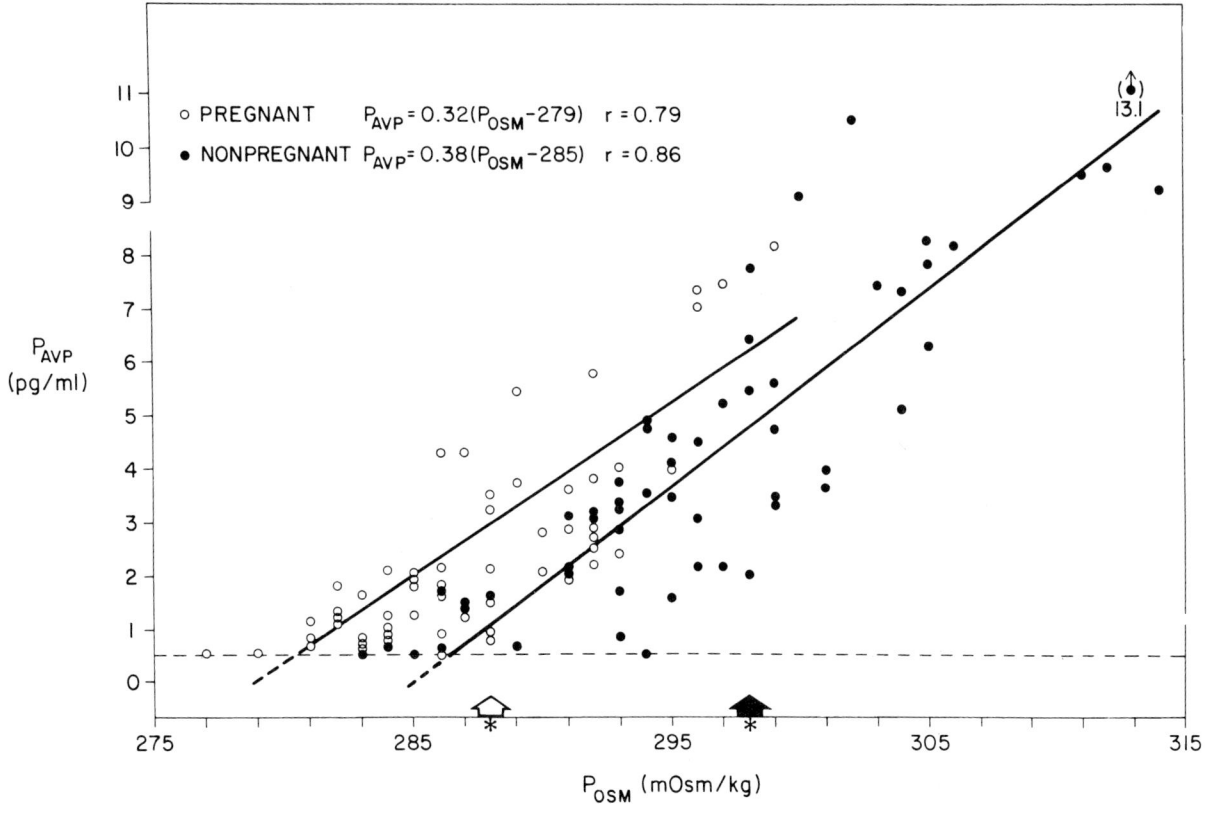

**Figure 36–2.** Relationship between $P_{osm}$ and $P_{AVP}$ when osmolality was altered by infusion of 5% saline in pregnant and nonpregnant women. Arrows represent thirst thresholds. (From Davison JM, Gilmore EA, Durr J, et al. Altered osmotic thresholds for vasopressin secretion and thirst in human pregnancy. Am J Physiol 246:F105, 1984.)

women lowered the osmotic thresholds for vasopressin release and thirst by 3 and 4 mOsm/kg $H_2O$, respectively.[70] In addition, in a patient with a hydatidiform mole and elevated serum chorionic gonadotropin level, abnormalities in the threshold for vasopressin release and thirst paralleled serum chorionic gonadotropin levels.[70] Although pregnant rats show similar changes in resetting of osmotic thresholds, pseudopregnant rats do not manifest these changes.[76] This contrasts to the previously cited findings of alterations in renal blood flow, GFR, and renal prostaglandin production that have been seen in pseudopregnant as well as in pregnant rats.[31, 32] Thus, the fetal-placental unit is apparently not necessary to induce changes in renal hemodynamics but is a necessary component of the osmoregulatory changes of pregnancy.

$K^+$ metabolism during pregnancy is generally unchanged, although the cumulative retention of approximately 350 mEq of $K^+$ is necessary for fetal-placental development as well as for expansion of maternal red blood cell mass.[9] Although plasma aldosterone levels are elevated in pregnancy, renal $K^+$ wasting does not occur.[25, 77, 78] This may be because elevated plasma progesterone in pregnancy inhibits the kaliuretic effect of mineralocorticoids.[79] On the other hand, pregnant women receiving high doses of the mineralocorticoid deoxycorticosterone acetate develop $Na^+$ retention.[78] Although some women with primary hyperaldosteronism may have a reversal of $K^+$ wasting, this is not a universal finding, and hypertension may remain severe during pregnancy.[80-83]

An interesting consequence of the pregnancy-induced antagonism of mineralocorticoid action is the occasional unmasking of otherwise insignificant defects in $K^+$ excretion. Two women with sickle cell anemia, a disease known to occasionally produce hyperkalemia by defective renal $K^+$ excretion, developed life-threatening hyperkalemia during pregnancy.[84] Other conditions that potentially predispose to the development of hyperkalemia during pregnancy include diabetes mellitus, renal insufficiency, and use of β-adrenergic antagonists. However, although these cases are interesting in terms of their pathophysiology, they are rare.

Pregnancy causes a compensated respiratory alkalosis. Arterial $PCO_2$ decreases by approximately 10 mm Hg, and arterial pH increases slightly to 7.44.[85, 86] Progesterone is a major factor in stimulating the respiratory center of the central nervous system.[87] Chronic respiratory alkalosis is accompanied by a decrease in plasma $HCO_3^-$ to 18 to 20 mEq/L. This reduction in total buffering capacity predisposes pregnant women to more severe acidosis with the development of either ketoacidosis or lactic acidosis. On the other hand, acid excretion by the kidney is unchanged during pregnancy. After the administration of an acid (ammonium chloride) load, pregnant women excreted normal amounts of both titratable acid and $NH_4^+$.[88]

The changes in renal hemodynamics during pregnancy also result in changes in the excretion of uric acid, glucose, and amino acids. Urate synthesis remains constant during pregnancy, whereas urate clearance increases, resulting in a decrease in serum uric acid to between 2.5 and 4 mg/dL early in pregnancy.[89] Late in pregnancy, uric acid clearance decreases in parallel with renal blood flow so that the serum uric acid level rises.

Glucosuria is common during pregnancy. The combination of an increase in the filtered load of glucose and a tendency to less efficient tubule reabsorption of glucose is the cause of glucosuria. Women with the least efficient tubule glucose reabsorption (determined before pregnancy) are the ones who develop glucosuria during pregnancy.[90-92]

The urinary excretion of some, but not all, amino acids is increased with diminished fractional amino acid reabsorption. In particular, excretion of glycine, histidine, threonine, serine, and alanine is increased.[93-95]

# HYPERTENSION AND PREECLAMPSIA

Hypertension is the most common medical complication of pregnancy; blood pressure of 140/90 mm Hg or higher occurs in approximately 10% of pregnant women. It has a bimodal frequency, being more common in young women in their first pregnancy and in older multiparous women. A rise in blood pressure in pregnancy virtually always indicates the presence of one of four conditions: 1) preeclampsia (toxemia), 2) preeclampsia superimposed on chronic hypertension or renal disease, 3) chronic essential hypertension, or 4) gestational hypertension.

The decrease in blood pressure observed in pregnancy makes the upper limit of normal blood pressure in nonpregnant women, 140/90 mm Hg, of little significance. The upper limit of blood pressure is determined in the nonpregnant population on epidemiologic evidence of subsequent development of vascular disease that has no relevance in pregnancy, in which hypertension is short-lived and virtually always disappears post partum. One relevant criterion is the level of blood pressure that adversely affects fetal survival. Data from a study of more than 24,000 pregnancies demonstrated that blood pressure in excess of 125/75 mm Hg before the 32nd week of gestation and 125/85 mm Hg thereafter was associated with a significant increase in fetal risk[96] (Fig. 36–3). In another report of 15,000 pregnant women, perinatal mortality rate rose progressively with each 5 mm Hg rise in mean arterial blood pressure (MAP), and those with MAP of 90 mm Hg or more during the second trimester had a higher risk of stillbirth, fetal growth retardation, and progression to preeclampsia.[97] A trend toward increased perinatal mortality is found when MAP is greater than 82 mm Hg at midpregnancy or greater than 92 mm Hg at the beginning of the third trimester. Because a blood pressure of 120/80 mm Hg indicates an MAP of 93 mm Hg, one can appreciate how values of blood pressure must be viewed differently in pregnancy.

Blood pressure in early pregnancy has value in detecting women in whom preeclampsia will ultimately develop in late pregnancy. The frequency of preeclampsia increases linearly with increase in systolic pressure in the first trimester from 100 to 134 mm Hg, and preeclampsia develops in late pregnancy in one third of women with MAP greater than 90 mm Hg in the second trimester, compared with only 2% of those with MAP less than 90 mm Hg.[98, 99] Blood pressure considered normal in nonpregnant women must be of concern in pregnancy.

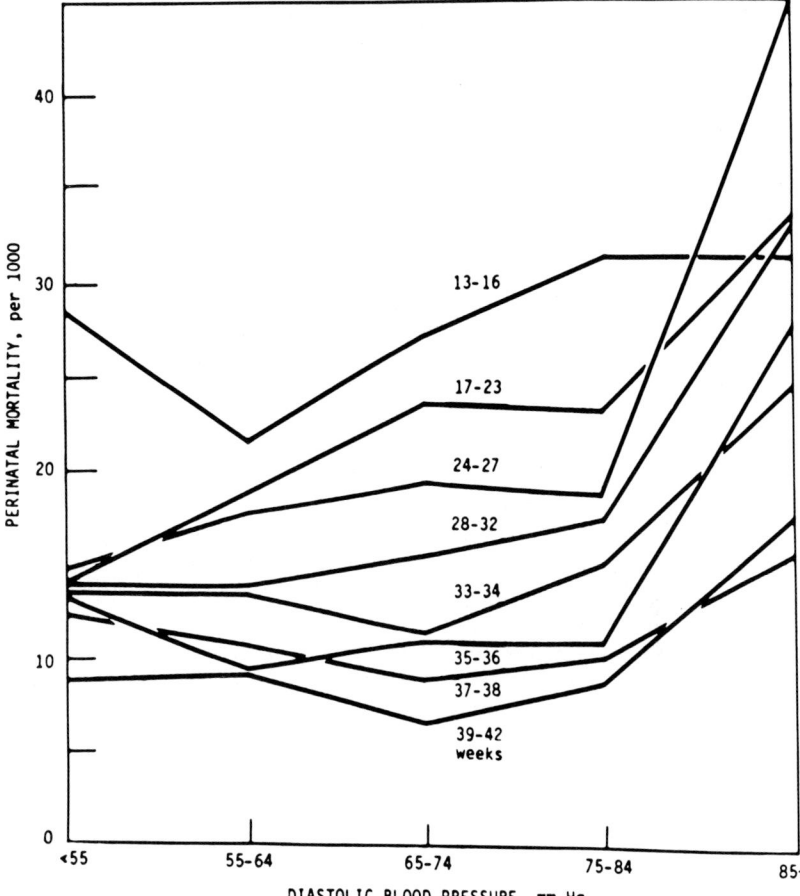

**Figure 36–3.** Relationship between blood pressure and perinatal mortality. Diastolic blood pressure is grouped by gestational age epochs. Note the uniformly increased mortality associated with pressures exceeding 84 mm Hg. (From Friedman EA, Neff RK: Pregnancy Hypertension: A Systemic Evaluation of Clinical Diagnostic Criteria. PSG Publishing, Littleton, MA, 1977, p 64. By permission of Mosby–Year Book, Inc.)

## Etiology and Pathogenesis of Preeclampsia

The term preeclampsia, which implies that eclampsia is the ultimate manifestation of the disease, is commonly used to describe the disease unique to pregnancy manifested by hypertension and multiple organ involvement. Historically, convulsions have been the most dramatic expression of the disease, but life-threatening preeclampsia may occur without seizures. The disease is not unique to humans; gorillas in the wild and in captivity may have convulsions in late pregnancy, and reducing uterine blood flow in monkeys causes hypertension with glomerular disease similar to preeclampsia.[100, 101]

The hypertension that develops with preeclampsia is caused by an increase in peripheral vascular resistance. Cardiac output measurements are variable, depending on the level of blood pressure, but renal blood flow and GFR fall 62% to 84%.[8] With preeclampsia, plasma urate rises, frequently before a measurable rise in the serum creatinine or urea nitrogen level.[89, 102, 103] Because there is no increase in urate production in preeclampsia, hyperuricemia indicates decreased renal clearance. Urate clearance is more dependent on plasma flow to the tubule secretory site than on glomerular filtration. When the filtration fraction increases (i.e., renal plasma flow is diminished more than GFR), urate clearance decreases.[104] Hyperuricemia occurs

with essential hypertension and volume depletion, both of which are associated with high filtration fraction.[105, 106] If increased sensitivity of the efferent arteriole to angiotensin II occurs in preeclampsia, a similar change in renal hemodynamics would occur. Measurements of filtration fraction in preeclampsia have been difficult because of small urine volumes. The decrease in urate clearance that occurs with volume depletion can be corrected by increasing sodium intake, whereas in preeclampsia, saline loading does not increase urate clearance.[107, 108] Hyperuricemia is a valuable marker to differentiate preeclampsia from other causes of hypertension in pregnancy when a decrease in urate clearance does not occur. A serum urate level greater than 5.5 mg/100 mL is a strong indicator of the presence of preeclampsia, and when it exceeds 6.0 mg/100 mL, the disease is usually severe. Hyperuricemia correlates well with the clinical severity of preeclampsia, with the histologic lesion found on renal biopsy, and with fetal survival.[103]

The majority of women with preeclampsia have sudden weight gain with development of edema, particularly of the face and upper extremities. The edema of preeclampsia has similarities to angioneurotic edema and probably has a different etiology from the common peripheral edema in pregnancy. There is evidence of a change in capillary permeability to protein in preeclampsia with increased disappearance of Evans blue dye and higher concentration of protein in edema fluid.[109–111] Although salt retention in pregnancy does not increase blood pressure, swelling with an increase in blood pressure suggests preeclampsia. Salt retention in the presence of hypertension increases blood pressure through several mechanisms including increasing sensitivity to angiotensin and altering arteriolar $Na^+$ and $Ca^{2+}$ concentration. It is imperative for physicians to appreciate the difference between benign peripheral edema and edema with a rise in blood pressure, which heralds the onset of preeclampsia.

$Na^+$ retention with preeclampsia is probably caused by the reduction in GFR that occurs. The urinary $Ca^{2+}$ level also falls, consistent with the reduction in GFR.[112, 113] In spite of $Na^+$ retention, plasma volume in preeclampsia is frequently, although not always, diminished when compared with that in normotensive pregnancy.[114] In all hypertension, extracellular volume is preferentially shifted from the vascular to the interstitial space because of loss of venous capacitance and increase in capillary hydraulic pressure. Severe volume depletion may occur with renal artery stenosis, pheochromocytoma, and malignant hypertension, and mild volume contraction is present in essential hypertension.[115, 116] The average contraction of plasma volume in preeclampsia is approximately 9%, which is the same as that reported in nonpregnant patients with essential hypertension.[116] However, unlike in other hypertensive states, the volume contraction in preeclampsia may precede the onset of hypertension, and plasma volume contraction correlates better with stillbirths and small-for-gestational-age infants than the severity of hypertension does.[108, 117] If plasma volume expansion in pregnancy is due to vasodilatation, diminished plasma volume may be due to decreased $PGI_2$ synthesis. An intriguing feature of preeclampsia is the greater antagonism to insulin that occurs compared with normal pregnancy.[118] Because insulin antagonism may occur with essential hypertension, the effect of insulin resistance on endothelial cell function is of obvious importance. It is known that hyperglycemia reduces endothelial cell $PGI_2$ synthesis and promotes generation of vasoconstrictor prostanoids in rabbit aortas.[119, 120] It is of interest that diabetic patients do not synthesize $PGI_2$ as well as nondiabetic patients do, and diabetic women have less volume expansion during pregnancy.[119, 120] Increased urinary thromboxane excretion occurs in diabetic patients, which may also be a factor in the increased incidence of preeclampsia in diabetic women.[121]

The decrease in plasma volume with preeclampsia should not be treated with volume expansion, which can lead to pulmonary edema. Although plasma volume is reduced, preeclampsia is accompanied by increased total exchangeable $Na^+$, normal venous pressure, and either a normal or a high pulmonary capillary wedge pressure.[122] When pulmonary edema occurs in women with preeclampsia, it is usually the result of administration of large volumes of fluid before and during delivery.[123] Plasma oncotic pressure falls after delivery because of rapid mobilization of fluid from the interstitial space and, when combined with elevated pulmonary wedge pressure, can also be a factor leading to pulmonary edema.[124]

There is evidence of a generalized endothelial cell dysfunction in preeclampsia with not only a fall in $PGI_2$ synthesis but also an increase in plasma cellular fibronectin and activation of von Willebrand factor, two proteins synthesized by endothelial cells.[125–128] Endothelin, a potent peptide synthesized in the endothelium with vasoconstricting and platelet-aggregating properties, is a potential factor in preeclampsia. However, measurements of plasma endothelin in preeclampsia have been conflicting.[129–134] As for all autacoids, plasma endothelin levels do not necessarily reflect concentration at the site of synthesis. The endothelium-derived vasodilating factor nitric oxide normally plays a role in regulating vascular resistance, and decreased synthesis of endothelium-derived relaxing factor in response to bradykinin has been demonstrated in umbilical vessels from women with preeclampsia.[135] Pregnant women and animals have decreased plasma L-arginine resulting, in part, from increased renal excretion of L-arginine during pregnancy. This may reduce the capacity of endothelial cells to synthesize nitric oxide during pregnancy and play a role in the propensity of pregnant animals to develop the Shwartzman reaction after administration of endotoxin.[135a]

Because a balance exists in pregnancy between the increased synthesis in platelets of thromboxane and endothelial cell synthesis of $PGI_2$, the rise in peripheral vascular resistance causing hypertension may be due to an imbalance in synthesis of these counteracting prostaglandins. Consistent with this hypothesis is the finding that in contrast to the fall in urinary $PGI_2$ metabolites with preeclampsia, urinary excretion of thromboxane metabolites increases.[136]

Serum from preeclamptic women demonstrates several effects on cultured endothelial cells. A cytotoxic effect occurs as evidenced by radioactive chromate release from endothelial cells, but the cells maintain viability and show no defect in attachment, spreading behavior, or proliferation during incubation. Also, preeclamptic serum reduces endothelin and $PGI_2$ synthesis and causes lipid accumulation within the cells similar to changes noted in glomerular and myocardial endothelial cells in preeclampsia.[125, 137, 138] The factor in preeclamptic sera causing these changes is unknown but may be released from the uterus and placenta in response to ischemia.

Because the uterus and placenta are rich sources of prorenin, which in experimental animals is released into the circulation with uterine hypoperfusion, one might speculate about its potential role in preeclampsia.[47, 48] There is evidence in diabetic patients that an elevated plasma prorenin level is associated with diabetic nephropathy and retinopathy.[139] Although plasma prorenin level does not increase with the development of preeclampsia, it does not fall as does plasma renin.[40] Plasma prorenin is elevated in the ovarian hyperstimulation syndrome, which is induced by gonadotropin administration and which has some similarities to preeclampsia. Capillary permeability to protein with ascites, pleural effusion, and severe volume depletion occurs, and coagulation abnormalities, hepatic failure, respiratory distress, and renal failure may also be features of the syndrome.[140] These patients have extraordinary concentration of prorenin in ascitic fluid compared with the low concentration found in ascites from other causes.[141]

The presence of a high concentration of prorenin in the uterus makes renin release an attractive hypothesis in causing hypertension, but plasma renin, angiotensin II, and aldosterone levels fall with the development of preeclampsia.

However, the concomitant reduction in $PGI_2$ synthesis increases sensitivity to angiotensin II, and pregnancy-associated insensitivity to angiotensin and norepinephrine disappears with the development of preeclampsia. A fall in urinary 6-keto-$PGF_{1\alpha}$ precedes the development of hypertension coinciding with the increased sensitivity to angiotensin II, which can also be demonstrated before hypertension.[61] Angiotensin insensitivity in human pregnancy is detectable as early as the 10th week of gestation, with a decrease occurring as early as the 18th week in women in whom preeclampsia is destined to develop. In contrast, normotensive women maintain insensitivity to angiotensin throughout pregnancy, with a slight increase in sensitivity after the 32nd week[142] (Fig. 36–4).

Increased sensitivity to angiotensin is probably the cause of the positive rollover test, in which pregnant women in whom preeclampsia ultimately develops are found to have an excessive rise in blood pressure when they turn from the lateral recumbent to a supine position.[143] Lying supine in pregnancy compresses the inferior vena cava and reduces cardiac output. The consequent fall in renal blood flow would increase renin secretion and serve as an endogenous test of angiotensin sensitivity. Although the clinical reliability of the test as a predictor of preeclampsia has not been validated in all studies, it probably does reflect angiotensin II sensitivity.

The fall in renin and aldosterone secretion with preeclampsia could be caused by decreased renal prostaglandin synthesis because a similar response occurs after administration of prostaglandin-inhibiting drugs in the nonpregnant patient. A decrease in $PGI_2$ synthesis in endothelial cells without concomitant reduction in thromboxane synthesis in platelets would predispose to widespread platelet aggregation and intravascular clotting. Urinary excretion of thromboxane metabolites increases in preeclampsia, which probably reflects platelet aggregation because it can be partially prevented with aspirin.[62] Several postpartum complications, such as renal failure, cardiomyopathy, and pituitary failure, may be caused by endothelial dysfunction with small-vessel thrombosis.

Striking changes in coagulation occur in pregnancy with an increase in most clotting factors and diminished fibrinolysin activity. Plasma fibrinogen and factors VII, VIII, X, and XIII increase with pregnancy, accompanied by a progressive decrease in plasminogen activator. Pregnancy is associated with a change in the balance of clotting toward a state of enhanced coagulability. Preeclampsia may be associated with thrombocytopenia, fibrin deposits in the kidney and liver, microangiopathic hemolytic anemia, and fulminant consumptive coagulopathy. Although overt evidence of a consumptive coagulopathy with reduction in clotting factors occurs in a minority of women with the disease, a great deal of evidence suggests mild intravascular coagulation.[144, 145] Studies of factor VIII consumption, estimated by the difference between the levels of factor VIII–related antigen and factor VIII clotting activity, show a high correlation with the severity of toxemia and the increase in plasma urate.[127] In some patients, the changes in factor VIII consumption precede hyperuricemia and are occasionally seen in the absence of hypertension. Studies of platelet function in preeclampsia reveal significantly lower maximal aggregation rates in response to collagen, vasopressin, and arachidonic acid, which may indicate that these platelets have undergone aggregation and disaggregation in the circulation. In one study, a fall in platelet count occurred as early as the 22nd week in women in whom preeclampsia developed.[146] Urinary and serum fibrin degradation products are elevated in preeclampsia and can remain elevated in the urine for up to 7 days post partum.

Uteroplacental hypoperfusion caused by inadequate trophoblastic invasion of the uterus with failure of normal development of the spiral arteries, which normally extend to the inner third of the myometrium, has been suggested as the cause of preeclampsia.[147, 148] These vessels are under-

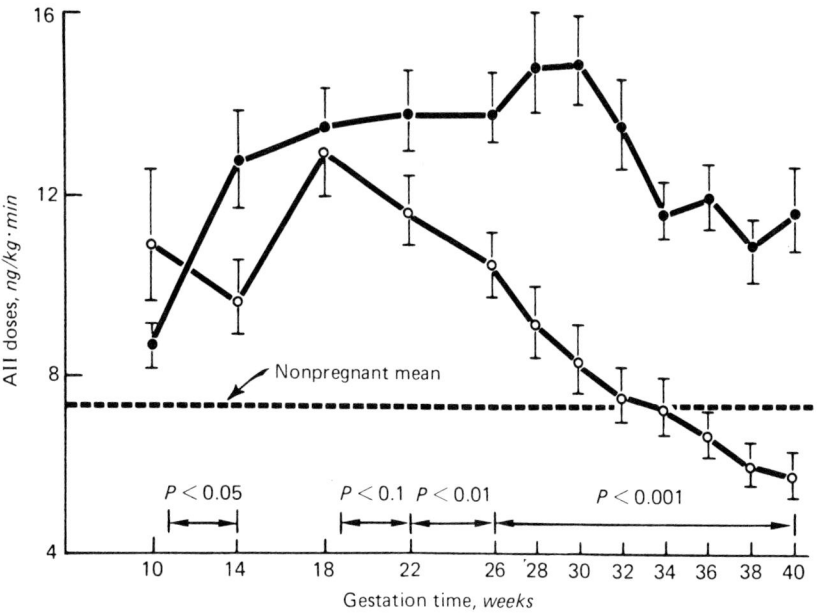

**Figure 36–4.** Effect of pregnancy on sensitivity to the pressor effects of angiotensin II. Ordinate displays the dose of angiotensin II needed to raise diastolic blood pressure 20 mm Hg. In normal pregnancy (*closed circles*; n = 120), a higher dose was required than for nonpregnant women (*broken line*); in women in whom preeclampsia ultimately developed (*open circles*; n = 72), insensitivity to angiotensin II was lost. (From Gant NF, Daley GL, Chand S, et al: A study of angiotensin II pressor response throughout primigravid pregnancy. Reproduced from the Journal of Clinical Investigation, 1973, vol 52, pp 2682–2689 by copyright permission of the American Society for Clinical Investigation.)

developed in preeclampsia but also when intrauterine growth retardation occurs without preeclampsia.[149] Women with the lupus anticoagulant, an immunoglobulin that binds to phospholipids and inhibits endothelial cell $PGI_2$ synthesis, have similar vascular changes of the placenta and spiral arteries.[150] These women have recurrent abortions in the first and second trimesters but can be carried through pregnancy if steroids or low-dose heparin is given. One would expect a higher occurrence of preeclampsia in these women, but clinical studies do not demonstrate an increase in preeclampsia in spite of placental atherosis with a high frequency of stillbirth and fetal growth retardation.[150–153]

Figure 36–5 depicts a hypothetic sequence of events occurring with preeclampsia based on the hypothesis that hypoperfusion of the uterus and placenta is the proximate cause of the disease. The increased occurrence of preeclampsia with twin pregnancies with a large placenta or with a hydatidiform mole suggests ischemia, and measurements of uterine blood flow in preeclampsia demonstrate reduction in flow.[154] Experimentally, reduction of uterine blood flow in pregnant monkeys causes hypertension with changes in the kidney similar to those in women with preeclampsia.[101]

## Pathology of Preeclampsia

### KIDNEY

Significant changes in the glomeruli in preeclampsia were first described in 1918 by Lohlein,[155] and in 1920 Fahr[156] called attention to the swelling of the capillary wall. The first electron microscopic study of the glomerulus in preeclampsia was reported in 1959 by Farquhar,[157] who demonstrated pronounced swelling of the glomerular endothelial cells and deposits of fibrin-like material within and under the endothelial cells. Spargo and co-workers[158] confirmed this report and called the lesion glomerular capillary endotheliosis (Fig. 36–6A) because of lipid accumulation within endothelial cells (Fig. 36–6B). In 1963, Pirani and colleagues[159] demonstrated with immunofluorescence staining that the deposits in the glomeruli were fibrinogen or one of its derivatives. Light microscopic studies of renal biopsy specimens demonstrate that the capillary lumen is bloodless and endothelial and mesangial cells are swollen. The lesion is generalized, involving all glomeruli. The basement membrane is not thickened, but there is proliferation of mesangial cells.[160] Complete resolution of these glomer-

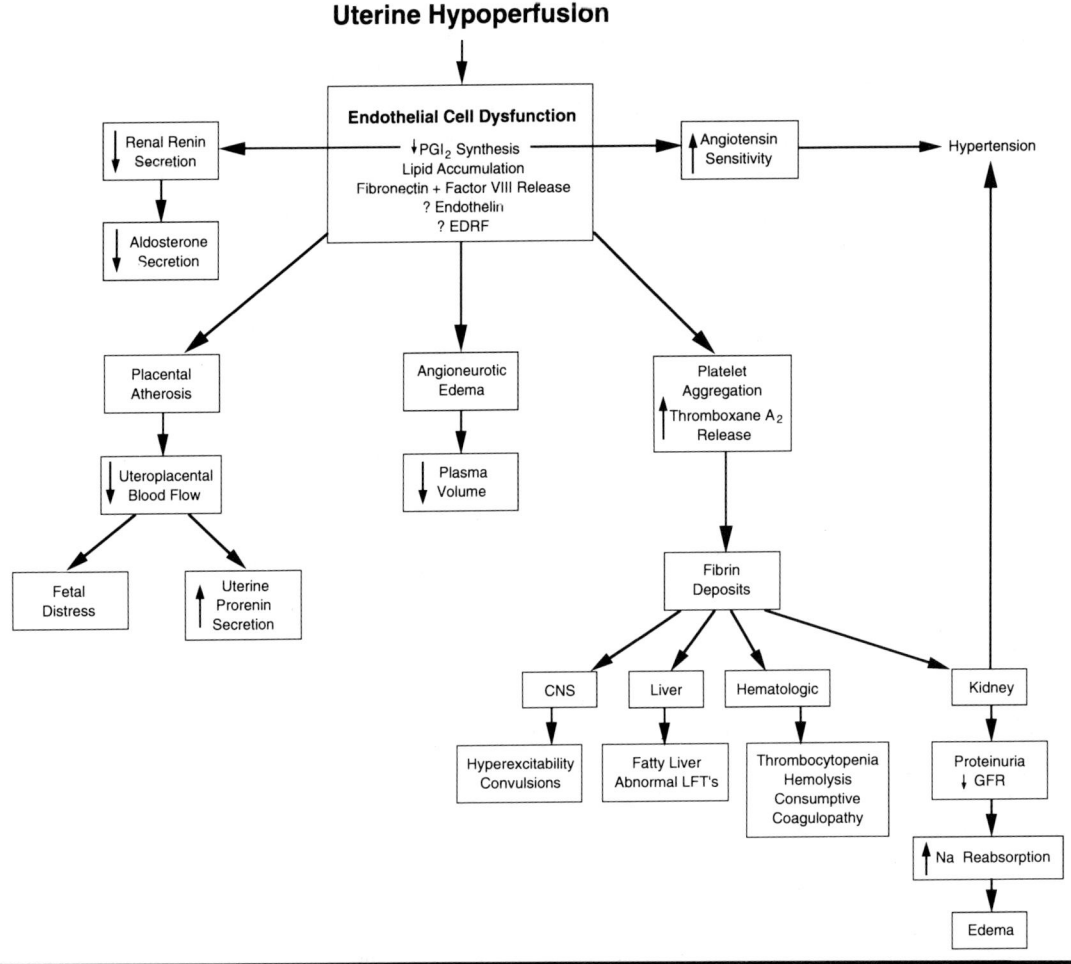

**Figure 36–5.** Hypothetic scheme for the pathogenesis of pre-eclampsia originating with uterine hypoperfusion and diffuse endothelial cell dysfunction. (From Ferris TF: Hypertension and pre-eclampsia. *In* Burrow GN, Ferris TF [eds]: Medical Complications During Pregnancy, 4th ed. WB Saunders, Philadelphia, 1995, pp 1–28.)

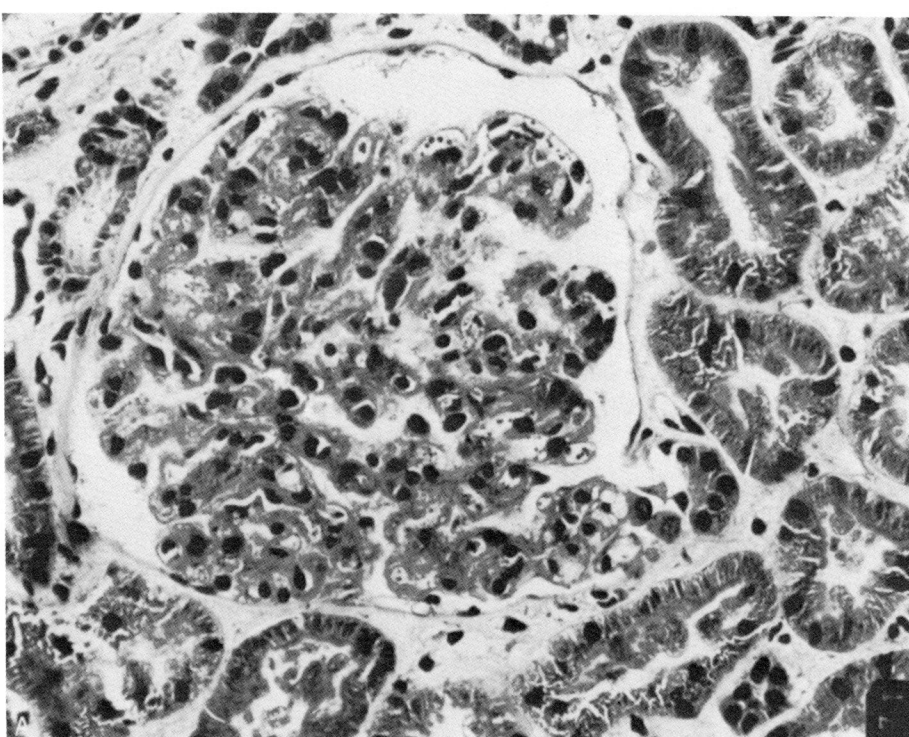

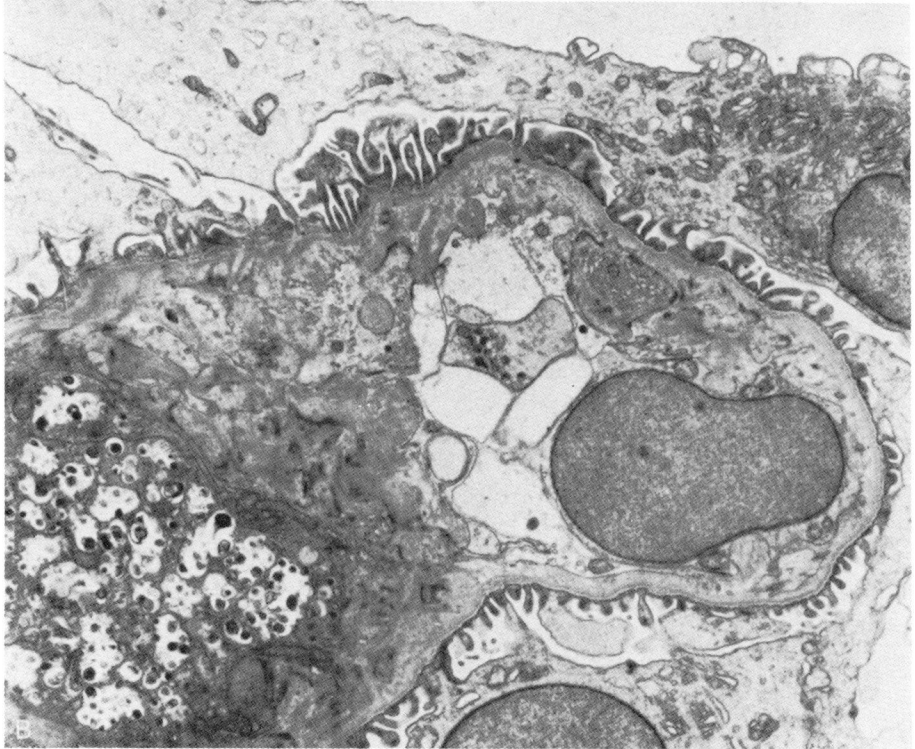

**Figure 36–6.** Renal histologic findings in preeclampsia. *A.* Light microscopic findings of glomerular endotheliosis. (Magnification × 500.) *B.* Electron micrograph of a glomerulus in preeclampsia. Note the swollen intracapillary cells with lipid-containing lysosomes in the mesangial cell. The endothelial cell contains vacuoles, and there is a trapped platelet. (Magnification × 10,000.) (*A* and *B* courtesy of Dr. B. Spargo.)

ular changes has been reported to occur as early as 4 weeks post partum. Kincaid-Smith[161] has emphasized the need for biopsy during pregnancy or immediately post partum to demonstrate the fibrin deposits that disappear quickly after delivery. Hypertension is not the cause of the glomerular disease; similar changes are seen in bovine toxemia, a disease similar to preeclampsia in which convulsions, protein-uria, and decreased GFR occur in the absence of hypertension.[51]

There is no evidence of immunologically mediated damage to the glomerulus. The swollen endothelial cells point to endothelial cell injury with resultant local activation of intravascular coagulation. When immunoglobulins have been noted by immunofluorescence in the glomeruli of patients with preeclampsia, they represent nonspecific trapping in injured glomeruli.

## LIVER

Before the advent of liver biopsy, studies of hepatic disease in preeclampsia were limited to patients with fatal disease. In these patients, large subcapsular hematomas were found, some of which had ruptured into the peritoneal cavity. The subcapsular hematomas arise either from deep within the liver or from the capsule.[162, 163] Sheehan and Lynch[164] postulated that the hemorrhagic changes in the liver were due to intense spasm of hepatic arterioles rather than to fibrin deposits. However, studies using percutaneous liver biopsies in patients with toxemia have demonstrated patchy areas of necrosis with fibrin deposits.[165] Of 12 preeclamptic women, 2 had focal areas of fibrinoid necrosis with either patchy or extensive necrosis of the liver cells. Immunofluorescence studies of all 12 biopsy specimens showed diffuse sinusoidal staining with antiserum to fibrinogen. In biopsy specimens from normal pregnant women, fibrin deposits were not demonstrated. Abnormalities in liver function with preeclampsia are usually manifested by elevations in lactate dehydrogenase and aspartate aminotransferase. In several patients with preeclampsia, histologic evidence of microvesicular fat, necrosis, and cholestasis has been found, which are the typical findings of acute fatty liver of pregnancy, a disease now thought to be a hepatic manifestation of preeclampsia.[166–170]

## PLACENTA

At 16 weeks' gestation in normal human pregnancy, the spiral arteries in the placental bed progressively lose their musculoelastic tissue and widen, thereby allowing the increase in blood supply required by the pregnant uterus. In preeclampsia, in infants born small for gestational age, and in women with chronic hypertension, necrosis and infiltration of these spiral vessels produce the picture of acute atherosis.[149, 171] The cause of these changes remains unclear, although an imbalance in $PGI_2$ and thromboxane synthesis with resultant platelet aggregation and fibrin deposition is an attractive hypothesis.

## CENTRAL NERVOUS SYSTEM

A common cause of death in preeclampsia is cerebral hemorrhage, which occurs in about 60% of patients who die after eclampsia. The hemorrhages are petechial as well as large hematomas.[164] Frequently, a large hemorrhage occurs in the white matter and may extend into the subarachnoid space or ventricles. Although cerebral edema may occur after eclampsia, it is unusual.[172] Cerebral edema occurs with malignant hypertension, but hypertension in preeclampsia seldom reaches the levels seen in malignant hypertension. Hypertension does not account for the central nervous system manifestations of preeclampsia, which are more likely due to endothelial cell dysfunction with platelet aggregation and fibrin deposition similar to that seen in glomeruli, liver, and heart. Fibrin deposits have been described in the brain of some patients dying of preeclampsia,

but because some had a consumptive coagulopathy, it is difficult to ascertain whether the cerebral disease is primary or secondary to the coagulopathy.

An unusual cause of postpartum headache and convulsion is central venous thrombosis. Thrombosis most commonly occurs in a vein over the parietal cortex and causes convulsions that may be indistinguishable from those of eclampsia. There are more than 396 recorded causes of postpartum central venous thrombosis with a mortality rate of approximately 40%.[173] Occasionally, central venous thrombosis may occur during pregnancy and mimic eclampsia. The absence of hypertension and proteinuria argues against preeclampsia in these women. Central venous thrombosis may be caused by the hypercoagulable state that occurs post partum.

## HEART

In 12 of 34 patients dying of eclampsia, postmortem examination revealed contraction band necrosis on myocardial sections.[174] In one woman with preeclampsia who underwent cardiac catheterization, an endocardial biopsy revealed narrowed capillary lumens. On electron microscopic studies, endothelial cell swelling and lipid accumulation similar to those noted in the glomeruli of preeclamptic women were seen.[175]

# Clinical Features and Epidemiology of Preeclampsia

The clinical onset of preeclampsia may be insidious and not accompanied by overt symptoms. Headache, visual disturbances, epigastric pain, and apprehension may occur. The usual sequence is rapid weight gain with edema, particularly of the hands and face, with rise in blood pressure and proteinuria. Rarely, proteinuria precedes the hypertension. Proteinuria in preeclampsia can range from minimal levels (500 mg/24 h) to levels seen in the nephrotic syndrome, but preeclampsia does not cause microscopic hematuria.[176] Some patients with preeclampsia have severe proteinuria with minimal hypertension, whereas in others the hypertension is prominent. Preeclampsia usually begins after the 32nd week of pregnancy but may begin earlier, particularly in women with pre-existing renal disease or hypertension. When it occurs in the first trimester, it is pathognomonic of a hydatidiform mole. The disease may be seen post partum, with hypertension and convulsions occurring within 24 to 48 hours after delivery, although it has been reported as late as 7 days post partum.[177]

The disease has a bimodal frequency, being more common in young primiparous and older multiparous women, but primiparous women are six to eight times more susceptible to preeclampsia than are multiparous women. The presence of underlying essential hypertension, diabetes mellitus, or renal disease increases the risk of preeclampsia, as do twin pregnancies, fetal hydrops, and hydatidiform mole. Preeclampsia has a familial prevalence.[178] In one series, the frequency of hypertension during pregnancy was 28% in daughters of preeclamptic mothers, compared with 13% in daughters of normotensive mothers.[179] Whether preeclampsia is more common in black women is unclear. The higher frequency of essential hypertension in black women makes it more common in multiparous women but probably not in primiparous black women.[180] In Chesley's[180] follow-up study of 270 white women with eclampsia, 26% of the daughters had preeclampsia in their first pregnancy compared with 8% of the daughters-in-law. In a series of 140 women in whom hypertension developed in their first pregnancy, 47% had a recurrence of hypertension with or without proteinuria in their second pregnancy.[181] Women who smoke have smaller infants compared with nonsmokers, and the frequency of toxemia is less in smokers.[182] However, the adverse effect of smoking on fetal size outweighs the protective effect on the development of preeclampsia.

The physical examination reveals puffy edema of the face and hands. Diastolic hypertension is prominent, with the systolic pressure usually below 160 mm Hg. Systolic blood pressure greater than 200 mm Hg points to preeclampsia superimposed on underlying chronic hypertension. Ophthalmoscopic examination shows segmental arteriolar narrowing with a wet glistening appearance indicative of retinal edema; hemorrhages and exudates are rare. Detachment of the retina may occur, with spontaneous reattachment occurring after diuresis and control of the hypertension.[183] Pulmonary edema is a common complication of preeclampsia, usually caused by left ventricular failure. It may occur with normal pulmonary capillary wedge pressure because of change in pulmonary capillary permeability.[8, 121, 184] Central nervous system excitability measures the severity of neurologic involvement, which is assessed by examination of the spinal reflexes.

Because preeclampsia is a multisystem disease, its presentation frequently mimics other diseases.[185] Thrombocytopenia may be prominent and suggest idiopathic thrombocytopenic purpura and, when accompanied by neurologic features, is reminiscent of thrombotic thrombocytopenic purpura. A microangiopathic anemia with hemolysis is frequent. Abdominal pain and elevated serum amylase level may suggest acute pancreatitis. The so-called HELLP syndrome comprises severe preeclampsia with hemolysis, elevated liver enzymes, and low platelet count.[186] Jaundice, which may be severe particularly when hemolysis occurs, and abnormalities of liver function tests suggest hepatitis.[168, 187] In some patients, hepatic abnormalities may be more prominent than either hypertension or proteinuria.

Acute fatty liver of pregnancy, which occurs in 1 in 13,000 pregnancies, may be an extreme hepatic manifestation of preeclampsia. More than 90% of cases occur in the third trimester (isolated cases occur in the second trimester or post partum).[188, 189] Nonspecific symptoms related to hepatic insufficiency, such as fatigue, malaise, nausea, and vomiting, are found; abdominal pain is often severe but is not invariably present. Laboratory findings suggest hepatic failure (marked elevation of bilirubin, lesser elevation of hepatic enzymes). A microangiopathic hemolytic anemia with thrombocytopenia and prolonged clotting times may develop.[190] In a review of 49 cases of acute fatty liver of pregnancy, 22% had evidence of preeclampsia preceding the onset of hepatic disease.[167] This may be an underestimation of the true occurrence of preeclampsia, because for many patients available information concerning blood pressure was not given. Liver biopsy results in preeclampsia show mild fatty infiltration of the liver even when hepatic involvement is not clinically apparent.[169, 191]

In as many as 60% of women with acute fatty liver of pregnancy, acute renal failure develops.[192] This has often been diagnosed clinically as acute tubule necrosis (ATN) and has occasionally been confirmed by renal biopsy.[193] In other cases, renal biopsy has revealed no abnormalities or fatty infiltration.[167, 194] Thus, the possibility that this is a form of hepatorenal syndrome should be considered. There is no specific treatment for this disease, and the prognosis appears to depend on the quality of supportive obstetric care because the mortality rate has decreased from greater than 80% to approximately 20%.[195]

A fascinating feature of a few patients with preeclampsia and hepatic involvement is the development of transient diabetes insipidus.[196, 197] Of the 16 cases reported in the literature, 12 patients had hypertension, and all had severe hyperuricemia and abnormal liver function. Vasopressinase activity, which is thought to be of placental origin, increases in pregnancy.[198] Whether higher vasopressinase activity occurs in preeclampsia is not known. The severe hepatic involvement in most of these patients suggests a combination of hepatic disease and increased vasopressinase activity as the cause of the diabetes insipidus. It can be treated with the synthetic arginine vasopressin analogue desmopressin (DDAVP), which is not metabolized by vasopressinase. Remission occurs post partum.

## Treatment of Preeclampsia

The first objective in the treatment of preeclampsia is its prevention. Proper prenatal care with attention to adequate but not excessive weight gain and careful monitoring of blood pressure and urinary protein concentration during pregnancy reduce the frequency and severity of the disease. There is no evidence of a nutritional basis for the disease, but in many countries, the poor suffer a higher frequency of preeclampsia. In Jerusalem, preeclampsia in illiterate women is twice that in control subjects, and in the United States, there is a higher frequency in the poor.[199] Because the poor are more likely to have children at early ages, this may be one factor explaining the increased occurrence.

The most important features to be recognized for the prevention of preeclampsia are that a rise in blood pressure greater than 30 mm Hg systolic or 15 mm Hg diastolic during pregnancy is significant in late pregnancy and that the development of proteinuria with a rise in blood pressure indicates preeclampsia.

In an attempt to correct a potential imbalance in endothelial $PGI_2$ and platelet thromboxane synthesis in preeclampsia, low-dose aspirin has been administered to women at high risk for preeclampsia. Low-dose aspirin inhibits platelet thromboxane synthesis more than endothelial $PGI_2$ synthesis. A meta-analysis of six published trials of low-dose aspirin up to 1992 demonstrated a significant reduction in preeclampsia but not hypertension in the aspirin-treated group.[200] In a National Institutes of Health study of 3135 healthy, nulliparous women randomly assigned to receive either 60 mg aspirin or a placebo daily throughout pregnancy, the incidence of preeclampsia was lower (4.7% versus 6.3%) in the treated group without a significant difference in gestational hypertension (6.7% versus 5.9%).[98] In women with a greater risk for preeclampsia (i.e., those with an initial systolic blood pressure of 120 to 134 mm Hg), aspirin reduced the incidence of preeclampsia from 11.9% to 5.6% (Fig. 36–7). However, the incidence of abruptio placentae was significantly higher, 0.7% in the aspirin-treated group versus 0.1% in the placebo group. The increased incidence of abruptio placentae cautions against the routine use of aspirin in all pregnant women, but in women at increased risk for preeclampsia (previous history of preeclampsia; twin pregnancies; MAP > 90 mm Hg in the second trimester; or underlying diabetes mellitus, essential hypertension, or renal disease), the use of low-dose aspirin seems warranted. The incidence of abruptio placentae of 0.1% in the placebo group is lower than the incidence of 0.5% to 1% reported in unselected pregnancies.[201] The 26% reduction in the incidence of preeclampsia outweighs the increased risk of abruptio placentae, which has not been reported in other studies evaluating the effect of aspirin in pregnant women.[202] Abruption is more likely to occur in hypertensive pregnant women, so the 0.7% incidence is not unduly high.

Calcium supplementation, 2 g daily, has been shown to lower blood pressure in most studies of nonpregnant hypertensive women and to reduce the frequency of hypertension in pregnancy.[203, 204] The mechanism of its antihypertensive effect is unknown, but in pregnant women it has been reported to decrease responsiveness to angiotensin II, which suggests an increase in endothelial cell synthesis of $PGI_2$.[205] The administration of calcium to pregnant women is not without potential risk because urinary excretion of $Ca^{2+}$ in pregnant women is about 300 mg/d compared with 100 mg/d in nonpregnant women. The hypercalciuria is caused by increased intestinal absorption of $Ca^{2+}$ induced by high plasma vitamin D levels.[206] The addition of 2 g of calcium to the diet increases urinary $Ca^{2+}$ excretion and might increase the risk of renal calculi, which occur in about 1 in 2000 pregnancies.

The physician must carefully evaluate all women with a rise in blood pressure in late pregnancy for evidence of preeclampsia because it is the most frequent cause of maternal mortality. Hypertension with clinical or laboratory evidence of systemic disease must be presumed to represent preeclampsia. Although all hypertension in pregnancy poses a risk to mother and child, preeclampsia poses a far greater risk. If the presumptive diagnosis is preeclampsia, hospitalization is indicated, whereas a rise in blood pressure without evidence of preeclampsia can be treated on an outpatient basis.

If the disease is mild (blood pressure < 140/90 mm Hg, proteinuria < 500 mg/24 h, normal renal function, serum urate level < 4.5 mg/100 mL, normal platelet count, no evidence of hemolysis or hepatic involvement), bed rest is usually sufficient therapy to lower the blood pressure and allow time for estimation of fetal size and maturity. If fetal size and maturation are thought to be adequate, delivery is the definitive treatment. If fetal size and maturation are of concern, management by an obstetrician and a physician with expertise in the treatment of hypertension is required. If there is no evidence of worsening of preeclampsia, the pregnancy can be continued. Any sign of worsening of the disease should be an indication for delivery, particularly if the pregnancy is of 32 weeks' duration or longer because fetal survival at that age in neonatal units is now close to 100%.

When blood pressure is above 140/95 mm Hg with decreased renal function, hyperuricemia, or proteinuria greater than 500 mg/24 h, delivery is indicated in pregnancies thought to be more than 32 weeks' duration. Blood pressure should be lowered to 140/90 mm Hg before delivery. Antihypertensive therapy lessens the likelihood of a rise in blood pressure during delivery with potential complications of congestive heart failure or cerebral hemorrhage. Hydrochlorothiazide, 25 mg daily, is often sufficient antihypertensive medication. The reluctance to use diuretics in treating pregnant women is because of the reduction in plasma volume that can occur with preeclampsia. However, thiazides have been used in pregnancy more extensively than any other antihypertensive drug. A meta-analysis of nine randomized trials comprising more than 11,000 pregnant women given diuretics throughout pregnancy revealed a decrease in the frequency of hypertension without adverse effects on the fetus.[207] Diuretics also potentiate the effect of all other antihypertensive drugs. Provided that dietary salt is not severely restricted, thiazides do not cause volume depletion. Alternatively, the $Ca^{2+}$ channel blocker nifedipine or the β-adrenergic antagonists atenolol or pindolol can be given orally.[208–211] There may be some advantage to pindolol because of its intrinsic sympathomimetic property that prevents the development of fetal bradycardia.[210] Atenolol has been demonstrated to reduce proteinuria and to

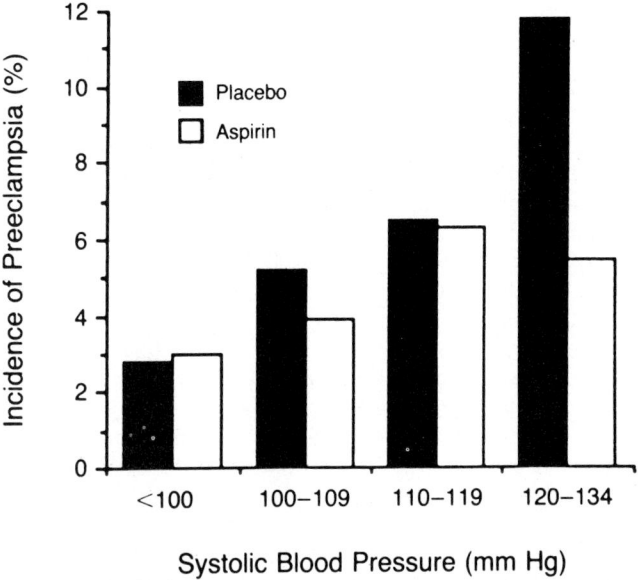

**Figure 36–7.** Incidence of preeclampsia among nulliparous pregnant women according to blood pressure at initiation of treatment. Low-dose aspirin reduced the incidence of preeclampsia in the subgroup of 519 women whose initial systolic blood pressure was 120 to 134 mm Hg (P = .01). (From Sibai BM, Caritis S, Thom E, et al: Prevention of preeclampsia with low dose aspirin in healthy, nulliparous pregnant women. Reprinted by permission from The New England Journal of Medicine, vol 329, page 1213, 1993.)

reduce the need for hospitalization in a group of women with preeclampsia.[211]

When blood pressure is above 160/100 mm Hg, parenteral therapy may be needed. Although intravenous hydralazine has been used extensively in pregnancy, its rapid duration of action and the reflex tachycardia it induces make it less effective than labetalol or a $Ca^{2+}$ channel blocker. Intravenous labetalol, a combined α- and β-adrenergic antagonist, has been used successfully to treat preeclampsia.[212–216] When rapid reduction in blood pressure is indicated, diazoxide is effective. Although sodium nitroprusside, a vasodilator, is frequently used for hypertensive emergencies in the nonpregnant patient, the possibility of fetal cyanide toxicity, which has been demonstrated in pregnant ewes, argues against its prolonged use in pregnancy.[217] Whether treatment of hypertension in preeclampsia affects the underlying disease is less clear, but it is not unreasonable to assume that hypertension is a factor adversely affecting endothelial cell function. Antihypertensive therapy can prevent pulmonary edema and cerebral hemorrhage, two severe complications of preeclampsia. However, convulsions (eclampsia) or the HELLP syndrome is always an indication for delivery.[218]

Obstetricians in the United States have relied on magnesium sulfate, a mild vasodilator, for the treatment of preeclampsia. At therapeutic serum levels of 4 to 6 mEq/L, $Mg^{2+}$ increases $PGI_2$ synthesis in cultured endothelial cells,[219] which may account for its efficacy. However, at therapeutic serum $Mg^{2+}$ levels, there is suppression of myoneuronal transmission, which can cause respiratory paralysis leading to maternal death.[220, 221] Vital capacity and maximal inspiratory and expiratory pressures fall in pregnant women receiving magnesium sulfate.[222] Care must be taken when magnesium sulfate is used in combination with a $Ca^{2+}$ channel blocker because a synergistic effect may occur and cause severe hypotension.[223] There is no convincing evidence that magnesium is an anticonvulsant in preeclampsia,[224–226] and most neurologists advocate the use of phenytoin to prevent seizures.[227] When hyperexcitability is severe and eclampsia is thought to be imminent, phenytoin may be given intravenously. Diazepam is the treatment of choice when convulsions occur.[228] Eclampsia may occur post partum, usually within 48 hours of delivery, and virtually always in women with preeclampsia.

When preeclampsia occurs in the second trimester, when delivery of the infant is not compatible with fetal survival, a difficult decision must be made by the mother and physician. In 109 preeclamptic women presenting in the second trimester, Sibai and co-workers[229] recommended termination of pregnancy if the pregnancy was less than 24 weeks' duration. Fifteen of the 25 women in this category refused termination, and there was only one surviving infant. The HELLP syndrome developed in three women, one woman had eclampsia, and two women had abruptio placentae. Fortunately, there were no maternal deaths, but all women were hospitalized in intensive care units. Of the 84 preeclamptic women thought to have pregnancies of longer duration than 24 weeks, 30 were delivered immediately; there were 20 fetal deaths, and the 10 living infants spent an average of 115 days in the neonatal intensive care unit. The 54 women not delivered immediately were treated with antihypertensives to maintain diastolic pressure below 100 mm Hg. There were 13 perinatal deaths. Pregnancy was prolonged in this group an average of 13 days, and there were 42 live infants who spent an average of 70 days in the neonatal intensive care unit. Thus, in women with preeclampsia in the second trimester with pregnancies longer than 24 weeks' duration, there was increased fetal survival by prolonging the pregnancy with treatment of the hypertension. Measurements of uterine blood flow in women with preeclampsia and in hypertensive pregnant animals usually demonstrate an increase in blood flow with antihypertensive therapy.[209, 210, 212, 214–216, 230] Although there is an appropriate reluctance to administer any drug during pregnancy, the burden of proof today is on the physician who does not treat hypertension during pregnancy.

# ESSENTIAL HYPERTENSION IN PREGNANCY

Although there has been reluctance to treat hypertension in pregnant women with essential hypertension, the evidence is overwhelming that antihypertensive therapy results in fewer exacerbations of hypertension, lowers the frequency of proteinuria, and improves perinatal outcome.[211, 231–237] The specific drug used to control hypertension reflects the experience of the physician caring for the patient. The only antihypertensive agents that are contraindicated in pregnancy are the angiotensin-converting enzyme inhibitors. They lower uterine and placental blood flow in pregnant animals and can cause renal failure, oligohydramnios, and failure of maturation in the human fetus.[54, 55, 238] With the number of effective agents available, it is possible to normalize blood pressure in the pregnant woman without undesirable side effects and without risk to the fetus. A meta-analysis of randomized trials of various antihypertensive drugs shows a lower risk of fetal or neonatal death in the treated group.[239] Hypertension must be considered a pathologic response, and lowering the blood pressure should be instituted in all pregnant women with hypertension.

As in the nonpregnant population, the beneficial effect of antihypertensive therapy is demonstrated best at higher levels of pressure. In one study of 44 pregnant women with severe essential hypertension primarily controlled by β-blockers and diuretics, all antihypertensive drugs and diuretics were stopped, and only methyldopa was given throughout pregnancy.[235] Preeclampsia developed in 52% of these women, 45% had a decrease in renal function, and malignant hypertension with encephalopathy developed in one woman. The perinatal mortality was 25%, and surviving children spent an average 39 days in the neonatal intensive care unit. These results are reminiscent of the experience of pregnant women with hypertension in the era before availability of antihypertensive therapy. For instance, in 1937, John P. Peters[240] reported a 13% maternal mortality in 203 women with hypertension in pregnancy. The evidence today indicates that maternal mortality from hypertensive complications can be eliminated in women with essential hypertension provided that hypertension is treated throughout pregnancy.

Before the availability of effective antihypertensive therapy, two thirds of women with chronic hypertension had a rise in blood pressure in late pregnancy, with proteinuria developing in half.[241] The hesitancy to treat maternal hypertension in the past has been based on unfounded assumptions concerning the beneficial effect of hypertension on uterine blood flow. The view that hypertension might increase perfusion of the uterus failed to recognize that an increase in pressure causes vasoconstriction in all vascular beds, the phenomenon of autoregulation. Pregnant rabbits autoregulate uterine blood flow over a wide range of blood pressure,[46] and when pregnant rats are made hypertensive by clipping the renal artery, uteroplacental blood flow is reduced to 68% of that in normotensive pregnant rats.[242]

Pregnant women with chronic essential hypertension have an increased risk of preeclampsia, abruptio placentae, intrauterine growth retardation, and second-trimester fetal death. However, those without proteinuria do well during pregnancy provided that blood pressure is controlled.[243–245] Approximately half of women with essential hypertension have a spontaneous reduction in pressure in the second trimester, which may allow lowering the dose or discontinuing antihypertensive medication. If blood pressure is taken for the first time in the second trimester, a subsequent rise in pressure in the third trimester is often diagnosed as gestational hypertension. Persistence of gestational hypertension post partum frequently indicates that chronic hypertension was present before the pregnancy. The higher frequency of preeclampsia in women with essential hypertension probably justifies giving 60 mg aspirin and 2 g of calcium supplementation daily throughout pregnancy. Because these women are usually taking antihypertensive medication before pregnancy, it is important to maintain whatever therapy has controlled their hypertension, with the exception of angiotensin-converting enzyme inhibitors. Thiazides can be continued throughout pregnancy. Although in one study plasma volume increased only 18% in women taking diuretics compared with 36% in hypertensive women not receiving diuretics, there was no difference in fetal survival or birth weight.[246]

Many women with chronic hypertension have been treated with β-adrenergic blockers throughout pregnancy.[247, 248] In randomized trials comparing atenolol and metoprolol, no adverse fetal effects were demonstrated with either drug.[211] One trial of atenolol given throughout pregnancy to a group of women with essential hypertension reported smaller infants in the treated group, although fetal survival was unchanged.[249]

The central α-adrenergic agonist methyldopa has been used extensively in pregnancy and has been shown to diminish second-trimester stillbirths with no untoward effects in the children who have been observed for up to 7 years of age.[250] Birth weights and fetal maturation with methyldopa treatment were similar to those of the control group. However, methyldopa causes somnolence, a frequent problem in pregnant women. Randomized trials comparing the use of β-blockers with methyldopa throughout pregnancy did not demonstrate significant differences in blood pressure control or the occurrence of preeclampsia with either agent.[236] However, methyldopa is not as effective in treating severe hypertension as are the β-blockers or Ca$^{2+}$ channel blockers.

Clonidine, another central α-adrenergic agonist, has been used throughout pregnancy in women with chronic hypertension.[251] Evidence of embryotoxicity in pregnant rats given low doses of clonidine and a report of behavioral changes in the offspring of women treated with clonidine make consideration of another agent during pregnancy reasonable.[252] Clonidine should not be stopped abruptly because severe hypertension may ensue; it should be gradually withdrawn in a period of 7 to 10 days.

A comparison of atenolol and nifedipine in one study reported no differences with either agent.[253] Birth weights, fetoplacental hemodynamics, and Apgar scores were similar in the two groups. The α-adrenergic receptor antagonist prazosin has also been used throughout pregnancy, and no untoward effects were reported.[254]

## GESTATIONAL HYPERTENSION

Hypertension that appears in late pregnancy, is not associated with signs of preeclampsia, and disappears post partum is termed gestational hypertension. Women with gestational hypertension are usually multiparous, are frequently overweight, and have a positive family history of hypertension; essential hypertension ultimately develops in many of them. For reasons not understood, pregnancy is a hypertensionogenic stress in susceptible women. The diabetogenic and hypertensionogenic effect of pregnancy may be related because although insulin resistance occurs in all pregnant women, greater insulin antagonism occurs in hypertensive pregnant women.[123] There is a genetic link among obesity, insulin resistance, and hypertension in many hypertensive populations, and Chesley[180] in his follow-up of white women with eclampsia found no higher frequency of hypertension in later life but a sevenfold higher occurrence of diabetes.

If gestational hypertension occurs in late pregnancy, the patient can be observed at weekly intervals as an outpatient. A β-adrenergic blocker such as atenolol or labetalol, methyldopa, nifedipine, or hydrochlorothiazide often controls the blood pressure. Frequently, obstetricians recommend bed rest for these women, which lowers blood pressure but is an inconvenience, particularly for a working woman or one with household responsibilities. Studies of women hospitalized or placed in a day care facility for treatment of gestational hypertension have not demonstrated advantages to either form of treatment.[255, 256]

## PREECLAMPSIA SUPERIMPOSED ON CHRONIC HYPERTENSION

Chronic essential hypertension may be associated with nephrosclerosis, particularly in multiparous black women. Because proteinuria in nephrosclerosis is minimal, it is often overlooked in routine urinalyses. With nephrosclerosis, as in all renal diseases, autoregulation of glomerular pressure is compromised so that any increase in blood pressure during pregnancy increases glomerular pressure, which may cause or worsen proteinuria (see later). When this occurs, the distinction between preeclampsia and increased proteinuria induced by glomerular hypertension is difficult.[257] Hyperuricemia or a rise in serum creatinine suggests preeclampsia.

# SECONDARY HYPERTENSION AND PREGNANCY

## Renal Artery Stenosis

Superimposed preeclampsia frequently develops in women with renal artery stenosis who become pregnant. Of the nine patients in the series of Landesman and co-workers,[258] five had exacerbation of hypertension during pregnancy, and preeclampsia developed in four. Interestingly, in one group of women with renal artery stenosis observed during pregnancy, plasma renin fell with the development of preeclampsia.[40] The presence of renal artery stenosis should be suspected in any woman with severe hypertension early in pregnancy, particularly if an abdominal bruit is present and there is no family history of hypertension. Because angiotensin-converting enzyme inhibitors are contraindicated in pregnancy, medical treatment for renal hypertension is complicated. Angioplasty has been carried out successfully in pregnant women to correct renal artery stenosis.[259, 260] If hypertension is refractory to other drugs and the lesion is not amenable to angioplasty, use of an angiotensin-converting enzyme inhibitor can be considered. Women have been carried through pregnancy successfully with use of converting enzyme inhibitors despite their potential to adversely affect the fetus.[261, 262]

## Primary Aldosteronism in Pregnancy

The original report of primary aldosteronism by Biglieri and Slaton[80] noted disappearance of hypokalemia and amelioration of hypertension in pregnancy, but these have not been uniform findings. Although increased progesterone secretion in pregnancy antagonizes the effect of aldosterone on the renal tubule, some pregnant patients have severe hypertension and hypokalemia.[263] The diagnosis can be difficult to make in pregnancy because plasma renin activity is not suppressed as in nonpregnant patients, and plasma aldosterone levels are high in all pregnant women. Treatment with spironolactone has been successful in some pregnant patients, but if an adenoma is identified in the first or second trimester, surgical therapy can be accomplished. One woman with hyperaldosteronism due to adrenal hyperplasia was treated with enalapril, which controlled blood pressure, but fetal distress necessitated early delivery.[83]

## Coarctation of the Aorta in Pregnancy

Coarctation of the aorta is a rare cause of hypertension and can be associated with preeclampsia. Of 10 patients requiring surgical repair for this condition during pregnancy, 9 underwent uncomplicated deliveries with live infants.[264] One patient died in her seventh month of pregnancy of an aneurysm of the aorta at the anastomotic site.

The major danger to the pregnant woman with an aortic coarctation is aortic rupture from the cystic medial necrosis often present in the aortic wall. These pathologic changes may be put under stress by the increase in cardiac output of pregnancy, the increase in blood pressure during preeclampsia, or the strain of labor.

## Pheochromocytoma

Although a rare cause of hypertension, pheochromocytoma is potentially lethal during pregnancy. Maternal mortality in pregnant women is 17% and fetal loss is 26% if the diagnosis is not made.[265–268] The cause of the maternal mortality is usually pulmonary edema, cerebral hemorrhage, or cardiovascular collapse. Treatment with α- and β-adrenergic blockers has eliminated maternal mortality, although fetal loss remains high (15%). Women with characteristic symptoms of paroxysmal hypertension, palpitations, diaphoresis, and headache should be evaluated with measurements of urinary catecholamine excretion. If catecholamine excretion is elevated, either a computed tomographic scan or magnetic resonance imaging should be done to localize the tumor. In the first or second trimester of pregnancy, most physicians would recommend surgical treatment, although some patients have been treated medically throughout pregnancy with surgical removal of the tumor post partum.[269]

# RENAL DISEASE COMPLICATING PREGNANCY

## Bacteriuria

Urinary tract infection occurs with the same frequency in pregnant as in nonpregnant women. However, the consequences of infection are far more serious during pregnancy, warranting the prompt diagnosis and treatment of infection. Women with diabetes or sickle cell trait or disease as well as those from lower socioeconomic groups have a higher prevalence of urinary tract infection in pregnancy.[270] When untreated, bacteriuria becomes symptomatic or evolves into pyelonephritis in approximately 30% of cases.[271] The increased capacity of the urinary collecting system with slowed emptying and vesicoureteral reflux is a major factor accounting for the increased occurrence of serious urinary tract infection in pregnancy. Glucosuria and aminoaciduria also aid bacterial growth.

Maternal risks associated with urinary tract infection are the development of bacteremia, septic shock, and decreases in renal function. Risks to the fetus may be even greater. Bacteriuria has been linked to an increased risk of mid-trimester abortions and to a twofold increase in perinatal mortality when urinary tract infection occurs within 2 weeks of delivery.[272] Acute pyelonephritis has been associated with an increased frequency of intrauterine growth retardation and prematurity.[273] Only half of pregnant women with bacteriuria are symptomatic,[270] which is the rationale for obtaining a screening urine culture at an initial prenatal visit. On the other hand, many pregnant women with symptoms suggestive of bacteriuria are not infected because nocturia, polyuria, and stress incontinence are common complaints during uncomplicated pregnancy.

Women with a history of asymptomatic bacteriuria during childhood also have an increased frequency of complications during pregnancy. These women had a significantly greater frequency of bacteriuria and pyelonephritis in pregnancy compared with pregnant women with no previous history of bacteriuria.[274] The possibility that asymptomatic bacteriuria during childhood results in subtle renal damage that can be unmasked during pregnancy is suggested by the finding that GFR and fractional reabsorption of glucose increased less in such women during pregnancy.[275] Those who were known to have sustained renal injury during childhood, as evidenced by the presence of renal scars on intravenous pyelograms, have an increased frequency of preeclampsia compared with normal pregnant women or women with a history of bacteriuria but no scars.[274] Women with subtle renal damage (but normal renal function) because of previous infection are more likely to require induction of labor or operative delivery than are those without such a history.[274] Apgar scores were also reported to be lower in children of women with a history of bacteriuria during childhood regardless of the presence or absence of renal scars.[274] Nevertheless, fetal outcome is generally satisfactory.

Because of the potential for fetal and maternal morbidity as a consequence of bacteriuria, infection, even if asymptomatic, should be treated. Short courses of therapy for 5 to 10 days result in long-term cure rates of approximately 65%.[276, 277] Single-dose therapy may be an effective alternative means of treating bacteriuria, but there is less experience with this approach.[277] Women in whom pyelonephritis develops usually require more prolonged therapy for eradication of the infection. In all women who have urinary tract infection, close follow-up during the remainder of pregnancy is essential. Urinary tract infection in pregnant women usually develops in the absence of underlying structural abnormalities. Only when urinary tract infection is difficult to eradicate or the history is suggestive of underlying disease should evidence for the presence of structural abnormalities be sought. As noted before, vesicoureteral reflux is seen in otherwise uncomplicated pregnancy and does not of itself indicate a urinary tract pathophysiologic process.

## Asymptomatic Urinary Abnormalities: Proteinuria and Hematuria

The development of proteinuria during pregnancy may be an indicator of unmasked kidney disease, worsening of pre-existent renal disease, the de novo development of renal disease, or the development of preeclampsia in which renal involvement is part of a systemic disorder. In normal pregnancy, both because of the increase in GFR and because of an increase in glomerular capillary permeability to albumin, there is increased urinary excretion of albumin. When corrected for GFR, fractional albumin excretion increases by approximately 80%.[278] Nevertheless, in otherwise healthy pregnant women, this should not result in a 24-hour urinary

excretion of protein of greater than 200 mg.[279] Urinary protein electrophoresis in normal pregnant women reveals that urinary proteins are not different from those observed in nonpregnant women.[280] When urinary protein is evaluated by dipstick testing of a concentrated urine specimen, trace-positive results can be seen despite quantitatively normal protein excretion. Whenever in doubt, 24-hour quantitation of urinary protein should be performed. As is true for renal disease in general, urinary protein excretion of greater than 2 g/d is suggestive of a glomerular process, whereas tubulointerstitial disease may produce less proteinuria. Although pregnancy does not predispose to the development of renal disease, the de novo development of glomerulonephritis, membranous nephropathy, focal glomerulosclerosis, minimal change nephropathy, diabetic nephropathy, systemic lupus erythematosus (SLE), and other renal diseases may occasionally occur in pregnant women.

The presence of red blood cells in the urine is almost always caused by an organic process. Although preeclampsia causes glomerular lesions and proteinuria, it does not cause hematuria. Therefore, the finding of hematuria, particularly with red blood cell casts, in a patient with preeclampsia suggests the presence of underlying renal disease.[176]

When pregnancy becomes complicated by the apparent development of glomerulonephritis or other renal disease, a biopsy of the kidney is often contemplated. The necessity of renal biopsies has been debated for years because most renal diseases have no specific therapy.[281, 282] Empirical trials of steroids have been recommended for patients with uncomplicated nephrotic syndrome by some clinicians because minimal-change nephropathy readily responds to that treatment.[282] For the rare case of rapidly progressive glomerulonephritis with onset during pregnancy, a renal biopsy can be diagnostic and suggest appropriate therapy (e.g., pulse methylprednisolone, cytotoxic agents, or plasmapheresis). In these cases, pregnancy is not likely to succeed. In most cases in which renal disease is first recognized during pregnancy, a renal biopsy can be postponed until after delivery. However, when a specific diagnosis is immediately required, renal biopsy can be safely performed in a pregnant patient. If the usual guidelines for renal biopsy are followed (control hypertension, avoid aspirin for 7 to 10 days before biopsy), complications are no more frequent than in the nongravid state.[283, 284]

## Acute Renal Failure

Acute renal failure is defined as impairment of renal function and reduction in urine output developing during a period of hours to days. Acute renal failure during pregnancy usually takes the form of one of three renal diseases—ATN, renal cortical necrosis, or postpartum acute renal failure. Rarely, fatty liver of pregnancy or obstructive uropathy also cause acute renal failure. Acute renal failure occurring during pregnancy should be approached in the same manner as in the nonpregnant state.[285] When acute renal failure develops, there are often clues as to what renal disease is responsible (see later). However, when diagnostic clues are not available and the history does not suggest the underlying process, a systematic approach should be taken. This approach requires evaluating the patient for the possibility of prerenal azotemia by a careful physical examination to observe for signs of volume depletion, evaluation of the urinary tract collecting system to rule out obstructive uropathy, and then careful physical and laboratory evaluation. When urinary tract obstruction is suspected, abdominal ultrasonography can be performed to rule out hydronephrosis. However, because of the physiologic hydronephrosis of pregnancy, this diagnosis can be difficult (see later).

## Acute Tubule Necrosis

ATN occurs as a complication of many conditions, most commonly sepsis or hypotension. This condition has become rare in industrialized nations as the frequency of septic abortion has dramatically diminished and occurs in about 1 in 20,000 pregnancies.[286] A variety of nephrotoxins can cause ATN (see Chapter 28), but exposure of pregnant women to these agents is limited. In the first trimester, septic abortion accounts for the majority of patients with acute renal failure. Septic abortion is particularly likely to cause ATN when shock develops. Sepsis due to any gram-negative organism, most commonly *Escherichia coli*, can cause hypotension leading to acute renal failure. When *Clostridium perfringens* is the responsible bacterium, toxin-induced hemolysis is an additional factor predisposing to ATN. *Clostridium*-induced myonecrosis of the uterus is a source of myoglobin, which is also a nephrotoxin, particularly in the setting of impaired renal perfusion as would occur during hypotension. Profound or prolonged volume depletion can also cause ATN. This may be the result of hemorrhage complicating spontaneous abortion or, rarely, a consequence of hyperemesis gravidarum.

In late pregnancy, acute renal failure is a complication of preeclampsia or of uterine bleeding in abruptio placentae. ATN is a rare complication of preeclampsia, occurring in 1% to 2% of cases.[286] It is not exactly clear how ATN develops in this condition, but the diffuse endothelial cell swelling is postulated to produce renal ischemia and ATN. The HELLP syndrome is a complication of preeclampsia, occurring in 2% to 12% of cases of preeclampsia.[286] In the largest series of patients with HELLP syndrome reported by Sibai and Ramadan,[286] acute renal failure occurred in 32 of 435 cases (7.4%). One case was due to renal cortical necrosis, whereas the rest were due to ATN. In this series, there were four maternal deaths (13%); disseminated intravascular coagulation was seen in 84%, and pulmonary edema complicated 44% of cases. Dialysis was required in one third of these cases of ATN. Fetal complications were also high: perinatal mortality occurred in 34%, premature delivery in 72%. Nevertheless, at follow-up averaging 4.5 years, maternal renal function and blood pressure were normal.

Abruptio placentae can cause ATN, but it is also the most common cause of renal cortical necrosis. Severe volume depletion due to hemorrhage resulting in renal ischemia is presumed to be the cause of ATN in this setting. The occurrence of oliguria and a rising creatinine level suggest ATN. Physical findings are usually not diagnostic, but urinalysis can be. In ATN, the urine contains renal tubule epithelial cells, debris derived from necrotic epithelial cells, and numerous dark or "muddy brown" granular casts.

## Renal Cortical Necrosis

Many of the risk factors for ATN are also risk factors for the development of renal cortical necrosis. The majority of cases of acute cortical necrosis are caused by abruptio placentae, but other obstetric complications including septic abortion, severe preeclampsia, amniotic fluid embolism, and retained fetus are also associated with the development of renal cortical necrosis.[287, 288] Initially, it may be difficult to distinguish renal cortical necrosis from ATN, although anuria suggests the former. Renal cortical necrosis should also be suspected when oliguria or anuria persists for more than 1 week. In addition, hematuria is more likely in renal cortical necrosis than in ATN. Definitive diagnosis may be made by renal biopsy or, preferably, by renal arteriogram. The renal arteriogram shows patchy blood flow or an absent nephrogram. The diagnosis has also been made by computed tomographic scan, on which a radiolucent rim in the cortex parallel to the capsule represents the ischemic zone.[289]

Activation of the coagulation system has been proposed as a predisposing factor in the development of renal cortical necrosis. Postpartum rats have markedly increased sensitivity to endotoxin infusion, which causes a generalized Shwartzman reaction with renal effects similar to postpartum hemolytic-uremic syndrome. Postpartum rats more readily develop glomerular hemodynamic changes and intraglomerular capillary deposition of fibrin.[290] However, increases in clotting factors V, VIII, and X are also seen in uncomplicated pregnancy.[291] In one study comparing ATN with renal cortical necrosis, only plasma fibrinogen level was lower in the latter group with no differences in platelet count, thrombin, or fibrin degradation productions between the two conditions.[288] Thus, it is not clear why ATN develops in some women whereas renal cortical necrosis develops in others during obstetric emergencies. In addition to obstetric complications, cortical necrosis is more frequent in older women and multigravida, although these may not be independent risk factors but merely factors associated with the development of obstetric complications.[288] In some series, maternal mortality in cortical necrosis has been high because of the severity of the underlying disease.[292] A large number of patients with cortical necrosis never recover renal function or recover renal function transiently with later development of end-stage renal disease.[288]

## Postpartum Acute Renal Failure

Postpartum acute renal failure is also known as postpartum hemolytic-uremic syndrome. This is a disease characterized by hypertension and coagulation abnormalities, particularly microangiopathic hemolytic anemia.[293] It occurs in otherwise uncomplicated pregnancies anywhere from 1 to 2 days to several months after delivery. A history of a preceding viral illness is often obtained. Symptoms are those related to renal insufficiency, such as headache, nausea, and vomiting. The signs include oliguria or anuria, evidence of a bleeding diathesis, and, in many cases, hypertension. The examination of the peripheral blood smear is remarkable for the presence of schistocytes and burr cells. Thrombocytopenia is usual. Bleeding times are not usually prolonged, although fibrin degradation products may be increased.[293] Neurologic symptoms, when present, suggest thrombotic thrombocytopenic purpura. Many believe that hemolytic-uremic syndrome and thrombotic thrombocytopenic purpura are different manifestations of the same general disease process (see Chapter 35).

Although the precise etiology of postpartum hemolytic-uremic syndrome is not known, the findings in this systemic disease are suggestive of diffuse vascular endothelial cell injury. A similar form of hemolytic-uremic syndrome has occurred in women taking oral contraceptives, which suggests a link with the hormonal changes of pregnancy.[294] Evidence of endothelial cell injury in the kidney obtained by renal biopsy includes glomerular thromboses and fibrin deposition as well as fibrinoid necrosis within arterioles.[293] Interstitial fibrosis becomes more prominent with chronicity of the disease.

Supportive therapy usually requires dialysis. Other therapies employed have derived from experience with thrombotic thrombocytopenic purpura in nonpregnant patients. In attempts to reduce intravascular clotting, anticoagulants, antiplatelet agents, and $PGI_2$ have all been administered. Because uncontrolled trials in thrombotic thrombocytopenic purpura have suggested beneficial effects of plasma exchange or the infusion of fresh frozen plasma, these therapies have also been employed.[295] However, there has not been substantial experience with any one of these therapies for a general recommendation to be provided for their use. Plasma exchange is most frequently employed currently, despite the imperfections in our database.

## Obstructive Uropathy

Fewer than 20 cases of acute renal failure due to bilateral ureteral obstruction from a gravid uterus have been reported.[296, 297] Although no specific predisposing cause has been identified, approximately one third of these cases have been multiple gestations and one third have been complicated by polyhydramnios.[296] Three quarters of the cases occurred in primigravidas. Amniotomy was a successful therapy in a patient with polyhydramnios.[296] Alternatively, there have been several cases successfully treated by ureteral stenting.[298] The diagnosis of obstructive uropathy due to ureteral obstruction by the gravid uterus is suggested by the finding of oliguria or anuria in the setting of moderate or severe dilatation of the urinary collecting system, particularly on the left. Ultrasound evaluation in uncomplicated pregnancy revealed moderate dilatation on the left in 14% of cases and severe dilatation on the left in only 1% of cases.[299] As noted previously, dilatation on the right side is far more common.

## Nephrolithiasis

Urinary calculi occur in pregnant women with the same frequency as in nonpregnant women.[300] This is perhaps surprising because urinary $Ca^{2+}$ excretion increases in pregnancy, a consequence of increased gut $Ca^{2+}$ absorption and intake.[301, 302] However, urinary calculi are probably the most common cause of hospitalization for abdominal pain during pregnancy.[303] In most series, more than 90% of women diagnosed as having urinary calculi during pregnancy presented with flank or abdominal pain.[304, 305] More than 95% also had microscopic or gross hematuria to suggest the cause of the pain. Ultrasonography is the recommended procedure for detection of urinary calculi to avoid the low risk of radiation required by intravenous pyelography. However, when it is essential for diagnosis and therapy, limited intravenous pyelography can be safely performed.

The effects of pregnancy on stone formation in women with a history of chronic stone formation has also been assessed. In 78 women, only urinary tract infection appeared to be a serious complication of chronic nephrolithiasis in pregnancy.[300] Pregnancy did not increase the rate of stone formation or the frequency of complications related to stones.[300] In 20 pregnancies in stone formers, urologic instrumentation and operations were not necessary.[300] On the other hand, selected reports of experiences with urinary tract calculi during pregnancy have suggested a higher rate of complication and the need for intervention. This suggests that case reports collect only the most serious problems. In the past, there was a high frequency of a need for surgical intervention. However, in those patients unable to pass a ureteral calculus spontaneously, it is possible to place an internal ureteral stent safely and efficaciously in a pregnant woman.[306] The presence of a ureteral stent does not present complications for subsequent vaginal delivery.[306]

## Renal Disease in the Fetus

It is beyond the scope of this chapter to discuss renal abnormalities of the fetus. However, there are rare instances when maternal renal disease may have a direct or indirect impact on fetal or neonatal renal function. One example is the effects of medications administered to the mother that affect fetal renal function after transplacental passage of the drug. Angiotensin-converting enzyme inhibitors, which are now contraindicated for use in pregnancy, are one such example. When these drugs were administered to pregnant women near term, there were several reports of neonatal acute renal failure or hyperkalemia.[307, 308] It was postulated that the immature neonatal kidney, which has impaired renal blood flow autoregulation in early life, was dependent on angiotensin II to maintain renal perfusion. Fetal accumulation of the angiotensin-converting enzyme inhibitor, therefore, resulted in a form of reversible but severe and sometimes prolonged prerenal azotemia. Several neonatal deaths were attributed to this complication.

An unlikely occurrence is the transmission of nonhereditary renal disease from mother to infant. However, there is at least one carefully evaluated report of the development of membranous nephropathy in a neonate due to transplacental passage of maternal immunoglobulin G resulting in neonatal glomerulopathy with anuria.[309] The rarity of such reports suggests that this phenomenon, although of great pathophysiologic interest, is not a major clinical consideration.

# PREGNANCY IN WOMEN WITH RENAL DISEASE

In women with renal disease, whether pre-existent or developing during pregnancy, there are several considerations relevant to the interaction between pregnancy and renal disease. Renal disease can have significant and serious consequences for both maternal health and fetal outcome. On the other hand, there is the risk that pregnancy will have an adverse effect on renal function that might be permanent. Although these topics are discussed individually, when the physician is counseling the patient with renal disease as to the advisability and risks of pregnancy, no simple recommendations can be given to a particular patient. Any pregnant woman with underlying renal disease should be managed jointly by an obstetrician experienced in high-risk pregnancies and by a nephrologist.

## Effects of Renal Disease on Fetal Outcome

Fertility is greatly diminished by renal insufficiency, particularly when the GFR is less than 50% of normal.[310] Nevertheless, pregnancy occasionally occurs in patients with severe renal insufficiency and even in patients on chronic dialysis. In one report of 907 women treated with chronic hemodialysis in Saudi Arabia, 7% of married women younger than 50 years had experienced at least one pregnancy between 1 month and 5 years after beginning hemodialysis.[311] Although a successful outcome was observed in only one third of pregnancies (see later), it is apparent that pregnancy occasionally occurs in women with even marginal renal function.

The important consequences of maternal renal disease include an increased frequency of fetal loss, intrauterine growth retardation, and prematurity. The major risk factor for these undesirable outcomes is hypertension. Renal insufficiency and the presence of the nephrotic syndrome are additional fetal risk factors. More than 30 years ago, Rauramo and colleagues[312] noted an inverse relationship between the interval between the onset of renal disease (when known) and pregnancy on the one hand, and the frequency of preeclampsia, perinatal mortality, and premature birth on the other. Therefore, those women with a more chronic and stable course (a longer interval between disease onset and pregnancy) had a lower risk of adverse outcome. Mackay[313] prospectively studied 150 women with renal disease complicating pregnancy during a 10-year period. This author observed that the overall rate of fetal wastage was 34%. However, in women with proteinuria and normal renal function, fetal loss depended on whether preeclampsia was superimposed on the pregnancy. Therefore, fetal loss was 10% in women in whom preeclampsia did not develop and

29% in those with superimposed preeclampsia. In women who had impaired renal function when they became pregnant, fetal outcome was even worse. When renal function was impaired, fetal loss was approximately 40%. In pregnancies in which renal insufficiency was accompanied by severe hypertension (blood pressure greater than 175/110 mm Hg), fetal loss was 60%.[313] It is often difficult to measure the severity of maternal renal disease other than by GFR. When Barceló and co-workers[314] analyzed their experience using the 24-hour excretion of protein as one indicator of the extent of renal disease in women with glomerulonephritis, they found an inverse relationship with birth weight (Fig. 36–8).

Katz and colleagues[315] reported the outcome of 121 pregnancies in 89 women with a variety of renal disorders treated at three medical centers. In their series, renal function was good in all women (serum creatinine level ≤ 1.4 mg/dL), hypertension was present before pregnancy in only 20%, and nephrotic syndrome was present in only four women. Superimposed preeclampsia developed in 12% of pregnancies. Perinatal mortality was 9%, a rate three to four times greater than that usual for the participating hospitals. Preterm deliveries occurred in 20% of pregnancies, and infants were small for gestational age in 24% of pregnancies (a fourfold increase). Thus, in women with a variety of glomerular diseases but preservation of renal function, there was still a considerable increase in the frequency of fetal morbidity and mortality.

In a retrospective review of 25 years' experience of pregnancy (398 pregnancies) in 238 Australian women with glomerulonephritis, Packham and associates[316] reported a fetal loss rate of 20% (three quarters in the second half of pregnancy). Twenty-four percent of infants were premature; only 50% of pregnancies resulted in live births at term. Infants were small for gestational age in 15% of live births. The presence of impaired renal function, pre-existing hypertension or the development of severe hypertension, or the nephrotic syndrome resulted in a perinatal mortality of 30%, whereas women without any of these features had only 5% perinatal mortality. Surian and co-workers[317] reported the course of 123 pregnancies in 86 patients with biopsy-proven glomerular disease. Their results were somewhat better. The perinatal death rate was 9%; 5.7% of infants were small for gestational age; 14% were premature.

One of the difficulties of evaluating the available literature is that obstetric outcomes in general have improved dramatically in the past 20 years. This makes it difficult to compare recent studies to older ones or to use historical control outcomes for comparisons. For example, Hou and colleagues[318] reported on the outcomes of 25 pregnancies in women with moderate renal insufficiency (creatinine level ≥ 1.4 mg/dL, a value that in earlier studies was associated with worse outcome). Fetal mortality rate was 16%, and 61% of live births were premature. Imbasciati and co-workers[319] reported their experience with a similar group of women in Italy. Fetal loss occurred in 21%, and 54% of the live births were preterm. Jungers and associates[320] retrospectively reviewed outcome in 148 pregnancies in women with a variety of biopsy-proven glomerulonephritides. As was seen in other studies, poor fetal outcome was associated with the presence of uncontrolled hypertension, ne-

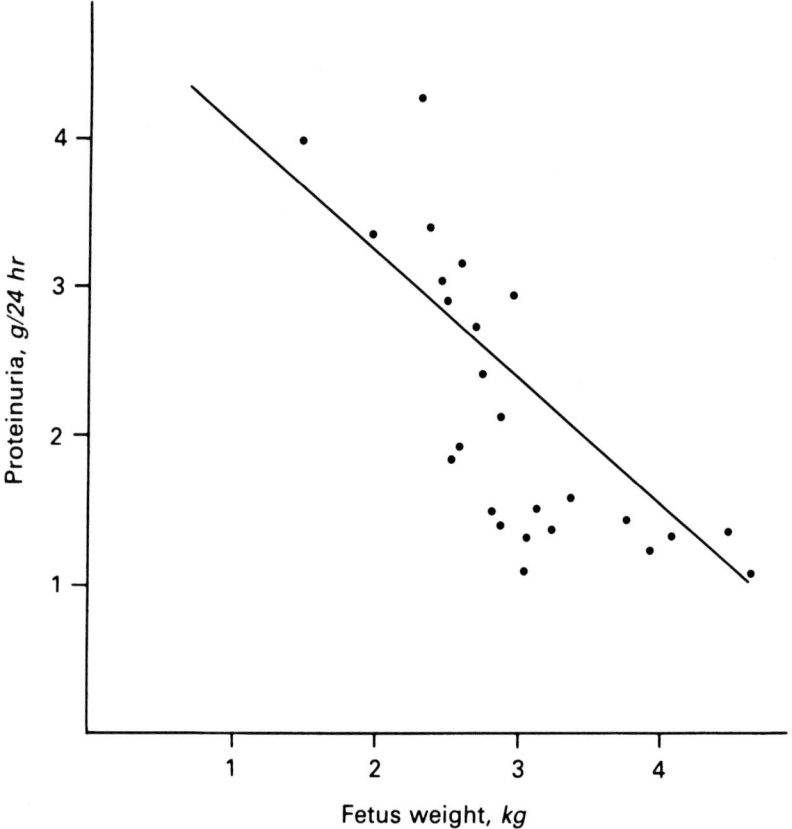

**Figure 36–8.** Inverse relationship between extent of proteinuria and fetal weight in women with primary glomerular disease ($r = .71$, $P < .01$). (From Barceló P, López-Lillo J, Cabero L, Del Río G: Successful pregnancy in primary glomerular disease. Used with permission from Kidney International, volume 30, p 914, 1986.)

phrotic range proteinuria, or renal insufficiency (creatinine level > 1.8 mg/dL). Similarly, in a report of the experience of 240 pregnancies in 166 Japanese women with renal disease, the live birth rate was 86% (perinatal deaths 6%, spontaneous abortion 8%).[321] Perinatal loss occurred with greater frequency in women with hypertension or a GFR less than 70 mL/min.

The signs and symptoms of renal disease influence the outcome of pregnancy rather than the specific renal diagnosis. Stettler and Cunningham[245] evaluated the outcome of 65 pregnancies in 53 women with proteinuria greater than 500 mg/24 h but no previously documented renal disease and normal renal function at the onset of pregnancy. Forty percent of the women had chronic hypertension, which suggests established but merely undiagnosed renal disease. Although the live birth rate was 93%, 45% of infants were preterm and 23% had intrauterine growth retardation. Two thirds of the women had superimposed preeclampsia. Twenty-one of these women eventually underwent renal biopsy and were found to have histologic evidence for renal disease.

Leppert and co-workers[322] assessed the outcome of pregnancy in women who had a history of childhood renal disease that had apparently resolved. These diseases included pyelonephritis or acute glomerulonephritis. The frequency of spontaneous abortion and perinatal mortality was not different between these women and concurrent control groups. However, the frequency of small-for-gestational-age infants was increased from 1.5% to 5.5%. Women in whom childhood renal disease resulted in sustained renal insufficiency (creatinine level > 1.5 mg/dL) had, not un-

expectedly, greater fetal mortality and a higher frequency of superimposed preeclampsia. In summary, even a history of previous renal disease represents a small but real risk factor for unfavorable fetal outcome. Renal insufficiency, hypertension, and heavy proteinuria are much more serious risk factors for an unfavorable pregnancy outcome.

As noted, the risk of developing superimposed preeclampsia during pregnancy varies between 20% and 40% in women with some form of underlying renal disease. When preeclampsia is associated with renal disease, multiparous as well as nulliparous women are affected, and the disease may manifest earlier than 32 weeks. In one study, 25% of all cases of preeclampsia had onset before 37 weeks of gestation. Ninety percent of these women had chronic renal disease or essential hypertension.[257] Because the chances for the development of superimposed preeclampsia are so great in women with renal disease, this high-risk group would seem to be most appropriate for intervention with therapeutic agents, such as low-dose aspirin or calcium. Most such trials have specifically excluded women with known or suspected renal disease. In the Italian study of aspirin in 1106 pregnant women, 232 had either chronic hypertension or nephropathy.[323] Low-dose aspirin therapy resulted in a nonsignificant increase in birth weight and percentage of infants below the 10th percentile for birth weight, but this subgroup was too small for any firm conclusions to be made regarding the benefit of aspirin therapy. The effects of aspirin therapy on blood pressure were not reported for this subgroup. Although the reported studies suggest overall that the greater risk for the development of preeclampsia or intrauterine growth retardation, the greater the likelihood of benefit of low-dose aspirin therapy, specific experience for patients with renal disease is inadequate. Although these patients are clearly in the highest risk group for the development of superimposed preeclampsia and intrauterine growth retardation, we can only extrapolate from the literature and surmise whether low-dose aspirin therapy would be beneficial. Conservative physicians will wait until a specific trial in this group of patients has been performed, whereas those with a more aggressive approach will prescribe low-dose aspirin for pregnant patients with renal disease because the risk of aspirin is relatively low and the potential benefits may be great.[324–327] Similarly, although calcium supplements have been advocated to reduce the frequency of preeclampsia in women at risk, there has been no experience with these supplements in women with renal disease.

## The Risk of Progression of Renal Disease in Pregnancy

Most renal diseases enter an inexorably deteriorating course once a threshold of initial renal injury has been reached, even if the initiating process resolves.[328, 329] In the last decade, there has been an explosive increase in the interest in and information about this process, in large part deriving from work in experimental renal disease. Brenner and Hostetter and their colleagues[328–330] proposed that the common feature in all chronic progressive renal disease is an increase in glomerular capillary blood flow and intraglomerular capillary pressure. Intraglomerular hypertension leads to progressive damage that is manifested by the histologic findings of glomerulosclerosis and subsequent interstitial fibrosis. Indeed, these are the features of chronic renal disease regardless of the initiating form of injury (see Chapter 44 for a more complete discussion of this subject).

The potential implication of pregnancy in women with chronic renal disease is that the development or worsening of hypertension during pregnancy will have a particularly detrimental effect on the disease. Because pregnancy, like chronic renal disease, is characterized by dilatation of the afferent arteriole of the glomerulus, systemic blood pressure would be more completely transmitted into the glomerulus and systemic hypertension would potentially be more damaging to the kidney than it would be in cases in which chronic renal disease or pregnancy did not exist. Animal studies suggest that in normotensive rats, afferent arteriolar dilatation results in increases in glomerular blood flow, but no change in intraglomerular pressure and consequently no renal damage despite repeated pregnancy.[18] Spontaneously hypertensive rats might be expected to develop accelerated renal injury when pregnant. However, of great interest, these rats have been observed not to develop afferent arteriolar relaxation during pregnancy and, therefore, no pregnancy-induced increase in GFR.[331] On the other hand, the absence of the normal renal vasodilatory response to pregnancy means that the kidneys of spontaneously hypertensive rats were not subjected to increased intraglomerular pressure during pregnancy, and repetitive pregnancies in spontaneously hypertensive rats did not lead to progressive renal insufficiency.[332] In a normotensive model of mild glo-

merulonephritis produced by injection of anti–glomerular basement membrane antibody, glomerular capillary hydraulic pressure did not increase during the first half of pregnancy, and there was no pregnancy-related worsening of proteinuria or glomerular morphologic features.[333] However, in another model of experimental glomerulonephritis produced by injection of rats with doxorubicin, pregnancy was associated with systemic hypertension and a marked increase in urinary protein excretion that presumably reflects an early adverse effect on the kidney.[334]

From these experiments, it is hard to predict what the effect of pregnancy would be in women with chronic renal disease, except that hypertension might adversely affect renal outcome. Women with mild renal insufficiency respond in a qualitatively normal way to pregnancy with an increase in GFR and renal blood flow in a pattern similar to that in Figure 36–1. When renal function is more severely impaired, the magnitude of the pregnancy-induced hyperfiltration is diminished.[315]

### RISK FACTORS FOR PROGRESSION OF RENAL DISEASE

Studies of the effects of pregnancy on renal outcome in women with renal disease in general bear out these predictions. For the most part, women with renal disease who become pregnant when renal function is normal or minimally depressed tolerate pregnancy without permanent deleterious effects on renal function. Conversely, as many as one third of women with moderate renal insufficiency experience a more rapid decline in renal function after pregnancy than would have been predicted on the basis of the natural history of their disease. The majority of observations of the effects of pregnancy on the course of renal disease were made before a complete understanding of the importance of systemic hypertension to the course of renal disease. Therefore, there has not been an adequate trial of vigorous control of hypertension during pregnancy in women with moderate renal insufficiency to see whether this would prevent an accelerated downhill course in some of these women.

In the study by Katz and colleagues[315] of pregnancy effects on renal disease in women with a variety of glomerulonephritides but normal renal function before conception, permanent impairment of renal function by pregnancy was rare. Sixteen percent of women developed transient decrements in renal function during pregnancy. In three patients, pregnancy occurred while glomerular filtration was already falling, but gestation did not appear to alter the time course. In 57 of the 121 pregnancies observed, there was severe or substantially increased proteinuria that was in the nephrotic range in 68% of these proteinuric cases.[101] As noted previously, superimposed preeclampsia developed in 12% of the women. However, after pregnancy, preeclampsia, by definition, resolved. Renal function returned to its previous level, except as noted, and proteinuria tended to return to prepartum levels. Other investigators studying several different populations have come to similar conclusions that in women with prepartum renal disease but preserved renal function, pregnancy does not appear to adversely affect the underlying renal disease.[314, 320, 321] Abe and colleagues[321] suggested that as long as the GFR was greater than 70 mL/min and that blood pressure remained below 140/90 mm Hg, the underlying glomerular disease was not adversely affected in 244 pregnancies. In another group of 148 women with chronic glomerulonephritis who became pregnant, the overall course of renal disease was not different from that of a control cohort of 172 women with the same types of glomerulonephritis who did not become pregnant.[320] Barceló and co-workers[314] evaluated 66 pregnancies in 48 women with glomerular disease. Although most patients had mild renal dysfunction, several had greater impairment of renal function, severe hypertension, or nephrotic range proteinuria. As a group, when evaluated 1 and 5 years after pregnancy, these women fared no worse in terms of their renal disease than did a control group of women who had not become pregnant. Individually, there were cases of apparent worsening of renal function in two women and the development of irreversible proteinuria in four, but these effects could not be differentiated from chance alone.[314]

Several studies do suggest, however, that if women become pregnant when they have moderate impairment of renal function, there is a greater chance of permanent deterioration in renal function as a consequence of pregnancy. Hou and associates[318] studied the effects of 25 pregnancies in 23 women with renal insufficiency before pregnancy (serum creatinine level $\geq$ 1.4 mg/dL). In seven of these women whose baseline creatinine level was between 1.7 and 2.7 mg/dL, pregnancy resulted in a decline in renal function that was greater than expected. In more than half of the pregnancies, hypertension developed or worsened; in 36% of the pregnancies, the diastolic blood pressure exceeded 110 mm Hg. Imbasciati and co-workers[319] studied a similar group of 18 women. In 14 pregnancies, there were sufficient data to plot reciprocal plasma creatinine values versus time before and after pregnancy. In 5 of these 14 women, there was an apparent acceleration in the rate of progression after pregnancy. These two studies found a remarkably similar frequency of approximately 33% of women with renal insufficiency that developed an accelerated course during pregnancy.

## PROGRESSION IN SPECIFIC RENAL DISEASES

In most studies, the number of women evaluated has been too small for conclusions to be made about the chance of progression of renal disease during pregnancy for a specific renal diagnosis. However, there is a suggestion that women with membranoproliferative glomerulonephritis, immunoglobulin A nephropathy, focal sclerosis, and reflux nephropathy are at a greater risk for the development of irreversible renal failure than are those with other diagnoses of renal disease. For example, although Barceló and colleagues[314] observed that pregnancy did not, in general, adversely affect renal disease, the few cases of renal deterioration they observed occurred in women with membranoproliferative glomerulonephritis. Similarly, Abe and colleagues[321] reported that the highest frequency of the development of hypertension or decreased renal function in pregnant women with glomerular disease occurred in those

with membranoproliferative glomerulonephritis. Jungers and associates[320] noted that several patients with membranoproliferative glomerulonephritis were among those who suffered deterioration in renal function during pregnancy, but these women also had impaired renal function before pregnancy.

Reflux nephropathy has been suggested as a specific diagnosis imparting increased risk for renal deterioration during pregnancy. Becker and co-workers[335] observed 20 women with reflux nephropathy and plasma creatinine levels between 2.3 and 4.5 mg/dL. Six women had a pregnancy lasting more than 12 weeks. All six experienced a rapid deterioration in renal function, and four of the six reached end-stage renal failure within 2 years of pregnancy. In the women who never became pregnant, renal function deteriorated slowly, and no patient reached end-stage renal failure within 7 years. By contrast, in women with reflux nephropathy and a serum creatinine level less than 1.5 mg/dL, renal deterioration was not observed and hypertension complicated pregnancy in only 11% of cases.[320]

Immunoglobulin A nephropathy is a common form of primary glomerulonephritis. In Japan, Abe[336] studied 168 pregnancies in 118 women with immunoglobulin A nephropathy during an 18-year period. Overall, the rate of spontaneous abortion was 9%, live birth rate 87%, and perinatal death rate 4%. When results were stratified by maternal renal function, if the GFR was lower than 70 mL/min before conception, the perinatal mortality rate was 14% versus 3%. Similarly, if the baseline blood pressure was consistently greater than 140/90 mm Hg, the perinatal mortality was 33% versus 1%. When the results were stratified by year of diagnosis, it was found that the perinatal death rate was 9% during the 1970s but 0% in the 1980s. More than half of the women were observed for 3 years or longer, and it was judged that their course was not different from the natural history of immunoglobulin A nephropathy. This study suggests that with the current excellent standards of obstetric care, complications should be minimal if renal function is preserved and hypertension is controlled before pregnancy.

One feature that seemed to predict a poor outcome was the presence on renal biopsy specimens of lesions in the arterioles, tubules, and interstitium, in addition to glomerular lesions.[336] This is of interest because Packham and colleagues[316] noted that the presence of vascular lesions on renal biopsy specimens from patients with glomerulonephritis also predicted a higher rate of fetal loss during pregnancy. In other series evaluating the outcome of pregnancy in women with glomerulonephritis, women with immunoglobulin A nephropathy have usually fared better than the mean. This was true in the series reported by Packham and colleagues[316] and by Barceló and co-workers.[314] Jungers and co-workers[320] found no effect of pregnancy on the course of immunoglobulin A nephropathy in 48 women experiencing at least one pregnancy compared with 44 who did not become pregnant.

SLE is not an uncommon disease affecting women of childbearing age. Historically, there were concerns that pregnancy induced exacerbations of SLE and that fetal wastage was extremely high in this disease.[337] Modern studies have not generally borne out these fears. Clinical exacerbations or relapses have been reported in between 9% and 60% of pregnancies.[337-339] However, the rate of disease exacerbations is not different in concurrent control groups and nonpregnant patients.[339] The major factor determining whether pregnancy results in an exacerbation of lupus is the stability of the disease before the pregnancy. Thus, when SLE is in remission or well controlled for a period of more than 6 months, the chance of a clinical flare during pregnancy is low.[337, 338] On the other hand, when pregnancy occurs in close temporal association with an exacerbation of SLE, exacerbations are also frequently seen during or shortly after pregnancy.

Fetal survival is also closely related to the clinical status of SLE before conception. Hayslett and Lynn[340] reported a fetal survival rate of 88% in women in remission at the onset of pregnancy compared with 64% when SLE was active at the beginning of pregnancy. Several other reports document a similar differential effect of lupus activity on fetal outcome in pregnancy.[338, 341] The presence of anticardiolipin antibodies is certainly related to an increased likelihood of spontaneous abortion.[150] However, it is controversial whether fetal outcome beyond the first trimester is adversely affected by the presence of antiphospholipid antibody. Permanent adverse effects on renal function are rare in women with lupus who have become pregnant. Packham and co-workers[342] found a 19% occurrence of reversible renal function deterioration during pregnancy, but only 1 case in 64 pregnancies of irreversible deterioration in renal function. As is true for all women with renal disease, hypertension may worsen during pregnancy. Packham and colleagues[342] observed the development of hypertension in 28% of their cases. The hypertension was severe in 13%. Similarly, proteinuria increased in 48% of pregnancies, but this increase was irreversible in only 5%. In the report of Bobrie and co-workers[338] of 213 pregnancies in 73 patients, irreversible deterioration in renal function was observed in 4 of the 53 pregnancies occurring in women whose SLE was not active at conception.

The effects of diabetes mellitus on fetal outcome are well known and include prematurity, congenital abnormalities, large-for-gestational-age infants, and the respiratory distress syndrome. Kitzmiller and associates[343] observed the effects of pregnancy on diabetic nephropathy. They studied 35 women with diabetes and nephropathy (defined as 24-hour urinary protein excretion > 400 mg) who became pregnant. Of 26 women whose pregnancy reached 24 weeks' gestation, the nephrotic syndrome developed in 69% in the third trimester (58% had 24-hour urinary protein excretion in excess of 6 g). Fifty-seven percent of the initially normotensive women (14 women) became hypertensive. Despite these pregnancy-induced exacerbations in proteinuria and hypertension, proteinuria decreased post partum in 60%, and the rate of decline of the GFR was not accelerated by pregnancy.

The group at Yale[344] studied a group of women with 31 pregnancies. One fourth of the patients had nephrotic syndrome at the beginning of pregnancy, and renal function was reduced in half of the pregnancies. One third of the pregnancies were complicated by further deterioration in renal function, and three fourths had nephrotic syndrome by the third trimester. Hypertension developed or worsened

in two thirds of the pregnancies. Nevertheless, fetal survival was 94%; after delivery, renal function, proteinuria, and hypertension returned to baseline levels.

Pregnancy appears to have a similar effect on nonglomerular renal disease, although this has been less well studied. In autosomal dominant polycystic kidney disease, pregnancy was frequently complicated by hypertension or preeclampsia (18% versus 1.6% in control subjects), although changes in renal function were not immediately apparent.[345] Despite the association of polycystic kidney diseases and infection, pregnancy did not increase the frequency of urinary tract infection.[345] On the other hand, in their broad survey of the risk factors associated with progression of renal disease in polycystic kidney disease, Gabow and co-workers[346] noted a positive association between women having experienced three or more pregnancies and worse renal function. However, because the number of pregnancies was not treated as a continuous variable in that study, it is not clear whether a smaller number of pregnancies also has an adverse consequence on polycystic kidney disease. This is one of the best available studies for evaluating the consequences of pregnancy in a renal disease that has a sufficiently slow and stable course to determine whether pregnancy represents an independent risk factor for renal disease progression. In this instance, pregnancy had the small but discernible effect of accelerating chronic renal injury.

Although it is often difficult to compare series of patients from different hospitals and different eras, it seems that differences in outcome are more heavily affected by the severity of the renal disease than by the histologic diagnosis or type of renal disease. Therefore, regardless of the specific type of glomerulonephritis or other renal disease, nearly every study has demonstrated that the presence of renal insufficiency, heavy proteinuria or nephrotic syndrome, or severe or uncontrollable hypertension represents an important risk factor for worsening of renal function during and after pregnancy.[347] Knowing the importance of these three risk factors for an adverse outcome in pregnancy associated with renal disease permits the counseling physician to relate this information to women contemplating pregnancy.

## PREVENTING PROGRESSION OF RENAL DISEASE

For many renal diseases, there is little that can be done therapeutically to restore renal function or to dramatically reduce proteinuria when chronically present (disease exacerbations in minimal-change glomerulopathy and SLE are two obvious exceptions). On the other hand, hypertension is treatable. Although prospective data are not available, it is probable that strict control of hypertension during pregnancy would have protective effects on the kidney as has been demonstrated in nonpregnant women and in men. An increase in proteinuria, even in the absence of increasing blood pressure, suggests the need for more aggressive blood pressure control. What is more controversial is the precise blood pressure goal for pregnant women. Recalling that pregnancy is a condition associated with afferent arteriolar vasodilatation and greater transmission of systemic blood pressure into the glomerulus, a nephrologist would generally recommend aggressive blood pressure control. However, these goals must be balanced with concerns for fetal well-being.

High levels of dietary protein intake are also associated with an adverse renal outcome in chronic progressive renal disease.[348] Dietary protein increases renal blood flow and stimulates renin secretion, factors that would lead to increased glomerular capillary flow and pressure.[349] In a prospective study of protein supplementation in women *without* renal disease, there was an increase in the frequency of premature birth, neonatal death, and intrauterine growth retardation.[350] Therefore, protein supplementation is not advisable for any pregnant woman and certainly not for women with renal disease. Women with renal disease who become pregnant should follow a normal or modestly restricted dietary protein intake rather than a high one.

## TREATMENT OF RENAL FAILURE IN PREGNANCY

### Dialysis

As noted earlier, although women undergoing chronic hemodialysis do occasionally become pregnant, most experience in the treatment of pregnant patients by hemodialysis has accrued with women who became pregnant with moderate renal insufficiency and progressed to end-stage renal disease during pregnancy. The general principle for treatment of chronic hemodialysis patients is that more dialysis is generally better.[351] This dictum has been empirically employed in cases complicated by pregnancy. This course of action has included instituting dialysis early (e.g., when the GFR is approximately 10 mL/min rather than waiting until it falls further) and treating with more frequent and longer hemodialysis sessions.[311, 352, 353] Among dialysis patients, the therapeutic abortion rate is higher than for the general population, which makes an unbiased assessment of the literature difficult. Most studies of dialysis in pregnancy consist of collections of case reports from several medical centers. It is not known whether the general trend to report only successful cases or those in which longer dialysis sessions were performed has biased these reports. The European Dialysis and Transplant Association reported pregnancy in 115 women. Of those not electively terminating pregnancy, 23% of pregnancies resulted in live birth.[354] Redrow and coworkers[352] reported cases of 13 pregnant women treated with hemodialysis. During pregnancy, hypertension worsened in most patients (77%). Premature labor complicated all but two pregnancies. Ninety percent of the infants were small for gestational age, but neither respiratory distress nor fetal abnormalities were problems during delivery. Souqiyyeh and colleagues[311] reported 8 live births in 27 cases of pregnancy in women on hemodialysis. Their patients did not have uncontrollable hypertension during pregnancy. In most reports of successful pregnancies, hemodialysis sessions were lengthened or their frequency was increased from three times to five or more times per week. Anemia has been more aggressively treated, now an easier task with the availability of erythropoietin, which has been successfully used in pregnant hemodialysis patients.[355] In addition,

hypotension has been carefully avoided to lessen the chance of fetal hypoperfusion.

As an alternative modality to provide continuous dialysis and to avoid the risks of intermittent hypotension and anticoagulation, chronic peritoneal dialysis has been employed. Both continuous ambulatory peritoneal dialysis and continuous cycling peritoneal dialysis have been reported to produce modest success.[353, 356] Interestingly, continuous ambulatory peritoneal dialysis was not technically difficult, and catheter leaks and inadequate peritoneal cavity volume were not problems. Most patients could tolerate at least 1500-mL exchanges.

In some cases of pregnancy occurring in women with advanced renal insufficiency (GFR < 10 mL/min), prophylactic dialysis has been employed on the basis of the reasoning that in normal pregnancy the GFR increases substantially to meet the needs of the mother and developing fetus, whereas in women with far-advanced renal disease this is not possible. Successful reports of this strategy are available, but controlled studies have not been performed.[357] It should be pointed out that there also exist a small number of case reports of pregnancy in women with advanced renal failure treated conservatively or with dietary protein restriction.[358, 359] These results were not apparently different from those reported for women more aggressively treated with hemodialysis. However, it is unlikely that such a conservative approach will gain wide acceptance or be subjected to a controlled trial.

### Transplantation

Outcomes of pregnancies that occur in women who are recipients of kidney transplants are dramatically different from the experience in hemodialysis patients. Davison[360] surveyed 2309 pregnancies in 1594 women who had previously received a kidney transplant. After therapeutic abortions and the 13% of pregnancies that ended in spontaneous abortion were accounted for, pregnancies were successful in 92%. When specifically evaluated, renal function increased in the transplanted kidney in a manner consistent with that observed in normal native kidneys.[361] Acute rejection episodes were seen in 9% of the patients, a frequency believed to be no greater than that in nonpregnant women.[360] Hypertension or preeclampsia developed in approximately 30% of pregnancies, representing the most important maternal complication. The most significant fetal complication was preterm delivery, which occurred in 45% to 60% of cases. Twenty percent to 30% of infants were small for gestational age. Vaginal delivery was not made difficult by the presence of the pelvic kidney. Therefore, cesarean sections should be reserved for the usual obstetric indications.

Although much of the experience with pregnancy in transplant recipients occurred before the general availability of cyclosporine, results in women treated with cyclosporine are similar. Muirhead and co-workers[362] reported their experience at a single transplant center and were able to compare results in women receiving cyclosporine with those not. In infants whose mothers received cyclosporine, mean birth weight was 2.1 versus 2.6 kg, mean gestational age was 34 versus 36 weeks, and the frequency of preterm delivery was 79% versus 50%. A preliminary report of the National Transplantation Pregnancy Registry of 154 pregnancies revealed similar outcomes in women treated with or without cyclosporine.[363]

Kidney allografts appear to tolerate pregnancy well. There was the fear that pregnancy-induced hyperfiltration could adversely affect long-term survival of allografts. Sturgiss and Davison[364] performed a case-control study of women with transplanted kidneys when they became pregnant and had a mean follow-up period of 12 years. At the end of the follow-up period, the GFR was similar whether pregnancy had occurred or not. Graft loss, chronic rejection, and death occurred with equal frequency whether pregnancy had occurred. Although this study encompassed only 36 patients, it suggests that there is no adverse effect of pregnancy on long-term outcome in kidney allograft recipients. The registry of the European Dialysis and Transplant Association also reported no adverse effect of successful pregnancy on graft function.[365] Renal function deteriorated in 18% of women experiencing a successful pregnancy and in 24% of control subjects during a similar period.

## REFERENCES

1. Garland HO, Green R, Moriarty RJ: Changes in body weight, kidney weight and proximal tubule length during pregnancy in the rat. Renal Physiol 1:42, 1978.
2. Christensen T, Klebe JG, Bertelsen V, et al: Changes in renal volume during normal pregnancy. Acta Obstet Gynecol Scand 68:541, 1989.
3. Guyer PB, Delany D: Urinary tract dilation and oral contraceptives. Br Med J 4:488, 1970.
4. Bozarki S, Lebay P, Gerber C: Prostaglandin inhibition of ureteral peristalsis. Invest Urol 4:9, 1966.
5. Sala NL, Rubi RA: Ureteral function in pregnant women. V. Incidence of vesicoureteral reflux and its effect upon ureteral contractility. Am J Obstet Gynecol 112:871, 1972.
6. MacGillivray I, Rose GA, Rowe B: Blood pressure survey in pregnancy. Clin Sci 37:395, 1969.
7. DeSwiet M: The cardiovascular system. In Hytten FE, Chamberlain GVP (eds): Clinical Physiology in Obstetrics. Blackwell Scientific Publications, Oxford, 1980, p 3.
8. Visser W, Wallenburg HCS: Central hemodynamic observations in untreated pre-eclamptic patients. Hypertension 17:1072, 1991.
9. Hytten FE, Leitch I: The Physiology of Human Pregnancy, 2nd ed. Blackwell Scientific Publications, Oxford, 1971.
10. Phippard AF, Horvath JS, Glynn EM, et al: Circulatory adaptation to pregnancy—serial studies of hemodynamics, blood volume, renin and aldosterone in the baboon (Papio hamadryas). J Hypertens 4:773, 1986.
11. Robertson EG: The natural history of oedema during pregnancy. J Obstet Gynaecol Br Commonw 78:520, 1971.
12. Thompson AM, Hytten RE, Billewecz WZ: The epidemiology of oedema during pregnancy. J Obstet Gynaecol Br Commonw 74:1, 1967.
13. Sims EAH, Krantz KE: Serial studies of renal function during pregnancy and the puerperium in normal women. J Clin Invest 37:1764, 1958.
14. Assali NS, Dignam WJ, Dasgupta K: Renal function in human pregnancy: Effects of venous pooling on renal hemodynamics and water, electrolyte and aldosterone excretion during normal gestation. J Lab Clin Med 54:394, 1959.
15. DeAlvarez RR: Renal glomerulotubular mechanisms during normal pregnancy: I. Glomerular filtration rate, renal plasma flow and creatinine clearance. Am J Obstet Gynecol 75:931, 1958.
16. Dunlop W: Renal physiology in pregnancy. Postgrad Med J 55:329, 1979.
17. Davison JM, Dunlop W: Renal hemodynamics and tubular function in normal human pregnancy. Kidney Int 18:152, 1980.
18. Baylis C, Reckelhoff JF: Renal hemodynamics in normal and hypertensive pregnancy: Lessons from micropuncture. Am J Kidney Dis 17:98, 1991.
19. Conrad KP: Renal hemodynamics during pregnancy in chronically catheterized, conscious rats. Kidney Int 26:24, 1984.
20. Baylis C, Brango C, Engels K: Renal effects of moderate hemorrhage in the conscious pregnant rat. Am J Physiol 259:F945, 1990.
21. Reckelhoff J, Samsell L, Baylis C: Dissociation between plasma volume expansion (PVE) and increases in GFR during pregnancy in the rat. Kidney Int 35:472, 1989.
22. Woods LL, Mizelle HL, Hall JE: Autoregulation of renal blood flow and glomerular filtration rate in the pregnant rabbit. Am J Physiol 252:R69, 1987.
23. Baylis C, Blantz RC: Tubuloglomerular feedback activity in virgin and 12 day pregnant rats. Am J Physiol 249:F169, 1985.
24. Baylis C: Effect of amino acid infusion as an index of renal vasodilatory capacity in pregnant rats. Am J Physiol 254:F650, 1988.
25. Bay WH, Ferris TF: Factors controlling plasma renin and aldosterone during pregnancy. Hypertension 1:410, 1979.
26. Lewis PJ, Boylan P, Friedman LA, et al: Prostacyclin in pregnancy. Br Med J 280:1581, 1980.
27. Brown GP, Venuto RE: In vitro renal eicosanoid production during pregnancy in rabbits. Am J Physiol 254:E687, 1988.
28. Conrad KP, Dunn MJ: Renal synthesis and urinary excretion of eicosanoids during pregnancy in rats. Am J Physiol 253:F1197, 1987.
29. Baylis C: Renal effects of cyclooxygenase inhibition in the pregnant rat. Am J Physiol 253:F158, 1987.
30. Conrad KP, Colpoys MC: Evidence against the hypothesis that prostaglandins are the vasodepressor agents of pregnancy. Serial studies in chronically instrumented, conscious rats. J Clin Invest 77:236, 1986.
31. Baylis C: Glomerular ultrafiltration in the pseudopregnant rat. Am J Physiol 243:F300, 1982.
32. Walker J, Garland HO: Single nephron function during prolactin-induced pseudopregnancy in the rat. J Endocrinol 107:127, 1985.
33. Conrad KP: Possible mechanisms for changes in renal hemodynamics during pregnancy: Studies from animal models. Am J Kidney Dis 9:253, 1987.
34. Baylis C, Badr K, Collins R: Effects of chronic prolactin administration on renal hemodynamics in the rat. Endocrinology 117:722, 1985.
35. Paller MS, Gregorini G, Ferris TF: Pressor responsiveness in pseudopregnant and pregnant rats. Am J Physiol 257:R866, 1989.
36. Bucht H, Werko L: Glomerular filtration rate and renal blood flow in hypertensive toxaemia of pregnancy. J Obstet Gynaecol Br Emp 60:157, 1953.
37. Shiffman RL, Tejani N, Verma U, et al: Effect of dietary protein on glomerular filtration rate in pregnancy. Obstet Gynecol 73:47, 1989.
38. Baylis C: The determinants of renal hemodynamics in pregnancy. Am J Kidney Dis 9:260, 1987.
39. Dal Canton A, Conte G, Esposito C, et al: Effects of pregnancy on glomerular dynamics: Micropuncture study in the rat. Kidney Int 22:608, 1982.
40. August P, Levy T, Ales KL, et al: Longitudinal study of the renin-angiotensin-aldosterone system in hypertensive pregnant women. Am J Obstet Gynecol 163:1612, 1990.
41. Brown MA, Zammit VC, Adsett D: Stimulation of active renin release in normal and hypertensive pregnancy. Clin Sci 79:505, 1990.
42. Hanssens M, Keirse MJ, Spitz B: Angiotensin II levels in pregnancy. Br J Obstet Gynaecol 98:155, 1991.
43. Weir RJ, Brown JJ, Fraser R, et al: Plasma renin, renin substrate, angiotensin II and aldosterone in hypertensive disease of pregnancy. Lancet 1:291, 1973.
44. Lenz T, Sealey JE, Happe RW, et al: Infusion of recombinant human pro-renin into rhesus monkeys. Am J Hypertens 3:257, 1990.
45. Sealey JE, Von Lutterotte N, Rubattu S, et al: The greater renin system. Its pro-renin directed vasodilator limb. Am J Hypertens 4:972, 1991.
46. Venuto R, Cox JW, Stein JH, et al: Regulation of uterine blood flow in the pregnant rabbit. J Clin Invest 57:938, 1976.
47. Woods LL, Brooks VL: Role of the renin-angiotensin system in

hypertension during reduced uteroplacental perfusion pressure. Am J Physiol 251:R204, 1989.

48. Ferris TF, Stein JH, Kauffman J: Uterine blood flow and uterine renin secretion. J Clin Invest 51:2828, 1972.

49. Franklin GO, Dowd AJ, Caldwell BV, et al: The effect of angiotensin II intravenous infusion on plasma renin activity and prostaglandins A₁, E, and F levels in the uterine vein of the pregnant monkey. Prostaglandins 6:271, 1974.

50. Sealey JE, Atlas SA, Laragh JH: Plasma pro-renin: Physiological and biochemical characteristics. Clin Sci 63:133, 1981.

51. Ferris TF, Herdson PB, Dunnill MS, et al: Toxemia of pregnancy in sheep: A clinical physiological and pathological study. J Clin Invest 48:1643, 1969.

52. Lardner CN, Brinkman CR III, Weston PV: Dynamics of uterine circulation in pregnant and non-pregnant sheep. Am J Physiol 218:257, 1970.

53. Fernandez LA, Twickler J, Mead A: Neovascularization produced by angiotensin II. J Lab Clin Med 105:141, 1985.

54. Broughton Pipkin F, Symonds EM, Turner SR: The effect of captopril (SQ14,225) upon mother and fetus in the chronically canulated ewe and in the pregnant rabbit. J Physiol (Lond) 323:415, 1982.

55. Ferris TF, Weir EK: The effect of captopril on uterine blood flow and prostaglandin synthesis in the rabbit. J Clin Invest 71:80, 1983.

56. Kawano M, Mori N: Prostacyclin producing activity of human umbilical, placental and uterine vessels. Prostaglandins 26:645, 1983.

57. Bussolino F, Benedetto C, Massobrio M, et al: Maternal vascular prostacyclin activity in pre-eclampsia. Lancet 2:702, 1980.

58. Dadak C, Kefalides A, Singinger H, et al: Reduced umbilical artery prostacyclin formation in complicated pregnancies. Am J Obstet Gynecol 144:792, 1982.

59. Koullapis EN, Nicolaides KH, Collins WP, et al: Plasma prostanoids in pregnancy-induced hypertension. Br J Obstet Gynaecol 89:617, 1982.

60. Remuzzi G, Marchesi D, Mecca G, et al: Reduction of fetal vascular prostacyclin activity in pre-eclampsia. Lancet 2:310, 1980. Letter.

61. Fitzgerald DJ, Entmann SS, Mulloy K, et al: Decreased prostacyclin biosynthesis preceding the clinical manifestations of pregnancy induced hypertension. Circulation 75:956, 1987.

62. Fitzgerald DJ, FitzGerald GA: Eicosanoids in pre-eclampsia. In Laragh JH, Brenner BM (eds): Hypertension. Pathophysiology and Diagnosis and Management. Raven Press, New York, 1990, p 1789.

63. Paller MS: Mechanism of decreased pressor responsiveness to Ang II, NE, and vasopressin in pregnant rats. Am J Physiol 247:H100, 1984.

64. Gill JR: Bartter's syndrome. Annu Rev Med 31:405, 1980.

65. Everett RB, Worley RJ, MacDonald PC, et al: Effect of prostaglandin synthesis inhibitors on pressor response to angiotensin II in human pregnancy. J Clin Endocrinol Metab 46:1007, 1978.

66. Chesley LC, Valenti C, Rein H: Excretion of sodium loads by nonpregnant and pregnant normal, hypertensive and pre-eclamptic women. Metabolism 7:575, 1958.

67. Katz AL: Urinary concentrating ability in pregnant women with asymptomatic bacteriuria. J Clin Invest 40:1331, 1961.

68. Lindheimer MD, Weston PV: Effect of hypotonic expansion on sodium, water and urea excretion in late pregnancy: The influence of posture on these results. J Clin Invest 48:947, 1969.

69. Davison JM, Gilmore EA, Durr J, et al: Altered osmotic thresholds for vasopressin secretion and thirst in human pregnancy. Am J Physiol 246:F105, 1984.

70. Davison JM, Shiells EA, Philips PR, et al: Serial evaluation of vasopressin release and thirst in human pregnancy: Role of human chorionic gonadotrophin in the osmoregulatory changes of gestation. J Clin Invest 81:798, 1988.

71. MacDonald HN, Good W: The effect of parity on plasma sodium, potassium, chloride and osmolality levels during pregnancy. Br J Obstet Gynaecol 72:173, 1972.

72. Lindheimer MD, Barron WM, Davison JM: Osmotic and volume control of vasopressin release in pregnancy. Am J Kidney Dis 17:105, 1991.

73. Barron WM, Stamoutsos BA, Lindheimer MD: Role of volume in the regulation of vasopressin secretion during pregnancy in the rat. J Clin Invest 73:923, 1984.

74. Davison JM, Shiells EA, Philips PR, et al: Influence of humoral and volume factors on altered osmoregulation of normal human pregnancy. Am J Physiol 258:F900, 1990.

75. Durr JA, Stamoutsos B, Lindheimer MD: Osmoregulation during pregnancy in the rat. J Clin Invest 68:337, 1981.

76. Barron WM, Lindheimer MD: Osmoregulation in pseudopregnant and prolactin-treated rats: Comparison with normal gestation. Am J Physiol 254:R478, 1988.

77. Ehrlich EN, Nolten WE, Oparil S, et al: Mineralocorticoids in normal pregnancy. In Lindheimer MD, Katz AL, Zuspan FP (eds): Hypertension in Pregnancy. John Wiley & Sons, New York, 1976, p 217.

78. Brown MA, Sinosich MJ, Saunders DM, et al: Potassium regulation and progesterone-aldosterone interrelationships in human pregnancy: A prospective study. Am J Obstet Gynecol 155:349, 1986.

79. Ehrlich EN, Lindheimer MD: Effect of administered mineralocorticoid or ACTH in pregnant women. Attenuation of kaliuretic influence of mineralocorticoids during pregnancy. J Clin Invest 51:1301, 1972.

80. Biglieri EG, Slaton PE Jr: Pregnancy and primary aldosteronism. J Clin Endocrinol 27:1628, 1967.

81. Hammond TG, Buchanan JD, Scoggins BA, et al: Primary hyperaldosteronism in pregnancy. Aust N Z J Med 2:537, 1982.

82. Lotgering FR, Derks FM, Wallenburg HC: Primary hyperaldosteronism in pregnancy. Am J Obstet Gynecol 155:986, 1986.

83. Merrill RH, Dombroski R, Mackenna JM: Primary hyperaldosteronism during pregnancy. Am J Obstet Gynecol 150:786, 1984.

84. Lindheimer MD, Richardson DA, Ehrlich EN, et al: Potassium homeostasis in pregnancy. J Reprod Med 32:517, 1987.

85. Lim VS, Katz AI, Lindheimer MD: Acid-base metabolism in pregnancy. Am J Physiol 231:1764, 1976.

86. Blechner JN, Cotter JR, Stenger VG, et al: Oxygen, carbon dioxide and hydrogen ion concentration in arterial blood during pregnancy. Am J Obstet Gynecol 100:1, 1968.

87. Lyons HA, Antonio R: The sensitivity of the respiratory center in pregnancy and after the administration of progesterone. Trans Assoc Am Physicians 72:173, 1959.

88. Assali NS, Herzig D, Singh BP: Renal responses to ammonium chloride acidosis in normal and toxemic pregnancies. J Appl Physiol 7:367, 1955.

89. Dunlop W, Davison JM: The effect of normal pregnancy upon the renal handling of uric acid. Br J Obstet Gynaecol 84:13, 1977.

90. Christensen PJ: Tubular reabsorption of glucose during pregnancy. Scand J Clin Lab Invest 10:364, 1958.

91. Welsh GW, Sims EAH: The mechanisms of renal glucosuria in pregnancy. Diabetes 9:363, 1960.

92. Davison JM, Hytten FE: The effect of pregnancy on the renal handling of glucose. Br J Obstet Gynaecol 82:374, 1975.

93. Christensen PJ, Date JW, Sconheyder F, et al: Amino acids in blood plasma and urine during pregnancy. Scand J Clin Lab Invest 9:54, 1957.

94. Wallraff EB, Brodie EC, Borden AL: Urinary excretion of amino acids in pregnancy. J Clin Invest 29:1542, 1950.

95. Hytten FE, Cheyne GA: The aminoaciduria of pregnancy. J Obstet Gynaecol Br Commonw 79:424, 1972.

96. Friedman EA, Neff RK: Pregnancy Hypertension: A Systemic Evaluation of Clinical Diagnostic Criteria. PSG Publishing, Littleton, MA, 1977.

97. Page EW, Christianson R: The impact of mean arterial pressure in the middle trimester upon the outcome of pregnancy. Am J Obstet Gynecol 125:740, 1976.

98. Sibai BM, Caritis S, Thom E, et al: Prevention of pre-eclampsia with low dose aspirin in healthy, nulliparous pregnant women. N Engl J Med 329:1213, 1993.

99. Oney T, Kaulhausen H: The value of the mean arterial blood pressure in the second trimester as a predictor of pregnancy-induced hypertension and pre-eclampsia. A preliminary report. Clin Exp Hypertens 2:211, 1983.

100. Thornton JG, Onerude MB: Convulsions in pregnancy in related gorillas. Am J Obstet Gynecol 167:240, 1992.

101. Combs CA, Katz MA, Kitzmiller JL, et al: Experimental pre-eclampsia produced by chronic constriction of the aorta in conscious rhesus monkeys. Am J Obstet Gynecol 169:215, 1993.

102. Hill LM: Metabolism of uric acid in normal and toxemic pregnancy. Mayo Clin Proc 53:743, 1978.

103. Redman CWG, Bonnar J: Plasma urate changes in pre-eclampsia. Br Med J 1:484, 1978.

104. Ferris TF, Gorden P: The effect of angiotensin and norepinephrine upon urate clearance in man. Am J Med 4:359, 1968.

105. Stander HJ, Cadden JF: Blood chemistry in pre-eclampsia and eclampsia. Am J Obstet Gynecol 28:856, 1934.
106. Steele TH: Evidence for altered renal urate reabsorption during changes in volume of the extracellular fluid. J Lab Clin Med 74:288, 1969.
107. Fadel HE, Northrop G, Misenheimer HR: Hyperuricemia in pre-eclampsia. A reappraisal. Am J Obstet Gynecol 125:640, 1976.
108. Gallery EDM: Volume homeostasis in normal and hypertensive human pregnancy. Semin Nephrol 4:221, 1984.
109. Brown MA, Zammit VC, Lowe SA: Capillary permeability and extracellular fluid volumes in pregnancy-induced hypertension. Clin Sci 77:599, 1989.
110. Brown MA, Zammit VC, Mitar DM: Extracellular fluid volume in pregnancy-induced hypertension. Hypertension 10:61, 1992.
111. Fadnes HO, Oian P: Transcapillary fluid balance and plasma volume regulation: A review. Obstet Gynecol Surv 44:769, 1989.
112. August P, Marcaccio B, Gertner JM, et al: Abnormal 1,25-dihydroxyvitamin D metabolism in pre-eclampsia. Am J Obstet Gynecol 166:1295, 1992.
113. Tanfield PA, Ales KL, Resnick LM, et al: Hypocalciuria in pre-eclampsia. N Engl J Med 316:715, 1989.
114. Hays PM, Cruikshank DP, Dunn LJ: Plasma volume determination in normal and pre-eclamptic pregnancies. Am J Obstet Gynecol 151:958, 1985.
115. Cohn JN: Relationship of plasma volume changes to resistance and capacitance vessel effects of sympathomimetic amine and angiotensin in man. Clin Sci 30:267, 1966.
116. Tarazi RC, Dustan HP, Frohlich ED: Relation of plasma to interstitial fluid volume in essential hypertension. Circulation 40:357, 1969.
117. Arias F: Expansion of intravascular volume and fetal outcome in patients with chronic hypertension and pregnancy. Am J Obstet Gynecol 123:610, 1975.
118. Bauman WA, Maimen M, Langer O: An association between hyperinsulinemia and hypertension during the third trimester of pregnancy. Am J Obstet Gynecol 159:446, 1988.
119. Ono H, Umeda F, Inoguch T, et al: Glucose inhibits prostacyclin production by cultured aortic endothelial cells. Thromb Haemost 60:174, 1988.
120. Tesformarian B, Brown ML, Deyhin D, et al: Elevated glucose promotes generation of endothelium derived vasoconstrictor prostanoids in rabbit aorta. J Clin Invest 85:929, 1990.
121. Van Assche FA, Spitz B, Hanssens M, et al: Increased thromboxane formation in diabetic pregnancy as a possible contribution to pre-eclampsia. Am J Obstet Gynecol 168:84, 1993.
122. Lang RM, Pridjian G, Feldman T: Left ventricular mechanics in pre-eclampsia. Am Heart J 121:1768, 1991.
123. Sibai BM, Mabie BC, Harvey CJ: Pulmonary edema in pre-eclampsia. Am J Obstet Gynecol 156:1174, 1987.
124. Zinaman M, Rubin J, Lindheimer MD: Serial plasma oncotic pressure levels during and after delivery in severe pre-eclampsia. Lancet 1:1245, 1985.
125. Downing I, Shepherd GL, Lewis PJ: Reduced prostacyclin production in pre-eclampsia. Lancet 2:1374, 1980.
126. Roberts JM, Taylor RM, Goldfein A: Clinical and biochemical evidence of endothelial cell dysfunction in pre-eclampsia. Am J Hypertens 4:700, 1991.
127. Redman CWG, Denson KW, Bellin LJ, et al: Factor-VII consumption in pre-eclampsia. Lancet 2:1249, 1977.
128. Taylor RN, Crombleholme WR, Friedman SA, et al: High plasma cellular fibronectin levels correlate with biochemical and clinical features of pre-eclampsia but cannot be attributed to hypertension alone. Am J Obstet Gynecol 165:895, 1991.
129. Benigni A, Orisio S, Gaspari F, et al: Evidence against a pathogenetic role for endothelin in pre-eclampsia. Br J Obstet Gynaecol 99:798, 1992.
130. Branch DW, Dudley DJ, Nutchell MD: Preliminary evidence for homeostatic mechanism regulating endothelin production in pre-eclampsia. Lancet 337:443, 1991.
131. Florijn KW, Derkx FH, Visser W, et al: Elevated plasma levels of endothelin in pre-eclampsia. J Hypertens 9:S166, 1991.
132. Ihara Y, Sagawa N, Hasegawa M, et al: Concentrations of endothelin-1 in maternal and umbilical cord blood at various stages of pregnancy. Cardiovasc Pharmacol 17:S443, 1991.
133. Taylor RN, Varma M, Teng NN, et al: Women with pre-eclampsia have higher plasma endothelin levels than women with normal pregnancies. J Clin Endocrinol Metab 71:1675, 1990.
134. Tsunoda K, Abe K, Yoshinaga K, et al: Maternal and umbilical venous levels of endothelin in women with pre-eclampsia. Hypertension 6:61, 1992.
135. Pinto A, Sorrentino R, Sorrentino P: EDRF (NO) released by endothelial cells of human umbilical vessels. Am J Obstet Gynecol 164:507, 1991.
135a. Raij L: Glomerular thrombosis in pregnancy: Role of the L-arginine–nitric oxide pathway. Kidney Int 45:775, 1994.
136. Fitzgerald DJ, Rocki W, Murray R, et al: Thromboxane A$_2$ synthesis in pregnancy-induced hypertension. Lancet 335:751, 1990.
137. Lorentzen B, Endresen MJ, Hovig T, et al: Effect of sera from pre-eclampsia in PGI$_2$ synthesis. Thromb Res 63:363, 1991.
138. Zammit VC, Whitworth JA, Brown MA: Endothelium-derived prostacyclin: Effect of serum from women with normal and hypertensive pregnancy. Clin Sci 82:383, 1992.
139. Wilson DM, Luetscher JA: Plasma pro-renin activity and complications in children with insulin dependent diabetes mellitus. N Engl J Med 323:110, 1990.
140. Ong ACM, Eisen V, Homburg RR, et al: The pathogenesis of the ovarian hyperstimulation syndrome: A possible role for ovarian renin. Clin Endocrinol 34:43, 1991.
141. Rosenberg ME, McKenzie JK, McKenzie IM, et al: Increased ascitic fluid pro-renin in the ovarian hyperstimulation syndrome. Am J Kidney Dis 23:427, 1994.
142. Gant NF, Daley GL, Chand S, et al: A study of angiotensin II pressor response throughout primigravid pregnancy. J Clin Invest 52:2682, 1973.
143. Gant NF, Chand S, Worley RJ, et al: A clinical test useful for predicting the development of acute hypertension in pregnancy. Am J Obstet Gynecol 120:1, 1974.
144. Leduc L, Wheeler JM, Kirshon B, et al: Coagulation profile in severe pre-eclampsia. Obstet Gynecol 79:14, 1992.
145. Schrocksnadel H, Sitte B, Steckel-Berger G, et al: Hemolysis in hypertensive disorders of pregnancy. Gynecol Obstet Invest 34:211, 1992.
146. Redman CWG, Bonnar J, Beilin L: Early platelet consumption in pre-eclampsia. Br Med J 1:467, 1978.
147. Pijnenborg R, Anthony J, Davey DA, et al: Placental bed spiral arteries in the hypertensive disorders of pregnancy. Br J Obstet Gynaecol 98:648, 1991.
148. Roberts JM, Redman CWG: Pre-eclampsia: More than pregnancy-induced hypertension. Lancet 341:1447, 1993.
149. Khong TY: Acute atherosis in pregnancies complicated by hypertension, small-for-gestational-age infants and diabetes mellitus. Arch Pathol Lab Med 115:722, 1991.
150. Branch DW, Scott JR, Kochenour NK, et al: Obstetric complications associated with the lupus anticoagulant. N Engl J Med 313:1322, 1985.
151. Milliez J, LeLong F, Bozani N, et al: The prevalence of autoantibodies during third trimester pregnancy complicated by hypertension of fetal growth retardation. Am J Obstet Gynecol 165:51, 1991.
152. Out HJ, Bruinse HW, Christiaens GC, et al: A prospective, controlled multicenter study on the obstetric risks of pregnant women with antiphospholipid antibodies. Am J Obstet Gynecol 167:26–32, 1992.
153. Taylor P, Sherrow S: Pre-eclampsia and anti-phospholipid antibody. Br J Obstet Gynaecol 98:604, 1991.
154. Lunell NO, Nylund L, Lewander R, et al: Uteroplacental blood flow in pre-eclampsia in measurements with indium 113. Clin Exp Hypertens 1:105, 1982.
155. Lohlein M: Zur Pathogenese der Nierenkrankheiten Nephritis und Nephrose mit besonderer Besichtigung der Nephropathia gravidarum. Dtsch Med Wochenschr 44:1187, 1918.
156. Fahr T; Über Marenveranderungen bei Eklampsie. Zentralbl Gynaekol 44:991, 1920.
157. Farquhar MG: Review of normal and pathologic glomerular ultrastructure. In Metcalf J (ed): Proceedings of the Tenth Annual Conference on the Nephrotic Syndrome. National Kidney Disease Foundation, New York, 1959.
158. Spargo B, McCartney CO, Winemiller R: Glomerular capillary endotheliosis in toxemia of pregnancy. Arch Pathol 68:593, 1959.
159. Pirani CL, Pollak VE, Lannigan R, et al: The renal glomerular lesions of pre-eclampsia. Am J Obstet Gynecol 87:1047, 1963.
160. Altchek A: Electron microscopy of renal biopsies in toxemia of pregnancy. JAMA 175:791, 1961.

161. Kincaid-Smith P: The renal lesion of pre-eclampsia revisited. Am J Kidney Dis 17:144, 1991.

162. Bis KA, Waxman B: Rupture of the liver associated with pregnancy: A review of the literature and report of 2 cases. Obstet Gynecol Surv 31:763, 1976.

163. Browne CH, Hanson GC, DeJude LR, et al: Rupture of subcapsular haematoma of the liver in a case of eclampsia. Br J Surg 62:237, 1975.

164. Sheehan HL, Lynch JB: Pathology of Toxemia of Pregnancy. Longman, New York, 1973.

165. Arias F, Mancilla-Jimenez R: Hepatic fibrinogen deposits in pre-eclampsia. N Engl J Med 295:578, 1976.

166. Amon E, Allen SR, Petrie RH, et al: Acute fatty liver of pregnancy associated with pre-eclampsia. Am J Perinatol 8:278, 1991.

167. Hatfield AK, Stein JH, Greenberger NJ, et al: Idiopathic acute fatty liver of pregnancy. Death from extrahepatic manifestations. Am J Dig Dis 17:167, 1972.

168. Killam AP, Dillard SH, Patton RC, et al: Pregnancy induced hypertension complicated by acute liver disease and disseminated intravascular coagulation. Am J Obstet Gynecol 123:823, 1975.

169. Minakami H, Oha N, Sato T, et al: Pre-eclampsia: A microvascular fat disease of the liver? Am J Obstet Gynecol 159:1043, 1988.

170. Riely CA, Lathan PS, Romero R: Acute fatty liver of pregnancy. Ann Intern Med 106:703, 1987.

171. Robertson WB, Khong TY, Brosens I, et al: The placental bed biopsy: A review of three European Centers. Am J Obstet Gynecol 155:401, 1986.

172. Brown CEL, Purdy P, Cunningham FG: Head computed tomographic scan in women with eclampsia. Am J Obstet Gynecol 159:915, 1988.

173. Donaldson JO: Neurologic complications. In Burrow GN, Ferris TF (eds): Medical Complications During Pregnancy, 3d ed. WB Saunders, Philadelphia, 1988, p 485.

174. Bauer TW, Moore GW, Hutchins GM: Morphologic evidence for coronary artery spasm in eclampsia. Circulation 65:255, 1982.

175. Barton JR, Hiett AK, O'Connor WN, et al: Endomyocardial ultrastructural findings in pre-eclampsia. Am J Obstet Gynecol 165:389, 1991.

176. Gallery ED, Ross M, Gyory AZ: Urinary red blood cell and cast excretion in normal and hypertensive human pregnancy. Am J Obstet Gynecol 168:67, 1993.

177. Miles JF, Martin JN, Blake PG: Post partum eclampsia a recurring perinatal dilemma. Obstet Gynecol 76:328, 1990.

178. Chesley LC, Cooper DW: Genetics of hypertension in pregnancy. Br J Obstet Gynaecol 93:898, 1986.

179. Humphries J: Occurrence of hypertensive toxemia of pregnancy in mother-daughter pairs. Bull Johns Hopkins Hosp 107:271, 1960.

180. Chesley LC: The remote prognosis of eclamptic women. Am Heart J 93:407, 1977.

181. Hargood JL, Brown MA: Pregnancy induced hypertension: Recurrence rate in second pregnancies. Med J Aust 154:376, 1991.

182. Marcoux S, Brisson J, Fabia J: The effect of cigarette smoking on the risk of pre-eclampsia and gestational hypertension. Am J Epidemiol 130:950, 1989.

183. Arulkumaran S, Gibb DM, Rauff M, et al: Transient blindness associated with pregnancy-induced hypertension. Case reports. Br J Obstet Gynaecol 92:847, 1985.

184. Hankins GDV, Wendel GD, Cunningham FG, et al: Longitudinal evaluation of hemodynamic changes in eclampsia. Am J Obstet Gynecol 150:506, 1984.

185. Goodlin RC: Pre-eclampsia as the great imposter. Am J Obstet Gynecol 164:1577, 1991.

186. Martin JN, Blake PG, Perry KG, et al: The natural history of HELLP syndrome. Am J Obstet Gynecol 164:1500, 1991.

187. Long RG, Scheuer PJ, Sherlock S: Pre-eclampsia presenting with deep jaundice. J Clin Pathol 30:212, 1977.

188. Holzbach RT: Jaundice in pregnancy. Am J Med 61:367, 1976.

189. Grunfeld JP, Ganeval D, Bournerias F: Acute renal failure in pregnancy. Kidney Int 18:179, 1980.

190. Kaplan MM: Acute fatty liver of pregnancy. N Engl J Med 313:367, 1985.

191. Mabie WC: Acute fatty liver of pregnancy. Gastroenterol Clin North Am 21:951, 1992.

192. Burroughs AK, Seong NGH, Dojcinov DM, et al: Idiopathic acute fatty liver of pregnancy in 12 patients. Q J Med 51:481, 1982.

193. Recant L, Lacy P: Clinicopathologic conference: Fulminating liver disease in a pregnant woman. Am J Med 35:231, 1963.

194. Ober WB, LeCompte PM: Acute fatty metamorphosis of the liver associated with pregnancy. A distinctive lesion. Am J Med 19:743, 1955.

195. Hou SH, Levin S, Ahola S, et al: Acute fatty liver of pregnancy: Survival with early caesarean section. Dig Dis Sci 29:449, 1984.

196. Durr JA, Haggard JG, Hunt JM, et al: Diabetes insipidus in pregnancy associated with high vasopressinase activity. N Engl J Med 316:1070, 1987.

197. Kreg J, Katz VL, Bower WA: Transient diabetes insipidus of pregnancy. Obstet Gynecol Surv 44:789, 1989.

198. Davison JM, Shiells EA, Barron WM: Changes in the metabolic clearance of AVP and plasma vasopressinase throughout human pregnancy. J Clin Invest 83:1313, 1989.

199. Davies AM: Geographical epidemiology of the toxemias of pregnancy. Isr J Med Sci 7:753, 1971.

200. Imperiale TF, Petrulis AS: A meta-analysis of low-dose aspirin for the prevention of pregnancy-induced hypertensive disease. JAMA 266:260, 1991.

201. Zuspan FP, Samuels P: Preventing preeclampsia. N Engl J Med 329:1265, 1993.

202. Hauth JC, Goldenberg RL, Parker CR, et al: Low dose ASA to prevent pre-eclampsia. Am J Obstet Gynecol 168:1083, 1993.

203. McCarron DA: Calcium metabolism and hypertension. Kidney Int 35:717, 1989.

204. Belizan JM, Villar J, Gonzalez L, et al: Calcium supplementation to prevent hypertension disorders of pregnancy. N Engl J Med 325:1399, 1991.

205. Kawasaki N, Matsui K, Ito M: Effect of calcium supplementation on the vascular sensitivity to angiotensin II in pregnant women. Am J Obstet Gynecol 153:576, 1985.

206. Gertner JM, Coustan DR, Kliger AS, et al: Pregnancy as a state of physiologic absorptive hypercalciuria. Am J Med 81:451, 1986.

207. Collins R, Yusuf S, Peto R: Overview of randomised trials of diuretics in pregnancy. Br J Med J 290:17, 1985.

208. Fenakel K, Fenakel G, Appelman Z: Nifedipine in the treatment of severe pre-eclampsia. Obstet Gynecol 77:331, 1991.

209. Moretti MM, Fairlie FM, Akl S: The effect of nifedipine on fetal and placental doppler wave forms in pre-eclampsia. Am J Obstet Gynecol 163:1844, 1990.

210. Montan S, Ingemarsson I, Marsal K, Sjoberg NO: Randomised controlled trial of atenolol and pindolol in human pregnancy: Effects on fetal haemodynamics. BMJ 304:946, 1992.

211. Rubin PC, Butters L, Clark DM, et al: Placebo-controlled trial of atenolol in treatment of pregnancy associated hypertension. Lancet 1:431, 1983.

212. Ahoha RA, Mabie WC, Sibai BM, et al: Labetalol does not decrease placental perfusion in the hypertensive term pregnant rat. Am J Obstet Gynecol 160:480, 1989.

213. Ashe RG, Moodley J, Richards AM: Comparison of labetalol and hydralazine in hypertensive emergencies of pregnancy. S Afr Med J 7:384, 1987.

214. Eisenach JC, Mandell G, Dervas DM: Maternal and fetal effects of labetalol in pregnant ewes. Anesthesiology 74:292, 1991.

215. Jouppila P, Kirkinen P, Koivula A, Ylikorkala O: Labetalol does not alter the placental and fetal blood flow or maternal prostanoids in pre-eclampsia. Br J Obstet Gynaecol 93:543, 1986.

216. Morgan MA, Silavrin SL, Donner KJ, et al: Effect of labetalol on uterine blood flow and cardiovascular hemodynamics in the hypertensive baboon. Am J Obstet Gynecol 168:1504, 1993.

217. Shoemaker CT, Meyers M: Sodium nitroprusside for control of severe hypertensive disease of pregnancy. Case report and discussion of potential toxicity. Am J Obstet Gynecol 149:171, 1984.

218. Sibai BM: Eclampsia. VI. Maternal-perinatal outcome in 254 consecutive cases. Am J Obstet Gynecol 163:1049, 1990.

219. Watson KV, Moldow CF, Ogburn PL, et al: Magnesium sulfate: Rationale for its use in pre-eclampsia. Proc Natl Acad Sci USA 83:1075, 1986.

220. McCubbin JM, Sibai BM, Ardella TN, Anderson GD: Cardiopulmonary arrest due to acute maternal hypermagnesaemia. Lancet 1:1058, 1981. Letter.

221. Richards A, Stather-Dunn L, Moodley J: Cardiopulmonary arrest after administration of MgSO₄. S Afr Med J 67:145, 1985.

222. Herpolsteimer A, Brady R, Yancey MK, et al: Pulmonary function

of pre-eclamptic women receiving intravenous $MgSO_4$ for seizure prophylaxis. Obstet Gynecol 78:241, 1991.

223. Waisman GD, Mayorga LM, Camera MI, et al: Magnesium plus nifedipine: Potentiation of hypotensive effect in pre-eclampsia? Am J Obstet Gynecol 159:308, 1988.

224. Appleton MP, Kuehl TJ, Raebel NM, et al: Magnesium sulfate versus phenytoin for seizure prophylaxis in pregnancy induced hypertension. Am J Obstet Gynecol 165:807, 1992.

225. Cotton DB, Janusey CA, Berman RF: Anti-convulsant effects of $MgSO_4$ in hippocampal seizures: Therapeutic implications in pre-eclampsia. Am J Obstet Gynecol 166:1127, 1992.

226. Densdale HB: Does $MgSO_4$ treat eclamptic seizures? Arch Neurol 45:1360, 1989.

227. Kaplan PW, Lesser RP, Fisher RS: Magnesium sulfate should not be used in treating eclamptic seizures. Arch Neurol 45:136, 1989.

228. Shannon RW, Frazer GP, Aitken RG, et al: Diazepam in pre-eclamptic toxaemia with special reference to its effect on the newborn infant. Br J Clin Pract 26:271, 1972.

229. Sibai BM, Ald S, Fairlie F: Management of severe pre-eclampsia in the second trimester. Am J Obstet Gynecol 163:773, 1990.

230. Pirkonen JP, Eskhole RV: Labetalol in pre-eclampsia: Effect on maternal hemodynamics and uterine and fetal flow velocity waveforms. J Perinat Med 19:167, 1991.

231. Blake S, MacDonald D: The prevention of the maternal manifestations of pre-eclampsia by intensive antihypertensive treatment. Br J Obstet Gynaecol 98:244, 1991.

232. Odendaal H, Pattinson RC, Dutoit R: Aggressive or expectant management with severe pre-eclampsia between 28–34 weeks. Obstet Gynecol 76:1070, 1991.

233. Phippard AF, Fischer WE, Horvath JS, et al: Early blood pressure control improves pregnancy outcome in primigravida women with mild hypertension. Med J Aust 154:378, 1991.

234. Redman CWG: Treatment of hypertension in pregnancy. Kidney Int 18:267, 1980.

235. Sibai BM, Anderson GD: Pregnancy outcome of intensive therapy in severe hypertension in the first trimester. Obstet Gynecol 67:517, 1986.

236. Sibai BM, Mabie BC, Shamsa F, et al: A comparison of no medication versus methyldopa or labetalol in chronic hypertension during pregnancy. Am J Obstet Gynecol 62:960, 1990.

237. Wichman K, Ryden G, Karlberg BE: A placebo controlled trial of metoprolol in the treatment of hypertension in pregnancy. Scand J Clin Lab Invest 169:80, 1984.

238. Schubiger G, Flury G, Nussberger J: Enalapril for pregnancy-induced hypertension: Acute renal failure in a neonate. Ann Intern Med 108:215, 1988.

239. Collins R, Wallenburg HCS: Pharmacological prevention and treatment of hypertensive disorders of pregnancy. In Chalmers I, Enkin M, Keirse MJ (eds): Effective Care in Pregnancy and Childbirth. Oxford University Press, Oxford, 1989, p 512.

240. Peters JP: Toxemias of Pregnancy. Yale J Biol Med 9:311, 1937.

241. Chesley LC, Annitto JE: Pregnancy in a patient with hypertensive disease. Am J Obstet Gynecol 53:372, 1947.

242. Karlson K, Ljungblad U, Lundgren Y: Blood flow of the reproductive system in renal hypertensive rats during pregnancy. Am J Obstet Gynecol 142:1039, 1982.

243. Chia S, Redman CWG: Prognosis for pre-eclampsia complicated by 5 gms or more of proteinuria/24 hrs. Eur J Obstet Gynecol Reprod Biol 43:9, 1992.

244. Ferrazzani S, Caruso A, DeCarolis S, et al: Proteinuria and outcome of 444 pregnancies complicated by hypertension. Am J Obstet Gynecol 162:366, 1990.

245. Stettler RW, Cunningham FG: Natural history of chronic proteinuria complicating pregnancy. Am J Obstet Gynecol 167:1219, 1992.

246. Sibai BM, Grossman RA, Grossman HG: Effects of diuretics on plasma volume in pregnancies with hypertension. Am J Obstet Gynecol 150:831, 1984.

247. Fabregues G, Alvarez L, Varas-Juri P, et al: Effectiveness of atenolol in the treatment of hypertension during pregnancy. Hypertension 19:II-129, 1992.

248. Lunell NO, Persson B, Aaron G, et al: Circulatory and metabolic effects of acute beta 1–blockade in severe pre-eclampsia. Acta Obstet Gynecol Scand 58:443, 1979.

249. Butters L, Kennedy S, Rubin PC: Atenolol in essential hypertension during pregnancy. Br Med J 301:587, 1990.

250. Ounsted M, Cockburn J, Moar VA, et al: Maternal hypertension with superimposed pre-eclampsia: Effects on child development at $7\frac{1}{2}$ years. Br J Obstet Gynaecol 90:644, 1983.

251. Horvath JS, Phippard A, Karda A: Clonidine: A safe and effective antihypertensive agent in pregnancy. Obstet Gynecol 66:634, 1985.

252. Huisjes HJ, Hadders-Algra M, Towwen BCI: Is clonidine a behavioral teratogen in the human? Early Hum Dev 14:43, 1986.

253. Ciraru-Vigneron C, Pruna A, Minta PH, et al: Comparison of nifedipine and atenolol in treatment of moderate pregnancy-hypertension. VII World Congress of Hypertension in Pregnancy, Perugia, Italy, 1990.

254. Rubin PC, Butters L, Low RA: Clinical pharmacological studies with prazosin during pregnancy complicated by hypertension. Br J Clin Pharmacol 16:543, 1983.

255. Crowther CA, Boumeester AM, Ashurst NM: Does admission to hospital for bed rest prevent disease progression or improve fetal outcome in pregnancy complicated by nonproteinuric hypertension? Br J Obstet Gynaecol 99:13, 1991.

256. Tuffnell DJ, Lilford RJ, Buchan PC, et al: Randomised controlled trial of day care for hypertension in pregnancy. Lancet 339:224, 1992.

257. Ihle BU, Long P, Oats J: Early onset pre-eclampsia: Recognition of underlying renal disease. Br Med J 294:79–81, 1987.

258. Landesman R, Halpern M, Knapp RC: Renal artery lesions associated with the toxemias of pregnancy. Obstet Gynecol 18:645, 1961.

259. Heyborne KD, Schultz MF, Goodlin RC, et al: Renal artery stenosis during pregnancy. Obstet Gynecol Surv 46:509, 1991.

260. Sellors L, Siamopoulous K, Wilkenson R: Prognosis for pregnancy after correction of renovascular hypertension. Nephron 39:280, 1985.

261. Coen G, Cugini P, Gerlini G, et al: Successful treatment of long-standing severe hypertension and captopril during a twin pregnancy. Nephron 40:498, 1985.

262. Millar JA, Wilson PD, Morrison N: Management of severe hypertension in pregnancy by a combined drug regimen including captopril: Case report. N Z Med J 96:796, 1983.

263. Neerhof MG, Shlossman PA, Poll DS, et al: Idiopathic aldosteronism in pregnancy. Obstet Gynecol 78:489, 1991.

264. Hillestad L: Aortic coarctation and pregnancy. Acta Obstet Gynecol Scand 51:95, 1972.

265. Easterling TR, Carlson K, Benedette TJ, et al: Hemodynamics associated with the diagnosis and treatment of pheochromocytoma in pregnancy. Am J Perinatol 9:462, 1992.

266. Feldman JM: Adult respiratory distress syndrome in a pregnant patient with a pheochromocytoma. J Surg Oncol 29:5, 1985.

267. Harper MA, Murnaghen GA, Kennedy L, et al: Pheochromocytoma in pregnancy. Br J Obstet Gynaecol 96:594, 1989.

268. Lyons CW, Colmargen GH: Medical management of pheochromocytoma in pregnancy. Obstet Gynecol 72:450, 1988.

269. Venuto R, Burnstein P, Schneider R: Pheochromocytoma: Antepartum diagnosis and management with tumor resection in the puerperium. Am J Obstet Gynecol 150:431, 1984.

270. Cunningham FG: Urinary tract infections complicating pregnancy. Baillieres Clin Obstet Gynaecol 1:891, 1987.

271. Whalley PJ: Bacteriuria of pregnancy. Am J Obstet Gynecol 47:723, 1967.

272. Kass EH: Infectious diseases and perinatal morbidity. Yale J Biol Med 55:231, 1982.

273. Gilstrap LC, Leveno KJ, Cunningham FG, et al: Renal infection and pregnancy outcome. Am J Obstet Gynecol 141:709, 1981.

274. Sacks SH, Jones KV, Roberts R, et al: Effect of symptomless bacteriuria in childhood on subsequent pregnancy. Lancet 2:991, 1987.

275. Davison JM, Sprott MS, Selkon JB: The effect of covert bacteriuria in schoolgirls on renal function at 18 years and during pregnancy. Lancet 2:651, 1984.

276. Hanis RE, Gilstcap LC: Cystitis during pregnancy: A distinct clinical entity. Obstet Gynecol 57:578, 1981.

277. Bailey RR, Peddie BA, Bishop V: Comparison of single dose with a five-day course of trimethoprim for asymptomatic (correct) bacteriuria of pregnancy. N Z Med J 99:501, 1986.

278. Wright A, Steele P, Bennett JR, et al: Urinary excretion of albumin in normal pregnancy. Br J Obstet Gynecol 94:408, 1987.

279. Kuo VS, Koumantakis G, Gallery ED: Proteinuria and its assessment in normal and hypertensive pregnancy. Am J Obstet Gynecol 167:723, 1992.

280. Nesselhut T, Rath W, Grospietsch G, et al: Urinary protein electro-

phoresis profile in normal and hypertensive pregnancies. Arch Gynecol Obstet 246:97, 1989.

281. Kassirer JP: Is renal biopsy necessary for optimal management of the idiopathic nephrotic syndrome? Kidney Int 24:561, 1983.

282. Levey AS, Lau J, Pauker SG, et al: Idiopathic nephrotic syndrome: Puncturing the biopsy myth. Ann Intern Med 107:697, 1987.

283. Packham D, Fairley KF: Renal biopsy: Indications and complications in pregnancy. Br J Obstet Gynaecol 94:935, 1987.

284. Lindheimer JD, Katz AI: Gestation in women with kidney disease: Prognosis and management. Baillieres Clin Obstet Gynaecol 1:921, 1987.

285. Paller MS: Pathophysiology of acute renal failure. In Greenberg A (ed): National Kidney Foundation Kidney Diseases Primer. National Kidney Foundation, Orlando, FL, 1994, p 126.

286. Sibai BM, Ramadan MK: Acute renal failure in pregnancies complicated by hemolysis, elevated liver enzymes, and low platelets. Am J Obstet Gynecol 168:1682, 1993.

287. Kelleher SP, Berl T: Acute renal failure in pregnancy. Semin Nephrol 1:61, 1981.

288. Kleinknecht D, Grunfeld JP, Cia Gomez P, et al: Diagnostic procedures and long-term prognosis in bilateral renal cortical necrosis. Kidney Int 4:390, 1973.

289. Papo J, Aviram A, Peer G, et al: Acute renal cortical necrosis as revealed by computerized tomography. Isr J Med Sci 21:862, 1985.

290. Conger JD, Falk SA, Guggenheim SJ: Glomerular dynamics and morphologic changes in the generalized Shwartzman reaction in postpartum rats. J Clin Invest 67:1334, 1981.

291. Bonar J: Blood coagulation and fibrinolytic systems during pregnancy. Clin Obstet Gynecol 2:321, 1975.

292. Chugh KS, Singhal PC, Kher VK, et al: Spectrum of acute cortical necrosis in Indian patients. Am J Med Sci 286:10, 1983.

293. Hayslett JP: Postpartum renal failure. N Engl J Med 312:1556, 1985.

294. Brown CB, Clarkson AR, Robson JS, et al: Haemolytic uraemic syndrome in women taking oral contraceptives. Lancet 1:1479, 1973.

295. Rock GA, Shumak KH, Buskard NA, et al: Comparison of plasma exchange with plasma infusion in the treatment of thrombotic thrombocytopenic purpura. N Engl J Med 325:393, 1991.

296. Brandes JC, Fritsche C: Obstructive acute renal failure by a gravid uterus: A case report and review. Am J Kidney Dis 18:398, 1991.

297. Homans DC, Blake GD, Harrington JT, et al: Acute renal failure caused by ureteral obstruction by a gravid uterus. JAMA 246:1230, 1981.

298. LaPata RE, McElin TW, Adelson BH: Ureteral obstruction due to compression by the gravid uterus. Am J Obstet Gynecol 106:941, 1970.

299. Peake SL, Roxbursh HB, Langlois SL: Ultrasonic assessment of hydronephrosis of pregnancy. Radiology 146:167, 1983.

300. Coe FL, Parks JH, Lindheimer MD: Nephrolithiasis during pregnancy. N Engl J Med 298:322, 1978.

301. Kumar R, Cohen WR, Epstein FH: Vitamin D and calcium hormones in pregnancy. N Engl J Med 302:1143, 1980.

302. Pitkin RM: Calcium metabolism in pregnancy and the perinatal period: A review. Am J Obstet Gynecol 151:99, 1985.

303. Folger GK: Pain and pregnancy. Obstet Gynecol 5:513, 1955.

304. Maikranz P, Coe FL, Parks J, et al: Nephrolithiasis in pregnancy. Am J Kidney Dis 9:354, 1987.

305. Stothers L, Lee LM: Renal colic in pregnancy. J Urol 148:1383, 1992.

306. Loughlin KR, Bailey RB Jr: Internal ureteral stents for conservative management of ureteral calculi during pregnancy. N Engl J Med 315:1647, 1986.

307. Schubiger G, Flury G, Nussberger J: Enalapril for pregnancy-induced hypertension: Acute renal failure in a neonate. Ann Intern Med 108:215, 1988.

308. Pryde PG, Sedman AB, Nugent CE, et al: Angiotensin-converting enzyme inhibitor fetopathy. J Am Soc Nephrol 3:1575, 1993.

309. Nanta J, de Heer E, Baldwin WM, et al: Transplacental induction of membranous nephropathy in a neonate. Pediatr Nephrol 4:111, 1990.

310. Lim VS: Reproductive function in patients with renal insufficiency. Am J Kidney Dis 9:363, 1987.

311. Souqiyyeh MZ, Huraib SO, Mohd AG, et al: Pregnancy in chronic hemodialysis patients in the kingdom of Saudia Arabia. Am J Kidney Dis 19:235, 1992.

312. Rauramo L, Kasanen A, Elfving K, et al: Fertility, pregnancy and labour in women with a history of nephritis or pyelonephritis. Acta Obstet Gynecol Scand 41:357, 1962.

313. Mackay EV: Pregnancy and renal disease. A ten-year survey. Aust N Z J Obstet Gynaecol 3:21, 1963.

314. Barceló P, López-Lillo J, Cabero L, Del Río G: Successful pregnancy in primary glomerular disease. Kidney Int 30:914, 1986.

315. Katz AI, Davison JM, Hayslett JP, et al: Pregnancy in women with kidney disease. Kidney Int 18:192, 1980.

316. Packham DK, North RA, Fairley KF, et al: Primary glomerulonephritis and pregnancy. Q J Med 71:537, 1989.

317. Surian M, Imbasciati E, Cosci P: Glomerular disease and pregnancy. A study of 123 pregnancies in patients with primary and secondary glomerular diseases. Nephron 36:101, 1984.

318. Hou SH, Grossman SD, Madias NE: Pregnancy in women with renal disease and moderate renal insufficiency. Am J Med 78:185, 1985.

319. Imbasciati E, Pardi G, Capetta P, et al: Pregnancy in women with chronic renal failure. Am J Nephrol 6:193, 1986.

320. Jungers P, Houillier P, Forget D, et al: Specific controversies concerning the natural history of renal disease in pregnancy. Am J Kidney Dis 17:116, 1991.

321. Abe S, Amagasaki Y, Konishi K, et al: The influence of antecedent renal disease on pregnancy. Am J Obstet Gynecol 153:508, 1985.

322. Leppert P, Risher CC, Cheng SS, et al: Antecedent renal disease and the outcome of pregnancy. Ann Intern Med 90:747, 1979.

323. Italian Study of Aspirin in Pregnancy: Low-dose aspirin in prevention and treatment of intrauterine growth retardation and pregnancy-induced hypertension. Lancet 341:396, 1993.

324. Slone D, Siskind V, Heinonen OP, et al: Aspirin and congenital malformations. Lancet 1:1373, 1976.

325. Shapiro S, Siskind V, Monson RR: Perinatal mortality and birthweight in relation to aspirin taken during pregnancy. Lancet 1:1375, 1976.

326. Werler MM, Mitchell AA, Shapiro S: The relation of aspirin use during the first trimester of pregnancy to congenital cardiac defects. N Engl J Med 321:1639, 1989.

327. Benigni A, Gregorini G, Frusca T, et al: Effect of low-dose aspirin on fetal and maternal generation of thromboxane by platelets in women at risk for pregnancy-induced hypertension. N Engl J Med 321:357, 1989.

328. Brenner BM, Meyer TW, Hostetter TH: Dietary protein intake and the progressive nature of kidney disease: The role of hemodynamically mediated glomerular injury in the pathogenesis of progressive glomerular sclerosis in aging, renal ablation, and intrinsic renal disease. N Engl J Med 307:652, 1982.

329. Hostetter TH, Rennke HG, Brenner BM: The case for intrarenal hypertension in the initiation and progression of diabetic and other glomerulopathies. Am J Med 72:375, 1982.

330. Neuringer JR, Brenner BM: Hemodynamic theory of progressive renal disease: A 10-year update in brief review. Am J Kidney Dis 22:98, 1993.

331. Baylis C: Immediate and long-term effects of pregnancy on glomerular function in the SHR. Am J Physiol 257:F1140, 1989.

332. Baylis C, Rennke HG: Renal hemodynamics and glomerular morphology in repetitively pregnant aging rats. Kidney Int 28:140, 1985.

333. Baylis C, Reese K, Wilson CB: Glomerular effects of pregnancy in a model of glomerulonephritis in the rat. Am J Kidney Dis 14:452, 1989.

334. Podjarny E, Bernheim J, Rathaus M, et al: Adriamycin nephropathy: A model to study effects of pregnancy on renal disease in rats. Am J Physiol 263:F711, 1992.

335. Becker GJ, Ihle BU, Fairley KF: Effect of pregnancy on moderate renal failure in reflux nephropathy. Br Med J 292:796, 1986.

336. Abe S: Pregnancy in IgA nephropathy. Kidney Int 40:1098, 1991.

337. Hayslett JP: Maternal and fetal complications in pregnant women with systemic lupus erythematosus. Am J Kidney Dis 17:123, 1991.

338. Bobrie G, Liote F, Houillier P: Pregnancy in lupus nephritis and related disorders. Am J Kidney Dis 9:339, 1987.

339. Mintz G, Rodriguez-Alvarez E: Systemic lupus erythematosus. Rheum Dis Clin North Am 15:255, 1989.

340. Hayslett JP, Lynn RI: Effect of pregnancy in patients with lupus nephropathy. Kidney Int 18:207, 1980.

341. Houser NT, Fish AJ, Tagatz GE, et al: Pregnancy and systemic lupus erythematosus. Am J Obstet Gynecol 138:409, 1980.

342. Packham DK, Lam SS, Nicolls K, et al: Lupus nephritis and pregnancy. Q J Med 83:315, 1992.

343. Kitzmiller JL, Brown ER, Phillippe M, et al: Diabetic nephropathy and perinatal outcome. Am J Obstet Gynecol 141:741, 1981.

344. Reece EA, Coustan DR, Hayslett JP, et al: Diabetic nephropathy: Pregnancy performance and feto-maternal outcome. Am J Obstet Gynecol 159:56, 1988.
345. Milutinovic J, Fialkow PJ, Agodoa LY, et al: Fertility and pregnancy complications in women with autosomal dominant polycystic kidney disease. Obstet Gynecol 61:566, 1983.
346. Gabow PA, Johnson AM, Kaehny WD, et al: Factors affecting the progression of renal disease in autosomal-dominant polycystic kidney disease. Kidney Int 41:1311, 1992.
347. Imbasciati E, Ponticelli C: Pregnancy and renal disease: Predictors for fetal and maternal outcome. Am J Nephrol 11:353, 1991.
348. Fouque D, Laville M, Boissel JP, et al: Controlled low protein diets in chronic renal insufficiency: Meta-analysis. Br Med J 304:214, 1992.
349. Hostetter TH, Olson JL, Rennke HG, et al: Hyperfiltration in remnant nephrons: A potentially adverse response to renal ablation. Am J Physiol 241:F85, 1981.
350. Rush D, Stein Z, Susser M: A randomized controlled trial of prenatal nutritional supplementation in New York City. Pediatrics 65:683, 1980.
351. Hakim RM, Depner TA, Parker TF III: Adequacy of hemodialysis. Am J Kidney Dis 20:107, 1992.
352. Redrow M, Cherem L, Elliott J, et al: Dialysis in the management of pregnant patients with renal insufficiency. Medicine (Baltimore) 67:199, 1988.
353. Hou S: Peritoneal dialysis and haemodialysis in pregnancy. Baillieres Clin Obstet Gynaecol 1:1009, 1987.
354. Registration Committee of EDTA: Successful pregnancies in women treated by dialysis and kidney transplantation. Br J Obstet Gynecol 87:839, 1980.
355. Hou S, Orlowski J, Pahl M, et al: Pregnancy in women with end-stage renal disease: Treatment of anemia and premature labor. Am J Kidney Dis 21:16, 1993.
356. Gadallah MF, Ahmad B, Karubian F, et al: Pregnancy in patients on chronic ambulatory peritoneal dialysis. Am J Kidney Dis 20:407, 1992.
357. Alcalay M, Blau A, Barkai G, et al: Successful pregnancy in a patient with polycystic kidney disease and advanced renal failure: The use of prophylactic dialysis. Am J Kidney Dis 19:382, 1992.
358. Vogt K, Keusch G, Baumann U, et al: Successful pregnancy in advanced renal failure without dialysis. Pediatr Nephrol 3:189, 1989.
359. Frohling PT: Successful pregnancy of a woman with advanced renal failure on nutritional treatment. Nephron 44:195, 1986.
360. Davison JM: Dialysis, transplantation, and pregnancy. Am J Kidney Dis 17:127, 1991.
361. Davison JM: The effect of pregnancy on kidney function in renal allograft recipients. Kidney Int 27:74, 1985.
362. Muirhead N, Sabharwal AR, Rieder MJ, et al: The outcome of pregnancy following renal transplantation—the experience of a single center. Transplantation 54:429, 1992.
363. Armenti VT, Ahlswede KM, Ahlswede BA, et al: National Transplant Pregnancy Registry—outcomes of 154 pregnancies in cyclosporine-treated female kidney transplant recipients. Transplantation 57:502, 1994.
364. Sturgiss SN, Davison JM: Effect of pregnancy on long-term function of renal allografts. Am J Kidney Dis 19:167, 1992.
365. Rizzoni G, Ehrich JH, Broyen M, et al: Successful pregnancies in women on renal replacement therapy: Report from the EDTA registry. Nephrol Dial Transplant 7:279, 1992.

# Inherited Disorders of the Renal Tubule

*R. Curtis Morris, Jr.*
*Harlan E. Ives*

## RENAL GLUCOSURIA

Under normal conditions, glucose is nearly quantitatively reabsorbed in the renal proximal tubule. The appearance of glucose in the urine is therefore due to either abnormal use of glucose with increased delivery to the kidney (diabetes mellitus) or abnormally reduced glucose reabsorption by the proximal tubule. Because primary renal glucosuria is generally a benign condition, the abnormality is clinically more important for what it is not than for what it is, and because diabetes mellitus is far more common than true renal glucosuria, diabetes mellitus should be rigorously ruled out before the diagnosis of renal glucosuria is made. In Marble's early work,[1, 2] renal glucosuria was defined as the presence of chemically identifiable glucose (as opposed to sucrose, galactose, or other sugars) in *all* urine specimens from a patient who is not hyperglycemic and who has a normal glucose tolerance test response. By use of these criteria, renal glucosuria was found in only about 0.2% of all patients who had a positive test response for sugar in the urine at any time.[1] However, these criteria are probably too strict. With less stringent criteria, Reubi estimated that between 0.5% and 1% of the entire population has glucosuria, albeit usually intermittently.[3] By use of this estimate, renal glucosuria is more common than type I diabetes mellitus (0.2% to 0.3% frequency) and less common than type II (2% to 4%) in the United States. Thus, in younger individuals, nondiabetic glucosuria is more common than diabetes[4]; in older individuals, this pattern is reversed.

## Normal Glucose Handling by the Nephron

Normal glucose handling by the kidney is covered in greater depth in Chapter 8.

Glucose is freely filtered at the glomerulus and is reabsorbed in the proximal tubule. Glucose concentration is reduced by 90% in the first 2 mm of the $S_1$ segment.[5] The remaining proximal nephron (particularly $S_3$) absorbs glucose more slowly than the $S_1$ segment but has a higher affinity for glucose, leading to virtually complete reabsorption. This bipartite system for reabsorption of glucose results in both rapid and complete removal of glucose from the filtered fluid. The presence of two distinct glucose transporters with different affinities has been firmly established from work with isolated perfused tubule segments,[6] membrane vesicles,[7] and molecular cloning (see later).

As for all membrane transport systems, the glucose transporters in the proximal tubule are "saturable." This means that as glucose concentration in the tubule fluid is increased, each transporting unit increases its rate of transport until its maximal rate ($V_{max}$) is achieved. Beyond this saturation point, transport is independent of further increases in tubule fluid glucose concentration. When the entire assemblage of transporters in the proximal nephron is considered, this translates to a maximal overall rate of glucose transport by the kidney. This maximal rate has been termed the "Tm" (or Tmax) for glucose[8, 9] (Fig. 37–1). In humans, determinations of Tm have varied from 260 to 350 mg/min/1.73 m², with a mean of approximately 300 mg/min/1.73 m².[10–14] When corrected for glomerular filtration rate (GFR), Tm can be expressed as a concentration—approximately 250 mg/dL.[10–14] At serum concentrations of glucose higher than this, glucose appears in the urine.

The maximal rate of transport for an isolated transporter in vitro is easier to comprehend and easier to determine than the Tm for the entire kidney, where factors like the tubule fluid flow rate and nephron heterogeneity may contribute to the overall pattern of glucose reabsorption. Much debate has been generated by the fact that glucose reabsorption by the kidney does not increase linearly until Tm is reached, but rather exhibits a significant "splay" in the curve after a certain Tmin is achieved[10, 15, 16] (see Fig. 37–1). In the region of splay, reabsorption does not match the filtered load, causing glucose to appear in the urine. Current understanding of the mechanisms of transport suggest that this splay is due to the expected shift from first-order kinetics (rate increases linearly with substrate concentration) to zero-order kinetics (rate independent of substrate concentration) as saturation of the individual transporters is approached.[17] The concept of splay became important in early observations of patients with glucosuria (see later).

## Molecular Mechanism of Glucose Transport

The brush border glucose transport system causes active uptake of glucose[18] and therefore must consume energy. The form of this energy consumption is not direct hydrolysis of ATP, but rather use of the energy in the electrochemical $Na^+$ gradient established by the $Na^+$ pump. Early studies with slices of renal cortex indicated that the uptake of sugars required $Na^+$[19] and later work with isolated brush border membranes showed that the uptake of glucose was actually driven by $Na^+$.[7, 20] Turner and Moran[21–23] found that the cortical proximal convoluted tubule has an $Na^+$/glucose stoichiometry of 1:1 but that the medullary $S_3$ segment exhibits $Na^+$/glucose stoichiometry of 2:1. Assuming a membrane potential of 70 mV, a 1:1 stoichiometry would predict a concentrative ability of 200:1, whereas a stoichiometry of 2:1 predicts a concentrative ability of 40,000:1. This difference in stoichiometry helps explain the ability of the $S_3$ segment to remove glucose nearly quantitatively from the tubule fluid.

In the past 15 years, much has been learned about the molecular details of the two proximal tubule transport systems responsible for glucose uptake. Work with isolated perfused tubules and membrane vesicles indicated that the $S_1$ and $S_2$ segments of the proximal tubule contain a high-capacity, low-affinity, phlorhizin-inhibitable[23] glucose transport system.[24, 25] The binding affinity (Michaelis constant, $K_m$) for glucose is of approximately 6 mM, and the transporter carries one $Na^+$ per glucose molecule.[22] The $S_3$ segment, on the other hand, has a high-affinity system with a $K_m$ for glucose of approximately 0.3 mM, carrying two $Na^+$ per glucose molecule.[21] The $S_3$ transporter has a greater than 10-fold higher affinity for D-galactose than the $S_1$ transporter does.[21]

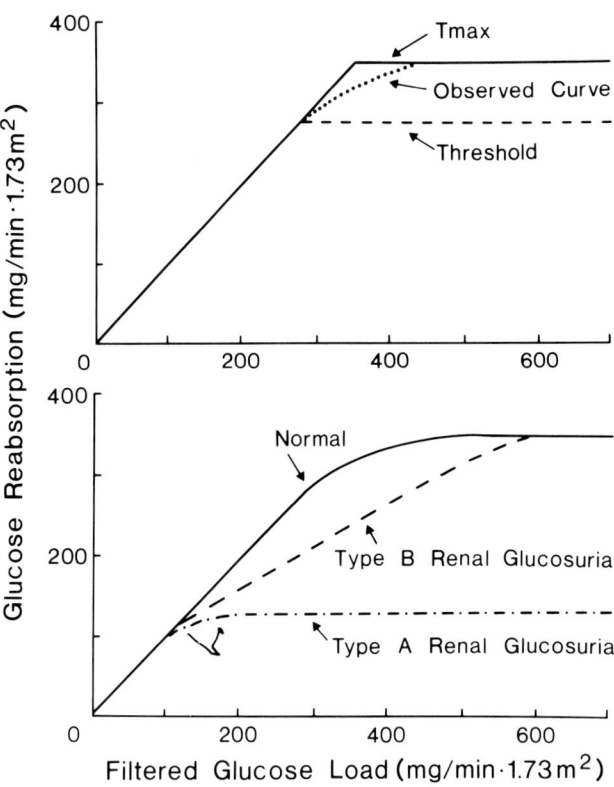

**Figure 37–1.** Normal renal glucose reabsorption as a function of the filtered load. Tmax = maximal rate of glucose absorption; Threshold = point at which glucose first appears in the urine. Two forms of abnormal glucose reabsorption are illustrated. In type A, the maximal rate of glucose reabsorption is reduced; in type B, the maximal rate of reabsorption is normal, but the "splay" is increased.

Patients with the rare congenital disorder of glucose/galactose malabsorption (see later) have a partial defect in renal absorption of glucose.[26, 27] This led to speculation that one of the renal glucose transporters might be identical with the intestinal glucose/galactose transporter. Indeed, when the intestinal $Na^+$/glucose transporter was cloned,[28] it was found to be a 665–amino acid protein expressed in both intestine and kidney.[29] Within the kidney, it was later shown to be expressed almost exclusively in the $S_3$ segment of the proximal tubule.[30] This transporter, termed SGLT1, has a $K_m$ for $Na^+$ of 0.4 mM and binds two $Na^+$,[30] properties virtually identical with those for the $S_3$ glucose transporter. A family has been identified in which a single base pair change in SGLT1 is responsible for classic intestinal glucose-galactose malabsorption.[31] Thus, SGLT1 is almost certainly the proximal tubule $S_3$ "high-affinity" glucose transporter.

A second glucose transporter, termed SGLT2, was cloned from a kidney library.[32, 33] This clone, coding for a 672–amino acid protein, is 59% homologous to SGLT1 and is expressed in kidney but not intestine.[32] SGLT2 confers phlorhizin-sensitive (1 to 5 mM) glucose transport with a $K_m$ for glucose of approximately 1.6 mM. One $Na^+$ is bound per glucose molecule. In situ hybridization shows that expression of SGLT2 is localized to the cortex, in $S_1$ proximal tubule segments. Thus, SGLT2 appears to be the $S_1$ segment "low-affinity" glucose transporter.

Whereas SGLT1 and SGLT2 are responsible for bringing glucose into the proximal tubule cell by secondary active transport, a different system is clearly needed to return this glucose from the cell to the blood. Early work with basolateral membrane vesicles showed this transporter to be a saturable glucose carrier that was inhibited by phloretin and cytochalasin B but not phlorhizin.[34, 35] This transporter has many characteristics in common with basolateral membranes of intestinal and liver epithelial cells and with transporters in red blood cells, muscle cells, and adipocytes.[36] The relationship between glucose transport in the proximal tubule basolateral membrane and glucose transport in other tissues has been clarified with the discovery of a large gene family termed the *GLUT* genes. There are now seven known members of the *GLUT* gene family.[37] Of these, two (*GLUT1* and *GLUT2*) are of interest for renal physiology.

The first member of the *GLUT* family to be discovered was *GLUT1*, which was cloned by use of an antibody to the red blood cell glucose transporter. This carrier has a high affinity for glucose (1 to 2 mM) and is found at variable levels in virtually all nephron segments.[38, 39] Its expression may correlate with nutritive requirements of the cell,[39] and it is probably also the mechanism for glucose exit in $S_3$.[40] *GLUT2* is a high-capacity, low-affinity (15 to 20 mM) basolateral transporter found in tissues with large glucose fluxes, such as the intestine, liver, pancreas, and $S_1$ segment of the proximal convoluted tubule.[39, 40]

## Abnormal Glucose Handling in Renal Glucosuria

In early work, analysis of the splay in the glucose reabsorption curve was considered important in separating two types of renal glucosuria.[41] In some individuals with glucosuria, the cause for the reduced capacity to reabsorb glucose is a simple reduction in the Tm for glucose. This has been referred to as a type A lesion.[41] Other individuals, referred to as type B, spill significant glucose in the urine but have a normal Tm for glucose. These individuals demonstrate an increase in the splay of the glucose reabsorption curve with a reduction in Tmin. Type B patients are thus capable of the same maximal rate of glucose transport as normal subjects are, but the rate at which they reabsorb glucose does not match the rate at which it is delivered to the absorbing site. There has been much debate about the explanation for the existence of these two forms of glucosuria coincident with the debate on the mechanism that causes the splay in the glucose reabsorption curve. Using kinetic principles, Woolf and co-workers[17] showed that the two types of glucosuria could arise from mutations that reduced (type A) the maximal velocity or the total number of transporters or that reduced (type B) the affinity of the transporter for glucose. In support of this idea, patients with glucose-galactose malabsorption, who lack the high-affinity SGLT1, generally exhibit type B glucosuria.[27, 42] Whether patients with a defect in SGLT2 further break down into types A and B or whether they are strictly type A is not known. As genetic analysis becomes more available in the future, analysis of splay in the reabsorptive curve will undoubtedly cede to

analysis of specific defects in the two glucose transport systems.

Abnormalities in glucose transport can also be caused by a generalized defect in proximal tubule transport. These generalized defects may be genetic or could arise in the course of renal disease or after toxin exposure. Genetic disorders leading to generalized proximal tubule dysfunction are discussed later.

## Clinical Features

Primary renal glucosuria is principally a laboratory abnormality. Whereas the disease could predispose to hypoglycemia during starvation, it is otherwise benign and not associated with renal or other organ dysfunction. Inasmuch as glucose transport is an essential function of virtually all cells, the benignity of renal glucosuria must reflect the renal specificity of the *SGLT2* gene. This was partially predicted by Elsas and Rosenberg,[43] who found that patients with renal glucosuria do not have abnormal intestinal glucose transport. The exception is the rarer defect in *SGLT1* (see later), with which patients do have diarrhea. Defects in the *GLUT* genes, which are responsible for glucose uptake in all other cells, have not yet been described.

As stated before, the most important clinical distinction to be made is between primary renal glucosuria and diabetes mellitus. It is important that a patient with primary renal glucosuria not inadvertently be given hypoglycemic therapy. The distinction is easily made with a fasting blood glucose determination and a glucose tolerance test. There have been several reports of the development of diabetes mellitus at a later date in patients with primary renal glucosuria.[44, 45] These authors argued that there might be a relationship between the two diseases. Others found no such relationship.[1, 2, 46] There is of course nothing that precludes the individual with primary glucosuria from having diabetes mellitus as well, and diabetes is a relatively common disease. Therefore, it is not unreasonable to check the fasting serum glucose concentration at some interval in patients with primary renal glucosuria.

## Genetics

The early literature on glucosuria suggested that the defect was inherited as an autosomal dominant trait.[47-49] However, assessment of penetrance is difficult with quantitative traits that can be affected by other variables. Because the disease is usually partial and presents in a variety of quantitative forms (see earlier), precise assessment of the magnitude of the defect must be made under identical conditions of serum glucose concentration before one can make a strong statement about the inheritance pattern. It has long been known that glucosuria varies in severity within families,[50] which suggests a recessive defect with variable penetrance. With quantitative assessment, it has been possible to show, at least in some families, that the Tm for glucose varies in proportion to the dose of the normal gene that the individual carries.[43, 51] Thus, homozygotes had a marked reduction in Tm, whereas heterozygotes had only a modest reduction in Tm. In other families, there may be individuals who have a reduction in Tm; others have exaggerated splay of the glucose titration curve. Thus, the relationship between zygosity and severity of the defect is not always straightforward.[43] It appears that one normal gene for the glucose transporter is probably not sufficient to give the individual a perfectly normal glucose transport curve. If a heterozygote has a small filtered load of glucose, glucose will not be spilled, and the disease may well appear to be recessive. On the other hand, if a heterozygote has a large filtered load of glucose, glucose will be spilled, and the defect will appear to be dominant. Without quantitation of the defect in glucose transport, the terms dominant and recessive are inadequate to describe the penetrance of the defect.

De Marchi and co-workers[52, 53] have found a number of immunologic abnormalities in patients with glucosuria and have also established some linkage between the genetic defect and the human leukocyte antigen locus. Because *SGLT2* was localized to chromosome 16[54] and human leukocyte antigen is on chromosome 6, it remains unclear what basis exists for this putative relationship.

## GLUCOSE-GALACTOSE MALABSORPTION SYNDROME

This rare disorder was first described by Lindquist and colleagues[26] in 1962 as a congenital diarrheal syndrome presenting in newborn infants. The stool was watery and acidic and contained both glucose and galactose. Diarrhea was completely relieved by feeding the infants a diet free of carbohydrate. Jejunal biopsy examinations showed that the mucosal membrane of homozygotes was completely deficient in glucose transport but exhibited normal transport of $Na^+$ and amino acids.[55–57] Homozygotes with glucose-galactose malabsorption have only a partial defect in renal glucose handling.[26, 27, 56, 57] Most of the patients examined have a normal Tm for glucose but an increased splay of the glucose reabsorption curve (type B).[27, 42] However, patients with homozygous renal glucosuria do not have a defect in intestinal absorption of glucose.[43] This is consistent with the molecular studies discussed before, which show that the kidney contains both SGLT1, the intestinal transporter, and SGLT2, which is specific to the kidney. Wright's group[31] has found a family in which a single base pair alteration in SGLT1 is responsible for classic intestinal glucose-galactose malabsorption. Abnormalities in SGLT2 are clearly more common than abnormalities in SGLT1, because primary renal glucosuria is far more common than the glucose-galactose malabsorption syndrome.

## AMINOACIDURIA

Because greater than 95% of filtered amino acids are reabsorbed by the normally functioning proximal tubule, the presence of more than 5% of the filtered load of any amino acid is abnormal and is termed "aminoaciduria." This abnormality could theoretically arise from one of several different metabolic or transport defects. First, the plasma concentration of an amino acid may be increased as a result of a metabolic defect, which increases the quantity filtered at the glomerulus. If the reabsorptive capacity of the tubule for that amino acid were exceeded, the patient would exhibit "overload aminoaciduria." Second, there could be a defect in the proximal tubule brush border amino acid transport system. Because the amino acid transport systems found in the proximal tubule are in some cases the same as those in the intestine, transport defects may be found simultaneously in both tissues. Third, the proximal tubule cell may take up the amino acid but fail to metabolize it or fail to return it to the blood because of a defect in basolateral membrane transport. Last, aminoaciduria could arise from a more generalized defect of the renal proximal tubule, as in some of the toxic nephropathies and in the Fanconi syndrome. For the purposes of this section, discussion is limited to specific inherited transport defects of the amino acids. For a thorough discussion of systemic metabolic defects leading to abnormal production of amino acids, the reader is referred to Scriver.[58] Toxic nephropathies causing aminoaciduria are discussed in Chapter 34, and the Fanconi syndrome is covered separately in this chapter.

## Overview of Amino Acid Transport

Dietary protein is degraded by pancreatic proteinases in the intestine to yield free amino acids and small peptides. Specific transport systems in the intestinal brush border transport these amino acids and small peptides from the intestinal lumen into the cytoplasm of the villus cell. The bulk of these amino acids is then secreted across the basolateral membrane into the blood. Because brush border and basolateral membranes from both kidney and intestine must transport amino acids in opposite directions (with respect to the cell cytoplasm), transporters on the two membranes are generally distinct molecular species (see later).

Amino acids delivered to the blood after intestinal absorption are available for uptake by other cells but are also freely filtered at the glomerulus. Circulating concentrations of the amino acids range from as low as 2 mM for L-aspartate to as high as 300 mM for L-alanine.[59] These concentrations of the amino acids are present in the glomerular filtrate and would be lost in the urine were it not for nearly quantitative reabsorption by the proximal tubule. Fractional clearances of the amino acids are all 1% or less, with a few notable exceptions. L-Aspartate and L-serine have a fractional clearance of 2%, L-glycine 3.5%, and L-histidine fully 6% of the filtered load.[59] The nonprotein β–amino acid L-taurine has a fractional clearance of 9% in humans.[60] Thus, normal urine is clearly not free of amino acids, but the quantities excreted are normally far below the filtered loads.

The site of amino acid reabsorption in the kidney was shown to be the proximal tubule on the basis of stop-flow experiments performed in the 1950s and 1960s.[61, 62] This was verified by direct microperfusion studies of Christopher and Deetjen[63] in 1967 and has subsequently been confirmed by numerous microperfusion studies and work with isolated tubules and membranes.

Absorption of amino acids by the proximal tubule epithelial cell is a two-step process. Amino acids enter the cell through the brush border and leave through the basolateral membrane. Amino acid transporters in these two membranes have different properties.[64-70] To accomplish uphill transport of amino acids into the proximal tubule cell, the brush border membrane carriers use what is called "secondary active" transport. Such transport is energized by the transmembrane $Na^+$ gradient established by the basolateral membrane $Na^+,K^+$-ATPase. Transport of virtually all amino acids, whether acidic,[71] neutral,[72] or basic,[73] is coupled to the $Na^+$ gradient. By lowering intracellular $Na^+$ concentration to approximately one-tenth the concentration found in blood or proximal tubule fluid, the $Na^+,K^+$-ATPase creates an energy source that is available to any transport system that couples transport of the desired substance to transport of $Na^+$. There are in vitro conditions under which transport of some amino acids can occur without $Na^+$, and with more careful analysis, other ionic dependencies have emerged for the transport of some of the amino acids.[74] Where relevant, these are discussed later. For more extensive discussion of this topic, the reader is referred to Chapter 8 and Silbernagl.[74]

## Classification of the Aminoacidurias

Because each of the amino acids has a unique structure that is easily recognizable by a variety of intracellular enzymes, it might have been predicted that each amino acid has its own transport system in the renal proximal tubule. This is not the case. Rather, groups of amino acids are transported by common carriers. With some important exceptions, amino acid transport is grouped in accordance with net charge of the amino acid at neutral pH. In most cases, the first evidence for the existence of these common carriers came from chemical analysis of the urine in patients with various clinical syndromes of amino acid transport. Thus, the inherited aminoacidurias are most readily classified by the net charge on the affected amino acids—neutral (no charge), basic (positive charge), or acidic (negative charge) (Table 37-1).

There are five distinct disorders of neutral amino acid transport. The first is Hartnup disease, an abnormality involving the transport of 12 neutral amino acids. Three additional neutral amino acids—glycine and the imino acids proline and hydroxyproline—are involved in a second disorder, termed "iminoglycinuria." Finally, the neutral amino acids methionine, tryptophan, and glycine are involved in distinct entities known as methioninuria, blue diaper syndrome, and glycinuria, respectively.

Cystine, a neutral amino acid, is transported along with the basic amino acids lysine, arginine, and ornithine, and all four are transported abnormally in the clinical entity known as cystinuria. Several rarer disorders involve only the basic amino acids. The reason for this distinction is discussed later. The final group, the acidic amino acids glutamate and aspartate, are involved in a single entity—acidic aminoaciduria. Thus, every amino acid found in proteins, and several that are not, are involved in at least one described disorder of amino acid transport. Although there are reports of other aminoacidurias involving single amino

**TABLE 37-1. Classification of the Aminoacidurias**

| Major Category | Forms | Amino Acids Involved |
|---|---|---|
| Neutral amino acids | Hartnup disease | Alanine, asparagine, glutamine, histidine, isoleucine, leucine, phenylalanine, serine, threonine, tryptophan, tyrosine, valine |
| | Blue diaper syndrome | Tryptophan |
| | Iminoglycinuria | Glycine, proline, hydroxyproline |
| | Glycinuria | Glycine |
| | Methioninuria | Methionine |
| Basic amino acids and cystine | Cystinuria | Cystine, lysine, arginine, ornithine |
| | Lysinuric protein intolerance | Lysine, arginine, ornithine |
| | Isolated cystinuria | Cystine |
| | Lysinuria | Lysine |
| Acidic amino acids | Acidic aminoaciduria | Glutamate, aspartate |

acids, the vast majority of patients fall into one of the three categories listed in Table 37-1.

## Neutral Aminoaciduria

### HARTNUP DISEASE

Hartnup disease is a rare familial disorder of neutral amino acid transport. Although there are suggestions that this disease occurred in Julius Caesar's family,[75] it was not recognized as a separate clinical entity until 1956. The disease was first reported by Baron and co-workers,[76] who performed an exhaustive analysis of the dietary content and urinary excretion of amino acids in the Hartnup family in London. The novel diagnosis was made when two sibs with a pellagra-like rash were found not to have dietary tryptophan insufficiency. Both sibs, and two others, exhibited a striking abnormality of amino acid excretion. More than 14 amino acids were found in excess on paper chromatograms of these patients' urine. Since that time, numerous cases of the disease have been reported.[77] Widespread screening of neonates indicates that the overall frequency of Hartnup disease is as high as 1 per 26,000 live births.[78]

### TRANSPORT DEFECT IN HARTNUP DISEASE

The urine of patients with Hartnup disease contains abnormal quantities of the L-forms of alanine, asparagine, glutamine, histidine, isoleucine, leucine, phenylalanine, serine, threonine, tryptophan, tyrosine, and valine. Small amounts of other amino acids are also usually found, although proline, hydroxyproline, methionine, and arginine are always spared. The vast majority of patients with this disorder have the same pattern of amino acid excretion.[77] On the basis of this observation, it is assumed that the proximal tubule brush border contains at least one transport system for all 12 of the involved amino acids. In vitro studies are not yet conclusive on this point.[74] A transporter was cloned from cultured pig kidney cells, which confers $Na^+$-dependent transport of many neutral amino acids, but the physiologic function of this transporter and its relationship to the Hartnup gene are still not known. Because of the large number of neutral amino acids, studies on transport of this group have been difficult to carry out and interpret. Some data raise the additional possibility that there are multiple neutral amino acid renal transport systems with overlapping specificities.[74] This, of course, could not explain the rather striking co-occurrence of defective transport of 12 amino acids in Hartnup disease unless expression of these different systems was coordinately regulated. The clinical signs and symptoms of Hartnup disease are due not to the renal transport defect or the number of amino acids involved but to the abnormal intestinal absorption of tryptophan. The existence of an associated intestinal disorder was suspected as early as the first report of Hartnup disease.[76] It was found that these individuals excrete indoles and indicans, breakdown products of tryptophan, in the stool. Milne and associates[79] carried out detailed studies of the intestinal defect in Hartnup disease and showed that ingestion of tryptophan led to the appearance of tryptophan breakdown products in the stool without increasing plasma concentration of tryptophan. Scriver[80] found that neutral amino acids were found in both urine and stool of affected patients. Later, Shih and colleagues[81] demonstrated abnormal transport of tryptophan in intestinal biopsy specimens of affected individuals. When tryptophan ethyl ester, a lipid-soluble form of tryptophan, is fed to children with Hartnup disease, serum tryptophan promptly increases, and the clinical signs of the disease are reversed.[82, 83] Hartnup disease is therefore clinically equivalent to pellagra, in which the essential amino acid tryptophan is deficient in the diet.

A separate intestinal transport defect of tryptophan, called the "blue diaper syndrome," has been identified.[84] These patients excrete indigo, an oxidation product of the tryptophan breakdown product indican. Indoles and indicans are absorbed after their production by bacterial metabolism of excess tryptophan that is not absorbed in the intestine. Unlike patients with Hartnup disease, patients with the blue diaper syndrome do not have an abnormality of the renal excretion of tryptophan. Tryptophan transport appears to be normal in a variety of nonrenal, nonintestinal tissues from patients with Hartnup disease. Placental transport of tryptophan appears to be unaffected, because the ratio of maternal to cord blood tryptophan is normal.[85] Tryptophan concentrations in sweat and saliva are likewise normal,[76] and transport of tryptophan in leukocytes is unaffected.[86] Taken together, these findings suggest that there are multiple transport systems for tryptophan and the other neutral amino acids. Hartnup disease involves only the system found in intestine and renal proximal tubule.

### CLINICAL FEATURES, GENETICS, AND TREATMENT

The clinical features of Hartnup disease are virtually identical to pellagra. However, Hartnup disease is often intermittent and usually less severe than pellagra. Patients present with a red, scaly rash that is exacerbated by exposure to sunlight. Cerebellar ataxia, psychiatric disturbances, and diarrhea are common. Intermittent dystonia, without ataxia, has also been reported.[87] "Attacks" of these clinical disturbances can frequently be associated with periods of dietary inadequacy.[88, 89] The Hartnup family had several members with mental retardation,[76] and mental retardation[77] or progressive encephalopathy[90] has been associated with the disease. However, careful analysis suggests normal or nearly normal IQ scores in most affected patients.[91] The differential diagnosis is straightforward, because patients with the classic symptoms must have either pellagra or Hartnup disease. Dietary history and chromatographic analysis of the urine readily distinguish the two processes. Careful genetic analysis of all the affected individuals revealed that it is an autosomal recessive disorder.[77] Heterozygotes exhibit no abnormality of amino acid excretion, although delayed rise in plasma tryptophan concentration has been found after oral tryptophan loading in heterozygotes.[92] As would be expected, Hartnup disease responds well to treatment with 40 to 200 mg of nicotinamide per day.[93] Some patients may respond well to diets rich in tryptophan.

## Iminoglycinuria

The use of new chromatographic techniques to study the composition of body fluids in the 1940s and 1950s[94] led to the discovery of several metabolic defects that had previously gone unrecognized because they are without significant clinical consequence. One of these is iminoglycinuria, the abnormal excretion of proline, hydroxyproline, and glycine. Excretion of glycine and the imino acids proline and hydroxyproline is ordinarily much greater in the newborn infant than in the adult.[95] As the appropriate transport system develops, these amino acids disappear from the urine by 6 months of age. Joseph and co-workers[96] were the first to describe iminoglycinuria as an inherited disorder of transport that persisted into adulthood in affected individuals. Scriver and co-workers[97] showed that a defect in proline excretion was always accompanied by abnormal excretion of hydroxyproline and glycine. Tada and colleagues[98] showed that this disorder was due to a transport defect in the kidney, because circulating levels of all three amino acids were normal. This rather simple picture was immediately clouded by the discovery that reabsorption of the imino acids in homozygotes was completely absent, whereas 50% of the filtered glycine was reabsorbed. This led to the conclusion that there may be a common transport system for the imino acids and glycine and a separate pure glycine transporter.[97, 99] Thus, as for cystine and the basic amino acids, the transport of glycine and the imino acids is complex.

### TRANSPORT OF THE IMINO ACIDS AND GLYCINE

Reabsorption of proline, hydroxyproline, and glycine is accomplished by distinct transporters on the apical and basolateral membranes of epithelial cells. Studies in isolated renal epithelial membranes have helped to characterize these transporters in detail. Brush border membranes from the proximal tubule have at least two distinct transport systems for these amino acids.[100–103] Both systems are driven by the transmembrane $Na^+$ gradient. One transports proline, hydroxyproline, and glycine; the second system transports only glycine. The brush border glycine transport systems may be further broken down into a high-affinity, low-capacity system, which requires both $Na^+$ and $Cl^-$, and a low-affinity, high-capacity system, which requires $Na^+$ only.[104] There may also be a separate system that is specific for the imino acids.[102, 103] Less information is available about the mechanism of the basolateral transport system for these amino acids, but what there is suggests that it is $Na^+$ independent.[100] In summary, the transport of these three amino acids is characterized by multiple transport systems, which makes genetic analysis of these disorders difficult. As is the case with most of the inherited disorders of transport, many patients with iminoglycinuria also exhibit an abnormality of intestinal transport.[105, 106] However, this abnormality is not uniformly found in homozygotes,[107] which suggests that multiple alleles or gene sites may be involved in this disorder. This is not surprising in view of the large number of different transport systems for the imino acids and glycine.

### CLINICAL ASPECTS, GENETICS, AND TREATMENT

Iminoglycinuria was originally thought to be associated with, or even to cause, mental retardation[105] or seizure disorders.[96, 108] Widespread screening has revealed that this is not the case.[109–111] In fact, the abnormality is relatively common, being found in approximately 1 per 15,000 live births.[109] The reason for the initial confusion is most likely that inborn errors of metabolism were often first sought in mental institutions. In reality, isolated iminoglycinuria is a benign condition and requires no treatment. Although iminoglycinuria is an autosomal recessive trait, the genetic analysis is complicated by the likelihood of multiple alleles and several gene loci for the transport of the imino acids and glycine. This is evidenced by the fact that some individuals have abnormal intestinal transport of imino acids,[105, 106] whereas others do not.[107]

### GLYCINURIA

Glycinuria as an isolated trait has been reported in a number of individuals.[112–114] Interestingly, this disorder appears to be inherited as an autosomal dominant trait. Isolated glycinuria is occasionally found in heterozygotes for iminoglycinuria.[113] Isolated glycinuria has also been reported in association with glucosuria, so-called glucoglycinuria.[115] These variants of the disease serve to further underscore the variety of alleles that can give rise to abnormalities in the renal handling of glycine and the imino acids.

## Methioninuria

Among the neutral amino acids, methionine is one of the few that is spared in Hartnup disease. It can be concluded

that methionine must have a separate transport system in the renal proximal tubule. This conclusion is supported by several case reports of individuals with isolated abnormal excretion of methionine or its metabolic breakdown products.[116, 117] These patients had seizures, mental retardation, and episodes of hyperventilation. Evidence of abnormal intestinal transport of methionine was discovered, with the production of α-hydroxybutyric acid by intestinal flora. $Na^+$-dependent transport of methionine has been identified in the bovine[118] and rat[119] intestine. In the proximal tubule, there is evidence that methionine may share transporters with other amino acids.[74, 120] However, these findings are not definitive.

## Cystine and Basic Aminoaciduria

### CYSTINURIA

The existence of cystinuria as a unique form of urinary stone disease has been recognized since 1810. Wollaston[121] and, later, Berzelius[122] mistakenly believed that the offending substance derived from the bladder, hence the names "cystic oxide" and "cystine." Further progress was not made until the turn of the century, when Archibald Garrod[123] identified cystinuria as one of the classic "inborn errors of metabolism." Technically speaking, Garrod's ideas were not correct either, because cystinuria is a defect in the transport and not the metabolism of cystine. This concept was not established until the studies of Yeh[124] and Dent[125, 126] and co-workers in the 1950s. These investigators discovered that cystinuria is accompanied by excess excretion of the basic amino acids lysine, arginine, and ornithine, but that serum levels of all four amino acids are normal. These observations led Dent to hypothesize that cystine, lysine, arginine, and ornithine were all transported by one carrier whose functional absence would lead to abnormal urinary excretion of all four amino acids. Whereas this conclusion was basically sound, subsequent examination of amino acid transport in the kidney and intestine has revealed a much more complicated picture of the mechanism by which these amino acids are transported than was originally anticipated.

### MECHANISM OF CYSTINE TRANSPORT

Early studies of basic amino acid transport in kidney slices appeared to refute Dent's hypothesis of a shared transport system for cystine, lysine, arginine, and ornithine. Although the basic amino acids competed with each other for uptake, they did not compete with cystine.[127] More surprisingly, uptake of cystine appeared normal in kidney tissue from individuals with cystinuria.[128] Other experiments clearly indicated that there are separate transport systems on the renal epithelial cell for lysine and cystine.[129, 130] Not only did these experiments fail to show competition between the amino acids, but there were also biochemical differences between the transport systems. For example, cystine transport was $Na^+$ dependent, but lysine transport was not.[129, 131] This and other work did not support the notion of a common carrier for cystine and the basic amino acids that derived from clinical observations.[132]

Subsequent work with isolated epithelial cell membranes has helped clarify the situation. As more was learned about the function of epithelia, it became clear that transepithelial transport is a two-step process. Solutes are first reabsorbed from the tubule fluid into the epithelial cell through the brush border membrane and then secreted from the epithelial cell into the blood through the basolateral membrane. The uptake studies with kidney slices discussed before had detected separate transport systems for cystine and the basic amino acids on the basolateral membrane but had failed to probe the common carrier for these amino acids, which is on the brush border membrane.

Working with isolated brush border membrane vesicles, Segal and co-workers[133] delineated two separate transport systems for cystine. The first is a high-affinity system ($K_m$ = 12 mM) on which lysine and cystine compete for transport. This is the common carrier that is presumably defective in cystinuria. The second cystine transporter is a low-affinity system ($K_m$ = 550 mM) that does not appear to bind lysine at all. The existence of these multiple transport systems has been confirmed in cultured renal epithelial cells.[134] A human complementary DNA (termed D2H) that confers transport of cystine and dibasic amino acids has been cloned by expression in *Xenopus* oocytes.[135] This clone is homologous to clones obtained from rabbit[136] and rat.[137] The $K_m$ for cystine transport is 30 mM, close to the $K_m$ for the high-affinity system. Furthermore, the D2H complementary DNA recognizes a message that is expressed abundantly in kidney. In situ hybridization of a related rat clone shows that this message is expressed in the $S_3$ segment of the proximal tubule.[138] Although there are some differences with previous physiologic descriptions of the proximal tubule cystine–dibasic amino acid transporter,[137] D2H appears to be a candidate for this system. Earlier work with patients demonstrated that there are multiple alleles of the cystine transport gene.[139] The various alleles exhibit different degrees of abnormality in the intestinal transport of cystine and the basic amino acids (Table 37–2). Additional work should soon determine whether D2H is the transporter that is defective in patients with cystinuria.

Basolateral membranes, like the membranes of nonepithelial cells, also have separate transport systems for cystine and the basic amino acids. Thus, the epithelial cell brush border contains the only common carrier for cystine and the basic amino acids, and this is the system that is defective in cystinuria. As would be predicted from this formulation, cystine and basic amino acid transport in nonepithelial cells is normal in cystinuria.[140, 141] The finding of multiple transport systems for cystine and the basic amino acids raises the possibility of separate disorders in which cystine or basic amino acid transport, but not both, would be abnormal. Indeed, such disorders have been reported in a few cases (see later).

## INTESTINAL TRANSPORT DEFECT IN CYSTINURIA

Although it was not appreciated at the time, evidence for an intestinal absorption defect in cystinuria was available before the turn of the century. Von Udransky and Baumann[142] found that the urine of patients with cystinuria contained large amounts of cadaverine and putrescine, the bacterial degradation products of lysine and arginine. The significance of this finding was not understood until Milne and co-workers[143, 144] showed that cadaverine and putrescine were produced from basic amino acids that escaped absorption in the intestine.

Demonstration of the abnormal transport system in the intestine was accomplished soon thereafter. Both Thier[145] and McCarthy[146] and co-workers were able to show that patients' intestinal mucosa in vitro exhibited abnormal transport of both cystine and the basic amino acids. Furlong and Stiel[147] showed that cystine transport in duodenal brush border vesicles obtained from cystinuric individuals is abnormal. Establishment of the intestinal defect was not confounded by the existence of the multiple cystine transport systems found in the kidney. The reason for this appears to be that the intestinal cell relies much more heavily on the common carrier than does the proximal tubule epithelial cell for the bulk of cystine transport.[148] Because patients with cystinuria clearly exhibit abnormal intestinal transport of cystine, the cystine and basic amino acid transporter of the intestinal epithelial cell must be coded by the same gene as that in the proximal tubule brush border. The D2H complementary DNA mentioned before is also expressed in the intestine.[135]

## GENETICS

Cystinuria is an autosomal recessive disorder. Heterozygotes demonstrate several different phenotypes, which were

**TABLE 37–2. Rosenberg Classification of Cystinuria**

| Category | Phenotype | Intestinal Transport Defect |
|---|---|---|
| **I** | | |
| Heterozygote | No abnormality | |
| Homozygote | Cystinuria, basic aminoaciduria, cystine stones | Cystine, basic amino acids |
| **II** | | |
| Heterozygote | Excess excretion of cystine and dibasic amino acids | |
| Homozygote | Cystinuria, basic aminoaciduria, cystine stones | Basic amino acids only |
| **III** | | |
| Heterozygote | Excess excretion of cystine and basic amino acids | |
| Homozygote | Cystinuria, basic aminoaciduria, cystine stones | None |

characterized in detail in the 1960s by Rosenberg.[139, 149] Rosenberg found that measurement of intestinal transport of cystine and the basic amino acids was critical in diagnosing the subtypes of the disease (see Table 37–2). In type I, intestinal transport of cystine and the basic amino acids is absent; in type III, it is normal. In type II, intestinal transport of cystine is normal, whereas intestinal transport of the basic amino acids is absent. It remains unclear precisely how the existence of these different forms of cystinuria can be rationalized with a common cystine–dibasic amino acid carrier in kidney and intestine. It is clear that the phenotypic variants are not due to defects in different genes. Rather, they represent different alleles of the same gene. This was proved by the discovery of fortuitous marriages between individuals with different forms of the disease. None of the offspring of these patients exhibited complementation consistent with cystinuria caused by two distinct genes. All were homozygous cystinurics, which shows that the defects in the various forms of cystinuria are all in the same gene.[139]

## CLINICAL FEATURES AND TREATMENT

Cystinuria is a relatively common inherited disorder, being found in approximately 1 per 7000 live births, although this figure varies widely with geographic region.[78] The disease is found equally in both sexes. The excretion of urine rich in cystine and basic amino acids does not give rise to any identifiable clinical symptoms. Thus, cystinuria would be nothing more than a curiosity were it not for the extreme insolubility of cystine in urine. Thus, patients are susceptible to the development of cystine calculi when their cystine excretion exceeds its solubility in urine (approximately 250 mg/L between pH 4.5 and 7.5). Although the disease is present from birth, it is rarely detected clinically until the second or third decades of life, when stone formation becomes significant. At that time, the disease usually presents with renal colic. If subclinical obstruction has occurred, cystinuria may also present with urinary tract infections, hypertension, or renal failure. Once suspected, the diagnosis of cystinuria is made easily by examination of the first morning urine specimen for the classic hexagonal crystals. The cyanide-nitroprusside test detects cystine in urine[150] but is nonspecific because it also reacts with acetone and homocystine. More recently, several automated tests have been described that are useful for screening large numbers of children.[151, 152] Definitive diagnosis and quantitation of the cystine excretion are made by chromatographic analysis of the urine.[153–155] Homozygous patients with cystinuria generally excrete 250 to 1000 mg of cystine per gram of creatinine in 24 hours, compared with a normal of 19 mg of cystine per gram of creatinine.[156] The radiographic appearance of cystine calculi is typically that of smooth, radiopaque stones or a smooth staghorn calculus.

The goal of treatment is to reduce the cystine concentration in the urine or to increase its solubility. Whereas reduced excretion could theoretically be accomplished by reducing metabolic production of cystine from methionine, this approach is only of limited usefulness.[157] Rather, three other approaches are of greater benefit. First, ingestion of large quantities of fluid will reduce the concentration of cystine in the urine. Because many patients may excrete 1000 mg of cystine per day,[156] excretion of 4 L of urine per day may be required to keep the concentration below the solubility limit of 250 mg/L. Second, cystine solubility can be greatly enhanced by maintenance of the urine pH at greater than 7.5 by ingestion of bicarbonate or citrate. Both fluid intake and alkalinization must be maintained around the clock to avoid stone formation when the urine is concentrated in the morning. Approximately two thirds of affected individuals respond to these conservative measures.

In patients who continue to form stones despite conservative therapy, the administration of large quantities of sulfhydryl-containing drugs, such as penicillamine,[158, 159] has proved particularly efficacious. These drugs form mixed disulfides with cystine that are considerably more soluble than cystine itself. Administration of 1 to 2 g/d of penicillamine is usually effective in reducing stone formation.[158] Unfortunately, penicillamine[111, 159, 160] and other sulfhydryl-containing compounds have a common spectrum of serious side effects.[161] These include severe rashes such as pemphigus,[162] membranous glomerulonephritis,[163, 164] and hematologic abnormalities including aplastic anemia. Therefore, although penicillamine is extremely effective, its use must be reserved for patients who are completely refractory to conservative measures. Mercaptopropionylglycine is another sulfhydryl agent that is efficacious in cystinuria.[165, 166] Unfortunately, it appears to exhibit the same spectrum of toxic effects as penicillamine does.[161, 167] Captopril also has a free sulfhydryl group, but its efficacy in treatment of cystinuria is still being debated.[168–170]

Once formed, cystine stones may require surgical therapy or ultrasonic lithotripsy.[166, 171] Patients with end-stage renal disease have successfully undergone kidney transplantation.

## Lysinuric Protein Intolerance

This disease, also termed basic aminoaciduria, is a rare disorder of lysine, arginine, and ornithine transport.[172–177] Cystine transport is normal. Almost half of the reported cases are from Finland. The patients usually present as children who reject dietary protein and have nausea, vomiting, lethargy, or seizures after protein intake. Symptoms are due to hyperammonemia. Hepatomegaly, muscle hypotrophy and hypotonia, and osteoporosis also develop.[178, 179] Children grow slowly, but there is no mental retardation. There is a high frequency of subclinical interstitial lung disease due to pulmonary hemorrhage and alveolar proteinosis. This process occasionally leads to respiratory insufficiency and death.[180, 181]

### TRANSPORT DEFECT IN LYSINURIC PROTEIN INTOLERANCE

As discussed in the section on cystinuria, the basolateral membrane transport system for basic amino acids does not involve cystine, which makes it a potential site for the defect in lysinuric protein intolerance. Indeed, studies of the renal clearance of lysine in these patients suggested that the defect is at the epithelial cell basolateral membrane.[175, 176, 182] A basolateral defect in lysinuric protein intolerance is also found in the intestine. Orally administered lysylglycine is taken up as a dipeptide and cleaved to lysine and glycine in the intestinal epithelial cell.[183, 184] Patients with lysinuric protein intolerance exhibit a normal rise in plasma glycine but no increase in plasma lysine. Thus, the defect is in transport of lysine from the cell to the blood through the basolateral membrane. Transport of lysine and arginine is also abnormal in fibroblasts from patients with lysinuric protein intolerance. Uptake of the basic amino acids is normal, but exit is diminished, leading to intracellular accumulation of the basic amino acids.[185]

The cause for the clinical hyperammonemia is a disturbance in the urea cycle,[186] in which arginine and ornithine play key roles. Precisely why the urea cycle is disturbed remains unclear. Because intracellular concentrations of lysine, arginine, and ornithine are actually increased in the disease,[187] it is possible that mitochondrial uptake, which is essential for urea cycle metabolism, is defective. Alternatively, increased intracellular lysine concentration may interfere with urea cycle activity.[177]

### TREATMENT

Elimination or reduction of episodes of hyperammonemia can be accomplished by limiting dietary protein to less than 0.8 g/kg/d in adults.[188] Whereas this is effective in most adults, it may lead to malnutrition in children. Arginine supplementation is effective when it is given intravenously, but because of the intestinal defect, it causes diarrhea and is only minimally useful when given orally. Provision of adequate urea cycle intermediates can apparently be accomplished by dietary administration of citrulline. Citrulline is a neutral amino acid and is transported separately from the basic amino acids, but it is converted to arginine and ornithine metabolically.[188] Oral citrulline is as effective as intravenous arginine in preventing hyperammonemia.

### ISOLATED CYSTINURIA AND LYSINURIA

Because the basolateral membranes of the proximal tubule cell and the enterocyte contain separate transport systems for the basic amino acids and cystine, it might be predicted that there could be an isolated defect in cystine excretion. Indeed, there has been a report of isolated cystinuria in two cases.[95] There is a single case report of isolated lysinuria, with normal transport of arginine, ornithine, and cystine.[189] The finding of these distinct clinical entities underlines the complexity of the transport systems for these amino acids in the renal and intestinal epithelia.

## Acidic Aminoaciduria

It has been recognized since the 1950s that the acidic, or dicarboxylic, amino acids L-glutamate and L-aspartate share a common carrier in the proximal tubule,[190, 191] which does not transport other amino acids. This was confirmed with the finding of two patients who exhibited abnormal excretion of both amino acids[192, 193] but normal excretion of the others. One of these patients also had abnormal intestinal absorption of the acidic amino acids. The disorder is probably autosomal recessive, because parents of the involved individuals had no abnormality. The disease appears to be without clinical consequence.

The mechanism of transport of the acidic amino acids in the proximal tubule is different from that of other amino acids. Sacktor and co-workers[194–196] clearly demonstrated that transport of L-glutamate is coupled to both the inwardly directed $Na^+$ gradient and the outwardly directed $K^+$ gradient in the proximal tubule cell. To achieve electroneutrality (uptake of the negatively charged acidic amino acids would be highly unfavorable thermodynamically), the complex transported into the cell probably consists of either two $Na^+$ and glutamate$^-$ or one $Na^+$, one $H^+$, and glutamate$^-$.[197]

## RENAL HYPOPHOSPHATEMIC RICKETS (AND OSTEOMALACIA)

This term refers to a group of disorders (Table 37–3) that have in common 1) persisting hypophosphatemia caused by a reduction in renal tubule reabsorption of $P_i$, expressed as an increased fractional excretion of filtered $P_i$ (or decreased TmP/GFR,[224] a nomogramic derivative of the fractional excretion of $P_i$), and 2) a metabolic bone disease, usually rickets in childhood or osteomalacia in adulthood.[225, 226] The term may imply the absence of impaired renal acidification and the complex dysfunction of the proximal renal tubule characteristic of the Fanconi syndrome. The etiologic bases of the renal disorders in this group have not been defined, although some are clearly genetically transmitted; in a small number of patients, the entire disorder can disappear with surgical removal of tumors of mesenchymal origin,[203, 213–219] fibrous dysplasia of bone,[220] or epidermal nevi.[221, 227]

**TABLE 37–3. Clinical Spectrum of Renal Hypophosphatemic Metabolic Bone Disease**

Sporadic
  Childhood onset[198]
  Adulthood onset[199]

Genetically transmitted
  X-linked dominant
    Childhood onset[198, 200–204]
    Adulthood onset[205]
  Autosomal recessive[206]
  Autosomal dominant[207]
  Apparently autosomal dominant[208, 209]
  "Hypophosphatemic nonrachitic bone disease"[209]
  Hereditary hypophosphatemic rickets with hypercalciuria[210–212]

Acquired (and often surgically reversible)
  Tumors of bone and soft tissue[203, 213–219]
  Fibrous dysplasia of bone[220]
  Epidermal nevus[220, 221]

Neurofibromatosis associated[222, 223]

## Overview of the Homeostatic Response to the Hypophosphatemia of Phosphate Depletion

The normal renal homeostatic response to dietary deprivation of phosphate and consequent hypophosphatemia includes not only increased reabsorption of $P_i$ by the proximal tubule but also this nephron segment's increased production of the hormone 1,25-dihydroxyvitamin D, $(1,25(OH)_2D_3)$.[228-235] This hormone is the most active metabolite of vitamin D known with respect to stimulating not only intestinal absorption of $Ca^{2+}$[236] and $P_i$[237] but also bone resorption.[238, 239] In most of the acquired and many of the inherited renal disorders expressed as renal hypophosphatemic rickets, the hormonal as well as the physiologic component of the renal homeostatic response appears to be impaired, and the attendant metabolic bone disease is "vitamin D resistant." Yet, it has become clear that in at least two inherited forms of renal hypophosphatemic rickets, hereditary hypercalciuric hypophosphatemic rickets in the human and in the *Gy* mouse (see later),[210-212] and in a probably inherited third form expressed as the Fanconi syndrome without renal tubular acidosis (RTA),[240] the physiologic derangement occurs unassociated with deranged renal metabolism of vitamin D, and the attendant metabolic bone and muscle disease is strikingly responsive to phosphate therapy alone. Accordingly, an understanding of the inherited and acquired syndromes of renal hypophosphatemic rickets, as well as of hypophosphatemic bone disorders that occur outside the setting of renal hypophosphatemic rickets, requires some consideration of both the physiologic and metabolic components of the normal renal homeostatic response to dietary phosphate deprivation and hypophosphatemia and also the potential of hypophosphatemia to induce metabolic bone disease and metabolic myopathy.

In normal subjects under normal metabolic conditions, the serum concentration of phosphorus undergoes a circadian variation: a decrease in the morning to a nadir shortly before noon, followed by a rapid increase to an extended plateau in the afternoon, and a modest further increase to a peak shortly after midnight.[201, 241] Employing spectral analysis, Portale and associates[242, 243] found that the normal circadian rhythm in serum concentration of phosphorus can be described as the sum of sinusoidal functions with periodicities of 24 and 12 hours. In men, dietary restriction of phosphorus, combined with orally administered aluminum hydroxide, induced within 10 days a striking change in the character of the circadian rhythm of serum phosphorus concentration. Although inducing only a modest decrease in the morning fasting value of serum phosphorus, such extreme restriction of dietary phosphorus (to less than 100 mg/d) abolished the 12-hour periodic component of the time series that normally includes the afternoon rise in serum phosphorus concentration and thus induced a 40% reduction in the 24-hour mean serum level of phosphorus. Indeed, the magnitude of reduction in the serum level of phosphorus induced throughout the afternoon was twice that induced at 8:00 AM, the values decreasing to 2.0 and 2.6 mg/dL, respectively. Even with phosphorus restriction, the nocturnal peak in phosphorus concentration persisted in

each subject, if at a lower level (i.e., the 24-hour periodicity was maintained). Substantial phosphorus supplementation (3 g/d for 10 days) that induced no persisting change in the morning fasting serum phosphorus level induced a 14% increase in the 24-hour mean serum level of phosphorus by exaggerating the afternoon rise in serum phosphorus concentration.[242]

When dietary phosphorus is even moderately restricted in normal humans, there rapidly occurs a reduction in the urinary excretion of $P_i$ attended by a modest reduction in the plasma concentration of $P_i$ that may not be demonstrable in the morning fasting period; the reduction in plasma concentration occurs only later during the day.[242, 243] In normal humans, substantial dietary restriction of phosphate that induces within a few days a modest reduction in the plasma concentration of $P_i$ demonstrable throughout the day induces the virtual disappearance of $P_i$ from the urine.[244] Such renal adaptation to phosphorus restriction in rats, mice, rabbits, and pigs is mediated by a marked increase in proximal tubule transport of $P_i$[245-249] and a parallel increase in $Na^+$-$P_i$ cotransport activity in isolated brush border vesicles.[245, 249, 250] In the rat, the enhancement of renal $P_i$ transport occurs in parallel with, and would appear to be mediated by, an increase in the proximal tubule level of a renal specific brush border $Na^+$-$P_i$ cotransporter protein and its encoding messenger RNA.[251]

In humans, dietary restriction of phosphorus that induces only a modest reduction in morning fasting serum concentration of $P_i$, but virtual disappearance of urinary $P_i$, induces within a few days a two-fold increase in the plasma concentration of $1,25(OH)_2D_3$ and striking hypercalciuria.[244, 252, 253] The change occurs with little if any change in serum concentration of immunoactive parathyroid hormone (PTH) or urinary excretion of cyclic AMP (cAMP), a marker of the renal physiologic response to increased circulating levels of PTH. In humans, dietary phosphorus physiologically regulates the plasma concentration of $1,25(OH)_2D_3$ by modulating its renal production,[244] presumably by modulating the renal activity of 25-hydroxyvitamin $D_3$ ($25(OH)D_3$) $1\alpha$-hydroxylase ("$1\alpha$-hydroxylase"),[254] a mitochondrial enzyme found in the proximal renal tubule. The modulation of $1\alpha$-hydroxylase by dietary phosphorus appears to be mediated by changes in some function of the plasma concentration of $P_i$. In normal humans, the mean 24-hour serum concentration of $P_i$ correlates strongly and inversely with the circulating concentration of $1,25(OH)_2D_3$.[242, 243] The correlation holds throughout the normal range of both values and beyond.[243] The mechanism by which dietary phosphate modulates $1\alpha$-hydroxylase activity and consequent synthesis of $1,25(OH)_2D_3$ is unknown but could not be related to changes in mitochondrial $P_i$ transport in the proximal tubule.[255]

## Hypophosphatemic Bone Disease

At least in part by stimulating bone resorption,[239] administered $1,25(OH)_2D_3$ increases the plasma concentration of phosphorus in phosphorus-depleted, hypophosphatemic vitamin D–deficient rats,[256] a state in which intestinal absorption of phosphorus is negligible and renal reabsorption of phosphorus virtually complete. Even moderate hypophosphatemia enhances bone resorption in the rat, and vitamin D deficiency mitigates this enhancement.[257] Insufficient intake of phosphorus in premature infants[258, 259] and excessive ingestion of the phosphorus-binding antacid aluminum hydroxide in adults[260–265] can induce hypophosphatemic metabolic bone disease in time. As induced experimentally in adult subjects by Bartter and colleagues,[260] this syndrome is characterized biochemically by severe hypophosphatemia, virtual disappearance of urinary phosphorus, striking hypercalciuria that is caused in part by bone resorption, and greatly increased values of serum alkaline phosphatase. However, in the index case, Bloom and Flinchum[263] observed that whereas the morning fasting value of serum phosphorus was hardly reduced at 2.9 mg/dL, the afternoon value was distinctly if not severely reduced at 2.0 mg/dL and remained so for as long as aluminum hydroxide was continued. Neither of two men with antacid-induced, histomorphometrically documented osteomalacia[264, 265] had severe hypophosphatemia, as judged by morning fasting values of serum phosphorus (3.2 and 2.0 mg/dL). Yet both had values of circulating $1,25(OH)_2D_3$ more than twice the upper limit of the normal range, as did phosphorus-deficient premature infants with metabolic bone disease.[258] Dietary supplementation of phosphorus rapidly normalized the serum concentrations of $P_i$ and $1,25(OH)_2D_3$, stopped bone pain, and healed the metabolic bone disease. Raisz and colleagues[258] proposed that the increased circulating concentration of $1,25(OH)_2D_3$ was an important pathogenetic determinant of hypophosphatemic rickets of prematurity.[258] Lemann and colleagues[266] have provided evidence that increased levels of $1,25(OH)_2D_3$ can induce bone resorption in healthy normal men.

## Hereditary Hypophosphatemic Rickets with Hypercalciuria

Hereditary hypophosphatemic rickets with hypercalciuria (HHRH), as described by Tieder and colleagues,[210–212] can be viewed as an instance of genetically transmitted renal hypophosphatemic rickets (and osteomalacia) in which only renal reabsorption of $P_i$ is impaired and the renal hormonal response to hypophosphatemia is not. Indeed, in those affected, the measured values of circulating $1,25(OH)_2D_3$ are apparently normally increased. The specific character of the genetic transmission of HHRH is uncertain, having been studied in a Bedouin tribe in which intermarriage is common. Those presumed to be homozygous for the trait have moderately severe hypophosphatemia, increased values of $1,25(OH)_2D_3$, striking hypercalciuria, clear-cut metabolic bone disease, and proximal muscle weakness. Those presumed to be heterozygous for the trait have values of plasma $P_i$, $1,25(OH)_2D_3$, and urinary $Ca^{2+}$ intermediate between those of presumed homozygotes and their unaffected relatives. In patients with HHRH, continued phosphorus therapy alone increases and decreases, respectively, the serum concentrations of $P_i$ and $1,25(OH)_2D_3$ toward normal values and, within months, stops the bone pain, reverses the radiographic signs of rickets, and accelerates linear growth in those children in whom the growth plate has remained

open. Phosphorus therapy alone also rapidly improves muscle strength and normalizes the urinary excretion of $Ca^{2+}$ and serum level of alkaline phosphatase. The bone disorder and the response to phosphorus supplementation in HHRH are then much like those of the hypophosphatemic metabolic disorder induced by ingestive abuse of aluminum hydroxide.

The genetically transmitted hypophosphatemic renal rickets of the *Gy* mouse,[267] like that of the *Hyp* mouse (see later), is X linked, and the mediating renal disorder of both, like that of HHRH, impairs reabsorption only of $P_i$.[268, 269] However, in the mediating renal disorder of the *Gy* mouse, as in that of HHRH, and in pointed distinction from that of the *Hyp* mouse (see later), the plasma concentration of $P_i$ normally modulates the renal production of $1,25(OH)_2D_3$. With graded degrees of hypophosphatemia and hyperphosphatemia, the extent of increase and decrease of circulating levels of $1,25(OH)_2D_3$ in the *Gy* mouse is not different from that in the normal mouse.[270] In further distinction from the X-linked *Hyp* mouse, the *Gy* mouse gyres, reflecting perhaps its abnormal inner ear.[267] Unlike the gyre of the falcon that cannot hear the falconer, the gyre of the *Gy* mouse does not widen.

## X-Linked Hypophosphatemic Rickets

### CLINICAL DESCRIPTION

The best characterized and apparently most common kind of renal hypophosphatemic rickets is that genetically transmitted as an X-linked dominant trait, X-linked hypophosphatemic rickets (XLH). A detailed map of the region around the *HYP* locus has been established, and closely linked flanking markers for XLH have been identified.[271] XLH is first expressed clinically in early childhood[200, 204, 225, 272, 273]; hypophosphatemia is detectable at 2 months, and rickets and reduced reabsorption of $P_i$ are noted by 6 months.[274] the severity of metabolic bone disease is greater in the affected boy (hemizygote) than in the affected girl (heterozygote), in whom the skeletal expression of the disease can be mild,[200] even though hypophosphatemia in the girl is not of lesser severity.[272] Growth impairment, which occurs in early childhood, appears to be of greater severity than can be accounted for by the characteristic leg bowing.[200, 275, 276] In the rachitic bone disease of XLH, in distinction from that of simple vitamin D deficiency or that of HHRH, the long bones (on x-ray examination) have coarse trabeculations, thickened cortices, evidence of periosteal new bone formation, and bone overgrowth at muscle attachments.[225] Bone pain is uncommon in children.[277] In affected adults, however, osteomalacia that causes bone pain is common, as is osteoarthritis affecting the ankles and knees and, in decreasing frequency, the sacroiliac joints and wrists.[278] Axial osteopenia has been found not to occur in adulthood; axial bone mass may in fact be increased.[279] A minor degree of peripheral bone loss may occur.[279] Fractures are rare.[278]

In sharp distinction from the increased levels in HHRH, circulating levels of $1,25(OH)_2D_3$ in XLH are not increased but abnormally "normal" or slightly reduced.[273, 280–283] The serum concentrations of $Ca^{2+}$ are normal[200, 225] or modestly reduced.[225] It is generally held that the circulating levels of immunoreactive PTH are increased only modestly if at all in XLH.[284-289] However, it has been reported that nocturnal levels of PTH are substantially increased in many of those affected, children and adults, treated and untreated.[290] Such nocturnal hyperparathyroidism is characterized by increased circulating levels of midmolecule fragments of PTH and is inferred to reflect their increased secretion and that of the intact molecule. Alkaline phosphatase activity can be either normal or increased. Net gut absorption of $Ca^{2+}$ is reduced.[291, 292]

Muscle weakness and other evidence of myopathy are conspicuously absent not only in children and adults with XLH[200, 204, 225] but in patients with most other forms of genetically transmitted renal hypophosphatemic rickets as well.[205-207, 209] By contrast, striking muscle weakness and general debility characteristically attend the hypophosphatemia and osteomalacia caused by the phosphate depletion induced in otherwise normal subjects by sustained restriction of $P_i$ absorption from the gut (ingested aluminum hydroxide).[260, 293-296] Furthermore, in children and adults with renal hypophosphatemic rickets that is not genetically transmitted, proximal muscle weakness is predictable,[203, 213-221, 227, 297-299] is often striking, and can be responsive to phosphate therapy alone,[297, 298] even though the hypophosphatemia of these patients is often no more severe than that of patients with XLH. In children with a genetically transmitted "hypophosphatemic nonrachitic bone disease" and no evidence of myopathy, Scriver and co-workers[209] noted that the bone disease is more benign than that of XLH despite "the same low concentration of phosphate anion in the extracellular fluid." Scriver and co-workers[209] suggested that this disease and XLH are "experiments of nature which may reveal a process regulating the distribution of inorganic phosphate between extracellular fluid and the bone compartment." In reported studies of patients with inherited, infant-onset hypophosphatemic rickets, magnetic resonance measurements[300] revealed no reduction of $P_i$ in somatic muscle, which suggests the possibility of an altered distribution of $P_i$ between extracellular fluid and somatic muscle cells.

## DISORDERED RENAL FUNCTION

In patients with XLH,[200, 225, 301-304] as in the X-linked analogue of this disease in the mouse, the *Hyp* mouse,[268, 269, 305] the renal response to hypophosphatemia and dietary deprivation of phosphorus is impaired. The physiologic impairment can be expressed as a reduced value of TmP/GFR.[226, 306] This value can be estimated from a nomogram relating the serum concentration of $P_i$ to the fractional excretion of $P_i$, as measured from determinations of the serum concentration of $P_i$ and urinary $P_i$ and creatinine concentrations. Expression of the defect has been demonstrated to be responsive to, but not requiring of, PTH.[307] In the *Hyp* mouse, the defect in renal $P_i$ transport occurs in the proximal tubule[307, 308] and involves the genetically determined high-affinity, low-capacity $Na^+$-$P_i$ cotransport system of the brush border membrane that occurs throughout the proximal tubule.[309] The reduction in the $Na^+$-$P_i$ cotransport on the *Hyp* mouse reflects a proportional reduction in

the abundance of $Na^+$-$P_i$ cotransporter messenger RNA and protein.[310] The renal-specific $Na^+$-$P_i$ cotransporter gene has been mapped to the human chromosome 5q35 by in situ hybridization using a full-length NaP$_i$-3 complementary DNA probe cloned from human kidney cortex.[311] The complementary DNA for renal-specific $Na^+$-$P_i$ cotransport isolated from human renal cortex (NaP$_i$-3) is highly homologous to that isolated from rat renal cortex (NaP$_i$-2); the complementary DNA-related cotransporter proteins are also highly homologous.[312] These findings exclude the renal-specific $Na^+$-$P_i$ cotransporter gene as a candidate gene for XLH in both the mouse and the human.[311, 312] Rather, a circulating substance in the *Hyp* mouse impairs its otherwise normal renal $P_i$ reabsorption as demonstrated in parabiotic experiments reported by Meyer and colleagues[313] and in cross-transplantation studies of Nesbitt and colleagues.[314] Transplanted into the *Hyp* mouse, the normal mouse kidney acquires an impairment of $P_i$ reabsorption as severe as that occurring in the original *Hyp* mouse.[314] Transplanted into the normal mouse, the kidney of the *Hyp* mouse loses its impairment of $P_i$ reabsorption.[314] Thus, it would appear that the genetic defect in the *Hyp* mouse gives rise to a circulating humor that is produced in amounts sufficient to account for the impairment in renal $P_i$ reabsorption characteristic of the *Hyp* mouse. It has been suggested that the putative phosphaturic humor might be identical to, or closely related to, that produced by certain tumors that cause surgically correctable renal hypophosphatemic metabolic bone disease, so-called oncogenic hypophosphatemic rickets/osteomalacia (see later).[315]

## DISORDERED VITAMIN D METABOLISM

In patients with XLH, the net increased circulating concentrations of 1,25(OH)$_2$D$_3$ are in fact reduced,[280, 281, 316-318] given the strength of the hypophosphatemic stimulus for increasing production and circulating concentrations of this hormone.[230, 243, 244, 252, 253, 319] Indeed, the capacity of patients with XLH to increase the plasma concentration of 1,25(OH)$_2$D$_3$ in response to either phosphorus restriction[303] or intravenous administration of parathyroid extract[283] is reported to be impaired. The issue with respect to hormonal responsiveness to PTH in humans with XLH would seem, however, to be unsettled. Two groups of investigators[320, 321] have now reported that the increase in circulating 1,25(OH)$_2$D$_3$ induced by intravenous administration of the 1-34 fragment of PTH was as great in patients with XLH as in control subjects. In the *Hyp* mouse, the frankly decreased plasma concentration of 1,25(OH)$_2$D$_3$ also does not increase normally with phosphorus restriction; rather, it decreases further.[322] Conversely, in the *Hyp* mouse, a high-phosphate diet induces an increase in both the serum levels of 1,25(OH)$_2$D$_3$[323] and the activity of 1α-hydroxylase.[324] Yamaoka and colleagues[325, 326] have also reported evidence of a similar P$_i$-1,25(OH)$_2$D$_3$ metabolic regulatory derangement in patients with XLH. In addition, the activity of 1α-hydroxylase in the *Hyp* mouse does not increase normally in response to hypocalcemia,[327, 328] PTH administration,[329] parathyroid-related peptide,[330, 331] or dietary depletion of vitamin D.[328] In the *Hyp* mouse, the abnormally unresponsive plasma concentration of $1,25(OH)_2D_3$ would seem to contribute to its impaired capacity to normally increase TmP/GFR in response to hypophosphatemia.[304] Increasing doses of $1,25(OH)_2D_3$ have been reported to mitigate this impairment.[332]

In the *Hyp* mouse, Tenenhouse and co-workers[333, 334] have found that the renal metabolism of $1,25(OH)_2D_3$ is abnormal in a way that involves more than a reduced mitochondrial synthesis from $25(OH)D_3$. They reported that the mitochondrial metabolism of $1,25(OH)_2D_3$ by the C-24 oxidation pathway to calcitroic acid is significantly increased. They suggest that increased renal catabolism of $1,25(OH)_2D_3$ through this pathway may "contribute to the clinical phenotype," that is, reduced plasma concentrations of $1,25(OH)_2D_3$.[333] In the *Hyp* mouse, it has been reported that the plasma clearance rate of high doses of intravenously administered $[^3H]1,25(OH)_2D_3$ is increased.[335] In a child deemed to have XLH, the finding of increased activity of $25(OH)D_3$ $1\alpha$-hydroxylase, in combination with a normal serum concentration of $1,25(OH)_2D_3$,[336] accords with the possibility of an increased metabolic clearance rate of $1,25(OH)_2D_3$. There are, however, no reported studies of the metabolic clearance rate of $1,25(OH)_2D_3$ in humans with XLH. The normal kidney has not been demonstrated to be an important metabolic "sink" for circulating $1,25(OH)_2D_3$; nephrectomy has not been demonstrated to reduce the metabolic clearance rate of $1,25(OH)_2D_3$.

The stimulation of renal $1,25(OH)_2D_3$ production in response to calcitonin infusion is reported to be intact in the *Hyp* mouse.[337] In the *Hyp* mouse, the differential response of $1\alpha$-hydroxylase with respect to its response to PTH and calcitonin accords with the demonstration by Kawashima and co-workers of two anatomically distinct, independently regulated $1\alpha$-hydroxylase systems in mammalian kidney, a PTH-responsive activity in the proximal convoluted tubule[338] and a calcitonin-responsive activity in the proximal straight tubule,[339] but in neither patients with XLH nor the *Hyp* mouse is the precise mechanism known for the observed abnormal regulation of $1\alpha$-hydroxylase.

## PATHOGENESIS OF BONE DISORDER

In patients with XLH, hypophosphatemia is an important determinant of both the rate of somatic growth and the rate of bone mineralization, but hypophosphatemia is not the only determinant.[200, 306, 340] Although the serum concentration of $P_i$ has been found to vary directly with the severity of bone deformity,[273] and phosphate supplementation of affected humans and mice can cure rickets, it does not cure osteomalacia.[341, 342] In adults with XLH, the severity of osteomalacia has been found to vary inversely with the serum level of $1,25(OH)_2D_3$[273, 343, 344] but not with the serum concentration of $P_i$ or $Ca^{2+}$.[273] A primary osteoblastic defect may contribute importantly to the bone disease of patients with XLH[340, 345] and could account for the supraphysiologic doses of $1,25(OH)_2D_3$ required to heal the bone disease.[345] Whereas *Hyp* kidneys reabsorb $P_i$ to a normal extent when transplanted into normal mice,[314] *Hyp* bone cells do not produce normal bone when transplanted into normal mice.[346, 347] The fate of normal bone cells transplanted into the *Hyp* mouse appears not to have been determined. The

failure of $1,25(OH)_2D_3$ to increase in response to hypophosphatemia restricts the intestinal absorption of $Ca^{2+}$. The chronically reduced plasma ion product of extracellular $Ca^{2+}$ and $P_i$ is clearly important to the pathogenesis of any metabolic bone disease. It is far from clear, however, how the disturbances in phosphorus and $Ca^{2+}$ metabolism, the disturbance of vitamin D metabolism, and the apparent dysfunction of the osteoblast give rise to the bone disease characteristic of XLH. It seems entirely possible that in patients with XLH, a genetic defect of bone-associated cells entrains both a "primary," "metabolic" bone disorder and excessive production of the putative phosphaturic humor.

## TREATMENT

Currently, there is no entirely satisfactory treatment for patients with XLH, particularly for those children whose growth is stunted.[226, 348] Yet, in many of those affected, the characteristically impaired rate of somatic growth, leg bowing, and attendant metabolic bone disease can be mitigated by oral phosphate given in combination with $1,25(OH)_2D_3$, which can be instituted in the first months of life.[274, 349, 350] In adults, such combined therapy may reduce bone pain and the histomorphometric severity of osteomalacia.[350] Phosphorus is administered as a neutral phosphate salt (Neutra-Phos-K), in four or five divided doses throughout the day at a daily dosage of 1.25 to 1.5 g. For this therapy to be effective in children, it must be started in early childhood and continued. Despite meticulous attention to the details of such combined therapy by both the physician and the patient, and careful monitoring of the clinical and metabolic response to this therapy, severely stunted children may grow little,[348] osteomalacia will not be completely corrected,[351] and the complications of recurrent hypercalcemia, nephrocalcinosis, and persisting $P_i$-induced hyperparathyroidism may not be prevented. Indeed, seemingly logical, aggressive phosphate therapy may predispose to nephrocalcinosis and "tertiary" hyperparathyroidism.[349, 352, 353] The optimal daily dose of $1,25(OH)_2D_3$ remains to be determined. Rasmussen and Tenenhouse[226] recommended an initial daily dose of 0.5 to 0.75 $\mu g/d$ and a gradual increase that is intended to achieve maximal suppression of PTH secretion without inducing hypercalcemia or hypercalciuria. When therapy induces rapid bone healing and growth spurting, the dose of $1,25(OH)_2D_3$ needed will be greater; at other times, that needed will be considerably less. Drezner and colleagues[354] recommended that $1,25(OH)_2D_3$ and phosphate therapy be initiated at higher doses, 2 to 3 $\mu g/d$ and 1 to 2 $g/d$, respectively, until bone healing occurs and then moderated as hypercalcemia and hypercalciuria attend bone healing.

## Oncogenic Hypophosphatemic Osteomalacia

In this rare hypophosphatemic disorder, there occurs a metabolic bone disease attended by a metabolic myopathy (expressed as muscle weakness) that can be corrected by the removal of a characteristically mesenchymal tumor.[203, 213–219, 355–361] Those affected with oncogenic hypophosphatemic osteomalacia (OHO), like patients with XLH, have a low TmP/GFR, have normal serum levels of PTH and Ca$^{2+}$, and may benefit from therapy with phosphate and 1,25(OH)$_2$D$_3$.[359] In patients with OHO, the value of 1,25(OH)$_2$D$_3$ is consistently, absolutely low[359, 361–366] or low-normal.[367] In a few patients, the impaired renal reabsorption of P$_i$ is part of a more complex renal dysfunction that can include generalized aminoaciduria,[219, 361, 368] renal glucosuria,[216, 355–357, 361] and perhaps RTA[368] (i.e., features of the Fanconi syndrome). A circulating humor mediating OHO has yet to be isolated. In opossum renal epithelial cells, Cai and co-workers[367] reported inhibition of Na$^+$-dependent P$_i$ transport with medium conditioned by sclerosing hemangioma cells obtained from a woman with OHO in whom only the renal reabsorption of P$_i$ appeared to be impaired. The conditioned medium did not inhibit transport of glucose or alanine, and its inhibitory effect on P$_i$ transport could not be ascribed to PTH or PTH-related peptide.[367] In cultured renal cells, an extract from an osteomalacia-causing hemangiopericytoma inhibited 25(OH)D$_3$ 1α-hydroxylase activity.[369] These observations raise the possibility that excessive production of a single gene product, or of closely related gene products, accounts for the phosphaturic renal disorders of both XLH and OHO.[315] The likelihood of this possibility, however, would seem to be lessened by the fact that severe muscle weakness is characteristic of patients with OHO but not of patients with XLH, who characteristically have little or none.

## PSEUDOHYPOPARATHYROIDISM

Pseudohypoparathyroidism is a heterogeneous group of hereditary disorders characterized by end-organ unresponsiveness to PTH. Normally, PTH exerts its major actions in kidney and bone. In kidney, PTH enhances Ca$^{2+}$ reabsorption and P$_i$ excretion and causes 1α-hydroxylation of vitamin D; in bone, PTH promotes mobilization of Ca$^{2+}$. In addition to the hypocalcemia and hyperphosphatemia associated with hypoparathyroidism, pseudohypoparathyroidism causes a group of developmental defects, including skeletal system abnormalities, short stature, and mental retardation. Patients with the developmental abnormalities but without overt hypoparathyroidism are termed pseudohypoparathyroid. The disease was first recognized as a distinct clinical entity in 1942, when Albright and co-workers[370] described three patients who exhibited certain clinical features of hypoparathyroidism but did not respond to infusion of PTH with the expected P$_i$ diuresis and increase in serum Ca$^{2+}$ concentration. Thus, Albright argued that this new entity, which he termed pseudohypoparathyroidism, was due to tissue unresponsiveness to PTH. Tashjian and co-workers[371] later demonstrated that patients with pseudohypoparathyroidism actually have elevated levels of PTH.

The next major breakthrough in understanding the pathophysiologic process of pseudohypoparathyroidism came in 1967 with the report by Chase and Aurbach[372] that unlike normal subjects, patients with pseudohypoparathyroidism failed to increase urinary excretion of cAMP in response to PTH infusion.[373] The role of cAMP became clear in 1972 with the demonstration that the phosphaturic action of PTH

could be mimicked by infusion of dibutyryl cAMP in patients with pseudohypoparathyroidism.[374] By cAMP-dependent protein kinase, cAMP depresses P$_i$ transport in the proximal tubule[375] (see Chapter 11). Shortly later, it became clear that not all patients with pseudohypoparathyroidism have a defective cAMP response to PTH. Patients who fail to elevate urinary excretion of cAMP after PTH infusion are termed type I, whereas those with normal cAMP responses are termed type II.[376] Expression of the type I and II phenotypes has been reported to vary within a family.[377] Furthermore, the severity of the type I phenotype was reported to progress with development in a young child.[378] Thus, the type I and II phenotypes may not always be distinct.

### Type I Pseudohypoparathyroidism

Failure of PTH to elicit an increase in urinary cAMP excretion in type I pseudohypoparathyroidism could be due to 1) a defective PTH receptor, 2) defective coupling of the receptor to adenylate cyclase, 3) defective adenylate cyclase, or 4) excessive breakdown of cAMP once formed. Mechanism 4 was unlikely because phosphodiesterase inhibitors failed to correct the defect.[379, 380] Mechanisms 1 and 3 were ruled out by the studies of Marcus[381] and Drezner[380] and co-workers, which indicated that there was no defect in the PTH receptor or in adenylate cyclase activity in renal cortical plasma membranes from patients with type I pseudohypoparathyroidism. These findings suggested that there was a failure of coupling between receptor and adenylate cyclase in patients with type I disease.

Coupling of the PTH receptor to adenylate cyclase is brought about through interaction with G$_s$, a member of the now extensively studied family of heterotrimeric GTP-binding, or G, proteins.[382–384] These proteins are involved in numerous macromolecular interactions within the cell. G$_s$ (which stimulates adenylate cyclase activity) has three subunits: α, β, and γ. Under resting conditions, these three subunits are joined, and GDP is bound to the α-subunit. Binding of PTH to its receptor causes a conformational change in the receptor that is transmitted to the G protein, causing GDP to be released from the guanine nucleotide binding site on the α-subunit. GDP is then replaced with the more abundant GTP, and α dissociates from βγ. Dissociated G$_{sα}$ then interacts with and activates the adenylate cyclase. GTP on the α-subunit is slowly (seconds to minutes) hydrolyzed to GDP, and the proteins revert to their basal state until the receptor is again occupied by PTH.

Farfel[385, 386] and Levine[387] and colleagues examined the activation of adenylate cyclase in erythrocytes of patients with pseudohypoparathyroidism. Erythrocytes from half of the patients exhibited a 50% reduction in G$_s$ activity. Likewise, G$_s$ activity was also significantly reduced in platelets,[388] fibroblasts,[389] and transformed lymphoblasts[389] from affected individuals. These data strongly suggested that the defect in PTH coupling in some of the patients was due to an inborn genetic defect in G$_s$. These individuals were labeled type Ia, whereas those with apparently normal G protein function were labeled type Ib. More recent work has shown that in type Ia pseudohypoparathyroidism, messenger RNA levels for the different molecular weight forms of $G_{s\alpha}$ (derived from alternative splicing of the primary RNA transcript) are all proportionally reduced.[390] This suggests that the defect is in the promoter region of the gene for $G_{s\alpha}$.

Because $G_s$ is involved in the coupling of multiple hormones to adenylate cyclase, it is expected that patients with type Ia pseudohypoparathyroidism should be unresponsive to other hormones. This is, in fact, the case. More than 50% of patients with pseudohypoparathyroidism have clinically evident hypothyroidism due to thyroid gland unresponsiveness to thyrotropin.[391] Gonadotropin resistance is also common,[392] although male patients are often spared. Diminished responses to other hormones, including glucagon and isoproterenol, have been described,[393] but they are usually subclinical. Phenotypic expression of this disorder appears to be variable, even within a single family.[394–396] Olfactory function, which also depends on adenylate cyclase activity,[397] has been reported to be abnormal in patients with type Ia pseudohypoparathyroidism.[398] This is surprising in view of the fact that $G_{olf}$, a G protein involved in olfactory signal transduction, is distinct from $G_s$.[399] Not all hormones that act through adenylate cyclase are affected in type Ia pseudohypoparathyroidism. For example, the antidiuretic response to vasopressin appears to be normal in type Ia patients.[400]

Skeletal abnormalities, which are found only in type Ia pseudohypoparathyroidism, still have an incompletely defined biochemical basis. Although some patients have bone disease similar to that seen in hyperparathyroidism,[401–403] the bone disease usually has a distinctive appearance that has been termed Albright hereditary osteodystrophy.[404] It has been proposed, but never proved, that bone resistance to the actions of PTH is less marked than the renal resistance to PTH in pseudohypoparathyroidism.[403] Thus, the bone defect in type Ia disease may arise from the elevated levels of PTH, coupled with diminished serum $Ca^{2+}$ and $1,25(OH)_2D_3$ concentrations.[405, 406]

The molecular defect in pseudohypoparathyroidism type Ib has not been defined. This entity may actually be a heterogeneous group of disorders causing resistance to PTH.[407] The disease has been described in both familial[408, 409] and sporadic[410] forms. Both $G_s$ activity[411] and adenylate cyclase[389] are normal, and hormone resistance is limited to PTH.[411] Some work suggests that PTH-mediated $Ca^{2+}$ signaling is abnormal specifically in type Ib patients.[412] Of note, type Ib patients appear to have more complete resistance to the action of PTH in bone and therefore do not have the skeletal abnormalities seen in type Ia disease. These observations raise the possibility that type Ib patients may produce a defective form of PTH that blocks the receptor[413] or that the PTH receptor itself is abnormal. Another group of patients may have a defective adenylate cyclase catalytic subunit.[414]

## Type II Pseudohypoparathyroidism

Type II pseudohypoparathyroidism is characterized by depressed phosphaturic response to PTH but normal activity of $G_s$ and normal production of nephrogenous cAMP.[385]

Even basal values of nephrogenous cAMP are significantly higher in type II patients, compared with those of type I patients.[415] The defect, which remains poorly defined, may be heterogeneous[404] and is often acquired. In some instances, the entity resembles vitamin D deficiency, and the phosphaturic response to PTH can be restored by treatment with vitamin D.[416, 417] Calcium infusion alone may also restore the response to PTH,[418] which suggests that the $Ca^{2+}$ dependence of the PTH response may be abnormal. There is at least one report of familial pseudohypoparathyroidism type II.[416] Studies with cultured epithelial cells suggest that protein kinase C may play an important role in the regulation of $P_i$ transport by PTH[419–421]; this signaling system could be involved in type II pseudohypoparathyroidism.

### Treatment

The main goal of treatment of pseudohypoparathyroidism is to correct the serum $Ca^{2+}$ concentration and to prevent the progression of hyperparathyroid bone disease, if it is present. This can generally be accomplished by oral supplementation with $1,25(OH)_2D$. By increasing intestinal absorption of $Ca^{2+}$, vitamin D raises serum $Ca^{2+}$ concentration and suppresses PTH secretion. Unfortunately, this approach is often fraught with difficulty, and serum $Ca^{2+}$ levels must be measured frequently to prevent the development of hypercalcemia due to vitamin D intoxication. One patient whose PTH was not suppressed with vitamin D therapy was successfully treated with total parathyroidectomy and autotransplantation of a remnant parathyroid gland.[422] In view of the high frequency of hypothyroidism, thyroid function should be checked regularly and corrected if it is abnormal.

## RENAL TUBULAR ACIDOSIS

RTA is a nonuremic syndrome of disordered renal acidification; if sufficiently severe, it is characterized by hyperchloremic acidosis. Its major cause is either a reduced urinary excretion of $NH_4^+$ or increased urinary excretion of $HCO_3^-$. In its classic clinical expression, RTA is further characterized by an inappropriately high urine pH and a reduced excretion of titratable acid[423–443] (Figs. 37–2 and 37–3). The syndrome reflects a disorder of renal acidification that can cause acidosis with no or only moderate reduction in renal mass. RTA can reflect several physiologically distinct disorders of renal acidification (Tables 37–4 to 37–6). In a number of diseases, RTA occurs as a predictable physiologic subtype. In several inherited diseases, RTA is the major clinically expressed trait, and in some cases, it is the only one.

## Overview of Renal Acidification and Basis of Classification of Subtypes of Renal Tubular Acidosis and Their Precursors

In normal humans, under physiologic conditions, the process of renal acidification maintains plasma $HCO_3^-$ at

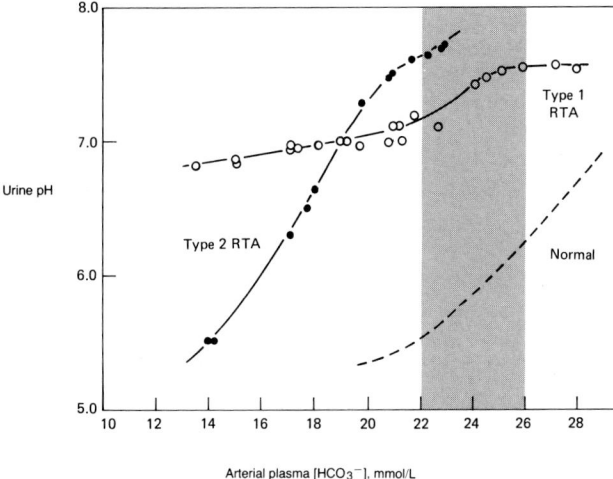

**Figure 37–2.** Relationship between urine pH and plasma $HCO_3^-$ concentration in patients with prototypic type I (classic) and type II (proximal) renal tubular acidosis (RTA). In patients with type II RTA, the urine pH may be inappropriately high or appropriately low, depending on the severity of systemic acidosis. (Shaded area represents range of normal plasma $HCO_3^-$ concentrations.)

normal concentrations by both reclaiming all filtered $HCO_3^-$ and effecting the excretion of an amount of acid that closely approximates the measured nonvolatile acid endogenously generated, approximately 1 mEq/kg of body weight per day in adults[581, 582] and 1 to 3 mEq/kg of body weight per day in infants and young children.[583] At normal plasma $HCO_3^-$ concentrations, under physiologic conditions, the proximal tubule secretes $H^+$ at a rate that reclaims 85% to 90% of filtered $HCO_3^-$,[584] a process that accounts for the great bulk of renal $H^+$ secretion. The capacity of the

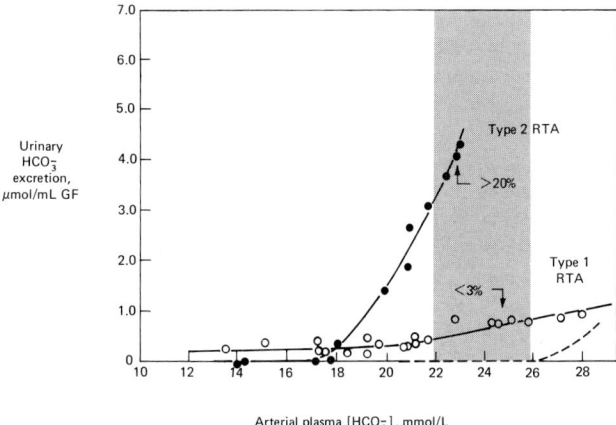

**Figure 37–3.** The relationship between urinary $HCO_3^-$ excretion and plasma $HCO_3^-$ concentration in patients with prototypic type I (classic) and type II (proximal) RTA. In patients with type I RTA, bicarbonaturia occurs during severe as well as mild degrees of acidosis, but in affected adult patients, the magnitude of bicarbonaturia is invariably small, predictably less than 5% of the filtered $HCO_3^-$ load. In patients with type II RTA, bicarbonaturia is absent during moderately severe acidosis but of large magnitude at normal plasma $HCO_3^-$ concentrations, often amounting to more than 15% of the filtered $HCO_3^-$ load. (Shaded area represents range of normal plasma $HCO_3^-$ concentrations.) (From Morris RC Jr, Sebastian A, McSherry E: Renal acidosis. Kidney Int 1:322–340, 1972.)

**TABLE 37–4. Clinical Spectrum of Type II (Proximal) Renal Tubular Acidosis**

**Associated with Multiple Dysfunction of Proximal Tubule (Fanconi Syndrome)**
Primary
    Genetically transmitted[444–448]
    Sporadic[449, 450]
Genetically transmitted systemic diseases
    Cystinosis[451]
    Lowe syndrome[452]
    Wilson disease[453, 454]
    Tyrosinemia[455]
    Hereditary fructose intolerance[432]
        (during fructose administration or ingestion)
    Mitochondrial phosphoenolpyruvate carboxykinase deficiency[456]
    Metachromatic leukodystrophy[457]
    Glycogen storage disorder[458, 459]
Disorders associated with chronic hypocalcemia and secondary hyperparathyroidism
    Vitamin D deficiency[436, 460–463]
    Vitamin D dependency[464]
Drug- or toxin-induced nephropathy
    Outdated tetracycline[465]
    3-Methylchromone[466]
    Streptozocin[467]
    Lead[468]
Other renal diseases
    Amyloidosis[469]
    Nephrotic syndrome[469–471]
    Renal transplantation[472]
    Sjögren syndrome[431]
    Medullary cystic disease[473]
    Paroxysmal nocturnal hemoglobinuria[474]
    Renal vein thrombosis[475]
Monoclonal light chain nephropathy[476–481]

**Unassociated with Multiple Dysfunction of Proximal Tuble**
Primary
    Sporadic
        Transient[482]
        Persisting[483]
    Genetically transmitted[484]
Pyruvate carboxylase deficiency[485, 486]
Glycogen storage disease, type I
Osteopetrosis[487]/carbonic anhydrase II deficiency[488, 489]
Carbonic anhydrase deficiency
    Acetazolamide[490, 491]
    Sulfanilamide[492]
York-Yendt syndrome[493]
Cyanotic congenital heart disease[494]

distal nephron to secrete $H^+$ is relatively small, but its capacity to generate a large gradient (lumen-peritubular)[585–587] enables the kidney to reduce urine pH to normal minimums (<5.3), reclaim all remaining filtered $HCO_3^-$, further titrate the major urinary buffers $NH_3$ and $Na_2HPO_4$ to $NH_4^+$ and $NaH_2PO_4$, and thereby excrete $NH_4^+$ and titratable acid at physiologic rates. $H^+$ excreted as $NaH_2PO_4$ accounts for most of so-called titratable acid. The combined excretion rates of $NH_4^+$ and titratable acid minus the normally negligible excretion rate of $HCO_3^-$ is termed "net acid excretion."[426] Net acid excretion normally accounts for no more than 3% of renal $H^+$ secretion at normal plasma $HCO_3^-$ concentrations. When the rate of excretion of $HCO_3^-$ exceeds that of the sum of titratable acid and $NH_4^+$, "net base excretion" is said to occur.

The proximal tubule generates all $NH_4^+$ excreted in the

**TABLE 37–5. Clinical Spectrum of Type I Renal Tubular Acidosis (Classic, Distal)**

Primary
    Hereditary[495–507]
    Sporadic[423–428, 432, 435, 436, 495, 508]

Genetically transmitted systemic diseases
    Ehlers-Danlos syndrome[509]
    Hereditary elliptocytosis[510]
    Sickle cell anemia[511, 512]
    Marfan syndrome[513]
    Inactive erythrocyte carbonic anhydrase B syndrome[514, 515]
    Carbonic anhydrase II deficiency syndrome with osteopetrosis, type I carnitine palmitoyltransferase deficiency[516]
    Sensorineural deafness[516–520]

Autoimmune disorders[521–537]
    Dysgammaglobulinemia
        Hyperglobulinemia purpura[521]
        Cryoglobulinemia[522]
    Sjögren syndrome[526–528, 532]
    Chronic active hepatitis[523, 533, 534]
    Primary biliary cirrhosis[534–536]
    Thyroiditis[530, 538]
    Fibrosing alveolitis[531]
    Polyarteritis nodosa[539]
    Disorders causing nephrocalcinosis
    Hypercalciuria
        Hereditary[506, 507]
        Sporadic[540, 541]
    Primary hyperparathyroidism[542, 543]
    Hyperthyroidism[544]
    Vitamin D intoxication[545]
    Medullary sponge kidney[546, 547]
    Hereditary fructose intolerance after long-term fructose ingestion[548]
    Wilson disease[549]
    Fabry disease[550]

Drug- or toxin-induced nephropathy
    Mercury[551]
    Amphotericin B[552, 553]
    Analgesics[554, 555]
    Lithium[556]
    Cyclamate[557]
    Toluene[558–560]
    Amiloride

Other renal diseases
    Pyelonephritis[561]
    Obstructive uropathy[562–565]
    Renal transplantation[566, 567]
    Leprosy[568]
    Hepatic cirrhosis[569–571]

Tubulointerstitial disease
    Balkan nephropathy[572]
    Chronic pyelonephritis[561]
    Obstructive uropathy[562–564, 573–575]
    Renal transplantation[472, 566, 567, 576–579]
    Jejunoileal bypass with hyperoxaluria[580]

urine. $NH_4^+$ is secreted into the proximal tubule,[588–590] apparently in exchange for luminal $Na^+$,[591–593] actively reabsorbed by the medullary thick ascending limb, and concentrated, along with ammonia, in the medullary interstitium by countercurrent multiplication.[594, 595] From the medullary interstitium, ammonia diffuses into the medullary collecting duct, which protonates it to $NH_4^+$ and thereby creates both a sink for its diffusion and a species, $NH_4^+$, so sparingly

diffusible that its excretion is compelled.[588, 596] The urinary excretion of $NH_4^+$ increases greatly in response to prolonged metabolic acidosis and reflects the major renal mechanism that moderates acidosis.[597] Acidosis induces the proximal tubule to generate and secrete increased amounts of $NH_4^+$ that are delivered to, and reabsorbed by, the thick ascending limb and concentrated in the medullary interstitium, along with increased amounts of ammonia.[595] Acidosis also augments the medullary collecting duct's secretion of $H^+$[598] and, hence, its protonation of ammonia to $NH_4^+$, thereby increasing the diffusion of ammonia from the medullary interstitium into the medullary collecting duct and, thus, the excretion of $NH_4^+$.[598] The increase in urinary excretion of $NH_4^+$ during acidosis reflects the proximal tubule's increased metabolic generation not only of $NH_4^+$ but also of $HCO_3^-$, which enters the systemic circulation and directly replenishes the plasma concentration of $HCO_3^-$ reduced by acidosis. In the mitochondria of the proximal tubule, glutamine extracted from the circulation is hydrolyzed to $NH_4^+$ and glutamate, which in turn is hydrolyzed to $NH_4^+$ and $\alpha$-ketoglutarate, the renal metabolism of a mole of which yields 2 mol of $HCO_3^-$.[599–602] In the normal renal response to metabolic acidosis, the increased $NH_4^+$ generated in the proximal tubule is entirely directed into the lumen of the proximal tubule and excreted.[596] That partitioning of the increased $NH_4^+$ generated is critical to the normal renal response to acidosis. Were any of the increased $NH_4^+$ generated delivered to the systemic circulation, it would consume $HCO_3^-$ when converted to urea and thus compromise the capacity of the kidney to moderate acidosis.[603]

Accordingly, RTA can give rise to metabolic acidosis in either of two general ways: 1) impaired reclamation of filtered $HCO_3^-$—"proximal" RTA; or 2) impaired excretion of $NH_4^+$ and titratable acid, and hence impaired generation of sufficient "new" $HCO_3^-$ to offset the normal amounts of nonvolatile acid endogenously produced—"distal" RTA. Impaired reclamation of $HCO_3^-$ in the proximal tubule, particularly when acutely induced, can so swamp the distal nephron with $HCO_3^-$ that excretion of $NH_4^+$ and titratable acid is severely reduced or absent. With such swamping, $NH_4^+$ may be shunted to the renal vein and systemic circulation.

Carlisle and colleagues[604, 605] and other investigators have rightly emphasized that reduced urinary excretion of $NH_4^+$ is a defining characteristic of all subtypes of fully expressed distal RTA and in most subtypes the major pathophysiologic determinant of acidosis. In proximal RTA, $NH_4^+$ is also usually reduced although not the major cause of acidosis. Thus, the finding of a normal or near-normal urinary excretion of $NH_4^+$ permits one to exclude distal RTA as a major cause of hyperchloremic acidosis and to deem as unlikely proximal RTA.[604–606] This finding, however, does not permit one to exclude a renal tubule disorder that can or might evolve into acidosis-causing distal RTA. Because that evolution might be susceptible to therapeutic interdiction, and because it is important to identify and treat acidosis-causing RTA as early in life as possible, it is important to identify precursors of acidosis-causing RTA.

Wrong and Davies[428] identified the first such nonacidotic precursor, "the incomplete syndrome of RTA,"[428] which is characterized by a brisk $NH_4^+$ excretion but a urine pH that

**TABLE 37–6. Hereditary Autosomally Transmitted Disorders of the Renal Tubule Expressed as Type I Renal Tubular Acidosis and Nephrocalcinosis***

| Syndrome | Acidification Defect (AD) | | | Nephrocalcinosis (N) | | Acidosis | | Hypercalciuria | | Hypocitraturia | |
|---|---|---|---|---|---|---|---|---|---|---|---|
| | Occurs in Children | Causes Acidosis in Children | Causes Acidosis with GFR >50 mL/min | Occurs in Children | Occurs Without AD | Occurs Without N | Attends N Invariably | Occurs Without Acidosis | Corrects with Alkali | Occurs | Corrects with Alkali |
| *Dominant* | | | | | | | | | | | |
| Primary RTA-I | | | | | | | | | | | |
| San Francisco[495-498] | + | + | + | + | 0 | + | + | 0 | + | + | + |
| Philadelphia[430, 505] | + | + | + | + | 0 | 0 | + | 0 | + | + | + and 0 |
| Hypercalciuric | | | | | | | | | | | |
| Atlanta[506] | + | 0 | 0 | + | + | 0 | 0 | + | – | 0 | – |
| Oklahoma City[507] | 0 | 0 | + | 0 | 0 | + | 0 | + | – | – | – |
| *Recessive, associated with* | | | | | | | | | | | |
| Sensorineural deafness[518-520] | + | + | + | + | 0 | + | + | – | – | – | – |
| Deficiency of B isoenzyme of carbonic anhydrase in erythrocytes[514, 515] | + | + | + | + | 0 | – | – | – | – | – | – |

*\* + = yes; − = unreported; 0 = nonoccurrence.*

is inappropriately high during $NH_4Cl$ loading.[428, 607, 608] Although not always a precursor, such incomplete RTA is an initial expression of a genetically transmitted renal disorder that is destined to cause acidosis by impairing distal $H^+$ and $NH_4^+$ excretion. But that impairment, although seemingly predictable, would seem only secondary, occurring only when medullary nephrocalcinosis supervenes and the distal nephron is damaged and the medullary interstitium disarrayed[505, 608, 609] (see later). Before that supervention, distal nephron $H^+$ secretion would seem to be largely intact: The capacity of the distal tubule to generate a normally steep $H^+$ gradient is indicated by a decrease in urine pH to values less than 5 during high urine flow,[609] and its capacity to secrete $H^+$ at a high rate is suggested by a robust increase in urine $PCO_2$ during $NaHCO_3$ loading.[608] In the normal rat, and presumably in the normal human, the increase in urine $PCO_2$ under this condition reflects, and varies directly with, $H^+$ secretion in the distal nephron.[610] According to DuBose and colleagues,[596] "If the urine $PCO_2$ minus the blood $PCO_2$ is below 25 mm Hg (after bicarbonate loading) and the plasma potassium is normal, a specific defect in the distal nephron $H^+$ pump is present." Halperin and colleagues[611, 612] and Sabatini and Kurtzman[443] and others have drawn a similar inference from their observations of this phenomenon in adult patients with acidosis-causing classic distal RTA.

However, distal $H^+$ secretion so inferred in the human during acute metabolic alkalosis may not reflect that distal $H^+$ secretory process that mediates increased excretion of $NH_4^+$ (and titratable acid) during sustained acidosis[606] and clearly cannot be the "gold standard" for diagnosing the renal basis of clinical hyperchloremic acidosis.[606] A reduced urine $PCO_2$ may not reflect only a decrease in distal $H^+$ secretion[606, 608, 613] (see later). Nevertheless, as proposed by Batlle and colleagues,[614] a reduction in so-inferred distal $H^+$ secretion during $HCO_3^-$ loading may permit the early identification of a subtle impairment that can evolve into a

defect that causes acidosis, and such an impairment might not otherwise be identified. Although such an evolution has not yet been documented in either a genetically transmitted or acquired renal tubule disorder, the possibility of such an evolution has not been widely investigated. The interpretation of the magnitude of increase in urine $PCO_2$ (after $HCO_3^-$ loading) as an index of distal $H^+$ secretion is an issue of active consideration and some controversy (see later), particularly in the clinical circumstance.[606, 608, 613] It seems clear, however, that under certain circumstances, the measurement of urine $PCO_2$ during $HCO_3^-$ loading provides a useful index of distal $H^+$ secretion.[596] A reduced value may yet characterize a second incomplete syndrome of RTA.[596, 614]

In addition to acidosis, RTA can cause clinically important hypokalemia and hyperkalemia, which can in turn further perturb the renal acidification process. Hyperkalemia in particular reduces the excretion of $NH_4^+$, in part by impairing its reabsorption in the medullary thick ascending limb.[594, 596] Characterization of the physiologic subtypes of RTA includes then not only that of the acidification defect but also that of the predictably associated disorders of the renal handling of $K^+$, particularly those causing hyperkalemia.

The RTAs can be classified according to the deranged nephron site and physiologic function. A disorder in resorption of filtered $HCO_3^-$ is called proximal (type II) RTA. A disorder causing acidosis because of impaired net acid excretion ($HCO_3^-$ regeneration) is called distal RTA. If impaired distal nephron secretion of $H^+$ causes acidosis without causing hyperkalemia, the disorder is called type I RTA. If impaired distal nephron secretion of both $K^+$ and $H^+$ causes hyperkalemia as well as acidosis, the disorder is called (type IV) RTA. There is no type III RTA; the term was once applied to type I RTA of infants and children whose excretion of large amounts of $HCO_3^-$ is the major determinant of their alkali requirement.

# Type II Renal Tubular Acidosis (Proximal)

## PHYSIOLOGIC CHARACTERISTICS

In patients with prototypic type II RTA (RTA-II), the identifying observation that the fractional excretion of $HCO_3^-$ is 15% or greater at normal plasma $HCO_3^-$ concentrations and under normal physiologic conditions implicates the acidification process of the proximal tubule[432, 434, 442] (Fig. 37–4; see Table 37–4 and Figs. 37–2 and 37–3). In prototypic RTA-II, the urine pH is inappropriately high, and bicarbonaturia occurs only during moderate or mild degrees of acidosis; the magnitude of bicarbonaturia varies directly with the plasma $HCO_3^-$ concentration[431, 433, 434] (see Figs. 37–3 and 37–4). During more severe degrees of acidosis, bicarbonaturia disappears, urine pH decreases to normal minima, and acid excretion is not reduced; this suggests that the acidification process of the distal nephron is intact[431, 433, 442] (see Figs. 37–3 and 37–4). With rare exception, RTA-II occurs as part of a Fanconi syndrome (see later) expressed as increased renal clearance of glucose, $P_i$, amino acids, and often uric acid at normal or reduced plasma concentrations of these solutes. When RTA-II is either prototypic or part of this complex dysfunction, the capacity of the proximal tubule to secrete $NH_4^+$ into its lumen and generate $HCO_3^-$ from glutamine for systemic export may well be impaired, as it is in acute experimental models of prototypic RTA-II (acetazolamide)[615] and in RTA-II combined with the Fanconi syndrome (RTA-II/FS) in animals.[616, 617] Renal vein $NH_4^+$ shunting has been demonstrated in these models. The acute massive bicarbonaturia in these models would be expected to impair the normal renal partitioning of $NH_4^+$.[603] Another characteristic of RTA-II/FS that is potentially pathogenetic of acidosis is increased urinary excretion of citrate[618, 619]; that excretion constitutes a systemic loss of base because retained citrate is normally metabolized to $HCO_3^-$.[620–622]

## CELLULAR AND PATHOGENETIC MECHANISMS

In the proximal tubule, most $H^+$ secretion is coupled to $Na^+$ reabsorption at the luminal cell membrane and is mediated by an electroneutral $Na^+/H^+$ antiporter that is driven

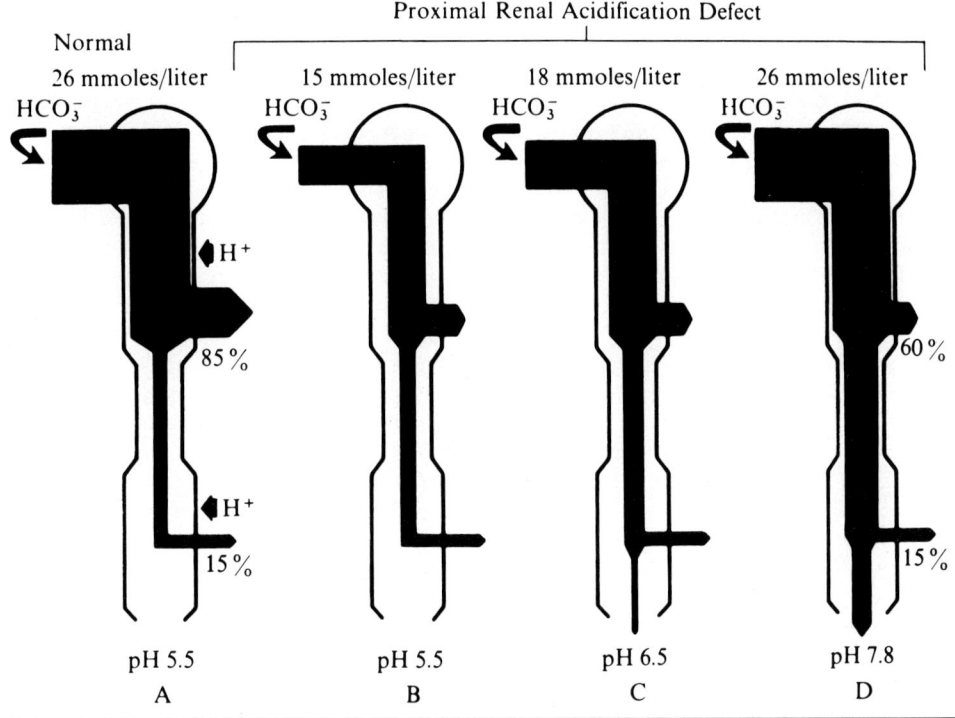

**Figure 37–4.** Schematic representation of the proximal renal acidification defect in type II RTA. Effect of changes in plasma $HCO_3^-$ concentration on delivery of $HCO_3^-$ to the distal nephron and, as a consequence, on urine pH and excretion of $HCO_3^-$ *A.* In normal subjects, at normal plasma $HCO_3^-$ concentrations, approximately 15% of the filtered $HCO_3^-$ load escapes reabsorption in the proximal tubule and is reabsorbed in the distal nephron; urinary $HCO_3^-$ excretion is nil, urine pH is appropriately low, and net acid excretion is normal. *B.* In patients with type II RTA, $HCO_3^-$ excretion may also be nil, urine pH may be appropriately low, and net acid excretion may not be reduced at reduced plasma $HCO_3^-$ concentration (metabolic acidosis). This is because the amount of $HCO_3^-$ escaping reabsorption proximally and delivered to the distal nephron is not supernormal when the amount of $HCO_3^-$ presented to the proximal tubule for reabsorption is sufficiently reduced. *C.* When, however, metabolic acidosis is somewhat mitigated (by administration of $NaHCO_3$), supernormal amounts of $HCO_3^-$ are delivered out of the proximal tubule because the defective proximal tubule cannot reabsorb the modest increase in filtered load of $HCO_3^-$. As a consequence, some $HCO_3^-$ escapes reabsorption in the distal nephron, urine pH becomes inappropriately high, and net acid excretion becomes reduced. *D.* If the plasma $HCO_3^-$ concentration and filtered $HCO_3^-$ load are increased to normal levels, the amount of $HCO_3^-$ escaping reabsorption proximally greatly exceeds the reabsorptive capacity of the normal distal nephron, and massive bicarbonaturia occurs. In the illustration of type II RTA, renal tubule reabsorption of $HCO_3^-$ at normal plasma $HCO_3^-$ concentration (26 mmol/L) is reduced by 25%. (*A to D* from Morris RC Jr, Sebastian A, McSherry E: Renal acidosis. Kidney Int 1:322–340, 1972.)

by the lumen-to-cell Na$^+$ concentration gradient.[623–628] The requisite low cell concentration of Na$^+$ is maintained by the activity of basolateral Na$^+$,K$^+$-ATPase. In the lumen, H$_2$CO$_3$ formed by the combination of secreted H$^+$ and filtered HCO$_3^-$ is catalytically dehydrated by the isoenzyme of carbonic anhydrase located at the luminal membrane (IV).[629] The catalysis facilitates H$^+$ secretion by reducing the steady-state concentration of luminal H$_2$CO$_3$ and hence luminal H$^+$. The intracellular isoenzyme of carbonic anhydrase (II)[630, 631] catalyzes the combination of OH$^-$ (derived from water) with CO$_2$ that has diffused from the lumen and thereby generates both HCO$_3^-$ that is reabsorbed into the peritubular blood and H$^+$ that is recycled (i.e., secreted). Some one third of the H$^+$ secreted in the proximal tubule is mediated by electrogenic secretion that is effected by a vacuolar H$^+$-ATPase located at the luminal plasma membrane.[626, 627, 632]

As depicted in Figure 37–5, impaired proximal HCO$_3^-$ reabsorption might result from a selective disorder of the acidification process affecting the apical Na$^+$/H$^+$ antiporter, which mediates the secretion of H$^+$ and probably that of NH$_4^+$ (labeled 1)[591, 592, 633]; the apical vacuolar H$^+$-ATPase, which also mediates the secretion of H$^+$ (labeled 2)[626, 627, 632]; the Na$^+$/HCO$_3^-$ symporter, which mediates HCO$_3^-$ exit from the proximal tubule cell (labeled 3)[634–636]; and the carbonic anhydrases (labeled 4 and 5).[629, 630, 637] An abnormality in the mechanism by which intracellular Na$^+$ concentration is maintained at a normally low level would dictate a diminished reabsorption of all solutes that depend on Na$^+$-coupled transport (including not only most of HCO$_3^-$ but also glucose, amino acids, P$_i$, and uric acid) and hence the expression of RTA-II/FS. Such a global abnormality might result from several mechanisms: a large increase in cell Na$^+$ permeability (labeled 6); diminished activity of the Na$^+$,K$^+$-ATPase pump itself (labeled 7);

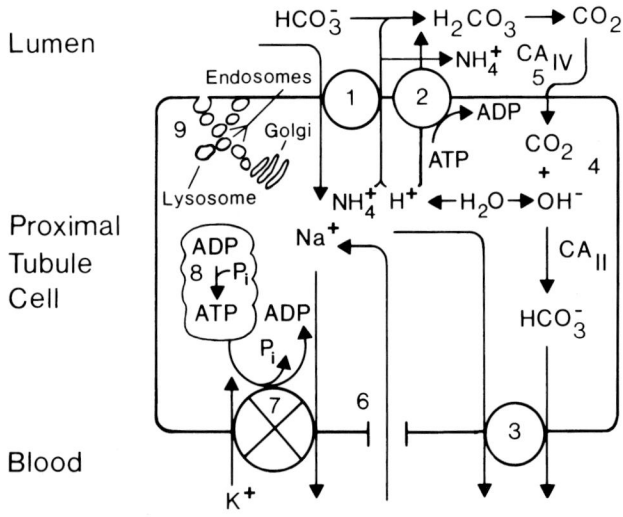

**Figure 37–5.** Potential cellular mechanisms of proximal (type II) RTA. The possible causes of impaired proximal acidification include defects in the luminal Na$^+$/H$^+$ antiporter, which may also impair NH$_4^+$ secretion (1); H$^+$-ATPase (2); the basolateral Na$^+$/HCO$_3^-$ symporter (3); the intracellular (4) or luminal (5) carbonic anhydrases (CA); Na$^+$ permeability (6); Na$^+$,K$^+$-ATPase (7); the intracellular generation of ATP (8); or membrane recycling, metabolism, or trafficking (9).

diminished availability of P$_i$ for mitochondrial metabolic generation of ATP needed to energize the pump (labeled 8)[638]; impaired membrane recycling, vacuolar transport, or trafficking (labeled 9)[639]; and loss of epithelial mass. The source of ATP needed to energize apical H$^+$-ATPase is unknown.

## ACUTE RTA-II/FS

### Hereditary Fructose Intolerance

The renal tubule disorder reversibly induced by either ingestion or intravenous administration of fructose in patients with hereditary fructose intolerance (HFI)[432, 640–646] can be a clinical cause of both acute and chronic RTA-II/FS[642, 643, 646, 647] and, uniquely, an acute, highly controllable experimental model of RTA-II/FS in humans.[432, 644–646] In both instances, the pathogenesis of RTA-II/FS is presumed to depend on an incapacity of the proximal tubule to generate the energy required to drive its Na$^+$-coupled resorptive transport processes. Aldolase B, the genetically defective enzyme in HFI,[648, 649] is a cytoplasmic enzyme that catalyzes the cleavage of fructose 1-phosphate and normally occurs only in the liver,[650, 651] small bowel,[652] and proximal renal tubule.[653–657] When patients with HFI are acutely exposed to fructose, their enzymatic defect[650, 651] dictates in the cells of these tissues a nearly immediate sequence of pathogenetic events: accumulation of fructose 1-phosphate → depletion of P$_i$ → depletion of ATP.[651, 658–661] In these tissues, the acute P$_i$ depletion both triggers a massive degradation of preformed total adenine nucleotides (ATP, ADP, and AMP), by activating cytoplasmic AMP deaminase,[658, 662, 663] and restricts the rate at which mitochondria can regenerate ATP.[663, 664] In the fructose-loaded rat, prior P$_i$ loading largely prevents the otherwise striking reduction of ATP and total adenine nucleotides in the renal cortex despite doubling its concentration of fructose 1-phosphate.[663]

In patients with HFI given fructose acutely, P$_i$ loading initiated shortly beforehand attenuates the severity of the RTA-II/FS[665] as well as that of the attendant hyperuricemia[665] and hyperinosinuria,[665] phenomena entrained by the P$_i$ depletion–dependent breakdown of preformed adenine nucleotides.[658, 659, 666] In a woman with HFI to whom fructose was administered intravenously for two 1-hour periods that were interrupted by a period of 100 minutes, P$_i$ loading initiated before the second period prevented the occurrence of RTA-II/FS.[665] Accordingly, and because fructose-induced depletion of hepatic adenine nucleotides in humans persists for at least 2 hours,[667] it seems likely that P$_i$ loading attenuated the renal tubule dysfunction despite continued, severely reduced concentrations of ATP and total ammonia nitrogen in the proximal renal tubule, possibly by enhancing this tissue's mitochondrial respiration and rate of regeneration of ATP.

For some time, the notion of phosphorylation potential and its determining ratio, log(ATP)/(ADP)(P$_i$), has been invoked to explain how disturbances of mitochondrial respiration and cytoplasmic concentrations of P$_i$, ATP, and ADP might be linked to disordered physiologic functions[668, 669] (e.g., maintaining a normally low intracellular concentration of $Na^+$). Employing nuclear magnetic resonance spectroscopy in studies of somatic muscle subjected to gradual ischemia, Blum and associates[670] found that "the sodium ion signal begins to increase at a certain point of energy depletion, marked not by exhaustion of high-energy phosphogens but by the fall to critical levels of the phosphorylation ratio, which more accurately measures the energy available to run the cellular machinery." Although the concentrations of "mobile" $P_i$ and ADP "seen" by nuclear magnetic resonance in both the liver[671] and the kidney[672] are much lower than those measured by chemical or enzymatic analysis, and uncertainties remain as to the cytoplasmic/mitochondrial apportionment of $P_i$, ATP, and ADP, employment of nuclear magnetic resonance to determine the phosphorylation ratio has proved fruitful in relating $Na^+$ transport in the kidney to renal energetics.[673] It is clear, however, that even a large reduction in the renal tissue concentration of ATP, specifically a reduction that is not caused by impaired mitochondrial respiration, is not necessarily attended by a discernible disorder in physiologic function.

## Experimental Model Induced by Maleic Acid

The experimental model of RTA-II/FS acutely induced by fructose in patients with HFI has striking parallels with the experimental model of RTA-II/FS acutely induced by parenterally administered maleic acid within minutes of initiation in the dog and rat.[674-683] On the basis of microperfusion and stop-flow studies in the rat, Bergeron and co-workers[682, 683] postulated that maleic acid induces in both proximal and distal tubules a "modification of cell membrane permeability" that gives rise to an increased luminal influx (cellular efflux) of normally reabsorbed solutes, and that only the proposed "modification" in the distal nephron gives rise to the hyperexcretion of these solutes. From clearance studies carried out during water diureses in the dog, however, Al-Bander and colleagues[683a] concluded that maleic acid induced the proximal tubule to reject greatly increased amounts of $HCO_3^-$ (and $Na^+$ and $Cl^-$) that accounted for the maleate-induced bicarbonaturia of RTA-II. In microperfusion studies of the proximal tubule in rats given maleate, Bank and associates[684] observed that both $HCO_3^-$ and NaCl were reabsorbed at reduced rates and that perfusion with an $HCO_3^-$-free solution did not increase the rate at which $HCO_3^-$ entered the lumen. Employing split droplet microperfusion of the proximal tubule, Reboucas and co-workers[685] made similar observations in rats given maleate and further determined that the rate of alkalinization of an acid perfusion solution was reduced, a finding not consistent with back-diffusion of luminal $H^+$. Both groups of investigators concluded that the maleate-induced acute reduction of net reabsorption of $HCO_3^-$ in the proximal tubule did not result from back-flux of $HCO_3^-$ through an abnormally leaky membrane but rather resulted from impaired active reabsorption of $HCO_3^-$ (i.e., impaired $H^+$ secretion).

In microperfusion studies of maleic acid–induced aminoaciduria, Gunther and co-workers[686] concluded that maleic acid inhibits the saturable reabsorption of amino acids along the proximal tubule; they showed that maleic acid does not induce a greater efflux of amino acid into the lumen at distal sites of the nephron. In brush border membrane vesicles, maleate does not affect $Na^+$-coupled transport of either glucose or amino acids.[687, 688]

Although not occurring in nature, maleic acid is the cis isomer of fumaric acid and, like that naturally occurring metabolite of the Krebs oxidative cycle, is readily metabolized by renal cortical mitochondria.[681, 689] At doses that induce RTA-II/FS, maleic acid induces in the proximal renal tubule striking structural abnormalities in the mitochondria,[677, 690, 691] an impairment in their oxidative metabolism,[678, 681, 692] and a reduced renal cortical concentration of ATP[676, 677, 693] and activity of $Na^+,K^+$-ATPase.[676] Presumably in part by impairing mitochondrial oxidation, maleic acid also induces in the renal cortex greatly increased rates of glucose uptake and glycolysis and increased concentrations of phosphorylated glycolytic intermediates.[679] That the increase in glycolysis induced by maleic acid might participate in the pathogenesis of its nephrotoxic effects is suggested by one of Berliner's[674] original observations. Whereas maleic acid administered alone induced only transient renal dysfunction, it induced persisting renal failure when administered in combination with previously initiated glucose loading.[674] The metabolic pathogenesis of RTA-II/FS acutely induced by maleic acid might then involve this pathogenetic sequence in cells of the proximal renal tubule: impaired mitochondrial oxidation → increased glucose uptake → increased glycolysis → increased production of lactic acid.[694] Consistent with this hypothesis and its possible relevance to the pathogenetic mechanism of chronic clinical RTA-II/FS is the observation by Jonas and colleagues[695] that urinary excretion of lactic acid and D-glyceraldehyde is greatly increased in patients with chronic RTA-II/FS in whom the plasma concentration of lactate or D-glyceraldehyde is not increased. The phenomenon was observed in a group of 16 patients affected with RTA-II/FS, most of whom had cystinosis; others had cytochrome c oxidase deficiency, tyrosinosis, glycogenesis, or Lowe syndrome; in one, the disorder was judged to be idiopathic. Hyperlacticaciduria without hyperlacticacidemia in combination with "tubule" proteinuria occurs in the RTA-II/FS acutely induced by fructose in patients with HFI[645] and as the earliest finding in young children affected with an autosomal dominant renal disorder that is expressed in early adulthood as RTA-II/FS[448] and sometime later as severe renal insufficiency as well. In those described with this disorder, the severity of aminoaciduria and hyperlacticaciduria has increased with age.

## Pathogenetic Implications of Lysozymuria and Lysosomal Enzymuria

Whether occurring as part of an acute experimental disorder or as a chronic clinical disorder, RTA-II/FS is attended by a reduction in renal tubule reabsorption of lysozyme and other low-molecular-weight proteins readily filtered by the normal glomerulus.[696-701] Normally, these low-molecular-weight proteins are almost completely reabsorbed in the proximal renal tubule by absorptive endocytosis of some selectivity.[702-704] Given the extensive system of clathrin-coated pits located at the base of the microvilli in the proximal tubule,[705] and the active participation of clathrin in the process of receptor-mediated endocytosis,[706–708] it seems likely that at least some of the selective reabsorption of low-molecular-weight proteins represents a form of receptor-mediated endocytosis.[703, 708, 709] The reabsorbed low-molecular-weight proteins, which also include $\beta_2$-microglobulin,[710] insulin,[711] immunoglobulin L chain,[697] and ribonuclease,[712] first attach to the luminal membrane, presumably in coated pits; are then internalized in apical endocytic vesicles; and thereafter are successively conveyed through "early" endosomes,[703] through "late" endosomes termed prelysosomal compartments,[713] and finally to lysosomes, where they are enzymatically degraded.[703] In the experimental model of RTA-II/FS induced acutely in the rat given maleic acid, Christensen and Maunsbach[690] reported the direct histochemical demonstration of impaired renal tubule uptake and vacuolar transport of lysozyme to lysosomes, an impairment that occurred restrictively in the proximal tubule and within 20 minutes of administration of maleic acid.[690]

Also observed whenever sought in either experimental or clinical RTA-II/FS is the phenomenon of increased urinary excretion of lysosomal enzymes, such as N-acetyl-$\beta$-glucosaminidase.[714, 715] Although too large to be filtered by the normal glomerulus, these proteins normally occur in the renal tubule, predominantly segregated in lysosomes of the proximal tubule,[716, 717] in whose cells they are synthesized in the endoplasmic reticulum.[713, 718] An increased urinary excretion of N-acetyl-$\beta$-glucosaminidase and other lysosomal enzymes is generally inferred to reflect "damage" or "injury" to the proximal tubule[719, 720] and simple leakage of lysosomal enzymes from its damaged lysosomes.

However, hyperexcretion of lysosomal enzymes can reflect much more complex mechanisms.[718, 721, 722] Because the process of endocytosis is dynamically coupled to that of exocytosis,[639, 704, 723–728] the combined hyperexcretion of lysozyme and lysosomal enzymes in RTA-II/FS could reflect a complex proximal tubule disorder of vacuolar transport affecting both endocytosis and exocytosis. In accordance with this hypothesis, Al-Bander and co-workers[729] observed in the dog that minutes after the onset of maleate-induced RTA-II/FS, the urinary excretion of lysosomal enzymes N-acetyl-$\beta$-glucosaminidase, $\beta$-glucuronidase, and $\beta$-galactosidase increased simultaneously with the anticipated increase in renal clearance of lysozyme. The severities of all these enzymurias increased rapidly and in parallel, all reaching a peak some 80 to 100 minutes after onset, then decreasing rapidly and in parallel. Sodium phosphate loading strikingly attenuated, and glucose loading exacerbated, the severities of both the RTA-II/FS and the hyperexcretion of lysozyme and lysosomal enzymes.[473, 694, 729, 730] These observations suggest that in the RTA-II/FS induced by maleic acid in the dog, a $P_i$-dependent disorder of carbohydrate metabolism in the cells of the proximal renal tubule underlies its dysfunction both of transepithelial transport of solute and processing of protein.[729] In the RTA-II/FS acutely induced by intravenous administration of fructose to patients with HFI, an acute, rapidly reversible hyperexcretion of lysozyme and lysosomal enzyme also occurs (see later).[473, 714]

The processes of endocytosis and exocytosis are coupled[639, 723, 725–728] such that they constitute opposing limbs of cyclic continua in which membrane fragments of endocytotic vacuoles are recycled to exocytotic vacuoles through endosomes[727] and to the plasma membrane, the recycling occurring within minutes.[639, 731, 732] The process is energy dependent,[733, 734] as is that of orderly clathrin assembly-disassembly.[735, 736] In the proximal renal tubule cells of the rat, just minutes after its receipt of maleate, large endocytic apical vacuoles accumulate; most of the apical tubules disappear[690]; coated pits lose their clathrin coat[737]; and the corresponding coated pit membrane, which normally remains restricted to the base of the microvilli during endocytosis, becomes internalized to the newly formed, large apical vacuoles.[737] The membrane incorporated into these vacuoles appears not to derive from either microvillar membranes or lysosomal membranes.[737] Because apical tubules function to return membrane material from the endocytic vacuoles to the luminal plasma membrane,[639, 704] the maleate-induced disappearance of these tubules indicates altered recycling of membrane to the luminal membrane.[639, 738]

Because a variety of cells can be induced to secrete newly synthesized lysosomal enzymes[718, 739–745] with enzymatic activity,[746, 747] the lysosomal enzymes hyperexcreted in RTA-II/FS may not be the mature, smaller enzymes normally segregated in renal lysosomes.[722, 747, 748] In both acquired and genetically transmitted human disease, increased amounts of newly synthesized, larger lysosomal enzymes exit affected cells and occur in "pathologic" urine.[722, 748] In fact, both newly synthesized and mature lysosomal enzymes occur in the urine of normal humans, the first apparently being secreted by a nonlysosomal pathway, the second by a lysosomal pathway.[722, 747]

After their synthesis in rough endoplasmic reticulum, enzymes destined for segregation in lysosomes traverse the Golgi complex.[749] There, most of these proteins gain phosphomannosyl residues that bind them to mannose 6-phosphate receptors and thereby "address" them to lysosomes.[750, 751] The ligand-receptor complexes exit the trans Golgi network, the last station along the Golgi pathway,[749] in clathrin-coated vesicles and proceed to a late endosome prelysosomal compartment[713, 750, 752] to some unknown extent by way of early endosomes.[753] The more acidic interior of the prelysosomal compartment[754] effects the dissociation of the ligand-receptor complexes, thus allowing released lysosomal enzymes to be segregated in lysosomes and unoccupied receptors to be recycled to the Golgi apparatus and plasma membrane.[743, 750, 751, 755] In normal rat kidney cells, the prelysosomal compartment appears to be stationed on the "main endocytic route" from the plasma membrane to the lysosome.[713] In consequence, both lysosomal enzymes liganded to mannose 6-phosphate receptors in the Golgi network and proteins endocytosed by absorptive endocytosis and receptor mediation accumulate in the prelysosomal compartment before they enter lysosomes.[713]

By rendering the late endosome prelysosomal compartment less acidic and thereby retarding the dissociation of ligand-receptor complexes, certain weak bases, like chloroquine and $NH_4Cl$,[739, 743] or genetically decreased activity of endosomal H⁺-ATPase[756–759] can restrict the recycling of unoccupied mannose 6-phosphate receptors to the Golgi apparatus and plasma membrane. Accordingly, these bases and this enzymatic disorder can effect the constitutive secretion of immature, mannose 6-phosphate–bearing lysosomal enzymes and impair their receptor-mediated endocytosis.[741, 743, 751] Caplan and colleagues[718] found that in canine renal tubule cells (Madin-Darby canine kidney), NH₄Cl induced secretion of newly synthesized cathepsin D, a lysosomal enzyme, into both apical and basolateral media. In abstract, chloroquine has been reported to inhibit endocytic reabsorption of protein in the isolated perfused rabbit proximal renal tubule.[760] Whereas it remains to be demonstrated that the lysosomal enzymes hyperexcreted in RTA-II/FS contain mannose 6-phosphate, Tager and colleagues[747] have demonstrated in urine of normal subjects the occurrence of a mannose 6-phosphate–bearing immature lysosomal enzyme, α-glucosidase, as well as a smaller, mature form of this enzyme that contains no mannose 6-phosphate residues. In acute RTA-II/FS, rapidly reversible, coordinate hyperexcretion of lysozyme and mannose 6-phosphate–bearing immature lysosomal enzymes could then result from a rapidly reversible loss of normal acidity in the late endosome prelysosomal compartment in cells of the proximal renal tubule caused by a reversible reduction in function of endosomal H⁺-ATPase consequent to impaired metabolic generation of ATP.

But, in the RTA-II/FS induced by fructose in patients with HFI, hyperexcretion of mannose 6-phosphate–bearing, immature lysosomal enzymes could result from another mechanism that restricts their access to mannose 6-phosphate receptors. When those affected are given fructose, their genetically defective aldolase B dictates in cells of the proximal tubule the cytoplasmic accumulation of fructose 1-phosphate and thereby depletion of Pᵢ → depletion of ATP. In the proximal renal tubule of the fructose-loaded rat, Pᵢ loading largely prevents the otherwise substantial decrease in ATP but doubles the already greatly increased concentration of fructose 1-phosphate.[663] In solution, fructose 1-phosphate and mannose 6-phosphate have similar stereochemical configurations and identically high affinities for the mannose 6-phosphate receptor.[761, 762] Thus, in patients with HFI given fructose, fructose 1-phosphate, at the high concentrations attained in cells of the proximal renal tubule, could competitively bind a large portion of the pool of mannose 6-phosphate receptors and render it unavailable for binding mannose 6-phosphate–bearing enzymes. If so, an increased number of immature, mannose 6-phosphate–bearing enzymes would fail to bind mannose 6-phosphate receptors in the Golgi apparatus and, hence, would not be sorted to the lysosomal pathway but would instead be secreted by default and excreted in the urine. In patients with HFI given fructose, Pᵢ loading initiated beforehand has been found to significantly mitigate the transepithelial transport dysfunction of RTA-II/FS but exacerbate the excretion of N-acetyl-β-glucosaminidase (as measured by its activity) and lysozyme.[763] Thus, Pᵢ loading could mitigate RTA-II/FS by attenuating the cellular depletion of ATP but exacerbate disordered renal protein handling by amplifying the cellular uptake of fructose 1-phosphate. Specifically, the exacerbated urinary excretion of N-acetyl-β-glucosaminidase with

Pᵢ loading could reflect not simple leakage of the mature enzyme from lysosomes but the increased constitutive secretion of its immature, mannose 6-phosphate–bearing form, which is known to have full enzymatic activity.[763] That the phenomenon of Pᵢ-induced exacerbation is one of some specificity is suggested by the observation that Pᵢ loading strikingly attenuated both the RTA-II/FS and hyperexcretion of lysosomal enzymes and lysozyme induced by maleic acid in the dog.

Whatever the details of its character and mechanism, the rapidly reversible lysozymuria/lysosomal enzymuria characteristic of acute RTA-II/FS, in conjunction with the loss of apical tubules in cells of the proximal tubule[639] and the accumulation there of large apical vacuoles containing membrane normally restricted to the base of microvilli,[737] reflects a severe if transient disordering of endocytosis and exocytosis and membrane recycling in the proximal tubule.[639, 729] This disordering could impair exocytotic replenishment of transport components of its luminal membrane (and the basolateral membrane) and thereby entrain varied and complex disturbances of its physiologic functions,[684, 700] somewhat as proposed by Bergeron and colleagues.[682] Such a disordering could impair exocytotic insertion into the luminal membrane not only of electrogenic H⁺-ATPase[764–766] and Na⁺,K⁺-ATPase in the basolateral membrane but also of water channels.[767] Impaired mitochondrial generation of ATP induced in the proximal tubule by maleic acid in animals, or by fructose in patients with HFI, might then be pathogenetically linked to RTA-II/FS through diminished availability of both basolateral Na⁺,K⁺-ATPase and apical H⁺-ATPase and water channels and consequent impairment not only of electroneutral H⁺/Na⁺ exchange, electrogenic H⁺ secretion, and fluid absorption but possibly also of reabsorptive transport of such solutes as Pᵢ[768] and glucose.

## CHRONIC RTA-II/FS

### Lysozyme and L-Chain Nephropathy

The hypothesis that chronic functional and structural disorders of the endocytic-endosomal-lysosomal system can cause RTA-II/FS is supported by observations made in patients with this group of renal disorders. Increased urinary excretion of the low-molecular-weight proteins lysozyme and immunoglobulin L chain can reflect their increased extrarenal production.[769–772] In patients in whom this occurs, increased reabsorption of these proteins by the proximal tubule seemingly induces in it the observed structural changes in lysosome-like structures[773] and the dysfunction of RTA-II/FS.[769–772] In patients with monocytic leukemia, the not uncommon syndrome of renal K⁺ wasting appears to be a consequence of lysozyme-induced renal dysfunction.[769–771] In patients ultimately diagnosed as having multiple myeloma, the occurrence of RTA-II in association with the renal findings of Fanconi syndrome may precede by years other evidence of the disease and reflect an immunoglobulin L chain–induced nephropathy.[479, 480, 774–777] Indeed, there are no reports of RTA-II/FS or isolated Fanconi syndrome occurring *after* myeloma has been diagnosed. Of particular note, with successful treatment with melphalan of a patient with multiple myeloma, both L-chainuria and RTA-II/FS disappeared.[778] L chain nephropathy also occurs in patients with chronic lymphocytic leukemia.[774, 775] In either instance, the immunoglobulin detected in the urine is presumably produced in excess by a single clone of cells and hence is of a single subtype, usually κ [479, 480] but sometimes λ.[774, 776] Thus, when patients with Fanconi syndrome excrete but one type of immunoglobulin L chain, monoclonal plasma cell dyscrasia or, less commonly, chronic lymphocytic leukemia can be inferred to be causal.[480] When increased urinary excretion of immunoglobulin L chain reflects a primary renal tubule dysfunction, that is, one unassociated with increased production of L chain, both κ- and λ-subtypes are characteristically excreted.[779, 780]

### Cystinosis

In patients with cystinosis, the most common cause of RTA-II/FS in children, "storage" of cystine in lysosomes is believed to be a primary pathogenetic event in the many tissues affected,[781–783] and the occurrence of this phenomenon in the proximal renal tubule might underlie RTA-II/FS.[783–786] In so-called nephropathic or infantile cystinosis, lysosomal accumulation of cystine occurs prenatally,[787] RTA-II/FS is expressed within the first 12 months of life, progressive reduction in GFR leads to uremia by middle childhood, and the free cystine content of leukocytes is 80 times normal.[788] In so-called benign cystinosis of adulthood, renal disease is absent,[789] and the free cystine content of leukocytes is 30 times normal.[790] So-called adolescent or intermediate cystinosis is intermediate in severity with respect to the renal lesion and cystine content of leukocytes.[791]

Cystine is the only amino acid stored in cystinotic lysosomes.[792, 793] A defect in carrier-mediated transport of cystine across lysosomal membrane accounts for its massive accumulation in the lysosomes of those homozygous for infantile cystinosis.[792, 794] Lysosomal accumulation of cystine occurs throughout the kidney, particularly in the interstitium and glomerulus, and apparently also in the cells of the proximal tubule.[795] The phenomenon of cystine storage would seem to be important to the pathogenesis of the glomerulopathy and progressive renal failure in childhood that is characteristic of cystinosis.[785, 796] Cysteamine depletes intracellular cystine stores.[797] In cystinotic children, early treatment with cysteamine that greatly reduces lysosomal cystine concentration in leukocytes[797] can moderate and perhaps prevent the otherwise predictable occurrence of both the progressive reduction of GFR and severe stunting of somatic growth characteristic of this disease.[785, 786, 796] Yet, with one apparent exception,[798] institution of cysteamine even in the first weeks of life has failed to either prevent the occurrence of RTA-II/FS or attenuate established RTA-II/FS.[796, 799, 800] Whereas this failure might reflect restricted access of cysteamine to lysosomes in the proximal renal tubule,[801] it also suggests that lysosomal storage of cystine is not the only or principal pathogenetic mechanism of the RTA-II/FS of cystinosis.

In the rat, Foreman, Segal, and co-workers[802] demonstrated that parenteral administration of cystine dimethyl ester for 4 days led to an increased urine volume and excretion of $P_i$, glucose, and various amino acids without affecting creatinine clearance. Incubation of cells with the permeable methyl ester derivative of an amino acid leads to accumulation of the amino acid in lysosomes.[803] In isolated perfused proximal renal tubules, Baum and associates[804, 805] have demonstrated that cystine dimethyl ester induces within 10 minutes large reductions in volume reabsorption ($J_v$), $HCO_3^-$ transport, and glucose transport that are associated with a reduction in ATP and oxygen consumption but not the activity of $Na^+,K^+$-ATPase. Somewhat similar observations have been made in LLC-PK$_1$ cells and in renal cortical tissue harvested from rats intraperitoneally injected with cystine dimethyl ester.[806, 807] Thus, the pathogenetic mechanism through which cystinosis gives rise to RTA-II/FS may involve impaired mitochondrial oxidative generation of ATP in the proximal renal tubule.[805, 807] Although it is not apparent how such a mitochondrial disorder might be causally linked to the lysosomal accumulation of cystine, such a mitochondrial mechanism has obvious parallels with that inferred in the RTA-II/FS induced by fructose in patients with HFI and that induced by maleate in experimental animals.

### Deficiency and Disordered Metabolism of Vitamin D

Vitamin D–reversible RTA-II/FS occurs in the clinical circumstances of dietary deficiency of vitamin D and genetically determined diminished synthesis of, or resistance to, $1,25(OH)_2D_3$.[462, 463, 808–812] Such disorders of vitamin D metabolism and their consequent attending hypocalcemia, secondary hyperparathyroidism, and hypophosphatemia may act in combination to suppress renal acidification in the proximal tubule.[813–816] Whereas circulating PTH can acutely dampen the normal renal acidification process in humans, rats, and dogs,[813, 817–819] PTH can inhibit $HCO_3^-$ reabsorption in the proximal tubule,[813] and primary hyperparathyroidism may lead to RTA-II that persists after surgical correction of hyperparathyroidism,[820] it seems unlikely that RTA-II is caused by the physiologic effect of increased levels of circulating PTH alone.[821, 822] In the rat studied at normal plasma $HCO_3^-$ concentrations, systemically administered PTH does not induce bicarbonaturia and decreased net acid excretion.[813] A reversible impairment in renal acidification severe enough to cause frank acidosis has been demonstrated in nonazotemic patients with hyperparathyroidism only when the hyperparathyroidism was secondary to hypocalcemia caused by either vitamin D deficiency or disordered metabolism of vitamin D in association with hypophosphatemia.

In the dog and rat, prolonged severe hypophosphatemia may be attended by a modest reduction in renal tubule reabsorption of $HCO_3^-$ at normal plasma $HCO_3^-$ concentrations and a slight decrease in plasma $HCO_3^-$ concentration.[823, 824] In humans, however, prolonged, severe hypophosphatemia does not give rise to RTA-II/FS in the absence of disordered metabolism of vitamin D. Specifically, RTA-II/FS or isolated RTA-II is not described in humans with the chronic hypophosphatemia caused by 1) continuing ingestion of aluminum hydroxide,[260, 263–265] 2) severe dietary calcium deficiency that gives rise to hypocalcemia and secondary hyperparathyroidism,[825, 826] or 3) genetically transmitted renal tubule defects that impair renal reabsorption only of $P_i$.[211, 226, 825] In familial Fanconi syndrome, severe symptomatic hypophosphatemia occurs unassociated with impaired renal acidification.[240]

In a patient with HFI who had undergone surgical parathyroidectomy and was maintained nearly eucalcemic with large doses of vitamin $D_2$, the experimental administration of fructose failed to induce fully expressed RTA-II/FS until a large amount of PTH was also administered.[827] If severe cellular depletion of $P_i$ in the proximal tubule is indeed critical to the pathogenesis of the fructose-induced RTA-II/FS in patients with HFI,[666] the absence of PTH may have attenuated its expression by enhancing $P_i$ reabsorption in the proximal tubule enough to prevent the otherwise severe cellular depletion of $P_i$ entrained by the fructose-induced cellular accumulation of fructose 1-phosphate. Such prevention might have been aided by the patient's having received large doses of vitamin $D_2$, which can be presumed to have been converted to some extent to $1,25(OH)_2D_3$. In the rat deprived of vitamin D, but not to the point of inducing a reduction in the serum concentration of either $Ca^{2+}$ or phosphorus, short-term administration of $1,25(OH)_2D_3$ induced an acute increase in $P_i$ reabsorption in the proximal tubule in situ and in brush border membrane vesicles prepared therefrom.[828] In several patients with idiopathic Fanconi syndrome unassociated with hypocalcemia,[829–831] large-dose vitamin D therapy has been attended by correction of RTA-II/FS; and, in one patient in whom the measurement was made, the plasma concentration of immunoreactive PTH was not increased.[831] Intracellular depletion of $P_i$ in the proximal tubule, possibly amplified by increased circulating concentration of PTH, may be critical to the vitamin D–reversible RTA-II/FS observed in disorders of vitamin D metabolism.

### Wilson Disease

RTA-II/FS of Wilson disease has not been extensively studied, in part because it appears to occur only occasionally in Wilson disease.[454, 687, 832, 833] Fanconi syndrome without RTA-II occurs, and the acidification may affect both the proximal and distal nephron. It is clear that Fanconi syndrome, including the acidification defect, and pathologic changes in the proximal tubule can disappear after sustained therapy with penicillamine and the attendant mobilization and urinary excretion of copper.[834, 835] Fanconi syndrome can recur after penicillamine therapy has been discontinued.[833] These and other observations are consistent with the view that the pathogenesis of Fanconi syndrome, as well as the hepatic and cerebral abnormalities of Wilson disease, depends on cellular deposition of copper.[836–840] The occurrence of Fanconi syndrome in patients with Wilson disease does not, however, appear to be related to the seriousness of the extrarenal disease.

Penicillamine therapy can be attended by a lessened impairment in renal acidification.[841, 842] However, in each of three patients with full-blown distal RTA studied by Leu and co-workers,[841] the renal acidification dysfunction persisted apparently unchanged despite penicillamine therapy and the finding in one of the three patients of a "normal"

copper concentration in the kidney post mortem. Wilson and Goldstein[453] also found that the physiologic characteristics of distal RTA could persist despite prolonged penicillamine therapy in patients with Wilson disease. The proximal disorder of renal acidification, as well as the complex dysfunction of Fanconi syndrome, may be more responsive to penicillamine therapy than is the distal disorder of acidification,[549] which may be a consequence more of sustained hypercalciuria and cellular deposition of $Ca^{2+}$ in the distal tubule than of deposition of copper.[549] Specifically, penicillamine therapy may act to reverse only those functional and structural lesions for which cellular deposition of copper is a requirement, as might be the case for disorders of the proximal tubule.

## PATHOPHYSIOLOGY

### Potassium, Sodium, and Water

In patients with RTA-II/FS, in contrast to patients with RTA-I, renal $K^+$ wasting and polyuria either occur or become more severe when the correction of acidosis is attempted with alkali therapy alone[476] (Fig. 37–6). Because the capacity of the proximal tubule to reabsorb $HCO_3^-$ is greatly reduced, the distal nephron is swamped with $HCO_3^-$ when the plasma $HCO_3^-$ concentration is increased from subnormal to normal levels with alkali therapy[476] (see Fig. 37–4). Furthermore, expanding an otherwise contracted extracellular fluid volume has the effect of further reducing proximal reabsorption of $Na^+$, $HCO_3^-$, and $Cl^-$.[843, 844] In the presence of a continued stimulus for $Na^+$ reabsorption in the distal nephron (e.g., hyperaldosteronism), the delivery

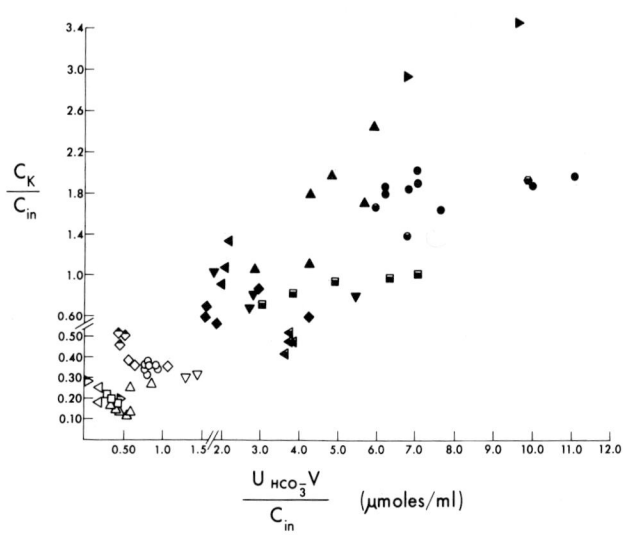

**Figure 37–6.** Relationship between fractional excretion of filtered $K^+$ ($C_K/C_{In}$) and urinary excretion of $HCO_3^-$ ($U_{HCO_3}V/C_{in}$) in patients with type II RTA associated with Fanconi syndrome (*closed* and *three-quarter–closed symbols*) in whom plasma $HCO_3^-$ concentration was maintained at normal levels (22 to 26 mmol/L for more than 2 months [*closed* and *open symbols*]) or was rapidly increased to normal levels (intravenous administration of sodium bicarbonate [*three-quarter–open symbols*]). Each geometric symbol represents measurements made in a single patient. (From Sebastian A, McSherry E, Morris RC Jr. On the mechanism of renal potassium wasting in renal tubular acidosis associated with the Fanconi syndrome [type 2 RTA]. J Clin Invest 50:231–243, 1971.)

of greatly supernormal amounts of $Na^+$, $HCO_3^-$, and $Cl^-$ out of the proximal nephron would be expected to augment net $K^+$ secretion in the distal nephron[476, 845] and thereby promote renal $K^+$ wasting (Fig. 37–7). During sustained correction of acidosis with alkali therapy, the fraction of the filtered load of $K^+$ excreted frequently exceeds 1.0 (which indicates net renal secretion of $K^+$) and varies directly with the fractional excretion of filtered $HCO_3^-$[476] (see Fig. 37–6). In at least some patients with RTA-II, as in some patients with RTA-I, hyperaldosteronism (and hyperreninemia) persists despite sustained correction of acidosis and the provision of normal or supernormal amounts of dietary sodium.[476] $K^+$ depletion causes not only an impairment in the renal concentrating function[846, 847] but also thirst and polydipsia as primary phenomena.[848] These phenomena, combined with the greatly increased delivery of solute and water out of the proximal tubule, may account for what is often strikingly severe polyuria. It is an important clinical point that in patients with RTA-II/FS, urine can be dilute (i.e., hypo-osmolar) despite dehydration.

In patients diagnosed as having RTA-II without associated Fanconi syndrome, both transient[482] and persisting,[483] hypokalemia and polyuria were not observed either before or during alkali therapy, and potassium supplements were

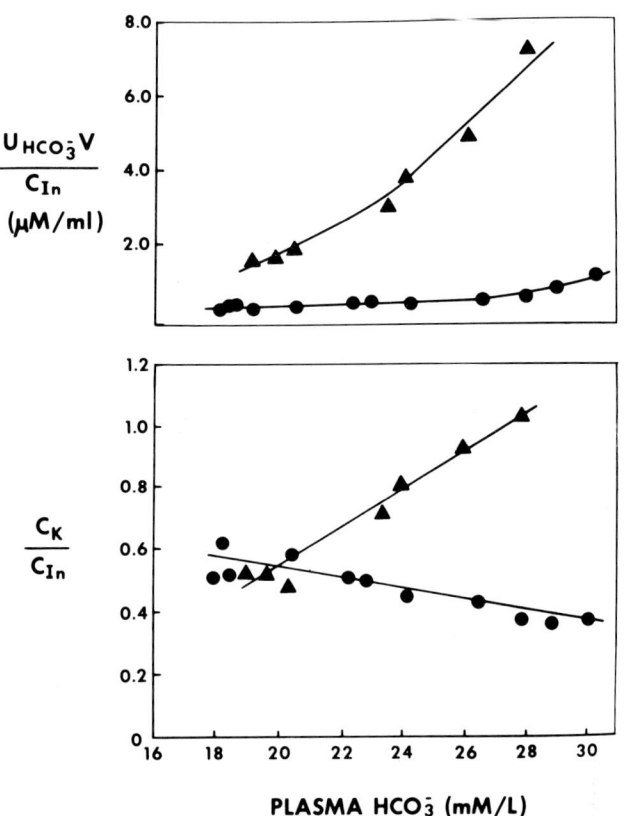

**Figure 37–7.** Effect of an acute, progressive increase in plasma $HCO_3^-$ concentration (intravenous administration of sodium bicarbonate) on the fraction of the filtered load of $K^+$ excreted in the urine ($C_K C_{In}$) and on the urinary excretion of $HCO_3^-$ ($U_{HCO_3}V/C_{In}$) in a patient with type I RTA *(circles)* and in a patient with type II RTA *(triangles)*. (From Morris RC Jr, Sebastian A, McSherry E: Renal acidosis. Kidney Int 1:322–340, 1972.)

not required. This finding suggests that the pathophysiologic basis of this acidification defect is different from that of RTA-II/FS.

## Phosphorus/Calcium/Metabolic Bone Disease and Vitamin D

In patients diagnosed as having RTA-II, either transient[482] or persisting,[483] in whom the renal dysfunction of the Fanconi syndrome was absent, hypocalcemia/hypercalciuria and hypophosphatemia/hyperphosphaturia did not occur, despite metabolic acidosis; rickets also did not occur. In the well-studied patients with genetically transmitted RTA-II reported by Brenes and co-workers,[484] metabolic bone disease was not apparent, but those affected were all stunted in somatic growth.

In patients with chronic RTA-II/FS or isolated Fanconi syndrome, metabolic bone disease is predictable. Indeed, in its classic definition, Fanconi syndrome is composed of two components, the characteristic complex dysfunction of the proximal renal tubule and metabolic bone disease, rickets in children and osteomalacia in adults. Indeed, painful, disfiguring metabolic bone disease often dominates the clinical picture of RTA-II/FS and isolated Fanconi syndrome in affected children. In adult patients with RTA-II/FS, metabolic bone disease can take years to become clinically apparent[448, 849] but may be diagnosed earlier by bone biopsy.[775] In RTA-II/FS or isolated Fanconi syndrome, sustained hypophosphatemia is a predictable consequence of the persisting impairment in renal reabsorption of $P_i$ and in most instances would appear to be the principal and sometimes sole pathogenic determinant of the metabolic bone disease.[240, 297, 850] Clinical and experimental chronic hypophosphatemia can cause metabolic bone disease.[257, 258, 260, 263–265] Phosphate therapy alone can heal hypophosphatemic metabolic bone disease.[211, 240, 263–265] In patients with RTA-II/FS, this therapeutic phenomenon would appear to have occurred most frequently in those with adult-onset disease,[297, 445, 775, 851] but it has been described in children with nephropathic cystinosis[852] and children with primary Fanconi syndrome.[240]

## Vitamin D Metabolism

$1,25(OH)_2D_3$ is the most biologically active metabolite of vitamin D known with respect to the stimulation of gut absorption of $Ca^{2+}$ and phosphorus. $1,25(OH)_2D_3$ is synthesized exclusively in mitochondria of the renal cortex[228, 229, 853–855] by the 1α-hydroxylation of $25(OH)D_3$, which is synthesized principally in the liver.[856] By impairing either the 1α-hydroxylation reaction or the accession of $25(OH)D_3$ to the mitochondrial site of the reaction, abnormalities of the renal cortical tubule capable of causing persisting Fanconi syndrome can reduce the renal synthesis of $1,25(OH)_2D_3$ and might thereby contribute to the pathogenesis of the bone disease of Fanconi syndrome.[857, 858] In animals, the experimental administration of maleic acid induces a reversible renal tubule dysfunction like that of Fanconi syndrome[674, 675] and metabolic and structural changes in the renal cortical tubule, particularly in the mitochondria.[674–681] In the vitamin D–deficient rat and chick, maleic acid induces a substantial reduction in the conversion of $25(OH)D_3$ to $1,25(OH)_2D_3$, and this reduction occurs without a significant decrease in GFR, when measured in the rat.[857] Frankly reduced [859-862] and "normal" levels of plasma $1,25(OH)_2D_3$ have been reported in RTA-II/FS.[858, 861-866] Because even modest hypophosphatemia is a potent stimulus for an increased renal production and plasma concentration of $1,25(OH)_2D_3$ in humans,[243, 244, 252] apparently normal plasma concentrations of $1,25(OH)_2D_3$ in hypophosphatemic patients with RTA-II/FS are in fact abnormally low. Interpretation of values of $1,25(OH)_2D_3$ is further complicated by the apparent dampening effect of metabolic acidosis on the capacity of hypophosphatemia to increase the plasma concentration of $1,25(OH)_2D_3$ in humans.[867] In one young girl with nephropathic cystinosis, treatment with a "physiologic" amount of $1,25(OH)_2D_3$ (1 μg/d) was attended by rapid healing of rickets and an increase in linear growth rate.[868] Gertner and colleagues[869] have also reported healing of rickets in three boys with cystinosis given $1\alpha(OH)D_3$. It remains unclear whether the administration of $1,25(OH)_2D_3$ has a primary effect on the bone in the healing of metabolic bone disease, as opposed to affecting bone indirectly by increasing the intestinal absorption and plasma concentrations of $Ca^{2+}$ and phosphorus.[870, 871]

In two sibling children with isolated Fanconi syndrome, the plasma concentration of $1,25(OH)_2D_3$ was about twice that of normal—an increase much like that observed in normal subjects rendered similarly hypophosphatemic with aluminum hydroxide.[240] With phosphate therapy alone in these two children, the circulating level of $1,25(OH)_2D_3$ decreased to normal values, the metabolic bone disease healed, and the proximal muscle weakness disappeared. Hypophosphatemia/phosphate depletion has been previously implicated in the pathogenesis of the proximal myopathy that can occur in RTA-II/FS.[445, 851, 872]

The renal dysfunction of RTA-II/FS usually does not give rise to hypocalcemia even after prolonged acidosis. Although hypercalciuria occurs[478, 851] and can disappear with alkali therapy,[449, 832] its occurrence is not predictably related to that of acidosis.[873] Hypercalciuria is characteristic of patients with Wilson disease,[454] regardless of Fanconi syndrome, and may reflect increased absorption of $Ca^{2+}$ from the gut[832] and may give rise to nephrocalcinosis.[454, 549, 832] In our experience, hypercalciuria is usual in patients with cystinosis, and its severity is unaffected by alkali therapy. In patients with RTA-II/FS, nephrocalcinosis (and nephrolithiasis) occurs only rarely, perhaps because urinary excretion of citrate is not reduced and is often increased in those affected.[618, 619]

## THERAPY

The therapy of RTA-II/FS can be dramatically successful when substances critical to its causation can be removed, as with fructose, galactose, and copper in patients with HFI,[643, 874] galactosemia,[875, 876] and Wilson disease,[834, 835] respectively. Cystinosis and tyrosinemia (type I) appear to be special cases. In children with cystinosis, it now seems clear that administration of cysteamine can greatly reduce the amount of cystine in lysosomes of some cells and, when

administered in early childhood, prevent or attenuate the otherwise progressive renal failure and severe growth stunting. Yet, even when it is initiated in the first 2 weeks of life, cysteamine would not appear to dramatically affect the course of RTA-II/FS.[785, 786] Conversely, in tyrosinemia, dietary restriction of tyrosine can greatly moderate the renal tubule dysfunction of Fanconi syndrome,[877-879] but this therapy does not prevent the occurrence of progressive liver damage, hepatoma, and cirrhosis of the liver, often in early childhood, or progressive renal insufficiency after childhood.[880, 881] Several reports document striking amelioration of the renal dysfunction of tyrosinemia after liver transplantation.[880-882] Furthermore, tyrosine loading no longer induced exacerbation of the renal dysfunction,[880] despite inducing a sharp increase in succinylacetone,[880, 881] a putative "toxic metabolite" of tyrosine.[883, 884] It has been proposed that metabolites of tyrosine made in the liver caused the renal disorder (even though the kidney can also make the same metabolites), and hence transplantation of a normal liver effected a cure of both the renal dysfunction and the hepatic disorder. In three children with glycogen storage disease caused by glucose-6-phosphatase deficiency (von Gierke disease), nocturnal glucose feeding induced within 2 weeks complete correction of a complex disorder of the proximal tubule like that of Fanconi syndrome; lactic acidosis precluded evaluation of an acidification defect.[885]

The treatment of RTA-II is directed toward amelioration of the fluid, electrolyte, and acid-base disturbance. Sustained correction of acidosis with alkali therapy requires the administration of alkali sufficient to offset the urinary excretion of net base plus the estimated endogenous production of nonvolatile acid, at normal plasma $HCO_3^-$ concentrations, net base excretion being essentially equal to $HCO_3^-$ excretion. As indicated, much of the alkali given to correct acidosis will have to be given as potassium bicarbonate (or an equivalent alkali-producing potassium salt), because sodium bicarbonate will predictably increase renal $K^+$ loss. When RTA-II occurs as part of the Fanconi syndrome, the mechanism of the acidosis and its treatment may be more complex. The large urinary excretion of citrate in Fanconi syndrome[618, 619] represents a further net base loss because it is normally combustible to $HCO_3^-$.[620-622] The magnitude of renal $HCO_3^-$ excretion at normal plasma $HCO_3^-$ concentrations can vary from as little as 2 to 3 mEq/kg body weight per day in patients with minimal impairment of proximal $HCO_3^-$ reabsorption, or great reductions in GFR, to values greater than 20 mEq/kg body weight per day in patients with more severe dysfunction or more nearly normal GFR. The alkali and potassium requirements must then be determined empirically for each patient. In some patients, it may not be possible to sustain correction of acidosis with alkali therapy. When the amount of alkali required to correct acidosis is prohibitively large, hydrochlorothiazide can be a useful therapeutic adjunct.[886-888] This agent may increase proximal $HCO_3^-$ reabsorption by inducing contraction of extracellular volume[844, 886, 887]; it may, however, increase $H^+$ secretion directly.[889] With hydrochlorothiazide, the severity of hypokalemia frequently increases. Restriction of dietary salt and water may also be useful in reducing the amount of alkali therapy required to correct acidosis and in reducing the severity of renal $K^+$ wasting and polyuria.[844, 890]

# Type I Renal Tubular Acidosis (Classic, Distal)

## PHYSIOLOGIC CHARACTERISTICS

In the classic expression of distal RTA, type I RTA (RTA-I), urine pH is inappropriately high during severe as well as mild degrees of acidosis (usually greater than 6) (see Fig. 37–2), and the complex dysfunction of the proximal tubule of the Fanconi syndrome (impaired renal reabsorption of glucose, $P_i$, and amino acids) is absent.[423, 427–437, 495, 891, 892] RTA-I can be the expression of a number of disease processes (see Table 37–5).

### Adults

In adults with RTA-I, the amount of $HCO_3^-$ excreted at both normal and reduced plasma $HCO_3^-$ concentrations is less than 5% of filtered $HCO_3^-$ over a broad range of normal and subnormal plasma $HCO_3^-$ concentrations (see Fig. 37–3). This finding permits the inference that reabsorption of $HCO_3^-$ in the proximal renal tubule (and the distal tubule) is not substantially reduced.[426, 427, 431–437, 495, 891, 892] In most adult patients with RTA-I, acidosis results principally from a modest impairment of acid excretion. Hence, correction of acidosis is characteristically sustained by an amount of alkali only a fraction more than the normal endogenous production of nonvolatile acid (i.e., a fraction more than 1 mEq/kg/d in adults).[429, 432, 433, 436, 437]

### Children

Renal $HCO_3^-$ wasting occurs in many prepubertal children with idiopathic or familial RTA-I who are given alkali therapy in amounts sufficient to sustain correction of acidosis.[435, 495, 508, 893] Renal $HCO_3^-$ wasting can be said to occur when the urinary excretion of net base exceeds the rate at which nonvolatile acid is endogenously produced.[435, 495] Because endogenous production of nonvolatile acid may be as high as 3 mEq/kg/d in rapidly growing children,[583] renal $HCO_3^-$ wasting can be defined arbitrarily as net base excretion of greater than 3 mEq/kg/d at normal (or reduced) plasma $HCO_3^-$ concentrations.[585] So defined, renal $HCO_3^-$ wasting is quantitatively more important in the causation of acidosis than is reduced excretion of acid (which predictably attends renal $HCO_3^-$ wasting because of the inappropriately high urine pH at which $HCO_3^-$ wasting occurs). Reduced excretion of acid leads to acidosis only to the extent that the endogenously produced, nonvolatile acid titrates body buffers, including plasma $HCO_3^-$. Such a loss of base is relatively minor and slowly developing compared with the loss of base that can result from a substantial fractional excretion of filtered $HCO_3^-$. (This statement assumes nonvolatile acid is not substantially greater than 3 mEq/kg/d, as in such conditions as lactic acidosis and diabetic ketoacidosis.)

In infants with RTA-I, renal $HCO_3^-$ wasting can be present from the outset of the disorder[435, 495, 508, 893] but usually occurs a few weeks after alkali therapy has been started.[495] In older affected children, renal $HCO_3^-$ wasting usually does not occur until several months after alkali therapy is begun, when growth velocity has greatly increased. In infants and children with RTA-I, the occurrence of renal $HCO_3^-$ wasting does not appear to reflect a qualitative change in the character of the renal acidification defect (Fig. 37–8), but when it occurs, its magnitude at normal plasma $HCO_3^-$ concentrations is the major determinant of the amount of alkali required to sustain correction of acidosis. This amount may range from 5 to 15 mEq/kg/d.[435, 436, 495, 508, 893] The persistence of renal $HCO_3^-$ wasting at reduced plasma $HCO_3^-$ concentrations accounts for the strikingly severe acidosis both before corrective alkali therapy is begun and soon after it is discontinued.[435]

## CELLULAR AND PATHOGENETIC MECHANISMS

In the distal nephron, specifically the cortical and medullary collecting ducts, $H^+$ secretion induces a decrease in the luminal fluid pH to 4.5 to 5.5, fully 2 to 3 pH units below that of the blood. The decrease in pH results mainly from $H^+$ secretion mediated by $H^+$-ATPase at the apical border of intercalated cells of the $\alpha$-subtype.[587, 632, 894, 895] $HCO_3^-$ generated during the process of luminal $H^+$ secretion exits the basolateral surface of the cell to enter the blood by means of an $HCO_3^-/Cl^-$ exchanger (with $Cl^-$ recycling)[895–897] (Figs. 37–9 and 37–10). Impaired $H^+$-ATPase may underlie the RTA-I that occurs in so many patients with Sjögren syndrome,[898] a renal biopsy sample from one of whom was devoid of any anti–$H^+$-ATPase staining in the intercalated cells.[899] Impaired $H^+$-ATPase would not, however, readily account for the hypokalemia characteristic of these patients.[900] The intercalated cells of the collecting tubule also contain an $H^+,K^+$-ATPase that effects secretion of $H^+$ and reabsorption of $K^+$.[901] The main physiologic function of this enzyme may not be $H^+$ secretion but $K^+$ reabsorption, when dietary potassium is restricted.[895] However, in the rat, long-term administration of vanadate that caused hypokalemic distal RTA induced a reduction in the activity of $H^+,K^+$-ATPase in the cortical and outer medul-

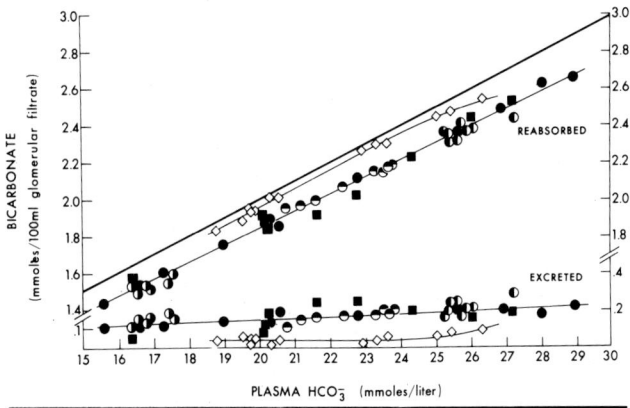

**Figure 37–8.** Relationship between arterial plasma concentration, renal tubule reabsorption, and urinary excretion of $HCO_3^-$ during the first year of life in three infants with apparently type I RTA, two with renal $HCO_3^-$ wasting (*circles* and *squares*), one without (*diamonds*). (From McSherry E, Sebastian A, Morris RC Jr: Renal tubular acidosis in infants: The several kinds, including bicarbonate-wasting, classic renal tubular acidosis. J Clin Invest 51:499–514, 1972.)

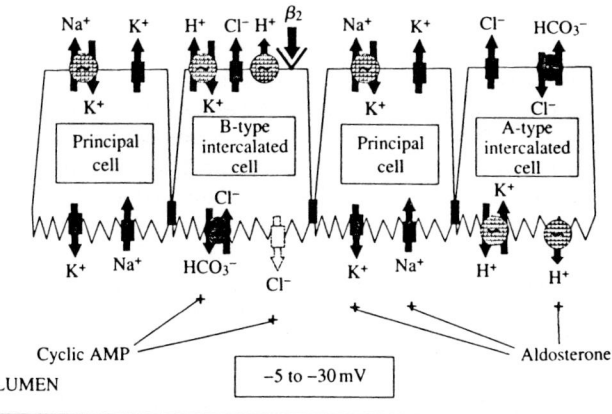

**Figure 37–9.** Diagram of cortical collecting tubule transport of $HCO_3^-$ and $H^+$ transport, and certain of their determinants; $\beta_2$ refers to $\beta_2$-adrenergic stimulus. (From Gluck S, Nelson R: The role of the V-ATPase in renal epithelial $H^+$ transport. J Exp Biol 172:205–218, 1992. © The Company of Biologists Ltd.)

lary collecting ducts but not in the activity of $H^+$-ATPase.[902] By inducing a reduction in the activity of this enzyme in the renal collecting tubule, environmental exposure to "toxic" amounts of vanadium may be critical to the pathogenesis of the hypokalemic distal RTA reported in such large numbers of people in Thailand.[903, 904]

A substantial portion of the intercalated cells in the cortical collecting duct are of the β-type, which secrete $HCO_3^-$ by means of an apical $Cl^-/HCO_3^-$ exchanger, at least during metabolic alkalosis,[905, 906] and $H^+$ by means of a vacuolar $H^+$-ATPase on the basolateral surface (see Fig. 37–9). A disorder of the $HCO_3^-/Cl^-$ exchanger in either α-cells or β-cells might cause RTA-I. Evidence in support of the former possibility has been presented.[906a] Other mechanisms can be postulated. An increase in the $H^+$ permeability of the luminal membrane of α-cells would allow $H^+$ backflux and prevent normal reduction in luminal fluid pH. In the cortical collecting tubule, electrogenic $Na^+$ reabsorption in principal cells adjacent to intercalated cells generates a lumen-negative potential difference. Because the $H^+$-ATPase is electrogenic, the lumen-negative potential difference generated by the principal cell potentiates $H^+$ secretion.[907–909]

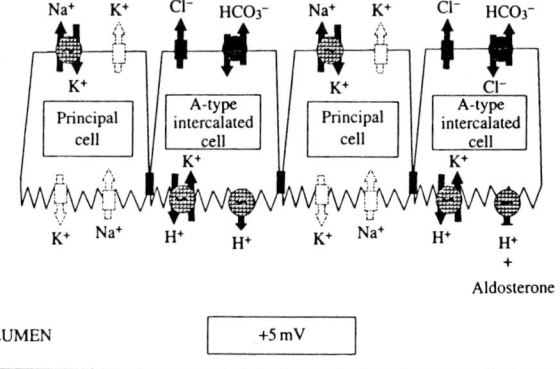

**Figure 37–10.** Diagram of outer medullary collecting tubule transport of $H^+$ and possibly of $Na^+$. (From Gluck S, Nelson R: The role of the V-ATPase in renal epithelial $H^+$ transport. J Exp Biol 172:205–218, 1992. © The Company of Biologists Ltd.)

and an impairment in its capacity to do so could impair renal acidification, as discussed in greater detail later.

In the medullary collecting tubule (see Fig. 37–10), principal cells also occur and might be involved in solute transport, but in this nephronal segment $H^+$ secretion by intercalated cells is the only solute transport demonstrated and accounts for a reduction in pH greater than that usually attained in the cortical collecting duct. Selective abolition of medullary collecting duct function (see Fig. 37–10) would leave intact the cortical collecting duct functions of $Na^+$ reabsorption, $K^+$ secretion, and $H^+$ titration of buffers not requiring a low luminal pH (such as protonation of $Na_2HPO_4$ to $NaH_2PO_4$) but would preclude attainment in the medulla of the low luminal pH required for normal $NH_4^+$ trapping and excretion.

A defect in the regulation of $H^+$ secretion, rather than one of the pump, exchanger, or luminal membrane, may underlie genetically transmitted RTA-I, at least in its early pristine expression. As depicted (see Figs. 37–9 and 37–10), vacuolar $H^+$-ATPase might seem fixed in deployment at the apex of α-type intercalated cells in the cortical and medullary collecting ducts, but the acidosis-induced increased secretion of $H^+$ in the distal nephron involves apical recruitment of this vacuolar enzyme from intracellular sites, rather than an increase in its activity or synthesized amount.[910–912] Thus, an impairment in the mechanism by which apical recruitment of $H^+$-ATPase is effected could impair $H^+$ secretion in the distal nephron. In an infant with RTA-I, initial treatment with arginine vasopressin for erroneously diagnosed diabetes insipidus resulted in severe metabolic alkalosis that immediately converted to hyperchloremic acidosis when the vasopressin was stopped (Morris RC Jr, unpublished observation). Vasopressin, like angiotensin II, can increase $HCO_3^-$ reabsorption in vivo in the distal tubule of the normal rat.[913, 914] An increased, unregulated secretion of $HCO_3^-$ by the β-cell could also give rise to RTA-I.[905, 906, 914, 915]

That medullary collecting duct function of $H^+$ secretion might be impaired in RTA-I is suggested not only by the inappropriately high urine pH during acidosis but also by the finding that the $PCO_2$ of the urine does not greatly exceed that of blood during loading with sodium bicarbonate.[612, 916] In normal subjects rendered bicarbonaturic by bicarbonate loading, the urine − blood $PCO_2$ ($U − B$ $PCO_2$) exceeds 20 mm Hg.[438, 612, 917, 918] To a major extent, the normal increment in urine $PCO_2$ stems from the delayed dehydration of carbonic acid ($H_2CO_3$) generated in the lumen of the collecting duct from the titration of $HCO_3^-$ by secreted $H^+$.[919] Luminal dehydration of $H_2CO_3$ in the collecting duct is normally uncatalyzed. Hence, a relatively slow luminal dehydration of $H_2CO_3$ continues throughout the collecting duct and beyond. Because neither the $H_2CO_3$ formed in the lumen nor the $CO_2$ generated from its dehydration readily diffuses out under normal circumstances, urine $PCO_2$ is a direct function of the amount of $H_2CO_3$ formed in the collecting duct, and the normally increased $U − B$ $PCO_2$ is an index of its rate of $H^+$ secretion.[610, 918] The model of RTA-I induced experimentally by amphotericin is characterized by a retained ability to increase $U − B$ $PCO_2$ normally, in sharp distinction from the acidification dysfunction of the great preponderance of patients with RTA-I who have been studied, including those in whom the dysfunction is the expression of either a genetically transmitted trait or an apparently "autoimmune" state. In the amphotericin model of RTA-I, it can be inferred that the ability of the collecting tubules to secrete $H^+$ at normal rates at normal or increased plasma $HCO_3^-$ concentrations is intact, whereas the permeability of the collecting duct with respect to $HCO_3^-$ may be impaired.[441, 920] However, although a reduced capacity to increase $U-B$ $P_{CO_2}$ suggests that the net rate of $H^+$ secretion in the collecting duct is reduced[438, 441, 612, 917, 920] and such a reduction might be the primary physiologic disorder in some patients with RTA-I,[438, 612, 920] the reduced increase of $U-B$ $P_{CO_2}$ might also result from impaired medullary trapping of $CO_2$ or increased backflux of either $H^+$ or $H_2CO_3$, or both, through an abnormally permeable epithelium of the medullary collecting duct.[441, 606, 608]

The physiologic character of an experimental model of RTA-I induced in animals is of uncertain relevance to the primary physiologic disorder underlying the chronic RTA-I occurring in most humans. Indeed, the physiologic disorder expressed as RTA-I in adult humans may be different from that expressed as RTA-I in young children, even when the same genetic defect gives rise to both disorders. In adult patients with genetically transmitted RTA-I, as in those in whom the disorder occurs as part of an apparent autoimmune disease or appears to be sporadic, medullary nephrocalcinosis and recurrent nephrolithiasis usually occur, and recurrent pyelonephritis commonly occurs. Thus, in some patients with RTA-I the phenomenon of impaired ability to normally increase $U-B$ $P_{CO_2}$ might be an epiphenomenon and only indirectly related to the primary physiologic disorder underlying RTA-I. As discussed later, in one genotype of RTA-I (the San Francisco genotype), the acidification defect is of a severity that causes acidosis virtually from birth, and that severity does not appear to increase when nephrocalcinosis occurs. Suppose that in non-nephrocalcinotic children affected with this genotype of RTA-I, $U-B$ $P_{CO_2}$ was not reduced, but it was so in their genetically affected nephrocalcinotic relatives. Until the value of $U-B$ $P_{CO_2}$ is observed to be clearly reduced in children with this genotype of RTA-I from the outset of its expression, specifically, long before the occurrence of nephrocalcinosis and pyelonephritis, the physiologic meaning of a reduced value of $U-B$ $P_{CO_2}$ remains unclear in humans affected with chronic RTA-I.

### Hypocitraturia

In most patients with RTA-I, the urinary excretion of citrate is reduced[500, 505, 912–930] and often increases only modestly with alkali therapy that corrects acidosis.[500, 505, 921–927, 930, 931] The hypocitraturia can occur unassociated with hypocitratemia,[926] hypokalemia,[932, 933] or any recognized basis for an intracellular depletion of $K^+$ that might cause hypocitraturia.[933] In those members of kindreds affected with genetically transmitted RTA-I in whom the acidification defect occurs in childhood without nephrocalcinosis, severe hypocitraturia would appear to be invariable, even when the acidification defect does not give rise to acidosis. The basis of the hypocitraturia is unknown, but its occurrence in

patients with RTA-I that is genetically transmitted, associated with presumably autoimmune hypergammaglobulinemia, or seemingly sporadic suggests that its pathogenesis might in some way be related to that of the acidification defect of RTA-I. This might seem an unlikely proposition, given that the acidification disorder of RTA-I is inferred to be distal and the great bulk of citrate reabsorbed in the kidney occurs in the proximal tubule.[934, 935] Yet, the physiologic evidence that might seem to exonerate the acidification process of the proximal tubule, a normal fractional reabsorption of $HCO_3^-$ at normal plasma $HCO_3^-$ levels, permits only the inference that $HCO_3^-$ reabsorption in the proximal tubule is not substantially reduced. Whatever its mechanism, hypocitraturia (and reduced renal content of citrate) apparently can be critical to the pathogenesis of nephrocalcinosis and nephrolithiasis[921, 924] that are characteristic of RTA-I, regardless of whether it is a genetic trait, acquired, or causal of acidosis.[936] Furthermore, hypocitraturia in patients with RTA-I has pathogenetic implications of its own, given its capacity to foster nephrocalcinosis that can amplify the acidification dysfunction (see later).[505] Citrate forms a soluble complex with $Ca^{2+}$[937] that can prevent the precipitation of $Ca^{2+}$ in the urinary tract as either calcium phosphate or calcium oxalate.[938]

### GENETICS OF RTA-I AND THE SYNDROME OF INCOMPLETE RTA

Primary RTA-I can occur as an autosomal dominant trait that is fully expressed as an unremitting, acidosis-causing renal acidification defect in the first months of life.[495, 497, 498] The genetic defect, which apparently can be intrinsic to the kidney,[503] can give rise to nephrocalcinosis but does not necessarily compel its occurrence[939] or that of two phenomena presumably critical to its pathogenesis, hypercalciuria and severe hypocitraturia (Fig. 37–11; see Table 37–6). In all seven affected members of generations I, II, and III of the kindred studied in San Francisco,[495–498, 939] and in the one affected member of generation IV who received low-dose alkali therapy (1 to 3 mEq/kg/d), nephrocalcinosis was radiographically demonstrable when first sought as early as 5 years of age, even though such alkali therapy had been started as early as 2.5 years of age. However, in the four affected members of generation IV[495] and in three other unrelated children with familial, apparently autosomal dominant RTA in whom high-dose alkali therapy (4 to 12 mEq/kg/d) was initiated before 4 years of age,[939] neither radiographically demonstrable nephrocalcinosis nor nephrolithiasis occurred in treatment periods ranging from 10 to 20 years, and the GFR remained normal. In these patients, and in other similarly treated children in whom autosomal dominant, acidosis-causing RTA-I has been fully expressed in early childhood without radiographically demonstrable nephrocalcinosis or reduction in GFR, somatic stunting of growth, hypercalciuria, and an otherwise severe hypocitraturia have been invariably corrected by high-dose alkali therapy.[939]

In proposing that a given genotype of RTA-I could be variably expressed with respect to the severity of impairment in renal acidification, Buckalew and co-workers[922] correctly predicted that a genetically transmitted trait of

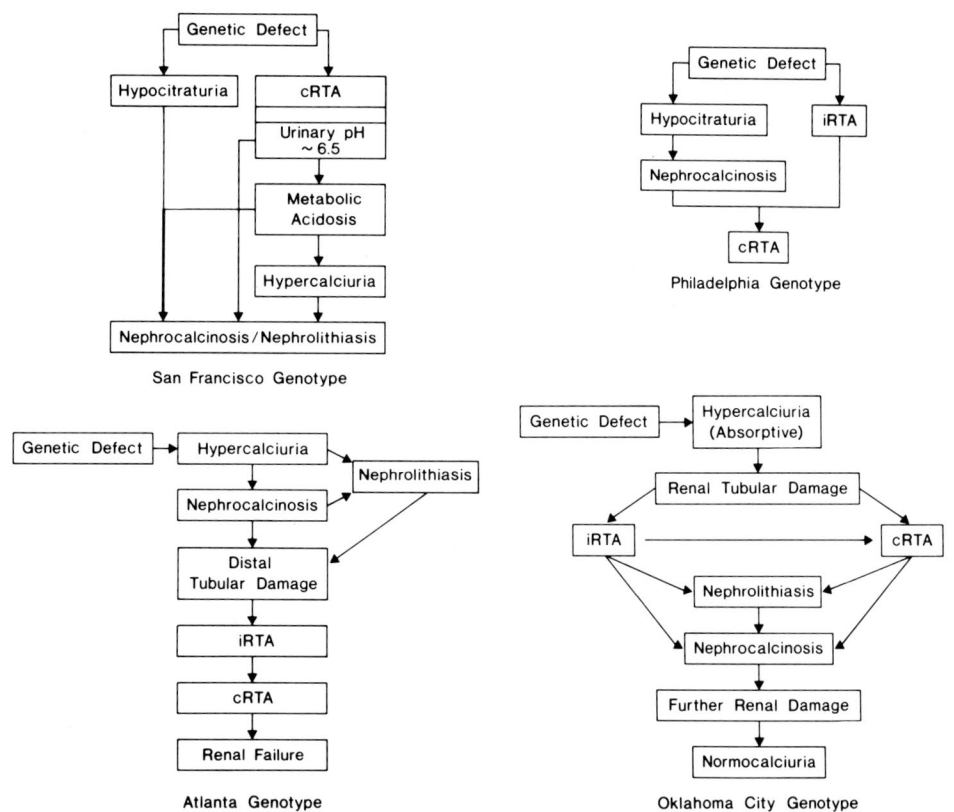

**Figure 37–11.** Proposed pathogenetic sequence through which genetic defects are linked to impaired renal acidification, nephrocalcinosis, and hypercalciuria (and, in two sequences, hypocitraturia) in patients in whom either RTA-I or hypercalciuria occurs as an autosomal dominant trait. RTA-I is qualified as incomplete RTA (iRTA) when the impairment in renal acidification does not give rise to acidosis and complete RTA-I (cRTA) when it does. The sequences depicted give rise to clinical syndromes that are separable from each other but variable (and sometimes similar) in physiologic and metabolic expression, depending on the age of those affected and, in at least two of the "genotypes" (San Francisco and Philadelphia), the likely mitigating effect of alkali therapy on hypercalciuria and hypocitraturia and, in one syndrome (Philadelphia), thereby on the apparently nephrocalcinosis-mediated progression of incomplete RTA-I to complete RTA. The genotypes are named after the city in which they were principally investigated. (From Morris RC Jr, Sebastian A: Renal tubular acidosis and Fanconi syndrome. *In* Stanbury JB, Wyngaarden JB, Fredrickson DS, et al [eds]: The Metabolic Basis of Inherited Disease, 5th ed. McGraw-Hill, New York, 1983, pp 1808–1866. Reproduced with permission of McGraw-Hill, Inc.)

RTA-I would be unaccompanied by frank acidosis in some affected members of some kindreds. Wrong and Davies[428] had earlier introduced the term incomplete syndrome of RTA to describe three nonacidotic patients with bilateral nephrocalcinosis who, like patients with the complete, acidotic syndrome of RTA, failed to decrease urine pH to normal minimums and to increase urinary excretion of titratable acid to normal maximums when they were challenged with NH₄Cl. Wrong and others have proposed that the renal disorder of those with incomplete RTA-I is a "milder" form of the acidosis-causing renal disorder of patients with complete RTA-I; the major difference is that in patients with incomplete RTA-I, functional renal mass and GFR are relatively well maintained, and as a consequence, excretion of $NH_4^+$ is great enough to prevent frank acidosis.[428, 607] Although this formulation may not always explain why acidosis occurs in some patients with RTA-I and not in others, the concept of an incomplete form of RTA has proved to be clinically useful.

In one apparently autosomal dominant genotype of RTA-I, it would appear that the phenotype invariably expressed initially is incomplete RTA in combination with severe hypocitraturia. Complete RTA predictably occurs in those affected with this genotype, but apparently only in progression from incomplete RTA, and apparently only after nephrocalcinosis has further restricted renal acidification. Norman and colleagues[505] studied three affected kindreds with the genotype in Philadelphia (see Table 37–6 and Fig. 37–11). In a woman in whom incomplete RTA-I had occurred at age 15 years without radiographically apparent nephrocalcinosis, they documented the occurrence at age 24 years of complete RTA in association with radiographically demonstrable nephrocalcinosis and a moderate reduction in GFR. In this woman's three affected first-order relatives, her father and an 8-year-old brother and son, RTA-I occurred in association with radiographically demonstrated nephrocalcinosis. In each of the other two kindreds they studied, Norman and colleagues also documented the occurrence of incomplete RTA unassociated with radiographically apparent nephrocalcinosis, in each instance in a 5-year-old girl. In each of the girls' three affected, older first-order relatives, including a parent of each, complete RTA occurred in association with radiographically demonstrated nephrocalcinosis. Whereas hypercalciuria occurred only in those with untreated complete RTA, hypocitraturia occurred in all affected members from all three kindreds and was invariably severe in each. The extent to which alkali therapy mitigated the hypocitraturia was, however, variable and unrelated to the severity of the acidification defect. Whereas alkali therapy readily corrected the hypocitraturia of one of the girls with incomplete RTA and one adult with complete RTA, the amount required by both boys with complete RTA (4 mEq/kg/d) was twice that needed to correct either acidosis or hypercalciuria. In one of the two girls with incomplete RTA-I, even such high-dose alkali therapy only slightly mitigated the hypocitraturia.[505] If, as proposed by Norman and colleagues, hypocitraturia in those with the "Philadelphia genotype" is critical to the pathogenesis of nephrocalcinosis that amplifies incomplete RTA into complete RTA, hypocitraturia would be not only a direct expression of that genotype but also a requirement for its full phenotypic expression.

In three children with familial RTA-I in whom nephrocalcinosis was radiographically nondemonstrable and in whom acidosis was of minimal severity, Coe and Parks[940] found that alkali therapy in amounts that raised plasma $HCO_3^-$ concentration to values well within the normal range had little effect on the strikingly severe hypocitraturia. Predictably, however, the alkali therapy did correct the hypercalciuria and appeared to reduce the frequency of nephrolithiasis. In a nonazotemic 24-year-old man with RTA-I, nephrocalcinosis, and nephrolithiasis, both hypercalciuria (on a low-calcium diet) and severe hypocitraturia occurred initially in the absence of acidosis. Buckalew and co-workers[922] described the occurrence in a 1-year period of progressively severe acidosis in association with repeated episodes of renal calculi. Nephrocalcinosis was radiographically demonstrated in the patient's older brother, who probably had RTA-I.[922] Their father had suffered from recurrent renal calculi. Apart from their obvious therapeutic implications, the observations of Norman, Coe, and Buckalew raise the important possibility that in some genotypes of RTA-I, either hypocitraturia or hypercalciuria or both can be primary expressions of the genetic defect and critical to the pathogenesis of nephrocalcinosis and nephrolithiasis and thereby lead to the progression of incomplete RTA to complete RTA. The observations of Norman and Coe and colleagues raise the additional possibility that severe hypocitraturia that is extremely resistant to alkali therapy may also be a particular primary expression of some genotypes of RTA-I.

Donnelly and co-workers[609] have proposed that the incomplete syndrome of RTA stems from intracellular acidosis in the proximal renal tubule. As a consequence of such a lesion, proximal tubule reabsorption of citrate is increased and its urinary excretion is reduced. Also, renal generation of $NH_4^+$ is increased. $NH_4^+$ excretion is thereby increased, and urine pH is inappropriately high during $NH_4Cl$ loading because buffering of distally secreted $H^+$ is increased by increased medullary ammonia. Donnelly and colleagues pointed out that $K^+$ depletion, which can cause intracellular acidosis in the kidney,[941] gives rise to urinary findings much like those of incomplete RTA. He suggested that in time, chronic hypocitraturia leads to nephrocalcinosis, and increased amounts of $NH_4^+/NH_3$ in the renal medulla lead to chronic tubulointerstitial disease. The formulation has a potentially important therapeutic implication.

In patients with incomplete RTA, particularly those in whom it is genetically transmitted and seemingly destined to evolve into acidosis-causing RTA-I, $KHCO_3$ might be a more effective therapy than $NaHCO_3$ as a way of increasing urinary citrate and decreasing urinary $Ca^{2+}$ excretion[929, 942–944] enough to possibly forestall or prevent that baleful evolution.

Hamed and co-workers[507] studied a large kindred in which RTA was an apparent consequence of hypercalciuria that occurred as an autosomal dominant trait in four successive generations (see Table 37–6 and Fig. 37–11). In this kindred, RTA-I was diagnosed in 8 members of the first three generations, in only those with hypercalciuria and in none of the 14 children studied (generation IV), including 3 with hypercalciuria. Nephrocalcinosis was radiographically demonstrable in only, but in each of, the five of seven members of generations I and II in whom RTA-I was diagnosed. Complete RTA was diagnosed in four members from generations I and II and in a 17-year-old girl from generation III in whom the GFR was normal. Incomplete RTA was diagnosed in three members, in two from generation III and in a 50-year-old woman from generation II. Hamed and co-workers proposed that in time, in those affected with the genotype ultimately expressed as RTA-I, hypercalciuria (which might reflect intestinal hyperabsorption) damaged the renal tubule so as to impair acidification and further the pathogenesis of nephrocalcinosis. These investigators reported neither measurements of urinary citrate nor results with alkali therapy.

Of considerable interest and exceptional potential importance is a described baby girl with $HCO_3^-$ wasting; apparently RTA-I; and reduced activity of type I carnitine palmitoyl transferase, which impairs mitochondrial β-oxidation of long-chain fatty acids but not that of medium-chain fatty acids.[945] After the girl ate a low-fat diet supplemented with medium-chain fatty acids for a period of 2.5 months, the RTA disappeared, as did intermittent episodes of nonketotic hypoglucosemic coma that were associated with transient hepatomegaly and increased plasma concentrations of hepatic enzymes, ammonia, and free fatty acids; her head circumference, height, and weight increased sharply. The parents of the affected girl are probably consanguineous. Thus, it seems likely that the severely reduced activity of type I carnitine palmitoyl transferase (measured in her fibroblasts) is genetically determined and in some way causal of both the renal and hepatic dysfunction she suffered. Only the diet-responsive, episodic hepatic disorder has previously been described in patients with this enzymatic defect,[946, 947] a defect demonstrated in the liver[946] but not yet in the kidney.

The RTA of the affected girl was demonstrably not associated with the proximal renal tubule dysfunctions characteristic of Fanconi syndrome. Despite severe hyperchloremic acidosis, the urine pH was 8.67, the fractional excretion of $HCO_3^-$, 6.4%. With dietary therapy, the initially reduced value of $U - B$ $PCO_2$ increased substantially, "indicating that the capacity to transport hydrogen ions had been restored"; the lowest value of urine pH recorded was 6.3. The investigators proposed that the RTA-I was a consequence of "an apparent energy shortage in the kidney" that was corrected by the dietary supplement of medium-chain fatty acids. This proposal, however, would require some revision if it were demonstrated that impaired renal acidification did not recur when the supplement was discontinued or did recur when dietary long-chain fatty acids were reinstituted, despite provision of the supplement. Specifically, a nephrotoxic metabolite of a long-chain fatty acid generated in either the kidney or liver, or both, could account for the reversible occurrence of RTA-I in the affected girl. Yet, with the apparent exception of the renal disorder of this patient, genetically determined RTA-I has not been reported to be a reversible, primary renal expression of a genetically determined enzymatic defect that occurs in both the liver and renal tubule. Rather, the reversible renal tubule dysfunction that occurs with an enzymatic defect of that distribution is predictably a complex dysfunction of the proximal tubule like that of Fanconi syndrome, which usually includes RTA-II.[642, 874, 876, 885, 948] Indeed, when mitochondrial β-oxidation of long-chain fatty acids is acutely, reversibly inhibited in the kidney and liver by intravenous administration of 4-pentenoate, there occurs within minutes a reversible complex dysfunction of the proximal tubule like that of Fanconi syndrome, including RTA-II.[617, 949] Although the possibility appears not to have been systematically investigated, 4-pentenoate might disorder both distal and proximal acidification simultaneously.[617] Long-chain fatty acids are preferred metabolic fuels of the kidney.[950]

Thus, in the affected girl, the occurrence of nutritionally reversible RTA-I without apparent dysfunction of the proximal tubule accords with the possibility that her presumed genetic renal defect of type I carnitine palmitoyl transferase involves only an isoform restricted to the distal tubule, or one occurring in both distal and proximal tubules but affecting only $H^+$ secretion mediated by $H^+$-ATPase. The $HCO_3^-$-wasting classic RTA-I of infants and children[435, 495, 893] may reflect impaired renal acidification of both proximal and distal nephrons.[893] By shunting metabolism of long-chain fatty acids to ω-hydroxylation–mediated formation of long-chain dicarboxylic acids that can uncouple mitochondrial oxidative phosphorylation,[951] defective type I carnitine palmitoyl transferase might disorder mitochondria-rich α-type intercalated cells in the cortical and outer medullary collecting duct and their $H^+$-ATPase[895, 911, 952] and possibly also $H^+,K^+$-ATPase.[901] In these cells, accumulation of so metabolized and nonmetabolized long-chain fatty acids might also disorder the basolateral $Cl^-$ channel[953] and thereby entrain the pathogenetic sequence of impaired basolateral $Cl^-$ exit → impaired basolateral $Cl^-/HCO_3^-$ exchange → impaired $HCO_3^-$ reabsorption.

Buckalew and co-workers[506] studied a large kindred of four generations in which hypercalciuria appeared to be the primary metabolic manifestation of an autosomal dominant genetic defect (see Table 37–6 and Fig. 37–11). Radiographically demonstrable nephrocalcinosis and hypercalciuria occurred in six affected members from the first three generations, including two children. Four of the six were diagnosed has having incomplete RTA-I. However, in the other two kindred members with nephrocalcinosis, an impairment in renal acidification was demonstrably absent, a combination not observed in other kindreds in which a renal disorder diagnosed as RTA-I has occurred in multiple members. Only one affected member of the kindred had acidosis, a 33-year-old man in whom the GFR was 6 mL/min and the serum creatinine concentration 7 mg/dL. In those with most severe hypercalciuria, there also occurred hyperexcretion of amino acids, lysozyme, and immunoglobulin L chain, phenomena that tend to implicate the proximal tubule and rarely accompany RTA-I. For the pathogenesis of this hereditary renal disorder, which would appear to be unique in the literature, Buckalew proposed that the sequence of hypercalciuria → nephrocalcinosis → renal damage was critical to the pathogenesis of the observed impairments in renal acidification. Hypocitraturia did not occur in those affected. In one of the hypercalciuric boys, bilateral nephrocalcinosis became radiographically apparent and incomplete RTA demonstrable 4 years after initiation of alkali therapy given to attenuate hypercalciuria.[506]

In a consideration of the classification, pathogenesis, and pathophysiology of genetically transmitted nonhyperkalemic distal RTA, certain questions arise. Has RTA so characterized ever been primarily expressed as a defect in distal $H^+$ secretion that impairs $NH_4^+$ excretion enough to cause acidosis but not its capacity to generate a high $H^+$ gradient and normally reduce urine pH during acidosis? One might think that such a genetically transmitted RTA would have been identified, given the increasing recognition of 1) the possibility of its occurrence, 2) the large numbers of patients reported with well-documented familial distal RTA and its clear genetic transmission in many, 3) the potential of hyperchloremic acidosis to impair growth, and 4) the importance of identifying all family members affected as early in life as possible to initiate appropriate alkali therapy. It can of course be argued that there is only a recent recognition of the possibility that genetically transmitted distal RTA might be of the type in question and that the long tradition of using urine pH as the litmus test for impaired renal acidification has worked to thwart its identification. Yet, the familial occurrence of persisting nonhyperkalemic hyperchloremic acidosis and $NH_4^+$ excretion reduced enough to cause it, despite an appropriately acid urine, is not such a subtle syndrome, particularly if it is associated with impaired somatic growth, as one might expect. Such a syndrome would presumably be recognized at least as a familial clinical disorder of renal acidification that might reflect a genetically transmitted disease. At this writing, there is no reported clear evidence of such a disorder.

However, observations reported by Strife and co-workers[953a] suggest that such a disorder may in fact occur. These investigations describe 11 quite young children with generally mild, chronic hyperchloremic acidosis in whom urine pH was normally reduced but in whom the capacity to increase $U - B$ $P_{CO_2}$ in response to $HCO_3^-$ loading was found to be impaired. Most of those affected were growth retarded. No patient had hyperkalemia. During 2 to 6 years of follow-up, the "rate-dependent dRTA" of none of these patients "evolved to a more severe impairment of distal acidification." Measurements of $NH_4^+$ excretion were not reported. The investigators stated that "the cousin of one of these patients is being treated for RTA at another medical center and the father and aunt of another patient have classic dRTA."

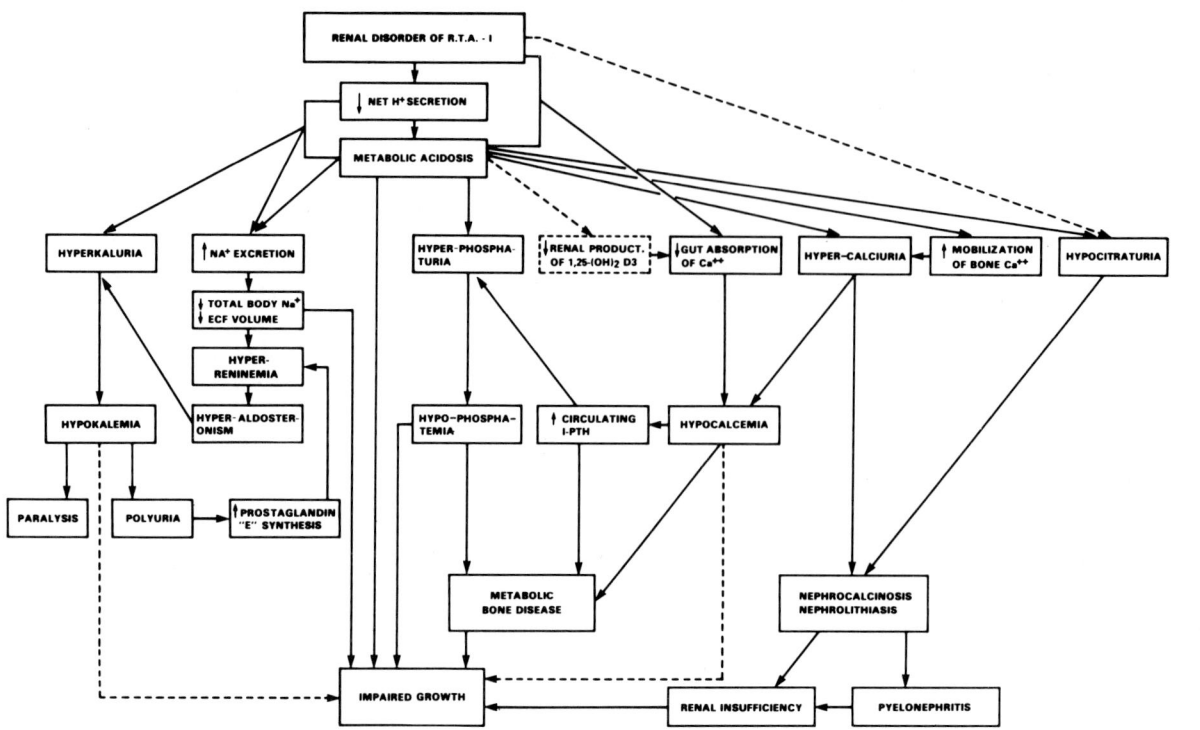

**Figure 37–12.** Pathogenetic basis of the metabolic and clinical expressions that can occur in patients with type I RTA. (From Morris RC Jr, Sebastian A: Renal tubular acidosis and Fanconi syndrome. *In* Stanbury JB, Wyngaarden JB, Fredrickson DS, et al [eds]: The Metabolic Basis of Inherited Disease, 5th ed. McGraw-Hill, New York, 1983, pp 1808–1866. Reproduced with permission of McGraw-Hill, Inc.)

## PATHOPHYSIOLOGY, METABOLIC DERANGEMENT, AND THE EFFECT OF ALKALI THERAPY

### Potassium and Sodium

Hypokalemia, renal $K^+$ wasting, and secondary hyperaldosteronism are common complications of both RTA-I and RTA-II* (Fig. 37–12). However, many and perhaps most patients with genetically transmitted RTA-I are not hypokalemic, which is more characteristic of RTA-I as part of an autoimmune disease.[900] Renal wasting of $K^+$ can be said to occur when urinary excretion of $K^+$ exceeds 40 mEq/d despite hypokalemia (and in the absence of more than moderate metabolic alkalosis)[956] (Fig. 37–13). In patients with RTA-I, but not in patients with RTA-II, correction of acidosis with alkali therapy is predictably attended by a reduction in the urinary excretion rate of $K^+$ (see Figs. 37–6 and 37–7), $Na^+$, and aldosterone; with sustained correction of acidosis, the external balances of $K^+$ and $Na^+$ may become sufficiently positive to correct hypokalemia and $Na^+$ depletion.[955] Correction of $Na^+$ depletion lessens the stimulus to hyperaldosteronism.[437, 955] In most patients with genetically transmitted RTA-I, potassium supplements are not required to maintain normokalemia when correction of acidosis is sustained with alkali therapy. However, in patients with type I RTA that occurs as part of an autoimmune disease, supplemental dietary potassium may be required to maintain normokalemia despite sustained correction of acidosis.[956]

*References 427–430, 433–435, 437, 476, 544, 821, 954–957.

### Calcium and Phosphorus

Hypercalciuria and increased renal clearance of $P_i$ predictably occur during metabolic acidosis.[423, 938, 958] Medullary nephrocalcinosis (Fig. 37–14) and recurrent nephrolithiasis are characteristic and presumably a consequence both of prolonged hypercalciuria[423, 437] and of greatly diminished urinary excretion of citrate (see earlier).[607, 924, 938] Calcium phosphate and calcium oxalate are the major constituents of urinary stones in patients with RTA-I.[936] Hypocalcemia and secondary hyperparathyroidism[423, 959, 960] are consequences of both hypercalciuria and impaired gut absorption of $Ca^{2+}$.[423, 437, 961] Hypocalcemia and hypophosphatemia are presumably causally related to the rickets and osteomalacia that can occur in patients with RTA-I,[423, 425, 962] if now uncommonly.[963] Caldas and co-workers[962] have suggested that the occurrence of rickets in RTA-I is causally related to vitamin D deficiency, not acidosis, which they believe may cause only osteopenia. Chronic metabolic acidosis titrates bone buffers and thereby promotes mobilization of skeletal $Ca^{2+}$.[958, 964] Metabolic acidosis can also stimulate osteoclastic activity and inhibit osteoblastic activity.[965–967] The plasma concentration of $1,25(OH)_2D_3$ has not been found to be reduced in acidotic patients with RTA-I.[863] Yet, metabolic acidosis can restrict the capacity of the kidney to respond to physiologic stimuli that normally increase its production rate of $1,25(OH)_2D_3$ and hence the plasma concentration of this hormone.[867] In growing children with RTA-I, metabolic acidosis may restrict the capacity of the kidney to sustain circulating concentrations of $1,25(OH)D_2$ at whatever increased levels may be needed for achieving optimal growth. Nephrocalcinosis combined with either rickets or osteomalacia is nearly specific for RTA-I when hypervitaminosis D is excluded by the patient's history.[968]

With sustained alkali therapy, hypercalciuria can disappear,[423, 495] citrate excretion can increase,[505, 925, 939] gut absorption of $Ca^{2+}$ can increase,[423, 961] the renal clearance of $P_i$ can decrease, and the serum concentrations of both $P_i$ and $Ca^{2+}$ can become normal.[423–426] Nephrocalcinosis and nephrolithiasis persist, but stones may be passed less frequently.[501, 940] Rickets, osteomalacia, and osteopenia can heal with alkali therapy alone.[962, 969, 970]

### Growth and Nephrocalcinosis of Children

In infants and young children with untreated RTA-I, impaired growth is characteristic, but normal growth is predictably attained and maintained with alkali therapy that maintains the plasma $HCO_3^-$ concentration well within normal limits.[495, 893, 962, 971] In stunted infants with RTA-I, the velocity of growth predictably increases strikingly within weeks of initiation of alkali therapy, and normal stature is predictably attained within 3 to 6 months.[495, 962] Older children may require several years to attain normal height. Renal $HCO_3^-$ wasting tends to occur or increase in severity when growth velocity increases sharply. When initiated before the age of 3 years, alkali therapy sufficient to maintain

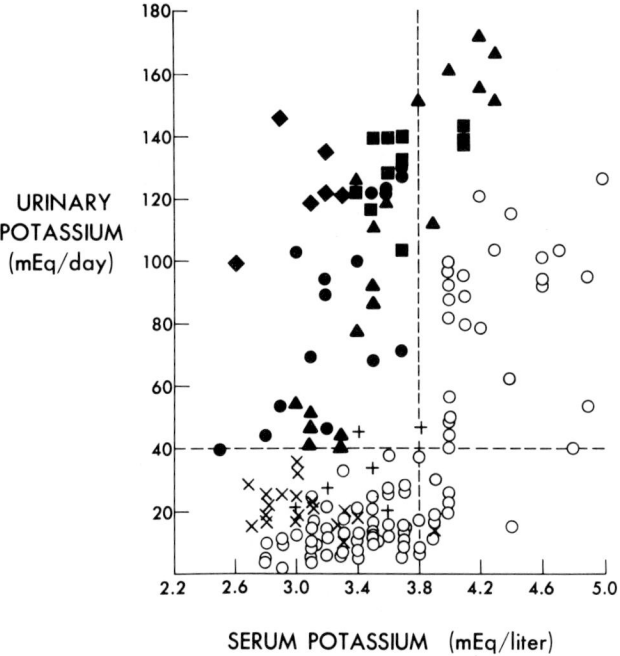

**Figure 37–13.** Relationship between urinary $K^+$ excretion and serum $K^+$ concentration in patients with RTA in whom correction of acidosis was sustained ( ◆, ●, ▲, ■) and in normal subjects experimentally depleted of $K^+$ by dietary restriction (○, +, ×). Some of the subjects represented by ○ were mildly alkalotic and were excreting significant amounts of urinary $HCO_3^-$; the subjects represented by + were moderately alkalotic and were excreting more than 50 mEq of urinary $HCO_3^-$ daily; the subjects represented by × were given large amounts of deoxycorticosterone after hypokalemia had supervened. (From Sebastian A, McSherry E, Morris RC Jr: Renal potassium wasting in renal tubular acidosis [RTA]: Its occurrence in types 1 and 2 RTA despite sustained correction of systemic acidosis. J Clin Invest 50:667–678, 1971.)

plasma $HCO_3^-$ concentration well within the normal limit (4 to 12 mEq/kg/d) can prevent nephrocalcinosis,[939] possibly by preventing the hypercalciuria and attenuating or correcting the severe hypocitraturia that are otherwise predictable without alkali therapy.[495, 505, 939, 940, 959] Accordingly, in many children with RTA-I, both impaired growth and nephrocalcinosis can be regarded as preventable.

## CLINICAL MANAGEMENT OF PATIENTS WITH RTA-I

In patients with previously undiagnosed RTA, hypokalemia, severe acidosis, and hypocalcemia often coexist and may require immediate therapeutic response. Management of hypokalemia-mediated muscle weakness and respiratory depression requires hospitalization and careful monitoring of ventilatory rate and depth, as well as facilities for airway maintenance and assisted ventilation. As described before, hypokalemia should be corrected rapidly with intravenously administered potassium—before correction of acidosis.[437, 891, 892]

Almost all children and infants are able to take $NaHCO_3$ in the amounts necessary to sustain correction of acidosis, even when these amounts are as great as 14 mEq/kg/d. In most children with RTA-I, the amount of alkali required will increase, usually when the rate of growth increases sharply. If dietary NaCl is restricted because of an $Na^+$-retaining state, the amount of alkali necessary to correct acidosis is decreased. In some patients, particularly those with autoimmune RTA, potassium supplements of 50 to 100 mEq/d may be required to maintain normokalemia even after acidosis has been corrected. One of the frequent complications (and conceivably a cause) of RTA-I is pyelonephritis, the optimal treatment of which has yet to be determined. Attempted eradication of the causal organism is rarely if ever successful and may be unrealistic, particularly in patients with nephrocalcinosis.

## PROGNOSIS

The prognosis of most well-managed adult patients with RTA-I is determined more by the usually accompanying autoimmune disease, Sjögren syndrome, or chronic liver disorder than by either the functional consequences of the renal disease or its complications—pyelonephritis, nephrocalcinosis, and nephrolithiasis. Morbidity, generally considered to be causally related to the autoimmune state, such as Raynaud phenomenon, recurrent purpura, and even the dry mouth of Sjögren syndrome, may disappear with alkali therapy. In the great majority of well-managed adult patients with RTA-I, the GFR and the severity of the acidification defect remain unchanged even when the GFR is reduced substantially when alkali therapy is started and despite continuing bacteriologic evidence of chronic pyelonephritis. For many patients in whom RTA-I occurs as part of Sjögren syndrome, life is long and vigorous. In patients in whom RTA-I occurs as an autosomal dominant trait that is not primarily expressed as hypercalciuria[506, 507] (see Table 37–6 and Fig. 37–11), the prognosis is good with continued alkali therapy.[972]

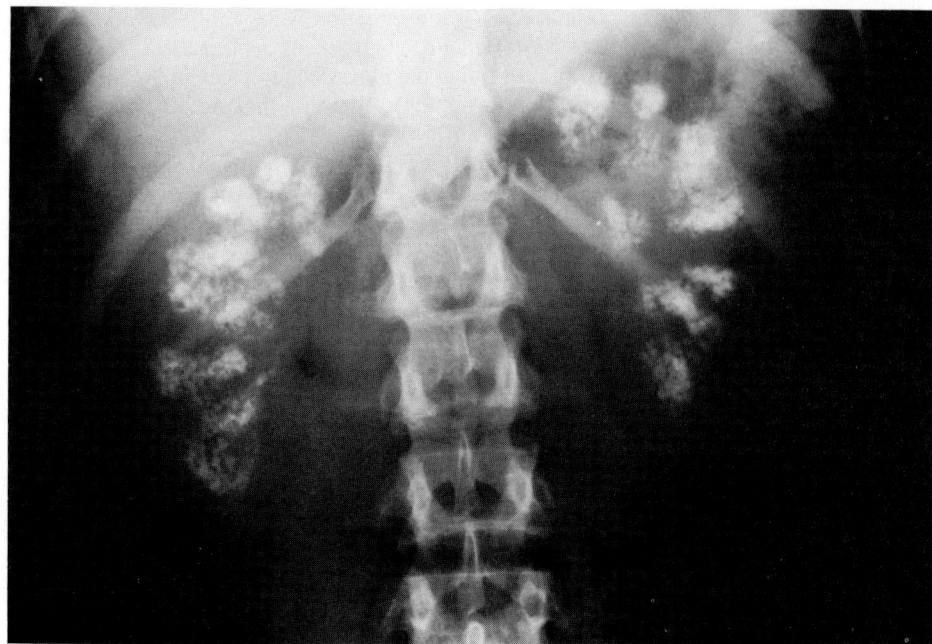

**Figure 37–14.** Bilateral nephrocalcinosis in a patient with type I RTA. (From Morris RC Jr, Sebastian A: Disorders of the renal tubule that cause disorders of fluid, acid-base, and electrolyte metabolism. *In* Maxwell MH, Kleeman CR [eds]: Clinical Disorders of Fluid and Electrolyte Metabolism, 3rd ed. McGraw-Hill, New York, 1980, p 883. Reproduced with permission of McGraw-Hill, Inc.)

## CLINICAL CONSIDERATIONS APPLICABLE TO BOTH RTA-I AND RTA-II

### "Autoimmune" RTA

Of 21 patients with autoimmune RTA we have studied, all have been women, and all but 1 have had Sjögren syndrome,[972] apparently the most common cause of acquired RTA-I. Eighteen have had prototypic RTA-I; in one, the disorder was a hybrid of RTA-I and RTA-II. One patient had prototypic RTA-II in association with the renal dysfunction of the Fanconi syndrome; in this patient, evidence of impaired distal acidification was demonstrably absent. Joint disease has not been apparent clinically or radiographically, and abnormal eye findings are usually minimal. Not all of these patients complained of dry mouth, but histologic changes in salivary ducts diagnostic of Sjögren syndrome have been invariable in buccal mucosa (except in 1 patient with autoimmune RTA and in none of 18 patients with familial, genetically transmitted RTA-I we have seen). In three patients, autoimmune RTA-I first became apparent in the immediate postpartum period, when severe proximal muscle weakness occurred acutely in association with striking hypokalemia and renal $K^+$ wasting.[972] Acute hypokalemia syndromes and renal $K^+$ wasting that persists despite alkali therapy appear to be much more common in autoimmune RTA-I than in familial or "idiopathic" RTA-I.

### Muscle Weakness and Metabolic Bone Disease

In patients with either RTA-I or RTA-II, the rapidly occurring, severe muscle weakness of severe hypokalemia is the most dramatic and acutely life-threatening abnormality[973]; in patients with autoimmune RTA-I, it is the all-too-common initial clinical expression, but this event is rare in patients with genetically transmitted RTA. In patients with RTA-II, muscle weakness is more commonly insidious in onset, less severe, and a consequence of the proximal myopathy that attends metabolic bone disease.[974] In adult patients in whom RTA-II occurs in the setting of intestinal malabsorption, hypocalcemia, secondary hyperparathyroidism, and hypophosphatemia, chronic weakness of the proximal muscles is often the major complaint.[423, 974–976] Those affected typically have difficulty rising unassisted from a seated position. The weakness is usually associated with bone pain; symmetric, often severe bone tenderness; and sometimes radiographic evidence of osteomalacia, most characteristically pseudofractures.[423, 968] The metabolic bone disease may be of such striking clinical severity that even modest pretibial pressure elicits excruciating pain. The gait is characteristically slow and waddling (like a duck). All muscle effort may be attended by great discomfort. Deep tendon reflexes remain active.[974] Electromyographic and histologic examinations usually reveal little, if any, objective evidence of muscle disease. The weakness is often mistaken for a psychoneurotic symptom. Although its pathogenetic mechanism is undefined, the myopathic disorder is responsive to therapy that heals the associated metabolic bone disease. The myopathy is rare in patients with RTA-I. In affected adults with RTA-I, normal muscle strength returns with alkali therapy alone, but often only after several weeks. In affected patients with RTA-II as part of the malabsorption syndrome, the myopathy responds dramatically and usually rapidly to therapy with alkali and vitamin D. By disturbing the metabolism of $Ca^{2+}$ and $P_i$ in muscles, a deficiency or disordered metabolism of vitamin $D^{977, 978}$ might be a pathogenetic factor in the myopathy that attends metabolic bone disease. Hyperparathyroidism and $P_i$ depletion might also be pathogenetic factors. In patients with renal osteodystrophy, striking and rapid amelioration of muscle weakness has been reported with the administration of $1,25(OH)_2D_3$.[979]

## pH-Dependent Urinary Excretion of Drugs

In patients with any type of RTA, corrective alkali therapy is invariably attended by intense alkalinity of the urine; the urine pH is frequently greater than 8. This has important implications with respect to the clinical pharmacology of certain drugs whose urinary excretion is pH dependent and an important mode of their disposition.[980, 981] As a group, the phenylalkylamines, including pseudoephedrine, have a high pK (greater than 8), and intense alkalinity of the urine greatly retards their excretion and acts to increase their blood level.[982, 983] The cinchona alkaloids, quinidine and quinine, which also have a pK greater than 8, and salicylates are affected similarly.[984, 985] Accordingly, in patients with any type of RTA, corrective alkali therapy predisposes them to certain kinds of drug intoxication. Frank psychosis has occurred in children with RTA who have received both a corrective dose of alkali therapy and the usual dose of pseudoephedrine for otitis media.

# Type IV Distal Renal Tubular Acidosis

Type IV distal RTA is a hyperkalemic, hyperchloremic metabolic acidosis associated with impaired $NH_4^+$ excretion and often some reduction in GFR.

## PHYSIOLOGIC CHARACTERISTICS

The physiologic characteristics of type IV RTA are those that would be predicted to occur in patients in whom aldosterone is reduced either in circulating amount or in renal physiologic effect[986, 987] (Table 37–7).

The effect of aldosterone deficiency on the acidification process of the mammalian nephron has been studied in adrenalectomized dogs and humans maintained with physiologic replacement doses of glucocorticoid and mineralocorticoid hormones.[987, 991, 1030, 1118, 1119] When the administration of mineralocorticoid hormones is discontinued, hyperkalemia and hyperchloremic acidosis occur, despite attainment of a normally reduced urine pH. A decrease in urinary excretion of $NH_4^+$ accounts for decreased net acid excretion. Renal $HCO_3^-$ reabsorption is reduced at normal plasma $HCO_3^-$ concentration (sustained by alkali therapy), but the magnitude of the reduction (<15%) is not sufficient to implicate the proximal tubule. Renal clearance of $K^+$ is greatly reduced, and the serum concentration of $K^+$ increases strikingly when dietary potassium is increased. Proximal tubule dysfunction does not occur as judged by the absence of hyperaminoaciduria or increased renal clearance of $P_i$.

## CELLULAR MECHANISM AND PATHOPHYSIOLOGY

In the cortical collecting duct, principal cells, unlike neighboring intercalated cells, do not secrete $H^+$ (see Fig. 37–9). Principal cells do, however, reabsorb $Na^+$ and generate thereby a lumen-negative potential difference that potentiates $H^+$ secretion in α-type intercalated cells and $K^+$ secretion in the principal cells. In the cortical collecting duct, transport of all of these ions is under exquisite tonic control of aldosterone.[1120, 1121] Aldosterone receptors are present in both principal and intercalated cells.[1122] In the principal cells, aldosterone increases 1) $Na^+$ absorption by increasing luminal $Na^+$ conductance[1123–1125] and by stimulating the activity of the basolateral $Na^+,K^+$-ATPase[1122, 1126–1129] and 2) $K^+$ secretion by increasing both the luminal[897, 1130] and basolateral[1131] membrane conductance of $K^+$ (in conjunction with the increased lumen negativity and activity of $Na^+,K^+$-ATPase). Aldosterone stimulates $H^+$ secretion directly by stimulating $H^+$-ATPase in the α-type intercalated cells in both the cortical collecting duct and outer medullary collecting duct.[1132–1135] Type IV RTA usually occurs as part of a global disorder of the distal nephron that impairs $Na^+$ absorption and $K^+$ secretion as well.

Type IV distal RTA can be caused by abnormalities in renin biosynthesis or release; angiotensin formation due to converting enzyme inhibition; aldosterone release, biosynthesis, or action; or luminal $Na^+$ permeability as can occur with diuretics such as triamterene or amiloride. In addition, shunting of the $Na^+$ transport potential by enhanced $Cl^-$ permeability or destruction by tubulointerstitial disease or other disorders of the cortical collecting tubule cell and $Na^+,K^+$-ATPase can globally affect transport in this nephron segment. The reduction in net acid excretion in type IV RTA results not only from diminished secretion of $H^+$ in the cortical collecting tubule but also from diminished excretion of $NH_4^+$, because in part hyperkalemia suppresses ammoniagenesis[1136] and $NH_4^+$ reabsorption in the medullary thick ascending limb.[594]

## HYPOALDOSTERONISM

### Animal Studies

In the dog and rat, aldosterone deficiency appears to impair the capacity of the distal nephron to secrete $H^+$ at normal rates, but not its ability to generate normally steep lumen-to-blood $H^+$ concentration gradients.[1119, 1137] Reduced urinary excretion of $NH_4^+$ occurs, apparently owing to a diminished renal production of ammonia, because it occurs in the absence of an increase in urine pH or a decrease in urine flow. The reduction in ammonia production is in part due to hyperkalemia,[1136] because the excretion rate of $NH_4^+$ varies inversely with the plasma $K^+$ concentration and does not decrease when mineralocorticoid is discontinued and hyperkalemia is prevented by restricting potassium intake. When measured at low luminal buffer concentrations (as when renal production and urinary excretion of ammonia are greatly reduced by hyperkalemia), the values of urine pH in mineralocorticoid-deficient dogs or rats are not higher than those in similarly acidotic mineralocorticoid-replete dogs or rats. However, when measured at increased luminal buffer concentrations (as when urinary $NH_4^+$ concentrations and excretion are increased), the urine pH is substantially greater in mineralocorticoid-deficient dogs than in mineralocorticoid-replete dogs, a finding indicating that in the former group the $H^+$ secretory capacity is blunted. In selec-

**TABLE 37–7. Clinical Spectrum of Disorders That Cause Type IV Renal Tubular Acidosis**

**Disorders That Cause Aldosterone Deficiency**
Combined deficiency of aldosterone and adrenal glucocorticoid hormones
    Addison disease[987-990]
    Bilateral adrenalectomy[987, 991]
    Inherited impairment of steroidogenesis: 21β-hydroxylase deficiency[992-994]
Aldosterone deficiency without glucocorticoid hormone deficiency
    Inherited impairment of aldosterone biosynthesis: corticosterone methyl oxidase deficiency[995-1006]
    Acquired impairment of aldosterone secretion
        Long-term heparin administration[1007-1011]
        Idiopathic zona glomerulosa defect[321, 1012-1015]
    Deficient renin secretion[573, 991, 1013, 1016-1031]
        Chronic, diffuse, histologically evident renal parenchymal disease and reduced GFR
            Diabetic nephropathy[1018, 1019]
            Tubulointerstitial nephritis[1016, 1023, 1032, 1033]
            Obstructive uropathy[1030]
            Renal transplantation[576]
            Systemic lupus erythematosus[1025, 1026, 1034]
        Impaired renal prostaglandin production
            Administration of prostaglandin synthesis inhibitors (indomethacin)[1035-1037]
            Renal disease[1038, 1039]
        Increased extracellular fluid volume due to impaired renal NaCl clearance associated with chronic, diffuse, histologically evident renal parenchymal disease and reduced GFR[1031]
        Increased extracellular fluid volume due to impaired renal NaCl clearance unassociated with chronic, diffuse, histologically evident renal parenchymal disease and reduced GFR (component of type II pseudohypoaldosteronism)
            Intrinsic defect of renal tubule?
            Atrial natriuretic peptide deficiency[1040, 1041]
        Associated with the acquired immunodeficiency syndrome[1042]
    Decreased angiotensin II production without renin deficiency
        Administration of converting enzyme inhibitors[1042, 1043]
        Endogenous impairment of angiotensin II production[1044]
    Acquired adrenal insensitivity to angiotensin II[1045]
    Impairment of angiotensinogen production[1046]
    Chronic idiopathic hypoaldosteronism in adults and children[993, 1047-1051]

**Attenunated Renal Responsiveness to Aldosterone and Consequent Hyperreninemia and Hyperaldosteronism: Pseudohypoaldosteronism**
Classic pseudohypoaldosteronism of infancy (type I pseudohypoaldosteronism)[995, 1000, 1052-1080]
Chronic tubulointerstitial disease with glomerular insufficiency, "salt-wasting nephritis"[1081-1086]
Drugs: spironolactone, amiloride, triamterene
Abnormally high levels of endogenous aldosterone antagonists (e.g., progesterone): 21β-hydroxylase deficiency[1087-1089]
Far-advanced or end-stage renal insufficiency

**Relative Aldosterone Deficiency and Attenuated Renal Responsiveness to Aldosterone**
Inherited impairment of steroidogenesis characterized by both aldosterone deficiency and increased levels of endogenous aldosterone antagonists: 21β-hydroxylase deficiency ("congenital adrenal hyperplasia")[1087-1089]
Selective transport defect of the renal tubule, often familial and accompanied by hypertension, characterized by both renal resistance to the kaliuretic and acid excretory effects of mineralocorticoid and subnormal renin secretion (type II pseudohypoaldosteronism[1040, 1041, 1090-1107]
Chronic, diffuse, histologically evident renal parenchymal disease and reduced GFR associated with deficient renin secretion[573, 1017, 1019, 1023, 1083, 1085, 1108-1110]
Obstructive uropathy with deficient renin secretion[573, 1030, 1111]
Renal transplantation with deficient renin secretion[576, 1112]
Lupus nephritis with deficient renin secretion[1022, 1026, 1109]
Sickle cell nephropathy[1113]
Cyclosporine nephrotoxicity[1114-1116]
Lead nephropathy[1117]

tively aldosterone-deficient rats studied during intravenous administration of bicarbonate, DuBose and Caflisch[1137] found that neither papillary nor urinary $CO_2$ increased to the same magnitude as observed in adrenal-intact control rats during similar $HCO_3^-$ loading.[1137] These investigations indicate that in the absence of aldosterone, the rate at which the distal tubule secretes $H^+$ is diminished. Robson[1138] had earlier demonstrated that administration of mineralocorticoid to adrenal-intact rabbits induced an increase in $U - B$ $P_{CO_2}$ relative to similarly hyperbicarbonaturic control animals.

## Human Studies

Of 31 hyperkalemic patients with apparently acquired renal parenchymal disease and chronic renal insufficiency investigated by Schambelan and co-workers,[1016] 14 had frank hypoaldosteronism and 23 had subnormal values. The degree of hyperkalemia was significantly greater in the patients with frank hypoaldosteronism, and the extent to which renal clearance of $K^+$ was decreased was directly related to the extent to which aldosterone secretion was decreased.

Sebastian and colleagues[1023] studied the pathogenetic role of aldosterone deficiency in the metabolic acidosis and hyperkalemia of patients with hyporeninemic hypoaldosteronism and chronic renal insufficiency as part of chronic tubulointerstitial nephritis. In some patients in whom GFR was greatly reduced, administration of a physiologic replacement dose (0.10 to 0.15 mg/d) of fludrocortisone induced a further decrease in an already reduced value of urine pH, an increase in net acid excretion and renal clearance of $K^+$, and a substantial amelioration of systemic acidosis and hyperkalemia. The reduction in urine pH suggests that mineralocorticoid replacement stimulated $H^+$ secretion. Presumably the pretreatment values of urine pH would have been considerably higher had the pretreatment rate of renal production of $NH_4^+$ not been restricted because of the reduction in renal mass. In those patients in whom GFR was not greatly reduced (i.e., when creatinine clearance is greater than 25 mL/min), the increase in net acid excretion observed during initial mineralocorticoid therapy was accounted for predominantly by increased titratable acid excretion (Fig. 37–15). When mineralocorticoid therapy was initiated, urine pH decreased, but with continued therapy, it increased in parallel with the observed increase in urinary

$NH_4^+$ excretion. These findings suggest that the rate of renal production of ammonia increased during mineralocorticoid therapy. A primary increase in ammonia production would result in an increase in the amount of ammonia diffusing into the tubule lumen, which would both augment the excretion of $NH_4^+$ and, by increasing the amount of luminal buffer, raise urine pH. Urinary $NH_4^+$ concentration correlated inversely with serum $K^+$ concentration and did not decrease on discontinuation of mineralocorticoid therapy, when hyperkalemia was prevented by reducing dietary intake of potassium; however, net titratable acid and net acid excretion did decrease.

Thus, in some patients with hypoaldosteronism and chronic renal insufficiency, administration of mineralocorticoid can augment both renal $H^+$ secretion and, by correcting hyperkalemia, renal ammonia production as well. Yet, in other patients with hyporeninemic hypoaldosteronism, administration of physiologic amounts of fludrocortisone has had little or no effect, but administration of "superphysiologic" amounts resulted in a substantial amelioration of hyperkalemia.[1023] This phenomenon raises the possibility that in some patients with hyporeninemic hypoaldosteronism, the kidney may be hyporesponsive to the action of aldosterone.

In some patients with mild renal failure and hypoaldosteronism, hyperkalemic distal RTA might result from an impaired capacity of the principal cell to generate an adequate lumen negativity (i.e., a voltage defect that secondarily impedes secretion of both $H^+$ and $K^+$). However, in a study of 18 patients with hyperkalemic RTA and hypoaldosteronism as part of a mild renal failure, Batlle and associates[1139] found no evidence for such a defect and concluded that the major acidification defect was most likely that of impaired $H^+$-ATPase in the collecting duct.

## TREATMENT

In addition to treatment with exogenous mineralocorticoid hormone (usually the orally effective steroid, fludrocortisone), hyperkalemia and acidosis can be ameliorated in patients with hyporeninemic hypoaldosteronism by oral administration of sodium bicarbonate and by oral administration of sodium polystyrene sulfonate, a resin that binds $K^+$ and releases $Na^+$ in the lumen of the gastrointestinal tract.[1108] Amelioration of hyperkalemia is mediated by movement of $K^+$ into cellular compartments due to increased plasma $HCO_3^-$ concentration (during sodium bicarbonate therapy), by increased excretion of $K^+$ (during resin therapy), and by stimulation of renal tubule secretion of $K^+$ (during fludrocortisone therapy). Despite impairment in renal $HCO_3^-$ reabsorption, administration of 1.5 to 2.0 mEq of sodium bicarbonate per day may be sufficient to sustain correction of acidosis, because GFR is usually somewhat reduced. Correction of acidosis usually mitigates the severity of hyperkalemia. Often, the serum $K^+$ concentration can be maintained at less than 5.0 mEq/L with combined alkali therapy and modest dietary potassium restriction.

Treatment of hyperkalemia and acidosis with those agents is not always effective and safe, however, particularly in those patients who are hypertensive and have increases in extracellular fluid volume and total exchangeable

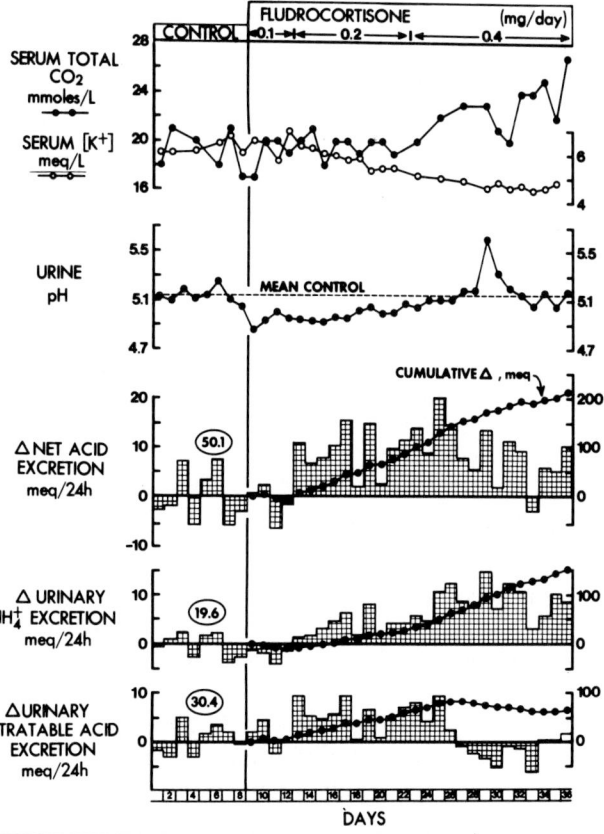

**Figure 37–15.** Effect of orally administered fludrocortisone on serum $CO_2$ and $K^+$ concentration, urine pH, urinary titratable acid, $NH_4^+$, and net acid excretion in a patient with hyporeninemic hypoaldosteronism and chronic renal insufficiency (creatinine clearance 35 mL/min/1.73 $m^2$). Systemic acidosis had not been previously treated. (From Sebastian A, Schambelan M, Lindenfeld S, Morris RC Jr: Amelioration of metabolic acidosis with fludrocortisone therapy in hyporeninemic hypoaldosteronism. N Engl J Med 297:576–583, 1977.)

$Na^+$ before treatment.[1031, 1140] Alternative therapeutic measures that can be considered in patients with hyporeninemic hypoaldosteronism include restriction of dietary potassium and administration of loop diuretics, such as furosemide.[1141] In dogs, long-term administration of furosemide is known to induce an increase in the urinary excretion of net acid and $K^+$ and a persisting hypokalemic metabolic alkalosis. Furosemide inhibits $Na^+$ and $Cl^-$ reabsorption in the loop of Henle, an effect that contracts extracellular fluid volume and causes secondary hyperaldosteronism. The kaliuretic response to furosemide can be attributed in part to inhibition of $K^+$ reabsorption in the loop of Henle. In addition, both the kaliuretic and acid excretory responses can be attributed to increased secretion of $K^+$ and $H^+$ in the distal nephron because of the combined effect of increased distal delivery of $Na^+$ and increased circulating levels of aldosterone.

In patients with chronic renal insufficiency and type IV RTA, administration of furosemide has been demonstrated to increase the urinary excretion of $K^+$ and net acid and to ameliorate substantially hyperkalemia and metabolic acidosis.[1141] The magnitude of the acid excretory and kaliuretic effect has been found to correlate directly with the level of endogenous aldosterone. In those patients with the most severe degree of hypoaldosteronism, the ameliorative effect of furosemide was greatly enhanced by pretreatment with small doses of fludrocortisone.

## PSEUDOHYPOALDOSTERONISM

Renal hyperkalemia and type IV RTA occur in several clinical disorders referred to by the term "pseudohypoaldosteronism" because the signs and symptoms suggest aldosterone deficiency, yet aldosterone levels are supernormal. Those disorders include classic pseudohypoaldosteronism of infancy*; chronic tubulointerstitial diseases usually associated with renal salt wasting[1081–1086]; and adrenal 21β-hydroxylase deficiency, a condition that produces abnormally high levels of endogenous aldosterone antagonists.[1087–1089] Pseudohypoaldosteronism is also associated with administration of so-called $K^+$-sparing diuretics (spironolactone, amiloride, triamterene).

### Type I Pseudohypoaldosteronism (Classic Pseudohypoaldosteronism of Infancy)

A clinically distinct form of pseudohypoaldosteronism occurs in infants as an apparently congenital and, in some cases, a familial disorder characterized by failure to thrive, dehydration and hyponatremia due to renal salt wasting, hyperkalemia due to renal $K^+$ retention, and RTA.† In those affected, plasma renin activity and plasma and urinary aldosterone concentrations are supernormal, and plasma deoxycorticosterone and corticosterone concentrations are normal. Parenteral administration of large amounts of deoxycorticosterone and aldosterone and oral administration of fludrocortisone have little effect on renal salt wasting and $K^+$ retention. Supplementing the diet with large

amounts of sodium chloride can greatly ameliorate hyponatremia and hyperkalemia, relieve symptoms, and permit normal or improved growth. Characteristically, the severity of renal salt wasting and $K^+$ retention so diminishes after infancy that sodium chloride supplements can be discontinued without recurrence of hyponatremia, hyperkalemia, or acidosis. Disordered renal handling of $Na^+$ and $K^+$ persists, however, as evidenced by recurrence of hyponatremia and hyperkalemia when dietary sodium chloride is restricted.[1079]

The pathophysiologic manifestations of the disorder are consistent with a cellular defect that interferes with the action of aldosterone in that segment of the renal tubule normally responsive to aldosterone, specifically the cortical collecting tubule. Generalized glomerular and tubule dysfunction is not present, and biopsy examination of renal tissue has usually revealed only the presence of mild hyperplasia of the juxtaglomerular apparatus. The patients are thus distinguishable from patients with pseudohypoaldosteronism associated with acquired generalized renal parenchymal destruction (e.g., salt-losing nephritis caused by methicillin nephritis, medullary cystic disease).

Armanini and co-workers[1144] demonstrated a decreased number of type I mineralocorticoid binding sites in monocytes obtained from three patients with pseudohypoaldosteronism of infancy, including the index case of Cheek and Perry.[1076] Because the steroid specificity of those receptors is indistinguishable from the renal mineralocorticoid receptor, it seems likely that a similar deficiency of type I receptors is present in the kidney. Bosson and colleagues[1054] likewise found no type I mineralocorticoid receptors in two siblings with classic pseudohypoaldosteronism. In biopsy specimens of rectal mucosal tissue from two children with classic pseudohypoaldosteronism, Popow[1052] found no reduction of binding capacity at the type I (high-affinity) binding site and a reduced binding capacity at the type II (low-affinity) binding site.

It is by no means certain that the same fundamental disorder underlies classic pseudohypoaldosteronism of infancy in all reported cases, nor is it certain that a genetic abnormality is present in all cases. The familial occurrence of the disorder has been documented in only a small fraction of the reported cases. The inheritance may perhaps be either autosomal dominant or autosomal recessive. Bosson and co-workers[1054] proposed that "PHA (pseudohypoaldosteronism) in which the end organ defect lies only in the renal tubule is an inherited disease different from PHA with generalized mineralocorticoid refractoriness of sodium conserving organs (e.g., salivary glands, sweat glands, etc.)."

### Type II Pseudohypoaldosteronism (Aldosterone Resistance Without Salt Wasting)

Renal tubule responsiveness to the action of aldosterone is impaired also in a rare syndrome characterized by hyperkalemia, hyperchloremic metabolic acidosis, hypertension, hyporeninemia, and abnormally low aldosterone levels.* GFR is usually normal. Mineralocorticoid resistance is apparent by persistence of hyperkalemia and a subnormal

*References 995, 1000, 1052–1061, 1063–1066, 1068–1080, 1142, 1143.
†References 488, 995, 1000, 1028, 1052–1065, 1069–1080, 1143.

*References 1040, 1041, 1090–1102, 1106, 1107, 1145–1147.

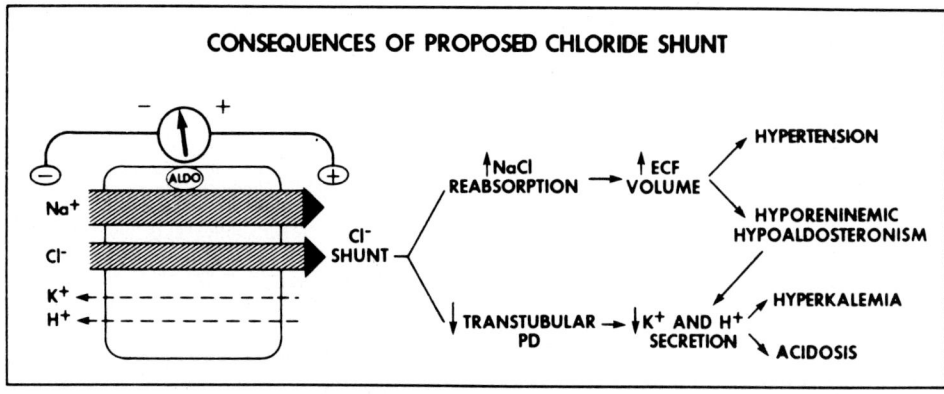

**Figure 37–16.** Pathophysiologic consequences of a defect of the distal nephron characterized by increased reabsorptive avidity for Cl⁻. ECF = extracellular fluid; PD = potential difference. (From Schambelan M, Sebastian A, Rector FC Jr: Mineralocorticoid-resistant renal hyperkalemia without salt wasting [type II pseudohypoaldosteronism]. Role of increased renal chloride reabsorption. Kidney Int 19:716–727, 1981.)

kaliuretic response to exogenously administered mineralocorticoid steroids. The antinatriuretic and antichloruretic responses to mineralocorticoid steroids appear intact. In one reported case, fractional renal K⁺ excretion was subnormal during normal sodium chloride intake despite administration of large amounts of mineralocorticoid steroids.[1098] However, K⁺ excretion increased greatly with the administration of either $Na_2SO_4$ or $NaHCO_3^-$.[1098]

These findings suggest that the primary abnormality is principally a defect of the collecting duct that increases its Cl⁻ reabsorptive avidity. That defect would 1) limit the Na⁺- and mineralocorticoid-dependent voltage driving force for K⁺ and H⁺ secretion, resulting in hyperkalemia and acidosis; and 2) augment distal sodium chloride reabsorption, resulting in hyperchloremia, extracellular fluid volume expansion, hyporeninemia, and hypertension (Fig. 37–16). Such a "Cl⁻ shunt" could result from an abnormally increased permeability of the distal nephron to Cl⁻. Consistent with the presence of such a Cl⁻ shunt, restriction of dietary sodium chloride or administration of a chloruretic diuretic (furosemide, thiazide) ameliorates hyperkalemia and acidosis in such patients.* Some workers believe that the finding of a kaliuretic response to exogenously administered mineralocorticoid and intravenously administered sodium chloride excludes the presence of a Cl⁻ shunt.[1040, 1041] However, a Cl⁻ shunt would be expected to attenuate, not necessarily abolish, the kaliuretic response to sodium chloride.

The hyperkalemia and acidosis in type II pseudohypoaldosteronism may be due in part to extracellular fluid volume expansion–induced hyporeninemia, which restricts angiotensin production and hence the secretion and the circulating concentration of aldosterone. The possibility that the primary abnormality is a defect in the transport mechanism for K⁺ cannot be entirely excluded. A defect in the active (electrogenic) component of K⁺ secretion in the collecting tubule would be expected to enhance lumen negativity and thereby increase the electrical driving force for Cl⁻ reabsorption.[1148, 1149] From a review of 28 reported cases, Gordon[1150] concluded that the disorder has a genetic

basis and that the mode of inheritance is dominant without sex linkage. It remains to be determined whether a single abnormality underlies the dysfunction in all cases.

## REFERENCES

1. Marble A: Renal glucosuria. Am J Med Sci 183:811, 1932.
2. Marble A: Non-diabetic melituria. *In* Joslin EP, Root HF, White P, Marble A (eds): The Treatment of Diabetes Mellitus. Lea & Febiger, Philadelphia, 1959.
3. Reubi FC: Renale familare Glukosurie. *In* Linneweh F (ed): Erbliche Stoffwechselkrankheiten. Urban & Schwarzenberg, Munich, 1962, p 234.
4. Lawrence RD: Symptomless glycosurias: Differentiation by sugar tolerance tests. Med Clin North Am 31:289, 1947.
5. Frohnert PP, Hohmann B, Zwiebel R, Baumann K: Free flow micropuncture studies of glucose transport in the rat nephron. Pflugers Arch 315:66–85, 1970.
6. Barfuss DW, Schafer JA: Differences in active and passive glucose transport along the proximal nephron. Am J Physiol 240:F322–F332, 1981.
7. Aronson PS, Sacktor B: The Na⁺ gradient–dependent transport of D-glucose in renal brush border membranes. J Biol Chem 250:6032, 1975.
8. Shannon J, Fisher S: The renal tubular reabsorption of glucose in the normal dog. Am J Physiol 122:765, 1938.
9. Shannon J, Farber S, Troast L: The measurement of glucose Tm in the normal dog. Am J Physiol 133:752, 1941.
10. Smith HW, Goldring W, Chasis H, et al: The application of saturation methods to the study of glomerular and tubular functions in the human kidney. J Mt Sinai Hosp 10:59, 1943.
11. Letteri JM, Weson LG: Glucose titration curves as an estimate of intrarenal distribution of glomerular filtrate in patients with congestive heart failure. J Lab Clin Med 65:387, 1965.
12. Brodehl J, Franken A, Gellissen K: Maximal tubular transport of glucose in infants and children. Acta Paediatr Scand 61:413–420, 1972.
13. Nielsen AL: On the mechanism of glycosuria. Acta Med Scand 130:219, 1948.
14. McPhaul JJ, Simonaitis JJ: Observations on the mechanisms of glucosuria during glucose loads in normal and non-diabetic subjects. J Clin Invest 47:702–711, 1968.
15. Oliver J, MacDowell M: The structural and functional aspects of the handling of glucose by the nephrons and the kidney and their correlation by means of structural-functional equivalents. J Clin Invest 40:1093, 1961.
16. Bradley SE, Laragh JH, Wheeler HO, et al: Correlation of structure and function in the handling of glucose by nephrons of the canine kidney. J Clin Invest 40:1113, 1961.
17. Woolf LI, Goodwin BL, Phelps CE: Tm-limited renal tubular reab-

*References 1090, 1094, 1095, 1097, 1098, 1106, 1107.

sorption and the genetics of renal glucosuria. J Theor Biol 11:10–21, 1966.

18. Tune BM, Burg MB: Glucose transport by proximal renal tubules. Am J Physiol 221:580–585, 1971.

19. Kleinzeller A, Kotyk A: Cations and the transport of galactose in kidney cortex slices. Biochim Biophys Acta 54:367–369, 1961.

20. Beck JC, Sacktor B: The sodium electrochemical potential–mediated uphill transport of D-glucose in renal brush border membrane vesicles. J Biol Chem 253:5531–5535, 1978.

21. Turner RJ, Moran A: Heterogeneity of sodium-dependent D-glucose transport sites along the proximal tubule: Evidence from vesicle studies. Am J Physiol 242:F406–F414, 1982.

22. Turner RJ, Moran A: Stoichiometric studies of renal outer cortical brush border membrane D-glucose transporter. J Membr Biol 67:73–80, 1982.

23. Turner RJ, Moran A: Further studies of proximal tubular brush border membrane D-glucose transport heterogeneity. J Membr Biol 70:37–45, 1982.

24. Moran A, Turner RJ, Handler JS: Regulation of sodium-coupled glucose transport by glucose in cultured epithelium. J Biol Chem 258:15087–15090, 1983.

25. Moran A, Turner RJ, Handler JS: Hexose regulation of sodium-hexose transport in LLC-PK1 epithelia: The nature of the signal. J Membr Biol 82:59–65, 1984.

26. Lindquist B, Meeuwisse G, Melin K: Glucose-galactose malabsorption. Lancet 2:666, 1962.

27. Elsas LJ, Hillman RE, Patterson JH, Rosenberg LE: Renal and intestinal hexose transport in familial glucose-galactose malabsorption. J Clin Invest 49:576–585, 1970.

28. Hediger MA, Coady MJ, Ikeda TS, Wright EM: Expression cloning and cDNA sequencing of the Na⁺/glucose co-transporter. Nature 330:379–381, 1987.

29. Ikeda TS, Hwang ES, Coady MJ, et al: Characterization of an Na⁺/glucose cotransporter cloned from rabbit small intestine. J Membr Biol 100:87–95, 1989.

30. Lee W-S, Kanai Y, Wells RG, Hediger MA: The high affinity Na⁺/glucose cotransporter. J Biol Chem 269:12032–12039, 1993.

31. Turk E, Zabel B, Mundlos S, et al: Glucose/galactose malabsorption caused by a defect in the Na⁺/glucose cotransporter. Nature 350:354–356, 1991.

32. Wells RG, Pajor AM, Kanai Y, et al: Cloning of a human kidney cDNA with similarity to the sodium-glucose cotransporter. Am J Physiol 263:F459–F465, 1992.

33. Kanai Y, Lee WS, You G, et al: The human kidney low affinity Na⁺/glucose cotransporter SGLT2. Delineation of the major renal reabsorptive mechanism for D-glucose. J Clin Invest 93:397–404, 1994.

34. Cheung PT, Hammerman MR: Na⁺-independent D-glucose transport in rabbit renal basolateral membranes. Am J Physiol 254:F711–F718, 1988.

35. Ling KY, Im WB, Faust RG: Na⁺-independent sugar uptake by rat intestinal and renal brush border and basolateral membrane vesicles. Int J Biochem 13:693–700, 1981.

36. Gliemann J, Rees WD: The insulin-sensitive hexose transport system in adipocytes. Curr Top Membr Transport 18:339, 1983.

37. Mueckler M: Facilitative glucose transporters. Eur J Biochem 219:713–725, 1994.

38. Takata K, Kasahara T, Kasahara M, et al: Localization of Na⁺-dependent active type and erythrocyte/HepG2-type glucose transporters in rat kidney: Immunofluorescence and immunogold study. J Histochem Cytochem 39:287–298, 1991.

39. Thorens B, Lodish HF, Brown D: Differential localization of two glucose transporter isoforms in rat kidney. Am J Physiol 259:C286–C294, 1990.

40. Dominguez JH, Camp K, Maianu L, Garvey WT: Glucose transporters of rat proximal tubule: Differential expression and subcellular distribution. Am J Physiol 262:F807–F812, 1992.

41. Reubi FC: Le mécanisme de la glycosurie au cours des deux variétés de diabete rénal (type A et type B). Mod Probl Paediatr 4:511, 1959.

42. Meeuwisse GW: Glucose-galactose malabsorption: Studies on renal glycosuria. Helv Paediatr Acta 25:13, 1970.

43. Elsas LJ, Rosenberg LE: Familial renal glycosuria: A genetic reappraisal of hexose transport by kidney and intestine. J Clin Invest 48:1845–1854, 1969.

44. Ackerman IP, Fajans SS, Conn JW: The development of diabetes mellitus in patients with nondiabetic glycosuria. Clin Res 6:251, 1958.

45. Tolosa Vilella C, Valles-Prats M, Simeon Aznar CP: Primary renal glycosuria and diabetes mellitus. Med Clin (Barc) 90:119–121, 1988.

46. McKiddie MJ, Scott RJ, Cole R: The insulin response to glucose in patients with nondiabetic glycosuria. Postgrad Med J 47:605, 1971.

47. Hjarne VA: Study of orthoglycemic glycosuria with particular reference to its heritability. Acta Med Scand 67:422, 1927.

48. Houston JC, Merivale WHH: Renal glycosuria in a family. Guys Hosp Rep 98:233, 1949.

49. Brown MS, Poleshuck R: Familial renal glycosuria. J Lab Clin Med 2:605, 1935.

50. Khachadurian AK, Khachadurian LA: The inheritance of renal glycosuria. Am J Hum Genet 16:189, 1964.

51. Elsas LJ, Busse D, Rosenberg LE: Autosomal recessive inheritance of renal glucosuria. Metabolism 20:968, 1971.

52. De Marchi S, Cecchin E: Immunological abnormalities and renal tubular disorders: A puzzling association. Am J Nephrol 6:327–328, 1986.

53. De Marchi S, Cecchin E, Basile A, et al: Close genetic linkage between HLA and renal glycosuria. Am J Nephrol 4:280–286, 1984.

54. Wells RG, Mohandas TK, Hediger MA: Localization of the Na⁺/glucose cotransporter gene SGLT2 to human chromosome 16 close to the centromere. Genomics 17:787–789, 1993.

55. Schneider AJ, Kinter WB, Stirling CE: Glucose-galactose malabsorption: Report of a case with autoradiographic studies of a mucosal biopsy. N Engl J Med 274:305, 1966.

56. Meeuwisse GW, Dahlquist A: Glucose-galactose malabsorption: A study with biopsy of the small intestinal mucosa. Acta Paediatr Scand 57:273, 1968.

57. Eggermont E, Loeb H: Glucose-galactose intolerance. Lancet 2:343, 1966.

58. Scriver CR: Disorders of amino acid metabolism. In Scriver CR, Beaudet AL, Sly WS, Valle D (eds): The Metabolic Basis of Inherited Disease, 6th ed. McGraw-Hill, New York, 1989, pp 495–771.

59. Cusworth D, Dent CE: Renal clearances of amino acids in normal adults and in patients with aminoaciduria. Biochem J 74:550, 1960.

60. Tizianello A, DeFerrari G, Garibotto G, et al: Renal metabolism of amino acids and ammonia in subjects with normal renal function and in patients with chronic renal insufficiency. J Clin Invest 65:1162, 1980.

61. Brown JL, Samiy AH, Pitts RF: Localization of amino-nitrogen reabsorption in the nephron of the dog. Am J Physiol 200:370, 1961.

62. Ruszkowski MC, Arasimowicz C, Knapowski J, et al: Renal reabsorption of amino acids. Am J Physiol 203:891, 1962.

63. Christopher W, Deetjen P: Mikroperfusionsuntersuchungen zum tubularen Transport von Glyzin. Pflugers Arch 297:R52, 1967.

64. Reynolds RA, Wald H, McNamara PD, Segal S: An improved method for isolation of basolateral membranes from rat kidney. Biochim Biophys Acta 601:92, 1980.

65. Wedeen RP, Thier SO: Intrarenal distribution of non-metabolized amino acids in vivo. Am J Physiol 200:507, 1971.

66. Wedeen RP, Weiner RP: The distribution of p-aminohippuric acid in rat kidney slices. I. Tubular localization. Kidney Int 3:205, 1973.

67. Ausiello DA, Segal S, Thier SO: Cellular accumulation of L-lysine in rat kidney cortex in vivo. Am J Physiol 222:1473, 1972.

68. Greth WE, Thier SO, Segal S: Transport of cystine in rat kidney cortex: Independent luminal and contraluminal mechanisms. Clin Res 19:742, 1971.

69. Foulkes EC, Bergeron M, Vadeboncoeur M: Cellular localization of amino acid carriers in renal tubules. Proc Soc Exp Biol Med 129:1032, 1972.

70. Bergeron M, Vadeboncoeur M: Antiluminal transport of L-arginine and L-leucine following microinjections in peritubular capillaries of the rat. Nephron 8:355, 1971.

71. Samarzija I, Fromter E: Electrophysiological analysis of rat renal sugar and amino acid transport. V. Acidic amino acids. Pflugers Arch 393:215–221, 1982.

72. Samarzija I, Fromter E: Electrophysiological analysis of rat renal sugar and amino acid transport. III. Neutral amino acids. Pflugers Arch 393:119–209, 1982.

73. Samarzija I, Fromter E: Electrophysiological analysis of rat renal sugar and amino acid transport. IV. Basic amino acids. Pflugers Arch 393:210–214, 1982.

74. Silbernagl S: The renal handling of amino acids and oligopeptides. Pharmacol Rev 68:911, 1988.

75. Dirckx JH: Julius Caesar and the Julian emperors. A family cluster with Hartnup disease? Am J Dermatopathol 8:351–357, 1986.

76. Baron DN, Dent CE, Harris H, et al: Hereditary pellagra-like skin rash with temporary cerebellar ataxia, constant renal aminoaciduria, and other bizarre biochemical features. Lancet 1:421, 1956.

77. Jepson JB: Hartnup disease. In Stanbury JB, Wyngaarden JB, Fredrickson DS (eds): The Metabolic Basis of Inherited Disease, 4th ed. McGraw-Hill, New York, 1978, p 1563.

78. Levy HL: Genetic screening. Adv Hum Genet 4:1–104, 1973.

79. Milne MD, Crawford MA, Girao CB, Loughridge L: The metabolic disorder in Hartnup disease. Am J Med 29:407, 1960.

80. Scriver CR: Hartnup disease: A genetic modification of intestinal and renal transport of certain neutral alpha-amino acids. N Engl J Med 273:530, 1965.

81. Shih VE, Bixby EM, Alpers DH, et al: Studies of intestinal transport defect in Hartnup disease. Gastroenterology 61:445, 1971.

82. Butler IJ: Circumvention of defective neutral amino acid transport in Hartnup disease using tryptophan ethyl ester. J Clin Invest 84:200–204, 1989.

83. Jonas AJ, Butler IJ: Circumvention of defective neutral amino acid transport in Hartnup disease using tryptophan ethyl ester. J Clin Invest 84:200–204, 1989.

84. Drummond KN, Michael AF, Ulstrom RA, Good RA: The blue diaper syndrome. Familial hypercalcemia with nephrocalcinosis and indicanemia. Am J Med 37:928, 1964.

85. Mahon BE, Levy HL: Maternal Hartnup disorder. Am J Med Genet 24:513–518, 1986.

86. Tada K, Morikawa T, Arakawa T: Tryptophan load and uptake of tryptophan by leukocytes in Hartnup disease. Tohoku J Exp Med 90:337, 1966.

87. Darras BT, Ampola MG, Dietz WH, Gilmore HE: Intermittent dystonia in Hartnup disease. Pediatr Neurol 5:118–120, 1989.

88. Henderson W: A case of Hartnup disease. Arch Dis Child 33:114, 1958.

89. Milne MD: Hartnup disease. Biochem J 111:3P, 1969.

90. Schmidtke K, Endres W, Roscher A, et al: Hartnup syndrome, progressive encephalopathy and allo-albuminaemia. A clinico-pathological case study. Eur J Pediatr 151:899–903, 1992.

91. Scriver CR, Mahon B, Levy HL, et al: The Hartnup phenotype: Mendelian transport disorder, multifactorial disease. Am J Hum Genet 40:401–412, 1987.

92. Wong PWK, Pillai PM: Clinical and biochemical observations in two cases of Hartnup disease. Arch Dis Child 41:383, 1966.

93. Halvorsen K, Halvorsen S: Hartnup disease. Pediatrics 31:29, 1963.

94. Dent CE: Detection of amino acids in urine and other fluids. Lancet 2:637, 1946.

95. Brodehl J, Gellissen K: Endogenous renal transport of free amino acids in infancy and childhood. Pediatrics 42:395, 1968.

96. Joseph R, Ribierre M, Job J, Girault M: Maladie familiale associant des convulsions à début très précoce, une hyperalbuminorachie et une hyperaminoacidurie. Arch Fr Pediatr 15:374–381, 1958.

97. Scriver CR, Wilson OH: Possible locations for a common gene product in membrane transport of amino acids and glycine. Nature 202:92, 1964.

98. Tada K, Morikawa T, Ando T, et al: Prolinuria: A new renal tubular defect in transport of proline and glycine. Tohoku J Exp Med 87:133, 1965.

99. Scriver CR, Wilson OH: Amino acid transport: Evidence for genetic control of two types in human kidney. Science 155:1428, 1967.

100. Slack EN, Liang C-C, Sacktor B: Transport of L-proline and D-glucose in luminal (brush border) and contraluminal (basal-lateral) membrane vesicles from the renal cortex. Biochem Biophys Res Commun 77:891–897, 1977.

101. Hammerman MR, Sacktor B: Transport of amino acids in renal brush border membrane vesicles. Uptake of L-proline. J Biol Chem 252:591–595, 1977.

102. McNamara PD, Ozegovic B, Pepe LM, Segal S: Proline and glycine uptake by renal brush border membrane vesicles. Proc Natl Acad Sci USA 73:4521–4525, 1976.

103. McNamara PD, Pepe LM, Segal S: Sodium gradient dependence of proline and glycine uptake in renal brush-border membrane vesicle. Biochim Biophys Acta 556:151–160, 1979.

104. Scalera V, Corcelli A, Frassanito A, Storelli C: Chloride dependence of the sodium-dependent glycine transport in pig kidney cortex brush-border membrane vesicles. Biochim Biophys Acta 903:1–10, 1987.

105. Morikawa T, Tada K, Ando T, et al: Prolinuria: Defect in intestinal absorption of amino acids and glycine. Tohoku J Exp Med 90:105, 1966.

106. Goodman SE, McIntyre CA, O'Brien D: Impaired intestinal transport of proline in a patient with familial aminoaciduria. J Pediatr 74:246, 1967.

107. Tancredi F, Guazzi G, Auricchio S: Renal aminoglycinuria without intestinal malabsorption of glycine and amino acids. J Pediatr 76:386, 1970.

108. Paine RS: Evaluation of familial mental retardation in children, with special reference to aminoaciduria. N Engl J Med 262:658, 1966.

109. Turner B, Brown DA: Amino acid excretion in infancy and early childhood: A survey of 200,000 infants. Med J Aust 1:62, 1972.

110. Rosenberg LE, Durant JL, Elsas LJ: Familial aminoglycinuria: An inborn error of renal tubular transport. N Engl J Med 278:1407, 1968.

111. Jones E, Sobkowski WW, Murray SJ, Walsh NM: Concurrent pemphigus and myasthenia gravis as manifestations of penicillamine toxicity. J Am Acad Dermatol 28:655–656, 1993.

112. DeVries A, Kochwa S, Lazebink J, et al: Glycinuria, a hereditary disorder associated with nephrolithiasis. Am J Med 23:408, 1957.

113. Greene ML, Lietman PS, Rosenberg LE, Seegmiller JE: Familial hyperglycinuria: New defect in renal tubular transport of glycine and the imino acids. Am J Med 54:265, 1973.

114. Oberiter V, Puretic Z, Fabecic-Sabadi V: Hyperglycinuria with nephrolithiasis. Eur J Pediatr 127:279–285, 1978.

115. Kaser H, Cottier P, Antener I: Glucoglycinuria, a new familial syndrome. J Pediatr 61:386, 1962.

116. Smith AJ, Strang LB: An inborn error of metabolism with the urinary excretion of α-hydroxybutyric acid and phenyl-pyruvic acid. Arch Dis Child 33:109, 1958.

117. Hooft C, Timmermans J, Snoeck J, et al: Methionine malabsorption syndrome. Ann Pediatr 205:73, 1965.

118. Guerino F, Baumrucker CR: Identification of methionine and lysine transport systems in cattle small intestine. J Anim Sci 65:630–640, 1987.

119. Brachet P, Alvarado F, Puigserver A: Kinetic evidence for separate systems in transport of D- and L-methionine by rat small intestine. Am J Physiol 252:G320–G324, 1987.

120. Stieger B, Stange G, Biber J, Murer H: Transport of L-lysine by rat renal brush border membrane vesicles. Pflugers Arch 397:106, 1983.

121. Wollaston WH: On cystic oxide: A new species of urinary calculus. Trans R Soc Lond 100:223, 1810.

122. Berzelius JJ: Calculus urinaries. Traite Chem 7:424, 1833.

123. Garrod A: The Croonian lectures. Lancet 2:21, 142, 173, 1908.

124. Yeh HL, Frankl W, Dunn MS, et al: The urinary excretion of amino acids by a cystinuric subject. Am J Med Sci 214:507–512, 1947.

125. Dent CE, Heathcote JG, Joron GE: The pathogenesis of cystinuria. I. Chromatographic and microbiological studies of the metabolism of sulphur-containing amino acids. J Clin Invest 33:1210, 1954.

126. Dent CE, Senior B, Walshe JM: The pathogenesis of cystinuria. II. Polarographic studies of the metabolism of sulphur-containing amino acids. J Clin Invest 33:1216, 1954.

127. Rosenberg L, Downing S, Segal S: Competitive inhibition of dibasic amino acid transport in rat kidney. J Biol Chem 237:2265, 1962.

128. Fox M, Thier SO, Rosenberg LE, et al: Evidence against a single renal transport defect in cystinuria. N Engl J Med 270:556, 1964.

129. Segal S, Crawhall JC: Characteristics of cystine and cysteine transport in rat kidney cortex slices. Proc Natl Acad Sci USA 59:231–237, 1968.

130. Segal S, Smith I: Delineation of separate transport systems in rat kidney cortex for L-lysine and L-cystine by developmental patterns. Biochem Biophys Res Commun 35:771–777, 1969.

131. Bowring MA, Foreman JW, Lee J, Segal S: Characteristics of lysine transport by isolated rat renal cortical tubule fragments. Biochim Biophys Acta 901:23–29, 1987.

132. Segal S, Thier SO: Cystinuria. *In* Stanbury JB, Wyngaarden JB, Fredrickson DS, et al (eds): The Metabolic Basis of Inherited Disease, 5th ed. McGraw-Hill, New York, 1983, pp 1774–1791.

133. Segal S, McNamara PD, Pepe LM: Transport interaction of cystine and dibasic amino acids in renal brush border vesicles. Science 197:169–171, 1977.

134. States B, Foreman J, Lee J, et al: Cystine and lysine transport in cultured human renal epithelial cells. Metabolism 36:356–362, 1987.

135. Lee WS, Wells RG, Sabbag RV, et al: Cloning and chromosomal localization of a human kidney cDNA involved in cystine, dibasic, and neutral amino acid transport. J Clin Invest 91:1959–1963, 1993.

136. Bertran J, Werner A, Moore ML, et al: Expression cloning of a cDNA from rabbit kidney cortex that induces a single transport system for cystine and dibasic and neutral amino acids. Proc Natl Acad Sci USA 89:5601–5605, 1992.

137. Tate SS, Yan N, Udenfriend S: Expression cloning of a Na⁺-independent neutral amino acid transporter from rat kidney. Proc Natl Acad Sci USA 89:1–5, 1992.

138. Kanai Y, Stelzner MG, Lee W-S, et al: Expression of mRNA (D2) encoding a protein involved in amino acid transport in the $S_3$ proximal tubule. Am J Physiol 263:F1087–F1093, 1992.

139. Rosenberg LE: Genetic heterogeneity in cystinuria. *In* Nyhan WL (ed): Amino Acid Metabolism and Genetic Variation. McGraw-Hill, New York, 1967.

140. Rosenberg LE, Downing SJ: Transport of neutral and dibasic amino acids by human leukocytes: Absence of defect in cystinuria. J Clin Invest 44:1382, 1965.

141. Gardner JD, Levy AG: Transport of dibasic amino acids by human erythrocytes. Metabolism 21:413, 1972.

142. von Udransky L, Baumann E: Über das Vorkommen von Diaminen, sogenannten Ptomainen, bei Cystinurie. Z Physiol Chem 13:562, 1899.

143. Milne MD, Asatoor AM, Edwards KDG, Loughridge LW: The intestinal absorption defect in cystinuria. Gut 2:323, 1961.

144. Asatoor AM, Lacey BW, London DR, Milne MD: Amino acid metabolism in cystinuria. Clin Sci 23:285, 1962.

145. Thier SO, Segal S, Fox M, et al: Cystinuria: Defective intestinal transport of basic amino acids and cystine. J Clin Invest 44:442, 1965.

146. McCarthy CF, Borland JL, Lynch HJ, et al: Defective uptake of basic amino acids and L-cystine by intestinal mucosa of patients with cystinuria. J Clin Invest 43:1518, 1964.

147. Furlong TJ, Stiel D: Decreased uptake of L-cystine by duodenal brush border membrane vesicles from patients with cystinuria. Aust N Z J Med 23:258–263, 1993.

148. Alpers DH, Thier SO: Role of the free amino acid pool of the intestine in protein synthesis. Biochim Biophys Acta 262:535, 1972.

149. Rosenberg LE, Downing SJ, Durant JL, Segal S: Cystinuria: Biochemical evidence for three genetically distinct diseases. J Clin Invest 45:365, 1966.

150. Hambraeus L: Comparative studies of the value of two cyanide-nitroprusside methods in the diagnosis of cystinuria. Scand J Lab Clin Invest 15:657, 1963.

151. Berg W, Pirlich W, Kilian O: Investigations on the early diagnosis of cystinuria in children. Eur Urol 14:458–463, 1988.

152. Larsen HF, Kisby M, Sampson DC, et al: Automated method for measuring cystine in urine. Clin Chem 34:2377–2378, 1988.

153. Sampson DC, Stewart PM, Hammond JW: Measurement of urinary cystine and cysteinyl-penicillamine in patients with cystinuria. Biomed Chromatogr 1:21–26, 1986.

154. Watanabe H, Sugahara K, Inoue K, et al: Liquid chromatographic–mass spectrometric analysis for screening of patients with cystinuria, and identification of cystine stone. J Chromatogr 568:445–450, 1991.

155. Birwe H, Hesse A: High-performance liquid chromatographic determination of urinary cysteine and cystine. Clin Chim Acta 199:33–42, 1991.

156. Crawhall JC, Purkiss P, Watts RWE, Young EP: The excretion of amino acids by cystinuric patients and their relatives. Ann Hum Genet 33:149–169, 1969.

157. Zinneman HH, Jones JE: Dietary methionine and its influence on cystine excretion in cystinuric patients. Metabolism 15:915, 1966.

158. Crawhall JC, Scowen EF, Watts RWE: Effect of penicillamine on cystinuria. Br Med J 1:588, 1963.

159. Halperin EC, Thier SO, Rosenberg LE: The use of D-penicillamine in cystinuria: Efficacy and untoward reactions. Yale J Biol Med 54:439–446, 1981.

160. Fries JF, Williams CA, Ramey D, Bloch DA: The relative toxicity of disease-modifying antirheumatic drugs. Arthritis Rheum 36:297–306, 1993.

161. Jaffe IA: Adverse effects profile of sulfhydryl compounds in man. Am J Med 80:471, 1986.

162. Benveniste M, Crouzet J, Homberg JC, et al: Pemphigus induced by D-penicillamine in rheumatoid arthritis and other diseases. Presse Med 4:3125, 1975.

163. Sadjadi SA, Seelig MS, Berger AR, Milstoc M: Rapidly progressive glomerulonephritis in a patient with rheumatoid arthritis during treatment with high dose D-penicillamine. Am J Nephrol 5:212–216, 1985.

164. Jaffe IA, Treser G, Suzuki Y, Ehrenreich T: Nephropathy induced by D-penicillamine. Ann Intern Med 69:549, 1968.

165. King JS: Treatment of cystinuria with alpha-mercaptopropionylglycine: A preliminary report. Proc Soc Exp Biol Med 129:927–932, 1968.

166. Martin X, Salas M, Labeeuw M, et al: Cystine stones: The impact of new treatment. Br J Urol 68:234–239, 1991.

167. Joost J, Jarosch E: Glutamine: A new anticystinuric drug? Eur Urol 7:363, 1981.

168. Dahlberg PJ, Jones JD: Cystinuria: Failure of captopril to reduce cystine excretion. Arch Intern Med 149:713–717, 1989. Letter.

169. Perazella MA, Buller GK: Successful treatment of cystinuria with captopril. Am J Kidney Dis 21:504–507, 1993.

170. Coulthard M, Richardson J, Fleetwood A: Captopril is not clinically useful in reducing the cystine load in cystinuria or cystinosis. Pediatr Nephrol 5:98, 1991.

171. Knoll LD, Segura JW, Patterson DE, et al: Long-term follow-up in patients with cystine urinary calculi treated by percutaneous ultrasonic lithotripsy. J Urol 140:246–248, 1988.

172. Kekkomaki M, Visakorpi JK, Perheentupa J, Saxen L: Familial protein intolerance with deficient transport of basic amino acids. Acta Paediatr Scand 56:617, 1967.

173. Whelan DT, Scriver CR: Hyperdibasicaminoaciduria: An inherited disorder of amino acid transport. Pediatr Res 2:525, 1968.

174. Brown JH, Fabre LF, Farrell GK, Adams ED: Hyperlysinuria with hyperammonemia. Am J Dis Child 124:127, 1972.

175. Desjeux J-F, Rajantie J, Simell O, et al: Lysine fluxes cross the jejunal epithelium in lysinuric protein intolerance. J Clin Invest 65:1382, 1980.

176. Simell O, Perheentupa J: Renal handling of diamino acids in lysinuric protein intolerance. J Clin Invest 54:9, 1974.

177. Simell O: Lysinuric protein intolerance and other cationic aminoacidurias. *In* Scriver CR, Beaudet AL, Sly WS, Valle D (eds): The Metabolic Basis of Inherited Disease, 6th ed. McGraw-Hill, New York, 1989, pp 2497–2514.

178. Parto K, Penttinen R, Paronen I, et al: Osteoporosis in lysinuric protein intolerance. J Inherit Metab Dis 16:441–450, 1993.

179. Svedstrom E, Parto K, Marttinen M, et al: Skeletal manifestations of lysinuric protein intolerance. A follow-up study of 29 patients. Skeletal Radiol 22:11–16, 1993.

180. Parto K, Svedstrom E, Majurin ML, et al: Pulmonary manifestations in lysinuric protein intolerance. Chest 104:1176–1182, 1993.

181. Kerem E, Elpelg ON, Shalev RS, et al: Lysinuric protein intolerance with chronic interstitial lung disease and pulmonary cholesterol granulomas at onset. J Pediatr 123:275–278, 1993.

182. Kato T, Mizutani N, Ban M: Renal transport of lysine and arginine in lysinuric protein intolerance. Eur J Pediatr 139:181–184, 1982.

183. Rajantie J, Simell O, Perheentupa J: Basolateral membrane transport defect for lysine in lysinuric protein intolerance. Lancet 1:1219, 1980.

184. Adibi SA: Intestinal transport of dipeptides in man: Relative importance of hydrolysis and intact absorption. J Clin Invest 50:2266, 1971.

185. Smith DW, Scriver CR, Tenenhouse HS, Simell O: Lysinuric protein intolerance mutation is expressed in the plasma membrane of cultured skin fibroblasts. Proc Natl Acad Sci USA 84:7711–7715, 1987.

186. Oynagi K, Sogawa H, Minawi R, et al: The mechanism of hyperammonemia in congenital lysinuria. J Pediatr 94:255, 1979.

187. Rajantie J, Simell O, Perheentupa J: "Basolateral" and mitochon-

drial membrane transport defect in the hepatocytes in lysinuric protein intolerance. Acta Paediatr Scand 72:65, 1983.

188. Rajantie J, Simell O, Rapola J, Perheentupa J: Lysinuric protein intolerance: A two year trial of dietary supplementation therapy with citrulline and lysine. J Pediatr 97:927, 1980.

189. Omura K, Yamanaka N, Higami S, et al: Lysine malabsorption syndrome: A new type of transport defect. Pediatrics 57:102, 1976.

190. Kamin H, Handler P: Effect of infusion of single amino acids upon excretion of other amino acids. Am J Physiol 164:654, 1951.

191. Webber WA: Characteristics of acidic amino acid transport in mammalian kidney. Can J Biochem Physiol 41:131, 1963.

192. Teijema HL, van Gelderen HH, Giesberts MAH, et al: Dicarboxylic aminoaciduria: An inborn error of glutamate and aspartate transport with metabolic implications, in combination with hyperprolinemia. Metabolism 23:115, 1974.

193. Melancon SB, Dallaire L, Lemieux B, et al: Dicarboxylic amino-aciduria: An inborn error of amino acid conservation. J Pediatr 91:422, 1977.

194. Schneider EG, Sacktor B: Sodium gradient–dependent L-glutamate transport in renal brush border membrane vesicles. Effect of an intravesicular > extravesicular potassium gradient. J Biol Chem 255:7645–7649, 1980.

195. Schneider EG, Hammerman MR, Sacktor B: Sodium gradient–dependent L-glutamate transport in renal brush border membrane vesicles. Evidence for an electroneutral mechanism. J Biol Chem 255:7650–7656, 1980.

196. Sacktor B: L-Glutamate transport in renal plasma membrane vesicles. Mol Cell Biol 39:239, 1981.

197. Lerner J: Acidic amino acid transport in animal cells and tissues. Comp Biochem Physiol 87:443, 1987.

198. Winters RW, McFalls VW, Graham JB: Sporadic hypophosphatemia in vitamin D resistant rickets. Pediatrics 25:959, 1960.

199. Dent CE, Stamp TCB: Hypophosphatemic osteomalacia presenting in adults. Q J Med 40:303–329, 1971.

200. Winters RW, Graham JB, Williams TF, et al: A genetic study of familial hypophosphatemia and vitamin D resistant rickets with a review of the literature. Medicine (Baltimore) 37:97, 1958.

201. Stanbury SW: Some aspects of disordered renal tubular function. Adv Intern Med 9:231–282, 1958.

202. Falkson G, Frame B: Phosphate diabetes: A review. Henry Ford Hosp Med Bull 6:244, 1958.

203. Prader A, Illig R, Uehlinger E, Stalder G: Rachitis in folge Knochentumors. Helv Paediatr Acta 14:544, 1959.

204. Greenberg BC, Winters RW, Graham JB: The normal range of serum inorganic phosphorus and its utility as a discriminant in the diagnosis of congenital hypophosphatemia. J Clin Endocrinol Metab 20:364, 1960.

205. Frymoyer JW, Hodgkin W: Adult-onset vitamin D–resistant hypophosphatemic osteomalacia. J Bone Joint Surg Am 59:101–106, 1977.

206. Stamp TCB, Baker LRI: Recessive hypophosphatemic rickets, and possible aetiology of the "vitamin D–resistant" syndrome. Arch Dis Child 51:360–365, 1976.

207. Bianchine JW, Stambler AA, Harrison HE: Familial hypophosphatemic rickets showing autosomal dominant inheritance. Birth Defects 7:287–293, 1971.

208. Wilson DR, York SE, Jaworski ZF, Yendt ER: Studies in hypophosphatemic vitamin D–refractory osteomalacia in adults. Medicine (Baltimore) 44:99–134, 1965.

209. Scriver CR, MacDonald W, Reade T, et al: Hypophosphatemic nonrachitic bone disease: An entity distinct from X-linked hypophosphatemia in the renal defect, bone involvement, and inheritance. Am J Med Genet 1:101–107, 1977.

210. Tieder M, Modai D, Samuel R, et al: Hereditary hypophosphatemic rickets with hypercalciuria. N Engl J Med 312:611–617, 1985.

211. Tieder M, Modai D, Shaked U, et al: "Idiopathic" hypercalciuria and hereditary hypophosphatemic rickets. N Engl J Med 316:125–129, 1987.

212. Tieder M, Arie R, Samuel R, et al: Hereditary hypophosphatemic hypercalciuria. Urol Res 16:212, 1988.

213. Dent CE, Friedman M: Hypophosphatemic osteomalacia with complete recovery. Br Med J 1:1676–1679, 1964.

214. Howard JE: Case records of the Massachusetts General Hospital (B. Castleman). N Engl J Med 273:494, 1965.

215. McCance RA: Osteomalacia with Looser's zones due to raised resistance to vitamin D acquired about the age of 15 years. Q J Med 16:33, 1947.

216. Olefsky J, Kempson R, Jones J, Reaven G: "Tertiary" hyperparathyroidism and apparent "cure" of vitamin D–resistant rickets after removal of an ossifying mesenchymal tumor of the pharynx. N Engl J Med 286:739–745, 1972.

217. Harrison HE: Oncogenous rickets: Possible elaboration by a tumor of a humoral substance inhibiting tubular reabsorption of phosphate. Pediatrics 52:432–434, 1973.

218. Linovitz RJ, Resnick D, Keissling P, et al: Tumor-induced osteomalacia and rickets: A surgically curable syndrome. J Bone Joint Surg Am 58:419, 1976.

219. Drezner MK, Feinglos MN: Osteomalacia due to 1,25-dihydroxycholecalciferol deficiency. J Clin Invest 60:1046–1053, 1977.

220. Dent CE, Gertner JM: Hypophosphataemic osteomalacia in fibrous dysplasia. Q J Med 179:411–420, 1976.

221. Aschinberg LC, Solomon LM, Zeis PM, et al: Vitamin D–resistant rickets associated with epidermal nevus syndrome: Demonstration of a phosphaturic substance in the dermal lesions. J Pediatr 91:56–60, 1977.

222. Albright F, Reifenstein EC Jr: The Parathyroid Glands and Metabolic Bone Disease. Williams & Wilkins, Baltimore, 1948.

223. Dent CE: Metabolic forms of rickets (and osteomalacia). In Bikel H, Stern J (eds): Inborn Errors of Calcium and Bone Metabolism. University Park Press, Baltimore, 1976, pp 124–149.

224. Bijvoet O: The importance of the kidney in phosphate homeostasis. In Avioli L, Bordier P, Fleisch H, et al (eds): Phosphate Metabolism, Kidney and Bone. Armour-Montague, Paris, 1976, p 421.

225. Williams TF, Winters RW: Familial (hereditary) vitamin D–resistant rickets with hypophosphatemia. In Stanbury JB, Wyngaarden JB, Fredrickson DS (eds): The Metabolic Basis of Inherited Disease, 3rd ed. McGraw-Hill, New York, 1972, pp 1465–1485.

226. Rasmussen H, Tenenhouse HS: Hypophosphatemias. In Scriver CR, Beaudet AL, Sly WS, Valle D (eds): The Metabolic Basis of Inherited Disease, 6th ed. McGraw-Hill, New York, 1989, pp 2581–2604.

227. Sugarman GI, Reeds WB: Two unusual neurocutaneous disorders with facial cutaneous signs. Arch Neurol 21:242–247, 1969.

228. Fraser DR, Kodicek E: Unique biosynthesis by kidney of a biologically active vitamin D metabolite. Nature 228:764–766, 1970.

229. Gray RW, Boyle I, DeLuca HF: Vitamin D metabolism: The role of kidney tissue. Science 172:1232–1234, 1971.

230. Tanaka Y, DeLuca HF: The control of 25-hydroxyvitamin D metabolism by inorganic phosphorus. Arch Biochem Biophys 154:566–574, 1973.

231. Norman AW: 1,25-Dihydroxyvitamin $D_3$: A kidney-produced steroid hormone essential to calcium homeostasis. Am J Med 57:21, 1974.

232. Haussler MR, Baylink DJ, Hughes MR, et al: The assay of 1-alpha, 25-dihydroxyvitamin $D_3$: Physiologic and pathologic modulation of circulating hormone levels. Clin Endocrinol 5:151s–161s, 1976.

233. Burnette MB, Chan M, Ferriere C, Roberts KD: Site of 1,25-(OH)$_2$ vitamin $D_3$ synthesis in the kidney. Nature 276:287–289, 1978.

234. Akiba T, Endou H, Koseki C, et al: Localization of 25-hydroxyvitamin $D_3$ 1α-hydroxylase activity in the mammalian kidney. Biochem Biophys Res Commun 94:313–318, 1980.

235. Kawashima H, Torikai S, Kurokawa K: Localization of 25-hydroxyvitamin $D_3$ 1α-hydroxylase and 24-hydroxylase along the rat nephron. Proc Natl Acad Sci USA 78:1199–1203, 1981.

236. Boyle IT, Miravet L, Gray RW, et al: The response of intestinal calcium transport to 25-hydroxy and 1,25-dihydroxy vitamin D in nephrectomized rats. Endocrinology 90:605–608, 1972.

237. Chen TC, Castillo L, Korycka-Dahl M, DeLuca HF: Role of vitamin D metabolites in phosphate transport of rat intestine. J Nutr 104:1056–1060, 1974.

238. Holick MF, Garabedian M, DeLuca HF: 1,25-Dihydroxycholecalciferol: Metabolite of vitamin $D_3$ active on bone in anephric rats. Science 176:1146–1147, 1972.

239. Raisz LG, Trummel CL, Holick MF, DeLuca HF: 1,25-Dihydroxycholecalciferol: A potent stimulator of bone resorption in tissue culture. Science 175:768–769, 1972.

240. Tieder M, Arie R, Modai D, et al: Elevated serum 1,25-dihydroxyvitamin D concentration in siblings with primary Fanconi's syndrome. N Engl J Med 319:845–849, 1988.

241. Markowitz M, Rotkin L, Rosen JF: Circadian rhythms of blood minerals in humans. Science 213:672–674, 1981.

242. Portale AA, Halloran BP, Morris RC Jr: Dietary intake of phosphorus modulates the circadian rhythm of serum concentration of phosphorus. J Clin Invest 80:1147–1154, 1987.

243. Portale AA, Halloran BP, Morris RC Jr: Physiologic regulation of the serum concentration of 1,25-dihydroxyvitamin D by phosphorus in normal men. J Clin Invest 83:1494–1499, 1989.

244. Portale AA, Halloran BP, Murphy MM, Morris RC Jr: Oral intake of phosphorus can determine the serum concentration of 1,25-dihydroxyvitamin D by determining its production rate in humans. J Clin Invest 77:7–12, 1986.

245. Gmaj P, Murer H: Cellular mechanism of inorganic phosphate transport in kidney. Physiol Rev 66:36–70, 1986.

246. Bonjour J, Caverzasio J: Phosphate transport in the kidney. Rev Physiol Biochem Pharmacol 100:162–214, 1984.

247. Brazy PC, McKeown JW, Harris RH, Dennis VW: Comparative effects of dietary phosphate, unilateral nephrectomy, and parathyroid hormone on phosphate transport by the rabbit proximal tubule. Kidney Int 17:788–800, 1980.

248. Knox FG, Haramati A: Renal regulation of phosphate excretion. In Seldin DW, Giebisch G (eds): The Kidney: Physiology and Pathophysiology. Raven Press, New York, 1985, p 1381.

249. Barrett PQ, Gertner JH, Rasmussen H: Effect of dietary phosphate on transport properties of pig renal microvillus vesicles. Am J Physiol 239:F352–F359, 1980.

250. Walker JJ, Yan TS, Quamme GA: Presence of multiple sodium-dependent phosphate transport processes in proximal brush-border membranes. Am J Physiol 252:F226–F231, 1987.

251. Werner A, Kempson SA, Biber J, Murer H: Increase of Na/$P_i$-cotransport encoding mRNA in response to low $P_i$ diet in rat kidney cortex. J Biol Chem 269:6637–6639, 1994.

252. Maierhofer WJ, Gray RW, Lemann J Jr: Phosphate deprivation increases serum 1,25-$(OH)_2$-vitamin D concentrations in healthy men. Kidney Int 25:571–575, 1984.

253. Gray RW, Wilz DR, Caldas AE, Lemann J Jr: The importance of phosphate in regulating plasma 1,25-$(OH)_2$-vitamin D levels in humans: Studies in healthy subjects, in calcium-stone formers and in patients with primary hyperparathyroidism. J Clin Endocrinol Metab 45:299–306, 1977.

254. Gray RW, Napoli JL: Dietary phosphate deprivation increases 1,25-dihydroxyvitamin $D_3$ synthesis in rat kidney in vitro. J Biol Chem 258:1152–1155, 1983.

255. Carpenter TO, Shiratori T: Renal 25-hydroxyvitamin D-1α-hydroxylase activity and mitochondrial phosphate transport in Hyp mice. Am J Physiol 22:E814–E821, 1990.

256. Castillo L, Tanaka Y, DeLuca HF: The mobilization of bone mineral by 1,25-dihydroxyvitamin $D_3$ in hypophosphatemic rats. Endocrinology 97:995–999, 1975.

257. Baylink D, Wergedal J, Stauffer M: Formation, mineralization and resorption of bone in hypophosphatemic rats. J Clin Invest 50:2519–2530, 1971.

258. Rowe JC, Wood DH, Rowe DW, Raisz LG: Nutritional hypophosphatemic rickets in a premature infant fed breast milk. N Engl J Med 300:293–296, 1979.

259. Greer FR, Steichen JJ, Tsang RC: Calcium and phosphate supplements in breast milk–related rickets. Am J Dis Child 136:581–583, 1982.

260. Lotz M, Zisman E, Bartter FC: Evidence for a phosphorus-depletion syndrome in man. N Engl J Med 278:409–415, 1968.

261. Lotz M, Ney R, Bartter FC: Osteomalacia and debility resulting from phosphorus depletion. Trans Assoc Am Physicians 77:281–395, 1964.

262. Baker LRI, Ackrill R, Cattell WR, et al: Iatrogenic osteomalacia and myopathy due to phosphate depletion. Br Med J 3:150–152, 1974.

263. Bloom WL, Flinchum D: Osteomalacia with pseudofractures caused by the ingestion of aluminum hydroxide. JAMA 174:1327–1330, 1960.

264. Carmichael KA, Fallon MD, Dalinka M, et al: Osteomalacia and osteitis fibrosa in a man ingesting aluminum hydroxide antacid. Am J Med 76:1137–1143, 1984.

265. Godsall JW, Baron R, Insogna KL: Vitamin D metabolism and bone histomorphometry in a patient with antacid-induced osteomalacia. Am J Med 77:747–750, 1984.

266. Maierhofer WJ, Gray RW, Cheung HS, Lemann J Jr: Bone resorption stimulated by elevated serum 1,25-$(OH)_2$ vitamin D concentrations in healthy men. Kidney Int 24:555–560, 1983.

267. Lyon MF, Scriver CR, Baker LRI, et al: The Gy mutation: Another cause of X-linked hypophosphatemia. Proc Natl Acad Sci USA 83:4899–4903, 1986.

268. Eicher EM, Southard JL, Scriver CR, Glorieux FH: Hypophosphatemia: Mouse model for human familial hypophosphatemic (vitamin D–resistant) rickets. Proc Natl Acad Sci USA 27:19, 1976.

269. Tenenhouse HS, Scriver CR, McInnes RR, Glorieux FH: Renal handling of phosphate in vivo and in vitro by the X-linked hypophosphatemic male mouse: Evidence for a defect in the brush border membrane. Kidney Int 14:236–244, 1978.

270. Davidai GA, Nesbitt T, Drezner MK: Normal regulation of calcitriol production in Gy mice; evidence for biochemical heterogeneity in the X-linked hypophosphatemic diseases. J Clin Invest 85:334–339, 1990.

271. Econs MJ, Fain PR, Norman M, et al: Flanking markers define the X-linked hypophosphatemic rickets gene locus. J Bone Miner Res 8:1149–1152, 1993.

272. Scriver CR, Tenenhouse HS, Glorieux FH: X-linked hypophosphatemia: An appreciation of a classic paper and a survey of progress since 1958. Medicine (Baltimore) 70:218–228, 1991.

273. Reid IR, Hardy DC, Murphy WA, et al: X-linked hypophosphatemia: A clinical, biochemical, and histopathologic assessment of morbidity in adults. Medicine (Baltimore) 68:336–352, 1989.

274. Moncrieff MW: Early biochemical findings in familial hypophosphatemic, hyperphosphaturic rickets and response to treatment. Arch Dis Child 57:70–72, 1982.

275. Harrison HE, Harrison HC, Lifshitz F, Johnson AD: Growth disturbance in hereditary hypophosphatemia. Am J Dis Child 112:290–297, 1966.

276. McNair SI, Stickler GB: Growth in familial hypophosphatemic vitamin D–resistant rickets. N Engl J Med 281:511–516, 1969.

277. Stickler GB, Beabout JW, Riggs BL: Vitamin D–resistant rickets: Clinical experience with 41 typical familial hypophosphatemic patients and 2 atypical nonfamilial cases. Mayo Clin Proc 45:197–218, 1970.

278. Hardy DC, Murphy WA, Siegel BA, et al: X-linked hypophosphatemia in adults: Prevalence of skeletal radiographic and scintigraphic features. Radiology 171:403–414, 1989.

279. Reid IR, Murphy WA, Hardy DC, et al: X-linked hypophosphatemia: Skeletal mass in adults assessed by histomorphometry, computed tomography, and absorptiometry. Am J Med 90:63–69, 1991.

280. Scriver CR, Reade TM, DeLuca HF, Hamstra AJ: Serum 1,25-dihydroxyvitamin D levels in normal subjects and in patients with hereditary rickets or bone disease. N Engl J Med 299:976–979, 1978.

281. Chesney RW, Mazess RB, Rose P, et al: Supranormal 25-hydroxyvitamin D and subnormal 1,25-dihydroxyvitamin D: Their role in X-linked hypophosphatemic rickets. Arch Dis Child 134:140–143, 1980.

282. Mason RS, Rohl PG, Lissner D, Posen S: Vitamin D metabolism in hypophosphatemic rickets. Am J Dis Child 136:909–913, 1982.

283. Lyles KW, Drezner MK: Parathyroid hormone effects on serum 1,25-dihydroxyvitamin D levels in patients with X-linked hypophosphatemic rickets: Evidence for abnormal 25-hydroxyvitamin D-1-hydroxylase activity. J Clin Endocrinol Metab 54:638–644, 1982.

284. Arnaud C: Serum parathyroid hormone in X-linked hypophosphatemia. Science 1730:845–847, 1971.

285. Roof BS, Piel CF, Gordan GS: Nature of defect responsible for familial vitamin D–resistant rickets (VDRR) based on radioimmunoassay for parathyroid hormone (PTH). Trans Assoc Am Physicians 85:172–180, 1972.

286. Lewy JE, Cabana EC, Repetto HA, et al: Serum parathyroid hormone in hypophosphatemic vitamin D–resistant rickets. J Pediatr 81:294–300, 1972.

287. Reitz RE, Weinstein RL: Parathyroid hormone secretion in familial vitamin-D–resistant rickets. N Engl J Med 289:941–945, 1973.

288. Fanconi A, Fisher JA, Prader A: Serum parathyroid hormone concentrations in hypophosphataemic vitamin D resistant rickets. Helv Paediatr Acta 29:187–194, 1974.

289. Short E, Morris RC Jr, Sebastian A, Spencer M: Exaggerated phosphaturic response to circulating parathyroid hormone in patients with familial X-linked hypophosphatemic rickets. J Clin Invest 58:152–163, 1976.

290. Carpenter TO, Mitnick MA, Ellison A, et al: Nocturnal hyperpara-

thyroidism: A frequent feature of X-linked hypophosphatemia. J Clin Endocrinol Metab 78:1378–1383, 1994.

291. Stickler GB: External calcium and phosphorus balances in vitamin D–resistant rickets. J Pediatr 63:942–948, 1963.

292. Soergel KH, Mueller KH, Gustke RF, Geenen JE: Jejunal calcium transport in health and metabolic bone disease: Effects of vitamin D. Gastroenterology 67:28, 1974.

293. Dent CE, Winter CS: Osteomalacia due to phosphate depletion from excessive aluminium hydroxide ingestion. Br Med J 1:551–552, 1974.

294. Cooke N, Teitelbaum S, Avioli LV: Antacid-induced osteomalacia and nephrolithiasis. Arch Intern Med 138:1007–1009, 1978.

295. Insogna KL, Bordley DR, Caro JF, Lockwood MD: Osteomalacia and weakness from excessive antacid ingestion. JAMA 244:2544–2546, 1980.

296. Saadeh G, Bauer T, Licata A, Sheeler L: Antacid-induced osteomalacia. Cleve Clin J Med 54:214–216, 1987.

297. De Deuxchaisnes CN, Krane SM: The treatment of adult phosphate diabetes and Fanconi syndrome with neutral sodium phosphate. Am J Med 43:508–543, 1967.

298. Schoot GD, Wills MR: Myopathy in hypophosphataemic osteomalacia presenting in adult life. J Neurol Neurosurg Psychiatry 38:297–304, 1975.

299. Teitelbaum SL, Rosenberg EM, Bates M, Avioli LV: The effects of phosphate and vitamin D therapy on osteopenic, hypophosphatemic osteomalacia of childhood. Clin Orthop 116:38–47, 1976.

300. Smith R, Newman RJ, Radda GK, et al: Hypophosphataemic osteomalacia and myopathy: Studies with nuclear magnetic resonance spectroscopy. Clin Sci 67:505–509, 1984.

301. Falls WFJ, Carter NW, Rector FC, Jr, Seldin DW: Familial vitamin D–resistant rickets: Study of six cases with evaluation of the pathogenetic role of secondary hyperparathyroidism. Ann Intern Med 68:553, 1968.

302. Scriver CR: Rickets and the pathogenesis of impaired tubular transport of phosphate and other solutes. Am J Med 57:43, 1974.

303. Insogna KL, Broadus AE, Gertner JM: Impaired phosphorus conservation and 1,25-dihydroxyvitamin D generation during phosphorus deprivation in familial hypophosphatemic rickets. J Clin Invest 71:1562–1569, 1983.

304. Tenenhouse HS, Martel J: Renal adaptation to phosphate deprivation: Lessons from the X-linked *Hyp* mouse. Pediatr Nephrol 7:312–318, 1993.

305. Sanjad SA, Kaddoura RE, Nazer HM, et al: Fanconi's syndrome with hepatorenal glycogenosis associated with phosphorylase *b* kinase deficiency. Am J Dis Child 147:957–959, 1993.

306. Harrison HE: Primary hypophosphatemic rickets and growth retardation. Growth 2:1, 1986.

307. Cowgill LD, Goldfarb S, Lau K, Slatopolsky E: Evidence for an intrinsic renal tubular defect in mice with genetic hypophosphatemic rickets. J Clin Invest 63:1203–1210, 1979.

308. Giasson SD, Brunetti MG, Danan G, et al: Micropuncture study of renal phosphorus transport in hypophosphatemic vitamin D resistant rickets mice. Pflugers Arch 371:33–38, 1977.

309. Custer M, Lotscher M, Biber J, et al: Expression of Na-P$_i$ cotransport in rat kidney: Localization by RT-PCR and immunohistochemistry. Am J Physiol 266:F767–F774, 1994.

310. Tenenhouse HS, Werner A, Biber J, et al: Renal Na$^+$-phosphate cotransport in murine X-linked hypophosphatemic rickets; molecular characterization. J Clin Invest 93:671–676, 1994.

311. Kos CH, Tihy F, Econs MJ, et al: Localization of a renal sodium-phosphate cotransporter gene to human chromosome 5q35. Genomics 19:176–177, 1994.

312. Magagnin S, Werner A, Markovich D, et al: Expression cloning of human and rat renal cortex Na/P$_i$ cotransport. Proc Natl Acad Sci 90:5979–5983, 1993.

313. Meyer RA Jr, Meyer MH, Gray RW: Parabiosis suggests a humoral factor is involved in X-linked hypophosphatemia in mice. J Bone Miner Res 4:493–500, 1989.

314. Nesbitt T, Coffman TM, Griffiths R, Drezner MK: Crosstransplantation of kidneys in normal and *Hyp* mice: Evidence that the *Hyp* mouse phenotype is unrelated to an intrinsic renal defect. J Clin Invest 89:1453–1459, 1992.

315. Econs MJ, Drezner MK: Tumor induced osteomalacia—unveiling a new hormone. N Engl J Med 330:1679–1681, 1994.

316. Drezner MK, Haussler MR: 1,25-Dihydroxyvitamin D in bone disease. N Engl J Med 300:435–436, 1979.

317. Delvin EE, Glorieux FH: Serum 1,25-dihydroxyvitamin-D concentration in hypophosphatemic vitamin-D resistant rickets. Calcif Tissue Int 33:173, 1981.

318. Lyles KW, Clark AG, Drezner MK: Serum 1,25-dihydroxyvitamin D levels in subjects with X-linked hypophosphatemic rickets and osteomalacia. Calcif Tissue Int 34:125–130, 1982.

319. Haussler M, Hughes M, Baylink D, et al: Influence of phosphate depletion on the biosynthesis and circulating level of 1α-25-dihydroxyvitamin D. Adv Exp Med Biol 81:233–250, 1977.

320. Yasuda T, Nakajima H: 1,25-Dihydroxyvitamin D production after stimulation with synthetic human parathyroid hormone (1–34) in hypoparathyroid and renal tubular disorders. Endocrinol Jpn 31:407–415, 1984.

321. McElduff A, Posen S: Parathyroid hormone sensitivity in familial X-linked hypophosphatemic rickets. J Clin Endocrinol Metab 69:386–389, 1989.

322. Meyer RA, Gray RW, Meyer MH: Abnormal vitamin D metabolism in the X-linked hypophosphatemic mouse. Endocrinology 107:1577–1581, 1980.

323. Yamamoto T, Seino Y, Tanaka H, et al: Effects of the administration of phosphate on nuclear 1,25-dihydroxyvitamin D$_3$ uptake by duodenal mucosal cells of *Hyp* mice. Endocrinology 122:576–580, 1988.

324. Yamaoka K, Seino Y, Satomura K, et al: Abnormal relationship between serum phosphate concentration and renal 25-hydroxycholecalciferol-1-α-hydroxylase activity in X-linked hypophosphatemic mice. Miner Electrolyte Metab 12:194–198, 1986.

325. Yamaoka K, Tanaka H, Kurose H, et al: Effect of single oral phosphate loading on vitamin D metabolites in normal subjects and in X-linked hypophosphatemic rickets. Bone Miner 7:159–169, 1989.

326. Seino Y, Shimotsuji T, Ishida M, et al: Vitamin D metabolism in hypophosphatemic vitamin-D resistant rickets. Contrib Nephrol 22:101–106, 1980.

327. Tenenhouse H: Metabolism of 25-hydroxyvitamin D$_3$ in renal slices from the X-linked hypophosphatemic (*Hyp*) mouse:Abnormal response to fall in serum calcium. Cell Calcium 5:43, 1984.

328. Tenenhouse HS: Abnormal renal mitochondrial 25-hydroxyvitamin D$_3$-1-hydroxylase activity in the vitamin D and calcium deficient X-linked *Hyp* mouse. Endocrinology 113:816–818, 1983.

329. Nesbitt T, Drezner MK, Lobaugh B: Abnormal parathyroid hormone stimulation of 25-hydroxyvitamin D-1-α-hydroxylase activity in the hypophosphatemic mouse: Evidence for a generalized defect of vitamin D metabolism. J Clin Invest 77:181, 1986.

330. Nesbitt T, Drezner MK: Abnormal parathyroid hormone–related peptide stimulation of renal 25-hydroxyvitamin D-1-hydroxylase in *Hyp* mice: Evidence for a generalized defect of enzyme activity in the proximal convoluted tubule. Endocrinology 127:843–848, 1990.

331. Henry HL, Norman AW: Vitamin D: Metabolism and biological actions. Annu Rev Nutr 4:493–520, 1984.

332. Muhlbauer RC, Bonjour J, Fleisch H: Abnormal tubular adaptation to dietary P$_i$ restriction in X-linked hypophosphatemic mice. Am J Physiol 242:F353–F359, 1982.

333. Tenenhouse HS, Yip A, Jones G: Increased renal catabolism of 1,25-dihydroxyvitamin D$_3$ in murine X-linked hypophosphatemic rickets. J Clin Invest 81:461–465, 1988.

334. Jones G, Yip A, Tenenhouse HS: Side chain oxidation of vitamin D$_3$ in mouse kidney mitochondria: Effect of the *Hyp* mutation and 1,25-dihydroxyvitamin D$_3$ treatment. Biochem Cell Biol 65:853, 1987.

335. Seino Y, Yamaoka K, Ishida M, et al: Plasma clearance for high doses of exogenous 1,25-dihydroxy [23,24(*n*)-3H] cholecalciferol in X-linked hypophosphatemic mice. Biomed Res 3:683–687, 1982.

336. Seino Y, Satomura K, Yamaoka K, et al: Activity of renal 25-hydroxyvitamin D$_3$-1-α-hydroxylase in a case of X-linked hypophosphatemic rickets. Eur J Pediatr 142:219–222, 1984.

337. Nesbitt T, Lobaugh B, Drezner MK: Calcitonin stimulation of renal 25-hydroxyvitamin D-1α-hydroxylase activity in hypophosphatemic mice. J Clin Invest 79:15–19, 1987.

338. Kawashima H, Torikai S, Kurokawa K: Localization of 25-hydroxyvitamin D$_3$-1-alpha-hydroxylase and 24-hydroxylase in the rat nephron. Proc Natl Acad Sci USA 78:1199, 1981.

339. Kawashima H, Torikai S, Kurokawa K: Calcitonin selectively stimulates 25-hydroxyvitamin D$_3$-1-α-hydroxylase in proximal straight tubule of rat kidney. Nature 291:327–329, 1981.

340. Ecarot B, Glorieux FH, Desbarats M, et al: Effect of dietary phosphate deprivation and supplementation of recipient mice on bone formation by transplanted cells from normal and X-linked hypophosphatemic mice. J Bone Miner Res 7:523–530, 1992.

341. Glorieux FH, Bordier PJ, Marie P, et al: Inadequate bone response to phosphate and vitamin D in familial hypophosphatemic rickets (FHR). *In* Massry SG, Ritz E, Rapado A (eds): Homeostasis of Phosphate and Other Minerals. Plenum Publishing, New York, 1978, pp 227–232.

342. Marie PJ, Travers R, Glorieux FH: Healing of rickets with phosphate supplementation in the hypophosphatemic male mouse. J Clin Invest 67:911–914, 1981.

343. Drezner MK, Lyles KW, Haussler MR, Harrelson JM: Evaluation of a role of 1,25-dihydroxyvitamin $D_3$ in the pathogenesis and treatment of X-linked hypophosphatemic rickets and osteomalacia. J Clin Invest 66:1020, 1980.

344. Glorieux FH, Insogna KL, Travers R, et al: Hypophosphatemic rickets with or without osteomalacia in correlation with circulating calcitriol levels. J Bone Miner Res 1:91, 1986.

345. Yamamoto T, Ecarot-Charrier B, Glorieux FH: Abnormal response of osteoblasts from *Hyp* mice to 1,25(OH)$_2$D$_3$. Bone 13:209–215, 1992.

346. Ecarot B, Glorieux FH, Desbarats M, et al: Defective bone formation by *Hyp* mouse bone cells transplanted into normal mice: Evidence in favor of an intrinsic osteoblast defect. J Bone Miner Res 7:215–220, 1992.

347. Ecarot-Charrier B, Glorieux FH, Travers R, et al: Defective bone formation by transplanted *Hyp* mouse bone cells into normal mice. Endocrinology 123:768–773, 1988.

348. Friedman NE, Lobaugh B, Drezner MK: Effects of calcitriol and phosphorus therapy on the growth of patients with X-linked hypophosphatemia. J Clin Endocrinol Metab 76:839–844, 1993.

349. Verge CF, Lam A, Simpson JM, et al: Effects of therapy in X-linked hypophosphatemic rickets. N Engl J Med 325:1843–1848, 1991.

350. Sullivan W, Carpenter T, Glorieux F, et al: A prospective trial of phosphate and 1,25-dihydroxyvitamin $D_3$ therapy in symptomatic adults with X-linked hypophosphatemic rickets. J Clin Endocrinol Metab 75:879–885, 1992.

351. Glorieux FH: Calcitriol treatment in vitamin D–dependent and vitamin D–resistant rickets. Metabolism 39:10–12, 1990.

352. Goodyer PR, Kronick JB, Jequier S, et al: Nephrocalcinosis and its relationship to treatment of hereditary rickets. J Pediatr 111:700–704, 1987.

353. Reusz GS, Hoyer PF, Lucas M, et al: X-linked hypophosphataemia: Treatment, height gain, and nephrocalcinosis. Arch Dis Child 65:1125–1128, 1990.

354. Harrell RM, Lyles KW, Harrelson JM, et al: Healing of bone disease in X-linked hypophosphatemic rickets/osteomalacia; induction and maintenance with phosphorus and calcitriol. J Clin Invest 75:1858–1868, 1985.

355. Evans DJ, Azzopardi JG: Distinctive tumours of bone and soft tissue causing acquired vitamin-D resistant osteomalacia. Lancet 1:353–354, 1972.

356. Moser CR, Fessel WJ: Rheumatic manifestations of hypophosphatemia. Arch Intern Med 134:674–678, 1974.

357. Daniels RA, Weisenfeld I: Tumorous phosphaturic osteomalacia; report of a case associated with multiple hemangiomas of bone. Am J Med 67:155–159, 1979.

358. Salassa RM, Jowsey J, Arnaud CD: Hypophosphatemic osteomalacia associated with "nonendocrine" tumors. N Engl J Med 283:65–70, 1970.

359. Ryan EA, Reiss E: Oncogenous osteomalacia; review of the world literature of 42 cases and report of two new cases. Am J Med 77:501–512, 1984.

360. Nuovo MA, Dorfman HD, Sun CJ, Chalew SA: Tumor-induced osteomalacia and rickets. Am J Surg Pathol 13:588–599, 1989.

361. Fukumoto Y, Tarui S, Tsukiyama K, et al: Tumor-induced vitamin D–resistant hypophosphatemic osteomalacia associated with proximal renal tubular dysfunction and 1,25-dihydroxyvitamin D deficiency. J Clin Endocrinol Metab 49:873–878, 1979.

362. Wener M, Cohen L, Bar RS, et al: Regulation of phosphate and calcium metabolism by vitamin D metabolites: Studies in a patient with oncogenic osteomalacia. Arthritis Rheum 22:672–673, 1979.

363. Camus JP, Crouzet J, Prier A, et al: Ostéomalacies hypophosphoré-

miques guéries par l'ablation de tumeurs bénignes du tissu conjonctif. Ann Med Interne (Paris) 131:422–426, 1980.

364. Sweet RA, Males JL, Hamstra AJ, DeLuca HF: Vitamin D metabolite levels in oncogenic osteomalacia. Ann Intern Med 47:523–528, 1980.

365. Parker MS, Klein I, Haussler MR, Mintz DH: Tumor-induced osteomalacia. JAMA 245:492–493, 1981.

366. Nortman DF, Coburn JW, Brautbar N, et al: Treatment of mesenchymal tumor associated osteomalacia (MTAO) with 1,25(OH)$_2$D$_3$: Report of a case. *In* Norman AW, Schaeffer K, Herrath DV, et al (eds): Vitamin D, Basic Research and its Clinical Application. Walter de Gruyter, Berlin, 1979, pp 1167–1168.

367. Cai Q, Hodgson SF, Kao PC, et al: Brief report: Inhibition of renal phosphate transport by a tumor product in a patient with oncogenic osteomalacia. N Engl J Med 330:1645–1649, 1994.

368. Leehey DJ, Ing TS, and Daugirdas JT: Fanconi syndrome associated with a non-ossifying fibroma of bone. Am J Med 78:708–710, 1985.

369. Miyauchi A, Fukase M, Tsutsumi M, Fujita T: Hemangiopericytoma-induced osteomalacia: Tumor transplantation in nude mice causes hypophosphatemia and tumor extracts inhibit renal 25-hydroxyvitamin D 1-hydroxylase activity. J Clin Endocrinol Metab 67:46–53, 1988.

370. Albright F, Burnett CH, Smith PH, Parson W: Pseudohypoparathyroidism, an example of Seabright-Bantam syndrome. Report of three cases. Endocrinology 30:922–932, 1942.

371. Tashjian AH Jr, Frantz AG, Lee JB: Pseudohypoparathyroidism: Assays of parathyroid hormone and thyrocalcitonin. Proc Natl Acad Sci USA 56:1138, 1966.

372. Chase LR, Aurbach GD: Parathyroid function and the renal excretion of 3′,5′-adenylic acid. Proc Natl Acad Sci USA 58:518, 1967.

373. Chase LR, Melson GL, Aurbach GD: Pseudohypoparathyroidism: Defective excretion of 3′-5′-AMP in response to parathyroid hormone. J Clin Invest 48:1832, 1969.

374. Bell NH, Sinha T, Clark LC Jr, et al: Effects of dibutyryl cyclic adenosine 3′-5′-monophosphate and parathyroid extract on calcium and phosphorus metabolism in hypoparathyroidism and pseudohypoparathyroidism. J Clin Invest 51:816–823, 1972.

375. Martin KJ, McConkey CL, Garcia JC, et al: Protein kinase-A and the effects of parathyroid hormone on phosphate uptake in opossum kidney cells. Endocrinology 125:295–301, 1989.

376. Drezner MK, Neelon FA, Lebovitz HE: Pseudohypoparathyroidism type II: A possible defect in the receptor of the cyclic AMP signal. N Engl J Med 289:1056, 1973.

377. Pollard AJ, Prendergast M, al-Hammouri F, et al: Different subtypes of pseudohypoparathyroidism in the same family with an unusual psychiatric presentation of the index case. Arch Dis Child 70:99–102, 1994.

378. Barr DG, Stirling HF, Darling JA: Evolution of pseudohypoparathyroidism: An informative family study. Arch Dis Child 70:337–338, 1994.

379. Wertznian R, Murad F: Effects of aminophylline, chlorpropamide, and parathyroid extract on plasma and urinary cyclic AMP in pseudohypoparathyroidism. Clin Res 21:89, 1973.

380. Drezner MK, Burch WM Jr: Altered activity of the nucleotide regulatory site in the parathyroid hormone–sensitive adenylate cyclase from the renal cortex of a patient with pseudohypoparathyroidism. J Clin Invest 62:1222, 1978.

381. Marcus R, Wilber JF, Aurbach GD: Parathyroid hormone–sensitive adenyl cyclase from the renal cortex of a patient with pseudohypoparathyroidism. J Clin Endocrinol Metab 33:537, 1981.

382. Casey PJ, Gilman AG: G protein involvement in receptor-effector coupling. J Biol Chem 263:2577, 1988.

383. Neer EJ: G proteins: Critical control points for transmembrane signals. Protein Sci 3:3–14, 1994.

384. Bourne HR, Sanders DA, McCormick F: The GTPase superfamily: A conserved switch for diverse cell functions. Nature 348:125–132, 1990.

385. Farfel Z, Brickman AS, Kaslow HR, et al: Defect of receptor-cyclase coupling in pseudohypoparathyroidism. N Engl J Med 303:237, 1980.

386. Farfel Z, Brothers VM, Brickman AS, et al: Pseudohypoparathyroidism: Inheritance of deficient receptor-cyclase coupling activity. Proc Natl Acad Sci USA 78:3098, 1981.

387. Levine MD, Downs RW Jr, Singer M, et al: Deficient activity of

guanine nucleotide regulatory protein in erythrocytes from patients with pseudohypoparathyroidism. Biochem Biophys Res Commun 34:1319, 1980.

388. Farfel Z, Bourne HR: Deficient activity of receptor-cyclase coupling protein in platelets of patients with pseudohypoparathyroidism. J Clin Endocrinol Metab 51:1202, 1980.

389. Bourne HR, Kaslow HR, Brickman AS, Farfel Z: Fibroblast defect in pseudohypoparathyroidism type I: Reduced activity of receptor-cyclase coupling protein. J Clin Endocrinol Metab 53:636, 1981.

390. Carter A, Bardin C, Collins R, et al: Reduced expression of multiple forms of the α subunit of the stimulatory GTP-binding protein in pseudohypoparathyroidism type Ia. Proc Natl Acad Sci USA 84:7266–7269, 1987.

391. Levine MA, Downs RX Jr, Moses AM, et al: Resistance to multiple hormones in patients with pseudohypoparathyroidism. Am J Med 74:545–556, 1983.

392. Kerr D, Hosking DJ: Pseudohypoparathyroidism: Clinical expression of PTH resistance. Q J Med 65:889–894, 1987.

393. Van Dop C: Pseudohypoparathyroidism: Clinical and molecular aspects. Semin Nephrol 9:168–178, 1989.

394. Schuster V, Eschenhagen T, Kruse K, et al: Endocrine and molecular biological studies in a German family with Albright hereditary osteodystrophy. Eur J Pediatr 152:185–189, 1993.

395. Izraeli S, Metzker A, Horev G, et al: Albright hereditary osteodystrophy with hypothyroidism, normocalcemia, and normal Gs protein activity: A family presenting with congenital osteoma cutis. Am J Med Genet 43:764–767, 1992.

396. Faull CM, Welbury RR, Paul B, Kendall-Taylor P: Pseudohypoparathyroidism: Its phenotypic variability and associated disorders in a large family. Q J Med 78:251–264, 1991.

397. Sklar PB, Anholt RRH, Snyder SH: The odorant-sensitive adenylate cyclase of olfactory receptor cells. J Biol Chem 261:15538, 1986.

398. Weinstock RS, Wright HN, Spiegel AM, et al: Olfactory dysfunction in humans with deficient guanine nucleotide–binding protein. Nature 322:635–636, 1986.

399. Jones DT, Reed RR: Golf: An olfactory neuron specific G protein involved in odorant signal transduction. Science 244:790, 1989.

400. Moses AM, Weinstock RS, Levine MA, Breslau NA: Evidence for normal antidiuretic responses to endogenous and exogenous arginine vasopressin in patients with guanine nucleotide–binding stimulatory protein-deficient pseudohypoparathyroidism. J Clin Endocrinol Metab 62:221–224, 1986.

401. Kolb FO, Steinbach HL: Pseudohypoparathyroidism with secondary hyperparathyroidism and osteitis fibrosa. J Clin Endocrinol Metab 22:59, 1962.

402. Kidd GS, Schaaf M, Adler RA, et al: Skeletal responsiveness in pseudohypoparathyroidism: A spectrum of clinical disease. Am J Med 68:772–781, 1980.

403. Burnstein MI, Kottamasu SR, Pettifor JM: Metabolic bone disease in pseudohypoparathyroidism: Radiologic features. Radiology 155:351, 1985.

404. Spiegel AM: Pseudohypoparathyroidism. In Scriver CR, Beaudet AL, Sly WS, Valle D (eds): The Metabolic Basis of Inherited Disease, 6th ed. McGraw-Hill, New York, 1989, pp 2013–2027.

405. Wilson JD, Hadden DR: Pseudohypoparathyroidism presenting with rickets. J Clin Endocrinol Metab 51:1148, 1980.

406. Metz SA, Baylink DJ, Hughes MR, et al: Selective deficiency of 1,25-dihydroxycholecalciferol: A cause of isolated skeletal resistance to parathyroid hormone. N Engl J Med 25:1084, 1977.

407. Hosking DJ, Kerr D: Mechanisms of parathyroid hormone resistance in pseudohypoparathyroidism. Clin Sci 74:561–566, 1988.

408. Winter JSD, Hughes JA: Familial pseudohypoparathyroidism without somatic abnormalities. Can Med Assoc J 123:26, 1980.

409. Carlson HE, Brickman AS, Bottazzo GF: Prolactin deficiency in pseudohypoparathyroidism. N Engl J Med 296:140, 1977.

410. Silve C, Santora A, Breslau N, et al: Selective resistance to parathyroid hormone in cultured skin fibroblasts from patients with pseudohypoparathyroidism type Ib. J Clin Endocrinol Metab 62:240, 1986.

411. Farfel Z, Bourne HR: Pseudohypoparathyroidism: Mutation affecting adenylate cyclase. Miner Electrolyte Metab 8:227–236, 1982.

412. Gupta A, Martin KJ, Miyauchi A, Hruska KA: Regulation of cytosolic calcium by parathyroid hormone and oscillations of cytosolic calcium in fibroblasts from normal and pseudohypoparathyroid patients. Endocrinology 128:2825–2836, 1991.

413. Fischer JA: Biologically inactive parathyroid hormone in pseudohypoparathyroidism type I (PHP-1). In Cohn DV, Talmage RV, Matthews LJ (eds): Hormonal Control of Calcium Metabolism. Excerpta Medica, Amsterdam, 1981.

414. Barrett D, Breslau NA, Wax MB, et al: New form of pseudohypoparathyroidism with abnormal catalytic adenylate cyclase. Am J Physiol 257:E277–E283, 1989.

415. Singhellakis P, Pappas A, Nicolou CH, Ikkos D: Separation of pseudohypoparathyroidism into types I and II using only basal nephrogenous cAMP determinations. Endocrinologie 29:67–71, 1991.

416. Rao DS, Parfitt AM, Kleerekoper M, et al: Dissociation between the effects of endogenous parathyroid hormone on adenosine 3′5′-monophosphate generation and phosphate reabsorption in hypocalcemia due to vitamin D depletion: An acquired disorder resembling pseudohypoparathyroidism type II. J Clin Endocrinol Metab 61:285–290, 1985.

417. Matsuda I, Takekoshi Y, Tanaka M, et al: Pseudohypoparathyroidism: Type II and anticonvulsant rickets. Eur J Pediatr 132:303, 1979.

418. Rodriguez HJ, Villareal H, Klahr S, Slatopolsky E: Pseudohypoparathyroidism type II. Restoration of normal renal responsiveness to parathyroid hormone by calcium administration. J Clin Endocrinol Metab 39:693, 1974.

419. Quamme G, Pfeilschifter J, Murer H: Parathyroid hormone inhibition of Na+/phosphate cotransport in OK cells: Requirement of protein kinase C–dependent pathway. Biochim Biophys Acta 1013:159–165, 1989.

420. Boneh A, Mandla S, Tenenhouse HS: Phorbol myristate acetate activates protein kinase C, stimulates the phosphorylation of endogenous proteins and inhibits phosphate transport in mouse renal tubules. Biochim Biophys Acta 1012:308–316, 1989.

421. Quamme G, Pfeilschifter J, Murer H: Parathyroid hormone inhibition of Na+/phosphate cotransport in OK cells: Generation of second messengers in the regulatory cascade. Biochem Biophys Res Commun 158:951–957, 1989.

422. Kinder BK, Rasmussen H: New applications of total parathyroidectomy and autotransplantation: Use in proximal renal tubular dysfunction. World J Surg 9:156–164, 1985.

423. Albright F, Burnett CH, Parson W, et al: Osteomalacia and late rickets: The various etiologies met in the United States with emphasis on that resulting from a specific form of renal acidosis, the therapeutic indications for each etiological sub-group, and the relationship between osteomalacia and Milkman's syndrome. Medicine (Baltimore) 25:399–479, 1946.

424. Pines KL, Mudge GH: Renal tubular acidosis with osteomalacia: Report of three cases. Am J Med 11:302–311, 1951.

425. Lightwood R, Payne WW, Black JA: Infantile renal acidosis. Pediatrics 12:628–644, 1953.

426. Smith LH Jr, Schreiner GE: Studies on renal hyperchloremic acidosis. J Lab Clin Med 43:347–358, 1954.

427. Reynolds TB: Observations on the pathogenesis of renal tubular acidosis. Am J Med 25:503–515, 1958.

428. Wrong O, Davies HEF: The excretion of acid in renal disease. Q J Med 28:259–313, 1959.

429. Relman AS: Renal acidosis and renal excretion of acid in health and disease. Adv Intern Med 12:295–347, 1964.

430. Elkinton JR, McCurdy DK, Buckalew VM Jr: Hydrogen ion and the kidney. In Black DAK (ed): Renal Disease, 2nd ed. FA Davis, Philadelphia, 1967, p 110.

431. Soriano JR, Boichis H, Edelmann CM Jr: Bicarbonate reabsorption and hydrogen ion excretion in children with renal tubular acidosis. J Pediatr 71:802–813, 1967.

432. Morris RC Jr: An experimental renal acidification defect in patients with hereditary fructose intolerance. II. Its distinction from classic renal tubular acidosis; its resemblance to the renal acidification defect associated with the Fanconi syndrome of children with cystinosis. J Clin Invest 47:1648–1663, 1968.

433. Rodriguez-Soriano J, Edelmann CM Jr: Renal tubular acidosis. Annu Rev Med 20:363–382, 1969.

434. Morris RC Jr: Renal tubular acidosis: Mechanisms, classification and implications. N Engl J Med 281:1405–1413, 1969.

435. McSherry E, Sebastian A, Morris RC Jr: Renal tubular acidosis in infants: The several kinds, including bicarbonate-wasting, classic renal tubular acidosis. J Clin Invest 51:499–514, 1972.

436. Sebastian A, McSherry E, Morris RC Jr: Metabolic acidosis with special reference to the renal acidoses. *In* Brenner BM, Rector FC Jr (eds): The Kidney, 1st ed. WB Saunders, Philadelphia, 1976.

437. Seldin DW, Wilson JD: Renal tubular acidosis. *In* Stanbury JB, Wyngaarden JB, Fredrickson DS (eds): The Metabolic Basis of Inherited Disease, 4th ed. McGraw-Hill, New York, 1978.

438. Arruda JAL, Kurtzman NA: Mechanisms and classification of deranged distal urinary acidification. Am J Physiol 239:F515–F523, 1980.

439. Buckalew VM Jr, Caruana RJ: The pathophysiology of distal (type I) renal tubular acidosis. *In* Gonick HC, Buckalew VMJ (eds): Renal Tubular Acidosis. Marcel Dekker, New York, 1985, pp 357–386.

440. Halperin ML, Goldstein MB, Richardson RMA, Stinebaugh BJ: Distal renal tubular acidosis syndromes: A pathophysiological approach. Am J Nephrol 5:1–8, 1985.

441. Dubose TD Jr, Alpern RJ: Renal tubular acidosis *In* Scriver CR, Beaudet AI, Sly WS, Valle, D (eds): The Metabolic Basis of Inherited Disease, 6th ed. McGraw-Hill, New York, 1989, pp 2539–2568.

442. Cogan MC, Rector FC Jr: Acid-base disorders. *In* Brenner BM, Rector FC Jr (eds): The Kidney, 4th ed. WB Saunders, Philadelphia, 1991, pp 737–804.

443. Sabatini S, Kurtzman NA: Pathophysiology of the renal tubular acidoses. Semin Nephrol 11:202–211, 1991.

444. Hunt DD, Stearns G, McKinley JB, et al: Long-term study of family with Fanconi syndrome without cystinosis (DeToni–Debre-Fanconi syndrome). Am J Med 40:492–510, 1966.

445. Smith R, Lindenbaum RH, Walton RJ: Hypophosphataemic osteomalacia and Fanconi syndrome of adult onset with dominant inheritance. Q J Med 45:387–400, 1976.

446. Friedman AL, Trygstad CW, Chesney RW: Autosomal dominant Fanconi syndrome with early renal failure. Am J Med Genet 2:225–232, 1978.

447. Patrick A, Cameron JS, Ogg CS: A family with a dominant form of idiopathic Fanconi syndrome leading to renal failure in adult life. Clin Nephrol 16:289–292, 1981.

448. Brenton DP, Isenberg DA, Cusworth DC, et al: The adult presenting idiopathic Fanconi syndrome. J Inherited Metab Dis 4:211–215, 1981.

449. Saville PD, Nassim JR, Stevenson H, et al: The effect of A.T. 10 on calcium and phosphorus metabolism in resistant rickets. Clin Sci 14:489–499, 1955.

450. Lee DBN, Drinkard JP, Rosen VJ, Gonick HC: The adult Fanconi syndrome. Medicine (Baltimore) 51:107–138, 1972.

451. Worthen HG, Good RA: The de Toni–Fanconi syndrome with cystinosis. Am J Dis Child 95:653–688, 1958.

452. Lamy M, Frezal J, Rey J, Larsen C: Étude métabolique du syndrome de Lowe. Rev Fr Etudes Clin Biol 7:271–283, 1962.

453. Wilson DM, Goldstein NP: Bicarbonate excretion in Wilson's disease (hepatolenticular degeneration). Mayo Clin Proc 49:394–400, 1974.

454. Litin RB, Randall RV, Goldstein NP, et al: Hypercalciuria in hepatolenticular degeneration (Wilson's disease). Am J Med Sci 238:614–620, 1959.

455. Gentz J, Jagenburg R, Zetterstrom R: Tyrosinemia. J Pediatr 66:670–696, 1965.

456. Clayton PT, Hyland K, Brand M, Leonard JV: Mitochondrial phosphoenolpyruvate carboxykinase deficiency. Eur J Pediatr 145:46–50, 1986.

457. Rodriguez-Soriano J, Rivera JM, Vallo A, et al: Proximal renal tubular acidosis in metachromatic leukodystrophy. Helv Paediatr Acta 33:45–52, 1978.

458. Carty R, Cooper M, Tabachnik E: The Fanconi syndrome associated with hepatic glycogenosis and abnormal metabolism of galactose. J Pediatr 850:821–823, 1974.

459. Brodehl J: The Fanconi syndrome. *In* Edelmann CM Jr (ed): Pediatric Kidney Disease. Little, Brown, Boston, 1978, pp 955–987.

460. Seo Y, Murakami M, Watari H, et al: Intracellular pH determination by a $^{31}$P-NMR technique. The second dissociation constant of phosphoric acid in a biological system. J Biochem 94:729–734, 1983.

461. Muldowney FP, Donhoe JF, Freaney R, et al: Parathormone-induced renal bicarbonate wastage in intestinal malabsorption and in chronic renal failure. Ir J Med Sci 3:221–231, 1970.

462. Vainsel M, Manderlier TH, Vis HL: Proximal renal tubular acidosis in vitamin D deficiency rickets. Biomedicine 22:35–40, 1975.

463. Scott J, Elias E, Moult PJA, et al: Rickets in adult cystic fibrosis with myopathy, pancreatic insufficiency and proximal renal tubular dysfunction. Am J Med 63:488–492, 1977.

464. Stoop JW, Schraagen MJC, Tiddens HAWM: Pseudo-vitamin D deficiency rickets. Acta Paediatr Scand 56:607–616, 1967.

465. Wegienka LC, Weller JM: Renal tubular acidosis caused by degraded tetracycline. Arch Intern Med 114:232, 1964.

466. Otten J, Vis HL: Acute reversible renal tubular dysfunction following intoxication with methyl-3-chromone. J Pediatr 73:422–425, 1968.

467. Sadoff L: Nephrotoxicity of streptozotocin. Cancer Chemother Rep 54:457–459, 1970.

468. Chisolm JJ Jr, Harrison HC, Eberlein WR, Harrison HE: Aminoaciduria, hypophosphatemia, and rickets in lead poisoning. Am J Dis Child 89:159–168, 1955.

469. Sebastian A, McSherry E, Ueki I, Morris RC Jr: Renal amyloidosis, nephrotic syndrome and impaired renal tubular reabsorption of bicarbonate. Ann Intern Med 69:541–548, 1968.

470. Stickler GB, Rosevear JW, Ulrich JA: Renal tubular dysfunction complicating the nephrotic syndrome: The disturbance in calcium and phosphorus metabolism. Mayo Clin Proc 37:376–388, 1962.

471. Tegelaers WHH, Tiddens HW: Nephrotic-glucosuric-aminoaciduric dwarfism and electrolyte metabolism. Helv Paediatr Acta 10:269–278, 1955.

472. Massry SG, Preuss HG, Maher JF, Schreiner GE: Renal tubular acidosis after cadaver kidney homotransplantation. Am J Med 24:284–292, 1967.

473. Morris RC Jr: The clinical spectrum of Fanconi's syndrome. Calif Med 108:225–231, 1968.

474. Riley AL, Ryan LM, Roth DA: Renal proximal tubular dysfunction and paroxysmal nocturnal hemoglobinuria. Am J Med 62:125–129, 1977.

475. Cade R, Spooner G, Juncos L, et al: Chronic renal vein thrombosis. Am J Med 63:387–397, 1977.

476. Sebastian A, McSherry E, Morris RC Jr: On the mechanism of renal potassium wasting in renal tubular acidosis associated with the Fanconi syndrome (type 2 RTA). J Clin Invest 50:231–243, 1971.

477. Engle RI Jr, Wallis LA: Multiple myeloma and the adult Fanconi syndrome. I. Report of a case with crystal-like deposits in the tumor cells and in the epithelial cells of the kidney. Am J Med 22:5–12, 1957.

478. Sirota JH, Hamerman D: Renal function studies in an adult subject with the Fanconi syndrome. Am J Med 16:138–152, 1954.

479. Harrison JF, Blainey JD: Adult Fanconi syndrome with monoclonal abnormality of immunoglobulin light chain. J Clin Pathol 20:42–48, 1967.

480. Maldonado JE, Velosa JA, Kyle RA, et al: Fanconi syndrome in adults: A manifestation of a latent form of myeloma. Am J Med 58:354–364, 1975.

481. Smithline N, Kassirer JP, Cohen JJ: Light-chain nephropathy: Renal tubular dysfunction associated with light-chain proteinuria. N Engl J Med 294:71–74, 1976.

482. Graziani G, De Vecchi A, Rosti D: Primary proximal renal tubular acidosis. Helv Paediatr Acta 31:427–434, 1976.

483. Donckerwolcke RA, Van Stekelenburg GJ, Tiddens HA: A case of bicarbonate-losing renal tubular acidosis with defective carboanhydrase activity. Arch Dis Child 45:769–773, 1970.

484. Brenes LG, Brenes JN, Hernandez MM: Familial proximal renal tubular acidosis: A distinct clinical entity. Am J Med 63:244–252, 1977.

485. Gruskin AB, Patel MS, Linshaw M, et al: Renal function studies and kidney pyruvate carboxylase in subacute necrotizing encephalomyelopathy (Leigh's syndrome). Pediatr Res 7:832–841, 1973.

486. Atkin BM, Buist NRM, Utter MF, et al: Pyruvate carboxylase deficiency and lactic acidosis in a retarded child without Leigh's disease. Pediatr Res 13:109–116, 1979.

487. Vainsel M, Fondu P, Cadranel S, et al: Osteopetrosis associated with proximal and distal tubular acidosis. Acta Paediatr Scand 61:429–434, 1972.

488. Sly WS, Whyte MP, Sundaram V, et al: Carbonic anhydrase II deficiency in 12 families with the autosomal recessive syndrome of osteopetrosis with renal tubular acidosis and cerebral calcification. N Engl J Med 313:139–145, 1985.

489. Ohlsson A, Cumming WA, Paul A, Sly WS: Carbonic anhydrase II deficiency syndrome: Recessive osteopetrosis with renal tubular acidosis and cerebral calcification. Pediatrics 77:371–381, 1986.

490. Leaf A, Schwartz WB, Relman AS: Oral administration of a potent carbonic anhydrase inhibitor ("Diamox"). N Engl J Med 250:759–764, 1954.

491. Seldin DW, Portwood RM, Rector FC Jr, Cade R: Characteristics of renal bicarbonate reabsorption in man. J Clin Invest 38:1663–1671, 1959.

492. Beckman WW, Rossmeisl EC, Pettingill RB, Bauer W: A study of the effect of sulfanilamide on acid-base metabolism. J Clin Invest 19:635–644, 1940.

493. York SE, Yendt ER: Osteomalacia associated with renal bicarbonate loss. Can Med Assoc J 94:1329–1342, 1966.

494. Rodriguez-Soriano J, Vallo A, Chouza M, Castillo G: Proximal renal tubular acidosis in tetralogy of Fallot. Acta Paediatr Scand 64:671–674, 1975.

495. McSherry E, Morris RC Jr: Attainment and maintenance of normal stature with alkali therapy in infants and children with classic renal tubular acidosis. J Clin Invest 61:509–527, 1978.

496. Pitts HH Jr, Schulte JW, Smith DR: Nephrocalcinosis in a father and three children. J Urol 73:208–211, 1955.

497. Randall RE Jr, Targgart WH: Familial renal tubular acidosis. Ann Intern Med 54:1108–1116, 1961.

498. Randall RE Jr: Familial renal tubular acidosis revisited. Ann Intern Med 66:1024–1025, 1967.

499. Schreiner GE, Smith LH Jr, Kyle LH: Renal hyperchloremic acidosis. Am J Med 15:122–129, 1953.

500. Gyory AZ, Edwards KDG: Renal tubular acidosis: A family with an autosomal dominant genetic defect in renal hydrogen ion transport, with proximal tubular and collecting duct dysfunction and increased metabolism of citrate and ammonia. Am J Med 45:43–62, 1968.

501. Wilansky DL, Schucher R: Familial acidosis of renal tubular origin. Can Med Assoc J 83:308–312, 1960.

502. Richards P, Wrong OM: Dominant inheritance in a family with familial renal tubular acidosis. Lancet 2:998–999, 1972.

503. Musgrave JE, Bennett WM, Campbelle RA, Eisemberg CS: Renal tubular acidosis. Lancet 2:1364, 1972.

504. Nebout T, Desaine C, Weil B, et al: Acidose tubulaire distale familiale. Sem Hop Paris 50:557–560, 1974.

505. Norman ME, Feldman NJ, Cohn RM, McCurdy DK: Urinary citrate excretion in the diagnosis of distal renal tubular acidosis. J Pediatr 92:394–400, 1978.

506. Buckalew VM Jr, Purvis ML, Shulman MG, et al: Hereditary renal tubular acidosis. Medicine (Baltimore) 53:229–254, 1974.

507. Hamed IA, Czerwinski AW, Coats B, et al: Familial absorptive hypercalciuria and renal tubular acidosis. Am J Med 67:385–391, 1979.

508. Rodriguez-Soriano J, Vallo A, Garcia-Fuentes M: Distal renal tubular acidosis in infancy: A bicarbonate wasting state. J Pediatr 86:524–532, 1975.

509. Levine AS, Michael AF Jr: Ehlers-Danlos syndrome with renal tubular acidosis and medullary sponge kidneys. J Pediatr 71:107–113, 1967.

510. Baehner RL, Gilchrist GS, Anderson EJ: Hereditary elliptocytosis and primary renal tubular acidosis in a single family. Am J Dis Child 115:414–419, 1968.

511. Goossens JP, Van Eps LWS, Schouten H, Giterson AL: Incomplete renal tubular acidosis in sickle cell disease. Clin Chim Acta 41:149–156, 1972.

512. Kong HH, Alleyne GAO: Defect in urinary acidification in adults with sickle-cell anaemia. Lancet 2:954–955, 1968.

513. Takeda R, Morimoto S, Kuroda M, Murakami M: Renal tubular acidosis, presenting as a syndrome resembling Bartter's syndrome, in a patient with arachnodactyly. Acta Endocrinol 73:531–542, 1973.

514. Shapira E, Ben-Yoseph Y, Eyal FG, Russell A: Enzymatically inactive red cell carbonic anhydrase B in a family with renal tubular acidosis. J Clin Invest 53:59–63, 1974.

515. Kondo T, Taniguchi N, Taniguchi K, et al: Inactive form of erythrocyte carbonic anhydrase B in patients with primary renal tubular acidosis. J Clin Invest 62:610–617, 1978.

516. Sly WS: The carbonic anhydrase II deficiency syndrome: Osteopetrosis with renal tubular acidosis and cerebral calcification. In

Scriver CR, Beaudet AL, Sly WS, Valle D (eds): The Metabolic Basis of Inherited Disease, 6th ed. McGraw-Hill, New York, 1989, pp 2857–2868.

517. Royer P, Broyer M: L'acidose rénale au cours des tubulopathies congénitales. In Actualités Néphrologiques de l'Hôpital Necker. Paris, Flammarion, 1967, p 73.

518. Donckerwolcke RA, Van Biervliet JP, Koorevaar G, et al: The syndrome of renal tubular acidosis with nerve deafness. Acta Paediatr Scand 65:100–104, 1976.

519. Dunger DB, Brenton DP, Cain AR: Renal tubular acidosis and nerve deafness. Arch Dis Child 55:221–225, 1980.

520. Cremers CWRJ, Monnens LAH, Marres EHMA: Renal tubular acidosis and sensorineural deafness. Arch Otolaryngol 106:287–289, 1980.

521. Cohen A, Way BJ: The association of renal tubular acidosis with hyperglobulinaemic purpura. Aust Ann Med 11:189–194, 1962.

522. LoSpalluto J, Dorward B, Miller W Jr, Ziff M: Cryoglobulinemia based on interaction between a gamma macroglobulin and 7S gamma globulin. Am J Med 32:142–147, 1962.

523. Seedat YK, Rain ER: Active chronic hepatitis associated with renal tubular acidosis and successful pregnancy. S Afr Med J 39:595–597, 1965.

524. McCurdy DK, Cornwell GG III, DePratti VJ: Hyperglobulinemic renal tubular acidosis: Report of the two cases. Ann Intern Med 67:110–117, 1967.

525. Morris RC Jr, Fudenberg HH: Impaired renal acidification in patients with hypergammaglobulinemia. Medicine (Baltimore) 46:57–69, 1967.

526. Talal N, Zisman E, Schur PH: Renal tubular acidosis, glomerulonephritis and immunologic factors in Sjögren's syndrome. Arthritis Rheum 11:774–786, 1968.

527. Shioji R, Furuyama T, Onodera S, et al: Sjögren's syndrome and renal tubular acidosis. Am J Med 48:456–463, 1970.

528. Mason AMS, Golding PL: Hyperglobulinaemic renal tubular acidosis: A report of nine cases. Br J Med 3:143–146, 1970.

529. Pasternack A, Linder E: Renal tubular acidosis: An immunopathological study on four patients. Clin Exp Immunol 7:115–123, 1970.

530. Mason AMS, Golding PL: Renal tubular acidosis and autoimmune thyroid disease. Lancet 2:1104–1107, 1970.

531. Mason AMS, McIllmurray MB, Golding PL, Hughes DT: Fibrosing alveolitis associated with renal tubular acidosis. Br J Med 4:596–599, 1970.

532. Talal N: Sjögren's syndrome, lymphoproliferation, and renal tubular acidosis. Ann Intern Med 74:633–634, 1971.

533. Bridi GS, Falcon PW, Brackett NC Jr, et al: Glomerulonephritis and renal tubular acidosis in a case of chronic active hepatitis with hyperimmunoglobulinemia. Am J Med 52:267–278, 1972.

534. Tsantoulas DC, McFarlane IG, Portmann B, et al: Cell-mediated immunity to human Tamm-Horsfall glycoprotein in autoimmune liver disease with renal tubular acidosis. Br Med J 4:491–494, 1974.

535. Golding PL: Renal tubular acidosis in chronic liver disease. Postgrad Med J 51:550–556, 1975.

536. Cochrane AMG, Tsantoulos DC, Moussouros A, et al: Lymphocyte cytotoxicity for kidney cells in renal tubular acidosis of autoimmune liver disease. Br Med J 2:276–278, 1976.

537. Andrassy K, Gebest J, Tan E, et al: Interstitial nephritis in a patient with atypical Sjögren's syndrome. Klin Wochenschr 58:563–567, 1980.

538. Jaeger P, Portmann L, Wauters J, et al: Distal renal tubular acidosis and lymphocytic thyroiditis with spontaneously resolving hyperthyroidism. Am J Nephrol 5:116–120, 1985.

539. Breedveld FC, Haanen HCM, Chang PC: Distal renal tubular acidosis in polyarteritis nodosa. Arch Intern Med 146:1009–1010, 1986.

540. Dent CE, Harper CM, Parfitt AM: The effect of cellulose phosphate on calcium metabolism in patients with hypercalcemia. Clin Sci 27:417–425, 1964.

541. Parfitt AM, Higgins BA, Nassim JR et al: Metabolic studies in patients with hypercalcemia. Clin Sci 27:463–482, 1964.

542. Cohen SI, Fitzgerald MG, Fourman P, et al: Polyuria in hyperparathyroidism. Q J Med 26:423–431, 1957.

543. Reynolds TB, Bethune JE: Renal tubular acidosis secondary to hyperparathyroidism. Clin Res 17:169, 1969.

544. Zisman E, Buccino RA, Gorden P, Barter FC: Hyperthyroidism and renal tubular acidosis. Arch Intern Med 121:118–122, 1968.

545. Ferris T, Kashgarian M, Levitin H, et al: Renal tubular acidosis and renal potassium wasting required as a result of hypercalcemic nephropathy. N Engl J Med 265:924–928, 1961.

546. Deck MDF: Medullary sponge kidney with renal tubular acidosis: A report of 3 cases. J Urol 94:330–335, 1965.

547. Morris RC Jr, Yamauchi H, Palubinskas AJ, Howenstine J: Medullary sponge kidney. Am J Med 38:883–892, 1965.

548. Mass RE, Smith WR, Walsh JR: The association of hereditary fructose intolerance and renal tubular acidosis. Am J Med Sci 251:516–523, 1966.

549. Fulop M, Sternlieb I, Scheinberg IH: Defective urinary acidification in Wilson's disease. Ann Intern Med 68:770–777, 1968.

550. Yeoh SA, Asan P: Fabry's disease with renal tubular acidosis. Singapore Med J 8:275–279, 1967.

551. Husband P, McKellar WJ: Infantile renal tubular acidosis due to mercury poisoning. Arch Dis Child 45:264–268, 1970.

552. McCurdy DK, Frederic M, Elkinton JR: Renal tubular acidosis due to amphotericin B. N Engl J Med 278:124–130, 1968.

553. Patterson RM, Ackerman GL: Renal tubular acidosis due to amphotericin B nephrotoxicity. Arch Intern Med 127:241–244, 1971.

554. Steele TW, Edwards KDG: Analgesic nephropathy: Changes in various parameters of renal function following cessation of analgesic abuse. Med J Aust 1:181–187, 1971.

555. Steele TW, Gyory AZ, Edwards KDG: Renal function in analgesic nephropathy. Br Med J 2:213–216, 1969.

556. Perez GO, Oster JR, Vaamonde CA: Incomplete syndrome of renal tubular acidosis induced by lithium carbonate. J Lab Clin Med 86:386–394, 1975.

557. Yong JM, Sanderson KV: Photosensitive dermatitis and renal tubular acidosis after ingestion of calcium cyclamate. Lancet 2:1273–1275, 1969.

558. Fischman CM, Oster JR: Toxic effects of toluene. JAMA 241:1713–1715, 1979.

559. Streicher HZ, Govow PA, Moss AH, et al: Syndromes of toluene sniffing in adults. Ann Intern Med 94:758–762, 1981.

560. Taher SM, Anderson RJ, McCartney R, et al: Renal tubular acidosis associated with toluene "sniffing." N Engl J Med 290:765–768, 1974.

561. Cochran M, Peacock M, Smith DA, Nordin BEC: Renal tubular acidosis of pyelonephritis with renal stone disease. Br Med J 2:721–729, 1968.

562. Berlyne GM: Distal tubular function in chronic hydronephrosis. Q J Med 30:339–355, 1961.

563. Better OS, Arieff AI, Massry SG, et al: Studies on renal function after relief of complete unilateral ureteral obstruction of three months' duration in man. Am J Med 54:234–240, 1973.

564. Hutcheon RA, Kaplan BS, Drummond KN: Distal renal tubular acidosis in children with chronic hydronephrosis. J Pediatr 89:372–376, 1976.

565. Wilson DR: Renal function during and following obstruction. Annu Rev Med 28:329–339, 1977.

566. Gyory AZ, Steward JH, George CRP, et al: Renal tubular acidosis, acidosis due to hyperkalemia, hypercalcemia, disordered citrate metabolism and other tubular dysfunctions following human renal transplantation. Q J Med 38:231–254, 1969.

567. Wilson DR, Siddigui AA: Renal tubular acidosis after kidney transplantation. Ann Intern Med 79:352–361, 1973.

568. Drutz DJ, Gutman RA: Renal tubular acidosis in leprosy. Ann Intern Med 75:475–476, 1971.

569. Better OS, Goldschmid Z, Chaimowitz C, Alroy GG: Defect in urinary acidification in cirrhosis. The role of excessive tubular reabsorption of sodium in its etiology. Arch Intern Med 130:77–83, 1972.

570. Oster JR, Hotchkiss JL, Carbon M, Vaamonde CA: Abnormal renal acidification in alcoholic liver disease. J Lab Clin Med 85:987–1000, 1975.

571. Shear L, Bonkowsky HL, Gabuzda GJ: Renal tubular acidosis in cirrhosis. N Engl J Med 280:1–7, 1969.

572. Hall PW III, Piscator M, Vasiljevic M, Popovic N: Renal function studies in individuals with the tubular proteinuria of endemic Balkan nephropathy. Q J Med 41:385–393, 1972.

573. Batlle DC, Arruda JAL, Kurtzman NA: Hyperkalemic distal renal tubular acidosis associated with obstructive uropathy. N Engl J Med 304:373–380, 1981.

574. Thirakomen K, Kozlov N, Arruda JAL, Kurtzman NA: Renal hydrogen ion secretion after release of unilateral ureteral obstruction. Am J Physiol 231:1233–1239, 1976.

575. Earley LE: Extreme polyuria in obstructive uropathy. N Engl J Med 255:600–605, 1956.

576. Batlle DC, Mozes MF, Manaligod J, et al: The pathogenesis of hyperchloremic metabolic acidosis associated with kidney transplantation. Am J Med 70:786–796, 1981.

577. Better OS, Chaimowitz C, Alroy GG, Sisman I: Spontaneous remission of the defect of urinary acidification after cadaver kidney homotransplantation. Lancet 1:110–112, 1970.

578. Better OS, Chaimowitz C, Naveh Y, et al: Syndrome of incomplete renal tubular acidosis after cadaver kidney transplantation. Ann Intern Med 71:39–46, 1969.

579. Mookerjee B, Gault MH, Dossetor JB: Hyperchloremic acidosis in early diagnosis of renal allograft rejection. Ann Intern Med 71:47–58, 1969.

580. Vainder M, Kelly J: Renal tubular dysfunction secondary to jejunoileal bypass. JAMA 235:1257–1260, 1969.

581. Relman AS, Lennon EJ, Lemann J Jr: Endogenous production of fixed acid and the measurement of the net balance of acid in normal subjects. J Clin Invest 40:1621–1630, 1961.

582. Lennon EJ, Lemann J Jr, Litzow JR: The effects of diet and stool composition on the net external acid balance of normal subjects. J Clin Invest 45:1601–1607, 1966.

583. Albert MS, Winters RW: Acid-base equilibrium of blood in normal infants. Pediatrics 37:728–732, 1966.

584. Bennett CM, Brenner BM, Berliner RW: Micropuncture study of nephron function in the rhesus monkey. J Clin Invest 47:203–216, 1968.

585. Rector FC Jr, Carter NW, Seldin DW: The mechanism of bicarbonate reabsorption in the proximal and distal tubules of the kidney. J Clin Invest 44:278–290, 1965.

586. Alpern RJ, Stone DK, Rector FC Jr. Renal acidification mechanisms. In Brenner BM, Rector FC Jr (eds): The Kidney, 4th ed. WB Saunders, Philadelphia, 1991, pp 318–379.

587. Steinmetz PR: Cellular organization of urinary acidification. Am J Physiol 251:F173–F187, 1986.

588. Knepper MA, Packer R, Good DW: Ammonium transport in the kidney. Physiol Rev 69:179–249, 1989.

589. Simon E, Martin D, Buerkert J: Contribution of individual superficial nephron segments to ammonium handling in chronic metabolic acidosis in the rat. J Clin Invest 76:855–864, 1985.

590. Good DW, Dubose TD Jr: Ammonia transport by early and late proximal convoluted tubule of the rat. J Clin Invest 79:684–691, 1987.

591. Nagami GT: Luminal secretion of ammonia in the mouse proximal tubule perfused in vitro. J Clin Invest 81:159–164, 1988.

592. Simon EE, Merli C, Herndon J, et al: Determinants of ammonia entry along the rat proximal tubule during chronic metabolic acidosis. Am J Physiol 256:F1104–F1110, 1989.

593. Preisig PA, Alpern RJ: Pathways for apical and basolateral membrane $NH_3$ and $NH_4^+$ movement in rat proximal tubule. Am J Physiol 259:F587–F593, 1990.

594. Good DW: Active absorption of $NH_4^+$ by rat medullary thick ascending limb; inhibition by potassium. Am J Physiol 255:F78–F87, 1988.

595. Good DW, Caflisch CR, DuBose TD Jr: Transepithelial ammonia concentration gradients in inner medulla of the rat. Am J Physiol 252:F491–F500, 1987.

596. DuBose TD Jr, Good DW, Hamm LL, Wall SM: Ammonium transport in the kidney: New physiological concepts and their clinical implications. J Am Soc Nephrol 1:1193–1203, 1991.

597. Tizianello A, DeFerrari G, Garibotto G, et al: Renal ammoniagenesis in an early stage of metabolic acidosis in man. J Clin Invest 69:240–250, 1982.

598. Graber ML, Bengele HH, Mroz E, et al: Acute metabolic acidosis augments collecting duct acidification rate in the rat. Am J Physiol 241:F669–F676, 1981.

599. Madison LL, Seldin DW: Ammonia excretion and renal enzymatic adaptations in human subjects, as disclosed by administration of precursor amino acids. J Clin Invest 37:1615–1627, 1958.

600. Goodman AD, Fuizy RE, Cahill GF: Renal gluconeogenesis in acidosis, alkalosis and potassium deficiency; its possible role in regulation and renal ammonia production. J Clin Invest 45:612–619, 1966.

601. Pitts RF, Pilkington LA, Macleod MB, Leal-Pinto E: Metabolism of glutamine by the intact functioning kidney of the dog. Studies in metabolic acidosis and alkalosis. J Clin Invest 51:557–565, 1972.

602. Pitts RF: Production of $CO_2$ by the intact functioning kidney of the dog. Med Clin North Am 59:507–622, 1975.

603. Kurtz I, Dass PD, Cramer S: The importance of renal ammonia metabolism to whole body acid-base balance: A reanalysis of the pathophysiology of renal tubular acidosis. Miner Electrolyte Metab 16:331–340, 1990.

604. Carlisle EJF, Donnelly SM, Halperin ML: Renal tubular acidosis (RTA): Recognize the ammonium defect and pHorget the urine pH. Pediatr Nephrol 5:242–248, 1991.

605. Carlisle EJF, Donnelly SM, Vasuvattakul S, et al: Glue-sniffing and distal renal tubular acidosis: Sticking to the facts. J Am Soc Nephrol 1:1019–1027, 1991.

606. Vasuvattakul S, Nimmannit S, Shayakul C, et al: Should the urine $P_{CO_2}$ or the rate of excretion of ammonium be the gold standard to diagnose distal renal tubular acidosis? Am J Kidney Dis 19:72–75, 1992.

607. Wrong OM, Feest TG: The natural history of distal renal tubular acidosis. Contrib Nephrol 21:137–144, 1980.

608. Wrong O: Distal renal tubular acidosis: The value of urinary pH, $P_{CO_2}$ and $NH_4^+$ measurements. Pediatr Nephrol 5:249–255, 1991.

609. Donnelly S, Kamel KS, Vasuvattakul S, et al: Might distal renal tubular acidosis be a proximal tubular cell disorder? Am J Kidney Dis 19:272–281, 1992.

610. DuBose TD Jr: Hydrogen ion secretion by the collecting duct as a determinant of the urine to blood $P_{CO_2}$ gradient in alkaline urine. J Clin Invest 69:145–156, 1982.

611. Halperin ML, Goldstein MB, Haig A, et al: Studies on the pathogenesis of type 1 (distal) renal tubular acidosis as revealed by the urinary $P_{CO_2}$ tensions. J Clin Invest 53:669–677, 1974.

612. Halperin ML, Carlisle EJF, Donnelly S, et al: Renal tubular acidosis. *In* Narins RG (ed): Maxwell & Kleemans's Clinical Disorders of Fluid and Electrolyte Metabolism, 5th ed. McGraw-Hill, New York, 1994, pp 875–910.

613. Morris RC Jr, Ives HE: Inherited disorders of the renal tubule. *In* Brenner BM, Rector FC Jr (eds): The Kidney, 4th ed. WB Saunders, Philadelphia, 1991, pp 1596–1656.

614. Batlle D, Grupp M, Gaviria M, Kurtzman NA: Distal renal tubular acidosis with intact capacity to lower urinary pH. Am J Med 72:751–758, 1982.

615. Gougoux A, Vinay P, Zizian L, et al: Effect of acetazolamide on renal metabolism and ammoniagenesis in the dog. Kidney Int 31:1279–1290, 1987.

616. Gougoux A, Vinay P, Duplain M: Maleate-induced stimulation of glutamine metabolism in the intact dog kidney. Am J Physiol 248:F585–F593, 1985.

617. Gougoux A, Zan N, Dansereau D, Vinay P: Experimental Fanconi's syndrome resulting from 4-pentenoate infusion in the dog. Am J Physiol 257:F959–F966, 1989.

618. Milne MD, Stanbury SW, Thomson AE: Observations on the Fanconi syndrome and renal hyperchloraemic acidosis in the adult. Q J Med 21:61–76, 1952.

619. De Toni E Jr, Nordio S: The relationship between calcium-phosphorus metabolism, the 'Krebs cycle' and steroid metabolism. Arch Dis Child 34:371–382, 1959.

620. Kaufman AM, Brod-Miller C, Kahn T: Role of citrate excretion in acid-base balance in diuretic-induced alkalosis in the rat. Am J Physiol 248:F796–F803, 1985.

621. Kaufman AM, Kahn T: Complementary role of citrate and bicarbonate excretion in acid-base balance in the rat. Am J Physiol 255:F182–F187, 1988.

622. Brown JC, Packer RK, Knepper MA: Role of organic anions in renal response to dietary acid and base loads. Am J Physiol 257:F170–F176, 1989.

623. Warnock DG, Reenstra WW, Yee VJ: $Na^+/H^+$ antiporter of brush border vesicles: Studies with acridine orange uptake. Am J Physiol 242:F733–F739, 1982.

624. Kinsella JL, Aronson PS: Properties of the $Na^+$-$H^+$ exchanger in renal microvillus membrane vesicles. Am J Physiol 238:F467–F469, 1980.

625. Ives HE, Rector FC Jr: Proton transport and cell function. J Clin Invest 73:285–290, 1984.

626. Preisig PA, Ives HE, Cragoe EJ Jr, et al: Role of the $Na^+/H^+$ antiporter in rat proximal tubule bicarbonate absorption. J Clin Invest 80:970–978, 1987.

627. Verkman AS, Alpern RJ: Kinetic transport model for cellular regulation of pH and solute concentration in the renal proximal tubule. Biophys J 51:533–546, 1987.

628. Aronson PS: Mechanisms of active $H^+$ secretion in the proximal tubule. Am J Physiol 245:F647–F659, 1983.

629. Wistrand PJ, Knuuttila K: Renal membrane-bound carbonic anhydrase. Purification and properties. Kidney Int 35:851–859, 1989.

630. Wistrand PJ: Human renal cytoplasmic carbonic anhydrase: Tissue levels and kinetic properties under near physiologic conditions. Acta Physiol Scand 109:239–248, 1980.

631. Preisig PA, Toto RD, Alpern RJ: Carbonic anhydrase inhibitors. Renal Physiol 10:136–159, 1987.

632. Brown D, Hirsch S, Gluck S: Localization of a proton-pumping ATPase in rat kidney. J Clin Invest 82:2114–2126, 1988.

633. Alpern RJ: Cell mechanisms of proximal tubular acidification. Physiol Rev 70:79–114, 1990.

634. Alpern RJ: Mechanism of basolateral membrane $H^+/OH^-/HCO_3^-$-transport in the rat proximal convoluted tubule. J Gen Physiol 86:613–636, 1985.

635. Lopes AG, Siebens AW, Giebisch G, Boron WF: Electrogenic $Na/HCO_3$ cotransport across basolateral membrane of isolated perfused *Necturus* proximal tubule. Am J Physiol 253:F340–F350, 1987.

636. Soleimani M, Grassi SM, Aronson PS: Stoichiometry of $Na^+$-$HCO_3^-$ cotransport in basolateral membrane vesicles isolated from rabbit renal cortex. J Clin Invest 79:1276–1280, 1987.

637. Lonnerholm G, Wistrand PJ: Carbonic anhydrase in the human kidney: A histochemical and immunocytochemical study. Kidney Int 25:886–898, 1984.

638. Soltoff SP, Mandel LJ: Active ion transport in the renal proximal tubule III. The ATP dependence of the Na pump. J Gen Physiol 84:643–662, 1984.

639. van Deurs B, Christensen EI: Endocytosis in kidney proximal tubule cells and cultured fibroblasts: A review of the structural aspects of membrane recycling between the plasma membrane and endocytic vacuoles. Eur J Cell Biol 33:163–173, 1984.

640. Levin B, Snodgrass GJAI, Oberholzer VG, et al: Fructosaemia: Observations on seven cases. Am J Med 45:826–838, 1968.

641. Morris RC Jr: An experimental renal acidification defect in patients with hereditary fructose intolerance. I. Its resemblance to renal tubular acidosis. J Clin Invest 47:1389–1398, 1968.

642. Odievre M, Gentil C, Gautier M, Alagille D: Hereditary fructose intolerance in childhood; diagnosis, management, and course in 55 patients. Am J Dis Child 132:605–608, 1978.

643. Baerlocher K, Gitzelmann R, Steinmann B, Gitzelmann-Cumarasamy N: Hereditary fructose intolerance in early childhood: A major diagnostic challenge. Helv Paediatr Acta 33:465–487, 1978.

644. Steiner G, Wilson D, Vranic M: Studies of glucose turnover and renal function in an unusual case of hereditary fructose intolerance. Am J Med 62:150–158, 1977.

645. Richardson RMA, Little JA, Patten RL, et al: Pathogenesis of acidosis in hereditary fructose intolerance. Metabolism 28:1133–1138, 1979.

646. Lamiere N, Mussche M, Baele G, et al: Hereditary fructose intolerance: A difficult diagnosis in the adult. Am J Med 65:416–423, 1978.

647. Gitzelmann R, Steinmann B, Van Den Berghe G: Disorders of fructose metabolism. *In* Scriver CR, Beaudet AL, Sly WS, Valle D (eds): The Metabolic Basis of Inherited Disease, 6th ed. McGraw-Hill, New York, 1989, pp 399–424.

648. Froesch ER: Essential fructosuria and hereditary fructose intolerance. *In* Stanbury JB, Wyngaarden JB, Fredrickson DS (eds): The Metabolic Basis of Inherited Disease, 2nd ed. McGraw-Hill, New York, 1966, p 124.

649. Ali M, Roosien U, Cox TM: DNA diagnosis of fatal fructose intolerance from archival tissue. Q J Med 86:25–30, 1993.

650. Hers H, Joassin G: Anomalie de l'aldolase hépatique dans l'intolérance au fructose. Enzymol Biol Clin 1:4–14, 1961.

651. Froesch ER: Essential fructosuria, hereditary fructose intolerance and fructose-1,6-diphosphatase deficiency. *In* Stanbury JB, Wyngaarden JB, Fredrickson DS (eds): The Metabolic Basis of Inherited Disease, 4th ed. McGraw-Hill, New York, 1978, p 121.

652. Nisell J, Linden L: Fructose-1-phosphate aldolase and fructose-1,6-

diphosphate aldolase activity in the mucosa of the intestine in hereditary fructose intolerance. Scand J Gastroenterol 3:80–82, 1968.

653. Morris RC Jr, Ueki I, Loh D, et al: Absence of renal fructose-1-phosphate aldolase activity in hereditary fructose intolerance. Nature 214:920–921, 1967.

654. Kranhold JF, Loh D, Morris RC Jr: Renal fructose-metabolizing enzymes: Significance in hereditary fructose intolerance. Science 165:402–403, 1969.

655. Wachsmuth ED, Thoner M, Pfleiderer G: The cellular distribution of aldolase isozymes in rat kidney and brain determined in tissue sections by the immuno-histochemical method. Histochemistry 45:143–161, 1975.

656. Burch HB, Cole B, Choi S, et al: Diversity of effects of fructose loads on different parts of the nephron. Int J Biochem 12:37–40, 1980.

657. Burch HG, Choi S, Dence CN, et al: Metabolic effects of large fructose loads in different parts of the rat nephron. J Biol Chem 255:8239–8244, 1980.

658. Maenpaa PH, Raivio KO, Kekomaki MP: Liver adenine nucleotides: Fructose-induced depletion and its effect on protein synthesis. Science 161:1253–1254, 1968.

659. Oberhaensli RD, Rajagopalan B, Taylor DJ, Radda GK: Study of hereditary fructose intolerance by use of $^{31}$P magnetic resonance spectroscopy. Lancet 2:931–934, 1987.

660. Gopher A, Vaisman N, Mandel H, Lapidot A: Determination of fructose metabolic pathways in normal and fructose-intolerant children: A $^{13}$C NMR study using [U-$^{13}$C]fructose. Proc Natl Acad Sci USA 87:5449–5453, 1990.

661. Hommes FA: Inborn errors of fructose metabolism. Am J Clin Nutr 58(suppl):788S–795S, 1993.

662. Woods HF, Eggleston LV, Krebs HA: The cause of hepatic accumulation of fructose-1-phosphate on fructose loading. Biochem J 119:501–510, 1970.

663. Morris RC Jr, Nigon K, Reed EB: Evidence that the severity of depletion of inorganic phosphate determines the severity of the disturbance of adenine nucleotide metabolism in the liver and renal cortex of the fructose-loaded rat. J Clin Invest 61:209–220, 1978.

664. Sestoft L: Regulation of fructose metabolism in the perfused rat liver: Interrelation with inorganic phosphate, glucose, ketone body and ethanol metabolism. Biochim Biophys Acta 343:1–16, 1974.

665. Morris RC Jr, Brewer ED, Brater C: Evidence of a severe phosphate depletion–dependent disturbance of cellular metabolism in patients with hereditary fructose intolerance (HFI). Clin Res 28:556A, 1980.

666. Fox IH, Kelley WN: Studies on the mechanism of fructose-induced hyperuricemia in man. Metabolism 21:713–721, 1972.

667. Hultman E, Nilsson LH, Sahlin K: Adenine nucleotide content of human liver: Normal values and fructose-induced depletion. Scand J Clin Lab Invest 35:245–251, 1975.

668. Veech RL, Raijman L, Krebs HA: Equilibrium relations between the cytoplasmic adenine nucleotide system and nicotinamide–adenine nucleotide system in rat liver. Biochem J 117:499–503, 1970.

669. Veech RL, Lawson JW, Cornell NW, Krebs HA: Cytosolic phosphorylation potential. J Biol Chem 254:6538–6547, 1979.

670. Blum H, Schnall MD, Chance B, Buzby GP: Intracellular sodium flux and high-energy phosphorus metabolites in ischemic skeletal muscle. Am J Physiol 255:C377–C384, 1988.

671. Iles RA, Stevens AN, Griffiths JR, Morris PG: Phosphorylation status of liver by $^{31}$P-n.m.r. spectroscopy, and its implications for metabolic control. Biochem J 229:141–151, 1985.

672. Stubbs M, Freeman D, Ross BD: Formation of n.m.r.-invisible ADP during renal ischaemia in rats. Biochem J 224:241–246, 1984.

673. Freeman D, Bartlett S, Radda G, Ross B: Energetics of sodium transport in the kidney. Saturation transfer $^{31}$P-NMR. Biochim Biophys Acta 762:325–336, 1983.

674. Berliner RW, Kennedy TJ, Hilton JG: Effect of maleic acid on renal function. Proc Soc Exp Biol Med 75:791–794, 1950.

675. Harrison HE, Harrison HC: Experimental production of renal glycosuria, phosphaturia, and aminoaciduria by injection of maleic acid. Science 120:606–608, 1954.

676. Kramer HJ, Gonick HC: Experimental Fanconi syndrome. I. Effect of maleic acid on renal cortical Na-K-ATPase activity and ATP levels. J Lab Clin Med 76:799–808, 1970.

677. Szczepanska M, Angielski S: Prevention of maleate-induced tubular dysfunction by acetoacetate. Am J Physiol 8:F50–F56, 1980.

678. Bassett DR, Duey WJ, Walder AJ, et al: Racial differences in maximal vasodilatory capacity of forearm resistance vessels in normotensive young adults. Am J Hypertens 5:781–786, 1992.

679. Rogulski J, Strzelecki T, Pacanis A, et al: Effects of maleate on renal carbohydrate metabolism in vivo and in vitro. In Angielski S, Dubach UC (eds): Biochemical Aspects of Renal Function. Hans Huber, Bern, 1975, pp 106–110.

680. Gmaj P, Hoppe A, Angielski S, Rogulski J: Acid-base behavior of the kidney in maleate-treated rats. Am J Physiol 222:1182–1186, 1972.

681. Angielski S, Rogulski J: Effect of maleic acid on the kidney. I. Oxidation of Krebs cycle intermediates by various tissues of maleate intoxicated rats. Acta Biochim Pol 9:357–365, 1962.

682. Bergeron M, Dubord L, Hausser C: Membrane permeability as a cause of transport defects in experimental Fanconi syndrome: A new hypothesis. J Clin Invest 57:1181–1189, 1976.

683. Bergeron M, Gougoux A: The renal Fanconi syndrome. In Scriver CR, Beaudet AL, Sly WS, Valle D (eds): The Metabolic Basis of Inherited Disease, 6th ed. McGraw-Hill, New York, 1989, pp 2569–2580.

683a. Al-Bander HA, Weiss RA, Humphreys MH, Morris RC Jr: Dysfunction of the proximal tubule underlies maleic acid–induced type II renal tubular acidosis. Am J Physiol 243:F604–F611, 1982.

684. Bank N, Aynedjian HS, Mutz BF: Microperfusion study of proximal tubule bicarbonate transport in maleic acid–induced renal tubular acidosis. Am J Physiol 250:F476–F482, 1986.

685. Reboucas NA, Fernandes DT, Elias MM, et al: Proximal tubular $HCO_3^-$, $H^+$ and fluid transport during maleate-induced acidification defect. Pflugers Arch 401:266–271, 1984.

686. Gunther R, Silbernagl S, Deetjen P: Maleic acid induced aminoaciduria studied by free flow micropuncture and continuous microperfusion. Pflugers Arch 382:109–114, 1979.

687. Bearn AG, Yu TF, Gutman AB: Renal function in Wilson's disease. J Clin Invest 36:1107–1114, 1957.

688. Silverman M: The mechanism of maleic acid nephropathy: Investigations using brush border membrane vesicles. Membr Biochem 4:63–69, 1981.

689. Angielski S, Rogulski J: Metabolic studies in experimental renal dysfunction resulting from maleate administration. In Angielski S, Dubach UC (eds): Biochemical Aspects of Renal Function. Hans Huber, Bern, 1975, pp 86–100.

690. Christensen EI, Maunsbach AB: Proteinuria induced by sodium maleate in rats: Effects on ultrastructure and protein handling in renal proximal tubule. Kidney Int 17:771–787, 1980.

691. Rosen VJ, Kramer HJ, Gonick HC: Experimental Fanconi syndrome: II. Effect of maleic acid on renal tubular ultrastructure. Lab Invest 28:446–455, 1973.

692. Rogulski J, Pacanis A, Adamowicz W, Angielski S: On the mechanism of maleate action on rat kidney mitochondria: Effect on oxidative metabolism. Acta Biochim Pol 21:403–413, 1974.

693. Scharer K, Yoshida T, Voyer L, et al: Impaired renal gluconeogenesis and energy metabolism in maleic acid induced nephropathy in rats. Res Exp Med 157:136–152, 1972.

694. Al-Bander HA, Etheredge SB, Paukert T, et al: Phosphate loading attenuates renal tubular dysfunction induced by maleic acid in the dog. Am J Physiol 248:F513–F521, 1985.

695. Jonas AJ, Lin S, Conley SB, et al: Urine glyceraldehyde excretion is elevated in the renal Fanconi syndrome. Kidney Int 35:99–104, 1989.

696. Barratt TM, Crawford R: Lysozyme excretion as a measure of renal tubular dysfunction in children. Clin Sci 39:457–465, 1970.

697. Mogielnicki RP, Waldmann TA, Strober W: Renal handling of low molecular weight proteins. I. L-chain metabolism in experimental renal disease. J Clin Invest 50:901–909, 1971.

698. Fredriksson A, Peterson PA: Effects of renal dysfunction on $\beta_2$-microglobulin metabolism. Scand J Urol Nephrol 26:61–76, 1975.

699. Fujita T, Itakura M: Renal handling of lysozyme in experimental Fanconi syndrome. J Lab Clin Med 92:135–140, 1978.

700. Morris RC Jr, Sebastian A: Renal tubular acidosis and Fanconi syndrome. In Stanbury JB, Wyngaarden JB, Frederickson DS, et al (eds): The Metabolic Basis of Inherited Disease, 5th ed. McGraw-Hill, New York, 1983, pp 1808–1866.

701. Hysing J, Ostensen J, Tolleshaug H, Kiil F: Effect of maleate on tubular protein reabsorption in dog kidneys. Renal Physiol 10:338–351, 1987.

702. Straus W: Occurrence of phagosomes and phago-lysosomes in different segments of the nephron in relation to the reabsorption, transport, digestion, and extrusion of intravenously injected horseradish peroxidase. J Cell Biol 21:295–308, 1964.

703. Wall DA, Maack T: Endocytic uptake, transport, and catabolism of proteins by epithelial cells. Am J Physiol 248:C12–C20, 1985.

704. Christensen EI, Nielsen S: Structural and functional features of protein handling in the kidney proximal tubule. Semin Nephrol 11:414–439, 1991.

705. Rodman JS, Kerjaschki D, Merisko E, Farquhar MG: Presence of an extensive clathrin coat on the apical plasmalemma of the rat kidney proximal tubule cell. J Cell Biol 98:1630–1636, 1984.

706. Bretscher MS, Thomson JN, Pearse BMF: Coated pits act as molecular filters. Proc Natl Acad Sci USA 77:4156–4159, 1980.

707. Brown MS, Anderson RGW, Goldstein JL: Recycling receptors: The round-trip itinerary of migrant membrane proteins. Cell 32:663–667, 1983.

708. Brown MS, Goldstein JL: A receptor-mediated pathway for cholesterol homeostasis. Science 232:34–47, 1986.

709. Verlander JW, Madsen KM, Larsson L, et al: Immunocytochemical localization of intracellular acidic compartments: Rat proximal nephron. Am J Physiol 257:F454–F462, 1989.

710. Peterson PA, Evrin P-E, Berggard I: Differentiation of glomerular, tubular, and normal proteinuria: Determination of urinary excretion of $\beta_2$-microglobulin, albumin, and total protein. J Clin Invest 48:1189–1198, 1969.

711. Chamberlain MJ, Stimmler L: The renal handling of insulin. J Clin Invest 46:911–919, 1967.

712. Harrison JF, Lunt GS, Scott P, Blainey JD: Urinary lysozyme, ribonuclease and low-molecular-weight protein in renal disease. Lancet 1:371, 1968.

713. Griffiths G, Hoflack B, Simons K, et al: The mannose 6-phosphate receptor and the biogenesis of lysosomes. Cell 52:329–341, 1988.

714. Morris RC Jr, Sandman R, McSherry E, Sebastian A: Urinary lysosomal enzymes in renal tubular disorders. Clin Res 18:460, 1970.

715. Kunin CM, Chesney RW, Craig WA, et al: Enzymuria as a marker of renal injury and disease: Studies of N-acetyl-beta-glucosaminidase in the general population and in patients with renal disease. Pediatrics 621:751–760, 1978.

716. Le Hir M, Dubach UC, Schmidt U: Quantitative distribution of lysosomal hydrolases in the rat nephron. Histochemistry 63:245–251, 1979.

717. Bauman R C, Bonvalet J, Farman N: Distribution of N-acetyl-β-D-glucosaminidase isoenzymes along the rabbit nephron. Kidney Int 25:636–642, 1984.

718. Caplan MJ, Stow JL, Newman AP, et al: Dependence on pH of polarized sorting of secreted proteins. Nature 329:632, 1987.

719. Dance N, Price RG: The excretion of N-acetyl-β-glucosaminidase and β-galactosidase by patients with renal disease. Clin Chim Acta 27:87–92, 1970.

720. Price RG: Urinary enzymes, nephrotoxicity and renal disease. Toxicology 23:99–134, 1982.

721. Koenig H, Goldstone A, Hughes C: Lysosomal enzymuria in the testosterone-treated mouse. A manifestation of cell defecation of residual bodies. Lab Invest 39:329–341, 1978.

722. Kress BC, Hirani S, Freeze HH, et al: Mucolipidosis III β-N-acetyl-D-hexosaminidase A. Purification and properties. Biochem J 207:421–428, 1982.

723. Schneider YJ, Tulkens P, De Duve C, Trouet A: Fate of plasma membrane during endocytosis. II. Evidence for recycling (shuttle) of plasma membrane constituents. J Cell Biol 82:466–474, 1979.

724. Besterman JM, Airhart JA, Woodworth RC, Low RB: Exocytosis of pinocytosed fluid in cultured cells: Kinetic evidence for rapid turnover and compartmentation. J Cell Biol 91:716–727, 1981.

725. Farquhar MG: Multiple pathways of exocytosis, endocytosis, and membrane cycling: Validation of a Golgi route. Fed Proc 42:2407–2413, 1983.

726. Steinman RM, Mellman IS, Muller WA, Cohn ZA: Endocytosis and the recycling of plasma membrane. J Cell Biol 96:1–27, 1983.

727. Helenius A, Mellman I, Wall D, Hubbard A: Endosomes. Trends Biochem Sci 8:245–250, 1983.

728. Mellman I, Fuchs R, Helenius A: Acidification of the endocytic and exocytic pathways. Ann Rev Biochem 55:663–700, 1986.

729. Al-Bander HA, Mock DM, Etheredge SB, et al: Coordinately increased lysozymuria and lysosomal enzymuria induced by maleic acid. Kidney Int 30:804–812, 1986.

730. Al-Bander HA, Morris RC Jr: Glucose loading exacerbates the renal tubular disorder induced by maleic acid in the dog. Kidney Int 29:296, 1986.

731. Steinman RM, Brodie SE, Cohn ZA: Membrane flow during pinocytosis. J Cell Biol 68:665–687, 1976.

732. Brown D: Membrane recycling and epithelial cell function. Am J Physiol 256:F1–F12, 1989.

733. Jamieson JD, Palade GE: Intracellular transport of secretory proteins in the pancreatic exocrine cell: IV. Metabolic requirements. J Cell Biol 39:589–603, 1968.

734. Tolleshaug H, Kolset SO, Berg H: The influence of cellular energy levels on receptor-mediated endocytosis and degradation of asialoglycoproteins in suspended hepatocytes. Biochem Pharmacol 34:1639–1645, 1985.

735. Schlossman DM, Schmid SL, Braell WA, Rothman JE: An enzyme that removes clathrin coats: Purification of an uncoating ATPase. J Cell Biol 99:723–733, 1984.

736. Rothman JE, Schmid SL: Enzymatic recycling of clathrin from coated vesicles. Cell 46:5–9, 1986.

737. Rodman JS, Seidman L, Farquhar MG: The membrane composition of coated pits, microvilli, endosomes, and lysosomes is distinctive in the rat kidney proximal tubule cell. J Cell Biol 102:77–87, 1986.

738. Maunsbach AB: Cellular mechanisms of tubular protein transport. Int Rev Physiol 11:145–167, 1976.

739. Hasilik A, Neufeld EF: Biosynthesis of lysosomal enzymes in fibroblasts. Synthesis as precursors of higher molecular weight. J Biol Chem 255:4937–4945, 1980.

740. Pohlmann R, Kruger S, Hasilik A, von Figura K: Effect of monensin on intracellular transport and receptor-mediated endocytosis of lysosomal enzymes. Biochem J 217:649–658, 1984.

741. Gonzalez-Noriega A, Grubb JH, Talkad V, Sly WS: Chloroquine inhibits lysosomal enzyme pinocytosis and enhances lysosomal enzyme secretion by impairing receptor recycling. J Cell Biol 85:839–852, 1980.

742. Brown JA, Novak EK, Swank RT: Effects of ammonia on processing and secretion of precursor and mature lysosomal enzyme from macrophages of normal and pale ear mice: Evidence for two distinct pathways. J Cell Biol 100:1894–1904, 1985.

743. von Figura K, Hasilik A: Lysosomal enzymes and their receptors. Annu Rev Biochem 55:167–193, 1986.

744. Rosenfeld MG, Kreibich G, Popov D, et al: Biosynthesis of lysosomal hydrolases: Their synthesis in bound polysomes and the role of co- and post-translational processing in determining their subcellular distribution. J Cell Biol 93:135–143, 1982.

745. Hasilik A, Von Figura K: Oligosaccharides in lysosomal enzymes. Distribution of high-mannose and complex oligosaccharides in cathepsin D and β-hexosaminidase. Eur J Biochem 121:125–129, 1981.

746. Hasilik A, von Figura K, Conzelman E, et al: Lysosomal enzyme precursors in human fibroblasts. Activation of cathepsin D precursor in vitro and activity of β-hexosaminidase A precursor towards ganglioside $GM_2$. Eur J Biochem 125:317–321, 1982.

747. Oude Elferink RPJ, Brouwer-Kelder EM, Surya I, et al: Isolation and characterization of a precursor form of lysosomal alpha-glucosidase from human urine. Eur J Biochem 139:489–495, 1984.

748. Zuhlsdorf M, Imort M, Hasilik A, von Figura K: Molecular forms of β-hexosaminidase and cathepsin D in serum and urine of healthy subjects and patients with elevated activity of lysosomal enzymes. Biochem J 213:733–740, 1983.

749. Griffiths G, Simons K: The trans Golgi network: Sorting at the exit site of the Golgi complex. Science 234:438–443, 1986.

750. Kornfeld S: Trafficking of lysosomal enzymes in normal and disease states. J Clin Invest 77:1–6, 1986.

751. Dahms NM, Lobel P, Kornfeld S: Mannose 6-phosphate receptors and lysosomal enzyme targeting. J Biol Chem 264:12115–12118, 1989.

752. Griffiths G, Matteoni R, Back R, Hoflack B: Characterization of the cation-independent mannose 6-phosphate receptor-enriched prelysosomal compartment in NRK cells. J Cell Sci 95:441–461, 1990.

753. Ludwig T, Griffiths G, Hoflack B: Distribution of newly synthesized lysosomal enzymes in the endocytic pathway of normal rat kidney cells. J Cell Biol 115:1561–1572, 1991.

754. Tycko B, Maxfield FR: Rapid acidification of endocytic vesicles containing $\alpha_2$-macroglobulin. Cell 28:643–651, 1982.

755. Brown WJ, Goodhouse J, Farquhar MG: Mannose 6-phosphate receptors for lysosomal enzymes cycle between the Golgi complex and endosomes. J Cell Biol 103:1235–1247, 1986.

756. Merion M, Schlesinger P, Brooks RM, et al: Defective acidification of endosomes in Chinese hamster ovary cell mutants "cross-resistant" to toxins and viruses. Proc Natl Acad Sci USA 80:5315–5319, 1983.

757. Robbins AR, Peng SS, Marshall JL: Mutant Chinese hamster ovary cells pleiotropically defective in receptor-mediated endocytosis. J Cell Biol 96:1064–1071, 1983.

758. Robbins AR, Oliver C, Bateman JL, Krag SS, Galloway CJ, and Mellman I: A single mutation in Chinese hamster ovary cells impairs both Golgi and endosomal functions. J Cell Biol 99:1296–1308, 1984.

759. Sly WS, Merion M, Schlesinger P, et al: Defective endosome acidification in mammalian cell mutants "cross-resistant" to certain toxins and viruses. In Abraham AK, Eikhom TS, Pryme IF (eds): Protein Synthesis. Humana Press, Clifton, NJ, 1983, pp 239–251.

760. Park CH, Clapp WL, Madsen KM, Tisher CC: Structure and function of endosomal-lysosomal (EL) system in the proximal tubule (PT). In Davison AM (ed): Xth International Congress of Nephrology. London, Baillière Tindall, 1987, p 589.

761. Tong PY, Kornfeld S: Ligand interactions of the cation-dependent mannose 6-phosphate receptor. J Biol Chem 264:7970–7975, 1989.

762. Tong PY, Gregory W, Kornfeld S: Ligand interactions of the cation-independent mannose 6-phosphate receptor: The stoichiometry of mannose 6-phosphate binding. J Biol Chem 264:7962–7969, 1989.

763. Morris RC Jr, Brewer E, Helms I, et al: Phosphate loading differentially modulates the renal tubular disorder induced by fructose in patients with hereditary fructose intolerance (HFI). J Am Soc Nephrol 5:315, 1994.

764. Schwartz GJ, Al-Awqati Q: Carbon dioxide causes exocytosis of vesicles containing H+ pumps in isolated perfused proximal and collecting tubules. J Clin Invest 75:1638–1644, 1985.

765. Gluck S, Cannon C, Al-Awqati Q: Exocytosis regulates urinary acidification in turtle bladder by rapid insertion of H+ pumps into the luminal membrane. Proc Natl Acad Sci USA 79:4327–4331, 1982.

766. Chambrey R, Paillard M, Podevin R: Enzymatic and functional evidence for adaptation of the vacuolar H+-ATPase in proximal tubule apical membrane from rats with chronic metabolic acidosis. J Biol Chem 269:3243–3250, 1994.

767. Verkman AS: Water channels in cell membranes. Annu Rev Physiol 54:97–108, 1992.

768. Kempson SA, Helmle C, Abraham MI, Murer H: Parathyroid hormone action on phosphate transport is inhibited by high osmolality. Am J Physiol 258:F1336–F1344, 1990.

769. Osserman EF, Lawlor DP: Serum and urinary lysozyme (muramidase) in monocytic and monomyelocytic leukemia. J Exp Med 124:921–952, 1966.

770. Muggia FM, Heinemann HO, Farhangi M, Osserman EF: Lysozymuria and renal tubular dysfunction in monocytic and myelomonocytic leukemia. Am J Med 47:351–366, 1969.

771. Pruzanski W, Platts ME: Serum and urinary proteins, lysozyme (muramidase), and renal dysfunction in mono- and myelomonocytic leukemia. J Clin Invest 49:1694–1708, 1970.

772. Rudders RA, Block KJ: Myeloma renal disease: Evaluation of the role of muramidase (lysozyme). Am J Med Sci 262:79–85, 1971.

773. Clyne DH, Brendstrup L, First MR, et al: Renal effects of intraperitoneal kappa chain injection. Induction of crystals in renal tubular cells. Lab Invest 31:131–142, 1974.

774. Thorner PS, Bedard YC, Fernandes BJ: λ-light-chain nephropathy with Fanconi's syndrome. Arch Pathol Lab Med 107:654–657, 1983.

775. Rao DS, Parfitt AM, Villanueva AR, et al: Hypophosphatemic osteomalacia and adult Fanconi syndrome due to light chain nephropathy; another form of oncogenous osteomalacia. Am J Med 82:333–338, 1987.

776. Yokota N, Yamamoto Y, Fujimoto S, Tanaka K: Acute renal failure presenting as Fanconi syndrome with lambda light chain proteinuria and interstitial nephritis. Clin Nephrol 31:277–278, 1989.

777. Sewell RL, Dorreen MS: Adult Fanconi syndrome progressing to multiple myeloma. J Clin Pathol 37:1256–1258, 1984.

778. Uchida S, Matsuda O, Yokota T, et al: Adult Fanconi syndrome secondary to κ–light chain myeloma: Improvement of tubular functions after treatment for myeloma. Nephron 55:332–335, 1990.

779. Walker BR, Alexander F, Tannenbaum PJ: Fanconi syndrome with renal tubular acidosis and light chain proteinuria. Nephron 8:103–107, 1971.

780. Kamm DE, Fischer MS: Proximal renal tubular acidosis and the Fanconi syndrome in a patient with hypergammaglobulinemia. Nephron 9:208, 1972.

781. Schulman JD, Bradley KH, Seegmiller JE: Cystine compartmentalization within lysosomes in cystinotic leukocytes. Science 166:1152–1154, 1969.

782. Schneider JA, Schulman JD: Cystinosis. In Stanbury JB, Wyngaarden JB, Fredrickson DS, et al (eds): The Metabolic Basis of Inherited Disease, 5th ed. McGraw-Hill, New York, 1983, pp 1844–1866.

783. Gahl WA, Renlund M, Thoene JG: Lysosomal transport disorders: Cystinosis and sialic acid storage. In Scriver CR, Beaudet AL, Sly WS, Valle D (eds): The Metabolic Basis of Inherited Disease, 6th ed. McGraw-Hill, New York, 1989, pp 2619–2648.

784. Schneider JA, Schulman JD, Seegmiller JE: Cystinosis and the Fanconi syndrome. In Stanbury JB, Wyngaarden JB (eds): The Metabolic Basis of Inherited Disease, 4th ed. McGraw-Hill, New York, 1978, p 1581.

785. Gahl WA: Cystinosis coming of age. Adv Pediatr 33:95–126, 1986.

786. Gahl WA: Cystinosis: Progress in a prototypic disease. Ann Intern Med 109:557–569, 1988.

787. Schneider JA, Verroust FM, Kroll WA, et al: Prenatal diagnosis of cystinosis. N Engl J Med 290:878–882, 1974.

788. Schneider JA, Wong V, Bradley K, Seegmiller JE: Biochemical comparisons of the adult and childhood forms of cystinosis. N Engl J Med 279:1253, 1968.

789. Lietman PS, Frazier PD, Wong VG, et al: Adult cystinosis—a benign disorder. Am J Med 40:511–517, 1966.

790. Cherrington AD, Wasserman DH, McGinnes OP: Renal contribution to glucose production after a brief fast: Fact or fancy? J Clin Invest 93:2303, 1994.

791. Goldman H, Scriver CR, Aaron K, et al: Adolescent cystinosis: Comparisons with infantile and adult forms. Pediatrics 47:979–988, 1971.

792. Gahl WA, Bashan N, Tietze F, et al: Cystine transport is defective in isolated leukocyte lysosomes from patients with cystinosis. Science 217:1263–1265, 1982.

793. Jonas AJ, Smith ML, Schneider JA: ATP-dependent lysosomal cystine efflux is defective in cystinosis. J Biol Chem 257:13185–13188, 1982.

794. Gahl WA, Tietze F, Bashan N, et al: Characteristics of cystine counter-transport in normal and cystinotic lysosome-rich leucocyte granular fractions. Biochem J 216:393–400, 1983.

795. Broyer M, Guillot M, Gubler MC, Habib R: Infantile cystinosis: A reappraisal of early and late symptoms. Adv Nephrol Necker Hosp 10:137–166, 1981.

796. Gahl WA, Reed GF, Thoene JG, et al: Cysteamine therapy for children with nephropathic cystinosis. N Engl J Med 316:971–977, 1987.

797. Thoene JG, Oshima RG, Crawhall JC, et al: Cystinosis: Intracellular cystine depletion by aminothiols in vitro and in vivo. J Clin Invest 58:180–189, 1976.

798. Da Silva VA, Zurbrugg RP, Lavanchy P, et al: Long-term treatment of infantile nephropathic cystinosis with cysteamine. N Engl J Med 313:1460–1463, 1985.

799. Yudkoff M, Foreman JW, Segal S: Effects of cysteamine therapy in nephropathic cystinosis. N Engl J Med 304:141–145, 1981.

800. Adamson M, Schneider JA, Bernardini I, et al: Attenuation but not prevention of renal Fanconi syndrome by cysteamine in nephropathic cystinosis. Pediatr Res 25:334A, 1989.

801. Pellett OL, Smith ML, Thoene JG, et al: Renal cell culture using autopsy material from children with cystinosis. In Vitro 20:53–58, 1984.

802. Foreman JW, Bowring MA, Lee J, et al: Effect of cystine dimethylester on renal solute handling and isolated renal tubule transport in the rat: A new model of the Fanconi syndrome. Metabolism 36:1185–1191, 1987.

803. Goldman R, Kaplan A: Rupture of rat liver lysosomes mediated by L–amino acid esters. Biochim Biophys Acta 318:205–216, 1973.

804. Salmon RF, Baum M: Intracellular cystine loading inhibits trans-

port in the rabbit proximal convoluted tubule. J Clin Invest 85:340–344, 1990.

805. Coor C, Salmon RF, Quigley R, et al: Role of adenosine triphosphate (ATP) and NaK ATPase in the inhibition of proximal tubule transport with intracellular cystine loading. J Clin Invest 87:955–961, 1991.

806. Ben-Nun A, Bashan N, Potashnik R, et al: Cystine loading induces Fanconi's syndrome in rats: In vivo and vesicle studies. Am J Physiol 34:F839–F844, 1993.

807. Ben-Nun A, Bashan N, Potashnik R, et al: Cystine dimethyl ester reduces the forces driving sodium-dependent transport in LLC-PK₁ cells. Am J Physiol 263:C516–C520, 1992.

808. Muldowney FP, Freaney R, McGeeney D: Renal tubular acidosis and amino-aciduria in osteomalacia of dietary or intestinal origin. Q J Med 38:517–539, 1968.

809. Arnaud C, Maijer R, Reade T, et al: Vitamin D dependency: An inherited postnatal syndrome with secondary hyperparathyroidism. Pediatrics 46:871–880, 1970.

810. Fraser D, Kooh SW, Kind HP, et al: Pathogenesis of hereditary vitamin D–dependent rickets: An inborn error of vitamin D metabolism involving defective conversion of 25-hydroxy-vitamin D to 1α,25-dihydroxy-vitamin D. N Engl J Med 289:817–822, 1973.

811. Sockalosky JJ, Ulstrom RA, DeLuca HF, Brown DM: Vitamin D–resistant rickets: End-organ unresponsiveness to 1,25(OH)₂D₃. J Pediatr 96:701–703, 1980.

812. Bell NH: Vitamin D–dependent rickets type II. Calcif Tissue Int 31:89–91, 1980.

813. Bank N, Aynedjian HS: A micropuncture study of the effect of parathyroid hormone on renal bicarbonate reabsorption. J Clin Invest 58:336–344, 1976.

814. Iino Y, Burg MB: Effect of parathyroid hormone on bicarbonate absorption by proximal tubules in vitro. Am J Physiol 236:F387, 1979.

815. McKinney TD, Myers P: Bicarbonate transport by proximal tubules: Effect of parathyroid hormone and dibutyryl cyclic AMP. Am J Physiol 238:F166–F174, 1980.

816. McKinney TD, Myers P: Effect of calcium and phosphate on bicarbonate and fluid transport by proximal tubules in vitro. Kidney Int 21:433, 1982.

817. Hellman DE, Au WY, Bartter FC: Evidence for a direct effect of parathyroid hormone on urinary acidification. Am J Physiol 209:643–650, 1965.

818. Crumb CK, Martinez-Maldonado M, Eknoyan G, Suki WN: Effects of volume expansion, purified parathyroid extract, and calcium on renal bicarbonate absorption in the dog. J Clin Invest 54:1287–1294, 1974.

819. Hermkens H, Nawar T, Caron C, Plante GE: Effect of parathyroid hormone on renal excretion of sodium and hydrogen ions. Can J Physiol Pharmacol 55:628–638, 1977.

820. Siddiqui AA, Wilson DR: Primary hyperparathyroidism and proximal renal tubular acidosis: Report of two cases. Can Med Assoc J 106:654–659, 1972.

821. Morris RC Jr, Sebastian A, McSherry E: Renal acidosis. Kidney Int 1:322–340, 1972.

822. Coe FL: Magnitude of metabolic acidosis in primary hyperparathyroidism. Arch Intern Med 134:262–265, 1974.

823. Gold LW, Massry SG, Arieff AI, Coburn JW: Renal bicarbonate wasting during phosphate depletion: A possible cause of altered acid-base homeostasis in hyperparathyroidism. J Clin Invest 52:2556–2561, 1973.

824. Emmett M, Goldfarb S, Agus ZS, Narins RG: The pathophysiology of acid-base changes in chronically phosphate-depleted rats. J Clin Invest 59:291–298, 1977.

825. Legius E, Prosemans W, Eggermont E, et al: Rickets due to dietary calcium deficiency. Eur J Pediatr 148:784–785, 1989.

826. Marie PJ, Pettifor JM, Ross P, Glorieux FH: Histological osteomalacia due to dietary calcium deficiency in children. N Engl J Med 307:584–588, 1982.

827. Morris RC Jr, McSherry E, Sebastian A: Modulation of experimental renal dysfunction of hereditary fructose intolerance by circulating parathyroid hormone. Proc Natl Acad Sci USA 68:132–135, 1971.

828. Kurnik BRC, Hruska KA: Effects of 1,25-dihydroxycholecalciferol on phosphate transport in vitamin D–deprived rats. Am J Physiol 247:F177–F182, 1984.

829. Salassa RM, Power MH, Ulrich JA, Hayles AB: Observations on the metabolic effects of vitamin D in Fanconi's syndrome. Mayo Clin Proc 29:214–224, 1954.

830. Bergstrom WH: The response of multiple renal tubular dysfunction to calciferol. Pediatr Res 2:408–409, 1968.

831. Huguenin M, Schacht R, David R: Infantile rickets with severe proximal renal tubular acidosis, responsive to vitamin D. Arch Dis Child 49:955–959, 1974.

832. Morgan HG, Stewart WK, Lowe KG, et al: Wilson's disease and the Fanconi syndrome. Q J Med 31:361–384, 1962.

833. Cooper AM, Eckhardt RD, Faloon WW, Davidson CS: Investigation of the aminoaciduria in Wilson's disease (hepatolenticular degeneration): Demonstration of a defect in renal function. J Clin Invest 29:265, 1950.

834. Elsas LJ, Hayslett JP, Spargo BH, et al: Wilson's disease with reversible renal tubular dysfunction: Correlation with proximal tubular ultrastructure. Ann Intern Med 75:427–433, 1971.

835. Holl DH, Troelstra JA: Renale tubulaire functiestoornissen bij de ziekte van Wilson. Ned T Geneeskd 112:2184–2188, 1968.

836. Goldfischer S, Sternlieb I: Changes in the distribution of hepatic copper in relation to the progression of Wilson's disease (hepatolenticular degeneration). Am J Pathol 53:883, 1968.

837. Walshe JM: The biochemistry of copper in man and its role in the pathogenesis of Wilson's disease (hepatolenticular degeneration). In Cumings JN (ed): Biochemical Aspects of Nervous Diseases. Plenum Publishing, New York, 1972, p 111.

838. Bearn AG: Wilson's disease. In Stanbury JB, Wyngaarden JB, Fredrickson DS (eds): The Metabolic Basis of Inherited Disease, 3rd ed. McGraw-Hill, New York, 1972, p 1033.

839. Sternlieb I, Scheinberg IH: Penicillamine therapy for hepatolenticular degeneration. JAMA 189:748, 1964.

840. Deiss A, Lynch RE, Lee GR, Cartwright GE: Long-term therapy of Wilson's disease. Ann Intern Med 75:57, 1971.

841. Leu ML, Strickland GT, Gutman RA: Renal function in Wilson's disease: Response to penicillamine therapy. Am J Med Sci 260:381–398, 1970.

842. Walshe JM: The effect of penicillamine on failure of renal acidification in Wilson's disease. Lancet 1:775, 1968.

843. Edelmann CM Jr, Houston IB, Rodriguez Soriano J, et al: Renal excretion of hydrogen ion in children with idiopathic growth retardation. J Pediatr 72:443–451, 1968.

844. Arant BS, Greifer I, Edelmann CM Jr, Spitzer A: Effect of chronic salt and water loading on the tubular defects of a child with Fanconi syndrome (cystinosis). Pediatrics 58:370–377, 1976.

845. Giebisch G: Some reflections on the mechanism of renal tubular potassium transport. Yale J Biol Med 48:315–336, 1975.

846. Rubini ME: Water excretion in potassium-deficient man. J Clin Invest 40:2215–2224, 1961.

847. Mannitius A, Levitin H, Beck D, Epstein FH: On the mechanism of impairment of renal concentrating ability in potassium deficiencies. J Clin Invest 39:684–692, 1960.

848. Berl T, Linas SL, Aisenbrey GA, Anderson RJ: On the mechanism of polyuria in potassium depletion. J Clin Invest 60:620–625, 1977.

849. Dent CE, Harris H: The genetics of cystinuria. Ann Eugen 16:60–87, 1951.

850. Leaf A: The syndrome of osteomalacia, renal glycosuria, aminoaciduria, and increased phosphorus clearance (the Fanconi syndrome). In Stanbury JB, Wyngaarden JB, Fredrickson DS (eds): The Metabolic Basis of Inherited Disease, 2nd ed. McGraw-Hill, New York, 1966, pp 1205–1220.

851. Wilson DR, Yendt ER: Treatment of the adult Fanconi syndrome with oral phosphate supplements and alkali. Am J Med 35:487–511, 1963.

852. Steendijk R: The effect of a continuous intravenous infusion of inorganic phosphate on the rachitic lesions in cystinosis. Arch Dis Child 36:321–324, 1961.

853. Midgett RJ, Speilvogel AM, Coburn JW, Norman AW: Studies on calciferol metabolism. VI. The renal production of the biologically active form of vitamin D, 1,25-dihydroxycholecalciferol; species, tissue, and subcellular distribution. J Clin Endocrinol Metab 36:1153–1161, 1973.

854. Norman AW, Henry H: 1,25-Dihydroxycholecalciferol: A hormonally active form of vitamin D₃. Recent Prog Horm Res 30:431–480, 1974.

855. Brommage R, DeLuca HF: Evidence that 1,25-dihydroxyvitamin

D$_3$ is the physiologically active metabolite of vitamin D$_3$. Endocr Rev 6:491–511, 1985.

856. Olson EB, Knutson JC, Bhattacharya MH, DeLuca HF: The effect of hepatectomy on the synthesis of 25-hydroxyvitamin D$_3$. J Clin Invest 57:1213–1220, 1976.

857. Brewer ED, Tsai HC, Szeto K, Morris RC Jr: Maleic acid–induced impaired conversion of 25(OH)D$_3$ to 1,25(OH)$_2$D$_3$: Implications for Fanconi's syndrome. Kidney Int 12:244–252, 1977.

858. Baran DT, Marcy TW: Evidence for a defect in vitamin D metabolism in a patient with incomplete Fanconi syndrome. J Clin Endocrinol Metab 59:998–1001, 1984.

859. Kitagawa T, Akatsuka A, Owada M, Mano T: Biologic and therapeutic effects of 1α-hydroxycholecalciferol in different types of Fanconi syndrome. Contrib Nephrol 22:107–119, 1980.

860. Chesney RW, Rosen JF, Hamstra AJ, DeLuca HF: Serum 1,25-dihydroxyvitamin D levels in normal children and in vitamin D disorders. Am J Dis Child 134:135–139, 1980.

861. Offermann G, Delling G, Haussler MR: 1,25-Dihydroxycholecalciferol in hypophosphatemic osteomalacia presenting in adults. Acta Endocrinol 88:408–416, 1978.

862. Colussi G, Surian M, Rombola G: Reduced 1α,25-dihydroxyvitamin D plasma levels in human Fanconi syndrome. In Norman AW, Schaefer K, Grigoleit HG, Herrath DV (eds): Vitamin D—Chemical, Biochemical and Clinical Update: Proceedings of the 6th Workshop on Vitamin D. Walter de Gruyter, New York, 1985, pp 1105–1106.

863. Chesney RW, Kaplan BS, Phelps M, DeLuca HF: Renal tubular acidosis does not alter circulating values of calcitriol (1,25(OH)$_2$D). J Pediatr 104:51–55, 1984.

864. Kruse K, Bartels H: Hypercalciuria in idiopathic Fanconi syndrome. Eur J Pediatr 131:247–254, 1979.

865. Chevalier RL: Hypercalciuria in a child with primary Fanconi syndrome and hearing loss. Int J Pediatr Nephrol 4:53–57, 1983.

866. Steinherz R, Chesney RW, Schulman JD, et al: Circulating vitamin D metabolites in nephropathic cystinosis. J Pediatr 102:592–594, 1983.

867. Portale AA, Halloran BP, Harris ST, et al: Metabolic acidosis reverses the increase in serum 1,25(OH)$_2$D in phosphorus-restricted normal men. Am J Physiol 263:E1164–E1170, 1992.

868. Etches P, Pickering D, Smith R: Cystinotic rickets treated with vitamin D metabolites. Arch Dis Child 52:661–664, 1977.

869. Gertner JM, Brenton DP, Dent CE, Demenech M: Treatment of the rickets of cystinosis with 1-α-hydroxy vitamin D$_3$. Calcif Tissue Res 521:63–67, 1977.

870. Underwood JL, DeLuca HF: Vitamin D is not directly necessary for bone growth and mineralization. Am J Physiol 246:E493–E498, 1984.

871. Weinstein RS, Underwood JL, Hutson MS, DeLuca HF: Bone histomorphometry in vitamin D–deficient rats infused with calcium and phosphorus. Am J Physiol 246:E499–E505, 1984.

872. Mallette LE, Patten BM: Neurogenic muscle atrophy and osteomalacia in adult Fanconi syndrome. Ann Neurol 1:131–137, 1977.

873. Rodriguez Soriano J, Houston IB, Boichis H, Edelmann CM Jr: Calcium and phosphorus metabolism in the Fanconi syndrome. J Clin Endocrinol Metab 28:1555–1563, 1968.

874. Lameire N, Mussche M, Baele G, et al: Hereditary fructose intolerance: A difficult diagnosis in the adult. Am J Med 65:416–423, 1978.

875. Komrower GM, Schwarz V, Holzel A, Goldberg L: A clinical and biochemical study of galactosaemia. A possible explanation of the nature of the biochemical lesion. Arch Dis Child 31:254–264, 1956.

876. Holzel A, Komrower GM, Schwarz V: Galactosemia. Am J Med 22:703–711, 1957.

877. Gentz J, Lindblad B, Lindstedt S, et al: Dietary treatment in tyrosinemia (tyrosinosis). Am J Dis Child 113:31–37, 1967.

878. Halvorsen S: Dietary treatment of tyrosinosis. Am J Dis Child 113:38–40, 1967.

879. Halvorsen S, Gjessing LR: Studies on tyrosinosis. I. Effect of low-tyrosine and low-phenylalanine diet. Br Med J 2:1171–1173, 1964.

880. Kvittingen EA, Jellum E, Stokke O, et al: Liver transplantation in a 23-year-old tyrosinemia patient: Effects on the renal tubular dysfunction. J Inherit Metab Dis 9:216–224, 1986.

881. Tuchman M, Freese DK, Sharp HL, et al: Persistent succinylacetone excretion after liver transplantation in a patient with hereditary tyrosinaemia type I. J Inherit Metab Dis 8:21–24, 1985.

882. Starzl TE, Zitelli BJ, Shaw BW Jr, et al: Changing concepts: Liver replacement for hereditary tyrosinemia and hepatoma. J Pediatr 106:604–606, 1985.

883. Fallstrom SP, Lindblad B, Steen G: On the renal tubular damage in hereditary tyrosinemia and on the formation of succinylacetoacetate and succinylacetone. Acta Paediatr Scand 70:315–320, 1981.

884. Spencer PD, Medow MS, Moses LC, Roth KS: Effects of succinylacetone on the uptake of sugars and amino acids by brush border vesicles. Kidney Int 34:671–677, 1988.

885. Chen Y, Scheinman JI, Park HK, et al: Amelioration of proximal renal tubular dysfunction in type 1 glycogen storage disease with dietary therapy. N Engl J Med 323:590–593, 1990.

886. Rampini S, Fanconi A, Illig R, Prader A: Effect of hydrochlorothiazide on proximal renal tubular acidosis in a patient with idiopathic "de Toni–Debre-Fanconi syndrome." Helv Paediatr Acta 23:13–21, 1967.

887. Oetliker O, Rossi E: The influence of extracellular fluid volume on the renal bicarbonate threshold: A study of two children with Lowe's syndrome. Pediatr Res 3:140–148, 1969.

888. Donckerwolcke RA, Van Stekelenburg GJ, Tiddens HA: Therapy of bicarbonate-losing renal tubular acidosis. Arch Dis Child 45:774–779, 1970.

889. Beyer KH: The mechanism of action of chlorothiazide. Ann N Y Acad Sci 71:363–379, 1958.

890. Van Biervliet JPGM, Donckerwolcke RAMG, Van Stekelenburg GJ, Wadman SK: Sodium chloride restriction and extracellular fluid volume contraction in hyperphosphaturic vitamin D resistant rickets in the Lowe syndrome. Helv Paediatr Acta 30:365–375, 1975.

891. Morris RC Jr, Sebastian A: Disorders of the renal tubule that cause disorders of fluid, acid-base, and electrolyte metabolism. In Maxwell MH, Kleeman CR (eds): Clinical Disorders of Fluid and Electrolyte Metabolism, 3rd ed. McGraw-Hill, New York, 1980, p 883.

892. Cogan MG, Rector FC Jr, Seldin DW: Acid-base disorders in the kidney. In Brenner BM, Rector FC Jr (eds): The Kidney, 2nd ed. WB Saunders, Philadelphia, 1981, pp 841–907.

893. Rodriguez-Soriano J, Vallo A, Castillo G, Oliveros R: Natural history of primary distal renal tubular acidosis treated since infancy. J Pediatr 101:669–676, 1982.

894. Brown D, Hirsch S, Gluck S: An H$^+$-ATPase in opposite plasma membrane domains in kidney epithelial cell subpopulations. Nature 331:622–624, 1988.

895. Gluck S, Nelson R: The role of the V-ATPase in renal epithelial H$^+$ transport. J Exp Biol 172:205–218, 1992.

896. Stone DK, Seldin DW, Kokko JP, Jacobson HR: Anion dependence of rabbit medullary collecting duct acidification. J Clin Invest 71:1505–1508, 1983.

897. Breyer MD, Jacobson HR: Functional evidence for parallel basolateral Na$^+$/H$^+$ and Cl$^-$/HCO$_3^-$ exchangers in the inner stripe, outer medullary collecting duct (OMCDi) of rabbit. Kidney Int 35:451, 1989.

898. Siamopoulos KC, Elisaf M, Drosos AA, et al: Renal tubular acidosis in primary Sjögren's syndrome. Clin Rheumatol 11:226–230, 1992.

899. Cohen EP, Bastani B, Cohen MR, et al: Absence of H(+)-ATPase in cortical collecting tubules of a patient with Sjögren's syndrome and distal renal tubular acidosis. J Am Soc Nephrol 3:264–271, 1992.

900. Wrong OM, Feest TG, Maciver AG: Immune-related potassium-losing interstitial nephritis: A comparison with distal renal tubular acidosis. Q J Med 86:513–534, 1993.

901. Wingo CS, Madsen KM, Smolka A, Tisher CC: H-K-ATPase immunoreactivity in cortical and outer medullary collecting duct. Kidney Int 38:985–990, 1990.

902. Dafnis E, Spohn M, Lonis B, et al: Vanadate causes hypokalemic distal renal tubular acidosis. Am J Physiol 262:F449–F453, 1992.

903. Nilwarangkur S, Nimmannit S, Chaovakul V, et al: Endemic primary distal renal tubular acidosis in Thailand. Q J Med 74:289–301, 1990.

904. Sitprija V, Tungsanga K, Leelhaphunt N, et al: Metabolic problems in Northeastern Thailand: Possible role of vanadium. Miner Electrolyte Metab 19:51–56, 1993.

905. McKinney TD, Burg MB: Bicarbonate secretion by rabbit cortical collecting tubules in vitro. J Clin Invest 61:1421–1427, 1978.

906. Schuster VL: Bicarbonate reabsorption and secretion in the cortical and outer medullary collecting tubule. Semin Nephrol 10:139–147, 1990.

906a. Schofield AE, Tanner MJA, Unwin RJ, Wrong OM: Alterations in the RBC anion transporter (BAND 3) associated with familial distal renal tubular acidosis (dRTA). J Am Soc Nephrol 5:372, 1994.

907. Levine DZ, Jacobson HR: The regulation of renal acid secretion: New observations from studies of distal nephron segments. Kidney Int 29:1099–1109, 1986.

908. Lombard WE, Kokko JP, Jacobson HR: Bicarbonate transport in cortical and outer medullary collecting tubules. Am J Physiol 244:F289–F296, 1983.

909. Star RA, Burg MB, Knepper MA: Luminal pH disequilibrium ammonia transport in outer medullary collecting duct. Am J Physiol 252:F1148–F1157, 1987.

910. Bastani B, Purcell H, Hemken P, et al: Expression and distribution of renal vacuolar proton-translocating adenosine triphosphatase in response to chronic acid and alkali loads in the rat. J Clin Invest 88:126–136, 1991.

911. Verlander JW, Madsen KM, Tisher CC: Structural and functional features of proton and bicarbonate transport in the rat collecting duct. Semin Nephrol 11:465–477, 1991.

912. Verlander JW, Madsen KM, Stone DK, Tisher CC: Ultrastructural localization of H⁺-ATPase in rabbit cortical collecting duct. J Am Soc Nephrol 4:1546–1557, 1994.

913. Tomita K, Pisano JJ, Burg MB: Effects of vasopressin and brady-kinin on anion transport by the rat cortical collecting duct. Evidence for an electroneutral sodium chloride transport pathway. J Clin Invest 77:136–141, 1986.

914. Levine DZ, Iacovitti M, Buckman S, Harrison V: In vivo modula-tion of rat distal tubule net HCO₃ flux by VIP, isoproterenol, angio-tensin II, and ADH. Am J Physiol 266:F878–F883, 1994.

915. McKinney TD, Burg MB: Bicarbonate transport by rabbit cortical collecting tubules. Effect of acid and alkali loads in vivo on trans-port in vitro. J Clin Invest 60:766–768, 1977.

916. Pak Poy RK, Wrong O: The urinary Pco₂ in renal disease. Clin Sci 19:631–639, 1960.

917. Batlle DC, Sehy JT, Roseman MK, et al: Clinical and pathophysi-ologic spectrum of acquired distal renal tubular acidosis. Kidney Int 20:389–396, 1981.

918. Arruda JAL, Nascimento L, Mehta PK, et al: The critical impor-tance of urinary concentrating ability in the generation of urinary carbon dioxide tension. J Clin Invest 60:922–935, 1977.

919. DuBose TD Jr: Urine to blood Pco₂ gradient (U-B Pco₂) is an index of hydrogen ion secretion by collecting duct. Clin Res 29:460A, 1981. Abstract.

920. DuBose TD Jr, Caflisch CR: Validation of the difference in urine and blood carbon dioxide tension during bicarbonate loading as an index of distal nephron acidification in experimental models of distal renal tubular acidosis. J Clin Invest 75:1116–1123, 1985.

921. Harrison HE, Chisolm JJ Jr, Harrison HC: Congenital renal tubular acidosis. Am J Dis Child 96:588–590, 1958.

922. Buckalew VM Jr, McCurdy DK, Ludwig GD, et al: Incomplete renal tubular acidosis. Physiologic studies in three patients with a defect in lowering urine pH. Am J Med 45:32–42, 1968.

923. Frick PG, Rubini ME, Meroney WH: Recurrent nephrolithiasis associated with an unusual tubular defect and hyperchloremic aci-dosis. Am J Med 25:590–599, 1958.

924. Dedmon RE, Wrong O: The excretion of organic anion in renal tubular acidosis with particular reference to citrate. Clin Sci 22:19–32, 1962.

925. Morrissey JF, Ochoa MJ, Lotspeich WD, Waterhouse C: Citrate excretion in renal tubule acidosis. Ann Intern Med 58:159–166, 1963.

926. Brodwall EK, Westlie L, Myhre E: The renal excretion and tubular reabsorption of citric acid in renal tubular acidosis. Acta Med Scand 192:137–139, 1972.

927. Purvis ML, Buckalew VM Jr: Lysozymuria in distal renal tubular acidosis. Nephron 13:472–478, 1974.

928. Konnak JW, Kogan BA, Lau K: Renal calculi associated with incomplete distal renal tubular acidosis. J Urol 128:900–902, 1982.

929. Preminger GM, Sakhaee K, Skurla C, Pak CYC: Prevention of recurrent calcium stone formation with potassium citrate therapy in patients with distal renal tubular acidosis. J Urol 134:20–23, 1985.

930. Harrington TM, Bunch TW, Van Den Berg CJ: Renal tubular aci-dosis. A new look at treatment of musculoskeletal and renal dis-ease. Mayo Clin Proc 58:354–360, 1983.

931. Nordin BEC, Smith DA: Citric acid excretion in renal stone disease and in renal tubular acidosis. Br J Urol 35:438–444, 1963.

932. Fourman P, Robinson JR: Diminished urinary excretion of citrate during deficiencies of potassium in man. Lancet 2:656–657, 1953.

933. Crawford MA, Milne MD, Scribner BH: The effects of changes in acid-base balance on urinary citrate in the rat. J Physiol (Lond) 149:413–423, 1959.

934. Simpson DP: Citrate excretion: A window on renal metabolism. Am J Physiol 244:F223–F234, 1983.

935. Brennan S, Hering-Smith K, Hamm LL: Effect of pH on citrate reabsorption in the proximal convoluted tubule. Am J Physiol 255:F301–F306, 1988.

936. Caruana RJ, Buckalew VM Jr: The syndrome of distal (type 1) renal tubular acidosis. Medicine (Baltimore) 67:84–99, 1988.

937. Neuman WF, Neuman MW: The Chemical Dynamics of Bone Mineral. University of Chicago Press, Chicago, 1958.

938. Bisaz S, Felix R, Newman WF, Fleisch H: Quantitative determina-tion of inhibitors of calcium phosphate precipitation in whole urine. Miner Electrolyte Metab 1:74–83, 1978.

939. McSherry E, Pokroy M: The absence of nephrocalcinosis in chil-dren with type 1 RTA on high dose alkali therapy since infancy. Clin Res 26:470A, 1978. Abstract.

940. Coe FL, Parks JH: Stone disease in hereditary distal renal tubular acidosis. Ann Intern Med 93:60–61, 1980.

941. Adam WR, Koretsky AP, Weiner MW: ³¹P-NMR in vivo measure-ment of renal intracellular pH: Effects of acidosis and K⁺ depletion in rats. Am J Physiol 251:F904–F910, 1986.

942. Sakhaee K, Alpern R, Jacobson HR, Pak CYC: Contrasting effects of various potassium salts on renal citrate excretion. J Clin Endo-crinol Metab 72:396–400, 1991.

943. Nicar MJ, Peterson R, Pak CYC: Use of potassium citrate as potas-sium supplement during thiazide therapy of calcium nephrolithiasis. J Urol 131:430–433, 1984.

944. Lemann J Jr, Gray RW, Pleuss JA: Potassium bicarbonate, but not sodium bicarbonate, reduces urinary calcium excretion and im-proves calcium balance in healthy men. Kidney Int 35:688–695, 1989.

945. Falik-Borenstein ZC, Jordan SC, Saudubray J, et al: Brief report: Renal tubular acidosis in carnitine palmitoyltransferase type 1 defi-ciency. N Engl J Med 327:24–27, 1992.

946. Bougneres P, Saudubray J, Marsac C, et al: Fasting hypoglycemia resulting from hepatic carnitine palmitoyl transferase deficiency. J Pediatr 98:742–746, 1981.

947. Demaugre F, Bonnefont J, Mitchell G, et al: Hepatic and muscular presentations of carnitine palmitoyl transferase deficiency: Two dis-tinct entities. Pediatr Res 24:308–311, 1988.

948. Berger R, van Faassen H, Smith GPA: Biochemical studies on the enzymatic deficiencies in hereditary tyrosinemia. Clin Chim Acta 134:129–141, 1983.

949. Yeoh HH, Rice LE, Maggio A, Levin ML: Effects of 4-pentenoic acid on renal phosphate and calcium excretion in the dog. Am J Physiol 231:216–221, 1976.

950. Gullans SR, Mandel LJ: Coupling of energy to transport in proxi-mal and distal nephron. In Seldin DW, Giebisch G (eds): The Kidney: Physiology and Pathophysiology, 2nd ed. Raven Press, New York, 1992, pp 1291–1337.

951. Tonsgard JH, Getz GS: Effect of Reye's syndrome serum on iso-lated chinchilla liver mitochondria. J Clin Invest 76:816–825, 1985.

952. Alper SL, Natale J, Gluck S, et al: Subtypes of intercalated cells in rat kidney collecting duct defined by antibodies against erythroid band 3 and renal vacuolar H⁺-ATPase. Proc Natl Acad Sci USA 86:5429–5433, 1989.

953. Matsuzaki K, Stokes JBI, Schuster VL: Inhibition of cortical col-lecting tubule chloride transport by organic acids. J Clin Invest 82:57–64, 1988.

953a. Strife CF, Clardy CW, Varade WS, et al: Urine-to-blood carbon dioxide tension gradient and maximal depression of urinary pH to distinguish rate-dependent from classic distal renal tubular acidosis in children. J Pediatr 122:60–65, 1993.

954. Chan JCM, Alon U: Tubular disorders of acid-base and phosphate metabolism. Nephron 40:257–279, 1985.

955. Gill JR Jr, Bell NH, Bartter FC: Impaired conservation of sodium and potassium in renal tubular acidosis and its correction by buffer anions. Clin Sci 33:577–592, 1967.

956. Sebastian A, McSherry E, Morris RC Jr: Renal potassium wasting in renal tubular acidosis (RTA): Its occurrence in types 1 and 2 RTA despite sustained correction of systemic acidosis. J Clin Invest 50:667–678, 1971.

957. Sebastian A, McSherry E, Morris RC Jr: Impaired renal conservation of sodium and chloride during sustained correction of systemic acidosis in patients with type 1, classic renal tubular acidosis. J Clin Invest 58:454–469, 1976.

958. Lemann J Jr, Litzow JR, Lennon EJ: The effects of chronic acid loads in normal man: Further evidence for participation of bone mineral in the defense against chronic metabolic acidosis. J Clin Invest 45:1608–1614, 1966.

959. Coe FL, Firpo JJ Jr: Evidence of mild reversible hyperparathyroidism in distal renal tubular acidosis. Arch Intern Med 135:1485–1489, 1975.

960. Coe FL, Firpo JJ, Hollandsworth DL, et al: Effect of acute and chronic metabolic acidosis on serum immunoreactive parathyroid hormone in man. Kidney Int 8:262–273, 1975.

961. Greenberg AJ, McNamara H, McCrory WW: Metabolic balance studies in primary renal tubular acidosis: Effects of acidosis on external calcium and phosphorus balances. J Pediatr 69:610–618, 1966.

962. Caldas A, Broyer M, Dechaux M, Kleinknecht C: Primary distal tubular acidosis in childhood: Clinical study and long-term follow-up of 28 patients. J Pediatr 121:233–241, 1992.

963. Brenner RJ, Spring DB, Sebastian A, et al: Incidence of radiographically evident bone disease, nephrocalcinosis, and nephrolithiasis in various types of renal tubular acidosis. N Engl J Med 307:217–221, 1982.

964. Bushinsky DA: Internal exchanges of hydrogen ions: Bone. In Seldin DW, Giebisch G (eds): The Regulation of Acid-Base Balance. Raven Press, New York, 1989, pp 69–88.

965. Teti A, Blair HC, Schlesinger P, et al: Extracellular protons acidify osteoclasts, reduce cytosolic calcium and promote expression of cell-matrix attachment structures. J Clin Invest 84:773–780, 1989.

966. Goldhaber P, Rabadjija L: H+ stimulation of cell-mediated bone resorption in tissue culture. Am J Physiol 253:E90–E98, 1987.

967. Krieger NS, Sessler NE, Buchinsky DA: Acidosis inhibits osteoblastic and stimulates osteoclastic activity in vitro. Am J Physiol 262:F442–F448, 1992.

968. Courey WR, Pfister RC: The radiographic findings in renal tubular acidosis. Radiology 105:497–503, 1972.

969. Foss GL, Perry CB, Wood FJ: Renal tubular acidosis. Q J Med 25:185–199, 1956.

970. Richards P, Chamberlain MJ, Wrong OM: Treatment of osteomalacia of renal tubular acidosis by sodium bicarbonate alone. Lancet 2:994, 1972.

971. Santos F, Chan JCM: Renal tubular acidosis in children; diagnosis, treatment and prognosis. Am J Nephrol 6:289–295, 1986.

972. Morris RC Jr, Sebastian A, McSherry E: Therapeutic experience in patients with classic renal tubular acidosis. In Proceedings of the VII International Congress of Nephrology. S Karger, Basel, 1978, pp 345–349.

973. Owen EE, Verner JW Jr: Renal tubular disease with muscle paralysis and hypokalemia. Am J Med 28:8–21, 1960.

974. Vicale CT: The diagnostic features of a muscular syndrome resulting from hyperparathyroidism, osteomalacia owing to renal tubular acidosis, and perhaps to related disorders of calcium metabolism. Trans Am Neurol Assoc 74:143–147, 1949.

975. Smith R, Stern G: Muscular weakness in osteomalacia and hyperparathyroidism. J Neurol Sci 8:511–520, 1969.

976. Mallette LE, Patten BM, Engel WK: Neuromuscular disease in secondary hyperparathyroidism. Ann Intern Med 82:474–483, 1975.

977. Curry OB, Basten JF, Francis MJO, Smith R: Calcium uptake by sarcoplasmic reticulum of muscle from vitamin D–deficient rabbits. Nature 249:83–84, 1974.

978. Birge SJ, Haddad JG: 25-Hydroxycholecalciferol stimulation of muscle metabolism. J Clin Invest 56:1100–1107, 1975.

979. Henderson RG, Ledingham JGG, Oliver DP, et al: Effects of 1,25-dihydroxycholecalciferol on calcium absorption, muscle weakness, and bone disease in chronic renal failure. Lancet 1:379–384, 1974.

980. Prescott LF: Metabolisms of renal excretion of drugs (with special reference to drugs used by anaesthetists). Br J Anaesth 44:246–251, 1972.

981. Mudge GH, Silva P, Stibitz GR: Renal excretion by nonionic diffusion: The nature of disequilibrium. Med Clin North Am 59:681–698, 1975.

982. Beckett AH, Rowland M: Urinary excretion kinetics of amphetamine in man. J Pharmacol Exp Ther 17:628, 1965.

983. Kuntzman RG, Tsai I, Brand L, Mark LC: The influence of urinary pH on the plasma half-life of pseudoephedrine in man and dog and a sensitive assay for its determination in human plasma. Clin Pharmacol Ther 12:62–67, 1971.

984. MacPherson CR, Milne MD, Evans BM: The excretion of salicylate. Br J Pharmacol 10:484–489, 1955.

985. Gerhardt RE, Knouss RF, Thyrum PT, et al: Quinidine excretion in aciduria and alkaluria. Ann Intern Med 71:927–933, 1969.

986. Sebastian A, Hernandez RE, Schambelan M: Disorders of renal handling of potassium. In Brenner BM, Rector FC Jr (eds): The Kidney, 3rd ed. WB Saunders, Philadelphia, 1986.

987. Sebastian A, Sutton JM, Hulter HN, et al: Effect of mineralocorticoid replacement therapy on renal acid-base homeostasis in adrenalectomized patients. Kidney Int 18:762–773, 1980.

988. Miller PD, Waterhouse C, Owens R, Cohen E: The effect of potassium loading on sodium excretion and plasma renin activity in addisonian man. J Clin Invest 56:346–353, 1975.

989. Smith SG, Markandu ND, Banks RA, et al: Evidence that patients with Addison's disease are undertreated with fludrocortisone. Lancet 1:11–14, 1984.

990. Giebisch G, Stanton B: Potassium transport in the nephron. Annu Rev Physiol 41:241–256, 1979.

991. Perez GO, Oster JR, Vaamonde CA: Renal acidification in patients with mineralocorticoid deficiency. Nephron 17:461–473, 1976.

992. Oetliker OH, Zurbrugg RP: Renal tubular acidosis in salt-losing syndrome of congenital adrenal hyperplasia (CAH). J Clin Endocrinol Metab 31:447–450, 1970.

993. Imai M, Igarashi Y, Sokabe H: Plasma renin activity in congenital virilizing adrenal hyperplasia. Pediatrics 41:897–904, 1968.

994. Oetliker OH, Zurbrugg RP: Renal regulation of fluid, electrolyte, and acid-base homeostasis in the salt-losing syndrome of congenital adrenal hyperplasia (SL-CAH). ECF volume: A compensating factor in aldosterone deficiency. J Clin Endocrinol Metab 46:543–551, 1978.

995. Rosler A: The natural history of salt-wasting disorders of adrenal and renal origin. J Clin Endocrinol Metab 59:689–700, 1984.

996. Stinebaugh B, Miller RB, Relman AS: The influence of non-reabsorbable anions on acid excretion. Clin Sci 36:53–65, 1969.

997. David R, Golan S, Drucker W: Familial aldosterone deficiency: Enzyme defect, diagnosis, and clinical course. Pediatrics 41:403–412, 1968.

998. Veldhuis JD, Kulin HE, Santen RJ, et al: Inborn error in the terminal step of aldosterone biosynthesis: Corticosterone methyl oxidase type II deficiency in a North American pedigree. N Engl J Med 303:117–121, 1980.

999. Veldhuis JD, James CM: Isolated aldosterone deficiency in man: Acquired and inborn errors in the biosynthesis or action of aldosterone. Endocr Rev 2:495–517, 1981.

1000. Rosler A, Theodor R, Boichis H, et al: Metabolic responses to the administration of angiotensin II, K and ACTH in two salt wasting syndromes. J Clin Endocrinol Metab 44:292–301, 1977.

1001. Rosler A, Rabinowitz D, Theodor R, et al: The nature of the defect in a salt-wasting disorder in Jews of Iran. J Clin Endocrinol Metab 44:279–291, 1977.

1002. Ulick S: Diagnosis and nomenclature of the disorders of the terminal portion of the aldosterone biosynthetic pathway. J Clin Endocrinol Metab 43:92–96, 1976.

1003. Rosler A, Gazit E, Theodor R, et al: Salt wastage, raised plasma-renin activity, and normal or high plasma-aldosterone. A form of pseudohypoaldosteronism. Lancet 1:959–962, 1973.

1004. Katznelson D, Sack J, Kraiem Z, Lunenfeld B: Congenital hypoaldosteronism. Thirteen year follow-up in identical twins. Horm Res 11:22–28, 1979.

1005. Globerman H, Rosler A, Theodor R, et al: An inherited defect in aldosterone biosynthesis caused by a mutation in or near the gene for steroid 11-hydroxylase. N Engl J Med 319:1193–1197, 1988.

1006. Lee PDK, Patterson BD, Hintz RL, Rosenfeld RG: Biochemical diagnosis and management of corticosterone methyl oxidase type II deficiency. J Clin Endocrinol Metab 62:225–229, 1986.

1007. Phelps KR, Oh MS, Carroll HJ: Heparin-induced hyperkalemia: Report of a case. Nephron 25:254–258, 1980.

1008. O'Kelly R, Magee F, McKenna TJ: Routine heparin therapy inhibits adrenal aldosterone production. J Clin Endocrinol Metab 56:108–112, 1983.

1009. Edes TE, Sunderrajan EV: Heparin-induced hyperkalemia. Arch Intern Med 145:1070–1072, 1985.

1010. Wilson ID, Goetz FC: Selective hypoaldosteronism after prolonged heparin administration. Am J Med 36:635–640, 1964.

1011. Durand D, Ader J-L, Rey J-P, et al: Inducing hyperkalemia by converting enzyme inhibitors and heparin. Kidney Int 34(suppl 25):S196–S197, 1988.

1012. Williams FA Jr, Schambelan M, Biglieri EG, Carey RM: Acquired primary hypoaldosteronism due to an isolated zona glomerulosa defect. N Engl J Med 309:1623–1628, 1983.

1013. Tuck ML, Mayes DM: Mineralocorticoid biosynthesis in patients with hyporeninemic hypoaldosteronism. J Clin Endocrinol Metab 50:341–347, 1980.

1014. Silver J, Rosler A, Friedlander M, Popovtzer MM: Unmasking of isolated hypoaldosteronism after renal allotransplantation in Mediterranean fever. Isr J Med Sci 18:495–498, 1982.

1015. Stern N, Beck FWJ, Sowers JR, et al: Plasma corticosteroids in hyperreninemic hypoaldosteronism: Evidence for diffuse impairment of the zona glomerulosa. J Clin Endocrinol Metab 57:217–220, 1983.

1016. Schambelan M, Sebastian A, Biglieri EG: Prevalence, pathogenesis, and functional significance of aldosterone deficiency in hyperkalemic patients with chronic renal insufficiency. Kidney Int 17:89–101, 1980.

1017. Perez GO, Oster JR, Vaamonde CA: Renal acidosis and renal potassium handling in selective hyperaldosteronism. Am J Med 57:809–816, 1974.

1018. Schambelan M, Stockigt JR, Biglieri EG: Isolated hypoaldosteronism in adults, a renin deficiency syndrome. N Engl J Med 287:573–578, 1972.

1019. Perez G, Siegel L, Schreiner GE: Selective hypoaldosteronism with hyperkalemia. Ann Intern Med 76:757–763, 1972.

1020. Weidmann P, Reinhart R, Maxwell MH, et al: Syndrome of hyporeninemic hypoaldosteronism and hyperkalemia in renal disease. J Clin Endocrinol Metab 36:965–977, 1973.

1021. Perez GO, Oster JR: Hyporeninemic hypoaldosteronism after renal transplantation. South Med J 70:363–364, 1977.

1022. DeFronzo RA: Hyperkalemia and hyporeninemic hypoaldosteronism. Kidney Int 17:118–134, 1980.

1023. Sebastian A, Schambelan M, Lindenfeld S, Morris RC Jr: Amelioration of metabolic acidosis with fludrocortisone therapy in hyporeninemic hypoaldosteronism. N Engl J Med 297:576–583, 1977.

1024. Matsuda O, Nonoguchi H, Tomita K, et al: Primary role of hyperkalemia in the acidosis of hyporeninemic hypoaldosteronism. Nephron 49:203–209, 1988.

1025. Lee FO, Quismorio FP Jr, Troum OM, et al: Mechanisms of hyperkalemia in systemic lupus erythematosus. Arch Intern Med 148:397–401, 1988.

1026. Kozeny GA, Hurley RM, Fresco R, et al: Systemic lupus erythematosus presenting with hyporeninemic hypoaldosteronism in a 10-year-old girl. Am J Nephrol 6:321–324, 1986.

1027. Brown JJ, Chinn RH, Fraser R, et al: Recurrent hyperkalaemia due to selective aldosterone deficiency correction by angiotensin infusion. Br Med J 1:650–653, 1973.

1028. Haverty TP, Neilson EG: Basement membrane gene expression in polycystic kidney disease. Lab Invest 58:245–248, 1988.

1029. Meyer MH, Meyer RA Jr, Gray RW, Irwin RL: Picric acid methods greatly overestimate serum creatinine in mice: More accurate results with high-performance liquid chromatography. Anal Biochem 144:285–290, 1985.

1030. Batlle DC: Hyperkalemic hyperchloremic metabolic acidosis associated with selective aldosterone deficiency and distal renal tubular acidosis. Semin Nephrol 1:260–274, 1981.

1031. Oh MS, Carroll HJ, Clemmons JE, et al: A mechanism for hyporeninemic hypoaldosteronism in chronic renal disease. Metabolism 23:1157–1165, 1974.

1032. Regan JJ Jr, Greenberg CS, Mooradian AD, et al: Reversible renal resistance to aldosterone associated with interstitial nephritis. West J Med 146:742–745, 1987.

1033. Kristjansson K, Laxdal T, Ragnarsson J: Type 4 renal tubular acidosis (sub-type 2) associated with idiopathic interstitial nephritis. Acta Paediatr Scand 75:1051–1054, 1986.

1034. Lim TK, Fong KY: Hyperkalemic distal renal tubular acidosis with hyporeninemic hypoaldosteronism in a patient with systemic lupus erythematosus—a case report. Singapore Med J 28:560–561, 1987.

1035. Tan SY, Shapiro R, Franco R, et al: Indomethacin-induced prostaglandin inhibition with hyperkalemia. Ann Intern Med 90:783–785, 1979.

1036. Schambelan M, Sebastian A: Pathogenesis of indomethacin-induced hyperkalemia and type 4 renal tubular acidosis. *In* Proceedings of the 5th International Conference on Prostaglandins, Florence, 1982.

1037. Kutyrina IM, Androsova SO, Tareyeva IE: Indomethacin-induced hyporeninaemic hypoaldosteronism. Lancet 1:785, 1979. Letter.

1038. Nadler JL, Lee FO, Hsueh W, Horton R: Evidence of prostacyclin deficiency in the syndrome of hyporeninemic hypoaldosteronism. N Engl J Med 314:1015–1020, 1986.

1039. Norby LH, Weidig J, Ramwell P, et al: Possible role for impaired renal prostaglandin production in pathogenesis of hyporeninaemic hypoaldosteronism. Lancet 2:1118–1122, 1978.

1040. Valimaki M, Pelkonen R, Tikkanen I, Fyhrqvist F: A deficient response of atrial natriuretic peptide to volume overload in Gordon's syndrome. Acta Endocrinol 120:331–336, 1989.

1041. Gordon RD, Ravenscroft PJ, Klemm SA, et al: A new Australian kindred with the syndrome of hypertension and hyperkalaemia has dysregulation of atrial natriuretic factor. J Hypertens 6:S323–S326, 1988.

1042. Sakemi T, Ohchi N, Sanai T, et al: Captopril-induced metabolic acidosis with hyperkalemia. Am J Nephrol 8:245–248, 1988.

1043. Warren SE, O'Connor DT: Hyperkalemia resulting from captopril administration. JAMA 344:2551–2552, 1980.

1044. Findling JW, Adams AH, Raff H: Selective hypoaldosteronism due to an endogenous impairment in angiotensin II production. N Engl J Med 316:1632–1635, 1987.

1045. Morimoto S, Kim KS, Yamamoto I, et al: Selective hypoaldosteronism with hyperreninemia in a diabetic patient. J Clin Endocrinol Metab 49:742–747, 1979.

1046. Landier F, Guyene TT, Boutignon H, et al: Hyporeninemic hypoaldosteronism in infancy: A familial disease. J Clin Endocrinol Metab 58:143–148, 1984.

1047. McGiff JC, Muzzarelli RE, Duffy PA, et al: Interrelationships of renin and aldosterone in a patient with hypoaldosteronism. Am J Med 48:247–253, 1970.

1048. Marieb NJ, Melby JC, Lyall SS: Isolated hypoaldosteronism associated with idiopathic hypoparathyroidism. Arch Intern Med 134:424–429, 1974.

1049. Mellinger RC, Petermann FL, Jurgenson JC: Hyponatremia with low urinary aldosterone occurring in an old woman. J Clin Endocrinol Metab 34:85–91, 1972.

1050. Russell A, Levin B, Sinclair L, Oberholzer VG: A reversible salt-wasting syndrome of the newborn and infant. Arch Dis Child 38:313–325, 1963.

1051. Vagnucci AH: Selective aldosterone deficiency. J Clin Endocrinol Metab 29:279–289, 1969.

1052. Popow C, Pollak A, Herkner K, et al: Familial pseudohypoaldosteronism. Acta Paediatr Scand 77:136–141, 1988.

1053. Speiser PW, Stoner E, New MI: Pseudohypoaldosteronism: A review and report of two new cases. Adv Exp Med Biol 196:173–195, 1986.

1054. Bosson D, Kuhnle U, Mees N, et al: Generalized unresponsiveness to mineralocorticoid hormones: Familial recessive pseudohypoaldosteronism due to aldosterone-receptor deficiency. Acta Endocrinol 279:376–380, 1986.

1055. Donnell GN, Litman N, Roldan M: Pseudohypoadrenalocorticism. Am J Dis Child 97:813–828, 1959.

1056. Lelong M, Alagille D, Philippe A, et al: Diabete salin par insensibilite congenitale du tubule a l'aldosterone "pseudo-hypo-adrenocorticisme." Rev Fr Etudes Clin Biol 5:558–565, 1960.

1057. Raine DN, Roy J: A salt-losing syndrome in infancy. Pseudohypoadrenocorticalism. Arch Dis Child 37:548–556, 1962.

1058. Royer P, Bonnette J, Mathieu H, et al: Pseudo-hypoaldosteronisme. Ann Pediatr (Paris) 54:596–605, 1963.

1059. Trung PH, Piussan C, Rodary C, et al: Etude du taux de sécrétion de l'aldosterone et de l'activité de la rénineplasmatique d'un cas de pseudo-hypoaldosteronisme. Arch Fr Pediatr 27:603–615, 1970.

1060. Barakat AY, Papadopoulou ZL, August GP: A hyperkalemic, salt-wasting syndrome in infancy. Pediatr Res 6:394, 1972.

1061. Savitt H, Molitch M, Kawaoka E, Leake R: Pseudohypoaldosteronism. Clin Res 23:165A, 1975.

1062. Roy C: Pseudohypoaldosteronisme familial. Arch Fr Pediatr 34:37–54, 1977.

1063. Bonnici F: Pseudohypoaldosteronisme familial. A transmission autosomique recessive. Arch Fr Pediatr 34:915–919, 1977.

1064. Kaufman E, Hayek A, Greenberg R: Pseudohypoaldosteronism in triplets. Pediatr Res 11:426, 1977.

1065. Lauras B, Ravussin JJ, David M, et al: Pseudo-hypoaldosteronisme chez l'enfant. A propos de quatre observations dont deux concernant des frères. Pediatrie 33:119–135, 1978.

1066. Lundberg JM, Franco-Cereceda A, Hua X, et al: Co-existence of substance P and calcitonin gene–related peptide–like immunoreactivities in sensory nerves in relation to cardiovascular and bronchoconstrictor effects of capsaicin. Eur J Pharmacol 108:315–319, 1985.

1067. Chan KW, Ho FCS, Chan MK: Adult Fanconi syndrome in κ light chain myeloma. Arch Pathol Lab Med 111:139–142, 1987.

1068. Limal JM, Rappaport R, Dechaux M, Morin C: Familial dominant pseudohypoaldosteronism. Lancet 1:51, 1978. Letter.

1069. Hanukoglu A, Fried D, Gotlieb A: Inheritance of pseudohypoaldosteronism. Lancet 1:1359–1360, 1978.

1070. Blacher Y, Kaplan BS, Griffel B, Levin S: Pseudohypoaldosteronism. Clin Nephrol 11:281–288, 1979.

1071. Rosenberg S, Franks RC, Ulick S: Mineralocorticoid unresponsiveness with severe neonatal hyponatremia and hyperkalemia. J Clin Endocrinol Metab 50:401–404, 1980.

1072. Hogg RJ, Frolich J, Marver D, Marks JF: The basic defect in pseudohypoaldosteronism. Clin Res 26:828A, 1978.

1073. Bierich JR, Schmidt U: Tubular Na,K-ATPase deficiency, the cause of the congenital renal salt-losing syndrome. Eur J Pediatr 121:81–87, 1976.

1074. Anand SK, Froberg L, Northway JD, et al: Pseudohypoaldosteronism due to sweat gland dysfunction. Pediatr Res 10:677–682, 1976.

1075. Petersen S, Giese J, Kappelgaard AM, et al: Pseudohypoaldosteronism. Clinical, biochemical and morphological studies in a long-term follow-up. Acta Paediatr Scand 67:255–261, 1978.

1076. Cheek DB, Perry JW: A salt wasting syndrome in infancy. Arch Dis Child 33:252–256, 1958.

1077. Proesmans W, Geussens H, Corbeel L, Eeckels R: Pseudohypoaldosteronism. Am J Dis Child 126:510–516, 1973.

1078. Oberfield SE, Levine LS, Carey RM, et al: Pseudohypoaldosteronism: Multiple target organ unresponsiveness to mineralocorticoid hormones. J Clin Endocrinol Metab 48:228–234, 1979.

1079. Postel-Vinay M-C, Alberti GM, Ricour C, et al: Pseudohypoaldosteronism: Persistence of hyperaldosteronism and evidence for renal tubular and intestinal responsiveness to endogenous aldosterone. J Clin Endocrinol Metab 39:1038–1044, 1974.

1080. Popovtzer MM, Rosler A, Cerasi E, et al: Na-K-ATPase deficiency: A possible mechanism of renal salt wasting in a newborn baby with "pseudohypoaldosteronism." Clin Res 28:536A, 1980.

1081. Cogan MC, Arieff AI: Sodium wasting, acidosis and hyperkalemia induced by methicillin interstitial nephritis. Am J Med 64:500–506, 1978.

1082. Popovtzer MM, Katz FH, Pinggera WF, et al: Hyperkalemia in salt-wasting nephropathy. Study of the mechanism. Arch Intern Med 132:203–208, 1973.

1083. Arruda JAL, Batlle DC, Sehy JT, et al: Hyperkalemia and renal insufficiency: Role of selective aldosterone deficiency and tubular unresponsiveness to aldosterone. Am J Nephrol 1:160–167, 1981.

1084. Stanbury SW, Mahler RF: Salt-wasting renal disease. Metabolic observations on a patient with salt-losing nephritis. Q J Med 28:425–447, 1959.

1085. Rado JP, Szende L, Szucs L: Hyperkalemia unresponsive to massive doses of aldosterone in a patient with renal tubular acidosis. Endocrinologie 68:183–188, 1976.

1086. Rodriguez-Soriano J, Vallo A, Oliveros R, Castillo G: Transient pseudohypoaldosteronism secondary to obstructive uropathy in infancy. J Pediatr 103:375–380, 1983.

1087. Horner JM, Hintz RL, Luetscher JA: The role of renin and angiotensin in salt-losing 21-hydroxylase–deficient congenital adrenal hyperplasia. J Clin Endocrinol Metab 48:776–783, 1979.

1088. Keenan BS, Holcombe JH, Kirkland RT, et al: Sodium homeostasis and aldosterone secretion in salt-losing congenital adrenal hyperplasia. J Clin Endocrinol Metab 48:430–436, 1979.

1089. Rodriguez-Soriano J, Vallo A, Castillo G, et al: Hyperkalemic distal renal tubular acidosis in salt-losing congenital adrenal hyperplasia. Acta Paediatr Scand 75:425–432, 1986.

1090. Farfel Z, Iaina A, Rosenthal T, et al: Familial hyperpotassemia and hypertension accompanied by normal plasma aldosterone levels. Arch Intern Med 138:1828–1832, 1978.

1091. Gordon RD, Geddes RA, Pawsey CGK, O'Halloran MW: Hypertension and severe hyperkalaemia associated with suppression of renin and aldosterone and completely reversed by dietary sodium restriction. Aust Ann Med 4:287–294, 1970.

1092. Stokes GS, Gentle JL, Edwards KDG, Stewart JH: Syndrome of idiopathic hyperkalaemia and hypertension with decreased plasma renin activity. Effects on plasma renin and aldosterone of reducing the serum potassium level. Med J Aust 2:1050–1054, 1968.

1093. Arnold JE, Healy JK: Hyperkalemia, hypertension and systemic acidosis without renal failure associated with a tubular defect in potassium excretion. Am J Med 47:461–472, 1969.

1094. Spitzer A, Edelmann CM Jr, Goldberg LD, Henneman PH: Short stature, hyperkalemia and acidosis: A defect in renal transport of potassium. Kidney Int 3:251–257, 1973.

1095. Weinstein SF, Allan DM, Mendoza SA: Hyperkalemia, acidosis, and short stature associated with a defect in renal potassium excretion. J Pediatr 85:355–358, 1974.

1096. Brautbar N, Levi J, Rosler A, et al: Familial hyperkalemia, hypertension, and hyporeninemia with normal aldosterone levels: A tubular defect in potassium handling. Arch Intern Med 138:607–610, 1978.

1097. Lee MR, Ball SG, Thomas TH, Morgan DB: Hypertension and hyperkalaemia responding to bendrofluazide. Q J Med 48:245–258, 1979.

1098. Schambelan M, Sebastian A, Rector FC Jr: Mineralocorticoid-resistant renal hyperkalemia without salt wasting (type II pseudohypoaldosteronism). Role of increased renal chloride reabsorption. Kidney Int 19:716–727, 1981.

1099. Soppi E, Viikari J, Seppala P, et al: Unusual association of hyperkalemia and hypertension. Hypertension 8:174–177, 1986.

1100. Biber TUL, Mylle M, Baines AD, et al: A study by micropuncture and microdissection of acute renal damage in rats. Am J Med 44:664–705, 1968.

1101. Licht JH, Amundson D, Hsueh WA, Lombardo JV: Familiar hyperkalaemic acidosis. Q J Med 54:161–176, 1985.

1102. Morell V: New light on writing in the Americas. Science 251:268–270, 1991.

1103. Appiani AC, Marra G, Tirelli SA, et al: Early childhood hyperkalemia: Variety of pseudohypoaldosteronism. Acta Paediatr Scand 75:970–974, 1986.

1104. Hansson R, Johansson S, Jonsson O, et al: Kidney protection by pretreatment with free radical scavengers and allopurinol: Renal function at recirculation after warm ischemia in rabbits. Clin Sci 71:245–251, 1986.

1105. Pines A, Kaplinsky N, Olchovsky D, et al: Anorexia nervosa, laxative abuse, hypopotassemia, and distal renal tubular acidosis. Isr J Med Sci 21:50–52, 1985.

1106. Sanjad SA, Mansour FM, Hernandez RH, Leighton Hill L: Severe hypertension, hyperkalemia, and renal tubular acidosis responding to dietary sodium restriction. Pediatrics 69:317–324, 1982.

1107. Sanjad SA, Keenan BS, Hill LL: Renal hypoprostaglandism, hypertension, and type IV renal tubular acidosis reversed by furosemide. Ann Intern Med 99:624–627, 1983.

1108. Szylman P, Better OS, Chaimowitz C, Rosler A: Role of hyperkalemia in the metabolic acidosis of isolated hypoaldosteronism. N Engl J Med 294:361–365, 1976.

1109. DeFronzo RA, Cooke CR, Goldberg M, et al: Impaired renal tubular potassium secretion in systemic lupus erythematosus. Ann Intern Med 86:268–271, 1977.

1110. Luke RG, Allison MEM, Davidson JF, Duguid WP: Hyperkalemia and renal tubular acidosis due to renal amyloidosis. Ann Intern Med 70:1211–1217, 1969.

1111. Pelleya R, Oster JR, Perez GO: Hyporeninemic hypoaldosteronism, sodium wasting and mineralocorticoid-resistant hyperkalemia in two patients with obstructive uropathy. Am J Nephrol 3:223–227, 1983.

1112. DeFronzo RA, Goldberg M, Cooke CR, et al: Investigations into the mechanisms of hyperkalemia following renal transplantation. Kidney Int 11:357–365, 1977.

1113. DeFronzo RA, Taufield PA, Black H, et al: Impaired renal tubular potassium secretion in sickle cell disease. Ann Intern Med 90:310–316, 1979.

1114. Bantle JP, Nath KA, Sutherland DER, et al: Effects of cyclosporine on the renin-angiotensin-aldosterone system and potassium excretion in renal transplant recipients. Arch Intern Med 145:505–508, 1985.

1115. Zazgornik J, Shaheen FAM, Kopsa H, et al: Severe hyperkalaemia, hyperchloraemia, hyporeninaemia and hyperaldosteronism in a cyclosporin-treated renal-transplant patient. Nephrol Dial Transplant 3:826–829, 1988.

1116. Stahl RAK, Kanz L, Maier B, Schollmeyer P: Hyperchloremic metabolic acidosis with high serum potassium in renal transplant recipients: A cyclosporine A associated side effect. Clin Nephrol 25:245–248, 1986.

1117. Ashouri OS: Hyperkalemic distal renal tubular acidosis and selective aldosterone deficiency. Combination in a patient with lead nephropathy. Arch Intern Med 145:1306–1307, 1985.

1118. Schambelan M, Sebastian A, Hulter HN: Mineralocorticoid excess and deficiency syndromes. *In* Brenner BM, Stein JH (eds): Contemporary Issues in Nephrology: Acid-Base and Potassium Homeostasis. Churchill Livingstone, New York, 1978, pp 232–268.

1119. Hulter HN, Ilnicki LP, Harbottle JA, Sebastian A: Impaired renal H$^+$ secretion and NH$_3$ production in mineralocorticoid-deficient glucocorticoid-replete dogs. Am J Physiol 232:F136–F146, 1977.

1120. Schwartz GJ, Burg MB: Mineralocorticoid effects on cation transport by cortical collecting tubules in vitro. Am J Physiol 238:F576–F585, 1978.

1121. O'Neil RG, Helman SI: Transport characteristics of renal collecting tubules: Influences of DOCA and diet. Am J Physiol 233:F544–F558, 1977.

1122. Katz AI: Renal Na-K-ATPase: Its role in tubular sodium and potassium transport. Am J Physiol 242:F207–F219, 1982.

1123. Garty H, Edelman IS: Amiloride-sensitive trypsinization of apical sodium channels. J Gen Physiol 81:785–803, 1983.

1124. O'Neil RG, Hayhurst RA: Sodium-dependent modulation of the renal Na-K-ATPase: Influence of mineralocorticoids on the cortical collecting duct. J Membr Biol 85:169–179, 1985.

1125. Palmer LG, Frindt G: Amiloride-sensitive Na channels from the apical membrane of the rat cortical collecting tubule. Proc Natl Acad Sci USA 83:2767–2770, 1986.

1126. Hayhurst RA, O'Neil RG: Time-dependent actions of aldosterone and amiloride on Na$^+$-K$^+$-ATPase of cortical collecting duct. Am J Physiol 254:F689–F696, 1988.

1127. Morel F, Doucet A: Hormonal control of kidney functions at the cell level. Physiol Rev 66:377–468, 1986.

1128. O'Neil RG: Adrenal steroid regulation of potassium transport. *In* Giebisch G (ed): Current Topics in Membranes and Transport. Academic Press, New York, 1987, pp 185–206.

1129. Garg LC, Knepper MA, Burg MB: Mineralocorticoid effects on Na-K-ATPase in individual nephron segments. Am J Physiol 240:F536–F544, 1981.

1130. Hunter M, Lopes AG, Boulpaep EL, Cohen B: Single channel recordings of calcium-activated potassium channels in the apical membrane of rabbit cortical collecting tubules. Proc Natl Acad Sci USA 81:4237–4239, 1984.

1131. Sansom SC, Agulian S, Muto S, et al: K activity of CCD principal cells from normal and DOCA-treated rabbits. Am J Physiol 256:F136–F142, 1989.

1132. Koeppen BM: Electrophysiology of collecting duct H$^+$ secretion: Effect of inhibitors. Am J Physiol 256:F79–F84, 1989.

1133. Stone DK, Xie X-S: Proton translocating ATPases: Issues in structure and function. Kidney Int 33:767–774, 1988.

1134. Stone DK, Seldin DW, Kokko JP: Mineralocorticoid modulation of rabbit medullary collecting duct acidification. A sodium-independent effect. J Clin Invest 72:77–83, 1983.

1135. Garg LC, Narang N: Effects of aldosterone on NEM-sensitive ATPase in rabbit nephron segments. Kidney Int 34:13–17, 1988.

1136. Tannen RL, McGill J: The influence of potassium on renal ammonia production. Am J Physiol 231:1178–1184, 1976.

1137. DuBose TD Jr, Caflisch CR: Effect of selective aldosterone deficiency on acidification in nephron segments of the rat inner module. J Clin Invest 82:1624–1632, 1988.

1138. Robson WLM, Halperin ML, Stinebaugh BJ, Goldstein MB: Effect of mineralocorticoids on collecting duct hydrogen ion secretion in the rabbit. Can J Physiol Pharmacol 59:235–238, 1981.

1139. Schlueter W, Keilani T, Hizon M, et al: On the mechanism of impaired distal acidification in hyperkalemic renal tubular acidosis: Evaluation with amiloride and bumetanide. J Am Soc Nephrol 3:953–964, 1992.

1140. Phelps KR, Lieberman RL, Oh MS, Caroll HJ: Pathophysiology of the syndrome of hyporeninemic hypoaldosteronism. Metabolism 29:186–199, 1980.

1141. Sebastian A, Schambelan M, Sutton JM: Amelioration of hyperchloremic acidosis with furosemide therapy in patients with chronic renal insufficiency and type 4 renal tubular acidosis. Am J Nephrol 4:287–300, 1984.

1142. Griendling KK, Berk BC, Alexander RW: Evidence that Na$^+$/H$^+$ exchange regulates angiotensin II–stimulated diacylglycerol accumulation in vascular smooth muscle cells. J Biol Chem 263:10620–10624, 1988.

1143. Alvarez MN, Barnes ND, Stickler GB: Salt wasting nephropathy of ''pseudohypoaldosteronism'' in twins. Pediatr Res 8:453–460, 1974.

1144. Armanini D, Kuhnle U, Strasser T, et al: Aldosterone-receptor deficiency in pseudohypoaldosteronism. N Engl J Med 313:1178–1181, 1985.

1145. Steele TH, DeLuca HF: Influence of dietary phosphorus on renal phosphate reabsorption in the parathyroidectomized rat. J Clin Invest 57:867–874, 1976.

1146. Freinkel N, Lewis NJ, Akazawa S, et al: The honeybee syndrome—implications of the teratogenicity of mannose in rat-embryo culture. N Engl J Med 310:223–230, 1984.

1147. Take C, Ikeda K, Kurasawa T, Kurokawa K: Increased chloride reabsorption as an inherited renal tubular defect in familial type II pseudohypoaldosteronism. N Engl J Med 324:472–476, 1991.

1148. Garcia-Filho E, Malnic G, Giebisch G: Effect of changes in electrical potential difference on tubular potassium transport. Am J Physiol 238:F235–F246, 1980.

1149. Boudry JF, Stoner LC, Burg MB: Effect of acid lumen pH on potassium transport in renal cortical collecting tubules. Am J Physiol 230:239–244, 1976.

1150. Gordon RD: Syndrome of hypertension and hyperkalemia with normal glomerular filtration rate. Hypertension 8:93–102, 1986.

# 38

# Cystic and Developmental Diseases of the Kidney

*Larry W. Welling*
*Jared J. Grantham*

## NOMENCLATURE AND PATHOGENESIS OF RENAL CYSTS

Renal cysts are abnormal, fluid-filled sacs that arise in the renal parenchyma. They begin as dilations or as outpouchings from existing nephrons or collecting ducts or from the developmental counterparts of those structures. The fluid they contain derives from their parent nephron or is a local secretion and may simulate that normally found in proximal or distal nephron segments.[1, 2] Cysts are usually lined by an epithelium that is probably continuous and usually has a primitive or simplified morphologic appearance.[3] Occasionally, however, the epithelium simulates that in normal proximal or distal nephron segments.[4] There is evidence that many cysts eventually lose all connection with their tubule of origin.[4] Although clinically important cysts are usually macroscopic in size, convention[5] requires only that they exceed 0.2 mm in diameter.

Renal cysts occur in a multitude of unrelated conditions and may be hereditary, developmental, or acquired. Renal involvement may be unilateral or bilateral and symmetric, localized, or irregular. Cysts may occur in cortex, in medulla, or in both regions of the kidney and may or may not be associated with other renal or systemic abnormalities. In general, only a small fraction of the total nephron population undergoes cystic change. Renal cystic disease may be defined as morbidity attributable to the presence of renal cysts, and a cystic kidney may be defined as one that contains three or more renal cysts. The classification of renal-

cysts given in Table 38–1 is based on listings that appear elsewhere.[6, 7]

The pathogenesis of renal cysts is not completely understood. Historically, a neoplastic origin was considered but generally discarded in favor of some form of urinary obstruction as an underlying mechanism. By the mid-1960s, emphasis shifted toward the possibility that varying degrees of dysfunction in the interacting anlagen of the developing kidney led eventually to several patterns of cyst formation in the nephrons and collecting ducts. Supported by extensive microdissection studies,[8] that view of a causal relationship between cysts and renal maldevelopment either rejected the earlier theories of cyst formation or refocused them into the context of developmental abnormalities. As a consequence, it was sometimes forgotten that many renal developmental abnormalities are not characterized by cyst formation and many renal cystic disorders are not associated with detectable renal maldevelopment. Finally, beginning in the mid-1970s, there occurred a virtual renaissance of new ideas. Renal cystic disease could be induced in normal animals by a variety of chemicals and was found to occur in humans as an acquired disorder. It was also observed in several patterns of inheritance in rats, mice, and other animals and could be simulated in cell culture and other in vitro systems. All of this allowed a new perspective and a new experimental approach that previously had not been possible.

In the past decade, there have been perhaps 100 publications that have contributed to our current understanding of

**TABLE 38–1. Classification of Renal Cysts**

Hereditary polycystic kidney disease
    Autosomal dominant polycystic kidney disease
        Polycystic disease in neonates and young children
        Polycystic disease in older children and adults (classic ''adult''
            polycystic disease with cystic involvement of liver and
            other organs)
    Autosomal recessive polycystic kidney disease
        Polycystic disease in neonates and infants (classic ''infantile''
            polycystic disease with severe renal involvement and mild
            hepatic fibrosis)
        Polycystic disease in young children and juveniles (with less
            severe renal involvement and more severe hepatic fibrosis,
            ''congenital hepatic fibrosis'')
Acquired cystic kidney disease (in azotemia and dialysis)
Cystic diseases of the renal medulla
    Medullary cystic disease
        Autosomal recessive, presenting mostly in children
        Autosomal dominant, presenting mostly in adults
        Renal-retinal dysplasia
    Medullary sponge kidney
Simple cysts
Cystic renal dysplasia
Miscellaneous renal cystic disorders
    Hereditary
        Tuberous sclerosis
        von Hippel–Lindau syndrome
    Nonhereditary
        Solitary multilocular cysts
        Pyelocalyceal cysts
        Renal lymphangiomatosis
        Hilar and perinephric pseudocysts

cyst formation. The reader is referred elsewhere for detailed reviews.[1, 9] For the present purpose, it is sufficient to list six important facts: 1) all cysts, whether acquired or inherited, develop from pre-existing renal tubule segments; 2) after achieving a size of perhaps a few millimeters, the majority of cysts lose their attachment to their parent nephron segment; 3) the cyst lining epithelium generally shows abnormal cellular differentiation and sustained proliferation; 4) the usually reabsorptive tubule epithelium is transformed into one capable of significant volume secretion that undoubtedly involves solute gradients and cyclic AMP mechanisms; 5) there must be appropriate remodeling of the extracellular matrix to accommodate the enlarging cysts; and 6) the proliferation, secretion, and matrix remodeling are undoubtedly modulated by yet to be discovered endocrine, paracrine, juxtacrine, and autocrine factors that would be important determinants of how fast the cysts grow and how rapidly renal insufficiency develops in cystic disease states. Clearly, although a great deal more work is required, it is probably not too far-fetched to suggest that our present, hard-won appreciation of the components of cyst pathogenesis will lead to new understanding and to new treatment strategies in the future.

# HEREDITARY POLYCYSTIC KIDNEY DISORDERS

Polycystic kidney disease is a subset of renal cystic disorders in which cysts are distributed throughout the cortex and medulla of both kidneys. It is usually the hallmark of a unique autosomal dominant or autosomal recessive disorder but may also be found in association with a variety of clinical conditions or be acquired at some point in the life of a patient with an underlying, noncystic renal disease. The hereditary disorders are considered first.

## Autosomal Dominant Polycystic Kidney Disease

This disease affects about 1 person per 1000 and is the most common of the polycystic kidney diseases. It has worldwide distribution, appears to affect all races, and affects males and females equally. It affects approximately 250,000 to 500,000 persons in the United States, where the incidence is about 6000 per year.[10] Although the process is usually not clinically apparent until the third or fourth decade of life, it has been found in infants and aborted fetuses. The commonly used term ''adult'' polycystic kidney disease is thus technically incorrect and misleading and should be abandoned. The more correct designation, autosomal dominant polycystic kidney disease (ADPKD), is used here.

ADPKD is inherited as an autosomal dominant trait with nearly complete penetrance but variable expression.[11] On the average, 50% of the offspring of one affected parent inherit the abnormal gene. In approximately 90% of cases, that abnormal gene or gene cluster (now known as *ADPKD1*) is linked to the α-globin cluster located on the short arm of chromosome 16.[12]* In some families, however, that linkage cannot be demonstrated,[13, 14] and new evidence has revealed a mutation (*ADPKD2*) on chromosome 4.[15, 16] The possibility of a third mutation unlinked to either chromosome 4 or 16 has also been suggested.

The disease probably begins in utero in most patients but, throughout its course, probably causes less than 1% of the total population of tubules to become cystic.[4] The kidneys increase in size and ultimately cause signs and symptoms in the fourth to fifth decade of life in most affected patients. Rarely, patients may be symptomatic in childhood or, conversely, may be unaware of their disorder until its chance discovery in the eighth or ninth decade. Siblings of a child presenting in the neonatal period have increased likelihood of also presenting in the neonatal period.[17] About 40% of patients are unable to give a family history consistent with ADPKD, and this has suggested the possibility of a high spontaneous mutation rate or, alternatively, the possibility that environmental or epidemiologic factors strongly affect the expression of ADPKD. Nonetheless, it has been projected that 100% of gene carriers will show evidence of the disease by the age of 80 years,[11] even though only about half of patients[18] progress to renal failure. An early study in Denmark indicated that patients within a family tree develop initial symptoms and signs and come to end-stage renal failure in a relatively consistent pattern.[11] However, more recent experience in the United States has found many exceptions to that rule, and it is now generally agreed that there is no way to predict when or whether renal failure will develop in a given patient. There is also no way to predict within a family the coincidence of liver cysts with ADPKD, but preliminary evidence indicates that intracra-

---
*See *Editor's note* at the end of the chapter.

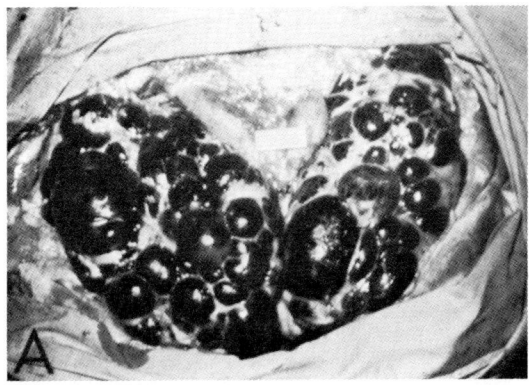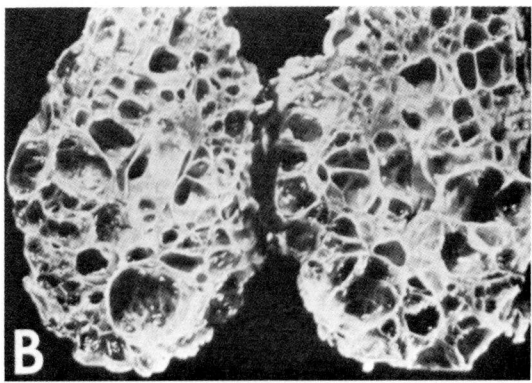

**Figure 38–1.** ADPKD in situ *(A)* and on cut section *(B)*. Note diffuse, bilateral distribution of cysts. *(A and B courtesy of FE Cuppage, Kansas City, KS.)*

nial aneurysms may cluster in certain families.[19, 20] Intrauterine testing for ADPKD has been reported, but the merits of this approach remain to be decided.[21]

## PATHOLOGY

Both kidneys are abnormal, although one of the pair may be considerably larger than the other and, even within one kidney, the extent of the process may be irregular.[22] The kidneys are usually diffusely cystic and, although enlarged, maintain their general reniform shape. Reported kidney weights in adult patients range from approximately normal to more than 4000 g, but mean weight has varied considerably from series to series and also as a function of circumstances. For example, in one series, the combined kidney weight was 943 ± 664 g (mean ± SD) in 19 patients without azotemia, 1143 ± 733 g in 11 patients with mild azotemia, and about 3500 ± 2000 g in 57 patients with moderate azotemia or with renal failure requiring dialysis.[22] Similar findings result from the use of computed tomography (CT) and indicate, in addition, that men are more likely to be azotemic and to have larger kidneys than are women of similar age. Mean single kidney volume was 1065 ± 723 $cm^3$ in 20 men aged 46 ± 16 years and 389 ± 134 $cm^3$ in 15 women aged 43 ± 13 years.[23] The normal combined volume of two kidneys by CT is 330 ± 30 $cm^3$. The point to be made is that football-sized kidneys should not be thought of as typical and that average kidney size in adult ADPKD is probably so much a function of the patient's age and sex, symptoms, and other factors that it cannot be defined.

Both the outer and the cut surfaces show numerous, usually spherical cysts ranging in size from barely visible to a few centimeters in diameter (Fig. 38–1). The papillae and pyramids are difficult or impossible to identify in severe examples, and the calyces and pelvis are often greatly distorted. The cysts usually appear to be distributed fairly homogeneously throughout both the cortical and medullary parenchyma, but they may be distributed irregularly. In children, the cysts average only a few millimeters in diameter and may be predominantly glomerular. Perhaps 50% of cases of so-called glomerulocystic disease can be accounted for by onset of this phenomenon in early infancy.

Nephron reconstruction and dissection studies have

shown the cysts to be, or at least to begin as, cylindric, fusiform, or spherical dilations of or outpouchings from pre-existing renal tubules.[1] With enlargement beyond a few millimeters in diameter, however, it appears that about 75% of cysts become totally detached from their tubule of origin.[4] In any case, the cysts always contain fluid, and analysis of that fluid has been taken as clear evidence of function in the cyst walls and possibly also of the expression of proximal or distal tubule characteristics in the cyst epithelium. As shown in Figure 38–2, about two thirds of cysts (termed "proximal" or "nongradient" cysts) contain fluid closely simulating that normally found in proximal tubules; its $Na^+$, $K^+$, $Cl^-$, $H^+$, creatinine, and urea concentrations are virtually equal to those in serum. In the other third of cysts (termed "distal" or "gradient" cysts), the fluid simulates that normally found in distal tubules; its $Na^+$ and $Cl^-$ concentrations are lower and its $K^+$, $H^+$, creatinine, and urea concentrations are greater than those in serum.[2] More recently, the question of function in the cyst wall has been answered in a most direct manner. In a study of carefully dissected individual cysts from adult ADPKD patients, cyst fluid was found to accumulate at rates of 0.1 to 1 mL/d, rates more than sufficient to account for the in vivo growth rate.[24] More important, however, was the finding that this secretion is largely dependent on a powerful, but as yet unidentified, secretagogue that is present in the cyst fluid and that apparently acts through cyclic AMP mechanisms.

On microscopic examination, normally formed renal tissue that may not be readily apparent grossly is always found among the cysts. It varies considerably in amount from area to area and often shows the effects of secondary glomerular sclerosis, tubule atrophy, and interstitial fibrosis on the basis of vascular sclerosis or pyelonephritis. Nevertheless, areas of normally formed tissue must be demonstrated if the diagnosis of ADPKD and a clear distinction from cystic dysplastic kidney are to be made. Cartilage or other dysplastic elements are not present. The walls of the cysts in the deeper portions of the collecting system are usually thin, whereas those in the terminal, subcapsular portions tend to be thicker and surrounded by zones of dense fibrotic connective tissue. Any segment of the nephron, including Bowman capsule, may be dilated or cystic but may be difficult to identify unless its normal position and epithelium are maintained. Most often, the epithelium

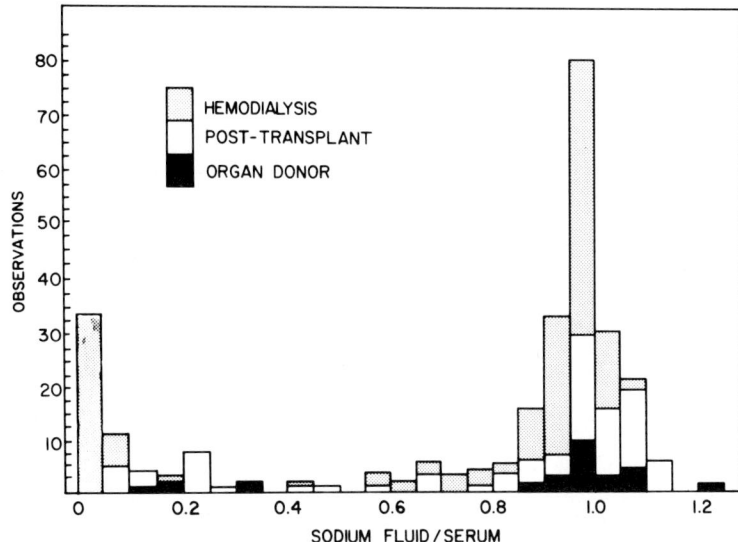

**Figure 38–2.** Distribution of Na$^+$ levels in renal cysts of eight patients with ADPKD. The cyst fluid Na$^+$ levels were determined after the kidneys had been removed surgically. Five patients were undergoing regular hemodialysis treatments; two patients had their kidneys removed several weeks after a successful renal allograft; one subject, a cadaver kidney donor, had a normal serum creatinine level before death. (From Huseman R, Grady A, Welling D, Grantham J: Macropuncture study of polycystic disease in adult human kidneys. Kidney Int 18:375, 1980.)

is of a nondescript, low cuboid type that by light microscopy alone cannot be ascribed to a specific segment. Microscopic polyps are common in the smaller cysts.[4, 22]

Transmission and scanning electron microscopy of cyst walls shows a generally single-layered, simple epithelium lying on a basement membrane that varies inconsistently from normal to thickened or extensively laminated.[4, 25] An adjacent collar of smooth muscle cells has been seen occasionally. The epithelium is found by electron microscopy to be of two types.[25, 26] One type is characteristic of cysts defined as proximal by the composition of their fluid (see earlier). It has smooth surfaces; indistinct cell margins; squamoid or low cuboid form; few apical microvilli, basal infoldings, mitochondria, or lysosomes; and relatively short (approximately 40 nm) apical zonulae occludens.[26] The other type is characteristic of distal cysts. This type has a "cobblestone" surface; distinct cell margins; taller cuboid cells; abundant microvilli, infoldings, mitochondria, and lysosomes; and relatively long (approximately 200 nm) zonulae occludens.

The appearance of the cyst epithelium by scanning electron microscopy contrasts somewhat with that by transmission electron microscopy. Several cell types and patterns are now identifiable (Fig. 38–3). However, in a large number of randomly selected cysts, the epithelial lining resembled proximal tubule, collecting tubule, or glomerular visceral epithelial cells in only about 10% and showed a curious pattern of micropolyps or cord-like hyperplasia in an additional 5%. The majority of cysts, about 85%, were lined by an apparently primitive epithelium that did not resemble that of normal tubule segments. It is not yet clear how the scanning and transmission electron microscopic patterns are related.

In contrast to persons with dysplastic kidneys, ADPKD patients rarely have associated congenital anomalies. However, about half of adults with ADPKD do have a few too many cysts of the liver, the prevalence increasing with age to perhaps 75% or even to 90% in patients whose life is prolonged by renal replacement therapy.[27, 28] Number and size also correlate with female sex and occurrence of pregnancy.[29] These cysts are spherical, usually unilocular, and rarely more than a few centimeters in diameter. They contain clear to viscid fluid that resembles serum in composition and are lined by a single layer of columnar epithelium resembling that of the biliary tract. (They are not, however, in communication with the biliary system.) In both children and adults, about two thirds have increased connective tissue in portal areas, and about half of these also have increased bile ducts.[8] Regardless of size and number of cysts and the extent of fibrosis, however, liver dysfunction and portal hypertension are rarely seen.[30] The usual situation is thus unlike that with liver involvement in congenital hepatic fibrosis and autosomal recessive polycystic kidney disease (ARPKD; see later). The liver cysts may continue to grow and to appear de novo after institution of renal replacement therapy and may calcify under those circumstances.[31, 32] They occasionally may become infected and have occasionally been the site of origin of cholangiocellular carcinoma.[30] There is rare association with congenital dilation of intrahepatic bile ducts.[33] There are also a few reported kindreds in which the hepatic change is indistinguishable from that seen in congenital hepatic fibrosis.[34]

Epithelial cysts in organs other than liver are less common. About 10% of patients have cysts, increased connective tissue, and duct proliferation in the pancreas. Less than 5% have cysts in the spleen. About 5% have arachnoid cysts.[35] Cysts of the thyroid, ovary, endometrium, seminal vesicle, and epididymis have been reported but are rare. One or more aneurysms of the cerebral arteries have been reported to occur in as many as 50% of patients with ADPKD.[36–38] However, two studies reported a frequency of only about 4% and questioned whether that is in fact greater than in the general population.[38, 39] Nevertheless, rupture of these aneurysms may account for 7% to 13% of deaths in ADPKD.[10, 11] About 6% of patients with berry aneurysm have polycystic kidney disease. Aneurysms of the abdominal aorta,[40, 41] primary dilation of the aortic root and annulus,[42] and mitral valve abnormalities[42] are also reported. Mitral valve prolapse or incompetence may occur in more than 30% of cases; aortic, tricuspid, and pulmonary valve

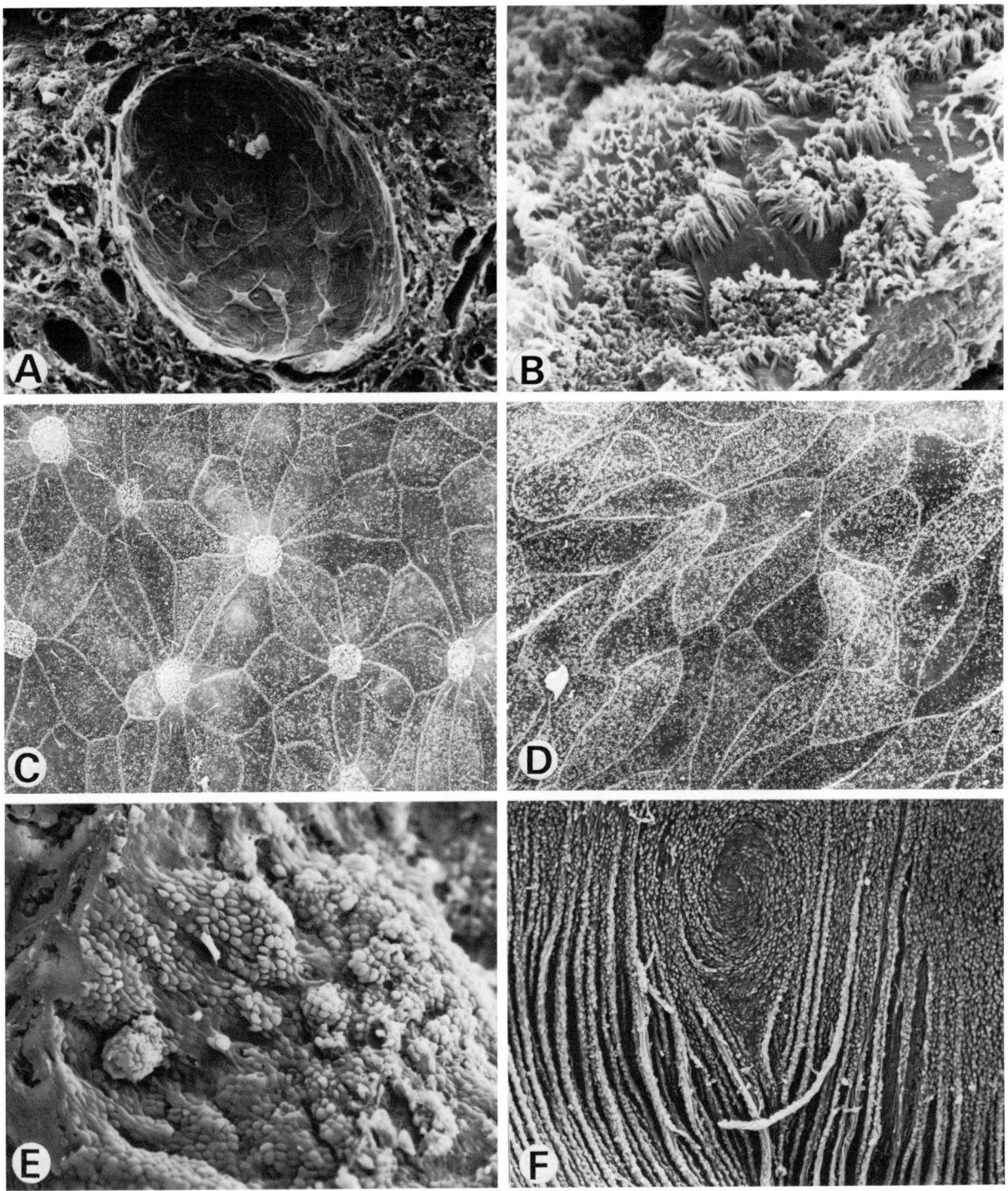

**Figure 38–3.** Scanning electron microscopy of cyst lining epithelium in ADPKD. *A.* Typical glomerular visceral layer. (Magnification × 250.) *B.* Typical of proximal tubule. (Magnification × 3000.) *C.* Typical of cortical collecting duct. (Magnification × 1000.) *D.* Epithelium not typical of any normal tubule segment. (Magnification × 1000.) *E.* Micropolyps. (Magnification × 250.) *F.* Cord-like hyperplasia. (Magnification × 80.) (*A* to *F* from Grantham JJ, Geiser JL, Evan AP: Cyst formation and growth in autosomal dominant polycystic kidney disease. Kidney Int 31:1145, 1987.)

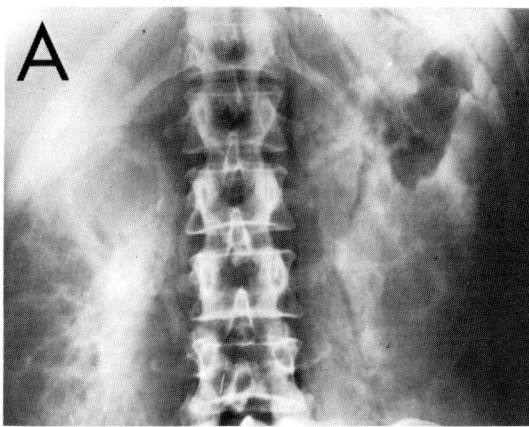
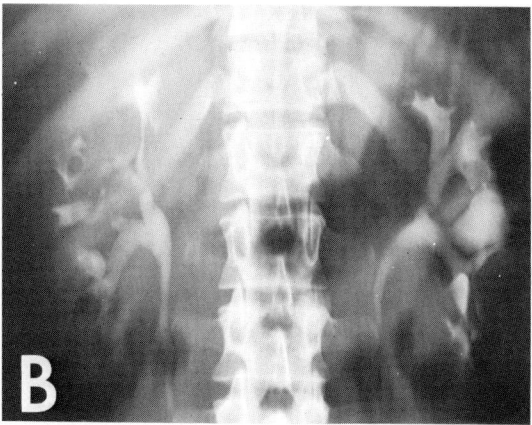

**Figure 38–4.** ADPKD seen by nephrotomography *(A)* and urography *(B).* The nephrotomogram was obtained a few seconds after intravenous injection of radiocontrast material and shows large and small cysts scattered throughout both kidneys. The urogram, taken several minutes after intravenous injection, reveals ADPKD by the distorted appearance of the collecting system. *(A* and *B* courtesy of GD Dixon, Kansas City, MO.)

incompetence is also increased in frequency.[43] In one autopsy series, the observed frequency of coexisting polycystic kidneys and dissecting thoracic aortic aneurysm was 7.3 times higher than expected by chance association.[44] Although it is the consensus that the frequency of renal cell carcinoma is not increased in ADPKD, that question is not entirely settled.[45, 46]

## DIAGNOSIS

In its fully developed form, ADPKD is not difficult to diagnose. Most polycystic kidneys are enlarged bilaterally and have irregular surfaces that can be felt on careful palpation. About 50% of patients have increased abdominal girth. An enlarged liver with palpable cysts adds further strength to the diagnosis. On careful questioning, a family history of or consistent with ADPKD can be obtained in about 60% of newly recognized cases. As described later, many patients report pain that may be associated with gross and microscopic hematuria. Hypertension is common, as are the signs and symptoms of renal infection and lithiasis. The early stages of ADPKD are not usually reflected in the urinalysis. There may be a defect in maximal concentrating ability, but urine dilution remains intact.[47–49] There is no salt wasting, except in the late stages of the disease, and urine acidification is normal.[50] Massive proteinuria is rare and, when found, should prompt a search for an additional renal disorder. In the middle to late stages of the disease (20 to 40 years of age), mild persistent proteinuria (>200 mg/d) may be found in 20% to 40% of cases. Patients with proteinuria may also excrete doubly refractile lipid bodies (oval fat bodies).[51] The erythrocyte count and hematocrit may be increased above normal, possibly owing to abnormal erythropoietin production by cysts, and patients with end-stage ADPKD do not have anemia as profound as that seen in other types of terminal renal disease. In the absence of complications, blood coagulation studies and leukocyte and platelet counts are normal.

Diagnosis can be confirmed by several radiologic tests. In more advanced cases, intravenous urography shows marked deformity of the collecting system with thinning of calyces and infundibula (Fig. 38–4). Ultrasonography reveals multiple echo-free areas in both kidneys (Fig. 38–5), but this is rarely used for diagnosis. In a comparative study, CT with contrast enhancement has been found to be more sensitive and is currently preferred by us for definitive diagnosis.[52] CT readily distinguishes between solid and liquid renal masses and portrays the diffuse distribution of large and small cysts (Fig. 38–6). In about 50% of patients, it reveals cysts in the liver as well (Fig. 38–7). When used in conjunction with intravenous iodinated radiocontrast material, it also allows an estimation of the relative volume of functioning renal tissue. Radioisotopic scanning methods using [131]I-labeled hippurate or technetium Tc 99m are not useful for diagnosis but are of value in assessing and comparing renal tubule function and glomerular filtration in each of the two affected kidneys.

Diagnosis in early cases of ADPKD is more difficult, and because of the ominous implications of the diagnosis, the

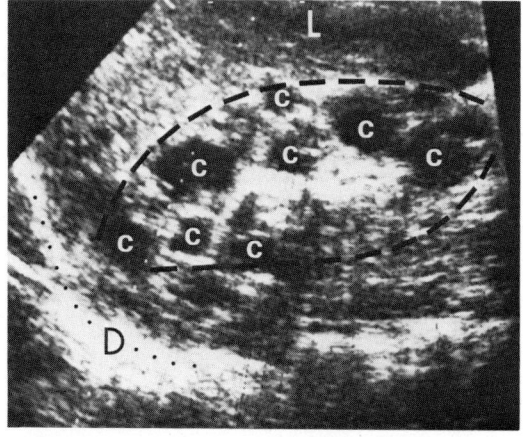

**Figure 38–5.** ADPKD seen in a parasagittal or longitudinal sonogram. This view of the right kidney was obtained with the patient in the right anterior oblique position. The approximate outline of the kidney is shown by the broken line. Some of the larger renal cysts are indicated by C. The liver (L) is at the top of the figure. The right dome of the diaphragm (D) is at the lower left. (Courtesy of E Levine, Kansas City, KS.)

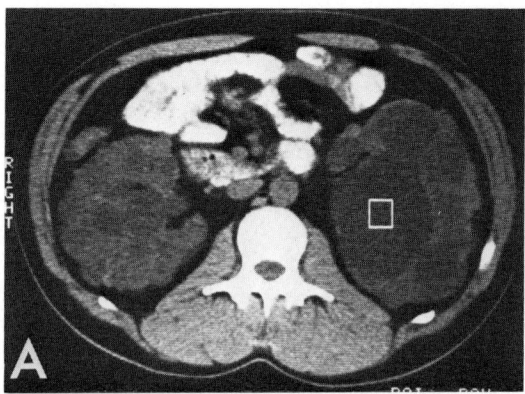
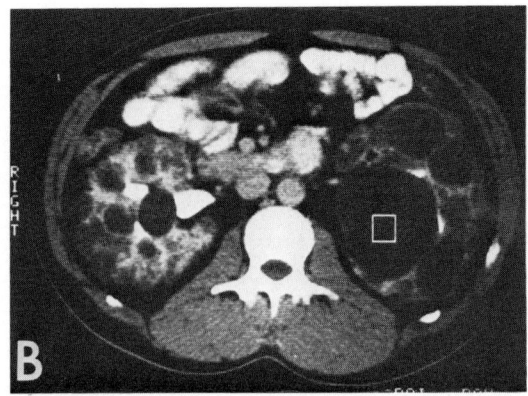

**Figure 38–6.** CT of polycystic kidneys. The patient (male) has ADPKD, and the serum creatinine level is within the normal range. Oral contrast medium was given to highlight the intestine. *A.* CT scan without contrast enhancement. *B.* CT scan at the same level as *A* but after intravenous infusion of iodinated radiocontrast material. Cursor (box) is used to determine relative density of cyst fluid, which in this case is equal to that of water. Contrast enhancement highlights functioning parenchyma, which here is concentrated primarily in the right kidney. The renal collecting system is also highlighted by contrast material in both kidneys.

most sensitive tests are indicated. In children at risk, the presence of even one renal cyst is considered suggestive of and the presence of three or more cysts distributed bilaterally is considered diagnostic for ADPKD.[21] For these reasons, the urogram is relatively insensitive unless it is combined with bolus intravenous nephrotomography. Ultrasonography is superior to nephrotomography in early cases[52] and has been used with good success in one large group of children younger than 18 years.[21] Nonetheless, it remains our opinion that CT is still the preferred method of establishing or ruling out ADPKD in the less obvious cases in which the disease is suspected. Ultrasonography is limited by its resolving power. In contrast, CT reveals diffusely cystic kidneys with individual lesions smaller than 1 cm in diameter[52, 53] (Fig. 38–8; see also Fig. 38–6). It is always important to define the diffuse cystic pattern. If one relies solely on calyceal attenuation and deformity, defined by urography, malrotation and other congenital renal deformities may be mistaken for ADPKD.

The primary and secondary criteria supporting the diagnosis of ADPKD are listed in Table 38–2. ADPKD must be differentiated from ARPKD in children and from tuberous sclerosis, multiple simple cysts, multicystic dysplastic kidney, von Hippel–Lindau syndrome, and acquired cystic kidney disease (ACKD).

In individuals, including fetuses, who are at risk but who have no radiographically defined cysts, genetic linkage analysis may be useful to identify those predisposed to the development of ADPKD.[54] The test, however, has practical limitation. At least two family members with unequivocal ADPKD must be willing to undergo testing for the marker alleles to be determined and thereby reveal the status of the unknown individual. Diagnosis by linkage analysis is also complicated by the fact that there is more than one genotype for ADPKD. Approximately 90% of cases can be ascribed to a mutation of chromosome 16 (*ADPKD1*). Others have a mutation of chromosome 4 (*ADPKD2*),[15, 16] and the possibility of a third mutation unlinked to either chromosome 4 or 16 has been suggested.

Although it is possible to diagnose ADPKD in asympto-

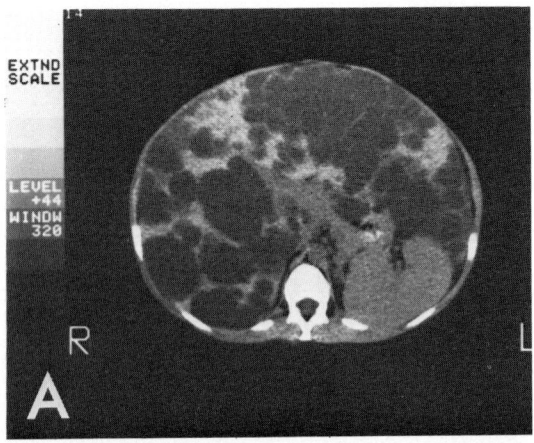
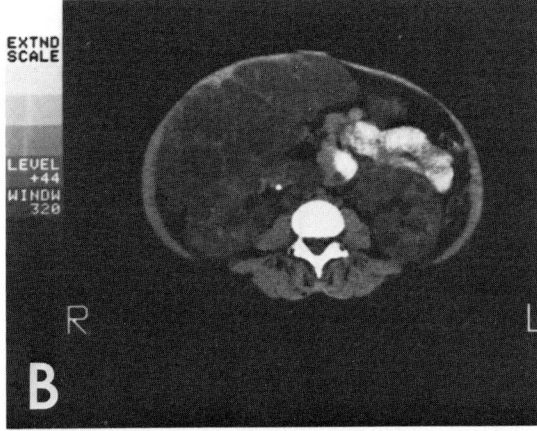

**Figure 38–7.** CT of polycystic liver and kidneys in female patient with ADPKD. The serum creatinine level and liver function tests were within the normal range. Oral contrast medium was given to highlight the intestine, but no intravenous contrast material was used. *A.* There is massive enlargement of the liver due to intraparenchymal cysts. *B.* CT at a lower level in the abdomen shows cystic kidneys and the lower portion of the cystic liver. (*A* and *B* courtesy of E Levine, Kansas City, KS.)

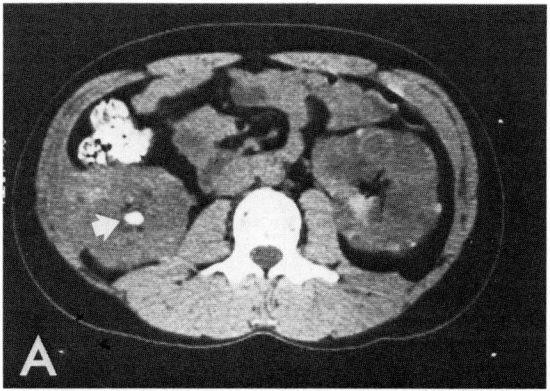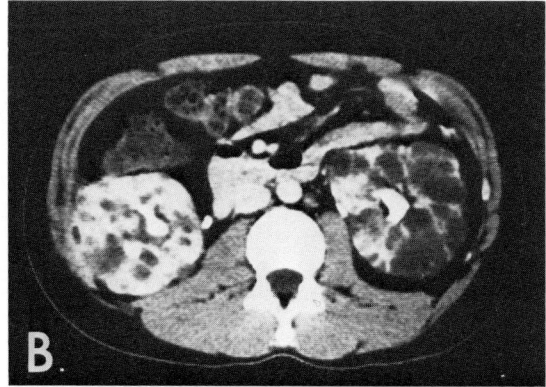

**Figure 38–8.** CT of polycystic kidneys in male patient with serum creatinine level within normal range. *A.* CT scan without contrast enhancement shows a radiopaque stone in the pelvis of the right kidney *(arrow). B.* CT scan after intravenous administration of iodinated radiocontrast material. The stone is now obscured by contrast medium in the renal pelvis. (*A* and *B* courtesy of E Levine, Kansas City, KS.)

matic individuals at risk, the wisdom of random testing may be questioned. Testing is appropriate only after the individual has been counseled about the risks and benefits of finding the disease before symptoms develop. Risks include difficulty of insurability and employment, and benefits include freedom from worry if the individual proves not to have the ADPKD genotype. Prenatal diagnosis by linkage analysis is not popular in this disease. Selection of unaffected family members in consideration of living related donor renal transplantation is useful.[55, 56]

## THERAPY

**Basic Fluid and Electrolyte Management.** Patients with early ADPKD may have a diminished ability to concentrate their urine maximally.[47] Nocturia may be the only symptom of this defect, and no specific therapy is indicated. Na[+] conservation is usually normal in the early stages of the disease, but some patients may pass through a stage of relative urinary salt wasting. Thus, it is important to monitor blood pressure and extracellular volume status (edema) carefully throughout the course of the disease and make appropriate adjustments in therapy. Water intake adequate to produce 1 to 2 L of urine is usually sufficient unless the patient has renal calculi or infection. Restriction of sodium intake is frequently necessary in those with arterial hyper-

tension, a complication that has been recognized to occur in children and young adults with this disease.[57]

The use of diuretics is a problem. On the one hand, diuretics may be helpful in the management of hypertension and calcium lithiasis; on the other hand, they have the potential to adversely alter the movement of fluid across the walls of the cysts. Hypokalemia, a common accompaniment of diuretic use, has been associated with the development of cysts in individuals with otherwise normal kidneys[58] and may, therefore, increase the growth of cysts in ADPKD.

**Physical Activity and Lifestyle.** Most patients with ADPKD require no modification in physical activity or lifestyle in the early stages of the disease. Evidence indicates that recurrent bouts of gross hematuria, usually related to direct trauma, are associated with a faster decline of renal function than otherwise[59, 60]; thus, avoidance of renal trauma seems prudent. Patients should probably not participate in strenuous athletics in which the abdomen may be traumatized repeatedly.

**Management of Pain.** Pain is the most common symptom in ADPKD. It may be a unilateral or bilateral vague sense of heaviness or a dull aching to knife-like and stabbing pain. When chronic, it may be disabling and lead to analgesic abuse. The cause is often unknown, but medium-sized blood vessels evidently do rupture occasionally and cause extravasation of blood either into cysts or into perinephric tissues. Perinephric hemorrhage may be associated with intense discomfort and obvious changes in the configuration of the abdomen detected on direct physical examination, but even these hemorrhages can usually be treated by simple bed rest and analgesics. After counseling, most patients recognize the problem as a transient disorder. When persistent pain occurs, however, one must consider the possibility of renal infection, stones, or tumors. Thus, renal pain that changes in character or that lasts more than a few days should be evaluated, especially when it is associated with gross or microscopic hematuria. Pain in association with fever, weight loss, anemia, and a striking change in the configuration of the kidney should raise the suspicion of renal malignant neoplasm (Fig. 38–9). The most reliable diagnostic signs of malignant change are speckled calcifications in the renal parenchyma,[61] the appearance of a solid

---

### TABLE 38–2. Clinical Criteria for Diagnosis of Autosomal Dominant Polycystic Kidney Disease

**Primary Criteria**
Innumerable fluid-filled cysts scattered diffusely throughout renal cortex and medulla
Definite history of polycystic kidney disease in genetically related family members

**Secondary Criteria**
Polycystic liver
Aneurysms of cerebral arteries
Cysts of pancreas
Renal insufficiency

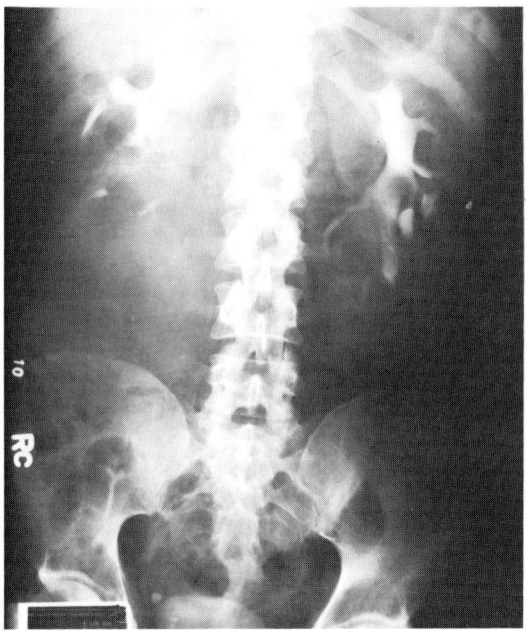

**Figure 38–9.** Urogram showing carcinoma in the cystic kidney of a patient with ADPKD. A large circular mass is evident extending from the lower pole of the right kidney. Note calcific densities within the tumor mass. (Courtesy of GD Dixon, Kansas City, MO.)

mass structure by ultrasonography, the appearance of tissue with a high CT number, and a typical arteriographic appearance after infusion of radiocontrast material into the renal artery. Fortunately, this complication is rare.

Pain may also be associated with the enlargement of one or more cysts in a kidney, and some relief may be obtained by the percutaneous aspiration of fluid combined with the instillation of a sclerosing agent.[62] Alternatively, surgical techniques may be of value for those with extremely large kidneys filled with innumerable cysts.[63–65] Surgical aspiration and unroofing of cysts has been reintroduced for the treatment of severe pain. When performed in specialized centers where large numbers of cases are treated, this radical therapy may produce relief that lasts for several years.

**Hematuria and Intrarenal Hemorrhage.** Hematuria is usually due to the rupture of a cyst into the pelvis of the kidney. It appears suddenly and persists as macroscopic or microscopic bleeding for several days. In addition to vascular rupture into cysts, hematuria may be caused by a renal stone, infection of cysts, or malignant tumors. On rare occasions, it may not be related to the cysts at all. Acute glomerulonephritis has been described to occur incidentally with ADPKD, so urine sediment should be examined carefully for casts at some point in all instances of bleeding. Reduced physical activity or bed rest is usually sufficient to control the bleeding. Transcatheter arterial infarction has been used to control recurrent hemorrhage in ADPKD[66] and would seem to be of some value in patients with severe renal blood loss and for whom dialysis is imminent or extant. It probably should not be used in kidneys with established infection. In patients who have reasonably normal renal function, every effort should be made to preserve that function. Bleeding may occur into cysts located near

the renal pelvis and thus cause obstruction to urine flow. Surgical removal of the clots and the dome of the cyst may permanently restore function in those cases.

**Renal Infection.** Parenchymal pyogenic bacterial infection is a major problem for patients with ADPKD, particularly for women.[67] One or more cysts may become infected, and like any deep-seated abscess, the condition may be difficult to treat. The infection is commonly unilateral and, unless accompanied by pyelonephritis, may not be associated with bacteriuria or bacteremia. With associated pain, fever, diaphoresis, bacteremia, and leukocytosis, the diagnosis of parenchymal infection is ensured, but unfortunately, a clear pattern of symptoms and signs is found only infrequently, and one must usually make empirical judgments. Infected cysts may be suspected from increased cyst wall thickness detected by CT,[52] and radioactive gallium or indium scanning has occasionally identified infected foci in polycystic kidneys.[68]

Little is known about the invading organisms in most cases of infected cysts. Coliform, staphylococcal, and *Bacteroides* organisms have been isolated from cyst fluid aspirates in occasional patients. In other cysts, the finding of a low oxygen tension ($Po_2 < 40$ mm Hg) has raised the possibility that anaerobic organisms might grow in such an environment.

There are several published studies of the penetration of antibiotics into cysts in ADPKD. In some cases, the cysts have been grouped into proximal (nongradient) and distal (gradient) varieties, depending on the $Na^+$ concentration of the fluid[69, 70] (see Fig. 38–2). Most antibiotics appear to enter nongradient cysts to some extent, and the occasional detection of cyst fluid drug levels approaching those in the plasma suggests that the drugs enter those cysts across their walls rather than by glomerular filtration. On the other hand, antibiotic levels have been vanishingly low in gradient cysts, except in the case of the highly lipid-soluble antibiotic clindamycin, which may be found in levels greater than in plasma[70, 71] (Fig. 38–10). It is suggested, therefore, that lipid-soluble drugs such as chloramphenicol, ciprofloxacin, erythromycin, tetracycline, and trimethoprim-sulfamethoxazole may be useful in infected distal cysts. Although these drugs would also enter proximal cysts, aminoglycosides, cephalosporins, and penicillin derivatives would still be the preferred agents for infected proximal cysts.

Infection in polycystic kidneys may be accompanied by intrapelvic urinary stones and may then be difficult or impossible to eradicate until the stones are removed (see Fig. 38–8). Urinary tract infections are more prevalent in women,[67] as is true in the non–polycystic kidney disease population, and for prevention we specifically recommend showers rather than tub baths, frequent voiding, good perineal hygiene, and voiding immediately after intercourse. All patients are advised in routine hygiene measures and are advised to refuse urinary tract instrumentation procedures unless absolutely necessary. Occasionally, renal infection will be so serious and intractable that nephrectomy is necessary. This should be a last resort, only in patients with good renal function, and only after parenteral antibiotics have been administered unsuccessfully. In patients who experience a decrease in signs and symptoms, some physi-

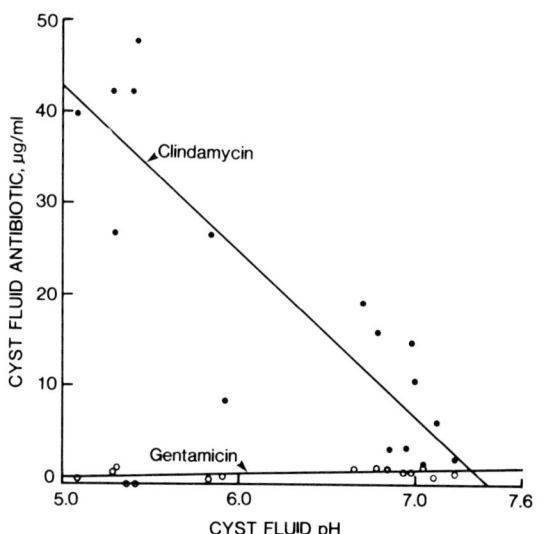

**Figure 38–10.** Antibiotic accumulation in renal cysts of a patient with ADPKD. Clindamycin and gentamicin were administered for several days preceding a unilateral nephrectomy. Clindamycin levels in cyst fluids were inversely proportional to cyst fluid pH. By contrast, gentamicin levels were uniformly low and independent of cyst fluid pH. (From Schwab S, Hinthorn D, Diederich D, et al: pH-dependent accumulation of clindamycin in a polycystic kidney. Am J Kidney Dis 3:63, 1983.)

cians would recommend oral antibiotics for an indefinite period.

**Hypertension.** Arterial hypertension develops in more than half of patients with ADPKD at some time in the course of their disease.[10, 60, 72] It often antedates measurable changes in renal function by several years and appears to accelerate renal destruction in some patients. Data indicate that blood pressure disproportionately high in relation to age may be a problem for young individuals with ADPKD.[21, 57] Left ventricular mass was greater than normal, and ambulatory daytime and nighttime blood pressures, although within the usually acceptable range of normal, were higher than in age- and sex-matched control subjects.

It is generally agreed that in ADPKD, as in other renal disorders, hypertension is one of the important risk factors for progression of renal insufficiency as well as a contributor to overall cardiovascular morbidity.[60] Current recommendations for blood pressure targets derive from studies of renal diseases in general. In view of the fact that ADPKD is present at birth and subtle hypertension may extend over decades, physicians should carefully monitor blood pressure and select a target value appropriate for the age and the sex of the patient. Salt restriction should be prescribed for most of the ADPKD patients with hypertension, as well as weight control and appropriate exercise.

A wealth of information indicates that the renin-angiotensin system has an important role in the pathogenesis of hypertension in ADPKD. A prominent view proposes that the cysts compromise the flow of blood through intrarenal vessels, thereby providing increased production and release of renin.[73, 74] This may explain why angiotensin-converting enzyme inhibitors are highly effective in the treatment of hypertension in patients with ADPKD.[75] Although angiotensin-converting enzyme inhibitor drugs are highly effec-

tive, especially in the early stages of the disease, they have been associated with severe renal hemorrhage and sudden renal failure in individuals with relatively large kidneys.[76] $Ca^{2+}$ channel blockers are highly effective in ADPKD, and $\alpha_2$-adrenergic blocking drugs may be helpful in refractory cases. In selected cases in which the volume component cannot be controlled by salt restriction, the cautious use of diuretics may be beneficial.

**Arterial Aneurysms.** Depending on the source of the report,[77] 0% to 41% of patients with ADPKD develop one or more intracranial saccular aneurysms (berry aneurysms). Three American studies, however, indicate that the overall prevalence of aneurysm may be closer to 5%.[19, 20, 39] The higher prevalence values cited in the older literature may be a consequence of the inclusion of patients with different racial or ethnic backgrounds, the use of different methods of diagnosis, and family clustering (i.e., the tendency for aneurysms to occur with greater frequency in certain families of ADPKD subjects).[19, 20]

ADPKD patients with symptoms consistent with intracranial aneurysm should be evaluated promptly by arteriography, with the fact borne in mind that this procedure carries a higher risk of morbid complication than in non-ADPKD subjects.[39] It seems reasonable to screen noninvasively for intracranial aneurysm in asymptomatic ADPKD patients with a positive family history or those with a history of previous aneurysm rupture. CT with 2-mm cuts in the axial and coronal planes[39] and magnetic resonance angiography[19] have proved reliable in specialized centers. The relative sensitivities of these methods for aneurysm detection undoubtedly vary from institution to institution. Individuals found to have obvious or suspicious aneurysms should undergo cerebral angiography. Current opinion recommends that lesions greater than 10 mm in diameter should be operated on, if that is possible.[20] Aneurysms less than 7 mm in diameter should be examined every 1 to 2 years, and those 7 to 10 mm in diameter should be observed yearly. In all cases, the blood pressure should be controlled rigorously.

**Nephrolithiasis.** Calcifications develop within the kidney parenchyma (nephrocalcinosis) and within the urinary collecting system (nephrolithiasis) of patients with ADPKD (see Fig. 38–8). The frequency of renal stone formation is approximately 20%.[78] CT is the most sensitive technique for the detection of renal stones and their differentiation from nephrocalcinosis.[79] The stones are most frequently composed of uric acid or calcium oxalate. Distal acidification defects, abnormal transport of $NH_4^+$, low urine pH, and hypocitraturia may be important factors in the pathogenesis of stones.

The treatment of urinary lithiasis is not different from that in patients without ADPKD. Adequate urine flow rate is a central element of therapy. Thiazide diuretics may be used for hypercalciuric states, and potassium citrate has a role when uric acid lithiasis, hypocitraturia, and a distal acidification defect are found in association with renal stones. Uric acid stones can be dissolved despite the anatomic distortion and local stasis of urine caused by cysts impinging on the collecting system. Extracorporeal shock wave lithotripsy and percutaneous nephrostolithotomy have been used safely for the removal of stones from polycystic kidneys.[79]

**Liver and Gastrointestinal Findings.** The development of hepatic cysts lags far behind that of renal cysts in ADPKD. Liver cysts are rarely found before puberty, but by the age of 50 years, 80% of patients have radiographically defined liver cysts.[80] Individuals with hepatic cystic disease appear to have worse renal function than those without hepatic cysts do. Women generally have greater liver involvement with cysts than do men, and it is not uncommon for the liver cysts to accelerate in size and number after pregnancy. The liver may become massively enlarged, although hepatocellular function remains amazingly intact.[81] Pain, distention, and inanition have been successfully alleviated by partial hepatectomy in extreme cases of liver enlargement.[82] Solitary, painful hepatic cysts can be drained percutaneously and fluid reaccumulation aborted by sclerotherapy.

Cysts are occasionally found in the pancreas and spleen. Diverticulosis is reported in 80% of cases and can be a source of complication after renal transplantation.[83] Hiatal hernia is a frequent complication, especially in children.[21]

**End-Stage Disease, Dialysis, and Transplantation.** ADPKD progresses to the end stage in approximately 45% of affected individuals by 60 years of age.[77, 84] Progression appears to be faster in those who have the *ADPKD1* as opposed to the *ADPKD2* genotype,[60, 84] although considerable variability is observed in the onset of end-stage renal failure within families of individuals with the same genotype. Consequently, comorbid factors (genetic and nongenetic) probably have strong modifying influences on the progression of the disease. In ADPKD patients with moderate to severe renal failure, the glomerular filtration rate appears to decline nearly twice as fast as in other types of progressive renal diseases (excluding diabetic nephropathy).[85] Women with ADPKD appear to progress to the end stage at a slower rate than do men.[60, 86]

In retrospective analyses,[10, 60] hypertension has been associated with a more rapid decline in renal function, whereas preliminary analysis of ADPKD subjects analyzed prospectively as a subgroup in the Modification of Diet in Renal Disease Study showed no discernible effect of mildly elevated blood pressure on the rate of decline in glomerular filtration rate.[87] Despite this finding, it is generally believed that arterial blood pressure should be maintained throughout the course of the disease within a range of normal as defined by age and sex.

Earlier onset of renal failure in both sexes has been related to a younger age at diagnosis, larger kidneys, episodes of gross and microscopic hematuria, and moderate to severe proteinuria.[68] A longitudinal study has indicated that women with more than three pregnancies experience an earlier onset of renal insufficiency.[60]

Dialysis has been used for more than two decades to treat patients with end-stage ADPKD. They generally have higher hematocrit values without erythropoietin supplementation than do individuals with other renal diseases. Complications associated with ADPKD subjects undergoing hemodialysis or peritoneal dialysis include rupture of cerebral artery aneurysm, abdominal and inguinal hernias, pyelonephritis, infected renal and hepatic cysts, and massive kidneys and livers requiring resection for symptomatic relief. Studies indicate that all in all, these patients do as well as or better than others with nondiabetic renal disorders.[88, 89]

Renal transplantation is used routinely to treat patients with end-stage ADPKD. Post-transplantation survival rates for the patient and kidney appear to be equal to those in patients with other renal disorders. Most ADPKD patients receive the allograft with their native kidneys in place. Indications for pretransplantation bilateral nephrectomy include severe pain, unrelenting infection, persistent bacteriuria, recurrent severe urinary tract hemorrhage, renal neoplasm, nephrolithiasis, and extreme kidney size with compression of intra-abdominal vessels and viscera leading to symptoms (Table 38–3). Routine pretransplantation nephrectomy, practiced in some centers, has not been critically examined vis-à-vis selective nephrectomy. Native kidneys appear to diminish in size in most patients, but persistent enlargement will occasionally necessitate nephrectomy. Other post-transplantation complications associated with ADPKD include cerebral vascular bleeding from aneurysms and peritonitis secondary to ruptured colonic diverticuli. Screening for aneurysm is discussed earlier. Colon complications can be diminished if patients are examined routinely by barium enema before transplantation and segments of bowel with heavy densities of diverticuli are resected.

## COUNSELING

Guilt and denial are prominent coping patterns in families with ADPKD.[90] Only approximately 60% of affected patients indicate knowledge of a family history of ADPKD at the time of diagnosis.[77] In patients with symptoms of ADPKD, a diagnosis should be established after informed consent. We recommend that screening be considered for asymptomatic adults (older than 18 years) only. If the patient has the rights of majority in the state in which counseling takes place and decides to undergo diagnostic studies to determine the presence or absence of ADPKD, it is reasonable to proceed with physical examination, a renal ultrasound examination, urinalysis, and measurement of serum creatinine and urea nitrogen concentrations. Ultrasound screening of those at risk for ADPKD should be performed only after the individual has been apprised of the benefits and the risks of diagnosis. Benefits that follow testing include the peace of mind that comes from not finding ADPKD, the opportunity for early management of treatable complications (hypertension, urinary tract infections, impaired renal function, and cerebral aneurysms), and family planning. Consequences that weigh against presymptomatic testing include the possibility of medical dis-

**TABLE 38–3. Indications for Pretransplantation Nephrectomy in Autosomal Dominant Polycystic Kidney Disease**

Intractable pain
Unrelenting pyelonephritis or infected cyst
Persistent bacteriuria
Recurrent urinary tract hemorrhage
Renal neoplasm
Nephrolithiasis
Extreme kidney size

qualification for certain careers, medical insurance, and life insurance; the loss of the psychologic denial defense; and the lack of a specific treatment or cure. In the experience of the authors, most asymptomatic individuals at 50% risk for ADPKD do not elect to undergo screening. We advise these individuals to have regular medical examinations that include blood pressure measurements and urinalysis. Those with a family history of cerebral aneurysms should probably be encouraged to have screening done for renal cysts, with the understanding that a positive finding would be reason to screen also for cerebral aneurysm.

Ultrasonography is the most cost-effective method of screening for ADPKD. In individuals older than 30 years, a diagnosis can be established in nearly all who have the mutated gene.[84] In individuals younger than 30 years, the probability of a diagnosis by ultrasound examination is estimated to be 22%, 66%, and 85% at ages 5, 15, and 25 years, respectively.[21] The probability of having ADPKD after normal ultrasonogram results is estimated at 46%, 28%, and 14% for persons at 50% risk in their first, second, and third decade, respectively.[18] Although the risk of a false-negative ultrasound diagnosis is low in this group, it seems prudent to examine kidneys found to be "negative" by ultrasonography with CT, with and without contrast enhancement, because this method appears to be more sensitive than ultrasonography.[52] We are unaware that anyone older than 30 years with a negative result of contrast-enhanced CT scan has been found to develop ADPKD.

## PROGNOSIS

Once a patient has begun to show a significant decrease in creatinine clearance, the prognosis for the progression of the disease can be judged relatively accurately from the relationship between the reciprocal of plasma creatinine concentration ($1/P_{cr}$) and time.[91] Barring intercurrent infections, ureteral obstruction, or other complications, a persistent loss of a fixed amount of creatinine clearance then usually occurs each year and is reflected in a linear decline in $1/P_{cr}$ versus time. This relationship is probably valid only when the serum creatinine level begins to rise appreciably. In other words, some patients may have normal glomerular filtration rates and plasma creatinine levels for up to 40 years and only then enter into a phase of relatively precipitous decline in $1/P_{cr}$ as their creatinine clearance begins to fall and their serum creatinine level to rise. For patients with ADPKD, the probability of being alive and not having end-stage renal disease is about 77% at age 50, 57% at age 58, and 52% at age 73 years.[92]

There is no therapy directed specifically at the polycystic disease process that is generally held to be of benefit. Surgical aspiration of surface cysts (Rovsing procedure) has been reported on several occasions to increase rather than decrease the progression to renal insufficiency. However, reports suggest that careful cyst aspiration or unroofing relieves pain and hypertension and has no untoward effect on renal function.[63, 93] Reduction in dietary protein intake has shown disappointing results on slowing progression of renal insufficiency.[85]

## Autosomal Recessive Polycystic Kidney Disease

ARPKD is a rare disorder that occurs once in 6000 to 55,000 live births.[94–96] It is inherited as an autosomal recessive trait and thus may be seen in siblings but almost never in the parents. Because both parents must carry the recessive gene, each of their offspring has one chance in four of having the disease. However, there is considerable variability in the expression of ARPKD such that siblings may or may not have disease of equal severity. Previously, this variability was taken to indicate as many as four separate but related gene defects.[95] It is now considered to indicate simply different manifestations of a single genetic defect.[96, 97] The actual genetic defect is not known but is not allelic to that in ADPKD.[98, 99]

In perhaps 75% of cases, ARPKD results is death within hours or days of birth. In the remainder, it presents in progressively milder forms in infancy, childhood, or early adult life and may have a reasonably good prognosis.[94, 96, 100] Those who survive the neonatal period have a 50% to 80% chance of surviving at least to age 15 years.[97, 101] The previously commonly used name for this disease, infantile polycystic kidney disease, thus does not accurately describe the nature of the disease, and the bleak prognosis that came to be associated with that term is not always justified.

## PATHOLOGY

ARPKD affects both the kidneys and the liver in approximately inverse proportions. That is, the disease may be viewed as a spectrum ranging from severe kidney damage and mild liver change at one end to mild kidney damage and severe liver change at the other. The form with severe kidney damage is the more common and is the form that presents itself at or near the time of birth. The form with less severe kidney damage and more severe liver damage is the less common and usually presents itself in infancy or later. It is now well recognized that siblings may present at different ages and with different forms of the disease.

When ARPKD presents in the perinatal period, it is usually rapidly fatal because of pulmonary hypoplasia, atelectasis, and insufficiency, with or without other features of the Potter sequence. The kidneys in such cases are symmetrically and bilaterally enlarged to some 10 times normal (Fig. 38–11B) and may have been the cause of dystocia because of their size. Average combined weight in one series was about 300 g (range, 240 to 563 g), versus a normal combined weight of about 25 g.[8] The cortical surfaces show innumerable 1- to 2-mm or smaller cysts, which on cut section (Fig. 38–11C) are seen to be continuous with radially oriented, 1- to 8-mm diameter, fusiform or cylindric channels that occupy the entire kidney. These channels are lined by nondescript cuboid epithelium and are found by microdissection[8, 102] and by histochemical and specific binding studies[103, 104] to be dilated terminal branches of collecting ducts. A few small saccular outpouchings from medullary collecting ducts are also found. Perhaps 60% to 90% of all collecting ducts are involved.[95] By careful microdissection, a few connecting tubules, distal convoluted tubules, and ascending limbs may also be found to be

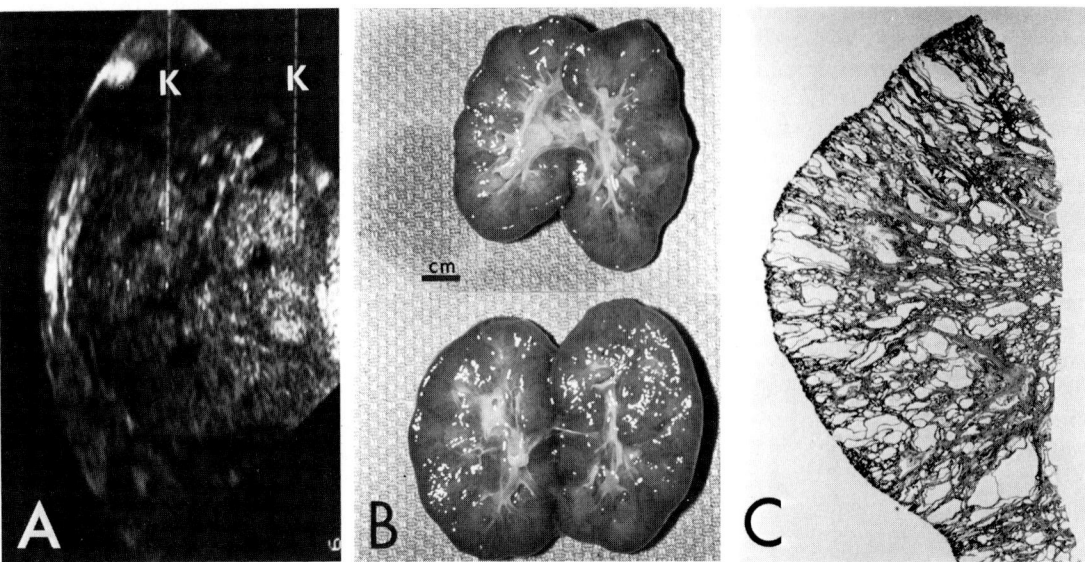

**Figure 38–11.** ARPKD in a 32-week fetus. *A.* Sonogram showing cystic kidneys (K) of fetus in utero. (Courtesy of E Levine, Kansas City, KS.) *B* and *C.* Gross and microscopic sections showing radially oriented cysts of collecting ducts. (*B* and *C* courtesy of FE Cuppage, Kansas City, KS.)

dilated; in some 30% of nephrons, the angle of the loop of Henle contains a small cyst.[8] Glomeruli and nephron segments proximal to the collecting tubules are generally normal in form and number but appear to be crowded into subcapsular wedges by the ectatic collecting ducts. The corticomedullary margin is obscured, and the renal papillae, although usually recognizable, contain spherically dilated ducts and are somewhat larger and less conic than normal. The calyces, pelvis, and ureter are normal or only mildly distorted. Connective tissue is not increased in the kidneys at this early age. Cartilage and other dysplastic elements should not be present and, when reported, cast doubt on diagnosis. The most striking feature in this young age group is the uniformity of the size and shape of the cortical cysts.

When clinical presentation occurs after the newborn period, the extent of the renal cystic involvement tends to be less in those who survive longer. The collecting duct cysts now tend to become more irregularly distributed, more spherical in shape, and larger (up to 2 cm diameter). Perhaps only 10% to 25% of the collecting ducts are involved.[95] Progressive glomerular obsolescence, tubule atrophy, and interstitial fibrosis are also found. The outer surface of the kidney may become bumpy and irregular, and the picture may be similar to that seen in ADPKD in children. An overall reduction in size may occur. Medullary ductal ectasia continues to be prominent and in kidneys from young adults may be the only obvious abnormality.[105] The picture thus also resembles, and may be confused with, that in medullary sponge kidney, a completely separate and distinct disease with a far different prognosis.

The hepatic lesion is diffuse but limited to the portal areas. The parenchyma is unremarkable, and there is no cirrhosis in the usual sense. The central portal bile ducts are absent or reduced in number, and there is hypoplasia of portal veins. The peripheral portal ducts, however, appear to be increased in number and have unusual shapes; particularly, they appear with surprising frequency to be cut lon-

gitudinally.[106] Bulbar protrusions from the walls of dilated ducts also occur, and sometimes bridges form. All of this is thought to result from an underlying hamartomatous abnormality, termed "ductal plate malformation," that represents an arrest in the normal organogenesis of the intrahepatic bile ducts.[107, 108] Evidently, there are few if any normal ducts. To date, this malformation has been found to occur occasionally as an isolated event (Caroli disease) but most often is associated with ARPKD.[106–109] The only histologic difference found in the liver in the various presentations of ARPKD is the degree of portal fibrosis with occasional formation of fibrous septa that bridge portal areas and tend to encircle hepatic lobules.[106, 110, 111] The spectrum of portal fibrosis is most often described as minimal in the youngest patients to marked in the oldest ones, the lesion in the latter case being indistinguishable from that originally described in the condition termed congenital hepatic fibrosis.[112, 113] However, the degree of fibrosis may not be so clearly a function of the patient's age and may or may not be progressive, depending, perhaps, on the presence or absence of complicating factors such as local biliary obstruction and recurrent cholangitis.[106] Whereas some bile ducts are dilated and a few may appear to be cystic, hepatic cysts are not a common or important feature in ARPKD. On the other hand, some patients have associated gross cystic dilation of the intrahepatic biliary tree, a condition otherwise known as Caroli disease.[108, 109] Some bile plugging may be apparent histologically, but significant ductal obstruction is not present, and free communication with extrahepatic ducts can be demonstrated. There may be inflammation and microabscesses associated with ascending cholangitis.

## DIAGNOSIS

The clinical presentation of ARPKD in the newborn infant is characterized by a history of oligohydramnios and often by a difficult delivery because of the enlarged fetal kidneys. Severely affected infants may also have Potter facies and respiratory distress on the basis of pulmonary hypoplasia and atelectasis. Pneumomediastinum and pneumothorax are common, and pneumonia may develop. Renal function is usually compromised, but death resulting from renal insufficiency is uncommon in the newborn period. Hypertension often develops in the first several months and may be complicated by cardiac hypertrophy, endocardial fibroelastosis, congestive heart failure, and the onset of renal failure. Older children and adolescents may present with symptoms and signs referable to their hepatic fibrosis and portal hypertension, including gastrointestinal bleeding from varices, portal thrombosis, and hepatosplenomegaly possibly complicated by hypersplenism with thrombocytopenia, anemia, and leukopenia. Liver function tests are usually normal. There may also be renal failure and concentrating defect with secondary effects including anemia, growth failure, and renal osteodystrophy.[94, 96]

The kidney changes in ARPKD can usually be diagnosed reliably by radiographic techniques. Intravenous nephrotomography may be of some value, but ultrasonography is the most important diagnostic tool for initial screening purposes as well as for prenatal diagnosis.[96, 114–118] The typical sonogram (see Fig. 38–11A) shows enlarged kidneys with increased echogenicity in the cortex and medulla. It also shows poor definition of the collecting system and fuzzy delineation of the kidneys from surrounding tissues. Macrocystic changes may be observed in the kidneys of older patients. CT has also been used with success for diagnostic purposes (Fig. 38–12) but is limited to those patients able to cooperate during the performance of the test.[119, 120] Thus, it is generally unsuitable for children younger than 3 years. CT can delineate fine details of renal architecture in patients with a doubtful diagnosis. Nonetheless, in children, it may still be difficult to distinguish between ARPKD and ADPKD. Particularly when there is no definitive family history of either recessive or dominant disease, a liver biopsy is probably essential for accurate diagnosis.[94] The presence of hepatic fibrosis with biliary dysgenesis strongly suggests the diagnosis of ARPKD. Ultrasonography of the liver and biliary tract may occasionally also show characteristic features of diagnostic value.[109] For prenatal diagnosis, an elevated maternal serum or amniotic fluid α-fetoprotein level has been suggested as a useful diagnostic adjunct.[121]

ARPKD has been reported in association with Ehlers-Danlos syndrome with cerebral berry aneurysms and dissecting aneurysms in the thoracic and abdominal aorta.[122] Glomerular cystic disease is a rare disorder that is virtually indistinguishable clinically from ARPKD except for the absence of abnormalities in the liver and spleen.[123, 124]

## THERAPY

The neonate with large kidneys and Potter sequence with a history of oligohydramnios is probably in a terminal phase. Neonates with pulmonary hypoplasia will probably succumb to pulmonary insufficiency within the first few days. Nonetheless, until the degree of the pulmonary insufficiency and its cause (pulmonary hypoplasia, pneumothorax, pneumomediastinum, atelectasis, pneumonia, abdominal mass, heart failure) can be assessed fully, artificial ventilation and aggressive resuscitative measures are indicated. Some of these infants, not otherwise distinguished from those with fatal outcome, have survived the neonatal period, and with appropriate therapy, survival past the neonatal period is an excellent prognostic sign.[100, 101, 125] Even when there has been anuria or oliguria, renal failure is not the usual cause of death in the neonatal period, and with improvement in respiratory status, renal status may improve as well.[125]

**Renal Insufficiency.** Patients with less severe ARPKD who survive the newborn period often have nearly normal renal function at the time of presentation and thereafter may show stable or even increasing creatinine clearance values during the first 36 months.[94] When they were observed for a mean of 60 ± 48 months in one series,[94] however, the subsequent course of 17 patients was remarkably variable. Nearly half continued to have an adequate glomerular filtration rate, whereas the other half proceeded to renal failure

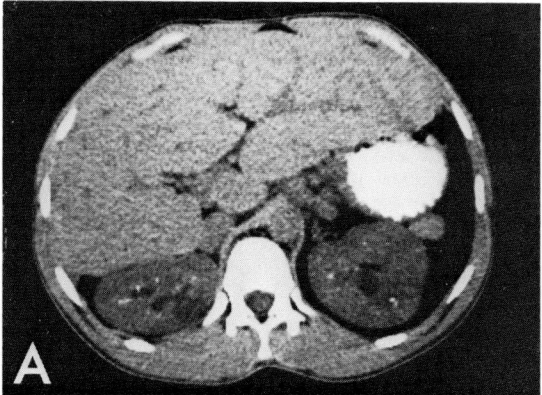 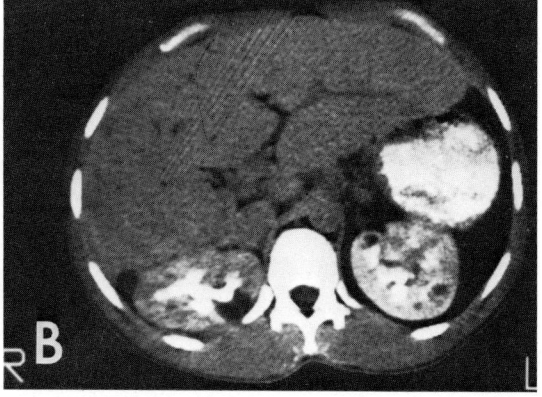

**Figure 38–12.** CT of an 18-year-old ARPKD patient with serum creatinine and liver function tests within normal ranges. The patient had clinical evidence of portal hypertension (gastric varices, enlarged spleen). Oral contrast medium was given to highlight intestines. *A.* CT scan without contrast enhancement. The liver is enlarged but not cystic. The kidneys are slightly enlarged and contain focal radiodense areas (nephrolithiasis). *B.* CT scan with intravenous administration of iodinated radiocontrast material showing cystic areas in both kidneys. The renal calcifications are now obscured by contrast medium in the collecting systems. (*A* and *B* courtesy of E Levine, Kansas City, KS.)

after 8 months to 16 years. In another series, the percentage of patients with severe renal insufficiency increased from 11% at 2 years of age to 32% at 5 years, 36% at 10 years, 43% at 15 years, and 100% at 20 years of age.[101]

The enlarged kidneys often appear to decrease in relative size, and this appears to be associated with slowly progressive renal insufficiency, anemia, renal osteodystrophy, and hypertension. As with most pediatric patients with renal insufficiency, growth is retarded but may improve in direct relation to improved renal function. Although no specific growth-promoting measures are known, increasing the calorie intake of children in chronic hemodialysis programs has resulted in linear growth rates that are more nearly normal. The management of chronic renal failure in children with ARPKD should follow the same general guidelines used for any patient with established chronic renal insufficiency. That is, children with ARPKD should probably be accepted for dialysis and transplantation on the same terms as other children with end-stage renal disease are. However, in view of the fact that the associated fibrosing liver disorder is progressive and untreatable except by liver transplantation, these patients must be classified as high-risk candidates for hemodialysis, peritoneal dialysis, and renal transplantation.[114] They also appear to have some increased susceptibility to infection and to show rather poor wound healing, probably as a consequence of their long-standing disease.

**Hypertension.** Arterial hypertension has been observed in many patients with ARPKD, either initially or later in the course. It appears to be persistent in most cases but occasionally may diminish or disappear.[94, 116] Although the proximate cause is not known, most patients respond favorably to salt restriction and the usual antihypertensive drugs (diuretics, vasodilators). There appear to be no unique requirements for specific types of antihypertensive drugs. The much improved prognosis for ARPKD in recent years has been attributed in large part to the control of hypertension.[101]

**Edema.** Edema is a frequent complication and is presumably due to impaired renal or hepatic function. It may be treated by a combination of salt restriction and diuretics but usually requires the more potent loop diuretics, such as furosemide, ethacrynic acid, and bumetanide.

**Hepatic Insufficiency.** Hepatocellular function is rarely deranged, and enzyme values are only occasionally mildly elevated. Elevated bilirubin or enzyme values suggest the possibility of cholangitis. Signs of portal hypertension usually develop between the ages of 5 and 10 years and must therefore be assessed relatively frequently. Esophageal and gastric varices have been observed frequently in these patients, and gastrointestinal hemorrhage may be life-threatening. Patients with splenomegaly secondary to portal hypertension may have hypersplenism with leukopenia, thrombocytopenia, and anemia. Portacaval and splenorenal shunts have been successful in such children,[126] but the frequency of surgical morbidity has been high. Postoperative renal failure may occur, and hemodialysis must then be available in that period. Splenectomy may be indicated in some cases but will increase susceptibility to overwhelming bacterial infections and may hinder post-transplantation immunosuppressive medication.[96] When intrahepatic bile duct

dilation is prominent (Caroli disease), recurrent cholangitis may be a problem.[108]

**Urinary Tract Infection.** As with patients with other renal cystic disorders, ARPKD patients are unusually susceptible to urinary tract infection and should not be subjected to unnecessary use of instrumentation. Retrograde ureteral and bladder catheterizations can usually be avoided by use of the new, noninvasive diagnostic techniques. Suprapubic bladder aspiration, rather than urethral catheterization, is the preferred method for culturing the urine. There have been no large series or even anecdotal clinical reports regarding specific treatment of urinary tract infection in these patients, but a therapeutic approach similar to that discussed in respect to ADPKD seems reasonable.

## COUNSELING

Parents who give birth to a child with ARPKD can be advised that on a statistical basis, each of their children will have one chance in four of having the disease and one in two of being a carrier of the abnormal gene. Persons with the disease who live long enough to become parents face a low risk of having children with the disease, provided that their mates are not relatives.

## ACQUIRED CYSTIC KIDNEY DISEASE

It was reported in 1977 that some patients maintained on hemodialysis for relatively long periods develop multiple cysts in their remnant kidneys.[127] Since that time, many additional cases have been reported and are the subject of several reviews.[128–134] The phenomenon is now more popularly known as "acquired cystic kidney disease" and is known to develop not only in patients undergoing hemodialysis but also, with approximately equal frequency and severity, in patients undergoing peritoneal dialysis. It occurs even in those patients, including children,[135] who are chronically azotemic without dialysis. It can affect native kidneys as well as chronically rejected transplant kidneys[136, 137] and has been described in all forms of chronic renal disease. Although there are exceptions,[128] the frequency of occurrence in most series is found not to be a function of the patient's age but rather of the duration of dialysis or end-stage renal failure. For example, acquired cysts are found in 7% to 22% of patients with renal failure and serum creatinine levels exceeding 3 mg/dL before dialysis, in 44% of patients with less than 3 years of dialysis, and in 75% of patients with more than 3 years of dialysis.[132] In another study, the frequency was 35% in patients with less than 2 years of dialysis, 58% in those with 2 to 4 years, 75% in those with 4 to 8 years, and 92% in patients with more than 8 years of dialysis.[138] Depending on the series, it may be more common in males than in females and somewhat more common in black than in white persons. The cysts are known to regress after successful renal transplantation.[129, 132]

An important additional feature in ACKD has been the occurrence of renal tumors.[139–149] In large cumulative series, 10% to 20% of acquired cystic kidneys have contained microscopic to grossly visible ''adenomas'' after $3 \pm 2$ (SD) years of dialysis, and another 3% to 6% have contained ''adenocarcinomas'' after $5 \pm 3$ years. In this context, however, adenocarcinomas are defined only as tumors greater than 1 to 3 cm in diameter or having demonstrable metastases, metastasis being the only definitive criterion for malignant neoplasm. Metastases have been present in 27%.[142] The mean age of all patients with ACKD has been $49 \pm 14$ years (range, approximately 17 to 75 years) and is not statistically different for those without tumors or for those with ''benign'' or with malignant tumors. Carcinoma in dialysis patients is three times more common in the presence than in the absence of acquired renal cysts and is six times more common in large cystic kidneys (single kidney weights more than 150 g) than in small cystic kidneys.[149] Overall, the frequency of renal malignant neoplasm in dialysis patients has sometimes been estimated to be 57 to 134 times greater than in the general population.[147] Elsewhere, however, it is argued that a frequency three to six times that in the age-adjusted general population is much more consistent with clinical experience.[148]

## PATHOLOGY

The kidneys are variable but, in a given patient, are generally equally involved. They may be small, large, or normal in size, even when totally involved by cysts. Most weigh less than 100 g, and about 30% of reported examples weigh less than 50 g. On the other hand, about 25% weigh more than 150 g, and a few exceptional specimens weigh more than 1000 g (Fig. 38–13). In nephrectomy and autopsy specimens, the cysts have varied in number and type from a few subcapsular cysts up to 2 to 3 cm in diameter

to numerous smaller cysts diffusely distributed. Perhaps 60% of cysts are smaller than 0.2 cm.[129] Bilateral involvement and a minimum of five cysts of detectable size in each kidney are reasonable requirements for diagnosis by appropriate imaging or radiologic techniques.[144] For gross and microscopic diagnosis, the replacement of 25% to 40% of the renal mass by cysts has been suggested as a minimal requirement,[141, 150] but, particularly in cases with numerous small cysts and at least a few adenomas (see later) on thorough gross examination, a smaller percentage involvement is probably acceptable. The cysts are sometimes visible on the external surface, may appear to concentrate near the pelvis or corticomedullary junction on cut section, and may be unilocular or multilocular. They may occupy a small portion of the renal mass or, occasionally, such a large portion that the appearance of ADPKD is simulated.[141, 150, 151] Microdissection studies have demonstrated the continuity of the cysts with both proximal and distal tubules and have suggested their origin both in the fusiform dilation of tubule segments and in multiple small tubule diverticula.[150, 151] Because the glomeruli serving the cystic tubule segments are often found to be sclerotic and presumably nonfunctional, the cyst fluid must arise predominantly by secretion rather than by glomerular filtration.

The cysts most often contain a clear fluid in which the cyst fluid/serum ratio for $Na^+$ is approximately 1 and that for creatinine is considerably greater than 1, a composition distinct from that in simple cysts or in the cysts of ADPKD.[129] The cyst fluid is occasionally hemorrhagic, and hemorrhage is sometimes the most prominent feature, with rupture into the pelvis or retroperitoneal area.

On microscopic examination, the original renal tissue is usually disorganized and contains sclerotic glomeruli, atrophic tubules, and interstitial fibrosis typical of most

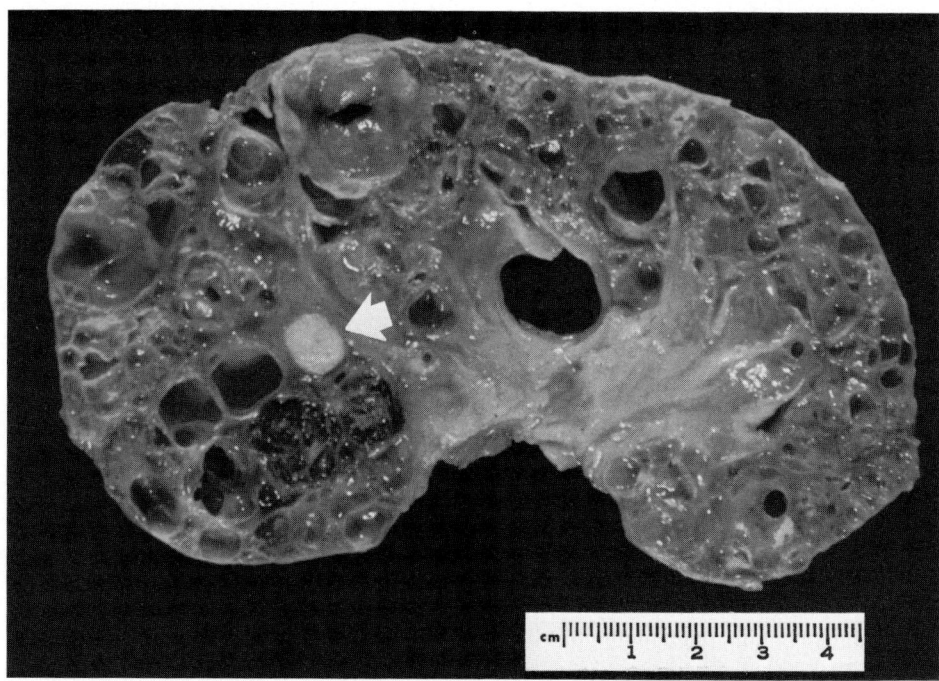

**Figure 38–13.** Acquired cystic disease in a 320-g kidney from a patient with a 10-year history of hemodialysis. There were bilateral, multifocal renal cell carcinomas *(arrow)* with multiple systemic metastases. (Courtesy of T Tomita, Kansas City, KS.)

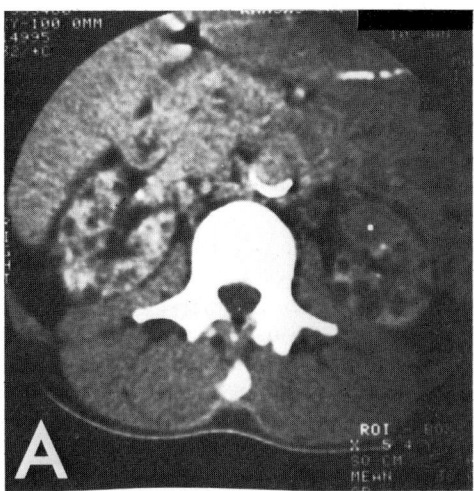 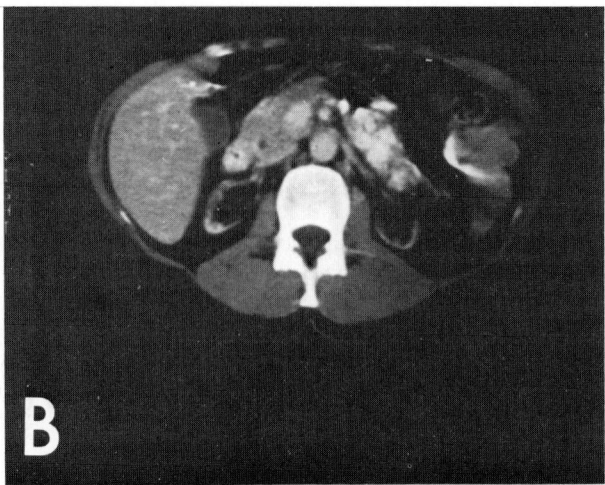

**Figure 38–14.** Acquired renal cystic disease. *A.* CT scan with intravenous administration of contrast medium. This male patient had renal failure due to diabetic nephropathy and had received hemodialysis for 6 years before this examination. There is bilateral renal enlargement with diffuse cysts in cortex and medulla. A solid tissue tumor is seen in the anterior part of the left kidney. *B.* CT scan of original kidneys in a patient with a functioning renal allograft. Note the marked atrophy of the renal parenchyma in contrast to the cystic changes seen in *A.* (*A* and *B* courtesy of E Levine, Kansas City, KS.)

end-stage renal diseases regardless of cause. Published series have specifically excluded known cases of hereditary polycystic disease. With long-term dialysis, there are the added features of smooth muscle nodules in necrotic arterioles and arteries; hyperplasia of Bowman capsule epithelium; small or microscopic "atypical" cysts lined by possibly malignant columnar cells, often forming multiple layers and small papillae; and remodeling of arteries and veins, often with marked intimal thickening and fibrosis of the arteries.[152, 153] Hemosiderin-laden macrophages and crystals (usually oxalate) may be prominent in the interstitium. The cyst walls themselves are often not impressive and, regardless of the location, are usually lined only by a flattened cuboid epithelium. Cyst lumens often contain golden yellow, gravel-like oxalate deposits.

In a significant fraction of reported cases, the cysts have contained single or, more often, multiple papillary, tubular, or solid neoplasms arising from the cyst lining and consistent with renal cell adenomas or adenocarcinomas. They are four to seven times more common in males than in females.[130, 147] The cytologic appearance of these tumors is usually not markedly anaplastic, even in the 20% of cases in which metastases have been documented.[153–155] Similar tumors apparently arising in the renal parenchyma have also been observed.[155] The relationship between these tumors and the atypical cysts in kidneys with long-term dialysis is not entirely clear, although renal cell tumors are found at a younger age in dialyzed patients than in nondialyzed patients.[154] Whether tumors are more common in the dialyzed patients than in the uremic, nondialyzed patients is also not clear, and conflicting reports have appeared.[156–158] There are rare reports of oncocytoma or of transitional cell carcinoma in addition to renal cell tumors in the same cystic kidney of a dialyzed patient.

The development of the cysts and tumors seems to be tied to the pronounced epithelial hyperplasia observed mi-

croscopically. The hyperplasia, in turn, seems to be due to the uremic state, even though there seems to be no relation between the occurrence of acquired cysts and the efficacy of dialysis.[138, 144] Patients with successful renal allografts do not seem to develop cystic disease in their native kidneys.[144] Furthermore, if acquired cystic disease already is present at the time of successful transplantation, that process seems to regress[159] or at least not to increase in severity.[144, 159, 160] Conceivably, the loss of renal mass causes the production of renotropic factors that stimulate hyperplasia.

## DIAGNOSIS

ACKD develops insidiously. Most patients have no symptoms, but when they do occur, gross hematuria, flank pain, renal colic, fever, palpable renal mass, and rising hematocrit are most common. Symptoms associated with renal neoplasm are also uncommon but again include gross hematuria, fever, and back or flank pain plus rising or falling hematocrit and the complications of metastases.[132] After the rupture of cysts, a large retroperitoneal or perirenal hemorrhage may produce acute pain, hypotension, and shock. Ultrasonography reveals the bilateral cystic process in advanced cases and is useful in the detection of neoplasms, particularly in patients with chronic renal failure not treated with dialysis and in whom contrast medium might cause a further deterioration in renal function.[148] However, CT, with or without contrast enhancement, is the preferred diagnostic technique and is more capable of distinguishing between kidneys with a few simple cysts and those with multiple acquired cysts (Fig. 38–14). Magnetic resonance imaging, with or without gadolinium enhancement, may also be useful, particularly for the diagnosis of neoplasms, as an alternative to contrast-enhanced CT in nondialyzed patients, and in those cases in which the CT findings are indeterminate.[148] Distinction from ADPKD and from multiple simple cysts is usually suggested by the generally smaller size of the kidneys and of the individual cysts in ACKD, by the usual absence of hepatic cysts, and by the family's and patient's histories.

## THERAPY

Bleeding episodes, either intrarenal or perirenal, may often be treated conservatively with bed rest and analgesics.[161] Persistent hemorrhage, however, may require nephrectomy or therapeutic renal embolization and infarction. Because the risk of undetected renal cell carcinoma is high in patients with retroperitoneal hemorrhage, nephrectomy is recommended in those cases if carcinoma cannot be ruled out.[141] When a few larger cysts are associated with flank pain, percutaneous aspiration (with cytologic examination) is a reasonable temporizing measure. ACKD may be prevented by, and certainly is known to regress after, successful renal transplantation[129, 132, 144] (see Fig. 38–14).

Because renal cell carcinoma is an important complication of ACKD, several authors have recommended CT screening for ACKD after 3 years of dialysis and then screening for neoplasm at 1- or 2-year intervals thereafter. However, because renal cell carcinoma is actually a relatively rare cause of death among dialysis patients, it has also been suggested that a more aggressive renal imaging program and, indeed, even an annual screening program would be unlikely to reduce the mortality of dialysis patients significantly and thus would not be justified from a financial standpoint.[162] In the end, the clinical decision must be based on the individual patient, with consideration given both to the known risk factors for carcinoma (including prolonged dialysis, the presence of ACKD, large kidneys, and male sex) and to the patient's age and general fitness.[129, 162] ACKD is known to regress after successful renal transplantation, and this, too, is a consideration even though it does not necessarily reduce the possibility for carcinoma. There are a number of reports of renal cell carcinoma developing in the native kidneys years after successful transplantation.[132, 148]

If renal cell carcinoma is detected in patients with ACKD, it is generally agreed that tumors larger than 3 cm should be treated by radical nephrectomy unless the patient is a poor operative risk.[148] For tumors smaller than 3 cm, some authors advise nephrectomy for the acceptable surgical candidate, whereas others recommend annual CT follow-up with resection if the lesions enlarge. Although metastases are statistically less likely to occur from small tumors than from large tumors, small size of tumor is not a guarantee against metastasis. Furthermore, in large kidneys with numerous small neoplastic foci, the total mass of the numerous small lesions might easily exceed that of a single lesion 3 cm or larger. It is not established whether it is tumor size or tumor load (total mass) that is the important determinant for the probability of metastasis in these cases.[149] Resection even of small neoplasms is probably mandatory in preparation for transplantation.[131, 141] Even though carcinoma is often multicentric and bilateral in ACKD, unilateral nephrectomy for tumor does not mandate the removal of an apparently tumor-free contralateral kidney. Instead, frequent monitoring of the contralateral kidney is advised.

# CYSTIC DISEASES OF THE RENAL MEDULLA

There are two distinct diseases that primarily involve structures of the renal medulla. Both are associated with variable enlargement of the distal tubules and collecting ducts and with interstitial fibrosis and inflammation of a variable extent. One of them, medullary cystic disease, progresses to end-stage renal failure, whereas the other, medullary sponge kidney, is a relatively benign condition.

## Medullary Cystic Disease

Medullary cystic disease has been described under two names, juvenile nephronophthisis and medullary cystic disease. Juvenile nephronophthisis is an autosomal recessive disorder that usually presents in childhood. The gene defect has been mapped to chromosome 2p.[163] Medullary cystic disease, on the other hand, is an autosomal dominant disorder that usually presents in older adults. Its gene defect is presently unknown. Aside from the hereditary features and ages of presentation, however, the two conditions are essentially identical. Although some authors wish to combine the two disorders under the name juvenile nephronophthisis–medullary cystic disease complex,[164] we believe that the single term "medullary cystic disease" is sufficient for practical use. Nonetheless, when medullary cystic disease occurs in association with retinal degeneration, familial retinitis pigmentosa, and pigmentary optic atrophy, the term "renal-retinal dysplasia" has been applied most often and seems appropriate.[165–169] Associated defects of the skeletal and central nervous system are seen less frequently.[167, 170]

## PATHOLOGY

The kidneys in these related disorders cannot be distinguished pathologically. They are moderately small with a finely but irregularly granular capsular surface. On cut section, the cortex and medulla are both thinned. The corticomedullary margin is indistinct but is the site of a variable number (5 to 50) of small to perhaps 2-cm diameter spherical, thin-walled cysts that contain fluid resembling normal urine (Fig. 38–15). Similar cysts may also be present in the deeper medulla and papilla.[171–173] Whereas most kidneys also have a variable number of minute cortical cysts, perhaps 25% have no grossly visible cysts.[164, 172] On microscopic examination, there is widespread but nonspecific glomerular hyalinization with basement membrane thickening and podocyte effacement, periglomerular fibrosis, tubule atrophy, and patchy and variable interstitial fibrosis. There may be intermixed compensatory hypertrophy and hyperplasia. Particularly at the corticomedullary junction, there is a sparse and sometimes nodular chronic inflammatory cell infiltrate. Tubule segments of a single nephron may be encompassed by dense sclerotic interstitium continuous with peritubular membranes. Microdissections have

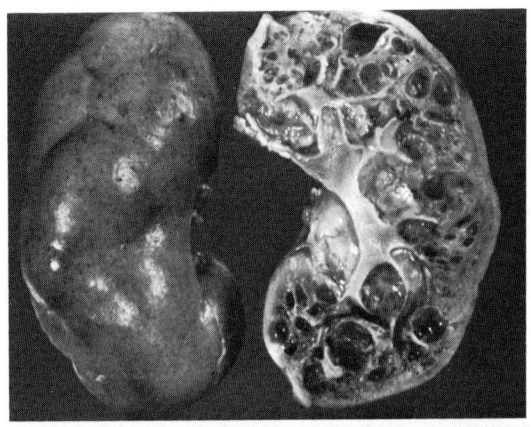

**Figure 38–15.** Outer and cut surface of kidney with severe medullary cystic disease.

shown the nephrons to be altered by numerous small diverticuli and to be highly variable in size. The cysts are separate objects not directly related to the diverticuli and are limited to the distal convoluted and collecting tubule segments.[171] Transmission and scanning electron microscopic studies show the cysts to be lined by a single layer of epithelium varying from cuboid or columnar cells that lack microvilli to squamous cells resembling those of the loop of Henle.[173] The tubule basement membranes frequently are excessively thickened, even fairly early in the course of the disease.[172, 174] Free communication is seen between cysts and nondilated tubules.

## DIAGNOSIS

The diagnosis of medullary cystic disease should be suspected in patients with end-stage renal disease in childhood and in azotemic adults with a familial history of renal disease. It is fairly common, at least in the sense that it may account for 1% to 5% of all patients who reach dialysis or transplantation and for 10% to 20% of cases of renal failure in childhood. Clinical presentation is usually in the first or second decades of life but may occur as late as the seventh decade.[164] Excretory urography shows the defect as inhomogeneous streaking confined to the medulla and due to the accumulation of contrast material in the collecting ducts.[175] Ultrasonography and CT may be helpful diagnostic procedures,[176] especially for those patients with relatively small medullary cysts that cannot be diagnosed unequivocally with the usual urographic procedures. Open renal biopsy may be the only certain way to make the diagnosis.

Within a family structure, the disease appears to be inherited in a relatively uniform way. For example, patients who manifest renal insufficiency in childhood usually have a form of the disease that is transmitted as an autosomal recessive trait and that presents in a 4- to 10-year-old child with a history of polydipsia, polyuria, pallor, lethargy, and growth retardation. Progression to the end stage of the disease then occurs before the age of 20 years. In the adult form, the clinical presentation is similar with the exceptions that growth retardation and a long history of anemia and other manifestations of end-stage renal disease are usually

not found and discovery may be delayed until the sixth or seventh decade of life. These adult patients may pass through a period in which they have urinary concentration defects sufficient to cause serious $Na^+$ wastage, hyponatremia, and extracellular fluid volume contraction. The authors remember one of these patients well for the fact that he ate approximately 20 g of rock salt and drank 5 to 6 L of fluid each day to maintain blood pressure in an acceptable range. Fractional excretion of $Na^+$ in the urine, estimated by $C_{Na}/C_{inulin}$, was approximately 50% in that patient.

It is unusual for patients with medullary cystic disease to have flank pain, hypertension, hematuria, or renal calculi. This is in contrast to patients with polycystic disease or medullary sponge kidney.

## THERAPY

**$Na^+$ Wasting.** It has been suggested that salt wasting is a cardinal sign of medullary cystic disease. Although this may be true during certain periods of a patient's life, it is usually a transient condition just preceding the development of end-stage renal disease. Presumably, the renal salt wasting is secondary to anatomic abnormalities in the distal collecting ducts and other nephron structures in the medulla, although the cysts themselves may not be directly responsible. It is occasionally associated with hyperreninemia and juxtaglomerular cell hyperplasia,[176] probably secondary to salt depletion. Salt wasting is managed by determining the amount of $Na^+$ replacement needed to maintain a stable upright position and blood pressure. Some patients require vast quantities of sodium chloride and water to maintain $Na^+$ balance. Should oral intake be interrupted for some reason, intravenous salt and water replacement is mandatory. On the other hand, as the disease progresses to end stage, it is not uncommon for patients to retain $Na^+$ and to become hypertensive as the number of residual functioning nephrons decreases. At this point, the sodium and water intake must be reduced to prevent expansion of the extracellular fluid volume. When acidosis occurs, the diet should be altered to reduce acid residues, and oral sodium bicarbonate should be given in addition to sodium chloride. The acidosis and hyperkalemia encountered in this disorder are probably due to a defect in distal tubule handling of $Na^+$, $K^+$, and $H^+$. These disorders are corrected by altering the dietary intake of $K^+$ and $H^+$ and by use of $K^+$-binding ion exchange resins.

**Anemia.** These patients may have profound anemia that appears earlier than is usual for other diseases leading to renal insufficiency. No specific therapy is known. Erythrocytosis has been described in one patient with medullary cystic disease.[176]

**Renal Insufficiency.** The onset of renal insufficiency in this disorder is usually insidious and not unique except for the occasional patient with salt wasting. In two patients with medullary cystic disease, the $1/P_{cr}$ relationship was linear for a period of 100 months and indicated that a constant amount of creatinine clearance was being lost per unit time.[177] Clinical infection of the kidney appears to be relatively uncommon in medullary cystic disease and does not appear to be a major factor in the development of chronic renal failure. Secondary hyperparathyroidism, renal osteodystrophy, and neuropathy may be observed. At the end stage, renal insufficiency can be managed by dialysis or renal transplantation.

## COUNSELING

The uncertain pattern of genetic transmission in medullary cystic disease is a severe obstacle in advising family members of the propensity for genetic transmission and in selecting donors for renal transplantation. It has been suggested that if the transplant recipient's renal morphologic appearance suggests chronic interstitial nephritis and a living related donor is considered, an extensive search should be made to detect renal disease within the family.[165] Unilateral nephrectomy of the recipient has even been advised to make sure that there are no cysts that might implicate a familial medullary cystic disorder.

The concept of genetic heterogeneity is well established for medullary cystic disease, and it has been emphasized that the patterns of presentation in children and in adults do not necessarily indicate different disorders. For example, in one study, the parents of 21 patients with childhood onset of medullary cystic disease also had renal disease in childhood, a situation suggesting autosomal dominant rather than recessive inheritance.[178] Thus, in dealing with medullary cystic disease, it would seem to be a good rule to consider the disorder to be dominantly inherited until proved otherwise by careful family study. Only when it is specifically warranted by family study should counseling be directed toward a recessive or dominant pattern.

## Medullary Sponge Kidney

Most authors consider medullary sponge kidney to be a congenital anomaly that is present at birth in its fully developed form. The diagnosis, however, is not usually made until the fourth or fifth decade, when secondary calcareous or infective complications emerge. Progression to renal failure is uncommon. The frequency of this disease is approximately 1 in 5000 in the general population and perhaps 1 in 1000 in patients studied in urology clinics.[179] In patients with nephrolithiasis, however, at least a mild degree of the condition may be found in about 20%, the frequency in males being about half that in females.[180] Although most cases appear sporadically, family tendencies have been reported. An occasional association with other congenital problems is reviewed elsewhere.[179] Curiously, as many as 25% of patients with medullary sponge kidney may have hemihypertrophy of the body, whereas about 10% of patients with hemihypertrophy also have medullary sponge kidney.[181, 182] Although the affected kidney does not closely resemble a sea sponge, the term "medullary sponge kidney" is common usage. Alternative terms, such as precalyceal canalicular ectasia or cystic dilation of renal collecting tubules, are more accurate but not widely accepted. Their use, however, would avoid confusion of this condition with other distinctly different conditions, such as ARPKD, that on occasion have also been called sponge kidneys.

## PATHOLOGY

The only visible abnormality in this disease is the marked spherical, oval, or irregular enlargement of the medullary and inner papillary portions of collecting ducts. One or several papillae may be affected, and the lesions are bilateral in 70% of cases. Unilateral involvement of only one pyramid is uncommon. The dilated ducts communicate proximally with collecting tubules of normal size and often show a relative constriction to approximately normal diameter at the point of their communication with the calyx.[7] Their diameter is often 1 to 3, occasionally 5, and rarely up to 7.5 mm.[179] They may contain clear, jelly-like, or dry brown material or, frequently, small calculi. Free calculi are found in about 60% of symptomatic patients. Intracystic communications are observed occasionally, as are entirely noncommunicating cysts. Except in the closed cysts, where the epithelium is usually atrophic and the lumen is filled with hyaline material positive for periodic acid–Schiff reaction, the lining cells of these cysts are cuboid to columnar and focally may be pseudostratified or even stratified squamous as a presumed response to intraductal calculi. Complications such as lithiasis with infection and intrarenal obstruction are common, and secondary changes of the cortex and medulla are seen accordingly. The kidney is otherwise normal in its architecture and development.

## DIAGNOSIS

The disease usually becomes apparent in the fourth or fifth decade of life. It is associated with gross and microscopic hematuria that may be recurrent and with urinary tract infections that are often the first signs of an underlying abnormality. Nephrolithiasis, with renal colic, loin pain, and excretion of small stones, is also a prominent feature. The disease seldom progresses to end-stage renal failure, although reduced glomerular filtration rates have been observed, and perhaps 10% of patients have relatively poor prognosis because of recurring urolithiasis, bacteriuria, septicemia, and probably pyelonephritis. The most commonly recognized functional abnormalities include defective urinary solute concentrating ability, inability to reduce the urine pH to a minimal value of 5.5, and systemic acidosis secondary to renal tubular acidosis. Diagnosis is by intravenous urography that shows radial, linear striations in the papillae or cystic collections of contrast medium in the ectatic collecting ducts[179, 180] (Fig. 38–16). Calcium precipitates also collect in the ectatic collecting duct segments to give, in some patients, a characteristic radiographic pattern that is obscured by radiocontrast material. Ultrasonography and CT are not usually necessary but may resolve confusion with papillary necrosis[183] or, rarely, even with polycystic disease[184] or transitional cell carcinoma.[185] In one report, however, even these techniques failed to distinguish between segmental sponge kidney and neoplasm.[186] On rare occasions, CT may reveal renal abscesses.[187]

## THERAPY

**Renal Tubular Acidosis.** The renal tubular acidosis in this condition has not been characterized beyond the rec-

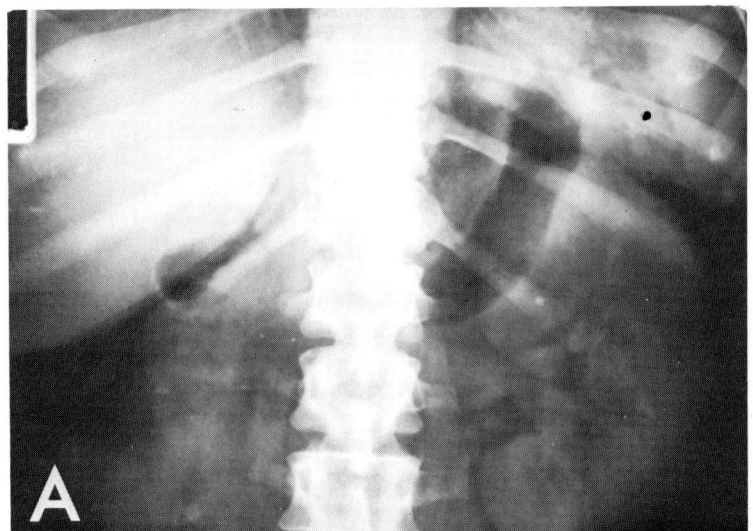

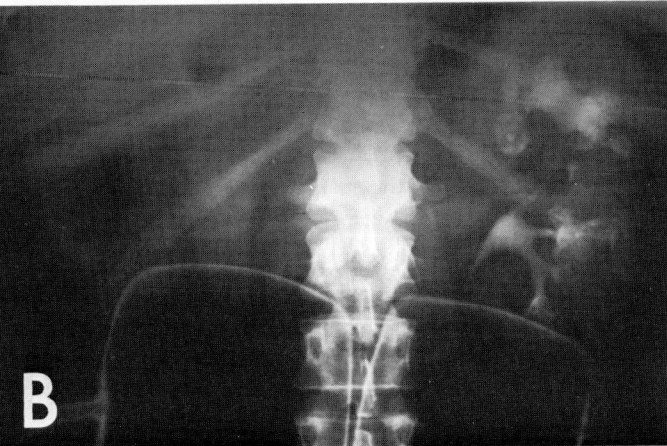

**Figure 38–16.** Medullary sponge kidney. *A.* Plain radiograph of a large solitary left kidney containing several calcific densities. *B.* Urogram showing the pronounced tubular ectasia of all papillae that is typical of medullary sponge abnormality. (*A* and *B* courtesy of GD Dixon, Kansas City, MO.)

ognition that it is of the classic distal type. The impact of bicarbonate therapy on the pathogenesis of nephrolithiasis has not been examined critically in patients with complete and incomplete renal tubular acidosis of this type. Because oral administration of alkali increases rather than decreases the urine pH, there might be some risk of promoting calculus formation in patients who have calcium phosphate stones in their ectatic tubules.

**Nephrolithiasis.** Renal stones consisting of calcium oxalate, calcium phosphate, and other types of calcium salts commonly form in the ectatic collecting ducts in this disease. Nephrolithiasis is thus a common clinical problem. In studies in which there are strict criteria for the quality of acceptable intravenous urograms, the frequency of medullary sponge kidney has been about 13% in patients with calcium urolithiasis but only about 2% in otherwise normal patients.[180, 188] Among all calcium stone formers, women have a greater frequency of medullary sponge kidney than do men.[189]

The possible relationship between hyperparathyroidism and medullary sponge kidney has been emphasized in numerous publications, and it has been postulated that renal $Ca^{2+}$ loss causes a reduction in plasma ionized $Ca^{2+}$ concentration that in turn stimulates the secretion of parathyroid hormone. It is thought that this process may ultimately cause the formation of parathyroid adenomas.

In a critical examination of the excretion of $Ca^{2+}$ in patients with medullary sponge kidney and other stone-forming disorders, absorptive hypercalciuria was the most common abnormality in medullary sponge kidney, occurring in 59% of patients, whereas only 18% had hypercalciuria due to renal $Ca^{2+}$ "leak."[190] It was the opinion of those authors and others,[191] therefore, that patients with medullary sponge kidneys and renal stones have the same spectrum of metabolic abnormalities as is found in the overall population of stone formers and should be so evaluated and treated. Asymptomatic patients found incidentally to have medullary sponge kidney require no specific therapy but should have yearly routine urinalysis. As a general rule, patients with nephrolithiasis should excrete about 2 L of urine each day to reduce the propensity for calcium salts to precipitate in the collecting ducts and renal pelvis. Patients with hypercalciuria may benefit from long-term therapy with thiazide diuretics, but this may elevate plasma $Ca^{2+}$ levels. For patients with calcium urolithiasis and normal urinary $Ca^{2+}$ excretion, oral phosphate therapy may be useful. There are no reports of an increased frequency of hyperuricosuria in patients with medullary sponge kidney, but, of course, this possibility should be kept in mind in the routine evaluation of such a patient. If hyperuricosuria is observed, a trial of allopurinol may slow the formation of urinary stones. In some instances, the persistence of renal stone formation in kidneys with medullary sponge disease has been associated with significant morbidity from the pain of urolithiasis and urinary tract infection with persistent bacteriuria. Renal abscesses are a rare complication that may require prolonged antibiotic therapy or surgical drainage.[187] In some cases, especially those in which the tubule ectasia is unilateral or segmental, a unilateral or partial nephrectomy has resulted in sustained freedom from nephrolithiasis, urolithiasis, and urosepsis. Because medullary sponge kidney is usually a bilateral disorder, however, partial or complete nephrectomy should be undertaken cautiously and only after careful evaluation indicates that sufficient function will remain to sustain life. Patients with medullary sponge kidney appear to be more susceptible to urinary tract infections, and routine preventive measures seem warranted, especially in female patients. Patients who recurrently form and pass stones may benefit from lithotripsy.[192]

## COUNSELING

Most patients discovered incidentally to have medullary sponge kidney can be advised that the disorder is benign and that they can anticipate no serious morbidity or mortality from the disorder. On the other hand, nephrolithiasis can be a difficult problem in symptomatic patients. A clear familial transmission of this disease has not been established. If there is a history of medullary sponge disease in the family, however, detailed investigation is advisable to determine a potential genetic pattern of transmission.

## SIMPLE CYSTS

Simple cysts are the most common cystic abnormality encountered in human kidneys. They may be solitary or multiple and are filled with a fluid chemically similar to an ultrafiltrate of plasma.[193] They are rare in children[194–196] and increase in frequency approximately linearly with age. In autopsy studies[197] and in incidental CT scans of the abdomen,[198] they are found in about 50% of patients at 40 years of age. Simple cysts do not appear to be associated with any decrease in renal function and, almost by definition, are not hereditary. Early work suggested that simple cysts develop in the renal parenchyma as a consequence of ischemia, but the exact mechanism remains obscure. Information indicates that as with other cystic structures in the cortex and medulla, simple cysts probably develop from pre-existing tubules and perhaps derive from tubule diverticula.[199, 200] In contrast to cysts in ADPKD, electrolyte gradients typical of proximal and distal cysts have not been found. The cyst walls also appear to be relatively impermeable to low-molecular-weight solutes and to antibiotics.[201] Nonetheless, the turnover of cyst fluid may be as great as 20 times per day as measured by $^3H_2O$ diffusion.[202]

## PATHOLOGY

Simple cysts may be unilateral or bilateral and are usually spherical and unilocular. There may be only one or a few per kidney, but, rarely, simple cysts may be so numer-

ous as to be confused with ADPKD or with ACKD. The cysts are often cortical and distort the renal contour but may be deep cortical or apparently medullary in origin. They do not communicate with the renal pelvis. Cyst diameters of 0.5 to 1 cm are common, but 3- to 4-cm cysts are not unusual. Rare cysts have been reported to contain many liters of fluid. The cyst fluid is usually urine-like in appearance but may occasionally be blood stained or, rarely, have the consistency of glazier's putty. Hydrostatic pressure within the cysts averages 15 mm Hg but has a wide range ($-1$ to $+42$ mm Hg), even among cysts in the same kidney.[203–205] The walls are typically thin and transparent but may become thickened, fibrotic, opaque, and even calcified as the presumed result of earlier infection. On microscopic examination, the cysts compress otherwise normal adjacent tissue and are lined by a single layer of simple, flattened epithelium that may appear to be discontinuous.

## DIAGNOSIS

Most simple cysts are found on routine urographic examinations (Fig. 38–17A) and, with increasing use of abdominal ultrasonography and CT (Fig. 38–17B), are being recognized more frequently. They are far more common in adults than in children. Patients, particularly children, occasionally may present with palpable abdominal mass, hematuria after abdominal trauma, or mild proteinuria. Simple cysts have also been associated with urethral valves or prostatic hyperplasia,[206, 207] calyceal obstruction,[208–210] hematuria and massive calycovenous reflux,[211] erythrocytosis,[212, 213] and intestinal or biliary obstruction.[214, 215] Hypertension has been attributed to simple cysts in a few cases,[216–218] and the occasional infected cyst may present with flank pain, pyuria, fever, and leukocytosis, and rarely by perforation with disastrous results.[219–222] In the vast majority of cases, however, the simple cysts are asymptomatic, and the major problem becomes one of differentiating between simple cyst and malignant mass.

With lesions as common as simple cysts, it is not surprising that the coincidence of simple cyst and tumor in the same kidney is 2% to 4%.[223] Nonetheless, it is uncommon to find neoplasm actually arising within a cyst, and with modern diagnostic techniques, the risk of failure to recognize cancer in association with a cyst is small.[224] Therefore, in asymptomatic patients with a few small and unequivocal simple cysts discovered at urography or CT, further evaluation, except perhaps for periodic follow-up with ultrasonography, is probably not indicated if there is no fever, leukocytosis, hematuria, or renal discomfort. On the other hand, if the renal mass discovered at urography is of questionable nature or indeterminate, ultrasonography is probably the next logical step. After that would be CT; suggested criteria for benign cyst include a homogeneous attenuation value near water density, no enhancement with intravenous contrast material, no measurable thickness of the cyst wall, and smooth interface with renal parenchyma.[225] If these criteria are not met, the cyst falls into an indeterminate or solid category, and surgical exploration is recommended. Magnetic resonance imaging may be of some help, as may be the finding of calcification.[226] Some 2% of simple cysts

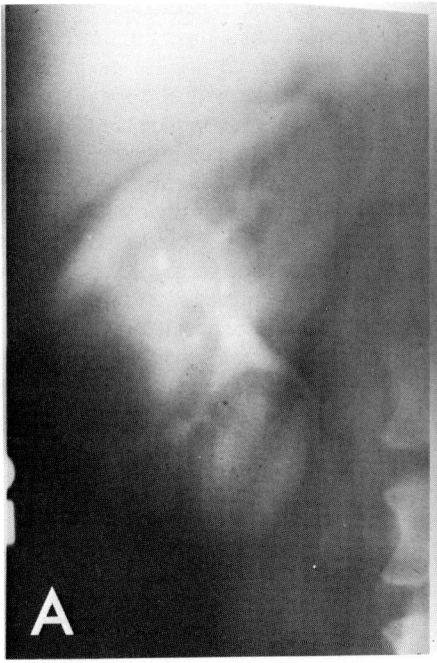
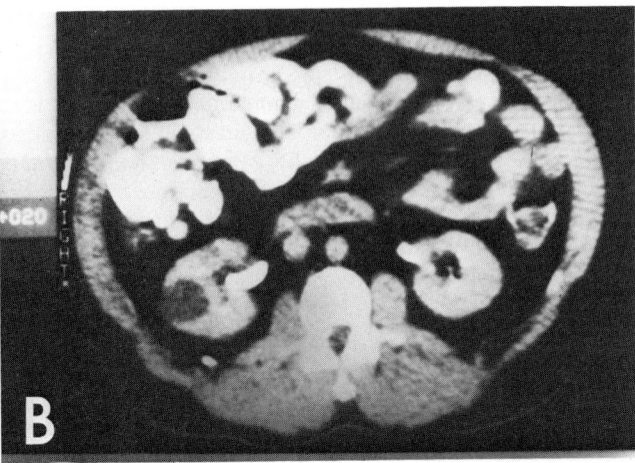

**Figure 38–17.** Simple renal cysts. *A.* Solitary cortical cyst of right kidney seen by intravenous urography. *B.* Solitary cyst of right renal cortex seen by CT with intravenous contrast enhancement. Oral contrast material was given to highlight the intestine. (*A* and *B* courtesy of E Levine, Kansas City, KS.)

and 10% of renal cell carcinomas contain calcium deposits, but calcification in simple cysts appears to be peripheral, whereas that in tumors is more central. Nonetheless, it has been said that calcification within a renal mass lesion should be considered to reflect malignant change until proved otherwise.

Percutaneous cyst puncture to confirm a benign cause has been advocated in the past but more recently has been argued to be unnecessary in view of the high probability of correct diagnosis by CT.[227] If cyst puncture is performed, however, the character of the aspirated fluid is of special importance. Simple cyst fluid is usually straw colored and clear and is free of erythrocytes, leukocytes, and atypical cells. By contrast, fluid aspirated from cystic malignant tumors is usually bloody or dark colored, has a high content of cholesterol and total lipids, and contains malignant cells on cytologic examination.

At present, it does not appear that rigid criteria have been adopted for the use of CT, ultrasonography, arteriography, magnetic resonance imaging, and cyst puncture in the evaluation of patients with questionable renal mass lesions. Clearly, all of these techniques have some value in their own right in selected cases. The quality and availability of the equipment and the expertise of the radiologist also figure prominently in the approach to the renal mass in individual institutions. There is insufficient information determined prospectively to decide whether CT can completely supplant ultrasound and angiographic evaluation of renal mass lesions. Until such studies are done, therefore, it seems reasonable to use arteriography, ultrasonography, and CT together in the evaluation of questionable cystic lesions of the kidney.

## THERAPY

A great diversity in the therapeutic approach to simple cysts has been reported, but with regard to the possibility of malignant neoplasm, it is now generally agreed that surgery is not usually indicated,[225] particularly if a malignant mass has in fact been ruled out by use of modern diagnostic tests. The management of symptomatic renal cysts can otherwise take several forms. Most intermediate-sized cysts can be aspirated percutaneously, and a sclerosing agent can be instilled into the cavity in an attempt to prevent recurrence. Cysts greater than 500 mL in volume are usually drained surgically.

Hypertension has been attributed to simple cysts in a few patients and has sometimes disappeared after successful aspiration of the cyst fluid or operative removal of the cyst. Plasma renin activity is usually elevated in such cases, and the mechanism is thought to be compression of adjacent vessels by cysts with selective renal ischemia and increased renin production.

Several examples of infected simple renal cysts have been reported in association with flank pain, pyuria, fever, and leukocytosis. Differentiation from renal abscess may be difficult, but it has been suggested that the clinical triad of acute pyelonephritis, a vascular mass lesion in the kidney, and ipsilateral pleural effusion is more characteristic of abscess. Enterobacteriaceae, staphylococci, and *Proteus* species have been encountered most frequently in infected cysts. An operative approach is usually taken, but percutaneous aspiration and drainage of infected cysts has also been used. Conservative treatment has not been specifically evaluated. When simple cysts cause calyceal obstruction, cyst drainage or enucleation is recommended to relieve the obstruction and the potential for urinary tract infection.

# RENAL DYSPLASIA*

The term "renal dysplasia" implies that the anlagen of the kidney, the ureteric bud and the metanephric blastema, have both formed embryologically but subsequently have failed to interact and develop in a normal way. In practice, it has come to mean any developmental abnormality resulting from anomalous metanephric differentiation and is applied to any kidney that contains structures that do not recapitulate any stage in the normal renal development. Renal dysplasia thus includes a spectrum of renal defects having certain features in common. Most dysplastic kidneys are associated either with an abnormally located ureteral orifice or with urinary tract anomalies expected to produce unilateral, bilateral, or segmental urinary obstruction. Many but not all are associated with renal cystic changes. In general, the most severely dysplastic kidneys are nonfunctional, have no patent connection to the urinary bladder, and remain asymptomatic if unilateral. Less severely dysplastic kidneys may have nearly normal function and present with clinical symptoms and signs related only to their size or to their increased susceptibility to infection. Renal dysplasia most often appears sporadically. A small minority of cases show a familial tendency.

There are three basic theories about the pathogenesis of renal dysplasia. The first and most traditional theory suggests that toxic or physical injury occurs to the interacting ureteric bud and nephrogenic blastema, the extent of the resulting damage being a function of the developmental stage of the kidney at that time.[8] Thus, injury beginning early in organogenesis would lead to altered development of the metanephric blastema and ducts, resulting in cartilaginous metaplasia and the formation of primitive ducts, and to abnormal nephron development. Injury occurring somewhat later would affect the nephrogenic zone more severely, leading to the formation of primitive ductules and nephronic elements in the peripheral cortex. The damaging insult is usually considered to be increased hydrostatic pressure, as would result from partial to complete obstruction of the ureter or bladder outlet, and the theory gains support from the fact that severely dysplastic kidneys are usually found to have atretic ureters. On the other hand, with partial obstruction by posterior valves, for example, the structure of the kidneys is found to vary from nearly normal to severely dysplastic.[228]

The second theory, like the first, suggests that the ureteral bud and metanephric components may have been normal initially but are injured secondarily. In this case, the insult occurs during the migration of the developing kidney from a sacral to a lumbar location and results from a failure of the shifting network of mesonephric vessels and capillaries to maintain an adequate blood supply to the rapidly elongating and migrating ureteral and renal structures. The result is ischemia with consequent atresia of a ureteral segment (long or short) and kidney damage ranging from extreme fibrosis and atrophy to severe dysplasia.[229] Because

renal migration takes place at a time early in renal organogenesis (4 to 6 weeks), this theory presumably could apply only to severely and totally dysplastic kidneys.

The third theory of renal dysplasia focuses on the precise location of the renal anlagen and implies an intrinsic deficiency or inadequacy of anlagen displaced even slightly from their normal positions. Thus, because dysplasia can be correlated with ectopia of the ureteral orifice and because ectopia of the orifice can be explained by an abnormal position of the ureteric bud along the distal wolffian duct, it is suggested that if the ureteric bud arises from the wolffian duct either proximal or distal to its normal point of origin, both the bud and the metanephric blastema that it encounters are defective and their interaction results in a dysplastic kidney.[230] The degree of bud and blastema deficiency and the extent of the dysplasia relate to the distance by which the ureteral orifice is displaced from its normal position in the trigone (either lateral or caudal). It is not closely correlated with the presence or absence of obstruction or reflux.

## PATHOLOGY

Although most dysplastic kidneys are grossly deformed in a fairly characteristic way, most authors accept only two absolute criteria for dysplasia, and both of those require histologic confirmation[231, 232] (Fig. 38–18). Of greater importance is the finding of primitive ducts encompassed by mantles of variably differentiated mesenchyme and lined by cuboid to columnar, sometimes ciliated, epithelium unlike that in any normally developing or mature duct. Somewhat less important because of its variable presence is the finding of metaplastic cartilage. Primitive or fetal glomeruli with cuboid epithelium, primitive tubules, and ductules surrounded by narrow collars of laminated connective tissue and cysts of glomerular, tubule, and ductal origin may also be present, but because they might represent either a maldevelopment or a histologically similar degenerative change in previously normal although immature structures, they do not provide absolute evidence of parenchymal maldevelopment.

The extent of the renal lesion in these cases is variable and represents a broad spectrum of changes. At one extreme are the approximately aplastic or slightly more developed kidneys in which the ureteric bud is represented by only a few generations of abnormal duct branches and the metanephric blastema by poorly organized connective tissue containing only a few structures suggestive of nephron induction. At the other extreme are kidneys in which the only evidence of maldevelopment is the presence of relatively aborted or otherwise abnormal glomerular tufts, often in cystically dilated capsules. In between is an overlapping series in which there is at least partly normal development such that the general architectural pattern of the kidney is preserved despite the presence of ductal and mesenchymal dysplasia in a medullary, cortical, segmental, or only focal distribution.

Cyst formation may accompany any dysplastic defect as an incidental feature. Microdissection studies have shown the cysts to occur most often at the terminal ends of short primitive ducts in the most severely dysplastic kidneys and at the ends or along the course of collecting tubules and

*See also Chapter 2.

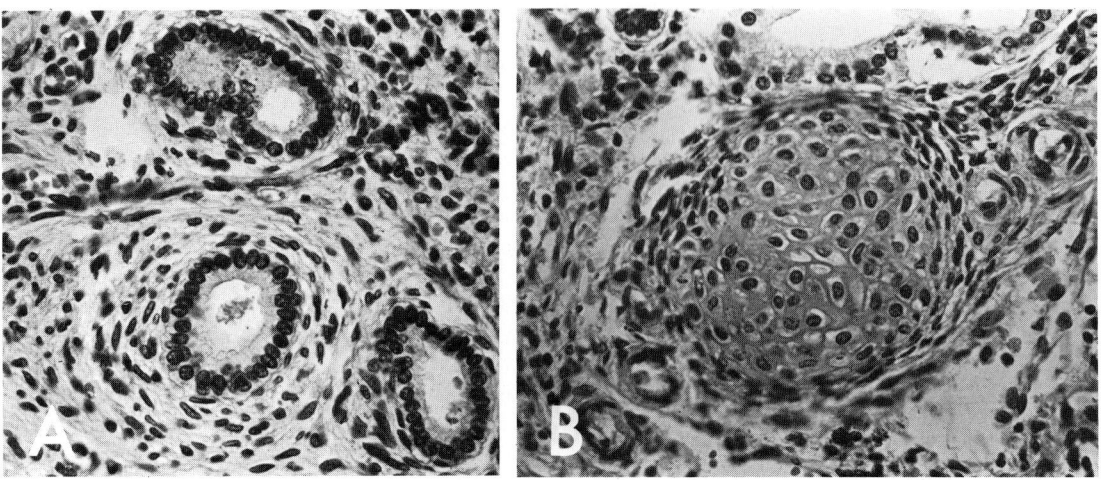

**Figure 38–18.** Renal dysplasia. The diagnostic microscopic features include primitive ducts *(A)* and metaplastic cartilage *(B)*.

terminal duct branches in less severe cases.[8] It must be emphasized, however, that cysts may or may not be present or, more accurately and with few exceptions, may range in size and number from small and few to large and numerous.

Because of the varying degrees and distributions of the dysplastic lesions as well as the varying sizes and distributions of incidental cysts, it is apparent that dysplastic kidneys will be found to be large or small, cystic or noncystic, and approximately normal in shape to grossly distorted. The most distorted cystic examples are said to resemble a bunch of grapes (Fig. 38–19).

## DIAGNOSIS

The clinical presentation and diagnosis of renal dysplasia are very much determined by the extent of the dysplastic involvement and by the degree of associated urinary obstruction. It is convenient, therefore, to consider two major clinicopathologic subsets of renal dysplasia, which for lack of a less confusing and more commonly accepted terminology, we call "total" and "subtotal" dysplasia. A third

uncommon subset of hereditary dysplasia is discussed separately.

**Total Dysplasia.** Kidneys with severe dysplasia involving both the cortex and the medulla (i.e., dysplasia affecting the total kidney) are nearly always, if not invariably, associated with ureteral or ureteropelvic absence or atresia. They contain solid areas consistent with rudimentary lobules but otherwise lack normal pyelocalyceal development and lobular organization.[231–233] A maldevelopment beginning in early gestation thus appears likely. Small, solid kidneys, termed "aplastic,"[234] and variably enlarged (up to several hundred grams) grossly cystic kidneys, termed "multicystic"[232, 235] (see Fig. 38–19), represent a spectrum ranging from small fibrotic nubbins at one end to large cystic masses at the other. All kidneys in this group are nonfunctional and are not visualized on excretory urograms, although high-dose urography may sometimes result in opacification of cyst walls and delayed films may demonstrate retention of contrast medium.[236] The ureter is found to be absent or atretic on a retrograde pyelogram. Cyst walls often calcify in older patients and may be seen as

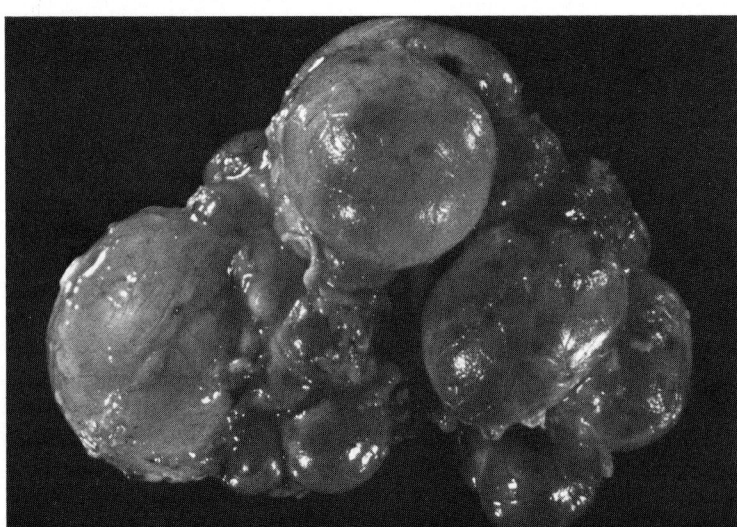

**Figure 38–19.** Severe renal cystic dysplasia (multicystic kidney). The renal architecture is markedly distorted.

ring-like densities in the region of the kidney.[237] The renal artery is usually small or absent. Ultrasonography and CT are also useful in diagnosis, and ultrasonography has revealed multicystic kidneys in fetuses in utero.[238–241]

Bilateral total dysplasia is fatal in the newborn period in association with Potter sequence of oligohydramnios and pulmonary insufficiency. When present as a unilateral isolated abnormality, however, a totally dysplastic kidney usually remains asymptomatic and is discovered incidentally during a renal or abdominal evaluation for unrelated reasons. In contrast to the less severely dysplastic kidneys that do have patent ureters (see later), these kidneys are not associated with hypertension or with infection.[235, 242] However, dysplastic kidneys are frequently ectopic, and a pelvic kidney is likely to be dysplastic. Furthermore, contralateral renal abnormalities are found in some 30% of cases and include, in addition to compensatory hypertrophy, an apparently increased susceptibility to hydronephrosis, lithiasis, and infection.[243] Particularly in autopsy series of newborns infants, there is a high frequency of bilateral defects (80%) and of other major anomalies in multiple organ systems that call attention to a diffuse embryonic defect.[8, 244]

The so-called multicystic variety of total renal dysplasia is about three times more common than the noncystic atrophic, or "hypodysplastic," variety and is the most common type of renal cystic disease throughout childhood. It is also the most common cause of abdominal mass in infancy and the most common type of bilateral cystic disease in neonates. The frequency is approximately 0.02 to 0.05 per 100,000 hospital admissions. Bilateral involvement is far less common than unilateral.[232] There is evidence that involution may occur after a maximal size has been reached and that so-called renal agenesis might in some cases actually represent an extreme form of involution of a multicystic kidney.[239, 245]

**Subtotal Dysplasia.** In contrast to the severely dysplastic kidneys with complete urinary obstruction, kidneys with partly normal development and dysplasia only in a medullary, cortical, or focal distribution are associated with evidence of less severe urinary obstruction in conditions such as ureteral narrowing, megaureter, megacystic megaureter,[246] posterior urethral valves or constriction, ectopic ureter with or without ureterocele,[228–230, 247] prune-belly syndrome,[248] and developmental neurospinal bladder dysfunction.[249] Segmental dysplasia is most common in the upper pole in association with ectopic ureterocele.[250–252] In general, urethral or other obstruction severe enough to be apparent shortly after birth is often accompanied by dysplasia of this type, whereas similar obstruction not manifest until later childhood is usually not.

In gross and radiographic appearance, subtotally dysplastic kidneys range from small with fewer than normal lobes to moderately large and normal or abnormal in shape, depending on the extent of the dysplasia and the incidental occurrence of cyst formation. They may be unilateral or bilateral. At the cost of some confusion with hypoplastic, secondarily atrophic, and aplastic dysgenetic kidneys, small kidneys in this subtotal dysplastic group are often referred to as hypoplastic dysplastic or hypodysplastic kidneys.

Kidneys with less than total dysplasia are functional to some extent and do appear on excretory urograms. Those with patent ureters also appear to be unusually liable to ascending infection. This has been attributed to an abnormal susceptibility of dysplastic tissue to infection,[234] to urinary stasis, or to concomitant, often asymmetric vesicoureteral reflux.[247, 253] Pyelonephritis is found in approximately 65% and lithiasis in 35% of cases[254] and, along with the progressive glomerular sclerosis, tubule atrophy, and interstitial fibrosis seen even in uncomplicated cases, may confuse the urologic and histopathologic picture. Hypertension is a complication in some 25%.[254] Prognosis is thus greatly influenced by secondary complications but, in general, is worse in patients with the most severe dysplasia. The frequency of contralateral and extra–urinary tract anomalies is high. The association in the literature of aplastic dysplastic kidneys with hypertension results mostly from a common failure to separate those cases from the small, hypoplastic dysplastic kidneys of the present group.

**Familial and Hereditary Dysplasia.** Not all dysplastic renal lesions are found in association with identifiable urinary tract obstruction. In addition to occasional examples of subtotal renal dysplasia indistinguishable from those just described, dysplastic changes are found in a wide variety of rare, often hereditary and familial disorders and multiple anomaly syndromes that presumably represent the expression of a nonspecific noxious, possibly metabolic stimulus at some critical time in renal development. Early interference with renal organogenesis would explain the occasionally severe dysplasias seen in Meckel and sometimes in Zellweger, Jeune, and oral-facial-digital syndromes. With these exceptions, however, the lesions tend to be mild, perhaps even limited to mildly abnormal glomeruli with cystic capsules (termed "peripheral cortical microcysts"), and usually produce no renal insufficiency.[255, 256] Terms such as micromulticystic, microcystic, pluricystic, multicystic, and even polycystic have been applied to these phenomena but should be read with great caution because the diseases bear no relationship to polycystic disease, either ARPKD or ADPKD. Excellent listings and discussions of these specific entities have appeared elsewhere.[7, 256–259]

## THERAPY

Bilateral totally dysplastic kidneys are rapidly fatal in the newborn period and require only supportive therapy. On the other hand, unilateral totally dysplastic, aplastic, or multicystic kidneys are usually asymptomatic and probably require only occasional follow-up. Neoplasms, both benign and malignant, have been reported in multicystic kidneys but are sufficiently rare that prophylactic nephrectomy is not warranted.

The subtotally dysplastic kidneys may be bilateral; unilateral subtotally dysplastic kidneys are associated with contralateral renal infection, lithiasis, or hydronephrosis. Renal failure may thus develop at some point and particularly in a growing child when the limited nephron population becomes insufficient to maintain adequate function in the face of increasing need. In general, treatment is directed first at relieving the often associated urinary obstruction and second at preventing infection. A subtotally dysplastic kidney should probably be removed when it is shown to be the probable cause of hypertension, hematuria, or recurrent infection. Partial nephrectomy may be effective in cases of segmental dysplasia. Particularly in infants, the renal status may be overshadowed by the multiple organ anomalies that frequently accompany renal dysplasia.

# MISCELLANEOUS RENAL CYSTIC DISORDERS

## Tuberous Sclerosis*

In this disease complex, hamartomatous tumors may develop in the skin, brain, retina, bone, liver, heart, lung, and kidney.[260] Renal angiomyolipomas are found in as many as 50% of cases[261–263] and must be distinguished from multiple renal cysts that occur less commonly. The tubule cysts in this disease are lined by a distinct, perhaps unique epithelium of markedly hypertrophic and hyperplastic cells with prominent eosinophilic cytoplasm bearing some resemblance to that of the proximal tubule. The combination of cystic kidneys and angiomyolipomas has been said to be virtually pathognomonic for tuberous sclerosis.[264, 265] The cysts may be large, and renal impairment, although relatively uncommon, may occur before other evidence of the syndrome.[256, 263, 266–268] Hypertension is a major manifestation of the renal abnormality. There have been several reports of associated renal carcinoma.[269–272]

Tuberous sclerosis has a frequency of approximately 1 per 10,000. It is inherited by autosomal dominant transmission; thus, family history is important in the diagnostic workup. Ultrasonography, CT, and arteriography are of value in distinguishing the multiple renal cysts from the more common angiomyolipomas in this disease and in ruling out ARPKD or ADPKD.

## von Hippel–Lindau Syndrome

This syndrome includes cerebellar and retinal hemangioblastomas, pancreatic cysts and carcinoma, and renal cysts and tumors. Numerous irregularly distributed renal cysts up to several centimeters in diameter are found in about 65% of cases. They occasionally are sufficiently numerous to simulate ADPKD.[273] The cyst lining is a flattened, nondescript or cuboid epithelium that focally may show nodular hyperplasia with apparent progression to clear cell carcinoma.[272, 274] These solid tumors are often multiple and bilateral.[275] Carcinomas occur in about one fourth of cases, metastasize in about half of those, and cause death in about one third.[272, 276, 277] Some of the renal cysts are surrounded by dense fibrous collars and appear to be involuting.

This disease is inherited by autosomal dominant transmission and usually presents in the third or fourth decade with visual or central nervous system complaints. The gene defect has been localized to the short arm of chromosome 3 and linked to an oncogene locus possibly involved in spontaneous renal cell carcinoma.[12] Because the chance for cancer to exist in a cyst wall or solid tumor is probably large, family screening and early diagnosis are imperative.

*See *Editor's note* at the end of the chapter.

CT is helpful in evaluating the renal lesions,[275, 278, 279] and in patients at risk, annual or semiannual examination is recommended, beginning in the second decade.[272, 280] A conservative approach has been advocated for the treatment of the associated renal adenocarcinomas.[272, 279, 281]

## Solitary Multilocular Cysts

Also termed benign cystic nephroma or papillary cystadenoma, these rare lesions are neoplasms arising from metanephric blastema.[282, 283] For proper diagnosis, the cystic lesions should be unilateral, solitary, and multilocular. The locules should not communicate with one another or with the pelvis and should be lined by flattened to cuboid epithelium. The septa dividing the locules should contain no fully developed nephrons, but the remainder of the kidney should be normal. On cut surface, the mass contains numerous individual cysts ranging from a few millimeters to a few centimeters in diameter and filled with clear fluid. Thin and delicate fibrous septa separate the locules and continue into a fibrous capsule that sharply circumscribes the lesion. Calcification, hemorrhage, and necrosis are usually absent. On microscopic examination, cysts and dilated tubules are surrounded by a loose mesenchymal stroma that contains clusters of small, poorly developed tubules. No cartilage or other strictly identifiable dysplastic structures are found within the lesion, although smooth muscle and cartilage have been described in the capsule.

Multilocular cysts have distinctive bimodal age and sex distributions.[283, 284] In one study, 88% of the lesions in males presented in the first 3 years of life, whereas in females 37% presented between ages 10 months and 15 years and 63% presented between 31 and 69 years, predominantly in the fifth and sixth decades. They are usually fairly large (5 to 10 cm in diameter) and often replace one pole. They are also capable of rapid growth and may be found in kidneys observed to be normal only a few years earlier. Even though these lesions are generally considered benign, extension beyond the renal capsule may be present. Furthermore, in 19 of the 200 or so reported cases, the multilocular mass has contained foci of nephroblastoma, sarcoma, or renal cell carcinoma. Three of four patients with sarcoma subsequently died of metastases.[283] Nonetheless, after angiographic and sonographic distinction from other potentially dangerous segmental renal lesions (particularly Wilms tumor and neuroblastoma in children), multilocular cysts require no specific therapy or, at most, partial nephrectomy. Occasionally, a locule of the cyst may prolapse into the renal pelvis to produce ureteropelvic obstruction.[285] Surgical relief may be required in such cases.

## Pyelocalyceal Cysts

Also termed pyelocalyceal diverticula or calyceal or pyelorenal cysts or diverticula, these lesions represent congenital, probably developmental saccular diverticula from a minor calyx (type I) or from the pelvis or adjacent major calyx (type II). Type I is more common, is usually located in the poles (especially the upper), and tends to be smaller and less often symptomatic than the centrally located type II variety. Both types are usually less than 1 cm in diameter but occasionally may be large. The cysts are encompassed by a muscularis, are lined by a usually chronically inflamed transitional epithelium, and usually contain cloudy fluid or frank pus that may be expressed with applied pressure. Transitional cell carcinoma arising in a pyelocalyceal cyst has been reported rarely.

Pyelocalyceal cysts occur sporadically, affect all age groups, and are almost always unilateral. They may be detected in as many as 0.5% of excretory urograms but are usually small and asymptomatic. Symptomatic lesions are more often of the larger or medium size and present with loin pain and evidence of recurrent pyelonephritis. Calculi are present within the cyst cavity in 10% to 40% of cases but are rarely passed. They may, however, be the cause of outlet obstruction and spontaneous cyst rupture into the perinephric space. Reviews of this subject, including radiographic diagnosis and the lithotripsy and surgical treatment of severe cases, are available.[286, 287]

## Renal Lymphangiomatosis

Also known as hilar lymphangiectasis, pericalyceal or paracalyceal lymphangiectasis, peripelvic or parapelvic lymphangiectasis, or polycystic disease of the renal sinus, renal lymphangiomatosis consists of cystically dilated renal lymphatic channels. They may be limited to the hilar region adjacent to major blood vessels or may extend approximately to the level of the corticomedullary junction.[288] Occasionally, they may also involve the renal capsule and adjacent areas and may simulate polycystic disease.[289] The cysts may be single and unilateral, multiple and unilateral, or multiple and bilateral. Their frequency is about 1% in autopsy series, and they usually occur in the fifth and sixth decades. The thin and collagenous cyst walls are lined by flattened cells having the histologic and electron microscopic characteristics of lymphatic endothelium.[289] The fluid contains albumin, lipid, and cholesterol and thus does not resemble urine.[290] Renal lymphangiomas are usually asymptomatic and are found incidentally. Sometimes, however, they present as a mass; as a cause of urinary obstruction, calculus formation, or infection; and perhaps even as a cause of renal ischemia and hypertension.[290–292] There is one report of association with nephrotic syndrome in an infant and one report of familial occurrence and of exacerbation during pregnancy.[293, 294] Diagnosis can be made by CT and ultrasonography.[295, 296]

## Hilar and Perinephric Pseudocysts

Hilar cysts are unlined spherical accumulations of clear, fat droplet–containing fluid within compressed fat of the renal sinus. They evidently result from atrophy of fat in debilitated patients.

Perinephric pseudocysts are unlined spaces filled with urine extravasated into the perirenal fascia after traumatic or spontaneous rupture of an underlying renal cyst. Some degree of chronic ureteral obstruction is probably also required, and extravasation may continue unless bleeding and clotting intervene.[295] There is a characteristic radiologic and CT appearance.[297] The most serious clinical complication is urinary obstruction requiring surgical intervention. Treatment is otherwise directed to the underlying cause. In one series, nephrectomy was eventually required in half of cases.[298]

# ANOMALIES OF RENAL POSITION, NUMBER, AND SIZE

## Renal Ectopia and Fusion

The metanephric kidneys begin their development as paired organs with blood supply from branches of the middle sacral and common iliac arteries. Disproportionate growth of the caudal region of the embryo then shifts their position to the approximate level of the first lumbar vertebra and their arterial supply to direct branches from the midabdominal aorta. This shift is accompanied by a change to the typical reniform shape and by a 90-degree rotation of the hilum from anterior to medial that brings the ureters to a more medial position. Failure to achieve normal position is termed "ectopia" and is found in approximately 1 in 800 urologic examinations. One or both kidneys may be involved. The ectopic kidney is usually lower than normal, anomalous in its blood supply (distinguishing it from simple ptosis), malrotated with hilum anterior or rarely lateral, and often disk shaped. In rare cases, it may be higher than normal and, with a frequency of perhaps 1 in 10,000, may be found in the thoracic cavity. Intrathoracic kidneys are about twice as common in males as in females and are about twice as common on the left side as on the right.[229, 299, 300] Their position is independent of that of the adrenal, which may be higher or lower. Bilateral examples have been reported. The function of intrathoracic kidneys is usually normal and their discovery incidental. An ectopic kidney may lie on the same side as its ureteral orifice (simple ectopia) or, with a frequency of 1 in 8000 postmortem studies, on the opposite side (crossed ectopia) where it lies below and is often fused with the kidney normal to that side (see duplex kidney).

Other urogenital and nonurogenital (particularly neural and cardiovascular) anomalies have been reported in a moderate to high percentage of cases of renal ectopia and are commonly the major source of complications.[301] A pelvic kidney is often associated with anorectal maldevelopment and is often dysplastic. The ureter of the ectopic kidney is usually short; frequently has an ectopic orifice in the vagina, urethra, or elsewhere along the course of the distal mesonephric duct; and may be compressed at the ureteropelvic junction by an artery to the malrotated renal hilum.

The most common form of ectopia (1 in 600) is fusion across the midline of the caudal portions only of bilateral kidneys (horseshoe kidney). Complete medial fusion or fusion at both caudal and cranial ends (ring kidney) is rare and at only the cranial ends exceptionally rare. The lower bridge of a horseshoe kidney often lies on the sacral promontory, where it is susceptible to trauma and may be palpated as an abdominal mass. Horseshoe kidneys are more common in males than in females (2:1) and have an increased frequency in persons with Turner and trisomy 18 syndromes.[302] In older children and adults, about one third have symptoms of infection, ureteral obstruction or reflux, or stone formation. ADPKD has been observed in horseshoe kidneys as an incidental feature.

# Supernumerary, Duplex, and Hyperplastic Kidneys

The presence of one or more supernumerary kidneys is rare. The supernumerary kidney is often small and nonfunctional and is usually located either caudal or cranial to a normal kidney. More rarely, it may be anterior or posterior. About half are served by a bifid ureter, the other ureter branch going to a normal kidney. The other half have a completely separate ureter that often has an ectopic orifice. In a review of 59 supernumerary kidneys in 58 patients (one bilateral), there was a significant frequency of hydronephrosis, pyelonephritis, and carcinoma in both the supernumerary and the ipsilateral kidney.[303] The diagnosis was usually made in the third or fourth decade.

Much more common (4% of the population) is a single unilateral (40%) or bilateral (60%) enlarged kidney mass with two pelves giving rise to two ureters (duplex kidney).[244] Associated extrarenal anomalies are common. The ureters may fuse at some point or have separate vesical orifices, an indication of premature ureteric bud division or of two separate buds. In the case of separate ureters, one ureteral orifice is often ectopic (usually urethral), and its intravesical portion is dilated to form a cyst or ureterocele (ectopic ureterocele). The ectopic ureter most often serves an upper renal pole that is hydronephrotic and often dysplastic.[230, 252] Ectopic ureterocele is seen mostly in children, is bilateral in 10% of cases, and presents with urinary tract infection. An intravesical ureterocele may obstruct the lower pole ureter or the bladder neck to produce ipsilateral or bilateral hydronephrosis. There is a marked female predominance.

In the sense that tubule and glomerular mass is in a developmental phase until adult size is achieved, any form of compensatory renal hyperplasia in childhood might legitimately be termed a developmental form of hyperplasia and is fairly common. On the other hand, if the definition of hyperplasia is restricted to kidneys with a demonstrably increased nephron population or number of lobes, its occurrence is exceptionally rare. Seven reported cases have been associated with gigantism of other organs.[304, 305]

# Renal Agenesis

The term "renal agenesis" implies that one of the renal anlagen, either the mesonephric duct and ureteric bud or the metanephric blastema, has failed to differentiate. Agenesis is thus distinct from dysplasia. Renal agenesis in the absence of a vesical hemitrigone or of a ureter alone thus indicates failure of the ductal or bud anlage, whereas a blind-end ureter but no kidney (a much less common finding) may indicate failure of the metanephric blastema. Renal agenesis may be unilateral or bilateral and occurs in approximately 1 per 1000 and 5000 births, respectively.[231, 306]

When the renal agenesis is unilateral, the initial defect evidently affects both the mesonephric duct and its adjacent structures, so that the ipsilateral vesical hemitrigone, adrenal, and ipsilateral fallopian tube and other genital tract structures may also be absent. Prognosis is affected by contralateral renal hypoplasia, dysplasia, and ureteral dilation in perhaps 50% of cases[244]; by an increased frequency of contralateral nephrolithiasis and infection in up to 70%[307]; and by associated anomalies of the cardiovascular, alimentary, respiratory, central nervous, genitourinary, or musculoskeletal systems in some 10%.[244, 308] Contralateral renal functional adaptation usually occurs but may be followed later by focal and segmental glomerulosclerosis with renal failure.[309]

In comparison to unilateral agenesis, bilateral renal agenesis reflects a greater suppression of structures arising from the posterior portion of the cloaca and the adjacent mesonephric and paramesonephric (müllerian) ducts that may be more widespread to affect the lower spine and legs (sirenomelus). The fallopian tubes are present, but the uterus and vagina are usually absent or abnormal.[8] Presumably owing to the lack of fetal micturition, there is usually oligohydramnios, amnion nodosum, postural deformities of the lower extremities, facial changes known as Potter facies, hypertrophic bladder, and pulmonary hypoplasia (Potter syndrome, also known as Potter sequence or oligohydramnios sequence).[8, 306] Death occurs in the perinatal period usually as a result of pulmonary maldevelopment and insufficiency rather than renal insufficiency.

Renal agenesis shows a 2:1 to 3:1 male predominance, particularly when bilateral. Although affected twins, affected siblings, and a familial tendency have been reported occasionally, and perhaps to the extent that other family members should be examined,[310] its occurrence is generally considered sporadic. There is an association with or an increased frequency in a variety of multiple anomaly syndromes.

# Renal Hypoplasia

During prenatal development, there are two or three phases of nephron induction resulting in kidneys weighing about 14 g each at birth and containing about 1,200,000 ± 200,000 nephrons.[311] During postnatal development, there is a further increase in kidney weight that correlates well with age and body size[312] and that comes about by an increase in tubule length and size, primarily in proximal tubules, and to a lesser extent by glomerular enlargement. Developmentally small kidneys might thus reflect one of four basic defects[313]: 1) an insufficient amount of metanephric blastema available for kidney production, 2) insufficient early duct branching resulting in less than the normal average number of renal lobes, 3) reduced nephron induction during the period of arcade and superficial nephron production resulting in a thin cortex, or 4) a retardation in the postnatal tubule and glomerular enlargement. In practice, however, kidneys that are hypoplastic on the basis of insufficient blastema have not been identified; hypoplastic kidneys due to a reduction in nephrogenesis have only rarely been seen in humans, and those attributable to postnatal developmental failure have been common only in autopsy series of young children with severe extra–urinary tract anomalies, particularly of the central nervous system.[244, 313] On the other hand, hypoplastic kidneys with only one or a few lobes are not uncommon as isolated anomalies and have been said to account for 10% of cases of renal failure in childhood.[314, 315]

Renal hypoplasia attributable to insufficient early branching of the ureteric bud, sometimes called true hypoplasia, is definitely identified by an abnormally small number of renal lobes, usually 1 to 5 in comparison to a normal complement of 9 or 10 lobes, and a weight less than 50% of that expected.[316] With greater technical difficulty, hypoplasia might also be confirmed by a measured reduction in the total nephron population. Hypoplasia is rare as a unilateral defect; statements to the contrary probably reflect an inappropriate inclusion of kidneys with secondary atrophy. Thus, reports that unilaterally hypoplastic kidneys are susceptible to lithiasis, infection, and vascular disease, or are the possible cause of hypertension, cannot be accepted without prejudice.

Bilateral true hypoplasia occurs in two forms. In a relatively small number of cases, the hypoplastic kidneys, at least initially, are histologically normal. These patients present in childhood with polyuria, salt wasting, and acidosis. Azotemia appears later or in association with stress, perhaps as the body mass or the renal demand increases relative to an insufficient renal mass.

The second form of true hypoplasia is a unique lesion termed ''oligomeganephronia'' or ''oligonephric hypoplasia'' and is the more common. These kidneys are small (combined weight as little as 20 g in children), usually have only a few lobes, and have a nephron population perhaps 20% of normal. At the same time, however, their glomeruli are as much as twice normal diameter, 5 times normal surface area, and 12 times normal volume. Their individual proximal tubules are disproportionally even larger, as great as 4 times normal length and 17 times normal volume.[317] There is often corresponding enlargement of the juxtaglomerular bodies, and the tubules may have small diverticula. Changes of this type have been described in a solitary kidney but not in the presence of a second normal kidney and may thus reflect an extreme attempt at compensation for a reduced nephron population, that is, a situation analogous to the effects of experimental subtotal nephrectomy. Later in the course, there develop progressive glomerular sclerosis, interstitial fibrosis, tubule atrophy, and a histologic picture that except for the enlarged glomeruli may be difficult to distinguish from end-stage glomerulonephritis or pyelonephritis. Oligomeganephronia appears not to be hereditary and, in contrast to other causes of bilaterally small kidneys (particularly dysplasia), is only rarely associated with urinary tract or other anomalies. There is a 3:1 male predominance.

Children with oligomeganephronia usually present in the first or second year of life with polyuria, polydipsia, vomiting, diarrhea, bouts of acute dehydration, and failure to thrive, all of which usually stabilize. The patients demonstrate defective $Na^+$ reabsorption, diminished creatinine

clearance, acidosis with low serum $HCO_3^-$ and high $Cl^-$ levels, and mild but persistent proteinuria. Renal insufficiency develops within 10 to 15 years as a possible consequence of both increasing body mass relative to kidney mass and the development of glomerular sclerosis with tubule atrophy and interstitial fibrosis. Hypertension is occasionally seen as a terminal feature. Treatment ultimately depends on dialysis and renal transplantation.

## Ask-Upmark Kidney

The problem of distinguishing among hypoplasia, dysplasia, and secondary change is well exemplified by a segmental renal abnormality referred to as the Ask-Upmark kidney or segmental atrophy.[318] As originally described, such a kidney, either unilateral or bilateral, had a reduced number of lobes (usually five) and was divided into upper and lower portions by a deep transverse groove. Subsequently, four different presentations have been described: 1) unilateral segmental atrophy with contralateral compensatory hypertrophy; 2) bilateral but asymmetrically segmental atrophy with one small kidney and contralateral normal-sized kidney with a single segmental lesion; 3) bilateral and nearly symmetric atrophy in small kidneys with one or several segmental lesions each; and 4) segmental atrophy in a normotensive latent period or with hypertension and superimposed renal dysplasia, oligomeganephronia, or urinary tract abnormality.[319]

Ask-Upmark kidney is seen predominantly in girls 5 to 14 years of age and presents most often after age 10 years. There is associated vesicoureteral reflux in 70% of cases.[320] Prognosis is related to the almost invariable appearance of hypertension, the successful treatment of which depends on the specific pattern of the defects.[319] Ophthalmoscopic changes, impairment of growth, proteinuria, and mild to severe renal insufficiency with decreased creatinine clearance and concentrating ability are seen in about half of cases. Intravenous urography usually shows calyces diverging on either side of a notch with decreased distance between the renal surface and the renal pelvis. CT may also aid in diagnosis. In addition to antihypertensive therapy, therapy is directed toward the often associated vesicoureteral reflux. Severe, persistent hypertension may require segmental or unilateral nephrectomy.

On the basis of the reduced number of renal lobes, the local abnormality of the pelvis, and the usual absence of glomeruli at the base of the groove, it was originally concluded that the Ask-Upmark lesions result from a diminution of early bud branching with subsequent local interference with further development of collecting tubules and nephron induction.[8, 318] In other words, the lesion was seen as a localized form of hypoplasia due to insufficient duct branching. Other authors, however, have pointed out that kidneys of similar gross and radiographic appearance may occur with dysplasia of papillary structures and with chronic pyelonephritis and have suggested that vesicoureteral reflux with intrarenal reflux may play an important role in development of all such defects.[321] Indeed, association with reflux is frequent,[320] and the development of typical renal lesions has been seen in sequential radiographic studies of these patients.[322] As a consequence, most authorities now consider Ask-Upmark kidney and segmental hypoplasia to be a condition identical with reflux nephropathy.

*Editor's note added in proof*

Genomic rearrangements, ascertained by cytogenetics or gel electrophoresis, have been identified in many genetic disorders. The tuberous sclerosis gene *TSC2* has been shown to be localized to a region on chromosome 16p13.3, which is deleted in patients affected with this disorder.[323] The European Chromosome 16 Tuberous Sclerosis Consortium, responsible for this discovery, also identified a pedigree in which two distinct phenotypes, TSC and ADPKD, are observed in different family members. Of interest, the two family members with ADPKD were shown to be carriers of chromosomal translocations with breakpoints within 16p13.3. This breakpoint has now been shown to contain a gene *(PKD1)* disrupted by this rearrangement, and the precise disruption has been defined.[324, 325] The European Consortium[324] and others[326–328] have shown that additional mutations of this gene occur in other ADPKD patients, thus establishing *PKD1* as the first gene recognized to cause ADPKD.

## REFERENCES

1. Grantham JJ: Fluid secretion, cellular proliferation, and the pathogenesis of renal epithelial cysts. J Am Soc Nephrol 3:1843, 1993.
2. Huseman R, Grady A, Welling D, Grantham J: Macropuncture study of polycystic disease in adult human kidneys. Kidney Int 18:375, 1980.
3. Evan AP, McAteer JA: Cyst cells and cyst walls. *In* Gardner KD Jr, Bernstein J: The Cystic Kidney. Kluwer Academic Publishers, Boston, 1990, pp 21–41.
4. Grantham JJ, Geiser JL, Evan AP: Cyst formation and growth in autosomal dominant polycystic kidney disease. Kidney Int 31:1145, 1987.
5. Gardner KD Jr: Cystic kidneys. Kidney Int 33:610, 1988.
6. Glassberg KI, Stephens FD, Lebowitz RL, et al: Renal dysgenesis and cystic disease of the kidney: A report of the committee on terminology, nomenclature and classification, section on urology. American Academy of Pediatrics. J Urol 138:1085, 1987.
7. Bernstein J: A classification of renal cysts. *In* Gardner KD Jr, Bernstein J (eds): The Cystic Kidney. Kluwer Academic Publishers, Boston, 1990, pp 147–170.
8. Potter EL: Normal and Abnormal Development of the Kidney. Year Book Medical Publishers, Chicago, 1972.
9. Gardner KD Jr, Bernstein J (eds): The Cystic Kidney. Kluwer Academic Publishers, Boston, 1990.
10. Iglesias CG, Torres VE, Offord KP, et al: Epidemiology of adult polycystic kidney disease. Olmsted Country, Minn: 1935–1980. Am J Kidney Dis 2:630, 1983.
11. Dalgaard OZ: Bilateral polycystic disease of the kidneys. A follow-up of two hundred and eighty four patients and their families. Acta Med Scand Suppl 328, 1957.
12. Reeders ST: The genetics of renal cystic disease. *In* Gardner KD Jr, Bernstein J: The Cystic Kidney. Kluwer Academic Publishers, Boston, 1990, pp 117–143.
13. Kimberling WJ, Fain PR, Kenyon JG, et al: Linkage heterogeneity of autosomal dominant polycystic kidney disease. N Engl J Med 319:913, 1988.
14. Romero G, Costa G, Catizone L, et al: A second genetic locus for autosomal dominant polycystic kidney disease. Lancet 2:7, 1988.
15. Peters DJM, Spruit L, Seris JJ, et al: Chromosome 4 localization of a second gene for autosomal dominant polycystic kidney disease. Nature Genet 5:359, 1993.
16. Kimberling WJ, Kumar S, Gabow PA, et al: Autosomal dominant polycystic kidney disease: Localization of the second gene to chromosome 4q13-q23. Genomics 18:467, 1993.
17. Kaariainen H: Polycystic kidney disease in children: A genetic and epidemiological study of 82 Finnish patients. J Med Genet 24:474, 1987.
18. Churchill DN, Bear JC, Morgan J, et al: Prognosis of adult onset polycystic kidney disease reevaluated. Kidney Int 26:190, 1984.
19. Huston J III, Torres VE, Sullivan PP, et al: Value of magnetic resonance angiography for detection of intracranial aneurysms in autosomal dominant polycystic kidney disease. J Am Soc Nephrol 3:1871, 1993.
20. Chapman AB, Johnson AM, Gabow PA: Intracranial aneurysms in patients with autosomal dominant polycystic kidney disease: How to diagnose and who to screen. Am J Kidney Dis 22:526, 1993.
21. Sedman A, Bell P, Manco-Johnson M, et al: Autosomal dominant polycystic kidney disease in childhood: A longitudinal study. Kidney Int 31:1000, 1987.
22. Gregoire JR, Torres VE, Holley KE, Farrow GM: Renal epithelial hyperplastic and neoplastic proliferation in autosomal dominant polycystic kidney disease (ADPKD). Am J Kidney Dis 9:27, 1987.
23. Levine E, Grantham JJ: High-density renal cysts in autosomal dominant polycystic kidney disease demonstrated by CT. Radiology 154:477, 1985.
24. Ye M, Grantham JJ: The secretion of fluid by renal cysts from patients with autosomal dominant polycystic kidney disease. N Engl J Med 329:310, 1993.
25. Cuppage FE, Huseman RA, Chapman A, Grantham JJ: Ultrastructure and function of cysts from human adult polycystic kidneys. Kidney Int 17:373, 1980.
26. Gardner KD Jr, Burnside JS, Skipper BJ, et al: On the probability that kidneys are different in autosomal dominant polycystic disease. Kidney Int 42:1199, 1992.
27. Grüfeld JP, Albouze G, Jungers P, et al: Liver changes and complications in adult polycystic kidney disease. Adv Nephrol 14:1, 1984.
28. Segal AJ, Spataro RF: Computed tomography of adult polycystic disease. J Comput Assist Tomogr 6:777, 1982.
29. Gabow PA, Johnson AM, Kaehny WD, et al: Risk factors for the development of hepatic cysts in autosomal dominant polycystic kidney disease. Hepatology 11:1033, 1990.
30. Levine E, Cook LT, Grantham JJ: Liver cysts in autosomal dominant polycystic kidney disease: Clinical and computed tomographic study. AJR 145:229, 1985.
31. Thomsen HS, Thaysen JH: Frequency of hepatic cysts in adult polycystic kidney disease. Acta Med Scand 224:381, 1988.
32. Coffin B, Hadengue A, Degos F, Benhamou JP: Calcified hepatic and renal cysts in adult dominant polycystic kidney disease. Dig Dis Sci 35:1172, 1990.
33. Terada T, Nakanuma Y: Congenital biliary dilation in autosomal dominant adult polycystic disease of the liver and kidneys. Arch Pathol Lab Med 112:1113, 1988.
34. Cobben JM, Breuning MH, Schoots C, et al: Congenital hepatic fibrosis in autosomal-dominant polycystic kidney disease. Kidney Int 38:880, 1990.
35. Torres VE, Wiebers DO, Forbes GS: Cranial computed tomography and magnetic resonance imaging in autosomal dominant polycystic kidney disease. J Am Soc Nephrol 1:84, 1990.
36. Levey AS, Pauker SG, Kassirer JP: Occult intracranial aneurysms in polycystic kidney disease. N Engl J Med 308:986, 1983.
37. Wiebers DL: General features of autosomal dominant polycystic kidney disease. L. Management of unruptured intracranial aneurysms. *In* Grantham JJ, Gardner KD (eds): Problems in Diagnosis and Management of Polycystic Kidney Disease. Proceedings of the First International Workshop on Polycystic Kidney Disease. PKR Foundation, Kansas City, MO, 1985, pp 145–153.
38. Schievink WI, Torres VE, Piepgras DG, Wiebers DO: Saccular intracranial aneurysms in autosomal dominant polycystic kidney disease. J Am Soc Nephrol 3:88, 1992.
39. Chapman AB, Rubinstein D, Hughes R, et al: Intracranial aneurysms in autosomal dominant polycystic kidney disease. N Engl J Med 327:916, 1992.
40. Montoliu J, Torras A, Revert L: Polycystic kidneys and abdominal aortic aneurysms. Lancet 1:1133, 1980. Letter.
41. Chapman JR, Hilson AJW: Polycystic kidneys and abdominal aortic aneurysms. Lancet 1:646, 1980. Letter.

42. Leier CV, Baker PB, Kilman JW, Wooley CF: Cardiovascular abnormalities associated with adult polycystic kidney disease. Ann Intern Med 100:683, 1984.

43. Hossack KF, Leddy CL, Schrier RW, Gabow PA: Incidence of cardiac abnormalities associated with autosomal dominant polycystic kidney disease (ADPKD). Kidney Int 31:203, 1987.

44. Torres EE, Holley KE, Offord KP: General features of autosomal dominant polycystic kidney disease. A. Epidemiology. *In* Grantham JJ, Gardner KD (eds): Problems in Diagnosis and Management of Polycystic Kidney Disease. Proceedings of the First International Workshop on Polycystic Kidney Disease. PKR Foundation, Kansas City, MO, 1985, pp 49–69.

45. Tan KH, Donner R, Oe PE: Renal carcinoma associated with polycystic kidneys: Occurrence after chronic hematuria and hypertension. J Urol 118:322, 1977.

46. Bernstein J, Evan AP, Gardner KD Jr: Epithelial hyperplasia in human polycystic kidney diseases. Its role in pathogenesis and risk of neoplasia. Am J Pathol 129:92, 1987.

47. Martinez-Maldonado M, Yium JJ, Eknoyan G, Suki WN: Adult polycystic kidney disease: Studies of the defect in urine concentration. Kidney Int 2:107, 1972.

48. D'Angelo A, Mioni G, Ossl E, et al: Alterations in renal tubular sodium and water transport in polycystic kidney disease. Clin Nephrol 3:99, 1975.

49. Martinez-Maldonado M, Yium JJ, Suki WN, Eknoyan G: Electrolyte excretion in polycystic kidney disease: Interrelationship between sodium, calcium, magnesium and phosphate. J Lab Clin Med 90:1066, 1977.

50. Preuss H, Geoly K, Johnson M, et al: Tubular function in adult polycystic kidney disease. Nephron 24:198, 1979.

51. Duncan KA, Cuppage FE, Grantham JJ: Urinary lipid bodies in polycystic kidney disease. Am J Kidney Dis 5:49, 1985.

52. Levine E, Grantham JJ: The role of computed tomography in the evaluation of adult polycystic kidney disease. Am J Kidney Dis 1:99, 1981.

53. Levine E, Grantham JJ: Radiology of cystic kidneys. *In* Gardner KD Jr, Bernstein J: The Cystic Kidney. Kluwer Academic Publishers, Boston, 1990, pp 171–206.

54. Kimberling WJ, Pieke-Dahl SA, Kumar S: The genetics of cystic diseases of the kidney. Semin Nephrol 11:596, 1991.

55. Sujanski E, Kreutzer SB, Johnson AM, et al: Attitudes of at-risk and affected individuals regarding presymptomatic testing for autosomal dominant polycystic kidney disease. Am J Med Genet 35:510, 1990.

56. Hannig VL, Hopkins JR, Johnson HK, et al: Presymptomatic testing for adult onset polycystic kidney disease in at-risk kidney transplant donors. Am J Med Genet 40:425, 1991.

57. Zeier M, Geberth S, Mandelbaum A, Ritz E: Elevated blood pressure profile and left ventricular mass in children and young adults with autosomal dominant polycystic kidney disease. J Am Soc Nephrol 3:1451, 1993.

58. Torres VE, Young WF Jr, Offord KP, Hattery RP: Association of hypokalemia, aldosteronism and renal cysts. N Engl J Med 322:345, 1990.

59. Gabow PA, Duley I, Johnson AM: Clinical profiles of gross hematuria in autosomal dominant polycystic kidney disease. Am J Kidney Dis 20:140, 1992.

60. Gabow PA, Johnson AM, Kaehny WD, et al: Factors affecting the progression of renal disease in autosomal dominant polycystic kidney disease. Kidney Int 41:1311, 1992.

61. Gernert JE, Stein J, Bischoff AJ: Solitary renal cysts: Experience with 100 cases. J Urol 100:251, 1968.

62. Umemasu J, Fujiwara M, Munemura C, et al: Effects of topical instillation of minocycline hydrochloride on cyst size and renal function in polycystic kidney disease. Clin Nephrol 39:140, 1993.

63. Elzinga LW, Barry JM, Torres VE, et al: Cyst decompression for autosomal dominant polycystic kidney disease. J Am Soc Nephrol 2:1219, 1992.

64. Elzinga LW, Barry JM, Lowe B, et al: Laparoscopic cyst decompression for refractory pain in polycystic kidney disease. *In* Gabow PA, Grantham JJ (eds): Proceedings of the Fifth International Workshop on Polycystic Kidney Disease. PKR Foundation, Kansas City, MO, 1993, p 134.

65. Grantham JJ: Renal pain in polycystic kidney disease: When the hurt won't stop. J Am Soc Nephrol 2:1161, 1992.

66. Harley JD, Shen FH, Carter SJ: Transcatheter infarction of a polycystic kidney for control of recurrent hemorrhage. AJR 134:818, 1980.

67. Schwab SJ, Bander SJ, Klahr S: Renal infection in autosomal dominant polycystic kidney disease. Am J Med 82:714, 1987.

68. Sfakianakis GB, Al-Sheikh W, Heal A, et al: Comparisons of sonography with In-111 leukocytes and Ga-67 in the diagnosis of occult sepsis. J Nucl Med 23:618, 1982.

69. Muther RS, Bennett WM: Cyst fluid antibiotic concentrations in polycystic kidney disease: Differences between proximal and distal cysts. Kidney Int 20:519, 1981.

70. Schwab S, Hinthorn D, Diederich D, et al: pH-dependent accumulation of clindamycin in a polycystic kidney. Am J Kidney Dis 3:63, 1983.

71. Elzinga LW, Golper TA, Rashad AL, et al: Trimethoprim-sulfamethoxazole in cyst fluid from autosomal dominant polycystic kidneys. Kidney Int 32:884, 1987.

72. Higashihara E, Aso Y, Shimazaka J, et al: Clinical aspects of polycystic kidney disease. J Urol 147:329, 1992.

73. Gabow PA, Chapman AB, Johnson AM, et al: Renal structure and hypertension in autosomal dominant polycystic kidney disease. Kidney Int 38:1177, 1990.

74. Chapman AB, Johnson A, Gabow PA, Schrier RW: The renin-angiotensin-aldosterone system and autosomal dominant polycystic kidney disease. N Engl J Med 323:1091, 1990.

75. Watson ML, Manicol AM, Allan PL, Wright AF: Effects of angiotensin converting enzyme inhibition in adult polycystic kidney disease. Kidney Int 41:206, 1992.

76. Chapman AB, Gabow PA, Schrier RW: Reversible renal failure associated with angiotensin-converting enzyme inhibition in polycystic kidney disease. Ann Intern Med 115:769, 1991.

77. Gabow PA: Autosomal dominant polycystic kidney disease. N Engl J Med 329:332, 1993.

78. Torres VE, Erickson SB, Smith LH, et al: The association of nephrolithiasis and autosomal dominant polycystic kidney disease. Am J Kidney Dis 11:318, 1988.

79. Torres VE, Wilson DM, Hattery RR, Segura JW: Renal stone disease in autosomal dominant polycystic kidney disease. Am J Kidney Dis 22:513, 1993.

80. Everson GT: Hepatic cysts in autosomal dominant polycystic kidney disease. Am J Kidney Dis 22:520, 1993.

81. Everson GT, Scherzinger A, Berger-Leff N, et al: Polycystic liver disease: Quantitation of parenchymal and cyst volume from computed tomography and clinical correlates of hepatic cysts. Hepatology 8:1627, 1988.

82. Newman KD, Torres VE, Rakela J, Nagorney D: The treatment of highly symptomatic polycystic liver disease. Preliminary evidence for a combined hepatic resection-fenestration procedure. Ann Surg 212:30, 1990.

83. Scheff RT, Zukerman G, Harter H, et al: Diverticular disease in patients with chronic renal failure due to polycystic kidney disease. Ann Intern Med 92:202, 1980.

84. Parfrey PS, Bear JC, Morgan J, et al: The diagnosis and prognosis of autosomal dominant polycystic kidney disease. N Engl J Med 323:1085, 1990.

85. Klahr S, Levey AS, Beck GJ, et al: The effects of dietary protein restriction and blood-pressure control on the progression of chronic renal disease. N Engl J Med 330:877, 1994.

86. Gretz N, Zeier M, Geberth S, et al: Is gender a determinant for evolution of renal failure? A study in autosomal dominant polycystic kidney disease. Am J Kidney Dis 14:178, 1989.

87. Klahr S, Breyer JA, Beck GJ, et al: Dietary protein restriction, blood pressure control and the progression of polycystic kidney disease. J Am Soc Nephrol (in press).

88. Gabow PA, Bennett WM: Renal manifestations: Complications, management and long-term outcome of autosomal dominant polycystic kidney disease. Semin Nephrol 11:643, 1991.

89. Ritz E, Seier M, Geberth S, et al: Dialysis and transplantation management in ADPKD. *In* Gabow PA, Grantham JJ (eds): Proceedings of the Fifth International Workshop on Polycystic Kidney Disease. PKR Foundation, Kansas City, MO, 1993, p 51.

90. Manjoney DM, McKegney FP: Individual and family coping with polycystic disease: The harvest of denial. Int J Psychiatry Med 9:19, 1978.

91. Grantham JJ: Polycystic kidney disease: A predominance of giant nephrons. Am J Physiol 244:F3, 1983.

92. Bear JC, McManamon P, Morgan J, et al: Age at clinical onset and at ultrasonographic detection of adult polycystic disease: Data for genetic counselling. Am J Med Genet 18:45, 1984.

93. Higashihara E, Nutahara K, Minowada S, et al: Percutaneous reduction of cyst volume of polycystic kidney disease: Effects on renal function. J Urol 147:1482, 1992.

94. Cole BR, Conley SB, Stapleton FB: Polycystic kidney disease in the first year of life. J Pediatr 111:693, 1987.

95. Blyth H, Ockenden BG: Polycystic disease of kidneys and liver presenting in childhood. J Med Genet 8:257, 1971.

96. Cole BR: Autosomal recessive polycystic kidney disease. In Gardner KD Jr, Bernstein J (eds): The Cystic Kidney. Kluwer Academic Publishers, Boston, 1990, pp 327–350.

97. Kaplan BS, Kaplan P, de Chadarevian JP, et al: Variable expression of autosomal recessive polycystic kidney disease and congenital hepatic fibrosis within a family. Am J Med Genet 29:639, 1988.

98. Wirth B, Zerres K, Fischbach M, et al: Autosomal recessive and dominant forms of polycystic kidney disease are not allelic. Hum Genet 77:221, 1987.

99. Ramsay M, Reeders ST, Thomson PD: Mutations for the autosomal recessive and the autosomal dominant form of polycystic kidney disease are not allelic. Hum Genet 79:73, 1988.

100. Kaariainen H, Koskimies O, Norio R: Dominant and recessive polycystic kidney disease in children: Evaluation of clinical features and laboratory data. Pediatr Nephrol 2:296, 1988.

101. Gagnadoux M-F, Habib R, Levy M, et al: Cystic renal diseases in children. Adv Nephrol 18:33, 1989.

102. Osathanondh V, Potter EL: Pathogenesis of polycystic kidneys. Type I due to hyperplasia of collecting tubules. Arch Pathol 77:466, 1964.

103. Faraggiana T, Bernstein J, Strauss L, Churg J: Use of lectins in the study of histogenesis of renal cysts. Lab Invest 53:575, 1985.

104. Verani R, Walker P, Silva FG: Renal cystic disease of infancy: Results of histochemical studies. Pediatr Nephrol 3:37, 1989.

105. Six R, Oliphant M, Grossman H: A spectrum of renal tubule ectasia and hepatic fibrosis. Radiology 117:117, 1975.

106. Bernstein J, Stickler GB, Neel IV: Congenital hepatic fibrosis: Evolving morphology. APMIS Suppl 4:17, 1988.

107. Jorgensen MJ: The ductal plate malformation. Acta Pathol Microbiol Scand Suppl 25:1, 1977.

108. Nakanuma Y, Terada T, Ohta G, et al: Caroli's disease in congenital hepatic fibrosis and infantile polycystic disease. Liver 2:346, 1982.

109. Marchal GJ, Desmet VJ, Proesmans WC, et al: Caroli disease: High-frequency US and pathologic findings. Radiology 158:507, 1986.

110. Gang DL, Herrin JT: Infantile polycystic disease of the liver and kidneys. Clin Nephrol 25:28, 1986.

111. Landing BH, Wells TR, Claireaux AE: Morphometric analysis of liver lesions in cystic diseases of childhood. Hum Pathol 11:549, 1980.

112. Kerr DNS, Harrison CV, Sherlock S, Walter RM: Congenital hepatic fibrosis. Q J Med 30:91, 1961.

113. Desmet VJ: What is congenital hepatic fibrosis? Histopathology 20:465, 1992.

114. Boal DK, Teele RL: Sonography of infantile polycystic kidney disease. AJR 135:575, 1980.

115. Habif DV Jr, Berdon WE, Yeh M-N: Infantile polycystic kidney disease: In utero sonographic diagnosis. Radiology 142:475, 1982.

116. Melson GL, Shackelford GD, Cole BR, McClennan BL: The spectrum of sonographic findings in infantile polycystic kidney disease with urographic and clinical correlations. J Clin Ultrasound 13:113, 1985.

117. Zerres K, Hansmann M, Mallmann R, Gembruch U: Autosomal recessive polycystic kidney disease. Problems of prenatal diagnosis. Prenat Diagn 8:215, 1988.

118. Reuss A, Wladimiroff JW, Stewart PA, Niermeijer MF: Prenatal diagnosis by ultrasound in pregnancies at risk for autosomal recessive polycystic kidney disease. Ultrasound Med Biol 16:355, 1990.

119. Howie JL, Nicholson RL: CT evaluation of infantile polycystic disease. J Can Assoc Radiol 31:202, 1980.

120. Berger PE, Munschauer RW, Kuhn JP: Computed tomography and ultrasound of renal and perirenal diseases in infants and children. Pediatr Radiol 9:91, 1980.

121. Townsend RR, Goldstein RB, Filly RA, et al: Sonographic identification of autosomal recessive polycystic kidney disease associated with increased maternal serum/amniotic fluid alpha-fetoprotein. Obstet Gynecol 71:1008, 1989.

122. Mauseth R, Lieberman E, Heuser ET: Infantile polycystic disease of the kidneys and Ehlers-Danlos syndrome in an 11-year-old patient. J Pediatr 90:81, 1977.

123. Vlachos J, Tsakraklidis V: Glomerular cysts, an unusual variety of "polycystic kidneys." Am J Dis Child 114:379, 1967.

124. Krous HF, Richie JP, Sellers B: Glomerulocystic kidney. Arch Pathol Lab Med 101:462, 1977.

125. McDonald RA, Avner ED: Inherited polycystic kidney disease in children. Semin Nephrol 11:632, 1991.

126. Alvarez F, Bernard O, Brunelle F, et al: Congenital hepatic fibrosis in children. J Pediatr 99:370, 1981.

127. Dunnill MS, Millard PR, Oliver D: Acquired cystic disease of the kidneys: A hazard of long-term intermittent maintenance haemodialysis. J Clin Pathol 30:868, 1977.

128. Miller LR, Soffer O, Nassar VH, Kutner MH: Acquired renal cystic disease in end-stage renal disease: An autopsy study of 155 cases. Am J Nephrol 9:322, 1989.

129. Ishikawa I: Acquired renal cystic disease. In Gardner KD Jr, Bernstein J (eds.): The Cystic Kidney. Kluwer Academic Publishers, Boston, 1990, pp 351–377.

130. Matson MA, Cohen EP: Acquired cystic kidney disease: Occurrence, prevalence, and renal cancers. Medicine (Baltimore) 69:217, 1990.

131. Ishikawa I: Uremic acquired renal cystic disease. Natural history and complications. Nephron 58:257, 1991.

132. Ishikawa I: Acquired cystic disease: Mechanisms and manifestations. Semin Nephrol 11:671, 1991.

133. Grantham JJ: Acquired cystic kidney disease. Kidney Int 40:143, 1991.

134. Mallofre C, Almirall J, Campistol JM, et al: Acquired renal cystic disease in HD: A study of 82 nephrectomies in young patients. Clin Nephrol 37:297, 1992.

135. Hogg RJ: Acquired renal cystic disease in children prior to the start of dialysis. Pediatr Nephrol 6:176, 1992.

136. Ishikawa I, Shikura N, Kitada H, et al: Severity of acquired renal cysts in native kidneys and renal allograft with long-standing poor function. Am J Kidney Dis 14:18, 1989.

137. Chung WY, Nast CC, Ettenger PB, et al: Acquired cystic disease in chronically rejected renal transplants. J Am Soc Nephrol 2:1298, 1992.

138. Mickisch O, Bommer J, Bachmann S, et al: Multicystic transformation of kidneys in chronic renal failure. Nephron 38:93, 1984.

139. Gardner KD Jr, Evan AP: Cystic kidneys: An enigma evolves. Am J Kidney Dis 3:403, 1984.

140. Grantham JJ, Levine E: Acquired cystic disease: Replacing one kidney disease with another. Kidney Int 28:99, 1985.

141. Gehrig JJ Jr, Gottheiner TI, Swenson RS: Acquired cystic disease of the end-stage kidney. Am J Med 79:609, 1985.

142. Hughson MD, Buckwald D, Fox M: Renal neoplasia and acquired cystic kidney disease in patients receiving long term dialysis. Arch Pathol Lab Med 110:592, 1986.

143. Bretan PN Jr, Busch MP, Hrick H, Williams RD: Chronic renal failure: A significant risk factor in the development of acquired renal cysts and renal cell carcinoma. Case reports and review of the literature. Cancer 57:1971, 1986.

144. Levine E, Grantham JJ, Slusher SL, et al: CT of acquired cystic kidney disease and renal tumors in long-term dialysis patients. AJR 142:125, 1984.

145. MacDougall ML, Welling LW, Wiegmann TB: Renal adenocarcinoma and acquired cystic disease in chronic hemodialysis patients. Am J Kidney Dis 9:166, 1987.

146. Boileau M, Folev R, Flechner S, Weinman E: Renal adenocarcinoma and end stage kidney disease. J Urol 138:603, 1987.

147. Ishikawa I, Saito Y, Shikura N, et al: Ten-year prospective study on the development of renal cell carcinoma in dialysis patients. Am J Kidney Dis 16:452, 1990.

148. Levine E: Renal cell carcinoma in uremic acquired renal cystic disease: Incidence, detection, and management. Urol Radiol 13:203, 1992.

149. MacDougall ML, Welling LW, Wiegmann TB: Prediction of carcinoma in acquired cystic disease as a function of kidney weight. J Am Soc Nephrol 1:828, 1990.

150. Feiner HD, Katz LA, Gallo GR: Acquired cystic disease of kidney in chronic dialysis patients. Urology 17:260, 1981.

151. Vandeursen H, Van Damme B, Baert J, Baert L: Acquired cystic disease of the kidney analyzed by microdissection. J Urol 146:1168, 1991.

152. McManus JF, Hughson MD, Henningar GR, et al: Dialysis enhances renal epithelial proliferations. Arch Pathol Lab Med 104:192, 1980.
153. Hughson MD, Henningar GR, McManus JFA: Atypical cysts, acquired renal cystic disease, and renal cell tumors in end stage dialysis kidneys. Lab Invest 42:475, 1980.
154. Ishikawa I, Saito Y, Onouchi Z, et al: Development of acquired cystic disease and adenocarcinoma of the kidney in glomerulonephritic chronic hemodialysis patients. Clin Nephrol 14:1, 1980.
155. Fayemi AO, Ali M: Acquired renal cysts and tumors superimposed on chronic primary kidney disease. Pathol Res Pract 168:73, 1980.
156. Krempien B, Ritz E: Acquired cystic transformation of the kidneys of hemodialyzed patients. Arch Pathol Anat Histol 386:189, 1980.
157. Miach PJ, Dawborn JK, Zipell J: Neoplasia in patients with chronic renal failure on long-term dialysis. Clin Nephrol 5:101, 1976.
158. Sutherland GA, Blass J, Babriel R: Increased incidence of malignancy in chronic renal failure. Nephron 18:182, 1977.
159. Ishikawa I, Yuri T, Kitada H, Shinoda A: Regression of acquired cystic disease of the kidney after successful renal transplantation. Am J Nephrol 3:310, 1983.
160. Vaziri ND, Darwish R, Martin DC, Hostetler J: Acquired renal cystic disease in renal transplant recipients. Nephron 37:203, 1984.
161. Levine E, Grantham JJ, MacDougall ML: Spontaneous subcapsular and perinephric hemorrhage in end-stage kidney disease: Clinical and CT findings. AJR 148:755, 1987.
162. Levine E, Slusher SL, Grantham JJ, Wetzel LH: Natural history of acquired renal cystic disease in dialysis patients: A prospective longitudinal CT study. AJR 156:501, 1991.
163. Antignac C, Arduy C, Beckman JS, et al: A gene for familial juvenile nephronophthisis (recessive medullary cystic kidney disease) maps to chromosome 2p. Nature Genet 3:342, 1992.
164. Gardner KD Jr: Juvenile nephronophthisis and renal medullary cystic disease. In Gardner KD Jr (ed): Cystic Diseases of the Kidney. John Wiley & Sons, New York, 1976, pp 173–185.
165. Avasthi PS, Erickson DG, Gardner KD: Hereditary renal-retinal dysplasia and the medullary cystic disease–nephronophthisis complex. Ann Intern Med 84:157, 1976.
166. Schimke RN: Hereditary renal-retinal dysplasia. Ann Intern Med 70:735, 1969.
167. Malnzer F, Saldino RM, Ozonoff MB, Minagi H: Familial nephropathy associated with retinitis pigmentosa, cerebral ataxia and skeletal abnormalities. Am J Med 49:556, 1970.
168. Senior B: Familial renal-retinal dystrophy. Am J Dis Child 125:442, 1973.
169. Collenberg JJM van Thompson MW, Huber JL: Clinical, pathological and genetic aspects of a form of cystic disease of the renal medulla: Familial juvenile nephronophthisis. Clin Nephrol 9:55, 1978.
170. Robins DG, French TA, Chakera TMH: Juvenile nephronophthisis associated with skeletal abnormalities and hepatic fibrosis. Arch Dis Child 51:799, 1976.
171. Sherman FE, Studnicki FM, Fetterman GH: Renal lesions of familial juvenile nephronophthisis examined by microdissection. Am J Clin Pathol 55:391, 1971.
172. Zollinger HU, Mihatsch MJ, Edfonti A, et al: Nephrolithiasis (medullary cystic disease of the kidney). A study using electron microscopy, immunofluorescence, and a review of the morphological findings. Helv Paediatr Acta 35:509, 1980.
173. Pascal RR: Medullary cystic disease of the kidney. Study of a case with scanning and transmission electron microscopy and light microscopy. Am J Clin Pathol 59:659, 1973.
174. Matsubara K, Susuki K, Lin YW, et al: Familial juvenile nephronophthisis in two siblings—histological findings at an early stage. Acta Paediatr Jpn 33:482, 1991.
175. Link DP, Hansen S, Palmer J: High dose excretory urography and medullary cystic disease of the kidney. AJR 133:303, 1979.
176. Fyhrquist FY, Klockars M, Gordin A, et al: Hyperreninemia, lysozymuria, and erythrocytosis in Fanconi syndrome with medullary cystic kidney. Acta Med Scand 207:359, 1980.
177. Mitch WE, Walser M, Buffington GA, Lemann J: A simple method of estimating progression of chronic renal failure. Lancet 2:1326, 1976.
178. Steele BT, Lirenman DS, Beattie CW: Nephronophthisis. Am J Med 68:531, 1980.
179. Kutper JJ: Medullary sponge kidney. In Gardner KD Jr (ed): Cystic Diseases of the Kidney. John Wiley & Sons, New York, 1976, pp 151–171.
180. Yendt ER: Medullary sponge kidney. In Gardner KD Jr, Bernstein J: The Cystic Kidney. Kluwer Academic Publishers, Boston, 1990, pp 379–391.
181. Sprayragen S, Strasberg Z, Naidich TP: Medullary sponge kidney and congenital total hypertrophy. N Y State J Med 73:2768, 1973.
182. Harrison AR, Rose GA: Medullary sponge kidney. Urol Res 7:197, 1979.
183. Zawada ET Jr, Sica DA: Differential diagnosis of medullary sponge kidney. South Med J 77:686, 1984.
184. Reed JR, Rutsky EA, Witten DM: Medullary sponge kidney presenting as polycystic renal disease. South Med J 77:909, 1984.
185. Choong M, Phillips GWL: Renal transitional cell carcinoma mimicking medullary sponge kidney. Br J Radiol 64:275, 1991.
186. Kaver I, Flanders EL, Kay S, Koontz WW Jr: Segmental medullary sponge kidney mimicking a renal mass. J Urol 141:1181, 1989.
187. Levine E: Computed tomography of renal abscesses complicating medullary sponge kidney. J Comput Assist Tomogr 3:440, 1989.
188. Ginalski JM, Portmann L, Jaeger P: Does medullary sponge kidney cause nephrolithiasis? AJR 155:299, 1990.
189. Parks JH, Coe FL, Strauss AL: Calcium nephrolithiasis and medullary sponge kidney in women. N Engl J Med 306:1088, 1982.
190. O'Neill M, Breslau NA, Pak CY: Metabolic evaluation of nephrolithiasis in patients with medullary sponge kidney. JAMA 245:1233, 1981.
191. Backman U, Danielson BG, Fellstrom B, et al: Clinical and laboratory findings in patients with medullary sponge kidney. In International Symposium on Urolithiasis. Plenum Publishing, New York, 1981.
192. Holmes SAV, Eardley I, Corry DA, et al: The use of extracorporeal shock wave lithotripsy for medullary sponge kidneys. Br J Urol 70:352, 1992.
193. Clarke BG, Hurwitz ES, Dudinsky E: Solitary serous cysts of the kidney. Biochemical, cytologic and histologic studies. J Urol 75:772, 1956.
194. Mir S, Rapola J, Koskimies O: Renal cysts in pediatric autopsy material. Nephron 33:189, 1983.
195. Orton KR, Smith JA Jr: Simple renal cysts in children. J Pediatr Surg 20:543, 1985.
196. McHugh K, Stringer AA, Hebert D, Babiak AA: Simple renal cysts in children: Diagnosis and follow-up with US. Radiology 178:383, 1991.
197. Sagel SS, Stanley RJ, Levitt RG, Geisse G: Computed tomography of the kidney. Radiology 124:359, 1977.
198. Tada S, Yamagishi J, Kobayashi H, et al: The incidence of simple renal cysts by computed tomography. Clin Radiol 34:437, 1983.
199. Baert L, Steg A: Is the diverticulum of the distal and collecting tubules a preliminary stage of the simple cyst in the adult? J Urol 118:707, 1977.
200. Baert L, Steg A: On the pathogenesis of simple renal cysts in the adult. Urol Res 5:103, 1977.
201. Muther RS, Bennett WM: Concentration of antibiotics in simple renal cysts. J Urol 124:596, 1980.
202. Jacobsson L, Lindqvist B, Michaelson G, Bjerle P: Fluid turnover in renal cysts. Acta Med Scand 202:327, 1977.
203. Bjerle P, Lindqvist G, Michaelson G: Pressure measurements in renal cysts. Scand J Clin Lab Invest 27:135, 1971.
204. Derezic D, Cecuk L: Hydrostatic pressure within renal cysts. J Urol 54:93, 1982.
205. Amis ES Jr, Coronan JJ, Yoder IC, et al: Renal cysts: Curios and caveats. Urol Radiol 4:199, 1982.
206. Gernert JD, Stein J, Bischoff AJ: Solitary renal cysts: Experience with 100 cases. J Urol 100:251, 1968.
207. Farkas A, Firstater M, Johnston JH: Neonatal solitary renal cysts associated with posterior urethral valves. J Pediatr Surg 14:132, 1979.
208. Reid RE: Pyelocalyceal obstruction due to a renal cyst. J Natl Med Assoc 58:342, 1966.
209. Evans AT, Coughlin JP: Urinary obstruction due to renal cysts. J Urol 103:277, 1970.
210. Notley RG: Calyceal obstruction due to parapelvic cyst. Proc R Soc Med 64:66, 1971.
211. Smith DC, Rich DH, Barnes RW: Hematuria and massive calycovenous reflux secondary to benign renal cyst. Urology 9:698, 1977.
212. Vertel RM, Morse BS, Prince JE: Remission of erythrocytosis after drainage of a solitary renal cyst. Arch Intern Med 120:54, 1967.

213. Weiner MA: Renal mass associated with polycythemia. JAMA 207:1229, 1969.

214. Bubrick MP, Hitchcock CR: Renal cyst causing afferent loop obstruction and acute pancreatitis. Am J Surg 41:440, 1975.

215. Becker JA, Schneider M: Simple cyst of the kidney. Semin Roentgenol 10:103, 1975.

216. Rockson SG, Stone RA, Gunnells JC: Solitary renal cyst with segmental ischemia and hypertension. J Urol 112:550, 1974.

217. Kala R, Fyhrquist F, Halttunen P, Rauste J: Solitary renal cyst, hypertension and renin. J Urol 116:710, 1976.

218. Churchill E, Kimoff R, Pinsky M, Gault MH: Solitary intrarenal cyst: Correctable cause of hypertension. Urology 6:485, 1978.

219. Limioco UR, Strauch AE: Infected solitary cyst of the kidney: Report of a case and review of the literature. J Urol 96:625, 1966.

220. Finlay DB, Lowe JS, Kaur K: Perforation of a suppurative solitary renal cyst. Br J Surg 68:585, 1981.

221. Sagalowsky A, Solotkin D: Infected renal mass successfully treated by ultrasound-guided needle aspiration. South Med J 73:957, 1980.

222. Stephenson BM, Evans AG: Sequelae of ruptured infected renal cysts. Br J Hosp Med 45:387, 1991.

223. Lang EK: Coexistence of cyst and tumor in the same kidney. Radiology 101:7, 1971.

224. Lang EK: Renal cyst puncture studies. Urol Clin North Am 14:91, 1987.

225. Steg A: Renal cysts in adults. III. Clinical aspect and diagnostical approach, based on the analysis of 1,342 cases. IV. Therapeutic problems. Eur Urol 2:209, 1976.

226. Marotti M, Hricak H, Fritzsche P, et al: Complex and simple renal cysts: Comparative evaluation with MR imaging. Radiology 162:679, 1987.

227. McClennan BL, Stanley RJ, Melson GL, et al: CT of the renal cyst: Is cyst aspiration necessary? AJR 133:671, 1979.

228. Schwarz RD, Stephens FD, Cussen LJ: The pathogenesis of renal dysplasia. III. Complete and incomplete urinary obstruction. Invest Urol 19:101, 1981.

229. Stephens FD: Congenital Malformations of the Urinary Tract. Praeger, New York, 1983.

230. Schwarz RD, Stephens FD, Cussen LJ: The pathogenesis of renal dysplasia. II. The significance of lateral and medial ectopy of the ureteric orifice. Invest Urol 19:97, 1981.

231. Bernstein J: The morphogenesis of renal parenchymal maldevelopment (renal dysplasia). Pediatr Clin North Am 18:395, 1971.

232. Piel CF: Congenital multicystic kidney. In Gardner KD Jr, Bernstein J (eds): The Cystic Kidney. Kluwer Academic Publishers, Boston, 1990, pp 393–411.

233. Ljungqvist A: Arterial vasculature of the multicystic dysplastic kidney: A microangiographical and histological study. Acta Pathol Microbiol Scand 64:309, 1965.

234. Nation EF: Renal aplasia: A study of sixteen cases. J Urol 51:570, 1944.

235. Spence HM: Congenital unilateral multicystic kidney. An entity to be distinguished from polycystic kidney disease and other cystic disorders. J Urol 74:693, 1955.

236. Leonidas JC, Strauss L, Krasna IH: Roentgen diagnosis of multicystic renal dysplasia in infancy by high dose urography. J Urol 108:936, 1972.

237. Kyaw MM, Koehler PR: Congenital multicystic kidney. In Gardner KD Jr (ed): Cystic Diseases of the Kidney. John Wiley & Sons, New York, 1976, pp 115–123.

238. Hashimoto BE, Filly RA, Callen PW: Multicystic dysplastic kidney in utero: Changing appearance on US. Radiology 159:107, 1986.

239. Avni EF, Thoua Y, Lalmand B, et al: Multicystic dysplastic kidney: Natural history from in utero diagnosis and postnatal followup. J Urol 138:1420, 1987.

240. Bronshtein M, Yoffe N, Brandes JM, Blumenfeld Z: First and early second-trimester diagnosis of fetal urinary tract anomalies using transvaginal sonography. Prenat Diagn 10:653, 1990.

241. Mandell J, Blyth BR, Peters CA, et al: Structural genitourinary defects detected in utero. Radiology 178:193, 1991.

242. Gur A, Siegel NJ, Davis CA, et al: Clinical aspects of bilateral renal dysplasia in children. Nephron 15:50, 1975.

243. Greene LF, Feinzaig W, Dahlin DC: Multicystic dysplasia of the kidney: With special reference to the contralateral kidney. J Urol 105:482, 1971.

244. Rubenstein M, Meyer R, Bernstein J: Congenital abnormalities of the urinary system. I. A postmortem survey of developmental anomalies and acquired congenital lesions in a children's hospital. J Pediatr 58:536, 1961.

245. Dungan JS, Fernandez MT, Abbitt PL, et al: Multicystic dysplastic kidney: Natural history of prenatally detected cases. Prenat Diagn 10:175, 1990.

246. Bodian M: Some observations on the pathology of congenital "idiopathic bladder-neck obstruction" (Marion's disease). Br Jr Urol 29:3, 1957.

247. Sommer JT, Stephens FD: Morphogenesis of nephropathy with partial ureteral obstruction and vesicoureteral reflux. J Urol 125:67, 1981.

248. Williams DI, Burkholder GF: The prune belly syndrome. J Urol 98:24, 1967.

249. Forbes M: Renal dysplasia in infants with neurospinal dysraphism. J Pathol 107:13, 1972.

250. Perrin EV: Renal dysplasia in anomalies of the urinary tract and in chronic pyelonephritis. Am J Pathol 43:18, 1963.

251. Williams DI, Woodard JR: Problems in the management of ectopic ureteroceles. J Urol 92:635, 1964.

252. Berdon WE, Baker DH, Recker JA, Uson AC: Ectopic ureterocele. Radiol Clin North Am 6:205, 1968.

253. Cussen LJ: Cystic kidneys in children with congenital urethral obstruction. J Urol 106:939, 1971.

254. Ekstrom T: Renal hypoplasia. A clinical study of 179 cases. Acta Chir Scand Suppl 203, 1955.

255. Bernstein J: Hereditary disorders of the kidney. Part I. Parenchymal defects and malformations. In Rosenberg HS, Rolande RP (eds): Perspectives in Pediatric Pathology. Year Book Medical Publishers, Chicago, 1973, pp 117–146.

256. Bernstein J, Brough AJ, McAdams AJ: The renal lesion in syndromes of multiple congenital malformations. Cerebrohepatorenal syndrome; Jeune asphyxiating thoracic dystrophy; tuberous sclerosis; Meckel syndrome. Birth Defects 10:35, 1974.

257. Bernstein J: Dysplasia and renal abnormalities associated with malformation syndromes. In Rubin MI, Barratt TM (eds): Pediatric Nephrology. Williams & Wilkins, Baltimore, 1975, pp 7–30.

258. Landing BH, Gwinn JL, Lieberman E: Cystic diseases of the kidney in children. In Gardner KD Jr (ed): Cystic Diseases of the Kidney. John Wiley & Sons, New York, 1976, pp 187–200.

259. Schimke RN: Genetics in cystic kidney disease. In Gardner KD Jr (ed): Cystic Diseases of the Kidney. John Wiley & Sons, New York, 1976, pp 83–90.

260. Bender BL, Yunis EJ: The pathology of tuberous sclerosis. Pathol Annu 17:339, 1982.

261. Wenzl JE, Lagos JC, Albers DD: Tuberous sclerosis presenting as polycystic kidneys and seizures in an infant. J Pediatr 77:673, 1970.

262. Chonko AM, Weiss SM, Stein JH, Ferris TF: Renal involvement in tuberous sclerosis. Am J Med 56:124, 1974.

263. Gomez MR: Tuberous Sclerosis. Raven Press, New York, 1979.

264. Bernstein J, Robbins TO, Kissane JM: The renal lesions of tuberous sclerosis. Semin Diagn Pathol 3:97, 1986.

265. Yu DT, Sheth JK: Cystic renal involvement in tuberous sclerosis. Clin Pediatr (Phila) 24:36, 1985.

266. Rosenberg JC, Bernstein J, Rosenberg B: Renal cystic disease associated with tuberous sclerosis complex: Renal failure treated by cadaveric kidney transplantation. Clin Nephrol 4:109, 1975.

267. Okada RD, Platt MA, Fleishman J: Chronic renal failure in patients with tuberous sclerosis: Association with renal cysts. Nephron 30:85, 1982.

268. Stapleton FB, Johnson D, Kaplan GW, Griswold W: The cystic renal lesion in tuberous sclerosis. J Pediatr 97:574, 1980.

269. Honey RJ, Honey RM: Tuberous sclerosis and bilateral renal carcinoma. Br J Urol 49:441, 1977.

270. Susiayich F, Older RA, Hinman CG: Calcified renal carcinoma in a patient with tuberous sclerosis. AJR 133:524, 1979.

271. Shapiro RA, Skinner DG, Stanley P, Edelbrock HH: Renal tumors associated with tuberous sclerosis: The case for aggressive surgical management. J Urol 132:1170, 1984.

272. Ibrahim RE, Weinberg DS, Weidner N: Atypical cysts and carcinomas of the kidneys in the phacomatoses. Cancer 63:148, 1989.

273. Frimodt-Moller PC, Nissen HM, Dyreborg U: Polycystic kidneys as the renal lesion in Lindau's disease. J Urol 125:861, 1981.

274. Richards RD, Mebust WK, Schimke RN: A prospective study on von Hippel–Lindau disease. J Urol 110:27, 1973.

275. Choyke PL, Glenn GM, McClellan MW, et al: The natural history of renal lesions in von Hippel–Lindau disease: A serial CT study in 28 patients. AJR 159:1229, 1992.
276. Horton WA, Wong V, Eldridge R: Von Hippel–Lindau disease. Clinical and pathological manifestations in nine families with 50 affected members. Arch Intern Med 136:769, 1976.
277. Solomon D, Schwartz A: Renal pathology in von Hippel–Lindau disease. Hum Pathol 19:1072, 1988.
278. Levine E, Collins DL, Horton WA, Schimke RN: CT screening of the abdomen in von Hippel–Lindau disease. AJR 139:505, 1982.
279. Levine E, Lee KR, Weigel JW, Farber B: Computed tomography in the diagnosis of renal carcinoma complicating Hippel-Lindau syndrome. Radiology 130:703, 1979.
280. Jennings AM, Smith C, Cole DR, et al: Von Hippel–Lindau disease in a large British family: Clinicopathological features and recommendations for screening and follow-up. Q J Med 66:233, 1988.
281. Pearson JC, Weiss J, Tanagho EA: A plea for conservation of kidney in renal adenocarcinoma associated with von Hippel–Lindau disease. J Urol 124:910, 1980.
282. Kissane JM: Multilocular cystic renal lesions—malformations, benign neoplasms or differentiated Wilms tumors? In Gardner KD Jr, Bernstein J (eds): The Cystic Kidney. Kluwer Academic Publishers, Boston, 1990, pp 413–436.
283. Madewell JE, Goleman SM, Davis CJ Jr, et al: Multilocular cystic nephroma: A radiologic-pathologic correlation of 58 patients. Radiology 146:309, 1983.
284. Baldauf MC, Schulz DM: Multilocular cyst of the kidney. Report of three cases with review of the literature. Am J Clin Pathol 65:93, 1976.
285. Uson AC, Melicow MM: Multilocular cysts of kidney with intrapelvic herniation of a ''daughter'' cyst: Report of four cases. J Urol 89:341, 1963.
286. Wulfsohn MA: Pyelocaliceal diverticula. J Urol 123:1, 1980.
287. Jones JA, Lingeman JE, Steidle CP: The roles of extracorporeal shock wave lithotripsy and percutaneous nephrostolithotomy in the management of pyelocaliceal diverticula. J Urol 146:724, 1991.
288. Henthorne J: Peripelvic lymphatic cysts of the kidney. A review of the literature on perinephric cysts. Am J Clin Pathol 1:28, 1938.
289. Lindsey JR: Lymphangiectasia simulating polycystic disease. J Urol 104:658, 1970.
290. Deliveliotis A, Kavadis C: Parapelvic cysts of the kidney: Report of seven cases. Br J Urol 41:386, 1969.
291. Androulakakis PA, Kirayianis B, Deliveliotis A: The parapelvic renal cyst. A report of 8 cases with particular emphasis on diagnosis and management. Br J Urol 52:342, 1980.
292. Chan JCM, Kodroff MB: Hypertension and hematuria secondary to parapelvic cyst. Pediatrics 65:821, 1980.
293. Mattoo TK, Giangreco AB, Afzal M, Akhtar M: Cystic lymphangiectasia of the kidneys in an infant with nephrotic syndrome. Pediatr Nephrol 4:228, 1990.
294. Murray KK, McLennan GL: Renal peripelvic lymphangiectasia: Appearance at CT. Radiology 180:455, 1991.
295. Meridith T, Ahlstrom N, Levine E, Grantham JJ: Familial renal lymphangiomatosis with exacerbation during pregnancy. AJR 151:965, 1988.
296. Hidalgo H, Dunnick NR, Rosenberg ER, et al: Parapelvic cysts: Appearance on CT and sonography. AJR 138:667, 1982.
297. Meyers MA: Uriniferous perirenal pseudocyst: New observations. Radiology 117:539, 1975.
298. Thompson IM, Ross G Jr, Habib EJ, Amoury RA: Experiences with 16 cases of pararenal pseudocyst. J Urol 116:289, 1976.
299. N'Guessen G, Stephens FG, Pick J: Congenital superior ectopic (thoracic) kidney. Urology 24:219, 1984.
300. Donat SM, Donat PE: Intrathoracic kidney: A case report with a review of the world literature. J Urol 140:131, 1988.
301. Kelalis PP, Malek RS, Segura JW: Observations on renal ectopia and fusion in children. J Urol 110:588, 1973.
302. Warkany J, Passarge E, Smith LB: Congenital malformations in autosomal trisomy syndromes. Am J Dis Child 112:502, 1966.
303. N'Guessan G, Stephens FD: Supernumerary kidney. J Urol 130:649, 1983.
304. Beckwith JB: Macroglossia, omphalocele, adrenal cytomegaly, gigantism, and hyperplastic visceromegaly. Birth Defects 5:188, 1969.
305. Roggensack G, McAlister WH: Bilateral nephromegaly in child with hemihypertrophy. AJR 110:546, 1970.
306. Potter EL: Bilateral absence of ureters and kidneys: A report of 50 cases. Obstet Gynecol 25:3, 1965.
307. Dees JE: Prognosis of the solitary kidney. J Urol 83:550, 1960.
308. Emanuel B, Nachman R, Aronson N, Weiss H: Congenital solitary kidney. A review of 74 cases. J Urol 111:394, 1974.
309. Kiprov DD, Colvin RB, McCluskey RT: Focal and segmental glomerulosclerosis and proteinuria associated with unilateral renal agenesis. Lab Invest 46:275, 1982.
310. McPherson E, Carey J, Kramer A, et al: Dominantly inherited renal adysplasia. Am J Med Genet 26:863, 1987.
311. Inke G: The Protolobular Structure of the Human Kidney. Its Biologic and Clinical Significance. AR Liss, New York, 1988.
312. Landing BH, Hughes ML: Analysis of weight of kidneys in children. Lab Invest 11:452, 1962.
313. Bernstein J, Meyer R: Some speculations on the nature and significance of developmentally small kidneys (renal hypoplasia). Nephron 1:137, 1964.
314. Gillerot Y, Koulischer L: Major malformations of the urinary tract. Anatomic and genetic aspects. Prenat Nephrol 53:186, 1988.
315. Broyer M: Chronic renal failure. In Royer P, Habib R, Mathieu H, Broyer M (eds): Pediatric Nephrology. WB Saunders, Philadelphia, 1974, pp 358–394.
316. Boissonnat P: What to call hypoplastic kidney? Arch Dis Child 37:142, 1962.
317. Fetterman GH, Habib R: Congenital bilateral oligonephronic renal hypoplasia with hypertrophy of nephrons (oligomeganephronia). Studies by microdissection. Am J Clin Pathol 52:199, 1969.
318. Liungqvist A, Lagergren C: The Ask-Upmark kidney: A congenital renal anomaly studied by microangiography and histology. Acta Pathol Microbiol Scand 56:277, 1962.
319. Royer P, Habib R, Broyer M, Nouaille Y: Segmental hypoplasia of the kidney in children. Adv Nephrol 1:145, 1971.
320. Arant BS Jr, Sotelo-Avila C, Bernstein J: Segmental ''hypoplasia'' of the kidney (Ask-Upmark). J Pediatr 95:931, 1979.
321. Habib R: Pathology of renal segmental corticopapillary scarring in children with hypertension: The concept of segmental hypoplasia. In Hodson J, Kincaid-Smith (eds): Reflux Nephropathy. Masson Publishing USA, New York, 1979, p 220.
322. Shindo S, Bernstein J, Arant BS Jr: Evolution of renal segmental atrophy (Ask-Upmark kidney) in children with vesicoureteric reflux: Radiographic and morphologic studies. J Pediatr 102:847, 1983.
323. European Chromosome 16 Tuberous Sclerosis Consortium: Identification and characterization of the tuberous sclerosis gene on chromosome 16. Cell 75:1305, 1993.
324. The European Polycystic Kidney Disease Consortium: The polycystic kidney disease 1 gene encodes a 14 kb transcript and lies within a duplicated region on chromosome 16. Cell 77:881, 1994.
325. The International Polycystic Kidney Disease Consortium: Polycystic kidney disease: The complete structure of the PKD1 and its protein. Cell 81:289–298, 1995.
326. Schnieder MC, Zhang F, Geng L, et al: Identification of the autosomal dominant polycystic kidney disease gene, PDK1. J Am Soc Nephrol 5:635, 1994. Abstract.
327. Geng L, Zhang F, Schnieder MC, et al: Gene structure, sequence, and a point mutation in the PKD1 gene, and search for point mutations. J Am Soc Nephrol 5:622, 1994. Abstract.
328. Qian F, Onuchic LF, Baldini A, et al: PKD1 gene is a unique member of a novel gene family. J Am Soc Nephrol 5:633, 1994. Abstract.

# 39

# Diabetic Nephropathy

*Hans-Henrik Parving*
*Ruth Østerby*
*Pamela W. Anderson*
*Willa A. Hsueh*

More than 2000 years ago, the Hindu medical texts Caraka and Sushruta noted the existence of two types of diabetes: one associated with emaciation, dehydration, polyuria, and lassitude, and the other associated with stout build, obesity, and sleepiness.[1] Diabetic patients are regarded as having insulin-dependent diabetes mellitus (IDDM, type I) if they are dependent on injected insulin to prevent ketosis and to preserve life.[2] Onset is usually in youth, but IDDM may occur at any age. Non–insulin-dependent diabetes mellitus (NIDDM, type II) can be diagnosed clinically if patients are treated by diet alone or diet combined with oral hypoglycemic agents, or if they are treated with insulin and had an onset of diabetes after the age of 40 years and a body mass index above normal at the time of diagnosis.[2, 3] If, for example, an insulin-treated patient with diabetic nephropathy cannot be correctly classified because of insufficient clinical data at the onset and during the course of diabetes, a correct diagnosis can be obtained even at this stage by measuring the endogenous insulin production with the glucagon/C peptide test.[4]

Although proteinuria had been demonstrated in diabetic patients since the 18th century,[5] it was Bright[6] who in 1836 postulated that albuminuria could reflect a serious renal disease specific to diabetes. A hundred years later, Kimmelstiel and Wilson[7] described the nodular glomerular intercapillary lesions in long-standing NIDDM patients suffering from the clinical syndrome of heavy proteinuria and renal failure accompanied by arterial hypertension. Persistent albuminuria (>300 mg/24 h or 200 µg/min) is the hallmark of diabetic nephropathy, which can be diagnosed clinically if the following additional criteria are fulfilled: presence of diabetic retinopathy and no clinical or laboratory evidence of kidney or urinary tract disease other than diabetic glomerulosclerosis.[8, 9] This clinical definition of diabetic nephropathy is valid in both IDDM and NIDDM.[8, 10]

During the last decade, several longitudinal studies have shown that raised urinary albumin excretion (based on a single measurement) below the level of clinical albuminuria (Albustix), so-called microalbuminuria, strongly predicts the development of diabetic nephropathy in both IDDM[11–14] and NIDDM.[15–17] Until recently, the definition of microalbuminuria has varied slightly from center to center; but consensus was obtained at a conference on early diabetic nephropathy, microalbuminuria being defined as urinary albumin excretion greater than 30 mg/24 h (20 µg/min) and less than or equal to 300 mg/24 h (200 µg/min), regardless of how the urine is collected.[18]

Nephropathy is a major cause of illness and death in diabetes. Indeed, the excess mortality of diabetes occurs mainly in proteinuric IDDM and NIDDM patients and results not only from end-stage renal disease (ESRD) but also from cardiovascular disease, particularly cardiovascular disease in NIDDM patients.[19–34] Diabetic nephropathy is the single most common cause of ESRD in the United States, with diabetic patients accounting for 33% of all patients enrolled in the Medicare ESRD program.[35, 36] The cost of caring for these diabetic patients with ESRD is currently $1.8 billion per year in the United States alone, and the amount is rapidly rising.[36]

# MORPHOLOGIC CHANGES

Morphologic changes, to a large extent, are the underlying cause of the functional abnormalities. The main purpose of morphologic studies is to project the information to knowledge about renal function. The first step is to describe the relationship between structure and function. At this basal level, some problems are already met. Discrepancy between morphologic and clinical features was stressed in an autopsy study, because marked structural changes were found in IDDM patients without persistent proteinuria.[37] However, in several extensive biopsy studies, the structural and functional derangements were found to correlate well.[38-44]

In overt diabetic nephropathy—and perhaps also in early stages—changes may be present in all renal compartments. Evidently, the sum of these various changes leads to the functional state. However, in our analyses of morphologic features as well as in systematic descriptions, the individual compartments have to be considered separately.

## Diabetic Glomerulopathy

In its advanced form, the diabetic glomerulopathy may have a distinctive appearance, as first perceived by Kimmelstiel and Wilson.[7] The description of the structural changes applies to NIDDM as well as to IDDM patients.

Light microscopy shows an increase in the solid spaces of the tuft, most frequently seen as a coarse branching of solid (positive periodic–acid Schiff reaction) material (i.e., the diffuse diabetic glomerulopathy). Large acellular accumulations may be seen within these areas, circular on section (i.e., the Kimmelstiel-Wilson nodules). Descriptions of these two classic types may be looked up in reviews or textbooks,[45-47] which also describe the exudative lesions. In the tuft, they occur in advanced stages as fibrinoid lesions. In Bowman capsule, they occur as capsular drops, which may be present in early stages.

The severity of lesions may be estimated as the volume fraction of the solid substance or described semiquantitatively by use of a scoring system. Such measures have been used in a number of studies.[37-39, 48-50]

Electron microscopy provides a more detailed definition of the structures involved. In a cross section of a glomerulus with advanced changes, the mesangial regions occupy a large proportion of the tuft, with a prominent content of matrix. Further, the basement membrane (BM) in the capillary walls (i.e., the peripheral BM) is thicker than normal. The dominating change is augmentation of the extracellular material (i.e., quantitative deviations from the normal). Severity of diabetic glomerulopathy is therefore estimated by the thickness of the peripheral BM and mesangium and matrix expressed as a fraction of appropriate spaces (e.g., volume fraction of mesangium/glomerulus, matrix/mesangium, or matrix/glomerulus). The sum of these

changes may be used as an index of glomerulopathy.[40] Another descriptor of matrix changes is the matrix star volume,[42, 51-53] which increases with increasing convexity and confluence of the individual matrix branches. Like the BM thickness, this is an absolute measure (estimated in cubic micrometers), in contradistinction to volume fractions, which are relative measures expressing glomerular composition. The relative as well as absolute measures are important in the description. The data, however, are valid only provided that proper sampling has been performed, which means unbiased and sufficiently extensive sampling. Concerning this point, the requirement is somewhat different for different structures and for different stages of disease. It was often not fulfilled in quantitative electron microscopic studies. The results for a given biopsy are given as a set of parameters for the individual structures. What is not apparent in these data is the variation within the biopsy sample. More attention should be paid to this condition in future studies.

## Diabetic Glomerulopathy in Relationship to Various Stages of Nephropathy

### OVERT NEPHROPATHY

As long as proteinuric IDDM patients are considered, the data by common assent indicate that this stage is associated with advanced glomerulopathy. Still, IDDM patients are not protected from other kidney diseases, and it may even be that the abnormal diabetic kidney is more susceptible to glomerulonephritis,[47] for example. Also, chronic pyelonephritis is likely to be overrepresented in diabetic patients.[54] These cases are relatively few but should be thought of in those with an atypical clinical course (e.g., fast development of proteinuria) or if hematuria is present.[55]

In proteinuric NIDDM patients, on the other hand, the association between affected renal function and diabetic glomerulopathy is less consistent. The prevalence of other renal diseases is likely to increase with increasing age. In a series of 35 proteinuric NIDDM patients, renal biopsy results were suggestive of alternative glomerulopathies in 8 cases.[10] Half these cases, however, were termed minimal lesions. Other light microscopic studies found a corresponding high frequency of alternative diagnosis in 22 of 46 cases[56] and 17 of 52 cases.[57] Not surprisingly, ischemic changes were frequently observed.[57] Whereas one publication concerned a population-based series,[10] other series may have been heavily biased by use of available biopsy results. It is noteworthy that the proteinuric patients with diabetic retinopathy all showed typical diabetic glomerulopathy.[10] Studies by electron microscopy [44, 58] have shown glomerular structural changes corresponding to those in IDDM patients. A remarkable variation among patients was seen (Table 39–1; Fig. 39–1). The patients with structural index within the normal range had no signs of retinopathy. A quantitative light microscopic study also failed to find a correlation between albuminuria and glomerular lesions.[50] Thus, the decisive difference between the two types of diabetes is that proteinuria in NIDDM patients may not reflect advanced glomerulopathy.

**TABLE 39–1. Structural Data\* in Nondiabetic, IDDM, and NIDDM Patients Grouped by Albumin Excretion Rate†**

| Parameter | Nondiabetic Patients | IDDM Patients | | | NIDDM Patients |
| | | *NA* | *MI* | *NP* | *NP* |
| --- | --- | --- | --- | --- | --- |
| n | 12 | 9 | 29 | 24 | 20 |
| Basement membrane thickness (nm) | 308 | 442 | 595 | 664 | 587 |
| | (0.09) | (0.25) | (0.15) | (0.15) | (0.27) |
| $V_v$ (mesangium/glomerulus) | 0.19 | 0.22 | 0.24 | 0.43 | 0.32 |
| | (0.10) | (0.14) | (0.22) | (0.22) | (0.41) |
| $V_v$ (matrix/mesangium) | 0.49 | 0.50 | 0.57 | 0.60 | 0.69 |
| | (0.19) | (0.13) | (0.09) | (0.09) | (0.17) |
| Matrix star volume ($\mu m^3$) | 14 | 22 | 34 | 195‡ | — |
| | (0.32) | (0.43) | (0.52) | (0.90) | |

\*Mean values and, in parentheses, CV = SD/mean are given.
†NA = normal albumin excretion; MI = microalbuminuria; NP = overt nephropathy; $V_v$ = volume fraction.
‡n = 11.

In kidneys with advanced lesions, a large variation among individual glomeruli in the expression of glomerulopathy may pertain,[59] and the mean values of structural parameters may not be a good reflection of the state of the kidney. This aspect is less decisive in earlier stages, although it should also be considered in such cases.

## STAGES OF NORMOALBUMINURIA AND MICROALBUMINURIA IN IDDM PATIENTS

With the knowledge that transition from normoalbuminuria to microalbuminuria signals a high risk of further progression to overt nephropathy, this stage has attracted much interest. A key question is, What conditions the appearance of abnormal urinary albumin excretion? In fact, this particular question has not been answered, nor have individual patients been observed with structural studies during this transition phase. As a substitute for this important but impracticable study, cross-sectional studies of dia-

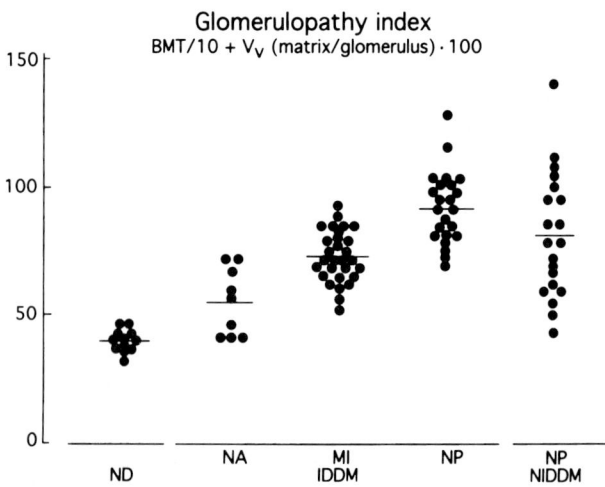

**Figure 39–1.** The glomerulopathy index is a sum of basement membrane thickness (BMT) and the volume fractions ($V_v$). ND = nondiabetic, living kidney donors. Diabetic patients are grouped as normoalbuminuric (NA), as microalbuminuric (MI), and with overt nephropathy (NP).

betic patients characterized by normoalbuminuria or microalbuminuria have been carried out. These studies all concern IDDM patients. From the first paper on this subject, some confusion arose.[60] No significant difference between diabetic patients with normal albumin excretion and microalbuminuric patients was found in BM thickness or in mesangial volume fraction. However, in grouping patients, the problems in defining microalbuminuria become important. Further, the structural data showed a large variation within groups. In later series,[61] more elaborate methods were applied to improve the precision in the estimates of mesangial volume fraction. These studies clearly showed the presence of early glomerulopathy in patients with microalbuminuria,[52, 53] and the glomerulopathy parameters were significantly increased compared with those in patients with normoalbuminuria (see Table 39–1 and Fig. 39–1). In the group with normoalbuminuria, there is no correlation between BM thickness and duration of diabetes,[52] which shows that some diabetic patients do not develop any signs of glomerulopathy even after many years of diabetes.[41, 42, 52]

Illustration of the expression of glomerulopathy and the changes in glomerular composition in clinically defined groups is given in Figures 39–1 and 39–2. The message that can be had in looking across the entire spectrum of patients is that more advanced functional abnormalities are associated with more advanced glomerulopathy. This holds true for IDDM as well as for NIDDM patients.[44]

## TIME COURSE OF DEVELOPMENT

Because diabetic patients who develop nephropathy pass the different stages in sequence, from normoalbuminuria to microalbuminuria and finally proteinuria, the data (see Table 39–1 and Figs. 39–1 and 39–2) may be taken as an expression of a time course, even if the groups shown had the same range of diabetes duration (5 to 36 years). This is conditioned by the large, and partly unexplained, variation in rate of development among different patients. Direct information on changes over time was obtained in a series of 20 patients with a low-level microalbuminuria.[62] Biopsy specimens before and after a 2- to 3-year period were analyzed. BM thickening had increased in all but one case, but

Glomerular compartments in nondiabetics (ND)
IDDM and NIDDM grouped by albumin excretion

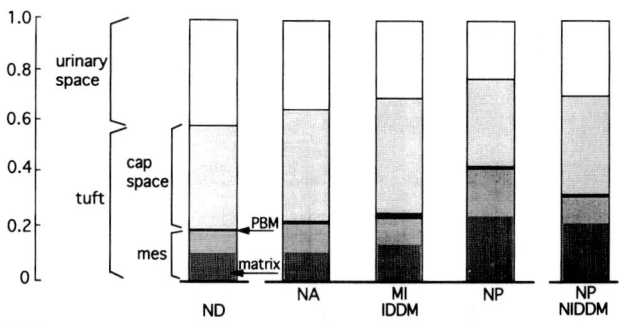

**Figure 39–2.** Graphic representation of the glomerular compartments as fractions of total glomerular volume in groups identified as in Figure 39–1. PBM = peripheral basement membrane.

with a wide variation among patients. The average increase was 44 nm/y. Also, the matrix/mesangium volume fraction and matrix star volume increased in the group of patients in this short period, whereas no change was detectable in the mesangium/glomerulus volume fraction.

## INTERRELATION OF CHANGES IN VARIOUS COMPARTMENTS

Over the full range of development, clear-cut correlations among the abnormalities in different compartments[41, 42] reflect that from the beginning, the structures are normal; in the long run, they are all grossly abnormal. For the initial stages, from normal to early glomerulopathy, significant correlations obtain between BM thickness and matrix parameters,[42, 52] an indication that the augmentation of extracellular material takes place in parallel at the two locations. An increase in the mesangial volume fraction becomes detectable only later. It has been suggested, on the basis of a poor correlation between BM thickness and mesangial volume fraction, that the two aspects of glomerulopathy are dissociate,[39] which has led to the often quoted opinion that the BM thickening detectable in early phases[63] has no significant clinical implications.

The available data indicate that the primary structural changes affect the extracellular material, BM, and matrix. The matrix changes, in configuration as well as constituents, may be responsible for the eventuating mesangial expansion.[64–66]

## Structural Modifications Associated with Glomerulopathy

Along with the developing glomerulopathy, modifications of glomerular composition may be identified. Some of them may be important in terms of glomerular function.

### VOLUME FRACTION OF TUFT/GLOMERULUS

An early change not previously noticed is an increase in the volume fraction of tuft/glomerulus (see Fig. 39–2). The

glomerular space encompasses the urinary space and the tuft, which is composed of capillaries and mesangium. In the normoalbuminuric group, the volume fraction of tuft/glomerulus is already increased, and it increases further in more advanced stages.

## GLOMERULAR SURFACES

The structure of relevance for the glomerular filtration rate (GFR) is the surface of the peripheral capillary wall. The loss of surface in advanced glomerulopathy is seen only when all structures are markedly abnormal, including an increase in the mesangial volume fraction. However, it is not the immediate consequence of the mesangial expansion, because the mesangial volume fraction does not correlate with total surface per glomerulus,[39, 40, 42] presumably owing to a concurrent enlargement of the glomerulus. Finally, compensation becomes insufficient, and loss of surface is the end result.

The capillary surface consists of two subsets: the peripheral part and the capillary-mesangial interface. With advancing glomerulopathy, the peripheral part makes up a smaller fraction of the total surface,[42, 44, 59] which presumably tends to decrease the filtration fraction. Also, the two subsets of mesangial surface show a shift: with increasing glomerulopathy, the surface facing the capillary makes up a larger fraction of the total mesangial surface,[42, 44, 58] which may favor mesangial accumulation of macromolecules.

## GLOMERULAR EPITHELIAL CELLS

Basic to the structural changes are alterations taking place at the cellular level. These are, however, to a large extent unexplored. The morphologic appearance of cells at the tissue level has been studied only as far as the epithelial cells are concerned.[40, 59, 67, 68] Widening of foot processes has been demonstrated in diabetic patients with albuminuria,[40, 59, 67] although it is not constantly recorded in those with proteinuria. The width of filtration slits between neighboring foot processes has been measured in diabetic patients with varying albumin excretion. The width was found to decrease with increasing albumin excretion.[68]

## INTRINSIC STRUCTURE OF EXTRACELLULAR MATERIAL

The ultrastructural appearance of the extracellular material in diabetic glomerulopathy often differs from the normal. The matrix is heterogeneous with vesicles, electron-dense inclusions, and membranous structures.[63] In particular, in the sharp angles of the urinary surface, accumulations of vesicles are often noted, also in the early stage of microalbuminuria. Such structural changes are not particular to diabetes.[69, 70] The membranes and vesicles have been shown to be associated with complement.[70] What is observed in the mesangial angles may be an expression of activity related to the "new capillary formation."

In the peripheral BM, loosening of the fibrillar meshwork may be seen in some capillary segments, and irregularities of the epithelial aspect with formation of spikes are not infrequent. Single loops with extremely thin and fluffy BM were suggested to represent new capillaries.[59, 71, 72]

## GLOMERULAR OCCLUSION

The occurrence of totally sclerosed, or occluded, glomeruli is of utmost importance in terms of renal function. The estimate of their frequency may be imprecise in kidney biopsy specimens. The distribution of occluded glomeruli within the kidney is nonrandom,[49] so that the biopsy specimen may not reflect the overall condition. This error may explain varying results; lack of correlation with renal function[39] as well as a positive correlation[48, 73, 74] has been reported. With regard to renal function, the percentage of occlusion should be combined with estimates of the glomerulopathy in open nephrons.[40]

The occlusion process is far from clarified. Most likely, extraglomerular as well as intraglomerular factors may condition the course.[74] The occluded profiles may appear as typical "ischemic" remnants of tufts or as large profiles with indications of a preceding, advanced glomerulopathy.[45, 57, 74] In the long run, the occluded glomeruli presumably disappear, being no longer identifiable.[75]

## Renal and Glomerular Hypertrophy

The hypertrophic changes have attracted much attention with emphasis on their possible role in the development of the ultimate structural destruction.[76]

In the early phase of IDDM, an increase in renal and glomerular size was found to accompany the elevated GFR.[77, 78] Although the increase is partly reversible after insulin treatment, the kidney may remain large for many years.[79, 80] In a series of IDDM patients in different functional stages, kidney size was found to be largest in patients with microalbuminuria and correlated closely with metabolic control.[80]

Information on glomerular volume during the course of diabetes is limited. Estimation of volume requires a large number of glomeruli,[81] a condition not always fulfilled in biopsy studies. The early enlargement of glomeruli may not as a general rule be persistent in the course of diabetes.[81, 82] However, with the increase in the volume fraction of tuft/glomerulus, the tuft may be larger than is immediately apparent.

The late phase of hypertrophy may appear in the stage of microalbuminuria as a compensation for the progressing glomerulopathy and sporadic glomerular closure. Whether this hypertrophy plays a role in the further progression of glomerulopathy is not known. The immediate effect is the preservation of total surface, regardless of the increase in mesangial volume fraction.[39, 40] Patients whose nephropathy developed after a long duration of diabetes were found to have larger glomeruli than those of patients whose nephropathy developed fast,[82] a finding compatible with a longer compensation period in those who have the best potential for enlargement.

In contrast to these findings, short-term NIDDM patients do not show an increase in renal or glomerular size.[50, 83] The elderly patients are capable of producing glomerular

hypertrophy. In patients with advanced glomerulopathy, the glomeruli are markedly enlarged in parallel with the expression of glomerulopathy,[44, 57] again indicating the compensatory nature.

## Extraglomerular Compartments

### TUBULE AND INTERSTITIAL CHANGES

With deterioration of glomerular function that ultimately results in closure, tubule degeneration is a necessary consequence. This change, including marked thickening of the BM, is therefore a prominent feature in advanced stages. Primary BM changes may also be considered.

Since the finding that expansion of the interstitial space correlates closely with renal function,[84] there has been some debate whether one or the other compartment was the most important. In advanced stages, the interstitium and the nephrons are greatly affected,[85] and there is probably no way of telling which is the most important. Presumably, the combination is what matters. Advanced glomerulopathy, including totally occluded glomeruli, must be linked to the increase in interstitium as a general expression of ischemia.[85, 86] The observation that an increase in the interstitial volume fraction is detectable in kidney biopsy specimens from IDDM patients in the early phase of microalbuminuria[53, 85] indicates a parallel development of interstitial and glomerular changes. The interstitial expansion is not solely a consequence of nephron loss.

### EXTRAGLOMERULAR VASCULATURE

The diabetic glomerulopathy is an integral part of the widespread diabetic angiopathy,[87] and concomitant structural abnormalities in the extraglomerular vessels are to be expected. The arteriolar hyalinosis, affecting the afferent as well as the efferent arterioles in the juxtaglomerular region,[45–47] is well known. Semiquantitative studies of the arteriolar wall structure showed a correlation between the degree of arteriolar involvement and the percentage of occluded glomeruli.[74, 85] In current quantitative studies by electron microscopy, it was found that the volume fraction of matrix/media is increased in young, normotensive IDDM patients with microalbuminuria (Østerby R and co-workers, unpublished data).

## Structure-Function Relationships

Questions about structure-function relationships are of somewhat different character, depending on whether broad or narrow ranges are studied. In the full range of structure and function from normal to end stages, many positive correlations are apparent.[39, 41]

In IDDM patients, good agreement between structure and function exists: The more advanced clinical stages are associated with more advanced lesions. A positive correlation between an index summing up structure and an index putting together clinical variables was found in a series of

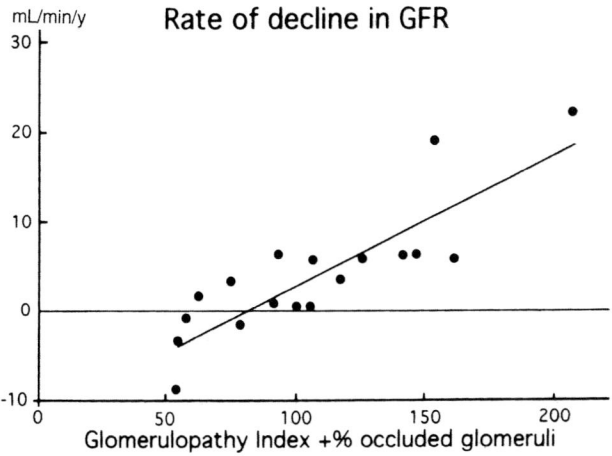

**Figure 39–3.** The correlation between glomerular structural involvement expressed as an index and the rate of decline in GFR over 5 to 84 months (median, 67 months) after the biopsy[95] is highly significant ($r = .85$, $P < .0001$). The series consists of NIDDM patients with proteinuria. (From Østerby R, Gall MA, Schmitz A: Glomerular structure and function in proteinuric type 2 [non–insulin-dependent] diabetic patients. Diabetologia 36:1064, 1993.)

IDDM patients with a broad range of functional involvement[40] and in the range of normal to slightly impaired glomerular function.[88]

Correlations have been studied with a more specific aim of elucidating possible interactions between structure and individual functional variables, GFR, albumin excretion rate, and systemic blood pressure. Findings of positive correlations between albumin excretion rate and some measures of glomerulopathy, whether over broad ranges[39, 41, 85] or narrower ones,[52, 68, 88] most likely indicate that the advancing glomerulopathy is accompanied by qualitative BM changes. An association between hypertension and the most advanced structural lesions is obvious, although hypertension is not a necessary condition for the development of glomerulopathy.[39, 74, 89] For each of the three functional variables, the interaction may be directed both ways.[74, 90, 91]

## STRUCTURE VERSUS GLOMERULAR FILTRATION RATE

The "coarse" structural determinant of GFR is the total area of peripheral capillary in the kidneys. Estimates are expressed as capillary surface per nephron. One disadvantage in this measure is a low precision; another is that the

number of nephrons shows a wide variation among individuals.[75] The good message, on the other hand, is that no systematic differences in nephron number exist between diabetic and nondiabetic cases.[75] Yet, with the limitations, positive correlations between biopsy estimates of capillary surface per nephron and current GFR were reported in the early hyperfunction phase[92, 93] as well as for the stage of declining GFR.[44, 73, 94] In the latter relationship, the glomerular occlusion is an important aspect.[40, 88] The close association between advanced glomerulopathy and loss of filtration surface, and thereby loss of GFR, was substantiated in a biopsy study of proteinuric NIDDM patients. The patients were observed with repeated kidney function tests for several months after the biopsy.[44, 95] Biopsy data showed a positive correlation with the ensuing rate of decline in GFR (Fig. 39–3).

The relationship between GFR and diabetic glomerulopathy in early stages, when markedly hyperfiltering patients are included, was studied to elucidate the possible impact of hyperfunction on the development of structural lesions. In our series (see Table 39–1), no tendency at all exists between current GFR and structural parameters, either current estimates or "normalized" by dividing with duration of diabetes. Also, the hyperfunction present in single kidneys does not necessarily lead to BM thickening.[96]

## EPIDEMIOLOGY OF MICROALBUMINURIA AND DIABETIC NEPHROPATHY

### Prevalence and Incidence

Table 39–2 displays the prevalence, incidence, and cumulative incidence of abnormal elevated urinary albumin excretion in IDDM and NIDDM. The overall prevalence of microalbuminuria and macroalbuminuria is about 30% to 35% in both types of diabetes. However, the range in prevalence of diabetic nephropathy is much wider in NIDDM patients. This is mainly explained by ethnic differences. The highest prevalence is found in Native Americans followed by American black, Mexican-American, Asian Indian, and European white patients.[118, 119] It should be stressed that good agreement has been documented between the clinic- and population-based studies. The cumulative incidence of persistent proteinuria in IDDM patients diagnosed before 1942 was about 40% to 50% after a 25- to 30-year duration, but it has declined to 25% to 30% in

**TABLE 39–2. Prevalence, Incidence, and Cumulative Incidence of Microalbuminuria and Nephropathy in Diabetes***

| | Clinic Based* | | Population Based* |
|---|---|---|---|
| **Parameter** | **IDDM** | **NIDDM** | **NIDDM** |
| Prevalence (%) | | | |
| Microalbuminuria[97–103] | 13 (9–20) | 25 (13–27) | 20 (17–21) |
| Macroalbuminuria[98, 100, 101, 103–116] | 15 (8–22) | 14 (5–48) | 16 (9–46) |
| Incidence of macroalbuminuria (%/y)[22, 28, 29, 31, 117] | 1.2 (0–3) | 1.5 (1–2) | — |
| Cumulative incidence of macroalbuminuria (%/25 y)[22, 28, 29, 31, 117] | 31 (28–34) | 28 (25–31) | — |

*Median and range are indicated.

**TABLE 39–3. Predictive Value of Microalbuminuria for the Development of Diabetic Nephropathy**

| Study | Number of Patients | Observation Period (y) | Cutoff Urinary Albumin Excretion (μg/min) | Patients with Nephropathy (%) |
|---|---|---|---|---|
| Parving et al.[11] | 23 IDDM | 6 | >28 | 75 |
| | | | <28 | 13 |
| Viberti et al.[12] | 63 IDDM | 14 | >30 | 87 |
| | | | <30 | 4 |
| Mogensen and Christensen[13] | 43 IDDM | 10 | >15 | 86 |
| | | | <15 | 0 |
| Mathiesen et al.[14] | 71 IDDM | 6 | >70 | 100 |
| | | | <70 | 5 |
| Mogensen[15] | 180 NIDDM | 9 | >30* | 22 |
| | | | <30* | 5 |
| Nelson et al.[16] | 439 NIDDM | 4 | >30† | 34 |
| | | | <30† | 4 |
| Ravid et al.[17] | 49 NIDDM | 5 | >20 | 42 |
| | | | <20 | — |
| Parving et al. (unpublished data) | 277 NIDDM | 5 | >20 | 21 |
| | | | <20 | 1 |

*Micrograms albumin per milliliter.
†Albumin/creatinine ratio (mg/g).

IDDM patients diagnosed after 1953.[23, 27, 28, 120] This so-called calendar effect is unfortunately not present in European white NIDDM patients.[31] The reason for the lower cumulative incidence of proteinuria in IDDM patients is unknown, but improved diabetes care and control have been suggested in addition to a general decline in nondiabetic glomerulopathies.

Diabetic nephropathy rarely develops before 10 years' duration of IDDM, whereas approximately 3% of newly diagnosed NIDDM patients have overt nephropathy.[100] The incidence peak (3%/y) is usually found between 10 and 20 years of diabetes; thereafter, a progressive decline in incidence takes place.[22, 26] Thus, the risk for development of diabetic nephropathy in a normoalbuminuric patient with a diabetes duration of greater than 30 years is low. This changing pattern of risk indicates that the magnitude of exposure to diabetes is not sufficient to explain the development of diabetic nephropathy and suggests that only a subset of patients are susceptible to kidney complications.

## Microalbuminuria Predicts Nephropathy

The IDDM subpopulation at risk may now be identified fairly accurately by the detection of microalbuminuria.[11–14] Several longitudinal studies have shown that microalbuminuria strongly predicts the development of diabetic nephropathy in IDDM patients (Table 39–3). These studies showed that 21 of 26 IDDM patients in whom diabetic nephropathy would develop could be identified by one measurement of urinary albumin excretion rate (predictive power of 80%). IDDM patients with microalbuminuria have a median risk ratio of 21 for the development of diabetic nephropathy (see Table 39–3). These conclusions were reached despite differences among centers in the procedure for collecting urine, the value of urinary albumin excretion designated microalbuminuria, and the duration of

follow-up. These confounders are also present in the longitudinal studies evaluating the predictive power of microalbuminuria in NIDDM patients (see Table 39–3). The risk ratio for development of diabetic nephropathy ranges from 4.4 to 21 (median, 8.5) in microalbuminuric NIDDM patients. In addition to microalbuminuria, several other risk factors or markers for development of diabetic nephropathy have been documented or suggested, as discussed in detail later (Table 39–4).

## Prognosis in Microalbuminuria

Several retrospective and prospective studies have demonstrated that microalbuminuria independently predicts cardiovascular morbidity and all causes of mortality in diabetes mellitus (Table 39–5). Microalbuminuria also predicts

**TABLE 39–4. Risk Factors or Markers for Development of Diabetic Nephropathy in IDDM and NIDDM Patients**

| Factor or Marker | IDDM Patients* | NIDDM Patients* |
|---|---|---|
| Microalbuminuria[11–17] | + | + |
| Sex[8, 22, 26, 31, 100] | M > F | M > F |
| Familial clustering[121–123] | + | + |
| Predisposition to arterial hypertension[124–128] | ± | ? |
| Increased Na+-Li+ countertransport[125–127, 129–132] | ± | − |
| Ethnicity[118, 119] | + | + |
| Onset of IDDM before 20 y[26, 28, 133] | + | |
| Glycemic control[110, 134, 135] | + | + |
| Hyperfiltration[136–140] | ± | ? |
| Prorenin[141–144] | + | ? |
| Smoking[140, 145–149] | + | ? |

*+ = present; − = not present; ? = no relevant information.

**TABLE 39–5. Microalbuminuria as Predictor of Mortality in Diabetes Mellitus**

| Study | Number of Patients | Observation Period (y) | Cutoff Urinary Albumin Excretion (μg/min) | Mortality (%) |
|---|---|---|---|---|
| Mogensen[15]* | 204 NIDDM | 9 | >30† | 78 |
| | | | <30† | 49 |
| Jarret et al.[150]* | 44 NIDDM | 14 | >10 | 91 |
| | | | <10 | 22 |
| Mattock et al.[151] | 141 NIDDM | 3.4 | >20 | 28 |
| | | | <20 | 4 |
| MacLeod et al.[152] | 400 NIDDM | 8 | >11 | 52 |
| | | | <11 | 30 |
| Atkinson et al.[153] | 216 NIDDM | 8 | >35† | 47 |
| | | | <35† | 21 |
| Gall et al.[154] | 328 NIDDM | 5 | >20 | 20 |
| | | | <20 | 8 |
| Stiegler et al.[155] | 290 NIDDM | 3 | >20† | 10 |
| | | | <20† | 5 |
| Parving et al. (unpublished data) | 768 IDDM | 7 | >20 | 16 |
| | | | <20 | 10 |

*Retrospective studies.
†Micrograms albumin per milliliter.

coronary and peripheral vascular disease and death from cardiovascular disease in the general nondiabetic population.[156, 157] The mechanisms of the link between microalbuminuria and death from cardiovascular disease are poorly understood. Several explanations have been proposed: microalbuminuria is a marker of widespread endothelial dysfunction, which might predispose to enhanced penetrations in the arterial wall of atherogenic lipoprotein particles[158]; microalbuminuria is a marker of established cardiovascular disease[159]; and microalbuminuria is associated with an excess of known and potential cardiovascular risk factors.[159] Raised blood pressure,[14, 133, 160, 161] dyslipoproteinemia,[162–166] increased platelet aggregability,[163] endothelial dysfunction,[167–170] and insulin resistance and hyperinsulinemia[171] have been found in microalbuminuric diabetic patients. Autonomic neuropathy, which is also associated with microalbuminuria, predicts death (often sudden) from cardiovascular disease in diabetic patients.[172] The prevalence of coronary heart disease based on electrocardiographic Minnesota codes is not increased in microalbuminuric NIDDM patients.[100] However, echocardiographic studies have revealed impaired diastolic function and cardiac hypertrophy in microalbuminuric IDDM and NIDDM patients.[173–175] Left ventricular hypertrophy predisposes the individual to ischemic heart disease, ventricular arrhythmia, sudden death, and heart failure.[176]

## Prognosis in Diabetic Nephropathy

In a cohort of 1030 IDDM patients diagnosed between 1933 and 1952, patients without proteinuria had a low and constant relative mortality, whereas patients with proteinuria on average had a 40 times higher relative mortality.[25, 26] IDDM patients with proteinuria showed the characteristic bell-shaped relationship between diabetes duration or age and relative mortality, with a maximal relative mortality in the age interval of 34 to 38 years of 110 in women and 80

in men. Several other studies have confirmed the poor prognosis in IDDM patients suffering from diabetic nephropathy, as reviewed by Borch-Johnsen.[26] In the three previous studies that described the natural course of diabetic nephropathy in IDDM patients,[22, 28, 33] the cumulative death rate 10 years after the onset of nephropathy ranged from 50% to 77% (Fig. 39–4).[177] The 50% figure is a minimal value because Krolewski and co-workers[28] included only death due to ESRD. Two studies have shown a decreasing relative mortality with increasing calendar year of diagnosis, the major decrease occurring between 1941 and 1955.[23, 28] The overall decrease in relative mortality from 1933 to 1972 was 40%. The decrease in the cumulative incidence of proteinuria explains the decreasing relative mortality observed during the past 50 years. Unfortunately,

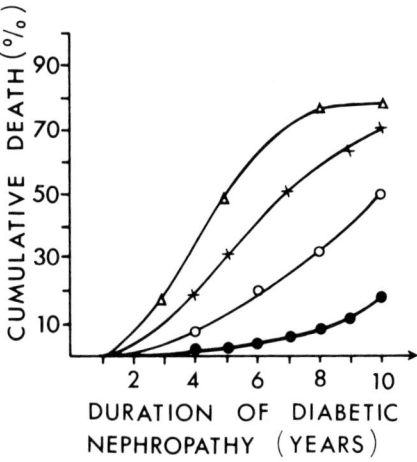

**Figure 39–4.** Deaths from diabetic nephropathy in IDDM patients: △, n = 45, Knowles[33]; ×, n = 360, Andersen and co-workers[22]; and ○, n = 67, Krolewski and co-workers[28] compared with those who had effective antihypertensive treatment (●, n = 45). (From Parving H-H, Hommel E: Prognosis in diabetic nephropathy. Br Med J 299:230, 1989.)

this calendar effect is lacking in proteinuric NIDDM patients, and subsequently no improved prognosis has been reported.[31] However, the prognostic importance of proteinuria in NIDDM patients is considerably less than in IDDM patients. Proteinuria confers a 3.5 times higher risk of death, and the concomitant presence of arterial hypertension increases this relative risk to 7 in Pima patients with NIDDM.[30] European NIDDM patients with proteinuria have a fourfold excess of premature death compared with patients without proteinuria.[178] The cumulative death rate 10 years after onset of abnormally elevated urinary albumin excretion in European NIDDM patients was 70% compared with 45% in normoalbuminuric NIDDM patients.[83, 179]

ESRD is the major cause of death (accounting for 59% to 66%) in IDDM patients with nephropathy.[21, 22, 26] The cumulative incidence of ESRD in proteinuric IDDM patients is 50% 10 years after onset of proteinuria,[28] compared with 3% to 11% after 10 years in proteinuric European NIDDM patients[180] and 65% after 10 years in proteinuric Pima patients with NIDDM.[181] However, renal insufficiency was defined as a serum creatinine level of 2.0 mg/dL or greater in the Pima study; 97% of the excess mortality associated with NIDDM in this population is found in patients with proteinuria: 16% of deaths were ascribed to ESRD, whereas 22% were due to cardiovascular disease.[30] Cardiovascular disease is also a major cause of death (15% to 25%) in IDDM patients with nephropathy, despite the relatively low age at death.[22, 26] Borch-Johnsen and Kreiner[24] studied a cohort of 2890 IDDM patients and demonstrated that the relative mortality from cardiovascular disease was 37 times higher in proteinuric IDDM patients compared with the general population. Abnormalities in well-established cardiovascular risk factors as described and discussed in the previous section cannot account for this finding alone. Several studies have shown abnormally raised levels of serum apolipoprotein A to be a strong independent risk factor for premature ischemic heart disease in nondiabetic subjects.[182] However, studies of IDDM and NIDDM patients with diabetic nephropathy have yielded conflicting results.[164–166] It has been demonstrated that a familial predisposition to cardiovascular disease is present in IDDM patients with diabetic nephropathy[183]; however, this finding has not been confirmed.[184]

## CLINICAL COURSE AND PATHOPHYSIOLOGY

A preclinical phase consisting of a normoalbuminuric and a microalbuminuric stage and a clinical phase characterized by albuminuria are well documented in both IDDM and NIDDM.

### Normoalbuminuria

In 1934, Cambier[185] suggested that the GFR is increased in some patients with diabetes mellitus. Numerous studies have confirmed and extended this observation in IDDM patients.[186–193] Approximately one third of IDDM patients have a GFR above the upper normal range of age-matched

**TABLE 39–6. Mediators of Hyperfiltration in Diabetes**

| |
|---|
| Glucose[186, 190, 199, 200] |
| Ketone bodies[201] |
| Insulin[202] |
| Growth hormone[203, 204] |
| Glucagon[205] |
| High protein intake[206] |
| Prostaglandins[207–209] |
| Atrial natriuretic peptide[210–212] |
| Nitric oxide[213] |
| Glomerulopressin[214] |
| $Na^+$-$Li^+$ countertransport[132] |
| Kidney and glomerular enlargement[77, 78, 92, 186, 191, 192, 215, 216] |

healthy nondiabetic subjects. The degree of hyperfiltration is less in NIDDM patients[194, 195] and reported lacking in some studies.[196] The GFR elevation is particularly pronounced in newly diagnosed IDDM and NIDDM patients and during other intervals with poor metabolic control. Intensified insulin treatment and near-normal blood glucose control reduce the GFR toward normal levels after a period of days to weeks in both IDDM and NIDDM patients.[186, 190, 192, 194, 197, 198] Additional metabolites, vasoactive hormones, and increased kidney and glomerulus size have been suggested as mediators of hyperfiltration in diabetes as reviewed by Christiansen[186] (Table 39–6).

Four factors govern the GFR.[217] First, the glomerular plasma flow influences the mean ultrafiltration pressure and thereby GFR. Enhanced renal plasma flow has been demonstrated in IDDM and NIDDM patients with an elevated GFR.[186, 190, 194, 198] The second factor is the systemic oncotic pressure, which is reported normal as calculated from plasma protein concentrations.[186, 190] The third determinant of the GFR is glomerular transcapillary hydraulic pressure difference, which cannot be measured in humans. However, the demonstrated increase in filtration fraction is compatible with an enhanced transglomerular hydraulic pressure difference.[186, 190] The last determinant of the GFR, the glomerular ultrafiltration coefficient $K_f$, is determined by the product of the hydraulic conductance of the glomerular capillary and the glomerular capillary surface area available for filtration. Total glomerular capillary surface area is clearly increased already at the onset of human diabetes.[78, 215]

Studies with insulin-treated experimental diabetic rats have revealed hyperfiltration, hyperperfusion, enhanced glomerular capillary hydraulic pressure, reduced proximal tubule pressure, unchanged systemic oncotic pressure, and unchanged or slightly elevated $K_f$.[218, 219] Several studies suggest that insulin-like growth factor-1 (IGF-1) plays a major role in the initiation of renal and glomerular growth in diabetic animals, as reviewed by Flyvbjerg.[220]

Longitudinal studies suggest that hyperfiltration is a risk factor for a subsequent increase in urinary albumin excretion and development of diabetic nephropathy in IDDM patients,[136, 137, 140] but conflicting results have also been reported.[138, 139] We have no information on the prognostic significance of hyperfiltration in NIDDM patients. Two prospective cohort studies investigating 148[221] and 501[140] normoalbuminuric IDDM patients for 4 and 7 years, respectively, revealed that minimal elevation of urinary albumin excretion, poor glycemic control, hyperfiltration, elevated arterial blood pressure, and smoking contribute to the development of persistent microalbuminuria and overt diabetic nephropathy. Because several of those risk factors are modifiable, intervention is feasible, as discussed later.

## Microalbuminuria

In 1969, Keen and co-workers[222] demonstrated elevated urinary albumin excretion in newly diagnosed NIDDM patients. The same phenomenon was also documented in newly diagnosed or short-term IDDM patients in poor glycemic control.[223] This abnormal but subclinical albumin excretion rate has been termed microalbuminuria, and it can be normalized by improved glycemic control. In addition to hyperglycemia, exercise can induce transient microalbuminuria in diabetic patients.[224] Furthermore, the day-to-day variation in urinary albumin excretion rate is high (30% to 50%)[225]; consequently, more than one urine sample is needed to determine whether the individual patient has persistent microalbuminuria. Urinary albumin excretion within the microalbuminuric range (30 to 300 mg/24 h) in at least two of three consecutive nonketotic sterile urine samples is the generally accepted definition of persistent microalbuminuria. Persistent microalbuminuria has not been detected in IDDM children younger than 12 years[97] and is exceptional in the first 5 years of IDDM.[226]

The annual rate of rise of urinary albumin excretion is about 20% in both NIDDM[17] and IDDM patients with persistent microalbuminuria.[227]

The excretion of albumin in the urine is determined by the amount filtered across the glomerular capillary barrier and the amount reabsorbed by the tubule cells. A normal urinary $\beta_2$-microglobulin excretion rate in microalbuminuria suggests that it derives from enhanced glomerular leakage rather than from reduced tubule reabsorption of protein. The transglomerular passage of macromolecules is governed by the size- and charge-selective properties of the glomerular capillary membrane and hemodynamic forces operating across the capillary wall.[228] Alterations in glomerular pressure and flows influence both the diffusive and the convecting driving forces for transglomerular passage of proteins.[229] Studies using renal clearance of endogenous plasma proteins or dextrans have not detected a simple size-selective defect.[190, 223, 230–234] Determination of immunoglobulin G/immunoglobulin G4 ratio suggests that a loss of glomerular charge selectivity precedes or accompanies the formation of new glomerular macromolecular pathways in the development of diabetic nephropathy.[232] Reduction in the negatively charged moieties of the glomerular capillary wall, particularly in sialic acid and heparan sulfate, has been suggested[159, 235] but not confirmed.[236, 237] Glomerular hydraulic pressure cannot be measured in humans, but filtration fraction is presumed to reflect the glomerular pressure. Microalbuminuric IDDM patients have an elevated filtration fraction both at rest and during exercise compared with normal control subjects.[238] A close correlation between filtration fraction and urinary albumin excretion has also been demonstrated. The demonstration that microalbuminuria diminishes promptly with short-term reduction in arterial blood pressure argues that reversible hemodynamic factors play an important role in the pathogenesis of microalbuminuria.[239] Finally, it should be mentioned that increased pressure has been demonstrated in the nail fold capillaries of microalbuminuric IDDM patients.[240]

GFR measured with the single-injection $^{51}$Cr-labeled ethylenediaminetetraacetic acid plasma clearance method or the renal clearance of inulin is normal or slightly elevated in IDDM patients with microalbuminuria.[241–243] Prospective studies have demonstrated that the GFR remains stable at normal or supranormal levels for at least 5 years if clinical nephropathy does not develop.[244] Nephromegaly is still present and even more pronounced in microalbuminuric compared with normoalbuminuric IDDM patients.[80]

Changes in tubule function take place early in diabetes and are related to the degree of glycemic control. The proximal tubule reabsorption of fluid, $Na^+$, and glucose is enhanced.[245] The process could diminish distal $Na^+$ delivery and thereby stimulate a tubuloglomerular feedback-mediated enhancement of GFR.[246–248] A direct effect of insulin to increase distal $Na^+$ reabsorption has also been demonstrated.[245, 249] The consequences of these alterations in tubule transport on overall kidney function are unknown.

Several studies have demonstrated blood pressure elevation in children and adults with IDDM and microalbuminuria.[14, 97, 133, 161] The prevalence of arterial hypertension (World Health Organization criterion, ≥160/95 mm Hg) in adult IDDM patients increases with albuminuria, being 19%, 30%, and 65% in subjects with normoalbuminuria, microalbuminuria, and macroalbuminuria, respectively.[133] The prevalence of hypertension in NIDDM patients (mean age, 60 years) was higher: 48%, 68%, and 85% in the normoalbuminuric, microalbuminuric, and macroalbuminuric groups, respectively.[100] A genetic predisposition to hypertension in IDDM patients in whom diabetic nephropathy develops has been suggested,[124] but much larger studies did not confirm the concept.[125, 127, 128, 250] Several studies have reported that retention of $Na^+$ and water plays a dominant role in the initiation and maintenance of systemic hypertension in microalbuminuria and diabetic nephropathy, whereas the contribution of the renin-angiotensin-aldosterone system is smaller.[242, 251–253]

## Diabetic Nephropathy

Diabetic nephropathy is a clinical syndrome characterized by persistent albuminuria (>300 mg/24 h), a relentless decline in GFR, and raised arterial blood pressure.[8, 254] Whereas albuminuria is the first sign, peripheral edema is the first symptom of diabetic nephropathy.[255] Fluid retention is frequently observed early in the course of this kidney disease, that is, at a stage with well-preserved renal function and only slight reduction in serum albumin.[255] A study suggests that capillary hypertension, increased capillary surface area, and reduced capillary reflection coefficient for plasma proteins contribute to the edema formation, whereas the washdown of subcutaneous interstitial protein tends to prevent the progressive edema formation in diabetic nephropathy.[256]

Most studies dealing with the natural history of diabetic nephropathy have demonstrated a relentless linear and highly variable rate of decline in GFR ranging from 2 to 20 mL/min/y (mean, 12 mL/min/y).[254, 257, 258] NIDDM patients with nephropathy display the same degree of variability in GFR.[95] Morphologic studies with both IDDM and NIDDM patients have demonstrated a close inverse correlation between the degree of glomerular and tubulointerstitial lesions on one side and the GFR level on the other side, as discussed in detail previously. Myers and co-workers[259–263] have demonstrated a reduction in the number of restrictive pores leading to loss of ultrafiltration capacity ($K_f$) and impairment of glomerular barrier size selectivity leading to progressive albuminuria and presence of immunoglobulin G in the urine of patients with diabetic nephropathy. Furthermore, the extent to which ultrafiltration capacity is impaired appears to be related to the magnitude of the defect in the barrier size selectivity. A defect in the glomerular barrier size selectivity has also been demonstrated in NIDDM patients with diabetic nephropathy.[264] The reduction in renal plasma flow is proportional to the reduction in GFR (filtration fraction unchanged), and the impact on GFR is partially offset by the diminished systemic colloid osmotic pressure.

Several putative promoters of progression in kidney function have been studied in IDDM[257, 265–268] and NIDDM[95] patients with nephropathy. Systemic blood pressure elevation and, to a lesser degree, albuminuria accelerate the progression of diabetic nephropathy in both IDDM and NIDDM patients.[95, 257, 265–268] Study of the impact of glycemic control[258, 269–271] and hyperlipidemia[95, 272, 273] has revealed conflicting results. No association between dietary protein intake and the rate of decline in GFR has been demonstrated in observational studies.[95, 274, 275]

Systemic blood pressure elevation to a hypertensive level is an early and frequent phenomenon in diabetic nephropathy.[100, 133, 254, 276, 277] Furthermore, nocturnal blood pressure elevation ("nondippers") occurs more frequently in IDDM and NIDDM patients with nephropathy.[278, 279] Exaggerated blood pressure response to exercise has also been reported in long-standing IDDM patients with microangiopathy.[280] Finally, the increase in glomerular pressure consequent to nephron adaptation may be accentuated with concomitant diabetes, as suggested by animal studies.[281]

## EXTRARENAL COMPLICATIONS IN DIABETIC NEPHROPATHY

Diabetic retinopathy is present in virtually all IDDM patients with nephropathy,[133] whereas only 50% to 60% of proteinuric NIDDM patients have retinopathy.[100, 282] Absence of retinopathy should require further investigation of nondiabetic glomerulopathies.[9, 10] Blindness due to severe proliferative retinopathy or maculopathy is approximately five times more common in IDDM and NIDDM patients with nephropathy than in normoalbuminuric patients.[100, 133] Macroangiopathy (e.g., stroke, carotid artery stenosis, coronary heart disease, and peripheral vascular disease)

is two to five times more common in nephropathic patients.[45, 100, 282–284]

Peripheral neuropathy is present in almost all patients with advanced nephropathy. Foot ulcers with sepsis leading to amputation occur frequently (>25%), probably because of a combination of neural and arterial disease.[285] Autonomic neuropathy may be asymptomatic and simply manifest as abnormal cardiovascular reflexes, or it may result in debilitating symptoms. Nearly all patients have grossly abnormal autonomic function tests. Grenfell and Watkins[285] reported that more than half of the patients with advanced nephropathy had symptoms of autonomic neuropathy: gustatory sweating, impotence, postural hypotension, and diarrhea. Diabetic cystopathy is also a frequent (>30%) problem in these patients.[286]

## PATHOGENESIS

Theories concerning the pathogenesis of diabetic nephropathy must explain its characteristic structural and functional changes. These changes include hyperfiltration, renal and glomerular hypertrophy, mesangial cell hypertrophy and matrix accumulation, glomerular BM thickening, and functional alterations in the glomerular filtration barrier.[287] In recent years, investigators have increasingly used animal models and cell culture to search for the factors responsible for causing these typical physiologic, structural, and biochemical changes. Hyperglycemia, advanced glycosylation end products (AGEs), and growth factors or cytokines have been identified, in addition to glomerular hypertension, as important participants in the pathogenesis of diabetic nephropathy.

### Hyperglycemia, Advanced Glycosylation End Products, and the Polyol Pathway

Despite disparate causes of their diabetes, patients with diabetes due to pancreatitis or hemochromatosis have nephropathy indistinguishable from that of IDDM and NIDDM patients, which suggests that risk factors for nephropathy are shared by all these groups. When normal human kidneys are transplanted into diabetic patients whose own kidneys have failed as a result of nephropathy, the normal kidneys develop typical lesions of diabetic nephropathy; this emphasizes the importance of the diabetic milieu in the development of diabetic nephropathy.[288]

Hyperglycemia may contribute to alterations in endothelial and mesangial cell structure, synthetic capacity, and function. For example, in endothelial cells, hyperglycemia leads to changes in cell shape, generalized BM thickening,[289, 290] vasoconstriction,[291–293] and reduction in endothelial cell life span.[294] Mesangial cells synthesize more extracellular matrix in response to hyperglycemia and become unresponsive to vasoconstrictors such as angiotensin II.[295, 296]

If hyperglycemia is sustained, AGEs may form. Hyperglycemia initially causes nonenzymatic glycation of proteins (through the Amadori reaction), resulting in products such as hemoglobin $A_{1c}$. Then, by a series of slowly occurring, irreversible chemical reactions, AGEs are produced, some of which are capable of forming covalent bonds with amino groups on other proteins, which results in the extensive cross-linking of proteins.[297] If AGEs form on long-lived molecules like collagen, the effect they exert can also be long-lived. Specific receptors for AGE compounds have been demonstrated on endothelial cells, mesangial cells, and monocyte-macrophages. AGE formation on collagens and matrix proteins tends to decrease endothelial cell adhesion and replication,[298] favor mesangial cell vasoconstriction and growth,[299, 300] and increase lipoprotein and immune complex adhesion to monocyte-macrophages.[301] Administration of aminoguanidine, an inhibitor of AGE formation, prevents increases in mesangial volume and decreases urinary albumin excretion in experimental animals with diabetes.[302] Preliminary studies with this drug in humans are currently being conducted.

Excess glucose is converted in the kidney to sorbitol through the polyol pathway by the enzyme aldose reductase. It is hypothesized that excess intracellular sorbitol leads to a reduction in intracellular *myo*-inositol, which initiates a cascade of events eventually leading to a loss of functional and structural integrity.[303] Whereas aldose reductase inhibitors have been touted as major therapeutic advances in the treatment of diabetic complications, their performance has been disappointing. Problems with toxicity have eliminated most of the drugs from the market.[304] Although modest clinical improvements in neuropathy have been noted with tolrestat,[305] and although it is effective in preventing or significantly reducing urinary albumin excretion in diabetic rats,[306] there are as yet no published studies that demonstrate any ability to alter the course of diabetic nephropathy in humans.

## Hemodynamic Alterations

Animals demonstrate glomerular hypertrophy and hyperfiltration almost immediately after the induction of diabetes.[218] The exact etiology of the hyperfiltration remains unknown, although many mechanisms have been proposed (see Table 39–6). Hyperfiltration has been proposed to cause or worsen diabetic nephropathy. Studies with nondiabetic rats with five-sixths nephrectomies (in which extreme increases in single-nephron GFR are seen in the remnant nephrons) show that the hyperfiltering glomeruli develop focal glomerulosclerosis with mesangial matrix expansion and glomerular BM thickening similar to that observed in diabetic glomerulosclerosis. When single-nephron GFR is reduced by administration of a low-protein diet, proteinuria and structural changes improve.[307] However, hyperfiltration may not be the etiologic agent in the development of diabetic nephropathy. In diabetic, hyperfiltering rats given the angiotensin-converting enzyme (ACE) inhibitor captopril, GFR remained supranormal, whereas blood pressure, glomerular capillary pressure, and the severity of glomerulosclerosis were reduced.[308] Similarly, in diabetic rats made hypertensive with a partially occluding clip on one renal artery (two-kidney one-clip Goldblatt model), glomerulosclerosis was more severe in the unclipped (hypertensive) kidney; the clipped (hypotensive) kidney

showed less severe nephropathy than in unclipped diabetic control animals.[309] This demonstrates that a reduction in blood pressure partially protects the kidney from developing the lesions of diabetic glomerulopathy. Taken together, these studies suggest that it is glomerular hypertension, not hyperfiltration, that is primarily responsible for the development of glomerulosclerosis.

Whether glomerular hypertension plays the primary role in the pathogenesis of diabetic nephropathy is still unclear. Although the bulk of the evidence indicates that hemodynamic changes play a major role in the initiation and the progression of diabetic nephropathy, this is clearly not the case in some nondiabetic models of glomerulosclerosis, which do not require the presence of hyperfiltration and intraglomerular hypertension for glomerulosclerosis to develop. Moreover, administration of captopril was associated with an attenuation in the development of glomerulosclerosis in these models, even though glomerular pressure was unaffected.[310] Additional questions have been raised about the applicability of rat models of diabetic glomerulopathy to human disease.[311]

## Growth Factors and Cytokines

Endothelial and mesangial cells manufacture a wide variety of factors capable of promoting or inhibiting growth in an autocrine or paracrine fashion.[312] Because glomerular endothelial and mesangial cells are separated by only a BM, passage of factors between these cells is easily accomplished. It has been proposed that many abnormalities encountered in diabetic nephropathy are due to the altered interaction between the glomerular endothelium and mesangium.[313] Whereas many growth factors and cytokines can induce mesangial cell growth and matrix protein synthesis in vitro,[314] the exact contribution of each of these factors in the development and progression of diabetic nephropathy remains unknown (Table 39–7). Messenger RNA (mRNA) levels for several growth factors are increased in diabetic rat glomeruli: 24 weeks after the induction of diabetes by streptozocin, messages for tumor necrosis factor-$\alpha$, platelet-derived growth factor B chain, transforming growth factor-$\beta$, and basic fibroblast growth factor are increased. In contrast, mRNAs for IGF-1, platelet-derived growth factor A chain, and epidermal growth factor are not altered.[315] However, it has not yet been determined whether the increase in mRNA for these growth factors is the cause or the result of diabetic nephropathy.

There is strong evidence that growth hormone or its effector molecule IGF-1 plays a pathogenic role in diabetic nephropathy. Levels of IGF-1 are elevated shortly after induction of diabetes in rats,[316] and treatment of humans with a somatostatin analogue (octreotide) that decreases growth hormone secretion reduces the initial renal hypertrophy and increased GFR associated with IDDM.[317] Nondiabetic mice made transgenic for growth hormone and growth hormone releasing hormone develop glomerulosclerosis associated with an increase in extracellular matrix.[318] Interestingly, mice transgenic for IGF-1 do not develop glomerulosclerosis; this may be because levels of IGF-1 are lower in these mice, or it may be that growth hormone has

**TABLE 39–7. Effect of Growth Factors on Mesangial Growth and Matrix Production**

| Agent | Promote or Inhibit Mesangial Growth | Effects on Mesangial Matrix Production | Manufactured by |
|---|---|---|---|
| Insulin-like growth factor-1 | + | + | Mesangium, collecting duct |
| Platelet-derived growth factor | + | Presumed + | Mesangium |
| Epidermal growth factor | + | Presumed + | Distal tubule, loop of Henle |
| Basic fibroblast growth factor | + | Presumed + | ? |
| Angiotensin II | + | + | Glomeruli |
| Endothelin | + | + | Mesangial cell |
| Interleukin-1 | + | ? | Monocyte-macrophages |
| Transforming growth factor-β | − | + | Glomeruli?, platelets, monocyte-macrophages, proximal tubule? |
| Atrial natriuretic peptide | − | ? | Unknown |
| Heparin and related substances | − | ? | Endothelium |
| Nitric oxide | − | ? | Endothelium, mesangium |

effects on the kidney apart from its ability to increase IGF-1. mRNA expression of transforming growth factor-β is increased in diabetic rat and human kidneys compared with that of nondiabetic control subjects.[319] In both experimental diabetic glomerulopathy and glomerulonephritis, transforming growth factor-β causes expansion of the extracellular matrix by inducing the synthesis of several matrix components.[320, 321] In mesangial cells in vitro, transforming growth factor-β also increases mesangial matrix production.[320] Alternatively, diabetic animals may not produce more systemic or local growth factors but may be more sensitive to the effects of normal amounts of growth factors. For example, fibroblasts from diabetic nephropathic patients, when cultured in vitro, have a greater growth response to growth factors than that of fibroblasts from diabetic patients without nephropathy or nondiabetic control patients.[322] Whether this increased sensitivity is genetically determined or acquired during the course of disease is unknown.

The finding that ACE inhibitors decrease proteinuria and reduce the rate of decline in GFR in diabetic nephropathy as well as in models of glomerulosclerosis associated with normal intraglomerular pressures has led investigators to examine the role of angiotensin II (and other vasoactive peptides) in the pathogenesis of nephropathy. Angiotensin II may contribute to diabetic nephropathy by inducing glomerular hypertension, but it has also been shown to promote mesangial cell growth in vitro,[323] increase the production of extracellular matrix proteins,[324] and alter the filtration properties of the glomerular barrier.[325] Other vasoactive peptides, such as arginine vasopressin and endothelin, both of which are vasoconstrictors, have also been shown to increase mesangial cell growth in vitro, but their role in diabetic nephropathy is not well defined.[326, 327] In contrast, vasodilators, such as atrial natriuretic peptide and nitric oxide, have been shown to inhibit mesangial cell growth in vitro and to modulate the effects of other vasoactive peptides and growth factors.[328, 329]

Cytokines, such as the interleukins, may also play a role in the pathogenesis of diabetic nephropathy. Macrophages have AGE receptors and bind AGE-modified proteins. This results in the release of a variety of factors from platelets, including nitric oxide and interleukins. Interleukin-1 has been shown to cause mesangial cell proliferation in vitro.[330] The role of interleukin-1 in glomerular injury is evident in immune-mediated models of glomerulonephritis; the role it plays in diabetic nephropathy is less clear.

In summary, growth factors and other cytokines produced by either the endothelium or mesangium may cause the abnormal growth, BM thickening, and mesangial matrix expansion seen in diabetic nephropathy. They may do this directly or by modulating actions of other factors. Whereas there are currently several strong candidates that may play a central etiologic role in the development of glomerulosclerosis in diabetes, their exact contribution to the process is unknown.

## Genetics

Inheritance plays an important role in the pathogenesis of diabetic nephropathy. This is demonstrated by the high concordance rate for diabetic nephropathy in families[121–123] and the fact that different rates of nephropathy exist in different racial groups.[331] Several studies with identical twins discordant for diabetes have shown that some nondiabetic twins have increases in muscle capillary BM thickness, which suggests that there may be an underlying disorder predisposing to abnormalities of the BM.[332, 333] In a long-term study of IDDM patients who received kidney transplants because of the development of ESRD due to diabetic nephropathy, only about 50% of the patients experienced a recurrence of nephropathy during a post-transplantation period of 6 to 14 years. This recurrence did not correlate with any potential transplant risk factor, and there was only a weak relationship with the degree of glycemia after transplantation. This suggests that there may be a difference in the donor kidney's resistance to the development of diabetic nephropathy.[334] Investigators have concentrated on identifying genetic markers that may underlie the heritable risk of nephropathy. It has been noted in some studies that there is a statistically significant increase in the $Na^+$-$Li^+$ countertransport mechanism in IDDM patients with nephropathy[126, 129] and their parents[125] compared with that in matched IDDM patients without nephropathy and their parents, but the data have not been confirmed.[127, 131]

**TABLE 39–8. Impact of Different Treatment Modalities on Initiation and Progression of Diabetic Nephropathy***

| Effect | Antihypertensive Drug | | | | Intensive Blood Glucose Control | Low-Protein Diet | Lipid Lowering |
| --- | --- | --- | --- | --- | --- | --- | --- |
| | *Diuretic* | *β-Blocker* | *Ca²⁺ Antagonist* | *ACEI* | | | |
| Retarded development of experimental diabetic glomerulopathy | ? | ? | +/0 | + | + | + | + |
| Reduced microalbuminuria | 0 | + | +/0/− | + | + | + | ? |
| Postponed development of diabetic nephropathy | ? | + | ? | + | + | ? | ? |
| Reduced macroalbuminuria | + | + | +/0/− | + | − | + | 0 |
| Postponed end-stage renal disease in diabetic nephropathy | + | + | ? | + | − | + | ? |
| Improved survival in diabetic nephropathy | + | + | ? | + | − | ? | ? |

*ACEI = angiotensin-converting enzyme inhibitor; ? = effect unknown; + = positive effect; − = negative effect; 0 = neutral effect.

Furthermore, enhanced $Na^+$-$Li^+$ countertransport activity has been demonstrated both in NIDDM patients with and without diabetic nephropathy (biopsy proven).[130] Findings suggest that insulin receptor gene polymorphism is associated with the development of proteinuria[335] and that type IV collagen mutations may be associated with an increased risk of nephropathy[336]; however, these findings are still preliminary.

## Other Potential Factors

Prostaglandins have been implicated in the pathogenesis of diabetic nephropathy. Early in the disease, increases in vasodilatory prostaglandins, such as prostacyclin, may contribute to hyperfiltration.[337] Production of the vasoconstrictor thromboxane is also increased in diabetes, with increases in urinary thromboxane excretion seen as early as 2 weeks after induction of diabetes in rats. Thromboxane and prostacyclin have been shown to have direct actions on matrix gene expression, with thromboxane causing increases in mRNA for collagen type IV, laminin, and fibronectin and decreases in heparan sulfate proteoglycan. Prostacyclin, in contrast, suppresses mRNA for type IV collagen and fibronectin, with stimulation of heparan sulfate proteoglycan and laminin B2.[338] In diabetic animals, treatment with a thromboxane inhibitor for 7 months from the time of induction of diabetes prevents increases in urinary albumin, mesangial volume, and glomerular BM thickening.[339]

Functional abnormalities of platelets play an important role in the etiology of vascular disease. Long-term studies with diabetic rats treated with aspirin show that the initial increase and subsequent fall in GFR, as well as BM thickening, can be prevented by aspirin.[340] In humans, short-term administration of aspirin to patients with diabetic nephropathy results in a reduction in proteinuria.[341] However, a small group of diabetic patients with nephropathy who were observed for 10 years while receiving aspirin showed a minimal long-term effect of aspirin on proteinuria, although there was some stabilization of renal function.[342]

In several animal models of progressive glomerular disease, treatment of hyperlipidemia with the hydroxymethylglutaryl–coenzyme A reductase inhibitor lovastatin reduced albuminuria and the magnitude of structural injury.[343, 344]

Experiments in vivo demonstrate that lovastatin can inhibit serum-stimulated cell proliferation, probably by its effects on mevalonate pathway products.[345] Whether lovastatin exerts its beneficial effects primarily by lowering lipid levels or by altering cell mevalonate product levels is currently unclear.

## TREATMENT

The major therapeutic interventions that have been investigated include near-normal blood glucose control, antihypertensive treatment, and restriction of dietary proteins (Table 39–8). The impact of these three treatment modalities on progression from normoalbuminuria to microalbuminuria (primary prevention), microalbuminuria to diabetic nephropathy (secondary prevention), and diabetic nephropathy to ESRD is described and discussed.

## Glycemic Control

### PRIMARY PREVENTION

Strict metabolic control achieved by insulin treatment or islet cell transplantation normalizes hyperfiltration, hyperperfusion, and glomerular capillary hypertension and reduces the rate of rise in urinary albumin excretion in experimental diabetic animals.[346–355] The treatment also mitigates the development of diabetic glomerulopathy, whereas the glomerular enlargement remains unaffected.[347, 356, 357] Short-term near-normal blood glucose control in normoalbuminuric IDDM patients reduces GFR, renal plasma flow, and urinary albumin excretion rate; in some[77, 216, 223, 358] but not all[186] investigations, this decrease was accompanied by a reduction in the enlarged kidney. Increased kidney size is associated with an exaggerated renal response to amino acid infusion, and studies suggest that both abnormalities can be corrected by 3 weeks of intensified insulin treatment.[359] A meta-analysis of long-term (8 to 60 months) intensive blood glucose control has documented a beneficial effect on the progression from normoalbuminuria to microalbuminuria in IDDM patients[360] (Fig. 39–5). The odds ratio for progressing from normoalbuminuria to microalbuminuria ranged

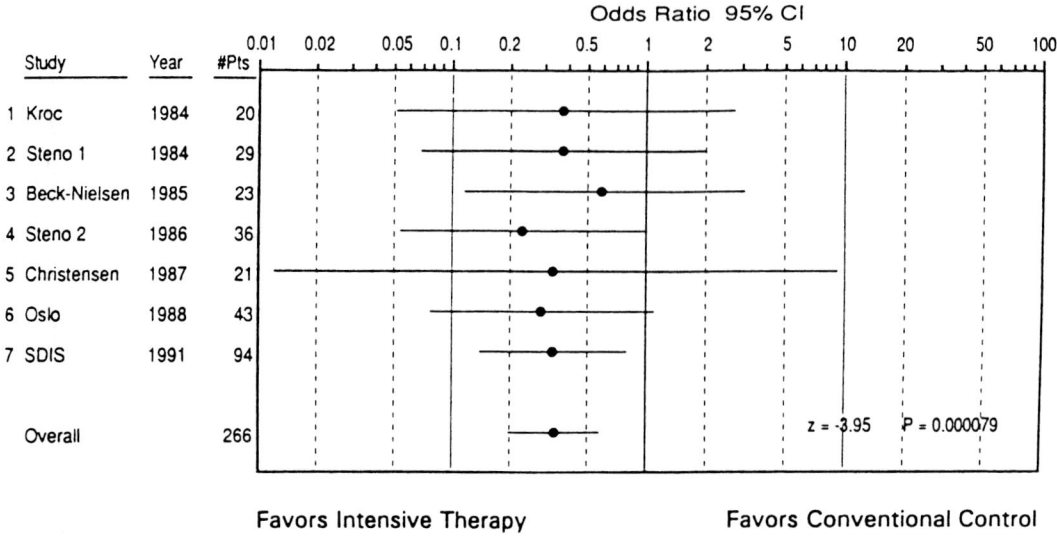

**Figure 39–5.** Effects of intensive blood glucose control on progression from normoalbuminuria to microalbuminuria and from microalbuminuria to nephropathy in IDDM patients. (From Wang PH, Lau J, Chalmers TC: Meta-analysis of effects of intensive blood-glucose control on late complications of type I diabetes. Lancet 441:1306, 1993.)

from 0.22 to 0.40 in the intensified treatment groups.[361–366] A worsening of diabetic retinopathy was observed during the initial months of intensive therapy, but in the longer term, the rate of deterioration was slower than it was in the conventionally treated IDDM patients.[367] Side effects are a major concern with intensive therapy, and the frequency of severe hypoglycemia and diabetic ketoacidosis was greater in several studies.[360] The Diabetes Control and Complications Trial[368] has confirmed and extended these clinical results: intensive insulin therapy reduced development of microalbuminuria in 35% of patients.

### SECONDARY PREVENTION

All long-term (8 to 96 months) randomized trials have documented a beneficial impact on the rate of rise in urinary albumin excretion and the development of overt diabetic nephropathy in IDDM patients with persistent microalbuminuria.[360, 368, 369] The odds ratio for progressing from microalbuminuria to overt nephropathy ranged from 0.3 to 0.6 in the groups receiving intensified treatment[361, 362, 366, 369, 370] (see Fig. 39–5). Part of this beneficial effect can possibly be of hemodynamic origin because a close correlation was found between the change in arterial blood pressure and the change in microalbuminuria.[370] A 10% to 15% reduction in GFR was observed at the initiation of strict metabolic control, after which no further reduction took place during the following 5 to 8 years if the patient remained microalbuminuric.[371] A progressive reduction in GFR was found in those patients who developed clinical diabetic nephropathy as defined in this chapter. These findings suggest that the development of clinical diabetic nephropathy is a valid principal end point.

### NEPHROPATHY

The impact of improved metabolic control on progression of kidney disease in IDDM patients with nephropathy

has been disappointing.[372, 373] The rate of decline in GFR and the rise in proteinuria and in systemic blood pressure were not affected by improved glycemic control. However, none of the trials were randomized, and the number of patients investigated was small.

## Blood Pressure Control

### PRIMARY PREVENTION

Originally, Zatz and colleagues[374] showed that prevention of glomerular capillary hypertension in normotensive insulin-treated streptozocin-induced diabetic rats effectively protects against the subsequent development of proteinuria and focal and segmental glomerular structural lesions. Jackson and associates[266] confirmed the beneficial effect of ACE inhibition in uninephrectomized rats made diabetic by streptozocin. Anderson and co-workers[375, 376] have demonstrated that antihypertensive therapy slows the development of diabetic glomerulopathy but that ACE inhibitors afford superior long-term protection compared with triple therapy with reserpine, hydralazine, and hydrochlorothiazide or a $Ca^{2+}$ channel blocker (nifedipine). Observations are consistent with the concept that glomerular hypertension is a factor in the pathogenesis of experimental diabetic glomerulopathy and indicate that lowering of systemic blood pressure without concomitant lessening of glomerular capillary pressure may be insufficient to prevent glomerular injury.[375–377] Lowering of systemic blood pressure by ACE inhibitors or conventional antihypertensive treatment affords significant renoprotection in spontaneously hypertensive streptozocin-induced diabetic rats.[378] No specific benefit of ACE inhibition was observed in this hypertensive model, in contrast to the normotensive models. The short-term renal effects of ACE inhibition have yielded conflicting results in normotensive normoalbuminuric IDDM patients.[379] No information is available regarding the long-term effects on kidney function and structure in normoalbuminuric IDDM and NIDDM patients.

## SECONDARY PREVENTION

Marre and co-workers[380, 381] assessed the effectiveness of ACE inhibition in preventing diabetic nephropathy in 20 normotensive diabetic (NIDDM and IDDM) patients with persistent microalbuminuria (30 to 300 mg/24 h) treated with enalapril or its matched placebo for 1 year. The group treated with ACE inhibition had a significant reduction in blood pressure and in microalbuminuria, whereas the opposite took place in the group left untreated. Furthermore, diabetic kidney disease developed in 3 of 10 patients taking placebo (urinary albumin excretion rates > 300 mg/24 h).

Whether early intervention works in the long term was tested in a 4-year prospective study by Mathiesen and colleagues.[382] They evaluated the effectiveness of ACE inhibition in preventing the development of diabetic nephropathy in 44 normotensive IDDM patients with persistent microalbuminuria (Fig. 39–6). Urinary albumin excretion was gradually reduced in the captopril-treated group, whereas an increase occurred in the group left untreated. Seven of the untreated patients progressed to diabetic nephropathy, whereas none of the 21 captopril-treated patients had clinically overt nephropathy. More important, in the seven patients who had persistent albuminuria, the GFR fell; in control patients who did not have overt nephropathy, it remained stable. A European Multicenter Study has confirmed and extended these observations.[383] Hallab and associates[384] found that enalapril effectively reduced microalbuminuria in normotensive and hypertensive IDDM patients, whereas hydrochlorothiazide was not effective.

Borch-Johnsen and co-workers[227] conducted a cost-benefit analysis of screening and antihypertensive treatment of early renal disease indicated by microalbuminuria in IDDM patients. The authors concluded that screening and intervention programs are likely to have life-saving effects and lead to considerable economic savings.

The impact of ACE inhibition in microalbuminuric NIDDM patients has also been evaluated.[385] A randomized study of diabetic patients with microalbuminuria treated with perindopril or nifedipine for 12 months was conducted. Both treatments significantly reduced mean arterial blood pressure and urinary albumin excretion rate. Unfortunately, the study was dealing with a heterogeneous group of hypertensive or normotensive IDDM or NIDDM patients. Ravid and colleagues[17] have conducted a double-blind randomized study in 94 normotensive microalbuminuric NIDDM patients receiving enalapril or placebo for 5 years. In the actively treated group, the kidney function remained stable, and diabetic nephropathy developed in only 12% of the patients; however, in the group receiving placebo, kidney function declined by 13%, and nephropathy developed in 42% of the patients. Chan and colleagues[386] have compared the efficacy, safety, and tolerance of enalapril and nifedipine in hypertensive NIDDM patients with normoalbuminuria (n = 44), microalbuminuria (n = 36), and macroalbuminuria (n = 22). The blood pressure reduction was equal in both treated groups, but albuminuria fell by 54% in the enalapril-treated group and by only 11%

in the nifedipine-treated group. Creatinine clearance fell (15%) similarly in both groups.

## NEPHROPATHY

Originally, Mogensen[387] demonstrated that long-term antihypertensive treatment reduced albuminuria and slowed the rate of decline in GFR from 15 to 6 mL/min/y in five hypertensive male IDDM patients with overt nephropathy. Parving and co-workers[388–390] confirmed and extended these observations by demonstrating that early and aggressive antihypertensive treatment with metoprolol, furosemide, and hydralazine reduces albuminuria, slows the decline in GFR, and postpones ESRD in young male and female IDDM patients with diabetic nephropathy. Figure 39–7 illustrates the mean values in nine patients receiving antihypertensive therapy for 10 years.[390] Hommel,[391] Parving,[392] and Björck[393, 394] and co-workers showed that long-term treatment with ACE inhibitors, usually combined with diuretics, reduces blood pressure and albuminuria and protects kidney function in hypertensive IDDM patients with nephropathy. Beneficial effects on kidney function have also been reported in normotensive IDDM patients with nephropathy.[395] Björck and colleagues[396] have reported that ACE inhibition can protect kidney function in IDDM patients with diabetic nephropathy more than treatment with a selective β-blocker can. This finding suggests that not all antihypertensive drugs are equally renoprotective. Other studies, in both IDDM[397–399] and NIDDM[400, 401] patients, have yielded conflicting results, which suggests that adequate blood pressure control by both ACE inhibitors and conventional antihypertensive drugs (diuretics and β-blockers) stabilizes GFR and reduces albuminuria to the same extent. Unfortunately, the observation period has been short (≤1.5 years) in all studies using $Ca^{2+}$ channel blockers, and the renoprotective effects differ importantly among the three main drug classes.[402–404] A multicenter randomized double-masked clinical trial comparing the effect of captopril (25 mg three times a day) versus placebo in normotensive and hypertensive IDDM patients (n = 407) with diabetic nephropathy has demonstrated an insignificant risk reduction (17%) in the time to doubling of the serum creatinine level in the 300 patients with a baseline creatinine concentration of less than 1.5 mg/dL.[405] In contrast, a significant risk reduction (67%) with ACE inhibition was demonstrated in patients with baseline serum creatinine concentration above 1.5 mg/dL. Furthermore, yearly GFR measurements with iothalamate confirmed the findings, which suggest that the beneficial effect of ACE inhibition is more pronounced in advanced diabetic nephropathy. The impact of antihypertensive treatment on diabetic retinopathy has not been evaluated properly in any of these trials. Furthermore, no controlled study has been conducted to evaluate whether antihypertensive therapy may delay or prevent the development or progression of diabetic retinopathy.[268]

The decline in GFR per unit of time early after the start of antihypertensive treatment is usually two to five times higher than during the remaining treatment period. It has been shown that the intrinsic vascular (arteriolar) mechanism underlying the normal autoregulation of GFR, that is,

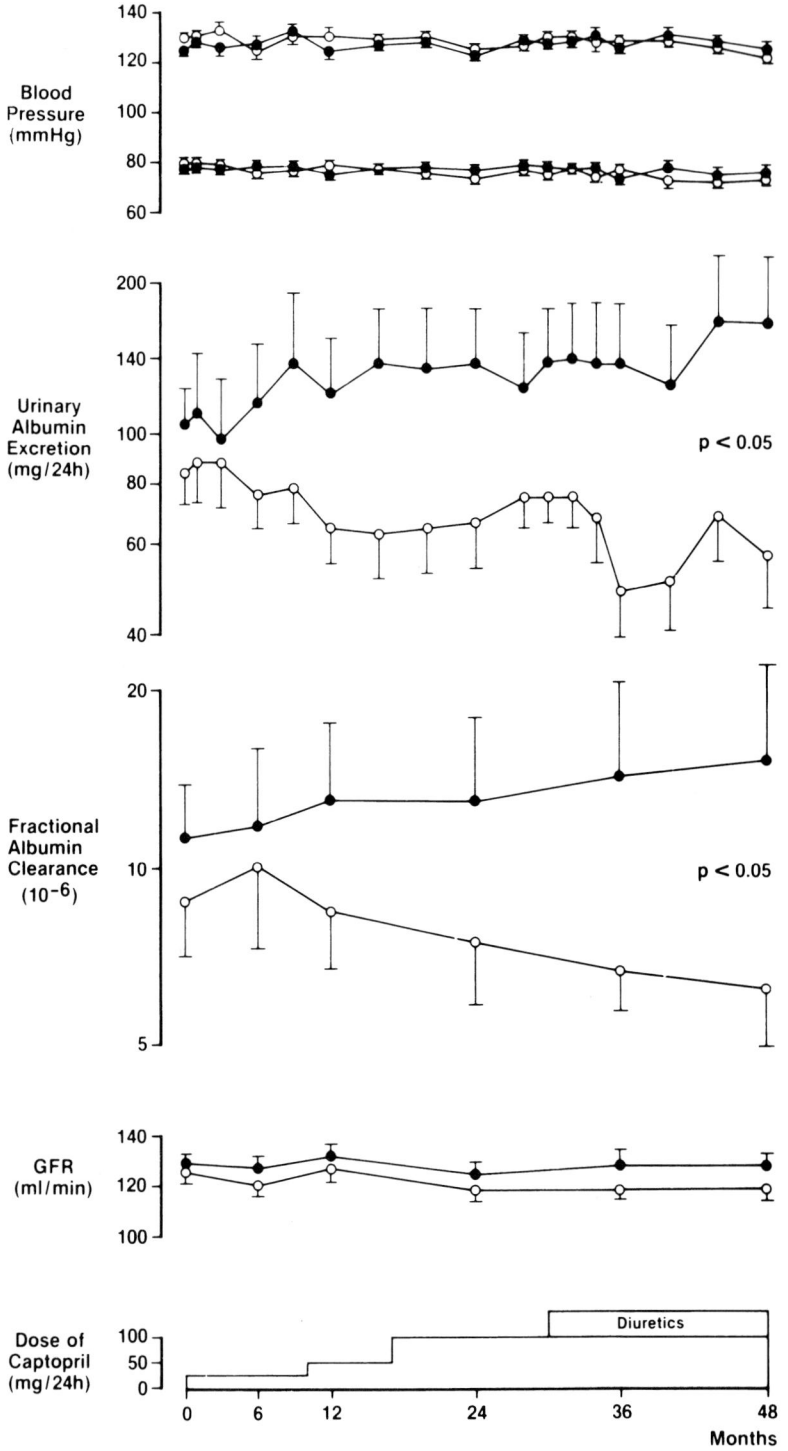

**Figure 39–6.** Time course of mean arterial blood pressure, urinary albumin excretion, fractional albumin clearance, and GFR in normotensive IDDM patients with microalbuminuria. Twenty-one patients received captopril (○), and 23 served as untreated control subjects (●). Ordinates of urinary albumin excretion and fractional albumin clearance are log scales. Bars are SEM. (From Mathiesen ER, Hommel E, Giese J, Parving H-H: Efficacy of captopril in postponing nephropathy in normotensive diabetic patients with microalbuminuria. Br Med J 300:81, 1991.)

the fairly constant GFR that occurs despite wide variations in perfusion pressure, is impaired in diabetic nephropathy.[406] In addition to this potentially reversible hemodynamic effect induced by antihypertensive treatment, closure of damaged glomeruli caused by ischemia induced by hypotension may also contribute.

Meta-analysis has documented that ACE inhibitors are superior to β-blockers, diuretics, and $Ca^{2+}$ channel blockers in reducing urinary albumin excretion in normotensive and hypertensive IDDM and NIDDM patients.[379] This superiority was more pronounced in the normotensive state; it diminished progressively with progressive blood pressure reduction.[379] Reduced glomerular capillary hydraulic pressure in combination with diminished size- and charge-selective properties of the glomerular capillary membrane is the most likely mechanism involved in the antiproteinuric effect of ACE inhibitors.[281, 325, 407–410] Rossing and colleagues[411, 412] have demonstrated that a decrease in albuminuria shortly

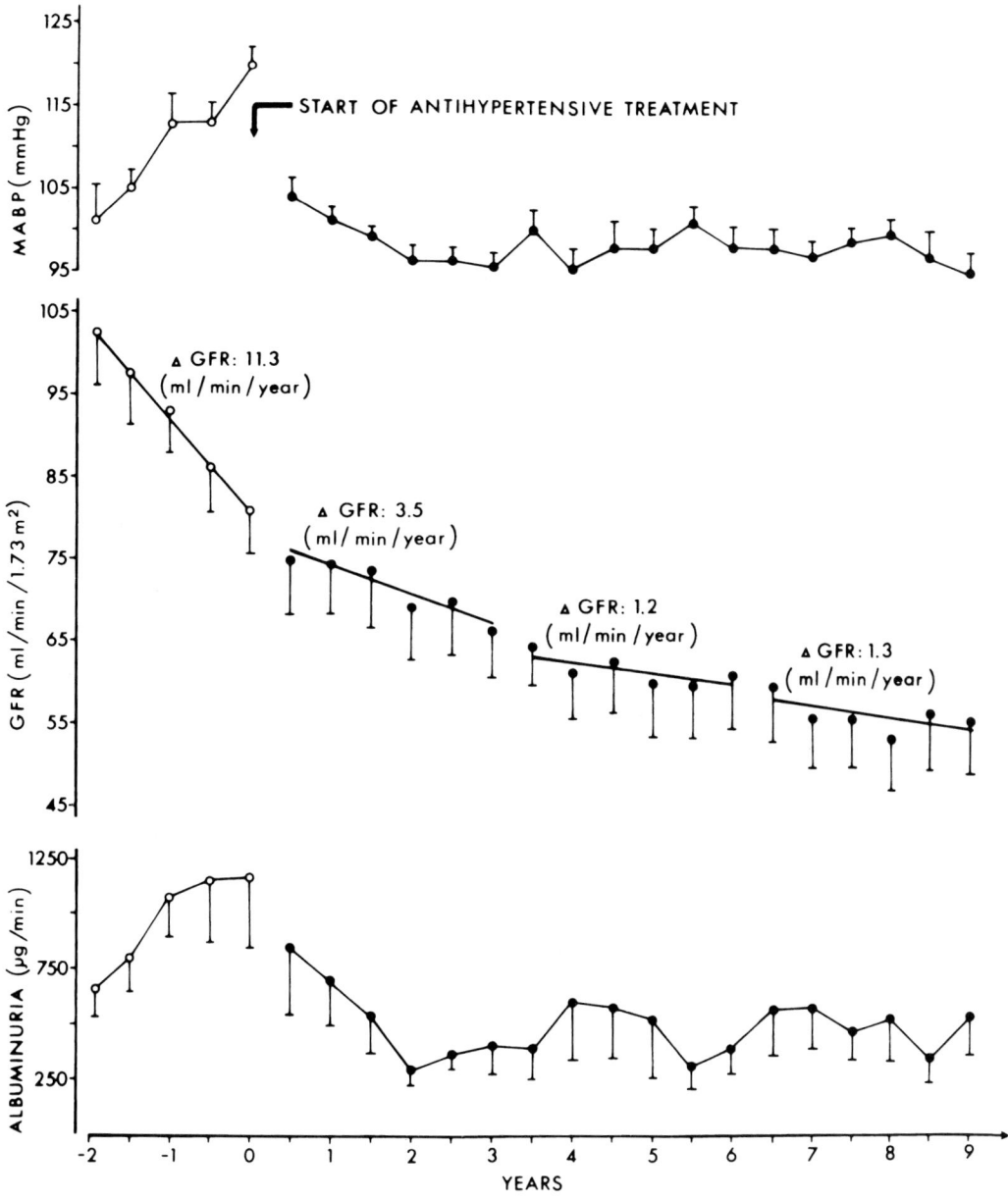

**Figure 39–7.** Average course of mean arterial blood pressure (MABP), GFR, and albuminuria before (○) and during (●) long-term effective antihypertensive treatment in nine IDDM patients with diabetic nephropathy. (From Parving H-H, Smidt UM, Hommel E, et al: Effective antihypertensive treatment postpones renal insufficiency in diabetic nephropathy. Am J Kidney Dis 22:188, 1993.)

after onset of antihypertensive treatment predicts an attenuated fall rate in GFR in diabetic nephropathy. The finding suggests a clinical application for monitoring the efficacy of antihypertensive treatment in diabetic nephropathy.

Parving and Hommel[412a] have assessed the effect of long-term antihypertensive therapy on prognosis in diabetic nephropathy (see Fig. 39–4). All IDDM patients with diabetic nephropathy between 1974 and 1978 at Steno Diabetes Center were enrolled. Forty-five patients were observed until death or for at least 10 years. The median follow-up was 13 (4 to 15) years. Mean blood pressure at start of antihypertensive treatment was 148/95 ± 15/15 mm Hg. Systolic blood pressure remained unchanged, whereas diastolic blood pressure decreased significantly (0.9 mm Hg/y) dur-

ing antihypertensive treatment. The cumulative death rate was 18% (95% confidence interval, 8% to 32%) 10 years after onset of proteinuria, in contrast to previous reports of 50% to 77% 10 years after onset of nephropathy.[412a] Uremia was the main cause of death (64%) in Parving and Hommel's study as in the three previous studies dealing with the natural course of diabetic nephropathy.[22, 28, 33] Mathiesen and co-workers[413] have shown that the survival of IDDM patients with nephropathy has improved substantially because early effective antihypertensive treatment has become routine treatment in their clinic. The Collaborative Study Group of Angiotensin Converting Enzyme Inhibition in diabetic nephropathy has demonstrated a risk reduction of 56% (95% confidence interval, 25% to 74%) for the occurrence of death or dialysis/transplantation in IDDM patients treated with captopril versus placebo.[405] All the hypertensive patients received conventional antihypertensive drugs and, in addition, captopril or placebo.

In conclusion, the prognosis of IDDM patients suffering from diabetic nephropathy has improved during the past decade, largely because of effective antihypertensive treatment with conventional drugs (β-blockers, diuretics) and ACE inhibitors. Unfortunately, no information on this important issue is available in NIDDM patients with diabetic nephropathy.

## Dietary Protein Restriction

Dietary protein restriction, which limits glomerular capillary pressures and flows in rats, was used by Zatz and colleagues[414, 415] to further clarify the role of hemodynamic factors in the pathogenesis of experimental diabetic glomerulopathy. After 14 months of streptozocin-induced diabetes, protein-restricted rats exhibited virtually no albuminuria or glomerular structural lesions, and glomerular capillary pressure was normalized. Short-term studies in normoalbuminuric and microalbuminuric IDDM patients have shown that low-protein diet (0.6 to 0.8 g/kg/d) reduces urinary albumin excretion and hyperfiltration, independently of changes in glucose control and blood pressure.[416, 417] Longer term trials in IDDM patients with diabetic nephropathy suggest that protein restriction reduces the progression of kidney injury,[418, 419] but the interpretation has been challenged.[420, 421] The potentially beneficial effect of dietary protein restriction in NIDDM patients with nephropathy will be analyzed in the Modification of Diet in Renal Disease study.

## Transplantation and Dialysis

Diabetic nephropathy is currently the leading cause of ESRD in the United States, accounting for 33% of all new cases. Diabetic nephropathy is more common in IDDM patients, but because of the greater number of NIDDM patients, the mean age of diabetic patients with ESRD is approximately 60 years.[422] The management of the diabetic patient with ESRD is challenging because the damage wrought by diabetes is rarely confined to the kidneys, as discussed previously. Currently, there are three therapeutic choices for ESRD diabetic patients: transplantation (kidney only or kidney and pancreas), continuous ambulatory peritoneal dialysis (CAPD), and hemodialysis. The choice of therapy is generally tailored to the patient's desires and abilities. Depending on the patient's condition and wishes, the refusal of treatment or the termination of dialysis is also a viable option.

## Transplantation

Kidney transplantation is the optimal treatment for diabetic patients with ESRD. Overall, approximately 20% of ESRD diabetic patients receive transplants. With improve-

ments in immunosuppressive protocols, statistics from the University of Minnesota demonstrate that the 1-year graft survival for diabetic patients receiving a cadaver kidney is as high as 93%.[423] The patients in this study are probably without other significant complications of diabetes because in a small study of patients with diabetes and underlying cardiovascular disease who received renal transplants, survival of patients after 1 year was only 48%; graft survival was 37%.[424]

Despite the encouraging statistics, survival of diabetic patients and grafts in diabetic patients is still inferior to that of nondiabetic patients. In a study of 1-year graft survivors, the survival rate for transplants to diabetic patients was 9 years; for nondiabetics, it was 13.6 years. However, when death with a functioning graft was excluded, there were no significant differences in graft survival between diabetic and nondiabetic patients.[425] In a longer term follow-up of patients receiving transplants, the overall 10-year survival of the patient and graft was 40% and 32%, respectively, for diabetic patients versus 61% and 51% for nondiabetic patients. Overall, the poorer graft survival in diabetic patients is primarily attributable to their excess mortality due to accelerated macrovascular disease. Because kidney transplantation will not alter the course of diabetic complications, such as macrovascular disease or retinopathy, simultaneous pancreas-kidney transplantation has been explored as a method of arresting the other complications of diabetes. With optimal human leukocyte antigen DR matching and immunosuppressive treatment, the 1-year graft survival for the pancreas in simultaneous pancreas-kidney transplants or pancreas-after-kidney transplants is approximately 71%.[426] Pancreas transplantation has been shown to reduce the recurrence of diabetic nephropathy in the transplanted kidney and has a positive impact on diabetic neuropathy. However, retinopathy initially worsens over the first several years, improving thereafter. The effect of euglycemia on the progression of macrovascular disease has not been closely examined. Currently, pancreas transplantation is viewed as an adjunct to kidney transplantation in diabetic patients with established nephropathy.

## Continuous Ambulatory Peritoneal Dialysis

In some centers, CAPD is considered the procedure of choice for the treatment of ESRD in diabetic patients,[427] although in the United States, only 10% to 20% of patients are treated with CAPD. CAPD offers several advantages to hemodialysis. Because the dialysis is continuous, there is more even correction of fluid overload and uremia, with better control of volume-dependent hypertension. There is less hypotension with CAPD, because fluid shifts are not as dramatic as with hemodialysis, an important consideration in patients with autonomic neuropathy who experience severe, prolonged hypotension during dialysis. Patients receiving CAPD have better preservation of hematocrits, because there is no blood loss associated with the procedure. Finally, patients may experience improved blood glucose control when insulin is added directly to the dialysate because the insulin is absorbed directly into the portal circulation from the peritoneum with immediate delivery to the liver.[428] On the other hand, the drawbacks of CAPD often restrict its use among diabetics; adequate vision and manual dexterity (often a problem for patients with retinopathy and sensory neuropathy) are necessary to perform CAPD, unless the patient has a full-time helper. Infection and catheter problems are common and often necessitate discontinuance of CAPD. In one study, survival of patients at 24 months was 60% (better than that of hemodialysis)[429]; however, in another study, survival of patients treated with CAPD or hemodialysis was similar.[430]

## Hemodialysis

Most ESRD diabetics in the United States (70%) are treated with hemodialysis, the majority in a center setting. As with transplantation and CAPD, survival rates for diabetic patients undergoing hemodialysis are lower than those for nondiabetic patients.[431] At the University of Wisconsin, overall survival for patients treated with hemodialysis was 65% at 1 year and 38% at 2 years[432]; other studies have documented better[433] or worse[434] statistics, depending on the condition and age of the patients participating. As with diabetic patients who receive kidney transplants and diabetic patients using CAPD, the leading cause of death in diabetic patients undergoing hemodialysis is cardiovascular in origin, followed by sepsis.[435] Hospitalizations for complications involving vascular access are frequent.[436] Hypotension during dialysis is common in patients with autonomic neuropathy and may be severe. Switching from acetate to a bicarbonate buffer may help reduce the severity of the hypertension, as may dialyzing against a bath with an $Na^+$ concentration of 140 to 144 mEq/dL.[437]

Like other treatment modalities, hemodialysis does not affect the natural history of the other macrovascular and microvascular complications, and retinopathy often progresses on dialysis, which emphasizes the need for frequent ophthalmologic follow-up and treatment.

## OTHER URINARY TRACT COMPLICATIONS ASSOCIATED WITH DIABETES

### Bladder Dysfunction

Objective testing demonstrates that approximately 26% to 87% of IDDM patients and 25% of NIDDM patients have neurogenic bladders,[438] although most are relatively asymptomatic. The primary clinical feature of cystopathy is decreased sensation of bladder fullness leading to increased residual urine, overflow incontinence, and infection. There may also be a feeling of straining to void. Evaluation by cystometrogram may demonstrate an enlarged bladder, hydroureter, and increased residual urine as well as abnormalities in detrusor, bladder neck, and external sphincter contractions.

Depending on the severity of the situation, therapy may include 1) scheduled voiding every 3 to 4 hours, with repetitive voiding to ensure that the bladder actually empties;

2) cholinergic therapy (bethanechol, 10 to 50 mg three times a day); 3) long-term catheterization, either intermittent or indwelling; and possibly 4) incision of the internal sphincter.

## Urinary Tract Infection

There is some dispute about whether urinary tract infections are more common in diabetic patients.[439] However, it is agreed that morbidity and mortality due to urinary tract infection are increased in diabetic patients because diabetic patients are more likely to have upper tract disease than are nondiabetic patients.[440] Pregnant diabetic women with bacteriuria experience a 50% perinatal mortality compared with a 15% rate among diabetic women without bacteriuria.[441]

The bacteriology of urinary tract infection is not significantly different in the diabetic patient; one study suggested that the frequency of *Klebsiella* species is higher than in nondiabetic patients.[442] In addition, fungal infection of the urinary tract is seen in diabetic patients; counts of greater than $1 \times 10^4$/mL on a catheterized specimen probably indicate primary infection.[443] Treatment consists of either local irrigation through a Foley catheter with an amphotericin solution or use of intravenous amphotericin.

## REFERENCES

1. Harris MJ, Zimmet P: Classification of diabetes mellitus and other categories of glucose intolerance. *In* Alberti KGMM, DeFronzo RA, Keen H, Zimmet P (eds): International Textbook of Diabetes Mellitus. John Wiley & Sons, Chichester, 1992, p 3.
2. Keen H: Diabetes diagnosis. *In* Alberti KGMM, DeFronzo RA, Keen H, Zimmet P (eds): International Textbook of Diabetes Mellitus. John Wiley & Sons, Chichester, 1992, p 19.
3. Hother-Nielsen O, Faber O, Sørensen NS, Beck-Nielsen H: Classification of newly diagnosed diabetic patients as insulin-requiring or non–insulin-requiring based on clinical and biochemical variables. Diabetes Care 11:531, 1988.
4. Faber OK, Binder C: C-peptide response to glucagon: A test for the residual β-cell function in diabetes mellitus. Diabetes 26:605, 1977.
5. Rollo J: Cases of Diabetes Mellitus, 2nd ed. Dilly, London, 1798.
6. Bright R: Cases and observations illustrative of renal disease accompanied with the secretion of albuminous urine. Guys Hosp Rep 1:338, 1836.
7. Kimmelstiel P, Wilson C: Intercapillary lesions in the glomeruli of the kidney. Am J Pathol 12:83, 1936.
8. Deckert T, Parving H-H, Andersen AR, et al: Diabetic nephropathy. A clinical and morphometric study. *In* Eschwege E (ed): Advances in Diabetes Epidemiology. Elsevier Biomedical Press, Amsterdam, 1982, p 235.
9. Grenfell A, Bewick M, Parsons V, et al: Non–insulin-dependent diabetes and renal replacement therapy. Diabetic Med 5:172, 1988.
10. Parving H-H, Gall M, Skøtt P, et al: Prevalence and causes of albuminuria in non–insulin-dependent diabetic patients. Kidney Int 41:758, 1992.
11. Parving H-H, Oxenbøll B, Svendsen PA, et al: Early detection of patients at risk of developing diabetic nephropathy. Acta Endocrinol 100:550, 1982.
12. Viberti GC, Hill RD, Jarrett RJ, et al: Microalbuminuria as a predictor of clinical nephropathy in insulin-dependent diabetes mellitus. Lancet 1:1430, 1982.
13. Mogensen CE, Christensen CK: Predicting diabetic nephropathy in insulin-dependent patients. N Engl J Med 311:89, 1984.
14. Mathiesen ER, Oxenbøll B, Johansen K, et al: Incipient nephropathy in type 1 (insulin-dependent) diabetes. Diabetologia 26:406, 1984.
15. Mogensen CE: Microalbuminuria predicts clinical proteinuria and

early mortality in maturity onset diabetes. N Engl J Med 310:356, 1984.

16. Nelson RG, Knowler WC, Pettitt DJ, et al: Assessing risk of overt nephropathy in diabetic patients from albumin excretion in untimed urine specimens. Arch Intern Med 151:1761, 1991.

17. Ravid M, Savin H, Jutrin I, et al: Long-term stabilizing effect of angiotensin-converting enzyme inhibition on plasma creatinine and on proteinuria in normotensive type II diabetic patients. Ann Intern Med 118:577, 1993.

18. Mogensen CE, Chachati A, Christensen CK, et al: Microalbuminuria: An early marker of renal involvement in diabetes. Uremia Invest 9:85, 1986.

19. Deckert T, Poulsen JE, Larsen M: Prognosis of diabetics with diabetes onset before the age of thirty-one. I. Survival, causes of death and complications. Diabetologia 14:363, 1978.

20. Deckert T, Poulsen JE, Larsen M: The prognosis of insulin-dependent diabetes mellitus and the importance of supervision. Acta Med Scand 624(suppl):48, 1979.

21. Andersen AR, Andersen JK, Christiansen JS, Deckert T: Prognosis for juvenile diabetics with nephropathy and failing renal function. Acta Med Scand 203:131, 1978.

22. Andersen AR, Christiansen JS, Andersen JK, et al: Diabetic nephropathy in type 1 (insulin-dependent) diabetes: An epidemiological study. Diabetologia 25:496, 1983.

23. Borch-Johnsen K, Kreiner S, Deckert T: Mortality of type 1 (insulin-dependent) diabetes mellitus in Denmark: A study of relative mortality in 2,930 Danish type 1 diabetic patients diagnosed from 1933 to 1972. Diabetologia 29:767, 1986.

24. Borch-Johnsen K, Kreiner S: Proteinuria: Value as predictor of cardiovascular mortality in insulin dependent diabetes mellitus. Br Med J 294:1651, 1987.

25. Borch-Johnsen K, Andersen PK, Deckert T: The effect of proteinuria on relative mortality in type 1 (insulin-dependent) diabetes mellitus. Diabetologia 28:590, 1985.

26. Borch-Johnsen K: The prognosis of insulin-dependent diabetes mellitus. An epidemiological approach. Dan Med Bull 36:336, 1989.

27. Green A, Borch-Johnsen K, Andersen PK, et al: Relative mortality of type 1 (insulin-dependent) diabetes in Denmark: 1933–1981. Diabetologia 28:339, 1985.

28. Krolewski AS, Warram JH, Christlieb AR, et al: The changing natural history of nephropathy in type 1 diabetes. Am J Med 78:785, 1985.

29. Nelson RG, Newman JM, Knowler WC, et al: Incidence of end-stage renal disease in type 2 (non–insulin-dependent) diabetes mellitus in Pima Indians. Diabetologia 31:730, 1988.

30. Nelson RG, Pettitt DJ, Carraher MJ, et al: Effect of proteinuria on mortality in NIDDM. Diabetes 37:1499, 1988.

31. Ballard DJ, Humphrey LL, Melton LJ III, et al: Epidemiology of persistent proteinuria in type II diabetes mellitus. Population-based study in Rochester, Minnesota. Diabetes 37:405, 1988.

32. Humphrey LL, Ballard DJ, Frohnert PP, et al: Chronic renal failure in non–insulin-dependent diabetes mellitus. A population-based study in Rochester, Minnesota. Ann Intern Med 111:788, 1989.

33. Knowles HC: Magnitude of the renal failure problem in diabetic patients. Kidney Int. 6(suppl 1):S2, 1974.

34. Breyer JA: Diabetic nephropathy in insulin-dependent patients. Am J Kidney Dis 20:533, 1992.

35. Eggers PW: Effect of transplantation on the Medicare end-stage renal disease program. N Engl J Med 318:223, 1988.

36. Striker GE, Agodoa LL, Held P, et al: Kidney disease of diabetes mellitus (diabetic nephropathy): Perspectives in the United States. J Diabetic Complications 5:51, 1992.

37. Frøkjær Thomsen O, Andersen AR, Christiansen JS, Deckert T: Renal changes in long-term type 1 (insulin-dependent) diabetic patients with and without clinical nephropathy: A light microscopic, morphometric study of autopsy material. Diabetologia 26:361, 1984.

38. Gellman DD, Pirani CI, Soothill JE: Diabetic nephropathy: A clinical and pathologic study based on renal biopsies. Medicine 38:321, 1959.

39. Mauer SM, Steffes MW, Ellis EN: Structural-functional relationships in diabetic nephropathy. J Clin Invest 74:1143, 1984.

40. Østerby R, Parving H-H, Hommel E, et al: Glomerular structure and function in diabetic nephropathy. Diabetes 39:1057, 1990.

41. Steffes MW, Bilous RW, Sutherland DER, Mauer SM: Cell and matrix components of the glomerular mesangium in type 1 diabetes. Diabetes 41:679, 1992.

42. Østerby R: Glomerular structural changes in type 1 (insulin-dependent) diabetes mellitus: Causes, consequences, and prevention. Diabetologia 35:803, 1992.

43. Fioretto P, Steffes MW, Mauer SM: Glomerular structure in nonproteinuric type 1 (insulin-dependent) diabetic patients with various levels of albuminuria. Diabetologia 36(suppl 1):A27, 1993.

44. Østerby R, Gall MA, Schmitz A: Glomerular structure and function in proteinuric type 2 (non–insulin-dependent) diabetic patients. Diabetologia 36:1064, 1993.

45. Thomsen C: The Kidney in Diabetes Mellitus. Munksgaard, Copenhagen, 1965.

46. Heptinstall RH: Pathology of the Kidney, 3rd ed. Little, Brown, Boston, 1983.

47. Olsen S: Light microscopy of diabetic glomerulosclerosis: Classic lesions and differential diagnosis. In Mogensen CE (ed): The Kidney and Hypertension in Diabetes Mellitus. Martinus Nijhoff Publishing, Boston, 1988, p 71.

48. Gundersen HJG, Østerby R: Glomerular size and structure in diabetes mellitus. II. Late abnormalities. Diabetologia 13:43, 1977.

49. Hørlyck A, Gundersen HJG, Østerby R: The cortical distribution pattern of diabetic glomerulopathy. Diabetologia 29:146, 1986.

50. Schmitz A, Gundersen HJG, Østerby R: Glomerular morphology by light microscopy in non–insulin-dependent diabetes mellitus: Lack of glomerular hypertrophy. Diabetes 37:38, 1988.

51. Gundersen HJG, Bendtsen TF, Korbo L: Some new, simple and efficient stereological methods and their use in pathological research and diagnosis. APMIS 96:379, 1988.

52. Walker JD, Close CF, Jones SL, et al: Glomerular structure in type 1 (insulin-dependent) diabetic patients with normo- and microalbuminuria. Kidney Int 41:741, 1992.

53. Bangstad H-J, Østerby R, Dahl-Jørgensen K, et al: Early glomerulopathy is present in young, type 1 (insulin-dependent) diabetic patients with microalbuminuria. Diabetologia 36:523, 1993.

54. Vejlsgaard R: Urinary tract infection and diabetes: Diagnosis and treatment. In Mogensen CE (ed): The Kidney and Hypertension in Diabetes Mellitus. Martinus Nijhoff Publishing, Boston, 1988, p 217.

55. Hommel E, Carstensen H, Skøtt P, Parving H-H: Prevalence and causes of microscopic haematuria in type 1 (insulin-dependent) diabetic patients with persistent proteinuria. Diabetologia 30:627, 1987.

56. Richards NT, Greaves I, Lee SJ: Increased prevalence of renal biopsy findings other than diabetic glomerulopathy in type II diabetes mellitus. Nephrol Dial Transplant 7:379, 1992.

57. Gambara V, Mecca G, Remuzzi G, Bertani T: Heterogeneous nature of renal lesions in type II diabetes. J Am Soc Nephrol 3:1458, 1993.

58. Hayashi H, Karasawa R, Inn H: An electron microscopic study of glomeruli in Japanese patients with non–insulin dependent diabetes mellitus. Kidney Int 41:749, 1992.

59. Østerby R, Gundersen HJG, Nyberg G, Aurell M: Advanced diabetic glomerulopathy. Quantitative structural characterization of non-occluded glomeruli. Diabetes 36:612, 1987.

60. Chavers BM, Bilous RW, Ellis EN, et al: Glomerular lesions and urinary albumin excretion in type 1 diabetes without overt proteinuria. N Engl J Med 320:966, 1989.

61. Østerby R, Bangstad H-J, Hanssen KF: Stereological studies of early phases of diabetic glomerulopathy. Diabetologia 33:A147, 1990.

62. Bangstad H-J, Østerby R, Dahl-Jørgensen K, et al: Improvement of blood glucose control in IDDM patients retards the progression of morphological changes in early diabetic nephropathy. Diabetologia 37:483, 1994.

63. Østerby R: Early phases in the development of diabetic glomerulopathy. A quantitative electron microscopic study. Acta Med Scand 574(suppl):1, 1975.

64. Kashgarian M: Mesangium and glomerular disease. Lab Invest 52:569, 1985. Editorial.

65. Kitamura M, Mitarai T, Maruyama N, et al: Mesangial cell behavior in a three dimensional extracellular matrix. Kidney Int 40:653, 1991.

66. Kashgarian M, Sterzel RB: The pathobiology of the mesangium. Kidney Int 41:524, 1992.

67. Ellis EN, Steffes MW, Chavers BM, Mauer SM: Observations of glomerular epithelial cell structure in patients with type 1 diabetes mellitus. Kidney Int 32:736, 1987.

68. Østerby R, Bangstad H-J, Hanssen KF: Interrelation of glomerular structure and abnormal albuminuria in IDDM. J Diabetic Complications 6:5, 1992.

69. Olsen S, Bohman S-O, Posborg Petersen V: Ultrastructure of the

glomerular basement membrane in long term renal allografts with transplant glomerular disease. Lab Invest 30:176, 1974.

70. Nakajima M, Hewitson TD, Mathews DC, Kincaid-Smith P: Localisation of complement components in association with glomerular extracellular particles in various renal diseases. Virchows Arch A 419:267, 1991.

71. Østerby R: Renal pathology in diabetes mellitus. Curr Opin Nephrol Hypertens 2:475, 1993.

72. Østerby R, Nyberg G: New vessel formation in the renal corpuscles in advanced diabetic glomerulopathy. J Diabetic Complications 1:122, 1987.

73. Østerby R, Parving H-H, Nyberg G, et al: A strong correlation between filtration rate and filtration surface in diabetic nephropathy. Diabetologia 31:265, 1988.

74. Harris RD, Steffes MW, Bilous RW, et al: Global glomerular sclerosis and glomerular arteriolar hyalinosis in insulin dependent diabetes. Kidney Int 40:107, 1991.

75. Bendtsen TF, Nyengaard JR: The number of glomeruli in type 1 (insulin-dependent) and type 2 (non–insulin-dependent) diabetic patients. Diabetologia 35:844, 1992.

76. Hostetter TH, Rennke HG, Brenner BM: The case for intrarenal hypertension in the initiation and progression of diabetic and other glomerulopathies. Am J Med 72:375, 1982.

77. Mogensen CE, Andersen MJF: Increased kidney size and glomerular filtration rate in early juvenile diabetes. Diabetes 22:706, 1973.

78. Østerby R, Gundersen HJG: Glomerular size and structure in diabetes mellitus. I. Early abnormalities. Diabetologia 11:225, 1975.

79. Ellis EN, Steffes MW, Goetz FC, et al: Relationship of renal size to nephropathy in type 1 (insulin-dependent) diabetes. Diabetologia 28:12, 1985.

80. Feldt-Rasmussen B, Hegedüs L, Mathiesen ER, Deckert T: Kidney volume in type 1 (insulin-dependent) diabetic patients with normal or increased urinary albumin excretion: Effect of long-term improved metabolic control. Scand J Clin Lab Invest 51:31, 1991.

81. Lane PH, Steffes MW, Mauer SM: Estimation of glomerular volume: A comparison of four methods. Kidney Int 41:1085, 1992.

82. Bilous RW, Mauer SM, Sutherland DER, Steffes MW: Mean glomerular volume and rate of development of diabetic nephropathy. Diabetes 38:1142, 1989.

83. Schmitz A: The kidney in non–insulin-dependent diabetes. Acta Diabetol Lat 29:47, 1992.

84. Bader R, Bader H, Grund KE: Structure and function of the kidney in diabetic glomerulosclerosis: Correlations between morphological and functional parameters. Pathol Res Pract 167:204, 1980.

85. Lane PH, Steffes MW, Fioretto P, Mauer SM: Renal interstitial expansion in insulin-dependent diabetes mellitus. Kidney Int 43:661, 1993.

86. Ziyadeh FN, Goldfarb S: The renal tubulointerstitium in diabetes mellitus. Kidney Int 39:464, 1991.

87. Lundæk K: Long-term Diabetes. Munksgaard, Copenhagen, 1953.

88. Østerby R, Bangstad H-J, Hanssen KF: Changes of glomerular structure versus the development of microalbuminuria in insulin-dependent diabetic patients. Pediatr Adolesc Endocrinol 22:1, 1992.

89. Mauer SM, Sutherland DER, Steffes MW: Relationship of systemic blood pressure to nephropathology in insulin-dependent diabetes mellitus. Kidney Int 41:736, 1992.

90. Remuzzi G, Bertani T: Is glomerulosclerosis a consequence of altered glomerular permeability to macromolecules? Kidney Int 38:384, 1990.

91. Fioretto P, Steffes MW, Mauer SM: Hypertension and diabetic renal disease. Clin Invest Med 14:630, 1991.

92. Kroustrup JP, Gundersen HJG, Østerby R: Glomerular size and structure in diabetes mellitus. III. Early enlargement of the capillary surface. Diabetologia 13:207, 1977.

93. Hirose K, Tsuchida H, Østerby R, Gundersen HJG: A strong correlation between glomerular filtration rate and filtration surface in diabetic kidney hyperfunction. Lab Invest 43:434, 1980.

94. Ellis EN, Steffes MW, Goetz FC, et al: Glomerular filtration surface in type 1 diabetes mellitus. Kidney Int 29:889, 1986.

95. Gall M-A, Nielsen FS, Smidt UM, Parving H-H: The course of kidney function in type 2 (non–insulin-dependent) diabetic patients with diabetic nephropathy. Diabetologia 36:1071, 1993.

96. Nyberg G, Andersson C, Persson H, Østerby R: Renal biopsy case. Twenty years of hyperfiltration without diabetic-type glomerulosclerosis. Am J Kidney Dis 13:345, 1989.

97. Mathiesen ER, Saurbrey N, Hommel E, Parving H-H: Prevalence of microalbuminuria in children with type 1 (insulin-dependent) diabetes mellitus. Diabetologia 29:640, 1986.

98. Mogensen CE: A complete screening of urinary albumin concentration in an unselected diabetic out-patient clinic population. Diabetic Nephropathy 2:11, 1983.

99. Viberti GC, Mackintosh D, Bilous RW, et al: Proteinuria in diabetes mellitus: Role of spontaneous and experimental variation of glycaemia. Kidney Int 21:714, 1982.

100. Gall M-A, Rossing P, Skøtt P, et al: Prevalence of micro- and macroalbuminuria, arterial hypertension, retinopathy and large vessel disease in European type 2 (non–insulin-dependent) diabetic patients. Diabetologia 34:655, 1991.

101. Fabre J, Balant LP, Dayer PG, et al: The kidney in maturity onset diabetes mellitus: A clinical study of 510 patients. Kidney Int 21:730, 1982.

102. Kunzelman CL, Knowler WC, Pettitt DJ, Bennett PH: Incidence of nephropathy in type 2 diabetes mellitus in the Pima Indians. Kidney Int 35:681, 1989.

103. Damsgaard EM, Mogensen CE: Microalbuminuria in elderly hyperglycaemic patients and controls. Diabetic Med 3:430, 1986.

104. Keiding NR, Root HF, Marble A: Importance of control of diabetes in prevention of vascular complications. JAMA 150:964, 1952.

105. Berglund J, Lins LE, Lins PE: Predictability in diabetic nephropathy. Acta Med Scand 215:263, 1984.

106. Rolfe M: Diabetic renal disease in Central Africa. Diabetic Med 5:630, 1988.

107. Ishihara M, Yukimura Y, Yamada T, et al: Diabetic complications and their relationships to risk factors in a Japanese population. Diabetes Care 7:533, 1984.

108. Haider Z, Obaidullah S, Din F: A prospective follow-up study of patients with newly diagnosed maturity onset diabetes mellitus. J Pakistan Med Assoc 31:35, 1981.

109. Paisey RB, Arredondo LN, Villalobos A, et al: Association of differing dietary, metabolic, and clinical risk factors with microvascular complications of diabetes: A prevalence study of 530 Mexican type II diabetic subjects. II. Diabetes Care 7:428, 1984.

110. Pirart J: Diabetes mellitus and its degenerative complications: A prospective study of 4,400 patients observed between 1947 and 1973. Diabetes Care 1:168, 1978.

111. Rate RG, Knowler WC, Morse HG, et al: Diabetes mellitus in Hopi and Navajo Indians. Diabetes 32:894, 1983.

112. Haffner SM, Mitchell BD, Pugh JA, et al: Proteinuria in Mexican Americans and non-Hispanic whites with non–insulin-dependent diabetes mellitus. Diabetes Care (in press).

113. Kamenetzky SA, Bennett PH, Dippe SE, et al: A clinical and histologic study of diabetic nephropathy in the Pima Indians. Diabetes 23:61, 1974.

114. Kawate R, Yamakido M, Nishimoto Y, et al: Diabetes mellitus and its vascular complications in Japanese migrants on the Island of Hawaii. Diabetes Care 2:161, 1979.

115. Klein R, Klein BEK, Moss SE, DeMets DL: Proteinuria in diabetes. Arch Intern Med 148:181, 1988.

116. West KM, Erdreich LJ, Stober JA: A detailed study of risk factors for retinopathy and nephropathy in diabetes. Diabetes 28:501, 1980.

117. Kofoed-Enevoldsen A, Borch-Johnsen K, Kreiner S, et al: Declining incidence of persistent proteinuria in type 1 (insulin-dependent) diabetic patients in Denmark. Diabetes 36:205, 1987.

118. Pugh JA: The epidemiology of diabetic nephropathy. Diabetes Metab Rev 5:531, 1989.

119. Cowie CC, Port FK, Wolfe RA, et al: Disparities in incidence of diabetic end-stage renal disease according to race and type of diabetes. N Engl J Med 321:1074, 1989.

120. Hirohata T, MacMahon B, Root HF: The natural history of diabetes. 1. Mortality. Diabetes 16:875, 1967.

121. Borch-Johnsen K, Nørgaard K, Hommel E, et al: Is diabetic nephropathy an inherited complication? Kidney Int 41:719, 1992.

122. Seaquist ER, Goetz FC, Rich S, Barbosa J: Familial clustering of diabetic kidney disease: Evidence of genetic susceptibility to diabetic nephropathy. N Engl J Med 320:1161, 1989.

123. Pettitt DJ, Saad MF, Bennett PH, et al: Familial predisposition to renal disease in two generations of Pima Indians with type 2 (non–insulin-dependent) diabetes mellitus. Diabetologia 33:438, 1990.

124. Viberti GC, Keen H, Wiseman MJ: Raised arterial pressure in parents of proteinuric insulin-dependent diabetics. Br Med J 295:515, 1987.

125. Walker JD, Tariq T, Viberti GC: Sodium-lithium countertransport activity in red cells of patients with insulin-dependent diabetes and nephropathy and their parents. BMJ 301:635, 1990.

126. Krolewski AS, Canessa H, Warram JH, et al: Predisposition to hypertension and susceptibility to renal disease in insulin-dependent diabetes mellitus. N Engl J Med 318:140, 1988.

127. Jensen JS, Mathiesen ER, Nørgaard K, et al: Increased blood pressure and erythrocyte sodium-lithium countertransport activity are not inherited in diabetic nephropathy. Diabetologia 33:619, 1990.

128. Molitch ME, Steffes MW, Cleary PA, Nathan DM: Baseline analysis of renal function in diabetes control and complications trial. Kidney Int 43:668, 1993.

129. Mangili R, Bending JJ, Scott G, et al: Increased sodium-lithium counter transport activity in red cells of patients with insulin dependent diabetes and nephropathy. N Engl J Med 318:146, 1988.

130. Gall M-A, Rossing P, Jensen JS, et al: Red cell Na$^+$/Li$^+$ countertransport in non–insulin-dependent diabetics with diabetic nephropathy. Kidney Int 39:135, 1991.

131. Elving LD, Wetzels JFM, de Nobel E, Berden JHM: Erythrocyte sodium-lithium countertransport is not different in type 1 (insulin-dependent) diabetic patients with and without diabetic nephropathy. Diabetologia 34:126, 1991.

132. Carr S, Mbanya J-C, Thomas T, et al: Increase in glomerular filtration rate in patients with insulin-dependent diabetes and elevated erythrocyte sodium-lithium countertransport. N Engl J Med 322:500, 1990.

133. Parving H-H, Hommel E, Mathiesen ER, et al: Prevalence of microalbuminuria, arterial hypertension, retinopathy and neuropathy in patients with insulin-dependent diabetes. Br Med J 296:156, 1988.

134. Feldt-Rasmussen B, Deckert T: Is metabolic control a determinant of renal disease progression in type I diabetic nephropathy? J Nephrol 2:58, 1993.

135. Hanssen KF, Dahl-Jørgensen K, Lauritzen T, et al: Diabetic control and microvascular complications. Diabetologia 29:677, 1986.

136. Mogensen CE: Early glomerular hyperfiltration in insulin-dependent diabetics and late nephropathy. Scand J Clin Lab Invest 46:201, 1986.

137. Rudberg S, Persson B, Dahlquist G: Increased glomerular filtration rate as a predictor of diabetic nephropathy—an 8-year prospective study. Kidney Int 41:822, 1992.

138. Lervang H-H, Jensen S, Bröchner-Mortensen J, Ditzel J: Early glomerular hyperfiltration and the development of late nephropathy in type 1 (insulin-dependent) diabetes mellitus. Diabetologia 31:723, 1988.

139. Jones SL, Wiseman MJ, Viberti GC: Glomerular hyperfiltration as a risk factor for diabetic nephropathy: Five year report of a prospective study. Diabetologia 34:59, 1991.

140. Rossing P, Borch-Johnsen K, Parving H-H: Risk factors for development of incipient and overt diabetic nephropathy in IDDM patients. J Am Soc Nephrol 4:308, 1993.

141. Luetscher JA, Kraemer FB, Wilson DM, et al: Increased plasma inactive renin in diabetes mellitus. A marker of microvascular complications. N Engl J Med 312:1412, 1985.

142. Wilson DM, Luetscher JA: Plasma prorenin activity and complications in children with insulin-dependent diabetes mellitus. N Engl J Med 323:1101, 1990.

143. Danser AHJ, van den Dorpel MA, Deinum J, et al: Renin, prorenin, and immunoreactive renin in vitreous fluid from eyes with and without diabetic retinopathy. J Clin Endocrinol Metab 68:160, 1989.

144. Franken AAM, Derkx FHM, Man in't Veld AJ, et al: High plasma prorenin in diabetes mellitus and its correlation with some complications. J Clin Endocrinol 71:1008, 1990.

145. Christiansen JS: Cigarette smoking and prevalence of microangiopathy in juvenile-onset insulin-dependent diabetes mellitus. Diabetes Care 1:146, 1978.

146. Telmer S, Christiansen JS, Andersen AR, et al: Smoking habits and prevalence of clinical diabetic microangiopathy in insulin-dependent diabetics. Acta Med Scand 215:63, 1984.

147. Nordén G, Nyberg G: Smoking and diabetic nephropathy. Acta Med Scand 215:257, 1984.

148. Mühlhauser I, Sawicki PT, Berger M: Cigarette smoking as a risk factor for macroproteinuria and proliferative retinopathy in type 1 (insulin-dependent) diabetes. Diabetologia 29:500, 1986.

149. Chase HP, Garg SK, Marshall G, et al: Cigarette smoking increases the risk of albuminuria among subjects with type 1 diabetes. JAMA 265:614, 1991.

150. Jarrett RJ, Viberti GC, Argyropoulos A, et al: Microalbuminuria predicts mortality in non–insulin-dependent diabetes. Diabetic Med 1:17, 1984.

151. Mattock MB, Morrish NJ, Viberti GC, et al: Prospective study of microalbuminuria as predictor of mortality in NIDDM. Diabetes 41:736, 1992.

152. MacLeod JM, Lutale J, Marshall SM: Excess mortality in type 2 diabetic patients with minimal elevation of albumin excretion. Diabetologia 35(suppl 1):A34, 1992.

153. Atkinson AB, Beatty OL, Ritchie CM, et al: Clinic urinary albumin concentration predicts both mortality and progression to nephropathy in NIDDM: Results of an 8 year prospective study. Diabetic Med 10(suppl 1):S4, 1993.

154. Gall M-A, Borch-Johnsen K, Nielsen FS, et al: Micro- and macroalbuminuria as predictors of mortality in non–insulin-dependent diabetes. Diabetologia 36(suppl 1):A207, 1993.

155. Stiegler H, Standl E, Schulz K, et al: Morbidity, mortality, and albuminuria in type 2 diabetic patients: A three-year prospective study of a random cohort in general practice. Diabetic Med 9:646, 1992.

156. Yudkin JS, Forrest RD, Jackson CA: Microalbuminuria as a predictor of vascular disease in non-diabetic subjects. Lancet 2:530, 1988.

157. Damsgaard EM, Frøland A, Jørgensen OD, Mogensen CE: Microalbuminuria as predictor of increased mortality in elderly people. BMJ 300:297, 1990.

158. Deckert T, Feldt-Rasmussen B, Borch-Johnsen K, et al: Albuminuria reflects widespread vascular damage. The Steno hypothesis. Diabetologia 32:219, 1989.

159. Winocour PH: Microalbuminuria. BMJ 304:1196, 1992.

160. Feldt-Rasmussen B, Borch-Johnsen K, Mathiesen ER: Hypertension as related to diabetic nephropathy. Hypertension 2(suppl):18, 1985.

161. Wiseman MJ, Viberti GC, Mackintosh D, et al: Glycaemia, arterial pressure and micro-albuminuria in type 1 (insulin-dependent) diabetes mellitus. Diabetologia 2:401, 1984.

162. Jensen T, Stender S, Deckert T: Abnormalities in plasma concentrations of lipoproteins and fibrinogen in type 1 (insulin-dependent) diabetic patients with increased urinary albumin excretion. Diabetologia 31:142, 1988.

163. Jones SL, Close CF, Mattock MB, et al: Plasma lipid and coagulation factor concentrations in insulin-dependent diabetics with microalbuminuria. BMJ 298:487, 1989.

164. Kapelrud H, Bangstad H-J, Dahl-Jørgensen K, et al: Serum Lp(a) lipoprotein concentrations in insulin dependent diabetic patients with microalbuminuria. BMJ 303:675, 1991.

165. Gall M-A, Rossing P, Hommel E, et al: Apolipoprotein(a) in insulin-dependent diabetic patients with and without diabetic nephropathy. Scand J Clin Lab Invest 52:513, 1992.

166. Nielsen FS, Voldsgaard AI, Gall M-A, et al: Apolipoprotein(a) and cardiovascular disease in type 2 (non–insulin-dependent) diabetic patients with and without diabetic nephropathy. Diabetologia 36:438, 1993.

167. Jensen T: Albuminuria—a marker of renal and generalized vascular disease in insulin-dependent diabetes mellitus. Dan Med Bull 38:134, 1991.

168. Jensen T, Feldt-Rasmussen B, Bjerre-Knudsen J, Deckert T: Features of endothelial dysfunction in early diabetic nephropathy. Lancet 1:461, 1989.

169. Jensen T: Increased plasma level of von Willebrand factor in type 1 (insulin-dependent) diabetic patients with incipient nephropathy. BMJ 298:27, 1989.

170. Feldt-Rasmussen B: Increased transcapillary escape rate of albumin in type 1 (insulin-dependent) diabetic patients with microalbuminuria. Diabetologia 29:282, 1986.

171. Groop L, Ekstrand A, Forsblom C, et al: Insulin resistance, hypertension and microalbuminuria in patients with type 2 (non–insulin-dependent) diabetes mellitus. Diabetologia 36:642, 1993.

172. Ewing DJ, Campbell IW, Clarke BF: The natural history of diabetic autonomic neuropathy. Q J Med 49:95, 1980.

173. Thuesen L, Christiansen JS, Mogensen CE, Henningsen P: Echocardiographic-determined left ventricular wall characteristics in insulin-dependent diabetic patients. Acta Med Scand 224:343, 1988.

174. Sampson MJ, Chambers JB, Sprigings DC, Drury PL: Abnormal diastolic function in patients with type 1 diabetes and early nephropathy. Br Heart J 64:266, 1990.

175. Sampson MJ, Chambers JB, Sprigings DC, Drury PL: Regression of

left ventricular hypertrophy with 1 year of antihypertensive treatment in type 1 diabetic patients with early nephropathy. Diabetic Med 8:106, 1991.

176. Frolich E, Apstein C, Chobanian AV, et al: The heart in hypertension. N Engl J Med 327:998, 1992.

177. Parving H-H, Hommel E: Prognosis in diabetic nephropathy. BMJ 299:230, 1989.

178. Morrish NJ, Stevens LK, Head J, et al: A prospective study of mortality among middle-aged diabetic patients (the London cohort of the WHO Multinational Study of Vascular Disease in Diabetics). II: Associated risk factors. Diabetologia 33:542, 1990.

179. Schmitz A, Vaeth M: Microalbuminuria: A major risk factor in non–insulin-dependent diabetes. A 10-year follow-up study of 503 patients. Diabetic Med 5:126, 1988.

180. Mogensen CE, Schmitz A, Christensen CK: Comparative renal pathophysiology relevant to IDDM and NIDDM patients. Diabetes Metab Rev 4:453, 1988.

181. Kunzelman CL, Nelson RG, Knowler WC, Pettitt DJ: Proteinuria determines prognosis in type 2 (non–insulin-dependent) diabetes. Kidney Int 33:197, 1988.

182. Rhoads GG, Dahlen G, Berg K, et al: Lp(a) lipoprotein as a risk factor for myocardial infarction. JAMA 256:2540, 1986.

183. Earle K, Walker J, Hill C, Viberti GC: Familial clustering of cardiovascular disease in patients with insulin-dependent diabetes and nephropathy. N Engl J Med 326:673, 1992.

184. Nørgaard K, Mathiesen E, Hommel E, et al: Lack of familial predisposition to cardiovascular disease in type 1 (insulin-dependent) diabetic patients with nephropathy. Diabetologia 34:370, 1991.

185. Cambier P: Application de la théorie de Rehberg à l'étude clinique des affections rénales et du diabète. Ann Med 35:273, 1934.

186. Christiansen JS: On the pathogenesis of the increased glomerular filtration rate in short-term insulin-dependent diabetes. Dan Med Bull 31:349, 1984.

187. Ditzel J, Schwartz M: Abnormally increased glomerular filtration rate in short-term insulin-treated diabetic subjects. Diabetes 16:264, 1967.

188. Mogensen CE: Glomerular filtration rate and renal plasma flow in short-term and long-term juvenile diabetes mellitus. Scand J Clin Lab Invest 28:91, 1971.

189. Mogensen CE: Kidney function and glomerular permeability to macromolecules in early juvenile diabetes. Scand J Clin Lab Invest 28:91, 1971.

190. Mogensen CE: Kidney function and glomerular permeability to macromolecules in juvenile diabetes. Dan Med Bull 19(suppl 3):1, 1972.

191. Christiansen JS, Gammelgaard J, Frandsen M, Parving H-H: Increased kidney size, glomerular filtration rate and renal plasma flow in short-term insulin-dependent diabetics. Diabetologia 20:451, 1981.

192. Christiansen JS, Gammelgaard J, Tronier B, et al: Kidney function and size in diabetics before and during initial insulin treatment. Kidney Int 21:683, 1982.

193. Stadler G, Schmid R: Severe functional disorders of glomerular capillaries and renal hemodynamics in treated diabetes mellitus during childhood. Ann Paediatr 193:129, 1959.

194. Nelson RG, Beck GJ, Bennett PH, et al: Changes in glomerular function with the onset of non–insulin-dependent diabetes in Pima Indians. Diabetologia 36:A27, 1993.

195. Vora J, Thomas DM, Dean J, et al: Renal function and albumin excretion rate in 62 newly presenting non–insulin-dependent diabetics (NIDDM). Kidney Int 37:245, 1990.

196. Schmitz A, Christensen T, Jensen FT: Glomerular filtration rate and kidney volume in normo-albuminuric non–insulin-dependent diabetics—lack of glomerular hyperfiltration and renal hypertrophy in uncomplicated NIDDM. Scand J Clin Lab Invest 49:103, 1989.

197. Schmitz A, Hansen HH, Christensen T: Kidney function in newly diagnosed type 2 (non–insulin-dependent) diabetic patients, before and during treatment. Diabetologia 32:434, 1989.

198. Vora J, Dolben J, Williams J, et al: Renal haemodynamics in newly presenting non-proteinuric normotensive non–insulin-dependent diabetic patients (NIDDMs): Changes over two years after diagnosis. Diabetic Med 10(suppl 1):S25, 1993.

199. Mogensen CE: Glomerular filtration rate and renal plasma flow in normal and diabetic man during elevation of blood sugar levels. Scand J Clin Lab Invest 28:177, 1971.

200. Christiansen JS, Frandsen M, Parving H-H: Effect of intravenous glucose infusion on renal function in normal man and in insulin-dependent diabetics. Diabetologia 21:368, 1981.

201. Trevisan R, Nosadini R, Fioretto P: Ketone bodies increase glomerular filtration rate in normal man and in patients with type 1 (insulin-dependent) diabetes mellitus. Diabetologia 30:214, 1987.

202. Christiansen JS, Frandsen M, Parving H-H: The effect of intravenous insulin infusion on kidney function in insulin-dependent diabetes mellitus. Diabetologia 20:199, 1981.

203. Christiansen JS, Gammelgaard J, Ørskov H, et al: Kidney function and size in normal subjects before and during growth hormone administration for one week. Eur J Clin Invest 11:487, 1981.

204. Christiansen JS, Gammelgaard J, Frandsen M, et al: Kidney function and size in type I diabetic patients before and during growth hormone administration for one week. Diabetologia 22:333, 1982.

205. Parving H-H, Christiansen JS, Noer I, et al: The effect of glucagon infusion on kidney function in short-term insulin-dependent juvenile diabetes. Diabetologia 19:350, 1980.

206. Kupin WL, Cortes P, Dumler F: Effect on renal function of change from high to moderate protein intake in type I diabetic patients. Diabetes 36:73, 1987.

207. Christiansen JS, Rasmussen JF, Parving H-H: Short-term inhibition of prostaglandin synthesis has no effect on the elevated glomerular filtration rate of early insulin-dependent diabetes. Diabetic Med 2:17, 1985.

208. Esmajtjes E, Fernandez MR, Halperin I, et al: Renal hemodynamic abnormalities in patients with short-term insulin-dependent diabetes mellitus: Role of renal prostaglandins. J Clin Endocrinol Metab 60:1231, 1985.

209. Jensen PK, Steven K, Blæhr H, et al: The effects of indomethacin on glomerular hemodynamics in experimental diabetes. Kidney Int 29:490, 1986.

210. Ortola FV, Ballermann BJ, Anderson S, et al: Elevated plasma arterial natriuretic peptide levels in diabetic rats. Potential mediators of hyperfiltration. J Clin Invest 80:670, 1987.

211. Sawicki PT, Heineman L, Rave K, et al: Atrial natriuretic factor in various stages of diabetic nephropathy. J Diabetic Complications 2:207, 1988.

212. Jones SL, Perico N, Benigni A, et al: Glomerular filtration rate, extracellular fluid volume and atrial natriuretic factor in insulin-dependent diabetics. Kidney Int 33:268, 1988.

213. Tilton RG, Chang K, Hasan KS, et al: Prevention of diabetic vascular dysfunction by guanidines. Diabetes 42:221, 1993.

214. del Castillo E, Fuenzalida R, Uranga J: Increased glomerular filtration rate and glomerulopressin activity in diabetic dogs. Horm Metab Res 2:46, 1977.

215. Mogensen CE, Østerby R, Gundersen HJG: Early functional and morphological vascular renal consequences of the diabetic state. Diabetologia 17:71, 1979.

216. Mogensen CE, Andersen MJF: Increased kidney size and glomerular filtration rate in untreated juvenile diabetes: Normalization by insulin treatment. Diabetologia 11:221, 1975.

217. Brenner BM, Humes HD: Mechanics of glomerular ultrafiltration. N Engl J Med 297:148, 1977.

218. Hostetter TH, Troy JL, Brenner BM: Glomerular hemodynamics in experimental diabetes mellitus. Kidney Int 19:410, 1981.

219. Michels LD, Davidman M, Keane WF: Determinants of glomerular filtration and plasma flow in experimental diabetic rats. J Lab Clin Med 98:869, 1981.

220. Flyvbjerg A: The role of insulin-like growth factor I in initial renal hypertrophy in experimental diabetes. *In* Flyvbjerg A, Ørskov H, Alberti KGMM (eds): Growth Hormone and Insulin-like Growth Factor I. John Wiley & Sons, Chichester, 1993, p 271.

221. Microalbuminuria Collaborative Study Group UK: Risk factors for development of microalbuminuria in insulin dependent diabetic patients: A cohort study. BMJ 306:1235, 1993.

222. Keen H, Chlouverakis C, Fuller JH, Jarrett RJ: The concomitants of raised blood sugar: Studies in newly detected hyperglycaemics. II. Urinary albumin excretion, blood pressure and their relation to blood sugar levels. Guys Hosp Rep 118:247, 1969.

223. Parving H-H, Noer I, Deckert T, et al: The effect of metabolic regulation on microvascular permeability to small and large molecules in short-term juvenile diabetics. Diabetologia 12:161, 1976.

224. Feldt-Rasmussen B, Baker L, Deckert T: Exercise as a provocative test in early renal disease in type 1 (insulin-dependent) diabetes: Albuminuric, systemic and renal haemodynamic responses. Diabetologia 28:389, 1985.

225. Feldt-Rasmussen B, Mathiesen ER: Variability of urinary albumin

excretion in incipient diabetic nephropathy. Diabetic Nephropathy 3:101, 1984.

226. Viberti GC, Walker JD, Pinto J: Diabetic nephropathy. *In* Alberti KGMM, DeFronzo RA, Keen H, Zimmet P (eds): International Textbook of Diabetes Mellitus. John Wiley & Sons, Chichester, 1992, p 1267.

227. Borch-Johnsen K, Wenzel H, Viberti GC, Mogensen CE: Is screening and intervention for microalbuminuria worthwhile in patients with insulin dependent diabetes? BMJ 306:1722, 1993.

228. Brenner BM, Hostetter TH, Humes HD: Molecular basis of proteinuria of glomerular origin. N Engl J Med 298:826, 1978.

229. Brenner BM, Bohrer MP, Baylis C, Deen WM: Determinants of glomerular permselectivity: Insights derived from observations in vivo. Kidney Int 12:229, 1977.

230. Viberti GC, Mackintosh D, Keen H: Determinants of the penetration of proteins through the glomerular barrier in insulin-dependent diabetes mellitus. Diabetes 32:92, 1983.

231. Deckert T, Feldt-Rasmussen B, Djurup R, Deckert M: Glomerular size and charge selectivity in insulin-dependent diabetes mellitus. Kidney Int 33:100, 1988.

232. Deckert T, Kofoed-Enevoldsen A, Vidal P, et al: Size- and charge selectivity of glomerular filtration in type 1 (insulin-dependent) diabetic patients with and without albuminuria. Diabetologia 36:244, 1993.

233. Scandling JD, Myers BD: Glomerular size-selectivity and microalbuminuria in early diabetic glomerular disease. Kidney Int 41:840, 1992.

234. Pietravalle P, Morano S, Christina G: Charge selectivity of proteinuria in type 1 diabetes explored by Ig subclass clearance. Diabetes 40:1685, 1991.

235. Shimomura S, Spiro RG: Studies on macromolecular components of human glomerular basement membrane and alterations in diabetes. Decreased levels of heparan sulfate proteoglycan and laminin. Diabetes 36:374, 1987.

236. Vernier RL, Steffes MW, Sisson-Ross S, Mauer SM: Heparan sulfate proteoglycan in the glomerular basement membrane in type 1 diabetes mellitus. Kidney Int 41:1070, 1992.

237. van den Born J, van Kraats AA, Bakker MAH, et al: No change in glomerular heparan sulfate despite albuminuria and altered renal hemodynamics in experimental diabetes. Diabetologia 36(suppl 1):A219, 1993.

238. Feldt-Rasmussen B: Microalbuminuria and clinical nephropathy in type 1 (insulin-dependent) diabetes mellitus: Pathophysiological mechanisms and intervention studies. Dan Med Bull 36:405, 1989.

239. Hommel E, Mathiesen ER, Edsberg B, et al: Acute reduction of arterial blood pressure reduces urinary albumin excretion in type 1 (insulin-dependent) diabetic patients with incipient nephropathy. Diabetologia 29:211, 1986.

240. Sandeman DD, Shore AC, Tooke JE: Relation of skin capillary pressure in patients with insulin-dependent diabetes mellitus to complications and metabolic control. N Engl J Med 327:760, 1992.

241. Christensen CK: The pre-proteinuric phase of diabetic nephropathy. Dan Med Bull 38:145, 1991.

242. Feldt-Rasmussen B., Mathiesen ER, Deckert T, et al: Central role for sodium in the pathogenesis of blood pressure changes independent of angiotensin, aldosterone and catecholamines in type 1 (insulin-dependent) diabetes mellitus. Diabetologia 30:610, 1987.

243. Mathiesen ER: Prevention of diabetic nephropathy. Microalbuminuria and perspectives for intervention in insulin-dependent diabetes. Dan Med Bull 40:273, 1993.

244. Mathiesen ER, Feldt-Rasmussen B, Hommel E, et al: A 5 year study of glomerular filtration rate in normotensive IDDM patients with microalbuminuria. Diabetologia 35(suppl 1):A60, 1992.

245. Skøtt P: Lithium clearance in the evaluation of segmental renal tubular reabsorption of sodium and water in diabetes mellitus. Dan Med Bull 41:23, 1994.

246. Ditzel J, Bröchner-Mortensen J, Kawahara R: Dysfunction of tubular phosphate reabsorption related to glomerular filtration and blood glucose control in diabetic children. Diabetologia 23:406, 1982.

247. Woods LL, Mizelle HL, Hall JG: Control of renal hemodynamics in hyperglycemia. Am J Physiol 252:F65, 1987.

248. Blantz RC, Peterson OW, Gushwa L, Tucker BJ: Effect of modest hyperglycemia on tubuloglomerular feedback activity. Kidney Int 22(suppl 12):S206, 1982.

249. DeFronzo RA: The effect of insulin on renal sodium metabolism. Diabetologia 21:165, 1981.

250. Stephenson J, Eurodiab IDDM Complications Study Group: Blood pressure and urinary albumin excretion in IDDM. Diabetes 42(suppl 1):29A, 1993.

251. Christlieb AR: Renin, angiotensin, and norepinephrine in alloxan diabetes. Diabetes 23:962, 1974.

252. Hommel E, Mathiesen ER, Giese J, et al: On the pathogenesis of arterial blood pressure elevation early in the course of diabetic nephropathy. Scand J Clin Lab Invest 49:537, 1989.

253. Parving H-H: Arterial hypertension in diabetes mellitus. *In* Alberti KGMM, DeFronzo RA, Keen H, Zimmet P (eds): International Textbook of Diabetes Mellitus. John Wiley & Sons, Chichester, 1992, p 1521.

254. Parving H-H, Smidt UM, Friisberg B, et al: A prospective study of glomerular filtration rate and arterial blood pressure in insulin-dependent diabetics with diabetic nephropathy. Diabetologia 20:457, 1981.

255. Malins JM: Clinical Diabetes Mellitus. Eyre & Spottiswoode, London, 1968.

256. Hommel E, Mathiesen ER, Auckland K, Parving H-H: Pathophysiological aspects of edema formation in diabetic nephropathy. Kidney Int 38:1187, 1990.

257. Mogensen CE: Progression of nephropathy in long-term diabetics with proteinuria and effect of initial antihypertensive treatment. Scand J Clin Lab Invest 36:383, 1976.

258. Viberti GC, Bilous RW, Mackintosh D, Keen H: Monitoring glomerular function in diabetic nephropathy. Am J Med 74:256, 1983.

259. Myers BD, Nelson RG, Williams GW, et al: Glomerular function in Pima Indians with non–insulin-dependent diabetes mellitus of recent onset. J Clin Invest 88:524, 1991.

260. Myers BD, Winetz JA, Chui F, Michaels AS: Mechanisms of proteinuria in diabetic nephropathy: A study of glomerular barrier function. Kidney Int 21:633, 1982.

261. Tomlanovich S, Deen WM, Jones HW III, et al: Functional nature of glomerular injury in progressive diabetic glomerulopathy. Diabetes 36:556, 1987.

262. Friedman S, Jones HW III, Golbetz HV, et al: Mechanisms of proteinuria in diabetic nephropathy II. A study of the size-selective glomerular filtration barrier. Diabetes 32(suppl 2):40, 1983.

263. Carrie BJ, Myers BD: Proteinuria and functional characteristics of the glomerular barrier in diabetic nephropathy. Kidney Int 17:669, 1980.

264. Gall M-A, Rossing P, Kofoed-Enevoldsen A, et al: Glomerular size- and charge selectivity in type 2 (non–insulin-dependent) diabetic patients with diabetic nephropathy. Diabetologia 37:195, 1994.

265. Watkins PJ, Blainey JD, Brewer DB, et al: The natural history of diabetic renal disease. A follow-up study of series of renal biopsies. Q J Med 41:437, 1972.

266. Jackson B, Debrevi L, Witty M, Johnson CF: Progression of renal disease: Effects of different classes of antihypertensive therapy. J Hypertens 4(suppl 5):S269, 1986.

267. Rossing P, Hommel E, Smidt UM, Parving H-H: Impact of arterial blood pressure and albuminuria on the progression of diabetic nephropathy in IDDM patients. Diabetes 42:715, 1993.

268. Parving H-H: Impact of blood pressure and antihypertensive treatment on incipient and overt nephropathy, retinopathy, and endothelial permeability in diabetes mellitus. Diabetes Care 14:260, 1991.

269. Nyberg G, Blohmé G, Nordén G: Impact of metabolic control on progression of clinical diabetic nephropathy. Diabetologia 30:82, 1987.

270. Viberti GC, Keen H, Dodds RA, Bending JJ: Metabolic control and progression of diabetic nephropathy. Diabetologia 30:481, 1987.

271. Berglund J, Lins L-E, Lins P-E: Metabolic and blood pressure monitoring in diabetic renal failure. Acta Med Scand 218:401, 1985.

272. Mulec H, Johnsen SA, Björck S: Relation between serum cholesterol and diabetic nephropathy. Lancet 335:1537, 1990.

273. Hommel E, Andersen P, Gall M-A, et al: Plasma lipoproteins and renal function during simvastatin treatment in diabetic nephropathy. Diabetologia 35:447, 1992.

274. Jameel N, Pugh JA, Mitchell BD, Stern MP: Dietary protein intake is not correlated with clinical proteinuria in NIDDM. Diabetes Care 15:178, 1992.

275. Nyberg G, Nordén G, Attman P-O, et al: Diabetic nephropathy—is dietary protein harmful? J Diabetic Complications 1:37, 1987.

276. Parving H-H, Andersen AR, Smidt UM, et al: Diabetic nephropathy and arterial hypertension. Diabetologia 24:10, 1983.

277. Drury PL: Diabetes and arterial hypertension. Diabetologia 24:1, 1983.

278. Nielsen FS, Rossing P, Gall M-A, Parving H-H: Impaired nocturnal decline in arterial blood pressure in type 2 (non–insulin-dependent) diabetic patients with nephropathy. J Am Soc Nephrol 3:337, 1992.

279. Torffvit O, Agardh C-D: Day and night variation in ambulatory blood pressure in type 1 diabetes mellitus with nephropathy and autonomic neuropathy. J Intern Med 233:131, 1993.

280. Karlefors T: Circulatory studies during exercise with particular reference to diabetics. Acta Med Scand 180(suppl 449):1, 1966.

281. Hostetter TH: Pathogenesis of diabetic glomerulopathy: Hemodynamic considerations. Semin Nephrol 10:219, 1990.

282. Marshall SM, Alberti KGMM: Comparison of the prevalence and associated features of abnormal albumin excretion in insulin-dependent and non–insulin-dependent diabetes. Q J Med 70:61, 1989.

283. Jensen T, Borch-Johnsen K, Kofoed-Enevoldsen A, Deckert T: Coronary heart disease in young type 1 (insulin-dependent) diabetic patients with and without diabetic nephropathy: Incidence and risk-factors. Diabetologia 30:144, 1987.

284. Jarrett RJ: Cardiovascular disease and hypertension in diabetes mellitus. Diabetes Metab Rev 5:547, 1989.

285. Grenfell A, Watkins PJ: Clinical diabetic nephropathy: Natural history and complications. Clin Endocrinol Metab 15:783, 1986.

286. Frimondt-Møller C: Diabetic cystopathy. Dan Med Bull 25:49, 1978.

287. Steffes MW, Østerby R, Chavers BM, Mauer SM: Mesangial expansion as a central mechanism for loss of kidney function in diabetic patients. Diabetes 38:1077, 1989.

288. Mauer SM, Steffes MW, Connett J, et al: The development of lesions in the glomerular basement membrane and mesangium after transplantation of normal kidneys to diabetic patients. Diabetes 32:948, 1983.

289. Cagliero E, Maiello M, Boeri D, et al: Increased expression of basement membrane components in human endothelial cells cultured in high glucose. J Clin Invest 82:735, 1988.

290. Cagliero E, Roth T, Roy S, Lorenzi M: Characteristics and mechanisms of high-glucose–induced overexpression of basement membrane components in cultured human endothelial cells. Diabetes 40:102, 1991.

291. Meraji S, Jayakody L, Senaratne MP, et al: Endothelium-dependent relaxation in aorta from diabetic rats. Diabetes 36:978, 1987.

292. Tesfamariam B, Brown ML, Cohen RA: Elevated glucose impairs endothelium-dependent relaxation by activating protein kinase C. J Clin Invest 87:1643, 1991.

293. Yamauchi T, Ohnaka K, Takayanagi R, et al: Enhanced secretion of endothelin-1 by elevated glucose levels from cultured bovine aortic endothelial cells. FEBS Lett 267:16, 1990.

294. Lorenzi M, Cagliero E, Toledo S: Glucose toxicity for human endothelial cells in culture: Delayed replication, disturbed cell cycle, and accelerated death. Diabetes 34:621, 1985.

295. Ayo SH, Radnik RA, Glass WF, et al: Increased extracellular matrix synthesis and mRNA in mesangial cells grown in high-glucose medium. Am J Physiol 260:F185, 1991.

296. Menè P, Pugliese G, Pricci F, et al: High glucose inhibits cytosolic calcium signalling in cultured rat mesangial cells. Kidney Int 43:585, 1993.

297. Brownlee M, Cerami A, Vlassara H: Advanced glycosylation end products in tissue and the biochemical basis of diabetic complications. N Engl J Med 318:1315, 1988.

298. Haitoglou CS, Tsilibary EC, Brownlee M, Charonis AS: Altered cellular interactions between endothelial cells and non-enzymatically glycosylated laminin/type IV collagen. J Biol Chem 267:12404, 1992.

299. Crowley ST, Brownlee M, Edelstein D, et al: Effects of nonenzymatic glycosylation on mesangial matrix on proliferation of mesangial cells. Diabetes 40:540, 1991.

300. Hogan M, Cerami A, Bucala R: Advanced glycosylation end products block the antiproliferative effect of nitric oxide. J Clin Invest 90:1110, 1992.

301. Brownlee M, Vlassara H, Cerami A: Nonenzymatic glycosylation products on collagen covalently trap low-density lipoproteins. Diabetes 34:938, 1985.

302. Soules-Liparota T, Cooper M, Papazoglou D, et al: Retardation by aminoguanidine of development of albuminuria, mesangial expansion, and tissue fluorescence in streptozotocin-induced diabetic rat. Diabetes 40:1328, 1991.

303. Greene D: The pathogenesis and prevention of diabetic neuropathy and nephropathy. Metabolism 37:25, 1988.

304. Tsai SC, Burnakis TG: Aldose reductase inhibitors: An update. Ann Pharmacol 27:751, 1993.

305. MacLeod AF, Boulton AJ, Owens DR, et al: A multicentre trial of the aldose-reductase inhibitor tolrestat, in patients with symptomatic diabetic peripheral neuropathy. Diabete Metab 18:14, 1992.

306. McCaleb ML, Sredy J, Millen J, et al: Prevention of urinary albumin excretion in 6-month streptozotocin-diabetic rats with the aldose reductase inhibitor tolrestat. J Diabetic Complications 2:16, 1988.

307. Brenner BM, Meyer TW, Hostetter TH: Dietary protein intake and the progressive nature of renal disease: The role of hemodynamically mediated glomerular injury in the pathogenesis of progressive glomerular sclerosis in aging, renal ablation, and intrinsic renal disease. N Engl J Med 307:652, 1982.

308. Anderson S, Meyer TW, Rennke HG, Brenner BM: Control of glomerular hypertension limits glomerular injury in rats with reduced renal mass. J Clin Invest 76:612, 1985.

309. Mauer SM, Steffes MW, Azar S, et al: The effects of Goldblatt hypertension on development of the glomerular lesions of diabetes mellitus in the rat. Diabetes 27:35, 1978.

310. Fogo A, Yoshida Y, Glick AD, et al: Serial micropuncture analysis of glomerular function in two rat models of glomerular sclerosis. J Clin Invest 82:322, 1988.

311. Anderson S, Brenner BM: Pathogenesis of diabetic glomerulopathy: Hemodynamic considerations. Diabetes Metab Rev 4:163, 1988.

312. Vallance P, Calver A, Collier J: The vascular endothelium in diabetes and hypertension. J Hypertens 10(suppl 1):S25, 1992.

313. Raij L: Mechanisms of vascular injury: The emerging role of the endothelium. J Am Soc Nephrol 2:S2, 1991.

314. Menè P, Simonson MS, Dunn MJ: Physiology of the mesangial cell. Physiol Rev 69:1347, 1989.

315. Nakamura T, Fukui M, Ebihara I, et al: mRNA expression of growth factors in glomeruli from diabetic rats. Diabetes 42:450, 1993.

316. Flyvbjerg A, Thorlacius-Ussing O, Naeraa R, et al: Kidney tissue somatomedin C and initial renal growth in diabetic and uninephrectomized rats. Diabetologia 31:310, 1988.

317. Serri O, Beauregard H, Brazeau P, et al: Somatostatin analogue, octreotide, reduces increased glomerular filtration rate and kidney size in insulin-dependent diabetes. JAMA 265:888, 1991.

318. Doi T, Striker LJ, Quaife C, et al: Progressive glomerulosclerosis develops in transgenic mice chronically expressing growth hormone and growth hormone releasing factor but not in those expressing insulin-like growth factor 1. Am J Pathol 131:398, 1988.

319. Yamamoto R, Nakamura R, Noble NA, et al: Expression of transforming growth factor β is elevated in human and experimental diabetic nephropathy. Proc Natl Acad Sci USA 90:1814, 1993.

320. Border WA, Okuda S, Languino LR, Ruoslahti E: Transforming growth factor-β regulates production of proteoglycans by mesangial cells. Kidney Int 37:689, 1990.

321. Border WA, Ruoslahti E: Transforming growth factor-beta 1 induces extracellular matrix formation in glomerulonephritis. Cell Differen Dev 32:425, 1990.

322. Trevisan R, Li LK, Messent J, et al: Na$^+$/H$^+$ antiport activity and cell growth in cultured skin fibroblasts of IDDM patients with nephropathy. Diabetes 41:1239, 1992.

323. Anderson PW, Do YS, Hsueh WA: Angiotensin II causes mesangial cell hypertrophy. Hypertension 21:29, 1993.

324. Wolf G, Haberstroh U, Neilson EG: Angiotensin II stimulates the proliferation and biosynthesis of type I collagen in cultured murine mesangial cells. Am J Pathol 140:95, 1992.

325. Morelli E, Loon N, Meyer T, et al: Effects of converting-enzyme inhibition on barrier function in diabetic glomerulopathy. Diabetes 39:76, 1990.

326. Ganz MB, Pekar SK, Perfetto MC, Sterzel RB: Arginine vasopressin promotes growth of rat glomerular mesangial cells in culture. Am J Physiol 255:F898, 1988.

327. Bakris GL, Re RN: Endothelin modulates angiotensin II induced mitogenesis of human mesangial cells. Am J Physiol 264:F937, 1993.

328. Johnson A, Lermioglu F, Garg UC, et al: A novel biological effect of atrial natriuretic hormone: Inhibition of mesangial cell mitogenesis. Biochem Biophys Res Commun 152:893, 1988.

329. Raij L, Shultz PJ: Endothelium-derived relaxing factor, nitric oxide: Effects on and production by mesangial cells and the glomerulus. J Am Soc Nephrol 3:1435, 1993.

330. Lovett DH, Ryan JL, Sterzel RB: Stimulation of rat mesangial cell

proliferation by macrophage interleukin I. J Immunol 131:2830, 1983.

331. Friedman EA: Race and diabetic nephropathy. Transplant Proc 19(suppl 2):77, 1987.

332. Ganda OP, Williamson JR, Soeldner JS, et al: Muscle capillary basement membrane width and its relationship to diabetes mellitus in monozygotic twins. Diabetes 32:549, 1983.

333. Steffes MW, Sutherland DER, Goetz FC, et al: Studies of kidney and muscle biopsy specimens from identical twins discordant for type I diabetes mellitus. N Engl J Med 312:1282, 1985.

334. Mauer SM, Goetz FC, McHugh LE, et al: Long-term study of normal kidneys transplanted into patients with type I diabetes. Diabetes 38:516, 1989.

335. Doria A, Warram JH, Krolewski AS: Insulin receptor gene polymorphism is associated with the development of overt proteinuria. J Am Soc Nephrol 3:756, 1992.

336. Krolewski AS, Tryggvarson K, Warram JH, et al: Diabetic nephropathy and polymorphism in the gene coding for the alpha I chain of collagen IV. Kidney Int 37:510, 1990.

337. Craven PA, Caines MA, DeRubertis FR: Sequential alterations in glomerular prostaglandin and thromboxane synthesis in diabetic rats: Relationship to hyperfiltration of early diabetes. Metabolism 36:95, 1987.

338. Bruggeman LA, Pellicoro JA, Horigan EA, Klotman PE: Thromboxane and prostacyclin differentially regulate murine extracellular matrix gene expression. Kidney Int 43:1219, 1993.

339. Craven PA, Melham MF, DeRubertis FR: Thromboxane in the pathogenesis of glomerular injury in diabetes. Kidney Int 42:937, 1992.

340. Moel DI, Safirstein RL, McEvoy RC, Hsueh WA: Effect of aspirin on experimental diabetic nephropathy. J Lab Clin Med 110:300, 1987.

341. Hopper AH, Tindall H, Davies JA: Administration of aspirin-dipyridamole reduces proteinuria in diabetic nephropathy. Nephrol Dial Transplant 4:140, 1989.

342. Donadio JV, Ilstrup DM, Holley KE, Romero JC: Platelet-inhibitor treatment of diabetic nephropathy: A 10-year prospective study. Mayo Clin Proc 63:3, 1988.

343. Kasiske BL, O'Donnell MP, Garvis WJ, Keane WF: Pharmacologic treatment of hyperlipidemia reduces glomerular injury in rat 5/6 nephrectomy model of chronic renal failure. Circ Res 62:367, 1988.

344. O'Donnell MP, Kasiske BL, Schmitz G, et al: Lovastatin but not enalapril reduces glomerular injury in Dahl salt-sensitive rats. Hypertension 20:651, 1992.

345. O'Donnell MP, Kasiske BL, Kin Y, et al: Lovastatin inhibits proliferation of rat mesangial cells. J Clin Invest 91:83, 1993.

346. Jensen PK, Christiansen JS, Steven K, Parving H-H: Strict metabolic control and renal function in the streptozotocin diabetic rat. Kidney Int 31:47, 1987.

347. Steffes MW, Mauer SM: Diabetic glomerulopathy in man and experimental animal models. Int Rev Exp Pathol 26:147, 1984.

348. Steffes MW, Vernier RL, Brown DM, et al: Diabetic glomerulopathy in the uninephrectomized rat resists amelioration following islet transplantation. Diabetologia 23:347, 1982.

349. Steffes MW, Brown DM, Basgen JM, Mauer SM: Amelioration of mesangial volume and surface alterations following islet transplantation in diabetic rats. Diabetes 29:509, 1980.

350. Steffes MW, Brown DM, Mauer SM: The development, enhancement, and reversal of the secondary complications of diabetes mellitus. Hum Pathol 10:293, 1979.

351. Rasch R: Prevention of diabetic glomerulopathy in streptozotocin diabetic rats by insulin treatment: Kidney size and glomerular volume. Diabetologia 16:125, 1979.

352. Rasch R: Prevention of diabetic glomerulopathy in streptozotocin diabetic rats by insulin treatment. Glomerular basement membrane thickness. Diabetologia 16:319, 1979.

353. Rasch R: Prevention of diabetic glomerulopathy in streptozotocin diabetic rats by insulin treatment. The mesangial regions. Diabetologia 17:243, 1979.

354. Rasch R: Prevention of diabetic glomerulopathy by careful insulin treatment, experimental studies of the mesangial regions. Diabetologia 15:264, 1978.

355. Hostetter TH, Meyer TW, Rennke HG, Brenner BM: Influence of strict control of diabetes on intrarenal hemodynamics. Kidney Int 23:215, 1983.

356. Mauer SM, Steffes MW, Sutherland DER: Studies of the rate of regression of the glomerular lesions in diabetic rats treated with pancreatic islet transplantation. Diabetes 24:280, 1974.

357. Mauer SM: Diabetic glomerulopathy in the uninephrectomized rat resists amelioration following islet transplantation. Diabetologia 23:347, 1982.

358. Wiseman MJ, Saunders AJ, Keen H, Viberti GC: Effect of blood glucose control on increased glomerular filtration rate and kidney size in insulin-dependent diabetes. N Engl J Med 312:617, 1985.

359. Tuttle KR, Bruton JL, Perusek M, et al: Effect of strict glycemic control on renal hemodynamic response to amino acid infusion. N Engl J Med 324:1626, 1991.

360. Wang PH, Lau J, Chalmers TC: Meta-analysis of effects of intensive blood-glucose control on late complications of type I diabetes. Lancet 441:1306, 1993.

361. The Kroc Collaborative Study Group: Diabetic retinopathy after two years of intensified insulin treatment. JAMA 260:37, 1988.

362. Deckert T, Lauritzen T, Parving H-H, et al: Effect of two years of strict metabolic control on kidney function in long-term insulin-dependent diabetics. Diabetic Nephropathy 2:6, 1983.

363. Beck-Nielsen H, Richelsen B, Mogensen CE: Effect of insulin pump treatment for one year on renal function and retinal morphology in patients with IDDM. Diabetes Care 8:585, 1985.

364. Christensen CK, Christiansen JS, Schmitz A: Effect of continuous subcutaneous insulin infusion on kidney function and size in IDDM patients: A 2 year controlled study. J Diabetic Complications 1:91, 1987.

365. Dahl-Jørgensen K, Hanssen KF, Kierulf P, et al: Reduction of urinary albumin excretion after 4 years of continuous subcutaneous insulin infusion in insulin-dependent diabetes mellitus. Acta Endocrinol 117:19, 1988.

366. Reichard P, Berglund B, Britz A, et al: Intensified conventional insulin treatment retards the microvascular complications of insulin-dependent diabetes mellitus (IDDM): The Stockholm Diabetes Intervention Study (SDIS) after 5 years. J Intern Med 230:101, 1991.

367. Brinchmann-Hansen O, Dahl-Jørgensen K, Hanssen KF, Sandvik L: The response of diabetic retinopathy to 41 months of multiple insulin injections, insulin pumps, and conventional insulin therapy. Arch Ophthalmol 106:1242, 1988.

368. The Diabetes Control and Complications Trial Research Group: The effect of intensive treatment of diabetes on the development and progression of long-term complications in insulin-dependent diabetes mellitus. N Engl J Med 329:977, 1993.

369. Reichard P, Nilsson BY, Rosenqvist U: The effect of long-term intensified insulin treatment on the development of microvascular complications of diabetes mellitus. N Engl J Med 329:304, 1993.

370. Feldt-Rasmussen B, Mathiesen ER, Deckert T: Effect of two years of strict metabolic control on progression of incipient nephropathy in insulin-dependent diabetes. Lancet 2:1300, 1986.

371. Feldt-Rasmussen B, Mathiesen ER, Jensen T, et al: Effect of improved metabolic control on loss of kidney function in type 1 (insulin-dependent) diabetic patients: An update of the Steno studies. Diabetologia 34:164, 1991.

372. Viberti GC, Bilous RW, Mackintosh D, et al: Long term correction of hyperglycaemia and progression of renal failure in insulin dependent diabetes. Br Med J 286:598, 1983.

373. Tamborlane WV, Puklin JE, Bergman M: Long-term improvement of metabolic control with the insulin pump does not reverse diabetic microangiopathy. Diabetes Care 5:58, 1982.

374. Zatz R, Dunn BR, Meyer TW, et al: Prevention of diabetic glomerulopathy by pharmacological amelioration of glomerular capillary hypertension. J Clin Invest 77:1925, 1986.

375. Anderson S, Rennke HG, Garcia DL, Brenner BM: Short and long term effects of antihypertensive therapy in the diabetic rat. Kidney Int 36:526, 1989.

376. Anderson S, Rennke HG, Brenner BM: Nifedipine versus fosinopril in uninephrectomized diabetic rats. Kidney Int 41:891, 1992.

377. Flyihara CK, Padilha RM, Zatz R: Glomerular abnormalities in long-term experimental diabetes. Diabetes 41:286, 1992.

378. Cooper ME, Allen TJ, O'Brien RC, et al: Nephropathy in model combining genetic hypertension with experimental diabetes. Diabetes 39:1575, 1990.

379. Kasiske BL, Kalil R, Ma JZ, et al: Effect of antihypertensive therapy on the kidney in patients with diabetes: A meta-regression analysis. Ann Intern Med 118:129, 1993.

380. Marre M, Leblanc H, Suarez L, et al: Converting enzyme inhibition and kidney function in normotensive diabetic patients with persistent microalbuminuria. Br Med J 294:1448, 1987.
381. Marre M, Chatellier G, Leblanc H, et al: Prevention of diabetic nephropathy with enalapril in normotensive diabetics with microalbuminuria. BMJ 297:1092, 1988.
382. Mathiesen ER, Hommel E, Giese J, Parving H-H: Efficacy of captopril in postponing nephropathy in normotensive diabetic patients with microalbuminuria. BMJ 300:81, 1991.
383. Viberti GC, Mogensen CE, Groop L, et al: Effect of captopril on progression to clinical proteinuria in patients with insulin-depentent diabetes mellitus and microalbuminuria. JAMA 271:275, 1994.
384. Hallab M, Gallois Y, Chatelier G, et al: Comparison of reduction in microalbuminuria by enalapril and hydrochlorothiazide in normotensive patients with insulin dependent diabetes. BMJ 306:175, 1993.
385. Melbourne Diabetic Nephropathy Study Group: Comparison between perindopril and nifedipine in hypertensive and normotensive diabetic patients with microalbuminuria. BMJ 302:210, 1991.
386. Chan JCN, Cockram CS, Nicholls MG, et al: Comparison of enalapril and nifedipine in treating non-insulin dependent diabetics associated with hypertension: One year analysis. BMJ 305:981, 1992.
387. Mogensen CE: Long-term antihypertensive treatment inhibiting progression of diabetic nephropathy. Br Med J 285:685, 1982.
388. Parving H-H, Andersen AR, Smidt UM, Svendsen PA: Early aggressive antihypertensive treatment reduces rate of decline in kidney function in diabetic nephropathy. Lancet 1:1175, 1983.
389. Parving H-H, Andersen AR, Smidt UM, et al: Effect of antihypertensive treatment on kidney function in diabetic nephropathy. Br Med J 294:1443, 1987.
390. Parving H-H, Smidt UM, Hommel E, et al: Effective antihypertensive treatment postpones renal insufficiency in diabetic nephropathy. Am J Kidney Dis 22:188, 1993.
391. Hommel E, Parving H-H, Mathiesen E, et al: Effect of captopril on kidney function in insulin-dependent diabetic patients with nephropathy. Br Med J 293:466, 1986.
392. Parving H-H, Hommel E, Smidt UM: Protection of kidney function and decrease in albuminuria by captopril in insulin dependent diabetics with nephropathy. BMJ 297:1086, 1988.
393. Björck S, Nyberg G, Mulec H, et al: Beneficial effect of angiotensin converting enzyme inhibition on renal function in patients with diabetic nephropathy. Br Med J 293:471, 1986.
394. Björck S, Johnsen SA: Contrasting effects of enalapril and metoprolol on proteinuria in diabetic nephropathy. BMJ 300:904, 1990.
395. Parving H-H, Hommel E, Nielsen MD, Giese J: Effect of captopril on blood pressure and kidney function in normotensive insulin dependent diabetics with nephropathy. BMJ 299:533, 1989.
396. Björck S, Mulec H, Johnsen SA, et al: Renal protective effect of enalapril in diabetic nephropathy. BMJ 304:339, 1992.
397. Parving H-H, Rossing P, Hommel E, Smidt UM: Renal protective effects of captopril and metoprolol in diabetic nephropathy. J Am Soc Nephrol 3:337, 1992.
398. Elving LD, Wetzels JFM, van Lier HJJ, et al: Captopril and atenolol are equally effective in retarding progression of diabetic nephropathy. Diabetologia 37:604, 1994.
399. Grönhagen-Riska C, Honkanen R, Metsärinne K, et al: ACE-inhibition versus conventional antihypertensive treatment (β-blockade) in diabetic nephropathy. Am J Hypertens 3:67A, 1990.
400. Walker WG, Hermann J, Anderson J, et al: Blood pressure (BP) control slows decline of glomerular filtration rate (GFR) in hypertensive NIDDM patients. J Am Soc Nephrol 3:339, 1992.
401. Lebovitz H, Cnaan A, Wiegmann T, et al: Enalapril slows the progression of renal disease in non–insulin dependent diabetes mellitus (NIDDM): Results of a 3-yr multicenter, randomized, prospective, double-blinded study. J Am Soc Nephrol 3:335, 1992.
402. Bakris GL: Effects of diltiazem or lisinopril on massive proteinuria associated with diabetes mellitus. Ann Intern Med 112:707, 1990.
403. Bakris GL, Barnhill BW, Sadler R: Treatment of arterial hypertension in diabetic humans: Importance of therapeutic selection. Kidney Int 41:912, 1992.
404. Parving H-H, Rossing P: Calcium antagonists and the diabetic hypertensive patient. Am J Kidney Dis 22(suppl 3):47, 1993.
405. Lewis EJ, Hunsicker LG, Bain RP, Rohde RD: The effect of angiotensin-converting-enzyme inhibition on diabetic nephropathy. N Engl J Med 329:1456, 1993.
406. Parving H-H, Kastrup J, Smidt UM: Reduced transcapillary escape rate of albumin during acute blood pressure–lowering in type 1 (insulin-dependent) diabetic patients with nephropathy. Diabetologia 28:797, 1985.
407. Anderson S, Rennke HG, Brenner BM: Therapeutic advantage of converting enzyme inhibitors in arresting progressive renal disease associated with systemic hypertension in the rat. J Clin Invest 77:1993, 1986.
408. Bank N, Klose R, Aynedjian HS: Evidence against increased glomerular pressure initiating diabetic nephropathy. Kidney Int 31:989, 1987.
409. Wiegmann TB, Herron KG, Chonko AM, et al: Effect of angiotensin-converting enzyme inhibition on renal function and albuminuria in normotensive type I diabetic patients. Diabetes 41:62, 1992.
410. Reddi AS, Ramamurthi R, Miller M, et al: Enalapril improves albuminuria by preventing glomerular loss of heparan sulfate in diabetic rats. Biochem Med Metab Biol 45:119, 1991.
411. Rossing P, Hommel E, Smidt UM, Parving H-H: Reduction in albuminuria predicts diminished progression in diabetic nephropathy. Kidney Int 45(suppl 45):S145, 1994.
412. Rossing P, Hommel E, Smidt UM, Parving H-H: Reduction in albuminuria predicts a beneficial effect on progression in diabetic nephropathy during antihypertensive treatment. J Am Soc Nephrol 3:338, 1992.
412a. Parving H-H, Hommel E: Prognosis in diabetic nephropathy. BMJ 299:230, 1989.
413. Mathiesen ER, Borch-Johnsen K, Jensen DV, Deckert T: Improved survival in patients with diabetic nephropathy. Diabetologia 32:884, 1989.
414. Zatz R, Meyer TW, Rennke HG, Brenner BM: Predominance of hemodynamic rather than metabolic factors in the pathogenesis of diabetic glomerulopathy. Proc Natl Acad Sci USA 82:5963, 1985.
415. Zatz R, Brenner BM: Pathogenesis of diabetic microangiopathy. The hemodynamic view. Am J Med 80:443, 1986.
416. Cohen D, Dodds R, Viberti GC: Effect of protein restriction in insulin-dependent diabetics at risk of nephropathy. Br Med J 294:795, 1987.
417. Dullaart PF, Beusekamp BJ, Meijer S, et al: Long-term effects of protein-restricted diet on albuminuria and renal function in IDDM patients without clinical nephropathy and hypertension. Diabetes Care 16:483, 1993.
418. Walker JD, Bending JJ, Dodds RA, et al: Restriction of dietary protein and progression of renal failure in diabetic nephropathy. Lancet 2:1411, 1989.
419. Zeller KR, Whittaker E, Sullivan L, et al: Effect of restricting dietary protein on the progression of renal failure in patients with insulin-dependent diabetes mellitus. N Engl J Med 324:78, 1991.
420. Parving H-H: Low-protein diet and progression of renal disease in diabetic nephropathy. Lancet 335:411, 1990.
421. Parving H-H: Protein restriction and renal failure in diabetes mellitus. N Engl J Med 324:1743, 1991.
422. US Renal Data System: USRDS 1991 Annual Data Report. The National Institutes of Health, National Institute of Diabetes and Digestive and Kidney Diseases, Bethesda MD, 1991.
423. Najarian JS, Canafax DM, Sutherland DER: Renal transplantation in diabetic patients is confirmed therapy while pancreas transplantation should be performed only in an investigational setting. J Diabetic Complications 2:158, 1988.
424. Rimmer JM, Sussman M, Foster R, Gennari FJ: Renal transplantation in diabetes mellitus. Influence of preexisting vascular disease on outcome. Nephron 42:304, 1986.
425. Fischel RJ, Matas AJ, Payne WD, et al: Long-term outcome in 1-year graft survivors: Comparison of diabetic and nondiabetic populations. Transplant Proc 23:1337, 1991.
426. Sutherland DER: Current status of pancreas transplantation. J Clin Endocrinol Metab 73:461, 1991.
427. Nolph KD, Lindblad AS, Novak JW: Current concepts: Continuous ambulatory peritoneal dialysis. N Engl J Med 1595, 1988.
428. Duckworth WC, Saudek CD, Henry RR: Why intraperitoneal delivery of insulin with implantable pumps in NIDDM? Diabetes 41:657, 1992.
429. Grefberg N, Danielson BG, Nilsson P: Continuous ambulatory peritoneal dialysis in the treatment of end-stage diabetic nephropathy. Acta Med Scand 215:427, 1984.
430. Maiorca R, Vonesh EF, Cavalli P, et al: A multicenter, selection-adjusted comparison of patient and technique survivals on CAPD and hemodialysis. Perit Dial Int 11:118, 1991.

431. Serkes KD, Blagg CR, Nolph KD, et al: Comparison of patient and technique survival in continuous ambulatory peritoneal dialysis and hemodialysis: A multicenter study. Perit Dial Int 10:15, 1990.

432. Zimmerman SW, Glass N, Sollinger H, et al: Treatment of end-stage diabetic nephropathy: Over a decade of experience at one institution. Medicine (Baltimore) 63:311, 1984.

433. Shapiro FL, Compty CM: Hemodialysis in diabetics—1981 update. *In* Friedman EA, L'Esperance FA (eds): Diabetic Renal-Retinal Syndrome, 2nd ed. Grune & Stratton, New York, 1983.

434. Cameron JS: Treatment of end-stage renal failure due to diabetes in the United Kingdom. Lancet 2:962, 1986.

435. American Diabetes Association: Consensus statement: Role of cardiovascular risk factors in prevention and treatment of macrovascular disease in diabetes. Diabetes Care 13(suppl 1):53, 1990.

436. Carlson DM, Duncan DA, Naessens JM, Johnson WJ: Hospitalization in dialysis patients. Mayo Clin Proc 59:769, 1984.

437. Markell MS, Friedman EA: Diabetic nephropathy. Management of the end-stage patient. Diabetes Care 15:1226, 1992.

438. Schiff HI: The neurogenic bladder in diabetes. N. Y. State J Med 82:922, 1982.

439. Wheat LJ: Infection and diabetes mellitus. Diabetes Care 3:187, 1980.

440. Forland M, Thomas V, Shelokov A: Urinary tract infections in patients with diabetes mellitus. JAMA 238:1924, 1977.

441. Schiff M, Glickman M, Weiss RM, et al: Antibiotic treatment of renal carbuncle. Ann Intern Med 87:305, 1977.

442. Lyne WC, Chan RKT, Lee EJC, Kumarasinghe G: Urinary tract infections in patients with diabetes mellitus. J Infect 24:169, 1992.

443. Goldberg PK, Kozinn PJ, Wise GJ, et al: Incidence and significance of candiduria. JAMA 241:582, 1979.

# Nephrolithiasis

*John R. Asplin*
*Murray J. Favus*
*Fredric L. Coe*

Renal stones generally consist of calcium salts, uric acid, cystine, or struvite (the triple salt of magnesium, ammonium, and phosphate). Calcium stones predominate[1-6] (Table 40–1) and are composed of calcium oxalate and calcium phosphate crystals. Calcium oxalate crystals are found in monohydrate and dihydrate forms, which have different lattice structures and microscopic appearances.[7] Calcium phosphate crystals are usually carbonate apatite or hydroxyapatite, and occasionally brushite (calcium hydrogen phosphate), whitlockite (calcium orthophosphate), and octocalcium phosphate.[5] Calcium phosphate crystals occur in stones as frequently as do calcium oxalate crystals (see Table 40–1), but the amount of calcium oxalate in mixed stones generally exceeds that of calcium phosphate, and pure calcium oxalate stones are more frequent than pure calcium phosphate stones. The data in Table 40–1 are based on findings at the present time in industrialized areas and relatively affluent cultures. In the past, lower urinary tract stones, arising mainly in the bladder, were far more frequent than upper tract stones[8, 9]; these were usually composed of ammonium acid urate and calcium oxalate and were more common in children than in adults. In less developed countries, such bladder stones are still the major form of urinary stone disease.[10] Our interest here, biased as it is by our own situation, focuses only on the stone types listed in Table 40–1. The incidence rate of upper tract stones has not been well defined in general, but between 1950 and the end of 1974, rates for one well-defined population were 36 cases/100,000 per year for women; for men, the rate increased from 78.5 cases/100,000 per year in 1950 to 123.6 cases/100,000 per year by 1974.[11]

Because calcium, uric acid, cystine, and struvite stones differ from one another in pathogenesis and treatment, each stone type is described separately. However, the clinical manifestations of the stones themselves, that is, the ways in which they disturb the urinary tract, are similar regardless of composition.

## CALCIUM STONES

Calcium oxalate and calcium phosphate stones make up the principal divisions of nephrolithiasis. Because they are so common, much is known about their natural history. Of the many causes of calcium stones, most are remediable.

### Natural History

The patient (usually young) who has formed a single stone tends to view with skepticism a lifetime of preventive efforts and invariably inquires about the likelihood of recurrence. The recurrent stone former usually wonders whether the stone disease will tend to wane with age or become worse.

#### RECURRENCE AFTER A SINGLE STONE

Many investigators have reported long-term prospective surveys of recurrence in patients who presented after forming their first stone.[12-15] Recurrence was the rule and was maximal at 2 to 3 years. Thereafter, cumulative recurrence was less dramatic, but 40% to 50% had recurred by 5 years and more than 50% to 60% by 10 years. Two of the studies reported follow-up of 20 to 30 years with recurrence rates of 75%.[12, 13] Although it has been said that recurrence is the exception and that a young patient who has formed a single stone is unlikely to form another,[16] these long-term studies suggest that recurrence is the rule, usually within 5 to 10

**TABLE 40–1. Types of Renal Stones Formed and Frequency of Occurrence***

| Reference | CaOx and CaP | CaOx | CaP | Uric Acid | CaOx and Uric Acid | Cystine | Struvite | Number of Stones |
|---|---|---|---|---|---|---|---|---|
| Nordin and Hodgkinson[1] | 46.0 | 14.7 | 8.0 | 2.9 | — | 3.3 | 25.1 | 243 |
| Lagergren[2] | 44.2 | 15.1 | 7.6 | 1.9 | 1.7 | 1.1 | 28.1 | 460 |
| Melick and Henneman[3] | 30.3 | 27.1 | 20.6 | 12.9 | — | 2.6 | 14.8 | 155 |
| Prien[4] | 34.3 | 32.7 | 5.3 | 4.7 | 1.1 | 2.9 | 19.0 | 1000 |
| Sutor et al.[5] | 35.9 | 28.5 | 7.4 | 1.1 | 1.4 | 1.6 | 24.1 | 810 |
| Mandel and Mandel[6] | 9.9 | 49.3 | 8.8 | 9.8 | 2.2 | 0.5 | 12.4 | 10163 |

*Numbers represent the percentage of each stone type in the series. CaOx = calcium oxalate; CaP = calcium phosphate.

years. Unfortunately, patients who will have stone recurrence cannot be distinguished by laboratory evaluation from those who will not have a recurrence.[14, 17, 18]

## COURSE OF UNTREATED RECURRENT NEPHROLITHIASIS

It is easy to believe that stones tend to abate with time. We have studied the pattern of stone occurrence in 460 patients before they entered our program and before systematic treatment.[17] For each patient, we estimated new stone occurrences using old records, radiographs, and the patient's recollection. When new stones were calculated per patient during each 5-year interval after the first stone (i.e., as recurrent stones per patient per 5 years), recurrence rate, adjusted for patients at risk, clearly fell. A similar pattern has been observed by Marshall and colleagues in a prospective study.[16]

The idea that stone recurrence decreases with time is identical to stating that the interval between successive stones increases, but this prediction is not true. Of the 460 stone formers, we selected those who had had two or more new stone events that were separated by an interval whose duration could be estimated precisely. Among these patients, "interevent" intervals fell with successive stones (Table 40–2). One hundred and sixty-eight patients had at least three separate intervals, so that the first and last intervals could be compared. The first interval was longer than the last in 115 of the 168 patients, indicating an accelerating pace of recurrence. In the remainder, the last interval was longer than the first.

Interevent intervals, unique to individuals, reveal a heterogeneous and complex pattern of recurrence. In a majority of patients, stone disease tends to accelerate; in a minority, it lessens. Thus far, it has been impossible to separate the two groups on the basis of their metabolic disorder, age, sex, or other characteristics.[17] The overall natural history of stone disease appears to be one of chronicity, and the hope of a waning of disease with age is, for a majority of patients, unrealistic.

Interevent intervals and stone occurrence data conflict; stone frequency seems to fall, even though the interval narrows with successive recurrence. The main reason is that stone counts in populations are a poor way of assessing stone activity. Retrospective studies are biased to the extent that referral to a program tends to occur after a given number of recurrences. More active stone formers are referred a shorter time after the onset of stones. Inactive stone formers contribute long intervals and are the only contributors of stone events in the later years. In a prospective study of recurrence, active stone formers, who have short interevent intervals, will all appear in the early segments of a recurrence graph, whereas the late segments can reflect only less active patients, who have long intervals and low recurrence rates. Recurrence in a population is misleading when it is extrapolated to the individual, because it depends on counting stones formed per year by a population whose composition with respect to active and less active stone formers is likely to vary with time.

## SPECIAL CLINICAL PROBLEMS

Within the large group of patients who form calcium stones, there exist small groups of patients who present unusual problems and deserve individual analysis. Women who form stones and become pregnant are often concerned that their disease may have a prejudicial effect on their pregnancy. Among women with renal stones, complications

**TABLE 40–2. Interevent Intervals* for 256 Calcium Stone Formers**

| Group | Number of Patients | Number of Stone Events | | | | |
|---|---|---|---|---|---|---|
| | | 2 | 3 | 4 | 5 | 6 |
| All patients | 256† | 4.48 | 4.02 | 2.05 | 2.05 | — |
| Last interval shorter | 115 | 5.03 | 3.23 | 2.08 | 2.10 | 1.67 |
| First interval shorter | 53 | 1.70 | 5.55 | 2.01 | 1.79 | 1.67 |

*Numbers represent mean intervals, in years, between each event and the preceding event.
†In 168 of the 256 patients, there were at least three separate events; of these, the last interval was shorter than the first in 115 patients. In 88 of these, there were only two separate stone events.

of pregnancy were not increased above those of the general population except for a slightly higher rate of urinary tract infection.[19] Furthermore, the rate of stone formation during their years of pregnancy was no higher than that observed in the same population during their years in the nonpregnant state. A less detailed retrospective analysis based only on hospital charts confirmed the conclusion that pregnancy and stone disease do not prejudicially affect each other.[20] Women with calcium stones are more likely to have medullary sponge kidneys than men are.[21]

A small fraction of patients who form calcium stones also form uric acid stones and occasionally form stones composed of both calcium oxalate and uric acid.[22] These patients display an unusually high recurrence rate; the average recurrence rate among 23 such patients was 67.8 stones/100 patient-years—nearly twice the average rate for calcium stone formers in general. These patients often have a mixture of metabolic disorders involving both calcium and uric acid, and when they do, both disorders must be treated or else stone recurrence will continue.

Another small group of patients, which appears to represent about 11% of calcium stone formers, produces large numbers of stones. Among 78 such patients, each of whom had formed at least 10 recurrent stones, the average recurrence rate was 172 stones/100 patient-years. Patients with such frequent recurrences usually display mild metabolic disorders and may easily be expected to harbor unusual causes of stones; however, in the one study published so far, the causes of their stones appeared to be the same as those usually encountered in calcium stone disease, and their response to treatment was excellent.[23] The mechanisms responsible for their "accelerated" nephrolithiasis have not been made clear.

## Pathogenesis

### SATURATION

Consider a beaker of water containing crystals of calcium oxalate, well mixed, and at a stable temperature. The crystals have been bathed in the solution for a long time and neither grow nor shrink. The $Ca^{2+}$ and oxalate concentrations in the solution must also be unchanging, because the crystals are of a stable mass. The system is at equilibrium. The product of the free $Ca^{2+}$ and oxalate concentrations in such a solution is called the equilibrium solubility product. A lower free ion activity product will cause the crystals to dissolve. Such a solution is called undersaturated. A higher free ion activity product will cause the crystals to grow.

Now, remove the crystals from the equilibrium system and raise the ion activity product by adding $Ca^{2+}$, oxalate, or both. The elevated activity product would have caused growth of preformed crystals, had they been left in the beaker, but in the absence of solid phase, nothing appears to happen: the solution remains clear and free of crystals. A solution that will cause growth of preformed crystals but not the appearance of new solid phase is called metastable. Raise the activity product sufficiently, however, and new crystals will appear. This point is often called the formation product, or the upper limit of metastability. Above the for-

mation product, a solution is unstable, tending to create new crystal nuclei. Urine may be undersaturated, metastable, or unstable with respect to calcium oxalate or the stone-forming calcium phosphate crystals (brushite, hydroxyapatite, and octocalcium phosphate).

## FACTORS INFLUENCING SATURATION

Renal excretion of $Ca^{2+}$, oxalate, $PO_4^{3-}$, and water is a primary determinant of saturation. However, binding of $Ca^{2+}$ and oxalate and urine pH, which influences the relative amounts of monohydrogen and dihydrogen phosphate, alter free ion concentrations drastically and have an importance in regulating saturation at least equal to that of the total concentrations. Ion binding also complicates the measurement of urine saturation; simple concentration measurements give little clue to the actual activity product. Citrate readily complexes $Ca^{2+}$, reducing the $Ca^{2+}$ levels[24]; a similar relationship exists for $Mg^{2+}$ and oxalate.[25] For this reason, among others, hypercalciuria, oxaluria, hypocitraturia, unduly alkaline urine, and long-term dehydration all seem to increase the risk of calcium stone formation but are not sufficient to ensure that stones will form.

## URINE SATURATION MEASUREMENTS

Using a computer, Robertson and associates[26] and Pak and colleagues[27] have calculated urine free ion activity for $Ca^{2+}$, oxalate, and $PO_4^{3-}$ from their concentrations and their known tendencies to form soluble complexes with each other and with other ligands such as citrate and sulfate. If a calculated free ion activity product, such as the calcium oxalate ion product, is divided by the corresponding equilibrium solubility product, estimated in the same way, the resulting activity product ratio (APR) estimates the degree of saturation. A ratio above 1 connotes oversaturation; below 1 is undersaturation. The upper limit of metastability can be determined by raising the activity product and noting the APR at which solid phase begins to appear. The APR at the formation product is called the formation product ratio (FPR).

Pak and colleagues[27] have taken a different approach. They add seed crystals to an aliquot of urine and incubate, at 37°C, with stirring, at constant pH, for 2 days. By that time, equilibrium is attained; the crystal mass has become stable. If the activity coefficients for $Ca^{2+}$, oxalate, and $PO_4^{3-}$—essentially the fractions of each that are free to react—remain stable throughout the incubation, the ratio of the concentration product at the start to the product after incubation, at equilibrium, must equal the APR even though the concentration products themselves do not equal the activity products. Pak has shown that the assumption of stable activity coefficients is valid, so the empirical concentration product ratio is a valid estimation of the APR, provided the $Ca^{2+}$ concentration is below 5.0 mM and the oxalate concentration is below 0.5 mM.[27, 28]

### OBSERVED URINE SATURATION

Robertson,[29-31] Pak,[32] and Weber[33] and their colleagues, using different measurements, have accumulated consider-

**TABLE 40–3. Urine Calcium Oxalate and Calcium Phosphate Activity Product Ratios in Normal Subjects and in Stone Formers**

| Group | Normal Subjects | Hypercalciuric Stone Formers | Normocalciuric Stone Formers | Hyperparathyroidism |
|---|---|---|---|---|
| Calcium oxalate monohydrate | | | | |
| Robertson* | 3 ± 1.2 | 5.5 ± 1.3 | — | — |
| | to 10.7 ± 1.3 | to 18.2 ± 1.3 | | |
| Pak† | 1.45 ± 0.70 | 2.8 ± 1.4 | 2.2 ± 6.1 | 2.4 ± 1.1 |
| Weber‡ | 1.97 ± 0.90 | 3.3 ± 2.2 | 2.2 ± 1.0 | — |
| Brushite | | | | |
| Pak† | 0.35 – 0.26 | 1.74 ± 0.79 | 0.9 ± 0.5 | 1.6 ± 1.1 |
| Marshall§ | 1.15 ± 0.60 | 1.35 ± 0.70 | 4 ± 1.4 | — |
| Octocalcium phosphate‖ | 63 | 79 | 200 | — |
| Hydroxyapatite‖ | $4.6 \times 10^5$ | $9.1 \times 10^5$ | $2.9 \times 10^8$ | — |

All values are means ± SD.

*From Robertson and co-workers[26, 29, 30] and Marshall and co-workers[31]; values of activity product ratios were calculated from activity products; the equilibrium solubility product ($K_{sp}$) was taken as $1.7 \times 10^{-9}$ m².

†From Pak and Holt[32]; values of activity product ratios were measured by experiments.

‡From Weber and co-workers[33]; values of concentration product ratios (see text) were measured by seeding experiments.

§From Marshall and co-workers[31]; $K_{sp}$ of brushite was taken as $9.32 \times 10^{-7}$ m²; values of activity product ratios were calculated.

‖From Marshall and co-workers[31]; $K_{sp}$ of octocalcium phosphate was taken as $2.3 \times 10^{-18}$ m² and of hydroxyapatite as $1.1 \times 10^{-56}$ m².

able evidence that urine from stone formers is more supersaturated than normal (Table 40–3). Probably because of the differences in methods, absolute values differ for the three investigative groups. However, stone formers, whether hypercalciuric, without detectable metabolic disorder (idiopathic), or hyperparathyroid, had higher average values of urine saturation than did normal people, whether saturation was measured with respect to calcium oxalate, brushite, octocalcium phosphate, or hydroxyapatite. In the Weber study,[33] supersaturation for calcium oxalate was higher among hypercalciuric than normocalciuric patients.

Another important observation common to both experimental approaches is that normal urine, on the average, is above the equilibrium solubility product and oversaturated, except with respect to brushite. In the case of the data of Pak and Holt[32] and of Weber and colleagues,[33] this is a visible fact: added crystals grow in urine from most normal persons.

The use of urinary measurements to assess supersaturation may be insufficient to reveal the full crystallization potential that exists in the renal tubule. Hautmann and colleagues[34] have studied the $Ca^{2+}$ and oxalate concentrations in tissue from cortex, medulla, and papilla of seven human kidneys. The $Ca^{2+} \times$ oxalate concentration product in the papillae ($1 \times 10^{-4}$ m²) exceeded that of urine ($5 \times 10^{-7}$ m²) and those of the medulla and cortex ($8 \times 10^{-7}$ m² and $6 \times 10^{-7}$ m², respectively).[34] If the high chemical concentration product in the papilla reflects a high free ion product in tubule fluid or interstitium, calcium oxalate crystallization in this region may occur more rapidly than would be predicted from the ion product of the final urine.

## LIMITS OF METASTABILITY

Urine APR describes whether pre-existent crystals, once formed, will grow or shrink while suspended in it, but the APR gives incomplete information about the ability of that urine to produce new crystals. In simple salt solutions, the upper limit of metastability for calcium oxalate has been found to occur at an APR of 8.5 by Pak and Holt[32] and 10.0 by Robertson and associates.[26] The small difference in upper limit is mainly methodologic in origin.

Pak and Holt[32] have measured the actual upper limits of APR for calcium oxalate and brushite in human urine samples from normal people and from hypercalciuric, normocalciuric, and hyperparathyroid stone formers and has found surprising variability (Fig. 40–1). The APR at the limit of metastability, that is, the FPR, is higher in normal urine than in a salt solution. The FPR in urine from stone formers is lower than normal, and in primary hyperparathyroidism, it may be below 8.5, the value observed in simple salt solution. So low an FPR value suggests facilitation of crystal formation. Comparable data have not been obtained for octocalcium phosphate and hydroxyapatite, so the likelihood of spontaneous precipitation is difficult to assess from APR values.

Despite their differences, the studies of Pak and Holt[32] and Robertson and colleagues[26] yield similar conclusions. Urine is abnormally saturated in stone formers. Values of APR lie close enough to the FPR, at least for calcium oxalate, that new crystal formation could be expected. Most urine, even from normal people, is metastable with respect to calcium oxalate, so growth of crystal nuclei into a significant mass is predictable.

## NUCLEATION

Homogeneous nucleation, the spontaneous formation of new crystal nuclei in an oversaturated solution, is uncommon. Usually, particles of dust or debris in solution, irregularities on the surface of the container, or other crystals furnish a surface on which crystal nuclei begin to form at a lower APR than is required for homogeneous nucleation. The very existence of the metastable zone reflects the greater free energy change required to create new nuclei than to enlarge preformed nuclei, so any surface that can serve as a substrate for ions in solution to organize on may act as a heterogeneous nucleus, abridge the costly process of creating a solid phase de novo, and lower the apparent FPR.

The efficiency of heterogeneous nucleation depends on the similarity between the spacing of charged sites on the preformed surface and in the lattice of the crystal that is to grow on that surface. This kind of matching is referred to as epitaxis, and its extent is usually referred to as a good or poor epitaxial relationship.[35] For homogeneous nucleation to be achieved, all potential heterogeneous nuclei must be excluded, an unreasonably difficult task when human urine is under study. So it is probable that the apparent urine FPR for any given crystal is conditioned by preformed heterogeneous nuclei and nuclei of other crystals that form as the APR is raised during the experimental determination itself.

A number of urine crystals have good epitaxial matching and behave toward one another as heterogeneous nuclei. Monosodium urate and uric acid are excellent heterogeneous nuclei for calcium oxalate,[36, 37] so uric acid or urate could, by crystallizing, lower the FPR for calcium oxalate. Heterogeneous nucleation may be the mechanism linking hyperuricosuria to calcium oxalate stones,[38–42] a matter discussed later in this chapter. Epitaxial overgrowth of calcium oxalate on a surface of uric acid has been experimentally documented.[43] Brushite can nucleate calcium oxalate,[44] but in vivo it is more likely to transform, above pH 6.9, to hydroxyapatite, which is also an effective nucleating surface for calcium oxalate.[45] The clinical correlate of this phenomenon is the frequent finding of apatite at the core of calcium oxalate stones.[46]

## CRYSTAL GROWTH AND AGGREGATION

Once present, crystal nuclei will grow if they are suspended in urine with an APR above 1. Growth and aggregation are critical to stone disease, because microscopic nuclei are too small to cause obstruction or produce symptoms. Crystals are regular lattices, composed of repeating subunits, and they grow by incorporation of $Ca^{2+}$ and oxalate, or $PO_4^{3-}$, into new subunits on their surfaces. In metastable solutions, at 37°C, growth rates of calcium oxalate and the stone-forming calcium phosphate crystals are rapid; appreciable changes in macroscopic dimensions occur over hours to days. Growth rate increases with the extent of oversaturation and tends to be most rapid in urine samples having the highest values of APR.

Small crystals aggregate into larger crystalline masses by electrostatic attraction from the charged surface of the crystals. This process can rapidly increase particle size, producing a crystal that can lodge in the urinary tract. Urine from stone formers contains larger crystal aggregates than does urine from non–stone formers.[47]

## CELL-CRYSTAL INTERACTIONS

Finlayson and Reid[48] have proposed that crystals cannot grow or aggregate fast enough to anchor in the urinary tract by obstruction of renal tubules during the normal transit time through the nephron. Crystals must anchor to the renal tubule epithelium or urothelium to grow large enough to be of clinical significance—the fixed particle theory. In vitro

studies have shown adherence of calcium oxalate crystals to rat collecting duct epithelial cells,[49] and adherence and subsequent endocytosis of calcium oxalate crystals by monkey kidney epithelial cells.[50] This new area of research proposes a mechanism for crystal anchoring in the urinary tract, a requirement for the formation of upper urinary tract stones.

## INHIBITORS OF GROWTH, NUCLEATION, AND AGGREGATION

In urine, the upper limit of metastability is higher and crystal growth rates are lower than in a salt solution with the same APR. This fact has provoked interest in the nature of the materials that confer on urine such unusual properties.

Inorganic pyrophosphate is present in urine[41] and is a significant inhibitor. It increases the formation products of calcium phosphate and calcium oxalate in salt solutions and, by adsorbing to their surfaces, retards the growth of hydroxyapatite[42] and calcium oxalate crystals.[51] The quantitative contribution it makes to urinary inhibition of calcium oxalate crystal growth seems small. Russell and Fleisch[42] have observed average urinary pyrophosphate concentrations of 20 to 40 μM in adults, a concentration sufficient to inhibit crystal growth.[52] However, Meyer and Smith[51] have found that 16 μM of pyrophosphate produced a 50% decrease in the rate constant for calcium oxalate

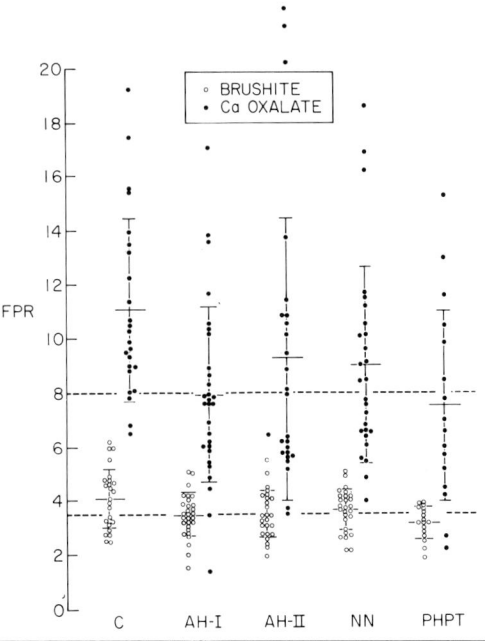

**Figure 40–1.** Urine formation product ratio (FPR) for calcium oxalate and brushite. Each point shows the value for a single urine sample. Dotted lines at 8 and 3.6 represent the values of APR at which spontaneous crystallization of calcium oxalate and brushite, respectively, occurs—the so-called formation product ratio. C = control subjects; AH-I and AH-II = severe and mild absorptive hypercalciuria; NN = normocalciuric stone formers; PHPT = primary hyperparathyroidism. Mean values and standard deviations are shown by horizontal lines. (From Pak CYC, Holt K: Nucleation and growth of brushite and calcium oxalate in urine of stone-formers. Metabolism 25:665, 1976.)

crystal growth in the same system in which whole urine, which contained 15 μM pyrophosphate, produced a 50% constant depression at a 62-fold dilution. From this, they concluded that urinary pyrophosphate contributes insignificantly to calcium oxalate crystal growth inhibition in whole urine. A similar conclusion was reached by others.[32, 53]

In their initial report, Fleisch and Bisaz[41] showed clearly that whole urine raised the formation product for calcium phosphate above the level expected from the pyrophosphate it contained, which suggests that other inhibitors accounted for about half the total effect. Smith and colleagues[54] observed considerable calcium phosphate growth inhibition from a 1.0:13.1 dilution of urine. Given the average of 16 μM/L in the urine, such a dilution would result in 1.2 μM/L of pyrophosphate; that concentration of pyrophosphate was able to produce a roughly comparable degree of inhibition in the assay system they used. Thus, for calcium phosphate crystal growth, as well as for elevation of the calcium phosphate formation product, urinary pyrophosphate appears to contribute half or more of the inhibitory effects of whole urine. This is in contrast to the much smaller role it appears to play in inhibiting calcium oxalate crystal growth.

Using a different assay for inhibition, in which samples did not need to be diluted, Bisaz and associates[55] found that pyrophosphate, citrate, and $Mg^{2+}$ ions all contributed to calcium phosphate crystal inhibition, and the three together accounted for 77% of the total activity in urine. Hallson and Rose[56] have suggested that the presence of certain materials in urine, which they refer to as "uromucoids," may promote calcium phosphate crystallization and aggregation. Samples of urine were evaporated to an osmolality of 1250 mOsm/kg. Ultrafiltration through a membrane that retained molecules above a molecular weight of 12,000 led to a smaller mass of crystals, which were not extensively aggregated, compared with those obtained from urine that was not passed through such a filter. The significance of these findings is still unclear.

Inhibitors of calcium oxalate crystal growth are somewhat better defined. Robertson has described a molecule above a molecular weight of 10,000 that is precipitated by cetylpyridinium chloride and was shown, by infrared spectrum analysis, to have carboxyl, hydroxyl, and sulfate groups. He postulates that this may be an acid mucopolysaccharide.[57] In support of this, inhibition by urine varies as a regular function of its acid mucopolysaccharide concentration, and heparin and chondroitin sulfate, both mucopolysaccharides, are known calcium oxalate crystal growth inhibitors.[47, 57]

Ito and Coe[52] have observed a seemingly different inhibitor system in urine. Strongly acidic peptides, such as poly-L-aspartic or poly-L-glutamic acids, inhibit calcium oxalate crystal growth, and urine appears to contain several glycopeptides that are unusually rich in these two amino acids and that inhibit crystal growth significantly at a low concentration. Treatment of urine with a nonselective proteinase reduced inhibition of calcium oxalate crystal growth in 17 of 19 instances, which supports an inhibitory role for protein in whole urine.[52]

Subsequent work has documented a urinary glycoprotein inhibitor of calcium oxalate crystal formation that contains γ-carboxyglutamic acid (Gla protein), forms strong air-water interfacial surface films (evidence of an amphiphilic molecule), and has a molecular weight of 14,000 but self-aggregates into a series of higher molecular weight polymers.[58, 59] This glycoprotein has been named nephrocalcin, by analogy with the bone Gla protein osteocalcin. Nephrocalcin inhibits crystal growth,[58] nucleation,[60] and aggregation.[61] Nephrocalcin from urine of some stone-forming patients[62] is abnormal, lacking Gla protein, forming weak air-water films, and having diminished growth and nucleation inhibition.[60] The possibility exists that Robertson may have been studying the nephrocalcin molecule. The glycopeptide is highly acidic and precipitates with cetylpyridinium chloride. The correlation between acid mucopolysaccharide concentration and inhibition by urine could be fortuitous, reflecting a generally higher inhibitor concentration in more concentrated urine.

Two other urinary proteins have been found to affect crystallization. Tamm-Horsfall protein, normally the most abundant urinary protein, inhibits calcium oxalate crystal aggregation[61] but does not alter growth[63] or nucleation.[60] Tamm-Horsfall protein from a group of patients with severe accelerated nephrolithiasis did not inhibit aggregation normally.[64] In addition, Tamm-Horsfall protein inhibits calcium oxalate crystal adherence to cultured renal epithelial cells.[65] Uropontin is a urinary glycoprotein that inhibits calcium oxalate crystal growth in vitro.[66] Abnormalities of uropontin in stone formers have not been documented at this time.

## OVERVIEW

Oversaturation is the force that drives calcium salts out of solution, into the solid phase. Heterogeneous nuclei may facilitate stone formation by bypassing the thermodynamically costly process of homogeneous nucleation. Inhibitors such as pyrophosphate and urinary macromolecules suppress nucleation, increase the supersaturation needed to produce a solid phase, and retard the growth and aggregation of nuclei already formed. In the main established stone-forming conditions, oversaturation, heterogeneous nucleation, and reduced inhibitors all have documented, or at least postulated, roles that vary from one disease to another[3, 15, 67–69] (Table 40–4). Treatment is often successful in reversing stone formation by eliminating those disturbances that enhance the risk of stones or, in some cases, by introducing secondary biochemical changes that compensate for the underlying defect.

Oversaturation occurs in idiopathic hypercalciuria, primary hyperparathyroidism, and hyperoxaluria because of overexcretion (see Table 40–4). Hypercalciuria and phosphaturia both occur in renal tubular acidosis (RTA); oversaturation with respect to calcium phosphate salts, which make up most stones in RTA, is also increased by an alkaline urine pH and by low levels of urinary citrate, an important $Ca^{2+}$-binding agent.

Evidence for heterogeneous nucleation in hyperparathyroidism is the finding of urinary formation products below those of simple salt solutions. The basis for this finding is not yet clear. Hyperuricosuria may engender urinary crystals of uric acid or sodium hydrogen urate, which are effi-

**TABLE 40–4. Occurrence Rates and Pathogenetic Mechanisms of Established Forms of Calcium Nephrolithiasis**

| Disorder | Mechanisms | | |
|---|---|---|---|
| | *Oversaturation* | *Heterogeneous Nucleation* | *Reduced Inhibition of Stone Formation* |
| Primary hyperparathyroidism | + | + | − |
| Idiopathic hypercalciuria | + | − | ? |
| Hyperuricosuria | − | + | + |
| Renal tubular acidosis | + | ? | ? |
| Hyperoxaluria | + | − | ? |
| Idiopathic lithiasis | − | − | + |

| Disorder | Occurrence in Selected Surveys* | | | | | |
|---|---|---|---|---|---|---|
| | *Coe*[67] | *Yendt*[68] | *Blacklock*[15] | *Melick and Henneman*[3] | *Hodgkinson and Pyrah*[69] | *Total* |
| | (460) | (408)† | (208)‡ | (189)§ | (344)‖ | (1658) |
| Primary hyperparathyroidism | 5.2¶ | 11.0 | 0.5 | 10.0 | X | 7.0 |
| Idiopathic hypercalciuria | 32.0 | 42.0 | 40.0 | 9.0 | 32.0 | 33.0 |
| Hyperuricosuria | 26.0 | X | X | X | X | 26.0 |
| Renal tubular acidosis | 3.7 | 0 | 0 | 3.0 | X | 3.4 |
| Hyperoxaluria | 4.6 | X | X | X | X | 4.6 |
| Idiopathic lithiasis | 20.2 | 25.8 | 50.0 | 53.6 | 68.0 | 34.1 |

*Numbers of patients in each survey are shown in parentheses at the top of each column; numbers in the table itself represent the percentage of patients in each survey with specific metabolic disorders. In most series, medullary sponge kidneys and infection or disorders of the upper urinary tract were listed as minor causes of stones and are not included here. X = the disorder was not sought.
†Thirty-one uric acid and cystine stone formers have been excluded from the table.
‡Only patients in whom urine studies were performed have been included.
§High frequency of bone disease and vitamin D excess; patients with uric acid lithiasis or cystinuria have been excluded from the table.
‖Selected for idiopathic lithiasis without obvious cause, with the exception of hypercalciuria.
¶Overall percentages apply only to the total number of patients in whom the disturbance was sought.

cient heterogeneous nuclei for calcium oxalate.[36, 37, 39] It is not certain whether these crystals are in a gel state.[57]

Robertson and co-workers[30] reported low levels of urinary inhibitors in some hypercalciuric and normocalciuric stone formers and that a urine supersaturation-inhibition index distinguished normal subjects from stone formers better than did either measurement alone. Other measurements of urinary inhibitors of calcium oxalate monohydrate crystal growth have shown that the lowest inhibitor levels occur in patients with hypercalciuria but no hyperuricosuria[70] and that samples from normal subjects can be distinguished from those of stone formers no more reliably by a combination of inhibitor and supersaturation measurements than by measurements of inhibition alone. The difference between these results and those of Robertson is probably related to differences in methodology. In general, the levels of crystallization inhibitors in the urine of stone formers differ from those in normal people, and in consequence of this, their urine samples can be distinguished from samples of normal people more reliably when inhibitor content is employed than by the use of supersaturation measurements alone. This fact highlights the presence of low inhibitor levels in stone-forming patients and suggests that inhibitors are important in preventing stones.

Table 40–4 also shows the frequencies of the main causes of calcium stones. Direct comparisons among the available surveys of patients are possible only when the diagnostic criteria and methods for selection of patients are similar. Hyperuricosuria and hyperoxaluria of intestinal origin were not sought in any survey other than our own. The survey by Hodgkinson and Pyrah[69] was based on patients

with idiopathic calcium lithiasis; patients with other types of stone disease were excluded. Nevertheless, all the surveys agree that idiopathic hypercalciuria and idiopathic calcium lithiasis are found frequently and that hyperparathyroidism and RTA are much less common. Hyperuricosuria is reported in 10% to 40% of calcium stone formers,[39, 71] and hypocitraturia in 15% to 60%.[72–76]

## Primary Hyperparathyroidism

All the known manifestations of primary hyperparathyroidism (see also Chapters 24 and 51) can be accounted for by chronic oversecretion of parathyroid hormone (PTH) and the resultant hypercalcemia. In the past, osteitis fibrosa cystica or renal calculi have been the basis for its detection,[77] although other organ systems may be involved.[78] Lately, hyperparathyroidism is being discovered mainly as a result of biochemical screening,[79] and the majority of such patients are asymptomatic. The frequency of primary hyperparathyroidism is now estimated to be 1 case/1000 adults, based on widespread screening of asymptomatic subjects.[79, 80]

A single parathyroid adenoma is responsible for hyperparathyroidism in 85% to 95% of patients. Four-gland hyperplasia is found in 5% to 15%, more often in association with familial hyperparathyroidism or as part of the multiple endocrine adenomatosis syndromes.[77, 81, 82] Parathyroid carcinoma is rare, being responsible for less than 1% of cases.[77, 81, 82]

## FORMS OF CIRCULATING PARATHYROID HORMONE

As judged by radioimmunoassay, PTH secretion is under negative feedback control by $Ca^{2+}$ and, to a lesser extent, $Mg^{2+}$ concentration in the serum. Fluctuations in $Ca^{2+}$ levels result in rapid changes in PTH secretion.[83, 84] Once secreted, the native hormone (molecular weight, 9500) is rapidly metabolized,[85] largely into two fragments, in the liver[86, 87] and kidney.[88] It has also been shown that fragments may be secreted from parathyroid glands in vitro.[89] The smaller fragment (molecular weight, 3500) is composed of the $NH_2$-terminal portion of the hormone and possesses biologic activity.[90] The larger fragment contains the middle and COOH-terminal portions of the hormone (molecular weight, 5500) and has no biologic activity.[90] The native hormone and the $NH_2$-terminal fragment undergo rapid clearance from the circulation; the larger middle and COOH-terminal fragment has a half-life 5 to 10 times as long as intact PTH and is excreted by the kidney.[91]

## NATURE OF THE PRIMARY DEFECT

There is no doubt that oversecretion of PTH is the basis of primary hyperparathyroidism, but the response of secretion to altered $Ca^{2+}$ levels in vivo is uncertain. In some patients, secretion seems unchanged despite the induction of increased hypercalcemia by calcium infusion—as if hormone secretion were autonomous. In others, secretion falls during calcium infusion but remains abnormally high—a set-point error. These two pathophysiologic models, autonomy versus set-point errors, are often juxtaposed as alternatives to each other but may, in fact, be the same thing. In vivo[92] and in vitro[93] basal PTH secretion per cell cannot be lowered below a distinct minimum. Given a large gland mass, PTH secretion will always be too high because of the aggregate output of an excessive number of cells, each producing a normal amount of PTH for the prevailing $Ca^{2+}$ concentration. As $Ca^{2+}$ concentration is raised, PTH secretion can fall until cells are secreting at their basal level. Thereafter, the gland will manifest autonomy. Attempts to distinguish parathyroid adenoma from four-gland hyperplasia preoperatively have yielded conflicting results regarding the suppressibility of parathyroid adenomas,[94–96] and these apparent differences may well be due to the use of antisera with affinity for different regions of the PTH molecule. Overall, in virtually all patients with parathyroid hyperplasia[94, 95] and in most with adenoma,[95, 96] serum immunoreactive PTH (iPTH) can be suppressed when the serum $Ca^{2+}$ concentration is raised by calcium infusion.

In vitro, PTH secretion by explants of surgically removed hyperplastic or adenomatous parathyroid glands can be suppressed by a high concentration of $Ca^{2+}$ in the medium.[97, 98] In general, the cells display a reduced sensitivity to $Ca^{2+}$.[99]

## CALCIUM ABSORPTION AND BALANCE

Negative $Ca^{2+}$ balance is common[100–107] (Fig. 40–2). Urinary $Ca^{2+}$ losses are offset, although not completely, by a variable increase in gastrointestinal $Ca^{2+}$ absorption as

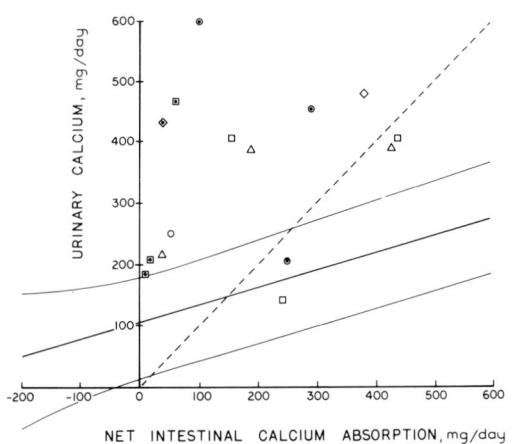

**Figure 40–2.** Relationship of urinary $Ca^{2+}$ excretion to net intestinal $Ca^{2+}$ absorption in patients with primary hyperparathyroidism. Each symbol represents individual patients from different sources: ■, Albright and co-workers[100]; ●, Aub and co-workers[101]; ◇, Hodgkinson[102]; □, Lafferty and Pearson[103]; △, Parfitt[105]; ○, Nassim and Higgins[106]; and ◆, Bauer and co-workers.[107] Solid lines represent the normal mean ± 2 SD. Normal data are derived from 6-day balance studies on 195 normal subjects, shown in Figure 40–6. The dotted line is the line of identity; points above the line indicate negative $Ca^{2+}$ balance. Data from reference 104 were not used in the figure.

measured by lower fecal $Ca^{2+}$ excretion.[100–107] Fractional $Ca^{2+}$ absorption (percentage of dietary intake absorbed) and the absorptive rate of $Ca^{2+}$ measured by double-isotope techniques or fecal excretion of an oral dose of $^{47}Ca$ provide more direct evidence that intestinal absorption is generally increased in hyperparathyroidism[108–112] (Table 40–5). In the few hyperparathyroid patients studied, the contribution of intestinal secretion of $Ca^{2+}$ to fecal $Ca^{2+}$ losses is variable and appears to be unrelated to the level of intestinal $Ca^{2+}$ absorption, $Ca^{2+}$ balance, or serum $Ca^{2+}$ levels.[103, 104] Because only 1% of total body $Ca^{2+}$ is extraosseous, the negative $Ca^{2+}$ balance in primary hyperparathyroidism is largely due to loss of bone mineral. Indeed, as fibrosis increases and osteoid accumulates and replaces normal bone, bone mineral content decreases, as measured by quantitative bone histology,[113] retention of $^{47}Ca$,[114] and photon absorptiometry.[115]

Vitamin D is required for intestinal hyperabsorption of $Ca^{2+}$,[116] and PTH is a known stimulator of the production of 1,25-dihydroxyvitamin $D_3$ (1,25$(OH)_2D_3$), the hormonal form of vitamin D known to stimulate $Ca^{2+}$ absorption (see Chapters 24 and 51). Kaplan and co-workers,[112] Brumbaugh and colleagues,[117] and Gray and associates,[118] using a chick intestinal cytosol receptor binding assay, have found increased blood levels of 1,25$(OH)_2D_3$ in some hyperparathyroid patients, and there is a correlation between 1,25$(OH)_2D_3$ blood levels and the absorption of an oral load of $^{47}Ca$. Thus, intestinal $Ca^{2+}$ absorption may be increased in primary hyperparathyroidism because of increased production of 1,25$(OH)_2D_3$. There is conflicting evidence regarding the site of enhanced $Ca^{2+}$ absorption along the intestinal tract. The duodenum normally has the highest rate of $Ca^{2+}$ absorption per unit length; in one study, hyperparathyroid patients absorbed $Ca^{2+}$ maximally in the duo-

**TABLE 40–5. Intestinal Calcium Absorption in Patients with Primary Hyperparathyroidism**

| Reference | Method | Calcium Intake (mg/24 h) | Dose Absorbed (%)* | |
|---|---|---|---|---|
| | | | *Normal Subjects* | *Hyperparathyroidism* |
| Birge et al.[108] | ⁴⁷Ca/⁴⁵Ca, PO/IV | 800 | 52.2 ± 13.2 (6) | 82.3 ± 15.6 (3) |
| Pak et al.[109] | Fecal ⁴⁷Ca | 400 | 50 ± 7 (20) | 68 ± 15 (26) |
| Reeve et al.[110] | ⁴⁷Ca/⁴⁵Ca, PO/IV | 850 ± 250 | None studied | 78.4 ± 16.0 (11)† |
| | | | | 68 ± 12 (5)‡ |
| Kaplan et al.[111] | Fecal ⁴⁷Ca | 400 | None studied | 71 ± 12 (12)† |
| | | | | 59 ± 12 (12)‡ |
| Kaplan et al.[112] | Fecal ⁴⁷Ca | 400 | 48 ± 8 (11) | 64 ± 14 (18) |

*Values are mean ± SD; numbers in parentheses represent number of patients studied.
†Preoperative.
‡After parathyroidectomy.

denum.[110] However, in another study, maximal absorption occurred in more distal segments,[108] not in the duodenum.

Dietary calcium contributes to hypercalcemia but is not completely responsible for its maintenance, because hypercalcemia and hypercalciuria persist during fasting.[109] Prolonged dietary calcium restriction, in the form of a low-calcium diet[119, 120] or binding of luminal $Ca^{2+}$ by cellulose phosphate,[105] lowers serum $Ca^{2+}$ concentration to normal in some, but not all, hyperparathyroid patients. Such calcium restriction will diminish urinary $Ca^{2+}$ excretion uniformly,[105, 119, 120] although efficient tubule reabsorption of $Ca^{2+}$ in some patients serves to maintain the hypercalcemia.[105] Concomitant phosphorus depletion enhances both hypercalcemia and hypercalciuria[121, 122] and may reverse the effects of calcium restriction.

## RENAL TUBULE CALCIUM REABSORPTION

The relative importance of bone mobilization to hypercalcemia appears to be small[105, 123]; intestinal overabsorption and enhanced renal conservation of filtered $Ca^{2+}$ appear to play the major role. Nordin and Peacock[123] have suggested that the PTH-stimulated increase in tubule reabsorption of filtered $Ca^{2+}$ (see Chapter 24) is quantitatively most important in the maintenance of hypercalcemia in hyperparathyroidism. A further increase in tubule $Ca^{2+}$ reabsorption occurs during calcium restriction and can maintain hypercalcemia despite a reduced net intestinal absorption of $Ca^{2+}$.[105, 124] Although technically difficult, measurement of tubule $Ca^{2+}$ reabsorption in hypercalcemic patients may be of diagnostic value.[124] Enhanced tubule reabsorption of $Ca^{2+}$ is responsible for normal urinary $Ca^{2+}$ excretion rates in some hyperparathyroid patients[77, 125] and for the observation that for any given level of serum $Ca^{2+}$, the urinary $Ca^{2+}$ excretion is lower in hyperparathyroidism than in other, nonparathyroid types of hypercalcemia (i.e., bone metastasis, sarcoidosis, vitamin D intoxication, multiple myeloma).[123, 125, 126]

Despite the fact that PTH stimulates tubule $Ca^{2+}$ reabsorption, urinary $Ca^{2+}$ excretion may be greatly elevated in those patients with primary hyperparathyroidism who form renal stones even when hypercalcemia is slight.[127] In a series of 1132 patients with nephrolithiasis, 48 had surgically documented hyperparathyroidism, and 30 of these had ex-

tremely mild hypercalcemia in the range of 10.1 to 11.0 mg/dL (Fig. 40–3). Urinary $Ca^{2+}$ excretion exceeded normal in a majority of the patients and was extremely high in a few in whom hypercalcemia was barely evident. Elevated levels of circulating $1,25(OH)_2D_3$ have been suggested as a cause of the marked hypercalciuria seen in patients such as these,[128] but no differences in serum $Ca^{2+}$, phosphorus, PTH, $1,25(OH)_2D_3$, or urinary $Ca^{2+}$ levels were found between hyperparathyroid stone formers and those without stones.[129]

## MECHANISM OF STONE FORMATION

Renal stones in hyperparathyroidism are usually composed of hydroxyapatite or calcium oxalate; more rarely, they are brushite or uric acid stones.[130] Stones composed of combinations of these basic types are also found. Stones often recur and become bilateral if the diagnosis is not made early in the course of the disease. Nephrocalcinosis may be the only renal manifestation of hyperparathyroidism. Less commonly, parenchymal calcification may be accompanied by calculi in the renal pelvis and ureters. The presence of nephrocalcinosis should prompt a diagnostic evaluation to exclude hyperparathyroidism, but there are other causes of that syndrome.

The physicochemical composition of urine is favorable to the nucleation and growth of calcium salts.[131] The APR for calcium oxalate and brushite is elevated in hyperparathyroid urine, mainly because of hypercalciuria.[32] Oxalate excretion is unremarkable; phosphorus excretion may not be elevated despite reduced $PO_4^{3-}$ reabsorption, because chronic phosphaturia tends to cause a negative phosphorus balance.[102] Nordin[132] has suggested that brushite stone formation may be enhanced by undue urine alkalinity. Although hyperchloremia and lowered blood carbon dioxide content are observed in some hyperparathyroid patients,[133] urine pH is not abnormally alkaline,[32] and the magnitude of the acidosis is negligible when renal glomerular function is normal,[134] which suggests that altered acid-base metabolism in hyperparathyroidism does not contribute to stone formation. Also unexplained are the low values of FPR for calcium oxalate and brushite (see Fig. 40–1).

## DIAGNOSIS

Despite advances in the measurement of iPTH and other adjunctive maneuvers, the diagnosis of primary hyperpara-

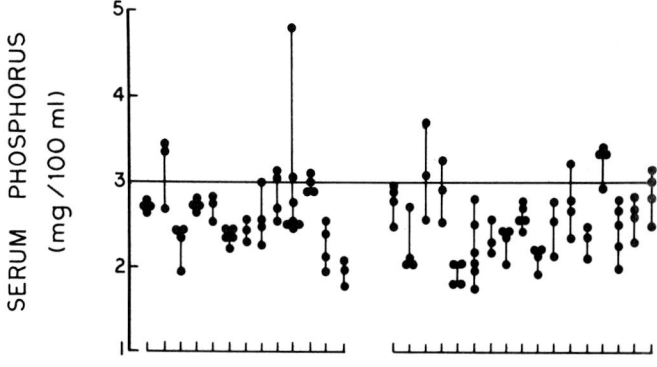

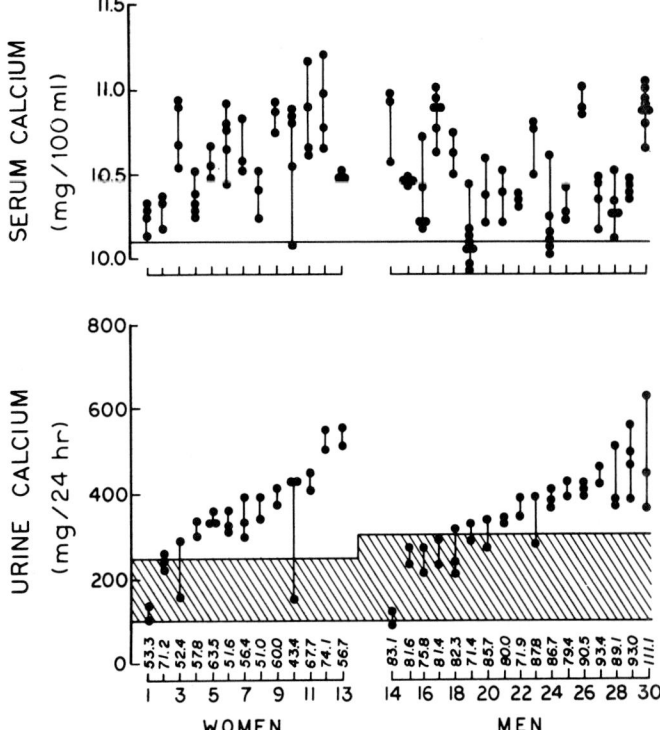

**Figure 40–3.** Selected characteristics of 30 patients with primary hyperparathyroidism, nephrolithiasis, and mild hypercalcemia. The lower limit for serum phosphorus and upper limit for serum $Ca^{2+}$ in the laboratory reporting the study[127] are shown by solid horizontal lines; the upper limits for urinary $Ca^{2+}$ excretion are crosshatched. Body weight is shown in kilograms for each subject.

thyroidism still depends on the demonstration of hypercalcemia and the exclusion of other causes (Table 40–6). In general, multiple serum samples should be studied, and even modest elevations of $Ca^{2+}$ concentration should be accorded considerable weight, if consistent.

The value of serum PTH levels depends on the assay that is used. Historically, radioimmunoassays using midmolecule, COOH-terminal antibodies have been used, with false-negative results in 10% to 20% of patients.[99, 135, 136] Also, radioimmunoassays often failed to show an appropriately suppressed PTH level in hypercalcemia of malignancy.[137] More recently developed immunometric assays recognize only the intact PTH molecule by using two antibodies directed against different sites of the PTH molecule.[138] The immunometric assays distinguish hyperparathyroidism and hypercalcemia of malignancy with a high level of reliability[137, 139] and show elevated PTH levels in 90% of

patients with hyperparathyroidism. The sensitivity of the immunometric assay is improved with the use of a nomogram relating PTH to serum $Ca^{2+}$ levels (Fig. 40–4), because PTH levels will not be appropriately suppressed in hyperparathyroidism.[137, 139]

Urinary excretion of cyclic AMP (cAMP) has also been used in the diagnostic evaluation of hyperparathyroid patients. PTH exerts its effects on the kidney through activation of the membrane-associated adenylate cyclase in cortical tubules[140, 141] and therefore increases cAMP levels in renal tissue and in the urine. The clinical utility of urinary cAMP determinations has been limited by overlap between normal and hyperparathyroid people[142–145] that arises, in part, from excretion of extrarenal cAMP in the urine. In normal subjects, approximately one third of urinary cAMP arises from the renal tubules; the remainder is derived from the plasma by glomerular filtration and is independent of

### TABLE 40–6. Causes of Hypercalcemia

Excessive parathyroid hormone secretion
  Primary hyperparathyroidism
  After renal transplant
  Lithium therapy
Malignant neoplasm
  Humoral hypercalcemia of malignancy
    Lung: squamous cell carcinoma
    Kidney: hypernephroma
    Other: pancreas, hepatoma, ovary, uterus, bladder, and others
  Bone invasion
    Metastasis from carcinoma: lung, breast, and others
    Multiple myeloma
    Leukemia, lymphoma
Excessive vitamin D activity
  Vitamin D supplementation
  Idiopathic hypercalcemia of infancy
  Granulomatous disease
    Sarcoidosis
    Tuberculosis
    Silicosis
    Leprosy
    Plasma cell granuloma
Excessive calcium intake
  Milk-alkali syndrome
Increased bone turnover
  Rapidly progressive osteoporosis of childhood
  Thyrotoxicosis
  Paget disease with immobilization
Other causes
  Familial hypocalciuric hypercalcemia
  Adrenal insufficiency
  Thiazide diuretic therapy
  Theophylline therapy
  Recovery phase of acute tubule necrosis
  Generalized periostitis
  Hypothyroidism
  Vitamin A intoxication
  Acquired immunodeficiency syndrome
  Pheochromocytoma

renal PTH effect.[146] The nephrogenous component, calculated as urinary cAMP excretion minus filtered load of cAMP, improves separation of mild hyperparathyroidism from normal.[147, 148] The test has limited utility because patients with familial hypocalciuric hypercalcemia and humoral hypercalcemia of malignancy may have elevated levels.[149]

Quantitative analysis of bone biopsy specimens reveals osteitis fibrosa cystica, porosity, and excessive rates of bone formation and resorption in a majority of hyperparathyroid patients[113, 150, 151] even at a time when x-ray films and serum alkaline phosphatase levels are normal.[150, 151] For example, Becker and colleagues[151] found hyperparathyroid changes on bone biopsy in 23 of 25 hyperparathyroid patients. Quantitative bone biopsy may contribute to the diagnostic evaluation of hypercalcemia, although bone biopsy results may be abnormal in patients with malignant tumors.[152]

Despite the measurement of serum iPTH level, diagnosis of the cause of hypercalcemia may be difficult in certain selected situations. Perhaps the most interesting of these is familial hypocalciuric hypercalcemia.[153] In this condition, hypercalcemia is associated with normal or subnormal urinary $Ca^{2+}$ excretion rates. Serum iPTH and urinary cAMP

levels may be elevated, but the hypocalciuria is not dependent on PTH.[154, 155] In one kindred, iPTH levels increased with age, becoming frankly elevated by age 30 years and making distinction from primary hyperparathyroidism difficult.[156] Patients with this disease do not form renal stones because urinary $Ca^{2+}$ levels are low. They are best separated from patients with primary hyperparathyroidism by having a urinary $Ca^{2+}$/creatinine clearance ratio of 0.01 or below.[154] Family members should be screened for hypercalcemia, when possible. Humoral hypercalcemia of malignancy may be difficult to distinguish from hyperparathyroidism because both present as hypercalcemia with hypercalciuria. PTH-related peptide has been identified as the mediator of humoral hypercalcemia of malignancy.[157–159] The PTH-related peptide has a high degree of homology with the first 13 amino acids at the biologically active $NH_2$-terminal end of PTH. The combination of an elevated PTH-related peptide by immunoassay and suppressed intact PTH should clearly separate humoral hypercalcemia of malignancy from hyperparathyroidism.

### TREATMENT

Removal of adenomatous or hyperplastic glands is indicated in patients with stone or bone disease; in those with

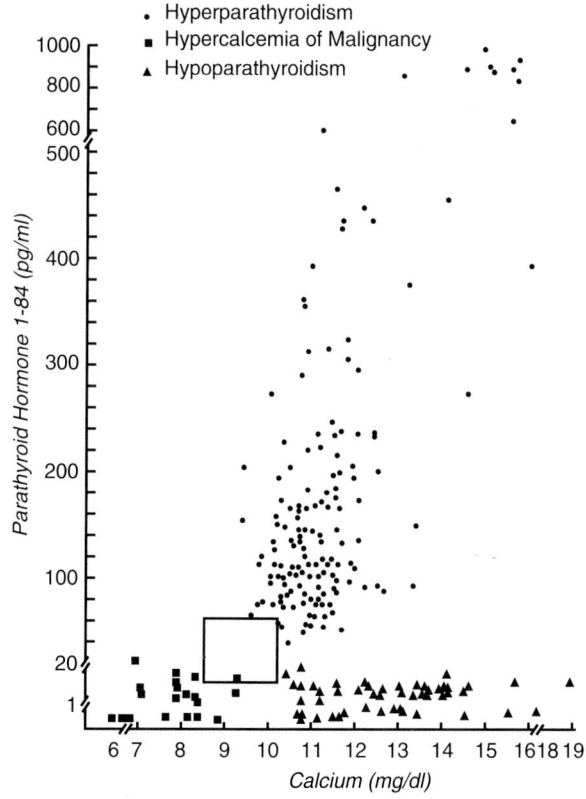

**Figure 40–4.** Results of PTH-(1–84) immunometric assay in 101 patients with surgically confirmed hyperparathyroidism, 79 patients with hypercalcemia of malignancy, and 23 patients with hypoparathyroidism. The area within the box represents normal serum $Ca^{2+}$ and serum PTH concentrations. (From Nussbaum S, Potts J: Immunoassays for parathyroid hormone 1–84 in the diagnosis of hyperparathyroidism. J Bone Miner Res 6[suppl 2]:S43–S50, 1991.)

pancreatitis, peptic ulcer, muscle weakness and fatigue, or changes in sensorium; and when serum $Ca^{2+}$ concentration exceeds 12 mg/100 mL.

However, many patients are asymptomatic and are discovered by routine screening; for them, the decision for surgery depends on the natural history of their disease. Purnell and associates[136] observed 147 patients with mild asymptomatic hyperparathyroidism for up to 5 years. Twenty percent eventually underwent surgery, but progression of the disease—increasing serum $Ca^{2+}$ levels, development of osteitis fibrosa, renal calculus formation—was responsible for only 14% of this 20%. The rest had surgery because of the inconvenience of yearly re-evaluation and anxiety about their uncured disease. Their anxiety may have some foundation, because renal function may deteriorate postoperatively[160] despite normalization of serum $Ca^{2+}$ levels after parathyroid surgery. A National Institutes of Health consensus conference has recommended surgery for asymptomatic patients with markedly elevated serum $Ca^{2+}$ concentration, low bone mineral density, reduced creatinine clearance, urinary $Ca^{2+}$ excretion greater than 400 mg/24 h, and age younger than 50 years and for patients with inadequate medical follow-up.[161]

At surgery, it is important to identify and perform biopsy of all four parathyroid glands; adenomas, although usually single, may be multiple, and four-gland hyperplasia may be difficult to distinguish from a single small adenoma.[77, 136] Preoperative localization of parathyroid glands has improved with the use of noninvasive techniques such as high-resolution ultrasonography, computed tomography, thallium/technetium subtraction scintigraphy, and magnetic resonance imaging.[162–164] However, these procedures do not improve outcome in first-time surgery performed by an experienced surgeon.[165] Preoperative localization is essential for patients undergoing re-exploration for recurrent hypercalcemia. If noninvasive techniques are inadequate, selective catheterization of thyroid veins with measurement of PTH levels may localize the parathyroid glands.[166]

In the immediate postoperative period, serum $Ca^{2+}$ concentration may fall to the hypocalcemic range, and calcium is required if the patient becomes symptomatic. It is important to distinguish the cause of the hypocalcemia. A massive shift of $Ca^{2+}$, $Mg^{2+}$, and phosphorus into bone can cause both serum $Ca^{2+}$ and serum phosphorus levels to be low; this occurs mainly in patients with osteitis fibrosa cystica, who often display the "hungry bones" syndrome postoperatively. Magnesium as well as calcium may be needed to prevent or treat tetany during the first 48 to 96 hours after surgery. Hypocalcemia with hyperphosphatemia indicates temporary or permanent hypoparathyroidism; calcium supplements and vitamin D may be required on a long-term basis. Postoperative phosphorus levels greater than 6 mg/dL strongly suggest permanent parathyroid gland damage.[145] Measurement of PTH can distinguish the cause of the hypocalcemia (i.e., low or undetectable in hypoparathyroidism and elevated in the hungry bones syndrome) and chart the subsequent course of recovery.[136]

Medical therapy may be used for patients deemed not to be surgical candidates. Estrogen or progestin therapy reduces serum $Ca^{2+}$ levels and may slow bone loss in postmenopausal women with primary hyperparathyroidism.[167–170]

Estrogens inhibit the action of PTH on bone but do not alter PTH secretion.[168, 169] Bisphosphonates, which inhibit osteoclast function, are effective in controlling hypercalcemia,[171] but the long-term effects of such treatment in hyperparathyroidism are unknown. Dietary salt restriction reduces urinary $Ca^{2+}$ excretion[172] and may be helpful in preventing stones in patients not having surgery.

## EFFECT OF TREATMENT

After successful surgery, serum $Ca^{2+}$ concentration becomes normal and $Ca^{2+}$ balance returns toward normal.[102–104] Gastrointestinal $Ca^{2+}$ absorption decreases,[104, 110] and hypercalciuria abates.[77, 102, 127] Cessation of hypercalciuria presumably accounts for the marked decrease in the rate of stone formation compared with that observed in the preoperative period.[127, 173, 174] It also results in a decline in calcium oxalate supersaturation from a concentration product ratio of 3.20 ± 0.56 to 1.53 ± 0.21 ($P < .05$) and an increase in the FPR for calcium oxalate from 7.19 ± 1.19 to 12.99 ± 1.69 ($P < .001$).[175] Pratley and colleagues[176] found 28 of their 54 patients well 1 to 10 years after successful parathyroidectomy; however, 8 of the 54 patients had residual renal disease in the form of persistent renal calculi, nephrocalcinosis, urinary tract infection, or increasing blood urea nitrogen level. Britton and associates[160] found 20 of 52 patients well, but the remaining 32 had continued renal and stone disease; in 9, blood urea nitrogen or creatinine level was elevated during postoperative follow-up. Parks and colleagues[127] observed recurrent stones in only 1 of 48 patients; this patient remained hypercalciuric despite curative parathyroidectomy.

Hypertension may accompany hyperparathyroidism, although the pathogenesis is not known.[77, 145] Britton and co-workers[160] found that of 20 patients with hyperparathyroidism and hypertension, only 1 became normotensive after parathyroidectomy, and 17 of 33 who were normotensive before surgery had hypertension in the follow-up period. Patients with osteitis fibrosa appear to suffer more severe renal damage than do those presenting with renal calculi alone as judged by creatinine clearance tests and nonprotein nitrogen.[174] However, renal damage in patients with nephrocalcinosis, as opposed to that in patients with calculi alone, was as severe as that in patients with osteitis fibrosa.[177]

## Idiopathic Hypercalciuria

Between 30% and 40% of calcium stone formers excrete in their urine more $Ca^{2+}$ than normal people customarily do—above 300 mg/24 h (men), 250 mg/24 h (women), or 4 mg/kg body weight per 24 hours (either sex)—and are therefore labeled hypercalciuric (see Table 40–4). Hypercalciuria is termed idiopathic if serum $Ca^{2+}$ concentration is normal and if sarcoidosis, RTA, hyperthyroidism, malignant tumors, rapidly progressive bone disease, immobilization, Paget disease, Cushing disease (or syndrome), and furosemide administration—the usual causes of normocalcemic hypercalciuria—can be excluded. Virtually all normocalcemic hypercalciuria encountered in patients with nephrolithiasis is idiopathic in origin.[67]

The frequency of idiopathic hypercalciuria is about 2% to 4% in otherwise normal adults, or 20 to 40 per 1000.[69] At most, stones occur in 5 per 1000 people, and if 40% of stone formers are hypercalciuric, stone formers account for 2 to 3 per 1000 instances of hypercalciuria. In other words, 80% to 90% of idiopathic hypercalciuria is silent. In a study of the families of nine patients with idiopathic hypercalciuria and nephrolithiasis, hypercalciuria was documented in 19 of 44 first-degree relatives.[178] The pattern of inheritance in consecutive generations and at a high frequency within generations (Fig. 40–5) is compatible with an inherited trait that has the broad characteristics of autosomal dominant transmission. A similar pattern of inheritance was demonstrated in another large family.[179] Idiopathic hypercalciuria has also been shown to occur in children at the same rate as that observed in adults.[180] Spontaneous hypercalciuria that resembles this condition in humans has been described in the laboratory rat,[181] and rats have been successfully bred for hypercalciuria.[182] Other distinct forms of genetic hypercalciuria include X-linked recessive nephrolithiasis with renal failure[183] and renal $PO_4^{3-}$ wasting with rickets.[184, 185]

The pathogenesis of idiopathic hypercalciuria involves excessive intestinal $Ca^{2+}$ absorption and depressed renal tubule $Ca^{2+}$ reabsorption. Excessive urinary $Ca^{2+}$ losses are offset by increased intestinal $Ca^{2+}$ absorption, but not always completely; $Ca^{2+}$ balance is negative in more than half the patients. Urinary $Ca^{2+}$ is increased without a rise in serum $Ca^{2+}$, which implies that renal tubule $Ca^{2+}$ reabsorption is depressed. Despite many attempts to assign primacy to the bowel or the kidney, the issue is still unresolved.

## INTESTINAL CALCIUM ABSORPTION

Net $Ca^{2+}$ absorption is the difference between the mucosal absorptive rate and the secretion of $Ca^{2+}$ in biliary, duodenal, and pancreatic fluids. Absorption rates may be measured by use of oral radiolabeled calcium, but only overall balance studies, in which fecal losses are measured, can measure net $Ca^{2+}$ absorption. The mucosal to serosal absorptive rate is higher in hypercalciuric people than in normal people (Table 40–7). In 10 studies, normal people absorbed an average of 27% to 52% of an oral dose of radioactive calcium, whereas 22% to 80% was absorbed by patients with idiopathic hypercalciuria. If one chooses only the six studies incorporating normal control subjects, the more efficient $Ca^{2+}$ absorption by hypercalciuric subjects is particularly evident. Increased mucosa-to-blood transport of $Ca^{2+}$ but not $Mg^{2+}$ has been demonstrated directly by in vivo jejunal perfusion in idiopathic hypercalciuria.[193]

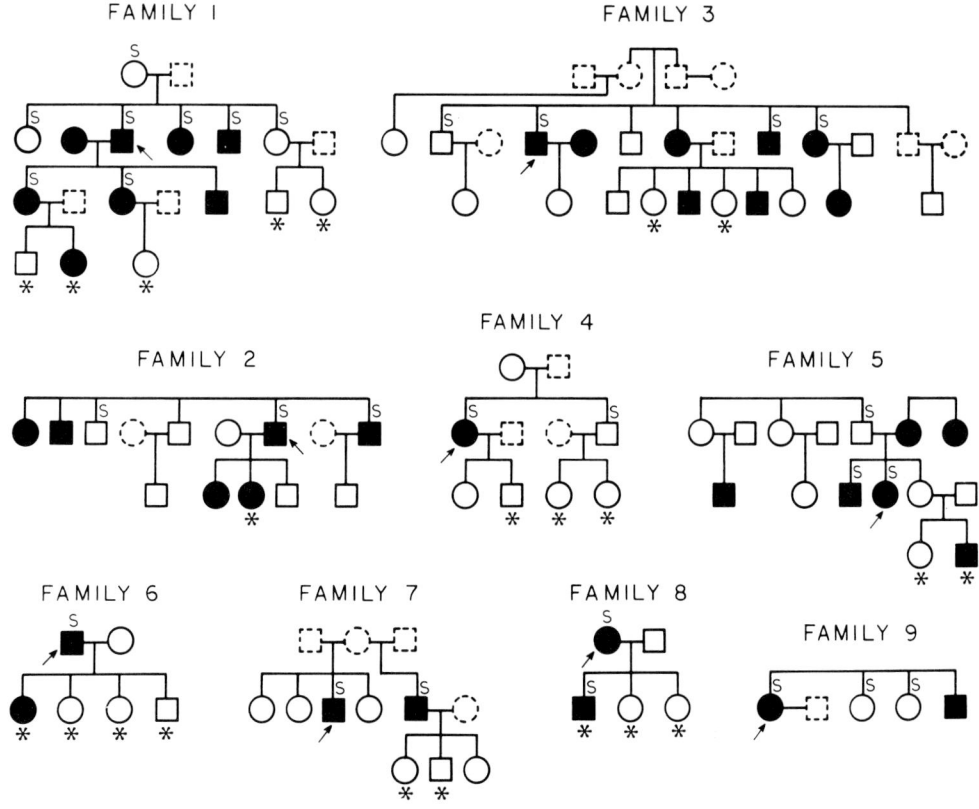

**Figure 40–5.** Family pedigrees of nine probands with idiopathic hypercalciuria. ● and ■ = family members with hypercalciuria; S = stone disease; * = children, defined here as younger than 20 years of age. Arrows indicate probands. Interrupted symbols represent relatives who were not studied but who are included to complete the pedigrees. Marginal hypercalciuria was present in four siblings, one each in families 1, 2, 3, and 5; in the mother of proband 4; in two aunts and one niece in family 5; and in one nephew in family 3. Altogether, hypercalciuria occurred in 11 of 24 siblings, 7 of 16 offspring, and 1 of 3 parents of the probands. (From Coe FL, Parks JH, Moore ES: Familial idiopathic hypercalciuria. N Engl J Med 300:337, 1979.)

**TABLE 40–7. Intestinal Calcium Absorption in Normal Subjects and Patients with Idiopathic Hypercalciuria**

| | | | Dietary Calcium Absorbed (%)* | |
| --- | --- | --- | --- | --- |
| Reference | Method | Calcium Intake (mg/24 h) | Normal Subjects | Idiopathic Hypercalciuria |
| Caniggia et al.[186] | Fecal $^{45}$Ca | Free diet† | None studied | 22.0 (1) |
| Birge et al.[108] | $^{47}$Ca, PO/IV | 800 | 52.2 ± 13.2 (6) | 58.5 ± 8.6 (4) |
| Wills et al.[187] | $^{47}$Ca, PO/IV | 400 | 49.0 ± 10.0 (4) | 76.0 ± 17.0 (5) |
| Pak et al.[188] | Fecal $^{47}$Ca | 400 | 45.6 ± 9.0 (29) | 69.7 ± 7.0 (9) |
| | | | | 58.1 ± 13.0 (11)‡ |
| Pak et al.[109] | Fecal $^{47}$Ca | 400 | 50.0 ± 7.0 (20) | 71.0 ± 7.0 (22)§ |
| | | | | 50.0 ± 17.0 (2)‖ |
| Ehrig et al.[189] | $^{47}$Ca/$^{45}$Ca, PO/IV | 462–952 | None studied | 47.8 ± 11.0 (22)¶ |
| | | | | 37.6 ± 11.0 (22)** |
| Kaplan et al.[112] | Fecal $^{47}$Ca | 400 | 48.0 ± 8.0 (11) | 80.0 ± 9.0 (211)§ |
| | | | | 73.0 ± 7.0 (3)‖ |
| Shen et al.[190] | $^{47}$Ca/$^{45}$Ca, PO/IV | Free diet† | 27.0 ± 9.0 (14) | 40.0 ± 9.0 (15) |
| Barilla et al.[191] | Fecal $^{47}$Ca | 400 | None studied | 69.5 ± 6.4 (10)§ |
| | | | | 70.1 ± 10.4 (8)‖ |
| Zerwekh and Pak[192] | Fecal $^{47}$Ca | 400 | None studied | 69.0 ± 7.0 (11)§ |
| | | | | 68.0 ± 9.0 (10)§ |

*Values are mean ± SD; numbers in parentheses represent numbers of patients studied.
†Usual diet but not measured.
‡Eleven patients listed as having normocalcemic primary hyperparathyroidism may be considered hypercalciuric.
§"Absorptive" idiopathic hypercalciuria.
‖"Renal" idiopathic hypercalciuria.
¶Before therapy.
**Three to 16 mo after administration of hydrochlorothiazide was begun.

In normal people, urinary $Ca^{2+}$ excretion rises slowly with net absorption (Fig. 40–6), and $Ca^{2+}$ balance is usually positive when absorption exceeds 200 mg/24 h. Average net intestinal $Ca^{2+}$ absorption for hypercalciuric patients is higher than in normal people, but overlap is extensive (see Fig. 40–6). At all levels of net absorption, urinary $Ca^{2+}$ excretion was higher in hypercalciuric than in normal subjects, so much so that none of the patients' data fell within the 95% confidence band derived from studies of normal people. For example, in the range of 200 to 300 mg of net $Ca^{2+}$ absorption, not 1 of 38 normal people excreted as much as 300 mg of $Ca^{2+}$ in the urine, whereas 15 of 16 hypercalciuric patients did (compare Figs. 40–6 and 40–7). In other words, hypercalciuric patients excreted in their urine an abnormally high percentage of the $Ca^{2+}$ they absorbed from the intestine. Net absorption exceeded 200 mg/24 h in 55 normal subjects (see Fig. 40–6). Urinary $Ca^{2+}$ excretion was less than net absorption, that is, $Ca^{2+}$ balance was positive, in 48. If we allow a generous margin for error

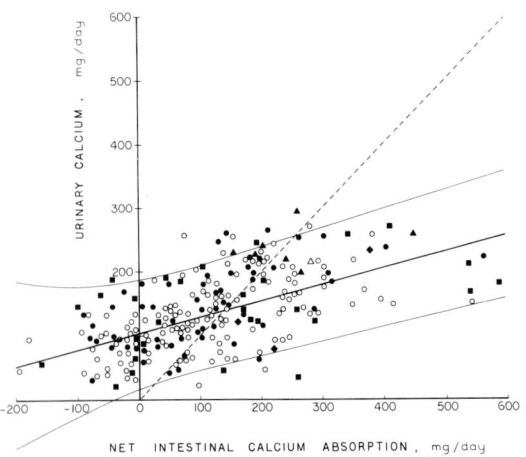

**Figure 40–6.** Urinary $Ca^{2+}$ excretion as a function of net intestinal $Ca^{2+}$ absorption. Data are derived from 6-day balance studies on 195 normal adults. Each symbol represents individual subjects from different sources: ○, Knapp[194]; □, Lafferty and Pearson[103]; ◇, Liberman and co-workers[195]; and △, Edwards and Hodgkinson.[196] Open symbols are women, and solid symbols are men. Solid lines represent mean and 2 SD. Dotted line is the line of identity; points above the line reflect negative $Ca^{2+}$ balance.

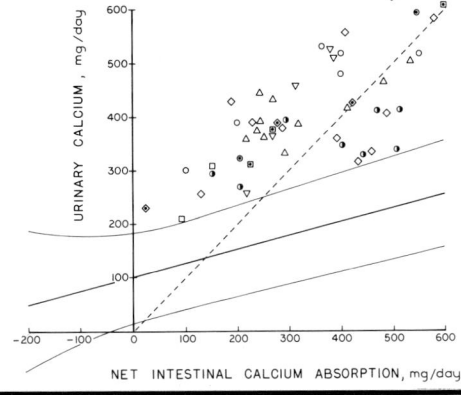

**Figure 40–7.** Urinary $Ca^{2+}$ excretion as a function of net intestinal $Ca^{2+}$ absorption from 6-day balance studies performed on 51 patients with idiopathic hypercalciuria reported as follows: ○, Nassim and Higgins[106]; □, Henneman and co-workers[197]; ■, Jackson and Dancaster[198]; ◆, Harrison[199]; ●, Dent and co-workers[200]; ▽, Parfitt and co-workers[201]; △, Edwards and Hodgkinson[196]; ◇, Liberman and co-workers[195]; and ◑, Lemann (personal communication, 1978). Solid lines represent mean and 2 SD derived from balance studies from 195 normal adults, shown in Figure 40–6. Dotted line is the line of identity, with positive $Ca^{2+}$ balance below the line.

**TABLE 40–8. Fraction of Filtered Calcium Excreted in the Urine by Normal and Hypercalciuric Subjects***

| Reference | Normal Subjects | Hypercalciuric Subjects† |
|---|---|---|
| Edwards and Hodgkinson[202] | 0.94% (7) | 2.94% (14) $P < .001$ |
| Peacock and Nordin[203] | 1.27% (5) | 4.25% (9) $P < .01$ |

*Number of subjects studied is shown in parentheses next to fractional excretion values.
†Urinary $Ca^{2+}$ excretion greater than 300 mg/24 h (men) or 250 mg/24 h (women).

(50 mg/24 h) in the balance data, none of the 55 normal people was in negative $Ca^{2+}$ balance. However, among 37 hypercalciuric patients with $Ca^{2+}$ absorption above 200 mg/24 h, $Ca^{2+}$ excretion exceeded net absorption in 23 patients by more than 50 mg/24 h (see Fig. 40–7). In other words, negative $Ca^{2+}$ balance was frequent in idiopathic hypercalciuric patients but not in normal people.

## RENAL TUBULE CALCIUM REABSORPTION

Two systematic studies have been made of overall fractional $Ca^{2+}$ reabsorption[202, 203] (Table 40–8). In both, the filtered load was calculated from inulin clearance or creatinine clearance and ultrafilterable serum $Ca^{2+}$ concentration, and the fraction of filtered load excreted was calculated for several clearance periods in normal and hypercalciuric people. Fractional $Ca^{2+}$ excretion was clearly high in the hypercalciuric subjects. Fractional $Ca^{2+}$ excretion is dependent on $Na^+$ excretion in normal people and in hypercalciuric people, increasing as dietary sodium increases.[204, 205] The effects of hydrochlorothiazide and acetazolamide on the tubule handling of $Na^+$, $Mg^{2+}$, and $Ca^{2+}$ in patients

with fasting hypercalciuria suggest a generalized defect in proximal tubule reabsorption of fluid and electrolytes.[206] Bianchi and colleagues[207] have shown increased activity of $Ca^{2+},Mg^{2+}$-ATPase in red blood cells from patients with idiopathic hypercalciuria as well as correlation between the enzyme activity and urinary $Ca^{2+}$ excretion in family studies. $Ca^{2+},Mg^{2+}$-ATPase is also present in the distal tubule and the intestine, which suggests that abnormalities in this enzyme activity may be involved in the pathogenesis of idiopathic hypercalciuria.

## BONE METABOLISM

There is an increasing body of evidence that the skeleton is involved in the pathogenesis of idiopathic hypercalciuria. Certainly, the high rate of negative $Ca^{2+}$ balance in patients with idiopathic hypercalciuria implicates bone involvement, because long-term negative $Ca^{2+}$ balance must involve bone mineral loss. A primary renal $Ca^{2+}$ leak might explain this phenomenon in some patients as a secondary response to PTH effect. However, negative $Ca^{2+}$ balance is more common than the high PTH, renal $Ca^{2+}$ leak subgroup of idiopathic hypercalciuria, which indicates active involvement of bone in many patients with idiopathic hypercalciuria.

Multiple studies have shown bone mineral density is lower in stone formers than in normal people[208–210] (Table 40–9). A variety of methods have been used, all showing at least some subgroup with decreased bone mineral density, even studies that included normocalciuric calcium stone formers.[208, 209] Lawoyin and co-workers[211] separated the patients into renal leak and absorptive hypercalciuria and noted low bone mineral density in only those with a renal $Ca^{2+}$ leak. However, Bataille and co-workers[212] found low bone mineral density in idiopathic hypercalciuric patients, including patients with type I absorptive hypercalciuria. Some of the differences between studies may be due

**TABLE 40–9. Bone Mineral Density and Histologic Studies in Patients with Nephrolithiasis**

| Reference | Number and Type of Patients* | Bone Area Studied | Technique | Results† |
|---|---|---|---|---|
| Lawoyin et al.[211] | RH 44<br>AH 117 | Distal radius | [125]I photon absorption | % Normal = 92.5, $P < .001$†<br>% Normal = 99.8, $P$ NS |
| Malluche et al.[216] | AH 15 | Iliac crest biopsy | Quantitative histomorphometry | Increased unmineralized osteoid, reduced matrix protein |
| Barkin et al.[208] | SF 109<br>N 115 | Trunk, thighs | Neutron activation | CBI 0.91 ± 0.13, $P < .01$ vs. normal<br>CBI 0.96 ± 0.13 |
| Borghi et al.[210] | DH 20<br>DIH 21 | Vertebral bone | Dual photon absorption | Z = −0.3 ± 1.19, $P$ NS‡<br>Z = −1.26 ± 1.18, $P < .02$ |
| Bataille et al.[212] | DH 18<br>DIH 24 | Vertebral bone | Computed tomographic densitometry | % Normal = 91, $P$ NS<br>% Normal = 69, $P < .01$ |
| Steiniche et al.[215] | IH 33 | Iliac crest biopsy | Quantitative histomorphometry | Increased mineralization lag time, reduced appositional rate |
| Alhava et al.[209] | MSF 54<br>FSF 21 | Distal radius | γ ray attenuation | % Normal 95.5, $P < .005$<br>% Normal 94.5, $P < .05$ |

*RH = renal hypercalciuria; AH = absorptive hypercalciuria; SF = unselected stone formers; DH = dietary hypercalciuria; DIH = dietary-independent hypercalciuria; IH = idiopathic hypercalciuria; MSF = male stone formers; FSF = female stone formers; N = normal.
†Percent normal is the bone mineral density in the study population expressed as a percentage of a normal control population. CBI = calcium bone index.
‡Results are normalized for age and sex by use of Z scores (value measured minus the mean from age- and sex-matched normal subjects divided by the standard deviation).

to variations in defining subgroups of patients. Bone turnover has been shown to be increased in idiopathic hypercalciuria. Urinary hydroxyproline is increased in unselected patients with idiopathic hypercalciuria,[213] whereas serum osteocalcin levels were found to be high in patients with renal leak hypercalciuria but not absorptive hypercalciuria.[214] Bone turnover studies using $^{47}$Ca show that idiopathic hypercalciuric patients have increased rates of bone formation and resorption.[195] Two studies have evaluated bone histologically.[215, 216] Malluche and colleagues[216] studied 15 patients with absorptive hypercalciuria and found reduced bone matrix apposition and delay of secondary mineralization of osteoid seams. Steiniche and colleagues[215] studied 33 idiopathic hypercalciuric patients and found prolonged mineralization lag time and a prolonged formation period, which suggested a mineralization defect possibly due to mild hypophosphatemia.

## MODELS OF HYPERCALCIURIA

A number of pathophysiologic mechanisms have been proposed as the cause of idiopathic hypercalciuria. Kidney, gut, skeleton, PTH, and vitamin D have all been implicated, and certainly no single theory can explain the etiology in every patient, because there are small numbers of patients with clearly defined abnormalities such as renal $PO_4^{3-}$ leak or renal $Ca^{2+}$ leak. However, the question of which mechanism is operative in the majority of patients is still a matter of debate.

**Renal Versus Absorptive Hypercalciuria.** In general, patients with idiopathic hypercalciuria have been separated into two groups, primary intestinal $Ca^{2+}$ overabsorption or primary renal tubule $Ca^{2+}$ leak, either of which could produce the findings summarized in Tables 40–7 and 40–8 and in Figures 40–6 and 40–7. Primary intestinal overabsorption would tend to raise postprandial serum $Ca^{2+}$ levels above normal and thereby increase the filtered load of $Ca^{2+}$ (Fig. 40–8, *left*). PTH secretion would be reduced by the hypercalcemia. Because PTH normally stimulates renal tubule $Ca^{2+}$ reabsorption (see Chapter 11), suppression of PTH secretion could reduce $Ca^{2+}$ reabsorption. Hypercalciuria would occur because of decreased reabsorption. A

**TABLE 40–10. Predictions of Absorptive and Renal Models of Idiopathic Hypercalciuria**

| Parameter | Absorptive Model | Renal Model |
|---|---|---|
| Fasting values | | |
| Serum iPTH | Low or normal | High |
| Urinary $Ca^{2+}$ | High or normal | High |
| Urinary cAMP | Low or normal | High |
| Serum 1,25(OH)$_2$D$_3$ | Uncertain | High |
| Response to thiazide | | |
| Serum iPTH | ± Fall | Fall |
| Urinary $Ca^{2+}$ | Fall | Fall |
| $Ca^{2+}$ absorption | No fall | Fall |
| Serum 1,25(OH)$_2$D$_3$ | Uncertain | Fall |
| Response to low-calcium diet | | |
| Serum iPTH | Increase or no change | Increase |
| Urinary $Ca^{2+}$ | Normal | High |
| $Ca^{2+}$ balance | Positive or neutral | Negative or neutral |
| $Ca^{2+}$ excreted ÷ absorbed | Normal | High |
| Risk of parathyroid adenoma | Normal | High |

renal leak (Fig. 40–8, *right*) would cause hypercalciuria. Secondary hyperparathyroidism, from excessive urinary $Ca^{2+}$ losses, would stimulate production of 1,25(OH)$_2$D$_3$ and produce intestinal hyperabsorption. Hyperabsorption would elevate postprandial serum $Ca^{2+}$ levels, raise the filtered load, and decrease the magnitude of the secondary hyperparathyroidism. The only way of distinguishing one mechanism from the other is by testing specific predictions, which differ for the two hypothetic models of hypercalciuria. Certain of these predictions are listed in Table 40–10.

Fasting iPTH, urinary $Ca^{2+}$ per gram creatinine or the calcium/creatinine ratio, and cAMP are interrelated and must be considered together. The overabsorption model permits low or normal fasting iPTH (see Fig. 40–8). If repeated bursts of postprandial hypercalcemia were to cause chronic hypoparathyroidism, fasting iPTH and urinary cAMP would be low and urinary calcium/creatinine ratio high (see Table 40–10). If PTH secretion were suppressed

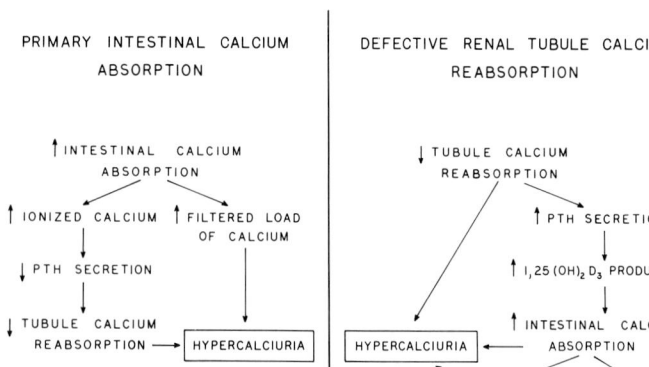

**Figure 40–8.** Proposed pathogenesis for two alternative models of idiopathic hypercalciuria. *Left.* Primary intestinal overabsorption. *Right.* Primary defective tubule $Ca^{2+}$ reabsorption. Dotted line indicates mechanisms tending to restore PTH secretion toward normal.

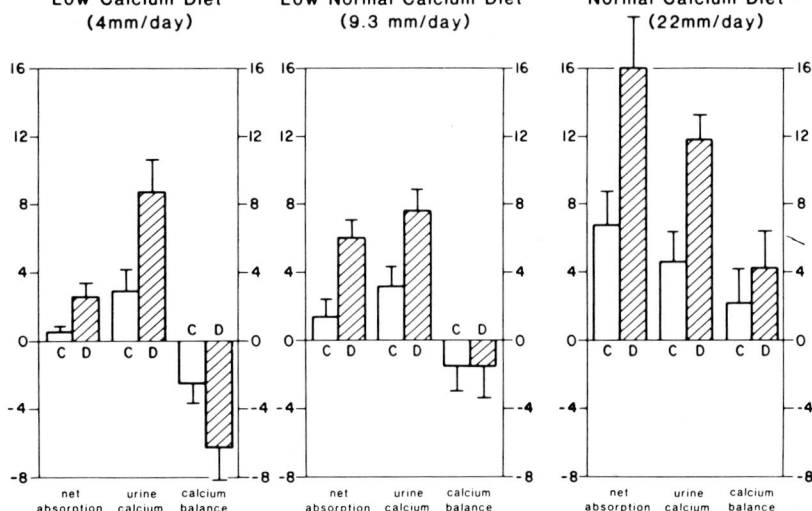

Low Calcium Diet
(4mm/day)

Low Normal Calcium Diet
(9.3 mm/day)

Normal Calcium Diet
(22mm/day)

**Figure 40–9.** Intestinal Ca$^{2+}$ absorption, urinary Ca$^{2+}$ excretion, and Ca$^{2+}$ balance in normal men receiving calcitriol *(crosshatched bars)* and in control subjects *(open bars)* at varying levels of calcium intake. (From Coe FL, Parks JH: Nephrolithiasis: Pathogenesis and Treatment, 2nd ed. Year Book Medical Publishers, Chicago, 1988, p 113. By permission of Mosby–Year Book.)

only transiently after calcium ingestion, all three fasting measurements would be normal. The absorptive hypothesis predicts a spectrum of fasting values, but it forbids the combination of elevated fasting urinary calcium/creatinine ratio with normal iPTH. The renal model requires elevated fasting urinary calcium/creatinine ratio and a high serum iPTH. Urinary cAMP excretion should also be elevated.

High PTH values have been reported in some patients[217, 218] as the renal model demands (see Fig. 40–8, *right*). The question of whether fasting PTH levels are reduced in some patients with idiopathic hypercalciuria is more difficult to answer because assays for PTH vary from one study to another, and many of the assays used had limited ability to detect low levels.[109, 190, 217, 219] Bataille and co-workers[212] studied 42 patients with idiopathic hypercalciuria using an intact PTH assay. They found only 1 of 16 patients with fasting hypercalciuria with an elevated PTH value. The 26 patients with absorptive hypercalciuria had PTH levels that were not different from those of normal people. In most studies of idiopathic hypercalciuric patients, renal leak hypercalciuria is found in the minority of patients.

The response of urinary Ca$^{2+}$ to a low-calcium diet or cellulose phosphate, a Ca$^{2+}$-binding ion exchange resin, has been described by Pak[220, 221] and Bordier[218] and colleagues. Both found a marked fall in absorptive hypercalciuria and, in fact, used this response—along with serum PTH—to classify the patients as absorptive. By hypothesis, urinary Ca$^{2+}$ must remain elevated in renal hypercalciuria despite low calcium intake. Bordier[218] and Pak[220, 221] observed this in patients with high PTH values, but the data are few.

Pak and associates[222] have developed a simplified outpatient protocol to distinguish renal and absorptive hypercalciuria. Patients are studied after 7 days of a low-calcium diet (400 mg of calcium, 100 mEq of sodium chloride per day). On the last day of the diet, a 24-hour urine specimen is collected. At the end of the study diet, urinary Ca$^{2+}$ excretion is measured in the fasting state and after a 1-g oral calcium load. Renal hypercalciuria is defined as elevated levels of fasting urinary Ca$^{2+}$ (>0.11 mg/100 mL glomerular filtration), urinary cAMP, and iPTH. Absorptive hypercalciuria type I is defined as normal fasting urinary

Ca$^{2+}$ level, high urinary Ca$^{2+}$ excretion after the oral calcium load, hypercalciuria on the calcium-restricted diet, and normal PTH and urinary cAMP values. Absorptive hypercalciuria type II is the same as type I except for normal urinary Ca$^{2+}$ excretion on the restricted calcium diet. In a study of 241 consecutive stone-forming patients, Pak and colleagues[222] found 24% had type I absorptive hypercalciuria, 30% had type II, and only 8% had a renal Ca$^{2+}$ leak.

**Calcitriol Excess.** When evaluated by the Pak method, the majority of idiopathic hypercalciuric patients fall into the absorptive group.[221, 222] However, intestinal hyperabsorption does not predict the high frequency of negative Ca$^{2+}$ balance seen in idiopathic hypercalciuric patients. An alternative hypothesis is that of vitamin D excess activity, a situation that would lead to intestinal overabsorption, increased bone resorption, and reduced renal Ca$^{2+}$ reabsorption.

Two studies in normal men have reproduced the clinical characteristics of idiopathic hypercalciuria by the administration of calcitriol. In one report, normal men were studied on a very low calcium diet (4.2 mmol/d) with and without calcitriol supplementation.[223] Calcitriol supplementation did not result in hypercalcemia. Urinary Ca$^{2+}$ levels and intestinal Ca$^{2+}$ absorption were significantly increased in the subjects taking calcitriol. Ca$^{2+}$ balance was more negative in the men taking calcitriol, indicating bone resorption as the source of Ca$^{2+}$ loss. In a second study,[224] normal men were studied on normal (22 mmol/d) and low-normal (9 mmol/d) calcium diets with and without calcitriol supplementation. Intestinal Ca$^{2+}$ absorption and urinary Ca$^{2+}$ excretion increased during calcitriol therapy, but Ca$^{2+}$ balance was unchanged. These two studies are summarized in Figure 40–9. Thus, elevated calcitriol increases urinary Ca$^{2+}$ levels and intestinal Ca$^{2+}$ absorption but leads to negative Ca$^{2+}$ balance only with extreme calcium restriction, findings similar to those in most idiopathic hypercalciuric patients. Breslau and co-workers[225] studied 19 patients with absorptive hypercalciuria using ketoconazole to suppress calcitriol production. Intestinal Ca$^{2+}$ absorption was measured by use of $^{47}$Ca. Twelve of the 19 subjects reduced Ca$^{2+}$ absorption and urinary Ca$^{2+}$ excretion significantly; the other 7 showed no response despite a degree of vitamin D

D suppression equal to that of the responders. These findings support the theory that a significant proportion of idiopathic hypercalciuric patients have a disorder of vitamin D regulation as the cause of their disease.

Multiple studies have reported serum $1,25(OH)_2D_3$ levels in hypercalciuric and normal subjects (Table 40–11). In hypercalciuric patients, the $1,25(OH_2)D_3$ levels, in general, are above normal. Some studies[112, 192, 229] have separated patients into renal leak and absorptive hypercalciuria, with higher levels seen in the apparent renal hypercalciuria. Even in the absence of elevated vitamin D levels, excess $1,25(OH_2)D_3$ activity may occur as has been shown in rats inbred for hypercalciuria; they have high levels of vitamin D receptor and normal levels of vitamin D but overabsorb dietary calcium and become hypercalciuric.[230]

**Renal Phosphate Leak.** Hypophosphatemia due to excess renal $PO_4^{3-}$ losses stimulates $1,25(OH_2)D_3$ production, producing hypercalciuria similar to that of primary $1,25(OH_2)D_3$ overproduction. This pattern of abnormalities has been shown in a large kindred from a Bedouin tribe.[184] In a study of 59 members, 9 had the characteristic syndrome of hypophosphatemic rickets, hypercalciuria, and markedly elevated levels of $1,25(OH_2)D_3$. Of the remaining 50 asymptomatic members of the tribe, 21 had "idiopathic hypercalciuria," with serum $PO_4^{3-}$ levels and $1,25(OH_2)D_3$ levels between those of normal members of the tribe and the patients with hypophosphatemic rickets. It appears that the magnitude of the hypophosphatemia, through control of $1,25(OH_2)D_3$ production, determines which subjects will have isolated hypercalciuria and which will have hypercalciuria and rickets. These findings indicate that a mild renal $PO_4^{3-}$ leak could produce the syndrome of idiopathic hypercalciuria.

The role of $PO_4^{3-}$ depletion in idiopathic hypercalciuria in a general stone-forming population has been studied in a group of stone formers with absorptive hypercalciuria and hypophosphatemia during outpatient evaluation.[231] The serum phosphorus level became normal, however, when the patients were studied as inpatients on a controlled diet. Three patients remained hypophosphatemic despite a controlled diet and had elevated levels of serum $1,25(OH)_2D_3$;

however, after 2 months of phosphate therapy, the serum $1,25(OH)_2D_3$ level was reduced to normal, yet intestinal $Ca^{2+}$ absorption remained elevated. The low phosphorus level observed in the outpatient setting probably reflected a high spontaneous phosphate intake rather than an intrinsic disorder of phosphorus metabolism in all but three patients; even in these three patients, hypophosphatemia could not be linked securely to the pathogenesis of increased intestinal $Ca^{2+}$ absorption. Although renal $PO_4^{3-}$ wasting can cause hypercalciuria, it seems to be a relatively uncommon cause of the disorder.

## AN ATTEMPT AT SYNTHESIS

Certainly there is controversy in the studies of the mechanism of idiopathic hypercalciuria. The frequency of any given subtype of hypercalciuria varies from one study to the next. Some of this may represent genetic heterogeneity of the populations studied, but often it is due to the criteria and conditions used to analyze the patients. PTH measurements have been made with a variety of antibodies, but only with the introduction of the intact molecule assay have low levels been reliably measured. Some of the earlier studies in which categorization of patients depended on the ability to distinguish low from normal PTH may not be accurate. Bataille and co-workers,[212] using an intact PTH assay, found more than one third of their hypercalciuric patients unclassifiable by the Pak criteria[222] because they had high fasting $Ca^{2+}$ levels with normal PTH levels. Studies of calcitriol supplementation in normal men show that calcitriol excess may cause fasting hypercalciuria[223] as well as intestinal hyperabsorption, blurring the distinctions of renal and absorptive hypercalciuria. In addition, a link has been shown between calcitriol levels and dietary calcium intake in hypercalciuric patients who have high intestinal absorption of $Ca^{2+}$.[232] However, the calcitriol levels also depend on the length of time of any set calcium intake, which makes it difficult to compare studies of patients consuming fixed diets unless the diets are used for similar lengths of time.

Separation of patients into absorptive and renal leak hy-

**TABLE 40–11. Serum $1,25(OH)_2D_3$ Levels in Normal Subjects and Patients with Idiopathic Hypercalciuria***

| Reference | Serum Calcium (mg/100 mL) | | Serum Phosphorus (mg/100 mL) | | Serum $1,25(OH)_2D_3$ (ng/100 mL) | |
|---|---|---|---|---|---|---|
| | *Normal Subjects* | *IH Subjects* | *Normal Subjects* | *IH Subjects* | *Normal Subjects* | *IH Subjects* |
| Shen et al.[190] | 10.2 ± 0.2 (8) | 10.2 ± 0.5 (7) | 3.8 ± 0.5 | 2.6 ± 0.3 | 3.2 ± 0.4 | 5.8 ± 2.3 |
| Haussler et al.[226] | — | | 3.8 ± 0.5 (18) | 2.6 ± 0.4 (18) | 3.3 ± 0.8 | 5.2 ± 1.9 |
| Kaplan et al.[112] | 9.7 ± 0.5 (11) | 9.6 ± 0.1 (3)† | 3.7 ± 0.7 | 3.6 ± 0.1† | 3.4 ± 0.9 | 6.9 ± 2.3† |
| | — | 9.4 ± 0.3 (21)‡ | — | 3.7 ± 0.5‡ | — | 4.5 ± 1.1‡ |
| Gray et al[118] | 9.6 ± 0.3 (48) | 9.6 ± 0.4 (26) | 4.0 ± 0.6 | 3.5 ± 0.6 | 3.6 ± 1.2 | 6.2 ± 3.1 |
| Shen et al.[190] | 10.0 ± 0.3 (15) | 9.9 ± 0.3 (16) | 3.7 ± 0.3 | 2.9 ± 0.6 | 3.4 ± 0.7 | 5.4 ± 1.9 |
| Zerwekh and Pak[192] | — | 9.6 ± 0.5 (11)‡ | — | 3.5 ± 0.3‡ | — | 4.5 ± 1.4‡ |
| | | 9.7 ± 0.4 (10)† | | 3.5 ± 0.6† | | 5.2 ± 2.2† |
| Broadus et al.[227] | 9.4 ± 0.2 (25) | 9.5 ± 0.3 (50) | — | — | 4.7 ± 1.4 | 7.7 ± 1.2 |
| Bataille et al.[212] | 9.6 ± 0.4 (12) | 9.5 ± 0.4 (24) | 3.1 ± 0.3 | 3.0 ± 0.3 | 5.0 ± 1.4 | 6.9 ± 2.4 |
| Coe et al.[228] | 9.2 ± 0.6 (9) | 9.3 ± 0.4 (24) | — | — | 3.5 ± 0.6 | 4.1 ± 0.7 |

*Values are mean ± SD; numbers in parentheses represent numbers of subjects. IH = idiopathic hypercalciuria.
†Renal idiopathic hypercalciuria.
‡Absorptive idiopathic hypercalciuria.

percalciuria gave promise of allowing therapy aimed at correcting the underlying pathophysiologic process. However, the high rate of negative $Ca^{2+}$ balance found in many hypercalciuric patients suggests that simple intestinal overabsorption cannot be the cause in the majority of patients, but rather some form of excess calcitriol activity. The commonly used outpatient evaluations cannot adequately separate these disorders.[223] Prescribing a low-calcium diet in patients with excess calcitriol activity would increase the risk of bone disease.[233] Additional studies are needed to further clarify the role of kidney, intestine, bone, PTH, and calcitriol in the pathogenesis of idiopathic hypercalciuria. Certainly some marker of calcitriol activity, in addition to calcitriol levels, is needed to clarify the pathogenesis of this disorder.

## TREATMENT

Hypotheses about pathogenesis, particularly the question of primacy, affect the choice of treatment or at least the conviction that a particular treatment is especially appropriate. If primary intestinal overabsorption is saturating the blood with $Ca^{2+}$ and the kidney is acting as a protective escape port—albeit at the price of an oversaturated urine—low-calcium diet or drugs that reduce $Ca^{2+}$ absorption are appropriate. In contrast, thiazide therapy, but not calcium restriction, is rational for renal hypercalciuria and, presumably, is superior to a low-calcium diet in states of $1,25(OH)_2D_3$ excess. Unfortunately, identifying the pathogenesis of any single patient's hypercalciuria is not easily done, which restricts the ability of the practicing physician to carefully tailor therapy.

**Diet.** Low-calcium diet has long been advocated in the treatment of hypercalciuric stone disease and has been shown to be effective in reducing urinary $Ca^{2+}$ excretion.[222] However, low-calcium diet may increase the intestinal absorption of oxalate, reducing the effectiveness of this therapy. No well-controlled studies of dietary calcium restriction have been performed to show efficacy of stone reduction, although open trials have reported reduction of stone formation of 29% to 47% with dietary manipulation alone.[234, 235] However, the low bone mineral density found in hypercalciuric patients[208, 210–212] and negative $Ca^{2+}$ balance seen with calcitriol excess[223] make calcium restriction a potentially dangerous therapy. Idiopathic hypercalciuric patients treated with low-calcium diets have shown bone mineral loss similar to that seen in patients with hyperparathyroidism.[233] If patients can be adequately evaluated before and during therapy to ensure that negative $Ca^{2+}$ balance is not induced by low-calcium diet, this may be effective in some patients. Calcium gluttony should certainly be avoided, but calcium restriction is a therapy that must be used with caution.

Dietary sodium restriction reduces urinary $Ca^{2+}$ excretion by reducing glomerular filtration rate and increasing distal $Ca^{2+}$ reabsorption.[204, 205] Salt restriction has been shown to be effective in reducing $Ca^{2+}$ excretion in patients with idiopathic hypercalciuria. High protein intake also increases urinary $Ca^{2+}$ excretion and causes negative $Ca^{2+}$ balance.[236, 237] We recommend low salt and reduced animal protein intake to our patients, although neither intervention

has been tested for efficacy in preventing stones by a randomized trial.

**Cellulose Phosphate.** Cellulose phosphate is a $Ca^{2+}$-binding ion exchange resin that has been recommended for the treatment of absorptive hypercalciuria. Pak and associates[220] have presented a careful study of 16 patients with severe recurrent calcium phosphate/calcium oxalate stone disease. Although the treatment interval was short, new stones formed during cellulose phosphate treatment were only 7.1% of the number predicted by multiplying the pretreatment recurrence rate, 376 stones/100 patients per year, by the 41 patient-years of follow-up.

It is not certain whether equally good results can be obtained in treatment of the more common calcium oxalate stone former. Although cellulose phosphate lowers urinary $Ca^{2+}$ excretion markedly, it induces a reciprocal increase in oxalate excretion. In one study, oxalate excretion rose from 30.1 to 60.3 mg/24 h,[238] and the hyperoxaluria offset the hypocalciuria, so that the mean APR for calcium oxalate fell only 20% from 2.75 to 2.19. In contrast, the mean APR for calcium phosphate fell dramatically to below 1.0 in 16 treated patients of Pak and colleagues.[220] Others have confirmed the development of hyperoxaluria[239, 240] in response to cellulose phosphate. One would expect such a drug to prevent calcium phosphate stones, whereas calcium oxalate stone disease might respond less impressively. Backman and colleagues[240] have described the clinical response of recurrent calcium oxalate stone disease to cellulose phosphate. Before treatment, 35 patients formed 120 stones during a total of 160 patient-years (75 stones/100 patients per year). If the first stone formed by each patient is subtracted and the data are omitted for one of their patients who formed several hundred stones before treatment, the pretreatment recurrence rate was 54 stones/100 patients per year. During approximately 70 patient-years of follow-up with cellulose phosphate treatment, stone recurrence averaged 20 stones/100 patients per year. Forty-seven percent of the patients had at least one recurrence. Stone recurrence in patients who received cellulose phosphate was comparable to that observed by the same authors in response to reduced dietary calcium and increased fluid intake.

It seems reasonable to say that cellulose phosphate as a treatment of the typical calcium stone former is unproved. Although the rationale for its use in primary intestinal hypercalciuria is excellent, it is flawed by a tendency toward reciprocal hyperoxaluria that blunts the effectiveness of the drug in lowering urine saturation with respect to calcium oxalate.[131] In the prevention of recurrent calcium oxalate stones, it has not proved very successful.[240] The high frequency of negative $Ca^{2+}$ balance in unselected, untreated patients with idiopathic hypercalciuria raises the same concern of bone mineral loss that may complicate low-calcium diets.

**Thiazide Diuretics.** Thiazide inhibits sodium chloride but not $Ca^{2+}$ reabsorption in the loop of Henle.[241] Overall, external $Na^+$ balance becomes normal after a few days of treatment, presumably because delivery of sodium chloride from more proximal nephron segments falls. $Ca^{2+}$ delivery may also fall, leading to decreased urinary $Ca^{2+}$ excretion. Thiazide directly stimulates $Ca^{2+}$ reabsorption by the distal convoluted tubule of the rat[242] and may also have this influence in humans. The studies of the effect of thiazides on intestinal $Ca^{2+}$ transport have shown mixed results of decreasing $Ca^{2+}$ absorption in some patients and causing no change in others.[106, 189, 191, 192, 243] Two studies from Pak's laboratory[191, 192] showed hydrochlorothiazide reduced intestinal $Ca^{2+}$ absorption in patients with high-PTH, presumably renal, hypercalciuria but failed to alter $Ca^{2+}$ absorption in patients with the absorptive form. In contrast, Ehrig and associates[189] showed $Ca^{2+}$ absorption fell from 59% to 42% in nine hypercalciuric patients with intestinal $Ca^{2+}$ hyperabsorption treated with thiazide. Reduction in urinary excretion in the setting of unchanged $Ca^{2+}$ absorption indicates the subject must be in positive $Ca^{2+}$ balance.

Whether thiazide does or does not change intestinal $Ca^{2+}$ absorption, it is likely that thiazide therapy improves $Ca^{2+}$ balance. Coe and associates[243] did formal $Ca^{2+}$ balance studies in seven hypercalciuric patients before and after 6 months of treatment with chlorthalidone. Intestinal $Ca^{2+}$ absorption decreased but $Ca^{2+}$ balance increased because urinary $Ca^{2+}$ excretion fell more than intestinal absorption. Studies have indicated that thiazide use in the hypertensive population increases bone mineral[244] and reduces the risk of hip fracture in the elderly.[245] Steiniche and co-workers[246] studied hypercalciuric patients before and 6 months after treatment with hydrochlorothiazide using histomorphometric analysis of iliac crest biopsy specimens. They found reduced bone turnover during treatment and reduced osteoid thickness, indications of improved mineralization during thiazide therapy.

Thiazide diuretics are the best studied of the treatment interventions for hypercalciuric stone formers. There have been numerous open trials that have suggested the efficacy of thiazides in the treatment of calcium stones. Supersaturation of calcium salts has been shown to fall in response to thiazide therapy as urinary $Ca^{2+}$ excretion falls; oxalate excretion is not affected. There have now been six randomized studies of thiazide diuretics in the treatment of recurrent calcium oxalate nephrolithiasis. Although these studies have been reported to show conflicting results, the conflicts are related to the duration of the therapy (Table 40–12). The two 1-year trials[247, 248] showed no difference between the placebo and thiazide groups. Both 3-year studies[249, 250] showed significant reduction in the number of patients with recurrent stones, but neither of these studies showed significant reductions in stone recurrence rate at the 1-year time

period. The other two studies of intermediate duration[251, 252] both showed reduction in the number of patients with stone recurrence, although the differences were just short of statistical significance. The study of Ohkawa[252] did show a significant reduction in the stone formation rate, 13 stones/100 patient-years in the thiazide group versus 31 stones/100 patient-years in the control group. The majority of these trials did not supplement potassium for the patients given thiazide, which would predispose the patients to hypocitraturia and reduce the effectiveness of the drug, nor were drug doses varied to get maximal reduction in urinary $Ca^{2+}$ excretion. Thiazides would be expected to be even more effective in clinical practice, with appropriate dosing to reach the desired response in urinary $Ca^{2+}$ excretion and potassium supplementation when needed. These randomized trials are the strongest evidence of effective therapy in the treatment of nephrolithiasis.

The two 3-year randomized trials included hypercalciuric and nonhypercalciuric calcium stone formers and still showed significant reduction in renal stone formation. The excellent overall therapeutic response suggests that the reduction of urinary calcium oxalate saturation is a general approach to calcium stone prevention that is useful even in normocalciuric patients, whose calcium oxalate stones must reflect their inability to excrete even normal amounts of $Ca^{2+}$ and oxalate without forming stones. Laerum and Larsen[249] analyzed hypercalciuric and normocalciuric patients separately, and thiazide was of equal efficacy in both groups of patients. The study by Ohkawa and colleagues[252] included both absorptive and renal hypercalciuric patients and showed similar reductions in stone formation rate. As well, the effectiveness of thiazide in the other studies, despite its certain use in some absorptive as well as renal hypercalciuric patients, suggests that as a practical matter, exact pathogenetic distinctions may not be crucial in determining choice of treatment.

## Hyperuricosuria

The usual upper limits of daily urinary uric acid excretion, 800 mg for men and 750 mg for women, are exceeded more frequently by calcium stone formers than by normal people (Table 40–13). In hyperuricosuric patients who form calcium stones, stone disease begins at a later average age

**TABLE 40–12. Summary of Six Randomized Trials of Thiazide Diuretics for Prevention of Calcium Nephrolithiasis**

| Reference | Drug Dose* | Number of Subjects | Year 1 Drug (%)† | Year 1 Placebo (%)† | D/P‡ | Year 2 Drug (%) | Year 2 Placebo (%) | D/P | Year 3 Drug (%) | Year 3 Placebo (%) | D/P | P Value at End of Study |
|---|---|---|---|---|---|---|---|---|---|---|---|---|
| Laerum and Larsen[249] | HCTZ 25 mg bid | 50 | 18 | 30 | 0.6 | 24 | 55 | 0.43 | 26 | 58 | 0.44 | $P = .04$ |
| Ettinger et al.[250] | CTD 25 or 50 mg qd | 73 | 10 | 20 | 0.5 | 10 | 48 | 0.21 | 20 | 50 | 0.4 | $P < .05$ |
| Mortensen et al.[251] | BFMT 2.5 mg tid | 22 | — | — | — | 0 | 40 | 0 | — | — | — | $.05 < P < .1$ |
| Ohkawa et al.[252] | TCM 4 mg qd | 175 | — | — | — | 8 | 14 | 0.57 | — | — | — | $.05 < P < .1$ |
| Scholz et al.[247] | HCTZ 25 mg bid | 51 | 24 | 23 | 1.04 | — | — | — | — | — | — | Not significant |
| Brocks et al.[248] | BFMT 2.5 mg tid | 62 | 15 | 17 | 0.88 | — | — | — | — | — | — | Not significant |

*HCTZ = hydrochlorothiazide; CTD = chlorthalidone; BFMT = bendroflumethiazide; TCM = trichlormethiazide.
†Percentage of subjects with recurrence of stones.
‡Ratio of drug-treated to placebo-treated subjects with recurrence of stones.

TABLE 40–13. Frequencies of Uric Acid Excretion Rates Among Calcium Oxalate Stone Formers and Normal Subjects*

| Urinary Urate (mg/24 h) | Men N (128) | Men P (1046) | Women N (77) | Women P (302) |
|---|---|---|---|---|
| <200 | 0 | 0 | 0 | 0 |
| 200–400 | 2 | 1 | 36 | 25 |
| 400–600 | 38 | 17 | 54 | 53 |
| 600–800 | 48 | 50 | 9 | 8 |
| 800–900 | 6 | 14 | 0 | 6 |
| 900–1000 | 4 | 11 | — | 5 |
| >1000 | 2 | 7 | — | 3 |

*Numbers represent the percentage of 24-h urine samples containing the amounts of urate indicated. The total number of urine samples in each group is shown in parentheses. P = stone formers; N = normal subjects.

than usual and is unusually active and severe.[67, 253] Complex mechanisms, not yet fully understood, link hyperuricosuria to calcium stones. Allopurinol treatment reduces stone formation, so detection of hyperuricosuria is important.

## FREQUENCY OF HYPERURICOSURIA

Of 460 calcium stone formers in our survey, 26.3% were hyperuricosuric.[67] Hyperuricosuria and idiopathic hypercalciuria coexisted in 11.7% of patients, close to what one might expect on the basis of independent occurrence rates of these two common disorders. Of our 121 hyperuricosuric patients, 40 men (39%) and 4 women (22%) were hyperuricemic; serum urate values were normal in the rest.

The usual upper limits of normal for uric acid excretion are arbitrary, because the distributions of daily uric acid excretion by normal men and women are continuous, not bimodal. However, even if higher limits are used, stone formers still differ from normal (see Table 40–13). The point two standard deviations above the normal mean could be used to replace these arbitrary limits, but patients who are most likely to benefit from treatment might not be selected with any greater precision. Saturation with respect to uric acid or its salt, not the amount excreted daily, is the property that can influence crystallization in the urine, so that the normal range should be defined in terms of saturation. In the meantime, given the indirect relationship between excretion rate and saturation, the usual limits, for all their inexactness, may be just as useful as higher ones. Simkin and colleagues[254] have suggested that "spot" mid-

TABLE 40–14. Purine and Calorie Intake by Patients and Normal Subjects*

| Group | Purine Intake (mg/24 h) | Calorie Intake (cal/24 h) |
|---|---|---|
| Patients (10) | 259 ± 29 | 2109 ± 161 |
| Normal men (5) | 155 ± 21 | 2104 ± 147 |

*F = 9.16, P < .01, for patients versus normal men; values are mean ± SEM.

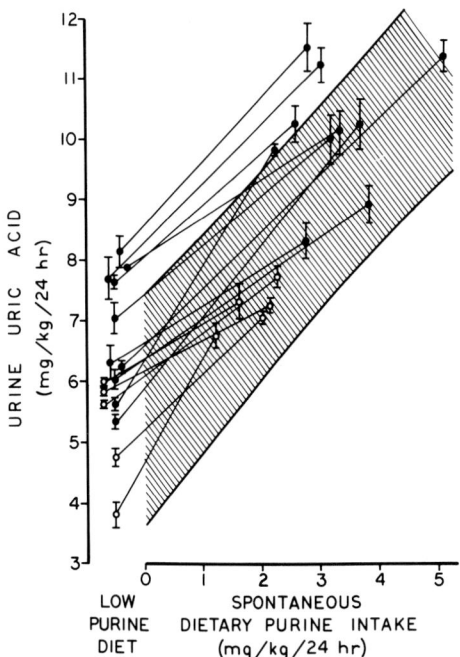

**Figure 40–10.** Relationship between purine intake and uric acid excretion in hyperuricosuric patients compared with that in normal subjects. Uric acid excretion in 3 of the 10 patients (solid circles) exceeded the upper limit of the normal range (hatched areas), indicating an abnormal rate of uric acid excretion. After 7 days of a purine-free diet, these three patients continued to excrete an abnormal amount of uric acid compared with five normal subjects (open circles). All values are mean ± 1 SEM of three separate determinations. (From Coe FL, Kavalach A: Hypercalciuria and hyperuricosuria in patients with calcium nephrolithiasis. N Engl J Med 291:1344, 1974.)

morning urine samples can substitute for 24-hour urine collections in diagnosing uric acid overexcretion, although the clinical utility of spot collections in stone disease has not been determined.

## CAUSE OF HYPERURICOSURIA

Coe and associates[255] studied purine consumption in hyperuricosuric stone formers and normal subjects. The patients habitually consumed a larger amount of purine than did five well-matched normal people whose calorie intake was nearly identical (Table 40–14). The patients preferred to eat more meat, fish, and poultry than normal people did and ate a correspondingly smaller amount of breads, grains, and starches.

Hyperuricosuria was not always due entirely to excessive consumption of purine. From a study of normal people, it was possible to construct a 95% confidence band relating urinary uric acid excretion to purine intake (Fig. 40–10). Three of the 10 patients studied excreted more uric acid than did normal subjects eating the same amount of purine. After 7 days of purine-free diet, these three patients continued to excrete more uric acid than the normal subjects did, and more than did the five normal people we studied. Presumably, this surplus uric acid arose from overproduction of uric acid during the course of endogenous purine metabolism.

**TABLE 40–15. Geometric Correspondence Between Naturally Occurring Faces of Uric Acid and Calcium Oxalate Crystals**

| Crystals | Face | Dimensions ($\mathring{A}$) |
|---|---|---|
| Uric acid | 100 | 6.21 × 7.40 |
| Uric acid • $2H_2O$ | 100 | 6.35 × 7.40 |
| CaOx • $H_2O$* | 001 | 6.28 × 14.57 |
| CaOx • $2H_2O$† | 101 | 12.30 × 7.34 |
| NaH urate • $H_2O$ | 100 | 3.567 × 8.693 |
| | 010 | 9.097 × 3.567 |

*Whewellite, or calcium oxalate monohydrate.
†Weddelite, or calcium oxalate dihydrate.

## MECHANISM OF STONE FORMATION

The network dimensions of calcium oxalate monohydrate or dihydrate crystals and uric acid crystals match closely enough, within a few percentage points either directly or as integral multiples of one another (Table 40–15), to permit epitaxial growth.[256, 257] Pak and Arnold[36] and we[37] have shown that seed crystals of sodium hydrogen urate or uric acid initiate calcium oxalate precipitation from a metastable solution. Sodium hydrogen urate is effective even though its dimensions[258] do not match those of calcium oxalate very well (see Table 40–15). Although Robertson[259] believed otherwise, Pak and we[28, 260] have shown that urine is metastably oversaturated with respect to sodium hydrogen urate and uric acid (Table 40–16), so that crystals could form.[260, 261] Crystals of the sodium salt are not found in fresh human urine, but uric acid crystals are commonplace in urine and could be a source of nuclei.

We measured urine supersaturation with respect to monosodium hydrogen urate[260] using a crystal seeding technique analogous to that employed for measurement of supersaturation with respect to calcium oxalate. Pak and col-leagues[261] have described similar measurements. When urine volume and urine pH are controlled experimentally,[261] hyperuricosuria increases urine supersaturation with respect to sodium hydrogen urate. However, when patients with hyperuricosuria are consuming their own free-choice diet, they produce a urine that has a lower pH than that of normal people (see Table 40–16). Because of the low pH, an abnormally high percentage of the total urinary uric acid in these patients is in the form of undissociated uric acid rather than urate. Consequently, supersaturation with respect to monosodium urate is not higher than normal, but urinary undissociated uric acid concentrations are. The solubility of undissociated uric acid in urine is 90 ± 5 mg/L; concentrations in hyperuricosuric patients exceed this solubility limit, whereas concentrations in urine from normal people and patients with idiopathic hypercalciuria do not. These findings suggest that undissociated uric acid rather than sodium hydrogen urate would be the favored solid phase in the urine of hyperuricosuric patients. The reason for the low urine pH in patients with hyperuricosuria may be the high intake of meat, fish, and poultry that characterizes their diet.[255]

The clinical role of heterogeneous nucleation is uncertain. Small nuclei of uric acid or urate could lodge in a calyceal niche or in the lumen of a collecting duct and be the center of a calcium oxalate stone. Uric acid itself certainly does plug renal collecting ducts,[262] and urate could do the same. The exposed end of such a plug, bathed perpetually by the flowing urine, is an attractive foundation for a stone. However, proof that heterogeneous nucleation is a link between hyperuricosuria and calcium stones is lacking.

Robertson and colleagues[57] have produced another mechanism: adsorption of certain urinary crystal growth inhibitors, acid mucopolysaccharides in particular, by urate or uric acid crystals. They suggested that hyperuricosuria may deplete urine of its inhibitors by increasing the mass of uric acid crystals and in this manner predispose to calcium stones. They found that increasing urinary uric acid concen-

**TABLE 40–16. Urinary Uric Acid Saturation***

| 24-Hour Urinary Values | Metabolic Group | | | | |
|---|---|---|---|---|---|
| | Normal (20) | IH (24) | HU (12) | Both (14) | Neither (17) |
| Number of samples | 24 | 69 | 36 | 42 | 51 |
| Total uric acid (mg/L) | 503 ± 32 | 421 ± 23 | 575 ± 28 | 616 ± 27‡[b] | 462 ± 32 |
| Urine volume (mL) | 1268 ± 65 | 1717 ± 133 | 1501 ± 79[a] | 1397 ± 70 | 1387 ± 90 |
| Urine pH | 6.22 | 5.92 | 5.62 | 5.74[b] | 5.67 |
| Undissociated uric acid (mg/L)‡ | 57 ± 8 | 84 ± 11 | 155 ± 21[c] | 150 ± 15[d] | 128 ± 18[b] |
| CPR, monosodium hydrogen urate | 2.8 ± 0.3§ | 2.2 ± 0.2 | 2.7 ± 0.2 | 3.1 ± 0.2 | 2.2 ± 0.2 |
| [Na][urate] ($m^2 \times 10^{-5}$), initial‖ | 37 ± 4 | 27 ± 3 | 35 ± 4 | 42 ± 3¶ | 29 ± 3 |
| Sodium concentration (mEq/L) | 131 ± 8 | 118 ± 7 | 130 ± 7 | 149 ± 7 | 132 ± 7 |

*All values except for the numbers of samples and the numbers of people in each metabolic group (in parentheses) are means ± SEM. IH = idiopathic hypercalciuria; HU = hyperuricosuria; CPR = concentration product ratio; [Na] = sodium concentration (mEq/L); [urate] = urate concentration (mM/L).
†Differs from control: [a]$P < .05$; [b]$P < .02$; [c]$P < .001$; [d]$P < .001$.
‡The mean equilibrium value, determined in 26 urine samples of pH below 5.6 after 48 h of incubation with crystals of uric acid, was 90 ± 5 (SEM) mg/L. Values were calculated by use of a p$K_a$ of 5.345.
§Based on the study of 16 of the 20 normal subjects who had CPR measurements.
‖Before incubation with crystals of sodium hydrogen urate.
¶Men differed from women, $P < .05$.
Adapted from Coe FL, Strauss AL, Tembe V, Le Dun S: Uric acid saturation in calcium nephrolithiasis. Kidney Int 17:662–668, 1980.

**TABLE 40–17. Effects of Allopurinol on Calcium Stone Formation in Hyperuricosuric Patients***

| Parameter | Hyperuricosuria | | Hyperuricosuria and Hypercalciuria | |
|---|---|---|---|---|
| | **P** | **T** | **P** | **T** |
| Number of patients | 48 | | 42 | |
| Time (patient-years) | 298 | 186 | 357 | 119 |
| Stone formed | 200 | 8 | 188 | 6 |
| Stones/patient | 4.17 | — | 4.48 | — |
| Years/patient | 6.21 | 3.90 | 8.50 | 2.83 |
| Stones/100 patients/y | 67.1 | 4.3 | 52.7 | 5.0 |
| New stones predicted | — | 124.8† | — | 62.7† |

*Patients with hyperuricosuria were treated with allopurinol; patients with hyperuricosuria and hypercalciuria were treated with allopurinol and thiazide. P and T refer to pretreatment and treatment intervals, respectively.

†$\chi^2$ for difference between predicted and observed values, 109.3 and 51.3, respectively; $P < .001$ for both.

tration lowers crystal growth inhibitor activity. However, the mechanism is far from established. Finlayson and DuBois[263] have shown that sodium hydrogen urate crystals can adsorb appreciable amounts of one particular acid mucopolysaccharide, heparin, when $Ca^{2+}$ or $Mg^{2+}$ is present at a 1 to 5 mM concentration. This is not directly relevant to human urine but does support Robertson's conjecture in a general way. On the other hand, we observed no reduction of urinary crystal growth inhibition in patients with hyperuricosuria.[70] Grover and co-workers[264] showed urate promotes crystallization of calcium oxalate independently of the presence of urinary macromolecules and proposed that urate "salts out" calcium oxalate from urine.[265]

## TREATMENT

Reduction of new stone formation during allopurinol administration is the most compelling evidence for a role of hyperuricosuria in calcium oxalate stone disease. Our treatment studies[38, 67, 266] rely on a comparison of stone production before and during treatment. Allopurinol reduced new

stones from the predicted 124.8 (Table 40–17 and Fig. 40–11) to 8. Dual treatment with thiazide and allopurinol was equally effective for patients with idiopathic hypercalciuria as well as hyperuricosuria (see Table 40–17).

Smith[267] has performed a prospective drug trial comparing allopurinol with placebo in treatment of calcium stone formers with a serum urate level above 6 mg/dL. The rationale for selecting patients was not clear because hyperuricemia by itself has no obvious pertinence to calcium renal stones. Still, there was a dramatic drug effect to 5 years of follow-up. The definitive study was performed by Ettinger and colleagues[268] in a randomized double-blind trial of allopurinol therapy in hyperuricosuric, normocalciuric calcium oxalate stone formers. There was a significant reduction in calculous events in the group receiving allopurinol, 0.26 stones per patient per year in the placebo group versus 0.12 in the allopurinol group. Actuarial analysis showed the allopurinol-treated patients to have a significantly longer time before stone recurrence (Fig. 40–12). The mechanism of allopurinol therapy must be due to decreased urate excretion because it has been shown that allopurinol or oxypurinol has no effect on growth or nucleation of calcium oxalate.[269]

It would seem that diet alone, that is, simple reduction of purine intake to a normal level, could be an ideal treatment for the majority of patients, but no published data support or deny this hypothesis. Changing a habit is difficult, especially when the change is quantitative and not the mere omission of a food category. Whether diet modification is a practical treatment, that is, one that can be accomplished, remains to be seen.

An alternative therapy was described by Pak and Peterson,[270] who have demonstrated reduced stone recurrence rates in hyperuricosuric stone formers treated with potassium citrate. The increased citrate lowers calcium oxalate supersaturation and may inhibit urate-induced crystallization of calcium oxalate.[271]

## Renal Tubular Acidosis

Type I, classic distal RTA, either the hereditary variety or that occurring sporadically without associated systemic

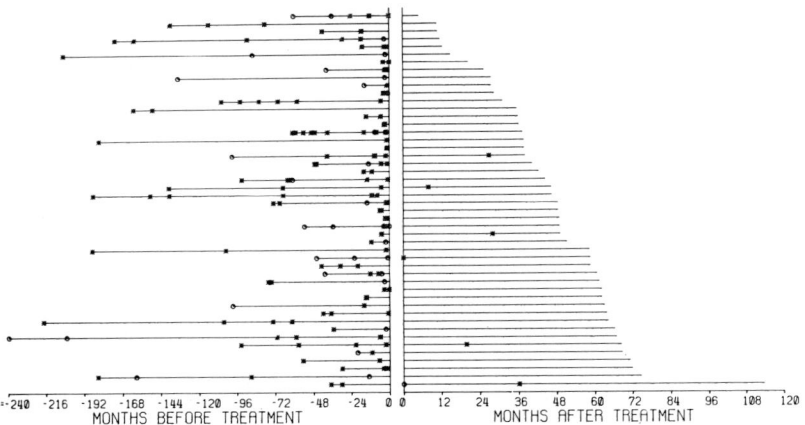

**Figure 40–11.** Calcium stone formation before and during treatment with allopurinol in 48 patients with hyperuricosuria. Each patient is represented by a horizontal line; new stones are represented by solid symbols and multiple stones by open symbols. (From Coe FL: Treated and untreated recurrent calcium nephrolithiasis in patients with idiopathic hypercalciuria, hyperuricosuria or no metabolic disorder. Ann Intern Med 87:404, 1977.)

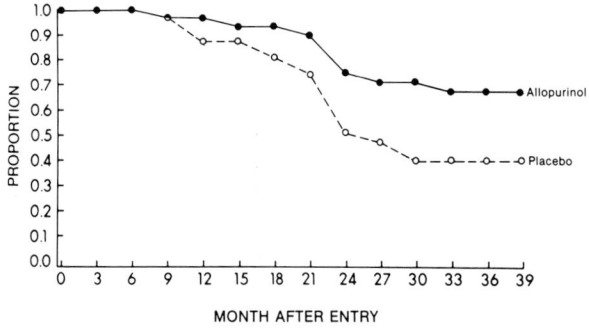

**Figure 40–12.** Life table plot showing proportion of patients without calculous events during treatment with allopurinol or placebo. (From Ethinger B, Tang A, Citron JT, et al: Randomized trial of allopurinol in the prevention of calcium oxalate calculi. Reprinted with permission from the New England Journal of Medicine, vol 315, pages 1386–1389, 1986.)

disease, is a cause of nephrocalcinosis and renal stone formation (see Chapter 22). When acquired because of another genetically transmitted disease, an autoimmune disorder, a primary renal disease, or a drug- or toxin-induced nephropathy, distal RTA usually does not cause stones, nor does proximal RTA (type II) or any other form of renal acidosis associated with renal disease. Stones can occur in the complete form of distal RTA with systemic acidosis or in the incomplete form, which expresses deficient renal acidification with acid loading. Stones in RTA result from hypercalciuria, hypocitraturia, and alkaline urine pH. Stones are most often calcium phosphate,[272] although one survey reported a high frequency of calcium oxalate and struvite stones as well as calcium phosphate stones.[273]

## HYPERCALCIURIA

In contrast to the situation in idiopathic hypercalciuria, intestinal $Ca^{2+}$ absorption is not elevated. It is normal or low[274–282] (Table 40–18), and bone mineral is lost into the urine. Metabolic acidosis, a result of the renal acidification defect that gives rise to the disease, causes the hypercalciuria. Normal people become hypercalciuric if an exogenous acid load, sufficient to produce metabolic acidosis, is administered for at least 7 days.[283] Net intestinal $Ca^{2+}$ absorption does not increase enough to balance urinary losses, and $Ca^{2+}$ balance becomes negative.[284] The surplus urinary $Ca^{2+}$ arises from bone, as in distal RTA. Alkali therapy at a dose that reverses acidosis reduces urinary $Ca^{2+}$ excretion in patients with RTA[285, 286] and improves $Ca^{2+}$ balance in some but not all cases (see Table 40–18); if alkali is discontinued, acidosis and hypercalciuria recur. Intestinal $Ca^{2+}$ absorption is low in these patients and inadequate to compensate for renal $Ca^{2+}$ losses. Preminger and colleagues[287] showed low intestinal $Ca^{2+}$ absorption in a group of patients with incomplete distal RTA that improved with citrate treatment. The changes in $Ca^{2+}$ absorption were independent of vitamin D.

Hypercalciuria is not always secondary to systemic acidosis in RTA. Hypercalciuria may predate RTA, apparently causing renal tubule damage through nephrocalcinosis. This has been shown in some families with hereditary distal RTA, in which there is also an autosomal dominant inheritance of hypercalciuria.[288]

## MECHANISM OF STONE FORMATION

Hypercalciuria and elevated urinary phosphorus excretion both tend to raise urine saturation with respect to calcium phosphate, but alkaline urine pH is more important than either one.[289] High pH increases the availability of $PO_4^{3-}$ and $HPO_4^{2-}$, which are incorporated into octocalcium phosphate and brushite, respectively. Urinary citrate excretion is reduced by metabolic acidosis, hypokalemia, and renal insufficiency.[290] The cause of low urinary citrate in incomplete RTA is unclear, but it has been suggested that there is a proximal tubule cell intracellular acidosis stimulating citrate use.[291] Reduction of urinary $Ca^{2+}$ binding by citrate raises urine supersaturation with calcium phosphate and calcium oxalate.

Alkali administration is said to reduce stone formation and slow the progress of nephrocalcinosis,[285, 292, 293] but details of the natural history of stones and nephrocalcinosis during treatment are not widely available. Nash and co-workers[285] found stable nephrocalcinosis in four patients. Perhaps the longest cohesive series of treated patients with nephrolithiasis due to hereditary distal RTA is one that describes six patients treated for 7 to 19 years.[272] During 43 patient-years of alkali treatment, only two new stones were formed, one by each of two patients, whereas the pretreatment stone recurrence rate for the group was 96 stones/100 patient-years. Nephrocalcinosis was present in three of the six patients; it lessened in one and remained unchanged in the other two.[272] A later study of nine patients with RTA showed no new stone formation during 3 years of potassium citrate therapy despite a pretreatment stone formation rate of 13 per patient per year.[293] Calcium oxalate supersaturation fell significantly during therapy, but there was not a significant fall in brushite supersaturation because the increase in citrate and decrease in $Ca^{2+}$ excretion were offset by the increase in urine pH.[293] Renal function tends to stabilize and linear skeletal growth in children tends to resume during alkali therapy.[294]

## Hypocitraturia

Hypocitraturia is found in 15% to 60% of stone formers.[72–76] It may occur as an isolated abnormality or be associated with some other stone-forming risk, such as hypercalciuria. Low urinary citrate levels are invariably found in distal RTA (see earlier), chronic diarrheal states, and diuretic-induced hypokalemia, or they may be found with no apparent cause (so-called idiopathic hypocitraturia).[24] One of the difficulties in determining the role of citrate in stone disease is that there is not a consensus as to what constitutes normal citrate levels. Some groups report differences in normal subjects related to age and sex,[73, 295–297] whereas others have not found such differences.[74, 75, 298, 299] The reason for these discrepancies in urinary citrate values is unclear.

**TABLE 40–18. Effect of Distal Renal Tubular Acidosis (Type I) or Experimental Acid Loading on Calcium Balance**

| Reference | Subject (Age and Sex) and Therapy | Calcium (mg/24 h) | | | | |
|---|---|---|---|---|---|---|
| | | Intake | Urine | Fecal | Net Absorption | Balance |
| Albright et al.[274] | 13, female | 80 | 163 | 137 | −57 | −220 |
| | | 530 | 125 | 460 | 70 | −600 |
| Baines et al.[275] | 29, female | 457 | 277 | 523 | −76 | −353 |
| Albright et al.[276] | 40, female | 76 | 264 | 39 | 37 | −227 |
| | Akali therapy | 604 | 475 | 174 | 430 | −45 |
| Pines and Mudge[277] | 28, female | 562 | 215 | 189 | 373 | 158 |
| | Akali therapy | 515 | 105 | 376 | 139 | 34 |
| | 28, female | 208 | 218 | 175 | 33 | −185 |
| | Akali therapy | 208 | 144 | 227 | −19 | −163 |
| Bauld et al.[278] | 29, female | 260 | 120 | 240 | 20 | −100 |
| | Akali therapy | 260 | 70 | 240 | 20 | −50 |
| Greenberg et al.[279] | 4, male | 743 | 123 | 640 | 103 | −20 |
| | Akali therapy | 760 | 26 | 406 | 354 | 327 |
| Wallach et al.[280] | 32, female | 458 | 138 | 434 | 24 | −114 |
| Weber et al.[281] | Normal subjects* | 1204† | 216 | 638 | 388 | 176 |
| | 18 days of acid loading‡ | 1000 | 580 | 480 | 520 | −72 |
| Lemann et al.[282] | Normal subjects§ | 1760‖ | 320 | 1520 | 240 | −80 |
| | 12–18 days of acid loading‡ | 1764 | 1016 | 1452 | 312 | −704 |

\* Three men and three women.
† Mean of six values.
‡ Acid loading was in the form of $NH_4Cl$.
§ Five men.
‖ Mean of five values.

## RENAL EXCRETION OF CITRATE

Citrate is freely filtered at the glomerulus, and 65% to 90% is reabsorbed in the proximal tubule.[290] It is a component of the tricarboxylic acid cycle, and the majority of citrate reabsorbed by the kidney is used in oxidative metabolism. Because the tubule does not secrete citrate, the final urinary excretion of citrate is determined by reabsorption in the proximal tubule. The most important regulator of citrate reabsorption is systemic acid-base status. Alkalosis increases and acidosis decreases renal citrate excretion.[290] In acidosis, there is increased citrate use by the mitochondria resulting in lower intracellular levels of citrate, which facilitates citrate reabsorption. Also, lower tubule fluid pH in acidosis converts more $citrate^{3-}$ to $citrate^{2-}$, which is the ionic species that is actively transported.[300] Hypokalemia also reduces urinary citrate, presumably by generating an intracellular acidosis in the proximal tubule cell.[301] Hypokalemia may prevent the increase in urinary citrate seen with alkalosis.[301]

## MECHANISM OF STONE FORMATION

Citrate binds $Ca^{2+}$ in the urine, reducing $Ca^{2+}$ activity and resulting in lower supersaturation of calcium salts.[24] Therefore, lowering urinary citrate levels is equivalent to increasing urinary $Ca^{2+}$ levels in producing supersaturation, the driving force of crystallization. Citrate also has direct effects on the crystallization of calcium salts, in addition to changes in supersaturation. Citrate has been found to have mild calcium oxalate crystal growth inhibition when correction is made for the changes in supersaturation.[302, 303] There are conflicting results concerning the effect of citrate on aggregation. Kok and colleagues[304] showed aggregation in-

hibition by citrate using an assay that measured growth and aggregation. Robertson and Scurr,[302] using a continuous crystallizer, showed minimal effects on aggregation by citrate, and Hess and co-workers[61] showed no aggregation inhibition by citrate using an assay that was at the calcium oxalate saturation point so crystal growth could not be a confounding factor. In total, citrate has a significant effect on calcium crystal formation, mainly by lowering supersaturation, and low levels of citrate in urine increase the risk of stone formation.

## TREATMENT

The basis of therapy for hypocitraturia is correction of any underlying disorder, such as acidosis or hypokalemia, that reduces urinary citrate or, if the patient has idiopathic hypocitraturia, induction of a mild metabolic alkalosis to increase urinary citrate levels. Any alkali supplement will raise urinary citrate levels. However, sodium alkali will increase urinary $Ca^{2+}$ excretion, which offsets the benefits of increased urinary citrate.[305] Either potassium bicarbonate or potassium citrate may be used. Citrate requires less frequent dosing because it is metabolized to bicarbonate in the liver.

Citrate is the most frequently used alkali for hypocitraturic patients. There are no double-blind, randomized studies documenting the efficacy of potassium citrate, but many studies show a reduction in stone formation rate after treatment with citrate. Pak and Fuller[306] treated 37 stone formers with idiopathic hypocitraturia with potassium citrate. Twelve of the 37 were also treated with allopurinol or thiazides for associated hyperuricosuria or hypercalciuria, respectively. They were able to show persistent improve-

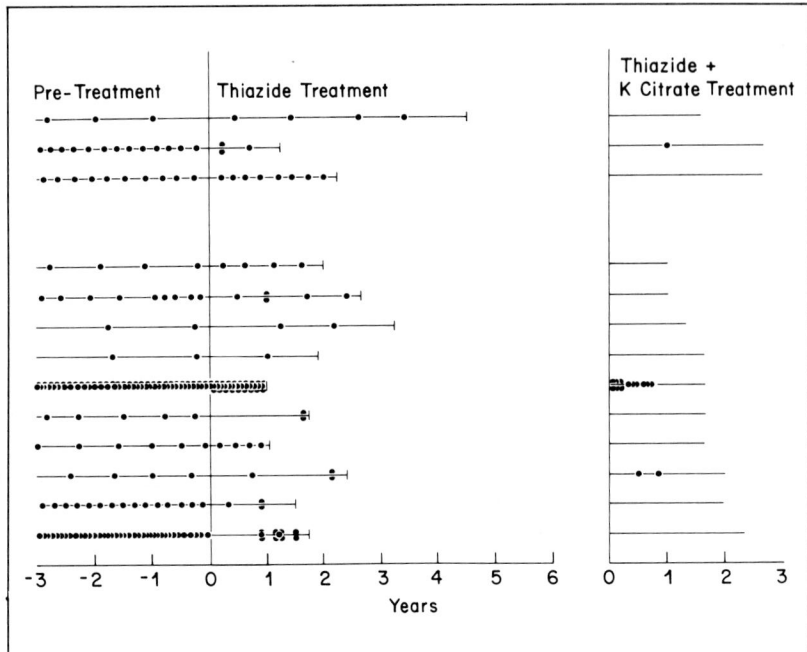

**Figure 40–13.** Effect of thiazide treatment and thiazide and potassium citrate treatment on new stone formation. Each patient is represented by a horizontal line, and each point indicates new stone formation. Combined thiazide and potassium citrate treatment was begun immediately after thiazide treatment. (From Pak CYC, Peterson R, Sakhaee K, et al: Correction of hypocitraturia and prevention of stone formation by combined thiazide and potassium citrate therapy in thiazide-unresponsive hypercalciuric nephrolithiasis. Am J Med 79:284–288, 1985.)

ment in urinary citrate levels during 2 years of follow-up as well as reduction in calcium oxalate supersaturation. Stone formation rate decreased from 2.11 ± 5.68 to 0.28 ± 1.3 with treatment. Pak and co-workers[307] also studied a group of 13 patients with idiopathic hypercalciuria and hypocitraturia who had failed to respond to thiazide treatment. Pretreatment stone formation rate was 4.69 ± 6.62 per patient-year and did not change with thiazide therapy (5.12 ± 10.87). When potassium citrate was added, stone formation rate fell to 0.57 ± 1.65 (Fig. 40–13). This study strongly supports the efficacy of citrate in calcium stone disease because it is not confounded by "the stone clinic effect," which is the tendency for stone formation rate to decrease after a visit to the stone center, regardless of treatment. These patients should have experienced any benefit of the stone clinic effect at the time they began use of thiazide.

We await a proper trial of citrate therapy, but at present, this therapy seems effective.

## Idiopathic Calcium Lithiasis

Despite a thorough evaluation, a remediable cause of stones will not be found in some patients. By definition, these patients are normocalciuric and free of identifiable metabolic abnormalities. For these patients, selective treatment cannot be fashioned. Hydration, a restriction of dietary calcium intake, and avoidance of foods that contain excessive oxalate are prudent measures but have limited effectiveness (Table 40–19). Ettinger[308] and Coe and Parks[309] have observed recurrence of stones in more than half of patients during 2 to 3 years of treatment with diet

**TABLE 40–19. Diet and Hydration and Orthophosphate Therapy for Idiopathic Calcium Stone Disease**

| Treatment | Patients Stone Free at Time of Follow-up* | | | | |
|---|---|---|---|---|---|
| | *6 Months* | *1 Year* | *2 Years* | *3 Years* | *4 Years* |
| Diet and hydration | | | | | |
| Coe and Parks[253] | 79 (34) | 71 (34) | 43 (28) | 47 (15) | 46 (13) |
| Ettinger[308] | 85 (26) | 77 (26) | 66 (15) | 46 (13) | — |
| Orthophosphate | | | | | |
| Ettinger[308] | 72 (25) | 63 (24) | 52 (23) | 53 (19) | — |
| Ettinger and Kolb[312] | 89 (47) | — | 74 (47) | — | 76 (37) |
| Smith et al.[310] | — | — | — | 91 (150) | — |
| Bernstein and Newton[313] | 78 (9) | 83 (6) | 83 (6) | — | — |

*Numbers represent the percentage of patients to be stone free on follow-up in each study; numbers of patients at the end of each follow-up interval are shown in parentheses.

and hydration. Pharmacologic therapy to further reduce urine supersaturation may be useful if hydration and diet fail to control stone formation.

## ORTHOPHOSPHATE

The rationale for using orthophosphate is that urinary $Ca^{2+}$ excretion may be reduced, by unknown mechanisms, and urinary excretion of inorganic pyrophosphate increases.[310] Supersaturation with respect to calcium oxalate is reduced.[311] Ettinger and Kolb[312] treated 47 patients who had idiopathic hypercalciuria with potassium acid phosphate (1 g of inorganic phosphorus daily) for up to 4 years (see Table 40–19). Stone formation rate and urinary $Ca^{2+}$ excretion did not fall below pretreatment values. A greater fraction of patients was stone free at 2 and 4 years of treatment than among patients treated by diet and hydration. Subsequently, Ettinger[308] compared acid phosphate, at a dose that provided 1 g of phosphorus daily, with placebo. The drug did not reduce new stone formation, and recurrence rates were above those observed during diet treatment (see Table 40–19). Smith and colleagues[310] treated idiopathic stone formers with twice the dose of orthophosphate daily and achieved a better result. In their report, data are presented for the population when the average treatment interval was 3 years (see Table 40–19) but not at the end of each year of the study. Urinary $Ca^{2+}$ excretion fell. Bernstein and Newton[313] reported a small sodium phosphate study involving patients with idiopathic hypercalciuria; their results were comparable to those of Smith (see Table 40–19).

Overall, the effectiveness of orthophosphate is uncertain. Ettinger[308] and Ettinger and Kolb[312] observed no therapeutic effect in two studies, one of which was placebo controlled. However, the dose they employed was only half as large as that used by Smith and colleagues[310] in their more encouraging study. Furthermore, Ettinger used acid phosphate, whereas Smith used neutral phosphate. Lau and associates[314] have shown that acid phosphate administration leads to higher levels of urinary $Ca^{2+}$ and lower levels of urinary citrate than does neutral phosphate. Therefore, it would not be expected to reduce urine supersaturation with respect to calcium oxalate as much as neutral phosphate does and might be ineffective in preventing calcium renal stones.

Orthophosphate is not always tolerated well. The drug is a cathartic. Symptoms range from mild abdominal discomfort to persistent diarrhea. With time, intestinal side effects may wane, and patients may adapt. If the drug is begun at half the full dose, symptoms are less prominent, and acceptance may be better.

There is also the problem of secondary hyperparathyroidism. Oral phosphate administration to normal people and patients with idiopathic hypercalciuria causes a prompt, transient rise in serum PTH and a decline in serum $1,25(OH)_2D_3$.[315, 316] Serum $PO_4^{3-}$ concentration rises, and $Ca^{2+}$ level falls. During long-term phosphate administration, serum $PO_4^{3-}$ level, measured in the postabsorptive state, is normal or low,[191, 220, 221] and serum PTH is normal.[312] Each dose of phosphate may, however, provoke transient release of PTH, as in the acute experiment of Reiss and colleagues.[315] Whether eventual parathyroid hyperpla-

sia results from cyclic stimulation is unknown, but in the rabbit, parathyroid bone disease can be produced by prolonged renal $PO_4^{3-}$ loading.[317]

## LOW-CALCIUM DIET

In the course of their studies of phosphorus treatment, Ettinger and Kolb[308, 312] obtained valuable information about the effects of a low-calcium diet. They treated 46 patients with a low-calcium diet and observed them for 6 years. During the first 3-year period, these patients were the control group for 25 additional patients treated with acid phosphate as well as low-calcium diet. During the first 3-year interval, they formed 43 new stones in 131 patient-years (33 stones/100 patients per year). Before treatment, they formed 164 stones in 243 patient-years (57 stones/100 patients per year). If their pretreatment stone recurrence rate had persisted during treatment, they should have formed 86.2 rather than 43 stones ($P < .001$). A low-calcium diet did appear to reduce stone recurrence, and acid phosphate appeared to offset the beneficial effects of the diet.

In the second 3-year period,[234] they discontinued acid phosphate treatment so that both groups of patients received low-calcium diet alone. The group that had previously had only diet therapy formed 35 stones in 130 patient-years (27 stones/100 patients per year), a rate that did not differ from that observed during the first 3-year period. When treated with diet alone, the patients who had received phosphate as well as diet formed 21 recurrent stones in 86 patient-years (24 stones/100 patients per year), a rate much below that observed while they received acid phosphate but virtually identical to that of the patients who had always been treated with diet alone. Of interest, Ettinger[234] calculated the average stone recurrence rate for both groups of patients during the two 3-year periods of observation, found a higher rate during the first 3-year period than during the second, and concluded that stone disease tends to wane with time. The higher rate during the first 3-year period derived, of course, from the high rate among acid phosphate–treated patients; among patients who received only a low-calcium diet throughout the 6-year period, the stone recurrence rate remained amazingly constant.

## THIAZIDE AND ALLOPURINOL

Because our experience with hydration and diet therapy was not encouraging (see Table 40–19), we treated 30 idiopathic stone formers with this combination of drugs to lower the calcium oxalate activity product and reduce the availability of heterogeneous nuclei. The results were only mildly encouraging[189, 309] (Fig. 40–14). More of the patients remained stone free compared with the 34 patients who were treated with diet and hydration (see Table 40–19), but the therapeutic response was much less evident than we observed when treating hypercalciuric and hyperuricosuric patients with the same drugs.[67] Either drug may have been sufficient to produce the modest decrease in new stone production, especially thiazide, which by itself appeared to reduce stone recurrence in idiopathic stone formers studied by Yendt.[68]

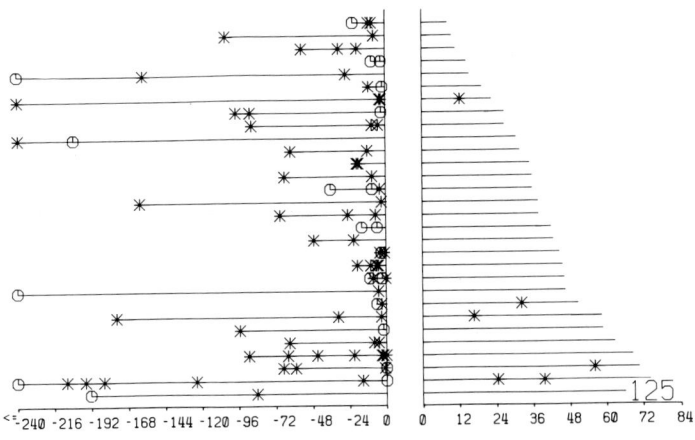

MONTHS BEFORE TREATMENT          MONTHS AFTER TREATMENT

**Figure 40–14.** Course of calcium stone disease in 30 patients with no metabolic disorder before and during combined thiazide and allopurinol administration. Symbols are as in Figure 40–11. (From Coe FL: Treated and untreated recurrent calcium nephrolithiasis in patients with idiopathic hypercalciuria, hyperuricosuria or no metabolic disorder. Ann Intern Med 87:404, 1977.)

## Hyperoxaluria

Even though oxalate occurs in most kidney stones, most stone formers excrete no more oxalate than do normal people. Excessive urinary oxalate excretion does occur in some people and causes stones by raising the saturation of the urine with respect to calcium oxalate.[29, 318] When severe, hyperoxaluria damages the kidneys. Nephrocalcinosis, tubulointerstitial nephritis, functional defects of the renal tubule, azotemia, and frank renal failure all have been reported.

### PRODUCTION OF OXALATE

Because humans cannot metabolize oxalate, renal excretion is the sole route of oxalate elimination. Urinary oxalate excretion decreases with deterioration of renal function, and calcium oxalate crystals may be deposited in the cardiac conduction system, renal parenchyma, joint spaces, blood vessel walls, bone, and elsewhere. The renal handling of oxalate is incompletely understood; it is freely filtered at the glomerulus, but there are conflicting results as to whether there is net secretion or reabsorption in the tubule.[319–322]

Oxalate is an end product of several metabolic pathways; the amount of oxalate in the urine reflects the sum total of intestinal absorption plus de novo synthesis. Hyperoxaluria may result from increased rates of oxalate production or intestinal hyperabsorption, and these processes serve as a useful basis for classification of both hereditary and acquired hyperoxaluric states (Table 40–20). The two main pathways for oxalate synthesis are from ascorbic acid and glyoxylate. The oxidation of ascorbic acid contributes about 35% of total oxalate production. Oral administration of large doses of ascorbic acid (4 g) increases urinary oxalate in some but not all subjects, which suggests that enzyme activity must be near maximum under usual conditions.[323] The significance of this finding has been questioned because ascorbic acid can be nonenzymatically converted to oxalate in alkaline urine.[324] However, a study in which urine was collected directly from nephrostomy tubes showed increased oxalate excretion when the subjects were given

greater than 1000 mg of ascorbic acid.[325] Thus, it appears that the ascorbic acid oxidation pathway usually plays little or no role in causing hyperoxaluria but may in people taking an excessive ascorbate load.

The oxidation of glyoxylate to oxalate represents the major source of oxalate production in humans.[323, 326] Several enzymes catalyze the irreversible oxidation reaction in vitro, but lactate dehydrogenase is probably responsible for most oxalate production (Fig. 40–15, steps I and II). Oxalate production can be further enhanced by the reoxidation of NADH to NAD by pyruvate or hydroxypyruvate. Glyoxylate is synthesized either from glycine by glycine oxidase (step IIIa) or from the oxidation of glycolate (step II). Glycine, in turn, arises from serine through ethanolamine and glycolaldehyde. Glyoxylate may be converted to glycine by a pyridoxine-dependent transaminase (step IIIb) or to α-hydroxy-β-keto-adipic acid by a thiamine-dependent carboligase that decarboxylates glyoxylate and α-ketoglutarate (step IV). Thiamine deficiency would be expected to cause hyperoxaluria; however, urinary oxalate levels are normal in thiamine-deficient humans.

### OVERPRODUCTION HYPEROXALURIA

Alterations in several of the steps of oxalate synthesis have been implicated in the overproduction hyperoxaluric

---

**TABLE 40–20. Classification of Hyperoxaluria**

Metabolic overproduction of oxalate
  Hereditary (types 1 and 2)
  Pyridoxine deficiency*
  Ethylene glycol ingestion
  Methoxyflurane anesthesia
Gastrointestinal overabsorption of oxalate
  Oxalate overingestion
  Ileal resection
  Celiac sprue
  Pancreatic insufficiency
  Small bowel bypass surgery
  Crohn disease
  Cellulose phosphate ingestion

---

*Occurs in experimental animals; not of proven clinical significance.

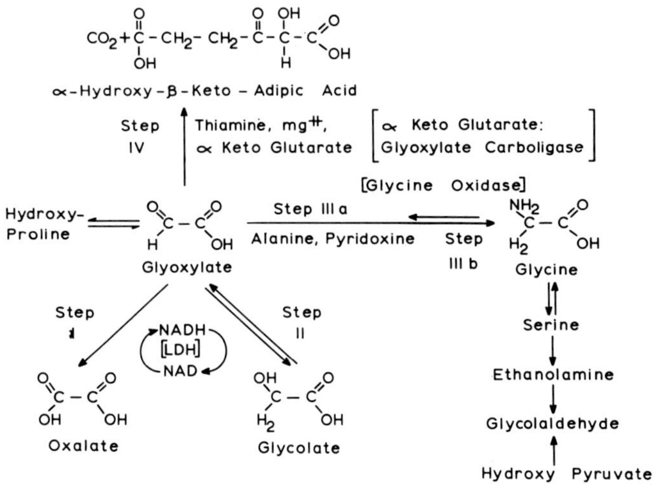

**Figure 40–15.** Glyoxylate production and metabolism and formation of oxalate. Steps I through IV are explained in the text. (From Coe FL: Nephrolithiasis: Pathogenesis and Treatment. Year Book Medical Publishers, Chicago, 1978, p 147.)

states. A deficiency in the activity of the peroxisomal enzyme alanine:glyoxylate aminotransferase (AGT) is responsible for hereditary hyperoxaluria type 1.[327] This enzyme converts glyoxylate to glycine; a reduction in activity allows more glyoxylate to be converted to oxalate in the cell cytosol. Type 1 primary hyperoxaluria is a heterogeneous disorder with multiple mechanisms for deficient enzyme activity. Sixty percent of patients completely lack hepatic enzyme activity, and most of these patients have no AGT immunoreactivity as shown by liver biopsy, although a small number have detectable amounts of peroxisome AGT that is inactive.[328] The other 40% have detectable levels of AGT activity, in the range of 3% to 48% of normal, but immunochemical localization shows AGT to be located in the mitochondria rather than the peroxisome.[329] This unusual error of enzyme trafficking places the AGT in an environment where the enzyme functions poorly. The disease is probably inherited as an autosomal recessive trait. Hyperoxaluria type 2 is due to a deficiency of D-glyceric dehydrogenase.[330] The defect leads to high levels of hydroxypyruvate, which is converted to L-glyceric acid. The reaction, catalyzed by lactate dehydrogenase, also generates NAD from NADH, making more NAD available for lactate dehydrogenase–driven oxidation of glyoxylate to oxalate (step 1). Low levels of glyoxylate reductase in addition to D-glyceric dehydrogenase have been found in one patient with type 2 hyperoxaluria.[331]

Urinary oxalate excretion is usually 150 to 300 mg/d in both disorders and declines as renal failure ensues. Both disorders may produce recurrent calcium oxalate calculi, progressive renal failure, and oxalosis, beginning as early as in childhood. Patients with type 1 disease overexcrete glyoxylate and glycolate as well as oxalate; those with type 2 disease overexcrete L-glyceric acid and oxalate.[332, 333] Once renal failure has developed, the diagnosis can be suspected from the history and evidence of systemic oxalosis. Liver biopsy for measurement of enzyme activity can make the diagnosis even in the presence of renal failure.[334]

Pyridoxine at dosages of 25 to 1000 mg/d reduces oxalate excretion in some patients with type 1 hyperoxaluria.[335] The patients who respond to pyridoxine will have some residual AGT activity in liver biopsy samples.[328] In the rat,

pyridoxine deficiency is associated with hyperoxaluria by virtue of the reduced transamination of glyoxylate to glycine, which makes more glyoxylate available for oxidation to oxalate. Pyridoxine deficiency in humans has not been associated with hyperoxaluria and stone formation, but subtle deficiencies in pyridoxine could contribute to some hyperoxaluric conditions. Neutral orthophosphate and magnesium supplements have been used with success,[336, 337] although no controlled trials exist. Potassium citrate was shown to reduce calcium oxalate supersaturation and stone formation rate in children with primary hyperoxaluria.[338]

Acquired overproduction of oxalate follows the ingestion of ethylene glycol, which is metabolized through glycolaldehyde to glycolate. The anesthetic methoxyflurane is converted to ethanolamine and then to oxalate. Nephrotoxic effects resulting from ethylene glycol and methoxyflurane are discussed in Chapter 22.

## GASTROINTESTINAL OVERABSORPTION OF OXALATE

Dietary intake of oxalate varies from 400 to 900 mg/d and largely depends on the consumption of green leafy vegetables. Hyperoxaluria due to excessive consumption of an oxalate-rich diet is rare and has been described as "rhubarb poisoning."[332]

Fractional absorption of oxalate is low, in the range of 2.0% to 4.5%.[339, 340] In rats, oxalate is absorbed by a nonsaturable, energy-independent process in duodenum, jejunum, ileum, and colon.[341] Experiments in monkeys and humans with ileostomies suggest that the colon is a major site of oxalate absorption.[342, 343] In the intestinal lumen, oxalate forms insoluble calcium salts that are unavailable for absorption. Dietary calcium restriction or cellulose phosphate administration increases oxalate absorption.[238] Calcium carbonate loading decreases oxalate excretion, probably by diminishing intestinal oxalate absorption.[344] Excessive luminal concentrations of bile salts and long-chain fatty acids also enhance oxalate absorption[345] by increasing the permeability of colon epithelium to oxalate.[346]

Several gastrointestinal disorders are associated with overabsorption of oxalate and consequent hyperoxaluria.[347, 348]

Hyperoxaluria with or without calcium oxalate calculi may complicate Crohn disease, celiac sprue, pancreatic insufficiency, and small intestinal bypass surgery for obesity.[349–351] Dietary fat malabsorption with steatorrhea is common to all conditions, and increased luminal free fatty acids may be critical in the development of oxalate overabsorption. There is a positive correlation between fecal fat and hyperoxaluria,[340, 352] whereas patients with jejunocolonic and jejunoileal bypass—procedures that virtually exclude the small intestine—absorb considerable oxalate from the colon. Therapy for "enteric hyperoxaluria" includes the control of steatorrhea by dietary restriction of fat, the reduction of oxalate intake, and the use of cholestyramine (a nonabsorbable anion exchange resin that binds oxalate in the bowel lumen). Restoration of small bowel continuity should be seriously considered if hyperoxaluria produces clinical manifestations in patients with intestinal bypass. Oral calcium carbonate, 1 to 4 g daily, may be useful in some patients.[344] In general, a low-fat, low-oxalate diet should be used first, followed by oral calcium carbonate or cholestyramine if diet is unsuccessful.

# URIC ACID STONES

Uric acid crystal formation in the urinary tract may manifest itself as crystalluria, stones, or obstruction. In addition, uric acid and its salt, sodium hydrogen urate, may produce intrarenal disease by initiating an inflammatory response to interstitial deposition as a consequence of hyperuricemia. Crystalluria often occurs in uric acid stone formers and is accompanied by dysuria and hematuria. It may occur in the absence of hyperuricemia or hyperuricosuria, and crystals may be present in the urine of normal subjects whenever urine pH is low.

## Natural History

### OCCURRENCE

Uric acid stones account for 5% to 10% of all renal stones in the United States, but this figure varies in other parts of the globe. Similar figures are found in Great Britain, and a slightly higher frequency occurs in Germany and France; the highest frequency is reported from Israel, where 75% of stones were of uric acid composition.[353]

### RELATIONSHIP TO GOUT

Uric acid stones are more frequent among gouty patients, and stone formation often develops before articular symptoms.[354] The chance of stone formation increases with increasing serum urate levels and urinary excretion rates. In one series, 35% of gouty patients with urinary uric acid levels of 700 to 1100 mg/24 h had stones.[355] In a retrospective analysis of patients' records, the incidence rate of stones for a patient with newly diagnosed gout was 1 per 114 patients per year.[356]

## Pathogenesis

Urine oversaturation with uric acid, and subsequent crystal formation, is determined largely by urine pH. Uric acid is a weak acid with two dissociable $H^+$ ions having pK values of 5.345[260] and 10. In biologic systems, only the first $H^+$ can be dissociated, so when we refer to the salt of uric acid as urate, we mean monohydrogen sodium urate. Urate is more soluble than is uric acid, and urate stones are rare, so that urine oversaturation is important only with respect to undissociated uric acid.

### EFFECTS OF URINE pH

Urine pH changes have a greater impact on uric acid stone formation than does a change in the amount of uric acid excreted. Urinary uric acid excretion may increase only twofold to threefold, up to 1500 mg/24 h, whereas a pH change between 5 and 6 alters the undissociated acid concentration sixfold. Therefore, uric acid stone formation is conditioned more by pH than by daily urinary uric acid excretion or urine volume. Normal uric acid excretion by adults is 500 to 600 mg/24 h in 1.0 to 1.5 L, or 330 to 600 mg/L. So at low urine pH, below 6.2, oversaturation (greater than 96 mg/L of free uric acid[260]) may occur even in normal subjects. The formation of clinically significant crystalluria or stone requires persistent and severe oversaturation due to hyperuricosuria, dehydration, or a markedly acid urine. Fortunately, such conditions are transient in most people.

### FACTORS THAT INFLUENCE URINE pH

The pH of the urine is determined mainly by the quantity of titratable acid excreted and the amount of $PO_4^{3-}$ available to buffer it. Titratable acid depends on the load of $H^+$ generated by body metabolism and the rate of ammonia production; ammonia permits the excretion of $H^+$ at a high pH, because it is a base. Generally, $NH_4^+$ constitutes more than half the total daily acid excretion. Renal acidification and $NH_4^+$ production are discussed fully in Chapter 10. Uric acid stone formers tend to excrete less $NH_4^+$, which contributes directly to low urine pH.[354, 357] In addition, gouty subjects and stone formers in particular have a reduced postprandial alkaline tide (alkaline urine pH).[358] Morning urine pH is generally low in gouty patients who form uric acid stones.[357] Defective $NH_4^+$ production due to a disturbance in renal glutamine deamination has been proposed as the reason for low $NH_4^+$ excretion in uric acid stone formers,[359] but direct measurement of the enzyme has not substantiated this hypothesis. Dehydration, by reducing urine volume, increases urinary uric acid concentration and also promotes a fall in urine pH.

### URIC ACID EXCRETION RATE

About two thirds of the daily uric acid load is excreted by the kidneys, and one third is degraded by intestinal uricolysis.[360] Renal handling of uric acid is discussed in Chapter 15. Hyperuricosuric states may derive from defective renal tubule handling of uric acid, which lowers blood uric acid levels and decreases intestinal uricolysis. Diminished uric acid excretion results in hyperuricemia and increased bowel uricolysis.

Either increased dietary purine ingestion or endogenous uric acid overproduction may increase the amount of uric acid that must be excreted daily. Dietary purine is contained mainly in meat, fish, and poultry in the form of nucleoproteins that are degraded by intestinal and pancreatic enzymes. Normally, dietary purine contributes about 50% of urinary uric acid. A high purine intake, about 4 mg/kg/d, causes an elevation of uric acid excretion that is roughly proportional to the amount of surplus purine ingested. Purine nucleosides from dietary sources are split by nucleoside phosphorylase into free purine bases and ribose 1-phosphate. Guanine is deaminated to form xanthine, which, along with hypoxanthine, is subsequently oxidized to uric acid by the enzyme xanthine oxidase. Some patients with gout, probably a minority, produce excess uric acid during the course of endogenous purine metabolism and for this reason have hyperuricosuria. Rarely, massive uric acid overproduction from hereditary deficiencies of enzymes that are critical for purine reuse is a cause of stones. The Lesch-Nyhan syndrome is a well-known example (Table 40–21).

## Clinical Classification of Uric Acid Lithiasis

Uric acid stone-forming conditions include a variety of disorders involving disturbances in purine metabolism, renal urate handling, and urine pH. These pathophysiologic mechanisms interact in a complex fashion in each entity, and each also serves as a means of classifying this diverse group of disorders (see Table 40–21).

### IDIOPATHIC URIC ACID STONES

Both sporadic and familial forms of this disorder occur. The familial form is inherited as an autosomal dominant trait, and stones are formed at an earlier age than in the sporadic form and are more likely to cause obstruction and subsequent loss of renal function.[361] Men and women are affected equally, and an ethnic predilection (Jewish, Italian) has been suggested.[3] In the sporadic variety, stone formation or crystalluria usually begins in middle age, with recurrence predictable if the disorder is not treated. Serum and urinary uric acid levels are normal in both forms, and urine pH and urinary $NH_4^+$ excretion are low. The mechanism for stone formation is related to the low urine pH due to reduced $NH_4^+$ excretion; the cause of the reduced $NH_4^+$ excretion remains unknown.

### GOUT

Patients with primary gout may also have uric acid stones. As described earlier, the frequency of uric acid stones is about 22% overall and is directly related to the degree of uricosuria. The disease may be heterogeneous, because uric acid overexcretion persists despite low-purine diet in some 21% to 28% of gouty subjects. This may be due to overproduction of endogenous purine.[362] In addition, urine pH tends to be low, which suggests a defect in $NH_4^+$ production. The majority of subjects also have a defect in renal uric acid excretion such that hyperuricemia is required to excrete even normal amounts of uric acid. Uric acid overproduction is incompletely understood; however, certain enzyme deficiency states involving the purine pathway and resulting in hyperuricemia have been described. These enzyme defects are most clearly expressed when they occur in infants and children with gout and uric acid stones and include the following: deficiency of hypoxanthine-guanine phosphoribosyltransferase (Lesch-Nyhan syndrome), adenine phosphoribosyltransferase deficiency, increased ribose-phosphate pyrophosphokinase synthetase activity, decreased phosphoribosylpyrophosphate substrate use, and type I glycogen storage disease. It has been estimated that

**TABLE 40–21. Etiologic and Pathophysiologic Classification of Uric Acid Stones***

| Etiology | Urine pH | Urine NH₃ | Source of Surplus Urinary Uric Acid | Urine Volume |
|---|---|---|---|---|
| Idiopathic | | | | |
|   Sporadic | Low | Low | NI | N |
|   Familial | Low | Low | NI | N |
| Associated with hyperuricemia | | | | |
|   Primary gout | Low | Low | Overproduction | N |
|   Lesch-Nyhan syndrome | N | N | Overproduction | N |
|   Glycogen storage disease | N | N | Overproduction | N |
|   Other enzyme defects | N | N | Overproduction | N |
|   Myeloproliferative and other neoplastic disorders | N | N | Overproduction | N |
| Associated with hyperuricosuria | | | | |
|   Purine gluttony | N | N | Diet | N |
|   Defects in tubule reabsorption | N | N | Reduced intestinal uricolysis | N |
|   Uricosuric drugs | N | N | Reduced intestinal uricolysis | N |
| Dehydration | | | | |
|   Gastrointestinal diseases | Low | N | NI | Reduced |
|   Losses through the skin | Low | N | NI | Reduced |

*N = normal; NI = not increased.

such enzyme defects, albeit in less severe forms, may be involved in the pathogenesis of up to 11% of cases of gout.

## MALIGNANT DISEASE

Myeloproliferative disease and chronic granulocytic leukemia in adults and acute leukemia in childhood are the common neoplastic disorders that cause hyperuricosuria. Massive cell necrosis in response to chemotherapy abruptly increases urinary uric acid excretion, which may cause extensive precipitation and urinary tract obstruction. In the absence of chemotherapy, less marked uricosuria may cause uric acid stones.

## GASTROINTESTINAL DISEASES

Acute diarrheal states and chronic inflammatory bowel disease may increase urinary uric acid concentration through excessive water loss and dehydration. Urine pH tends to fall with extracellular volume contraction, increasing the possibility of stone formation.[363] Patients with ileostomy are particularly at risk, and associated small bowel disease (proximal ileum) may contribute to the lowered urine pH through significant $HCO_3^-$ loss.[364] Hyperoxaluria may also be present in patients with ileal resection, leading to mixed stones composed of both uric acid and calcium oxalate.[363]

## DRUG-INDUCED STONES

Probenecid and aspirin in large doses are both common uricosuric drugs. Hyperuricemic patients respond to these agents with a transient increase in uric acid excretion. Excretion then falls but remains higher than pretreatment levels owing to reduced intestinal uricolysis.[365] In patients with high dietary purine intake, the efficient excretion of uric acid induced by the drugs may increase the risk of uric acid stone formation or calcium oxalate stone formation.

# Treatment

## GENERAL MEASURES

The goals of therapy are regression in the size of preformed stones and prevention of new ones. These objectives can be achieved only by lowering urinary uric acid concentration below levels of saturation. A combination of reducing uric acid excretion, increasing urine volume, and increasing urine pH will be effective. The available therapeutic tools include fluids, alkali, diet, and allopurinol. Urine volume can be increased to about 2 L/d with minimal inconvenience.

## ALKALI AND DIET

Urine pH should be maintained within the range of 6.0 to 6.5. During the day, this can be achieved by ingestion of alkali, as either bicarbonate or citrate. Citrate may be preferred over bicarbonate because it requires less frequent dosing.[271] With either preparation, 0.5 to 1.5 mEq/kg/d in divided doses is effective. If nocturnal urine pH falls, a single dose of 250 mg of acetazolamide at bedtime usually maintains an alkaline urine. Dietary purine may be reduced to avoid periods of transient excessive uric acid excretion.

## ALLOPURINOL

Allopurinol (4-hydroxypyrazolo[3,4-*d*]pyrimidine) is an isomer of hypoxanthine and competes with this purine base as a substrate for xanthine oxidase, thus blocking the oxidation of xanthine or hypoxanthine to uric acid. Also, the drug lowers overall purine synthesis by decreasing the availability of phosphoribosylpyrophosphate and by inhibiting the enzyme phosphoribosylpyrophosphate amidotransferase.[366] Allopurinol is converted to a biologically active metabolite, oxypurinol, which has a long half-life (18 to 30 hours) compared with that of the parent compound (60 to 90 minutes). Oxypurinol is, itself, soluble only to the extent of 350 mg/L. A single case report describes the formation of oxypurinol stones in a woman with regional enteritis and an ileostomy who was treated with a large dose of allopurinol (600 mg/d).[367]

Allopurinol should be used if stones recur despite fluid and alkali or when uric acid excretion is above 1000 mg/d. Allopurinol is also indicated in the dissolution or reduction in size of existing stones and when large, nonobstructing renal pelvic stones are too large to pass. If given before chemotherapy for myeloproliferative or lymphoproliferative malignant disease, allopurinol prevents widespread uric acid precipitation. When allopurinol is used for treatment of patients with massive uric acid overproduction, excellent hydration must be maintained. Xanthine kidney stone formation and acute renal failure from intrarenal xanthine crystal deposition have been described in patients with overproduction of uric acid.[368, 369]

# CYSTINURIA

Cystinuria (see also Chapter 37) is a rare hereditary disorder of amino acid transport involving the intestinal epithelia and renal tubule cells. As a result of renal tubule transport disorders, abnormally large amounts of cystine are excreted in the urine. The solubility of cystine in urine is approximately 300 mg/L. When overexcretion leads to higher concentrations than the solubility limit, cystine stones tend to form. The inheritance of cystinuria is complex; it results from allelic mutations and follows an autosomal recessive pattern. Renal stones begin to form in the first to fourth decades. Urinary tract obstruction, infection, and even renal failure are common, especially in men. Calculi tend to occur as staghorns or as multiple and bilateral separate stones and are visible on radiographs because of the density of the sulfur in the cystine molecule. Without treatment, recurrence is the rule. This disease is not to be confused with cystinosis, in which intracellular cystine accumulation leads to widespread tissue damage, including renal failure. In cystinuria, the amino acid accumulates only in the lumen of renal tubules.

## Pathogenesis

Cystine overexcretion raises urinary cystine concentration above the limits of solubility for this most insoluble amino acid. Characteristic hexagonal crystals may be identified in cystinuria, particularly in the first-voided morning urine, which is concentrated and usually acid. The normal adult excretes less than 19 mg of cystine per gram of creatinine in 24 hours,[370] whereas homozygous stone formers usually excrete more than 250 mg per gram of creatinine; intermediate values occur among heterozygotes.[371] Urinary excretion of the dibasic amino acids arginine, ornithine, and lysine is also increased in homozygous cystinuria and, to a variable extent, in the heterozygous form.

Amino acids are filtered and normally almost completely reabsorbed by the proximal tubule. Excessive urinary excretion of cystine and the dibasic amino acids in cystinuria occurs with normal or subnormal blood levels, which indicates a tubule reabsorption defect in the common transport mechanism for the dibasic amino acids.[372–375] A similar transport defect exists in intestinal epithelial cells. After oral administration of cystine, urinary excretion of cystine does not rise, as it does in normal subjects; urinary excretion of orally ingested arginine, lysine, or ornithine is variable and often low.[376, 377] Jejunal perfusion studies have shown defects in arginine as well as cystine absorption,[376] and in vitro studies of specimens of jejunal mucosa obtained by peroral biopsy have confirmed the presence of defects in intestinal transport of these amino acids.

Family studies have revealed heterogeneity in the transport of dibasic amino acids, and these observations plus the urinary excretion patterns of the four dibasic amino acids permit the classification of homozygous cystinuria into three types (Table 40–22). In addition, one patient has been described in whom defects in dibasic amino acid transport occurred in the presence of normal cystine transport.[378] Another family study has revealed cystinuria accompanied by only slight defects in arginine, ornithine, and lysine transport; this may represent a fourth type of cystinuria, although no intestinal transport studies were performed.[379] Thus, it appears that the in vitro study of intestinal transport of cystine and the other three dibasic amino acids is a sensitive

method for classifying homozygous cystinuria. Urinary excretion patterns are a less sensitive means of classification.

In addition to pure cystine stones, homozygous cystinuric patients are susceptible to calcium oxalate and uric acid stones, as well as cystine stones mixed with other solid phases.[380] This appears to be due to a higher rate of metabolic stone-forming risks than in normal people. In a study of 27 cystinuric patients, 18% had hypercalciuria, 22% had hyperuricosuria, and 44% had hypocitraturia.[381] Heterozygous cystinuria may have an increased risk of calcium oxalate stone formation.[382]

## Treatment

Therapy is designed to reduce the excretion and increase the solubility of cystine. Lowering urinary cystine concentration by increasing urine volume reduces the likelihood of precipitation and is the basis for clinical treatment. An intake of 4 L/d or more may be required, because patients may excrete up to 1 g of cystine daily, and the solubility limit for cystine is about 300 mg/L unless the urine pH is above 7.5. At most, alkali can raise urine pH to 7.9, so this measure confers only a marginal benefit. Methionine is the precursor of cystine, and dietary restriction of methionine has been recommended as treatment.[383] However, the reduction in cystine excretion was only 20% in seven patients fed a high-protein diet (140 g/d) and then switched to a low-protein diet (54 g/d).[384] Because methionine is an essential amino acid, long-term restriction may also lead to sulfur amino acid deficiencies. Martensson and co-workers[385] have found low leukocyte glutathione and taurine levels and low urinary sulfate, taurine, and thiosulfate levels, which suggests a mild intracellular cystine deficiency in homozygous cystinuric patients. Long-term methionine restriction might cause a clinically significant cystine deficiency. Cystine excretion is linked to $Na^+$ excretion, and low-sodium diets have been shown to reduce cystine excretion by 40%.[386, 387] Glutamine has been reported to reduce cystine excretion,[388] but this effect is present only with high salt intake and is of little clinical benefit.[386]

Pharmacologic therapy is required when patients have not responded to diet, fluid, and alkali therapy. Drug ther-

### TABLE 40–22. Functional Classification of Cystinuria

| Transport Defects | Type I | Type II | Type III |
|---|---|---|---|
| **Intestine** | | | |
| In vitro transport | No transport of cystine, lysine, or arginine; normal cysteine transport | No transport of lysine; markedly reduced cystine transport | Transport of cystine reduced but may be normal; lysine variably reduced |
| Oral cystine | No plasma cystine elevation | No plasma cystine elevation | Slow increase in plasma cystine to normal elevation |
| **Kidney** | | | |
| In vitro transport | Normal cystine and cysteine; reduced lysine transport | — | Normal cystine; reduced lysine transport |
| Urinary amino acid excretion | Increased cystine, lysine, arginine, and ornithine | Increased cystine, lysine, arginine, and ornithine | Increased cystine, lysine, arginine, and ornithine |
| Urinary amino acid excretion in heterozygotes | Normal | Cystine and lysine above normal | Cystine and lysine above normal |

apy increases cystine solubility by creating a thiol-cysteine disulfide, which is more soluble than cystine. D-Penicillamine and tiopronin are the most commonly used drugs, but they have significant side effects including rash, proteinuria, nausea, and fever that often force discontinuation of the drug.[389] Tiopronin appears to be better tolerated than D-penicillamine.[389] Acetylcysteine is not recommended for therapy because it increases the excretion of cystine.[385] Captopril, a thiol, has been reported to reduce stone formation in some patients with cystinuria and is well tolerated.[390, 391]

Treatment of large cystine stones can be difficult. The stones are difficult to fragment by extracorporeal shock wave lithotripsy and percutaneous lithotripsy.[392] Stone fragments remain after these procedures in approximately 50% of patients.[393, 394] Irrigation of the renal pelvis with alkaline solutions can be used to dissolve remaining fragments after percutaneous or extracorporeal lithotripsy.[393]

## STRUVITE (INFECTION) STONES

Struvite ($MgNH_4PO_4 \cdot 6H_2O$) stones form in the renal pelvis and calyces only when the urinary tract is infected by a urea-splitting bacterium, usually *Proteus* species.[395] Struvite stones tend to branch and enlarge, and their growth is rapid. Often, they fill the renal collecting systems and assume a staghorn configuration. They frequently grow back after surgical removal because infected chalky fragments have been left behind. Kidneys are often damaged by obstruction and infection. Because of the size of these calculi, pyelolithotomy is difficult. Bleeding is common, and the kidney can be lost because of a need for emergency nephrectomy. Infection stones are most destructive and difficult to control.

The actual composition of struvite stones in humans is variable in that carbonate apatite ($Ca_{10}(PO_4)_6 \cdot CO_3$) is usually present along with struvite and may even predominate.[396] However, the presence of struvite always implicates urinary tract infection with urea-splitting organisms, whatever the apatite concentration in the stone.

### Urea Splitting

Bacterial urease hydrolyzes urea as follows: $H_2NCONH_2 \rightarrow H_2O + 2NH_3 + CO_2$. The ammonia hydrolyzes spontaneously to form $NH_4OH$, whereas the carbon dioxide hydrates to form $H_2CO_3$ and then $HCO_3^-$. Urine pH increases because ammonia hydrolyzes, just as it would if ammonia were bubbled through it from a storage tank. At a high pH, $HCO_3^-$ loses its $H^+$ to become $CO_3^{2-}$.

The urinary conditions produced by ureolysis are unique. Normally, urinary $NH_4^+$ concentration rises only with an acid load or $K^+$ depletion, conditions of low urine pH and negligible urinary carbonate concentration (see Chapter 10). In RTA type I, the urine is alkaline and may contain $HCO_3^-$, especially during alkali treatment, but urinary $NH_4^+$ levels, although relatively high for the prevailing pH, are low in absolute concentration (see Chapter 37). In other conditions of alkaline urine, such as antacid abuse, the urinary $NH_4^+$ concentration is also low.

It is only in infection that urease is present in urine, and only urease can elevate $NH_4^+$, pH, and carbonate concentration at the same time. So it is not surprising that struvite stones arise only from infection and always contain carbonate apatite. All normal urine is undersaturated with respect to struvite,[397, 398] so one could expect dissolution of an infection stone during prolonged antimicrobial treatment, if the treatment were successful in eradicating infection. However, normal urine need not be undersaturated with respect to carbonate apatite,[397] only metastable. So whether an infection stone will dissolve depends on its apatite concentration.

### Bacteriology

*Proteus* and *Providencia* species possess urease in more than 90% of isolates.[399] Other common urinary pathogens that frequently contain urease include *Klebsiella, Pseudomonas,* and enterococci. *Escherichia coli* rarely possesses urease activity.[400] *Ureaplasma urealyticum,* a fastidious bacterium that requires special culture techniques for isolation, has been shown to cause struvite stones.[401]

The bacteria produce oversaturation in their own immediate environment, so crystals tend to form around clusters of bacteria. As a result, bacteria permeate every crevice of a struvite-apatite stone. The stone becomes like a harbor; it keeps the bacteria from washing away in the flowing urine. Every fragment of the stone is infected and therefore can enlarge in urine. Bits of a growing stone swept into an uninvolved calyx, or into the bladder, can create a metastatic focus if they adhere to the urothelium. It has been proposed that the high urinary ammonia concentration interferes with the ability of glycosaminoglycans to prevent bacterial adhesion to the urothelium, thus increasing the risk for struvite crystals to anchor in the collecting system.[399]

### Predisposing Factors

Calcium, uric acid, or cystine stones can become infected, especially as a result of cystoscopy or retrograde ureteral catheterization or because of renal or ureteral surgery. These patients tend to have underlying metabolic abnormalities, such as idiopathic hypercalciuria, and maintain relatively well preserved renal function.[402] Long-term bladder catheterization promotes infection, and *Proteus* or *Pseudomonas* species can predominate despite the use of antimicrobial agents. Patients with spinal cord injury or another form of neurogenic bladder or in whom ileal diversion of the ureter has been performed are especially likely to form struvite stones. However, struvite stones also occur without any predisposing cause. They are three times as common in women as in men, presumably because urinary tract infection is much more common in women.[399] Often they grow silently. Radiographic studies performed because of recurrent symptoms of urinary infection, hematuria, or pyuria or because of symptoms not related to the urinary system can disclose a staghorn calculus so large that it fills the renal collecting system and provokes a sense of amazement that its symptoms could be so meager.

## Treatment

A natural reaction to the size of a staghorn calculus and the damage and obstruction that it produces is surgical removal. Untreated staghorn calculi ultimately require nephrectomy in 50% of cases.[403, 404] Open surgical removal had been the procedure of choice and often led to improved renal function if obstruction was present. However, Griffith and colleagues[396] estimated that after 435 such operations, there were recurrences in 118 cases (27%) within 6.3 years, and urinary tract infection persisted after surgery in 129 of 315 cases, or 41%. A later study by Silverman and Stamey[405] showed only a 2.2% stone recurrence rate during 7 years of follow-up, when open surgery was followed by aggressive lavage of the renal pelvis with hemiacidrin to ensure no stone fragments remained.

Newer procedures have reduced the morbidity of struvite stone removal with reasonably low rates of stone recurrence. Percutaneous nephrolithotomy can completely remove struvite stones in 85% to 90% of kidneys,[406, 407] with only a 10% relapse rate in those kidneys rendered stone free.[408] Extracorporeal shock wave lithotripsy with ureteral stenting has been used as monotherapy for large-volume struvite stones, resulting in stone-free rates of 50% to 75%.[409, 410] Combination procedures of percutaneous debulking followed by extracorporeal shock wave lithotripsy have resulted in stone-free rates similar to those seen with percutaneous nephrolithotomy alone.[410, 411] No matter which approach is taken, the best long-term results depend on clearing the urinary tract of stones and sterilizing the urine.

Antibiotic treatment and conservative measures may well be preferable to surgery in selected cases. Any metabolic disorder should be treated. Antibiotic use should be based on antibiotic resistance patterns of the infecting organism. Culture of stone material may allow more specific antibiotic therapy directed against the organism producing the stone.[405] Although hope of cure is remote, stone growth can be slowed by reducing the bacterial population. Stamey[412] has reported the partial dissolution of stones during long-term antibiotic treatment.

Acetohydroxamic acid, a compound that inhibits bacterial urease, provides another therapy as an alternative to surgery or as an adjunct after surgical reduction of stone mass.[413] Three randomized, double-blind clinical trials have been performed using acetohydroxamic acid.[414–416] In all three studies, a significant reduction in the rate of stone growth or formation was found. There is a high rate of side effects, which has led to significant rates of withdrawal of patients from treatment in all three trials. The most common side effects are headache, tremulousness, and anemia. Higher rates of deep venous thrombosis have been reported in patients receiving the active drug in these trials, but the difference has not been significant.

Between medical management and surgical removal of the stone, there is the complex treatment of irrigation with solutions that can dissolve struvite. Hemiacidrin, a commonly used acid citrate solution, can be used to irrigate the intact unobstructed renal pelvis, although the procedure is potentially hazardous.[417] The procedure can lead to renal and ureteral damage and sepsis and must be carried out with great caution. It can be used, however, even in such complex settings as infection stone with ileal conduit urinary diversion.[418] The use of this treatment is usually as an adjunct to open or percutaneous surgery, although it has been used as monotherapy.

Although many improvements have been made in the medical and surgical approach to struvite stones, a cure may still be difficult to obtain. The correct surgical approach is not always clear, and many patients require multiple procedures. Struvite stones often recur, and patients need long-term follow-up and surveillance for urinary tract infections. The burden of infection stone weighs on the patient heavily.

## REFERENCES

1. Nordin BEC, Hodgkinson A: Urolithiasis. Adv Intern Med 13:155–182, 1967.
2. Lagergren C: Biophysical investigations of urinary calculi. Acta Radiol Scand Suppl 133:1, 1956.
3. Melick RA, Henneman PH: Clinical and laboratory studies of 207 consecutive patients in a kidney-stone clinic. N Engl J Med 259:307–314, 1958.
4. Prien EL: Studies in urolithiasis. J Urol 61:821, 1949.
5. Sutor DJ, Wooley SE, Illingworth JJ: Some aspects of the adult urinary stone problem in Great Britain and Northern Ireland. Br J Urol 46:275, 1974.
6. Mandel NS, Mandel GS: Urinary tract stone disease in the United States veteran population. II. Geographical analysis of variations in composition. J Urol 142:1516–1521, 1989.
7. Berenyi M, Frang D, Legrady J: Theoretical and clinical importance of the differentiation between the two types of calcium oxalate hydrate. Int Urol Nephrol 4:341, 1972.
8. Ellis H: A History of Bladder Stones. Blackwell Scientific Publications, Oxford, 1969.
9. Sutor DJ, Wooley SE, Illingworth JJ: A geographical and historical survey of the composition of urinary stones. Br J Urol 46:393, 1974.
10. Anderson DA: Historical and geographical differences in the pattern of incidence of urinary stones considered in relation to possible aetiological factors. *In* Hodgkinson A, Nordin BEC (eds): Renal Stone Research Symposium. JA Churchill, London, 1969, p 7.
11. Johnson CM, Wilson DM, O'Fallon WM, et al: Renal stone epidemiology: A 25-year study in Rochester, Minnesota. Kidney Int 16:624–631, 1979.
12. Sutherland JW, Parks JH, Coe FL: Recurrence after a single renal stone in a community practice. Miner Electrolyte Metab 11:267–269, 1985.
13. Williams RE: Long-term survey of 538 patients with upper urinary tract stones. Br J Urol 35:416, 1963.
14. Ljunghall S, Danielson BG: A prospective study of renal stone recurrences. Br J Urol 56:122–124, 1984.
15. Blacklock NJ: The pattern of urolithiasis in the Royal Navy. *In* Hodgkinson A, Nordin BEC (eds): Renal Stone Research Symposium. JA Churchill, London, 1969, p 33.
16. Marshall V, White RH, Chaput DE, et al: The natural history of renal and ureteric colic. Br J Urol 47:117, 1975.
17. Coe FL, Keck J, Norton ER: The natural history of calcium urolithiasis. JAMA 238:1519–1523, 1977.
18. Strauss AL, Coe FL, Parks JH: Formation of a single calcium stone of renal origin. Clinical and laboratory characteristics of patients. Arch Intern Med 142:504–507, 1982.
19. Coe FL, Parks JH, Lindheimer MD: Nephrolithiasis during pregnancy. N Engl J Med 298:324–326, 1978.
20. Jones WA, Correa RJ Jr, Ansell JS: Urolithiasis associated with pregnancy. J Urol 122:333, 1979.
21. Parks JH, Coe FL, Strauss AL: Calcium nephrolithiasis and medullary sponge kidney in women. N Engl J Med 306:1088–1091, 1982.

22. Coe FL: Calcium–uric acid nephrolithiasis. Arch Intern Med 138:1090–1093, 1978.

23. Coe FL, Parks JH, Strauss AL: Accelerated calcium nephrolithiasis. JAMA 244:809–810, 1980.

24. Pak CYC: Citrate and renal calculi. Miner Electrolyte Metab 13:257–266, 1987.

25. Hallson PC, Rose GA, Sulaiman S: Magnesium reduces calcium oxalate crystal formation in human whole urine. Clin Sci 62:17–19, 1982.

26. Robertson WG, Peacock M, Nordin BEC: Activity products in stone-forming and non–stone-forming urine. Clin Sci 34:579–594, 1968.

27. Pak CYC, Hayashi Y, Finlayson B, Chu S: Estimation of the state of supersaturation of brushite and calcium oxalate in urine: A comparison of three methods. J Lab Clin Med 89:891–909, 1977.

28. Millman S, Strauss AL, Parks JH, Coe FL: Pathogenesis and clinical course of mixed calcium oxalate and uric acid nephrolithiasis. Kidney Int 22:366–370, 1982.

29. Robertson WG, Peacock M, Nordin BEC: Calcium oxalate crystalluria and urine saturation in recurrent renal stone formers. Clin Sci 40:365–374, 1971.

30. Robertson WG, Peacock M, Marshall RW, et al: Saturation-inhibition index as a measure of the risk of calcium oxalate stone formation in the urinary tract. N Engl J Med 294:249–252, 1976.

31. Marshall RW, Cochran M, Robertson WG, et al: The relation between the concentration of calcium salts in the urine and renal stone composition in patients with calcium-containing renal stones. Clin Sci 43:433–441, 1972.

32. Pak CYC, Holt K: Nucleation and growth of brushite and calcium oxalate in urine of stone formers. Metabolism 25:665–673, 1976.

33. Weber DV, Coe FL, Parks JH, et al: Urinary saturation measurements in calcium nephrolithiasis. Ann Intern Med 90:180–184, 1979.

34. Hautmann R, Lehmann A, Komor S: Calcium and oxalate concentrations in human renal tissue: The key to the pathogenesis of stone formation. J Urol 123:317–319, 1980.

35. Nielson AE: Kinetics of Precipitation. Pergamon Press, New York, 1964.

36. Pak CY, Arnold LH: Heterogeneous nucleation of calcium oxalate by seeds of monosodium urate. Proc Soc Exp Biol Med 149:930–932, 1975.

37. Coe FL, Lawton RL, Goldstein RB, Tembe V: Sodium urate accelerates precipitation of calcium oxalate in vitro. Proc Soc Exp Biol Med 149:926–929, 1975.

38. Coe FL, Raisen L: Allopurinol treatment of uric-acid disorders in calcium-stone formers. Lancet 1:129–131, 1973.

39. Coe FL: Hyperuricosuric calcium oxalate nephrolithiasis. Kidney Int 13:418–426, 1978.

40. Coe FL: Hyperuricosuric calcium oxalate nephrolithiasis. In Coe FL, Brenner BM, Stein JH (eds): Contemporary Issues in Nephrology, Vol VI, Nephrolithiasis. Churchill Livingstone, New York, 1980, p 116.

41. Fleisch H, Bisaz S: Isolation from urine of pyrophosphate, a calcification inhibitor. Am J Physiol 203:671–675, 1962.

42. Russell RGG, Fleisch H: Inhibitors in urinary stone disease: Role of pyrophosphate in urinary calculi. In Cifuentes-Delatte L, Rapado A, Hodgkinson A (eds): Urinary Calculi. S Karger, Basel, 1973, p 307.

43. Deganello S, Coe F: Epitaxy between uric acid and whewellite: Experimental verification. Neues Jahrb Mineral Monatsh 6:270–276, 1983.

44. Meyer JL, Bergert JH, Smith LH: Epitaxial relationships in urolithiasis: The brushite-whewellite system. Clin Sci Mol Med 52:143–148, 1977.

45. Meyer JL, Bergert JH, Smith LH: Epitaxial relationships in urolithiasis: The calcium oxalate monohydrate–hydroxyapatite system. Clin Sci Mol Med 49:369–374, 1975.

46. Herring LC: Observations on the analysis of ten thousand urinary calculi. J Urol 88:545–555, 1962.

47. Robertson WG, Peacock M, Nordin BEC: Inhibitors of the growth and aggregation of calcium oxalate crystals in vitro. Clin Chim Acta 43:31–37, 1973.

48. Finlayson B, Reid F: The expectation of free and fixed particles in urinary stone disease. Invest Urol 15:442–448, 1978.

49. Riese RJ, Riese JW, Kleinman JG, et al: Specificity in calcium oxalate adherence to papillary epithelial cells in cultures. Am J Physiol 255:F1025–F1032, 1988.

50. Lieske JC, Walsh-Reitz MW, Toback FG: Calcium oxalate monohydrate crystals are endocytosed by renal epithelial cells and induce proliferation. Am J Physiol 262:F622–F630, 1992.

51. Meyer JL, Smith LH: Growth of calcium oxalate crystals. II. Inhibition by natural urinary crystal growth inhibitors. Invest Urol 13:36–39, 1975.

52. Ito H, Coe FL: Acidic peptide and polyribonucleotide crystal growth inhibitors in human urine. Am J Physiol 233:F455–F463, 1977.

53. Welshman SG, McGeown MG: A quantitative investigation of the effects on the growth of calcium oxalate crystals on potential inhibitors. Br J Urol 44:677, 1972.

54. Smith LH, Meyer JL, McCall JT: Chemical nature of crystal inhibitors isolated from human urine. In Cifuentes-Delatte L, Rapado A, Hodgkinson A (eds): Urinary Calculi. S Karger, Basel, 1973, p 310.

55. Bisaz S, Felix R, Neuman WF, Fleisch H: Quantitative determination of inhibitors of calcium phosphate precipitation in whole urine. Miner Electrolyte Metab 1:74–83, 1978.

56. Hallson PC, Rose GA: Uromucoids and urinary stone formation. Lancet 1:1000–1001, 1979.

57. Robertson WG, Knowles F, Peacock M: Urinary acid mucopolysaccharide inhibitors of calcium oxalate crystallisation. In Fleisch H, Robertson WG, Smith LH, Vahlensieck W (eds): Urolithiasis Research. Plenum Publishing, London, 1976, pp 331–340.

58. Nakagawa Y, Margolis HC, Yokoyama S, et al: Purification and characterization of a calcium oxalate monohydrate crystal growth inhibitor from human kidney tissue culture medium. J Biol Chem 256:3936–3944, 1981.

59. Nakagawa Y, Abram V, Kezdy FJ, et al: Purification and characterization of the principal inhibitor of calcium oxalate monohydrate crystal growth in human urine. J Biol Chem 258:12594–12600, 1983.

60. Asplin J, Deganello S, Nakagawa YN, Coe FL: Evidence that nephrocalcin and urine inhibit nucleation of calcium oxalate monohydrate crystals. Am J Physiol 261:F824–F830, 1991.

61. Hess B, Nakagawa Y, Coe FL: Inhibition of calcium oxalate monohydrate crystal aggregation by urine proteins. Am J Physiol 257:F99–F106, 1989.

62. Nakagawa Y, Abram V, Parks JH, et al: Urine glycoprotein crystal growth inhibitors. Evidence for a molecular abnormality in calcium oxalate nephrolithiasis. J Clin Invest 76:1455–1462, 1985.

63. Worcester EM, Nakagawa Y, Wabner CL, et al: Crystal adsorption and growth slowing by nephrocalcin, albumin, and Tamm-Horsfall protein. Am J Physiol 255:F1197–F1205, 1988.

64. Hess B, Nakagawa Y, Parks JH, Coe FL: Molecular abnormality of Tamm-Horsfall glycoprotein in calcium oxalate nephrolithiasis. Am J Physiol 260:F569–F578, 1991.

65. Lieske JC, Toback FG: Regulation of renal epithelial cell endocytosis of calcium oxalate monohydrate crystals. Am J Physiol 264:F800–F807, 1993.

66. Shiraga H, Min W, VanDusen WJ, et al: Inhibition of calcium oxalate crystal growth in vitro by uropontin: Another member of the aspartic acid–rich protein superfamily. Proc Natl Acad Sci USA 89:426–430, 1992.

67. Coe FL: Treated and untreated recurrent calcium nephrolithiasis in patients with idiopathic hypercalciuria, hyperuricosuria, or no metabolic disorder. Ann Intern Med 87:404–410, 1977.

68. Yendt ER: Renal calculi. Can Med Assoc J 102:479, 1970.

69. Hodgkinson A, Pyrah LN: The urinary excretion of calcium and inorganic phosphate in 344 patients with calcium stones of renal origin. Br J Surg 46:10, 1958.

70. Coe FL, Margolis HC, Deutsch LH, Strauss AL: Urinary macromolecular crystal growth inhibitors in calcium urolithiasis. Miner Electrolyte Metab 3:268–275, 1980.

71. Hodgkinson A: Uric acid disorders in patients with calcium stones. Br J Urol 48:1–5, 1976.

72. Rudman D, Kutner MH, Redd SC 2d, et al: Hypocitraturia in calcium nephrolithiasis. J Clin Endocrinol Metab 55:1052–1057, 1982.

73. Minisola S, Rossi W, Pacitti MT, et al: Studies on citrate metabolism in normal subjects and kidney stone patients. Miner Electrolyte Metab 15:303–308, 1989.

74. Menon M, Mahle CJ: Urinary citrate excretion in patients with renal calculi. J Urol 129:1158–1160, 1983.

75. Hosking DH, Wilson JWL, Liedtke RR, et al: Urinary citrate excretion in normal persons and patients with idiopathic calcium urolithiasis. J Lab Clin Med 106:682–689, 1985.

76. Nicar MJ, Skurla C, Sakhaee K, Pak CYC: Low urinary citrate excretion in nephrolithiasis. Urology 21:8–13, 1983.

77. Pyrah LN, Hodgkinson A, Anderson CK: Primary hyperparathyroidism. Br J Surg 53:245–316, 1966.

78. Aurbach GD, Mallette LE, Pattern BM, et al: Hyperparathyroidism: Recent studies. Ann Intern Med 79:566, 1973.

79. Keating FR: The clinical problem of primary hyperparathyroidism. Med Clin North Am 54:511, 1970.

80. Boonstra CE, Jackson CE: Hyperparathyroidism detected by routine serum calcium analysis. Ann Intern Med 63:468, 1965.

81. Yendt ER: Disorders of calcium, phosphorus and magnesium metabolism. *In* Maxwell MG, Kleeman CR (eds): Clinical Disorders of Fluid and Electrolyte Metabolism. McGraw-Hill, New York, 1972, p 401.

82. Golden A, Canary JJ: The parathyroid gland. *In* Bloodworth JMB Jr (ed): Endocrine Pathology. Williams & Wilkins, Baltimore, 1968, p 181.

83. Sherwood LM, Mayer GP, Care AD, et al: Evaluation by radioimmunoassay of factors controlling the secretion of parathyroid hormone. Nature 209:52, 1966.

84. Sherwood LM, Mayer GP, Romberg CF Jr, et al: Regulation of parathyroid hormone secretion: Proportional control by calcium, lack of effect of phosphate. Endocrinology 83:1043, 1968.

85. Martin IJ, Hruska KA, Freitag JJ, et al: The peripheral metabolism of parathyroid hormone. N Engl J Med 301:1092, 1979.

86. Canterbury JM, Bricker LA, Levey GS, et al: Metabolism of bovine parathyroid hormone. J Clin Invest 55:1245, 1975.

87. D'Amour P, Segre GV, Roth SI, Potts JT, Jr: Analysis of parathyroid hormone and its fragments in rat tissues: Chemical identification and microscopical localization. J Clin Invest 63:89, 1979.

88. Catherwood B, Singer FR: Generation of a carboxy terminal fragment of bovine parathyroid hormone by canine renal plasma membrane. Biochem Biophys Res Commun 57:496, 1974.

89. Hanley DA, Takatsuki K, Sultan JM, et al: Direct release of parathyroid hormone fragments from functioning bovine parathyroid glands in vitro. J Clin Invest 62:1247, 1978.

90. Canterbury JM, Levey GS, Reiss E: Activation of renal cortical adenylate cyclase by circulating immunoreactive parathyroid hormone fragments. J Clin Invest 52:524, 1973.

91. Segre JV, D'Amour P, Hultman A, Potts JT Jr: Effects of hepatectomy, nephrectomy and nephrectomy/uremia on the metabolism of parathyroid hormone in the rat. J Clin Invest 67:439–448, 1981.

92. Mayer GP, Habener JF, Potts JT Jr: Parathyroid hormone–secretion in vivo: Demonstration of a calcium independent, nonsuppressible component of secretion. J Clin Invest 57:678, 1976.

93. Targevnik JH, Rodman JS, Sherwood LM: Regulation of parathyroid hormone secretion in vitro: Quantitative aspects of calcium and magnesium ion control. Endocrinology 88:1477, 1971.

94. Reiss E, Canterbury JM: Application of radioimmunoassay to differentiation of adenoma and hyperplasia and to preoperative localization of hyperfunctioning parathyroid glands. N Engl J Med 280:1381, 1969.

95. Potts JT Jr, Murray TM, Peacock M, et al: Parathyroid hormone: Sequence, synthesis, immunoassay studies. Am J Med 50:639, 1971.

96. Murray TM, Peacock M, Powell D, et al: Non-autonomy of hormone secretion in primary hyperthyroidism. Clin Endocrinol 1:235, 1972.

97. Sherwood LM, Lundberg WB, Targevnik JH, et al: Synthesis and secretion of parathyroid hormone in vitro. Am J Med 50:658, 1971.

98. Birnbaumer ME, Schneider AB, Palmer D, et al: Secretion of parathyroid hormone by abnormal human parathyroid glands in vitro. J Clin Endocrinol Metab 45:105, 1977.

99. Coe FL, Parks JH: Nephrolithiasis: Pathogenesis and Treatment, 2nd ed. Year Book Medical Publishers, Chicago, 1988, pp 59–99.

100. Albright F, Bauer W, Claflin D, et al: Studies in parathyroid physiology. III. The effect of phosphate ingestion in clinical hyperparathyroidism. J Clin Invest 11:411, 1932.

101. Aub MC, Tibbets DM, McLean R: The influence of parathyroid hormone, urea, sodium chloride, fat and intestinal activity upon calcium balance. J Nutr 13:635, 1937.

102. Hodgkinson A: Biochemical aspects of primary hyperparathyroidism: Analysis of 50 cases. Clin Sci 25:231, 1963.

103. Lafferty FW, Pearson OH: Skeletal, intestinal, and renal calcium dynamics in hyperparathyroidism. J Clin Endocrinol Metab 23:891, 1963.

104. Anderson J, Osborn SC, Tomlinson RWS, Wall M: Calcium dynamics of the gastrointestinal tract and bone in primary hyperparathyroidism. Q J Med 33:421, 1964.

105. Parfitt AM: Effect of cellulose phosphate and dietary calcium restriction in primary hyperparathyroidism. Clin Sci Mol Med 49:91, 1975.

106. Nassim JR, Higgins BA: Control of idiopathic hypercalciuria. Br Med J 1:675–681, 1965.

107. Bauer W, Albright F, Aub JC: A case of osteitis fibrosa cystica (osteomalacia?) with evidence of hyperactivity of the parathyroid bodies. Metabolic study II. J Clin Invest 8:229, 1930.

108. Birge SJ, Peck WA, Berman M, et al: Study of calcium absorption in man: A kinetic analysis and physiologic model. J Clin Invest 48:1705–1713, 1969.

109. Pak CYC, Ohata M, Lawrence EC, Snyder W: The hypercalciurias: Causes, parathyroid functions, and diagnostic criteria. J Clin Invest 54:387–400, 1974.

110. Reeve J, Hesp R, Veall N: Effects of therapy on rate of absorption of calcium from gut in disorders of calcium homeostasis. Br Med J 3:310, 1974.

111. Kaplan RA, Snyder WH, Stewart A, Pak CYC: Metabolic effects of parathyroidectomy in asymptomatic primary hyperparathyroidism. J Clin Endocrinol Metab 42:415, 1976.

112. Kaplan RA, Haussler MR, Deftos LJ, et al: The role of 1,25 dihydroxyvitamin D in the mediation of intestinal hyperabsorption of calcium in primary hyperparathyroidism and absorptive hypercalciuria. J Clin Invest 59:756–760, 1977.

113. Jowsey J: Bone histology and hyperparathyroidism. Clin Endocrinol Metab 3:267, 1974.

114. Mallette LE, Sode JE, Marx SJ, et al: Total body retention of orally administered $^{47}$Ca in primary hyperparathyroidism. J Clin Endocrinol Metab 50:582, 1975.

115. Warner J, Clifton-Bligh P, Posen S, et al: Longitudinal changes in forearm bone mineral content in primary hyperparathyroidism. J Bone Miner Res 6:S91–S95, 1991.

116. Woodhouse NJY, Doyle FH, Joplin GF: Vitamin-D deficiency and primary hyperparathyroidism. Lancet 2:283, 1971.

117. Brumbaugh PF, Haussler DH, Bressler R, Haussler MR: Radioreceptor assay for 1,25-dihydroxy vitamin $D_3$. Science 183:1089, 1974.

118. Gray RW, Wilz DR, Caldas AE, LeMann J Jr: The importance of phosphate in regulating plasma 1,25(OH)$_2$ vitamin D levels in humans: Studies in healthy subjects, in calcium stone formers, and in patients with primary hyperparathyroidism. J Clin Endocrinol Metab 45:299–306, 1977.

119. Bauer W, Albright F, Aub JC: Studies of calcium and phosphorous metabolism. II. The calcium excretion of normal individuals on a low-calcium diet; also data on a case of pregnancy. J Clin Invest 7:75, 1929.

120. McGeown MG: Calcium and phosphorus metabolism in the diagnosis of hyperparathyroidism. Urol Int 19:83, 1965.

121. Pronove P, Bell NH, Bartter FC: Production of hypercalciuria by phosphorus deprivation on a low-calcium diet. A new clinical test for hyperparathyroidism. Metabolism 10:364, 1961.

122. Wibell L, Werner I: Serum phosphate and calcium phosphate excretion at different levels of serum calcium. Acta Med Scand 193:161, 1973.

123. Nordin BEC, Peacock M: Role of kidney in regulation of plasmacalcium. Lancet 2:1280, 1969.

124. Transbol I, Hornum I, Hahnemann S, et al: Tubular reabsorption of calcium in the differential diagnosis of hypercalcemia. Acta Med Scand 188:505, 1970.

125. Transbol I, Hahnemann S, Hornum I: The tubular reabsorption of calcium in primary hyperparathyroidism and non-parathyroid hypercalcemia. Acta Med Scand 184:33, 1968.

126. Kleeman CR, Bernstein D, Rockney R, et al: Studies on the renal clearance of diffusible calcium and the role of the parathyroid glands in its regulation. Yale J Biol Med 34:1, 1961.

127. Parks JH, Coe FL, Favus MJ: Hyperparathyroidism in nephrolithiasis. Arch Intern Med 140:1479, 1980.

128. Broadus AE, Horst EL, Lang R, et al: The importance of circulating 1,25-dihydroxyvitamin D in the pathogenesis of hypercalciuria and renal-stone formation in primary hyperparathyroidism. N Engl J Med 302:421, 1980.

129. Pak CYC, Nicar MJ, Peterson R, et al: A lack of unique pathophysiologic background for nephrolithiasis of primary hyperparathyroidism. J Clin Endocrinol Metab 53:536–542, 1981.

130. Hodgkinson A, Marshall RW: Changes in the composition of urinary tract stones. Invest Urol 13:131, 1975.

131. Nicar MJ, Hill K, Pak CY: A simple technique for assessing the

propensity for crystallization of calcium oxalate and brushite in urine from the increment in oxalate or calcium necessary to elicit precipitation. Metabolism 32:906–910, 1983.

132. Nordin BEC: Metabolic Bone and Stone Disease. Churchill Livingstone, London, 1973.

133. Muldowney FP, Donohoe JF, Carroll DV, et al: Parathyroid acidosis in uremia. Q J Med 163:321, 1972.

134. Coe FL: Magnitude of metabolic acidosis in primary hyperparathyroidism. Arch Intern Med 134:262–265, 1974.

135. Berson SA, Yalow PS: Parathyroid hormone in plasma in adenomatous hyperparathyroidism, uremia and bronchogenic carcinoma. Science 154:907, 1966.

136. Purnell DC, Scholz DA, Smith LH, et al: Treatment of primary hyperparathyroidism. Am J Med 56:800, 1974.

137. Nussbaum SR, Potts JT Jr: Immunoassays for parathyroid hormone 1–84 in the diagnosis of hyperparathyroidism. J Bone Miner Res 6:S43–S50, 1991.

138. Brown RC, Aston JP, Weeks I, Woodhead JS: Circulating intact parathyroid hormone measured by a two-site immunochemiluminometric assay. J Clin Endocrinol Metab 65:407–414, 1987.

139. Blind E, Schmidt-Gayk H, Scharla S, et al: Two-site assay of intact parathyroid hormone in the investigation of primary hyperparathyroidism and other disorders of calcium metabolism compared with a midregion assay. J Clin Endocrinol Metab 67:353–360, 1988.

140. Chase LR, Aurbach GD: Renal adenyl cyclase: Anatomically separate sites for parathyroid hormone and vasopressin. Science 159:545, 1968.

141. Melson GL, Chase LR, Aurbach GD: Parathyroid hormone sensitive adenyl cyclase in isolated renal tubules. Endocrinology 86:511, 1970.

142. Kaminsky NI, Broadus AE, Hardman JG, et al: Effects of parathyroid hormone on plasma and urinary adenosine 3′,5′ monophosphate in man. J Clin Invest 49:2387, 1970.

143. Dohan PH, Yamashita K, Larsen PR, et al: Evaluation of urinary cyclic 3′,5′-adenosine monophosphate excretion in the differential diagnosis of hypercalcemia. J Clin Endocrinol Metab 35:775, 1972.

144. Neelon FA, Drezner M, Birch BM, Lebovitz HE: Urinary cyclic adenosine monophosphate as an aid in the diagnosis of hyperparathyroidism. Lancet 1:631, 1973.

145. Mallette LE, Bilezikian JP, Heath DA, Aurbach GD: Primary hyperparathyroidism: Clinical and biochemical features. Medicine (Baltimore) 53:127, 1974.

146. Broadus AE, Kaminsky NI, Hardman JG, et al: Kinetic parameters and renal clearances of plasma adenosine 3′,5′-monophosphate and guanosine 3′,5′-monophosphate in man. J Clin Invest 49:2222, 1970.

147. Babka JC, Bower RH, Sode J: Nephrogenous cyclic AMP levels in primary hyperparathyroidism. Arch Intern Med 136:1140, 1976.

148. Broadus AE, Mahaffey JE, Bartter FC, Neer RM: Nephrogenous cyclic adenosine monophosphate as a parathyroid function test. J Clin Invest 60:771, 1977.

149. Lafferty FW: Differential diagnosis of hypercalcemia. J Bone Miner Res 6:S51–S59, 1991.

150. Byers PD, Smith R: Quantitative histology of bone in hyperparathyroidism: Its relation to clinical features, x-ray, and bone biochemistry. Q J Med 40:471, 1971.

151. Becker FO, Eisenstein R, Schwartz TB, Economou SG: Needle bone biopsy in primary hyperparathyroidism. Arch Intern Med 131:651, 1973.

152. Buckle R: Ectopic PTH syndrome, pseudohyperparathyroidism; hypercalcemia of malignancy. J Clin Endocrinol Metab 3:237, 1974.

153. Marx SJ, Spiegel AM, Brown EM, et al: Divalent cation metabolism: Familial hypocalciuric hypercalcemia vs typical primary hyperparathyroidism. Am J Med 65:235–242, 1978.

154. Marx SJ, Stock JL, Attie MF, et al: Familial hypocalciuric hypercalcemia: Recognition among patients referred after unsuccessful parathyroid exploration. Ann Intern Med 92:351, 1980.

155. Attie MF, Gill JR, Stock JL, et al: Urinary calcium excretion in familial hypocalciuric hypercalcemia. J Clin Invest 72:667, 1983.

156. McMurtry CT, Schranck FW, Walkenhorst DA, et al: Significant developmental elevation in serum parathyroid hormone levels in a large kindred with familial benign (hypocalciuric) hypercalcemia. Am J Med 93:247–258, 1992.

157. Suva LJ, Winslow GA, Wettenhall REH, et al: A parathyroid hormone–related protein implicated in malignant hypercalcemia: Cloning and expression. Science 237:893–896, 1987.

158. Broadus AE, Mangin M, Ikeda K, et al: Humoral hypercalcemia of cancer. N Engl J Med 319:556–563, 1988.

159. Strewler GJ, Stern PH, Jacobs JW, et al: Parathyroid hormonelike protein from human renal carcinoma cells. J Clin Invest 80:1803–1807, 1987.

160. Britton DC, Thompson MH, Johnston IDA, Fleming LB: Renal function following parathyroid surgery in primary hyperparathyroidism. Lancet 2:74, 1971.

161. Potts JT Jr, Ackerman IP, Barker CF, et al: Diagnosis and management of asymptomatic primary hyperparathyroidism: Consensus development conference statement. Ann Intern Med 114:593–597, 1991.

162. Krubsack AJ, Wilson SD, Lawson TL, et al: Prospective comparison of radionuclide, computed tomographic, sonographic, and magnetic resonance localization of parathyroid tumors. Surgery 106:639–646, 1989.

163. Reading CC, Charboneau JW, James EM, et al: High-resolution parathyroid sonography. AJR 139:539–546, 1982.

164. Auffermann W, Gooding GAW, Okerlund MD, et al: Diagnosis of recurrent hyperparathyroidism: Comparison of MR imaging and other imaging techniques. AJR 150:1027–1033, 1988.

165. Doppman JL, Miller DL: Localization of parathyroid tumors in patients with asymptomatic hyperparathyroidism and no previous surgery. J Bone Miner Res 6:S153–S158, 1991.

166. Eisenberg H, Pallotta J, Sherwood LM: Selective arteriography, venography and venous hormone assay in diagnosis and localization of parathyroid lesions. Am J Med 56:810, 1974.

167. Marcus R: Estrogens and progestins in the management of primary hyperparathyroidism. J Bone Miner Res 6:S125–S129, 1991.

168. Marcus R, Madvig P, Crim M, et al: Conjugated estrogens in the treatment of postmenopausal women with hyperparathyroidism. Ann Intern Med 100:633–640, 1984.

169. Selby PL, Peacock M: Ethinyl estradiol and norethindrone in the treatment of primary hyperparathyroidism in postmenopausal women. N Engl J Med 314:1481–1509, 1986.

170. Wishart J, Horowitz M, Need A, et al: Treatment of postmenopausal hyperparathyroidism with norethindrone. Arch Intern Med 150:1951–1953, 1990.

171. Schmidli RS, Wilson I, Espiner EA, et al: Aminopropylidine diphosphonate (APD) in mild primary hyperparathyroidism: Effect on clinical status. Clin Endocrinol 32:293–300, 1990.

172. Muldowney FP, Freaney R, Muldowney WP, Murray F: Hypercalciuria in parathyroid disorders: Effect of dietary sodium control. Am J Kidney Dis 17:323–329, 1991.

173. McGeown MG: Effect of parathyroidectomy on the incidence of renal calculi. Lancet 1:586, 1961.

174. Edvall CA: Renal function in hyperparathyroidism. A clinical study of 30 cases with special reference to selective renal clearance and renal vein catheterization. Acta Chir Scand Suppl 299, 1958.

175. Pak CYC: Effect of parathyroidectomy on crystallization of calcium salts in urine of patients with primary hyperparathyroidism. Invest Urol 17:146–148, 1979.

176. Pratley SK, Posen S, Reeve TS: Primary hyperparathyroidism: Experience with 60 patients. Med J Aust 1:421, 1973.

177. Hellstrom J, Ivemark BI: Primary hyperparathyroidism. Acta Chir Scand Suppl 294, 1962.

178. Coe FL, Parks JH, Moore ES: Familial idiopathic hypercalciuria. N Engl J Med 300:337–340, 1979.

179. Hamed IA, Czerwinski AW, Coats B, et al: Familial absorptive hypercalciuria and renal tubular acidosis. Am J Med 67:385–391, 1979.

180. Moore ES, Coe FL, McMann BJ, Favus MJ: Idiopathic hypercalciuria in children: Prevalence and metabolic characteristics. J Pediatr 92:906–910, 1978.

181. Favus MJ, Coe FL: Evidence for spontaneous hypercalciuria in the rat. Miner Electrolyte Metab 2:150–154, 1979.

182. Bushinsky DA, Favus MJ: Mechanism of hypercalciuria in genetic hypercalciuric rats: Inherited defect in intestinal calcium transport. J Clin Invest 82:1585–1591, 1988.

183. Frymoyer PA, Scheinman SJ, Dunham PB, et al: X-linked recessive nephrolithiasis with renal failure. N Engl J Med 325:681–686, 1991.

184. Tieder M, Modai D, Shaked U, et al: "Idiopathic" hypercalciuria and hereditary hypophosphatemic rickets. N Engl J Med 316:125–129, 1987.

185. Tieder M, Arie R, Modai D, et al: Elevated serum 1,25-dihydroxy-

vitamin D concentrations in siblings with primary Fanconi's syndrome. N Engl J Med 319:845–849, 1988.

186. Caniggia A, Gennari C, Cesari L: Intestinal absorption of $^{45}$Ca in stone-forming patients. Br Med J 1:427, 1965.

187. Wills MR, Zisman E, Wortsman J, et al: The measurement of intestinal calcium absorption by external radioisotope counting: Application to study of nephrolithiasis. Clin Sci 39:95–106, 1970.

188. Pak CYC, East DA, Sanzenbacher LJ, et al: Gastrointestinal calcium absorption in nephrolithiasis. J Clin Endocrinol Metab 35:261–270, 1972.

189. Ehrig U, Harrison JE, Wilson DR: Effect of long-term thiazide therapy on intestinal calcium absorption in patients with recurrent renal calculi. Metabolism 23:139–149, 1974.

190. Shen FH, Baylink DJ, Nielsen RL, et al: Increased serum 1,25-dihydroxyvitamin D in idiopathic hypercalciuria. J Lab Clin Med 90:955–962, 1977.

191. Barilla DE, Tolentino R, Kaplan RA, Pak CYC: Selective effects of thiazide on intestinal absorption of calcium in absorptive and renal hypercalciurias. Metabolism 27:125–131, 1978.

192. Zerwekh JE, Pak CYC: Selective effects of thiazide therapy on serum 1-alpha, 25-dihydroxyvitamin D and intestinal calcium absorption in renal and absorptive hypercalciurias. Metabolism 29:13–17, 1980.

193. Brannan PG, Morawski S, Pak CYC, Fordtran JS: Selective jejunal hyperabsorption of calcium in absorptive hypercalciuria. Am J Med 66:425, 1979.

194. Knapp EL: Studies on the Urinary Excretion of Calcium. Department of Chemistry, State University of Iowa, 1943. PhD thesis.

195. Liberman UA, Sperling O, Atsmonia A, et al: Metabolic and calcium kinetic studies in idiopathic hypercalciuria. J Clin Invest 47:2580, 1968.

196. Edwards NA, Hodgkinson A: Metabolic studies in patients with idiopathic hypercalciuria. Clin Sci 29:143–157, 1965.

197. Henneman PH, Benedict PH, Forbes AP, Dudley HR: Idiopathic hypercalciuria. N Engl J Med 259:802–807, 1958.

198. Jackson WPU, Dancaster C: A consideration of the hypercalciuria in sarcoidosis, idiopathic hypercalciuria, and that produced by vitamin D. A new suggestion regarding calcium metabolism. J Clin Endocrinol Metab 19:658, 1959.

199. Harrison AR: Some results of metabolic investigations in cases of renal stone. Br J Urol 31:398, 1959.

200. Dent CE, Harper CM, Parfitt AM: The effect of cellulose phosphate on calcium metabolism in patients with hypercalciuria. Clin Sci 27:417–425, 1964.

201. Parfitt AM, Higgins BA, Nassim JR, et al: Metabolic studies in patients with hypercalciuria. Clin Sci 27:463–482, 1964.

202. Edwards NA, Hodgkinson A: Studies of renal function in patients with idiopathic hypercalciuria. Clin Sci 29:327, 1965.

203. Peacock M, Nordin BEC: Tubular reabsorption of calcium in normal and hypercalciuric subjects. J Clin Pathol 21:355, 1968.

204. Phillips MJ, Cooke JNC: Relation between urinary calcium and sodium in patients with idiopathic hypercalciuria. Lancet 1:1354–1357, 1967.

205. Kleerman CR, Bohannan J, Bernstein D, et al: Effect of variations in sodium intake on calcium excretion in normal humans. Proc Soc Exp Biol Med 115:29–32, 1964.

206. Sutton RAL, Walker VR: Responses to hydrochlorothiazide and acetazolamide in patients with calcium stones. N Engl J Med 302:709–713, 1980.

207. Bianchi G, Vezzoli G, Cusi D, et al: Abnormal red-cell calcium pump in patients with idiopathic hypercalciuria. N Engl J Med 319:897–901, 1988.

208. Barkin J, Wilson DR, Manuel MA, et al: Bone mineral content in idiopathic calcium nephrolithiasis. Miner Electrolyte Metab 11:19–24, 1985.

209. Alhava EM, Juuti M, Karjalainen P: Bone mineral density in patients with urolithiasis. Scand J Urol Nephrol 10:154–156, 1976.

210. Borghi L, Meschi T, Guerra A, et al: Vertebral mineral content in diet-dependent and diet-independent hypercalciuria. J Urol 146:1334–1338, 1991.

211. Lawoyin S, Sismilich S, Browne R, Pak CYC: Bone mineral content in patients with calcium urolithiasis. Metabolism 28:1250–1254, 1979.

212. Bataille P, Achard JM, Fournier A, et al: Diet, vitamin D and vertebral mineral density in hypercalciuric calcium stone formers. Kidney Int 39:1193–1205, 1991.

213. Sutton RAL, Walker VR: Bone resorption and hypercalciuria in calcium stoneformers. Metabolism 35:485–488, 1986.

214. Urivetzky M, Anna PS, Smith AD: Plasma osteocalcin levels in stone disease. A potential aid in the differential diagnosis of calcium nephrolithiasis. J Urol 139:12–14, 1988.

215. Steiniche T, Mosekilde L, Christensen MS, Melsen F: A histomorphometric determination of iliac bone remodeling in patients with recurrent renal stone formation and idiopathic hypercalciuria. APMIS 97:309–316, 1989.

216. Malluche HH, Tschoepe W, Ritz E, et al: Abnormal bone histology in idiopathic hypercalciuria. J Clin Endocrinol Metab 50:654–658, 1980.

217. Coe FL, Canterbury JM, Firpo JJ, Reiss E: Evidence for secondary hyperparathyroidism in idiopathic hypercalciuria. J Clin Invest 52:134–142, 1973.

218. Bordier P, Ryckewart A, Gueris J, Rasmussen H: On the pathogenesis of so-called idiopathic hypercalciuria. Am J Med 63:398, 1977.

219. Burckhardt P, Jaeger P: Secondary hyperparathyroidism in idiopathic renal hypercalciuria: Fact or theory? J Clin Endocrinol Metab 55:550, 1981.

220. Pak CY, Delea CS, Bartter FC: Successful treatment of recurrent nephrolithiasis (calcium stones) with cellulose phosphate. N Engl J Med 290:175–180, 1974.

221. Pak CYC, Kaplan R, Bone H, et al: A simple test for the diagnosis of absorptive, resorptive and renal hypercalciurias. N Engl J Med 292:497, 1975.

222. Pak CYC, Britton F, Peterson R, et al: Ambulatory evaluation of nephrolithiasis: Classification, clinical presentation and diagnostic criteria. Am J Med 69:19–30, 1980.

223. Maierhofer WJ, Gray RW, Cheung HS, Lemann J Jr: Bone resorption stimulated by elevated serum 1,25(OH) vitamin D concentrations in healthy men. Kidney Int 24:555–560, 1983.

224. Adams ND, Gray RW, Lemann J Jr, Cheung HS: Effects of calcitriol administration on calcium metabolism in healthy men. Kidney Int 21:90–97, 1982.

225. Breslau NA, Preminger GM, Adams BV, et al: Use of ketoconazole to probe the pathogenetic importance of 1,25-dihydroxyvitamin D in absorptive hypercalciuria. J Clin Endocrinol Metab 75:1446–1452, 1992.

226. Haussler MR, Baylink DJ, Hughes MR, et al: The assay of 1,25-dihydroxy vitamin D$_3$: Physiologic and pathologic modulation of circulating hormone levels. Clin Endocrinol Metab 5:151, 1976.

227. Broadus AE, Insogna KL, Lang R, et al: A consideration of the hormonal basis and phosphate leak hypothesis of absorptive hypercalciuria. J Clin Endocrinol Metab 58:161, 1984.

228. Coe FL, Favus MJ, Crockett T, et al: Effects of low-calcium diet on urine calcium excretion, parathyroid function and serum 1,25(OH)$_2$D$_3$ levels in patients with idiopathic hypercalciuria and in normal subjects. Am J Med 72:25–32, 1982.

229. Bataille P, Bouillon R, Fournier A, et al: Increased plasma concentrations of total and free 1,25-(OH)$_2$D$_3$ in calcium stone formers with idiopathic hypercalciuria. Contrib Nephrol 58:137–142, 1987.

230. Li X, Tembe V, Horwitz GM, et al: Increased intestinal vitamin D receptor in genetic hypercalciuric rats. J Clin Invest 91:661–667, 1993.

231. Barilla DE, Zerwekh JE, Pak CYC: A critical evaluation of the role of phosphate in the pathogenesis of absorptive hypercalciuria. Miner Electrolyte Metab 2:302, 1979.

232. Broadus AE, Insogna KL, Lang R, et al: Evidence for disordered control of 1,25 dihydroxyvitamin D production in absorptive hypercalciuria. N Engl J Med 311:73–80, 1984.

233. Fuss M, Pepersack T, Bergman P, et al: Low calcium diet in idiopathic urolithiasis: A risk factor for osteopenia as great as in primary hyperparathyroidism. Br J Urol 65:560–563, 1990.

234. Ettinger B: Recurrence of nephrolithiasis: A six-year prospective study. Am J Med 67:245, 1979.

235. Hosking DH, Erickson SB, Van Den Berg CJ, et al: The stone clinic effect in patients with idiopathic calcium urolithiasis. J Urol 130:1115–1118, 1983.

236. Walker RM, Linkswiler HM: Calcium retention in the adult human male as affected by protein intake. J Nutr 102:1297–1302, 1972.

237. Allen LH, Oddoye EA, Margen S: Protein-induced hypercalciuria: A longer term study. Am J Clin Nutr 32:741–749, 1979.

238. Hayashi Y, Kaplan RA, Pak CYC: Effect of sodium cellulose phosphate therapy on crystallization of calcium oxalate in urine. Metabolism 24:1273–1278, 1975.

239. Hautmann R, Hering FJ, Lutzeyer W: Calcium oxalate stone disease: Effects and side effects of cellulose phosphate and succinate in long-term treatment of absorptive hypercalciuria or hyperoxaluria. J Urol 120:712–715, 1978.

240. Backman U, Danielson BG, Johansson G, et al: Treatment of recurrent calcium stone formation with cellulose phosphate. J Urol 123:9–13, 1980.

241. Edwards BR, Baer PG, Sutton RA, Dirks JH: Micropuncture study of diuretic effects on sodium and calcium reabsorption in the dog nephron. J Clin Invest 52:2418–2427, 1973.

242. Costanzo LS, Windhager EE: Calcium and sodium transport by the distal convoluted tubule of the rat. Am J Physiol 235:F492, 1978.

243. Coe FL, Parks JH, Bushinsky DA, et al: Chlorthalidone promotes mineral retention in patients with idiopathic hypercalciuria. Kidney Int 33:1140–1146, 1988.

244. Wasnich RD, Benfante RJ, Yano K, et al: Thiazide effect on the mineral content of bone. N Engl J Med 309:344–347, 1983.

245. LaCroix AZ, Wienpahl J, White LR, et al: Thiazide diuretic agents and the incidence of hip fracture. N Engl J Med 322:286–290, 1990.

246. Steiniche T, Mosekilde L, Christensen MS, Melsen F: Histomorphometric analysis of bone in idiopathic hypercalciuria before and after treatment with thiazide. APMIS 97:302–308, 1989.

247. Scholz D, Schwille PO, Sigel A: Double-blind study with thiazide in recurrent calcium lithiasis. J Urol 128:903–907, 1982.

248. Brocks P, Dahl C, Wolf H: Do thiazides prevent recurrent idiopathic renal calcium stones? Lancet 2:124–125, 1981.

249. Laerum E, Larsen S: Thiazide prophylaxis of urolithiasis: A double-blind study in general practice. Acta Med Scand 215:383–389, 1984.

250. Ettinger B, Citron JT, Livermore B, Dolman LI: Chlorthalidone reduces calcium oxalate calculous recurrence but magnesium hydroxide does not. J Urol 139:679–684, 1988.

251. Mortensen JT, Schultz A, Ostergaard AH: Thiazides in the prophylactic treatment of recurrent idiopathic kidney stones. Int Urol Nephrol 18:265–269, 1986.

252. Ohkawa M, Tokunaga S, Nakashima T, et al: Thiazide treatment for calcium urolithiasis in patients with idiopathic hypercalciuria. Br J Urol 69:571–576, 1992.

253. Coe FL, Parks JH: Nephrolithiasis: Pathogenesis and Treatment, 2nd ed. Year Book Medical Publishers, Chicago, 1988, pp 205–231.

254. Simkin PA, Hoover PL, Paxson CS, Wilson WF: Uric acid excretion: Quantitative assessment from spot, midmorning serum and urine samples. Ann Intern Med 91:44, 1979.

255. Coe FL, Moran E, Kavalach AG: The contribution of dietary purine over-consumption to hyperuricosuria in calcium oxalate stone formers. J Chronic Dis 29:793–800, 1976.

256. Lonsdale K: Human stones. Science 159:1199, 1968.

257. Lonsdale K: Epitaxy as a growth factor in urinary calculi and gallstones. Nature 217:56–58, 1968.

258. Mandel NS, Mandel GF: Monosodium urate monohydrate, the gout culprit. J Am Chem Soc 98:2319–2323, 1976.

259. Robertson WG, Marshall RW, Peacock M, Knowles F: The saturation of urine in recurrent, idiopathic stone formers. In Fleisch H, Robertson WG, Smith LH, Vahlensieck W (eds): Urolithiasis Research. Plenum Publishing, London, 1976, p 335.

260. Coe FL, Strauss AL, Tembe V, Le Dun S: Uric acid saturation in calcium nephrolithiasis. Kidney Int 17:662–668, 1980.

261. Pak CYC, Waters O, Arnold L, et al: Mechanism for calcium urolithiasis among patients with hyperuricosuria. J Clin Invest 59:426–431, 1977.

262. Emmerson BT, Graham-Row P: Pathogenesis of the gouty kidney. Kidney Int 8:65, 1975.

263. Finlayson B, DuBois L: Adsorption of heparin on sodium acid urate. Clin Chim Acta 84:203–206, 1978.

264. Grover PK, Ryall RL, Marshall VR: Effect of urate on calcium oxalate crystallization in human urine: Evidence for a promotory role of hyperuricosuria in urolithiasis. Clin Sci 79:9–15, 1990.

265. Grover PK, Ryall RL, Marshall VR: Calcium oxalate crystallization in urine: Role of urate and glycosaminoglycans. Kidney Int 41:149–154, 1992.

266. Coe FL, Kavalach AG: Hypercalciuria and hyperuricosuria in patients with calcium nephrolithiasis. N Engl J Med 291:1344–1350, 1974.

267. Smith MJV: Placebo versus allopurinol for renal calculi. J Urol 117:690–692, 1977.

268. Ettinger B, Tang A, Citron JT, et al: Randomized trial of allopurinol in the prevention of calcium oxalate calculi. N Engl J Med 315:1386–1389, 1986.

269. Finlayson B, Burns J, Smith A, Du Bois L: Effect of oxipurinol and allopurinol riboside on whewellite crystallization: In vitro and in vivo observations. Invest Urol 17:227–229, 1979.

270. Pak CYC, Peterson R: Successful treatment of hyperuricosuric calcium oxalate nephrolithiasis with potassium citrate. Arch Intern Med 146:863–867, 1986.

271. Pak CYC, Sakhaee K, Fuller C: Successful management of uric acid nephrolithiasis with potassium citrate. Kidney Int 30:422–428, 1986.

272. Coe FL, Parks JH: Stone disease in hereditary distal renal tubular acidosis. Ann Intern Med 93:60–61, 1980.

273. Caruana RJ, Buckalew VM Jr: The syndrome of distal (type 1) renal tubular acidosis. Clinical and laboratory findings in 58 cases. Medicine (Baltimore) 67:84–99, 1988.

274. Albright F, Consolazio WV, Coombs FS, et al: Metabolic studies and therapy in a case of nephrocalcinosis with rickets and dwarfism. Bull Johns Hopkins Hosp 66:7, 1940.

275. Baines GH, Barclay JA, Cooke WT: Nephrocalcinosis associated with hyperchloremia and low plasma bicarbonate. Q J Med 14:113, 1945.

276. Albright F, Burnett CH, Parson W, et al: Osteomalacia and late rickets: The various etiologies met in the United States with emphasis on that resulting from a specific form of renal acidosis, the therapeutic indications for each etiological subgroup, and the relationship between osteomalacia and milkman's syndrome. Medicine (Baltimore) 25:399, 1946.

277. Pines KL, Mudge GH: Renal tubular acidosis with osteomalacia. Am J Med 11:302, 1951.

278. Bauld WS, MacDonald SA, Hill MC: Effect of renal tubular acidosis on calcium excretion. Br J Urol 30:285, 1958.

279. Greenberg AJ, McNamara H, McCrory WW: Metabolic balance studies in primary renal tubular acidosis: Effects of acidosis on external calcium and phosphorus balances. J Pediatr 69:610, 1966.

280. Wallach S, Baker RK, Nicastri A: Primary renal tubular acidosis and secondary hyperparathyroidism. Am J Med 52:809, 1972.

281. Weber HP, Gray RW, Dominguez JH, Lemann J Jr: The lack of effect of chronic metabolic acidosis on 25-OH-vitamin D metabolism and serum parathyroid hormone in humans. J Clin Endocrinol Metab 43:1047, 1976.

282. Lemann J Jr, Litzow JR, Lennon EJ: The effects of chronic acid loads in normal man: Further evidence for the participation of bone mineral in the defense against chronic metabolic acidosis. J Clin Invest 45:1608–1614, 1966.

283. Lemann J Jr, Litzow JR, Lennon EJ: Studies of the mechanism by which chronic metabolic acidosis augments urinary calcium excretion in man. J Clin Invest 46:1318–1328, 1967.

284. Lemann J Jr, Lennon EJ, Goodman AD, et al: The net balance of acid in subjects given large loads of acid or alkali. J Clin Invest 44:507–517, 1965.

285. Nash MA, Torrado AD, Greifer I, et al: Renal tubular acidosis in infants and children. J Pediatr 80:738, 1972.

286. Coe FL, Firpo JJ Jr: Evidence for mild reversible hyperparathyroidism in distal renal tubular acidosis. Arch Intern Med 135:1485–1489, 1975.

287. Preminger GM, Sakhaee K, Pak CYC: Hypercalciuria and altered intestinal calcium absorption occurring independently of vitamin D in incomplete distal renal tubular acidosis. Metabolism 36:176–179, 1987.

288. Buckalew VM Jr, Purvis ML, Shulman MG, et al: Hereditary renal tubular acidosis. Medicine (Baltimore) 53:229–254, 1974.

289. Robertson WG, Peacock M, Nordin BEC: Measurement of activity products in urine from stone-formers and normal subjects. In Finlayson B, Hench LC, Smith LH (eds): Urolithiasis: Physical Aspects. National Academy of Science, Washington, DC, 1972, p 79.

290. Hamm LL: Renal handling of citrate. Kidney Int 38:728–735, 1990.

291. Donnelly S, Kamel KS, Vasuvattakul S, et al: Might distal renal tubular acidosis be a proximal tubular cell disorder? Am J Kidney Dis 19:272–281, 1992.

292. Wilansky DC, Schneiderman C: Renal tubular acidosis with recurrent nephrolithiasis and nephrocalcinosis. N Engl J Med 257:399, 1957.

293. Preminger GM, Sakhaee K, Skurla C, Pak CY: Prevention of recurrent calcium stone formation with potassium citrate therapy in patients with distal renal tubular acidosis. J Urol 134:20–23, 1985.

294. McSherry E, Morris RC Jr: Attainment and maintenance of normal stature with alkali therapy in infants and children with classic renal tubular acidosis. J Clin Invest 61:509, 1978.

295. Hodgkinson A: Citric acid excretion in normal adults and in patients with renal calculus. Clin Sci 23:203–212, 1962.

296. Parks JH, Coe FL: A urinary calcium-citrate index for the evaluation of nephrolithiasis. Kidney Int 30:85–90, 1986.

297. Sarada B, Satyanarayana U: Urinary composition in men and women and the risk of urolithiasis. Clin Biochem 24:487–490, 1991.

298. Nikkila M, Koivula T, Jokela H: Urinary citrate excretion in patients with urolithiasis and normal subjects. Eur Urol 16:382–385, 1989.

299. Marangella M, Bianco O, Grande ML, et al: Patterns of citrate excretion in healthy subjects and patterns with idiopathic stone disease. Contrib Nephrol 58:34–38, 1987.

300. Wright EM: Transport of carboxylic acids by renal membrane vesicles. Annu Rev Physiol 47:127–141, 1985.

301. Evans BM, MacIntyre I, MacPherson CR, Milne MD: Alkalosis in sodium and potassium depletion. Clin Sci 16:53–64, 1957.

302. Robertson WG, Scurr DS: Modifiers of calcium oxalate crystallization found in urine. I. Studies with a continuous crystallizer using an artificial urine. J Urol 135:1322–1326, 1986.

303. Nicar MJ, Hill K, Pak CY: Inhibition by citrate of spontaneous precipitation of calcium oxalate in vitro. J Bone Miner Res 2:215–220, 1987.

304. Kok DJ, Papapoulos SE, Bijvoet OLM: Crystal agglomeration is a major element in calcium oxalate urinary stone formation. Kidney Int 37:51–56, 1990.

305. Lemann J Jr, Gray RW, Pleuss JA: Potassium bicarbonate, but not sodium bicarbonate, reduces urinary calcium excretion and improves calcium balance in healthy men. Kidney Int 35:688–695, 1989.

306. Pak CY, Fuller C: Idiopathic hypocitraturic calcium-oxalate nephrolithiasis successfully treated with potassium citrate. Ann Intern Med 104:33–37, 1986.

307. Pak CYC, Peterson R, Sakhaee K, et al: Correction of hypocitraturia and prevention of stone formation by combined thiazide and potassium citrate therapy in thiazide-unresponsive hypercalciuric nephrolithiasis. Am J Med 79:284–288, 1985.

308. Ettinger B: Recent nephrolithiasis: Natural history and effect of phosphate therapy. Am J Med 61:200, 1976.

309. Coe FL, Parks JH: Nephrolithiasis: Pathogenesis and Treatment, 2nd ed. Year Book Medical Publishers, Chicago, 1988, pp 1–37.

310. Smith CH, Thomas WC, Arnaud CD: Orthophosphate therapy in calcium renal lithiasis. In Cifuentes-Delatte L, Rapado A, Hodgkinson A (eds): Urinary Calculi. S Karger, Basel, 1973, p 188.

311. Pak CYC, Holt K, Zerwekh J, Barilla DE: Effects of orthophosphate therapy on the crystallization of calcium salts in urine. Miner Electrolyte Metab 1:147, 1978.

312. Ettinger B, Kolb FO: Inorganic phosphate treatment of nephrolithiasis. Am J Med 55:32, 1973.

313. Bernstein OS, Newton R: The effect of oral sodium phosphate on the formation of renal calculi and on idiopathic hypercalciuria. Lancet 1:1105, 1966.

314. Lau K, Wolf C, Nussbaum P, et al: Differing effects of acid versus neutral phosphate therapy of hypercalciuria. Kidney Int 16:736, 1979.

315. Reiss E, Canterbury JM, Bercovitz MA, Kaplan EL: The role of phosphate in the secretion of parathyroid hormone in man. J Clin Invest 49:2146, 1970.

316. Van Den Berg CJ, Kumar R, Wilson DM, et al: Orthophosphate therapy decreases urinary calcium excretion and serum 1,25-dihydroxyvitamin D concentration in idiopathic hypercalciuria. J Clin Endocrinol Metab 51:998, 1980.

317. Jowsey J, Balasubramanian P: Effects of phosphate supplements on soft tissue calcification and bone turnover. Clin Sci 42:289, 1971.

318. Hodgkinson A: Relations between oxalic acid, calcium, magnesium and creatinine excretion in normal men and male patients with calcium oxalate kidney stones. Clin Sci Mol Med 46:357–367, 1974.

319. Wilson DM, Smith LH, Erickson SB, et al: Renal oxalate handling in normal subjects and patients with idiopathic renal lithiasis: Primary and secondary hyperoxaluria. In Walker VR, Sutton RAL, Cameron ECB, et al (eds): Urolithaisis. Plenum Publishing, New York, 1989, pp 453–455.

320. Schwille PO, Manoharan M, Rumenapf G, et al: Oxalate measurement in the picomol range by ion chromatography: Values in fasting plasma and urine of controls and patients with idiopathic calcium urolithiasis. J Clin Chem Clin Biochem 27:87–96, 1989.

321. Hodgkinson A, Wilkinson R: Plasma oxalate concentration and renal excretion of oxalate in man. Clin Sci Mol Med 46:61–73, 1974.

322. Williams HE, Johnson GA, Smith LH Jr: The renal clearance of oxalate in normal subjects and patients with primary hyperoxaluria. Clin Sci 41:213–218, 1971.

323. Hagler L, Herman RH: Oxalate metabolism. I. Am J Clin Nutr 26:758–765, 1973.

324. Lemann J Jr, Hornick LJ, Pleuss JA, Gray RW: Oxalate is overestimated in alkaline urine collected during administration of bicarbonate with no specimen pH adjustment. Clin Chem 35:2107–2110, 1989.

325. Urivetzky M, Kessaris D, Smith AD: Ascorbic acid overdosing: A risk factor for calcium oxalate nephrolithiasis. J Urol 147:1215–1218, 1992.

326. Hagler L, Herman RH: Oxalate metabolism. II. Am J Clin Nutr 26:882–889, 1973.

327. Danpure CJ: Molecular and clinical heterogeneity in primary hyperoxaluria type I. Am J Kidney Dis 17:366–369, 1991.

328. Cooper PJ, Danpure CJ, Wise PJ, Guttridge KM: Immunocytochemical localization of human hepatic alanine: glyoxylate aminotransferase in control subjects and patients with primary hyperoxaluria type 1. J Histochem Cytochem 36:1285–1294, 1988.

329. Danpure CJ, Cooper PJ, Wise PJ, Jennings PR: An enzyme trafficking defect in two patients with primary hyperoxaluria type 1: Peroxisomal alanine/glyoxylate aminotransferase rerouted to mitochondria. J Cell Biol 108:1345–1352, 1989.

330. Williams HE, Smith LH: L-Glyceric aciduria. A new genetic variant of primary hyperoxaluria. N Engl J Med 278:233–239, 1968.

331. Mistry J, Danpure CJ, Chalmers RA: Hepatic D-glycerate dehydrogenase and glyoxalate reductase deficiency in primary hyperoxaluria type 2. Biochem Soc Trans 16:626–627, 1988.

332. Williams HE, Smith LH Jr: Primary hyperoxaluria. In Stanbury JP, Wyngaarden JB, Fredrickson DS (eds): The Metabolic Basis of Inherited Disease, 5th ed. McGraw-Hill, New York, 1972, p 196.

333. Hockaday TDR, Frederick EW, Clayton JE, Smith LH Jr: Studies on primary hyperoxaluria II: Urinary oxalate, glycolate, and glyoxylate measurement by isotope dilution methods. J Lab Clin Med 65:677–687, 1965.

334. Danpure CJ, Jennings PR, Watts RWE: Enzymological diagnosis of primary hyperoxaluria type 1 by measurement of hepatic alanine:glyoxalate aminotransferase activity. Lancet 1:289–291, 1987.

335. Yendt ER, Cohanim M: Response to a physiologic dose of pyridoxine in type I primary hyperoxaluria. N Engl J Med 312:953–957, 1985.

336. Watts RWE, Chalmers RA, Gibbs DA, et al: Studies on some possible biochemical treatments of primary hyperoxaluria. Q J Med 48:259–272, 1979.

337. Smith LH Jr, Williams HE: Treatment of primary hyperoxaluria. Mod Treat 4:522–530, 1967.

338. Leumann E, Hoppe B, Neuhaus T: Management of primary hyperoxaluria: Efficacy of oral citrate administration. Pediatr Nephrol 7:207–211, 1993.

339. Zarembski PM, Hodgkinson A: The oxalic acid content of English diets. Br J Nutr 16:627, 1962.

340. Dobbins JW, Binder HJ: Importance of colon in enteric hyperoxaluria. N Engl J Med 296:298, 1977.

341. Binder HJ: Intestinal oxalate absorption. Gastroenterology 67:441–446, 1974.

342. Chadwick VS, Elias E, Bell GD, Dowling RH: The role of bile acids in the increased intestinal absorption of oxalate after ileal resection. In Matern S, Hackenschmidt J, Bach P, Gerok W (eds): Advances in Bile Acid Research, III, Bile Acid Meeting. FK Schattauer Verlag, Stuttgart, 1975, p 435.

343. Fairclough PD, Feest TG, Chadwick VS, Clark ML: Effect of sodium chenodeoxycholate on oxalate absorption from the excluded human colon—a mechanism for "enteric" hypercalciuria. Gut 18:240, 1977.

344. Earnest DL, Gaucher S, Admirand WH: Treatment of enteric hyperoxaluria with calcium and aluminum. Gastroenterology 70:881A, 1976.

345. Saunders DR, Sillery J, McDonald GB: Regional differences in oxalate absorption by rat intestine: Evidence for excessive absorption by the colon in steatorrhoea. Gut 16:543–554, 1975.

346. Kathpalia SC, Favus MJ, Coe FL: Evidence for size and charge permselectivity of rat ascending colon: Effects of ricinoleate and bile

salts on oxalic acid and neutral sugar transport. J Clin Invest 74:805–811, 1984.

347. Chadwick VS, Modha K, Dowling RH: Mechanism for hyperoxaluria in patients with ileal dysfunction. N Engl J Med 289:172, 1973.

348. Smith LH: Enteric hyperoxaluria and other hyperoxaluric states. *In* Coe FL, Brenner BM, Stein JH (eds): Contemporary Issues in Nephrology, Vol VI, Nephrolithiasis. Churchill Livingstone, New York, 1980, p 136.

349. Dowling RH, Rose GA, Sutor DJ: Hyperoxaluria and renal calculi in ileal disease. Lancet 1:1103, 1971.

350. Smith LH, Fromm H, Hoffman AF: Acquired hyperoxaluria, nephrolithiasis and intestinal disease. N Engl J Med 286:1371, 1972.

351. Stauffer JQ, Stewart RJ, Bertand G: Acquired hyperoxaluria: Relationship to dietary calcium content and severity of steatorrhea. Gastroenterology 66:783A, 1974.

352. Earnest DL, Johnson G, Williams HE, Admirand WH: Hyperoxaluria in patients with ileal resection: An abnormality in dietary oxalate absorption. Gastroenterology 77:1114, 1974.

353. Atsman A, DeVries A, Frank M: Uric Acid Lithiasis. Elsevier Publishing, Amsterdam, 1963.

354. Yu TF, Gutman AB: Uric acid nephrolithiasis in gout. Predisposing factors. Ann Intern Med 67:1133, 1967.

355. Hall AP, Berry PE, Dawber TR, McNamara PM: Epidemiology of gout and hyperuricemia. A long-term population study. Am J Med 42:27, 1967.

356. Fessel WJ: Renal outcomes of gout and hyperuricemia. Am J Med 67:74, 1979.

357. Gutman AB, Yu TF: Urinary ammonium excretion in primary gout. J Clin Invest 44:1474, 1965.

358. Elliot JS, Sharp RF, Lewis L: Urinary pH. J Urol 81:339, 1959.

359. Gutman AB, Yu TF: An abnormality in glutamine metabolism in primary gout. Am J Med 35:820, 1963.

360. Sorensen LB: The elimination of uric acid in man studied by means of $^{14}$C-labelled uric acid. Scand J Clin Lab Invest 12(suppl 54):1, 1960.

361. DeVries A, Frank M, Atsman A: Inherited uric acid lithiasis. Am J Med 33:880, 1962.

362. Seegmiller JE, Grayzel AI, Laster L, Liddle L: Uric acid production in gout. J Clin Invest 40:1304, 1961.

363. Bambach CP, Robertson WG, Peacock M, Hill GL: Effect of intestinal surgery on the risk of stone formation. Gut 22:257–263, 1981.

364. Clarke AM, McKenzie RG: Ileostomy and the risk of urinary uric acid stones. Lancet 2:395–397, 1969.

365. Crane C, Lassen UV: The action of probenecid (p-[di-N-propylsulphamylbenzoic acid]) on uric acid excretion and plasma uric acid level in normal human subjects. Acta Pharmacol (KBH) 11:295, 1955.

366. Fox IH, Wyngaarden JB, Kelley WN: Depletion of erythrocyte phosphoribosylpyrophosphate in man. A newly observed effect of allopurinol. N Engl J Med 283:1177, 1970.

367. Stote RM, Smith LH, Dubb JW, et al: Oxypurinol nephrolithiasis in regional enteritis secondary to allopurinol therapy. Ann Intern Med 92:384–385, 1980.

368. Gomez GA, Stutzman L, Chu TM: Xanthine nephropathy during chemotherapy in deficiency of hypoxanthine-guanine phosphoribosyltransferase. Arch Intern Med 138:1017, 1978.

369. Kranen S, Keough D, Gordon RB, Emmerson BT: Xanthine-containing calculi during allopurinol therapy. J Urol 133:658–659, 1985.

370. Crawhall JC, Purkiss P, Watts RWE, Young EP: The excretion of amino acids by cystinuric patients and their relatives. Ann Hum Genet 33:149, 1969.

371. Hambraeus L: Comparative studies of the value of two cyanide-nitroprusside methods in the diagnosis of cystinuria. Scand J Clin Lab Invest 15:657, 1963.

372. Dent CE, Senior B, Walshe JM: The pathogenesis of cystinuria. II. Polarographic studies of the metabolism of sulfur-containing amino acids. J Clin Invest 33:1216, 1954.

373. Arrow VK, Westall RG: Amino acid clearance in cystinuria. J Physiol (Lond) 142:141, 1958.

374. Rosenberg LE, Downing SJ, Segal S: Competitive inhibition of dibasic amino acid transport in rat kidney. J Biol Chem 237:2265, 1962.

375. Fox M, Thier SO, Rosenberg LE, et al: Evidence against a single renal transport defect in cystinuria. N Engl J Med 270:556, 1964.

376. Hellier MD, Holdsworth CD, Perrett D: Dibasic amino acid absorption in man. Gastroenterology 65:613, 1973.

377. Rosenberg LE, Downing S, Durant JL, Segal S: Cystinuria: Biochemical evidence for three genetically distinct diseases. J Clin Invest 45:365, 1966.

378. Whelan DT, Schriver CR: Hyperdibasicaminoaciduria, an inherited disease of amino acid transport. Pediatr Res 2:525, 1968.

379. Stephens AD, Perrett D: Cystinuria: A new genetic variant. Clin Sci Mol Med 51:27, 1976.

380. Evans WP, Resnick MI, Boyce WH: Homozygous cystinuria—evaluation of 35 patients. J Urol 127:707–709, 1982.

381. Sakhaee K, Poindexter JR, Pak CYC: The spectrum of metabolic abnormalities in patients with cystine nephrolithiasis. J Urol 141:819–821, 1989.

382. Resnick MJ, Goodman HO, Boyce WH: Heterozygous cystinuria and calcium oxalate urolithiasis. J Urol 122:52, 1979.

383. Kolb FO, Earle JM, Harper HA: Disappearance of cystinuria in a patient treated with prolonged low methionine diet. Metabolism 16:378, 1967.

384. Rodman JS, Blackburn P, Williams JJ, et al: The effect of dietary protein on cystine excretion in patients with cystinuria. Clin Nephrol 22:273–278, 1984.

385. Martensson J, Denneberg T, Lindell A, Textorius O: Sulfur amino acid metabolism in cystinuria: A biochemical and clinical study of patients. Kidney Int 37:143–149, 1990.

386. Jaeger P, Portman L, Saunders A, et al: Anticystinuric effects of glutamine and of dietary sodium restriction. N Engl J Med 315:1120–1123, 1986.

387. Norman RW, Manette WA: Dietary restriction of sodium as a means of reducing urinary cystine. J Urol 143:1193–1195, 1990.

388. Miyagi K, Nakada F, Ohshiro S: Effect of glutamine on cystine excretion in a patient with cystinuria. N Engl J Med 301:196, 1979.

389. Pak CYC, Fuller C, Sakhaee K, et al: Management of cystine nephrolithiasis with alpha-mercaptopropionylglycine. J Urol 136:1003–1008, 1986.

390. Perazella MA, Buller GK: Successful treatment of cystinuria with captopril. Am J Kidney Dis 21:504–507, 1993.

391. Sloand JA, Lizzo JL Jr: Captopril reduces urinary cystine excretion in cystinuria. Arch Intern Med 147:1409–1412, 1987.

392. Dretler SP: Stone fragility—a new therapeutic distinction. J Urol 139:1124, 1988.

393. Singer A, Das S: Cystinuria: A review of the pathophysiology and management. J Urol 142:669–673, 1989.

394. Martin X, Salas M, Laebeeuw M, et al: Cystine stones: The impact of new treatment. Br J Urol 68:234–239, 1991.

395. Chute R, Suby HI: Prevalence and importance of urea-splitting bacterial infections of the urinary tract in the formation of calculi. J Urol 44:590, 1943.

396. Griffith DP, Gibson JR, Clinton C, Musher DM: Acetohydroxamic acid: Clinical studies of a urease inhibitor in patients with staghorn renal calculi. J Urol 119:9, 1978.

397. Robertson WG, Peacock M: Calcium oxalate crystalluria and inhibitors of crystallization in recurrent renal stone formers. Clin Sci 43:499–506, 1972.

398. Elliot JS, Sharp RF, Lewis L: The solubility of struvite in urine. J Urol 80:169, 1959.

399. Griffith DP, Osborne CA: Infection (urease) stones. Miner Electrolyte Metab 13:278–285, 1977.

400. Farmer JJ, Davis BR, Hickman-Brenner FW: Biochemical identification of new species and biogroups of Enterobacteriaceae isolated from clinical specimens. J Clin Microbiol 21:46–76, 1985.

401. Hedelin H, Brorson JE, Grenabo L, et al: *Ureaplasma urealyticum* and upper urinary tract stones. Br J Urol 56:244–249, 1984.

402. Kristensen C, Parks JH, Lindheimer M, Coe FL: Reduced glomerular filtration rate and hypercalciuria in primary struvite nephrolithiasis. Kidney Int 32:749–753, 1987.

403. Wojewski A, Zajaczkowski T: The treatment of bilateral staghorn calculi of the kidneys. Int Urol Nephrol 5:249, 1974.

404. Singh M, Chapman R, Tressider GC, Blandy J: The fate of the unoperated staghorn calculus. Br J Urol 45:581, 1973.

405. Silverman DE, Stamey TA: Management of infection stones: The Stanford experience. Medicine (Baltimore) 62:44–51, 1983.

406. Kerlan RK, Kahn RK, Laberge JM, et al: Percutaneous removal of renal staghorn calculi. AJR 145:797–801, 1985.

407. Segura JW, Patterson DE, LeRoy AJ, et al: Percutaneous removal of kidney stones: Review of 1000 cases. J Urol 134:1077–1081, 1985.

408. Patterson DE, Segura JW, LeRoy AJ: Long-term follow-up of pa-

tients treated by percutaneous ultrasonic lithotripsy for struvite stag-horn calculi. J Endourol 1:177, 1987.

409. Michaels EK, Fowler JE Jr: Extracorporeal shock wave lithotripsy for struvite renal calculi: Prospective study with extended followup. J Urol 146:728–732, 1991.

410. Miller K, Bachor R, Sauter T, Hautmann R: ESWL monotherapy for large stones and staghorn calculi. Urol Int 45:95–98, 1990.

411. Segura JW: The role of percutaneous surgery in renal and ureteral stone removal. J Urol 141:780–781, 1989.

412. Stamey TA: Urinary Infections. Williams & Wilkins, Baltimore, 1972, p 213.

413. Griffith DP, Musher DM: Acetohydroxamic acid: Potential use in urinary infections caused by urea-splitting bacteria. Urology 5:299, 1975.

414. Griffith DP, Khonsari F, Skurnick JH, James KE: A randomized trial

of acetohydroxamic acid for the treatment and prevention of infec-tion-induced urinary stones in spinal cord injury patients. J Urol 140:318–324, 1988.

415. Williams JJ, Rodman JS, Peterson CM: A randomized double blind study of acetohydroxamic acid in struvite nephrolithiasis. N Engl J Med 311:760–764, 1984.

416. Griffith DP, Gleeson MJ, Lee H, et al: Randomized, double-blind trial of Lithostat (acetohydroxamic acid) in the palliative treatment of infection-induced urinary calculi. Eur Urol 20:243–247, 1991.

417. Jacobs SP, Gittes RF: Dissolution of residual renal calculi with hemiacidrin. J Urol 115:2, 1976.

418. Brock WA, Nachtscheim DA, Parsons CL: Hemiacidrin irrigation of renal pelvic calculi in patients with ileal conduit urinary diversion. J Urol 123:345, 1980.

# Urinary Tract Obstruction

*Gary C. Curhan*
*Mark L. Zeidel*

Adequate elimination of soluble wastes and toxins from the body through the urinary tract is essential to survival. On average, 1.5 to 2 L of urine flows daily from the renal papilla to the exterior in an uninterrupted, unidirectional flow, which necessitates the proper interactions of ureter, bladder, and urethra. Any obstruction that interrupts this orderly flow of urine may cause a build-up of urine volume and pressure that may damage the kidney and interfere with its integral functions of waste excretion and fluid and electrolyte homeostasis. Early recognition and treatment are essential because recovery of renal function is inversely related to both the duration and completeness of the obstruction. Fortunately, urinary tract obstruction represents a potentially curable form of kidney disease.

Although several terms are commonly applied in the presence of urinary obstruction, their definitions vary.[1, 2] Hydronephrosis is a dilatation of the renal calyces and pelvis proximal to the point of obstruction. Obstructive uropathy refers to the presence of an impediment to urine flow due to any structural or functional change occurring anywhere from the renal pelvis to the tip of the urethra that necessitates an increase in proximal pressure to transport the urine past the point of obstruction, with or without associated renal parenchymal damage. Obstructive nephropathy describes any functional and pathologic changes in the kidney that result from urinary tract obstruction.

## PREVALENCE AND INCIDENCE

The frequency of occurrence of urinary tract obstruction depends on many factors, including age, sex, and concurrent medical conditions. Unfortunately, few studies define true incidence (the number of new cases that occur during a specified period of time) or prevalence (the proportion of people with urinary tract obstruction at a specific point in time). Reported frequencies have been based on selected populations, such as autopsy series and high-risk pregnancies. However, no data are available for an unselected population.

In a retrospective review of 59,064 autopsy studies of patients ranging in age from birth to 80 years, the frequency of hydronephrosis was 3.1% (2.9% in female patients and 3.3% in male patients).[3] No great differences by sex were found until age 20 years. Between the ages of 20 and 60 years, urinary tract obstruction was more common in women than in men owing predominantly to pregnancy and uterine cancer. Above the age of 60 years, urinary tract obstruction was more common in men because of prostatic disease. In the group younger than 10 years of age, representing 1.5% of the autopsy examinations, the principal causes of urinary tract obstruction were stricture of the ureters or urethra and neurologic abnormalities. However, it is unclear what proportion of these findings were clinically recognized or merely incidental discoveries.

In an autopsy series of 15,919 children ranging in age from birth to 15 years, the frequency of obstruction was 2%.[4] Hydronephrosis was demonstrated in 2.2% of the boys and 1.5% of the girls, and 80% of the patients with hydronephrosis were younger than 12 months of age. As in the preceding study, the proportion of clinically recognized cases remains unknown.

The overall proportion of individuals who have urinary tract obstruction is probably higher than these reports suggest. Several common but temporary causes of obstruction, such as renal calculi and pregnancy, contribute to this underestimate.

## CLASSIFICATION

Urinary tract obstruction may be classified by duration, location, and degree.[5] Duration may be acute, subacute, or chronic. Acute obstruction is characterized by its short duration of hours to days and typically abrupt onset, such as with obstruction due to a kidney stone or unintentional surgical ligation of the ureter. Subacute urinary tract obstruction develops over a period of days to weeks and may be characterized by an insidious onset, such as in the case of pregnancy. In contrast, chronic obstruction, frequently due to bladder outlet obstruction secondary to benign prostatic hyperplasia or prostate cancer, develops over many months to years.

In addition, the location of the obstruction influences the clinical presentation and course. Obstruction may occur anywhere from the level of the renal tubules to the urethral meatus. Finally, the severity of urinary tract obstruction may be classified as high grade, denoting complete occlusion of the lumen with no passage of urine, or low grade, denoting incomplete or partial obstruction.

## ETIOLOGY

To understand urinary tract obstruction, it is useful to discuss etiology in terms of congenital and acquired (intrinsic and extrinsic) causes.

### Congenital Causes of Obstruction

Any site along the urinary tract from the ureteropelvic junction to the urethral meatus may be obstructed by a congenital abnormality, with resultant unilateral or bilateral obstruction (Table 41–1). Although each individual lesion is rare, as a group these abnormalities constitute an important cause of urinary tract obstruction, particularly in young patients in whom they represent a major cause of end-stage renal disease.[6]

**TABLE 41–1. Congenital Causes of Urinary Tract Obstruction by Location**

**Ureteropelvic Junction**
Ureteropelvic junction obstruction

**Proximal and Middle Ureter**
Ureteral folds
Ureteral valves
Strictures
Benign fibroepithelial polyps
Retrocaval ureter

**Distal Ureter**
Ureterovesical junction obstruction
Vesicoureteral reflux
Prune-belly syndrome
Ureteroceles

**Bladder**
Bladder diverticula
Neurologic conditions (e.g., meningomyelocele)

**Urethra**
Posterior urethral valves
Urethral diverticula
Anterior urethral valves
Urethral atresia

Ureteropelvic junction obstruction is the most common cause of hydronephrosis in fetuses[7] and young children,[8] with a reported incidence of 5 cases/100,000 population per year,[9] and may be seen in adults[10, 11] as well. In fact, at the Mayo Clinic, it was found that more than 50% of patients with congenital ureteropelvic junction obstruction were older than 20 years.[9] Although most cases of ureteropelvic junction obstruction appear to develop spontaneously, familial forms exist as well.[12] Two thirds of the cases occur in males, and about 60% are on the left side. In the age group younger than 1 year, 20% of cases are bilateral.[13] Whereas the majority are now diagnosed prenatally by ultrasonography,[13] the most common clinical presentation in neonates is as an abdominal or flank mass.[14] In contrast, adults generally present with flank pain.[10, 11] Symptoms of intermittent obstruction can mimic gastrointestinal disease and thus delay diagnosis. In any age group, ureteropelvic junction obstruction may also be associated with hematuria, recurrent urinary tract infection, kidney stones, and hypertension.[9–11]

A frequently found defect in patients with congenital ureteropelvic junction obstruction is an aperistaltic segment of the ureter with an inability to propagate the urine distally from the renal pelvis.[15] Less commonly, the obstruction is due to a ureteral stricture.[15] On histopathologic examination, a spectrum of abnormalities at the ureteropelvic junction is seen. By light microscopy, the findings range from no identifiable abnormality to decreased muscle bulk, malorientation of the muscle fibers, and infiltration by inflammatory cells.[16] Electron microscopy typically demonstrates an abundance of collagen.[16] An apparent association between abnormal angulation of the ureter and aberrant renal vessels suggests that the functional defect may be a secondary process,[13, 17] but this remains controversial.[18]

Obstruction may also occur at several points between the proximal and middle ureter. Obstruction due to a ureteral fold, a noncircumferential area of redundant mucosa, is generally asymptomatic and usually disappears as the child grows.[19] Ureteral valves, consisting of transverse folds of redundant mucosa that contain smooth muscle, are an uncommon cause of obstruction and may be associated with other genitourinary anomalies.[20, 21] Congenital strictures[22] and benign fibroepithelial polyps[23] may also be obstructive. Abnormal development of the venous system with obstruction of the right ureter by the inferior vena cava may occur.[24] A retrocaval ureter produces the classic "reversed J" sign or "fishhook" deformity on the intravenous urogram. It is usually right sided, partial, and initially asymptomatic; thus, it is generally undetected until adult life. Diagnosis is usually made after the fourth decade and occurs three times more frequently in men. These patients experience chronic urinary tract infections and usually present with intermittent abdominal pain that often mimics renal colic.

Congenital anomalies of the distal ureter also represent important causes of obstruction. Ureterovesical junction obstruction, a functional defect similar to ureteropelvic junction obstruction, is the second most common cause of congenital ureteral obstruction.[25] This entity often results in enormous enlargement of the involved ureter and is one cause of congenital megaureter.[26, 27] Vesicoureteral reflux, an anatomic abnormality of the ureterovesical junction, may also cause a congenitally enlarged ureter and may be due to a dysmorphic ureter or an abnormally positioned ureteral orifice or may be secondary to bladder outflow obstruction.[28] Megaureter is also associated with the prune-belly syndrome, a triad of the absence of abdominal musculature, ureteral dilatation, and bilateral cryptorchidism.[29, 30] A ureterocele, a congenital cystic dilatation of the terminal portion of the ureter, may obstruct the ureteral orifice.[31] Ureteroceles can be ectopic, with the ureter emptying at a site other than the lateral angle of the trigone, and are most commonly associated with a duplicated collecting system.[31, 32] Less commonly, a ureterocele may be orthotopic.[33] Orthotopic ureteroceles that cause obstruction during childhood tend to be large enough to obstruct both ureters; thus, their prognosis is worse than for those discovered in adults.[33]

Bladder outlet obstruction may be mechanical, such as a congenital bladder diverticulum that obstructs one or both ureters,[34] or functional, as a result of congenital neurologic conditions.[35, 36] Myelodysplasias, typically myelomeningocele with or without hydrocephalus, are associated with a 10% frequency of hydronephrosis at birth. Because hydronephrosis develops in an additional 15% of these patients in the period of the next few years,[37] careful follow-up is imperative.[35]

At the level of the urethra, posterior urethral valves, seen exclusively in boys, are the most common congenital cause of obstruction.[38] Because of the highly variable presentation of this lesion, its exact prevalence is unknown. Although posterior urethral valves usually present during childhood,[39] they may also be discovered in adults.[40] Diagnosis is best made by voiding cystourethrogram, and in cases of severe obstruction, early surgical intervention may prevent the development of renal failure.[39] Urethral diverticula, another cause of urethral obstruction, occurs most commonly in girls.[41]

The role of fetal[42, 43] and newborn[43, 44] surgery for the relief of obstruction remains controversial,[45] with reports of a high frequency of operative complications by some[46] but not all[47] centers. Although bilateral obstruction requires intervention, the simple presence of unilateral hydronephrosis does not necessitate surgery. The primary indications for surgery are symptoms of obstruction or impaired function in a presumably salvageable hydronephrotic kidney (see later).

## Acquired Causes of Obstruction

### INTRINSIC CAUSES

Acquired causes of obstruction may be intrinsic or extrinsic to the urinary tract (Table 41–2). Intrinsic causes may result from intraluminal or intramural processes.

Intraluminal processes that cause obstruction may be intrarenal, involving the formation of crystals or casts, or extrarenal. Intrarenal causes include uric acid nephropathy,[48] sulfonamide[49] or acyclovir[50] crystal deposition, and multiple myeloma.[51] Uric acid nephropathy is usually seen as a complication of the use of alkylating agents in the treatment of patients with hematologic malignant neo-

plasms, and the risk of its development is directly related to the plasma uric acid concentration[48] (see Chapter 28). It may also occur with disseminated adenomatous carcinoma of the gastrointestinal tract.[52] Newer sulfonamides are more soluble in acid urine than were earlier preparations, so that sulfonamide crystal deposition is now rarely seen. However, sulfadiazine is often used in high doses for the treatment of toxoplasmosis in patients with acquired immunodeficiency syndrome and has been associated with intrarenal crystallization and acute renal failure.[49, 53] The obstructive effects of casts composed of Bence Jones proteins or their toxic effect on tubule epithelium results in a high mortality rate in patients with multiple myeloma and acute renal failure.[51] In fact, as a result of renal damage due to the Bence Jones proteins and other concomitant abnormalities frequently seen in patients with multiple myeloma, such as hypercalcemia and amyloidosis, renal failure is the second most common cause of death in these patients.[51] Multiple myeloma may also present as obstructive uropathy with proteinaceous precipitates within the renal pelvis causing unilateral hydronephrosis.[54]

Several extrarenal, or intraureteral, processes may also result in obstruction. Nephrolithiasis is the most common cause of ureteral obstruction in younger men (Fig. 41–1). Twelve percent of the U.S. population will form a stone at some time,[55] with a male/female ratio of 3:1. Calcium oxalate stones are the most common type formed, and when they cause obstruction, it tends to be acute and intermittent with no long-term effect on renal function. A stone obstructing a solitary kidney, however, can cause anuric acute renal failure. Less common types of stones, such as struvite and cystine stones, are more frequently associated with renal damage. Typical sites at which a stone can obstruct the flow of urine include the ureteropelvic junction, the pelvic brim (where the ureter begins to arch over the iliac vessels), and the ureterovesical junction.

Other processes that cause ureteral obstruction include papillary necrosis[56] resulting from sickle cell trait or disease, analgesic abuse, amyloidosis, acute pyelonephritis, and diabetes mellitus. Blood clots, such as those that may accompany hematuria in patients with polycystic kidney disease, may also cause obstruction.

In addition, several intramural processes may be classified as acquired intrinsic causes of obstruction. Functional abnormalities, such as those associated with neurologic dysfunction[57] seen in diabetes mellitus, multiple sclerosis, spinal cord injury, cerebrovascular disease, and Parkinson disease, can be caused by upper motor neuron damage that produces involuntary micturition (spastic bladder dysfunction) or lower spinal tract injury that results in a flaccid, atonic bladder. Various drugs have been associated with extrarenal obstructive uropathy. Functional obstruction may be caused by anticholinergic agents,[58] which decrease bladder contractility, or by levodopa[59] because of its α-adrenergic–mediated increase in bladder outlet resistance. Renal damage may then result as a consequence of recurrent urinary tract infections and back-pressure produced by the accumulation of residual urine. Anatomic abnormalities include ureteral strictures, urethral strictures, and malignant and benign tumors of the renal pelvis, ureter, and bladder. Ureteral strictures may occur as a result of radiation therapy

**TABLE 41–2. Acquired Causes of Urinary Tract Obstruction**

| | |
|---|---|
| **Intrinsic Processes** | **Extrinsic Processes** *Continued* |
| ***Intraluminal*** | ***Malignant Neoplasms*** |
| Intrarenal | Genitourinary tract |
|   Uric acid nephropathy |   Tumors of the kidney, ureter, bladder, or urethra |
|   Sulfonamides | Other sites |
|   Acyclovir |   Metastatic spread |
|   Multiple myeloma |   Direct extension |
| Extrarenal (intraureteral) | ***Gastrointestinal System*** |
|   Nephrolithiasis | Crohn disease |
|   Papillary necrosis | Appendicitis |
|   Blood clots | Diverticulitis |
|   Fungus balls | Chronic pancreatitis with pseudocyst formation |
| ***Intramural*** | Acute pancreatitis |
| Functional (e.g., neurogenic bladder) | ***Vascular System*** |
|   Diseases | Arterial aneurysms |
|     Diabetes mellitus |   Abdominal aortic aneurysm |
|     Multiple sclerosis |   Iliac artery aneurysm |
|     Cerebrovascular disease | Venous |
|     Spinal cord injury |   Ovarian vein thrombophlebitis |
|     Parkinson disease | Vasculitides |
|   Drugs |   Systemic lupus erythematosus |
|     Anticholinergic agents |   Polyarteritis nodosa |
|     Levodopa (α-adrenergic properties) |   Wegener granulomatosis |
| Anatomic |   Schönlein-Henoch purpura |
|   Ureteral strictures | ***Retroperitoneal Processes*** |
|     Schistosomiasis | Fibrosis |
|     Tuberculosis |   Idiopathic |
|     Drugs (e.g., nonsteroidal anti-inflammatory agents) |   Drug-induced |
|     Ureteral instrumentation |   Inflammatory |
|   Urethral strictures |     Ascending lymphangitis of the lower extremities |
|   Benign or malignant tumors of the renal pelvis, ureter, or bladder |     Chronic urinary tract infection |
| **Extrinsic Processes** |     Tuberculosis |
| ***Reproductive Tract*** |     Sarcoidosis |
| Females |   Iatrogenic |
|   Uterus |     Multiple abdominal surgical procedures |
|     Pregnancy | Enlarged retroperitoneal nodes |
|     Tumor | Tumor invasion |
|       Fibroids | Tumor mass |
|       Endometrial adenocarcinoma | Hemorrhage |
|       Carcinoma of the cervix | Urinoma |
|     Endometriosis | ***Biologic Agents*** |
|     Uterine prolapse | Actinomycosis |
|     Ureteral ligation (surgical) | |
|   Ovary | |
|     Tubo-ovarian abscess | |
|     Tumor | |
|     Cyst | |
| Male | |
|   Benign prostatic hyperplasia | |
|   Adenocarcinoma of the prostate | |

in patients with cervical cancer[60] or a result of analgesic abuse.[61] In addition, ureteral strictures may occur as a complication of ureteral instrumentation or surgery, such as cystoscopy, ureteroscopy, or ureterolithotomy.

Certain biologic agents may produce intrinsic obstruction of the urinary tract. Around the world, nearly 100 million people may be infected with *Schistosoma haematobium*; in 10 to 40 million, it may cause obstructive uropathy.[62] Active schistosomal infection is readily treatable, and the obstructive uropathy may resolve. Left untreated, chronic schistosomiasis (also known as bilharziasis) can lead to irreversible ureteral or bladder fibrosis and obstruction.[63] Five percent of patients with tuberculosis have genitourinary involvement,[64] with predominantly unilateral tubercu-

lous stricture of the ureter.[65] Mycoses, such as *Candida albicans* infection, have increasingly been associated with obstruction due to invasion of the ureteral wall or intraluminal obstruction (fungus ball).[66]

## EXTRINSIC CAUSES

Acquired extrinsic causes of urinary tract obstruction are many and varied (see Table 41–2). Processes affecting the female reproductive tract are a frequent cause of obstructive uropathy. In fact, urinary tract obstruction occurs with greater frequency in young adult women than in men primarily because of the obstructive processes associated with pregnancy and pelvic malignant neoplasms.[2] More than two

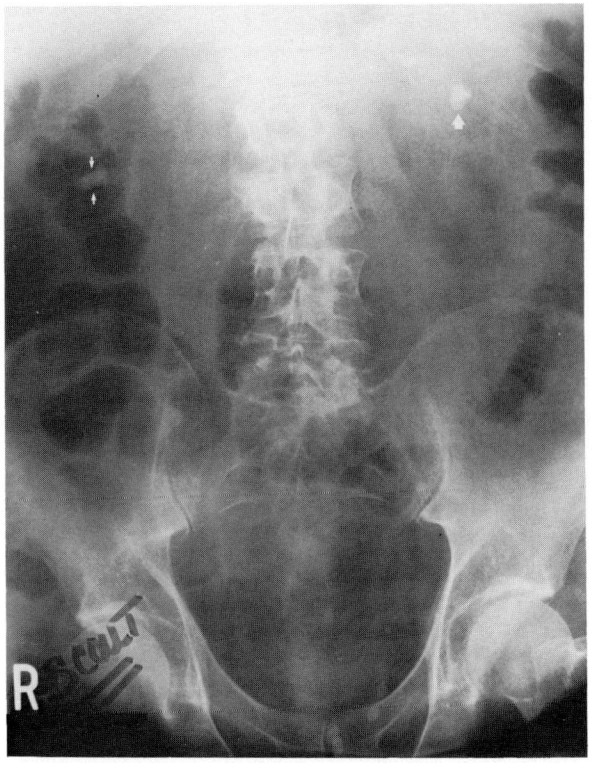

**Figure 41–1.** Kidney, ureter, and bladder film of a man presenting with left flank pain and a fever. The film reveals a calcification overlying the left kidney *(large arrow)*, which was found to be obstructing the left ureter by intravenous urogram. An asymptomatic stone was also seen in the right kidney *(small arrows)*.

thirds of pregnant women entering their third trimester display some degree of dilatation of the collecting system,[67, 68] most likely due to mechanical ureteral compression[69] usually at the pelvic brim and affecting the right side more often than the left.[67] The vast majority resolve soon after delivery.[70] Clinically significant obstruction is almost always accompanied by flank pain.[71] In these cases, ultrasonography may be a useful screening test; if obstruction is suspected, a diuresis renogram (see later) will result in less radiation exposure to the fetus than an intravenous urogram will.[72] Although bilateral obstruction during pregnancy can cause acute renal failure, it is rare.[55, 71] Those pregnancies most often associated with obstructive acute renal failure are characterized by the presence of polyhydramnios, twins, incarcerated gravid uterus, or a solitary kidney.[73]

Pelvic malignant neoplasms represent the second most common cause of extrinsic obstructive uropathy in women, particularly adenocarcinoma of the cervix.[74] In older women, uterine prolapse is another gynecologic cause of obstruction, with hydronephrosis developing in approximately 5% of patients.[75] A possible mechanism may be compression of the ureter by uterine blood vessels. Urinary tract infection, sepsis, pyonephrosis, and renal insufficiency have all been reported in association with uterine prolapse. Posthysterectomy vaginal prolapse may result in obstruction as well.[76] Benign pelvic masses, such as fibroid uterus or cystic ovary, may cause obstruction with increasing frequency as the size of the mass increases.[77] Pelvic inflam-

matory disease, particularly a tubo-ovarian abscess, may result in obstruction as well.[78]

Although endometriosis only rarely causes ureteral obstruction, it should be suspected in any premenopausal woman presenting with obstruction. The onset may be subtle, and the process is usually confined to the pelvic portion of the ureter.[79] Ureteral involvement may be intrinsic or extrinsic; extrinsic compression is primarily due to adhesions associated with endometriosis. Because ureteral obstruction is often unsuspected, the routine use of excretory urography is advisable for earlier diagnosis,[80] particularly in patients with advanced endometriosis undergoing surgery.[79] Notably, whereas many forms of abdominal or retroperitoneal surgery may result in inadvertent ligation of the ureter or ureteral injury, 52% of these cases occur during gynecologic procedures.[81]

Processes involving the genitourinary system, particularly the prostate, result in greater occurrence of obstructive uropathy in men than in women older than 60 years. Benign prostatic hyperplasia is the most common cause of urinary tract obstruction in men and results in some symptoms of bladder outlet obstruction in 75% of men age 50 years and older.[82] Presenting symptoms of benign prostatic hyperplasia include decreased force of urine stream, difficulty starting or stopping micturition, incomplete bladder emptying, and nocturia. The diagnosis may be established by urodynamic studies and measurement of the postvoid residual urine volume.

Malignant genitourinary tumors frequently result in obstruction of the urinary tract, particularly bladder cancer, which is the second most common cause of malignant obstruction after cervical cancer,[2] and adenocarcinoma of the prostate, the second leading cause of cancer death in U.S. men. Prostate cancer may result in obstruction at the bladder neck, invasion of the ureteral outlets, or metastatic involvement of the ureter or pelvic nodes.[83] Although urothelial tumors of the renal pelvis, ureter, bladder, and urethra are more rare, they often cause obstruction when they arise.[84]

Several gastrointestinal processes may also cause obstructive uropathy. Obstruction related to Crohn disease may be due to retroperitoneal extension of the inflammatory process,[85] usually on the right side,[86] or the associated nephrolithiasis.[87] Retroperitoneal scarring or abscess formation due to inflammatory disease of the appendix,[88] particularly in children, and large bowel diverticulitis,[89] typically seen in patients older than 50 years and involving the left ureter, are less common causes of obstruction. Chronic pancreatitis with pseudocyst formation may cause left-sided ureteral obstruction,[90] whereas right-sided obstruction may occur with acute pancreatitis.[91]

Obstructive uropathy due to vascular abnormalities and diseases may also occur. The most common vascular cause of obstruction is an abdominal aortic aneurysm[92] from the associated retroperitoneal fibrosis or direct pressure of the aneurysm. Aneurysms of the iliac vessels may also cause obstruction.[93] A rare cause of right ureteral obstruction is thrombophlebitis of the ovarian venous system.[94] Rarely, several vasculitides may directly or indirectly cause obstruction, including systemic lupus erythematosus,[95] polyarteritis nodosa,[96, 97] Wegener granulomatosis,[98] and Schönlein-Henoch purpura.[99]

Retroperitoneal processes that may result in obstruction include tumor invasion and fibrosis. Seventy percent of extrinsic malignant causes of retroperitoneal obstruction are due to tumors of the cervix, prostate, bladder, colon, ovary, and uterus.[2, 100] Retroperitoneal fibrosis may be idiopathic,[101] usually involves the middle third of the ureter, and affects men and women equally, predominantly in the fifth and sixth decades. Retroperitoneal fibrosis may be drug induced (e.g., methysergide); may be associated with a wide variety of conditions, including Schönlein-Henoch purpura, gonorrhea, biliary tract disease, chronic urinary tract infections, tuberculosis, sarcoidosis, and inflammatory processes of the lower extremities with ascending lymphangitis; or may occur as a consequence of multiple abdominal surgical procedures.

Various malignant neoplasms may cause urinary tract obstruction, both by metastases, with an overall frequency of 1% in one large autopsy series,[102] and by direct extension. Cervical cancer is the most common, with 30% of patients having obstruction,[103, 104] followed by cancer of the bladder.[2] Rare childhood tumors include pelvic neurofibromas, which cause upper tract obstruction in 60% of patients,[105] and Wilms tumor, which causes local compression of the renal pelvis.[106] In addition to the vasculitides described, other inflammatory processes may also result in obstruction. Granulomatous causes include sarcoidosis[107] and chronic granulomatous disease of childhood.[108] Amyloid deposits may also produce isolated involvement of the ureter.[109] Furthermore, a pelvic mass associated with actinomycosis may cause external ureteral compression.[110]

There are several mechanisms by which hematologic abnormalities may cause obstruction of the urinary tract. Extrinsic compression may result from enlarged retroperitoneal nodes or a tumor mass.[111] Alternatively, intrinsic obstruction may occur by precipitation of cellular breakdown products and paraproteins, such as in multiple myeloma. Blood clots or hematomas in patients with clotting abnormalities or sloughed papillae in patients with sickle-cell disease may obstruct as well. Whereas leukemic infiltrates are a rare cause in adults, they cause obstruction in 5% of pediatric patients.[112] Lymphomatous infiltration of the kidney affects 33% of patients, and obstruction related to ureteral involvement occurs in approximately 6%.[113]

## CLINICAL ASPECTS

Patients with urinary tract obstruction may present with a variety of symptoms referable to the urinary tract. However, even patients with severe obstruction may be asymptomatic, especially if the obstruction develops gradually.

Pain is commonly associated with obstruction of sudden onset, such as with a kidney stone, blood clot, or sloughed papilla, and is thought to result from stretching of the renal capsule or collecting system. The severity of the pain appears to correlate with the rate rather than the degree of distention. The pain may be typical renal colic, or, in patients with reflux, it may radiate to the flank only during micturition. With ureteropelvic junction obstruction, flank pain may develop after the patient ingests large amounts of

fluid or receives diuretics.[114] An ileus or other gastrointestinal symptoms may accompany the pain.

Urinary symptoms may or may not occur along with changes in urine output. Mild episodes of polyuria may alternate with periods of oliguria. Urinary tract obstruction is one of the few conditions that can cause anuria. Anuria implies complete bilateral obstruction, commonly with an enlarged bladder secondary to bladder outlet obstruction, or obstruction of a solitary kidney at any level. Enuresis, nocturia, and recurrent urinary tract infections are especially common in children. Difficulty initiating urination, decrease in the size or force of the urine stream, postvoid dribbling, and incomplete emptying are seen with bladder outlet obstruction typically due to prostatic disease.[115] A spastic bladder or irritative symptoms such as dysuria, frequency, and urgency may result from urinary tract infection.

On physical examination, a number of signs suggest urinary tract obstruction. A palpable abdominal mass may be due to hydronephrosis, perhaps the most common cause of a palpable abdominal mass in children. A palpable mass in the suprapubic region may be due to a distended bladder. On laboratory examination, proteinuria, if present, is generally less than 2 g/d. Microscopic hematuria is a common finding, but gross hematuria occasionally occurs.[116] The urine sediment is often unremarkable.

Less common manifestations of urinary tract obstruction include deterioration of renal function without apparent cause, renin-dependent[117] or $Na^+$-dependent[118] hypertension, polycythemia, and abnormal urine acidification and concentration.

## DIAGNOSTIC APPROACHES

A thorough history and physical examination may often lead to the diagnosis of urinary tract obstruction and may also suggest the cause and thereby direct the evaluation. Thus, the time and number of tests performed before selection of the appropriate treatment can be minimized.

### History and Physical Examination

Important information obtainable by history should include type and duration of symptoms (e.g., voiding difficulties in older men that may suggest lower urinary tract obstruction), number of urinary tract infections, pattern of urine output, history of stone disease, recent surgery, and drug use.

The physical examination should begin with an assessment of the patient's extracellular volume status because this will guide fluid therapy. Volume depletion is suggested by dry mucous membranes, absence of axillary sweat, and orthostatic changes in pulse rate and blood pressure. Volume-depleted patients may require intravenous saline. In contrast, elevated jugular venous pressure, pulmonary rales, and peripheral edema suggest volume overload. The abdominal examination may reveal a hydronephrotic kidney presenting as a mass in the flank or a distended bladder presenting as a suprapubic mass. Features of chronic renal failure, such as pallor (anemia), drowsiness (uremia), neuromuscular irritability (metabolic abnormalities), or pericardial friction rub (uremic pericarditis), may also be present. Finally, a complete pelvic examination in women and a rectal examination in all patients are mandatory; these evaluations often reveal many causes of obstruction.

## Laboratory Evaluation

The laboratory evaluation must include a urinalysis with examination of the sediment by an experienced observer. Whenever an unremarkable urinalysis is associated with a case of unexplained renal failure, the presence of urinary tract obstruction should be strongly considered. The finding of microscopic hematuria alone suggests a calculus or tumor. The presence of white blood cells and bacteria may indicate pyelonephritis, whereas bacteriuria alone suggests stasis. Crystals in a freshly voided specimen should prompt an evaluation for nephrolithiasis or intrarenal crystal deposition.

Hematologic evaluation should include the white blood cell count (to assess the possibility of a hematologic malignant neoplasm) and the hematocrit (to look for anemia due to chronic renal disease). Serum electrolytes ($Na^+$, $Cl^-$, $K^+$, and $HCO_3^-$), blood urea nitrogen concentration, and creatinine as well as $Ca^{2+}$, phosphorus, $Mg^{2+}$, uric acid, and albumin levels should be measured. If chronic tubule damage is present, urinary chemistry tests may be consistent with acute tubule necrosis (urinary $Na^+$ > 20 mEq/L, fractional excretion of $Na^+$ [$FE_{Na}$] > 1%, and osmolality < 350 mOsm). Alternatively, acute obstruction may be suggested by urinary chemistry values consistent with prerenal azotemia (urinary $Na^+$ < 20 mEq/L, $FE_{Na}$ < 1%, and osmolality > 500 mOsm).[5]

## Radiologic Procedures

The radiologic evaluation of suspected urinary tract obstruction should be guided by the results of the history, physical examination findings, and laboratory data. The presence of pain, evidence of renal dysfunction, or urinary tract infection should dictate the speed and nature of the evaluation. A variety of radiologic techniques are available, each with advantages and disadvantages. The ability to identify the site and cause of obstruction and to separate functional obstruction from mere dilatation of the urinary system varies by technique. When an approach is chosen for a patient with renal insufficiency, the risks associated with the use of radiocontrast agents need to be considered.[119, 120] In addition, in pregnant patients, radiation exposure should be limited.

### PLAIN FILM OF THE ABDOMEN (KIDNEY, URETER, AND BLADDER)

Abdominal or flank pain with normal or mildly impaired renal function suggests the presence of a renal calculus. In this setting, a plain film of the abdomen (kidney, ureter, and bladder) provides information on the size and gross contour of the kidneys. It may reveal calculi, 90% of which

are radiopaque, in the renal pelvis, along the course of the ureter, or in the bladder (see Fig. 41–1). Calcification of the renal parenchyma may also be noted.

## ULTRASONOGRAPHY

When obstruction is suspected, ultrasonography is the preferred screening modality[121] because of its high sensitivity for detecting hydronephrosis,[122] safety, low cost, and lack of radiation exposure. Moreover, it is often used in patients with an elevated or rising serum creatinine level to rule out obstruction as the cause of the diminished renal function.[123] Ultrasonography can determine renal size and reveal dilatation of the calyces, the renal pelvis, and occasionally the proximal ureter (Fig. 41–2). With severe longstanding obstruction and hydronephrosis, the renal cortex may be thinned.

Ultrasonography has both high sensitivity (the probability that the test result will be positive when the condition is present) and specificity (the probability that a test result will be negative when the condition is absent) for detecting hydronephrosis. These are both approximately 90%,[122, 124] even in azotemic patients,[124] with the intravenous urogram as the "gold standard." Whereas ultrasonography may be used to evaluate the size and shape of the collecting system and thus diagnose hydronephrosis, it can only suggest but not diagnose the presence of obstruction. Although ultrasonography is a highly sensitive and specific test, its positive predictive value (the probability that the disease is present when the test result is positive) is still critically dependent on the prevalence, or pretest probability, of the disease.[125]

The false-positive rate for a finding of apparent hydronephrosis is between 10%[126] and 20%.[127] False-positive results by ultrasound examination are primarily due to the presence of an extrarenal pelvis (normal variant), congenital megacalyces, calyceal diverticula, diuresis, an easily distensible renal pelvis, or renal cysts.[126] A dilated collecting system without obstruction is seen in more than 50% of patients with urinary drainage through an ileal conduit.[128]

In some instances, obstruction may not be associated

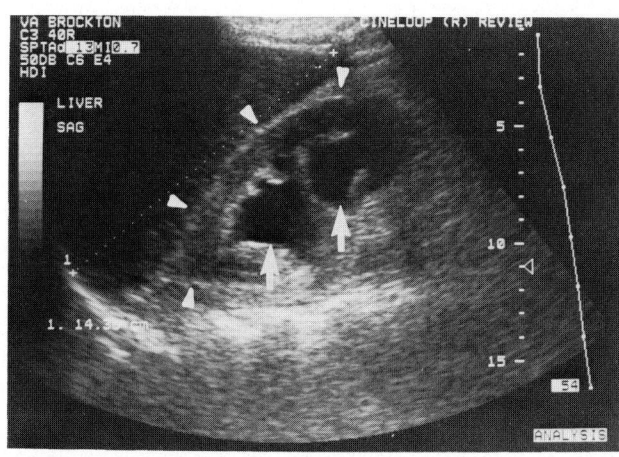

**Figure 41–2.** Ultrasound image of the right kidney in a male patient presenting with urinary retention. Marked pyelocalyceal dilatation is present *(large arrows)*. The kidney is of normal size (outlined by the arrowheads) with slightly thinned cortex.

with significant dilatation of the collecting system, even in patients with severe azotemia and anuria,[129, 130] and thus would be undetectable by ultrasonography. These may include the presence of staghorn calculi, nephrocalcinosis,[124] retroperitoneal fibrosis,[131] or bilateral obstruction in a volume-contracted patient. Occasionally, the presence of hydronephrosis may be misinterpreted as renal cystic disease.[126]

Thus, whereas ultrasonography remains a useful screening test, it cannot completely rule out the presence of obstruction in a patient with a high likelihood of disease. Consequently, the diagnosis of obstruction must still be considered in patients with chronic azotemia or acute changes in renal function or urine output despite the absence of hydronephrosis by ultrasonography.[132]

## ANTENATAL ULTRASONOGRAPHY

The introduction of maternal ultrasonography has resulted in a fourfold increase in antenatal detection of congenital urinary tract obstruction.[25] Early identification of prenatal urinary tract obstruction by ultrasound examination followed by prophylactic use of antibiotics can decrease the risk of urinary tract infections and urosepsis in infants.[133] Although obstruction suspected prenatally is not confirmed postnatally in as many as 30% of cases,[134] some patients will develop obstructive uropathy later in life.[135] Therefore, long-term follow-up of these children is necessary.

## INTRAVENOUS UROGRAPHY

If upper tract obstruction is suggested by history, physical examination, or ultrasonography, intravenous urography, also known as intravenous pyelography, is the procedure of choice for defining the anatomy, particularly of the ureter, and the location of the obstruction. However, there are drawbacks to this procedure. The nephrotoxicity of the contrast material should be considered, particularly in high-risk patients such as those with diabetes or impaired renal function.[119, 120] Furthermore, the kidneys may not be well visualized in patients with a low glomerular filtration rate (GFR) because of delayed excretion of the contrast agent; hence, adequate films may not be obtainable until 12 to 24 hours after injection of the radiocontrast agent.[136] Moreover, in cases of severe obstruction, insufficient contrast material may be excreted by the affected side for adequate identification of the site of obstruction. Still, because of its ready availability and ability to identify a significant proportion of causes of obstruction, intravenous urography remains a useful and informative diagnostic tool.

## INVASIVE PYELOGRAPHY

When the risks of intravenous urography are considered to be too great or when it does not provide adequate anatomic detail, more invasive techniques may be required. Antegrade pyelography entails the percutaneous injection of contrast material through a needle or nephrostomy tube placed in the renal pelvis, typically under sonographic guidance (Fig. 41–3). Retrograde pyelography is performed by cystoscopically guided ureteral catheterization followed by

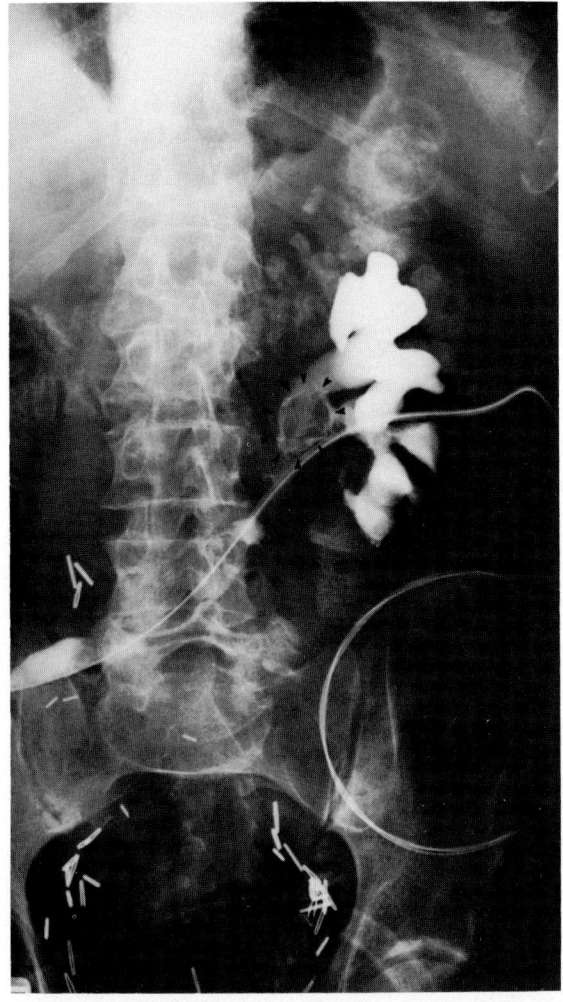

**Figure 41–3.** Antegrade pyelogram through a left nephrostomy tube in a patient with ureteropelvic junction obstruction due to a struvite stone *(arrowheads)*. Note the dilated calyces. (This patient has an ileal conduit after a radical cystectomy.)

injection of the contrast agent. Whereas this method demonstrates the distal site of obstruction,[137] the contrast agent may not reach the kidney in cases of complete obstruction. In addition, retrograde pyelography may not distinguish between obstruction and a nonobstructed dilated collecting system. Finally, the risk of introducing infection proximal to the obstruction, which may be difficult to eradicate with conventional therapy, cannot be ignored.

## COMPUTED TOMOGRAPHY

Computed tomography is a sensitive test for diagnosing the cause of hydronephrosis and is useful when the cause remains uncertain after ultrasonography or intravenous urography.[136, 138] A particular advantage is that a dilated collecting system can still be seen even if it is necessary to perform the procedure without contrast enhancement. Computed tomography is particularly good for identifying extrinsic obstruction (e.g., retroperitoneal fibrosis, lymphadenopathy, hematoma) and may also detect intraluminal problems of the ureter, such as a stone or tumor (Fig. 41–4).

## ISOTOPIC RENOGRAPHY

Isotopic renography, also known as a nuclear medicine renal scan, can be used to diagnose upper urinary tract obstruction while avoiding the risk of radiocontrast agent administration.[139, 140] It is performed by the intravenous injection of a radioisotope and the recording of images with a gamma scintillation camera. Although this method provides a functional assessment of the obstructed kidney, there is poor anatomic definition. In the past, there has been only a poor correlation between the results of standard radiologic procedures and the postoperative return of renal

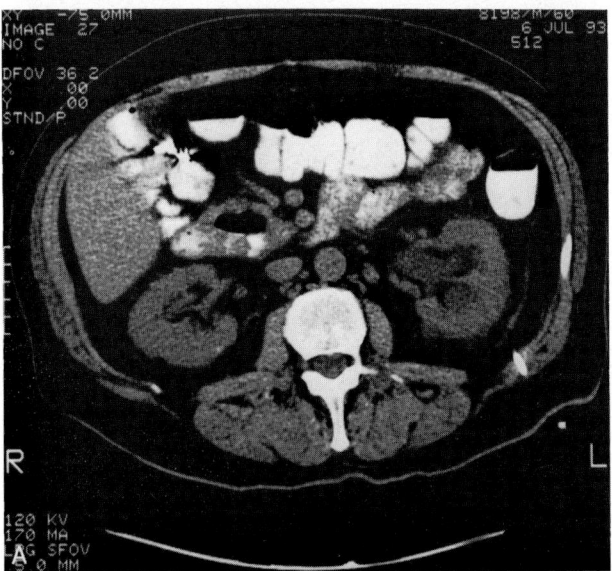

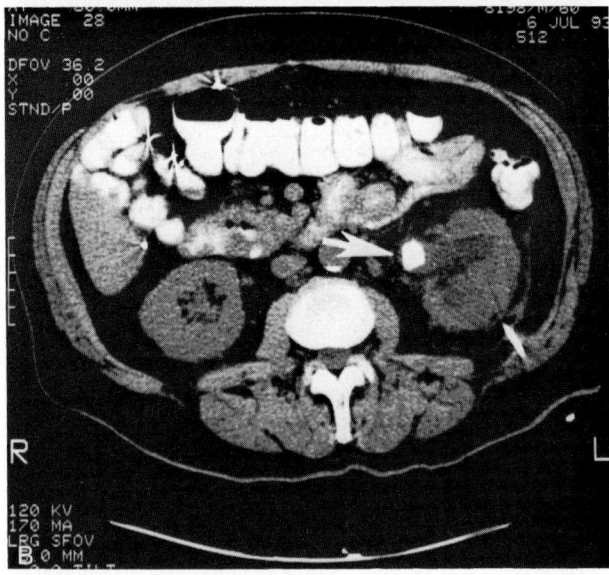

**Figure 41–4.** Computed tomograms (without radiocontrast enhancement) of the same patient as in Figure 41–3. *A.* Computed tomogram demonstrates renal pelvic and calyceal dilatation of the left kidney. *B.* The next level just distal demonstrates the cause of the hydronephrosis: a large calculus *(arrow)* at the ureteropelvic junction.

function. Whereas isotopic renography is increasingly becoming the method employed to assess renal function when surgical repair as opposed to nephrectomy is being considered,[141] its ultimate utility in this capacity remains to be defined.

Diuresis renography can be used to distinguish dilatation with obstruction from that without obstruction (Fig. 41–5). An intravenous loop diuretic, such as furosemide, is given 20 to 30 minutes after the injection of an isotope[142] or when the tracer first appears in the renal pelvis. If stasis alone is responsible for the dilatation, the induced diuresis leads to a rapid washout of collected radioactivity. With true obstruction, there is no washout but rather a persistence of radioactivity proximal to the obstruction. An absent or blunted response to the diuretic resulting from decreased renal function limits the usefulness of diuresis renography because interpretation of the test may be difficult.[143]

## MAGNETIC RESONANCE IMAGING

Thus far, magnetic resonance imaging remains a research tool for the evaluation of urinary tract obstruction. Advantages of magnetic resonance imaging include improved spatial resolution and the avoidance of ionizing radiation and iodinated contrast agents. However, it currently provides no substantial diagnostic advantages over combined ultrasonography and computed tomography. Although no single radiologic method currently provides detailed anatomic and functional information, magnetic resonance imaging may meet these goals with the development of paramagnetic contrast agents.[144, 145]

# PATHOPHYSIOLOGY OF OBSTRUCTIVE NEPHROPATHY

Although obstructive uropathy in humans is often partial and of long duration, most studies of the mechanisms of renal dysfunction in this condition have used models of complete obstruction for relatively short periods, such as 24 hours. These models avoid such issues as the degree of obstruction and the effects of long-term changes in renal architecture brought on by fibrosis or inflammation. Complete obstruction of short duration results in profound alterations in renal hemodynamics and glomerular filtration, as well as in tubule function, with minimal anatomic changes.[2, 17] Thus, acute complete obstruction provides an excellent model of regulation of renal function.

## Effects of Obstruction on Glomerular Filtration

Obstructive uropathy alters several aspects of glomerular function, depending on the severity and duration of the obstruction, whether the obstruction is bilateral or unilateral, and the extent to which the obstruction has been relieved or remains in effect.[2, 17] Whole kidney GFR is determined by the proportion of glomeruli actually receiving blood flow and filtering as well as the filtration rate of

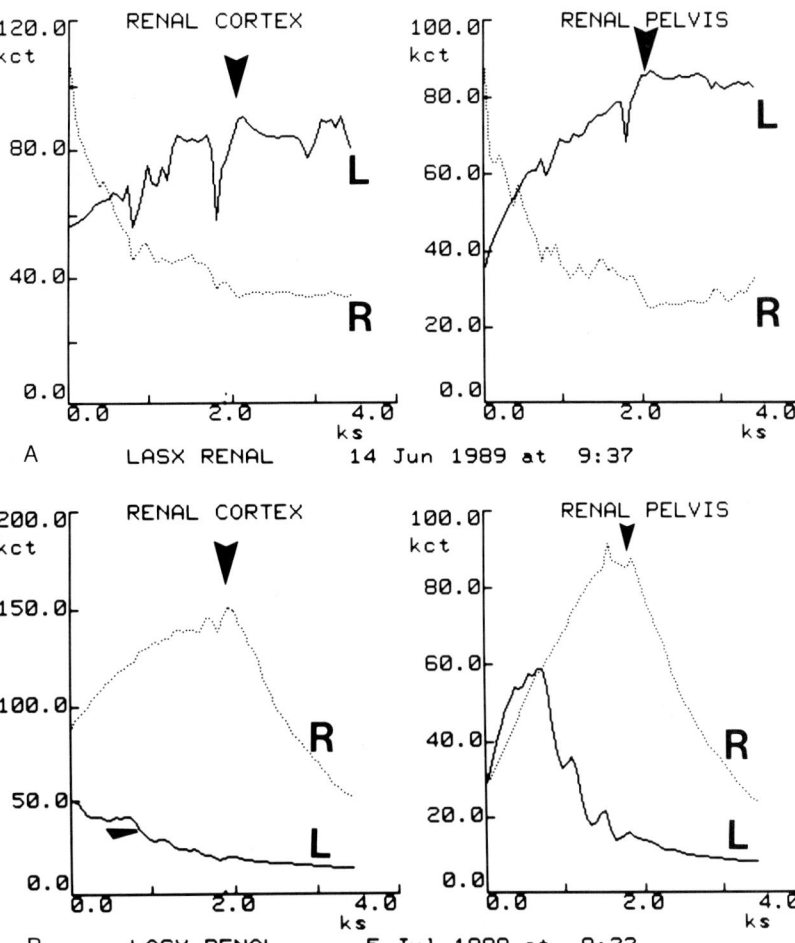

**Figure 41–5.** Diuresis renograms from two different patients. Furosemide was given intravenously at approximately 2 ks *(arrowheads)*. *A.* In the tracing of this patient, excretion of the tracer is rapid on the right but slow on the left. The radionuclide does not "wash out" after furosemide administration, which suggests urinary tract obstruction. *B.* In a different patient, excretion is rapid on the left but delayed on the right. The administration of furosemide results in a prompt and rapid excretion of the radionuclide, which suggests dilatation of the collecting system without significant obstruction.

functional glomeruli. The GFR of individual glomeruli, or single-nephron GFR (SNGFR), is determined by the glomerular blood flow rate; the net ultrafiltration pressure across the glomerular capillary, which is governed by the hydraulic pressure in the glomerular capillary ($P_{GC}$), the hydraulic pressure of Bowman space (or of the proximal tubule), and the differences in oncotic pressure between glomerular capillary and Bowman space; and the ultrafiltration coefficient ($K_f$), which depends on the surface area available for filtration and the permeability properties of this filtering surface (see Chapter 7). Glomerular blood flow rate and $P_{GC}$, in turn, are governed by the resistances of the afferent ($R_A$) and efferent ($R_E$) arterioles. The effects of obstruction on these determinants of glomerular filtration are discussed in detail later.

## EARLY, HYPEREMIC PHASE

During the first 2 to 3 hours of unilateral ureteral obstruction, the lack of antegrade urine flow results in striking increases in proximal tubule hydraulic pressure ($P_T$). Such increases, transmitted back into Bowman space, would be expected to reduce GFR.[146–148] However, during this early phase, $P_{GC}$ also increases markedly, resulting in relative preservation of GFR. The increase in $P_{GC}$ is due to dilatation of the afferent arteriole leading to reduced $R_A$.[146, 147] Because this "hyperemic response" is observed in dener-

vated as well as in isolated perfused kidneys,[149, 150] it is thought to result from intrarenal mechanisms. Indeed, a similar response is observed in individual nephrons when antegrade urine flow is retarded by placement of a wax block in the tubules.[151]

This afferent vasodilatation has several potential mechanisms, including a direct myogenic reflex, regulation by the macula densa, and increases in vasodilatory hormones, such as prostaglandins.[2] Because the hyperemic response is not reduced by infusion of catecholamines or electrical stimulation of renal nerves,[152] it is possible that it is caused by an increase in interstitial pressure, which reduces the transmural pressure gradient in the afferent arteriolar wall that leads to reduced contractility of the smooth muscle cells of the vessel wall.[149, 153] Because obstruction reduces the flow of urine past the macula densa, it is possible that this structure mediates increased afferent blood flow, as is observed in the tubuloglomerular feedback response,[151] wherein decreasing rates of distal tubule flow past the macula densa increase SNGFR by decreasing $R_A$ and increasing $P_{GC}$. However, micropuncture studies have provided evidence that the signal arises from obstruction of the nephron itself and not from decreased flow past the macula densa.[147] Thus, the increase in $P_{GC}$ observed after tubule obstruction did not occur in nephrons that were obstructed proximal to the macula densa but in which tubule pressures were maintained at normal levels by placement of a hole in the tubule proximal to the blockage. Therefore, $P_{GC}$ was elevated not by reduced flow of urine past the macula densa but by obstruction to urine flow itself.[147] In several studies, this hyperemic response was inhibited by treatment with indomethacin, which suggests that vasodilatory prostaglandins may mediate it.[148, 154, 155]

Interestingly, the early hyperemic response is absent or markedly attenuated during bilateral obstruction.[2, 17, 153] A possible mechanism for this difference was provided in studies of unilateral obstruction in which the ipsilateral or contralateral kidney was denervated.[153] Obstruction of the left kidney increased afferent nerve traffic from that kidney and efferent nerve traffic to the right kidney, resulting in reduced blood flow to the right kidney. When either the left or right kidney was denervated, the contralateral vasoconstrictor response to obstruction was abolished. These results suggest that in bilateral obstruction, increased renal nerve activity may counteract the early vasodilatory effects of obstruction.[153]

## LATE, VASOCONSTRICTIVE PHASE

Because it is difficult to study regulation of glomerular filtration during complete obstruction, most data on the mechanisms involved in regulation of GFR at this stage have been obtained soon after the release of obstruction.[2, 156] After 3 hours of unilateral obstruction, and progressing to 12 to 24 hours of obstruction, renal blood flow declines.[157–159] Initially, tubule pressures remain elevated, but these, too, decline; by 24 hours, renal plasma flow and GFR are reduced to 25% of normal, and intratubule pressures are also decreased.[146, 148, 158–161] Examination of regional renal blood flow by use of silicone rubber injection reveals that there are large unperfused and underperfused areas of the cortex.[2, 148, 158, 159, 162] Depending on the species, different vascular beds in the outer and juxtamedullary cortex receive larger or reduced proportions of blood flow. Thus, a major reason for reduced whole kidney GFR is the lack of perfusion of many glomeruli.

In addition, SNGFR is also decreased markedly owing to afferent vasoconstriction, which reduces $P_{GC}$.[160, 163] Interestingly, identical changes in $P_{GC}$ occur if the individual nephron is blocked with oil for 24 hours before micropuncture measurements.[164] These results indicate that the late vasoconstrictive response to obstruction, like the early hyperemic phase, is due primarily to intrarenal mechanisms.

In bilateral obstruction, renal blood flow is decreased to 40% to 70% of normal, an indication that the vasoconstriction is not nearly as severe as is observed in unilateral obstruction[2, 160, 163, 165] (Table 41–3). SNGFR is reduced to a similar degree in bilateral and unilateral obstruction, but the mechanisms differ. In unilateral obstruction, reduced $P_{GC}$ lowers the driving pressure for filtration, despite near normalization of intratubule pressures.[163] By contrast, in bilateral obstruction, $P_{GC}$ is at normal levels, and the reduction in GFR is due to persistence of high intratubule pressures.[160] These results point to the activity of systemic factors, such as renal nerve activity, accumulation of volume and urea, and increase in natriuretic substances, in modulating the vasoconstrictive effect of obstruction on the affected kidney.[165] The factors involved in regulation of GFR after

**TABLE 41–3. Glomerular Hemodynamics in Ureteral Obstruction***

| Condition | $P_T$ | $R_A$ | $P_{GC}$ | SNGFR |
|---|---|---|---|---|
| 1- to 2-h unilateral | ↑↑ | ↓ | ↑ | = |
| 24-h unilateral | = | ↑↑ | ↓ | ↓↓ |
| 24-h bilateral | ↑↑ | = | = | ↓↓ |
| Release 24-h unilateral | ↓ | ↑↑ | ↓↓ | ↓↓ |
| Release 24-h bilateral | = | ↑↑ | ↓ | ↓↓ |

*See text for discussion and references. The = denotes unchanged; ↑ or ↓ denotes increased or decreased, respectively; ↑↑ or ↓↓ denotes marked increases or reductions, respectively.

release of 24-hour obstruction have been studied in detail and are discussed in the following.

## REGULATION OF GLOMERULAR FILTRATION RATE IN THE POSTOBSTRUCTIVE PERIOD

The degree of impairment of renal blood flow and GFR after release of obstruction depends on the duration of the obstruction and the species studied.[148, 159, 166, 167] However, after release of 24 hours of unilateral obstruction, GFR is reduced to 25% of normal in rats and to less than 50% of normal in dogs, whereas renal blood flow is markedly decreased in both species. After release of bilateral obstruction, renal blood flow is less impaired than in unilateral obstruction, but GFR is markedly reduced. The reduction in GFR is caused by the lack of perfusion or underperfusion of many glomeruli, as reflected in silicone rubber injections.[148, 158, 159] In functioning nephrons, tubule pressures fall after release of obstruction, but $P_{GC}$ falls markedly also, which reduces the net transcapillary filtration pressure.[160, 163] The fall in $P_{GC}$ is due to intense preglomerular vasoconstriction, which appears to be similar in both unilateral and bilateral obstruction. Moreover, it appears likely that $K_f$ is also decreased in both conditions.[160, 163, 168]

Several mechanisms, probably acting in concert, contribute to this intense vasoconstriction and decline in $K_f$ (see Fig. 41–3). First, during release of obstruction, the rate of flow of filtrate past the macula densa increases dramatically. Although the rate of flow is far below normal, it is possible that the macula densa senses the change in the rate of flow and stimulates vasoconstriction of the afferent arteriole.[2] Indeed, the sensitivity of the tubuloglomerular feedback mechanism was found to be enhanced in unilateral but not in bilateral obstruction, which suggests that depending on the extrarenal hormonal milieu, this system may play a role in the vasoconstriction after release of obstruction.[169]

Increased levels of angiotensin II may also contribute to the intense vasoconstriction and reduction in $K_f$. Although several studies showed that ureteral obstruction rapidly increased renal vein renin levels, this increase occurred early in the obstruction, when renal blood flow was normal or elevated.[170–172] At later time points, renal vein renin levels were not elevated.[170, 172] Infusion of saralasin, an angiotensin II antagonist, also did not improve GFR after obstruction,[170, 172] but this agent has agonist properties as well, as reflected in its ability to decrease renal blood flow in obstruction.[170] By contrast, captopril has been shown to blunt or reverse the decline in renal blood flow and GFR observed in both unilateral and bilateral obstruction.[168, 170, 173] Because captopril can also act by increasing the level of kinins, studies were performed to determine the role of kinins in the salutary response to captopril. Infusions of either carboxypeptidase B, which destroys kinins, or aprotinin, which blocks kinin synthesis, did not alter the response to captopril, which indicates that this agent reduced $R_A$ by reducing the generation of angiotensin II.[170] Because angiotensin II also increases the contractility of mesangial cells, an effect that reduces $K_f$, it can be anticipated that any reduction in $K_f$ observed during the postobstructive period is partially due to increased angiotensin II levels.[168]

Thromboxane $A_2$ ($TXA_2$) has also been implicated as a major vasoconstrictor in the postobstructive period.[170, 174] Early studies demonstrated that the hydronephrotic kidney is capable of synthesizing high levels of $TXA_2$ (measured in the form of its more stable metabolite, thromboxane $B_2$).[174] However, the kidneys in these studies were removed from the animals and exposed to nonphysiologic solutions for prolonged periods.[174] Administration of high concentrations of imidazole, a thromboxane synthase inhibitor, into the renal artery,[170] but not systemically,[175] ameliorated the vasoconstrictive effects of release of obstruction, increasing both renal blood flow and whole kidney GFR. In a subsequent study, more specific and potent inhibitors, such as UK-37248 and UK-38485, were infused into renal arteries and markedly improved renal blood flow and GFR.[173, 176, 177] Under these conditions, the agents markedly reduced $TXA_2$ generation by kidneys excised and immediately perfused in vitro.[177] Glomerular micropuncture of kidneys after relief of obstruction revealed that another thromboxane synthase inhibitor, OKY-1581, reduced renal vasoconstriction and increased $K_f$.[168] Thus, a significant portion of the vasoconstriction observed on release of obstruction is mediated by $TXA_2$.

However, the source of $TXA_2$ remains unclear. Glomeruli isolated from obstructed kidneys have been shown to be capable of increased $TXA_2$ generation by some,[178] but not all[179, 180] investigators. Such generation may mediate changes in $K_f$ but is unlikely to play a major role in increases in $R_A$, because the afferent arteriole is upstream to the glomerulus. Studies of inflammatory cells have suggested that they may be the source of $TXA_2$ and other vasoconstrictors in obstruction. During the first 24 hours of obstruction, leukocytes, predominantly macrophages and suppressor T cells, infiltrate the renal cortex and medulla, reaching levels up to 15-fold higher than baseline values.[181] Interestingly, the density of glomerular macrophages diminishes sharply. Release of obstruction results in reversal of these changes over several days. It is notable that inulin clearance decreases and $TXA_2$ generation increases in conjunction with the appearance of these mononuclear cells.[181] Moreover, irradiation of obstructed kidneys, which markedly reduced the extent of the cellular infiltration, also resulted in clear-cut reduction in urinary thromboxane $B_2$ levels and improvement in GFR.[182] These results suggest that obstruction stimulates infiltration of inflammatory mononuclear cells that generate vasoconstrictors, among

them $TXA_2$.[181, 182] These vasoconstrictors probably contribute to the increases in $R_A$ observed in obstructed kidneys.

Because irradiation only partially prevented the release of $TXA_2$ and the decrease in GFR, it is likely that renal tissues themselves also generate important mediators. Indeed, the reduction in glomerular macrophage counts is consistent with synthesis of mediators by glomerular cells, possibly mesangial cells.[181] Glomerular eicosanoid synthesis in obstruction is stimulated in part by angiotensin II.[183] Treatment of obstruction in animals with converting enzyme inhibitors enhanced GFR and reduced $TXA_2$ generation by isolated glomeruli[183] (see Fig. 41–3).

As noted before, there are clear-cut differences in the hemodynamic response of the obstructed kidney in the presence of unilateral and bilateral obstruction, with somewhat reduced vasoconstriction observed in bilateral obstruction. A number of extrarenal factors have been identified that by modifying intrarenal signaling pathways probably mediate these differences. In the studies of early postobstruction vasodilatation, we have already noted that renal nerves might reduce vasodilatation in bilateral obstruction. Several factors, including accumulation of solutes such as urea, atrial natriuretic peptide (ANP) and urodilatin, and other natriuretic substances, may tend to reduce the effect of obstructive vasoconstriction on GFR in bilateral obstruction. In 24-hour obstruction, GFR was preserved somewhat if the contralateral kidney was also obstructed, or if the contralateral kidney was removed.[184] Moreover, if 24-hour unilateral obstruction was released and the urea, salt, and water content of the urine from the contralateral kidney was reinfused into the animal, there was a striking increase in GFR.[184, 185] Because the plasma urea levels were similar among groups with widely differing GFR, it appears that the infusion of urea and not the urea level was responsible for the improvement in GFR.[184] Moreover, urine reinfusion in intact animals also increased GFR.[185] Similarly, volume expansion itself can ameliorate the reduction in GFR to some extent. These results suggest that factors that are normally excreted by the kidney, including volume, can stimulate GFR in obstructed kidneys.

ANP is a major factor that probably reduces the vasoconstrictive effect of obstruction. In animals with bilateral obstruction in which no volume restriction is imposed, as well as in most patients, volume expansion occurs. This expansion stimulates ANP release.[186] Moreover, because the kidney represents a major site of degradation of ANP, it is likely that the obstructed kidney does not degrade ANP at normal rates.[186] Indeed, it has been shown that ANP levels increase in bilateral but not in unilateral obstruction whether or not the animal's access to food and water is restricted.[186, 187] Changes in volume and ANP degradation contribute to the known increase in plasma ANP levels in animals and patients with bilateral obstruction.

In normal kidneys, ANP has several effects that promote increased renal blood flow and GFR. These include direct vasodilatation of afferent arterioles, vasoconstriction of efferent arterioles, and increase in $K_f$.[186] Moreover, ANP reduces renin release by the macula densa, an effect that would be expected to reduce circulating levels of angiotensin II.[186] It is therefore not surprising that infusions of ANP can improve GFR in unilateral and bilateral obstruction.[173, 187]

Additional vasodilatory factors that may ameliorate the vasoconstrictive effect of obstruction include arachidonate derivatives such as prostaglandin $E_2$ ($PGE_2$) and nitric oxide. Renal $PGE_2$ levels increase markedly in states of volume expansion (such as can occur during bilateral obstruction) and obstruction itself (see later). These increases may reduce the level of vasoconstriction occurring in obstruction. Although there have been few studies of nitric oxide in obstructive nephropathy to date, preliminary data suggest that in bilateral obstruction, circulating levels of L-arginine (the precursor of nitric oxide) are decreased, potentially reducing the levels of this vasodilator in the kidney.[188]

In summary, the interplay of intrarenal and extrarenal factors results in profound decreases in GFR during and immediately after obstruction. The decrease in GFR is caused by a sharp reduction in the number of functioning glomeruli due to reduction and redistribution of renal blood flow as well as by a reduction in the SNGFR of functioning nephrons. The reductions in SNGFR are brought about by increased $R_A$ and reduced $K_f$. Increased angiotensin II activity and release of $TXA_2$, in part by inflammatory cells, contribute to these hemodynamic effects. In bilateral obstruction, retention of urea and other substances and increases in plasma levels of ANP help offset these vasoconstrictive influences, but only partially.

## RECOVERY OF GLOMERULAR FUNCTION AFTER RELIEF OF OBSTRUCTION

The duration and the degree of obstruction as well as the presence or absence of a functioning contralateral kidney determine the extent to which GFR recovers.[166] In dogs subjected to 1 week of complete unilateral ureteral obstruction, GFR was 25% of normal on release of the obstruction, with gradual partial restoration of function up to 50% of normal levels at 2 years after the obstruction.[189] In rats, unilateral obstruction of 7 and 14 days' duration resulted in residual GFR of 17% and 9% of normal, respectively, if the contralateral kidney was left in place, and 31% and 14%, respectively, if the contralateral kidney was removed at the time of release of the obstruction.[161] A similar salutary effect of contralateral nephrectomy was obtained in a model of chronic partial obstruction in the rat.[161] This beneficial effect probably results from the accumulation of solutes, urea, and other vasodilatory substances such as ANP when the normal contralateral kidney is absent.

Although some recovery of total kidney GFR from chronic obstruction is observed, micropuncture studies demonstrate that this recovery is uneven; some nephrons never regain function, whereas others exhibit striking hyperfiltration.[166] Thus, in chronic partial obstruction, near-normal values of the SNGFR of surface nephrons would have predicted near-normal total kidney GFR, although the measured value was only 18% of normal.[190] These results indicate that deep cortical and juxtamedullary nephrons are selectively damaged in chronic partial obstruction.[158, 166, 190] In animal studies of the long-term sequelae of complete 24-hour ureteral obstruction, total kidney GFR was restored to normal levels by 14 and 60 days after release of the obstruction. However, 15% of glomeruli were found to be

nonfiltering, with evidence of hyperfiltration of remnant nephrons, as measured by the entrapment of labeled ferricyanide within functioning nephrons. In this model of relatively short-term obstruction, the long-term function of superficial and deep nephrons was affected similarly.[166]

## Effects of Obstruction on Tubule Function

Obstruction profoundly reduces the ability of renal tubules to reabsorb $Na^+$, $K^+$, and $H^+$ and reduces the ability to concentrate and dilute the urine[2, 191] (Table 41–4). The resulting failure to reabsorb solutes contributes to the syndrome of postobstructive diuresis. The extent of the defects depends on the duration and severity of the obstruction. With prolonged obstruction, profound tubule atrophy and chronic inflammatory changes are observed; whereas at earlier time points, such as 24 hours, there are only modest structural and ultrastructural changes.[192, 193] These changes include slight mitochondrial swelling and a reduction in

**TABLE 41–4. Segmental Reabsorption in Superficial and Juxtamedullary Nephrons and in Collecting Ducts in Normal Rats and After Release of Bilateral or Unilateral Ureteral Obstruction**

| Site* | Water Remaining (%) | Na+ Remaining (%) |
|---|---|---|
| *Normal* | | |
| $S_1$ | 100 | 100 |
| $S_2$ | 44 | 44 |
| $S_3$ | 26 | 14 |
| $S_4$ | 9.4 | 5 |
| $J_1$ | 100 | 100 |
| $J_2$ | 12 | 40 |
| $CD_1$ | 3.3 | 2 |
| $CD_2$ | 0.4 | 0.6 |
| *After Bilateral Obstruction* | | |
| $S_1$ | 100 | 100 |
| $S_2$ | 45 | 45 |
| $S_3$ | 40 | 22 |
| $S_4$ | 25 | 7 |
| $J_1$ | 100 | 100 |
| $J_2$ | 42 | 62 |
| $CD_1$ | 8 | 6 |
| $CD_2$ | 16.7 | 12 |
| *After Unilateral Obstruction* | | |
| $S_1$ | 100 | 100 |
| $S_2$ | 26 | 26 |
| $S_3$ | 21 | 12 |
| $S_4$ | 3.2 | 1.9 |
| $J_1$ | 100 | 100 |
| $J_2$ | 42 | 52 |
| $CD_1$ | 4.2 | 3.8 |
| $CD_2$ | 2.9 | 2.5 |

*$S_{1-4}$, values found in superficial nephrons: $S_1$ = Bowman space; $S_2$ = end of proximal convoluted tubule; $S_3$ = earliest portion of distal tubule; $S_4$ = end of distal tubule/beginning of collecting duct. $J_{1-2}$, values found in juxtamedullary nephrons: $J_1$, Bowman space; $J_2$ = tip of loop of Henle. $CD_1$ = collecting duct at base of papilla, first accessible portion of inner medullary collecting duct; $CD_2$ = end of collecting duct as it opens into renal pelvis.
Data compiled from references, 146, 158, 160, 162, 165, 194–196, and 226–228.

**TABLE 41–5. Function of Isolated Perfused Tubules in Obstructive Nephropathy***

|  | $J_v$ SPCT (nL/mm/min) | $J_v$ PST (nL/mm/min) | $\Delta Cl^-$ mTAL (mEq/L) | $^{22}Na^+$ Flux (pmol/mm/min) | $J_v$ CCT (+ ADH) (nL/mm/min) |
|---|---|---|---|---|---|
| Control | $0.75 \pm 0.08$ | $0.25 \pm 0.02$ | $-37 \pm 3$ | $38.2 \pm 4.0$ | $0.90 \pm 0.08$ |
| Unilateral obstruction | $0.73 \pm 0.11$ | $0.12 \pm 0.03$ | $-9 \pm 1$ | $26.2 \pm 3.3$ | $0.22 \pm 0.04$ |
| Bilateral obstruction | $0.80 \pm 0.08$ | $0.16 \pm 0.02$ | $-10 \pm 1$ |  | $0.23 \pm 0.04$ |

*$J_v$ = volume reabsorption; SPCT = superficial proximal convoluted tubule; PST = proximal straight tubule; $\Delta Cl^-$ = change in $Cl^-$ concentration; mTAL = medullary thick ascending limb; CCT = cortical collecting tubule; ADH = antidiuretic hormone.
    Data from references 197, 198, and 200.

basolateral interdigitations in the medullary thick ascending limb (mTAL), and flattening of epithelium and some widening of intercellular spaces in the collecting duct.[192, 193] Aside from the tip of the papilla, where there is focal necrosis of epithelial cells, there is little or no cell death.[192] The lack of severe structural changes, plus the relative simplicity of the model, has led most investigators to confine their studies to 24 hours of complete obstruction. In general, the defects in tubule transport are due to both damage to the tubules' intrinsic transport capability and the actions of extratubule hormones, which may arise from the kidney or from extrarenal sources.

## EFFECTS OF OBSTRUCTION ON TUBULE REABSORPTION OF Na$^+$

After release of 24-hour unilateral obstruction, volume excretion by the postobstructed kidney has been found to be normal or mildly elevated[2, 165, 184, 194] (see Table 41–4). However, given the marked impairment of GFR to levels of only about 20% of control values, the excretion of normal urine volume indicates a striking increase in $FE_{Na}$. In bilateral obstruction, there is a striking increase in Na$^+$ and water excretion, with values of five to nine times normal often reported.[165, 195, 196] In this setting, GFR is also decreased, so that the $FE_{Na}$ may be 20-fold higher than normal. Micropuncture studies, which are summarized in Table 41–4, reveal a similar localization of the Na$^+$ reabsorption defect in both unilateral and bilateral obstruction. Proximal tubule reabsorption ($S_1$ to $S_2$) appeared to be normal in superficial nephrons in bilateral obstruction and may have been enhanced in unilateral obstruction. However, in juxtamedullary nephrons, the proportion of filtered salt and water delivered to the loop of Henle ($J_1$ to $J_2$ in Table 41–4) was increased, indicating reduced reabsorption. The delivery of salt and water to the first accessible portion of the papillary collecting duct ($CD_1$) was increased, and net reabsorption in the papillary collecting duct ($CD_1$ to $CD_2$) was diminished in both forms of obstruction. Indeed, in bilateral obstruction, net addition of salt and water to the papillary collecting duct was noted.[195] These results indicate that between the loop of Henle and the beginning of the papillary collecting duct, there was diminished net reabsorption of salt and water. This implicates the mTAL; the distal convoluted tubule; and the entire length of the collecting duct, including the cortical collecting duct (CCD), outer medullary collecting duct (OMCD), and inner medullary collecting duct (IMCD) portions.

These results have been confirmed and extended by a series of studies from several laboratories in isolated perfused tubule and cell suspension preparations, which are summarized in part in Table 41–5. Volume reabsorption in isolated perfused superficial proximal convoluted tubules was normal in both unilateral and bilateral obstruction.[197] By contrast, volume reabsorption in proximal straight tubules, which arise from juxtamedullary nephrons, was sharply diminished in obstruction.[197] An estimate of active reabsorption in the mTAL was obtained by measuring the ability of the perfused tubule to lower the $Cl^-$ concentration of the perfusate. As shown in Table 41–5, mTALs from obstructed kidneys exhibited striking decreases in active reabsorption of NaCl.[197] This interpretation was confirmed in studies of freshly prepared suspensions of mTAL cells from obstructed nephrons, in which transport-dependent oxygen consumption was markedly reduced.[198] The reabsorptive capacity of the collecting duct in unilateral obstruction was determined in measurements of isotopic Na$^+$ fluxes from lumen to bath, and these revealed a striking decrease in Na$^+$ reabsorption.[197] Measurements of transepithelial voltages revealed marked decreases in unilateral and bilateral obstruction,[199] and these decreases occurred whether or not the animal was pretreated with mineralocorticoid.[197, 199, 200] Because it is difficult to perfuse the IMCD in vitro, studies of the function of freshly isolated IMCD are best performed in cell suspensions. In these studies, transport-dependent oxygen consumption was strikingly reduced in cells from animals with bilateral obstruction.[201]

Taken together, the in vivo micropuncture and in vitro tubule studies demonstrate striking impairment of volume reabsorption in the proximal straight tubule, the mTAL, and the CCD and IMCD. Despite the lack of major ultrastructural damage, the cellular mechanisms of active transport are strikingly impaired in obstructive nephropathy. Interestingly, both unilateral and bilateral obstruction resulted in identical impairment of function.[197, 200] Thus, the impaired active transport in these cells is due primarily to tubule cell injury rather than to the continuous action of natriuretic substances.

Studies of tubule function in obstructive nephropathy have focused on the mechanisms leading to impairment of active transport in these cells. Active Na$^+$ transport in tubule epithelial cells requires an apical entry pathway, such as the apical Na$^+$-K$^+$-2Cl$^-$ cotransporter in mTAL or the Na$^+$ channel in CCD and IMCD, coupled to the basolateral Na$^+$,K$^+$-ATPase. In addition, the cell must be capable of generating sufficient metabolic energy to power the Na$^+$,K$^+$-ATPase. In mTAL suspensions from obstructed kidneys, furosemide- and ouabain-sensitive oxygen consumption (QO$_2$) was markedly reduced.[198] Because the reduction in furosemide-sensitive QO$_2$ indicated reduced activity of the apical Na$^+$-K$^+$-2Cl$^-$ cotransporter, the amount of cotransporter protein was measured by use of [$^3$H]bumetanide binding. These studies revealed a marked reduction in the number of binding sites, with no change in the affinity of binding, which suggests that obstruction down-regulates the expression of cotransporter protein.[198] Because ouabain-sensitive QO$_2$ was also reduced, the activity of Na$^+$,K$^+$-ATPase was examined. As has been shown previously, ouabain-sensitive ATPase was markedly reduced in mTAL from obstructed kidneys.[198] The mechanism of this decrease was investigated with immunoblots, which revealed a marked decrease in the levels of both α- and β-subunits.[198] To define the mechanism underlying this decreased expression of pump subunit proteins, levels of Na$^+$,K$^+$-ATPase messenger RNA (mRNA) were measured.[202] After 12 hours of obstruction, levels of β- but not α-subunit mRNA were sharply reduced. Interestingly, levels of mRNA of both subunits were normal at 24 hours, when the levels of both subunit proteins are markedly reduced. These results indicate that down-regulation of Na$^+$,K$^+$-ATPase is mediated both by reduced transcription of subunit mRNA and by post-transcriptional mechanisms.[202]

In the IMCD, similar studies revealed a striking decrease in amiloride-sensitive QO$_2$, indicating reduced activity of apical Na$^+$ channels.[201] In addition, measurement of amiloride-sensitive Na$^+$ uptake in hyperpolarized cells revealed clear-cut decreases in Na$^+$ channel activity.[201] This reduction in channel activity corresponds with results in isolated perfused CCD from obstructed animals, which revealed clear-cut decreases in apical membrane conductance compared with control tubules.[199] To determine whether this reduction in channel activity was due to reduced expression of Na$^+$ channel protein or to reduced activity of channel proteins in the membrane, immunoblot studies were again performed. These studies revealed that levels of Na$^+$ channel protein were unchanged by obstruction, which suggests that the reduced channel activity is due to reduced open time of channels within the membrane.[201] Studies of Na$^+$,K$^+$-ATPase in IMCD gave results that closely paralleled those obtained in the mTAL. Thus, ouabain-sensitive QO$_2$, ouabain-sensitive ATPase, and the levels of both α- and β-subunit proteins were strikingly reduced. The pattern of mRNA expression was also similar, with a transient dip in levels of β-subunit mRNA at 12 hours that reached normal levels at 24 hours and no drop in the levels of α-subunit mRNA.[198, 201, 202]

These results indicate selective down-regulation of transporter activities and the levels of expression of transporter proteins after 24 hours of obstruction. Metabolic studies have revealed reductions in several enzymes of the oxidative and glycolytic pathways in obstruction (see later), which suggests a reduced capacity for metabolic energy generation. Indeed, examination of mTAL after obstruction reveals reduced basolateral infolding and reduced density of mitochondria.[192] However, studies of mTAL and IMCD cells in suspension reveal decreases in the basal rates of ouabain-sensitive QO$_2$, and not of ouabain-insensitive QO$_2$,

which suggests that the ability to generate ATP is not rate limiting for active transport in these cells.[198, 201] Rather, it appears more likely that the metabolic machinery is down-regulated in response to a decrease in active transport.

The mechanisms whereby obstruction down-regulates transporter activity and expression in tubule epithelial cells remain unclear. Possibilities include the halting of urine flow, increased interstitial pressure, alterations in blood flow to the tubules, and the generation of natriuretic substances in the kidney that lead to long-lasting changes in transporter function.

When obstruction occurs, urine flow ceases or slows dramatically. The reduction of delivery of solutes to the tubule cells reduces the rate at which Na$^+$ enters the cells, because the gradients for Na$^+$ entry between the stationary apical fluid and the interior of the cell become increasingly unfavorable. Reduction in Na$^+$ entry would then down-regulate the activity or expression of transporter proteins. Such a mechanism has indeed been shown to regulate the activity of Na$^+$,K$^+$-ATPase, because reduction of Na$^+$ entry by amiloride in IMCD cells[203, 204] or by furosemide in mTAL cells promptly reduces ouabain-sensitive QO$_2$.[198, 205] Moreover, in adrenalectomized animals given exogenous mineralocorticoid, long-term inhibition of Na$^+$ entry by administration of furosemide or amiloride reduces the levels of ouabain-sensitive ATPase activity in microdissected mTAL[206] and CCD,[207] respectively. These results suggest that cessation of urine flow might be a major mechanism by which obstruction down-regulates Na$^+$ transporter activity.[204]

There is strong evidence that changes in intrarenal hormones are responsible for at least some of the down-regulation of transporters observed in obstruction. Numerous studies have demonstrated that obstruction markedly stimulates the already high generation of PGE$_2$ in the renal medulla.[174, 177, 179, 208, 209] PGE$_2$ has been shown to inhibit Na$^+$ reabsorption acutely in mTAL, CCD, and IMCD, with inhibition of Na$^+$,K$^+$-ATPase being at least one mechanism of action.[210–215] Interestingly, preliminary studies have shown that PGE$_2$ can act by reducing deployment of Na$^+$,K$^+$-ATPase to the plasma membrane in the CCD.[216] Moreover, long-term treatment of animals with indomethacin increases Na$^+$,K$^+$-ATPase activity, which suggests that renal levels of PGE$_2$ regulate expression of Na$^+$,K$^+$-ATPase chronically.[217] From these results, it is possible that obstruction reduces Na$^+$,K$^+$-ATPase by elevating renal levels of PGE$_2$.

As noted before, obstruction induces a mononuclear cell infiltrate.[181] Interestingly, in obstruction, macrophages localize in a peritubular distribution.[181] Irradiation of kidneys during obstruction reduced the level of medullary inflammation, and this reduction corresponded with a modest improvement in FE$_{Na}$.[182] It is possible that the mononuclear infiltrate stimulates PGE$_2$ generation, although the levels of PGE$_2$ in obstruction in the presence and absence of irradiation were not measured.

In summary, obstruction reduces net reabsorption of Na$^+$ at several nephron sites, including the proximal straight tubule, mTAL, CCD, and IMCD, by down-regulating the activities and expression of specific transporter proteins. The mechanisms by which obstruction reduces the activity of these transporters remain unclear.

In the setting of bilateral obstruction, extrarenal factors markedly enhance the salt-wasting tendency of the affected kidney. Such factors include volume expansion, which reduces the activity of volume-retentive influences (such as the sympathetic nervous system and aldosterone) and, along with reduced renal clearance, increases levels of ANP. In addition, accumulation of solutes, such as urea, and other urinary natriuretic substances may augment the natriuretic effects of obstruction. In 24-hour obstruction, renal $Na^+$ excretion was markedly enhanced if the contralateral kidney was also obstructed or if the contralateral kidney was removed.[184] Moreover, if 24-hour unilateral obstruction was released and the urea, salt, and water content of the urine from the contralateral kidney was reinfused into the animal, there was a striking increase in $Na^+$ excretion in both the obstructed and contralateral kidney,[184, 185] an effect that occurred when the urine was infused into normal animals.[185] These studies indicate that natriuretic substances normally present in the urine may accumulate in bilateral obstruction, enhancing natriuresis when the obstruction is released.

As discussed before, ANP levels are markedly increased in bilateral but not in unilateral obstruction.[187] Because ANP can reduce angiotensin II–stimulated proximal volume reabsorption and can markedly inhibit collecting duct $Na^+$ reabsorption, increased levels of this hormone may mediate a significant portion of the postobstructive natriuresis observed in bilateral obstruction.[173, 186, 187] In line with this view, infusions of ANP into postobstructive animals markedly increased $Na^+$ and water excretion.[187] Moreover, reduction in circulating ANP levels with heparin reduced $Na^+$ excretion after bilateral obstruction.[187]

## EFFECTS OF OBSTRUCTION ON URINE CONCENTRATION AND DILUTION

The urine osmolality in patients and animals with obstructive uropathy approaches that of plasma, denoting reduced capacity to concentrate and dilute the urine.[2, 17] Dilution of urine requires reabsorption of $Na^+$ without water in the thick ascending limb and maintenance of dilute urine in the collecting duct despite the increasing osmolality in the medullary interstitium[218, 219] (see Chapter 13). Concentration of urine requires active solute reabsorption in the thick ascending limb for generation of a high osmolality in the medullary interstitium as well as the ability of the collecting duct to insert water channels into the apical membrane in response to antidiuretic hormone.[218, 219]

Several of these mechanisms are disrupted in obstructive nephropathy. First, as noted before, active $Na^+$ reabsorption is markedly reduced in the mTAL of obstructed kidneys, which reduces the ability to dilute the urine and to generate a high osmolality in the interstitium. Indeed, measured interstitial osmolality is reduced in obstruction.[2] Studies of water transport by CCD isolated from obstructed and control kidneys have revealed similar water permeabilities in the basal state but marked impairment in the ability of the tubule to increase water permeability in response to both antidiuretic hormone and cyclic AMP.[197, 200] As was the case with $Na^+$ transport, these defects were similar whether the animal was subjected to unilateral or bilateral obstruction.[197, 200]

These results indicate that the defect in urine dilution results from a reduction in the ability of the mTAL to remove solute without water from the urine, not from a failure of the collecting duct to maintain osmotic gradients. The reduction in urine concentrating ability results from reduced ability of the mTAL to generate a concentrated interstitium and reduced ability of the collecting duct to increase water permeability in response to antidiuretic hormone. Because cyclic AMP did not restore the collecting duct response, the defect must be at some point beyond the receptor–adenylate cyclase step,[200] perhaps involving reduced numbers of water channels or defective trafficking of water channel–containing vesicles.[219, 220] With the availability of antibody and complementary DNA probes to antidiuretic hormone–regulated water channels, the mechanisms underlying these defects can be examined (see Chapter 12).

## EFFECTS OF RELIEF OF OBSTRUCTION ON URINE ACIDIFICATION

Obstruction results in significant impairment of urine acidification, in both humans and experimental animals. In humans, release of obstruction is not accompanied by bicarbonaturia, which indicates relative preservation of proximal tubule $HCO_3^-$ reabsorption. However, patients and experimental animals exhibit reduced ability to lower urine pH in response to acid loading, which indicates a defect in the ability of the distal nephron to acidify the urine after relief of the obstruction.[2, 17, 221, 222] These results indicate that the site of the acidification defect is the collecting duct.[221, 222] In the CCD and medullary collecting duct, acidification of the urine is mediated by apical $H^+$-ATPase and $H^+,K^+$-ATPase coupled to basolateral $Cl^-/HCO_3^-$ exchangers; these transporters are located in the membranes of intercalated cells. Interestingly, some intercalated cells are oriented with apical $Cl^-/HCO_3^-$ exchangers and apical $H^+$-ATPase. In the CCD, a lumen-negative voltage regulates $H^+$ secretion by the electrogenic $H^+$-ATPase; in the medullary collecting duct, the voltage is of less importance because of negligible to positive luminal voltage. Thus, reduced acidification by the collecting duct may result from defective $H^+$ or $HCO_3^-$ transport pathways; back-leakage of $H^+$ from the lumen into the interstitium; or, in the CCD, a failure to generate adequate lumen negativity.[221–223] The last mechanism has been demonstrated in studies revealing a marked inhibition of acidification in the presence of the $Na^+$ channel inhibitor amiloride. As discussed before, several studies have demonstrated that obstruction reduces the ability of the CCD to generate a negative luminal voltage, establishing this defect as a potential cause of defective acidification.[197, 200, 221, 222] However, studies of CCD acidification in obstruction have not demonstrated an acidification defect. In the rabbit, CCD acidification was not altered at 1 to 2 days of obstruction, whereas inner stripe OMCD acidification was reduced at 2 to 4 days but not at 1 day.[222] By contrast, in the rat OMCD, 24-hour obstruction markedly reduced acidification.[221] These results suggest that the lack of effect of obstruction on CCD acidification in the rabbit may be unique to that species.

In the isolated perfused rat and rabbit OMCD and in rat IMCD by micropuncture, obstruction induces a significant acidification defect.[221] Given the lack of importance of $Na^+$ transport in governing acidification in these segments, these results indicate a defect in transporter pathways or a failure of the epithelial barrier to $H^+$ back-flux.[223] Measurements of acidification in OMCD perfused at low rates indicated no defect in the ability of the tubule to generate a steep pH gradient.[221] However, at high perfusion rates, acidification was strikingly decreased in the tubules from obstructed kidneys.[221] These results indicate that obstruction reduces the maximal rate at which the tubule can acidify but does not damage the ability of the tubule to maintain pH gradients.

Because the major transport pathways in collecting duct acidification are the $H^+$-ATPase and $Cl^-/HCO_3^-$ exchanger, the effects of obstruction on these two proteins were studied with use of specific antisera directed against them.[223] By use of immunofluorescence to localize the $H^+$-ATPase, the frequency and orientation of intercalated cells were shown to be the same in obstructed, contralateral, and control kidneys. Moreover, the amount of $H^+$-ATPase protein present in extracts of cortex and medulla was not altered by obstruction. However, the distribution of $H^+$-ATPase within the intercalated cells was altered in obstructed kidneys.[223] Along the apical membranes of up to 30% of intercalated cells, there were discontinuities or gaps in labeling for $H^+$-ATPase. Moreover, the proportion of intercalated cells exhibiting a plasma membrane or "rim" labeling pattern was diminished.[223] These results suggest that obstruction interferes with the ability of the intercalated cell to deploy $H^+$-ATPase to the apical membrane. However, this alteration in cellular trafficking of the enzyme cannot alone account for the disturbance in acid secretion.[223] First, the reduction in cells with the rim pattern and the appearance of gaps in apical membrane labeling resolve as obstruction is prolonged, whereas the acidification defect persists. Second, it seems unlikely that a reduction in apical $H^+$-ATPase in 30% of intercalated cells could account for the magnitude of the acidification defect observed. These considerations indicate that additional mechanisms must be responsible for the defective acidification observed in obstructed kidneys.

In addition to defects in distal nephron acid transport, reduced ammoniagenesis in the proximal tubule may contribute to reduced acid excretion in obstruction. Studies in cortical slices from obstructed kidneys revealed a reduced capacity to generate ammonia from glutamine at several steps along the pathway, including decreased glutamine uptake and oxidation, reduced generation of glucose and ammonia, and reduced oxygen consumption.[224, 225]

## EFFECT OF RELIEF OF OBSTRUCTION ON EXCRETION OF $K^+$

$K^+$ excretion is markedly increased after release of bilateral obstruction, in parallel with the increase in $Na^+$ excretion.[226, 227] Micropuncture and microcatheterization studies have shown that proximal $K^+$ reabsorption is normal but that additional $K^+$ is added to the urine in the collecting duct, probably because of increased distal delivery of $Na^+$ and volume in this setting.[195, 226] In unilateral obstruction, $K^+$ excretion is reduced, roughly in proportion to the fall in GFR.[228] This reduction may be due to reduced net distal delivery of volume. However, administration of sodium sulfate does not stimulate $K^+$ excretion normally, which suggests an intrinsic defect in distal $K^+$ secretion.[229]

## EFFECT OF RELIEF OF OBSTRUCTION ON EXCRETION OF $PO_4^{3-}$ AND DIVALENT CATIONS

In bilateral ureteral obstruction, $PO_4^{3-}$ excretion is increased in parallel with $Na^+$ excretion.[230] This increment in excretion can be blocked by dietary phosphate restriction to prevent the accumulation of $PO_4^{3-}$ that normally accompanies bilateral obstruction.[230] Moreover, $PO_4^{3-}$ loading of animals to achieve blood levels similar to those seen in bilateral obstruction results in phosphaturia of similar magnitude.[230] By contrast, in unilateral obstruction, $PO_4^{3-}$ excretion is markedly reduced in the obstructed kidney, probably because of the striking decrease in GFR, which results in avid proximal tubule $PO_4^{3-}$ reabsorption.[231] $Ca^{2+}$ excretion may be increased or decreased, depending on the species studied and whether the obstruction is unilateral or bilateral.[230, 232] $Mg^{2+}$ excretion is markedly increased in both unilateral and bilateral obstruction, probably because its reabsorption is closely linked to that of $Na^+$ in the mTAL, a site at which obstruction markedly reduces $Na^+$ reabsorption[232] (see earlier).

## Effects of Obstruction on Metabolic Pathways and Gene Expression

Obstruction reduces oxidative and increases anaerobic respiration, accompanied by decreases in tissue ATP levels and corresponding increases in levels of ADP and AMP.[225, 233, 234] In addition, a wide variety of metabolic enzymes and the expression of various gene products are altered in obstructed kidneys.[193, 225, 234–236] These are summarized in Table 41–6. In many cases, it is difficult to link these changes in enzyme activities to known defects in tubule or glomerulus function. However, as discussed before, reduced ability to generate ATP may contribute to defective $Na^+$ reabsorption. Moreover, as noted, the reduction in $Na^+,K^+$-ATPase activity in several nephron segments probably contributes to natriuresis in obstruction.

## TREATMENT OF URINARY TRACT OBSTRUCTION AND RECOVERY OF RENAL FUNCTION

Once the diagnosis of obstruction is established, surgical or instrumental procedures may be indicated. In general, the location of the obstruction dictates the most effective therapy. For example, passage of a urethral catheter may be sufficient to alleviate an obstruction distal to the bladder.

**TABLE 41–6. Effects of Urinary Tract Obstruction on Renal Enzymes and Renal Gene Expression**

**Changes in Energy and Substrate Metabolism**
Decreased oxygen consumption
Decreased substrate uptake
Increased anaerobic glycolysis
Decreased ATP/(ADP + AMP)
Decreased ammoniagenesis

**Changes in Enzyme Activity**
Decreased
  Alkaline phosphatase
  $Na^+,K^+$-ATPase
  Glucose-6-phosphatase
  Succinate dehydrogenase
  NADH/NADPH dehydrogenase
  Glycerol-3-phosphate dehydrogenase
Increased
  Glucose-6-phosphate dehydrogenase
  Phosphogluconate dehydrogenase

**Changes in Gene Expression**
Reduction in glomerular $G_{\alpha s}$ and $G_{\alpha q/11}$ proteins
Reduction in pre-pro–epidermal growth factor and Tamm-Horsfall
  protein
Transient induction of growth factors FOS and MYC
Striking induction of cellular damage (TRPM2) genes

Data from references 193, 225, 234–236.

Rarely, suprapubic cystostomy may be required. Alternatively, the insertion of nephrostomy tubes at the time of the diagnostic ultrasound examination is indicated in cases of upper tract obstruction. The urgency of any intervention depends on the degree of renal dysfunction, the presence of infection, and the overall risk of the procedure. Obstruction that presents as acute renal failure or urosepsis requires emergent relief of the obstruction. Urosepsis also requires treatment with intravenous antibiotics.

Calculi, the most common cause of acute unilateral ureteral obstruction, may initially be treated conservatively with intravenous fluids to increase urine flow and with narcotics for analgesia. Although approximately 90% of stones less than 5 mm pass spontaneously, the likelihood of passage decreases with increasing stone size. Surgery or instrumentation of the urinary tract is indicated when there is persistent obstruction, uncontrollable pain, or urinary tract infection. At this point, possible interventions include placement of a nephrostomy tube for drainage, nephroscopy to attempt stone removal from the renal pelvis or proximal ureter under direct vision, and fragmentation by extracorporeal shock wave lithotripsy. Distal ureteral stones can be removed cystoscopically by use of a loop or basket or fragmented by ultrasonic or laser lithotripsy. The introduction of these newer techniques has markedly reduced the need for open surgical procedures.

Intramural or extrinsic ureteral obstruction may be relieved by placement of a ureteral stent through a cystoscope. Because partial obstruction due to benign prostatic hyperplasia does not always progress, surgery can be safely delayed or completely avoided in a patient with minimal symptoms, no infection, and an anatomically normal upper urinary tract. Either dilatation or internal urethrotomy with direct visualization may be effective in the treatment of urethral strictures. However, external bladder drainage through suprapubic cystostomy may be necessary in patients with an impassable urethral stricture or urethral injury.

A variety of approaches are used for treatment of obstruction due to a neurogenic bladder, including frequent voiding, pharmacologic agents, and clean intermittent catheterization. If possible, long-term indwelling bladder catheters should be avoided because of the increased risk of infection.

Once the patient's condition is stabilized, the next decision is whether to continue observation or to proceed with reparative surgery or nephrectomy. This decision is based on the likelihood that renal function will improve with repair of the obstruction. Factors that influence this surgical decision include the age of the patient, the appearance and function of the contralateral kidney, and the presence of symptoms or infection. Because better recovery of renal function presumably occurs with early diagnosis and treatment, the shorter the duration of obstruction, the greater the likelihood that renal damage will be reversible. In addition, urinary tract infection, hypercalcemia, acute tubule necrosis, and parenchymal infiltration may contribute to renal damage.

Indications for surgery for lower urinary tract obstruction include progressive loss of renal function despite conservative therapy, intractable incontinence, and a small contracted bladder. For patients with obstruction due to a malignant neoplasm, the decision to proceed with urinary diversion should be made on an individual basis. In a patient with lower urinary tract obstruction, the ileal conduit is the procedure of choice for permanent diversion. A detailed discussion of the available techniques used to treat urinary tract obstruction is beyond the scope of this chapter; the reader is referred to other sources.[237, 238]

## Estimate of Renal Damage and Potential for Recovery

An estimate of the degree of functional damage to the obstructed kidney is necessary to determine whether surgical repair of a severely hydronephrotic kidney should be attempted or a nephrectomy should be performed. Because the degree of anatomic distortion of the renal collecting system demonstrated by ultrasonography or intravenous urography does not correlate well with the degree of functional damage,[141] isotopic renography, a functional test, should be performed. Several different isotopes with varying ability to predict recoverable renal function have been used.[141] It has been suggested that relief of the obstruction by nephrostomy tube drainage for several weeks before the performance of isotopic renography improves the predictive value of the test.[141]

## Recovery of Renal Function with Prolonged Obstruction

The potential for recovery of renal function depends on the duration and completeness of the obstruction as well as the number of urinary tract infections. Studies in dogs found no recovery of renal function after 40 days of unilateral ureteral ligation. In contrast, case reports in humans have demonstrated some recovery 69 days[239] or longer[240] after the relief of unilateral ureteral obstruction. Because the recovery of renal function cannot be predicted with confidence at the time of diagnosis, temporary drainage procedures (such as placement of a nephrostomy tube) with sequential functional evaluations of renal function should be performed to better assess the potential for recovery before a decision on surgery is made. Chronic bilateral obstruction, typically due to benign prostatic hyperplasia, can cause chronic renal failure,[241, 242] particularly in men with long duration of obstruction and multiple urinary tract infections.[242] Progressive loss of renal function can usually be prevented in these patients by relief of the obstruction and aggressive treatment of urinary tract infections.

## POSTOBSTRUCTIVE DIURESIS

A marked natriuresis and diuresis can occur after the release of bilateral ureteral obstruction.[243–247] Postobstructive diuresis is characterized by polyuria with the excretion of large amounts of electrolytes and water. In addition to the potential danger of severe volume depletion due to $Na^+$ wasting, other serious disorders such as hypokalemia, hyponatremia, hypernatremia, and hypomagnesemia may be seen.

### Etiology

Several factors associated with bilateral obstruction may contribute to postobstructive diuresis, including volume expansion, urea accumulation, tubule damage, and accumulation of natriuretic factors. Whereas volume expansion may occur during the period of obstruction,[245] the retained $Na^+$ is usually appropriately excreted after the obstruction is relieved. Urea and other relatively nonreabsorbable solutes accumulate during the period of obstruction[244] and may contribute to the water and solute loss after relief of the obstruction. However, urea accumulation alone is not responsible for the entire volume of fluid loss,[248] and patients with a significant postobstructive diuresis may still have an initially normal blood urea nitrogen level.[246] Tubule damage as a consequence of obstruction may occur in one or more nephron segments and may result in decreased reabsorption of filtrate. This is associated with significant $Na^{+197}$ and water[200] loss despite a marked decrease in GFR and a deficient response to exogenous mineralocorticoid and vasopressin.[246] Furthermore, the natriuresis may be augmented by the accumulation of natriuretic factors during the period of obstruction, such as ANP.[249]

### Treatment

Postobstructive diuresis is usually self-limited in duration, lasting several days to a week. Rarely, it may persist for several months.[243] Massive polyuria of short duration or

persistent postobstructive diuresis may result in clinical deficiencies of $Na^+$, $K^+$, $Cl^-$, and water as well as of $Mg^{2+}$, $Ca^{2+}$, $PO_4^{3-}$, and $HCO_3^-$. Fluid replacement is justified only when excessive losses of $Na^+$ and water occur and result in volume or water depletion. Postobstructive diuresis will be perpetuated and prolonged by excessive fluid replacement. Initially, the urine is isosthenuric with a urinary $Na^+$ concentration of approximately 80 mEq/L. Thus, an appropriate starting fluid is 0.45% saline at a rate slightly less than the urine output. Close monitoring of volume status, vital signs, urine output, and chemistry values is imperative. Assessment of the need for ongoing fluid replacement may be based on the results of frequent measurements of weight, urine volume, and serum and urinary electrolytes. In cases of massive diuresis, these measurements may be necessary at least every 6 hours. Moreover, it may be necessary to add $K^+$, $Mg^{2+}$, $Ca^{2+}$, $PO_4^{3-}$, and $HCO_3^-$ to the intravenous fluid to replace any deficits.

## REFERENCES

1. Bricker NS, Klahr S: Obstructive nephropathy. In Strauss MB, Welt LG (eds): Diseases of the Kidney. Little, Brown, Boston, 1971, pp 997–1037.
2. Yarger WE: Urinary tract obstruction. In Brenner BM, Rector FC (eds): The Kidney, 4th ed. WB Saunders, Philadelphia, 1991, pp 1768–1808.
3. Bell ET: Renal Diseases. Lea & Febiger, Philadelphia, 1950.
4. Campbell MF: Urinary obstruction. In Campbell MF, Harrison JH (eds): Urology. WB Saunders, Philadelphia, 1970, pp 1772–1793.
5. Klahr S, Buerkert J, Morrison A: Urinary tract obstruction. In Brenner BM, Rector FC Jr (eds): The Kidney, 3rd ed. WB Saunders, Philadelphia, 1986, pp 1443–1490.
6. US Renal Data System: USRDS 1993 Annual Data Report. The National Institutes of Health, National Institute of Diabetes and Digestive and Kidney Diseases, Bethesda, MD, March 1993.
7. Snyder HM, Lebowitz RL, Colodny AH: Ureteropelvic junction obstruction in children. Urol Clin North Am 7:273–290, 1980.
8. Young DW, Lebowitz RL: Congenital abnormalities of the ureter. Semin Roentgenol 21:172–187, 1986.
9. Graverson HP, Tofte T, Genster HG: Ureteropelvic stenosis. Int Urol Nephrol 19:245–251, 1987.
10. Lowe FC, Marshall FF: Ureteropelvic junction obstruction in adults. Urology 23:331–335, 1984.
11. Clark WR, Malek RS: Ureteropelvic junction obstruction. I. Observations on the classic type in adults. J Urol 138:276–279, 1987.
12. Buscemi M, Shanske A, Mallet E, et al: Dominantly inherited ureteropelvic junction obstruction. Urology 26:568–571, 1985.
13. Elder JS, Duckett JW: Perinatal urology. In Gillenwater JY, Grayhack JT, Howards SS, Duckett JW (eds): Adult and Pediatric Urology. Mosby–Year Book, St. Louis, 1991, pp 1711–1810.
14. Murphy JP, Holder TM, Ashcraft KW, et al: Ureteropelvic junction obstruction in the newborn. J Pediatr Surg 19:642–648, 1984.
15. Novick AC, Streem SB: Surgery of the kidney. In Walsh PC, Retik AB, Stamey TA, Vaughan ED Jr (eds): Campbell's Urology. WB Saunders, Philadelphia, 1992, pp 2413–2500.
16. Hanna MK, Jeffs RD, Sturgess JM, Barkin M: Ureteral structure and ultrastructure. Part II. Congenital ureteropelvic junction obstruction and primary obstructive megaureter. J Urol 116:725–729, 1976.
17. Klahr S, Harris KPG: Obstructive uropathy. In Seldin DW, Giebisch G (eds): The Kidney: Physiology and Pathophysiology, 2nd ed. Raven Press, New York, 1992, pp 3327–3369.
18. Hanna MK: Some observations on congenital ureteropelvic junction obstruction. Urology 12:151–159, 1978.
19. Stephens FD: Primary obstructing megaureter. In Stephens FD (ed): Congenital Malformations of the Urinary Tract. Praeger, New York, 1983, pp 267–281.
20. Wall B, Wachter HE: Congenital ureteral valve: Its role as a primary obstructive lesion: Classification of the literature and report of an authentic case. J Urol 129:1222–1224, 1983.

21. Sant GR, Barbalias GA, Klauber GT: Congenital ureteral valves: An abnormality of ureteral embryogenesis? J Urol 133:427–431, 1985.
22. Ayyat FM, Adams G: Congenital midureteral strictures. Urology 26:170–172, 1985.
23. Macksood MJ, Roth DR, Chang CH, Perlmutter AD: Benign fibro-epithelial polyps as a cause of intermittent ureteropelvic junction obstruction in a child: A case report and review of the literature. J Urol 134:951–952, 1985.
24. Eidelman A, Yuval E, Simon D, Sibi Y: Retrocaval ureter. Eur Urol 4:279–281, 1978.
25. Brown T, Mandell J, Lebowitz RL: Neonatal hydronephrosis in the era of sonography. AJR 148:959–963, 1987.
26. Tanagho EA, Pugh RCB: The anatomy and function of the uretero-vesical junction. Br J Urol 35:151–165, 1963.
27. Woodburne RT: Anatomy of the ureterovesical junction. J Urol 92:431–435, 1964.
28. Lockhart JL, Singer AM, Glenn JF: Congenital megaureter. J Urol 122:310–314, 1979.
29. Welch KJ, Kearney GP: Abdominal musculature deficiency syndrome: Prune belly. J Urol 111:693–700, 1974.
30. Snow BW, Duckett JW: Prune belly syndrome. In Gillenwater JY, Grayhack JT, Howards SS, Duckett JW (eds): Adult and Pediatric Urology. Mosby–Year Book, St. Louis, 1991, pp 1921–1938.
31. Fenelon MJ, Alton DJ: Prolapsing ectopic ureteroceles in boys. Radiology 140:373–376, 1981.
32. Newman LB, McAlister WH, Kissane J: Segmental renal dysplasia associated with ectopic ureteroceles in childhood. Urology 3:23–26, 1974.
33. Snyder HM, Johnston JH: Orthotopic ureteroceles in children. J Urol 119:543–546, 1978.
34. Livne PM, Gonzales ET Jr: Congenital bladder diverticula causing ureteral obstruction. Urology 25:273–276, 1985.
35. Bauer SB: Neurogenic vesical dysfunction in children. In Walsh PC, Retik AB, Stamey TA, Vaughan ED Jr (eds): Campbell's Urology. WB Saunders, Philadelphia, 1992, pp 1634–1668.
36. McLorie GA, Perez-Marero R, Csima A, Churchill BM: Determinants of hydronephrosis and renal injury in patients with myelomeningocele. J Urol 140:1289–1292, 1988.
37. Shochat SJ, Perlmutter AD: Myelodysplasia with severe neonatal hydronephrosis: The value of urethral dilatation. J Urol 107:146–148, 1972.
38. Glassberg KI: Current issues regarding posterior urethral valves. Urol Clin North Am 12:175–185, 1985.
39. Kurth KH, Alleman ER, Schroder FH: Major and minor complications of posterior urethral valves. J Urol 126:517–519, 1981.
40. Martin J, Anderson J, Raz S: Posterior urethral valves in adults: A report of 2 cases. J Urol 118:978–979, 1977.
41. Freeny PC: Congenital anterior urethral diverticulum in the male. Radiology 111:173–174, 1974.
42. Fine RN: Diagnosis and treatment of fetal urinary tract abnormalities. J Pediatr 121:333–341, 1992.
43. Crombleholme TM, Harrison MR, Longaker MT, Langer JC: Prenatal diagnosis and management of bilateral hydronephrosis. Pediatr Nephrol 2:334–342, 1988.
44. Mandell J, Peters CA, Retik AB: Current concepts in the perinatal diagnosis and management of hydronephrosis. Urol Clin North Am 17:247–262, 1990.
45. Allen TD: The swing of the pendulum. J Urol 148:534–535, 1992. Editorial.
46. Thorup J, Mortensen T, Diemer H, et al: The prognosis of surgically treated congenital hydronephrosis after diagnosis in utero. J Urol 134:914–917, 1985.
47. Wolpert JJ, Woodard JR, Parrott TS: Pyeloplasty in the young infant. J Urol 142:573–575, 1989.
48. Conger JD: Acute uric acid nephropathy. Semin Nephrol 1:69–74, 1981.
49. Simon DI, Brosius FC, Rothstein DM: Sulfadiazine crystalluria revisited. The treatment of Toxoplasma encephalitis in patients with acquired immunodeficiency syndrome. Arch Intern Med 150:2379–2384, 1990.
50. Sawyer MH, Webb DE, Balow JE, Straus SE: Acyclovir-induced renal failure. Clinical course and histology. Am J Med 84:1067–1071, 1988.
51. DeFronzo RA, Humphrey RL, Wright JR, Cooke CR: Acute renal failure in multiple myeloma. Medicine (Baltimore) 54:209–223, 1975.
52. Crittenden DR, Ackerman GL: Hyperuricemic acute renal failure in disseminated carcinoma. Arch Intern Med 137:97–99, 1977.
53. Molina JM, Belenfant X, Doco-Lecompte T, et al: Sulfadiazine-induced crystalluria in AIDS patients with Toxoplasma encephalitis. AIDS 5:587–589, 1991.
54. Waugh DA, Ibels LS: Multiple myeloma presenting as obstructive uropathy. Aust N Z J Med 10:555–558, 1980.
55. Johnson CM, Wilson DM, O'Fallon WM, et al: Renal stone epidemiology: A 25-year study in Rochester, Minnesota. Kidney Int 16:624–631, 1979.
56. Eknoyan G, Quinibi WY, Grissom RT, et al: Renal papillary necrosis: An update. Medicine (Baltimore) 61:55–73, 1982.
57. Wein AJ: Neuromuscular dysfunction of the lower urinary tract. In Walsh PC, Retik AB, Stamey TA, Vaughan ED Jr (eds): Campbell's Urology. WB Saunders, Philadelphia, 1992, pp 573–642.
58. Novicki DE, Willscher MK: Case profile: Anticholinergic-induced hydronephrosis. Urology 13:324–325, 1979.
59. Murdock MI, Olsson CS, Sac DS, Krane RJ: Effects of levodopa on the bladder outlet. J Urol 113:803–805, 1975.
60. Graham JB, Abad RS: Ureteral obstruction due to radiation. Am J Obstet Gynecol 99:409–412, 1967.
61. MacGregor GA, Jones NF, Barraclough MA, et al: Ureteric stricture with analgesic nephropathy. Br Med J 2:271–272, 1973.
62. Smith JH, von Lichtenberg F, Lehman JS: Parasitic diseases of the genitourinary system. In Walsh PC, Retik AB, Stamey TA, Vaughan ED Jr (eds): Campbell's Urology. WB Saunders, Philadelphia, 1992, pp 883–927.
63. Nash TE, Cheever AW, Ottesen EA, Cook JA: Schistosome infections in humans: Perspectives and recent findings. NIH conference. Ann Intern Med 97:740–754, 1982.
64. Christensen WJ: Genitourinary tuberculosis. Review of 102 cases. Medicine (Baltimore) 53:377–390, 1974.
65. Murphy DM, Fallon B, Lane V, O'Flynn JD: Tuberculous stricture of the ureter. Urology 20:382–384, 1982.
66. Aragona F, Glazel GP, Povanello L, et al: Upper urinary tract obstruction in children caused by Candida fungal balls. Eur Urol 11:188–191, 1985.
67. Badr M: Renography in normal pregnant patients. Acta Obstet Gynecol Scand 52:69–76, 1973.
68. Murao F: Ultrasonic evaluation of hydronephrosis during pregnancy and puerperium. Gynecol Obstet Invest 35:94–98, 1993.
69. Lapata RE, Adelson BH: Ureteral obstruction due to compression by gravid uterus. Am J Obstet Gynecol 106:941–942, 1970.
70. Klein EA: Urologic problems of pregnancy. Obstet Gynecol Surv 39:605–615, 1984.
71. Bennett AH, Adler S: Bilateral ureteral obstruction causing anuria secondary to pregnancy. Urology 20:631–633, 1982.
72. Muller-Suur R, Tyden O: Evaluation of hydronephrosis in pregnancy using ultrasound and renography. Scand J Urol Nephrol 19:267–273, 1985.
73. D'Elia FL, Brennan RE, Brownstein PK: Acute renal failure secondary to ureteral obstruction by a gravid uterus. J Urol 128:803–804, 1982.
74. Beach EW: Urologic complications of cancer of uterine cervix. J Urol 68:178–189, 1952.
75. Kontogeorgos L, Vassilopoulos P, Tentes A: Bilateral severe hydro-ureteronephrosis due to uterine prolapse. Br J Urol 57:360–361, 1985.
76. Melser M, Miles BJ, Kastan D, et al: Chronic renal failure secondary to post-hysterectomy vaginal prolapse. Urology 38:361–363, 1991.
77. Resnick MI, Kursh ED: Extrinsic obstruction of the ureter. In Walsh PC, Retik AB, Stamey TA, Vaughan ED Jr (eds): Campbell's Urology. WB Saunders, Philadelphia, 1992, pp 533–569.
78. Philips JC: Spectrum of radiologic abnormalities due to tubo-ovarian abscess. Radiology 110:307–311, 1974.
79. Klein RS, Cattolica E: Ureteral endometriosis. Urology 13:477–482, 1979.
80. Kane C, Drouin P: Obstructive uropathy associated with endometriosis. Am J Obstet Gynecol 151:207–211, 1985.
81. Dowling RA, Corrier JN, Sandler CM: Iatrogenic ureteral injury. J Urol 135:912–915, 1986.
82. Peters CA, Walsh PC: The effect of nafarelin acetate, a luteinizing-hormone–releasing agonist, on benign prostatic hyperplasia. N Engl J Med 317:599–604, 1987.
83. Marks LS, Gallo DA: Ureteral obstruction in the patient with prostatic carcinoma. Br J Urol 44:411–416, 1972.

84. Batata MA, Whitmore WF, Hilaris BS, et al: Primary carcinoma of the ureter, a prognostic study. Cancer 35:1626–1632, 1975.

85. Present DH, Rabinowitz JG, Banks PA, Janowitz HD: Obstructive hydronephrosis in regional ileitis. N Engl J Med 280:523–528, 1963.

86. Schofield PF, Staff WG, Moose T: Ureteral involvement in regional ileitis. J Urol 99:412–416, 1968.

87. Shield DE, Lytton B, Weiss RM, Schiff M Jr: Urologic complications of inflammatory bowel disease. J Urol 115:701–706, 1976.

88. Cook GF: Appendiceal abscess causing urinary obstruction. J Urol 101:212–215, 1969.

89. Bissada M, Redman J: Ureteral complications in diverticulitis of the colon. J Urol 112:454–456, 1974.

90. Kiviat MD, Miller EV, Ansell JS: Pseudocysts of the pancreas presenting as renal mass lesions. Br J Urol 43:257–262, 1971.

91. Morehouse HL, Thornhill BA, Alterman DD: Right ureteral involvement associated with pancreatitis. Urol Radiol 7:150–152, 1985.

92. Loughlin K, Kearney G, Helfrich W, Carey R: Ureteral obstruction secondary to perianeurysmal fibrosis. Urology 24:332–336, 1984.

93. Safran R, Sklenicka R, Kay H: Iliac artery aneurysms: A common cause of ureteral obstruction. J Urol 113:605–609, 1975.

94. Mitty HA: Ovarian vein septic thrombophlebitis causing ureteral obstruction. J Urol 112:451–453, 1974.

95. Weisman MH, McDonald EC, Wilson CB: Studies of the pathogenesis of interstitial cystitis, obstructive uropathy, and intestinal malabsorption in a patient with systemic lupus erythematosus. Am J Med 70:875–881, 1981.

96. Melin JP, Lemaire P, Birembaut P, et al: Polyarteritis nodosa with bilateral ureteric involvement. Nephron 32:87–89, 1982.

97. Lie JT: Retroperitoneal polyarteritis nodosa presenting as ureteral obstruction. J Rheumatol 19:1628–1631, 1992.

98. Adelizzi RA, Shockley FK, Pietras JR: Wegener's granulomatosis with ureteric obstruction. J Rheumatol 13:448–451, 1986.

99. Kher KK, Sheth KJ, Makker SP: Stenosing ureteritis in Henoch-Schönlein purpura. J Urol 129:1040–1042, 1983.

100. Wagenknecht LV, Hardy JC: Value of various treatments for retroperitoneal fibrosis. Eur Urol 7:193–200, 1981.

101. Keith DS, Larson TS: Idiopathic retroperitoneal fibrosis. J Am Soc Nephrol 3:1748–1752, 1993.

102. Cohen WM, Freed SZ, Hasson J: Metastatic cancer to the ureter: A review of the literature and case presentations. J Urol 112:188–189, 1974.

103. Goldman SM, Fishman EK, Rosenshin NB, et al: Excretory urography and computed tomography in the initial evaluation of patients with cervical carcinoma: Are both examinations necessary? AJR 143:991–996, 1984.

104. Jones CR, Woodhouse CRJ, Hendry WF: Urologic problems following treatment of carcinoma of the cervix. Br J Urol 56:609–613, 1984.

105. Blum MD, Bahnson RR, Carter MF: Urologic manifestations of von Recklinghausen neurofibromatosis. Urology 26:209–217, 1985.

106. David HS, Lavengood RW: Bilateral Wilms' tumor: Treatment, management and review of the literature. Urology 3:71–74, 1974.

107. Schoenfeld RH, Belville WD, Buck A, et al: Unilateral ureteral obstruction secondary to sarcoidosis. Urology 25:57–59, 1985.

108. Bloomberg SD, Neu HC, Erhlick RM, Blank WA: Chronic granulomatous disease of childhood. Urology 4:193–197, 1974.

109. Robinson CR, Fowler JE: Localized amyloidosis of the ureter. J Urol 131:112–113, 1984.

110. Brown R, Bancewicz J: Ureteric obstruction due to pelvic actinomycosis. Br J Surg 69:156, 1982.

111. Talreja D, Slater LM, Dara P, et al: Multiple myeloma complicated by myelomatous obstructive uropathy. Cancer 46:1893–1895, 1980.

112. Gore RM, Shkolnik A: Abdominal manifestations of pediatric leukemias: Sonographic assessment. Radiology 143:207–210, 1982.

113. Richmond J, Sherman RS, Diamond HD, Craver LF: Renal lesions associated with malignant lymphomas. Am J Med 32:184–207, 1962.

114. Covington T, Reeser W: Hydronephrosis associated with overhydration. J Urol 63:438–445, 1950.

115. Chute CG, Panser LA, Girman CJ, et al: The prevalence of prostatism: A population based survey of urinary symptoms. J Urol 150:85–89, 1993.

116. Shimada K, Katsumi T, Fujita H: Appendiceal granuloma causing bilateral hydronephrosis and macroscopic haematuria. Br J Urol 48:418, 1976.

117. Weidmann P, Beretta-Piccoli C, Hirsch D, et al: Curable hypertension with unilateral hydronephrosis. Studies on the role of circulating renin. Ann Intern Med 87:437–440, 1977.

118. Whiting JC, Stanisis TH, Drach GW: Congenital ureteral valves: Report of 2 patients including one with a solitary kidney and associated hypertension. J Urol 129:1222–1224, 1983.

119. Parfrey PS, Griffiths SM, Barrett BJ, et al: Contrast material–induced renal failure in patients with diabetes mellitus, renal insufficiency, or both. N Engl J Med 320:143–149, 1989.

120. Coggins CH, Fang LST: Acute renal failure associated with antibiotics, anesthetic agents and radiographic contrast agents. In Brenner BM, Lazarus JM (eds): Acute Renal Failure. Churchill Livingstone, New York, 1988, pp 295–352.

121. Coleman BG: Ultrasound of the upper genitourinary tract. Urol Clin North Am 12:633–644, 1985.

122. Rao KG, Hackler RH, Woodlief RM, et al: Real-time renal sonography in spinal cord injury patients: Prospective comparison with excretory urography. J Urol 135:72, 1986.

123. Stuck KJ, White GM, Granke DS, et al: Urinary obstruction in azotemic patients: Detection by sonography. AJR 149:1191–1193, 1987.

124. Talner LB, Scheible W, Ellenbogen PH, et al: How accurate is ultrasonography in detecting hydronephrosis in azotemic patients? Urol Radiol 3:1–6, 1981.

125. Weinstein MC, Fineberg HV: Clinical Decision Analysis. WB Saunders, Philadelphia, 1980.

126. Amis ES, Cronan JJ, Pfister RC, Yoder IC: Ultrasonic inaccuracies in diagnosing renal obstruction. Urology 19:101, 1982.

127. Scheible W, Talner LB: Gray scale ultrasound and the genitourinary tract: A review of clinical applications. Radiol Clin North Am 17:281–300, 1979.

128. Cronan JJ, Amis ES, Scola FH, Schepps B: Renal obstruction in patients with ileal loops: US evaluation. Radiology 158:647–648, 1986.

129. Maillet PJ, Pelle-Francoz D, Laville M, et al: Nondilated obstructive acute renal failure: Diagnostic procedures and therapeutic management. Radiology 160:659–662, 1986.

130. Currey ND, Gobien RP, Schabel SI: Minimal-dilatation obstructive nephropathy. Radiology 143:531–534, 1982.

131. Lalli AF: Retroperitoneal fibrosis and inapparent obstructive uropathy. Radiology 122:339–342, 1977.

132. Charasse C, Camus C, Darnault P, et al: Acute nondilated anuric obstructive nephropathy on echography: Difficult diagnosis in the intensive care unit. Intensive Care Med 17:387–391, 1991.

133. Winters WD, Lebowitz RL: Importance of prenatal detection of hydronephrosis of the upper pole. AJR 155:125–129, 1990.

134. Corteville JE, Gray DL, Crane JP: Congenital hydronephrosis: Correlation of fetal ultrasonographic findings with infant outcome. Am J Obstet Gynecol 165:384–388, 1991.

135. Dejter SW Jr, Gibbons MD: The fate of infant kidneys with fetal hydronephrosis but initially normal postnatal sonography. J Urol 142:661–662, 1989.

136. Kaye AD, Pollack HM: Diagnostic imaging approach to the patient with obstructive uropathy. Semin Nephrol 2:55–73, 1982.

137. Davidson AJ: Radiologic contrast studies. In O'Reilly PH, George NJR, Weiss RM (eds): Diagnostic Techniques in Urology. WB Saunders, Philadelphia, 1990, pp 1–12.

138. Bosniak MA, Megibow AJ, Ambos MA, et al: Computed tomography of ureteral obstruction. AJR 138:1107–1113, 1982.

139. Testa HJ: Nuclear Medicine. In O'Reilly PH, George NJR, Weiss RM (eds): Diagnostic Techniques in Urology. WB Saunders, Philadelphia, 1990, pp 99–118.

140. English PJ, Testa HJ, Lawson RS, et al: Modified method of diuresis renography for the assessment of equivocal pelviureteric junction obstruction. Br J Urol 59:10–14, 1987.

141. Gillenwater JY: The pathophysiology of urinary tract obstruction. In Walsh PC, Retik AB, Stamey TA, Vaughan ED Jr (eds): Campbell's Urology. WB Saunders, Philadelphia, 1992, pp 499–532.

142. O'Reilly PH, Lawson RS, Shields RA, Testa HJ: Idiopathic hydronephrosis—the diuresis renogram: A new non-invasive method of assessing equivocal pelvioureteral junction obstruction. J Urol 121:153–155, 1979.

143. Upsdell SM, Leeson SM, Brooman PJC, O'Reilly PH: Diuretic-induced urinary flow rates at varying clearances and their relevance to the performance and interpretation of diuresis renography. Br J Urol 61:14–18, 1988.

144. Kikinis R, von Schulthess GK, Jager P, et al: Normal and hydronephrotic kidney: Evaluation of renal function with contrast-enhanced MR imaging. Radiology 165:837–842, 1987.
145. Semelka RC, Hricak H, Tomei E, et al: Obstructive nephropathy: Evaluation with dynamic Gd-DTPA–enhanced MR imaging. Radiology 175:797–803, 1990.
146. Dal Canton A, Stanziale R, Corradi A, et al: Effects of acute ureteral obstruction on glomerular hemodynamics in rat kidney. Kidney Int 12:403–411, 1977.
147. Ichikawa I: Evidence for altered glomerular hemodynamics during acute nephron obstruction. Am J Physiol 242:F580–F585, 1982.
148. Gaudio KM, Siegel NJ, Hayslett JP, Kashgarian M: Renal perfusion and intratubular pressure during ureteral occlusion in the rat. Am J Physiol 238:F205–F209, 1980.
149. Vaughan ED, Shenasky JH, Gillenwater JY: Mechanism of acute hemodynamic response to ureteral occlusion. Invest Urol 9:22–26, 1971.
150. Navar LG, Baer PG: Renal autoregulatory and glomerular filtration responses to graduated ureteral obstruction. Nephron 7:301–316, 1970.
151. Wright FS, Briggs JP: Feedback control of glomerular blood flow, pressure, and filtration rate. Physiol Rev 55:958–996, 1979.
152. Schramm LP, Carlson DE: Inhibition of renal vasoconstriction by elevated ureteral pressure. Am J Physiol 228:1126–1133, 1975.
153. Francisco LL, Hoversten LG, DiBona GF: Renal nerves in the compensatory adaptation to ureteral occlusion. Am J Physiol 238:F229–F234, 1980.
154. Allen JT, Vaughan ED Jr, Gillenwater JY: The effect of indomethacin on renal blood flow and ureteral pressure in unilateral ureteral obstruction in awake dogs. Invest Urol 15:324–327, 1978.
155. Blackshear JL, Wathen RL: Effects of indomethacin on renal blood flow and renin secretory responses to ureteral occlusion in the dog. Miner Electrolyte Metab 1:271–278, 1978.
156. Harris RH, Gill JM: Changes in glomerular filtration rate during complete ureteral obstruction in rats. Kidney Int 19:603–608, 1981.
157. Moody TE, Vaughan ED Jr, Gillenwater JY: Relationship between renal blood flow and ureteral pressure during 18 hours of total unilateral ureteral occlusion. Invest Urol 13:246–251, 1975.
158. Harris RH, Yarger WE: Renal function after release of unilateral ureteral obstruction in rats. Am J Physiol 227:806–815, 1974.
159. Yarger WE, Griffith LD: Intrarenal hemodynamics following chronic unilateral ureteral obstruction in the dog. Am J Physiol 227:816–826, 1974.
160. Dal Canton A, Corradi A, Stanziale R, et al: Glomerular hemodynamics before and after release of 24-hour bilateral ureteral obstruction. Kidney Int 17:491–496, 1980.
161. Prevoost AP, Molenaar JC: Renal function during and after a temporary complete unilateral ureter obstruction in rats. Invest Urol 18:242–246, 1981.
162. Jaenike JR: The renal functional defect of postobstructive nephropathy: The effects of bilateral ureteral obstruction in the rat. J Clin Invest 51:2999–3006, 1972.
163. Dal Canton A, Corradi A, Stanziale R, et al: Effects of 24-hour unilateral ureteral obstruction on glomerular hemodynamics in rat kidney. Kidney Int 15:457–462, 1979.
164. Tanner GA: Effects of kidney tubule obstruction on glomerular function in rats. Am J Physiol 237:F379–F385, 1979.
165. Yarger WE, Aynedjian HS, Bank N: A micropuncture study of postobstructive diuresis in the rat. J Clin Invest 51:625–637, 1972.
166. Bander SJ, Buerkert JE, Martin D, Klahr S: Long-term effects of 24-hr unilateral ureteral obstruction on renal function in the rat. Kidney Int 28:614–620, 1985.
167. Ichikawa I, Brenner BM: Local intrarenal vasoconstrictor-vasodilator interactions in mild partial ureteral obstruction. Am J Physiol 236:F131–F140, 1979.
168. Ichikawa I, Purkerson ML, Yates J, Klahr S: Dietary protein intake conditions the degree of renal vasoconstriction in acute renal failure caused by ureteral obstruction. Am J Physiol 249:F54–F61, 1985.
169. Wahlberg J, Stenberg A, Wilson DR, Persson AE: Tubuloglomerular feedback and interstitial pressure in obstructive nephropathy. Kidney Int 26:294–301, 1984.
170. Yarger WE, Schocken DD, Harris RH: Obstructive nephropathy in the rat: Possible roles for the renin-angiotensin system, prostaglandins, and thromboxanes in postobstructive renal function. J Clin Invest 65:400–412, 1980.
171. Vaughan ED, Sweet RC, Gillenwater JY: Peripheral renin and blood pressure changes following complete unilateral ureteral occlusion. J Urol 104:89–93, 1970.
172. Moody TE, Vaughan ED, Wyker AT, Gillenwater JY: The role of intrarenal angiotensin II in the hemodynamic response to unilateral obstructive nephropathy. Invest Urol 14:390–397, 1977.
173. Purkerson ML, Klahr S: Prior inhibition of vasoconstrictors normalizes GFR in postobstructed kidneys. Kidney Int 35:1306–1314, 1989.
174. Morrison AR, Benabe JE: Prostaglandins in vascular tone in experimental obstructive nephropathy. Kidney Int 19:786–790, 1981.
175. Strand JC, Edwards BS, Anderson ME, et al: Effect of imidazole on renal function in unilateral ureteral-obstructed rat kidneys. Am J Physiol 240:F508–F514, 1981.
176. Loo MH, Egan D, Vaughan ED, et al: The effect of the thromboxane $A_2$ synthesis inhibitor OKY-046 on renal function in rabbits following release of unilateral ureteral obstruction. J Urol 137:571–576, 1987.
177. Klotman PE, Smith SR, Volpp BD, et al: Thromboxane synthetase inhibition improves function of hydronephrotic rat kidneys. Am J Physiol 250:F282–F287, 1986.
178. Yanagisawa H, Morrissey J, Morrison AR, Klahr S: Eicosanoid production by isolated glomeruli of rats with unilateral ureteral obstruction. Kidney Int 37:1528–1535, 1990.
179. Folkert VW, Schlondorff D: Altered prostaglandin synthesis by glomeruli from rats with unilateral ureteral ligation. Am J Physiol 241:F289–F299, 1981.
180. Schlondorff D, Folkert VW: Prostaglandin synthesis in glomeruli from rats with unilateral ureteral obstruction. Adv Prostaglandin Thromboxane Res 7:1177–1179, 1980.
181. Schreiner GF, Harris KPG, Purkerson ML, Klahr S: Immunological aspects of acute ureteral obstruction: Immune cell infiltrate in the kidney. Kidney Int 34:487–493, 1988.
182. Harris KPG, Schreiner GF, Klahr S: Effect of leukocyte depletion on the function of the postobstructed kidney in the rat. Kidney Int 36:210–215, 1989.
183. Yanagisawa H, Morrissey J, Morrison AR, et al: Role of ANG II in eicosanoid production by isolated glomeruli from rats with bilateral ureteral obstruction. Am J Physiol 258:F85–F93, 1990.
184. Harris RH, Yarger WE: The pathogenesis of postobstructive diuresis: The role of circulating natriuretic and diuretic factors, including urea. J Clin Invest 56:880–887, 1975.
185. Harris RH, Yarger WE: Urine-reinfusion natriuresis: Evidence for potent natriuretic factors in rat urine. Kidney Int 11:93–105, 1977.
186. Brenner BM, Ballermann BJ, Gunning ME, Zeidel ML: The diverse actions of atrial natriuretic peptide. Physiol Rev 70:665–688, 1990.
187. Purkerson ML, Baline EH, Stokes TJ, Klahr S: Role of atrial peptide in the natriuresis and diuresis that follows relief of obstruction in rat. Am J Physiol 256:F583–F589, 1989.
188. Reyes AA, Karl IE, Klahr S: Bilateral ureteral obstruction decreases plasma and tissue L-arginine, the substrate for EDRF synthesis. J Am Soc Nephrol 3:551, 1992.
189. Kerr WS Jr: Effect of complete ureteral obstruction for one week on kidney function. J Appl Physiol 6:762–772, 1954.
190. Wilson DR: Micropuncture study of chronic obstructive nephropathy before and after release of obstruction. Kidney Int 2:119–130, 1972.
191. Stone DK, Seldin DW, Kokko JP, Jacobson HR: Mineralocorticoid modulation of rabbit medullary collecting duct acidification. A sodium independent effect. J Clin Invest 72:2050–2059, 1983.
192. Nagle RB, Bulger RE, Cutler RE, et al: Unilateral obstructive nephropathy in the rabbit: Early morphologic, physiologic and histochemical changes. Lab Invest 28:456–467, 1973.
193. McDougal WS, Rhodes RS, Persky L: A histochemical and morphologic study of postobstructive diuresis in the rat. Invest Urol 14:169–176, 1976.
194. Wilson DR: The influence of volume expansion on renal function after relief of chronic unilateral ureteral obstruction. Kidney Int 5:402–410, 1974.
195. Sonnenberg H, Wilson DR: The role of the medullary collecting ducts in postobstructive diuresis. J Clin Invest 57:1564–1574, 1976.
196. Buerkert J, Martin D, Head M, et al: Deep nephron function after release of acute unilateral ureteral obstruction in the young rat. J Clin Invest 62:1228–1239, 1978.
197. Hanley MJ, Davidson K: Isolated nephron segments from rabbit models of obstructive nephropathy. J Clin Invest 69:165–174, 1982.
198. Hwang S, Haas M, Harris HW Jr, et al: Transport defects of rabbit

medullary thick ascending limb cells in obstructive nephropathy. J Clin Invest 91:21–28, 1993.

199. Miyata Y, Muto S, Ebata S, et al: Sodium and potassium transport properties of the cortical collecting duct following unilateral ureteral obstruction. J Am Soc Nephrol 3:815, 1992.

200. Campbell HT, Bello-Reuss E, Klahr S: Hydraulic water permeability and transepithelial voltage in the isolated perfused rabbit cortical collecting tubule following acute unilateral ureteral obstruction. J Clin Invest 75:219–225, 1985.

201. Hwang S, Harris HW Jr, Otuechere G, et al: Transport defects of rabbit inner medullary collecting duct cells in obstructive nephropathy. Am J Physiol 264:F808–F815, 1993.

202. Hwang S, Hu G, Charness ME, et al: Regulation of Na/K-ATPase expression in obstructive nephropathy. Clin Res 41:141A, 1993.

203. Zeidel ML, Seifter JL, Lear S, et al: Atrial peptides inhibit oxygen consumption in kidney medullary collecting duct cells. Am J Physiol 251:F379–F383, 1986.

204. Zeidel ML: Hormonal regulation of inner medullary collecting duct sodium transport. Am J Physiol 265:F159–173, 1993. Review.

205. Eveloff J, Bayerdoerffer E, Silva P, Kinne R: NaCl transport in the thick ascending limb of Henle's loop. Oxygen consumption studies in isolated cells. Pflugers Arch 389:263–270, 1981.

206. Grossman EB, Hebert SC: Modulation of Na-K-ATPase activity in the mouse medullary thick ascending limb of Henle. Effects of mineralocorticoids and sodium. J Clin Invest 81:885–892, 1988.

207. Petty KJ, Kokko JP, Marver D: Secondary effect of aldosterone on Na-KATPase activity in the rabbit cortical collecting tubule. J Clin Invest 68:1514–1521, 1981.

208. Okegawa T, Jonas PE, DeSchryver K, et al: Metabolic and cellular alterations underlying the exaggerated renal prostaglandin and thromboxane synthesis in ureter obstruction in rabbits: Inflammatory response involving fibroblasts and mononuclear cells. J Clin Invest 71:81–90, 1983.

209. Smith WL, Bell TG, Needleman P: Increased renal tubular synthesis of prostaglandins in the rabbit kidney in response to ureteral obstruction. Prostaglandins 18:269–277, 1979.

210. Lear S, Silva P, Kelley VE, Epstein FH: Prostaglandin E$_2$ inhibits oxygen consumption in rabbit medullary thick ascending limb. Am J Physiol 258:F1372–F1378, 1990.

211. Jabs K, Zeidel ML, Silva P: Prostaglandin E$_2$ inhibits Na/K-ATPase in rabbit inner medullary collecting duct cells. Am J Physiol 257:F424–F430, 1989.

212. Stokes JB, Kokko JP: Inhibition of sodium transport by prostaglandin E$_2$ across the isolated, perfused rabbit collecting tubule. J Clin Invest 59:1099–1104, 1977.

213. Stokes JB: Sodium and potassium transport by the collecting duct. Kidney Int 38:679–686, 1990.

214. Stokes JB: Effect of prostaglandin E$_2$ on chloride transport across the rabbit thick ascending limb of Henle. J Clin Invest 64:495–502, 1979.

215. Strange K: Ouabain-induced cell swelling in rabbit cortical collecting tubule: NaCl transport by principal cells. J Membr Biol 107:249–261, 1989.

216. Marver D, Bernabe J: Inhibition of Na/K-ATPase by PGE$_2$. J Am Soc Nephrol 3:500A, 1992.

217. Cordova HR, Kokko JP, Marver D: Chronic indomethacin increases rabbit cortical collecting tubule Na/K-ATPase activity. Am J Physiol 256:F570–F576, 1989.

218. Zeidel ML, Strange K, Emma F, Harris HW Jr: Mechanisms and regulation of water transport in the kidney. Semin Nephrol 13:155–167, 1993.

219. Harris HW Jr, Strange K, Zeidel ML: Current understanding of the cellular biology and molecular structure of the antidiuretic hormone–stimulated water transport pathway. J Clin Invest 88:1–8, 1991.

220. Holmgren K, Danielson BG, Fellstrom B, et al: The relation between urinary tract infections and stone composition in renal stone formers. Scand J Urol Nephrol 23:131–136, 1989.

221. Ribeiro C, Suki WN: Acidification in the medullary collecting duct following ureteral obstruction. Kidney Int 29:1167–1171, 1986.

222. Laski ME, Kurtzman NA: Site of the acidification defect in the perfused postobstructed collecting tubule. Miner Electrolyte Metab 15:195–200, 1989.

223. Purcell H, Bastani B, Harris KPG, et al: Cellular distribution of H$^+$ ATPase following acute unilateral ureteral obstruction in rats. Am J Physiol 261:F365–F376, 1991.

224. Blondin J, Purkerson ML, Rolf D, et al: Renal function and metabolism after relief of unilateral ureteral obstruction. Proc Soc Exp Biol Med 150:71–76, 1975.

225. Klahr S, Schwab SJ, Stokes TJ: Metabolic adaptations of the nephron in renal disease. Kidney Int 29:80–89, 1986.

226. Buerkert J, Head M, Klahr S: Effects of acute bilateral ureteral obstruction on deep nephron and terminal collecting duct function in the young rat. J Clin Invest 59:1055–1065, 1977.

227. McDougal WS, Wright FS: Defect in proximal and distal sodium transport in post-obstructive diuresis. Kidney Int 2:304–317, 1972.

228. Buerkert J, Martin D, Head M: Effect of acute ureteral obstruction on terminal collecting duct function in the weanling rat. Am J Physiol 236:F260–F267, 1979.

229. Thirakomen K, Kozlov N, Arruda JAL, Kurtzman NA: Renal hydrogen ion secretion after release of unilateral ureteral obstruction. Am J Physiol 231:1233–1239, 1976.

230. Beck N: Phosphaturia after release of bilateral ureteral obstruction in rats. Am J Physiol 237:F14–F19, 1979.

231. Purkerson ML, Rolf DB, Chase LR, et al: Tubular reabsorption of phosphate after release of complete ureteral obstruction in the rat. Kidney Int 5:326–336, 1974.

232. Purkerson ML, Slatopolsky E, Klahr S: Urinary excretion of magnesium, calcium, and phosphate after release of unilateral ureteral obstruction in the rat. Miner Electrolyte Metab 6:182–189, 1981.

233. Stecker JF Jr, Vaughan ED Jr, Gillenwater JY: Alteration in renal metabolism occurring in ureteral obstruction in vivo. Surg Gynecol Obstet 133:846–848, 1971.

234. Nito H, Descoeudres C, Kurokawa K, Massry SG: Effects of unilateral ureteral obstruction on renal cell metabolism and function. J Lab Clin Med 91:60–71, 1978.

235. Storch S, Saggi S, Megyesi J, et al: Ureteral obstruction decreases renal prepro-epidermal growth factor and Tamm-Horsfall expression. Kidney Int 42:89–94, 1992.

236. Sawczuk IS, Hoke G, Olsson CA, et al: Gene expression in response to acute unilateral ureteral obstruction. Kidney Int 35:1315–1319, 1989.

237. Walsh PC, Retik AB, Stamey TA, Vaughan ED Jr (eds): Campbell's Urology. WB Saunders, Philadelphia, 1992.

238. Gillenwater JY, Grayhack JT, Howards SS, Duckett JW (eds): Adult and Pediatric Urology. Mosby–Year Book, St. Louis, 1991.

239. Lewis HY, Pierce JM: Return of function after relief of complete ureteral obstruction of 69 days' duration. J Urol 88:377–379, 1962.

240. Shapiro SR, Bennett AL: Recovery of renal function after prolonged unilateral ureteral obstruction. J Urol 115:136–140, 1976.

241. Bishop MC: Diuresis and renal function recovery in chronic retention. Br J Urol 57:1–5, 1985.

242. Sarmina I, Resnick MI: Obstructive uropathy in patients with benign prostatic hyperplasia. J Urol 141:866–869, 1989.

243. Bricker NS, Shwayri EI, Readan JB, et al: An abnormality in renal function resulting from urinary tract obstruction. Am J Med 23:554–564, 1957.

244. Massry SG, Schainuck LI, Goldsmith C, Schreiner GE: Studies on the mechanism of diuresis after relief of urinary-tract obstruction. Ann Intern Med 66:149–158, 1967.

245. Muldowney FP, Duffy GJ, Kelly DG, et al: Sodium diuresis after relief of obstructive uropathy. N Engl J Med 274:1294–1298, 1966.

246. Peterson LJ, Yarger WE, Schocken DD, Glenn JF: Post-obstructive diuresis: A varied syndrome. J Urol 113:190–194, 1975.

247. Vaughan ED Jr, Gillenwater JY: Diagnosis, characterization and management of post-obstructive diuresis. J Urol 109:286–292, 1973.

248. Purkerson ML, Klahr S: Protein intake conditions the diuresis seen after relief of bilateral ureteral obstruction in the rat. Proc Soc Exp Biol Med 177:62–68, 1984.

249. Gulmi FA, Mooppan UMM, Chou SY, Kim H: Atrial natriuretic peptide in patients with obstructive uropathy. J Urol 142:268–272, 1989.

# 42

# Renal Neoplasia

*Marc B. Garnick*
*Jerome P. Richie*

Malignant neoplasms involving the renal parenchyma and renal pelvis may be primary or secondary in origin. Although in the kidney the frequency of metastatic neoplasms is higher than that of primary tumors, the secondary lesions are usually asymptomatic and most are discovered at postmortem examination.

Renal cell carcinoma accounts for approximately 85% of all primary renal neoplasms. Primary neoplasm of the renal pelvis or ureter, the second most common, accounts for 7% to 8% of renal neoplasms. Nephroblastoma (Wilms tumor) accounts for 5% to 6%, and various sarcomas of renal origin account for the remainder of primary tumors. In this chapter we consider primarily renal cell carcinoma and Wilms tumor.

## RENAL CELL CARCINOMA

Renal cell carcinoma, known as the internist's tumor because of its diverse and often obscure presenting signs and symptoms, challenges the most astute diagnostician. Subtle presenting symptoms, physical findings, and laboratory abnormalities may produce manifestations as protean as those of syphilis or tuberculosis. The numerous endocrine effects have given rise to the use of detailed laboratory investigations, and the promise of spontaneous regression and prolonged survival have led to intensive investigation by immunologists.

These tumors have existed for centuries, but specific attention was drawn to them in the 19th century, when Grawitz[1] named them hypernephromas because it had previously been proposed that they arose from adrenal rests. It took 25 years to dispel this belief, but the term is still used, inappropriately, in everyday parlance. The site of origin is probably the proximal tubule cells, as it has been shown that renal cell carcinomas react positively with fluorescein-labeled anti–human kidney serum.[2] Most of the fluorescence is found in the normal proximal tubule epithelium and in the neoplastic areas. Thus, the term favored by Mostofi,[3] renal cell carcinoma, is preferred.

Controversy still exists over the relationship of renal cell carcinoma to renal adenoma. There are no gross histologic, immunologic, or ultrastructural features that readily distinguish between renal cell carcinoma and renal adenoma. Both types of cells have been demonstrated by immunologic and electron microscopic techniques to arise from the proximal convoluted tubule.[4] Adenoma and renal cell carcinoma arise in the same age groups, and the frequencies of both are observed to increase among tobacco users. A distinction between adenoma and adenocarcinoma is important, as many renal adenomas are incidental findings at autopsy, usually as a small, well-circumscribed lesion of the renal cortex. The frequency of renal adenoma ranges from 7% to 22% of all kidneys examined.[5] In a large autopsy series reported by Bell,[6] size was used as a criterion of malignancy, and a correlation was found between the size of the adenoma and the presence or absence of metastases. Tumors greater than 3 cm in diameter more frequently had metastases; still, small renal cell carcinomas have been reported, as have large renal adenomas. Perhaps it is prudent to consider larger lesions as renal cell adenocarcinomas when they are recognized clinically. Careful nuclear cytologic and histologic studies may enable us to distinguish between the two entities, but clinical similarities will persist.

### Incidence

In 1993, 10,000 people died of renal cell carcinoma in the United States. The overall incidence is 7.5 cases/100,000 population, and it is estimated that there will be 25,000 newly diagnosed cases yearly. Renal cell carcinoma is twice as common in males as in females.[7, 8]

Studies indicate that renal cell carcinoma is somewhat more common in Scandinavians and North Americans and that the frequency is distinctly lower in Asians and Africans. Most patients are found to have the disease when they are between 55 and 60 years old. A moderate association between tobacco use and the incidence of renal cell carcinoma has been found,[9] and a variety of chemical and biologic agents have produced renal tumors in animals. These agents include lead phosphate, demethylnitrosamine, estrogen (prolonged administration to male hamsters), aflatoxin $B_1$, viruses (infections in leopard frogs),[9–12] and streptozocin.[13–17] No conclusive evidence has established a causal link to renal cell carcinoma in humans, although preliminary work has indicated a potentially higher risk in cadmium workers who smoke.[18] Von Hippel–Lindau disease, which is transmitted in an autosomal dominant fashion, is associated with retinal angiomas and hemangioblastomas of the central nervous system and may be associated with renal cell carcinoma.[19] The *VHL* gene has been identified.[20] More recently, constitutional chromosome translocations between chromosomes 3 and 8 and 3 and 11 have been found in a kindred in which many persons had advanced renal cell carcinoma.[21, 22] Other cytogenetic abnormalities have been described, including abnormalities in chromosomes 1, 11, and 17. If abnormal chromosomes can be used as markers, family members at risk can be screened at an early, asymptomatic stage.

## Presenting Signs and Symptoms

The classic presenting triad of renal cell carcinoma has been described as flank pain, gross hematuria, and palpable renal mass. Unfortunately, this triad represents far advanced disease and is seen in only 5% to 10% of patients at presentation. More frequently, renal tumors are discovered incidentally during the course of various diagnostic studies. In a review of 309 consecutive patients undergoing nephrectomy for renal cell carcinoma, Skinner and Gibbons and their associates[23, 24] reported that hematuria was the most common presenting symptom, followed by abdominal mass, pain, and weight loss (Table 42–1).

Hematuria, gross or microscopic, is usually observed only if the tumor has invaded the collecting system. Gibbons and associates[24] reported the absence of gross or microscopic hematuria in 63% of their patients with proven renal cell carcinoma. Substantial bleeding may lead to clot formation and clot colic. An abdominal or a flank mass is

**TABLE 42–1. Presenting Symptoms and Signs in Patients with Renal Cell Carcinoma in Two Series**

| Symptom or Sign | In 309 Patients* (%) | In 110 Patients† (%) |
|---|---|---|
| Hematuria | 59 | 37 |
| Abdominal or flank mass | 45 | 21 |
| Pain | 41 | 21 |
| Weight loss | 28 | 30 |
| Symptom from metastases | 10 | |
| Classic triad | 9 | |
| Acute varicocele | 2 | |

*Data from Skinner and colleagues.[23]
†Data from Gibbons and colleagues.[24]
From Richie JP, Garnick MB: Primary renal and ureteral cancer. *In* Rieselbach RE, Garnick MB (eds): Cancer and the Kidney. Lea & Febiger, Philadelphia, 1982, p 662.

**TABLE 42–2. Frequency of Systemic Effects in Patients with Renal Cell Carcinoma***

| Symptom | Incidence (%) |
|---|---|
| Elevated erythrocyte sedimentation rate | 362/651 (55.6) |
| Anemia | 409/991 (41.3) |
| Hypertension | 89/237 (37.6) |
| Cachexia | 338/979 (34.5) |
| Pyrexia | 164/954 (17.2) |
| Abnormal liver function tests | 60/400 (15.0) |
| Elevated alkaline phosphatase level | 64/434 (14.7) |
| Hypercalcemia | 33/577 (5.7) |
| Polycythemia | 33/903 (3.7) |
| Neuromyopathy | 13/400 (3.3) |
| Amyloidosis | 12/573 (2.1) |

*Modified from Chisholm and Roy.[26]
From Richie JP, Garnick MB: Primary renal and ureteral cancer. *In* Rieselbach RE, Garnick MB (eds): Cancer and the Kidney. Lea & Febiger, Philadelphia, 1982, p 662.

more commonly palpated in pediatric patients or thin adults, and tumors of the lower pole of the kidney are more easily palpable. The mass is generally firm, homogeneous, and nontender and moves with respiration. Occasionally, hemorrhage into a tumor may cause exquisite pain and, on palpation of the mass, tenderness.

Pain in association with renal cell carcinoma is usually a constant dull ache in either the flank or the abdomen. Bleeding within the tumor may cause acute pain. Passage of clots in the urine may be associated with clot colic. More frequently, local extension of tumor or tumor metastases may be manifested as diffuse pain with systemic symptoms and inanition.

Sudden onset of a scrotal varicocele has been reported in up to 11% of patients with renal cell carcinoma.[25] This manifestation should always raise the possibility of an associated renal cell neoplasm. The majority of patients have had varicoceles on the left side, acute in onset, that failed to empty in the recumbent position. These symptoms are most compatible with obstruction by tumor thrombus of the left gonadal vein at its entry point into the left renal vein.

## Paraneoplastic Findings

Renal cell carcinoma may masquerade as a variety of symptom patterns suggestive of other illnesses. More obscure problems are common, such as fever of unknown origin, erythrocytosis, weight loss, anemia, or symptoms of hypercalcemia. The numerous systemic and humoral manifestations of renal cell carcinoma have become known collectively as the paraneoplastic syndromes. These manifestations may be divided into systemic, hematologic, gastrointestinal, and endocrine categories. The frequency of some of these systemic effects in combined series of more than 900 patients is detailed in Table 42–2.[26]

### FEVER

Fever is one of the more common systemic manifestations of renal cell carcinoma, occurring in up to 20% of patients.[27] It is usually intermittent and not of any consistent degree or pattern. Usually noted in conjunction with other symptoms, the fever normally abates when the primary tumor is removed. The etiology of the fever is unknown; however, endogenous pyrogens released from the tumor have been demonstrated in patients with renal cell carcinoma.[28]

## ANEMIA

Anemia, seen in 30% to 40% of patients, is usually out of proportion to any hematuria from the tumor. Although hematuria may be secondary to blood loss, hemolysis, or bone marrow replacement, the anemia usually resembles the normochromic and normocytic anemia of chronic renal failure. Chisholm and Roy[26] have postulated a lack of erythropoietin resulting from renal tissue destruction or toxic effects of the renal cell cancer on the bone marrow. The anemia is generally associated with low serum iron titer and low total iron-binding capacity.

## ERYTHROCYTOSIS

Erythrocytosis (defined as a hematocrit value greater than 55 mL/dL or hemoglobin value greater than 15 g/100 mL) occurs in almost 4% of patients with renal cell carcinoma. The white blood cell count and platelet count are not elevated. Damon and associates[29] reported that 39% of patients with erythrocytosis and hematuria are eventually proved to have renal cell carcinoma. Extracts of renal cell carcinoma may elaborate erythropoietin.[30] Increased levels of erythropoietin may also be seen secondary to hypoxia of the normal renal parenchyma as a result of compression. Because current assays for erythropoietin rely on biologic techniques, their accuracy is limited; radioimmunoassays for erythropoietin may help establish the site of origin of erythropoietin elevation in patients with renal cell carcinoma. A human renal cell line has been established that secretes erythropoietin activity into the growth medium, which is consistent with the biologic behavior of the tumor in vivo.[31]

## HEPATIC DYSFUNCTION

Reversible hepatic dysfunction, manifested by abnormal liver function tests, has been reported in up to 15% of patients with renal cell carcinoma,[32] but the overall prevalence is probably much lower. Hepatosplenomegaly may be present, but the most striking findings are increased retention of sulfobromophthalein (Bromsulphalein) and elevation of serum alkaline phosphatase, prothrombin time, alpha$_2$-globulin, and bilirubin values. The cause of abnormal liver function tests is unknown, but in the absence of hepatic metastases, the abnormal results often revert to normal after nephrectomy. Even if the hepatic function returns to normal after nephrectomy, few patients survive 5 years without evidence of disease.[33] Prognosis is certainly ominous if the results of liver function tests remain elevated. Such findings may herald a Budd-Chiari–like syndrome with venous obstruction secondary to tumor thrombus in the inferior vena cava and hepatic veins.

## HYPERCALCEMIA

Hypercalcemia, occurring in 10% to 15% of patients with renal cell carcinoma, may be secondary to osseous metastases, but other patients may have hypercalcemia without bone involvement. In such instances, ectopic production of material resembling parathyroid hormone by the renal cell tumor has been documented.[34–37] Immunoreactive parathyroid hormone fragments have been demonstrated by immunologic methods in tissue culture of renal cell tumors.[38] In other patients with hypercalcemia, elevated prostaglandin levels may contribute and may be suppressed by indomethacin.[39] Prostaglandins A and E have been demonstrated in venous effluent of a kidney bearing a renal cell carcinoma.[40] In patients with marked hypercalcemia, intensive medical management may include use of indomethacin, aspirin, mithramycin, furosemide, or calcitonin. In rare cases, surgical removal of the majority of the tumor may be necessary to control hypercalcemia.[41] Ectopic corticotropin may rarely be produced by renal cell carcinoma.[42] Several patients have been identified with Cushing syndrome, usually with marked hypercalcemia as a major component of the disease.

## AMYLOIDOSIS

Secondary amyloidosis occurs in 1% to 3% of patients with renal cell carcinoma.[43] The amyloidosis itself, rather than direct tumor involvement, may be responsible for renal failure. In some cases, nephrotic syndrome as well as hepatosplenomegaly may be present. The prognosis of patients with amyloidosis secondary to renal cell carcinoma is dismal.[44]

## OTHER EFFECTS

Other systemic or endocrine effects may rarely be seen in patients with renal cell carcinoma. A polyneuromyopathy manifested by neurologic complaints may be present in 3% to 4% of patients with renal cell carcinoma. Thrush[45] has postulated an antigen-antibody reaction specifically directed against nerve tissue. A rare case of enteropathy causing protein loss has been documented in a patient with renal cell carcinoma that produced glucagon.[46] Twenty-five percent of patients with renal cell carcinoma have some degree of hypertension. Some may be secondary to arteriovenous fistula, but renin-secreting adenocarcinoma of the kidney has been described.[47] Sufrin and associates[48] reported peripheral serum renin levels in an advanced-stage renal cell carcinoma. Nephrectomy resulted in a decreased serum renin level, but it is unclear whether the renin was produced by the tumor itself, by compression of adjacent normal renal parenchyma, or by a decreased rate of renin degradation.

Elevation of serum human chorionic gonadotropin (hCG) level in patients with renal cell carcinoma, with the clinical picture of gynecomastia, areolar pigmentation, and diminished libido, has been detected by radioimmunoassay.[49] Syncytiotrophoblastic cells found in the tumor have been shown by immunoperoxidase staining to produce hCG. Production of hCG by renal cell carcinoma is apparently rare;

Sufrin and associates[48] studied 57 patients with renal cell carcinoma and failed to demonstrate elevation of intact hCG or β-hCG by radioimmunoassay techniques.

## Diagnosis

A variety of uroradiographic techniques are available to aid in the detection and delineation of renal masses. It has been estimated that 8% of all patients examined by intravenous urography have a space-occupying lesion, and in patients with suggestive clinical symptoms the frequency of renal masses increases to more than 60%.[50] Numerous diagnostic studies, both invasive and noninvasive, are available for characterization of the presence or absence of cancer in renal masses. Our systematized approach for the evaluation of renal masses is depicted in Figure 42–1.

### PLAIN ABDOMINAL FILM

The plain abdominal film (kidneys, ureters, and bladder, or KUB) may show a mass effect that alters the renal profile or may suggest generalized unilateral enlargement of the kidney. The presence of calcification may be associated with a benign or a neoplastic process. The calcification within a renal cell carcinoma usually appears as a local or diffuse flocculation within the mass. Less frequently, curvilinear calcification may be noted in the periphery of the lesion, but this pattern of calcification is more commonly associated with a benign process, such as calcified hematoma or cyst. Calcifications may be classified as peripheral or nonperipheral. In a study of more than 2000 renal masses reviewed at the Mayo Clinic, 4.1% were calcified.[51] Nonperipheral calcification was associated with renal cell carcinoma in the majority of patients; however, even when peripheral ("eggshell") calcification was the only finding, 20% of the patients were found to have renal cell carcinoma. Therefore, findings of calcification in the renal area are suggestive, but certainly not diagnostic, of renal cell carcinoma.

### INTRAVENOUS UROGRAPHY WITH NEPHROTOMOGRAPHY

The first step in the diagnosis of renal cell carcinoma is usually intravenous urography. The diagnosis of most renal tumors is suspected on the basis of this technique, which for many decades was the principal modality of radiologic diagnosis. The most striking diagnostic criterion is splaying or distortion of the collecting system (Fig. 42–2), but other signs, such as lack of visualization of a portion of the collecting system or distortion of the renal outline, may suggest a space-occupying lesion in the kidney. The lack of specificity in this examination and the difficulty of interpretation owing to overlying bowel gas requires additional studies to differentiate between benign and malignant lesions.

Nephrotomography performed 1 to 2 minutes after injection of contrast material during the nephrogram phase of intravenous urography eliminates distortion from bowel gas and can clearly delineate the lateral border of the kidney.

This examination is critical in differentiating between cysts and renal cell carcinoma. A benign cyst on a nephrotomogram should have a sharply defined border with the contrast medium–filled renal parenchyma, should have a pencil-thin wall projecting outside the renal parenchyma, and should form a cortical spur or "beak" sign where the normal renal parenchyma is expanded by a subcortical cyst. The avascular mass should be radiographically translucent and uniform. The findings in a patient with renal cell carcinoma include indistinct margins of the mass from the renal parenchyma, a thick wall outside the renal parenchyma, and some degree of opacification within the mass. Opacification may be homogeneous (viable mass without necrosis) or uneven with "puddling" (partial necrosis), or it may even have a central radiolucency surrounded by a thick opacified wall (extensive central necrosis).[52] The important addition of nephrotomography should provide a clinical impression of a cyst or tumor, but other diagnostic techniques should be utilized judiciously to increase the diagnostic accuracy.

Modifications of nephrotomography have been suggested to allow better definition of renal lesions. Greene and associates[53] at the Mayo Clinic introduced bolus nephrotomography, a technique involving rapid intravenous injection of large amounts of contrast medium. The vascular phase is recorded in a multilevel tomographic cassette, allowing tomographic filming of the kidney while contrast medium is present in the renal artery and its branches. Infusion nephrotomography (parenchymal phase) may identify a renal cell carcinoma by its decreased or mottled staining characteristics.[54] The late phase of nephrotomography may show prominent capsular veins, indicating collateral venous circulation from increased flow through the carcinoma or obstruction of the major renal vein.

### RETROGRADE PYELOGRAPHY

Cystoscopy and occlusive retrograde pyelography aid in opacification of portions of the collecting systems that are not filled by standard intravenous urography. A washing for cytology may indicate the presence of a renal adenocarcinoma, although, because the majority of these tumors do not involve the collecting system, the yield of cytology is minimal. In patients with hematuria as the presenting symptom, cystoscopy is an important adjunct to rule out an unsuspected urothelial tumor, such as carcinoma of the bladder.

### ULTRASONOGRAPHY

Ultrasound scanning is a simple, inexpensive modality that has improved the ability to differentiate between a simple benign cyst and a solid tumor.[55] The advent of real-time and gray-scale ultrasonography has improved the ability of sonar techniques to delineate homogeneous (sonolucent) from heterogeneous lesions from internal echoes. Smith and Bennett[56] found that ultrasonography alone had a sensitivity of 97%, a specificity of 97%, and a false-negative rate of only 1% in 413 patients. Thus, when the modalities of nephrotomography and ultrasonography support the diagnosis of a benign cyst, the accuracy rate approaches 97% to 98%. Ultrasonography and radionuclide

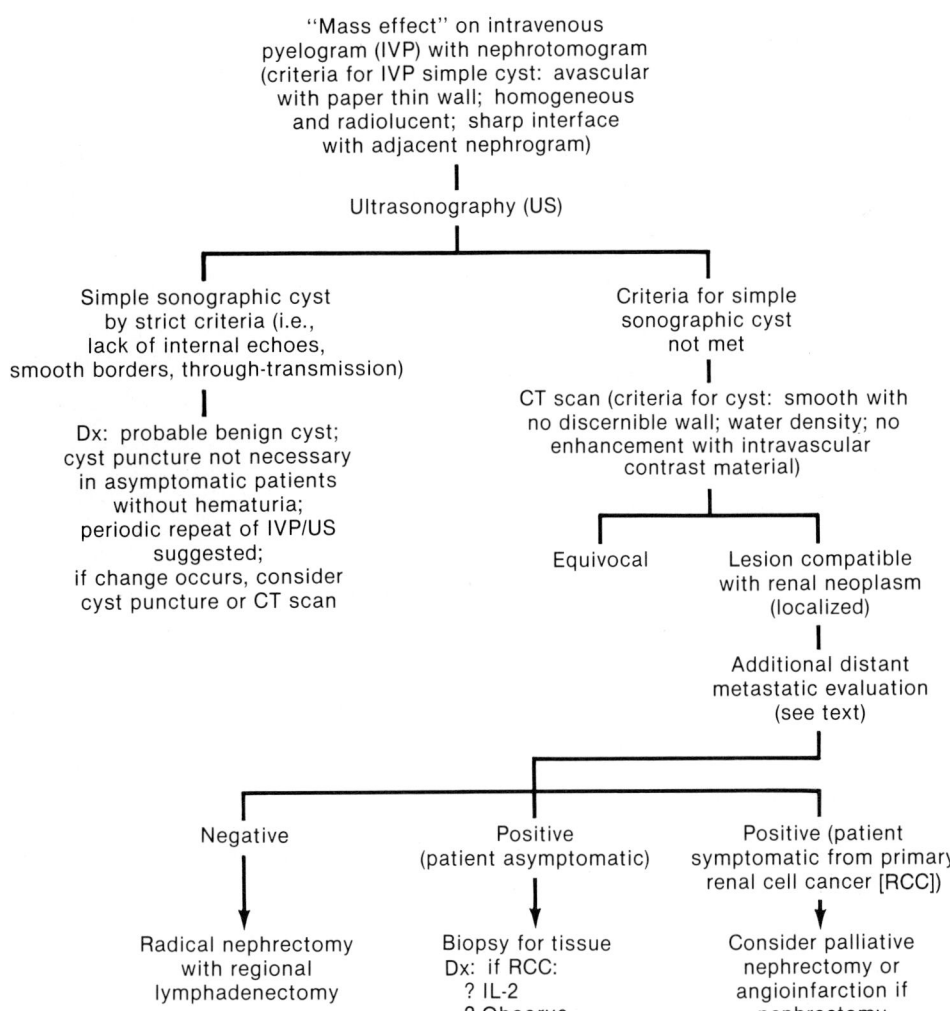

**Figure 42–1.** Flow chart for the diagnostic evaluation and therapeutic approach to patients with mass lesions of the kidney.

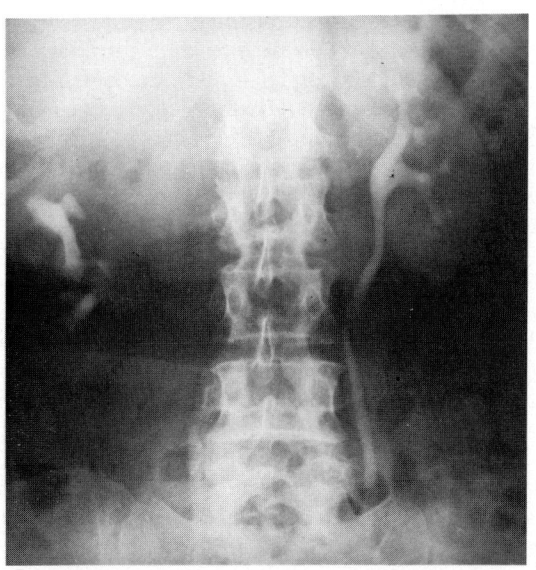

**Figure 42–2.** A plain abdominal (KUB) film made 10 minutes after injection of contrast medium shows a normal left kidney and distortion of the right collecting system caused by renal cell carcinoma.

scanning in combination have been recommended by one group as the definitive modalities for the diagnosis of simple renal cyst.[57] The coexistence of a renal cyst and tumor is rare.[58] A simple serous cyst and renal carcinoma may coexist in the same kidney, but the frequency is less than 1%.[59]

## CYST PUNCTURE

Nephrotomography and ultrasonography may be adequate to diagnose a renal cyst in the majority of patients. If there is any suspicion on clinical or radiographic grounds or if the physician wishes to increase diagnostic accuracy beyond 97%, percutaneous needle puncture of the lesion may be performed. With ultrasonographic guidance, needle aspiration is a relatively low-risk procedure. It consists of localization under radiographic or ultrasonographic guidance; percutaneous placement of the needle into the cyst cavity with local anesthesia; aspiration of cyst contents for cytology and assay of fat and lactate dehydrogenase; and instillation of contrast material to outline the contours of the cyst wall. Bloody aspirate is strongly suggestive of cancer, even without abnormal cytologic results.[60] The potential risks of percutaneous puncture include sepsis, violation and seeding of renal cell carcinoma, and false-negative diagnosis.

The dilemma of whether to aspirate all cysts becomes more critical with the increased delineation of asymptomatic space-occupying lesions of the kidney. It has been estimated that more than 50% of the population older than age 50 years have at least one renal cyst. With increased use of intravenous urography, ultrasonography, and computed tomography (CT), more of these lesions will be diagnosed. We believe that for an asymptomatic patient without hematuria and with nephrotomographic and ultrasonographic evidence of a classic benign cyst the addition of cyst puncture is an unnecessary risk. If, however, any clinical suspicion exists, this procedure should be considered, as detailed in the flow chart in Figure 42–1.

## ARTERIOGRAPHY

Selective renal arteriography via percutaneous femoral artery catheter has been the mainstay for diagnosis and staging of renal cell carcinoma. The typical renal cell carcinoma is a well-vascularized lesion that exhibits tumor vessels, venous lakes within the tumor, puddling of contrast medium in vascular spaces or necrotic areas of the tumor, and shunting of contrast medium rapidly into the renal vein (Fig. 42–3). A useful adjunct has been epinephrine arteriography, which causes normal vessels to constrict and preferentially opacifies the nonresponsive (and hence abnormal) tumor vasculature[61] (Fig. 42–4). With careful angiographic technique and the addition of pharmacologic agents, selective renal arteriography has an accuracy rate of 95% to 98% in differentiating renal cell carcinoma from benign cyst.[62, 63] The false-negative rate is approximately 3%, and the false-positive rate is similar. A small number of renal cell carcinomas outgrow their blood supply and become necrotic. These tumors may be difficult or impossible to diagnose by arteriography. Furthermore, up to 10% of renal cell carcinomas, usually the papillary type, may be hypovascular or

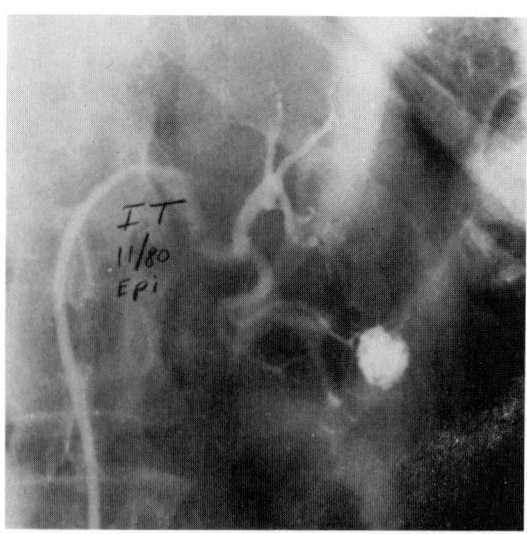

**Figure 42–4.** Selective left epinephrine arteriogram demonstrates discrete tumor blush from renal cell carcinoma in the lower pole of the kidney. (From Richie JP, Garnick MB: Primary renal and ureteral cancer. *In* Rieselbach RE, Garnick MB [eds]: Cancer and the Kidney. Lea & Febiger, Philadelphia, 1982, p 662.)

avascular. Abscess, granuloma, xanthogranulomatous pyelonephritis, or angiomyolipoma may mimic a neoplasm on an arteriogram.[64, 65] Renal arteriography is tolerated well. The risk of major complications was 0.71% and that of minor complications was 2.9% in more than 11,000 procedures.[66]

## COMPUTED TOMOGRAPHY

CT has added a new dimension to the diagnosis and staging of renal cell carcinoma by allowing visualization of cross-sectional anatomy and of the relationship of mass lesions of the kidney to surrounding structures (see later). A reproducible and less invasive technique than arteriography, CT with infusion of contrast medium demonstrates normal renal parenchyma and associated mass lesions (Fig. 42–5). Although delineation of a cyst may be adequate with nephrotomography and ultrasonography, CT may be preferable for definitive diagnosis in patients with suspicious mass lesions. The use of an attenuation coefficient allows determination of a water density or solid density (Fig. 42–6). Weyman and associates[67] compared the diagnostic accuracy of CT and arteriography in 62 patients with proven renal cell carcinoma. CT confirmed the diagnosis in 59 of 62 patients, whereas results of arteriography were diagnostic in 44 of 49 others and questionable in 2 of 49 patients. In a study from our own institutions, CT was more accurate than arteriography in the diagnosis of renal cell cancer. The modalities were equally accurate in determining renal vein involvement, but CT was superior in determining regional node involvement.[68] These findings would support the use of CT as the preferred modality for the diagnosis and staging of renal cell carcinoma. If the findings are questionable, however, arteriography and inferior or superior venacavography, or both, should complement CT.

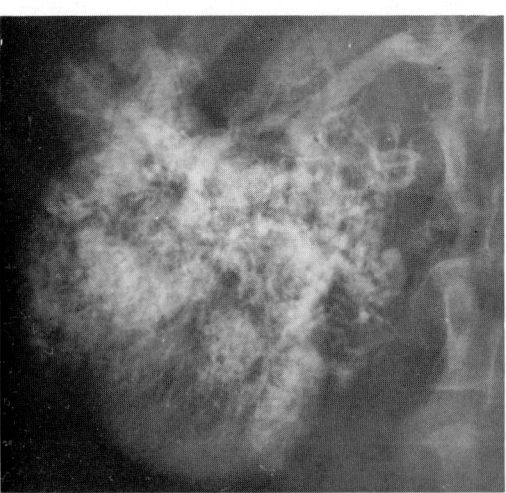

**Figure 42–3.** Selective right renal arteriogram demonstrates typical tumor hypervascularity with puddling in a patient with renal cell carcinoma.

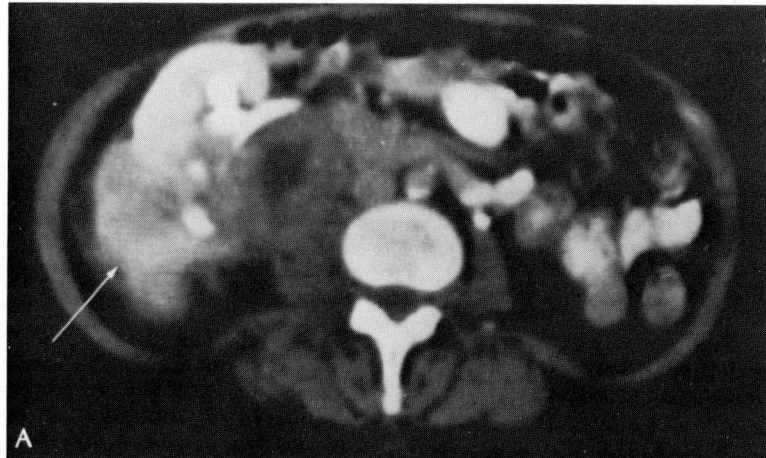

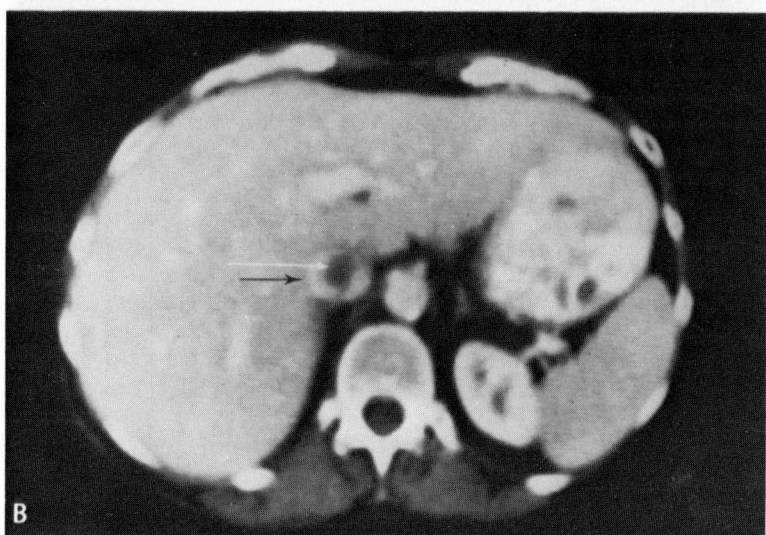

**Figure 42–5.** *A.* CT scan reveals massive renal cell carcinoma arising from the right kidney *(arrow)* and pushing the kidney anteriorly. Note the distortion of the collecting system. *B.* CT scan of the same patient demonstrates tumor thrombus *(white arrow)* in the center of the inferior vena cava *(black arrow).* This section was taken at the upper pole of the left kidney and craniad to the right kidney. (From Richie JP, Garnick MB: Primary renal and ureteral cancer. *In* Rieselbach RE, Garnick MB [eds]: Cancer and the Kidney. Lea & Febiger, Philadelphia, 1982, p 662.)

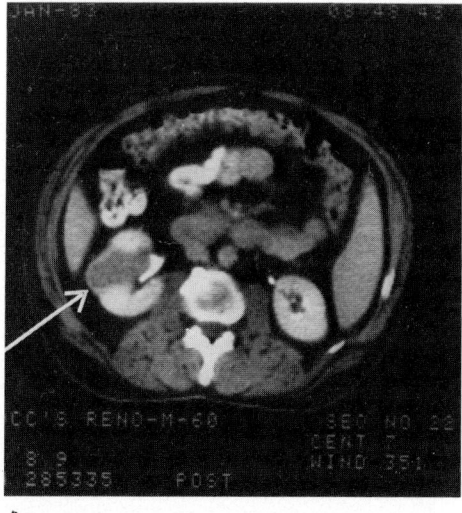

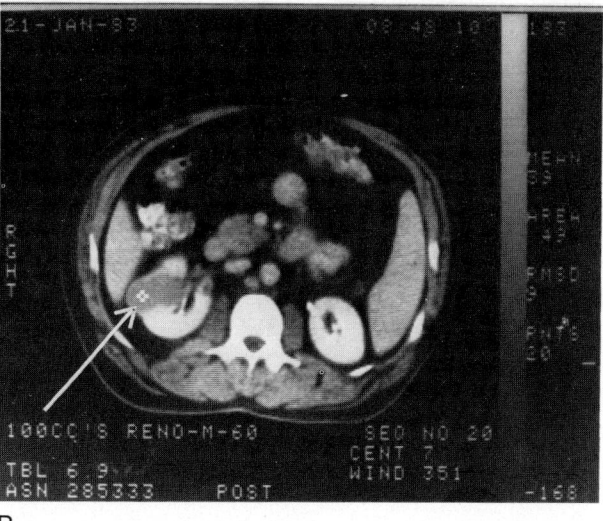

**Figure 42–6.** *A.* CT scan discloses a mass lesion distorting the right kidney *(arrow)* and a normal left kidney. *B.* Similar CT scan with density-attenuation cursor *(arrow).* The readout from the cursor demonstrated in the right-hand aspect of the figure shows a mean of 39 Hounsfield units. This reading is consistent with a solid tumor and not with water density, as in a cyst, which would be less than 20 Hounsfield units.

## MAGNETIC RESONANCE IMAGING

Magnetic resonance imaging has proved useful in the evaluation of renal masses.[69] It is also a useful modality for evaluation of renal vein or inferior vena cava involvement in patients with renal cell cancer. The ability to produce a three-dimensional picture of the tumor can be invaluable with both cross-sectional and parasagittal scans. Most important, magnetic resonance imaging, especially with new techniques such as the GRASS technique, can visualize flow through the major vessels and accurately depict the presence or absence of a thrombus in the inferior vena cava. Although ultrasonography may be able to show tumor thrombus in the vena cava, magnetic resonance imaging has become the procedure of choice for staging of involvement of the renal vein and vena cava.[70]

## Staging and Grading

### CLINICAL STAGING

After the diagnosis of renal cell carcinoma has been established, attention must be turned to delineation of the extent of involvement of regional and distant sites. The most common sites are the lymph vessels, lungs, skeleton, liver, and the ipsilateral adrenal gland and the contralateral kidney. The search for evidence of metastatic disease should include a radionuclide bone scan utilizing technetium Tc 99m radiopharmaceutical. Any areas of suspicious

uptake should be confirmed by plain radiography, and a solitary lesion may be considered for biopsy.

In the past, renal arteriography served as the main preoperative radiologic procedure for diagnosing renal cancer and assessing the degree of local spread. Because of the propensity of renal cell carcinoma to extend into the renal veins and inferior vena cava, careful scrutiny of this area on the arteriogram may yield valuable information. Unless the renal vein is adequately visualized at the time of renal arteriography, inferior venacavography with selective renal venography should be performed (Fig. 42–7A). In patients with complete occlusion of the inferior vena cava by tumor thrombus, a superior venacavogram is necessary to delineate the superior aspect of the tumor thrombus (Fig. 42–7B). The importance of preoperative knowledge of the extent of renal vein or inferior vena cava involvement is essential for proper planning of the surgical removal of the tumor.

Improvements in CT have made it more accurate than arteriography for both diagnosis and staging of renal cancer. If the CT study provides adequate information on hepatic, lymph node, renal vein, and vena cava involvement, arteriography is unnecessary. If, however, CT provides equivocal or suboptimal information on these anatomic areas, arteriography, inferior venacavography with selective renal venography, superior venacavography, or magnetic resonance imaging may become a necessary part of the preoperative workup.

Because of the frequent hematogenous dissemination of renal cell carcinoma to the lungs, chest radiography and whole lung tomography are important studies for detection

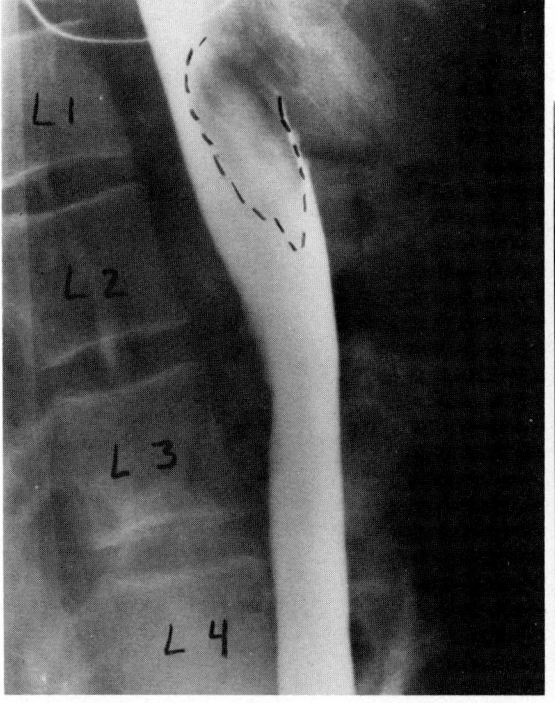
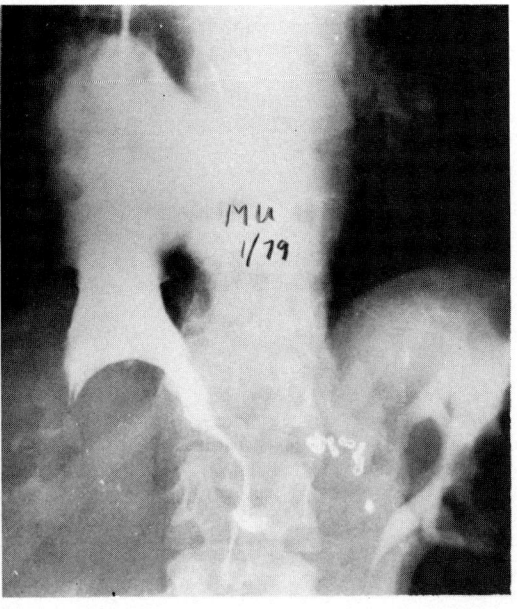

A B

**Figure 42–7.** *A.* Lateral view inferior venacavogram demonstrates tumor thrombus at the L1-2 level *(dotted line).* *B.* Superior venacavogram demonstrates superior extent of vena cava tumor thrombus that completely occludes the lower inferior vena cava to the level of the highest hepatic veins just at the level of the diaphragm. (From Richie JP, Garnick MB: Primary renal and ureteral cancer. *In* Rieselbach RE, Garnick MB [eds]: Cancer and the Kidney. Lea & Febiger, Philadelphia, 1982, p 662.)

of unsuspected pulmonary metastases. Whole lung tomography shows lesions less than 1 cm in diameter that may be missed on plain chest films. In addition, chest tomography demonstrates mediastinal involvement.

Cerebral metastases from renal cell carcinoma are uncommon. Radioisotopic brain scanning and CT of the head region are reserved for patients with symptoms of central nervous system involvement.

## PATHOLOGIC GRADING

Histologic features of the primary tumor have some bearing on prognosis; however, the extent of tumor at the time of resection tends to be the most important prognostic determinant. Microscopic features such as papillary pattern, usually hypovascular on arteriograms, are associated with a better prognosis, even stage for stage.[71] Tumors composed of clear cells are associated with a slightly better 5-year survival rate than those composed of granular cells: 58%

compared with 46%.[72] Spindle cell carcinoma, a much more anaplastic tumor, has the worst prognosis: only 23% of patients survive 5 years.[72]

Evaluation of nuclear characteristics has some bearing on prognosis. More anaplastic nuclear characteristics are associated with diminished 5-year survival.

## PATHOLOGIC STAGING

The single most important determinant of prognosis of a patient with renal cell carcinoma is the pathologic stage of the tumor when it is initially diagnosed and treated. Preoperative studies can give some indication of the extent of involvement, especially distant involvement, but accurate staging depends primarily on histologic evaluation of the resected tumor. A pathologic staging system that has been in general use was proposed by Flocks and Kadesky[73] and modified by Robson and colleagues.[74]

Stage I. Tumor is confined to within the kidney capsule.

# RENAL CELL CARCINOMA

### STAGE I
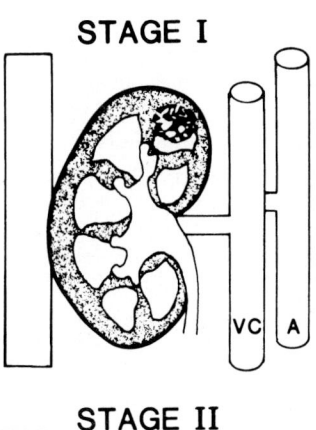

### STAGE II
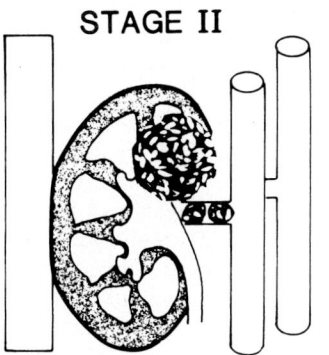

### STAGE III
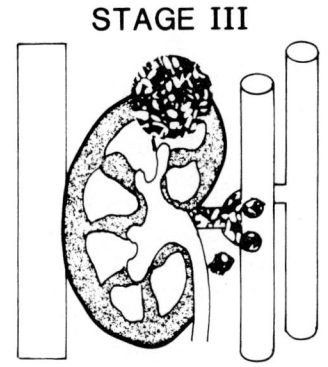

### STAGE IV
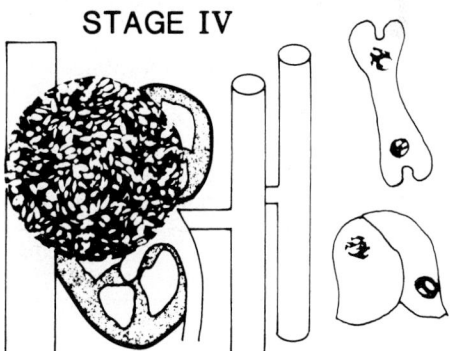

**Figure 42–8.** Staging of renal adenocarcinoma. (Modified from Brodsky GL, Garnick MB: Neoplasms in the adult patient. *In* Tisher CC, Brenner BM [eds]: Renal Pathology. JB Lippincott, Philadelphia, 1989, p 1479.)

STAGE I : CONFINED TO KIDNEY
STAGE II : INCLUDING RENAL
VEIN INVOLVEMENT
STAGE III : LYMPHNODE & CAVAL
INVOLVEMENT
STAGE IV : ADJACENT ORGAN
METASTASES

**TABLE 42–3. TNM Staging System for Renal Cell Carcinoma**

| Tumor | |
|---|---|
| T1 | Small tumor with minimal calyceal distortion |
| T2 | Large tumor with calyceal deformity |
| T3a | Tumor extension to perirenal fat |
| T3b | Renal vein involvement |
| T3c | Inferior vena cava involvement below diaphragm |
| T4a | Spread to contiguous organs except adrenal |
| T4b | Caval involvement above the diaphragm |
| **Nodes** | |
| N0 | Nodes negative |
| N1 | Single homolateral regional node involved |
| N2 | Multiple regional or bilateral nodes involved |
| N3 | Fixed regional nodes |
| N4 | Juxtaregional nodes involved |
| **Metastases** | |
| M0 | Lack of distant metastasis |
| M1 | Distant metastasis |

Stage II. Tumor invades through the renal capsule but is confined to within Gerota fascia.

Stage III. Tumor has invaded the regional lymph nodes, ipsilateral renal vein, or inferior vena cava.

Stage IV. Distant metastases or involvement of adjacent organs other than the ipsilateral adrenal gland is documented.

This staging system is represented in Figure 42–8. An international TNM classification has been proposed with an extensive breakdown into four or five categories for tumor, node, and metastases (Table 42–3).

The effect on prognosis of renal vein involvement or even extension to the inferior vena cava in the absence of regional lymphatic involvement is a subject of controversy. Waters and Richie[75] have shown that involvement of the renal vein alone carries a prognosis similar to that for stage II tumors, a finding that would seem to justify inclusion of renal vein involvement as a subset of stage II (Table 42–4).

## Surgical Treatment

The treatment of choice for renal cell carcinoma is surgical removal. Radical nephrectomy is accomplished by

**TABLE 42–4. Correlation of 5-Year Survival Rate with Pathologic Stage in Patients with Renal Cell Carcinoma***

| Pathologic Stage | Patients (No.) | Survival (%) |
|---|---|---|
| I | 36 | 51.0 |
| II | 54 | 58.5 |
| With renal vein involvement† | 21 | 64.0 |
| With inferior vena cava involvement† | 7 | 25.4 |
| III | 8 | 12.3 |
| IV | 32 | 0 |

*Modified from Waters and Richie.[75]

†Prior series have classified patients with renal vein and inferior vena cava involvement as stage III (see text).

From Richie JP, Garnick MB: Primary renal and ureteral cancer. *In* Rieselbach RE, Garnick MB (eds): Cancer and the Kidney. Lea & Febiger, Philadelphia, 1982, p 662.

early ligation of the renal artery and renal vein and removal en bloc of the kidney with the surrounding Gerota fascia. The concept of radical nephrectomy with excision en bloc of Gerota envelope was advocated by Robson,[76] who reported a 5-year survival rate of 66% compared with a previous cumulative surgical survival rate of 48% for simple nephrectomy. Thus, radical nephrectomy has become the procedure of choice.

Various surgical approaches are available for the effective performance of this procedure. The thoracoabdominal approach described by Chute and associates[77] offers the distinct advantage of palpation of the ipsilateral lung cavity and mediastinum and the opportunity to resect solitary pulmonary metastases. Alternative approaches include an extrapleural supracostal incision or an anterior transabdominal incision. Regardless of which approach is utilized, the principle of early ligation of the vascular pedicle is important to prevent dissemination of tumor at the time of operation.

### REGIONAL LYMPHADENECTOMY

Involvement of the regional lymphatics and periaortic lymph nodes has been noted in almost 25% of patients with renal cell carcinoma,[78] so there is a rationale for performing regional lymphadenectomy in conjunction with radical nephrectomy. The major value of identifying regional lymph node involvement would seem to be its prognostic import, although an occasional patient with one or two involved nodes has survived a long time.[75] Nevertheless, because the 5-year survival of patients with regional nodal involvement is substantially less than that of patients with stage I and II tumors, this factor may be important in the design of trials for adjuvant therapy. Regional lymphadenectomy adds little in terms of operative time or risk and should be performed with radical nephrectomy.

### RENAL VEIN OR INFERIOR VENA CAVA INVOLVEMENT

Approximately 5% of patients with renal cell carcinoma have inferior vena cava involvement. Tumor invasion of the renal vein and inferior vena cava usually occurs as a well-vascularized thrombus covered with its own intimal surface, and this is important for surgical planning and approach. In such instances, and in the absence of demonstrable metastases, radical nephrectomy is performed with early ligation of the renal artery but no manipulation of the renal vein. Vascular control of the inferior vena cava is obtained above and below the tumor thrombus (occasionally up to the right atrium, if necessary, with cardiopulmonary bypass) and closure of the vena cava.[79] An occasional tumor may actually invade the inferior vena cava, necessitating inferior vena caval resection, as described by McCullough and Gittes,[80] but the survival rate of patients with invasion of the inferior vena cava wall is poor in the absence of effective adjuvant therapy.

### PROGNOSIS

The 5-year survival rate after radical nephrectomy for patients with stage I renal cell carcinoma ranges from 60%

to 75%, and that for patients with stage II lesions is 47% to 65%.[23, 74, 75] Patients with renal vein or inferior vena cava involvement have a survival rate of 25% to 50%, and patients with regional lymph node involvement or extracapsular extension, 12% to 25%. For patients who undergo effective surgical removal of renal vein or inferior vena cava thrombus, 5-year survival rates of 25% to 50% have been reported.[75, 81]

## TUMORS IN THE SOLITARY KIDNEY OR SIMULTANEOUS BILATERAL TUMORS

More than 90 cases of renal cell carcinoma arising in a solitary kidney have been reported,[78] and the subject has been reviewed extensively by Wickham.[82] The only techniques that had previously been available for management of the tumor in a solitary kidney were partial nephrectomy (preferably for polar lesions) and radical nephrectomy and institution of dialysis with possible later renal transplantation. More recent advances in transplantation and renal preservation, as well as more aggressive surgical techniques, have allowed management of larger or more centrally located tumors by two additional methods: partial nephrectomy in vivo with local hypothermia and "workbench" surgery ex vivo with subsequent autotransplantation. The majority of tumors in solitary kidneys can be managed adequately by partial nephrectomy techniques in vivo, but occasionally workbench surgery with autotransplantation is necessary.

Wickham[82] concluded that if the contralateral kidney had been removed for previous renal cell carcinoma, the chance of survival was not as good as if the contralateral kidney had been removed for benign disease or was congenitally absent. However, a review of his own data showed that within each category survival rates were better for patients who underwent partial nephrectomy as primary therapy than for those who got no treatment. Novick and associates,[83] in a review of 64 patients reported in the literature with tumor in a solitary kidney, found no difference in overall survival when the contralateral kidney was removed for carcinoma. The results of intensive therapy by partial nephrectomy in a patient with a solitary kidney support the contention that a potentially resectable tumor can be excised whenever the patient's medical condition and physical status permit.

Patients with bilateral synchronous renal cell carcinoma often have evidence of other disseminated disease.[84] Few such patients survive 2 years even with radical nephrectomy or partial nephrectomy. Nonetheless, if distant metastases have been excluded, the most reasonable approach would be to treat the contralateral renal involvement as a solitary metastasis and to excise by partial nephrectomy when feasible. Simultaneous surgical management may be achieved through an anterior abdominal (chevron) incision.[85]

The option of complete radical nephrectomy and maintenance hemodialysis is one that can be considered for certain patients. The risks of long-term hemodialysis are considerable, and transplantation with immunosuppression raises the risk of tumor recurrence. However, satisfactory long-term results can be achieved.

## PREOPERATIVE ARTERIAL EMBOLIZATION

Percutaneous transaortic embolization of the main renal artery has been advocated as a procedure to diminish blood loss, especially in patients with large or locally invasive tumors.[86] This approach helps simplify the radical nephrectomy by allowing ligation of the main renal vein initially rather than dissection more posteriorly to ligate the renal artery first. Several investigators have hypothesized that infarction of the tumor enhances the immune response. The procedure of arterial embolization has been associated with complications, including potential distal emboli, pain, fever, and generalized malaise. Because renal cell carcinomas parasitize other vessels, infarction of tumors is seldom complete. Furthermore, numerous venous collaterals must still be dealt with intraoperatively, and blood loss has been reduced only minimally. In general, angioinfarction should be reserved for special conditions.

## Adjuvant Therapy

Surgical excision is the procedure of choice for treatment of renal cell carcinoma, but adjunctive therapies may include surgical excision of distant metastases (usually solitary), radiotherapy, chemotherapy, and immunotherapy. Metastatic renal cell carcinoma tends to be resistant to most forms of adjunctive therapy, but newer techniques and modalities offer some promise.

### ADJUVANT RADIOTHERAPY

The role of radiotherapy remains controversial in the treatment of renal cell carcinoma. Renal cell carcinoma is a relatively radioresistant tumor, although Riches[87] has advocated both preoperative and postoperative radiotherapy in conjunction with radical nephrectomy. He recommended postoperative radiotherapy in instances of incomplete removal of tumor or in cases of extrarenal spread and regional lymphatic invasion. Others have documented regression of renal cell carcinoma after radiotherapy.[88] Van der Werf-Messing[89] conducted a randomized study of 141 patients; half received 3000 rad in a period of 3 weeks followed by immediate radical nephrectomy and half received radical nephrectomy alone. Preoperative radiotherapy had no influence on the 5-year survival rate, although it did reduce recurrence of tumor in the renal fossa.

## Treatment of Metastatic Disease

### HORMONE THERAPY

Induction of renal tumors in male Syrian hamsters by stilbestrol administration and subsequent regression of tumor growth on discontinuation of stilbestrol or the administration of a progestational agent served as the basis for hormone therapy in patients with advanced renal cell carcinoma. The initial studies of hormone therapy in more than 100 patients so treated reported an overall objective re-

**TABLE 42–5. Hormone Therapy in Advanced Renal Cell Carcinoma***

| Therapy | Patients (No.) | % Response (Range) |
|---|---|---|
| Progestational agents | 695 | 5 (0–17) |
| Androgenic agents | 190 | 3 (0–14) |
| Hormonal responses by year of reporting | | |
| 1967–1971 | 228 | 17 |
| 1971–1976 | 415 | 2 |

*Modified from Bodey.[95]
From Richie JP, Garnick MB: Primary renal and ureteral cancer. *In* Rieselbach RE, Garnick MB (eds): Cancer and the Kidney. Lea & Febiger, Philadelphia, 1982, p 662.

sponse rate of 16%.[90, 91] Unfortunately, these data were not universally reproducible. When strict criteria for defining objective responses were employed, the overall response rates for most hormonal agents (progestational, androgenic, and glucocorticoid) were less than 5%[92–95] (Table 42–5). The majority of patients with advanced renal cell carcinoma do not exhibit a meaningful response to hormonal manipulation.

More recently, attempts have been made to select patients for hormone therapy on the basis of hormone receptors identified in the primary renal cancer. Both estradiol and progesterone receptors have been demonstrated in the cytosol fraction of renal adenocarcinomas in 23 patients.[96] Estrogen receptors (ER) were found in 61% and progesterone receptors (PR) in 61% of the carcinomas studied. Thirty-nine percent of the tumors were positive for both ER and PR, and 17% were negative for both. The effect of progestational or androgenic therapy was then assessed and related to the ER and PR activity of the primary renal

**TABLE 42–6. Single-Agent Activity in Renal Cell Cancer**

| Agent | Patients (No.) | Response No. | Response % Range |
|---|---|---|---|
| Vinblastine | 296 | 47 | 16 (8–25) |
| 5-Fluorouracil | 201 | 10 | 5 (0–8) |
| 6-Mercaptopurine | 73 | 5 | 7 (0–17) |
| Hydroxyurea | 140 | 16 | 11 (5–20) |
| Cyclophosphamide | 132 | 12 | 9 (0–21) |
| Doxorubicin | 65 | 0 | 0 |
| Nitrogen mustard | 45 | 2 | 4 (4–10) |
| CCNU* | 59 | 4 | 7 |
| BCNU† | 11 | 0 | 0 |
| Streptozocin | 15 | 0 | 0 |
| Methyl GAG‡ | 54 | 4 | 7 (0–16) |
| Cisplatin | 60 | 0 | 0 |
| Chlorambucil | 37 | 6 | 16 (14–17) |
| Actinomycin D | 37 | 1 | 3 (0–11) |
| Mitomycin C | 28 | 4 | 14 (11–50) |

*CCNU = 1-(2-chloroethyl)-3-cyclohexyl-1-nitrosourea (lomustine).
†BCNU = 1,3-bis-(2-chloroethyl)-1-nitrosourea (carmustine).
‡Methyl GAG = methylglyoxal-bis-guanylhydrazone.
Modified from Richie JP, Garnick MB: Primary renal and ureteral cancer. *In* Rieselbach RE, Garnick MB (eds): Cancer and the Kidney. Lea & Febiger, Philadelphia, 1982, p 662.

**TABLE 42–7. Combination Chemotherapy and Hormone Therapy for Advanced Renal Adenocarcinoma**

| Agents | Patients (No.) | Response (%) |
|---|---|---|
| Vinblastine + CCNU | 29 | 24 |
| Vinblastine + methyl CCNU* | 38 | 10 |
| Vinblastine + hydroxyurea | 15 | 15 |
| Vinblastine + MPA† | 38 | 8 |
| Vinblastine + methyl GAG‡ | 15 | 6 |
| Vinblastine + 5FU§ + MPA | 20 | 0 |
| Adriamycin + vincristine + MPA + BCG‖ | 31 | 33 |
| Methyl CCNU + MPA | 38 | 11 |
| Tamoxifen + vinblastine + MTX¶ + bleomycin | 14 | 36 |
| Vinblastine + MTX + bleomycin | 14 | 36 |

*Methyl CCNU = methyl-1-(2-chloroethyl)-3-cyclohexyl-1-nitrosourea.
†MPA = medroxyprogesterone acetate.
‡Methyl GAG = methylglyoxal-bis-guanylhydrazone.
§5FU = 5-fluorouracil.
‖BCG = bacillus Calmette-Guérin.
¶MTX = methotrexate.
From Richie JP, Garnick MB: Primary renal and ureteral cancer. *In* Rieselbach RE, Garnick MB (eds): Cancer and the Kidney. Lea & Febiger, Philadelphia, 1982, p 662.

cancer. Six of nine patients who tested positive for both ER and PR demonstrated a therapeutic effect; four of five patients with ER positivity and PR negativity had temporary control of cancer, as did three of five patients who were ER negative and PR positive. Only one of four patients who were ER negative and PR negative had a therapeutic result. These data require cautious interpretation. Many patients were being treated with hormone therapy as an adjunct to nephrectomy, so the response rate and evaluation are difficult to interpret.

In two related studies using the antiestrogen tamoxifen, little if any benefit resulted.[97, 98] In one review, 148 patients with advanced renal cell cancer were treated with antiestrogens; the overall response rate was 7%.[98]

## CHEMOTHERAPY

Tables 42–6 and 42–7 summarize the evaluation of chemotherapeutic agents that have been utilized in advanced renal cell carcinoma.[92–95, 99–104] Although vinblastine has been associated with response rates as high as 25%, other investigators have reported lower rates. Part of this discrepancy reflects the dose chosen, as some investigators have used extremely low doses. Because of a lack of meaningful remissions with both single and combination therapies, most investigators are employing investigational approaches in well-designed phase I (toxicity) and phase II (activity-seeking) studies for advanced renal cancer. A summary of programs currently under way is presented in Table 42–8, and it underscores the fact that active investigation is ongoing in chemotherapy, immunotherapy, hormone therapy, and combinations of such programs.

## INTERFERON

In preliminary work, the use of human leukocyte ($\alpha$) interferon resulted in a partial response rate of 26% of 19

**TABLE 42–8. Selected Investigational Approaches Under Evaluation for Advanced Renal Cancer**

Interleukin-2
Interleukin-2 + lymphokine-activated killer cells
Warfarin and hormonal agents
Interleukin-2 and cisplatin
Tumor necrosis factor
Tumor necrosis factor and interleukin-2
Interferons (alfa and gamma)
Combination therapy: interferon plus interleukin-2
Interleukin-2 + vinblastine
Chronochemotherapy regimens
Tumor necrosis factor + interferon alfa
Interleukin-2, interferon, and 5-fluorouracil
Interleukin-4
Interleukin-6
Interleukin-12

patients.[105] All objective responses were seen in lung or mediastinal areas. A correlation was established between antitumor activity and interferon-induced leukopenia and granulocytopenia. Other studies have also demonstrated limited effectiveness of leukocyte interferon in patients with both pulmonary and subcutaneous metastases. Toxicity is tolerable; symptoms include fever, lethargy, leukopenia, and anorexia. These preliminary data support a potential role for further investigation of interferon in renal neoplasia.

Given the large number of investigative trials of chemotherapeutic agents, it is important to realize that there is no standard therapy for patients with advanced renal cancer. Only through carefully designed protocols will headway be made in this most refractory disease. Programs utilizing new drugs or altering schedules of currently existing chemotherapeutic agents hold the promise for advances in treatment of this disease.

## IMMUNOTHERAPY

A wide spectrum of biologic agents have been utilized for metastatic renal cell carcinoma. These agents include relatively nonspecific immune modulators used as adoptive immunotherapy as well as combinations of biologic agents. More recently, recombinant human interleukin (IL)-2 has gained approval by the U.S. Food and Drug Administration for treatment of metastatic renal cell carcinoma in patients with a good performance status. This approval was based on multiple studies including 255 patients, 37 of whom had a response—an overall response rate of 15%, including a 4% complete response rate and an 11% partial response rate. The median duration of the response was 23.2 months. Of the patients completely responding, 85% had a durable response lasting longer than 12 months, as did 79% of the patients who had a partial response. Although the toxicity of various IL-2 programs is prohibitive, the response rate was deemed important by the U.S. Food and Drug Administration and to warrant approval. Since introduction of IL-2, studies have been published with response rates ranging from 10% to 35%. The latter figure represents patients who have an excellent performance status, minimal pulmonary

disease, minimal lymph node disease, and previous nephrectomy.

More recently, studies of combinations of immune modulators including interferon alfa plus IL-2, or interferon alfa plus IL-2 plus 5-fluorouracil or interferon gamma have resulted in some promising responses. Data from the University of Texas M.D. Anderson Cancer Center have suggested that the combination of IL-2, interferon alfa, and 5-fluorouracil may have achieved the highest response rates yet.

Metastatic renal cell carcinoma seems to be an excellent target for immunotherapeutic agents, as many of the tumors are immunogenic and may respond to biologic agents. On the horizon are clinical studies using IL-4, IL-6, and IL-12. An excellent monograph on the immunotherapy and cellular biology of renal cell carcinoma has been published.[106]

## SURGICAL CONSIDERATIONS FOR METASTATIC DISEASE

Almost 25% of patients with newly diagnosed renal cell carcinoma have evidence of metastases at presentation.[23] In the absence of distant metastatic disease but with locally extensive and invasive tumors, adjacent structures such as bowel, spleen, or psoas muscle may be excised en bloc at the time of radical nephrectomy. This radical approach is justified by a reasonable survival rate for complete resection; the survival after incomplete resection is notoriously poor. Response to radiotherapy, percutaneous arterial occlusion, or arterial injection of radioactive seeds is variable but may allow resolution of symptoms in selected patients.

Treatment of patients with disseminated disease is contingent on location of the metastatic involvement, whether the metastasis appears to be solitary or multiple, and whether the patient has symptoms from the primary tumor.[107, 108]

### Solitary Metastasis

Because of the dismal results with adjunctive therapy, an aggressive surgical approach has been advocated for patients with a solitary metastasis from renal cell carcinoma. In a series of 40 patients who underwent removal of a metastatic focus from renal cell carcinoma, 13 (33%) survived longer than 5 years after removal of the solitary metastasis.[23] The prognosis is more favorable for patients with an isolated pulmonary metastasis. In an evaluation of patients who underwent pulmonary resection for metastatic renal cell carcinoma, Katzenstein and co-workers[109] found that a favorable prognosis was associated with 1) a greater interval from removal of the primary lesion until appearance of the metastatic focus, 2) evidence of a solitary lesion on radiographic examination (even if multiple nodules were found at operation), and 3) demonstration of extensive necrosis in the resected specimen.

Galicich and associates[110] evaluated patients with solitary cerebral metastases from renal cell carcinoma. For patients whose cerebral metastases appeared more than 1 year after excision of the primary lesion, the 1-year survival rate after local excision and radiotherapy was almost twice that (36% versus 19%) of patients whose cerebral metastases appeared less than 1 year after primary tumor excision. Results of excision of isolated metastases (both pulmonary and cerebral) are better for patients whose disease-free interval after resection of the primary tumor is longer. This finding suggests that the doubling time of the primary tumor and various host-tumor interactions have a profound effect on prognosis in patients with metastases.

### Multiple Metastases

Individualization is essential for the treatment of patients with multiple metastases from renal cell carcinoma. Palliative nephrectomy has been advocated to alleviate symptoms attributable to the primary tumor and possibly to induce spontaneous regression of metastatic foci. Nephrectomy for symptoms of local pain, for hemorrhage, or for severe hormone-related and paraneoplastic symptoms secondary to the primary tumor is rational for the patient who has a reasonable chance of surviving at least several months. For a patient with an asymptomatic primary lesion, however, palliative nephrectomy is simply not justified. DeKernion and associates[111] have compared survival of patients with metastatic renal cell carcinoma, stratifying those who underwent adjunctive radical nephrectomy. As delineated in Figure 42–9, the survival for the two groups was identical. In a collected series of 474 cases, Montie and associates[112] could find only four examples (0.8%) of spontaneous regression of various metastases after radical nephrectomy. Furthermore, in a series of almost 1700 cases reviewed by Mostofi,[3] all but 2 of the patients with metastases at initial presentation died from metastatic disease within 2 years, regardless of therapy. In more than 500 patients with renal cell cancer treated by radical nephrectomy, Myers and associates[113] reported no patient whose metastatic lesions resolved after nephrectomy. Because the operative mortality approaches 10%, nephrectomy should be reserved for patients with significant local symptoms from the primary tumor or with significant systemic symptoms secondary to the tumor. An exception to this caveat would include de-

velopment of effective adjuvant therapy for patients with only a few metastases.

Spontaneous regression of metastatic renal cell carcinoma, often after removal of the primary lesion, has been documented in sporadic reports.[114, 115] In 1977, Freed and associates[116] reviewed the literature and collected approximately 50 cases of spontaneous regression. The majority of patients had pulmonary metastases, and 80% of the patients were male. Many, but certainly not all, were treated with radical nephrectomy. In fewer than 20 cases was histologic documentation available. Furthermore, the term ''regression'' does not equate with cure; the majority of patients with regression suffer a relapse within 1 or 2 years. Nevertheless, the fact that spontaneous regression of metastases has occurred (even after radiotherapy for a dominant metastasis)[117] is evidence for a host-tumor interaction in patients with renal cell carcinoma.

## SARCOMAS OF RENAL ORIGIN

Sarcomas of primary renal origin are relatively rare; they are estimated to constitute 1% to 3% of all primary malignant tumors of the kidney.[118] The most common histologic type is fibrosarcoma, usually arising from the renal capsule. The tumor is manifested by rapid growth, with invasion of the renal vein in nearly half the cases. The presenting symptoms may be a palpable abdominal mass, hematuria, or pain, but these are usually late symptoms. Five-year survival rates are generally poor and have been reported to be as low as 10%.[119]

The second most common renal sarcoma is leiomyosarcoma, with approximately 40 cases reported in the literature.[120] These tumors are more common in females. Pain is the usual initial symptom, and metastases are often present at diagnosis. Long-term survival is unusual.

Other rare histologic types include rhabdomyosarcoma, osteogenic sarcoma, and liposarcoma. In general, all of these sarcomas are highly malignant and often have local or distant metastatic involvement at the time of diagnosis. Angiographic studies disclose various degrees of vascularity, and CT may allow better resolution of the extent of involvement. Surgical excision with wide margins is the treatment of choice, as sarcomas are relatively radioresistant and, in general, respond poorly to chemotherapeutic regimens.

## WILMS TUMOR (NEPHROBLASTOMA)

Wilms tumor, or nephroblastoma, is an embryonal neoplasm initially described in the early 1800s that was described in its definitive form and characteristics in an extensive monograph in 1899.[121] Various other terms, including embryoma or adenomyosarcoma, have been utilized, but nephroblastoma and Wilms tumor are the preferred terms. Wilms tumor, one of the more common tumors of childhood, has a dramatic story of therapeutic success by the combination of modalities of surgery, radiotherapy, and chemotherapy. This tumor accounts for 6% to 30% of ma-

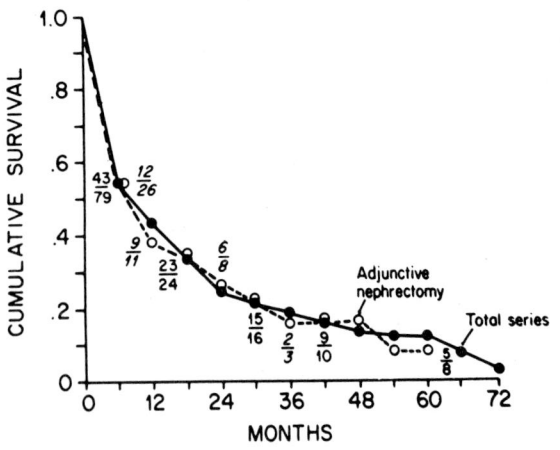

**Figure 42–9.** Survival rates in a series of 86 patients with metastatic renal cell carcinoma treated by various modalities are compared with the survival of patients treated with adjunctive nephrectomy. (From DeKernion JB, Ramming KP, Smith RB: Natural history of metastatic renal cell carcinoma: Computer analysis. J Urol 120:148, 1978.)

lignant solid abdominal tumors in children and is second only to neuroblastoma in overall prevalence.[122] Wilms tumor is the most common malignant renal tumor of childhood, involving approximately 1 child in every 13,500 live births, with an incidence of 2 new cases per million population per year.[123]

## Clinical Findings

Many patients with Wilms tumor have no symptoms, and an abdominal mass is usually discovered incidentally by the parent or the examining physician. Systemic symptoms, such as fatigue, malaise, weight loss, and fever, are usually late characteristics. Approximately 50% of patients have abdominal pain as a presenting symptom. One third of patients with Wilms tumor are younger than 2 years of age at presentation, and almost two thirds are younger than 4 years of age.

Tumors vary markedly in size, from small tumors several centimeters in diameter to extremely large ones that almost completely fill the abdomen and cause respiratory embarrassment. The tumor is easily palpable, firm, immobile, and smooth, but it may on occasion feel nodular. The firmness and immobility tend to distinguish it from hydronephrosis and renal cysts.

Hematuria may be seen in 10% to 20% of patients and has no prognostic significance. The incidence of hypertension varies, although Sukarochana and associates[124] reported a rate of 63% in patients with Wilms tumor. Hypertension may be secondary to excessive renin production by the tumor[125] or to subcapsular hemorrhage. The Wilms tumor gene *WT1* has been identified on chromosome 11.[126, 127]

## Evaluation and Staging

When a diagnosis of Wilms tumor is probable, few studies are needed for confirmation, and surgical intervention should not be delayed unduly. The differential diagnosis of Wilms tumor includes hydronephrosis, cystic disease of the kidney, adrenal tumor, and hematoma. Intravenous urography is the most helpful radiologic procedure for differentiation of these causes of abdominal masses and is diagnostic of Wilms tumor in the majority of patients. There is usually distortion of the calyces with splaying of contrast medium around the mass. There may be obstruction by a large tumor, or a small tumor may cause intrarenal distortion of the kidney in the calyceal system. Ultrasonography or CT can delineate whether the mass lesion is solid or cystic and can also indicate other organ involvement. CT seems to be the most effective means of imaging the contralateral kidney to exclude bilateral involvement.

Arteriography is usually not indicated and may be unreliable in differentiating Wilms tumor from neuroblastoma.[128] Furthermore, arteriography may be associated with increased complications, especially in infants and young children. Although there is a need to determine bilaterality (in approximately 5% to 10% of cases), surgical exploration is usually better and more effective than arteriography. Arteriography may be considered, however, if bilateral disease

is suspected. Inferior venacavography is usually not indicated and only rarely contributes important findings.

The most common site of metastasis from Wilms tumor is the lung; therefore, chest radiography and lung tomography are indicated to exclude metastases, although the latter method may not be helpful in young patients. Other studies that could be considered during clinical evaluation include bone and liver scans, but these are not mandatory before surgery unless clinical symptoms indicate.

There is no place for needle biopsy of a flank mass in a child with a suspected Wilms tumor. Surgical exploration may still be necessary, and needle biopsy serves only to increase the risk of tumor spillage.

Wilms tumor is staged according to the National Wilms Tumor Study,[129] a combined clinical and pathologic staging system (Table 42–9). Almost half the patients are classified as group I, approximately 25% as group II, approximately 20% as group III, and the remainder as groups IV and V.

Bilaterality, with concurrent or asynchronous tumor in the opposite kidney, occurs in approximately 5% to 10% of patients (group V). Sonley[130] reported that 5 of 211 patients with Wilms tumors had bilateral involvement at the time of original diagnosis. The National Wilms Tumor Study Group[129] reported that 5% of the children had bilateral tumors.

Several factors influence prognosis. The most recognized, and probably the most significant, is histopathology.[131] Wilms tumors have been classified histopathologically as favorable or unfavorable. The former group represents about 90% of tumors and has an overall cure rate of 85% to 90%, whereas the latter group represents 10% to 15% of patients and has only a 25% cure rate. Other prognostic factors include tumor size, capsular invasion, lymph node or distant metastases, and collecting system or vascular invasion.

## Treatment

The treatment of a child with Wilms tumor has been expanded considerably by the adoption of a multimodality approach involving oncologist, radiotherapist, and surgeon. Treatment should be aggressive and, in general, limited to large centers where all components of therapy are readily available. The majority of patients' disease is curable, even widely disseminated disease; however, the course of treatment may require surgical excision, precise radiotherapy,

### TABLE 42–9. Staging of Wilms Tumor

| Group | Characteristics |
|---|---|
| I | Tumor is limited to one kidney and is completely resectable |
| II | Tumor extends outside the kidney but is completely resectable |
| III | Tumor is incompletely resected with residual intra-abdominal involvement |
| IV | Hematogenous metastases |
| V | Bilateral Wilms tumor involves both kidneys (either synchronous or metachronous) |

and chemotherapy. Specific aspects of each modality are considered separately.

## SURGICAL TECHNIQUE

The transabdominal transperitoneal approach, utilizing a chevron incision, is preferred for removal of tumor with minimal manipulation and adequate access to the renal vasculature. Complete exploration of the abdomen should be performed, with particular attention to the affected kidney and the opposite kidney and regional and para-aortic lymph nodes. The uninvolved kidney should be carefully palpated and visually inspected by opening Gerota fascia to rule out metastases. If an unsuspected nodule is delineated, excision or partial nephrectomy should be performed. Likewise, excision or biopsy of suspicious nodules should be performed.

In mobilizing the primary tumor, the surgeon should attempt to ligate the renal pedicle before manipulating the specimen, just as for a radical nephrectomy for renal cell carcinoma. The renal vein should be carefully palpated to exclude tumor thrombus before ligation. The primary tumor should be mobilized carefully, as many Wilms tumors are soft and friable and may rupture at the time of manipulation. Because intraoperative spillage has been associated with a poorer prognosis, this complication should be avoided if at all possible. Cassady and co-workers[132] have shown that tumor spillage requires additional whole abdominal radiotherapy, which does prevent local abdominal recurrence. Gerota fascia, with the ipsilateral kidney and usually the ipsilateral adrenal gland, is removed en bloc, along with regional lymph nodes.

If the tumor is adherent to adjacent organs such as spleen, tail of the pancreas, or psoas muscle, these may be removed with the specimen, but if the tumor is involved with vital structures such as the duodenum, body of the pancreas, or root of the mesentery, the incision should be closed after biopsy is performed. Radical resection is recommended only if the tumor can be removed completely at the time of the operative procedure.

## RADIOTHERAPY

Wilms tumor is a relatively radioresponsive tumor, and radiotherapy has increased the local control rate over that of surgical excision alone. Radiotherapy has remained an essential part of the overall plan for therapy. Chemotherapy and radiotherapy seem to be additive in antitumor effect.

Routine postoperative radiotherapy is used for patients in groups II, III, and IV and for those older than 2 years of age with group I disease. Radiotherapy is usually instituted 48 hours after surgical extirpation. Although it can be delayed until bowel function returns to normal, the National Wilms Tumor Study[133] found that postoperative delay beyond 10 days is an adverse prognostic factor. The field of irradiation should be adequate to encompass the tumor as indicated by preoperative studies and as demonstrated at surgery by clips placed around the tumor. In general, the radiation field encompasses the renal bed well across the midline to include the entire vertebral bodies, and it extends superiorly to the diaphragm and inferiorly to the anterior superior iliac spine (or lower for lower pole lesions). The

opposite kidney should be shielded to prevent radiation damage. In the past, the radiation dose was based on the age of the patient,[129] but some believe that dose should not vary with age. With higher doses, the shrinking-field technique is used to diminish complications.

For patients with group I disease who are younger than 2 years of age, radiotherapy of the tumor bed is not necessary. The National Wilms Tumor Study showed a disease-free survival rate of 89%, with or without radiotherapy, if prophylactic chemotherapy was administered.[129] There have been no local recurrences among nonirradiated patients. Radiotherapy does seem to be beneficial for group I patients who are older than 2 years.

Preoperative radiotherapy is frequently used in Europe but, in the United States, chemotherapy has generally replaced this modality for preoperative therapy. Both chemotherapy and radiotherapy may complicate proper histopathologic evaluation.

## CHEMOTHERAPY

Chemotherapy has resulted in a dramatic improvement in survival rate of patients with Wilms tumor. The tumor is clearly chemosensitive, and actinomycin D and vincristine are both active agents for therapy. They can reduce the size of a tumor before surgery, reduce pulmonary metastases, and prolong survival. Although actinomycin D was traditionally administered in small daily intravenous doses (15 $\mu$g/kg body weight for a 5-day cycle),[134] understanding of the mechanisms of actinomycin D action suggests that it may be better used at a dosage of 1.2 mg/m$^2$ every 3 weeks.[135] Vincristine is given in combination with actinomycin D at 1.5 mg/m$^2$ (maximal single dose, 2.0 mg) intravenously at the time of diagnosis and weekly for 12 weeks.

The addition of chemotherapy has changed the dismal overall survival rate of patients with Wilms tumor. Before chemotherapy, survival rates ranged from 25% to 40%.[136] Curability for patients with group II and III disease treated with surgery and chemotherapy now approaches 86%; survival of patients with group I disease ranges from 92% to 97%.[129]

At the present time, the combination of surgery, radiotherapy, and chemotherapy has resulted in survival rates and presumed cure for approximately 80% of patients with Wilms tumor.[133] There is some morbidity associated with combined therapy, and studies are under way by the National Wilms Tumor Study Group to see whether equally good survival rates can be achieved with less therapy.

## REFERENCES

1. Grawitz P: Die sogennaneten Lipoma der Niere. Virchows Arch Pathol Anat 93:39, 1883.
2. Nairn RC, Ghose T, Tannenberg AEG: Kidney-specific antigen depletion in human renal carcinomas. Br J Cancer 20:756, 1967.
3. Mostofi FK: Pathology and spread of renal cell carcinoma. *In* King JS Jr (ed): Renal Neoplasia. Little, Brown, Boston, 1967, p 41.
4. Fisher ER, Horva B: Comparative ultrastructural study of so-called renal adenoma and carcinoma. J Urol 108:382, 1972.
5. Kipell JM: The incidence of benign renal nodules (a clinicopathologic study). J Urol 106:503, 1971.
6. Bell ET: Renal Disease, 2nd ed. Lea & Febiger, Philadelphia, 1950, p 435.

7. Boring CC, Squires TS, Tong T, et al: Cancer statistics, 1993. CA 43:7, 1993.
8. See WA, Williams RD. Tumors of the kidney, ureter and bladder. West J Med 156:523, 1992.
9. Kantor AF, Meigs JW, Heston JF, Flannery T: Epidemiology of renal cell carcinoma in Connecticut. J Natl Cancer Inst 57:495, 1976.
10. Richie JP, Skinner DG: Renal neoplasia. *In* Brenner BM, Rector F (eds): The Kidney, 2nd ed. WB Saunders, Philadelphia, 1981, p 2109.
11. Kantor AF: Current concepts in the epidemiology and etiology of primary renal cell carcinoma. J Urol 117:415, 1977.
12. Wynder EL, Mabuschi K, Whitmore WF Jr: Epidemiology of adenocarcinoma of the kidney. J Natl Cancer Inst 53:1619, 1974.
13. Arison RN, Feudale EL: Induction of renal tumor by streptozotocin in rats. Nature 214:1254, 1967.
14. Rakieten N, Gordon BS, Cooney DA, et al: Renal tumorigenic action of streptozotocin (NSC-85998) in rats. Cancer Chemother Rep 52:563, 1968.
15. Mauer SM, Lee CS, Najarian JS, Brown DM: Induction of malignant kidney tumors in rats with streptozotocin. Cancer Res 34:158, 1974.
16. Berman LD, Hayes JA, Sibay RM: Effect of streptozotocin on Chinese hamsters (*Cricetulus giseus*). J Natl Cancer Inst 51:1287, 1973.
17. Myerowitz RL, Sartiano GP, Cavallo T: Nephrotoxic and cytoproliferative effects of streptozotocin. Cancer 38:1550, 1976.
18. Kolonel LN: Association of cadmium with renal cancer. Cancer 38:1782, 1976.
19. Horton WA, Wong V, Eldridge R: Von Hippel–Lindau disease: Clinical and pathological manifestations in 9 families with 50 affected members. Arch Intern Med 136:769, 1976.
20. Seizinger BR, Rouleau GA, Lzelius LJ, et al: Von Hippel–Lindau disease maps to the region of chromosome 3 associated with renal cell carcinoma. Nature 332:268, 1988.
21. Cohen AJ, Li FP, Berg S, et al: Hereditary renal cell carcinoma associated with a chromosomal translocation. N Engl J Med 301:592, 1979.
22. Pathak S, Strong LC, Ferrell RE, Trindade A: Familial renal cell carcinoma with a 3:11 chromosome translocation limited to tumor cells. Science 217:939, 1982.
23. Skinner DG, Calvin RB, Vermillion CD, et al: Diagnosis and management of renal cell carcinoma. A clinical and pathologic study of 309 cases. Cancer 28:1165, 1971.
24. Gibbons RP, Monte JE, Correa RJ Jr, Mason JT: Manifestations of renal cell carcinoma. Urology 8:201, 1976.
25. Pinals RS, Krane SK: Medical aspects of renal carcinoma. Postgrad Med J 38:507, 1962.
26. Chisholm GD, Roy RR: The systemic effects of malignant renal tumors. Br J Urol 43:687, 1971.
27. Berger L, Sinkoff MW: Systemic manifestations of hypernephroma. A review of 273 cases. Am J Med 22:791, 1957.
28. Cranston WI, Luff RH, Owen D, Rawlins MD: Studies on the pathogenesis of fever in renal carcinoma. Clin Sci Mol Med 45:459, 1973.
29. Damon A, et al: Polycythemia and renal carcinoma. Am J Med 25:182, 1958.
30. Murphy GP, Kenny GM, Mirand EA: Erythropoietin levels in patients with renal tumor or cysts. Cancer 26:191, 1970.
31. Sytkowski AJ, Richie JP, Bicknell KA: New human renal carcinoma cell line established from a patient with erythrocytosis. Cancer Res 43:1415, 1983.
32. Walsh P, Kissane J: Non-metastatic hypernephroma with reversible hepatic dysfunction. Arch Intern Med 122:214, 1968.
33. Boxer RJ, Waisman J, Lieber MM, et al: Non-metastatic hepatic dysfunction associated with renal carcinoma. J Urol 119:468, 1978.
34. O'Grady AS, Morse LJ, Lee JB: Parathyroid hormone–secreting renal carcinoma associated with hypercalcemia and metabolic alkalosis. Ann Intern Med 63:858, 1965.
35. Lytton B, Rosof B, Evans J: Parathyroid hormone–like activity in a renal carcinoma producing hypercalcemia. J Urol 93:127, 1965.
36. Goldberg MF, Tashjian AH Jr, Order SE, et al: Renal adenocarcinoma containing a parathyroid hormone–like substance and associated with marked hypercalcaemia. Am J Med 36:805, 1964.
37. Buckle RM, McMillan M, Mallinson C: Ectopic secretion of parathyroid hormone by a renal adenocarcinoma in a patient with hypercalcaemia. Br Med J 4:724, 1970.
38. Greenberg AB, Martin JJ, Sutcliff HS: Synthesis and release of parathyroid hormone by a renal carcinoma in cell culture. Clin Sci Mol Med 45:183, 1973.
39. Brereton HD, Halushka PV, Alexander RW, et al: Indomethacin-responsive hypercalcemia in a patient with renal-cell adenocarcinoma. N Engl J Med 291:83, 1974.
40. Cummings KB, Robertson RP: Prostaglandin: Increased production by renal cell carcinoma. J Urol 118:720, 1977.
41. Goldberg RS, Pilcher DB, Yates JW: The aggressive surgical management of hypercalcemia due to ectopic parathormone production. Cancer 45:2652, 1980.
42. Riggs BL Jr, Sprague RG: Association of Cushing's syndrome and neoplastic disease. Arch Intern Med 109:841, 1961.
43. Spencer D: Secondary amyloidosis in relation to carcinoma of the kidney. Postgrad Med J 47:820, 1971.
44. Cline MJ, Williams HE: Extra-renal manifestations of hypernephroma. Calif Med 109:35, 1968.
45. Thrush DC: Neuropathy, IgM paraproteinaemia, and autoantibodies in hypernephroma. Br Med J 4:474, 1970.
46. Gleeson MH, Bloom SR, Polak JM, et al: An endocrine tumour in kidney affecting small bowel structure, motility, and function. Gut 11:1060, 1970.
47. Hollifield JW, Page DL, Smith C, et al: Renin-secreting clear cell carcinoma of the kidney. Arch Intern Med 135:859, 1975.
48. Sufrin G, Mirand EA, Moore RH, et al: Hormones in renal cancer. J Urol 117:433, 1977.
49. Turkington RW: Ectopic production of prolactin. N Engl J Med 285:1455, 1971.
50. Lang EK: Diagnosis of renal parenchymal tumors. *In* Skinner DG, DeKernion JB (eds): Genitourinary Cancer. WB Saunders, Philadelphia, 1978, p 40.
51. Daniel WW Jr, Hartman GW, Witten DM, et al: Calcified renal masses. A review of 10 years experience at the Mayo Clinic. Radiology 103:503, 1972.
52. Pfister RC, Shea TE: Nephrotomography: Performance and interpretation. Radiol Clin North Am 9:41, 1971.
53. Greene LF, et al: Bolus nephrotomography in the diagnosis of mass lesions of the kidney. Presented at the annual meeting of the American Urological Association; 1974; St. Louis, MO.
54. Chynn KY, Evans JA: Nephrotomography in differentiation of renal cyst from neoplasm: Review of 500 cases. J Urol 83:21, 1960.
55. Schreck WR, Holmes JH: Ultrasound as a diagnostic aid for renal neoplasms and cysts. J Urol 103:281, 1970.
56. Smith EH, Bennett AH: The usefulness of ultrasound in the evaluation of renal masses in adults. J Urol 113:525, 1975.
57. O'Reilly PH, Osborn DE, Testa HJ, et al: Renal imaging: A comparison of radionuclide, ultrasound, and computed tomographic scanning in investigation of renal space-occupying lesions. Br Med J Clin Res 282:943, 1981.
58. McFarland WL, Wallace S, Johnson DE: Renal carcinoma and polycystic disease. J Urol 107:530, 1972.
59. Emmett JL, Levine SR, Woolner LB: Co-existence of renal cyst and tumour: Incidence in 1,007 cases. Br J Urol 35:403, 1963.
60. Harris RD, Goergen TG, Talner LB: The bloody renal cyst aspirate: A diagnostic dilemma. J Urol 114:832, 1975.
61. Abrams HL: Response of neoplastic renal vessels to epinephrine in man. Radiology 82:217, 1964.
62. Watson RC, Fleming RJ, Evans JA: Arteriography in the diagnosis of renal carcinoma. Radiology 91:188, 1968.
63. Weinerth JL, Johnsrude IS, Anderson EE, Hendrix PC: Surgical validation of angiographic studies in renal lesions. J Urol 116:550, 1976.
64. Lang EK: Roentgenographic assessment of asymptomatic renal lesions. Radiology 109:257, 1973.
65. Goodman M, Curry T, Russell T: Xanthogranulomatous pyelonephritis (XGP): A local disease with systemic manifestations. Report of 23 patients and review of the literature. Medicine (Baltimore) 58:171, 1979.
66. Lang EK: Complications of retrograde percutaneous arteriography. J Urol 90:604, 1963.
67. Weyman PJ, McClennan BL, Stanley RJ, et al: Comparison of computed tomography and angiography in the evaluation of renal cell carcinoma. Radiology 137:417, 1980.
68. Richie JP, Garnick MB, Seltzer S, Bettman MA: Computerized tomography scan for diagnosis and staging of renal cell carcinoma. J Urol 129:1114, 1983.

69. Hricak H: Detection and staging of renal neoplasms: A reassessment of MR imaging. Radiology 166:643, 1988.
70. Karstaedt N, McCullough DL, Wolfman NT, et al: Magnetic resonance imaging of the renal mass. J Urol 136:566, 1986.
71. Mancilla-Jimenez R, Stanley RJ, Blath RA: Papillary renal cell carcinoma: A clinical, radiologic and pathologic study of 34 cases. Cancer 38:2469, 1976.
72. Colvin RB, Dickersin GR: Pathology of renal tumors. In Skinner DG, DeKernion JB (eds): Genitourinary Cancer. WB Saunders, Philadelphia, 1978, p 84.
73. Flocks RH, Kadesky MC: Malignant neoplasms of the kidney: An analysis of 353 patients followed five years or more. J Urol 79:196, 1958.
74. Robson CJ, Churchill BM, Anderson W: The results of radical nephrectomy for renal cell carcinoma. Trans Am Assoc Genitourin Surg 60:122, 1968.
75. Waters WB, Richie JP: Aggressive surgical approach to renal cell carcinoma: Review of 130 cases. J Urol 122:306, 1979.
76. Robson CJ: Radical nephrectomy for renal cell carcinoma. J Urol 89:37, 1963.
77. Chute R, Soutter L, Kerr W: The value of the thoracoabdominal incision in removal of kidney tumors. N Engl J Med 241:951, 1949.
78. Skinner DG, DeKernion JB: Clinical manifestations and treatment of renal parenchymal tumors. In Skinner DG, DeKernion JB (eds): Genitourinary Cancer. WB Saunders, Philadelphia, 1978, p 107.
79. Freed SZ, Gliedman ML: The removal of renal carcinoma thrombus extending into the right atrium. J Urol 113:163, 1975.
80. McCullough DL, Gittes RF: Ligation of the renal vein in the solitary kidney: Effects on renal function. J Urol 113:295, 1975.
81. Schefft P, Novick AC, Straffon RA, Stewart BH: Surgery for renal cell carcinoma extending into inferior vena cava. J Urol 120:28, 1978.
82. Wickham JEA: Conservative renal surgery for adenocarcinoma. The place of bench surgery. Br J Urol 47:25, 1975.
83. Novick AC, Stewart BH, Straffon RA, Banowsky LH: Partial nephrectomy in the treatment of renal adenocarcinoma. J Urol 118:932, 1977.
84. Vermillion CD, Skinner DG, Pfister RC: Bilateral renal cell carcinoma. J Urol 108:219, 1972.
85. Finkbeiner A, Moyad R, Herwig K: Bilateral simultaneously occurring adenocarcinoma of the kidney. J Urol 116:26, 1976.
86. Goldstein HM, Medellin H, Beydoun MT, et al: Transcatheter embolization of renal cell carcinoma. AJR 123:557, 1975.
87. Riches EW: The place of radiotherapy in the management of parenchymal carcinoma of the kidney. J Urol 95:313, 1966.
88. Malkin RB: Regression of renal carcinoma following radiation therapy. J Urol 114:782, 1975.
89. Van der Werf-Messing B: Carcinoma of the kidney. Cancer 32:1056, 1973.
90. Bloom HJG: Medroxyprogesterone acetate (Provera) in the treatment of renal cell carcinoma. Br J Cancer 25:250, 1971.
91. Samuels ML, Sullivan P, Howe CD: Medroxyprogesterone acetate in the treatment of renal cell carcinoma (hypernephroma). Cancer 22:525, 1968.
92. Tally RW: Chemotherapy of adenocarcinoma of the kidney. Cancer 32:1062, 1973.
93. Alberto P, Senn HJ: Hormonal therapy of renal carcinoma alone and in association with cytostatic drugs. Cancer 33:1226, 1974.
94. Lokich JJ, Harrison JH: Renal cell carcinoma: Natural history and chemotherapeutic experience. J Urol 114:371, 1975.
95. Bodey GP: Current status of chemotherapy in metastatic renal carcinoma. In Johnson DE, Samuels ML (eds): Cancer of the Genitourinary Tract. Raven Press, New York, 1979, p 67.
96. Concolino G, Marocchi A, Conti C, et al: Human renal cell carcinoma as a hormone-dependent carcinoma. Cancer Res 38:4340, 1978.
97. Glick JL, et al: Tamoxifen in metastatic prostate and renal cancer. Proc Am Soc Clin Oncol 20:311, 1979.
98. Weiselberg L, Budman D, Vinciguerra V, et al: Tamoxifen in unresectable hypernephroma: A phase II trial and review of literature. Cancer Clin Trials 4:195, 1981.
99. Mittleman A, Albert DJ, Murphy GP: Lomustine treatment of metastatic renal cell carcinoma. JAMA 225:32, 1973.
100. Kiruluta G, Morales A, Lott S: Response of renal adenocarcinoma to cyclophosphamide. Urology 6:557, 1975.
101. Davis TE, Manolo FB: Combination chemotherapy of advanced renal cell cancer with CCNU and vinblastine. Proc Am Soc Clin Oncol 19:316, 1978.
102. Ishmael DR, Burpo LJ, Bottomley RH: Combination therapy of advanced hypernephroma with medroxyprogesterone, BCG, Adriamycin, and vincristine. Proc Am Soc Clin Oncol 19:407, 1978.
103. Katakkar SB, Franks CR: Chemo-hormonal therapy for metastatic renal cell carcinoma with Adriamycin, hydroxyurea, vinblastine and medroxyprogesterone acetate. Cancer Treat Rep 62:1379, 1978.
104. Hahn RG, Temkin NR, Savlov ED, et al: Phase II study of vinblastine, methyl-CCNU, and medroxyprogesterone in advanced renal cell cancer. Cancer Treat Rep 62:1093, 1978.
105. Quesada JR, Swanson DA, Trindade A, Gutterman, JU: Renal cell carcinoma: Antitumor effects of leukocyte interferon. Cancer Res 43:940, 1983.
106. Klein EA, Bukowski RM, Finke JH (eds): Renal Cell Carcinoma: Immunotherapy and Cellular Biology. Marcel Dekker, New York, 1993.
107. Richie JP, Garnick MB: Primary renal and ureteral cancer. In Rieselbach RE, Garnick MB (eds): Cancer and the Kidney. Lea & Febiger, Philadelphia, 1982, p 662.
108. Garnick MB: Advanced renal cell. Kidney Int 20:127, 1981.
109. Katzenstein AL, Purvis R Jr, Gmelich J, Askin F: Pulmonary resection for metastatic renal adenocarcinoma: pathologic findings and therapeutic value. Cancer 41:712, 1978.
110. Galicich JH, Sundaresan N, Arbit E, Passe S: Surgical treatment of single brain metastasis: Factors associated with survival. Cancer 45:381, 1980.
111. DeKernion JB, Ramming KP, Smith RB: Natural history of metastatic renal cell carcinoma: Computer analysis. J Urol 120:148, 1978.
112. Montie JE, Stewart BH, Straffon RA, et al: The role of adjunctive nephrectomy in patients with metastatic renal cell carcinoma. J Urol 117:272, 1977.
113. Myers GH, Fehrenbaker LG, Kelias PP: Prognostic significance of renal vein invasion by hypernephroma. J Urol 100:420, 1968.
114. Goodwin WE, et al: Under what circumstances does "regression" of hypernephroma occur? In King JS Jr (ed): Renal Neoplasia. Little, Brown, Boston, 1967.
115. Bloom HJG: Hormone-induced and spontaneous regression of metastatic renal cancer. Cancer 32:1066, 1973.
116. Freed SZ, Halperin JP, Gordon M: Idiopathic regression of metastases from renal cell carcinoma. J Urol 118:538, 1977.
117. Fairlamb DJ: Spontaneous regression of metastases of renal cancer. A report of two cases including the first recorded regression following irradiation of a dominant metastasis and a review of the world literature. Cancer 47:2102, 1981.
118. Gupta OP, Dube MK: Rare primary renal sarcoma. Br J Urol 43:546, 1971.
119. Demming CL, Harvard BM: Tumors of the kidney. In Campbell MF, Harrison JH (eds): Urology, 3rd ed. WB Saunders, Philadelphia, 1970, p 884.
120. Loomis RC: Primary leiomyosarcoma of the kidney. Report of a case and review of the literature. J Urol 107:557, 1972.
121. Wilms M: Die Misgeschwulste der Nieren. Leipzig, Arthur Georgi, 1899.
122. Koop CE: Abdominal tumors in infants and children. Arch Dis Child 35:1, 1960.
123. Glenn JF, Rhamy RC: Wilms' tumor—epidemiological experience. J Urol 85:911, 1961.
124. Sukarochana K, Tolentino W, Kiesewetter WB: Wilms' tumor and hypertension. J Pediatr Surg 5:573, 1972.
125. Ganguly A, Gribble J, Tune B, et al: Renin-secreting Wilms' tumor with severe hypertension. Report of a case and brief review of renin-secreting tumors. Ann Intern Med 79:835, 1973.
126. Koo HP, Hensle TW: Molecular biology of Wilms' tumor. Urol Clin North Am 20:323, 1993.
127. Velasco S, D'Amico D, Schneider NR, et al: Molecular and cellular heterogeneity of Wilms' tumor. Int J Cancer 53:672, 1993.
128. Grossman H: The evaluation of abdominal masses in children with emphasis on noninvasive methods. A roentgenographic approach. Cancer 35:884, 1975.
129. Tournade MF, Com-Nougue C, Voute PA, et al: Results of the Sixth International Society of Pediatric Oncology Wilms' Tumor Trial and Study: A risk-adapted therapeutic approach in Wilms' tumor. J Clin Oncol 11:1014, 1993.

130. Sonley MJ: Wilms' tumor: A review of the Toronto experience. *In* Golden JD (ed): Cancer in Childhood. Holt, Rinehart & Winston, Toronto, 1973, p 29.
131. Beckwith JB, Palmer NF: Histopathology and prognosis of Wilms' tumor—results from the first National Wilms' Tumor Study. Cancer 41:1937, 1978.
132. Cassady JR, Tefft M, Filler RM, et al: Considerations in the radiation therapy of Wilms' tumor. Cancer 32:598, 1973.
133. D'Angio GJ, Beckwith JB, Breslow NE, et al: Wilms' tumor: An update. Cancer 45:1791, 1980.
134. Wolff JA, et al: Long-term evaluation of single versus multiple course of actinomycin-D therapy of Wilms' tumor. N Engl J Med 290:84, 1974.
135. Green DM, Jaffe N: The role of chemotherapy in the treatment of Wilms' tumor. Cancer 44:52, 1979.
136. Snyder WH Jr, Hastings TN, Pollack W: Wilms' tumor: Embryoma of the kidney. *In* Benson CD et al (eds): Pediatric Surgery, Vol. 2. Year Book Medical Publishers, Chicago, 1962, p 281.

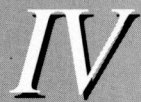

# IV

# PATHOPHYSIOLOGY OF RENAL DISEASE

# Renal and Systemic Manifestations of Glomerular Disease

*Sharon Anderson*
*Thomas M. Kennefick*
*Barry M. Brenner*

## PROTEINURIA

Proteinuria characterizes most forms of glomerular injury and causes or contributes to all of the complications of the nephrotic syndrome. This section reviews the physiology and pathophysiology of glomerular permselectivity in clinical and experimental glomerular diseases. Extensive discussion of the mechanisms of proteinuria may also be found in several reviews,[1-6] and immunologic mechanisms are discussed in Chapter 29.

## Physiologic Basis of Permselectivity

The glomerular capillary wall is extremely permeable to water and small solutes, yet it imposes a barrier to passage of plasma proteins. This permselectivity has been characterized by examination of the extent to which the glomerular capillary wall discriminates among molecules of different size, charge, and configuration. Classically, measurement of the Bowman space/plasma concentration ratio (the sieving coefficient, $\theta$) for various proteins in the rat has been determined by direct sampling with use of micropuncture techniques.[1] These studies indicate that inulin and smaller substances appear in the glomerular filtrate and in plasma water in similar concentrations, whereas serum albumin is filtered to a lesser extent ($>0.1\%$ that of inulin).

The most extensively used method for quantitation of glomerular capillary permselectivity involves measurement of fractional clearances of test macromolecules. For a particular macromolecular test solute (m), the fractional clearance is defined as the urinary clearance of m divided by the glomerular filtration rate (GFR). With the clearance of inulin used to measure GFR, fractional clearance of m is calculated from the urine and plasma concentrations of inulin (I) and m as follows:

$$\text{Fractional clearance of m} = \frac{C_{mu}C_{Ia}}{C_{ma}C_{Iu}}$$

where C refers to solute concentration and the second subscript denotes urine (u) or afferent arteriolar (systemic) plasma (a). If, like inulin, the test macromolecule is not reabsorbed or secreted, its fractional clearance exactly equals its Bowman space/plasma concentration ratio, $\theta$.[7]

Proteins are not ideal test macromolecules for such studies because of variations in size, charge, and shape as well as in tubule reabsorption of protein. These practical difficulties may be circumvented by use of a variety of exogenous nonprotein polymers, including dextran, dextran sulfate, diethylaminoethyldextran, polyvinylpyrrolidone, Ficoll, and polyethylene glycol.[1] Much of the available permselectivity data relates to use of dextran. However, as discussed in the following, Ficoll has been evaluated and may be the better marker.[8]

## Permselectivity Based on Molecular Size

The use of neutral dextran to analyze glomerular size selectivity is illustrated in the middle curve of Figure 43–1.[9-11] Measurement of the molecular radii of discrete dextran fractions is based on their elution from gel chromatographic columns calibrated with several proteins of known

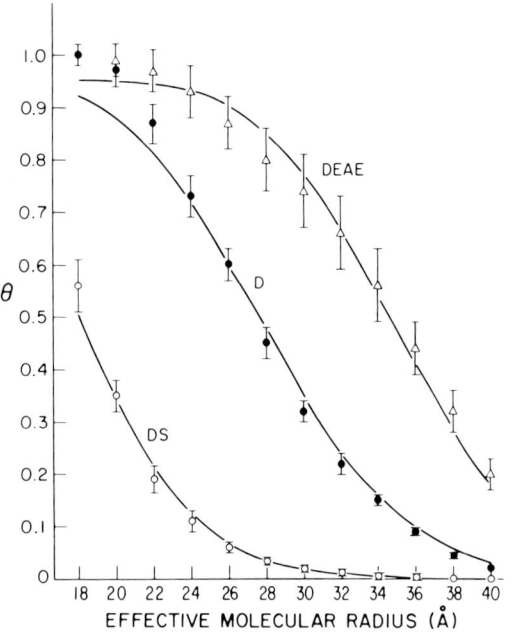

**Figure 43–1.** Filtrate/plasma concentration ratio (θ) as a function of molecular size for tritiated dextran sulfate (DS), neutral dextran (D), and diethylaminoethyldextran (DEAE). Data points are means ± SE measured in the normal Munich-Wistar rat.[9, 10] All three curves were calculated theoretically by use of the membrane parameters $K_f$ = 4.8 nL/min/mm Hg, $r_p$ = 47 Å, and $C_m$ = 165 mEq/L. (From Deen WM, Satvat B, Jamieson JM: Theoretical model for glomerular filtration of charged solutes. Am J Physiol 238:F126, 1980.)

Stokes-Einstein radius.[7] A value of 1.0 on the ordinate denotes a dextran clearance equal to that of inulin, indicating no measurable resistance to filtration of dextran. Measurable restriction to filtration of neutral dextran does not occur until the effective dextran radius exceeds about 20 Å. As dextran size increases, the fractional dextran clearance ($θ_D$) decreases progressively, approaching zero as dextran radii exceed about 40 Å.

## THEORETIC INTERPRETATION OF SIZE SELECTIVITY

**Isoporous Models.** The most useful theoretic descriptions of macromolecular transport across the glomerular capillary wall are based on the concept of hindered movement of solutes through water-filled pores, as modeled by Pappenheimer.[12] With use of such theoretic analysis, the dextran filtration data, such as those in Figure 43–1, are accurately predicted by models that envision transport as taking place through numerous, identical cylindric pores with a radius of approximately 55 Å. Solutes are regarded as solid spheres whose movements through pores occur by diffusion and convection. Fluxes are hindered both by a partitioning phenomenon (whereby the macromolecule is partially excluded by virtue of its shape, size, or charge) and by a hydrodynamic effect related to the nearby presence of the pore wall.[13] For uncharged spherical molecules, interactions between solute and membrane depend on a single parameter, λ, the ratio of solute molecule radius to

pore radius. Solute flux declines toward 0 as solute size approaches that of the pore, whereas no hindrance is attributable to the pore if the pore is relatively large.

By use of these concepts, the flux, $J_T$, of an uncharged solute (T) across the glomerular capillary wall may be expressed mathematically in terms of $C_T$, the concentration of T in the glomerular capillary plasma; $J_v$, the local glomerular transcapillary volume flux; $D_T$, the diffusivity of T in bulk solution; f, the fraction of the capillary surface area occupied by pores; l, the length of the pores; and hindrance factors that are each unique functions of l. For relatively high fluid flow rates through the pore and for large solutes that diffuse poorly, solute movement is primarily by convection. For lower fluid flow rates or small solutes that diffuse rapidly, solute movement is governed primarily by diffusion.

The rate of filtration of solute T is dependent on two independent glomerular membrane properties: $K_f$, the glomerular capillary ultrafiltration coefficient; and $r_p$, the apparent glomerular pore radius. This term is evaluated by fitting experimentally observed values of θ into the model. A complete discussion of the theories of partitioning and particle motion may be found in several reviews.[1, 14, 15]

Application of this theoretic model to the data depicted in Figure 43–1 results in calculated values of $r_p$ that are relatively independent of molecular size, averaging about 47 Å. Presumably all molecules "see" the same pores, so the finding that the "best fit" value of $r_p$ is independent of molecular size confirms that the theory successfully correlates most of the available data. Values of θ calculated with use of the theory for neutral dextran are shown by the middle curve in Figure 43–1. In this case, a pore radius of 47 Å provides an excellent fit to the data presented (mean ± 1 SEM), except for molecular radii less than about 24 Å, for which the isoporous theory appears to underestimate dextran transport.

An additional parameter that may be derived from values of $K_f$ and $r_p$ is the ratio of total pore area to pore length, fS/l, where f is the fraction of the capillary surface area (S) occupied by pores, and l represents pore length. For pores of a given radius and length, this is a measure of "pore density," the apparent number of pores per unit area of the capillary wall. Assuming that l corresponds roughly to the thickness of the glomerular basement membrane (GBM), the dextran data yield an estimate of f to be about 0.1,[16] which suggests that some 10% of the glomerular capillary surface area is perforated by pores.

**Heteroporous Models.** Theoretic calculations (based on fractional clearance of neutral dextrans) indicate that the normal glomerular capillary wall behaves approximately like an isoporous filter with a pore radius of about 50 to 55 Å.[10, 17] This approach has proved most useful in interpreting data for dextrans with effective molecular radii of approximately 20 to 45 Å. However, in some human proteinuric disorders, the available results were found to be incompatible with the isoporous theory. In these proteinuric patients, $θ_D$ was enhanced for the largest dextrans (>45 Å) but often decreased for the smallest dextrans, compared with clearances in normal subjects[18] (Fig. 43–2). These observations suggested that the selective increases in the filtration of large dextrans could be explained by the emergence of a

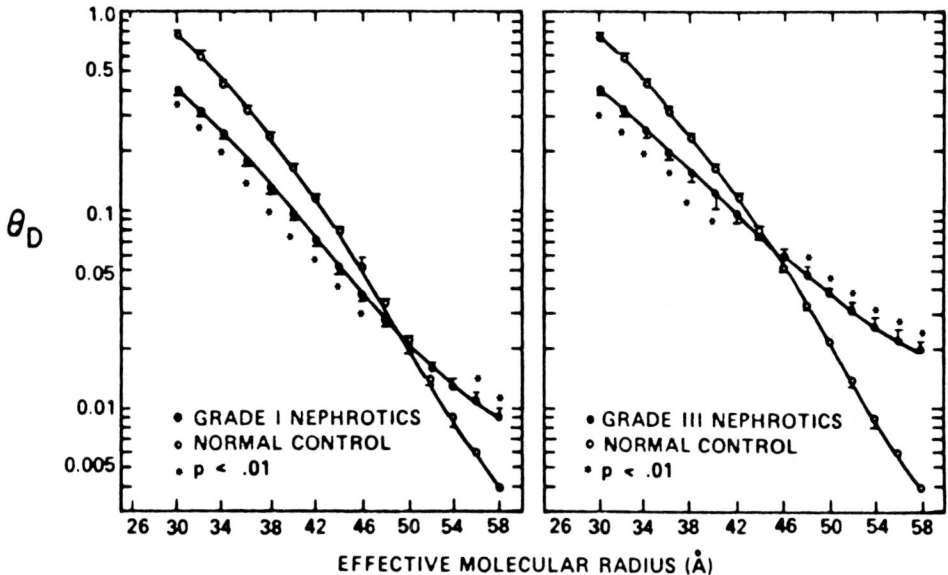

**Figure 43–2.** Fractional dextran clearances ($\theta_D$) plotted as a function of molecular radius. Grade I *(left)* and grade III *(right)* nephrotic patients are compared with normal control subjects. Values are means ± SE. (From Deen WM, Bridges CR, Brenner BM, Myers BD: Heteroporous model of glomerular size selectivity: Application to normal and nephrotic humans. Am J Physiol 249:F374, 1985.)

second population of pores, relatively few in number but of larger radius, and thus suggested the need for a heteroporous description of the functional characteristics of the capillary barrier. Accordingly, Deen and co-workers[18] formulated a heteroporous model of size selectivity designed to account for the experimental observations cited before.

The rationale for this model can be appreciated from a consideration of fractional immunoglobulin G (IgG) clearances obtained in subjects with extensive proteinuria.[18] The large size of IgG (r = 55 Å) makes it likely that its passage into Bowman space is most directly related to the extent to which the size-selective properties of the glomerular capillary wall are impaired. A study of 70 nephrotic patients showed considerable variability in IgG excretion; fractional IgG clearances were found to span three orders of magnitude, which were used to arbitrarily define three grades of increasing barrier injury.[18] Minimal IgG leakage (grade I) was associated with a low selectivity index ($C_{IgG}/C_{alb}$), indicating that the glomerular capillary wall was highly permeable to albumin but still relatively impermeable to IgG. At the opposite extreme (grade III), high rates of IgG leakage were associated with a high selectivity index approaching unity, indicating that the glomerular capillary wall did not discriminate between the smaller albumin and the larger IgG molecule.

Fractional clearances of neutral dextrans for normal subjects and for patients with various grades of injury are depicted in Figure 43–2. Similarities in the sieving curves were noted in all three grades of injury, with depressed values of $\theta_D$ for smaller and relatively impermeant dextrans and enhanced values for $\theta_D$ for larger macromolecules. However, the curves differed in the point at which the dextran sieving curve intersected that of the normal subjects, occurring earlier with increasing IgG leakage and thus appearing at r = 54 Å in grade I and at r = 46 Å in grade III. In addition, the large radius end of the sieving curve

deviated more prominently from normal with increasing grades of injury. These findings are inconsistent with the concept of the glomerular capillary wall as an isoporous filter, because no single population of pores of identical size could simultaneously account for restricted transport of smaller dextrans and enhanced transport of larger dextrans.

Rather, the data fit more closely to a model of solute transport through a heteroporous membrane, with a subpopulation of large pores. This model assumes that the major portion of the glomerular capillary wall is perforated by cylindric pores of radius $r_o$, and that a smaller portion of the capillary wall is permeated by large, nondiscriminatory "shunt" pores so large that they exhibit no size selectivity. The portion of the capillary wall permeated by shunt pores is denoted $\omega_o$, and this parameter provides a quantitative measure of the magnitude of the size selectivity defect in injured glomeruli. The fractional area of the membrane occupied by this shunt pathway, although small, increases with each successive grade of barrier injury. This subpopulation of large pores is presumed to allow passage of IgG and probably of most of the filtered albumin. Therefore, nonselective heavy proteinuria appears to result from loss of barrier size selectivity, which renders the glomerular membrane more porous to large plasma proteins.[4, 18]

**Lognormal Models.** In some cases, the isoporous plus shunt model has not accurately fit the experimental data, and better results have been obtained with use of a lognormal model, which assumes a lognormal distribution of pore radii.[8, 19] This distribution is characterized by two parameters, u and s, which correspond respectively to the mean pore radius and the spread of the distribution.[19] The model has been further refined by calculation of the theoretic fraction of filtrate volume passing through the largest pores of the pore population. Remuzzi and colleagues[19] have used this model to define an index of the size of the largest pores in the glomerular membrane. By definition, 5% of the glomerular filtrate passes through pores with radii greater than r*(5%), and 1% passes through pores with radii greater than r*(1%).

Whereas the majority of the data examining glomerular permselectivity has been obtained by use of dextran as a marker, a consistent problem has been the finding that θ for normal subjects tends to be large, given the absence of proteinuria. Thus, dextran appears to overestimate the true θ. Oliver and co-workers[8] have proposed that Ficoll, which behaves more like an ideal spherical molecule than does dextran, is a better probe of glomerular pore size. In normal rats, the θ for dextran significantly exceeded that of Ficoll at all molecular sizes, being nearly 10 times that of Ficoll for $r_s$ greater than 30 Å, and values of θ for Ficoll approximated previously reported values for uncharged glomerular proteins. For Ficoll, a lognormal plus shunt pathway model was found to be the most effective[8] (Fig. 43–3).

## Permselectivity Based on Molecular Charge

The charge-selective characteristics of the glomerular capillary wall can be evaluated by use of negatively charged markers, such as dextran sulfate. In the normal kidney, the fractional dextran sulfate clearance ($\theta_{DS}$) is lower than that for neutral dextran at any given molecular radius[7, 11] (see Fig. 43–1). Conversely, positively charged molecules pass through more freely, as was shown with use of diethylaminoethyldextran, a cationic form.[10] Fractional clearances of diethylaminoethyldextran are significantly enhanced relative to neutral dextran for a wide range of molecular radii (see Fig. 43–1).

The importance of molecular charge is further demonstrated in proteinuric glomerular diseases. In a model of nephrotoxic serum nephritis, Chang and co-workers[7, 10, 20–23] noted that $\theta_D$ for neutral dextran was less than that seen in normal rats (Fig. 43–4), and thus these molecules could not account for the observed proteinuria; if albumin behaved like neutral dextran, albumin excretion would be predicted to decrease rather than increase. Similarly, fractional clearances of cationic diethylaminoethyldextran were reduced and therefore could not explain the proteinuria. However, for any molecular size, $\theta_{DS}$ in rats with nephrotoxic serum nephritis was substantially greater than that observed in normal animals.[23] These observations suggested that albuminuria in this disorder was a specific consequence of the reduction in fixed negative charge of the diseased capillary wall.

## THEORETIC INTERPRETATION OF CHARGE SELECTIVITY

Analysis of electrical charge has been incorporated into the expression for solute flux by assuming that the glomerular capillary wall may be represented as a barrier containing a uniform concentration, $C_m$, of fixed negative charges.[11] The fixed charges cause the intramembrane electrical potential to be negative with respect to that in the capillary lumen or Bowman space. Partitioning of charged solutes between the membrane and external solutions is influenced both by molecular size and by these potential differences, the negative intramembrane potential tending to exclude anions and enhance cation entry. This effect is enhanced as the molecular charge increases.

This model predicts that for charged macromolecules, solute flux will be strongly dependent on $C_m$, because $C_m$ is the primary determinant of the negative intramembrane potential. With values of $K_f$ and $r_p$ determined from GFRs of water and neutral macromolecules, values of $C_m$ may be estimated from measured values of θ for charged macro-

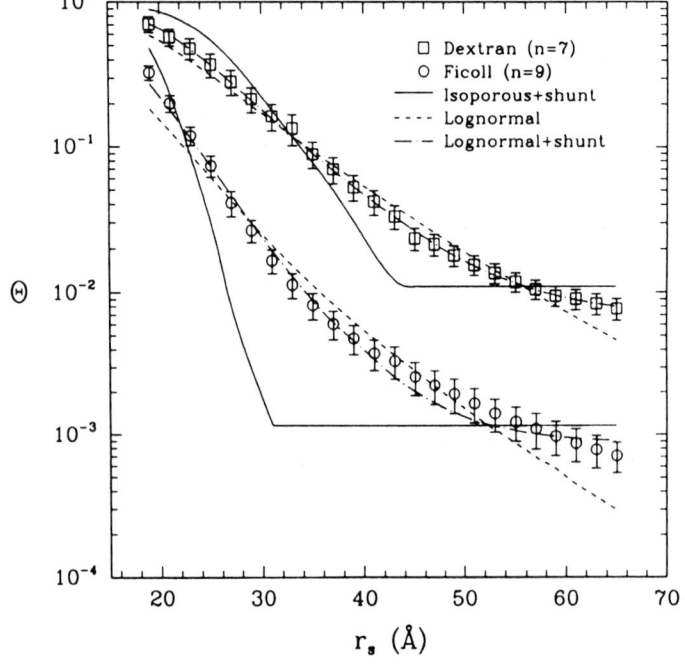

**Figure 43–3.** Sieving coefficient (θ) of dextran and Ficoll as a function of molecular radius ($r_s$) in normal rats. Experimental values are means ± SE; curves represent the best fits to the data obtained with the three types of pore size distributions. (From Oliver JD III, Anderson S, Troy JL, et al: Determination of glomerular size-selectivity in the normal rat with Ficoll. J Am Soc Nephrol 3[2]:214–228, 1992.)

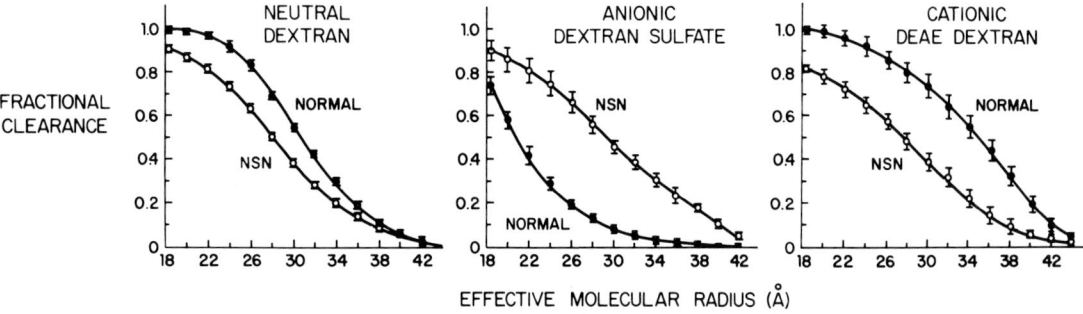

**Figure 43–4.** Fractional clearances of neutral dextran *(left)*, anionic dextran sulfate *(middle)*, and cationic diethylaminoethyldextran *(right)* plotted as functions of effective molecular radii for normal rats and those with nephrotoxic serum nephritis (NSN). Data from references 9, 12, 25, 27, and 28. (From Brenner BM, Hostetter TH, Humes HD: Molecular basis of proteinuria of glomerular origin. N Engl J Med 298:826, 1978.)

molecules. The glomerular barrier is thus fully characterized by the membrane properties $K_f$, $r_p$, and $C_m$.

## Permselectivity Based on Molecular Configuration

To compare sieving results for macromolecules of different conformations (i.e., a relatively linear coil for dextran) with those for lobular proteins, the potential effects of molecular shape or configuration must be taken into account. The effect of molecular configuration in the rat was studied by Bohrer and associates[24] by comparison of fractional clearances of neutral dextran with those of Ficoll, an uncharged cross-linked copolymer of sucrose and epichlorohydrin. At any given effective radius, the flexible coil dextran was filtered more readily than was Ficoll, a nearly rigid sphere; the superior accuracy of Ficoll was subsequently confirmed, as described before.[8] These studies suggest that protein configuration also plays a role in filtration, although size and charge appear to be more important.[1]

## The Anatomic and Functional Barrier to Filtration of Macromolecules

The extensive body of work aimed at determining the anatomic barrier to filtration of macromolecules, as well as the changes that result in pathologic proteinuria, has been reviewed by Kanwar and co-workers.[2, 3] Early studies by Farquhar and colleagues[25] using native ferritin to probe the filtration barrier found that intravenous ferritin was restricted at the endothelial fenestrae and lamina rara interna of the GBM; it was concluded that the GBM was the component of the filtration barrier that restricts the passage of macromolecules. Subsequent studies were consistent with this "single-barrier" hypothesis,[2] until examination of the behavior of peroxidative tracers suggested otherwise. Horseradish peroxidase was found to readily cross the filtration barrier,[26] whereas lactoperoxidase and myeloperoxidase were localized under the slit diaphragms,[26, 27] which suggests that the slit diaphragms are an effective barrier to filtration. Later studies indicated that catalase displayed a decreasing gradient across the GBM with minimal concen-

tration under the slit diaphragm,[28] leading to the "double-barrier" hypothesis that the GBM restricts passage of larger macromolecules, whereas slit diaphragms regulate the passage of smaller macromolecules. However, this hypothesis also failed to explain the observations that some relatively large tracers were restricted just beneath the slit diaphragms, whereas some were completely restricted at the level of the inner layers of the GBM, and accordingly the potential contribution of molecular charge needed to be addressed. This question was partially resolved in studies of Caulfield and Farquhar,[29] who infused neutral dextrans into normal rats and found urinary concentration to decrease with increasing molecular size; none of the dextrans was found under the slit diaphragm, further supporting the single-barrier hypothesis and implicating the GBM as the important barrier.[29, 30] To further examine this question, Rennke and co-workers[31] used several ferritin fractions of similar size with varying isoelectric points (pI) ranging from 4.5 to 11.5. Infusion studies indicated that a stepwise increase in the pI of ferritin resulted in a proportionate increase in the molecule's permeation into the GBM, with the more negatively charged particles penetrating the farthest. Thus, these studies pointed to the existence of an intrinsic electrical charge in the GBM, imparted by fixed anionic sites.[31]

The existence of these anionic sites has been confirmed by histochemical studies; the sites are found on the surfaces of endothelial and epithelial cells as well as in the GBM interposed between these cells.[2, 32, 33] The glomerular epithelial cell and its foot processes are covered with a surface coat of acidic glycoproteins (sialoproteins or glomerular polyanion), which are highly negatively charged. Stainable polyanion has been identified to be podocalyxin, a sialoprotein that carries most of the glomerular sialic acid.[34] The epithelial slit diaphragm also consists, in part, of glycosialoproteins,[35, 36] as does the endothelial cell coat.

The biochemical composition of the GBM has been extensively studied in recent years.[2–6] The GBM consists of two classes of glycopeptides: a nonpolar collagen-like component, and another more polar noncollagen fraction of asparagine-linked polysaccharide units. Glomerular epithelial cells indicate that these cells are capable of synthesizing all major GBM components. Integral components of the GBM include type IV collagens and various proteoglycans, including chondroitin sulfate proteoglycan and heparan sulfate proteoglycan (HSPG). HSPG has proved particularly important in imparting charge selectivity to the GBM.[2, 3, 5, 37] HSPGs are distributed throughout the GBM but concentrated in the lamina rara interna and externa.[38] The importance of these anionic polymers in retarding passage of negatively charged molecules is demonstrated when the anionic charge of HSPG is neutralized. Infusion of polycations[39–41] or enzymatic degradation of heparan sulfate with heparinase or heparitinase[42, 43] results in increased urinary excretion of albumin and IgG as well as enhanced permeation of native (anionic) ferritin into the substance of the GBM. Further experiments demonstrated that when the electrical charge of the GBM was rendered neutral, anionic proteins were adsorbed onto the GBM, thus reducing the flow of water and solute across the glomerular capillary.[44] Normally, the polyanions (particularly HSPG) act as "anticlogging" agents, which prevents the adsorption of plasma protein so that ultrafiltration may proceed.[2, 3, 44, 45]

Many studies have confirmed the importance of anionic sites, as well as of heparan sulfate specifically, in the defense against proteinuria. The number of anionic sites is reduced in patients with congenital nephrotic syndrome[46] as well as in some experimental models of proteinuria[29] and after acute infusion of protamine sulfate.[47] Proteinuric states are characterized by abnormalities in the synthesis, composition, and charge density as well as in the total number of stainable anionic sites. In some models, the content of HSPG is reduced.[48, 49] In others, although the total number of anionic sites[50, 51] and HSPG content[52–54] may be normal, the incorporation of sulfate into heparan sulfate[54] as well as the biochemical structure and charge density[52, 54] may be abnormal and thereby contribute to proteinuria.

## NEW IN VITRO MODELS FOR PERMEABILITY STUDIES

Macromolecular tracer studies as described in the preceding are often unable to differentiate the effects of hemodynamic and hormonal influences from those properties intrinsic to glomerular filtration. Innovative models have been developed to assess glomerular permeability in vitro. Daniels and colleagues[55, 56] have examined diffusion of fluorescent macromolecules across individual glomerular capillaries in intact glomeruli using confocal microscopy; the relative contribution of glomerular cells may be assessed by comparison of intact glomeruli with acellular glomeruli, in which cells have been removed, leaving GBM with some residual mesangial matrix. When placed in a filtration cell, these intact and acellular glomeruli can also be used to assess dextran sieving. Using these techniques, these investigators found that $\theta_D$ in intact glomeruli is much less than that for GBM alone, which suggests that most of the size selectivity of the glomerular barrier resides in the cells rather than in the GBM and that this effect is particularly prominent at larger molecular sizes. Savin and co-workers[57] have also demonstrated the utility of isolated glomeruli for assessment of albumin permeability under various experimental conditions.

## Influence of Hemodynamic Factors on Filtration of Macromolecules

Hemodynamic factors influence the filtration of macromolecules. In many cases, $\theta$ varies inversely with the single-nephron GFR (SNGFR).[1, 58] Thus, filtration of macromolecules is influenced not only by the intrinsic membrane properties of the glomerular capillary wall ($r_p$, $C_m$, and $K_f$) but also by the other determinants of SNGFR: $Q_A$, the glomerular capillary plasma flow rate; $\Delta P$, the glomerular transcapillary hydraulic pressure difference; and $C_A$, the afferent arteriolar plasma protein concentration.

The absolute single-nephron clearance of a macromolecule is given by the product $\theta \times$ SNGFR.[11, 15] Absolute clearance usually increases as $Q_A$ is elevated, but less than in proportion to SNGFR; hence, $\theta$ decreases. The effect of $Q_A$ may be explained by considering that at a high flow rate, a given amount of filtrate produces a smaller increase in the capillary plasma concentration of the test solute, making the increased filtration of neutral molecules somewhat less than that of water and thereby decreasing $\theta$. Absolute macromolecular clearance rates also increase as $\Delta P$ rises. For neutral and anionic macromolecules, this increase is less than the increase in SNGFR, and thus $\theta$ decreases. For highly anionic molecules, at sufficiently high $\Delta P$, this trend reverses, and $\theta$ may increase. The opposite behavior is observed for positively charged macromolecules, with $\theta$ increasing with $\Delta P$. The theoretic effects of $C_A$ on $\theta$ are similar to those for inverse changes in $\Delta P$, because $C_A$ and $\Delta P$ exert opposing effects on SNGFR. The actual effects of changes in $C_A$ are likely to be more complicated because of parallel changes in $K_f$.[59] Hemodynamic factors may also influence the rate of volume flux through the shunt pathway (see later).

## Evaluation of the Filtration Barrier in Glomerular Disease

### ANIMAL MODELS OF GLOMERULAR DISEASE

Tracer macromolecules have been used extensively to characterize the glomerular permeability defects that result in proteinuria, as well as the permeability response to therapeutic interventions, in a number of experimental glomerular diseases characterized by proteinuria. Not surprisingly, all proteinuric models exhibit impaired glomerular size selectivity, with passage of large molecules through the glomerular barrier. This defect has been noted in diverse animal models, including renal ablation,[60–62] diabetes,[63, 64] puromycin nephrosis,[65, 66] doxorubicin (Adriamycin) nephrosis,[19, 67, 68] nephrotoxic serum nephritis,[23, 69–72] Heymann nephritis,[73] renal vein constriction,[74] normal aging,[75] protein overload,[76] the fawn-hooded rat,[77] and the MWF/Ztm rat model.[78] In some models, a charge-selective defect has been documented as well. As one example, extensive reduction in renal mass leads to systemic hypertension and progressive proteinuria together with elevated SNGFR, $Q_A$, and $\Delta P$ and reduced $K_f$.[60–62] Permselectivity studies indicate that proteinuria results from defects in both size and charge selectivity,[60–62] with increased flux through the shunt pathway.[62] Peak pore size (u) is decreased, whereas the width of the pore size distribution (s) is increased; both r*(5%) and r*(1%) increase as well.[62] Another prominent example is diabetic nephropathy, a model with similar hemodynamic changes (see also Chapter 39). Studies using Ficoll in diabetic rats found impaired size selectivity at all molecular sizes tested (Fig. 43–5); in addition, the pore size distribution was shifted toward larger sizes, as reflected by increases in u, $\omega_o$, and r*(1%).[64] Multiple factors play a role in this process. Nonenzymatically glycosylated ferritin is transported through the GBM more readily than is nonglycosylated ferritin; the glycosylated form is more anionic than is the nonglycosylated form, which suggests that plasma protein abnormalities in diabetes may alter glomerular permeability characteristics independent of changes in the GBM.[79, 80] The biochemistry of the GBM is also altered in diabetes, with impaired HSPG synthesis, reduced GBM HSPG content, and decreased HSPG anionic sites.[81]

Another model is administration of puromycin aminonucleoside into rats, which induces massive proteinuria in association with predominant epithelial cell injury. Ultrastructural studies indicate focal permeability to tracer macromolecules, particularly in areas of epithelial detachment from the GBM,[28, 82] with altered distribution of anionic sites and sulfation of heparan sulfate.[50–53] In a puromycin aminonucleoside regimen that results in diminution of $K_f$ with relative preservation of $\Delta P$, $Q_A$, and $K_f$, the $\theta_D$ for neutral dextrans 38 Å and smaller is decreased, whereas $\theta_{DS}$ is enhanced. Because hemodynamics are normal in this model, these data suggested a functional loss of the electrostatic barrier.[65] The $\theta_D$ of neutral dextrans larger than 38 Å is also increased, which suggests that a size-selective defect

also contributes to the increased permeability in this model.[66] In another proteinuric model, injection of neutral dextrans into rats with doxorubicin nephrosis results in increased clearances of molecules larger than 40 Å.[19, 68] The lognormal model indicates increases in u and s as well as in r*(1%) and r*(5%).[19] The role of a charge-selective defect is controversial.[19, 67, 68]

Another model used to investigate glomerular permselectivity is nephrotoxic serum nephritis, which is characterized by decreased $\theta_D$ for neutral dextrans smaller than 40 Å[22] and enhanced clearances of anionic dextrans.[28] Inducing hypertension in this model with saline in the drinking water results in substantial elevations in $\Delta P$.[71] Superimposition of hypertension is also associated with increased $\theta_D$, particularly for those molecules larger than 40 Å.[72] Acutely reducing renal perfusion pressure, as well as renal plasma flow and $\Delta P$, returned the sieving curve toward normal, with enhanced clearance found only with molecules larger than 55 Å. The calculated fraction of glomerular filtrate traversing the nondiscriminatory shunt pathway was elevated during the hypertensive period and reduced toward normal at lower perfusion pressures. These observations suggested that hemodynamic factors play an important role in the pathogenesis of the size-selective defect in this model.[72]

## EFFECTS OF HEMODYNAMIC PERTURBATIONS ON GLOMERULAR PERMSELECTIVITY

The influence of hemodynamic perturbations on glomerular permselectivity has been extensively examined in both normal and diseased animal models. Acute hypertension induced by angiotensin II (AII) enhances protein filtration,[9]

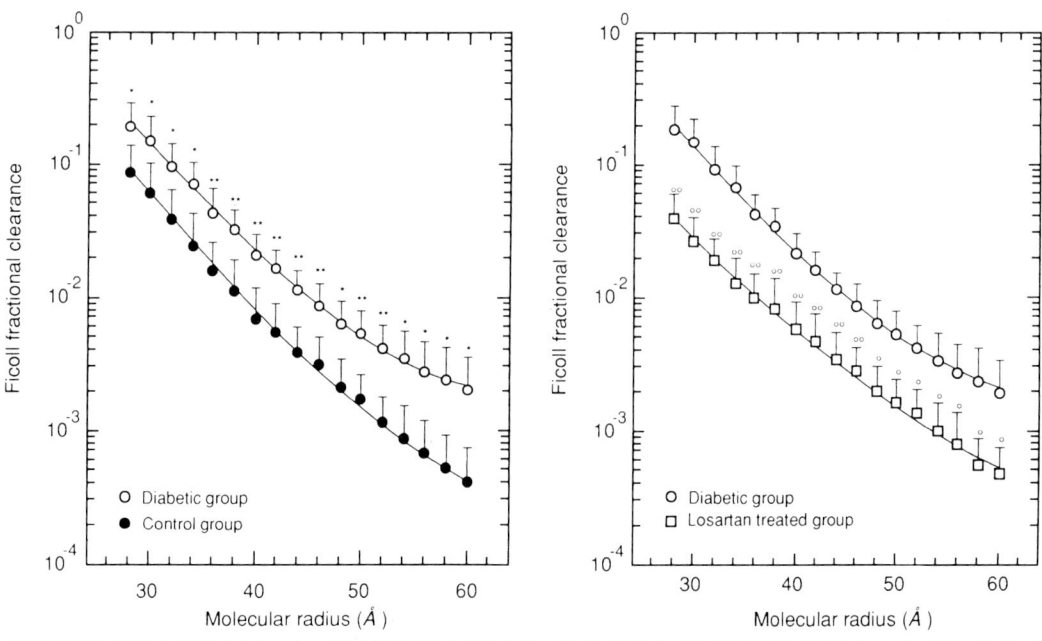

**Figure 43–5.** Fractional clearance of Ficoll as a function of molecular radius (Å) in diabetic and nondiabetic control rats *(left)* and in diabetic rats and diabetic rats treated with losartan *(right)*. Values are means ± SE. *$P < .05$, **$P < .01$ versus control subjects; °$P < .05$, °°$P < .01$ versus diabetic group. (From Remuzzi A, Perico N, Amuchastegui CS, et al: Short- and long-term effect of angiotensin II receptor blockade in rats with experimental diabetes. J Am Soc Nephrol 4[1]:40–49, 1993.)

and the role of AII in chronic proteinuria has been characterized in the model of partial renal vein constriction by Yoshioka and co-workers.[74] This perturbation was associated with a marked decrease in $Q_A$ with a proportionally lesser decrease in SNGFR and an increase in $\Delta P$. These hemodynamic changes were associated with an increase in $\theta_D$ for dextrans larger than 44 Å, with no discernible changes in the clearances of dextrans smaller than 42 Å. Infusion of the AII receptor antagonist saralasin led to normalization of the glomerular hemodynamic profile. Fractional clearances of dextrans larger than 46 Å fell toward normal with saralasin; clearances of dextrans smaller than 40 Å were unaffected. The radius of the small selective pores and the index for fractional volume flux through these pores were relatively unaffected by either renal vein constriction or saralasin. However, renal vein constriction induced a 10-fold increase in the fraction of filtrate passing through larger, nonselective pores. About half of this increase was reversed with saralasin. Thus, these observations suggested that AII may enhance proteinuria by inducing reversible changes in the sieving properties of the glomerular capillary wall, specifically by increasing flow through the shunt pathway, and that these changes might relate to perturbations of $\Delta P$.[74] The action of AII is somewhat variable, however. Clinical studies have not found such an effect with AII in nephrotic subjects. AII did increase fractional neutral dextran clearances in normal subjects, but the effect could be attributed solely to hemodynamic factors.[83] Studies of AII antagonism are discussed later.

The role of $\Delta P$ in mediating proteinuria was subsequently examined by these investigators in rats with Heymann nephritis.[73] Induction of Heymann nephritis resulted in a significant increase in $\Delta P$ and a significantly enhanced $\theta_D$ of dextrans larger than 50 Å. Short-term administration of AII further increased both $\Delta P$ and $\theta_D$ for dextrans larger than 26 Å. Conversely, administration of acetylcholine resulted in a reduction in $\Delta P$ together with a shift in the $\theta_D$ of larger dextrans toward the normal range. Values for $r_o$ were similar in all groups, whereas marked changes in the shunt pathway occurred in parallel with the changes in $\Delta P$. These observations suggested that changes in $\Delta P$ play an important role in glomerular permselectivity, with increased $\Delta P$ recruiting previously unexposed pores of the nonselective shunt pathway.[73]

## HUMAN GLOMERULAR DISEASE

**Protein Clearances and Selectivity Index.** Proteinuria in the nephrotic range is associated with passage of large plasma proteins into the urine. The permselective characteristics of such diseased glomeruli have been determined by measurement of urinary clearances of proteins of graded size.[84] The smallest proteins, usually albumin (36 Å) or transferrin (38 Å), have been used as reference markers. When the clearance ratio of larger test proteins to that of the reference protein is plotted as a function of the molecular mass, an inverse relationship is observed; this suggests that the diseased glomerulus continues to discriminate among proteins of increasing size, but that the pore size distribution is shifted to pores of larger size. Thus, two categories of clinical proteinuria have been designated "se-

lective" and "nonselective." Selective proteinuria is characterized by a relatively sharp molecular size cutoff; proteinuria consists primarily of relatively small albumin molecules. Nonselective proteinuria contains a large proportion of larger plasma proteins, particularly IgG. When the selectivity index (the clearance ratio of a large protein such as IgG to that of a smaller protein such as albumin) is less than 0.2, proteinuria is considered to be selective; values greater than 0.2 indicate nonselective proteinuria.

This method, although relatively simple, has some theoretic limitations. The test proteins used have different isoelectric points in physiologic solution, and this technique is unable to take into account changes in glomerular charge selectivity. Similarly, this technique cannot account for changes in tubule reabsorption of proteins, protein catabolic capacity, or a potential selective increase in the glomerular filtration of one or more proteins.

**Studies of Glomerular Barrier Function in Clinical Glomerular Disease.** In view of these limitations, dextran clearance techniques have been used to more accurately characterize clinical alterations in glomerular permselectivity. The defective permselectivity in patients with various forms of proliferative glomerulonephritis was examined by use of fractional dextran and IgG clearances.[85] The $\theta_D$ values of smaller dextrans were similar regardless of the magnitude of IgG excretion, whereas those of larger dextrans were elevated in patients excreting larger amounts of IgG. These data could not be explained on the basis of a single population of pores, but they could be explained by the existence of a second population of larger pores (i.e., the shunt pathway). This model predicted that passage of macromolecules such as IgG may be totally unrestricted in this damaged segment; and in fact, the filtered load of IgG was of sufficient magnitude to account for the urinary IgG content. Thus, it was conceivable that the passage of IgG was entirely through the larger pores, whereas that of the smaller albumin molecule was more likely due to a charge-selective defect in the small pore component of the glomerular capillary wall. The estimated radius of small pores was similar in the two groups; the radius of larger pores was increased in those patients with greater urinary loss of IgG.[85] These observations suggested that when glomerulonephritis is associated with selective proteinuria, the major abnormality is in the charge-selective barrier to smaller proteins; in glomerulonephritis associated with nonselective proteinuria and massive IgG loss, the glomerular membrane exhibits a subpopulation of enlarged pores that are highly permeable toward proteins of large size and variable charge.

Subsequent studies have indicated that in a variety of human clinical diseases, the permselectivity defect consists of a combination of impaired size selectivity, impaired charge selectivity, and an increase in volume through the shunt pathway. This pattern has been documented or strongly suggested in patients with minimal change disease,[17, 86–88] membranous nephropathy,[88–90] and diabetic nephropathy.[91–97] In proliferative lupus nephritis, there appears to be loss of size selectivity and increased traffic through the shunt pathway, although lesser evidence of a charge-selective defect.[98–100]

In diabetes, the dextran clearance profile has been examined in the context of the various stages of clinical diabetic nephropathy.[91] In patients with microalbuminuria (<300 mg/d), studies with IgG[92, 93] and with neutral dextrans[94] both confirm the presence of a size-selective defect. The dextran studies indicate increased filtration of dextrans smaller than 48 Å and enhanced filtration of larger dextrans, with increased filtrate volume through the shunt pathway.[94] Studies in overt nephropathy (persistent proteinuria) indicate qualitatively similar changes, but enhanced in magnitude.[92, 94–96] Although it is not yet directly confirmed, the available evidence is also most consistent with the presence of a concomitant charge-selective defect. Indeed, a study of both size and charge in patients with various stages of diabetes suggests that the charge defect may even precede the size defect.[97] In diabetic patients, glycosylation of proteins may contribute to the abnormality, because glycosylated proteins including albumin appear in the urine more readily than do nonglycosylated forms,[79] and nonenzymatic glycation of albumin increases its permeability through GBM in vitro.[80] Analytic electrofocusing of glycosylated albumin indicates the appearance of bands of pI above and below those observed for nonglycosylated albumin, with only the lower pI isoforms appearing in the urine,[101] which suggests diminished restriction of anionic albumin isoforms as a primary defect in diabetic proteinuria. Similarly, the fractional clearance of immunoreactive anionic IgG4 is enhanced relative to that of total IgG.[93] In addition, it is conceivable that configurational changes contribute to diabetic proteinuria, or the density of sites that attract polyanions may be increased in diabetic patients.[102] The current data suggest that the primary abnormality in diabetes is a loss of size selectivity but that charge and perhaps shape selectivity defects also contribute.[91, 95]

## INTERVENTIONS OR MODULATION OF PERMSELECTIVITY IN GLOMERULAR DISEASES

A variety of pathophysiologic and therapeutic interventions, known to influence proteinuria, have been studied by permselectivity techniques to ascertain potential effects on determinants of proteinuria. Most of the studies have assessed size, but not charge, permselectivity. Interventions such as plasma volume expansion,[7, 103, 104] dietary protein restriction,[19, 60, 105] and use of acetylcholine,[73] verapamil,[61] and indomethacin[70, 106] have been found to restore neutral dextran sieving curves toward normal (i.e., to restore normal glomerular size selectivity). Of note, whereas some antihypertensive regimens tend to reverse size-selective defects, others do not; for example, limited evidence suggests absence of such a beneficial effect with prazosin[107] or clonidine.[93] Moreover, interventions that restore size selectivity do not do so in a uniform manner. Although many interventions reduce permeability only for larger dextrans, drugs that block AII formation (angiotensin-converting enzyme inhibitors and the AII receptor antagonist losartan) appear in some cases to reduce clearances of neutral dextrans of all sizes[64, 78, 108] (as shown in Fig. 43–5). In other cases, however, the same interventions reduced clearances of only the largest molecules.[62, 109, 110] Further studies are needed to clarify these interesting but conflicting findings.

## CLINICAL CONSEQUENCES OF PROTEINURIA

Loss of albumin and other plasma proteins into the urine is the hallmark of the nephrotic syndrome and a proximate or contributing cause to virtually all of the systemic complications of this disorder. As depicted in Figure 43–6, increased filtration of plasma proteins contributes to hypoalbuminemia and its complications; to hyperlipoproteinemia; to alterations in coagulation factors; and to alterations in cellular immunity, hormonal status, and mineral and electrolyte metabolism.

### Hypoalbuminemia

#### PATHOGENESIS OF HYPOALBUMINEMIA

The hypoalbuminemia that characterizes the nephrotic syndrome results from multiple abnormalities of albumin homeostasis and is only partially explained by urinary albumin loss.[4, 111–113] Normal albumin metabolism is schematized in Figure 43–7A. The liver normally synthesizes 12 to 14 g/d of albumin, 90% of which is catabolized in extrarenal sites, primarily the vascular endothelium.[114–116] About 10% of the albumin synthesized daily is catabolized in the kidney, probably by proximal tubule reabsorption of filtered albumin.[117] Normally, about 150 g of albumin (or 30% to 50% of the total exchangeable pool) is located intravascularly, with the remainder being in the interstitial fluid.[116, 118] The fractional catabolic rate, or percentage of the plasma pool that is catabolized, is about 6% to 10%.[114, 119, 120] Thus, abnormalities predisposing to nephrotic hypoalbuminemia could include extracorporeal losses (primarily urinary), decreased or insufficiently increased hepatic albumin synthesis, increased albumin catabolism, and altered albumin distribution.[4, 111–113]

**Extracorporeal Losses.** The magnitude of hypoalbuminemia tends to increase with increasing proteinuria, but significant hypoalbuminemia may occur in the presence of urinary loss of only a few grams of albumin per day.[121] Extracorporeal losses alone should not necessarily lead to hypoalbuminemia, because the liver possesses ample ability to augment albumin synthesis and thus compensate for such losses, as occurs in patients on continuous ambulatory peritoneal dialysis.[115] Evidence for enhanced intestinal albumin loss, or increased albumin catabolism, in the nephrotic syndrome is inconsistent and therefore not compelling.[122–125] Little is known of the consequences of the nephrotic syndrome on other potential sites of albumin catabolism. As discussed later, renal albumin catabolism is increased in the nephrotic syndrome, thereby contributing to the greater tendency to hypoalbuminemia in the nephrotic syndrome than in peritoneal dialysis.

**Hepatic Albumin Synthesis.** Hepatic albumin synthesis is not impaired in the nephrotic syndrome; studies of nephrotic patients indicate that hepatic albumin synthesis is in fact increased.[126–128] In nephrotic rats, hepatic release of both albumin and total secretory protein is enhanced,[129] and there is a marked increase in the rate of albumin synthesis

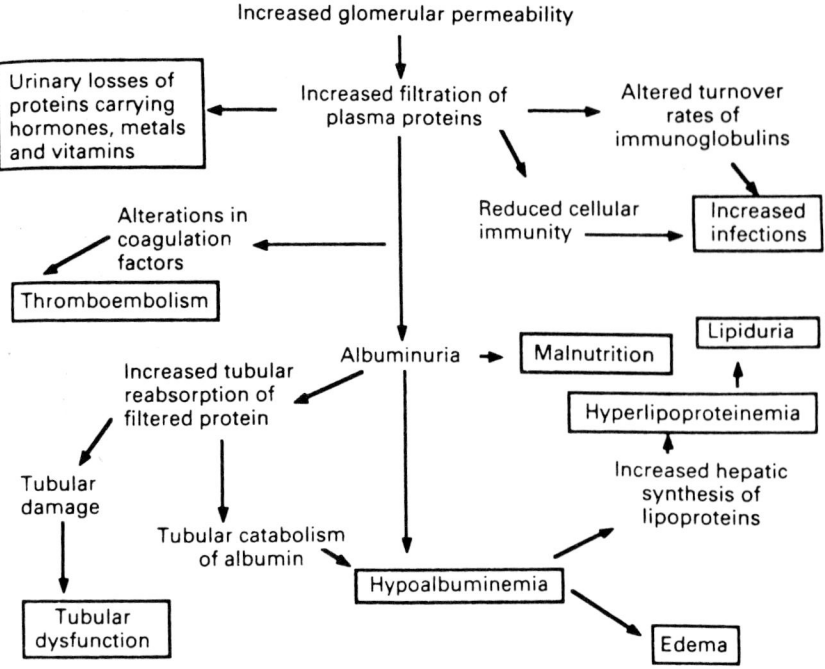

**Figure 43–6.** Pathophysiology of nephrotic syndrome. All abnormalities originate from increased glomerular permeability to plasma proteins; hypoalbuminemia initiates the major manifestations. (From Bernard DB: Extrarenal complications of the nephrotic syndrome. Kidney Int 33:1184, 1988.)

relative to total hepatic protein synthesis accompanied by a relative increase of the same magnitude in albumin messenger RNA (mRNA). The relative amounts of several other mRNAs are increased, including those encoding for β-fibrinogen, haptoglobin, and metallothionein II, whereas the amount of mRNA encoding for $\alpha_1$-acid glycoprotein is decreased.[130, 131] Oncotic pressure may play a role in regulation of hepatic albumin synthesis, because albumin gene expression varies inversely with oncotic pressure in experimental models.[132] That a transcriptional process is mainly responsible for the increased albumin mRNA level is suggested in studies of nephrotic rats indicating that in the presence of hypoalbuminemia and massive proteinuria, both the level of albumin mRNA and the transcription rate of the albumin gene in the liver are higher than in livers

from normal rats. Significant correlations were found between the transcription rate of the albumin gene and the ratio of albumin mRNA to mRNA levels of noninducible control rats.[133, 134]

However, the increase in hepatic albumin synthesis is not maximal in the nephrotic state and is inadequate for the degree of hypoalbuminemia; thus, the albumin synthetic response rate is relatively impaired.

**Albumin Catabolism.** In certain hypoalbuminemic states, both absolute and fractional rates of albumin catabolism are reduced.[135] In contrast to those conditions, the possibility that nephrotic hypoalbuminemia might be exacerbated by a maladaptive *increase* in albumin catabolism was suggested by Katz and co-workers,[136, 137] who reasoned that the massive urinary albumin load might lead to exces-

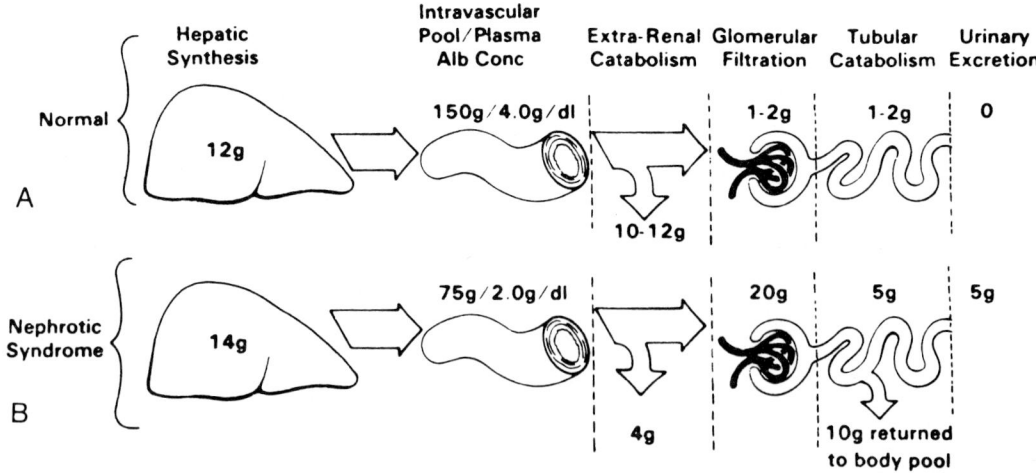

**Figure 43–7.** Daily albumin turnover in normal individuals and in patients with nephrotic syndrome. (*A* and *B* from Bernard DB: Metabolic complications in nephrotic syndrome: Pathophysiology and complications. *In* Brenner BM, Stein JH [eds]: The Nephrotic Syndrome. Churchill Livingstone, New York, 1982, p 85.)

sive tubule albumin catabolism. Accordingly, most of the filtered albumin would be catabolized, and urinary albumin would thus represent only a small fraction of the filtered load. Certain observations are consistent with an increase in the fractional albumin catabolic rate. In rats with nephrotoxic serum nephritis, tubule albumin reabsorptive rates increase, although variably.[138] Nephrotic rats exhibit protein reabsorption droplets containing both albumin and globulin in proximal and distal tubule cells,[139] and lysosomal activity (cathepsins B and L) in tubule cells increases in response to an increased urinary protein load.[140] Additional support for an increase in catabolic capacity comes from the demonstration of a dual transport system for albumin uptake in the isolated perfused proximal tubule of the rabbit. There exist both a low-capacity system, which saturates once the protein load exceeds physiologic levels, and a high-capacity, low-affinity system, which permits tubule albumin reabsorptive rates to rise as the filtered load increases.[141] Thus, an increase in the fractional catabolic rate may occur in the nephrotic syndrome.

Micropuncture studies indicate that albumin reabsorption may in fact be saturated at near-physiologic levels so that most of the urinary albumin is excreted rather than catabolized,[138, 142, 143] so urinary albumin excretion does not markedly underestimate overall albumin loss. Whether fractional catabolism is normal or increased, total body albumin stores are markedly decreased in the nephrotic syndrome. The net result is that absolute catabolic rates are normal or decreased.[126, 136, 144, 145] As discussed later, nutritional considerations affect this process markedly. In nephrotic rats, absolute catabolic rates are decreased in animals fed adequate dietary protein but increased in animals receiving a low-protein diet.[145] Whereas decreased catabolism may serve to preserve total albumin stores in the face of massive urinary losses, it is obviously insufficient to maintain albumin homeostasis.

**Albumin Distribution.** In the nephrotic syndrome, the extravascular albumin pool is even more depleted than is the intravascular pool,[144, 146] mechanisms of which are detailed in the following. However, although this mobilization of extravascular albumin represents an early response to acute albumin loss, this compensatory mechanism is clearly inadequate in the face of continuing albumin loss.

## REGULATION OF ALBUMIN METABOLISM IN THE NEPHROTIC SYNDROME

Several factors are known to contribute to regulation of albumin metabolism and may contribute to the abnormalities seen in the nephrotic syndrome.[113, 147] The most important factors regulating albumin synthesis are the serum oncotic pressure and nutritional status (particularly dietary protein intake).

Whereas albumin synthesis in the isolated perfused liver preparation is inversely proportional to the oncotic pressure of the bathing solution,[148] albumin synthetic rates do not correspond to either serum albumin concentration or oncotic pressure in nephrotic patients.[127, 136] It has been postulated that the hepatic albumin synthetic rate is more directly determined by changes in a hepatic extravascular interstitial albumin pool than by plasma characteristics and that this hepatic interstitial pool is not depleted in the nephrotic syndrome, and so albumin synthesis is not stimulated.[148, 149]

Dietary factors also play a role. The potential interaction between plasma oncotic pressure and nutritional status has been suggested by the work of Kaysen and associates,[134] who found that albumin synthesis and serum albumin were not correlated in nephrotic rats fed a low-protein diet, but in the presence of a high protein intake, albumin synthetic rates varied inversely with serum albumin concentration. Increasing dietary protein intake in nephrotic rats results in increased hepatic albumin mRNA content as well as increased transcription of albumin message, whereas dietary protein intake limits hepatic albumin synthesis.[134, 150] Although less well studied, hepatic albumin synthesis may also respond to changes in dietary fat intake[151] as well as to the relative proportion of protein to nonprotein calories.

These observations suggest that in the nephrotic syndrome, the optimal diet would include an adequate calorie intake with a moderate to high amount of protein. However, increasing dietary protein intake has not been successful in augmenting serum albumin concentration or body albumin pools in nephrotic animals[145, 152] or patients.[127] As depicted in Figure 43–8, feeding a high-protein diet markedly stimulates hepatic albumin synthesis in nephrotic rats.[134, 145] As is also demonstrated in Figure 43–8, this beneficial effect does not ameliorate the abnormal albumin homeostasis because dietary protein supplementation also increases urinary protein loss. This unfortunate consequence of dietary protein supplementation also occurs in nephrotic patients; compared with patients ingesting a low-protein diet, those eating a high-protein diet exhibit increases in the albumin synthetic rate but also increased urinary albumin excretion, which results in net constancy of serum albumin levels.[127]

Factors contributing to enhanced proteinuria in the setting of a high-protein diet may include increased renal blood flow and GFR, with enhanced fractional renal clearance of albumin[153] and stimulation of the renin-angiotensin system.[154] The exact dietary component of protein that stimulates albumin synthesis is unknown but does not appear to be either arginine[155] or branched chain amino acids.[156] However, the net result is that despite the enhanced albumin synthesis, increased urinary losses predominate so that serum albumin concentration and body albumin pools may in fact be further reduced.[152] Experimentally, blockade of the renin-angiotensin system in the setting of a high-protein diet allows increased hepatic synthesis but limits proteinuria, allowing some amelioration of hypoalbuminemia.[150, 152] In nephrotic patients, both dietary protein restriction and angiotensin-converting enzyme inhibition reduce proteinuria; however, protein restriction also reduces hepatic albumin synthesis, whereas albumin synthetic rates are maintained with converting enzyme inhibitor therapy.[157]

Hormones such as insulin,[158–160] thyroid hormone,[161] growth hormone,[162, 163] and glucocorticoids[164] are all required to maintain normal albumin synthesis, but their importance in the pathogenesis of nephrotic hypoalbuminemia is not well understood. Albumin synthesis is suppressed in the presence of inflammation[165]; it is also possible that in the nephrotic syndrome, elevated levels of lymphokines such as tumor necrosis factor[166] interfere with albumin synthesis.

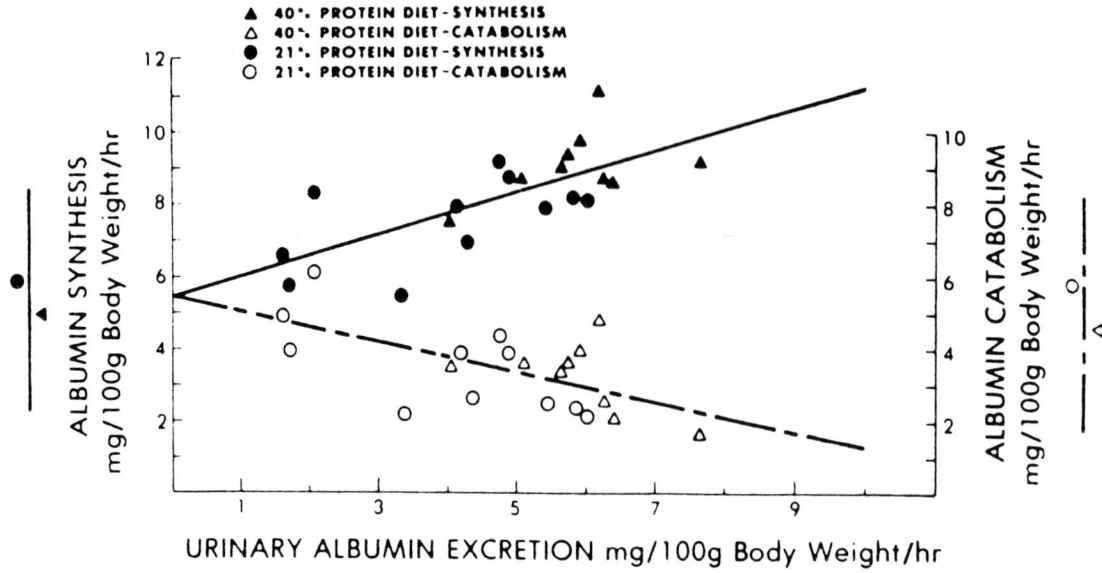

**Figure 43–8.** Relationship between albumin synthesis and catabolism and albuminuria in nephrotic rats fed 21% or 40% protein diets. (From Kaysen GA, Kirkpatrick WG, Couser WG: Albumin homeostasis in the nephrotic rat: Nutritional considerations. Am J Physiol 247:F192, 1984.)

In summary, nephrotic hypoalbuminemia is characterized by large urinary albumin losses and a marked reduction in the total exchangeable albumin pool. Mechanisms tending to counteract these forces are mobilization of extravascular pools, increases in albumin synthesis, and decreases in albumin catabolism. However, in contrast to other protein-losing states, these compensatory mechanisms are insufficient to correct the hypoalbuminemia. Comparisons between normal and nephrotic albumin homeostasis are schematized in Figure 43–7*B*. Hepatic synthesis normally equals the amount catabolized, yielding 1 to 2 g of albumin that undergoes glomerular filtration, after which it is catabolized in the proximal tubule. In the nephrotic state, hepatic synthesis may be slightly increased, and the plasma albumin pool is smaller; however, extrarenal catabolism is proportionally enhanced. Larger amounts are presented to the glomerulus, resulting in both urinary losses and enhanced tubule catabolism.

## CONSEQUENCES OF HYPOALBUMINEMIA

Hypoalbuminemia causes or exacerbates numerous complications of the nephrotic syndrome. As described in the following, these include altered blood volume and composition, edema formation, compromised renal function, increased platelet aggregability, enhanced potential for drug toxicity, and hyperlipidemia.

### Edema Formation and Blood Volume Homeostasis

Given the multiple mechanisms that defend against edema formation, the accumulation of edema in nephrotic states is not solely a result of the lowered serum albumin concentration. As reviewed,[167] transcapillary fluid flux ($J_v$) across a membrane is defined by the Starling relationship:

$J_v = L_p(\Delta P - \sigma\Delta\pi)$, where $\Delta P$ and $\Delta\pi$ are the transmembrane hydraulic and oncotic pressure gradients, respectively; $L_p$ is the hydraulic conductivity of the membrane; and $\sigma$ is the reflection coefficient for plasma proteins, mainly albumin. The balance of Starling forces prevailing at the arteriolar end of the capillary ($\Delta P > \Delta\pi$) favors net filtration of fluid into the interstitium.[168] However, ongoing fluid transudation (edema accumulation) is normally limited by at least three protective mechanisms. First, the lymphatics are able to expand and proliferate, and the ability of lymphatic flow to increase in response to increased interstitial fluid formation provides one protective mechanism. Second, transudation of protein-tree filtration into the interstitium tends to reduce interstitial fluid oncotic pressure ($\pi_{IF}$), thereby decreasing $\Delta\pi$ and slowing ultrafiltration. Third, fluid flux tends to increase interstitial fluid hydraulic pressure ($P_{IF}$), thereby reducing $\Delta P$ and further slowing filtration.[169]

Furthermore, the compliance characteristics of the interstitium resist fluid accumulation.[170, 171] The interstitium consists of collagen fibers in a relatively acellular matrix or ground substance composed of glycosaminoglycans (GAGs). The collagen fibers resist changes in tissue volume and partially immobilize the GAGs; the high negative charge density of the GAGs sets up a Gibbs-Donnan distribution of diffusible counterion species that accounts for the osmotic pressure exerted by the GAGs. This osmotic pressure rises steeply and out of proportion to the concentration of polysaccharide and is extremely nonideal. The negative charge density also contributes to the sieving characteristics of the GAGs, which retard negatively charged dextrans more than dextrans of comparable size.[170] Compartmentalization within the interstitial space prevents rapid local translocation of fluid in subcutaneous and subserosal tissues.

Accordingly, the appearance of edema in the setting of glomerulonephritis implies a substantial disruption in the normal defenses against edema formation. Generalized edema in glomerulonephritis therefore implies substantial and ongoing renal $Na^+$ retention, which further supports the concept that intrarenal mechanisms prevail in the pathogenesis of $Na^+$ retention associated with glomerular disease.[172-174]

**Relation of Edema Formation to Reduced Plasma Oncotic Pressure.** According to the traditional view of nephrotic edema formation, hypoalbuminemia results in a reduction in the colloid π of the blood, favoring movement of water from the vascular to the interstitial space. However, continued edema formation would require disruption of normal defenses against edema, and evidence for such derangement is not clearly found. For example, in nephrotic patients, hypoalbuminemia has been shown to be accompanied by a fall in $\pi_{IF}$ sufficient to substantially retard interstitial fluid accumulation.[175] Measurements of interstitial colloid osmotic pressures in nephrotic animals and patients also indicate that $\pi_{IF}$ falls virtually in parallel with the fall in plasma colloid osmotic pressure as serum albumin levels fall, thus maintaining the net transcapillary $\Delta\pi$ in the normal range.[175-178] Studies of the same patients during relapse and remission showed almost equivalent changes in interstitial and plasma colloid osmotic pressures.[178] The reduction in interstitial colloid osmotic pressure results in part from acceleration of lymphatic flow, which in turn returns interstitial protein to the intravascular space.[178-180] It has been suggested that this "wash-down" phenomenon is triggered by a slight increase in interstitial volume and hydraulic pressure induced by the initial loss of fluid into the interstitium. Body albumin pools are thus redistributed so that a greater fraction than normal is located in the intravascular space; interstitial albumin concentration may be as low as 5% of that in the plasma in nephrotic patients.[144, 181] These events thus serve to maintain blood volume and to defend against edema formation.[4, 112]

Accordingly, it appears that a substantial disruption of renal mechanisms for extracellular fluid homeostasis, rather than the level of hypoalbuminemia, is the primary determinant of the severity of edema formation. In assessing the relative contribution of hypoalbuminemia to edema formation, it is necessary to take into consideration the prevailing intravascular volume as well.

**Relation of Edema Formation to Prevailing Intravascular Volume.** One postulated scenario linking hypoalbuminemia to edema formation relates to "underfill" mechanisms,[167, 174, 182-185] as depicted in Figure 43-9. According to this scenario, reduced serum albumin and the resultant decrease in plasma π lead to edema formation but also to hypovolemia. The reduced plasma volume then triggers compensatory mechanisms (such as nonosmotic vasopressin release, the renin-angiotensin-aldosterone system, and the sympathetic nervous system), which stimulate renal $Na^+$ and water retention. These serve to restore intravascular volume but also exacerbate hypoalbuminemia, such that edema formation continues. However, as reviewed,[167, 182] some experimental observations are at odds with this hypothesis. First, the clinical syndrome of congenital analbuminemia is not necessarily associated with edema,[186] nor is the transcapillary $\Delta\pi$ abnormal in analbuminemic rats.[187] Second, the presence of hypovolemia is questionable. The evidence against hypovolemia as the proximate cause of

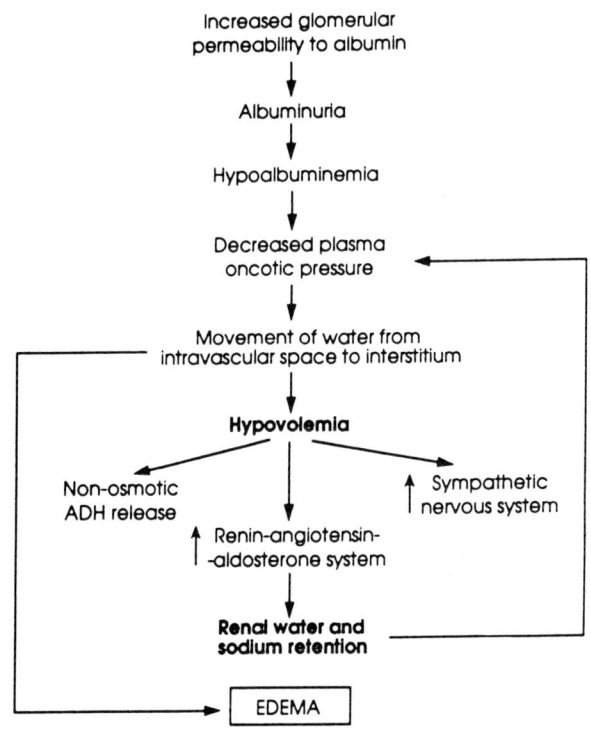

**Figure 43-9.** The underfill mechanism of edema formation. Hypovolemia (resulting from hypoalbuminemia and decreased plasma oncotic pressure) is viewed as the key event promoting $Na^+$ and water retention by the kidney. (From Perico N, Remuzzi G: Edema of the nephrotic syndrome: The role of the atrial peptide system. Am J Kidney Dis 22:355, 1993.)

$Na^+$ retention comes from three lines of evidence: inability to document hypovolemia by direct measurements; inability to consistently find changes in hormonal modulators consistent with hypovolemia, or after maneuvers designed to alter blood volume acutely; and failure of predicted changes after remission of nephrotic syndrome or diuretic therapy of edema. In patients with nephrotic syndromes, plasma and blood volumes are not usually reduced; in fact, they are usually normal or even expanded.[173, 176, 188-196] However, many of the available studies actually note a range of plasma volumes among patients studied. Moreover, methodologic differences and limitations in measurements of blood and plasma volume may interfere with the interpretation of these studies.[174, 192]

Nonetheless, in addition to direct measurements of blood and plasma volumes, it should be possible to estimate these parameters by measurement of vasoactive hormones that change in response to alterations in prevailing intravascular volume. Thus, a diminished intravascular volume should be reflected in elevated values for hematocrit and plasma renin, aldosterone, arginine vasopressin, and norepinephrine concentrations and reduced values for atrial natriuretic peptide (ANP). Such functional evidence of hypovolemia is not consistently found in the nephrotic syndrome.[112, 167, 174, 182, 192] Plasma renin activity and aldosterone concentrations tend to be reduced and not always well correlated with changes in blood volume.[188, 190, 193, 196] Similarly, plasma levels of norepinephrine, arginine vasopressin, and ANP tend to be normal (or inconsistently changed) in nephrotic patients.[192, 195, 197, 198] Moreover, maneuvers that expand plasma volume, including infusion of hyperoncotic plasma,[199] salt-poor albumin,[200] and head-out water immersion,[201, 202] do not regularly result in diuresis or natriuresis. However, despite the lack of a uniform response, some studies have found evidence consistent with hypovolemia and a natriuretic response to these maneuvers.[174, 197, 203]

Evidence from patients undergoing remission from the nephrotic syndrome is likewise not clear. In responsive patients, steroid therapy leads to diuresis and natriuresis before any change in serum albumin. Plasma renin and aldosterone levels were initially high and fell during natriuresis. After resolution of edema, plasma renin and aldosterone levels again rose to high levels, whereas plasma albumin levels and blood volumes remained low; yet, $Na^+$ retention did not occur, and $Na^+$ balance was maintained.[193] Thus, it was concluded that the absence of $Na^+$ retention in the face of evidence of hypovolemia and hypoalbuminemia during remission pointed to an intrarenal defect as the likely cause of edema during the nephrotic syndrome. Resolution of this intrarenal defect is characterized by an increase in filtration fraction, which again suggests that natriuresis results from renal repair rather than from changes in blood volume.[204]

Taken together, these observations suggest a wide spectrum in prevailing plasma volumes. In support of this concept, one study found a suggestion of two populations of patients. Those with steroid-responsive minimal-change disease tended to have volume contraction and stimulation of the renin-angiotensin-aldosterone axis; patients with more advanced steroid-resistant disease exhibited volume expansion and suppression of the renin axis.[188] In head-out water immersion studies, the natriuretic response to this maneuver was correlated with the preimmersion state of salt balance.[202] Studies with experimental animals further support this concept. Kaysen and co-workers[205] studied nephrotic rats in the presence or absence of plasma volume expansion induced by reduction of renal mass. Rats with chronic renal failure exhibited plasma volume expansion that was further expanded when they became nephrotic; edema formation did not occur in the presence of chronic renal failure or nephrotic syndrome alone, but only when nephrotic rats were plasma volume expanded.[205] These observations have important therapeutic implications. The evidence suggests that edema is not necessary to maintain blood volume and, by corollary, that vigorous treatment of edema with diuretics does not result in failure to maintain blood volume.[195, 206]

**Role of Intrarenal Mechanisms.** It now appears that no single mechanism accounts for edema formation in all nephrotic patients. However, changes in blood volume, although perhaps contributory in some patients, are generally insufficient to explain the avid $Na^+$ retention that characterizes the nephrotic syndrome. The majority of the available evidence tends to implicate a primary intrarenal defect in this disorder. This alternative hypothesis, termed the "overfill" theory,[174, 185] is schematized in Figure 43–10. According to this hypothesis, a primary increase in renal $Na^+$ retention leads to extracellular fluid volume expansion, altered Starling forces, and edema formation. Interesting evidence in support of such a mechanism comes from ob-

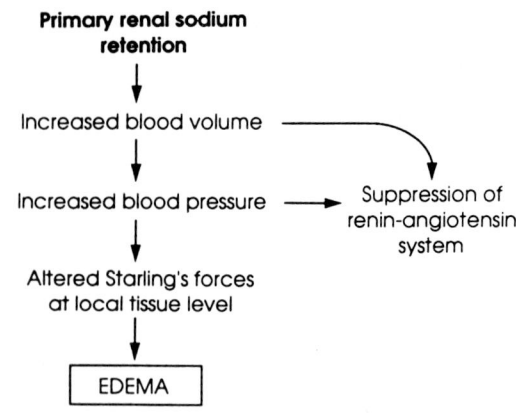

**Figure 43–10.** The overfill mechanism of edema formation. The abnormal renal $Na^+$ retention is viewed as the primary event, which through the increased plasma volume leads to alteration of Starling forces at the local tissue level. (From Perico N, Remuzzi G: Edema of the nephrotic syndrome: The role of the atrial peptide system. Am J Kidney Dis 22:355, 1993.)

servations that $Na^+$ retention occurs only in the ipsilateral kidney of dogs[207] and rats[172, 208] with unilateral glomerulonephritis. Micropuncture studies, as well as indirect observations, have localized the primary $Na^+$ handling abnormality to the distal nephron.[172] Moreover, the reduction in GFR that characterizes many forms of glomerulonephritis would further limit urinary $Na^+$ excretion and thus also contribute to renal $Na^+$ retention.

The mechanism by which $Na^+$ handling is altered in the distal tubule is not entirely understood, although attention has focused on the role of ANP. As reviewed,[167, 182] clinical[209, 210] and experimental[211, 212] studies have documented renal ANP resistance (i.e., blunted or absent natriuretic responses to ANP) in the nephrotic syndrome. This ANP resistance is confined to the ipsilateral kidney in unilateral glomerulonephritis,[212] which suggests a role for this hormone in mediating the primary renal $Na^+$ retention. Although the mechanisms of ANP resistance are still being unraveled, there is evidence relating this abnormality to heightened efferent sympathetic nervous activity.[213] At the level of the tubule cell, evidence suggests that the problem is accelerated breakdown of normally produced cyclic GMP[214] or altered levels of intrarenal genes that influence $Na^+$ handling.[215]

### Alterations in Renal Function

The Starling equation predicts that hypoalbuminemia, and thus reduced plasma colloid $\pi$, would tend to reduce the forces opposing ultrafiltration of water and solutes, thereby increasing glomerular filtration. However, clinical[216] and experimental[59, 217, 218] studies indicate that this is not the case and that values for GFR are in fact lower than normal in conditions of reduced plasma protein levels. To examine the influence of plasma protein concentration on the determinants of glomerular ultrafiltration, Baylis and colleagues[59] acutely changed plasma protein concentration in normal rats. When plasma protein concentration was reduced, observed values for SNGFR were lower than values predicted by the Starling relationship; this failure of SNGFR to rise resulted from a concomitant reduction in $K_f$.[59]

Reduced values for SNGFR, due primarily to a reduction in $K_f$, have subsequently been observed in some[218] but not all[219] experimental models of the nephrotic syndrome; these differences in SNGFR derive, in part, from the presence or absence of compensatory elevations in the glomerular capillary $\Delta P$. Studies in a unique strain of rats with no circulating albumin, the Nagase analbuminemic rat,[220] have yielded further insight into the role of serum albumin in the regulation of GFR. Plasma $\pi$ are modestly reduced in this strain, but a comparable reduction in $\pi_{IF}$ yields a fairly normal transcapillary $\Delta\pi$ and normal extracellular fluid volume.[187, 221] Values for GFR and renal plasma flow are normal; constancy of GFR relates in part to elevation of values for $K_f$, because glomerular capillary pressure is somewhat reduced.[187, 221] These observations suggest that serum albumin does not directly affect $K_f$ or that other factors mitigate the effects of hypoalbuminemia on $K_f$ in the chronic setting.

Calculations of plasma $\pi$ are generally performed by use of the equation of Landis and Pappenheimer, in which the albumin/globulin ratio slightly exceeds unity.[1] In the presence of severe hypoalbuminemia, the Landis-Pappenheimer equation tends to overestimate values for colloid osmotic pressure and therefore to underestimate values for the ultrafiltration pressure used to calculate $K_f$. Accordingly, Miller and Meyer[222] have derived the equations required to modify the Landis-Pappenheimer relationship in this setting.

## Alterations in Drug Pharmacokinetics

Uremia is associated with changes in all aspects of drug handling, including changes in bioavailability, volume of distribution, renal drug metabolism, and renal excretion of a drug or its metabolites.[223] Principles and guidelines for modification of drug dosage in renal insufficiency are readily available[224, 225] and are detailed in Chapter 60. The nephrotic syndrome poses special problems in drug handling and enhanced potential for both drug resistance and drug toxicity.

Hypoalbuminemia limits the sites available for protein binding, thereby increasing the amount of circulating free drug and potentially increasing first-pass hepatic drug removal. In addition, binding of organic acids and bases is altered in hypoalbuminemic states; the effect on organic acids is the more prominent.[226] In nephrotic patients, reduced protein binding results from both a lower serum albumin concentration and a decrease in albumin's affinity for drugs. Accordingly, the unbound fraction of acidic drugs, including salicylate and phenytoin, may be markedly increased, and protein binding for many drugs is altered in renal failure.[225] The clinical consequences of altered protein binding may be difficult to predict: decreased binding allows a higher concentration of free drug, but this effect may be counteracted by a larger volume of distribution or faster metabolism of the drug. Furthermore, protein binding may enhance tubule drug secretion; the lesser protein binding in the nephrotic syndrome may result in delayed renal excretion of some drugs.[223] Thus, in nephrotic patients, phenytoin is less protein bound, but the available free drug

is more rapidly metabolized in the liver, so plasma levels are not elevated and dosage need not be adjusted. In contrast, other protein-bound drugs, including prednisone and benzodiazepines, achieve significantly higher drug levels in nephrotic patients, with enhanced risk for toxic effects.[225] Edema and ascites may increase the apparent volume of distribution of drugs that are highly water soluble or protein bound, thereby resulting in inadequate plasma levels in nephrotic patients; this effect appears to be particularly prominent with aminoglycoside antibiotics.[223]

The actions of diuretics are substantially altered in renal insufficiency and in the nephrotic syndrome, thereby contributing to the observed resistance to these drugs in this state.[227–230] The unbound fraction of furosemide increases markedly in severely hypoalbuminemic patients.[231] Nephrotic patients without impairment in GFR deliver loop diuretics into the urine in amounts equivalent to those in normal subjects; the delivery of the drug into the urine is decreased in the setting of renal insufficiency.[232] When proteinuria is also present, a substantial amount of furosemide may bind to urinary proteins, thereby reducing the amount of active, unbound drug in the urine, and urinary binding increases with increasing amounts of proteinuria.[233, 234] Tubule albumin blunts the inhibitory effects of furosemide on fractional loop $Cl^-$ reabsorption,[235] whereas agents that block albumin-furosemide binding in the proximal tubule partially restore diuretic responsiveness.[236] Nephrotic patients exhibit abnormal pharmacodynamic responses to furosemide in addition to the binding effects,[232] so that the renal response to the drug is diminished even when adequate amounts of unbound, active drug reach the site of action. In addition, animal studies indicate that furosemide is less potent in inhibiting $Cl^-$ reabsorption in the loop in nephrotic rats.[237] Thus, both pharmacodynamics and pharmacokinetics of loop diuretics are altered in the nephrotic syndrome. Single intravenously administered doses of 80 to 120 mg may be needed to attain therapeutic levels of furosemide in the urine, but higher doses are unlikely to achieve any added therapeutic response.[228]

That hypoalbuminemia, and consequent altered protein binding, is an important factor in resistance to diuretics is further supported by studies in a strain of analbuminemic rats.[238] Compared with normal rats, these animals exhibited resistance to furosemide, with more rapid plasma disappearance of the drug and a larger total plasma clearance and volume of distribution, although no differences in these parameters were found for the unbound fraction. Injection of furosemide bound to albumin resulted in a natriuresis, with normalization of the plasma disappearance rate and increased urinary excretion of furosemide. Thus, binding to plasma albumin appeared to be necessary for efficient delivery of drug into the urine. These investigators then examined hypoalbuminemic patients with furosemide resistance, finding that injections of furosemide as an admixture with equimolar albumin produced a substantial diuresis, whereas administration of either alone was without effect. Whether natriuresis occurred in these patients was not specifically mentioned, but a later study confirmed a natriuretic response to salt-free albumin mixed with bumetanide.[239] Because administration of large amounts of albumin alone is both ineffective and expensive, this therapeutic combination deserves further study.

Therapy for glomerular disease or the nephrotic syndrome may also be associated with drug interactions that need to be recognized.[225] For example, corticosteroids may inhibit hepatic microsomal enzymes, thereby altering metabolism of other drugs. Cyclophosphamide is not associated with significant drug interactions, but clinically important drug interactions may be seen with other immunosuppressive drugs, including cyclosporine and azathioprine, as well as with diuretics and antihypertensive agents.[225]

### Alterations in Platelet Function

Hypoalbuminemia may contribute to abnormal platelet function in nephrotic patients, because conversion of arachidonic acid into metabolites that aggregate platelets is regulated by albumin.[240] In the presence of hypoalbuminemia, arachidonic acid may be metabolized into platelet-aggregating substances, such as endoperoxides and thromboxane $A_2$.[241] In support of this notion, the degree of platelet dysfunction tends to correlate with severity of hypoalbuminemia and proteinuria.[242] In addition, blood from hypoalbuminemic patients displays hypersensitivity to platelet aggregation induced by arachidonic acid in vitro, and this hyperaggregability is corrected as serum albumin concentration increases.[243] Platelets from nephrotic patients are refractory to adenylate cyclase stimulation by prostaglandin $E_1$, further promoting increased platelet aggregation.[244] However, a firm correlation between plasma albumin concentration and platelet aggregability is not well established clinically.[245]

# Hyperlipidemia

Hypoalbuminemia also contributes to another important consequence of the nephrotic syndrome, which is hyperlipidemia. Atherosclerotic heart disease is the foremost cause of morbidity and mortality in patients with end-stage renal disease (see Chapter 56). Chronic renal disease features various abnormalities of lipid metabolism, which result in an exceedingly atherogenic profile. Although most striking in the nephrotic syndrome, hyperlipidemia characterizes renal diseases of every cause, as has been reviewed.[246, 247]

## NORMAL LIPOPROTEIN METABOLISM

The metabolism of cholesterol and lipoprotein may be summarized as follows.[248, 249] Lipoproteins transport nonpolar lipids (primarily triglycerides and cholesterol esters) through the bloodstream. Each lipoprotein is composed of a hydrophobic core containing triglycerides and cholesterol esters surrounded by a polar surface layer containing unesterified cholesterol, phospholipids, and apolipoproteins (apo). Apolipoproteins are proteins with various specific functions including actions as ligands for receptors and cofactors for enzymatic reactions. Lipoproteins are categorized by density into chylomicrons, very low density (VLDL), intermediate-density (IDL), low-density (LDL), and high-density (HDL) lipoproteins.

Lipid transport is a two-compartment process involving processing of dietary lipids as well as hepatic lipid synthesis.[248] In the exogenous pathway, dietary cholesterol and free fatty acids are re-esterified in the endoplasmic reticulum of intestinal mucosal epithelial cells, packaged into chylomicrons (containing apo B-48, apo A-I, apo A-II, and apo A-IV), and transported through the lymphatics into the bloodstream. In the bloodstream, apo C and apo E are acquired from HDL. Next, chylomicrons are hydrolyzed by lipoprotein lipase (LPL) located on vascular endothelium in adipose and skeletal muscle, a reaction activated by apo C-II within the chylomicron. Hydrolysis results in the release of free fatty acids and monoglycerides, which are transported to the tissues. Apo A-I and apo A-II are transferred to HDL, and the remainder of the chylomicron re-enters the circulation as a chylomicron remnant particle that is enriched in cholesterol esters and apo B-48 and apo E. Chylomicron remnants are taken up in the liver by a specific apo E receptor and then degraded. In the liver, cholesterol esters from the remnant particle are catabolized to free cholesterol and either secreted into bile or reincorporated into endogenous lipoproteins.

The endogenous pathway of lipoprotein transport and metabolism consists of hepatic lipoprotein synthesis and secretion. Newly synthesized triglyceride originates from the liver as VLDL, with apo B-100 serving as the secretory protein. Once secreted, VLDL is hydrolyzed by LPL at the endothelial cell surface. This hydrolysis allows the progressive removal of triglyceride from VLDL, creating IDL. In the liver, some IDL particles are taken up directly by LDL receptors, but other IDL particles are reduced further to cholesterol-rich LDL by hepatic lipase.

LDL is taken up by LDL receptors both in peripheral tissues and in the liver, where it is used to supply cholesterol for membrane and steroid precursor synthesis. Hepatic LDL uptake down-regulates both hydroxymethylglutaryl–coenzyme A reductase and LDL receptor expression.[4, 250] Thus, hepatic uptake of LDL represents a key regulatory step in hepatic lipid metabolism.

As cell membranes undergo turnover, cholesterol is released into the circulation, where it is esterified through the action of lecithin-cholesterol acyltransferase (LCAT) and incorporated into nascent HDL particles. As cholesterol ester is added, the disk-shaped nascent HDL is converted to a spherical HDL particle, which then carries cholesterol ester to the liver where it is hydrolyzed and either excreted into bile or recycled into endogenous lipoproteins.

## LIPOPROTEINS AND ATHEROGENESIS

Hypercholesterolemia has long been recognized as a significant risk factor for atherosclerosis. LDL-cholesterol and apo B levels correlate directly with risk of heart disease; levels of HDL-cholesterol and apo A-I are inversely correlated with risk.[251] The $HDL_2$ subfraction appears to confer the protective effect.[252] Lp(a) is a unique low-density lipoprotein containing a protein similar to plasminogen covalently linked to apo B-100. Lp(a) is thought to be highly atherogenic and possibly thrombogenic.[253, 254]

## LIPID ABNORMALITIES IN CHRONIC RENAL FAILURE (see also Chapter 56)

Patients with chronic renal failure exhibit a number of lipid abnormalities that together comprise an especially atherogenic profile. These abnormalities characterize uremia in general and occur regardless of the underlying cause of renal disease.[246, 247] Hypertriglyceridemia, which is not an independent risk factor for atherogenesis, is found in 33% to 70% of patients with chronic renal failure,[255–257] and hypercholesterolemia is found in up to 20% of patients. HDL levels are decreased in 50% to 75%, whereas LDL-cholesterol tends to be in the normal range, resulting in a high LDL/HDL ratio.[247, 255–259] Lp(a) levels are also elevated.[259, 260] In a study of 346 nondiabetic patients receiving hemodialysis, rates of cardiovascular mortality were found to be higher in white men than in black men. This higher mortality rate in white men was associated with lower levels of HDL, apo A-I (the major apolipoprotein of HDL), and apo A-II as well as a more abnormal distribution of subfractions.[261] Whether Lp(a) is an independent risk factor for cardiovascular death in hemodialysis patients is currently controversial.[262, 263] Both IDL and chylomicron remnant levels are also elevated in chronic renal failure, representing further derangement of normal lipid metabolism.[259, 264]

Several abnormalities in lipoprotein metabolism contribute to the altered lipid profile associated with chronic renal disease. In addition to abnormalities in serum total lipoprotein concentrations, uremic patients exhibit potentially atherogenic abnormalities in lipoprotein composition.[259, 264–266] Most notable is an elevated concentration of apo C-III. In addition, most authors have found decreased concentrations of apo A-I and apo A-II. Apo C-III and apo E are also abnormally distributed. These apolipoproteins are usually found in HDL, but in chronic renal failure, 60% to 80% of apo C-III and apo E are found in VLDL and LDL. The shift of apo C-III from predominantly HDL particles to predominantly triglyceride-rich particles represents a catabolic defect in triglyceride metabolism that results in the accumulation of a variety of remnant particles including IDL.[267–270] This defect is found in chronic renal failure even in patients with seemingly normal lipid profiles.[262, 270] Moreover, LPL, hepatic triglyceride lipase, and LCAT all have decreased activity in renal failure.[271, 272] Dysfunction of the LPL receptor has also been reported in end-stage renal disease.[272]

Observations in predialysis patients suggest that abnormalities in lipid metabolism occur early in the course of renal failure. LPL activity has been found to be reduced in patients with a GFR value of 50 mL/min,[273] although triglycerides do not increase until GFR reaches the range of 15 to 30 mL/min.[274] Contributing factors are frequently present in uremia; hormonal abnormalities (such as insulin resistance and hypothyroidism), diabetes, and drugs may also adversely influence lipid metabolism.

## LIPID ABNORMALITIES IN DIABETIC GLOMERULOPATHY

Lipid abnormalities resulting in adverse LDL/HDL ratios also characterize type I and type II diabetes mellitus.[275–278]

These abnormalities are accentuated by factors such as poor metabolic control, advanced renal failure, and hypertension[275–278] and are somewhat ameliorated with intensive hypoglycemic therapy.[279, 280] Diabetic patients without glomerulopathy and good metabolic control have no differences in total cholesterol, triglyceride, or lipoprotein cholesterol compared with control subjects; but abnormalities of lipid and apolipoprotein content similar to those seen in other forms of chronic renal failure develop when glomerulopathy is present and are correlated with GFR.[278] In addition, poor metabolic control results in worsening of the lipid profile. Thus, patients without albuminuria may exhibit elevations in serum VLDL levels, and reduced HDL-cholesterol levels, when metabolic control is not optimal. Patients with incipient nephropathy (albuminuria of 30 to 300 mg/d) exhibit a pattern similar to those without albuminuria in poor metabolic control; patients with overt nephropathy exhibit marked increases in total cholesterol, VLDL, and triglyceride levels, with reductions in HDL.[281, 282] Lp(a) levels are also high in diabetes, particularly in periods of poor metabolic control.[283, 284]

## LIPID ABNORMALITIES IN THE NEPHROTIC SYNDROME

Hyperlipidemia is a significant adverse component of the nephrotic syndrome, which may feature prominent lipid abnormalities even in the absence of a marked reduction in GFR. In nephrotic patients, cholesterol and phospholipid levels rise early in the course of the disease and continue to rise as the severity of the nephrotic syndrome increases.[285–287] Triglyceride levels are more variable, particularly early in the disease, but they also increase as the disease progresses.[285, 288] Typically, LDL, VLDL, and IDL levels are elevated early in the course of the disease. Although total HDL levels may be variable, subtype analysis demonstrates a significant reduction in the protective subtype $HDL_2$.[289] Lp(a) is also elevated in nephrotic syndrome[290–292] but has not been correlated with proteinuria or albumin. However, remission of nephrotic syndrome after treatment with immunosuppressants has been associated with reduction in Lp(a) levels.[291] Lipoproteins from nephrotic patients also exhibit altered composition. The cholesterol/triglyceride ratio is elevated in all classes of lipoproteins. Apolipoprotein content is also abnormal, with elevated levels of apo B, C-II, C-III, and E.[287] Taken together, these abnormalities result in an increased atherogenic profile.[287, 293, 294]

## PATHOGENESIS OF NEPHROTIC HYPERLIPIDEMIA

Hyperlipidemia may result from increased synthesis or impaired degradation of serum lipids. Hepatic VLDL synthesis is markedly increased in clinical and experimental nephrotic syndromes,[295–297] whereas impaired conversion of VLDL and IDL to LDL results in accumulation of large cholesterol-rich lipoprotein particles.[298, 299]

In general, the severity of hyperlipidemia tends to correlate with the severity of hypoalbuminemia.[286] In addition, remission from nephrotic syndrome is usually associated with a decrease in the serum cholesterol level as the albumin level rises, whereas albumin infusion into nephrotic rats or humans acutely raises serum albumin and lowers serum cholesterol levels.[112, 285, 300, 301] Because hepatic synthetic rates for albumin and lipoproteins appear to react to similar stimuli and to follow the same synthetic pathways, it has been hypothesized that increased VLDL synthesis is simply a side effect of increased albumin synthesis. However, although many data suggest that albumin synthesis is increased, studies have failed to find a clear correlation between hyperlipidemia and the rate of albumin synthesis in nephrotic patients. Kaysen and co-workers[302] performed simultaneous measurements of albumin synthesis and of plasma and urinary protein and lipid parameters in nephrotic patients. With a low-protein diet, these patients exhibited normal albumin synthetic rates and yet marked hypercholesterolemia and triglyceridemia; with a high-protein diet, albumin synthesis increased, but plasma lipids showed little change. Regression analysis showed that serum cholesterol levels were dependent only on the renal clearance of albumin and totally independent of albumin synthetic rates, whereas serum triglyceride levels showed some dependence on albumin synthesis.[302] In nephrotic rats, serum lipid levels are not closely correlated with either the albumin synthetic rate or the transcription of albumin mRNA.[303] In a similar experiment, nephrotic rats given a high-protein diet and an angiotensin-converting enzyme inhibitor had lower lipid levels than did protein-fed control rats, demonstrating that proteinuria and not albumin synthesis rate is correlated with hyperlipidemia.[304] Thus, the relationship between albumin synthetic rate and hyperlipidemia is not all direct. Subjects may exhibit marked hyperlipidemia in the presence of near-normal serum albumin levels or normal total cholesterol levels when hypoalbuminemia is present.

An alternative stimulus may be the reduction in plasma π rather than the hypoalbuminemia. Infusion of either albumin or dextrans into nephrotic patients and animals reduces serum lipid levels, which suggests that low plasma π may stimulate hepatic lipoprotein synthesis.[304-307] Experimental support for this concept also comes from the observation that levels of apo B mRNA are reduced in cultured liver cells when albumin or dextran is added to the medium and increased in the presence of hypo-oncotic medium.[130, 308] Studies of nephrotic patients indicate that there is a significant inverse correlation between total plasma cholesterol concentration and both plasma albumin concentration and plasma π.[309]

Another factor contributing to enhanced liver synthesis may relate to greater availability of the cholesterol precursor mevalonate in the nephrotic state. In normal animals, circulating mevalonate is metabolized in the kidney, but both renal excretion and renal metabolism of this substance are impaired in the nephrotic state,[310] thus allowing more delivery to the liver, in which cholesterogenesis from circulating mevalonate is enhanced.[311] Furthermore, nephrotic rats exhibit enhanced activity of the enzyme hydroxymethylglutaryl–coenzyme A reductase, which catalyzes the production of mevalonate, a major feedback inhibitor of cholesterol synthesis.[311]

Diminished activity of the enzyme LPL also appears to play a role in the nephrotic syndrome; LPL activity may be reduced by as much as 30% to 60%, thereby substantially retarding VLDL removal.[312-314] One mechanism contributing to the decreased LPL activity relates to the increased levels of circulating free fatty acids, which are the result of hypoalbuminemia and therefore lowered protein-binding capacity of the plasma. The increased level of circulating free fatty acids contributes by providing the lipid substrate for increased hepatic lipoprotein synthesis and by leading to a decrease in the activity of LPL.[315, 316]

It has also been suggested that LPL is inhibited by a circulating plasma factor or that its action is retarded by deficiency in apo C-II or other activator peptides (such as heparan sulfate) that result from the abnormal synthetic rates and urinary losses.[4, 307, 308, 317] LPL is attached to the endothelium by ionic bonding to a negatively charged matrix of heparan sulfate.[4, 315] Of the GAGs found in the urine, only heparan sulfate stimulates the LPL reaction, and urinary excretion of HSPG is markedly increased in nephrotic patients.[316] Because urinary GAGs are probably derived from plasma GAGs, it has been hypothesized that levels of this cofactor for LPL are also reduced in nephrotic plasma, thus further contributing to the decrease in LPL activity.[4] In support of this concept, studies with nephrotic rats indicate that the markedly delayed plasma disappearance of radiolabeled chylomicrons may be completely normalized by injections of minute amounts of purified urinary heparan sulfate.[4, 317] Defective chylomicron clearance appears to be correlated with proteinuria, or urinary loss of a liporegulatory substance, rather than with hypoalbuminemia, because the serum half-life of chylomicrons remains normal in analbuminemic rats whereas it is markedly impaired in hypoalbuminemic animals with nephrotic syndrome.[304] The deficiency of heparan sulfate in the nephrotic syndrome may in turn result from deficient hepatic synthesis of GAGs. The nephrotic syndrome is characterized by excessive urinary losses of orosomucoid; this plasma glycoprotein is synthesized by the liver, and excessive urinary losses may lead to an increase in hepatic synthesis with resultant excessive drain of key sugar intermediates from liver parenchymal cells, thus limiting the substrates available for heparan sulfate synthesis.[4]

Diminished activity of the enzyme LCAT also appears to contribute to lipoprotein abnormalities in the nephrotic syndrome.[318-320] LCAT is normally responsible for catalyzing the synthesis of HDL, which removes cholesterol from the circulation and transports it to the liver for catabolism; it is also responsible for catalyzing the peripheral esterification of cholesterol in plasma, rendering it more amenable for transfer by HDL. In the nephrotic syndrome, the decreased LCAT activity results from increased levels of free (unbound) lysolecithin, an inhibitor of LCAT.[4, 319] The increase in free lysolecithin results from hypoalbuminemia. In addition, urinary losses of LCAT may contribute to its reduced plasma activity.[321]

Defective hepatic removal of IDL may also contribute to hyperlipidemia in this setting, and experiments with nephrotic rats suggest that there may be a metabolic defect in the recognition and removal of IDL by the liver.[4, 322] The signal for recognition of IDL by a liver ''receptor site'' may be LPL, an associated cofactor such as heparan sulfate, or certain apolipoproteins; it has been hypothesized that the observed deficiencies in LPL or heparan sulfate may be responsible for failure of recognition and hence defective removal of these particles in the nephrotic syndrome.[4]

Accordingly, the nephrotic syndrome is characterized by abnormalities in virtually every aspect of lipid and lipoprotein metabolism,[323] as depicted in Figure 43–11. Many of these derangements can, in turn, be blamed on proteinuria,[293] as schematized in Figure 43–12.

## CLINICAL CONSEQUENCES OF NEPHROTIC HYPERLIPIDEMIA

Several features of the nephrotic syndrome, including hypertension, abnormal lipoprotein metabolism, and hypercoagulability, may contribute to the risk of atherosclerotic cardiovascular disease, and nephrotic patients may exhibit multiple cardiovascular risk factors.[294] However, evidence that these features do in fact heighten coronary risk is somewhat controversial. Studies that have tried to define the cardiovascular risk in the nephrotic syndrome have been flawed by inclusion of patients with minimal-change disease (which typically remits), diabetes (which is inherently atherogenic), and the presence of hypertension or corticosteroid therapy. These studies, which included relatively young patients with nephrotic syndrome, contained small numbers, and were retrospectively designed, have not uniformly found an increased risk of coronary events.[324–327] However, 157 patients with nephrotic range proteinuria

without diabetes were observed for 5 years. In this group, the relative risk of cardiovascular death was 5.5, that of myocardial infarction was 5.3, and that of all coronary artery disease was 2.5 compared with non-nephrotic control subjects.[328] In addition to the short duration of hyperlipidemia in some cases, the HDL profile may be a protective factor. Total HDL levels are variable in the nephrotic syndrome.[287, 289, 293, 300, 301] The profile of the HDL subfractions has not been extensively studied, although one study found that levels of $HDL_2$ tended to be low in nephrotic patients with normal total HDL levels.[289] Overall, the magnitude of the risk, and thus the need for aggressive hypolipidemic therapy, remains unclear.[293]

## THERAPY FOR NEPHROTIC HYPERLIPIDEMIA

These observations notwithstanding, attempts to modify the lipoprotein profile may be worthwhile in patients with unremitting nephrotic syndrome, particularly if other risk factors for cardiovascular disease are present. Moderate reduction of dietary cholesterol intake is generally ineffective, although a low-protein vegetarian soy diet has been associated with beneficial improvements in serum cholesterol, LDL, and apo B in patients with chronic renal disease and long-standing proteinuria.[329] Pharmacologic therapy of nephrotic hyperlipidemia has also been examined. Early stud-

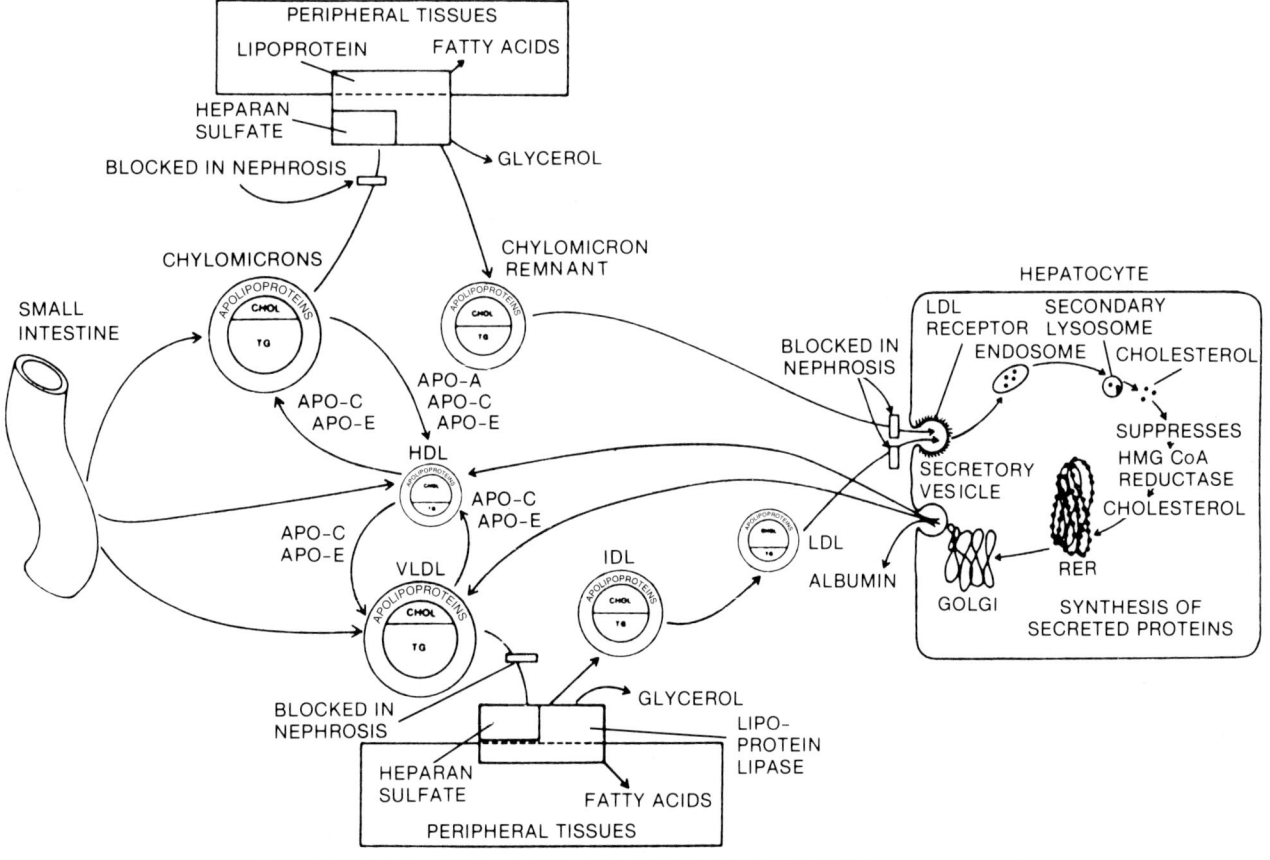

**Figure 43–11.** Normal pathways of lipoprotein metabolism and potential derangements occurring in the nephrotic syndrome. (From Kaysen GA: Hyperlipidemia in the nephrotic syndrome. Am J Kidney Dis 12:548, 1988.)

Abnormality

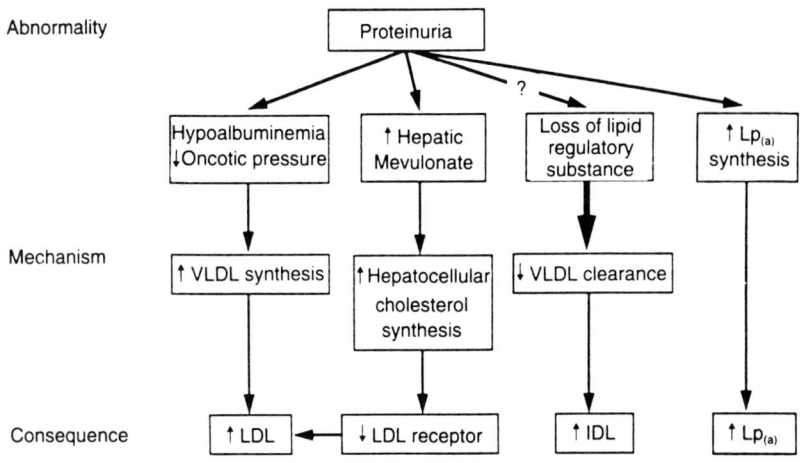

**Figure 43–12.** Potential effects of proteinuria on dyslipidemia in the nephrotic syndrome. ↑ = increase; ↓ = decrease; ? = questionable. (From Keane WF, St Peter JV, Kasiske BL: Is the aggressive management of hyperlipidemia in nephrotic syndrome mandatory? Used with permission from Kidney International, volume S-38, page S-134, 1992.)

ies of clofibrate therapy found a frequent complication of toxic muscle effects.[330] Controlled prospective studies have indicated that colestipol or probucol may offer effective hypolipidemic therapy.[331] In seven patients treated with colestipol, levels of total cholesterol and LDL were reduced while HDL remained stable, resulting in a decreased LDL/HDL ratio. In eight patients treated with probucol, levels of total cholesterol, LDL, and HDL all fell, although not significantly; however, the LDL/HDL ratio was reduced.[331] In 11 patients treated with gemfibrozil, triglyceride levels were reduced and HDL levels rose, but little change in total cholesterol or LDL levels was noted.[332] Studies using the hydroxymethylglutaryl–coenzyme A reductase inhibitors lovastatin[333, 334] and simvastatin[335, 336] have shown reductions in total cholesterol, LDL, apo B-100, and triglycerides, with elevation of HDL. Interventions that reduce proteinuria may also indirectly improve serum lipid profiles, as has been shown with angiotensin-converting enzyme inhibitor therapy.[337]

## OTHER CONSEQUENCES OF NEPHROTIC HYPERLIPIDEMIA

Hyperlipidemia may contribute to several other adverse consequences of the nephrotic syndrome. The increased platelet aggregation observed in the nephrotic syndrome tends to correlate with the magnitude of hyperlipidemia.[241] Two additional potential adverse consequences of hyperlipidemia are worthy of mention. Hyperlipidemia may contribute to the increased susceptibility of nephrotic patients to infection. It has been reported that hyperlipidemic serum from nephrotic patients inhibits lymphocyte proliferation in response to specific and nonspecific antigen stimulation,[338] although the clinical significance of this observation remains to be determined. Finally, the role of hyperlipidemia as a risk factor for progression of glomerular injury is discussed in detail in Chapter 44.

## Hypertension (see also Chapter 48)

Hypertension frequently accompanies glomerular diseases with a nephritic pattern and may accompany nephrotic diseases as well. Exceptions exist, but hypertension

in the absence of renal insufficiency is more likely to be present in primary glomerular diseases than in diseases of tubulointerstitial origin. The relationship between hypertension and glomerular disease has been the subject of several reviews[339–341] and is discussed in detail in Chapter 48.

Hypertension is almost universally present during the active stages of acute glomerulonephritis, although the frequency varies slightly with the type of glomerulonephritis. The frequency of hypertension has been reported to be as high as 86% in patients with acute poststreptococcal glomerulonephritis.[342] Hypertension is a frequent presenting symptom, and the frequency of hypertension at the time of presentation or biopsy in several large series of patients with biopsy-proven glomerular disease ranges from about 23% to 61%.[339–345] Differences in classification among these studies make direct comparisons imprecise, but overall it appears that hypertension is a fairly frequent presenting symptom in patients with acute poststreptococcal glomerulonephritis,[342] immunoglobulin A nephropathy,[339, 340, 346–348] membranoproliferative glomerulonephritis, fibrillary glomerulonephritis,[349, 350] and focal sclerosis.[340, 343, 351, 352] Hypertension less frequently characterizes the onset of glomerular disease associated with vasculitis (unless hypertension was previously present) or anti-GBM disease.[340] The frequency of occurrence in membranous nephropathy is intermediate.[340] Proteinuria and hematuria frequently precede the onset of hypertension,[339, 341] and a number of additional cases of hypertension develop in the course of glomerular disease. Hypertension almost invariably occurs during the course of chronic glomerulonephritis[341] and in end-stage renal disease.[351] In general, the degree of hypertension tends to correlate with the severity of morphologic injury[353] and possibly the degree of proliferation[345] found on renal biopsy.

Multiple factors are likely to play a role in the pathogenesis of hypertension associated with glomerular disease.[354] In patients with severe renal functional impairment, and with an acute nephritic syndrome with extracellular volume expansion, hypertension is generally volume dependent and responsive to interventions that ameliorate the volume overload.[173, 355] In addition, elevated peripheral vascular resistance may contribute to hypertension, even in the presence of volume expansion. Whereas absolute values for plasma renin and AII in such patients may be normal, they

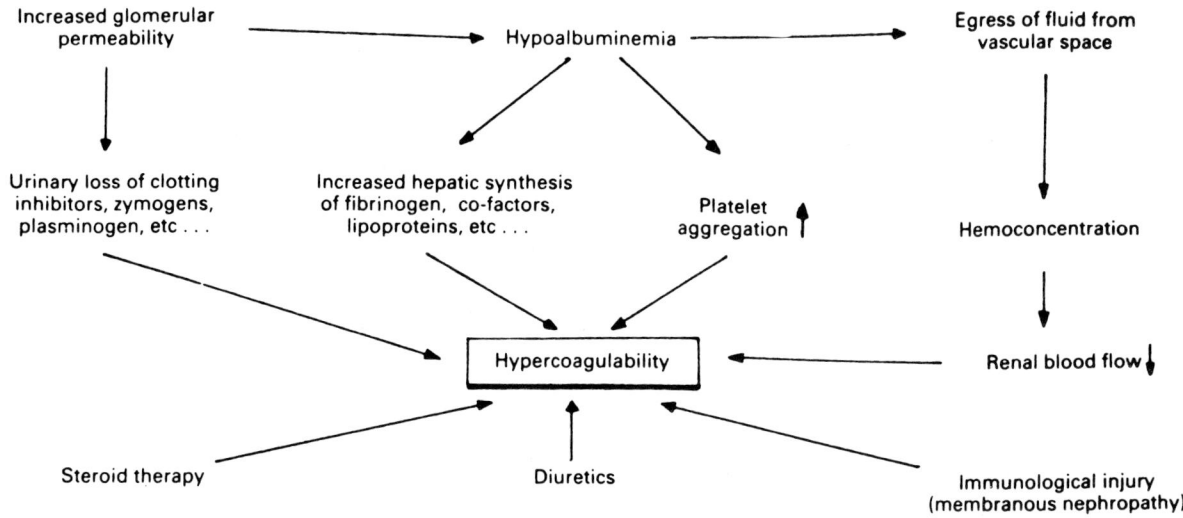

**Figure 43–13.** Schematic representation of pathogenetic factors leading to hypercoagulability, thromboembolic phenomena, and renal vein thrombosis in nephrotic syndrome. (From Llach F: Hypercoagulability, renal vein thrombosis, and other thrombotic complications of nephrotic syndrome. Kidney Int 28:429, 1985.)

are also inappropriately high for the degree of volume expansion, which suggests resetting of the $Na^+$-volume-renin feedback mechanism.[354, 356] In the nephrotic syndrome, hypertensive patients also appear to fall in the group with plasma volume expansion,[188, 190] with blood pressures falling after remission or diuretic therapy.

## Hematologic Abnormalities
(see also Chapter 50)

### HYPERCOAGULABLE STATE AND RENAL VEIN THROMBOSIS

An enhanced tendency for intravascular coagulation, with consequent risk for thromboembolic complications, also characterizes the nephrotic syndrome. The most common manifestation of this tendency is development of renal vein thrombosis, which is most frequently associated with membranous glomerulonephritis. Prospective studies of the frequency of renal vein thrombosis in patients with this disease indicate an average of about 35%, with individual studies finding a range from 5% to 62%.[241, 357, 358] The frequency is much lower in membranoproliferative glomerulonephritis, amyloidosis, minimal-change disease, and all other causes of the nephrotic syndrome. Renal vein thrombosis is now thought to represent a complication of the nephrotic syndrome related to the generalized hypercoagulable state, although a definite cause-and-effect relationship between hypercoagulability and renal vein thrombosis is not firmly established.[241] The predominant association with membranous glomerulonephritis is unexplained.

Thrombosis is not limited to the renal venous circulation, although this site predominates. The frequency of thrombotic complications at other sites ranges from 8.5% to 44%, with an average of about 20%.[357, 359] Of these, pulmonary embolism is the most frequent and serious complication. In a study of 204 children and 116 adults with nephrotic syndrome, children exhibited a lower frequency of events than

did adults. However, the complications tended to be more severe in children, almost half of whom exhibited arterial thromboses.[360]

## PATHOGENESIS OF HYPERCOAGULABILITY

The numerous abnormalities in the coagulation and hemostasis systems that accompany the nephrotic syndrome have been extensively reviewed,[111, 241, 357, 361] are discussed in detail in Chapter 50, and are briefly summarized here. These abnormalities include alterations in the levels and activities of factors in the intrinsic and extrinsic coagulation cascades, levels of antithrombotic and fibrinolytic components of plasma, platelet counts and platelet function, blood viscosity, and other factors. A pathogenetic mechanism for these abnormalities is depicted in Figure 43–13, and reported abnormalities are summarized in Table 43–1.

As reviewed by Llach,[241] abnormalities of coagulation in the nephrotic syndrome may relate to each of the five major functional classes of coagulation components: 1) zymogens (factors II, V, VII, IX, X, XI, and XII), which are activated to enzymes, and cofactors (factors V and VIII), which accelerate conversion of zymogens; 2) fibrinogen; 3) the fibrinolytic system; 4) clotting inhibitors; and 5) components of platelet reaction and thrombogenesis.

### ALTERATIONS IN ZYMOGENS AND COFACTORS

Most studies have noted deficiencies in levels of factors IX, XI, and XII,[362–367] which are likely to relate to loss of these low-molecular-weight proteins in the urine. Deficient levels of factor XII are of particular importance, because this factor regulates coagulation activity as well as the fibrinolytic and kinin-kallikrein pathways. Increases in levels of factor II and combined factors VII and X have also been

**TABLE 43–1. Coagulation Abnormalities in the Nephrotic Syndrome**

Alterations in zymogens and cofactors
  Deficiency in factors IX, XI, and XII
  Increased levels of factor II and combined factors VII and X
  Increased levels of factors V and VIII
Increased plasma fibrinogen levels
Alterations in the fibrinolytic system
  Deficiency in plasma plasminogen
  Low antiplasmin activity ($\alpha_1$-antitrypsin)
  Increased antiplasmin activity ($\alpha_2$-macroglobulin fraction)
  Increased $\alpha_2$-antiplasmin
Alterations in coagulation inhibitors
  Deficiency of antithrombin III
  Deficiency of protein S
  Deficiency of protein C (possible)
Alterations in platelet function
  Enhanced platelet aggregability
  Increased levels of $\beta$-thromboglobulin

Adapted from Llach F: Hypercoagulability, renal vein thrombosis, and other thrombotic complications of nephrotic syndrome. Used with permission from Kidney International, volume 28, page 429, 1985.

noted.[368] These zymogen abnormalities usually normalize with clinical remission from the nephrotic syndrome.[362]

The nephrotic syndrome is also characterized by increased levels of the cofactors factors V and VIII,[368–370] which may correlate inversely with the level of serum albumin.[364, 369, 370] The increased serum levels appear to result from increased hepatic synthesis, perhaps in response to the decreased $\pi$ or decreased serum albumin levels. These abnormalities in zymogens and cofactors, although present in the nephrotic syndrome, have not been clearly associated with thrombotic events.[241]

## ALTERATIONS IN FIBRINOGEN LEVELS

The nephrotic syndrome is associated with elevated plasma fibrinogen levels,[360, 368–372] which most likely result from increased hepatic synthesis with normal catabolic rates.[373] Fibrinogen levels correlate directly with urinary protein levels[373] and serum cholesterol levels and inversely with serum albumin levels.[369, 370] Fibrinogen is an important determinant of plasma viscosity, and the increased levels may be of pathogenetic importance in the hypercoagulability of the nephrotic syndrome. Indeed, a study suggests that hyperfibrinogenemia may be a major factor determining thrombotic risk by inducing fibrin deposition.[374]

## ALTERATIONS IN THE FIBRINOLYTIC SYSTEM

The data on fibrinolytic abnormalities, which are associated with thrombosis in other conditions, are somewhat conflicting in the nephrotic syndrome. Several studies have found deficiencies in plasma levels of plasminogen, with the decrease correlating with the magnitude of hypoalbuminemia and proteinuria.[375–377] Other reported abnormalities include low antiplasmin activity ($\alpha_1$-antitrypsin)[370] and increased antiplasmin activity ($\alpha_2$-macroglobulin fraction),

which is the primary plasmin inhibitor and which may be the most reliable marker of renal vein thrombosis.[378, 379]

## ALTERATIONS IN COAGULATION INHIBITORS

Nephrotic patients exhibit increased urinary losses and decreased plasma levels of the protease inhibitor antithrombin III, the most important inhibitor of coagulation and of thrombin.[360, 371, 380] Deficient serum levels of antithrombin III are sometimes[380] but not always[381] correlated with thromboembolic phenomena in nephrotic patients as well as in patients with an inherited deficiency of antithrombin III.[382] Antithrombin III deficiency occurs commonly although not universally in the nephrotic syndrome,[241] a defect that is reversible with steroid therapy.[383]

Abnormalities in other coagulation inhibitors, including protein C and protein S, may also occur in the nephrotic syndrome; congenital deficiencies of each of these are associated with recurrent venous thrombosis.[384, 385] Both of these proteins are found in the urine of nephrotic patients[386, 387]; levels of total protein S and protein C antigens are elevated, but activity of protein S is reduced owing to significant reduction in free (active) protein S levels, a consequence of elevated urinary losses.[387] Protein C anticoagulant activity is elevated, although a marked reduction in specific activity has been noted. Values for proteins C and S are not reduced in patients with nephrotic syndrome due to diabetic nephropathy.[388]

## ALTERATIONS IN PLATELET FUNCTION

Platelet counts in nephrotic patients tend to be normal[389] or elevated.[368, 369] Platelet aggregability may be increased[381, 390]; the potential contributions of hyperlipidemia and hypoalbuminemia to this abnormality are discussed elsewhere in this chapter. In addition, nephrotic patients may exhibit elevated levels of $\beta$-thromboglobulin, a specific protein released by platelets on aggregation.[391, 392]

In summary, numerous abnormalities of coagulation are found in the nephrotic syndrome. In addition to the factors described, increased blood viscosity[392, 393] due to both hyperlipidemia and increased fibrinogen may characterize the nephrotic syndrome. Steroid therapy may also exacerbate hypercoagulability in nephrotic patients.[394]

The specific role of each of these abnormalities in the pathogenesis of thromboembolic complications remains incompletely defined.[241] An increased tendency toward thrombotic events has been correlated with increased $\alpha_2$-antiplasmin levels,[379] and the presence of factor XII and prekallikrein in subepithelial deposits of patients with membranous glomerulonephritis has been noted.[395] However, a prospective study of nephrotic adults observed for an average of 21 months found significant increases in factor I, factor VIIIc, factor VIIIr:Ag, $\alpha_1$-antitrypsin and $\alpha_2$-macroglobulin, and platelet hyperaggregability in the group as a whole, but no correlation was made between these abnormalities and thromboembolic events. Low levels of antithrombin III and severe hypoalbuminemia were of no predictive value for thromboembolic events.[381] Of five patients with three potential risk factors (severe hypoalbuminemia, low antithrombin III levels, and platelet hyperaggregability), none had thromboembolic complications during the course of the study. Thus, whereas the nephrotic syndrome features various and diverse hematologic abnormalities as well as a tendency toward thromboembolic events, the relationship between these problems remains to be completely defined.

## Hormonal and Other Systemic Manifestations

Other systemic manifestations of glomerular disease, which are covered in detail elsewhere in this volume, include enhanced susceptibility to infection,[112, 361] possibly because of urinary loss of components of the alternative complement pathway (including factor B) and IgG.[396] Deficiencies of trace metals such as copper,[397] iron,[398] and zinc[397, 399] may occur. Urinary losses of thyroxine-binding globulin, triiodothyronine, and thyroxine have been noted, although patients remain euthyroid.[400] Urinary levels of corticosteroid-binding globulin[401] and insulin-like growth factor-1[402] are elevated, although the clinical consequences are unclear. Abnormalities of $Ca^{2+}$ and vitamin D metabolism also characterize the nephrotic syndrome, with hypocalcemia, hypocalciuria, and low serum levels of vitamin D.[112, 403] Urinary levels of erythropoietin are increased, and plasma levels fail to rise despite anemia.[404] Finally, extrarenal protein loss in the presence of inadequate protein intake may be associated with negative nitrogen balance and protein malnutrition.[113]

## REFERENCES

1. Maddox DA, Deen WM, Brenner BM: Glomerular filtration. *In* Windhager EE (ed): Handbook of Physiology, Sec 8, Renal Physiology. Oxford University Press, New York, 1992, p 545.
2. Kanwar YS, Liu ZZ, Kashihara N, Wallner EI: Current status of the structural and functional basis of glomerular filtration and proteinuria. Semin Nephrol 4:390, 1991.
3. Kanwar YS, Venkatachalam MA: Ultrastructure of glomerulus and juxtaglomerular apparatus. *In* Windhager EE (ed): Handbook of Physiology, Sec 8, Renal Physiology. Oxford University Press, New York, 1992, p 3.
4. Kaysen GA, Myers BD, Couser WG, et al: Mechanisms and consequences of proteinuria. Lab Invest 54:479, 1986.
5. Timpl R: Recent advances in the biochemistry of glomerular basement membrane. Kidney Int 30:293, 1986.
6. Symposium on cell and molecular biology of basement membranes in health and disease. Kidney Int 43:1, 1993.
7. Chang RL, Ueki IF, Troy JL, et al: Permselectivity of the glomerular capillary wall to macromolecules. II. Experimental studies in rats using neutral dextran. Biophys J 15:887, 1975.
8. Oliver JD III, Anderson S, Troy JL, et al: Determination of glomerular size-selectivity in the normal rat with Ficoll. J Am Soc Nephrol 3:214, 1992.
9. Bohrer MP, Deen WM, Robertson CR, Brenner BM: Mechanism of angiotensin II–induced proteinuria in the rat. Am J Physiol 233:F13, 1977.
10. Bohrer MP, Baylis C, Humes HD, et al: Permselectivity of the glomerular capillary wall. Facilitated filtration of circulating polycations. J Clin Invest 61:72, 1978.
11. Deen WM, Satvat B, Jamieson JM: Theoretical model for glomerular filtration of charged solutes. Am J Physiol 238:F126, 1980.
12. Pappenheimer JR: Passage of molecules through capillary walls. Physiol Rev 33:387, 1953.
13. Anderson JL, Quinn JA: Restricted transport in small pores. A model for steric exclusion and hindered particle motion. Biophys J 14:130, 1974.
14. Brenner BM, Baylis C, Deen WM: Transport of molecules across renal glomerular capillaries. Physiol Rev 56:502, 1976.
15. Deen WM, Bridges CR, Brenner BM: Biophysical basis of glomerular permselectivity. J Membr Biol 71:1, 1983.
16. Deen WM, Bohrer MP, Brenner BM: Macromolecule transport across glomerular capillaries. Application of pore theory. Kidney Int 16:353, 1979.
17. Winetz JA, Robertson CR, Golbetz HV, et al: The nature of the glomerular injury in minimal change and focal sclerosing glomerulopathies. Am J Kidney Dis 1:91, 1981.
18. Deen WM, Bridges CR, Brenner BM, Myers BD: Heteroporous model of glomerular size selectivity: Application to normal and nephrotic humans. Am J Physiol 249:F374, 1985.
19. Remuzzi A, Battaglia C, Rossa L, et al: Glomerular size selectivity in nephrotic rats exposed to diets with different protein contents. Am J Physiol 253:F318, 1987.
20. Chang RL, Deen WM, Robertson CR, Brenner BM: Permselectivity of the glomerular capillary wall. III. Restricted transport of polyanions. Kidney Int 8:212, 1975.
21. Brenner BM, Hostetter TH, Humes HD: Molecular basis of proteinuria of glomerular origin. N Engl J Med 298:826, 1978.
22. Chang RLS, Deen WM, Robertson CR, et al: Permselectivity of the glomerular capillary wall: Studies of experimental glomerulonephritis in the rat using neutral dextran. J Clin Invest 57:1272, 1976.
23. Bennett CM, Glassock RJ, Chang RLS, et al: Permselectivity of the glomerular capillary wall: Studies of experimental glomerulonephritis in the rat using dextran sulfate. J Clin Invest 57:1287, 1976.
24. Bohrer MP, Deen WM, Robertson CR, et al: Influence of molecular configuration on the passage of macromolecules across the glomerular capillary wall. J Gen Physiol 74:583, 1979.
25. Farquhar MG, Wissig SL, Palade GE: Glomerular permeability. I. Ferritin transfer across the normal glomerular capillary wall. J Exp Med 113:47, 1961.
26. Graham RC, Karnovsky MJ: Glomerular permeability: Ultrastructural cytochemical studies using peroxidases as protein tracers. J Exp Med 124:1123, 1966.
27. Graham RC, Kellermeyer RW: Bovine lactoperoxidase as a cytochemical protein tracer for electron microscopy. J Histochem Cytochem 16:275, 1968.
28. Venkatachalam MA, Cotran RS, Karnovsky MJ: An ultrastructural study of glomerular permeability in aminonucleoside nephrosis using catalase as a tracer protein. J Exp Med 132:1168, 1970.
29. Caulfield JP, Farquhar MG: The permeability of glomerular capillaries to graded dextrans. J Cell Biol 63:883, 1974.
30. Farquhar MG: The primary glomerular filtration barrier: Basement membrane or epithelial slits? Kidney Int 8:197, 1975.
31. Rennke HG, Cotran RS, Venkatachalam MA: Role of molecular charge in glomerular permeability: Tracer studies with cationized ferritins. J Cell Biol 67:638, 1975.
32. Venkatachalam MA, Rennke HG: The structural and molecular basis of glomerular filtration. Circ Res 43:337, 1978.
33. Caulfield JP, Farquhar MG: Distribution of anionic sites in glomerular basement membranes: Their possible role in filtration and attachment. Proc Natl Acad Sci USA 73:1646, 1976.
34. Kerjaschki D, Sharkey DJ, Farquhar MG: Identification and characterization of podocalyxin—the major sialoprotein of the renal glomerular epithelial cell. J Cell Biol 98:1591, 1984.
35. Spiro RG: Studies on the renal glomerular basement membrane: Preparation and chemical composition. J Biol Chem 242:1915, 1967.
36. Dekan G, Gabel CA, Farquhar MG: Sulfate contributes to the negative charge of podocalyxin—the major sialoglycoprotein of the filtration slits. Proc Natl Acad Sci USA 88:5398, 1991.
37. Kanwar YS, Farquhar MG: Presence of heparan sulfate in the glomerular basement membrane. Proc Natl Acad Sci USA 76:1303, 1979.
38. Kanwar YS, Veis A, Kimura JH, Jakubowski ML: Characterization of heparan sulfate proteoglycan of glomerular basement membranes. Proc Natl Acad Sci USA 81:762, 1984.
39. Kelley VE, Cavallo T: Glomerular permeability: Transfer of native ferritin in glomeruli with decreased anionic sites. Lab Invest 39:547, 1978.

40. Hunsicker LG, Shearer TP, Shaffer SJ: Acute reversible proteinuria induced by infusion of the polycation hexadimethrine. Kidney Int 20:7, 1981.

41. Barnes JL, Radnik RA, Gilchrist EP, Venkatachalam MA: Size and charge selective permeability defects induced in glomerular basement membrane by a polycation. Kidney Int 25:11, 1984.

42. Kanwar YS, Linker A, Farquhar MG: Increased permeability of the glomerular basement membrane to ferritin after removal of glycosaminoglycans (heparan sulfate) by enzyme digestion. J Cell Biol 86:688, 1980.

43. Rosenzweig LJ, Kanwar YS: Removal of sulfated (heparan sulfate) or nonsulfated (hyaluronic acid) glycosaminoglycans results in increased permeability of the glomerular basement membrane to [125]I-bovine serum albumin. Lab Invest 47:177, 1982.

44. Kanwar YS, Rosenzweig LJ: Clogging of the glomerular basement membrane. J Cell Biol 93:489, 1982.

45. Kanwar YS, Rosenzweig LJ: Altered glomerular permeability as a result of focal detachment of visceral epithelium. Kidney Int 21:565, 1982.

46. Vernier RL, Klein DJ, Sisson SP, et al: Heparan sulfate–rich anionic sites in the human glomerular basement membrane. Decreased concentration in congenital nephrotic syndrome. N Engl J Med 309:1001, 1983.

47. Vehaskari VM, Root ER, Germuth FG Jr, Robson AM: Glomerular charge and urinary protein excretion: Effects of systemic and intrarenal polycation infusion in the rat. Kidney Int 22:127, 1982.

48. Kasinath BS, Singh AK, Kanwar YS, et al: Effect of aminonucleoside puromycin on the heparan sulfate–proteoglycan core protein content of glomerular epithelial cells. Am J Physiol 255:F590, 1988.

49. Mynderse LA, Hassell JR, Kleinman HK, et al: Loss of heparan sulfate proteoglycan from glomerular basement membrane of nephrotic rats. Lab Invest 48:292, 1983.

50. Grond J, Elema JD: Localization and distribution of anionic charges in the glomerular mesangium of normal and nephrotic rats. Virchows Arch B 48:135, 1985.

51. Kanwar YS, Jakubowski ML: Unaltered anionic sites of glomerular basement membrane in aminonucleoside nephrosis. Kidney Int 25:613, 1984.

52. Lelongt B, Makino H, Kanwar YS: Status of glomerular proteoglycans in aminonucleoside nephrosis. Kidney Int 31:1299, 1987.

53. Groggel GC, Hovingh P, Border WA, Linker A: Changes in glomerular heparan sulfate in puromycin aminonucleoside nephrosis. Am J Pathol 128:521, 1987.

54. Groggel GC, Stevenson J, Hovingh P, et al: Changes in heparan sulfate correlate with increased glomerular permeability. Kidney Int 33:517, 1988.

55. Daniels BS, Hauser EB, Deen WM, Hostetter TH: Glomerular basement membrane: In vitro studies of water and protein permeability. Am J Physiol 262:F919, 1992.

56. Daniels BS, Deen WM, Mayer G, et al: Glomerular permeability barrier in the rat. Functional assessment by in vitro methods. J Clin Invest 92:929, 1993.

57. Savin VJ, Sharma R, Lovell HB, Welling DJ: Measurement of albumin reflection coefficient with isolated rat glomeruli. J Am Soc Nephrol 3:1260, 1992.

58. Chang RLS, Robertson CR, Deen WM, Brenner BM: Permselectivity of the glomerular capillary wall to macromolecules: I. Theoretical considerations. Biophys J 15:861, 1975.

59. Baylis C, Ichikawa I, Willis WT, et al: Dynamics of glomerular ultrafiltration. IX. Effects of plasma protein concentration. Am J Physiol 232:F58, 1977.

60. Olson JL, Hostetter TH, Rennke HG, et al: Altered glomerular permselectivity and progressive sclerosis following extreme ablation of renal mass. Kidney Int 22:112, 1982.

61. Yoshioka T, Shiraga H, Yoshida Y, et al: "Intact nephrons" as the primary origin of proteinuria in chronic renal disease. Study in the rat model of subtotal nephrectomy. J Clin Invest 82:1614, 1988.

62. Mayer G, Lafayette RA, Oliver J, et al: Effects of angiotensin II receptor blockade on remnant glomerular permselectivity. Kidney Int 43:346, 1993.

63. Michels LD, Davidman M, Keane WF: Glomerular permeability to neutral and anionic dextrans in experimental diabetes. Kidney Int 21:699, 1982.

64. Remuzzi A, Perico N, Amuchasteugui CS, et al: Short- and long-term effect of angiotensin II receptor blockade in rats with experimental diabetes. J Am Soc Nephrol 4:40, 1993.

65. Bohrer MP, Baylis C, Robertson CR, Brenner BM: Mechanism of the puromycin-induced defects in the transglomerular passage of water and macromolecules. J Clin Invest 60:152, 1977.

66. Olson JL, Rennke HG, Venkatachalam MA: Alterations in the charge and size selectivity barrier of the glomerular filter in aminonucleoside nephrosis in rats. Lab Invest 44:271, 1981.

67. Bertolatus JA, Abuyousef M, Hunsicker LG: Glomerular sieving of high molecular weight proteins in proteinuric rats. Kidney Int 31:1257, 1987.

68. Weening JJ, Rennke HG: Glomerular permeability and polyanion in adriamycin nephrosis in the rat. Kidney Int 24:152, 1983.

69. Alfino PA, Neugarten J, Schacht RG, et al: Glomerular size-selective barrier dysfunction in nephrotoxic serum nephritis. Kidney Int 34:151, 1988.

70. Neugarten J, Kozin A, Cook K: Effect of indomethacin on glomerular permselectivity and hemodynamics in nephrotoxic serum nephritis. Kidney Int 36:51, 1989.

71. Neugarten J, Kaminetsky B, Feiner H, et al: Nephrotoxic serum nephritis with hypertension: Amelioration by antihypertensive therapy. Kidney Int 28:135, 1985.

72. Neugarten J, Alfino P, Langs C, et al: Nephrotoxic serum nephritis with hypertension: Perfusion pressure and permselectivity. Kidney Int 33:53, 1988.

73. Yoshioka T, Rennke HG, Salant DJ, et al: Role of abnormally high transmural pressure in the permselectivity defect of glomerular capillary wall: A study in early passive Heymann nephritis. Circ Res 61:531, 1987.

74. Yoshioka T, Mitarai T, Kon V, et al: Role for angiotensin II in overt functional proteinuria. Kidney Int 30:538, 1986.

75. Baylis C, Fredericks M, Leypoldt J, et al: The mechanisms of proteinuria in aging rats. Mech Ageing Dev 45:111, 1988.

76. Lemley KV: Glomerular size selectivity during protein overload in the rat. Am J Physiol 264:F1046, 1993.

77. Simons JL, Oliver JD, Provoost AP, et al: Reduction of glomerular hypertension prevents development of focal glomerular sclerosis, and preserves glomerular charge-selectivity in uninephrectomized fawn-hooded rats: Effects of $N^\omega$-nitro-L-arginine methyl ester (L-NAME) and enalapril. Proc Int Congr Nephrol 51, 1993. Abstract.

78. Remuzzi A, Puntorieri S, Battaglia C, et al: Angiotensin converting enzyme inhibition ameliorates glomerular filtration of macromolecules and water and lessens glomerular injury in the rat. J Clin Invest 85:541, 1990.

79. Williams SK, Siegal RK: Preferential transport of non-enzymatically glucosylated ferritin across the kidney glomerulus. Kidney Int 28:146, 1985.

80. Daniels BS, Hauser EB: Glycation of albumin, not glomerular basement membrane, alters permeability in an in vitro model. Diabetes 41:1415, 1992.

81. Vernier RL, Steffes MW, Sisson-Ross S, Mauer SM: Heparan sulfate proteoglycan in the glomerular basement membrane in type I diabetes mellitus. Kidney Int 41:1070, 1992.

82. Ryan GB, Karnovsky MJ: An ultrastructural study of the mechanisms of proteinuria in aminonucleoside nephrosis. Kidney Int 8:219, 1975.

83. Loon N, Shemesh O, Morelli E, Myers BD: Effect of angiotensin II infusion on the human glomerular filtration barrier. Am J Physiol 257:F608, 1989.

84. Joachim GR, Cameron JS, Schwartz M, Becker EL: Selectivity of protein excretion in patients with the nephrotic syndrome. J Clin Invest 43:2332, 1964.

85. Myers BD, Okarma TB, Friedman S, et al: Mechanisms of proteinuria in human glomerulonephritis. J Clin Invest 70:732, 1982.

86. Carrie BJ, Myers BD: Proteinuria and functional characteristics of the glomerular barrier in diabetic nephropathy. Kidney Int 17:669, 1980.

87. Carrie BJ, Salyers WR, Myers BD: Minimal change nephropathy: An electrochemical disorder of the glomerular membrane. Am J Med 70:262, 1981.

88. Guasch A, Deen WM, Myers BD: Charge selectivity of the glomerular filtration barrier in healthy and nephrotic humans. J Clin Invest 92:2274, 1993.

89. Shemesh O, Ross JC, Deen WM, et al: Nature of the glomerular capillary injury in human membranous glomerulopathy. J Clin Invest 77:868, 1986.

90. Guasch A, Sibley RK, Huie P, Myers BD: Extent and course of

glomerular injury in human membranous glomerulopathy. Am J Physiol 263:F1034, 1992.

91. Meyer TW: Mechanisms of proteinuria in diabetic renal disease. Semin Nephrol 10:194, 1990.

92. Viberti GC, Mackintosh D, Keen H: Determinants of the penetration of proteins through the glomerular barrier in insulin-dependent diabetes mellitus. Diabetes 32(suppl 2):92, 1983.

93. Di Mario U, Bacci S, Morano S, et al: Selective decrement of anionic immunoglobulin clearance after induced renal hemodynamic changes in diabetic patients. Am J Physiol 262:F381, 1992.

94. Scandling JD, Myers BD: Glomerular size-selectivity and microalbuminuria in early diabetic glomerular disease. Kidney Int 41:840, 1992.

95. Nakamura Y, Myers BD: Charge selectivity of proteinuria in diabetic glomerulopathy. Diabetes 37:1202, 1988.

96. Austin SM, Lieberman JS, Newton LD, et al: Slope of glomerular filtration rate and the progression of diabetic glomerular disease. J Am Soc Nephrol 3:1358, 1993.

97. Deckert T, Kofoed-Enevoldsen A, Vidal P, et al: Size- and charge selectivity of glomerular filtration in type I (insulin-dependent) diabetic patients with and without albuminuria. Diabetologia 36:244, 1993.

98. Chagnac A, Kiberd BA, Fariñas MC, et al: Outcome of the acute glomerular injury in proliferative lupus nephritis. J Clin Invest 84:922, 1989.

99. Myers BD, Chagnac A, Golbetz H, et al: Extent of glomerular injury in active and resolving lupus nephritis: A theoretical analysis. Am J Physiol 260:F717, 1991.

100. Myers BD: Pathophysiology of proteinuria in immune glomerular injury. Am J Nephrol 10(suppl 1):19, 1990.

101. Ghiggeri GM, Candiano G, Delfino G, Queirolo C: Electrical charge of serum and urinary albumin in normal and diabetic humans. Kidney Int 28:168, 1985.

102. Melvin T, Kim Y, Michael AF: Selective binding of IgG₄ and other negatively charged plasma proteins in normal and diabetic human kidneys. Am J Pathol 115:443, 1984.

103. Shemesh O, Deen WM, Brenner BM, et al: Effect of colloid volume expansion on glomerular barrier size-selectivity in humans. Kidney Int 29:916, 1986.

104. Loon N, Chagnac A, Parra L, et al: Filtration dynamics and natriuretic response to volume expansion in humans. Am J Physiol 263:F284, 1992.

105. Rosenberg ME, Swanson JE, Thomas BL, Hostetter TH: Glomerular and hormonal responses to dietary protein intake in human renal disease. Am J Physiol 253:F1083, 1987.

106. Golbetz H, Black V, Shemesh O, Myers BD: Mechanism of the antiproteinuric effect of indomethacin in nephrotic humans. Am J Physiol 256:F44, 1989.

107. Rosenberg ME, Hostetter TH: Comparative effects of antihypertensives on proteinuria: Angiotensin-converting enzyme versus α₁-antagonist. Am J Kidney Dis 18:472, 1991.

108. Morelli E, Loon N, Meyer T, et al: Effects of converting-enzyme inhibition on barrier function in diabetic glomerulopathy. Diabetes 39:76, 1990.

109. Remuzzi A, Perticucci E, Ruggenenti P, et al: Angiotensin converting enzyme inhibition improves glomerular size-selectivity in IgA nephropathy. Kidney Int 39:1267, 1991.

110. Remuzzi A, Ruggenenti P, Mosconi L, et al: Effect of low-dose enalapril on glomerular size-selectivity in human diabetic nephropathy. J Nephrol 6:36, 1993.

111. Bernard DB: Extrarenal complications of the nephrotic syndrome. Kidney Int 33:1184, 1988.

112. Bernard DB: Metabolic complications in nephrotic syndrome: Pathophysiology and complications. In Brenner BM, Stein JH (eds): The Nephrotic Syndrome. Churchill Livingstone, New York, 1982, p 85.

113. Kaysen GA: Albumin metabolism in the nephrotic syndrome: The effect of dietary protein intake. Am J Kidney Dis 12:461, 1988.

114. Rothschild MA, Oratz M, Schreiber SS: Albumin synthesis. N Engl J Med 286:748, 1972.

115. Kaysen GA, Schoenfeld PY: Albumin homeostasis in patients undergoing continuous ambulatory peritoneal dialysis. Kidney Int 25:107, 1984.

116. Waldmann TA: Albumin catabolism. In Rosemoer M, Oratz M, Rothschild A (eds): Albumin Structure, Function and Use. Pergamon, New York, 1977, p 255.

117. Sellers AL, Katz J, Bonorris G, et al: Determination of extravascular albumin in the rat. J Lab Clin Med 68:177, 1966.

118. Katz J, Bonorris G, Okuyama S, Sellers AL: Albumin synthesis in perfused liver of normal and nephrotic rats. Am J Physiol 212:1255, 1967.

119. Katz J, Rosenfeld S, Sellers AL: Role of the kidney in plasma albumin catabolism. Am J Physiol 198:814, 1960.

120. Yedgar S, Carew TW, Pittman RC, et al: Tissue sites of catabolism of albumin in rabbits. Am J Physiol 244:E101, 1983.

121. Earley LE, Havel RJ, Hopper J, et al: Nephrotic syndrome. Calif Med 115:23, 1971.

122. Jensen H, Jarnum S, Hart Nansen JP: Gastrointestinal protein loss and intestinal function in the nephrotic syndrome. Nephron 3:209, 1966.

123. Yssing M, Jensen H, Jarnum S: Albumin metabolism and gastrointestinal protein loss in children with nephrotic syndrome. Acta Paediatr Scand 58:109, 1969.

124. Johansson SV, Odar-Cederlog I, Plantin LO, Strandberg PO: Albumin metabolism and gastrointestinal loss of proteins in chronic renal failure. Acta Med Scand 201:353, 1977.

125. Schultze G, Ahuja S, Faber U, Molzahn M: Gastrointestinal protein loss in the nephrotic syndrome studied with ⁵¹Cr-albumin. Nephron 25:227, 1980.

126. Gitlin D, Janeway CA, Farr LE: Studies on the metabolism of plasma proteins in the nephrotic syndrome. I. Albumin, gamma-globulin, and iron-binding globulin. J Clin Invest 35:44, 1956.

127. Kaysen GA, Gambertoglio J, Jimenez I, et al: Effect of dietary protein intake on albumin homeostasis in nephrotic patients. Kidney Int 29:572, 1986.

128. Ballmer PE, Weber BK, Roy-Chaudhury P, et al: Elevation of albumin synthesis rates in nephrotic patients measured with [1-¹³C]leucine. Kidney Int 41:132, 1992.

129. Lewandowski AE, Liao WSL, Stinson-Fisher CA, et al: Effects of experimentally induced nephrosis on protein synthesis in rat liver. Am J Physiol 254:C634, 1988.

130. Yamauchi A, Fukuhara Y, Yamamoto S, et al: Oncotic pressure regulates gene transcriptions of albumin and apolipoprotein B in cultured rat hepatoma cells. Am J Physiol 263:C397, 1992.

131. Sun X, Martin V, Weiss RH, Kaysen GA: Selective transcriptional augmentation of hepatic gene expression in the rat with Heymann nephritis. Am J Physiol 264:F441, 1993.

132. Pietrangelo A, Panduro A, Chowdhury JR, Shafritz DA: Albumin gene expression is down-regulated by albumin or macromolecule infusion in the rat. J Clin Invest 89:1755, 1992.

133. Yamauchi A, Imai E, Noguchi T, et al: Albumin gene transcription is enhanced in liver of nephrotic rats. Am J Physiol 254:E676, 1988.

134. Kaysen GA, Jones H Jr, Martin V, Hutchison FN: A low protein diet restricts albumin synthesis in nephrotic rats. J Clin Invest 81:1623, 1989.

135. Hoffenberg R: Control of albumin degradation in vivo and in the perfused liver. In Rothschild MA, Waldmann T (eds): Plasma Protein Metabolism Regulation of Synthesis, Distribution, and Degradation. Academic Press, New York, 1970, p 239.

136. Katz J, Sellers AL, Bonorris G: Effect of nephrectomy on plasma albumin catabolism in experimental nephrosis. J Lab Clin Med 63:680, 1964.

137. Katz J, Bonorris G, Sellers AL: Albumin metabolism in aminonucleoside nephrotic rats. J Lab Clin Med 62:910, 1963.

138. Galaske RG, Baldamus CA, Stolte H: Plasma protein handling in the rat kidney: Micropuncture experiments in the acute heterologous phase of anti-GBM–nephritis. Pflugers Arch 375:269, 1978.

139. Exaire E, Pollak VE, Pesce AJ, Ooi BS: Albumin and gamma-globulin in the nephron of the normal rat and following the injection of aminonucleoside. Nephron 9:42, 1972.

140. Olbricht CJ, Cannon JK, Tisher CC: Cathepsin B and L in nephron segments of rats with puromycin aminonucleoside nephrosis. Kidney Int 32:354, 1987.

141. Park CH, Maack T: Albumin absorption and catabolism by isolated perfused proximal convoluted tubules of the rabbit. J Clin Invest 73:767, 1984.

142. Eisenbach GM, van Liew JB, Boylan JW: Effect of angiotensin on the filtration of protein in the rat kidney. A micropuncture study. Kidney Int 8:80, 1975.

143. Landwehr DM, Carvallo JS, Oken DE: Micropuncture studies of the filtration and absorption of albumin by nephrotic rats. Kidney Int 11:9, 1977.

144. Jensen H, Rossing N, Anderson SB, Jarnum S: Albumin metabolism in the nephrotic syndrome in adults. Clin Sci 33:445, 1967.

145. Kaysen GA, Kirkpatrick WG, Couser WG: Albumin homeostasis in the nephrotic rat: Nutritional considerations. Am J Physiol 247:F192, 1984.

146. Sellers AL, Katz J, Bonorris G: Albumin distribution in the nephrotic rat. J Lab Clin Med 71:511, 1968.

147. Kaysen GA, Al-Bander H: Metabolism of albumin and immunoglobulins in the nephrotic syndrome. Am J Nephrol 10(suppl 1):36, 1990.

148. Oratz M: Oncotic pressure and albumin synthesis. *In* Bianchi R, Mariani AS, McFarlane AS (eds): Plasma Protein Turnover. University Park Press, Baltimore, 1976, p 223.

149. Rothschild MA, Oratz M, Evans CD, et al: Role of hepatic interstitial albumin in regulating albumin synthesis. Am J Physiol 210:57, 1966.

150. Kaysen GA, Jones H Jr, Hutchison FN: High protein diets stimulate albumin synthesis at the site of albumin mRNA transcription. Kidney Int 36(suppl 27):S-168, 1989.

151. Castro CE, Sevall JS: Hepatic level of rat albumin messenger RNA is influenced by factors other than dietary protein. J Nutr 115:491, 1985.

152. Hutchison FN, Schambelan M, Kaysen GA: Modulation of albuminuria by dietary protein and converting enzyme inhibition. Am J Physiol 253:F192, 1987.

153. Kaysen GA, Rosenthal C, Hutchison FN: GFR increases before renal mass or ODC activity increase in rats fed high protein diets. Kidney Int 36:441, 1989.

154. Paller MS, Hostetter TH: Dietary protein increases plasma renin and reduces pressor activity to angiotensin II. Am J Physiol 251:F34, 1986.

155. Kaysen GA, Martin VI, Jones H Jr: Arginine augments neither albuminuria nor albumin synthesis caused by high-protein diets in nephrosis. Am J Physiol 263:F907, 1992.

156. Kaysen GA, Al-Bander H, Martin VI, et al: Branch chain amino acids augment neither albuminuria nor albumin synthesis in nephrotic rats. Am J Physiol 260:F177, 1991.

157. Don B, Kaysen GA, Hutchison FN, Schambelan M: The effect of angiotensin-converting enzyme inhibition and dietary protein restriction in the treatment of proteinuria. Am J Kidney Dis 17:10, 1991.

158. Peavey DE, Taylor JM, Jefferson LS: Correlation of albumin production rates and albumin mRNA levels in livers of normal, diabetic and insulin-treated diabetic rats. Proc Natl Acad Sci USA 75:5879, 1978.

159. Lloyd CE, Kalinyak JE, Hutson SM, Jefferson LS: Time course of changes in albumin synthesis and mRNA in diabetic and insulin-treated diabetic rats. Am J Physiol 252:C205, 1987.

160. De Feo P, Gaisano MG, Haymond MW: Differential effects of insulin deficiency on albumin and fibrinogen synthesis in humans. J Clin Invest 88:833, 1991.

161. Siddiqui UA, Goldflam T, Goodridge AG: Nutritional and hormonal regulation of the translatable levels of malic enzyme and albumin mRNAs in avian liver cells in vivo and in culture. J Biol Chem 256:4544, 1981.

162. Keller GH, Taylor JM: Effect of hypophysectomy on the synthesis of rat liver albumin. J Biol Chem 251:3768, 1976.

163. Kernoff LM, Pimstone BL, Solomon J, et al: The effect of hypophysectomy and growth hormone replacement on albumin synthesis and catabolism in the rat. Biochem J 124:529, 1971.

164. Moshage HJ, Haard HJW, Princen HMG, et al: The influence of glucocorticoid on albumin synthesis and its messenger RNA in rat in vivo and in hepatocyte suspension culture. Biochim Biophys Acta 824:27, 1985.

165. Moshage HJ, Janssen JAM, Franssen JH, et al: Study of the molecular mechanism of decreased liver synthesis of albumin in inflammation. J Clin Invest 79:1635, 1987.

166. Suranyi MG, Guasch A, Hall BM, Myers BD: Elevated levels of tumor necrosis factor-α in the nephrotic syndrome in humans. Am J Kidney Dis 21:251, 1993.

167. Humphreys MH: Mechanisms and management of nephrotic edema. Kidney Int 45:266, 1994.

168. Intaglietta M, Zweifach BW: Microcirculatory basis of fluid exchange. Adv Biol Med Phys 15:11, 1974.

169. Bradley SE: The pathophysiology of hypoproteinemic edema. Contrib Nephrol 21:75, 1980.

170. Aukland K, Nicolaysen G: Interstitial fluid volume: Local regulatory mechanisms. Physiol Rev 61:556, 1981.

171. Brace RA, Guyton A: Effect of hindlimb isolation procedure on isogravimetric capillary pressure and transcapillary fluid dynamics in dogs. Circ Res 38:192, 1976.

172. Ichikawa I, Rennke HG, Hoyer JR, et al: Role for intrarenal mechanisms in the impaired salt excretion of experimental nephrotic syndrome. J Clin Invest 71:91, 1983.

173. Glassock RJ: Sodium homeostasis in acute glomerulonephritis and the nephrotic syndrome. Contrib Nephrol 23:181, 1980.

174. Schrier RW: Pathogenesis of sodium and water retention in high-output and low-output cardiac failure, nephrotic syndrome, cirrhosis, and pregnancy. N Engl J Med 319:1065, 1988.

175. Noddeland H, Riisnes SM, Fadnes HO: Interstitial fluid colloid osmotic and hydrostatic pressures in subcutaneous tissue of patients with nephrotic syndrome. Scand J Clin Lab Invest 42:139, 1982.

176. Reed RK: Interstitial fluid volume, colloid osmotic and hydrostatic pressure in rat skeletal muscle. Effect of hypoproteinemia. Acta Physiol Scand 112:141, 1981.

177. Golden MHN, Golden BE, Jackson AA: Albumin and nutritional oedema. Lancet 1:114, 1980.

178. Koomans HA, Kortlandt W, Geers AB, Dorhout Mees EJ: Lowered protein content of tissue fluid in patients with the nephrotic syndrome: Observations during disease and recovery. Nephron 40:391, 1985.

179. Fadnes HO, Pape JF, Sundsfjord JA: A study on oedema mechanism in nephrotic syndrome. Scand J Clin Lab Invest 46:533, 1986.

180. Fadnes HO, Reed RK, Aukland K: Mechanisms regulating interstitial fluid volume. Lymphology 11:165, 1978.

181. Crockett DJ: The protein levels of oedema fluids. Lancet 2:1179, 1956.

182. Perico N, Remuzzi G: Edema of the nephrotic syndrome: The role of the atrial peptide system. Am J Kidney Dis 22:355, 1993.

183. Squire JR: The nephrotic syndrome. Adv Intern Med 7:201, 1955.

184. Brown E, Hopper J Jr, Wennesland R: Blood volume and its regulation. Annu Rev Physiol 19:231, 1957.

185. Bernard DB, Alexander EA: Edema formation in the nephrotic syndrome: Pathophysiologic mechanisms. Cardiovasc Med 4:605, 1979.

186. Benhold H, Klaus D, Scheurlen PG: Volume regulation and renal function in analbuminemia. Lancet 2:1169, 1960.

187. Joles JA, Willekes-Koolschijn N, Braam B, et al: Colloid osmotic pressure in young analbuminemic rats. Am J Physiol 245:H284, 1983.

188. Meltzer JL, Keim HJ, Laragh JH, et al: Nephrotic syndrome: Vasoconstriction and hypervolemic types indicated by renin-sodium profiling. Ann Intern Med 91:688, 1979.

189. Brown EA, Markandu ND, Roulston JE, et al: Is the renin-angiotensin-aldosterone system involved in the sodium retention in the nephrotic syndrome? Nephron 32:102, 1982.

190. Dorhout Mees EJ, Roos JC, Boer P, et al: Observations on edema formation in the nephrotic syndrome in adults with minimal lesions. Am J Med 67:378, 1979.

191. Geers AB, Koomans HA, Boer P, Dorhout Mees EJ: Plasma volume measurements in patients with nephrotic syndrome. Kidney Int 23:123, 1983.

192. Dorhout Mees EJ, Geers AB, Koomans HA: Blood volume and sodium retention in the nephrotic syndrome: A controversial pathophysiological concept. Nephron 36:201, 1984.

193. Brown EA, Markandu N, Sagnella GA, et al: Sodium retention in nephrotic syndrome is due to an intrarenal defect: Evidence from steroid-induced remission. Nephron 39:290, 1985.

194. Koomans HA, Braam B, Geers AB, et al: The importance of plasma protein for blood volume and blood pressure homeostasis. Kidney Int 30:730, 1986.

195. Koomans HA, Geers AB, Dorhout Mees EJ, Kortlandt W: Lowered tissue-fluid oncotic pressure protects the blood volume in the nephrotic syndrome. Nephron 42:317, 1986.

196. Shapiro MD, Nicholls KM, Groves BM, Schrier RW: Role of glomerular filtration rate in the impaired sodium and water excretion of patients with the nephrotic syndrome. Am J Kidney Dis 8:81, 1986.

197. Tulassay T, Rascher W, Lange RE, et al: Atrial natriuretic peptide and other vasoactive hormones in nephrotic syndrome. Kidney Int 31:1391, 1987.

198. Usberti M, Federico S, Meccariello S, et al: Role of plasma vasopressin in the impairment of water excretion in nephrotic syndrome. Kidney Int 25:422, 1984.

199. Koomans HA, Geers AB, van der Meiracker AH, et al: Effects of

plasma volume expansion on renal salt handling in patients with the nephrotic syndrome. Am J Nephrol 4:227, 1984.

200. Brown EA, Markandu ND, Sagnella GA, et al: Evidence that some mechanism other than the renin system causes sodium retention in nephrotic syndrome. Lancet 2:1237, 1982.

201. Berlyne GM, Sutton J, Brown C, et al: Renal salt and water handling in water immersion in the nephrotic syndrome. Clin Sci 61:605, 1981.

202. Krishna GG, Danovitch GM: Effects of water immersion on renal function in the nephrotic syndrome. Kidney Int 21:395, 1982.

203. Rascher W, Tulassay T, Seyberth HW, et al: Diuretic and hormonal responses to head-out water immersion in nephrotic syndrome. J Pediatr 109:609, 1986.

204. Koomans HA, Boer WH, Dorhout Mees EJ: Renal function during recovery from minimal lesions nephrotic syndrome. Nephron 47:173, 1987.

205. Kaysen GA, Pukert TT, Menke DJ, et al: Plasma volume expansion is necessary for edema formation in the rat with Heymann nephritis. Am J Physiol 248:F247, 1985.

206. Fauchald P, Noddeland H, Norseth J: An evaluation of ultrafiltration as treatment of diuretic-resistant oedema in nephrotic syndrome. Acta Med Scand 217:127, 1985.

207. Wagnild JP, Gutmann FD: Functional adaptation to nephrons in dogs with acute progressing to chronic experimental glomerulonephritis. J Clin Invest 57:1575, 1976.

208. Chandra M, Hoyer JR, Lewy JE: Renal function in rats with unilateral proteinuria produced by renal perfusion with aminonucleoside. Pediatr Res 15:340, 1976.

209. Peterson C, Madsen B, Perlmann A, et al: Atrial natriuretic peptide and renal response to hypervolemia in nephrotic humans. Kidney Int 34:825, 1988.

210. Shapiro MD, Hasbargen J, Hensen J, Schrier RW: Role of aldosterone in the sodium retention of patients with nephrotic syndrome. Am J Nephrol 10:44, 1990.

211. Perico N, Delaini F, Lupini C, Remuzzi G: Renal response to atrial peptides is reduced in experimental nephrosis. Am J Physiol 252:F654, 1987.

212. Perico N, Delaini F, Lupini C, et al: Blunted excretory response to atrial natriuretic peptide in experimental nephrosis. Kidney Int 36:57, 1989.

213. DiBona GF, Herman PJ, Sawin LL: Neural control of renal function in edema-forming states. Am J Physiol 254:R1017, 1988.

214. Valentin J-P, Qiu CQ, Muldowney WP, et al: Cellular basis for blunted volume expansion natriuresis in experimental nephrotic syndrome. J Clin Invest 90:1302, 1992.

215. Orisio S, Perico N, Benatti L, et al: Renal cyclophilin-like protein gene expression parallels changes in sodium excretion in experimental nephrosis and is positively modulated by atrial natriuretic peptide. J Am Soc Nephrol 3:746, 1992. Abstract.

216. Klahr S, Alleyne GAO: Effects of chronic protein-calorie malnutrition on the kidney. Kidney Int 3:129, 1973.

217. Vereerstraeten P, Toussaint C: Effects of plasmapheresis on renal hemodynamics and sodium excretion in dogs. Pflugers Arch 306:92, 1969.

218. Anderson S, Diamond JR, Karnovsky MJ, Brenner BM: Mechanisms underlying transition from acute glomerular injury to late glomerular sclerosis in a rat model of nephrotic syndrome. J Clin Invest 82:1757, 1988.

219. Meyer TW, Rennke HG: Increased single-nephron protein excretion after renal ablation in nephrotic rats. Am J Physiol 255:F1243, 1988.

220. Nagase S, Shimamune K, Shumiya S: Albumin-deficient rat mutant. Science 205:590, 1979.

221. Sanfelice NFT, Fujihara CK, Marcondes M, et al: Glomerular hemodynamics and fluid compartments in the analbuminemic rat. Kidney Int 35:473, 1989. Abstract.

222. Miller PL, Meyer TW: Plasma protein concentration and colloid osmotic pressure in nephrotic rats. Kidney Int 34:220, 1988.

223. Aronoff GR, Abel SR: Principles of administering drugs to patients with renal failure. *In* Bennett WM, McCarron DA, Brenner BM, Stein JH (eds): Pharmacotherapy of Renal Disease and Hypertension. Churchill Livingstone, New York, 1987, p 1.

224. Bennett WM, Aronoff GR, Golper TA, et al: Drug Prescribing in Renal Failure, 2nd ed. American College of Physicians, Philadelphia, 1991.

225. Morrison G, Audet PR, Singer I: Clinically important drug interac-

tions for the nephrologist. *In* Bennett WM, McCarron DA, Brenner BM, Stein JH (eds): Pharmacotherapy of Renal Disease and Hypertension. Churchill Livingstone, New York, 1987, p 49.

226. Reidenberg MN: The biotransformation of drugs in renal failure. Am J Med 62:482, 1977.

227. Brater DC: Resistance to diuretics: Emphasis on a pharmacological perspective. Drugs 22:477, 1981.

228. Brater DC, Voelker JR: Use of diuretics in patients with renal disease. *In* Bennett WM, McCarron DA, Brenner BM, Stein JH (eds): Pharmacotherapy of Renal Disease and Hypertension. Churchill Livingstone, New York, 1987, p 115.

229. Ellison DH: The physiological basis of diuretic synergism: Its role in treating diuretic resistance. Ann Intern Med 114:886, 1991.

230. Kirchner KA: Mechanisms of diuretic resistance in nephrotic syndrome. *In* Puschett JB, Greenberg A (eds): Diuretics IV: Chemistry, Pharmacology and Clinical Applications. Elsevier Science Publishing, Amsterdam, 1993, p 435.

231. Andreasen F: Determination of furosemide in blood plasma and its binding to proteins in normal plasma and in plasma from patients with acute renal failure. Acta Pharmacol Toxicol 32:417, 1973.

232. Keller E, Hoppe-Seyler G, Schollmeyer P: Disposition and diuretic effect of furosemide in the nephrotic syndrome. Clin Pharmacol Ther 32:442, 1982.

233. Smith DE, Hyneck ML, Berardi RR, Port FK: Urinary protein binding, kinetics and dynamics of furosemide in nephrotic patients. J Pharm Sci 74:603, 1985.

234. Voelker JR, Jameson DM, Brater DC: In vitro evidence that urine composition affects the fraction of active furosemide in the nephrotic syndrome. J Pharmacol Exp Ther 250:772, 1989.

235. Kirchner KA, Voelker JR, Brater DC: Intratubular albumin blunts the response to furosemide—a mechanism for diuretic resistance in nephrotic syndrome. J Pharmacol Exp Ther 252:1097, 1990.

236. Kirchner KA, Voelker JR, Brater DC: Binding inhibitors restore furosemide potency in tubule fluid containing albumin. Kidney Int 40:418, 1991.

237. Kirchner KA, Voelker JR, Brater DC: Tubular resistance to furosemide contributes to the attenuated diuretic response in nephrotic rats. J Am Soc Nephrol 2:1201, 1992.

238. Inoue M, Okajima K, Itoh K, et al: Mechanism of furosemide resistance in analbuminemic rats and hypoalbuminemic patients. Kidney Int 32:198, 1987.

239. Fernandez J, Roth D, Bourgoignie J: Treatment of refractory edema in hypoalbuminemic patients with bumetanide and albumin. Am J Kidney Dis 20:A4, 1992. Abstract.

240. Yoshida A, Aoki N: Release of arachidonic acid from human platelets: A key role for the potentiation of platelet aggregability in normal subjects as well as in those with the nephrotic syndrome. Blood 52:969, 1978.

241. Llach F: Hypercoagulability, renal vein thrombosis, and other thrombotic complications of nephrotic syndrome. Kidney Int 28:429, 1985.

242. Bang N, Tygstad C, Schroeder J, et al: Enhanced platelet function in glomerular renal disease. J Lab Clin Med 81:651, 1973.

243. Remuzzi G, Mecca G, Marchest D, et al: Platelet hyperaggregability and the nephrotic syndrome. Thromb Res 16:345, 1979.

244. Kreusser W, Andrassy K, Wietasch A: Gestorte Thrombozymenfunktion beim nephrotischen Syndrome. Verh Dtsch Ges Inn Med 87:704, 1981.

245. Bennett A, Cameron JS: Platelet hyperaggregability in the nephrotic syndrome which is not dependent on arachidonic acid metabolism or on plasma albumin concentration. Clin Nephrol 27:182, 1987.

246. Appel G: Lipid abnormalities in renal disease. Kidney Int 39:169, 1991.

247. Attman P-O, Samuelsson O, Alaupovic P: Lipoprotein metabolism in renal failure. Am J Kidney Dis 21:573, 1993.

248. Scanu AM: Physiopathology of plasma lipoprotein metabolism. Kidney Int 39(suppl 31):S-3, 1991.

249. Illingworth DR: Lipoprotein metabolism. Am J Kidney Dis 22:90, 1993.

250. Hobbs HH, Russell DW, Brown MS, Goldstein JL: The LDL receptor locus in familial hypercholesterolemia: Mutational analysis of a membrane protein. Annu Rev Genet 24:133, 1990.

251. The National Pooling Project Research Group: Relationship of blood pressure, serum cholesterol, smoking habits, relative weight and electrocardiographic abnormalities to the incidence of major coronary events. J Chronic Dis 31:201, 1978.

252. Ballantyne FC, Clark RS, Simpson HS, et al: High density and low density lipoprotein fractions in survivors of myocardial infarction and in control subjects. Metabolism 31:433, 1982.

253. Sato H, Suzuki S, Ueno M, et al: Localization of apolipoprotein(a) and B-100 in various renal diseases. Kidney Int 43:430, 1993.

254. Loscalzo J, Weinfeld M, Fless GM, Scanu AM: Lipoprotein(a), fibrin binding and plasminogen activation. Arteriosclerosis 10:240, 1990.

255. Bagdade JD, Porte D, Bierman EL: Hypertriglyceridemia: A medical consequence of chronic renal failure. N Engl J Med 279:181, 1968.

256. Chan MK, Varghese Z, Moorhead JF: Lipid abnormalities in uremia, dialysis, and transplantation. Kidney Int 19:625, 1981.

257. Hahn R, Oette M, Mondorf H, et al: Analysis of cardiovascular risk factors in chronic hemodialysis patients with special attention to the hyperlipoproteinemias. Atherosclerosis 48:279, 1983.

258. Rappaport J, Aviram M, Chaimovitz C, Brook JM: Defective high density lipoprotein composition in patients on chronic hemodialysis. N Engl J Med 29:1326, 1978.

259. Cheung AK, Wu LL, Kablitz C, Leypoldt JK: Atherogenic lipids and lipoproteins in hemodialysis patients. Am J Kidney Dis 22:271, 1993.

260. Barbagallo CM, Averna MR, Sparacino V, et al: Lipoprotein(a) levels in end-stage renal failure and renal transplantation. Nephron 64:560, 1993.

261. Goldberg AP, Harter HR, Patsch W, et al: Racial differences in plasma high-density lipoproteins in patients receiving hemodialysis. A possible mechanism for accelerated atherosclerosis in white men. N Engl J Med 308:1245, 1983.

262. Cressman MD, Hoogwerf BJ, Schreiber MJ, Cosentino FA: Lipid abnormalities and end-stage renal disease: Implications for atherosclerotic cardiovascular disease? Miner Electrolyte Metab 19:180, 1993.

263. Goldwasser P, Michel M-A, Collier J, et al: Prealbumin and lipoprotein(a) in hemodialysis: Relationships with patient and vascular access survival. Am J Kidney Dis 22:215, 1993.

264. Weintraub M, Burstein A, Rassin T, et al: Severe defect in clearing postprandial chylomicron remnants in dialysis patients. Kidney Int 42:1247, 1992.

265. Joven J, Vilella E, Ahmad S, et al: Lipoprotein heterogeneity in end-stage renal disease. Kidney Int 43:410, 1993.

266. Senti M, Romero R, Pedro-Botet J, et al: Lipoprotein abnormalities in hyperlipidemic and normolipidemic men on hemodialysis with chronic renal failure. Kidney Int 41:1394, 1992.

267. Nestel PJ, Fidge NH, Tan MH: Increased lipoprotein-remnant formation in chronic renal failure. N Engl J Med 307:329, 1982.

268. Mordasini R, Frey F, Flury W, et al: Selective deficiency of hepatic triglyceride lipase in uremic patients. N Engl J Med 297:1362, 1977.

269. Goldberg A, Sherrard DJ, Brunzell JD: Adipose tissue lipoprotein lipase in chronic hemodialysis: Role in plasma triglyceride metabolism. J Clin Endocrinol Metab 47:1173, 1978.

270. Attman P-O, Alaupovic P: Abnormalities of lipoprotein composition in renal insufficiency. Prog Lipid Res 30:275, 1991.

271. Goldberg AP, Applebaum-Bowden DM, Bierman EL, et al: Increase in lipoprotein lipase during clofibrate treatment of hypertriglyceridemia in patients on hemodialysis. N Engl J Med 301:1073, 1979.

272. Portman RJ, Scott RC III, Rogers DD, et al: Decreased low-density lipoprotein receptor function and mRNA levels in lymphocytes from uremic patients. Kidney Int 42:1238, 1992.

273. McCosh EJ, Solangi K, Rivers JM, Goodman A: Hypertriglyceridemia in patients with chronic renal insufficiency. Am J Clin Nutr 28:1036, 1975.

274. Attman P-O, Alaupovic P: Lipid and apolipoprotein profiles of uremic dyslipoproteinemia—relation to renal function and dialysis. Nephron 57:401, 1991.

275. Garg A, Grundy SM: Management of dyslipidemia in NIDDM. Diabetes Care 13:153, 1990.

276. Sosenko JM, Breslow JL, Miettinen OS, Gabbay KH: Hyperglycemia and plasma lipid levels. A prospective study of young insulin-dependent diabetic patients. N Engl J Med 302:650, 1980.

277. Dall'aglio E, Strata A, Reaven G: Abnormal lipid metabolism in treated hypertensive patients with non–insulin dependent diabetes mellitus. Am J Med 84:899, 1988.

278. Attman P-O, Nyberg G, William-Olsson T, et al: Dyslipoproteinemia in diabetic renal failure. Kidney Int 42:1381, 1992.

279. Rosenstock J, Vega GL, Raskin P: Effect of intensive diabetes treatment on low-density lipoprotein apolipoprotein B kinetics in type I diabetes. Diabetes 37:393, 1988.

280. The Diabetes Control and Complications Trial Research Group: The effect of intensive treatment of diabetes on the development and progression of long-term complications in insulin-dependent diabetes mellitus. N Engl J Med 329:977, 1993.

281. Jensen T, Stender S, Deckert T: Abnormalities in plasma concentrations of lipoproteins and fibrinogen in type 1 (insulin-dependent) diabetic patients with increased urinary albumin excretion. Diabetologia 31:142, 1988.

282. Winocour PH, Durrington PN, Ishola M, et al: Influence of proteinuria on vascular disease, blood pressure, and lipoproteins in insulin dependent diabetes mellitus. Br Med J 294:1645, 1987.

283. Ramirez LC, Arauz-Pacheco C, Lackner C, et al: Lipoprotein (a) levels in diabetes mellitus: Relationship to metabolic control. Ann Intern Med 117:42, 1992.

284. Haffner SM, Morales PA, Stern MP, Gruber MK: Lp(a) concentrations in NIDDM. Diabetes 41:1267, 1992.

285. Baxter JH: Hyperlipoproteinemia in nephrosis. Arch Intern Med 109:742, 1962.

286. Gherardi E, Rota E, Calandra S, et al: Relationship among the concentrations of serum lipoproteins and changes in their chemical composition in patients with untreated nephrotic syndrome. Eur J Clin Invest 7:563, 1977.

287. Joven J, Villabona C, Vilella E, et al: Abnormalities of lipoprotein metabolism in patients with the nephrotic syndrome. N Engl J Med 323:579, 1990.

288. Jensen H: Plasma protein and lipid pattern in the nephrotic syndrome. Acta Med Scand 182:465, 1967.

289. Short CD, Durrington PN, Mallick NP, et al: Serum and urinary high density lipoproteins in glomerular disease with proteinuria. Kidney Int 29:1224, 1986.

290. Thomas ME, Freestone AL, Varghese Z, et al: Lipoprotein (a) in proteinuric patients. Nephrol Dial Transplant 7:597, 1992.

291. Wanner C, Rader D, Bartens W, et al: Elevated plasma lipoprotein(a) in patients with the nephrotic syndrome. Ann Intern Med 119:263, 1993.

292. Faucher C, Doucet C, Baumelou A, et al: Elevated lipoprotein (a) levels in primary nephrotic syndrome. Am J Kidney Dis 22:808, 1993.

293. Keane WF, St Peter JV, Kasiske BL: Is the aggressive management of hyperlipidemia in nephrotic syndrome mandatory? Kidney Int 42(suppl 38):S-134, 1992.

294. Radhakrishnan J, Appel AS, Valeri A, Appel GB: The nephrotic syndrome, lipids, and risk factors for cardiovascular disease. Am J Kidney Dis 22:135, 1993.

295. Marsh JB, Sparks CE: Hepatic secretion of lipoproteins in the rat and the effect of experimental nephrosis. J Clin Invest 64:1229, 1979.

296. Tarugi P, Calandra S, Chan L: Changes in apolipoprotein A-I mRNA level in the liver of rats with experimental nephrotic syndrome. Biochim Biophys Acta 868:51, 1986.

297. Calandra S, Gherardi E, Fainaru M, et al: Secretion of lipoproteins, apolipoprotein A-I and apolipoprotein E by isolated perfused liver of rat with experimental nephrotic syndrome. Biochim Biophys Acta 665:331, 1981.

298. Garber DW, Gottlieb BA, Marsh JB, Sparks CE: Catabolism of very low density lipoproteins in experimental nephrosis. J Clin Invest 74:1375, 1984.

299. Warwick GL, Packard CJ, Demant T, et al: Metabolism of apolipoprotein B–containing lipoproteins in subjects with nephrotic-range proteinuria. Kidney Int 40:129, 1991.

300. Appel GB, Blum CB, Chien S, et al: The hyperlipidemia of the nephrotic syndrome: Relation to plasma albumin concentration, oncotic pressure, and viscosity. N Engl J Med 312:1544, 1985.

301. Muls E, Rosseneu M, Daneels R, et al: Lipoprotein distribution and composition in the human nephrotic syndrome. Atherosclerosis 54:225, 1985.

302. Kaysen GA, Gambertoglio J, Felts J, Hutchison FN: Albumin synthesis, albuminuria, and hyperlipemia in nephrotic patients. Kidney Int 31:1368, 1987.

303. Davies RW, Jones H Jr, Hutchison FN, Kaysen GA: Hyperlipemia is coupled neither to the rate of albumin synthesis nor to albumin gene transcription in nephrotic rats. Clin Res 37:165A, 1989. Abstract.

304. Allen JC, Baxter JH, Goodman HC: Effects of dextran, polyvinyl-pyrrolidone and gamma globulin on the hyperlipidemia of experimental nephrosis. J Clin Invest 40:499, 1961.

305. Baxter JH, Goodman HC, Allen JC: Effects of albumin infusion on serum lipids and lipoproteins in nephrosis. J Clin Invest 40:490, 1961.

306. Heymann W, Nash G, Gilkey C, Lewis M: Studies on the causal role of hypoalbuminemia in experimental nephrotic hyperlipemia. J Clin Invest 37:808, 1958.

307. de Mendoza SG, Kashyap ML, Chen CY, Lutmer RF: High density lipoproteinuria in nephrotic syndrome. Metabolism 25:1143, 1976.

308. Pullinger CR, de Brito AER, Rifici VA, et al: Effects of albumin on Apo-B mRNA levels on the secretion of triglyceride-rich lipoprotein by HepG2 cells. Proc Xth Int Congr Nephrol 514, 1987. Abstract.

309. Davies RW, Staprans I, Hutchison FN, Kaysen GA: Proteinuria, not altered albumin metabolism, affects hyperlipidemia in the nephrotic rat. J Clin Invest 86:600, 1990.

310. Golper TA, Schwartz SH: Impaired renal mevalonate metabolism in nephrotic syndrome: A stimulus for increased hepatic cholesterogenesis independent of GFR and hypoalbuminemia. Metabolism 31:471, 1982.

311. Golper TA, Feingold KR, Fulford MH, Siperstein MD: The role of circulating mevalonate in nephrotic hypercholesterolemia in the rat. J Lipid Res 27:1044, 1986.

312. Chan MK, Persaud J, Varghese Z, Moorhead JF: Pathogenic roles of post-heparin lipases in lipid abnormalities in hemodialysis patients. Kidney Int 25:812, 1984.

313. Chan MK, Varghese Z, Persaud JM, Moorhead JF: Post-hepatic and lipoprotein lipase activities in nephrotic syndrome. Aust N Z J Med 14:841, 1984.

314. Roullet JB, Lacour B, Yvert JP, et al: Factors of increase in serum triglyceride-rich lipoproteins in uremic rats. Kidney Int 27:420, 1985.

315. Olivecrona T, Bengtsson G, Markland SE, et al: Heparin-lipoprotein lipase interactions. Fed Proc 36:60, 1977.

316. Staprans I, Garon SJ, Hooper J, Felts JM: Characterization of glycosaminoglycans in urine from patients with nephrotic syndrome and control subjects, and their effects on lipoprotein lipase. Biochim Biophys Acta 678:414, 1981.

317. Staprans I, Felts JM, Couser WG: Glycosaminoglycans and chylomicron metabolism in control and nephrotic rats. Metabolism 36:496, 1987.

318. Dixit VM, Hettiaratchi ESG: The mechanism of hyperlipidemia in the nephrotic syndrome. Med Hypotheses 5:1327, 1979.

319. Cohen L, Cramp DG, Lewis AD, Tickner TR: The mechanism of hyperlipidaemia in nephrotic syndrome: Role of low albumin and the LCAT reaction. Clin Chim Acta 104:393, 1980.

320. Moorhead JF, El Nahas AM, Harry D, et al: Focal glomerulosclerosis and nephrotic syndrome with partial lecithin:cholesterol acetyltransferase deficiency and discoidal high density lipoprotein in plasma and urine. Lancet 1:936, 1983.

321. Gherardi E, Vecchia L, Cashandra S: Experimental nephrotic syndrome in the rat induced by puromycin aminonucleoside. Plasma and urinary lipoproteins. Exp Mol Pathol 32:128, 1980.

322. Felts JM, Gould MC, Gorman RA, Frank A: The quantitative separation of chylomicrons and chylomicron remnants by column chromatography. Physiologist 26:A61, 1983.

323. Kaysen GA: Hyperlipidemia in the nephrotic syndrome. Am J Kidney Dis 12:548, 1988.

324. Berlyne GM, Mallick NP: Ischaemic heart disease as a complication of nephrotic syndrome. Lancet 2:399, 1969.

325. Wass VJ, Jarrett RJ, Chilvers C, Cameron JS: Does the nephrotic syndrome increase the risk of cardiovascular disease? Lancet 2:664, 1979.

326. Wass V, Cameron JS: Cardiovascular disease and the nephrotic syndrome: The other side of the coin. Nephron 27:58, 1981.

327. Mallick NP, Short CD: The nephrotic syndrome and ischaemic heart disease. Nephron 27:54, 1981.

328. Ordonez JD, Hiatt R, Killebrew E, Fireman B: The risk of coronary artery disease among patients with the nephrotic syndrome. Kidney Int 37:243, 1990. Abstract.

329. D'Amico G, Gentile MG: Influence of diet on lipid abnormalities in human renal disease. Am J Kidney Dis 22:151, 1993.

330. Langer T, Levy RI: Acute muscular syndrome associated with administration of clofibrate. N Engl J Med 279:856, 1968.

331. Valeri A, Gelfand J, Blum C, Appel GB: Treatment of the hyperlipidemia of the nephrotic syndrome: A controlled trial. Am J Kidney Dis 8:388, 1986.

332. Groggel GC, Cheung AK, Ellis-Benigni K, Wilson D: Treatment of the nephrotic hyperlipoproteinemia with gemfibrozil. Kidney Int 36:266, 1989.

333. Golper TA, Illingworth DR, Morris CD, Bennett WM: Lovastatin in the therapy of multifactorial hyperlipidemia associated with proteinuria. Am J Kidney Dis 13:312, 1989.

334. Vega GL, Grundy SM: Lovastatin therapy in nephrotic hyperlipidemia: Effects on lipoprotein metabolism. Kidney Int 33:1160, 1988.

335. Rabelink AJ, Hene RJ, Erkelens DW, et al: Effects of simvastatin and cholestyramine on lipoprotein profile in hyperlipidaemia of nephrotic syndrome. Lancet 2:1335, 1988.

336. Thomas ME, Harris KPG, Ramaswamy C, et al: Simvastatin therapy for hypercholesterolemic patients with nephrotic syndrome or significant proteinuria. Kidney Int 44:1124, 1993.

337. Keilani T, Schlueter WA, Levin ML, Batlle DC: Improvement of lipid abnormalities associated with proteinuria using fosinopril, an angiotensin converting enzyme inhibitor. Ann Intern Med 118:246, 1993.

338. Lenorsky C, Jordan SC, Ladisch S: Plasma inhibition of lymphocyte proliferation in nephrotic syndrome: Correlation with hyperlipidemia. J Clin Immunol 2:276, 1982.

339. Kincaid-Smith P, Whitworth JA: Pathogenesis of hypertension in chronic renal disease. Semin Nephrol 8:155, 1988.

340. Cameron JS: Hypertension in glomerulonephritis. Contrib Nephrol 54:103, 1987.

341. Baldwin DS, Neugarten J: Hypertension and renal diseases. Am J Kidney Dis 10:186, 1987.

342. Baldwin DS, Gluck MC, Schacht RG, et al: The longterm course of poststreptococcal glomerulonephritis. Ann Intern Med 80:342, 1974.

343. Orofino L, Quereda C, Lamas S, et al: Hypertension in primary chronic glomerulonephritis. Analysis of 288 biopsied patients. Nephron 45:22, 1987.

344. Danielsen H, Kornerup HJ, Olsen S, Posborg V: Arterial hypertension in chronic glomerulonephritis. An analysis of 310 cases. Clin Nephrol 19:284, 1983.

345. Kheder MA, Maïz HB, Abderrahim E, et al: Hypertension in primary chronic glomerulonephritis: Analysis of 359 cases. Nephron 63:140, 1993.

346. Zucchelli P, Zuccala A, Santoro A, et al: Characteristics of hypertension in primary IgA glomerulonephritis. Contrib Nephrol 40:174, 1984.

347. Wyatt RJ, Julian BA, Bathena DB, et al: IgA nephropathy: Presentation, clinical course, and prognosis in children and adults. Am J Kidney Dis 4:694, 1984.

348. D'Amico G, Vendemia F: Hypertension in IgA nephropathy. Contrib Nephrol 54:113, 1987.

349. Korbet SM, Schwartz MM, Rosenberg B, et al: Immunotactoid glomerulopathy. Medicine (Baltimore) 64:228, 1985.

350. Alpers CE, Rennke HG, Hopper J Jr, Biava CG: Fibrillary glomerulonephritis: An entity with unusual immunofluorescence features. Kidney Int 31:781, 1987.

351. Vendemia F, Fornasieri A, Velis O, et al: Different prevalence rates of hypertension in various reno-parenchymal diseases. *In* Blaufox MD, Bianchi C (eds): Secondary Forms of Hypertension: Current Diagnosis and Management. Grune & Stratton, New York, 1981, p 89.

352. Korbet SM, Schwartz MM, Lewis EJ: The prognosis of focal segmental glomerular sclerosis of adulthood. Medicine (Baltimore) 65:304, 1986.

353. Jennings RB, Earle DP: Post-streptococcal glomerulonephritis: Histopathologic and clinical studies of the acute subsiding, acute and early chronic latent phases. J Clin Invest 40:1525, 1961.

354. Herrera Acosta J: Hypertension in chronic renal disease. Kidney Int 22:702, 1982.

355. Power HR, Rosenberg E, Williams AL, McCredie DA: Plasma renin activity in acute poststreptococcal glomerulonephritis and the hemolytic-uraemic syndrome. Arch Dis Child 49:802, 1974.

356. Weidmann P, Beretta-Piccoli C, Steffen F, et al: Hypertension in terminal renal failure. Kidney Int 9:294, 1976.

357. Llach F: Hypercoagulability, renal vein thrombosis, and other thromboembolic complications. *In* Brenner BM, Stein JH (eds): The Nephrotic Syndrome. Churchill Livingstone, New York, 1982, p 121.

358. Hoyer PF, Gonda S, Barthels M, et al: Thromboembolic complications in children with nephrotic syndrome. Acta Paediatr Scand 75:804, 1986.

359. Sullivan MJ, Hough DR, Agodga L: Peripheral arterial thrombosis due to the nephrotic syndrome: The clinical spectrum. South Med J 76:1011, 1983.

360. Mehls O, Andrassy K, Koderisch J, et al: Hemostasis and thromboembolism in children with nephrotic syndrome: Differences from adults. J Pediatr 110:862, 1987.

361. Cameron JS: Coagulation and thromboembolic complications in the nephrotic syndrome. Adv Nephrol 13:75, 1984.

362. Handley DA, Lawrence JR: Factor IX deficiency in the nephrotic syndrome. Lancet 1:1079, 1967.

363. Natelson EA, Lynch EC, Hetting RA, Alfrey CP: Acquired factor IX deficiency in the nephrotic syndrome. Ann Intern Med 73:373, 1970.

364. Green D, Arruda H, Honig G, Muehrcke RC: Urinary loss of clotting factor due to hereditary membranous nephropathy. Am J Clin Pathol 65:376, 1976.

365. Honig GR, Lindley A: Deficiency of Hageman factor (factor XII) in patients with nephrotic syndrome. J Pediatr 78:633, 1971.

366. Saito H, Goodnough LT, Makker SP, Kallen RJ: Urinary excretion of Hageman factor (factor XII) and the presence of nonfunctional Hageman factor in the nephrotic syndrome. Am J Med 70:531, 1981.

367. Vaziri ND, Ngo J-CT, Ibsen KH, et al: Deficiency and urinary loss of factor XII in adult nephrotic syndrome. Nephron 32:342, 1982.

368. Kendall AG, Lohmann RE, Dossetor JB: Nephrotic syndrome: A hypercoagulable state. Arch Intern Med 127:1021, 1971.

369. Kanfer A, Kleinknecht D, Broyer M, Josso F: Coagulation studies in 45 cases of nephrotic syndrome without uremia. Thromb Diathes Haemorh 24:562, 1970.

370. Thomson C, Forbes CD, Prentice CRM, Kennedy AC: Changes in blood coagulation and fibrinolysis in the nephrotic syndrome. Q J Med 43:399, 1974.

371. Andrassy K, Ritz E, Bonner J: Hypercoagulability in the nephrotic syndrome. Klin Wochenschr 58:1029, 1980.

372. Alkjaersig N, Fletcher AP, Narayanan M, Robson AM: Course and resolution of the coagulopathy in nephrotic children. Kidney Int 31:772, 1987.

373. Takeda Y, Chen A: Fibrinogen metabolism and distribution in patients with the nephrotic syndrome. J Lab Clin Med 70:678, 1967.

374. Zwaginga JJ, Koomans HA, Sixma JJ, Rabelink TJ: Thrombus formation and platelet-vessel wall interaction in the nephrotic syndrome under flow conditions. J Clin Invest 93:204, 1994.

375. Edward N, Young DP-G, MacLeod M: Fibrinolytic activity in plasma and urine in chronic renal disease. J Clin Pathol 17:365, 1964.

376. Wu KK, Koak JC: Urinary plasminogen and chronic glomerulonephritis. Am J Clin Pathol 60:915, 1973.

377. Lau SO, Tkachuk JY, Hasegawa DK, Edson JR: Plasminogen and antithrombin III deficiencies in the childhood nephrotic syndrome associated with plasminogenuria and antithrombinuria. J Pediatr 96:390, 1980.

378. Jacobbson K: Studies on the trypsin and plasmin inhibitors in human blood serum. Scand J Clin Lab Invest 7:91, 1955.

379. Du XH, Glas-Greenwalt P, Kant KS, et al: Nephrotic syndrome with renal vein thrombosis: Pathogenetic importance of a plasmin inhibitor (α-2-antiplasmin). Clin Nephrol 24:186, 1985.

380. Kauffman RH, Veltkamp JJ, Van Tilburg NC, Van Es LE: Acquired antithrombin III deficiency and thrombosis in the nephrotic syndrome. Am J Med 65:607, 1978.

381. Robert A, Olmer M, Sampol J, et al: Clinical correlation between hypercoagulability and thrombo-embolic phenomena. Kidney Int 31:830, 1987.

382. Egebert O: Inherited antithrombin deficiency causing thrombophilia. Thromb Haemost 13:516, 1974.

383. Thaler E, Blazar E, Kopsa H, Pinggera W: Acquired anti-thrombin III deficiency in patients with glomerular proteinuria. Haemostasis 7:257, 1978.

384. Griffin JH, Evati B, Zimmerman TS, et al: Deficiency of protein C in congenital thrombotic disease. J Clin Invest 68:1370, 1981.

385. Comp PC, Esmon DT: Recurrent venous thromboembolism in patients with a partial deficiency of protein S. N Engl J Med 311:1525, 1984.

386. Mannucci PM, Valsecchi C, Bottaso B, et al: High plasma levels of protein C activity and antigen in the nephrotic syndrome. Thromb Haemost 55:31, 1986.

387. Vigano-D'Angelo S, D'Angelo A, Kaufman CE Jr, et al: Protein S deficiency occurs in the nephrotic syndrome. Ann Intern Med 107:42, 1987.

388. Garcia-Maldonado M, Comp PC, Kaufman CE: Proteins C and S are not low in the diabetic nephropathy. Kidney Int 35:226, 1989. Abstract.

389. Boneu B, Boissou F, Abbal M, et al: Comparison of progressive antithrombin activity and concentration of three thrombin inhibitors in nephrotic syndrome. Thromb Haemost 46:623, 1981.

390. Bang N, Tygstad C, Schroeder J, et al: Enhanced platelet function in glomerular renal disease. J Lab Clin Med 81:651, 1973.

391. Andrassy K, Depperman D, Walter E, et al: Is beta thromboglobulin a useful indicator of thrombosis in nephrotic syndrome? Thromb Haemost 42:486, 1979.

392. McGinley E, Lowe GDO, Boulton-Jones M, et al: Blood viscosity and hemostasis in the nephrotic syndrome. Thromb Haemost 49:155, 1983.

393. Ozanne P, Francis RB, Meiselman HJ: Red blood cell aggregation in nephrotic syndrome. Kidney Int 23:519, 1983.

394. Mukherjee AP, Toh BH, Chan GL, et al: Vascular complications in nephrotic syndrome. Relationship to steroid therapy and accelerated thromboplastin generation. Br Med J 4:273, 1970.

395. Berger J, Yaneva H: Hageman factor deposition in membranous nephropathy. Transplant Proc 3:472, 1982.

396. McLean RH, Forsgren A, Bjorksten B, et al: Decreased serum factor B concentration associated with decreased opsonization of *Escherichia coli* in idiopathic nephrotic syndrome. Pediatr Res 11:910, 1977.

397. Stec J, Podracká L, Pavkovceková O, Kollár J: Zinc and copper metabolism in nephrotic syndrome. Nephron 56:186, 1990.

398. Ellis D: Anemia in the course of the nephrotic syndrome secondary to transferrin depletion. J Pediatr 90:953, 1977.

399. Pedraza-Chaverrí J, Torres-Rodríguez GA, Cruz C, et al: Copper and zinc metabolism in aminonucleoside-induced nephrotic syndrome. Nephron 66:87, 1994.

400. Afrasiabi MA, Vaziri ND, Gwinup G, et al: Thyroid function studies in the nephrotic syndrome. Ann Intern Med 90:335, 1979.

401. Musa BU, Seal US, Doe RP: Excretion of corticosteroid-binding globulin, thyroxine-binding globulin and total protein in adult males with nephrosis: Effect of sex hormones. J Clin Endocrinol 27:768, 1967.

402. Haffner D, Töshoff B, Blum WF, et al: Disturbance of IGF's and their carrier protein (IGF-BP3) in patients with nephrotic syndrome. J Am Soc Nephrol 3:276, 1993. Abstract.

403. Khamiseh G, Vaziri N, Oveisi F, et al: Vitamin D absorption, plasma concentration and urinary excretion of 25(OH) vitamin D in nephrotic syndrome. Proc Soc Exp Biol Med 196:210, 1991.

404. Vaziri ND, Kaupke CJ, Barton CH, Gonzales E: Plasma concentration and urinary excretion of erythropoietin in adult nephrotic syndrome. Am J Med 92:35, 1992.

# 44

# Nephron Adaptation to Renal Injury

*Timothy W. Meyer*
*Keshwar Baboolal*
*Barry M. Brenner*

Approximately 180 L of fluid is ultrafiltered at the glomerulus each day and then transformed by successive nephron segments so that the final urine volume and composition are matched to the water and solute load imposed by the daily intake of fluid and food. Yet patients with chronic renal disease and major reductions in glomerular filtration rate (GFR) continue to accomplish these vital functions and to excrete water, nitrogenous wastes, and mineral solutes without notable alterations in their diet. Patients with GFR values of about one-fourth normal are free from symptoms and may seek medical attention only for mild hypertension. Patients with GFR values reduced to 10% of normal are still able to excrete average dietary loads of water and of Na$^+$, K$^+$, and other solutes. Before dialysis became available, life was often sustained in patients with GFR values as low as 4 L/d, or about 2% of the normal value, albeit with many of the debilitating signs and symptoms of uremia.

Patients survive renal insufficiency in part because modern living habits do not test the capacity of the renal excretory mechanisms. The structure of the normal kidney allows excretion of the daily solute load (~600 mOsm) in as little as 0.5 L of water. Body fluid hypertonicity can thus be prevented when water is scarce. Similarly, the rate of Na$^+$ excretion can be reduced to as little as 1 or 2 mEq/d. Extracellular fluid (ECF) volume can thus be maintained when sodium intake is limited and be repaired rapidly after extrarenal Na$^+$ losses. However, in chronic renal insuffi-

ciency, the ability of the kidney to *conserve* important body fluid constituents is limited, as illustrated for Na$^+$ and water in Figure 44–1. Thus, if patients with chronic renal insufficiency were obliged to undergo water and salt deprivation, their disease would become apparent at an earlier stage. As illustrated in Figure 44–1, renal insufficiency not only limits the ability to conserve water and solute but also impairs excretion of large water and solute loads.

Given the limited range of water and solute intake in usual daily diets, the ability of the diseased kidney to maintain external balance of water and solutes still represents a remarkable biologic adaptation. As GFR declines, the fraction of the filtered load excreted must increase for each solute and for water. Increased fractional excretion of water and solutes by the whole kidney is an expression of increased fractional water and solute excretion by each remnant nephron. If the initial complement of approximately 2 million nephrons in humans is reduced by disease while the diet remains constant, the rate of excretion of water and solutes per nephron must increase. Bricker[1, 2] originally employed the term "intact nephron hypothesis" to describe the dependence of altered kidney function on parallel alterations in remnant nephron function. The intact nephron hypothesis does not imply that each nephron is either untouched by disease or totally destroyed. Experimental studies have shown that whereas disease processes reduce the GFR in some nephrons, compensatory mechanisms elevate the GFR and enlarge the tubules of less damaged neph-

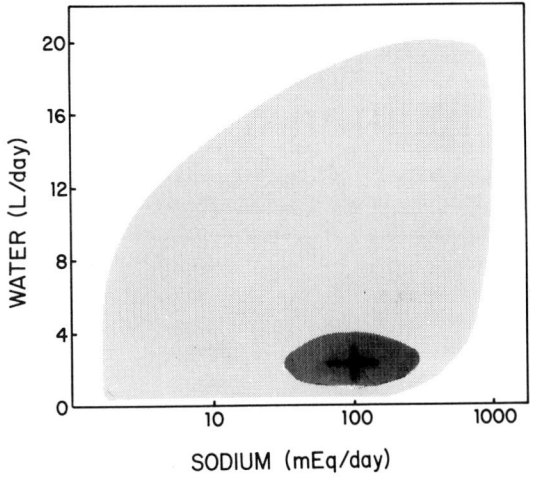

**Figure 44–1.** Limitation of the ability to vary Na⁺ and water excretion imposed by renal insufficiency. The large lightly shaded area represents the capacity of a normal subject to excrete 0.5 to 20 L of water and 2 to 1000 mEq of Na⁺ per day. The smaller darkly shaded area represents the much more limited range of water and Na⁺ excretion that can be achieved when the GFR is reduced to about 10% of the normal value. External balance is still maintained because the water and sodium content of the "usual" daily diet in U.S. society varies over an even more narrow range, represented by the central cross.

rons.[3–5] The first aim of this chapter is to describe the compensatory changes in function and structure of remnant nephrons caused by reduction in functioning nephron number. Specific alterations in handling of individual solutes and water by these adapted remnant nephrons are then described. Finally, evidence suggesting that maintenance of excretory function by a reduced complement of nephrons has a biologic price is examined. The adaptive mechanisms that increase fractional solute excretion may contribute to the systemic toxicity of the uremic state, as reviewed in Chapters 5 and 49. Studies have shown, moreover, that adaptive changes in remnant nephron function may eventually cause sclerosis of remnant glomeruli and thus contribute to the progression of renal disease.

## ALTERATIONS IN GLOMERULAR STRUCTURE AND FUNCTION ACCOMPANYING REDUCTION IN NEPHRON NUMBER

### Increases in Single-Nephron Glomerular Filtration Rate and Renal Blood Flow

The simplest model of reduction in nephron number is afforded by surgical ablation of renal tissue. In human subjects donating a kidney for transplantation[6–9] and in rats subjected to experimental uninephrectomy,[10–13] the GFR in the remnant kidney has generally been shown to increase from 40% to 60% above its preoperative value; slightly lesser increases in remnant kidney GFR have been observed in uninephrectomized dogs.[14, 15] The response to nephron loss has been studied less extensively in nonmammals, but an increase in the GFR of the remnant kidney has been

reported in chickens subjected to partial renal ablation.[16] Studies in mammals suggest that most of the increase in remnant kidney GFR is apparent within 4 to 6 days and that the response is complete within 2 to 4 weeks after nephrectomy. Early studies suggesting more prolonged increase in remnant kidney GFR after uninephrectomy in young rodents failed to take into account the increases in GFR and kidney weight that occur with normal growth in these animals.[17, 18] A report showing a further modest increase in GFR of young adult human kidney donors more than 3 years after uninephrectomy remains to be confirmed.[19]

An increase in single-nephron GFR (SNGFR) of remnant nephrons, an increase in number of nephrons within remnant renal tissue, or a combination of these processes could theoretically account for the observed increase in remnant kidney GFR after uninephrectomy. It is generally agreed that new nephrons are not formed in mature animals and that the increases in remnant kidney GFR that follow nephrectomy in adulthood are thus entirely due to increases in SNGFR. Studies by Bonvalet and co-workers[20–22] employing both micropuncture and glomerular counting techniques suggested that when nephrectomy was performed during the first few weeks of life, the increase in remnant kidney GFR in rats and mice, but not in guinea pigs, could be attributed in part to generation of new glomeruli. It was argued that in guinea pigs (as in humans), nephrogenesis is complete at the time of birth, so that formation of new nephrons cannot be induced by nephrectomy, whereas in neonatal mice and in rats, kidneys still contain nephrogenic zones capable of evoking an additional complement of glomeruli.[23, 24] Later studies of rats subjected to uninephrectomy at an equally early age have cast doubt on this hypothesis.[25–27] These studies have confirmed that the magnitude of the increase in GFR is greater in young than in mature animals but showed that glomerular number did not increase after nephrectomy at any age, which suggests that the relatively larger increase in GFR in young animals is due to a greater compensatory response on the part of individual remnant nephrons. Renal ablation in chickens also fails to increase nephron number in the remnant kidney, even when the ablation procedure is carried out before the formation of new nephrons from embryonic foci is complete.[16]

The increases in SNGFR that must accompany postnephrectomy increases in whole kidney GFR if no new nephrons are formed have been demonstrated by micropuncture in rats.[11, 28] Micropuncture measurements in rats after removal of two thirds to five sixths of their total renal mass have further shown that the magnitude of the adaptive increase in SNGFR is similar in superficial and juxtamedullary nephrons.[29, 30] These studies confirm earlier results obtained with the ferrocyanide technique showing that the SNGFR of juxtamedullary nephrons remains approximately twice that of superficial nephrons, with both increasing after uninephrectomy.[14, 21]

The increase in GFR in the remaining kidney of uninephrectomized animals and humans is associated with an increase in renal blood flow (RBF) of similar magnitude.[7, 11, 14] Just as the increase in whole kidney GFR represents an increase in GFR of individual nephrons, the increase in total

RBF represents increased perfusion of individual glomeruli. Micropuncture measurements in the rat have further identified the glomerular hemodynamic determinants of the increase in SNGFR after uninephrectomy.[11–13] In this species, in which SNGFR exhibits marked plasma flow dependence, the majority of the increase in SNGFR is due to elevation of glomerular plasma flow; a smaller portion of the increase may be due to elevation of the mean glomerular transcapillary hydraulic pressure ($\overline{\Delta P}$) and the glomerular ultrafiltration coefficient ($K_f$). The tubuloglomerular feedback mechanism remains intact, with its set-point altered in a way that permits remnant nephron hyperfiltration.[31, 32]

The 40% to 60% increase in SNGFR that follows uninephrectomy does not represent the limit of the glomerular functional response to reduction in nephron number. When a greater portion of renal mass is removed, SNGFR of remnant nephrons increases further. Elevation of SNGFR to values approximately 2.5 times normal has been observed in rats after ablation of 75% to 90% of their initial renal mass.[28, 33, 34] Micropuncture studies show that these remarkable increases in SNGFR are associated with equally prominent increases in glomerular plasma flow owing to further dilation of afferent and efferent arterioles.[33, 34] Whereas systemic blood pressure does not increase after uninephrectomy, blood pressure is usually elevated in rats subjected to more extensive renal ablation.[33–35] Elevation of mean glomerular hydraulic pressure ($\overline{P}_{GC}$) accompanies elevation of blood pressure in this setting. Because tubule pressure increases little if at all after renal ablation, increasing $\overline{P}_{GC}$ results in an increase in $\overline{\Delta P}$. This increase in $\overline{\Delta P}$ contributes notably to the remarkable increases in SNGFR observed after extensive renal ablation in the rat.[33, 34] In contrast, most but not all studies indicate that $K_f$ is not increased in rats subjected to renal ablation.[33, 34, 36, 37] The apparent stability of $K_f$ in the setting of prominent glomerular hypertrophy is a surprising finding, as discussed in the following section. The hemodynamic determinants of remnant nephron hyperfiltration in the dog differ somewhat from those in the rat. In the dog, extensive ablation of renal mass is not accompanied by systemic hypertension and $\overline{\Delta P}$ is only modestly elevated, whereas $K_f$ is markedly increased.[38, 39]

The stimuli responsible for glomerular hypertension, hyperperfusion, and hyperfiltration after extensive renal ablation in the rat remain to be identified. Glomerular hypertension has been attributed to impaired afferent arteriolar autoregulation by remnant nephrons in the setting of systemic hypertension.[40, 41] The mechanisms responsible for impaired remnant nephron autoregulation have not been elucidated; the mechanisms responsible for systemic hypertension after extensive renal ablation are reviewed in Chapter 48. The finding that chronic inhibition of angiotensin I–converting enzyme normalizes $\overline{P}_{GC}$ in rats subjected to renal ablation suggests that angiotensin II (AII) could cause capillary hypertension in remnant glomeruli.[34] Whether acute AII blockade can rapidly reduce remnant glomerular pressure is not settled.[42–44] It may be that AII increases remnant glomerular pressure by promoting $Na^+$ retention and causing systemic hypertension rather than by direct action on the renal microcirculation.[44] A number of studies have sought to identify the source of the AII activity that contributes to remnant glomerular hypertension. These studies have shown that in rats with nephron number reduced by partial renal infarction, renin activity is concentrated in areas adjacent to the infarcted tissue.[45, 46] The production of renin by hypoperfused nephrons adjacent to infarcted tissue could explain why blood pressure is increased when nephron number is halved by uninephrectomy.[13] The production of renin by such hypoperfused nephrons could also explain why blood pressure tends to be higher when extensive renal ablation is accomplished by partial renal infarction than when a similar degree of renal ablation is accomplished by surgical removal of renal tissue.[47]

Whereas sustained blockade of AII activity reduces glomerular pressure, it does not reduce remnant kidney plasma flow or GFR.[34, 48] Other factors, therefore, must account for remnant glomerular hyperperfusion and hyperfiltration. The most promising candidate among the vasomotor hormones is atrial natriuretic peptide (ANP), which contributes to elevation of remnant nephron GFR after reduction in nephron number in rats maintained on a liberal salt intake.[49] Endothelin-1 activity in the remnant kidney has been found to remain constant for the first week after renal ablation and then to rise[50, 51]; the activity of nitric oxide has not been well characterized. There is evidence of altered prostanoid activity in the remnant kidney. Synthesis of prostaglandin $E_2$, prostaglandin $I_2$, and thromboxane $A_2$ is increased in glomeruli isolated from subtotally nephrectomized rats, and *per nephron* excretion of prostaglandin $E_2$ and thromboxane $A_2$ is increased in these animals.[52–55] These findings suggest that remnant glomerular hemodynamic function may be altered by increased intrarenal production of both vasodilator and vasoconstrictor prostanoids. Short-term inhibition of prostaglandin synthesis has been shown to reduce remnant nephron plasma flow and GFR without reducing glomerular capillary pressure in rats subjected to renal ablation, whereas long-term inhibition of thromboxane synthesis has been shown to decrease vascular resistance and increase plasma flow and GFR.[53, 54] Prostaglandin synthesis inhibition has also been shown to reduce renal plasma flow and GFR in rabbits subjected to 75% reduction in renal mass and in patients with renal insufficiency.[56–59] The possibility of species variation in the determinants of remnant glomerular hemodynamic function is again raised by the observation that prostaglandin synthesis inhibitors had no effect on renal plasma flow or GFR in dogs subjected to 85% ablation of renal mass.[60]

## Alterations in Glomerular Structure

Thomas Addis and Jean Oliver[61, 62] first described increases in glomerular volume after uninephrectomy in rabbits. Similar increases in glomerular volume have since been observed after nephrectomy in rats and dogs.[13, 34, 63, 64] Serial morphologic and functional studies in the rat suggest that glomerular volume and SNGFR increase in parallel after uninephrectomy.[64, 65] The contribution of constituent parts of the glomerulus to its expansion after nephrectomy has been debated. In one study, glomeruli isolated by sieving from kidneys of uninephrectomized mice were found to be no larger than those of control animals.[66] This led the authors to suggest that expansion of the glomerular tuft observed in studies of remnant kidney tissue sections may in part reflect capillary dilation due to high in vivo perfusion pressures and flows before tissue fixation. In this same study, however, an increase in glomerular RNA content was observed after nephrectomy, which suggests true glomerular hypertrophy. Later morphometric studies have demonstrated an increase in the total volume occupied by cellular constituents in the remnant glomeruli of nephrectomized rats.[63, 67, 68] Overall, these studies indicate that the fractions of the glomerular volume occupied by different structural components, including capillary lumens, endothelial cells, epithelial cells, and mesangium, remain constant as the glomerulus enlarges. Further morphometric studies are required to settle remaining questions concerning the pattern of compensatory glomerular growth. It is not clear to what extent different glomerular cell types increase in number and in volume after renal ablation. The original study by Olivetti and co-workers[67] noted a prominent increase in the number of glomerular endothelial, mesangial, and epithelial cells after uninephrectomy in young rats. Subsequent studies, however, have found that visceral epithelial cell number remains constant when the glomerulus grows both after uninephrectomy and after more extensive renal ablation.[69, 70] The effect of glomerular hypertrophy on endothelial and mesangial cell number has not been evaluated in equal detail. The pattern of expansion of capillary lumens in compensatory glomerular hypertrophy also remains to be fully defined. Olivetti and co-workers[63, 67] found that capillary growth after uninephrectomy was largely the result of elongation and duplication of capillary segments, so that the capillary surface increased in proportion to glomerular tuft volume while the capillary radius was significantly increased. Subsequent studies have confirmed these findings and shown that there is a larger increase in capillary segment number after uninephrectomy in young rats than in mature rats.[70, 71] After more extensive renal ablation, there is greater glomerular hypertrophy and a different pattern of capillary growth, in that capillary radius increases as well as capillary length.[72, 73]

Attempts have been made in these morphologic studies to estimate the filtering capacity of the enlarged remnant glomeruli. Certain difficulties are inherent in the calculations on which these estimates are based. The glomerular capillary ultrafiltration coefficient $K_f$ is the product of the surface area available for filtration S and the hydraulic permeability of the glomerular capillary wall per unit surface area k. It is uncertain which anatomic boundary constitutes the surface corresponding to S. Attempts to estimate S by measuring the glomerular capillary area in direct apposition to epithelial foot processes have suggested that S increases after nephrectomy, albeit to a slightly lesser degree than total glomerular volume.[63, 64] Whereas these morphologic studies suggest an increase in the filtering surface area of remnant glomeruli, most physiologic studies have not demonstrated a proportional increase in the $K_f$ of remnant glomeruli after extensive renal ablation in rats.[33, 34, 36, 37, 54] It is possible that k is reduced in remnant glomeruli. Morphometric studies have revealed an increase in the average width of epithelial cell foot processes in rats subjected to extensive renal ablation.[64, 74] Theoretically, an increase in

average foot process width must cause a decrease in the length of filtration slit overlying each unit area of peripheral capillary surface. Because it is generally accepted that fluid leaving the glomerular capillaries passes through the filtration slits, an increase in average foot process width could cause a decrease in k in remnant glomeruli. It is also possible that the filtering surface estimated by morphologic techniques in remnant glomeruli does not represent effective area available for filtration in vivo. Theoretic studies by Shea and Raskova[75] suggest that much of the glomerular capillary network is relatively underperfused in rats subjected to extensive renal ablation. It is notable that no increase in S was found after uninephrectomy in rats when infusion of glomerular basement membrane antibody was used to estimate capillary surface area in vivo.[76] An increase in capillary surface area has been demonstrated with this technique during growth in young rats, a circumstance in which $K_f$ has also been shown by micropuncture measurements to increase.[77, 78]

## ALTERATIONS IN TUBULE STRUCTURE AND FUNCTION ACCOMPANYING REDUCTION IN NEPHRON NUMBER

An increase in remnant kidney mass accompanies the increases in remnant kidney blood flow and GFR that follow reduction in nephron number. Oliver[62] first showed that the majority of the increase in renal mass after uninephrectomy in mammals is accounted for by growth of the proximal nephron, whereas proportionally lesser growth is observed in other nephron segments. Of note, a similar increase in the mass of remnant pronephric tubules is observed after unilateral pronephrectomy in larval amphibians.[79] Changes in tubule structure after partial removal of renal tissue in other nonmammalian species have not been studied. The magnitude of nephron hypertrophy after uninephrectomy in the rat was carefully measured by Hayslett and co-workers,[80] who found that the proximal convoluted tubule enlarges by about 15% in luminal and outside diameter and 35% in length; the distal convoluted tubule enlarges by about 10% in luminal and outside diameter and by 17% in length. Slightly larger increases in the diameter and length of the proximal convoluted tubule along with lesser increases in the diameter of thick ascending limb and collecting duct segments have been noted in uninephrectomized rabbits.[62, 81] Further studies have demonstrated that the increase in remnant proximal tubule size, like the increase in remnant nephron GFR, is proportional to the extent of reduction in nephron number.[82]

### PROXIMAL NEPHRON

Enlargement of the proximal nephron is associated with increased proximal reabsorption of glomerular filtrate. Studies in animals subjected to renal ablation[83] and in human kidney donors[8] indicate that the increase in proximal reabsorption is approximately proportional to the increase in remnant nephron GFR, so that glomerulotubular balance is preserved. The operation of peritubular Starling forces presumably contributes to preservation of glomerulotubular balance after reduction in nephron number. Increases in remnant glomerular plasma flow and filtration rate result in increased perfusion of peritubular capillaries by efferent arteriolar plasma, favoring fluid reabsorption. In vitro studies, however, have shown that increased proximal fluid reabsorption after reduction in nephron number also reflects intrinsic adaptation of tubule transport mechanisms. Fluid reabsorption by segments of isolated proximal straight tubule increases within 24 hours after nephrectomy.[84] This early increase in tubule fluid reabsorption is associated with an increase in GFR but precedes detectable increase in tubule size. These findings have been taken to suggest that increased delivery of filtrate triggers increased proximal fluid reabsorption and that increased fluid reabsorption then stimulates proximal tubule hypertrophy.[84, 85] When remnant kidney hypertrophy is complete, increases in isolated proximal tubule fluid reabsorption are approximately proportional to increases in the size and protein content of tubule cells.[86–88] The folding in the basolateral membrane is increased, so that basolateral surface area increases in proportion to tubule cell volume; there is an accompanying increase in the activity of the basolateral membrane $Na^+,K^+$-ATPase, which provides the motive force for most proximal nephron solute transport processes.[81] Energy for increased transport is provided by an increase in mitochondrial volume that parallels the increase in proximal tubule volume.[81, 89]

The increase in remnant nephron GFR after reduction in nephron number increases the tubule load of glucose, amino acids, and other solutes that are normally reabsorbed entirely by the proximal nephron. Although detailed segmental studies have not been performed, proximal reabsorption of these solutes appears to increase in proportion with remnant nephron GFR and with proximal tubule size. Thus, maximal reabsorptive capacity for glucose increases in proportion to SNGFR in dogs subjected to varying degrees of renal ablation.[90] Normal values for activity of $Na^+$-glucose and $Na^+$–amino acid cotransport have been obtained in membrane vesicles from the brush border remnant nephrons.[91, 92] These findings suggest that proximal glucose and amino acid reabsorption, like proximal fluid reabsorption, is increased in proportion to tubule mass. Some proximal tubule metabolic functions also increase in proportion to tubule mass. Filtered citrulline is converted to arginine by the proximal tubule, and the activity of the responsible enzymes is increased in proportion to total protein content in enlarging remnant nephrons. This increase in enzyme activity, together with an increase in plasma citrulline levels, maintains renal arginine synthesis and plasma arginine levels constant even when functioning nephron number is severely reduced.[93] A comparable increase in the capacity of remnant nephrons to convert glycine to serine may help maintain near-normal plasma serine levels after renal ablation.[94]

Other proximal tubule functions are altered out of proportion to tubule mass after reduction in nephron number. Decreased fractional proximal reabsorption of $PO_4^{3-}$ in remnant nephrons is associated with decreased $PO_4^{3-}$ reabsorption per unit tubule mass in isolated proximal nephron segments and with decreased activity of $Na^+$-$PO_4^{3-}$ cotransport in membrane vesicles from the brush border of remnant nephrons.[91, 95] Reduction in proximal capacity for $PO_4^{3-}$ reabsorption presumably facilitates the increase in fractional excretion of $PO_4^{3-}$ that must accompany reduction in nephron number in the face of constant dietary phosphate intake. Likewise, increased activity of proximal nephron enzymes required for ammonia production presumably facilitates the increase in remnant nephron $NH_4^+$ excretion that must accompany reduction in nephron number in the face of a constant acid load imposed by metabolism of the daily diet.[96–98] The physiologic significance of a prominent increase in $Na^+/H^+$ exchange activity of the brush border membrane of remnant proximal nephrons is less clear.[92, 99, 100] This increase in $Na^+/H^+$ exchange activity cannot be attributed to a requirement for increased remnant nephron acid excretion, because it is disproportionate to the increased proximal $HCO_3^-$ reabsorption in remnant nephrons and cannot be prevented by long-term administration of sodium bicarbonate to reduce acid excretion.[92, 101] It may be that increased $Na^+/H^+$ exchange is a general manifestation of tubule cell hypertrophy rather than an expression of the necessity to increase reabsorption of some specific solute.[102] The physiologic significance of an increase in alkaline phosphatase activity out of proportion to the increase in remnant tubule mass after nephrectomy also remains unexplained.[103]

## LOOP OF HENLE AND DISTAL NEPHRON

Relatively few studies have examined the structure and function of the loop of Henle after reduction in nephron number. Oliver[62] found little increase in the cross-sectional area of thick ascending limb segments after uninephrectomy in the rabbit. Functional studies, however, suggest that fluid reabsorption in the thick ascending limb increases in proportion to remnant nephron GFR after reduction in nephron number in rats.[80, 104] A mechanism to account for the increase in fluid reabsorption out of proportion to tubule mass in the remnant thick ascending limb remains to be established. An increase in the activity of $Na^+,K^+$-ATPase, an enzyme closely linked to active solute transport, has been observed after nephrectomy in some but not all studies of this segment.[105, 106]

The cross-sectional area of both the lumen and epithelium is increased in distal convoluted tubules and cortical collecting ducts after reduction in nephron number, but the volume of these segments increases less than the volume of the proximal tubule.[62, 80, 107] The cross-sectional area of the medullary collecting duct is increased after renal ablation in the rabbit but not in the rat; the length of the remnant medullary collecting duct has not been measured but presumably increases as the thickness of the medulla increases in the hypertrophied remnant kidney.[108, 109] The most extensively studied transport function in the distal remnant nephron is $K^+$ secretion. Increased $K^+$ secretion in distal remnant nephrons is necessary to increase remnant nephron $K^+$ excretion as nephron number decreases. Studies in cortical collecting duct segments isolated from uremic rabbits have established that increased distal $K^+$ secretion is facilitated by an increase in tubule $K^+$ secretion.[107] A similar increase in $K^+$ secretion by cortical collecting duct segments can be induced by dietary potassium loading in intact animals. In both circumstances, increased collecting duct $K^+$ secretion is accompanied by increased $Na^+$ reabsorption and associated with an increase in the basolateral membrane surface area of principal cells and with a local increase in $Na^+,K^+$-ATPase activity.[105, 106, 110–115] The dependence of these functional and structural changes on aldosterone is controversial.[116, 117] The close similarity of the changes observed with $K^+$ loading and renal ablation suggests, however, that the increase in $K^+$ secretion observed in isolated remnant collecting ducts is the result of a long-term increase in dietary potassium load *per nephron*. Studies by Fine and co-workers[107] showed directly that increased $K^+$ secretion by remnant cortical collecting ducts could be prevented by reducing dietary potassium intake in proportion to nephron number. Of particular note, reducing dietary potassium intake did not prevent hypertrophy of the remnant collecting ducts. These observations indicate that changes in the structure and function of remnant tubules reflect the combination of a general hypertrophic response associated with remnant nephron hyperfiltration and specific structural adaptations required for increased remnant nephron excretion of individual solutes. Besides the increase in remnant cortical collecting duct $K^+$ transport capacity, the decrease in $Na^+$-$PO_4^{3-}$ cotransport activity and increase in ammonia synthetic capacity observed in remnant proximal nephrons may represent examples of structural adaptations required for increased remnant nephron excretion of individual solutes. The general hypertrophic response to reduction in nephron number is considered further in the following section; specific adaptations in the handling of individual solutes are described more thoroughly in subsequent sections.

## MECHANISMS OF COMPENSATORY RENAL HYPERTROPHY

The phenomenon of renal enlargement after uninephrectomy has been studied extensively in an effort to identify the mechanism by which renal cells are induced to increase in size and number. In studies of this phenomenon, the designation "compensatory renal hypertrophy" has generally been used to describe the aggregate changes in nephron structure and function, including both cellular hypertrophy and hyperplasia, that follow loss of renal mass. Extensive work in this area was presented at symposia held in 1968 and in 1974, proceedings of which were edited by Nowinski and Goss[118] and by Peters and associates.[119] One more symposium has been devoted to this subject,[120] and further summaries of the literature are available in an early review by Malt[121] and in later reviews by Fine[122] and Wesson.[123] The observation that compensatory changes in nephron function may contribute to ultimate loss of renal function when nephron number is reduced has rekindled interest in this area and stimulated new efforts to identify the mechanisms responsible for remnant nephron hypertrophy.

### Biochemical Changes

Early workers noted that the "dry" or desiccated kidney weight increases in proportion to the "wet" or fresh kidney weight after nephrectomy, which implies an increase in the mass of tissue solids composed largely of protein.[124] Subsequent studies have verified that the ratio of kidney protein to kidney wet weight remains constant during renal hypertrophy. A 10% increase in renal protein content has been demonstrated as early as 24 hours after uninephrectomy in the mouse, whereas a 15% increase in renal protein content has been found 48 hours after uninephrectomy in the rat.[125, 126] Radiolabeled amino acid incorporation studies suggest that the rate of renal protein synthesis is increased as early as 3 hours after uninephrectomy in the mouse.[127]

Synthesis of new RNA has been shown to precede synthesis of new protein. The quantity of RNA is notably increased within 12 hours after uninephrectomy, and radiolabeled nucleotide incorporation studies have demonstrated an increased rate of RNA synthesis within 1 to 4 hours after nephrectomy.[121, 127, 128] Studies employing nucleic acid hybridization techniques have established that this early increase in RNA synthesis reflects largely increased production of ribosomal RNA.[129] Decreased degradation of RNA may also contribute to the increase in RNA levels after nephrectomy.[128, 130] The peak in the RNA content of individual cells is reached within 2 days after uninephrectomy.[121] Levels decline thereafter as kidney weight reaches a plateau and protein synthetic rate, expressed per unit kidney weight, declines to normal levels.

DNA content begins to increase after RNA and protein content in renal growth after uninephrectomy. Radionucleotide incorporation studies suggest that increased DNA synthesis does not begin before 9 to 18 hours after nephrectomy; a notable increase in mitotic figures, largely among proximal tubule cells, is apparent only after 1 to 2 days.[127, 131–133] Like the rate of protein synthesis, the prevalence of tubule mitotic figures declines to normal levels in a period of 1 to 2 weeks after uninephrectomy as the process of compensatory renal enlargement is completed.[131] The lag of DNA synthesis behind RNA synthesis may reflect stimulation of mitosis by increases in cell size.[127] According to this view, the renal hypertrophic stimulus causes cell enlargement, and cells reaching the largest size are stimulated to divide.

The ratio of increases in protein and DNA content has been used to estimate the relative contributions of cellular hypertrophy and increased cell number, or hyperplasia, to compensatory renal hypertrophy. In uninephrectomized adult animals, these estimates suggest that an increase in cell number of between 10% and 25% accounts for one quarter to one half of the net increase in remnant kidney size.[126, 127, 134] In young animals and in adult animals subjected to more extensive renal ablation, remnant nephron enlargement is more pronounced than it is after uninephrectomy in adult animals. In these circumstances, cellular hyperplasia plays a proportionally greater role in the compensatory process.[135–138]

The activities of most renal enzymes increase in parallel with protein content of the hypertrophying kidney. Specific activities of various enzymes thus remain constant as the kidney grows, with exceptions that may be grouped in two important categories. First, remnant nephron excretion of individual solutes is increased out of proportion to remnant nephron mass after reduction in nephron number. Increased specific activity of enzymes required to excrete these solutes may therefore be observed in the remnant kidney. For example, increased activity of Na$^+$,K$^+$-ATPase is presumably required for increased secretion of K$^+$ in remnant collecting ducts.[105–107] Similarly, an increase in the specific activity of enzymes required for ammonia synthesis after uninephrectomy presumably reflects increased ammonia synthesis per gram of renal tissue, because ammonia excretion by the remnant kidney must double whereas kidney weight increases by only about 50%.[96–98]

A second category of enzymes that exhibit increased activities after nephrectomy consists of those involved in cell growth. An increase in the activity of ornithine decarboxylase presumably contributes to increasing renal content of the aliphatic polyamines putrescine and spermidine after nephrectomy.[134–142] These substances are thought to play a role in the synthesis and accumulation of both nucleic acids and proteins. An early increase in the activity of guanylate cyclase has been related to an increase in tissue content of cyclic GMP, and early increases have also been observed in the activities of protein kinase C and of enzymes of the pentose phosphate pathway.[143–147] An increase in $^{14}$C-labeled choline incorporation into cortical phospholipid noted within 5 minutes after uninephrectomy has been associated with an almost equally rapid increase in the activity of choline kinase.[148, 149] An increase in the activity of choline phosphotransferase, which is also important in cellular membrane synthesis, has been observed after 24 hours.[150]

All the enzymatic changes described are nonspecific concomitants of tissue growth and have been noted during hypertrophy of organs other than the kidney. Developments in cell biology have shifted the focus of investigation of the hypertrophic process from enzymes to genes. Particular attention has been devoted to the participation of "early response" genes in renal hypertrophy. The protein products of these genes regulate transcriptional control of large numbers of other genes, and the activation of early response genes is an early step in cell proliferation and differentiation evoked by mitogens and growth factors. To date, studies of the expression of early response genes in the remnant kidney after uninephrectomy have not yielded clear results.[129, 151–156] It has been found that expression of early response genes involved in cell proliferation is more marked during folic acid–induced renal hypertrophy than after uninephrectomy.[151, 153] This result is not surprising in that folic acid administration induces florid proximal tubule cell proliferation, whereas uninephrectomy induces only modest cell proliferation. Other findings are more controversial. For instance, remnant kidney activity of *FOS* after uninephrectomy has been found to increase in some studies and to remain constant in other studies.[151, 153–155] Increases in the renal activity of some early response genes induced by sham surgery and catecholamine exposure may make it hard to define the role of these genes in compensatory renal hypertrophy.[156, 157] Ultimately, delineation of changes in known early response gene activity after nephron loss should facilitate comparison of compensatory renal hypertrophy with growth in other organs but may not identify stimuli responsible for selective renal growth after nephrectomy. Isolation of new genes whose activities in the remnant kidney increase after nephrectomy could provide a better means of identifying stimuli that trigger renal growth in this setting.[158]

## Growth Factors: The Search for a Renotrophic Hormone

Compensatory renal hypertrophy does not require renal innervation. Anephric humans receiving an isograft kidney from identical twins show a prompt increase in GFR equivalent to that observed in the remnant kidney of the donors, although the nerve supply to the donated kidney is interrupted by operation and is not re-established for at least a month.[159, 160] Single kidneys transplanted into anephric rats and dogs hypertrophy as much as remnant kidneys in uninephrectomized animals do, again despite surgical denervation.[161]

Exclusion of a neural signal as the mediator of compensatory hypertrophy has prompted an extensive search for a circulating agent, or "renotrophic hormone," that controls renal growth. Fractions of urine, serum, and liver from uninephrectomized animals and urine and serum from humans have been shown to stimulate biochemical changes, such as incorporation of radiolabeled nucleotides into DNA in isolated renal tissue preparations, and to stimulate growth in cultures of kidney-derived cells.[162–168] Such properties do not establish that these fractions do induce growth of the whole kidney, however, and no truly renotrophic hormone has so far been isolated.[130, 132] Although no factor that causes selective kidney growth has been identified, a large number of factors have been shown to cause hypertrophy or hyperplasia of kidney cells. The list of factors shown to promote growth, usually in cultured proximal tubule or mesangial cells, includes insulin, insulin-like growth factor-1 (IGF-1), epidermal growth factor (EGF), hepatocyte growth factor (HGF), platelet-derived growth factor, prostaglandin E$_2$, and hormones including hydrocortisone, thyroxine, arginine vasopressin, and angiotensin.[122, 145, 169] In general, these factors promote growth in many cell types. It seems likely that, like early response gene products, they participate in compensatory renal hypertrophy in a nonspecific manner, after growth has been triggered by some unidentified kidney-specific signal. Once growth has been triggered, sequential production of different growth factors, whose activity has not been detectably altered in whole kidney assays, is presumably required to achieve coordinated growth of specific kidney cell types. Moreover, some factors that cause growth of kidney cells in culture may not contribute significantly overall growth of the remnant kidney after nephron loss. For instance, AII has been shown to cause growth of proximal tubule and mesangial cells in culture.[170] Yet prolonged administration of exogenous AII does not cause kidney growth in intact rats, and blockade of AII activity does not prevent remnant kidney hyperfiltration or hypertrophy in rats subjected to renal ablation.[34, 171]

There is stronger evidence for the participation of IGF-1 in compensatory renal hypertrophy. Administration of IGF-1 causes an increase in GFR and kidney weight in intact rodents; reports differ as to whether the increase in kidney weight is slightly greater than or only proportional to the IGF-1–induced increase in body weight.[172–175] After uninephrectomy, there is an increase in renal levels of IGF-1, whereas IGF-1 receptor levels remain constant.[172, 176–179] There is disagreement concerning the time course of the increase in IGF-1 activity, however, and some studies have found that renal IGF-1 levels begin to increase only after compensatory hypertrophy is already detectable.[172, 176–178] Whether the increase in remnant kidney IGF-1 activity is associated with an increase in IGF-1 message is also controversial, and levels of the IGF-1 binding proteins remain to be assessed.[172, 177] Attempts to identify changes in IGF-1 activity after more extensive renal ablation have been complicated by the finding that partial renal infarction increases IGF-1 activity in the adjacent renal tissue.[180] Taken together, available studies are consistent with the hypothesis that IGF-1 participates in renal hypertrophy but does not initiate the hypertrophic process. Increased IGF-1 production is not unique to renal hypertrophy, and increased local IGF-1 levels have been observed during growth of other tissues.

The participation of other growth factors in compensatory renal hypertrophy has been less extensively studied. The distal nephron produces a large amount of the precursor protein for EGF. Renal content of EGF, distribution of EGF, and receptor levels for EGF, however, all remain constant over the first few days after uninephrectomy.[181–183] An increase in EGF content and a reduction in EGF receptor levels have been observed only after compensatory renal hypertrophy is established.[182, 183] In contrast, there is an early increase in remnant kidney HGF and HGF message after uninephrectomy.[184] However, uninephrectomy and operative stress also increase HGF expression in distant organs, such as the lung.[185] Thus, whereas there is solid evidence that HGF is an important morphogen for growing tubule cells, the significance of the early nephrectomy-induced increase in remnant kidney HGF content remains unclear.[186]

## The Relation of Structural to Functional Changes After Nephrectomy: The Work Hypothesis

The earliest hypothesis advanced to explain renal enlargement after nephrectomy was the ''work hypertrophy'' theory of Addis.[187] Addis believed that excretion of urea required consumption of energy. He therefore suggested that renal enlargement after nephrectomy and during long-term feeding of protein-rich diets represents a response to an increase in renal workload imposed by the necessity to excrete more urea. When Addis tested this hypothesis, however, he found that an increase in urea load does not cause renal hypertrophy in intact rats.[188] It remains possible that the remnant kidney grows in response to increased demand for other forms of renal ''work.'' The possibility that increased demand for substances synthesized by the kidney causes kidney growth has received limited attention. However, studies have indicated that addition of exogenous 1,25-dihydroxyvitamin $D_3$, erythropoietin, or arginine does not prevent remnant kidney hypertrophy and hyperfiltration after renal ablation.[189–191] Since the realization that renal energy consumption is devoted largely to cation reabsorption rather than urea excretion, the phrase work hypertrophy has most often been employed to suggest that renal hypertrophy is a tubule response to the increased reabsorption of solutes necessitated by an increase in GFR. However, if hypertrophy is indeed the result of hyperfiltration, the stimulus to remnant nephron hyperfiltration after reduction in nephron number remains to be identified. Nor is it possible at present to exclude the alternative hypothesis that nephron loss first stimulates growth of remnant tubules, which then causes an increase in remnant nephron GFR.

## RELATION OF RENAL MASS TO GLOMERULAR FILTRATION RATE IN OTHER CIRCUMSTANCES

Renal mass and GFR usually remain closely matched during kidney growth, whereas nephron number remains normal just as it does during kidney growth after nephrectomy. After the early neonatal period, RBF, GFR, and renal mass increase in proportion so that RBF and GFR expressed per unit kidney weight remain approximately constant.[77, 78, 192] Further parallel increases in RBF and GFR and in renal mass occur not only in response to nephrectomy but with sustained feeding of protein-rich diets[193, 194] and in diabetes mellitus.[195, 196] It is tempting to speculate that some feature of altered metabolism common to protein catabolism and diabetes causes increased renal perfusion and renal growth in these circumstances. Presumably, such a metabolic signal could also govern the increase in renal function and size during normal body growth and could moreover be related to the stimulus causing renal hypertrophy after nephrectomy. It is interesting that kidneys of animals subjected to nephrectomy, fed protein, or made diabetic cannot clearly be distinguished from kidneys that have achieved the same increase in mass through continued normal growth. Tubule enlargement is most prominent in the proximal nephron in each circumstance. More detailed segmental analyses of tubule structure and function, which may reveal differences between these forms of renal growth, have yet to be performed.

## RELATION OF TUBULE BIOCHEMICAL CHANGES TO GLOMERULAR FILTRATION RATE AFTER NEPHRECTOMY

At present, the question of whether hypertrophy causes hyperfiltration or whether hyperfiltration causes hypertrophy remains unanswered. One approach for deciding this issue has been to examine whether growth-related biochemical changes develop in remnant tubules before remnant nephron GFR increases. Some studies have found that tubule biochemical changes do precede any detectable increase in GFR.[197, 198] These studies, however, cannot be considered to prove that hyperfiltration is not the cause of hypertrophy. One difficulty in accepting this conclusion is that studies of biochemical changes have been performed in animals nephrectomized under light anesthesia, allowed to recover, and then quickly killed for biochemical assays, whereas measurements of renal function after nephrectomy have usually been performed during a prolonged second operative procedure requiring barbiturate anesthesia. Thus, it is possible that failure to detect early functional changes may in part reflect fluid losses and other effects of the second operation. Increases in GFR have been noted within 1 day after uninephrectomy in dogs, in which postoperative fluid losses may be smaller than in rats, and in rats studied without anesthesia.[14, 199] GFR has usually been found not to increase in the first several hours after nephrectomy, but increases in GFR were observed at 90 minutes after nephrectomy in a study in which rats were given large volumes of fluid during postnephrectomy functional studies.[200, 201]

Tubule biochemical changes observed within 1 hour after nephrectomy, as described in the preceding section, presumably cannot be mediated by an increase in remnant nephron GFR. Some of these early biochemical changes, however, are known not to be essential to remnant nephron hypertrophy. For instance, the early increase in proximal $Na^+/H^+$ antiport activity after nephrectomy is blocked by renal denervation, but this maneuver has no effect on compensatory renal hypertrophy.[202] Likewise, the early increase in ornithine decarboxylase activity after nephrectomy can be blocked pharmacologically without preventing remnant kidney growth.[142]

Some changes in tubule function, as well as changes in tubule biochemistry, precede a detectable increase in GFR after uninephrectomy. The most prominent of these changes are decreases in tubule $Na^+$ and $K^+$ reabsorption, which cause approximately twofold increases in remnant kidney $Na^+$ and $K^+$ excretion within 1 hour after nephrectomy.[199, 203–208] Micropuncture studies suggest that acute postnephrectomy natriuresis and kaliuresis reflect decreased solute reabsorption by the proximal nephron.[204, 207] Studies by Humphreys and co-workers[209, 210] suggest that the early increase in $Na^+$ excretion after nephrectomy can be prevented by renal denervation and by abolition of ANP activity. Their finding that the early postnephrectomy increase in $Na^+$ excretion depends on intact renal innervation indicates that the mechanisms responsible for this phenomenon are different from those that cause compensatory renal hyperfiltration and hypertrophy. Presumably, the mechanisms responsible for acute postnephrectomy natriuresis could also cause some of the early biochemical changes observed in the remnant kidney.

A further difficulty in relating biochemical changes in the remnant kidney to compensatory renal hypertrophy is presented by the observation that a number of biochemical parameters exhibit a biphasic response after renal ablation. Included in this category are ornithine decarboxylase activity and polyamine levels,[139, 140] ribosomal RNA synthesis,[211] protein synthetic rate,[125, 212] and hexose monophosphate shunt enzyme activity.[117] In general, these parameters exhibit an early increase after uninephrectomy, followed by a decline over the second postoperative day and then an increase in activity on the third to fifth postoperative day. It should be emphasized that some of the early biochemical changes seen after uninephrectomy are also induced by maneuvers that do not lead ultimately to kidney growth. Incorporation of radiolabeled nucleotide into DNA and the prevalence of tubule mitotic figures are greater in obstructed kidneys than in remnant kidneys of uninephrectomized animals.[131, 213] Increased tubule mitotic activity has also been noted during long-term saline loading, which does not cause an increase in renal mass.[131]

## EFFECTS OF URETERAL DIVERSION COMPARED WITH THOSE OF NEPHRECTOMY

A long-standing question has been whether compensatory renal hypertrophy is triggered by loss of excretory function or whether it occurs only when renal tissue is destroyed. The original study of this problem compared renal mass after anastomosis of one ureter to the vena cava with renal mass after unilateral nephrectomy.[214] Subsequent studies have compared renal mass after uninephrectomy with renal mass after drainage of one ureter into the gut,[215] peritoneal cavity,[216–218] or venous circulation.[219, 220] It has generally been concluded that the kidney with normal ureteral drainage does not undergo hypertrophy as long as the kidney with the diverted ureter continues to be perfused. In many of these studies, patency of the diverted ureter has not been confirmed. However, because unilateral ureteral ligation leads to hypertrophy of the contralateral kidney, inadvertent ureteral obstruction cannot account for the failure of intact kidneys to enlarge after unilateral ureteral diversion.[221, 222] Inflammatory complications of the diversion procedure, including peritonitis and sepsis, may present a more serious difficulty. Reduced food intake and poor weight gain have generally been observed in animals subjected to ureteral diversion. Starvation as well as operative trauma and infection can impair kidney growth. These complications may be avoided by the technique of daily reinfusion of half the urine volume, so that excretory function is effectively reduced while both kidneys are left intact. Animals reinfused with half their urine volume have been shown to exhibit increases in kidney weight and GFR when compared with animals infused with saline.[223]

## RENAL "HYPOTROPHY"

The suggestion that kidney growth is conditioned by some metabolic "load" is consistent with the observation that renal perfusion and GFR increase rapidly shortly after birth.[192] In humans born with unilateral renal agenesis or with unilateral multicystic renal disease, the structurally intact kidney is of normal size for a two-kidney neonate at birth but then enlarges rapidly after delivery.[224, 225] These observations suggest that before birth, the excretory requirements of the fetus are met by the maternal kidney. If this were the case, uninephrectomy or unilateral renal obstruction in utero would not be expected to cause compensatory hypertrophy of the remnant fetal kidney. Experimental studies of this question have produced conflicting results.[226–229] Maternal uninephrectomy has been found not to cause fetal kidney hypertrophy in a single study.[230]

If enhanced renal function serves to limit renal size, compensatory renal hypertrophy might be reversible. Reversal of kidney growth (hypotrophy) has in fact been demonstrated when a second kidney is transplanted into a uninephrectomized rat,[231, 232] when ureteral obstruction is released after 1 week,[233] and when a rat with intact kidneys is disconnected from an anephric rat to which it had been joined by cross-circulation.[234] In contrast to these findings, an early study in which a third kidney was transplanted into a rat with two intact kidneys revealed that neither the native kidneys nor the transplanted kidney decreased in size and that the GFR was maintained at levels approximately 50% greater than those seen in two-kidney animals.[231] The authors suggested that whereas compensatory renal hypertrophy and hyperfunction are reversible, increases in renal mass and GFR with normal aging are "obligatory" and cannot decline even when clearance function is supranormal. Subsequent studies in a similar three-kidney preparation found, in contrast, that the GFR declined proportionally in each of the three kidneys so that the total GFR was equivalent to that of a two-kidney animal.[235] Studies in humans suggest that the GFR may decline in adult human kidneys transplanted into children but are difficult to evaluate because of the potential contribution of rejection to reduction in GFR.[236, 237]

## Factors That Influence Compensatory Hypertrophy

**Dietary Protein.** Feeding a low-protein diet to rats subjected to renal ablation limits remnant kidney GFR and weight.[238, 239] This finding has often been taken to suggest that dietary protein restriction prevents compensatory renal hypertrophy. Renal function in rats subjected to uninephrectomy and placed on a low-protein diet, however, must be compared with renal function in rats with intact kidneys maintained on the same diet. Such comparisons reveal that dietary protein restriction lowers baseline GFR and kidney weight in intact animals but does not prevent compensatory increases in GFR and kidney weight after nephrectomy.[238, 239] It has further been shown that feeding a protein-rich diet increases GFR and kidney weight in uninephrectomized rats. These observations suggest that the stimuli to hyperfiltration and hypertrophy associated with nephrectomy and protein feeding are additive. Similar observations suggest that the stimuli to hyperfiltration and hypertrophy associated with nephrectomy, diabetes mellitus, and pregnancy are also additive. Thus, in women with only one kidney, the already supranormal GFR increases further with pregnancy,[240, 241] and induction of diabetes leads to a further increase in GFR and size of the remnant kidney of uninephrectomized rats.[242]

**Endocrine Hormones.** The finding that renal function and size increase in altered metabolic states such as diabetes and pregnancy led to the suggestion that endocrine hormones might cause renal growth. Early observations showed that renal mass was diminished in rats subjected to pituitary ablation and was increased in patients with acromegaly.[243, 244] Further studies have shown that GFR declines after hypophysectomy in humans despite glucocorticoid and thyroid hormone replacement therapy and increases when normal subjects are given exogenous growth hormone.[245–248] Some early studies suggested that compensatory renal hypertrophy did not occur in rats subjected to

pituitary ablation.[249] Careful examination of these studies reveals that kidney weight remained stable only when pituitary ablation and uninephrectomy were performed at about the same time. Later studies have shown that pituitary ablation, like dietary protein restriction, lowers kidney weight in intact rats but does not prevent an increase in remnant kidney weight above the low basal value after uninephrectomy.[250] Use of recombinant growth hormone to increase stature in children has prompted evaluation of the amount of growth hormone required to cause renal hypertrophy. Available studies suggest that doses of exogenous growth hormone sufficient to normalize increases in stature do not increase GFR in pediatric patients with transplant kidneys or primary renal disease.[251, 252] Increases in kidney weight after uninephrectomy equivalent to those seen in control animals have been observed not only in rats subjected to pituitary ablation[142, 250, 253] but in rats and mice with congenital growth hormone deficiency.[254–256]

Similar results have been obtained in rats subjected to thyroidectomy[257] and adrenalectomy.[258] Both these maneuvers reduce kidney weight and GFR in rats with two kidneys,[258–260] but despite complete lack of thyroid and corticosteroid hormones, the proportional increase in renal mass after uninephrectomy is nearly equivalent to that observed in animals with normal endocrine function. The magnitude of compensatory renal hypertrophic changes is similarly unaffected by androgens. Administration of androgens increases kidney weight in female mice and rats.[261–263] In the rat, this change appears to be in large part the result of body growth, because castration only modestly reduces kidney weight in fully grown male rats.[262] In the mouse, androgens stimulate more marked renal hypertrophy by a direct action on the kidney.[264–266] Equivalent increases in renal mass, however, are observed after nephrectomy in female rats, in intact male rats, in castrated male rats, and in male rats and mice with congenital end-organ unresponsiveness to androgens.[262, 264–267] The magnitude of increases in remnant kidney GFR and size after kidney donation for transplantation in human subjects has similarly been noted not to depend on the sex of the donor.[7, 8]

**Age.** In contrast to endocrine manipulations, age has a definite effect on the magnitude of compensatory kidney growth.[27, 268] The studies of Addis and co-workers[269] showed that kidney weight in rats increased about 70% when contralateral nephrectomy was performed shortly after birth but only by about 30% to 40% when uninephrectomy was performed after maturity. Later studies have confirmed these findings and shown that postnephrectomy increases in GFR are also proportionally greater in young animals.[25, 26, 270] In human subjects born with one functioning kidney or subjected to uninephrectomy early in life, values for GFR of the solitary functioning kidney are nearly equal to those seen in normal individuals with two kidneys, whereas in adults subjected to uninephrectomy, the contralateral kidney GFR increases only about 50% above preoperative levels so that the total GFR is about 75% of normal when the compensatory response is complete.[7, 8, 271] The increased magnitude of compensatory renal hypertrophy in youth may reflect generally greater responsiveness of young tissue to stimuli responsible for organ growth. Thus, increases in lung size after unilateral pneumonectomy and in adrenal size after unilateral adrenalectomy are also greater in young than in mature rats.[272, 273]

## FUNCTION OF SURVIVING NEPHRONS IN DIFFUSE RENAL DISEASE: THE INTACT NEPHRON HYPOTHESIS AND THE MAINTENANCE OF GLOMERULOTUBULAR BALANCE

Experimental studies have shown that when diffuse disease processes reduce the GFR in some nephrons, compensatory mechanisms elevate the GFR in less damaged nephrons.[3–5] The normal nephron population is thus replaced by a reduced nephron population in which neighboring structures exhibit different patterns of form and function.[274] Maintenance of body fluid homeostasis by the diseased kidney depends on the ability of this heterogeneous nephron population to control water and solute excretion. The intact nephron hypothesis proposed by Bricker[1, 2] suggests that despite distortion of renal architecture and a widened range of values for SNGFR, glomerular function and tubule function remain as closely integrated in the diseased kidney as they do in the normal organ. Thus, the physiologically appropriate behavior of the diseased kidney is the result of physiologically appropriate behavior of each remnant nephron unit.

Support for the intact nephron hypothesis was originally derived from clearance studies in animals with unilateral renal disease.[2] In these experiments, the diseased kidney contained many damaged nephrons and had a markedly reduced GFR. Excretion of most of the daily load of water and solutes was accomplished by the intact contralateral kidney. Yet remarkably, when factored for the reduced GFR, excretion of Na$^+$,[275] phosphorus,[276] K$^+$,[277] net acid,[278] and other solutes by the diseased kidney proceeded at rates comparable to those measured in the intact kidney. It is highly unlikely that the physiologically appropriate handling of these different solutes by the diseased kidney represents a fortuitous combination of elevated solute excretion by some remnant nephrons and reduced solute excretion by others. Rather, as suggested by the intact nephron hypothesis, each remnant nephron presumably transports water and solutes in proportion to its individual GFR, whether reduced by disease processes or elevated by compensatory hypertrophy.

A crucial feature of physiologically appropriate remnant nephron function is maintenance of glomerulotubular balance. Compensatory elevation of SNGFR must be accompanied by increased proximal water and solute reabsorption, or increased delivery of filtrate would overwhelm the distal nephron's transport capacity and prevent it from contributing to elaboration of urine of appropriate volume and composition. Similarly, primary reduction in SNGFR must be matched by reduction in proximal volume reabsorption, or fluid delivery to the distal portion of the altered nephron would cease and again make fine regulation of solute excretion impossible.

Micropuncture studies by Gottschalk and colleagues[3, 4] first confirmed that glomerulotubular balance is maintained over a wide range of SNGFR values in both tubulointerstitial and glomerular diseases. Subsequent studies by Ichikawa and co-workers[279] elucidated the mechanism by which this remarkable adaptation is accomplished. In the chronic phase of experimental membranous glomerulonephritis, SNGFR values were found to vary from approximately one half to twice normal. Proximal fluid reabsorption was correlated closely with SNGFR in individual nephron units, so that fractional reabsorption was the same in hypofiltering and hyperfiltering nephrons. Alterations in Starling forces governing peritubular capillary fluid reabsorption were shown to account for this appropriate coupling of proximal Na$^+$ and water reabsorption to glomerular filtration. Efferent arteriolar oncotic pressure varied directly with SNGFR, whereas hydraulic pressure was similar throughout the peritubular capillary network. The net force favoring fluid reabsorption by capillaries surrounding each proximal nephron thus varied in proportion to the SNGFR of the same nephron unit.

Structural changes in the proximal tubule and peritubular capillary network presumably act in concert with alterations in Starling forces to promote glomerulotubular balance. In the studies of experimental glomerulonephritis described before, the net hydraulic permeability of the peritubular capillary network surrounding severely damaged nephrons was shown to be reduced, which suggests loss of capillary surface area available for fluid reabsorption.[279] Morphologic studies have further shown that nephrons whose glomeruli are severely damaged by experimental immune injury exhibit proximal tubule atrophy, presumably associated with decreased tubule reabsorptive capacity. In contrast, proximal tubules of less damaged nephrons increase in diameter and in length. Hypertrophy of these tubule segments is presumably associated with an increase in tubule reabsorptive capacity.

Mechanisms by which glomerular function is matched to tubule function in primary tubulointerstitial disease are less clear. A widened range of values for SNGFR similar to that observed in chronic glomerulonephritis has been demonstrated in tubule disease induced by administration of salts of heavy metals.[4] Filtration was markedly reduced in glomeruli of the most severely damaged nephrons so that glomerulotubular balance was again maintained. Morphologic studies have shown that a similarly wide range of values for glomerular volume is observed in rats with tubulointerstitial disease caused by administration of lithium.[280] As would be predicted by the intact nephron hypothesis, small glomeruli are attached to atrophic tubules and larger glomeruli to intact tubules; in a subpopulation of small "atubule" glomeruli, tubule attachment is no longer discernible. In some cases, glomerular dysfunction after tubule injury may be the result of obstruction. Studies by Tanner and co-workers[281, 282] have shown that obstruction of single proximal tubules causes reduction of blood flow to the attached glomeruli followed by atrophy of both glomeruli and tubules. In other cases, however, obstruction appears not to account for glomerular dysfunction after tubule injury. In experimental disease caused by heavy metals and by experimental pyelonephritis, glomeruli attached to damaged tubules appear initially "compressed" and later

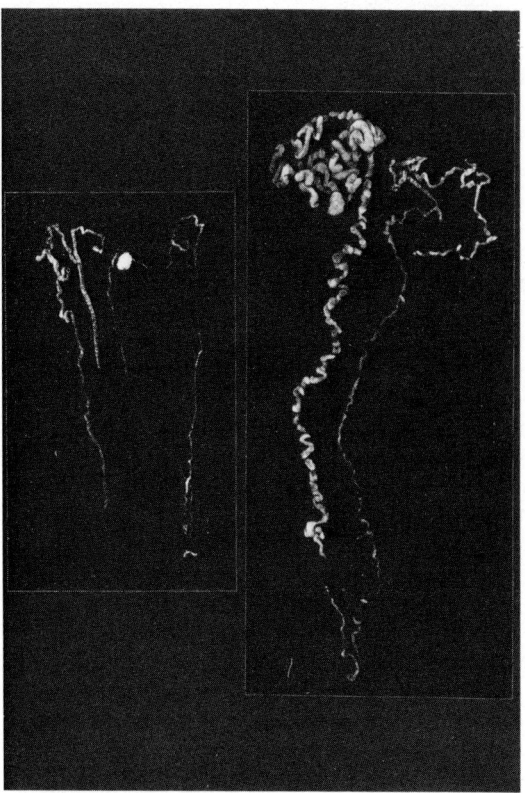

**Figure 44–2.** Nephrons microdissected from the kidney of a patient with chronic glomerulonephritis. The nephron on the left exhibits marked atrophy of the proximal convolution, presumably reflecting a reduction in SNGFR. The nephron on the right exhibits hypertrophy of the proximal convolution, presumably reflecting an adaptive increase in SNGFR in a glomerulus less damaged by the primary disease process. (From Oliver J: Architecture of the Kidney in Chronic Bright's Disease. Paul B Hoeber, New York, 1939, with permission from Harper & Row.)

become sclerotic.[4, 283] Arteriolar vasoconstriction could account for the reduction in filtration by glomeruli of damaged nephrons, but the mechanism remains to be established.

Studies in human renal disease, although necessarily less complete, are in general agreement with the intact nephron hypothesis. Thus, as illustrated in Figure 44–2, hypertrophied tubules are most often attached to hypertrophied glomeruli and shrunken tubules to shrunken glomeruli. Other patterns of structural changes are observed, however, and their functional significance remains unclear.[284] The finding of atubule glomeruli may represent continued perfusion at a reduced rate of glomeruli that have lost their tubule attachment, as suggested by Marcussen.[280] The pathophysiologic significance of occasional hypertrophied ''aglomerular tubules'' remains to be determined.

## TUBULE HANDLING OF WATER AND SOLUTES BY THE ADAPTED NEPHRON

As nephron number is reduced, radical increases in excretion of water and of individual solutes by each remnant

nephron are required to maintain external balances in the face of continued food and fluid intake. The balanced changes in SNGFR and proximal reabsorption that ensure adequate distal fluid delivery in altered nephrons must therefore be assisted by *specific* mechanisms that enhance single-nephron excretion of water and ions. In general, these mechanisms are not unique to renal insufficiency but are the same as those described in Volume I that enable normal individuals, when challenged, to excrete extraordinarily large quantities of water and solutes. With a 90% reduction in GFR, for example, each remnant nephron must function as would a normal nephron in a subject whose water and solute intake was increased 10-fold. In general, as has been emphasized, this adaptation is accomplished with remarkable success, and external balances are maintained. There are limits to the adaptive process, however. Rapid elimination of large water and solute loads may not be achieved by a reduced number of nephrons already operating near their excretory capacity. The patient with renal insufficiency is therefore notably susceptible to iatrogenic hyperkalemia, acidosis, and volume overload. Similarly, fully efficient conservation of water and salt cannot be achieved by the diseased kidney. Patients with chronic renal insufficiency are therefore also susceptible to dehydration and volume depletion.

## Sodium Excretion and the Regulation of Extracellular Fluid Volume

ECF volume is maintained remarkably close to normal in patients with chronic renal insufficiency.[285] As depicted in Figure 44–3, this is accomplished by an increase in fractional excretion of $Na^+$ proportional to the decline in GFR.[286] The capacity to excrete a large fraction of filtered $Na^+$ with little if any increase in ECF or plasma volume is characteristic of the normal as well as of the diseased kidney. The patient with a GFR of 10 mL/min excreting 100

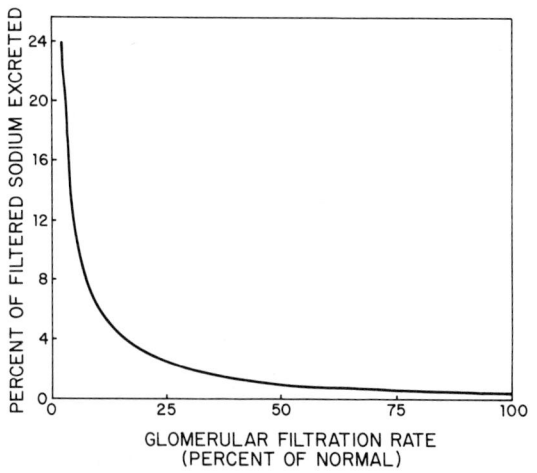

**Figure 44–3.** The relation between steady-state GFR and the fraction of filtered $Na^+$ excreted on a diet containing 7 g of salt. (Adapted from Slatopolsky E, Elkan IO, Weerts C, Bricker NS: Studies on the characteristics of the control system governing sodium excretion in uremic man. J Clin Invest 47:521, 1968.)

mEq of $Na^+$ per day may be thought of as comparable to a normal individual with a GFR of 120 mL/min given a diet containing 1200 mEq of sodium per day. Normal subjects will in fact excrete such large quantities of $Na^+$ with only a slight increase in systemic blood pressure and without a clinically detectable increase in ECF volume.[287, 288]

The mechanisms responsible for increased $Na^+$ excretion by remnant nephrons after reduction in GFR have been widely studied.[289, 290] An important object of these studies has been to determine in which nephron segments fractional $Na^+$ reabsorption is decreased. Some micropuncture studies have suggested that the fraction of filtered fluid and $Na^+$ reabsorbed by the proximal nephron falls when GFR is reduced by renal ablation[291, 292] and by glomerulonephritis.[3] Other studies in rats with comparable reductions in GFR, however, have failed to detect any reduction in proximal reabsorption.[80, 283, 293] When observed, a fall in fractional proximal reabsorption does not necessarily represent an adaptation to the increased $Na^+$ excretory load placed on remnant nephrons. Thus, in rats subjected to 85% renal ablation, Weber and colleagues[292] found that the fraction of filtrate reabsorbed in the proximal nephron remained low even when fractional excretion of $Na^+$ was normalized by restricting salt intake. Taken together, cortical micropuncture studies suggest that in moderate renal insufficiency, adaptive changes in $Na^+$ excretion are accomplished by more distal portions of the nephron. Results obtained by use of more direct techniques further support this view. Microcatheterization[294] and micropuncture[30] studies have shown that $Na^+$ reabsorption in the terminal collecting duct practically ceases when fractional $Na^+$ excretion is increased to only about three times normal values by renal ablation in the rat. These findings are in accord with the general principle, as reviewed in Chapters 8 and 20, that fine control of $Na^+$ excretion is localized in the distal nephron.

A number of mechanisms have been suggested to account for decreased $Na^+$ reabsorption in the setting of renal insufficiency. Early workers considered the possibility that increased $Na^+$ excretion might reflect reduced mineralocorticoid hormone activity.[295] However, later studies have shown that aldosterone levels are normal or increased in the majority of patients with renal insufficiency.[288, 296–298] Moreover, in patients with advanced renal failure, administration of the mineralocorticoid antagonist spironolactone generally causes natriuresis and reduction in body weight.[297] This finding suggests that endogenous aldosterone contributes to $Na^+$ retention in uremia and may account for the observation that exogenous mineralocorticoid often does not cause further $Na^+$ retention in uremic patients.[286, 299, 300]

The finding that increased fractional excretion of $Na^+$ in renal insufficiency cannot be attributed to low aldosterone levels has prompted extensive efforts to identify a circulating natriuretic hormone responsible for reducing avidity of distal $Na^+$ reabsorption when GFR is reduced. Fractions isolated from serum and urine of patients and animals with renal failure were shown to induce natriuresis in rats.[301, 302] Similar natriuretic isolates were obtained from urine and serum of normal subjects undergoing natriuresis induced by water immersion or increased salt intake.[303, 304] These various natriuretic fractions not only increased $Na^+$ excretion

in intact rats but also limited $Na^+$ reabsorption by isolated toad bladders[305] and rabbit cortical collecting tubules,[306] which suggests a distal site of action. Despite intensive effort, the chemical structure responsible for natriuretic activity in these isolates proved difficult to identify. One line of evidence suggests that elevated levels of factors with cardiac glycoside–like activity contribute to the response to volume expansion both in normal and in uremic animals.[307, 308] Such factors, which exhibit digoxin-like immunoreactivity and suppress "ouabain-sensitive" cellular $Na^+,K^+$-ATPase, could cause not only increased $Na^+$ excretion but also cellular electrolyte abnormalities and contribute to uremic toxicity.

The discovery of ANP brought new direction to the study of humoral control of $Na^+$ excretion in renal insufficiency. Attempts to isolate a novel natriuretic compound have largely been abandoned in favor of studies of ANP action. Rats subjected to renal ablation exhibit increases in ANP levels that are related to dietary sodium intake and to fractional $Na^+$ excretion.[309, 310] Similar increases in ANP levels in patients with renal insufficiency have been related to increased blood volume and to increased blood pressure.[311–314] Interpretation of these studies may be complicated by the presence of heart failure and by errors in the assay of plasma ANP caused by related peptides that are retained in renal failure. Studies with a recently developed ANP antagonist, however, suggest that increased ANP levels make a major contribution to increased fractional $Na^+$ excretion in experimental renal insufficiency.[315]

Guyton and co-workers have emphasized that systemic hypertension may contribute to increased fractional $Na^+$ excretion in renal insufficiency.[316, 317] According to this view, maintenance of constant sodium intake when functioning nephron number is reduced leads to $Na^+$ retention and expansion of ECF and blood volumes. The increase in blood volume causes an increase in blood pressure, which in turn causes an increase in fractional $Na^+$ excretion. A new steady state is reached when the pressure-mediated increase in fractional $Na^+$ excretion allows the diseased kidney to excrete the daily $Na^+$ load. Dependence of $Na^+$ excretion on blood pressure could account for the observation that attempts to control hypertension with vasodilator drugs lead to marked $Na^+$ retention in uremic patients.[318] Further studies have shown, however, that blood pressure does not increase as much in normal subjects consuming a high-salt diet as it does in patients with renal insufficiency consuming a "standard" diet.[287, 288, 319] These studies have confirmed that blood pressure is dependent on blood volume in uremic patients but have also shown that blood pressure is higher in uremic patients than in normal subjects whose blood volumes have been increased by salt loading. Finally, it has been shown that reducing dietary salt intake does not prevent hypertension in rats with reduced nephron number.[320] Together, these observations suggest that fractional $Na^+$ excretion in renal insufficiency is regulated by factors other than systemic blood pressure.

## LIMITATION OF SODIUM EXCRETION IN CHRONIC RENAL FAILURE

Whereas excretion of the normal daily sodium intake is effectively accomplished in renal insufficiency, the immediate natriuretic response to a large $Na^+$ challenge may be impaired.[291] Studies have documented reduction in the portion of an intravenous $Na^+$ load excreted over 5 hours after renal ablation in dogs.[38, 321] Of note, the natriuresis evoked by $Na^+$ loading is generally reduced less than is the GFR.[60, 291, 321] Thus, as emphasized by earlier studies, acute volume expansion actually causes a greater increase in fractional $Na^+$ excretion in uremic animals than in normal control subjects.[322] This "magnification" of the natriuretic response to volume expansion is observed not only in animals with renal insufficiency but in the damaged kidneys of patients and animals with unilateral renal disease.[275, 291, 322–324] The increased natriuretic response of unilaterally diseased kidneys clearly cannot be attributed to alterations in systemic blood pressure or circulating hormone levels. Wen and associates[291] suggested that this phenomenon reflects decreased $Na^+$ reabsorption by the loop of Henle, the mechanism of which remains unknown.

The ability to conserve $Na^+$ is also impaired in renal insufficiency. When sodium intake is reduced, most patients with serious chronic renal disease are unable to lower $Na^+$ excretion below 20 to 30 mEq/d,[299, 325] and occasional patients continue to excrete much larger amounts of $Na^+$.[325–330] Modest obligate $Na^+$ losses in uremic patients were initially related to an inability to lower luminal $Na^+$ concentration in the terminal nephron below a fixed value.[299] This defect has in turn been attributed to an increased per nephron load of urea and other solutes. Greater obligate $Na^+$ losses in patients with so-called salt wasting have generally been attributed to structural damage to the distal nephron.[325–327, 330] These explanations for the inability of uremic patients to conserve $Na^+$ have been questioned by Danovitch and associates.[329] These workers found that in severely uremic patients, including salt wasters, $Na^+$ excretion could be reduced to less than 10 mEq/d if dietary sodium intake was lowered gradually during a period of 4 to 14 weeks. They suggested that the ability of uremic patients to adapt to a gradual reduction in sodium intake was related to slow suppression of circulating natriuretic hormone levels. No other plausible explanation for this remarkable phenomenon has been advanced.

## Water Excretion and the Regulation of Body Fluid Tonicity

### THE DILUTING MECHANISM

The capacity of the kidney to excrete water loads has traditionally been expressed in terms of solute-free water generation. In the normal kidney, about 12 mL of solute-free water can be generated for each 100 mL of glomerular filtrate. This is equivalent to about 18 L of water for a normal GFR of 150 L/d. The urine volume under conditions of maximal water diuresis may be viewed as consisting of 18 L of solute-free water and 2.0 L of "isotonic urine" containing the average daily solute load of 600 mOsm at a concentration of 30 mOsm/L. In normal subjects, this large volume of water may be consumed and excreted without a

measurable decline in ECF osmolality. Minimal urine osmolality is approximately

$$\text{Minimal } U_{osm} = \frac{\text{total osmoles excreted}}{\text{total volume excreted}} \approx \frac{600 \text{ mOsm}}{20 \text{ L}} \approx 30 \text{ mOsm/L}$$

Normal generation of solute-free water depends on dilution of tubule fluid in the thick ascending limb and on maintenance of low water permeability in the distal nephron in the absence of antidiuretic hormone (ADH). The excretion of maximally dilute urine is further facilitated by decreased hypertonicity of the medullary interstitium during water diuresis, as described in Chapter 13. Given the complexity of the diluting mechanism, the capacity to generate solute-free water expressed as a fraction of the GFR is remarkably well maintained when renal function is impaired. The capacity to dilute the urine remains nearly normal in humans and rats subjected to uninephrectomy.[8, 331] Even patients with advanced renal disease can usually generate a normal volume of solute-free water from each milliliter of glomerular filtrate, and dogs subjected to five-sixths renal ablation can actually generate an increased volume of solute-free water from each milliliter of glomerular filtrate.[332–335]

Overall reduction in the GFR, however, impairs the capacity of the kidney to excrete a water load even while solute-free water generation by functioning remnant nephrons remains normal. For example, with a GFR of 15 L/d (10 mL/min), generation of 12 mL of solute-free water per 100 mL of GFR gives the diseased kidney the capacity to excrete only about 1.8 L of solute-free water in addition to the 2.0 L of isotonic urine containing the average daily osmolar load. This limitation in ability to excrete water in excess of solute finds expression in a reduction in the minimal urine osmolality that can be attained by the diseased kidney:

$$\text{Minimal } U_{osm} = \frac{\text{total osmoles excreted}}{\text{total volume excreted}} \approx \frac{600 \text{ mOsm}}{3.8 \text{ L}} \approx 160 \text{ mOsm/L}$$

Reduction in the ability to excrete solute-free water puts patients with renal insufficiency at risk for water intoxication. A patient with a GFR of 10 mL/min can safely take in no more than about 3.5 L of fluid per day. Ill-planned administration of intravenous fluid or psychogenic polydipsia, which would cause only polyuria in normal individuals, may thus precipitate hyponatremia in patients with renal insufficiency.

In an occasional patient, inability to dilute the urine appears to result from disproportionate disturbance of ascending limb function by disease processes. Thus, a patient with pyelonephritis described by Kleeman and associates[333] had a GFR of 8 mL/min but was unable to dilute his urine below 300 mOsm. A much more common cause of impaired ascending limb function is administration of loop diuretic agents, such as furosemide. These drugs are often required to promote $Na^+$ excretion and treat hypertension in renal insufficiency but can further impair the ability of the diseased kidney to excrete water loads by inhibiting sodium chloride reabsorption and tubule fluid dilution in the thick ascending limb.

## THE CONCENTRATING MECHANISM

Concentration of the urine requires maintenance of hypertonicity of the medullary interstitium and normal water transport across distal nephron segments in response to ADH. Maintenance of medullary interstitial hypertonicity in turn requires structural preservation of the countercurrent system. It is not surprising, therefore, that limitation of concentrating ability may occur early in the course of renal insufficiency. Figure 44–4 illustrates the maximal urine osmolality attained by patients with a variety of renal diseases and by normal subjects, plotted as a function of GFR. Maximal urine osmolality, normally about 1200 mOsm, may be reduced to 600 mOsm when the GFR is reduced by only one third. When the GFR is reduced to 15 mL/min, maximal urine osmolality is commonly about 400 mOsm. Excretion of the normal daily solute load of 600 mOsm thus requires a urine volume of about 1.5 L in the patient with renal disease, whereas the normal subject with maximal urine osmolality of 1200 mOsm can excrete the same daily solute load in a urine volume of 500 mL.

Part of the defect in urine concentration in patients with chronic renal disease may be attributed to the high load of urea and other solutes imposed on each nephron. As demonstrated by Dorhout-Mees,[336] however, the osmotic effect of urea does not fully account for the reduction in maximal urine osmolality profiled in Figure 44–4. Not surprisingly, renal diseases that profoundly disturb the medullary architecture may cause disproportionate impairment of concentrating ability at any given level of GFR. Patients with tubulointerstitial diseases therefore tend to have high obligate water excretion as well as high obligate salt excretion when compared with patients with primary glomerular diseases. Maximal urine osmolalities in patients with polycystic kidney disease, in which the majority of early cysts form in the collecting ducts, are compared with maximal urine osmolalities in unselected patients in Figure 44–4.[334] Other tubulointerstitial diseases that cause pronounced impairment of concentrating ability include sickle cell nephropathy,[337, 338] analgesic nephropathy,[339] medullary cystic disease,[340] obstructive nephropathy,[341] multiple myeloma,[342] and nephrocalcinosis.[343] Of note, disproportionate reduction in concentrating ability has also been demonstrated in experimental animals with renal disease induced by surgical excision of the papilla.[344] Derangement of countercurrent flow in medullary vasa recta may result in inability to maintain medullary interstitial hypertonicity and thus contribute to limitation of concentrating ability in these conditions.

Tubulointerstitial disease processes cannot, however, reliably be distinguished from glomerular disease processes by the pattern of renal functional impairment. Pronounced defects in urine concentration and in $K^+$ and acid excretion may be more common in tubulointerstitial diseases, but similar defects may be seen in the glomerulopathies. This overlap may be explained by the eventual development of tubulointerstitial injury in diseases that begin in the glomerulus. Indeed, the urine specific gravity has been shown to be inversely correlated with the severity of medullary fibrosis in patients with primary glomerulonephritis.[345]

Concentration of the urine with reduced nephron number requires that an increased amount of water be reabsorbed across the distal epithelium of each remnant nephron. Before dialysis was routinely available, it was observed that in patients with severe reductions in nephron number (GFR < 10 mL/min), the maximal urine osmolality that could be attained was less than plasma osmolality in spite of injection of large doses of ADH.[346, 347] Micropuncture and microcatheterization studies indicate that further impaired concentrating ability in renal insufficiency may be caused by the limitation of ADH-stimulated water reabsorption in the distal nephron.[29, 348] Limited ADH responsiveness of the distal nephron may in turn be caused by two factors. First, ADH-stimulated adenylate cyclase activity and water permeability in the distal nephron may be impaired in uremia, as shown by some[349] but not all[350] studies of perfused collecting duct segments isolated from rabbits subjected to renal ablation. Second, increased tubule fluid flow rates may limit the fraction of water that can be reabsorbed by the distal nephron in response to ADH when nephron number is reduced.[351]

Because concentrating ability is impaired early in the course of renal insufficiency, dehydration would probably be the earliest symptom of chronic renal failure, were it not for the ready availability of water and the stimulation of thirst in response to even slight elevations in ECF tonicity. Patients therefore usually suffer not dehydration but *nocturia*, which results from inability to concentrate the urine sufficiently to permit a full night's sleep. Inability to conserve water, combined with the inability to conserve $Na^+$ described before, can contribute to rapid dehydration and volume depletion if water intake is interrupted during intercurrent illness.

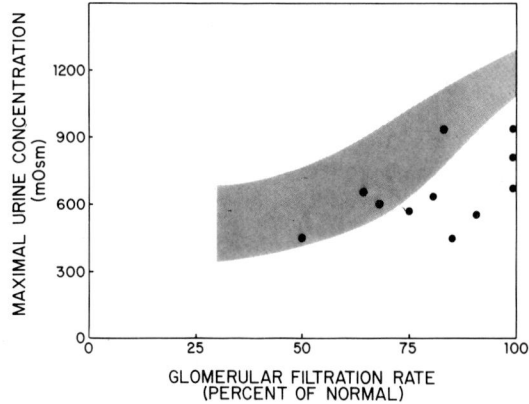

**Figure 44–4.** Concentrating capacity in chronic renal insufficiency. The shaded area illustrates the reduction in maximal urine concentration that may be attained as the GFR falls in patients with a variety of renal diseases. The plotted points from a study of sickle cell nephropathy illustrate the early impairment of concentrating ability that characterizes this condition. (Adapted from Martinez-Maldonado M, Yium JJ, Eknoyan G, Suki WN: Adult polycystic kidney disease: Studies of the defect in urine concentration. Kidney Int 2:107, 1972; and Dorhout-Mees EJ: Relation between maximal urine concentration, maximal water reabsorption capacity and mannitol clearance in patients with renal disease. Br Med J 1:1159, 1959.)

## Potassium Excretion

In diseased as well as in normal kidneys, the majority of filtered $K^+$ is reabsorbed in the proximal tubule and loop of Henle, and urinary $K^+$ excretion is determined largely by secretion of $K^+$ in the distal nephron.[277, 352-355] $K^+$ secretion per nephron must increase to maintain $K^+$ balance with reduced nephron number. Increased distal nephron flow rates and anion concentrations may facilitate $K^+$ excretion but are not essential to the maintenance of $K^+$ balance in renal failure. The major factors responsible for increased $K^+$ excretion per nephron appear to be transient elevation of plasma and intracellular $K^+$ concentrations after potassium ingestion and an adaptive tubule process that augments $K^+$ secretion. In addition, reduction of $K^+$ reabsorption by the loop of Henle may facilitate excretion of acute $K^+$ loads in renal insufficiency.[356]

After ingestion of 50 mEq of potassium, serum $K^+$ concentration increases by about 1 mEq/L in both normal subjects and most patients with moderate renal insufficiency.[357] Slightly greater increases in serum $K^+$ levels may be seen in some patients, particularly those with low aldosterone levels and those with more severe renal insufficiency.[358-360] In both normal and uremic subjects, postload increases in serum $K^+$ levels cause an increase in distal $K^+$ secretion and thus in $K^+$ excretion. When factored for GFR, the rise in $K^+$ excretion rate in patients with moderate renal insufficiency (GFR, 20 to 60 mL/min) is the same as in normal subjects.[357, 359] That is, a patient with a GFR value approximately one third of normal will respond to a rise in serum $K^+$ level of 1 mEq/L with a maximal $K^+$ excretion rate about one third of that achieved in a normal subject. Because the patient with renal failure excretes $K^+$ more slowly than the normal subject does, there will be prolonged elevation of serum $K^+$ concentration after an oral load (or meal). The daily $K^+$ load will eventually be excreted, but more slowly than in the normal subject. The role of small increases in serum $K^+$ concentration in regulating $K^+$ excretion has been verified in dogs with GFR reduced to about one third of normal by uninephrectomy and partial infarction of the remaining kidney.[361, 362] Fasting $K^+$ levels were the same as in normal dogs. Relatively large dietary potassium loads could be excreted by the diseased kidney but at the expense of a prolonged postprandial elevation of serum $K^+$ concentration.

$K^+$ excretion in severe renal insufficiency depends not only on episodic elevations in serum $K^+$ concentration but on an adaptive process whereby distal nephron secretion of $K^+$ is increased at any given level of serum $K^+$. This adaptive process can be demonstrated not only in patients with renal failure but in normal subjects ingesting large amounts of potassium. Excretion of 60 mEq/d of $K^+$ with a GFR of 12 mL/min may be thought of as equivalent to excretion of 600 mEq/d of $K^+$ with a GFR of 120 mL/min. Excretion of such amounts of $K^+$ can be accomplished by normal subjects without notable elevation of the serum $K^+$ level. The adaptive process responsible for increased distal $K^+$ secretion in $K^+$-loaded normal subjects is characterized by increased activity of $Na^+,K^+$-ATPase and basolateral surface area in principal cells of the cortical collecting duct.[110, 111, 115] Similar changes appear to be responsible for increased dis-

tal $K^+$ secretion in animals subjected to renal ablation.[113, 114] Both these alterations in collecting duct structure and the increase in $K^+$ secretion by collecting ducts isolated from uremic animals can be blocked by reducing potassium intake in proportion to the reduction in nephron number.[107, 114]

## ROLE OF ALDOSTERONE IN CHRONIC RENAL FAILURE

The adaptation of tubule secretory processes to handle large $K^+$ loads can be accomplished in adrenalectomized animals maintained on fixed doses of mineralocorticoid.[355] Increased mineralocorticoid synthesis is therefore not necessary for maintenance of $K^+$ balance in most cases of renal failure. Administration of the aldosterone antagonist spironolactone to patients with renal failure, however, often results in dangerous hyperkalemia.[363] Hyperkalemia has also been observed when aldosterone levels are reduced by the administration of converting enzyme inhibitors or, less frequently, by heparin in patients with renal insufficiency.[364, 365] Thus, it appears that "normal" levels of aldosterone are required to facilitate increased $K^+$ secretion per nephron.

Hyperkalemia, often in association with metabolic acidosis, may occur relatively early in the course of renal failure in patients who have low plasma aldosterone levels.[366-368] These cases further suggest a facilitative role for aldosterone in the increased excretion of $K^+$ per remnant nephron. They were at first considered examples of a single metabolic disorder, the syndrome of hyporeninemic hypoaldosteronism or type IV renal tubular acidosis. It has since become clear that no single pathophysiologic mechanism can explain the subnormal mineralocorticoid levels in these patients. A survey of patients with renal failure and hyperkalemia by Schambelan and associates[366] revealed that in some patients, aldosterone levels were low whereas plasma renin activity was normal. In the majority of cases, however, low aldosterone levels were associated with suppression of plasma renin activity. As described in Chapter 9, $K^+$ acts directly on the adrenal gland, and elevation of the serum $K^+$ concentration stimulates aldosterone release even in anephric patients. The association of hypoaldosteronism with hyporeninemia is thought to result from a reduction in the magnitude of the adrenal response to hyperkalemia when renin activity is chronically suppressed and circulating AII levels are continually low. No one mechanism appears to account for the suppression of plasma renin activity usually observed in renal failure patients who exhibit hyperkalemia and low aldosterone levels. Case reports have suggested that renin release in these patients is reduced by long-term volume expansion,[369] use of nonsteroidal anti-inflammatory drugs,[370] destruction of the renin secretory cells of the juxtaglomerular apparatus,[371] and release of an inactive renin precursor.[372] Damage to the juxtaglomerular apparatus may be pronounced in diabetic nephropathy, explaining the apparent prevalence of hyperkalemic metabolic acidosis associated with low plasma renin and aldosterone levels in this disorder.

Incomplete understanding of the pathophysiologic process of hyperkalemia associated with low aldosterone levels in renal insufficiency does not prevent effective therapy.

Prescription of synthetic mineralocorticoid will reverse the electrolyte abnormality in many patients but often causes $Na^+$ retention and exacerbates hypertension. More appropriate initial therapy is prescription of furosemide, which facilitates $K^+$ secretion by increasing distal delivery of sodium chloride and which may also stimulate renin release by reducing ECF volume. Furosemide alone is sufficient to lower $K^+$ levels in most patients with hyporeninemic hypoaldosteronism, but addition of mineralocorticoid is required in occasional patients.[373] Furosemide is also effective when hyperkalemia and metabolic acidosis occur in association with normal or elevated circulating mineralocorticoid levels. "Mineralocorticoid-resistant" hyperkalemia in these cases is presumably the result of distal nephron damage by prominent tubulointerstitial injury in disease processes such as sickle cell nephropathy and interstitial nephritis.[374-378] In such patients, impaired $K^+$ excretion may be combined with unusually severe concentrating defects, as described in the preceding section.

Finally, excessive potassium intake will cause hyperkalemia in any patient with advanced renal insufficiency. With severe reductions in nephron number, the normal dietary intake of approximately 60 to 80 mEq of potassium per day taxes the adaptive capacity of remnant distal nephrons. Elimination of $K^+$ by the colon increases slightly with severe reductions in GFR but is insufficient to allow excretion of increased $K^+$ loads. Ingestion of salt substitutes or "health food" diets containing large amounts of fruit and nuts therefore commonly leads to hyperkalemia in patients with renal failure.

## Acid-Base Regulation

Reduction of the GFR in patients with renal insufficiency is accompanied by a parallel reduction in serum $HCO_3^-$ concentration, reflecting development of systemic acidosis.[379-382] This acidosis is caused by a reduction in the diseased kidney's capacity to excrete acid, because the total daily production of metabolic acids is not increased in uremia. Careful studies have shown that the acidosis of renal insufficiency is caused by impairment of each of the processes required for normal acid excretion, including ammonia synthesis, $HCO_3^-$ reabsorption in the proximal nephron, and luminal fluid acidification in the distal nephron. Unequal impairment in these processes in individual patients presumably accounts for the varying severity of acidosis encountered at any given level of renal function,[382] as illustrated in Figure 44–5.

The major limitation of net acid excretion in renal insufficiency is imposed by reduction of the kidney's capacity to synthesize ammonia. With compensatory tubule hypertrophy, the ammonia synthetic capacity of individual proximal nephrons increases.[97, 383] However, the increased capacity of individual remnant nephrons to synthesize ammonia cannot compensate for severe reductions in nephron number, so that when GFR is markedly reduced, the portion of net acid excreted as ammonia decreases.[379-381, 384] Concentrations of ammonia in the urine are less than normal when plotted against urine pH, as illustrated in Figure 44–6. Initially, modest reductions in the serum $HCO_3^-$ concentration result in maintenance of an acid urine pH

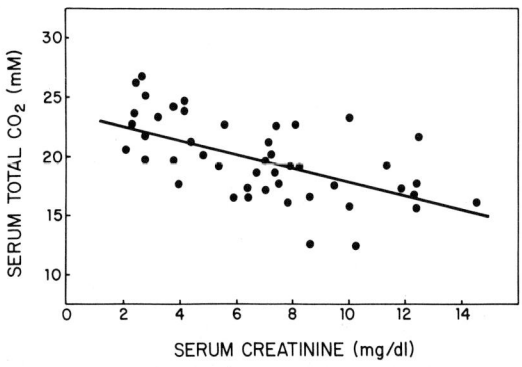

**Figure 44–5.** Serum carbon dioxide level plotted against serum creatinine concentration in patients with a variety of renal diseases. (From Widmer B, Gerhardt RE, Harrington JT, Cohen JJ: Serum electrolyte and acid base composition. The influence of graded degrees of chronic renal failure. Arch Intern Med 139:1099, 1979.)

throughout the day. This prolonged stimulus to $NH_4^+$ excretion results in near-normal daily acid excretion in moderate renal insufficiency, just as the prolonged postprandial hyperkalemia provides a stimulus to normal daily $K^+$ excretion in spite of reduced $K^+$ secretory capacity. Eventually, however, $NH_4^+$ excretion falls in spite of continued urine acidification, and metabolic acidosis becomes more severe.

Micropuncture studies in rats with renal insufficiency have shown that urinary ammonia excretion may be impaired even before ammonia synthetic capacity is exhausted.[96] Impaired excretion of ammonia in these animals was originally attributed to impairment of countercurrent mechanisms that were thought to increase $NH_4^+$ concentration in the medulla and facilitate "trapping" of ammonia by acidified luminal fluid in the collecting duct. Derangement of medullary countercurrent mechanisms was also held responsible for impaired excretion of $NH_4^+$ in animals subjected to ablation of the papilla[344] and for the frequent,[385] although not invariable,[386] finding that acidosis is particu-

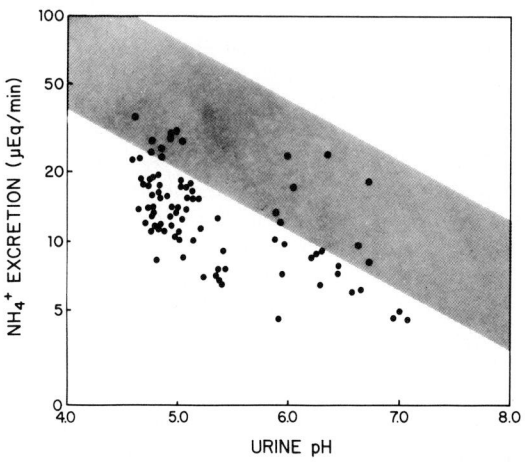

**Figure 44–6.** $NH_4^+$ excretion in chronic renal insufficiency. The data points show that $NH_4^+$ excretion increases as urine pH falls but remains, on average, below the level expected in normal subjects as represented by the shaded area. (From Wrong O, Davies HEF: Excretion of acid in renal disease. Q J Med 28:259, 1959, by permission of Oxford University Press.)

larly severe in patients with tubulointerstitial disease. This explanation for reduced $NH_4^+$ excretion, however, may require modification in light of the discovery that ammonia enters tubule fluid by active secretion as well as by trapping.

In addition to ammonia synthesis, acid excretion requires reabsorption of filtered $HCO_3^-$, accomplished largely in the proximal nephron, and generation of a 100- to 1000-fold $H^+$ gradient in the distal nephron. Either of these processes can be impaired independently of the defect in ammonia synthesis. Studies in animals suggest that proximal $HCO_3^-$ reabsorption is well maintained when nephron number is reduced by surgical ablation of renal tissue. Thus, many[101, 387, 388] but not all[96] micropuncture studies in rats and dogs subjected to renal ablation have demonstrated slight increases in fractional reabsorption of $HCO_3^-$, whereas clearance studies in dogs subjected to renal ablation have demonstrated an increased threshold for $HCO_3^-$ excretion.[389, 390] Clinical studies, however, have shown that the threshold for $HCO_3^-$ excretion is often low in patients with chronic renal failure, which suggests impairment of the proximal $HCO_3^-$ reabsorptive mechanism.[391] In some patients, impaired proximal $HCO_3^-$ reabsorption may be a manifestation of selective damage to the proximal tubule epithelium during the course of renal disease. Patients with multiple myeloma and increased immunoglobulin light chain excretion, for example, have been noted to have bicarbonaturia in association with phosphaturia and aminoaciduria.[392] The threshold for $HCO_3^-$ reabsorption may also be reduced early in the course of renal insufficiency in patients with the nephrotic syndrome[393, 394] and in patients with early renal allograft rejection.[395, 396] These patients can be said to have a component of proximal or type II renal tubular acidosis. In severe renal insufficiency, the threshold for $HCO_3^-$ reabsorption may be reduced regardless of the nature of the renal disease.[390, 391] Physiologic stimuli including hyperkalemia, hyperparathyroidism, and ECF volume expansion may decrease proximal $HCO_3^-$ reabsorption in this setting.[397–400]

Distal acidification is generally better maintained than proximal $HCO_3^-$ reabsorption in chronic renal failure. Notable exceptions are seen in chronic allograft rejection[396] and in the nephropathy associated with Sjögren syndrome,[401] in which urine pH may never be reduced below 6, thus satisfying the usual definition of type I or distal renal tubular acidosis. The pathophysiologic mechanism of the acidification defect in these conditions is not certain, but they provide striking examples of how immune inflammatory diseases can interfere with a specific tubule function. A list of other conditions in which early renal insufficiency may be associated with marked impairment of distal acidification is presented in Chapter 22. In most patients with chronic renal insufficiency, however, urine pH is about 5. Whereas this represents successful generation of an $H^+$ gradient of more than 100 to 1, it is not as low a urine pH as is achieved in normal subjects with experimentally induced acidemia.[379] Thus, a relative decrease in distal $H^+$ pump capacity may contribute to acidosis in renal failure. Failure to attain normal minimal pH prevents optimal titration of nonammonia buffers, such as $PO_4^{3-}$, urate, and creatinine, and thus reduces the excretion of the titratable

acid on which net acid excretion becomes increasingly dependent as ammonia production is impaired. Restriction of dietary phosphate intake may further contribute to reduced excretion of titratable acid in uremic patients.

As described in detail in Chapter 22, metabolic acidosis associated with hyperkalemia may develop early in renal insufficiency in patients with low mineralocorticoid levels.[366] This defect, often referred to as type IV renal tubular acidosis, usually does not reflect a limitation of the attainable distal $H^+$ gradient. Urine pH in these subjects is about the same as in other patients with renal insufficiency. Studies in dogs have suggested that the defect is due to limitation of the maximal distal $H^+$ secretion rate.[402] Measures aimed at correcting the hyperkalemia usually also tend to correct the acidosis in mineralocorticoid-deficient patients with renal insufficiency.[403, 404]

## Phosphate and Calcium

Abnormalities of $PO_4^{3-}$ and $Ca^{2+}$ metabolism in uremia are caused not only by impaired capacity of the kidney to excrete these solutes but by complex abnormalities in parathyroid hormone (PTH) and vitamin D metabolism. The complex relationships among these metabolic abnormalities and their contributions to renal osteodystrophy are discussed in Chapter 51. The discussion in this chapter is limited to alterations in remnant nephron reabsorption of $PO_4^{3-}$ and $Ca^{2+}$ observed in kidney disease.

### PHOSPHATE

$PO_4^{3-}$ absorbed in the gut must be excreted by the kidney to maintain $PO_4^{3-}$ balance. In normal individuals, this is accomplished by excretion into the urine of about 10% of the filtered load of $PO_4^{3-}$. Several early studies showed that a progressive increase in the fractional excretion of $PO_4^{3-}$ maintains $PO_4^{3-}$ balance as GFR is reduced in patients with renal insufficiency.[405–408] These studies were performed before restriction of phosphate intake and absorption became a routine part of the treatment of renal failure. The increase in fractional excretion of $PO_4^{3-}$ observed was sufficient to maintain normal serum $PO_4^{3-}$ levels until the GFR fell below about 25 mL/min. In more advanced renal insufficiency, $PO_4^{3-}$ excretion was maintained by a further increase in the fractional excretion of $PO_4^{3-}$ along with an increase in serum $PO_4^{3-}$ levels.

Initial studies by Slatopolsky and Bricker and their coworkers[406, 409–412] suggested that the increasing levels of PTH caused the increase in fractional excretion of $PO_4^{3-}$ that accompanies reduction of the GFR when phosphate intake remained normal. These studies showed that dogs subjected to renal ablation exhibited an increase in fractional excretion of $PO_4^{3-}$ similar to that observed in patients with renal insufficiency. The magnitude of the increase in fractional excretion of $PO_4^{3-}$ was correlated with the magnitude of the increase in circulating PTH levels. Finally, restriction of phosphate intake in proportion to the reduction in nephron number was shown to prevent both an increase in PTH levels and an increase in fractional $PO_4^{3-}$ excretion after renal ablation.[410–412] These observations formed the basis for the ''tradeoff hypothesis,'' as initially proposed by Bricker.[413] According to this hypothesis, the adverse consequences of hyperparathyroidism represented the biologic price paid to maintain excretion of a constant dietary phosphate intake when nephron number was reduced. This adverse tradeoff could be avoided by reducing phosphate intake as renal function declined.

Later studies have established that the increase in fractional excretion of $PO_4^{3-}$ that accompanies reduction in nephron number does not depend on an increase in PTH levels or tubule responsiveness to PTH.[414] Thus, increases in fractional excretion of $PO_4^{3-}$ are proportional to the reduction in GFR after renal ablation in animals previously subjected to thyroparathyroidectomy or parathyroidectomy.[415–418] These results do not indicate that PTH is without effect on $PO_4^{3-}$ excretion in the remnant kidney. They suggest, rather, that PTH and renal ablation have separate and additive effects on $PO_4^{3-}$ excretion.[416] Serum $PO_4^{3-}$ levels are higher in parathyroidectomized rats with two kidneys than in normal rats with two kidneys. Fractional excretion of $PO_4^{3-}$ increases after renal ablation in both parathyroidectomized and normal rats. Serum $PO_4^{3-}$ levels are therefore not perceptibly increased after renal ablation in either setting and remain higher in parathyroidectomized rats subjected to renal ablation than in rats with intact parathyroid glands subjected to renal ablation. Although elevated PTH levels are no longer considered responsible for maintaining $PO_4^{3-}$ excretion when nephron number is reduced, an unrestricted intake of phosphate does contribute to hyperparathyroidism in patients with renal insufficiency.[419] Reduction of phosphate intake is thus an important part of modern therapy for prevention of renal osteodystrophy, as described in Chapter 51.

At present, it seems reasonable to assume that the increase in fractional excretion of $PO_4^{3-}$ observed after renal ablation is achieved by the same mechanism responsible for the increase in fractional excretion of $PO_4^{3-}$ observed in intact animals maintained on a high-phosphate diet. The increase in $PO_4^{3-}$ excretion induced by feeding a high-phosphate diet has also been shown not to depend on an increase in PTH levels.[420–422] Micropuncture studies have shown that increased fractional excretion of $PO_4^{3-}$ in both settings is largely the result of decreased $PO_4^{3-}$ reabsorption in the proximal nephron.[423, 424] The mechanism whereby proximal $PO_4^{3-}$ reabsorption is decreased by renal ablation and by feeding a high-phosphate diet remains to be elucidated. $PO_4^{3-}$ uptake per unit tubule mass has been shown to be reduced in proximal nephron segments isolated from uremic rabbits, and $Na^+$-$PO_4^{3-}$ cotransport activity has been shown to be reduced in brush border membrane vesicles from uremic dogs.[91, 95] The reductions in $PO_4^{3-}$ transport observed in isolated proximal nephron tissue, however, have not been of sufficient magnitude to fully account for the reduction in proximal $PO_4^{3-}$ reabsorption observed in vivo.

Whereas reduced proximal reabsorption accounts for most of the increase in fractional excretion of $PO_4^{3-}$ after reduction in nephron number, there is also some evidence of altered distal $PO_4^{3-}$ transport. As described in Chapter 25, studies in intact animals have shown the fractional delivery of $PO_4^{3-}$ to the distal nephron exceeds fractional

excretion of $PO_4^{3-}$ in the urine. The magnitude of the difference between distal delivery and urinary excretion of $PO_4^{3-}$ was found to be reduced in a study in uremic dogs, whereas excretion of $PO_4^{3-}$ was found actually to exceed distal delivery of $PO_4^{3-}$ in a study in uremic rats.[423, 424] As noted by the authors of these studies, their findings could have been accounted for by a difference in superficial and deep nephron reabsorption of $PO_4^{3-}$ rather than by an alteration in distal nephron $PO_4^{3-}$ transport.

## CALCIUM

Absorption of $Ca^{2+}$ from the gut is controlled by the active vitamin D metabolite 1,25-dihydroxycholecalciferol ($1,25(OH)_2D_3$), which is produced in the kidney. $Ca^{2+}$ is thus unique among solutes in that its absorption into the ECF as well as its excretion into the urine is controlled by the kidney. As renal disease advances, the production of $1,25(OH)_2D_3$ is impaired, so that the amount of $Ca^{2+}$ absorbed from the gut is reduced as the GFR is reduced. Reduced absorption of dietary calcium presumably accounted for the reduced excretion of $Ca^{2+}$ observed in early studies of patients with renal insufficiency.[407, 408, 425] These studies showed that fractional excretion of $Ca^{2+}$ as well as total urinary excretion of $Ca^{2+}$ was reduced in patients with moderate renal insufficiency receiving no calcium or vitamin D supplementation. As renal insufficiency advanced, fractional excretion of $Ca^{2+}$ was shown eventually to increase. Differences in diet, heterogeneity in the impairment of $1,25(OH)_2D_3$ production, and a tendency toward impaired renal reabsorption of $Ca^{2+}$ in patients with tubulointerstitial disease may account for the wide variability in $Ca^{2+}$ excretion rates that has been observed in patients with renal insufficiency.[419, 425]

Because the chief problem in patients with renal insufficiency has been to increase calcium intake rather than to facilitate $Ca^{2+}$ excretion, there have been relatively few experimental studies of $Ca^{2+}$ excretion in animals subjected to renal ablation.[426–429] In contrast to clinical studies, these experimental studies have shown urinary $Ca^{2+}$ excretion remains constant whereas fractional excretion of $Ca^{2+}$ increases when the GFR is reduced to about one third of normal.[426, 429] This difference may be accounted for by better maintenance of $1,25(OH)_2D_3$ production in remnant kidneys of animals subjected to renal ablation than in human kidneys damaged by disease, or by liberal provision of calcium and vitamin D in standard laboratory chows. The mechanism responsible for the increase in fractional excretion of $Ca^{2+}$ associated with reduction of GFR in animals with renal insufficiency remains to be elucidated. As described in Chapter 24, $Ca^{2+}$ excretion in normal animals subjected to $Ca^{2+}$-loading is increased by suppression of PTH-mediated $Ca^{2+}$ reabsorption in the distal nephron and also by inhibition of $Ca^{2+}$ reabsorption in the thick ascending limb and distal nephron by PTH-independent mechanisms. The increase in fractional excretion of $Ca^{2+}$ observed in animals subjected to renal ablation cannot be attributed to suppression of PTH-mediated $Ca^{2+}$ reabsorption, because PTH levels are elevated after reduction in nephron number. The mechanism responsible for increased fractional excretion of $Ca^{2+}$ in patients with advanced renal insufficiency is even less well defined. These patients often exhibit increases in fractional excretion of $Ca^{2+}$ in the presence of low serum $Ca^{2+}$ levels.[407] Such increases in fractional $Ca^{2+}$ excretion cannot be attributed to the same mechanism that promotes increased $Ca^{2+}$ excretion in normal humans subjected to $Ca^{2+}$ loading. Possible factors contributing to increased $Ca^{2+}$ excretion in advanced renal failure included acidosis, marked suppression of vitamin D production, increased distal nephron flow rates, and ECF volume expansion. Studies in rats subjected to renal ablation suggest that the increase in remnant nephron $Ca^{2+}$ excretion associated with ECF expansion may be mediated by ANP.[429]

## Organic Solutes

Given the presumed contribution of organic compounds to uremic toxicity, there have been remarkably few studies of organic solute excretion by the diseased kidney. Among the organic cations excreted by the kidney, creatinine has been studied most extensively. The aim of these studies has been to determine whether creatinine clearance provides an accurate measure of the GFR in renal insufficiency. In rats, tubule reabsorption and secretion of creatinine make creatinine clearance an inaccurate measure of GFR even when renal function is normal.[430] In humans with normal renal function, however, tubule reabsorption of creatinine is observed only at low urine flow rates, and tubule secretion of creatinine accounts for only a small part of creatinine excretion.[431] Thus, creatinine clearance provides a useful measure of GFR in humans with normal renal function. The contribution of tubule secretion to creatinine excretion is increased, however, when the GFR is reduced and the serum creatinine level is elevated. Creatinine clearance has thus been found to exceed inulin clearance in most although not all studies in patients with renal insufficiency.[432–439] In a large series of patients with glomerular disease, tubule creatinine was shown to account for an average of one third of the total creatinine excretion when the inulin clearance was reduced to 40 mL/min and for half of the total creatinine excretion when the inulin clearance was reduced to 10 to 15 mL/min.[435] These results suggest that reduction of the creatinine clearance to half of normal reflects reduction of the GFR to about one-third normal, whereas reduction of creatinine clearance to one-fifth normal reflects reduction of the GFR to about one-tenth normal. Thus, the severity of chronic renal disease may be underestimated by the use of creatinine clearance to assess GFR. As discussed in Chapter 26, serial determinations of serum creatinine level and creatinine clearance may still provide useful clinical information but may not provide sufficiently accurate indices of GFR for use in studies of the progression of renal disease.[431, 438]

In contrast to creatinine, urea clearance decreases roughly in proportion to GFR in patients with moderate renal insufficiency. To date, there is no evidence that any intrinsic change in remnant tubules reduces urea reabsorption in renal insufficiency. In severe renal disease, the fractional clearance of urea may increase slightly, presumably reflecting decreased fractional fluid reabsorption in the proximal nephron.[440] Urea clearance remains lower than inulin clearance, however, whereas creatinine clearance is elevated above inulin clearance by creatinine secretion. It has been suggested, therefore, that values for GFR may be obtained by averaging values for creatinine clearance and urea clearance in uremic patients. GFR values calculated in this manner have proved unreliable, however, because the relations of both creatinine clearance and urea clearance to inulin clearance are variable in uremia.[435, 438, 440]

Proximal nephron reabsorption of glucose and amino acids is generally well maintained in human and experimental renal insufficiency, with modest aminoaciduria usually reflecting an insignificant portion of the filtered load of amino acids.[441, 442] Occasional patients with prominent proximal nephron injury exhibit marked aminoaciduria or glucosuria, often in association with $HCO_3^-$ or $PO_4^{3-}$ wasting.[392, 393] Studies in animals subjected to renal ablation have shown that the proximal reabsorption of glucose and amino acids is maintained by increasing $Na^+$-glucose and $Na^+$–amino acid cotransport activities in proportion to proximal tubule size.[91, 92] Studies in humans and animals with diffuse renal disease have established that glucose reabsorptive capacity varies with SNGFR in functioning nephrons, so that glomerulotubular balance is well maintained.[443–446] In the most detailed of these studies, heavy metal toxins were administered to rats to produce a heterogeneous pattern of intrarenal injury, characterized by atrophy of the most severely injured nephrons and hypertrophy of less injured nephrons.[446] Glucose reabsorption rates were shown to be well correlated with SNGFR and proximal tubule size in individual remnant nephrons.

Among the organic anions excreted by the kidney, only urate has been extensively studied in renal insufficiency. A progressive increase in the fractional excretion of urate is largely responsible for maintaining urate balance as GFR is reduced.[447–451] This increase in fractional excretion of urate is sufficient to maintain near-normal urate levels until the GFR is reduced below about 50 mL/min. A further increase in fractional excretion of urate, along with a modest reduction in urate load due to increased intestinal degradation of urate, maintains urate levels at about twice normal when the GFR is reduced to 10 to 15 mL/min. Drugs that block urate secretion and reabsorption have been employed to elucidate the mechanism responsible for the increase in fractional excretion of urate in renal insufficiency.[449, 451] These studies have variously been interpreted as showing that the urate secretion is increased or that postsecretory reabsorption of urate is decreased in moderate renal insufficiency. Competition by other organic ions for proximal reabsorptive sites may reduce presecretory urate reabsorption and further contribute to increased fractional excretion of urate in advanced renal insufficiency.[451–457]

## THE BIOLOGIC PRICE OF ADAPTATION TO REDUCTION IN NEPHRON NUMBER: THE ULTIMATE DETERIORATION OF ADAPTED NEPHRONS

Patients with established renal insufficiency regularly exhibit progressive loss of renal function. Progressive reduction of the GFR in these patients is often characterized by a steady decline in the reciprocal of serum creatinine plotted against time, as illustrated in Figure 44–7 and further described in Chapter 26. Patients whose GFR has been reduced to about one fourth of normal can expect eventually to require dialysis or transplantation. These observations suggest that after a certain point, reduction in functioning nephron numbers leads to failure of the remaining units. Hope of interrupting this process has stimulated investigation into the mechanisms responsible for injury to functioning nephrons in kidneys damaged by disease.[194, 458]

## Remnant Glomerular Injury

### ADVERSE EFFECTS OF GLOMERULAR CAPILLARY HYPERTENSION

Increased glomerular filtration in remnant nephrons has generally been regarded as adaptive because it partially offsets the loss of function that would otherwise follow reduction in nephron number. Mounting evidence suggests, however, that the hemodynamic changes that cause remnant nephron hyperfiltration eventually prove injurious to residual glomeruli. More than 60 years ago, Chanutin and Ferris[459] showed that removal of three fourths of the renal mass in rats led to a syndrome of proteinuria and progressive glomerular sclerosis, ultimately resulting in uremic death. The development of pathologic changes in remnant glomeruli after five-sixths renal ablation was later profiled by Shimamura and Morrison.[460] Early glomerular hypertrophy was accompanied by ultrastructural changes including vacuolization of epithelial cells and "fusion" of epithelial cell foot processes. These changes were followed by focal detachment of endothelial and epithelial cells from the glomerular basement membrane. Progressive accumulation of subendothelial hyaline material and collapse of capillary lumens eventually resulted in the appearance of focal and segmental glomerular sclerosis. Further studies have shown that the prevalence of segmental sclerotic lesions increases with time and that progression to global sclerosis is observed. Moreover, the pace of glomerular injury, like

the magnitude of remnant glomerular hemodynamic changes, increases in proportion to the loss of renal mass.[13, 33, 34, 36, 460, 461]

Micropuncture studies by Hostetter and co-workers[33] provided direct evidence that increases in glomerular pressure and flow that serve to elevate remnant nephron GFR are responsible for progressive glomerular injury after reduction in nephron number. Restriction of dietary protein intake, which lowers GFR in normal animals, was used to blunt increases in glomerular pressure and flow after extensive renal ablation. Limitation of glomerular pressure and flow largely prevented proteinuria and early glomerular morphologic changes seen in ablated animals maintained on standard chow. Further studies have shown that dietary protein restriction also lowers remnant kidney GFR and retards development of proteinuria and glomerular sclerosis in rats subjected to less extensive renal ablation.[462-464] The beneficial effects of protein restriction have been demonstrated not only by these functional and morphologic studies but by studies showing that reduction of protein intake increases the life span of rats subjected to renal ablation.[465]

In the initial studies showing that dietary protein restriction reduces remnant glomerular injury, protein restriction was instituted near the time of, or before, reduction in nephron number. Subsequent studies showed that later institution of protein restriction limits the progression of established remnant glomerular injury.[36, 466] These studies further suggested that protein restriction protects the remnant glomerulus largely by lowering glomerular capillary hydraulic pressure. Whereas early institution of protein restriction blunts increases in remnant glomerular capillary pressure and in glomerular plasma flow and filtration rate after renal ablation, late institution of protein restriction reduces glomerular capillary pressure without reducing remnant glomerular hyperperfusion and hyperfiltration. The hypothesis that capillary hypertension is the hemodynamic factor responsible for remnant glomerular injury has received further support from the observation that injury is absent in a remnant kidney rat model that develops glomerular hyperfiltration without glomerular hypertension.[467]

Studies in experimental hypertension are consistent with the hypothesis that capillary hypertension is the hemodynamic derangement most responsible for glomerular injury

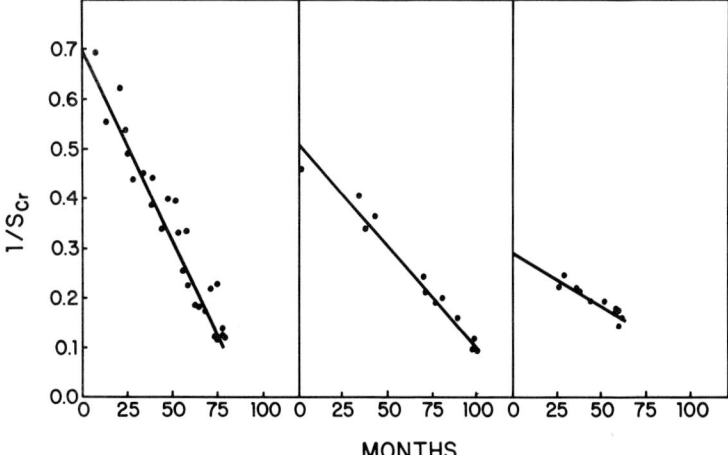

**Figure 44–7.** Time plots of the reciprocal of serum creatinine ($1/S_{cr}$) in three patients with renal insufficiency illustrating the occurrence of a predictable decline in renal function. (Adapted from Mitch WE, Walser M, Buffington GA, Lemann J Jr: A simple method for estimating progression of chronic renal failure. Lancet 2:1326, 1976.)

after reduction in nephron number. These studies indicate that systemic hypertension causes glomerular sclerosis only when the increase in systemic blood pressure is transmitted to the glomerulus.[459, 468] Studies have shown that sustained blockade of nitric oxide synthesis causes both systemic and glomerular capillary hypertension and rapid development of glomerular sclerosis in intact rats with normal nephron number.[469, 470] Sustained infusion of AII also increases systemic and glomerular pressure and causes glomerular sclerosis in intact rats.[171] Heptinstall and Hill[471] initially proposed that elevated glomerular capillary pressure caused glomerular injury in rats with mineralocorticoid-salt hypertension, whereas Azar and colleagues[472, 473] related increased glomerular capillary pressure to early glomerular sclerosis in rats with ''post-salt'' hypertension. Other studies have shown that rats with two-kidney one-clip hypertension exhibit elevation of glomerular capillary pressure and rapid development of glomerular lesions only in the unclipped kidney.[474, 475] In contrast, early glomerular sclerosis is not prominent in spontaneously hypertensive rats and Milan hypertensive rats, in which glomerular capillary pressures remain nearly normal despite elevation of systemic blood pressure.[476-478]

The hypothesis that capillary hypertension causes remnant glomerular injury is further supported by studies of antihypertensive drug therapy in rats subjected to renal ablation. Use of an angiotensin I–converting enzyme inhibitor to control systemic blood pressure has been shown to normalize glomerular capillary pressure and to prevent glomerular injury in rats subjected to renal ablation.[34, 36] In contrast, a combination drug regimen that was equally effective in controlling systemic blood pressure but did not reduce glomerular capillary pressure did not prevent glomerular injury in rats subjected to the same ablation procedure.[479] A number of other antihypertensive drug regimens have been tested in the remnant kidney model; effects of these regimens have been reviewed by Anderson.[480] In many cases, including that of thromboxane synthesis inhibition,[53] drug regimens have been shown to normalize systemic blood pressure and protect against remnant glomerular injury, but their effect on glomerular pressure has not been assessed.

Other studies suggest that increased glomerular pressure accelerates glomerular injury when the kidney is damaged by diffuse disease as well as when nephron number is reduced by renal ablation. Antihypertensive therapy that lowers glomerular capillary pressure has been shown to retard glomerular injury in hypertensive rats with nephrotoxic serum nephritis,[481] rats with doxorubicin (Adriamycin) nephrosis,[482] spontaneously hypertensive rats subjected to uninephrectomy,[483] and rats recovering from the proteinuric phase of puromycin nephrosis.[484] Dietary protein restriction has been shown to reduce glomerular capillary pressure and protect against glomerular injury in rats with mineralocorticoid-salt hypertension and in spontaneously hypertensive rats subjected to uninephrectomy.[468, 485] Although micropuncture measurements are not available, reduction of glomerular capillary pressure could also account for the observation that dietary protein restriction slows the progression of nephrotoxic serum nephritis in rats,[486, 487] lupus-like ne-

phropathy in NZB/NZW mice,[488, 489] and age-related glomerular sclerosis in intact rats and hamsters.[490, 491] Acceleration of glomerular injury by increased glomerular pressure can also account for the findings of studies in which experimental immune diseases have been exacerbated by superimposed systemic hypertension.[492-496]

Evidence that capillary hypertension causes glomerular injury has stimulated interest in the mechanisms that alter glomerular hemodynamic function after reduction in nephron number. The observation that sustained AII blockade normalizes $\overline{P}_{GC}$ in rats subjected to renal ablation suggests that AII could cause capillary hypertension in remnant glomeruli.[34, 48] Studies of the contribution of AII and other vasomotor hormones to altered remnant glomerular hemodynamic function are described earlier. The mechanism by which protein restriction lowers glomerular capillary pressure remains to be elucidated. An intriguing suggestion is that protein restriction alters remnant kidney function by decreasing urea production and ADH levels.[497] Studies have shown that food restriction,[498] thyroid deficiency,[499] growth hormone deficiency,[500] and castration in male rats[501] all protect against the development of remnant glomerular injury after renal ablation. Thyroid deficiency has been shown to result in a reduction in remnant glomerular pressure similar to that caused by protein restriction, whereas the effects of the other maneuvers on remnant glomerular hemodynamic function have not been studied in detail.

Different mechanisms may contribute to glomerular capillary hypertension in other models of renal disease. This is suggested by the observation that a given antihypertensive regimen can have different effects on glomerular capillary pressure in different disease models. The combination antihypertensive regimen that does not reduce capillary pressure or prevent injury in remnant glomeruli[479] also does not reduce capillary pressure or prevent glomerular injury in rats with mineralocorticoid-salt hypertension[502] but does lower glomerular capillary pressure and reduce glomerular injury in hypertensive rats with nephrotoxic serum nephritis[481] and in spontaneously hypertensive rats subjected to uninephrectomy.[483] Of note, converting enzyme inhibitors have so far been shown to afford some protection against glomerular injury in every model of renal disease in which they have been tested.[34, 36, 482, 484, 503]

Taken together, results of experimental studies are consistent with the hypothesis that capillary hypertension precipitates glomerular injury after renal ablation and accelerates glomerular injury in other renal disease models. The great majority of these studies have been performed in rats, and only limited information is available in other species. Dogs subjected to renal ablation develop proteinuria and progressive glomerular sclerosis, but at a slower pace than do rats subjected to a similar degree of renal ablation.[504, 505] The observation that systemic pressure remains constant and glomerular transcapillary hydraulic pressure is only moderately elevated in dogs subjected to renal ablation may account for the slow pace of glomerular injury in this model.[38, 39] Long-term studies of primates subjected to renal ablation have not been completed, but baboons subjected to renal ablation have been shown to develop marked systemic hypertension.[506]

## OTHER FACTORS CONTRIBUTING TO REMNANT NEPHRON INJURY

A number of factors other than glomerular capillary hypertension have been considered to account for progressive glomerular sclerosis after surgical nephrectomy and in diffuse renal disease. One early hypothesis was that an immune response directed against renal antigens caused progressive renal injury after surgical nephrectomy. Immune complexes have not been found in damaged glomeruli of remnant kidneys, however. Furthermore, accelerated glomerular damage does not occur when part of one kidney is infarcted and the contralateral kidney is left intact rather than excised.[35, 507] The hypothesis that remnant glomerular injury is immune mediated has therefore been largely abandoned. There is persuasive evidence, however, that a number of other nonhemodynamic mechanisms contribute to remnant nephron injury after reduction in nephron number.

## GLOMERULAR HYPERTROPHY

It has been suggested that glomerular injury may be precipitated by glomerular hypertrophy as well as by glomerular capillary hypertension.[508–510] Glomerular hypertrophy could contribute to glomerular injury in many of the disease models in which glomerular hypertension has been associated with development of glomerular sclerosis. Thus, both glomerular volume and glomerular capillary pressure are increased in rats with renal ablation, mineralocorticoid-salt hypertension, and diabetes mellitus.[34, 468, 511] Similarly, increases in both glomerular volume and glomerular pressure could contribute to the acceleration of glomerular injury regularly observed after uninephrectomy in experimental renal disease.[485, 487, 491, 512] Reduction of glomerular volume could contribute to the protective effect of protein restriction in rats with renal disease.[513] A protective effect of low glomerular volume could also account for the observation that a strain of rats with unusually small glomeruli exhibits less glomerular injury after uninephrectomy[514] and puromycin administration[515] than does a strain of rats with larger glomeruli.

The studies cited are consistent with the hypothesis that glomerular hypertrophy accelerates development of glomerular injury but do not distinguish the effects of glomerular hypertrophy from those of glomerular hypertension. Several reports suggest that glomerular hypertrophy makes a contribution to glomerular injury that is additional to that of glomerular hypertension. Two of these reports have shown that dietary sodium restriction reduces glomerular volume and limits glomerular injury without altering glomerular capillary pressure in rats subjected to five-sixths renal ablation.[73, 508] Another study compared rats having partial ablation of one kidney and contralateral ureteral diversion with rats in which a similar reduction in functioning nephron number was accomplished by partial ablation of one kidney and contralateral surgical nephrectomy.[509] Glomerular capillary pressure was elevated in both groups, but glomeruli were smaller and glomerular injury was less extensive in rats whose renal function was reduced in part by ureteral diversion. These studies suggest that glomerular hypertrophy exacerbates remnant glomerular injury but do

not establish that capillary hypertension is not by itself injurious. A study comparing rats subjected to segmental infarction of both kidneys with rats subjected to surgical uninephrectomy has established that glomerular hypertension causes glomerular injury independent of glomerular hypertrophy.[13] Rats subjected to segmental infarction of both kidneys developed glomerular capillary hypertension and notable glomerular sclerosis. Rats subjected to uninephrectomy exhibited little elevation of glomerular pressure and less glomerular sclerosis despite a larger increase in glomerular volume. A study of the effects of long-term AII infusion and uninephrectomy has suggested that glomerular hypertension and hypertrophy exert synergistic injurious influences on the glomerulus.[171] Intact rats receiving AII developed glomerular hypertension and progressive glomerular sclerosis, whereas glomerular volume remained normal. An increase in glomerular volume induced by uninephrectomy was associated with an increase in the extent of glomerular injury.

The mechanism by which glomerular hypertrophy contributes to remnant glomerular injury remains to be established. It has been proposed that glomerular hypertrophy exacerbates glomerular injury by increasing capillary wall tension. This hypothesis provides an attractive explanation for the observation that glomerular hypertension and glomerular hypertrophy have additive effects in promoting glomerular injury. Studies have established that the number of visceral epithelial cells remains constant during glomerular growth after renal ablation.[69, 70] Impaired ability of a limited number of epithelial cells to maintain permselective function in enlarged glomeruli could therefore contribute to glomerular injury associated with glomerular hypertrophy.[69, 70, 513] The important question of whether increases in glomerular pressure or flow stimulate glomerular growth requires further investigation. Available studies suggest that normalizing glomerular capillary pressure may limit but cannot prevent glomerular hypertrophy after renal ablation. These studies indicate that the protective effect of reducing glomerular pressure cannot be attributed to reduction in glomerular volume.

## HYPERLIPIDEMIA AND GLOMERULAR LIPID DEPOSITION

It has also been suggested that glomerular deposition of circulating lipids contributes to progressive glomerular injury in renal disease.[516] This hypothesis was originally based on the finding of lipid droplets in glomerular sclerotic lesions in humans and in experimental animals.[516, 517] Subsequent studies showed that glomerular injury could be precipitated by lipid feeding in rabbits and guinea pigs.[518, 519] More recently, hyperlipidemia has been associated with progressive glomerular injury in rats with hereditary obesity and in rats subjected to renal ablation. Agents that lower serum lipid levels have been shown to limit development of glomerular sclerosis in these disease models.[520, 521] These observations have prompted the suggestion that the pathogenesis of glomerular sclerosis is analogous to that of systemic atherosclerosis, with hypertension and hyperlipidemia constituting additive risk factors in both processes.[516, 522] An incomplete feature of this attractive hy-

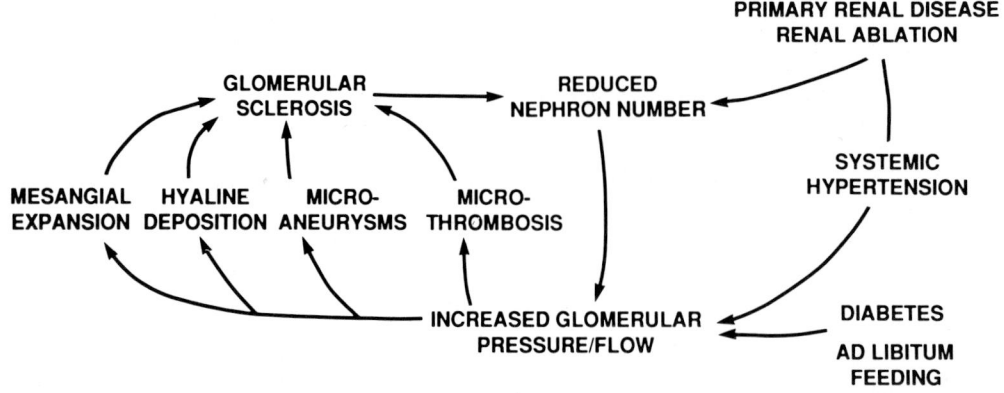

**Figure 44–8.** Hypothetic scheme detailing the progression of renal disease. Reductions in renal mass, systemic hypertension (whether primary or secondary to reduced renal mass), diabetes mellitus, and ad libitum feeding all increase glomerular pressures and flows. The mechanisms by which these hemodynamic changes can cause glomerular injury, including mesangial expansion, hyaline deposition, development of microaneurysms, and microthrombosis, are described by Rennke.[528]

pothesis is that the lipoprotein constituents that cause glomerular injury remain to be identified. In humans, an increased risk of atherosclerosis has been most closely associated with increased levels of low-density lipoproteins. Low-density lipoprotein levels generally remain low in hyperlipidemic rats, however, and rabbits with hereditary low-density lipoprotein receptor deficiency do not develop accelerated glomerular sclerosis.[523–525] The difficulty in establishing the contribution of circulating lipids to glomerular injury has been emphasized by findings that cholesterol feeding can increase glomerular pressure and that antilipemic drugs may prevent glomerular injury by mechanisms that are independent of changes in lipid levels.[526, 527]

## GLOMERULAR CAPILLARY THROMBOSIS

Development of capillary microthrombi is a notable feature of glomerular injury after reduction in nephron number.[528] It has been suggested that capillary thrombosis is precipitated by early endothelial cell injury in the remnant glomeruli and that capillary microthrombi contribute to glomerular sclerosis by direct occlusion of capillary lumens and by release of platelet-derived factors that aggravate glomerular injury.[528–530] The finding of microthrombi in injured glomeruli provided the impetus to study the effect of anticoagulant drugs in rats subjected to renal ablation. Purkerson and co-workers[35] showed that heparin largely prevented early development of glomerular sclerosis in this disease model, and this finding has been confirmed in subsequent studies.[531, 532] The protection against remnant glomerular injury afforded by thromboxane synthesis inhibition has also been attributed to prevention of capillary thrombosis, whereas sodium warfarin (Coumadin) and aspirin have been shown to be less effective than heparin in preventing remnant glomerular injury.[53, 533, 534] These findings are consistent with the hypothesis that anticoagulant agents prevent remnant glomerular injury by inhibiting formation of capillary microthrombi. Heparin, however, may also protect remnant glomeruli by other mechanisms, including reduction of blood pressure in rats subjected to

renal ablation.[531, 532, 535] Studies of nonanticoagulant heparin fractions have yielded mixed results and thus have not settled the question of whether heparin protects the glomerulus by preventing capillary thrombosis.[531, 532, 536]

## CELLULAR MECHANISMS RESPONSIBLE FOR REMNANT GLOMERULAR INJURY

The different mechanisms proposed to account for remnant injury should not be regarded as mutually exclusive. Morphologic studies suggest that there is extensive interaction among the mechanisms responsible for remnant glomerular injury.[528] Given the close apposition and functional interdependency of glomerular cell types, such interaction among mechanisms of glomerular injury should be expected.

As illustrated in Figure 44–8, a number of mechanisms have been proposed to account for the link between increased glomerular pressure and ultimate glomerular injury. An early suggestion was that glomerular hypertension increases movement of circulating macromolecules into the mesangium. Studies in intact rats suggest that maneuvers that increase glomerular capillary pressure cause increased movement of macromolecules into the mesangium, and early deposition of circulating macromolecules in the mesangium has been demonstrated in rats subjected to renal ablation.[537–539] The presence of circulating macromolecules in the mesangium may stimulate proliferation of mesangial cells, recruitment of monocytes into the mesangium, and altered production of mesangial matrix constituents.[540, 541] In particular, the injurious effect of mesangial deposition of lipoproteins could account for the association of glomerular sclerosis and hyperlipidemia described in the preceding section. Another suggestion has been that increased glomerular pressure, by stretching mesangial cells, directly causes cell growth and matrix proliferation.[542] The contribution of mesangial expansion to ultimate obliteration of remnant glomeruli is controversial. Morphometric studies have detected no increase in the average volume fraction of the mesangium early in the course of remnant kidney disease in rats subjected to renal ablation.[543] This suggests that mesangial expansion occurs as part of focal and segmental injury in the remnant glomerulus and is not a diffuse response to glomerular hyperfiltration and hypertrophy.

Glomerular hypertension and hypertrophy may also cause glomerular sclerosis by promoting movement of circulating macromolecules through the glomerular capillary wall. The development of proteinuria in rats subjected to renal ablation results from defects in both the charge- and size-selective properties of the glomerular capillary wall.[539, 544, 545] These permselective defects are associated with abnormalities of epithelial cell structure, including retraction of epithelial cell foot processes and focal detachment of epithelial cells from the underlying basement membrane. Epithelial cell injury in remnant glomeruli may reflect increased capillary wall tension and the inability of highly differentiated epithelial cells to replicate as glomerular volume increases after reduction in nephron number.[69, 70] Subendothelial deposition of large macromolecules in areas where macromolecule passage through the capillary wall is increased may result in hyalinosis, eventually proceeding to occlusion of capillary lumens.[70, 528]

Other processes of glomerular injury depicted in Figure 44–8 have been described in the preceding section. Increased wall tension in enlarging remnant loops of the glomerular capillary wall may cause development of microaneurysms.[70, 528] These lesions have been shown to progress to form areas of segmental capillary collapse. Microthrombosis may be precipitated by hemodynamically mediated injury to glomerular endothelial cells. As noted before, microthrombi may contribute to glomerular sclerosis by occlusion of capillary lumens and by release of factors causing further cell injury or cell proliferation and matrix production. Serial studies in rats subjected to renal ablation suggest all these processes of remnant glomerular injury proceed in parallel. At present, it is not possible to distinguish any feature of structural injury as initiatory or as predominant in the development of remnant glomerular sclerosis.

Similarly, it is not possible at present to identify a single cell type or cell product as having a predominant role in remnant glomerular injury. Macrophages accumulate in the mesangium of injured remnant glomeruli and platelets are deposited in microthrombi. The list of cytokines that may participate in glomerular injury thus includes not only those made by native glomerular cells but all those produced by macrophages and platelets.[528, 530, 546–548] Identification of the role of these factors will become possible as specific inhibitors for individual factors are developed. Among the factors considered most likely to contribute to remnant glomerular injury are platelet-derived growth factor, transforming growth factor-β, and endothelin.[51, 530, 549, 550] Increased intraglomerular activity of each of these factors has been detected during the course of remnant glomerular injury. Of particular note, increased activity of transforming growth factor-β in remnant glomeruli has been associated with local activity of the renin-angiotensin system.[550, 551] These findings suggest that transforming growth factor-β may mediate injurious effects of AII on the glomerulus and that a reduction in glomerular transforming growth factor-

β activity could contribute to the protective effects of AII blockade.

## Tubulointerstitial Injury After Reduction in Nephron Number

Glomerular injury in rats subjected to renal ablation is associated with development of extensive tubulointerstitial injury.[34, 459, 463] Tubulointerstitial injury in this setting may be caused by proteinuria and thus be a consequence of glomerular injury. The appearance of protein casts suggests that remnant nephron proteinuria causes tubule obstruction and dilatation. Luminal fluid protein may also injure proximal tubule cells in the absence of tubule obstruction.[552, 553] In addition to these injurious effects of glomerular protein leakage, several primary tubulointerstitial processes may contribute to remnant nephron destruction after renal ablation.

**Altered Phosphate Metabolism and Renal Calcium Deposition.** Studies by Alfrey and co-workers[554, 555] provided the first evidence that intrarenal $Ca^{2+}$ deposition contributes to progressive loss of renal function in experimental renal disease. These studies showed that restricting phosphate intake reduced renal $Ca^{2+}$ content, preserved renal function, and prolonged life span in rats subjected to renal ablation and in rats with nephrotoxic serum nephritis. Subsequent studies have shown that the protective effect of dietary phosphate restriction is not attributable to reduction of protein or calorie intake or to reduction in PTH levels.[556–558] It is not clear, however, that dietary phosphate restriction protects the remnant kidney by preventing intrarenal deposition of calcium phosphate salts. Only stringent dietary phosphate restriction that reduces serum $PO_4^{3-}$ levels below normal has so far been shown to be protective in rats subjected to renal ablation.[554, 556] Phosphorus restriction of this degree may protect remnant nephrons by lowering circulating lipid levels, reducing tubule energy consumption, altering remnant glomerular hemodynamic function, or reducing glomerular volume.[556, 559–561] Likewise, the beneficial effects of parathyroidectomy and hypocalcemia may be attributable to reduction of lipid levels and prevention of remnant kidney growth rather than to reduction of intrarenal $Ca^{2+}$ deposition.[562]

**Tubule Metabolism.** It has been shown that remnant nephron oxygen consumption is increased out of proportion to remnant nephron GFR after renal ablation.[563–567] The physiologic significance of this observation is unclear, and it is notable that oxygen consumption does not increase out of proportion to renal mass. It has been suggested, however, that increased energy consumption may increase oxidant injury in remnant tubule cells, and nonspecific maneuvers that reduce oxygen consumption have been shown to limit remnant kidney disease.[563, 564, 568, 569] In addition to increased oxygen consumption, increased ammonia production by remnant nephrons has been associated with intrarenal complement activation and interstitial inflammation.[570] Long-term administration of sodium bicarbonate, which reduces remnant nephron ammonia production, also limits tubule injury and interstitial inflammation in rats subjected to renal ablation.

## Progression of Human Renal Insufficiency

The experimental studies described in the preceding have demonstrated progressive injury to remnant nephrons after reduction in nephron number. Clinical studies suggest that remnant nephrons in diseased human kidneys are also subject to progressive injury. Morphologic studies in patients with a variety of renal diseases have demonstrated hypertrophy (presumably reflecting hyperperfusion and hyperfiltration) of those nephrons least damaged by disease[274, 571] (see Fig. 44–2). Other clinical studies have demonstrated progressive loss of renal function associated with increasing glomerular sclerosis in patients whose initiating disease process has either remitted spontaneously or been controlled therapeutically. Patients with bilateral cortical necrosis may temporarily recover stable albeit reduced renal function before proceeding to end-stage renal failure.[572] Recovery of renal function is frequently incomplete in acute renal failure of other causes, and progressive loss of renal function also follows initial recovery in some of these cases.[573] Patients with vesicoureteric reflux who have significant impairment of renal function and glomerular disease manifested by proteinuria may progress to renal failure despite control of systemic hypertension, prevention of urinary tract infection, and surgical correction of the reflux.[574] Likewise, patients with analgesic nephropathy, sometimes said to exhibit stable renal insufficiency, in fact often progress to renal failure despite discontinuation of analgesic medications.[575] Progressive glomerular sclerosis in the absence of continuing immunologic injury has been demonstrated in certain patients after initial recovery from acute poststreptococcal glomerulonephritis.[576] Progressive renal failure in these conditions is characterized by development of proteinuria and glomerular segmental sclerosis, which suggests that the mechanisms responsible for the failure of remnant nephrons in patients with kidneys damaged by disease are the same as those responsible for sclerosis of remnant glomeruli in animals subjected to renal ablation.

**Renal Disease in Humans with a Solitary Kidney.** Renewed interest in glomerular injury after reduction in nephron number in animals has prompted re-examination of the consequences of uninephrectomy in humans. Assurance that uninephrectomy in adult humans is without long-term adverse effects is of particular importance to individuals donating a kidney for transplantation. Several studies of kidney donors observed for more than 10 years after nephrectomy have been presented.[577–582] Overall, mean values for serum creatinine were no different from those in studies conducted in the first few years after donation, and the prevalence of hypertension was not clearly greater than in control populations. Perhaps of most importance, few transplant donors have had heavy proteinuria or renal failure not clearly attributable to causes other than nephrectomy.[583–586]

The chief limitation of available studies of transplant donors is that they do not extend for a sufficient period after nephrectomy. Because transplantation is a relatively new procedure, these studies include few individuals observed for more than 20 years. A study of American servicemen subjected to uninephrectomy for trauma during World War II, however, suggests that uninephrectomy in young adults has few major adverse consequences after 45 years.[587] The subjects in this study were adult men of European ancestry, and the long-term consequences of uninephrectomy performed at an earlier age, in women, or in subjects of other ethnic backgrounds could differ. Uninephrectomy could also have more serious adverse consequences when it is performed in subjects at risk for later development of renal disease, such as those subjects with a hereditary predisposition to diabetes.

Nephrectomy may have significant adverse consequences when it is performed to remove a diseased kidney. Survival of longer than 40 years after nephrectomy has been documented in such cases, but late development of remnant kidney disease has also been reported.[588–592] Remnant kidney disease in these patients may, however, be a consequence of kidney abnormalities that were not noted at the time of operation. Studies documenting an increased risk of renal failure in patients with unilateral renal agenesis present the same difficulty in interpretation.[593–597] Malformations of the solitary kidney are common in cases of unilateral renal agenesis, and progressive renal disease may be caused by these anomalies as well as by reduced nephron number.[593] Moreover, early loss of a kidney causes a greater degree of remnant glomerular hyperfiltration and hypertrophy than is observed after uninephrectomy in adults.[597, 598] Patients with unilateral renal agenesis may thus be more subject to hemodynamically mediated remnant glomerular injury than are adult kidney donors. Similarly, marked remnant nephron hyperfiltration and associated hemodynamically mediated injury could account for development of focal glomerular sclerosis in patients subjected to surgical removal of greater than 50% of their renal mass.[599, 600]

**Efforts to Arrest the Progression of Renal Insufficiency.** If glomerular capillary hypertension contributes to progressive glomerular sclerosis in patients with renal insufficiency, therapies aimed at reducing glomerular pressure should help preserve residual renal function. One possible therapy is restriction of dietary protein intake, implemented early in the course of intrinsic renal disease. Results of clinical trials of dietary protein restriction are reviewed in Chapter 55. Antihypertensive therapy directed toward reduction of glomerular capillary pressure may ultimately prove more efficacious than dietary protein restriction. As described in Chapter 39, systemic hypertension is a regular feature of progressive renal insufficiency, and elevation of blood pressure appears to accelerate loss of renal function. Reduction of mean arterial pressure to 95 to 100 mm Hg has been shown to slow the progression of diabetic nephropathy, and studies suggest that converting enzyme inhibitors may have a greater beneficial effect than other antihypertensive agents in this disorder.[601, 602] As described in Chapter 48, increasing evidence suggests that blood pressure reduction will also slow the progression of other renal diseases.

The variety of mechanisms of remnant nephron injury suggests that other therapeutic maneuvers may also slow the progression of renal disease. Few clinical trials to assess the benefit of these potential therapies have been performed. Anticoagulant agents have been shown in some studies to retard the progression of membranoproliferative glomerulonephritis, as discussed in Chapter 30. As reviewed in Chapter 55, dietary phosphate restriction has so far not been shown to slow the progression of renal insufficiency. The protective effect of agents that lower serum lipid levels remains to be assessed. It is hoped that better understanding of the mechanisms responsible for progression of renal insufficiency will facilitate development of therapies to preserve renal function.

## REFERENCES

1. Bricker NS: On the meaning of the intact nephron hypothesis. Am J Med 46:1, 1969.
2. Bricker NS, Fine LG: The renal response to progressive nephron loss. In Brenner BM, Rector FC Jr (eds): The Kidney, 2nd ed. WB Saunders, Philadelphia, 1981, p 1056.
3. Allison MEM, Wilson CB, Gottschalk CW: Pathophysiology of experimental glomerulonephritis in rats. J Clin Invest 53:1402, 1974.
4. Kramp RA, MacDowell M, Gottschalk CW, Oliver JR: A study by microdissection and micropuncture of the structure and function of the kidneys and the nephrons of rats with chronic renal damage. Kidney Int 5:147, 1974.
5. Hostetter TH, Brenner BM: Glomerular adaptations to renal injury. In Brenner BM, Stein JH (eds): Contemporary Issues in Nephrology, Vol 7, Chronic Renal Failure. Churchill Livingstone, New York, 1981, p 1.
6. Krohn AG, Ogden DA, Holmes JH: Renal function in 29 healthy adults before and after nephrectomy. JAMA 196:110, 1966.
7. Ogden DA: Donor and recipient function 2–4 years after renal homotransplantation. A paired study of 28 cases. Ann Intern Med 67:998, 1967.
8. Pabico RC, McKenna BA, Freeman RB: Renal function before and after unilateral nephrectomy in renal donors. Kidney Int 8:166, 1975.
9. Anderson RG, Bueschen AJ, Lloyd LK, et al: Short-term and long-term changes in renal function after donor nephrectomy. J Urol 145:11, 1991.
10. Kaufman JM, DiMeola HJ, Siegel NJ, et al: Compensatory adaptation of structure and function following progressive renal ablation. Kidney Int 6:10, 1974.
11. Deen WM, Maddox DA, Robertson CR, Brenner BM: Dynamics of glomerular ultrafiltration in the rat. VII. Response to reduced renal mass. Am J Physiol 227:F556, 1974.
12. Finn WF: Compensatory renal hypertrophy in Sprague-Dawley rats: Glomerular ultrafiltration dynamics. Renal Physiol 5:222, 1982.
13. Meyer TW, Rennke HG: Progressive glomerular injury following limited renal infarction in the rat. Am J Physiol 254:F856, 1988.
14. Rous SN, Wakim KG: Kidney function before, during and after compensatory hypertrophy. J Urol 98:30, 1967.
15. Carriere S, Gagnon-Brunette M: Compensatory renal hypertrophy in dogs: Single nephron glomerular filtration rate. Can J Physiol Pharmacol 55:105, 1977.
16. Gregg CM, Wideman RF Jr: Morphological and functional comparisons of normal and hypertrophied kidneys of adult domestic fowl (Gallus gallus). Am J Physiol 258:F403, 1990.
17. Hutson JM, Holt AB, Egami K, et al: Compensatory renal growth in the mouse. I. Allometric approach to the effect of age. Pediatr Res 15:1370, 1981.
18. Harsing L, Baranyi K, Posch E: Pattern of renal growth and compensatory hypertrophy during development in rats: A mathematical approach. Kidney Int 22:398, 1982.
19. Boner G, Shelp WD, Newton M, Rieselbach RE: Factors influencing the increase in glomerular filtration rate in the remaining kidney of transplant donors. Am J Med 55:169, 1973.
20. Bonvalet JP, Champion M, Wanstok F, Berjal G: Compensatory renal hypertrophy in young rats: An increase in the number of nephrons. Kidney Int 1:391, 1972.
21. Imbert MJ, Berjal G, Moss N, et al: Number of nephrons in hyper-

22. trophic kidneys after unilateral nephrectomy in young and adult rats. Pflugers Arch 346:279, 1974.
22. Bonvalet JP, Champion M, Courtalon A, et al: Number of glomeruli in normal and hypertrophied kidneys of mice and guinea pigs. J Physiol (Lond) 269:627, 1977.
23. Canter CE, Goss RJ: Induction of extra nephrons in unilaterally nephrectomized immature rats (38525). Proc Soc Exp Biol Med 148:294, 1975.
24. Bonvalet JP: Evidence of induction of new nephrons in immature kidneys undergoing hypertrophy. Yale J Biol Med 51:315, 1978.
25. Kaufman JM, Hardy R, Hayslett JP: Age-dependent characteristics of compensatory renal growth. Kidney Int 8:21, 1975.
26. Larsson L, Aperia A, Wilron P: Effect of normal development on compensatory renal growth. Kidney Int 18:29, 1980.
27. Hayslett JP: Effect of age on compensatory renal growth. Kidney Int 23:599, 1983.
28. Kaufman JM, Siegel NJ, Hayslett JP: Functional and hemodynamic adaptation to progressive renal ablation. Circ Res 36:286, 1975.
29. Buerkert J, Martin D, Prasad J, et al: Response of deep nephrons and the terminal collecting duct to a reduction in renal mass. Am J Physiol 236:F454, 1979.
30. Pennel JP, Bourgoignie JJ: Adaptive changes of juxtamedullary glomerular filtration in the remnant kidney. Pflugers Arch 389:131, 1981.
31. Salmond R, Seney FD Jr: Reset tubuloglomerular feedback permits and sustains glomerular hyperfunction after extensive renal ablation. Am J Physiol 260:F395, 1991.
32. Pollock CA, Bostrom TE, Dyne M, et al: Tubular sodium handling and tubuloglomerular feedback in compensatory renal hypertrophy. Pflugers Arch 420:159, 1992.
33. Hostetter TH, Olson JL, Rennke HG, et al: Hyperfiltration in remnant nephrons: A potentially adverse response to renal ablation. Am J Physiol 241:F85, 1981.
34. Anderson S, Meyer TW, Rennke HG, Brenner BM: Control of glomerular hypertension limits glomerular injury in rats with reduced renal mass. J Clin Invest 76:612, 1985.
35. Purkerson ML, Hoffsten PE, Klahr S: Pathogenesis of the glomerulopathy associated with renal infarction in rats. Kidney Int 9:407, 1976.
36. Meyer TW, Anderson S, Rennke HG, Brenner BM: Reversing glomerular capillary hypertension stabilizes established glomerular injury. Kidney Int 31:752, 1987.
37. Kasiske BL, O'Donnell MP, Garvis WJ, Keane WF: Pharmacologic treatment of hyperlipidemia reduces glomerular injury in rat 5/6 nephrectomy model of chronic renal failure. Circ Res 62:367, 1988.
38. Langston JB, Guyton AC, Douglas BH, Dorsett PE: Effect of changes in salt intake on arterial pressure and renal function in nephrectomized dogs. Circ Res 12:508, 1963.
39. Brown SA, Finco DR, Crowell WA, et al: Single-nephron adaptations to partial renal ablation in the dog. Am J Physiol 258:F495, 1990.
40. Pelayo JC, Westvott JY: Impaired autoregulation of glomerular capillary hydrostatic pressure in the rat remnant nephron. J Clin Invest 88:101, 1991.
41. Bidani AK, Schwartz MM, Lewis EJ: Renal autoregulation and vulnerability to hypertensive injury in remnant kidneys. Am J Physiol 252:F1003, 1987.
42. Rosenberg ME, Kren SM, Hostetter TH: Effect of dietary protein on the renin-angiotensin system in subtotally nephrectomized rats. Kidney Int 38:240, 1990.
43. Pelayo JC, Quan AH, Shanley PF: Angiotensin II control of the renal microcirculation in rats with reduced renal mass. Am J Physiol 258:F414, 1990.
44. Baboolal K, Meyer T: Acute angiotensin II receptor blockade does not reverse systemic or glomerular capillary hypertension in remnant kidney rats. J Am Soc Nephrol 3:557, 1992.
45. Rosenberg ME, Correa-Rotter R, Inagami T, et al: Glomerular renin synthesis and storage in the remnant kidney in the rat. Kidney Int 40:677, 1991.
46. Pupilli C, Chevalier RL, Carey RM, Gomez RA: Distribution and content of renin and renin mRNA in remnant kidney of adult rat. Am J Physiol 263:F731, 1992.
47. Terzi F, Beaufils H, Laouari D, et al: Renal effect of anti-hypertensive drugs depends on sodium diet in the excision remnant kidney model. Kidney Int 42:354, 1992.

48. Lafayette RA, Mayer G, Park SK, Meyer TW: Angiotensin II receptor blockade limits glomerular injury in rats with reduced renal mass. J Clin Invest 90:766, 1992.

49. Zhang PL, Mackenzie HS, Troy JL, et al: Effects of a natriuretic peptide receptor antagonist in rats with reduced renal mass. J Am Soc Nephrol 4:591, 1993.

50. Benigni A, Perico N, Gaspari F, et al: Increased renal endothelin production in rats with reduced renal mass. Am J Physiol 260:F331, 1991.

51. Orisio S, Benigni A, Bruzzi I, et al: Renal endothelin gene expression is increased in remnant kidney and correlates with disease progression. Kidney Int 43:354, 1993.

52. Stahl RA, Kudelka S, Paravicini M, Schollmeyer P: Prostaglandin and thromboxane formation in glomeruli from rats with reduced renal mass. Nephron 42:252, 1986.

53. Purkerson ML, Joist JH, Yates J, et al: Inhibition of thromboxane synthesis ameliorates the progressive kidney disease of rats with subtotal ablation. Proc Natl Acad Sci USA 82:193, 1985.

54. Nath KA, Chmielewski DH, Hostetter TH: Regulatory role of prostanoids in glomerular microcirculation of remnant nephrons. Am J Physiol 252:F829, 1987.

55. Griffin KA, Bidani AK, Picken M, et al: Prostaglandins do not mediate impaired autoregulation or increased renin secretion in remnant rat kidneys. Am J Physiol 263:F1057, 1992.

56. Kirschenbaum MA, Serros ER: Effect of prostaglandin inhibition on glomerular filtration rate in normal and uremic rabbits. Prostaglandins 22:245, 1981.

57. Arisz L, Donker AJM, Brentjens JRH, van der Hem GK: The effect of indomethacin on proteinuria and kidney function in the nephrotic syndrome. Acta Med Scand 199:121, 1976.

58. Michielsen P, Vanrenterghem Y: Proteinuria and nonsteroid anti-inflammatory drugs. Adv Nephrol 12:139, 1983.

59. Ciabattoni G, Cinotti GA, Pierucci A, et al: Effects of sulindac and ibuprofen in patients with chronic glomerular disease. N Engl J Med 310:279, 1984.

60. Altsheler P, Klahr S, Rosenbaum R, Slatopolsky E: Effects of inhibitors of prostaglandin synthesis on renal sodium excretion in normal dogs and dogs with decreased renal mass. Am J Physiol 235:F338, 1978.

61. Addis T, Meyers BA, Oliver J: The regulation of renal activity. IX. The effect of unilateral nephrectomy on the function and structure of the remaining kidney. Arch Intern Med 34:243, 1924.

62. Oliver J: The regulation of renal activity. X. The morphologic study. Arch Intern Med 34:258, 1924.

63. Olivetti G, Anversa P, Rigamonti W, et al: Morphometry of the renal corpuscle during normal postnatal growth and compensatory hypertrophy. A light microscope study. J Cell Biol 75:573, 1977.

64. Shea SM, Raskova J, Morrison AB: A stereologic study of glomerular hypertrophy in the subtotally nephrectomized rat. Am J Pathol 90:201, 1978.

65. Seyer-Hansen K, Hansen J, Gundersen HJG: Renal hypertrophy in experimental diabetes. A morphometric study. Diabetologia 18:501, 1980.

66. Vancura P, Miller WL, Little JW, Malt RA: Contribution of glomerular and tubular RNA synthesis to compensatory renal growth. Am J Physiol 219:F78, 1970.

67. Olivetti G, Anversa P, Melissari M, Loud AV: Morphometry of the renal corpuscle during postnatal growth and compensatory hypertrophy. Kidney Int 17:438, 1980.

68. Schwartz MM, Bidani AK: Mesangial structure and function in the remnant kidney. Kidney Int 40:226, 1991.

69. Fries JWU, Sandstrom DJ, Meyer TW, Rennke HG: Glomerular hypertrophy and epithelial cell injury modulate progressive glomerulosclerosis in the rat. Lab Invest 60:205, 1989.

70. Nagata M, Schärer K, Kriz W: Glomerular damage after uninephrectomy in young rats. I. Hypertrophy and distortion of capillary architecture. II. Mechanical stress on podocytes as a pathway to sclerosis. Kidney Int 42:136, 1992.

71. Nyengaard JR: Number and dimensions of rat glomerular capillaries in normal development and after nephrectomy. Kidney Int 43:1049, 1993.

72. Daniels BS, Hostetter TH: Adverse effects of growth in the glomerular microcirculation. Am J Physiol 258:F1409, 1990.

73. Lax DS, Benstein JA, Tolbert E, Dworkin LD: Effects of salt restriction on renal growth and glomerular injury in rats with remnant kidneys. Kidney Int 41:1527, 1992.

74. Schwartz MM, Bidani AK: Role of glomerular epithelial cell injury in the pathogenesis of glomerular scarring in the rat remnant kidney model. Am J Pathol 142:209, 1993.

75. Shea SM, Raskova J: Glomerular hemodynamics and vascular structure in uremia: A network analysis of glomerular path lengths and maximal blood transit times computed for a microvascular model reconstructed from serial ultrathin sections. Microvasc Res 28:37, 1984.

76. Knutson DW, Chieu F, Bennett CM, Glassock RJ: Estimation of relative glomerular capillary surface area in normal and hypertrophic rat kidneys. Kidney Int 14:437, 1978.

77. Tucker BJ, Blantz RC: Factors determining superficial nephron filtration in the mature, growing rat. Am J Physiol 232:F97, 1977.

78. Ichikawa I, Maddox DA, Brenner BM: Maturational development of glomerular ultrafiltration in the rat. Am J Physiol 236:F465, 1979.

79. Fox H: Compensation in the remaining pronephros of *triturus* after unilateral pronephrectomy. J Embryol Exp Morphol 4:139, 1956.

80. Hayslett JP, Kashgarian M, Epstein FH: Functional correlates of compensatory renal hypertrophy. J Clin Invest 47:774, 1968.

81. Salehmoghaddam S, Bradley T, Mikhail N, et al: Hypertrophy of basolateral Na-K pump activity in the proximal tubule of the remnant kidney. Lab Invest 53:443, 1985.

82. Oliver J: New direction in renal morphology. A method, its results and its future. Harvey Lect 40:102, 1945.

83. Hayslett JP, Kashgarian M, Epstein FH: Mechanism of change in the excretion of sodium per nephron when renal mass is reduced. J Clin Invest 48:1002, 1969.

84. Tabei K, Levenson DJ, Brenner BM: Early enhancement of fluid transport in rabbit proximal straight tubules after loss of contralateral renal excretory function. J Clin Invest 72:871, 1983.

85. Fine LG, Bradley T: Adaptation of proximal tubular structure and function: Insights into compensatory renal hypertrophy. Fed Proc 44:2723, 1985.

86. Fine LG, Trizna W, Bourgoignie JJ, Bricker NS: Functional profile of the isolated uremic nephron. Role of compensatory hypertrophy in the control of fluid reabsorption by the proximal straight tubule. J Clin Invest 60:1508, 1978.

87. Trizna W, Yanagawa N, Bar-Khayim Y, et al: Functional profile of the isolated uremic nephron. Evidence of proximal tubular "memory" in experimental renal disease. J Clin Invest 68:760, 1981.

88. Johnson JR, Brenner BM, Herbert SC: Uninephrectomy and dietary protein affect fluid absorption in rabbit proximal straight "tubules." Am J Physiol 253:F222, 1987.

89. Hwang S, Bohman R, Navas P, et al: Hypertrophy of renal mitochondria. J Am Soc Nephrol 1:822, 1990.

90. Mitchell AD, Valk WL: Compensatory renal hypertrophy. J Urol 88:11, 1962.

91. Hruska KA, Klahr S, Hammerman MR: Decreased luminal membrane transport of phosphate in chronic renal failure. Am J Physiol 242:F17, 1982.

92. Harris RC, Seifter JL, Brenner BM: Adaptation of Na$^+$-H$^+$ exchange in renal microvillus membrane vesicles: The role of dietary protein and uninephrectomy. J Clin Invest 74:1979, 1984.

93. Bouby N, Hassler C, Parvy P, Bankir L: Renal synthesis of arginine in chronic renal failure: In vivo and in vitro studies in rats with 5/6 nephrectomy. Kidney Int 44:676, 1993.

94. Wang M, Vyhmeister I, Kopple JD, Swendseid ME: Effect of protein intake on weight gain and plasma amino acid levels in uremic rats. Am J Physiol 230:1455, 1976.

95. Yanagawa N, Nissenson RA, Edwards B, et al: Functional profile of the isolated uremic nephron: Intrinsic adaptation of phosphate transport in the rabbit proximal tubule. Kidney Int 23:674, 1983.

96. Buerkert J, Martin D, Trigg D, Simon E: Effect of reduced renal mass on ammonium handling and net acid formation by the superficial and juxtamedullary nephron of the rat. Evidence of impaired re-entrapment rather than decreased production of ammonium in the acidosis of uremia. J Clin Invest 71:1661, 1983.

97. Schoolwerth AC, Sandler RS, Hoffsten PM, Klahr S: Effects of nephron reduction and dietary protein content on renal ammoniagenesis in the rat. Kidney Int 7:397, 1975.

98. Lotspeich WD: Metabolic aspects of acid-base change. Science 155:1066, 1967.

99. Cohn DE, Hruska KA, Klahr S, Hammerman MR: Increased Na$^+$-H$^+$ exchange in brush border vesicles from dogs with renal failure. Am J Physiol 243:F293, 1982.

100. Nord EP, Hafezi A, Kaunitz JD, et al: pH gradient–dependent increased Na⁺-H⁺ antiport capacity of the rabbit remnant kidney. Am J Physiol 249:F90, 1985.

101. Maddox DA, Horn JF, Famiano FC, Gennari FJ: Load dependence of proximal tubule fluid and bicarbonate reabsorption in the remnant kidney of the Munich-Wistar rat. J Clin Invest 77:1639, 1986.

102. Fine LG: The biology of renal hypertrophy. Kidney Int 29:619, 1986.

103. Nowinski WW, Carpentieri U, Mahaffey WC: Glutamic dehydrogenase and alkaline phosphatase in compensatory hypertrophy of the rat kidney. Proc Soc Exp Biol Med 129:26, 1968.

104. Bank N, Aynedjian HS: Individual nephron function in experimental bilateral pyelonephritis. II. Distal tubular sodium and water reabsorption and the concentrating defect. J Lab Clin Med 68:728, 1966.

105. Mujais SK, Kurtzman NA: Regulation of renal Na-K-ATPase in the rat: Effect of uninephrectomy. Am J Physiol 251:F506, 1986.

106. Scherzer P, Wald H, Czaczkes JW: Na-K-ATPase in isolated rabbit tubules after unilateral nephrectomy and Na⁺ loading. Am J Physiol 248:F565, 1985.

107. Fine LG, Yanagawa N, Schultze RG, et al: Functional profile of the isolated uremic nephron. Potassium adaptation in the rabbit cortical collecting duct. J Clin Invest 64:1033, 1979.

108. Vehaskari VM, Hering-Smith KS, Klahr S, Hamm LL: Increased sodium transport by cortical collecting tubules from remnant kidneys. Kidney Int 36:89, 1989.

109. Zalups RK, Henderson DA: Cellular morphology in outer medullary collecting duct: Effect of 75% nephrectomy and K⁺ depletion. Am J Physiol 263:F1119, 1992.

110. Kaissling B: Structural aspects of adaptive changes in renal electrolyte excretion. Am J Physiol 243:F211, 1982.

111. Stanton BA, Biemesderfer D, Wade JB, Giebisch G: Structural and functional study of the rat distal nephron: Effects of potassium adaptation and depletion. Kidney Int 19:36, 1981.

112. Wade JB, O'Neil RG, Pryor JL, Boulpaep EL: Modulation of cell membrane area in renal collecting tubules by corticosteroid hormones. J Cell Biol 81:439, 1979.

113. Zalups RK, Stanton BA, Wade JB, Giebisch G: Structural adaptation in initial collecting tubule following reduction in renal mass. Kidney Int 27:636, 1985.

114. Schon DA, Silva P, Hayslett JP: Mechanism of potassium excretion in renal insufficiency. Am J Physiol 227:F1323, 1974.

115. Finkelstein FO, Hayslett JP: Role of medullary Na-K-ATPase in renal potasium adaptation. Am J Physiol 229:F524, 1975.

116. Vehaskari VM, Herndon J: Role of mineralocorticoids in adaptation of rabbit cortical collecting duct after loss of renal mass. Am J Physiol 260:F793, 1991.

117. Ebata S, Muto S, Asano Y: Effects of uninephrectomy on electrical properties of the cortical collecting duct from rabbit remnant kidneys. J Clin Invest 90:1547, 1992.

118. Nowinski WW, Goss RJ (eds): Compensatory Renal Hypertrophy. Academic Press, New York, 1969.

119. International Symposium on Renal Adaptation to Nephron Loss. Yale J Biol Med 51:235, 1978.

120. Preuss HG (ed): Symposium on compensatory renal growth. Kidney Int 23:569, 1983.

121. Malt R: Compensatory growth of the kidney. N Engl J Med 280:1446, 1969.

122. Fine LG: The biology of renal hypertrophy. Kidney Int 29:619, 1986.

123. Wesson LG: Compensatory growth and other growth responses of the kidney. Nephron 51:149, 1989. Editorial.

124. Nowinski WW: Early history of renal hypertrophy. In Nowinski WW, Goss RJ (eds): Compensatory Renal Hypertrophy. Academic Press, New York, 1969, p 1.

125. Coe FL, Korty PR: Protein synthesis during compensatory renal hypertrophy. Am J Physiol 213:F1585, 1967.

126. Halliburton IW, Thomson RY: Chemical aspects of compensatory renal hypertrophy. Cancer Res 25:1882, 1967.

127. Johnson HA, Roman JMV: Compensatory renal enlargement. Hypertrophy versus hyperplasia. Am J Pathol 49:1, 1966.

128. Ouellette AJ: Messenger RNA regulation during compensatory renal growth. Kidney Int 23:575, 1983.

129. Ouellette AJ, Moonka R, Zelenetz AD, Malt RA: Regulation of ribosome synthesis during compensatory renal hypertrophy in mice. Am J Physiol 253:C506, 1987.

130. Melvin WT, Kumar A, Malt RA: Conservation of ribosomal RNA during compensatory renal hypertrophy. A major mechanism in RNA accretion. J Cell Biol 59:548, 1976.

131. Goss RJ, Rankin M: Physiological factors affecting compensatory renal hyperplasia in the rat. J Exp Zool 145:209, 1960.

132. Williams GEG: Effect of starvation and of adrenalectomy on compensatory hyperplasia of the kidney. Nature 196:1221, 1962.

133. Argyris TS, Trimble ME, Janicki R: Control of induced kidney growth. In Nowinski WW, Goss RJ (eds): Compensatory Renal Hypertrophy. Academic Press, New York, 1969, p 45.

134. Threlfall G, Taylor DM, Buck AT: Studies of changes in growth and DNA synthesis in the rat kidney during experimentally induced renal hypertrophy. Am J Pathol 50:1, 1967.

135. Dicker SE, Shirley DG: Compensatory renal growth after unilateral nephrectomy in the new-born rat. J Physiol (Lond) 228:193, 1973.

136. Barrows CH Jr: Aging in the kidney. In Nowinski WW, Goss RJ (eds): Compensatory Renal Hypertrophy. Academic Press, New York, 1969, p 283.

137. Zumoff B, Pachter MR: Studies of rat kidney and liver growth using total nuclear counts. Am J Anat 114:479, 1964.

138. Celsi G, Jakobsson B, Aperia A: Influence of age on compensatory renal growth in rats. Pediatr Res 20:347, 1986.

139. Austin HA, Goldin H, Gaydos D, Preuss HG: Polyamine metabolism in compensatory renal growth. Kidney Int 23:581, 1983.

140. Brandt JT, Pierce DA, Fausto N: Ornithine decarboxylase activity and polyamine synthesis during kidney hypertrophy. Biochem Biophys Acta 279:184, 1972.

141. Desiderio MA, Sessa A, Perin A: Induction of diamine oxidase activity in rat kidney during compensatory hypertrophy. Biochem Biophys Acta 714:243, 1982.

142. Humphreys MH, Etheredge SB, Lin S-Y, et al: Renal ornithine decarboxylase activity, polyamines, and compensatory renal hypertrophy in the rat. Am J Physiol 255:F270, 1988.

143. Schlondorff D, Weber H: Cyclic nucleotide metabolism in compensatory renal hypertrophy and neonatal kidney growth. Proc Natl Acad Sci USA 73:524, 1976.

144. Dicker SE, Greenbaum AL: Changes in renal cyclic nucleotide content as a possible trigger to the initiation of compensatory renal hypertrophy in rats. J Physiol (Lond) 271:505, 1977.

145. Caramelo C, Tsai P, Okada K, Schrier RW: Protein kinase C activity in compensatory renal growth. Biochem Biophys Res Commun 152:315, 1988.

146. Farquhar JK, Scott WN, Coe FL: Hexose monophosphate shunt activity in compensatory renal hypertrophy. Proc Soc Exp Biol Med 129:809, 1968.

147. Steer KA, Sochor M, Gonzales AM, McLean P: Regulation of pathways of glucose metabolism in kidney. Specific linking of pentose phosphate pathway activity with kidney growth in experimental diabetes and unilateral nephrectomy. FEBS Lett 150:494, 1982.

148. Toback FG, Smith PD, Lowenstein LM: Phospholipid metabolism in the initiation of renal compensatory growth after acute reduction of renal mass. J Clin Invest 54:91, 1974.

149. Toback FG: Phosphatidylcholine metabolism during renal growth and regeneration. Am J Physiol 246:F249, 1984.

150. Hise MK, Harris RH, Mansbach CM II: Regulation of de novo phosphatidylcholine biosynthesis during renal growth. Am J Physiol 247:F260, 1984.

151. Norman JT, Bohman RE, Fischmann G, et al: Patterns of mRNA expression during early cell growth differ in kidney epithelial cells destined to undergo compensatory hypertrophy versus regenerative hyperplasia. Proc Natl Acad Sci USA 85:6768, 1988.

152. Beer DG, Zweifel KA, Simpson DP, Pitot HC: Specific gene expression during compensatory renal hypertrophy in the rat. J Cell Physiol 131:29, 1987.

153. Ouellette AJ, Malt RA, Sukhatme VP, Bonventre JV: Expression of two "immediate early" genes, Egr-1 and c-fos, in response to renal ischemia and during compensatory renal hypertrophy in mice. J Clin Invest 85:766, 1990.

154. Sawczuk IS, Olsson CA, Hoke G, Buttyan R: Immediate induction of c-fos and c-myc transcripts following unilateral nephrectomy. Nephron 55:193, 1990.

155. Nakamura T, Ebihara I, Tomino Y, et al: Gene expression of growth-related proteins and ECM constituents in response to unilateral nephrectomy. Am J Physiol 262:F389, 1992.

156. Kujubu DA, Norman JT, Herschman HR, Fine LG: Primary response gene expression in renal hypertrophy and hyperplasia: Evidence for different growth initiation processes. Am J Physiol 260:F823, 1991.

157. Rosenberg ME, Hostetter TH: Effect of angiotensin II and norepi-

nephrine on early growth response genes in the rat kidney. Kidney Int 43:601, 1993.

158. Kojlma R, Troy J, Brenner BM, Gullans SR: Identification and characterization of novel genes induced by uninephrectomy. J Am Soc Nephrol 4:774, 1993.

159. Flanagan WS, Burns RO, Takacs FJ, Merrill JP: Serial studies of glomerular filtration rate and renal plasma flow in kidney transplant donors, identical twins and allograft recipients. Am J Surg 116:788, 1968.

160. Gazdiar AF, Dammin GJ: Neural degeneration and regeneration in human renal transplants. N Engl J Med 283:222, 1970.

161. Malt RA: Humoral factors in regulation of compensatory renal hypertrophy. Kidney Int 23:611, 1983.

162. Lowenstein LM, Stern A: Serum factor in renal compensatory hyperplasia. Science 142:1479, 1963.

163. Preuss HG, Glodin H: A renotropic system in rats. J Clin Invest 57:94, 1976.

164. Gaydos DS, Goldin H, Jenson B, et al: Partial characterization of a renotropic factor. Renal Physiol 6:139, 1983.

165. Harris RH, Hise MK, Best CF: Renotropic factors in urine. Kidney Int 23:616, 1983.

166. Yamamoto H, Kanetake H, Yamada J: In vitro evidence from tissue cultures to prove existence of rabbit and human renotropic growth factor. Kidney Int 23:624, 1983.

167. Kanda S, Nomata K, Saha PK, et al: A study of growth regulators of renal cortical tubular cells in the rabbit liver. Kidney Int 37:875, 1990.

168. Nomura K, Puett D, Nicholson WE, Liddle GW: Partial purification and characterization of a renotropic fraction from ovine pituitaries. Proc Natl Acad Sci USA 79:6675, 1982.

169. Igawa T, Kanetake H, Saitoh Y, et al: Hepatocyte growth factor is a potent mitogen for cultured rabbit renal tubular epithelial cells. Biochem Biophys Res Commun 174:831, 1991.

170. Wolf G, Neilson EG: Angiotensin II as a renal growth factor. J Am Soc Nephrol 3:1531, 1993.

171. Miller PL, Rennke HG, Meyer TW: Glomerular hypertrophy accelerates hypertensive glomerular injury in rats. Am J Physiol 261:F459, 1991.

172. Lajara R, Rotwein P, Bortz JD, et al: Dual regulation of insulin-like growth factor I expression during renal hypertrophy. Am J Physiol 257:F252, 1989.

173. Miller SB, Hansen VA, Hammerman MR: Effects of growth hormone and IGF-I on renal function in rats with normal and reduced renal mass. Am J Physiol 259:F747, 1990.

174. Quaife CJ, Mathews LS, Pinkert CA, et al: Histopathology associated with elevated levels of growth hormone and insulin-like growth factor I in transgenic mice. Endocrinology 124:40, 1989.

175. Mehls O, Irzynjec T, Ritz E, et al: Effects of rhGH and rhIGF-1 on renal growth and morphology. Kidney Int 44:1251, 1993.

176. Stiles AD, Sosenko IR, Dercole AJ, Smith BT: Relation of kidney tissue somatomedin-C/insulin-like growth factor I to postnephrectomy renal growth in the rat. Endocrinology 117:2397, 1985.

177. Fagin JA, Melmed S: Relative increase in insulin-like growth factor I messenger ribonucleic acid levels in compensatory renal hypertrophy. Endocrinology 120:718, 1987.

178. Flyvbjerg A, Thorlacius Ussing O, Naeraa R, et al: Kidney tissue somatomedin C and initial renal growth in diabetic and uninephrectomized rats. Diabetologia 31:310, 1988.

179. Hise MK, Lahn JS, Shao ZM, et al: Insulin-like growth factor-I receptor and binding proteins in rat kidney after nephron loss. J Am Soc Nephrol 4:62, 1993.

180. Rogers SA, Miller SB, Hammerman MR: Enhanced renal IGF-I expression following partial kidney infarction. Am J Physiol 264:F963, 1993.

181. Behrens MT, Corbin AL, Hise MK: Epidermal growth factor receptor regulation in rat kidney: Two models of renal growth. Am J Physiol 257:F1059, 1989.

182. Sack EM, Arruda JA: Epidermal growth factor binding to cortical basolateral membranes in compensatory renal hypertrophy. Regul Pept 33:339, 1991.

183. Miller SB, Rogers SA, Estes CE, Hammerman MR: Increased distal nephron EGF content and altered distribution of peptide in compensatory renal hypertrophy. Am J Physiol 262:F1032, 1992.

184. Nagaike M, Hirao S, Tajima H, et al: Renotropic functions of hepatocyte growth factor in renal regeneration after unilateral nephrectomy. J Biol Chem 266:22781, 1991.

185. Yanagita K, Nagaike M, Ishibashi H, et al: Lung may have an endocrine function producing hepatocyte growth factor in response to injury of distal organs. Biochem Biophys Res Commun 182:802, 1992.

186. Montesano R, Matsumoto K, Nakamura T, Orci L: Identification of a fibroblast-derived epithelial morphogen as hepatocyte growth factor. Cell 67:901, 1991.

187. Addis T: The ratio between the urea content of the urine and of the blood after the administration of large quantities of urea: An approximate index of the quantity of actively functioning kidney tissue. J Urol 1:263, 1917.

188. MacKay LL, MacKay E, Addis T: Factors which determine renal weight. J Nutr 4:379, 1932.

189. Matthias S, Busch R, Merke J, et al: Effects of $1,25(OH)_2D_3$ on compensatory renal growth in the growing rat. Kidney Int 40:212, 1991.

190. Garcia DL, Anderson S, Rennke HG, Brenner BM: Anemia lessens and its prevention with recombinant human erythropoietin worsens glomerular injury and hypertension in rats with reduced renal mass. Proc Natl Acad Sci USA 85:6142, 1988.

191. Reyes AA, Purkerson ML, Karl I, Klahr S: Dietary supplementation with L-arginine ameliorates the progression of renal disease in rats with subtotal nephrectomy. Am J Kidney Dis 20:168, 1992.

192. Yared A, Kon V, Ichikawa I: Functional development of the kidney. In Tune BM, Mendoza SA, Brenner BM, Stein JH (eds): Contemporary Issues in Nephrology, Vol 12, Pediatric Nephrology. Churchill Livingstone, New York, 1984, p 61.

193. Moise TS, Smith AH: The effect of high protein diet on the kidneys. Arch Pathol Lab Med 4:530, 1927.

194. Brenner BM, Meyer TW, Hostetter TH: Dietary protein intake and the progressive nature of renal disease. N Engl J Med 307:652, 1982.

195. Hostetter TH, Rennke HG, Brenner BM: The case for intrarenal hypertension in the initiation and progression of diabetic and other glomerulopathies. Am J Med 72:375, 1982.

196. Seyer-Hansen K: Renal hypertrophy in experimental diabetes mellitus. Kidney Int 23:643, 1983.

197. Katz AI, Epstein FH: Relation of glomerular filtration rate and sodium reabsorption to kidney size in compensatory renal hypertrophy. Yale J Biol Med 40:222, 1967.

198. Katz AI, Toback FG, Lindheimer MD: Independence of onset of compensatory kidney growth from changes in renal function. Am J Physiol 230:1067, 1976.

199. Peters G: Compensatory adaptation of renal functions in the unanesthetized rat. Am J Physiol 205:F1042, 1963.

200. Blantz RC, Peterson OW, Thomson SC: Tubuloglomerular feedback responses to acute contralateral nephrectomy. Am J Physiol 260:F749, 1991.

201. Potter DE, Leumann EP, Sakai T, Holliday MA: Early responses of glomerular filtration rate to unilateral nephrectomy. Kidney Int 5:131, 1974.

202. Mackovic-Basic M, Fan R, Kurtz I: Denervation inhibits early increase in Na⁺-H⁺ exchange after uninephrectomy but does not suppress hypertrophy. Am J Physiol 263:F328, 1992.

203. Diezi J, Michoud-Hausel P, Nicolas-Buxcel N: Studies on possible mechanisms of early functional compensatory adaptation in the remaining kidney. Yale J Biol Med 51:265, 1978.

204. Dirks JH, Wong NLM: Acute functional adaptation to nephron loss: Micropuncture studies. Yale J Biol Med 51:255, 1978.

205. Guignard JP, Filioux B: Studies on compensatory adaptation of renal function. Yale J Biol Med 51:247, 1978.

206. Humphreys MH, Ayus JC: Role of hemodynamic changes in the increased cation excretion after acute unilateral nephrectomy in the anesthetized dog. J Clin Invest 61:590, 1978.

207. Allison NEM, Lipham EM, Kassiter WE, Gottschalk CW: The acutely reduced kidney. Kidney Int 3:354, 1973.

208. Ayus JC, Humphreys MH: Hemodynamic and renal functional changes after acute unilateral nephrectomy in the dog: Role of carotid sinus baroreceptors. Am J Physiol 242:F181, 1982.

209. Humphreys MH, Lin SY, Wiedemann E: Renal nerves and the natriuresis following unilateral renal exclusion in the rat. Kidney Int 39:63, 1991.

210. Valentin J-P, Ribstein J, Neuser D, et al: Effect of monoclonal anti-ANP antibodies on the acute functional adaptation to unilateral nephrectomy. Kidney Int 43:1260, 1993.

211. Malt RA, Miller WL: Sequential changes in classes of RNA during compensatory growth of the kidney. J Exp Med 126:1, 1967.

212. Tomashefsky P, Tannenbaum M: Macromolecular metabolism in renal compensatory hypertrophy. II. Protein turnover. Lab Invest 21:358, 1969.

213. Benitez L, Shaka JA: Cell proliferation in experimental hydronephrosis and compensatory renal hyperplasia. Am J Pathol 44:961, 1964.

214. Reid MR: Uretero-venous anastomosis. Bull Johns Hopkins Hosp 29:55, 1918.

215. Block MA, Wakim KG, Mann FC: Appraisal of certain factors influencing compensatory renal hypertrophy. Am J Physiol 172:60, 1953.

216. Bugge-Asperheim B, Kiil F: Examination of growth-mediated changes in hemodynamics and tubular transport of sodium, glucose and hippurate after nephrectomy. Scand J Clin Lab Invest 22:255, 1968.

217. Gittes GK, Gittes RF: The effect of uretero-peritoneostomy on renal mass in rats with porto-caval shunts. J Urol 128:411, 1982.

218. Weinman EJ, Renquist K, Stroup R, et al: Increased tubular reabsorption of sodium in compensatory renal growth. Am J Physiol 224:F565, 1973.

219. Eckert D, Kountz SL, Cohn R: Inhibition of compensatory renal growth by uretero-caval fistula. J Surg Res 9:187, 1969.

220. Morris GCR: Growth of rats' kidneys after unilateral uretero-caval anastomosis. J Physiol (Lond) 258:755, 1976.

221. Dicker SE, Shirley DG: Compensatory hypertrophy of the contralateral kidney after unilateral ureteral ligation. J Physiol (Lond) 220:199, 1972.

222. Zelman SJ, Zenser TV, Davis BB: Renal growth in response to unilateral ureteral obstruction. Kidney Int 23:594, 1983.

223. Harris RH, Best CF: Circulatory retention of urinary factors as a stimulus to renal growth. Kidney Int 12:305, 1977.

224. Laufer I, Griscom NT: Compensatory renal hypertrophy. Absence in utero and development in early life. Am J Roentgenol 113:464, 1971.

225. Dinkel E, Britscho J, Dittrich M, et al: Renal growth in patients nephrectomized for Wilms tumour as compared to renal agenesis. Eur J Pediatr 147:54, 1988.

226. Rollason HD: Mitotic activity in the fetal rat kidney following maternal and fetal nephrectomy. *In* Nowinski WW, Goss RJ (eds): Compensatory Renal Hypertrophy. Academic Press, New York, 1969, pp 61–67.

227. Goss RJ, Walker MJ: Compensatory renal hypertrophy in fetal rats. J Urol 106:360, 1971.

228. Moore ES, deLeon LB, Weiss LS, et al: Compensatory renal hypertrophy in fetal lambs. Pediatr Res 13:1125, 1979.

229. Peters CA, Carr MC, Lais A, et al: The response of the fetal kidney to obstruction. J Urol 148:503, 1992.

230. Goss RJ: Effects of maternal nephrectomy on foetal kidneys. Nature 198:1108, 1963.

231. Silber S, Malvin RL: Compensatory and obligatory renal growth in rats. Am J Physiol 226:F114, 1974.

232. Churchill M, Churchill PC, Schwartz M, et al: Reversible compensatory hypertrophy in transplanted brown Norway rat kidneys. Kidney Int 40:13, 1991.

233. Shankel SW, McDaniel J: Reversible uremia and its effect on the glomerular filtration rate. Nephron 32:359, 1982.

234. Dijkhuis CM, van Urk H, Malamud D, Malt RA: Rapid reversal of compensatory renal hypertrophy after withdrawal of the stimulus. Surgery 78:476, 1975.

235. Gittes RF, Rist M, Treves S, Biewiner A: Autoregulation in rats with transplanted supernumerary kidneys. Nature 284:618, 1980.

236. Silber SJ: Renal transplantation between adults and children. Differences in renal growth. JAMA 228:1143, 1974.

237. Bohlin A-B, Berg U: Renal functional adaptation of the adult kidney following transplantation to the child. Kidney Int 39:129, 1991.

238. Dicker SE, Shirley DG: Mechanism of compensatory renal hypertrophy. J Physiol (Lond) 219:507, 1971.

239. Hostetter TH, Meyer TW, Rennke HG, Brenner BM: Chronic effects of dietary protein on renal structure and function in the rat with intact and reduced renal mass. Kidney Int 30:509, 1986.

240. Davison JM: Changes in renal function in early pregnancy in women with one kidney. Yale J Biol Med 51:347, 1978.

241. Absy M, Metreweli C, Matthews C, Al Khader A: Changes in transplanted kidney volume measured by ultrasound. Br J Radiol 60:525, 1987.

242. Steffes MW, Brown DM, Mauer SM: Diabetic glomerulopathy following unilateral nephrectomy in the rat. Diabetes 27:35, 1978.

243. Ross J, Goldman JK: Compensatory renal hypertrophy in hypophysectomized rats. Endocrinology 87:620, 1970.

244. Gershberg H, Heinemann HO, Stumpf HH: Renal function studies and autopsy report in a patient with giganticism and acromegaly. J Clin Endocrinol 17:377, 1957.

245. Falkheden T: Renal function following hypophysectomy in man. Acta Endocrinol 42:571, 1963.

246. Corvilain J, Abramow M, Bergans A: Some effects of human growth hormone on renal hemodynamics and on tubular phosphate transport in man. J Clin Invest 41:1230, 1962.

247. Christiansen JS, Gammelgaard J, Ørskov H, et al: Kidney function and size in normal subjects before and during growth hormone administration for one week. Eur J Clin Invest 11:487, 1981.

248. Hirschberg R, Rabb H, Bergamo R, Kopple JD: The delayed effect of growth hormone on renal function in humans. Kidney Int 35:865, 1989.

249. McQueen-Williams M, Thompson KW: The effect of ablation of the hypophysis upon the weight of the kidney of the rat. Yale J Biol Med 12:531, 1940.

250. Dicker SE, Greenbaum AL, Morris CA: Compensatory renal hypertrophy in hypophysectomized rats. J Physiol (Lond) 273:241, 1977.

251. Ogle GD, Rosenberg AR, Kainer G: Renal effects of growth hormone. I. Renal function and kidney growth. Pediatr Nephrol 6:394, 1992.

252. Tonshoff B., Haffner D, Mehls O, et al: Efficacy and safety of growth hormone treatment in short children with renal allografts: Three year experience. Members of the German Study Group for Growth Hormone Treatment in Children with Renal Allografts. Kidney Int 44:199, 1993.

253. Poffenbarger PL, Prince MJ: The role of serum nonsuppressible insulin-like activity (NSILA) in compensatory renal growth. Growth 40:83, 1976.

254. Basinger GT, Gittes RF: Compensatory renal hypertrophy in male dwarf mice. Invest Urol 13:165, 1975.

255. Hutson JM, Graystone JE, Egami R, et al: Compensatory renal growth in the mouse. II. The effect of growth hormone deficiency. Pediatr Res 15:1375, 1981.

256. El Nahas AM, Le Carpentier JE, Bassett AH: Compensatory renal growth: Role of growth hormone and insulin-like growth factor-I. Nephrol Dial Transplant 5:123, 1990.

257. Bradley SE, Coelho JB: Glomerulotubular dimensional readjustments during compensatory renal hypertrophy in the hypothyroid rat. Yale J Biol Med 51:327, 1978.

258. Reiter RJ: The endocrines and compensatory renal enlargement. *In* Nowinski WW, Goss RJ (eds): Compensatory Renal Hypertrophy. Academic Press, New York, 1969, p 183.

259. Bradley SE, Stéphan F, Coelho JB, Réville P: The thyroid and the kidney. Kidney Int 6:346, 1974.

260. Conger JD, Falk SA: Glomerular dynamics in the hypothyroid rat and the role of the renin-angiotensin system. Am J Physiol 253:F170, 1987.

261. Selye H: The effect of testosterone on the kidney. J Urol 42:637, 1939.

262. Schlondorff D, Trizna W, DeRosis E, Korth-Schutz S: Effect of testosterone on compensatory renal hypertrophy in the rat. Endocrinology 101:1670, 1977.

263. Blantz RC, Peterson OW, Blantz ER, Wilson CB: Sexual differences in glomerular ultrafiltration: Effect of androgen administration in ovariectomized rats. Endocrinology 122:767, 1988.

264. Jean-Faucher C, Berger M, Gallon C, et al: Sex-related differences in renal size in mice: Ontogeny and influence of neonatal androgens. J Endocrinol 115:241, 1987.

265. Catterall JF, Kontula KK, Watson CS, et al: Regulation of gene expression by androgens in murine kidney. Recent Prog Horm Res 42:71, 1986.

266. Shukla A, Shukla GS, Radin NS: Control of kidney size by sex hormones: Possible involvement of glucosylceramide. Am J Physiol 262:F24, 1992.

267. Malt RA, Ohnu S, Paddock JK: Compensatory renal hypertrophy in the absence of androgen binding. Endocrinology 96:806, 1975.

268. Galla JH, Klein-Robbenhaar T, Hayslett JP: Influence of age on the compensatory response in growth and function to unilateral nephrectomy. Yale J Biol Med 47:218, 1974.

269. MacKay EM, Mackay LL, Addis T: The degree of compensatory renal hypertrophy following unilateral nephrectomy. I. The influence of age. J Exp Med 56:225, 1932.

270. Barrows CH Jr, Roeder LM, Olewine DA: Effect of age on renal compensatory hypertrophy following unilateral nephrectomy in the rat. J Gerontol 17:148, 1962.

271. Simon J, Zamora I, Mendizabal S, et al: Glomerulotubular balance and functional compensation in nephrectomized children. Nephron 37:203, 1982.

272. Verzár F: Compensatory hypertrophy in old age. In Nowinski WW, Goss RJ (eds): Compensatory Renal Hypertrophy. Academic Press, New York, 1969, p 291.

273. Buhain WJ, Brody JS: Compensatory growth of the lung following pneumonectomy. J Appl Physiol 35:898, 1973.

274. Gottschalk CW: Function of the chronically diseased kidney: The adaptive nephron. Circ Res 28(suppl 2):1, 1971.

275. Wagnild JP, Gutmann FD, Rieselbach RE: Functional characterization of chronic unilateral glomerulonephritis in the dog. Kidney Int 5:422, 1974.

276. Reiss E, Bricker NS, Kime SW Jr, Morrin PAF: Observations on phosphate transport in experimental renal disease. J Clin Invest 41:1303, 1962.

277. Schultze RG, Taggert DD, Shapiro H, et al: On the adaptation in potassium excretion associated with nephron reduction in the dog. J Clin Invest 50:1061, 1971.

278. Morrin PAF, Bricker NS, Kime SW Jr, Klein C: Observations on the acidifying capacity of the experimentally diseased kidney in the dog. J Clin Invest 41:1297, 1962.

279. Ichikawa I, Hoyer JR, Seiler MW, Brenner BM: Mechanism of glomerulotubular balance in the setting of heterogeneous glomerular injury. Preservation of a close functional linkage between individual nephrons and surrounding microvasculature. J Clin Invest 69:185, 1982.

280. Marcussen N: Biology of disease. Atubular glomeruli and the structural basis for chronic renal failure. Lab Invest 66:265, 1992.

281. Tanner GA, Knopp LC: Glomerular blood flow after single nephron obstruction in the rat kidney. Am J Physiol 250:F77, 1986.

282. Tanner GA, Evan AP: Glomerular and proximal tubular morphology after single nephron obstruction. Kidney Int 36:1050, 1989.

283. Bank N, Aynedjian HS: Individual nephron function in experimental bilateral pyelonephritis. I. Glomerular filtration rate and proximal tubular sodium, potassium, and water reabsorption. J Lab Clin Med 68:713, 1966.

284. Oliver J: Architecture of the Kidney in Chronic Bright's Disease. Paul B. Hoeber, New York, 1939.

285. Mitch WE, Wilcox CS: Disorders of body fluids, sodium and potassium in chronic renal failure. Am J Med 72:536, 1982.

286. Slatopolsky E, Elkan IO, Weerts C, Bricker NS: Studies on the characteristics of the control system governing sodium excretion in uremic man. J Clin Invest 47:521, 1968.

287. Luft FC, Rankin LI, Bloch R, et al: Cardiovascular and humoral responses to extremes of sodium intake in normal black and white men. Circulation 60:697, 1979.

288. Koomans HA, Roos JC, Dorhout-Mees EJ, Delawi IM: Sodium balance in renal failure. A comparison of patients with normal subjects under extremes of sodium intake. Hypertension 7:714, 1985.

289. Hayslett JP: Functional adaptation to reduction in renal mass. Physiol Rev 59:137, 1979.

290. Bricker NS: Sodium homeostasis in chronic renal disease. Kidney Int 21:886, 1982.

291. Wen S-F, Wong NLM, Evanson RL, et al: Micropuncture studies of sodium transport in the remnant kidney of the dog. J Clin Invest 52:386, 1973.

292. Weber H, Lin K, Bricker NS: Effect of sodium intake on single nephron glomerular filtration rate and sodium reabsorption in experimental uremia. Kidney Int 8:14, 1975.

293. Lubowitz H, Mazumdar DC, Kawamura J, et al: Experimental glomerulonephritis in the rat: Structural and functional observations. Kidney Int 5:356, 1974.

294. Wilson DR, Sonnenberg H: Medullary collecting duct function in the remnant kidney before and after volume expansion. Kidney Int 15:487, 1979.

295. Thorn GW, Koepf GF, Clinton MC: Renal failure simulating adrenocortical insufficiency. N Engl J Med 231:76, 1944.

296. Schrier RW, Regal EM: Influence of aldosterone on sodium, water and potassium metabolism in chronic renal disease. Kidney Int 1:156, 1972.

297. Berl T, Katz FH, Heinrich WL, et al: Role of aldosterone in the control of sodium excretion in patients with advanced chronic renal failure. Kidney Int 14:228, 1978.

298. Hene RJ, Boer P, Koomans HA, Dorhout-Mees EJ: Plasma aldosterone concentrations in chronic renal disease. Kidney Int 21:98, 1982.

299. Coleman AJ, Arias M, Carter NW, et al: The mechanism of salt wastage in chronic renal disease. J Clin Invest 45:116, 1966.

300. Hene RJ, Koomans HA, Boer P, Dorhout-Mees EJ: Effect of high-dose aldosterone infusions on renal electrolyte excretion in patients with renal insufficiency. Am J Nephrol 7:33, 1987.

301. Schmidt RW, Bourgoignie JJ, Bricker NS: On the adaptation in sodium excretion in chronic uremia. The effects of ''proportional reduction'' of sodium intake. J Clin Invest 53:1736, 1974.

302. Bourgoignie JJ, Hwang KH, Ipakchi E, Bricker NS: The presence of a natriuretic factor in urine of patients with chronic uremia. The absence of the factor in nephrotic uremic patients. J Clin Invest 53:1559, 1974.

303. Epstein M, Bricker NS, Bourgoignie JJ: Presence of a natriuretic factor in urine of normal men undergoing water immersion. Kidney Int 13:152, 1978.

304. Favre H, Hwang KH, Schmidt RW, et al: An inhibitor of sodium transport in the urine of dogs with normal renal function. J Clin Invest 56:1302, 1975.

305. Bourgoignie JJ, Klahr S, Bricker NS: Inhibitor of transepithelial sodium transport in the frog skin by a low molecular weight fraction of uremic serum. J Clin Invest 50:303, 1971.

306. Fine LG, Bourgoignie JJ, Hwang KH, Bricker NS: On the influence of the natriuretic factor from patients with chronic uremia on the bioelectric properties and sodium transport of the isolated mammalian collecting tubule. J Clin Invest 58:590, 1976.

307. Kelly RA, O'Hara DS, Mitch WE, et al: Endogenous digitalis-like factors in hypertension and chronic renal insufficiency. Kidney Int 30:723, 1986.

308. Kelly RA, Canessa ML, Steinman TI, Mitch WE: Hemodialysis and red cell cation transport in uremia: Role of membrane free fatty acids. Kidney Int 35:595, 1989.

309. Jackson B, Hodsman P, Johnston CI: Changes in the renin-angiotensin system, exchangeable body sodium, and plasma and atrial content of atrial natriuretic factor during evolution of chronic renal failure in the rat. Am J Hypertens 1:298, 1988.

310. Smith S, Anderson S, Ballerman BJ, Brenner BM: Role of atrial natriuretic peptide in adaptation of sodium excretion with reduced renal mass. J Clin Invest 77:1395, 1986.

311. Yamamoto Y, IIiga T, Kitamura K, ct al: Plasma conccntration of human atrial natriuretic polypeptide in patients with impaired renal function. Clin Nephrol 27:84, 1987.

312. Predel HG, Backer A, Kipnowski J, et al: Relationship of plasma concentrations of human atrial natriuretic peptide to renal function and blood pressure in patients with progressive chronic renal failure. Klin Wochenschr 65(suppl 8):127, 1987.

313. Ogawa K, Smith AI, Hodsman GP, et al: Plasma atrial natriuretic peptide: Concentrations and circulating forms in normal man and patients with chronic renal failure. Clin Exp Pharmacol Physiol 14:95, 1987.

314. Suda S, Weidman P, Saxenhoffer H, et al: Atrial natriuretic factor in mild to moderate chronic renal failure. Hypertension 11:483, 1988.

315. Zhang PL, Mackenzie HS, Troy JL, et al: Effects of a natriuretic peptide receptor antagonist in rats with reduced renal mass. J Am Soc Nephrol 4:591, 1993.

316. Langston JB, Guyton AC, Douglas BH, Dorsett PE: Effects of changes in salt intake on arterial pressure and renal function in partially nephrectomized dogs. Circ Res 12:508, 1966.

317. Guyton AC, Coleman TG, Young DB, et al: Salt balance and long-term blood pressure control. Annu Rev Med 31:15, 1980.

318. Dormois JC, Young JL, Nies AS: Minoxidil in severe hypertension: Value when conventional drugs have failed. Am Heart J 90:360, 1975.

319. Koomans HA, Braum B, Geers AB, et al: The importance of plasma protein for blood volume and blood pressure homeostasis. Kidney Int 30:730, 1986.

320. Daniels BS, Hostetter TH: Adverse effects of growth in the glomerular microcirculation. Am J Physiol 258:F1409, 1990.

321. Bourgoignie JJ, Kaplan M, Gavellas G, Jaffe D: Sodium homeostasis in dogs with chronic renal insufficiency. Kidney Int 21:820, 1982.

322. Schultze RG, Shapiro HS, Bricker NS: Studies on the control of sodium excretion in experimental uremia. J Clin Invest 48:869, 1969.

323. Ghani M, Kahn T, Stein RM: Effects of saline loading in hypertensive and normotensive azotemic men. Clin Res 20:603A, 1972. Abstract.

324. Gutmann FD, Rieselbach RE: Disproportionate inhibition of sodium reabsorption in the unilaterally diseased kidney of dog and man after an acute saline load. J Clin Invest 50:422, 1971.

325. Gonick HC, Maxwell MH, Rubini ME, Kleeman CR: Functional impairment in chronic renal disease. I. Studies on sodium conserving ability. Nephron 3:137, 1966.

326. Stanbury SW, Mahler RF: Salt wasting renal disease: Metabolic observations on a patient with "salt-losing nephritis." Q J Med 28:425, 1959.

327. Kahn T, Levitt MF: Salt wasting in myeloma. Arch Intern Med 126:664, 1970.

328. Polack A: Sodium depletion in chronic renal failure. J R Coll Physicians Lond 51:333, 1971.

329. Danovitch GM, Bourgoignie JJ, Bricker NS: Reversibility of the "salt-losing" tendency of chronic renal failure. N Engl J Med 296:14, 1977.

330. Chagnac A, Zevin D, Weinstein T, et al: Combined tubular dysfunction in medullary cystic disease. Arch Intern Med 146:1007, 1986.

331. Emmanouel DS, Lindheimer MD, Katz AI: Urinary concentration and dilution after unilateral nephrectomy in the rat. Clin Sci Mol Med 49:563, 1975.

332. Bricker NS, Dewey RR, Lubowitz H, et al: Observations on the concentrating and diluting mechanisms of the diseased kidney. J Clin Invest 38:516, 1959.

333. Kleeman CR, Adams DA, Maxwell MH: An evaluation of maximal water diuresis in chronic renal disease. 1. Normal solute intake. J Lab Clin Med 58:169, 1961.

334. Martinez-Maldonado M, Yium JJ, Eknoyan G, Suki WN: Adult polycystic kidney disease: Studies of the defect in urine concentration. Kidney Int 2:107, 1972.

335. Coburn JW, Gonick HC, Rubini ME, Kleeman CR: Studies of experimental renal failure in dogs. I. Effect of 5/6 nephrectomy on concentrating and diluting capacity of residual nephrons. J Clin Invest 44:603, 1965.

336. Dorhout-Mees EJ: Relation between maximal urine concentration, maximal water reabsorption capacity and mannitol clearance in patients with renal disease. Br Med J 1:1159, 1959.

337. Keitel HG, Thompson D, Itano HA: Hyposthenuria in sickle cell anemia: A reversible renal defect. J Clin Invest 35:998, 1956.

338. Hatch FE, Culberston JW, Diggs LW: Nature of the renal concentrating defect in sickle cell disease. J Clin Invest 46:336, 1967.

339. Duback UC, Rosner B, Müller A, et al: Relationship between regular intake of phenacetin-containing analgesics and laboratory evidence for uro-renal disease in a working female population of Switzerland. Lancet 1:539, 1975.

340. Gardner KD Jr: Juvenile nephronophthisis and renal medullary cystic disease. In Gardner KD Jr (ed): Cystic Diseases of the Kidney. John Wiley & Sons, New York, 1976, pp 173–187.

341. Arruda JAL: Obstructive uropathy. In Cotran RS, Brenner BM, Stein JH (eds): Contemporary Issues in Nephrology, Vol 10, Tubulo-Interstitial Nephropathy. Churchill Livingstone, New York, 1983, p 243.

342. DeFronzo RA, Humphrey RL, Wright JR, Cooke CR: Renal function in patients with multiple myeloma. Medicine (Baltimore) 57:151, 1978.

343. Gill JR, Bartter FC: On the impairment of renal concentrating ability in prolonged hypercalcemia and hypercalciuria in man. J Clin Invest 40:716, 1961.

344. Finkelstein FO, Hayslett JP: Role of medullary structures in the functional adaptation of renal insufficiency. Kidney Int 6:419, 1974.

345. Conte G, Dal Canton A, Fuiano G, et al: Mechanism of impaired urinary concentration in chronic primary glomerulonephritis. Kidney Int 27:792, 1985.

346. Holliday MA, Egan TJ, Morris CR, et al: Pitressin-resistant hyposthenuria in chronic renal disease. Am J Med 42:378, 1967.

347. Tannen RL, Regal EM, Dunn MJ, Schrier RW: Vasopressin-resistant hyposthenuria in advanced chronic renal disease. N Engl J Med 280:1135, 1969.

348. Wilson DR, Sonnenberg H: Medullary collecting duct function in the remnant kidney before and after volume expansion. Kidney Int 15:487, 1979.

349. Fine LG, Schlondorff D, Trizna W, et al: Functional profile of the isolated uremic nephron. Impaired water permeability and adenylate

cyclase responsiveness of the cortical collecting tubule to vasopressin. J Clin Invest 61:1519, 1978.

350. Bonilla-Felix M, Hamm LL, Herndon J, Vehaskari VM: Response of cortical collecting ducts from remnant kidneys to arginine vasopressin. Kidney Int 41:1150, 1992.

351. Pennell JP, Bourgoignie JJ: Water reabsorption by papillary collecting ducts in the remnant kidney. Am J Physiol 242:F657, 1982.

352. Leaf A, Camara AA: Renal tubular secretion of potassium in man. J Clin Invest 28:1526, 1949.

353. Bank N, Aynedjian HS: A micropuncture study of potassium excretion by the remnant kidney. J Clin Invest 52:1480, 1973.

354. Bengele HH, Evan A, McNamara ER, Alexander EA: Tubular sites of potassium regulation in the normal and uninephrectomized rat. Am J Physiol 234:F146, 1978.

355. Van Ypersele de Strihou C: Potassium homeostasis in renal failure. Kidney Int 11:491, 1977.

356. Milanes CL, Jamison RL: Effect of acute potassium load on reabsorption in Henle's loop in chronic renal failure in the rat. Kidney Int 27:919, 1985.

357. Gonick HC, Kleeman CR, Rubini ME, Maxwell MH: Functional impairment in chronic renal disease. III. Studies of potassium excretion. Am J Med Sci 261:281, 1971.

358. Bia MJ, DeFronzo RA: Extrarenal potassium homeostasis Am J Physiol 240:F257, 1981.

359. Perez GO, Pelleya R, Oster JR, et al: Blunted kaliuresis after an acute potassium load in patients with chronic renal failure. Kidney Int 24:656, 1983.

360. Stemmer CL, Perez GO, Oster JR: Impairment of $beta_2$-adrenoceptor–stimulated potassium uptake in end-stage renal disease. J Clin Pharmacol 27:628, 1987.

361. Tuck ML, Davidson MB, Asp N, Schultze RG: Augmented aldosterone and insulin responses to potassium infusion in dogs with renal failure. Kidney Int 30:883, 1986.

362. Bourgoignie JJ, Kaplan M, Pincus J, et al: Renal handling of potassium in dogs with chronic renal insufficiency. Kidney Int 20:482, 1981.

363. Greenblatt DJ, Koch-Weser J: Adverse reactions to spironolactone. A report from the Boston Collaborative Drug Surveillance Program. JAMA 225:40, 1973.

364. Rimmer JM, Horn JF, Gennari FJ: Hyperkalemia as a complication of drug therapy. Arch Intern Med 147:867, 1987.

365. Edes TE, Sunderrajan EV: Heparin-induced hyperkalemia. Arch Intern Med 145:1070, 1985.

366. Schambelan M, Sebastian A, Biglieri EG: Prevalence, pathogenesis, and functional significance of aldosterone deficiency in hyperkalemic patients with chronic renal insufficiency. Kidney Int 17:89, 1980.

367. DeFronzo RA: Hyperkalemia and hyporeninemic hypoaldosteronism. Kidney Int 17:118, 1980.

368. Batlle DC, Arruda JAL, Kurtzman NA: Hyperkalemic distal renal tubular acidosis associated with obstructive uropathy. N Engl J Med 304:373, 1981.

369. Oh MS, Carroll HJ, Clemmons JE, et al: A mechanism for hyporeninemic hypoaldosteronism in chronic renal disease. Metabolism 23:1157, 1974.

370. Norby LH, Weidig J, Ramwell P, et al: Possible role for impaired renal prostaglandin production in pathogenesis of hyporeninaemic hypoaldosteronism. Lancet 2:1118, 1978.

371. Sparagana M: Hyporeninemic hypoaldosteronism with diabetic glomerulosclerosis. Biochem Med 14:93, 1975.

372. DeLeiva A, Christlieb R, Melby J, et al: Big renin and biosynthetic defect of aldosterone in diabetes mellitus. N Engl J Med 295:639, 1976.

373. Sebastian A, Schambelan M., Sutton JM: Amelioration of hyperchloremic acidosis with furosemide therapy in patients with chronic renal insufficiency and type 4 renal tubular acidosis. Am J Nephrol 4:287, 1984.

374. DeFronzo RA, Tanfield PA, Black H, et al: Impaired renal tubular potassium secretion in sickle cell disease. Ann Intern Med 86:268, 1977.

375. Luke RG, Allison MEM, Davidson JF, Duguid WP: Hyperkalemia and renal tubular acidosis due to renal amyloidosis. Ann Intern Med 70:1211, 1969.

376. Cogan MG, Arieff AI: Sodium wasting, acidosis and hyperkalemia induced by methicillin interstitial nephritis. Evidence for selective distal tubular dysfunction. Am J Med 64:500, 1978.

377. Morris RC, Fudenberg HH: Impaired renal acidification in patients with hypergammaglobulinemia. Medicine (Baltimore) 46:57, 1967.

378. Tu WH, Shearn MA: Systemic lupus erythematosus and latent renal tubular dysfunction. Ann Intern Med 67:100, 1967.

379. Wrong O, Davies HEF: Excretion of acid in renal disease. Q J Med 28:259, 1959.

380. Elkington JR: Hydrogen ion turnover in health and in renal disease. Ann Intern Med 57:660, 1962.

381. Simpson DP: Control of hydrogen ion homeostasis and renal acidosis. Medicine (Baltimore) 50:503, 1971.

382. Widmer B, Gerhardt RE, Harrington JT, Cohen JJ: Serum electrolyte and acid base composition. The influence of graded degrees of chronic renal failure. Arch Intern Med 139:1099, 1979.

383. Klahr S, Schwab SJ, Stokes TJ: Metabolic adaptations of the nephron in renal disease. Kidney Int 29:80, 1986.

384. Dourhout-Mees EJ, Machado M, Slatopolsky E, et al: The functional adaptation of the diseased kidney. III. Ammonium excretion. J Clin Invest 45:289, 1966.

385. Johnson CW, Morgan JM: Acidosis: A clue to the etiology of renal failure. South Med J 58:1513, 1965.

386. Gonick HC, Kleeman CR, Rubini ME, Maxwell MH: Functional impairment in chronic renal disease. II. Studies of acid excretion. Nephron 6:28, 1969.

387. Bank N, Su W-S, Aynedjian HS: A micropuncture study of $HCO_3$ reabsorption by the hypertrophied proximal tubule. Yale J Biol Med 51:275, 1978.

388. Wong NLM, Quamme GA, Dirks JH: Tubular handling of bicarbonate in dogs with experimental renal failure. Kidney Int 25:912, 1984.

389. Schmidt RW, Bricker NS, Gavellas G: Bicarbonate reabsorption in the dog with experimental renal disease. Kidney Int 10:287, 1976.

390. Arruda JAL, Carrasquillo T, Cubria A, et al: Bicarbonate reabsorption in chronic renal failure. Kidney Int 9:481, 1976.

391. Muldowney FP: Renal acidosis. In Black D, Jones NF (eds): Renal Disease, 4th ed. Blackwell Scientific Publications, Oxford, 1979, p 588.

392. Maldonado JE, Velosa JA, Kyle RA, et al: Fanconi syndrome in adults: A manifestation of a latent form of myeloma. Am J Med 58:354, 1975.

393. Stanbury SW, Macaulay D: Defects of renal tubular function in the nephrotic syndrome. Q J Med 26:7, 1957.

394. Sebastian A, McSherry E, Ueki I, Morris RC: Renal amyloidosis, nephrotic syndrome, and impaired renal tubular reabsorption of bicarbonate. Ann Intern Med 69:541, 1968.

395. Györy AZ, Stewart JH, George CRP, et al: Renal tubular acidosis, acidosis due to hyperkalemia, hypercalcemia, disordered citrate metabolism and other tubular dysfunctions following human renal transplantation. Q J Med 38:231, 1969.

396. Wilson DR, Siddiqui AA: Renal tubular acidosis after kidney transplantation. Ann Intern Med 79:352, 1973.

397. Slatopolsky E, Hoffsten P, Purkerson M, Bricker NS: On the influence of extracellular fluid volume expansion on bicarbonate reabsorption in the rat. J Clin Invest 48:1754, 1969.

398. Sastrasinh S, Tanen RL: Effect of potassium on renal $NH_3$ production. Am J Physiol 244:F383, 1983.

399. Muldowney FP, Donohoe JF, Carroll DV, et al: Parathyroid acidosis in uremia. Q J Med 41:321, 1972.

400. Dennis VW: Influence of bicarbonate on parathyroid hormone–induced changes in fluid absorption by the proximal tubule. Kidney Int 10:373, 1976.

401. Shioji R, Furuyama T, Onodera S, et al: Sjögren's syndrome and renal tubular acidosis. Am J Intern Med 48:456, 1970.

402. Hulter HN, Ilnicki LP, Harbottle JA, Sebastian A: Impaired renal $H^+$ secretion and $NH_3$ production in mineralocorticoid-deficient glucocorticoid-replete dogs. Am J Physiol 232:F136, 1977.

403. Maher T, Schambelan M, Kurtz I, et al: Amelioration of metabolic acidosis by dietary potassium restriction in hyperkalemic patients with chronic renal insufficiency. J Lab Clin Med 103:432, 1984.

404. Matsuda O, Nonoguchi H, Tomita K, et al: Primary role of hyperkalemia in the acidosis of hyporeninemic hypoaldosteronism. Nephron 49:203, 1988.

405. Goldman R, Bassett SH: Phosphorous excretion in renal failure. J Clin Invest 33:1623, 1954.

406. Slatopolsky E, Robson AM, Elkan I, Bricker NS: Control of phosphate excretion in uremic man. J Clin Invest 47:1865, 1968.

407. Coburn JW, Popovtzer MM, Massry SG, Kleeman CR: The physicochemical state and renal handling of divalent ions in chronic renal failure. Arch Intern Med 124:302, 1969.

408. Popovtzer MM, Schainuck LI, Massry SG, Kleeman CR: Divalent ion excretion in chronic kidney disease: Relation to degree of renal insufficiency. Clin Sci 38:297, 1970.

409. Slatopolsky E, Gradowska L, Kashemsant C, et al: The control of phosphate excretion in uremia. J Clin Invest 45:672, 1966.

410. Slatopolsky E, Caglar S, Pennell JP, et al: On the pathogenesis of hyperparathyroidism in chronic experimental renal insufficiency in the dog. J Clin Invest 50:492, 1971.

411. Slatopolsky E, Caglar S, Gradowska L, et al: On the prevention of secondary hyperparathyroidism in experimental chronic renal disease using "proportional reduction" of dietary phosphorus intake. Kidney Int 2:147, 1972.

412. Kaplan MA, Canterbury JM, Bourgoignie JJ, et al: Reversal of hyperparathyroidism in response to dietary phosphorus restriction in the uremic dog. Kidney Int 15:43, 1979.

413. Bricker NS: On the pathogenesis of the uremic state. An exposition of the "trade off hypothesis." N Engl J Med 286:1093, 1972.

414. Milanes CL, Pernalete N, Starosta R, et al: Altered response of adenylate cyclase to parathyroid hormone during compensatory renal growth. Kidney Int 36:802, 1989.

415. Caverzasio J, Gloor HJ, Fleisch H, Bonjour JP: Parathyroid hormone–independent adaptation of the renal handling of phosphate in response to renal mass reduction. Kidney Int 21:471, 1982.

416. Kraus E, Briefel G, Cherry L, et al: Phosphate excretion in uremic rats: Effects of parathyroidectomy and phosphate restriction. Am J Physiol 248:F175, 1985.

417. Swenson RS, Weisinger JR, Ruggeri JL, Reaven GM: Evidence that parathyroid hormone is not required for phosphate homeostasis in renal failure. Metabolism 24:199, 1975.

418. Isaac J, Berndt TJ, Thothathri V, et al: Catecholamines and phosphate excretion by the remnant kidney. Kidney Int 43:1021, 1993.

419. Feinfeld DA, Sherwood LM: Parathyroid hormone and $[1,25(OH)_2D_3]$ in chronic renal failure. Kidney Int 33:1049, 1988.

420. Steele TH, DeLuga HF: Influence of dietary phosphorus on renal phosphate reabsorption in the parathyroidectomized rats. J Clin Invest 57:867, 1976.

421. Tröhler U, Bonjour JP, Fleisch H: Inorganic phosphate homeostasis. Renal adaptation to the dietary intake in intact and thyroparathyroidectomized rats. J Clin Invest 57:264, 1976.

422. Stoll R, Kinne R, Murer H, et al: Phosphate transport by rat renal brush border membrane vesicles: Influence of dietary phosphate, thyroparathyroidectomy and 1,25-dihydroxyvitamin $D_3$. Pflugers Arch 380:47, 1979.

423. Bank N, Su WS, Aynedjian HS: A micropuncture study of renal phosphate transport in rats with chronic renal failure and secondary hyperparathyroidism. J Clin Invest 61:884, 1978.

424. Wen SF, Stoll RW: Renal phosphate adaptation in uraemic dogs with a remnant kidney. Clin Sci 60:273, 1981.

425. Better OS, Kleeman CR, Gonick HC, et al: Renal handling of calcium, magnesium and inorganic phosphate in chronic renal failure. Isr J Med Sci 3:60, 1967.

426. Finkelsteine FO, Kliger AS: Medullary structures in calcium reabsorption in rats with renal insufficiency. Am J Physiol 233:F197, 1977.

427. Wong NLM, Quamme GA, Dirks JH, Sutton RAL: Divalent ion transport in dogs with experimental chronic renal failure. Can J Physiol Pharmacol 60:1296, 1982.

428. Suk Han D, Bank N: Phosphorus and cadmium homeostasis in chronic subtotally nephrectomized parathyroidectomized rats. Yonsei Med J 26:8, 1985.

429. Ortola FV, Ballermann BJ, Brenner BM: Endogenous ANP augments fractional excretion of $P_i$, Ca, and Na in rats with reduced renal mass. Am J Physiol 255:F1091, 1988.

430. Namnum P, Insogna K, Baggish D, Hayslett JP: Evidence for bidirectional net movement of creatinine in the rat kidney. Am J Physiol 244:F719, 1983.

431. Levey AS, Perrone RD, Madias NE: Serum creatinine and renal function. Annu Rev Med 39:465, 1988.

432. Berlyne GM: Endogenous creatinine clearance and the glomerular filtration rate. Am Heart J 70:143, 1965.

433. Skov PE: Glomerular filtration rate in patients with severe and very severe renal insufficiency. Acta Med Scand 187:419, 1970.

434. Bauer JH, Brooks CS, Burch RN: Clinical appraisal of creatinine clearance as a measurement of glomerular filtration rate. Am J Kidney Dis 2:337, 1982.

435. Shemesh O, Golbetz H, Kriss JP, Myers BD: Limitations of creatinine as a filtration marker in glomerulopathic patients. Kidney Int 28:830, 1985.

436. Rosenberg ME, Swanson JE, Thomas BL, Hostetter TH: Glomerular and hormonal responses to dietary protein intake in human renal disease. Am J Physiol 253:F1083, 1987.

437. Norden G, Bjorck S, Granerus G, Nyberg G: Estimation of renal function in diabetic nephropathy. Comparison of five methods. Nephron 47:36, 1987.

438. Walser M, Drew HH, LaFrance ND: Creatinine measurements often yield false estimates of progression in chronic renal failure. Kidney Int 34:412, 1988.

439. Tomlanovitch S, Goldbetz H, Perlroth M, et al: Limitations of creatinine in quantifying the severity of cyclosporine-induced chronic nephropathy. Am J Kidney Dis 8:332, 1986.

440. Lubowitz H, Slatopolsky E, Shankel S, et al: Glomerular filtration rate. Determination in chronic renal disease. JAMA 199:100, 1967.

441. Nádorniková H, Schück O, Malý J, et al: Renal clearance of amino acids in patients with severe chronic renal failure. Nephron 20:83, 1978.

442. Perez G, Epstein M, Reitberg B, et al: Uptake and release of amino acids by normal and remnant kidneys: Studies in the isolated perfused rat kidney. Am J Clin Nutr 33:1373, 1980.

443. Rieselbach RE, Shankel SW, Slatopolsky E, et al: Glucose titration studies in patients with chronic progressive renal disease. J Clin Invest 46:157, 1967.

444. Bricker NS, Orlowski T, Kime SW Jr, Morris PAF: Observations on the functional homogeneity of the nephron population in the chronically diseased kidney of the dog. J Clin Invest 39:1771, 1960.

445. Shankel SW, Robson AM, Bricker NS: On the mechanism of the splay in the glucose titration curve in advanced experimental renal disease in the rat. J Clin Invest 46:164, 1967.

446. Kramp RA, Lorentz WB: Glucose transport in chronically altered rat nephrons. Am J Physiol 243:F393, 1982.

447. McPhaul JJ: Hyperuricemia and urate excretion in chronic renal disease. Metabolism 17:430, 1968.

448. Danovitch GM, Weinberger J, Berlyne GM: Uric acid in advanced renal failure. Clin Sci 43:331, 1972.

449. Steele TH, Rieselbach RE: The contribution of residual nephrons within the chronically diseased kidney to urate homeostasis in man. Am J Med 43:876, 1967.

450. Sorensen LB: Role of the intestinal tract in the elimination of uric acid. Arthritis Rheum 8:694, 1965.

451. Garyfallos A, Magoula I, Tsapas G: Evaluation of the renal mechanisms for urate homeostasis in uremic patients by probenecid and pyrazinamide test. Nephron 46:273, 1987.

452. Boumendil-Podevin EF, Podevin RA, Richet G: Uricosuric agents in uremic sera. Identification of indoxyl sulfate and hippuric acid. J Clin Invest 55:1142, 1975.

453. Porter RD, Cathcart-Rake WF, Wan SH, et al: Secretory activity and aryl acid content of serum, urine and cerebrospinal fluid in normal and uremic man. J Lab Clin Med 85:723, 1975.

454. White AG: Uremic serum inhibition of renal paraaminohippurate transport. Proc Soc Exp Biol Med 123:309, 1966.

455. Preuss HG, Massry SG, Maher JF, et al: Effects of uremic sera on renal tubular *p*-aminohippurate transport. Nephron 3:265, 1966.

456. Depner TA: Suppression of tubular anion transport by an inhibitor of serum protein binding in uremia. Kidney Int 20:511, 1981.

457. Rieselbach RE, Todd L, Rosenthal M, Bricker NS: The functional adaptation of the diseased kidney. II. Maximum rate of transport of PAH and the influence of acetate. J Lab Clin Med 64:725, 1964.

458. Olson JL, Heptinstall RH: Nonimmunologic mechanisms of glomerular injury. Lab Invest 59:564, 1988.

459. Chanutin A, Ferris EB: Experimental renal insufficiency produced by partial nephrectomy. I. Control diet. Arch Intern Med 49:767, 1932.

460. Shimamura T, Morrison AB: A progressive glomerulosclerosis occurring in partial five-sixths nephrectomized rats. Am J Pathol 79:95, 1975.

461. Striker GE, Nagle RB, Kohnen PW, Smuckler EA: Response to unilateral nephrectomy in old rats. Arch Pathol 87:439, 1969.

462. El Nahas AM, Paraskevakou H, Zoob S, et al: Effect of dietary protein restriction on the development of renal failure after subtotal nephrectomy in rats. Clin Sci 65:399, 1983.

463. Kenner CH, Evan AP, Blomgren P, et al: Effect of protein intake on renal function and structure in partially nephrectomized rats. Kidney Int 27:739, 1985.

464. Hostetter TH, Meyer TW, Rennke HG, Brenner BM: Chronic effect of dietary protein on renal structure and function in the rat with intact and reduced renal mass. Kidney Int 30:509, 1986.

465. Kleinknecht C, Salusky I, Broyer M, Gubler MC: Effect of various protein diets on growth, renal function, and survival of uremic rats. Kidney Int 15:534, 1979.

466. Nath KA, Kren SM, Hostetter TH: Dietary protein restriction in established renal injury in the rat: Selective role of glomerular capillary pressure in progressive glomerular dysfunction. J Clin Invest 78:1199, 1986.

467. Bidani AK, Michell KD, Schwartz MM, et al: Absence of glomerular injury or nephron loss in a normotensive rat remnant kidney model. Kidney Int 38:28, 1990.

468. Dworkin LD, Hostetter TH, Rennke HG, Brenner BM: Hemodynamic basis for glomerular injury in rats with desoxycorticosterone-salt hypertension. J Clin Invest 73:1448, 1984.

469. Baylis C, Mitruka B, Deng A: Chronic blockade of nitric oxide synthesis in the rat produces systemic hypertension and glomerular damage. J Clin Invest 90:278, 1992.

470. Ribeiro MO, Antune E, de Nucci G, et al: Chronic inhibition of nitric oxide synthesis. A new model of arterial hypertension. Hypertension 20:298, 1992.

471. Heptinstall RM, Hill GS: Steroid-induced hypertension in the rat. Lab Invest 16:751, 1967.

472. Azar S, Johnson MA, Hertel B, Tobian L: Single-nephron pressures, flows and resistances in hypertensive kidneys with nephrosclerosis. Kidney Int 12:28, 1977.

473. Azar S, Johnson MA, Iwai J, et al: Single-nephron dynamics in "post-salt" rats with chronic hypertension. J Lab Clin Med 91:156, 1978.

474. Schweitzer G, Gertz KH: Changes in hemodynamics and glomerular ultrafiltration in renal hypertensive rats. Kidney Int 15:134, 1979.

475. McQueen EG, Hodge JV: Modification of secondary lesions in renal hypertensive rats by control of the blood pressure with reserpine. Q J Med 30:213, 1961.

476. Arendshorst WJ, Beierwaltes WH: Renal and nephron hemodynamics in spontaneously hypertensive rats. Am J Physiol 236:F246, 1979.

477. Feld LG, VanLiew JB, Galaske RG, et al: Selectivity of renal injury and proteinuria in the spontaneously hypertensive rat. Kidney Int 12:332, 1977.

478. Brandis A, Bianchi G, Reale E, et al: Age-dependent glomerulosclerosis and proteinuria occurring in rats of the Milan normotensive strain and not in rats of the Milan hypertensive strain. Lab Invest 55:234, 1986.

479. Anderson S, Rennke HG, Brenner BM: Therapeutic advantage of converting enzyme inhibitors in arresting progressive renal disease associated with systemic hypertension in the rat. J Clin Invest 77:1993, 1986.

480. Anderson S: Antihypertensive therapy in experimental renal disease. *In* El Nahas AM, Mallick MP, Anderson S (eds): Prevention of Progressive Chronic Renal Failure. Oxford University Press, Oxford, 1993, p 173.

481. Neugarten J, Kaminetsky B, Feiner H, et al: Nephrotoxic serum nephritis with hypertension. Amelioration by antihypertensive therapy. Kidney Int 28:135, 1985.

482. Scholey JW, Meyer TW: Reducing glomerular capillary pressure does not reduce proteinuria in rats with Adriamycin nephrosis. Kidney Int 31:393, 1987.

483. Dworkin L, Grosser M, Feiner H, et al: Both converting enzyme inhibitors and vasodilators reduce glomerular capillary pressure and injury in uninephrectomized spontaneously hypertensive rats (SHR). Kidney Int 31:383, 1987.

484. Anderson S, Diamond JR, Karnovsky MJ, Brenner BM: Mechanisms underlying transition from acute glomerular injury to late glomerular sclerosis in a rat model of nephrosis. J Clin Invest 82:1757, 1988.

485. Dworkin LD, Feiner HD: Glomerular injury in uninephrectomized spontaneously hypertensive rats. A consequence of glomerular capillary hypertension. J Clin Invest 77:797, 1986.

486. Farr LE, Smadel JE: The effect of dietary protein on the course of nephrotoxic nephritis in rats. J Exp Med 70:615, 1939.

487. Neugarten J, Feiner HD, Schacht RG, Baldwin DS: Amelioration of experimental glomerulonephritis by dietary protein restriction. Kidney Int 24:595, 1983.

488. Friend PS, Fernandes G, Good RA, et al: Dietary restrictions early and late: Effects on the nephropathy of the NZB/NZW mouse. Lab Invest 38:629, 1978.

489. Beyer MM, Steinberg AD, Nicastri AD, Friedman EA: Unilateral nephrectomy: Effect on survival in NZB/NZW mice. Science 198:511, 1977.

490. Feldman DB, McConnell EE, Knapka JJ: Growth, kidney disease and longevity of Syrian hamsters (Mesocricetus auratus) fed varying levels of protein. Lab Anim Sci 32:613, 1982.

491. Iwasaki K, Gleiser CA, Masoro EJ, et al: The influence of dietary protein source on longevity and age-related disease processes of Fischer rats. J Gerontol 43:B5, 1988.

492. Teoduru CV, Saifer A, Frankel H: Conditioning factors influencing evolution of experimental glomerulonephritis in rabbits. Am J Physiol 196:457, 1959.

493. Raij L, Azar S, Keane WF: Mesangial immune injury, hypertension, and progressive glomerular damage in Dahl rats. Kidney Int 26:137, 1984.

494. Tikkanen I, Fyhrquist F, Miettinin A, Tornroth T: Autologous immune complex nephritis and DOCA-NaCl load: A new model of hypertension. Acta Pathol Microbiol Scand 88:241, 1980.

495. Neugarten J, Feiner HD, Schacht RG, et al: Aggravation of experimental glomerulonephritis by superimposed clip hypertension. Kidney Int 22:257, 1982.

496. Baldwin DS, Neugarten J: Role of hypertension in the evolution of renal diseases. Contrib Nephrol 54:63, 1987.

497. Bouby N, Bachmann S, Bichet D, Bankir L: Effect of water intake on the progression of chronic renal failure in the 5/6 nephrectomized rat. Am J Physiol 258:F973, 1990.

498. Kobayashi S, Venkatachalam MA: Differential effects of calorie restriction on glomeruli and tubules of the remnant kidney. Kidney Int 42:710, 1992.

499. Falk SA, Buric V, Hammond WS, Conger JD: Serial glomerular and tubular dynamics in thyroidectomized rats with remnant kidneys. Am J Kidney Dis 17:218, 1991.

500. El Nahas AM, Bassett AH, Cope GH, Le Carpentier JE: Role of growth hormone in the development of experimental renal scarring. Kidney Int 40:29, 1991.

501. Sakemi T, Baba N: Castration attenuates proteinuria and glomerular injury in unilaterally nephrectomized male Sprague-Dawley rats. Lab Invest 69:51, 1993.

502. Dworkin LD, Feiner HD, Randazzo J: Glomerular hypertension and injury in deoxycorticosterone-salt rats on antihypertensive therapy. Kidney Int 31:718, 1987.

503. Zatz R, Dunn BR, Meyer TW, et al: Prevention of diabetic glomerulopathy by pharmacological amelioration of glomerular capillary hypertension. J Clin Invest 77:1925, 1986.

504. Bourgoignie JJ, Garellas G, Martinez E, Pardo V: Glomerular function and morphology after renal mass reduction in dogs. J Lab Clin Med 109:380, 1987.

505. Polzin DJ, Leininger JR, Osborne CA, Jeraj K: Development of renal lesions in dogs after 11/12 nephrectomy. Lab Invest 58:172, 1988.

506. Bourgoignie JJ, Gavellas G, Sabnis SG, Antonovych TT: Effect of protein diets on the renal function of baboons (Papio hamadryas) with remnant kidneys: A 5-year follow-up. Am J Kidney Dis 23:199, 1994.

507. White FN, Grollman A: Autoimmune factors associated with infarction of the kidney. Nephron 1:93, 1964.

508. Daniels B. S., Hostetter T. H.: Adverse effects of growth in the glomerular microcirculation. Am J Physiol 258:F1409, 1990.

509. Yoshida Y, Fogo A, Ichikawa I: Glomerular hemodynamic changes vs. hypertrophy in experimental glomerular sclerosis. Kidney Int 35:654, 1989.

510. Fogo A, Ichikawa I: Evidence for a pathogenic linkage between glomerular hypertrophy and sclerosis. Am J Kidney Dis 17:666, 1991.

511. Hirose K, Osterby R, Nozaqa M: Development of glomerular lesions in experimental long-term diabetes in the rat. Kidney Int 21:689, 1982.

512. Velosa JA, Glasser RJ, Nevins TE, Michael AF: Experimental model of focal sclerosis. II. Correlation with immunopathologic changes, macromolecular kinetics, and polyanion loss. Lab Invest 36:527, 1977.

513. Miller PL, Rennke HG, Meyer TW: Dietary protein restriction reduces glomerular volume and proteinuria in rats with established Adriamycin nephrosis. Kidney Int 33:380, 1988.

514. Grond J, Beukers JYB, Schilthuis MS, et al: Analysis of renal structural and functional features in two rat strains with a different susceptibility to glomerular sclerosis. Lab Invest 54:77, 1986.

515. Grond J, Van Goor H, Weening JJ, et al: Glomerular sclerosis in nephrotic rats. Interstrain differences in response to puromycin aminonucleoside. Kidney Int 31:1043, 1987.

516. Keane WF, Kasiske BL, O'Donnell MP: Hyperlipidemia and the progression of renal disease. Am J Clin Nutr 47:157, 1988.

517. Grond J, Schilthuis MS, Koudstaal J, Elema JD: Mesangial function and glomerular sclerosis in rats after unilateral nephrectomy. Kidney Int 22:338, 1982.

518. Wellman KF, Volk BW: Renal changes in experimental hypercholesterolemia in normal and subdiabetic rabbits. II. Long term studies. Lab Invest 24:144, 1971.

519. Al-Shebeb T, Frohlich J, Magil AB: Glomerular disease in hypercholesterolemic guinea pigs: A pathogenic study. Kidney Int 33:498, 1988.

520. Kasiske BL, O'Donnell MP, Cleary MP, Keane WF: Treatment of hyperlipidemia reduces glomerular injury in obese Zucker rats. Kidney Int 33:667, 1988.

521. Kasiske BL, O'Donnell MP, Garvis WJ, Keane WF: Pharmacologic treatment of hyperlipidemia reduces glomerular injury in rat 5/6 nephrectomy model of chronic renal failure. Circ Res 62:367, 1988.

522. Diamond JR, Karnovsky MJ: Focal and segmental glomerulosclerosis: Analogies to atherosclerosis. Kidney Int 33:917, 1988.

523. Schonfeld G, Felski C, Howald MA: Characterization of the plasma lipoproteins of the genetically obese hyperlipoproteinemic Zucker fatty rat. J Lipid Res 15:457, 1974.

524. Bagdade JD, Yee E, Wilson De, Shafrir E: Hyperlipidemia in renal failure: Studies of plasma lipoproteins, hepatic triglyceride production, and tissue lipoprotein lipase in a chronically uremic rat model. J Lab Clin Med 91:176, 1978.

525. Raij L, Tolins JP, Luscher T: Hyperlipemia and renal injury. Studies in atherosclerosis prone Watanabe rabbits with hereditary hyperlipemia. Kidney Int 33:383, 1988.

526. Kasiske BL, O'Donnell MP, Schmitz PG, et al: Renal injury of diet-induced hypercholesterolemia in rats. Kidney Int 37:880, 1990.

527. O'Donnell MP, Kasiske BL, Kim Y, et al: Lovastatin inhibits proliferation of rat mesangial cells. J Clin Invest 91:83, 1993.

528. Rennke HG: Structural alterations associated with glomerular hyperfiltration. In Mitch WE, Brenner BM, Stein JH (eds): The Progressive Nature of Renal Disease. Churchill Livingstone, New York, 1986, p 111.

529. Ganz MB, Sterzel RB: Effects of PDGF on growth, intracellular pH, and calcium of cultured rat mesangial cells. Kidney Int 33:156, 1988.

530. Floege J, Burns MW, Alpers CE, et al: Glomerular cell proliferation and PDGF expression precede glomerulosclerosis in the remnant kidney model. Kidney Int 41:297, 1992.

531. Olson JL: Role of heparin as a protective agent following reduction of renal mass. Kidney Int 25:376, 1984.

532. Purkerson ML, Tollefsen DM, Klahr S: N-Desulfated/acetylated heparin ameliorates the progression of renal disease in rats with subtotal renal ablation. J Clin Invest 81:69, 1988.

533. Purkerson ML, Joist JH, Greenberg JM, et al: Inhibition of anticoagulant drugs of the progressive hypertension and uremia associated with renal infarction in rats. Thromb Res 26:227, 1982.

534. Zoja C, Benigni A, Livio M, et al: Selective inhibition of platelet thromboxane generation with low-dose aspirin does not protect rats with reduced renal mass from the development of progressive disease. Am J Pathol 134:1027, 1989.

535. Castello JJ Jr, Hoover RL, Harper PA, Karnovsky MJ: Heparin and glomerular epithelial cell–secreted heparin-like species inhibit mesangial-cell proliferation. Am J Pathol 120:427, 1985.

536. Diamond JR, Karnovsky MJ: Non-anticoagulant protective effect of heparin in chronic aminonucleoside nephrosis. Renal Physiol 9:366, 1988.

537. Keane WF, Raij L: Relationship between altered glomerular barrier permselectivity, angiotensin II and mesangial uptake of macromolecules. Kidney Int 25:247, 1984.

538. Stein HD, Feddergreen W, Kashgarian M, Sterzel RB: Role of angiotensin II–induced renal functional changes in mesangial deposition of exogenous ferritin in rats. Lab Invest 49:270, 1983.

539. Olson JL, Hostetter TH, Rennke HG, et al: Altered glomerular perm-selectivity and progressive sclerosis following extreme ablation of renal mass. Kidney Int 22:112, 1982.

540. Seiler MW, Terrell CH, Finnegan A, et al: Studies of glomerular mesangial uptake and processing of macromolecules. I. Effect of polyvinyl alcohol–induced macrophages on uptake of iron dextran. Lab Invest 54:616, 1986.

541. Schlondorff D: The glomerular mesangial cell: An expanding role for a specialized pericyte. FASEB J 1:272, 1987.

542. Riser BL, Cortes P, Zhao X, et al: Intraglomerular pressure and mesangial stretching stimulate extracellular matrix formation in the rat. J Clin Invest 90:1932, 1992.

543. Schwartz MM, Bidani AK: Mesangial structure and function in the remnant kidney. Kidney Int 40:226, 1991.

544. Robson AM, Mor J, Root ER, et al: Mechanism of proteinuria in nonglomerular disease. Kidney Int 16:416, 1979.

545. Mayer G, Lafayette RA, Oliver J, et al: Effects of angiotensin II receptor blockade on remnant glomerular permselectivity. Kidney Int 43:346, 1993.

546. Van Goor H, van der Horst MLC, Fidler V, Grond J: Glomerular macrophage modulation affects mesangial expansion in the rat after renal ablation. Lab Invest 66:564, 1992.

547. Floege J, Alpers CE, Burns MW, et al: Glomerular cells, extracellular matrix accumulation, and the development of glomerulosclerosis in the remnant kidney model. Lab Invest 66:485, 1992.

548. Lovett DH, Martin M, Bursten S, et al: Interleukin 1 and the glomerular mesangium. III. IL-1–dependent stimulation of mesangial cell protein kinase activity. Kidney Int 34:26, 1988.

549. Border WA, Ruoslahti E: Transforming growth factor-β in disease: The dark side of tissue repair. J Clin Invest 90:1, 1992.

550. Junaid A, Rosenberg ME, Hostetter TH: Interaction of angiotensin II and transforming growth factor β in the remnant kidney. J Am Soc Nephrol 4:772, 1993.

551. Lee LK, Meyer TW, Pollock AS, Lovett DH: Endothelial cell injury initiates the onset of glomerular sclerosis following subtotal renal ablation. J Am Soc Nephrol 4:614, 1993.

552. Remuzzi G, Bertani T: Is glomerulosclerosis a consequence of altered glomerular permeability to macromolecules? Kidney Int 38:384, 1990.

553. Takahashi K, Kato T, Schreiner GF, et al: Essential fatty acid deficiency normalizes function and histology in rat nephrotoxic nephritis. Kidney Int 41:1245, 1992.

554. Ibels LS, Alfrey AC, Haut L, Huffer WE: Preservation of function in experimental renal disease by dietary restriction of phosphate. N Engl J Med 298:122, 1978.

555. Karlinsky ML, Haut L, Buddington B, et al: Preservation of renal function in experimental glomerulonephritis. Kidney Int 17:293, 1982.

556. Lumlertgl D, Burket J, Gillum DM, et al: Phosphate depletion arrests progression of chronic renal failure independent of protein intake. Kidney Int 29:658, 1986.

557. Tomford RC, Karlinsky ML, Buddington B, Alfrey AC: Effect of thyroparathyroidectomy and parathyroidectomy on renal function and the nephrotic syndrome in rat nephrotoxic serum nephritis. J Clin Invest 68:655, 1981.

558. Lau K: Phosphate excess and progressive renal failure: The precipitation-calcification hypothesis. Kidney Int 36:918, 1989.

559. Harris DC, Chan L, Schrier RW: Remnant kidney hypermetabolism and progression of chronic renal failure. Am J Physiol 254:F267, 1988.

560. Carter HR, Merado A, Rutherford WE, et al: Effects of phosphate depletion and parathyroid hormone on glucose reabsorption. Am J Physiol 227:1422, 1974.

561. Shimamura T: Prevention of 11-deoxycorticosterone-salt–induced glomerular hypertrophy and glomerulosclerosis by dietary phosphate binder. Am J Pathol 136:549, 1990.

562. Shigematsu T, Caverzasio J, Bonjour J-P: Parathyroid removal prevents the progression of chronic renal failure induced by high protein diet. Kidney Int 44:173, 1993.

563. Nath KA, Croatt AJ, Hostetter TH: Oxygen consumption and oxidant stress in surviving nephrons. Am J Physiol 258:F1354, 1990.

564. Harris DC, Chan L, Schrier RW: Remnant kidney hypermetabolism and progression of chronic renal failure. Am J Physiol 254:F267, 1988.

565. Schrier RW, Harris DC, Chan L, et al: Tubular hypermetabolism as

a factor in the progression of chronic renal failure. Am J Kidney Dis 12:243, 1988.

566. Fine A: Remnant kidney metabolism in the dog. J Am Soc Nephrol 2:70, 1991.

567. Culpepper RM, Schoolwerth AC: Remnant kidney oxygen consumption: Hypermetabolism or hyperbole? J Am Soc Nephrol 3:151, 1992.

568. Harris DCH, Hammond WS, Burke TJ, Schrier RW: Verapamil protects against progression of experimental chronic renal failure. Kidney Int 33:41, 1987.

569. Shapiro JI, Harris DCH, Schrier RW, Chan L: Attenuation of hypermetabolism in the remnant kidney by dietary phosphate restriction in the rat. Am J Physiol 258:F183, 1990.

570. Nath KA, Hostetter MK, Hostetter TH: Pathophysiology of chronic tubulo-interstitial disease in rats. Interactions of dietary acid load, ammonia, and complement component C3. J Clin Invest 76:667, 1985.

571. El-Khatib MT, Becker GJ, Kincaid-Smith PS: Morphometric aspects of reflux nephropathy. Kidney Int 32:261, 1987.

572. Kleinknecht D, Grunfeld J-P, Gomez PC, et al: Diagnostic procedures and long-term prognosis in bilateral renal cortical necrosis. Kidney Int 4:390, 1973.

573. Finn WF: Recovery from acute renal failure. In Brenner BM, Lazarus JM (eds): Acute Renal Failure. WB Saunders, Philadelphia, 1983, p 753.

574. Torres VE, Velosa JA, Holley KE, et al: The progression of vesicoureteral reflux. Ann Intern Med 92:776, 1980.

575. Kincaid-Smith P: Analgesic abuse and the kidney. Kidney Int 17:250, 1980.

576. Baldwin DA: Poststreptococcal glomerulonephritis: A progressive disease? Am J Med 62:1, 1977.

577. Vincenti F, Amend WJC, Kaysen G, et al: Long-term renal function in kidney donors. Transplantation 36:626, 1983.

578. Hakim RM, Goldszer RC, Brenner BM: Hypertension and proteinuria: Long-term sequelae of uninephrectomy in humans. Kidney Int 25:930, 1984.

579. Torres VE, Offord KP, Anderson CF, et al: Blood pressure determinants in living-related renal allograft donors and their recipients. Kidney Int 31:1383, 1987.

580. Talseth T, Fauchald P, Skrede S, et al: Long-term blood pressure and renal function in kidney donors. Kidney Int 29:1072, 1986.

581. Williams SL, Oler J, Jorkasky DK: Long-term renal function in kidney donors: A comparison of donors and their siblings. Ann Intern Med 105:1, 1986.

582. Schmitz A, Christensen CK, Christensen T, Sølling K: No microalbuminuria or other adverse effects of long-standing hyperfiltration in humans with one kidney. Am J Kidney Dis 13:131, 1989.

583. Miller JJ, Suthanthiran M, Riggio RR, et al: Impact of renal donation: Long-term clinical and biochemical follow-up of living donors in a single center. Am J Med 79:201, 1985.

584. Dean S, Rudge CJ, Joyce M, et al: Live related renal transplantation: An analysis of 141 donors. Transplant Proc 14:65, 1982.

585. Paul LC, Mandin H, Benediktsson H: Nephrotic-range proteinuria after donor nephrectomy and transplantation in a monozygous twin recipient. Transplantation 48:348, 1989.

586. Ladefoged J: Renal failure 22 years after kidney donation. Lancet 339:124, 1992. Letter.

587. Narkun-Burgess DM, Nolan CR, Norman JE, et al: Forty-five year follow-up after uninephrectomy. Kidney Int 43:1110, 1993.

588. Kohler B: The prognosis after nephrectomy: A clinical study of early and late results. Acta Chir Scand 91(suppl 94):1, 1944.

589. Goldstein AE: Longevity following nephrectomy. J Urol 76:31, 1956.

590. Zucchelli P, Cagnoli L, Casanova S, et al: Focal glomerulosclerosis in patients with unilateral nephrectomy. Kidney Int 24:649, 1983.

591. Ingelfinger JR: Case records of the Massachusetts General Hospital (CPC). N Engl J Med 312:1111, 1985.

592. Drash A, Sherman F, Hartman WH, Blizzard RM: A syndrome of pseudohermaphrodism, Wilms' tumor, hypertension, and degenerative renal disease. J Pediatr 76:585, 1970.

593. Ashley DJB, Mostofi FK: Renal agenesis and dysgenesis. J Urol 83:211, 1960.

594. Kiprov DD, Colvin RB, McCluskey RT: Focal and segmental glomerulosclerosis and proteinuria associated with unilateral renal agenesis. Lab Invest 46:275, 1982.

595. Thorner PS, Arbus GS, Celermajer DS, Baumal R: Focal segmental glomerulosclerosis and progressive renal failure associated with a unilateral kidney. Pediatrics 73:806, 1984.
596. Weinstein T, Gafter U, Levi J, et al: Proteinuria and chronic renal failure associated with unilateral renal agenesis. Isr J Med Sci 21:919, 1985.
597. Bhathena DB, Julian BA, McMorrow RG, Baehler RW: Focal sclerosis of hypertrophied glomeruli in solitary functioning kidneys of humans. Am J Kidney Dis 5:226, 1985.
598. Simon J, Zamora I, Mendizabal S, et al: Glomerulotubular balance and functional compensation in nephrectomized children. Nephron 37:203, 1982.
599. Novick AC, Gephardt G, Guz B, et al: Long-term follow-up after partial removal of a solitary kidney. N Engl J Med 325:1058, 1991.
600. Foster MH, Sant GR, Donohoe JF, Harrington JT: Prolonged survival with a remnant kidney. Am J Kidney Dis 17:261, 1991.
601. Rossing P, Hommel E, Parving HH: Impact of arterial blood pressure and albuminuria on the progression of diabetic nephropathy in IDDM patients. Diabetes 42:715, 1993.
602. Lewis EJ, Hunsicker LG, Bain RP, Rohde RD: The effect of angiotensin-converting–enzyme inhibition on diabetic nephropathy. N Engl J Med 329:1456, 1993.

# Biology of the Vascular Wall in Hypertension

*Bradford C. Berk*
*R. Wayne Alexander*

The structural changes of the human vascular wall in response to the development of hypertension are well characterized. They include appearance of intimal smooth muscle cells, thickening of the media as a result of increases in smooth muscle cell number and/or size as well as matrix deposition, and increased vasa vasorum in the adventitia.[1–5] In the pathogenesis of hypertension, however, how these structural alterations are related to underlying functional abnormalities and elevated blood pressure remains unclear. Substantial new data suggest that, in the setting of altered hemodynamic forces, genetically determined functional alterations in vessel wall components cause these structural alterations. In turn, the alterations in vessel structure then contribute to increased vascular resistance.

In this chapter, the structural and functional abnormalities of the vessel wall in hypertension are discussed. Figure 45–1 illustrates the conceptual framework for this discussion. In this scheme, a variety of pathogenic stimuli (environmental, genetic, and pathologic) contribute to alterations in vessel structure. The appearance of these alterations is enhanced locally by hemodynamic forces. For example, turbulence and loss of steady flow cause increased atherosclerosis in the carotid bulb.[6] These primary changes lead to increased vascular resistance, which, if left uncorrected, contributes to vessel wall growth and remodeling. This creates a vessel whose structure is permanently altered so that vascular resistance increases and thereby raises blood pressure. Simultaneously, there are functional alterations in the cellular components of the vessel wall (endothelial cells, smooth muscle cells, inflammatory cells, and fibroblasts)

that lead to characteristic features of the hypertensive vessel such as altered reactivity and elasticity. The multiple mechanisms for regulation of these structural and functional changes are apparent in the heterogeneity of responses that have been shown for hypertensive vessels in different tissues (e.g., brain, coronary, kidney) and of different sizes (conduit, resistance, microvascular).

The structural and functional abnormalities that have been observed in hypertensive vessels are described first, followed by discussion of the role of specific functional alterations (e.g., increased growth factor production) in causing specific structural changes (e.g., increased smooth muscle cell mass). Finally, the cellular mechanisms that are responsible for these functional alterations are described. In this way, adaptive changes that occur in response to hypertension (e.g., maintenance of cerebral autoregulation) may be analyzed separately from maladaptive changes (e.g., increased atherogenesis). Ultimately, an understanding of the fundamental cellular and molecular abnormalities in hypertension should provide insight into the features of the disease that are genetic and predetermined versus those that are environmental and a consequence of the disease process itself.

## VASCULAR MORPHOLOGY AND STRUCTURE IN HYPERTENSION
### Morphology

The morphologic changes that occur in vessels during chronic hypertension vary according to vessel size and tis-

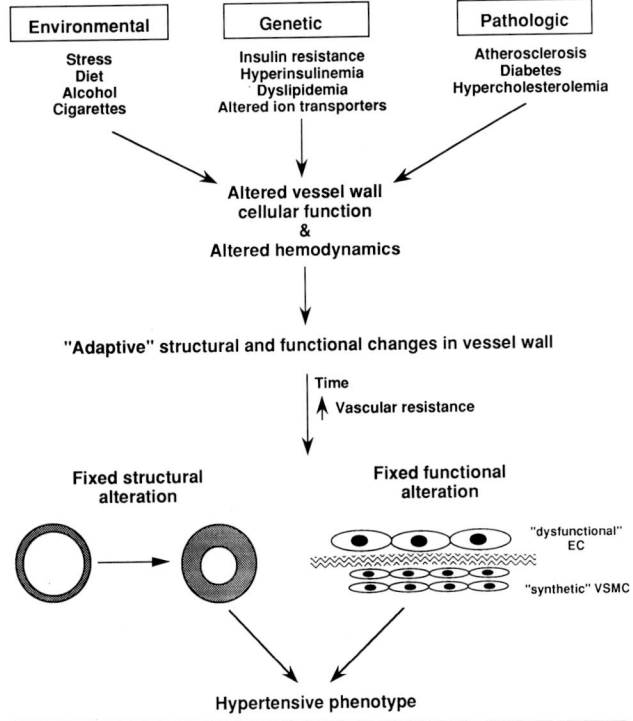

**Figure 45–1.** Model for development of structural and functional alterations characteristic of the hypertensive vessel wall. EC = endothelial cell; VSMC = vascular smooth muscle cell.

sue type.[4, 5, 7, 8] The arterioles are the physical sites for the largest increase in vascular resistance (Fig. 45–2A) and thus the most important from a functional point of view. It is clear that the relative proportion of smooth muscle cells to endothelium decreases as vessels become smaller (Fig. 45–2B), implying less contractile power. However, as the cross-sectional area of the vessel diminishes the resistance

rises to the fourth power. Thus, a small change in surface area of a small vessel causes a large increase in its resistance. These physical properties explain the fact that arterioles are the most important regulators of blood pressure.

Most of our knowledge of the progression of hypertensive changes in the vessel wall comes from animal models. Among the most important are the rat models of genetic hypertension: the spontaneously hypertensive rat (SHR); its related strain, the stroke-prone SHR; and its normotensive control, the Wistar-Kyoto (WKY) rat. Other common models are the Dahl salt-resistant and salt-sensitive strains and salt-induced hypertensive rats (the one-kidney, one-clip deoxycorticosterone salt rats, which are referred to as one-kidney one-clip hypertensive rats).

The earliest change after onset of hypertension observed in the arterioles of these rat models is a thickening of the media.[9–11] This is due to at least three processes: matrix deposition, smooth muscle cell hypertrophy (increase in cell size without division), and smooth muscle cell hyperplasia (increase in cell number). In arterioles and smaller vessels, hyperplasia is more prominent than hypertrophy.[10, 11] In addition, remodeling has been commonly found in these smaller vessels.[2, 3, 7, 12] Remodeling of the vessel occurs when the smooth muscle cells of the media rearrange to create a smaller (rarely larger) lumen without change in number or size (Fig. 45–3). Next, there may be development of a neointima with appearance of smooth muscle cells inside the internal elastic lamina. Other morphologic features include local areas of endothelial cell denudation and inflammatory cell infiltration. Finally, there may be resorption and loss of blood vessels in the tissue, a process termed "rarefaction." In human hypertension, less is known regarding the time course of these events, but similar processes are apparent in autopsy specimens and in biopsies of patients with essential hypertension.[4, 5, 7, 13]

In conduit vessels, many of the same events occur except that smooth muscle cell hypertrophy and endoreduplication

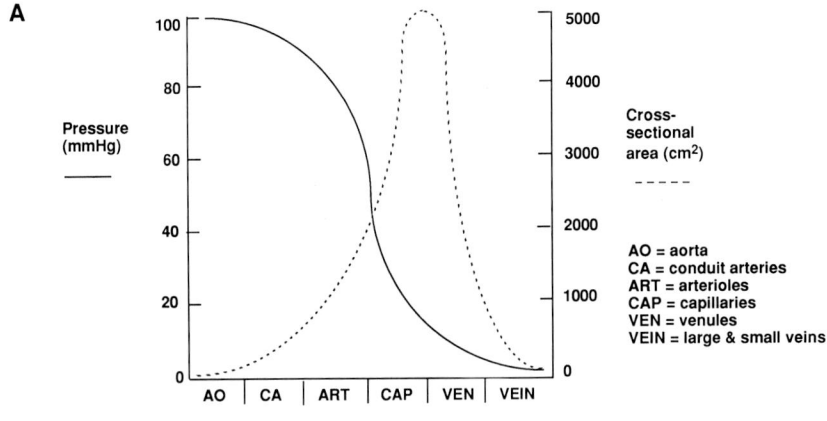

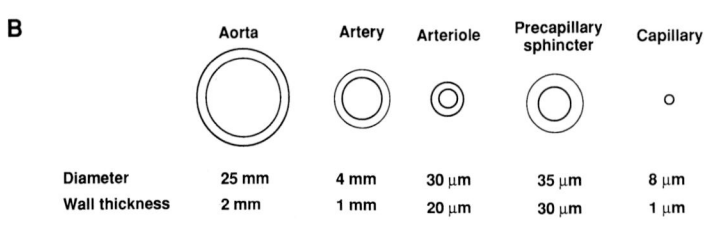

**Figure 45–2.** A. Pressure and cross-sectional area of the blood vessels of the normal human systemic circulation. The important features are that the major pressure drop occurs across the arterioles and the maximal cross-sectional area is represented by the capillaries. (A from Berne RM, Levy MN [eds]: Cardiovascular Physiology, 5th ed. CV Mosby, St. Louis, 1992, p 2.) B. Internal diameter and wall thickness of the various blood vessels that constitute the circulatory system. Cross sections of the vessels are not drawn to scale because of the large range in size from aorta to capillary. (B modified from Burton AC: Relation of structure to function of the tissues of the wall of blood vessels. Physiol Rev 34:619, 1954.)

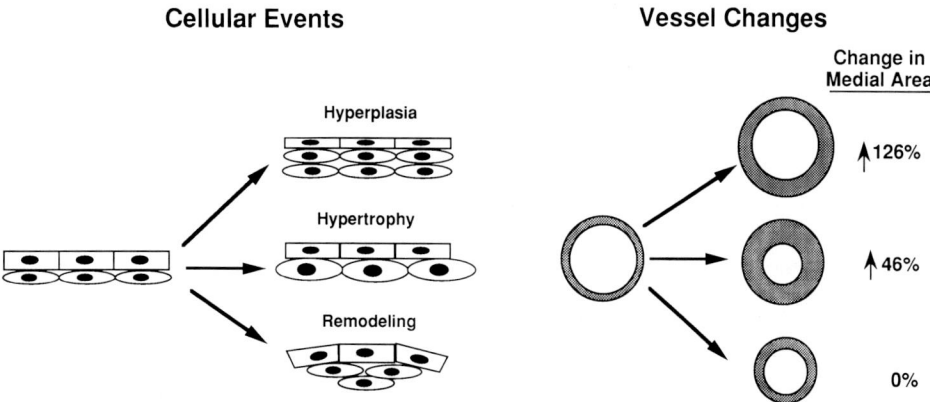

**Figure 45–3.** Model for changes in vessel wall cellular architecture in hypertension. On the left, smooth muscle cell hyperplasia, hypertrophy, and remodeling are shown. On the right, combinations of smooth muscle cell hypertrophy and remodeling are shown. Progressive increases in media area from bottom to top occur with a small decrease in lumen *(bottom)*, large decrease in lumen *(middle)*, and small increase in lumen *(top)*. These changes would be characteristic of an adaptive response to increased pressure by remodeling only without smooth muscle cell hypertrophy *(bottom)*, a maladaptive response to increased pressure with smooth muscle cell hypertrophy and/or remodeling *(middle)*, and an adaptive response to increased pressure and/or flow with smooth muscle cell hypertrophy and/or remodeling *(top)*.

are more common. Endoreduplication refers to synthesis of DNA and increase in chromosome number (e.g., 2n to 4n) without cell division. In most studies, hypertrophy and polyploidy have been documented in the aorta and other large vessels of hypertensive rats to a greater extent than hyperplasia.[10, 11] Owens and Schwartz[10, 11] showed that about 25% of the cells in SHR aorta had undergone S phase with synthesis of DNA, yet had failed to divide. These cells appeared hypertrophied because of their increase in size but also had a DNA content that was twice or occasionally four times the normal content. Similar processes have been demonstrated in human hypertensive aorta. The dominant change in hypertensive conduit vessels, however, is a loss of elasticity. In elderly humans, this is a major cause of systolic hypertension, often referred to as ''stiff'' arteries. This correlates with vessel morphology in which elastin and collagen contents are increased and the more elastic smooth muscle cells decrease in number because of the death of smooth muscle cells (medial atrophy or necrosis). An important feature of conduit vessels, not found in smaller vessels, is the vasa vasorum, tiny vessels in the adventitia that supply nutrients and oxygen to the deeper layers of the media. Significant increases in size and number of vasa vasorum occur during chronic hypertension. This process, termed ''angiogenesis,'' is part of the hypertensive response in conduit vessels and is probably adaptive in the sense that the increased smooth muscle cell mass in the hypertensive vessel requires more oxygen and nutrients.

In microvessels, the ratio of endothelial cells to smooth muscle cells is approximately 1:1. Alterations in endothelial cell structure and function therefore have a major impact on hypertensive changes in these vessels. Although chronic hypertension causes little change in the number of smooth muscle cells present in microvessels and no significant increase in the matrix surrounding the smooth muscle cells, there is increased subendothelial matrix. Most important, the morphology of the endothelial cell is altered. This morphologic change is associated with increased vascular permeability. Electron microscopy shows decreased endothelial cell tight junctions to be the cause.

In summary, morphologic analysis of hypertensive vessels shows alterations in all cellular components as well as matrix. These changes vary depending on vessel size and the duration of hypertension. The hypertensive vessel wall is generally characterized by increased medial thickness or an increased media/lumen ratio of the resistance arterioles. This structural change in the hypertensive vessel causes it to have a mechanical advantage over the normotensive vessel (greater contractile force). Functionally, this means that there is greater resistance for a given contractile stimulus. In the next section, the etiologic interaction between smooth muscle cell growth and contractile function is examined.

## Vascular Structure and Hypertension: Cause or Consequence?

In long-standing essential hypertension, the fundamental abnormality is an increase in peripheral vascular resistance in the setting of normal cardiac output.[14] The increase in resistance occurs even when vessels are fully dilated, indicating that the altered structure of the vessel is the cause, rather than a functional ''overactivity.''[15] Two processes may contribute to the structural increase in resistance: 1) increased mass of the vascular wall causing a narrowing of the lumen[15] or 2) rarefaction of the vasculature causing a decrease in the number of parallel circuits[16] or both. Two questions must be answered to understand whether the structural increase in vessel resistance is a cause or consequence of hypertension. First, which vessels are responsible? Second, is there a correlation between vascular structure and blood pressure and, if so, what is the nature of this relationship?

The answers to these questions have been provided during the past 10 years by the work of many investigators.[3–5, 10–12, 15, 17, 18] To summarize their important findings:

1. Resistance vessels are the site of the structural changes. These vessels include both the microvasculature

(arterioles and precapillary sphincters with lumen diameters < 100 μm) and small arteries (lumen diameters of 100 to 300 μm).

2. There is a strong correlation between vascular structure and blood pressure in a variety of hypertensive models in these resistance vessels.

3. Altered vascular structure is not simply a consequence of increased blood pressure but is due to primary functional changes in the cellular components of the vessel wall mediated by genetic and environmental influences that control cell growth and the neurohormonal milieu.

## RESISTANCE VESSELS: THE PRIMARY SITE OF STRUCTURAL CHANGE

Analysis of changes in blood pressure across various vascular beds in the SHR and renal hypertensive rats demonstrates increased vascular resistance in both the microvasculature and small arteries (100 to 300 μm). Figure 45–4 shows that these vessels are the site of pressure regulation in the hypertensive animal. These measurements are supported by the morphologic analysis of media thickness and media/lumen ratios, which shows the greatest changes in vessels of this size. In a variety of human hypertensive states, structural changes in these vessels also correlate with blood pressure (e.g., in women with preeclampsia,[19] patients with uremia,[20] and patients with essential hypertension[7, 13, 21]).

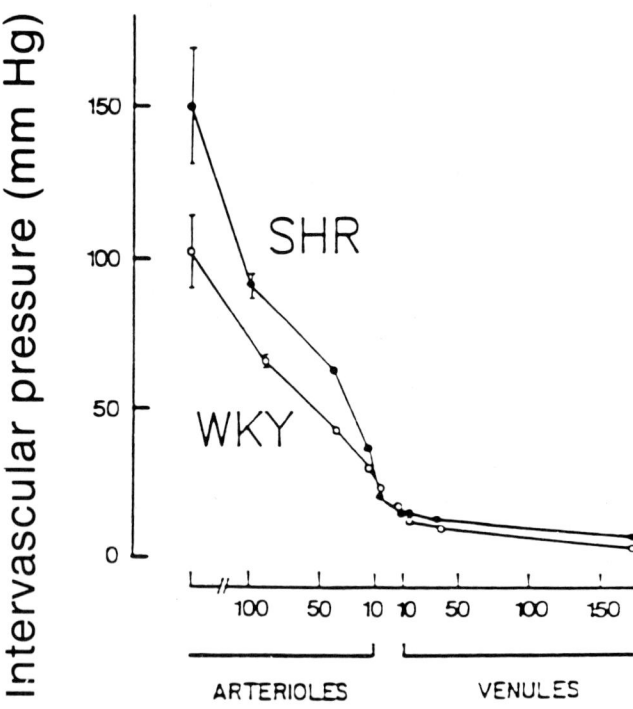

**Figure 45–4.** Pressure profile in the vasculature of the hypertensive SHR and normotensive WKY rat. The relationship between intravascular pressure and vessel diameter in micrometers shows a significantly greater pressure at any diameter in the SHR. (Modified from Mulvany MJ: Vascular structure and smooth muscle contractility in experimental hypertension. J Cardiovasc Pharmacol 6[suppl]:S79, 1987.)

Rarefaction appears to be confined to microvessels in humans and animals.[16, 22] Its importance in different vascular beds remains to be determined. In particular, because it is difficult to study the microvasculature in humans, the discussion focuses on changes in small arteries.

## POSITIVE CORRELATION BETWEEN VESSEL STRUCTURE AND BLOOD PRESSURE

In both human patients and hypertensive animals the fundamental structural abnormality in chronic hypertension is a decrease in the lumen diameter of the resistance vessel. This is explained by an increase in the media thickness and media cross-sectional area. In addition, this change is associated with increased contractile force generation when assayed in vitro. However, when the force generated is expressed relative to the medial mass there is no inherent difference in the contractile ability of the smooth muscle in the hypertensive vessel compared with the normotensive vessel.[21, 23, 24] Thus, the increased contractile force associated with hypertension is accounted for primarily by the altered structure of the resistance vessels (i.e., improved mechanical advantage relative to normotensive vessels).

A caveat to this last statement is required. As discussed in the following section, many functional alterations in the endothelial cells and smooth muscle cells of hypertensive vessels may modulate the contractile response. This is particularly true for agonists such as α-adrenergic agents, angiotensin II, and vasopressin, whose receptor number and signal transduction coupling to the contractile machinery may be altered. Nonetheless, structural change in resistance vessels is the primary abnormality that characterizes the chronic hypertensive state. It is also clear that underlying genetic and environmental stimuli are responsible for altered endothelial and smooth muscle cell function leading to this structural change (see Fig. 45–1).

The relation between media area and lumen size for SHR and WKY resistance vessels is shown in Figure 45–5. It is clear from these studies by Mulvany and co-workers,[8, 9, 25-27] as assembled in a review,[24] that for lumen sizes between 100 and 300 μm the SHR media area is relatively greater. This is most apparent in vessels larger than 200 μm. As discussed in the following, this alteration in media area is a consequence of vessel remodeling and increased smooth muscle cell size.

There is a strong correlation between the media/lumen ratio and the magnitude of blood pressure increase in hypertension. Data from a variety of hypertensive models (SHR, stroke-prone SHR, one-kidney one-clip) show a clear relation between higher blood pressure and greater media/lumen ratio (Fig. 45–6), suggesting cause and effect. Thus, the elevation of blood pressure in the chronic hypertensive state is due to a permanent change in vessel structure. Several elegant experiments[5, 9, 28] indicate that the primary abnormality is in medial growth and/or remodeling and that the increase in blood pressure is secondary rather than primary.

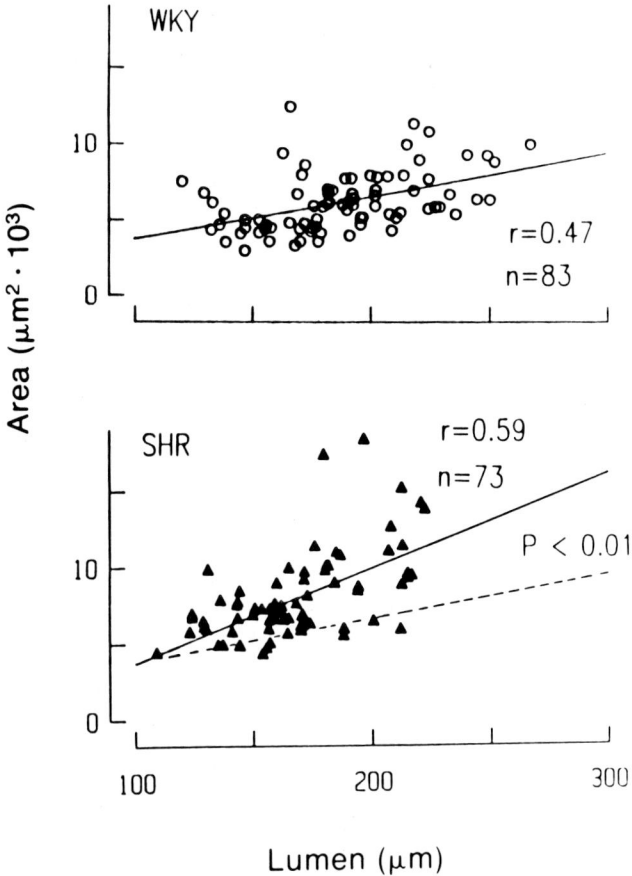

**Figure 45–5.** Relation of cross-sectional area of the media to the normalized luminal diameter of the mesenteric resistance vessels of 83 WKY rats *(top)* and 73 SHRs *(bottom)*. In the lower panel, the dashed line shows the regression line for the WKY data redrawn from the top panel. The slopes of the regression lines are different (*P* < .01). (From Mulvany MJ: Vascular structure and smooth muscle contractility in experimental hypertension. J Cardiovasc Pharmacol 6[suppl]:S79, 1987.)

## STRUCTURAL ABNORMALITIES RESULTING FROM FUNCTIONAL CHANGES IN SMOOTH MUSCLE CELLS CAUSED BY GENETIC AND ENVIRONMENTAL STIMULI

Three lines of evidence support the proposal that abnormalities of the smooth muscle cells in the media (in particular, vessel remodeling and smooth muscle cell growth) rather than blood pressure per se cause the hypertensive phenotype:

1. Lowering blood pressure of the SHR with hydralazine fails to normalize the media/lumen ratio in mesenteric arterioles[25] (Fig. 45–7).
2. Treatment of the SHR with inhibitors of the renin-angiotensin system, such as the angiotensin-converting enzyme (ACE) inhibitor captopril,[11, 29] causes much greater reduction in media growth for a given decrease in blood pressure compared with hydralazine or β-blockers (see Fig. 45–7). Conversely, subpressor doses of angiotensin II promote smooth muscle cell hypertrophy.[30]
3. The vessel response to hypertension differs in different tissues and vascular beds. Thus, controlling systolic

blood pressure has lowered the incidence of stroke by about 50% but has had much less benefit in hypertensive cardiomyopathy and coronary artery disease.

The functional abnormalities in the cells that make up the vessel wall and the cellular mechanisms by which medial growth is stimulated are discussed in the following section.

## The Smooth Muscle Response: Hypertrophy, Hyperplasia, and Remodeling

### HYPERTROPHY

The most characteristic feature of hypertension is an increase in media mass, known as medial hypertrophy. Medial hypertrophy occurs in almost all vascular beds during chronic hypertension and may be viewed as adaptive because it returns wall stress to normal. This is accomplished by increasing wall thickness or reducing vessel diameter (see Fig. 45–4). Increases in wall thickness result from both increases in smooth muscle cell size (cell hypertrophy) and increases in smooth muscle cell number (cell hyperplasia), as well as deposition of matrix. Decreasing vessel diameter requires remodeling, a rearrangement of the vessel wall components. Among the causes of medial hypertrophy, pulse pressure may be more important than mean arterial pressure, as shown by Heistad and Baumbach.[18, 31] Hypertrophy is a reversible mechanism when unaccompanied by endoreduplication. However, when DNA synthesis occurs, the change in cell size is probably irreversible. Thus, cell hypertrophy caused by protein synthesis is adaptive, whereas hypertrophy associated with DNA synthesis is maladaptive in the sense that the increase in cell size (and increase in media/lumen ratio) cannot be returned to normal. Because endoreduplication is such a common finding in hypertension and so little is known regarding its mechanisms, this should be an area of future research focus.

As discussed later, several mechanisms have been estab-

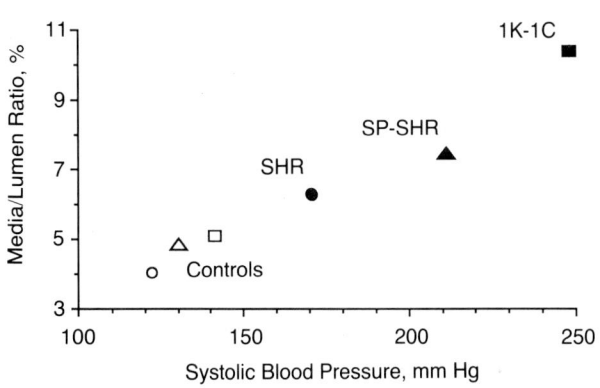

**Figure 45–6.** The media/lumen ratio correlates with the systolic blood pressure in hypertensive rats. Both genetic models of hypertension (SHR and stroke-prone [SP] SHR) and induced models (one-kidney one-clip [1K-1C]) show a positive correlation between the blood pressure and the percentage of the media relative to the lumen. (Modified from Mulvany MJ: Vascular structure and smooth muscle contractility in experimental hypertension. J Cardiovasc Pharmacol 6[suppl]:S79, 1987.)

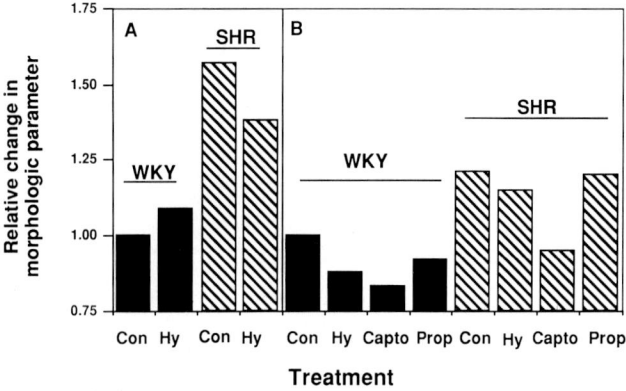

**Figure 45–7.** Captopril, an ACE inhibitor, causes the greatest change in vessel morphology. SHR and WKY rats were treated between 2 and 5 months of age with hydralazine (Hy, 40 mg/L in drinking water), captopril (Capto, 375 mg/L), and propranolol (Prop, 1.5 mg/L). The changes in media/lumen ratio *(A)* and media area *(B)* were measured at 5 months. (Modified from Owens GK: Influence of blood pressure on development of aortic medial smooth muscle hypertrophy in spontaneously hypertensive rats. Hypertension 9:178, 1987.)

lished for smooth muscle cell hypertrophy, including stimulation by angiotensin II[32, 33] and transforming growth factor-β (TGF-β).[34] In particular, there is a strong correlation between blood pressure and the frequency of polyploid smooth muscle cell and medial smooth muscle content. Conversely, the efficacy of drugs (captopril and hydralazine) in preventing the development of smooth muscle cell polyploidism and medial hypertrophy in the SHR was the same as their efficacy in lowering blood pressure.[11] Of interest, propranolol caused no decrease in smooth muscle hypertrophy despite a decrease in blood pressure of 26 mm Hg (see also Fig. 45–7). These findings suggest that the primary cause of smooth muscle cell polyploidy and hypertrophy associated with endoreduplication is blood pressure itself. However, important secondary roles are suggested by the greater efficacy of captopril (an ACE inhibitor) than of hydralazine and propranolol.

## HYPERPLASIA

Hyperplasia also appears to be an important element in human hypertension. This is suggested by the significant increase in smooth muscle cell proliferative rate and the number of cell layers in the media of vessels from animals with chronic hypertension.[35, 36] As described earlier, there is also medial necrosis or atrophy in conduit vessels associated with loss of smooth muscle cells. Thus, if cell death precedes smooth muscle cell growth, hyperplasia could be viewed as an adaptive change. However, the reverse appears to be true: smooth muscle cell proliferation precedes medial necrosis. Hyperplasia is a slow process in chronic human hypertension. Normal rat aortic smooth muscle cell growth is 0.01%/d.[37] In hypertensive models, this increases to a maximum of 1%/d. Simple calculations indicate that if this rate persisted, an arteriole 30 μm in diameter would occlude in 40 days, based on a medial thickness of 20 μm and cell diameter of 5 μm. This implies that only a certain percentage of cells may be able to replicate (smooth muscle

cell heterogeneity) or there must be only brief periods of proliferation (e.g., environmental stimuli) followed by inhibition of cell growth. Both processes appear to occur and contribute to the proliferation of smooth muscle cells in hypertension. Alternatively, there may be programmed cell death of some proliferating cells, a process termed "apoptosis."

Although smooth muscle cells in the vessel wall appear morphologically similar, it is likely that they are functionally heterogeneous. Several mechanisms could explain this. 1) There may be embryonic cells ("progenitors") left from development[38] similar to those isolated from fetal animals. For example, Schwartz and colleagues[39] have shown that proliferating smooth muscle cells isolated from the aorta express unique cytochrome P-450 enzymes that are typical of embryonic smooth muscle cells. 2) There may be two types of smooth muscle cells: one that can undergo a dedifferentiation process recapitulating development and hence proliferation and another that is terminally differentiated and therefore able to migrate but not proliferate. These two types could be genetically determined or a consequence of environmental modification. For example, inflammatory cells or oxidized low-density lipoproteins may stimulate expression of growth factor receptors in smooth muscle cells, which could then respond to release of growth factors by proliferating. Because smooth muscle cells are sources of many autocrine growth factors, they may be constantly exposed to potential mitogens. 3) There may be heterogeneity within the vessel wall that modifies the local environment. To take three examples: a) Variations in hemodynamic forces may cause local gradients in nutrients (e.g., increased residence time of oxidized lipids) or local metabolic requirements (e.g., increased energy metabolism or altered cytoskeleton arrangements).[6, 40, 41] Hemodynamic forces are sensed by the vessel, because atherosclerosis develops in regions of low shear stress. Data show that endothelial cell production and release of growth factors are regulated by shear stress.[40–42] b) Variation in matrix composition may be important, as illustrated by the fact that fibronectin is thought to be growth promoting and laminin growth inhibiting.[43–45] c) Variations in uptake of circulating cells (e.g., leukocytes) or materials (e.g., low-density lipoprotein) may create different local environments. In summary, multiple mechanisms may account for the appearance of smooth muscle cell hyperplasia compared with hypertrophy in different vascular beds.

## REMODELING

Remodeling is a complex process that involves changes in smooth muscle cell growth and migration as well as alterations in vessel matrix. It occurs primarily in resistance vessels. The process appears to be fundamentally dependent on the presence of an intact endothelium. This has been best shown in growing vessels. In young rats, if one carotid is ligated to decrease flow (but pressure maintained constant via collateral circulation) the ligated vessel fails to grow and after 10 weeks has a diameter only 50% of that of the control carotid.[46, 47] If the endothelium is removed, the normal vessel also fails to grow, establishing the endothelium as critical to vessel growth. In a similar manner, if flow is increased by a graft anastomosis, the subsequent downstream increase in vessel size is dependent on an intact endothelium.[48] Thus remodeling in response to flow appears to be an endothelium-dependent process.

Remodeling appears to be important in the changes in arteriolar structure in humans with essential hypertension. In small arteries (200 μm in diameter) obtained from gluteal biopsies of skin and subcutaneous fat of patients with essential hypertension, there was a significant decrease in lumen diameter (17%) and increase in media/lumen ratio (31%) compared with arteries of normotensive subjects.[28] Most important, there was no significant change (10% decrease) in the media volume per segment length (media cross-sectional area). This suggests that the dominant change in vessel structure was a rearrangement or remodeling of the lumen without increase in the media mass. It should be noted that a small increase in smooth muscle cell volume (16%) and decrease in smooth muscle cell number (26%) occurred in the hypertensive vessels, values that were not statistically significant. These results suggest a minor role for smooth muscle cell hypertrophy in human essential hypertension and a predominant role for remodeling. Similar results were shown by Short[13] in chronic human hypertension.

Analyses of mesenteric resistance arteries of hypertensive rats suggest that remodeling is predominant in genetic models and hypertrophy predominant in induced models of hypertension. In both SHR[8] and transgenic rats containing the mouse *REN2* gene,[49] there was no change in smooth muscle cell volume despite an increased media/lumen ratio, indicating that remodeling had occurred. In contrast, in one-kidney one-clip hypertensive rats[7] and rats infused with subpressor doses of angiotensin II,[30] smooth muscle cell volume was increased. Thus, both remodeling and smooth muscle cell hypertrophy are important in the altered structure of the hypertensive arteriole. Remodeling must involve matrix dissolution, cell migration, and matrix resynthesis. Little is known regarding the mechanisms underlying regulation of these processes, making this an important area for future studies.

## Functional Consequences of Vessel Wall Hypertrophy, Hyperplasia, and Remodeling

Increases in vessel wall thickness caused by hypertrophy, hyperplasia, and remodeling are adaptive responses to hypertension in that they decrease wall stress. Increases in blood pressure increase wall stress, which increases smooth muscle cell work and oxygen consumption. In large vessels this may drive oxygen tension to zero, causing tissue hypoxia and smooth muscle cell dysfunction or death.[50–52] As discussed previously, increases in wall thickness and reductions in vessel diameter both act to return wall stress to normal (see Fig. 45–4). Furthermore, if increases in pressure during hypertension were transmitted unabated to arterioles and capillaries, the microcirculation would be damaged. This is especially critical in the cerebral circulation,

where increased vascular permeability would rapidly lead to cerebral edema. Thus, medial hypertrophy may be viewed as adaptive.

Both vascular hypertrophy and remodeling increase the media/lumen ratio. This increases the apparent responsiveness to vasoconstrictor stimuli in that the same increase in smooth muscle cell tone causes a much larger increase in resistance because the proportionate decrease in lumen diameter is much greater. In larger vessels, there is no significant effect on minimal resistance because the diameter is so large. However, in smaller vessels, the passive properties of the vessel are changed and resting resistance may be substantially increased. It is in this setting that the adaptive compensatory increase in vessel wall thickness (relative to lumen) becomes maladaptive and contributes to hypertension.

# FUNCTIONAL ABNORMALITIES IN HYPERTENSION: LINK TO STRUCTURAL ALTERATIONS

The functional abnormalities that have been observed in hypertension are of two types: those related to the passive properties of the vessel and those related to the dynamic properties. Passive properties include the features related to the tissue composition of the vessel. Dynamic or active properties refer to the characteristics determined by cellular mechanisms that require energy and change on a moment-to-moment basis.

## Alterations in the Passive Properties of Hypertensive Vessels

The most characteristic feature of the passive properties in hypertension is a decrease in compliance or elasticity. It should be noted that the contribution of arterial compliance is dependent on the blood pressure. For example, at high levels of pressure, vessels have active tone and arterial compliance may make little contribution to vascular resistance. At low levels of pressure, vessels have little active tone, so arterial compliance is likely to contribute more to vascular resistance. Such shifts in cerebral vessels of hypertensive rats have been shown by Heistad and Baumbach.[18]

## Alterations in the Active Properties of Hypertensive Vessels: Overview

The changes in hypertensive vessels in response to agonists that stimulate relaxation or contraction can be divided into processes associated with impaired vessel relaxation and those associated with augmented vessel contraction. Impaired relaxation has been attributed primarily to dysfunctional endothelium, and augmented contraction has been attributed to enhanced smooth muscle cell vasoreactivity. As discussed later, the endothelium secretes a variety of vasoactive substances including both vasodilators and vasoconstrictors. Decreased relaxation could therefore be due to impaired production of vasodilating substances or to increased production of vasoconstricting substances or both. Increased smooth muscle cell responsiveness may be due to alterations in the ability of these vasodilating substances to exert their effects or changes in the ability of smooth muscle cells to respond to the vasodilators. Conversely, there may be increased responsiveness to vasoconstrictors because of increased numbers of receptors or an augmented contractile machinery. All of these disturbances have been observed in different models of hypertension, with different mechanisms being prevalent in different vascular beds and in vessels of different size.

## Examples of Altered Active Vessel Properties

### ENDOTHELIUM-DEPENDENT ALTERATIONS

There is strong evidence for multiple alterations in endothelial function in hypertension with increased production of constricting factors and decreased production of relaxing factors.

**Endothelium-Derived Relaxing Factor.** Perhaps the most important endothelium-derived regulator of vascular tone is endothelium-derived relaxing factor (EDRF). The best known EDRF is nitric oxide (NO). Two abnormalities of endothelial function related to NO have been described by Dohi and colleagues[53]: reduced basal release of NO and impaired endothelium-dependent relaxation to acetylcholine. The defects in endothelial function in rat hypertensive models are complex, as shown by the fact that impairment of endothelium-dependent relaxations occurs only with certain agonists. For example, in the SHR aorta, the response to acetylcholine is markedly reduced, whereas the response to thrombin is normal and to histamine slightly enhanced.[54] In mesenteric resistance arteries of the SHR, the relaxations to acetylcholine are impaired although relaxations to endothelium-independent vasodilators such as the NO-donating 3-morpholinosydnonimine (SIN-1) are normal, suggesting reduced formation of endothelium-derived NO.[53, 55, 56] In perfused mesenteric resistance arteries, intraluminal administration of acetylcholine is markedly impaired but extraluminal application of acetylcholine stimulates a normal response.[55] These findings suggest that the luminal surface of the endothelium is selectively impaired in hypertension. A possible mechanism might be the presence of a more oxidizing environment in the luminal surface that more rapidly degrades NO[57-59] or a physical barrier in the luminal subendothelial space.

**Endothelium-Derived Vasoconstrictors.** The endothelium may also be a source of vasoconstrictors. In the SHR aorta, high concentrations of acetylcholine ($>10^{-6}$ M) cause an endothelium-dependent contraction that is prevented by phospholipase $A_2$ inhibitors (e.g., quinacrine) or by cyclooxygenase inhibitors (e.g., indomethacin or meclofenamate).[54] These factors have been termed "endothelium-derived constricting factors." The composition of these factors is unknown. Likely candidates include cyclooxygenase products of arachidonic acid and other cis-unsaturated fatty acids.[60]

## CHANGES IN SMOOTH MUSCLE CELL–MEDIATED TONE

The changes in contractile tone of smooth muscle cells in vessels exposed to chronic hypertension present a paradox. On the one hand, some of these cells undergo phenotypic modulation to a "synthetic" as opposed to a "contractile" phenotype with loss of α-1-actin and smooth muscle myosin.[12, 61] These synthetic growing cells would be expected to be less contractile than normal. On the other hand, there is increased tone in hypertension. This is in part explained by the mechanical advantage of an increased media/lumen ratio. However, it is well established that there is increased sensitivity to vasopressors as well. For example, the dose response for contraction of mesenteric arteries to norepinephrine showed enhanced sensitivity in the SHR compared with the WKY rat.[62] This was thought to be due to depressed endothelium-dependent vasodilation. In the absence of endothelium, there is controversy regarding the sensitivity to norepinephrine. Some investigators have reported no difference in the sensitivity of mesenteric resistance vessels of the SHR and WKY rat to norepinephrine as measured by contractile response.[25] Other investigators have reported increased receptor affinity for norepinephrine and increased contractile sensitivity in the SHR.[63] The discrepancy in results obtained may be due to differences in the strains examined (the WKY and SHR strains are no longer homogeneous genetically), the ages of the animals examined, and the extent to which endothelial cell function is preserved under the conditions used for the contraction studies.

Even receptor-independent vasoconstricting mechanisms are enhanced in the SHR. If vessels are first depleted of $Ca^{2+}$ and then repleted, there is a marked increase in tone in the SHR compared with the WKY rat.[26] In the stroke-prone SHR vessels, there are frequently oscillations of isolated vessels with increased tone.[64, 65] Experiments that bypass membrane receptors and target intracellular mediators such as protein kinase C indicate that there are intracellular defects in the SHR.[66, 67] For example, phorbol esters, which directly stimulate protein kinase C, provoke greater contractions at lower concentrations in the SHR than the WKY rat. In summary, it appears that both receptor-coupled and receptor-independent mechanisms are augmented in several hypertensive models.

## CHANGES IN NERVOUS SYSTEM– MEDIATED TONE

Several features of the sympathetic nervous system suggest that it contributes to the medial hypertrophy of hypertension. First, norepinephrine and epinephrine are both vasoconstrictors. Vasoconstrictors are generally growth factors for smooth muscle cells,[68] as discussed subsequently. Second, a number of studies have shown that sympathectomy markedly diminishes medial hypertrophy in the SHR model. Lee and colleagues[36] demonstrated that neonatal sympathectomy (anti–nerve growth factor antibody and sympathectomy) prevented development of SHR hypertension. In these rats, the arteries showed hypertrophy but no evidence of hyperplasia. In another study, infusion of epinephrine increased polyploidy of vascular smooth muscle cells in the absence of an increase in blood pressure.[69] These authors also showed that both epinephrine and norepinephrine stimulated polyploidy in vitro. In addition, propranolol has been shown in the deoxycorticosterone acetate salt hypertensive rat model to prevent the development of polyploidy even when it failed to lower blood pressure.[70] Finally, during development of vessels, sympathectomy inhibits the increase in DNA mass of the vessel, suggesting an important role for the sympathetic nervous system in the formation of blood vessels.[71, 72] Thus, it appears that sympathectomy and other inhibitors of the sympathetic nervous system inhibit smooth muscle cell growth in hypertensive vessels.

Functional vessel abnormalities in hypertension exist alongside structural abnormalities that are in part adaptive. The next issue to be addressed regards the fundamental pathogenetic mechanisms that underlie these processes. Specifically, what unifying pathogenetic processes could cause both increased media/lumen ratios and altered vascular responsiveness, two nearly universal features of the hypertensive vessel?

## THE ENDOTHELIUM IN HYPERTENSION

### Endothelium-Derived Vasoactive Mediators

The endothelium has become a focus for research in hypertension because of the expanding knowledge regarding its importance as a source of vasoactive mediators and its dysfunction during chronic hypertension. The best-characterized alteration in hypertension is diminished endothelium-dependent relaxation in response to acetylcholine. This has been demonstrated in both mesenteric resistance arteries of hypertensive rats and in the forearm circulation of hypertensive patients.[54, 73–75] In a study by Panza and colleagues,[73] increased forearm blood flow during intrabrachial infusion of acetylcholine was markedly diminished in hypertensive subjects compared with normotensive individuals, but dilation to nitroprusside (a direct smooth muscle cell vasodilator) was unchanged.

This dysfunction is related to a decrease in the effective concentration of EDRF. Furchgott and Zawadzki[76] were the first to establish that the endothelium was the source of an acetylcholine-stimulated vasorelaxing factor by showing that acetylcholine was a vasodilator in the presence of intact endothelium and a vasoconstrictor in the absence of endothelium. The properties of this factor were initially puzzling, as it was characterized as a small (<1000 daltons), rapidly diffusing, rapidly degraded (half-life < 10 seconds) substance. The finding that its rate of degradation could be accelerated by superoxide and by hemoglobin suggested that EDRF was a free radical. The discovery that nitrovasodilators stimulated cyclic GMP–dependent kinase in smooth muscle cells and hence stimulated relaxation suggested that an endogenous substance might be present that performed a similar function. A major advance was made by Moncada's group,[77, 78] who showed that NO could be produced from L-arginine in endothelium. NO is produced in endothelial cells by the enzyme NO synthase (Fig. 45–8), which is a $Ca^{2+}$- and calmodulin-dependent enzyme of the flavin-biopterin class. This enzyme is dynamically regulated and can increase production of NO by more than 20-fold within seconds. Stimuli that have been shown to increase NO synthesis include fluid shear stress (increased flow) and a variety of vasomediators including bradykinin, histamine, norepinephrine, substance P, serotonin, thrombin, and vasopressin. All these factors probably work by increasing intracellular $Ca^{2+}$ levels and activating the enzyme. There does not seem to be any control of NO release, as NO rapidly diffuses out of the cell. However, before it reaches target cells, it may be inactivated by factors such as oxygen radicals ($O_2^-$ and $OH^-$) and iron-containing compounds (e.g., hemoglobin). As already discussed, NO stimulates soluble guanylate cyclase, which increases cyclic GMP. In smooth muscle cells, increased cyclic GMP causes relaxation, and in platelets it inhibits adhesion and aggregation.[79] Elevation of cyclic GMP also appears to be growth inhibitory for smooth muscle cells.[80] Thus, if NO production is diminished, this would lead to decreased cyclic GMP in smooth muscle cells and remove a growth-inhibiting and vasodilating mechanism. This might contribute to increased smooth muscle cell growth in conditions of impaired NO production such as hypercholesterolemia, oxidative stress, and homocystinuria.

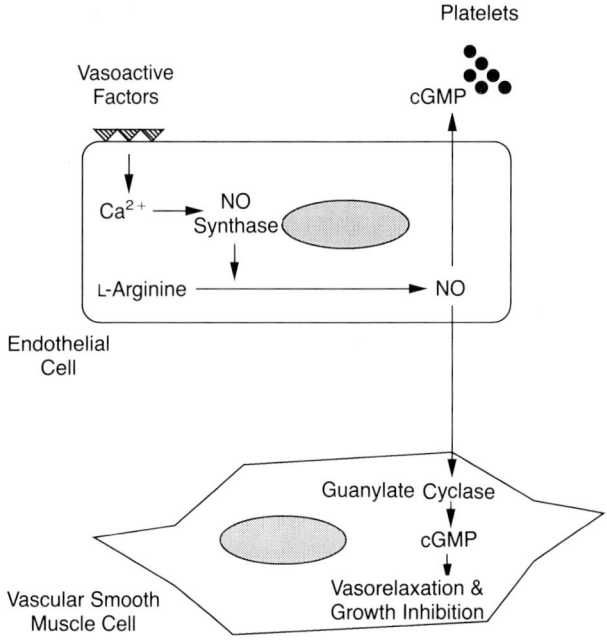

**Figure 45–8.** NO is an important regulator of vessel wall function. In response to a variety of vasoactive factors including increased fluid shear stress, endothelial cells activate NO synthase, which generates NO from L-arginine. NO diffuses rapidly from the cell and activates guanylate cyclase in target cells. In platelets this inhibits aggregation; in smooth muscle it causes vasorelaxation and growth inhibition.

## Abnormalities in Nitric Oxide Action (Function) in Hypertension

Two abnormalities of endothelial function related to NO have been described by Dohi and colleagues[53]: reduced basal release of NO and impaired endothelium-dependent relaxation to acetylcholine. Three mechanisms appear most likely to explain decreased NO responsiveness. 1) Increased destruction: NO is readily destroyed by a wide variety of oxygen-derived free radicals as well as by advanced glycosylation end products.[81] Substantial evidence has accumulated that there are increased oxygen radicals in atherosclerosis and hypertension.[50, 51] In fact, administration of superoxide dismutase (an enzyme that destroys the superoxide radical) decreased blood pressure in the SHR.[59] 2) Decreased production: NO production by NO synthase requires arginine, which appears to be present in excess within the cell. However, it is possible that alterations in activation of NO synthase may limit NO production in response to physiologic stimuli such as increased flow. 3) Impaired smooth muscle cell responsiveness: As illustrated in Figure 45–8, NO exerts its vasodilating effects by increasing cyclic GMP, which activates cyclic GMP–dependent kinase, inhibiting myosin phosphorylation. It appears that this series of intracellular events may be altered in smooth muscle cells exposed to chronic hypertension, as shown by decreased relaxation in the aorta and carotid of SHR on administration of a variety of compounds that donate NO (e.g., nitroprusside and SIN-1) and thereby stimulate cyclic GMP.[74, 82] In summary, the decrease in endothelium-dependent relaxation is one of the fundamental abnormalities in the vessel wall in chronic hypertension.

## Several Endothelium-Dependent Functions Are Abnormal in Hypertension

Several other aspects of endothelial dysfunction contribute to the altered function of the vessel wall:

1. There is disruption of the permeability barrier of the endothelium allowing transudation of lipids and serum proteins. In particular, oxidized lipids may contribute in several ways to abnormal smooth muscle cell growth and endothelial cell dysfunction. For example, low-density lipoprotein induces expression of chemotactic proteins such as monocyte chemotactic peptide-1 that may stimulate transmigration of monocytes and promote residence in the subendothelial space.[83] Subsequent macrophage activation and generation of inflammatory cytokines and active oxygen species may cause a more oxidizing vessel environment. This environment would shorten the half-life of NO.

2. There is increased adhesion of circulating blood elements. In particular, there may be expression of leukocyte adhesion molecules such as vascular cell adhesion molecule and endothelial leukocyte adhesion molecule-1 by the endothelium. These inflammatory cells may release a variety of smooth muscle cell growth factors and vasoconstrictors that alter vasoreactivity and promote smooth muscle cell growth.

3. The endothelium may release increased amounts of constricting factors not normally present.[60] Two important endothelium-derived constricting factors are endothelin (ET) and cyclooxygenase-dependent contracting factors. ET-1 is a 21–amino acid peptide that is produced in endothelial cells by many stimuli including thrombin, TGF-β, norepinephrine, and phorbol esters. ET-1 is extremely potent on a molar basis and appears to play an important role in local regulation of vessel tone. Responses to ET are regulated by processing of a 212–amino acid precursor molecule, secretion of mature ET-1, and receptor expression by smooth muscle cells.[84] Of interest, in many vessels NO and nitrovasodilators are able to inhibit the release of ET, suggesting a self-regulating mechanism.[85]

4. Decreased production of other vasodilating substances such as prostacyclin and endothelium-derived hyperpolarizing factor. The production of prostacyclin is stimulated in endothelium by fluid shear stress and many of the same agonists that release NO. However, inhibition of prostacyclin formation shows that it is normally much less important than NO in mediating vasorelaxation.[76, 86] The nature of endothelium-derived hyperpolarizing factor remains unclear, but in certain vessels an endothelium-dependent hyperpolarization of smooth muscle cells has been demonstrated that is mediated by a diffusible substance.[87]

In summary, alterations in EDRFs (especially NO) appear to be critical to the altered function of the hypertensive vessels. Other vasoactive substances derived from the endothelium, including constrictors such as ET-1, cyclooxygenase-derived fatty acids, and platelet-derived growth factor (PDGF), may also be abnormal.[60] However, the evidence that these factors are important in altering resistance vessel function is limited at the present time. Future work should establish the importance of EDRF (and the mechanisms for its dysfunction) in human patients with essential hypertension.

## SMOOTH MUSCLE IN HYPERTENSION

Smooth muscle cells have been the focus of research related to the vessel wall response to hypertension for many years. The morphologic changes in the smooth muscle cells described in the following section indicate their ability to respond to the hemodynamic environment. Despite a clear description of the morphologic changes associated with hypertension, the biochemical changes responsible for the altered phenotype remain largely unknown. That these morphologic changes are biochemical in nature was suggested by the use of the terms contractile and synthetic phenotype.[61] As outlined in Table 45–1, contractile cells are spindle shaped, are located in the media, contract in response to agonists, and express high levels of contractile proteins such as α-actin and smooth muscle cell–specific myosin. Most important, these cells do not proliferate initially when placed in tissue culture. In contrast, synthetic phenotype smooth muscle cells are round, may be present in the intima, do not contract, and do not express α-actin and smooth muscle cell–specific myosin. These cells are characterized by large amounts of rough endoplasmic reticulum

**TABLE 45–1. Synthetic and Contractile Smooth Muscle Cells**

| Property | Contractile | Synthetic |
|---|---|---|
| Shape | Spindle | Round |
| Location | Media | Media and intima |
| Contractile | Yes | Probably not |
| Proteins | $\alpha$-1 actin | $\beta$ and $\gamma$ actin |
| Growth factors | No response to PDGF | Proliferate in response to PDGF |
| | Do not secrete PDGF | Secrete PDGF |

and secretion of large quantities of tissue matrix proteins. Most important, these cells proliferate when placed in culture. In fact, upon being placed in culture, contractile smooth muscle cells undergo a process of phenotypic modulation in which they take on the appearance of synthetic cells and begin to proliferate in response to mitogens. In the following sections, the smooth muscle cell growth response and the biochemical mechanisms unique to hypertension are discussed.

## Smooth Muscle Cells: Phenotypic Plasticity

One of the distinguishing features of smooth muscle cells is the plasticity of their growth responses. As shown in Figure 45–3, smooth muscle cells can respond in three ways to alterations in hemodynamic stress: hyperplasia, hypertrophy, and remodeling. In chronic hypertension, all three responses may be observed in different-sized vessels or even within the same vessel. Although smooth muscle cell plasticity offers an advantage in terms of its adaptability, in hypertensive humans this process may be pathologic. In particular, although hypertrophy and remodeling appear to be reversible, hyperplasia and endoreduplication are not. At this time, the mechanisms controlling hyperplasia have been best studied, so they are the focus of the ensuing discussion. Our knowledge of hypertrophy is limited[88] and information regarding mechanisms for remodeling scant.[2, 3, 28]

## Smooth Muscle Cell Growth Factors in Hypertension

Growth factors have been isolated and characterized by their ability to stimulate growth of cultured cells. This research approach has caused us to think of growth factors as circulating materials that are released by platelets during injury (e.g., PDGF) or generated from circulating prohormones (e.g., angiotensin I to angiotensin II, prothrombin to thrombin). However, this concept may be the exception rather than the rule. In fact, temporal and spatial expression of growth factors and their receptors is dynamically regulated locally within the vessel wall. New techniques such as in situ hybridization and gene transfer, as well as the availability of antibodies to specific vascular growth fac-

tors, have helped define the growth factors that are important in vessel growth. Because several excellent reviews detail the range of growth factors that may stimulate smooth muscle cell growth in the hypertensive vessel wall,[89–92] the following discussion focuses on specific examples of mechanisms that are probably important in human essential hypertension. Table 45–2 provides a summary for those interested in greater detail.

## VASOCONSTRICTORS AS GROWTH FACTORS

Agonists that act as vasoconstrictors frequently stimulate smooth muscle cell growth and, conversely, many growth factors have vasoconstrictor activity. This paradigm has been proved many times over.[32, 33, 68, 93–97] For example, PDGF is a vasoconstrictor[68] and angiotensin II is a potent smooth muscle cell growth factor.[32, 33] Shared initial signal transduction events activated by vasoconstrictors and growth factors probably account for activation of the growth response. Examples of shared signaling events include activation of phospholipase C, mobilization of intracellular $Ca^{2+}$, activation of protein kinase C, stimulation of $Na^+/H^+$ exchange, and stimulation of *FOS* messenger RNA (mRNA) expression.[98, 99] These shared initial events are modified by later downstream regulatory mechanisms that determine the nature of the growth response: hypertrophy, hyperplasia, or remodeling.

**Angiotensin II.** The importance of angiotensin II in the smooth muscle cell growth response in hypertension was suggested by the findings that ACE inhibitors have special beneficial effects on vessel wall function in the SHR,[29] that angiotensin II induces smooth muscle cell growth at subpressor concentrations,[30, 100] and that ACE inhibitors block neointimal proliferation after balloon injury of the rat carotid.[101]

Two caveats to the interpretation of these data should be made. 1) ACE inhibitors also block kinin metabolism and therefore increase the concentration of kinins.[90, 102] The presence of a local vessel wall kinin system is suggested by the findings that both arteries and veins contain a kallikrein-like enzyme and cultured smooth muscle cells express mRNA for glandular kallikrein.[103] In addition, cultured smooth muscle cells have been shown to release both glandular kallikrein and kininogen.[104] These kinins (e.g., bradykinin) may be important smooth muscle cell growth inhibitors. For example, after rat carotid injury, the inhibition of smooth muscle cell growth observed with ACE inhibitors is significantly reduced by coadministration of Hoe 140, an antagonist for the bradykinin B2 receptor.[102] These findings suggest that increases in bradykinin as well as decreases in angiotensin II are important in the growth-inhibiting effects of ACE inhibitors. 2) Much of the effect of angiotensin II may be due to facilitated release of norepinephrine from nerve terminals as $\alpha_1$-adrenergic blockade also decreases angiotensin II–induced DNA synthesis after injury.[105]

In the past 5 years it has become clear that the entire renin-angiotensin system is present within the vessel wall and can act as an autocrine growth mechanism for smooth muscle cells.[106] All the components of a local vascular wall renin-angiotensin system appear to be present in normal

TABLE 45–2. Smooth Muscle Cell Growth Factors in Essential Hypertension

| Growth Factor | Cell Source* | Regulated by | Comments |
|---|---|---|---|
| Angiotensin II | SMC | ACE<br>Angiotensinogen<br>Renin | ACE inhibition, ↓ SHR media<br>↑ TGF-β, ↑ PDGF A<br>↑ PDGF β-receptor |
| Endothelin | EC | TGF-β and thrombin<br>Angiotensin<br>Arginine vasopressin<br>Shear stress<br>PDGF AA | ↑ SMC growth |
| Vasopressin | Nerves | Autonomic activity | ↑ SMC growth |
| Epidermal growth factor | Platelets<br>Salivary gland | Unknown, ? testosterone | Synergistic with thrombospondin |
| Fibroblast growth factor | EC<br>SMC | Unknown | Extracellular matrix<br>Binds to heparans<br>Angiogenic<br>Multiple receptors<br>↑ Insulin-like growth factor |
| Thrombin | Liver | EC prothrombotic state | ↑ PDGF A, ↑ SMC growth |
| Insulin-like growth factor | SMC | Angiotensin II ↑<br>Stimulated by PDGF and epidermal growth factor | Regulated by insulin-like growth factor binding proteins<br>Synergistic with PDGF |
| PDGF | EC<br>SMC | Shear stress<br>Angiotensin II | ↑ Thrombospondin synthesis<br>Receptor-specific interactions for AA, AB, BB forms<br>↑ IGF |
| TGF-β | SMC<br>Platelets | Angiotensin II | Can both ↑ and ↓ SMC proliferation<br>Multiple receptors<br>Regulated by bonding protein<br>Must be activated by proteases<br>Down-regulates PDGF receptor α-subunits |
| Norepinephrine and catecholamines | Nerves | Central nervous system | Chemical sympathectomy<br>↓ SHR media |
| Serotonin | Platelets<br>Nerves | EC prothrombotic state | Stimulates endothelial cells to release EDRF<br>Directly ↑ SMC growth |

*SMC = smooth muscle cell; EC = endothelial cell.

vessels,[107] and their activity is dynamically regulated. For example, angiotensinogen mRNA is present in the endothelium, medial smooth muscle, and periadventitial fat of normal rat arteries,[108] suggesting that several cell types in the vessel can synthesize angiotensinogen.[107] After balloon injury, the ratio of medial to adventitial angiotensinogen mRNA increases, implying increased production of this angiotensin II precursor in the media. Renin is also present in the vascular wall and cleaves angiotensinogen to angiotensin I. ACE then generates the vasoconstrictor and growth factor angiotensin II. Furthermore, ACE is highly regulated,[109] and increased expression of ACE by endothelial and smooth muscle cells may then increase the amounts of angiotensin II present locally in the vessel wall.

It has been suggested that angiotensin II exerts its trophic effects in part through stimulation of PDGF A chain mRNA and protein production.[51, 110] This has been supported most strongly by experiments in which transfection into vascular smooth muscle cells of antisense PDGF A chain oligomers (to prevent PDGF A chain translation) inhibited angiotensin II–stimulated protein synthesis by more than 50%.[111, 112] As discussed in the following, angiotensin II also induces TGF-β mRNA in smooth muscle cells. Gibbons and

colleagues[111, 112] observed that, in the presence of a neutralizing antibody to TGF-β, angiotensin II stimulated DNA synthesis and cell division of smooth muscle cells from normotensive rats. Based on this finding, they hypothesized that angiotensin II was a bifunctional growth factor. Angiotensin II stimulated hyperplasia when PDGF A chain activity was the dominant growth factor expressed, and angiotensin II–stimulated cell hypertrophy occurred when TGF-β activity was dominant.[92, 111, 112] Hahn's group[113] obtained similar findings regarding PDGF A chain and TGF-β induction by angiotensin II in cultured aortic smooth muscle cells from the SHR. However, other investigators[34] have found that angiotensin II induction of TGF-β was associated with enhanced PDGF-stimulated mitogenesis. Although most investigators agree that PDGF A chain is a weak mitogen for cultured smooth muscle cells by itself, it appears to be critical to the hypertrophic response stimulated by angiotensin II in normotensive smooth muscle cells.[114] The increase in cell volume after exposure to angiotensin II follows a time course similar to that for induction of PDGF A chain expression, and antibodies against the PDGF A chain prevent hypertrophy. These studies indicate that smooth muscle cell growth in hypertension that is mediated by angiotensin II actually involves complex regulation of multiple hormones and their receptors. The mechanisms by which angiotensin II alters long-term expression of smooth muscle cell growth factors are likely to be clarified in the near future, given the cloning of the angiotensin II type 1 receptor.[115, 116]

**Catecholamines.** Classic vasoconstrictors such as catecholamines are potent smooth muscle cell mitogens in certain settings.[94–96] In vitro, it has been shown that norepinephrine stimulates both endoreduplication[96] and hyperplasia.[94] In carotid injury models, Majesky and colleagues[117] showed that $\alpha_1$-adrenergic stimulation caused PDGF A chain expression. The importance of this finding was emphasized by the discovery that $\alpha_1$-adrenergic receptor blockade with prazosin inhibited balloon injury–induced smooth muscle cell proliferation.[105] It appears that norepinephrine may be part of an autocrine growth loop because $\alpha_1$-stimulation induced both PDGF A chain expression[117] and PDGF receptor expression.[118]

**Endothelin.** ET-1, the most potent vasoconstrictor yet identified, is a growth factor derived from endothelial cells. It stimulates several proto-oncogenes as well as cell cycle progression.[119, 120] ET-1 is induced by several other smooth muscle cell growth factors including angiotensin II, vasopressin, and PDGF. However, when administered in serum-free conditions, ET-1 is a weak mitogen, suggesting that its importance is as a comitogen with other growth factors present in the vessel wall.[89, 121]

**Vasopressin.** Both hypertrophy[93] and hyperplasia[97, 122] have been reported for vasopressin. These different results may have an explanation similar to that for angiotensin II: both positive and negative growth events are stimulated by vasopressin. For example, vasopressin stimulates many of the same early growth events as classic growth factors including ET-1. However, it also increases production of prostaglandin E$_2$ and prostacyclin,[123, 124] which are known to inhibit vascular smooth muscle cell growth.[125, 126]

## PEPTIDE GROWTH FACTORS

A focus of research has been on the peptide growth factors synthesized locally in the vessel in an autocrine or paracrine fashion. The role of these growth factors in hypertension has been extensively reviewed.[89, 92, 107, 110–112] Tables 45–2 and 45–3 summarize the growth factors shown to be involved in smooth muscle cell growth. In the following discussion, we address specifically the issue of autocrine or paracrine growth mechanisms, focusing on both positive and negative growth regulatory mechanisms.

**Platelet-Derived Growth Factor.** PDGF has been the center of focus because it is made by many cells present in the vessel wall. Endothelial cells and macrophages produce both PDGF A and B chains, whereas adult smooth muscle cells and fibroblasts produce only PDGF A chain.[127] In the hypertensive vessel it appears that the dominant PDGF isoform expressed is the AA homodimer. This isoform can bind only to the $\alpha$-$\alpha$ PDGF receptor.[128] However, the dominant PDGF receptor type appears to be the $\beta$-$\beta$–receptor, which does not bind PDGF AA homodimers.[129, 130] Thus there is a mismatch between hormone and receptor. This suggests that the source of PDGF for smooth muscle cell

**TABLE 45–3. Growth Inhibitors in the Vessel Wall**

| Growth Inhibitor | Cell Source* | Regulates† |
|---|---|---|
| Heparinoids | EC | FGF availability |
| | SMC | Inhibits SMC growth |
| NO | EC | ↑ Cyclic GMP, inhibits SMC |
| | SMC | ↓ Platelet aggregation |
| Prostacyclin | EC | ↑ Cyclic AMP, inhibits SMC |
| Atrial natriuretic peptide | SMC | ↑ Cyclic GMP, inhibits SMC |
| | Atria | |
| | EC | |
| Kinins | Kininogen | ↓ SMC growth |

*EC = endothelial cell; SMC = smooth muscle cell.
†FGF = fibroblast growth factor.

growth is likely to be either platelets (which contain all three PDGF isoforms) or macrophages (which have been shown to express PDGF BB). Alternatively, PDGF A chain may not be that important in smooth muscle cell growth in hypertension. It is unclear what role the PDGF $\alpha$-$\alpha$–receptor may play.

**Insulin-like Growth Factor.** The insulin-like growth factors (IGF-1 and IGF-2) are a family of growth factors whose importance in hypertension is increasingly evident. IGF-1 has been the best studied in the vasculature and is thought to be regulated by endocrine, autocrine, and paracrine mechanisms.[131] Work by Delafontaine and colleagues[132] has established that IGF-1 is increased in hypertension. These investigators observed a specific increase in IGF-1 mRNA in the aorta above the coarctation after infrarenal aortic coarctation. Because the cellular actions of IGF-1 are also determined by its protein binding and receptor expression, the precise effect of this increase remains to be determined. However, these investigators have further demonstrated that IGF-1 mRNA is induced by angiotensin II, suggesting that IGF-1 participates in the angiotensin II growth pathway.[133] IGF-1 is also likely to play an important role in vascular remodeling, as it has been shown to stimulate expression of extracellular matrix components such as collagens I and II and elastin.[134, 135] Of great interest is the apparent relationship in some essential hypertensive patients of insulin resistance, hyperinsulinemia, and the development of hypertension.[81] There appears to be a strong genetic predisposition in these patients to develop hypertension. Whether insulin acts as a growth factor by stimulating its own receptors or by relatively weak interactions with IGF-1 receptors remains to be determined.

**Transforming Growth Factor.** The variety of smooth muscle cell responses to TGF-β is daunting. It appears clear that TGF-β expression is increased in hypertension. Aortic smooth muscle cells from the SHR have higher levels than those from WKY control rats,[136] and both the SHR and one-kidney one-clip hypertensive rats have increased TGF-β expression.[130, 137] In addition, infusion of TGF-β into animals after carotid injury promoted neointimal proliferation, suggesting a mitogenic effect.[138] However, the significance of increased mRNA expression is unclear. TGF-β is secreted in a latent form and then must be proteolyzed to be active. In addition, there is extensive binding of TGF-β to extracellular matrix proteins such as decorin.[139] Thus, fur-

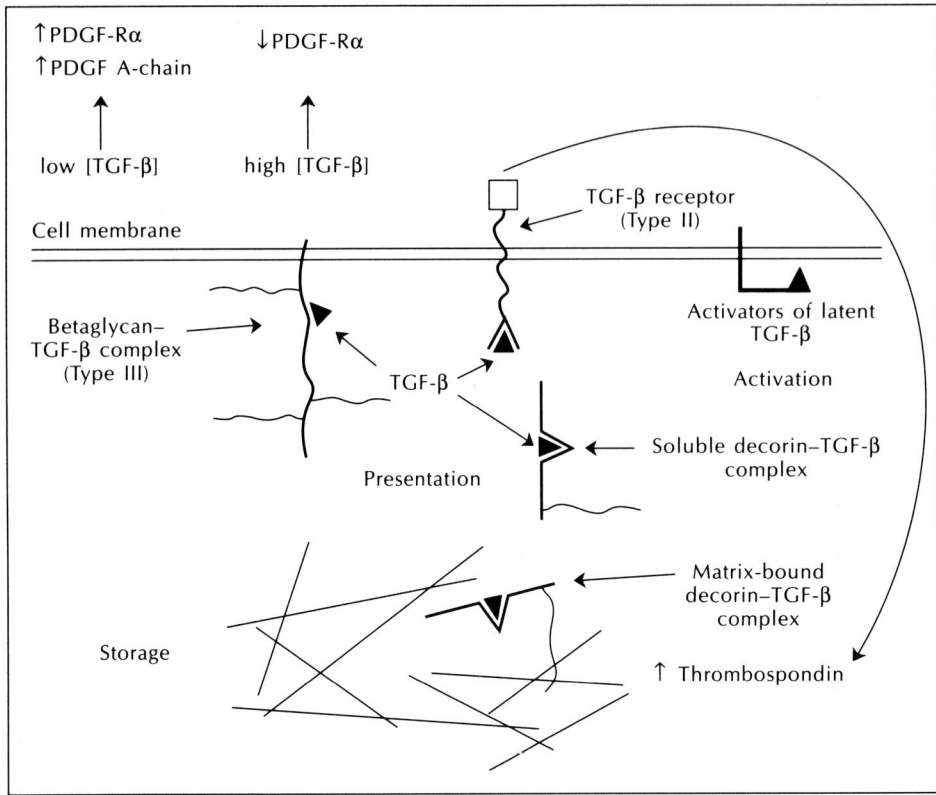

**Figure 45–9.** Interactions of TGF-β with extracellular matrix and activator proteases. TGF-β binds to low-affinity sites, including betaglycan and decorin, that determine availability for signal-transducing membrane-associated receptors. TGF-β binding is associated with positive growth stimulation (PDGF A chain, PDGF α-receptor, and thrombospondin synthesis) and negative growth effects, particularly at high concentrations (decreased PDGF α-receptor expression and inhibition of activation by plasminogen activator inhibitor-1). (Modified from Ruoslahti E, Yamaguchi Y: Proteoglycans as modulators of growth factor activities. Cell 64:867, 1991. Copyright by Cell Press.)

ther work is required to demonstrate that there is increased functional TGF-β in hypertensive vessels.

In vitro experiments suggest that TGF-β can be both growth promoting and growth inhibiting for smooth muscle cells. At low concentrations (<0.1 ng/mL), TGF-β is growth promoting, which is thought to be due to increased expression of PDGF A chain and the PDGF α-receptor,[140–142] as well as thrombospondin.[142, 143] At higher concentrations, TGF-β is growth inhibiting, which may be due to decreased PDGF A chain and PDGF α-receptor expression.[140, 141] Other investigators have found that TGF-β induces a delayed increase in DNA synthesis associated primarily with cell hypertrophy.[144] The complexity of TGF-β growth effects is compounded when combinations of growth factors are examined (e.g., PDGF and TGF-β or angiotensin II and TGF-β). For example, smooth muscle cells from the SHR show different growth responses to angiotensin II than those of WKY animals.[34, 145] In SHR smooth muscle cells, angiotensin II is mitogenic, and this correlates with relatively diminished TGF-β expression[145] compared with WKY cells, where angiotensin II is primarily hypertrophic. As already discussed, TGF-β neutralizing antibody inhibited angiotensin II–induced increases in DNA synthesis.[34, 111, 112] However, exogenous TGF-β, at concentrations similar to those induced by angiotensin II, failed to elicit a mitogenic response in the SHR.[34]

Several new findings may explain these contradictory results. As discussed in detail later (in the section on extracellular matrix and growth factors), it is now clear that TGF-β is a family of growth factors with several receptors.[146, 147] In particular, because TGF-β is synthesized and secreted in a latent form, storage of this latent molecule by matrix-bound receptors such as decorin[139] and activation of the latent molecule by proteases such as plasmin are critical regulatory steps. In addition, the system that activates TGF-β is highly regulated: TGF-β itself stimulates production of the protease inhibitor plasminogen activator inhibitor-1.[148] Thus, as shown in Figure 45–9, post-translational regulation of TGF-β (activation, storage, and presentation) contributes significantly to its physiologic effects in the vessel wall. Because of the complexity of TGF-β actions,[110, 138, 143, 148, 149] its role in the blood vessel in hypertension requires further investigation.

**Fibroblast Growth Factor.** The importance of fibroblast growth factor (FGF) as an autocrine or paracrine mediator of smooth muscle cell growth in hypertensive vessels is supported by its diverse actions on other smooth muscle cell growth factors (see Table 45–2). For example, FGF stimulates PDGF A chain expression,[150] it induces ACE expression in endothelial cells[151] and in smooth muscle cells (Berk BC, unpublished data), and PDGF-stimulated smooth muscle cell migration is inhibited by anti-FGF antibody.[152]

**Atrial Natriuretic Peptides.** The family of atrial natriuretic peptides, also known as atrial natriuretic factors, have been increasingly recognized as important regulators of smooth muscle cell growth in hypertension. There are at least three peptides and their cognate receptors: A type or ANP which is produced by atrial myocardium; B type or BNP, which is produced mainly by the myocardium and also found in brain; and C type or CNP, which is produced by endothelial cells.[153] The three atrial natriuretic peptide receptors that have been described are the A receptor, which binds ANP and BNP and contains intrinsic guanylate cyclase activity; the B receptor, which is structurally related to the A receptor but is activated by CNP; and the C or "clearance" receptor, which has no intrinsic cyclase activity and appears to be involved in clearance of circulating forms of natriuretic peptides.[153–155] ANP and CNP appear to be the most important in regulation of smooth muscle cell growth and hence may be important in the hypertensive vessel wall.

ANP is a vasodilator and inhibits growth of cultured smooth muscle cells.[154, 155] In addition, ANP prevents the hypertrophy of cultured smooth muscle cells stimulated by angiotensin II and TGF-β.[156] Because ANP activates guanylate cyclase, cyclic GMP levels rise. As discussed earlier for NO, elevations in guanylate cyclase appear to be growth inhibitory, suggesting that ANP exerts its antiproliferative effects by increasing guanylate cyclase activity.[80] When smooth muscle cells are placed in culture they rapidly lose guanylate cyclase activity, which may be one form of loss of growth inhibition. Because the intact vessel expresses ANP mRNA,[157] it is possible that the family of atrial natriuretic peptides may be a local autocrine growth-regulating system analogous to the renin-angiotensin system. The potential importance of this system in hypertension is suggested by the demonstration that long-term infusion of low concentrations of ANP in the SHR (insufficient to lower blood pressure) decreased carotid artery media thickness and also inhibited smooth muscle cell hypertrophy (endoreduplication) as measured by nuclear size.[158]

Although less studied, CNP appears to be critical for the ANP autocrine growth loop as it is highly regulated in endothelial cells. It has been demonstrated that the normally low level of endothelial cell CNP expression is dramatically increased by TGF-β.[159] Receptors for CNP have been demonstrated in both cultured smooth muscle cells[154] and aorta.[160] Activation by CNP increases cyclic GMP, suggesting a hormonally activated receptor that is functionally coupled. In vitro growth inhibition studies show that CNP may be more potent than ANP at inhibiting smooth muscle cell proliferation.[161] In summary, this peptide family is emerging as another autocrine or paracrine growth regulatory system for smooth muscle cells that may have special importance in hypertension.

## EXTRACELLULAR MATRIX, WITH EMPHASIS ON TISSUE REMODELING

The extracellular matrix is a critical regulator of vessel wall function. As already described, changes in conduit vessel elasticity are a hallmark of the chronic hypertensive state. However, the importance of the extracellular matrix has become more evident with the new knowledge that its structure and interactions with growth factors are regulated by many factors. Two concepts are widespread regarding the role of extracellular matrix in hypertension. 1) Dynamic alterations in vessel structure such as occur with remodeling are mediated by interactions between extracellular matrix and cellular components. 2) Changes in extracellular matrix composition and growth factor binding may alter the phe-

notypic expression of smooth muscle cells, thereby regulating cell proliferation.

**Extracellular Matrix Composition and Changes with Hypertension.** The extracellular matrix is a complex protein-carbohydrate network consisting of collagens, elastin(s), proteoglycans, and glycopeptides.[162] Among the proteins that appear to be most highly regulated during vessel growth and remodeling are collagen, elastin, laminin, thrombospondin, fibronectin, and tenascin. During development of hypertension there are significant increases in both elastin and fibronectin.[44, 45] It has become clear that the interactions between these molecules are regulated by a variety of enzymes produced both by smooth muscle cells and endothelial cells that alter the structure of the extracellular matrix. For example, collagenase is highly regulated in smooth muscle cells. Expression of collagenase is stimulated by growth factors via a phorbol ester response element; heparin inhibits its induction.[163] Expression of proteases such as urokinase and tissue plasminogen activator is stimulated during smooth muscle cell mitogenesis and their induction is also blocked by heparin.[164–166] Conversely, TGF-β stimulates production of the protease inhibitor, plasminogen activator inhibitor-1.[148] This would act as a negative feedback mechanism for production of active TGF-β by inhibiting the proteases required for activation of latent TGF-β.[110, 148] The relative composition of the extracellular matrix is likely to be important as well. For example, fibronectin promotes the phenotypic modulation of smooth muscle cells to a synthetic proliferative phenotype when cells are placed in culture.[167] In contrast, laminin maintains smooth muscle cells in a contractile form for a prolonged time.[167] At this time, the mechanisms responsible for the ordered dissolution of matrix and its reassembly during vessel remodeling remain to be defined.

**Extracellular Matrix and Growth Factors.** Although many growth factors may have interactions with the extracellular matrix, TGF-β and FGF have the most clearly defined regulatory mechanisms. TGF-β binds to two matrix proteoglycans: betaglycan (type III TGF-β receptor) and decorin.[139] Competition for TGF-β among these receptors may regulate its activity. Because decorin neutralizes TGF-β and its synthesis is stimulated by TGF-β, it may function as a negative regulatory component.

As with TGF-β, binding of FGF to heparan sulfate proteoglycans has been established for several years[168] (Fig. 45–10). This interaction has been thought to serve as both a reservoir of FGF and a proteolytic protective mechanism. It has become clear that heparan sulfate proteoglycans are required for binding of basic FGF to cells, even in the presence of the FGF receptor.[169] Presentation of basic FGF by heparan sulfates may involve its oligomerization or conformational changes. Finally, the membrane heparan sulfate proteoglycan that appears to maintain FGF in an inactive form may be cleaved by glycosylphosphatidylinositol phospholipase C to yield a free heparan sulfate–basic FGF complex.[170] This complex appears to be a powerful mediator of FGF signal transduction.

In summary, the extracellular matrix is a critical regulator of vessel growth and structure by virtue of its own dynamic regulation and because it modulates the activity of both growth-promoting and growth-inhibiting factors.

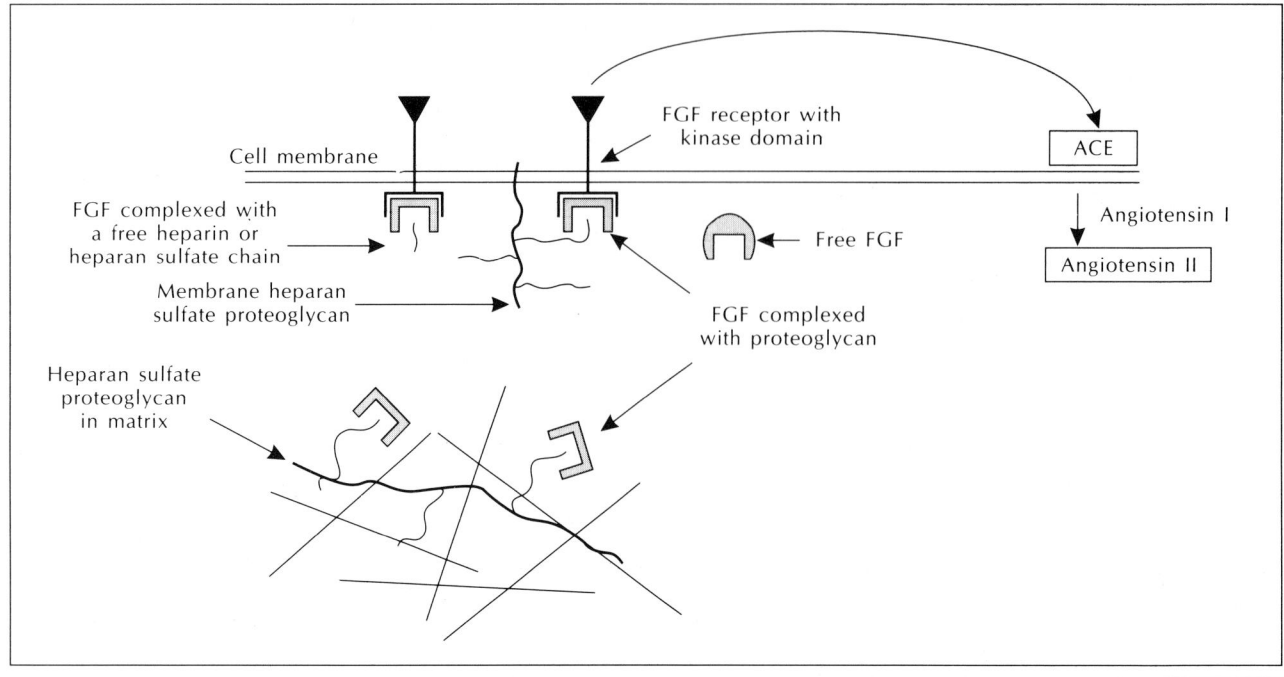

**Figure 45–10.** Interactions of FGF with extracellular matrix and activation by heparan sulfates. FGF is shown in a complex with proteoglycans in an inactive form. Free heparin or heparan sulfate (generated from either matrix or cell membrane) presents FGF in a different conformation that is recognized by the cell-associated FGF receptor. Interactions with other growth factors include induction of ACE. (Modified from Ruoslahti E, Yamaguchi Y: Proteoglycans as modulators of growth factor activities. Cell 64:867, 1991. Copyright by Cell Press.)

## INCREASED GROWTH FACTOR RESPONSIVENESS: SIGNAL TRANSDUCTION AND ION TRANSPORT

### Signal Transduction

The foregoing discussion suggests that the hypertensive vessel exists in a state of increased growth responsiveness that, over time, results in increased numbers and/or size of vascular smooth muscle cells. In addition, these cells appear to have both increased and decreased contractile responses to a variety of factors (measured by median effective concentrations, $EC_{50}$, for a given contractile force). This is puzzling when one considers that if some of these cells have undergone phenotypic modulation they may have relatively less contractile machinery. In addition, it appears that the alterations in sensitivity to contractile agonists (e.g., norepinephrine) include both increases and decreases. This has led to the general hypothesis that alterations in the coupling of vasoactive hormones to intracellular events may be a fundamental genetic abnormality of hypertension. Numerous examples of such alterations exist at all steps of agonist signal transduction, from hormone-receptor binding to stimulation of gene expression. For example, increased contractile responsiveness may be secondary to up-regulation of receptor number as observed with the epidermal growth factor[171] and angiotensin II receptors.[172] Altered agonist affinity, as has been described for norepinephrine,[63] may be a consequence of expression of a different receptor subtype or modulation of receptor affinity by intracellular

receptor modulators such as GTP-binding proteins (G proteins). Decreased contractile responses could be explained by decreased amounts of contractile proteins (myosin and actin). However, this mechanism would primarily cause a decrease in maximal tone rather than sensitivity to constrictors. Thus, the decrease in contractile sensitivity is better explained by alterations in hormone-receptor coupling such as those mediated by G proteins and downstream effectors like phospholipases and protein kinases.

In fact, many alterations in downstream effectors have been demonstrated in SHR-derived cells compared with WKY-derived cells. For example, phospholipase C–mediated phosphoinositide turnover is stimulated by significantly lower concentrations of thrombin and angiotensin II in the SHR.[173] This would have consequences for downstream events mediated by the two second messengers generated by phospholipase C: inositol trisphosphate, which mobilizes intracellular $Ca^{2+}$, and diacylglycerol, which stimulates protein kinase C. In fact, increased protein kinase C activity[66, 67] and increased intracellular $Ca^{2+}$ [174, 175] have been demonstrated in smooth muscle cells from the SHR. The fact that these abnormalities persist in culture suggests that there may be a genetic abnormality in the regulation of these enzymes.

### Ion Transport

Many investigators have suggested that a generalized abnormality in membrane function, especially ion transport, may explain the abnormal contractility and growth of smooth muscle cells from SHR vessels.[176, 177] Increases in cellular $Ca^{2+}$ fluxes, intracellular $Na^+$ concentration, and agonist-induced $Ca^{2+}$ mobilization have been shown in the SHR. In addition, $Na^+$ uptake and the activity of $Na^+$-regulating ion transporters such as the $Na^+,K^+$-ATPase[178, 179] and the $Na^+/H^+$ exchanger[171, 180, 181] have been demonstrated in the SHR. As discussed in the following, the most consistent abnormality in both human essential hypertension and animal models of hypertension has been enhanced $Na^+/H^+$ exchange.

The growth-activated $Na^+/H^+$ exchanger (NHE-1) is a member of a multigene family[75, 134, 135, 179] whose activity is increased in tissues of hypertensive humans and animals. The exchanger extrudes $H^+$ in exchange for one $Na^+$ when decreases in intracellular pH occur. In addition, it is an important regulator of cell volume: when cell shrinkage occurs, $Na^+/H^+$ exchange is activated and restores cell volume by increasing intracellular $Na^+$ (via obligate water entry[182–184]). Rapid increases in $Na^+/H^+$ exchange activity occur on exposure to growth factors and vasoconstrictors.[76, 159] Both activation of protein kinase C and elevation of intracellular $Ca^{2+}$ have been reported to mediate the stimulatory effects of $Na^+/H^+$ exchange.[98, 185–187] This stimulation is characterized by a change in affinity for intracellular $H^+$ and extracellular $Na^+$.[98, 186]

Evidence indicates that the $Na^+/H^+$ exchanger participates in signal transduction pathways by which vasoactive agents modulate vascular tone and regulate smooth muscle cell proliferation.[180, 181, 186, 188] The effect of increased $Na^+/H^+$ exchange on growth would likely be an enhanced sensitivity to mitogens.[181] Increased activity of the $Na^+/H^+$ exchanger could lead to increased vascular tone by two mechanisms. First, increased $Na^+$ entry would activate $Na^+/Ca^{2+}$ exchange, leading to increased intracellular $Ca^{2+}$.[186] Second, increased intracellular pH would enhance the $Ca^{2+}$ sensitivity of the contractile apparatus, leading to an increase in contractility for a given intracellular $Ca^{2+}$ concentration.[186] Because of the activation of the $Na^+/H^+$ exchanger by both hyperplastic and hypertrophic agents, it has been proposed that abnormal function of this protein may be involved in the pathophysiology of hypertension.[177, 186]

Evidence for dysfunction of the $Na^+/H^+$ exchanger in hypertension is provided by observations that its activity is increased in neutrophils, lymphocytes, and platelets from SHRs and in platelets and lymphocytes from hypertensive patients.[177, 186, 189] Data from several laboratories[171, 181] indicate that both cultured smooth muscle cells and intact mesenteric arteries from SHRs[180] have a greater capacity for $Na^+/H^+$ exchange and altered kinetic characteristics compared with those from WKY rats. The report that immortalized lymphoblasts from patients with a family history of essential hypertension had greater $Na^+/H^+$ exchange than lymphoblasts from normotensive patients further suggests that this is a genetic property of hypertension. Yet, restriction fragment length polymorphism[190] and sequence polymorphism[191] analyses demonstrated that the $Na^+/H^+$ exchanger gene itself is not a candidate gene for hypertension. There is no evidence for mutations or altered regulation in several hypertensive populations of this gene. Studies with the SHR have demonstrated increased activity of the

$Na^+/H^+$ exchanger[180, 181] but no change in regulation at the mRNA level.[191a] This suggests that the abnormality in $Na^+/H^+$ exchange is a consequence of a post-translational mechanism. It has become clear that the $Na^+/H^+$ exchanger is regulated by several post-translational mechanisms that may alter its activity. These include phosphorylation, glycosylation, binding of calmodulin, and binding of an accessory protein that may mediate interactions with the cytoskeleton and integrins.[192] Thus alterations in any of these mechanisms might increase $Na^+/H^+$ exchange activity in the SHR.

## UNIFYING HYPOTHESIS

To account for the hypertensive phenotype, several mechanisms of abnormalities in signal transduction and ion transport have been proposed as etiologic. For example, in the SHR, many new insights into the regulation of the kinases and phosphatases responsible for activating and inactivating these patterns suggest that a common regulatory factor or "integrator" may account for multiple changes in hypertensive cells. Unifying hypotheses for this integrator have been based on alterations in ion transport (regulation of intracellular $Na^+$ and $Ca^{2+}$) or alterations in signal transduction mechanisms (kinases and phosphatases).[172, 176, 193, 194] As evidence mounts that many ion transporters are regulated by phosphorylation,[192, 195, 196] these two hypotheses have come together. In particular, genes for many of the ion transporters have been cloned and sequenced. Comparison of normotensive and hypertensive strains of rats has uniformly failed to identify significant differences in the coding sequences of these transport molecules.[189, 197] This has focused attention on the enzymes that regulate the transporters rather than the transporters themselves. Specifically (Fig. 45–11), it is proposed that intracellular signal mediators that are integrators of extracellular stimuli are enhanced in hypertensive smooth muscle cells and these

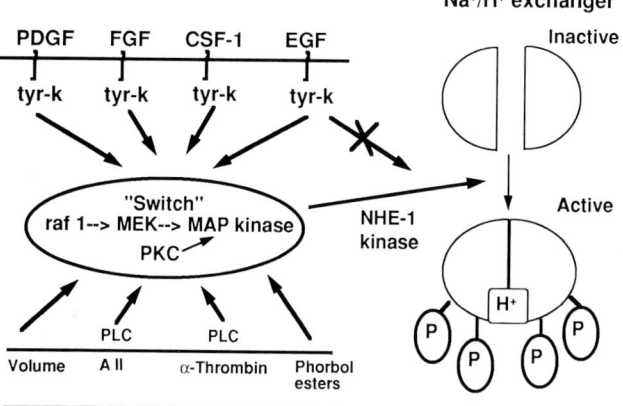

**Figure 45–11.** Model for activation of $Na^+/H^+$ exchanger by receptor-coupled kinase cascade. Multiple stimuli including both tyrosine kinases (tyr-k) coupled to growth factor receptors and vasoactive mediators (volume, angiotensin II [AII], α-thrombin, and phorbol esters) activate the MAP kinase. The MAP kinase now stimulates downstream effector kinases (e.g., the $Na^+/H^+$ exchanger [NHE-1] kinase), which activate intracellular ion transporters such as the exchanger.

mediators in turn affect common regulatory events such as ion fluxes and cell cycle genes that cause both increased tone and growth.[66, 67]

By using the $Na^+/H^+$ exchanger as an example, an alteration in phosphorylation of the exchanger would be a likely mechanism as it would explain both increased smooth muscle cell growth and function. A variety of growth factors phosphorylate the $Na^+/H^+$ exchanger and this increases its affinity for intracellular $H^+$.[195] It is now known that these growth factors activate a cascade of intracellular kinases that include Raf kinase, the mitogen-activated protein kinase (MAP kinase), and the MAP kinase kinase (or MEK-1, MAP kinase/ERK [extracellular-regulated kinase] kinase).[198, 199] Inhibiting these kinases by overexpressing a dominant negative mutant of MAP kinase inhibits growth factor–stimulated mitogenesis and $Na^+/H^+$ exchange activity.[200] Conversely, an increase in the activity of one of these kinases would increase activity of many growth factors because it acts as a convergence or integration point for multiple stimuli. The increase in kinase activity could arise by several mechanisms: a primary abnormality in its structure that causes increased activity, an abnormality in its regulation that causes it to be overexpressed (increased synthesis or decreased degradation), and a change in the enzymes that regulate its activity (e.g., a phosphatase that inactivates the kinase or a kinase that activates it). Future work in this rapidly developing field should yield many candidate kinases and phosphatases to mediate these effects. Based on these findings, it appears reasonable that alterations in the function of these intracellular enzymes may cause the multiple abnormalities in smooth muscle cell ion transport and growth that are the hallmarks of hypertension at the cellular level.

## SUMMARY

The hypertensive vessel wall is typified by abnormalities in structure and function. These alterations include increased smooth muscle cell mass relative to lumen size with an increase in vascular resistance mediated at the level of the resistance arterioles. This appears to be due to a primary abnormality in smooth muscle cell growth regulation that is caused by genetic, environmental, and hemodynamic factors. Genetic analysis suggests that five or six genes are responsible for essential hypertension.[201] The establishment of transgenic mice and rats[202] that express candidate gene abnormalities should enable the role of these genes to be studied in a tissue-specific manner. Ultimately, defining the specific events that alter vascular cell–specific function to a hypertensive phenotype will permit therapy that is more effective in preventing chronic end-organ damage.

## REFERENCES

1. Chobanian AV: Corcoran lecture: Adaptive and maladaptative responses of the arterial wall to hypertension. Hypertension 15:666, 1990.
2. Mulvany MJ, Aalkjaer C: Structure and function of small arteries. Physiol Rev 70:921, 1990.
3. Mulvany MJ: Abnormalities of resistance vessel structure in essential hypertension. Clin Exp Pharmacol Physiol 18:13, 1991.
4. Heagerty AM: Changes in vascular morphology in essential hypertension. J Hum Hypertens 1:3, 1991.
5. Heagerty AM, Aalkjaer C, Bund SJ, et al: Small artery structure in hypertension. Dual processes of remodeling and growth. Hypertension 21:391, 1993.
6. Ku DN, Giddens DP, Zarins CK, Glagov S: Pulsatile flow and atherosclerosis in the human carotid bifurcation. Positive correlation between plaque location and low oscillating shear stress. Arteriosclerosis 5:293, 1985.
7. Korsgaard N, Mulvany MJ: Cellular hyertrophy in mesenteric resistance vessels from renal hypertensive rats. Hypertension 12:162, 1988.
8. Mulvany MJ, Baadrup U, Gundersen HJG: Evidence for hyperplasia in mesenteric resistance vessels of spontaneously hypertensive rats using a three-dimensional dissector. Circ Res 57:794, 1985.
9. Mulvany MJ, Hansen PK, Aalkjaer C: Direct evidence that the greater contractility of resistance vessels in spontaneously hypertensive rats is associated with a narrower lumen, a thicker media and a greater number of smooth muscle cell layers. Circ Res 43:854, 1978.
10. Owens G, Schwartz S: Alterations in vascular smooth muscle mass in the spontaneously hypertensive rat. Role of cellular hypertrophy, hyperploidy and hyperplasia. Circ Res 51:280, 1982.
11. Owens GK: Influence of blood pressure on development of aortic medial smooth muscle hypertrophy in spontaneously hypertensive rats. Hypertension 9:178, 1987.
12. Schwartz SM, Majesky MW, Dilley RJ: Vascular remodeling in hypertension and atherosclerosis. In Laragh J, Brenner BM (eds): Hypertension: Pathophysiology, Diagnosis and Management. Raven Press, New York, 1990, p 521.
13. Short D: Morphology of the intestinal arterioles in chronic human hypertension. Br Heart J 28:184, 1966.
14. Lund-Johansen P: Haemodynamics in essential hypertension. State of the art review. Clin Sci 59:343, 1980.
15. Folkow B, Grimby G, Thulesius O: Adaptive structural changes of the vascular walls in hypertension and their relation to the control of peripheral resistance. Acta Physiol Scand 44:255, 1958.
16. Harper RN, Moore MA, Marr MC, et al: Arteriolar rarefaction in the conjunctiva of human essential hypertensives. Microvasc Res 16:369, 1978.
17. Harrison DG, Treasure CB, Mugge A, et al: Hypertension and the coronary circulation. With special attention to endothelial regulation. Am J Hypertens 4:454, 1991.
18. Heistad DD, Baumbach GL: Cerebral vascular changes during chronic hypertension: Good guys and bad guys. J Hypertens Suppl 10:S71, 1992.
19. Aalkjaer C, Danielsen H, Johannesen P, et al: Abnormal vascular function and morphology in preeclampsia: A study of isolated resistance vessels. Clin Sci 69:477, 1985.
20. Aalkjaer C, Pedersen EB, Danielsen H, et al: Morphological and functional characteristics of isolated resistance vessels in advanced uraemia. Clin Sci 71:657, 1976.
21. Aalkjaer C, Heagerty AM, Peterson KK, et al: Evidence for increased media thickness, increased neuronal amine uptake, and depressed excitation-contraction coupling in isolated resistance vessels from essential hypertensives. Circ Res 61:181, 1987.
22. Bohlen HG, Gore RW, Hutchins PM: Comparison of micro vascular pressures in normal and spontaneously hypertensive rats. Microvasc Res 13:125, 1977.
23. Schiffrin EL, Deng LY, Larochelle P: Blunted effects of endothelin upon small subcutaneous resistance arteries of mild essential hypertensive patients. J Hypertens 10:437, 1992.
24. Mulvany MJ: Vascular structure and smooth muscle contractility in experimental hypertension. J Cardiovasc Pharmacol 6(suppl):S79, 1987.
25. Jespersen LT, Nyborg NCB, Pedersen OL, et al: Cardiac mass and peripheral vascular structure in hydralazine-treated spontaneously hypertensive rats. Hypertension 7:734, 1985.
26. Mulvany MJ, Nyborg N: An increased calcium sensitivity of mesenteric resistance vessels in young and adult spontaneously hypertensive rats. Br J Pharmacol 71:585, 1980.
27. Mulvany MJ, Nilsson H, Nyborg N, Mikkelsen E: Are isolated femoral resistance vessels or tail arteries good models for the hindquarter vasculature of spontaneously hypertensive rats? Acta Physiol Scand 116:275, 1982.
28. Korsgaard N, Aalkjaer C, Heagerty AM, et al: Histology of subcu-

taneous small arteries from patients with essential hypertension. Hypertension 22:523, 1993.

29. Owens GK: Differential effects of antihypertensive drug therapy on vascular smooth muscle cell hypertrophy, hyperploidy and hyperplasia in the spontaneously hypertensive rat. Circ Res 56:525, 1985.

30. Griffin SA, Brown WC, MacPherson F, et al: Angiotensin II causes vascular hypertrophy in part by a non-pressor mechanism. Hypertension 17:626, 1991.

31. Christensen KL: Reducing pulse pressure in hypertension may normalize small artery structure. Hypertension 18:722, 1991.

32. Geisterfer AAT, Peach MJ, Owens GK: Angiotensin II induces hypertrophy, not hyperplasia, of cultured rat aortic smooth muscle cells. Circ Res 62:749, 1988.

33. Berk BC, Vekshtein V, Gordon HM, Tsuda T: Angiotensin II–stimulated protein synthesis in cultured vascular smooth muscle cells. Hypertension 13:305, 1989.

34. Stouffer GA, Owens GK: Angiotensin II–induced mitogenesis of spontaneously hypertensive rat–derived cultured smooth muscle cells is dependent on autocrine production of transforming growth factor-beta. Circ Res 70:820, 1992.

35. Halpern W, Warshaw DM, Mulvany MJ: Mechanical and morphological properties of arterial resistance vessels in young and old spontaneously hypertensive rats. Circ Res 45:250, 1979.

36. Lee RMKW, Triggle CR, Cheung DWT, Coughlin MD: Structural and functional consequence of neonatal sympathectomy on the blood vessels of spontaneously hypertensive rats. Hypertension 10:328, 1987.

37. Thomas WA, Lee KT, Kim DN: Cell population kinetics in atherogenesis. Cell births and losses in intimal cell mass-derived lesions in the abdominal aorta of swine. Ann N Y Acad Sci 454:305, 1985.

38. Schwartz SM, Reidy MR, Clowes A: Kinetics of atherosclerosis: A stem cell model. Ann N Y Acad Sci 454:292, 1985.

39. Majesky MW, Giachelli CM, Reidy MA, Schwartz SM: Rat carotid neointimal smooth muscle cells reexpress a developmentally regulated mRNA phenotype during repair of arterial injury. Circ Res 71:759, 1992.

40. Davies PF: Endothelial cells, hemodynamic forces, and the localization of atherosclerosis. *In* Ryan US (ed): Endothelial Cells, Vol II. CRC Press, Boca Raton, FL, 1988, p 123.

41. Davies PF: How do vascular endothelial cells respond to flow? News Physiol Sci 4:22, 1989.

42. Mitsumata M, Fishel RS, Nerem RM, et al: Fluid shear stress stimulates platelet-derived growth factor expression in endothelial cells. Am J Physiol 265:H3, 1993.

43. Howard PS, Myers JC, Gorfien SF, Macarak EJ: Progressive modulation of endothelial phenotype during in vitro blood vessel formation. Dev Biol 146:325, 1991.

44. Saouaf R, Takasaki I, Eastman E, et al: Fibronectin biosynthesis in the rat aorta in vitro: Changes due to experimental hypertension. J Clin Invest 88:1182, 1991.

45. Takasaki I, Chobanian AV, Sarzani P, Brecher P: Effects of hypertension on fibronectin expression in the rat aorta. J Biol Chem 265:21935, 1990.

46. Langille BL, O'Donnell F: Reductions in arterial diameter produced by chronic decreases in blood flow are endothelium-dependent. Science 231:405, 1986.

47. Langille BL, Brownlee RD, Adamson SL: Perinatal aortic growth in lambs: Relation to blood flow changes at birth. Am J Physiol 259:H1247, 1990.

48. Kohler TR, Kirkman TR, Kraiss LW, et al: Increased blood flow inhibits neointimal hyperplasia in endothelialized vascular grafts. Circ Res 69:1557, 1991.

49. Thybo NK, Korsgaard N, Mulvany MJ: Morphology and function of mesenteric resistance arteries in transgenic rats with low-renin hypertension. J Hypertens 10:1191, 1992.

50. Crawford DW, Blankenhorn DH: Arterial wall oxygenation, oxyradicals, and atherosclerosis. Atherosclerosis 89:97, 1991.

51. Halliwell B: Free radicals, reactive oxygen species and human disease: A critical evaluation with special reference to atherosclerosis. Br J Exp Pathol 70:737, 1989.

52. Crawford DW, Back LH, Cole MA, et al: In vivo oxygen transport in the normal rabbit femoral arterial wall. J Clin Invest 65:1498, 1980.

53. Dohi Y, Thiel MA, Buhler FR, Lüscher TF: Activation of endothelial L-arginine pathway in resistance arteries: Effect of age and hypertension. Hypertension 15:170, 1990.

54. Lüscher TF, Vanhoutte PM: Endothelium-dependent contractions to acetylcholine in the aorta of the spontaneously hypertensive rat. Hypertension 8:344, 1986.

55. Dohi Y, Lüscher TF: Endothelin in hypertensive resistance arteries. Intraluminal and extraluminal dysfunction. Hypertension 18:543, 1991.

56. Diederich D, Yang Z, Buhler FR, Lüscher TF: Impaired endothelium-dependent relaxations in hypertensive resistance arteries involve the cyclooxygenase pathway. Am J Physiol 258:H445, 1990.

57. Hunter GC, Dubick MA, Keen CL, Eskelson CD: Effects of hypertension on aortic antioxidant status in human abdominal aneurysmal and occlusive disease. Proc Soc Exp Biol Med 196:273, 1991.

58. Cuccurullo F, Porreca E, Lapenna D, et al: Aortic glutathione-related antioxidant defenses in rabbits subjected to suprarenal aortic coarctation hypertension. J Mol Cell Cardiol 23:727, 1991.

59. Nakazono K, Watanabe N, Matsuno K, et al: Does superoxide underlie the pathogenesis of hypertension? Proc Natl Acad Sci USA 88:10045, 1991.

60. Lüscher TF, Boulanger CM, Dohi Y, Yang ZH: Endothelium-derived contracting factors. Hypertension 19:117, 1992.

61. Campbell-Chamley JH, Campbell GR: What controls smooth muscle phenotype? Atherosclerosis 40:347–357, 1981.

62. Falloon BJ, Bund SJ, Tulip JR, Heagerty AM: In vitro perfusion studies of resistance artery function in genetic hypertension. Hypertension 22:486, 1993.

63. Nyborg NCB, Bevan JA: Increased alpha-adrenergic receptor affinity in resistance vessels from hypertensive rats. Hypertension 11:635, 1988.

64. Webb RC, Schreur KD, Papadopoulos SM: Oscillatory contractions in vertebral arteries from hypertensive subjects. Clin Physiol 12:69, 1992.

65. Lamb FS, Webb RC: Potassium conductance and oscillatory contractions in tail arteries from genetically hypertensive rats. J Hypertens 7:457, 1989.

66. Takaori K, Itoh S, Kanayama Y, Takeda T: Protein kinase C activity in platelets from spontaneously hypertensive rats (SHR) and normotensive Wistar Kyoto rats (WKY). Biochem Biophys Res Commun 141:769, 1986.

67. Silver PJ, Lepore RE, Cumiskey WR, et al: Protein kinase C activity and reactivity to phorbol ester in vascular smooth muscle from spontaneously hypertensive rats (SHR) and normotensive Wistar Kyoto rats (WKY). Biochem Biophys Res Commun 154:272, 1988.

68. Berk BC, Alexander RW, Brock TA, et al: Vasoconstriction: a new activity for platelet-derived growth factor. Science 232:87, 1986.

69. Yamori Y, Mano M, Nara Y, Horie R: Catecholamine-induced polyploidization in aortic smooth muscle cells of hypertensive rats. Circulation 75:I92, 1987.

70. Leitschuh M, Chobanian AV: Inhibition of nuclear polyploidy by propranolol in aortic smooth muscle cells of hypertensive rats. Hypertension 9(suppl III):III106, 1987.

71. Bevan RD, Tsuru H: Functional and structural changes in the rabbit ear artery after sympathetic denervation. Circ Res 49:478, 1981.

72. Bevan RD: Effect of sympathetic denervation on smooth muscle cell proliferation in the growing rabbit ear artery. Circ Res 37:14, 1975.

73. Panza JA, Quyyumi AA, Brush JE, Epstein SE: Abnormal endothelium-dependent vascular relaxation in patients with essential hypertension. N Engl J Med 323:22, 1990.

74. Lüscher TF, Diederich D, Weber E, et al: Endothelium-dependent responses in carotid and renal arteries of normotensive and hypertensive rats. Hypertension 11:573, 1988.

75. Linder L, Kiowski W, Buhler FR, Lüscher TF: Indirect evidence for the release of endothelium-derived relaxing factor in human forearm circulation in vivo: Blunted response in essential hypertension. Circulation 81:1762, 1990.

76. Furchgott RF, Zawadzki JV: The obligatory role of endothelial cells in the relaxation of arterial smooth muscle by acetylcholine. Nature 288:373, 1980.

77. Palmer RMJ, Ashton DS, Moncada S: Vascular endothelial cells synthesize NO from L-arginine. Nature 333:664, 1988.

78. Palmer RMJ, Ferrige AG, Moncada S: Nitric oxide accounts for the biological activity of endothelium-derived relaxing factor. Nature 327:524, 1987.

79. Radomsky MW, Palmer RMJ, Moncada S: The anti-aggregatory properties of vascular endothelium: Interactions between prostacyclin and nitric oxide. Br J Pharmacol 92:639, 1987.

80. Garg UC, Hassid A: Nitric oxide–generating vasodilators and 8-bromo-cyclic guanosine monophosphate inhibit mitogenesis and proliferation of cultured rat vascular smooth muscle cells. J Clin Invest 83:1774, 1989.

81. Sowers JR: Insulin resistance, hyperinsulinemia, dyslipidemia, hypertension, and accelerated atherosclerosis. J Clin Pharmacol 32:529, 1992.

82. Lüscher TF, Vanhoutte PM, Raij L: Antihypertensive treatment normalizes decreased endothelium-dependent relaxations in rats with salt-induced hypertension. Hypertension 9:III-193, 1987.

83. Navab M, Imes SS, Hama SY, et al: Monocyte transmigration induced by modification of low density lipoprotein in cocultures of human aortic wall cells is due to induction of monocyte chemotactic protein 1 synthesis and is abolished by high density lipoprotein. J Clin Invest 88:2039, 1991.

84. Fabbrini MS, Vitale A, Patrano C, et al: Heterologous in vivo processing of human preproendothelin 1 into bioactive peptides. Proc Natl Acad Sci USA 88:8939, 1991.

85. Boulanger C, Lüscher TF: Release of endothelin from the porcine aorta: Inhibition by endothelium-derived nitric oxide. J Clin Invest 85:587, 1990.

86. Yang Z, Stulz P, von Segesser L, et al: Different activation of the endothelial L-arginine and cyclooxygenase pathway in the human internal mammary artery and saphenous vein. Circ Res 68:52, 1991.

87. Feletou M, Vanhoutte PM: Endothelium-dependent hyperpolarization of canine coronary smooth muscle. Br J Pharmacol 93:352, 1988.

88. Owens GK: Control of hypertrophic versus hyperplastic growth of vascular smooth muscle cells. Am J Physiol 257:H1755, 1989.

89. Scott-Burden T, Hahn AW, Buhler FR, Resink TJ: Vasoactive peptides and growth factors in the pathophysiology of hypertension. J Cardiovasc Pharmacol 20 (suppl 1):S55, 1992.

90. Carretero OA, Scicli AG: Local hormonal factors (intracrine, autocrine, and paracrine) in hypertension. Hypertension 18(suppl):I58, 1991.

91. De Mey JG, Schiffers PM: Effects of the endothelium on growth responses in arteries. J Cardiovasc Pharmacol 21(suppl 1):S22, 1993.

92. Dzau VJ, Gibbons GH: Endothelium and growth factors in vascular remodeling of hypertension. Hypertension 18(suppl III):III-115, 1991.

93. Geisterfer AAT, Owens GK: Arginine vasopressin–induced hypertrophy of cultured rat aortic smooth muscle cells. Hypertension 14:413, 1989.

94. Blaes N, Boissel JP: Growth stimulating effect of catecholamines on rat aortic smooth muscle cells in culture. J Cell Physiol 116:167, 1983.

95. Nakaki T, Nakayama M, Yamamoto S, Kato R: $\alpha_1$-Adrenergic stimulation and $\beta_2$-adrenergic inhibition of DNA synthesis in vascular smooth muscle cells. Mol Pharmacol 37:30, 1990.

96. Printseva OY, Tjurmin AV, Rudchenko SA, Repin VS: Noradrenaline induces the polyploidization of smooth muscle cells: The synergism of second messengers. Exp Cell Res 184:342, 1989.

97. Hamada M, Nishio I, Baba A, et al: Enhanced DNA synthesis of cultured vascular smooth muscle cells from spontaneously hypertensive rats: Difference of response to growth factor, intracellular free calcium concentration and DNA synthesizing cell cycle. Atherosclerosis 81:191, 1990.

98. Berk BC, Aronow MS, Brock TA, et al: Angiotensin II-stimulated $Na^+/H^+$ exchange in cultured vascular smooth muscle cells. Evidence for protein kinase C–dependent and –independent pathways. J Biol Chem 262:5065, 1987.

99. Taubman MB, Berk BC, Izumo S, et al: Angiotensin II induction of c-*fos* mRNA in aortic smooth muscle involves $Ca^{2+}$ mobilization and protein kinase C activation. J Biol Chem 264:526, 1989.

100. Daemen MJAP, Lombardi DM, Bosman FT, Schwartz SM: Angiotensin II induces smooth muscle cell proliferation in the normal and injured rat arterial wall. Circ Res 68:450, 1991.

101. Powell JS, Clozel JP, Muller RKM, et al: Inhibitors of angiotensin-converting enzyme prevent myointimal proliferation after vascular injury. Science 245:186, 1989.

102. Farhy RD, Carretero OA, Ho K-L, Scicli AG: Role of kinins and nitric oxide in the effects of angiotensin converting enzyme inhibitors on neointima formation. Circ Res 72:1202, 1993.

103. Saed GM, Carretero OA, MacDonald RJ, Scicli AG: Kallikrein messenger RNA in rat arteries and veins. Circ Res 67:510, 1990.

104. Oza NB, Schwartz JH, Goud HD, Levinsky NG: Rat aortic smooth muscle cells in culture express kallikrein, kininogen, and bradykininase activity. J Clin Invest 85:597, 1990.

105. van Kleef EM, Smits JFM, De Mey JGR, et al: Alpha 1–adrenergic blockade reduces the angiotensin II–induced vascular smooth muscle cell DNA synthesis in the rat thoracic aorta and carotid artery. Circ Res 70:1122, 1992.

106. Dzau VJ: Circulating versus local renin-angiotensin system in cardiovascular homeostasis. Circulation 77:4, 1988.

107. Dzau VJ, Gibbons GH, Pratt RE: Molecular mechanisms of vascular renin-angiotensin system in neointimal hyperplasia. Hypertension 18(suppl II):II-100, 1991.

108. Naftilan AJ, Zuo WM, Inglefinger J, et al: Localization and differential regulation of angiotensinogen mRNA expression in the vessel wall. J Clin Invest 87:1300, 1991.

109. Dasarathy Y, Fanburg BL: Involvement of second messenger systems in stimulation of angiotensin converting enzyme of bovine endothelial cells. J Cell Physiol 148:327, 1991.

110. Berk BC, Corson MA: Autocrine and paracrine growth mechanisms in vascular smooth muscle. Curr Opin Cardiol 7:739, 1992.

111. Gibbons GH, Pratt RE, Dzau VJ: Vascular smooth muscle cell hypertrophy vs. hyperplasia. Autocrine transforming growth factor beta expression determines growth response to angiotensin II. J Clin Invest 90:456, 1992.

112. Koibuchi Y, Lee WS, Gibbons GH, Pratt RE: Role of transforming growth factor-beta1 in the cellular growth response to angiotensin II. Hypertension 21:1046, 1993.

113. Hahn AW, Resink TJ, Bernhardt J, et al: Stimulation of autocrine platelet-derived growth factor AA homodimer and transforming growth factor β in vascular smooth muscle cells. Biochem Biophys Res Commun 178:1451, 1991.

114. Berk BC, Rao GN: Angiotensin II–induced vascular smooth muscle cell hypertrophy: PDGF A-chain mediates the increase in cell size. J Cell Physiol 154:368, 1993.

115. Murphy TJ, Alexander RW, Griendling KK, et al: Isolation of a cDNA encoding the vascular type-1 angiotensin II receptor. Nature 351:233, 1991.

116. Sasaki K, Yamamo Y, Bardham S, et al: Cloning and expression of a complementary DNA encoding a bovine adrenal angiotensin type-1 receptor. Nature 351:230, 1991.

117. Majesky MW, Daemen MJAP, Schwartz SM: Alpha 1-adrenergic stimulation of platelet-derived growth factor A-chain gene expression in aorta. J Biol Chem 265:1082, 1990.

118. Bobik A, Grinpukel S, Little PJ, et al: Angiotensin II and noradrenaline increase PDGF BB receptors and potentiate PDGF BB stimulated DNA synthesis in vascular smooth muscle. Biochem Biophys Res Commun 166:580, 1990.

119. Hirata Y, Takagi Y, Fukuda Y, Maruma F: Endothelin is a potent mitogen for rat vascular smooth muscle cells. Atherosclerosis 78:225, 1989.

120. Bobik A, Grooms A, Millar JA, et al: Growth factor activity of endothelin on vascular smooth muscle. Am J Physiol 258:C409, 1990.

121. Scott-Burden T, Resink TJ, Hahn AW, Vanhoutte P: Induction of endothelin secretion by angiotensin II: effects on growth and synthetic activity of vascular smooth muscle cells. J Cardiovasc Pharmacol 17(suppl 7):S96, 1991.

122. Murase T, Kozawa O, Miwa M, et al: Regulation of proliferation by vasopressin in aortic smooth muscle cells: function of protein kinase C. Hypertension 10:1505, 1992.

123. Vallotton MB, Wthrich RP, Lew PD, Capponi AM: Effects of vasopressin and its analogues on rat aortic smooth muscle and renal medullary tubular cells: Characterization of receptor subtypes. J Cardiovasc Pharmacol 1986:S5, 1986.

124. Hassid A, Williams C: Vasoconstrictor-evoked prostaglandin synthesis in cultured vascular smooth muscle cells. Am J Physiol 245:C278, 1983.

125. Loesberg C, van Wijk R, Zandvergen J, et al: Cell cycle–dependent inhibition of human vascular smooth muscle cell proliferation by prostaglandin $E_1$. Exp Cell Res 160:117, 1985.

126. Morisaki N, Kanzaki T, Motoyama N, et al: Cell cycle–dependent inhibition of DNA synthesis by prostaglandin $E_2$ in cultured rabbit aortic smooth muscle cells. Atherosclerosis 71:165, 1988.

127. Libby P, Warner SJC, Salomon RN, Birinyi LK: Production of platelet-derived growth factor–like mitogen by smooth-muscle cells from human aorta. N Engl J Med 318:1493, 1988.

128. Seifert RA, Hart CE, Philiphs PE, et al: Two different subunits associate to create isoform-specific platelet-derived growth factor receptors. J Biol Chem 264:8771, 1989.

129. Sarzani R, Arnaldi G, Chobanian AV: Hypertension-induced changes of platelet-derived growth factor receptor expression in rat aorta and heart. Hypertension 17:888, 1991.

130. Sarzani R, Arnaldi G, Takasaki I, et al: Effects of hypertension and aging on platelet-derived growth factor receptor expression in rat aorta and heart. Hypertension 18(suppl III):III-93, 1991.

131. Sara VR, Hall K: Insulin-like growth factors and their binding proteins. Physiol Rev 70:591, 1990.

132. Fath KA, Alexander RW, Delafontaine P: Abdominal coarctation increases insulin-like growth factor I mRNA levels in rat aorta. Circ Res 72:271, 1993.

133. Delafontaine P, Lou H: Angiotensin II regulates insulin-like growth factor I gene expression in vascular smooth muscle cells. J Biol Chem 268:16866, 1993.

134. Badesch DB, Lee PDK, Parks WC, Stenmark KR: Insulin-like growth factor stimulates elastin synthesis by bovine pulmonary arterial smooth muscle cells. Biochem Biophys Res Commun 160:382, 1989.

135. Goldstein RH, Polliks CF, Pilch PF, et al: Stimulation of collagen formation by insulin and insulin-like growth factor I in culture of human lung fibroblasts. Endocrinology 124:964, 1989.

136. Hamet P, Hadrava V, Kruppa V, Tremblay J: Transforming growth factor beta 1 expression and effect in aortic smooth muscle cells from spontaneously hypertensive rats. Hypertension 17:896, 1991.

137. Sarzani R, Brecher P, Chobanian AV: Growth factor expression in aorta of normotensive and hypertensive rats. J Clin Invest 83:1404, 1989.

138. Majesky MW, Linder V, Twardzik DR, et al: Production of transforming growth factor beta-1 during repair of arterial injury. J Clin Invest 88:904, 1991.

139. Ruoslahti E, Yamaguchi Y: Proteoglycans as modulators of growth factor activities. Cell 64:867, 1991.

140. Battegay EJ, Raines EW, Seifert RA, et al: TGF-B1 induces bimodal proliferation of connective tissue cells via complex control of an autocrine PDGF loop. Cell 63:515, 1990.

141. Gronwald RGK, Seifert RA, Bowen-Pope DF: Differential regulation of expression of two platelet-derived growth factor receptor subunits by transforming growth factor-beta. J Biol Chem 264:8120, 1989.

142. Janat MF, Liau G: Transforming growth factor beta 1 is a powerful modulator of platelet-derived growth factor action in vascular smooth muscle cells. J Cell Physiol 150:232, 1992.

143. Majack RA, Majesky MW, Goodman LV: Role of PDGF-A expression in the control of vascular smooth muscle cell growth by transforming growth factor-beta. J Cell Biol 111:239, 1990.

144. Owens GK, Geisterfer AAT, Yang Y, Komoriya A: Transforming growth factor beta induced growth inhibition and cellular hypertrophy in cultured vascular smooth muscle cells. J Cell Biol 107:771, 1988.

145. Hahn AW, Resink TJ, Scott BT, et al: Stimulation of endothelin mRNA and secretion in rat vascular smooth muscle cells: A novel autocrine function. Cell Regul 1:649, 1990.

146. Cheifetz S, Hernandez H, Laiho M, et al: Determinants of cellular responsiveness to the three transforming growth factor-β isoforms. J Biol Chem 265:20533, 1990.

147. Wang X-F, Lin HY, Ng-Eaton E, et al: Expression cloning and characterization of the TGF-β type III receptor. Cell 67:797, 1991.

148. Sato Y, Tsuboi R, Lyons R, et al: Characterization of the activation of latent TGF-beta by co-cultures of endothelial cells and pericytes or smooth muscle cells: A self-regulating system. J Cell Biol 111:757, 1990.

149. Chen JK, Hoshi H, McKeehan WL: Transforming growth factor type beta specifically stimulates synthesis of proteoglycan in human adult arterial smooth muscle cells. Proc Natl Acad Sci USA 84:5287, 1987.

150. Winkles JA, Gay CG: Regulated expression of PDGF A-chain mRNA in human saphenous vein smooth muscle cells. Biochem Biophys Res Commun 180:519, 1991.

151. Okabe T, Yamagata K, Fujisawa M, et al: Induction by fibroblast growth factor of angiotensin converting enzyme in vascular endothelial cells in vitro. Biochem Biophys Res Commun 145:1211, 1987.

152. Sato Y, Hamanaka R, Ono J, et al: The stimulatory effect of PDGF on vascular smooth muscle cell migration is mediated by the induction of endogenous basic FGF. Biochem Biophys Res Commun 174:1260, 1991.

153. Koller KJ, Goeddel DV: Molecular biology of the natriuretic peptides and their receptors. Circulation 86:1081, 1992.

154. Suga S-I, Nakao K, Kishimoto I, et al: Phenotype-related alteration in expression of natriuretic peptide receptor in aortic smooth muscle cells. Circ Res 71:34, 1992.

155. Nakao K, Ogawa Y, Suga S-I, Imura H: Molecular biology and biochemistry of the natriuretic peptide system. II: Natriuretic peptide receptors. J Hypertens 10:1111, 1992.

156. Itoh H, Pratt IH, Dzau VJ: Atrial natriuretic polypeptide inhibits hypertrophy of vascular smooth muscle cells. J Clin Invest 86:1690, 1990.

157. Gardner DG, Deschepper CF, Baxter JD: The gene for the atrial natriuretic factor is expressed in the aortic arch. Hypertension 9:103, 1987.

158. Mourlon-Le Grand MC, Poitevin P, Benessiano J, et al: Effect of a nonhypotensive long-term infusion of ANP on the mechanical and structural properties of the arterial wall in Wistar-Kyoto and spontaneously hypertensive rats. Arterioscler Thromb 13:640, 1993.

159. Suga S-I, Nakao K, Itoh H, et al: Endothelial production of C-type natriuretic peptide and its marked augmentation by transforming growth factor B. J Clin Invest 90:1145, 1992.

160. Komatsu Y, Nakao K, Itoh H, et al: Vascular natriuretic peptide. Lancet 340:622, 1992.

161. Porter JG, Catalano R, McEnroe G, et al: C-type natriuretic peptide inhibits growth factor-independent synthesis in smooth muscle cells. Am J Physiol 263:C1001, 1992.

162. Wagner WD: Proteoglycan structure and function as related to atherosclerosis. Ann N Y Acad Sci 454:52, 1985.

163. Au YP, Montgomery KF, Clowes AW: Heparin inhibits collagenase gene expression mediated by phorbol ester–responsive element in primate arterial smooth muscle cells. Circ Res 70:1062, 1992.

164. Au YP, Kenagy RD, Clowes AW: Heparin selectively inhibits the transcription of tissue-type plasminogen activator in primate arterial smooth muscle cells during mitogenesis. J Biol Chem 267:3438, 1992.

165. Clowes AW, Clowes MM, Au YP, et al: Smooth muscle cells express urokinase during mitogenesis and tissue-type plasminogen activator during migration in injured rat carotid artery. Circ Res 67:61, 1990.

166. Clowes AW, Clowes MM, Kirkman TR, et al: Heparin inhibits the expression of tissue-type plasminogen activator by smooth muscle cells in injured rat carotid artery. Circ Res 70:1128, 1992.

167. Hedin U, Bottger BA, Forsberg E, et al: Diverse effects of fibronectin and laminin on the phenotypic properties of cultured arterial smooth muscle cells. J Cell Biol 107:307, 1988.

168. Burgess WH, Maciag T: The heparin-binding (fibroblast) growth factor family of proteins. Annu Rev Biochem 58:575, 1989.

169. Yayon A, Klagsbrun M, Esko JD, et al: Cell surface, heparin-like molecules are required for binding of basic fibroblast growth factor to its high affinity receptor. Cell 64:841, 1991.

170. Bashkin P, Neufeld G, Gitay GH, Vlodavsky I: Release of cell surface–associated basic fibroblast growth factor by glycosylphosphatidylinositol-specific phospholipase C. J Cell Physiol 151:126, 1992.

171. Scott-Burden T, Resink TJ, Baur U, et al: Epidermal growth factor responsiveness in smooth muscle cells from hypertensive and normotensive rats. Hypertension 13:295, 1989.

172. Berk BC, Vallega G, Muslin AJ, et al: Spontaneously hypertensive rat vascular smooth muscle cells in culture exhibit increased growth and Na⁺/H⁺ exchange. J Clin Invest 83:822, 1989.

173. Koutouzov S, Remmal A, Marche P, Meyer P: Hypersensitivity of phospholipase C in platelets of spontaneously hypertensive rats. Hypertension 10:497, 1987.

174. Bhalla RC, Webb RC, Singh D, et al: Calcium fluxes, calcium binding, and adenosine cyclic 3′,5′-monophosphate–dependent protein kinase activity in the aorta of spontaneously hypertensive and Kyoto Wistar normotensive rats. Mol Pharmacol 14:468, 1978.

175. Oshima T, Young EW, Bukoski RD, McCarron DA: Abnormal calcium handling by platelets of spontaneously hypertensive rats. Hypertension 15:606, 1990.

176. Resnick LM, Gupta RK, Lewanczuk RZ, et al: Intracellular ions in salt-sensitive essential hypertension: Possible role of calcium-regulating hormones. Contrib Nephrol 90:88, 1991.

177. Rosskopf D, Dusing R, Siffert W: Membrane sodium-proton exchange and primary hypertension. Hypertension 21:607, 1993.

178. Friedman SM: Evidence for enhanced sodium transport in the tail artery of the spontaneously hypertensive rat. Hypertension 1:572, 1979.

179. Tamura H, Hopp L, Kino M, et al: Na⁺-K⁺ regulation in cultured vascular smooth muscle cells of the spontaneously hypertensive rat. Am J Physiol 250:C939, 1986.

180. Foster CD, Hill WAG, Honeyman TW, Scheid CR: Characterization of Na⁺-H⁺ exchange in segments of rat mesenteric artery. Am J Physiol 262:H1651, 1992.

181. Berk BC, Vallega G, Muslin AJ, et al: Spontaneously hypertensive rat vascular smooth muscle cells in culture exhibit increased growth and Na⁺/H⁺ exchange. J Clin Invest 83:822, 1989. (Erratum in J Clin Invest 84:2029, 1989.)

182. Brayden JE, Halpern W, Brann LR: Biochemical and mechanical properties of resistance arteries from normotensive and hypertensive rats. Hypertension 5:17, 1983.

183. Fridovich I: Hypoxia and oxygen toxicity. Adv Neurol 26:256, 1979.

184. Back LH: Analysis of oxygen transport in the vascular region of arteries. Math Biosci 31:285, 1976.

185. Berk BC, Taubman MT, Cragoe EJ Jr, et al: Thrombin signal transduction mechanisms in rat vascular smooth muscle cells: Calcium and protein kinase C–dependent and –independent pathways. J Biol Chem 265:17334, 1990.

186. Hogue D, Michalak M, Fliegel L: The role of ion antiporters in the maintenance of intracellular pH in rat vascular smooth muscle cells. Mol Cell Biochem 102:125, 1991.

187. Little PJ, Weissberg PL, Cragoe EJ Jr, Bobik A: Dependence of Na⁺/H⁺ antiport activation in cultured rat aortic smooth muscle on calmodulin, calcium, and ATP. Evidence for the involvement of calmodulin-dependent kinases. J Biol Chem 263:16780, 1988.

188. Mitsuka M, Nagae M, Berk BC: Na⁺-H⁺ exchange inhibitors decrease neointimal formation after rat carotid injury. Effects on smooth muscle cell migration and proliferation. Circ Res 73:269, 1993.

189. Rosskopf D, Fromter E, Siffert W: Hypertensive sodium-proton exchanger phenotype persists in immortalized lymphoblasts from essential hypertensive patients. J Clin Invest 92:2553, 1993.

190. Lifton RP, Hunt SC, Williams RR, et al: Exclusion of the Na⁺-H⁺ antiporter as a candidate gene in human essential hypertension. Hypertension 17:8, 1991.

191. Dudley CRK, Taylor DJ, Ng LL, et al: Evidence for abnormal Na⁺/H⁺ antiport activity detected by phosphorus nuclear magnetic resonance spectroscopy in exercising skeletal muscle of patients with essential hypertension. Clin Sci 79:491, 1990.

191a. Lucchesi PA, DeRoux N, Berk BC: Na⁺/H⁺ exchanger expression in vascular smooth muscle of spontaneously hypertensive and Wistar Kyoto rats. Hypertension (in press).

192. Grinstein S, Rothstein A: Mechanisms of regulation of the Na⁺/H⁺ exchanger. J Membr Biol 90:1, 1986.

193. Ashida T, Kuramochi M, Omae T: Increased sodium-calcium exchange in arterial smooth muscle of spontaneously hypertensive rats. Hypertension 13:890, 1989.

194. Berk BC, Elder E, Mitsuka M: Hypertrophy and hyperplasia cause differing effects on vascular smooth muscle cell Na⁺/H⁺ exchange and intracellular pH. J Biol Chem 265:19632, 1990.

195. Sardet C, Fafournoux P, Pouysségur J: α-Thrombin, epidermal growth factor, and okadaic acid activate the Na⁺/H⁺ exchanger, NHE-1, by phosphorylating a set of common sites. J Biol Chem 266:19166, 1991.

196. Bianchini L, Woodside M, Sardet C, et al: Okadaic acid, a phosphatase inhibitor, induces activation and phosphorylation of the Na⁺/H⁺ antiport. J Biol Chem 266:15406, 1991.

197. Simonet L, St-Lezin E, Kurtz TW: Sequence analysis of the alpha 1 Na⁺,K⁺-ATPase gene in the Dahl salt-sensitive rat. Hypertension 18:689, 1991.

198. Lange-Carter CA, Pleiman CM, Gardner AM, et al: A divergence in the MAP kinase regulatory network defined by MEK kinase and Raf. Science 260:315, 1993.

199. Boulton TG, Nye SH, Robbins DJ, et al: ERKs: A family of protein-serine/threonine kinases that are activated and tyrosine phosphorylated in response to insulin and NGF. Cell 65:663, 1991.

200. Pages G, Lenormand P, L'Allemain G, et al: Mitogen-activated protein kinases p42mapk and p44mapk are required for fibroblast proliferation. Proc Natl Acad Sci USA 90:8319, 1993.

201. Jacob HJ, Lindpaintner K, Lincoln SE, et al: Genetic mapping of a gene causing hypertension in the stroke-prone spontaneously hypertensive rat. Cell 67:213, 1991.

202. Mullins JJ, Peters J, Ganten D: Fulminant hypertension in transgenic rats harbouring the mouse Ren-2 gene. Nature 344:541, 1990.

# 46

# Essential Hypertension

*John H. Laragh*
*Jon D. Blumenfeld*

The phenomenon of hypertension was first characterized at the turn of the century, when Riva-Rocci[1] developed the prototype of the modern sphygmomanometer and so allowed the routine measurement of blood pressure. Korotkov[2] then perfected the sphygmomanometric technique by describing the sounds heard over the brachial artery as the pressure in the cuff is reduced. In general, the upper limits of normal blood pressure in older persons have been considered to be a systolic value of 160 mm Hg and a diastolic value of 95 mm Hg. These figures may be adjusted downward for younger patients to the point that a 20-year-old person with readings in excess of 120/80 mm Hg may be considered hypertensive. As pointed out by Pickering,[3] population studies suggest that blood pressure is a continuous variable, with no absolute dividing line between normal and abnormal values. This situation has resulted in an inevitable continuous debate over borderline readings that focuses on whether people with such pressures are normal and on what in fact constitutes normalcy. Moreover, studies using 24-hour monitoring techniques have revealed that significant fractions of patients who appear hypertensive in the office setting do not have hypertension at other times.[4]

Early on, however, life insurance studies indicated that relatively higher blood pressures that are casually recorded, even those that are within the normal range, are statistically associated with increased mortality from cardiovascular complications[5–7] (Table 46–1). The Veterans Administration established through a subsequent trial of therapy (principally with diuretics, which are often combined with other agents) that antihypertensive treatment could provide a sig-

nificant degree of protection against such complications—notably congestive heart failure, renal failure, and stroke but not coronary artery disease.[8, 9] From such demonstrations sprang the concept of a medical obligation to treat all cases of hypertension.

Nonetheless, the risks of death and disability associated with hypertension are increased only in the broad statistical sense; a large majority of patients with clearly elevated blood pressures live lives of normal longevity and health. Not only are the risks variable from one person to another, but also great variability has been found among hypertensive patients in their responses to antihypertensive treatments, a phenomenon that also suggests no single cause. Thus, risks are apparently not distributed randomly but are concentrated in subgroups that have been difficult to identify. For these and other reasons, hypertension cannot yet be considered a discrete disease entity but must rather be considered a marker common to the course of perhaps several pathologic developments. Thus, hypertension is a physical sign and a risk factor to be assessed in conjunction with other physiologic and environmental factors.

Variant patterns may be recognized. Hypertension may be purely systolic and accompanied by normal or even lowered diastolic pressure. Systolic hypertension usually occurs in the elderly and may be a manifestation of atherosclerosis, the increased systolic pressure resulting from decreased arterial elasticity. Often in the elderly, diastolic pressure is either normal or low, which suggests less or no arteriolar vasoconstriction and a different pathophysiologic process involving changes in the large vessels rather than

**TABLE 46–1. Ratio (Percentage) of Actual to Expected Mortality**

| Systolic Blood Pressure (mm Hg) | Ratio for Diastolic Blood Pressure of (mm Hg) | | | | |
|---|---|---|---|---|---|
| | 68–82 | 83–87 | 88–92 | 93–97 | 98–102 |
| Men (ages 15–69) | | | | | |
| 128–137 | 109 | 127 | 140 | 168 | 197 |
| 138–147 | 141 | 153 | 170 | 199 | 224 |
| 148–157 | — | 180 | 191 | 224 | 269 |
| 158–167 | — | 215 | 240 | 268 | 289 |
| Women (ages 15–69) | | | | | |
| 128–137 | 101 | 107 | 123 | 110 | — |
| 138–147 | 118 | 122 | 120 | 195 | 220 |
| 148–157 | — | 120 | 160 | 163 | 232 |
| 158–167 | — | 214 | 228 | 287 | 362 |

From Kaplan NM: Systemic hypertension: Mechanisms and diagnosis. *In* Braunwald E (ed): Heart Disease. WB Saunders, Philadelphia, 1980, pp 852–921.

in the arterioles. Systolic hypertension may also occur as part of a hyperdynamic cardiovascular state, such as that occurring in hyperthyroidism or in younger people who appear to have increased β-adrenergic activity.

Labile hypertension describes an intermittent form of hypertension, also sometimes referred to as prehypertension, neurocirculatory asthenia, or hyperkinetic heart syndrome. This term lacks definition, for investigators have not yet determined whether such patients go on to sustained hypertension with consequent secondary cardiovascular damage. Borderline hypertension defines blood pressure readings close to the upper limits of the normal range or only slightly elevated. Diastolic hypertension is usually accompanied by systolic hypertension. If persistent and severe, it may result in so-called hypertensive vascular disease, a condition involving the arterioles, most frequently of the kidneys, eyes, and brain, and also producing cardiac enlargement and left ventricular failure. The sustained hypertension induces a thickening of the walls and occlusion of the lumens of the small arteries and arterioles and may favor the development of atherosclerotic changes in larger arteries.

Malignant hypertension, a syndrome defined originally by Volhard and Fahr[10] in 1914, is characterized clinically by severe accelerating hypertension with neuroretinopathy or papilledema of the optic nerves and by evidence of renal damage. Clinically, it is almost always associated with massive oversecretion of renin and aldosterone[11] and is strikingly relieved by binephrectomy or antirenin drugs but not by total adrenalectomy (see later). On pathologic examination, it is characterized by fibrinoid and necrotizing arteriolitis. This syndrome can occur de novo, but most often it follows pre-existing milder forms of hypertension. Malignant hypertension may occur as a complication of essential hypertension and of virtually every form of secondary hypertension, with the notable exception of coarctation of the aorta,[3] a condition in which the renal circulation is protected from the high pressures that occur proximally to the coarctation. Accelerated hypertension is a term often used synonymously with malignant hypertension, but sometimes only to imply a significant increase in the pace or severity of the hypertensive process.

Fortunately, the heterogeneity of pattern, risk, survival, and etiology in hypertension is better recognized today than

it was in the past. Differential diagnosis of hypertension is coming into its own; the practice of considering hypertension a single, uniform disease entity remains without a firm theoretic basis.

Some causes of hypertension may now be identified, and some may even be corrected. By definition, these primary conditions give rise to "secondary hypertension"; however, the pathophysiologic mechanism of by far the largest portion of the hypertensive population, about 85%, resists hard description. Members of this group are classified as having "primary hypertension" or "essential hypertension," signifying that no cause for their disorder has been found. Thus, essential hypertension is a diagnosis (if indeed a confession of ignorance can be called a diagnosis) reached only after known causes of hypertension have been excluded. The diagnostic exclusion process is of vital importance, however, because cure or effective treatment is available for some of the known causes.

Even when known causes have been excluded, the enormous residue defaulted as essential hypertension suggests etiologic variability, reflected by heterogeneity not only in morbidity and mortality but also in the response or lack of it to different classes of drugs. Moreover, much of this considerable variability is not well correlated with the level of hypertension. Converging clinical and pharmaceutical research is providing clues to physiologic mechanisms that might explain this variability. In this chapter, we discuss this evidence and its implications for diagnosis and treatment.

## EPIDEMIOLOGY

### Prevalence

Current rough estimates of the prevalence of hypertension in the United States range from 40 to 60 million persons, or a fifth to a quarter of all adult Americans. A frequently cited screening program found hypertension in 18% of the population when 160/95 mm Hg was used as the criterion, and 38% when the benchmark was dropped to 140/90 mm Hg.[12] The frequency of high blood pressure increases with age, predictably enough to support the time-honored, age-related reference standard for systolic pressure of 100 plus one's age. At every age, high blood pressure is more common among black men and women, who can also be more vulnerable than whites to hypertension-induced vascular damage[13–15] (Fig. 46–1). In general, women receive more treatment for hypertension than do men; however, for the majority of their life span, men may surpass women in prevalence of hypertensive disorders and their cardiovascular consequences.[16, 17] In cross-sectional studies of systolic blood pressure, a crossover appears to take place from approximately age 45 to 55 years, but the higher pressures among women older than 55 years may in part reflect the greater mortality among men with high blood pressure.[16]

Observations in England and the United States show a strong familial aggregation for blood pressure strata, which could be the result of a genetic basis as well as of common environmental factors.[3, 18] Dietary salt has been implicated because of observations that hypertension and its sequelae are more common in societies with high sodium chloride intake. Correlation of sodium intake with blood pressure within societies, such as those in the United States, Japan, or New Zealand, has not been possible, however.[19] This lack of correlation has been most convincingly demonstrated by the Intersalt study, which found no correlation between sodium intake and blood pressure in 48 centers around the world.[20] Some primitive tribal societies, however, have low sodium intake and low blood pressures.[21]

Possibly more convincing is the association between high blood pressure and certain psychosocial and behavioral factors. Studies of cross-cultural variation have shown that blood pressures are higher and tend to rise more steeply with age in groups who are more involved in a money economy, engage in more economic competition, and have more contact with people of different cultures, attitudes, or beliefs.[22]

## Natural History of Untreated Essential Hypertension

Life insurance statistics have well established that hypertensive individuals, as a population, have shortened survival

and that this vulnerability correlates broadly with increasing levels of arterial blood pressure.[23] The long-term, ongoing studies conducted at Framingham, Massachusetts,[24, 25] confirmed these findings and demonstrated that high blood pressure is the leading risk factor predisposing to stroke, heart failure, heart attack, and kidney failure. Whether these complications occur in a specific hypertensive patient, however, and how soon, appear to be matters strongly determined by the concurrence of other risk factors, such as cardiac hypertrophy, glucose intolerance, smoking, hypercholesterolemia, and obesity. One must remember that hypertension—as a risk factor, not as a cause—does not inevitably predict stroke or heart attack. In fact, only a minority of hypertensive patients experience a vascular calamity, whereas many people with normal blood pressure (and thus without the pressure risk factor) can still suffer such cardiovascular events. Therefore, in a seeming paradox, although hypertension is associated with 35% to 45% of all cardiovascular disease, most cardiovascular events probably occur in individuals with normal blood pressure because more people are normotensive than hypertensive.[26]

In the 1950s, Perera[27] observed 500 untreated patients, 150 from before the onset of their hypertension until their death, and another 350 from the uncomplicated phase until their death. The mean survival of these patients after discovery of their hypertension was 20 years. Perera also noted that the height of the casually obtained blood pressure had little prognostic value. Some patients with readings above 200 mm Hg systolic survived untreated for more than 35 years. In general, according to Perera,[27] the disease process could be said to consist of an uncomplicated phase lasting about 15 years followed by a phase in which organ complications, largely arteriolosclerotic and atherosclerotic, became apparent. Of these complications, 74% were cardiac in nature, 42% were renal, and 32% were retinal. More than half the subjects died of heart disease (principally congestive heart failure), 10% to 15% died of cerebral accidents, and about 10% died of renal failure. Malignant hypertension occurred in less than 5% of these patients (Fig. 46–2).

Patients with untreated essential hypertension (those with known causes of hypertension having been excluded) usu-

**Figure 46–1.** Prevalence of hypertension in the United States defined as the percentage of people with systolic blood pressure of at least 140 mm Hg or diastolic blood pressure of at least 90 mm Hg. (From Kaplan NM: Systemic hypertension: Mechanisms and diagnosis. *In* Braunwald E [ed]: Heart Disease, 3rd ed. WB Saunders, Philadelphia, 1988, pp 819–861.)

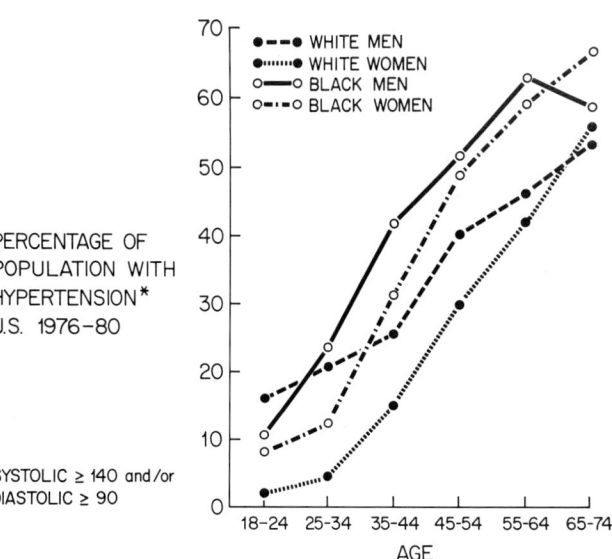

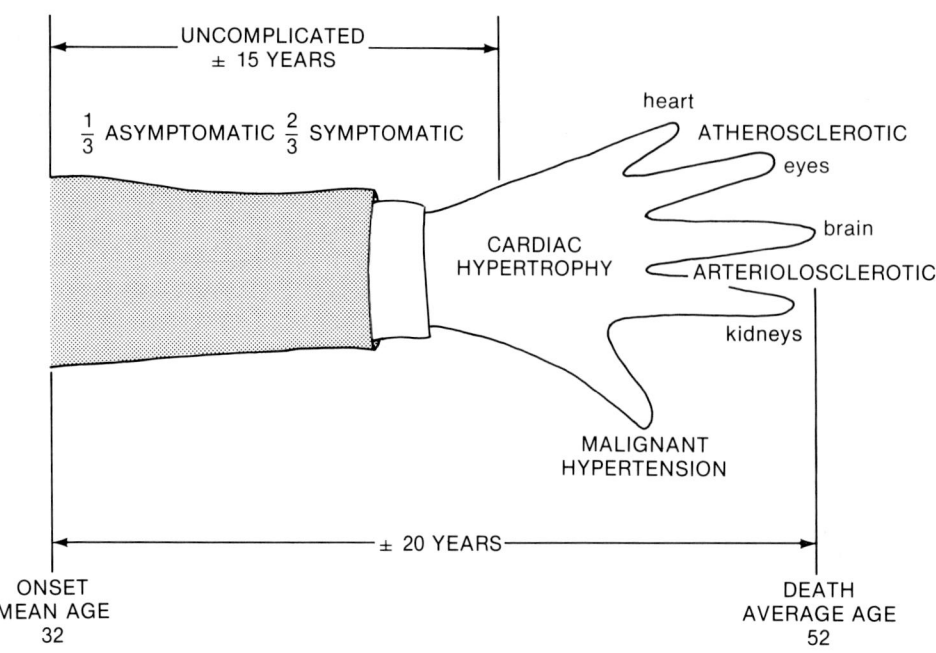

**Figure 46–2.** The average natural history of untreated so-called essential or primary hypertension. (Reprinted from J Chronic Dis [now J Clin Epidemiol], Volume 1, Perera GA, Hypertensive vascular disease: Description and natural history, Page 33, Copyright 1955, with kind permission from Elsevier Science Ltd, The Boulevard, Langford Lane, Kidlington OX5 1GB, UK.)

ally experience a long and almost entirely asymptomatic course that is responsible for the possibly overoptimistic term "benign essential hypertension." Symptoms believed to be characteristic of this form of hypertension (headache, fainting, tinnitus, and dizziness) may occur just as frequently in normotensive persons.[28]

## Benefits of Treatment

The Veterans Administration Cooperative Trial[9] of the 1960s was the first major American effort to evaluate the impact of antihypertensive therapy in a group of patients with essential hypertension. Compliant veterans were randomly assigned to placebo or medication, and treatment was rapidly found to result in great improvement of cardiovascular morbidity and mortality in patients with diastolic blood pressures of 115 to 129 mm Hg. A statistically favorable outcome was shown after 3.3 years of follow-up in patients of the treated group whose diastolic blood pressure was between 105 and 115 mm Hg. The benefit was manifested by a reduced frequency of strokes, congestive heart failure, and dissection of the aorta but not of ischemic cardiac events. The benefits of treating patients with moderate to severe hypertension were thus clearly shown.

No benefit was achieved, however, among the patients with diastolic blood pressure below 105 mm Hg. Furthermore, a particularly relevant finding was that the major benefit in the group with diastolic blood pressures between 105 and 115 mm Hg was realized by those patients who had displayed evidence of pre-existing cardiovascular disease on entering the study or who were 50 years of age or older. Among patients who had no pre-existing end-organ disease or who were younger than 50 years, no difference in benefit was found between the treated and untreated groups.

One of the first attempts to address some of the issues left unresolved by the original Veterans Administration study was undertaken by the U.S. Public Health Service Hospital Study Group.[29] Although the study was inconclusive—largely because it involved a small sample of 389 subjects whose diastolic pressures were below 104 mm Hg and who had shown no evidence of target organ disease—no differences in mortality were found between the two groups. Increased blood pressure levels, however, and the beginning of left ventricular hypertrophy were evident in the untreated control subjects. The study's chief value was its demonstration that blood pressure levels in a general population could be controlled.

The benefits of treatment were studied in the early 1970s by the National Institutes of Health in a far broader population (approximately 11,000 subjects screened from 158,000 in 14 communities), which included women and a higher proportion of asymptomatic patients.[30] This study was the so-called Hypertension Detection and Follow-up Program. Patients were randomly allocated to "stepped-care" intervention or to "referred care." The stepped-care group received systematic chemotherapy without cost, whereas patients in the referred group were simply referred to their own physicians. Diastolic blood pressure was substantially reduced in both groups but to a significantly greater degree, with a difference of 5 mm Hg, in the stepped-care group. Because the study did not control for such factors as compliance (in the first group, compliance was encouraged by gratis treatment), distinguishing the benefits of the nature and quality of medical care from the benefits of specific pharmacologic therapy is difficult. The fact that the stepped-care group had a 17% reduction in mortality from all causes (e.g., a significant reduction in cancer mortality was found) supports the notion that aspects of care other than antihypertensive treatment, such as consistent, enthusiastic, and cost-defrayed general care, may have contributed to the observed outcome.[30]

One must also recognize that death rates in both groups

were extremely small and that the incremental gain realized by intervention was limited. One reason for these results may have been that most subjects had only mild (90 to 104 mm Hg diastolic) hypertension. Five-year survivorship in the referred-care group was slightly less than 93%, whereas that in the stepped-care group was slightly more than 94%, a difference of about 0.3%. Thus, 1000 people would need to be treated continuously for 5 years to derive a similar benefit in 8 patients.

Under more careful scrutiny, even this study of mild hypertension demonstrates the underlying heterogeneity of hypertension. For example, black persons of both sexes had high rates of cardiovascular events and benefited substantially from treatment, whereas white women had low mortality rates and did not seem to benefit from treatment.[31]

The implication of these findings is that one should be absolutely certain that the drugs employed, which might be given for life rather than for just 5 years, have less inherent risk than that posed by the untreated hypertension itself.[32] Who is the patient at minimal risk, and who will benefit most from treatment? The blood pressure reading is crude and nonspecific regarding these questions, and important fallacies result from extrapolating statistics derived from large populations of undifferentiated patients to individuals.

Each patient must be considered in terms of all available clinical, demographic, and pathophysiologic information for an appropriate course of management to be determined. In patients with mild to moderate hypertension and with small risk of cardiovascular sequelae, watchful waiting could be the most prudent course.[32]

Prudence suggests vigorous antihypertensive therapy, however, for patients with diastolic blood pressures equal to or greater than 105 mm Hg. For patients with diastolic pressures between 90 and 105 mm Hg, treatment is justified when cardiovascular end-organ damage is evident. For uncomplicated patients in this lower range, intervention is favored for patients who are older than 50 years, who are black, or who are white men. Young persons and white women in this milder range are probably best managed by careful observation, with treatment being initiated if the blood pressure begins to rise.

Two large controlled studies support such a course. In the Australian study[33] of community residents with mild hypertension, 78% of placebo-treated patients whose diastolic blood pressures ranged between 100 and 104 mm Hg experienced a decline in pressure into the normal range in the 4 years of the project. Morbid events were confined almost entirely to those untreated patients whose pressures remained above 100 mm Hg. The untreated group of men with mild hypertension studied in the Oslo trial[34] did not differ after 5 years from the treated patients in terms of mortality. The treated group in the Oslo study did show a significant reduction in cerebrovascular events, but it also showed an increase in coronary events, which supports the general finding that stroke prevention is easier to demonstrate than is prevention of heart attack.

Although only 62% of the subjects in the Multiple Risk Factor Intervention Trial[35] had hypertension, this randomized primary prevention study of 13,866 men at high risk for cardiovascular events (assessed by blood pressure level, cigarette smoking, and cholesterol levels) is, by virtue of

its size, worth mentioning. After an average of 7 years, individuals in the treatment group (which offered counseling with regard to smoking and diet as well as antihypertensive therapy) experienced reduction in all three risk factors, but cardiovascular or total mortality rates did not differ significantly between the groups. In fact, within the treated group, some increase in mortality occurred in relation to the untreated subjects. The study thus underlines the hypothesis that some people with mild hypertension may be placed in jeopardy by certain kinds of drug treatment.[36]

In the Medical Research Council treatment trial for mild hypertension,[37] a significant reduction in the rate of strokes was observed, but no difference was observed between rates of coronary events for treated and placebo groups. The estimate of this study's authors that giving 850 mildly hypertensive patients active antihypertensive therapy for 1 year may prevent one stroke lends support to the idea that for many hypertensive people, the best treatment may be no treatment at all. Even more disturbing evidence was presented in a later study, which revealed that after 5 years of continuous diuretic therapy, the subjects of the Medical Research Council trial exhibited not only hypokalemia and hyperuricemia but also a 12% frequency of impotence and a 14% frequency of abnormal glucose tolerance.[38] Again, drug therapy is apparently never free of risk; the risks of the untreated disease must always be weighed against the possible risks of long-term drug therapy itself before any continuing or lifetime commitments are made.

Altogether, then, these four major trials have demonstrated conclusively that diuretic-based stepped-care drug regimens can reduce blood pressure and that 5 years of such therapy will produce statistically significant partial protection from stroke. However, none of these four major studies shows any protection from coronary events related to hypertension, a great disappointment because coronary events compose about 80% of the added cardiovascular risk burden of hypertension. However, notwithstanding the general failure of diuretic-based regimens to achieve protection from cardiac morbid events, three clinical trials involving elderly hypertensive patients reported more encouraging results. These are the Systolic Hypertension in the Elderly Program[39] sponsored by the National Institutes of Health, the Swedish Trial in Old Patients with Hypertension,[40] and the Medical Research Council trial.[41] All three trials reported significant reductions in stroke. The Systolic Hypertension in the Elderly Program reported significant reductions in nonfatal but not in fatal cardiovascular events. In the Swedish Trial in Old Patients with Hypertension, the myocardial infarction rate was not reduced. In the Medical Research Council trial, coronary events were not reduced; an interesting anomalous finding of this study was that diuretic monotherapy produced significantly better all-cause outcome than did β-blocker therapy.

These findings, although more promising than heretofore, require confirmation and should not be extrapolated to apply to younger patients with diastolic (essential) hypertension. Thus, the mean diastolic pressure at entry in the Systolic Hypertension in the Elderly Program was 78 mm Hg. Systolic hypertension of the elderly person probably involves the larger arteries and may also involve a larger $Na^+$-volume factor associated with nephron loss of aging.

This is in keeping with the known lower renin levels and the overall better performance of diuretics in these three trials of the elderly. Another factor in the improved diuretic performance may have been the use of lower doses than heretofore.

## ABNORMAL PHYSIOLOGY

Essential hypertension is characterized by sustained diastolic blood pressure in excess of 95 mm Hg and by some of the characteristics listed in Table 46–2. Many of these features, however, can be found in other known forms of hypertension with widely different causes. As already discussed, several etiologic factors may also possibly exist within the large category referred to as essential hypertension. The diagnosis of essential hypertension is made purely on a manometric basis after exclusion of the known causes listed in Table 46–3.

In essential hypertension, the column of blood in the arterial tree between the aortic valves and the capillaries moves at abnormally high pressure throughout the cardiac cycle of contraction and relaxation. Cardiac output, however, is usually normal or close to normal; thus, the main determinant of the sustained elevated blood pressure is an increase in peripheral resistance, usually ascribed to a narrowing of the small arterioles strategically located throughout the arterial system. The increase in vascular resistance, a cardinal characteristic of diastolic hypertension, is commonly related to excessive vasoconstriction of arteriolar smooth muscle, although it can also result, at least in part, from structural changes in these arterioles, from increased blood viscosity,[42] or even perhaps from increased extravascular (interstitial) pressure.

The total peripheral resistance (TPR) cannot be measured. It is a calculated value obtained by dividing the blood pressure (BP) by the cardiac output (CO), a transposition of the basic equation $BP = CO \times TPR$. The generalized vasoconstriction presumed responsible for the elevated total peripheral resistance in essential hypertension may be functional, as evidenced by its reversibility by various drugs

### TABLE 46–2. Pathophysiologic Characteristics of Essential Hypertension

No known cause
Diastolic pressure repeatedly >95 mm Hg
Total peripheral resistance usually increased
Pulse pressure possibly increased or decreased
Cardiac output normal, or elevated in some, possibly early in the disease
Cardiac work increased
Altered renal physiology, with accelerated natriuresis and reduced renal blood flow
Normal blood flow to most regions; diminished renal and skin blood flow and increased muscle flow may develop
Plasma volume reduced (may be inversely related to diastolic pressure)
Hyperreactivity of pressure to stress, abnormal vascular reactivity, and impaired circulatory homeostasis

From Laragh JH, Niarchos AP, Sealey JE: Arterial hypertension. *In* Stein JA (ed): Internal Medicine. Little, Brown, Boston, 1983, p 13.

### TABLE 46–3. Known Causes of Hypertension

**Renal Disorders**

*Renal Parenchymal*
Acute and chronic glomerulonephritis; pyelonephritis; nephrocalcinosis; neoplasms; glomerulosclerosis; interstitial, hereditary, or radiation nephritis
Obstructive uropathies and hydronephrosis
Renin-secreting renal tumors (hemangiopericytoma, Wilms or renal cell, pancreatic, ovarian tumors)
Renal trauma

*Renovascular*
Renal arterial lesions, occlusions, stenoses, aneurysms, thromboses, vasculitis
Connective tissue or autoimmune disease with renal vasculitis or glomerulitis
Coarctation of the aorta with renal ischemia
Aortitis with renal ischemia

**Adrenocortical Disorders**
Cushing syndrome (cortisol excess)
Primary aldosteronism due to adenoma (Conn syndrome)
Pseudoprimary aldosteronism (bilateral adrenocortical hyperplasia)
Congenital adrenal hyperplasias due to enzymatic defects with excess precursor Na$^+$-retaining steroids (11β-hydroxylase, Bongiovanni; 17α-hydroxylase, Biglieri)
Adrenal carcinomas
Ectopic corticotropin-secreting tumors

**Pheochromocytoma**
(adrenal medullary or chromaffin tumors secreting norepinephrine or epinephrine)

**Other Endocrine Causes**
Hypothyroidism (diastolic hypertension)
Hyperthyroidism (systolic hypertension)
Hypercalcemic states, hyperparathyroidism
Acromegaly

**Toxemias of Pregnancy**

**Neurogenic Factors**
Increased intracranial pressure
Familial dysautonomia
Acute porphyria
Buffer denervation, poliomyelitis, spinal cord injuries
Psychogenic?

**Iatrogenic Causes**
Oral contraceptive or estrogen therapy
Licorice ingestion or mineralocorticoid or glucocorticoid therapies
Sympathomimetic drugs (decongestant or systemic abuse)
Tricyclic antidepressants
Alcohol abuse
Lead poisoning
Monoamine oxidase inhibitors plus tyramine ingestion
Excessive salt appetite?

Blumenfeld JD, Mann SJ, Laragh JH: Clinical evaluation and differential diagnosis of the individual hypertensive patient. *In* Laragh JH, Brenner BM (eds): Hypertension Pathophysiology, Diagnosis, and Management, 2nd ed. Raven Press, New York, 1995, pp 1897–1911.

and procedures and by the wide fluctuations in diastolic blood pressure and the vasomotor instability so often observed in these patients. Some investigators have reported that in perhaps a fourth of hypertensive patients who are in an early stage of their disease, the elevated blood pressure is related instead to increased cardiac output. Whether this finding represents an earlier stage of the same disease or a separate, more labile form of hypertension remains to be determined.

The basis for the generalized vasoconstriction of the arteriolar bed in common forms of hypertension is not completely understood. Two known pressor substances, norepinephrine and angiotensin II, can produce constrictive changes in the arterioles that resemble the changes occurring in established hypertension, but the arteriolar bed, responding to changes in blood pressure or flow or to various local chemical transmitters or alterations in tissue metabolism, can undergo vasoconstriction independently of these two substances. The likelihood that mechanisms other than those mediated by norepinephrine and angiotensin could be involved in the long-term vasoconstriction characteristic of hypertension provides an interesting research problem. In considering all possible mechanisms, however, one must appreciate that the arteriolar vasoconstriction of hypertension is generalized and that it *always* involves the renal vasculature, both physiologically and pathologically. Therefore, the initiating event, if it does not reflect a generalized intrinsic arteriolar lesion, is most likely to be humorally induced or to result from a diffuse neural, endocrine, or metabolic signal.

Besides the size of the vascular bed between the aortic valves and the capillaries, the second critical determinant of arterial blood pressure is the volume of liquid that fills this bed on each heart beat.[43-45] This plasma volume factor is largely determined by the amount of $Na^+$ in the body; $Na^+$ constitutes the major osmotic factor regulating the amount of water in the bloodstream and extracellular space. Available $Na^+$ thus serves to determine the fluid pressure of the circulating blood. Clearly, plasma protein and red blood cell mass are also key elements in determining circulating whole blood volume, but these factors appear normal and fixed in most patients with uncomplicated hypertension. Accordingly, "sodium balance," reflecting dietary intake minus the amount of $Na^+$ eliminated or retained by the kidneys, contributes crucially to the volume factor that is involved to some extent in all blood pressure phenomena. Thus, when normal cardiac performance is assumed, arteriolar vasoconstriction and the arterial filling volume become the two dynamic final determinants of blood pressure.

$Na^+$ appears to affect both sides of this equation, however. Besides a hydraulic contribution to the volume factor, $Na^+$ may also affect peripheral resistance by increasing the arteriolar vasoconstrictive factor. This increase could occur by autoregulation-induced changes in arteriolar constriction or as a consequence of changes in the transport or distribution of $Na^+$ across cell membranes and between the intravascular and interstitial compartments, inducing changes in arteriolar tone or resistance. This topic is discussed further in a later section in which the etiologic features of essential hypertension are described.

At this point, however, in considering hypertensive disease and its pathophysiologic basis, one must bear in mind that hypertension appears to be a generalized or systemic disorder of perhaps the entire arteriolar vasculature but essentially involving the renal vessels. Early in the disease, no structural changes in the arterioles may be detectable, but with time, hypertrophy of arteriolar smooth muscle and then characteristic hyaline changes in arteriolar walls may develop.[46-48] Thus, any theory of causation must invoke a generalized target organ defect of vascular smooth muscle

or, alternatively, a normal target organ response to abnormal neural, hormonal, or metabolic signals. The latter possibility, which we favor, suggests that high blood pressure should be viewed as a disorder of normal regulatory control systems. Such a hypothesis, of course, supposes the existence of coordinated control systems that have the basic purpose of ensuring adequate blood pressure and tissue perfusion. This matter, too, is discussed further in the following pages.

In early uncomplicated essential hypertension, no clear-cut abnormalities in regional distribution of blood flow are noted, although some investigators claim to have demonstrated increased flow to muscle and reduced flow in skin. The earliest convincing abnormality in regional flow appears to occur in the kidneys.[49-53] Thus, a reduction in renal blood flow—that is, renal vasoconstriction—may be considered the earliest established physiologic change to develop.

## Altered Renal Physiology

In essential hypertension, physiologic and pathologic renal changes often precede changes identifiable in other organs, but whether they precede or follow the onset of the hypertension itself has not been determined. Early hypertensive patients may exhibit no renal structural changes observable by light microscopy.[46-48] Renal vein catheterization has indicated that the earliest physiologic lesion of essential hypertension is vascular: glomerular filtration rate (GFR) is maintained, whereas total renal blood flow is reduced (increased filtration fraction).[49-53] This pattern may be explained by diffuse, predominantly efferent but also afferent vasoconstriction of all nephrons or, alternatively, by selective afferent vasoconstriction with diversion of blood away from some nephrons to maintain near-normal GFR. That renal vasoconstriction can be reversible is shown by the depressor response to pyrogens or to antihypertensive drugs. The renal vasoconstriction of essential hypertension could lead to reduced pressure and flow in the postglomerular circulation, and this change might predispose to increased tubule $Na^+$ reabsorption. A normal reading for *p*-aminohippurate extraction suggests that renal parenchymal cell function remains normal in uncomplicated hypertension.[49-51]

This process is unlike that of malignant hypertension, in which gross pathologic change is accompanied by major disruption of renal function.[54] Renal blood flow and GFR may be greatly reduced, and *p*-aminohippurate extraction can be markedly impaired, indicating damaged parenchymal cell function. *p*-Aminohippurate and inulin studies suggest hyperemia of both functioning and nonfunctioning nephrons.[51] The renal vasculature in malignant hypertension, unlike that in essential hypertension, may no longer respond to pyrogens or vasodilators. Indeed, in the more advanced forms of hypertensive disease, sodium deprivation may be contraindicated, because it may further reduce renal blood flow by inducing more renal vasoconstriction. This observation provides a rationale for administering adequate amounts of dietary sodium to azotemic patients who express the so-called uremia par manque du sel.[55]

## Abnormal Renal Sodium Transport in Essential Hypertension

**Accelerated Natriuresis.** Patients with systemic high blood pressure, whatever its type (with the possible exception of coarctation of the aorta), respond to saline or other types of infusions with much more rapid natriuresis than is induced by similar infusions in normotensive people.[56-61] Impressively, rejection fractions may reach 10% to 15% of the filtered load within a half hour. In contrast, normotensive individuals continue to reabsorb about 99% of the filtrate and eliminate the excess salt slowly the following day.[56] Accelerated natriuresis can be induced in normal subjects by prehydration or by raising their blood pressure with metaraminol. The condition may be corrected by effective hypotensive drug therapy and may be attenuated by sodium deprivation.

The phenomenon has intrigued some observers, who thought that it might offer some keys to understanding hypertension.[62] Some have believed that it is due to increased venous tone or reduced venous capacity, so that the excess fluid is immediately pushed through the central circulation rather than allowed to leak into interstitial space.[63] Hypertensive patients appear to behave as though there were a tighter fit of the blood volume so that the vascular bed tolerates no further expansion.

**Reduced Sodium Excretion of Renal Artery Occlusion.** Many studies have established that the kidney's $Na^+$-excreting capacity is highly sensitive to slight changes in renal blood flow.[64] The slightest reduction of renal blood flow leads to a relatively greater fall in renal $Na^+$ and water excretion. Indeed, the phenomenon has been exploited to screen hypertensive patients for unilateral renal ischemia.[65] The marked reduction in $Na^+$ excretion in the ipsilateral kidney, as revealed by differential ureteral catheterization, provided a physiologic basis for identifying surgically curable unilateral hypertension. The test has now been superseded by technically simpler but equally relevant procedures, such as renin-$Na^+$ profiling and renal vein renin assays, but from a theoretic standpoint, the sensitive relationship between renal blood flow and $Na^+$ excretion is of basic importance.

In patients with essential hypertension, which presumably involves both kidneys equally, such a defect of $Na^+$ excretion might be present bilaterally but escape detection in the compensated state. Evidence for this phenomenon has been reported.[66] Chronic but mild hypervolemia and continued hypertension could be the long-term consequences of such a defect. This kind of hypertension, involving an overfilling of the circulation due to an inability to excrete $Na^+$, is the form most common in patients with azotemic renal failure. In addition, as explained in the following pages, it could be the basic defect in patients in the medium-renin subgroup of essential hypertension.

## Nephron Heterogeneity with Unsuppressible Renin Secretion and Impaired Natriuresis as a Cause of Essential Hypertension

Within the kidney there exists a structural and functional basis for the abnormal renin secretion with impaired $Na^+$ excretion characteristic of hypertensive states. Our research[67] indicates that there are two functionally abnormal nephron populations in essential hypertension: 1) a minor subgroup of ischemic hypofiltering nephrons with impaired $Na^+$ excretion and with unabated renin secretion that is not turned off by sodium feeding; and 2) a larger subgroup of normal but adapting, hyperfiltering nephrons that excrete the added $Na^+$ burden and exhibit chronically suppressed renin secretion with increased GFR and distal $Na^+$ supply. The two populations thus resemble what happens in the interaction between the two kidneys of animals with two-kidney one-clip Goldblatt hypertension.

With this nephron heterogeneity,[68] the normal nephrons cannot fully compensate by natriuresis; the unwanted renin secretion coming from the neighboring ischemic nephrons acts to promote $Na^+$ retention in the adapting normal nephrons by causing afferent constriction and enhancing proximal reabsorption. This internephron discord results in too much $Na^+$ in the body in the face of unsuppressible plasma renin levels—a hallmark hypertensive situation in which total GFR and mean renal renin secretion remain normal. Yet, blockade of this "normal" plasma renin level by converting enzyme inhibitors enables correction of salt balance and normalization of blood pressure.[67]

## Abnormalities in Plasma and Extracellular Fluid Volumes

In established forms of hypertension, plasma volume is often subnormal, and the reduction is inversely proportional to the increase in diastolic pressure.[69] The relative hypovolemia may result from sustained arterial vasoconstriction, which promotes transudation of fluid from vascular space. The concept is supported by findings indicating that the extracellular fluid volume of hypertensive patients is normal or slightly decreased. Research indicates that plasma volumes differ in equally hypertensive patients within renin subgroups; the presence or absence of renin activity and its attendant vasoconstriction may be associated with lower rather than higher blood volumes in patients with similar degrees of hypertension.[69]

Such space measurements pose interpretive problems because of errors inherent in the techniques and because the critical arterial volume in question is an unmeasurable fraction of the measured total blood volume. Another difficulty with space measurements is the lack of a meaningful reference standard. When space measurements are related to height, weight, or surface area, extremely broad normal ranges are found, which lead to ambiguity in identifying possible abnormalities.

## Impaired Circulatory Homeostasis

Several studies suggest that patients with essential hypertension have impaired circulatory homeostasis with abnormal vascular reactivity. When monitored for 24 hours, these patients generally show a resetting of their diurnal blood pressure profile to a higher level, with somewhat wider than normal fluctuations in blood pressure.[70] They may also have a wider blood pressure response to various psychic or physical stimuli.[71] They may exhibit abnormal responses (fainting) to venous occlusion of the legs and can exhibit such other vasomotor phenomena as increased flushing, tachycardia,[72] and sweating in response to various stimuli.

These phenomena are not necessarily or consistently related to the hypertension itself. They may reflect a relative instability of the individual's circulation compared with that of normotensive people, whose blood pressure level is closer to the midpoint of defensive buffering systems that protect against assaults on the circulation.

## ETIOLOGIC FACTORS

### The Nervous System and Catecholamines

A popular belief is that hypertension may arise from persistent vasomotor alarm reactions.[73, 74] Hypertensive patients have been reported to respond to such noxious stimuli as mental arithmetic and psychic trauma with increased blood pressure, visceral and skin vasoconstriction, and increased blood flow to muscles.[75] The hemodynamic pattern resembles that occurring after exercise, and investigators believe that it reflects an abnormal conditioned reflex arising in the central nervous system, which suggests that hypertension is an expression of a central nervous system disorder.

In apparent support of this view are animal studies demonstrating severe hypertension with renal damage in a strain of mice subjected to the psychosocial stress of overcrowding.[76] Hypertension has been induced by operant conditioning in primates and dogs, although this type of hypertension is not severe and tends to subside when the stimulus is withdrawn.[77]

Nearly all observers agree that the nervous system may participate importantly in the pathogenesis or maintenance of hypertension. The beneficial effects of tranquilizers, anesthetics, autonomic blocking drugs, and sympathectomy are well recognized. The rare tumors of chromaffin tissue (pheochromocytoma), which secrete excessive norepinephrine or epinephrine, constitute a surgically curable cause of hypertension.

With the identification of the buffer nerve system,[78] the catecholamines, the autonomic nervous system, and the subcortical regions of the brain are understood to function in a coordinated way to defend the arterial circulation against acute changes in pressure. Any decrease in arterial blood pressure perceived in the carotid sinus or aortic body results in reduced traffic transmitted by the 9th and 10th nerves to the nucleus tractus solitarius in the medulla. This change causes reduced inhibition of neurogenic activity and a consequent increased sympathetic outflow leading to systemic vasoconstriction and tachycardia. The reverse phenomena (bradycardia and systemic vasodilatation) occur with an increase in pressure or flow to baroreceptors in the carotid and aortic regions. The system thus provides instant defense of the circulation and undoubtedly accounts for much of the short-term regulation of blood pressure and tissue perfusion in response to a variety of physiologic stimuli, including posture and exercise.

Can abnormalities in baroreceptor activity chronically affect blood pressure? Dock and associates[79] showed that pithing of the brain could correct Goldblatt hypertension in experimental animals. McCubbin and associates[80] postulated a "resetting" of baroreceptor activity in human hypertension, permitting a new level of blood pressure to become the midpoint for the buffer nerve activity. The human counterpart of buffer nerve hypertension, produced experimentally by denervation of the carotid–aortic body network has not been convincingly demonstrated, however, and some investigations cast serious doubt on the persistence of buffer nerve hypertension in animals.[81] Such experimental hypertension, rather than resulting in a sustained average increase in mean pressure throughout the day, appears merely to increase upward and downward lability, that is, to produce an *un*buffering.[81] Significantly, neither cardiac hypertrophy nor other target organ vascular disease occurs in these animal models.

Research by Nathan and Reis[82] showed that in experimental animals, bilateral destruction of the nucleus tractus solitarius can produce acute fulminant hypertension that is sustained in a milder form resembling buffer nerve hypertension. Similar bilateral lesions in dogs have been shown by Carey and co-workers[83] to result in only transient hypertension associated with a sustained increase in peripheral resistance. Thus, the possibility that a central or peripheral disorder of neural behavior may be involved in established human hypertension, although still unproved, remains an extremely attractive subject for future research. The characterization of an interaction of this rapidly acting, centrally controlled system with other, more prolonged pressor mechanisms, such as the renin system, may be fundamental to a complete understanding of blood pressure regulation and the pathogenesis of hypertension.

Nevertheless, despite the attractiveness of these possibilities, numerous biochemical measurements and indirect testing procedures have failed to reveal any convincing evidence that abnormal catecholamine secretion or metabolism, or abnormal nervous system function, participates significantly in the established forms of chronic human hypertension.[84] What does seem clear is that the autonomic nervous system and the subcortical region of the brain coordinate the defense of blood pressure in response to acute stimuli. This defense appears for the most part to be transient, lasting from a few minutes to several hours or until longer term mechanisms take over. The operation of this system does not seem to be markedly altered in hypertensive patients, except that their diurnal blood pressure patterns may possibly be more labile. Furthermore, investigators have not been able to measure differences in circulating levels of catecholamines or to predict consistently the responses or lack of response to $\alpha$- or $\beta$-blocking drugs in individual hypertensive patients.

### The Kidneys

As indicated before, abnormal renal physiology plays a central role in virtually all sustained hypertensive states. Actually, the key role of the kidneys in blood pressure phenomena was pointed out in 1826 when Richard Bright[85] called attention to a group of patients who had bounding pulse and edema and, at autopsy, demonstrated hardened, contracted kidneys and cardiac hypertrophy. The central role of the kidneys in blood pressure was later reinforced by numerous investigations, particularly those of Tigerstedt and Bergmann[86] in 1898. Their elegant experiments revealed a humoral substance, which they called renin, in saline extracts of rabbit kidneys. This substance had a powerful capacity to raise blood pressure when injected into another rabbit. Goldblatt's[87] landmark experiment in 1934, in which hypertension similar to the human form was produced hemodynamically by constricting the renal artery of the dog, further documented the kidney's vital role. The organ's importance in physiologic and pathologic blood pressure events was reconfirmed by studies in the 1960s that showed renin and aldosterone to be key elements in a normal servocontrol system that simultaneously regulates electrolyte balance and blood pressure.[11, 88, 89]

Clearly, the kidneys play a dual role in all blood pressure phenomena. First, under modulation by the adrenocortical $Na^+$-retaining hormone aldosterone, they determine the amount of $Na^+$ retained by the kidneys and hence the balance of $Na^+$ and water retained in the body. Second, they provide the site and cybernetics for a critical endocrine function, the secretion of renin, and thereby the generation of angiotensin II, the major long-term regulator of arteriolar vasoconstriction and an important stimulus for aldosterone secretion. (See also preceding sections on altered renal physiology and nephron heterogeneity.)

## Dietary Sodium

Populations with high salt intakes appear to have more hypertension, whereas less hypertension seems to prevail in those societies with little or no access to dietary sodium.[20, 90, 91] The meaning of such observations is clouded by a number of considerations, however, especially the observation that among individuals in the same society, no relationship exists between the level of salt intake and the height of the blood pressure.[21] Dietary sodium appears to induce changes in blood pressure only at the extremes of high and low intake. Manipulations of salt intake within the ranges usually ingested in industrialized countries (2 to 30 g/d) produce little or no observable change for the population as a whole.[19]

Strains of rats that are especially sensitive to the pressor effects of a high-sodium diet have been developed. Parallel studies of such animal models verify the amplifying effect of extremely high sodium diets on blood pressure and the blunting effect of sodium deprivation. The pressor action of a high-sodium diet (equivalent to 250 g/d in human beings) and, conversely, the depressor influence of a low-sodium diet underline the important role of the kidneys, because the kidneys are the only route for eliminating dietary sodium. In the same context, the greater occurrence of hypertension in chronic renal disease can largely be attributed to a failure to excrete appropriate dietary amounts of sodium.

Sodium intake and $Na^+$ balance are basic determinants of blood pressure and flow, influencing extracellular fluid and plasma volumes and their viscosity. For this reason, dietary salt provides a reserve for undue losses that may occur with exercise, fever, trauma, and alimentary losses. However, the relevance of variations in dietary intake to blood pressure levels within the usual ranges of dietary intake prevailing among human subjects remains to be clarified. Clearly, sodium deprivation can greatly improve high blood pressure in certain subgroups, but the evidence so far does not support the blanket recommendation of sodium deprivation for all hypertensive patients. In addition, there is even less reason to believe that sodium deprivation of normal people would prevent the occurrence of hypertensive disease.[21]

## Aldosterone: Primary Aldosteronism

An important role of the adrenocortical $Na^+$-retaining hormones in hypertensive phenomena was first defined by the research of Selye and colleagues,[92] which established that the administration of the adrenal prototype $Na^+$-retaining and kaliuretic (mineralocorticoid) hormone deoxycorticosterone consistently produces hypertension in rats when dietary sodium is adequate. The human counterpart of this hypertensive model is known as primary aldosteronism or Conn syndrome, which is caused by the autonomous oversecretion of aldosterone by an adrenocortical adenoma in an otherwise healthy subject.[93] The condition is highly curable by adrenalectomy, which makes its diagnosis an important part of the initial evaluation. The syndrome is characterized by mild, often long-standing hypertension, $Na^+$ and volume expansion identifiable by suppressed plasma renin activity, and chronic $K^+$ wastage reflected in hypokalemia and excessive urinary $K^+$ excretion.

Other adrenocortical steroids secreted in excess can produce similar syndromes (see Table 46–3 and later discussion). Investigators also recognize that high or borderline rates of aldosterone secretion support various forms of human hypertension besides primary aldosteronism. As an example, patients with low-renin essential hypertension who are treated with the aldosterone antagonist spironolactone consistently exhibit improvement in blood pressure.[94, 95]

## The Renin-Angiotensin-Aldosterone System in Malignant and Renovascular Hypertension as Opposed to Primary Aldosteronism

### DESCRIPTION

An important contribution to the modern understanding of hypertension was the discovery of the involvement of the renin system in high blood pressure states.[96, 97] A short description of the mechanics of the renin system is in order here. Figure 46–3 illustrates the normal operation of the renin system. The kidney secretes renin in response to changes in renal perfusion (e.g., shock, hemorrhage, heart failure, or renal damage) or in renal flow (e.g., $Na^+$ and volume depletion).[98] Renin's role is immediately realized in its stimulation of angiotensin II production, which quickly raises blood pressure by constricting the arterioles. At the

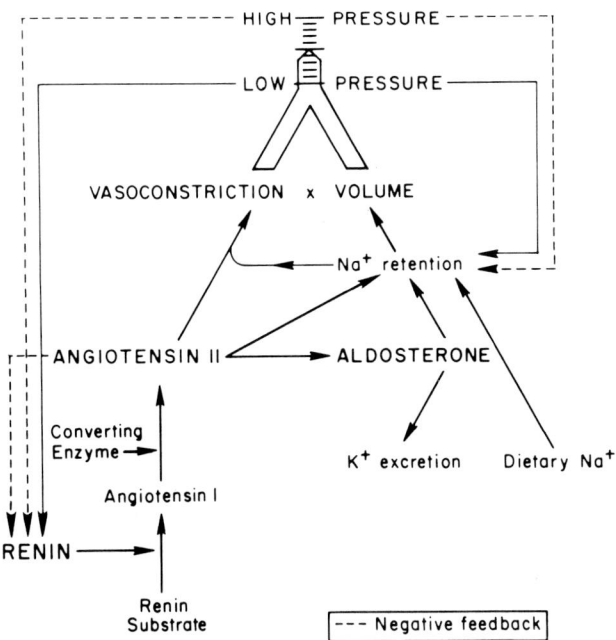

**Figure 46–3.** Renin-angiotensin-aldosterone system. Renin, secreted in response to reduced arterial pressure or reduced renal tubule Na$^+$, cleaves angiotensin I from circulating angiotensinogen (renin substrate). Angiotensin-converting enzyme then converts angiotensin I to angiotensin II. Angiotensin II raises pressure, by direct arteriolar vasoconstriction, and stimulates adrenal aldosterone secretion; together, aldosterone and angiotensin II cause renal Na$^+$ retention. The resultant fluid accumulation leads to improved flow. These pressure and volume effects in turn lead to suppression of renin release. Dashed line indicates negative feedback. (From Laragh JH, Letcher RL, Pickering TG: Renin profiling for modern diagnosis and treatment of hypertension. JAMA 241:151–156, 1979. Copyright 1979, American Medical Association.)

same time, angiotensin II stimulates the adrenocortical production of aldosterone, which at a slower pace expands the extracellular fluid by means of Na$^+$ retention at the cost of K$^+$ release. The retained Na$^+$ adds its own vasoconstrictive effect. The increased volume results in restored flow in the kidney, shutting off the signal for renin release.

Clinical studies in normal volunteers demonstrated that prolonged infusion of angiotensin for 10 days or more could produce sustained hypertension with Na$^+$ retention.[89] Moreover, this effect could be achieved with diminishingly small doses. Neither the sustained hypertension nor the Na$^+$ retention could be produced by norepinephrine infusion. These studies established that angiotensin, which was effective at low concentrations, was unique among known pressor agents in that it could produce and sustain chronic hypertension that was indistinguishable from human essential hypertension. By contrast, norepinephrine infusions do not produce sustained hypertension in normal humans or animals.

A typical study illustrating angiotensin's hypertensionogenic effect in a normal volunteer is shown in Figure 46–4. Here, an initial state of angiotensin-induced vasoconstriction is gradually replaced by increased aldosterone secretion and concomitant Na$^+$ retention. In the face of the resulting volume expansion and Na$^+$-induced vasoconstriction, less and less angiotensin is required to maintain the hypertension. This means that as the angiotensin-induced

Na$^+$ retention develops, less angiotensin (values approaching the normal range) is needed to sustain the hypertension. By contrast, norepinephrine induces paroxysms of pressure natriuresis, and the hypertension is not sustained.

This research indicated that the renin system, like other endocrinologic control systems, did not function in isolation but was reactive to other forces, both internal and external, affecting blood pressure and electrolyte balance. Just as a normal level of serum insulin may be defined only in relationship to the concurrent influence of glucose, so a normal level of plasma renin may be defined only in relationship to the concurrent influence of Na$^+$.

This point was demonstrated by the development of a protocol of renin-Na$^+$ profiling, in which plasma renin levels were indexed to the current state of sodium intake as determined by a 24-hour Na$^+$ excretion analysis.[99–102] The nomograms obtained from normal subjects (Fig. 46–5; values inside dotted lines define the normal range according to Na$^+$ excretion used as an index of intake) display a range of renin values that depend on sodium intake. This pattern follows the classic reactive behavior of an endocrinologic control system responding to that which it has been assigned to control. With this index of normalcy, the role of the renin system in the various types of hypertension could be examined with the potential for stratifying patients

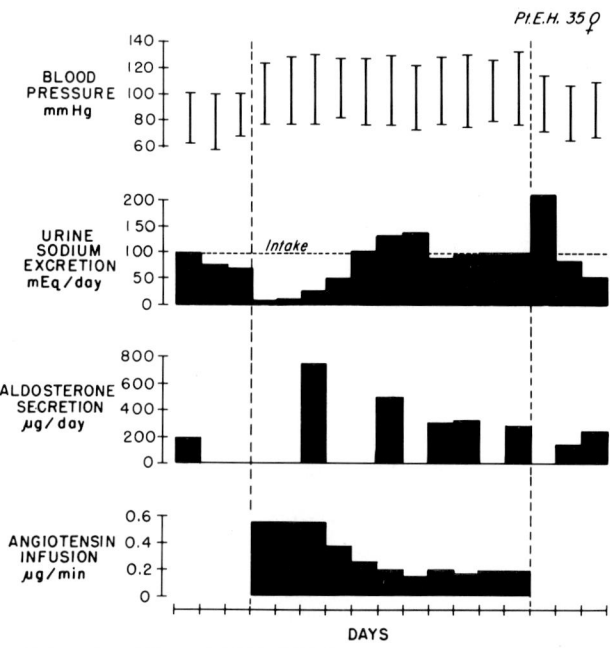

**Figure 46–4.** Prolonged continuous angiotensin infusion in a normal subject for 11 days. The dose of angiotensin was adjusted to keep a mildly pressor response. Angiotensin II induced a marked and selective increase in the adrenocortical secretion of aldosterone together with consequent Na$^+$ retention. As Na$^+$ was retained, angiotensin became more pressor. Because of this increasing pressor sensitivity to angiotensin, the dose was serially reduced to a point at which aldosterone secretion returned to control levels. Thus, the pressor sensitivity to angiotensin increased as Na$^+$ retention progressed. The results indicate that angiotensin, unlike norepinephrine, can produce and thus sustain hypertension in diminishingly small amounts as Na$^+$-volume gain turns off the need for angiotensin. (From Laragh JH, Sealey JE, Niarchos AP, Pickering TG: The vasoconstriction-volume spectrum in normotension and pathogenesis of hypertension. Fed Proc 41:2415, 1982.)

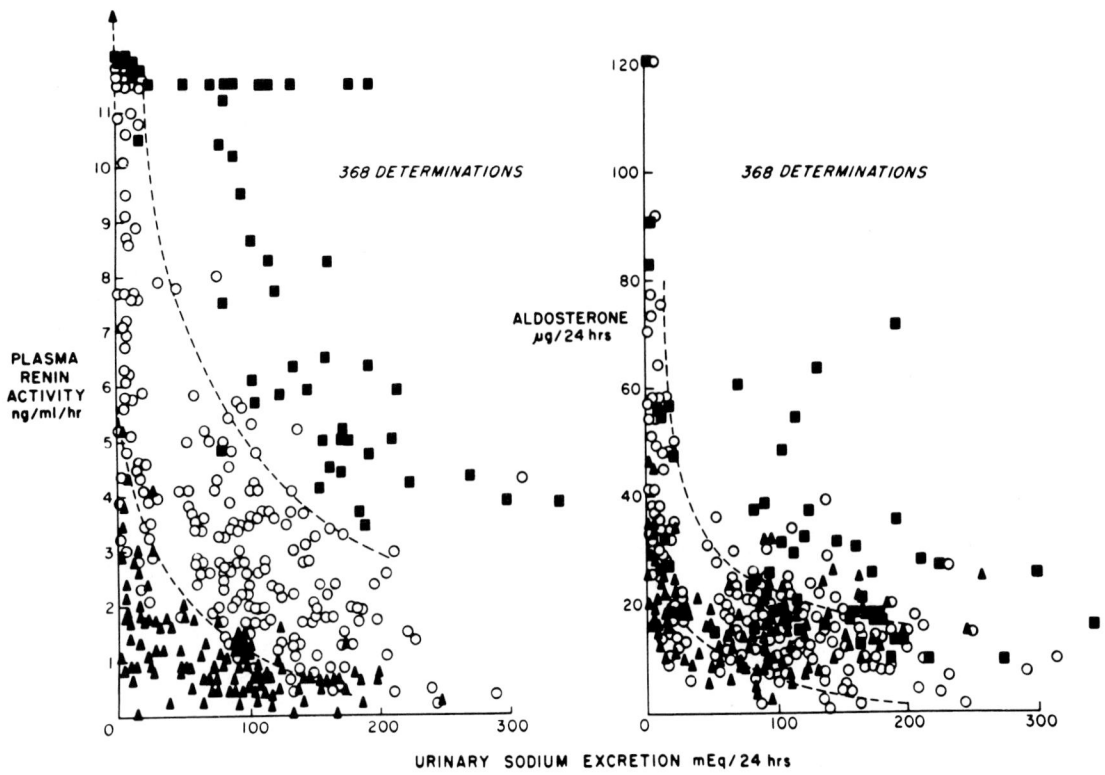

**Figure 46–5.** Relation of the noon ambulatory plasma renin activity *(left)* and the corresponding daily urinary aldosterone excretion *(right)*. The dashed lines define the normal channel derived from the study of normotensive people. A total of 219 patients with untreated essential hypertension were studied, some on several occasions at different levels of sodium intake. ▲ = low renin; ○ = normal renin; ■ = high-renin essential hypertension. Three major subgroups are defined by the appropriateness or normalcy of the plasma renin activity to the rate of Na⁺ excretion, which is used as an index of dietary intake and of Na⁺ balance. Additional normal subgroups are defined when aldosterone *(right)* is included in the analysis. Plasma renin activity results are expressed as nanograms angiotensin I formed per milliliter per hour. Multiply these plasma renin activity values by 0.65 to conform to the National Bureau of Standards angiotensin I reference standard used by Metpath Laboratories. (From Brunner HR, Laragh JH, Baer L, et al: Essential hypertension: Renin and aldosterone, heart attack and stroke. N Engl J Med 286:441, 1972.)

pathophysiologically according to their renin system patterns.

## MALIGNANT HYPERTENSION

The process of malignant hypertension begins with a critical degree of renovascular damage due to causes that are not always clear but are generally associated with severe hypertension[11, 88, 103] (Fig. 46–6). The deficit in renal perfusion produces an artifactual local hypotension in the kidneys, which triggers a massive release of renin. In its joint vasoconstrictive and Na⁺-retentive effects, the system produces a massive increase of pressure. This change normally shuts off the renin production, but the compromised kidney cannot participate in the systemic hypertension; it continues to pour out renin as though the local hypotension were systemic. Possibly, either because of local damage or because of the overwhelming effect of the renin, the kidney cannot muster enough natriuresis to tame the blood pressure surge; thus, it increases the Na⁺ contribution to the blood pressure.

A vicious circle results (see Fig. 46–6). More renin causes more hypertension, which causes more renal and systemic arteriolar necrosis, which again causes more renin, and so on to the inevitable end.

This description of the processes of malignant hypertension is supported by several observations. Diffuse vasculitis and death result within 1 or 2 days in rats overloaded by simultaneous injections of renin and aldosterone.[104] Also, the experience from dialysis wards shows that the blood pressure of malignant hypertensive patients can be lowered to virtually normal values and their arteriolar necrosis reversed by bilateral nephrectomy.[96]

An equally convincing demonstration of the causal role of the renin system can be made by pharmacologic blockade.[105] Renin system blockers, such as propranolol[106] and captopril,[107, 108] can alone normalize and maintain the blood pressure of an impressive proportion of malignant hypertensive patients, some in encephalopathic crises. In other such patients, the addition of diuretics may be required for normalization of blood pressure, illustrating the joint participation of renin and Na⁺ retention.

## RENOVASCULAR HYPERTENSION

Investigators have defined two general types of renovascular hypertension, a category accounting for possibly up to 5% of all clinical diastolic hypertension,[109] which is discussed in more detail in Chapter 47. The first type is typical unilateral renovascular disease, which, if the contra-

## The Renal-Adrenal Axis in Malignant Hypertension

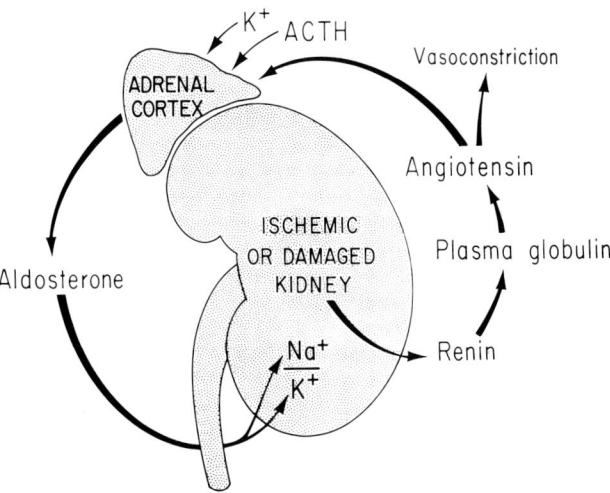

**Figure 46–6.** The renal-adrenal axis for normal regulation of blood pressure and $Na^+$ balance was originally discovered by studies of patients with the most severe form of hypertension, that is, malignant hypertension. These patients uniformly exhibit massive oversecretion of aldosterone[103] with hypokalemia. The high aldosterone level is not the primary cause of the hypertension because total adrenalectomy fails to arrest the syndrome. Because of major renal disease, a renin-angiotensin signal to the adrenals was suspected and proved.[11, 88] Proof of its pathogenic role in the malignant syndrome emerged from subsequent demonstrations that deleting or blocking the runaway renin secretion by binephrectomy or by giving β-blockers or converting enzyme inhibitors strikingly relieves the syndrome. Malignant hypertension is thus the ultimate expression of excess plasma renin-angiotensin-aldosterone causing hypertension with severe vasculitis and damage to the vasculature of the heart, brain, and kidneys. This model provided the basis for analyzing and relating milder instances of plasma renin excess to the causation of cardiac, renal, and cerebrovascular damage that occurs more often in hypertensive patients. (Adapted from Laragh JH: The role of aldosterone in man: Evidence for regulation of electrolyte balance and arterial pressure by renal-adrenal system which may be involved in malignant hypertension. JAMA 174:293–295, 1960. Copyright 1960, American Medical Association.)

lateral kidney can be demonstrated to be unaffected, is curable by surgery or balloon angioplasty. The second type, bilateral renovascular disease, is now often treatable by balloon angioplasty. These two types may involve equal levels of hypertension. Differentiation between the two is greatly aided by preliminary study of the renin system followed by definitive angiography.

**Unilateral Renovascular Disease.** An experimental analogue of human unilateral renovascular disease can be found in the two-kidney Goldblatt model, in which one renal artery of the animal is clipped and the other is left intact.[110] In general, plasma renin activity levels are excessively high. The affected kidney, suffering a perfusion deficit beyond a stenotic renal artery, reacts to the situation as if there were systemic hypotension and thus releases renin. The conversion to angiotensin II results in vasoconstriction, which raises blood pressure. The raised systemic blood pressure shuts off all renin release in the unaffected contralateral kidney but not in the affected kidney, where the perfusion deficit and reduced filtration continue beyond the arterial stenosis. Thus, a high amount of renin coming from the affected kidney vein and a low to absent amount of

renin from the contralateral kidney are classic diagnostic findings.

Although the affected ischemic kidney cannot respond with appropriate natriuresis, the contralateral kidney can, which cancels aldosterone's $Na^+$-retaining effect and causes fluid volume to be maintained at relatively normal levels, although without reduction of blood pressure. Thus, fully appropriate suppression of renin in the contralateral kidney does not counterbalance the uncontrolled release of renin in the affected kidney, because the contralateral kidney is exposed to high angiotensin II levels from the ischemic kidney. This angiotensin II promotes inappropriate $Na^+$ retention in the uninvolved normal kidney and thereby interferes with that kidney's capacity to eliminate $Na^+$. It does this by enhancing proximal tubule $Na^+$ reabsorption and also by enhancing afferent tone mediated by tubuloglomerular feedback.[67]

The renin dependency of unilateral renovascular hypertension can be demonstrated in animals or in patients by a prompt depressor response to renin system blockade. In a patient with high peripheral renin, such a response, particularly to the specific antiangiotensin agent captopril,[111] is highly suggestive and provides sound reason for pursuing the possibility of curable renovascular hypertension. A second renal vein study after the administration of captopril in the radiology suite[112] provides even greater precision, because converting enzyme inhibition produces a pronounced increase in renin release from the ischemic kidney.

The renin system is so clearly involved in unilateral renovascular hypertension that it provides the basis for definitive diagnosis and for the making of management decisions. Normally, each renal vein renin level is about 25% higher than the renal arterial level,[113] and this determines the normal peripheral level. With renin totally suppressed in the contralateral kidney in unilateral renal disease, the affected kidney must produce at least a 50% increment to sustain the peripheral level. If it does so, the fully suppressed contralateral kidney is behaving normally and so would most probably be capable of good function in the event of nephrectomy.

The ability to use such relatively innocuous measurements to define curable renovascular hypertension, together with the development of balloon angioplasty as an alternative to surgery,[112] has helped in identifying a greater frequency of cases of curable renovascular disease than was ever supposed. Many such patients, now cured by an outpatient procedure, would in earlier days have been deemed to have essential hypertension and might have been given antihypertensive drugs for the rest of their lives.

**Bilateral Renovascular Disease.** In the patient with bilateral renovascular disease, peripheral renin levels are either "normal" or even slightly reduced.[112] This finding also prevails in the experimental one-kidney Goldblatt model, in which one kidney is clipped and the other removed. In the model or the human with two compromised kidneys, the perfusion defect initially stimulates renin production, but at the same time, it results in an inability to excrete $Na^+$ and water freely or to react properly with natriuresis to the increased pressure. Because of the absence of a functioning contralateral kidney, as in unilateral renal disease, adequate run-off of $Na^+$ and water is not provided.

The result is a build-up of $Na^+$ and volume to the point at which pressure is restored beyond the stenosis in the compromised kidneys, and renin production is thus depressed to normal or even subnormal levels. This restoration of equilibrium in the kidney is accomplished at the cost of systemic volume expansion and systemic hypertension. The hypertension is sustained by the influence of $Na^+$ retention rather than of angiotensin,[114] because total GFR and nephron number are seriously compromised.

The $Na^+$ dependence in the presence of a masked or suppressed renin factor can be demonstrated in experimental animals with the two forms of renovascular hypertension. Infusion of an angiotensin blocker produces no fall in blood pressure[115, 116] in the one-kidney one-clip model when dietary salt is not curtailed. Neither does sodium depletion produce a fall in blood pressure, although it does raise the renin level sharply, converting the $Na^+$-dependent hypertension to renin-dependent hypertension, in which anti–renin system drugs now become dramatically effective. Altogether, the system appears to be tending toward maintenance of blood pressure equilibrium in the compromised organ by whatever means are available, either renin- or $Na^+$-dependent hypertension. The behavior of the renin system, participating in or reacting to this goal, provides the clue to the underlying mechanism.

Other patients with bilateral renovascular disease show a marked decrease of blood pressure and exacerbation of azotemia when they are given a converting enzyme inhibitor. Furthermore, renal vein renin patterns may be similar for patients with unilateral disease, with all of the renin coming from the most ischemic kidney.[117] Thus, these patients may also have renin-dependent hypertension. Possibly, in such patients, both renin and volume factors play a role. Acute pulmonary edema is much more common in patients with bilateral disease than it is in those with unilateral disease. This phenomenon may reflect an inability to handle acute volume loads; the same patients may become azotemic when given a converting enzyme inhibitor.[118] Further evidence for volume factors is provided by the observations that such patients typically have a higher cardiac output than do patients with unilateral disease[119] and that natriuresis occurs after angioplasty.

## PRIMARY AND PSEUDOPRIMARY ALDOSTERONISM

Primary aldosteronism, or Conn syndrome, is due to autonomous overproduction of aldosterone by a solitary adrenocortical adenoma.[93] The term pseudoprimary aldosteronism describes a subgroup characterized instead by diffuse bilateral adrenocortical hyperplasia.[120, 121] Together, these conditions are underdiagnosed and account for at least 1% to 2% of all hypertension. In both disorders, overproduction of aldosterone is sustained, producing a clinical syndrome manifested by $Na^+$ and volume retention, low plasma renin activity, hypokalemia with excess kaliuresis, and a $Cl^-$ unresponsive metabolic alkalosis. "Escape" from the $Na^+$-retaining effects of aldosterone accounts for the enhanced natriuresis of an exogenous $Na^+$ load and renal $K^+$ wasting.[122] Plasma renin activity levels are suppressed to nearly zero because of the $Na^+$-volume expansion, increased renal

perfusion pressure, and enhanced sodium chloride delivery to the macula densa.[123, 124] The magnitude of the hypertension and metabolic abnormalities tends to be more marked when an adenoma is identified as the cause of hyperaldosteronism.[124a]

Unilateral adrenalectomy can cure primary aldosteronism when it is caused by a functioning adenoma or, in some cases, by adrenal hyperplasia when aldosterone secretion is comparably autonomous and is confined to one adrenal gland.[124a, 124b] By contrast, adrenalectomy does not cure hypertension in most patients with bilateral hyperplasia. Diagnostic tests that discriminate between primary and pseudoprimary aldosteronism are based on the 1) greater degree of autonomy of aldosterone secretion from renin-angiotensin by the adenoma (i.e., postural stimulation test), 2) the elevated plasma levels of 18-hydroxycorticosterone and urinary excretion of novel metabolites of cortisol metabolism (18-hydroxycortisol, 18-oxocortisol) by the adenoma, and 3) lateralization of aldosterone secretion.[125, 125a] Results of adrenal imaging studies are often inconclusive. Despite the potential for cure, 50% to 60% of patients with an adenoma have persistent hypertension requiring medication after unilateral adrenalectomy.[124a] Those most likely to become normotensive are younger than 50 years and have a maximally suppressed plasma renin activity before surgery.

Some rare, interesting variations on this pathophysiologic theme have been observed. Glucocorticoid remediable aldosteronism, a congenital form of hyperaldosteronism, is caused by a chimeric gene that is formed by unequal crossing over between the genes that encode for $11\beta$-hydroxylase and 18-hydroxylase.[125b] This syndrome and the more common aldosteronoma are the only disorders associated with excess production of C-18–methyloxygenated metabolites.[125c] In other syndromes, such as ectopic corticotropin and excessive ingestion of licorice (which contains glycyrrhizic acid), acquired mineralocorticoid excess occurs because the normal mechanisms of cortisol inactivation are either overwhelmed or attenuated.[125d, 125e] Cortisol is thus allowed to bind to the type I mineralocorticoid receptor with an affinity similar to that of aldosterone. Mineralocorticoid excess syndromes can also be produced by overproduction of deoxycorticosterone[126] and adrenal androgens.[127] In many of these syndromes, $Na^+$-volume expansion and hypertension suppress renin secretion, and consequently endogenous aldosterone production is markedly decreased. By contrast, in hypertension associated with other forms of Cushing syndrome and chronic oral contraceptive use, the renin-angiotensin-aldosterone system may be inappropriately activated as a consequence of increased production of angiotensinogen[128] or by direct augmentation of vascular reactivity.[129]

## TWO FORMS OF VASOCONSTRICTION: WET AND DRY

### Secondary Renal or Adrenal Hypertension

The mechanisms of the more extreme forms of hypertension described so far suggest a spectrum of etiology and of renin system involvement. At one pole of the spectrum is hypertension sustained (and possibly caused) by the vasoconstrictive forces of the renin system's active agent, angiotensin II. At the other pole is the hypertension sustained by nonrenin vasoconstrictive forces, which mainly involves the pressor influence of $Na^+$ retention and the possible joint participation of norepinephrine. The predominance of activity at either pole depresses activity at the other, whereas both vasoconstrictive forces may well assert their influence in the middle regions of the spectrum.

Either polar force is capable of producing the exalted peripheral resistance that is the common characteristic of all hypertension. The similarity ends there, however, for the conditions imposed by these two agents are radically different in their implications for risk, survival, and treatment.

As may be inferred from Figure 46–7, the vasoconstriction generated by angiotensin II, the active component evoked from excess renin secretion, results in a "dry"

| HIGH RENIN | | LOW RENIN |
|---|---|---|
| (Dry vasoconstriction) | | (Wet vasoconstriction) |

### PATHOPHYSIOLOGIC DIFFERENCES

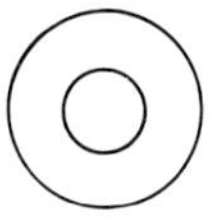

Arterioles

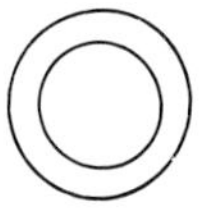

| Higher | Peripheral resistance | High |
|---|---|---|
| High | Aldosterone | Low to High |
| Low | Plasma volume | High |
| Low | Cardiac output | High |
| High | Hematocrit | Low |
| High | Blood urea | Low |
| High | Blood viscosity | Low |
| Low | Tissue perfusion | High |
| Yes | Postural hypotension | No |

### CLINICAL EXAMPLES

| High-renin essential hypertension | Low-renin essential |
|---|---|
| Renovascular and | hypertension |
| malignant hypertension | Primary aldosteronism |

### VASCULAR SEQUELAE

| (+) | Stroke | (−) |
|---|---|---|
| (+) | Heart attack | (−) |
| (+) | Renal damage | (−) |
| (+) | Retinopathy-encephalopathy | (−) |

### TREATMENTS

| (+) | Converting enzyme inhibitors | (−) |
|---|---|---|
| (+) | Beta blockers | (−) |
| | | |
| (−) | Calcium channel blockers | (+) |
| (−) | Diuretics | (+) |
| (−) | Alpha blockers | (+) |

**Figure 46–7.** High blood pressure mechanisms. (Adapted from Laragh JH: Role of the renin-angiotensin-aldosterone axis in human hypertensive disorders. *In* Kaplan NM, Brenner BM, Laragh JH [eds]: Perspectives in Hypertension, Vol 1, The Kidney in Hypertension. Raven Press, New York, 1987, pp 35–52.)

hypertension.[130] It is characterized by a peripheral resistance generally higher than that imposed by the $Na^+$ volume–induced form. Because angiotensin stimulates aldosterone production even while it directly constricts arterioles, aldosterone secretion is correspondingly high. Nevertheless, plasma volume is reactively low (given a reasonable renal capacity for pressure natriuresis), as is cardiac output. By-products of this reactive pressure diuresis are an elevation of blood viscosity, blood urea, and hematocrit. Understandably, tissue perfusion is low, and the patient is susceptible to postural hypotension. The extreme of this dry hypovolemic, ischemic, hemodynamic-rheologic pattern is typical of malignant or renovascular hypertension.

In nonrenin-imposed hypertension, a category in which $\alpha$-adrenergic influences can be circumstantially implicated, peripheral resistance is generally less dramatically elevated. Plasma renin activity ranges from low to absent, whereas aldosterone production varies from low to high. This condition can be called "wet" hypertension because it is associated with higher plasma volumes and cardiac outputs and with lower hematocrit, blood urea, and viscosity. Tissue perfusion is relatively high, and postural hypotension is absent. Primary aldosteronism is the ultimate expression of wet salty hypertension, and low-renin essential hypertension is another good example.

Renin-mediated, or dry, hypertension has been shown to have a higher frequency of vascular sequelae: stroke, heart attack, renal damage, retinopathy, and encephalopathy.[101, 130, 131] The reasons for this finding are probably the poor perfusion and tissue nourishment associated with further vasoconstriction and hemoconcentration. Rheologic study suggests that the friction generated by the viscous blood may contribute to the greater blood pressures associated with this type of hypertension. The relative cardiac protection afforded by low-renin wet hypertension, with its luxurious blood volume and cardiac output, may stem from more congenial rheologic factors and better flow and tissue nourishment (see Fig. 46–7).

The differences between the two major types of hypertension and the role of renin are demonstrated dramatically by the most extreme pathologic conditions. Soaring plasma renin values with reduced blood flow and cardiac output can readily be shown in such dry hypertensions as malignant hypertension or malignant scleroderma; indeed, in the latter, the extremities are black because of poor perfusion. That renin-induced vasoconstriction is the source of the trouble is shown by the dramatic and prompt reversal of these effects by renin system blockade. On the other hand, in primary aldosteronism, wet hypertension finds its paradigm: the runaway $Na^+$ retention builds up massive fluid accumulations, with abundant flow and cardiac output, and causes a reactive shutdown of the renin system. Temporary easing of the situation can be achieved with diuretics, and permanent cure can be achieved by surgically removing the offending adrenocortical tumor. Renin blockade is conspicuously ineffective in this case, for which the source of the vasoconstriction must be sought in other mechanisms.

Interestingly, the existence of the two vasoconstrictive mechanisms, one mediated by renin and the other by $Na^+$-volume forces, is also expressed by Goldblatt's two experimental models. In the animal, when renin secretion is stimulated by clipping a single kidney while leaving the other intact, dry hypertension results because the properly functioning unclipped kidney is able to attempt compensation for the renin-induced vasoconstriction by diuresing $Na^+$ and water. If the unclipped kidney is removed (or both kidneys are clipped), effective glomerular filtration is compromised, and the resultant renal inability to excrete $Na^+$ and water causes accumulation of fluid and then a reactive shutdown of renin secretion; this condition becomes an $Na^+$-volume–induced hypertension. If the animal is deprived of salt and thus the ability to retain fluid, however, renin secretion increases reciprocally to sustain the hypertension. In short, this animal converts its hypertension from $Na^+$ dependence to renin dependence, moving from one pole of the hypertensive vasoconstrictive spectrum to the other.

The clipped kidney behaves as though it *requires* hypertension proximal to the clip and will maintain it by one means or the other. More than one mechanism must then be available to the animal or human host. Considering that vasoconstriction is the common characteristic of all hypertension, expressed universally in increased peripheral resistance, one must conclude that more than one vasoconstrictive mechanism is available for sustaining hypertension. One mechanism is related to renin secretion; the other is related in some way to nonrenin pressor mechanisms, a complex of forces in which $Na^+$, $Ca^{2+}$, and $\alpha$-adrenergic receptors now appear to be in some way linked or interactive.

These animal models find their human counterparts in unilateral and bilateral renovascular disease. Here, too, the level of renin activity in the periphery and renal veins helps make the diagnosis. Like the animal, the human patient with normal- or low-renin bilateral renal artery disease is $Na^+$ retentive but may be converted by salt deprivation to renin-mediated hypertension.

An interesting demonstration of this kind of reciprocation between renin- and $Na^+$-mediated types of vasoconstriction has been made in patients with congestive heart failure who demonstrate a broad splay of renin values, from low to high.[132] Administration of diuretics was stopped in an attempt to manage the patients only by manipulating dietary salt. A high-salt diet promptly converted the high-renin patients to a low-renin state, and a low-salt diet was able to reverse the condition. In some cases, the change in renin values approached 20-fold. The significant finding is that whatever the renin state, blood pressure remained the *same*. Indeed, peripheral resistance, measured with cardiac catheterization before and after salt feeding, remained virtually unchanged even though the means of blood pressure support was switched from $Na^+$ to renin to $Na^+$.

## Two Forms of Vasoconstriction in Essential Hypertension

A reasonable speculation is that the spectral patterns of vasoconstriction demonstrated in the more extreme forms of hypertension might also operate in essential hypertension. Indeed, when renin profiling is correctly performed and indexed in patients with essential hypertension, about 20% are found to have high renin values and about 30% to have low renin values, with the remaining half distributed between these extremes.[101] Does this finding indicate that renin has nothing to do with essential hypertension, or does it instead suggest a vasoconstrictive spectrum like the one identified in the model hypertensive forms described previously?

The question has aroused some controversy in the past, mainly owing to lack of agreement regarding proof of renin blockade. The conflicts have been settled, however, with the advent of converting enzyme inhibitors, which demonstrably interfere with the conversion of angiotensin I to its active vasoconstrictive octapeptide form. These agents are especially effective as depressors in high-renin patients with essential hypertension. They also help in identifying a renin factor or an $Na^+$-volume factor in patients with medium renin levels. In such patients, a brisk depressor response points to a renin factor, and the total lack of depressor response suggests instead an $Na^+$-volume factor that might well be treated long term with diuretic monotherapy. The same guidelines apply to interpreting the responses of low-renin patients, except that a significant renin factor is much less likely in them.

$Na^+$ retention obviously plays a dominant role in low-renin essential hypertension, given the impressive performance of diuretics and $Na^+$ depletion in this category compared with their spotty results in high-renin patients.[133] The diuretic correction of this hypertension is associated with a reactive rise of renin levels, sometimes to normal values. Moreover, in all studies, hypertensive patients with low renin values have been found to exhibit larger blood and extracellular fluid volumes than do the normal or high-renin patients.[69]

The means by which $Na^+$ retention exerts its pressor effects are still not completely understood, however. In just the last few years, the possibility that there may be more than one pathway to the source of low-renin hypertension has become apparent. The first of these indications has come from the worldwide experience showing that $Ca^{2+}$ influx antagonists act most predictably as depressors in low-renin patients with essential hypertension.[134, 135] Resnick and co-workers[136] have shown that serum $Ca^{2+}$ concentration is directly related to plasma renin activity, whereas serum $Mg^{2+}$ concentration is inversely related to plasma renin activity. A high-salt diet has also been demonstrated to reduce plasma $Ca^{2+}$ (most probably because of influx to the cell) to levels similar to those seen in low-renin essential hypertension, and salt restriction has been shown to do the reverse.[137] One may consider the possibility that the influence of dietary sodium on blood pressure may be mediated by companion or induced changes in these divalent cations.

The significance of the $Na^+$-$Ca^{2+}$ relationship takes on additional dimensions when one realizes that cytosolic $Ca^{2+}$ is a critical actor in the neural theater,[138] and that neural blockade is yet another avenue through which vasopressor phenomena may be influenced. What makes this avenue especially attractive now is the availability of the newer $\alpha_1$-adrenergic blockers doxazosin and terazosin, which selectively engage postsynaptic $\alpha_1$-receptors with a specificity unconnected with the widespread side effects associated with the earlier ganglionic blockers.

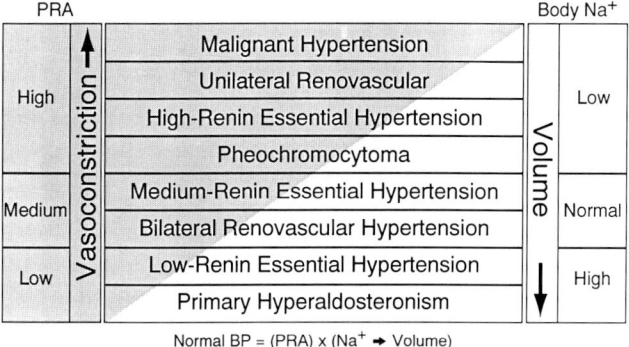

**The Laragh Vasoconstriction-Volume Spectrum of Clinical Hypertension**

Normal BP = (PRA) x (Na⁺ ➡ Volume)

**Figure 46–8.** Normal subjects, as indicated by the equation, maintain and defend normotension by curtailing renal renin secretion in reaction to a rise in sodium intake or autonomic vasoconstriction, or by proportionally increasing renin secretion in the face of either $Na^+$ depletion or hypotension from fluid or blood loss or a neurogenic fall in blood pressure. Hypertensive subjects sustain their higher blood pressures by renal secretion of too much renin for their $Na^+$-volume states, or by renal retention of too much $Na^+$ ($\rightarrow$ volume) for their renin level, which often fails to fully turn off as it does in normal subjects. High-renin hypertensive patients are proportionately more vasoconstricted with poorer tissue perfusion and therefore most susceptible to cardiovascular tissue ischemic damage (see text). BP = blood pressure; PRA = plasma renin activity.

Significantly, the depressor effects of these agents are particularly selective among low-renin hypertensive patients, those also preferred by $Ca^{2+}$ channel blockers and diuretics. This form of vasoconstriction is related to antecedent $Na^+$-volume retention. Nicholson and associates[139] have demonstrated marked orthostatic decreases in blood pressure as a first-dose response to prazosin, the degree of which was inversely correlated with baseline plasma renin activity. Furthermore, this α-antagonism stimulated reactive renin secretion when it lowered pressure, again demonstrating reciprocation between renin and nonrenin pressor phenomena. Also, the antihypertensive effectiveness of a $Ca^{2+}$ channel blocking drug is apparently not helped by $Na^+$ depletion and may actually be enhanced by the concurrent liberalization of salt intake.[140–142] Because this suppresses renin levels, these drugs, too, appear to be most effective in reversing $Na^+$-volume–related arteriolar vasoconstriction.

## Human Hypertensive Disorders as a Spectrum of Abnormal Plasma Renin–Sodium-Volume Products

From the foregoing it is apparent that just as normotension is sustained and defended by fluctuation of plasma renin activity according to salt intake and $Na^+$ balance, human hypertensive states are characterized instead by too much renal renin secretion and thus plasma renin activity for the concurrent state of $Na^+$ balance (i.e., by a spectrum of abnormally high plasma renin levels) for the $Na^+$-volume status or vice versa. At the renal level, this situation arises from a failure to turn off renin secretion normally in the face of abnormal $Na^+$ retention caused by nephron

heterogeneity with a subpopulation of hypofiltering nephrons with unabated renin secretion; this interferes with the adaptive natriuresis of the neighboring normal nephrons[67, 68] (see earlier).

The higher renin states (Fig. 46–8, top four disorders) have the most severe vascular disease, with damage to the heart, brain, and kidneys. Even pheochromocytoma is associated with high renin levels consequent to norepinephrine-induced renal ischemia. By contrast, the $Na^+$-retaining high-volume forms of hypertension have suppressed renin secretion and present with much less vascular disease and better tissue perfusion associated with an $Na^+$-volume excess. The ultimate examples are low-renin hypertension and primary aldosteronism, both of which are typically benign long-standing conditions because of better tissue perfusion. The intermediate forms with a mixed renin-$Na^+$ excess develop intermediate degrees of cardiovascular damage. Bilateral renal artery stenosis (or a coarctation) have $Na^+$-volume retention, which only partially suppresses renin secretion distal to the destruction. This category can present with pulmonary edema when $Na^+$-volume is not controlled.[143]

## EXCESS PLASMA RENIN ACTIVITY IN HYPERTENSIVE CARDIOVASCULAR INJURY AND THE POTENTIAL FOR PHARMACOLOGIC CONTAINMENT

The foregoing defines a key role for excess plasma renin activity in causing the vascular damage of malignant and renovascular hypertension. A large literature has now accumulated characterizing the vasculotoxic effects of renin or angiotensin I administration and relating high renin levels in humans to situations associated with encephalopathy, stroke, myocardial infarction, and renal damage. This has been extensively reviewed.[144]

Accordingly, there is now special promise for this concept of blocking or curtailing excessive plasma renin activity in hypertensive people to prevent, or reverse, the vascular disease in the heart, brain, and kidneys that accounts for premature morbidity and mortality in hypertension. Thus, clinical studies in both moderate to severe[101] and mild hypertension[102] confirm that the baseline plasma renin level is a powerful predictor of a subsequent heart attack. Conversely, too, the lowness of the renin level in low-renin patients (values <0.65 ng/mL/h) is directly related to the absence of subsequent myocardial infarction. The plasma renin level is an even more potent predictor of heart attack in patients with no other risk factors. In this large group, the heart attack rate was directly related to the height of the renin level, and in 241 consecutive low-renin patients observed for 8 years, no heart attacks occurred.[102] These relationships hold even though low-renin patients have at least as much hypertension and are often older, two factors that would work to increase heart attack and stroke rates in them. On the other side of the coin, too, it has been recognized that high-renin states in general (e.g., malignant scleroderma, renovascular and malignant hypertensions) are associated with the most severe cardiovascular damage and premature death.[144]

New evidence also supports the idea that the plasma renin level is pathogenically involved in human heart attack. Thus, an unexpected finding in both the SAVE[145] (captopril) and SOLVD[146] (enalapril) trials of congestive heart failure was that addition of either of these two anti–renin system drugs produced impressive reductions in the myocardial infarction rates in these patients. In the Consensus Trial of heart failure, both the effectiveness of enalapril and the mortality rates with treatment were favorably correlated to the entry plasma renin activity value.[147] Another converting enzyme inhibitor has also produced protection from all causes of death in patients with heart failure.[148] When this evidence is combined with other studies showing that β-blocker therapy also protects impressively against myocardial reinfarction,[149] it becomes apparent that it is the anti–renin system agents (either angiotensin-converting enzyme inhibitors or β-blockers) that have special value for protection from progression of coronary artery disease. Furthermore, angiotensin-converting enzyme inhibition therapy has been shown to protect against ventricular remodeling when it is given soon after an acute myocardial infarction.[150] All of this is to be contrasted with the negative or even worsening effects obtained in older trials involving diuretics or later trials using dihydropyridine calcium antagonists,[151, 152] agents that deplete volume and increase plasma renin activity.

There is also a large literature in animals defining the coronary cerebral and renal vascular damage caused by renin or angiotensin II administration.[144] However, three animal studies seem especially relevant. One study confirmed that potassium feeding to stroke-prone spontaneously hypertensive rats dramatically reduces the stroke rate.[153] This prevention was associated with potassium feeding–induced prevention of the usual prestroke rises in plasma renin activity. In two other studies,[154, 155] administration of the specific type I angiotensin receptor blocker losartan dramatically protected against development of cerebral cardiac and renal vascular disease in both stroke-prone spontaneously hypertensive[155] and Dahl salt-sensitive[154] rats, even when the blood pressure was *not* reduced. Thus, it appears that excessive plasma angiotensin II formation may be directly involved in causation of experimental hypertensive cardiovascular disease with ischemic stroke, myocardial infarction, and fibrinoid renal vascular disease.

## EVALUATION AND TREATMENT OF THE INDIVIDUAL PATIENT

### General Principles

The evaluation of a new patient with high blood pressure embraces all the principles of good medical practice. It relies on a complete history and physical examination and the routine application of appropriately chosen laboratory tests. A thorough initial evaluation can avoid the prescription of needless or inappropriate drugs for the lifetime commitment that hypertension may often require, and at the

start, it can reveal surgically curable hypertension or other important medical diseases.

For most hypertensive patients, the pretreatment evaluation is most efficiently accomplished in the office setting. Multiple visits have the advantage of defining the persistence or lability of the hypertensive process. In general, the milder or more labile the hypertension is, the longer the evaluation period will be before commitment to therapy.[32] Except when the hypertension is severe or complications are impending or present, treatment should be withheld throughout the evaluation. For patients already on ineffective therapy, cautious withdrawal of the drugs during the initial evaluation is worthwhile to determine whether the hypertension is persistent or even drug induced and, in the case of multiple drug therapy, whether all or any of the agents are in fact necessary. In this general approach, hospitalization is reserved for those patients with severe hypertensive disease, those with impending complications, and those for whom the outpatient data suggest the need for specialized diagnostic procedures.

For some patients receiving relatively simple and well-tolerated therapy, the physician may decide that the program already in force is adequate and need not be disturbed. However, the physician should not hesitate to stop medications in those in whom the regimen appears even slightly unsatisfactory or unpalatable. A repeated observation at The New York Hospital–Cornell Medical Center is that when hypertension persists in patients receiving multiple drug therapy, which sometimes involves as many as four or five different agents, stopping medications gradually and serially usually does not lead to any further rise in blood pressure. Surprisingly often, the blood pressure may actually improve as the medical regimen is simplified. In the Veterans Administration study of severe hypertension (diastolic pressure greater than 110 mm Hg), 15% of those patients in whom all drugs were stopped remained normotensive for the ensuing 18 months of observation.[156] Serial withdrawal of drugs in patients who are poorly controlled with multiple drug therapy puts the physician in the best position for re-evaluating the disease process and setting up new therapeutic strategies.

The foregoing portions of this chapter have suggested that two clinically quantifiable mechanisms for long-term arteriolar vasoconstriction can be identified in individual patients. The first, renin-mediated vasoconstriction, is directly related to the height of the plasma renin level. The second, $Na^+$-volume–related hypertension, is marked by a subnormal renin level and involves abnormal $Na^+$-volume retention and $Ca^{2+}$ transport. The baseline renin-$Na^+$ profile permits the diagnosis of two curable forms that fully express one of these two mechanisms—renovascular hypertension and primary aldosteronism. Renovascular hypertension, which is more common than once thought, can often be cured by balloon angioplasty. Thus, ruling out these two possibilities before beginning long-term therapy is especially important.

Converting enzyme inhibitors or β-blockers given alone are, by themselves, often fully effective in high- or medium-renin patients, whereas $Ca^{2+}$ antagonists or diuretics given alone are most effective against the low-renin form of vasoconstriction. In the large middle zone of renin values, both mechanisms may operate. The renin-Na$^+$ profile, used in conjunction with baseline serum K$^+$ and creatinine measurements, is useful for screening patients with curable forms of hypertension and for stratifying the remaining patients according to the pathophysiologic mechanism that underlies the hypertension. This simplifies the drug selection process and also indicates the likelihood of cardiovascular complications.

## Goals of the Initial Evaluation

There are five major goals of the initial evaluation:

1. To establish whether the hypertension is sustained and might benefit from treatment
2. To define coexisting diseases
3. To characterize other risk factors
4. To identify the presence and extent of target organ damage
5. To identify or exclude curable causes of the hypertension

A rational method for selecting drugs for the individual hypertensive patient must be based on an individual pathophysiologic evaluation. The diagnostic workup, aside from the routine blood count and urinalysis, includes serum K$^+$, blood urea nitrogen, and serum creatinine concentrations; an electrocardiogram and a baseline echocardiogram for full evaluation of left ventricular mass; and the renin-Na$^+$ profile, which is described in the next section. The first goal of this process (see Table 46–3) is to identify or exclude definable and curable causes for the hypertensive disorder. Doing so may spare many patients a lifetime of needless, costly, and intrusive drug therapy, for often a cure can be effected by relatively simple, nonsurgical techniques.

The remaining 90% or so of patients, for whom no definable cause for the hypertension can be found but who can be stratified pathophysiologically by the renin-Na$^+$ test, are candidates for long-term drug therapy. This statistic assumes, of course, that their hypertension is significant ($\geq$150/95 mm Hg) and sustained, is possibly causing target organ strain, and is not responsive to simple nonpharmacologic forms of therapy (weight reduction, exercise, low-salt diet, and alcohol and tobacco withdrawal). For these individuals, the baseline evaluation process informs the selection of the most effective and least counterproductive non-drug or drug regimen from the diversity of modern antihypertensive agents available.

With the initial workup in hand, today's practitioner can arrive more directly at the primary goal of any long-term drug therapy: to give each patient the fewest number of drugs in the smallest effective amounts and with the lowest possible frequency. This goal is particularly important in hypertension, because every antihypertensive drug presents a problem of toxicity of one degree or another, and because the commitment to such a drug may be long term and possibly lifelong. Effective monotherapy of hypertension is now more possible than many physicians think, and this advance is significant in a field so characterized in the past by additive and multiple drug therapy.

## Medical History

Evaluation of the severity and pace of the hypertensive disorder is important to allow planning of the pace of the medical workup and treatment. Normally, the workup is accomplished in an unhurried manner during several visits spaced at weekly or biweekly intervals. The initial examination, however, should bring out enough information so that the workup can be accelerated for more critically ill patients.

Accordingly, after learning of any current symptoms, the physician should record the duration of the hypertension, the circumstances of its onset, and the highest known readings. Was the blood pressure elevation merely discovered on routine examination? Has loss of well-being, decline in general vigor, or weight loss occurred? What drugs has the patient tried, and what effect have they produced? Has the patient taken oral contraceptives?

The neurologic history may disclose headaches. Classically, headaches in hypertensive patients are said to be occipital and pulsatile, most prominent on awakening, and gradually lessening during the day. In some patients, however, the headaches may be constricting and nonpulsatile, the so-called tension headaches. Possibly, this symptom is no more common in hypertensive patients than in normotensive people. Moreover, studies indicate that when headaches do occur in hypertensive patients, they are not well correlated with the degree of elevation of blood pressure.

Signs and symptoms of autonomic nervous system vasomotor instability seem more common among hypertensive patients. These signs include a tendency for flushing, and the patient may report excessive sweating or even a lack of sweating. In a previous era, patients with flushing phenomena associated with high blood pressure were termed "diencephalic"; although flushing can occur in hypertensive patients, its cause remains unexplained.

Other neurologic symptoms include blurred vision, unsteadiness of gait, depression, insomnia, sluggishness, and in some patients, a decreased libido. Whereas some of these symptoms may be nonspecific, blurred vision may reflect vascular changes in the fundi. More advanced hypertensive disease may also be accompanied by more defined focal sensory or motor neurologic changes, occurring paroxysmally and associated with either transient ischemic attacks or more sustained attacks presaging the onset of hypertensive encephalopathy or stroke.

The cardiovascular system may be symptom free in early or uncomplicated hypertensive disease. Early signs of dysfunction are expressed by palpitations signifying either tachycardia or a forceful heart beat, by increased fatigability, or by shortness of breath on effort, which probably reflect the increased cardiac work of hypertension or impending heart failure. Young patients with labile or largely systolic hypertension may exhibit tachycardia and signs of an unstable or hyperdynamic circulation. This sort of vasomotor instability (also called neurocirculatory asthenia, or soldier's heart) can occur in normotensive people. On the other hand, it could at times reflect higher cardiac output and stroke volume, which are described in some patients with early hypertensive disease. Palpitations may also reflect dysrhythmia. Evidence that cardiac arrhythmias are more common in hypertensive than in normotensive people, especially in the presence of demonstrable left ventricular hypertrophy, has been obtained.[157–159] Because coronary artery disease and myocardial infarction occur more frequently in hypertensive patients, a history of angina pectoris, and even of a documented myocardial infarction, may be elicited. Hypertensive patients with left ventricular hypertrophy have been reported to have a higher mortality despite apparent control of blood pressure.[159]

The renal history may reveal antecedent acute glomerulonephritis, proteinuria, hematuria, nocturia, polyuria, or recurrent urinary tract infections. Renal colic or renal trauma should be noted, and the physician should suspect that the hypertension has a renal basis whenever it can be established that the urinary tract symptoms or the proteinuria preceded the hypertension. An abrupt onset of hypertension with rapid progression, especially in young or old patients, should lead the physician to a strong suspicion of renovascular hypertension due to either fibromuscular hyperplasia or an atherosclerotic plaque. This suspicion is reinforced by retinopathy or by cardiac or renal involvement, all of which are likely to be more prominent in renovascular (renin-dependent) hypertension. Renin-secreting tumors (hemangiopericytoma) of the juxtaglomerular apparatus[160] and Wilms tumor represent rare diseases that are more common in childhood and also may be associated with abrupt and severe hypertension.

Polyuria or nocturia may indicate more severe renal hypertension or a metabolic abnormality such as hypokalemia or hypercalcemia. Inability to concentrate the urine, with polydipsia, polyuria, and nocturia, commonly occurs in patients with primary aldosteronism or malignant hypertension or in patients with such chronic renal disorders as glomerulonephritis, polycystic disease, pyelonephritis, or diabetic nephropathy. Muscle weakness may accompany hypokalemia or hypercalcemia.

Patients should be interrogated about their smoking, drinking, exercise, and dietary habits. Obesity is certainly an important factor in producing or amplifying hypertension, especially when body weight exceeds 20% or more of the norm. Excessive regular consumption of alcohol can also induce or aggravate hypertension, and in some patients, cessation of the habit may correct the hypertensive process. Tobacco, because of its known vasoconstrictive action, is especially contraindicated in hypertensive subjects, even though no causal relationship between smoking and the development of essential hypertension has been defined. Physical exercise purportedly reduces blood pressure in previously untrained subjects, but more research on this relationship and its claimed benefits is needed. Also, an estimate should be made of the adjustment of the patient to his or her life situation and of any emotional or psychiatric factors that seem relevant. The risk factor analysis is completed by the identification of any target organ damage and of any other coexisting diseases.

## Physical Examination

**Special Aspects.** The general appearance is unrevealing in most patients with hypertension. However, a florid facies—with or without a tendency for rapid color changes, which would suggest vasomotor instability—may signify an underlying metabolic process, perhaps pheochromocytoma, a hyperdynamic circulation, hyperthyroidism, or, alternatively, the anxiety or the vasomotor instability characteristic of some patients with essential hypertension. Chronic alcoholism may also produce some of these signs, and it can also cause hypertension characterized by β-adrenergic activity on withdrawal from alcohol use. A ruddy complexion with a bluish tinge characterizes some patients with essential hypertension and reactive polycythemia (Gaisböck syndrome). High-renin patients with essential hypertension may also present with a dusky appearance associated with vasoconstriction and a higher hematocrit.

Truncal obesity with moon facies, frontal baldness, atrophic extremities with abdominal striae, atrophy of the skin, and spontaneous ecchymoses suggests Cushing syndrome. Multiple neurofibromas or café au lait discoloration of the skin suggests a familial basis for an associated pheochromocytoma. Also, mucosal neuromas may be associated with other components of the syndrome of multiple endocrine adenomatosis with hypertension. Renal failure may be expressed by a pale yellowish skin, periorbital and peripheral edema, and uremic breath.

**Blood Pressure.** In the majority of hypertensive patients, elevated blood pressure is the only abnormal finding. Hence, the way in which the blood pressure is measured assumes great importance. The patient should be seated quietly, and a cuff size appropriate to the arm diameter should be chosen.[161] Several readings should be taken, and it is generally recommended that phase 5 of Korotkoff sounds be taken as diastolic pressure. Establishing a diagnosis of hypertension often requires more than one visit, because the pressure tends to fall with repeated measurement. Even after several visits, however, a fairly sizable group of patients show a persistently elevated pressure in the clinic although they are normotensive at other times.[4] This phenomenon, often referred to as "white coat hypertension," can be detected only by including measurements made outside the clinic; these measurements can be obtained by having the patient measure his or her blood pressure at home or by ambulatory monitoring.[162] A knowledge of the patient's blood pressure in these circumstances can be of great value in deciding on the need for treatment and in evaluating its efficacy.

**Fundus.** Ophthalmoscopic examination of the optic fundi is one of the most valuable clinical tools for assessing target organ damage, the severity and duration of the hypertension, and the urgency for applying treatment. The degree of changes observed in the retina is rated from grade 0 to grade IV according to the classification of Wagener and Barker.

Grade 0 represents normal optic fundi. Grade I is minimal lesion disease, characterized by spasm or by the so-called copper or silver wire appearance of the arterioles, with some tortuosity and perhaps segmental constriction. Spasm can be visualized as a subnormal lumen wall/ratio. When spasm occurs with little or no sclerosis, it may be interpreted as representing angiospastic disease, which suggests the recent onset of hypertension.

With grade II retinopathy, there is evidence of arteriolar

sclerosis including heightened light reflex, or arteriovenous nicking, in addition to generalized or local focal spasm. These sclerotic changes usually indicate that the disease has been present for at least several months and probably for several years.

Grade III changes in the fundi are characterized by all of the foregoing alterations with the addition of overt hemorrhage or exudates. Hemorrhage may be diffuse and asymmetric, or it may take the shape of a flame radiating from the optic disk along the vascular tree. To some extent, the color of the hemorrhage suggests the age of the process. Exudates may be described as soft or hard. Hard exudates are shiny and circumscribed, reflecting an older and healing process. They are the result of deposition of lipid material from older extravasations and may be diffusely scattered or arranged in prominent lines emanating from the macular area. Soft exudates are cottony or wool-like spots reflecting fibrinoid change. Soft exudates and hemorrhage suggest ongoing severe or accelerated hypertension requiring urgent treatment.

Grade IV retinopathy is characterized by papilledema or edema of the optic disk margins, especially on the temporal side. (Blurring of the nasal margin may occasionally occur without disease.) Elevation of the optic nerve is generally considered to be characteristic of malignant hypertension. It is usually accompanied by hemorrhage and fresh exudates and is especially prominent when the hypertension is associated with overt vasoconstriction. The vasoconstriction is usually caused by renin excess, but it can also be observed in patients with pheochromocytoma.

When hypertension is of more recent onset, papilledema may occur without grade III changes. It can occur in the various low-renin states, in which volume excess and water intoxication figure as the largest factors in pathogenesis. Papilledema without attendant vascular changes may also suggest pseudomotor cerebri or central nervous system disease with increased intracranial pressure. The presence of attendant neurologic signs, especially seizures, may help diagnosis. Whenever neurologic signs appear, the physician should look for microemboli in the retinal arterioles and increased ocular pressure; these findings could indicate an ulcerated plaque in the internal carotid artery on the ipsilateral side.

**Heart.** In hypertensive disease, the heart is frequently more affected than either the brain or kidneys. Hypertension in adults is a leading cause of cardiac hypertrophy and dilatation as well as congestive heart failure.

The mechanical effects on the heart of sustained increase of pressure work may be reflected in the physical findings. A forceful apical thrust is common even in early hypertensive disease and may be exaggerated in the so-called hyperdynamic state. In contrast, a sustained, heaving left ventricular pulse indicates significant hypertrophy due to pressure overload. Probably the earliest physical sign of cardiac involvement is the fourth heart sound (S₄), the "atrial gallop" occasionally heard in normal patients; it is usually audible before cardiac enlargement is detectable, and it is said to reflect a reduced ventricular compliance leading to a more forceful atrial contraction. The fourth heart sound may correlate with the finding of P wave abnormalities on the electrocardiogram. The third heart sound, the "ventricular

gallop," may occur in young subjects with rapid ventricular filling. In older patients, it may be a late manifestation of hypertensive heart disease and reflects the early diastolic compliance abnormality of left ventricular failure.

In severe hypertension, an accentuated aortic second sound may be accompanied by an aortic insufficiency murmur. This soft diastolic murmur may be heard in the second right interspace and along the left sternal border. It suggests dilatation of the aortic ring and may indicate the need for more urgent therapy.

The aforementioned murmur should not be confused with the diastolic murmur of calcific aortic disease, which is more commonly found in hypertensive patients older than 60 years. When associated with primary aortic regurgitation disease, hypertension in elderly patients is usually systolic, with a wider pulse pressure. This form of systolic hypertension is best treated with agents that reduce peripheral resistance, such as vasodilators, α-adrenergic blocking drugs, and antiangiotensin agents. Diuretics and β-adrenergic blockers are relatively contraindicated in this syndrome. Aortic stenosis in the elderly, usually from calcific valvular disease, is associated with a systolic murmur, a narrow pulse pressure, and a slow carotid upstroke. Diastolic hypertension is rare or mild in this situation.

Finally, the syndrome of a hyperkinetic or hyperdynamic circulation may occasionally be encountered in adolescents and young adults with or without hypertension. If present, the hypertension is labile, largely systolic, and accompanied by tachycardia at rest, a forceful apical thrust, and occasional pulsation in the carotid arteries. Whenever this syndrome is encountered, the possibility of metabolic or psychiatric factors should be pursued.

In a younger patient, a harsh systolic murmur over the precordium or midscapular area of the back suggests coarctation of the aorta. This finding should lead the physician to compare the blood pressures in the arms and legs and obtain an echocardiographic examination of the aortic valve, because bicuspid aortic valves commonly occur in association with coarctation of the aorta.

**Vascular System.** Bruits and thrills, evidencing occlusive disease, are increased in hypertensive patients and may occur throughout the arterial tree. Accordingly, the physician should examine the peripheral arteries, the carotid arteries in the neck, the abdominal aorta, the renal arteries, and the femoral arteries. A diastolic component to a bruit or palpable thrill over a peripheral vessel usually suggests a tighter stenosis. Systolic bruits without diastolic components tend to be less significant; when they occur in the abdomen, they may have no particular importance.

A systolic bruit over the carotid artery can be significant, however. Carotid auscultation should be performed in every patient. The stethoscope is placed over the external carotid in the supraclavicular region as close to the angle of the jaw as possible. Particularly when a precordial bruit is also heard, this approach may help distinguish a transmitted sound from an intrinsic sound.

Bruits can be unilateral or bilateral. They may be audible throughout the cardiac cycle or only during systole. In our experience, although bruits are likely to occur with equal frequency in normotensive and hypertensive subjects (about 5%), they have far graver prognostic significance in the hypertensive person. Although the carotid bruit is a marker for subsequent cardiovascular disease, it does not predict the location of the lesion. Indeed, our experience suggests that patients with carotid bruits are more likely to have heart attacks than cerebrovascular accidents.

A systolic bruit over the femoral artery suggests atherosclerotic disease but does not necessarily imply occlusion. When pulses in the lower extremities are absent or dampened, coarctation of the aorta should be suspected in a young person, and occlusive aortic femoral disease should be suspected in an older one.

**Abdomen.** The aorta should be palpated carefully in all patients inasmuch as aortic dilatation or aneurysm is a highly treatable condition best identified in the initial physical examination. A systolic and diastolic bruit in the upper epigastrium or in one or both upper quadrants of the abdomen suggests renal artery stenosis and should encourage the physician to pursue this diagnosis if other criteria are compatible. A palpable enlargement of one or both kidneys can suggest polycystic renal disease, hydronephrosis, or a renal tumor. Rarely is a pheochromocytoma large enough to be palpable.

**Neurologic Examination.** Gross neurologic deficits in sensory or motor function, mentation, or mood are not likely to be ignored. More subtle deficits suggesting transient cerebral ischemia or autonomic dysfunction may be overlooked and should be sought for clinically, especially when the history is suggestive.

## Laboratory Evaluation

### INITIAL LABORATORY EXAMINATION

The initial laboratory workup should include complete blood count and hematocrit together with complete urinalysis; blood urea nitrogen, serum creatinine, serum uric acid, fasting blood glucose, and serum electrolyte measurements; and a lipid profile. If the serum $K^+$ level is borderline or low (i.e., $\leq 3.6$ mEq/L), the test should be repeated on two or three separate occasions. The serum $K^+$ concentration serves as a baseline value for the subsequent response to thiazide diuretics and often provides the first laboratory clue to the presence of aldosterone excess.

With the current widespread use of automated laboratory testing, a variety of other relevant tests may be added at little or no extra cost. Serum $Ca^{2+}$ and circulating thyroid hormone levels may point to parathyroid or thyroid disease, which can sometimes exist without clear-cut clinical evidence.

Tests of lipid, cholesterol, and triglyceride metabolism are usually offered as part of these automated testing profiles. Even the advocates of this group of tests, however, agree that in patients older than 60 and probably older than 50 years, blood lipids have little or no prognostic value except when they are markedly abnormal.

When pheochromocytoma is suspected, measurements of catecholamines in plasma or in urine, or in both, or measurements of their urinary metabolites can be extremely helpful. Similarly, measurement of urinary free cortisol or urinary 17-hydroxycorticosteroids can help to confirm the diagnosis. Sometimes, the dexamethasone suppression test may be necessary to define the nature of the Cushing syndrome.

Urinary aldosterone levels are extremely valuable for revealing the rate of adrenal aldosterone secretion and thus for establishing the diagnosis of primary or pseudoprimary aldosteronism, and they help in evaluating other hypertensive situations associated with either high renin levels or $K^+$ wastage or with both.

In some major centers, excretory urography has been included routinely in the basic workup, primarily to screen patients who might have surgically curable renovascular disease. Clearly, however, the test has too many shortcomings for this purpose. Various studies show that false-negative results occur in 10% to 30% of patients who are subsequently treated surgically.[163] False-positive results of a similar degree also occur. At best, a positive test result is merely an indication for more specific testing, and a negative test result should not deter the physician from more specific tests when renovascular disease is strongly suspected.

In patients diagnosed as having renal disease, excretory urography remains useful for defining renal architecture and for revealing discrepancies in the size of the kidneys and their capacity for concentrating dye. The test may also help define renal anatomy in patients slated for surgery. Because the procedure is relatively expensive, invasive, and not without hazard, its replacement by such simpler and more specific screening tests as the peripheral plasma renin and renal vein studies constitutes a practical advance. The introduction of digital subtraction angiography has made it possible to perform renal arteriograms safely on an outpatient basis. However, this procedure can fail to identify significant arterial lesions detectable by traditional arteriography. This approach as well as other newer methods of vascular visualization (ultrasonography, Doppler ultrasonography, and nuclear magnetic resonance) hold promise for the near future.

A chest x-ray examination is highly desirable as part of every initial workup, particularly in patients older than 50 years. It can reveal coarctation of the aorta and can be useful in assessing cardiac hypertrophy. Moreover, it still has value for pulmonary screening of smokers.

### ELECTROCARDIOGRAPHY

A routine electrocardiogram is highly desirable for all new patients with established high blood pressure. Manifestations of hypertensive heart disease include T wave abnormalities, expressed either by notching or by a biphasic form, particularly in the precordial leads. As left ventricular hypertrophy progresses, voltage of the R waves increases, and then a characteristic strain pattern involving ST segment depressions and T wave inversion occurs.

Cardiac hypertrophy has relevance for identifying patients at risk. Studies show that at any level of blood pressure elevation, patients with electrocardiographic or radiographic abnormalities had twofold or greater increases in premature mortality rates.[164, 165] Electrocardiography and chest radiography are of limited efficiency, however, in detecting left ventricular hypertrophy; they have been shown to detect this feature in approximately only 5% or fewer of unselected hypertensive patients.[164]

## ECHOCARDIOGRAPHY

Significantly greater sensitivity has been demonstrated by echocardiography, which enabled Savage and associates[166] to detect left ventricular hypertrophy in nearly 50% of hypertensive patients. Other studies showed that among patients with essential hypertension, left ventricular performance was best in the low-renin group[167, 168] (Fig. 46–9).

Despite the greater sensitivity of echocardiography, left ventricular hypertrophy may occasionally be identifiable by electrocardiographic criteria even when echocardiographic results are normal. This situation may occur when cardiac mass is still not greatly increased, although myocardial ischemia may be sufficient to produce the inverted T waves of the so-called strain pattern.[169]

With the advent of echocardiography and its application to the development of highly sensitive methods for examining cardiac structure and function,[170, 171] investigators have been able to study the evolution of cardiac hypertrophy in hypertensive patients with greater precision than before. An increased left ventricular mass is much more common than earlier methods indicated, involving 20% or more of unselected patients with established hypertension. Moreover, the presence of left ventricular hypertrophy has powerful prognostic value.[171] In fact, it now appears more relevant than blood pressure itself for predicting morbid events. The development of left ventricular hypertrophy is, in general, directly related to blood pressure,[172] and especially to the blood pressure level during activity.[170, 173] It is also directly related to whole blood viscosity.[174] These associations notwithstanding, some patients with severe established hypertension do not demonstrate left ventricular hypertrophy. Moreover, among those in whom left ventricular hypertro-

phy does develop, one of two different patterns is observed—concentric or eccentric hypertrophy.

Further research is required to determine whether this heterogeneity in the cardiac response to hypertension is in fact related to different mechanisms of hypertension. Based on preliminary evidence, a particularly attractive theory implicates activity of the renin-angiotensin system in some situations and perhaps an $Na^+$-volume, $Ca^{2+}$-mediated stimulus in others. This possible linkage between cardiac and hormonal heterogeneity in hypertensive diseases may also provide a basis for understanding differences in effectiveness of various antihypertensive drugs in reversing left ventricular hypertrophy.

## Identifying Curable Forms of Hypertension

As pointed out earlier in this chapter, curable and definable forms of hypertension should be identified before long-term drug therapy is contemplated. Rarer causes of chronic hypertension aside, the baseline evaluation has much to offer in detecting the presence or absence of kidney disease, including such surgically curable forms of hypertension as renovascular hypertension, coarctation of the aorta, pheochromocytoma, and primary aldosteronism.

The renin-$Na^+$ profile, which shows either high-normal or increased renin levels in curable renovascular disease and suppressed levels in primary aldosteronism, is a valuable primary screen in this endeavor.[111] It is no more expensive or complicated than the cholesterol assays so common nowadays, and it is potentially far more relevant, not only because it can enable the absolute diagnosis of curable forms, but also because it can be used for physiologic evaluation and treatment planning. The test originally involved the collection of a 24-hour urine specimen for $Na^+$ measurement; a venous blood sample for renin measurement is collected while the patient is seated quietly in the office. The 24-hour urine collection has been replaced by a casual urinary $Na^+$/creatinine measurement to exclude the influence of drastic salt depletion. The plasma renin activity level is plotted against the 24-hour urinary $Na^+$ level and in this way provides correction for the fact that renin, as a regulatory hormone, rises normally in response to a low-salt diet and declines in response to a high-salt diet (see Fig. 46–5). As with most laboratory tests, the renin-$Na^+$ profile is most powerful when its deviations from normal are great. Low or high values lead one to suspect, respectively, adrenocortical or curable renovascular disease. Indeed, the baseline plasma renin and serum $K^+$ measurements are the essential tools for the exclusion or diagnosis of these types of hypertension.

The matter of excluding curable hypertension has a special meaning and urgency these days, for the possibilities of cure of renovascular disease have multiplied dramatically with the advent of balloon angioplasty, and the number of cases being detected by a simple and inexpensive captopril test (see later) has increased. At The New York Hospital–Cornell Medical Center, balloon dilatation has been successfully employed in treating well over 1000 patients. More than two thirds of those patients with normal renal

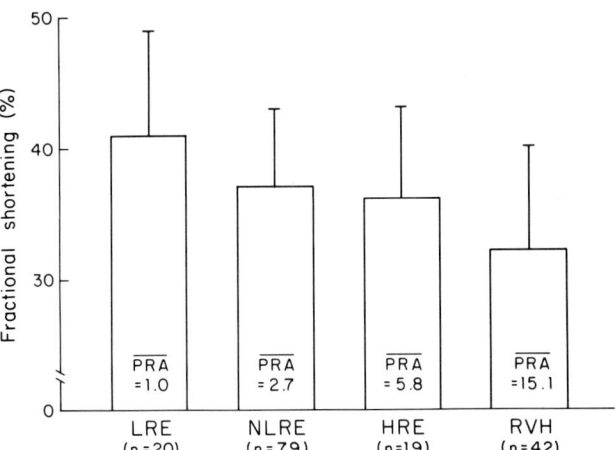

**Figure 46–9.** An inverse relation is observed between left ventricular performance as measured by fractional shortening and plasma renin activity (PRA) level in groups of patients with low-renin (LRE), normal-renin (NLRE), and high-renin (HRE) forms of essential hypertension and with renovascular hypertension (RVH). (Data from Devereux et al[167] and Vensel et al.[168])

function were able to stop taking drugs completely or had greatly improved blood pressure. If not for today's advanced testing protocols, a large proportion of these patients would be on a lifetime regimen of drugs and would be incorrectly thought to have essential hypertension.

The committing of a new patient to long-term drug therapy before the diagnosis of curable renovascular disease has been duly considered and excluded demonstrates poor judgment. Diagnosis no longer requires waiting for the autopsy, which has historically shown structural renovascular disease to be even more common than coronary artery disease. The steps necessary to accomplish this goal are now simple and precise. Formerly, the excretory urogram proved neither sensitive nor specific, and renin assays were often technically inadequate. Today, however, peripheral blood renin assays are uncomplicated and reliable.

Any untreated hypertensive patient with an ambulatory plasma renin value greater than 1.6 ng/mL/h is a candidate for further evaluation for unilateral renal artery stenosis. A study of 52 consecutive patients showed no patient with proven unilateral renal disease whose renin level was less than that value.[111] Any patient with an abnormal serum creatinine value, regardless of plasma renin values, is also a candidate for further workup, because renin is usually not elevated in bilateral renal artery stenosis. Moreover, renin levels can actually be reduced somewhat in reaction to impaired Na$^+$ excretion. Even in this group, however, a renin value under 1 ng/mL/h is unusual.

Patients with plasma renin values greater than 1.6 ng/mL/h, with a normal serum creatinine concentration, are given the diagnostically powerful captopril test.[111] This test, best performed in untreated patients (or possibly in patients receiving only a β-blocker), is based on the remarkable specificity of captopril to wipe out the formation of angiotensin II and induce a reactive increase in renin secretion from the ischemic kidney. Patients who are Na$^+$ depleted, because of either a low-salt diet or a diuretic, are ineligible for the test because they start with high renin levels and may show a false-positive increase.[111]

In this test, a single dose of 25 mg captopril is given orally to a quietly seated patient. Captopril is rapidly absorbed, blockading the renin system within 1 hour. Patients with renovascular hypertension react to this blockade with an unusually vigorous rise in renin secretion from the ischemic kidney, whereas those hypertensive patients without renal artery obstruction show little or no plasma renin response. With the angiotensin effect eliminated by the captopril, the kidney with renovascular disease abruptly loses its intense efferent constriction, and its filtration is threatened. In reaction, renin secretion from the stenotic kidney soars, in an apparent attempt to restore the situation.

Table 46–4 lists the procedures for performing the captopril test, and Table 46–5 displays the criteria for interpreting the test. *The 60-minute plasma renin response, rather than the blood pressure response, is the discriminator for the diagnosis of renovascular hypertension.* Although a substantial blood pressure decline usually but not always accompanies soaring of the plasma renin level, this finding is not altogether a reliable indicator of renin dependency or of renovascular hypertension because other transient defenses of the blood pressure level may operate acutely.

**TABLE 46–4. How to Do a Captopril Test**

Maintain the patient on normal salt intake; give no diuretics.
If possible, withdraw all antihypertensive medications 3 weeks before the test.
Allow the patient to sit quietly for at least 30 minutes.
Measure blood pressure at 20, 25, and 30 minutes (average the three readings to obtain baseline reading).
Draw a venous blood sample for measurement of baseline renin activity.
Administer 25 mg captopril, orally.
Measure blood pressure 15, 30, 40, 45, 50, 55, and 60 minutes after administration of captopril.
At 60 minutes draw a second venous blood sample for measurement of stimulated plasma renin activity.

From Laragh JH: Issues and goals in the selection of first-line drug therapy for hypertension. Hypertension 13(suppl 1):103, 1989.

A positive test result that meets the criteria listed in Table 46–5 strongly suggests the possibility of renovascular disease. In a series comparing 56 patients with proven renovascular disease with 112 patients with essential hypertension, the captopril test was found to be 95% sensitive and 95% specific for renin-dependent hypertension related to renal artery stenosis. The real value of the test is its function as a primary screen, because although some false-positive results are inevitable, false-negative results are uncommon.

Thus, a positive captopril test result does not discriminate between unilateral and bilateral kidney disease, nor does it discriminate between a parenchymal and an arteriolar lesion. In patients with a positive captopril test result, these questions can be definitively resolved by digital subtraction angiography or arteriography of the renal vessels and by a renal vein renin study. In typical unilateral renovascular disease, renin is secreted from only one kidney; a simple arithmetic analysis of the concentration of renin in each renal vein can be used to identify the renin-secreting kidney and assess its degree of ischemia. At the same time, the peripheral blood level of renin reflects the secretion rate of renin from that kidney.[175, 176]

Curable primary aldosteronism is characterized typically by the following diagnostic triad: 1) serum K$^+$ level is less than 3.5 mEq/L; 2) plasma renin activity is markedly suppressed—plasma renin levels are typically less than 0.65

**TABLE 46–5. Criteria for the Captopril Test That Together Distinguish Patients with Renovascular Hypertension from Those with Essential Hypertension**

1. Stimulated plasma renin activity of 12 ng/mL/h or more by 60 min*

*and*

2. Absolute increase in plasma renin activity of 10 ng/mL/h or more*

*and*

3. Percent increase in plasma renin activity of 150% or more, or 400% or more if baseline plasma renin activity is less than 3 ng/mL/h

*To conform to the National Bureau of Standards angiotensin I reference standard, multiply plasma renin activity values shown by 0.65.
From Laragh JH: Issues and goals in the selection of first-line drug therapy for hypertension. Hypertension 13(suppl 1):103, 1989.

ng/mL/h but occasionally may be as high as 1.0; and 3) hyperaldosteronism is revealed by 24-hour urinary or plasma aldosterone measurements. These aldosterone values may not be very high, but they should be assessed in relation to the degree of hypokalemia, which markedly suppresses aldosterone secretion even in primary aldosteronism. Special radiographic studies, scanning by computed tomography, and, in some instances, adrenal vein hormone measurements then enable definitive diagnosis of either adenoma or bilateral hyperplasia.

Chronic bilateral renal disease or bilateral renal artery stenosis is possible when the creatinine value is greater than 2.0 mg/dL, or between 1.5 and 2.0 mg/dL when the blood urea concentration exceeds 25.0 mg/dL. In the former hypertensive state, plasma $K^+$ values tend to be high, and renin is often suppressed because of impaired $Na^+$ excretion and volume expansion. Proteinuria may also be present. In bilateral renovascular disease, however, parenchymal function is less impaired, and $Na^+$-volume expansion dampens activation of the renin system. Proteinuria may occasionally be pronounced in such patients, particularly when one renal artery is totally occluded.[177]

Of course, to complete the initial pretreatment evaluation, special tests for other uncommon curable forms, such as pheochromocytoma, Cushing syndrome, and thyroid disease, should also be performed whenever suggested by the clinical picture.

## Algorithm for the Modern Analysis and Diagnosis of the Hypertensive Patient

Figure 46–10 displays the basic steps involved in the initial laboratory evaluation of the individual hypertensive patient. It is apparent, especially in the untreated patient, that the initial plasma renin value and serum $K^+$ level play a central role in a process designed to either rule out or diagnose the curable adrenal or renal forms. Thus, hypokalemia with a plasma renin activity less than 0.65 ng/mL/h raises the possibility of surgically curable primary aldosteronism, whereas higher values make it unlikely. Conversely, higher plasma values of 1.6 ng/mL/h or greater, especially when accompanied by hypokalemia, make cure of renovascular hypertension by either angioplasty or surgery a likely possibility.

For all those not meeting these criteria, the plasma renin test remains useful as an indicator of 1) the presence and degree of renin-related vasoconstriction for values above 0.65 and 2) the $Na^+$-volume factor for values below 0.65.[3] The plasma renin activity is also a determinant of the likelihood (values >0.65) or unlikelihood (values <0.65) of subsequent cardiac and vascular sequelae.[4] Finally, the plasma renin activity simplifies and hastens the drug selection process and finding of the best single drug or combination for the long term.

## Drug Therapy for Essential Hypertension

After performing the initial evaluation, in which the diagnosis or exclusion of curable renovascular disease has been accomplished, the clinician should find the same baseline renin data of additional use for deciding which treatment to give the patient whose hypertension is not curable but essential. With the renin participation in blood pressure maintenance already well defined, the pathway to simpler and more specific drug treatments can be considerably clearer for patients without renovascular disease and for those in whom balloon dilatation is either impractical or technically unsuccessful.

When plasma renin values are extremely low (≤0.65 ng/mL/h), converting enzyme inhibitors usually are ineffective or produce little depressor effect.[107, 178–180] When plasma renin values are high (>3.2 ng/mL/h), converting enzyme inhibitors are almost always effective in lowering pressure. Baseline renin measurements in the middle ranges, however, are less consistently predictive for choosing the first-line drug in therapy for patients in whom curable disease has been excluded. The reason, as shown in Figure 46–11, is that considerable overlap of blood pressure responses to converting enzyme inhibitor occur in the middle region (between 1 and 10 ng/mL/h) of the plasma renin spectrum. Some patients in this range exhibit little or no depressor response to anti–renin system agents, whereas others respond impressively. In this region, the renin test is like many other commonly used and valuable tests, such as the electrocardiogram and blood glucose assay. In all of these tests, normal or near-normal values may not be helpful or conclusive, but as deviations become more extreme, they often redirect therapeutic strategy.

Possibly, those hypertensive patients with middle zone renin values have a mixed vasoconstrictive signal involving both renin and $Na^+$ factors. In other patients, for reasons still unclear, the $Na^+$-related vasoconstriction mechanism may have actually displaced the renin mechanism. In either case, the success of combination therapy indicates that one or both of the two mechanisms are still involved in some reciprocal manner.

A few other general guidelines for selecting drugs, some so well known or obvious as to appear trivial, should be mentioned here because of their practical value. By statistical measurement, elderly, black, or obese patients are susceptible to lower renin levels, and these individuals are somewhat more likely to respond to diuretics or $Ca^{2+}$ antagonists. Diabetic patients should not be given thiazide diuretics or β-blockers, and β-blockers should also be avoided in the presence of bradycardia, airway disease, or peripheral vascular disease. In addition, converting enzyme inhibitors and $Ca^{2+}$ antagonists, because of their putative positive effects on the renal circulation, may be preferred in hypertensive patients with diabetes or with chronic renal disease. β-Blockers and $Ca^{2+}$ antagonists may be preferred in cases of coronary insufficiency.

**The High-Renin Patient.** For those patients with a medium to high renin profile (>1.6 ng/mL/h) in whom the captopril test confirms renin dependence but who turn out not to have curable renovascular disease, the modern choice for first-line therapy is most certainly a converting enzyme inhibitor, either captopril or enalapril. This choice is based on the specificity of these drugs; they eliminate the possibility that the overwhelming portion of their depressor effect is due to their inhibition of angiotensin II formation.

## Laboratory Evaluation of the Hypertensive Patient

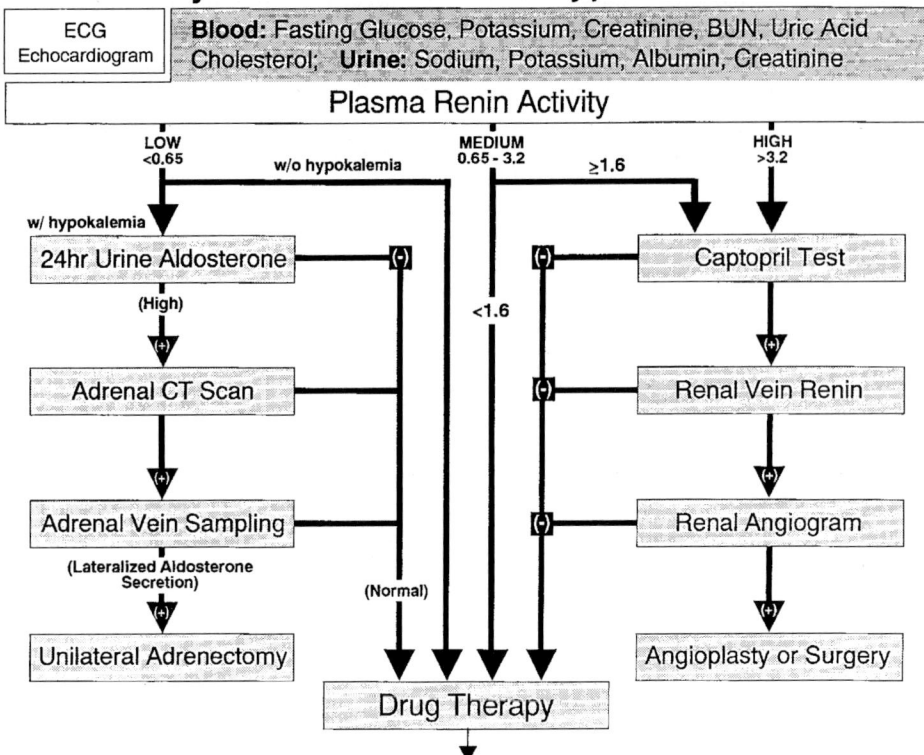

**Figure 46–10.** Working algorithm for the initial laboratory evaluation of the individual hypertensive patient, which enables the diagnosis or exclusion of curable adrenal or renovascular forms; the identification and quantitation of one or both of the two long-term pressor mechanisms, the renin and the $Na^+$-volume factors; and the characterization of the risk of subsequent cardiac or vascular damage (plasma renin activity > 0.65) or the lack of risk (plasma renin activity < 0.65). The level of plasma renin activity also simplifies and speeds the drug selection process and maximizes the possibility of long-term monotherapy with the best-fit drug type (see text).

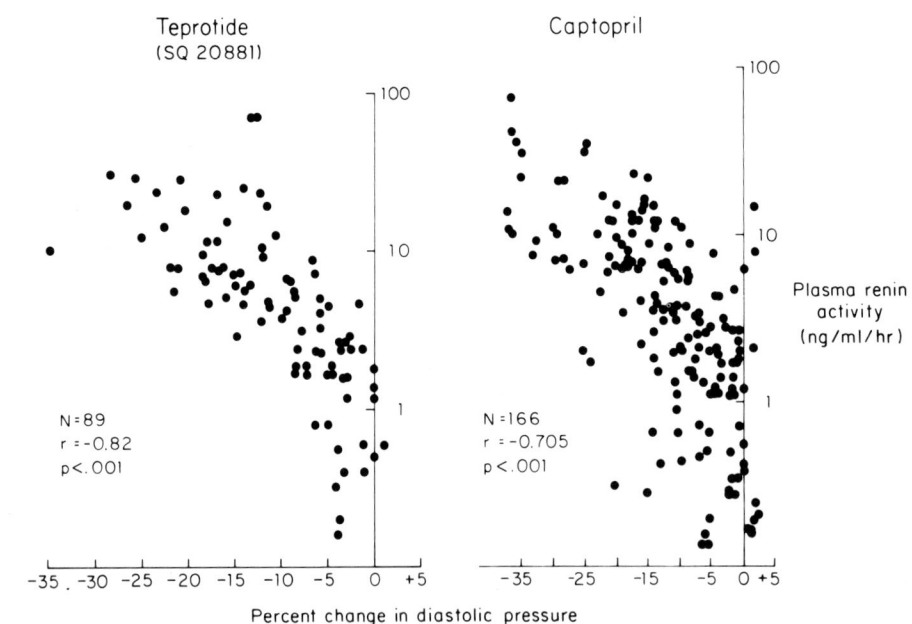

**Figure 46–11.** The acute effects (at 90 minutes) of intravenous and oral converting enzyme inhibitors on diastolic blood pressure. With both drugs, the percentage fall in blood pressure is closely related to the pretreatment levels of plasma renin activity in quietly seated, untreated hypertensive patients. The left panel illustrates the effects of the intravenous administration of the nonapeptide isolated from snake venom, teprotide (SQ 20881), to 89 patients; data are replotted from Case et al.[178, 179] The right panel shows changes in seated diastolic blood pressure in 166 patients 90 minutes after a single oral dose of 25 mg captopril; data are replotted from Case et al.[107, 180] Notwithstanding the errors in cuff pressure measurements, the data reveal remarkable and extremely similar correlations between the height of the pretreatment plasma renin values and the degree of induced fall in blood pressure. Note that patients with plasma renin values below 1.0 ng/mL/h usually exhibited no change in pressure. The data in both panels also provide strong indirect evidence that a plasma renin value closely reflects the active role of renin in supporting arterial pressure in hypertensive individuals. Plasma renin activity values are expressed as nanograms angiotensin I formed per milliliter per hour. Multiply these values by 0.65 to conform to the National Bureau of Standards angiotensin I reference standard now adopted by our laboratory and commercial laboratories.

The effectiveness of converting enzyme inhibition is well illustrated in Figure 46–11, which depicts the relationship of intravenous teprotide, the first converting enzyme inhibitor,[178] and teprotide's oral analogue, captopril,[107] to the pretreatment plasma renin level. The higher the baseline renin is, of course, the more dramatic is the blood pressure correction—and vice versa. Not illustrated in this plot of the acute response to the drug is the additional long-term effect achieved by the accompanying blockade of aldosterone's $Na^+$ retention.

A reasonable alternative for first-drug therapy in the high-renin group is a β-blocker.[106] Although they are not as potent as converting enzyme inhibitors, β-blockers are extremely effective in lowering renal renin secretion, and in certain subgroups of patients (e.g., those with tachycardia or coronary disease), they have the added value of reducing cardiac work and perhaps offering protection against future coronary events.

**The Low-Renin Patient.** A low renin profile ($<0.65$ ng/mL/h) suggests a nonrenin, $Na^+$-dependent factor in the hypertension; in such a situation, the choice of first-line therapy is somewhat broader. Historically, a strict low-sodium diet or a diuretic, the first choice for this group, has been the cornerstone of the old-fashioned stepped-care empirical approach to treating essential hypertension. This treatment mode was necessary in the past because all of the older drugs caused reactive fluid retention. Now, even in low-renin patients, the ground occupied by diuretics is under sharp challenge by the newer $Ca^{2+}$ channel antagonists and $α_1$-adrenergic blockers.[181] These agents appear most effective in low-renin patients, who have the $Na^+$-dependent type of vasoconstriction.

The specificity of $Ca^{2+}$ antagonists for this group is by no means absolute. These drugs may also produce significant depressor responses in medium-renin and even in high-renin patients, possibly because a vascular smooth muscle cytosolic $Ca^{2+}$ increase may be the final pathway for all forms of vasoconstriction.[45] Their greater effectiveness against low-renin hypertension, however, may be exploited in an interesting way. Investigators have shown that sodium administration may actually enhance the antihypertensive action of these agents.[140] Feeding the patient salt reduces renin and shifts the patient to the $Na^+$-dependent type of vasoconstriction, against which $Ca^{2+}$ antagonists are most effective. On the other hand, in verification of the same principle, $Na^+$ depletion and high renin secretion induced by diet or diuretic therapy may rob these agents of their depressor power while enhancing the antihypertensive effect of converting enzyme inhibitors. This relationship is of practical interest because patients can liberalize their sodium intake and thereby improve volume and flow without an adverse effect on blood pressure.

The $Ca^{2+}$ channel blockers are theoretically more attractive than diuretics; like the converting enzyme inhibitors, as they reduce blood pressure, they actually improve blood flow to the heart, brain, and kidneys. They are not associated, as the diuretics are, with dehydration, hemoconcentration, impotence, abnormal lipid profiles, hypokalemia, hyperuricemia, and azotemia. Indeed, it may be for these reasons that long-term clinical trials using a diuretic-based regimen have failed to show protection against coronary

artery disease.[182] Converting enzyme inhibitors and $Ca^{2+}$ channel blockers may demonstrate such cardiac protection in long-term controlled trials.

All of these factors suggest that the effect of antirenin therapy, with either converting enzyme inhibitors or β-blockers, might be significantly enhanced (when enhancement appears to be needed) by adding a $Ca^{2+}$ antagonist instead of a diuretic. Such enhancement has been demonstrated.[183] Such a two-pronged approach, when necessary, is likely to be effective in a large majority of patients.

Some cautionary considerations are as follows. When combination therapy is indicated, the foregoing suggests combination of antirenin and antisodium agents. The data that provide the rational basis for such combinations, however, also indicate that hypotension and possibly renal failure may occur when full-dosage antirenin therapy is given to patients undergoing states that already involve excessive $Na^+$ depletion. In fact, in both animal models and humans, previous $Na^+$ depletion with high renin activity can set the stage for converting enzyme inhibitors to produce marked hypotension and acute renal failure.[184] For this reason, administration of converting enzyme inhibitors should probably always be commenced in $Na^+$-replete patients; $Na^+$ depletion should be superimposed only in resistant patients, and only gradually. Such precautionary guidelines do not apply when β-blockers are used as the antirenin agent, because their antirenin effect is weaker.

Another flow-conserving alternative is provided by such α-blockers as prazosin and its longer acting analogues, doxazosin and terazosin. As with $Ca^{2+}$ channel blockade, the best responders to prazosin are low-renin patients.[136, 185] The $α_1$-blockers and $Ca^{2+}$ channel blockers appear to affect the same vasoconstrictor mechanism, perhaps because of the proximity of α-receptors and $Ca^{2+}$ receptors on the cell membrane.[138]

**The Medium-Renin Patient.** As can be seen in Figures 46–10 and 46–11, plasma renin activity values greater than 3.2 ng/mL/h and less than 0.65 ng/mL/h point reliably to selective and effective monotherapy, but intermediate values show far less accuracy. (Values shown should be corrected to conform with the National Bureau of Standards angiotensin I reference standard. Plasma renin activity values shown should be multiplied by 0.65.) Possibly, in this range, renin-mediated and $Na^+$-mediated mechanisms of vasoconstriction may overlap or function reciprocally. Unfortunately, this is the range in which the majority of patients with essential hypertension are to be found, and the clinician is left to draw on the technique called diagnosis ex juvantibus, the deductive process of defining causal pressor mechanisms from observing a depressor response or lack of response to specifically acting pharmacologic probes. Five major drug types are now available for this exercise (Fig. 46–12).

This process need not be as blind as it was formerly. For one thing, the renin profile may be available to add its weight to other tests in the baseline evaluation. Values on the high-medium side or the low-medium side suggest which type of drug should be tried first. In general, unless the renin profile is extremely low or borders between low and medium, the trial-and-error strategy is best begun with a converting enzyme inhibitor.

## Single Antihypertensive Drug Efficacy Related to Plasma Renin Activity

| | Low | Medium | High |
|---|---|---|---|
| ACE Inhibitors | + | +++ | ++++ |
| β-Blockers | + | +++ | ++++ |
| α-Blockers | +++ | ++ | + |
| Diuretics | ++++ | ++ | + |
| Ca²⁺ Antagonists | ++++ | ++ | + |
| **PRA** | **Low** | **Medium** | **High** |

**Figure 46–12.** A schematized representation of the selective action of major types of antihypertensive drugs. About 30% of people with essential hypertension have low levels (<0.65) of plasma renin activity (PRA), about 50% have medium levels (0.65 to 3.2 ng/mL/h), and about 20% have high levels (>3.2 ng/mL/h). β-Blockers and angiotensin-converting enzyme (ACE) inhibitors are most effective in patients with the renin-dependent type of vasoconstriction and have little or no effect in low-renin states. Conversely, the Ca²⁺ antagonists, diuretics, and α-receptor blockers are most effective in people with the renin-independent, Na⁺-volume–mediated type of vasoconstriction and may become ineffective in higher renin patients.

The rationale for this choice is that of all the medications available, the converting enzyme inhibitor is the most specific, so that a negative result is as informative as a positive one. The strongest effect of converting enzyme inhibition is its counteraction of angiotensin's direct vasoconstriction. Over the long term, however, converting enzyme inhibitors also block aldosterone secretion, thus working on the Na⁺-related side as well, albeit more slowly. If they fail after a few weeks, one should seek a purely Na⁺-related solution, and the next alternatives are, in sequence, the Ca²⁺ channel blockers, α₁-adrenergic blockers, and diuretics. The reason for this ranking is that the first two of these agents, when bringing about a successful depressor result, do so without affecting the blood flow, which is so vital to cardiovascular health and which may be compromised by diuretics. Of course, exceptions to this sequence must sometimes be made. Diuretics may be a first choice in patients with overt hemodilution or fluid retention, phenomena that are often present in obese and low-renin hypertensive subjects.

Perhaps the most efficient and conceptually attractive approach to patients in whom converting enzyme or calcium antagonist monotherapy fails involves a combination of the two agents, thereby blocking both major vasoconstrictive mechanisms. With a liberalized salt intake, this strategy may maintain or improve tissue blood flow as blood pressure is reduced.

In addition, a rational basis exists for combining an antirenin drug with a diuretic to block both vasoconstrictive mechanisms. In low-renin and some medium-renin patients with an underlying Na⁺ excess, in whom converting enzyme inhibitors alone are ineffective, diuretic therapy may arouse a reactive renin release, iatrogenically introducing an element of renin-dependent vasoconstriction and thus enabling the converting enzyme inhibitor to work to achieve full control. As previously indicated, however, the full exploitation of this dual blockade of both vasoconstric-

tive mechanisms can be hazardous in the more severely Na⁺-depleted patients.

Two important caveats should be observed in applying the empirical evaluation-treatment process to patients in the medium-renin range. First, the clinician should restrain the temptation to begin adding other drugs when, at first, converting enzyme monotherapy seems inadequate. Converting enzyme inhibitors also curtail aldosterone secretion, but because the full expression of this effect is reached slowly (endogenous aldosterone activity accounts for only 1% to 2% of the daily renal Na⁺ reabsorption), several weeks may pass before the full benefits of converting enzyme inhibitors are felt in patients in whom both an Na⁺ dependence and a renin dependence are factors in the hypertension. This component of the converting enzyme inhibitor's antihypertensive action resembles that of spironolactone in the delayed onset of what eventually can be a considerable depressor force, often greater than full-dose thiazides.

Second, the clinician must be willing to pursue the objective of monotherapy, trying only one drug at a time. Unless a rigorous, systematic trial of various types of monotherapy makes it the last resort, additive therapy provides few clues to the nature of the basic hypertensive lesion, little advance in an understanding of the pathophysiologic process of hypertension, and less than optimal service to the patient. Superimposition of one drug on the other, which is so often done in the stepped-care regimen, renders the entire pursuit impossible to analyze and leaves many patients taking nontherapeutic and possibly detrimental drugs for life. As a review of 1486 clinical trials shows, the finding that a larger number of patients were controlled by combination therapy rather than by monotherapy most likely represents a summing of patients, not of drug effectiveness.[186] These patients, responding separately and specifically to the effective components in their antihypertensive recipe, would have been better served had there been an orderly effort to discover the specific component of the combination to which they were responding.

Other possible combinations of the five major drug types work against either the renin-related or the Na⁺-related type of vasoconstriction. The addition of a β-blocker can counter the reflex tachycardia and headache that sometimes accompanies the use of the dihydropyridine types of Ca²⁺ antagonists and α-blockers. Caution should be exercised, however, when combining β-blockade with verapamil or diltiazem, drugs that slow atrioventricular nodal conduction; converting enzyme inhibition is the safer antirenin additive in this case.

The older antihypertensive agents—hydralazine, minoxidil, and guanethidine—are often effective. The reflex tachycardia and reactive fluid retention of the first two agents, however, render their use almost impossible except in combination with two other types of drugs—a β-blocker and a diuretic. Today, this type of triple therapy is rarely needed, inasmuch as converting enzyme inhibitors or Ca²⁺ blockers, even when given alone, are usually simpler alternatives. Similarly, guanethidine is an extremely potent agent but is too often associated with an array of unpleasant side effects consequent to broad autonomic blockade. Accordingly, these agents are now used only as back-up therapy.

Furthermore, drugs that lower pressure by acting on the

brain should be the last choice for treating hypertension, because such drugs (e.g., reserpine, methyldopa, clonidine, and guanabenz) interfere with mood, mentation, and sexual function. Surely, however, situations exist in which these side effects do not occur or are not an issue. In addition, these drugs can be useful as primary agents or adjuvants in some special but rare situations.

Figure 46–12 is a summary representation of the antihypertensive effectiveness, or lack of effectiveness, of each of the five major classes of agents according to the baseline plasma renin profile of the individual patient. The anti–renin system drugs—β-blockers, converting enzyme inhibitors, and (not shown) the new type 1 angiotensin II receptor blockers—are effective according to the height of the renin level, and they have no antihypertensive action whatever in zero plasma renin states (such as binephrectomized humans or animals) or in primary aldosteronism or deoxycorticosterone-salt hypertension. Conversely, diuretics and $Ca^{2+}$ antagonists and α-receptor blockers are most effective in low-renin $Na^+$-retaining forms of hypertension, and they exhibit little or no antihypertensive action in high-renin states.[105, 106, 108, 133, 178, 179]

# RECAPITULATION AND SYNTHESIS

Hypertension afflicts 20% or more of the adult populations of the world, depending on the arbitrary cutoffs used to define what is hypertension and what is normotension. About 85% to 90% of hypertension is classified, after exclusion of the known and curable causes (usually kidney or adrenal disorders), as essential hypertension. Historically, adult blood pressure levels of 150/95 mm Hg or above were widely used to define the presence of hypertension, often supplemented by the general guide of 100 plus age for systolic pressure to define the limits of normalcy.

Clinical trials since 1970 of diuretic-based stepped-care regimens, in which drug on drug is added until the blood pressure is subdued, have established the feasibility and reasonable safety of long-term oral drug regimens. Statistically significant protection has been shown for stroke but, unfortunately, not for cardiac events (e.g., myocardial infarction, left ventricular hypertrophy, congestive heart failure, and sudden death), the sequelae that collectively compose 80% or so of the added risk burden of being hypertensive.

Possibly in an effort to improve on these results, it has become popular to redefine adult hypertension as any blood pressure above the region or 120 to 130/80 or 85 mm Hg and advise more intensive drug regimens in more "hypertensive" people to achieve these new target pressure levels. However, there is no evidence as yet, even preliminary, to suggest that this strategy will improve the poor results in protecting from cardiac sequelae and thus prolong useful life. Meanwhile, it is already clear that more intensive treatment with use of more drugs or larger doses can reduce pressure more but may produce more side effects (some serious), increase cost, and reduce the quality of life.

A serious problem with all clinical trials to date is that their design and analyses have conveniently assumed that all essential hypertension is alike and is a single process amenable to a single drug treatment recipe. Unfortunately, this is not the case. Essential hypertension is heterogeneous, prognostically and in its individual response or lack of response to particular drug types and in its hormonal and biochemical patterns. Thus, clinicians have long known that patients with similar degrees of hypertension, left untreated, differ greatly in their prognoses; many live a normal life span without cardiac or cerebral sequelae, whereas others, sometimes with less hypertension, can die prematurely of a cardiac event or stroke. Furthermore, practicing physicians are well aware of gross differences in individual responses to the six major drug classes (diuretics, β-blockers, α-blockers, converting enzyme inhibitors, $Ca^{2+}$ antagonists, and the centrally acting α-agonists). Each of these drug types, given alone, will correct hypertension in about 40% of patients[187]; but for each drug class, *different* subpopulations will respond. Thus, for example, about the same percentage of patients (~40% of the whole) will respond to either a diuretic alone or a β-blocker alone. However, they are largely not the *same* people. Confirming this, when the two agents are given, their effects summate, with the combination controlling 80% or so of patients. This being the case, many physicians, including those at our center, have chosen to ignore the government guidelines (which still advocate diuretic-based stepped-care regimens for all) in favor of one-at-a-time prototype drug trials with the goal of achieving for every patient the "best fit" single drug to control hypertension over the long term, using for all patients the fewest number of drugs in the lowest amount and frequency possible.

Future large-scale clinical trials are not likely to improve understanding of hypertension and its treatments unless every patient is given a prototype of every drug class and then classified as a nonresponder or responder to each prototype drug studied. It does not make sense to proceed to long-term therapy with drug combinations without this information in hand. This is especially so because now that we have available many different drugs and many more possible drug combinations, the primary goal of drug treatment is no longer blood pressure correction. This is usually easy to achieve. Now, the *main goal* of antihypertensive drug therapy is to design a drug strategy that will protect against the cardiovascular morbid and mortal events that shorten useful life. However, for this goal, only two drug classes have been convincingly shown to protect against cardiac events (notably myocardial infarction); these two drug classes, the β-blockers and converting enzyme inhibitors, both lower blood pressure largely by opposing renin system activity by suppressing renal renin secretion or angiotensin II formation, respectively.

This information takes on more relevance when one considers the growing evidence indicating that excess plasma renin activity damages the heart and blood vessels both in animals and in humans. Thus, the height of the renin level in medium- and high-renin hypertensive patients is directly related to the likelihood of a subsequent myocardial infarction in both severe[101] and mild[102] hypertension with a follow-up of 8 years. Conversely, too, in the low-renin patients, the *lowness* of the plasma renin activity (reflecting $Na^+$-volume suppression of renal renin secretion) conveys the statistically significant unlikeliness of subsequent cardiac and vascular damage.

The concept that a plasma renin excess is vasculotoxic and that hypertensive disorders, including essential hypertension, involve a disordered hormonal control system began in 1960 with the discovery of massive oversecretion of aldosterone in 14 patients with malignant hypertension (value up to 10,000 times normal).[103] This striking abnormality seemed causally relevant because no pathogenic biochemical abnormality had been identified in hypertensive patients. Bilateral adrenalectomy was performed in 12 patients in the hope of reversing this uniformly fatal syndrome. It was learned, however, that the aldosterone excess and hypokalemia of this syndrome were related to marked bilateral adrenal hyperplasia, which suggested an extra-adrenal site for the adrenal stimulation. The search for the source led directly to the kidneys, the main site of injury in malignant hypertension, and to the suspicion of a renin-angiotensin factor even though earlier research failed to show a role for renin in human biology. Accordingly, angiotensin II was infused into normal volunteers, and this produced consistent, striking increases in aldosterone secretion.[88] This research thus revealed a new hormonal servo-control involving a renin-angiotensin-aldosterone hormonal cascade, and it defined a massive derangement of the system with runaway renin secretion as the cause of the malignant hypertension.[11] Subsequent research has defined this renin axis as the major long-term regulator of both blood pressure and Na$^+$ balance in normal people.[97] At the same time, this research implicated overactivity of the renin system in the pathogenesis not only of malignant vasculitis but also of other hypertensive conditions in which plasma renin activity is inappropriately high.

## Contrasting Pathophysiologies of Malignant Hypertension and Primary Aldosteronism and the Vasoconstriction-Volume Analytic Model

If one considers the contrasting pathophysiologic processes of two prototypical hypertensive syndromes, that is, human malignant hypertension (or renal artery and aortic banding in animals) as opposed to primary aldosteronism (or the deoxycorticosterone-salt animal model), it becomes apparent that the two disorders represent the ultimate expressions of two different, normally reciprocating pressor mechanisms. Thus, renin excess with aldosterone excess causes and characterizes malignant hypertensive vasculitis, whereas massive Na$^+$-volume excess with reciprocal suppression of renal renin secretion characterizes a primary aldosterone excess arising from an autonomous adrenal tumor in an otherwise healthy subject. The renin excess state presents with severe vasoconstriction; acrocyanosis; ravaging ischemic vascular injury to the heart, brain, and kidneys; and early demise. By contrast, primary aldosteronism, with similar or even higher blood pressures, is characterized instead by a marked suppression of renin secretion with much better tissue perfusion and a generally benign long-standing course with little evidence of fulminant vasculitis.

These two syndromes are the polar extremes of a spectrum of abnormal plasma renin–Na$^+$-volume products that sustain human hypertensive states. Those with an Na$^+$-volume excess (e.g., low-renin essential hypertension) can often be effectively treated by sodium deprivation or diuretic therapy alone to reduce body Na$^+$ content. Conversely, those with a primary plasma renin excess (medium- or high-renin patients) respond well to drugs that block renin secretion or angiotensin II formation (β-blockers or converting enzyme inhibitors), which allows blood pressure to fall and Na$^+$-volume status to be restored. The plasma renin level in untreated patients plays the central role in identifying which of the two pressor mechanisms predominates.

The data thus indicate that hypertensive patients compose a spectrum of abnormal plasma renin–Na$^+$-volume products. Medium- to high-renin patients secrete too much renin for their high blood pressure or Na$^+$-volume status. (Normal subjects exposed to such high pressure would promptly turn off renal renin secretion.[67, 68]) Conversely, low-renin patients are attempting unsuccessfully to suppress their renal renin secretion to zero, which is what the normal kidney does when blood pressure rises or the Na$^+$-volume status rises above normal.

Accordingly, hypertensive states are characterized by inappropriate renal renin secretion and by an inability to suppress renin secretion normally. The hypertensive kidney is characterized by nephron heterogeneity.[67] Structural afferent vascular lesions in a minor subpopulation of nephrons account for the characteristic unsuppressible renin secretion, the abnormal Na$^+$ retention, and the prototypical paradoxical accelerated natriuresis, which provides the renal basis for the abnormal plasma renin–Na$^+$-volume products. In this concept, there is a minor fraction of hypofiltering ischemic nephrons with afferent arteriolar narrowing that unabatedly secrete renin and fail to excrete Na$^+$. In response, a major fraction of normal nephrons are in adaptive hypernatriuresis. However, this adaptation fails because the unabated renin secretion from neighboring nephrons works to impair Na$^+$ excretion in the adapting normal nephrons. Blockade of this renin by converting enzyme inhibitors in patients with normal or even slightly low plasma renin levels can correct the hypertension.

## Evaluation and Treatment of the Individual Hypertensive Patient

The baseline plasma renin activity plays a central role in analysis, diagnosis, and treatment of individual hypertensive patients. At the Hypertension Center at The New York Hospital where we see more than 11,000 patients a year, we routinely perform 2000 or more plasma renin activity assays every month. The delay in broad adoption of the plasma renin activity test can be related to an early debate about how to perform the assay and how to interpret it. This has been resolved. The plasma renin activity test is extremely sensitive, accurate, and reproducible. Our method[188] has been scaled up for widespread use (at modest price) by a major national laboratory.

We collect blood for the plasma renin determination and other baseline tests in seated ambulatory patients. The baseline hypertension assessment profile[189] consists of a complete blood count plus hematocrit; serum Na$^+$, K$^+$, creatinine, urea, and uric acid concentrations plus the plasma renin level; and a casual urinalysis that includes a sample for urinary Na$^+$, K$^+$, microalbumin, and creatinine measurements. The casual urinary Na$^+$/creatinine value, an index of intake, is used to determine the normalcy of the plasma renin level for the rate of Na$^+$ excretion. A fasting blood glucose measurement and lipid pattern complete the cardiovascular risk factor profile. A baseline electrocardiogram and echocardiogram define cardiac function and left ventricular wall thickness.

The plasma renin value is central to the initial evaluation of the patient. 1) At the outset, it rules in or out the diagnostic possibilities of curable renovascular disease (values ≥1.6 ng/mL/h make it possible) or of primary aldosteronism due to an adrenal tumor (values that fall below 0.65 ng/mL/h make it possible). 2) Physiologically, the height of the renin level is a direct measure of the participation of renin–angiotensin II vasoconstriction in the hypertension. Conversely, too, for values less than 0.65, the lowness of the renin is a measure of the presence and degree of the Na$^+$-volume factor in sustaining the hypertension.[3] Furthermore, for those patients with medium to high renin levels (>60% of the whole), the height of the renin level defines the likelihood of subsequent coronary disease; its lowness (for values <0.65 ng/mL/h) implicates an Na$^+$ mechanism and indicates an unlikelihood of future cardiovascular damage.[4] The baseline renin value simplifies and speeds the drug selection process, guiding the physician to begin with a monotherapy targeted for the renin factor (converting enzyme inhibitor or β-blocker) or, in the low-renin patient, to start with a drug targeted against the Na$^+$ factor (diuretics, Ca$^{2+}$ antagonists, or α-blockers).

What has given this strategy its greatest impetus is burgeoning clinical and experimental evidence that defines renin excess as a potent risk factor for causing cardiovascular damage.[101] Besides the report[102] verifying that plasma renin is a risk factor for myocardial infarction in mild hypertension too, there are demonstrations that the anti–renin system drugs (β-blockers, converting enzyme inhibitors, and the new type 1 angiotensin II receptor blockers [e.g., losartan]) all provide impressive protection from cardiovascular damage to the brain, heart, and kidneys in stroke-prone spontaneously hypertensive rats and Dahl salt-sensitive rats[154, 155] even when blood pressure is not reduced.

In human studies, the only two drug classes that have been shown to convincingly reduce myocardial reinfarction rates are anti–renin system agents: the β-blockers, which sharply curtail renin secretion; and converting enzyme inhibitors, which prevent angiotensin II formation. Converting enzyme inhibitor treatment as reported in two major trials of congestive heart failure[145, 146] produced impressive reductions in myocardial infarction rates. Thus, it is no longer a question of whether you can get along without renin testing. Of course you can. But is this the best way to analyze, diagnose, and treat hypertension in the 1990s when protection from hypertensive sequelae that shorten useful life has become the major goal of therapy?

## REFERENCES

1. Riva-Rocci S: Un nuovo sfigmomanometro. Gaz Med Torino 47:981, 1896.
2. Korotkov NS: A contribution to the problem of methods for the determination of the blood pressure. Izv Imperatorskoi Voenno-Meditsinskoy Akad 11:365, 1905.
3. Pickering G: High Blood Pressure. Churchill, London, 1968.
4. Pickering TG, James GD, Boddie C, et al: How common is white coat hypertension? JAMA 259:225, 1988.
5. Blood Pressure Study 1925. Actuarial Society of America and Association of Life Insurance Medical Directors, New York, 1925.
6. Build and Blood Pressure Study 1959, Vols I and II. Society of Actuaries, New York, 1959.
7. Lew EA: Hypertension and longevity. In Laragh JH, Brenner BM (eds): Hypertension: Pathophysiology, Diagnosis, and Management. Raven Press, New York, 1990, pp 175–190.
8. Veterans Administration Cooperative Study Group on Antihypertensive Agents: Return of elevated blood pressure after withdrawal of antihypertensive drugs. Circulation 51:1107, 1975.
9. Freis ED: Veterans Administration Cooperative Study Group on Antihypertensive Agents: Effects of treatment on morbidity in hypertension. JAMA 213:1143, 1970.
10. Volhard E, Fahr T: Die Brightsche Nierenkrankheit Klinik: Pathologie und Atlas. Springer, Berlin, 1914.
11. Laragh JH: The role of aldosterone in man: Evidence for regulation of electrolyte balance and arterial pressure by renal-adrenal system which may be involved in malignant hypertension. JAMA 174:293, 1960.
12. Itskovitz HS, Kochar MS, Anderson AJ, Rimm AA: Patterns of blood pressure in Milwaukee. JAMA 238:864, 1977.
13. Gillum RF: Pathophysiology of hypertension in blacks and whites. Hypertension 1:468, 1979.
14. Messerli FH, DeCarvalho JG, Christie B, Frohlich ED: Essential hypertension in black and white subjects. Am J Med 67:27, 1969.
15. Kaplan NM: Systemic hypertension: Mechanisms and diagnosis. In Braunwald E (ed): Heart Disease: A Handbook of Cardiovascular Medicine, Vol 1. WB Saunders, Philadelphia, 1980, p 852.
16. Detre KM: Hypertension in women—review. In Gold EB (ed): The Changing Risk of Disease in Women: An Epidemiological Approach. DC Heath, Lexington, MA, 1984, p 243.
17. Rice DP, Hing E, Kovar MG, Prager K: Sex differences in disease risk. In Gold EB (ed): The Changing Risk of Disease in Women: An Epidemiological Approach. DC Heath, Lexington, MA, 1984, p 1.
18. De Faire U, Iselius L, Lundman T: Biological and cultural determinants of blood pressure. Hypertension 4:725, 1982.
19. Simpson EO, Paulin J: Sodium and blood pressure: A New Zealand study. In Laragh JH (ed): Frontiers in Hypertension Research. Springer-Verlag, New York, 1981, p 54.
20. Intersalt Cooperative Research Group: Intersalt: An international study of electrolyte excretion and blood pressure: Results for 24-hour urinary sodium and potassium excretion. Br Med J 297:319, 1988.
21. Laragh JH, Pecker MS: Dietary sodium and essential hypertension: Some myths, hopes, and truths. Ann Intern Med 98:735, 1983.
22. Waldron I, Nowotarski M, Freimer M, et al: Cross-cultural variation in blood pressure: A quantitative analysis of the relationships of blood pressure to cultural characteristics, salt consumption and body weight. Soc Sci Med 16:419, 1982.
23. Lew EA: High blood pressure, other risk factors and longevity: The insurance viewpoint. In Laragh JH (ed): Hypertension Manual. Yorke Medical Books, New York, 1974.
24. Kannel WB: Hypertension and the risk of cardiovascular disease. In Laragh JH, Brenner BM (eds): Hypertension: Pathophysiology, Diagnosis, and Management. Raven Press, New York, 1990, pp 107–117.
25. Kannel WB: Some lessons in cardiovascular epidemiology from Framingham. Am J Cardiol 37:269, 1976.
26. Kannel WB: Hypertension and other risk factors in coronary artery disease. Am Heart J 114:918, 1987.
27. Perera GA: Hypertensive vascular disease: Description and natural history. J Chronic Dis 1:33, 1955.
28. Weiss, NS: Relation of high blood pressure to headache, epistaxis, and selected other symptoms. N Engl J Med 287:631, 1972.
29. Smith WM: Treatment of mild hypertension: Results of a ten-year intervention trial. Circ Res 40(suppl 1):I98, 1977.
30. Hypertension Detection and Follow-Up Program Cooperative Group: Five-year findings of the hypertension detection and follow-up program. I. Reduction of mortality in persons with high blood pressure,

including mild hypertension. II. Mortality by race, sex, and age. JAMA 242:2562, 1979.

31. Schnall PL, Alderman MH, Kern R: An analysis of the HDFP trial: Evidence of adverse effects of antihypertensive treatment on white women with moderate and severe hypertension. N Y State J Med 84:299, 1984.

32. Alderman MH, Marantz PR: Clinical trials as a guide to when and in whom to intervene. In Laragh JH, Brenner BM (eds): Hypertension: Pathophysiology, Diagnosis, and Management. Raven Press, New York, 1990, pp 1941–1953.

33. The Management Committee: The Australian therapeutic trial in mild hypertension. Lancet 1:261, 1980.

34. Helgeland A: Treatment of mild hypertension: A five-year controlled drug trial. The Oslo Study. Am J Med 69:725, 1980.

35. Multiple Risk Factor Intervention Trial Research Group: Multiple risk factor intervention trial: Risk factor changes and mortality results. JAMA 248:1465, 1982.

36. Multiple Risk Intervention Trial Research Group: Coronary heart disease death, nonfatal acute myocardial infarction and other clinical outcomes in the multiple risk factor intervention trial. Am J Cardiol 58:1, 1986.

37. MRC Working Party on Mild to Moderate Hypertension: Randomised controlled trial of treatment for mild hypertension: Design and pilot trial. Br Med J 2:1427, 1977.

38. Medical Research Council Working Party on Mild to Moderate Hypertension: Adverse reactions to bendrofluazide and propranolol for the treatment of mild hypertension. Lancet 2:539, 1981.

39. SHEP Cooperative Research Group: Prevention of stroke by antihypertensive drug treatment in older persons with isolated systolic hypertension: Final results of the Systolic Hypertension in the Elderly Program (SHEP). JAMA 265:3255–3264, 1991.

40. Dahlof B, Lindholm LH, Hansson L, et al: Morbidity and mortality in the Swedish Trial in Old Patients with Hypertension (STOP-Hypertension). Lancet 338:1281–1285, 1991.

41. MRC Working Party: Medical Research Council trial of treatment of hypertension in older adults: Principal results. BMJ 304:405–412, 1992.

42. Chabanel A, Chien S: Blood viscosity as a factor in human hypertension. In Laragh JH, Brenner BM (eds): Hypertension: Pathophysiology, Diagnosis, and Management. Raven Press, New York, 1990, pp 329–337.

43. Laragh JH: Vasoconstriction-volume analysis for understanding and testing hypertension: The use of renin and aldosterone profiles. Am J Med 55:261, 1973.

44. Laragh JH, Sealey JE, Niarchos AP, Pickering TG. The vasoconstriction-volume spectrum in normotension and pathogenesis of hypertension. Fed Proc 41:2415, 1982.

45. Laragh JH, Resnick LM: Recognizing and treating two types of longterm vasoconstriction in hypertension. Kidney Int 34(suppl 25):S-162, 1988.

46. Sommers SC, Relman AS, Smithwick RH: Histologic studies of kidney biopsy specimens from patients with hypertension. Am J Pathol 34:685, 1958.

47. Sommers SC, McLaughlin RJ, McAuley RL: Pathology of diastolic hypertension as a generalized vascular disease. Am J Cardiol 9:653, 1962.

48. Sommers SC: Hypertension and kidney disease. Prog Cardiovasc Dis 8:210, 1965.

49. Bradley SE: Physiology of essential hypertension. Am J Med 4:398, 1948.

50. Chasis H, Goldring W, Breed E, et al: Effects of salt and protein restriction on blood pressure and renal hemodynamics in hypertensive patients. J Clin Invest 28:775, 1949. Abstract.

51. Goldring W, Chasis H, Ranges HA, Smith HW: Effective renal blood flow in subjects with essential hypertension. J Clin Invest 20:637, 1941.

52. Hollenberg NR, Adams DF, Soloman H, et al: Renal vascular tone in essential and secondary hypertension: Hemodynamic and angiographic responses to vasodilators. Medicine (Baltimore) 54:29–44, 1975.

53. de Leeuw PW, Kho TL, Falke HE, et al: Hemodynamic and endocrinological profile of essential hypertension. Acta Med Scand Suppl 622:9–85, 1978.

54. Bradley SE, Bradley GP, Tyson CJ, et al: Renal function in renal diseases. Am J Med 9:766, 1950.

55. Nickel JE, Lawrence PB, Leifer E, Bradley SE: Renal function, electrolyte excretion and body fluids and patients with chronic renal insufficiency before and after sodium deprivation. J Clin Invest 32:68, 1953.

56. Farnsworth EB: Renal reabsorption of chloride and phosphate in normal subjects and in patients with essential arterial hypertension. J Clin Invest 25:897, 1946.

57. Grim CE, Luft EC, Fineberg NS, Weinberger MH: Responses to volume expansion and contraction in categorized hypertensive and normotensive man. Hypertension 1:476, 1979.

58. Cottier PT, Weller JM, Hoobler SW: Effect of an intravenous sodium chloride load on renal hemodynamics and electrolyte excretion in essential hypertension. Circulation 17:750, 1958.

59. Luft E, Weinberg MH: Determinants of exaggerated natriuresis in arterial hypertension. In Messerli FH (ed): Kidney in Essential Hypertension. Martinus Nijhoff, Boston, 1984, p 105.

60. Hollander W, Judson WE: Electrolyte and water excretion in arterial hypertension. I. Studies in non-medically treated subjects with essential hypertension. J Clin Invest 36:1460, 1957.

61. Papper S, Belsky JL, Bleifer KH: The response to the administration of an isotonic sodium chloride–lactate solution in patients with essential hypertension. J Clin Invest 39:876, 1960.

62. Smith HW: Salt and water volume receptors: An exercise in physiologic apologetics. Am J Med 23:623, 1957.

63. Ulrych M, Hofman J, Hejl Z: Cardiac and renal hyperresponsiveness to acute plasma volume expansion in hypertension. Am Heart J 68:193, 1964.

64. Mueller CB, Surtshin A, Carlin MR, White HL: Glomerular and tubular influences on sodium and water excretion. Am J Physiol 165:411, 1951.

65. Howard JE, Berthrong M, Goiuld DM, Yendt ER: Hypertension resulting from unilateral renal vascular disease and its relief by nephrectomy. Bull Johns Hopkins Hosp 94:51, 1954.

66. Baldwin DS, Gombos EA, Chasis H: Urinary concentrating mechanism in essential hypertension. Am J Med 38:864, 1965.

67. Sealey JE, Blumenfeld JD, Bell GM, et al: On the renal basis for essential hypertension: Nephron heterogeneity with discordant renin secretion and sodium excretion causing a hypertensive vasoconstriction-volume relationship. J Hypertens 6:763–777, 1988.

68. Sealey JE, Blumenfeld JD, Bell GM, et al: Nephron heterogeneity with unsuppressible renin secretion: A cause of essential hypertension. In Laragh JH, Brenner BM (eds): Hypertension: Pathophysiology, Diagnosis, and Management, 2nd ed. Raven Press, New York, 1995.

69. Laragh JH, Letcher RL, Pickering TG. Renin profiling for modern diagnosis and treatment of hypertension. JAMA 241:151, 1979.

70. Pickering TG, Harshfield GA, Kleinert HD, et al: Blood pressure during normal daily activities, sleep and exercise: Comparison of values in normal and hypertensive subjects. JAMA 247:992, 1982.

71. Pickering TG, Gerin W: Cardiovascular reactivity in hypertension: A critical review. Ann Behavior Med (in press).

72. Julius S: Hemodynamic, pharmacologic and epidemiologic evidence for behavioral factors in human hypertension. In Julius S, Bassett DR (eds): Handbook of Hypertension, Vol 9, Behavioral Factors in Hypertension. Elsevier, Amsterdam, 1987.

73. Laragh JH, Cannon PJ, Meltzer JI, et al: Recent advances in hypertension: Combined staff clinic. Am J Med 39:616, 1965.

74. Folkow B: Psychosocial and central nervous influences in primary hypertension. Circulation 76(suppl I):I-10, 1987.

75. Brod J, Fenci V, Hejl Z, et al: General and regional haemodynamic pattern underlying essential hypertension. Clin Sci 23:339, 1962.

76. Henry JP, Meehan JP, Stephans PM: The use of psychosocial stimuli to induce prolonged systolic hypertension in mice. Psychosom Med 29:408, 1967.

77. Herd JA, Morse WH, Kelleher RT, Jones LG: Arterial hypertension in the squirrel monkey during behavioral performances. Am J Physiol 217:24, 1969.

78. Heymans C, Neil E: Reflexogenic Areas of the Cardiovascular System. Little, Brown, Boston, 1958.

79. Dock W, Shidler E, Moy B: The vasomotor center essential in maintaining renal hypertension. Am Heart J 23:513, 1942.

80. McCubbin JW, Green JW, Page IH: Baroreceptor function in chronic renal hypertension. Circ Res 4:205, 1956.

81. Cowley AW Jr, Guyton AC: Baroreceptor reflex effects on transient and steady-state hemodynamics of salt-loading hypertension in dogs. Circ Res 36:536, 1975.

82. Nathan MA, Reis DJ: Chronic labile hypertension produced by lesions of the nucleus tractus solitarii in the cat. Circ Res 40:72, 1977.
83. Carey RM, Dacey RG, Jane JA, et al: Production of sustained hypertension by lesions in the nucleus tractus solitarii of the American foxhound. Hypertension 1:246, 1979.
84. Kopin IJ, Goldstein DS, Feuerstein GZ: The sympathetic nervous system and hypertension. In Laragh JH, et al (eds): Frontiers in Hypertension Research. Springer-Verlag, New York, 1981.
85. Bright R: Reports of Medical Cases, Selected with a View of Illustrating the Symptoms and Cure of Diseases by a Reference to Morbid Anatomy. Longman, Rees, London, 1827.
86. Tigerstedt R, Bergmann PG: Niere und Kreislauf. Scand Arch Physiol 8:223, 1898.
87. Goldblatt HJ, Lynch RE, Hanzai RE, et al: Studies on experimental hypertension: Production of persistent elevation of systolic blood pressure by means of renal ischemia. J Exp Med 59:347, 1934.
88. Laragh JH, Angers M, Kelly WG, Lieberman S: Hypotensive agents and pressor substances: The effect of epinephrine, norepinephrine, angiotensin II and others on the secretory rate of aldosterone in man. JAMA 174:234, 1960.
89. Ames RP, Borkowski AJ, Sicinski AM, Laragh JH: Prolonged infusions of angiotensin II and norepinephrine and blood pressure, electrolyte balance, aldosterone and cortisol secretion in normal man and in cirrhosis with ascites. J Clin Invest 44:1171, 1965.
90. Oliver WJ, Cohen EL, Neel JV: Blood pressure, sodium intake, and sodium related hormones in the Yanomamo Indians, a ''no-salt'' culture. Circulation 52:146, 1975.
91. Prior IA, Evans JG, Davidson R, Lindsey M: Sodium intake and blood pressure in two Polynesian populations. N Engl J Med 279:515, 1968.
92. Selye H, Hall CE, Rowley EM: Malignant hypertension produced by treatment with desoxycorticosterone acetate and sodium chloride. Can Med Assoc J 49:88, 1943.
93. Conn JW, Knopf RE, Nesbit RM: Clinical characteristics of primary aldosteronism from an analysis of 145 cases. Am J Surg 107:157, 1964.
94. Vaughan ED Jr, Laragh JH, Gavras I, et al: Volume factor in low and normal renin essential hypertension: Treatment with either spironolactone or chlorthalidone. Am J Cardiol 32:523, 1973.
95. Laragh JH: Spironolactone for Treatment of Hypertension or Congestive Heart Failure: A Review. Excerpta Medica, Princeton, NJ, 1987.
96. Laragh JH, Baer L, Brunner HR, et al: Renin, angiotensin and aldosterone system in pathogenesis and management of hypertensive vascular disease. Am J Med 52:633, 1972.
97. Laragh JH, Sealey JE: Renin-angiotensin-aldosterone system and the renal regulation of sodium, potassium, and blood pressure homeostasis. In Windhager EE (ed): Handbook of Physiology, Sect 8, Renal Physiology. Oxford University Press, New York, 1991, pp 1409–1541.
98. Sealey JE, Laragh JH: The integrated regulation of electrolyte balance and blood pressure by the renin system. In Seldin DW, Giebisch G (eds): The Regulation of Sodium and Chloride Balance. Raven Press, New York, 1990, pp 133–193.
99. Ledingham JG, Bull MB, Laragh JH: The meaning of aldosteronism in hypertensive disease. Circ Res 21(suppl 2):177, 1967.
100. Laragh JH, Sealey JE, Sommers SC: Patterns of adrenal secretion and urinary excretion of aldosterone and plasma renin activity in normal and hypertensive subjects. Circ Res 18 and 19(suppl I):I-158, 1966.
101. Brunner HR, Laragh JH, Baer L, et al: Essential hypertension: Renin and aldosterone, heart attack and stroke. N Engl J Med 286:441, 1972.
102. Alderman MH, Madhavan S, Ooi WL, et al: Association of renin/sodium profile with risk of myocardial infarction in patients with hypertension. N Engl J Med 324:1098–1104, 1991.
103. Laragh JH, Ulick S, Januszewicz V, et al: Aldosterone secretion and primary and malignant hypertension. J Clin Invest 39:1091, 1960.
104. Masson GM, Kashii C, Matsunaga M, Page IH: Hypertensive vascular disease induced by heterologous renin. Circ Res 18:219, 1966.
105. Laragh JH: The meaning of plasma renin measurements: Renin and sodium volume–mediated (low renin) forms of vasoconstriction in experimental and human hypertension and in the oedematous states of nephrosis and heart failure. J Hypertens 2(suppl 1):141, 1984.
106. Bühler FR, Laragh JH, Baer L, et al: Propranolol inhibition of renin

secretion: A specific approach to diagnosis and treatment of renin-dependent hypertensive diseases. N Engl J Med 287:1209, 1972.
107. Case DB, Atlas SA, Laragh JH, et al: Clinical experience with blockade of the renin-angiotensin-aldosterone system by an oral converting-enzyme inhibitor (SQ 14,225, captopril) in hypertensive patients. Prog Cardiovasc Dis 21:195, 1978.
108. Laragh JH, Case DB, Atlas SA, Sealey JE: Captopril compared with other anti–renin system agents in hypertensive patients: Its triphasic effects on blood pressure and its use to identify and treat the renin factor. Hypertension 2:586, 1980.
109. Laragh JH: Renovascular hypertension: A paradigm for all hypertension. J Hypertens 4(suppl):S79, 1986.
110. Laragh JH, Sealey JE, Bühler FR, et al: The renin axis and vasoconstriction volume analysis for understanding and treating renovascular and renal hypertension. Am J Med 58:4, 1975.
111. Müller FB, Sealey JE, Case DB, et al: The captopril test for identifying renovascular disease in hypertensive patients. Am J Med 80:633, 1986.
112. Pickering TG, Sos TA, Vaughan ED Jr, et al: Predictive value and changes of renin secretion in hypertensive patients with unilateral renovascular disease undergoing successful renal angioplasty. Am J Med 76:398, 1984.
113. Sealey JE, Bühler FR, Laragh JH, Vaughan ED Jr: The physiology of renin secretion in essential hypertension: Estimation of renin secretion rate and renal plasma flow from peripheral and renal vein renin levels. Am J Med 55:391, 401, 1973.
114. Tobian L, Coffee K, McCrea P: Contrasting exchangeable sodium in rats with different types of Goldblatt hypertension. Am J Physiol 217:458, 1969.
115. Brunner HR, Kirshman JD, Sealey JE, Laragh JH: Hypertension of renal origin: Evidence for two different mechanisms. Science 174:1344, 1971.
116. Gavras H, Brünner HR, Vaughan ED Jr, Laragh JH: Angiotensin-sodium interaction in blood pressure maintenance of renal hypertensive and normotensive rats. Science 180:1369, 1973.
117. Pickering TG, Sos TA, James GD, et al: Comparison of renal vein renin activity in hypertensive patients with stenosis of one or both renal arteries. J Hypertens 3(suppl 3):S-291, 1985.
118. Pickering TG, Devereux RB, James GD, et al: Recurrent pulmonary edema in hypertension due to bilateral renal artery stenosis: Treatment by angioplasty or surgical revascularization. Lancet 2:551, 1988.
119. Vensel LA, Devereux RB, Pickering TG, et al: Cardiac structure and function in renovascular hypertension produced by unilateral and bilateral renal artery stenosis. Am J Cardiol 58:575, 1986.
120. Laragh JH, Ledingham JG, Sommers SC: Secondary aldosteronism and reduced plasma renin in hypertensive disease. Trans Assoc Am Physicians 80:168, 1967.
121. Baer L, Sommers SC, Krakoff LR, et al: Pseudo-primary aldosteronism: An entity distinct from true primary aldosteronism. Circ Res 26 and 27(suppl I):203, 1970.
122. Biglieri EG, Forsham PH: Studies on the expanded extracellular fluid and the responses to various stimuli in primary aldosteronism. Am J Med 34:564, 1961.
123. Laragh JH, Cannon PJ, Ames RP: Aldosterone secretion and various forms of hypertensive vascular disease. Ann Intern Med 59:117, 1963.
124. Conn JW: Plasma renin activity in primary aldosteronism: Importance in differential diagnosis and in research on essential hypertension. JAMA 190:222, 1964.
124a. Blumenfeld JD, Sealey JE, Schlussel Y, et al: Diagnosis and treatment of primary aldosteronism. Ann Intern Med 121:877–885, 1994.
124b. Fontes R, Kater C, Biglieri EG, Irony II: Reassessment of the predictive value of the postural stimulation test in primary aldosteronism. Am J Hypertens 4:786–791, 1991.
125. Biglieri EG, Lopez JM: Clinical and laboratory diagnosis of adrenocortical hypertension. Cardiovasc Med 1:335, 341, 1976.
125a. Ulick S, Blumenfeld JD, Atlas SA, et al: The unique steroidogenesis of the aldosteronoma in the differential diagnosis of primary aldosteronism. J Clin Endocrinol Metab 76:873–878, 1992.
125b. Lifton RP, Dluhy RG, Powers M, et al: A chimeric 11β-hydroxylase/aldosterone synthase gene causes glucocorticoid remediable aldosteronism and human hypertension. Nature 16:262–265, 1992.
125c. Ulick S, Chan CK: Physiologic insights derived from the search for

unknown steroids in low renin essential hypertension. *In* Mantero F, Takeda R, Scoggins BA, et al (eds): The Adrenal and Hypertension: From Cloning to Clinic. Serono Symposia, No. 57. Raven Press, New York, 1989, pp 313–322.

125d. Farese RV, Biglieri EG, Shackleton CHL, et al: Licorice-induced hypermineralocorticoidism. N Engl J Med 325:1223–1227, 1991.

125e. Ulick S, Wang JZ, Blumenfeld JD, Pickering TG: Cortisol inactivation overload: A mechanism of mineralocorticoid hypertension in the ectopic adrenocorticotropin syndrome. J Clin Endocrinol Metab 74:963–967, 1992.

126. Biglieri EG, Stockigt JR, Schambelan M: Adrenal mineralocorticoids causing hypertension. Am J Med 52:523, 1972.

127. Ulick S, Ramirez LC: Adrenocortical factors in hypertension. II. The significance of 16-oxygenated C-19 steroids. J Steroid Biochem 7:953, 1976.

128. Krakoff LR: Plasma renin substrate: Measurement by radioimmunoassay of angiotensin I concentration in syndromes associated with steroid excess. J Clin Endocrinol Metab 37:110, 1973.

129. Dalakos TG, Anderson GH, Streeten DH: Mechanism of the hypertension in Cushing's syndrome. Clin Res 24:271A, 1976. Abstract.

130. Laragh JH, Sealey JE: The renin-angiotensin-aldosterone system in hypertensive disorders: A key to two forms of arteriolar vasoconstriction and a possible clue to risk of vascular injury (heart attack and stroke) and prognosis. *In* Laragh JH, Brenner BM (eds): Hypertension: Pathophysiology, Diagnosis, and Management. Raven Press, New York, 1990, pp 1239–1348.

131. Laragh JH: Hypertension, vasoconstriction, and the causation of cardiovascular injury: The renin-sodium profile as an indicator of risk. *In* Laragh JH (ed): Frontiers in Hypertension Research. Springer-Verlag, New York, 1981, p 383.

132. Cody RJ, Covit AB, Schaer GL, et al: Sodium and water balance in chronic congestive heart failure. J Clin Invest 77:1441, 1986.

133. Laragh JH: The renin system in high blood pressure, from disbelief to reality: Converting-enzyme blockade for analysis and treatment. Prog Cardiovasc Dis 21:159, 1978.

134. Erne P, Bolli P, Bertel O, et al: Factors influencing the hypotensive effects of calcium antagonists. Hypertension 5(suppl II):5-II-97, 1983.

135. Resnick LM, Nicholson JP, Sealey JE, Laragh JH: Acute and long-term effects of calcium channel blockade on divalent ions, blood pressure, and plasma renin activity. Clin Res 31:253A, 1983. Abstract.

136. Resnick LM, Laragh JH, Sealey JE, Alderman MH: Divalent cations in essential hypertension: Relations between serum ionized calcium, magnesium, and plasma renin activity. N Engl J Med 309:888, 1983.

137. Resnick LM, Nicholson JP, Laragh JH: Alterations in calcium metabolism mediate dietary salt sensitivity in essential hypertension. Trans Assoc Am Physicians 98:313, 1985.

138. Van Zweiten PA, van Meel JC, Timmermans PB: Pharmacology of calcium entry blockers' interaction with vascular alpha-adrenoceptors. Hypertension 5(suppl II):II-8, 1983.

139. Nicholson JP, Resnick LM, Pickering TG, et al: Relationship of blood pressure response and the renin-angiotensin system to first-dose prazosin. Am J Med 78:241, 1985.

140. Nicholson JP, Resnick LM, Laragh JH: The antihypertensive effect of verapamil at extremes of dietary sodium intake. Ann Intern Med 107:329, 1987.

141. Nicholson JP, Resnick LM, James GD, et al: Sodium restriction and the antihypertensive effect of nitrendipine. Clin Res 34:404A, 1986. Abstract.

142. Nicholson JP, Resnick LM, Laragh JH: Hydrochlorothiazide is not additive to verapamil in treating essential hypertension. Arch Intern Med 149:125, 1989.

143. Pickering TG, Devereux RB, James GD, et al: Recurrent pulmonary oedema in hypertension due to bilateral renal artery stenosis: Treatment by angioplasty or surgical revascularization. Lancet 2:551–552, 1988.

144. Laragh JH, Sealey JE: Renin system analysis for treatment of individual hypertensive patients: A means to quantify vasoconstrictor components, diagnose curable renal and adrenal causes, assess risk of cardiovascular morbid events, and find the best-fit drug regimen. *In* Laragh JH, Brenner BM (eds): Hypertension: Pathophysiology, Diagnosis, and Management, 2nd ed. Raven Press, New York, 1995.

145. Pfeffer MA, Braunwald E, Moye L, et al: Effects of captopril on mortality and morbidity in patients with left ventricular dysfunction after myocardial infarction. Results of the survival and ventricular enlargement trial. The SAVE Investigators. N Engl J Med 327:669–677, 1992.

146. Anonymous: Effect of enalapril on mortality and the development of heart failure in asymptomatic patients with reduced left ventricular ejection fractions. The SOLVD Investigators. N Engl J Med 327:685–691, 1992. (Erratum in N Engl J Med 327:1768, 1992.)

147. Swedberg K, Eneroth P, Kjekshus J, Wilhelmsen L: Hormones regulating cardiovascular function in patients with severe congestive heart failure and their relation to mortality. CONSENSUS Trial Study Group. Circulation 82:1730–1736, 1990.

148. The Acute Infarction Ramipril Efficacy (AIRE) Study Investigators: Effect of ramipril on mortality and morbidity of survivors of acute myocardial infarction with clinical evidence of heart failure. Lancet 342:821–828, 1993.

149. Yusuf S, Wittles J, Friedman L: Overview of results of randomized clinical trials in heart disease. I. Treatments following myocardial infarction. JAMA 260:2088–2093, 1988.

150. Sharpe N, Smith H, Murphy J, et al: Early prevention of left ventricular dysfunction after myocardial infarction with angiotensin-converting-enzyme inhibition. Lancet 337:872–876, 1991.

151. Held P, Yusuf S, Furberg C: Calcium channel blockers in acute myocardial infarction and unstable angina: An overview. BMJ 299:1187–1192, 1989.

152. Goldbourt U, Behar S, Reicher-Reiss H, et al: Early administration of nifedipine in suspected acute myocardial infarction. Arch Intern Med 153:345–352, 1993.

153. Volpe M, Camargo MJ, Mueller FB, et al: Relation of plasma renin to end organ damage and to protection of K$^+$ feeding in stroke-prone hypertensive rats. Hypertension 15:318–326, 1990.

154. Lutterotti N von, Camargo MJF, Campbell WG Jr, et al: Angiotensin II receptor antagonist delays renal damage and stroke in salt-loaded Dahl salt-sensitive rats. J Hypertens 10:949–957, 1992.

155. Camargo MJF, Lutterotti N von, Campbell WG Jr, et al: Control of blood pressure and end-organ damage in maturing salt-loaded stroke-prone spontaneously hypertensive rats by oral angiotensin II receptor blockade. J Hypertens 11:31–40, 1993.

156. Freis ED: Effects of treatment on morbidity in hypertension: Results in patients with diastolic blood pressure averaged 115–129 mm Hg. Veterans Administration Cooperative Study Group on Antihypertensive Agents. JAMA 202:1028, 1967.

157. Messerli FH, Ventura HO, Elizardi DJ, et al: Hypertension and sudden death: Increased ventricular ectopic activity in left ventricular hypertrophy. Am J Med 77:18, 1984.

158. McLenachan JM, Henderson E, Morris KI, Dargie HJ: Ventricular arrhythmias in patients with hypertensive left ventricular hypertrophy. N Engl J Med 317:787, 1987.

159. Dunn FG, Isles CG, Brown I, et al: The influence of left ventricular hypertrophy on mortality in the Glasgow Blood Pressure Clinic. Circulation 72(pt II):III-133, 1985. Abstract.

160. Corvol P, Pinet E, Plouin PF, et al: Primary reninism. *In* Laragh JH, Brenner BM (eds): Hypertension: Pathophysiology, Diagnosis, and Management, 2nd ed. Raven Press, New York, 2nd ed. 1995.

161. Frohlich ED, Grim C, Labarthe DR, et al: Recommendations for human blood pressure determination by sphygmomanometer: Report of a special task force appointed by the Screening Committee, American Heart Association. Hypertension 11:209A, 1988.

162. Pickering TG, Harshfield GA, Devereux RB, Laragh JH: What is the role of ambulatory blood pressure monitoring in the management of hypertensive patients? Hypertension 7:171, 1985.

163. Thornburg JR, Stanley JC, Fryback DG: Hypertensive urogram: A nondiscriminatory test for renovascular hypertension. AJR 138:43, 1982.

164. Sokolow M, Perloff D: The prognosis of essential hypertension treated conservatively. Circulation 23:697, 1961.

165. Breslin DJ, Gifford RW Jr, Fairbairn JF II: Essential hypertension: A twenty-one year follow-up study. Circulation 33:87, 1966.

166. Savage DD, Drayer JI, Henry WL, et al: Echocardiographic assessment of cardiac anatomy and function in hypertensive subjects. Circulation 59:623, 1979.

167. Devereux RB, Savage DD, Drayer JI, Laragh JH: Left ventricular hypertrophy and function in high, normal, and low-renin forms of essential hypertension. Hypertension 4:524, 1982.

168. Vensel LA, Devereux RB, Pickering TG, et al: Cardiac structure and function in renovascular hypertension produced by unilateral and bilateral renal artery stenosis. Am J Cardiol 58:575, 1986.

169. Devereux RB, Reichek N: Repolarization abnormalities of left ventricular hypertrophy: Clinical, echocardiographic and hemodynamic correlates. J Electrocardiol 15:47, 1982.
170. Hammond IW, Alderman MH, Devereux RB, et al: The prevalence and correlates of echocardiographic left ventricular hypertrophy among employed patients with uncomplicated hypertension. J Am Coll Cardiol 7:639, 1986.
171. Devereux RB, Caseal PN, Kligfield P, et al: Performance of primary and derived M-mode echocardiographic measurements for detection of left ventricular hypertrophy in necropsied subjects and in patients with systemic hypertension, mitral regurgitation and dilated cardiomyopathy. Am J Cardiol 57:1388, 1986.
172. Devereux RB, Savage DD, Sachs I, Laragh JH: Relation of hemodynamic load to left ventricular hypertrophy and performance in hypertension. Am J Cardiol 51:171, 1983.
173. Devereux RB, Pickering TG, Harshfield GA, et al: Left ventricular hypertrophy in patients with hypertension: Importance of blood pressure response to regularly recurring stress. Circulation 68:470, 1983.
174. Devereux RB, Drayer JI, Chien S, et al: Whole blood viscosity as a determinant of cardiac hypertrophy in systemic hypertension. Am J Cardiol 54:592, 1984.
175. Vaughan ED Jr, Bühler FR, Laragh JH, et al: Renovascular hypertension: Renin measurements to indicate hypersecretion and contralateral suppression, estimate renal plasma flow, and score for surgical curability. Am J Med 55:402, 1973.
176. Pickering TG, Sos TA, Laragh JH: Role of balloon dilatation in the treatment of renovascular hypertension. Am J Med 77:61, 1984.
177. Zimbler MS, Pickering TG, Sos TA, Laragh JH: Proteinuria in renovascular hypertension and the effects of renal angioplasty. Am J Cardiol 59:406, 1987.
178. Case DB, Wallace JM, Keim HR, et al: Possible role of renin in hypertension as suggested by renin-sodium profiling and inhibition of converting enzyme. N Engl J Med 296:641, 1977.
179. Case DB, Wallace JM, Keim HJ, et al: Estimating renin participation in hypertension: Superiority of converting enzyme inhibitor over saralasin. Am J Med 61:790, 1976.
180. Case DB, Atlas SA, Laragh JH: Physiologic effects and diagnostic relevance of acute converting enzyme blockade. In Laragh JH (ed): Frontiers in Hypertension Research. Springer-Verlag, New York, 1981, p 541.
181. Laragh JH: Issues and goals in the selection of first-line drug therapy for hypertension. Hypertension 13(suppl I):I-103, 1989.
182. Laragh JH: Modification of stepped care approach to antihypertensive therapy. Am J Med 77:78, 1984.
183. Müller FB, Bolli P, Linder L, et al: Calcium antagonists and the second drug for hypertensive therapy. Am J Med 81(suppl):25, 1986.
184. Grossman A, Eckland D, Price P, Edwards CR: Captopril: Reversible renal failure with severe hyperkalaemia. Lancet 1:7, 1980.
185. Bolli P, Amann FW, Bühler FR: Antihypertensive response to postsynaptic alpha blockade with prazosin in low and normal renin hypertension. J Cardiovasc Pharmacol 2(suppl):S399, 1980.
186. Laragh JH, Lamport B, Sealey J, Alderman MH: Diagnosis ex juvantibus: Individual response patterns to drugs reveal hypertension mechanisms and simplify treatment. Hypertension 12:223, 1988.
187. Materson BJ, Reda DJ, Cushman WC, et al: Single-drug therapy for hypertension in men: A comparison of six antihypertensive agents with placebo. N Engl J Med 328:914–921, 1993.
188. Sealey JE, James GD, Laragh JH: Interpretation and guidelines for the use of plasma and urine aldosterone and plasma angiotensin II, angiotensinogen, prorenin, peripheral and renal vein renin tests. In Laragh JH, Brenner BM (eds): Hypertension: Pathophysiology, Diagnosis, and Management, 2nd ed. Raven Press, New York, 1995.
189. Blumenfeld JD, Mann SJ, Laragh JH: Clinical evaluation and differential diagnosis of the individual hypertensive patient. In Laragh JH, Brenner BM (eds): Hypertension: Pathophysiology, Diagnosis, and Management, 2nd ed. Raven Press, New York, 1995.

# Renovascular Hypertension and Ischemic Nephropathy

*Thomas G. Pickering*
*Jon D. Blumenfeld*
*John H. Laragh*

## RENOVASCULAR HYPERTENSION

The exact prevalence of renovascular hypertension in the general population is not known, and the diagnosis is probably missed in many patients. It is an important diagnosis to make clinically because, first, it is the most common curable form of hypertension at any age and, second, it is one of the few potentially reversible causes of chronic renal failure.

The demonstration of a renal artery stenosis in a hypertensive patient does not necessarily establish a diagnosis of renovascular hypertension because essential hypertension may accelerate the development of atheromatous plaques, which may occur in the renal arteries and elsewhere. Ideally, it is necessary to demonstrate that there is also renal ischemia; this is thought to be the stimulus that raises the blood pressure, acting mainly through the renin-angiotensin system.

## PATHOPHYSIOLOGY OF RENOVASCULAR HYPERTENSION IN ANIMALS

The classic experiments on the production of renovascular hypertension were published in 1934 by Goldblatt and co-workers,[1] who demonstrated that persistent hypertension could be produced in dogs by constricting both renal arteries or one artery if the other kidney was removed. Goldblatt postulated that a humoral mechanism could be responsible for the hypertension, which was later confirmed by numerous other workers.

Despite the early work suggesting that hypersecretion of renin by the ischemic kidney was directly responsible for the raised blood pressure, later studies indicated that other factors were responsible for the maintenance of the hypertension because the hyperreninemia often did not persist. Nevertheless, the overwhelming bulk of evidence favors a predominant role for the two limbs of the renin-angiotensin system: vasoconstriction and $Na^+$ retention.[2] The reciprocal action of these two pressor mechanisms in the two models is illustrated in Figure 47–1.

### Stages in the Development of Renovascular Hypertension

Although clipping a renal artery produces an immediate and sustained rise of blood pressure, the mechanism by which the hypertension is produced changes over time. The relative importance of the different factors involved varies

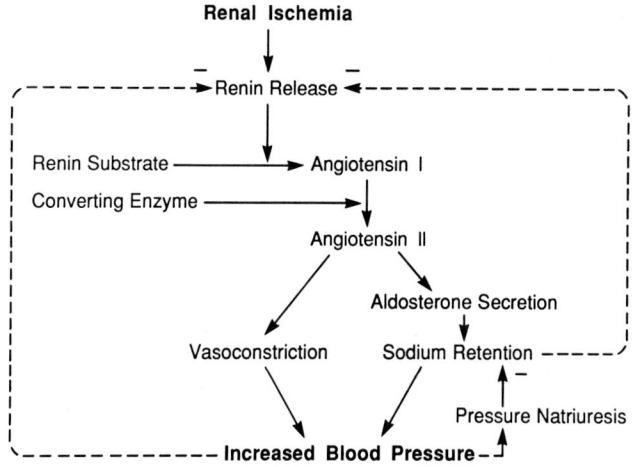

**Figure 47–1.** The effects of renal ischemia on the renin-angiotensin-aldosterone system in renovascular hypertension.

according to the species, the duration of hypertension, and the state of Na$^+$ balance.

The time course of the evolution of the hypertension is well illustrated by Figure 47–2, which shows an experiment performed in dogs by Anderson and colleagues.[3] Constriction of one renal artery causes an immediate rise of blood pressure, which in hemodynamic terms is the result of vasoconstriction, which is sustained. Sixty percent of the increased vascular resistance is attributable to generalized vasoconstriction, 25% to the stenosed kidney, and 15% to vasoconstriction in the intact kidney.

In the first few days, there is a dramatic increase in plasma renin activity (PRA), and interruption of the renin-angiotensin system by angiotensin-converting enzyme (ACE) inhibitors can completely obliterate the hypertension.[4, 5] Later, renin levels fall toward the baseline level and the hypertension becomes less angiotensin dependent, although ACE inhibitors still have an effect.[3]

In the third and final phase, the hypertension may persist despite removal of the stenosis or ischemic kidney.[6] In this situation, the hypertension is presumably maintained as a result of damage to the contralateral kidney.[7]

## Two Experimental Models of Renovascular Hypertension

The physiologic mechanisms underlying renovascular hypertension in experimental animal models differ according to whether the contralateral kidney is intact (two-kidney one-clip model) or removed (one-kidney one-clip model), as summarized in Table 47–1.

### TWO-KIDNEY ONE-CLIP HYPERTENSION

In the two-kidney one-clip model, PRA is high. Blockade of the renin-angiotensin system, whether by angiotensin antibody, saralasin, or ACE inhibitors, produces a bigger fall of pressure in two-kidney one-clip rats than in one-

kidney rats, which suggests a greater degree of renin dependency in two-kidney hypertension.[2, 5, 8, 9] The simplest explanation for the difference between one- and two-kidney hypertension is that in the two-kidney model, the contralateral kidney can excrete Na$^+$ normally, thereby preventing Na$^+$ retention. The contralateral kidney does not function entirely normally, however; experiments using saralasin indicate that there is an angiotensin-mediated vasoconstriction.[10]

Several other mechanisms have been implicated, but their role is at best secondary. Possible pressor mechanisms include increased sympathetic nerve activity and increased vasopressin and thromboxane synthesis. Depressor mechanisms might include increased synthesis of vasodilator prostaglandins, atrial natriuretic factor, renomedullary vasodepressor substance, and kallikrein.[11]

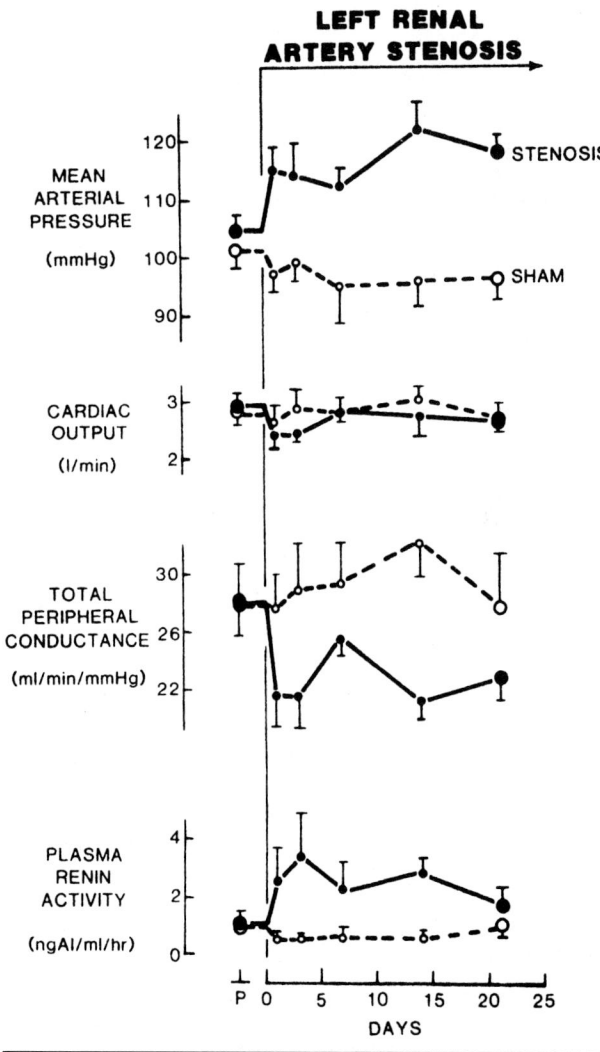

**Figure 47–2.** Development of experimental renovascular hypertension (two-kidney one-clip) in the dog. Stenosis *(solid lines)* was induced without surgery and anesthesia. Note the initial sharp increase of plasma renin activity with subsequent return toward normal but persistent elevation of blood pressure. (From Anderson WP, Ramsey DE, Takata M: Development of hypertension from unilateral renal artery stenosis in conscious dogs. Hypertension 16:441–451, 1990.)

**TABLE 47–1. Comparison of Animal and Human Models of Renovascular Hypertension**

| Parameter | Animal | Human |
|---|---|---|
| | *Two-Kidney One-Clip* | *Unilateral Stenosis* |
| Renin level | High | High |
| Plasma volume | Normal | Normal |
| Blood pressure response to angiotensin-converting enzyme inhibitors | Decrease | Decrease |
| | *One-Kidney One-Clip* | *Bilateral Stenosis* |
| Renin level | Normal | Normal/high |
| Plasma volume | High | ? High |
| Blood pressure response to angiotensin-converting enzyme inhibitors | No change | Decrease |

## ONE-KIDNEY ONE-CLIP HYPERTENSION

In this model, there is an expansion of the plasma volume occurring as a result of $Na^+$ retention, with normal plasma renin levels. If an ACE inhibitor is given, blood pressure falls little if at all.[4] If the animals are maintained on a low-sodium diet throughout, the rise of pressure still takes place, but the mechanism is different: renin levels remain elevated, but there is no $Na^+$ retention or increase of plasma volume.[12] These findings are consistent with experiments done in rats by Gavras and co-workers,[13] who found that short-term saralasin infusion lowered the blood pressure of one-kidney one-clip hypertensive rats only if they were depleted of $Na^+$. Thus, it appears that this type of hypertension may be either renin dependent or volume dependent according to the sodium intake. Prolonged administration of captopril has a modest blood pressure–lowering effect, which is accompanied by a natriuresis; this effect is more pronounced if the animals are in the malignant phase.[5]

A role for the sympathetic nervous system in one-kidney one-clip hypertension has been suggested by several workers, but this remains controversial.[14, 15]

As the blood pressure rises after clipping, there is also a rise of peripheral PRA, but there is a closer correlation between renal vein renin activity from the ischemic kidney and blood pressure than between peripheral PRA and pressure.[16] The renin content of the contralateral kidney is correspondingly diminished.[17] These changes occurring in rats appear to parallel what has been observed in humans (see later).

## EFFECTS OF UNCLIPPING THE ISCHEMIC KIDNEY

Although the majority of studies of renovascular hypertension have investigated its development after a renal artery is clipped, studies of its reversal when the clip is removed are of greater relevance to the treatment of human renovascular hypertension by surgery or angioplasty. Once again, the response differs according to whether the contralateral kidney is present or absent, but in both cases there is a remarkably prompt fall of blood pressure after unclipping.

**One-Kidney One-Clip Hypertension.** After unclipping the stenosed renal artery in one-kidney one-clip Goldblatt hypertensive rats, Liard and Peters[18] found that the fall of pressure correlated with the degree of natriuresis and also that the pressure did not fall if the ureter was ligated beforehand. On this basis, they attributed the fall of pressure to the loss of excess $Na^+$. Other work, however, has not supported this theory. Thus, replacement of the $Na^+$ loss, either by reinfusion or by ureterocaval anastomosis,[19] did not prevent the fall of pressure. In the dog, the fall of blood pressure may be more gradual, occurring for a period of about 3 days.[20] As in the rat, however, removal of the clip produces a negative $Na^+$ balance.

**Two-Kidney One-Clip Hypertension.** Removal of the clip in this model of hypertension produces an acute fall of blood pressure to normal within 24 hours associated with a fall of renin and a markedly positive $Na^+$ balance.[21] Decreased activity of the renin-angiotensin system thus seems to be the most important mechanism, although the authors raised the possibility that the unclipped kidney might release a vasodepressor substance into the plasma.[21]

The possibility that active vasodilatation might contribute to the fall of pressure receives some support from hemodynamic studies, which have shown that the fall of pressure is due to an immediate fall of peripheral resistance to normal levels, with an increase of cardiac output.[22, 23] From these studies it is argued that because there are structural changes contributing to the raised peripheral resistance in animals with renovascular hypertension that are not rapidly reversible, merely withdrawing vasoconstrictor influences by unclipping would not in itself be sufficient to normalize peripheral resistance. Muirhead and associates[24] have demonstrated increased quantities of an antihypertensive neutral renomedullary lipid, derived from renomedullary interstitial cells, after unclipping. Ablation of the renal medulla has also been shown to diminish the fall of pressure that results from removal of the clip.[25]

Russell and co-workers[26] sought to test the contribution of the renin-angiotensin system to the fall of pressure after unclipping by blocking the system with either saralasin or captopril before the clip was removed. Although administration of both agents lowered the pressure to some extent, subsequent removal of the clip produced a much bigger fall of pressure, the extent of which was similar whether or not the renin-angiotensin system had previously been blocked. These authors concluded that some other factors were responsible for the fall of pressure, again invoking the possibility of a vasodepressor substance released at the time of unclipping.

# PATHOPHYSIOLOGY OF RENOVASCULAR HYPERTENSION IN HUMANS

An important question is whether the pathophysiologic mechanisms of the two common human patterns can be equated with the two animal models described. The resemblance between unilateral human renal artery stenosis and the two-kidney one-clip model is close; both are clearly dependent on increased secretion of renin by the ischemic kidney. What is much less clear is what occurs with bilateral stenoses. Relatively little information is available concerning peripheral renin levels, although two studies have reported that renin levels may be high in patients with both unilateral and bilateral disease.[27, 28] Consistent with this finding, patients with bilateral renal artery stenosis are just as likely to show a decrease of blood pressure when given ACE inhibitors.[28] The pattern of renal vein renin is also the same as in unilateral disease, and in patients with bilateral renal artery stenosis, the renins tend to lateralize to the most ischemic kidney.[29]

In addition to this evidence of hypersecretion of renin in patients with bilateral renovascular disease, a number of circumstantial pieces of evidence suggest that there may also be an increased effective blood volume. First, in patients with bilateral disease, the cardiac output is usually higher than in patients with unilateral disease.[30] Second, as described in more detail later, we have found that recurrent pulmonary edema is more common in patients with bilateral than unilateral disease.[31] Third, successful revascularization by angioplasty in a patient with bilateral renal artery stenosis or a solitary kidney is frequently followed by a diuresis, which is not seen in patients with unilateral disease[32] (Fig. 47–3).

The overall picture in patients with bilateral renal artery stenosis is thus a mixed one, with both renin and volume factors typically being involved (see Table 47–1). In this respect it differs from the one-kidney animal model, which is more highly dependent on volume factors. The most likely reason for this is that bilateral disease almost never develops symmetrically in the two kidneys, as witnessed by the common finding of unequal kidney sizes and asymmetric renal vein renin patterns. All bilateral cases presumably start out with unilateral disease. During the early stages of unilateral involvement, there may well be parenchymal disease developing in the contralateral kidney, which would impair the pressure natriuresis by which the contralateral kidney normally maintains the classic high-renin–normal volume pattern of unilateral renal artery stenosis. This volume retention would be further exacerbated when the second stenosis develops in the contralateral renal artery.

Plasma catecholamine levels are usually normal in human renovascular hypertension,[33] unless there is azotemia.[34] It has been suggested that the sympathetic nervous system contributes to short-term fluctuations of blood pressure, because a positive correlation has been observed for 24 hours

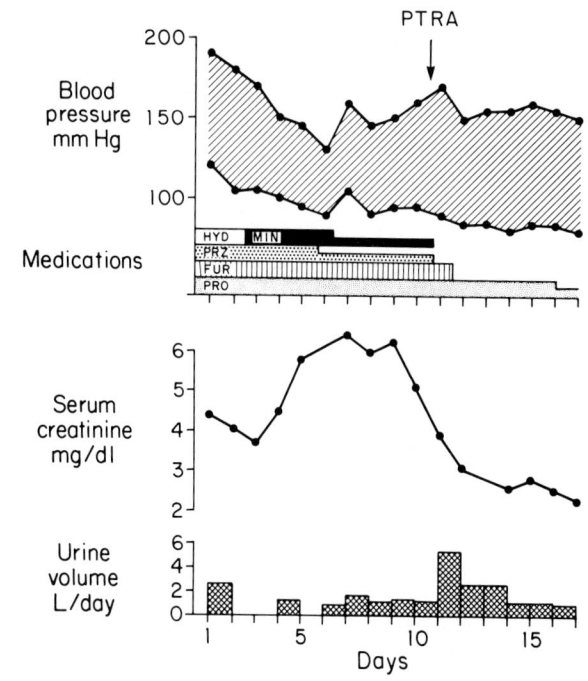

**Figure 47–3.** The effects of percutaneous transluminal renal angioplasty (PTRA) in a patient with bilateral renal artery stenosis, showing an improvement in serum creatinine level and a diuresis.

between plasma norepinephrine and blood pressure and between plasma norepinephrine and renin.[34]

The ischemic kidney produces increased amounts of prostaglandins (particularly E$_2$) as well as renin, and both may be suppressed by nonsteroidal anti-inflammatory drugs such as aspirin.[35] These agents may lower blood pressure in patients with renovascular hypertension, whereas they tend to raise it in patients with essential hypertension.

## The Renin-Angiotensin System and the Control of Intrarenal Hemodynamics in Renovascular Hypertension

The clinical observation that ACE inhibitors may cause a deterioration of renal function in some patients with renovascular hypertension can be accounted for by animal studies that have demonstrated the important effects of angiotensin on intrarenal hemodynamics.[36] One of the most important intrarenal effects of angiotensin II is to decrease renal blood flow, with a smaller decrease of glomerular filtration rate (GFR). Thus, filtration fraction increases.[37] It has been proposed that these changes are brought about by a vasoconstriction of both afferent and efferent arterioles, with the predominant effect being on the efferent arterioles (Fig. 47–4). Thus, in the normal kidney, particularly when renin levels are high, angiotensin blockade increases renal blood flow, with less consistent changes of GFR.[38] In the ischemic kidney, GFR is maintained by angiotensin II–mediated efferent vasoconstriction, so that angiotensin blockade lowers it. This effect provides the rationale for captopril renography.

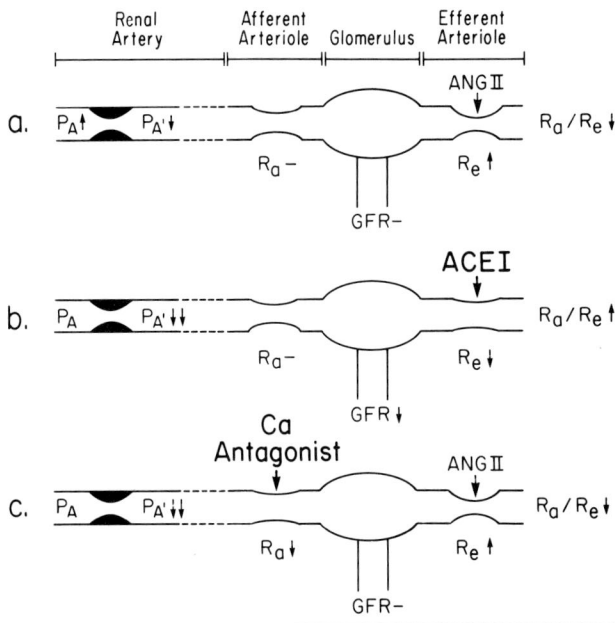

**Figure 47–4.** Hypothetic effects of angiotensin (ANG II), ACE inhibitors (ACEI), and $Ca^{2+}$ antagonists in renovascular hypertension. $P_A$ = blood pressure in renal artery proximal and distal ($P_{A'}$) to a stenosis; $R_a$ and $R_e$ = afferent and efferent arteriolar resistance, respectively.

## Pathology of Renal Arteries

### ATHEROMATOUS LESIONS

Atheromatous plaques occur most commonly in the proximal third of the renal artery; in many cases, plaques in the wall of the aorta may encroach the ostium of the renal artery. Differentiation between proximal and ostial lesions is important because of their different response to renal angioplasty (see later). If atheromatous lesions are left untreated, there is a high probability of progression to complete occlusion. In one series, the average rate of progression of the percentage of transluminal diameter stenosis was estimated to be about 1.5% per month.[39] It has been estimated that 15% of patients with end-stage renal disease have renovascular disease as the primary cause.[40]

### FIBROMUSCULAR DYSPLASIA

Fibromuscular dysplasia of the renal arteries is the most common cause of renovascular hypertension in younger patients and has been classified into four types according to the pathologic differences in the lesions.[41] Medial fibroplasia is the most common variety in adults (accounting for at least 70% of cases) but is rare in children; it produces the classic beaded appearance on angiograms because of areas of thickening of the media interspersed by areas of aneurysmal dilatation. This type of lesion may also occur in the carotid and cerebral arteries. Progression of these lesions to complete occlusion almost never occurs.[42]

### ARTERITIS

Takayasu arteritis, a rare disease mainly affecting young women, can cause discrete stenosis of the aorta and major arteries, including the renal arteries.[41]

## CHOLESTEROL EMBOLI

In patients who have diffuse atheroma, fragments of plaque may break off and cause embolization in the kidneys and other vascular beds. This may occur spontaneously or after aortic surgery and renal arteriography.[43] On pathologic examination, the lesions are characterized by microemboli of cholesterol crystals and amorphous debris, which are later replaced by foreign body giant cells and fibrosis. Clinically, the emboli are manifested by a deterioration of renal function and an exacerbation of the hypertension.[44] Other features include symptoms of mesenteric vascular insufficiency, acute pancreatitis, and gangrene or livedo reticularis in the feet. The diagnosis may be suspected if these manifestations develop after an invasive procedure in a patient with known atheromatous disease but can be established with certainty only if the microemboli are visualized on a tissue biopsy specimen.

## CLINICAL FEATURES

### Prevalence

The prevalence of renovascular hypertension is unknown but is probably anywhere between 0.2% and 5% of the general hypertensive population,[45–48] although it may be much higher in patients with more severe hypertension. In patients with accelerated or malignant hypertension (grade III or IV retinopathy), a prevalence of 43% in white patients and 7% in black patients has been reported.[49] Other studies have also reported a lower prevalence in black than in white patients.[50]

These results were all based on clinical studies, which, with one exception,[49] did not use arteriography in all patients. The prevalence rates are therefore almost certainly an underestimate. However, the situation is complicated by the fact that the demonstration of an anatomic stenosis in the renal artery of a hypertensive patient does not imply that the lesion is causing the hypertension; renal artery stenosis has been reported to occur not infrequently in normotensive subjects.[51, 52]

### Clinical Signs and Symptoms

Clues to the presence of renal artery stenosis may be derived from the history and clinical examination. Some of the most important features that distinguish it from essential hypertension, and also the differences between the two most common types, atheroma and fibromuscular dysplasia, are shown in Table 47–2.

In younger patients, and particularly in women, fibromuscular disease is the most common cause, but it is relatively rare in black patients. A family history of hypertension is less likely to be present than in cases of essential hypertension, although a familial occurrence of fibromuscular dysplasia has occasionally been described.[53] Thus, in a young white woman with a recent onset of hypertension and a negative family history, there should be a high index of suspicion for fibromuscular disease. Women with fibro-

**TABLE 47–2. Clinical Characteristics\* of Renovascular Hypertension**

| Characteristic | Essential Hypertension (%) | Renovascular Hypertension (%) | |
| --- | --- | --- | --- |
| | | *Atheroma* | *Fibromuscular Dysplasia* |
| Race (black) | 29 | 7 | 10 |
| Family history | 67 | 58 | 41 |
| Age at onset | | | |
| <20 y | 12 | 2 | 16 |
| >50 y | 7 | 39 | 13 |
| Duration > 1 y | 10 | 23 | 19 |
| Obese | 38 | 17 | 11 |
| Abdominal bruit | 7 | 41 | 57 |
| High-renin profile | 15 | 80 | 80 |
| Hypokalemia (K$^+$ < 3.4 mEq/L) | 7 | 14 | 17 |
| Smoking | 42 | 88 | 71 |

\*Based on the U.S. Cooperative Study.[53]

muscular dysplasia tend to be taller than those with essential hypertension or atheromatous renal artery stenosis.[54]

Conversely, the finding of hypertension in a middle-aged man with other evidence of atheromatous disease, such as coronary heart disease, should raise the possibility of atheromatous renovascular hypertension. In patients undergoing coronary angiography, a significant and previously unsuspected renal artery stenosis was reported in 17% of hypertensive patients but was equally common in normotensive patients.[55] In patients referred for investigation of peripheral vascular disease, 59% had stenosis (of 50% or more) of at least one renal artery.[56] Again, the presence or absence of a stenosis was unrelated to hypertension.

A history of smoking is another potential clue to the presence of renovascular hypertension. In our series of patients with atheromatous renal artery stenosis, 88% were smokers, compared with only 42% of patients with essential hypertension.[57] Smoking is also a risk factor for fibromuscular disease.[57, 58]

Abdominal bruits are present in about 40% of patients and usually signify the presence of renal artery stenosis, although they may originate from other vessels. Such bruits are of course most likely to be heard in thin patients.

Retinopathy may be particularly pronounced in patients with renovascular hypertension, perhaps because of its more brief and stormy course. In our experience, pulmonary edema in a hypertensive patient should raise consideration of bilateral renal artery stenosis.

## Pulmonary Edema

We have been impressed by the relatively frequent occurrence of pulmonary edema in patients with advanced renovascular hypertension.[31] In a series of 55 consecutive patients who were also azotemic, pulmonary edema had occurred in 13 (23%). In the majority of these cases (92%), the renal artery stenosis was bilateral, or there was a solitary kidney with a stenosed artery. Successful revascularization of even one of the ischemic kidneys prevented further occurrence of the pulmonary edema. The occurrence of pulmonary edema was not related to the severity of the hypertension or renal failure. Although it was more common in

patients who had associated coronary heart disease, it could also occur in patients with normal coronary arteries. Others have reported similar cases.[59, 60]

## Laboratory Investigations

Evidence of impaired renal function on routine biochemical tests, such as an elevated blood urea nitrogen or creatinine level, suggests either that there is parenchymal disease or, if there is renovascular disease, that it is bilateral. In the U.S. Cooperative Study,[53] 15% of patients with atheromatous renal artery stenosis had an elevated serum creatinine level compared with 11% of patients with essential hypertension and only 2% of patients with fibromuscular dysplasia.

A low serum K$^+$ concentration is an occasional marker of renovascular disease. In the U.S. Cooperative Study, about 15% of patients had a K$^+$ level below 3.4 mEq/L. This occurs because hyperreninemia stimulates angiotensin and aldosterone.

Urinalysis may show a slightly increased frequency of bacteriuria. Proteinuria is not uncommon[61] and may occasionally be sufficiently pronounced to present as a nephrotic syndrome.[62] In our experience, proteinuria in excess of 500 mg/24 h usually signifies complete occlusion of a renal artery in patients with renovascular hypertension.[63] This proteinuria may be reversed by surgery or angioplasty.

## Renal Segmental Infarction

In occasional patients who present with acute accelerated hypertension, the underlying abnormality may be renal segmental infarction.[64] Clinically, it is characterized by abdominal or flank pain sometimes associated with nausea, vomiting, and fever. Hematuria and proteinuria may also occur. Although there may be high blood pressure with retinopathy, the electrocardiogram and renal function may both be normal. Investigations show hyperreninemia with lateralizing renal vein renins. Excretory urography and renal scans may demonstrate a decreased kidney size on one side, but the diagnosis is confirmed by arteriography, which shows characteristic defects in the nephrogram phase. The patients are typically young (e.g., 30 to 50 years old), and the underlying pathologic process is usually fibromuscular dysplasia with thrombosis occurring in an aneurysm. The hypertension is renin dependent and may respond dramatically to treatment with ACE inhibitors. Surgery may therefore not be necessary.

## Renovascular Hypertension in Children

Fibromuscular dysplasia is the most common cause of renovascular hypertension in children and is usually of the intimal or perimedial type.[65, 66] In contrast to adults, children rarely have medial fibroplasia. The lesions are commonly ostial and bilateral and may be associated with neurofibromatosis or coarctation of the abdominal aorta.

## DIAGNOSIS

Renovascular hypertension is almost certainly underdiagnosed in clinical practice. Extensive screening of all hypertensive patients is impractical, but a number of clinical clues should increase the clinician's suspicion of its presence. Some of these are listed in Table 47–3.

There is no perfect screening test for its detection. Many tests have been proposed, which can be classified in two categories. First are those that can be done in a physician's office, which are relatively simple to perform and inexpensive but do not indicate which kidney is involved. Measurement of peripheral PRA and the captopril test are in this category. Second are tests that provide anatomic or functional information about each kidney. Ideally, one or more of these tests should be done after the first-stage test.

## Peripheral Plasma Renin Activity

A high PRA, measured in the morning in the seated position and indexed against $Na^+$ excretion, is present in

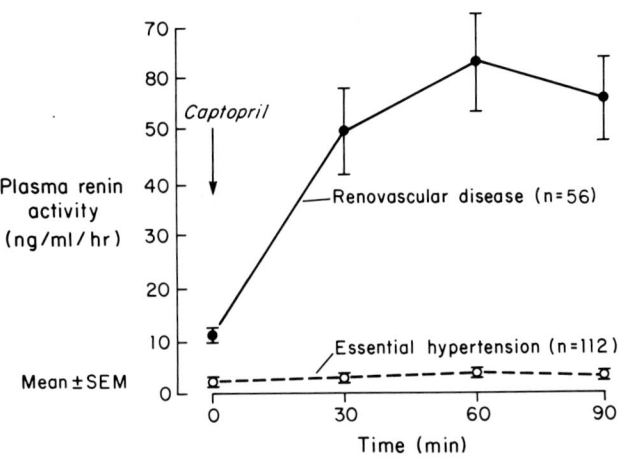

**Figure 47–5.** Comparison of reactive hyperreninemia in patients with renovascular and essential hypertension during the captopril test.

about 75% of patients with proven renovascular hypertension.[67, 68] However, its predictive value in the absence of clinical clues of renovascular hypertension is low. PRA is normal in some patients with renovascular hypertension but rarely, if ever, low.

## Captopril Test

Case and Laragh[69] were the first to show that the reactive rise of renin after administration of captopril is greater in patients with renovascular hypertension than in patients with essential hypertension (Fig. 47–5). The criteria that we found to be the most reliable for distinguishing patients with renovascular hypertension are a post–captopril test renin level of more than 12 ng/mL/h; an absolute increase of 10 ng/mL/h or more; and a percentage increase of 150% or more, or 400% if the baseline renin level is below 3. In a series of more than 200 patients, we found that the sensi-

---

**TABLE 47–3. Testing for Renovascular Hypertension: Index of Clinical Suspicion as a Guide to Selecting Patients for Workup**

*Low* (should not be tested)
Borderline, mild, or moderate hypertension in the absence of clinical clues

*Moderate* (noninvasive tests recommended)
Severe hypertension (diastolic blood pressure > 120 mm Hg)
Hypertension refractory to standard therapy
Abrupt onset of sustained moderate to severe hypertension at age <20 or >50 y
Hypertension with a suggestive abdominal bruit (long, high-pitched, and localized to the region of the renal artery)
Moderate hypertension (diastolic blood pressure > 105 mm Hg) in a smoker, a patient with evidence of occlusive vascular disease
  (cerebrovascular, coronary, peripheral vascular), or a patient with unexplained but stable elevation of serum creatinine level
Normalization of blood pressure by an ACE inhibitor in a patient with moderate or severe hypertension (particularly in a smoker or patient with
  recent onset of hypertension)

*High* (may consider proceeding directly to arteriography)
Severe hypertension (diastolic blood pressure > 120 mm Hg) with either progressive renal insufficiency or refractoriness to aggressive treatment
  (particularly in a patient who has been a smoker or has other evidence of occlusive arterial disease)
Accelerated or malignant hypertension (grade III or IV retinopathy)
Hypertension with recent elevation of serum creatinine level, either unexplained or reversibly induced by an ACE inhibitor
Moderate to severe hypertension with incidentally detected asymmetry of renal size

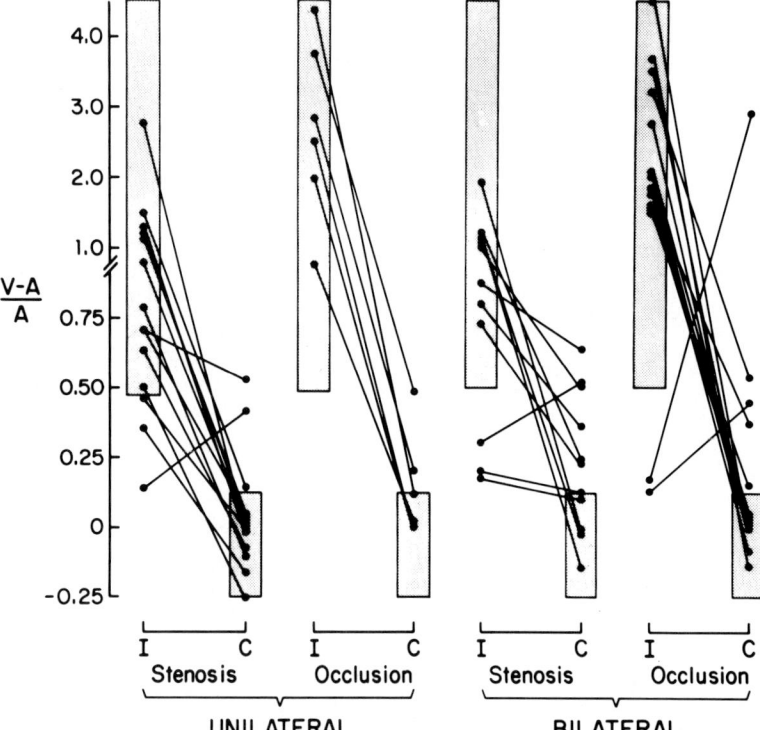

**Figure 47–6.** Renal vein renin patterns in patients with unilateral and bilateral renal artery stenosis. I = ischemic kidney; C = contralateral kidney. (From Pickering TG, Sos TA, James GD, et al: Comparison of renal vein renin activity in hypertensive patients with stenosis of one or both renal arteries. J Hypertens 3[suppl 3]:S291–S293, 1985.)

tivity and specificity of this test with these criteria were greater than 95%.[70]

Subsequent studies have confirmed the value of the captopril test but have also found lower sensitivity and specificity.[70–79] The overall sensitivity is approximately 74%, and specificity is 89%. Differences in the reported accuracy of the test may be attributed to a number of factors, including the assay used, the varying criteria for defining renovascular hypertension, and the position of the patient during the test.

Most investigators have found the test to be less reliable in patients who are azotemic. It does not discriminate between unilateral and bilateral disease; both groups of patients usually show a positive response,[28, 70] although others have found that it is still reliable.[71]

## Renal Vein Renin Determinations

In patients with unilateral renal artery stenosis, the ischemic kidney typically secretes an increased amount of renin, causing an elevation in the systemic levels and suppression of renin secretion by the contralateral kidney. This results in a marked asymmetry in PRA in the two renal veins, which can be expressed either as the ratio of PRA in the two renal veins (with an upper limit of normal or 1.5:1 or 2:1) or as the increment of PRA between the renal vein (V) and renal artery (A) compared separately on each side, expressed as $(V - A)/A$.[67] In practice, the PRA measured in the inferior vena cava distal to the renal veins can be substituted for the arterial level. The normal increment is 25%; in patients with renovascular hypertension, it is typi-

cally 50% or more in the ischemic kidney and zero in the contralateral kidney.

In patients with stenoses of both renal arteries, the pattern of renal vein renins often shows the same degree of asymmetry as in patients with unilateral stenosis and usually lateralizes to the kidney that shows the greatest degree of stenosis on the arteriogram[29] (Fig. 47–6). The most marked asymmetry is seen in patients who have complete occlusion of one renal artery. Extreme elevations of renal vein renin may represent low flow through the kidney rather than hypersecretion of renin.

## Renal Scintigraphy

The use of renal scintigraphy (isotope renography) was based on the finding that iodohippurate sodium I 131 (Hippuran I 131) is selectively taken up by the kidney, and the technique has been used to measure both renal size and blood flow. However, the test has an unacceptably high rate of both false-positive and false-negative results and is relatively expensive.[80] Another isotope that has been used is technetium Tc 99m diethylenetriaminepentaacetic acid, which measures GFR. The sensitivity and specificity are around 70% and 79%, which is not much better than those for excretory urography.[81] Its use as a routine screening procedure is therefore not recommended, unless captopril is given first.

## Captopril Renography

Comparison of renograms obtained before and after administration of a single dose of captopril may improve their diagnostic accuracy. The rationale for this is that the GFR and renal blood flow of an ischemic kidney are dependent on the effects of angiotensin on the efferent glomerular arterioles and hence fall markedly with ACE inhibition. Thus, the characteristic effect of captopril in a kidney with a renal artery stenosis is to cause a decrease of diethylenetriaminepentaacetic acid or Hippuran I 131 uptake.[82, 83] It has been suggested that prior furosemide administration may augment the sensitivity of the test.[84]

Captopril renography has been found to have a high sensitivity (92%) and specificity (93%), which has led to its becoming one of the most popular noninvasive diagnostic tests.[71, 83–88] The test has been performed with two main isotopes: diethylenetriaminepentaacetic acid as a measure of GFR,[88] and Hippuran I 131 of renal blood flow.[89, 90] More recently, [99mTc]-mercaptoacetyltriglycine has become popular.[91–93]

Several different diagnostic criteria have been proposed for evaluating captopril renography. Two different approaches have been used: comparison of the two kidneys in the scintiscans performed after injection of captopril, and examination of the effects of captopril on each kidney individually by comparison of the scintiscans taken before and after captopril administration. The uptake of isotope is usually maximal between 1.5 and 2.5 minutes after injection, and an asymmetry of uptake of more than 60%:40% is a commonly used criterion for defining an abnormality (Fig. 47–7). A second criterion is the time to peak activity, which may be delayed in the presence of a renal artery stenosis; a third is the percentage of the peak activity that remains at 15 or 20 minutes after injection. When the stenosis is mild, a delayed excretion of isotope may be the only renographic abnormality.

The changes induced by captopril, when present, are highly specific for renovascular disease and are helpful in distinguishing it from unilateral renal parenchymal disease. Their sensitivity, however, is relatively low (43% to 80%), and they may be difficult to detect when the stenosis is severe because the uptake of isotope may already be low on the scintiscan taken before captopril injection.[85, 94–97] It may therefore be more appropriate to obtain a single scintiscan after captopril injection, which of course greatly reduces the cost.

## Excretory Urography

The sensitivity of the excretory urogram for detecting renovascular hypertension is around 75%, and the specificity is 85%.[98] The excretory urogram is unreliable for detecting either branch stenoses or bilateral stenoses, and its low level of accuracy, together with the high doses of dye and radiation that it necessitates, has rendered it obsolete as a routine screening test.

## Intravenous Digital Subtraction Angiography

When it was first introduced, intravenous digital subtraction angiography was regarded as a great step forward; it enabled visualization of the renal arteries directly while avoiding many of the hazards of arteriography.[99–102] Today, however, it is little used, for several reasons. First, it requires a relatively large dye load, which must be injected centrally. This reduces its convenience and poses hazards for patients with impaired renal function. Second, its resolution is significantly less than that obtained with arteriography; proximal stenoses may be obscured by overlapping mesenteric vessels, and branch stenoses may be missed. The resolution may also be impaired in obese patients or in the presence of impaired cardiac function. It has a sensitivity of about 88% and a specificity of 90%.[98]

## Magnetic Resonance Angiography

This is a new technique that has the ability to visualize arteries noninvasively. In one study of its use for diagnos-

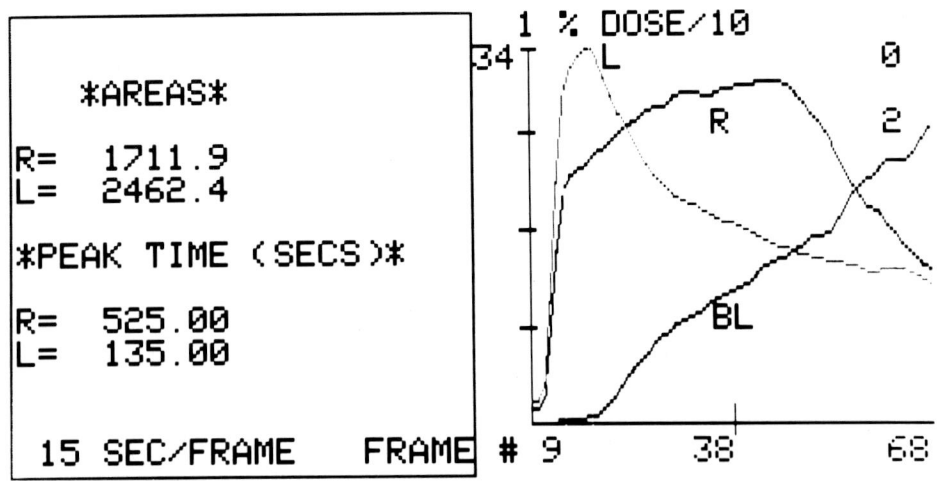

**Figure 47–7.** Diethylenetriaminepentaacetic acid renogram obtained after captopril administration. A normal time-activity curve is demonstrated for the left kidney (L), and an abnormal curve results from stenosis of the renal artery in the right kidney (R). The normal curve (L) is characterized by a rapid initial uptake phase, a function of blood flow, with continued accumulation of radioactive counts until, at the peak, excretion begins to exceed uptake. The area under the curve for the uptake at 1.5 to 2.5 minutes is represented numerically by the counts displayed to the left of the figure and correlates well with GFR. The time to peak, also displayed to the left of the figure, and the percentage of the peak uptake retained at 15 minutes are derived from the time-activity curve. In the abnormal curve (R), uptake at 1.5 to 2.5 minutes is reduced; because of reduced excretion, total counts continue to increase, resulting in a delayed peak. The curve labeled BL is a measure of bladder uptake. (Modified from Mann SJ, Pickering TG, Sos TA, et al: Captopril renography in the diagnosis of renal artery stenosis: Accuracy and limitations. Am J Med 90:30–40, 1991.)

ing renovascular hypertension, eight of nine renal artery stenoses were detected.[103] There were no false-positive responses, and the single false-negative result was a failure to detect a branch stenosis. It may exaggerate the severity of a stenosis, and given its high cost and questionable accuracy, it cannot be recommended for routine use at present.

## Exercise Renography

A development of the conventional renal scan has been the recording of Hippuran I 131 scans before and after exercise.[104, 105] In normal subjects, there is some delay in Hippuran I 131 transport during exercise, probably as a result of neurogenically mediated renal vasoconstriction. In patients with essential hypertension, there is a much more pronounced delay, which may be indicative of a transient cortical perfusion disturbance. Patients with curable renovascular hypertension show a normal response to exercise. This test is potentially of interest because it may be able to detect irreversible parenchymal changes, but it requires further evaluation.

## Ultrasound Scans

Another relatively new technique is the Doppler ultrasound scan to record velocity profiles from the renal arteries.[106, 107] In patients with renal artery stenosis, the flow profile is abnormal, with an acceleration of flow across the stenosis.

There are several problems with this technique, which have so far limited its widespread adoption as a routine diagnostic procedure. The number of reported studies is still relatively small; whereas some authors have claimed to be able to visualize the renal artery in 80% to 90% of cases,[108, 109] for others this figure was only 60%.[110] Problems may occur because of obesity, bowel gas, recent surgery, and the presence of multiple renal arteries. The technique cannot reliably detect branch renal artery stenoses. One area where it finds greater application is in the detection of transplant renal artery stenoses; the superficial location of the artery to the transplanted kidney may make it easier to detect.[111]

## Arteriography

To cause renal ischemia and hypertension, a stenosis must occlude at least 75% of the arterial lumen, but the correlation between the arteriographic appearance and the degree of ischemia is poor.[112, 113] Advances in arteriographic techniques have led to considerable improvements in its safety and convenience. Digital subtraction technology enables the acquisition of high-resolution pictures with significantly reduced dye loads,[114] and the use of smaller lumen catheters has helped reduce the problems associated with the arterial puncture and cholesterol emboli.[115] In uncomplicated cases, it can now be done as an outpatient procedure.

## Approaches to the Detection of Patients with Renovascular Hypertension

The low prevalence of renovascular hypertension in the general population of hypertensive individuals, together with the cost and imperfect accuracy of the available screening tests for its diagnosis, means that universal screening of all hypertensive patients is inappropriate. This raises the question of when it is appropriate to perform these diagnostic tests. We have suggested a triage approach, based on the level of clinical suspicion,[116] as summarized in Table 47–3.

With a low index of suspicion, no further evaluation is needed (Fig. 47–8). This includes the majority of patients with mild or borderline hypertension, in whom clinical clues favoring the presence of renovascular disease are absent, and patients with low-renin hypertension. In such

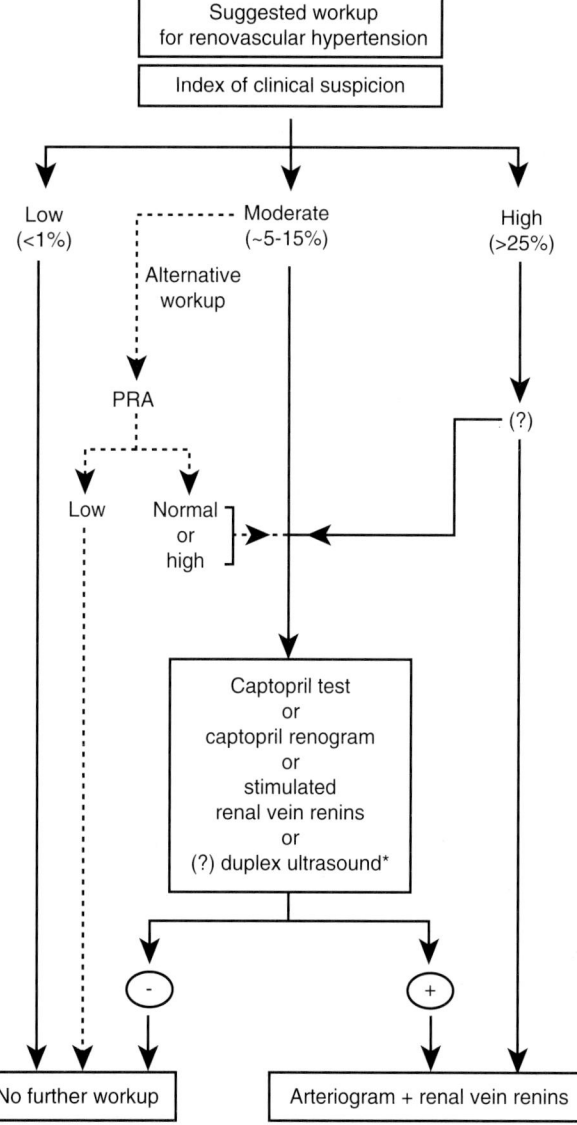

**Figure 47–8.** Suggested workup for patients with suspected renovascular hypertension. PRA = plasma renin activity.

cases, the prevalence of renovascular disease is likely to be less than 1%, and most of the positive test results will turn out to be falsely positive.

With a moderate index of suspicion, that is, clinical clues are present but the evidence for renovascular disease is not overwhelming, the prevalence is likely to be between 5% and 15%. In such cases, the predictive value of a negative result of a diagnostic test with a sensitivity and specificity of 90% would exceed 98%, and the predictive value of a positive test result would be 32%, which would justify proceeding to an arteriogram.

Finally, there is a third group of patients for whom the index of clinical suspicion is so high that an arteriogram would be justified even if the noninvasive diagnostic test results turn out to be negative. Examples are patients with severe hypertension whose renal function deteriorates when they are treated with an ACE inhibitor and patients with accelerated hypertension, who have been reported to have a prevalence of renovascular disease of more than 30%. In such patients, the presence of azotemia may impair the reliability of the noninvasive tests, and it may be appropriate to proceed directly to arteriography.

## TREATMENT

There are in principle three modes of treatment for renovascular hypertension—medical, surgical, and angioplasty. Because renal artery stenoses tend to lead to impairment of renal function as well as hypertension, some type of revascularization is to be preferred. Whereas surgery is the traditional treatment of choice, angioplasty has gained greatly in popularity in the past few years and is now often attempted in preference to it.

### Surgery

The first curative treatment of renovascular hypertension was unilateral nephrectomy, which today is rarely performed except when there is no prospect of the preservation of renal function by revascularization, usually because the kidney is atrophic. The role of surgical revascularization was first established by the U.S. Cooperative Study, the results of which were published 20 years ago.[117, 118]

The blood pressure response to surgery (or angioplasty) is usually classified as cured (i.e., a diastolic pressure below 90 mm Hg without medication), improved (a decrease of at least 15% but still requiring medication), or failed (a decrease of less than 15%), according to the criteria originally developed for the U.S. Cooperative Study of surgery for renovascular hypertension. By today's standards, the results were not good: 51% of patients were cured, 15% improved, and 34% failed. The mortality was high: 5.5% in patients with normal renal function, and 22.5% in those with a creatinine level above 1.4 mg/dL.[117] Since then, a number of large series have been reported with much better results.[119–124] Lawrie and co-workers[124] described a series of 919 patients observed for up to 31 years. Most had atherosclerotic disease and were treated with a Dacron bypass graft or endarterectomy. The combined cure and improvement rate was 82% and the mortality 1.1%.

The major determinant of the results of surgical revascularization is the underlying diagnosis. In patients with fibromuscular dysplasia, the cure rate is as high as 80% and the morbidity is low. Although these results are excellent, they are not significantly better than what can be achieved by renal angioplasty at less cost and inconvenience. However, there are some situations in which surgery is clearly preferable, for example, when there is a fusiform stenosis from intimal hyperplasia that may be resistant to angioplasty. Some lesions may be complex, with multiple branch stenoses and aneurysmal areas distal to the stenosis that may preclude the use of angioplasty.

In patients with atherosclerotic renal artery stenosis, the results are less favorable (Fig. 47–9). There are three main reasons for this. First, in contrast to fibromuscular diseases, there is less certainty that the renal artery stenosis is the cause of the hypertension. Second, the prognosis may be determined more by the extent of atherosclerosis elsewhere in the body. The third potential problem is the release of cholesterol emboli during the operation. In Lawrie's series,[124] the 10-year survival rate was approximately 90% in patients with fibromuscular dysplasia, 70% in those with isolated atherosclerosis, and 30% when there was diffuse atherosclerosis. It is noteworthy that the majority of deaths were due to the consequences of atheroma elsewhere in the body (e.g., from myocardial infarction).

Several studies have demonstrated that neither age nor impaired renal function need exclude the possibility of surgical revascularization. In one series[125] of patients older than 60 years, surgical mortality was 2.8% and was not significantly higher in those with a baseline creatinine level above 1.4 mg/dL.

### Renal Angioplasty

There are now several published series of clinical results obtained with angioplasty,[126–130] but as with surgery, it is appropriate to consider the results with atheroma and fibromuscular dysplasia separately.

The results for the patients with fibromuscular dysplasia are uniformly good (about 58% cured, 35% improved, and 7% failed) and comparable to those obtained with surgery. Restenosis is uncommon in these patients, and follow-up angiograms (up to 5 years after angioplasty) often show no trace of any stenosis at all.

When the stenosis is caused by atheroma, the results of revascularization are not as good (22% cured, 57% improved, and 21% failed), whichever modality (angioplasty or surgery) is used. Furthermore, in patients with diffuse atheromatous disease, the complication rate with both surgery and angioplasty is relatively high, and medical therapy may be preferred.

In those patients in whom the procedure is technically successful, there is usually a prompt fall of blood pressure. In our series, the eventual benefit rate (defined as an improvement or cure of the hypertension 3 months after angioplasty) was 87% in the atheromatous patients with unilateral stenoses and 92% in the fibromuscular patients.[126]

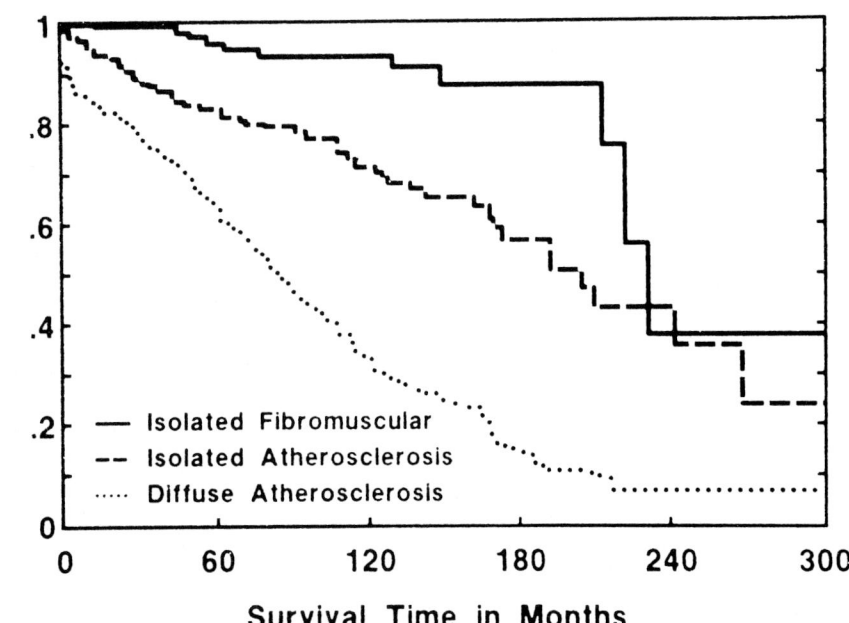

**Figure 47–9.** Survival probability (Kaplan-Meier curves) of patients after surgery for renovascular hypertension according to preoperative diagnosis. (From Lawrie GM, Morris GC, Glaeser DH, DeBakey ME: Renovascular reconstruction: Factors affecting long-term prognosis in 919 patients followed up to 31 years. Am J Cardiol 63:1085–1092, 1989.)

The rate of restenosis in patients with atheromatous disease has been reported to be 19% after 9 months and 35% if the lesion was ostial.[131] The latter figure may be an underestimate.

**Complications of Angioplasty.** The complications of angioplasty, including hematoma at the puncture site, azotemia from the dye load, and cholesterol emboli, tend to be more common in older patients with diffuse atheromatous disease. Dissection or occlusion of the renal artery may also occur but is rare.

**Surgery and Angioplasty for the Preservation of Renal Function.** In patients with renal failure, both surgical revascularization and angioplasty can result in a significant improvement in renal function. We have seen this either in patients who have a critical stenosis of a solitary kidney or in patients who have severe bilateral stenoses. Such patients are notoriously difficult to treat with medications because a reduction of blood pressure is associated with a dramatic deterioration of renal function. This is most common when ACE inhibitors are used.[132] If angioplasty can be achieved, it is particularly rewarding because it can both improve renal function and make the blood pressure easier to control (Fig. 47–10). However, we have seen other patients in whom renal function has not improved or has deteriorated despite a technically successful angioplasty. In our series of patients, all of whom had baseline serum creatinine levels

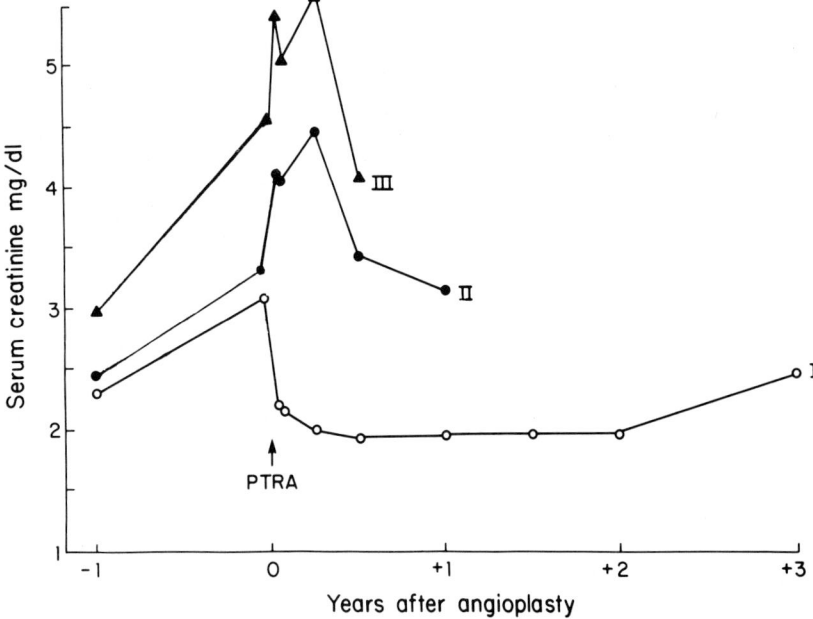

**Figure 47–10.** Effects of percutaneous transluminal renal angioplasty (PTRA) in azotemic patients. Patients were divided into three groups: group I = angioplasty successful, with improved creatinine levels at 3 months; group II = successful angioplasty but no improvement in renal function; group III = angioplasty unsuccessful. (Data from Jenni R, Vieli A, Lüscher TF, et al: Combined two-dimensional ultrasound Doppler technique. New possibilities for the screening of renovascular and parenchymatous hypertension? Nephron 44[suppl 1]:2–4, 1986.)

above 2 mg/dL, 43 (75%) had successful dilatation; 27 (63%) of these showed a decrease of creatinine, 5 (17%) no change, and 11 (26%) an increase.[133]

Several studies, reviewed by Rimmer and Gennari,[40] have reported the effects of surgical revascularization on renal function in azotemic patients. In many cases, the surgery involved aortic replacement as well as repair of the renal artery stenosis. The mortality rate was 6%, and 55% had improved renal function postoperatively. Rimmer and Gennari[40] compared the published results of surgery (eight studies) and angioplasty (six studies) performed in azotemic patients and concluded that improvement in renal function was seen in 55% of patients with surgery and 43% with angioplasty.

Another advantage of angioplasty over surgery is that it can be undertaken in patients who would be turned down for surgery because of associated conditions, such as coronary artery disease or cerebrovascular disease, both of which are of course common in patients with atheromatous renovascular hypertension.

## Medical Management

The two main concerns with medical treatment of patients who are judged to be ineligible for surgery or angioplasty are the progression of the renal artery stenosis and the hemodynamic effects of blood pressure reduction on renal function. In 1974, Hunt and co-workers[134] compared the results of medically and surgically treated patients and reported mortality for a period of 7 to 14 years of 70% in the medically treated patients and 30% in the surgically treated patients. Most of the deaths were due to complications of atheroma, such as myocardial infarction or stroke, with only a minority dying of uremia. In another series, Dean and colleagues[135] observed 41 medically treated patients with atheromatous renovascular disease. Twelve percent progressed to complete occlusion, and 41% had deterioration of renal function.

There have as yet been no randomized trials comparing medical and surgical treatment, but these studies merely serve to underline the high probability of progression of atheromatous disease. Both of these studies were reported nearly 20 years ago, however; it seems likely that just as with coronary artery disease, the prognosis of medically treated patients with renal artery disease should be better today. Introduction of the ACE inhibitors and $Ca^{2+}$ channel blockers has greatly facilitated blood pressure control without seriously compromising the patient's quality of life.

The long-term use of ACE inhibitors in patients with known renovascular disease is controversial. Whereas animal experiments have indicated that ischemic atrophy of the ischemic kidney can be accelerated by ACE inhibitors,[136–138] comparable data in humans are inconclusive. In patients with bilateral renal artery stenosis or with a stenosed renal artery and a solitary kidney, treatment with ACE inhibitors may cause a dramatic increase in the serum creatinine and blood urea nitrogen levels[132] for reasons described before. These acute changes are generally thought to be reversible. One retrospective analysis suggested a marginally significant association between the use of ACE

inhibitors and the development of renal artery occlusion,[139] but another reported no adverse effects on creatinine clearance or kidney size in patients with unilateral renal artery stenosis treated with captopril for 1 year.[140]

In short-term studies, dihydropyridine $Ca^{2+}$ channel blockers have been shown to lower blood pressure with less impairment of function of the ischemic kidney than that with ACE inhibitors.[141, 142] It has been suggested that they may have beneficial long-term effects, but this remains uncertain.[143]

## ISCHEMIC NEPHROPATHY

Apart from its role in the pathogenesis of hypertension, renal artery stenosis is also increasingly recognized as an important cause of chronic renal insufficiency and end-stage renal disease.[40, 144] The term "ischemic nephropathy" refers to the reduction in GFR that is caused by hemodynamically significant renal artery obstruction.[144] The most common cause of ischemic renal disease in adults is bilateral atheromatous disease when both kidneys are present or unilateral stenosis in a solitary kidney. The major clinical questions confronting the nephrologist in considering the diagnosis of ischemic nephropathy include 1) What is its prevalence in the population with end-stage renal disease? 2) What is the natural history in patients with less severe renal insufficiency? 3) Which clinical and laboratory features are most useful in its detection? 4) What are the indications for renal artery revascularization? and 5) Which method of revascularization is more effective?

## EPIDEMIOLOGY

Hypertension is reportedly a common cause of end-stage renal disease, second only to diabetic nephropathy.[145] During the past decade, the frequency of end-stage renal disease attributed to hypertension has increased fivefold, and during the past 5 years, its prevalence has increased by more than 10%/y. The median age of this group is 67 years at the time of the initiation of dialysis, which is among the oldest for all causes of end-stage renal disease. The age-adjusted mortality rate for hypertensive nephropathy is 30% at 2 years and 60% after 5 years; for patients older than 65 years, the mortality rate is 20% to 30%/y.[40, 145] This proliferation of hypertensive end-stage renal disease is occurring at a time when high blood pressure is being adequately controlled in an increasing proportion of patients in the general population and malignant hypertension is uncommon.[146] Although the U.S. Renal Data System report did not stratify end-stage renal disease patients according to the causes of hypertension, data from local dialysis registries and nephrology clinics suggest that ischemic nephropathy may contribute importantly to the increasing frequency of end-stage renal disease attributed to hypertension.[147–150]

In a retrospective study, Mailloux and co-workers[147] found that atheromatous renovascular disease was present in 16.5% of 182 dialysis patients observed between 1982 and 1985. This rate increased from 7% of the 350 patients presenting with end-stage renal disease at their center from

1970 to 1981.[147] In that population, the mortality rate was highest among those with ischemic renal disease compared with other causes of end-stage renal disease. The median survival for patients with ischemic nephropathy was 27 months, compared with 56 months for the other diagnostic groups. Furthermore, the 5-year survival was 12% compared with 39% for the other groups. This poor outcome was attributed to the increasing age of the patients at the time of initiation of dialysis (46 to 60 years) and their advanced systemic atherosclerosis.

Results from several prospective studies also indicate that ischemic nephropathy is a common cause of end-stage renal disease. Scoble and colleagues[150] found high-grade renovascular stenoses in 14% of patients older than 50 years in whom renal replacement therapy was indicated. In another study,[148] angiographic evidence of hemodynamically significant renal artery occlusion was found in more than half of the elderly patients in whom creatinine clearance was less than 50 mL/min. Bilateral stenosis was severe in 20%, and in another 10% with severe unilateral stenosis, the contralateral renal artery also had a relatively minor lesion. Compared with a group in whom other causes of chronic renal disease were found, those with ischemic nephropathy were older, had more systemic atherosclerosis, and had a threefold higher frequency of deterioration of GFR after treatment with an ACE inhibitor. The magnitude of hypertension was comparable in both groups.

Data from a variety of sources indicate that hemodynamically significant renovascular stenoses are often found incidentally and are not suspected clinically.[51, 151–153] In a series of 295 autopsies, renal narrowing exceeded 50% of the intraluminal diameter in 17% of normotensive patients and in 56% of hypertensive patients.[51] In that study, the stenoses were bilateral in 7% of normotensive patients and in 41% of the hypertensive patients. These lesions were invariably located at the aortic orifice or within the proximal third of the renal artery.

Renovascular stenosis is often found unexpectedly during the evaluation of occlusive disease of the aorta and lower extremities.[151–153] In a prospective study, Olin and co-workers[153] discovered renal arteries with greater than 50% narrowing as an incidental finding during angiography in 38% of patients with aortic aneurysm, 33% with aorto-occlusive disease, and 39% with lower extremity occlusive disease. In another prospective study of patients referred for angiographic evaluation of occlusive peripheral vascular disease, renal artery stenosis was present in 45%, of whom 16% had a high-grade lesion.[152] Bilateral stenoses were present in 12% to 20% of the patients in these two studies, but others have reported a prevalence of 27% to 61%.[40, 148, 149, 152, 153]

## NATURAL HISTORY

There is compelling evidence that ischemic nephropathy is the consequence of progressive renal artery stenosis and occlusion.[39, 40] Angiographic progression of renal artery narrowing was found in 49% of 237 patients in five studies in which the follow-up period ranged from 6 to 180 months.[40] However, there was considerable variability in the rate at which renal artery lesions progressed, ranging from approx-

imately 1.5% to 5.0%/y.[39, 40, 151] Nevertheless, one consistent finding in those studies was that when progression occurred, it was apparent soon after the lesion was initially detected. Schreiber and co-workers[39] reported that approximately half of the stenoses that progressed did so within 2 years of the initial angiogram. The rate of progression in that study appeared to be similar for all renal arteries, regardless of the severity of stenosis during the initial angiogram. In a prospective study of patients in whom serial renal hemodynamic measurements were obtained with duplex ultrasonography, progression of stenosis from less than 60% to 60% or greater occurred in 23% of the arteries after 1 year and in 42% after 2 years.[154] Bilateral progression was found in 20% to 30% of patients with atherosclerotic renovascular disease.[40]

Progression to complete occlusion has been observed in approximately 15% of patients with renal artery stenosis.[39, 40, 154] However, occlusion was more likely to occur in arteries with high-grade lesions. Angiographic evidence of occlusion occurred within 13 months in 39% of patients in whom the initial angiogram showed more than 75% stenosis.[39] In another series in which duplex ultrasonography was employed, progression to total occlusion was found exclusively in arteries with greater than 60% stenosis during the initial measurement.[154] The cumulative incidence of occlusion in that study was 5% at 1 year and 11% at 2 years. In contrast to these observations in patients with atheromatous lesions, fibromuscular dysplasia did not commonly progress to complete occlusion.[39]

## DETECTION

Few clinical signs or noninvasive laboratory tests point to the diagnosis of ischemic nephropathy or signal its progression to occlusion.[39, 144, 151] Clinical suspicion should be high in elderly patients with progressive renal insufficiency when it is associated with an inactive urine sediment, protein excretion less than 1 g/d, hypertension, and peripheral vascular disease.[144] With these criteria, hemodynamically significant renal artery stenosis was detected angiographically in more than half of the patients in a prospective study.[148] However, the sensitivity of these clinical and laboratory signs is relatively poor for identifying patients with ischemic nephropathy. Olin and co-workers[153] reported that renal artery stenosis was not present in 30% of patients with these features who underwent angiography because ischemic nephropathy was strongly suspected.

Progression of renal artery stenosis to complete occlusion often occurs without an accompanying sign or symptom. In some patients, a reduction in kidney length heralds progressive stenosis and occlusion, but this is neither a sensitive nor a specific marker.[135, 151] Schreiber and co-workers[39] reported a 1.5 cm difference in kidney size measured angiographically in 70% of patients with progressive stenosis. However, a similar reduction in kidney size was also observed in approximately 30% of those in whom progressive stenosis did *not* occur. Duplex ultrasonography detected a decrease in length greater than 1 cm in only 26% of those with progressive stenosis.[155] Similarly, excretory urography

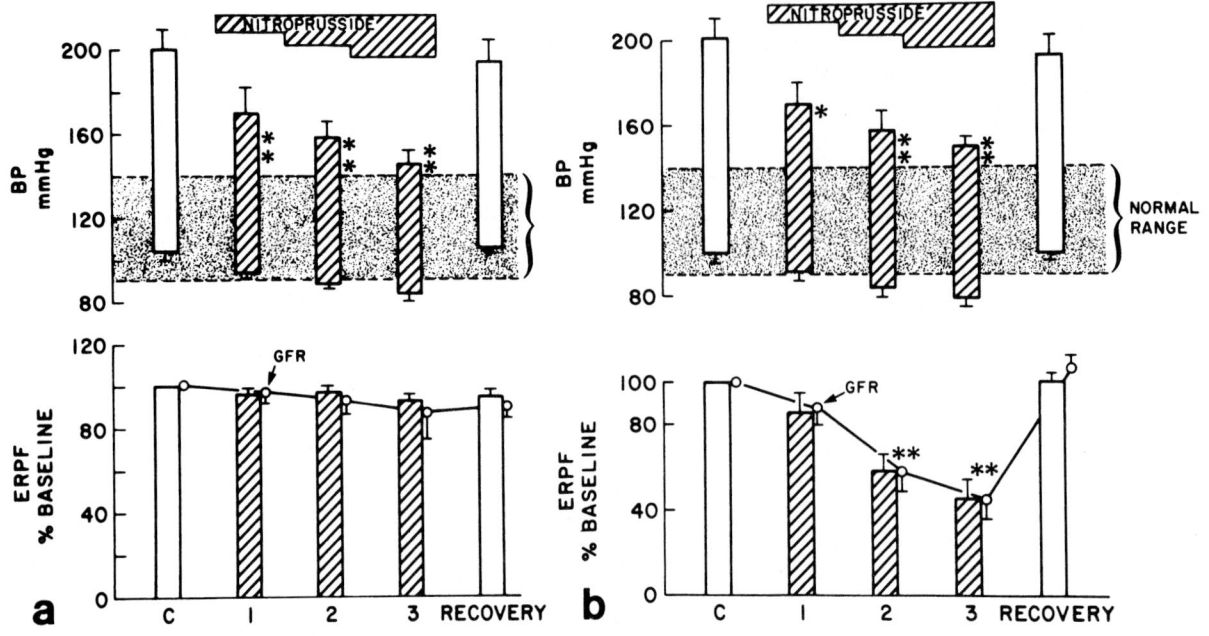

**Figure 47–11.** Changes in blood pressure (BP), effective renal plasma flow (ERPF), and GFR during infusion of nitroprusside. *a.* In eight patients with unilateral renal artery stenosis, effective renal plasma flow and GFR were relatively constant despite reduction in blood pressure. *b.* In eight patients with bilateral renal artery stenosis, effective renal plasma flow and GFR fell progressively during successive reductions in blood pressure. \*\**P* < .01 and \**P* < .05 versus preinfusion values. (*a* and *b* from Textor SC, Novick AG, Tarazi RC, et al: Critical perfusion pressure for renal function in patients with bilateral atherosclerotic renal vascular disease. Ann Intern Med 102:308–314, 1985.)

and renal scintigraphy are inadequate for identifying patients with ischemic nephropathy.[148]

Changes in biochemical measurements are often unsatisfactory for detecting progressive disease. Although Schreiber and co-workers found that serum creatinine concentration increased more commonly in patients with ongoing stenosis, this was not the case in other series.[39, 144, 151, 154] PRA, when measured during the captopril test or renal vein renin sampling, is less reliable for identifying bilateral renovascular stenosis than for unilateral lesions.[29, 70]

## THERAPEUTIC STRATEGIES FOR PRESERVATION OF RENAL FUNCTION

### Medical Therapy

Several features of ischemic nephropathy discussed in this chapter indicate that conservative management with antihypertensive medication is often unsuccessful. Medical treatment does not reliably prevent the progression of renal artery stenosis, and it is associated with a high mortality rate after initiation of dialysis. Furthermore, the rate of progression of renal insufficiency often accelerates during antihypertensive drug treatment in patients with ischemic renal disease.[123, 148, 156] This is a well-recognized complication of ACE inhibitor therapy, especially in the setting of $Na^+$ depletion when the GFR is especially dependent on angiotensin II.[8, 9, 157] Accordingly, acute deterioration is most likely to be provoked by ACE inhibitors during diuretic therapy, dietary sodium restriction, or excessive extrarenal losses (e.g., vomiting, diarrhea).

Other classes of antihypertensive agents can also cause acute renal failure. Textor and colleagues[156] demonstrated that in patients with hemodynamically significant bilateral renal artery stenosis, acute blood pressure reduction with nitroprusside (to approximately 145/85 mm Hg) caused significant decrements in GFR and renal plasma flow. By contrast, renal function did not deteriorate when the nitroprusside infusion was repeated in these patients after unilateral surgical revascularization. Furthermore, in patients with unilateral renal artery stenosis, GFR and effective renal plasma flow remained stable when blood pressure was lowered by nitroprusside[156] (Fig. 47–11). Thus, a clinically significant impairment in renal function occurs when blood flow to the entire renal mass is compromised by renal artery stenosis and a concomitant reduction in systemic pressure.[123, 156] This adverse outcome reflects the fall in transcapillary hydraulic pressure below the critical level required to maintain GFR.

There are individual patients for whom medical therapy is selected because more invasive procedures may pose unacceptable risks. In this group, renal function should be observed closely while the patient is receiving antihypertensive medication, especially when ACE inhibitors are used. Diuretics should not be used routinely in combination with ACE inhibitors in patients with ischemic nephropathy because of the increased risk of acute renal failure.

## RENAL REVASCULARIZATION

### Surgery

Reports from uncontrolled retrospective studies have clearly documented that surgical revascularization can im-

**TABLE 47–4. Outcome of Surgical Revascularization**

| Reference | No. of Patients | Outcome | | | |
|---|---|---|---|---|---|
| | | Improved (%) | Stable (%) | Worse (%) | Death (%) |
| Luft et al.[166] | 12 | 8 (67) | 2 (17) | 2 (17) | 2 (17) |
| Jamieson et al.[167] | 23 | 15 (65) | 0 (0) | 8 (35) | 4 (17) |
| Novick et al.[159] | 153 | 93 (61) | 50 (33) | 10 (6) | 5 (3) |
| Hansen et al.[170] | 25 | 12 (48) | 11 (44) | 2 (8) | 2 (8) |
| Dean et al.[172] | 58 | 31 (59) | 15 (28) | 7 (13) | 5 (9) |
| Messina et al.[163] | 17 | 12 (71) | 2 (12) | 3 (18) | 1 (6) |
| Bredenberg et al.[168] | 25 | 9 (36) | 12 (48) | 4 (16) | NA* |
| Libertino et al.[169] | 97 | 45 (46) | 31 (32) | 21 (22) | 6 (6) |
| Fergany et al.[158] | 18 | 4 (22) | 13 (72) | 1 (6) | 0 (0) |
| Total | 428 | 229 (54) | 136 (32) | 58 (14) | 25 (6) |

*NA = data not available.
Adapted from Rimmer JM, Gennari FJ: Atherosclerotic renovascular disease and progressive renal failure. Ann Intern Med 118:712–719, 1993.

prove renal function in patients with ischemic nephropathy.[40, 158] Postoperative improvement, generally defined as a 20% decrease in serum creatinine concentration, was reported in more than half of the patients in nine studies[40] (Table 47–4). This success accounts for the higher proportion of patients being referred for surgical revascularization for preservation of renal function rather than for correction of hypertension (74% versus 26%).[159]

One unresolved issue is how to determine whether revascularization will salvage renal function from a kidney in which the artery is totally occluded.[144, 160, 161] Some features that may predict successful restoration of renal function include collateral circulation and nephrogram on angiography, renal length greater than 9.0 cm, lateralization of renin secretion, differential concentration of urine on split-function studies, spontaneous back-bleeding on arteriotomy during surgery, and viable nephrons on biopsy examination.[144] However, these should serve only as general guidelines because they lack sufficient specificity and sensitivity to determine outcome.

An aggressive approach toward the totally occluded renal artery, including bilateral surgical revascularization, has been advocated by some investigators.[40, 144] Geyskes and co-workers[160] found that when a totally occluded artery and a contralateral high-grade stenosis were both present, renal function improved when ipsilateral nephrectomy was combined with angioplasty of the contralateral renal artery.

There have been several reports describing recovery of renal function after unilateral revascularization in selected patients requiring dialysis.[144, 162–164] Those who presented with acute pulmonary edema were included in these reports, indicating that benefit can be achieved in patients who appear to have prohibitive risks for perioperative complications. This striking potential for surgically remediable disease is particularly important in view of the high mortality rate of hypertensive end-stage renal disease.[145, 147] However, these provocative studies have not adequately defined the criteria necessary for identifying patients with end-stage renal disease who are most likely to respond to surgical revascularization.

## Renal Angioplasty

As discussed earlier, angioplasty is effective for treating renovascular hypertension associated with atheromatous lesions. This is highlighted by the reported decreased rate of referral for surgical revascularization of atheromatous renovascular hypertension by the early 1980s (41% to 26%).[159] Furthermore, there has been increasing interest in the role of renal angioplasty for treatment of ischemic nephropathy. In our series of patients (see Fig. 47–10), all of whom had serum creatinine levels above 2 mg/dL, 45 (82%) could have successful dilatation.[133] Of those, creatinine levels decreased in 26 (47%). This response rate is comparable to that described by others (Table 47–5). An

**TABLE 47–5. Outcome of Renal Angioplasty**

| Reference | No. of Patients | Outcome | | | |
|---|---|---|---|---|---|
| | | Improved (%) | Stable (%) | Worse (%) | Death (%) |
| Luft et al.[166] | 12 | 3 (25) | 5 (42) | 4 (43) | 0 (0) |
| Pickering et al.[133] | 55 | 26 (47) | 19 (35) | 10 (18) | NA* |
| Bell et al.[171] | 20 | 7 (35) | 10 (50) | 3 (15) | 0 (0) |
| O'Donovan et al.[164] | 17 | 9 (53) | 2 (12) | 6 (35) | 5 (29) |
| Total | 104 | 45 (43) | 36 (35) | 23 (22) | 5 (10) |

*NA = data not available.
Adapted from Rimmer JM, Gennari FJ: Atherosclerotic renovascular disease and progressive renal failure. Ann Intern Med 118:712–719, 1993.

important exception is the report by O'Donovan and colleagues,[164] in which the mortality rate was 29%. This poor outcome is most likely a consequence of the patients' advanced age (mean, 73 years) and severe renal insufficiency (mean serum creatinine level, 7 mg/dL).

Once the decision is made to revascularize the kidney, an important issue is how one determines whether surgery or angioplasty is preferable. Previous assessments of the relative efficacy of renal angioplasty and surgery for the treatment of ischemic renal disease have been limited to comparisons of retrospective, uncontrolled clinical series.[40, 144] Therefore, the criteria for determining which revascularization procedure to select for an individual patient are not well established. However, one potential advantage of angioplasty over surgery is that it can be undertaken in patients who have prohibitively high surgical risks that are related to systemic atherosclerosis, such as coronary artery disease or cerebrovascular disease.

A prospective, randomized study compared the responses to angioplasty and surgery in patients with hypertension and unilateral atherosclerotic renovascular disease.[165] Although this study was not designed to assess recovery of renal function in ischemic nephropathy, some of the findings may have important implications in this regard. Compared with the surgery group, the angioplasty group had a lower technical success rate (83% versus 97%). A repeated intervention was required to correct restenosis in 25% of the angioplasty group but in only one patient of the surgery group. Another important finding was that contralateral stenosis occurred in 14% of the patients within a median period of 9 months; this event was equally likely to occur in both groups. More important, hypertension signaled the presence of the contralateral stenosis in only half of these patients; the remainder were asymptomatic and were discovered during a scheduled follow-up angiogram. Blood pressure was equally well controlled in both groups, and there was no change in renal function in either group after unilateral renal revascularization. Although these data cannot be extrapolated to patients with ischemic nephropathy, this is a good experimental model for comparing the efficacy of surgery and angioplasty in that population. Regardless of the method of revascularization, the high rate of asymptomatic progression reported in this and other studies clearly indicates that follow-up angiography is required.[39, 40]

## SUMMARY

Renovascular disease often causes hypertension that can be cured or improved by renal revascularization. Another important consequence of renal artery stenosis is ischemic nephropathy. This refers to the progressive deterioration in GFR that occurs when renal blood flow is impaired. Ischemic nephropathy is increasingly recognized as an important cause of end-stage renal disease that has a high mortality rate when treated conservatively. By contrast, clinical improvement is reported commonly after renal revascularization. There are few reliable clinical or laboratory markers for ischemic nephropathy, so that angiography is usually required to confirm the diagnosis. However, the diagnosis is likely in the elderly patient with systemic atherosclerosis

and hypertension in whom a rapid rise in serum creatinine concentration is associated with decreased renal length. Revascularization by either renal angioplasty or surgery can successfully preserve renal function in selected patients.

## REFERENCES

1. Goldblatt H, Lynch J, Hanzal RF, Summerville WW: Studies on experimental hypertension. I. The production of persistent elevation of systolic blood pressure by means of renal ischemia. J Exp Med 59:347–378, 1934.
2. Laragh JH, Sealey JE, Buhler FR, Vaughan ED Jr, et al: The renin axis and vasoconstriction volume analysis for understanding and treating renovascular and renal hypertension. Am J Med 58:4–13, 1975.
3. Anderson WP, Ramsey DE, Takata M: Development of hypertension from unilateral renal artery stenosis in conscious dogs. Hypertension 16:441–451, 1990.
4. Miller ED, Samuels AI, Haber E, Barger AC: Inhibition of angiotensin conversion and prevention of renal hypertension. Am J Physiol 228:448–453, 1975.
5. Bengis RG, Coleman TG: Antihypertensive effect of prolonged blockade of angiotensin formation in benign and malignant one- and two-kidney Goldblatt hypertensive rats. Clin Sci 57:53–62, 1979.
6. Brown JJ, Davies DL, Morton JJ, et al: Mechanism of renal hypertension. Lancet 1:1219–1221, 1976.
7. Floyer MA: Role of the kidney in experimental hypertension. Br Med Bull 13:29–32, 1957.
8. Brunner HR, Kirshman JD, Sealey JE, Laragh JH: Hypertension of renal origin: Evidence for two different mechanisms. Science 174:1344–1346, 1971.
9. Gavras H, Brunner HR, Vaughan ED Jr, Laragh JH: Angiotensin-sodium interaction in blood pressure maintenance of renal hypertensive and normotensive rats. Science 180:1369–1372, 1973.
10. Huang W-C, Ploth DW, Bell PD, et al: Bilateral renal function responses to converting enzyme inhibitor (SQ 20,881) in two-kidney, one clip Goldblatt hypertensive rats. Hypertension 3:285–293, 1981.
11. Martinez-Maldonado M: Pathophysiology of renovascular hypertension. Hypertension 17:707–719, 1991.
12. Rocchini AP, Barger AC: Renovascular hypertension in sodium-depleted dogs: Role of renin and carotid sinus reflex. Am J Physiol 236:H101–H107, 1979.
13. Gavras H, Brunner HR, Thurston H, Laragh JH: Reciprocation of renin dependency in renal hypertension. Science 188:1316–1317, 1979.
14. Dargie JH, Franklin SS, Reid JL: Plasma noradrenaline concentrations in experimental renovascular hypertension in the rat. Clin Sci Mol Med 52:477–483, 1977.
15. Katholi RE, Winthlow PL, Winternitz S, Oparil S: Importance of the renal nerves in established two-kidney, one-clip Goldblatt hypertension in the rat. Hypertension 4(suppl II):II-166–II-174, 1982.
16. Leenen FHH, DeJong W, DeWied D: Renal venous and peripheral plasma renin activity in renal hypertension in the rat. Am J Physiol 225:1513–1518, 1973.
17. Jong W de: Release of renin by rat kidney slices; relationship to plasma renin after desoxycorticosterone and renal hypertension. Proc Soc Exp Biol Med 130:85–88, 1969.
18. Liard JF, Peters G: Mechanism of the fall in blood pressure after "unclamping" in rats with Goldblatt-type hypertension. Experientia 26:743–745, 1980.
19. Neubig RR, Hoobler SW: Reversal of chronic renal hypertension: Role of salt and water excretion. Proc Soc Exp Biol Med 150:254–256, 1975.
20. Liard JF, Cowley AW, McCaa RE, et al: Renin, aldosterone, body fluid volumes, and the baroreceptor reflex in the development and reversal of Goldblatt hypertension in conscious dogs. Circ Res 34:549–560, 1974.
21. Thurston H, Bing RF, Swales JD: Reversal of two-kidney one-clip hypertension in the rat. Hypertension 2:256–265, 1980.
22. Hallbäck-Nordlander M, Noresson E, Lundgren Y: Haemodynamic alterations after reversal of renal hypertension in rats. Clin Sci 57:15s–17s, 1979.
23. Russell GI, Brice JM, Bing RF, et al: Haemodynamic changes after

surgical reversal of chronic two-kidney, one-clip hypertension in the rat. Clin Sci 61:117s–119s, 1981.

24. Muirhead EE, Byers LW, Pitcock JA, et al: Denervation of neutral antihypertensive lipid from renal venous effluent in rats. Clin Sci 61:331s–333s, 1981.

25. Russell GI, Bing RF, Tavener D, et al: The role of the renal medulla in experimental renovascular hypertension. *In* Glorioso N, Laragh JH, Rappelli A, et al (eds): Renovascular Hypertension. Raven Press, New York, 1987, pp 53–60.

26. Russell GI, Bing RF, Thurston H, Swales JD: Surgical reversal of two-kidney one clip hypertension during inhibition of the renin-angiotensin system. Hypertension 4:69–76, 1982.

27. Bianchi C, Bonadio M, Andriole VT: Influence of postural changes on the glomerular filtration rate in nephroptosis. Nephron 16:161–172, 1976.

28. Derkx RHM, Tan-Tjiong HL, Wenting GJ, et al: Captopril test for diagnosis of renal artery stenosis. *In* Glorioso N, Laragh JH, Rappelli A, et al (eds): Renovascular Hypertension. Raven Press, New York, 1987, pp 295–315.

29. Pickering TG, Sos TA, James GD, et al: Comparison of renal vein renin activity in hypertensive patients with stenosis of one or both renal arteries. J Hypertens 3(suppl 3):S291–S293, 1985.

30. Vensel LA, Devereux RB, Pickering TG, et al: Cardiac structure and function in renovascular hypertension produced by unilateral and bilateral renal artery stenosis. Am J Cardiol 58:575–582, 1986.

31. Pickering TG, Herman L, Sotelo JE, et al: Recurrent pulmonary edema as a manifestation of renovascular hypertension and its treatment by renal revascularization. Circulation 76(suppl IV):274, 1987.

32. Sutters M, Al-Kutoubi MA, Mathias CJ, Peart S: Diuresis and syncope after renal angioplasty in a patient with one functioning kidney. Br Med J 295:527–528, 1987.

33. Maslowski AH, Nicholls MG, Espiner EA, et al: Mechanisms in human renovascular hypertension. Hypertension 5:597–602, 1983.

34. Lake CR, Chernow B, Goldstein DS, et al: Plasma catecholamine levels in normal subjects and in patients with secondary hypertension. Fed Proc 43:52–56, 1984.

35. Imanishi M, Ohta M, Kawamura M, et al: Aspirin test for differentiation of unilateral renovascular hypertension from hyperreninemic essential hypertension. Am J Hypertens 4:761–768, 1991.

36. Navar LG, Rosivall L: Contribution of the renin-angiotensin system to the control of intrarenal hemodynamics. Kidney Int 25:857–868, 1984.

37. Lohmeier TE, Cowley AW: Hypertensive and renal effects of chronic low level intrarenal angiotensin infusion in the dog. Circ Res 44:154–160, 1979.

38. Hollenberg NK, Swartz SL, Passan DR, Williams GA: Increased glomerular filtration rate after converting-enzyme inhibition in essential hypertension. N Engl J Med 301:9–12, 1979.

39. Schreiber MJ, Pohl MA, Novick AC: The natural history of atherosclerotic and fibrous renal artery disease. Urol Clin North Am 11:383–392, 1984.

40. Rimmer JM, Gennari FJ: Atherosclerotic renovascular disease and progressive renal failure. Ann Intern Med 118:712–719, 1993.

41. Ratliff NB: Renal vascular disease: Pathology of large blood vessel disease. *In* Porush JG, Chou SY, Ferris TF, et al (eds): Hypertension and the Kidney. Grune & Stratton, Orlando, FL, 1985, pp A93–A103.

42. Goncharenko V, Gerlock AJ, Schaff MI, Hollifield SW: Progression of renal artery fibromuscular dysplasia in 42 patients as seen on angiography. Radiology 139:45–51, 1981.

43. Harrington JT, Sommers SC, Kassirer JP: Atheromatous emboli with progressive renal failure. Renal arteriography as the probable inciting factor. Ann Intern Med 68:152–160, 1968.

44. Kassirer JP: Atheroembolic renal disease. N Engl J Med 280:812–817, 1969.

45. Gifford R: Evaluation of the hypertensive patient with emphasis on detecting curable causes. Millbank Mem Fund Q 47:170–186, 1969.

46. Lewin A, Blaufox MD, Castle H, et al: Apparent prevalence of curable hypertension in the Hypertension Detection and Follow-Up Program. Arch Intern Med 145:424–472, 1985.

47. Danielson M, Dammstrom BG: The prevalence of secondary and curable hypertension. Acta Med Scand 209:451–455, 1981.

48. Berglund G, Andersson O, Wilhelmsen L: Prevalence of primary and secondary hypertension: Studies in a random population sample. Br Med J 2:554–556, 1976.

49. Davis BA, Crook JE, Vestal RE, Oates JA: Prevalence of renovascular hypertension in patients with grade III or IV hypertensive retinopathy. N Engl J Med 301:1273–1276, 1979.

50. Keith TA: Renovascular hypertension in black patients. Hypertension 4:438–443, 1982.

51. Holley KE, Hunt JC, Brown AL, et al: Renal artery stenosis. A clinical-pathologic study in normotensive and hypertensive patients. Am J Med 37:14–22, 1964.

52. Eyler WR, Clark MD, Garman JE, et al: Angiography of the renal areas including a comparative study of renal arterial stenoses in patients with and without hypertension. Radiology 78:879–891, 1962.

53. Maxwell MH, Bleifer KH, Franklin SS, Varady P: Cooperative Study of Renovascular Hypertension. Demographic analysis of the study. JAMA 220:1195–1204, 1972.

54. Goldman AG, Varady PD, Franklin SS: Body habitus and serum cholesterol in essential hypertension and renovascular hypertension. Cooperative study of renovascular hypertension. JAMA 221:378–383, 1972.

55. Harding MB, Smith LR, Himmelstein SI, et al: Renal artery stenosis: Prevalence and associated risk factors in patients undergoing routine cardiac catheterization. J Am Soc Nephrol 2:1608–1616, 1992.

56. Choudri AH, Cleland JGF, Rowlands PL, et al: Unsuspected renal artery stenosis in peripheral vascular disease. BMJ 301:1197–1198, 1990.

57. Nicholson JP, Teichman SL, Alderman MH, et al: Cigarette smoking and renovascular hypertension. Lancet 2:765–766, 1983.

58. Sang CN, Whelton PK, Hamper UM, et al: Etiologic factors in renovascular fibromuscular dysplasia. A case-control study. Hypertension 14:472–479, 1989.

59. Diamond JR: Flash pulmonary edema and the diagnostic suspicion of occult renal artery stenosis. Am J Kidney Dis 21:328–330, 1993.

60. Missouris CG, Buckenham T, Vallance PJT, MacGregor GA: Renal artery stenosis masquerading as congestive heart failure. Lancet 341:1521–1522, 1993.

61. Simon N, Franklin SS, Bleifer KH, Maxwell MH: Clinical characteristics of renovascular hypertension. JAMA 220:1209–1218, 1972.

62. Berlyne GW, Tarill AS, Baker SBC: Renal artery stenosis and the nephrotic syndrome. Q J Med 33:325–335, 1964.

63. Zimbler MS, Pickering TG, Sos TA, Laragh JH: Proteinuria in renovascular hypertension and the effects of renal angioplasty. Am J Cardiol 59:406–408, 1987.

64. Elkik F, Corvol P, Idatte JM, Menard J: Renal segmental infarction: A cause of reversible malignant hypertension. J Hypertens 2:149–156, 1984.

65. Stanley JC, Fry WJ: Pediatric renal artery occlusive disease and renovascular hypertension. Etiology, diagnosis, and operative treatment. Arch Surg 116:669–676, 1981.

66. Novick AL, Straffon RA, Stewart BH, Benjamin S: Surgical treatment of renovascular hypertension in the pediatric patient. J Urol 119:794–799, 1978.

67. Vaughan ED Jr, Bühler FR, Laragh JH, et al: Renovascular hypertension: Renin measurements to indicate hypersecretion and contralateral suppression, estimate renal plasma flow, and score for surgical curability. Am J Med 55:402–414, 1973.

68. Vaughan ED Jr, Carey RM, Ayers CR, et al: A physiologic definition of blood pressure response to renal revascularization in patients with renovascular hypertension. Kidney Int 15:S83–S92, 1979.

69. Case DB, Laragh JH: Reactive hyperreninemia in renovascular hypertension after angiotensin blockade with saralasin or converting enzyme inhibitor. Ann Intern Med 91:153–160, 1979.

70. Müller FB, Sealey JE, Case CB, et al: The captopril test for identifying renovascular disease in hypertensive patients. Am J Med 80:633–644, 1986.

71. Elliott WJ, Martin WB, Murphy MB: Comparison of two noninvasive screening tests for renovascular hypertension. Arch Intern Med 153:755–764, 1993.

72. Frederickson ED, Wilcox CS, Bucci M, et al: A prospective evaluation of a simplified captopril test for the detection of renovascular hypertension. Arch Intern Med 150:569–572, 1990.

73. Postma CT, Van der Steen PH, Hoefragels WH, et al: The captopril test in the detection of renovascular disease in hypertensive patients. Arch Intern Med 150:625–628, 1990.

74. Hansen PD, Garsdal P, Fruergaard P: The captopril test for identification of renovascular hypertension: Value and immediate adverse effects. J Intern Med 228:159–163, 1990.

75. Idrissi A, Fourmier A, Renaud H, et al: The captopril challenge test as a screening test for renovascular hypertension. Kidney Int 34(suppl 25):S138–S141, 1988.

76. Thibonnier M, Sassano P, Joseph A, et al: Diagnostic value of a single dose of captopril in renin- and aldosterone-dependent, surgically curable hypertension. Cardiovasc Rev Rep 3:1659–1667, 1982.

77. Gosse P, Dupas JY, Reynaud P, et al: Captopril test in the detection of renovascular hypertension in a population with low prevalence of the disease. A prospective study. Am J Hypertens 2:191–193, 1989.

78. Svetkey LP, Himmelstein SI, Dunnick NR, et al: Prospective analysis of strategies for diagnosing renovascular hypertension. Hypertension 14:247–257, 1989.

79. Kutkuhn B, Godehardt E, Kunert J, et al: Validity of the captopril test for identifying correctable unilateral renovascular hypertension. Clin Exp Hypertens A 13:143–156, 1991.

80. Maxwell MH, Lupu AN, Taplin GV: Radioisotope renogram in renal arterial hypertension. J Urol 100:376–383, 1968.

81. Schalekamp MADH, Derkx FHM: Functional diagnosis of renovascular hypertension, with special reference to renin measurements. *In* Schilfgaarde RV, Stanley JC, Van Brummelen P, Overbosch EH, et al (eds): Clinical Aspects of Renovascular Hypertension. Martinus Nijhoff Publishing, Boston, 1983, pp 62–73.

82. Geyskes GG, Oei HY, Puylaert CBAJ, Dorhout Mees EJ: Unilateral renal failure after captopril in patients with renovascular hypertension. *In* Glorioso N, Laragh JH, Rappelli A, et al (eds): Renovascular Hypertension. Raven Press, New York, 1987, pp 281–294.

83. Fommei E, Ghione S, Palla L, et al: Renal scintigraphic captopril test in the diagnosis of renovascular hypertension. Hypertension 10:212–220, 1987.

84. Kopecky RT, Thomas FD, McAfee JG: Furosemide augments the effects of captopril on nuclear studies in renovascular stenosis. Hypertension 10:181–188, 1987.

85. Mann SJ, Pickering TG, Sos TA, et al: Captopril renography in the diagnosis of renal artery stenosis: Accuracy and limitations. Am J Med 90:30–40, 1991.

86. Chen CC, Hoffer PB, Vahjen G, et al: Patients at high risk for renal artery stenosis: A simple method of scintigraphic analysis with Tc-99m DPTA and captopril. Radiology 176:365–370, 1990.

87. Dondi M, Franchi R, Levorato M, et al: Evaluation of hypertensive patients by means of captopril enhanced renal scintigraphy with technetium-99m DTPA. J Nucl Med 30:615–621, 1989.

88. Dunnick AR, Sfakianakis GN: Screening for renovascular hypertension. Radiol Clin North Am 29:497–510, 1991.

89. Dubovsky EV, Russell CD: Quantitation of renal function with glomerular and tubular agents. Semin Nucl Med 12:308–329, 1982.

90. Schlegel JV, Hamway SA: Individual renal plasma flow determinations in two minutes. J Urol 116:282–285, 1976.

91. Dondi M, Monetti N, Fanti S, et al: Use of technetium-99m-MAG₃ for renal scintigraphy after angiotensin-converting enzyme inhibition. J Nucl Med 32:424–428, 1991.

92. Russell DC, Thorstad B, Yester MV, et al: Comparison of technetium-99m-MAG₃ with iodine-131 hippuran by a simultaneous dual channel technique. J Nucl Med 29:1189–1193, 1988.

93. Al-Nahhas AA, Jafri RA, Britton KE, et al: Clinical experience with ⁹⁹ᵐTc-MAG₃, mercaptoacetyltriglycine, and a comparison with ⁹⁹ᵐTc-DTPA. Eur J Nucl Med 14:453–462, 1988.

94. Sfakianakis GN, Bourgoignie JJ, Jaffe D, et al: Single-dose captopril scintigraphy in the diagnosis of renovascular hypertension. J Nucl Med 28:1383–1892, 1987.

95. Erbsloh-Moller B, Dumas A, Roth C, et al: Furosemide–¹³¹I-hippuran renography after angiotensin-converting enzyme inhibition for the diagnosis of renovascular hypertension. Am J Med 90:23–29, 1991.

96. Geyskes GG, Oei HY, Puylaert CB, Mees EJ: Renovascular hypertension identified by captopril-induced changes in the renogram. Hypertension 9:451–458, 1987.

97. Geyskes GG, Puylaert CBA, Oei HY, Mees EJ: Follow up study of 70 patients with renal artery stenosis treated by percutaneous transluminal dilatation. Br Med J Clin Res 287:333–336, 1983.

98. Havey RJ, Krumlovsky F, del Greco F, Martin HG: Screening for renovascular hypertension. JAMA 254:388–393, 1985.

99. Buonocore E, Meaney TF, Borkowsky GP, et al: Digital subtraction angiography of the abdominal aorta and renal arteries. Radiology 139:281–286, 1981.

100. Clark RA, Alexander ES: Digital subtraction angiography of the renal arteries—prospective comparison with conventional arteriography. Invest Radiol 18:6–10, 1983.

101. Hillman BJ, Ovitt TW, Capp MP, et al: The potential impact of digital video subtraction angiography on screening for renovascular hypertension. Radiology 142:577–579, 1982.

102. Zabbo A, Novick AC: Digital subtraction angiography for noninvasive imaging of the renal artery. Urol Clin North Am 11:409–416, 1984.

103. Debatin JF, Grist T, Svetkey L, et al: MR angiography: Screening examination for renovascular hypertension? Am J Hypertens 4:38A, 1991.

104. Clorius JH, Allenberg J, Hupp T, et al: Predictive value of exercise renography for presurgical evaluation of nephrogenic hypertension. Hypertension 10:280–286, 1987.

105. Clorius JH, Mann J, Schmidlin P, et al: Clinical evaluation of patients with hypertension and exercise-induced renal dysfunction. Hypertension 10:287–293, 1987.

106. Jenni R, Vieli A, Lüscher TF, et al: Combined two-dimensional ultrasound Doppler technique. New possibilities for the screening of renovascular and parenchymatous hypertension? Nephron 44(suppl 1):2–4, 1986.

107. Kohler TR, Zierler E, Martin RL, et al: Noninvasive diagnosis of renal artery stenosis by ultrasonic duplex scanning. J Vasc Surg 4:450–456, 1986.

108. Hoffman V, Edwards JM, Carer S, et al: Role of duplex scanning for the detection of atherosclerotic renal artery disease. Kidney Int 39:1232–1239, 1991.

109. Robertson R, Murphy A, Dubbins PA: Renal artery stenosis: The use of duplex ultrasound as a screening technique. Br J Radiol 61:196–201, 1988.

110. Lewis BD, James EM: Current applications of duplex and color Doppler ultrasound imaging: Abdomen. Mayo Clin Proc 643:1158–1169, 1984.

111. Taylor KJ, Morse SS, Rigsby CM, et al: Vascular complications in renal allografts. Detection and duplex Doppler US. Radiology 162:31–38, 1987.

112. Shipley RE, Gregg DE: The effect of external constriction of a blood vessel on blood flow. Am J Physiol 141:289–296, 1944.

113. Levin DC, Beckmann CF, Serur JR: Vascular resistance changes distal to progressive arterial stenosis: A critical re-evaluation of the concept of vasodilator reverse. Invest Radiol 14:120–128, 1980.

114. Talierco CP, Vlietstra RE, Fisher LD, Burnett JC: Risks for renal dysfunction with cardiac angiography. Ann Intern Med 104:501–504, 1986.

115. Saint-Georges G, Aube M: Safety of outpatient angiography: A prospective study. AJR 144:235–236, 1985.

116. Mann SJ, Pickering TG: Detection of renovascular hypertension. State of the art: 1992. Ann Intern Med 117:845–853, 1992.

117. Franklin SS, Young JD, Maxwell MH, et al: Operative morbidity and mortality in renovascular disease. JAMA 231:1148–1153, 1975.

118. Foster JH, Maxwell MJ, Franklin SS, et al: Renovascular occlusive disease: Results of operative treatment. JAMA 231:1043–1048, 1975.

119. Lankford NS, Donohue JP, Grim CE, Weinberger MH: Results of surgical treatment of renovascular hypertension. J Urol 122:439–441, 1979.

120. Novick AC, Straffon RA, Stewart BH, et al: Diminished operative morbidity and mortality in renal revascularization. JAMA 246:749–753, 1981.

121. Novick AC, Textor SC, Bodie B, Khauh RB: Revascularization to preserve renal function in patients with atherosclerotic renovascular disease. Urol Clin North Am 11:477–490, 1984.

122. Thevenet A, Mary H, Boennec M: Results following surgical correction of renovascular hypertension. J Cardiovasc Surg 21:517–528, 1980.

123. Ying CY, Tifft CP, Gavras H, Chobanian AV: Renal revascularization in the azotemic hypertensive patient resistant to therapy. N Engl J Med 311:1070–1075, 1984.

124. Lawrie GM, Morris GC, Glaeser DH, DeBakey ME: Renovascular reconstruction: Factors affecting long-term prognosis in 919 patients followed up to 31 years. Am J Cardiol 63:1085–1092, 1989.

125. Bedoya L, Ziegelbaum M, Vidt DG, et al: Baseline renal function and surgical revascularization in atherosclerotic renal arterial disease in the elderly. Cleve Clin J Med 56:415–421, 1989.

126. Sos TA, Pickering TG, Sniderman K, et al: Percutaneous translumi-

nal renal angioplasty in renovascular hypertension due to atheroma or fibromuscular dysplasia. N Engl J Med 309:274–279, 1983.

127. Tegtmeyer CJ, Elson J, Glass TA: Percutaneous transluminal angioplasty: The treatment of choice for renovascular hypertension due to fibromuscular dysplasia. Radiology 143:631–637, 1982.

128. Martin ED, Mattern RF, Baer L: Renal angioplasty for hypertension: Predictive factors for long-term success. AJR 137:921–924, 1981.

129. Grim CE, Luft FC, Yune HY: Percutaneous transluminal dilatation in the treatment of renal vascular hypertension. Ann Intern Med 95:439–442, 1981.

130. Tegtmeyer CG, Dyer R, Teates CD: Percutaneous transluminal dilatation of renal arteries. Radiology 135:589–599, 1980.

131. Plouin P-F, Darne B, Chatellier G, et al: Restenosis after a first percutaneous transluminal renal angioplasty. Hypertension 21:89–96, 1993.

132. Hricik DE, Browning PJ, Kapelman R, et al: Captopril-induced functional renal insufficiency in patients with bilateral renal-artery stenoses or renal-artery stenosis in a solitary kidney. N Engl J Med 308:373–376, 1983.

133. Pickering TG, Sos TA, Saddekni S, et al: Renal angioplasty in patients with azotemia and renovascular hypertension. J Hypertens 4(suppl 6):S667–S669, 1986.

134. Hunt JC, Sheps SG, Harrison EG, et al: Renal and renovascular hypertension: A reasoned approach to diagnosis and management. Arch Intern Med 133:988–999, 1974.

135. Dean RH, Kieffer RW, Smith BW, et al: Renovascular hypertension. Anatomic and renal functional changes during drug therapy. Arch Surg 116:1408–1415, 1981.

136. Michel JB, Dussaule JC, Choudat L, et al: Effects of antihypertensive treatment in one-clip, two kidney hypertension in rats. Kidney Int 29:1011–1020, 1986.

137. Jackson B, Franze L, Sumithran E, Johnston CI: Pharmacologic nephrectomy with chronic angiotensin converting enzyme inhibitor treatment in renovascular hypertension in the rat. J Lab Clin Med 115:21–27, 1990.

138. Grone HJ, Helmchen U: Impairment and recovery of the clipped kidney in two kidney, one clip hypertensive rats during and after antihypertensive therapy. Lab Invest 54:645–655, 1986.

139. Postma CT, Hoefnagels WHL, Barentz JO, et al: Occlusion of unilateral stenosed renal arteries—relation to medical treatment. J Hum Hypertens 3:185–190, 1989.

140. Arzilli F, Giovannetti R, Meola M, et al: ACE-inhibition vs surgical treatment in the outcome of ischemic kidney of renovascular patients: A one year follow-up. High Blood Press 1:47–50, 1992.

141. Ribstein J, Mourad G, Mimran A: Contrasting acute effects of captopril and nifedipine on renal function in renovascular hypertension. Am J Hypertens 1:239–244, 1988.

142. Miyamori I, Yasuhara S, Matsubara T, et al: Comparative effects of captopril and nifedipine on split renal function in renovascular hypertension. Am J Hypertens 1:359–363, 1988.

143. Epstein M: Calcium antagonists and renal protection. Current status and future perspectives. Arch Intern Med 152:1572–1584, 1992.

144. Jacobson H: Ischemic renal disease. Kidney Int 34:729–743, 1988.

145. USRDS Coordinating Center: United States Renal Data System 1993 Annual Data Report. Am J Kidney Dis 22:1–118, 1993.

146. The Fifth Report of the Joint National Committee on Detection, Evaluation, and Treatment of Hypertension. National Institutes of Health publication, Washington, DC, 1993, pp 93–108.

147. Mailloux LU, Bellucci AG, Mossey RT, et al: Predictors of survival in patients undergoing dialysis. Am J Med 84:855–862, 1988.

148. Corradi B, Malberti F, Farina M, et al: Chronic renal failure due to atheromatous renovascular disease in the elderly. Contrib Nephrol 105:167–171, 1993.

149. Zucchelli P, Zucchala A: Ischemic nephropathy in the elderly. Contrib Nephrol 105:13–24, 1993.

150. Scoble JE, Maher ER, Hamilton G, et al: Atherosclerotic renovascular disease causing renal impairment—a case for treatment. Clin Nephrol 31:119–122, 1989.

151. Tollefson DFJ, Ernst CB: Natural history of atherosclerotic renal artery stenosis associated with aortic disease. J Vasc Surg 14:327–331, 1991.

152. Missouris CG, Buckenham T, Cappuccio FP, MacGregor GA: Renal artery stenosis: A common and important problem in patients with peripheral vascular disease. Am J Med 96:10–14, 1994.

153. Olin JW, Melia M, Young JR, et al: Prevalence of atheroslerotic renal artery stenosis in patients with atherosclerosis elsewhere. Am J Med 88(suppl I):46N–51N, 1990.

154. Zierler RE, Bergelin RO, Isaacson JA, Strandness DE: Natural history of atherosclerotic renal artery stenosis: A prospective study with duplex ultrasonography. J Vasc Surg 19:250–258, 1994.

155. Guzman RP, Zierler RE, Isaacson JA, et al: Renal atrophy and renal artery stenosis: A prospective study with duplex ultrasound. Hypertension 23:346–350, 1994.

156. Textor SC, Novick AG, Tarazi RC, et al: Critical perfusion pressure for renal function in patients with bilateral atherosclerotic renal vascular disease. Ann Intern Med 102:308–314, 1985.

157. Hall JE, Guyton AC, Jackson TE, et al: Control of glomerular filtration rate by the renin-angiotensin system. Am J Physiol 233:F366–F372, 1977.

158. Fergany A, Novick AC, Goldfarb D: Management of atherosclerotic renal artery disease in younger patients. J Urol 151:10–12, 1994.

159. Novick AC, Ziegelbaum M, Vidt DG, et al: Trends in surgical revascularization for renal artery disease: Ten years' experience. JAMA 257:498–501, 1987.

160. Geyskes GG, Oei HY, Klinge J, et al: Renovascular hypertension: The small kidney updated. Q J Med 251:203–217, 1988.

161. Dean RH, Englund R, Dupont WD, et al: Retrieval of renal function by revascularization. Study of outcome predictors. Ann Surg 202:367–375, 1985.

162. Ascer E, Gennaro M, Rogers D: Unilateral renal artery revascularization can salvage renal function and terminate dialysis in selected patients with uremia. J Vasc Surg 18:1012–1018, 1993.

163. Messina LM, Zelenock GB, Yao KA, Stanley JC: Renal revascularization for recurrent pulmonary edema in patients with poorly controlled hypertension and renal insufficiency: A distinct subgroup of patients with arteriosclerotic renal artery occlusive disease. J Vasc Surg 15:73–82, 1992.

164. O'Donovan RM, Gutierrez OH, Izzo JL: Preservation of renal function by percutaneous renal angioplasty in high-risk elderly patients: Short-term outcome. Nephron 60:187–192, 1992.

165. Weibull H, Bergqvist D, Bergentz S-E, et al: Percutaneous transluminal renal angioplasty versus surgical reconstruction of atherosclerotic renal artery stenosis: A prospective randomized study. J Vasc Surg 18:841–852, 1993.

166. Luft FC, Grim CE, Weinberger MH: Intervention in patients with renovascular hypertension and renal insufficiency. J Urol 130:654–656, 1983.

167. Jamieson CG, Clarkson AR, Woodroff AJ, Faris I: Reconstructive vascular surgery for chronic renal failure. Br J Surg 71:338–340, 1984.

168. Bredenberg CE, Sampson LN, Ray FS, et al: Changing patterns in surgery for renal artery occlusive diseases. J Vasc Surg 15:1018–1023, 1992.

169. Libertino JA, Bosco PJ, Ying CY, et al: Renal revascularization to preserve and restore renal function. J Urol 147:1485–1487, 1992.

170. Hansen KJ, Ditesheim JA, Metropol SH, et al: Management of renovascular hypertension in the elderly population. J Vasc Surg 10:266–273, 1989.

171. Bell GM, Reid J, Buist TA: Percutaneous transluminal angioplasty in management of atherosclerotic renovascular hypertension. Q J Med 63:393–403, 1987.

172. Dean RH, Tribble RW, Hansen K, et al: Evolution of renal insufficiency in ischemic nephropathy. Ann Surg 213:446–455, 1990.

# Hypertension in Renal Parenchymal Disease

*John H. Galla*
*Robert G. Luke*

UNILATERAL RENAL DISEASE

BILATERAL RENAL DISEASE
Acute Renal Disease
Chronic Renal Disease

END-STAGE RENAL DISEASE
Post-transplantation Hypertension
Hypertension in Dialysis Patients

The association between Bright disease and high blood pressure or at least cardiac enlargement has been known since the 1830s.[1] Hypertension does not develop in the presence of normal kidneys, which are free from nonphysiologic factors influencing NaCl reabsorption and are able to sense changes in systemic blood pressure[2]; in the presence of hypertension a natriuresis develops that reduces plasma volume and restores normotension. These relationships are disturbed in the presence of acute and chronic kidney disease, and hypertension is a common complication of such diseases. Primary hypertension itself is an important cause of progressive renal disease and, when hypertension develops as a result of renal disease, is the predominant risk factor for accelerated loss of renal function. "Vicious circle" hypertension is said to occur when hypertension and kidney disease compound one another, leading to both systemic cardiovascular disease and progressive renal disease. Therapeutic interruption of this cycle is mandatory. It is anticipated that by the end of the century there will be more than 300,000 patients who are alive in the United States because of renal replacement therapy (dialysis and/or renal transplantation). Cardiovascular disease, including myocardial infarction, cardiac failure, and cerebrovascular accident, remains by far the most important cause of mortality in these patients. Early and effective treatment of hypertension in patients with underlying kidney disease is the most important therapeutic intervention, not only to slow the rate of progression of renal disease[3] but also to reduce morbidity and mortality of cardiovascular causes in patients with chronic renal failure both before and after renal replacement therapy.[4]

Essential hypertension constitutes approximately 90% of all hypertension. Hypertension associated with renal parenchymal disease is second, and renovascular hypertension (Chapter 47) is the most important type of curable hypertension. Related syndromes such as renovascular renal failure (Chapter 47) and atheroembolic renal disease (Chapter 35) are discussed elsewhere. Hypertension associated with

acute renal failure (Chapter 28) and with diabetes mellitus (Chapter 39 is discussed here briefly.

## UNILATERAL RENAL DISEASE

When a decision is made to investigate a patient for renovascular hypertension, the possibility of unilateral parenchymal renal disease must be kept in mind (Table 48–1). Thus, although the excretory urogram is not an ideal screening test for renal artery stenosis, it has the advantage of showing structural change of the causes listed[5] in Table 48–1, except for a juxtaglomerular apparatus tumor, which is often small. Many of these conditions are discovered because of renal pain, hematuria, or a palpable abdominal mass with hypertension as an incidental finding. Especially in the adult, documentation that a lesion such as unilateral hydronephrosis is a cause of hypertension rather than an incidental finding in a patient with essential hypertension is difficult. This was pointed out by Smith.[6] When he defined "cure" as a fall in blood pressure to 140/90 mm Hg or less for at least 1 year after nephrectomy, this standard was met in only 26% of patients. If the only indication for removing a kidney is to cure or improve hypertension, a healthy skepticism as to the likelihood of benefit is indicated. Nev-

**TABLE 48–1. Unilateral Renal Parenchymal Disease as a Cause of Hypertension**

| |
|---|
| Renin-secreting tumor |
|     Juxtaglomerular apparatus |
|     Wilms tumor |
|     Adenocarcinoma (unusual) |
| Hydronephrosis |
| Reflux nephropathy |
| Renal tuberculosis |
| Adenocarcinoma |

ertheless, with careful selection, patients can benefit markedly from this procedure.

The best chance of cure in patients with hypertension and unilateral renal disease probably lies with a tumor of the juxtaglomerular apparatus and with Wilms tumor. The renin-producing tumor of the juxtaglomerular apparatus, sometimes termed hemangiopericytoma, was first described by Robertson and colleagues.[7] It is quite rare, is more common in young adults, and does not recur, and its removal is associated with cure of hypertension.[8, 9] It is usually discovered because of workup of a patient for renovascular hypertension or for hyperreninemic hyperaldosteronism with hypokalemia. It can be seen with selective renal arteriography[10] but is often as small as 2 cm. When renal vein renins are supportive of unilateral production of renin in the absence of ipsilateral renal artery stenosis, computed tomography may be helpful if no lesion is seen by angiography, because the lesions are typically not associated with increased vascularity. An alternative to surgery in treatment of tumors of the juxtaglomerular apparatus is conservative management with converting enzyme inhibitors.[11]

About half of patients with Wilms tumor, two thirds of whom are children younger than 4 years of age, are hypertensive.[12] Hypertension may be due to either renin production by the tumor[12] or renin secretion caused by compression of intrarenal vessels by the tumor. Appropriate treatment is now associated with an 80% cure rate, which rises to nearly 100% when the tumor is confined to the kidney.

Hypertension occurs in up to 38% of patients with adenocarcinoma of the kidney.[13] This tumor, however, occurs in older patients in whom essential hypertension is also common. Renin production by the tumor has been documented[14] but is rare. In general, correction of hypertension would be an incidental occurrence in a patient in whom treatment was directed to managing the cancer. On the other hand, patients may be found to have renal carcinoma during the workup for an underlying renal cause of hypertension.

Reflux nephropathy, the term now preferred to chronic pyelonephritis, is usually asymmetric in its effect on the kidneys but much more frequently bilateral than unilateral. Cortical scarring and calicectasis are acquired in the first few years of life (Chapter 32) and, if the disease is truly unilateral, compensatory hypertrophy of the remaining kidney should be evident. Significant proteinuria is usually associated with acquired focal glomerular sclerosis[15, 16] secondary to hypertrophy and hemodynamic changes in the adapted nephrons of the unscarred areas. Such proteinuria would contraindicate nephrectomy. The degree of scarring correlates with the frequency and severity of hypertension.[15, 17, 18] Kincaid-Smith and colleagues[18] found that hypertension was the presenting feature of reflux nephropathy in approximately 20% of patients; overall, approximately 50% of adult patients were hypertensive. Initial presentation was during pregnancy for 20% of patients, with first-semester hypertension or with persistent hypertension after pregnancy. In all of these circumstances, bilateral disease is more common than unilateral disease. Nevertheless, there is clear evidence of potential benefit of nephrectomy for reflux nephropathy in carefully selected patients.[19–21] In a personal series,[21] benefit was most likely in younger patients with a shorter history of hypertension, contralateral

hypertrophy with no caliceal damage or cortical scarring, and when the affected kidney contributed less than 25% to overall renal function. Bailey and co-workers[22] similarly demonstrated significant benefit of nephrectomy for blood pressure in patients with unilateral reflux nephropathy in whom the contralateral kidney was normal radiologically as well as hypertrophied and the diseased kidney had a measured glomerular filtration rate (GFR) of 10 mL/min or less. In patients with mild to moderate hypertension, antihypertensive drug therapy is an alternative[19] unless there are additional indications for surgery, such as frequent episodes of pyelonephritis in the affected kidney. Because, especially in young female patients, fibromuscular dysplasia may coexist in the contralateral kidney,[23] selective renal arteriography should be considered before nephrectomy. If the serum creatinine level is elevated above normal or measured GFR is less than 70 to 80 mL/min, the disease should be assumed to be bilateral and nephrectomy avoided.

Especially when relief of hypertension is the sole reason for removing a kidney with unilateral parenchymal renal disease such as reflux nephropathy, an elevation of renal vein renin on the ipsilateral side with suppression of renal renin release on the contralateral side is a helpful indication of likelihood of improvement in hypertension.[24–26] As with renal vein renin measurements for renal artery stenosis, not all agree with the predictive value of this test.[20] Embolization of the kidney is an alternative to nephrectomy, especially if the kidney is quite small.[27]

Unilateral pelviureteric obstruction (hydronephrosis) can cause hypertension. This has been demonstrated in experimental animals and is renin dependent at least in the acute experimental situation.[28, 29] Acute hypertension has also been seen with acute hydronephrosis in humans[30] in association with enhanced renin secretion by the obstructed kidney. In both the acute experimental and human situations, blood pressure usually returns to normal in the succeeding several weeks or months. In chronic hypertension associated with unilateral hydronephrosis, elevation of peripheral plasma renin activity and of ipsilateral renal vein renin has been inconsistent.[31, 32] Further concern about the etiologic relationship between unilateral obstruction and hypertension is raised by two series in which prevalence of hypertension was not above that in a control population.[33, 34] Nevertheless, operative intervention was associated with 80% cure or improvement in the study by Wanner and colleagues[33] and about 50% in the study by Clark and Malek.[34] Enhanced renin secretion in the ipsilateral kidney and suppression of renin in the contralateral kidney may provide evidence about the hemodynamic significance of the lesion, but the usefulness of this test is again controversial.[31, 33] A decision about surgery in such cases must depend on the severity of the hypertension; the likelihood in terms of family history, age, and so forth that the patient has essential hypertension; convincingly normal function in the contralateral kidney; and, perhaps, measurement of renal vein renins. The variability of the hypertension in unilateral hydronephrosis is probably related to variation in the degree and duration of obstruction and perhaps the degree of renal ischemia produced by the obstruction. The decision is easier if the patient has related pain or the obstruction can be relieved surgically with preservation of function on that side. Significant hypertension is unlikely to be related to mild degrees of unilateral hydronephrosis.

The frequency of hypertension in renal tuberculosis in one large series was 4%.[35] Occasional cures by unilateral nephrectomy have, however, been reported.[36] Because tuberculosis can be a bilateral disease, care must be taken that the contralateral kidney is free of disease and that active renal tuberculosis is treated before nephrectomy. Urinary tract obstruction caused by strictures of the ureter may be present at diagnosis or develop during or after antituberculosis chemotherapy. Again, renal vein renin measurements may be helpful in predicting response to nephrectomy.[37]

Other rare causes of unilateral renal disease associated with hypertension, such as radiation nephritis, the Page kidney, renal cysts, and the Ask-Upmark kidney, are discussed in a review.[38]

## BILATERAL RENAL DISEASE

### Acute Renal Disease

An overall frequency of 40% for hypertension was noted in one large series of patients with acute renal failure.[39] Hypertension is much more common in acute renal failure caused by glomerular-vascular disease than in that caused by acute tubule necrosis or by acute interstitial nephritis. For example, in the series of Bonomini and colleagues[39] 15% was the frequency of hypertension in tubulointerstitial disease and 73% in glomerular-vascular disease. In acute tubule necrosis, hypertension reflects salt and water retention or pre-existing essential hypertension.

Accelerated or malignant hypertension may cause renal failure.[40, 41] Initial antihypertensive treatment in patients with severe hypertension may also cause an acute reduction in renal function secondary to an impaired renal autoregulatory capacity for GFR[42] secondary to preglomerular arteriolar injury. When severe hypertension accompanies acute renal failure, it should be treated appropriately by antihypertensive drugs and by diuretics or dialysis if necessary. Reduction of blood pressure to normal levels in these circumstances should, however, be more cautious and gradual. Angiotensin-converting enzyme (ACE) inhibitors can precipitate a form of prerenal failure in patients whose nephrons are all distal to a functionally active renal artery stenosis.[43] This is not a specific effect and can occur in other circumstances in which maintenance of GFR is highly dependent on angiotension II–induced efferent arteriolar constriction.[44–46] These events are particularly likely in patients with severe hypertensive nephrosclerosis or in severe congestive heart failure. ACE inhibitors should not necessarily be avoided in such circumstances, but the physician should be aware of the possibility of acute renal failure and measure serum creatinine concentration weekly for a few weeks after their introduction.

Scleroderma renal crisis is usually, but not invariably, associated with severe hypertension.[47] ACE inhibitors are urgently indicated and have vastly improved the prognosis for such patients.[48] Other examples of glomerular-vascular disease often associated with severe hypertension are the vasculitides, especially classic polyarteritis nodosa, hemo-

lytic-uremic syndrome, and atheroembolic renal disease. The hemolytic-uremic syndrome is characterized by microangiopathic hemolytic anemia, and hypertension is present in the majority of patients.[49] Hypertension can be quite severe in atheroembolic renal disease, may precede the development of the syndrome as a risk factor for diffuse atherosclerosis, or may be exacerbated or develop de novo because of occlusion of small intrarenal vessels and resulting renal ischemia.[50] In acute poststreptococcal glomerulonephritis, hypertension occurs in 80% of patients and is substantially due to an acute reduction of GFR with retention of NaCl and water.[51, 52]

## Chronic Renal Disease

### PREVALENCE

Hypertension secondary to underlying renal parenchymal disease accounts for about 5% of all hypertension.[53] As patients progress toward end-stage renal disease, hypertension becomes more frequent until nearly all patients are hypertensive before requiring renal replacement therapy.[54, 55] Hypertension occurs earlier in the course of chronic renal failure in polycystic kidney disease (PKD) and in the proliferative glomerulonephritides than it does in tubulointerstitial disorders.[55–57] In "malignant" focal glomerulosclerosis, it may also occur earlier, although the lesion is not proliferative, because of related hyaline arteriosclerosis of the preglomerular vessels.[58] In tubulointerstitial diseases, when salt wasting occurs even with a normal salt intake, hypertension may not occur before end-stage renal disease—for example, in medullary cystic kidney disease. Hypertension can occur before an elevation of serum creatinine concentration or even a reduction in GFR in PKD and in chronic glomerulonephritis.[56, 59] Blood pressure increases as renal function deteriorates and with increasing age and body mass index.[57]

Underlying kidney disease is a risk factor for cardiovascular events, left ventricular hypertrophy, and further progression of the kidney disease; for any given level of blood pressure retinopathy is more marked in patients with renal parenchymal hypertension.[60] Renal hypertension is more likely to progress to an accelerated or malignant phase than is essential hypertension.[61] The mechanism of hypertension in glomerulonephritis with a normal or nearly normal GFR and a quiescent renin-angiotension system is not clear.[59] Possibilities include activation of renal afferent reflexes that stimulate the sympathetic nervous system,[62] and alterations in intrinsic renal vasoactive agents.

### MECHANISMS OF HYPERTENSION

The pathogenetic mechanisms are complex and interactive (Fig. 48–1). As GFR falls, there is a tendency for retention of NaCl; the normal guytonian natriuretic response is impaired by activation of the sympathetic nervous system secondary to renal afferent reflexes, an inappropriately stimulated renin-angiotensin-aldosterone system, and an impaired nitrovasodilatation system in the renal vas-

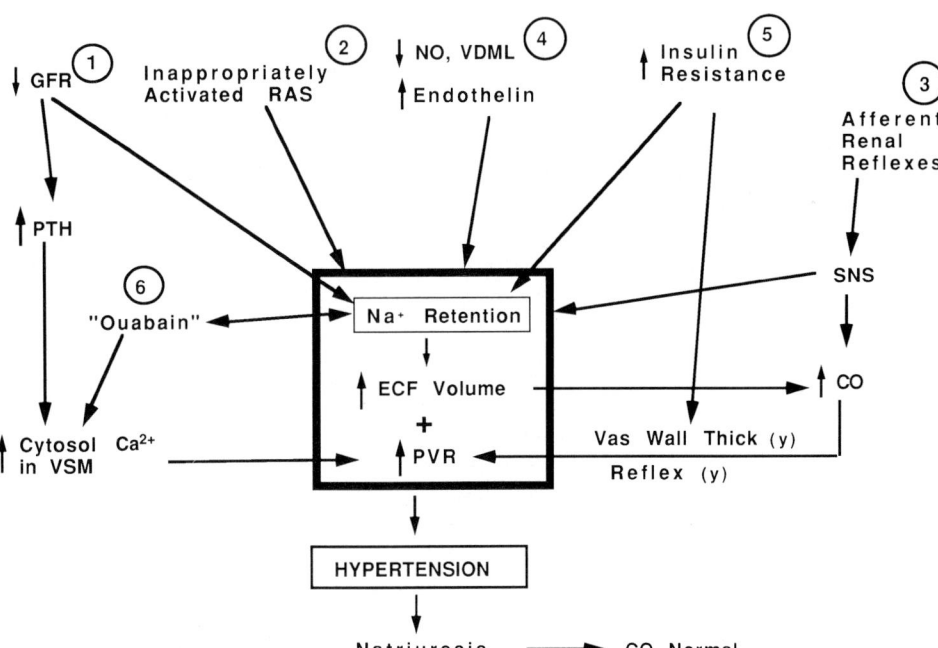

**Figure 48–1.** Mechanisms by which primary renal disease may lead to hypertension. Arrows to box perimeter indicate effects on all mechanisms contained within. Double-headed arrow indicates a feedback loop. GFR = glomerular filtration rate; RAS = renin-angiotensin-aldosterone system; NO = nitric oxide; VDML = vasodepressor medullary lipids; SNS = sympathetic nervous system; CO = cardiac output; PTH = parathyroid hormone; VSM = vascular smooth muscle; ECF = extracellular fluid; PVR = peripheral vascular resistance; Vas wall thick = vascular wall thickening.

culature. Extracellular fluid (ECF) volume expansion leads to release of endogenous ouabain-like factors[63] that impair renal tubule reabsorption of NaCl in an attempt to normalize ECF volume, but the inhibition of $Na^+,K^+$-ATPase in vascular smooth muscle leads to an increase in cytosolic $Ca^{2+}$ with resulting vasoconstriction and increased sensitivity to circulating vasoactive agents. Peripheral resistance is also increased by reflex vasoconstriction secondary to increased organ flow,[64] increased vascular responsiveness secondary to thickening of the vascular wall,[65] and impairment of the endothelial–vascular smooth muscle paracrine system. Insulin resistance develops in chronic renal failure, but the higher insulin levels can lead to hypertrophy of vascular smooth muscle and renal NaCl retention.[66] Chronic renal failure is associated with progressive elevations of parathyroid hormone levels that also increase the cytosolic $Ca^{2+}$ concentration in vascular smooth muscle cells.

In serial studies of almost 100 patients with early chronic renal failure, Brod and colleagues[67] demonstrated progression over several years from a normotensive state characterized by ECF volume expansion, increased cardiac output, and reduced peripheral resistance to a hypertensive state associated with a normal ECF volume and increased peripheral resistance. Moderate renal insufficiency is associated with ECF volume expansion and increased total exchangeable $Na^+$ compared with essential hypertension or normotensive control subjects.[68] There is a direct correlation between the degree of plasma volume expansion and $Na^+$ retention and the degree of hypertension.[69] Suppression of the renin-angiotensin-aldosterone system in chronic renal failure by ECF volume expansion appears to be impaired.[67–70] Thus plasma renin activity levels are inappropriately high for the degree of ECF volume expansion. As in accelerated essential hypertension, malignant hypertension associated with underlying renal parenchymal disease occurs with high levels of activity of the renin-angiotensin system. It is probably overly simplistic to divide renal parenchymal hyper-

tension into volume-mediated and renin-dependent hypertension[71]; in most patients there is a spectrum of importance of these two factors. As GFR falls, increased salt intake produces a larger increase in the degree of salt retention and in blood pressure.[72]

The sympathetic nervous system is activated in renal failure.[62, 73] Ishii and associates[73] showed that plasma norepinephrine levels are increased in hypertensive patients with early renal failure compared with normal control subjects or normotensive patients with the same degree of renal insufficiency. There is also an increased sensitivity of the pressor response to norepinephrine in patients with early renal failure.[70] An activated sympathetic nervous system could increase cardiac output, enhance renal NaCl retention, interfere with pressure natriuresis, and enhance systemic and renal vasoconstriction (see Fig. 48–1). To date, these measurements of sympathetic activation have been made only in dialysis patients[62]; we do not know at what stage of progression of chronic renal failure they develop. However, afferent renal sympathetic responses have been noted in experimental hypertension of renovascular causes,[74] and it seems plausible that the damaged kidney can initiate these reflexes in the earlier stages of chronic renal failure.

In essential hypertension, there is evidence for release from the brain of a ouabain-like inhibitor of $Na^+,K^+$-ATPase,[63] which tends to restore normal salt balance in the presence of a high salt intake in genetically predisposed subjects at the expense of inhibition of the $Na^+,K^+$-ATPase in vascular smooth muscle with a resultant increase in cytosolic $Ca^{2+}$.[75] A similar phenomenon may occur in chronic renal failure.[76] An increase in such a ouabain-like factor would facilitate increased NaCl excretion per nephron as the number of nephrons diminishes in progressive renal disease. Inhibition of $Na^+,K^+$-ATPase in vascular smooth muscle could increase cytosolic $Ca^{2+}$ by diminishing $Na^+/Ca^{2+}$ exchange or by depolarization of voltage-dependent $Ca^{2+}$ channels. Peripheral vascular sensitivity to circulating vasoconstrictors would also be enhanced in chronic renal failure by increasing parathyroid hormone levels and by structural changes and hypertrophy in arteriolar walls.[65] The latter may also be enhanced by the insulin resistance of chronic renal failure.[66]

The hypothesis that in both essential hypertension and chronic renal failure there is defective regulation of systemic and renal vascular tone because of diminished production of endothelium-relaxing factor (nitric oxide) and increased production of endothelium-constricting factor (endothelin) is attractive. Blockade of endogenous nitric oxide formation leads in animals[77, 78] to both acute and sustained hypertension. Increased synthesis of nitric oxide from L-arginine via an inducible enzyme, nitric oxide synthase, is necessary for a normal natriuretic response to a high NaCl intake.[79] In Dahl salt-sensitive hypertensive rats, inhibition of nitric oxide production leads rapidly to severe hypertension and renal failure, which can be prevented by oral or intravenous administration of L- but not D-arginine.[80, 81] In normal humans, short-term blockade of nitric oxide production produces hypertension,[82] and there is evidence of defective nitrovasodilatation in essential hypertension.[83] Impairment of the renal nitric oxide system also interferes with pressure natriuresis.[84] Thus, impairment of nitric oxide formation in the peripheral and renal vasculature or elevation of plasma endothelin levels would impair NaCl excretion and enhance renal and systemic vasoconstriction.

Muirhead[85] described a vasodepressor medullary lipid that may have an important role in the regulation of blood pressure. Whether reduced production of this substance is important in the pathogenesis of renal parenchymal hypertension is unknown. Because it is possible to maintain normal blood pressure by control of ECF volume in patients who are anephric, it seems unlikely that this medullary lipid is of fundamental importance in renal parenchymal hypertension.

There is an important difference between essential hypertension and renal parenchymal hypertension in terms of the behavior of blood pressure at night.[86] In contrast to patients with essential hypertension, in whom blood pressure falls at night as in normal subjects, patients with chronic renal failure have a nocturnal rise in blood pressure. This phenomenon could explain, at least in part, increased cardiovascular morbidity and left ventricular hypertrophy associated with the same levels of blood pressure in patients with chronic renal failure compared with those with essential hypertension.

## ROLE OF HYPERTENSION IN PROGRESSION

Important findings on the role of hypertension in progression of parenchymal disease and benefits of reduction in blood pressure by therapy were obtained by the Modification of Diet and Renal Disease study.[3] In this study, approximately 600 patients with GFR values of 25 to 55 mL/min were randomly assigned to the usual protein diet or a low-protein diet and to a usual mean arterial pressure (MAP) (107 mm Hg) or a low MAP (92 mm Hg) treatment group (group A). An additional 250 patients with GFR values of

13 to 24 mL/min (group B) were randomly assigned to a low-protein diet or a very low protein diet and the same two blood pressure treatment groups. The mean follow-up period was 2.2 years. Drug regimens were based on the stepped-care approach, but ACE inhibitors and Ca$^{2+}$ channel blockers were encouraged as first choice. Insulin-requiring diabetic patients were excluded, and only 3% of the patients had non–insulin-dependent diabetes. The most common renal diagnoses were glomerular diseases and PKD. Patients with an MAP greater than 125 mm Hg were excluded. MAP was calculated as the diastolic blood pressure plus one third of the pulse pressure.

Overall, a higher mean follow-up MAP was significantly related to a faster decline of GFR during the period of the study in both groups. Nearly all patients required antihypertensive therapy to achieve blood pressure goals. In group A, the fall in GFR in the low-MAP treatment group was greater in the first 4 months of the study[87]; this decrease was hypothesized to be induced hemodynamically by the fall in blood pressure. Thereafter, the fall of GFR was significantly less rapid than in the higher MAP group. The effect of levels of both MAP and systolic blood pressure correlated better with progression than did diastolic blood pressure.

An effect of the degree of proteinuria on the frequency of hypertension and the beneficial effect of treatment was noted. Increased baseline proteinuria was associated with an increased level of hypertension before treatment. The degree of reduction in mean proteinuria in the first 4 months after treatment predicted the long-term efficacy of the low-MAP treatment. For example, a decline in this period of proteinuria by 1 g/d was associated with a decline in the rate of progression of GFR by 0.9 mL/min/y in the first study and by 1.3 mL/min/y in the second study. In patients with proteinuria value greater than 3 g/24 h, there was a clear-cut beneficial effect of reducing MAP to 92 mm Hg or less. Proteinuria value greater than 1 g/24 h has been noted to be a marker of progression.[88]

Although the number of black patients in the study was small (52 in group A), these patients have increased proteinuria at entry and the rate of fall of GFR was greater than in white patients if MAP was greater than 98 mm Hg. This suggests a greater sensitivity of renal function in black persons to superimposed hypertension in parenchymal disease. In keeping with this, there was an overall greater effect of the lower MAP control in black than in white patients. Thus, both the risk of hypertension-induced acceleration of decline in GFR and the benefits of controlling MAP to a low normal blood pressure range are greater in black than in white persons. It is already well established that black persons are much more likely to develop progressive renal disease caused by primary hypertensive nephrosclerosis than are white persons, especially in the age group 30 to 50 years.[89] The U.S. Renal Data System for end-stage renal disease[89] also shows a three- to fourfold increase in end-stage renal disease of virtually all causes except for PKD in black compared with white persons. The Modification of Diet and Renal Disease study data suggest that one of the mechanisms by which primary renal disease more often progresses to end stage in black compared with white persons may be increased susceptibility of the kidney to hypertensive damage when hypertension is secondary to renal parenchymal disease or to hypertensive nephrosclerosis.

Because virtually all common antihypertensive agents were used in this study, which was not planned to compare the relative effects of these agents, the Modification of Diet and Renal Disease study provides no evidence for the beneficial effect of any specific class of antihypertensive drugs. ACE inhibitors are most efficient in reducing proteinuria in nondiabetic renal disease,[90–93] and because the degree of reduction of proteinuria correlates with the beneficial effect and rate of reduction in GFR, it is plausible, although not established, that ACE inhibitors may be especially beneficial in patients with proteinuria value greater than 3 g/24 h. For the most beneficial antihypertensive effect, modest reduction of dietary NaCl is also needed.[93] The overall value of reduction in blood pressure in patients with chronic renal failure, probably to a blood pressure less than 140/90 mm Hg has also been emphasized by the National High Blood Pressure Program.[94] Other retrospective and prospective studies of patients with hypertension and parenchymal renal disease have also supported these findings.[88, 91–93, 95, 96]

The greater beneficial effect of lowering blood pressure in patients with significant proteinuria may be related to a more important effect of hypertension on progression in primarily glomerular compared with primarily interstitial renal diseases, perhaps because of a synergistic injurious effect of increased glomerular capillary pressure and immune damage to the glomerulus in glomerulonephritis.[97, 98] As nephron dropout progresses in renal parenchymal disease, nephron adaptation in the remaining less severely damaged nephrons may produce hemodynamically mediated additional glomerular damage (focal glomerulosclerosis) associated with preglomerular arteriolar dilatation.[99] If systemic arterial blood pressures were thereby transmitted to the glomerular capillary bed, hypertension could accelerate this process.[100–102] ACE inhibitors might therefore, at least in part, also exert their beneficial effect on both proteinuria and loss of nephron function because of their predominant effect on the efferent arteriole and the resulting reduction in glomerular capillary hydraulic pressure. An outline of these proposed mechanisms is shown in Figure 48–2.

## INDIVIDUAL RENAL DISEASES

### Autosomal Dominant Polycystic Kidney Disease

The prevalence and pathogenesis of hypertension and its role in the progression of PKD have been well studied.[56, 103–106] Hypertension occurs in at least 50% of such patients before elevation of serum creatinine.[105] Indeed, postpubertal children with PKD had higher blood pressure than their nonaffected siblings or appropriate age-matched control subjects.[102, 103] Young adults have an early absence of fall in blood pressure at night and an increase in left ventricular mass as measured by ultrasonography.[104] Thus, before established hypertension, blood pressure levels are increased within the normal range, blood pressure fall at night is diminished, and left ventricular mass is elevated but still within the upper limits of normal.

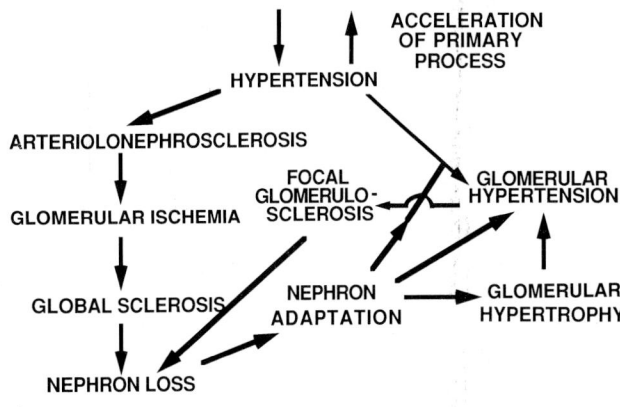

**Figure 48–2.** Mechanisms by which hypertension accelerates rate of progression of primary renal disease.

In a comparison with essential hypertensive patients, matched for level of blood pressure and for normal GFR values, those with PKD had an activated renin-angiotensin-aldosterone system; in the same subjects treatment for 6 weeks with an ACE inhibitor increased plasma flow and reduced renal vascular resistance only in the PKD patients.[56] These investigators also demonstrated that hypertensive PKD patients had greater renal volumes (larger cysts) than did normotensive PKD patients.[106] The authors argued reasonably that renin production in the areas of cyst enlargement is increased because of renal ischemia at these sites.[56, 103, 106, 107] There is, however, evidence for renin production, not only in arterioles adjacent to cysts but also by cyst wall epithelial cells.[103, 108] Abnormal $Na^+$ handling, with diminished pressure natriuresis, has also been demonstrated in PKD patients.[109, 110]

Hypertension is an especially important factor in the progression of PKD to the end stage.[103, 104] Careful study of the histology of early versus late renal failure in PKD patients demonstrated that the major mechanism of progression was afferent arteriolosclerosis and global glomerulosclerosis, a lesion consistent with glomerular ischemia; there was little evidence of focal glomerulosclerosis, the marker of the adapted nephron syndrome. Tubulointerstitial and vascular changes were more prominent overall than glomerular disease as a factor in progression.

### Diabetic Glomerulopathy

There is now firm evidence that ACE inhibitors slow the progression of renal disease in diabetic patients with established glomerulopathy (urinary protein excretion > 500 mg/d).[111] This effect is independent of control of blood pressure as demonstrated by its absence in control subjects in whom blood pressure was treated to the same level by other antihypertensive medications. These observations were made in patients with insulin-dependent diabetes and cannot necessarily be extended to patients with non–insulin-dependent diabetes, although it seems reasonable to treat hypertension in subjects with non–insulin-dependent diabetes with an ACE inhibitor in the absence of contraindications. In the study by Lewis and colleagues,[111] the fall of creatinine clearance was slowed by approximately 40%. The authors proposed that the beneficial effect may be related to the reduction of glomerular capillary pressures. In this study, for which patients with a serum creatinine value of 2.5 mg/dL or less were selected, hyperkalemia developed in only 3 of 200 subjects.

Beneficial effects of ACE inhibitors in normotensive patients with insulin-dependent diabetes and microalbuminuria have also been observed in the absence of blood pressure reduction.[112, 113] In a randomized double-blind placebo-controlled trial in which normotensive subjects with non–insulin-dependent diabetes and microalbuminuria were observed for 5 years, ACE inhibitors stabilized the level of microalbuminuria, compared with an increase in the control subjects, and preserved renal function as measured by the reciprocal of serum creatinine, a less accurate measure of GFR.[114] The evidence is thus suggestive, but not yet fully convincing, that normotensive subjects with non–insulin-dependent diabetes and microalbuminuria should be treated with ACE inhibitors. The important role of vigorous treatment of hypertension in all diabetic patients has been emphasized by the National High Blood Pressure Education Program.[115]

Especially with an initially elevated serum creatinine level, serum creatinine (and serum $K^+$) should be monitored weekly for a period after institution of ACE inhibitor therapy to detect deterioration of renal function related to bilateral renal artery stenosis or severe diabetic afferent arteriolar disease.

## TREATMENT

We have emphasized the important role of reduction in blood pressure to less than 140/90 mm Hg, and in selected patients close to or in the normal range, in all patients with parenchymal renal disease. This concept is now widely supported.[94, 116] We believe that this is the best-documented and most important therapeutic measure, short of curative interventions aimed at the primary renal disease, for slowing progression of chronic renal failure. Hypertension secondary to underlying parenchymal disease, compared with essential hypertension, is more likely to progress to an accelerated state and more likely to be associated with cardiovascular morbidity and mortality. Virtually all antihypertensive medications can be used except for the $K^+$-sparing diuretics.

Loop diuretics are necessary in almost all patients with a serum creatinine concentration of 2.0 mg/dL or more, because of the important role of NaCl retention in the pathogenesis of hypertension. Even more than in patients with essential hypertension, however, the physician should be on guard for volume depletion, hyperuricemia, and gout.

We have discussed the strong indications for the use of ACE inhibitors in diabetic glomerulosclerosis, PKD, and scleroderma and in nondiabetic patients with proteinuria value greater than 3 g/24 h. ACE inhibitors are also valuable for reducing nephrotic level proteinuria independent of blood pressure reduction.[44, 92] They may also have benefits in improving lipid abnormalities that are common in

chronic renal failure and may also be related to the reduction in proteinuria.[117] These effects of ACE inhibitors (independent of the blood pressure–lowering effect) on proteinuria and, at least in experimental animals, on the vascular lesions of chronic renal failure[118] are probably related to inhibition of the intrarenal renin-angiotensin system.[119] The effects of a low-protein diet and of ACE inhibitors on nephrotic level proteinuria in nondiabetic renal disease are additive.[120] It is not established, however, that ACE inhibitors are the drugs of choice for all patients with hypertension related to underlying parenchymal renal disease, especially in those patients with minimal proteinuria.

$Ca^{2+}$ channel blockers may also provide renal protective effects independent of their antihypertensive action, but the evidence overall is less strong than that for ACE inhibitors.[121–124]

Because of the role of activation of the sympathetic nervous system in chronic renal disease, central or peripherally acting adrenergic antagonists are also useful. Hypertension complicating parenchymal renal disease can be extremely difficult to control, and minoxidil is sometimes necessary, usually as a fourth drug. When it is used, it is usually essential to increase considerably the dose of loop diuretic being employed and to add a β-blocker to inhibit reflex tachycardia.

In the absence of specific indications or contraindications, we prefer a loop diuretic and then addition of an ACE inhibitor followed by a $Ca^{2+}$ channel blocker for the management of hypertension associated with parenchymal renal disease.

# END-STAGE RENAL DISEASE
## Post-transplantation Hypertension
### COURSE

Many, if not most, patients with end-stage renal disease who undergo organ transplantation are already receiving antihypertensive therapy. In carefully managed patients with a live related donor, transplantation is possible without preparative dialysis treatment. In most cases, however, and especially for cadaveric transplantation, prior dialysis for a period of some weeks or months is required. In either case, previous antihypertensive therapy is generally continued if blood pressure has been satisfactorily controlled. Adequate control of blood pressure is essential before transplantation because the blood pressure response to the procedure is unpredictable. If nearly normal excretory function is quickly established, blood pressure in most cases is substantially easier to control, although loop diuretics may continue to be required, especially if large doses of steroids are being given.

The severity of hypertension before transplantation does not predict post-transplantation blood pressure because of the initially variable excretory function after the insertion of the allograft and the now virtually routine long-term administration of the hypertensinogenic immunosuppressive agent cyclosporine.

Post-transplantation hypertension is frequently multifac-

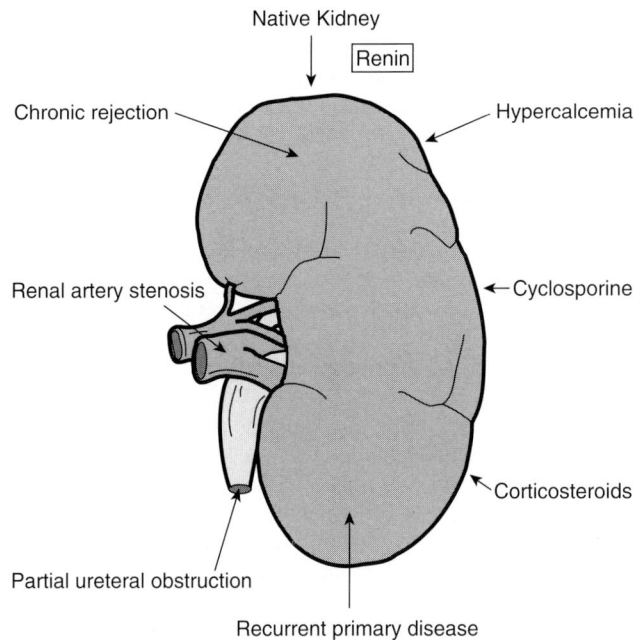

**Figure 48–3.** Intrarenal causes are indicated by arrow ending inside kidney, in contrast to extrinsic causes.

torial[125–129] in origin (Fig. 48–3). It generally tends to become less severe if the allograft is well tolerated, steroid and cyclosporine dosages are gradually reduced, and careful attention is given to controlling trough cyclosporine blood levels. Even so, by 1 year after transplantation, the prevalence of hypertension remains around 50% to 60%.[125–129] Because of the dynamic nature of the pathophysiologic mechanisms causing post-transplantation hypertension, unlike essential hypertension, the physician should attempt to reduce blood pressure medications after immunosuppressive treatment has been lowered to maintenance levels. One possible exception to this approach is to continue to use dihydropyridine $Ca^{2+}$ channel blockers for their beneficial effects on cyclosporine-induced renal vasoconstriction, independent of their effects on blood pressure. Suggestive but not yet conclusive data showing the benefits of this prophylactic approach for improving allograft function have been obtained.[130–134]

## MECHANISMS

Before the introduction of cyclosporine in the United States in 1983, post-transplantation hypertension was mainly renin dependent.[128, 135, 136] Blood pressure did not respond to a low-salt diet.[137] The common feature in all such hypertension is allograft vasoconstriction[137]; relevant mechanisms are given in Table 48–2. In a study of 33 hypertensive transplant recipients chosen in an effort to exclude chronic rejection and before the use of cyclosporine,[137] we attributed hypertension in 64% to native kidneys, in 18% to renal artery stenosis, and in 15% to occult chronic rejection, which was established by the subsequent clinical course and/or by renal biopsy. All these causes persist, but the pathogenesis is now complicated by the pervasive effects of cyclosporine.

Compared with a group of azathioprine-treated recipients, matched cyclosporine-treated transplant recipients had a hypotensive response to, and conserved NaCl more efficiently after, a low-NaCl diet, excreted an NaCl load less efficiently, and had a blood pressure unresponsive to captopril.[138] Renal hemodynamic response to the same 10% plasma volume contraction also differed: GFR fell in cyclosporine-treated patients but not in the other allograft recipients.[139] In additional studies of hypertensive cyclosporine-treated patients, nifedipine and captopril in crossover experiments produced a similar fall in blood pressure but a contrasting renal hemodynamic response[130]: GFR and renal plasma flow increased and renal vascular resistance decreased after nifedipine but not after captopril. Nifedipine acts predominantly to dilate the afferent arterioles and captopril to dilate the efferent[45, 140, 141] arterioles. These responses to plasma volume contraction and to a reduction in blood pressure are consistent with a predominant preglomerular arteriolar action of cyclosporine with resulting impaired ability to autoregulate GFR[142] by both afferent arteriolar dilatation and, in the presence of captopril, efferent vasoconstriction.

There is additional evidence for a predominant renal effect of cyclosporine on the afferent arteriolar vessels in experimental animals[143–145] and in histologic studies in humans.[146–149] The morphometric studies of Remuzzi's group[146] revealed that the predominant pattern of initial glomerular damage was glomerular ischemia with global sclerosis, akin to hypertensive arterionephrosclerosis.

Cyclosporine causes systemic as well as, albeit more marked, renal vasoconstriction.[150] It has become increasingly difficult to separate the adverse renal hemodynamic and hypertensinogenic effects of the drug from the beneficial and relatively specific immunosuppressive effects, which partially block the T cell cascade. Cyclosporine interferes with several $Ca^{2+}$-dependent mechanisms after binding to cyclophilins in the cytosol, nucleus, and endoplasmic reticulum.[151] The major immunologic effect is to interfere with calcineurin, a phosphatase enzyme important in the proliferative signals for increased interleukin-2 production.[151] The precise mechanism by which cyclosporine activates vascular smooth muscle remains to be established, but the net effect probably involves increased cytosolic $Ca^{2+}$,[152] increased sensitivity to most vasoconstrictors,[153] and altered endothelial and arteriolar smooth muscle functions to favor the vasoconstrictive response over the vasodilatory pathway.[144, 154–159] Responses to, or levels of, endothelin are enhanced[160–162] and nitric oxide levels or

**TABLE 48–2. Mechanisms of Increased Allograft Vascular Resistance as a Cause of Post-transplantation Hypertension**

| Condition | Mechanism |
|---|---|
| Chronic rejection | Intrarenal narrowing of small blood vessels |
| Renal artery stenosis | Obstruction of major vessel |
| Cyclosporine | Predominantly preglomerular vasoconstriction |
| Native kidneys | Angiotensin-induced vasoconstriction of allograft |

responses reduced.[163, 164] FK 506, an entirely different molecular structure (macrolide compared with cyclic peptide structure of cyclosporine) has similar immunosuppressive effects, binds to another cyclophilin that inhibits calcineurin, and also causes "salt-dependent" hypertension with renal vasoconstriction.[165]

Cyclosporine, short term[166] in animals and long term in humans,[167] stimulates the sympathetic nervous system. This sympathetic stimulation is not essential for the production of post-transplantation hypertension because cyclosporine-induced hypertension occurs within 2 weeks of transplantation from a live related donor at a time when allograft reinnervation has not occurred.[150] Nevertheless, the allograft denervation may explain the higher percentage of hypertension after cardiac (90%) compared with renal (50% to 60%) transplantation.

There is substantial evidence for enhanced proximal reabsorption of the glomerular filtrate in cyclosporine-treated patients compared with normal subjects. Diminished free water clearance factored by GFR, diminished excretion fraction of $Na^+$, diminished urea clearance at the same high urine flow rates, and an increased incidence of hyperuricemia and gout all support this view.[159, 166, 168, 169] This probably occurs via a hemodynamic effect to reduce proximal peritubular capillary pressure and, if sympathetic reinnervation occurs in the allograft, by direct stimulation of $Na^+$ transport via sympathetic receptors on proximal tubule epithelial cells.

Three types of hypertension are associated with the use of cyclosporine,[170] which is now used not only for solid organ and bone marrow transplantation but also for a wide variety of presumed immunologic diseases.[171] The first and most common type is related to renal vasoconstriction but not to impaired GFR[150, 168] and is $Na^+$ dependent.[138] The second type is due to chronic renal failure secondary to cyclosporine vasculopathy. For example, Myers and Newton[149] described a 10% renal failure rate after 10 years of cyclosporine treatment for cardiac transplantation. Vasoconstriction is initially reversible,[150] as is the vasculopathy.[148] Eventually, however, ischemic glomerulopathy, interstitial fibrosis, and chronic renal failure result. The third type is rare but usually requires withdrawal of cyclosporine: hemolytic-uremic syndrome related to severe endothelial damage induced by cyclosporine. This appears to be an idiosyncratic reaction except for the patients who developed end-stage renal disease because of a primary hemolytic-uremic syndrome.[172]

Before the introduction of cyclosporine, chronic rejection was the most common cause of hypertension after renal transplantation. This is probably still true, but the differential diagnosis between cyclosporine vasculopathy and chronic rejection is difficult[173] because both are associated with arteriopathy in small intrarenal vessels. Although cyclosporine has substantially reduced the occurrence of acute rejection, which is a major risk factor for chronic rejection,[174] it produces renal small vessel disease. Some have argued that cyclosporine-induced arteriopathy and nephropathy do not progress even when serum creatinine levels are in the range 3 to 3.5 mg/dL. This would be atypical for chronic renal failure because of the expected development of the adapted nephron syndrome[99] with hypertrophy and

hyperperfusion of the remaining undamaged nephrons. Indeed, there is morphologic evidence for this with cyclosporine.[146] Serum creatinine concentration may, initially at least, remain constant despite the loss of nephrons because of hypertrophy of the remaining nephrons.

## DIAGNOSIS AND THERAPY

There is a real conflict between the goal of reducing cyclosporine dosage to the minimal possible level to decrease nephropathy and hypertension and the potential danger of diminishing the persistent and important immunosuppressive effect of the drug even at doses as low as 2 to 3 mg/kg body weight.[174–176] A better case can be made for cautiously discontinuing cyclosporine 6 to 12 months after well-tolerated transplantation from a live related donor. In both cadaveric and live related donor transplantations, episodes of acute cyclosporine nephrotoxicity should be minimized by carefully monitoring the trough blood level and avoiding drug-induced reduction in the hepatic metabolism via the P-450 enzyme system.[174]

Among the extrinsic causes (see Fig. 48–3), steroid therapy is only a minor contributor to hypertension[177] but may act synergistically with cyclosporine[168, 178] on blood pressure. In general, cyclosporine is gradually reduced to a 2 to 5 mg/kg daily dose but often still causes hypertension, usually mild, at that level. If renal function is then stable and serum creatinine is less than about 2.5 mg/dL, hypertension requiring multiple antihypertensive drugs should suggest consideration of native kidney or renovascular hypertension.

Native kidney hypertension is probably an underdiagnosed entity[107, 179] and has become more difficult to diagnose now than before the use of cyclosporine. Then, an increase in allograft blood flow after administration of the ACE inhibitor associated with a fall in systemic blood pressure was an indication of possible dependence of hypertension on the native kidneys.[179] It certainly showed the capacity of allograft renal blood flow to increase, in contrast to fixed intrarenal small vessel disease. Cyclosporine, however, causes a non–renin-dependent[150, 180] allograft vasoconstriction and inhibits the vasodilatory response to ACE inhibitors, so that the diagnostic vasodilatory response is not observed. Discontinuing cyclosporine to establish a new baseline allograft effective renal plasma flow is a possible approach. Even in a stable situation, however, this must be done with caution.[175] Bilateral nephrectomy of native kidneys can be done by a retroperitoneal approach and its consequences if return to dialysis is later required are much less severe now that erythropoietin is available.

For the diagnosis of allograft renal artery stenosis, the renal functional response to an ACE inhibitor plus a diuretic was also more useful before cyclosporine.[43, 181] Distal to a functionally significant stenosis, GFR is often dependent on angiotension II–induced efferent arteriolar vasoconstriction. A prerenal form of acute renal failure then results from the use of these drugs.[142] Unfortunately, the specificity of this response is now much less because cyclosporine may impair afferent arteriolar vasodilatation when blood pressure is reduced even in the absence of allograft renal artery stenosis. Such responses have been observed.[182, 183]

Nevertheless, any such fall in renal function after introduction of an ACE inhibitor should be looked for and should lead to careful consideration of a diagnosis of allograft artery stenosis.

This stenosis can be atherogenic in origin in the native vessel proximal to the allograft, at the anastomosis, or due to rejection or atherosclerotic injury in the allograft major arteries. Cyclosporine itself can also cause stenosis of major renal vessels by its endothelial and smooth muscle effects.[184]

Transluminal angioplasty is usually the preferred initial therapeutic approach.[185] Reconstructive vascular surgery is much more difficult than surgery for native renovascular hypertension because of fibrosis resulting from the transplantation procedure. Renal vein renins have not proved useful in this clinical situation,[107] and collateral vessels usually do not develop. Renovascular renal failure (ischemic nephropathy) can develop in allograft as well as native kidneys and should be considered when neither the clinical circumstances nor the presence of proteinuria nor typical changes in the renal biopsy support chronic rejection, cyclosporine nephropathy, or recurrent primary renal disease. Renal arteriograms, angioplasty, and renovascular surgery all put the allograft at risk, and considerable clinical judgment is necessary before embarking on such diagnostic and therapeutic procedures. Especially when blood pressure is difficult to control with multiple drugs, it is well worth looking for renovascular hypertension.

Hypercalcemia caused by recurrent or persistent tertiary hyperparathyroidism may contribute to hypertension but rarely requires subtotal parathyroidectomy. Post-transplantation erythrocytosis may also contribute and often responds to an ACE inhibitor[186] to inhibit erythropoietin production, which is usually from the native kidneys. Recurrent focal glomerulosclerosis may occur in the early postoperative period because of a circulating endogenous factor in the transplant recipient.[187] Recurrent disease is more likely in malignant focal glomerulosclerosis[58] that progresses to end-stage renal disease in a relatively short time.

### DRUG TREATMENT

Virtually all of the various classes of antihypertensive drugs may be needed from time to time. This is not surprising in view of the multiple mechanisms of hypertension after renal transplantation. When cyclosporine is probably the major cause, use of modest NaCl restriction and the dihydropyridines is now the favored approach, although β-adrenergic blockers[168] and labetalol[188] have also been used successfully. Loop diuretics are useful but must be used with caution to avoid volume depletion because, as noted, cyclosporine interferes with the renal autoregulatory response that maintains GFR in such circumstances. If $Ca^{2+}$ channel blockers with or without diuretics are insufficient, β-adrenergic blockers may be useful for the renin-inhibiting effect. ACE inhibitors are more efficient for inhibiting renin-induced hypertension, but their use can precipitate acute renal failure because of either a cyclosporine–ACE inhibitor hemodynamic interaction or a functionally significant renal artery stenosis.

Both cyclosporine[167] and chronic renal failure[62] stimulate the sympathetic nervous system; hence, β-blockers, α- and β-blockers, and peripheral $\alpha_1$-antagonists or central $\alpha_2$-agonists may all be useful. Cyclosporine can occasionally contribute to hyperkalemia,[189] and the serum $K^+$ concentration should be checked carefully when cyclosporine and ACE inhibitors are used together. In post-transplantation situations with heavy proteinuria or nephrotic syndrome, ACE inhibitors reduce the proteinuria significantly.[190]

Treatment of hypertension is an important part of the long-term management of renal transplant patients both because cardiovascular events remain the major late cause of mortality and because treatment of hypertension is the most important factor in slowing the rate of deterioration of renal function in chronic rejection,[191] as it is in primary parenchymal disease.

## Hypertension in Dialysis Patients

### PREVALENCE

Hypertension is estimated to be present in 80% to 90% of patients with end-stage renal disease.[192–196] This percentage can be deduced from the proportions of various etiologies of renal disease in patients receiving dialysis[197]; 78% in chronic glomerulonephritis,[198] 100% in hypertensive nephrosclerosis, and about 80% in diabetic nephropathy[199] are representative.

Although recombinant human erythropoietin (rHuEPO) has benefited dialysis patients considerably,[200–202] associated hypertension has also increased. Within the first year of treatment when the hematocrit exceeds 30%, multicenter trials[203–206] have consistently shown an increased prevalence of about 33%. After more than 3 years of rHuEPO therapy, 50% of patients who had been maintained normotensive required antihypertensive medications.[202]

### CHARACTERISTICS

Two general patterns of blood pressure response have been recognized in hemodialysis patients. About 85% of well-dialyzed patients achieve sustained normal blood pressure when free of edema and become hypotensive with further volume removal (volume responsive); this pattern is more common in black patients.[207] The remainder have sustained hypertension in the apparently euvolemic state or become more hypertensive with volume removal (volume unresponsive or renin dependent). This group may develop sudden hypotension during dialysis; in these instances, modest volume repletion promptly restores blood pressure often to hypertensive levels. These two patterns are likely to represent the ends of a spectrum in which the individual presentation is dependent on multiple variables.

During rHuEPO therapy, seizures with a clinical picture resembling hypertensive encephalopathy have developed infrequently, usually after a rapid increase in hematocrit[208] but unrelated to the absolute hemoglobin concentration or its rate of increase or to the level of blood pressure. The rapid increase of blood pressure has been postulated to be an initiating factor possibly because of a failure of cerebral autoregulation.[209]

Blood pressure typically falls at night in normotensive subjects and in those with essential hypertension with or without treatment. This diurnal variation is absent in dialysis patients, as it is in patients with chronic renal failure.[210]

## HEMODYNAMICS

In uremic patients with no clinically apparent heart disease, cardiac output is generally higher than normal because of increased heart rates accompanying normal stroke volumes[211, 212] but does not differ between normotensive and hypertensive patients (Fig. 48–4). Increased resistance accounts for hypertension.

During hemodialysis in hypertensive patients in whom blood pressure and heart rate do not change, ultrafiltration produces a reduction in stroke volume and ejection fraction and no change in contractility, whereas dialysis—with or without ultrafiltration—is accompanied by an increase in contractility and ejection fraction[213] with an increase in serum $Ca^{2+}$ without a change in $HCO_3^-$ concentration, which may explain this improvement.[214] Similarly, during hemodialysis in normotensive patients, ventricular filling decreases without a change in systolic or diastolic blood pressure or heart rate, suggesting that increased contractility compensates to maintain blood pressure.[215]

With severe anemia, tissue hypoxia produces peripheral vasodilatation and blood viscosity is reduced; in turn, cardiac output is increased.[216] However, differences in hematocrit do not explain the differences in blood pressure in hemodialysis patients.[211, 217] Arteriovenous fistulas contrib-ute slightly to the increased cardiac output, but the blood flow rates are likely to be similar between normotensive and hypertensive dialysis patients and not a factor in accounting for hypertension.[218]

The observed hemodynamic responses to changes in fluid volume in hemodialysis patients are diverse.[219] In patients who were never known to be hypertensive, volume expansion produced no change in blood pressure; cardiac output rose and peripheral resistance fell reciprocally. Hypertensive patients showed three distinct patterns in response to volume expansion–induced increases in blood pressure: 1) no change in cardiac output with an increase in peripheral resistance, 2) an increase in cardiac output with no change in peripheral resistance, and 3) increased cardiac output followed by increased peripheral resistance. Thus, the pathogenesis of hypertension in dialysis patients is multifactorial and is not simply explained by the autoregulatory hypothesis,[64] as discussed later.

Bilateral nephrectomy produces no changes in peripheral resistance, cardiac output, or blood pressure in normotensive patients,[220] whereas patients with nonmalignant hypertension experience a decrease in total peripheral resistance with no change in cardiac output and a decrease—at times delayed—in blood pressure (Fig. 48–5). Patients with malignant hypertension have a more marked decrease in resistance with an increase in cardiac output with augmentation of stroke volume but also a decrease in blood pressure. Anephric hypertensive patients showed a progressive increase in diastolic blood pressure with increasing exchangeable body $Na^+$ and blood volume,[220, 221] whereas previously normotensive patients showed no such change in blood pressure (Fig. 48–6). The hemodynamic data suggest that,

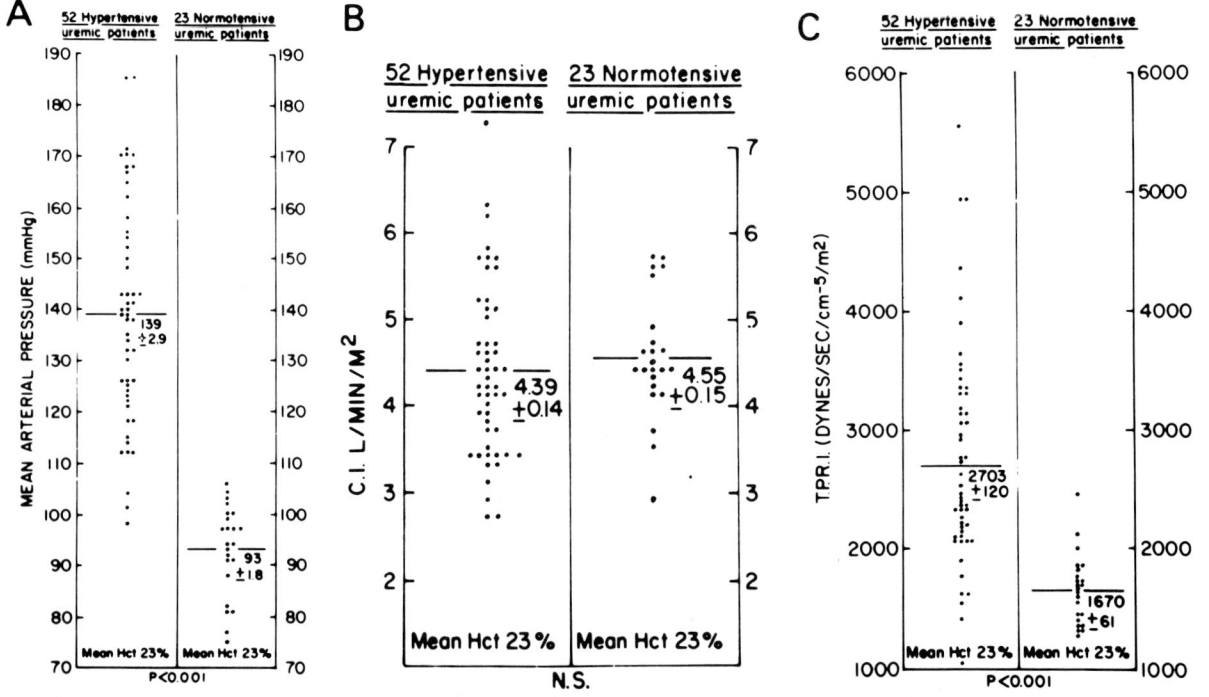

**Figure 48–4.** Hypertensive compared with normotensive hemodialysis patients *(A)* have similar cardiac indices *(B)* but increased peripheral vascular resistance *(C)*. *(A to C* from Kim KE, Onesti G, Schwartz AB, et al: Hemodynamics of hypertension in chronic end-stage renal disease. Circulation 46:456–464, 1972. Reproduced with permission. Circulation. Copyright 1972 American Heart Association.)

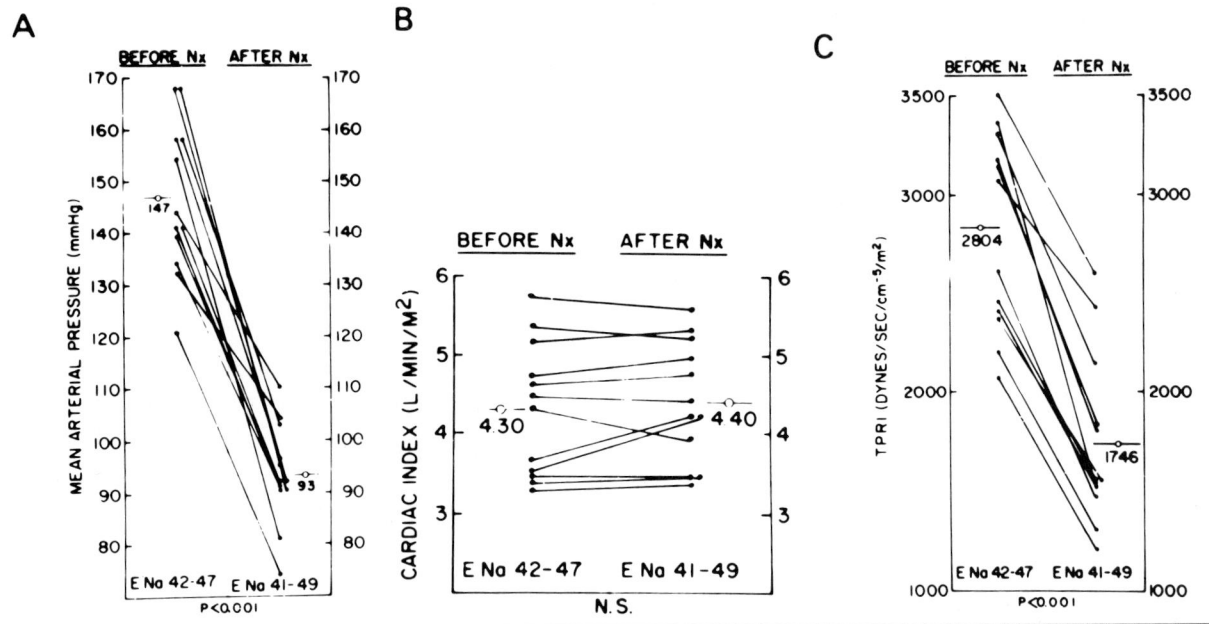

**Figure 48–5.** In hypertensive hemodialysis patients at dry weight and taking no antihypertensive medications, bilateral nephrectomy decreases peripheral vascular resistance *(C)* and lowers blood pressure *(A)* with no change in cardiac index *(B)*. Exchangeable Na⁺ was similar before and after nephrectomy. *(A to C from Kim KE, Onesti G, Schwartz AB, et al: Hemodynamics of hypertension in chronic end-stage renal disease. Circulation 46:456–464, 1972. Reproduced with permission. Circulation. Copyright 1972 American Heart Association.)*

in addition to volume, some pressor function of the kidney is important in maintaining hypertension.

## MECHANISMS

From the preceding hemodynamic observations, excess intravascular volume, the persistence of vasoconstriction, or the absence of a vasodilator all can be, to varying degrees,

implicated as mechanisms of hypertension in dialysis patients.

### Volume

Removal of excess volume by hemodialysis as well as peritoneal dialysis unquestionably decreases blood pressure in most patients,[71, 194, 222] but the mechanism by which this occurs is not established.

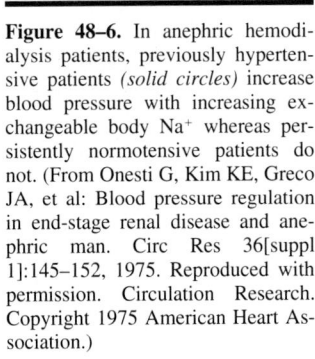

**Figure 48–6.** In anephric hemodialysis patients, previously hypertensive patients *(solid circles)* increase blood pressure with increasing exchangeable body Na⁺ whereas persistently normotensive patients do not. (From Onesti G, Kim KE, Greco JA, et al: Blood pressure regulation in end-stage renal disease and anephric man. Circ Res 36[suppl 1]:145–152, 1975. Reproduced with permission. Circulation Research. Copyright 1975 American Heart Association.)

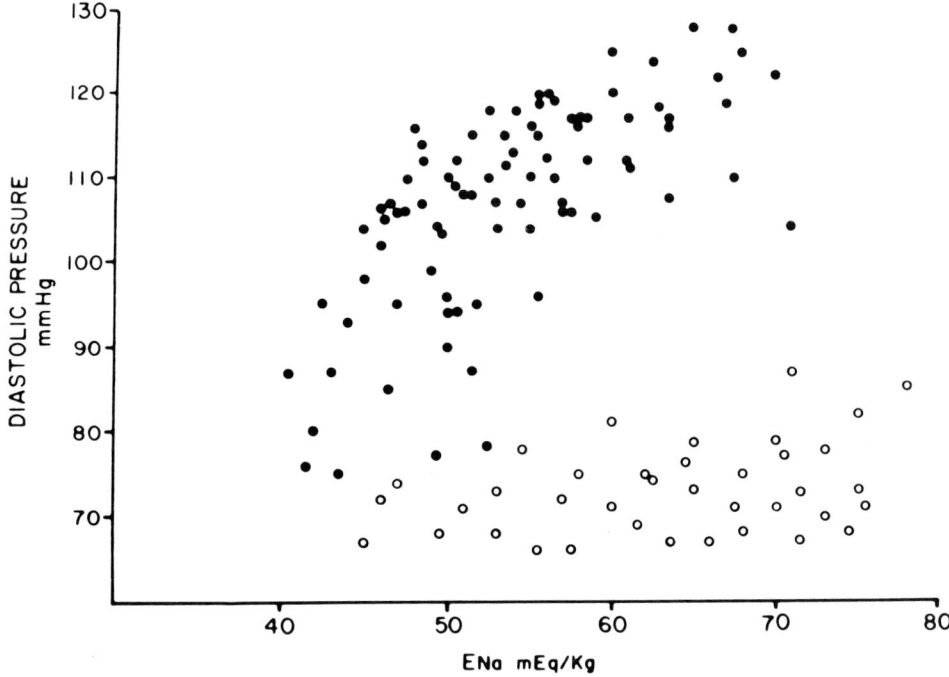

Studies of the correlations between blood pressure and body fluid volumes do not present a consistent picture. In maintenance hemodialysis, MAP, which was controlled by volume removal in 25 of 26 patients, did not correlate with fluid volumes or renin.[223] Cangiano and colleagues[218] observed greater blood and plasma volume but not ECF volume in hypertensive dialysis patients. Of 52 hemodialysis patients, none of whom were anephric, 37 were hypertensive despite volume removal.[224] Plasma volumes were elevated compared with those of normal subjects, whereas blood and ECF volumes were normal. Moreover, blood pressure did not correlate with any ECF space, consistent with earlier observations.[225, 226] After bilateral nephrectomy in hypertensive patients,[219, 220, 225] blood pressure correlated with blood volume and exchangeable Na+; patients normotensive before and after nephrectomy showed no such correlation.[220]

The study by Dathan and co-workers[223] suggests that excess NaCl in dialysis patients may distribute preferentially to the intravascular space rather than the interstitial space. Similarly, with rapid NaCl loading, blood volume increased more in patients with end-stage renal disease than in normal subjects despite similar increases in ECF volume.[227]

In the autoregulatory theory of the pathogenesis of hypertension,[64] fluid volume expansion leads initially to increased cardiac output. Metabolic needs are thus exceeded by organ hyperperfusion, thereby eliciting myogenic vasoconstriction and a consequent decrease in cardiac output but with increased blood pressure. Although Coleman and colleagues[221] described this sequence of events in three anephric hemodialysis patients, Kim and co-workers[219] observed it in only one of eight hypertensive patients. Five of those patients, two of whom were anephric, showed an increase in peripheral resistance with no change in cardiac output when exchangeable Na+ was increased. Thus, mechanisms other than that advanced by the autoregulatory hypothesis apply in many dialysis patients.

With the conflicting evidence regarding body fluid volume and its relationship to blood pressure, it seems likely that a complex interrelationship among volume, renin, and blood pressure exists, as proposed by several investigators.[223, 225, 228–230]

## Renin-Angiotensin System

Vertes and associates[71] found elevated circulating renin in dialysis patients with intractable hypertension and introduced the term "renin-dependent" hypertension. Since then, several lines of evidence have strongly implicated the renin-angiotensin system, but it appears to be the dominant factor in a minority of these instances.

In general, plasma renin levels are higher in patients who remain hypertensive despite optimal dialysis to achieve "dry weight,"[194, 224, 228, 230–235] and approximately 30% of patients have plasma renin activities above the upper limit of normal. Weidmann and co-workers[194] found normal plasma renin activity in 31 of 33 patients with volume-responsive hypertension in contrast to elevated renin activity in 17 of 18 patients with volume-unresponsive hypertension (Fig. 48–7); the latter group had predominantly glomerulonephri-

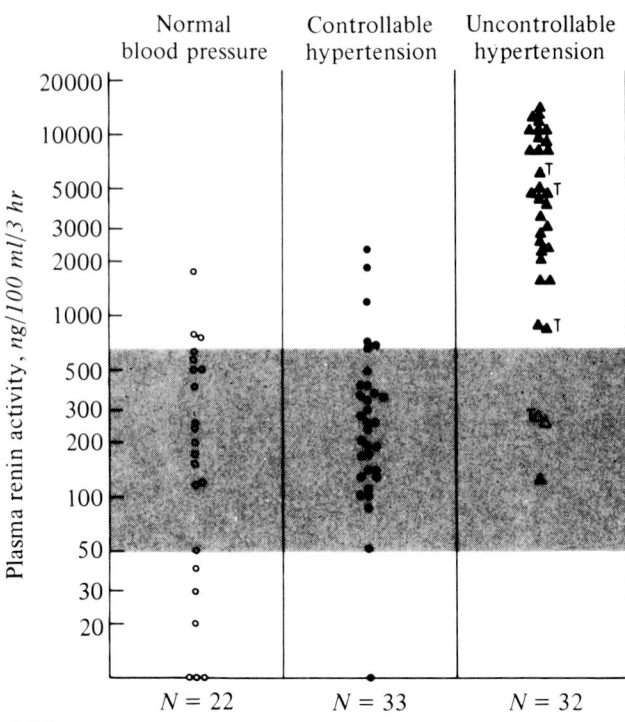

**Figure 48–7.** Basal plasma renin activity in hemodialysis patients with normal blood pressure and with volume-responsive and volume-unresponsive hypertension. T indicates patients taking antihypertensive medications. (From Weidmann P, Maxwell MH: The renin-angiotensin-aldosterone system in terminal renal failure. Used with permission from Kidney International, volume 8, suppl 5, pages S-219–S-234, 1975.)

tis or nephrosclerosis. Patients with nephrosclerosis usually had hyperreninemia with volume-responsive hypertension, whereas only 66% of patients with glomerular diseases had volume-responsive hypertension, and only half of them had elevated plasma renin activity.[236] Malignant nephrosclerosis has been associated with extremely high renin concentrations.[232] Plasma renin has also been detected in low concentrations in 29 of 33 anephric patients without relation to sex or to time elapsed since nephrectomy.[232]

Renin or angiotensin II has been shown to correlate with blood pressure in some studies[232] but not in others.[224, 230, 237] Plasma renin activity in the interdialytic period correlated with dietary and plasma Na+ but not with diastolic blood pressure in 89 hemodialysis patients, 10 of whom maintained a pressure greater than 100 mm Hg.[237] In 31 dialysis patients with normal ECF and blood volumes, some were hypertensive with a normal plasma renin activity and others were normotensive with an elevated plasma renin activity.[238] These contradictions may be due in part to differences in the responses of renin to volume in different groups of patients. In dialysis patients with volume-responsive hypertension, the rise in renin in response to volume depletion is small[71, 232, 234, 239, 240]; indeed, a fall in renin may be seen.[239, 240] In most patients with intractable or volume-unresponsive hypertension,[194, 232, 236, 240] plasma renin concentration usually rises as exchangeable Na+ is removed (Fig. 48–8). However, others have found that relative increases in plasma renin concentration with decreases in blood volume were similar in both volume-responsive and

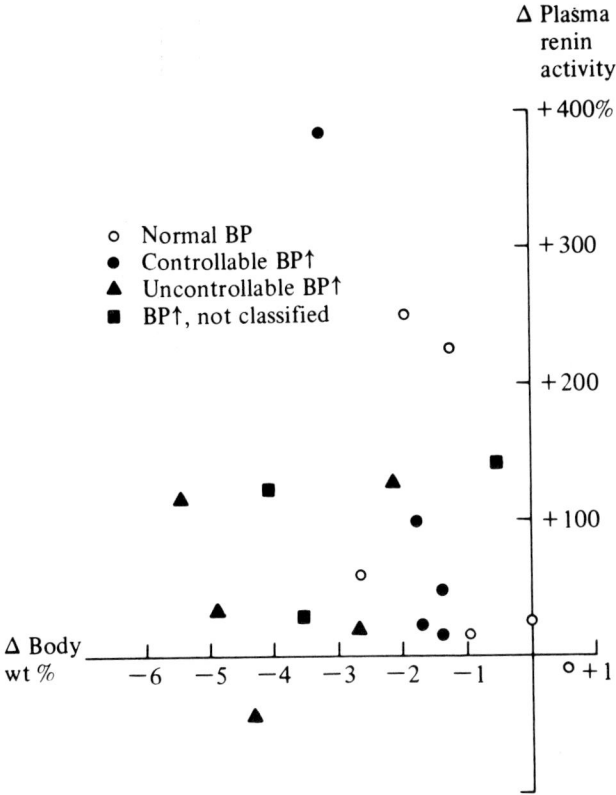

**Figure 48–8.** Reduction in fluid volume with hemodialysis did not correlate with a change in plasma renin activity regardless of the response of blood pressure (BP) to volume removal. (From Weidmann P, Maxwell MH: The renin-angiotensin-aldosterone system in terminal renal failure. Used with permission from Kidney International, volume 8, suppl 5, pages S-219–S-234, 1975.)

volume-unresponsive patients[229] or have found an inverse relationship between plasma renin concentration and exchangeable Na+ in patients with volume-responsive hypertension but not in patients with "resistant" hypertension.[230] Schultze and colleagues[224] found high plasma renin activity in only 7 of 34 patients and no correlation with blood pressure or body fluid volumes. Thus, on the basis of only plasma renin levels under various conditions, evidence for a primary pathogenetic role of renin in most hypertensive dialysis patients is not conclusive.

Infusion of saralasin, an angiotensin II antagonist, decreased blood pressure in only 9 of 27 hypertensive patients[241] while plasma renin activity increased sharply; in the remaining patients, blood pressure was unaffected and plasma renin activity was stable. Others have found a consistent decrease in blood pressure with saralasin in patients with volume-unresponsive hypertension.[242] The interpretation is confounded by the agonist (hypertensive) effect of saralasin, which may result in underestimation of the hypertensive effect of angiotensin II, particularly if it occurs principally with low or normal plasma renin activity. Herrera Acosta[54] studied hemodialysis patients after 20% volume depletion with no resultant change in MAP and a slight increase in plasma renin; when captopril was added, MAP decreased with a marked rise in renin. A similar response to captopril has been noted by others.[243, 244] Because ACE

also degrades bradykinin and an increase in bradykinin could conceivably explain the decrease in blood pressure, the interpretation should be cautious. Although the arterial wall possesses all of the requisite factors for local production of angiotensin II,[245] the potential role of this tissue renin-angiotensin system has not been studied in dialysis patients.

After bilateral nephrectomy in most reported experiences,[195, 212, 229, 234] high plasma renin concentrations fall to low or undetectable levels and blood pressure usually becomes more manageable. Del Greco and colleagues[195] showed that hypertension improved markedly after nephrectomy in 115 of 145 patients but not in the remainder; 74 of 79 patients with high plasma renin activity but only 13 of 29 with normal plasma renin became normotensive. Verniory and co-workers[232] found that blood pressure decreased in 5, increased in 5, and was unchanged in the remaining 13 patients after bilateral nephrectomy in patients with normal plasma renin concentration. The effect of bilateral nephrectomy on blood pressure occurs without a necessary decrease in blood volume in patients with volume-unresponsive[212] or volume-responsive[234] hypertension. Thus, although these studies after bilateral nephrectomy do not establish a definitive pathogenetic role for renin in all instances, they clearly show the presence of a pressor effect of the kidneys regardless of the severity or controllability of hypertension by volume depletion.

## Sympathetic Nervous System

Sympathetic nervous system stimulation augments cardiac output and increases peripheral resistance. β-Adrenergic stimulation promotes renin release, whereas angiotensin II stimulates the sympathetic system. Although autonomic insufficiency in uremia[246] may confound the interpretation, the role of the sympathetic nervous system in the hypertension of dialysis patients has been examined in several ways.

Plasma norepinephrine concentrations have been shown to be elevated in hypertensive hemodialysis patients[247] and may correlate with blood pressure. Plasma epinephrine concentrations may also be higher in hypertensive patients.[248] In patients with frequent episodes of intradialytic hypotension or hypertension unrelated to plasma volume and renin, compared with those with few hypotensive episodes and normotension, a decreased response to amyl nitrate inhalation (a test of the entire reflex arc) and a normal cold pressor response (a test of the efferent limb) suggest a defect localized to the afferent limb of the baroreceptor or cardiopulmonary reflexes; plasma dopamine β-hydroxylase (a purportedly better reflector of adrenergic activity) was also higher in hypertensive patients.[249] Blockade with guanethidine, phentolamine, propranolol, and atropine produced a fall in blood pressure in hypertensive hemodialysis patients even if volume expanded.[250] Similarly, blockade with debrisoquin, a postganglionic blocker, decreased blood pressure in hypertensive patients but not in normotensive hemodialysis patients or normal subjects.[251]

Sympathetic nerve discharge has been determined directly to examine the hypothesis that intrarenal accumulation of uremic toxins or ischemic metabolites may act as the afferent signal in the sympathetic involvement in uremic hypertension. Nerve discharge rates in skeletal muscle in hypertensive hemodialysis patients with native kidneys were 2.5 times those in hemodialysis patients who had had bilateral nephrectomy or in normal subjects[62] (Fig. 48–9). Among the patients with native kidneys, the results did not depend on the intake of antihypertensive medications at any time; normotensive hemodialysis patients were not specifically compared. Nerve discharge rate was also unrelated to plasma renin activity, angiotensin II or norepinephrine levels, or rHuEPO dose. Thus, the increased discharge rate is not caused by hemodialysis, stimulation of arterial chemoreceptors, or permanent alterations in the sympathetic nervous system. Cumulatively, these data provide consistent support for a pathogenetic role of afferent renal adrenergic reflexes in activation of the sympathetic nervous system.

### Other Vasoactive Factors

Both endothelin-1 and endothelin-3 are increased in hemodialysis patients compared with healthy control subjects,[252] but the relationship to blood pressure in these subjects was not reported.

Endogenous asymmetric dimethylarginine, which inhibits nitric oxide synthesis, accumulates in patients with end-stage renal disease—about eight times higher than normal—and decreases during hemodialysis. Increased asymmetric dimethylarginine, which would prevent vasodilatation, may contribute to hypertension in these patients.[253]

Antihypertensive substances—renomedullary lipids,[254] prostaglandins, and kinins[255]—that may emanate from the kidney have not been studied in dialysis patients with hypertension but, in patients with scarred shrunken kidneys or anephric patients, their potential role is not difficult to envision.

Plasma atrial natriuretic factor concentrations are high, increase with volume expansion, and decrease with volume contraction in hemodialysis patients.[256] These changes are appropriate but in the direction opposite to that expected for a potent vasodilator. Thus, a role, if any, for atrial natriuretic factor would be to modulate other pressors.

Whatever their actual blood pressure at the start of dialysis, most patients receiving hemodialysis have had chronic hypertension that results in structural alterations in the vascular wall and consequent narrowing.[257] The elasticity of large arteries is decreased in uremia because of calcification and fibroelastic intimal thickening, which are not necessarily related to an altered lipid profile or hypertension but are related to uremia per se.[258] This decrease in compliance results in increased pulse pressure and systolic hypertension, which begets further damage.[259, 260]

### Erythropoietin

Several observations suggest that rHuEPO does not directly induce hypertension. rHuEPO-related hypertension has not been observed in normal volunteers or patients with multiple myeloma, rheumatoid arthritis, or acquired immunodeficiency syndrome[209] and does not correlate with the dose of rHuEPO or the rate of increase in hematocrit.[203–205] Furthermore, the half-life of rHuEPO is short and hypertension is not seen in response to intravenous boluses.[261]

Pre-existing hypertension appears to predispose hemodialysis patients to increased blood pressure in some studies[203, 205] but not others[204, 206] and an increased severity of prior anemia may also be a risk factor.[200, 262]

With correction of an anemia, peripheral vascular resistance increases as hypoxic vasodilatation is reversed and produces a baroreflex-mediated decrease in cardiac output.[216, 263] Because blood viscosity appears to remain lower than normal in dialysis patients, higher viscosity does not contribute greatly to the increased peripheral vascular resis-

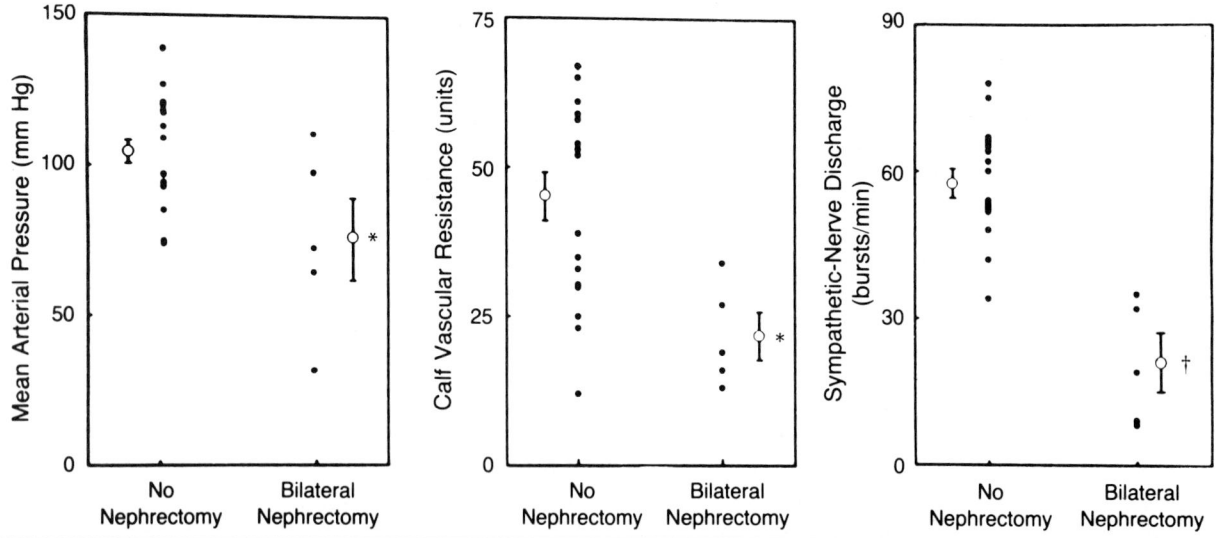

**Figure 48–9.** Mean blood pressure, vascular resistance, and sympathetic nerve discharge in hemodialysis patients with or without bilateral nephrectomy. Means ± standard error are indicated by the open circles and vertical bars. *$P < .05$; †$P < .01$. (From Converse RL, Jacobsen TN, Toto RD, et al: Sympathetic overactivity in patients with chronic renal failure. N Engl J Med 327:1912–1918, 1992. Reprinted by permission of The New England Journal of Medicine. Copyright 1992, Massachusetts Medical Society.)

tance.[261] Elevated endothelin-1 concentrations have not been observed consistently in hypertensive hemodialysis patients treated with intravenous rHuEPO.[264, 265] Cardiac output may not decrease but remains inappropriately high in hemodialysis patients as anemia is corrected.[266, 267] Thus, impaired baroreflex[268] or myocardial compliance[269] may account for the increased cardiac output and hypertension.

## MANAGEMENT

Dialysis has long been recognized to control hypertension in uremic patients.[192] Indeed, hypertension requiring drug therapy is strikingly less frequent (about 3%) in patients receiving long slow hemodialysis than in those having conventional hemodialysis, particularly high flux (20% to 50%).[270–272] Whether this is related to "better" dialysis or more effective volume removal is conjectural. However, intensive hemodialysis—mean dialysis clearance of 1.67—can result in normal blood pressure without the need for antihypertensive drugs in 98% of patients 6 months after the initiation of treatment; survival in this group of patients was 87% at 5 years and 75% at 10 years.[270]

Adequate control of hypertension is probably not achieved in many dialysis populations. Ambulatory blood pressure monitoring has shown that blood pressure in volume-responsive hypertensive hemodialysis patients returned to control hypertensive levels within the first 12 to 24 hours in the interdialytic period.[207]

Reduction of fluid volume is the first and most effective treatment, as is evident from the foregoing discussion. When maintenance dialysis is started, antihypertensive agents that are being employed should be reduced in dosage and discontinued as blood pressure is brought under control with volume depletion and establishment of dry weight. Even with optimal fluid management, some patients require antihypertensive drugs to achieve acceptable control of blood pressure. The practice of omitting these agents on the day of dialysis should probably be amended to prescribe antihypertensive agents to be taken regularly in the evening. Fortunately, most of these agents except diuretics are effective in dialysis patients.

β-Adrenergic blockers have been shown to be effective in hemodialysis patients with renin-dependent hypertension.[273] They should be used with caution in patients with dialysis hypotension, severe peripheral vascular disease, and diabetes mellitus. Conversely, patients with angina pectoris or a recent myocardial infarction may clearly benefit. Agents with intrinsic sympathomimetic activity—for example, pindolol or acebutolol—are preferred in patients with low resting heart rates or peripheral vasoconstriction. Dialyzable β-blockers such as nadolol or acebutolol may be required after dialysis. Nadolol and acebutolol require a 75% reduction in dose in dialysis patients, whereas the doses of propranolol, metoprolol and atenolol are reduced modestly. Labetolol, a combined nonselective β- and peripheral α₁-adrenergic blocker, is useful in severe hypertension and may be given once daily to patients with end-stage renal disease.

Clonidine, an α₂-adrenergic agonist, has been shown to lower blood pressure in hemodialysis patients, but only six patients were studied, all of whom were volume respon-

sive.[274] Because these agents decrease cardiac output and peripheral vascular resistance, they should also be used with caution in patients with dialysis hypotension. Abrupt withdrawal can cause severe hypertension, so these agents are ill-advised for patients prone to noncompliance or forgetfulness; clonidine, as a transdermal patch, may be useful in this setting. Doses of clonidine and methyldopa should be reduced and guanabenz and guanfacine given at the low end of the useful dose range.

Prazosin, an α₁-adrenergic antagonist, has been shown to be effective to a limited degree but additional agents were frequently required.[275] The dose of doxazosin is unchanged but the dose of prazosin and terazosin should be reduced.

The direct vasodilators hydralazine and minoxidil are potent agents that relax vascular smooth muscle by an unknown mechanism. Because the normal sympathetic response is not altered, induced tachycardia usually requires the concomitant use of a β-adrenergic blocker. Minoxidil can be given once daily, but because it is dialyzable it is best taken after dialysis; the risk of pericardial effusion in dialysis patients is not established. Hydralazine dose is unchanged.

ACE inhibitors can be effective in low-renin hypertension and even in anephric patients,[276] suggesting an effect on the tissue renin-angiotensin system.[245] Their vasodilatory and cardioprotective actions are particularly beneficial to the patient with congestive heart failure and left ventricular hypertrophy. A potential added benefit of these agents is a reduction in polydipsia, which may present a particularly difficult management problem in some patients[277]; the control of polydipsia may be accompanied by the control of blood pressure.[278] The dose of captopril should be reduced by 50% and, because captopril is dialyzable, it should be given after dialysis. With enalapril, lisinopril, benazepril, quinapril, or ramipril, it is prudent to begin at the low end of the recommended dose range. The half-life of fosinopril is not affected by renal failure.

The most serious side effects of ACE inhibitors are hypersensitivity reactions and neutropenia. Anaphylactoid reactions have been reported in patients for whom polyacrylonitrile membranes are used in dialysis[279] (because of generation of bradykinin at high rates[280]) and have been associated with polysulfone dialyzers prepared for reuse with peracetic acid and hydrogen peroxide solution.[281] The inhibition of kininase and the resultant persistence of bradykinin may have an important role in this phenomenon.[280]

Ca²⁺ channel blockers are negative inotropes, the most potent being verapamil; they should be used with caution for patients with congestive heart failure. On the other hand, verapamil has been shown to be useful for patients with left ventricular hypertrophy with diastolic dysfunction. Verapamil and diltiazem decrease sinoatrial and atrioventricular node conduction and can cause bradycardia and arrhythmias precipitated by conduction delay. In contrast, dihydropyridines may accelerate the heart rate; these are the most potent as peripheral vasodilators. In renal failure, the dose of nicardipine should be reduced; the others, including felodipine, nifedipine, verapamil, and diltiazem, require no adjustment. As a class, these agents have particular benefit for patients with coronary artery disease or peripheral vascular disease.

Because dialysis patients usually take numerous medications, once-daily dosing may be an important factor in achieving compliance. In this regard, $Ca^{2+}$ channel blockers and ACE inhibitors are often the best initial choice because they have few side effects and do not promote hemodynamic instability.

If rHuEPO-induced hypertension persists despite volume removal or drug therapy, the dose should be reduced or discontinued for 2 to 4 weeks and then reinstituted at a lower maintenance dose. If hypertensive encephalopathy or seizures develop or prodromal symptoms such as severe headache or visual disturbances occur, rHuEPO should be stopped and the patient hospitalized for observation and intensive antihypertensive therapy.[209] The net impact of rHuEPO therapy also appears to reduce left ventricular end-diastolic diameter,[282] and cardiovascular-related deaths and overall mortality appear to be decreased.[202]

Left ventricular hypertrophy can be reversed in hypertensive hemodialysis patients with strict blood pressure control—systolic less than 140 mm Hg and diastolic between 75 and 85 mm Hg—achieved by dialytic volume removal and a combination of drugs including $Ca^{2+}$ channel blockers, ACE inhibitors, and β-adrenergic antagonists.[283] Interventricular septum thickness and left ventricular mass indices did not differ from those in normotensive hemodialysis control patients.

# REFERENCES

1. Bright R: Tabular view of morbid appearance in 100 cases connected with albuminous urine. Guys Hosp Rev 1:380–410, 1836.
2. Guyton AC, Coleman TG, Cowley AW Jr, et al: Arterial pressure regulation: Overriding dominance of the kidneys in long-term regulation and in hypertension. Am J Med 52:584–594, 1972.
3. Klahr S, Levey AS, Beck GJ, et al: The effects of dietary protein restriction and blood-pressure control on the progression of chronic renal disease. N Engl J Med 330:877–884, 1994.
4. Kasiske BL: Risk factors for accelerated atherosclerosis in renal transplant recipients. Am J Med 84:985–992, 1988.
5. Cameron HA, Close CF, Yeo WW, et al: Investigation of selected patients with hypertension by the rapid-sequence intravenous urogram. Lancet 339:658–661, 1992.
6. Smith HW: Unilateral nephrectomy in hypertensive disease. J Urol 76:685–701, 1956.
7. Robertson PW, Klidjian A, Harding LK, et al: Hypertension due to a renin-secreting renal tumor. Am J Med 43:963–976, 1967.
8. Corvol P, Pinet F, Galen FX, et al: Seven lessions from seven renin secreting tumors. Kidney Int Suppl 25:S38–S44, 1988.
9. Conn JW, Cohen EL, Lucas CP, et al: Primary reninism: Hypertension, hyperreninemia and secondary aldosteronism due to renin-producing juxtaglomerular cell tumors. Arch Intern Med 130:682–696, 1972.
10. Dunnick NR, Hartman DS, Ford KK, et al: The radiology of juxtaglomerular tumors. Radiology 147:321–326, 1983.
11. Newrick PG, Miller N, Corral RJM: Primary renal renin secretion responding to angiotensin converting enzyme inhibition. Postgrad Med J 68:686–688, 1992.
12. Ganguly A, Gribble J, Tune B, et al: Renin-secreting Wilms' tumor with severe hypertension. Report of a case and a brief review of renin-secreting tumors. Ann Intern Med 79:835–837, 1973.
13. Chisholm GD, Roy RR: The systemic effects of malignant renal tumours. Br J Urol 43:687–700, 1971.
14. Hollifield JW, Page DL, Smith C, et al: Renin-secreting clear cell carcinoma of the kidney. Arch Intern Med 135:859–864, 1975.
15. Torres VE, Velosa JA, Holley KE, et al: The progression of vesico-ureteral reflux nephropathy. Ann Intern Med 92:776–784, 1980.
16. Bhathena DB, Weiss JH, Holland NH, et al: Focal and segmental glomerular sclerosis in reflux nephropathy. Am J Med 68:886–892, 1980.
17. Smellie JM, Normand C: Reflux nephropathy in childhood. In Hodson J, Kincaid-Smith P (eds): Reflux Nephropathy. Masson, New York, 1978, p 14.
18. Kincaid-Smith PS, Bastos MG, Becker GJ: Reflux nephropathy in the adult. Contrib Nephrol 39:94–101, 1984.
19. Wanner C, Luscher T, Groth H, et al: Unilateral parenchymatous kidney disease and hypertension: results of nephrectomy and medical treatment. Nephron 41:250–257, 1985.
20. Bailey RR, McRae CR, Maling MJ, et al: Renal vein renin concentration in the hypertension of unilateral reflux nephropathy. J Urol 120:21–23, 1978.
21. Luke RG, Kennedy AC, Briggs JD, et al: Results of nephrectomy in hypertension associated with unilateral renal disease. Br Med J 3:764–768, 1978.
22. Bailey RR, Lynn KL, McRae CU, Smith A: Proceedings of Second CJ Hodson Symposium on Reflux Nephropathy. Design Printing Services, Christchurch, UK, 1991.
23. deJong PE, van Bockel JH, de Zeeuw D: Unilateral renal parenchymal disease with contralateral renal artery stenosis of the fibrodysplasia type. Ann Intern Med 110:437–445, 1989.
24. Vaughan ED, Bühler FR, Laragh JH, et al: Hypertension and unilateral renal parenchymal disease: Evidence for abnormal vasoconstriction-volume interaction. JAMA 233:1177–1183, 1975.
25. Delin K, Aurell M, Granerus G: Renin-dependent hypertension in patients with unilateral kidney disease not caused by renal artery stenosis. Acta Med Scand 201:345–351, 1977.
26. Gordon RD, Tunny TJ, Evans EB, et al: Unstimulated renal venous renin ratio predicts improvement in hypertension following nephrectomy for unilateral renal disease. Nephron 44(suppl 1):25–28, 1986.
27. Peregrin JH, Zabka J, Boruvka V, et al: Embolization of the kidney in secondary renal hypertension as an alternative to surgical nephrectomy. An experimental study. Int Urol Nephrol 18:19–25, 1986.
28. Vaughan ED, Sweet RC, Gillenwater JW: Peripheral renin and blood pressure changes following complete unilateral ureteral occlusion. J Urol 104:89–92, 1970.
29. Vaughan ED, Shenasky JH, Gillenwater JY: Mechanism of acute hemodynamic response to ureteral occlusion. Invest Urol 9:109–118, 1971.
30. Klein LA, Lupa A, Brosman SA: Hypertension due to traumatic ureteral occlusion. Invest Urol 10:327–330, 1973.
31. Weidmann P, Beretta-Piccoli C, Hirsch D, et al: Curable hypertension with unilateral hydronephrosis. Studies on the role of circulating renin. Ann Intern Med 87:437–440, 1977.
32. Palmer JM, Zweiman FG, Assaykeen TA: Renal hypertension due to hydronephrosis with normal plasma renin activity. N Engl J Med 283:1032–1033, 1970.
33. Wanner C, Luscher TF, Schollmeyer P, Vetter W: Unilateral hydronephrosis and hypertension: Cause or coincidence? Nephron 45:236–241, 1987.
34. Clark WR, Malek RS: Ureteropelvic junction obstruction. I. Observations on the classic type in adults. J Urol 138:276–279, 1987.
35. Schwartz DT, Lattimer JK: Incidence of arterial hypertension in 540 patients with renal tuberculosis. J Urol 98:651–652, 1968.
36. Marks LS, Poutasse EF: Hypertension from renal tuberculosis: Operative cure predicted by renal vein renin. J Urol 109:149–151, 1974.
37. Kelly JF, Atkinson AB, Adgey AA: Renal tuberculosis and accelerated hypertension: The use of renal vein renin sampling to predict the outcome after nephrectomy. Int J Cardiol 16:318–320, 1987.
38. Stair DC, Rios WA, Black HR: Atypical causes of curable renovascular hypertension: A review. Prog Cardiovasc Dis 33:185–210, 1990.
39. Bonomini V, Campieri C, Scolari MP, Vangelista A: Hypertension in acute renal failure. Contrib Nephrol 54:152–158, 1987.
40. Woods JS, Blythe WB: Management of malignant hypertension complicated by renal insufficiency. N Engl J Med 277:57–61, 1967.
41. Woods JW, Blythe WB, Wuffines WD: Management of malignant hypertension complicated by renal insufficiency. A follow-up study. N Engl J Med 291:10–14, 1974.
42. Almeida JB, Saragoca MA, Tavares A, et al: Severe hypertension induces disturbances of renal autoregulation. Hypertension 19(suppl):279–283, 1992.
43. Curtis JJ, Luke RG, Whelchel JD, et al: Inhibition of angiotensin-converting enzyme in renal transplant recipients with hypertension. N Engl J Med 308:377–381, 1983.

44. Keane WF, Anderson S, Aurell M, et al: Angiotensin converting enzyme inhibitors and progressive renal insufficiency. Ann Intern Med 111:503–516, 1989.

45. Hall JE, Guyton AC, Trippodo NC: Control of glomerular filtration rate by renin angiotensin system. Am J Physiol 233:F366–F372, 1977.

46. Toto RD, Mitchell HC, Lee HC, et al: Reversible renal insufficiency due to angiotensin converting enzyme inhibitors in hypertensive nephrosclerosis. Ann Intern Med 115:513–519, 1991.

47. Traub YM, Shapiro AP, Rodnan GP, et al: Hypertension and renal failure (scleroderma renal crisis) in progressive systemic sclerosis. Review of a 25-year experience with 68 cases. Medicine (Baltimore) 62:335–352, 1983.

48. Steen VD, Constantino JP, Shapiro AP, Medsger TAJ: Outcome of renal crisis in systemic sclerosis: relation to availability of angiotensin converting enzyme (ACE) inhibitors. Ann Intern Med 113:352–357, 1990.

49. Hammond D, Lieberman E: The hemolyticuremic syndrome. Renal cortical thrombotic microangiopathy. Arch Intern Med 126:816–822, 1970.

50. Dalakos TG, Streeten DPH, Jones D, et al: "Malignant" hypertension resulting from atheromatous embolization predominantly of one kidney. Am J Med 57:135–138, 1974.

51. Rodriguez-Iturbe B, Parra G: Loop diuretics and angiotensin enzyme inhibitors in acute nephritic syndrome. *In* Puschett JB, Greenberg A (eds): Chemistry, Pharmacology and Clinical Applications. Elsevier, New York, 1987, pp 536–541.

52. Rodriguez-Iturbe B, Baggio B, Colina-Chourio J, et al: Studies on the renin-aldosterone system in the acute nephritic syndrome. Kidney Int 19:445–453, 1981.

53. Sinclair AM, Isles CG, Brown I, et al: Secondary hypertension in a blood pressure clinic. Arch Intern Med 147:1289–1293, 1987.

54. Herrera Acosta J: Hypertension in chronic renal disease. Kidney Int 22:702–712, 1982.

55. Blythe WB: Natural history of hypertension in renal parenchymal disease. Am J Kidney Dis 5:A50–A56, 1985.

56. Chapman AB, Johnson A, Gabor PA, Schrier RW: The renin-angiotensin-aldosterone system and autosomal dominant polycystic kidney disease. N Engl J Med 323:1091–1096, 1990.

57. Kheder MA, Ben Maiz H, Abderrahim E, et al: Hypertension in primary chronic glomerulonephritis analysis of 359 cases. Nephron 63:140–144, 1993.

58. Brown CB, Cameron JS, Turner DR, et al: Focal segmented glomerulosclerosis with rapid decline in renal function ("malignant FSGS"). Clin Nephrol 10:51–61, 1978.

59. Zucchelli P, Zuccalà A, Mancini E: Hypertension in primary glomerulonephritis without renal insufficiency. Nephrol Dial Transplant 4:605–610, 1989.

60. Heidland A, Heidbreder E: Retinopathy in hypertension. Increased incidence in renoparenchymal disease. Contrib Nephrol 54:144–151, 1987.

61. Luke RG, Curtis JJ: Nephrosclerosis. *In* Schrier RW, Gottschalk CW (eds): The Diseases of the Kidney. Little, Brown, Boston, 1993, pp 1433–1450.

62. Converse RL, Jacobsen TN, Toto RD, et al: Sympathetic overactivity in patients with chronic renal failure. N Engl J Med 327:1912–1918, 1992.

63. de Wardener HE: The primary role of the kidney and salt intake in the etiology of essential hypertension. Clin Sci 79:193–200, 1990.

64. Ledingham JM, Cohen RD: The role of the heart in the pathogenesis of renal hypertension. Lancet 2:979–981, 1963.

65. Schiffrin EL: Reactivity of small blood vessels in hypertension: Relation with structural changes. Hypertension 19:SII-1–SII-9, 1992.

66. Reaven GM: Banting Lecture 1988: Role of insulin resistance in human disease. Diabetes 37:1595–1607, 1988.

67. Brod J, Bahlmann J, Cachovan M, Pretschner P: Development of hypertension in renal disease. Clin Sci 64:141–152, 1983.

68. Davies DL, Beever DG, Briggs JD, et al: Abnormal relation between exchangeable sodium and the renin-angiotensin system in malignant hypertension in hypertension with chronic renal failure. Lancet 1:683–686, 1973.

69. Beretta-Piccoli C, Weidmann P, de Chatel R, Reubi F: Hypertension associated with early stage kidney disease. Complementary roles of circulating renin, the body sodium/volume state and duration of hypertension. Am J Med 61:739–746, 1976.

70. Beretta-Piccoli C, Weidmann P, Schiffl H, et al: Enhanced cardiovascular pressor reactivity to norepinephrine in mild renal parenchymal disease. Kidney Int 28:814–822, 1985.

71. Vertes V, Cangiano JL, Berman LB, Gould A: Hypertension in end-stage renal disease. N Engl J Med 280:978–981, 1969.

72. Koomans HA, Roos JC, Boer P, et al: Salt sensitivity of blood pressure in chronic renal failure, evidence for renal control of body fluid distribution in man. Hypertension 4:190–197, 1982.

73. Ishii M, Ikeda T, Takagi M, et al: Elevated plasma catecholamines in hypertensives with primary glomerular diseases. Hypertension 5:545–551, 1983.

74. Katholi RE, Winthlow PL, Winternitz S, Oparil S: Importance of the renal nerves in established two-kidney, one-clip Goldblatt hypertension in the rat. Hypertension 4:166–174, 1982.

75. Blaustein MP: Sodium ions, calcium ions, blood pressure regulation and hypertension: A reassessment and a hypothesis. Am J Physiol 232:C165–C173, 1977.

76. Huot SJ: The role of sodium intake, the $Na^+$-$K^+$ pump and a ouabain-like humoral agent in the genesis of reduced renal mass hypertension. Am J Nephrol 3:92–99, 1983.

77. Baylis C, Mitruka B, Deng A: Chronic blockade on nitric oxide synthesis in the rat produces systemic hypertension and glomerular damage. J Clin Invest 90:278–281, 1992.

78. Salazar FJ, Alberola A, Pinilla JM, et al: Salt-induced increase in arterial pressure during nitric oxide synthesis inhibition. Hypertension 22:49–55, 1993.

79. Schultz PJ, Tolins JP: Adaptation to increased dietary salt intake in the rat. J Clin Invest 91:642–650, 1993.

80. Chen PY, Sanders PW: L-Arginine abrogates salt-sensitive hypertension in Dahl/Rapp rats. J Clin Invest 88:1559–1567, 1992.

81. Chen PY, Sanders PW: Role of nitric oxide synthesis in salt-sensitive hypertension in Dahl/Rapp rats. Hypertension 22:812–818, 1993.

82. Rees DD, Palmer RMJ, Moncada S: Role of endothelium-derived nitric oxide in the regulation of blood pressure. Proc Natl Acad Sci USA 86:3375–3378, 1989.

83. Panza JA, Quyyumi AA, Brush JE, Epstein SE: Abnormal endothelium-dependent vascular relaxation in patients with essential hypertension. N Engl J Med 323:22–27, 1990.

84. Patel A, Layne S, Watts D, Kirchner KA: L-Arginine administration normalizes pressure natriuresis in hypertensive Dahl rats. Hypertension 22:863–869, 1993.

85. Muirhead EE: Antihypertensive functions of the kidney. Hypertension 2:444–464, 1980.

86. Portaluppi F, Montanari L, Massari M, et al: Loss of nocturnal decline of blood pressure in hypertension due to chronic renal failure. Am J Hypertens 4:20–26, 1914.

87. Levey AS, Beck GJ, Caggiula AW, et al: A hypothesis for the results of the modification of diet in renal disease (MDRD) study. J Am Soc Nephrol 4:253, 1993. Abstract.

88. Wright JP, Salzano S, Brown CB, El Nahas AM: Natural history of chronic renal failure: A reappraisal. Nephrol Dial Transplant 7:379–383, 1992.

89. United States Renal Data System: 1993 Annual Report. Am J Kidney Dis 22:21–57, 1993.

90. Praga M, Hernandez E, Montoyo C, et al: Long-term beneficial effects of angiotensin-converting enzyme inhibition in patients with nephrotic proteinuria. Am J Kidney Dis 20:240–248, 1992.

91. Kamper AL, Strandgaard S, Leyssac PP: Effect of enalapril on the progression of chronic renal failure. A randomized controlled trial. Am J Hypertens 5:423–430, 1992.

92. Apperloo AJ, deZeeuw D, deJong PE: Short-term antiproteinuric response to antihypertensive treatment predicts long-term GFR decline in patients with non-diabetic renal disease. Kidney Int 45:S174–S178, 1994.

93. Gansevoort RT, deZeeuw D, deJong PE: Long-term benefits on the antiproteinuric effect of angiotensin-converting enzyme inhibition in non-diabetic renal disease. Am J Kidney Dis 22:202–206, 1993.

94. National High Blood Pressure Education Program: National High Blood Pressure Education Program Working Group report on hypertension and chronic renal failure. Arch Intern Med 151:1280–1287, 1991.

95. Brazy PC, Stead WW, Fitzwilliam JF: Progression of renal insufficiency: Role of blood pressure. Kidney Int 35:670–674, 1989.

96. Wright JP, Brown CB, El Nahas AM: Effect of control of hypertension on progressive renal failure. Clin Nephrol 39:305–311, 1993.

97. Blantz RC, Gabbai F, Gushwa LC, Wilson CB: The influence of concomitant experimental hypertension and glomerulonephritis. Kidney Int 32:652–663, 1987.

98. Neugarten J, Kaminetsky B, Feiner H, et al: Nephrotoxic serum nephritis with hypertension: Amelioration by antihypertensive therapy. Kidney Int 28:135–139, 1985.

99. Brenner BM, Meyer TW, Hostetter TH: Dietary protein intake and the progressive nature of kidney disease: The role of hemodynamically mediated glomerular injury in the pathogenesis of progressive glomerular sclerosis in aging, renal ablation and intrinsic renal disease. N Engl J Med 307:652–659, 1982.

100. Dworkin LD, Hostetter TH, Rennke HG, Brenner BM: Hemodynamic basis for glomerular injury in rats with desoxycorticosterone-salt hypertension. J Clin Invest 73:1448–1461, 1984.

101. Meyer TW, Anderson S, Rennke HG, Brenner BM: Reversing glomerular hypertension stabilizes established glomerular injury. Kidney Int 31:752–759, 1987.

102. Dworkin LD, Feiner HD, Randazzo J: Glomerular hypertension and injury in desoxycorticosterone-salt rats on antihypertensive therapy. Kidney Int 31:718–724, 1987.

103. Zeier M, Fehrenbach P, Geberth S, et al: Renal histology in polycystic kidney disease with incipient and advanced renal failure. Kidney Int 42:1259–1265, 1992.

104. Zeier M, Geberth S, Schmidt KG, et al: Elevated blood pressure profile and left ventricular mass in children and young adults with autosomal dominant polycystic kidney disease. J Am Soc Nephrol 3:1451–1457, 1993.

105. Gabow PA, Ikle DW, Holmes JH: Polycystic kidney disease: Prospective analysis of non-azotemic patients and family members. Ann Intern Med 101:238–247, 1984.

106. Gabow PA, Chapman AB, Johnson AM, et al: Renal structure and hypertension in autosomal dominant polycystic kidney disease. Kidney Int 38:1177–1180, 1990.

107. Curtis JJ, Lucas BA, Kotchen TA, Luke RG: Surgical therapy for persistent hypertension after renal transplantation. Transplantation 31:125–128, 1981.

108. Torres VE, Donovan KA, Scicli G, et al: Synthesis of renin by tubulocystic epithelium in autosomal dominant polycystic kidney disease. Kidney Int 42:364–373, 1992.

109. Harrap SB, Davies DL, Macnicol AN, Watson ML: Renal, cardiovascular and hormonal characteristics of young adults with autosomal dominant polycystic kidney disease. Kidney Int 40:501–508, 1991.

110. Schmid M, Mann J, Stein G, et al: Natriuresis-pressure relationship in polycystic kidney disease. J Hypertens 3:277–283, 1990.

111. Lewis EJ, Hunsicker LG, Bain RP, Rohde RD: The effect of angiotensin-converting-enzyme inhibition on diabetic nephropathy. N Engl J Med 329:1456–1462, 1993.

112. Bakris GL: Angiotensin-converting enzyme inhibitors and progression of diabetic nephropathy. Ann Intern Med 118:643–644, 1993.

113. Kasiske BL, Kalil RSN, Ma JZ, et al: Effect of antihypertensive therapy on the kidney in patients with diabetes: A meta-regression analysis. Ann Intern Med 118:129–138, 1993.

114. Ravid M, Savin H, Jutrin I, et al: Long-term stabilizing effect of angiotensin-converting enzyme inhibition of plasma creatinine and on proteinuria in normotensive type II diabetes patients. Ann Intern Med 118:577–581, 1993.

115. National High Blood Pressure Education Program Working Group: National High Blood Pressure Education Program Working Group report on hypertension in diabetes. Hypertension 23:145–158, 1994.

116. Joint National Committee on Detection, Evaluation and Treatment of High Blood Pressure: The fifth report of the Joint National Committee on Detection, Evaluation, and Treatment of High Blood Pressure (JNC V). Arch Intern Med 153:154–183, 1993.

117. Keilani T, Schleuter WA, Levin ML, Batlle DC: Improvement of lipid abnormalities associated with proteinuria using fosinopril, an angiotensin-converting enzyme inhibitor. Ann Intern Med 118:246–254, 1993.

118. Kakinuma Y, Kawamura T, Bills T, et al: Blood pressure–independent effect of angiotensin inhibition on vascular lesions of chronic renal failure. Kidney Int 42:46–55, 1992.

119. Paul M, Wagner J, Dzau VJ: Gene expression of the renin-angiotensin system in human tissues. J Clin Invest 91:2058–2064, 1993.

120. Ruilope LM, Casal MC, Praga M, et al: Additive antiproteinuric effect of converting enzyme inhibition and a low protein intake. J Am Soc Nephrol 3:1307–1311, 1992.

121. Rodicio JL, Morales JM, Alcazar JM, Ruilope LM: Calcium antagonists and renal protection. J Hypertens 11:S49–S53, 1993.

122. Brazy PC, Fitzwilliam JF: Progressive renal disease: Role of race and antihypertensive. Kidney Int 37:1113–1119, 1990.

123. Eliahou HL, Cohen D, Hellberg B, et al: Effect of the calcium channel blocker nisoldipine on the progression of chronic renal failure in man. Am J Nephrol 8:285–290, 1988.

124. Zucchelli P, Zuccala A, Gaggi R: Calcium channel blockers; effects on progressive renal disease. Am J Kidney Dis 17(suppl 1):94–97, 1991.

125. Luke RG: Hypertension in renal transplant recipients. Kidney Int 31:1024–1037, 1987.

126. Curtis JJ: Hypertension and kidney transplantation. Am J Kidney Dis 7:181–196, 1986.

127. Van Ypersele de Strihou C, Vereerstraeten P, Wauthier M, et al: Prevalence, etiology and treatment of last post-transplant hypertension. Adv Nephrol Necker Hosp 12:41–60, 1983.

128. Luke RG: Pathophysiology and treatment of post-transplant hypertension. J Am Soc Nephrol 2:S37–S44, 1991.

129. First MR, Neylan JF, Rocher LL, Tejani A: Hypertension after renal transplantation. J Am Soc Nephrol 4:S30–S36, 1994.

130. Curtis JJ, Laskow DA, Jones PA, et al: Captopril-induced fall in glomerular filtration rate in cyclosporine-treated hypertension patients. J Am Soc Nephrol 3:1570–1574, 1993.

131. Ruggenenti P, Perico N, Mosconi L, et al: Calcium channel blockers protect transplant patients from cyclosporine-induced daily renal hypoperfusion. Kidney Int 43:706–711, 1993.

132. Abu-Romeh SH, el-Khatib D, Rashid A, et al: Comparative effects of enalapril and nifedipine on renal hemodynamics in hypertensive renal allograft recipients. Clin Nephrol 37:183–188, 1992.

133. Morales JM, Andres A, Hernandez E, et al: Long-term protective effect of calcium antagonist on renal function in hypertensive renal transplant patients on cyclosporine therapy. A 5 year randomized study. J Am Soc Nephrol 4:950, 1993. Abstract.

134. Kirk AJ, Omar I, Dark JH: Long term improvement in renal function using nifedipine in cyclosporine-associated hypertension. Transplantation 50:1061, 1990.

135. Curtis JJ: Hypertension following kidney transplantation. Am J Kidney Dis 23:471–475, 1994.

136. Porter GA, Bennett WM, Sheps SG: Cyclosporine-associated hypertension. Arch Intern Med 150:280–283, 1990.

137. Curtis JJ, Luke RG, Jones P, et al: Hypertension after successful renal transplantation. Am J Med 79:193–200, 1985.

138. Curtis JJ, Luke RG, Jones P, Diethelm AG: Hypertension in cyclosporine-treated renal transplant recipients is sodium dependent. Am J Med 85:134–138, 1988.

139. Laskow DA, Curtis J, Luke R, et al: Cyclosporine impairs the renal response to volume depletion. Transplant Proc 20:568–571, 1988.

140. Carmines P, Navar L: Disparate effects of $Ca^{2+}$ channel blockade on afferent and efferent arteriolar responses to ANG II. Am J Physiol 256:F1015–F1020, 1989.

141. Epstein M: Calcium antagonists and the kidney: Implications for renal protection. Kidney Int 41(suppl 36):66s–72s, 1992.

142. Badr KR, Ichikawa I: Prerenal failure: A deleterious shift from renal compensation to decompensation. N Engl J Med 319:623–629, 1988.

143. Thomson SC, Tucker BJ, Gabbai F, Blantz RC: Functional effects on glomerular hemodynamics of short-term chronic cyclosporine in male rats. J Clin Invest 83:960–969, 1989.

144. Lanese DM, Conger JD: Effects of endothelin receptor antagonist on cyclosporine-induced vasoconstriction in isolated rat renal arterioles. J Clin Invest 91:2144–2149, 1993.

145. English J, Evan A, Houghton D, Bennett W: Cyclosporine-induced acute renal dysfunction in the rat. Transplantation 44:135–141, 1987.

146. Bertani T, Ferrazzi P, Schieppati A, et al: Nature and extent of glomerular injury induced by cyclosporine in heart transplant patients. Kidney Int 40:243–250, 1991.

147. Feutren G, Mihatsch MJ: Risk Factors for cyclosporine-induced nephropathy in patients with autoimmune diseases. N Engl J Med 326:1654–1660, 1992.

148. Morozumi K, Thiel G, Albert FW, et al: Studies on morphological outcome of cyclosporine-associated arteriolopathy after discontinuation of cyclosporine in renal allografts. Clin Nephrol 38:1–8, 1992.

149. Myers BD, Newton L: Cyclosporine-induced chronic nephropathy: An obliterative microvascular renal injury. J Am Soc Nephrol 2:S45–S52, 1991.

150. Curtis JJ, Luke RG, Dubovsky E, et al: Cyclosporine in therapeutic dose increases renal allograft vascular resistance. Lancet 2:477–479, 1986.

151. Swanson S, Born T, Zydowsky LD, et al: Cyclosporin-mediated inhibition of bovine calcineurin by cytophilins A and B. Proc Natl Acad Sci USA 89:3741–3745, 1992.

152. Pfeilschifter J, Ruegg UT: Cyclosporin A augments angiotensin II–stimulated rise in intracellular free calcium in vascular smooth muscle cells. Biochem J 248:883–887, 1987.

153. Garr MD, Paller MS: Cyclosporine augments renal but not systemic vascular reactivity. Am J Physiol 258:F211–F217, 1990.

154. Coffman T, Carr D, Yarger W, Klotman P: Evidence that renal prostaglandin and thromboxane production is stimulated in chronic cyclosporine nephrotoxicity. Transplantation 43:282–285, 1986.

155. Fogo A, Hellings SE, Inagami T, Kon V: Endothelin receptor antagonism is protective in in vivo acute cyclosporine toxicity. Kidney Int 42:770–774, 1992.

156. Kon V, Sugiura M, Inagami T, et al: Role of endothelin in cyclosporine-induced glomerular dysfunction. Kidney Int 37:1487–1491, 1990.

157. Lüscher TF, Seo B, Bühler FR: Potential role of endothelin in hypertension. Hypertension 21:752–757, 1993.

158. Perico N, Benigni A, Zoja C, et al: Functional significance of exaggerated renal thromboxane $A_2$ synthesis induced by cyclosporin A. Am J Physiol 20:F581–F587, 1986.

159. Conte G, Canton AD, Sabbatini M, et al: Acute cyclosporine renal dysfunction reversed by dopamine infusion in healthy subjects. Kidney Int 36:1086–1092, 1989.

160. Bloom ITM, Bentley FR, Garrison RN: Acute cyclosporine-induced renal vasoconstriction is mediated by endothelin-1. Surgery 114:480–488, 1993.

161. Gaston RS, Schlessinger SD, Sanders PW, et al: Cyclosporine inhibits the renal vasodilatory response to L-arginine in human renal allograft recipients. J Am Soc Nephrol 4:550, 1993. Abstract.

162. Perico N, Ruggenenti P, Gaspari F, et al: Daily renal hypoperfusion induced by cyclosporine in patients with renal transplantation. Transplantation 54:56–60, 1992.

163. Richards NT, Poston L, Hilston PJ: Cyclosporin A inhibits endothelium-dependent, prostanoid-induced relaxation in human subcutaneous resistance vessels. J Hypertens 8:159–163, 1990.

164. Diederich D, Yang Z, Luscher F: Chronic cyclosporine therapy impairs endothelium-dependent relaxation in the renal artery of the rat. J Am Soc Nephrol 2:1291–1297, 1992.

165. Curtis JJ, Laskow DA, Jones PA: Sodium sensitivity of blood pressure: FK 506 compared to CSA treated cadaveric renal transplant recipients. American Society Transplant Physicians Meeting; 1994; Chicago. Abstract.

166. Moss NG, Powell SL, Falk RJ: Intravenous cyclosporine activates afferent and efferent renal nerves and causes sodium retention in innervated kidneys in rats. Proc Natl Acad Sci USA 82:8222–8226, 1985.

167. Scherrer R, Vissing SF, Morgan BJ, et al: Cyclosporine-induced sympathetic activation and hypertension after heart transplantation. N Engl J Med 323:693–699, 1990.

168. Deray G, Benhmida M, Hoang PL, et al: Renal function and blood pressure in patients receiving long-term, low-dose cyclosporine therapy for idiopathic autoimmune uveitis. Ann Intern Med 117:578–583, 1992.

169. Lin HY, Rocher LL, McQuillan MA, et al: Cyclosporine-induced hyperuricemia and gout. N Engl J Med 321:287–292, 1989.

170. Luke RG: Mechanism of cyclosporine-induced hypertension. Am J Hypertens 4:468–471, 1991.

171. Hannedouche TP, Delgado AG, Gnionsahe AD, et al: Nephrotoxicity of cyclosporine in autoimmune diseases. Adv Nephrol Necker Hosp 19:169–185, 1990.

172. Remuzzi G, Bertani T: Renal vascular and thrombotic effects of cyclosporine. Am J Kidney Dis 13:261–272, 1989.

173. Solez K, Axelsen RA, Benediktsson H, et al: International standardization of criteria for the histologic diagnosis of renal allograft rejection: The Banff working classification of kidney transplant pathology. Kidney Int 44:411–422, 1993.

174. First MR: Renal allograft survival after 1 and 10 years: Comparison between pre-cyclosporin and cyclosporin data. Nephrol Dial Transplant 9:90–97, 1994.

175. Sanders SE, Curtis JJ, Julian BA, et al: Tapering or discontinuing cyclosporine for financial reasons—a single-center experience. Am J Kidney Dis 21:9–15, 1993.

176. Kasiske BL, Heim-Duthoy K, Ma JZ: Elective cyclosporine withdrawal after renal transplantation: A meta-analysis. JAMA 269:395–400, 1993.

177. Luke RG, Curtis JJ, Jones P, et al: Mechanisms of post-transplant hypertension. Am J Kidney Dis 5:A79–A84, 1985.

178. Hricik DE, Lautman J, Bartucci MR, et al: Variable effects of steroid withdrawal on blood pressure reduction in cyclosporine-treated renal transplant recipients. Transplantation 53:1232–1235, 1992.

179. Curtis JJ, Luke RG, Diethelm AG, et al: Benefits of removal of native kidneys in hypertension after renal transplantation. Lancet 2:739–742, 1985.

180. Bantle JP, Coudreau RJ, Ferris TF: Suppression of plasma renin activity by cyclosporine. Am J Med 83:59–64, 1987.

181. Dubovsky E, Curtis J, Luke R, et al: Captopril as a predictor of curable hypertension in renal transplant recipients. Contrib Nephrol 56:117–123, 1987.

182. Murray BM, Venuto RC, Kohli R, Cunningham EE: Enalapril-associated acute renal failure in renal transplants: Possible role of cyclosporine. Am J Kidney Dis 16:66–69, 1990.

183. Ahmad T, Coulthard M, Eastham E: Reversible renal failure due to the use of captopril in a renal allograft recipient treated with cyclosporin. Nephrol Dial Transplant 4:311–312, 1989.

184. Sawaya B, Provenzano R, Kupin W, Venkat KK: Cyclosporine-induced renal macroangiopathy. Am J Kidney Dis 12:534–737, 1988.

185. Matalon TA, Thompson MJ, Patel SK, et al: Percutaneous transluminal angioplasty for transplant renal artery stenosis. J Vasc Interv Radiol 3(1):55–58, 1992.

186. Gaston RS, Julian BA, Diethelm AG, Curtis JJ: Effects of enalapril on erythrocytosis after renal transplantation. Ann Intern Med 115:954–955, 1991.

187. Dantal J, Bigot E, Rogers W, et al: Effect of plasma protein adsorption on protein excretion in kidney-transplant recipients with recurrent nephrotic syndrome. N Engl J Med 330:7–14, 1994.

188. Textor SC: De novo hypertension after liver transplantation. Hypertension 22:257–267, 1993.

189. Gupta AK, Rocher LL, Schmaltz SP, et al: Short-term changes in renal function, blood pressure, and electrolyte levels in patients receiving cyclosporine for dermatologic disorders. Arch Intern Med 151:356–362, 1991.

190. Traindl O, Falger S, Reading S, et al: The effects of lisinopril on renal function in proteinuric renal transplant recipients. Transplantation 44:1309–1313, 1993.

191. Brazy PC, Pirsch JD, Belzer FO: Factors affecting renal allograft function in long-term recipients. Am J Kidney Dis 14:558–566, 1992.

192. Hegstrom RM, Murray JS, Pendras JP, et al: Hemodialysis in the treatment of chronic uremia. Trans Am Soc Artif Intern Organs 7:136–144, 1961.

193. Brown JJ, Dusterdieck G, Fraser R, et al: Hypertension and chronic renal failure. Br Med Bull 27:128–135, 1971.

194. Weidmann P, Maxwell MH, Lupu AN, et al: Plasma renin activity and blood pressure in terminal renal failure. N Engl J Med 285:757–762, 1971.

195. del Greco F, Davies WA, Simon NM, et al: Hypertension of chronic renal failure: Role of sodium and the renal pressor system. Kidney Int 7(suppl 1):S176–S183, 1975.

196. Zucchelli P, Santoro A, Zuccala A: Genesis and control of hypertension in hemodialysis patients. Semin Nephrol 8:163–168, 1988.

197. Blythe WB: Natural history of hypertension in renal parenchymal disease. Am J Kidney Dis 5:A50–A56, 1985.

198. Danielsen H, Kornerup HJ, Olsen S, Posborg V: Arterial hypertension in chronic glomerulonephritis. An analysis of 310 cases. Clin Nephrol 19:284–287, 1983.

199. Parving H-H, Hommel E, Mathiesen E, et al: Prevalence of microalbuminuria, arterial hypertension, retinopathy and neuropathy in patients with insulin-dependent diabetes. Br Med J 296:156–160, 1988.

200. Buckner FS, Eschbach JW, Haley NR, et al: Hypertension following erythropoietin therapy in anemic hemodialysis patients. Am J Hypertens 3:947–955, 1990.

201. Nonnast-Daniel B, Deschodt G, Brunkhorst R, et al: Long-term effects of treatment with recombinant human erythropoietin on haemodynamics and tissue oxygenation in patients with renal anemia. Nephrol Dial Transplant 5:444–448, 1990.

202. Eschbach JW, Aquiling T, Haley NR, et al: The long-term effects of recombinant human erythropoietin on the cardiovascular system. Clin Nephrol 38:S98–S103, 1992.
203. Akizawa T, Koshikawa S, Takaku F, et al: Clinical effect of recombinant human erythropoietin on anemia associated with chronic renal failure: A multi-institutional study in Japan. Int J Artif Organs 11:343–350, 1988.
204. Samtleben W, Baldamus CA, Bommer J, et al: Blood pressure changes during treatment with recombinant human erythropoietin. Contrib Nephrol 66:114–122, 1988.
205. Eschbach JW, Abdulhadi MH, Browne JK, et al: Recombinant human erythropoietin in anemic patients with end-stage renal disease: Results of a phase III multicentre clinical trial. Ann Intern Med 111:992–1000, 1989.
206. Sundal E, Kaeser U: Correction of anaemia of chronic renal failure with recombinant human erythropoietin: Safety and efficacy of one year's treatment in a European multicentre study of 150 haemodialysis-dependent patients. Nephrol Dial Transplant 4:979–987, 1989.
207. Cheigh JS, Milite C, Sullivan JF, et al: Hypertension is not adequately controlled in hemodialysis patients. Am J Kidney Dis 19:453–459, 1992.
208. Edmunds ME, Walls J, Tucker B, et al: Seizures in haemodialysis patients treated with recombinant human erythropoietin. Nephrol Dial Transplant 4:1065–1069, 1989.
209. Raine AEG, Roger SD: Effects of erythropoietin on blood pressure. Am J Kidney Dis 18(suppl 1):76–83, 1991.
210. Baumgart P, Walger P, Gemen S, et al: Blood pressure elevation during the night in chronic renal failure, hemodialysis and after renal transplantation. Nephron 57:293–298, 1991.
211. Kim KE, Onesti G, Schwartz AB, et al: Hemodynamics of hypertension in chronic end-stage renal disease. Circulation 46:456–464, 1972.
212. Kim KE, Onesti G, Swartz C: Hemodynamics of hypertension in uremia. Kidney Int 7(suppl 1):S155–S162, 1975.
213. Nixon JV, Mitchell JH, McPhaul JJ Jr, Henrich WL: Effect of hemodialysis on left ventricular function: Dissociation of changes in filling volume and in contractile state. J Clin Invest 71:377–384, 1983.
214. Henrich WL, Hunt JM, Nixon JV: Increased ionized calcium and left ventricular contractility during hemodialysis. N Engl J Med 310:19–23, 1984.
215. Sadler DB, Brown J, Nurse H, Roberts J: Impact of hemodialysis on left and right ventricular Doppler diastolic filling indices. Am J Med Sci 304:83–90, 1992.
216. Varat MA, Adolph RJ, Fowler NO: Cardiovascular effects of anemia. Am Heart J 83:415–426, 1972.
217. Kim KE, Onesti G, Neff MD, et al: Hemodynamic alterations in hypertension of chronic end-stage renal disease. In Onesti G, Kim KE, Moyer JH (eds): Hypertension: Mechanisms and Management. Grune & Stratton, New York, 1973, pp 606–616.
218. Cangiano JL, Ramirez-Muxo O, Ramirez-Gonzalez R, et al: Normal renin uremic hypertension. Arch Intern Med 136:17–23, 1976.
219. Kim KE, Onesti G, DelGuercio ET, et al: Sequential hemodynamic changes in end-stage renal disease and the anephric state during volume expansion. Hypertension 2:102–110, 1980.
220. Onesti G, Kim KE, Greco JA, et al: Blood pressure regulation in end-stage renal disease and anephric man. Circ Res 36(suppl 1):145–152, 1975.
221. Coleman TG, Bower JD, Langford HG, Guyton AC: Regulation of arterial pressure in the anephric state. Circulation 42:509–514, 1970.
222. Mion C, Slingeneyer A, Canaud B: Pathophysiology and management of hypertension in continuous ambulatory peritoneal dialysis patients. Contrib Nephrol 54:202–209, 1987.
223. Dathan JRE, Johnson DB, Goodwin FJ: The relationship between body fluid compartment volumes, renin activity and blood pressure in chronic renal failure. Clin Sci Mol Med 445:77–88, 1973.
224. Schultze G, Piefke S, Molzahn M: Blood pressure in terminal renal failure. Fluid spaces and the renin-angiotensin system. Nephron 25:15–24, 1980.
225. Wilkinson R, Scott DF, Uldall PR, et al: Plasma renin and exchangeable sodium in the hypertension of chronic renal failure. The effect of bilateral nephrectomy. Q J Med 39:377–394, 1970.
226. Weidmann P, Beretta-Piccoli C, Steffen F, et al: Hypertension in terminal renal failure. Kidney Int 9:294–301, 1976.
227. Koomans HA, Geers AB, Boers P, et al: A study of the distribution of body fluids after rapid saline expansion in normal subjects and in patients with renal insufficiency: Preferential intravascular deposition in renal failure. Clin Sci 64:153–160, 1983.
228. Schalekamp MA, Beevers DG, Briggs JD, et al: Hypertension in chronic renal failure. An abnormal relation between sodium and the renin-angiotensin system. Am J Med 55:379–390, 1973.
229. Schalekamp MADH, Schalekamp-Kuyken MPA, de Moor-Furytier M, et al: Interrelationships between blood pressure, renin, renin substrate, and blood volume in terminal renal failure. Clin Sci Mol Med 45:417–428, 1973.
230. Rosen SM, Robinson PJA: Interdependence of exchangeable sodium and plasma renin concentration in determining blood pressure in patients treated by maintenance dialysis. Br Med J 4:139–143, 1973.
231. Chrysanthakopoulos SG, Kastagir BK, Jubiz W, Kolff WJ: Hypertension in patients on maintenance hemodialysis: Evaluation of peripheral renin activity and bilateral nephrectomy. Am J Med Sci 264:9–21, 1972.
232. Verniory A, Potvliege P, Van Geertrudyden JJ, et al: Renin and control of arterial blood pressure during terminal renal failure treated by hemodialysis and by transplantation. Clin Sci 42:685–700, 1972.
233. Gutkin M, Levinson GE, King AS, Lasker N: Plasma renin activity in end-stage kidney disease. Circulation 40:563–574, 1969.
234. Bianchi G, Ponticelli C, Bardi U, et al: Role of the kidney in 'salt and water dependent hypertension' of end-stage renal disease. Clin Sci 42:47–55, 1972.
235. Kornerup HJ: Hypertension in end-stage renal disease. Acta Med Scand 200:257–261, 1976.
236. Weidmann P, Maxwell MH: The renin-angiotensin-aldosterone system in terminal renal failure. Kidney Int 8:S219–S234, 1975.
237. Craswell PW, Hird VM, Judd PA, et al: Plasma renin activity and blood pressure in 89 patients receiving maintenance haemodialysis therapy. Br Med J 4:749–752, 1972.
238. Boer P, Koomans HA, Dourhout Mees EJ: Renin and blood volume in chronic renal failure: A comparison with essential hypertension. Nephron 45:7–15, 1987.
239. Brown JJ, Curtis JR, Lever AF, et al: Plasma renin concentration and the control of blood pressure in patients on maintenance hemodialysis. Nephron 6:329–349, 1969.
240. Stokes GS, Mani MK, Stewart JH: Relevance of salt, water, and renin to hypertension in chronic renal failure. Br Med J 3:126–129, 1970.
241. Fadem SZ, Lifschitz MD: Use of saralasin in end-stage renal disease. Kidney Int 15:S93–S100, 1979.
242. Mimran A, Shaldon S, Barjon P, Mion C: The effect of an angiotensin antagonist on arterial pressure and plasma aldosterone in hemodialysis-resistant hypertensive patients. Clin Nephrol 9:63–67, 1978.
243. Vaughan ED Jr, Carey RM, Ayers CR, Peach MJ: Hemodialysis-resistant hypertension: control with an orally active inhibitor of angiotensin-converting enzyme. J Clin Endocrinol Metab 48:869–871, 1979.
244. Wauters J-P, Waebner B, Brunner HR, et al: Uncontrollable hypertension in patients on hemodialysis: Long-term treatment with captopril and salt subtraction. Clin Nephrol 16:86–92, 1981.
245. Campbell DJ: Circulating and tissue angiotensin systems. J Clin Invest 79:1–6, 1987.
246. Kersh ES, Kronfield SJ, Unger A, et al: Autonomic insufficiency in uremia as a cause of hemodialysis-induced hypotension. N Engl J Med 290:650–653, 1974.
247. Zucchelli P, Zuccala A, Degli Esposti A, et al: Pathophysiology and management of hypertension in hemodialysis patients. Contrib Nephrol 54:209–217, 1987.
248. McGrath BP, Ledingham JGG, Benedict CR: Catecholamines in peripheral venous plasma in patients on chronic hemodialysis. Clin Sci Mol Med 55:89–96, 1978.
249. Lilley JJ, Golden J, Stone RA: Adrenergic regulation of blood pressure in chronic renal failure. J Clin Invest 57:1190–1200, 1976.
250. McGrath BP, Tilder DJ, Bune A, et al: Autonomic blockade and the Valsalva maneuver in patients on maintenance hemodialysis: A hemodynamic study. Kidney Int 12:294–302, 1978.
251. Schohn D, Weidemann P, Jahn H, Beretta-Piccoli C: Norepinephrine-related mechanism in hypertension accompanying renal failure. Kidney Int 28:814–822, 1985.
252. Suzuki N, Matsumto H, Miyauchi T, et al: Endothelin-3 concentrations in human plasma: The increased concentrations in patients undergoing haemodialysis. Biochem Biophys Res Commun 169:809–815, 1990.

253. Vallance P, Leone A, Calver A, et al: Accumulation of an endogenous inhibitor of nitric oxide synthesis in chronic renal failure. Lancet 339:572–575, 1992.

254. Muirhead EE: Vasodepressor renal medullary lipids. *In* Dunn MJ (ed): Renal Endocrinology. Williams & Wilkins, Baltimore, 1983, pp 75–95.

255. Smith MC, Dunn MJ: Renal kallikrein, kinins, and prostaglandins in hypertension. *In* Brenner BM, Stein JH (eds): Contemporary Issues in Nephrology: Hypertension. Churchill Livingstone, New York, 1981, pp 168–202.

256. Needleman P, Greenwald JE: Atriopeptin: A cardiac hormone intimately involved in fluid, electrolyte and blood pressure homeostasis. N Engl J Med 314:828–834, 1986.

257. Folkow B: Physiological aspects of primary hypertension. Physiol Rev 62:347–504, 1982.

258. Ibels LS, Alfrey AC, Huffer WE, et al: Arterial calcification and pathology in uremic patients undergoing dialysis. Am J Med 66:790–796, 1979.

259. London GM, Marchais SJ, Safar ME, et al: Aortic and large artery compliance in end-stage renal failure. Kidney Int 37:137–142, 1990.

260. London GM, Guerin AP, Pannier B, et al: Increased systolic pressure in chronic uremia. Role of arterial wave reflections. Hypertension 20:10–19, 1992.

261. Brunkhorst R, Nonnast-Daniel B, Koch KM, Frei U: Hypertension as a possible complication of recombinant erythropoietin therapy. Contrib Nephrol 88:118–125, 1991.

262. Raine AEG: Seizures and hypertension events. Semin Nephrol 10(suppl):40–47, 1990.

263. Duke M, Abelmann W: The haemodynamic response to chronic anaemia. Circulation 39:503–515, 1969.

264. Brunet P, Lorec AM, Roubicek C, et al: Erythropoietin does not increase endothelin in hemodialysis patients. Proceedings of the 12th International Congress of Nephrology, International Society of Nephrology; June 1993; Jerusalem; p 358.

265. Carlini RG, Obialo CI, Rothstein M: Intravenous erythropoietin (rHuEPO) administration increases plasma endothelin and blood pressure in hemodialysis patients. Am J Hypertens 6:103–107, 1993.

266. Vallance P, Benjamin N, Collier J: Erythropoietin, haemoglobin and hypertensive crises. Lancet 1:107, 1988.

267. Hori K, Onoyama K, Iseki K, et al: Hemodynamic changes by recombinant human erythropoietin (rHuEPO) in the treatment of anemic hemodialysis patients. Clin Nephrol 33:293–298, 1990.

268. Pickering TG, Gribben B, Oliver DO: Baroreflex sensitivity in patients on long-term hemodialysis. Clin Sci 43:645–657, 1972.

269. Schwartz AB, Mintz GS, Kim KE, et al: Recombinant human erythropoietin increases MAP, TPRI and systolic and diastolic dysfunction with increased impedance to LV ejection due to increased HCT and rbc mass in patients with CRF. Kidney Int 35:334A, 1989. Abstract.

270. Charra B, Calemard E, Ruffet M, et al: Survival as an index of adequacy of dialysis. Kidney Int 41:1286–1291, 1992.

271. Charra B: How can the mortality rate of chronic dialysis patients be reduced? Semin Dial 6:91–93, 1993.

272. Wizemann V, Kramer W: Short-term dialysis, long-term complications: Ten years experience with short duration renal replacement therapy. Blood Purif 5:193–201, 1987.

273. Lindner A, Douglas SW, Adamson JA: Propranolol effects in long-term hemodialysis patients with renin-dependent hypertension. Ann Intern Med 88:457–462, 1978.

274. Hulter HN, Licht JH, Ilnicki LP, Singh S: Clinical efficacy and pharmacokinetics of clonidine in hemodialysis and renal insufficiency. J Lab Clin Med 94:223–231, 1979.

275. Harter HR, Delmez JA: Effects of prazosin in the control of blood pressure in hypertensive dialysis patients. J Cardiovasc Pharmacol 1:S43–S55, 1979.

276. Wenting GJ, Blankenstijin PJ, Poldermans D, et al: Blood pressure response of nephrectomized subjects and patients with essential hypertension to ramipril. Am J Cardiol 59:92D–97D, 1987.

277. Graziani G, Badalamenti S, Del Bo A, et al: Abnormal hemodynamics and elevated angiotensin II plasma levels in polydipsic patients on regular hemodialysis treatment. Kidney Int 44:107–114, 1993.

278. Oldenburg B, Macdonald GJ, Shelley S: Controlled trial of enalapril in patients with chronic fluid overload undergoing dialysis. Br Med J 296:1089–1091, 1988.

279. Parnes EL, Shapiro WB: Anaphylactoid reactions in hemodialysis patients treated with the AN69 dialyzer. Kidney Int 40:1148–1152, 1991.

280. Schulman G, Hakim R, Arias R, et al: Bradykinin generation by dialysis membranes: Possible role in anaphylactoid reaction. J Am Soc Nephrol 3:1563–1569, 1993.

281. Pegues DA, Beck-Sague CM, Woollen SW, et al: Anaphylactoid reactions associated with reuse of hollow-fiber hemodialyzers and ACE inhibitors. Kidney Int 42:1232–1237, 1992.

282. Zehnder C, Zuber M, Sulzer M, et al: Influence of long-term amelioration of anemia and blood pressure control on left ventricular hypertrophy in hemodialyzed patients. Nephron 61:21–25, 1992.

283. Cannella G, Paoletti E, Delfino R, et al: Regression of left ventricular hypertrophy in hypertensive dialyzed uremic patients on long-term antihypertensive therapy. Kidney Int 44:881–886, 1993.

# Pathophysiology of Uremia

*Robert C. May*
*William E. Mitch*

The term "uremia" was first coined in 1840 by Piorry[1] to indicate a condition caused by "contaminating the blood with urine." It is a complex condition with distinctive signs and symptoms resulting from renal insufficiency, which causes the accumulation of unexcreted waste products. Obviously not all patients with renal failure are uremic. This distinction is important as well as practical because a diagnosis of uremia is an indication for initiation of dialysis.

Important manifestations of the uremic syndrome are listed in Table 49–1. It is not our intention to review all components of the uremic syndrome because they are covered thoroughly in monographs.[2] Instead, we focus on the pathophysiology of the uremic state. Nevertheless, certain inferences pertinent to uremia may be drawn from Table 49–1. First, involvement of multiple organs suggests that several factors are required to produce uremia or that a small number of substances can disturb cellular metabolism by affecting one or more functions that are basic to different cells. These alternatives are not mutually exclusive. Second, the symptoms of uremia do not lend themselves to studies using in vitro systems; consequently, unequivocal identification of any uremic toxins has been a problem. Finally, the central nervous system manifestations are reminiscent of intoxication, which constitutes a strong argument in favor of uremia's being a state of systemic intoxication. Because patients with marginal but stable renal function can become uremic if protein catabolism is accentuated or if they are fed a high-protein diet, uremia can be considered a state of intoxication from protein-derived waste products.

## UREMIC TOXINS

The notion that unexcreted substances accumulate and cause uremia dates back to the early 1900s, when it was noted that removal of kidneys led to a rise in blood urea concentration.[3] The strongest argument for the systemic intoxication concept rests on the repeated finding that symptoms promptly abate on institution of effective dialysis to remove low-molecular-weight substances. Indeed, the impressive, long-term survival of dialysis patients attests to the importance of low- to middle-molecular-weight molecules in causing uremia. Many investigators have attempted to ascertain the identity of uremic "toxins"; with rare exception, these efforts have been unsuccessful.

The difficulty in identifying a specific toxin arises from several factors. Even though protein intake (or catabolism) is closely linked to the severity of symptoms, it is not protein but rather the products of protein degradation plus the ions that always accumulate when foods rich in protein are eaten. In short, the rate of accumulation of nitrogenous compounds varies with dietary protein intake. Because the major end product of amino acid catabolism is urea, it follows that the rate of urea accumulation provides an excellent index of the accumulation of all waste products. Another difficulty with specifying a compound or ion as a toxin is that any list of potential toxins includes compounds arising from metabolism of ingested or secreted proteins by bacteria, and there is evidence of bacterial overgrowth in the small intestines of patients with chronic renal failure.[4, 5] To complicate matters further, combinations of compounds (e.g., urea, magnesium, acetoin, 2,3-butylene glycol, sulfate, creatinine, cresol, and guanidine) impair oxidative metabolism in slices of cerebral cortex, even though separately each agent at the same concentration is nontoxic.[6]

Besides a direct effect on metabolism, waste products could exert a cumulative toxic effect through nonenzymatic modification of proteins. Indeed, carbamylation of hemoglobin by nitrogen from urea has been uncovered in patients with chronic renal failure by use of either high-performance liquid chromatography[7] or enzyme-linked immunosorbent assays.[8] Likewise, Maillard reaction–mediated damage to the extracellular matrix and tissue proteins has been reported in uremia.[9] Because so many substances accumulate

**TABLE 49–1. Manifestations of the Uremic Syndrome**

**Neurologic**

*Central*
Daytime drowsiness and a tendency to sleep progressing to increasing obtundation and eventual coma
Decreased attentiveness and cognitive tasking
Imprecise memory
Slurred speech
Asterixis and myoclonus
Seizures
Disorientation and confusion

*Peripheral*
Sensorimotor peripheral neuropathy, often with burning dysesthesia
Singultus
Restless leg syndrome
Increased muscle fatigability and muscle cramps

**Cardiovascular**
Accelerated atherosclerosis
Cardiomyopathy
Pericarditis

**Pulmonary**
Atypical pulmonary edema
Pneumonitis
Fibrinous pleuritis

**Gastrointestinal**
Anorexia progressing to nausea and vomiting
Stomatitis and gingivitis
Parotitis
Peptic ulcer diathesis
Gastritis and duodenitis
Enterocolitis
Pancreatitis
Ascites

**Dermatologic**
Pruritus
Dystrophic calcification
Changes in skin pigmentation

**Hematologic**
Anemia
Altered neutrophilic chemotaxis
Depressed lymphocyte function
Bleeding diathesis with platelet dysfunction

**Endocrinologic**
Secondary hyperparathyroidism
Carbohydrate intolerance due to insulin resistance
Type IV hyperlipidemia
Altered peripheral thyroxine metabolism
Testicular atrophy
Ovarian dysfunction with amenorrhea, dysmenorrhea, dysfunctional uterine bleeding, cystic ovarian disease

**Ophthalmic**
Conjunctival or corneal calcifications

logic fluids; 2) its concentration in tissue or plasma from uremic subjects should exceed that present in nonuremic subjects; 3) its concentration should correlate with specific uremic symptoms that disappear when the concentration is reduced to normal; and 4) toxic effects of the compound in a test system should be demonstrable at the concentration found in tissue or fluids from uremic patients. All of these criteria have rarely been met, often for technical reasons. First, accurate quantitation of a compound in a fluid as chemically complex as plasma requires separation techniques with exacting precision, such as high-performance liquid chromatography, gas chromatography–mass spectroscopy, or capillary zone electrophoresis.[13–15] Second, there are no specific means of lowering the concentration of a single putative toxin, or even a small group of toxins. Limiting dietary protein or dialysis treatments reduces the concentrations of a host of compounds. With these caveats in mind, we discuss certain proposed uremic toxins.

Before organic compounds are discussed, it should be emphasized that features of uremia can be related to accumulation or depletion of inorganic ions. Changes in ions could cause symptoms directly by impairing cell metabolism or indirectly by provoking other responses, frequently hormonal ones. Evidence for the indirect response is discussed subsequently in the context of the tradeoff hypothesis. In view of the critical role of the kidney in regulating water balance, it is surprising that water intoxication is not more prevalent in patients with renal failure.[16] This is a prime example of the adaptive capacity of the kidney; if adaptation does not occur (e.g., in acute renal failure), hyponatremia occurs frequently, and severe water intoxication can mimic or exacerbate the central nervous system symptoms of uremia.[17] As another example, positive $Na^+$ balance occurring when intake exceeds the limits of excretion aggravates hypertension and can cause pulmonary edema, which may be the major factor causing the pneumonitis of uremia.[18] Fortunately, the adaptive capacity of the damaged kidney generally maintains neutral $Na^+$ balance, even in advanced cases of renal insufficiency[16] (Fig. 49–1).

Metabolic acidosis often accompanies uremia because of the limited capacity to augment renal ammoniagenesis.[19] If not corrected, acidosis can cause nausea, vomiting, anorexia, exercise intolerance,[20] and changes in mental status. Studies with rats have established that metabolic acidosis accelerates skeletal muscle protein catabolism both in vitro[21, 22] and in vivo[23] and stimulates branched chain amino acid oxidation.[24] Correction of the acidosis accompanying uremia largely corrects these abnormalities.[22, 25] These studies have been confirmed in patients. Both ammonium chloride–induced acidemia and the acidemia of chronic renal failure accelerate degradation of whole body proteins and the oxidation of amino acids.[26, 27] The relevance of these findings to patients with chronic renal failure is underscored by the close relationship between predialytic plasma $HCO_3^-$ and muscle valine concentration.[28] They could also blunt or block the metabolic responses that are necessary for preserving lean body mass (Chapter 55). Finally, acidosis can exacerbate renal osteodystrophy by accelerating skeletal mineral loss[29, 30] and contribute to glucose intolerance by causing insulin resistance.[31]

Abnormal trace metal metabolism may contribute to

in body fluids in renal failure, the number of combinations of compounds that could act together to produce toxic reactions is enormous.

Studies aimed at identifying toxins either have attempted to reproduce various aspects of the uremic syndrome in experimental animals by administering an alleged toxin or have used an in vitro system (e.g., cerebral cortex slices or lymphocytes).[10, 11] To prevent uncritical acceptance of conclusions from such studies, Bergstrom and Furst[12] proposed that a toxin should satisfy the following criteria: 1) it should be chemically identified and accurately quantifiable in bio-

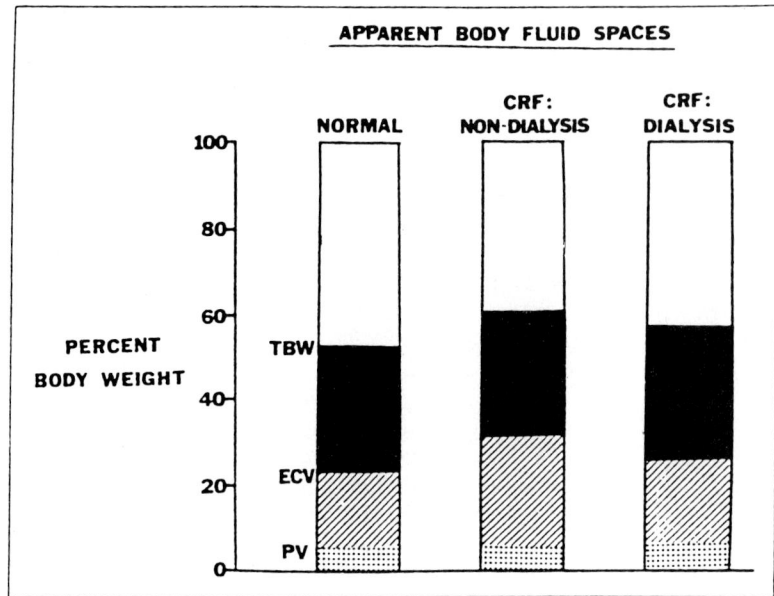

**Figure 49–1.** Diagrammatic representation of the distribution of body water as a percentage of body weight in normal subjects and in patients with chronic renal failure not receiving dialysis or receiving dialysis. Among patients not receiving dialysis, intracellular fluid volume (*dark shaded area*, calculated from the difference between total body water [TBW] and extracellular fluid volume [ECV]) remains normal, yet there is an increase in the extracellular volume because of increases in the plasma volume (PV, *dotted area*) and more especially in the interstitial fluid volume (*cross-hatched area*). These apparent abnormalities in body water distribution are diminished in patients receiving regular dialysis. (From Mitch WE, Wilcox CS: Disorders of body fluids, sodium, and potassium in chronic renal failure. Am J Med 72:536, 1982.)

the uremic syndrome.[32] Oxidized vanadium can inhibit ATPases, including $Na^+,K^+$-ATPase,[33] and the level of serum vanadium is high in chronically uremic patients.[34] Aluminum intoxication from contamination of dialysate with aluminum or ingestion of too much aluminum-containing $PO_4^{3-}$-binding gels can exacerbate renal osteodystrophy and rarely cause mental status changes mistakenly attributed to uremia.[35, 36] Zinc deficiency has been noted in some patients with uremia and has been implicated in testicular atrophy, abnormal taste, and other phenomena frequently present in uremia.[37]

## Products of Protein Metabolism

Several lines of evidence indicate that many symptoms of uremia result from accumulation of products of protein metabolism. For example, a decrease in blood urea nitrogen (BUN) and in the severity of uremic symptoms when dietary protein is restricted has been known for more than 100 years.[38] The production of other putative toxins besides urea (Table 49–2) increases as protein breakdown rises; when renal function is impaired, these compounds accumulate.[39] The importance of waste nitrogen accumulation in mediating symptoms of uremia was underscored by the results of the National Cooperative Dialysis Study, which prospectively compared the clinical outcome of various dialysis regimens. The goal was to maintain BUN at various levels between dialyses (time-averaged concentration of urea [$TAC_{urea}$]) and to determine whether the level of waste nitrogen accumulation resulted in different clinical outcomes.[40] Patients who were maintained at higher $TAC_{urea}$ values had more hospitalizations and more morbid complications of uremia. Moreover, electroencephalogram abnormalities were seen with greater frequency in the groups with higher $TAC_{urea}$, as were such trends in neurobehavioral symptoms as impaired concentration and wakefulness.[41] These results have led to refinements in prescribing dialysis

therapy. The amount of dialysis is based on the need to eliminate urea and can be calculated from mathematic models of urea metabolism.[42] Still, prescriptions based on urea kinetics rely on urea as a substitute for or index of the accumulation of all products of protein metabolism.

The most elegant demonstration of the importance of excess dietary protein in producing uremia was provided by Knochel and colleagues. They found that when patients had uremic symptoms, the resting membrane potential of their skeletal muscles became less negative.[43, 44] However, when they studied patients who had received intensive dialysis for at least 6 weeks, not only were there fewer symptoms of uremia, but skeletal muscle resting membrane potentials were within the normal range[45] (Fig. 49–2). For six hemodialysis patients, the experiment was extended. They had normal muscle membrane potential while eating a diet containing 1 g/kg/d protein, but when the frequency of dialysis was reduced gradually, the membrane potential became abnormal and anorexia, nausea, and vomiting appeared in four patients. At this stage, dietary protein was reduced to 0.5 g/kg/d plus a supplement of essential amino acids.[46] Without a change in the frequency of dialysis treatments, five of the six patients had a return of muscle potential to normal and resolution of their symptoms; the sixth patient did not comply with the restricted diet. There can be little doubt that many symptoms of uremia are due to accumulation of

**TABLE 49–2. Potentially Toxic Compounds That Accumulate in Renal Failure**

| | |
|---|---|
| Urea | Pyridine derivatives |
| Phenols | Guanidino compounds |
| Indoles | $\beta_2$-Microglobulin |
| Skatoles | Aliphatic amines |
| Hormones | Hippurate esters |
| Polyamines | Middle molecules |
| Trace elements | Aromatic amines |
| Serum proteineases | |

## MEMBRANE POTENTIAL MEASUREMENT

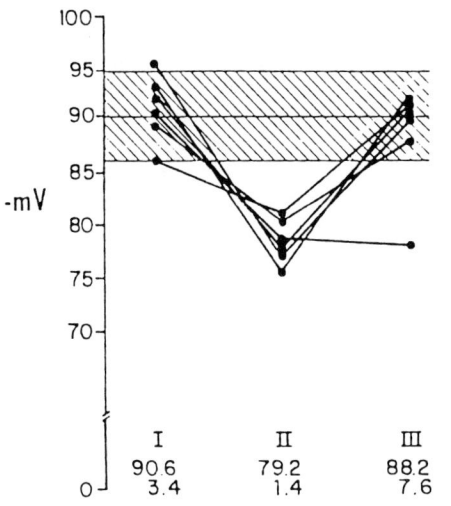

**Figure 49–2.** Transmembrane electrical potential values in six patients with end-stage renal disease were almost all within normal limits ($\pm 5.0$) after they had undergone 6 hours of hemodialysis three times weekly for a long time (I). Successive reduction of dialysis time eventually resulted in a decline of membrane potential to abnormally low values (II). Although dialysis was continued at the same reduced rate, dietary protein intake was reduced from 1.0 to 0.5 g/kg/d, but the diet was supplemented with 6.5 g of mixed essential amino acids. In five patients, membrane potential returned to normal; the remaining patient did not comply with the diet (III).

byproducts of protein metabolism. Some of the leading candidates for uremic toxins are reviewed.

### UREA

The possibility that urea itself might be toxic was initially raised by Richard Bright[47] in 1831. Since then, a large number of studies have examined the toxicity of urea, but the results are inconclusive. In part, conclusions are speculative because of experimental design and the difficulty of measuring the degree of uremia objectively. Administration of urea to normal animals causes rapid but transient shifts in fluid across cell membranes and an osmotic diuresis. Because the half-life of urea is only about 7 hours, it is difficult to sustain a high level of urea in animals or humans with normal kidney function.[48] Consequently, the toxicity of urea has been studied in patients or animals with renal failure, generally by examining the consequences of a dialysis regimen that fails to eliminate urea. Bilaterally nephrectomized dogs were treated by peritoneal dialysis for 4 to 10 days with use of a dialysate supplemented with urea.[49] Within several days, all dogs with BUN values between 173 and 224 mg/dL had weakness, anorexia, and decreased attentiveness. Continued therapy resulted in vomiting, hemorrhagic diarrhea, and hypothermia; eventually, in two of the six dogs, stupor, coma, and death followed. These results contrast with those obtained when both ureters of dogs with normal kidneys were implanted into the gastrointestinal tract.[50] In one dog, a BUN level as high as 808 mg/dL was maintained for weeks without toxic signs. In humans, Merrill and co-workers[51] found no apparent toxic effect

when long-term dialysis patients were dialyzed against urea-supplemented dialysate. In sharp contrast, Johnson and associates[52] gradually increased the urea concentration in the dialysate of stable, long-term hemodialysis patients so that their BUN levels were sustained between 140 and 200 mg/dL for several weeks. Even though ions and other compounds were removed by dialysis, the patients experienced malaise, weakness, lethargy, and a bleeding diathesis after 2 weeks when the BUN level was greater than 190 mg/dL. One patient, however, maintained a BUN level above 130 mg/dL for 90 days yet remained essentially asymptomatic. However, when her BUN level was raised above 190 mg/dL, she also complained of lethargy, malaise, nausea, and vomiting but never had confusion, uremic fetor, or stomatitis. It would appear, therefore, that at least some of the symptoms of uremia—especially nausea, vomiting, malaise, and possibly bleeding—are partly due to intoxication with urea or a product of its metabolism (e.g., ammonia). Because many of the symptoms of uremia cannot be provoked even at extremely high concentrations of BUN, there must be other products resulting from protein breakdown that are uremic toxins. In summary, urea appears to fulfill criteria for a uremic toxin but seems to be clinically important only at extreme concentrations.

In vitro assays of urea toxicity generally use urea concentrations that exceed those in vivo.[53] At such concentrations, urea inhibits argininosuccinate lyase and could exert feedback inhibition of urea production,[54] possibly channeling waste nitrogen into more toxic compounds.[55] A metabolic product that is toxic is ammonia, but systemic blood ammonia levels are normal or minimally elevated in uremia.[56] In aqueous solutions, urea spontaneously decomposes to ammonia, carbonate, or cyanate. Cyanate is potentially important because it can condense with $NH_2$-terminal amino or lysine amide groups in proteins to alter the tertiary structure or change enzyme activity. Indeed, chronic renal failure is associated with excessive carbamylation of hemoglobin.[57] High-performance liquid chromatography and enzyme-linked immunosorbent assays for detecting carbamylated amino acids should expand the investigation as to the importance of protein carbamylation in the uremic syndrome.[7, 8] All steps in the urea cycle, except arginase, are reversible, but the clinical relevance of this feature is unclear. With regard to arginine, its concentration is elevated in hepatocytes of patients with chronic renal failure[58] and could contribute to the production and accumulation of guanidino compounds in uremic patients.[59]

A potential method of redirecting waste nitrogen from the urea cycle would be to take advantage of the amino acid acylation reaction. For example, administration of sodium benzoate to patients with chronic renal failure increased the synthesis of hippurate from glycine by the benzoyl–coenzyme A glycine transferase reaction.[60] Because hippurate is eliminated by both filtration and secretion, it accumulates to a lower degree than urea does. Moreover, benzoate administration sharply reduces urea production. Because plasma glycine and serine levels remained unchanged during benzoate therapy, it was concluded that nitrogen destined for urea must have been redirected toward synthesis of these nonessential amino acids. This strategy has also been used to treat children with inherited disorders of urea cycle enzymes.[61]

## GUANIDINO COMPOUNDS AND ARGININE

Guanidino compounds are strong organic bases that bear the amidino group NCNH; monosubstituted guanidines give a red color in the Sakaguchi reaction with α-naphthol, thymine, sodium hydroxide, sodium hypochlorite, and sodium thiosulfate. Much of the early work on guanidines was flawed by technical problems. The assays had low sensitivity, and the different compounds were incompletely separated.[62] Later studies have identified multiple guanidino compounds in the serum of uremic patients.[59, 63] To date, approximately 120 naturally occurring guanidino compounds have been described; some 27 of them have been identified or isolated from ureotelic animals.[64] DeDeyn and co-workers[59] used a sensitive fluorometric assay after separation by high-performance liquid chromatography and were able to measure the concentration of 13 different guanidino compounds. They found striking elevations in many of these compounds (Table 49–3) and have extended their techniques to measure guanidino compounds from multiple tissues in a variety of animals. There were striking differences in the concentrations among different species.[64] For instance, there is a 100-fold difference in serum concentration of α-keto-δ-guanidinovaleric acid in humans compared with that in dogs.[64] These species differences are also reflected in the urinary excretion of many of the guanidino compounds. Hence, the impact of renal disease on the accumulation of guanidino compounds must vary considerably among species, depending on the compound being studied. In short, conclusions based on experiments in animals must be validated for humans.

High plasma guanidino levels result from an increase in the production rate or a decrease in the renal or extrarenal clearance of the compound. For example, a guanidino compound, such as creatinine, is cleared mainly by the kidney, so decreased renal function leads to high plasma levels. Curiously, the urinary excretion of guanidino compounds in the steady state is actually increased in patients with renal failure, even when dietary protein intake is the same as that of control subjects.[63, 65] This means that in uremia, the renal secretory rate of guanidino compounds is increased because extrarenal clearance of these compounds is negligible. It also implies that the production of these compounds exceeds that of subjects with normal renal function.

The biochemical pathways for synthesis of many of the guanidino compounds are largely unknown. Certain aspects of the metabolism of guanidino compounds are understood. Urinary excretion of both methylguanidine (MG) and guanidinosuccinic acid (GSA) is increased when dietary protein is increased.[63, 65] Indeed, GSA excretion varies linearly with urea production and dietary protein intake.[65] Kopple and associates[65] have reported increased urinary GSA excretion coincident with the catabolism due to a superimposed illness in three uremic patients who had no change in their dietary protein intake. In two of the three, the increase in GSA excretion was paralleled by an increase in urea excretion. Marescau and colleagues[66] compared serum GSA levels in patients who had high plasma arginine levels (hyperargininemia) from urea cycle enzyme defects with those in patients who had chronic renal failure. In the uremic patients, there was a striking linear relationship between GSA and urea levels; in contrast, plasma GSA levels in patients with hyperargininemia were below the level of detection. Nevertheless, even in that group, the urinary GSA level was related to plasma urea concentration, an indication that urea must be the precursor for GSA rather than arginine. Consequently, with low arginine levels that accompany other inherited disorders of urea cycle enzymes, there is a low production rate of both MG and GSA.[67] This relationship between urea production and guanidino synthesis raises another possibility: arginine availability may be an important determinant of the synthetic rate of guanidino compounds. Indeed, feeding an arginine-rich diet increases MG production, but only in patients with renal failure.[68] Similarly, when rats with acute renal failure were given an exogenous load of creatinine, plasma and tissue levels of MG rose.[69] This is thought to reflect the increased production of 5-hydroxycreatinine, the probable precursor of MG.[70]

Although many tissues express certain enzymes that are present in the urea cycle, it is likely that most guanidines

**TABLE 49–3. Levels (Mean ± SD) of Guanidino Compounds and Urea in Serum of Uremic Patients Receiving Maintenance Hemodialysis Before and After a Single Treatment**

| Substance | Control Group (n = 24) | Total Group (n = 30) Before Hemodialysis | Total Group (n = 30) After Hemodialysis |
|---|---|---|---|
| Guanidino compound (μmol/L) | | | |
| Guanidinosuccinic acid | 0.36 ± 0.18 | 13.1 ± 5.99 | 3.58 ± 1.87 |
| Creatine | 57.8 ± 24.5 | 62.7 ± 51.7 | 38.1 ± 22.2 |
| Guanidinoacetic acid | 1.96 ± 0.72 | 2.90 ± 0.76 | 1.37 ± 0.39 |
| N-α-Acetylarginine | 0.16 ± 0.08 | 0.87 ± 0.28 | 0.52 ± 0.22 |
| Arginic acid | 0.08 ± 0.04 | 0.40 ± 0.17 | 0.17 ± 0.09 |
| Creatinine | 73.9 ± 25.0 | 1225 ± 324 | 551 ± 186 |
| γ-Guanidinobutyric acid | <0.025 | 0.23 ± 0.11 | 0.08 ± 0.04 |
| Arginine | 115 ± 25.4 | 127 ± 42.4 | 104 ± 26.4 |
| Homoarginine | 1.86 ± 0.75 | 1.05 ± 0.41 | 0.63 ± 0.25 |
| Guanidine | <0.20–0.40 | 1.85 ± 0.66 | 1.01 ± 0.29 |
| Methylguanidine | <0.10 | 5.24 ± 2.42 | 2.99 ± 1.54 |
| Urea (mmol/L) | 3.3–7.7 | 24.8 ± 4.51 | 9.5 ± 3.2 |

are synthesized in the liver. This may be related to the high activity of glycine transamidinase in liver[71] or to the low rate of arginine export by hepatocytes.[72] In support of a major role of the liver, GSA excretion is undetectable in patients with hepatorenal syndrome.[73] Perez and colleagues[74] used perfused rat livers to demonstrate a progressive increase in the release of [14]C-labeled GSA when the perfusate contained L-[guanidino-[14]C]arginine. Conversely, no [14]C-GSA release was detected if livers were perfused with DL-[guanidino-[14]C]canavanine. They concluded that there is no ''guanidine cycle'' and postulated that creatinine could be synthesized from canavanine in a series of condensation products yielding GSA as a byproduct[73, 75] (Fig. 49–3). This metabolic scheme could explain the close correlation between urea and GSA concentrations, but it seems unlikely that this pathway is a major source of guanidines because canavanine has never been isolated or identified in mammalian tissues and must arise from bacterial metabolism. If a guanidine cycle were active in mammals, one would predict that GSA production should fall when broad-spectrum oral antibiotics are administered. However, GSA excretion was unaffected by the use of antibiotics.[73] Tissue

MG levels are highest in the liver, which suggests that metabolic precursors are produced in hepatocytes.[76] In line with this conclusion, ingestion of L-[guanidino-[15]N]arginine by uremic patients yielded [15]N-MG at levels that initially exceeded those present in creatinine.[74] Thus, arginine may be metabolized to MG and γ-aminobutyric acid. Other evidence for production of guanidines in the liver is that GSA and MG production is high in chronic renal failure patients compared with that in control subjects eating the same amount of protein, which suggests that uremia-induced changes in hepatocyte metabolism are at least partly responsible for the increased production of guanidino compounds. Potential precursors for GSA (arginine, aspartic acid, and urea) are increased in hepatocytes from uremic patients and could raise GSA production by mass action. On the basis of these relationships, Cohen[73] has postulated an inhibitory effect of high concentrations of creatinine or its immediate precursor, guanidinoacetic acid, which leads to a decreased use of arginine to form guanidinoacetic acid. This effect would increase the availability of arginine. In this scheme, arginine donates its amidino group to form other compounds, such as GSA, MG, γ-guanidinobutyric acid, and

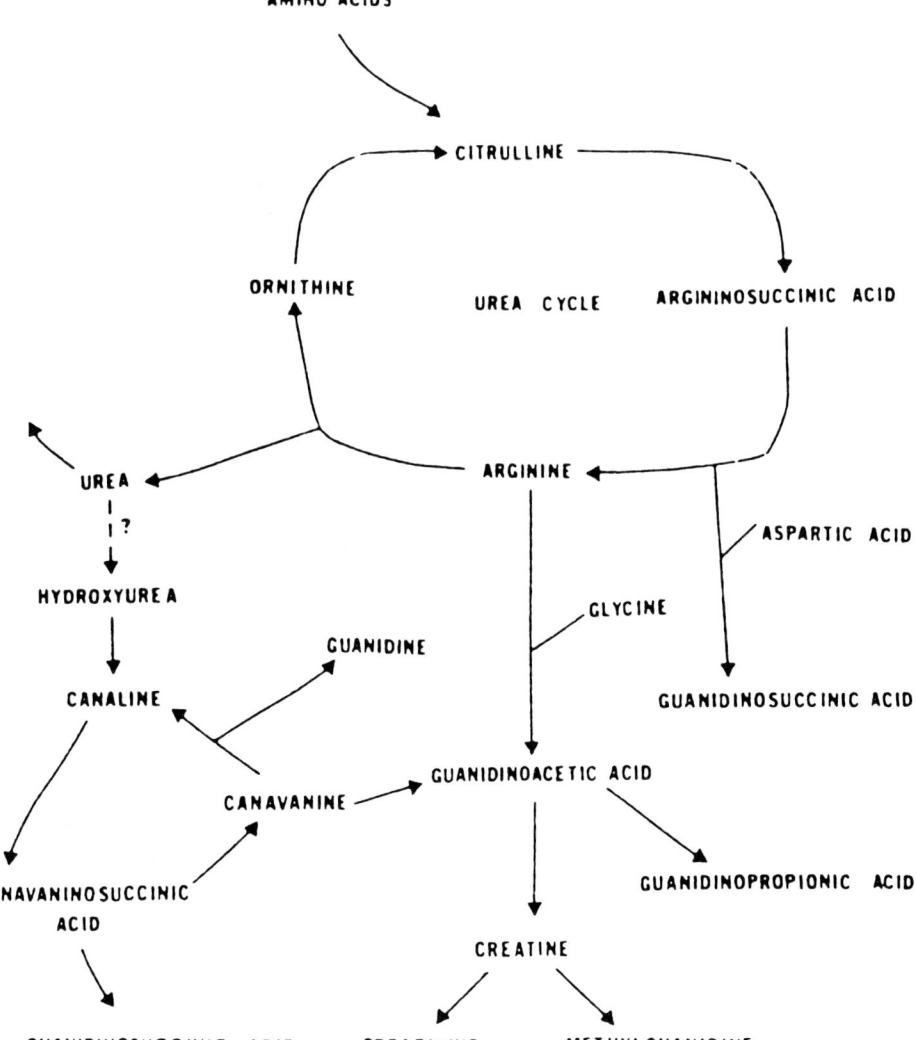

**Figure 49–3.** Proposed relationships between urea metabolism and the production of guanidino compounds. (From Kelly RA, Mitch WE: Creatinine, uric acid, and other nitrogenous waste products: Clinical implication of the imbalance between their production and elimination in uremia. Semin Nephrol 3:286, 1983.)

guanidinopropionic acid. Whether this mechanism or others are correct, there is little doubt that the concentration of guanidino compounds in tissue and plasma increases as renal function declines; their concentrations are best correlated with the level of dietary protein.

Much of the controversy surrounding guanidino compounds as uremic toxins has centered on measurements of plasma and tissue concentrations, especially that of MG. Early studies using the method of Yatzidis and co-workers[77] to measure guanidines noted plasma MG levels as high as 40 μM in uremic patients; these studies were flawed, possibly because creatinine was converted to MG in vitro. Later measurements documented lower levels (8 to 10 μM), but the paucity of MG measurements in human tissues makes the interpretation of MG toxicity in renal failure difficult. Moreover, there can be marked differences in guanidino metabolism among species.[64] For example, Giovannetti and co-workers[76] injected 12 normal dogs with 10 mg of MG three times daily for 20 days. Weight loss and anemia developed in all dogs, and neurologic symptoms (primarily hypertonia and myoclonus) plus decreased nerve conduction velocity were seen in about half of the dogs. However, plasma MG levels in these dogs far exceeded those present in patients. Although the concentration of MG in tissues of uremic patients could be far higher than normal[78] (MG accumulates intracellularly in uremia), it is not known whether intracellular levels would match those in intoxicated dogs. MG has been detected in the cerebrospinal fluid of uremic patients but not in that of normal subjects.[79] The pathophysiologic relevance of this finding is uncertain because others have failed to detect elevated brain MG levels in experimental animal models of renal failure.[78] Other in vitro effects of MG include autohemolysis,[80] inhibition of salivary and exocrine pancreatic secretion,[81] inhibition of $^{59}$Fe uptake by bone marrow cultures,[82] and inhibition of DNA synthesis from lymphocytes.[83] With the possible exception of toxic effects on bone marrow function, MG concentrations used in these studies far exceeded levels likely to be present in vivo. In summary, the evidence for an important role of MG in the toxicity of uremia at present is unconvincing; the compound is undoubtedly toxic in vitro but only at levels unlikely to occur in vivo.

The relationship between symptoms of uremia and the concentrations of GSA in tissues and plasma remains undefined. Rabbits injected with GSA did not show signs of uremia, such as anemia, neurobehavioral changes, or platelet dysfunction.[84] GSA infusion in dogs caused depression of cardiac function[85]; similar effects were not present in guinea pigs.[86] A similar controversy exists regarding GSA and the inhibition of normal platelet function. It has been reported that GSA interferes with ADP activation of platelet factor III and with platelet aggregation in vitro in response to ADP, epinephrine, or collagen[87]; as with cardiac abnormalities, there are reports to the contrary.[79]

Besides MG and GSA, guanidinopropionic acid has been shown to cause autohemolysis of red blood cells and to inhibit glucose-6-phosphate dehydrogenase in vitro.[88, 89] In uremic patients, plasma levels of this compound correlate inversely with red blood cell glutathione concentration, which suggests loss of the protective effect of glutathione

against autohemolysis. Guanidinoacetic acid and γ-guanidinobutyric acid can induce autohemolysis in vitro.[80] Other guanidino compounds may have neurotoxic effects: guanidine and MG have been related to peripheral neuropathy,[90] and infusion of large quantities of γ-guanidinobutyric acid, taurocyamine, homoarginine, and α-keto-δ-guanidinovaleric acid may lower the seizure threshold of experimental animals.[91–94] Changes in the seizure threshold may be relevant; levels of both guanidine and taurocyamine are elevated in the cerebrospinal fluid of rabbits with experimental renal failure.[79] Moreover, DeDeyn and MacDonald[95] have shown that guanidine, MG, GSA, and creatinine, when applied to mouse neurons cultured in vitro, inhibited the response to γ-aminobutyric acid and glycine, most likely by blocking Cl$^-$ channels. These observations may explain the apparent lowering of the seizure threshold in patients with chronic renal failure. Nevertheless, there is no compelling evidence implicating any specific guanidino compound or group of compounds as neurotoxins, at least at the concentrations likely to exist in uremic patients.

Abnormalities in the metabolism of arginine could exert toxic effects because of changes in the nitric oxide pathway in chronic renal failure.[96] Not only is nitric oxide an endogenous vasorelaxant, it also acts as a mediator of cell signaling in macrophages and other cells. For instance, Remuzzi and colleagues[97] reported that the prolonged bleeding time of experimental uremia in rats could be corrected by N-monomethyl-L-arginine, a reversible inhibitor of nitric oxide synthase. These effects were overcome by infusion of L-arginine, but not D-arginine, which attests to the specificity of the inhibition. Endogenous dimethylated derivatives of arginine can inhibit nitric oxide synthase and reduce the production of nitric oxide.[98] It is postulated that different species of dimethylarginines accumulate in uremic patients because of impaired elimination by the kidney.[98, 99] MacAllister and colleagues[99] tested several guanidine-containing compounds for inhibitory action and found that only aminoguanidine, MG, and asymmetric dimethylarginine blunted nitrite production; creatinine, GSA, monomethylarginine, and guanidinopropionate exerted little effect. Within the inhibitory group, only asymmetric dimethylarginine inhibited nitric oxide synthase at concentrations that might be found in vivo. Another potential method of inhibiting nitric oxide synthesis could involve intracellular interactions among amino acids because high concentrations of L-glutamine reduce the production of L-arginine in endothelial cells.[100] This change could also reduce nitric oxide production. The physiologic relevance of inhibiting nitric oxide production is controversial, but it has been suggested that reduced nitric oxide production could contribute to the high prevalence of arterial hypertension in patients with chronic renal failure.[98] Moreover, studies in rats suggest that feeding large amounts of arginine could slow the progressive loss of renal function.[101] However, administration of large quantities of L-arginine to achieve a benefit would undoubtedly increase the production of guanidines. The toxicity of these compounds would have to be controlled by other means. The importance of nitric oxide synthase underscores why a thorough understanding of the metabolism and potential toxicity of guanidino compounds is needed.

## Products of Bacterial Metabolism

Uremic toxins are not limited to products of mammalian metabolism. Exogenous toxins could be ingested or synthesized by gut bacteria and accumulate in renal failure patients because of impaired renal clearance. For instance, potential carcinogens including a variety of heterocyclic amines and tryptophan pyrolysis products are reported to be elevated in plasma of patients with chronic renal failure.[102, 103] Aliphatic amines are high in the plasma of patients with chronic renal failure owing largely to production by gut bacteria.[104] For example, monomethylamine is thought to be derived from bacterial metabolism of creatinine through sarcosine[104] (Fig. 49–4). Bacterial metabolism of choline and lecithin can also produce tertiary methylamines, which are absorbed and either oxidized or demethylated to form secondary methylamines that are excreted in urine or bile.[104] Gastrointestinal absorption of these compounds could lead to toxic effects if they are poorly excreted by the kidney. Trimethylamine-*N*-oxide has been found in the plasma of patients with renal failure[105] and could contribute to the "fishy" smell of these patients. Trimethylamine-*N*-oxide is readily absorbed after a meal of fish and promptly excreted when renal function is normal. Secondary methylamines are at supranormal concentrations in blood, cerebrospinal fluid, and brain tissue of uremic patients[106] and in duodenal aspirates of uremic patients.[104] This may reflect the greater density of bacteria in the small intestines of uremic patients[5] or the higher choline levels in plasma of uremic patients.[107] Alternatively, increased absorption of bacterial products might be related to increased permeability of the gastrointestinal mucosa[108]; this would become more important in patients eating a high-protein diet.[109]

It has been proposed that secondary methylamines contribute to the altered mental state of uremia. Administration of nonabsorbable antibiotics to two patients with uremic encephalopathy resulted in marked improvement in asterixis, myoclonus, mental alertness, and electroencephalographic abnormalities; these benefits coincided with a decline in serum amine levels.[104] However, a decrease in intestinal bacteria could influence a number of compounds. In fact, the survival time of anephric, germ-free rats is nearly twice that of conventionally raised rats.[110]

Secondary methylamines can inhibit neuronal oxidative metabolism, although these in vitro observations have required concentrations of methylamines that far exceed those described in vivo.[111] Understanding the contribution of gastrointestinal bacteria to the uremic syndrome awaits a more detailed taxonomic analysis of bacteria in the small intestine and characterization of nitrogenous byproducts of their metabolism.

Aromatic amines, resulting from bacterial metabolism of tyrosine and phenylalanine, are also elevated in the plasma of uremic patients. These amino acids as well as tryptophan exist in free and conjugated forms,[112, 113] and it is possible that they or other aromatic amines such as tyramine contribute to uremic encephalopathy by serving as false neurotransmitters. There has been no formal demonstration of this possibility. Using mass fragmentographic analysis and gas chromatography, Niwa and associates[112] measured and identified different hydroxyphenolic acids that were markedly elevated in serum from patients undergoing maintenance hemodialysis. The plasma concentrations of *p*-hydroxybenzoic acid and *p*-hydroxyphenylacetic acid, precursors of phenol and *p*-cresol, respectively, were increased to the highest level. As expected, both plasma phenol and *p*-cresol concentrations were increased in uremic patients; the con-

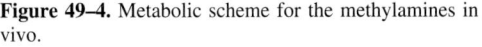

**Figure 49–4.** Metabolic scheme for the methylamines in vivo.

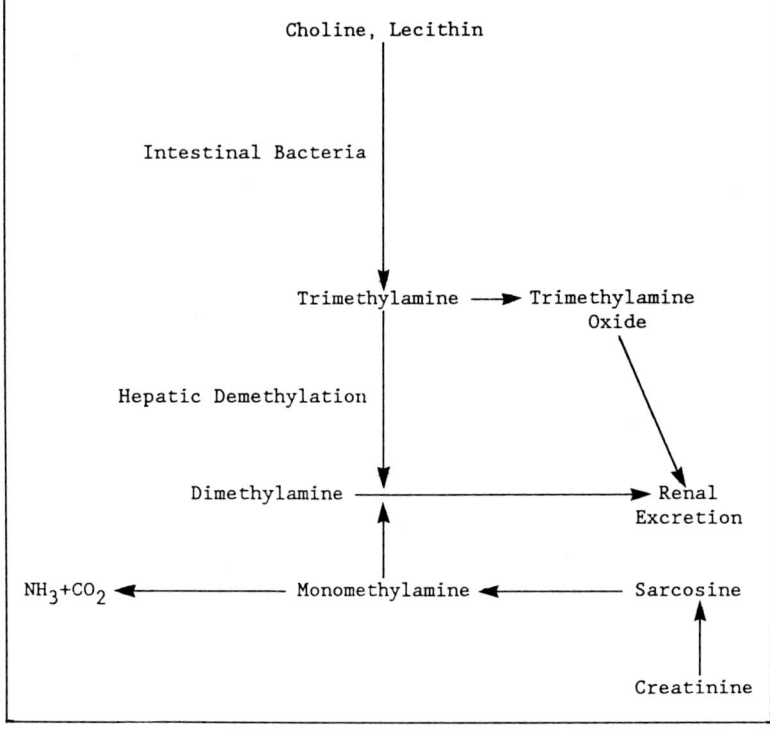

centration of p-cresol (but not of phenol) was found to be proportional to dietary protein.[114] Infusion of phenol or p-cresol into dogs results in a variety of neurologic symptoms,[115] and phenolic acids at concentrations present in serum of uremic patients can change the activity of membrane-bound ATPases.[116] Likewise, conjugated phenols can inhibit ATPases and ion transport systems in different tissues and change the intracellular ionic composition to inhibit normal cellular metabolism.

Another aromatic amino acid, tryptophan, has been implicated in the production of uremic symptoms. Tryptophan undergoes deamination and decarboxylation by gut bacteria, yielding a variety of metabolites that include indole, indoxyl, skatole, skatoxyl, indican, and indoleacetic acid. Several of these compounds are found to be increased in the plasma of uremic subjects and have been suggested as inhibitors of brain slice oxidation.[117] Moreover, patients with uremic encephalopathy have supranormal concentrations of tryptophan, 5-hydroxyindoleacetic acid, and homovanillic acid in their cerebrospinal fluid. Although the pathogenetic importance of high levels of these metabolites is unclear, 5-hydroxyindoleacetic acid is a precursor of the neurotransmitter serotonin,[118] so tryptophan or its metabolites could contribute to uremic encephalopathy. Another byproduct, indoxyl sulfate, may interfere with thyroxine uptake into hepatocytes by competing for binding proteins.[119] Niwa and colleagues[120] were able to show that the ingestion of the activated charcoal adsorbent AST-120 greatly reduced plasma and urinary indoxyl sulfate in rats with chronic renal failure. There was no change in the degree of azotemia, but there were benefits to lowering indoxyl sulfate. When chronically fed rats with chronic renal failure after subtotal nephrectomy were given AST-120, there was a reduced rate of segmental sclerosis and delay in the loss of glomerular filtration.[121] Similarly, Motojima and colleagues[122] reported that AST-120 significantly reduced the degree of glomerular sclerosis in an animal model of progressive renal failure. Micropuncture results revealed that despite higher dietary protein intake, the group receiving the adsorbent had lower transglomerular pressures. Whether AST-120 exerted a protective effect by removing one or more toxic compounds or through lowering transglomerular pressure could not be delineated. An interesting and potentially important observation was that rats receiving AST-120 ate better. Perhaps bacterial products contribute to the anorexia so prevalent among patients with uremia. AST-120 has been licensed for use in Japan, and it is hoped that these provocative animal experiments will be extended to patients with progressive renal failure.

Polyamines are strongly basic, low-molecular-weight compounds that are necessary for cell growth.[123] Putrescine, spermidine, and spermine are synthesized in mammalian tissues, whereas cadaverine and putrescine are formed by decarboxylation of lysine and ornithine by intestinal bacteria. In vitro, spermine is an inhibitor of erythropoiesis, and serum spermine levels vary inversely with the hematocrit of patients undergoing maintenance hemodialysis.[124] The concentration of unconjugated spermidine and spermine in red blood cells is elevated in uremic patients,[125] and plasma levels of free and conjugated spermidine, spermine, cadav-

erine, and putrescine are supranormal in uremic patients even with dialysis treatment.[126] In one study,[126] serum putrescine and spermidine levels were directly correlated with serum creatinine concentration. The significance of these reports is unknown; Bagdade and colleagues[127] hypothesized that a high serum polyamine level in dialysis patients might contribute to accelerated atherogenesis by promoting proliferation of arterial smooth muscle cells. Results of direct testing of this hypothesis are not available.

From this review, it should be obvious why there is so much confusion surrounding what are uremic toxins. Much of the available information is based on correlations between blood or plasma concentrations and changes in symptoms that are difficult to measure. The indirectness of methods used for analyses also creates problems. For example, postulating that uremic encephalopathy can be reversed by broad-spectrum antibiotics could reflect modification of tryptophan metabolites as well as a change in aliphatic amines. Similarly, the renal sparing effect of AST-120 might be due to the adsorption of compounds other than bacterially derived indoles. Although a number of candidates have been suggested as uremic toxins, none has been identified as the cause of uremia. Certain general principles have emerged, however. First, the degree of uremic toxicity is directly related to protein intake (the most severe symptoms occur in patients with the highest dietary protein intake, and most symptoms decline in severity when dietary protein intake is reduced). Second, uremia must involve an impairment of a cell function because there is impairment of multiple tissues in patients with renal failure. The nature of this fundamental defect is obscure; it might be linked to a defect in energy metabolism common to all cells or to an abnormality in intracellular ions leading to secondary metabolic defects.

## MIDDLE MOLECULE HYPOTHESIS

There is a poor correlation between the severity of the uremic syndrome and serum creatinine concentrations. This discrepancy seems most marked in patients who are treated with maintenance peritoneal dialysis. Despite high BUN and creatinine levels, they have few uremic symptoms, and some researchers have claimed that peritoneal dialysis patients are at less risk for the development of peripheral neuropathy than are hemodialysis patients.[128] This suggestion has been disputed.[129] Such observations led Scribner and associates[130] to postulate that the toxic effect was related to accumulation of higher molecular weight substances, which were cleared more readily by peritoneal dialysis than by hemodialysis.

In comparing the permeability characteristics of peritoneal and cellulose-based hemodialysis membranes, it is clear that the peritoneal membrane is more permeable to solutes of middle molecular mass (approximately 500 to 3000 daltons).[131] The middle molecule scheme proposes that molecules within this range are inadequately removed by hemodialysis, which leads to uremic toxicity. The middle molecule hypothesis predicts that shortening the duration of dialysis by using more permeable membranes will jeopardize the adequacy of treatment, even though reducing the concentration of urea and other small solutes might be unaffected. It also predicts that increasing the surface area of dialysis membranes would eliminate more middle molecules than smaller solutes, such as urea, because the concentration gradients of middle molecules would be relatively unaffected. These predictions were tested formally in the prospective National Cooperative Dialysis Study sponsored by the National Institutes of Health. Patients were divided into two groups, each of which received 4.5-hour treatments with dialysis regimens to maximize clearance of small solutes or to provide a lower clearance of small solutes. Two other groups received only 3-hour treatments but the same two levels of solute clearance. Unfortunately, the results are equivocal. Patients with higher BUN values throughout the week (high $TAC_{urea}$) did less well than did groups with low $TAC_{urea}$.[40] In fact, clinical outcomes could be generally predicted by the dimensionless parameter Kt/V, where K is the dialyzer urea clearance, t is the treatment time, and V is the volume of distribution for urea. The probability of developing clinical manifestations of uremia was high (approximately 60%) when Kt/V values were between 0.4 and 0.8 and declined sharply to 13% when Kt/V values were between 0.9 and 1.5.[132] In fact, these results demonstrate the major pathophysiologic role of low-molecular-weight solutes rather than of middle molecules in causing uremia. As discussed earlier, the relationship between outcome and differences in $TAC_{urea}$ may simply be that urea production closely reflects protein intake and thus the production of all protein-derived waste products. The study did not exclude an additional (albeit small) benefit from more efficient clearing of middle molecules with the longer dialysis regimens. In both the high and low $TAC_{urea}$ groups, there was a greater likelihood of uremic complications among patients given the short treatment.[40] Unfortunately, $TAC_{urea}$ values were imperfectly matched between groups treated for different times; $TAC_{urea}$ values were higher in groups whose treatment times were shorter, so it remains possible that middle molecules may play some role in mediating the uremic syndrome.

Few hypotheses in nephrology have generated more controversy than middle molecules. Undoubtedly much of the controversy stems from difficulties in separating and identifying compounds present in small amounts of fluid as chemically complex as plasma. Much of the earlier literature relied on relatively crude separation techniques, so plasma fractions still contained a complex mixture of compounds.

Several approaches have been taken to study middle molecules in plasma. One has been to separate plasma into fractions that contain compounds of different molecular size (e.g., size-exclusion chromatography or ultrafiltration across filters excluding molecules above defined molecular sizes). Furst and co-workers[133] used size-exclusion chromatography to fractionate plasma from patients with renal failure and found ultraviolet-absorbing compounds at apparently greater concentrations than the comparable fractions isolated from normal subjects. Certain of these peaks migrated with molecular masses of middle molecules. Further fractionation using ion exchange chromatography revealed that each peak could be resolved into several peaks[134]; even further fractionation using more sophisticated

methods, such as high-performance liquid chromatography and gas chromatography–mass spectroscopy, has revealed these subpeaks to be heterogeneous mixtures of molecules.[135] Clearly, identifying a single toxin causing a uremic symptom would be a major undertaking.

Another approach to studying middle molecules is to isolate a specific compound with a molecular mass expected to be in the middle molecule range. Since 1938, it has been known that the concentration of certain small polypeptides is increased in plasma from uremic patients.[136] At least 38 Ninhydrin-positive peptides have been isolated from the dialysate,[137] and peptide-bound, N-substituted amino acids are present in high amounts in plasma of patients with chronic renal failure; the level increases as azotemia worsens.[138] The identity of most of these peptides is unknown. Abiko and associates[139–141] isolated four peptides from the plasma of patients with severe uremia and determined their amino acid sequences. The amino acid sequences were identical to those known to be present in other proteins, which led to the conclusion that circulating peptides represent fragments of plasma proteins ordinarily eliminated or metabolized by the kidney. The toxicity of these peptides has not been established, but $\beta_2$-microglobulin, which accumulates in the plasma of patients with renal failure, is the major constituent of amyloid-like deposits present in dialysis-related secondary amyloidosis.[142, 143]

A third approach to identifying toxic middle molecules is to analyze plasma for known compounds with molecular masses in the middle molecule range. For example, a number of hormones or fragments of hormones accumulate in renal failure. Increased parathyroid hormone (PTH) levels are due in part to impaired renal degradation. In animal models of uremia, PTH is implicated in the cause of anemia,[144] platelet dysfunction,[145] encephalopathy,[146] neuropathy,[147] cardiomyopathy,[148] and glucose intolerance.[149] It remains controversial whether similar toxic effects occur in humans with renal disease.

Aside from the indirect nature of this type of evidence, the middle molecule hypothesis has several shortcomings. First, the amazing efficacy with which dialysis removes low-molecular-weight solutes and repairs the uremic syndrome is a powerful argument in favor of low-molecular-weight solutes playing a pathophysiologically pre-eminent role. Second, newer analytic techniques have called into serious question the hypothesis that plasma can be partitioned on the basis of molecular weight by use of only size-exclusion chromatography or ultracentrifugation membranes. In fact, more rigorous investigations of middle molecule fractions of plasma revealed that most solutes are of low molecular mass rather than 500 to 3000 daltons.[135, 150] For example, chemically identified middle molecules include glucuronyl-O-hydroxyhippurate,[151] ascorbic acid 2-sulfate,[152] phenylacetylglutamine,[153] and 3-carboxy-4-methyl-5-propyl-2-furanpropionic acid,[154] but there is little or no evidence that these compounds are toxic. It may be more fitting to think of middle molecules as compounds with a renal or dialyzer clearance similar to that of compounds with a molecular mass between 500 and 3000 daltons. Even this characterization would be too simple because it blurs the distinction between dialyzability and elimination. For instance, MG is easily cleared across cuprophane dialysis

**TABLE 49–4. Endocrine Dysfunction in Chronic Renal Failure**

| Nature of Defect | Hormonal Defects |
| --- | --- |
| Diminished production of renal hormones | Decreased erythropoietin production |
| | Decreased conversion of 25-hydroxyvitamin $D_3$ to 1,25-dihydroxyvitamin $D_3$ |
| Hormonal hypersecretion to re-establish homeostasis | Hyperparathyroidism |
| | Secretion of the "natriuretic hormone" |
| Decreased metabolic clearance of hormones | Follicle-stimulating hormone, luteinizing hormone, prolactin, growth hormone, melanocyte-stimulating hormone, gastrin |
| Blunted feedback response causing increased hormone secretion | Luteinizing hormone, corticotropin, prolactin |
| Defective tissue conversion of prohormone to hormone | Thyroxine to triiodothyronine |
| | 25-Hydroxyvitamin $D_3$ to 1,25-dihydroxvitamin $D_3$ |
| Decreased hormone production | Testosterone |
| End-organ unresponsiveness | Insulin, parathyroid hormone |
| Increased circulating inhibitors of hormones | Somatomedin inhibitory factor |

From May RC, Mitch WE: Chronic renal failure. *In* Branch WT (ed): Office Practice of Medicine, 2nd ed. WB Saunders, Philadelphia, 1987, p 608.

membranes, yet it is poorly removed by dialysis because of its large volume of distribution, its high transcellular concentration gradient, and the slow release of MG from intracellular stores into the plasma pool. Inorganic phosphorus has similar properties: it is readily dialyzable but poorly removed by dialysis. A final problem in identifying a toxic middle molecule is that in vitro toxicity assays are highly sensitive to pH, ionic strength, trace elements, or other factors that vary considerably among fractions obtained from size-exclusion chromatography.[144] Thus, assays of middle molecule toxicity must be carefully controlled to prevent misidentification. Partly on the basis of these complexities, Vanholder and colleagues,[155, 156] have proposed that dialysis adequacy be more extensively defined in terms of a variety of simultaneously determined plasma solutes.

In summary, the middle molecule hypothesis remains controversial and unproven, despite a great deal of research. Regardless, investigation of the hypothesis has led to considerable improvements in artificial membrane design. It is paradoxical that innovations in membrane design have yielded a high-flux membrane that maximizes clearance of small solutes rather than middle molecules. A better understanding of the toxicity of middle molecules awaits newer separation techniques.

## ENDOCRINE CONTRIBUTION TO UREMIC SYNDROME

A large number of hormonal systems are affected by chronic renal failure,[157] yet it remains unclear to what extent endocrine perturbations are responsible for manifestations of the uremic syndrome. On the one hand, it is clear that secondary hyperparathyroidism may be responsible for certain complications (e.g., osteodystrophy; see Chapter 51). On the other hand, end-organ resistance to certain hormones (e.g., insulin) results from uremia rather than altered hormone production or elimination. In evaluating an endocrinopathy, it is important to realize that prohormones (e.g., proinsulin, proglucagon)[158, 159] or fragments of hormones (e.g., COOH-terminal fragment of PTH) accumulate in chronic renal failure and cross-react with the antibodies used in immunoassays. These fragments or prohormones

may be far less biologically active than the intact hormone, and high levels can lead to the erroneous diagnosis of endocrine system hyperfunction. To avoid this problem, it is crucial to know the specificity of antibodies used in a specific hormone assay.

There can be several defects in endocrine dysfunction in chronic renal failure (Table 49–4). First, the production of a hormone produced by the kidneys, such as erythropoietin or 1,25-dihydroxycholecalciferol, can be inadequate, resulting in anemia and osteomalacia, respectively. Second, the kidneys are responsible for the metabolic clearance of several peptide hormones, and loss of kidney mass prolongs their half-lives. Ordinarily, this would elevate the plasma levels and decrease production of the hormones through classic feedback loops. Because there appears to be an additional defect in the feedback response of a number of hormonal systems (see Table 49–4), suppression of production may not occur, leading to a sustained increase in the hormone concentration. For example, Sievertsen and co-workers[160] reported that the plasma prolactin level was high in 70% of 73 patients receiving maintenance hemodialysis. The pharmacokinetics of prolactin in these patients indicated a prolonged half-life (180% of control subjects) due to delayed clearance as well as an increase in pituitary production. The higher secretion rate is most likely caused by a lactotroph unresponsive to the inhibitory effects of dopamine, because prolactin disappearance was markedly prolonged even during a dopamine infusion of 4 μg/kg/min. Third, uremia may exert toxic effects on endocrine glands. This effect is prominent in the gonads, resulting in deficiencies in gonadol steroid production.[161] Besides limited gonadal function, hormonal deficiencies can cause other abnormalities, such as deficiencies in androgen-dependent hepatic cytochrome P-450 oxidases.[162] Fourth, uremia may be associated with an increase in circulating inhibitors of hormone action. For example, there are inhibitors of the action of somatomedin or insulin-like growth factors.[163] Finally, uremia can induce target tissues' resistance to a hormone. Unfortunately, characterization of the biochemical mechanism causing hormonal resistance awaits a better understanding of the intracellular events that mediate the action of the hormone.

One of the most intensively studied examples of end-organ resistance is that involving insulin. Despite a prolonged half-life due to impaired renal clearance[164] and a higher plasma level of insulin, patients with chronic renal failure typically exhibit glucose intolerance. This is not due to excessive hepatic gluconeogenesis but results from an impaired response of target organs to insulin.[165] Westervelt[166] reported a decrease in forearm glucose uptake in response to infused insulin in patients with chronic renal failure and concluded that the glucose intolerance of renal failure was due to insulin resistance in skeletal muscle. Smith and DeFronzo[167] evaluated insulin resistance in seven patients with chronic renal failure (average plasma creatinine level, 7.1 mg/dL) using the euglycemic insulin clamping technique at different infusion rates of insulin. With this technique, the amount of glucose required to maintain plasma glucose at the preinfusion level provides a direct measure of the quantity of glucose metabolized in response to each level of insulin infused. Patients with renal failure metabolized less glucose at each insulin level and had a lower maximal rate of glucose metabolism than did normal subjects (Fig. 49–5). The insulin concentration required for half-maximal response in uremic patients was nearly twice that of control subjects (187 versus 96 $\mu$U/mL). They also found that the amount of [125]I-labeled insulin specifically bound to monocytes from patients with chronic renal failure was similar to control values and concluded that uremia must cause insulin resistance by affecting a postbinding event to alter intracellular hormone action. The mediation of the postreceptor defect has not been identified,[168] but the defect is undoubtedly present in skeletal muscle[169] and involves $K^+$ and glucose uptake.[170]

On binding to its ligand, the insulin receptor undergoes an activation step that requires phosphorylation of certain tyrosine residues in the $\beta$-subunit of the receptor. Phosphorylation confers on the receptor tyrosine kinase activity toward other substrates.[171–173] A well-defined substrate of the receptor tyrosine kinase activity is insulin receptor substrate-1. On phosphorylation, this protein may serve a docking function bringing together enzymes critical for subsequent events in the insulin cascade, such as an insulin-specific phosphatidylinositol kinase activity.[174] The activated insulin receptor is rapidly deactivated by a member of the poorly characterized tyrosine phosphoprotein phosphatase family.[175] To date, published studies examining postbinding steps inhibited by uremia have focused on either the in vitro rate of autophosphorylation of the receptor or the tyrosine kinase properties of the receptor with use of a variety of artificial substrates. Studies using insulin receptors from skeletal muscle of uremic rats[176] or humans[177] have failed to reveal any abnormalities. Whether uremia affects other steps (e.g., impaired activity of protein phosphatases, or the phosphorylation of insulin receptor substrate-1) is not known with certainty, but preliminary data suggest that uremia decreases phosphatase activity.[178] Thorough understanding of the insulin resistance of uremia depends on better delineation of subsequent intracellular cascade events mediated by insulin.

Another complex example of end-organ resistance in uremia involves thyroid hormone. Patients with uremia are often intolerant of cold and have low body temperatures. A large prospective study involving more than 300 dialysis patients revealed a high frequency of goiters (43% versus 6% in control subjects) that could not be attributed to antithyroid medications.[179] In animal models of uremia, the presence of goiter appears to be related to accumulation of iodide caused by impaired renal excretion.[180] Patients undergoing dialysis have a high frequency of subnormal plasma levels of total thyroxine ($T_4$), triiodothyronine ($T_3$), and free thyroid hormones and higher levels of thyroid-stimulating hormone. There appears to be decreased peripheral conversion of $T_4$ to $T_3$,[181] as seen in other states of euthyroid sick syndrome,[182] plus an additional end-organ resistance to $T_3$. For example, the basal rate of oxygen uptake by uremic patients was normal but there was a blunting of stimulation by administration of $T_3$.[183] Despite impaired peripheral conversion of $T_4$ to $T_3$, the pituitary-hypothalamic axis appears to be intact because supplements of $T_3$ suppress thyroid-stimulating hormone release whereas ipodate administration (to suppress peripheral conversion of $T_4$ to $T_3$) results in normal stimulation of thyroid-stimulating hormone release. Thus, there is evidence for abnormal thyroid metabolism at several levels in uremia: inefficient iodination in the thyroid gland, depressed $T_4$ to $T_3$ conversion, and suppressed thermogenic response to $T_3$.

These examples of endocrine abnormalities highlight the complex nature of the defects in cellular metabolism induced by uremia. The mediators of or toxins responsible for these defects are unknown.

## TRADEOFF HYPOTHESIS

The accumulation of ions or waste products stimulates responses to the loss of functional renal mass that appear to act to preserve homeostasis. However, the responses, in turn, may exert toxic effects with severe loss of renal mass. Thus, there is a tradeoff for effector systems; homeostasis is achieved, but at the expense of systemic intoxication.

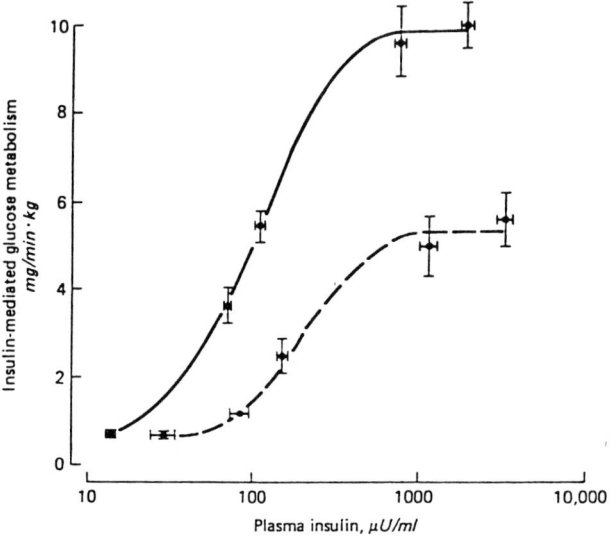

**Figure 49–5.** Dose-response relationship between the plasma insulin concentration and insulin-mediated glucose metabolism in seven uremic subjects *(dashed line)* and nine control subjects *(solid line)*. (From Smith D, DeFronzo RA: Insulin resistance in uremia mediated by postbinding defects. Kidney Int 22:54, 1982.)

The hypothesis that certain aspects of uremia may result from a tradeoff of activation of adaptations has been eloquently presented by Bricker.[184] The most persuasive example of the tradeoff hypothesis involves increasing PTH-mediated control of $PO_4^{3-}$ homeostasis as renal function deteriorates. Because there is no adaptive decrease in gastrointestinal $PO_4^{3-}$ absorption with progressive renal insufficiency, a greater proportion of filtered $PO_4^{3-}$ must be excreted ($FE_{PO_4}$). At least part of the increase in $FE_{PO_4}$ is related to the increase in circulating PTH stimulated by hypocalcemia (attributed to retention of $PO_4^{3-}$). Despite declining renal function, PTH is able to re-establish $PO_4^{3-}$ homeostasis by increasing $FE_{PO_4}$ until the glomerular filtration rate falls below 25% that of normal subjects.[184] One consequence of prolonged hyperparathyroidism is renal osteodystrophy (see Chapter 51). If aspects of the uremic syndrome are due to tradeoff of higher levels of a hormone for homeostasis, it would be expected that these same physiologic events would be alleviated by reducing intake in proportion to the reduction in glomerular filtration rate. Rutherford and associates[185] investigated this issue by reducing phosphate intake in proportion to the loss of renal function in a group of dogs; dogs receiving the low-phosphate diet maintained normal $FE_{PO_4}$, and renal osteodystrophy was prevented. Because the groups of dogs were well matched for the degree of azotemia, glomerular filtration rate, and filtered $PO_4^{3-}$ load, it appears that $PO_4^{3-}$ homeostasis was achieved in the group not receiving low phosphate diet by PTH, which in turn led to the development of renal osteodystrophy. Although studies of patients with early renal insufficiency have failed to reveal hyperphosphatemia, this may, in fact, be an early manifestation of hyperparathyroidism.[186, 187] However, in vitro studies examining the solubility of calcium phosphate have cast doubt on the tradeoff hypothesis. Adler and associates[188] noted that serum $PO_4^{3-}$ concentrations would have to increase by 3.7 mg/dL before serum $Ca^{2+}$ would be lowered to a level sufficient to stimulate PTH release. Although details of the tradeoff hypothesis as originally formulated may change, it remains an intriguing concept that underscores the complexity of achieving electrolyte homeostasis in the setting of progressive renal failure.

Bricker[184] extended the tradeoff hypothesis to more speculative effector hormones or factors that lead to $Na^+$ homeostasis despite a reduction of renal function. If an increase in the fractional excretion of $Na^+$ ($FE_{Na}$) that occurs regularly in advancing renal insufficiency were due exclusively to mechanisms confined to the kidney, they argued, $FE_{Na}$ should remain high in severe renal failure regardless of dietary sodium intake. Yet, $FE_{Na}$ was found to be normal if dietary sodium was reduced gradually, which led to the postulate that $FE_{Na}$ was increased by a circulating factor that inhibits tubule $Na^+$ reabsorption.[189] This factor could cause uremic symptoms by interfering with $Na^+$ transport in other tissues (e.g., blood vessels; see later). Schmidt and colleagues[190] used a dog model of chronic renal failure to show that reducing dietary sodium in proportion to the loss of glomerular filtration rate restores $FE_{Na}$ to normal and prevents the appearance of bioassayable natriuretic factor in the serum of dogs with renal failure. Although the tradeoff hypothesis is intriguing, it draws largely on indirect

results and an inability to identify effector compounds unequivocally (see later).

## ION TRANSPORT ABNORMALITIES IN UREMIA

Although our understanding of the complex metabolic derangements that compose the uremic syndrome has improved, there are many unanswered questions about defects in specific cellular and subcellular functions. Some of the most fundamental derangements relate to observations that plasmalemma ion transport in a number of tissues is affected by renal failure in both animals and humans with renal insufficiency. The result of such transport abnormalities might change membrane potential as measured by Knochel and colleagues (see previous discussion) and intracellular ions. Such a change would have a major impact on cellular metabolism, especially the metabolism of substrates that require transmembrane ion gradients for their uptake.

### Abnormal Active Sodium-Potassium Transport in Erythrocytes

The initial observation that cellular ion homeostasis is abnormal in uremia was made in the early 1960s by Welt and colleagues.[191] They reported that 25% of patients with end-stage renal disease had a high red blood cell $Na^+$ content. Using ouabain as a specific inhibitor of $Na^+,K^+$-ATPase, they showed that red blood cell $Na^+,K^+$-ATPase activity was reduced in 50% of the uremic patients they studied. Patients with a high cell $Na^+$ content also exhibited low $Na^+,K^+$-ATPase activity in red blood cells and were clinically more ill than the patients with normal cell $Na^+$ content. Although there was no correlation between red blood cell $Na^+$ content and BUN level, both the cell $Na^+$ concentration and $Na^+,K^+$-ATPase activity were improved by hemodialysis. Finally, red blood cells from normal subjects acquired a similar defect in active cation transport when they were incubated in serum obtained from patients with elevated cell $Na^+$ content, but not when they were incubated in serum from patients with normal red blood cell $Na^+$ content.[192]

Since this initial observation, there has been a reasonably consistent characterization of the red blood cell ion transport abnormalities due to uremia. A number of reports have confirmed Welt's original observations to a various extent[193–198] and have extended these observations to leukocytes,[199] intestinal epithelia,[200] and skeletal muscle[45] from uremic subjects. Finding $Na^+,K^+$-ATPase defects in other tissues is important because red blood cells have a uniquely low rate of $Na^+$ transport by $Na^+,K^+$-ATPase and permeability to $Na^+$. In contrast, $Na^+$ transport by leukocytes is similar to that by cells in other tissues (approximately 50-fold higher than in red blood cells). $Na^+$ transport in leukocytes correlates with $Na^+$ transport in smooth muscle from resistance vessels, at least in hypertension.[201] Although others fail to demonstrate a significantly higher red blood cell $Na^+$ content, the difference may lie in the intensity of the dialysis treatments.[197, 198, 202–206] Such an explanation is consistent with the finding by Cheng and colleagues,[197] who reported that the subset of patients with elevated red blood cell $Na^+$ concentration also had higher serum creatinine levels. Using high-resolution nuclear magnetic resonance, Monti and colleagues[207] confirmed that in a subgroup of uremic patients with elevated red blood cell $Na^+$ content, there was depressed $Na^+,K^+$-ATPase activity. They could not find abnormalities in membrane lipids to explain their findings. Few investigators have controlled for the relatively younger average age of red blood cells in patients with renal failure; this may be important because young red blood cells, on average, have a lower intracellular $Na^+$ concentration, owing at least in part to a greater number of $Na^+$ pumps per cell.[208] It is also not known how the absence or low levels of erythropoietin might alter cell $Na^+$ content.

In contrast to the reasonably consistent findings of high red blood cell $Na^+$ content in a subgroup of patients with chronic renal failure, studies examining the density of red blood cell $Na^+$ pumps or $Na^+,K^+$-ATPase–mediated cation flux appear contradictory. For example, both Izumo[198] and Kelly[206] and colleagues reported that the number of $Na^+$ pumps per cell (measured by $^3H$-ouabain binding) is normal in dialysis patients and does not correlate with cell $Na^+$ content. Cheng and co-workers[197] found a striking reduction in red blood cell $^3H$-ouabain binding in patients with high cell $Na^+$ content; the degree of reduced ouabain binding was correlated with red blood cell $Na^+$ concentration. Most investigators measure $Na^+$ pump–mediated cation flux by measuring either ouabain-inhibitable $K^+$ influx ($^{86}Rb$ is usually substituted for the more unstable $^{42}K$) or $Na^+$ efflux from erythrocytes. Under physiologic conditions, the intracellular $Na^+$ concentration is near the level that results in half-maximal stimulation of the pump (about 7 mEq/L). To measure cation flux rates, the cells are studied without manipulating intracellular $Na^+$ or after treatment with ionophores to set the intracellular $Na^+$ at a predetermined level yielding maximal activity (usually $>30$ mEq/L). In general, cation flux rates in $Na^+$-loaded cells correlate well with the total number of $Na^+$ pumps measured by $^3H$-ouabain binding even when the red blood cells are from dialysis patients.[197, 206] Corry and co-workers[209] found that cation transport was normal in $Na^+$-loaded cells, which was consistent with their failure to detect differences in either red blood cell $Na^+$ concentration or $^3H$-ouabain binding. Izumo and associates[198] reported that ouabain-inhibitable $^{86}Rb$ influx rates were lower in non–$Na^+$-loaded red blood cells from dialysis patients; $^3H$-ouabain binding was unaffected. Unfortunately, they did not report any observations on $Na^+$-loaded cells. Likewise, Cheng and colleagues[197] examined cation flux in red blood cells of dialysis patients with high cell $Na^+$ values and increased $^3H$-ouabain binding. Ouabain-sensitive $^{42}K$ influx was normal in cells freshly isolated from such patients, whereas maximal $^{42}K$ influx determined in $Na^+$-loaded cells was reduced; the degree of this change correlated well with the degree to which $^3H$-ouabain binding was reduced. They concluded that the $Na^+$ pump turnover rates were normal in patients with elevated red blood cell $Na^+$ content because the higher intracellular $Na^+$ concentration stimulates $Na^+,K^+$-ATPase, thereby leading to normal $^{42}K$ influx rates from fresh cells.

If maximal $Na^+,K^+$-ATPase activity is reduced in some patients with renal failure, what defects could explain such findings? Virtually all reports suggest that the abnormality improves with long-term aggressive dialysis,[210–212] which indicates reversibility of the defect (unless it is limited only to older red blood cells). Potential mechanisms for inhibition of $Na^+,K^+$-ATPase in uremia include 1) accumulation of uremic factors that inhibit the $Na^+$ pump; 2) alteration of the lipid composition of cell membranes to change pump activity; 3) impairment of the action of hormones that change pump activity (e.g., insulin); and 4) change in the activity of other ion transporters to affect the $Na^+$ pump indirectly. These potential explanations are not mutually exclusive (see later).

## TOXINS AND ENDOGENOUS INHIBITORS

The mature red blood cell is incapable of protein synthesis and cannot respond to increased intracellular $Na^+$ concentration or to a circulating inhibitor of the $Na^+$ pump by synthesizing additional pumps. Still, short-term interventions can change the activity of the pump. For example, hemodialysis or transplantation results in a prompt improvement in $Na^+,K^+$-ATPase activity,[194, 198, 203, 204, 211, 213, 214] although the degree of improvement correlates better with the net fluid removed than with changes in BUN.[198, 210, 214, 215] In one such study, Izumo and co-workers[198] reported that a hemodialysis treatment led to a 21% increase in ouabain-sensitive $^{86}Rb$ influx without affecting $^3H$-ouabain binding. In the absence of any changes in the red blood cell electrolyte content, dialysis must have removed an inhibitor of the $Na^+,K^+$-ATPase. Likewise, Kelly and associates[206] found that hemodialysis-related changes in ouabain-sensitive $Na^+$ efflux were correlated with dialysis-related changes in intracellular $Na^+$ concentration. On the other hand, hemodialysis does not appear to change cationic flux when $Na^+$-loaded cells are used.[197, 202, 206] These findings would suggest that the inhibitor is not dialyzable.

Putative inhibitors of the $Na^+$ pump have been described[216, 217]; the heterogeneity of these factors underscores the difference in assay systems. In general, the presence of an inhibitor is detected as $Na^+,K^+$-ATPase activity measured in vitro or as cross-reactivity in radioreceptor assays[218, 219] with use of antibodies directed against cardiac glycosides; radioimmunoassays based on $^3H$-ouabain displacement have also detected inhibitors.[219–222] Both ouabain[223, 224] and a compound chemically similar to digoxin[225] have been isolated from human sources. Whether these factors are pathophysiologically important as inhibitors of $Na^+,K^+$-ATPase in uremia is not certain. Certain observations suggest that the uremic factor differs from digoxin and ouabain because digoxin-like immunoreactive factors are highly protein bound, unlike either digoxin or ouabain.[226] Indeed, Dasgupta and Peng[226] reported that digoxin-like factors are bound to unidentified proteins between 30,000 and 40,000 daltons and thus are not albumin (67,000 daltons). Others report that $Na^+$ pump inhibition does not correlate with the natriuretic or the pressor activities partially purified from human urine.[227] Thus, distinguishing natriuretic factors such as those acting in the tradeoff hypothesis of Bricker from inhibitors of the $Na^+$ pump is difficult.[228–232]

## ABNORMALITIES OF MEMBRANE COMPOSITION AND FUNCTION

At least a portion of the digitalis-like activity present in normal human plasma is due to polar lipids, including non-esterified fatty acids (NEFAs) and certain lysophospholipids.[233–236] These findings have generated renewed interest in the possibility that intrinsic abnormalities of the plasma membrane could affect transmembrane cation flux in uremia. Kelly and associates[206] demonstrated that only patients who have a relatively large decrease in the NEFA content of red blood cell membranes during dialysis have an immediate improvement in ouabain-sensitive $Na^+$ efflux rates. Indeed, among patients with at least a 10% drop in red blood cell content after dialysis, improvement in $Na^+$ pump activity was correlated with the degree to which NEFAs were reduced. The same improvement was confirmed by simply incubating the red blood cells in delipidated albumin to reduce membrane NEFA content. It is unlikely that NEFAs or lysophospholipids directly and specifically inhibit the pump; more likely, these compounds affect the pump by altering physical characteristics within the lipid bilayer or at least within lipid domains that affect the function of $Na^+$ pumps. Reduced red blood cell membrane fluidity has been described in uremia; it was ascribed to a decline in the molar ratio of phosphatidylcholine to sphingomyelin.[237] Changes in membrane permeability are consistent with the findings of altered permeability to both creatinine and uric acid in red blood cells from uremic patients.[238]

## ABNORMAL HORMONAL MILIEU AND ERYTHROPOIESIS IN UREMIA

Another potential explanation for the decrease in red blood cell $Na^+$ pump activity in some uremic patients is impaired synthesis of $Na^+,K^+$-ATPase by immature red blood cell precursors in the bone marrow. Consistent with this possibility, Cheng and co-workers[197] separated red blood cells by age gradient density centrifugation and found that patients with chronic renal failure tended to have fewer $Na^+$ pumps in the youngest cells. The difference could be due to local factors within the marrow that reduce the synthesis or translocation of pumps to the membrane. For example, the resistance to insulin might change pump number because insulin stimulates the $Na^+$ pump in a variety of tissues.[239, 240] Uremia-induced changes in thyroid hormone, mineralocorticoids, or catecholamines affect active $Na^+$ and $K^+$ transport in other tissues as well as in red blood cells.[237–244] Unfortunately, no definitive studies allow firm conclusions about the identity of an $Na^+,K^+$-ATPase inhibitor.

## ABNORMALITIES IN OTHER ERYTHROCYTE CATION TRANSPORT PATHWAYS

In addition to impaired $Na^+$ pump–mediated cation flux, defects in bumetanide-sensitive $Na^+$-$K^+$-$2Cl^-$ cotransport

and $Na^+/Li^+$ exchange and depressed $Ca^{2+}$-ATPase activity have been described in red blood cells of patients with chronic renal failure. Most investigators have reported that $Na^+$ efflux through $Na^+$-$K^+$-$2Cl^-$ transporters is reduced in red blood cells of dialysis patients[202, 206, 209, 210]; some investigators have found virtually no $Na^+$-$K^+$-$2Cl^-$ activity.[202, 206] Kelly and colleagues[206] found that cotransport rates increased acutely after a hemodialysis treatment, similar to stimulation of the $Na^+$ pump.[245] The decrease in cotransporter activity cannot be explained by changes in the affinity of the cotransporter for intracellular $Na^+$,[209] nor was the decrease due to high plasma $K^+$ values[246, 247] or changes in cell volume.[209] Woods and co-workers[248] first reported that $Na^+/L^+$ exchange was increased in red blood cells of black persons treated by dialysis relative to that of normal white persons; the rate was decreased by a dialysis treatment. Such an effect could be seen when red blood cells from normal subjects were incubated in either normal saline or predialysis plasma, but not with incubation in postdialysis plasma. Although the authors infer the presence of a circulating digitalis-like factor, others cannot reproduce these findings.[202, 205, 214, 245, 249, 250] A report also noted that $Na^+/H^+$ exchange activity is increased in red blood cells of dialysis patients but concluded that $Na^+/Li^+$ exchange activity is normal in uremic patients, which casts doubt on this transport function as an index of uremia.[251] Finally, Zidek and co-workers[252] observed that the intracellular $Ca^{2+}$ level was elevated in red blood cells from patients on maintenance hemodialysis, and this was due to depression in both basal and maximal $Ca^{2+}$-ATPase activity. As with other transport systems, the abnormalities could be reproduced in red blood cells from normal subjects by incubating the cells in plasma from uremic patients.

All of these reports revealing changes in cation transport pathways in red blood cells were carried out in the last decade in studies of patients who were well dialyzed by other criteria. The more marked and consistent abnormalities reported in earlier descriptions of defective ouabain-sensitive cation flux in red blood cells of uremic patients might not have been present if those patients had had more vigorous dialysis. Consequently, the condition of the groups of patients being studied must be carefully defined and the methods used to measure transport should be rigorously standardized to facilitate comparisons of data from different laboratories. The notion that the $Na^+$ pump activity is abnormal in only a cohort of patients with chronic renal failure raises the possibility that the measurement could be used to define the adequacy of dialysis, but prospective studies to show prognostic significance are needed.

## Abnormal Membrane Potential in Skeletal Muscle

Aside from red blood cells, the only tissue from uremic humans in which transmembrane ion flux has been studied is skeletal muscle. As discussed earlier, Knochel and colleagues[45] observed a significant fall in membrane potential in patients whose creatinine clearance had fallen below 6 mL/min. If this defect were due to a primary abnormality in the $Na^+$ pump, they should have found high intracellular

Na$^+$ and Cl$^-$ concentrations and low intracellular K$^+$ concentration, which they did. They also found that the resting membrane potential returned to normal with regular hemodialysis or when a less frequent dialysis schedule was accompanied by a low-protein essential amino acid–supplemented diet. These studies have been extended by Aparicio and co-workers,[253] who observed a decrease in leukocyte Na$^+$,K$^+$-ATPase activity from predialysis patients with chronic renal failure; this impairment was fully reversed by treating the patients with a 0.3 g/kg/d protein diet plus a supplement of amino and keto acids. Taken together, these data strongly suggest that abnormal membrane ion flux could result from the accumulation of some dialyzable uremic toxin derived from dietary protein.[254]

## ION TRANSPORT ABNORMALITIES IN EXPERIMENTAL RENAL FAILURE

Insights into mechanisms underlying the pathophysiologic process of uremia have been gained by use of animal models of renal failure, usually the adult rat.[255] Early studies of rats with acute renal failure uncovered a generalized defect in Na$^+$,K$^+$-ATPase activity.[256, 257] Fraser and colleagues[258] studied Na$^+$ transport in synaptosomes obtained from homogenized cerebral cortex. When synaptosomes from acutely uremic rats were incubated with veratridine, a toxin that induces persistent activation of voltage-sensitive Na$^+$ channels, there was a substantial increase in Na$^+$ uptake compared with that of synaptosomes from control rats. To determine whether the result was due to enhanced Na$^+$ influx or decreased Na$^+$,K$^+$-ATPase activity, they examined both $^{86}$Rb influx into synaptosomes and ATP-stimulated Na$^+$ uptake into K$^+$-loaded inverted synaptosomes. With both techniques, there was a lower Na$^+$ pump activity but no depletion of ATP. The uremic milieu was also excluded because all experiments were carried out in physiologic buffers. Subsequently, Arieff and Massry investigated Ca$^{2+}$ transport across synaptosomal membranes from acutely uremic rats because brain Ca$^{2+}$ content is high in dogs with acute renal failure.[259] Rates of Na$^+$/Ca$^{2+}$ exchange and Ca$^{2+}$-ATPase activity in synaptosomes were measured with use of $^{45}$Ca as a tracer. Both initial and maximal rates of Ca$^{2+}$ flux were found to be higher in synaptosomes from acutely uremic rats relative to those from control rats.[260] Because both pathways account for Ca$^{2+}$ efflux from neurons, enhanced extrusion could lead to a higher extracellular brain Ca$^{2+}$ content. In contrast, Verkman and Fraser[261] were unable to detect any difference in synaptosomal permeability to either water or urea.

A connection between depressed monovalent cation flux and an abnormal accumulation of Ca$^{2+}$ intracellularly is not limited to the pathophysiologic process of uremia. Inhibition of Na$^+$,K$^+$-ATPase in vascular smooth muscle from arteriolar resistance vessels has been suggested to cause partial depolarization and enhanced Ca$^{2+}$ entry. These events would lead to vasoconstriction and systemic arterial hypertension.[262] Alternatively, Blaustein[263] hypothesized that Na$^+$ pump inhibition leads to a rise in cytosolic Ca$^{2+}$

concentration because Ca$^{2+}$ efflux through the Na$^+$/Ca$^{2+}$ exchanger is reduced. Indeed, if there is a natriuretic Na$^+$,K$^+$-ATPase inhibitory factor causing salt retention, the presence of enhanced smooth muscle vasoconstriction would contribute to the high prevalence of hypertension in chronic renal failure.

A decrease in Na$^+$,K$^+$-ATPase activity in uremic rats appears to be present in tissues besides blood cells. Druml and colleagues[264] measured ouabain-sensitive $^{86}$Rb influx in skeletal muscle and adipocytes from uremic rats and found decreased activity in both. As expected, the intracellular Na$^+$ content was increased in muscle and adipocytes. Consistent with results from human red blood cells, there was reduced furosemide-sensitive Na$^+$-K$^+$-2Cl$^-$ cotransport. A surprising finding was that the apparent mechanism for a decrease in Na$^+$ pump activity differed between the two tissues. In adipocytes, the number of Na$^+$ pumps as assessed by $^3$H-ouabain binding was reduced in proportion to the decline in Na$^+$ flux; in skeletal muscle, $^3$H-ouabain binding was unchanged by uremia. The activity normalized to the number of Na$^+$ pumps must be reduced in skeletal muscle, whereas the pump turnover rate in adipocytes remained unaffected by uremia. Moreover, when normal muscle was incubated with uremic serum, there was an immediate drop in ouabain-sensitive $^{86}$Rb uptake; in identical experiments with adipocytes, uremic serum failed to change Na$^+$ pump function. These results have been extended to myocardial slices from acutely or chronically uremic rats and their respective control groups.[265] In contrast to its effect in skeletal muscle, uremia did not change myocardial ouabain-sensitive $^{86}$Rb uptake, and intracellular Na$^+$ concentration remained normal (even though intracellular Na$^+$ content was high in skeletal muscle of the same rats). Surprisingly, myocardial $^3$H-ouabain binding was reduced 45% by chronic renal failure. Although maximal Na$^+$ pump–mediated ionic fluxes were not measured in these experiments, the reduced $^3$H-ouabain binding is consistent with data from other studies using cardiac sarcolemmal vesicles, which indicates that maximal Na$^+$,K$^+$-ATPase–associated ionic fluxes are depressed in chronic uremia.[266, 267] A potential explanation for decreased activity of Na$^+$,K$^+$-ATPase in uremia is impaired expression of genes regulating production of the α- and β-subunits of the enzyme. Several hormones (e.g., thyroid hormone, glucocorticoids, and others) influence the expression of Na$^+$,K$^+$-ATPase subunits, and because the action of these hormones is abnormal in uremia, gene expression could be altered. In fact, Jones and co-workers[268] reported low levels of the messenger RNA for α-subunits in soleus muscle of chronically uremic rats. However, Greiber and colleagues[269] could find no differences in the messenger RNA of α- or β-subunits in different types of skeletal muscle of uremic rats. Because they also found no change in the content of immunoreactive subunits in muscle, they concluded that uremia-induced defects in Na$^+$,K$^+$-ATPase could not be attributed to defects in gene expression.

In summary, a number of transport systems appear to be affected by uremia. The mechanisms for these defects vary with the tissue, and the cause of these changes is likely to be multifactorial.[270–272] This conclusion seems reasonable because tissue-specific responses of Na$^+$ pump number and

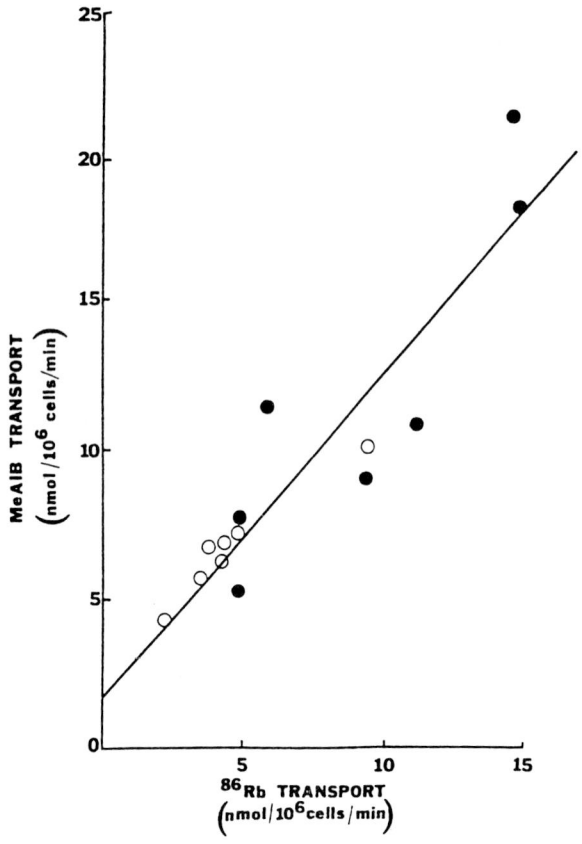

**Figure 49–6.** The rate of uptake of a nonmetabolizable amino acid probe specific for the Na$^+$-dependent amino acid uptake pathway system A, MeAIB, is plotted against the ouabain-sensitive influx of $^{86}$Rb into adipocytes from both uremic *(open circles)* and pair-fed, sham-operated control animals *(closed circles)*. The correlation between these two parameters is highly significant ($r = .91$; $P < .001$). (From Druml W, Kelly RA, May RC, Mitch WE: Abnormal cation flux in uremia: Mechanism in adipocytes and skeletal muscle from uremic rats. J Clin Invest 81:1197, 1988.)

activity are well documented in conditions other than uremia. For example, the number of Na$^+$ pumps on the basolateral membranes of renal tubules or cardiac myocytes in K$^+$-depleted animals changes in an opposite direction to that of skeletal muscle.[241, 273, 274] In contrast to defects in basal transport, $^{86}$Rb influx stimulated by insulin was unchanged by uremia in adipocytes, skeletal muscle, and myocardium,[264, 265] which suggests that at least the insulin-responsive subset of Na$^+$ pumps is not affected by uremia. A defect in basal Na$^+$ pump activity could be important in initiating or sustaining abnormalities in protein and amino acid metabolism in uremia. First, a decrease in ouabain-sensitive $^{86}$Rb influx rates in adipocytes is correlated directly with impaired Na$^+$-dependent amino acid uptake[264] (Fig. 49–6). Second, a generalized impairment in membrane ion transport could affect intracellular pH or Ca$^{2+}$ concentration, yielding marked changes in the control of amino acid and protein metabolism. Finally, abnormal depolarization of the plasma membrane in skeletal muscle, and probably in other tissues as well, suggests that metabolic characteristics of the uremic syndrome might be direct consequences of a generalized defect in monovalent cation transport.

## REFERENCES

1. Piorry PA, l'Heritier D: Traite des Altérations du Sang. Bury & JB Baillière, Paris, 1840.
2. Schreiner GE, Maher JF: Uremia: Biochemistry, Pathogenesis and Treatment. Charles C Thomas, Springfield, IL, 1961.
3. Prevost JL, Dumas JA: Examen du sang et de son action dans les divers phenomenes de la vie. Ann Chim Phys 23:90, 1921.
4. Muting D: Studies on the pathogenesis of uremia. Comparative determinations of glucuronic acid, indican, free and bound phenols in the serum, cerebrospinal fluid, and urine of renal diseases with and without uremia. Clin Chim Acta 12:551, 1965.
5. Simenhoff ML, Saukkonen JJ, Burke JF, et al: Bacterial populations of the small intestine in uremia. Nephron 22:63, 1978.
6. Lascelles PT, Taylor WH: The effect upon tissue respiration in vitro of metabolites which accumulate in uremic coma. Clin Sci 31:403, 1966.
7. Kwan JTC, Carr EC, Bending MR, Barron JL: Determination of carbamylated hemoglobin by high-performance liquid chromatography. Clin Chem 36:607, 1990.
8. Kraus LM, Miyamura S, Pecha BR, Kraus AP Jr: Carbamoylation of hemoglobin in uremic patients determined by antibody specific for homocitrulline (carbamolyated ε-N-lysine). Mol Immunol 28:459, 1991.
9. Monnier VM, Sell DR, Nagaraj RH, et al: Maillard reaction–mediated molecular damage to extracellular matrix and other tissue proteins in diabetes, aging, and uremia. Diabetes 41(suppl 2):36, 1992.
10. Quastel JH, Wheatley AHM: The effects of amines on oxidations of the brain. Biochem J 27:1609, 1933.
11. Ota K, Sanaka T, Agishi T, Nakajama O: Influence of uremic middle molecules on blood cells. Artif Organs 4:113, 1980.
12. Bergstrom J, Furst P: Uremic toxins. In Drukker W, Parsons FM, Maher JF (eds): Replacement of Renal Function by Dialysis. Martinus Nijhoff Publishers, Boston, 1983, p 354.
13. Gallice P, Monti JP, Crevat A, et al: A compound from uremic plasma and from normal urine isolated by liquid chromatography and identified by nuclear magnetic resonance. Clin Chem 31:30, 1985.
14. Pinkston D, Spiteller G, von Henning H, Matthaei D: High-resolution gas chromatography–mass spectrometry of the methyl esters of organic acids from uremic hemofiltrates. J Chromatogr 223:1, 1981.
15. Schoots AC, Verheggen TPEM, De Vries PMJM, Evaeraerts FM: Ultraviolet absorbing organic ions in uremic serum separated by capillary zone electrophoresis and quantification of hippuric acid. Clin Chem 36:435, 1990.
16. Mitch WE, Wilcox CS: Disorders of body fluids, sodium and potassium in chronic renal failure. Am J Med 72:536, 1982.
17. Bluemle CW Jr, Potter HP, Elkington JR: Changes in body composition in acute renal failure. J Clin Invest 35:1094, 1951.
18. Bush A: The lungs in uremia. Semin Respir Med 9:273, 1988.
19. Goodman AD, Lemann J, Lennon EJ, Relman AS: Production, excretion, and net balance of fixed acid in patients with renal acidosis. J Clin Invest 44:495, 1965.
20. Spriet LL, Matsos CG, Peters SJ, et al: Effects of acidosis on rat muscle metabolism and performance during heavy exercise. Am J Physiol 248:C337, 1985.
21. May RC, Kelly RA, Mitch WE: Metabolic acidosis stimulates protein degradation in rat muscle by a glucocorticoid-dependent mechanism. J Clin Invest 77:614, 1986.
22. May RC, Kelly RA, Mitch WE: Mechanisms for defects in muscle protein metabolism in rats with chronic uremia: Influence of metabolic acidosis. J Clin Invest 79:1099, 1987.
23. May RC, Masud T, Logue B, et al: Chronic metabolic acidosis accelerates whole body proteolysis and leucine oxidation in awake rats. Kidney Int 41:1535, 1992.
24. May RC, Hara Y, Kelly RA, et al: Branched-chain amino acid metabolism in rat muscle: Abnormal regulation in acidosis. Am J Physiol 252:E712, 1987.
25. Papadoyannakis NJ, Stefandis CJ, McGeown M: The effect of the correction of metabolic acidosis on nitrogen and potassium balance of patients with chronic renal failure. Am J Clin Nutr 40:623, 1986.
26. Reich D, Channon SM, Scrimgeour CM, Goodship THJ: Ammonium chloride–induced acidosis increases protein breakdown and amino acid oxidation in humans. Am J Physiol 263:E735, 1992.

27. Reaich D, Channon SM, Scrimgeour CM, et al: Correction of acidosis in humans with CRF decreases protein degradation and amino acid oxidation. Am J Physiol 265:E230, 1993.

28. Bergstrom J, Alvestrand A, Furst P: Plasma and muscle free amino acids in maintenance hemodialysis patients without protein malnutrition. Kidney Int 38:108, 1990.

29. Litzow JR, Lemann J, Lennon EJ: The effect of treatment of acidosis on calcium balance in patients with chronic azotemic renal disease. J Clin Invest 46:280, 1967.

30. Bushinsky DA, Lam BC, Nespeca R, et al: Decreased bone bicarbonate content in response to metabolic, but not respiratory, acidosis. Am J Physiol 265:F530, 1993.

31. DeFronzo RA, Beckles AD: Glucose intolerance following chronic metabolic acidosis in man. Am J Physiol 236:E328, 1979.

32. Gilmour ER, Hartley GH, Goodship THJ: Trace elements and vitamins in renal disease. *In* Mitch WE, Klahr S (eds): Nutrition and the Kidney. Little, Brown, Boston, 1993, p 114.

33. Balfour WE, Grantham JS, Glynn IM: Vanadate-stimulated natriuresis. Nature 275:768, 1978.

34. Bello-Reuss EN, Grady T, Mazumdar EC: Serum vanadium levels in chronic renal disease. Ann Intern Med 91:743, 1979.

35. Ott SM, Maloney NA, Coburn JW, et al: The prevalence of aluminum in renal osteodystrophy and its relationship to response to calcitriol therapy. N Engl J Med 307:709, 1982.

36. Parkinson IS, Ward MK, Feest TG, et al: Fracturing dialysis osteodystrophy and dialysis encephalopathy. An epidemiological survey. Lancet 1:406, 1979.

37. Mahajan SK, Abbasi AA, Prasad AS, et al: Effect of oral zinc therapy on gonadal function in hemodialysis patients: A double-blind study. Ann Intern Med 97:357, 1982.

38. Richet G: Early history of uremia. Kidney Int 33:1013, 1988.

39. Ludwig GD, Senesky D, Bluemle LW Jr, Elkinton JR: Indoles in uremia: Identification by countercurrent distribution and paper chromatography. Am J Clin Nutr 21:436, 1968.

40. Lowrie EG, Laird NM, Parker TF, Sargent JA: Effect of hemodialysis prescription on patient morbidity: Report from the National Cooperative Dialysis Study. N Engl J Med 305:1176, 1981.

41. Teschan PE, Bourne JR, Reed RB, Ward JW: Electrophysiological and neurobehavioral response to therapy: The National Cooperative Dialysis Study. Kidney Int 23(suppl 13):S58, 1983.

42. Levine J, Bernard DB: The role of urea kinetic modeling, TAC$_{urea}$ and Kt/V in achieving optimal dialysis: A critical reappraisal. Am J Kidney Dis 15:285, 1990.

43. Bilbrey GL, Carter NW, White MG, et al: Potassium deficiency in chronic renal failure. Kidney Int 4:423, 1973.

44. Cunningham JN, Carter NW, Rector FC, Seldin DW: Resting transmembrane potential difference of skeletal muscle in normal subjects and severely ill patients. J Clin Invest 50:49, 1971.

45. Cotton JR, Woodard T, Carter NW, Knochel JP: Resting skeletal muscle membrane potential as an index of uremic toxicity. J Clin Invest 63:501, 1979.

46. Cotton JR, Knochel JP: Correction of uremic cellular injury with a protein-restricted, amino acid–supplemented diet. Am J Kidney Dis 5:233, 1985.

47. Bright R: Reports of Medical Cases, Selected with a View of Illustrating the Symptoms and Cure of Disease by a Reference to Morbid Anatomy, Vol 2. Longman, Rees, Orme, Brown & Green, London, 1831.

48. Walser M, Bodenlos LJ: Urea metabolism in man. J Clin Invest 38:1617, 1959.

49. Grollman EF, Grollman A: Toxicity of urea and its role in the pathogenesis of uremia. J Clin Invest 38:749, 1959.

50. Bollman JL, Mann FC: Nitrogenous constituents of blood following transplantation of ureters into different levels of intestine. Proc Soc Exp Biol Med 24:923, 1927.

51. Merrill JP, Legrain M, Hoigne R: Observations on the role of urea in uremia. Am J Med 14:519, 1953.

52. Johnson WJ, Hagge WW, Wagoner RD, et al: Effects of urea loading in patients with far-advanced renal failure. Mayo Clin Proc 47:21, 1972.

53. Kajogopalan KV, Fridovich I, Handler P: Inhibition of enzyme activity by uremia. Fed Proc 19:49, 1960.

54. Menyhart J, Grof J: Urea as a selective inhibitor of argininosuccinate lyase. Eur J Biochem 75:405, 1977.

55. Davis JW, Field MC Jr, Phillips PE, Graham BA: Effects of exoge-
nous urea, creatinine, and guanidinosuccinic acid on human platelet aggregation in vitro. Blood 39:388, 1972.

56. Walser M: Urea metabolism in chronic renal failure. J Clin Invest 53:1385, 1974.

57. Oimoni M, Ishikawa K, Kawasaki T, et al: Carbamylation of hemoglobin in renal failure and clinical aspects. Metabolism 33:999, 1984.

58. Tizianello A, Deferrari G, Garibotto G, Robaudo C: Amino acid metabolism and the liver in renal failure. Am J Clin Nutr 33:1354, 1980.

59. DeDeyn P, Marescau B, Lornoy W, et al: Guanidino compounds in uremic dialyzed patients. Clin Chim Acta 157:143, 1986.

60. Mitch WE, Brusilow S: Benzoate-induced changes in glycine and urea metabolism in patients with chronic renal failure. J Pharmacol Exp Ther 222:572, 1982.

61. Batshaw ML, Brusilow S, Waber L, et al: Treatment of inborn errors of urea synthesis. N Engl J Med 306:1387, 1982.

62. Jones JD, Giovannetti S: Charcoal-catalyzed oxidation of creatinine to methylguanidine. Biochem Med 5:281, 1971.

63. Ando A, Orita Y, Nakata K, et al: Effect of low protein diet and surplus of essential amino acids on the serum concentration and the urinary excretion of methylguanidine and guanidinosuccinic acid in chronic renal failure. Nephron 24:161, 1979.

64. Marescau B, Deshumkh DR, Kockx M, et al: Guanidino compounds in serum, urine, liver, kidney, and brain of man and some ureotelic animals. Metabolism 41:526, 1992.

65. Kopple JD, Gordon SI, Wang M, Swendseid ME: Factors affecting serum and urinary guanidinosuccinic acid levels in normal and uremic subjects. J Lab Clin Med 90:303, 1977.

66. Marescau B, DeDeyn PP, Qureshi IA, et al: The pathobiochemistry of uremia and hyperargininemia further demonstrates a metabolic relationship between urea and guanidinosuccinic acid. Metabolism 41:1021, 1992.

67. Marescau B, Qureshi IA, DeDeyn P, et al: Guanidino compound in plasma, urine and cerebrospinal fluid of hyperargininemic patients during therapy. Clin Chim Acta 146:21, 1985.

68. Orita Y, Tsubakihara Y, Ando A, et al: Effect of arginine or creatinine administration on the urinary excretion of methylguanidine. Nephron 22:328, 1978.

69. Yokozawa T, Fujitsuka N, Oura H: Studies on the precursor of methylguanidine in rats with renal failure. Nephron 58:90, 1991.

70. Nakamura K, Ienaga K: Creatol (5-hydroxycreatinine), a new toxin candidate in uremic patients. Experientia 46:470, 1990.

71. Brusilow S, Tinker T, Batshaw ML: Amino acid acylation: A mechanism of nitrogen excretion in inborn errors of urea synthesis. Science 207:659, 1980.

72. Windmueller HG, Spaeth AE: Source and fate of circulating citrulline. Am J Physiol 241:E473, 1981.

73. Cohen BD: Guanidinosuccinic acid in uremia. Arch Intern Med 126:846, 1970.

74. Perez G, Rey A, Schiff E: The biosynthesis of guanidinosuccinic acid by perfused rat liver. J Clin Invest 57:807, 1976.

75. Kelly RA, Mitch WE: Creatinine, uric acid, and other nitrogenous waste products: Clinical implication of the imbalance between their production and elimination in uremia. Semin Nephrol 3:286, 1983.

76. Giovannetti S, Balestri PL, Barsotti G: Methylguanidine in uremia. Arch Intern Med 131:709, 1973.

77. Yatzidis H, Oreopoulos D, Tsaparas N, et al: Colorimetric determination of guanidines in blood. Nature 212:1498, 1966.

78. Orita Y, Ando A, Tsubakihara Y: Tissue and blood cell concentration of methylguanidine in rats and patients with chronic renal failure. Nephron 27:35, 1981.

79. Yamamoto Y, Saito A, Manji T, et al: A new automated analytical method for guanidino compounds and their cerebrospinal fluid levels in uremia. Trans Am Soc Artif Organs 24:61, 1978.

80. Giovannetti S, Cioni L, Balestri PL, Biagini M: Evidence that guanidines and some related compounds cause hemolysis in chronic uremia. Clin Sci 34:141, 1974.

81. Wizeman V: Exocrine pancreatic function in chronic renal failure. Proc Eur Dial Transplant Assoc 13:585, 1977.

82. Lamperi S, Bandiani G, Fiorio P, et al: Effects of some substances retained in uremia on erythropoiesis: The effect on bone marrow cell cultures. Nephron 13:278, 1974.

83. Touraine JL, Touraine F, Revillard JB: T lymphocytes and serum inhibition of cell-mediated immunity in renal insufficiency. Nephron 14:195, 1975.

84. Dobbelstein H, Grunst J, Schubert G, Edel HH: Guanidinosuccinic acid and uremia. II. Result of animal experiments. Klin Wochenschr 49:1077, 1971.

85. Scheuer J, Stezoski SW: The effect of uremic compounds on cardiac function and metabolism. J Mol Cell Cardiol 5:287, 1973.

86. Penpargkul S, Kuziak J, Scheuer J: Effect of uremia upon carbohydrate metabolism in isolated perfused rat heart. J Mol Cell Cardiol 7:499, 1975.

87. Horowitz HI, Stein IM, Cohen RD, White JG: Further studies on the platelet-inhibitory effect of guanidinosuccinic acid and its role in uremic bleeding. Am J Med 49:336, 1970.

88. Shainkin R, Giatt V, Berlyne GM: The presence and toxicity of guanidinopropionic acid in uremia. Kidney Int 75:302, 1975.

89. Shainkin R, Biatt V, Berlyne GM: The toxicity of guanidino compounds in the red blood cell in uremia and the effects of hemodialysis. Nephron 31:20, 1982.

90. Minot A, Dodd K: Guanidino intoxication. Am J Dis Child 46:522, 1933.

91. Mori A, Watanabe U, Akagi M: Guanidino compound abnormalities in epilepsy. In Akimoto H, Kazamatsuri H, Seino M, Ward A (eds): Advances in Epileptology. Raven Press, New York, 1982.

92. Jinnai D, Sawai A, Mori A: Gamma-guanidinobutyric acid as a convulsive substance. Nature 212:617, 1966.

93. Yokoi I, Toma J, Mori A: The effect of homoarginine on the EEG of rats. Neurochem Pathol 2:295, 1984.

94. Marescau B, Hiramatsu M, Mori A: Alpha-keto-δ-guanidinovaleric acid induced electroencephalographic, epileptiform discharges in rabbits. Neurochem Pathol 1:203, 1983.

95. DeDeyn PP, MacDonald RL: Guanidino compounds that are increased in cerebrospinal fluid and brain of uremic patients inhibit GABA and glycine responses on mouse neurons in cell culture. Ann Neurol 28:627, 1990.

96. Palmer RMJ, Ashto DS, Moncada S: Vascular endothelial cells synthesize nitric oxide from L-arginine. Nature 333:664, 1988.

97. Remuzzi G, Perico N, Zoja C, et al: Role of endothelium-derived nitric oxide in the bleeding tendency of uremia. J Clin Invest 86:1768, 1990.

98. Vallance P, Leone A, Calver A, et al: Accumulation of an endogenous inhibitor of nitric oxide synthesis in chronic renal failure. Lancet 339:572, 1992.

99. MacAllister RJ, Whitley STJ, Vallance P: Effects of guanidino and uremic compounds on nitric oxide pathways. Kidney Int 45:737, 1994.

100. Sessa WC, Hecker M, Mitchell JA, Vane JR: The metabolism of L-arginine and its significance for the biosynthesis of endothelium-derived relaxing factor: L-Glutamine inhibits the generation of L-arginine by cultured endothelial cells. Proc Natl Acad Sci USA 87:8607, 1990.

101. Reyes AA, Purkerson ML, Karl I, Klahr S: Dietary supplementation with L-arginine ameliorates the progression of renal disease in rats with subtotal nephrectomy. Am J Kidney Dis 20:168, 1992.

102. Yanagisawa H, Wada O: Significant increase of IQ-type heterocyclic amines, dietary carcinogens in the plasma of patients with uremia just before induction of hemodialysis treatment. Nephron 52:6, 1989.

103. Manabe S, Suszuke M, Kusano E, et al: Elevation of levels of carcinogenic tryptophan pyrolysis products in plasma and red blood cells of patients with uremia. Clin Nephrol 37:23, 1992.

104. Simenhoff ML, Burke JF, Saukkonen JJ, et al: Amine metabolism and the small bowel in uraemia. Lancet 2:818, 1976.

105. Bell JD, Lee JA, Lee HA, et al: Nuclear magnetic resonance studies of blood plasma and urine from patients with chronic renal failure: Identification of trimethylamine-N-oxide. Biochim Biophys Acta 1096:191, 1991.

106. Simenhoff ML, Milne MD, Asatoor AM, Zilva JF: Retention of aliphatic amines in uremia. Clin Sci 25:65, 1963.

107. Rennick B, Acara M, Hysert P, Mookerjee B: Choline loss during hemodialysis: Homeostatic control of plasma choline concentrations. Kidney Int 10:329, 1976.

108. Magnusson M, Magnusson KE, Sundqvist T, Denneberg T: Increased intestinal permeability to differently sized polyethylene glycols in uremic rats: Effects of low- and high-protein diets. Nephron 56:306, 1990.

109. Magnusson M, Magnusson KE, Sundqvist T, Denneberg T: Urinary excretion of differently sized polyethylene glycols after intravenous administration in uremic and control rats: Effects of low- and high-protein diets. Nephron 56:312, 1990.

110. Einheber A, Carter D: The role of the microbial flora in uremia. I. Survival times of germ-free limited-flora, and conventionalized rats after bilateral nephrectomy and fasting. J Exp Med 123:239, 1966.

111. Young DS, Wootton IDP: The retention of amines as a factor in uremic toxaemia. Clin Chim Acta 9:503, 1964.

112. Niwa T, Ohki T, Maeda K, et al: A gas chromatographic–mass spectrometric assay for nine hydroxyphenolic acids in uremic serum. Clin Chim Acta 96:247, 1979.

113. Walser M, Hill SB: Free and protein-bound tryptophan in serum of untreated patients with chronic renal failure. Kidney Int 44:1366, 1993.

114. Wengle B, Hellstrom K: Volatile phenols in serum of uremic patients. Clin Sci 43:493, 1972.

115. Mason MF, Resnik H, Mino AS, et al: Mechanism of experimental uremia. Arch Intern Med 60:312, 1937.

116. Wardle EN: Phenols, phenolic acids, and sodium-potassium ATPases. J Mol Med 3:319, 1978.

117. Byrd DJ, Berthold HW, Trefz KZ, et al: Indolic tryptophan metabolism in uremia. Proc Eur Dial Transplant Assoc 12:347, 1976.

118. Siassi F, Wang M, Chan W, Swendseid ME: Brain serotonin metabolism in experimental uremia. Fed Proc 33:651, 1974.

119. Lim C, Bernard BF, De Jong M, et al: A furan fatty acid and indoxyl sulfate are the putative inhibitors of thyroxine hepatocyte transport in uremia. J Clin Endocrinol Metab 76:318, 1993.

120. Niwa T, Yazawa T, Ise M, et al: Inhibitory effect of oral sorbent on accumulation of albumin-bound indoxyl sulfate in serum of experimental uremic rats. Nephron 57:84, 1991.

121. Niwa T, Miyazaki T, Hashimoto N, et al: Suppressed serum and urine levels of indoxyl sulfate by oral sorbent in experimental uremic rats. Am J Nephrol 12:201, 1992.

122. Motojima M, Nishijima F, Ikoma M, et al: Role for "uremic toxin" in the progressive loss of intact nephrons in chronic renal failure. Kidney Int 40:461, 1991.

123. Janne J, Poso H, Raina A: Polyamines in rapid growth and cancer. Biochim Biophys Acta 473:242, 1978.

124. Radtke HW, Rege AB, LaMarche MB, Bartos D: Identification of spermine as an inhibitor of erythropoiesis in patients with chronic renal failure. J Clin Invest 67:1623, 1981.

125. Swendseid ME, Panagua M, Kopple JD: Polyamine concentrations in red cells and urine of patients with chronic renal failure. Life Sci 26:533, 1980.

126. Saito A, Takagi T, Chung TG, Ohta K: Serum levels of polyamines in patients with chronic renal failure. Kidney Int 24(suppl 16):S234, 1985.

127. Bagdade JD, Subbaiah PY, Bartos D, et al: Polyamines: An unrecognized cardiovascular risk factor in chronic dialysis? Lancet 1:412, 1979.

128. Tenckhoff H, Curtis FK: Experience with maintenance peritoneal dialysis in the home. Trans Am Soc Artif Intern Organs 11:11, 1970.

129. Lowrie EG, Steinberg SM, Galen MA, et al: Factors in the dialysis regimen which contribute to alterations in the abnormalities of uremia. Kidney Int 10:409, 1976.

130. Scribner BH: Discussion. Trans Am Soc Artif Intern Organs 11:29, 1965.

131. Babb AL, Johansen PJ, Strand MJ, et al: Bidirectional permeability of the human peritoneum to middle molecules. Proc Eur Dial Transplant Assoc 10:247, 1973.

132. Gotch FA: Dialysis of the future. Kidney Int 33(suppl 24):S100, 1988.

133. Furst P, Zimmerman L, Bergstrom J: Determination of endogenous middle molecules in normal and uremic body fluids. Clin Nephrol 5:178, 1976.

134. Asabu H, Alvestrand A, Furst P, Bergstrom J: Clinical implications of uremic middle molecules in regular hemodialysis patients. Clin Nephrol 19:179, 1983.

135. Schoots AC, Mikkers FEP, Claessens HA, et al: Characterization of uremic "middle molecular" fractions by gas chromatography, mass spectrometry, isotachophoresis, and liquid chromatography. Clin Chem 28:45, 1982.

136. Cristol P, Jeanbrau E, Monnier P: La polypeptidémie en pathologie rénale. J Med France 27:24, 1938.

137. Lubash GD, Stenzel KH, Rubin AL: Nitrogenous compounds in hemodialysate. Circulation 30:848, 1964.

138. Czerniak E: N-Substituted amino acids in serum of patients with chronic renal insufficiency. Clin Chim Acta 28:403, 1970.

139. Abiko T, Kumikawa M, Ishizaki M, et al: Identification and synthesis of a tripeptide in coecum fluid of a uremic patient. Biochem Biophys Res Commun 83:357, 1978.

140. Abiko T, Kunikawa M, Higuchi H, Sekono H: Identification and synthesis of a heptapeptide in uremic fluid. Biochem Biophys Res Commun 84:184, 1978.

141. Abiko T, Onodera I, Sekono H: Isolation, structures and biological activity of the Trp-containing pentapeptide from uremic fluid. Biochem Biophys Res Commun 89:813, 1979.

142. Gejyo F, Yamada T, Odani S, et al: A new form of amyloid protein associated with chronic hemodialysis was identified as beta₂-microglobulin. Biochem Biophys Res Commun 129:701, 1985.

143. Gejyo F, Homma N, Arakawa M: Long-term complications of dialysis: Pathogenic factors with special reference to amyloidosis. Kidney Int 43(suppl 41):S78, 1993.

144. Meytes D, Bogin E, Ma A, et al: Effect of parathyroid hormone on erythropoiesis. J Clin Invest 67:1263, 1981.

145. Massry SG: The toxic effects of parathyroid hormone in uremia. Semin Nephrol 3:306, 1983.

146. Goldstein DA, Feinstein EI, Chui LA, et al: The relationship between the abnormalities in electroencephalogram and blood levels of parathyroid hormone in dialysis patients. J Endocrinol Metab 61:130, 1980.

147. Avram MM, Feinfeld DA, Huatuco AH: Search for the uremic toxin: Decreased motor-nerve conduction velocity and elevated parathyroid hormone in uremia. N Engl J Med 298:1000, 1978.

148. Bogin E, Massry SG, Harary I: Effect of parathyroid hormone on heart cells. J Clin Invest 67:1215, 1981.

149. Fadda GZ, Hajjar SM, Perna AF, et al: On the mechanism of impaired insulin secretion in chronic renal failure. J Clin Invest 87:255, 1991.

150. Shoots A, Mikkers F, Cramers C, et al: Uremic toxins and the elusive middle molecules. Nephron 38:1, 1984.

151. Zimmerman L, Jornvall H, Bergstrom J, et al: Characterization of a double conjugate in uremic body fluids. FEBS Lett 129:237, 1981.

152. Gallice PM, Monti JP, Braguer DL, et al: Identification of an ascorbic acid metabolite among "uremic middle molecules." Clin Chem 36:1369, 1990.

153. Zimmerman L, Jornvall H, Bergstrom J: Phenylacetylglutamine and hippuric acid in uremic and healthy subjects. Nephron 55:265, 1990.

154. Henderson SJ, Lindup WE: Interaction of 3-carboxy-4-methyl-5-propyl-2-furanpropanoic acid, an inhibitor of plasma protein binding in uremia, with human albumin. Biochem Pharmacol 40:2543, 1990.

155. Vanholder RC, Ringoir SM: Adequacy of dialysis: A critical analysis. Kidney Int 42:540, 1992.

156. Vanholder RC, De Smet RV, Ringoir SM: Assessment of urea and other uremic markers for quantification of dialysis efficacy. Clin Chem 38:1429, 1992.

157. May RC, Mitch WE: Chronic renal failure. In Branch WT (ed): Office Practice of Medicine. WB Saunders, Philadelphia, 1987, p 608.

158. Katz AI, Rubenstein AH: Metabolism of proinsulin, insulin, and C-peptide in the rat. J Clin Invest 52:1113, 1973.

159. Bilbrey GL, Faloona GR, White MG, Knochel JP: Hyperglucagonemia of renal failure. J Clin Invest 53:841, 1974.

160. Sievertsen GD, Lim VS, Nakawatase C, Frohman LA: Metabolic clearance and secretion rates of human prolactin in normal subjects and in patients with chronic renal failure. J Clin Endocrinol Metab 50:846, 1980.

161. Lim VS, Fang VS: Gonadal dysfunction in uremic men. A study of the hypothalamo-pituitary-testicular axis before and after renal transplantation. Am J Med 58:555, 1975.

162. Ikemoto S, Imaoka S, Hayahara N, et al: Expression of hepatic microsomal cytochrome P450s is altered by uremia. Biochem Pharmacol 43:2407, 1992.

163. Phillips LS, Fusco AC, Unterman TG, del Greco F: Somatomedin inhibitor in uremia. J Clin Endocrinol Metab 59:764, 1984.

164. Navalesi R, Pilo A, Lenzi S, Donato L: Insulin metabolism in chronic uremia and in the anephric state: Effect of the dialytic treatment. J Clin Endocrinol Metab 40:70, 1975.

165. DeFronzo RA, Tobin JD, Rowe JW, Andres R: Glucose intolerance in uremia. Quantification of pancreatic beta cell sensitivity to glucose and tissue sensitivity to insulin. J Clin Invest 62:425, 1980.

166. Westervelt FB: Insulin effect in uremia. J Lab Clin Med 74:79, 1969.

167. Smith D, DeFronzo RA: Insulin resistance in uremia mediated by postbinding defects. Kidney Int 22:54, 1982.

168. Maloff BL, McCaleb ML, Lockwood DH: Cellular basis of insulin resistance in chronic uremia. Am J Physiol 245:E178, 1983.

169. May RC, Clark AS, Goheer A, Mitch WE: Identification of specific defects in insulin-mediated muscle metabolism in acute uremia. Kidney Int 28:490, 1985.

170. Alvestrand A, Wahren J, Smith D, DeFronzo RA: Insulin-mediated potassium uptake is normal in uremic and healthy subjects. Am J Physiol 246:E174, 1984.

171. Haring HU: The insulin receptor: Signalling mechanism and contribution to the pathogenesis of insulin resistance. Diabetologia 34:848, 1991.

172. Saltiel AR, Cuatrecasas P: In search of a second messenger for insulin. Am J Physiol 255:C1, 1988.

173. Kasuga M, Fujita-Yamaguchi Y, Blithe DL, et al: Characterization of the insulin receptor kinase purified from human placental membranes. J Biol Chem 258:10973, 1983.

174. Saad MJA, Araki E, Miralpeix M, et al: Regulation of insulin receptor substrate-1 in liver and muscle of animal models of insulin resistance. J Clin Invest 90:1839, 1992.

175. Hashimoto N, Zhang W, Goldstein BJ: Insulin receptor and epidermal growth factor receptor dephosphorylation by three major liver protein–tyrosine phosphatases expressed in a recombinant bacterial system. Biochem J 284:569, 1992.

176. Cecchin F, Ittoop O, Sinha MK, Caro JF: Insulin resistance in uremia: Insulin receptor kinase activity in liver and muscle from chronic uremic rats. Am J Physiol 254:E394, 1988.

177. Bak JF, Schmitz O, Sorensen SS, et al: Activity of insulin receptor kinase and glycogen synthase in skeletal muscle from patients with chronic renal failure. Acta Endocrinol (Copenh) 121:744, 1989.

178. Bai C, Bailey JL, May RC: Tyrosine phosphorylation of skeletal muscle proteins is reduced in uremic rats. J Am Soc Nephrol 4:763, 1993.

179. Kaptein EM, Quion-Verde H, Chooljian CJ, et al: The thyroid in end-stage renal disease. Medicine (Baltimore) 67:187, 1988.

180. Robertson BF, Prestwich S, Ramirez G, et al: The role of iodine in the pathogenesis of thyroid enlargement in rats with chronic renal failure. Endocrinology 101:1272, 1977.

181. Kaptein EM, Feinstein EI, Nicoloff JT, Massry SG: Serum reverse tri-iodothyronine and thyroxine kinetics in patients with chronic renal failure. J Clin Endocrinol Metab 57:181, 1983.

182. Wartofsky L, Burman KD: Alterations in thyroid function in patients with systemic illnesses: The "euthyroid sick syndrome." Endocr Rev 3:164, 1982.

183. Lim VS, Zavala DC, Flanigan MJ, Freeman RM: Blunted peripheral tissue responsiveness to thyroid hormone in uremic patients. Kidney Int 31:808, 1987.

184. Bricker NS: On the pathogenesis of the uremic state: An exposition of the "trade-off" hypothesis. N Engl J Med 286:1093, 1972.

185. Rutherford WE, Bordier P, Marie P, et al: Phosphate control and 25-hydroxycholecalciferol administration in preventing experimental renal osteodystrophy in the dog. J Clin Invest 60:332, 1977.

186. Prince RS, Hutchinson BG, Kent JC, et al: Calcitriol deficiency with retained synthetic reserve in chronic renal failure. Kidney Int 33:722, 1988.

187. Wilson L, Felsenfeld A, Drezner MK, Llach F: Altered divalent ion metabolism in early renal failure: Role of 1,25(OH)₂D. Kidney Int 27:565, 1985.

188. Adler AJ, Ferran N, Berlyne GM: Effect of inorganic phosphate on serum ionized calcium concentration in vitro: A reassessment of the "trade-off" hypothesis. Kidney Int 28:932, 1985.

189. Danovitch GM, Bourgoignie J, Bricker NS: Reversibility of the "salt-losing" tendency of chronic renal failure. N Engl J Med 296:14, 1977.

190. Schmidt RW, Bourgoignie JJ, Bricker NS: On the adaptation in sodium excretion in chronic uremia: The effects of "proportional reduction" of sodium intake. J Clin Invest 53:1736, 1974.

191. Welt LG, Smith EKM, Dunn MJ, et al: Membrane transport defect: The sick cell. Trans Assoc Am Physicians 80:217, 1967.

192. Cole CH, Balfe JW, Welt LG: Induction of a ouabain-sensitive ATPase defect by uremic plasma. Trans Assoc Am Physicians 81:213, 1968.

193. Cole CH: Decreased ouabain-sensitive adenosine triphosphatase activity in the erythrocyte membrane of patients with chronic renal disease. Clin Sci Mol Med 45:775, 1973.

194. Kramer HJ, Gospodinov D, Kruck F: Functional and metabolic stud-

ies on red blood cell sodium transport in chronic uremia. Nephron 16:344, 1976.

195. Jessop S, Eales L: Erythrocyte electrolyte content and sodium efflux in chronic renal failure. Nephron 18:82–87, 1977.

196. Villamil MF, Rettori V, Kleeman CR: Sodium transport by red blood cells in uremia. J Lab Clin Med 72:308, 1968.

197. Cheng JT, Kahn T, Kaji DM: Mechanism of alteration of sodium potassium pump of erythrocytes from patients with chronic renal failure. J Clin Invest 74:1811, 1984.

198. Izumo H, Izumo S, DeLuise M, Flier JS: Erythrocyte Na,K pump in uremia. Acute correction of a transport defect by hemodialysis. J Clin Invest 74:581, 1984.

199. Edmundson RPS, Hilton PJ, Jones NF, et al: Leucocyte transport in uremia. Clin Sci Mol Med 49:213, 1975.

200. Nene RJ, Boer P, Koomans HA, Dorhout Mees EJ: Sodium potassium ATPase activity in human rectal mucosa with and without renal insufficiency. Am J Kidney Dis 5:177, 1985.

201. Aalkjaer C, Heagerty AM, Parvin SD, et al: Cell membrane sodium transport: A correlation between human resistance vessels and leucocytes. Lancet 1:649, 1986.

202. Corry DB, Tuck ML, Brickman AS, et al: Sodium transport in red blood cells from dialyzed uremic patients. Kidney Int 20:1197, 1986.

203. Swaminathan R, Clegg G, Cumberbatch M, et al: Erythrocyte sodium transport in chronic renal failure. Clin Sci 62:489, 1982.

204. Zannad F, Royer RJ, Kessler M, et al: Cation transport in erythrocytes of patients with renal failure. Nephron 32:347, 1982.

205. DeSanto NG, Trevisan M, Decolle S, et al: Intraerythrocytic cation metabolism in children with uremia undergoing hemodialysis. J Lab Clin Med 110:231, 1987.

206. Kelly RA, Canessa ML, Steinman TI, Mitch WE: Hemodialysis and red cell cation transport in uremia: Role of membrane free fatty acids. Kidney Int 35:595, 1989.

207. Monti JP, Baz M, Elsen R, et al: High-resolution NMR studies of transmembrane cation transport in uremic patients. Biochim Biophys Acta 1027:31, 1990.

208. Kaji D, Kahn T: Na+-K+ pump in chronic renal failure. Am J Physiol 252:F785, 1987.

209. Corry DB, Lee DBN, Tuck ML: A kinetic study of cation transport in erythrocytes from uremic patients. Kidney Int 32:256, 1987.

210. Zannad F, Kessler M, Royer RJ, Robert J: Effect of hemodialysis on red blood cell Na+-K+-ATPase activity in terminal renal failure. Nephron 40:127, 1985.

211. Brod J, Schaeffer J, Hengstenberg JH, Kleinschmidt TG: Investigations on the Na+,K+-pump in erythrocytes of patients with renal hypertension. Clin Sci 66:351, 1984.

212. Cole CH: Erythrocyte sodium transport in patients on chronic hemodialysis. Proc Dial Transplant Forum 7:152, 1977.

213. Cole CH, Steinberg R, Guttmann R: Altered erythrocyte sodium efflux following renal transplantation. Nephron 20:248, 1978.

214. Quarello F, Boero R, Guarena C, et al: Acute effects of hemodialysis on erythrocyte sodium fluxes in uremic patients. Nephron 41:22, 1985.

215. Krzisinski JM, Du F, Pequeux ML, Rorive GL: Plasma Na+-K+ ATPase inhibitor activity and intracellular ions during hemodialysis. Int J Artif Organs 16:23, 1993.

216. Cornelis R, Versieck J: Serum vanadium levels. Ann Intern Med 92:710, 1980.

217. Mikami H, Ando A, Fujii M, et al: Effect of methylguanidine on erythrocyte membranes. In Mori A, Cohen BD, Lowenthal A (eds): Guanidines. Plenum Publishing, New York, 1985, p 205.

218. Kelly RA, O'Hara DS, Canessa ML, et al: Characterization of digitalis-like factors in human plasma: Interactions with NaK-ATPase and cross-reactivity with cardiac glycoside–specific antibodies. J Biol Chem 260:11396, 1985.

219. Kelly RA, O'Hara DS, Mitch WE, et al: Endogenous digitalis-like factors in hypertension and chronic renal insufficiency. Kidney Int 230:723, 1986.

220. Graves SW, Brown B, Valdes R: An endogenous digoxin-like substance in patients with renal impairment. Ann Intern Med 99:604, 1983.

221. Deray G, Pernollet MG, Devynck MA, et al: Plasma digitalislike activity in essential hypertension or end-stage renal disease. Hypertension 8:632, 1986.

222. Kramer JH, Penning J, Klingmuller D, et al: Digoxin-like immunoreacting substance(s) in the serum of patients with chronic uremia. Nephron 40:297, 1985.

223. Ludens JH, Clark MS, DuCharme DW, et al: Purification of an endogenous digitalis-like factor from human plasma for structural analysis. Hypertension 17:923, 1991.

224. Mathews WR, DuCharme DW, Hamlyn JM, et al: Mass spectral characterization of an endogenous digitalis-like factor from human plasma. Hypertension 17:930, 1991.

225. Goto A, Ishiguro T, Yamada K, et al: Isolation of a urinary digitalis-like factor indistinguishable from digoxin. Biochem Biophys Res Commun 173:1093, 1990.

226. Dasgupta A, Peng Y: Dialyzability and binding of digoxin-like immunoreactive factors (DLIF) with serum macromolecules in uremic patients on hemodialysis. Life Sci 49:1603, 1991.

227. Benaksas EJ, Murray ED, Rodgers CL, et al: Endogenous natriuretic factors I: Sodium pump inhibition does not correlate with natriuretic or pressor activities from uremic urine. Life Sci 52:1045, 1993.

228. Bricker NS, Bourgoignie JJ, Klahr S: A humoral inhibitor of sodium transport in uremic serum. Arch Intern Med 126:860, 1970.

229. Kelly RA: Endogenous cardiac glycosidelike compounds. Hypertension 10:I87, 1987.

230. Graves SW, Williams GH: Endogenous digitalis-like natriuretic factors. Annu Rev Med 38:433, 1987.

231. deWardener HE, Clarkson EM: Concept of a natriuretic hormone. Physiol Rev 65:658, 1985.

232. Buckalew VM, Gruber KA: Natriuretic hormone. In Epstein M (ed): The Kidney in Liver Disease, 2nd ed. Elsevier Press, New York, 1983, p 479.

233. Tamura M, Kuwano H, Kinoshita T, Inagami I: Identification of linoleic and oleic acids on endogenous NaK-ATPase inhibitors from acute volume-expanded hog plasma. J Biol Chem 260:9672, 1985.

234. Kelly RA, O'Hara DS, Mitch WE, Smith TW: Identification of Na+,K+-ATPase inhibitors in human plasma as nonesterified fatty acids and lysophospholipids. J Biol Chem 261:11704, 1986.

235. Tamura M, Harris TM, Higashimori K, et al: Lysophosphatidylcholines containing polyunsaturated fatty acids were found as Na+,K+-ATPase inhibitors in acutely volume-expanded hog. Biochemistry 26:2797, 1987.

236. Hamyln JM, Schenden JA, Zyren J, Baczynsky L: Purification and characterization of digitalis-like factors from human plasma. Hypertension 10:I71, 1987.

237. Komidori K, Kamada T, Yamashita T, et al: Erythrocyte membrane fluidity decreased in uremic hemodialyzed patients. Nephron 40:185, 1985.

238. Langsdorf LJ, Zydney AL: Effect of uremia on the membrane transport characteristics of red blood cells. Blood 81:820, 1993.

239. Rosie NK, Standnert ML, Pollet RJ: The mechanism of insulin stimulation of (Na+-K+)-ATPase transport activity in muscle. J Biol Chem 260:6202, 1985.

240. Lytton J: Insulin affects the sodium affinity of the rat adipocyte (Na+-K+)-ATPase. J Biol Chem 260:10075, 1985.

241. Clausen T: Regulation of active Na+-K+ transport in skeletal muscle. Physiol Rev 66:542, 1986.

242. Edelman IS, Pressley TA, Hiatt A: Regulation of mammalian Na,K-ATPase. In Glynn I, Ellory C (eds): The Sodium Pump. Company of Biologists, Cambridge, England, 1985, p 153.

243. Kim D, Smith TW: Effect of thyroid hormone on sodium pump sites, sodium content, and contractile response to cardiac glycosides in cultured chick ventricular cells. J Clin Invest 74:1481, 1984.

244. Brown MJ, Brown DC, Murphy MB: Hypokalemia from beta2 stimulation by circulating epinephrine. N Engl J Med 309:1414, 1983.

245. Trevisan M, DeSanto N, Laurenzi M, et al: Intracellular ion metabolism in erythrocytes and uremia: The effect of different dialysis treatments. Clin Sci 71:545, 1986.

246. Duhm J, Globel DO: Role of the furosemide-sensitive Na+-K+ transport system in determining the steady state Na+ and K+ content and volume of human erythrocyte in vitro and in vivo. Membr Biol 77:243, 1984.

247. Korff JM, Siebes AW, Gill JR Jr: Correction of hypokalemia corrects the abnormality in erythrocyte sodium transport in Bartter's syndrome. J Clin Invest 74:1724, 1984.

248. Woods JW, Parker JC, Watson BS: Perturbation of sodium-lithium countertransport in red cells. N Engl J Med 308:1258, 1983.

249. Bluckelmann D, Erdmann E: perturbation of sodium-lithium countertransport in red cells. N Engl J Med 312:1193, 1985.

250. Smith JB, Owen Ash K, Gregory MC, et al: Hemodialysis does not affect erythrocyte sodium-lithium countertransport. Clin Chim Acta 143:275, 1984.

251. Corry DB, Ruck ML, Nicholas S, Weinman EJ: Increased Na/H antiport activity and abundance in uremic red blood cells. Kidney Int 44:574, 1993.

252. Zidek W, Rustemeyer T, Schluter W, et al: Isolation of an ultrafilterable $Ca^{2+}$-ATPase inhibitor from the plasma of uraemic patients. Clin Sci 82:659, 1992.

253. Aparicio M, Vincendeau P, Combe C, et al: Improvement of leucocytic $Na^+$ $K^+$ pump activity in uremic patients on low protein diet. Kidney Int 40:238, 1991.

254. Bolte HD, Riecke G, Rohl D: Measurements of membrane potential of individual muscle cells in normal men and patients with renal insufficiency. *In* Proceedings of the Second International Congress on Nephrology. S Karger, Basel, 1963, p 114.

255. Mitch WE: Amino acid release from the hindquarter and urea appearance in acute uremia. Am J Physiol 241:E415, 1981.

256. Minkoff L, Gaertner G, Darab M, et al: Inhibition of brain sodium-potassium ATPase in uremic rats. J Lab Clin Med 80:71, 1972.

257. Kramer HJ, Backer A, Kruck F: Inhibition of intestinal $Na^+$-$K^+$-ATPase in experimental uremia. Clin Chim Acta 50:13, 1974.

258. Fraser CL, Sarnacki P, Arieff AI: Abnormal sodium transport in synaptosomes from brain of uremic rats. J Clin Invest 75:2014, 1985.

259. Arieff AI, Massry SG: Calcium metabolism of brain in acute renal failure: Effects of uremia, hemodialysis and parathyroid hormone. J Clin Invest 53:387, 1974.

260. Fraser CL, Sarnacki P, Arieff AI: Calcium transport abnormality in uremic rat brain synaptosomes. J Clin Invest 76:1789, 1985.

261. Verkman AS, Fraser CL: Water and nonelectrolyte permeability in brain synaptosomes isolated from normal and uremic rats. Am J Physiol 250:R306, 1986.

262. Haddy FJ, Overbeck HW: The role of humoral agents in volume expanded hypertension. Life Sci 19:935, 1976.

263. Blaustein MP: Sodium ions, calcium ions, blood pressure regulation and hypertension: A reassessment and a hypothesis. Am J Physiol 232:C165, 1977.

264. Druml W, Kelly RA, May RC, Mitch WE: Abnormal cation flux in uremia: Mechanisms in adipocytes and skeletal muscle from uremic rats. J Clin Invest 81:1197, 1988.

265. Kelly RA, England BK, Druml W, Mitch WE: Specificity of abnormal cation transport in uremia: Differences in myocardium from skeletal muscle. Kidney Int 37:510, 1990.

266. Huot SJ, Pamnani MB, Clough DL, et al: Sodium-potassium pump activity in reduced renal-mass hypertension. Hypertension 5:I94, 1983.

267. Penpargkul S, Bhan AK, Scheuer J: Studies of subcellular control factors in hearts of uremic rats. J Lab Clin Med 88:563, 1976.

268. Bonilla S, Goecke IA, Bozzo S, et al: Effect of chronic renal failure on $Na^+$,$K^+$-ATPase $\alpha_1$ and $\alpha_2$ mRNA transcription in rat skeletal muscle. J Clin Invest 88:2137, 1991.

269. Greiber S, England BK, Price SR, et al: Na pump defects in chronic uremia cannot be attributed to changes in Na-K-ATPase mRNA or protein. Am J Physiol 266:F536, 1994.

270. Grimes AJ, Mansel M: Annotation: Red and white cell abnormalities in chronic renal failure. Br J Haematol 42:169, 1979.

271. Van Der Noort S, Eckel RE, Brine K, Hrdlicka JT: Brain metabolism in uremic and adenosine-infused rats. J Clin Invest 47:2133, 1968.

272. Mansell MA, Grimes AJ, Jones NF: Leucocyte ATP and renal failure. Clin Sci 61:43, 1981.

273. Doucet A, Katz AI: Renal potassium adaptation: Na-K-ATPase activity along the nephron after chronic potassium loading. Am J Physiol 238:F380, 1980.

274. Werdan K, Schneider G, Krawietz W, Erdmann E: Chronic exposure to low $K^+$ increases in cardiac glycoside receptors in cultured cardiac cells: Different responses of cardiac muscle and non-muscle cells from chicken embryos. Biochem Pharmacol 33:1161, 1984.

# 50

# Hematologic Consequences of Renal Failure

*Giuseppe Remuzzi*
*Ennio C. Rossi*

Hematologic manifestations associated with renal failure were first noted by Richard Bright in 1836 when he observed pallor in the development of Bright disease.[1] In 1907, Riesman[2] documented its hemorrhagic diathesis and cited the description by Morgagni (1682–1771) of epistaxis and hematemesis in a patient who "had the odor of urine on the breath." By 1922, Brown and Roth[3] had concluded that the anemia of chronic nephritis was due to decreased bone marrow production, and by 1933 Parsons and Ekola-Strolberg[4] had observed that the hemoglobin concentration in azotemia had roughly the same prognostic significance as the creatinine level. Hematologic changes had been firmly linked to renal failure. The elucidation of the complexities of this relationship would occupy many investigators for the remainder of the century.

## THE ANEMIA OF RENAL FAILURE

The anemia of renal failure is characterized by normocytic and normochromic red blood cells.[5] On blood smears, occasional deformed, spiculed red blood cells (burr cells) can be seen. A large number of schistocytes (helmet cells) suggests the possibility of hemolytic-uremic syndrome—a unique condition that is discussed separately. The bone marrow shows erythroid hypoplasia with little or no interference with leukopoiesis or megakaryocytopoiesis.[5] Anemia, initially mild and inconsequential, is virtually a constant feature of acute or chronic renal failure. However, as renal function progressively deteriorates, the hematocrit continues to decline and may reach levels as low as 15% to 20%. At that point, the patient usually experiences symptoms and transfusions may be necessary.

## Pathophysiology of Anemia

The anemia of renal failure is a complex disorder determined by a variety of factors. Although the primary defect is decreased erythropoiesis, a number of other factors may play contributory roles. Some degree of hemolysis is frequently present, bleeding can occur, and a superimposed iron or folic acid deficiency can complicate the problem. Finally, fluctuations in plasma volume caused by the disease or its treatment (i.e., hemodialysis) produce alterations in hematocrit that are spurious if the red blood cell mass has remained constant.

If the blood volume is constant and bleeding is absent, anemia must be explained by the decreased production or increased destruction of red blood cells. In the anemia of renal failure, both processes appear to be involved. The presence of anemia is evidence per se of failed production under existing conditions. However, if marrow is operating at maximal capacity, failure is relative to the presumptively overwhelming rate of red blood cell destruction that must dominate the clinical picture. Definition of the balance between red blood cell production and destruction in chronic renal failure was the subject of many early studies.

## Erythropoiesis and Hemolysis

In 1949, Finch and colleagues[6] showed that the utilization of iron in erythropoiesis was decreased in uremia. This observation was confirmed by others[7–10] and established decreased production as an important determinant of the anemia of chronic renal failure. The role of hemolysis was more ambiguous. Chaplin and Mollison[11] performed red blood cell survival studies on nine anemic patients with chronic nephritis. Three patients had normal survival times, indicating that anemia was due exclusively to a production defect. Six patients, of whom five had terminal disease, had decreased survival times indicative of increased red blood cell destruction. Hemolysis in the terminal stages of nephritis was also observed by others. Joske[7] and Loge[10] and their colleagues noted diminished red blood cell life span as a late complication of nephritis, and Shaw[12] demonstrated an inverse correlation between red blood cell survival time and serum blood urea nitrogen concentration. The frequency of hemolysis was variable and may be explained by differences in the population of patients or methodology. Using $^{51}$Cr, Kurtides and co-workers[13] observed decreased red blood cell survival in only 3 of 18 patients, and Eschbach and associates[14] using $^{32}$P-labeled diisopropyl flurophosphate observed a diminished red blood cell life span in 13 of 14 patients. Nonetheless, there was common agreement that decreased red blood cell production was the predominant defect in the anemia of chronic renal failure.[7–12] In the presence of normal erythropoiesis, increased marrow production can easily offset the mild to moderate hemolysis that occurs in uremia.[15] The hemolytic defect in uremia is extracorpuscular. Cross-transfusion studies have shown that normal red blood cells have a shortened life span in uremic patients, and uremic red blood cells have a normal survival in normal subjects.[8–10]

## Uremic Toxins

The inverse correlations between hemoglobin concentration[8] and red blood cell survival,[12] on the one hand, and blood urea concentration on the other drew attention to a potential direct effect of uremic waste products on red blood cells. With the advent of dialysis, azotemia could be controlled and its effect on anemia could be monitored. Both hemodialysis[14] and continuous ambulatory peritoneal dialysis[16] ameliorated the anemia. However, the mechanism of improvement was not lengthened red blood cell life span because red blood cell survival times were unchanged by hemodialysis.[14] Rises in hematocrit were ascribable instead to increases in iron utilization[13, 14] and red blood cell production.[17] The improved ferrokinetics and diminished transfusion requirement after dialysis now focused attention on uremic toxins as possible inhibitors of erythropoiesis.

Markson and Rennie[18] were the first to propose that a substance contained in uremic serum might inhibit erythropoiesis. Since that time, workers in a number of laboratories have sought such an inhibitor.[19] Wallner and Vautrin[20] reported that uremic serum inhibited heme synthesis by rabbit and mouse marrow cells. The level of inhibitor increased as the hematocrit fell and decreased as the hematocrit rose after dialysis. McGonigle and co-workers showed that the formation of erythroid colony-forming units in fetal mouse liver cell culture was inhibited by serum from uremic adults[21] and uremic children.[22] The effect appeared to be specific for the erythroid line in that granulocytic progenitor cell growth (granulocyte-macrophage colony-forming units) was not inhibited by uremic serum. However, these studies have not been totally confirmed. Although Delwiche and colleagues[23] confirmed the presence of inhibitors, they could not substantiate erythroid specificity. Brunati and co-

workers[24] were unable to demonstrate inhibition of erythroid burst-forming units by uremic serum. A number of specific compounds initially offered as inhibitors of erythropoiesis were subsequently challenged. The proposal that the polyamine spermine might be an inhibitor[25] was disputed by a report that polyamines are not elevated in uremic serum.[26] The data indicating that parathyroid hormone (PTH) is a uremic toxin responsible for erythropoietic inhibition[27] could not be reproduced with purified preparations of the hormone.[28] The latter conclusion is supported by a study that correlated resistance to erythropoietin and increased PTH with marrow fibrosis.[29]

The data concerning uremic toxins are confusing, and specific waste products demonstrably active as hemolysins or inhibitors of erythropoiesis remain to be identified.[30] However, the kidney is not limited to an excretory function.[31] It is also an endocrine organ that elaborates a number of hormones, including erythropoietin.

## Erythropoietin

In 1893, Miescher suggested that low oxygen pressure acted directly on the bone marrow to stimulate the production of red blood cells. However, in 1906 Carnot and Deflandre produced an increase in red blood cell count by injecting serum from anemic rabbits into normal rabbits. They suggested that the serum contained a substance called ''hémopoietine'' that was capable of stimulating the bone marrow.[32] In 1943, Krumdieck[33] documented reticulocytosis in normal rabbits after injection of anemic serum. Bonsdorff and Jalavisto[34] induced erythropoiesis in rabbits with plasma derived from patients with congestive heart failure and coined the term ''erythropoietin.'' A linkage between a humoral erythropoietic factor and hypoxia was fashioned by Reissmann[35] in 1950 with an ingenious experiment on parabiotic rats. He produced hypoxemia in one animal enclosed in a special breathing chamber containing 7.6% oxygen and augmented erythropoiesis in the parabiotic partner breathing normal air. Thus, hypoxemia was shown to act indirectly through an intermediary substance. Erslev[36, 37] confirmed the presence of an erythropoietic factor in the blood of anemic animals, and Stohlman and colleagues[38] associated increased erythropoiesis and secondary polycythemia with regional hypoxia in a patient with patent ductus arteriosus. In 1957, Jacobson and associates[39] demonstrated that bilaterally nephrectomized animals subjected to bleeding failed to elaborate increased erythropoietin. The following year, Gurney and co-workers[40] reported that patients with renal disease and anemia lacked erythropoietic stimulating factor (ESF) in their plasma.

### ERYTHROPOIETIN AND RENAL DISEASE

Many investigators attempted to clarify the kidney's role in erythropoiesis. The lack of an adequate ESF response in patients with chronic renal disease was confirmed in a number of laboratories.[41–43] However, in vivo bioassays of ESF were relatively insensitive and the detection of any measurable ESF in chronic renal disease was uncommon. Nonetheless, some erythropoiesis was clearly taking place. Decrease in the hematocrit after total nephrectomy demonstrated some residual ESF-secreting capacity in diseased kidneys.[44] Moreover, hemoglobin concentrations between 7 and 9 g/dL in anephric patients strongly suggested that ESF production was not completely dependent on renal tissue.[45] Extrarenal sources of erythropoietin were identified when ESF production in anephric rats was abolished by hepatectomy[46] and enhanced in partially hepatectomized animals as hepatic regeneration took place.[47] It was ultimately shown that 10% to 15% of all erythropoietin is produced by the liver and accounts for the residual red blood cell production observed in anephric patients.[48]

Modifications in technique increased the sensitivity of bioassays for erythropoietin. Adamson[49] measured urinary erythropoietin in normal subjects and patients with polycythemia. He noted the logarithmic increase in erythropoietic activity associated with decreasing hematocrit, the diminished erythropoietin secretion after transfusion, and the lack of increased erythropoietin in polycythemia vera. Radtke and co-workers[50] used in vitro bioassays in fetal mouse liver cell culture to obtain measurable erythropoietin levels in patients with chronic renal failure. Thus, they were able to demonstrate increasing erythropoietic activity in the serum of uremic patients as creatinine clearance and hematocrit declined. This suggested that the regulatory feedback mechanism between hematocrit and serum erythropoietin, with a lower set-point, remained operative in chronic renal failure. Caro and associates,[51] using concentrated plasma in a bioimmunoassay, noted detectable levels of erythropoietin in anephric patients, affirming the existence of the extrarenal sources.

## CHARACTERIZATION OF ERYTHROPOIETIN

In 1977, Miyake and co-workers[52] purified human erythropoietin and in 1986 Lai and colleagues[53] characterized its molecular structure. Several reviews summarize current knowledge regarding the structure and function of erythropoietin[54, 55] and its receptor.[56, 57] Erythropoietin is a sialylglycoprotein composed of 165 amino acids[55] with an estimated molecular mass of 34,000 daltons.[54] The carbohydrate moiety, rich in sialic acid, is critical to in vivo reactivity in that the asialo form is rapidly sequestered in the liver.[58] Erythroid colony-forming units are responsive to erythropoietin and are considered its main target cells.[55]

Purification of human erythropoietin led to the development of radioimmunoassay,[59–61] which replaced the more laborious and cumbersome bioassays. Normal human plasma contains 15 to 25 mU/mL erythropoietin. Under normal conditions, this concentration is increased by bleeding and decreased by transfusion.[60, 61] In the nonuremic anemic patient, the erythropoietin level may increase 100-fold.[60, 61] In uremia, erythropoietin may increase but not to the same degree[62] (Fig. 50–1). Despite the lack of a normal erythropoietic response, the erythropoietin-hematocrit feedback circuit is still operative in chronic renal failure. Studies have shown that erythropoietin levels in chronic uremic and anephric patients decline after transfusion[63, 64] and measurably increase after hemorrhage[64] or hypoxic crisis.[65]

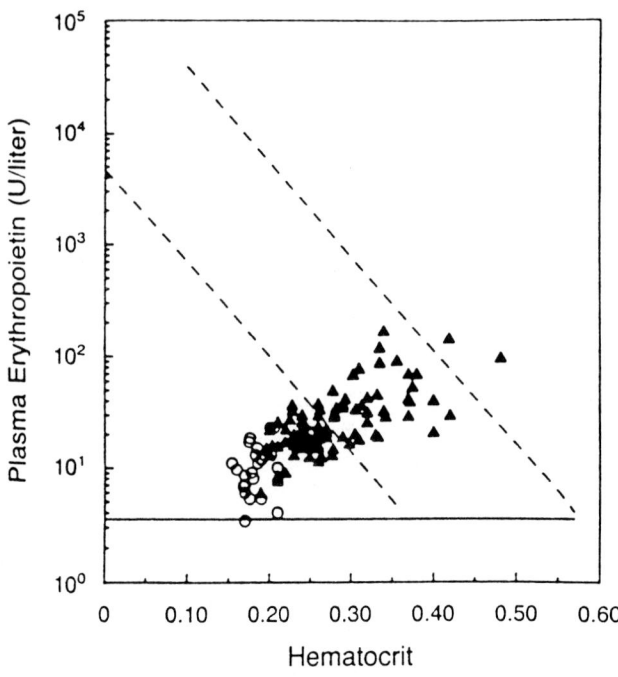

**Figure 50–1.** Plasma erythropoietin levels in 120 patients receiving dialysis, according to hematocrit. Open circles denote anephric patients and triangles, patients with kidneys. The broken lines represent 95% confidence limits for 175 normal blood donors and patients with anemia. The solid line represents the limit of detection of the assay. (From Erslev AJ: Erythropoietin. N Engl J Med 324:1339–1344, 1991. Reprinted by permission of The New England Journal of Medicine. Copyright 1991 Massachusetts Medical Society.)

Purification and structural definition of erythropoietin also permitted the cloning of the human erythropoietin gene.[66, 67] This led to the development of human recombinant erythropoietin[68] and the first truly effective treatment for the anemia of chronic renal failure.

## Management of Anemia

Before the development of recombinant human erythropoietin (rHuEPO), transfusions and androgens were the primary forms of treatment for the anemia of chronic renal failure. Although the hematocrit may be quite low, particularly in anephric patients transfusions should be used sparingly. Iron overload, transmission of infectious disease, suppression of residual erythropoietic stimulus, and the development of transfusion dependence are all inherent risks of chronic transfusion therapy in any patient with refractory, hypoproliferative anemia. The decision to transfuse should be based on a careful clinical assessment and judgment that the benefits of transfusion outweigh the risks. If transfusion can be avoided, it should be.

Androgens have been employed since 1970 with only modest success.[69] The injectable preparations nandrolone and testosterone enanthate are superior to the orally administered oxymetholone and fluoxymesterone. Only 50% of patients respond with an average increase in hematocrit of only 5%. Anephric patients and patients with an established transfusion requirement do not, as a rule, benefit from the administration of androgens. Balanced against potential benefits are the untoward effects of liver toxicity, acne, and virilization in women.[70]

## Recombinant Human Erythropoietin

The first clinical trials of rHuEPO were performed in England[71] and the United States.[72] The results were remarkable. Winearls and colleagues[71] gave rHuEPO by intravenous bolus to nine patients three times per week and raised the mean hemoglobin concentration from 6.1 to 10.3 g/dL within 12 weeks. Eschbach and co-workers[72] gave rHuEPO intravenously to 25 patients in doses ranging from 15 to 500 U/kg body weight and demonstrated a dose-dependent response (Fig. 50–2). Anephric transfusion-dependent patients responded equally well to rHuEPO, and the need for transfusion was eliminated. Other clinical trials in the United States,[73] Europe,[74, 75] and Japan[76] confirmed these favorable results. Concerns that the effectiveness of rHuEPO might be dependent on concomitant hemodialysis were dispelled by the equally favorable results obtained with predialysis patients[73, 77, 78] and patients receiving continuous ambulatory peritoneal dialysis.[79] A large multicenter trial reported in 1989[80] greatly expanded the number of favorable responses to rHuEPO. By 1990,[81] an estimated 2000 patients had been treated, and a 1991 review placed at 175,000 the number of patients who had been treated with this remarkable drug.[82]

A number of adverse effects have been documented in patients receiving rHuEPO. Myalgias and influenza-like symptoms of unknown etiology have occasionally been noted. They occur within 1 to 2 hours of rHuEPO infusion[71, 74, 80] and subside spontaneously after 10 to 12 hours. Six percent of patients (25 of 450) have experienced seizures during the first 3 months of rHuEPO therapy. However, this incidence is similar to that observed in a control dialysis population and may be unrelated to treatment with rHuEPO.[83] Thrombotic events are not increased by rHuEPO,[80, 83] although clotting within the dialyzer because of a rising hematocrit may require a slight increase in the dose of heparin.[84] An increasing hematocrit may also be associated with diminished dialyzer clearance, and minimal increases in creatinine, $K^+$, and phosphorus have been documented.[80] Although $K^+$ and phosphorus changes may be due to dietary increases, monitoring of these parameters in patients receiving rHuEPO is probably warranted.[83] Accelerated glomerular injury after correction of anemia has been observed in an animal model.[85] Concerns that this might occur in patients treated with rHuEPO have not held true.[86]

## ERYTHROPOIETIN AND HYPERTENSION

Hypertension occurs in approximately 30% to 35% of patients and is the most important adverse effect associated with rHuEPO therapy.[87] Its occurrence appears related to an accompanying defect in uremia in that increased blood pressure has not been observed in normal subjects who have received rHuEPO. Hypertension usually occurs during the first 4 months of treatment while the hematocrit is increasing. Thereafter, blood pressure stabilizes and is more easily controlled. Despite the temporal relationship with rHuEPO administration, hypertension is not correlated with the dose of rHuEPO or the rate of hematocrit increase. In addition, previously hypertensive patients do not appear to be at greater risk. Although dialysis patients are prone to seizures, an occasional patient receiving rHuEPO may demonstrate a clinical picture of hypertensive encephalopathy with headache, visual disturbances, seizures, and hypertension.[87]

The mechanism of hypertension is not clear. Neff and colleagues[88] noted increased peripheral vascular resistance in uremic patients rendered hypertensive by transfusion. Increased resistance induced by hematocrit-related changes of increased blood viscosity and loss of hypoxic vasodilatation may explain the hypertension observed with rHuEPO. Roger and colleagues[89] have shown that rHuEPO and 60% $O_2$ produce greater reversal of hypoxic vasodilatation in hypertensive than in normotensive uremic patients. Other possibilities have also been suggested. The plasma concentration of endothelin, an endothelium-derived vasoconstrictive peptide, is elevated in uremia.[90] Carlini and associates[91] have shown that rHuEPO increases endothelin-1 release from bovine pulmonary artery endothelial cells. Further studies are needed to clarify the etiology of rHuEPO-associated hypertension. In the interim, close monitoring of blood pressure changes during treatment with rHuEPO is essential.

## TREATMENT GUIDELINES

As experience in the use of rHuEPO increased, there was a growing awareness of the problems that could occur dur-

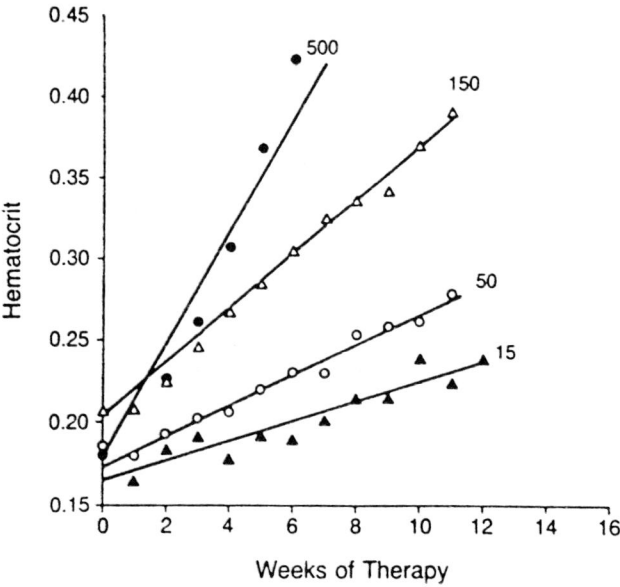

**Figure 50–2.** Slopes of the rates of increase in hematocrit associated with various doses of erythropoietin (U/kg body weight) given three times per week. (From Eschbach JW, Egrie JC, Downing MR, et al: Correction of the anemia of end-stage renal disease with recombinant human erythropoietin: Results of a combined phase I and II clinical trial. N Engl J Med 316:73–78, 1987. Reprinted by permission of The New England Journal of Medicine. Copyright 1987 Massachusetts Medical Society.)

ing therapy and the measures that might prevent them. Because rHuEPO is extraordinarily effective, the response must be carefully observed. A target hematocrit must be set, an appropriate rHuEPO dose selected, and schedules for monitoring the patient established. The guidelines suggested by an Ad Hoc Committee of the National Kidney Foundation[92] (Table 50–1) deal with safety and evaluation of the patient required to ensure an adequate response. Selection of an appropriate rHuEPO dose is a more complex issue.

During early clinical trials, Bommer and co-workers[93] noted that the dose of rHuEPO could be decreased 50% if given subcutaneously rather than intravenously. Other investigators[78, 79, 94–98] have made the same observation. Although intravenous doses give large peak concentrations, slow release from subcutaneous sites provides lower but more sustained concentrations that may stimulate erythropoiesis more efficiently. Besarab and colleagues[99] prepared concentration-time simulations for different dosing strategies and concluded that a total weekly rHuEPO dose of 110 to 120 U/kg divided into two or three subcutaneous injections is an effective and cost-efficient treatment for most dialysis patients. It is important to obtain maximal benefit from rHuEPO dosage schedules because costs are enormous[100] and highly dependent on rHuEPO dose.[101]

## Iron Balance and Other Deficiencies

Iron balance is maintained as long as iron intake equals iron loss. In chronic renal failure, this equilibrium can be displaced in either direction. Frequent, periodic transfusions constitute an excessive ''intake'' and inevitably lead to iron overload. Conversely, repeated loss of red blood cells during hemodialysis may lead to iron deficiency unless supplemental iron is prescribed.[102] Thus, the iron stores in a patient given chronic hemodialysis who receives an occasional transfusion are difficult to predict. They must be assessed and therapy instituted, preferably with oral ferrous sulfate, if a deficiency is found.[103] The estimation of iron stores before and during rHuEPO therapy is particularly

### TABLE 50–1. Guidelines for Treatment with Recombinant Human Erythropoietin

Patients with renal failure and hematocrits less than 30% are candidates for rHuEPO therapy.
Before therapy, iron stores should be assessed by determination of serum ferritin, serum iron, and total iron-binding capacity (TIBC).
Patients with microcytic anemia and normal iron stores should be evaluated for aluminum toxicity and thalassemia.
Uncontrolled hypertension is a contraindication for initiation of rHuEPO therapy.
Patients must be urged to adhere to pre-rHuEPO dietary restriction.
The hemoglobin level or hematocrit should be measured each week during induction of therapy and every 2 wk thereafter.
Serum iron, TIBC, and serum ferritin should be measured monthly for 3 mo and every 2–3 mo thereafter.

Adapted from Ad Hoc Committee for the National Kidney Foundation: Statement on the clinical use of recombinant erythropoietin in anemia of end-stage renal disease. Am J Kidney Dis 14:163–169, 1989.

important (see Table 50–1). Erythropoietin-induced red blood cell production may rapidly deplete even normal iron stores and necessitate oral or parenteral replacement. Response to rHuEPO therapy should be monitored with periodic serum iron, ferritin, and iron-binding capacity determinations. If transferrin saturation falls below 16% to 20% or the serum ferritin value below 30 μg/L, iron therapy should be initiated.[92, 104] If iron overload is the problem, the combination of rHuEPO and phlebotomy can produce impressive decreases in serum ferritin.[105]

Various deficiencies or complications can aggravate the anemia of chronic renal failure or be unmasked by an erythropoietin stimulus. Folate supplementation may be needed to offset the loss of folic acid during chronic hemodialysis,[106] and vitamin $B_{12}$ deficiency in the course of rHuEPO therapy has been noted in one patient.[107] Hemolysis caused by accidental formalin intoxication during hemodialysis[108, 109] and resistance to erythropoietin because of residual formaldehyde in dialyzers[110] have been described. Aluminum in antacids or in the dialysate may superimpose an aluminum-induced microcytosis on the anemia of chronic renal failure.[111] Patients with microcytosis but normal iron stores should be evaluated for aluminum toxicity to anticipate the potential for erythropoietin resistance.[92, 112]

## Quality of Life

The correction of anemia with rHuEPO has virtually eliminated the need for transfusion in most patients with the anemia of chronic renal failure. It has also improved quality of life as measured by several different parameters. Exercise capacity and tolerance have been measurably increased,[113–115] and surveys of both objective and subjective quality of life indicators have shown significant improvement.[116–118] rHuEPO has had a truly extraordinary impact on the treatment of the anemia of chronic renal failure.

## EFFECT OF RENAL FAILURE ON HEMOSTASIS

Bleeding in uremia[119, 120] is more easily controlled since the introduction of dialysis. Ecchymoses and epistaxis are the major bleeding manifestations seen today, with gastrointestinal bleeding, hemopericardium, or subdural hematoma occurring only occasionally.[121] However, the underlying bleeding diathesis remains. Uremic patients who undergo surgery or invasive procedures are always at risk for serious bleeding.

### Causes of Uremic Bleeding

In the past 20 years, research has clarified in part the nature of uremic bleeding. The pathogenesis is multifactorial and the major defects involve platelet–vessel wall and platelet-platelet interactions. The skin bleeding time is the best predictor of clinical bleeding.[122–124] It depends on the platelet number and function, vascular integrity, and hematocrit and thus gives an excellent overall assessment of primary hemostasis.[123] The platelet count in uremia is usually normal[125, 126] but platelet function is impaired. Dense granule content is decreased,[127, 128] and a storage pool defect with reduction in platelet ADP and serotonin is present. Decreased subnormal platelet ATP release in response to stimuli[127] indicates a defect in granule secretion.[129] $Ca^{2+}$ content is increased in uremic platelets,[130] which also mobilize $Ca^{2+}$ abnormally in response to stimulation.[131] Elevation in platelet cyclic AMP[132] and abnormal $Ca^{2+}$ mobilization[131] drew attention to the possibility that PTH plays a role in uremic platelet dysfunction. This speculation was supported by the observation that PTH inhibits platelet aggregation in vitro.[133, 134] However, the bleeding time does not correlate with serum concentrations of intact PTH or PTH fragments.[135] This suggests that elevated PTH in patients with renal failure is not likely to play a major role in the uremic platelet defect.

Several abnormalities of platelet-platelet interaction have also been reported in uremia. They include defective platelet aggregation in vitro in response to various stimuli[127, 136, 137, 138] and defective platelet thromboxane $A_2$ production in response to endogenous and exogenous stimuli[139, 140] not correctable by thrombin.[140] In a subpopulation of uremic patients, irreversible platelet aggregation does not occur in response to platelet-activating factor.[141, 142] This abnormality is independent of plasma factor(s) but is probably due to the platelets' reduced capacity to form thromboxane $A_2$ in response to platelet-activating factor. Animal experiments have suggested that the bleeding tendency in uremia is associated with excessive formation of nitric oxide (NO),[143] an endogenous vasoactive molecule that also inhibits platelet function.[144] This is supported by the observation that the prolonged bleeding time returns completely to normal when uremic rats are given N-monomethyl-L-arginine, a competitive inhibitor of NO synthesis. Data have indicated that in patients with chronic renal failure defective platelet aggregation is associated with increased platelet NO synthesis.[145] The same study also found significantly higher plasma levels of L-arginine, the substrate for NO synthesis, in uremic patients compared with healthy volunteers. Increased substrate availability cannot be expected to increase NO by upregulating a constitutive enzyme whose Michaelis constant, $K_m$, is already saturated by the levels of L-arginine found in control plasma. Rather it has been documented[146] that the inducible NO-forming enzyme, which has a $K_m$ around 30 $\mu$M, is dependent on the availability of extracellular arginine.

Two adhesive proteins, fibrinogen and von Willebrand factor (vWF), and two adhesion receptors, glycoprotein (gp) Ib and the gpIIb-IIIa complex, play a vital role in the formation of platelet thrombi at sites of injury.[147] The activation-dependent receptor function of the gpIIb-IIIa complex is defective in uremia, as shown by decreased binding of both vWF and fibrinogen to stimulated platelets.[148] The number of gpIIb-IIIa receptors expressed on the platelet membrane is normal but their activation is impaired. In contrast, the vWF-binding activity of gpIb is normal. Removal of substances present in uremic plasma markedly improved the gpIIb-IIIa defect. Thus, a reversible abnor-

mality of the activation-dependent binding activity of gpIIb-IIIa caused by a dialyzable toxic substance is probably a major component of the altered platelet function in uremia. The impaired gpIIb-IIIa activation in uremia may explain aggregation defects as well as reduced vWF-dependent adhesion and thrombus formation.[149–151]

The evidence that several dialyzable "toxins" (e.g., urea, creatinine, phenol, phenolic acids, or guanidinosuccinic acid) may be involved in the genesis of the uremic platelet dysfunction[152–154] is not compelling. Guanidinosuccinic acid, which accumulates in uremic plasma, inhibits the second wave of platelet aggregation to ADP when added to normal platelet-rich plasma.[153] Phenolic acid, at the concentrations found in uremic plasma, also impairs primary aggregation to ADP.[152] All these observations suggest that reducing the blood levels of these compounds may partially correct the abnormal hemostasis of patients with renal failure. However, no correlation has been found between bleeding time or platelet adhesion and the serum level of the dialyzable metabolites that mainly accumulate in uremia.[154]

Platelet adherence to foreign surfaces is impaired in uremia,[154–156] but this does not fully explain the prolonged bleeding time.[126, 154] Formation of vascular prostacyclin ($PGI_2$), a potent vasodilator and inhibitor of platelet function, is increased in both uremic patients[157, 158] and rats with experimental uremia.[159, 160] Plasma of uremic patients contains higher than normal amounts of a factor that stimulates vascular $PGI_2$.[161] This could be PTH, in view of findings that PTH increases urinary excretion of the $PGI_2$ metabolite, 6-keto-prostaglandin $F_{1\alpha}$.[162] In an investigation of vWF and platelet adhesion using blood from uremic patients with bleeding tendency, evidence was found of both platelet and plasma abnormalities.[149]

Quantitative and qualitative abnormalities of the vWF molecule, which promotes platelet adhesion and aggregation to subendothelial collagen,[163] have been reported. They may alter the platelet–vessel wall interaction and contribute to the hemorrhagic tendency of uremia.[164] Kazatchkine and colleagues[165] reported elevated vWF antigen levels but reduced ristocetin cofactor activity in uremic patients. However, other investigators have reported increased vWF functional activity.[166–168] Studies of the multimeric structure of vWF have not disclosed abnormalities.[169, 170]

The observation that cryoprecipitate,[169] a plasma derivative rich in factor VIII and vWF, and desmopressin,[170] a synthetic derivative of antidiuretic hormone that releases autologous vWF from storage sites, significantly shorten the bleeding time of uremic patients suggests that a functional defect in the vWF-platelet interaction may indeed play a role in the abnormal hemostasis of these patients.

Platelet adhesion and aggregation in flowing systems[171, 172] are markedly potentiated by red blood cells. Red blood cells enhance platelet function by releasing ADP,[173] by inactivating $PGI_2$,[174] and by increasing platelet–vessel wall contact by displacing platelets away from the axial flow and toward the vessel wall.[171] The independent role of anemia in the bleeding tendency of uremia has been extensively investigated. A significant negative correlation was found between bleeding time and packed cell volume (PCV) in 52 patients receiving chronic hemodialysis.[175] The bleeding time was longer than 270 seconds in 90% of patients with PCV less than 30% but in only 45% of patients with PCV greater than 30%. Despite a shorter bleeding time, a significant negative correlation between hematocrit and bleeding time was still demonstrable in 15 nonuremic anemic patients. These results were subsequently confirmed by other studies[176, 177] that found that anemia was the main determinant of the prolonged bleeding time in uremic patients. Uremic bleeding time has been shortened and symptomatic hemostatic improvement achieved by treatment with rHuEPO.[178, 179] In one randomized study,[180] the bleeding time became normal in all patients receiving erythropoietin as hematocrits increased to 27% to 32%. Thus, partial correction of anemia was sufficient to correct defective primary hemostasis in uremia (Table 50–2).

## Consequences of the Bleeding Tendency in Uremia

Gastrointestinal bleeding occurs with greater frequency and higher mortality in uremic patients than in the general population.[181, 182] Upper gastrointestinal bleeding is the second leading cause of death in acute renal failure.[183] The most common causes of bleeding are peptic ulcers, hemorrhagic esophagitis, gastritis, duodenitis, and gastric telangiectasias.[184–186] Angiodysplasia with gastrointestinal bleeding has been observed in the stomach, duodenum, jejunum, and colon.[187, 188] This abnormality, affecting the microcirculation of the gastrointestinal mucosa and submucosa, occurs most often in hemodialysis patients.[189] Finally, dialysis patients

---

**TABLE 50–2. Guidelines for the Management of Hemorrhagic Complications of Uremia**

For all patients with hemorrhagic complications or undergoing major surgery the adequacy of dialysis should be appropriately checked. It is also advisable to change the dialysis schedule for 1 or 2 mo in patients who have experienced severe hemorrhages (such as major gastrointestinal bleeding, hemorrhagic pericarditis, subdural hematomas) or who have undergone recent cardiovascular surgery, so that heparin can be avoided.

Acute bleeding episodes may be treated with desmopressin at a dose of 0.3 μg/kg, intravenously (added to 50 mL of saline over 30 min) or subcutaneously. Intranasal administration of this drug at a dose of 3 μg/kg is also effective and well tolerated. Because the favorable effect of cryoprecipitate on bleeding time has not been uniformly observed, we do not recommend its use. The effect of desmopressin lasts only a few hours, a major limitation to its use in treating severe hemorrhage, and desmopressin appears to lose efficacy when repeatedly administered.

The ideal treatment of persistent chronic bleeding should have a long-lasting effect. Conjugated estrogen treatment given by intravenous infusion in a cumulative dose of 3 mg/kg as daily divided doses (i.e., 0.6 mg/kg for 5 consecutive days) is the most appropriate way to achieve long-lasting hemostatic competence.

Severely anemic patients should receive blood or red blood cell transfusions to improve hematocrit values. Red blood cell transfusion is hemostatically effective only when the hematocrit rises above 30%. As an alternative, bleeding in patients with renal failure and hematocrit less than 30% can be treated successfully with erythropoietin (see Table 50–1).

---

suffering from human immunodeficiency virus nephropathy may have specific lesions such as Kaposi sarcoma, cytomegalovirus colitis, and non-Hodgkin lymphoma[190] that contribute to gastrointestinal bleeding. Although now rare, hemorrhagic pericarditis with cardiac tamponade can occur in uremia.[191, 192] The clinical features of this condition include normal cardiac shadow, increased jugular venous distention with hypotension, shortness of breath, and a pericardial friction rub. Deaths caused by hemorrhagic pericarditis have been reported to be as high as 3% to 5% among dialysis patients.[193, 194]

Subdural hematoma has been reported to occur in 5% to 15% of hemodialysis patients.[195] It usually overlies the frontal or parietal lobe and is bilateral in approximately 15% of cases. Headache, vomiting, seizures, hypertension, drowsiness, confusion, and coma are usual symptoms. Head trauma, hypertension, and systemic anticoagulation are risk factors.[195] Prognosis is at least partly related to the stage of diagnosis, and the mortality rate may be as high as 90% in patients requiring emergency surgery.

Anticoagulation during dialysis may be a major risk factor in causing bleeding in patients with fibrinous pleuritis.[196, 197] Spontaneous retroperitoneal bleeding is a rare complication in patients having chronic hemodialysis.[198, 199] Trauma, anticoagulation, and the presence of polycystic kidneys are predisposing factors. The symptoms and signs include sudden onset of pain in the abdomen, flank, back, or hip, with an associated drop in blood pressure. The hematocrit drops in the absence of any obvious blood loss. Computed tomography is useful in the diagnosis of retroperitoneal bleeding.

Spontaneous subcapsular hematoma of the liver is a newly recognized complication in uremia.[200] Typically patients have right upper quadrant pain, fever, and sometimes elevated bilirubin and alkaline phosphatase levels accompanied by a falling hematocrit.

Intraocular hemorrhage can also occur in uremia, and spontaneous hyphema has been reported during dialysis.[201] There is no visual loss and the hemorrhage generally resolves without any therapy. Intraocular bleeding with only temporary visual loss has also been reported in a large percentage of transplantation and dialysis patients after cataract surgery.

Another risk of bleeding in uremic patients is associated with aspirin given to prevent vascular access thrombosis[202] or platelet activation on dialyzer membranes.[203] The beneficial effect of aspirin on vascular access thrombosis can be achieved with the moderate dose of aspirin (160 mg/d) that inhibits platelet thromboxane $A_2$ generation without affecting vascular $PGI_2$ formation.[202] However, even a moderate dose of aspirin prolongs the bleeding time[204] and may explain the frequency of gastrointestinal bleeding in uremic patients.[188, 205] Thus, the use of aspirin for uremic patients treated with rHuEPO to prevent thrombotic complications associated with an increasing hematocrit is highly questionable.

## Abnormalities of Coagulation and Fibrinolysis

Activated partial thromboplastin, prothrombin, and thrombin times are generally normal in uremia.[155, 156, 165,]

[206–212] Fibrinogen and factor VIII are usually increased. Changes in the major natural inhibitors of coagulation have been reported and include increased antithrombin III,[206, 213–215] decreased protein C anticoagulant activity with normal protein C amidolytic activity and antigen,[216, 217] and decreased protein S.[218] Fibrinolytic activity has been reported to be decreased in uremia either absolutely[219–225] or relative to the extent of activation of coagulation.[215] This decrease is apparently due to a reduction in plasminogen activator coupled with an increase in antiplasmin and plasminogen activator inhibitor. In addition, desmopressin-induced release of tissue plasminogen activator from vascular endothelium is blunted in uremia.[226]

These abnormalities of coagulation or fibrinolysis partially corrected by dialysis[219, 226] predispose the uremic patient to thrombosis rather than bleeding.

Of interest, protein C and its cofactor protein S are further and significantly decreased in association with erythropoietin therapy, a finding that might contribute to the increased risk of thrombosis of the vascular access in patients receiving long-term erythropoietin treatment.

## Thrombotic Complications

Thrombosis of the arteriovenous shunt is a frequent occurrence in uremic patients undergoing hemodialysis. Because platelet aggregation plays a major role in thrombus formation, antiplatelet agents have been used, with encouraging results. Sulfinpyrazone, aspirin, and dipyridamole have proved useful in several studies.[227] Fibrinolytic agents, such as streptokinase[228, 229] or urokinase,[230] have produced contrasting results. More studies are needed to determine the most effective treatment for this complication.

## Therapeutic Strategies

Although hemodialysis may improve some aspects of the platelet functional environment,[231] it also can contribute to dysfunction and bleeding by inducing platelet–artificial surface interactions. Heparin may also present a problem. "Regional" heparinization has been used to minimize the effects of systemic anticoagulation.[232–234] Heparin is given by constant infusion through the inlet line of the dialyzer. Simultaneously, protamine sulfate is infused into the outlet port before the blood returns to the patient. Even this schedule of heparin administration, however, may be associated with a high incidence of bleeding.[235] As an alternative, frequent injections of low-dose heparin can be given during dialysis to maintain a lower and more constant level.[236] Usually, heparin at 40 to 50 IU/kg is given at the beginning of hemodialysis, followed by 60% of the initial dose after 1 and 2 hours and 30% of the initial dose after 3 hours.[236] The activated partial thromboplastin time is measured hourly and should be maintained at 1.5 to 2 times the basal value. Patients at high risk of bleeding can use an ethylene-vinyl alcohol copolymer hollow-fiber dialysis membrane that does not require systemic anticoagulation provided blood flow is maintained at greater than 200 mL/min.[237] Low-molecular-weight heparin has been proposed as an alternative to unfractionated heparin in patients having chronic hemodialysis who are at high risk of bleeding.[238] Aspirin and dipyridamole analogues reduce fibrin and cellular deposition on the filter membrane but increase the risk of gastrointestinal bleeding.[203, 239] $PGI_2$ shows some promise as an alternative.[240–242] Given in a continuous infusion during dialysis at a mean dose of 5 ng/kg/min, $PGI_2$ completely inhibited platelet aggregation without causing bleeding.[240] However, $PGI_2$ was associated with headache, flushing, tachycardia, and chest and abdominal pain, which required careful monitoring and a physician's supervision.[242–244] Thus, the use of $PGI_2$ should be limited to patients at high risk of hemorrhage. Peritoneal dialysis, when applicable, avoids the risk of bleeding associated with heparin or anticoagulants.

Anemia can contribute to the prolongation of bleeding time in uremia.[175–177] The progressive increase in hematocrit associated with rHuEPO therapy was accompanied by a significant decrease in the bleeding time[179, 180, 245] (Fig. 50–3). No consistent changes were found in platelet number, platelet aggregability, or platelet thromboxane $A_2$ formation.[179, 245] Only one study[246] observed a significant increase in the levels of vWF and ristocetin cofactor activity. In another study, 20 dialysis patients with prolonged bleeding time ($\geq 15$ minutes) were randomly allocated to receive rHuEPO or no specific treatment. Erythropoietin was given intravenously at the dose of 50 U/kg three times a week; every 4 weeks the dose was increased by 25 U/kg until bleeding time became normal. An erythropoietin dose of 150 to 300 U/kg/wk increased PCV to a range of 27% to 32% and normalized bleeding times in all patients (Fig. 50–4). A significant negative correlation was found between PCV and bleeding time.[180] Thus, the correction of anemia with rHuEPO may contribute significantly to the prevention and control of bleeding in uremic patients.

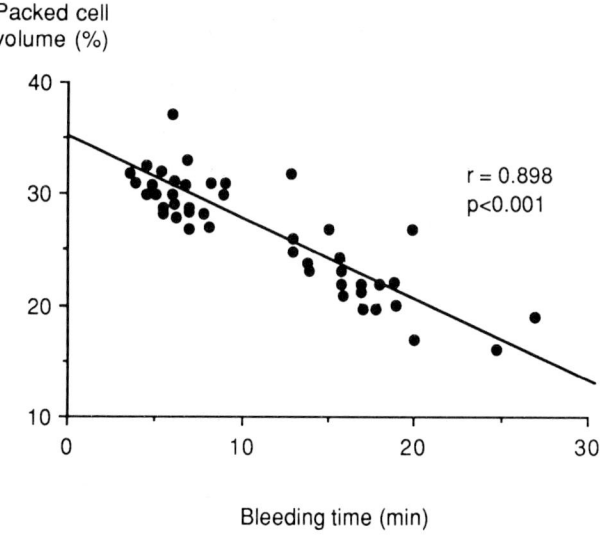

**Figure 50–3.** Correlation between bleeding time and PCV in patients treated with erythropoietin. This relationship was obtained when basal values and values obtained during erythropoietin therapy were pooled. (From Vigano G, Benigni A, Mendogni D, et al: Recombinant human erythropoietin to correct uremic bleeding. Am J Kidney Dis 18:44–49, 1991.)

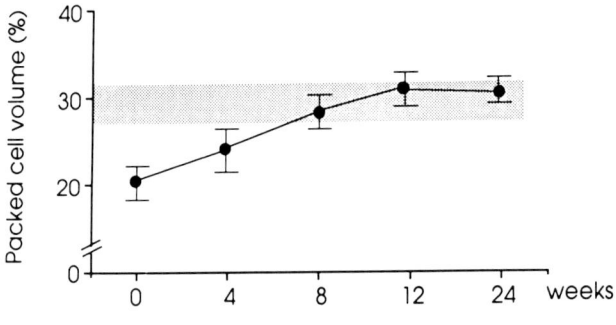

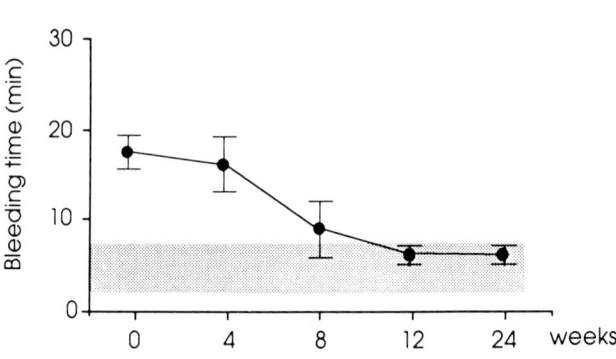

**Figure 50–4.** Effect of rHuEPO therapy on PCV and bleeding time in uremic patients. Dotted areas indicate the threshold of PCV to be reached for normalization of bleeding time values (up) and the normal range of bleeding time test (down).

Cryoprecipitate is a plasma derivative rich in vWF, fibrinogen, and fibronectin that has traditionally been used in the treatment of hemophilia A, von Willebrand disease, hypofibrinogenemia, and dysfibrinogenemia. Cryoprecipitate corrects prolonged bleeding in uremic patients within 4 to 12 hours, and the effect lasts 24 to 36 hours.[169] The mechanism of action of cryoprecipitate is not known. A small rise in platelet levels of fibrinogen and vWF-related properties were the only changes noted after cryoprecipitate infusion. Different preparations of cryoprecipitate, however, had different effects on bleeding time.[247]

The poor reproducibility of results and the risk of disease transmission prompted the search for alternatives to cryoprecipitate. Desmopressin (1-desamino-8-D-arginine vasopressin)—a synthetic derivative of the antidiuretic hormone—induces the release of autologous vWF from storage sites.[248] In a randomized, double-blind, crossover trial, desmopressin given intravenously at a dose of 0.3 μg/kg body weight in 50 mL of physiologic saline during a period of 30 minutes temporarily corrected the prolonged bleeding time in patients with chronic renal failure.[170] The shortening of bleeding time was significant 1 hour after the end of the infusion and the effect lasted 6 to 8 hours (Fig. 50–5). Desmopressin loses efficacy with repeated administration.[249] Desmopressin can also be given by the intranasal route,[250, 251] which is well tolerated and quite safe. At 10 to 20 times the intravenous dose, intranasal desmopressin (3 μg/kg) shortened the bleeding time[250, 251] and decreased clinical bleeding. Desmopressin has also been given subcutaneously,[252] in the same dose used for intravenous administration. Peak responses are achieved after a 30- to 90-

minute delay when the subcutaneous route is used. Adverse effects include facial flushing, mild transient headache, nausea, abdominal cramps, and mild tachycardia. In one case report, an elderly uremic patient with atherosclerosis suffered a stroke immediately after desmopressin infusion.[253] Nonetheless, desmopressin is useful in the treatment of bleeding and prophylactically in the prevention of bleeding during surgery or invasive procedures.

The anecdotal observation of diminished gastrointestinal bleeding in uremic patients treated with conjugated estrogens and the improved hemostasis in von Willebrand disease during pregnancy led to investigations of the effect of estrogens on bleeding in uremia.[254–256] One oral dose of 25 mg of conjugated estrogen normalized the bleeding time for 3 to 10 days with no apparent ill effects.[254] A controlled study showed that conjugated estrogens, given intravenously at the cumulative dose of 3 mg/kg divided over 5 consecutive days, produced a long-lasting reduction in the bleeding time in uremic patients. At least 0.6 mg/kg estrogen was needed to reduce the bleeding time,[256] and four or five infusions spaced 24 hours apart were needed to reduce the bleeding time by at least 50% (Fig. 50–6). The effect of estrogens on bleeding time in an animal model of chronic uremia was completely reversed by the NO precursor L-arginine,[257] suggesting that the effect of estrogens might be mediated by changes in NO synthesis. Thus, estrogens may be a reasonable alternative to cryoprecipitate or desmopressin in the treatment of uremic bleeding, especially when a long-lasting effect is required.

## EFFECT OF RENAL FAILURE ON GRANULOCYTES

Renal failure is associated with increased susceptibility to infections. This has stimulated research on the effect of uremia on leukocyte function. In cell-mediated defense against infectious agents, granulocytes and monocytes move by chemotaxis to the site of injury. Cells then phagocytose microorganisms through complex processes that in-

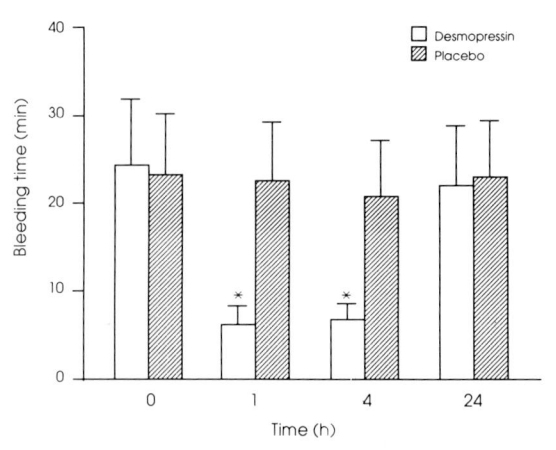

**Figure 50–5.** Effect of desmopressin (0.3 μg/kg) or placebo infusion on bleeding time measurements in uremic patients. *$P < .01$ versus basal values.

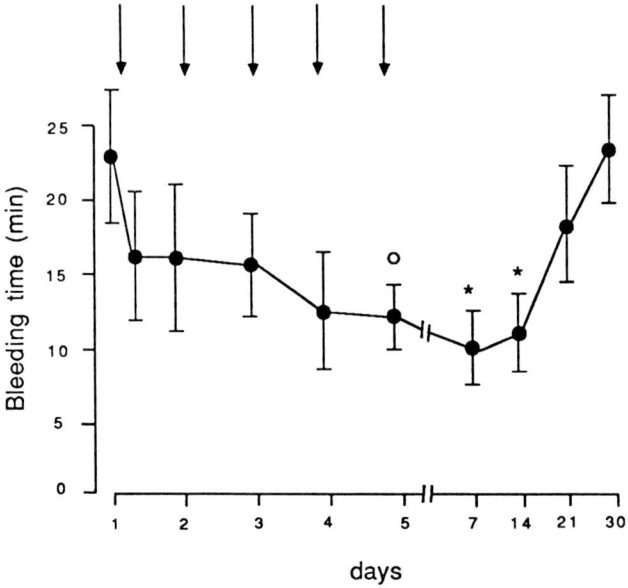

**Figure 50–6.** Effect of five infusions of conjugated estrogens (0.6 mg/kg each) on bleeding time in seven patients with uremia. Arrows indicate estrogen infusions ($^\circ P < .05$ and $*P < .01$ versus basal values). Data are expressed as means ± SD. (From Viganò G, Gaspari F, Locatelli M, et al: Dose-effect and pharmacokinetics of estrogens given to correct bleeding time in uremia. Used with permission from Kidney International, volume 34, pages 853–858, 1988.)

clude cell adhesion and the formation of oxygen free radicals (particularly hydrogen peroxide) from oxygen.

Many studies have found that leukocyte chemotaxis is impaired in uremia.[258–263] Impairment of chemotactic function may be associated with a circulating inhibitor of chemotaxis,[260, 263] decreased intracellular cyclic GMP/cyclic AMP ratio,[264, 265] or a plasma factor blocking granulocyte membrane receptors. Interestingly, the chemotactic activity of granulocytes is diminished further rather than corrected by hemodialysis.[266]

Studies of granulocyte phagocytosis and respiratory burst in uremia are conflicting. Abrutyn and co-workers[267] found normal phagocytic and bactericidal activities in uremic granulocytes together with normal serum opsonizing activity for staphylococci. Hydrogen peroxide formation and oxygen consumption during phagocytosis were also normal. Other investigators found depressed phagocytic activity[268] and respiratory burst.[269] A subsequent study[270] reported reduced phagocytosis related to decreased expression of Fc receptors on polymorphonuclear leukocytes. Hydrogen peroxide production by phorbol myristate acetate–stimulated polymorphs was impaired but normalized with hemodialysis. Because the subjects of the latter study had virtually no renal function, conflicting results might be reconciled by the speculation that uremic granulocytes retain the capacity to generate hydrogen peroxide until the late stages of renal failure. In another study,[271] reduced phagocytosis by granulocytes was associated with increased intracellular $Ca^{2+}$ concentration and reduced ATP. The last two findings suggest that the activity of the ATP-dependent $Ca^{2+}$ pump is reduced in uremia. A possible explanation might be that elevated PTH augments leukocyte $Ca^{2+}$ which inhibits mi-

tochondrial oxygen consumption and reduces ATP. A protein that inhibited chemotaxis, oxidative metabolism, and bacterial killing by granulocytes has been isolated from uremic serum.[272] Studies of leukocyte function during peritoneal dialysis are of particular interest because of the recurrent peritoneal infections that occur in these patients. Circulating and peritoneal neutrophils from patients having chronic ambulatory peritoneal dialysis showed various abnormalities including defects in the phagocytosis and intracellular killing of *Staphylococcus epidermidis*, the most common causative agent of peritonitis in chronic ambulatory peritoneal dialysis patients.[273]

Hemodialysis has a profound effect on granulocyte kinetics. During the first 2 hours of hemodialysis, all patients develop peripheral neutropenia mediated by complement activation on the dialysis membrane[274] and sequestration of granulocytes in the lung. In the hours following hemodialysis the release of neutrophils from the bone marrow and sites of sequestration produces rebound neutrophilia. Thus, pulmonary dysfunction occurring within the first hours of hemodialysis may be the result of endothelial injury caused by massive granulocyte adherence to pulmonary vessels. The normal interaction between dialysis membrane and plasma complement components is diminished as the dialyzer is reused.[275]

Workers in several laboratories have studied the effects of hemodialysis on white blood cell integrins, a family of transmembrane glycoproteins that interact with endothelial cell ligands as well as with complement components.[276–278] Mac-1, an integrin expressed primarily on granulocytes and macrophages, is a receptor for C3b1[278–280] and is involved in the adhesion of white blood cells to dialysis membranes.[281–284] During cuprophane hemodialysis, there is a rapid increase in the surface expression of Mac-1 associated with a consistent decrease in granulocyte counts,[285] which suggests that Mac-1 probably plays a role in the increased adhesion of leukocytes to dialysis membranes.[282, 285] By contrast, the use of hemophan or polysulfone membranes produced less Mac-1. Morever, during cuprophane hemodialysis the surface expression of Mac-1 remains elevated even as the granulocyte count normalizes. This suggests that more than one molecule may be implicated in the mechanism of granulocytopenia during cellulose membrane dialysis. A new family of leukocyte adhesion molecules has been described and the structure of one of them, leukocyte adhesion molecule-1 (LAM-1), has been elucidated.[286] LAM-1 is shed during leukocyte activation by chemotactic factors. LAM-1 shedding associated with decreased endothelial cell binding has also been exhibited by granulocytes harvested early during the first use of a cellulose dialysis membrane. This suggests that during cellulose hemodialysis complement activation up-regulates Mac-1, producing cell adhesion and sequestration. This is followed by LAM-1 shedding. Possibly the increased susceptibility to infection exhibited by hemodialysis patients is the consequence of low–LAM-1 granulocytes and the loss of their capacity to transmigrate to sites of infection. This suggestion is concordant with the higher incidence of infection in patients who have long-term cuprophane compared with polysulfone hemodialysis.[287]

Study of the adhesive properties of circulating cells can

be misleading because the most adhesive cells are likely to adhere and be unobtainable for study. Up-regulation of Mac-1 during cuprophane hemodialysis was slower and less pronounced for monocytes than for granulocytes even though the degree of monocytopenia during the first 15 minutes of hemodialysis was comparable to that observed for granulocytes. This may reflect a lesser amount of Mac-1 on monocytes[288] or the involvement of different molecules in monocyte adhesion.

Monocytes are markedly activated by contact with dialysis membranes, as documented by transient increases in plasma levels of interleukin-1 (IL-1) and tumor necrosis factor (TNF)[289] during hemodialysis.[290–294] Thus, within 5 minutes of cuprophane hemodialysis monocytes initiate transcription of IL-1 and TNF in large amounts.[295] In addition, macrophage colony-stimulating factor[296]—the growth factor for monocytes—accumulates in uremia and provides a further stimulus for the synthesis and secretion of IL-1 and TNF, by monocytes.

Because IL-1 and TNF up-regulate cell metabolism in different systems and increase the expression of genes encoding various biologically active proteins,[297] the functional consequences of monocyte activation during hemodialysis may be of some importance. The possibility that cytokines released by activated monocytes augment susceptibility to infections, immune dysfunction, and atherosclerosis has been investigated.[298] However, attempts to modify these abnormalities with IL-1 receptor antagonist or soluble TNF receptors have been inconclusive. Other studies have indicated that IL-1 and TNF may mediate hemodialysis-associated hypotension.[299, 300] A review[301] advanced the theory that both chronic and acute hypotension during dialysis may be the consequence of cytokine-induced activation of NO synthesis by endothelial cells and macrophages. This possibility is consistent with data[302] showing that NO production is elevated in patients having chronic hemodialysis. The same study demonstrated that uremic plasma is a potent inducer of NO synthesis by cultured human endothelial cells. Thus, hemodialysis-associated hypotension is probably the consequence of cytokine-activated vascular NO synthesis[301] that produces elevation in vascular smooth muscle cell cyclic GMP and vascular relaxation.

It has been known for many years that uremic patients have an acquired form of immunodeficiency characterized by abnormal T cell proliferation in response to antigenic challenges. This defect could well be the consequence of monocyte dysfunction, because T cell activation is monocyte dependent. The monocytes in uremic nonresponders to hepatitis B vaccination are unable to deliver to T lymphocytes the signal required to trigger IL-2 synthesis. Consistently, exogenous IL-2 normalizes the proliferative response of uremic T lymphocytes. Other studies[303, 304] have shown that purified IL-1, the monocyte-derived signal for T cell activation, is unable to normalize the T cell proliferative response. However, exogenous IL-2 eliminates the defect.[303] This observation is consistent with other studies[304, 305] showing reduced IL-2 production by uremic T cells.

Normal T cell activation is followed by the release of a soluble form of IL-2 receptor (IL-2R) into the circulation.[306] Uremic serum markedly inhibits the release of IL-2R.[304]

Because the release of IL-2R is IL-2 dependent and improved by dialysis, uremic serum may contain a "toxin" that inhibits IL-2 production. IL-2 exerts its biologic effect by binding to a high-affinity receptor that consists of two different α- and β-polypeptide chains. The α-subunit is expressed de novo and is an index of lymphocyte activation.[307] The β-subunit is constitutively expressed on resting T cells.[308] Both subunits have low affinity for IL-2, but the association of the two generates a receptor complex, IL-2R, with high affinity for IL-2. This receptor complex mediates IL-2 binding and internalization, thus triggering IL-2–dependent T cell proliferation,[309] which serves as a marker for specific, high-affinity, cell membrane receptors. The normal proliferative response of activated lymphocytes to recombinant IL-2 in the presence of uremic serum[304] could be taken as indirect evidence that uremia does not inhibit IL-2 binding to its high-affinity receptors or IL-2 internalization. Moreover, in the same set of experiments uremic serum up-regulated cell surface expression of biologically active high-affinity IL-2R. Chronic dialysis with a cuprophane membrane increased the expression of IL-2R α- and β-subunits but reduced the lymphocytes' expression of high-affinity receptors after stimulation with mitogens in vitro.[298] This abnormality is evident after 2 weeks of cuprophane membrane hemodialysis and persists thereafter. The same phenomenon has been reported in other immunodeficiency states such as acquired immunodeficiency syndrome.[310] In cuprophane hemodialysis, this observation could be explained by the assumption that lymphocytes activated by contact with cuprophane membrane become refractory to subsequent stimulation. However, further studies are needed to clarify the true clinical impact of reduced surface expression of IL-2R on the immunodeficiency of uremic patients.

### *Acknowledgments*

The authors are grateful to Dr. Gianluigi Viganò and Dr. Marina Noris for their invaluable cooperation. Ms. Laura Piccoli helped to prepare the manuscript.

## REFERENCES

1. Bright R: Cases and observations illustrative of renal disease accompanied with the secretion of albuminous urine. Guy's Hosp Rep 1:338–400, 1836.
2. Riesman D: Hemorrhages in the course of Bright's disease, with especial reference to the occurrence of a hemorrhagic diathesis of nephritic origin. Am J Med Sci 134:709–716, 1907.
3. Brown GE, Roth GM: The anemia of chronic nephritis. Arch Intern Med 30:817–840, 1922.
4. Parsons L, Ekola-Strolberg M: Anemia in azotemia. Am J Med Sci 185:181–190, 1933.
5. Callen IR, Limarzi LR: Blood and bone marrow studies in renal disease. Am J Clin Pathol 20:3–23, 1950.
6. Finch CA, Gibson JG, Peacock WC, Fluharty RG: Iron metabolism: Utilization of intravenous radioactive iron. Blood 4:905–927, 1949.
7. Joske RA, McAlister JM, Prankerd TAJ: Isotope investigations of red cell production and destruction in chronic renal disease. Clin Sci 15:511–522, 1956.
8. Kaye M: The anemia associated with renal disease. J Lab Clin Med 52:83–100, 1958.
9. Desforges JF, Dawson JP: The anemia of renal failure. Arch Intern Med 101:326–332, 1958.
10. Loge JP, Lange RD, Moore CV: Characterization of the anemia

associated with chronic renal insufficiency. Am J Med 24:4–18, 1958.
11. Chaplin H Jr, Mollison PL: Red cell life-span in nephritis and in hepatic cirrhosis. Clin Sci 12:351–360, 1953.
12. Shaw AB: Haemolysis in chronic renal failure. BMJ 2:213–216, 1967.
13. Kurtides ES, Rambach WA, Alt HL, del Greco F: Effect of hemodialysis on erythrokinetics in anemia of uremia. J Lab Clin Med 63:469–479, 1964.
14. Eschbach JW Jr, Funk D, Adamson J, et al: Erythropoiesis in patients with renal failure undergoing chronic dialysis. N Engl J Med 276:653–658, 1967.
15. Crosby WH, Akeroyd JH: The limit of hemoglobin synthesis in hereditary hemolytic anemia. Am J Med 13:273–283, 1952.
16. Zappacosta AR, Caro J, Erslev A: Normalization of hematocrit in patients with end-stage renal disease on continuous ambulatory peritoneal dialysis. Am J Med 72:53–57, 1982.
17. Eschbach JW, Adamson JW, Cook JD: Disorders of red blood cell production in uremia. Arch Intern Med 126:812–815, 1970.
18. Markson JL, Rennie JB: The anemia of chronic renal insufficiency. The effect of serum from azotaemic patients on the maturation of normoblasts in suspension cultures. Scott Med J 1:320, 1956.
19. Fisher JW: Mechanism of the anemia of chronic renal failure. Nephron 25:106–111, 1980.
20. Wallner SF, Vautrin RM: Evidence that inhibition of erythropoiesis is important in the anemia of chronic renal failure. J Lab Clin Med 97:170–178, 1981.
21. McGonigle RJS, Wallin JD, Shadduck RK, Fisher JW: Erythropoietin deficiency and inhibition of erythropoiesis in renal insufficiency. Kidney Int 25:437–444, 1984.
22. McGonigle RJS, Boineau FG, Beckman B, et al: Erythropoietin and inhibitors of in vitro erythropoiesis in the development of anemia in children with renal disease. J Lab Clin Med 105:449–458, 1985.
23. Delwiche F, Segal GM, Eschbach JW, Adamson JW: Hematopoietic inhibitors in chronic renal failure: Lack of in vitro specificity. Kidney Int 29:641–648, 1986.
24. Brunati C, Cappellini MD, DeFeo T, et al: Uremic inhibitors of erythropoiesis: A study during treatment with recombinant human erythropoietin. Am J Nephrol 12:9–13, 1992.
25. Radtke HW, Rege AB, LaMarche MB, et al: Identification of spermine as an inhibitor of erythropoiesis in patients with chronic renal failure. J Clin Invest 67:1623–1629, 1981.
26. Spragg BP, Bently AP, Coles GA: Anemia of chronic renal failure: Polyamines are not raised in uremic serum. Nephron 38:65–66, 1984.
27. Meytes D, Bogin E, Ma A, et al: Effect of parathyroid hormone on erythropoiesis. J Clin Invest 67:1263–1269, 1981.
28. Delwiche F, Garrity MJ, Powell JS, et al: High levels of the circulating form of parathyroid hormone do not inhibit in vitro erythropoiesis. J Lab Clin Med 102:613–620, 1983.
29. Rao DS, Shih M-S, Mohini R: Effect of serum parathyroid hormone and bone marrow fibrosis on the response to erythropoietin in uremia. N Engl J Med 328:171–175, 1993.
30. Bergstrom J, Furst P: Uremic toxins. Kidney Int 13(suppl 8):S9–S12, 1978.
31. Eschbach JW, Adamson JW: Anemia of end-stage renal disease (ESRD). Kidney Int 28:1–5, 1985.
32. Erslev A: Blood and mountains. In Wintrobe MM (ed): Blood Pure and Eloquent. McGraw-Hill, New York, 1980, pp 257–280.
33. Krumdieck N: Erythropoietic substance in the serum of anemic animals. Proc Soc Exp Biol Med 54:14–17, 1943.
34. Bonsdorff E, Jalavisto E: A humoral mechanism in anoxic erythrocytosis. Acta Physiol Scand 16:150–170, 1948.
35. Reissmann KR: Studies on the mechanism of erythropoietic stimulation in parabiotic rats during hypoxia. Blood 5:372–380, 1950.
36. Erslev A: Humoral regulation of red cell production. Blood 8:349–357, 1953.
37. Erslev A: Physiologic control of red cell production. Blood 10:954–961, 1955.
38. Stohlman F Jr, Rath CE, Rose JC: Evidence for a humoral regulation of erythropoiesis. Blood 9:721–733, 1954.
39. Jacobson LO, Goldwasser E, Fried W, Plzak L: Role of the kidney in erythropoiesis. Nature 179:633–634, 1957.
40. Gurney CW, Jacobson LO, Goldwasser E: The physiologic and clinical significance of erythropoietin. Ann Intern Med 49:363–370, 1958.
41. Gallagher NI, McCarthy JM, Lange RD: Observations on erythropoietic-stimulating factor (ESF) in the plasma of uremic and non-uremic anemic patients. Ann Intern Med 52:1201–1212, 1960.
42. Naets J-P, Heuse AF: Measurement of erythropoietic stimulating factor in anemic patients with or without renal disease. J Lab Clin Med 60:365–373, 1962.
43. Mann DL, Donati RM, Gallagher NI: Erythropoietin assay and ferrokinetic measurements in anemic uremic patients. JAMA 194:153–154, 1965.
44. Kominami N, Lowrie EG, Ianhez LE, et al: The effect of total nephrectomy on hematopoiesis in patients undergoing chronic hemodialysis. J Lab Clin Med 78:524–532, 1971.
45. Nathan DG, Schupak E, Stohlman F Jr, Merrill JP: Erythropoiesis in anephric man. J Clin Invest 43:2158–2165, 1964.
46. Fried W: The liver as a source of extrarenal erythropoietin production. Blood 40:671–677, 1972.
47. Anagnostou A, Schade S, Barone J, Fried W: Effects of partial hepatectomy on extrarenal erythropoietin production in rats. Blood 50:457–462, 1977.
48. Erslev A: Erythropoietin coming of age. N Engl M Med 316:101–103, 1987.
49. Adamson JW: The erythropoietin/hematocrit relationship in normal and polycythemic man: Implications of marrow regulation. Blood 32:597–609, 1968.
50. Radtke HW, Claussner A, Erbes PM, et al: Serum erythropoietin concentration in chronic renal failure: Relationship to degree of anemia and excretory renal function. Blood 54:877–884, 1979.
51. Caro J, Brown S, Miller O, et al: Erythropoietin levels in uremic nephric and anephric patients. J Lab Clin Med 93:449–458, 1979.
52. Miyake T, Kung CK-H, Goldwasser E: Purification of human erythropoietin. J Biol Chem 252:5558–5564, 1977.
53. Lai P-H, Everett R, Wang F-F, et al: Structural characterization of human erythropoietin. J Biol Chem 261:3116–3121, 1986.
54. Krantz SB: Erythropoietin. Blood 77:419–434, 1991.
55. Jelkmann W: Erythropoietin: Structure, control of production and function. Physiol Rev 72:449–489, 1992.
56. D'Andrea AD, Zon LI: Erythropoietin receptor: Subunit structure and activation. J Clin Invest 86:681–687, 1990.
57. Youssoufian H, Longmore G, Neumann D, et al: Structure, function and activation of the erythropoietin receptor. Blood 81:2223–2236, 1993.
58. Spivak JL, Hogans BB: The in vivo metabolism of recombinant human erythropoietin in the rat. Blood 73:90–99, 1989.
59. Sherwood JB, Goldwasser E: A radioimmunoassay for erythropoietin. Blood 54:885–893, 1979.
60. Garcia JF, Sherwood J, Goldwasser E: Radioimmunoassay for erythropoietin. Blood Cells 5:405–419, 1979.
61. Cotes PM: Immunoreactive erythropoietin in serum. Br J Haematol 50:427–438, 1982.
62. Erslev AJ: Erythropoietin. N Engl M Med 324:1339–1344, 1991.
63. Naets JP, Garcia JF, Toussaint C, et al: Radioimmunoassay of erythropoietin in chronic uraemia or anephric patients. Scand J Haematol 37:390–394, 1986.
64. Walle AJ, Wong GY, Clemons GK, et al: Erythropoietin-hematocrit feedback circuit in the anemia of end-stage renal disease. Kidney Int 31:1205–1209, 1987.
65. Chandra M, Clemons GK, McVicar MI: Relation of serum erythropoietin levels to renal excretory function: Evidence for lowered set point for erythropoietin production in chronic renal failure. J Pediatr 113:1015–1021, 1988.
66. Jacobs K, Shoemaker C, Rudersdorf R, et al: Isolation and characterization of genomic and cDNA clones of human erythropoietin. Nature 313:806–810, 1985.
67. Lin F-K, Suggs S, Lin C-H, et al: Cloning and expression of the human erythropoietin gene. Proc Natl Acad Sci USA 82:7580–7584, 1985.
68. Egrie JC, Strickland TW, Lane J, et al: Characterization and biological effects of recombinant human erythropoietin. Immunobiology 172:213–224, 1986.
69. Androgens in the anaemia of chronic renal failure. BMJ 2:417–418, 1977. Editorial.
70. Neff MS, Goldberg J, Slifkin RF, et al: A comparison of androgens for anemia in patients on hemodialysis. N Engl J Med 304:871–875, 1981.
71. Winearls CG, Oliver DO, Pippard MJ, et al: Effect of human eryth-

ropoietin derived from recombinant DNA on the anaemia of patients maintained by chronic haemodialysis. Lancet 2:1175–1178, 1986.

72. Eschbach JW, Egrie JC, Downing MR, et al: Correction of the anemia of end-stage renal disease with recombinant human erythropoietin. N Engl J Med 316:73–78, 1987.

73. Stone WJ, Graber SE, Krantz SB, et al: Treatment of the anemia of predialysis patients with recombinant human erythropoietin: A randomized, placebo-controlled trial. Am J Med Sci 296:171–179, 1988.

74. Casati S, Passerini P, Campise MR, et al: Benefits and risks of protracted treatment with human recombinant erythropoietin in patients having haemodialysis. BMJ 295:1017–1020, 1987.

75. Bommer J, Kugel M, Schoeppe W, et al: Dose-related effects of recombinant human erythropoietin on erythropoiesis: Results of a multicenter trial in patients with end-stage renal disease. Contrib Nephrol 66:85–93, 1988.

76. Akizawa T, Koshikawa S, Takaku F, et al: Clinical effect of recombinant human erythropoietin on anemia associated with chronic renal disease. A multiinstitutional study in Japan. Int J Artif Organs 11:343–350, 1988.

77. Lim VS, DeGowin RL, Zavala D, et al: Recombinant human erythropoietin treatment in pre-dialysis patients. Ann Intern Med 110:108–114, 1989.

78. Eschbach JW, Kelly MR, Haley NR, et al: Treatment of the anemia of progressive renal failure with recombinant human erythropoietin. N Engl J Med 321:158–163, 1989.

79. Steinhauer HB, Lubrich-Birkner I, Dreyling KW, Schollmeyer P: Effect of human recombinant erythropoietin on anaemia and dialysis efficiency in patients undergoing continuous ambulatory peritoneal dialysis. Eur J Clin Invest 21:47–52, 1991.

80. Eschbach JW, Abdulhadi MH, Browne JK, et al: Recombinant human erythropoietin in anemic patients: Results of a phase III multicenter clinical trial. Ann Intern Med 111:992–1000, 1989.

81. Adamson JW, Eschbach JW: Treatment of the anemia of chronic renal failure with recombinant human erythropoietin. Annu Rev Med 41:349–360, 1990.

82. Eschbach JW: Erythropoietin 1991—an overview. Am J Kidney Dis 18(suppl 1):3–9, 1991.

83. Eschbach JW, Adamson JW: Guidelines for recombinant human erythropoietin therapy. Am J Kidney Dis 14(suppl 1):2–8, 1989.

84. Eschbach JW, Adamson JW: Recombinant human erythropoietin: Implication for nephrology. Am J Kidney Dis 11:203–209, 1988.

85. Garcia DL, Anderson S, Rennke HG, Brenner BM: Anemia lessens and its prevention with recombinant human erythropoietin worsens glomerular injury and hypertension in rats with reduced renal mass. Proc Natl Acad Sci USA 85:6142–6146, 1988.

86. Lim VS, Fangman J, Flanigan MJ, et al: Effect of recombinant human erythropoietin on renal function in humans. Kidney Int 37:131–136, 1990.

87. Raine AEG, Roger SD: Effects of erythropoietin on blood pressure. Am J Kidney Dis 18(suppl 1):76–83, 1991.

88. Neff MS, Kim KE, Persoff M, et al: Hemodynamics of uremic anemia. Circulation 43:876–883, 1971.

89. Roger SB, Grasty MS, Baker LRI, Raine AEG: Effects of oxygen breathing and erythropoietin on hypoxic vasodilation in uremic anemia. Kidney Int 42:975–980, 1992.

90. Shichiri M, Hirata Y, Ando K, et al: Plasma endothelin levels in hypertension and chronic renal failure. Hypertension 15:493–496, 1990.

91. Carlini RG, Dusso AS, Obialo CI, et al: Recombinant human erythropoietin (rHuEPO) increases endothelin-1 release by endothelial cells. Kidney Int 43:1010–1014, 1993.

92. Ad Hoc Committee for the National Kidney Foundation: Statement on the clinical use of recombinant erythropoietin in anemia of end-stage renal disease. Am J Kidney Dis 14:163–169, 1989.

93. Bommer J, Ritz E, Weinreich T, et al: Subcutaneous erythropoietin. Lancet 2:406, 1988.

94. Hughes RT, Cotes PM, Pippard MJ, et al: Subcutaneous administration of recombinant human erythropoietin to subjects on continuous ambulatory peritoneal dialysis: An erythrokinetic assessment. Br J Haematol 75:268–273, 1990.

95. Lui SF, Chung WWM, Leung CB, et al: Pharmacokinetics and pharmacodynamics of subcutaneous and intraperitoneal administration of recombinant human erythropoietin in patients on continuous ambulatory peritoneal dialysis. Clin Nephrol 33:47–51, 1990.

96. Muirhead N, Churchill DN, Goldstein M, et al: Comparison of subcutaneous and intravenous recombinant human erythropoietin for anemia in hemodialysis patients with significant comorbid disease. Am J Nephrol 12:303–310, 1992.

97. Montini G, Zacchello G, Perfumo F, et al: Pharmacokinetics and hematologic response to subcutaneous administration of recombinant human erythropoietin in children undergoing long-term peritoneal dialysis: A multicenter study. J Pediatr 122:297–302, 1993.

98. Ateshkadi A, Johnson CA, Oxton LL, et al: Pharmacokinetics of intraperitoneal, intravenous and subcutaneous recombinant human erythropoietin in patients on continuous ambulatory peritoneal dialysis. Am J Kidney Dis 21:635–642, 1993.

99. Besarab A, Flaharty KK, Erslev AJ, et al: Clinical pharmacology and economics of recombinant human erythropoietin in end-stage renal disease: The case for subcutaneous administration. J Am Soc Nephrol 2:1405–1416, 1992.

100. Doolittle RF: Biotechnology—the enormous cost of success. N Engl J Med 324:1360–1362, 1991.

101. Powe NR, Griffiths RI, Bass EB: Cost implications to Medicare of recombinant erythropoietin therapy for the anemia of end-stage renal disease. J Am Soc Nephrol 3:1660–1671, 1993.

102. Eschbach JW, Cook JD, Scribner BH: Iron balance in hemodialysis patients. Ann Intern Med 87:710–713, 1977.

103. Parker PA, Izard MW, Maher JF: Therapy of iron deficiency anemia in patients on maintenance dialysis. Nephron 23:181–186, 1979.

104. Van Wyck DB, Stivelman JC, Ruiz J, et al: Iron status in patients receiving erythropoietin for dialysis-associated anemia. Kidney Int 35:712–716, 1989.

105. McCarthy JT, Johnson WJ, Nixon DE, et al: Transfusional iron overload in patients undergoing dialysis: Treatment with erythropoietin and phlebotomy. J Lab Clin Med 114:193–199, 1989.

106. Hampers CL, Streiff R, Nathan DG, et al: Megaloblastic hematopoiesis in uremia and in patients on long-term hemodialysis. N Engl J Med 276:551–554, 1967.

107. Zachee P, Chew SL, Daelemans R, Lins RL: Erythropoietin resistance due to vitamin $B_{12}$ deficiency. Am J Nephrol 12:188–191, 1992.

108. Orringer EP, Mattern WD: Formaldehyde-induced hemolysis during chronic hemodialysis. N Engl J Med 294:1416–1420, 1976.

109. Pun KK, Yeung CK, Chan TK: Acute intravascular hemolysis due to accidental formalin intoxication during hemodialysis. Clin Nephrol 21:188–190, 1984.

110. Ng Y-Y, Chow M-P, Lyou J-Y, et al: Resistance to erythropoietin: Immunohemolytic anemia induced by residual formaldehyde in dialyzers. Am J Kidney Dis 21:213–216, 1993.

111. Touam M, Martinez F, Lacour B, et al: Aluminium-induced, reversible microcytic anemia in chronic renal failure: Clinical and experimental studies. Clin Nephrol 19:295–298, 1983.

112. Ponticelli C, Casati S: Correction of anemia with recombinant human erythropoietin. Nephron 52:201–208, 1989.

113. Mayer G, Thum J, Cada EM, et al: Working capacity is increased following recombinant human erythropoietin treatment. Kidney Int 34:525–528, 1988.

114. Robertson HT, Haley NR, Guthrie MR, et al: Recombinant erythropoietin improves exercise capacity in anemic hemodialysis patients. Am J Kidney Dis 15:325–332, 1990.

115. Guthrie M, Cardenas D, Eschbach JW, et al: Effects of erythropoietin on strength and functional status of patients on hemodialysis. Clin Nephrol 39:97–102, 1993.

116. Evans RW, Rader B, Manninen DL, et al: The quality of life of hemodialysis recipients treated with recombinant human erythropoietin. JAMA 263:825–830, 1990.

117. Evans RW: Recombinant human erythropoietin and the quality of life of end-stage renal disease patients: A comparative study. Am J Kidney Dis 18(suppl 1):62–70, 1991.

118. McMahon LP, Dawborn JK: Subjective quality of life assessment in hemodialysis patients at different levels of hemoglobin following use of recombinant human erythropoietin. Am J Nephrol 12:162–169, 1992.

119. Morgagni GB: Opera Omnia. Ex Typographia Remondiniana, Venezia, 1764.

120. Bright R: Reports of Medical Cases. London, 1827.

121. Watson AJ, Gimenez LF: The bleeding diathesis of uremia. Semin Dial 4:86–93, 1991.

122. Steiner RW, Coggins C, Carvalho ACA: Bleeding time in uremia. A

useful test to assess clinical bleeding. Am J Hematol 7:107–117, 1979.

123. Lind SE: Prolonged bleeding time. Am J Med 77:305–312, 1984.

124. Kumar R, Ansell JE, Conoso RT, Deykin D: Clinical trial of a new bleeding time device. Am J Clin Pathol 70:642–645, 1978.

125. Lindsay RM, Moorthy AV, Koens F, Linton AL: Platelet function in dialyzed and non-dialyzed patients with chronic renal failure. Clin Nephrol 4:52–57, 1975.

126. Eknoyan G, Wacksman SJ, Glueck HI, Will JJ: Platelet function in renal failure. N Engl J Med 280:677–681, 1969.

127. Di Minno G, Martinez J, McKean M, et al: Platelet dysfunction in uremia. Multifaceted defect partially corrected by dialysis. Am J Med 79:552–559, 1985.

128. Eknoyan G, Brown CH: Biochemical abnormalities of platelets in renal failure. Evidence for decreased platelet serotonin, adenosine diphosphate and Mg-dependent adenosine triphosphatase. Am J Nephrol 1:17–23, 1981.

129. Kyrle PA, Stockenhuber F, Brenner BM, et al: Evidence for an increased generation of prostacyclin in the microvasculature and an impairment of the platelet alpha-granule release in chronic renal failure. Thromb Haemost 60:205–208, 1988.

130. Gura V, Creter D, Levi J: Elevated thrombocyte calcium content in uremia and its correction by $1\alpha(OH)$ vitamin D treatment. Nephron 30:237–239, 1982.

131. Ware JA, Clark BA, Smith M, Salzman EW: Abnormalities of cytoplasmic $Ca^{2+}$ in platelets from patients with uremia. Blood 73:172–176, 1989.

132. Vlachoyannis J, Schoeppe W: Adenylate cyclase activity and cAMP content of human platelets in uremia. Eur J Clin Invest 12:379–381, 1982.

133. Remuzzi G, Benigni A, Dodesini P, et al: Parathyroid hormone inhibits human platelet function. Lancet 2:1321–1323, 1981.

134. Benigni A, Livio M, Dodesini P, et al: Inhibition of human platelet aggregation by parathyroid hormone: Is cyclic AMP implicated? Am J Nephrol 5:243–247, 1985.

135. Viganò G, Gotti E, Comberti E, et al: Hyperparathyroidism does not influence the abnormal primary haemostasis in patients with chronic renal failure. Nephrol Dial Transplant 4:971–974, 1989.

136. Rabiner SF: Uraemic bleeding. In Spaet TH (ed): Progress in Hemostasis and Thrombosis. Grune & Stratton, New York, 1972, pp 233–250.

137. Remuzzi G, Benigni A, Dodesini P, et al: Platelet function in patients on maintenance hemodialysis: Depressed or enhanced? Clin Nephrol 17:60–63, 1982.

138. Zicker MB: Biological aspects of heparin action. Heparin and platelet function. Fed Proc 36:47–49, 1977.

139. Smith MC, Dunn MJ: Impaired platelet thromboxane production in renal failure. Nephron 29:133–137, 1981.

140. Remuzzi G, Benigni A, Dodesini P, et al: Reduced platelet thromboxane formation in uremia. Evidence for a functional cyclooxygenase defect. J Clin Invest 71:762–768, 1983.

141. Macconi D, Viganò G, Bisogno G, et al: Defective platelet aggregation in response to platelet-activating factor in uremia associated with low platelet thromboxane $A_2$ generation. Am J Kidney Dis 19:318–325, 1992.

142. Livio E, Benigni A, Remuzzi G: Coagulation abnormalities in uremia. Semin Nephrol 5:82–90, 1985.

143. Remuzzi G, Perico N, Zoja C, et al: Role of endothelium-derived nitric oxide in the bleeding tendency of uremia. J Clin Invest 86:1768–1771, 1990.

144. Ignarro LJ: Endothelium-derived nitric oxide: Actions and properties. FASEB J 3:31–36, 1988.

145. Noris M, Benigni A, Boccardo P, et al: Enhanced nitric oxide synthesis in uremia: Implications for platelet dysfunction and dialysis hypotension. Kidney Int 44:445–450, 1993.

146. Yui Y, Hattori R, Kosuga K, et al: Purification of nitric oxide synthase from rat macrophages. J Biol Chem 266:12544–12547, 1991.

147. Schmitt GW, Moake JL, Rudy CK, et al: Alterations in hemostatic parameters during hemodialysis with dialyzers of different membrane composition and flow design. Am J Med 83:411–418, 1987.

148. Benigni A, Boccardo P, Galbusera M, et al: Reversible activation defect of the platelet glycoprotein IIb-IIIa complex in patients with uremia. Am J Kidney Dis 22:668–676, 1993.

149. Castillo R, Lozano T, Escolar G, et al: Defective platelet adhesion on vessel subendothelium in uremic patients. Blood 65:337–342, 1986.

150. Zwaginga JJ, Ijsseldijk MJW, Beeser-Visser N, et al: High von Willebrand factor concentration compensates a relative adhesion defect in uremic blood. Blood 75:1498–1508, 1990.

151. Escolar G, Cases A, Bastida E, et al: Uremic platelets have a functional defect affecting the interaction of von Willebrand factor with glycoprotein IIb-IIIa. Blood 76:1336–1340, 1990.

152. Rabiner SF, Molinas F: The role of phenol and phenolic acids on the thrombocytopathy and defective platelet aggregation of patients with renal failure. Am J Med 49:346–351, 1970.

153. Horowitz HI, Stein IM, Cohen BD, White JG: Further studies on the platelet inhibitory effect of guanidinosuccinic acid and its role in uremic bleeding. Am J Med 49:336–345, 1970.

154. Remuzzi G, Livio E, Marchiaro G, et al: Bleeding in renal failure: Altered platelet function in chronic uraemia only partially corrected by haemodialysis. Nephron 22:347–353, 1978.

155. Larsson SO: On coagulation and fibrinolysis in renal failure. Scand J Haematol 15(suppl):1–59, 1971.

156. Rabiner SF: Bleeding in uremia. Med Clin North Am 56:221–233, 1972.

157. Remuzzi G, Cavenaghi AE, Mecca G, et al: Prostacyclin-like activity and bleeding in renal failure. Lancet 2:1195–1197, 1977.

158. Remuzzi G, Marchesi D, Livio M, et al: Prostaglandins, plasma factors and haemostasis in uraemia. In Remuzzi G, Mecca G, De Gaetano G (eds): Hemostasis, Prostaglandins and Renal Disease. Raven Press, New York, 1980, pp 273–281.

159. Leithner H, Winter M, Sibauer K, et al: Enhanced prostacyclin availability of blood vessels in uraemic humans and rats. Proc Eur Dial Transplant Assoc 15:418–423, 1978.

160. Zoja C, Viganò G, Bergamelli A, et al: Prolonged bleeding time and increased vascular prostacyclin in rats with chronic renal failure: Effects of conjugated estrogens. J Lab Clin Med 112:380–386, 1988.

161. Defreyn G, Dauden MV, Machin SJ, Vermylen J: A plasma factor in uraemia which stimulates prostacyclin release from cultured endothelial cells. Thromb Res 19:695–699, 1980.

162. Saglikes Y, Massry SG, Iseki K, et al: Effect of PTH on blood pressure and response to vasoconstrictor agonists. Am J Physiol 248:F674–F681, 1985.

163. Ruggeri ZM, Zimmerman TS: von Willebrand factor and von Willebrand disease. Blood 70:895–904, 1987.

164. Gordge MP, Neild GH: Platelet function in uremia. Platelets 2:115–123, 1991.

165. Kazatchkine N, Sultan V, Caen JP, Bartiety J: Bleeding in renal failure: A possible cause. BMJ 2:612–615, 1976.

166. Nerrmann RP, Marshall LR, Hurst PE: Bleeding in renal failure: A possible cause. BMJ 1:1601–1602, 1977.

167. Remuzzi G, Livio M, Roncaglioni MC, et al: Bleeding in renal failure: Is von Willebrand factor implicated? BMJ 2:359–361, 1977.

168. Warrell RP Jr, Hultin MB, Coller BS: Increased factor VIII/von Willebrand factor antigen and von Willebrand factor activity in renal failure. Am J Med 66:226–228, 1979.

169. Janson PA, Jubelirer SJ, Weinstein MJ, Deykin D: Treatment of the bleeding tendency in uremia with cryoprecipitate. N Engl J Med 303:1318–1322, 1980.

170. Mannucci PM, Remuzzi G, Pusineri F, et al: Deamino-8-D-arginine vasopressin shortens the bleeding time in uremia. N Engl J Med 308:8–12, 1983.

171. Turitto VT, Weiss HJ: Red blood cells; their dual role in thrombus formation. Science 207:541–543, 1980.

172. Sakariassen KS, Bolhuis PA, Sixma JJ: Platelet adherence to subendothelium of human arteries in pulsatile and steady flow. Thromb Res 19:547–559, 1980.

173. Gaarder A, Jonsen J, Lland S, et al: Adenosine diphosphate in red cells as a factor in the adhesiveness of human blood platelets. Nature 192:531–532, 1961.

174. Willems C, Stel HV, van Aken WG, van Mourik JA: Binding and inactivation of prostacyclin ($PGI_2$) by human erythrocytes. Br J Haematol 54:43–52, 1983.

175. Livio M, Gotti E, Marchesi D, et al: Uraemic bleeding: Role of anaemia and beneficial effect of red cell transfusions. Lancet 2:1013–1015, 1982.

176. Fernandez F, Goudable C, Sie P, et al: Low hematocrit and prolonged bleeding time in uraemic patients: Effect of red cell transfusions. Br J Haematol 59:139–148, 1985.

177. Howard AD, Moore J Jr, Welch PG, Gouge SF: Analysis of the quantitative relationship between anemia and chronic renal failure. Am J Med Sci 297:303–313, 1989.
178. Gordge MP, Leaker BR, Patel A, et al: Recombinant human erythropoietin shortens the uraemic bleeding time without causing intravascular haemostatic activation. Thromb Res 57:71–182, 1990.
179. Moia M, Mannucci PM, Vizzotto L, et al: Improvement in the haemostatic defect of uraemia after treatment with recombinant human erythropoietin. Lancet 2:1227–1229, 1987.
180. Viganò G, Benigni A, Mendogni D, et al: Recombinant human erythropoietin to correct uremic bleeding. Am J Kidney Dis 18:44–49, 1991.
181. Eiser AR: Gastrointestinal bleeding in maintenance dialysis patients. Semin Dial 1:198–202, 1988.
182. Dinoso VP, Murthy SNS, Saris AL, et al: Gastric and pancreatic function in patients with end-stage renal disease. J Clin Gastroenterol 4:321–324, 1982.
183. Kleinknecht D, Jungers P, Chanard J, et al: Uremic and non-uremic complications in acute renal failure: Evaluation of early and frequent dialysis on prognosis. Kidney Int 1:190–196, 1972.
184. Shepherd AM, Stewart WK, Wormsley KG: Peptic ulceration in chronic renal failure. Lancet 1:1357–1359, 1973.
185. Margolis DM, Saylor JL, Geisse G, et al: Upper gastrointestinal disease in chronic renal failure: A prospective evaluation. Arch Intern Med 138:1214–1217, 1978.
186. Dave PB, Romeu J, Antonelli A, Eiser AR: Gastrointestinal telangiectasias. A source of bleeding in patients receiving hemodialysis. Arch Intern Med 144:17810, 1984.
187. Boley SJ, Sammartano R, Adams A, et al: On the nature and etiology of vascular ectasias of the colon. Degenerative lesions of aging. Gastroenterology 72:652–660, 1977.
188. Zuckerman GR, Cornette GL, Clouse RE, Harter HR: Upper gastrointestinal bleeding in patients with chronic renal failure. Ann Intern Med 102:588–592, 1985.
189. Cunningham JT: Gastric telangiectasis in chronic hemodialysis patients: A report of six cases. Gastroenterology 81:1131–1133, 1981.
190. Doroty CC: Gastrointestinal bleeding in dialysis patients. Nephron 63:132–139, 1993.
191. Kumar S, Lesch M: Pericarditis in renal disease. Prog Cardiovasc Dis 22:357–369, 1980.
192. Rutsky EA, Rostand SG: Treatment of uraemic pericarditis and pericardial effusion. Am J Kidney Dis 10:2–8, 1987.
193. Comty CM, Shapiro FL: Cardiac complications of regular dialysis therapy. In Mather J (ed): Replacement of Renal Function by Dialysis. Kluwer Academic Publishers, Dordrecht, 1983, pp 33–70.
194. Drueke T, Le-Pailleur C, Zingraff J, Jungers P: Uraemic cardiomyopathy and pericarditis. Adv Nephrol Necker Hosp 9:33–70, 1980.
195. Bechar M, Lakke JP, van der Hem GK, et al: Subdural hematoma during long-term hemodialysis. Arch Neurol 26:513–516, 1972.
196. Berger HW, Rammohan G, Neff MS, Buhain WJ: Uraemic pleural effusion: A study in 14 patients on chronic dialysis. Ann Intern Med 82:362–364, 1975.
197. Galen MA, Steinberg SM, Lowrie FG, et al: Hemorrhagic pleural effusion in patients undergoing chronic dialysis. Ann Intern Med 82:359–361, 1975.
198. Bhasin HK, Dana CL: Spontaneous retroperitoneal hemorrhage in chronically hemodialyzed patients. Nephron 22:322–327, 1978.
199. Milutinovich J, Follette WC, Scribner BH: Spontaneous retroperitoneal bleeding in patients on chronic hemodialysis. Ann Intern Med 86:189–192, 1977.
200. Borra S, Kleinfeld M: Subcapsular liver hematomas in a patient on chronic hemodialysis. Ann Intern Med 93:574–575, 1980.
201. Slusher MN, Hamilton RW: Spontaneous hyphema during hemodialysis. N Engl J Med 293:561, 1975.
202. Harter HR, Burch JW, Majerus PW, et al: Prevention of thrombosis in patients on hemodialysis by low dose aspirin. N Engl J Med 301:577–579, 1979.
203. Lindsay RM, Ferguson D, Prentice CR, et al: Reduction of thrombus formation on dialyser membranes by aspirin and RA233. Lancet 2:1287–1290, 1972.
204. Livio M, Benigni A, Viganò G, et al: Moderate doses of aspirin and risk of bleeding in renal failure. Lancet 1:414–416, 1986.
205. Boyle JM, Johnston B: Acute upper gastrointestinal hemorrhage in patients with chronic renal disease. Am J Med 75:409–412, 1983.
206. Gross R, Nieth H, Mammen E: Blutungsbereitschaft und Gerinnungsstorungen bei Uraemie. Klin Wochenschr 136:107–109, 1958.
207. Lewis J, Zucher MB, Ferguson JH: Bleeding tendency in uremia. Blood 11:1073–1076, 1956.
208. Rath CD, Mailliard JA, Schreiner GE: Bleeding tendency in uremia. N Engl J Med 257:808–811, 1957.
209. Cheney K, Bonnin JA: Haemorrhage, platelet dysfunction and other coagulation defects in uraemia. Br J Haematol 8:215–222, 1962.
210. Panicucci F, Sagripanti A, Pinori E, et al: Comprehensive study of haemostasis in chronic uremia. Nephron 33:5–8, 1983.
211. Ruggeri ZM, Ponticelli C, Mannucci PM: Factor VIII and chronic renal failure. BMJ 1:1085, 1977.
212. Quereda C, Pardo A, Lamas S, et al: Lupus-like anticoagulant activity in end-stage renal disease. Nephron 49:39–44, 1988.
213. von Kaulla E, von Kaulla KN: Antithrombin III and diseases. Am J Clin Pathol 48:69–75, 1976.
214. Jorgensen KA, Stoffersen E: Antithrombin III in uremia. Scand J Urol Nephrol 13:299–303, 1979.
215. Tomura S, Nakamura Y, Deguchi F, et al: Coagulation and fibrinolysis in patients with chronic renal failure undergoing conservative treatment. Thromb Res 64:81–90, 1991.
216. Sorensen PJ, Knudsen F, Nielsen AH, Dyerberg J: Protein C assays in uremia. Thromb Res 54:301–310, 1989.
217. Faioni EM, Franchi F, Krachmalnicoff A, et al: Low levels of the anticoagulant activity of protein C in patients with chronic renal insufficiency: An inhibitor of protein C is present in uremic plasma. Thromb Haemost 66:420–425, 1991.
218. D'Angelo A, Vigano-D'Angelo SV, Esmon CT, Comp PC: Acquired deficiencies of protein S. Protein S activity during oral anticoagulation, in liver disease and in disseminated intravascular coagulation. J Clin Invest 81:1445–1454, 1988.
219. Bennett NB, Ogston D: Inhibitors of the fibrinolytic enzyme system in renal disease. Clin Sci 39:549–557, 1970.
220. Ito T, Niwa T, Matsui E: Fibrinolytic activity in renal disease. Clin Chim Acta 36:145–151, 1972.
221. Homma T, Ichikawa T: Studies of fibrinolytic activity of uremic and longterm hemodialysis patients with special reference to fibrinolytic inhibitor. Biochem Exp Biol 15:229–236, 1979.
222. Canavese C, Stratta P, Pacitti A, et al: Impaired fibrinolysis in uremia: Partial and variable correction by four different dialysis regimens. Clin Nephrol 17:82–89, 1982.
223. Lane DA, Ireland H, Knight I, et al: The significance of fibrinogen derivatives in plasma in human renal failure. Br J Haematol 56:251–260, 1984.
224. Tomura S, Oono Y, Kuriyama R, Takeuchi J: Plasma concentrations of fibrinopeptide A and fibrinopeptide Bβ15–42 in glomerulonephritis and the nephrotic syndrome. Arch Intern Med 145:1033–1035, 1985.
225. Nishimoto K, Yamagami S, Katoh Y, et al: Coagulation and fibrinolysis in chronic renal failure. Change in tissue-type plasminogen activator activity. Trans Am Soc Artif Intern Organs 32:478–481, 1986.
226. Brommer EJP, Schicht I, Wijngaards G, et al: Fibrinolytic activators and inhibitors in terminal renal insufficiency and in anephric patients. Thromb Haemost 52:311–314, 1984.
227. Del Greco F, Soper WS, Krumlovsky FA, et al: Thrombosis of vascular access for haemodialysis. In Remuzzi G, Rossi EC (eds): Haemostasis and the Kidney. Butterworth, London, 1989, pp 303–308.
228. Rodkin RS, Bookstein JJ, Heeney DJ, Davis GB: Streptokinase and transluminal angioplasty in the treatment of acutely thrombosed hemodialysis access fistulas. Radiology 149:425–428, 1983.
229. Young AT, Hunter DW, Castaneda-Zuniga WR, et al: Thrombosed synthetic hemodialysis access fistulas: Failure of fibrinolytic therapy. Radiology 154:639–642, 1985.
230. Mangiarotti G, Canavese C, Thea A, et al: Urokinase treatment for arteriovenous fistulae declotting in dialyzed patients. Nephron 36:60–64, 1984.
231. Remuzzi G, Marchesi D, Livio M, et al: Altered platelet and vascular prostaglandin-generation in patients with renal failure and prolonged bleeding times. Thromb Res 13:1007–1015, 1978.
232. Gordon LA, Somon ER, Rukes JM, et al: Studies in regional heparinization. N Engl J Med 255:1063–1066, 1956.
233. Maher JF, Lapierre L, Schreiner GE, et al: Regional heparinization for hemodialysis. N Engl J Med 268:451–456, 1963.
234. Lindholm DD, Murray S: A simplified method of regional heparinization during hemodialysis according to a predetermined dosage formula. Trans Am Soc Artif Intern Organs 10:92–97, 1964.

235. Blaufox MD, Hampers CL, Merril JP: Rebound anticoagulation occurring after regional. Heparinization for hemodialysis. Trans Am Soc Artif Intern Organs 12:207–209, 1966.

236. Lohr YW, Schwab S: Minimizing hemorrhagic complications in dialysis patients. J Am Soc Nephrol 2:961–975, 1991.

237. Tolkoff-Rubin NE, Nardini J, Fang LST, Rubin RH: Successful hemodialysis of patients at high risk of hemorrhage using the Ex Val dialyzer. Dial Transplant 15:125–126, 1986.

238. Ljungberg B: A low molecular heparin fraction as an anticoagulant during hemodialysis. Clin Nephrol 25:15–20, 1985.

239. Morring K, Sinn H, Schuler HW, et al: Comparative evaluation of iatrogenic sources of blood loss during maintenance dialysis. *In* Proceedings of the 13th Congress of the European Dialysis and Transplant Association, Vienna, 1976, p 233.

240. Turney JH, Williams LC, Fewell MR, et al: Platelet protection and heparin sparing with prostacyclin during regular therapy. Lancet 2:219–222, 1980.

241. Arze RS, Ward MK: Prostacyclin safer than heparin in haemodialysis. Lancet 2:50, 1981.

242. Zusman RM, Rubin RH, Cato AE, et al: Hemodialysis using prostacyclin instead of heparin as the sole antithrombotic agent. N Engl J Med 304:934–939, 1981.

243. Swartz RD, Flamenbaum W, Dubrow A, et al: Epoprostenol (PGI, prostacyclin) during high risk hemodialysis: preventing further bleeding complications. J Clin Pharmacol 28:818–825, 1988.

244. Dubrow A, Flamenbaum W, Mittman N, et al: Safety and efficacy of epoprostenol (PGI$_2$) versus heparin H in hemodialysis HD. Trans Am Soc Artif Intern Organs 30:52–54, 1984.

245. Zwaginga JJ, Ijsseldijk MJW, de Groot PG, et al: Treatment of uremic anemia with recombinant erythropoietin also reduces the defects in platelet adhesion and aggregation caused by uremic plasma. Thromb Haemost 66:638–647, 1991.

246. van Geet C, Hauglustaine D, Verresen L, et al: Haemostatic effects of recombinant human erythropoietin in chronic haemodialysis patients. Thromb Haemost 61:117–121, 1989.

247. Triulzi DJ, Blumberg N: Variability in response to cryoprecipitate treatment for hemostatic defects in uremia. Yale J Biol Med 63:1–7, 1990.

248. Mannucci PM, Ruggeri ZM, Pareti FI, Capitanio A: 1-Deamino-8-D-arginine vasopressin: A new pharmacological approach to the management of haemophilia and von Willebrand's diseases. Lancet 1:869–872, 1977.

249. Canavese C, Salomone M, Pacitti A, et al: Reduced response of uraemic bleeding time to repeated doses of desmopressin. Lancet 1:867–868, 1985.

250. Shapiro MD, Kelleher SP: Intranasal deamino-8-D-arginine vasopressin shortens the bleeding time in uremia. Am J Nephrol 4:260–261, 1984.

251. Rydzewski A, Rowinski M, Mysliwiec M: Shortening of the bleeding time after intranasal administration of 1-deamino-8-D-arginine vasopressin to patients with chronic anemia. Folia Haematol Int Mag Klin Morphol Blutforsch 113:823–830, 1986.

252. Viganò G, Mannucci PM, Lattuada A, et al: Subcutaneous injection of desmopressin (DDAVP) shortens the bleeding time in uremia. Am J Hematol 31:32–35, 1989.

253. Byrnes JJ, Larcada A, Moake JL: Thrombosis following desmopressin for uremic bleeding. Am J Hematol 28:63–65, 1988.

254. Liu YK, Kosfeld RE, Marcum SG: Treatment of uraemic bleeding with conjugated oestrogen. Lancet 2:887–890, 1984.

255. Livio M, Mannucci PM, Viganò GL, et al: Conjugated estrogens for the management of bleeding associated with renal failure. N Engl J Med 315:731–735, 1986.

256. Viganò G, Gaspari F, Locatelli M, et al: Dose-effect and pharmacokinetics of estrogens given to correct bleeding time in uremia. Kidney Int 34:853–858, 1988.

257. Zoja C, Noris M, Corna D, et al: L-Arginine, the precursor of nitric oxide, abolishes the effect of estrogens on bleeding time in experimental uremia. Lab Invest 65:479–483, 1991.

258. Salant DJ, Galver AM, Anderson R, et al: Depressed neutrophil chemotaxis in patients with chronic renal failure and after renal transplantation. J Lab Clin Med 88:536–545, 1976.

259. Clark RA, Hamory BH, Ford GH, Kimball HR: Chemotaxis in acute renal failure. J Infect Dis 126:460–463, 1972.

260. Baum J, Cestero RV, Freeman RB: Chemotaxis of the polymorphonuclear leukocyte and delayed hypersensitivity in uremia. Kidney Int 7(suppl 2):S147–S153, 1975.

261. Bjorksten B, Mauer SM, Mills EL, Quie PG: The effect of hemodialysis on neutrophil chemotactic responsiveness. Acta Med Scand 203:67–70, 1978.

262. Siriwatratananonta P, Sinsakul V, Stern K, Slavin RG: Defective chemotaxis in uremia. J Lab Clin Med 92:402–407, 1978.

263. Martin RR, Eknoyan G, Saenz C, et al: Effects of renal failure on leukotaxis. J Med 10:267–278, 1979.

264. Anderson R, Glover A, Koornhof HJ, Rabson AR: In vitro stimulation of neutrophil motility by levamisole: Maintenance of cGMP levels in chemotactically stimulated levamisole-treated neutrophils. J Immunol 117:428–432, 1976.

265. Hogan NA, Hill HR: Enhancement of neutrophil chemotaxis and alteration of levels of cellular cyclic nucleotides by levamisole. J Infect Dis 138:437–444, 1978.

266. Greene WH, Ray C, Mauer SM, Quie PG: The effect of hemodialysis on neutrophil chemotactic responsiveness. J Lab Clin Med 88:971–974, 1976.

267. Abrutyn E, Solomons NW, Clair L St, et al: Granulocyte function in patients with chronic renal failure: Surface adherence, phagocytosis, and bactericidal activity in vitro. J Infect Dis 135:1–8, 1977.

268. Burleson RL: Reversible inhibition of phagocytosis in anephric uremic patients. Surg Forum 24:75–77, 1973.

269. Davidson WD, Tanaka KR: Effect of uremia on phagocytosis-stimulated glucose oxidation (PSGO) in human granulocytes. Clin Res 19:416, 1971.

270. Hirabayashi Y, Kobayashi T, Nishikawa A, et al: Oxidative metabolism and phagocytosis of polymorphonuclear leukocytes in patients with chronic renal failure. Nephron 49:305–312, 1988.

271. Alexiewicz JM, Smogorzewski M, Fadda GZ, Massry SG: Impaired phagocytosis in dialysis patients: Studies on mechanisms. Am J Nephrol 11:102–111, 1991.

272. Horl WH, Haag-Weber M, Georgopoulos A, Block LH: Physicochemical characterization of a polypeptide present in uremic serum that inhibits the biological activity of polymorphonuclear cells. Proc Natl Acad Sci USA 87:6353–6357, 1990.

273. Harvey DM, Sheppard KJ, Morgan AG, Fletcher J: Neutrophil function in patients on continuous ambulatory peritoneal dialysis. Br J Haematol 68:273–278, 1988.

274. Craddock PR, Fehr J, Dalmasso AP, et al: Hemodialysis leukopenia. Pulmonary vascular leukostasis resulting from complement activation by dialyzer cellophane membranes. J Clin Invest 59:879–888, 1977.

275. Stroncek DF, Keshaviah P, Craddock PR, Hammerschmidt DE: Effect of dialyzer reuse on complement activation and neutropenia in hemodialysis. J Lab Clin Med 104:304–311, 1984.

276. Cohen MS, Elliott DM, Chaplinski T, et al: A defect in oxidative metabolism in human polymorphonuclear leukocytes that remain in circulation early in hemodialysis. Blood 60:1283–1289, 1982.

277. Skubitz KM, Craddock PR: Reversal of hemodialysis granulocytopenia and pulmonary leukostasis: A clinical manifestation of selective down-regulation of granulocyte responses to C5a$_{desarg}$. J Clin Invest 67:1383–1391, 1981.

278. Larson RS, Springer TA: Structure and function of leukocyte integrins. Immunol Rev 114:181–217, 1990.

279. Arnaout MA: Leukocyte adhesion molecules deficiency: Its structural basis, pathophysiology and implications for modulating the inflammatory response. Immunol Rev 114:145–180, 1990.

280. Miller LJ, Bainton DF, Borregard N, Springer TA: Stimulated mobilization of monocyte Mac-1 and p150,95 adhesion proteins from an intracellular vesicular compartment to the cell surface. J Clin Invest 80:535–544, 1987.

281. Roccatello D, Mazzucco G, Coppo R, et al: Functional changes of monocytes due to dialysis membranes. Kidney Int 35:622–631, 1989.

282. Arnaout MA, Hakim RM, Todd III RF, et al: Increased expression of an adhesion-promoting surface glycoprotein in the granulocytopenia of hemodialysis. N Engl J Med 312:457–462, 1985.

283. Jacobs AA, Ward RA, Wellhausen SR, McLeish KR: Polymorphonuclear leukocyte function during hemodialysis: Relationship to complement activation. Nephron 52:119–124, 1982.

284. Lundahl J, Hed J, Jacobson SH: Dialysis granulocytopenia is preceded by an increased surface expression of the adhesion-promoting glycoprotein Mac-1. Nephron 61:163–169, 1992.

285. Thylén P, Lundahl J, Fernvik E, et al: Mobilization of an intracellular glycoprotein (Mac-1) on monocytes and granulocytes during hemodialysis. Am J Nephrol 12:393–400, 1992.

286. Ord DC, Ernst TJ, Zhou LJ, et al: Structure of the gene encoding of the human leukocyte adhesion molecule-1 (TQ1, Leu-8) of lymphocytes and neutrophils. J Biol Chem 265:7760–7767, 1990.
287. Vanholder R, Ringoir S, Dhondt A, Hakim RM: Phagocytosis in uremic and hemodialysis patients: A prospective and cross sectional study. Kidney Int 39:320–327, 1991.
288. Miller LJ, Bainton DF, Borregaard N, Springer TA: Stimulated mobilization of monocyte Mac-1 and p150,95 adhesion proteins from an intracellular vesicular compartment to the cell surface. J Clin Invest 74:1280–1290, 1984.
289. Dinarello CA, Lonnemann G, Bingel M, et al: Biological consequences of monocyte activation during hemodialysis. In Koch KM, Streicher E (eds): Contribution to Nephrology. S Karger, Basel, 1987, p 1.
290. Descamps-Latscha B, Herbelin A, Nguyen AT, et al: Hemodialysis-membrane–induced phagocyte oxidative metabolism activation and interleukin-1 production. Life Support Syst 4:349–353, 1986.
291. Lonnemann G, Bingel M, Koch KM, et al: Plasma interleukin-1 activity in humans undergoing hemodialysis with regenerated cellulosic membranes. Lymphokine Res 6:63–70, 1987.
292. Luger A, Kovarik J, Stummvoll HK, et al: Blood-membrane interaction in hemodialysis leads to increased cytokine production. Kidney Int 32:84–88, 1987.
293. Bingel M, Lonnemann G, Koch KM, et al: Plasma interleukin-1 activity during hemodialysis: The influence of dialysis membranes. Nephron 50:273–276, 1988.
294. Herbelin A, Nguyen AT, Zingraff J, et al: Influence of uremia and hemodialysis on circulating interleukin-1 and tumor necrosis factor alpha. Kidney Int 37:116–125, 1990.
295. Schindler R, Dinarello CA, Shaldon S, Koch KM: Induction of IL-1β during hemodialysis in vivo. Proc Eur Dial Transplant Assoc (in press).
296. Lamperi S, Carozzi S: Monocyte-macrophage mediated suppression of erythropoiesis in renal anemia. Nephrol Dial Transplant 2:86–92, 1987.
297. Dinarello CA: Interleukin-1 and interleukin-1 antagonism. Blood 77:1627–1652, 1991.
298. Dinarello CA: Interleukin-1 and tumor necrosis factor and their naturally occurring antagonists during hemodialysis. Kidney Int 42:S68–S77, 1992.
299. Henderson LW, Koch KM, Dinarello CA, Shaldon S: Hemodialysis hypotension: The interleukin hypothesis. Blood Purif 1:3–8, 1983.
300. Shaldon S, Deschodt G, Branger B, et al: Haemodialysis hypotension: The interleukin hypothesis restated. Proc Eur Dial Transplant Assoc 22:229–243, 1985.
301. Beasley D, Brenner BM: Role of nitric oxide in hemodialysis hypotension. Kidney Int 42:S96–S100, 1992.
302. Noris M, Benigni A, Boccardo P, et al: Enhanced nitric oxide synthesis in uremia: Implications for platelet dysfunction and dialysis hypotension. Kidney Int 44:445–450, 1993.
303. Ladefoged J, Langhoff E: Accessory cell functions in mononuclear cell cultures from uremic patients. Kidney Int 37:126–130, 1990.
304. Donati D, Degiannis D, Raskova J, Raska K Jr: Uremic serum effects on peripheral blood mononuclear cell and purified T lymphocyte responses. Kidney Int 42:681–689, 1992.
305. Beaurain G, Naret C, Marcon L, et al: In vivo T-cell preactivation in chronic uremic hemodialyzed and nonhemodialyzed patients. Kidney Int 36:636–644, 1989.
306. Rubin LA, Kurman CC, Fritz ME, et al: Soluble interleukin-2 receptors are released from activated human lymphoid cells in vitro. J Immunol 135:3172–3177, 1985.
307. Uchiyama T, Broder S, Waldmann TA: A monoclonal antibody (anti-Tac) reactive with activated and functionally mature human T cells. I. Production of anti-Tac monoclonal antibody and distribution of Tac (+) cells. J Immunol 126:1393–1397, 1981.
308. Dukovich M, Wano Y, Thyu L, et al: A second human IL-2 binding protein that may be a component of high affinity IL-2 receptors. Nature 327:518–522, 1987.
309. Reed JC, Robb RJ, Greene WC, Nowell PC: Effect of wheat germ agglutinin on the interleukin pathway of human T lymphocyte activation. J Immunol 134:314–323, 1985.
310. Gupta S: Interleukin-2 receptor and transferrin receptor expression on T cells and production of interleukin-2 in patients with acquired immune deficiency syndrome (AIDS) and AIDS-related complex. Clin Immunol Immunopathol 38:93–100, 1986.

# 51

# Renal Osteodystrophy

*Francisco Llach*
*Jordi Bover*

The presence of renal bone disease in patients with chronic renal failure (CRF) has been known for years. The studies of Stanbury and Lumb[1] as well as those of Dent and colleagues[2] were of great importance in linking abnormalities of divalent ion metabolism, parathyroid hormone (PTH), and vitamin D with the bone abnormalities observed in CRF. With better management of patients with end-stage renal disease, the long-term course of these bone abnormalities and their clinical features have changed. Moreover, new entities have been recognized. Thus, in addition to secondary hyperparathyroidism (HPTH), aluminum (Al) bone disease and adynamic bone disease (ABD) have emerged as clinically relevant problems. In the last decade, significant pathogenetic and therapeutic advances have been made in the management of these disorders.

Today, the term renal osteodystrophy is used to include various bone lesions. They include osteitis fibrosa (a reflection of secondary HPTH), osteomalacia (often related to Al toxicity), and ABD. In children, rickets and skeletal deformities may also be present. Osteosclerosis and osteoporosis are less commonly observed. Of these lesions, osteitis fibrosa is characterized by a high bone turnover, whereas in osteomalacia and ABD bone turnover is low.

## PATHOGENESIS

### Secondary Hyperparathyroidism (High-Turnover Bone Disease)

Since the first descriptions of "late rickets associated with albuminuria" by Lucas in 1883[3] and "tumor of the parathyroid gland" by MacCallum in 1905,[4] it was not until 1933 that Langmead and Orr[5] suggested that parathyroid hyperplasia was secondary to advanced CRF. In the following years, the development of secondary HPTH in CRF was demonstrated in several studies and was also related to the presence of bone disease[6–9] as well as to the abnormalities of divalent ion metabolism.[1, 2, 10] With the advent of radio-immunoassays (RIAs) for PTH measurement,[11–13] high circulating levels of PTH have been detected at earlier stages of CRF[14–18] (Fig. 51–1) and the consequences of the increased PTH levels have been demonstrated in bone biopsies of patients with mild to moderate CRF.[19, 20]

Because of the pathogenic implications of these findings, considerable effort has been made to define the factors that may contribute to the development of parathyroid hyperplasia and/or secondary HPTH. These factors are (Table 51–1)

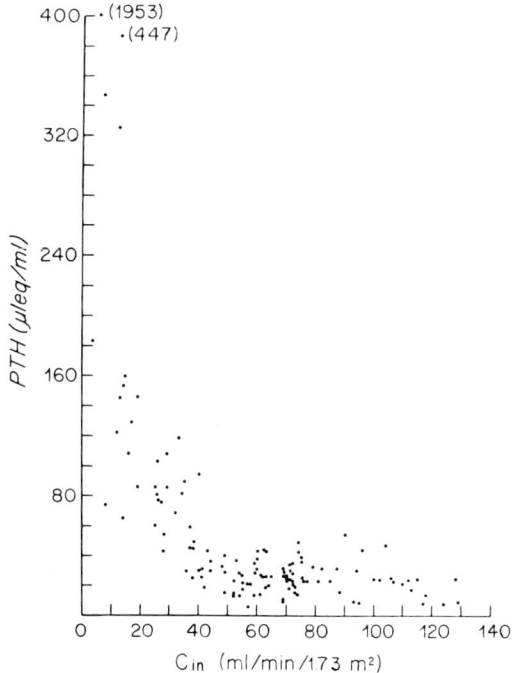

**Figure 51–1.** Relationship between serum immunoreactive PTH and the renal clearance of inulin in patients with varying levels of renal function. The immunoassay of PTH was done utilizing an antiserum believed to react with 1–84 PTH as well as with its midregion and terminal fragments. (From Arnaud CD: Hyperparathyroidism and renal failure. Used with permission from Kidney International, volume 4, pages 89–95, 1973.)

1) hypocalcemia, 2) phosphorus (P) retention, 3) impaired calcemic response to PTH, 4) altered vitamin D metabolism and resistance to calcitriol, 5) altered degradation of PTH by the kidney, 6) abnormal regulation of $Ca^{2+}$-controlled PTH release (shift in the set-point of $Ca^{2+}$, and 7) calcitonin (CT). These pathogenic factors are not mutually exclusive but rather interrelated; thus, the problem of isolating the importance of each factor often arises. Furthermore, it is likely that one factor may play a more prominent role than others at certain stages of CRF.

## HYPOCALCEMIA

The main factor increasing PTH secretion and causing hyperplasia of the parathyroid glands in uremic patients has been thought to be the presence of hypocalcemia. In the

**TABLE 51–1. Factors Contributing to the Development of Secondary Hyperparathyroidism**

Hypocalcemia
Phosphorus retention
Impaired calcemic response to parathyroid hormone (PTH) (skeletal resistance to PTH)
Altered vitamin D metabolism and resistance to calcitriol
Autonomous parathyroid cell proliferation
Altered degradation of PTH
Abnormal regulation of $Ca^{2+}$-controlled PTH release
Calcitonin (?)

1960s, Bricker[21] and Slatopolsky[22] and their colleagues emphasized its importance in the genesis of secondary HPTH. Hypocalcemia has been shown to increase both synthesis and secretion of PTH.[23–25] Moreover, some of the factors already mentioned may lead to hypocalcemia and thus increase PTH production.

Observations in the past decade suggest that other factors may also be at work. First, studies of patients with early CRF have shown increases in serum PTH not associated with hypocalcemia.[16, 17, 26–28] Also, when oral physiologic doses of calcitriol were given to seemingly normocalcemic patients, a significant increase in serum $Ca^{2+}$ was observed.[28] Furthermore, Lopez-Hilker and co-workers[29] have demonstrated that hypercalcemia did not prevent the development of secondary HPTH in azotemic dogs when calcitriol deficiency was present. Kaplan and colleagues[30] also demonstrated increases in serum $Ca^{2+}$ levels in uremic dogs with secondary HPTH compared with control dogs. Similar results have also been obtained by others after bilateral nephrectomy.[31, 32] The presence of increased PTH levels together with stable or even increased $Ca^{2+}$ concentrations observed in these studies also suggest a defective regulation of PTH secretion at the parathyroid gland level. This issue is discussed further later.

## PHOSPHORUS RETENTION

The role of P retention as a major factor in the pathogenesis of secondary HPTH has been demonstrated by Slatopolsky and associates.[33–35] As the P retention theory was initially proposed, a transient and possibly undetectable increase in serum P concentration was believed to occur in moderate CRF as a result of a small decrement in renal function.[34] The transient hyperphosphatemia would temporarily reduce the concentration of blood $Ca^{2+}$, which in turn would stimulate PTH secretion. The high levels of PTH would reduce tubule reabsorption of P, cause phosphaturia, and return both serum P and $Ca^{2+}$ levels toward normal, but at the expense of a higher circulating PTH level. This theory was formulated by Bricker[36] and Slatopolsky and colleagues[22] as the "trade-off" hypothesis.

Considerable evidence supports an important role of P retention in the development of secondary HPTH. Reiss and co-workers[37] demonstrated that a large oral P load led to an increase in serum P, a fall in $Ca^{2+}$, and an increase in serum PTH level in normal subjects. Others have shown that the long-term feeding of a high-P diet to animals caused parathyroid hyperplasia, high PTH, and mild hypocalcemia.[38, 39] Also, serum PTH levels correlated positively with the degree of hyperphosphatemia in dialysis patients.[40, 41] Furthermore, in experimentally induced CRF a reduction of dietary P intake in proportion to the decrease in glomerular filtration rate (GFR) largely prevented the development of secondary HPTH in dogs with CRF[33, 34] (Fig. 51–2). Nevertheless, when dietary P intake was reduced and an aluminum hydroxide gel was given to patients with CRF, serum PTH fell substantially but the values remained greater than normal. Also, only a mild reduction of PTH levels has been occasionally observed after P restriction in dialysis patients.[41]

The available data suggest that although P retention is

important in the development of secondary HPTH in advanced CRF, it may not be a factor in early CRF. Because of these significant differences, it may be appropriate to discuss 1) the role of P in the development of secondary HPTH in early CRF and 2) P retention in advanced CRF.

### Early Renal Failure

New data suggest that hyperphosphatemia may not play a role in early CRF. Thus, low serum P levels have been reported in these patients.[15, 26, 42] To explain the hypophosphatemia, it was initially suggested that postprandial hyperphosphatemia and subsequent hypocalcemia may occur; then, hypocalcemia would stimulate PTH secretion, leading to low fasting serum P levels,[35] so serum P concentration should be higher in azotemic patients than in normal subjects after a P-containing meal. However, Portale and colleagues[27] measured serum P and PTH concentrations hourly in children with early CRF; they were unable to detect any postprandial increment in serum P concentration. Furthermore, patients with a GFR of 40 to 80 mL/min receiving an oral P load displayed, rather than hyperphosphatemia and P retention, low serum P and a more rapid excretion of P compared with control subjects[28] (Fig. 51–3). Interestingly, these patients excreted a P load in a manner similar to patients with primary HPTH.[43] Nonetheless, despite the absence of P retention in early CRF, P restriction resulted in a significant decrease in PTH levels both in children[27] and in adults.[26] This was accompanied by a significant increment in calcitriol levels[26, 27] (Fig. 51–4). This issue is discussed further later.

### Advanced Renal Failure

As CRF progresses, P retention eventually occurs. Thus, in more advanced CRF there is an impairment in P excretion after an oral P load.[44] The fact that patients had a tendency to remain in P balance until the GFR was less than 20 to 25 mL/min was observed in 1954.[45] A decade later, Slatopolsky and colleagues[46, 47] noted that fractional excretion of P rises progressively in CRF as renal function worsens, and it is proportional to the level of PTH.[48] Some of the factors that aggravate the degree of hyperphosphatemia in these patients are noted in Table 51–2.

P retention can induce secondary HPTH through several mechanisms. As mentioned earlier, the reciprocal decrease in serum $Ca^{2+}$ after an increase in serum P was considered the mechanism by which P retention induced secondary HPTH. Thus, in advanced CRF and during dialysis, hypocalcemia may be related to the marked elevation of serum P.[44] However, the increase of P concentration in vitro within the usual range observed in dialysis patients did not reduce the $Ca^{2+}$ concentration.[49] In fact, in normal subjects, only a large increase in serum P (2.2 mM) reduced total serum $Ca^{2+}$ by 0.18 mM.[50] P retention can also be at work through an indirect mechanism such as inhibiting the activity of the renal enzyme 1α-hydroxylase, which is responsible for the conversion of 25-hydroxyvitamin D (25(OH)D) to its active metabolite 1,25-dihydroxyvitamin D, 1,25(OH)$_2$D (calcitriol).[51, 52] P retention can also decrease the calcemic response to PTH.[53, 54]

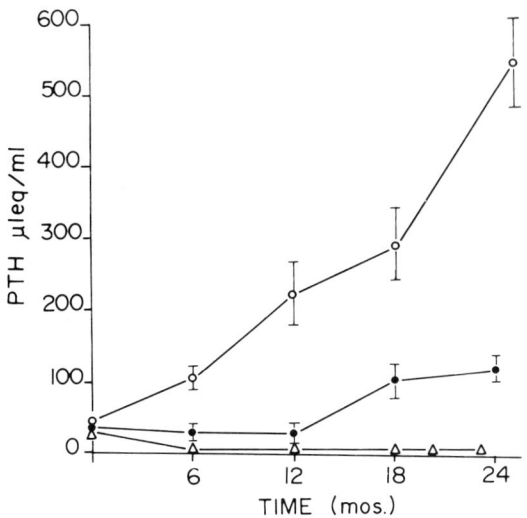

**Figure 51–2.** Serial values of immunoreactive PTH (mean ± SE) in dogs with chronic renal insufficiency. The dogs received a normal constant phosphate intake (○), a phosphate intake reduced in proportion to the decrease in GFR (●), or a proportional reduction in phosphate intake and 25(OH)D₃, 20 μg twice a week (△), for 2 years. (Modified from Rutherford WE, Bordier P, Marie P, et al: Phosphate control and 25-hydroxycholecalciferol administration in preventing experimental renal osteodystrophy in the dog. Reproduced from The Journal of Clinical Investigation, 1977, vol 60 pp 332–341 by copyright permission of The American Society for Clinical Investigation.)

A direct effect of P on the parathyroid gland has also been suggested. Lucas and co-workers[55] administered a low-P diet to patients with advanced CRF during 3 months; although $Ca^{2+}$ and calcitriol levels did not increase, an important decrease in serum PTH was observed. Similar results have been reported by others.[56, 57] These findings suggest an effect of a low-P diet in the control of PTH secretion. Lopez-Hilker and colleagues[58] have shown in dogs that P restriction in advanced CRF improves secondary HPTH by a mechanism that may be independent of changes in serum $Ca^{2+}$ and calcitriol (Fig. 51–5). The authors suggested that "P may affect the phospholipid composition of the parathyroid cell membrane, Ca fluxes in the

**TABLE 51–2. Factors That Influence Serum Phosphorus Levels in Patients with Renal Failure**

Residual renal function
Dietary P intake
Ingestion of P-binding compounds
Intake of large amounts of supplemental $Ca^{2+}$
Degree of intestinal malabsorption of $PO_4^{3-}$
Extent of vitamin D deficiency and treatment with active vitamin D compounds
Secretion of PTH; responsiveness of the skeleton to PTH
Rate of skeletal accretion (i.e., healing of osteomalacia or osteitis fibrosa)
Balance between degradation and synthesis of protoplasm
Translocation of $PO_4^{3-}$ from extracellular to intracellular locations (glucose, insulin, parenteral alimentation)
Hypomagnesemia
P-containing enemas
Frequency, duration, and efficiency of dialysis

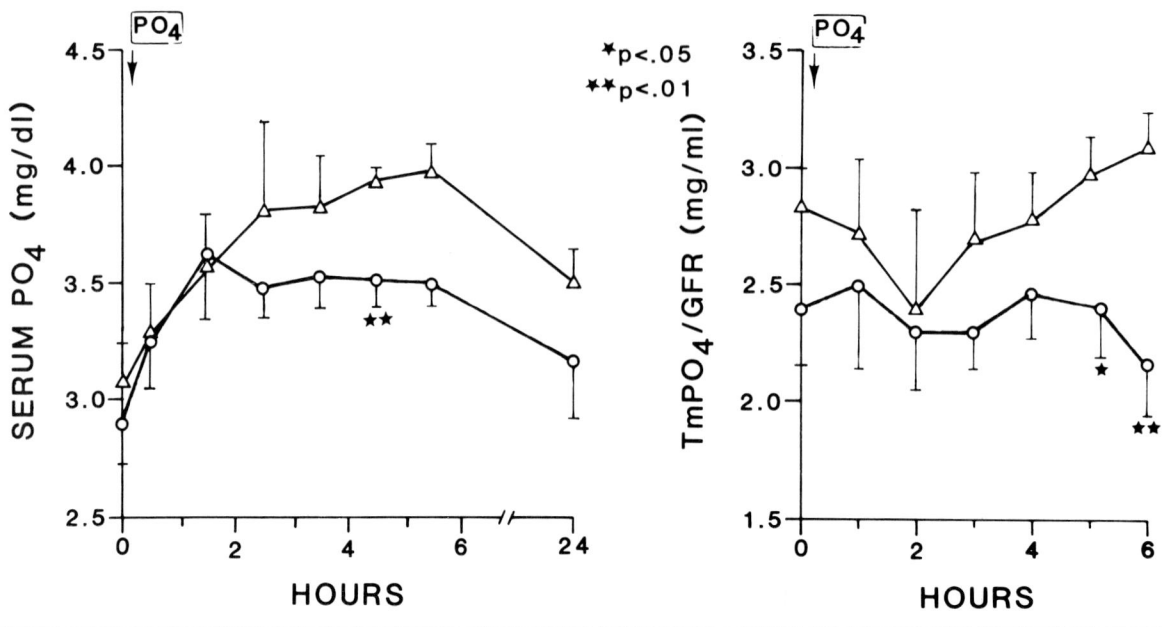

**Figure 51–3.** Mean values (± SE) of serum phosphorus (PO₄) and tubule reabsorption of P (TmPO₄/GFR) during a P loading test in patients with early renal failure *(open circles)* and in normal subjects *(open triangles).* (From Wilson L, Felsenfeld A, Drezner MK, Llach F: Altered divalent ion metabolism in early renal failure: Role of 1,25-(OH)₂D. Used with permission from Kidney International, volume 27, pages 565–573, 1985.)

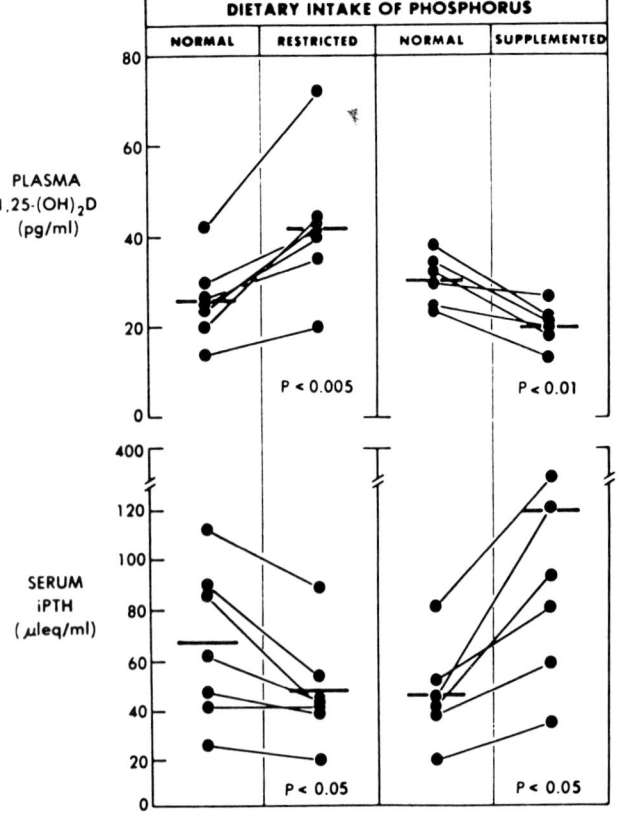

**Figure 51–4.** Different effects of dietary P restriction and dietary P loading on plasma levels of immunoreactive PTH and 1,25(OH)₂D in children with moderate renal failure. (From Portale AA, Booth BE, Haloran BP, Morris RC Jr: Effect of dietary phosphorus on circulating concentrations of 1,25-dihydroxyvitamin D and immunoreactive parathyroid hormone in children with moderate renal insufficiency. Reproduced from The Journal of Clinical Investigation, 1984, vol 73, pp 1580–1589 by copyright permission of The American Society for Clinical Investigation.)

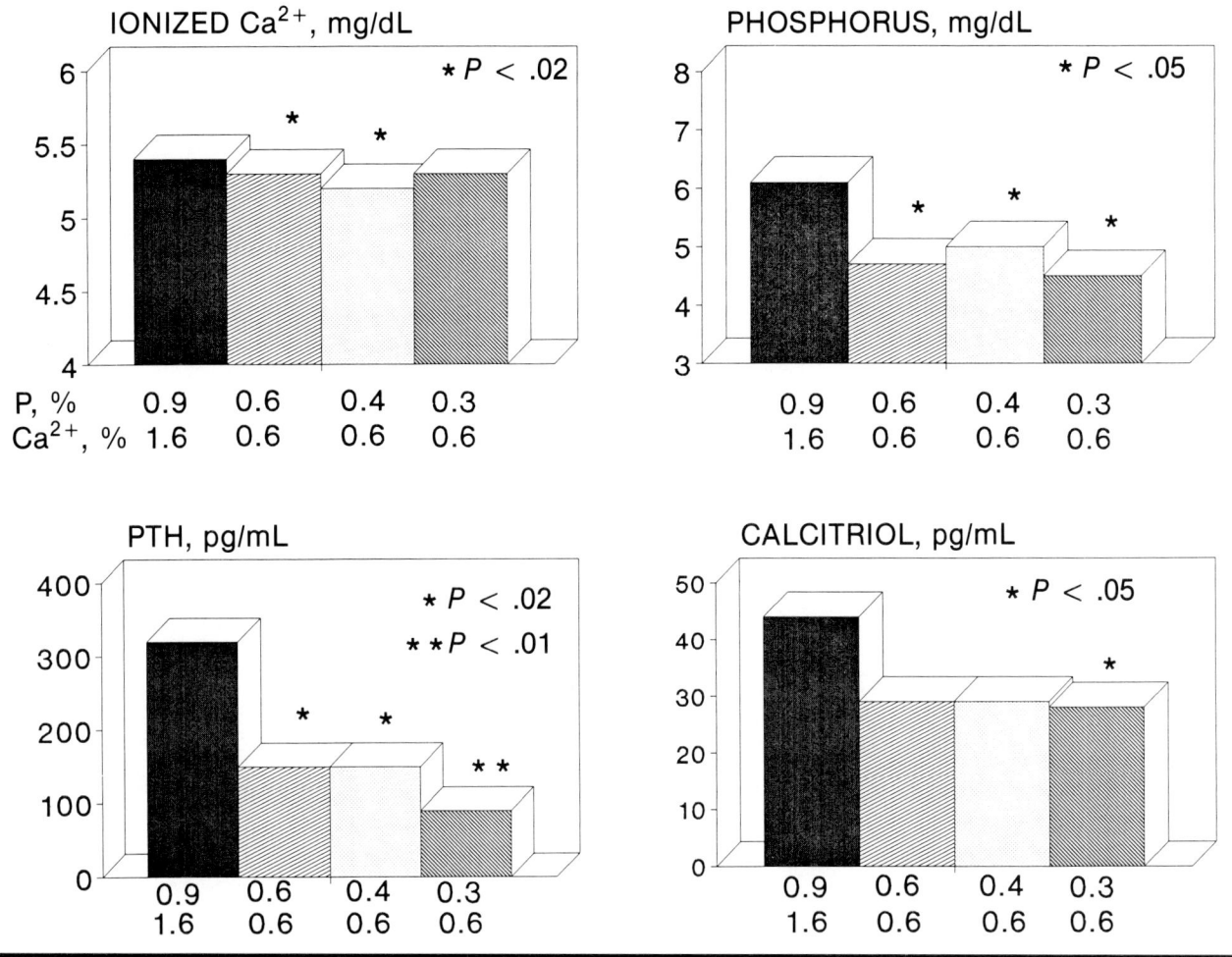

**Figure 51–5.** Effects of dietary P on plasma Ca$^{2+}$, plasma P, NH$_2$-terminal PTH, and calcitriol in five uremic female dogs. (Modified from Lopez-Hilker S, Dusso AS, Rapp NS, et al: Phosphorus restriction reverses hyperparathyroidism in uremia independent of changes in calcium and calcitriol. Am J Physiol 259:F432–F437, 1990.)

parathyroid cells, and/or regulation of calcitriol receptors in the parathyroid cell.'' Similarly, hemodialysis patients may have P-related changes in PTH without changes in serum Ca$^{2+}$ and calcitriol.[59, 60] We have also observed severe hyperphosphatemia worsening the secondary HPTH in dialysis patients receiving intravenous calcitriol.[61] Finally, Yi and associates[62] have shown, using Northern blot techniques, that moderate P restriction decreased the levels of PTH messenger RNA (mRNA) in rats with mild CRF independently of Ca$^{2+}$ and calcitriol.

## IMPAIRED CALCEMIC RESPONSE TO PTH

A decreased calcemic response to the action of PTH is another cause of hypocalcemia in CRF. It was first described by Evanson in 1966[63]; he noted that the calcemic response to an infusion of parathyroid extract was significantly lower in hypocalcemic patients with CRF than in normal subjects or in patients with primary hypoparathyroidism. Subsequently, Massry and associates[64] observed that the calcemic response to a parathyroid extract in patients with moderate and advanced CRF was significantly

lower than in normal individuals. This reduced calcemic response was unrelated to the initial levels of serum Ca$^{2+}$, P, or PTH. Llach and colleagues[15] noted a delayed recovery from ethylenediaminetetraacetic acid (EDTA)-induced hypocalcemia in patients with early CRF (creatinine clearances of 34 to 93 mL/min) compared with normal subjects, despite higher PTH levels in the former (Fig. 51–6). A later study confirmed these results.[28] Such observations indicate that the impaired calcemic response to PTH appears early in the course of CRF. Thus, a greater concentration of circulating PTH may be required to maintain a normal serum Ca$^{2+}$ level in patients with CRF.

Factors linked to the impaired calcemic response of CRF include P retention, decreased calcitriol levels, down-regulation of PTH receptors, CT, and uremia per se.

Phosphorus retention decreases the calcemic response to PTH in CRF.[53, 54] Somerville and Kaye[53] reinfused urine in the rat, inducing acute uremia and calcemic resistance to PTH after 5 hours of PTH infusion. Removing the P by treating the urine with zirconium oxide restored the calcemic response to PTH.[53] An improvement in the calcemic response to PTH was noted in rats fed a low-P diet during the infusion of PTH[54]; moreover, rats with both moderate

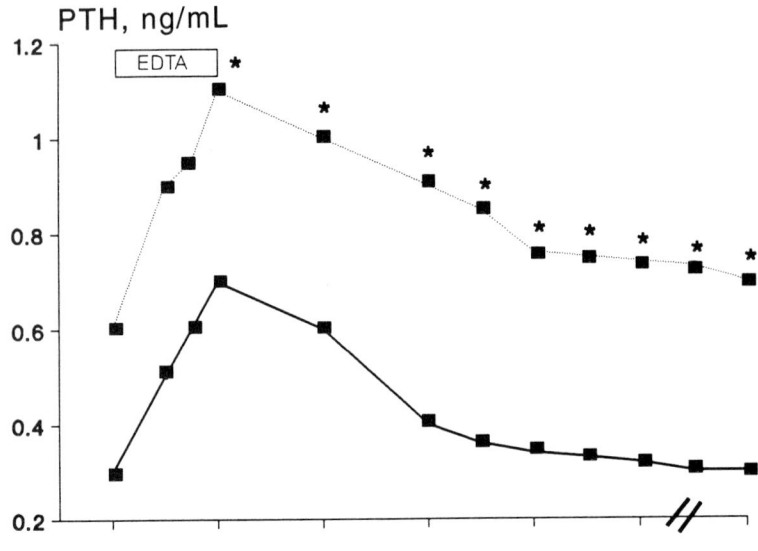

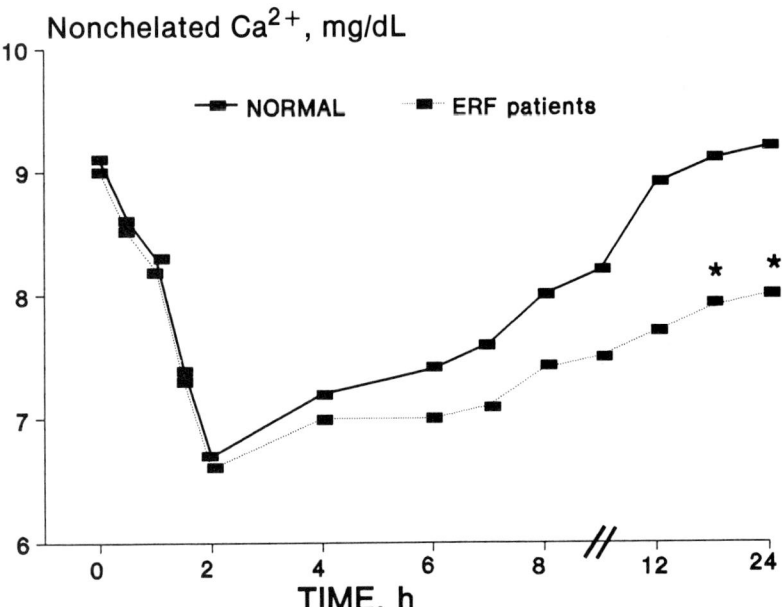

**Figure 51–6.** Mean values ( ± SE) of PTH and nonchelated $Ca^{2+}$ in relation to time during and after the infusion of EDTA before calcitriol therapy. The closed square–dotted line represents values for patients with early renal failure (ERF). The closed square–continuous line represents values for normal subjects. *$P < .01$. (From Llach F, Massry SG, Singer FR, et al: Skeletal resistance to endogenous parathyroid hormone in patients with early renal failure. A possible cause for secondary hyperparathyroidism. J Clin Endocrinol Metab 41[2]:339–345, 1975. © The Endocrine Society.)

and advanced CRF had an impaired calcemic response to PTH and low levels of calcitriol compared with control rats. The low-P diet improved the calcemic response to PTH in both groups of rats. Whereas rats with advanced CRF had no increase in calcitriol levels during the PTH infusion, those with moderate CRF had a significant increment. Thus, in moderate CRF, P restriction improved the calcemic response to PTH and this effect could be, at least in part, due to higher levels of calcitriol. However, in advanced CRF, because calcitriol levels were not influenced by P restriction, the improvement in the calcemic response to PTH may have been independent of calcitriol. In patients with mild CRF, Llach and Massry[26] observed that dietary P restriction improved the calcemic response to a standardized infusion of PTH. In addition to the effect of P on calcitriol, the ambient P concentration in bone may also affect the amount of exchangeable $Ca^{2+}$ that can be mobilized by PTH. Thus, higher inorganic P leads to reduced $Ca^{2+}$ release from bone both in the perfused rat tail preparation[65] and in osteoclasts.[66]

Decreased calcitriol levels have also been related to the impaired calcemic response to PTH in CRF.[67, 68] Thus, animals with experimental CRF exhibited a blunted calcemic response to PTH; the administration of calcitriol partly corrected it.[69, 70] Similarly, the administration of calcitriol at 0.5 μg/d for 6 weeks improved the calcemic response to PTH in patients with early CRF[28] (Fig. 51–7). Studies of experimental animals have shown correction of the calcemic response to PTH after administration of calcitriol together with 24,25(OH)$_2$D.[68] Such data support the possibility that altered vitamin D metabolism plays a role in the impaired calcemic response to PTH. However, other investigators have not been able to confirm these findings.[69, 71]

Although both P retention and calcitriol supplementation

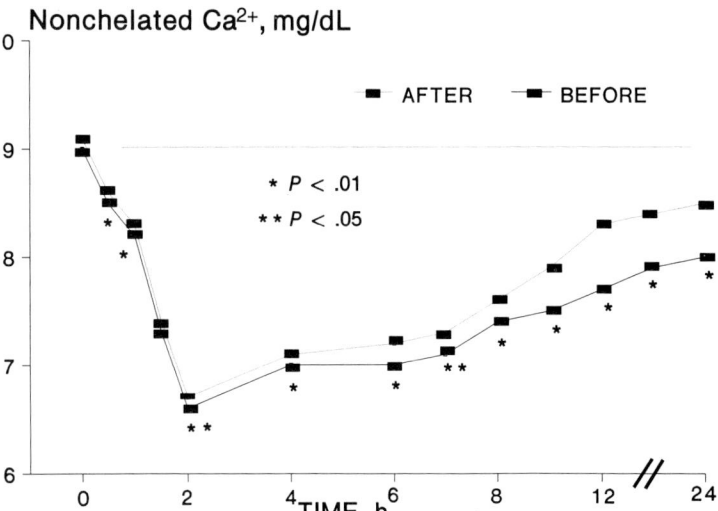

**Figure 51–7.** Mean values (± SE) of PTH and nonchelated $Ca^{2+}$ during the EDTA test in patients before *(closed square–continuous line)* and after *(closed square–dotted line)* calcitriol therapy. (From Wilson L, Felsenfeld AJ, Drezner MK, Llach F: Altered divalent ion metabolism in early renal failure: Role of 1,25-$(OH)_2$D. Used with permission from Kidney International, volume 27, pages 565–573, 1985.)

have been shown to improve the calcemic response to PTH, alone or together they do not correct it. Conversely, Galceran and associates[71] in thyroparathyroidectomized dogs and our group[70] in parathyroidectomized rats have noted that removal of circulating PTH restores to normal the calcemic response to PTH. These findings suggested that the presence of high PTH levels in the uremic animal may induce down-regulation of bone receptors to PTH and that the removal of PTH would restore the responsiveness of these receptors. Likewise, in isolated perfused bones obtained from uremic dogs with acute renal failure[72] and CRF[73] blunted release of cyclic AMP (cAMP) has been shown in response to PTH, whereas it was restored when dogs underwent thyroparathyroidectomy. However, a direct relationship between parathyroidectomy (PTX) and down-regulation of PTH receptors has not been established. We have noted that although PTX corrected the calcemic response to PTH in CRF, the maintenance of PTH levels in the normal range in rats with CRF did not correct the calcemic response to PTH.[74] This is in agreement with clinical studies in which subtotal PTX, almost resulting in normalization of PTH levels, did not improve the calcemic response to PTH.[64] Moreover, PTX normalizes the calcemic response to PTH, surmounting inhibitory factors such as hyperphosphatemia and probably calcitriol deficiency.[70, 74] These results suggest that the mechanism by which PTX restored the calcemic response to PTH in uremia may include factors other than down-regulation of PTH receptors.

The role of endogenous CT production in the calcemic response to PTH in rats with CRF may be of importance.[75] Thus, in the absence of CT, the calcemic response to PTH increased in rats with or without CRF; in the presence of secondary HPTH and hypercalcemia, CT was an important modifier of the calcemic response to PTH in the rat, especially in CRF. The importance of CT in the decreased calcemic response to PTH of CRF remains to be determined.

We have also observed[76] a decreased calcemic response to PTH despite normal levels of serum P and calcitriol, suggesting that factors intrinsic to uremia may impair the

calcemic response to PTH. Similarly, Wills and Jenkins[77] have shown that serum from uremic patients inhibited PTH-induced bone resorption in an in vitro model, and this effect was not observed with serum obtained after dialysis. Whether resistance to calcitriol induced by uremia may be at least partly responsible for these observations remains to be elucidated.

## ALTERED VITAMIN D METABOLISM AND RESISTANCE TO CALCITRIOL

Abnormal conversion of vitamin D to its active form, calcitriol, probably plays a fundamental role in the development of secondary HPTH in early CRF (Fig. 51–8). The evidence that vitamin D metabolism is altered in advanced CRF is most convincing.[78–80] Thus, intestinal absorption of $Ca^{2+}$ is diminished and poorly responsive to vitamin D. Liu and Chu[7] found no improvement of osteomalacia or $Ca^{2+}$ balance in uremic patients treated with usual oral doses of vitamin D. These authors, for the first time, clearly enunciated renal disease as a vitamin D–resistant state. Also, in patients with advanced CRF, metabolic balance studies revealed that fecal $Ca^{2+}$ excretion is equal to or even greater than dietary intake of calcium.[1, 2, 81] Radioisotopic methods indicate that intestinal absorption of $Ca^{2+}$ is reduced in most patients with advanced uremia.[82] It was also shown that the intestinal malabsorption of $Ca^{2+}$ could be overcome by the administration of vitamin D in doses of 100,000 to 300,000 IU/d.[1, 2] With such treatment, $Ca^{2+}$ absorption increased and rickets or osteomalacia healed.

The kidney is the principal organ responsible for converting 25(OH)D to 1,25-$(OH)_2$D (calcitriol)[83, 84]; this conversion is also the rate-limiting step in the production of calcitriol. This discovery provided the framework for the hypothesis that vitamin D metabolism is altered in uremia. Anephric rats are unable to produce calcitriol from its precursor,[85] an observation that led to speculation that impaired renal production of calcitriol accounts for impaired $Ca^{2+}$ absorption and osteomalacia in uremia. Several observations support this premise. Mawer and colleagues[86] and

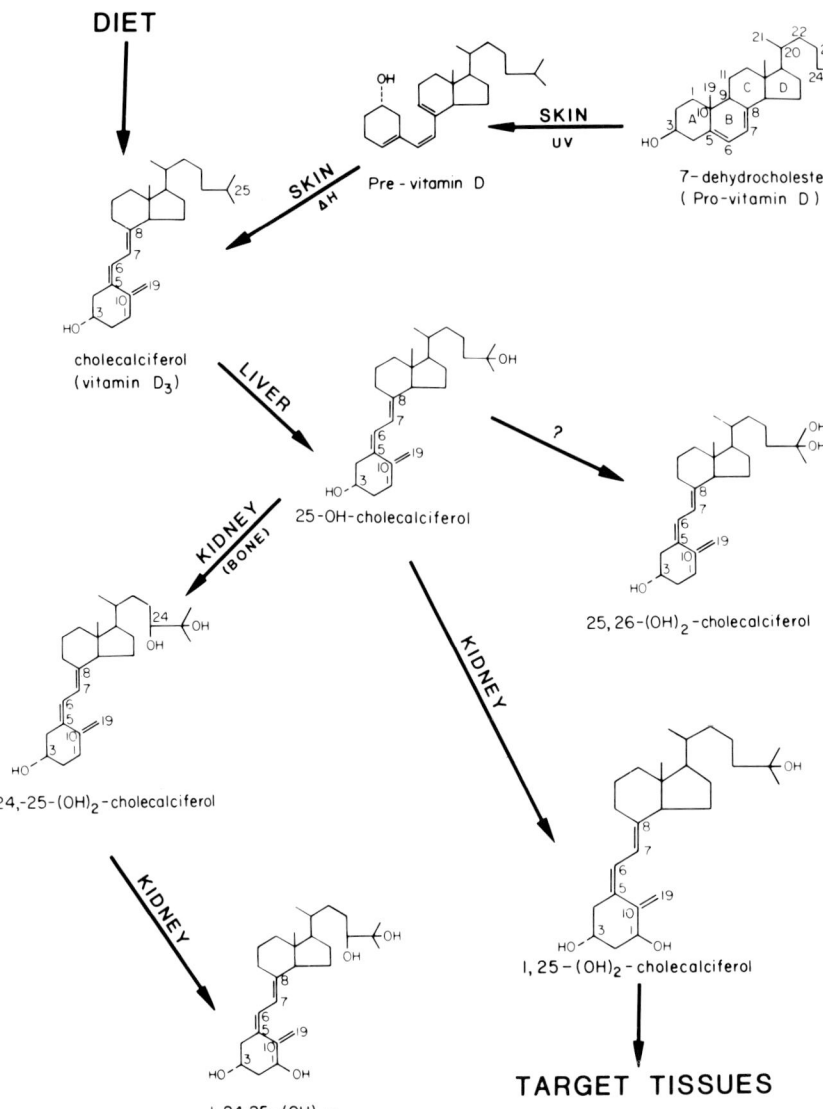

**Figure 51–8.** Schematic illustration of the bioactivation of vitamin D that may arise either from the skin, via 7-dehydrocholesterol, or from the diet. UV = ultraviolet light; ΔH = increased temperature.

Schaefer and colleagues[87] have shown data providing indirect evidence for the failure to hydroxylate (see Fig. 51–8) 25(OH)D at the C-1 position and thus convert it to calcitriol. Moreover, the serum levels of calcitriol have been uniformly noted to be decreased in patients with advanced CRF.[78, 79, 88–90]

The nature of the response to replacement with various vitamin D derivatives also supports the view that impaired conversion of 25(OH)D to calcitriol is of importance in CRF. Thus, calcitriol in doses of 0.6 to 1.0 μg/d can increase $^{47}Ca^{2+}$ absorption to normal in uremic patients,[91, 92] whereas the quantity of 25(OH)D needed to augment $Ca^{2+}$ absorption in uremia is 100 to 500 μg[93]; the amount of vitamin D needed, as stated before, is even greater.[1, 2, 42] The relative effect of different vitamin D sterols on $Ca^{2+}$ absorption is shown in Figure 51–9. Although the levels of calcitriol have been found to be low in patients with advanced uremia, data indicate that abnormalities in calcitriol production may occur even in early CRF.[28] Moreover, because the 1α-hydroxylase is present in the mitochondria of

proximal tubule cells,[94] calcitriol synthesis may be more impaired in patients with tubulointerstitial renal disease. Thus, such patients have been described to have lower plasma levels of calcitriol even at early stages of CRF.[95] Patients with chronic pyelonephritis developed a greater parathyroid gland mass than those with chronic glomerulonephritis. Vitamin D–deficient osteomalacia is also more frequently observed in the former than in the latter.[96] However, in other studies,[18, 26, 89] the presence or absence of tubulointerstitial disease did not appear to affect calcitriol levels.

The pathophysiologic consequences of reduced generation of calcitriol in renal insufficiency deserve further consideration. They include, as stated earlier, decreased intestinal absorption of $Ca^{2+}$[82, 97] and a reduced calcemic response to PTH on the skeleton,[67, 68] thereby contributing to hypocalcemia. Moreover, Lopez-Hilker and co-workers[29] have shown that despite the presence of hypercalcemia, secondary HPTH develops when calcitriol deficiency is present. As discussed shortly, low serum calcitriol levels

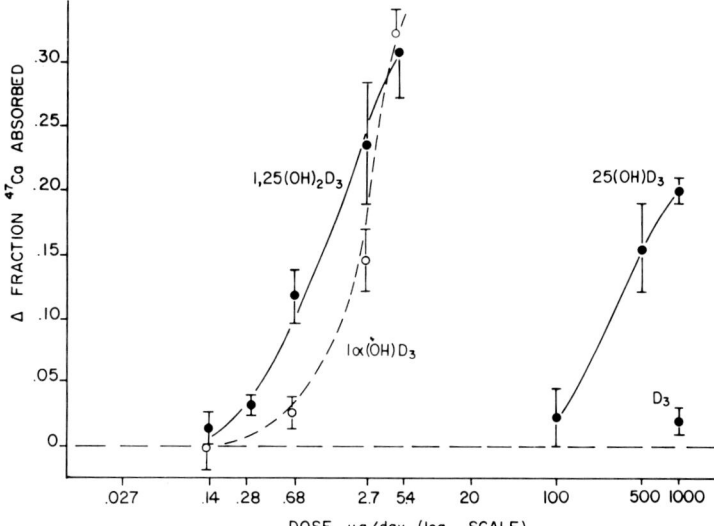

**Figure 51–9.** Changes (Δ) in the fraction of $^{47}Ca^{2+}$ absorbed by patients with advanced renal failure who were studied before and 8 to 10 days after they received a vitamin D sterol in the daily dosage indicated. Values are mean ± SE. (From Coburn JW, Llach F: Renal osteodystrophy. *In* Maxwell MH, Kleeman CR [eds]: Clinical Disorders of Fluid and Electrolyte Metabolism. McGraw-Hill, New York, 1979, pp 850–899. Reproduced with permission of McGraw-Hill, Inc.)

may lead to an increase in the synthesis and secretion of PTH.[98–102]

When in the course of progressive CRF does a decrease in calcitriol occur? Martinez and associates[18] have noted, in 150 patients with various degrees of renal function, that calcitriol may be reduced with creatinine clearances of 70 mL/min (Fig. 51–10). Chesney and colleagues[95] have also observed low levels of calcitriol in patients with creatinine clearances greater than 75 to 80 mL/min. In addition, a significant correlation was found between creatinine clearance rates and calcitriol levels. Wilson and colleagues[28] have also noted low levels of calcitriol in patients with GFR between 50 and 80 mL/min. Other studies have also noted a significant decrease in mean serum calcitriol levels in early CRF.[57, 103] Detailed observations by Portale and coworkers[104] in children with moderate CRF (GFR between 25 and 50 mL/min/1.73 m$^2$) have indicated that calcitriol levels are reduced by 40%. When analyzed over the range from normal to severely impaired renal function, the PTH values in these children correlated inversely with their calcitriol levels. Thus, the available data suggest that patients with early CRF have low levels of calcitriol. Conversely, few authors have noted normal or elevated levels of calcitriol in early CRF.[26, 79, 89, 105, 106] These differences in calcitriol levels could be related to the measurement of calcitriol in different populations, differences in the PTH and calcitriol assays used, or simply heterogeneity in the ability of the renal hydroxylase in early CRF to convert 25(OH)D at the C-1 position to calcitriol. However, such seemingly normal levels of calcitriol in the presence of elevated PTH suggest the presence of a relative calcitriol deficiency, because PTH is a potent stimulus for calcitriol production.[107, 108] Thus, the normal levels of calcitriol are inappropriately low.

Do the low levels of calcitriol have pathogenic importance regarding the abnormal divalent ion metabolism in patients with mild CRF? This hypothesis was tested by Wilson and colleagues[28] by giving patients with early CRF physiologic doses of oral calcitriol. Thus, the calcemic response to PTH and the handling of an oral P load were studied in 12 patients with early CRF and 6 normal volunteers both before and after 6 weeks of therapy with calci-

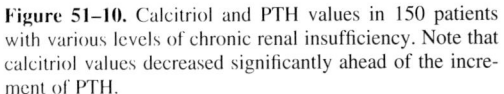

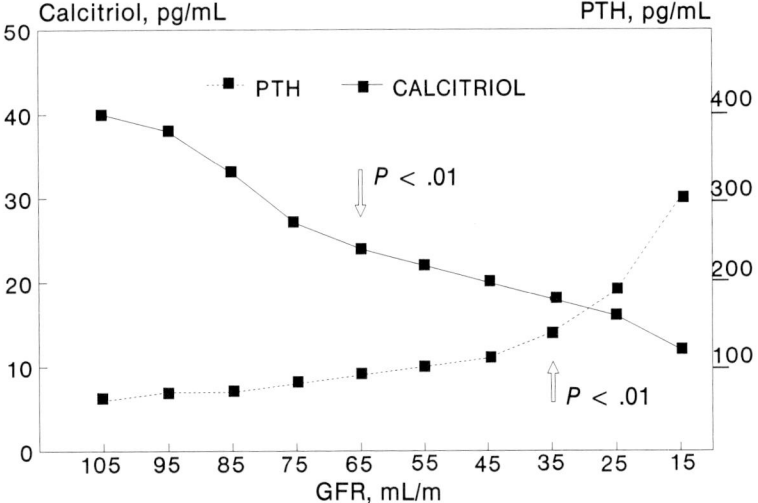

**Figure 51–10.** Calcitriol and PTH values in 150 patients with various levels of chronic renal insufficiency. Note that calcitriol values decreased significantly ahead of the increment of PTH.

triol. Compared with normal subjects, patients with mild renal disease had lower serum P concentrations and lower urinary $Ca^{2+}$ excretion, lower serum calcitriol, and higher PTH levels, as well as higher levels of urinary cAMP. With EDTA infusion, an impaired calcemic response to PTH was observed in patients with early CRF but not in normal individuals. These patients demonstrated an increased ability to excrete a P load. After therapy with calcitriol, significant increases in serum P concentration and urinary $Ca^{2+}$ excretion and a decrease in urinary cAMP were observed. Furthermore, the impaired calcemic response to PTH improved significantly (see Fig. 51–7), the renal handling of P became normal, and the low baseline levels of plasma calcitriol increased to normal after the sterol. In addition, a significant correlation between levels of plasma calcitriol and creatinine clearances was observed in both patients and normal subjects. These data suggest that a mild deficiency of calcitriol is present in patients with early CRF and that administration of this sterol results in substantial improvement in divalent ion metabolism.

The cause of reduced calcitriol synthesis has not yet been fully evaluated. As mentioned earlier, because 1α-hydroxylase is present in the mitochondria of proximal tubule cells, it is possible that calcitriol synthesis by the kidney is related to the functional state of the proximal renal tubules. As the GFR reasonably reflects functional renal mass, a decrement in calcitriol may occur slowly and progressively as GFR declines. In support of this hypothesis are the observations by Kawaguchi and colleagues,[109] who noted a progressive decline in calcitriol synthesis after graded reductions in the renal mass of rats. Similarly, in P-deprived rats, in vitro calcitriol synthesis was a linear function of the wet weight of renal tissue slices.[110]

The proximal tubule concentration of P may be an important determinant of 1α-hydroxylation. Thus, Tanaka and DeLuca[51] have demonstrated that the intracellular P content of kidney cortical cells is a major control mechanism for the renal hydroxylation of $25(OH)_2D$. Portale and co-workers[27] postulated that the intracellular concentration of P in the proximal tubules may increase in early CRF. This, in turn, may reduce the activity of the 1α-hydroxylase and decrease the synthesis of calcitriol. Our observations in four patients with early CRF ingesting a P-restricted diet support such a hypothesis.[26] In these patients, after P restriction, renal P excretion decreased, intestinal absorption of $Ca^{2+}$ increased, and PTH concentration decreased. Most important, there was a significant increase in the plasma calcitriol level after P restriction. These events occurred in the absence of significant changes in serum P concentration and net external balance of P (Fig. 51–11). Because there were no changes in serum $Ca^{2+}$ or P, it is likely that the increment in calcitriol may have been due to a decrease in tubule P concentration, which may have stimulated the 1α-hydroxylation. Thus, an increased P concentration in the renal tubule cells may lead to decreased synthesis of calcitriol and high PTH levels (Fig. 51–12). Such elevation of PTH may induce a compensatory synthesis of calcitriol in the remaining nephrons.[107, 108] Kawaguchi and associates[109] have shown the important role of PTH in stimulating the production of calcitriol in rats fed normal or high-P diets in the presence of CRF. Prince and co-workers[111] have also

noted a decrease in the renal ability of patients with moderate CRF to synthesize calcitriol; however, when the calcitriol/GFR ratio was calculated, no difference in maximal calcitriol production was observed between normal subjects and patients.

Factors other than secondary HPTH may also play a role in the observed levels of calcitriol. Thus, calcitriol levels were not different between unilaterally nephrectomized rats and sham-operated rats with or without PTX.[112] Hsu and colleagues[113, 114] have shown that both the production rate and the metabolic clearance rate of calcitriol are decreased in uremic rats. However, in uremic dogs, Dusso and co-workers[115] noted only a decreased production rate of calcitriol but not a decreased metabolic clearance rate. Later, Hsu and colleagues[116] observed in patients with moderate CRF (clearance of creatinine $34 \pm 6$ mL/min) that uremic plasma contains inhibitory factors that suppress not only the synthesis but also the degradation of calcitriol. They also noted that uremic toxins suppress the genomic synthesis of the 24-hydroxylase, thereby reducing the metabolic clearance rate of calcitriol.[117] This mechanism would appear to be a way to minimize the decrease in serum calcitriol in CRF.

Interestingly, an increase in serum calcitriol levels after administration of 25(OH)D has also been observed in anephric patients undergoing hemodialysis.[118, 119] This effect was not observed in normal humans or in dogs with moderate CRF.[115] These results suggest extrarenal production of calcitriol in the presence of low calcitriol levels; moreover, they suggest that physiologic levels of calcitriol may regulate its production.[120] However, this source of calcitriol is not enough to correct the calcitriol deficit observed in CRF.

Regardless of the cause of decreased secretion of calcitriol, an important pathophysiologic consequence of this deficiency may be the absence of a modulating inhibitory action of this hormone on PTH synthesis and secretion, leading to secondary HPTH. A number of studies have shown that calcitriol exerts a negative feedback on the parathyroid glands. Booth and colleagues[121] have provided evidence that parathyroid activity is increased and stimulation of 1α-hydroxylase activity diminished in early vitamin D deficiency. Observations of Oldham and co-workers[100] of vitamin D–deficient puppies suggest that parenteral administration of calcitriol could enhance the suppression of serum PTH by increasing blood $Ca^{2+}$ levels. Results of these in vitro and experimental studies were confirmed for hemodialysis patients by Slatopolsky and colleagues.[101] Thus, these authors have provided evidence for a direct suppressive effect of intravenously administered calcitriol on PTH secretion in hemodialysis patients. In these patients, after the administration of intravenous calcitriol, serum PTH started to decrease before any change in blood $Ca^{2+}$ level was detected. However, increased levels of serum $Ca^{2+}$ were observed later and were a contributory factor in the additional decrement of PTH. Delmez and associates[122] also evaluated the inhibitory effect of intravenous calcitriol in dialysis patients with secondary HPTH. Serum $Ca^{2+}$ and PTH ($NH_2$-terminal fragment) were determined before and after 2 weeks of intravenous calcitriol. Despite no significant changes in $Ca^{2+}$, PTH levels fell by

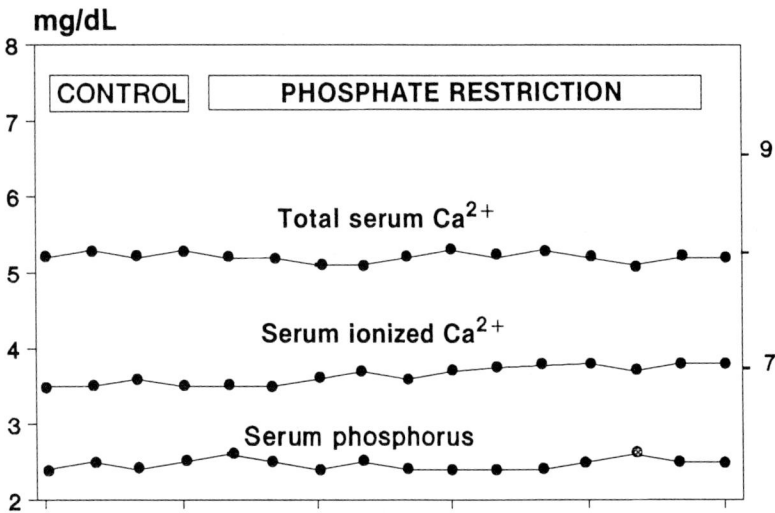

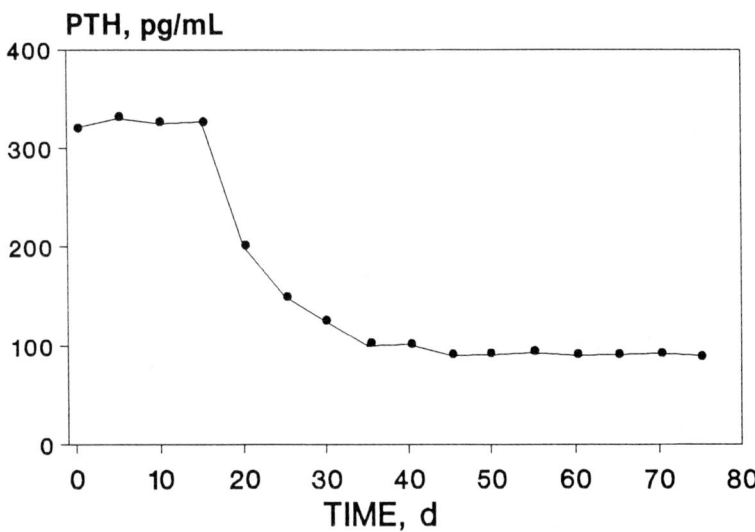

**Figure 51–11.** Total serum calcium, Ca²⁺, P, and PTH in five patients with early renal failure before and during the P restriction. Note that with P restriction PTH decreased significantly without changes in the other parameters. (Modified from Llach F, Massry SG: On the mechanism of secondary hyperparathyroidism in moderate renal insufficiency. J Clin Endocrinol Metab 61[4]:601–606, 1985. © The Endocrine Society.)

22%. We have also evaluated the direct inhibitory effect of calcitriol on parathyroid function in nine dialysis patients with severe hyperparathyroidism.[123] They received 2 μg of calcitriol intravenously at the end of each dialysis for 10 weeks. To avoid hypercalcemia, the dialysate Ca²⁺ concentration was reduced to 2.5 mEq/L. The basal PTH (intact molecule) fell from 902 ± 126 to 466 ± 152 pg/mL after 10 weeks of therapy. This occurred in the absence of any significant changes in total serum Ca²⁺ concentration (Fig. 51–13).

A significant suppression by calcitriol of mRNA coding for pre-pro-PTH (PTH mRNA) in bovine parathyroid cell cultures has been observed.[98] This reduction in PTH mRNA occurs primarily at the transcriptional level.[124, 125] Silver and colleagues[126] have also shown that administration of calcitriol to rats had a profound suppressive effect on in vivo PTH synthesis. Elevated PTH mRNA levels have also been demonstrated in experimental CRF and were attributed to reduced plasma levels of calcitriol.[127] Thus, it seems that the major action of calcitriol on PTH secretion may occur

by inhibiting transcription of DNA, thereby decreasing the synthesis of PTH available for secretion. Conversely, a decrease in the level of calcitriol would increase the synthesis and secretion of hormone by the parathyroid cell.

Finally, as with other steroid hormones, the biologic actions of calcitriol appear to be mediated through a hormone–cytoplasmic receptor complex. The activated hormone-receptor complex then interacts with nuclear chromatin and binds a specific regulatory region of the 5′-flanking sequence of affected genes, altering DNA transcription of specific precursor mRNA molecules.[125, 128, 129] This vitamin D receptor (VDR) is widespread in different tissues including intestine and parathyroid gland. Reduced density and binding of VDRs have been observed in parathyroid glands of both animals[130, 131] and patients with CRF.[132] Because the biologic response to calcitriol is proportional to the density of VDRs within the cell,[133] a reduction in the number of VDRs or inhibition of the VDR interaction with DNA may diminish the biologic response to calcitriol. It is possible that reduced VDR number or

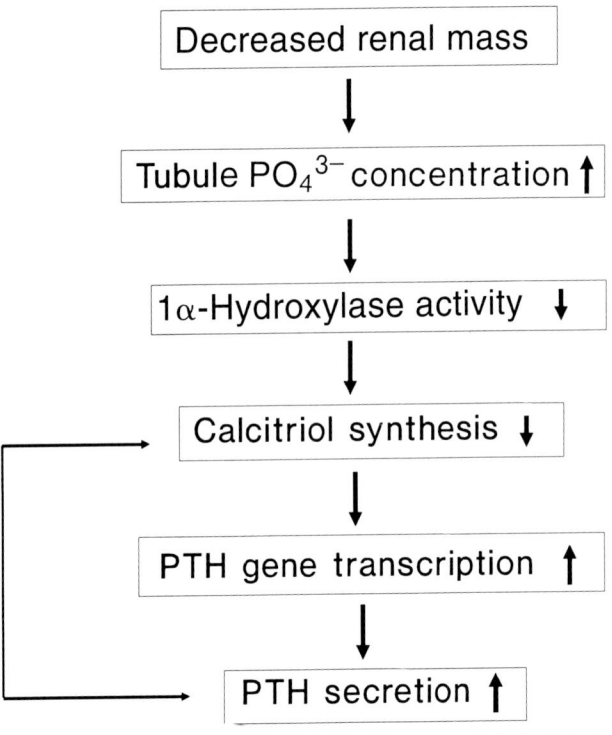

| Decreased renal mass |
| :---: |

↓

| Tubule PO$_4^{3-}$ concentration ↑ |
| :---: |

↓

| 1α-Hydroxylase activity ↓ |
| :---: |

↓

| Calcitriol synthesis ↓ |
| :---: |

↓

| PTH gene transcription ↑ |
| :---: |

↓

| PTH secretion ↑ |
| :---: |

**Figure 51–12.** Schematic representation of a hypothetic mechanism by which calcitriol may decrease in patients with early renal failure.

function renders the parathyroid glands less responsive to the inhibitory action of calcitriol. In addition, in dispersed bovine parathyroid cells, it was observed that near-physiologic amounts of calcitriol induced an increase in the concentration of cytosolic Ca$^{2+}$; thus, this nongenomic action of calcitriol would also contribute to decreased synthesis and secretion of PTH.[134]

In dialysis patients, physiologic serum levels of calcitriol may not suppress severe secondary HPTH, but the higher peak levels that occur after intermittent administration of intravenous calcitriol[135] could decrease PTH levels. Data of

Fukagawa and colleagues[136] and our own data[76] have shown that normal Ca$^{2+}$, P, and calcitriol levels do not preclude the development of secondary HPTH in an experimental rat model (Fig. 51–14), suggesting resistance to physiologic levels of calcitriol in uremia as a new pathogenic mechanism to explain the secondary HPTH. Fukagawa and associates[136] also noted that treatment with calcitriol and oxacalcitriol, a noncalcemic analogue of calcitriol, were able to normalize the PTH mRNA levels measured by Northern blot techniques. These data suggest that transient supraphysiologic levels of calcitriol may lead to binding of calcitriol to its receptor and suppress PTH; this, in turn, would explain the resistance of parathyroid cells to physiologic levels of calcitriol in uremia. In support of this hypothesis, Hsu and co-workers,[117] using intestine as a source of VDR, have shown that uremic ultrafiltrate reduced the receptor interaction with DNA in vitro. Furthermore, infusion of uremic ultrafiltrate in normal rats reduced the intestinal VDR concentration and also suppressed the calcitriol-induced up-regulation of the receptor; they concluded that uremic toxins may reduce the biologic action of calcitriol in CRF by inhibiting receptor synthesis and the interaction of the hormone-receptor complex with nuclear chromatin.[137] Also, De Francisco and colleagues,[138] studying the expression of VDRs in peripheral blood mononuclear cells, observed in a preliminary study that in addition to reduced VDRs in uremia, the correction of uremia by successful kidney transplantation reversed that abnormality independently of calcitriol. Finally, dietary calcium, calcitriol, and PTH have been shown to regulate the tissue content of VDRs.[137, 139–141] However, the interrelationship among these factors in the regulation of the VDRs remains unclear.

### Autonomous Proliferation

Secondary HPTH is characterized by marked enlargement of the parathyroid glands, which can be defined histologically as diffuse and/or nodular hyperplasia, the latter being a more severe histologic form.[142–144] In 1963 the term "tertiary hyperparathyroidism," describing the formation

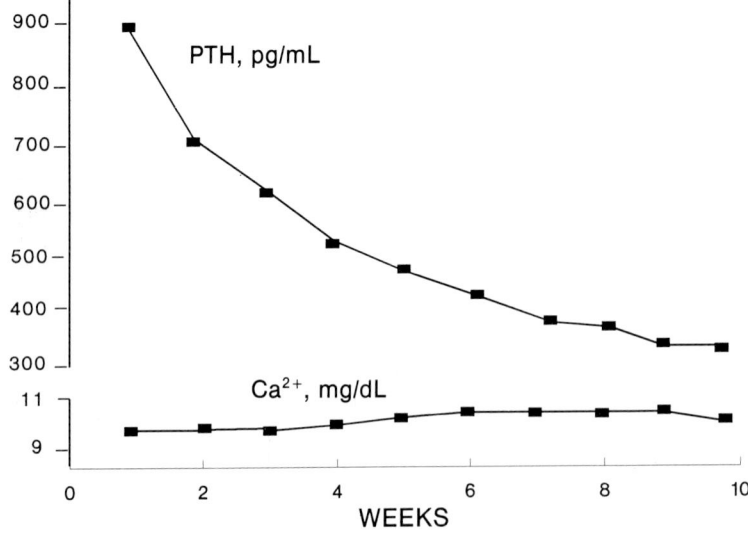

**Figure 51–13.** Baseline intact PTH and total serum calcium levels in patients with significant secondary HPTH during 10 weeks of intravenous calcitriol. Note the significant decrease in PTH ($P < .01$) in the absence of changes in serum calcium. (Data from Dunlay R, Rodriguez M, Felsenfeld AJ, Llach F: Direct inhibitory effect of calcitriol on parathyroid function [sigmoidal curve] in dialysis patients. Kidney Int 36:1093–1098, 1989.)

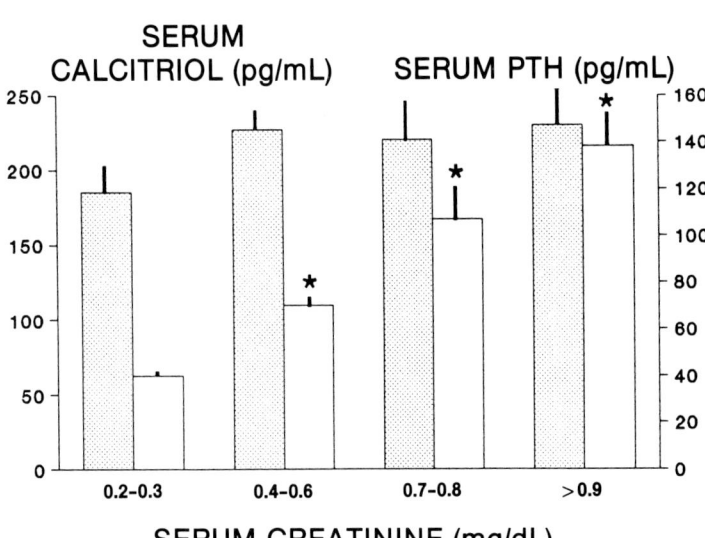

**Figure 51–14.** *Top.* Serum Ca²⁺ *(solid bars)* and serum P *(hatched bars)* in rats with different degrees of renal failure maintained on a normal 0.6% Ca²⁺, 0.6% P diet. Serum calcitriol *(stippled bars)* and serum PTH *(open bars)* are represented on the bottom. Serum PTH progressively increased at each level of renal failure even though serum Ca²⁺, P, and calcitriol did not change significantly. Resistance to calcitriol or the observed decreased calcemic response to PTH may be the putative factor. (From Bover J, Rodriguez M, Trinidad P, et al: Factors in the development of secondary hyperparathyroidism in graded renal failure in the rat. Used with permission from Kidney International, volume 45, pages 953–961, 1994.)

of an adenoma superimposed on diffuse hyperplasia, was introduced.[145] Also, this term has frequently been applied to describe the condition in which hypercalcemia develops in secondary HPTH.[146–148] It is known that residual or transplanted parathyroid tissue containing nodular hyperplasia has a higher rate of recurrent hyperparathyroidism than that with diffuse hyperplasia.[149–151] These areas of nodular hyperplasia may consist of cells with high secretory activity that are not normally suppressed by hypercalcemia. Furthermore, in parathyroid glands from hemodialysis patients, nodular hyperplasia is associated with a decrease in VDR density compared with that in diffuse hyperplasia.[152] Whether glands with nodular hyperplasia are less responsive to calcitriol treatment remains to be proved.

Finally, Kremer and co-workers[153] have shown in vitro that calcitriol and not extracellular Ca²⁺ may directly modulate parathyroid cell proliferation by altering the expression of specific replication-associated oncogenes (*MYC* and *FOS*). Falchetti and associates[154] have also reported an allelic loss on chromosome 11 in dialysis patients with marked secondary HPTH; they concluded that autonomous monoclonal parathyroid cell proliferation may develop in uremic patients through inactivation of a tumor suppressor

gene on chromosome 11. The relationship between autonomous proliferation, nodular hyperplasia, and resistance to calcitriol remains to be determined.

## ALTERED DEGRADATION OF PTH

An increased rate of secretion of PTH is the major mechanism responsible for high plasma levels of PTH in CRF. Considerable evidence demonstrates that the kidney plays an important role in the degradation of PTH and that the metabolic clearance of PTH is reduced in CRF[155]; thus, reduced renal degradation of PTH may contribute to the hyperparathyroid state in uremia. Berson and Yalow[156] reported immunochemical heterogeneity of PTH in the plasma of uremic patients; they suggested that the presence of more than one peptide fragment of PTH and altered metabolism of the hormone could account for the observed heterogeneity. This initial discovery was followed by extensive research into the biochemistry and metabolism of PTH.[157, 158]

Intact PTH is secreted from the parathyroid gland into the circulation mainly as a 9500-dalton, 84–amino acid peptide chain. It is secreted in a pulsatile fashion in both

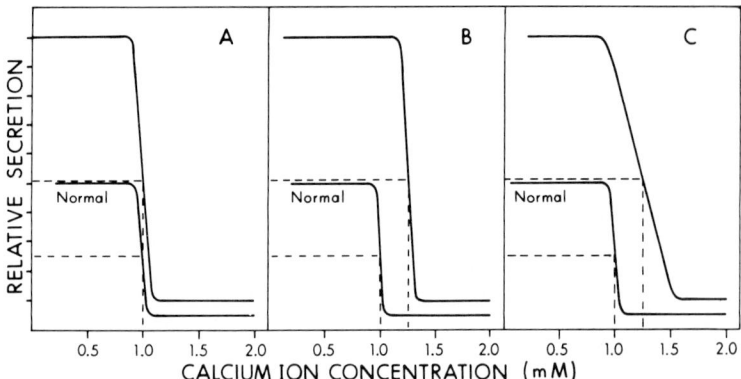

**Figure 51–15.** Diagrammatic representation of the relative rates of PTH secretion in relation to $Ca^{2+}$ concentrations in the normal state and with secondary hyperparathyroidism, with three different schemes to account for increased secretion of PTH. The set-point, or $Ca^{2+}$ concentration with 50% reduction in PTH, release is indicated by the interrupted line. For complete description, see text. (From Morrisey J, Martin K, Slatopolsky E: *In* Massry SG, Maschio G [eds]: Phosphate and Other Minerals. Plenum Publishing, New York, 1983, p 389.)

normal subjects[159] and patients with CRF.[160] The first 34 $NH_2$-terminal residues bind to PTH receptors, activate cellular responses, and mimic all the $Ca^{2+}$-regulating actions of the intact hormone in animals.[161, 162] Lacking a clear extracellular function, the COOH-terminal fragment of PTH seems to be essential for hormone processing (efficient transport across the endoplasmic reticulum) and secretion.[163] Although intact PTH is the main source of secreted PTH, it is also known that the gland can secrete PTH fragments 37–84 and 34–84 (COOH-terminal fragments) and that the relative secretion of these fragments increases or decreases in the presence of hyper- or hypocalcemia.[164]

Once intact PTH is secreted, the hormone is rapidly degraded, the $NH_2$-terminal portion is cleaved, and several inactive fragments from the COOH-terminal fraction of the peptide appear in the serum. Because of the shorter half-life of both intact PTH and the $NH_2$-terminal fragment, the COOH-terminal fragments become the predominating PTH peptide in the circulation. The intact parent peptide is rapidly degraded in the peripheral tissues, particularly in the kidney and the liver.[165] The liver has a large capacity to degrade the peptide, but it may not play an important role in degradation of either the COOH- or $NH_2$-terminal fragments.[166] By contrast, the kidney can extract and degrade the intact 84-residue molecule and both the COOH- and $NH_2$-terminal fragments.[167–169] Cathepsin D has been identified as one of the factors responsible for the intrarenal cleavage of intact PTH.[170] In the presence of CRF, PTH metabolism is altered and the renal excretion of PTH and its fragments is decreased.[171, 172] Such altered PTH metabolism may also account for the elevated PTH levels observed in CRF; this was particularly relevant when PTH was measured with immunoassays that used an antiserum directed to the middle or, especially, the COOH-terminal region. Also, different specificities of antisera probably accounted for the variability of PTH levels reported from various laboratories.

The advent of more advanced techniques such as immunoradiometric and immunochemiluminescence assays has improved the diagnosis and management of patients with renal osteodystrophy.[13, 173] These new techniques use antibodies directed toward the intact PTH molecule and, thus, avoid measurement of the various PTH fragments. At present, there are data correlating levels of intact PTH and various bone histomorphometric parameters characteristic of osteitis fibrosa.[174]

## ABNORMAL REGULATION OF CALCIUM-CONTROLLED PTH SECRETION (SET-POINT OF CALCIUM)

Studies of the regulation of PTH secretion by $Ca^{2+}$ indicate a sigmoid relationship between PTH secretion and ionized $Ca^{2+}$ over a narrow range of $Ca^{2+}$ concentration.[175] It has been shown that, to suppress the secretion of PTH, parathyroid cells from uremic patients require higher extracellular $Ca^{2+}$ concentrations than normal cells.[176] Moreover, the adenylate cyclase of hyperplastic parathyroid glands is less susceptible to $Ca^{2+}$-mediated inhibition.[177] Thus, the set-point for $Ca^{2+}$ is shifted toward the right. This abnormality may be an important factor in the abnormal secretion of PTH noted in uremia.

Uremia may alter the release of PTH from parathyroid cells by several mechanisms: 1) increasing tissue mass via hypertrophy and/or hyperplasia; 2) altering the set-point of $Ca^{2+}$, that is, the concentration of $Ca^{2+}$ required to inhibit 50% of maximal PTH secretion[178]; and 3) changing the slope of the sigmoid curve. These mechanisms are illustrated diagrammatically in Figure 51–15.[179] Thus, with each cell operating in a normal manner, the increased number of cells can cause hyperparathyroidism without any alteration in the $Ca^{2+}$ set-point (see Fig. 51–15A). The facts that PTH secretion is not totally blunted during hypercalcemia and that it is possible to induce hypercalcemia by transplantation of multiple normal parathyroid glands[180] suggest that a persistent basal secretion of PTH can have physiologic implications when the parathyroid mass, as in uremia, increases. A second possibility is that an increase in parathyroid gland size and a change in the secretion rate, as a result of an increased set-point for $Ca^{2+}$, occur (see Fig. 51–15B); the slope of the curve for $Ca^{2+}$ suppression then remains normal. Thus, the degree of hyperparathyroidism is higher as a result of both increased tissue mass and failure to suppress PTH secretion normally when extracellular $Ca^{2+}$ concentration is in the normal range. A third possibility is the existence of an increase in tissue mass, an increase in the set-point of $Ca^{2+}$, and a change in the slope of the PTH-$Ca^{2+}$ curve (see Fig. 51–15C). Because the slope of the PTH-$Ca^{2+}$ curve reflects the relation between PTH production and a change in serum $Ca^{2+}$, and maximal PTH is transformed to 100% to factor for differences in absolute values of maximal PTH, a decrease in the slope would

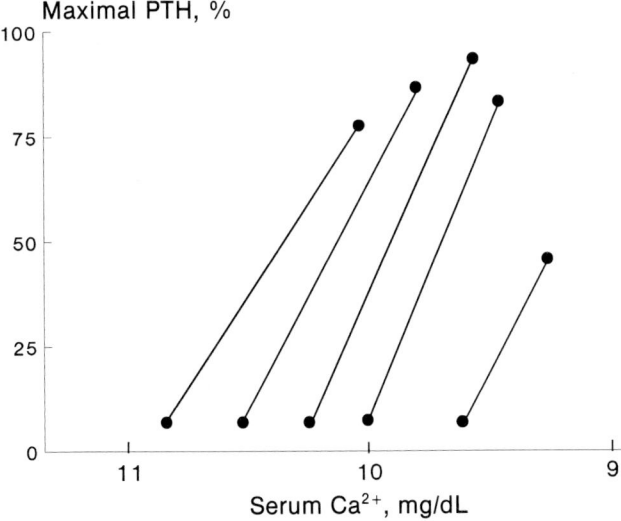

**Figure 51–16.** Serum Ca$^{2+}$ and percent maximal PTH in five patients after 30 minutes of zero Ca$^{2+}$ dialysis. Plasma Ca$^{2+}$ was greater than 9 mg/dL, yet all five patients responded with marked increases in PTH. (From Voigts A, Felsenfeld AJ, Andress DL, Llach F: Parathyroid hormone and bone histology: Response to hypocalcemia in osteitis fibrosa. Used with permission from Kidney International, volume 25, pages 445–452, 1984.)

reflect decreased sensitivity of the individual parathyroid cell (PTH production per parathyroid cell).[178] This might occur because of heterogeneity of the set-points for suppressibility by Ca$^{2+}$ among different populations of parathyroid cells. From the available data it seems that PTH secretion in hyperplastic parathyroid cells would behave similarly to the mechanism represented in Figure 51–15C.

The earliest evidence suggesting an abnormal set-point of Ca$^{2+}$ in CRF was presented by Voigts and colleagues[181] in a report on dialysis patients with significant secondary HPTH. During acute hypocalcemia produced by a low-Ca$^{2+}$ dialysate (Fig. 51–16), patients exhibited a marked increase in PTH levels as the serum Ca$^{2+}$ level decreased but was still within the normal range (more than 9 mg/dL). Later, Delmez and associates[122] demonstrated that the ad-

ministration of calcitriol for 2 weeks to dialysis patients returned the abnormal set-point for Ca$^{2+}$ toward normal. Thus, calcitriol appeared to have increased the sensitivity of the gland to changes in serum Ca$^{2+}$ concentration. However, the set-point of Ca$^{2+}$ was estimated as a 50% decrease from basal levels of PTH, rather than from maximal PTH stimulation.[122] We have assessed parathyroid gland function in nine patients with significant secondary HPTH.[123] This was evaluated by inducing hypo- and hypercalcemia using a low- and a high-Ca$^{2+}$ dialysate during two separate dialyses performed 1 week apart. PTH values after dialysis-induced hypo- and hypercalcemia were plotted against Ca$^{2+}$ for each patient, and the set-point for Ca$^{2+}$ was determined. As can be appreciated in Figure 51–17, the PTH-Ca$^{2+}$ sigmoid curve was shifted toward the right, resembling the curve observed by Brown and colleagues[176] in in vitro studies. After 10 weeks of intravenous calcitriol therapy (2 μg at the end of each dialysis), the curve was shifted to the left. Basal PTH levels fell from 902 ± 126 to 466 ± 152 pg/mL ($P < .01$) after calcitriol without any significant change in the serum total Ca$^{2+}$ concentration. The maximal PTH response during hypocalcemia decreased, after calcitriol therapy, from 1661 ± 485 to 1031 ± 280 pg/mL ($P < .05$). The PTH level at maximal inhibition during hypercalcemia decreased from 281 ± 76 to 192 ± 48 pg/mL. Although calcitriol reduced the PTH level at any Ca$^{2+}$ concentration, neither the set-point of Ca$^{2+}$ nor the slope of the PTH-Ca$^{2+}$ curve was significantly different after 10 weeks of calcitriol. However, if a noncompliant patient who had persistent hyperphosphatemia is excluded, a significant change in the set-point of Ca$^{2+}$ was observed (see Fig. 51–17). We have also evaluated the effect of long-term intravenous calcitriol administration in six patients who received calcitriol treatment during 42 weeks.[61] At the end of the study, the slope of the PTH-Ca$^{2+}$ curve was decreased ($P < .05$) compared with both 0 and 10 weeks (Fig. 51–18). Malberti and co-workers[102] obtained similar results for patients with secondary HPTH refractory to oral calcitriol. These patients received 2 μg of intravenous calcitriol three times a week for 4 months. A shift in the set-point of Ca$^{2+}$ and a decrease in the slope of the curve were observed.

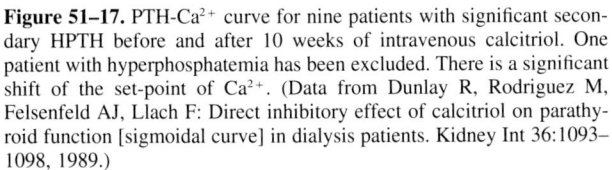

**Figure 51–17.** PTH-Ca$^{2+}$ curve for nine patients with significant secondary HPTH before and after 10 weeks of intravenous calcitriol. One patient with hyperphosphatemia has been excluded. There is a significant shift of the set-point of Ca$^{2+}$. (Data from Dunlay R, Rodriguez M, Felsenfeld AJ, Llach F: Direct inhibitory effect of calcitriol on parathyroid function [sigmoidal curve] in dialysis patients. Kidney Int 36:1093–1098, 1989.)

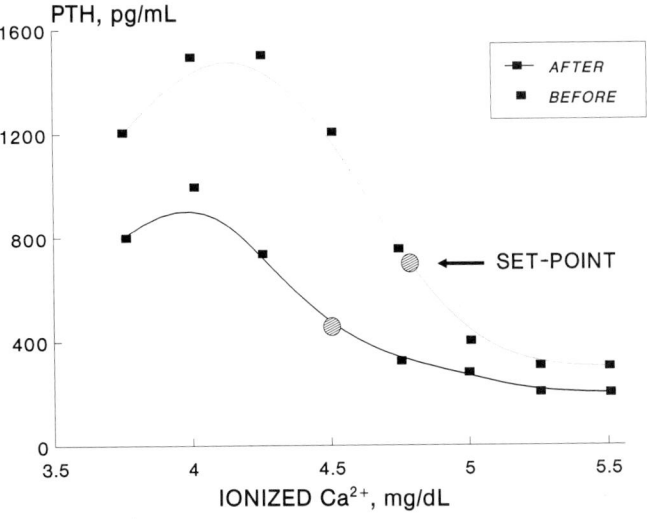

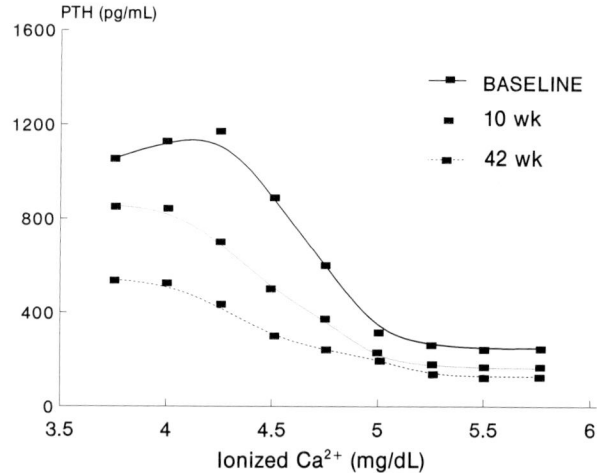

**Figure 51–18.** Effect of calcitriol treatment on the PTH-Ca²⁺ curve. The baseline (0 weeks) PTH-Ca²⁺ curve is before calcitriol therapy, and the other two PTH-Ca²⁺ curves are after 10 and 42 weeks of intravenous calcitriol. Between 0 weeks and both 10 and 42 weeks, significant differences were present in the hypocalcemic segment of the PTH-Ca²⁺ curves. *$P < .05$ versus 42 weeks. (From Rodriguez M, Felsenfeld AJ, Williams C, et al: The effect of long-term calcitriol administration on parathyroid function in hemodialysis patients. J Am Soc Nephrol 2[5]:1014–1020, 1991.)

These findings suggest that calcitriol 1) reduced the functional mass of parathyroid cells (based on the significant decrease in maximal and minimal PTH) and 2) decreased the sensitivity of parathyroid cells. Malberti and co-workers[102] also evaluated the PTH-Ca²⁺ curve for a patient before and after subtotal PTX and compared the curve with that before and after intravenous calcitriol treatment. PTX not only reduced the basal PTH levels but also resulted in an increased slope of the PTH-Ca²⁺ curve. This may indicate that increased sensitivity of the parathyroid cell followed PTX. Thus, it is possible that secretion of PTH decreased more with intravenous calcitriol (medical PTX) than with a decrease in the mass of parathyroid cells (surgical PTX).[178] A comprehensive editorial review of parathyroid gland function in CRF has been published.[178]

## ROLE OF CALCITONIN

Plasma levels of CT measured by RIA have been noted to be increased in patients with acute or CRF.[182, 183] Evidence exists for immunologic heterogeneity of circulating plasma CT, which may account for wide differences in values reported from different laboratories. Lee and colleagues[183] suggested that a different chromatographic pattern of CT may be observed in patients with CRF compared with individuals with medullary carcinoma of the thyroid. Thus, some immunoassays may detect inactive forms of CT and these forms are probably detected in CRF. The biologic significance of increased levels of CT in uremia remains to be established. Some observations suggest that there is a different relationship between serum CT and PTH levels in uremic patients with features of renal osteodystrophy and those without.[184, 185] Thus, dialysis patients were separated into two groups on the basis of a bimodal distribution of plasma alkaline phosphatase activity. Patients with normal

alkaline phosphatase activity had lower mean serum PTH and higher serum CT than patients with elevated alkaline phosphatase; serum levels of Ca²⁺ and P did not differ in the two groups. In uremic patients with normal alkaline phosphatase levels and in normal subjects a positive correlation was noted between plasma PTH and plasma CT. In the patients with elevated alkaline phosphatase activity, serum PTH and CT were negatively correlated, with higher serum PTH levels and lower CT values; the result was a higher ratio of PTH to CT. These authors suggested that high CT levels in patients with normal alkaline phosphatase levels may have inhibited or blocked the action of PTH on bone. Thus, normal alkaline phosphatase activity may be the result of the ability of CT to block the high bone turnover associated with high PTH levels. Patients with elevated alkaline phosphatase levels and overt renal osteodystrophy may have high levels of circulating PTH accompanied by a relative deficiency of CT. The reason for such deficiency is unclear; the authors suggested that it may represent either a lack of adequate stimulus for CT secretion or a failure of normal CT synthesis and secretion in response to an appropriate stimulus. Thus, high levels of CT may protect against the effects of excess PTH.[184, 185]

Kanis and associates[186] noted in dialysis patients after bilateral nephrectomy a fall in plasma alkaline phosphatase activity, a decrease in the number of osteoblasts in bone biopsy specimens, a decrease in plasma P concentration, and a rise in plasma CT level; plasma Ca²⁺ and PTH concentrations were unchanged. The authors suggested that the rise in plasma CT may be responsible for the transient decrease in bone turnover observed after nephrectomy. Such observations provide additional support for their contention that low levels of CT may contribute to increased bone turnover in uremic patients. Similarly, we have shown that CT is an important factor in the decreased calcemic response to PTH.[75] We have also shown a sigmoid relationship between CT and Ca²⁺.[187] The presence of a stimulus for CT in the physiologic range of serum Ca²⁺ suggested that endogenous CT may decrease the calcemic response in CRF. Whether these observations have any clinical relevance remains to be shown.

In summary, the relative contribution of the foregoing factors, including P retention, altered vitamin D metabolism and resistance to calcitriol, impaired calcemic response to PTH, altered metabolism of PTH, decreased sensitivity to ambient Ca²⁺ levels, and CT in the pathogenesis of secondary HPTH is uncertain. In early CRF, serum Ca²⁺ levels and intestinal Ca²⁺ absorption have generally been normal and serum P concentrations either normal or low. Rather than P retention, these patients have an increased ability to excrete a P load, similar to that noted in patients with primary hyperparathyroidism. However, serum PTH levels are commonly increased, and restriction of dietary P intake early in the course of CRF reduces the magnitude of secondary HPTH and improves the calcemic response to PTH. These observations suggest that P, through mechanisms other than P retention and hyperphosphatemia, may be an important pathogenic factor in the development of secondary HPTH. A hypothetic sequence of events is displayed in Figure 51–12. It is possible that an increase in intracellular P concentration in proximal tubule cells may lead to a decrease in the synthesis of calcitriol, which in turn may lead to increased PTH synthesis and secretion by releasing the transcription of PTH mRNA. With more advanced CRF, P retention and hyperphosphatemia play an important additional role in the development of severe secondary HPTH. A P load has a cumulative action on the mechanisms that increase PTH production; P may induce hypocalcemia, decreases the calcemic response to PTH, and decreases calcitriol production. Thus, a P load blocks all counter-regulatory mechanisms that minimize the increase in PTH. Moreover, increasing evidence supports a direct effect of P on the parathyroid gland.

PTH increases despite the absence of P retention, hypocalcemia, and low calcitriol levels; this suggests that other mechanisms may be involved in secondary HPTH in early stages of CRF. Resistance of parathyroid cells to the physiologic serum concentration of calcitriol, perhaps because of reduced density or responsiveness of calcitriol receptors in the parathyroid gland, may be another contributory factor. Similarly, because a decreased calcemic response to PTH has been observed without any known cause of skeletal resistance, unknown factors intrinsic to uremia may contribute to this abnormality. Hypothetically, a uremia-induced generalized defect of receptors or postreceptor events could contribute to the development of secondary HPTH in the early stages of CRF. This concept may be supported by studies of uremic patients, in whom resistance to other hormones such as growth hormone[188, 189] and insulin[190] has been observed even in early stages of CRF.[191]

## Osteomalacia and Adynamic Bone Disease (Low-Turnover Bone Disease)

Another skeletal lesion in patients with CRF is that represented by states of low bone turnover. The main bone features include a low bone formation rate and a defect in bone mineralization, which, in severe cases, leads to osteomalacia. A new low-bone-turnover entity has been identified: ABD or aplastic bone disease. There are few data on the pathogenesis of the low-bone-turnover states. Earlier, it was thought that these states characterized by impaired mineralization resulted from altered vitamin D metabolism; later, other pathogenic factors, including Al accumulation, were implicated. The factors that may impair bone formation, mineralization, and bone turnover are given in Table 51–3.

### ROLE OF VITAMIN D

Despite the observations that plasma levels of calcitriol are low in most uremic patients and that intestinal $Ca^{2+}$ absorption is decreased in uremia,[80, 82, 97] overt osteomalacia or even histologic features suggestive of impaired mineralization are noted rarely.[192, 193] Moreover, osteomalacia is often absent in anephric patients.[194]

Defective skeletal mineralization may have been more common in the United Kingdom than in North America. Eastwood and associates[195] noted that uremic osteomalacia correlated with decreased plasma levels of 25(OH)D, the latter reflecting decreased vitamin D intake. Thus, relative

**TABLE 51–3. Factors That May Contribute to a Low Bone Formation Rate in Patients with Renal Failure**

Decreased vitamin D (when nutritional vitamin D deficiency coexists with renal failure)
Al accumulation (mechanism: Al on forming surface, Al in osteoblasts, increased serum Al)
Low serum PTH levels (mechanism: PTX, diabetes mellitus, high serum $Ca^{2+}$, continuous ambulatory peritoneal dialysis, calcitriol treatment, Al loading)
Diabetes mellitus (multifactorial)
Iron accumulation
Age
Hypothyroidism
Corticosteroid treatment and Cushing syndrome
Fluoride (at toxic doses)
Reduced plasma $Ca^{2+}$ or P levels (low $Ca^{2+}$ × P product)
(?) Altered collagen synthesis and maturation
(?) $Mg^{2+}$ accumulation
(?) Pyrophosphate accumulation
(?) Acidosis
(?) Heparin therapy
Unidentified factors (e.g., immobilization)

vitamin D deficiency is more common in the United Kingdom and Scandinavian countries than in the United States because of less sunlight exposure and because fortification of foods with vitamin D is not extensive in the former areas.

Because calcitriol production is impaired in CRF, it is not surprising that vitamin D deficiency leads to greater impairment of skeletal mineralization in patients with CRF. As patients with advanced CRF are often malnourished, low plasma levels of 25(OH)D are also not infrequent.[196] Plasma levels of 25(OH)D have also been correlated with the protein content of the diet.[196] Furthermore, enhanced renal losses of this sterol may occur in patients with nephrotic syndrome[197]; this mechanism may contribute to the low levels of 25(OH)D observed in azotemic nephrotic patients.

The mechanism whereby the absence of calcitriol impairs the mineralization of bone is not well understood. Whether vitamin D or calcitriol directly stimulates bone mineralization or merely leads to bone mineralization by maintaining the appropriate milieu of $Ca^{2+}$ and P remains controversial.[198, 199] Other vitamin D derivatives such as 25(OH)D or $24,25(OH)_2D$ may have an independent beneficial effect on bone mineralization.[200–202]

### ALUMINUM ACCUMULATION

Convincing data indicate that accumulation of Al in patients with CRF can cause osteomalacia, hypercalcemia, encephalopathy, and hypochromic microcytic anemia.[203, 204] Outbreaks of fracturing "dialysis osteomalacia" were first reported from dialysis centers in the United Kingdom; encephalopathy was also common in those patients.[205, 206] It was first postulated that this bone disease arose from fluoride accumulation[207] or from P depletion,[208] despite the rarity of hypophosphatemia in patients with advanced CRF. Then Al levels were noted to be increased in the brain of patients dying with dialysis encephalopathy,[209] and epidemiologic data showed a correlation between the incidence of osteomalacia, dialysis encephalopathy, and high concentrations of Al in water used for dialysis.[206]

The Al content of bone was noted to be increased in most dialysis patients, whether measured by neutron activation,[210] electron probe,[211] atomic absorption spectroscopy,[212] or a histochemical staining method.[213] Bone Al levels were markedly elevated in patients with refractory osteomalacia, and the Al content of bone correlated directly with the extent of osteomalacia in these patients.[212] Moreover, Al deposits were noted along the mineralization front.[213, 214] Little or no tetracycline was incorporated along the surfaces with heavy Al staining, indicating absent bone formation; the extent of surface Al staining correlated inversely with bone formation rate.[213] In dialysis patients showing bone biopsy features of osteitis fibrosa, mixed features of osteomalacia plus osteitis fibrosa, or "mild" disease (mild secondary HPTH), bone Al content has often been noted to be above normal, but the values were generally less than those in patients with pure dialysis osteomalacia.[213–215]

Rarely, other metals can also produce a low-turnover bone disease. Staining at the mineralization front for iron and Al[216] as well as for iron alone[217, 218] has been observed in some patients receiving dialysis treatment. The standard aluminon stain (auryltricarboxylic acid) to detect Al in bone can also stain iron, and thus bone samples with iron deposits in bone may be erroneously identified as having Al.[219] Silicon and sulfur may also accumulate at the mineralization front and may cause osteomalacia.

Refractoriness to treatment with the active vitamin D sterols is another feature of Al-related osteomalacia. When dialysis patients with symptomatic Al bone disease were treated with calcitriol or 1α(OH)D, they generally had no change in symptoms or improvement of bone disease, and hypercalcemia often developed after low doses of the vitamin D derivatives.[220–222]

The clinical features of Al bone disease include progressive bone pain, especially affecting the axial skeleton; proximal muscle weakness; and fractures of the ribs, vertebrae, pelvis, and hips. Severe disability and skeletal deformities may occur.[222] Serum $Ca^{2+}$ levels are usually normal or slightly increased; serum P concentrations do not differ from those of other patients with advanced CRF and plasma levels of 25(OH)D are not depressed (excluding the coexistence of nutritional deficit of vitamin D). Some patients develop spontaneous hypercalcemia; in others hypercalcemia occurs during immobilization, while vitamin D derivatives or $Ca^{2+}$-containing P binders are taken, or with the use of a high dialysate $Ca^{2+}$ concentration.[220] Tumor-like calcifications have been reported in association with severe Al intoxication,[223] and improvement of a tumor-like calcification has been observed after appropriate therapy of Al intoxication and despite aggravation of secondary HPTH.[149] In patients with Al intoxication, PTX has been performed because these patients presented with hypercalcemia, fractures, bone pain, and sometimes tumoral calcifications; thus, they were erroneously diagnosed as having secondary HPTH.[224] These patients may also have abnormal skeletal surveys suggestive of secondary HPTH that actually represent old erosions that were not mineralized as Al toxicity developed. Normal or elevated plasma alkaline phosphatase

levels were reported.[212, 222, 225] These differences may be related to the country of origin or the source of Al. Thus, plasma alkaline phosphatase levels are usually lower when the source of Al is parenteral intoxication[226] and are usually high when the source is intestinal absorption of Al-containing P binders.[212, 222, 225] Serum levels of calcitriol are low, as expected in end-stage renal disease. Serum levels of PTH are often lower than usual for dialysis patients[212, 222] and fail to increase normally after the induction of hypocalcemia.[227, 228] Serum PTH levels are low because of Al accumulation in the parathyroid gland, or the increase in blood $Ca^{2+}$ concentration caused by an effect of Al on bone or $Ca^{2+}$-binding to serum proteins, or a combination of these effects. Shown in Table 51–4 are the features that can help distinguish patients with Al-related bone disease from those with secondary HPTH.

The parathyroid glands can accumulate Al preferentially compared with other tissues.[229] Al, in vitro, can inhibit PTH release by parathyroid cells and this effect is dose related.[230] It is possible that Al itself inhibits PTH release, thereby lowering bone turnover and rendering the bone more susceptible to osteomalacia.[231]

Al-related bone disease may appear after parathyroid surgery and after high PTH levels are reduced by treatment with vitamin D sterols.[232–234] Bone surface Al deposits often increase after PTX,[233] and the decrease in PTH levels predisposes to the appearance of osteomalacia. There is clinical and experimental evidence suggesting that high PTH levels may "protect" against Al-induced osteomalacia. Thus, in dialysis units with a high dialysate Al content, patients with severe osteitis fibrosa and high PTH levels rarely developed osteomalacia.[235] We have noted that, in the azotemic rat, high PTH levels appeared to protect against the development of low-turnover Al bone disease and that secondary HPTH changed the histologic expression of Al-related bone disease.[236] Conversely, in Al-loaded uremic animals bone is substantially less responsive to PTH than that of uremic animals not given Al.[237, 238] We have also noted that the administration of PTH increases osteoblasts and osteoblast surface even in the presence of Al, but mineralization of osteoid was not improved.[239] These results suggest the presence of a bidirectional relationship between Al and PTH.

Also, the pattern of localization of Al in osteitis fibrosa may differ from that observed in osteomalacia. In the former, the Al is diffusely distributed in bone; in the latter, it is localized at the bone surface.[214] However, Al-related bone disease may occasionally occur in patients with markedly elevated serum PTH levels.[225] Also, the clinical and histologic features of Al-related osteomalacia can improve substantially when only modest amounts of Al are removed after infusions of deferoxamine and with only small increments in serum PTH levels.[240] Removal of accumulated Al from dialysis patients leads to an increase in serum levels of both PTH and calcitriol.[241] Thus, the mechanism whereby PTH modifies the features of Al-related bone disease remains unclear, but it is likely that if bone turnover is reduced because of a decrease in PTH, Al may be redistributed in the bone predominantly in the mineralization front, leading to abnormal bone matrix synthesis and mineralization.

Several experiments in animals have shown that paren-

**TABLE 51–4. Features That Can Help Distinguish Patients with Aluminum-Related Bone Disease from Those with Hyperparathyroid Bone Disease**

| Feature | Hyperparathyroid Bone Disease | Aluminum-Related Bone Disease |
|---|---|---|
| Fractures | Not characteristic | Common |
| Proximal muscle weakness | Can occur | Common |
| Periarthritis | Occurs | Not characteristic |
| Tendon rupture | Occurs | Not characteristic |
| Extraskeletal calcifications | Common | Not characteristic |
| Serum $Ca^{2+}$ | Low to high; often > 10.0 mg/dL | Low to high; often > 10.5 mg/dL |
| Serum P | Variable; often > 6.5 mg/dL | Variable; often < 5.5 mg/dL |
| Alkaline phosphatase | 80%–800% of normal | 30%–300% of normal |
| Serum PTH | | |
|   Intact or N assay | >3–4 times normal* | <4–5 times normal* |
|   Midregion assay | >15–20 times normal* | <40–60 times normal* |
| Plasma Al† | Rarely > 150 μg/L; often < 90 μg/L | Generally > 75 μg/L; rarely < 40 μg/L |
| Increment of plasma Al after deferoxamine† | Rarely > 350 μg/L; often < 100 μg/L | Generally > 180 μg/L; rarely < 90 μg/L |
| Microcytic anemia | Unusual | Common in epidemics (dialysate Al), rare in endemic cases (oral Al) |
| Risk factors | Younger age, noncompliance | Prior PTX, diabetes mellitus, earlier kidney transplant, earlier binephrectomy |

*Increment above PTH range for normal subjects.
†After exposure to Al is withdrawn (stopping Al-containing drugs and eliminating dialysate Al), values are often lower.
Modified from Crooks PW, Coburn JW: Management of bone disease in the dialysis patient. Blood Purif 3:27–41, 1985. S Karger AG, Basel, publisher.

teral Al loading can impair bone formation and produce osteomalacia. Ellis and associates[210] first reported that parenteral injections of Al inhibited mineralization in the epiphyseal cartilage of rats. Typical lesions of osteomalacia in trabecular bone of rats, dogs, and pigs have been induced after parenteral Al.[242–245] It has also been shown that a reduction of renal function can increase the susceptibility to osteomalacia, because the kidney is the major route of Al excretion.[242, 244] In addition, low-bone-turnover disease and bone Al deposits have been observed in patients with normal renal function who received long-term parenteral nutrition solutions containing Al-contaminated casein hydrolysate.[246, 247]

The view that Al itself is toxic to bone has been challenged.[248, 249] Quarles and colleagues[248] observed Al deposits at the mineralization front in vitamin D–deficient dogs; however, they suggested that the deposits may not be pathogenic but rather may represent an epiphenomenon related to the osteomalacic state. In these dogs, the administration of Al led to its deposition at the mineralization front, but when the animals were treated with vitamin D the skeletal abnormalities reversed despite continued administration of Al, albeit at a lower dose. However, it is worth emphasizing that the osteomalacia of vitamin D deficiency with normal renal function may differ from that occurring in either Al-loaded animals or dialysis patients with Al-related bone disease. Other studies by the same authors have shown that low-dose Al may stimulate osteogenesis in normal beagles.[249] Nevertheless, the importance of such observations and the findings observed in patients with Al intoxication is unclear.

The mechanism whereby Al produces its effect on bone is uncertain. The finding of Al along the mineralization front has led to the view that Al interferes with bone mineralization[213, 214, 250]; it inhibits mineralization even when osteoblasts are not decreased.[239] Al added in vitro can both

prevent the generation of hydroxyapatite crystals and retard their growth.[251] Others suggested that aluminum citrate inhibits crystal formation.[252] Conversely, the presence of Al staining on the cement lines of bone indicates that mineralization has occurred over sites with earlier deposition of Al.[213] As stated before, osteomalacia caused by vitamin D deficiency and bone Al deposits can be healed by administering vitamin D, indicating that Al deposition at the mineralization front per se does not necessarily impair mineralization.[248] Other observations indicate that Al can inhibit the activity of osteoblasts,[253] and inclusion bodies containing Al have been noted within active osteoblasts.[211] Al may also directly inhibit PTH secretion[228, 230] and can reduce the synthesis of calcitriol.[243] Both features may contribute to abnormal mineralization. These possible pathogenic mechanisms of impaired mineralization or reduced osteoblast function are not mutually exclusive. Inhibition of the osteoblast may be a first step that reduces matrix synthesis; it may be followed by inhibition of crystal growth and mineralization as increased amounts of Al are localized at the mineralization front. Also, Al may be more toxic when PTH levels are low and osteoblasts are inactive or absent.

What are the sources of Al intoxication in patients with CRF? Although Al is ubiquous in nature, the Al concentration is low in biologic systems[254] because Al does not cross the skin and only small amounts are absorbed through the gastrointestinal tract.[255] The first cases of Al-induced osteomalacia occurred in dialysis units using water with Al concentrations above 100 μg/L[206]; however, a high incidence of bone disease has occurred in units using a dialysate Al concentration near 50 μg/L.[256] Because 80% to 95% of Al in plasma is bound to transferrin[257] and albumin,[258] Al is transferred into the patient from the dialysate when the dialysate Al concentration exceeds the level of ultrafilterable Al in blood. Al may also come from other sources: the cartridges used in the past for the regeneration of dialysate (sorbent system) released Al into dialysate[259]; occasionally, preparations of peritoneal dialysate have had high concentrations of Al.[260] Sorbent cartridges currently in use have proved to be safe and have not added Al to the dialysate, with either acetate[261] or $HCO_3^-$ [262] as dialysis buffer. Similarly, samples of peritoneal dialysate have been shown to be low in Al content (<7 μg/L). On the basis of the available evidence, we recommend that dialysate Al levels be lower than 10 μg/L and preferably below 5 μg/L. Significant amounts of Al have also been noted in albumin solutions[263] and in certain other constituents of parenteral solutions,[264] including vesical irrigations with alum.[265, 266] As mentioned earlier, if the parenteral load of Al is high enough, osteomalacia can develop even in patients with normal renal function.[246]

Al can accumulate in the body by not only the parenteral but also the oral route. This was first noted by Berlyne and associates,[267] but the evidence was largely ignored. Studies of normal subjects ingesting aluminum hydroxide indicate that small amounts of Al are absorbed[255]; because the kidney is the sole route for the excretion of Al, the absorbed Al accumulates in patients with CRF. The Al-related bone disease in uremic patients who have never undergone dialysis but who ingest aluminum hydroxide clearly indicates that Al toxicity can result from an accumulated oral source.[268–270] Moreover, close correlation has been noted between plasma Al concentration, which indicates recent Al loading,[271] and the amount of ingested Al-containing P binders.[272, 273] Finally, after the Al-containing P binders were discontinued for dialysis patients, plasma Al levels fell substantially, which provided additional evidence for the contribution from an oral source.[273–275] Al toxicity and intestinal absorption can occur also with the ingestion of sucralfate.[276, 277] Evidence of brain accumulation of Al was noted in premature infants who had ingested a low-protein, low-phosphate formula that is often recommended for infants with CRF,[278] although a subsequent prospective study failed to find any evidence of Al accumulation in 14 children who ingested this formula for up to 18 months.[279]

The knowledge that oral absorption of Al is a major factor leading to Al accumulation in CRF has led to a consideration of the factors that augment its intestinal uptake. Many CRF patients can ingest Al gels for long periods with little accumulation, whereas others develop Al overload within a few months after they are given large doses of Al gels. The presence of uremia increases Al absorption,[280] although the mechanism for this effect is uncertain. Both PTH and calcitriol have been implicated as causing an increase in the intestinal absorption of Al[281, 282]; however, in other studies their effects were small or could not be detected.[283] As mentioned earlier, patients with high PTH levels seem to be protected from the toxic effects of Al.[234] The ingestion of Al compounds in conjunction with sodium citrate or citric acid—present in common drinks such as orange juice—may significantly enhance Al absorption.[284, 285] Severe and fatal Al toxic reactions have developed before dialysis in patients receiving Al gels and citric acid plus sodium citrate (Shohl solution) to correct acidosis.[286, 287] Marked enhancement of Al absorption has also been shown during ingestion of calcium citrate[288] and certain over-the-counter compounds (e.g., Alka-Seltzer),

which contain citrate and can thus augment Al absorption.[289, 290] All these compounds should be used with caution if not completely avoided in patients with CRF who are ingesting Al gels. The solubility of Al compounds increases substantially as the pH falls, indicating that gastric pH may modify Al absorption substantially. Thus, ranitidine, a histamine $H_2$-receptor inhibitor, has been suggested to reduce Al toxicity in patients with CRF.[291]

Iron stores may also modify Al kinetics because Al and iron share common pathways for intestinal absorption, serum transport, and cellular uptake. Thus, in rats with normal renal function or CRF, short- or long-term oral Al administration is followed by a greater increase in serum, urinary, and brain Al in iron-depleted animals.[292] Also, the degree of iron transferrin saturation may regulate the transport of Al by transferrin as well as cellular uptake.[219, 293] Thus, iron deficiency may increase the risk of Al toxicity, and appropriate iron stores seem to offer some protection against Al toxicity.[219, 294] Al overload may interfere with iron absorption[219] and be a causal factor in iron-resistant anemia[295] and resistance to erythropoietin.[296] The state of iron stores should also be considered when interpreting the deferoxamine test to diagnose Al overload, as discussed later.[219, 297, 298]

Finally, certain host factors, mostly associated with low bone remodeling and/or low PTH, may make certain individuals susceptible to the toxic effects of Al. These include 1) prior PTX,[232–234] 2) glucocorticoid treatment for a rejected renal transplant,[225] 3) diabetes mellitus,[299–301] 4) decreasing PTH after calcitriol therapy,[302] and 5) bilateral nephrectomy.[225]

## LOW SERUM PTH, "IDIOPATHIC" ADYNAMIC BONE DISEASE

ABD has been described in uremic patients receiving chronic dialysis.[303, 304] This entity has been termed "aplastic"[305] or "adynamic" bone disease,[306] but because the main diagnostic criterion is an abnormally low bone formation rate, the term adynamic is preferred. Subsequently, it has been noted with increasing frequency in dialysis patients.[307–309] It was reported that 60% of patients undergoing peritoneal dialysis and 36% of hemodialysis patients were found to have ABD.[308] Although this unusually high prevalence of the disease may be due to the inclusion of idiopathic and secondary forms of ABD and a greater awareness of the disease, specific regional and local factors may also play a role. The afflicted patients have a low bone formation rate without osteoid accumulation.[309, 310] This latter finding is a major feature that distinguishes this entity from osteomalacia. However, the diagnostic criteria of ABD may vary among different investigators and this could partially account for the observed differences in the prevalence of ABD. In addition to the osteoid surface, decreased osteoblast number and osteoblastic surfaces are also noted; osteoclast number and osteoclastic surfaces are usually normal or low.[311, 312]

In some patients, serial bone biopsy specimens have shown the evolution from an aplastic state to osteomalacia, suggesting that the aplastic lesion may be a precursor of more typical osteomalacia. Conversion of the aplastic lesion to true osteomalacia suggests that the earliest abnormality may be inhibition of osteoid synthesis (a cellular insufficiency to form bone matrix) and that this is impaired to a greater extent than bone mineralization.[311, 312]

In previous observations, patients with histologic features of ABD were noted to have significant Al deposits and were thought to have Al-related bone disease. Thus, reduced bone mineralization without wide osteoid was observed in rats after short-term, high-dose Al loading.[313] Also, administration of low-dose Al to dogs resulted in a decreased bone formation rate without changes in mineralization.[314] For some investigators, the main etiologic difference between Al-induced osteomalacia and ABD is the presence of a smaller Al burden in ABD as reflected by a lesser increase in plasma Al after a deferoxamine test. Thus, ABD has been described mainly in patients with relatively low Al overload; these patients were dialyzed with a dialysate not contaminated with Al and the main Al source was the ingestion of Al-containing P binders.[315, 316] However, as discussed later, Al is not the only cause of ABD.

An association among osteomalacia, ABD, and the presence of low serum PTH was noted a decade ago.[307, 317] A smaller Al overload was observed in ABD by Andress and colleagues.[315] However, we have shown experimental data suggesting an important role of PTH in favoring osteomalacia rather than ABD.[318] We noted in uremic parathyroidectomized rats that Al administration produced a bone lesion resembling that of ABD; the osteoid volume was higher when the parathyroid glands were present than when they were absent despite similar Al exposure. Thus, a potential contribution of low serum PTH values to an excessive reduction in bone turnover and the development of ABD has been raised.[306, 309]

A growing fraction of patients with ABD have been identified without Al deposits.[308–310, 312, 319] Unlike that of Al bone disease, its incidence seems to be increasing, and it is more frequently observed in the absence of Al accumulation.[309] Furthermore, no difference in the incidence of ABD has been observed in the presence or absence of Al deposits.[308] Thus, factors other than Al have to be considered, including age,[309, 312] hypothyroidism,[320] corticosteroid treatment and Cushing syndrome,[321] fluoride at toxic doses,[322] iron,[323, 324] hypophosphatemia,[325] and acidosis.[326] Also, diabetic patients receiving chronic hemodialysis have been shown to have lower plasma PTH concentrations and lower bone formation and resorption than their matched nondiabetic control subjects,[300, 327–330] and diminished parathyroid gland responsiveness to an acute hypocalcemic challenge.[331] In fact, diabetes has been associated with low PTH secretion and osteopenia even in the absence of CRF.[332–334] Sugimoto and co-workers[335] demonstrated in an in vitro model that glucose and insulin independently modulate PTH release. Moreover, when CRF is present the associated low bone formation may be the cause or the consequence of the higher bone accumulation of Al observed in diabetic patients.[299, 301] ABD has also been described without the presence of any of the foregoing factors in both children[336] and adults.[309, 310]

The real incidence of ABD is not known. The percentage of afflicted patients has varied from 10% to as high as 48% among those treated with continuous ambulatory peritoneal dialysis (CAPD); it has also been observed in 17% of hemodialysis patients.[337] Thus, ABD seems to be more common in patients treated with CAPD.[308, 309, 312, 338] The continuous peritoneal exposure to a high $Ca^{2+}$ concentration in the dialysate increases serum $Ca^{2+}$,[339, 340] which may inhibit PTH secretion, leading to a decrease in bone formation rate. This hypothesis, although plausible, is not proved, because older patients and a higher prevalence of diabetic patients are commonly encountered among those treated with CAPD. However, a decrease in the peritoneal dialysate $Ca^{2+}$ concentration to 2.0 mEq/L results in increased serum PTH, suggesting that the "high" dialysate $Ca^{2+}$ contributes to the suppressed PTH levels.[309]

Ingestion of large doses of calcium carbonate or acetate as a P binder and excessive parathyroid suppression with calcitriol may also be contributing factors in the development of ABD.[308, 309, 311] ABD has also been associated with overtreatment with vitamin D derivatives even in predialysis patients.[302, 310] Serum intact PTH levels have ranged from normal to three times the upper limit of normal in patients with ABD.[308–310, 341] Several authors[174, 309, 342, 343] have observed that a normal bone formation rate in uremia corresponded to plasma intact PTH levels between 1.5 and 3 times the upper limit of normal, suggesting that mild secondary HPTH may be necessary to maintain a normal bone formation rate. Until more is known about the natural history of ABD, it would seem prudent not to oversuppress intact PTH levels in dialysis patients to values lower than 1.5 times the upper limit of normal.

Biochemically, ABD is characterized by normal or low alkaline phosphatase and osteocalcin. Measurement of bone alkaline phosphatase may be also useful because levels below 20 U/L have been shown to have a sensitivity of 66% and a specificity of 86% in the diagnosis of ABD.[344] Serum PTH levels are often above the normal range[309, 316, 345] but lower than those observed in patients with osteitis fibrosa. More than 50% of patients with biopsy-proven ABD may have normal intact PTH levels.[341] Intact PTH levels greater than 200 pg/mL yield a positive predictive value of 88% for the diagnosis of mild and severe secondary HPTH, and a value below 65 pg/mL had a positive predictive value of 78% for ABD.[346] Plasma $Ca^{2+}$ concentration tends to be high and/or increase rapidly when oral $Ca^{2+}$, calcitriol, or high dialysate $Ca^{2+}$ concentrations are used.[308, 309, 319]

Although Al-related ABD may be a symptomatic disease with afflicted patients having more frequent bone pain, fractures, and decreased bone density, patients with idiopathic ABD are often asymptomatic and without radiologic abnormalities at the time of diagnosis. Thus, idiopathic ABD at present is a histologic finding rather than a disease. Moreover, no bone-fracturing disease has been described in either primary or secondary hypoparathyroidism. Finally, in dialysis patients, ABD may reverse to a hyperparathyroid state; persistence of this bone lesion is more likely after kidney transplantation because of the suppressive effect of corticoids on bone.

## REDUCED PLASMA PHOSPHORUS LEVELS

A low plasma P concentration may be the cause of low bone turnover.[325] However, severe hypophosphatemia is rare in uremic patients. As early as 1966, Stanbury and Lumb[347] observed an association between the presence of osteomalacia and a low plasma $Ca^{2+} \times P$ product in patients with moderate to advanced CRF. In the United Kingdom, Kanis and colleagues[348] noted an inverse relationship between the number of osteoid lamellae, an index of osteomalacia, and the predialysis plasma P levels in a large group of hemodialysis patients (Fig. 51–19). Evidence for a mineralization defect was common in patients whose mean plasma P concentration was below the limit of normality. Because coexisting nutritional vitamin D deficiency could also be present, it is possible that the development of osteomalacia may require both a vitamin D deficiency and hypophosphatemia.

## ALTERED COLLAGEN SYNTHESIS AND MATURATION

Formation of bone requires both synthesis and maturation of collagen. Without maturation of collagen and the development of specific cross-linkages between collagen molecules, mineral deposition may not proceed normally. There is evidence of abnormal collagen synthesis and maturation in uremia; rats with experimental uremia fail to develop mature, insoluble collagen and exhibit a preponderance of immature and soluble collagen that fails to mineralize normally.[195] The underlying mechanism is unknown, but similarities exist between the abnormalities of collagen maturation observed in uremia and those noted in vitamin D deficiency.[349, 350] Russell and Avioli[351] found that treatment of uremic animals with 25(OH)D largely restored

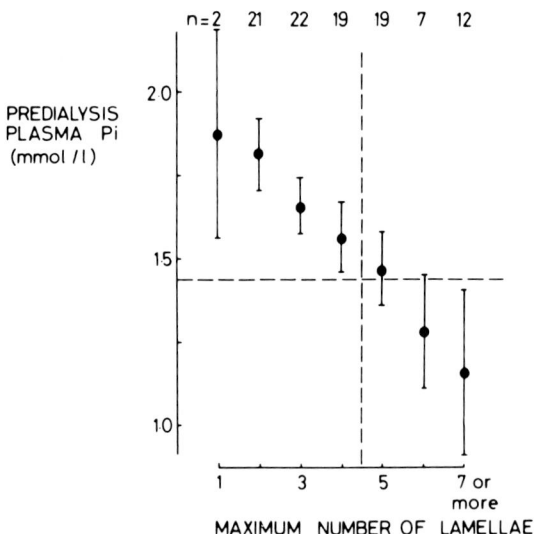

**Figure 51–19.** Relationship between mean predialysis plasma phosphorus (Pi) level and the maximal number of lamellae seen on bone biopsy (an index of osteomalacia) in a large number of patients treated with regular hemodialysis. Osteomalacia (five or more lamellae) was uncommon in patients with high plasma P levels, whereas there was evidence of defective mineralization in many patients whose plasma P levels were below the upper limits of normal (*horizontal dashed line*). (From Kanis JA, Adams ND, Earnshaw M: Vitamin D, osteomalacia and chronic renal failure. *In* Norman AW, Schaefer K, Coburn JW, et al [eds]: Vitamin D: Biochemical, Chemical and Clinical Aspects Related to Calcium Metabolism. Walter de Gruyter, Berlin, 1977, p 671.)

collagen maturation toward normal, providing additional evidence that altered vitamin D metabolism plays a role in defective collagen maturation. Whether these mechanisms are affected in uremic patients remains to be determined.

## MATURATION OF BONE CRYSTALS

Formation of mineralized bone involves the initial precipitation of amorphous calcium phosphate and its subsequent transformation into crystalline hydroxyapatite. This transformation and maturation of bone are required for the formation of bone of high structural quality. One characteristic of immature bone is the presence of large quantities of amorphous calcium phosphate, and the evaluation of animals with CRF has revealed a correlation between the skeletal content of amorphous calcium phosphate and the quantity of immature, soluble collagen.[352]

The reason for the delay in maturation of bone mineral in uremia is uncertain; several factors may contribute. Thus, an increased bone $Mg^{2+}$ content, correlated with serum $Mg^{2+}$ levels[353, 354]; an elevated pyrophosphate content,[355] which may impair the normal conversion of amorphous calcium phosphate to crystalline apatite[356]; and/or a diminished carbonate content may be causative factors.[354, 357] It has been suggested that pyrophosphate may exist in the form of a magnesium salt and hence may be less susceptible to degradation by naturally occurring pyrophosphatases[355] or may slow the normal conversion of amorphous calcium phosphate to crystalline hydroxyapatite.[356] In support of a role of $Mg^{2+}$ is the observation that the rate of bone crystal maturation can be modified by altering the intake of $Mg^{2+}$.[358] However, other authors observed that bone $Mg^{2+}$ content positively correlated with bone $Ca^{2+}$ content and that bone $Mg^{2+}$ did not consistently reflect serum $Mg^{2+}$ levels.[359, 360]

## ROLE OF ACIDOSIS

The contribution of metabolic acidosis to the pathogenesis of mineral abnormalities in patients with CRF has yet to be clarified. A number of metabolic studies of patients with uremia implicate acidosis in leading to negative $Ca^{2+}$ balance and thereby contributing to skeletal disease in CRF. Patients with stable CRF can maintain a stable serum $HCO_3^-$ level despite continued dietary acid loading and reduction in renal acid excretion[361]; this suggests that $H^+$ continues to be buffered by the body, particularly in bone. Litzow and colleagues[362] noted that alkali treatment of azotemic patients with chronic acidosis reduced both urinary and fecal losses of $Ca^{2+}$, causing a zero $Ca^{2+}$ net balance but failing to induce $Ca^{2+}$ retention.

It has also been shown that during acidosis there is a net $Ca^{2+}$ efflux from bone, resulting in a loss of bone carbonated apatite.[363] During both short- and long-term studies, the $Ca^{2+}$ efflux is greater when the medium is acidified by decreasing the concentration of $HCO_3^-$ than when acidosis is induced by increasing the partial pressure of carbon dioxide (a model of respiratory acidosis).[364] Thus, during metabolic acidosis, release of bone mineral was induced in both in vivo[365] and in vitro[366–368] studies. In vitro acidosis produces $Ca^{2+}$ release from bone through both physicochemical and cell-mediated mechanisms.[366, 367] Acidosis has also been shown to stimulate osteoclastic and to inhibit osteoblastic function.[368, 369] Furthermore, metabolic acidosis induces an increase in bone resorption and a decrease in bone formation in parathyroidectomized rats[370]; however, there is more bone buffering during acidosis in animals with intact parathyroid glands than in those with PTX, presumably because of more rapid bone turnover in the former.[371]

Pellegrino and Biltz[372] noted the reduction in carbonate and $Ca^{2+}$ content in uremic bone at autopsy to be proportional to the duration of uremia, and Burnell and colleagues[354] reported no correlation between the degree of acidosis and the quantity of bone carbonate in dialysis patients. They also observed an increase in P content of bone in patients treated with dialysis,[372] but Burnell and colleagues[354] found no change in P content except a decrease in P in patients with marked osteitis fibrosa. Kaye and co-workers[373] observed an increase in P content of bone in association with a decrease in carbonate. On the basis of the reciprocal relationship between changes in P and $HCO_3^-$ content, they suggested that a carbonate-deficient apatite is formed in uremia, where P is substituted by carbonate. The failure of Burnell and co-workers[354] to detect an increase in P despite reduced carbonate content suggests that the loss of carbonate may not require P replacement; the data may also reflect a different degree of uremia and duration of dialysis treatment in the patients studied. The role of bone in the regulation of acid-base status is discussed extensively in an excellent editorial review.[374]

Certain observations suggest only a minor role of acidosis in leading to bone disease in uremia. Alkali therapy of patients suffering from overt renal osteodystrophy failed to produce healing of the bone lesion.[2, 375] Also, pharmacologic doses of vitamin D led to healing even in the presence of acidosis.[376] Moreover, long-term acid feeding of animals produced skeletal lesions similar to osteoporosis[377] or osteomalacia[378] rather than osteitis fibrosa. However, a combination of uremia and acidosis may have effects different from those of acidosis per se. The situation may be more complex in dialysis patients, because restoration of body and bone buffer may be incomplete with the usual dialysate concentration of acetate as a buffer. As mentioned earlier, bone carbonate content is generally reduced and the carbonate in bone may affect crystal growth and maturation, providing a mechanism whereby acidosis indirectly affects the skeleton.[354]

In normal individuals with metabolic acidosis there is evidence of increased bone resorption[379] but no evidence of increased PTH secretion.[379–381] Lefebvre and colleagues,[326] in a prospective study done to evaluate the role of acidosis in dialysis patients, noted that lower doses of a vitamin D sterol were required to maintain normal serum $Ca^{2+}$ levels in patients whose mild metabolic acidosis was corrected. In this study, a control group of dialysis patients with a dialysate $HCO_3^-$ of 33 mEq/L was followed and compared with an "acidosis-correlated" group, with dialysate $HCO_3^-$ increased by 7 to 15 mEq/L to maintain the predialysis plasma $HCO_3^-$ level at 24 mEq/L. In the control group, midregion PTH rose progressively, but the PTH values were stable in the corrected group. Bone biopsies done before the study and after 18 months revealed a progressive

increase of osteoid and osteoblast surface in the control patients, but these alterations did not worsen in the acidosis-corrected group. In patients who entered the study with an elevated bone formation rate, the basal high plasma osteocalcin levels increased further in the control group but were stable in the acidosis-corrected group. Thus, there was evidence of progressive secondary HPTH in the group with a standard dialysate $HCO_3^-$ level, and the disease process was arrested with correction of metabolic acidosis. The investigators suggested that acidosis might enhance bone resorption and thereby release more P into extracellular fluid, with the latter being responsible for the worsening of secondary HPTH.

Krapf and associates[382] have provided new insights in other metabolic pathways through which chronic metabolic acidosis can affect divalent ion metabolism. They observed that metabolic acidosis results in graded increases in serum calcitriol by stimulating its production rate in humans. This increased production rate was explained by acidosis-induced hypophosphatemia, which resulted, in part, from decreased tubule P reabsorption. These observations apparently contradict previous observations of metabolic acidosis inducing decreases in calcitriol; however, in the latter studies an increase in plasma $Ca^{2+}$ concentration was usually present.[383–385] Krapf and co-workers[382] have also shown that intact PTH did not change in mild metabolic acidosis (mean $HCO_3^-$ 20.8 ± 0.4 mEq/L) or even decreased in more severe acidosis (mean $HCO_3^-$ 16.4 ± 4); they suggested that this decrease could be due to the induced hypophosphatemia and/or increased serum calcitriol concentrations observed especially in that range of metabolic acidosis.

Increased,[386] unchanged,[380] or decreased[379] serum PTH has been reported in association with chronic metabolic acidosis. Although different assays could be responsible for these differences, it was also observed that elevated levels of PTH do not significantly correlate with low plasma $HCO_3^-$ concentrations.

Finally, we do not know how the effects of metabolic acidosis that have been induced in normal individuals translate to the more complex context of the patient with CRF, with a limited ability to excrete P and synthesize calcitriol. Further studies are needed to address the effect of mild metabolic acidosis on divalent ion metabolism and to clarify how acidosis can modify the course of the various types of uremic bone disease.

## BIOCHEMICAL FEATURES

Despite evidence that pathophysiologic alterations in divalent ion metabolism develop early in the course of CRF, the related signs and symptoms generally appear only in patients with advanced and/or prolonged uremia. Most often, they develop while patients are already receiving maintenance dialysis. In part, this may occur because symptoms, such as muscle weakness, are so insidious in their appearance that they are not even noticed by the patient. Moreover, many symptoms are usually attributed to the uremic syndrome per se. In contrast to the late onset of symptoms, a number of biochemical alterations appear earlier in the course of progressive CRF; thus, the initial evaluation of altered divalent ion homeostasis and renal osteo-dystrophy can often be made from the measurement of biochemical parameters long before symptoms develop. Hence, these biochemical parameters are reviewed first and the clinical signs and symptoms are considered thereafter.

## Serum Phosphorus Levels

Serum P levels are usually slightly lower than normal[15, 97] or normal in early stages of CRF.[45, 387] Hyperphosphatemia is generally absent until renal function falls to 20% to 30% of normal.[45, 388] However, in patients with creatinine clearances below 20 mL/min, although hyperphosphatemia is common, serum P levels show wide variation, ranging from 2.5 to 15 mg/dL, and are mainly affected by dietary P intake.

Dietary P is absorbed along the entire intestinal tract both by passive diffusion through the paracellular route—usually the main pathway—and by active transcellular absorption.[389, 390] Passive P absorption is not saturable and increases linearly with intake.[391] Some factors that can affect the serum P levels in patients with renal insufficiency are shown in Table 51–2. Thus, dietary P intake and fraction of P absorbed from the intestinal tract have an important effect on blood P levels, particularly in advanced CRF. The relationship between daily net absorption of P and dietary P intake in both patients with advanced CRF and normal subjects is shown in Figure 51–20. Many observations of net absorption of P in patients with CRF lie below the normal limits. The factors responsible for this mildly impaired P absorption include altered calcitriol metabolism and increased endogenous fecal P losses. Although it was thought that the latter may arise because of hyperphospha-temia, Kopple and Coburn[81] found no relationship between fecal P excretion and serum P levels; such observations suggest that endogenous fecal losses of P are so small in relation to total fecal P that the total loss is not modified by changes in the serum P levels. Calcitriol stimulates active P absorption in the intestine[392]; thus, impaired absorption of P in uremia may arise from the same abnormality that impairs $Ca^{2+}$ absorption. However, as shown in Figure 51–

20, net intestinal absorption of P is minimally reduced in advanced CRF, as determined by metabolic balance studies and studies using radiophosphate,[7, 42, 375, 393] rendering the patient with markedly decreased renal function unprotected against the development of hyperphosphatemia.

The administration of vitamin D derivatives and the status of body stores of vitamin D (i.e., vitamin D deficiency) can also affect serum P levels. Vitamin D derivatives can change serum P directly by influencing P homeostasis or indirectly through PTH. Because a major effect of calcitriol on P homeostasis is to enhance intestinal P absorption,[375, 389, 392, 394] serum P may increase after administration of calcitriol, especially in noncompliant patients with an unrestricted P diet.[123] Administration of calcitriol often suppresses secondary HPTH in uremic patients; this may lead to reduced bone resorption with increased net deposition of $Ca^{2+}$ and P in bone. Thus, serum P levels sometimes decrease and the need for P binders is less during the first 2 to 3 months of treatment with calcitriol; later, when the period of rapid skeletal mineralization is complete, serum P may increase.[395] However, increased serum P levels after calcitriol have also been reported[396]; differences in the dietary intake of P and calcitriol dosages could account for these differences. Treatment of osteomalacia is sometimes also associated with a transient fall in serum P, presumably because bone formation and the deposition of $Ca^{2+}$ and P in the skeleton are increased out of proportion to the rate of bone resorption. Finally, vitamin D may affect serum P by enhancing the intracellular flux of inorganic P; thus, in vitamin D–deficient animals the administration of either vitamin D or 25(OH)D leads to movement of P into cells.[397] Whether this effect is important in uremic patients is unknown.

Compliant patients, not taking vitamin D derivatives, can also have high P levels because of increased bone resorption in severe secondary HPTH. Thus, serum P levels are often higher in patients with overt secondary HPTH.[212, 398] Similarly, not only may patients with severe secondary HPTH be resistant to PTH inhibition by oral calcitriol, but it may also further increase P absorption and aggravate the hyperphosphatemia, further aggravating secondary HPTH.

The ingestion of $PO_4^{3-}$-binding compounds and the intake of large amounts of supplemental $Ca^{2+}$ can also lead

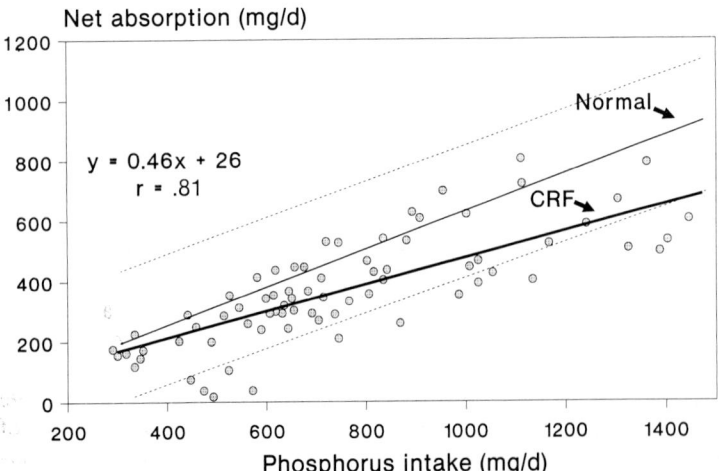

**Figure 51–20.** Relationship between net absorption of P and dietary P in patients with advanced renal failure. Solid regression line for normal subjects adapted from Stanbury and colleagues.[916] Dashed lines indicate the 95% confidence limits for data in normal subjects. Solid heavy line indicates the regression line of data for patients with CRF. (From Kopple JD, Coburn JW: Metabolic studies of low protein diets in uremia. II. Calcium, phosphorus and magnesium. Medicine [Baltimore] 52[6]:597–607, 1973.)

to changes in serum P concentration. Serum P may be influenced by the balance between synthesis and degradation of body proteins. Thus, marked hyperphosphatemia may appear during hypercatabolic states. Such an effect is magnified in a patient with markedly decreased renal function; thus, even a mild infection may be associated with disproportionate increases in serum urea nitrogen and P levels. Alternatively, periods of increased protein anabolism may be associated with the development of hypophosphatemia caused by intracellular shift of P. Hypophosphatemia may also occur with refeeding after starvation or protein depletion. Because dietary P is linked to the dietary protein content, diets markedly restricted in proteins and not supplemented with essential amino acids may be associated with the appearance of marked hypophosphatemia.[399] However, uremic patients ingesting a natural protein-restricted diet rarely develop hypophosphatemia, despite the limitation of P intake to 300 to 400 mg/d.[81] Thus, the ingestion of essential amino acids may stimulate protein anabolism to a greater extent than that observed in patients receiving natural protein-restricted diets; this may usually result in more significant hypophosphatemia. Infusion of amino acids and hypertonic glucose for total parenteral nutrition may also lead to substantial hypophosphatemia unless P is added to the parenteral solution.

Few uremic or dialysis patients exhibit normal or slightly low levels of plasma P although they ingest a normal diet and are not taking P binders.[400] The reason for this is uncertain; some patients may have a greater degree of malabsorption of P than others.[401] As osteomalacia may be more common in uremic patients ingesting a low-P diet[402] serum P levels must be monitored during P (or protein) restriction to avoid hypophosphatemia. Patients with stable CRF and those undergoing dialysis may be in a negative P balance and yet exhibit modest hyperphosphatemia.[81] This negative balance does not correlate with the balance of either nitrogen or $Ca^{2+}$, suggesting that excess P is deposited in soft tissues.[81] Body composition data from neutron activation studies support this view.[403, 404] Whether changes in acid-base status have significant effects on serum P level in uremic patients is unknown.

## Serum Calcium Levels

### HYPOCALCEMIA

A detectable fall in total serum $Ca^{2+}$ concentration occurs, but not invariably, in patients with advanced CRF. The factors underlying the hypocalcemia have already been discussed as they are of importance in the genesis of secondary HPTH. They may include decreased intestinal $Ca^{2+}$ absorption, as a result of a reduced calcitriol synthesis or resistance to its action, hyperphosphatemia, and a decreased calcemic response to PTH.

Although both the mean total serum calcium level and the $Ca^{2+}$ level are significantly lower in patients with advanced CRF (creatinine clearance 5 to 20 mL/min) than in normal subjects, total serum calcium levels were below the lower limits of normal in only 40% of uremic patients.[388] Moreover, levels below 7.5 mg/dL are noted infrequently.

The complexed calcium fraction is increased in advanced uremia because of increased binding of $Ca^{2+}$ to various anions.[405] If the fraction of complexed calcium increases substantially, the level of blood $Ca^{2+}$ may be low despite a normal total serum calcium level. A similar phenomenon may occur immediately after hemodialysis as hemoconcentration increases the protein-bound $Ca^{2+}$ component.[406] On the other hand, acidosis can decrease the degree of protein binding, and marked acidosis—present in some uremic patients—may induce this effect in vivo.

Low levels of total calcium and $Ca^{2+}$ are observed in uremic patients; however, the range of individual values is wide. Initiation of maintenance hemodialysis is often associated with an increase in total serum $Ca^{2+}$ concentration toward normal.[399, 407] This increase in serum $Ca^{2+}$ has been observed despite persistent hyperphosphatemia and during the use of a dialysate $Ca^{2+}$ of 2.5 mEq/L.[399] Such an observation, made several years ago when the control of hyperphosphatemia was poor, suggests the existence of some unknown factor, related to uremia and dialysis, that promotes correction of hypocalcemia. It may also be due to an improvement in the calcemic action of PTH, because intestinal absorption of $Ca^{2+}$ is either unchanged or only slightly improved in regular hemodialysis.[97, 408–410] When dialysis is carried out with more modern techniques and with the current therapeutic regimens to control renal osteodystrophy, the incidence of hypocalcemia is low and hypercalcemia becomes a more common problem.

### HYPERCALCEMIA

Hypercalcemia also occurs in patients with CRF. Measurement of $Ca^{2+}$ increases the sensitivity for recognizing hypercalcemia, particularly in patients undergoing peritoneal dialysis,[340] because their serum albumin levels are often below normal and lower than those observed in hemodialysis patients.

In general, it is known that the defect in intestinal $Ca^{2+}$ absorption can be surmounted with an increase in calcium intake or with calcitriol supplementation. The former increases $Ca^{2+}$ absorption, probably through simple ionic diffusion, a process not considered to be affected by uremia; the latter increases the carrier-mediated transport of $Ca^{2+}$ across the intestinal mucosa.

The recognized causes of hypercalcemia in patients with CRF are listed in Table 51–5. They must always be carefully delineated; in particular, Al toxicity and in general low-bone-turnover states should be distinguished from overt secondary HPTH, because management is different. Thus, hypercalcemia in patients with overt secondary HPTH may appear within weeks to months after hemodialysis has been initiated. Such hypercalcemia is usually related to a large mass of parathyroid tissue not inhibited by the presence of high serum $Ca^{2+}$. As mentioned earlier, this condition has also been termed tertiary HPTH. Hypercalcemia may also result from Al accumulation or, in general, a low-bone-turnover state. Moreover, radiographs can show only "osteopenia," although subperiosteal erosions may persist from earlier secondary HPTH that failed to mineralize when PTH synthesis was inhibited by Al accumulation.[411] We have evaluated the mechanism for the hy-

**TABLE 51–5. Conditions Associated with Hypercalcemia in Patients with Renal Failure**

Severe secondary HPTH (tertiary HPTH?)
Al-related bone disease
High dietary calcium uptake
Treatment with vitamin D metabolites
Use of high-$Ca^{2+}$ dialysate (3.5 mEq/L or higher)*
P restriction and hypophosphatemia
Immobilization*
Administration of thiazide diuretics
Use of $Ca^{2+}$ exchange resins
Use of low-protein diets (usually low in P)
Coexistence of other diseases causing hypercalcemia (e.g., multiple myeloma, sarcoidosis, tuberculosis, malignancy)
Recovery phase of acute renal failure
After successful kidney transplantation

*Often in association with the first two items above.

percalcemia of Al-related bone disease; Al increases the protein-bound fraction of calcium and decreases $Ca^{2+}$. This, in turn, mobilizes $Ca^{2+}$ from bone and interstitium into the vascular space, leading to an increase in total calcium concentration.[412] In addition, a low bone formation rate and Al deposition along the mineralization front prevent the absorbed intestinal $Ca^{2+}$ from being incorporated into the bone.

Transient hypercalcemia can develop during therapy with large doses of oral calcium, especially in patients with advanced CRF,[413, 414] in those treated with vitamin D derivatives, after prolonged use of a high dialysate $Ca^{2+}$ concentration (3.0 to 4.0 mEq/L), or because of the combined effect of these therapies. The hypercalcemia associated with low-bone-turnover states may appear or become worse when any of these treatments, even in small doses, is used.[220, 225] Hypercalcemia may occur during treatment with calcium carbonate,[274, 415] calcium acetate,[416] or $Ca^{2+}$-containing ion exchange resins,[417] in association with marked P restriction and hypophosphatemia,[399] immobilization, and thiazide diuretics.[418] Uremic patients may also develop hypercalcemia because of associated illnesses, such as multiple myeloma or malignancy. They may also develop hypercalcemia because of extrarenal synthesis of calcitriol, mostly in granulomatous diseases such as sarcoidosis or tuberculosis.[419, 420] The hypercalcemia is usually prolonged and more marked in uremic patients because the loss of renal function eliminates the body's ability to excrete $Ca^{2+}$ mobilized from bone, absorbed through the intestine, or entering from the dialysate.

## Serum Magnesium Levels

Serum $Mg^{2+}$ levels are commonly elevated in patients with advanced CRF. The homeostasis of $Mg^{2+}$ in CRF has received less attention than that of $Ca^{2+}$ or P. Normally the kidney is the main organ regulating body $Mg^{2+}$; hence, the loss of renal excretory function leads to altered $Mg^{2+}$ homeostasis. Whether intestinal handling of $Mg^{2+}$ may be altered in uremia is controversial. Its net absorption is normal, yet the jejunal and ileal transport of $Mg^{2+}$ has been reported to be reduced in uremic patients, as studied by perfusion of different intestinal segments. Treatment with calcitriol restores the $Mg^{2+}$ transport of a perfused intestine to normal,[421] yet there has been no detectable effect of either calcitriol or $1\alpha(OH)D$ on net intestinal absorption.[42] The reasons for discrepancies between results obtained with intestinal perfusion and those from metabolic balance studies have not been determined. It is possible that $Mg^{2+}$ transport is impaired in one portion of the intestine while it is normal or even increased in others, resulting in normal net $Mg^{2+}$ absorption through the entire gut. In general, in patients with advanced CRF, studies of $Mg^{2+}$ balance suggest that its net absorption is not markedly different from normal,[42] although the intestinal absorption may be modestly decreased.[422] With normal absorption and reduced renal excretion, a tendency to develop hypermagnesemia can be understood.

Serum $Mg^{2+}$ levels are generally normal until the creatinine clearance rate is below 30 mL/min.[388] With further impairment in renal function, a larger number of uremic patients exhibit hypermagnesemia. A small increase in magnesium intake in advanced CRF generally leads to an equal increase in urinary excretion of $Mg^{2+}$, suggesting that $Mg^{2+}$ accumulates slowly.[81] Approximately 20% of $Mg^{2+}$ is bound to albumin, a fraction that is unchanged in CRF despite an increase in total serum $Mg^{2+}$ level.[353, 388] The increase in serum $Mg^{2+}$ levels is associated with an increase in skeletal $Mg^{2+}$ content,[353, 388] and this may have an adverse effect on crystal bone formation[423] and the development of an osteomalacia-like picture.[424] Other authors do not support this view.[359, 360]

In the patient with advanced CRF who is not receiving maintenance dialysis, the major factor that affects serum $Mg^{2+}$ levels is an increase in dietary magnesium intake. With $Mg^{2+}$-containing antacids, cathartics, or enemas, abrupt and marked hypermagnesemia may occur.[425] In uremic patients undergoing dialysis, the dialysate $Mg^{2+}$ concentration is a major factor influencing serum $Mg^{2+}$. Most dialysis centers have used 1.5 mEq/L, a level similar to the non–protein-bound or diffusible $Mg^{2+}$ level in normal serum. With the use of this concentration, mildly elevated blood $Mg^{2+}$ levels of 2.5 to 4.0 mEq/L are common.[388] The use of dialysate containing 0.5 to 0.8 mEq/L results in serum $Mg^{2+}$ concentrations in the upper range of normal or only slightly elevated in most dialysis patients.[426] Centers using magnesium-containing calcium salts as P binders should monitor serum $Mg^{2+}$ frequently and/or use a dialysate with low or no $Mg^{2+}$ to avoid hypermagnesemia.[427, 428]

The clinical consequences of hypermagnesemia and increased skeletal content of this cation in uremia are not known. Most uremic patients exhibit no known sequelae of the moderate hypermagnesemia, although the hypothermia of uremia has been attributed, in part, to $Mg^{2+}$ retention.[429] When the serum $Mg^{2+}$ concentration is increased to levels above 3.5 to 5.0 mEq/L, flushing and burning of the skin may occur. Such symptoms have developed when the water purification system used for preparing dialysate fails.[430] It has also been shown that an abrupt and marked elevation of serum $Mg^{2+}$ can suppress the secretion of PTH.[431, 432] However, no data are available to suggest that long-standing hypermagnesemia can reduce PTH secretion; moreover, any suppressive effect of hypermagnesemia on PTH secretion would be offset by the stimulation of the parathyroid glands produced by the ensuing hypocalcemia.

On the other hand, hypomagnesemia may develop in uremic patients with an intestinal malabsorptive disease, poor nutritional intake, or marked renal $Mg^{2+}$ wasting. Severe hypomagnesemia impairs the secretion and biologic action of PTH and increases the metabolism of PTH resulting in marked hypocalcemia.[433, 434] $Mg^{2+}$ depletion may also cause a decrease in both osteoblast and osteoclast activity and lead to ABD.[424]

## Biologic Markers of Bone Formation

### SERUM ALKALINE PHOSPHATASE

Serum alkaline phosphatase is made up of isoenzymes produced by the intestine, liver, kidney, and bone. Despite the heterogeneity of this enzyme, the measurement of total alkaline phosphatase activity provides a rough indication of increased osteoblastic activity; moreover, isoenzyme studies have shown that the increased alkaline phosphatase noted in uremia arises mainly from bone.[435, 436] Although high levels are observed in osteitis fibrosa, osteomalacia, or mixed lesions, markedly elevated levels are more characteristic of osteitis fibrosa.[226] Moreover, serial measurements of plasma alkaline phosphatase activity usually identify the slow progression of skeletal disease in a uremic patient even if the rise is observed within the normal range.[337] Serial measurements may also provide a useful clinical guide for monitoring the therapy of secondary HPTH with calcitriol. Thus, values that decrease over weeks or months usually indicate bone remineralization. However, uremic patients may have overt skeletal disease and normal plasma alkaline phosphatase levels; thus, a normal alkaline phosphatase activity does not exclude significant skeletal disease in an individual patient.

Plasma alkaline phosphatase levels correlate with histologic features of secondary HPTH, such as percentage of osteoblastic and active resorption surface.[437, 438] Plasma alkaline phosphatase also frequently correlates with serum PTH levels.[439] In low-bone-turnover states (osteomalacia or aplastic bone disease), the plasma alkaline phosphatase level is usually not elevated.[311] Normal alkaline phosphatase levels are more common in severe Al toxicity resulting from Al-contaminated dialysate.[226] It may reflect the toxic effect of Al on the osteoblast.[239] Nevertheless, elevated alkaline phosphatase activity has been noted,[222, 440] especially if Al toxicity resulted from the ingestion of Al-containing P binders.[212] Serum alkaline phosphatase levels may also increase early in the course of treatment with the chelating agent deferoxamine. In pediatric patients undergoing peritoneal dialysis, plasma alkaline phosphatase levels have been a poor predictor of histologic characteristics.[336] Thus, the alkaline phosphatase does not discriminate accurately between low- and high-turnover bone disease.

Because hepatic abnormalities are common in dialysis patients, liver disease should be excluded as a cause of elevated alkaline phosphatase levels. Isoenzyme measurements often allow the identification of the source.[436, 441, 442] Also, preliminary observations have noted a low bone alkaline phosphatase activity in ABD; low phosphatase activity had a sensitivity of 66% and a specificity of 86% when a value of 20 U/L or less was used as a cutoff.[344] However, these determinations are not widely available and further studies are needed. A practical clinical approach is to measure the γ-glutamyltransferase or 5'-nucleotidase when the alkaline phosphatase is elevated. The finding of normal values for these enzymes can largely exclude hepatic disturbances as the source of an elevated alkaline phosphatase level.

## OSTEOCALCIN (BONE GLA PROTEIN)

Osteocalcin (bone Gla protein, BGP, or γ-carboxyglutamic acid–containing protein) is a vitamin K–dependent protein produced by the osteoblast.[443] It is the most abundant noncollagenous protein of bone and is delivered in the interstitial bone tissue, from which it reaches the circulation fluids. Although osteocalcin levels reflect bone formation,[444–446] they are increased in CRF because of reduced renal clearance of the protein.[447] Unlike total alkaline phosphatase, osteocalcin levels are normal in disorders not involving bone provided that renal function is normal.[448]

Although absolute values are increased in patients with CRF, it has been suggested that osteocalcin can be helpful in separating patients with high-turnover from those with low-turnover bone lesions such as osteomalacia and ABD.[446, 449, 450] In a study of 30 patients undergoing maintenance dialysis, a correlation was observed between the plasma level of osteocalcin, histologic parameters of bone turnover, and the degree of peritrabecular fibrosis.[446] The osteocalcin level averaged 8 times the normal value in dialysis patients with low-turnover bone disease, but the values were more than 40 times normal in patients with high bone turnover. The level of osteocalcin provided a better separation of the two disorders than either alkaline phosphatase or $NH_2$-terminal PTH. In another study of 42 patients with mild to severe chronic CRF (serum creatinine $4.3 \pm 2.0$ mg/dL) the levels of osteocalcin were above normal in more than 80% of the patients.[451] There was a direct relationship between serum osteocalcin and serum creatinine levels, indicating the important role of renal function in determining the level of this peptide. In addition, there was a progressive rise in osteocalcin in patients not treated with calcitriol. In the treated group the osteocalcin levels either stabilized or fell. These observations indicate that the levels of osteocalcin may identify different conditions affecting bone in patients with CRF but, because the degree of CRF affects the osteocalcin level, it is not yet possible to identify an individual renal patient as having a specific condition from the results of this measurement. In the same preliminary study mentioned before,[344] low levels of osteocalcin had a sensitivity of 72% and a specificity of 77% in the diagnosis of ABD in dialysis patients.

Preliminary data obtained with an immunoradiometric assay (IRMA)[452, 453] or an enzyme immunoassay,[454] both of which recognize the intact molecule of osteocalcin, have been more discriminant than measurements by conventional RIA. This is probably because these new assays exclude fragment forms that are present in uremic sera. Because the residues of γ-carboxyglutamic acid are responsible for the affinity of osteocalcin for bone mineral, measurement of the biologically active carboxylated osteocalcin has been suggested to be more suitable for evaluating bone turnover in patients with end-stage renal disease.[455]

### TYPE I PROCOLLAGEN PROPEPTIDE

Type I collagen is the major component (90%) of bone matrix, and its circulating precursor levels may reflect type I collagen synthesis in tissues and have been developed as an index to investigate, among others, metabolic bone diseases, including renal osteodystrophy.[456, 457]

In the latter study, type I procollagen did not correlate with intact PTH, osteocalcin, alkaline phosphatase, or static histomorphometric parameters in the bone biopsy. However, and unlike osteocalcin, this marker correlated significantly with all dynamic parameters.[457] The meaning of these observations is not clear.

## Biologic Markers of Bone Resorption

### COLLAGEN BREAKDOWN PRODUCTS

Total hydroxyproline and free hydroxyproline are released with the degradation of bone collagen and, normally, both are excreted in the urine.[458] In patients with impaired urinary excretion associated with CRF, the plasma levels of total and free hydroxyproline are increased. With an increase in bone resorption and collagen degradation, plasma levels of hydroxyproline increase even further.[459] Thus, total plasma hydroxyproline may be a valuable index of the extent of bone resorption and the response to therapy.[460] Plasma hydroxyproline usually decreases in association with improvement of skeletal disease after partial PTX or treatment with calcitriol. Plasma concentration of free hydroxyproline correlates with bone histologic features suggestive of increased bone resorption.[461] Despite the claims for its utility, the determination of hydroxyproline has not gained popularity. The measurement of collagen breakdown products such as hydroxylysyl pyridinoline and lysyl pyridinoline may prove more useful in the future.[462]

### TARTRATE-RESISTANT ACID PHOSPHATASE

Isoenzyme 5b of this bone resorption marker is synthesized by the osteoclast[463, 464] and released into the circulation. Plasma tartrate-resistant acid phosphatase is increased in a variety of metabolic bone disorders with increased bone turnover.[465, 466] Preliminary studies seem to indicate that this marker, like the others, does not add further information and does not predict satisfactorily bone histology findings.

## Other Bone Biologic Markers

### CYCLIC AMP

cAMP is an important regulator of cell function, acting as a second messenger within the cell. Plasma levels of cAMP are increased in uremic patients; normally, the plasma levels of cAMP reflect PTH biologic activity.[467] However, no correlation has been noted between plasma cAMP levels and the degree of secondary HPTH. Also, the levels can remain elevated for some time after PTX.[467] The reason for the elevated levels of cAMP in patients with CRF is unknown; they may be related to catecholamines or other peptide hormones for which cAMP is also the second messenger.

### SERUM PTH

Serum PTH levels are elevated in most patients with CRF. A given PTH RIA can react with the $NH_2$-terminal region, the middle region, the COOH-terminal region, or both the middle and COOH-terminal regions. Serum PTH levels are dramatically elevated when measured with an antiserum directed primarily against the middle or the COOH-terminal region, but the degree of elevation is less when measured with an antiserum directed against the $NH_2$-terminal region.[155] Thus, the conventional RIA of PTH was limited by the measurement of biologically inactive midterminal and COOH-terminal fragments generated by the metabolism of the hormone; this was even more important in patients with CRF, because these fragments are cleared by the kidney. With the advent of IRMA, which exclusively detects the intact PTH molecule, the evaluation of dialysis patients with secondary HPTH is more precise and in many instances the performance of bone biopsy may be avoided. Moreover, the IRMAs have high specificity and sensitivity as well as excellent precision, allowing accurate measurements above, below, and within the normal range. In addition to the diagnostic value, IRMAs have been instrumental in the dynamic evaluation of parathyroid gland function in dialysis patients, measuring acute changes in PTH levels.[123, 178]

A large number of commercially available conventional RIAs for serum PTH provide no information about the predictive value of a given serum PTH level in regard to the severity of osteitis fibrosa. Thus, the discrimination between RIA-measured PTH levels in normal subjects and values in patients with primary hyperparathyroidism[345] provides little or no information about the meaning of a PTH level so measured in a patient with end-stage renal disease. Despite limitations, good correlations have been reported between the results of both midregion–COOH-terminal and COOH-terminal PTH assays[181, 336, 341, 439, 449, 468] and several histologic features of secondary HPTH in biopsies of hemodialysis patients; however these findings are not uniform.[181, 336] Furthermore, it has often been difficult to compare the results from different laboratories, so clinicians have had to use their experience in recognizing the clinical significance of a specific PTH level. Because the $NH_2$-terminal fragment of PTH is difficult to detect in plasma, this assay may reflect intact PTH. Thus, Voigts[181] and Andress[345] and their colleagues noted slightly better correlations with histologic features of secondary HPTH with the $NH_2$-terminal assay than with the midregion or COOH-terminal PTH.

Preliminary data suggest that IRMAs correlate with histologic features of bone disease in dialysis patients.[13, 341]

Moreover, these studies show a reasonably good separation of one type of bone disorder from another. Thus, Solal and colleagues[341] compared intact, midregion, and COOH-terminal assays of PTH for the diagnosis of histologic type of bone disease; they showed that the intact PTH measurement had the best correlation with the bone formation rate and was superior to the other assays for separating patients with secondary HPTH from those with adynamic lesions. The IRMA PTH assays also reveal remarkably similar ranges of normal values from one laboratory to another,[469] allowing comparisons of different reports. Available evidence indicates that serum values 1.5 to 3 times above normal, based on an intact PTH assay, correspond to a relatively normal bone formation rate from bone biopsies in patients with CRF.[174, 309, 341–343] In summary, with IRMA the diagnosis of secondary HPTH can be made accurately provided that Al toxicity is ruled out and the therapeutic response to calcitriol therapy can be appropiately monitored.[61, 341]

Serum PTH levels are sometimes normal or undetectable in patients with CRF. Such a finding may occur with hypomagnesemia,[433] low-turnover bone disease,[307, 341] and excessive dosage of calcitriol,[302] and in parathyroidectomized patients.

An immunochemiluminiscent assay also directed toward intact PTH has become available.[470] Its main advantage is that it avoids the radioisotopic hazard. A good correlation ($r = .93$) was noted between an IRMA and an immunochemiluminiscent assay in 104 dialysis patients.[173]

## Plasma Aluminum and the Deferoxamine Infusion Test

Electrothermal atomic absorption spectroscopy provides an accurate way to measure plasma Al levels. The use of an international quality assessment program has improved the precision, accuracy, and reproducibility of Al measurements.[471] Tissue and plasma Al levels are substantially above normal in most patients with end-stage renal disease, particularly those who have taken Al-containing P binders or have been exposed to Al-contaminated dialysate.[203, 472] The plasma Al concentration largely reflects a recent "load" of Al rather than Al toxicity,[473] because plasma Al concentration does not correlate highly with tissue stores.[271, 474] However, most patients with Al-related bone disease have markedly elevated plasma Al concentrations (e.g., >75 to 100 μg/L compared with <10 μg/L in normal individuals). Also, patients with markedly elevated plasma Al levels (e.g., above 150 to 200 μg/L) are likely to develop Al-related bone disease and/or encephalopathy if the exposure to Al is maintained.[271] In a large population study, higher alkaline phosphatase levels and lower erythrocyte cell volume were observed in dialysis patients with plasma Al levels above 100 μg/L compared with the group with levels below 100 μg/L.[475] In another study, electroencephalographic features of encephalopathy were noted in 8 of 27 patients with plasma Al levels above 100 μg/L and none were noted among 24 patients with plasma Al below 50 μg/L.[476] It is of interest that only five of the eight patients had any clinical manifestations of encephalopathy. In the former group, with plasma Al levels above 100 μg/L, the 8

patients with abnormal electroencephalograms (EEGs) had higher plasma levels than the 19 patients with normal EEGs.

In patients who have been withdrawn from Al-containing P binders, plasma Al levels fall during the next 2 to 6 months, so they are far less helpful in identifying those with clinically significant Al accumulation (e.g., greater than 25% surface-stainable Al and subnormal bone formation rate). Plasma Al levels as low as 21 μg/L were observed in a patient with biopsy evidence of Al-related bone disease when the ingestion of all Al-containing P binders was discontinued 18 months earlier.[477]

It is important to monitor the Al content of dialysate. The maximal concentration permitted according to the American National Standard for HD Systems (Arlington, VA, AAMI, 1992 [RD-5-1992]) is 10 μg/L. Also, plasma Al concentrations should be measured at regular intervals in dialysis patients; we recommend every 4 months. Marked elevation of plasma Al levels in the majority of patients in a dialysis unit indicates that there has been exposure to unacceptably high concentrations of Al in the dialysate. This may indicate malfunctioning of the water treatment system or a dramatic increase in Al concentration in the water, which may overwhelm the purification system. When only an isolated patient exhibits high concentrations of Al (e.g. >40 μg/L), ingestion of excessive amounts of Al-containing P binders is usually present.

Bone, brain, heart, and liver are major sites of Al deposition within the body[203] but, as mentioned before, the degree of Al retention in these tissues does not correspond tightly to measurements in plasma. Measurement of the increment in plasma Al concentration after a standardized infusion of the chelating agent deferoxamine has been proposed as a method for recognizing dialysis patients with increased Al stores and a greater risk of Al-related bone disease.[473] The relationship between the increment in plasma Al after deferoxamine and the total Al content in bone is closer than that between the basal plasma Al and the bone Al content. However, it has been noted that the magnitude of the rise in plasma Al after deferoxamine was not specific in all cases.[212, 478] Hodsman and colleagues[212] demonstrated that dialysis patients with secondary HPTH may have substantial increases in plasma Al after infusions of deferoxamine despite little evidence of stainable Al in bone biopy specimens. Such patients with secondary HPTH and a positive deferoxamine infusion test may be at increased risk for the development of Al-related bone disease after PTX or if Al contamination is not avoided. Moreover, Al may not be distributed in tissues similarly in all patients, and a certain total quantity of Al in a tissue may not always be pathogenic. When patients are protected from any Al exposure for several months (dialysate Al concentration below 10 μg/L and all Al-containing P binders avoided), both basal plasma Al and the increment in plasma Al after deferoxamine decrease substantially, even in the presence of Al staining at the bone mineralization front. Thus, a certain pool of bone Al may be resistant to removal or removed slowly.[264] The latter is particularly likely in a patient who has had prior PTX.

Several factors may account for the variable results with use of the deferoxamine infusion test in the recognition of

Al toxicity. The initial studies were done in patients with marked Al loading and severe symptomatic Al toxicity; moreover, the patients continued either to be exposed to inappropriately elevated dialysate Al levels or to ingest Al-containing P binders. Studies of patients with mild Al toxicity indicate that the rise in plasma Al after deferoxamine correlates well with bone Al content but it is not a good predictor of the bone histologic picture.[479]

It appears that Al bone disease is decreasing in frequency and severity.[308] Thus, patients with Al bone disease are fewer but more difficult to diagnose. Some investigators have attempted to develop noninvasive strategies for the identification and serial monitoring of these patients. Thus, for Al values less than 30 to 40 µg/L, Al-related bone disease is unlikely but possible, especially if the patient has been totally withdrawn from Al exposure for 6 to 8 months or longer. As long as serum Al levels remain less than 30 µg/L, it is also unlikely that such a patient could develop de novo Al toxicity. For Al levels between 40 and 100 µg/L, the presence of this disease is likely, especially if associated with low PTH values, hypercalcemia, or a positive deferoxamine test; for Al levels greater than 100 µg/L Al-related bone disease is probable but is not invariably present, especially if serum PTH levels are high. Using the combination of an intact PTH assay (IRMA) and the deferoxamine infusion test, Pei and colleagues[480] found that an intact PTH level below 200 pg/mL and an increment of plasma Al after deferoxamine infusion of 150 µg/L or more provided the best positive predictive value (≥95%) for Al bone disease in both peritoneal dialysis and hemodialysis patients; however, the sensitivity was only 35% to 45%. Moreover, this test cutoff would remain highly predictive even if the prevalence of the disorder decreased to as low as 5% for CAPD patients and 10% for hemodialysis patients. The sensitivity of the combined PTH-deferoxamine test evaluation was substantially lower in patients who had Al gels withdrawn for more than 6 months compared with those still ingesting Al-containing P binders. Other authors, using COOH-terminal PTH, found that the combination of deferoxamine test and PTH was helpful not to recognize but to exclude Al-related bone disease.[481] "Low-dose" deferoxamine tests (0.5 g, 5 mg/kg) have been reported as useful in the diagnosis of Al-related bone disease.[298, 482] Thus, it is apparent that a bone biopsy may often be required for the diagnosis of Al toxicity in borderline and uncertain cases.

The state of iron stores may influence the deferoxamine test, so the status of iron stores should be considered in the interpretation of this test.[219, 483] Thus, patients with iron deficiency have higher increments of serum Al after deferoxamine than those with iron overload. This may occur because deferoxamine mobilizes iron in addition to Al; thus, the more iron, the smaller the increment in serum Al after deferoxamine. This may explain some of the frequent false-negative responses observed in patients with obvious Al-induced bone disease.

Finally, Al determination in the skin by inductively coupled plasma optical emission spectrometry has been suggested for the evaluation of body Al content,[484] although there is no uniform agreement about its utility.[485]

## Vitamin D Levels

Under normal circumstances, serum calcitriol levels are either undetectable or below the normal range in patients with advanced CRF. Thus, the measurement of serum calcitriol is not usually helpful in the differential diagnosis of hypercalcemia in dialysis patients. However, if the cause of hypercalcemia is not identified and the patient is not receiving calcitriol treatment, extrarenal production of calcitriol, as in a granulomatous or lymphoproliferative disorder,[419, 420] should be suspected when calcitriol is in the normal range or higher.

## CLINICAL SIGNS AND SYMPTOMS OF OSTEODYSTROPHY

By the time symptoms appear, the patient usually has significant biochemical abnormalities and histologic evidence of bone disease. Thus, symptoms appear late in the course of renal osteodystrophy, are rather nonspecific, and are usually subtle and insidious in their onset. The severity of symptoms often does not correlate closely with radiologic or histologic changes. Severely abnormal skeletal radiographs or bone biopsy specimens may be observed in patients who are totally asymptomatic. So far, only the idiopathic form of ABD has not been associated with clinical signs or symptoms. Although the subject is beyond the scope of this chapter, the manifestations of dialysis-related amyloidosis may be confused with other forms of renal osteodystrophy; therefore, we include a brief mention of this disorder and refer the interested reader to excellent reviews.[486–489]

## Bone Pain

Although not common, bone pain may develop and progress slowly to produce total disability.[490] This can occur independently of skeletal disease, whether primarily osteitis fibrosa, osteomalacia, or a mixture of both. However, the most common cause of bone pain is osteomalacia and it is most often observed in Al-related bone disease. Pain is generally vague and deep-seated and may be diffuse or located in the low back, hips, knees, or legs. It often varies in intensity and is aggravated by weight bearing or by sudden movement or pressure. Occasionally, pain is localized around the knee, ankle, or heel, and it may be of such sudden appearance as to suggest acute arthritis. Pain in the low back may arise from collapse of a vertebral body; sharp chest pain may be the first indication of a rib fracture that has occurred during a cough, sneeze, or even normal breathing. A change in position, such as sitting up from the supine position or spontaneous rolling over during sleep, may evoke generalized pain throughout the back, hips, and chest. Pain is not relieved by massage or local heat, and the patient usually perceives it as being more deeply seated than in the joints or muscles. Patients undergoing regular hemodialysis who are normally active and asymptomatic may develop, within several weeks to months, such severe pain as to make walking across a room difficult. Others experience such a slow and gradual progression of symptoms that little notice is given until total debility has occurred.

Physical findings are frequently lacking; occasionally, localized tenderness may be apparent with pressure on the chest wall or lateral compression of the pelvis; tenderness may also be localized over the vertebral spinous processes or ribs. Spontaneous fractures can also be present. Commonly, the fractures involve the ribs, but any bone can be affected; the majority of fractures have been observed in low-bone-turnover Al-related bone disease.

Bone pain can also develop in association with dialysis-related amyloidosis.

## Periarthritis and Arthritis

These are manifested by acute pain, redness, stiffness, and swelling around one or more joints. Rarely, pain may occur in the ankle or foot without local signs except for vague tenderness and can be associated with radiographic changes of subperiosteal resorption and/or periosteal new bone formation.[491] Thus, this disorder may reflect overt secondary HPTH. The affected patients usually have higher levels of serum alkaline phosphatase activity, $Ca^{2+} \times P$ product, and PTH levels than other dialysis patients.[492] Further evidence that such symptoms are related to secondary HPTH is provided by the observation that such discomfort can disappear completely within 1 to 2 weeks after subtotal PTX. Occasionally, $Ca^{2+}$ deposits may be observed radiographically about the affected joints. Synovial biopsy may reveal crystals that, when studied by x-ray diffraction, are characteristic of hydroxyapatite. This syndrome must be differentiated from pseudogout or gouty arthritis; the last two are characterized by a true monarticular arthritis and can be differentiated by the identification of specific crystals of either calcium pyrophosphate or urate, respectively, within the synovial fluid.[493]

In general, periarthritis or arthritis responds well to treatment with anti-inflammatory agents such as indomethacin; medical treatment of secondary HPTH or PTX, as already mentioned, may lead to marked improvement.[491, 494]

Erosive arthritis and joint effusions can be also skeletal manifestations of dialysis-related amyloidosis. Metacarpophalangeal or interphalangeal joints, shoulders, wrists, and knees can be involved.[495]

## Myopathy and Muscle Weakness

Muscle weakness is largely limited to the proximal musculature and can be a serious and debilitating problem even in patients without end-stage renal disease. This myopathy resembles in many ways the muscle weakness reported in vitamin D deficiency in patients without CRF or in patients with primary HPTH.[397, 496] Plasma levels of muscle enzymes, such as creatine kinase, are usually normal, and electromyographic abnormalities are either absent or nonspecific. The muscle weakness appears slowly, with the patient unable to climb stairs easily or to rise from a sitting position without help. The gait may become abnormal so

that the patient waddles from side to side in a "penguin" style. The afflicted patient may be confined to a wheelchair or may be unable to hold his or her arms above the head or to comb the hair because of shoulder girdle weakness.

Proximal muscle weakness can be caused by secondary HPTH,[497] P depletion,[498] abnormal metabolism of vitamin D,[499] or Al loading.[500] Striking improvement in muscle weakness has been observed in some uremic children and adults after administration of either calcitriol (1 to 5 μg/d) or 25(OH)D (10 to 100 μg/d).[501–503] Muscle biopsy, in selected patients, has revealed mild, nonspecific myopathic alterations by light microscopy and severe degenerative changes by electron microscopy.[504, 505] After treatment with 25(OH)D, some findings have reverted to normal.[505] Muscle weakness in uremic patients can promptly improve after treatment with calcitriol even before serum PTH levels fall or with doses that are too low to reduce serum PTH[501, 502]; this suggests a role of vitamin D rather than secondary HPTH in certain patients. Muscle weakness may also be profound in patients with Al-related bone disease; furthermore, striking improvement has occurred after Al removal with deferoxamine, with little change in PTH status and without vitamin D therapy.[506]

Other causes of muscle weakness can be noted in uremia, such as peripheral neuropathy, electrolyte disturbances, iron overload, and carnitine deficiency. Thus, not all muscle abnormalities present in uremia can be attributed to altered divalent ion metabolism. However, in patients with prominent symptoms of muscle pain and weakness, an empirical therapeutic trial of calcitriol or 25(OH)D is warranted and the presence of Al intoxication or severe secondary HPTH must be excluded.[337]

## Spontaneous Tendon Rupture

Spontaneous tendon rupture also occurs in patients with long-standing CRF and is usually associated with evidence of marked secondary HPTH.[507] The syndrome has been reported in association with primary HPTH and other causes of secondary HPTH.[508–510] It had been suggested that an abnormality of collagen metabolism, which also affected the bone, may occur in tendons and cause weakening[508, 511]; an effect of systemic acidosis causing elastosis of tendons was also proposed as a pathogenic mechanism.[512] However, the histologic finding on biopsy specimens of excised quadriceps suggested that repeated minor fractures of the bone cortex had occurred at the site of tendon insertion and preceded the final total tendon rupture. It was concluded that osteitis fibrosa was responsible for the minor fractures[513]; the slow progressive rise in alkaline phosphatase in the preceding 4 to 5 years provided additional evidence for uncontrolled secondary HPTH as the most likely pathogenic factor in those ruptures.

Rupture occurs most commonly in the quadriceps or triceps tendons or in extensor tendons of the fingers. Typically, the quadriceps tendon ruptures while the patient is walking or descending stairs or after stumbling. Patients are usually unable to extend the affected leg and a palpable gap and ecchymoses above the tendon are characteristic. Surgical treatment with slow rehabilitation has yielded satisfactory results.[509] The presence of tendon ruptures should alert the clinician to inappropriate control of secondary HPTH, although it has also been described in dialysis-related amyloidosis.[514]

## Calciphylaxis

Calciphylaxis is characterized by peripheral ischemic tissue necrosis, vascular calcifications, and cutaneous ulcerations.[493, 515] Ischemic necrosis can also affect muscles and/or subcutaneous fat.[515] This syndrome usually appears in patients with end-stage renal disease and is associated with a long-standing history of CRF, although patients have developed the syndrome after successful kidney transplantation.[516, 517] The syndrome has been observed in association with renal diseases of varying causes and there is no predilection for a specific sex or age.

The skin lesions make their appearance as painful superficial violaceous discolorations in a mottled, circumscribed pattern involving the tips of the toes or fingers or occurring about the ankles, thighs, or buttocks. As these lesions progress, they become hemorrhagic with ischemic, "dry" necrosis. Frequently, boring nonhealing ulcerations and eschars occur; lesions of the terminal phalanges are often clearly demarcated and toe or fingertips may even fall off (Fig. 51–21). Such lesions resemble those that accompany vasculitis; however, biopsy specimens fail to show fibrinoid necrosis or granulomatous formation. All patients with calciphylaxis have demonstrated evidence of medial calcinosis of small and medium-sized arteries; skin biopsies generally reveal the presence of medial calcification and intimal thickening.[515, 516] Ischemic myolysis, ischemic cardiac disease, and hemorrhagic panniculitis have been reported in individual cases.

The pathogenesis of this syndrome is uncertain. Extensive medial calcinosis of arteries can occur in patients with CRF and yet not lead to gangrene and ulceration; however, the possibility has been considered that $Ca^{2+}$ deposition may give rise to mechanical obstruction. The favorable response of some patients within several days of PTX suggests that mechanical obstruction cannot totally explain the ischemia. Vascular spasms related to either hypercalcemia[518] or an effect of PTH itself[519] may be implicated. The occurrence of such lesions after kidney transplantation in patients receiving glucocorticoid raises the possibility that steroids may play a role.[515, 516] Thus, Selye[520] showed in an animal model of this syndrome that calciphylaxis was more common in animals if they had been given large doses of glucocorticoid.

Most uremic patients presenting with this syndrome either previously had or now have evidence of overt secondary HPTH[515] and most have shown substantial improvement after partial PTX.[521] Nevertheless, calciphylaxis has been described after subtotal PTX, suggesting other physiopathologic pathways at work as well.[522] With no treatment, the lesions often progress with varying degrees of rapidity and a number of afflicted patients have died, usually from secondary uncontrollable sepsis.[515, 521] Because of the poor prognosis, urgent partial PTX is recommended when such lesions appear in conjunction with overt secondary

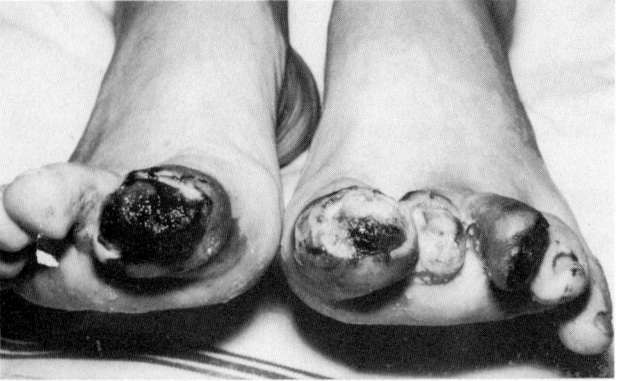
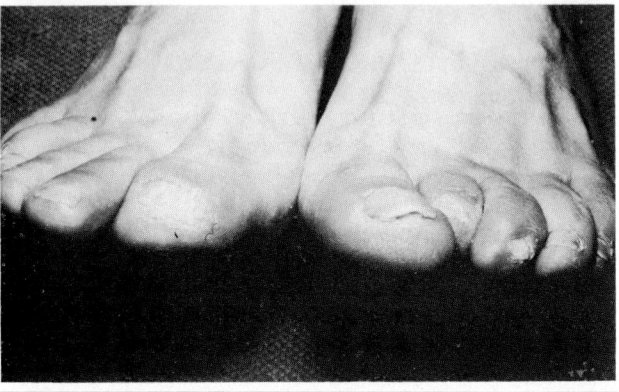

**Figure 51–21.** Ischemic and necrotic lesions of the feet that appeared after successful renal transplantation *(top)* in a patient with hypercalcemia caused by secondary HPTH. The lesions healed witin 3 to 4 months after partial PTX *(bottom)*. (From Massry SG, Gordon A, Coburn JW: Vascular calcification and peripheral necrosis in a renal transplant recipient: Reversal of lesion following subtotal parathyroidectomy. Reprinted from American Journal of Medicine: 49:3; September, 1970; 416 to 422.)

HPTH.[515, 521] In some patients, serum PTH levels are not high; severe P restriction may reverse this syndrome.[515] Patients with diabetes mellitus and CRF may also develop ischemic lesions, medial vascular calcifications, and a similar clinical picture. However, the lesions observed in diabetic patients rarely improve after PTX.

## Corneal-Conjunctival Calcification

This frequently occurs when the $Ca^{2+} \times P$ product is high. The corneal calcification can even take a band-like configuration in the interpalpebral area, called band keratopathy.[523] Usually asymptomatic, it can also result in ocular inflammation ("red eye" syndrome) and decreased visual acuity.[524] A rise in local pH because of loss of carbon dioxide into the air has been suggested to predispose to ocular calcifications.

## Pruritus

Itching is a common symptom in patients with advanced CRF, and it often improves and disappears after initiation of regular hemodialysis. However, pruritus may persist and can be of such intensity that it prevents sleep and interferes with the patient's normal activities. Pruritus may reflect the presence of high PTH levels, hypercalcemia, high $Ca^{2+} \times P$ product ($>70$ mg$^2$/dL$^2$) or metastatic calcifications. It may improve or, indeed, totally disappear within a few days after partial PTX.[525] Thus, the presence of refractory pruritus in a patient with CRF should alert the clinician to the possibility of secondary HPTH; if a patient with intractable itching has high PTH levels, PTX should be considered, especially if refractoriness to appropriate medical treatment (i.e., intravenous calcitriol) is present.

The mechanism whereby secondary HPTH can lead to pruritus is uncertain. Elevated levels of $Ca^{2+}$ in the skin have been reported in such patients.[525] However, the increased $Ca^{2+}$ content in the skin is probably not responsible for the itching, because the symptom improves within a few hours after surgery, whereas much more time is required before the skin $Ca^{2+}$ content decreases. Itching may develop in uremic patients with administration of pharmacologic doses of vitamin D and during infusions of calcium; such observations suggest that an elevated concentration of $Ca^{2+}$ in the extracellular fluid may be an important factor contributing to pruritus.

Observations that uremic pruritus may be relieved after intravenous injection of lidocaine,[526] irradiation with ultraviolet light,[527, 528] ingestion of activated charcoal,[529] or erythropoietin therapy[530] point to the fact that uremic pruritus is multifactorial in nature. Thus, xerosis of the skin,[531] peripheral neuropathy,[532] or the presence of increased histamine levels has been noted.[530, 533] In some cases severe pruritus did not improve after PTX; thus, in the absence of specific evidence of secondary HPTH—high levels of PTH, radiographic evidence of erosions, and/or bone biopsy features of osteitis fibrosa—parathyroid surgery should not be performed.

## Skeletal Deformities

True deformities of bone are common in uremic children with long-standing CRF in whom the bone undergoes rapid growth, but skeletal deformities occasionally occur in adults. Such deformities arise from abnormalities of skeletal remodeling and from recurrent fractures. The deformities commonly observed in children include bowing of the long bones, especially tibia and femur, and defects arising from slipped epiphyses.[534] Most commonly, slipped epiphyses become manifest in preadolescence. The hip is the most common site afflicted, followed by the radius and ulna; lower humeral, femoral, and tibial sites are more rarely involved.[535] With hip involvement a limp is common and pain is often absent. When the radius and ulna are involved, local swelling and ulnar deviation of the hands appear. The histologic abnormalities associated with slipped epiphyses are those of secondary HPTH.[536]

The pattern of bone deformity varies with age, and in patients younger than 3 to 4 years changes of secondary HPTH often exhibit the typical radiographic findings of vitamin D deficiency.[537] They include rachitic rosary, Harrison grooves, and enlargement of the wrists and ankles caused by widening of the metaphysis beneath the growth plate in long bones.[536] A rickets-like lesion observed in uremic children has additional histologic features of secondary HPTH.[534] Craniotabes and frontal bossing of the skull occur in children who develop CRF in the first 2 years of life.[536] Uremia is a common cause of "knock-knee" or genu valgum at any age.[538] This can appear within a few months; the presenting symptoms are difficulty in walking and pain in the knees.

In adults with CRF, particularly those with Al-related osteomalacia, skeletal deformities can be marked. They are usually confined to the axial skeleton. Lumbar scoliosis, thoracic kyphosis, and recurrent rib fracture may cause marked deformities to develop during 1 to 2 years in dialysis patients.

## Retardation of Growth

Growth retardation is an almost invariable finding in children with chronic renal insufficiency, both before and during management with maintenance hemodialysis or with CAPD.[539, 540] Growth can be impaired even without evidence of renal osteodystrophy. Before dialysis, one third to one half of children with a "preterminal" stage of chronic CRF had heights below the third percentile[540]; growth velocity was below normal limits for age in two thirds of children under treatment with dialysis.[541] Providing caloric supplements has been reported to improve growth,[542] although this is not always successful.[543, 544] Studies showing that correction of acidosis can improve growth in children with renal tubular acidosis provide support for the idea that long-standing acidosis could have a deleterious effect on growth.[545] Low levels of somatomedin have also been implicated in this complex problem.[546] Improved or even catch-up growth has been observed in a few children after treatment with calcitriol.[547] During treatment with calcitriol, catch-up growth did not occur during the early period of treatment when the serum PTH levels were still elevated and renal osteodystrophy was still evident, but it began after the apparent healing of the secondary HPTH. Nevertheless, the number of patients studied is small, and consistent increases in growth rate in subsequent reports on larger numbers of patients have not been observed in the majority of children undergoing maintenance dialysis during treatment with vitamin D, 1α(OH)D, or calcitriol.[541, 548]

The observations of strikingly improved growth velocity of children with CRF during therapy with supraphysiologic amounts of human growth hormone are of interest.[549] Resistance to the action of the growth hormone[188, 189] as well as other hormones (PTH, insulin)[64, 191] has been described in CRF. The response to growth hormone is more pronounced when it is given before ages 8 to 10 years, and such treatment is associated with markedly increased plasma alkaline phosphatase, suggesting that there is increased osteoblastic activity.[549–551] The long-term results and potential side effects of such therapy are not known.

## Anemia

Refractoriness to recombinant human erythropoietin treatment can be observed both in severe secondary HPTH and in Al-related bone disease. The former is discussed later. The anemia of Al toxicity is usually mild and can be overcome by increasing the erythropoietin dose. At least two mechanisms seem to be involved: impaired iron uptake from transferrin into the erythrocyte precursor and inhibition of iron incorporation into heme.[552] Al-induced resistance to erythropoietin therapy should be considered in patients with microcytic anemia and normal iron stores and in patients with refractory normochromic-normocytic anemia with low-turnover bone disease. Therapy with deferoxamine may ameliorate the anemia but secondary iron deficiency should be avoided.

## Central Nervous System Disturbances

Although central nervous system involvement is the most severe manifestation of Al intoxication,[209] it is decreasing in frequency. Symptoms and signs of brain and bone involvement may not occur together, and the absence of findings in one does not preclude severe involvement in the other. Early symptoms are intermittent speech disturbances like stuttering and stammering; later, personality changes, apraxia, asterixis, seizures, and global dementia can appear. Signs and symptoms may be exacerbated by dialysis and by deferoxamine administration. The EEG may show characteristic multifocal bursts of delta and theta activity.

Central nervous system disturbances have also been related to secondary HPTH, as discussed shortly. A variety of symptoms may accompany even mild hypercalcemia in uremic patients, including mental confusion and lethargy.[553]

## Myocardial Function Abnormalities

Uremic patients often have cardiomyopathy. Uremia is associated with an increase in the $Ca^{2+}$ content of the myocardium; these changes may be due to excess PTH. PTH may also play an ancillary role in mitral annulus calcification.[554] Bogin and colleagues[555] examined the in vitro effects of PTH on cultured isolated heart cells. Both PTH fragments caused a significant increase in number of beats per minute, and the cells died earlier than control cells. In addition, serum from uremic parathyroidectomized rats did not affect heart rate, but serum from uremic rats had effects similar to those of PTH. Furthermore, London and co-workers[556] noted, in dialysis patients studied by echocardiography, that left ventricular hypertrophy was associated with the severity of secondary HPTH. Also, these patients had an increased heart rate, higher systolic pressure and end-systolic stress, increased velocity of fiber shortening, and shorter left ventricular ejection time.[557] These authors, as well as others, have shown a marked improvement in left ventricular function after PTX.[558, 559]

Al may also affect myocardial function in patients with end-stage CRF. Thus, high mortality resulting from cardiac failure, often accompanied by cardiac arrhythmias, has been noted in dialysis patients with evidence of Al overload, as determined by bone biopsy[307] or the deferoxamine infusion test.[560] Preferential accumulation of Al has been noted in the myocardium of uremic patients,[203] and an association

between left ventricular dysfunction or myocardial hypertrophy and the ultrastructural findings of myocardial Al accumulation has been observed.[561, 562] London and colleagues[563] evaluated left ventricular function in hemodialysis patients by echocardiography in relation to Al stores, as assessed by a bone biopsy and the increment in plasma Al after deferoxamine. The patients without Al accumulation had significantly lower left ventricular mass and an increased velocity of myocardial fiber shortening compared with those with evidence of Al accumulation. Moreover, for the entire hemodialysis population Al stores correlated with increased left ventricular mass. Thus, these observations suggest that in uremic patients, left ventricular hypertrophy may sometimes be linked to increased Al stores.

## Other Uremic Signs and Symptoms Related to Secondary Hyperparathyroidism

A number of nonskeletal symptoms that commonly coexist in uremic patients with overt renal osteodystrophy may arise as a consequence of a common pathogenic mechanism leading to both the skeletal disease and the nonskeletal manifestations. PTH and the PTH-induced increase in intracellular $Ca^{2+}$ may be uremic toxins.[564–567] Some features of the uremic state that may be related to the marked secondary HPTH are shown in Table 51–6.

There is evidence that the secondary HPTH of experimental acute renal failure may lead to increased $Ca^{2+}$ content of the brain in association with an abnormal EEG.[568, 569] Probable relevance of these animal experiments to humans has been established by Cooper and associates,[570] who noted that EEG abnormalities, increased levels of PTH, and increased brain $Ca^{2+}$ content occurred early in the course of acute renal failure. During the diuretic and recovery phases, serum PTH decreased to normal and the EEG became normal. A role for high PTH levels in altering central nervous system function in CRF and dialysis patients is less

---

**TABLE 51–6. Symptoms, Signs, and Other Features in Uremic Patients Possibly Related to Parathyroid Hormone**

Bone pain and fractures
Acute periarthritis and pseudogout
Myopathy and muscle weakness
Spontaneous tendon rupture
Calciphylaxis
Corneal-conjunctival calcification: band keratopathy, red eye syndrome
Pruritus
Skeletal deformities and retardation of growth
Anemia, pancytopenia, platelet dysfunction
Immunologic abnormalities
Central nervous system disturbances and abnormal EEG
(?) Peripheral neuropathy
(?) Impotence
(?) Myocardial failure
Abnormal carbohydrate metabolism: insulin resistance, hyperglycemia, hyperglucagonemia
(?) Hyperlipidemia and arteriosclerosis
Hypertension

well established. The EEG abnormalities of uremia may revert toward normal with regular and adequate dialysis[571]; moreover, brain $Ca^{2+}$ levels were normal in most patients with CRF who were tested.[570] Anecdotal experience has shown rather striking improvement of behavioral abnormalities after partial PTX in some uremic patients with secondary HPTH, suggesting a neurotoxic role of PTH in some patients.[572] Moreover, neural mechanisms of behavior and motor functions are affected by the cholinergic system, and CRF is associated with these abnormalities.[573] Thus, it has been shown that uremia causes derangements in acetylcholine metabolism mainly because of reduced activity of choline kinase mediated, at least partly, by secondary HPTH.[574]

Although it has been suggested that peripheral neuropathy may occur with greater frequency in patients with secondary HPTH,[575] this supposition has been challenged.[576] Arieff and Schmidt[576] noted that motor nerve conduction velocity was not associated with PTH levels. In acute uremia, increased nerve content of $Ca^{2+}$ and decreased motor nerve conduction velocity were related to increased parathyroid activity.[577] Available information provides support for the view that PTH acts as a neurotoxin in the central nervous system abnormalities observed in acute CRF; whether it plays a role in peripheral neuropathy remains unclear.[576]

The possibility that secondary HPTH contributes to impotence in patients with end-stage CRF has been suggested.[564] In one prospective study, administration of calcitriol was associated with an increase in potency in two of seven dialysis patients; a concomitant fall in plasma luteinizing hormone occurred in one of the two and a rise in plasma testosterone in the other.[578] However, another study showed no benefit after calcitriol administration.[579] Thus, the impotence of chronic uremia is probably of multifactorial origin, but excess PTH may play a role in certain cases.

Extensive marrow fibrosis and sclerosis of bone can develop in uremic patients as a consequence of secondary HPTH; such alterations may contribute to the hematologic abnormalities present in uremia. An association among renal osteodystrophy, myelofibrosis, and abnormal hematopoiesis has been noted[580]; thus, patients with leukopenia, thrombocytopenia, and severe anemia are more likely to have overt bone disease than other dialysis patients. It has been suggested that splenomegaly may arise in certain uremic patients as a compensatory mechanism in response to the replacement of normal erythroid tissue by osteitis fibrosa. An increased incidence of anemia has been reported in patients with primary HPTH[581] and correlates with the extent of marrow fibrosis. Refractoriness to recombinant erythropoietin treatment has also been related to the presence of bone marrow fibrosis.[582] It has been also observed that the hematocrit may increase in uremic patients with severe secondary HPTH after partial PTX.[583] It appears that PTH may suppress erythropoietic function through local factors produced by marrow fibrosis. However, a direct effect of PTH on erythrocytes is also possible. Meytes and colleagues[584] examined the in vitro effects of intact PTH and some of its fragments on erythroid colony formation in human peripheral blood and mouse bone marrow. They observed that intact PTH and its COOH-terminal fragment exert an inhibitory effect on erythropoiesis that might be overcome by increased erythropoietin levels. These observations are complemented by others demonstrating inhibition of RNA and heme synthesis by PTH extracts.[585] In addition, the $NH_2$-terminal PTH fragment has been shown to induce hemolysis of erythrocytes.[586] Thus, an excess of PTH could contribute to the shortened life span of erythrocytes in uremia.

Inhibition of platelet function occurs in uremia, and an inhibitory effect of PTH on platelet aggregation has also been noted.[587] Thus, it is possible that excess PTH may be a contributing factor in the bleeding tendency of uremia.

PTH has also been implicated in the immunologic abnormalities present in uremia.[588–591]

Hypertriglyceridemia has been noted in a fraction of patients with uremia.[592] Furthermore, PTX partially inhibits the increase in lipids observed after bilateral nephrectomy, and the administration of parathyroid extract restores the hyperlipidemia in parathyroidectomized uremic rats.[593] Such data provide support for the possibility that the hyperlipidemia of uremia may be related to an excess of PTH. Other observations suggest that insulin secretion is impaired after chronic excess of PTH.[594] PTH increases intracellular $Ca^{2+}$ of pancreatic islets through both stimulation of cAMP generation and activation of protein kinase C.[595] Thus, insulin resistance and hyperglycemia observed in uremia may be related to secondary HPTH.

## DIALYSIS-RELATED AMYLOIDOSIS

This entity is observed in patients receiving long-standing maintenance dialysis and is characterized by generalized arthralgias, bone cysts, scapulohumeral periarthritis, pathologic fractures, carpal tunnel syndrome (CTS), and sometimes visceral involvement.[596–600] The accumulation of a unique type of amyloid protein made up of $\beta_2$-microglobulin ($\beta$-chain of the human leukocyte antigen class I molecule), normally degraded by the kidney, is most likely responsible for this disorder.[601] Although the pathophysiology of the process is not completely understood, these amyloid fibrils have a strong predilection to deposit in tendons, periarticular structures, at the end of long bones, and within the intervertebral disks.[487, 602, 603] The clinical manifestations of this entity almost never appear before 5 years of dialysis therapy and are more common in patients who begin regular dialysis after the age of 50 years.[495, 604] The fraction of afflicted patients increases with the duration of dialysis therapy; thus, 70% to 80% of patients treated with hemodialysis for 10 years or more accumulate $\beta_2$-amyloid in tissues.[604]

CTS is the most prominent and usually first symptom of dialysis-related amyloidosis.[597] Thus, CTS is not common in patients who have had less than 5 years of dialysis and the incidence increases with the duration of maintenance dialysis. The reported incidence ranges from 30% to 100% in patients with more than 10 years of hemodialysis. CTS results from entrapment of the median nerve by amyloid tissue deposits in the wrist, and the symptoms of CTS are not different between uremic and nonuremic patients.[495] It is usually bilateral and progressive, accompanied by numbness, paresthesias, and hyperesthesia of the thumb, index and middle fingers, and radial aspect of the fourth finger. As the CTS progresses, amyotrophy may develop. In contrast to osteitis fibrosa, pain often worsens at night and during dialysis. Amyloid fibril deposits have been noted in the transverse carpal ligament in 50% of patients affected by CTS. Surgical decompression is the treatment of choice because the response to local anesthetic agents and corticosteroids is only transient.

Severe arthralgias are also common in patients with dialysis-related amyloidosis. The affected joints are usually shoulders, knees, wrists, hip, ankle, elbow, small joints of the hand, and occasionally the intervertebral disks. Scapulohumeral involvement with shoulder pain is a common clinical presentation. Joint effusion is reported to be as high as 50% of patients who have hemodialysis for more than 10 years.[605] Aspiration of the joint reveals a clear, sterile fluid without inflammatory characteristics; the cell count ranges from 50 to 5000 cells/mm³, and normal glucose levels and a low protein content are usually observed. Sometimes, centrifuged joint fluid stained with Congo red reveals the typical green birefringence of amyloid proteins. These findings strongly suggest dialysis-related amyloidosis, especially if they are associated with CTS, bone cysts, and pathologic fractures. This arthropathy involves large and medium-sized joints. The lesion can start unilaterally, but usually the contralateral joint is affected. A pathologic fracture may be the first manifestation of an affected joint.[596] The spine can also be affected,[606–608] with destructive spondyloarthropathy or pseudotumor of the craniocervical junction, causing serious spinal neurologic complications.[609] However, destructive spondyloarthropathy can also be due to secondary HPTH with or without brown tumors, Al intoxication, and apatite crystal deposition.[609, 610] The distinction between dialysis-related amyloidosis and the different forms of renal osteodystrophy can be difficult. Furthermore, $\beta_2$-amyloidosis may coexist with either high- or low-turnover lesions of renal osteodystrophy.

Overall, the management of dialysis-related amyloidosis in patients with CRF is unsatisfactory. In the acute setting, treatment with nonsteroidal anti-inflammatory drugs, corticosteroids, and physical therapy is rarely useful. Shoulder arthroscopic synovectomy has been shown to induce pain relief, and more radical open surgery may be of value in patients who do not respond to conservative therapy.[611] It has been shown that the use of highly permeable dialysis membranes can lower serum $\beta_2$-amyloid levels, but there is limited evidence that this has any effect on the progression of established disease; however, patients treated with polyacrylonitrile dialysis membranes from the onset of the regular dialysis seem to have a lower incidence of the disease than patients treated with standard cellulosic membranes.[604] A specific adsorbent column has also been developed to be used in direct hemoperfusion, but there is not enough experience to evaluate its effectiveness.[612] Kidney transplantation is the only alternative treatment, although the effectiveness of this modality for treating clinical manifestations of dialysis-related amyloidosis has rarely been reported.[613, 614] After successful kidney transplantation, rapid normalization of $\beta_2$-microglobulin levels occurs and the symptoms often disappear[615]; however, the histologic features of amyloidosis may persist.[614]

# RADIOGRAPHIC FEATURES OF RENAL OSTEODYSTROPHY

Both the types of radiographic abnormality encountered and the incidence of specific bone radiographic alterations of dialysis patients vary considerably in reports from different centers.[538] Such differences probably reflect some variation in the type of skeletal disease observed. Also, it is likely that differences in both the radiographic techniques employed, including type of film used, and knowledge of the radiologist are important. Thus, the apparent bone density in plain films is voltage dependent; the higher the voltage, the more "washed out" the bone appears.[616] Also, the x-ray film and automatic film-developing procedures currently in use result in radiographs of much poorer quality than those available 30 to 40 years ago.[617] Sensitive radiographs are particularly useful for views of the hands and so should be made with fine-grain film; manual rather than automatic film developing should be used, and grid or screen techniques should be omitted. Magnification techniques can add further to the sensitivity. Meema and associates[618] noted the phalanges to be normal in 67% of uremic patients using conventional techniques for x-ray films and only 8% showed subperiosteal erosions. With the introduction of better films and use of magnification techniques, only 26% appeared normal and 29% exhibited subperiosteal erosions. In our experience, there is a danger of over-reading films when using these magnification techniques; familiarity with normal variation is required.[619] It should also be mentioned that more than 50% of bone can be lost without any evidence in a radiograph because only the cortical bone is clearly noted, and an important loss of cancellous bone can occur before it is appreciated.[616]

## Radiographic Features of Secondary Hyperparathyroidism

One of the principal radiographic features of secondary HPTH is the presence of bone resorption and erosions, which may occur on the subperiosteal, intracortical, and endosteal surfaces of cortical bone. Another radiographic feature is the presence of new bone formation at the periosteal surface, a process termed periosteal neostosis.[620] Alterations of the trabecular volume of spongy bone may lead to both osteosclerosis and osteopenia.

Erosions occurring in conjunction with new bone formation may take the form of cysts or osteoclastomas (brown tumors), although these occur less commonly in secondary than in primary HPTH.[538] They may require a differential diagnosis with malignant tumors, metastasis, or cysts related to dialysis amyloidosis. Occasionally, these brown tumors are accompanied by pain, which does not increase during dialysis as it does for amyloidosis-related cysts. Although they can appear elsewhere, brown tumors develop most frequently in the maxillary region and may alter the configuration of the teeth. Subperiosteal erosions almost invariably accompany such lesions. With healing, the cystic areas may be replaced by areas of sclerosis.

Subperiosteal erosions of the phalanges identified with the use of fine-grain radiographs of the hands are the single most sensitive radiographic sign of secondary HPTH.[621] Abnormalities have been noted on radiographs in approximately 40% to 50% of patients who show increased resorptive surfaces on bone biopsy specimens[618, 621, 622]; this frequency is increased with magnification of radiographs. The appearance of bone erosions has been shown to correlate well with serum PTH levels.[619] The earliest lesions usually appear on the radial surface of the middle phalanges of the second or third digits of the dominant hand; they first appear as slight irregularities near either the proximal or the distal shoulder formed by the metaphysis of the phalanx.[538] As the lesions progress the erosions extend along a greater length of the radial surface of the phalanx (Fig. 51–22) and involve other digits and adjacent proximal and distal phalanges; erosions eventually appear on the ulnar border. The evolution of such lesions has been described in detail by Parfitt.[538] Although such erosions are generally asymptomatic, they occasionally produce erosive synovitis, which leads to soft tissue swelling, pain, and stiffness.

The tufts of the terminal phalanges of the second or third digit commonly show areas of resorption. Because of the natural occurrence of irregularities of the tuft, recognition of loss of the cortical margin may be difficult. Nonetheless, it has been possible to quantify and grade the extent of such

erosions.[619] When the erosion of a terminal tuft is severe, marked loss of its structure may result, leading to collapse of the soft tissues; this can change the contour of the fingers to such an extent that they appear to show clubbing.[623] Healing of erosions of the tuft and phalanges is believed to occur initially with replacement of poorly mineralized fibrous tissue and woven bone. Despite successful treatment and healing, the shape of the bone may not revert to normal.[624] When Al overload occurs in conjunction with the presence of significant subperiosteal erosions, remineralization and normalization of radiographs may not occur when secondary HPTH is reversed by treatment with an active vitamin D sterol or by PTX.[411] Thus, some caution must be exercised in interpreting the presence of subperiosteal erosions as a specific radiologic sign of osteitis fibrosa.

Other skeletal sites commonly showing subperiosteal erosions include the upper end of the tibia, the neck of the femur and humerus, the lower end of the radius and ulna, the ischium and pubis, the sacroiliac joints, the junction of the metaphysis and diaphysis of long bones, and the distal end of the clavicles.[538, 617] The predilection for subperiosteal erosions to occur near the junction of the metaphysis with the shaft is believed to occur because bone modeling during

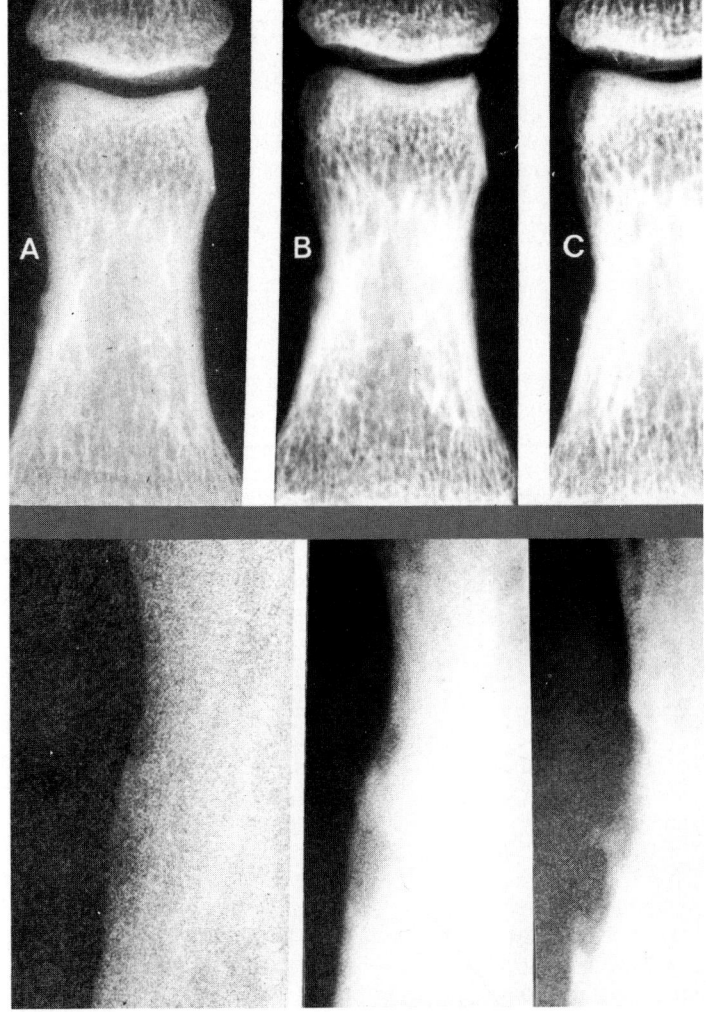

**Figure 51–22.** Serial radiographs of the right index finger of a 43-year-old man with CRF under treatment with peritoneal dialysis. These views illustrate the value of fine-grain film and the use of simple magnification techniques to detect changes in periosteal resorption. The upper panels are magnified ×3, the lower ×12. *A.* Periosteal resorption at the midshaft is poorly identified owing to the large-grain film (Kodak dental film). *B.* The radiolucent areas in the cortex are more clearly visualized, but only the higher magnification shows convincingly that there is an intact periosteal layer of bone covering these juxtaperiosteal resorption cavities. *C.* Six months later, juxtaperiosteal resorption had progressed to periosteal resorption. (*B* and *C,* Kodak M-film.) (*A* to *C* from Meema HE, Meema S: Microradioscopic quantitation of periosteal resorption in secondary hyperparathyroidism of chronic renal failure. Clin Orthop [130]:297–302, 1978.)

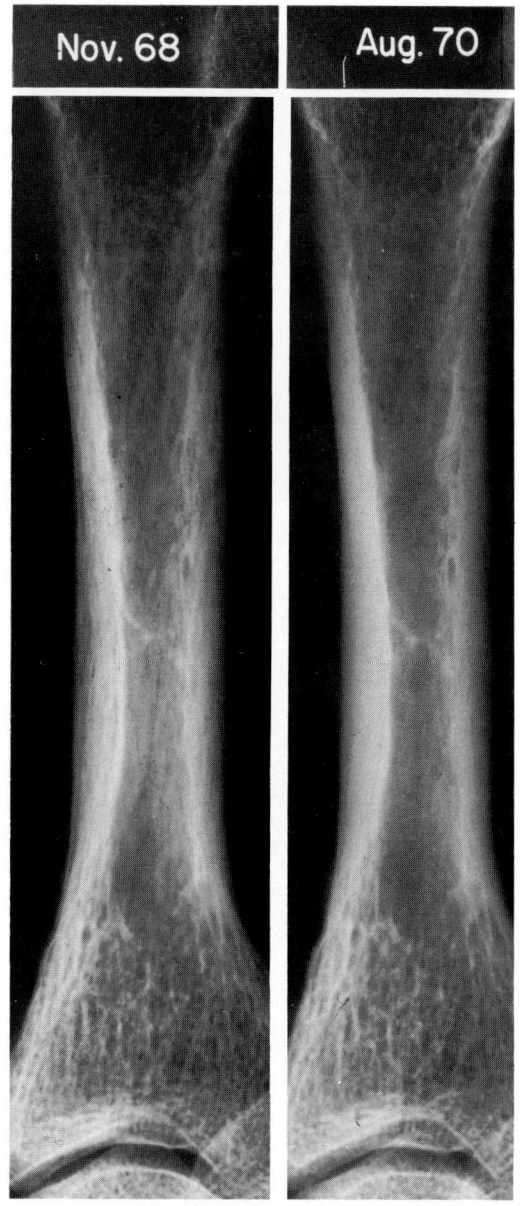

**Figure 51–23.** Magnification view of a digit obtained with fine-grain film shows increased intracortical resorption (grade +3) in a 30-year-old uremic woman before her treatment with dialysis *(left)*. Approximately 2 years later *(right)*, the intracortical resorptive tunnels had disappeared, indicating that net bone formation exceeded net resorption. (From Meema HE, Oreopoulos DG, Meema S: A roentgenologic study of cortical bone resorption in chronic renal failure. Radiology 126:67–74, 1978.)

growth into a normal triangular shape with typical metaphyseal flaring requires that surplus bone on the outer cortex be removed. Consequently, the precursor cells of mesenchymal origin are more prone to differentiate into osteoclast at this site. Such areas are often the first site of subperiosteal resorption in uremic children.[535] Typical resorption of the phalanges may be uncommon in young children, but it does occur in older adolescents and young adults; it is also less common in uremic patients older than 40 years.[625] Resorption can be seen in the skull, leading to a mottled, lucent appearance; this is commonly associated with areas of osteosclerosis.

Erosions in the lamina dura are frequently noted in primary HPTH but are less commonly observed in uremic secondary HPTH.[626] In the latter, increased resorption of bone also occurs in intracortical bone or in the haversian canals and results in increased intracortical striations on radiographs (Fig. 51–23). These cortical striations occur in a number of pathophysiologic processes associated with increased bone turnover: hyperthyroidism, acromegaly, and rapid growth spurt at adolescence. The striations are less specific for secondary HPTH than are subperiosteal erosions.[627]

Periosteal neostosis, new woven bone arising within fibrous tissue overlying the periosteum, is separated from existing bone by a radiolucent area that represents the interposed area of fibrous tissue.[620] As the process progresses, the fibrous tissue may calcify and the lucent zone disappear, and the existence of such new bone formation may be distinguished from an increased outer bone diameter.

Osteosclerosis arises because of an increase in the thickness and number of trabeculae in spongy bone. It is generally apparent only in skeletal areas composed largely of cancellous bone with little contribution of compact bone; these areas include the vertebrae, pelvis, skull, clavicle, proximal humerus, and proximal and distal femur and tibia. Patchy osteosclerosis may lead to a characteristic "rugger jersey" appearance on lateral views of the vertebrae and a "salt-and-pepper" appearance of the skull.

Radiographic alterations of the skull have been classified into four types[628]: 1) a diffuse "ground glass" appearance, with loss of sharp margins at the vascular grooves and diploic venous channels; 2) a diffuse mottled or granular appearance (the most frequent type), probably arising from a network of enlarged resorption spaces within the tables of the skull; 3) focal lucent defects, 1 to 3 cm in diameter, which may be present with or without a ground glass or mottled appearance of surrounding areas; and 4) focal areas of sclerosis. The lesions may be confused with those of Paget disease or multiple myeloma. These abnormalities of the skull may disappear after appropriate treatment (Fig. 51–24).

Radiographic changes do not correlate well with histologic characteristics.[629] Such lack of association may be related, in part, to the fact that radiographic abnormalities are most easily noted in cortical bone, whereas the bone biopsy evaluates primarily trabecular bone. Also, the presence of Al-related osteomalacia may prevent healing of erosions as secondary HPTH is reversed.[411]

## Radiographic Features of Osteomalacia

The radiographic features of osteomalacia are far less distinctive than those of secondary HPTH. Once the epiphyses have closed, the typical radiographic findings of rickets, that is, widening and splaying of the epiphyseal growth plate, do not occur. The only pathognomonic findings of osteomalacia present in adults are Looser zones or pseudofractures. These are straight, wide bands of radiolucency that abut the cortex and are usually perpendicular to the long axis of the bone; they may be bilateral and symmetric and may or may not be accompanied by a narrow area of

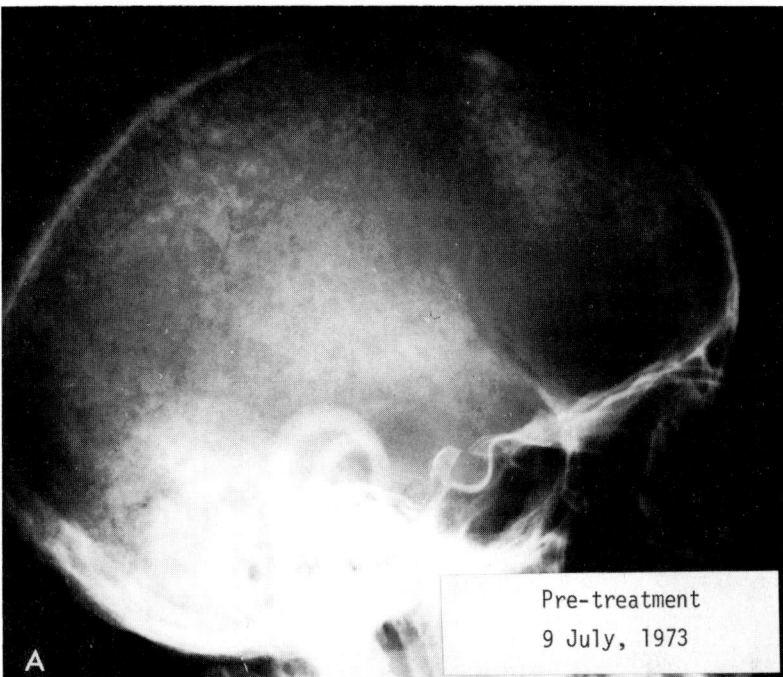

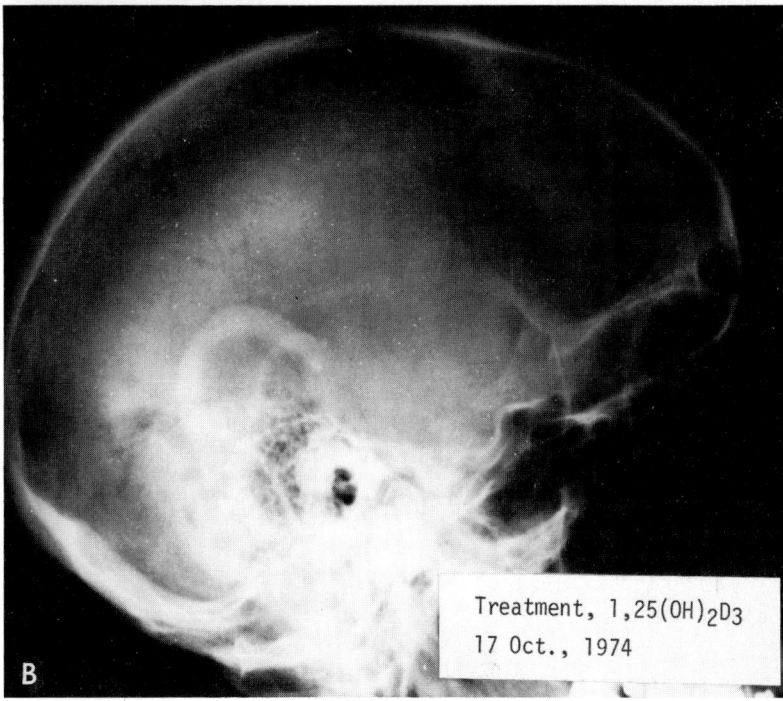

**Figure 51–24.** Abnormalities in the skull radiograph of a patient with renal osteodystrophy and bone biopsy findings of osteitis fibrosa. *A.* Bone has diffuse granular appearance with focal areas of sclerosis. *B.* After 1,25(OH)₂D treatment for 14 months, the bone appearance is improved.

sclerosis or a small, poorly mineralized callus.[538, 630] Healing or callus formation is usually minimal unless specific treatment is given. The means of distinguishing a Looser zone from a stress fracture have been outlined by Parfitt.[538] One important difference is that the initial hairline break of a stress fracture does not enlarge but heals with minimal callus formation. In uremic patients, spontaneous stress fractures commonly occur in the metatarsals or ribs with variable degrees of pain; these fractures tend to heal spontaneously but slowly with good callus formation. With mechanical stress or when vitamin D deficiency is severe and prolonged, the Looser zone, like stress fractures, may ex-

tend across the full width of bone to produce a true fracture with displacement of the fragments.[630] Looser zones have appeared remarkably infrequently in the authors' experience. Less than 2% of German dialysis patients exhibited Looser zones,[631] although they were reported in 20% of uremic patients with symptomatic osteodystrophy in Australia.[538] They can occur with osteomalacia related to Al accumulation but are infrequent; true fractures may be seen more commonly. True fractures of the ribs and hips and compression fractures of the vertebral bodies are more common in dialyzed patients with osteomalacia than in those with osteitis fibrosa.[307]

Protrusio acetabuli, identified as a convex bulging into the pelvis over the acetabulum, may be a specific feature of osteomalacia.[632] Skeletal demineralization occurs with osteomalacia but is nonspecific. Features such as increased haziness or coarsening of the trabeculae, biconcavity of the vertebral bodies (particularly in association with normal bone density), and bending deformities of long bones are said to be typical of osteomalacia; however, few radiologists can make such distinctions.[617] Uremic patients with osteomalacia may also have secondary HPTH; thus, bone erosions may coexist with osteomalacic features. In conclusion, because the features of osteomalacia are predominantly microscopic, this diagnosis can be verified only by bone histology.

## Extraskeletal Calcifications

Soft tissue calcifications of several distinct types are common in patients with end-stage renal disease. The factors that predispose to their development include serum P levels greater than 8 to 9 mg/dL and/or an increase in the $Ca^{2+} \times P$ product of plasma (greater than 70 mg$^2$/dL$^2$), overt secondary HPTH, Al toxicity, high dialysate $Ca^{2+}$ concentration, the presence of alkalosis, and local tissue injury.[633] Three major clinical varieties of extraskeletal calcifications occur in uremia: 1) calcification of medium-sized arteries; 2) periarticular calcifications; and 3) visceral calcifications, which can involve the heart, lung, and kidney. Periarticular calcifications have also been separated into three types[633]: 1) periarticular chondrocalcinosis, which can occur in both primary and secondary HPTH; 2) calcific periarthritis, with associated calcifications similar to those of typical dystrophic calcification; and 3) tumoral calcinosis, which was previously common in hemodialysis patients but is still reported.[149, 223, 634] Periarticular calcifications remain a problem in dialysis patients. Early reports of dialysis patients noted a prevalence as high as 52%.[634] Although more effective control of hyperphosphatemia and secondary HPTH may have ameliorated this problem, it is still observed in 7% to 45% of hemodialysis patients.[635–639] Table 51–7 shows some observations regarding the frequency of periarticular calcifications. This is also a problem in CAPD patients, who have a frequency varying from 12% to 22%.[637, 638] As mentioned before, tumoral or periarticular calcifications may occasionally be associated with acute periarticular inflammation with pain, stiffness, and soft tissue swelling resembling acute arthritis.

**TABLE 51–7. Frequency of Periarticular Calcifications in Dialysis Patients**

| Author | Patients (n) | Age (Range or Mean) | Calcifications n | % |
|---|---|---|---|---|
| Rubin et al[637] | 59 | 54 | 7 | 12 |
| Chou et al[636] | 68 | 51 | 5 | 7.5 |
| Benhamou et al[635] | 72 | 56 | 32 | 44 |
| Bardin et al[638] | 37 | 32–70 | 17 | 45 |
| Kessler et al[639] | 171 | 59 | 33 | 19 |

The most frequent form of vascular calcification in patients with CRF is localized in the medial layer of small and medium-sized arteries (Mönckeberg type of arterial calcification); the calcifications are diffuse and continuous along the contour of the vessel wall. Involvement is most common in diabetic patients and the radiologic appearance contrasts with the dense, irregular, and discrete appearance of calcified plaques of the intimal layer of the vessel. Vascular calcifications may be first detected as a "ring" or "tube" in the dorsalis pedis artery where it descends between the first and second metatarsals.[625] Other common sites are the ankles, feet, pelvis, hands, and wrists (Fig. 51–25). Calcifications of the medial layer often occur without any symptoms; however, the consequent rigidity and lack of compressibility of the vessel may make it difficult to palpate pulses or hear the Korotkoff sounds; also, vascular access for dialysis may be difficult to achieve. Vascular calcifications are better detected by lateral views of the ankle or anteroposterior views of the hands or feet using magnification techniques.[640] Occasionally, extensive vascular calcifications are associated with ischemic lesions and the syndrome of calciphylaxis.[515]

An evaluation of the frequency of vascular calcifications suggests that they are age related; vascular calcifications were noted in 50% of dialysis patients aged 40 to 50 years, compared with 30% in the 15- to 30-year age group. Vascular calcifications are quite uncommon but can occur in children with end-stage renal disease.[641] Meema and colleagues[642] documented the occurrence of calcifications in 36% of uremic patients not treated with dialysis, 13% of patients who had received a kidney transplant, and 8% of those undergoing hemodialysis.

The pathogenesis of these different types of extraskeletal calcification may vary; thus, visceral calcifications can occur in patients totally lacking arterial and periarticular calcification, and the converse also occurs. Most authors agree that periarticular or tumoral calcifications can be reversed by P restriction with a reduction of the $Ca^{2+} \times P$ product in plasma. However, in other series of dialysis patients, the serum $Ca^{2+} \times P$ product did not correlate with the extent of periarticular calcifications.[633] Although such calcifications may be related to the solubility product of $Ca^{2+}$ and P, other possibilities exist; thus, PTH may enhance the accumulation of $Ca^{2+}$ in soft tissues[525, 643] or poorly identified inhibitors of crystallization may be lacking. A direct role of PTH is difficult to assess, because overt secondary HPTH is usually associated with a high $Ca^{2+} \times P$ product. Furthermore, although PTX may lead to improvement of soft tissue calcification,[644] regression of this calcification does not always occur.[644]

Zins and co-workers[223] observed that overt secondary HPTH appeared not to be a prerequisite for the occurrence of tumoral calcification in hemodialysis patients. Eight of 10 patients had evidence of Al overload; thus, Al intoxication may play a pathogenic role in the development of some tumoral calcifications. Furthermore, the tumoral calcifications may regress during Al chelation therapy despite aggravation of the concomitantly present secondary HPTH.[149] Duration of dialysis may play a role; Tatler and colleagues[625] noted that the frequency of calcification increased with time during a 10-year period of hemodialysis treat-

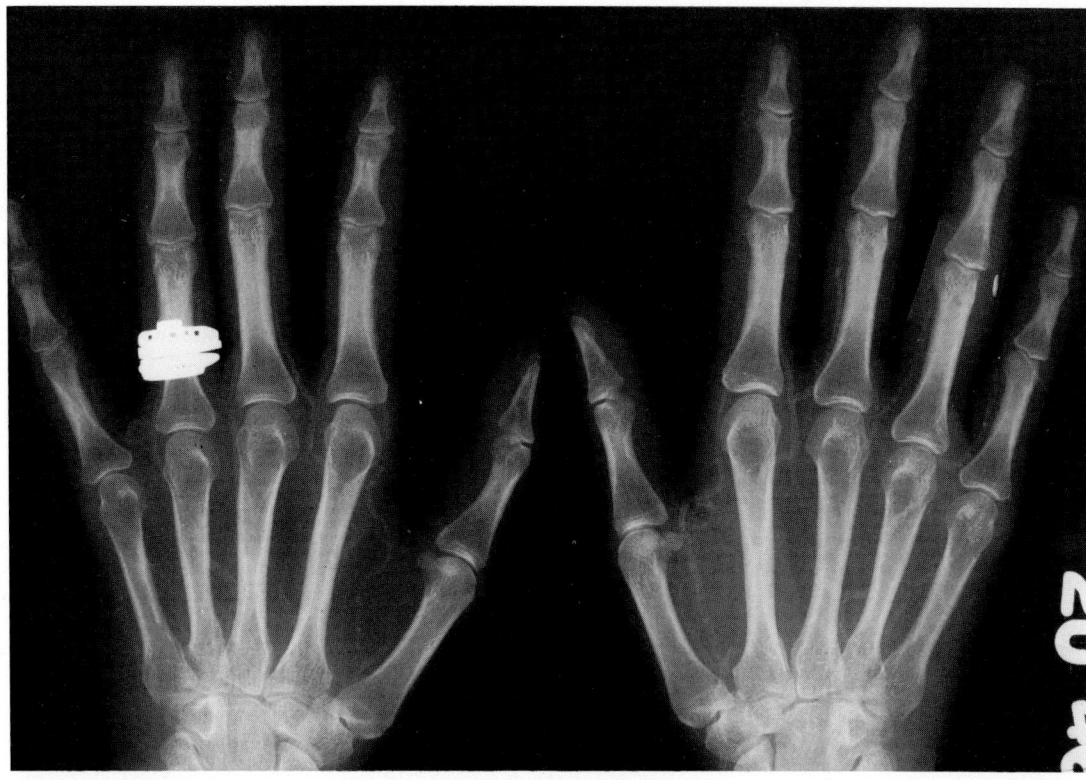

**Figure 51–25.** Radiographs show extensive calcification of the arteries of the hands; the fine, lacy appearance, resembling an arteriogram, is characteristic of calcification involving the media of arteries.

ment, despite the maintenance of an average serum P concentration and a $Ca^{2+} \times P$ product below 70 $mg^2/dL^2$.

It is our strong impression that the dialysate $Ca^{2+}$ concentration may be an important factor in the development of soft tisue calcifications. During the past two decades, a dialysate $Ca^{2+}$ concentration of 3.5 mEq/L has been commonly used. The prevalence of soft tissue calcifications has been shown to decrease only from 68% in the period 1981 to 1983 to 57% in 1991 to 1992.[645] The intradialytic $Ca^{2+}$ concentration dramatically increases in patients dialyzed with a 3.5 mEq/L dialysate $Ca^{2+}$. Furthermore, the rate of $Ca^{2+}$ loss from the dialysate to the patient is significant. The intradialytic $Ca^{2+}$ increment totally disappears 1 hour after dialysis (Fig. 51–26). It is quite possible that this decrement in serum $Ca^{2+}$ may represent rapid deposition of $Ca^{2+}$ into soft tissues.

Visceral calcifications are rather infrequent and may differ from arterial and periarticular calcifications in chemical characteristics and pathogenesis[633, 646]; thus, visceral calcifications are associated with factors such as tissue dystro-

**Figure 51–26.** Intradialytic changes in serum $Ca^{2+}$ in five patients undergoing standard hemodialysis session of 4 hours (dialysate $Ca^{2+}$, 3.5 mEq/L). Note the increase in serum $Ca^{2+}$ and the fall to baseline values by 1 hour after dialysis. (Courtesy of F Llach.)

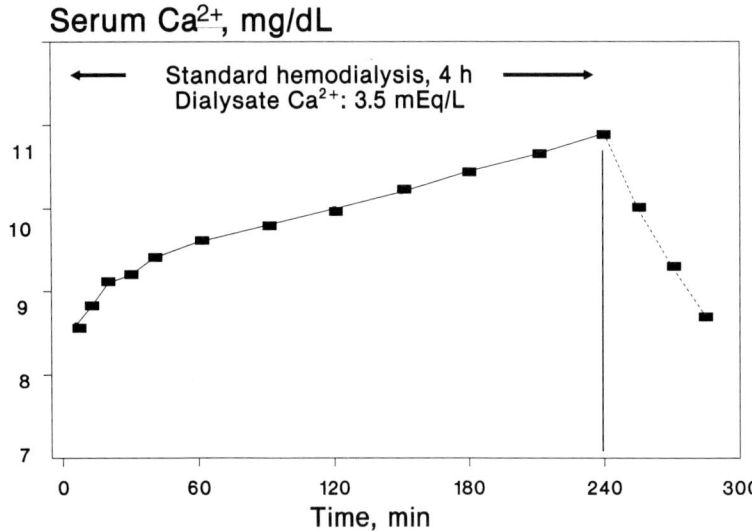

**Serum $Ca^{2+}$, mg/dL**

Standard hemodialysis, 4 h
Dialysate $Ca^{2+}$: 3.5 mEq/L

Time, min

phy.[633] Visceral calcification exists as amorphous calcium phosphate. Usually, amorphous calcium phosphate is rapidly converted to apatite at a physiologic pH; the lack of such conversion led to the inference that increased pyrophosphate content of bone and serum might account for the occurrence of visceral calcifications.[355, 423] Contrary to the idea that soft tissue calcification may be associated with secondary HPTH, Contiguglia and colleagues[646] noted that the degree of secondary HPTH, based on either parathyroid size at autopsy or serum $Ca^{2+} \times P$ product, was not related to the extent of soft tissue calcifications observed in uremic patients at autopsy. Kuzela and associates[647] observed morphologic evidence of visceral calcification in 6 of 56 patients who died with CRF. Lungs, heart, kidneys, skeletal muscle, and stomach are the organs mainly involved, and visceral calcification may give rise to serious symptoms. Thus, atrioventricular block may occur because of deposition of $Ca^{2+}$ in the cardiac conduction system; intractable cardiac failure has been related to the extensive replacement of myocardium with calcifications.[646, 648, 649] Extensive pulmonary calcifications may lead to diffuse thickening of alveolar septa. Such calcifications are rarely extensive enough to be seen by radiography.[650] Various alterations of pulmonary function, including reduced vital capacity, reduced carbon monoxide diffusion, and low $Po_2$ have been observed after death in patients subsequently shown to have severe pulmonary calcifications. Such pulmonary calcifications may be detected with the technetium pyrophosphate scan,[651] but the disorder can often persist even after successful kidney transplantation and/or PTX.

Finally, an increased $Ca^{2+} \times P$ product may lead to increased $Ca^{2+}$ deposition in the kidney, and this may play a role in either accelerating or aggravating the progression of CRF.[652, 653] In the study by Lumlertgul and co-workers,[653] P absorption was reduced by giving dihydroxyaluminum aminoacetate to P-restricted rats while the P-replete group received glycine; the groups were pair-fed to ensure similar intakes of total calories, protein, carbohydrate, vitamins, and minerals. The tissue content of $Ca^{2+}$ in the heart, aorta, and kidneys was higher in the P-replete than in the P-restricted group; the P-replete rats had more glomerular sclerosis, interstitial inflammation with fibrosis, and greater tubule atrophy. Thus, P independent of protein restriction can retard the progression of renal insufficiency in rats after partial nephrectomy.[653] Also, the use of a low-P diet in partially nephrectomized rats was associated with little or no progression of renal insufficiency, whereas CRF progressed in animals receiving normal dietary levels of P.[652] In clinical studies, Barsotti and co-workers[654] prospectively compared two groups of patients with moderate renal CRF who were given low-protein diets; one group received a low-P diet that provided P at 6.5 mg/kg/d, and the other group consumed a diet with 12 mg/kg/d. The rate of progression of CRF was greater with the higher protein intake. The data suggest that some benefit may be obtained in reducing P intake to decrease the rate of progression of CRF.

## Osteopenia or Osteoporosis

A common radiographic feature of patients with advanced CRF is decreased density of bone, which can arise from either secondary HPTH or osteomalacia and therefore is nonspecific. Parfitt and colleagues[655] applied the term dialysis osteopenia to a syndrome characterized by a substantial reduction in bone density with an incidence of bone pain and fractures that is increased out of proportion to the radiographic and histologic evidence for either osteomalacia or osteitis fibrosa. The radiographic findings have been likened to those noted in the idiopathic osteoporosis of young adults. Features include loss of cortical bone from the endosteal surface, periarticular rarefaction, loss of trabecular bone with a honeycomb or fishnet pattern, and fractures that are somewhat intermediate in appearance between stress fractures and typical Looser zones. Unfortunately, detailed biochemical and histologic studies with radiologic correlations in patients described two decades ago with this syndrome are not available; it is most likely that it represents the radiologic counterpart of Al-related bone disease with osteomalacia or ABD.

## Dialysis-Related Amyloidosis

Radiologic findings of dialysis-related amyloidosis are usually present before the onset of pain. A periarticular cystic bone lesion located in sites such as carpal and tarsal bones, femoral head, humeral head, distal radius, acetabulum, pubic symphysis, and tibial plateau strongly suggests dialysis-related amyloidosis.[597–599, 656] Although these lesions can be characteristic, they are not pathognomonic and it is necessary to demostrate the presence of $\beta_2$-amyloid deposit.[657]

As mentioned before, brown tumors should be distinguished from amyloid-related cysts; the former usually appear in the metaphysis and epyphysis of tubular bones and are rarely located in carpal bones (Fig. 51–27). The amyloid-related cysts involve large joints and are restricted to the vicinity of synovial joints, without correlation with subperiosteal resorption. Thus, the occurrence of subchondral cysts appears to be specific to dialysis-related amyloidosis.[658] The presence of multiple rather than solitary cysts also suggests amyloid deposition. Fractures can develop in bones weakened by such cysts.[495, 596] Also, bone cysts have been shown to persist even after successful kidney transplantation.[602] Magnetic resonance imaging seems to be a technique well suited to show the extent and distribution of articular disease,[659] including the upper cervical spine.[660] Finally, ultrasonography has been helpful in the diagnosis of this disorder.[661]

## SCINTISCAN AND ULTRASONOGRAPHY

Skeletal scintigraphy using $^{99m}$Tc-labeled pyrophosphate provides a sensitive method for the detection of skeletal alterations in patients with CRF. The technique allows a noninvasive follow-up evaluation of the response to treatment. Although the mechanism responsible for the accumulation of pyrophosphate in bone has not been elucidated, evidence indicates that the pyrophosphate accumulates in areas of increased bone turnover.[662] Rosenthal and Kaye[663]

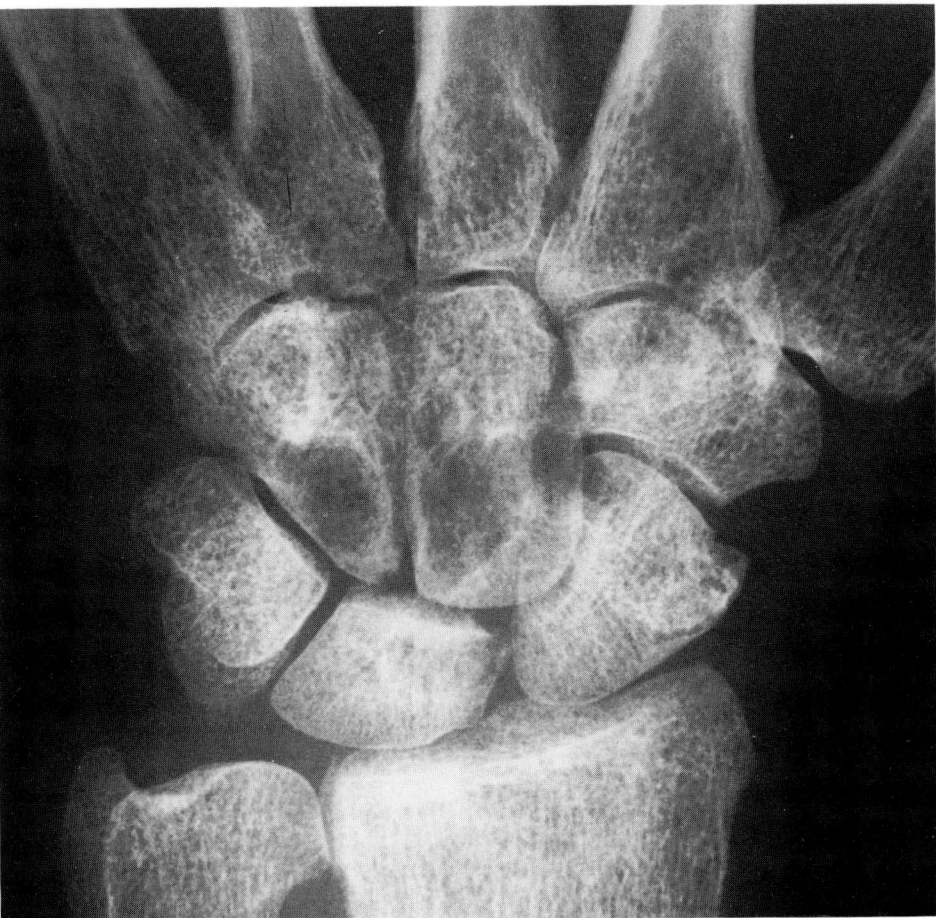

**Figure 51–27.** Radiograph of the wrist of a patient with dialysis amyloidosis; there are multiple cysts in the carpal bones. (From Fenves AZ, Emmett M, White MG, et al: Carpal tunnel syndrome with cystic bone lesions secondary to amyloidosis in chronic hemodialysis patients. Am J Kidney Dis 7:130, 1986.)

suggested that pyrophosphate accumulates in skeletal areas with abnormal collagen metabolism, including either osteitis fibrosa or osteomalacia. From evaluation of the uptake of the isotopes over the distal femur, Lien and associates[664] calculated the bone/soft tissue ratio of isotope uptake. Abnormal uptake was found in 78% of long-term dialysis patients and in a similar proportion of patients with chronic CRF who were not undergoing regular dialysis. On the basis of a correlation between bone uptake of $^{99m}$Tc-labeled pyrophosphate and urinary excretion of hydroxyproline, the authors concluded that increased skeletal uptake in uremia is related to the presence of immature collagen.[664] Others have noted abnormal scintiscans in 13 of 14 patients undergoing dialysis.[665] Symmetrically increased activity was noted over the skull, mandible, sternum, shoulders, vertebrae, and distal aspects of the femur and tibia. Uptake of the labeled pyrophosphate over certain areas, such as the mandible, was pronounced and appeared before radiographic abnormalities. Olgaard and co-workers[666] noted that 90% of patients undergoing regular dialysis had pathologic pyrophosphate accumulation on scintiscans, and radiographic abnormalities were present in only one third (Fig. 51–28). The scintiscan can also be used to detect soft tissue calcifications, particularly in the lungs.[651] Finally, abnormal scintiscans are more common in dialysis patients who previously received renal homografts; intensive glucocorticoid treatment may aggravate the abnormalities responsible for an abnormal scintiscan.

In the presence of low-turnover bone disease, bone scintiscans may reveal increased uptake at sites of either true fractures or pseudofractures, particularly the ribs, pelvis, and scapulae (Fig. 51–29); these may be seen on scintiscans at a time when they cannot be detected by radiography.[490] In general, however, pyrophosphate uptake is usually less in patients with Al-related osteomalacia than in those with osteitis fibrosa; the uptake may increase strikingly during chelation therapy. Thus, it is possible to differentiate between patients with osteitis fibrosa and osteomalacia from Al intoxication by the uptake in a bone scan.[667] However, patients with mixed lesions on biopsy specimens may be difficult to identify. Other authors noted that bone scans do not agree closely with the type or severity of renal osteodystrophy.[668] Timing the hemodialysis sessions before scintigraphic imaging has been suggested, because they seem to reduce nonspecific high soft tissue activity, allowing bone uptake to be assessed more accurately.[669] It appears that although the bone scintiscan may help to establish the severity and/or type of bone disease in some patients, at present this technique is of limited value in the clinical evaluation of skeletal abnormalities in CRF.

Subtraction thallium 201–technetium 99m ($^{201}$Tl-$^{99m}$Tc) scintigraphy has been suggested as a valuable technique in the diagnosis of the localization of enlarged parathyroid glands. Thallium is a potassium analogue and distributes in relation to blood flow and state of the Na$^+$,K$^+$-ATPase system.[670] Both thyroid and parathyroid glands exhibit in-

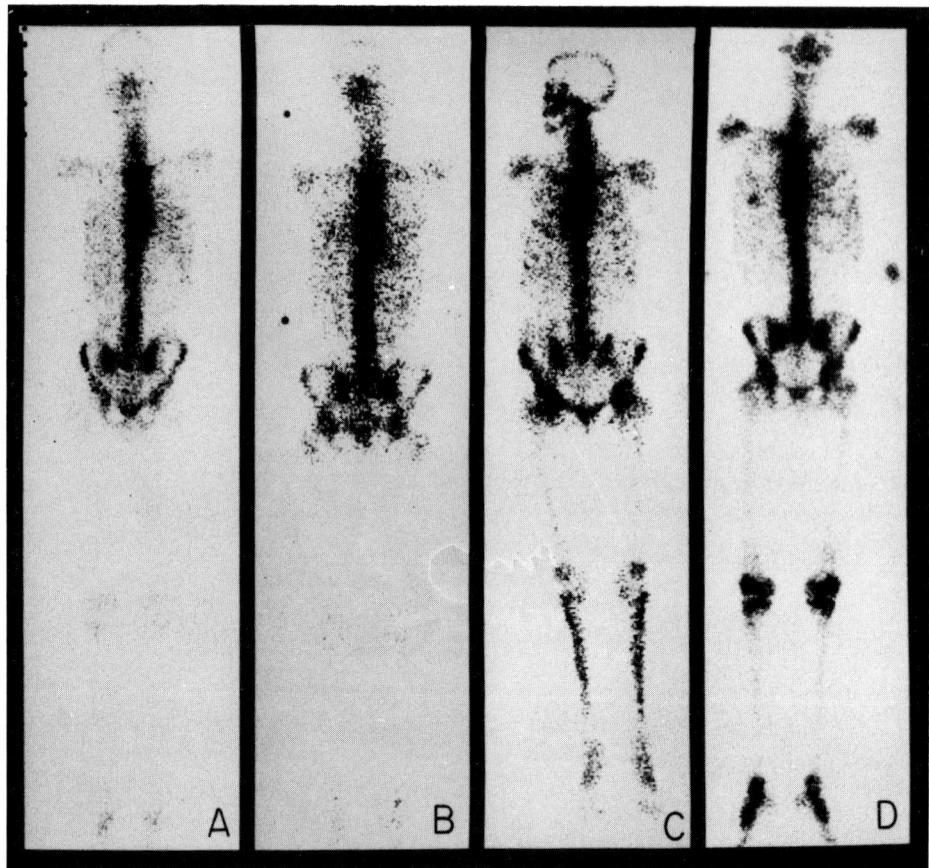

**Figure 51–28.** Scintiscans of bone, obtained with technetium-labeled diphosphonate, in a normal subject *(A)* and in selected patients with renal failure *(B, C,* and *D).* The severity of the abnormality has been graded 0 through 3; *A* represents grade 0, a normal scintiscan; *B* shows grade 1, with normal uptake in the femoral head but extension into the femoral neck and trochanteric region; *C* illustrates grade 2, showing abnormal uptake in the femoral head and neck and in the proximal half of the tibial shaft; *D* represents grade 3, with extensive uptake of technetium in the femoral head, the femoral and tibial condyles, the tarsi, and the proximal part of the metatarsi. (*A* to *D* from Ølgaard K, Heerfordt J, Madsen S: Scintigraphic skeletal changes in uremic patients on regular hemodialysis. Nephron 17:325–334, 1976. S Karger AG, Basel, publisher.)

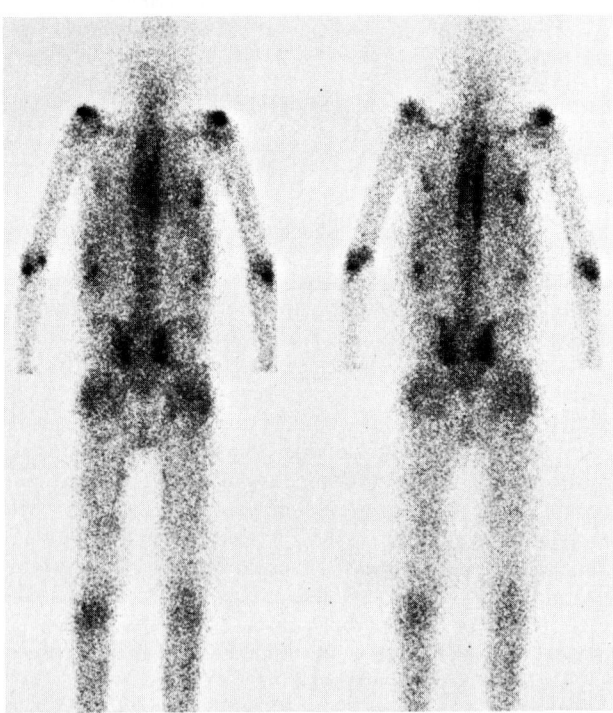

**Figure 51–29.** Scintiscan of bone utilizing $^{99m}$Tc-labeled pyrophosphate in a dialysis patient with osteomalacia arising from Al accumulation. There is only modest uptake of radioisotope at metaphyseal sites and in the skull; prominent uptake is observed in ribs at sites of pseudofractures, and there is a generalized increase in background uptake.

creased uptake of thallium relative to the surrounding tissue. By contrast, technetium is taken up only by the thyroid; thus, an image of the parathyroid gland can be obtained by subtracting the technetium from the thallium image. Subtraction $^{201}$Tl-$^{99m}$Tc scintigraphy is most useful before reoperation in patients with a failed initial surgery because the scan may aid in locating an ectopic gland or an abnormal gland in a patient with surgically altered anatomy.[670, 671] Scintigraphy with $^{201}$Tl plus iodine 131 or 123 can also be used to locate abnormal parathyroid glands with an efficacy at least similar than that with $^{201}$Tl-$^{99m}$Tc.[672]

Other scintigraphic techniques have been developed as noninvasive procedures for assessing bone pathology in dialysis patients. It has been noted that serum PTH and the severity of subperiosteal resorption correlated with the $^{51}$Cr-EDTA/$^{99m}$Tc-medronate ratio.[673] EDTA and medronate are handled identically by the body except that the latter is taken up by osteoblasts; thus, a low ratio indicates increased osteoblastic activity.

Finally, a radiodiagnostic test using serum amyloid P component labeled with $^{123}$I has been shown to detect the amyloid fibril ligand for this protein.[674] Similarly, a $^{131}$I-labeled $\beta_2$-microglobulin has also been developed to assist in the diagnosis of dialysis-related amyloidosis.[675] The relative value of these techniques needs further evaluation.[669]

Ultrasonography has been suggested as a useful noninvasive method in evaluating the size of the parathyroid glands in secondary HPTH. Patients with enlarged glands had a higher frequency of radiologic features of secondary

HPTH than did those with undetected glands. Bone and joint pains and higher levels of serum alkaline phosphatase and intact PTH have also been noted in these patients.[676] Ultrasonography has also been used to monitor the treatment of secondary HPTH with calcitriol; a decrease of the size of the glands has been reported after calcitriol therapy.[677] Preliminary data also suggest that ultrasonography may be useful in the recognition and localization of graft-dependent recurrent secondary HPTH.[678] However, there is not enough experience with this technique in the diagnosis of secondary HPTH to reach a final conclusion. Ultrasonography has been also valuable in the diagnosis of dialysis-related amyloidosis; it can detect and quantify the swelling of articular and periarticular soft tissue such as joint capsules, synovia, and tendons usually seen in this disease.[661, 679, 680] In a study using high-resolution ultrasonography of the shoulder, the presence of rotator cuffs greater than 8 mm in thickness and/or echogenic pads between muscle groups of the rotator cuff had a sensitivity of 72% and a specificity of 97% in the diagnosis of dialysis-related amyloidosis.[661]

## QUANTITATIVE MEASUREMENTS OF BONE MINERAL CONTENT

### Metacarpal Index

The metacarpal index can be obtained by measuring the dimensions of the cortex of a metacarpal bone on x-ray film using magnification and a special caliper.[681] Normal data are available for the second left metacarpal, and the metacarpal index is the ratio of cortical to total bone width. On the basis of the assumption that this bone is a perfect cylinder, the ratio of cross-sectional cortical area to total cross section can be calculated.[682] The metacarpal index has been validated by direct comparison with measurement of bone ash.[683] Observations of patients with primary HPTH have suggested that total bone area is increased while the cortical area is reduced.[684] In patients with CRF not treated with dialysis, the metacarpal index was found to be reduced in 20% to 40%.[618, 627] One study suggested that the metacarpal index progressively decreases with duration of dialysis.[685] Sugisaki and co-workers,[686] monitoring the metacarpal index, performed long-term observations of 44 hemodialysis patients for 9 years to assess the combined effects of changes in therapeutic modality during this period. They observed that from 1980 to 1984, bone mineral content deteriorated significantly, but it improved from 1984 on. The combined effect of $HCO_3^-$ dialysate, the use of active derivatives of vitamin D, and removal of Al are suggested explanations.

### Photon Absorptiometry

Another noninvasive method for the serial evaluation of the skeleton is single-photon absorptiometry,[687, 688] in which the absorption of photons emitted from an isotopic source is used to assess the mineral content of bone. The isotopes employed, iodine 125 and americium 241, emit photons of specific, narrow wavelengths and low energy.[689] Such measurements are taken over the phalanges, the radius and ulna, and the femur. Hahn and Hahn[690] measured both the distal radius, which is primarily trabecular bone, and the midshaft of the radius, which is compact bone; this has enabled them to evaluate the ratio of these two types of bone, which have different turnover rates. Griffiths and colleagues[691] noted the mineral content of the midradius and ulna to be lower in dialysis patients than in age-matched control subjects; they also observed a progressive loss of bone with increasing duration of dialysis treatment. In a subsequent study they reported that most women receiving dialysis maintained a stable bone mineral content, whereas 44% of men lost bone mass.[692] No significant correlation was noted between single-photon absorptiometry scores and histomorphometric parameters.[346]

Photon absorptiometry appears to be more accurate than the methods that measure bone density from radiographs; however, the measurements are limited to certain sites of the skeleton that are primarily cortical bone. It should be noted that bone mineral content can be reduced as a result of several causes: 1) primary reduction in volume of bone tissue, 2) increase in intracortical porosity as a consequence of enlarged haversian canals, or 3) replacement of normally mineralized bone by unmineralized osteoid or poorly mineralized woven bone.[538] The measurement of bone density by photon absorptiometry does not allow distinction between these causes; the technique is best used when serial measurements are obtained for quantifying bone mineral and the results are evaluated in conjunction with findings on fine-detail radiographs.

Dual-beam photon absorptiometry uses two separate isotopes or a dual-photon source (gadolinium 153), permitting the subtraction of overlying soft tissue mass from that of bone. The technique can thus be used to measure the mineral content of sites of the skeleton lying deep within tissues; it is useful for assessing the mineral content of vertebral bodies and the femoral neck.[693–696] With the advent of dual-energy x-ray bone absorptiometry, a more precise and complete evaluation of bone mineral content can be obtained. Instead of a radioactive source of energy it uses x-rays at two energy levels. Preliminary observations with this more advanced technique suggest that it may be valuable in the follow-up of dialysis patients with bone disease rather than diagnosis.[697] However, the presence of normal bone density shown by noninvasive techniques does not exclude the presence of bone disease.[346, 698]

### Neutron Activation

Neutron activation provides a more accurate method for measuring total $Ca^{2+}$ or bone mineral content either in the entire body or in isolated parts of the skeleton. This technique requires the availability of a neutron source to activate $Ca^{2+}$ and other elements in the skeleton and immediate access to a whole body counter to measure the short-lived radionuclides. This technique has proved useful mainly in research studies of bone mineral content in uremic patients, and it may be particularly helpful when serial measurements are used to evaluate the effects of a specific treatment modality.[699]

## Quantitative Computed Tomography

Computed tomography has been applied to measure the mineral content of the vertebral bodies.[346, 700–702] Several computed tomographic "cuts" of vertebrae are compared with a standard. It is of value in conditions, such as osteoporosis, that affect primarily the trabecular bone and axial skeleton. It also has the theoretic advantage that is less affected by volume than dual-photon absorptiometry or the newest dual-energy x-ray bone absorptiometry[703] but it gives a high radiation dose. It has not been applied widely to renal osteodystrophy, but, no significant correlation was noted between quantitative computed tomography and histomorphometric parameters.[346]

## HISTOLOGIC FEATURES OF RENAL OSTEODYSTROPHY

The systematic performance of bone biopsy and histologic evaluation of bone in dialysis patients has advanced significantly the understanding of the various bone lesions and established appropiate guidelines in the management of renal osteodystrophy. The techniques for sampling, preparing, and interpreting microscopic sections of bone have improved, and laboratories that are specialized for processing and preparing undecalcified sections of bone are now available. The use of tetracycline labeling has allowed the evaluation of bone formation rate, mineral apposition rate, and other dynamic parameters of bone. The development of a staining method by Maloney and colleagues[213] to determine bone Al deposits has helped in the understanding of Al-induced bone disease. Bone biopsy has now been performed safely in many patients with various bone diseases studied in centers throughout the world.[235, 704] For more detailed information, the reader is referred to excellent reviews regarding technique and processing of bone biopsy specimens as well as a comprehensive exposition of the histologic features of renal osteodystrophy.[705, 706]

Renal osteodystrophy is a term used to include a wide spectrum of histologic lesions ranging from high- to low-bone-turnover states, as defined by dynamic parameters, such as the bone formation rate. It has been shown that bone formation rate is increased in patients with osteitis fibrosa but is decreased in patients showing a mineralizing defect of osteomalacia or aplastic bone disease (ABD).[193, 705]

The majority of untreated patients with advanced renal disease have high-turnover bone disease caused by the effect of high serum PTH levels on bone. Its histologic lesion is osteitis fibrosa (Figs. 51–30 and 51–31). This lesion is characterized by increased bone resorption, extensive osteoclastic and osteoblastic activity, and progressive increase in endosteal fibrosis. Osteoblastic activity is extensive; it is represented by excess unmineralized osteoid and correlates with active bone resorption. The number of osteoclasts is markedly increased in osteitis fibrosa; the osteoclasts are frequently multinucleate and large. In addition to exten-

sively increased surface resorption, there are numerous dissecting cavities through which the osteoclasts tunnel into individual trabeculae (see Fig. 51–30B).

The presence of endosteal fibrosis is also characteristic of osteitis fibrosa; the fibrosis can first be appreciated in the resorption lacunae. With continued stimulation, the endosteal fibrosis extends beyond the resorption cavities in a narrow band along the peritrabecular surface. The next stage of extension is represented by bridging of fibrosis between spicules. Finally, the fibrosis may occupy a large, contiguous area of marrow space. Bone mineralization, as assessed by tetracycline labeling, may be increased or normal, although there may be abundant osteoid containing many active osteoblasts. Active resorption surface, number of osteoclasts, and increased fibrosis have been correlated with parathyroid gland weight and serum levels of PTH.[704, 707]

Another feature of osteitis fibrosa is the alignment of strands of collagen in the bone matrix (osteoid) in an irregular, haphazard, woven pattern, which contrasts with the normal parallel alignment of strands of collagen in lamellar bone. This disorganized structure of collagen in woven bone may lead to defective physical properties of bone in response to stress. Woven osteoid is capable of becoming mineralized in the absence of vitamin D; however, the $Ca^{2+}$ is often deposited as amorphous calcium phosphate rather than as hydroxyapatite. Such deposition in woven osteoid may explain the presence of osteosclerosis.[708]

Mild features of osteitis fibrosa may be already present in early CRF. Malluche and colleagues[19] carried out bone biopsies in 22 patients with creatinine clearances between 40 and 117 mL/min. Among the patients having a creatinine clearance rate above 60 mL/min, 40% exhibited an increase in woven osteoid, which probably indicates the previous existence of increased osteoclastic resorption and high bone turnover. Both the fraction of surface showing active osteoclast and osteoid volume were normal in these patients. Evidence of a mineralization defect, although present in some patients with creatinine clearance rates above 40 mL/min/1.73 m², was unusual; moreover, a severe mineralizing defect was noted only in patients with more advanced CRF. The authors interpreted their findings in early CRF as consistent with excess PTH acting on bone.[19]

On the other side of the spectrum of the renal osteodystrophies are osteomalacia and ABD, which represent the low-bone-turnover states. Osteomalacia is characterized by an excess of unmineralized lamellar osteoid, providing wide osteoid seams (see Figs. 51–30C and 51–31C). The osteoid arises from impaired mineralization of the bone protein matrix. A marked decrease or absence of bone mineralization is present. Other features of osteomalacia include the absence of cell activity and endosteal fibrosis. The presence of increased unmineralized osteoid does not itself imply the presence of a mineralization defect (as in osteomalacia); increased quantities of unmineralized osteoid appear in conditions associated with high rates of skeletal turnover, and mineralization can lag behind the synthesis of matrix (as in secondary HPTH). In these situations, tetracycline labeling can identify the presence of increased or decreased mineralization.

The frequency of osteomalacia appears to have a marked

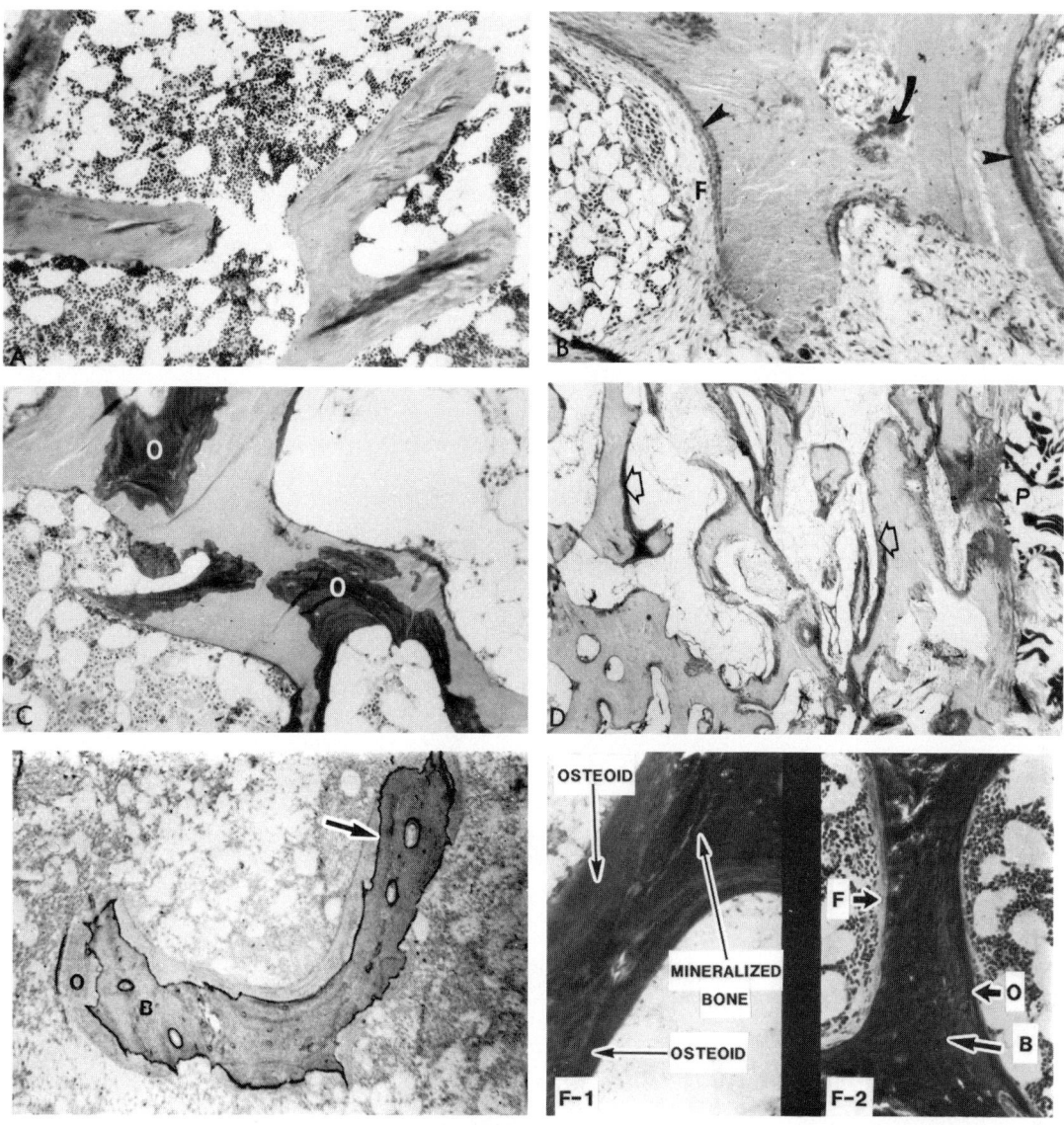

**Figure 51–30.** Black-and-white prints of photomicrographs showing the same areas of bone as those appearing in color in Figure 51–31. *A.* Normal trabecular bone (undecalcified Goldner stain; original magnification × 100). *B.* Osteitis fibrosa in a patient with renal failure, with excess unmineralized osteoid covered by osteoblasts *(arrow)* and peritrabecular marrow fibrosis *(F)* (undecalcified Goldner stain; original magnification × 100). *C.* Osteomalacia in a patient with renal failure, showing wide osteoid seams (undecalcified Goldner stain; original magnification × 100). *D.* Low-power view of cortical and trabecular bone in a patient with long-standing renal failure and osteosclerosis. There is a loss of distinction between cortical and trabecular bone, and wide osteoid seams are present *(arrows).* The periosteum (P) is in the right-hand corner (undecalcified, modified Masson stain; original magnification × 40). *E.* Low-power view of trabecular bone from a patient with Al-related osteomalacia. Al is stained as a dark band along the mineralizing front between mineralized bone (B) and areas of widened osteoid (undecalcified aluminon stain according to Maloney et al[709]; original magnification × 100). *F.* Views of two separate bone biopsy specimens in a patient with Al-related osteomalacia before *(F-1)* and after *(F-2)* weekly infusions of deferoxamine. Before treatment there are wide osteoid seams surrounding the mineralized bone; features of osteitis fibrosa are absent. On the right, there is substantial reduction in the width of the osteoid seams and there is the development of modest peritrabecular fibrosis *(arrow)* (undecalcified Goldner stain; original magnification × 160). (*A, B, C, D,* and *F* courtesy of SL Teitelbaum; *E* courtesy of DJ Sherrard.)

geographic variation. Osteomalacia was initially observed in patients receiving maintenance dialysis.[206, 307] More recently, patients with osteomalacia have been reported before the initiation of maintenance dialysis.[269, 270] As discussed earlier, epidemiologic evidence has implicated the presence of Al in the water[472] and, by removing Al by pretreatment of water with reverse osmosis, the incidence of osteomalacia has been dramatically reduced. With the advent of the Maloney stain for Al (aluminon), it has been

shown that the great majority of osteomalacic dialysis patients have large deposits of Al in the bone.[213, 709] The characteristic pattern is linear deposition of Al along the interface between trabecular bone and osteoid[213] (see Figs. 51–30*E* and 51–31*E*). The degree of osteomalacia has been noted to correlate closely with bone Al content, whether the latter is analyzed biochemically or histologically.[86, 213] Also, stainable Al has been shown to be more sensitive than total bone Al in identifying Al toxicity.[250] Others[214] have noted

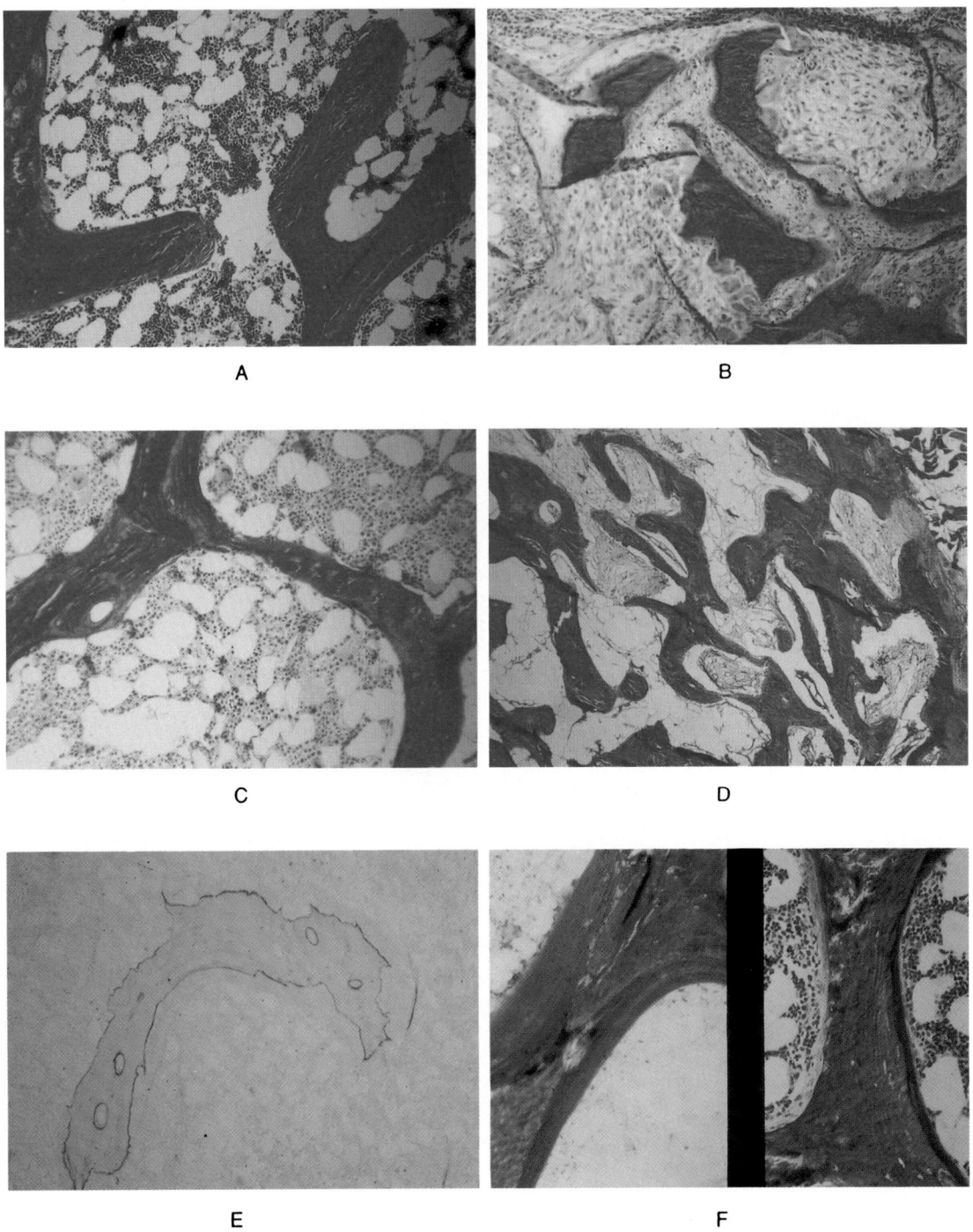

**Figure 51–31.** Color photomicrographs showing representative features of renal osteodystrophy. *A.* Normal trabecular bone. Mineralized bone matrix is stained blue; there is little unmineralized osteoid (undecalcified, modified Masson stain; original magnification × 100). *B.* Osteitis fibrosa in renal failure. There is an excess of unmineralized osteoid, which is stained red and lined by osteoblasts, and numerous multinucleate osteoclasts are present. Note that marrow fibrosis is evident (undecalcified, modified Masson stain; original magnification × 100). *C.* Osteomalacia with wide osteoid seams (red-staining material) in a patient with renal failure (undecalcified, modified Masson stain; original magnification × 100). *D.* Low-power view of cortical and trabecular bone in a patient with long-standing renal failure and osteosclerosis. There is a loss of distinction between cortical and trabecular bone, and wide osteoid seams are present (red material). The periosteum can be seen in the upper right-hand corner. (Undecalcified, modified Masson stain; original magnification × 40.) *E.* Low-power view of trabecular bone stained for Al. The Al stains as a bright red band at the junction between mineralized bone (the pale blue in the center) and wide osteoid seams (paler area surrounding the bone). In this patient with Al-related osteomalacia, nearly all the forming surface is positive for Al (undecalcified, modified aluminon stain according to Maloney et al.[709]) *F.* Higher power views of two separate bone biopsies in a dialysis patient with Al-related osteomalacia before *(left)* and after *(right)* chelation therapy with weekly infusions of deferoxamine. Before therapy, there are widened osteoid seams (red) surrounding mineralized bone (blue). After therapy, there is a marked reduction in the osteoid thickness and there is the appearance of peritrabecular fibrosis. Normal marrow elements are seen to the right of the trabeculum (undecalcified, Goldner stain; original magnification × 160). Except for the area shown in *B,* these figures show findings similar to those labeled in black and white in Figure 51–30. (*A, B, C, D,* and *F* courtesy of SL Teitelbaum; *E* courtesy of DJ Sherrard.)

that Al localized on the bone surface correlates better with evidence of osteoblastic toxicity than Al at other sites. Furthermore, the standard aluminon stain correlates strongly with total bone Al, suggesting that this stain accurately reflects Al toxicity.[213, 304] However, although some authors suggest that any amount of Al deposited in bone is toxic,[710, 711] others believe that bone formation is usually normal until bone surface Al is more than 25%, and thus this is the arbitrary cutoff often used to distinguish symptomatic bone disease.[712] Other authors even consider Al deposits no more than an epiphenomenon.[713] A new and more sensitive stain (acid solochrome azurine) has been developed,[714] raising further questions about the toxic role of Al at low levels of exposure.[711] However, clinicopathologic correlations are still lacking.

Another type of low-bone-turnover lesion observed in dialysis patients is ABD.[308, 309] This entity is characterized histologically by features similar to those observed in osteomalacia; the major difference is the absence of large osteoid seams.[310–312] These patients also have a deficiency of cellular activity; thus osteoblasts and osteoclasts are also commonly decreased. Al deposits can be present both at the osteoid-bone interface and on the surface of trabecular bone. However, as discussed earlier, ABD is being increasingly noted without the presence of Al staining in bone. The histologic features of this entity are similar to those of Al-related ABD; however, Al deposits are not present. This lesion has been observed with increasing frequency in the elderly, diabetic patients, CAPD patients, and patients switched from Al gels to calcium salts for serum P control.[309, 310, 312, 715]

Serial bone biopsies have shown that the adynamic state may evolve to osteomalacia as well as to secondary HPTH.[615] In fact, each bone lesion may evolve to another in an individual patient, depending on the clinical setting. This fact reflects the dynamic nature of renal osteodystrophy.

Mixed uremic osteodystrophy displays features of both high-turnover and low-turnover bone lesions in the same patient. It usually refers to patients with mixed features of secondary HPTH and Al-related bone disease.

There appears to be considerable variation in the incidence, type, and severity of skeletal disease from one part of the world to another. In the 1980s, whereas in Israel, Italy, and certain parts of the United Kingdom the preponderant bone disease was osteomalacia,[716–718] investigators in Germany,[708] the Netherlands,[719] and the United States[720] noted lesions of secondary HPTH to be more common. Different dietary P intake, differences in latitude and climate (which are known to have major effects on vitamin D production),[494] different policies of food fortification with vitamin D, and, more important, different exposure to Al-containing P binders or high dialysate Al levels may contribute to differences in the types of bone lesion observed in various parts of the world. Dietary calcium intake varies depending on cultural circumstances, providing yet another possible factor. Another factor is the criteria for selection of patients which undergo bone biopsies, because these can be an important source of bias when incidence and prevalence of the different types of bone disease are reported.

Do patients undergoing regular dialysis have a different bone disease than patients with end-stage renal disease not yet in dialysis? From their observations, Ritz and co-workers[708] concluded that there were no qualitative differences between the findings in bones of patients undergoing dialysis and patients with stable advanced uremia. Certain investigators have suggested that differences do occur. Other authors believe that dialysis merely prolongs the lives of patients with end-stage CRF, exposing them to the various pathogenic factors for a longer period. Certain incriminating factors are unique to dialysis patients, such as administration of heparin,[721] exposure to fluoridated water, exposure to high concentrations of acetate, periodic removal of $HCO_3^-$, exposure to varying concentrations of $Ca^{2+}$ and $Mg^{2+}$ in dialysate, and the presence of Al, trace elements, and other substances in dialysate. The most important and toxic factor may be increased Al exposure.

It has become apparent that the incidence of the different bone lesions has been changing over time. Although osteitis fibrosa was a common finding in patients during the early years of maintenance dialysis, Al-related osteomalacia was increasingly diagnosed after workers in Newcastle identified a subgroup of dialysis patients exhibiting osteomalacia resistant to vitamin D treatment. In 1986, Llach and co-workers[307] evaluated the prevalence of the type of bone lesions in a large and unselected dialysis population from the same geographic region; osteitis fibrosa was present in 88 of the 131 patients studied. Osteomalacia was present in 31 patients (24%) and aplastic bone disease with Al deposits was present in 12 patients (9%). Other studies have shown that patients with osteomalacic lesions are less common.[308, 309] Largely because of Al, this lesion has become less frequent as the use of Al-containing P binders decreases. Thus, the pattern of bone lesions observed in our dialysis population has been changing in the past decade. In a largely unselected population, ABD was the most common histopathologic pattern in peritoneal dialysis, and it was as frequent as osteitis fibrosa in hemodialysis patients.[308] Nevertheless, the distribution was different for both types of dialysis; low-turnover disorders constituted 66% of the lesions seen in peritoneal dialysis and high-turnover disorders accounted for 62% of the findings in hemodialysis.[308] These investigators also reported that ABD was present in half of their dialysis patients, and Al toxicity was present in only one third.[309] The increasing percentage of diabetic and older patients and the widespread use of high-$Ca^{2+}$ dialysate and calcium carbonate are some of the factors that may influence the prevalence of bone disease.

## PREVENTION AND MANAGEMENT

The management of altered divalent ion metabolism and osteodystrophy in patients with CRF is directed toward correcting the pathogenic factors already discussed. As such, important objectives in the clinical management of patients with renal osteodystrophy include 1) maintaining $Ca^{2+}$ and P as normal as possible; 2) preventing the development of parathyroid hyperplasia or, if it has already occurred, suppressing parathyroid secretion and reducing hyperplasia; 3) avoiding exposure to toxic agents such as Al, iron, or excess fluoride; 4) restoring the skeleton to normal as much as possible; 5) preventing and reversing extraskeletal calcifications; and 6) avoiding the hazards inherent in the different treatment modalities.

The intensity of treatment and the specific treatment modality must vary depending on the stage of renal insufficiency, the presence or absence of overt bone disease, and whether regular dialysis has been initiated. Some specific means for the management of renal osteodystrophy are given in Table 51–8, with details provided in the text.

# TREATMENT OF SECONDARY HYPERPARATHYROIDISM

## Prevention of Phosphorus Retention and Hyperphosphatemia

As already discussed, P retention and hyperphosphatemia are major factors in the development and maintenance of secondary HPTH in CRF. High serum P is also an important factor in causing soft tissue calcifications. Therefore, the goal of therapy must be to reduce serum P levels to normal or as near normal as possible. In dialysis patients, predialysis serum P levels should ideally be maintained between 4.0 and 5.5 mg/dL.

The available options for reducing the P burden include 1) reducing the intake of dietary P, 2) preventing the absorption of P with P-binding agents, and 3) enhancing the removal of P from the body through more efficient dialysis in patients undergoing maintenance dialysis.[722] Moreover, it is possible that with the improvement of secondary HPTH associated with P restriction[22, 26, 27, 34] the control of hyperphosphatemia may become easier because the P efflux from bone decreases when PTH levels are lower. Conversely, compliant patients can show severe hyperphosphatemia that may be directly related to resistant secondary HPTH and/or increased individual susceptibility to P absorption.

## DIETARY PHOSPHORUS RESTRICTION

Dietary P restriction is the main and first step in the control of hyperphosphatemia. The dietary intake of P depends primarily on consumption of meat and dairy products. Poultry, fish, most soft drinks (especially colas), whole grain breads and cereals, nuts, and legumes are also foods especially high in P content. The usual intake of P by normal adults in the United States varies between 1 and 1.8 g/d.[723] Theoretically, the dietary intake of P could be reduced in proportion to the decrease in GFR in patients with mild CRF. With elimination of dairy products and limitation to 40 g of protein per day, the dietary intake of P ranged from 650 to 1000 mg/d, a quantity that is approximately 60% of normal intake.[81] With a more restricted protein diet (e.g., 20 g of high-biologic-value protein per day), the dietary P intake ranged from 450 to 700 mg/d. With the preparation of special diets, utilizing pasta products made from starch and egg white, and with prolonged boiling and washing of certain foods to remove P, Barsotti and associates[654, 724] lowered the P intake to 350 to 450 mg/d (6 mg/kg of body weight). With a diet of vegetal

origin supplemented with essential amino acids and their keto analogues, Lafage and colleagues[725] provided P at 3 to 5 mg/kg/d without the development of malnutrition in uremic patients. Thus, it is possible to reduce P intake substantially by modifying dietary intake, but this is difficult to achieve in practice without compromising the palatability of the diet, which may affect adherence to it. Consequently, restriction of dietary P intake in proportion to the decrease in GFR as the sole measure for avoiding P retention is feasible only in patients with moderate CRF.

When patients begin maintenance dialysis and are prescribed diets with greater protein intake, the P intake also rises. The National Cooperative Dialysis Study suggested

**TABLE 51–8. Guidelines for Management of Renal Osteodystrophy**

**Control of Serum Phosphorus (4.0 to 5.5 mg/dL)**
Restrict maximally dietary P within an adequate protein intake.
Give P-binding agents: calcium carbonate or calcium acetate.
 Individual dosage should be proportional to the amount of P contained in the meals.
Avoid Al-containing P binders whenever possible.
Avoid hypophosphatemia and marked elevation of serum Al.

**Dietary Calcium Supplements**
Give oral $Ca^{2+}$ to supply 1 g/d in dialysis patients, but only if the serum P concentration is controlled.

**Dialysate Calcium Concentration**
Use a 2.5 mEq/L dialysate $Ca^{2+}$ concentration with $Ca^{2+}$ containing P binders and vitamin D metabolites.

**Vitamin D Metabolites**
Adequate control of serum P and any of the following:
 Hypocalcemia
 Secondary HPTH (intact PTH > two to three times normal) with serum $Ca^{2+}$ < 11–12 mg/dL
 Osteomalacia (with nutritional vitamin D deficiency or coexisting with secondary HPTH)
 CRF in children
 Concurrent anticonvulsant therapy
 Myopathy and muscle weakness

 ? Prophylaxis in dialysis patients

 25(OH)D (calcifediol), 25–100 μg/d
 1α(OH)D, 0.5–4 μg/d
 1,25(OH)$_2$D (calcitriol), 0.25–1 μg/d; intravenous calcitriol 0.5–5 μg three times weekly; oral pulses 2–5 μg twice weekly

**Parathyroidectomy**
Ineffective medical treatment, evidence of severe secondary HPTH, exclusion of Al-related bone disease and any of the following:
 Persistent hypercalcemia (serum $Ca^{2+}$ > 12 mg/dL)
 Progressive extraskeletal calcifications
 Persistent elevation of serum $Ca^{2+}$ × P product
 Severe and intractable pruritus
 Symptomatic hypercalcemia after kidney transplantation (including secondary deterioration of renal function)
Calciphylaxis (urgent PTX may be necessary)

**Other Factors**
Dialysate $Mg^{2+}$ concentrations of 0.6–1 mg/dL (0.5–0.7 mEq/L). Decrease if $Mg^{2+}$-containing P binders are used.
Water treatment: maintain Al < 5–10 μg/L and remove excess fluoride, $Ca^{2+}$, and $Mg^{2+}$ in dialysate.
Infuse deferoxamine for Al chelation (5–15 mg/kg/wk or every 10 d).
Avoid concurrent treatment with barbiturates, phenytoin, glutethimide, or corticosteroids.
Normalize or improve acid-base status.

that with commencement of dialytic therapy, patients should ingest a diet with a protein level of at least 0.8 g/kg/d.[726] The average dietary intake of P in 162 hemodialysis patients who entered this study was $879 \pm 248$ mg/d.[727] Although metabolic balance studies suggest that a minimal protein intake of 1 g/kg/d is necessary to maintain positive nitrogen balance, studies of CAPD patients noted a nearly neutral balance with a protein intake of 1 g/kg/d, and a positive balance was always achieved with 1.4 g/kg/d.[728] Moreover, with a protein intake of 1 g/kg/d, the measured P intake ranged from 920 to 1200 mg/d, and when dietary protein was increased to 1.4 g/kg/d, the P intake was 1700 to 2400 mg/d.

## PHOSPHORUS-BINDING AGENTS

Because it is difficult to achieve adequate dietary restriction of P, particularly in dialysis patients ingesting appropriate dietary protein, P-binding agents are required by most patients with end-stage CRF and by many patients with advanced CRF when the GFR decreases to 25% to 30% of normal.[40, 41] A mathematic consideration of the mass balance for P in dialysis patients is given in Table 51–9. The fraction of P that is absorbed by dialysis patients is only slightly lower than the fraction absorbed by normal subjects. Thus, Ramirez and co-workers[729] noted that 70% of the P was absorbed from a single meal, and Kaye and colleagues[730] estimated that $61 \pm 9\%$ was absorbed, based on fecal recovery. Even with the intake of aluminum hydroxide in doses ranging from 3.4 to 15 g/d, Blumenkrantz and colleagues[728] noted that the net absorption of P was $55 \pm 14\%$ of the intake in 13 long-term metabolic balance studies of CAPD patients.

P-binding agents lower intestinal P absorption by creating poorly soluble complexes of P in the intestinal tract. They can be mainly divided into Al-containing and $Ca^{2+}$-containing P binders, although other types are also used.

### Aluminum-Containing Phosphorus Binders

Al-containing P binders were the standard treatment prescribed for patients with end-stage CRF before 1985, and

**TABLE 51–9. Considerations Regarding Phosphorus Removal and Balance in Dialysis Patients with Three Different Diets\***

| Intake (mg/d) | 900 | 1200 | 1500 |
|---|---|---|---|
| Absorbed (60%)† | 540 | 720 | 900 |
| Hemodialysis removal (mg/d) (700 mg/4 h dialysis three times a week)‡ | 300 | 300 | 300 |
| Balance (mg/d) | +240 | +420 | +600 |
| Binder needed for "zero" balance (calcium acetate tablets per day)§ | 8 | 14 | 20 |

*P intake 900 mg/d (moderate compliance with P diet), 1200 mg/d (occasional noncompliance with dialysis diet), and 1500 mg/d ("normal" North American diet).
†May be as high as 75% or as low as 50%; augmented slightly by vitamin D metabolites.
‡With serum P of 6.0 mg/dL; increases moderately as serum P rises.
§These figures are only approximate.

then the risk of Al toxicity from oral Al was appreciated. As discussed earlier, Al toxicity is especially important in high-risk conditions such as diabetes, postparathyroidectomy, and ABD.[232, 319, 731]

Are there any safe quantities of Al gels that can be used? It was suggested that there was little or no risk with the ingestion of up to six capsules or tablets of aluminum hydroxide per day in adult uremic patients.[271] It was also suggested that doses below 30 mg/kg of body weight had little risk in children with end-stage CRF.[732] However, in children undergoing peritoneal dialysis, Al accumulation was noted even though the dosage of Al gels did not exceed 30 mg/kg of body weight.[733] A progressive increase of mean plasma Al from 22 to 59 µg/L was observed in the children and young adults assigned to aluminum hydroxide, compared with a significant fall of plasma Al in the patients ingesting calcium carbonate. Moreover, one patient developed histologic evidence of skeletal Al toxicity after receiving this supposedly low dose of Al for 1 year. The control of hyperphosphatemia and secondary HPTH was poorer with the restricted doses of Al gel than in the group given calcium carbonate. Jenkins and co-workers[734] noted, in adults limited to six tablets of aluminum hydroxide per day or 30 mL/d of a liquid suspension (maximum, 2.85 g/d), significant Al staining on bone biopsies in 2 of 16 adult hemodialyzed patients. Thus, a certain fraction of dialysis patients who ingest aluminum hydroxide, even in modest doses, may develop clinical evidence of Al toxicity. Larger doses are generally required for adult patients; thus, the doses required to prevent serum P from rising in the National Cooperative Dialysis Study ranged from 3.5 to 4.9 g/d in the two major treatment groups with dialysis treatment schedules that resulted in the best survival and least morbidity.[735] For the reasons noted earlier, we recommend that Al gels should not be the primary P-binding agents prescribed for patients with CRF. They may be needed for patients who have side effects with calcium carbonate or calcium acetate or when a calcium salt alone is not effective. The latter patients often require a combination of either calcium carbonate or calcium acetate with an Al-based P binder.[415]

When Al gels are needed, considerable data indicate that capsules or tablets are less effective than liquid suspensions[736]; however, compliance is generally better with capsules than with the liquid forms. Constipation, which commonly accompanies their ingestion, is the most troublesome side effect limiting compliance with these agents. Because of wide variation in the individual patient's preference for different preparations, it is difficult to identify one preparation that satisfies all patients. Hence, efforts should be made to find a specific preparation that is suitable for each patient. Nevertheless, if Al-containing P binders need to be given, doses must be kept as low as possible, the duration of the treatment limited, the concurrent administration of citrate salts or citric acid discontinued, and plasma Al levels monitored at regular intervals.

### Calcium-Containing Phosphorus Binders

It was known many years ago that large doses of calcium carbonate were effective in reducing the absorption of P from the gastrointestinal tract.[737] A number of clinical studies have subsequently shown that calcium carbonate is an effective P-binding agent.[274, 415, 738–740] However, calcium carbonate had side effects such as hypercalcemia and gastrointestinal symptoms such as constipation, diarrhea (less common), changes in bowel habits, vague abdominal discomfort, and dyspepsia. Occasionally these symptoms are so profound that patients have difficulty complying with the prescribed dosages. The long-term side effects of $Ca^{2+}$-containing P binders are unknown; nevertheless, no difference in the incidence or extent of progression of extraskeletal calcifications was noted in adult patients treated with $Ca^{2+}$-containing P binders for as long as 2[741] or 3 years.[742]

Episodes of hypercalcemia have occurred in a substantial fraction of patients[274, 415, 740]; occasionally the hypercalcemia is severe enough to cause symptoms that require the withdrawal of the calcium salt. When serum $Ca^{2+}$ was measured serially in dialysis patients started on calcium carbonate, the mean level increased significantly.[743] In the United States, most patients undergo dialysis with a dialysate $Ca^{2+}$ concentration of 3.0 to 3.5 mEq/L, and a positive balance for $Ca^{2+}$ is induced by dialysis with a dialysate $Ca^{2+}$ level of 3.0 mEq/L or higher.[744, 745] Because of the development of hypercalcemia, the dialysate $Ca^{2+}$ concentration has been reduced as calcium carbonate is widely used as a P binder.[275, 746–748] Thus, dialysate $Ca^{2+}$ level was lowered from 3.5 to 2.5 mEq/L by Slatopolsky and co-workers[275] in a group of dialysis patients receiving 1.5 to 18 g/d of calcium carbonate; they successfully managed hyperphosphatemia, and the incidence of hypercalcemia was substantially reduced compared with a historical group receiving calcium carbonate and a dialysate $Ca^{2+}$ value of 3.5 mEq/L. Sawyer and colleagues[747] utilized a stepwise reduction in dialysate $Ca^{2+}$ concentration based on the serum $Ca^{2+}$ when they initiated therapy with calcium carbonate; they lowered the dialysate $Ca^{2+}$ concentration first to 2.7 mEq/L and then, if necessary, to 2.1 mEq/L. In a large group of hemodialysis patients, they avoided hypercalcemia, achieved adequate P control, and noted a significant fall in intact PTH levels. In general, calcium carbonate has proved effective as the sole P binder in 70% to 90% of adult and pediatric dialysis patients. However, others have observed only 50% of dialysis patients attaining adequate control of serum P levels when calcium carbonate was used as the sole P binder.[738]

Calcium carbonate has been used together with strict dietary P restriction in the treatment of renal osteodystrophy. Thus, in patients with a GFR of 20 mL/min or less Lafage and colleagues[725] evaluated the efficacy of a low-protein diet (0.3 g protein per kilogram of body weight per day) supplemented with essential amino acids, their keto analogues, and 1 g of calcium carbonate—without pharmacologic doses of vitamin D or physiologic doses of 1α-hydroxylated derivatives—for a year. Despite the progression of CRF, they observed that P and PTH levels decreased significantly and low plasma $HCO_3^-$ returned to normal. Moreover, bone biopsies performed before and after 1 year showed an improvement of histodynamic parameters of osteitis fibrosa. In five of nine patients histologic changes were not different from normal and bone improved in the other four patients. Furthermore, in four patients with mixed osteodystrophy, the osteomalacic component was cured, and the component of secondary HPTH was cured in two and improved in the remaining two. Only a noncompliant patient developed severe osteitis fibrosa during the follow-up.

Finally, it should be emphasized that although the ingestion of calcium salts can reduce the blood level of P, in severe hyperphosphatemia $Ca^{2+}$-containing P binders must be avoided because the $Ca^{2+} \times P$ product can increase above 70 $mg^2/dL^2$, predisposing to soft tissue calcification. In such patients, Al-containing P binders should be used first to lower the plasma P to a safer level (e.g., <5.5 to 6 mg/dL) before calcium salts are initiated. Administration of large quantities of oral calcium should also be done cautiously when the serum $Ca^{2+}$ value is in the upper range of normal and vitamin D derivatives are given. Under such circumstances, it is wise to use a dialysate $Ca^{2+}$ concentration of 2.5 mEq/L to reduce the risk of hypercalcemia.

## Quantitation and Comparison of Phosphorus Binders

Calcium carbonate contains 40% and calcium acetate 25% of elemental calcium. Calcium lactate contains 12% and calcium gluconate 8%. Calcium chloride should be avoided in uremic patients because it causes metabolic acidosis.

Most observations with P binders have been done in clinical trials with dosage adjustment to achieve adequate serum P levels; controls have been either patients receiving aluminum hydroxide or a relatively brief control period with no binder ingested. Only a few studies have addressed the issue of the amount of a P binder required to bind the P in a diet. In metabolic balance studies, the administration of aluminum hydroxide gel at 100 mL/d caused a decrease in net absorption of P from 463 ± 108 to 128 ± 68 mg/d in five patients who ingested a diet containing 1135 ± 246 mg of P per day.[749] In two other patients with dietary P intake below 700 mg/d, the dietary fecal losses of P exceeded the amount in the diet. In a few studies with the dosage of Al gel at 75 or 150 mL/d, the reduction of P absorption was similar to that with 100 mL/d.[749]

Single-meal studies have been used to evaluate the effect of various P binders on intestinal P absorption.[729, 750–752] In normal subjects the ingestion of 50-mEq amounts of aluminum carbonate, calcium carbonate, calcium citrate, and calcium acetate was compared, with the doses of calcium salts or Al-containing preparations based on the dosage of $Ca^{2+}$ or Al provided. In normal subjects, the administration of calcium carbonate containing 1000 mg of $Ca^{2+}$ decreased the average net absorption from a meal with 342 mg of P from 263 to 151 mg, an average reduction in net absorption of 112 mg. The reduction of absorption with calcium acetate was 174 mg; with aluminum carbonate suspension, 202 mg; and with calcium citrate, 92 mg. The degrees of reduction with calcium acetate and aluminum carbonate were not different, but each was more effective than both calcium citrate and calcium carbonate[752] (Fig. 51–32). In yet another study of normal subjects, administration of 50 mEq of calcium acetate reduced the mean net absorption of P from a similar meal by 150 to 170 mg[751] when the

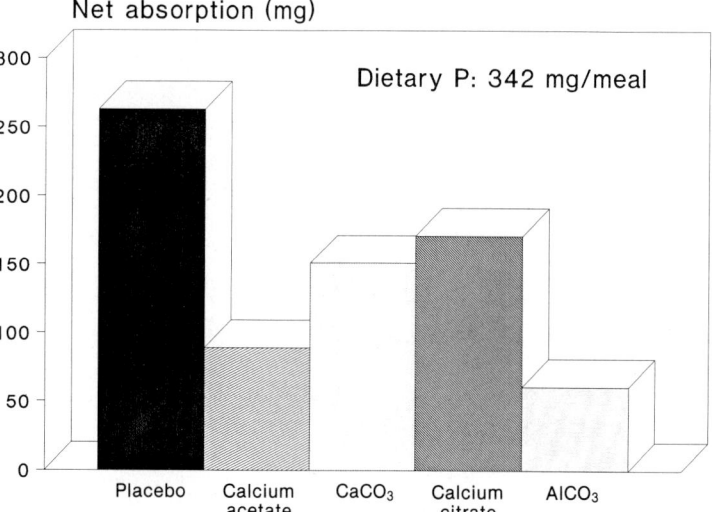

Net absorption (mg)

Dietary P: 342 mg/meal

**Figure 51–32.** Effect of various P binders on net intestinal absorption of P after a standarized meal containing 342 mg of P. (Modified from Sheikh M, Maguire J, Emmett M, et al: Reduction of dietary phosphorus absorption by phosphorus binders. Reproduced from The Journal of Clinical Investigation, 1989, vol 83 pp 66–73 by copyright permission of The American Society for Clinical Investigation.)

agent was taken either immediately before or immediately after a meal. However, there was a significant reduction of the amount of P bound when the calcium acetate was taken 2 hours after the meal. Ramirez and co-workers[729] compared the effect of either calcium carbonate or aluminum hydroxide capsules (75 mEq) in patients with end-stage renal failure; they observed mean reductions of P absorption of 45 and 55 mg per meal. In a separate comparison of calcium carbonate and calcium acetate, 50 mEq per dose, there were mean reductions of P absorption of 43 and 106 mg per meal, respectively[750]; moreover, the calcium acetate was more effective on the basis of its $Ca^{2+}$ content. In addition, these authors observed less $Ca^{2+}$ absorption from the calcium acetate than from calcium carbonate. Thus, although calcium acetate may be more efficient in in vitro and short-term in vivo studies[416, 752, 753] only limited data are available for patients undergoing long-term dialysis.

In a report comparing patients receiving calcium acetate with those receiving calcium carbonate, serum P was controlled similarly by either binder. Although the daily amount of elemental calcium ingested by the patients taking calcium acetate was half that of those ingesting calcium carbonate, the number of hypercalcemic episodes was small and comparable in both groups.[416, 754] Others, in comparing the efficacy and side effects of calcium acetate and calcium carbonate in hemodialysis patients, have not been able to identify a major advantage of calcium acetate over calcium carbonate.[748, 755] Thus, calcium carbonate still remains the most commonly used $Ca^{2+}$-containing binder. Calcium acetate is more expensive, the size of tablets is rather large, and it is less palatable and less tolerated.[753] In addition, calcium acetate is not widely available.

It is important to titrate the dose appropriately to the amount of P ingested in each meal. Large doses of binders may be required, particularly if there is an increase in dietary P. The average daily doses of calcium carbonate employed in trials in dialysis patients have been 8.5 g/d (range 2.5 to 17 g),[415] 5.1 ± 2.5 g/d,[279] and 5.8 ± 2.5 g/d[274] in trials in the United States; reports in Europe described adequate control with use of 2.48 g/d (range 1 to 6 g)[747] and 2.57 g/d (range 1 to 6 g).[739] It is likely that such variations

exist because of differences in dietary intake of P. In individual patients, the dose should be adjusted empirically according to the levels of serum P.[274, 415, 738] It must be emphasized that P binders, both Al and $Ca^{2+}$ based, are most effective when the dietary intake of P is below 1.0 g/d. With P intake greater than 2.0 g/d, their effectiveness is markedly reduced and hyperphosphatemia can persist despite their use. Finally, variable efficacy of calcium carbonate tablets has been observed; preparations with inadequate solubility can render calcium carbonate ineffective.[756]

### Other Phosphorus Binders

Several other P-binding agents have been used in patients with CRF, but they have certain disadvantages or have not been widely used. These include calcium citrate, 21% elemental calcium[757]; magnesium carbonate or hydroxide[425, 428]; and salts of polyuronic acid.[758] Although calcium citrate is as effective a P binder as calcium carbonate, its use should be limited to certain specific situations, because calcium citrate, like other citrate salts,[284, 285] markedly augments intestinal absorption of Al.[288] As some dialysis patients may need a small dose of Al gel with the calcium salt,[415] there is a risk of acute Al toxicity, a condition with a high mortality.[286, 287] Magnesium carbonate in conjunction with $Mg^{2+}$-free dialysate in patients undergoing regular hemodialysis was effective in controlling serum P[428]; serum $Mg^{2+}$ levels did not change. However, other trials using magnesium hydroxide have proved this salt ineffective or poorly tolerated.[425, 759] When constipation accompanies the use of either Al-based P binders or calcium salts, the use of an $Mg^{2+}$-free or lower-$Mg^{2+}$ dialysate combined with a modest ingestion of magnesium salt may be effective. Thus, Moriniere and associates[760] have had success combining calcium carbonate with small doses of magnesium hydroxide in long-term management of their patients.[427] However, they were unsuccessful using magnesium hydroxide as the sole P binder in the treatment of secondary HPTH with intravenous $1\alpha(OH)D$. The polyuronic acid derivatives have also been shown to be effective P binders.[758] They are not available in the United States and have not been widely used in Europe. The use of these agents may be advisable for patients who are intolerant of calcium acetate, calcium carbonate, or any of the P-binding Al gels.

Finally, it is important to consider that the fall in serum P level during dietary P restriction and therapy with P binders is often associated with a rise in serum $Ca^{2+}$.[398, 749] If the magnitude of the rise in serum $Ca^{2+}$ is adequate, the blood levels of PTH may further decrease.[749] It is equally important to avoid lowering the concentration of serum P to levels lower than normal. A few patients require no P-binding agents; others require larger doses. Overzealous use of P binders may result in hypophosphatemia, P depletion, and osteomalacia.[498, 761]

## DIALYSANCE OF PHOSPHORUS

Although removal of P by dialysis would seem appropriate to control hyperphosphatemia, the various dialytic techniques available cannot achieve this goal. The amount of P removed during hemodialysis varies mainly with the predialysis serum P level and also with the efficiency of the dialyzer being used. Kaye and colleagues[730] noted that the net P removal was 600 to 750 mg during 4 hours of dialysis utilizing a 1.2-$m^2$ cuprophane dialyzer when the predialysis serum P level varied from 5.0 to 7.0 mg/dL. Hou and co-workers[762] observed a high rate of P removal throughout the dialysis treatment (blood flow of 300 mL/min, dialysate flow of 500 mL/min, mean predialysis P level 6.8 mg/dL); however, the amount removed steadily declined during the 4 hours of treatment. Overall, 1 g of P was removed with each dialysis, and this value was not affected by dialyzer membrane type, dialysis technique, or dialysate $Ca^{2+}$ concentration in this particular study. Other studies observed that P removal was 587 ± 61 mg during 4 hours of dialysis and 721 ± 53 mg with high-flux hemodiafiltration carried out for 2 hours with a blood flow of 500 mL/min.[763, 764] With dialysis treatment targeted to achieve optimal urea removal, Shinaberger and colleagues[765] noted a 500- to 600-mg net removal of P during 4 hours of conventional dialysis; removal of P increased only to 600 to 700 mg per dialysis during 3 hours of high-efficiency or high-flux dialysis using cellulose acetate, polysulfone, and other highly permeable membranes. Interestingly, correction of anemia with erythropoietin resulted in a P removal decreased by 18%.

Several explanations account for the low mass transfer of P. First, the dialyzer clearances of P are somewhat lower than those of urea (40% to 50% of the rate for urea), and although this difference is less with polysulfone dialyzers the differences become greater when blood flow is increased. Second, there is little or no removal of P from the erythrocyte and only plasma P is cleared by the dialyzer; and third, the excess of P that accumulates between two dialysis treatments has a volume of distribution well beyond the extracellular space so that the equilibration between the plasma P and extravascular compartment is delayed. Thus, serum P levels fall rapidly in the first 30 to 45 minutes of dialysis to values below 3.0 mg/100 mL.[744, 763, 766] This results in a low P gradient between plasma and dialysate, with less efficient mass transfer as the length of dialysis is extended. Moreover, the steady decrease in P removal efficiency during treatment is associated with an efflux of P from intracellular space and bone to the extracellular space as a result of the early decrease in serum P.[762] In most patients, postdialysis serum P rapidly rebounds to predialysis values within 2 to 3 hours after completion of dialysis. In CAPD patients, the clearance of P is approximately 4.7 mL/min, and with each dialysate exchange 65 mg is removed, resulting in a daily removal of 307 mg.[767] Thus, the net removal of P may be slightly higher in CAPD, and this may explain some observations that serum P is easier to control during CAPD.[768, 769]

With the widespread use of calcitriol, the control of hyperphosphatemia is of paramount importance. New dialyzer membranes have been used to improve P removal. The clearance ratios of plasma P to urea when a cellulose or a polycarbonate membrane is used are similar, 64% and 78%, respectively.[770] High-flux hemodiafiltration improves the ratio to only 30%.[763] However, the mass removal rates of P are similar regardless of the membrane used. For example, the total P removed during 4 hours of hemodialysis using a cuprophane membrane with a mean blood flow of 227 mL/min was 597 ± 61 mg per dialysis, and high-flux hemodiafiltration, at a blood flow of 504 mL/min, removed 721 ± 53 mg per dialysis. As mentioned before, the main factor in P removal is the predialysis serum P and the sharp decrease occurring during the first hour of dialysis,[744] which precludes higher P removal. It has been suggested that $HCO_3^-$-based dialysate, compared with acetate, may increase the intracellular P pool and decrease serum P concentration; however, no differences in P transfer from the patient were noted in a preliminary comparison of dialysate solutions containing each of the two buffers.[771] From all these observations and the mass balance calculations (see Table 51–9), it is apparent that although dialysis removes substantial amounts of P, additional efforts to control hyperphosphatemia are required in 80% to 90% of dialysis patients.

## FAILURE TO CONTROL HYPERPHOSPHATEMIA

The most common cause of hyperphosphatemia is poor compliance with both dietary P restriction and P binders. Dietary training and support from the dietitian and nursing staff are of utmost importance. Reduced effectiveness of the P binder may be another cause.[756] Also, the patients with the most severe secondary HPTH present the most severe hyperphosphatemia; they may also have a more rapid rebound of serum P to higher levels during the interdialytic interval.[772] The high serum P levels probably arise because bone resorption is markedly increased and P is released from bone into the blood. These patients may present a marked fall in serum P after PTX or when PTH is decreased by intravenous calcitriol.

## Nutritional Calcium Supplements

Calcium carbonate and calcium acetate are usually given, as described earlier, as P binders but they can also be used as a nutritional supplement. When either calcium carbonate or calcium acetate is given orally as a P binder, some $Ca^{2+}$ is inevitably absorbed. However, if $Ca^{2+}$ supplements are prescribed to reverse the negative $Ca^{2+}$ balance, they should be administered between meals as opposed to prescription as P binders. Similarly, to maximize $Ca^{2+}$ absorption the amount prescribed should be ingested in several small doses throughout the day rather than one large dose.

Addition of $Ca^{2+}$ is important in patients with advanced CRF and those undergoing dialysis because intestinal absorption of $Ca^{2+}$ is impaired in these patients and because the diets generally consumed by uremic patients contain reduced amounts of dairy products and, consequently, low quantities of $Ca^{2+}$. The dietary calcium intake in patients with advanced CRF was noted to be 400 to 700 mg/d[81]; a neutral or positive balance for $Ca^{2+}$ can be achieved in uremic patients by supplementation of the diet with calcium carbonate, calcium citrate, or calcium lactate,[773] to increase the total intake of $Ca^{2+}$ to 1.5 g or more per day.[81, 737, 774] When, during the course of CRF, is the best time to add $Ca^{2+}$ supplements has not been resolved. Coburn and coworkers[97] observed normal intestinal $Ca^{2+}$ absorption in male patients with serum creatinine levels below 2.5 mg/dL, and Malluche and colleagues[775] observed intestinal $Ca^{2+}$ absorption to be decreased in certain patients with a GFR of 20 to 50 mL/min. Patients with more advanced CRF are more prone to develop hypercalcemia with oral $Ca^{2+}$ supplements, because they lack the renal route for $Ca^{2+}$ excretion.

Effects of long-term $Ca^{2+}$ supplementation for patients with advanced CRF have been reported. Makoff and coworkers[776] gave 4 to 10 g of calcium carbonate per day to uremic patients not yet receiving dialysis. They observed a reduction of serum P, a slight rise in serum $Ca^{2+}$, and a small increase in serum $HCO_3^-$. Meyrier and associates[414] gave 5 to 20 g of calcium carbonate per day to hemodialysis patients and compared them to other patients not receiving calcium carbonate. In the former group, bone biopsy specimens showed less resorptive activity, radiographs showed less evidence of skeletal disease and fewer fractures, and fewer episodes of pseudogout and extraskeletal calcifications were noted. Hypercalcemia, which was sometimes profound, resolved on reduction of the calcium salt dosage. Plasma alkaline phosphatase and serum PTH concentrations may decrease in uremic patients with overt secondary HPTH given supplements of either calcium carbonate or, in those with low serum P, calcium phosphate.[413] Eastwood and colleagues[623, 777] compared bone biopsies of uremic patients with renal osteodystrophy treated with vitamin D with those of similar patients treated with calcium carbonate. In patients receiving calcium carbonate, diffuse patchy deposition of $Ca^{2+}$ in osteoid was observed and a distinct calcification front did not develop, whereas a calcification front was regularly observed in patients given vitamin D. This study provides evidence that vitamin D is more effective than $Ca^{2+}$ supplements in reversing overt uremic skeletal disease.

As mentioned before, treatment with oral $Ca^{2+}$ supplements is not free of risk. Large amounts of oral $Ca^{2+}$ compounds should be used cautiously in patients with marked hyperphosphatemia, because of the risk of elevating the $Ca^{2+} \times P$ product and thereby predisposing to extraskeletal calcification. Hypercalcemia may develop in uremic patients, as in patients with normal renal function, during therapy with large quantities of oral calcium salts.[414, 778] Hypercalcemia may be more common in patients with serum P concentrations below 3 mg/dL.[399] Mild hypercalcemia (11 to 12 mg/dL) is usually associated with no symptoms[273]; occasionally, uremic patients may exhibit symptoms despite only modestly elevated serum $Ca^{2+}$ levels. In addition to nausea, anorexia, vomiting, mental confusion, and lethargy, patients with advanced CRF may develop pruritus, red eye syndrome, band keratopathy, and even a sharp elevation in blood pressure, which can be clues for the suspicion of hypercalcemia.

## Initiation of Dialysis and Dialysate Calcium Concentration

Within a few months after initiation of regular hemodialysis, the basal concentration of serum $Ca^{2+}$ generally increases to between 9.0 and 10.0 mg/dL. This increase in serum $Ca^{2+}$ levels generally occurs in patients who were previously hypocalcemic; little or no change occurs in patients with initial serum $Ca^{2+}$ levels near normal.[407, 779] Such increments in serum $Ca^{2+}$ may occur despite hyperphosphatemia or the use of a dialysate $Ca^{2+}$ concentration lower than that in blood.[399] The mechanism responsible for this increase in serum $Ca^{2+}$ is unknown; no improvement of the calcemic response to PTH has been detected with the initiation of dialysis,[64] although uremic toxins have been shown to alter the calcemic response.[77] Initiation of regular hemodialysis produces little or no change in intestinal $Ca^{2+}$ absorption,[97] although a transient increase immediately after dialysis has been noted.[780] With regular dialysis using the standard dialysate $Ca^{2+}$ content (3.5 mEq/L), there is a positive balance of $Ca^{2+}$ during the dialysis procedure; thus, it can explain the correction of hypocalcemia in some patients and the fact that predialysis serum $Ca^{2+}$ levels are sometimes normal. In a few patients, overt and persistent hypercalcemia appears some time after the initiation of hemodialysis.[779]

The total serum $Ca^{2+}$ level almost invariably increases during the dialysis procedure. This may occur because of an increase in albumin level as a consequence of the ultrafiltration and hemoconcentration that accompany hemodialysis; the affinity of plasma albumin for $Ca^{2+}$ may also be increased as a result of a rise in blood pH. Earlier studies carried out with $Ca^{2+}$-specific electrodes indicate that the blood $Ca^{2+}$ concentration can fall during hemodialysis with a dialysate $Ca^{2+}$ of 2.5 mEq/L even though total blood $Ca^{2+}$ level increases.[406] However, other studies have failed to show a specific effect of hemoconcentration or change in pH on $Ca^{2+}$ binding to serum albumin.[412] When the same evaluation is made during dialysis with a dialysate $Ca^{2+}$ level of 3.0 to 3.5 mEq/L, the $Ca^{2+}$ level increases.[744, 762]

It is likely that with a dialysate $Ca^{2+}$ concentration of either 3.0 or 3.5 mEq/L, patients receive inappropriately large amounts of $Ca^{2+}$ too rapidly with each dialysis. Argiles and colleagues[744] have shown dramatic increments in intradialytic serum $Ca^{2+}$ when a dialysate $Ca^{2+}$ concentration of 3.5 mEq/L was used; no significant intradialytic changes in serum $Ca^{2+}$ were observed with a dialysate $Ca^{2+}$ concentration of 2.5 mEq/L (Fig. 51–33). Furthermore, significant intradialytic flux of $Ca^{2+}$ from dialysate to patient was observed with both 3.5 and 3.0 mEq/L dialysate $Ca^{2+}$ and none with 2.5 mEq/L.[744] These observations are similar to those of Hou and co-workers,[762] who evaluated $Ca^{2+}$ fluxes across the hemodialysis membrane in seven patients treated with 3.5, 2.5, and 1.5 mEq/L dialysate $Ca^{2+}$. Whereas dramatic positive $Ca^{2+}$ influx from dialysate to patients was observed in patients dialyzed against a 3.5 mEq/L dialysate $Ca^{2+}$, only moderate $Ca^{2+}$ influxes were observed with a dialysate $Ca^{2+}$ value of 2.5 mEq/L. Surprisingly, a dialysate $Ca^{2+}$ level of 1.5 mEq/L resulted only in a moderate negative cumulative $Ca^{2+}$ efflux. Thus, these data strongly suggest that the standard 3.5 mEq/L dialysate $Ca^{2+}$ induces significant unwarranted intradialytic hypercalcemia. Our own observations support these results. As we dialyzed patients with a standard dialysate $Ca^{2+}$ of 3.5 mEq/L for 4 hours, we measured serum $Ca^{2+}$ during dialysis at 1, 2, 3, and 4 hours, as well as 1, 2, and 3 hours after dialysis. There was the expected dramatic increase in serum $Ca^{2+}$ during dialysis; however, by the first hour after dialysis the high serum $Ca^{2+}$ returned to predialysis values (see Fig. 51–26). Thus, the important question is, What is the

fate of the acute and marked positive $Ca^{2+}$ balance induced during dialysis? It is likely that most of the intradialytic increment in serum $Ca^{2+}$ may be rapidly deposited in soft tissues. In our view, the current use of 3.5 mEq/L dialysate $Ca^{2+}$ may be an important factor in the development of soft tissue calcifications.

The importance of a significant gradient of $Ca^{2+}$ as a factor in soft tissue calcifications is demonstrated by the observations of E Fernandez and J Montoliu (personal communication). They evaluated a patient receiving dialysis with massive tumoral right shoulder calcifications. Serum PTH (IRMA) was in the low-normal range, calcitriol was below normal, and serum Al was consistently less than 20 μg/L. As can be noted in Figure 51–34, once the patient was given daily hemodialysis with a dialysate $Ca^{2+}$ concentration of 1 mEq/L, the predialysis serum $Ca^{2+}$ increased to a hypercalcemic range that lasted about 6 weeks. At the same time, the postdialysis serum $Ca^{2+}$ concentration steadily decreased with each dialysis; however, each time by the next dialysis the $Ca^{2+}$ values were back to the hypercalcemic range. Eight weeks later, because of the low postdialysis $Ca^{2+}$, the patient was changed to five dialysis sessions per week and a dialysate $Ca^{2+}$ of 1.5 mEq/L. During the 12 months of frequent dialysis therapy, the tumoral

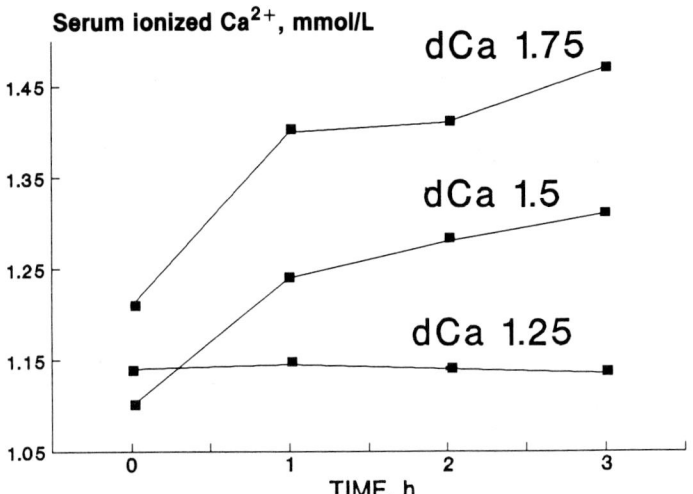

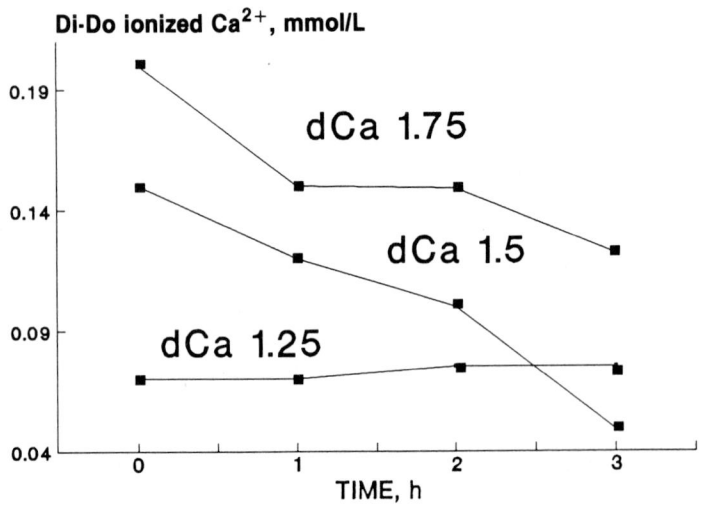

**Figure 51–33.** *Top.* Intradialytic $Ca^{2+}$ changes during regular hemodialysis with three different dialysate $Ca^{2+}$ concentrations (dCa) of 1.75, 1.5 and 1.25 mmol/L (3.5, 3, and 2.5 mEq/L). *Bottom.* Loss of $Ca^{2+}$ from dialysate (Di-Do) during hemodialysis using the same dialysate $Ca^{2+}$ concentrations. Di = dialysate inlet $Ca^{2+}$; Do = dialysate outlet $Ca^{2+}$. (*Top* and *bottom* modified from Argiles A, Kerr PG, Canaud B, et al: Calcium kinetics and the long-term effects of lowering dialysate calcium concentration. Used with permission from Kidney International, volume 43, pages 630–640, 1993.)

**Serum Ca²⁺, mg/dL**

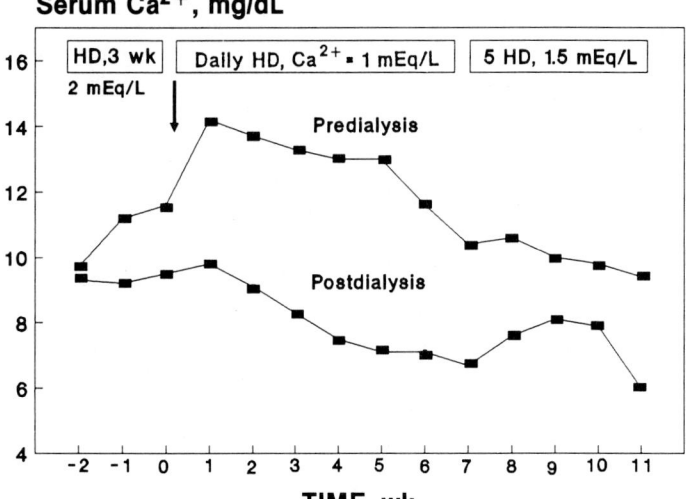

**Serum P, mg/dL**

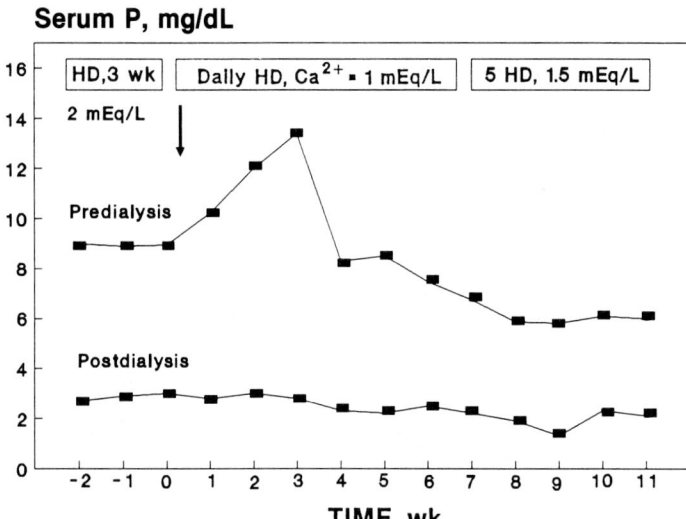

**Figure 51–34.** *Top.* Pre- and postdialysis serum Ca²⁺ changes in a patient with tumoral calcifications of the shoulder. He was treated three times a week with a 2 mEq/L Ca²⁺ dialysate, and then switched to daily dialysis (for 8 weeks) using a 1 mEq/L dialysate Ca²⁺. Finally, because of postdialysis hypocalcemia, the patient was treated five times a week with a dialysate Ca²⁺ of 1.5 mEq/L. *Bottom.* Serum P during the treatment sequence. (*Top* and *bottom* courtesy of E Fernandez and J Montoliu.)

calcification of the right shoulder progressively and dramatically disappeared and the patient's shoulder became functional. Moreover, during this period PTH levels remained below 20 pg/mL. In summary, this case exemplifies that a significant Ca²⁺ gradient between dialyzer and patient resulted in massive removal of Ca²⁺ and P and disappearance of large soft tissue calcifications. Conversely, it is likely that prolonged exposure to a positive Ca²⁺ gradient may lead to soft tissue calcifications.

Furthermore, a dialysate Ca²⁺ of 2.5 mEq/L together with calcium carbonate may be effective in ameliorating secondary HPTH. Thus, studies evaluating the long-term effect of calcium carbonate and 2.5 mEq/L dialysate Ca²⁺ in 21 hemodialysis patients noted not only that serum P was well controlled and serum Al fell significantly but also that serum Ca²⁺ increased and PTH decreased by 20% after 7 months of therapy[407]; this suggests the presence of a positive Ca²⁺ balance during this regimen. Moreover, the use of calcitriol promoted a more positive Ca²⁺ balance. Thus, there is growing evidence that when calcium salts or calcitriol is used to treat secondary HPTH, the dialysate Ca²⁺ should be reduced to 2.5 mEq/L.[275, 415, 746] In addition,

such a dialysate Ca²⁺ concentration usually allows patients to receive more appropriate doses of calcium salts and vitamin D derivatives, which may result in better control of the secondary HPTH (Fig. 51–35). Fewer patients may develop hypercalcemia with the dialysate Ca²⁺ level of 2.5 mEq/L; in some patients with persistent hypercalcemia a dialysate Ca²⁺ as low as 2.0 mEq/L may be used.[746, 747] Furthermore, a dialysate Ca²⁺ of 2.5 mEq/L was not associated with clinical intolerance[744] and may even decrease hypertension and/or make blood pressure easier to control. However, a greater reduction of the dialysate Ca²⁺ may increase the risk of hypotension as a direct consequence of the lowered Ca²⁺ level.[781]

In patients not taking calcium salts as a P binder or vitamin D, a number of earlier studies evaluated the effect of various levels of Ca²⁺ in dialysate.[782] The use of dialysate Ca²⁺ below 3.0 to 3.25 mEq/L was associated with more rapid loss of bone mineral than the use of dialysate Ca²⁺ levels of 3.25 to 3.5 mEq/L.[685, 699, 783] Under these circumstances, serum PTH levels have often slowly risen despite the increase in serum Ca²⁺ concentration. Thus, there is little information to indicate that a dialysate Ca²⁺

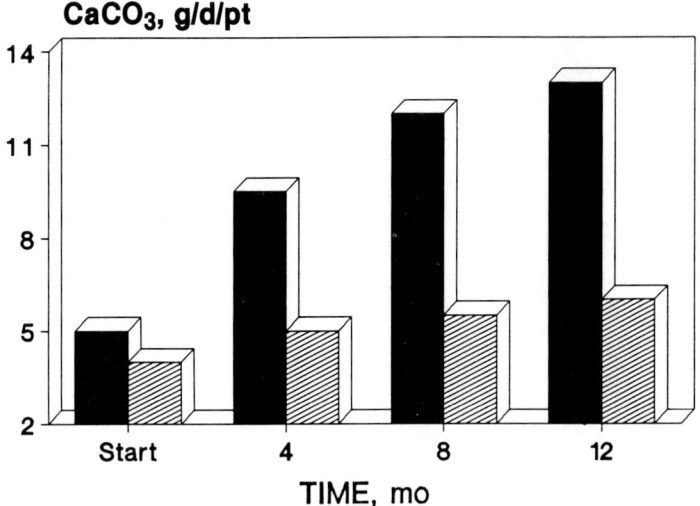

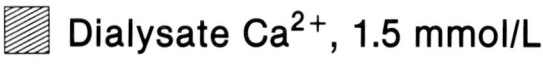

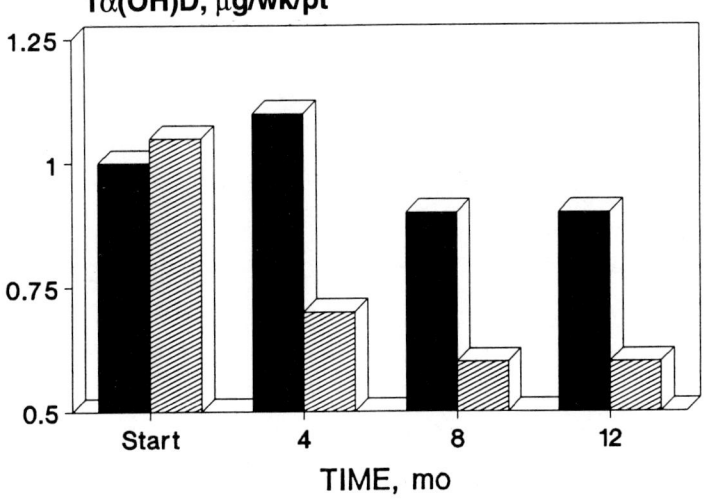

**Figure 51–35.** Calcium carbonate and oral 1α(OH)D treatments during 1 year follow-up. Open bars correspond to the control group maintained with dialysate Ca²⁺ of 1.5 mmol/L (3 mEq/L) for 1 year; solid bars correspond to the study group (switched to a dialysate Ca²⁺ of 1.25 mmol/L, or 2.5 mEq/L). (Modified from Argiles A, Kerr PG, Canaud B, et al: Calcium kinetics and the long-term effects of lowering dialysate calcium concentration. Used with permission from Kidney International, volume 43, pages 630–640, 1993.)

of 3.25 to 3.5 mEq/L per se may prevent the development of bone disease.[625, 784] Earlier, the use of a lower concentration of 2.5 mEq/L was associated with progression of the bone disease; however, none of these patients received calcium salts or calcitriol.[785, 786] In nine patients given hemodiafiltration, it was noted that intact PTH increased (from 94 ± 40 to 296 ± 99 pg/mL) after 1 year of treatment with a dialysate Ca²⁺ of 2.5 mEq/L, whereas a dialysate Ca²⁺ of 3.0 mEq/L resulted in no changes in PTH; this occurred even though the former group had an oral calcium intake almost double that of the latter.[744] However, when patients were treated for 4 months with intravenous 1α(OH)D, similar PTH reduction (72% and 75%) was noted in both groups. Thus, when a dialysate Ca²⁺ of 2.5 mEq/L is used, efforts should be made to ascertain that patients remain compliant with their prescribed Ca²⁺-containing P binders and a vitamin D metabolite is added to avoid a negative Ca²⁺ balance. Regular measurements of

intact PTH should also be performed. With the availability of vitamin D derivatives, an increase in gut absorption of Ca²⁺, as well as a direct suppression of PTH secretion, can be effectively achieved. In this situation, a lower dialysate Ca²⁺ concentration may be advisable to avoid repeated episodes of hypercalcemia.

It has also been reported that CAPD patients with the use of a dialysate Ca²⁺ of 3.5 mEq/L may have more sustained and higher Ca²⁺ levels than patients given hemodialysis[339, 340]; this may result in more effective PTH suppression than the intermittent Ca²⁺ loading of hemodialysis. As mentioned before, the higher serum Ca²⁺ may at least partly explain the high incidence of low-turnover bone lesions observed in peritoneal dialysis.[308, 309] Peritoneal dialysates with Ca²⁺ of 2.5 mEq/L are now commercially available, and there is growing evidence that, as is already happening in hemodialysis patients, they may be desirable for patients treated with CAPD.[787]

## Use of Vitamin D Derivatives

Despite dietary compliance with appropriate intake of $Ca^{2+}$ and restriction of P, the use of P binders, and a dialysate $Ca^{2+}$ of 3.5 mEq/L, a significant number of patients develop secondary HPTH. Because a deficit in calcitriol is important in the genesis of secondary HPTH, the use of calcitriol and other derivatives has become a widely accepted therapy. It is likely that the widespread and appropriate use of vitamin D derivatives is the most important single factor in the markedly decreased number of PTXs performed in the past decade.

When uremic patients exhibit evidence of overt secondary HPTH with bone erosions and significantly high levels of PTH and plasma alkaline phosphatase, treatment with vitamin D derivatives usually leads to clinical improvement. Pharmacologic doses of vitamin $D_2$,[2, 788, 789] dihydrotachysterol,[789, 790] 25(OH)D,[789, 791, 792] $1\alpha$(OH)D,[793, 794] and $1\alpha,25(OH)_2D$,[91, 92, 788] have led to improvement of symptoms and of radiographs toward normality, amelioration of bone pathology, and a fall in serum alkaline phosphatase and PTH concentrations.

Although vitamin $D_2$, vitamin $D_3$, and dihydrotachysterol have been available for a long time, there are only a few well-documented reports on their efficacy.[7, 795] Vitamin $D_2$ or $D_3$ has been reported to induce more normal bone mineralization than $Ca^{2+}$ supplementation alone.[7] Stanbury and Lumb[375] and Dent and colleagues[2] have shown that vitamin $D_2$ at a dosage of 50,000 to 200,000 IU/d improves overt skeletal disease in patients with advanced CRF. However, the responsiveness of individual patients varied greatly. Similarly, Witmer and colleagues[791] reported improvement of radiographic evidence of bone disease in children given 30,000 to 50,000 IU/d vitamin D for 5 to 13 months.

Several highly active, naturally occurring forms of vitamin D—25(OH)D (calcifediol), $1\alpha,25(OH)_2D$ (calcitriol), and $24,25(OH)_2D$—have been evaluated in clinical trials.[788, 789] Also, several synthetic vitamin D derivatives that bypass the need for renal $1\alpha$-hydroxylation have been introduced, including $1\alpha$(OH)D; 5,6-*trans*-25(OH)D; and 5,6-*trans*-D. Also, various synthetic analogues with some of the beneficial properties of vitamin D, such as inhibition of the synthesis of PTH mRNA, but lacking inherent side effects, such as hypercalcemic activity, are being developed experimentally. Of all the mentioned compounds, calcifediol, calcitriol, and $1\alpha$(OH)D have had the widest use. Few data comparing the efficacy of different vitamin D sterols are available.[796–798]

### CALCIFEDIOL

Despite the availability of 25(OH)D (calcifediol) for research purposes since 1969, there are few reports of its use in patients with renal osteodystrophy.[347] Intestinal absorption of $Ca^{2+}$ can be increased with 100 μg of calcifediol per day, and 20 μg/d is enough to augment $Ca^{2+}$ absorption in normal subjects.[799] However, some data indicate that uremic patients may respond favorably to treatment with doses below 100 μg/d. Teitelbaum and co-workers[800] treated five patients with 40 μg/d for 3 to 9 months; serum PTH and alkaline phosphatase levels decreased, and serial

bone biopsy specimens showed decreased numbers of osteoclasts, size of osteoid surface covered with active osteoblasts, and marrow fibrosis. Witmer and associates[791] treated nine uremic children with calcifediol. Five had severe osteodystrophy that previously failed to respond to 13,000 to 27,000 IU/d of vitamin D before calcifediol was given. Osteitis fibrosa improved and the number of osteoblasts and marrow fibrosis decreased in these five children receiving 25 to 200 μg/d of calcifediol. Other children with normal or near-normal skeletal radiographs at the initiation of hemodialysis were given either 25 to 50 μg/d of calcifediol plus an oral $Ca^{2+}$ supplement or oral $Ca^{2+}$ alone. Bone lesions progressively worsened in the group receiving only oral $Ca^{2+}$, but skeletal biopsies showed improved mineralization and decreased fibrosis in those given calcifediol. Fournier and colleagues[798] noted a rise in plasma alkaline phosphatase activity and an increase in the active formation surface area of trabecular bone in three patients given 200 to 300 μg of calcifediol three times per week for 4 to 8 weeks. These effects differed from those observed in other patients given $1\alpha$(OH)D for the same time, suggesting that calcifediol may have a specific effect on bone different from that of other vitamin D derivatives. Results of a five-center study have been summarized by Recker and co-workers.[792] These hemodialysis patients received 200 μg of calcifediol three times weekly for 29 weeks, with the dose adjusted to avoid hypercalcemia; the final dose averaged 46 μg/d. As a group, the patients noted a significant improvement in musculoskeletal-related symptoms and a better overall clinical status. Small increases in serum $Ca^{2+}$ and P concentrations were noted, and serum alkaline phosphatase activity fell. Plasma PTH concentration for the entire group did not change, although it decreased in individual patients. Bone biopsy specimens showed an increased resorption surface area in conjunction with decreased fibrosis. Plasma levels of calcifediol rose to 200 to 300 μg/dL concurrently with the maximal elevation of serum $Ca^{2+}$ concentration. In each of the series reported, several patients developed hypercalcemia. The major disadvantages of calcifediol are that it is less potent than calcitriol and it has a greater half-life; thus, a greater number of days is also required for the episodes of hypercalcemia to resolve.

### CALCITRIOL

#### Oral Calcitriol

In multiple clinical trials, calcitriol has proved highly efficacious in the treatment of patients with renal osteodystrophy. In an early study, Brickman and colleagues[92] reported observations in eight patients given 0.14 to 0.68 μg/d of oral calcitriol for 2 to 4 months. Patients with secondary HPTH and osteitis fibrosa showed decreases in serum PTH concentration, resorption surface area, and marrow fibrosis.[796, 801] Those afflicted by muscle weakness improved their muscle strength. There was some improvement in the abnormal mineralization front in those with osteomalacia. Similar observations were reported by other authors.[502, 802] Eastwood and co-workers[803] gave 0.54 to 1.35 μg/d of calcitriol to five patients for 4 weeks and noted an improvement in bone mineralization in three of them. Similarly, in a series of 40 patients treated with calcitriol at an average dose of 0.62 μg/d for 4 to 90 weeks,[395] bone pain improved in 71% and muscle weakness in 85% of the patients. In patients with elevated serum PTH levels, these levels often decreased and alkaline phosphatase activity declined toward normal. Bone biopsy results improved and a close correlation was observed between improvement in the degree of osteitis fibrosa and reduction in serum PTH.[804] A subgroup of patients with refractory osteomalacia developed hypercalcemia while receiving low doses of calcitriol; these patients were subsequently identified as having Al-related bone disease.[304]

In many patients showing a favorable response, serum P concentration usually decreased within 1 to 3 months of treatment; subsequently, this often increased (Fig. 51–36). Sherrard and co-workers[804] evaluated pre- and post-treatment bone biopsy samples of uremic patients treated with calcitriol and two control groups of patients undergoing dialysis using a dialysate $Ca^{2+}$ of either 3.0 or 4.0 mEq/L. Pretreatment bone biopsies showed more extensive osteitis fibrosa in the calcitriol group. Nonetheless, there was a marked decrease in fibrosis in 10 of 11 patients with osteitis fibrosa and increased mineralization in 16 of 17 patients treated with calcitriol. The patients treated with high dialysate $Ca^{2+}$ showed little or no improvement. Thus, the authors concluded that calcitriol was more effective than $Ca^{2+}$ added to the dialysate in both improving mineralization and reversing secondary HPTH.

The studies just reviewed were carried out in patients with advanced CRF and overt secondary HPTH. Several controlled prospective studies have also been carried out in dialysis patients, including those who were asymptomatic. Thus, in a controlled double-blind study of 31 dialysis patients, Berl and co-workers[796] gave either calcitriol, at an average dose of 0.82 μg/d, or vitamin D, at a dose of 400 IU/d, for 12 weeks. They noted an increase in serum $Ca^{2+}$

from 9.05 ± 0.15 to 10.25 ± 0.20 mg/dL in those receiving calcitriol; serum $Ca^{2+}$ concentration did not change in those receiving vitamin D. Serum PTH fell significantly in 11 of 13 patients receiving calcitriol; this response was not observed after vitamin D. Bone biopsy specimens showed improvement of osteitis fibrosa in patients given calcitriol but no change in those receiving vitamin D; osteomalacia failed to improve in patients receiving calcitriol. Maxwell and colleagues[797] followed a similar protocol in a controlled study. They noted a significant decrease in plasma alkaline phosphatase activity in those receiving calcitriol but no change in those receiving vitamin D. Hypercalcemia in patients taking calcitriol rapidly reversed after drug withdrawal.

In a double-blind trial, Memmos and co-workers[805] gave either 0.5 μg/d of calcitriol or a placebo to asymptomatic patients who had had hemodialysis for at least 1 year; the trial lasted 1 or 2 years. At the end of 1 year, 16 of the 30 patients receiving placebo but only 1 of 27 patients receiving calcitriol showed deterioration in hand radiographs. Among the patients who entered the trial with abnormal skeletal radiographs, none receiving placebo showed improvement after 2 years, compared with 5 of 11 given calcitriol. Serum PTH levels, which were closely related to the severity of radiologic secondary HPTH, and alkaline phosphatase levels showed a slight increase or no change, respectively, in the placebo group, whereas both fell after calcitriol.

In a controlled study of asymptomatic dialysis patients with normal skeletal radiographs and good biochemical control of $Ca^{2+}$ and P levels, the frequency of new or worsened erosions was lower in patients given up to 1.0 μg/d of calcitriol compared with placebo-treated patients.[805] Serum PTH concentration was suppressed in a larger fraction of the patients treated with calcitriol, and PTH concentration more often increased in the control subjects. Analy-

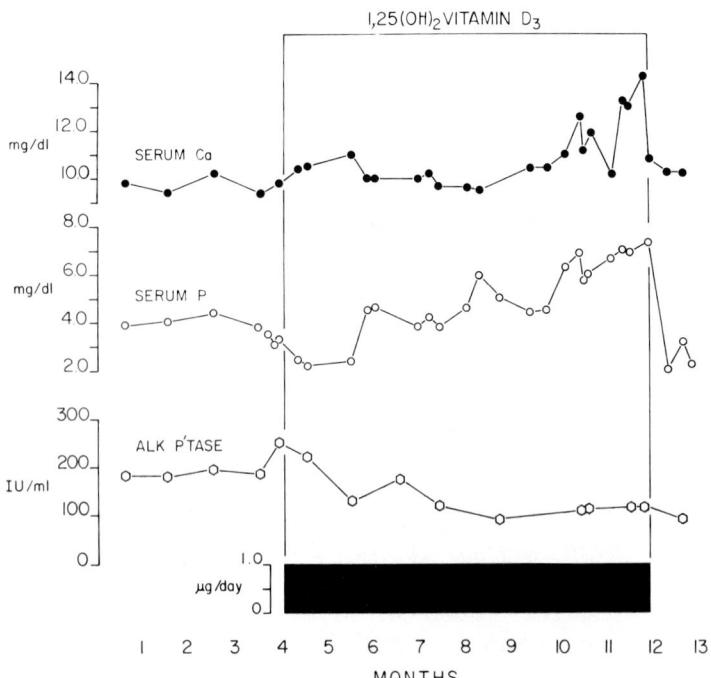

**Figure 51–36.** Changes in serum $Ca^{2+}$, P, and alkaline phosphatase as a 56-year-old man undergoing regular hemodialysis was treated with $1,25(OH)_2D$. Serum immunoreactive PTH fell from 1580 to 220 pg/mL during this period (normal, 400 pg/mL). The early drop and subsequent rise in serum P level are notable. The rise occurred after the alkaline phosphatase level fell and coincident with the development of hypercalcemia. The prominent decrease in both serum $Ca^{2+}$ and P levels after withdrawal of treatment is evident. (From Coburn JW, Brickman AS, Sherrard DJ, et al: Clinical efficacy of 1,25 dihydroxy vitamin $D_3$ in renal osteodystrophy. In Norman AW, Schaefer K, Coburn JW, et al [eds]: Vitamin D: Biochemical, Chemical and Clinical Aspects Related to Calcium Metabolism. Walter de Gruyter, Berlin, 1977, pp 657–666.)

sis of the data for these patients disclosed considerable heterogeneity in the suppressibility of the parathyroid glands; a serum $Ca^{2+}$ value of 10.0 to 10.8 mg/dL was needed in many patients to reduce serum PTH levels.[806] Such observations are consistent with an increase in the set-point of $Ca^{2+}$; that is, in uremic patients a higher $Ca^{2+}$ concentration is required to suppress parathyroid gland activity.

In children with advanced CRF, overt skeletal disease has a high frequency compared with adults; those who received calcitriol have responded favorably. As mentioned before, improvement in growth or catch-up growth was initially reported in children receiving calcitriol,[547] although subsequent observations have not confirmed such a beneficial effect.[807] Observations in children undergoing treatment with CAPD suggest that the maintenance of normal serum $Ca^{2+}$ concentration during treatment with calcitriol may not invariably lead to reversal of the features of secondary HPTH.[215] Indeed, it may be necessary to raise the serum $Ca^{2+}$ concentration to levels slightly above normal to achieve a more consistent reversal of secondary HPTH.[548]

In general, the trials with calcitriol and $1\alpha(OH)D$ suggest that these sterols are the most effective in secondary HPTH, particularly when serum $Ca^{2+}$ concentration is normal or decreased; when osteomalacia and secondary HPTH coexist, a favorable response also occurs. Overall, oral calcitriol and $1\alpha(OH)D$ appear to be similarly effective. Under some circumstances the bone can be restored largely to normal, but in other settings the elevated serum PTH levels persist and treatment with oral calcitriol is not successful in reversing the secondary HPTH. In this situation, as we discuss later, intravenous calcitriol may be helpful.

Administration of calcitriol may help to predict the underlying bone disease. Thus, patients with low-turnover bone disease are prone to develop hypercalcemia with low doses of calcitriol within the first several weeks of treatment, as well as patients with severe secondary HPTH and marked parathyroid gland hyperplasia.[147, 304] When hypercalcemia develops after many weeks or months of treatment and alkaline phosphatase levels have returned to normal, it is likely that osteitis fibrosa has substantially regressed.

As shown, administration of oral calcitriol to dialysis patients—in many studies from 0.25 to 2 μg/d—is effective in reducing serum PTH levels and improving bone disease. In a study by Seidel and associates,[808] a single oral dose of 2 μg of calcitriol induced a delayed (between 24 and 48 hours) but long-lasting (>96 hours) decrease of intact PTH levels, even though calcitriol levels returned to baseline levels earlier. Thus, new information on the kinetics of intact PTH after treatment with calcitriol may provide new insights into the treatment schedules used, eventually improving results with less secondary effects.

Prophylactic treatment of dialysis patients with calcitriol may prevent the development of secondary HPTH. Preliminary data have suggested that administration of calcitriol, or $1\alpha(OH)D$, in daily doses of 0.25 to 0.50 μg to patients with early to moderate CRF may reverse and/or prevent secondary HPTH and is rarely associated with hypercalcemia, hyperphosphatemia, or impairment of renal function.[20, 283, 809, 810] Moreover, careful monitoring is advised, and if such complications arise they are usually reversible.

It should also be mentioned that there is evidence that calcitriol impairs creatinine secretion by the renal tubule; thus, serum creatinine levels may increase and the clearance of creatinine decrease without any change in true GFR.[811] Thus, calcitriol therapy in early stages of CRF may prevent secondary HPTH. Moreover, patients such as children or those with slow progression of CRF such as in interstitial diseases may greatly benefit from early calcitriol therapy.

### Intravenous Calcitriol

The observation that calcitriol has a direct inhibitory effect on the parathyroid cell and that this effect is dose related makes the use of intravenous calcitriol an important alternative in the control of secondary HPTH. Thus, intravenous calcitriol administered three times weekly at the end of regular dialysis, by inducing a higher peak in serum calcitriol concentration, results in a greater suppression of PTH and fewer undesirable hypercalcemic episodes.[101, 123, 812] Slatopolsky and co-workers[101] compared the effects of oral and intermittent intravenous calcitriol administration on the circulating plasma levels of calcitriol as well as on PTH secretion. They observed that oral administration of calcitriol in doses adequate to maintain serum $Ca^{2+}$ in the upper limits of normal did not alter PTH levels, whereas a marked suppression of PTH levels (70.1% ± 3.2%) was observed in 20 patients receiving intravenous calcitriol. Norris and colleagues[813] also treated 10 patients with overt secondary HPTH with intravenous calcitriol. These patients received from 1 to 5 μg of calcitriol at the end of each dialysis for a period of 13 months. They observed a significant decrease in serum PTH (42% ± 4%) and alkaline phosphatase (62% ± 4%); serum $Ca^{2+}$ increased from 10.1 to 11.2 mg/dL. Intravenous calcitriol has also been shown to improve histologic features of secondary HPTH; thus, Andress and colleagues[814] studied 12 hemodialysis patients with severe secondary HPTH refractory to oral calcitriol therapy. They were treated with intravenous calcitriol, 1 to 2.5 μg three times a week given at the end of each dialysis, for 1 year or longer. The authors noted a mild increase in serum $Ca^{2+}$, from 2.5 to 2.6 mmol/L; a significant decrease in PTH, from 172 ± 34 to 69 ± 16 pg/L; and a marked improvement in bone histologic features.

Although higher $Ca^{2+}$ levels per se may have been a factor in the observed PTH suppression, Slatopolsky and colleagues[101] observed that PTH started to decrease before any increment in serum $Ca^{2+}$ was detected. After this study, we evaluated the direct inhibitory effect of calcitriol on parathyroid function, avoiding the presence of hypercalcemia, in nine hemodialysis patients with marked secondary HPTH.[123] After a baseline evaluation of parathyroid function, we administered 2 μg of intravenous calcitriol after each hemodialysis for a 10-week period. Parathyroid gland function was assessed by inducing hypo- and hypercalcemia using a low- and a high-$Ca^{2+}$ dialysate during two separate dialyses performed a week apart. To avoid the previously observed hypercalcemia during calcitriol administration, the dialysate $Ca^{2+}$ was reduced to 2.5 mEq/L. Parathyroid hormone values after dialysis-induced hypo- and hypercalcemia were plotted against serum $Ca^{2+}$ for each patient, and the sigmoid relationship between PTH and $Ca^{2+}$ was evaluated. A sigmoid relationship was established for each patient and the set-point of $Ca^{2+}$, as previously defined, was determined. The basal PTH levels fell from $902 \pm 126$ to $466 \pm 152$ pg/mL ($P < .01$) after 10 weeks of calcitriol therapy. This occurred in the absence of any significant changes in serum $Ca^{2+}$ concentration (see Fig. 51–13). The PTH-$Ca^{2+}$ sigmoid curve shifted to the left and downward after calcitriol therapy. Moreover, after calcitriol therapy, the maximal PTH response during hypocalcemia decreased from $1661 \pm 485$ to $1031 \pm 280$ pg/mL ($P < .05$) and the minimal PTH level from $281 \pm 76$ to $192 \pm 48$ pg/mL ($P < .05$). However, neither the set-point of $Ca^{2+}$ nor the slope of the PTH-$Ca^{2+}$ curve was significantly different after 10 weeks of calcitriol. If a noncompliant patient with persistent hyperphosphatemia was excluded, a significant shift of the set-point of $Ca^{2+}$ to the left was noted (see Fig. 51–17).

Later, six patients continued to receive intravenous calcitriol and were re-evaluated after 42 weeks of treatment.[61] The continued treatment with calcitriol resulted in a progressive decrease in serum PTH levels for a similar serum $Ca^{2+}$ concentration. In addition, the slope of the PTH-$Ca^{2+}$ curve was decreased at 42 weeks ($P < .05$) compared with both 0 and 10 weeks. These findings suggest that calcitriol 1) reduced the functional mass of parathyroid cells (based on the lower maximal PTH) and 2) decreased the sensitivity of parathyroid cells (difference in the slope of PTH-$Ca^{2+}$ curve with PTH as a percentage of maximal PTH) as a result of long-term calcitriol treatment. Malberti and colleagues[102] have reported similar results.

Hamdy and associates[815] evaluated the effect of intravenous calcitriol in four patients with persistent hypercalcemia and marked secondary HPTH. These patients had been shown to be intolerant to oral administration of calcitriol. After each dialysis, calcitriol was administered intravenously in doses of 0.5 to 2.5 µg for 2 months. Calcitriol therapy continued for 7 and 8 months, respectively, in two of the four patients. After 4 weeks of therapy, a significant decrease in serum $Ca^{2+}$ was observed that was maintained throughout treatment as the dosage of intravenous calcitriol was increased. This was associated with a decrease in PTH levels. During the long-term administration of calcitriol, serum $Ca^{2+}$ values increased but lower concentrations of PTH were maintained. The authors concluded that the increment in serum $Ca^{2+}$ is not a prerequisite for the suppression of PTH secretion by calcitriol and that the presence of hypercalcemia does not preclude the use of intravenous calcitriol.

Finally, although the average dose has varied in different studies, most have used 0.5 to 1 µg per dialysis as a starting dose. Gallieni and co-workers[396] used an average dose of 0.87 µg per dialysis in a large multicenter study that included 76 patients. Dressler and associates[816] have evaluated 12 symptomatic hemodialysis patients with severe overt secondary HPTH (half of patients had PTH values ranging from 1500 to 3400 pg/mL). Patients were selected for the presence of persistent or progressive secondary HPTH nonresponsive to oral calcitriol therapy; some patients were being considered for PTX. They received intravenous calcitriol at the end of each dialysis for a mean period of 14 months. From a starting dose of 1 µg, calcitriol

was dosed up to a maximum of 8 µg; the mean intravenous calcitriol dose administered was 4.4 µg. By the end of the study, there was significant clinical improvement in all patients. In addition, PTH decreased from 1179 to 159 pg/mL. Serum $Ca^{2+}$ increased from 9.2 to 10.8 mg/dL. Hypercalcemic episodes were infrequently noted (mostly in two patients), and only three patients were given a dialysate $Ca^{2+}$ of 2.5 mEq/L. No changes in serum P were observed except in a noncompliant patient. These observations suggest that the severity of secondary HPTH may be an important factor in deciding what dose of intravenous calcitriol to use. Thus, the higher the levels of PTH, the higher the dose of calcitriol to be administered.

In summary, the available data on intravenous calcitriol suggest that it is an alternative in patients who may develop hypercalcemia or hyperphosphatemia after oral therapy, as well as in those with overt secondary HPTH and in noncompliant patients.

### Oral Pulse Therapy with Calcitriol

Because the efficacy of intermittent intravenous calcitriol is most likely related to the high peak of serum calcitriol achieved, the use of intermittent "oral pulses" of calcitriol, ranging from 2 to 5 µg two or three times a week, has been evaluated.[677, 817–820] Good results have been observed with such an approach to the treatment of secondary HPTH.[817, 818] Fukagawa and colleagues[677] noted in patients with moderate secondary HPTH that 4 µg of oral calcitriol twice weekly not only reduced the PTH levels but also the size of the parathyroid glands by 41% as measured by ultrasonography. This therapeutic regimen has also proved effective in patients having CAPD with mild to moderate secondary HPTH.[819] The efficacy of calcitriol in reduction of PTH mRNA and serum PTH levels was assessed when the calcitriol was administered as intermittent bolus or continuously by an osmotic minipump in an experimental model.[821] Preliminary results showed that although the total increment (area under the curve) of serum calcitriol was smaller in the bolus group, the bolus administration was more efficient, probably in relation to a higher peak calcitriol levels. Thus, the response of parathyroid glands to calcitriol seems to be more influenced by short-term calcitriol peak levels than by long-term steady-state calcitriol levels. Similarly, a comparison of serum calcitriol levels after a single oral versus an intravenous dose revealed serum levels exceeding the normal range for a period of up to 24 hours with both routes,[135] but the overall area under the curve after intravenous calcitriol was 62% greater.

### Other Routes of Administration

Intraperitoneal calcitriol administration has also proved effective in adult patients undergoing CAPD[822, 823] as well as in children.[824] The subcutaneous route has also been successfully tested in a few patients in both CAPD and hemodialysis.[825, 826]

### 1α(OH)D

This synthetic form of calcitriol undergoes 25-hydroxylation in the liver to be converted to calcitriol before exerting its action (see Fig. 51–8). It is active in patients with advanced uremia; the dose required to increase intestinal $Ca^{2+}$ absorption is only 1.5- to 2-fold of that needed for calcitriol.[827] The improvement of hyperparathyroid bone disease and reversal of other features of secondary HPTH after its use are also similar to those with calcitriol, although the required dosage is 50% to 75% higher.[828] Both short-term and long-term clinical trials have shown $1\alpha(OH)D$ to be effective in patients with CRF.[793, 796, 827] Not surprisingly, patients subsequently shown to have Al-related osteomalacia also failed to respond to $1\alpha(OH)D$,[829] as did those treated with calcitriol.[830]

The $1\alpha(OH)D$ is widely used in Europe, Canada, and Japan, but only short-term trials have been carried out in the United States.[827] The importance of concurrent use of P binders to control serum P concentration has been stressed by Davison and associates.[831] Twenty patients receiving $1\alpha(OH)D$ were compared with a group given aluminum hydroxide to reduce serum P to below 5.0 mg/dL before treatment with $1\alpha(OH)D$ was initiated. In the former group, the frequency of corneal calcifications, pruritus, and radiographic evidence of soft extraskeletal calcifications were higher. Bone erosions resolved in a similar number of patients in both groups, but there was a higher incidence of periosteal new bone formation in the group not given P binders.

Brandi[832] and Lind[833] and their colleagues have described the effect of intravenous administration of $1\alpha(OH)D$ in patients having hemodialysis. They observed a marked suppression of PTH and only a slight increase in serum $Ca^{2+}$. Thus, intravenous $1\alpha(OH)D$ has an inhibitory effect on PTH secretion similar to that of calcitriol. Ljunghall and co-workers[834] studied normocalcemic patients treated for 12 weeks with an increasing dose of the sterol, but because of hypercalcemic episodes, the dose had to be reduced in most patients and withdrawn in three. At the end of the study, only 6 patients were receiving the maximal dose (4 μg per dialysis session) and in 17 patients the dose used was 1 μg per dialysis session. Significant reductions of PTH were observed after 1 week of treatment, and maximal suppression was obtained after 4 weeks. However, a mild increase in PTH levels was observed at the end of the study as a result of the dose adjustment to avoid hypercalcemic episodes.

Long-term suppression of secondary HPTH by intravenous $1\alpha(OH)D$ has also been evaluated. Brandi and colleagues[835] also reported on 13 patients who received intravenous $1\alpha(OH)D$, 6 of them up to 96 weeks. At the end of the study, PTH levels were still suppressed by 78% ± 4% after 300 days, 78% ± 9% after 550 days, and 85% ± 7% after 720 days.

Finally, in the choice of either $1\alpha(OH)D$ or any vitamin D derivative lacking the 25-OH group it should be kept in mind that hepatic 25-hydroxylation is necessary before they become biologically active. Thus, simultaneous treatment with a drug such as phenobarbital, phenytoin, or glutethimide, as well as the presence of concomitant liver disease, may impair the hepatic 25-hydroxylation and may result in impaired action of the vitamin D sterol.[836, 837]

## OTHER VITAMIN D DERIVATIVES

In addition to the sterols just discussed, several other synthetic vitamin D derivatives have been used in short-term trials. Several of these sterols have the A ring of the steroid molecule rotated 180 degrees about the 5,6 double bond; this converts the molecule from a cis to a trans configuration, with the normal 3-hydroxyl group assuming a geometric position equivalent to that of the $1\alpha$-hydroxyl moiety of calcitriol. This may be referred to as a "pseudo–$1\alpha$-hydroxyl" configuration. Several such compounds can enhance $Ca^{2+}$ absorption in uremic patients[838, 839]; these include 5,6-trans-D and 5,6-trans-25(OH)D.[838, 839] These agents have been given to dialysis patients in Europe but it is not clear that these compounds have any advantage over calcitriol.

Another naturally occurring vitamin D sterol is $24,25(OH)_2D$. It appears that there are qualitative differences between the effect of this sterol and that of calcitriol in patients with CRF.[200, 201] A small number of patients whose osteomalacia was refractory to calcitriol alone responded to $24,25(OH)_2D$ combined with calcitriol.[840] Subsequently these patients were found to have Al-related osteomalacia,[212] and their favorable responses have not been confirmed.[841] Other studies have suggested that $24,25(OH)_2D$ may have a suppressive effect on the parathyroid glands[126, 842]; however, other studies of patients with secondary HPTH and dogs with experimental uremia failed to demonstrate this effect.[843, 844] Nevertheless, observations strongly suggest that this sterol, unlike calcitriol, specifically inhibits bone resorption and that this effect is independent of PTH.[845] Thus, a study of 29 dialysis patients treated with either calcitriol or $24,25(OH)_2D$ alone or both together showed that calcitriol inhibited PTH secretion and that $24,25(OH)_2D$ decreased bone resorption and formation without any change in PTH levels. More important, administration of both sterols together resulted in greater improvement in the abnormal bone resorption. Popovtzer and colleagues[202, 846] have evaluated the effect of $24,25(OH)_2D$ together with $1\alpha(OH)D$ in dialysis patients. Osteoclastic parameters and bone mineralization improved significantly after 10 to 16 months only in the group receiving both sterols. Thus, these studies strongly suggest that combined treatment with $24,25(OH)_2D$ and $1\alpha(OH)D$ or calcitriol may result in a greater improvement in bone histology.

Calcitriol analogues, mainly oxacalcitriol, are promising for the treatment of secondary HPTH. Thus, oxacalcitriol suppressed PTH synthesis and showed no hypercalcemic activity in experimental studies.[847–849] However, such a dissociative effect is not always present.[850] The apparent discrepancy between these studies may be explained by the fact that in the later study oxacalcitriol was administered in rats with more severe secondary HPTH. At present, it is doubtful that oxacalcitriol offers any real advantage over calcitriol.

## GENERAL CONSIDERATIONS IN RELATION TO VITAMIN D USE

The principal hazard in the use of vitamin D derivatives is hypercalcemia, and when it occurs its resolution may require several weeks. The time required for the resolution of undesired hypercalcemia is related to the half-life of the vitamin D metabolite. One major feature of calcitriol and 1α(OH)D is their rapid turnover compared with vitamin D itself. Kanis and Russell[851] evaluated the rate of reversal of hypercalcemia or hypercalciuria induced by vitamin D, dihydrotachysterol, 1α(OH)D, and calcitriol. The half-time for reversal of the effects was shorter after discontinuing calcitriol than was the case for 1α(OH)D, vitamin D, or dihydrotachysterol; the differences were independent of the dose given or the length of treatment. Similar results were reported by Brickman and co-workers[827] when comparing 1α(OH)D and calcitriol. Thus, calcitriol shows the most rapid reversal of hypercalcemia, a useful feature should toxicity occur. Hypercalcemia has been suggested to be less frequent when oral calcitriol is given at night.[852]

Likewise, intestinal absorption of P increases after calcitriol therapy[853]; thus, hyperphosphatemia is not uncommon after oral calcitriol.[102, 396] The magnitude of this increment seems to be lower with intravenous than with oral calcitriol. However, Gallieni and colleagues[396] have reported the effects of low-dose intravenous calcitriol (<1 μg) in hemodialysis patients with significant secondary HPTH (mean intact PTH 767 ± 76 pg/mL); 58 of 76 patients had a significant reduction of PTH levels. Although asymptomatic hypercalcemia was observed in 30% of the patients, hyperphosphatemia developed in 60%. In 12 of 22 patients who were taking calcium carbonate as the only P binder at the beginning of treatment, an Al-containing P binder had to be used to control their serum P levels.

Although vitamin D derivatives, either orally or intravenously, are effective in decreasing synthesis and secretion of PTH,[101, 126] improving bone histology, suppressing parathyroid cell proliferation,[854] decreasing the size of the hyperplastic parathyroid glands,[677] and even triggering the apoptotic process (programmed cell death) of hyperplastic parathyroid cells,[855] it should also be mentioned that a few patients do not experience such improvement. Factors responsible for such therapeutic failures are not well known. Endogenous resistance to normal levels of calcitriol[136] and decreased vitamin D receptor density in nodular hyperplasia[152] could account for such failures. It has also been shown by in situ hybridization and cytometric DNA analysis that although there were no differences in the amount of PTH mRNA in the cells from either diffuse or nodular hyperplastic glands, the recurrence of secondary HPTH may be due not to enhanced PTH synthetic activity but to the abnormal growth rate of the transplanted nodular graft.[150, 151]

A known cause of failure in the treatment with calcitriol is irregular administration of the sterol because of repeated episodes of hypercalcemia. Parathyroid size, in preliminary studies, was noted to be critical for long-term prognosis of calcitriol therapy in dialysis patients.[856] It is our impression that the larger the gland, the more severe the secondary HPTH and the more likely the presence of resistance to treatment. In this regard, the use of higher doses of intravenous calcitriol may correct the calcitriol resistance and avoid the need for PTX even in patients with severe secondary HPTH.[816]

Another emerging cause of failure to control secondary

HPTH despite appropriate calcitriol therapy is the presence of significant hyperphosphatemia. Of particular interest is the observation in our previous study[123] of two patients, in whom we observed a decreased basal and maximal PTH levels after 10 weeks of calcitriol treatment. These patients later developed severe hyperphosphatemia and simultaneously the serum PTH levels increased despite continued calcitriol therapy (Fig. 51–37). These findings suggest that P per se may lead to worsening of secondary HPTH and resistance to the inhibitory effect of calcitriol on PTH synthesis. E. Fernandez and J. Montoliu (personal communication) have evaluated parathyroid function and hyperphosphatemia in dialysis patients. As shown in Figure 51–38, the presence of hyperphosphatemia displaced the PTH-$Ca^{2+}$ curve toward the right in only 3 days. Figure 51–39 shows a schematic representation of the deleterious effects of hyperphosphatemia on PTH secretion and inhibitory action on calcitriol. Thus, hyperphosphatemia in the presence of calcitriol therapy not only may lead to an increase in the risk of soft tissue calcification through an increase in the $Ca^{2+} \times P$ product,[857] but also may render calcitriol therapy ineffective and aggravate the secondary HPTH.

Finally, despite appropriate therapy with calcitriol, bone histologic features do not always return to normal in a substantial number of patients, clearly indicating the presence of factors other than calcitriol in the pathogenesis of secondary HPTH. In an experimental model calcitriol failed to reverse hyperplasia completely once the latter had been established.[854] Also, parathyroid gland weights tend to be increased even after successful kidney transplantation. We have observed that despite good clinical responses to calcitriol, a significant number of patients have a rebound in PTH to previous values once calcitriol is discontinued. Moreover, calcitriol did not have the same effect on the PTH-$Ca^{2+}$ sigmoid curve as PTX.[102] Thus, medical PTX with intravenous calcitriol is not equivalent to surgical PTX. It is possible that with calcitriol the secretion of PTH decreases proportionally more than with a decrease in the mass of parathyroid cells.[178]

Useful guidelines to therapy with calcitriol and other active vitamin D derivatives in patients on dialysis are the following: 1) In patients with intact PTH levels five- to sixfold greater than the upper limit of normality, calcitriol should almost always be initiated; 2) in patients with intact PTH levels three- to fivefold normal, therapy at low doses might be considered, especially if serial determinations show a PTH increase; 3) in patients with intact PTH levels two- to threefold normal, calcitriol may not be advisable because of the risk of inducing low-turnover bone disease unless the cause is a rare severe malnutrition with nutritional vitamin D deficiency.

Patients who may benefit from intravenous calcitriol are 1) noncompliant patients; 2) patients with overt secondary HPTH who cannot be treated with oral calcitriol therapy because of induced hypercalcemia; 3) patients who develop hyperphosphatemia immediately after oral administration of calcitriol (they may respond to intravenous calcitriol with a lesser degree of hyperphosphatemia); and 4) patients with marked secondary HPTH who are considered for PTX (in some cases the administration of intravenous calcitriol may avoid surgery; the dosage of calcitriol may be increased as long as serum $Ca^{2+}$ and P are adequately controlled).

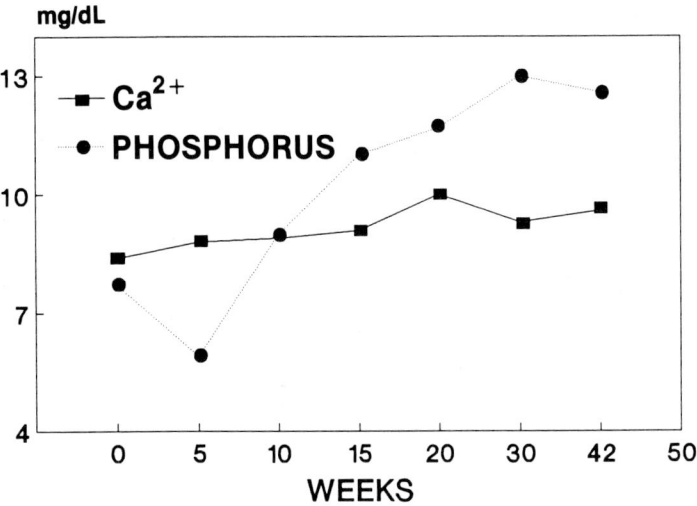

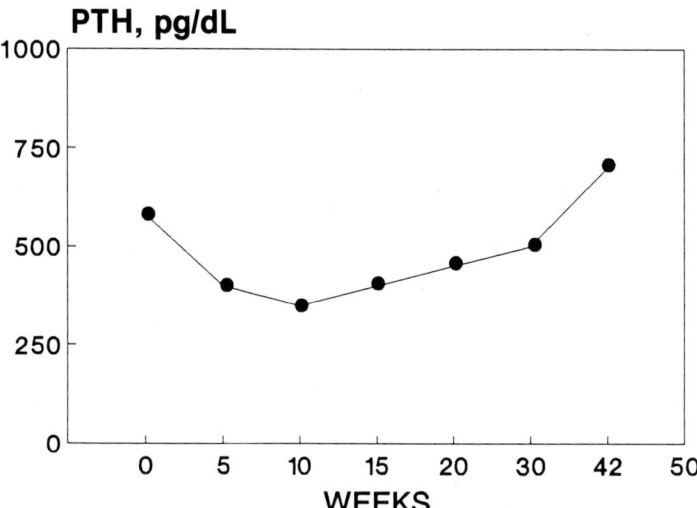

**Figure 51–37.** A patient with secondary HPTH treated with intravenous calcitriol for 42 weeks. *Top.* Serum $Ca^{2+}$ and P during this period. *Bottom.* Serum PTH. Note that although the patient developed severe hyperphosphatemia (dietary noncompliance) and despite appropriate intravenous calcitriol treatment and serum $Ca^{2+}$ in the upper limit of normal, PTH progressively increased after the fifth week.

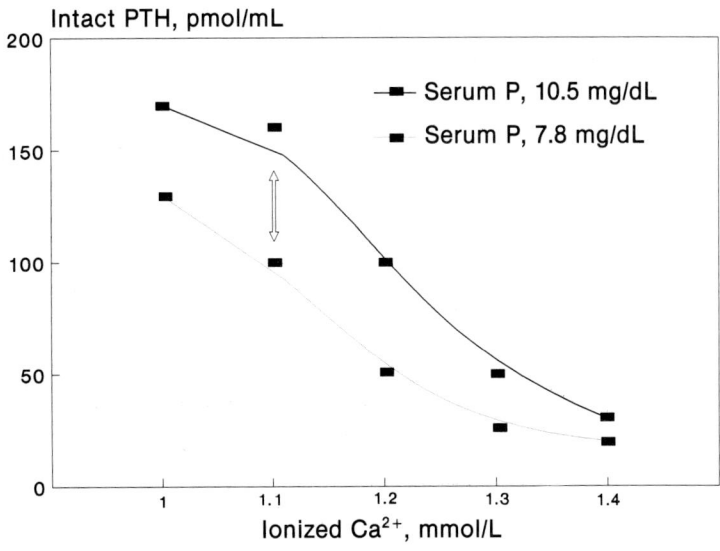

**Figure 51–38.** Sigmoid PTH-$Ca^{2+}$ relationship in a noncompliant patient with severe hyperphosphatemia. The continuous line displays the PTH-$Ca^{2+}$ curve in the presence of severe hyperphosphatemia (10.5 mg/dL). The dotted line displays the PTH-$Ca^{2+}$ curve 3 days later after lowering serum P to 7.8 mg/dL. (Courtesy of E Fernandez and J Montoliu.)

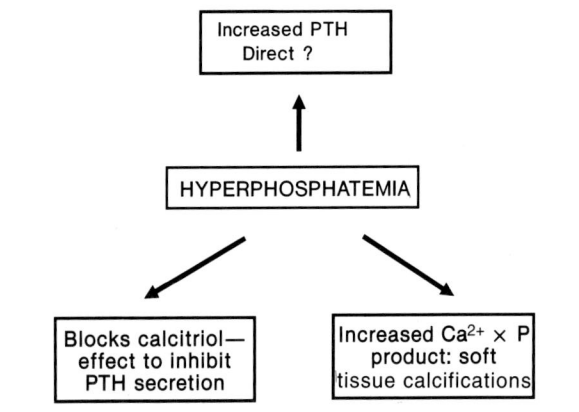

**Figure 51–39.** Schematic representation of the deleterious effects of hyperphosphatemia.

## Parathyroid Surgery

The medical management just described may not succeed, and the progression of overt secondary HPTH may necessitate PTX. Thus, the clinical indications for parathyroid surgery include unequivocal evidence of secondary HPTH (high levels of serum PTH and the presence of osteitis fibrosa on bone biopsy), exclusion of Al toxicity, and any of the following: 1) persistent hypercalcemia not attributable to other causes, especially if hypercalcemia is symptomatic; 2) severe and intractable pruritus; 3) serum $Ca^{2+} \times P$ product that consistently exceeds 70 to 80 $mg^2/dL^2$ together with progressive extraskeletal calcifications; 4) progressive skeletal and articular pain, fractures, or deformities; 5) symptomatic hypercalcemia after successful kidney transplantation; and 6) calciphylaxis. When a patient does not have a refractory hypercalcemia or hyperphosphatemia, a therapeutic trial with intravenous calcitriol should be tried before PTX.

Since Stanbury and co-workers[858] carried out the first PTX in a patient with severe secondary HPTH, three surgical procedures for management of overt secondary HPTH have been developed. They are subtotal PTX, total PTX with autotransplantation, and total PTX without autotransplantation. Each procedure has its advocates[859, 860]; however, the most important factor is a surgeon who is highly skilled and experienced with parathyroid surgery and/or a particular technique. Some groups advocate the superiority of PTX with autotransplantation,[861, 862] because a reoperation in the forearm is technically simpler than in the neck. However, malignant degeneration of the autografted tissue has been reported[863] as well as muscle invasion by benign parathyroid hyperplasia.[864] Observations of several hundred patients after PTX seem to indicate that similar results are obtained with subtotal PTX and total PTX with autotransplantation.[859]

Substantial numbers of patients may have recurrence of secondary HPTH after PTX regardless of the procedure. Gagne and colleagues[144] noted that one third of the patients who underwent subtotal PTX or total PTX with autotransplantation had elevated intact levels of PTH. Because of the high rate of recurrence, Kaye and colleagues[860] favor total PTX without autotransplantation. In a long-term post-PTX follow-up (mean 3.8 years), seven of nine patients had measurable levels of intact PTH and one even mild secondary HPTH. All patients improved clinically and bone mineral density increased even in two patients.[860] Total PTX without autotransplantation remains controversial, especially considering the propensity of these patients to develop Al-related bone disease and the unknown evolution of bone disease after an eventual kidney transplantation and corticosteroid treatment.

At surgery, it is imperative that all the parathyroid glands be identified. The number of glands normally varies from two to six[865]; failure to recognize sites of normal fifth and sixth glands is a common cause of failure of parathyroid surgery.[866] Good judgment and, even more important, extensive experience of the parathyroid surgeon are clearly important for the identification and management of these atypical cases. When subtotal PTX is being performed, it is important that the most suitable gland be identified. Usually the gland that appears least hyperplastic but has an adequate blood supply is the best to partially resect; 40 to 60 mg of tissue should be left. After visually ascertaining that a satisfactory blood supply is preserved in the remaining parathyroid tissue, the surgeon can excise the other glands. The residual parathyroid tissue sometimes undergoes hyperplasia, necessitating a second surgical procedure; therefore, it is recommended that the remaining gland be marked by a metal clip and/or a long, black silk suture.[867] When only two or three parathyroid glands in the neck or the upper anterior thorax are accessible at the time of neck exploration, removal of all three glands is recommended under the assumption that the fourth gland is located elsewhere. Tissues should be maintained by cryopreservation in case permanent hypoparathyroidism develops.[868]

For parathyroid autotransplantation, parathyroid tissue, which has been identified by frozen section, is placed in chilled culture medium; then slices are implanted in multiple pockets in muscle on the lateral aspect of the flexor surface of the forearm of the nondominant arm.[868] Nonabsorbable suture is used to secure the slices in the muscle pockets and to provide a marker for subsequent identification should surgical resection be required. Presternal subcutaneous implantation of the autograft has also been shown to be safe and effective.[869] Finally, technical problems during the PTX should be few and blood loss minimal. A dialysis patient should be treated with dialysis 1 day before the elective PTX, and the hematocrit should be higher than 30% to ensure the best possible coagulation. Usually the patient can leave the hospital within a week.

The most important problem in the postoperative period is hypocalcemia. Blood $Ca^{2+}$ levels almost invariably fall after removal of parathyroid tissue; the degree of hypocalcemia is related to the severity of histologic parameters of osteitis fibrosa.[870] It is the so-called hungry bone syndrome because, in the absence of PTH, $Ca^{2+}$ influx to the bone dramatically increases and the resulting hypocalcemia is usually significant. The magnitude of $Ca^{2+}$ administration correlates closely with the severity of skeletal disease.[871] Because of it, hypocalcemia is often more marked and prolonged than that observed in patients with primary HPTH after PTX. To minimize the postoperative hypocalcemia, 0.5 to 1.0 μg/d of oral calcitriol or 1.5 to 2 μg per dialysis of intravenous calcitriol may be given for 4 to 6 days before PTX and immediately after it; also, oral calcium carbonate is given to provide 1 to 2 g of elemental calcium. Significant and often prolonged hypophosphatemia also develops after surgery because of the "hungry bone."

Tetany may occur during the postoperative period and usually occurs during the first hemodialysis sessions; this is most likely related to the pH increase induced by dialysis. The amount of oral $Ca^{2+}$ needed is often quite large; it can be increased 0.5 to 1.0 g/d at intervals of 3 to 7 days until the serum $Ca^{2+}$ concentration begins to increase. If the concentration of serum $Ca^{2+}$ falls below 7.5 mg/dL or if tetany appears, intravenous $Ca^{2+}$ should be given as well. Thus, after PTX careful monitoring of serum $Ca^{2+}$ is mandatory. Tetany occurring in a uremic patient with severe bone disease may be catastrophic; the simultaneous fracture of scapula, clavicle, and both femoral necks has been reported during an episode of tetany during dialysis.[872] These major fractures have usually been observed 1 to 3 weeks after surgery. Interestingly, they often occurred late during the hemodialysis procedure. Seizures can also cause fractures and tendon avulsion. Such seizures may occur from 1 to 2 days up to 4 weeks after the surgery. In the postoperative management of patients with marked periarticular calcifications, it may be wise to maintain a modest hypocalcemia—serum $Ca^{2+}$ concentration of 8.0 to 9.0 mg/dL—until the ectopic calcifications have resolved. Similarly, administration of $Ca^{2+}$-containing P binders may be indicated to maintain serum P concentration in the range of 3.5 to 5.0 mg/dL.

In patients with marked skeletal disease, hypocalcemia may occasionally persist for 2 to 3 months after PTX. Large amounts of oral $Ca^{2+}$ supplements and appropriate doses of calcitriol usually are also successful in correcting hypocalcemia. Serum levels of P and $Mg^{2+}$ may also decrease during this time. If serum $Mg^{2+}$ falls below 1.5 mg/dL (1.2 mEq/L), oral supplemental $Mg^{2+}$ should be given. Administration of P salts aggravates hypocalcemia; thus, patients should not receive P unless the serum P falls to extremely low levels (<1.5 to 2 mg/dL). An increase in the calcitriol dosage may be needed. If the serum P concentration falls below 2.5 mg/dL, administration of P binders should be reduced or stopped, but no effort should be made to increase the P concentration above 3.5 to 4.0 mg/dL. Calcium carbonate or acetate is the agent of choice, and Al salts should be avoided.[232, 233]

During the period of hypocalcemia, remineralization of the skeleton is usually occurring; blood $Ca^{2+}$ concentration starts to rise and the requirement for $Ca^{2+}$ and calcitriol decreases markedly once bone remineralization is completed. If the doses of $Ca^{2+}$ and calcitriol are not reduced, hypercalcemia may ensue. The fall of a markedly elevated plasma alkaline phosphatase level to near normal may indicate that the bone is reaching a stage at which healing is largely completed; when this occurs, the $Ca^{2+}$ supplements and vitamin D dosage should be reduced.

Failure of serum $Ca^{2+}$ concentration to decrease significantly after surgery may indicate either that too much residual parathyroid tissue was left behind or that missed, ectopic, or supernumerary glands were present. Thus, several techniques such as echography, computed tomography, $^{201}Tl$-$^{99m}Tc$ scintigraphy, or a combination of these have been used for presurgical localization of parathyroid glands.[671, 672, 678] Another cause of failure of serum $Ca^{2+}$ to decrease after PTX may be that severe osteitis fibrosa was not responsible for the hypercalcemia present before PTX. In this situation, Al toxicity or a granulomatous or neoplastic disorder, among other causes, has to be excluded (see Table 51–5).

Hyperkalemia is another preventable complication after PTX.[873] This is in agreement with information demonstrating an important role of PTH in regulating $K^+$ homeostasis. When even modest hyperkalemia occurs in a dialysis patient during the immediate postoperative period, substantial electrocardiographic abnormalities may occur because of the rise in $K^+$ concentration and the concomitant hypocalcemia.

Another postoperative complication of PTX is the development of Al-related osteomalacia.[232, 233] The mechanism responsible for this is unclear; most likely, substantial accumulation of Al in bone had developed before the PTX, and the presence of high PTH levels with an increased bone turnover rate may have protected the bone from the deleterious effect of Al. After PTX, bone turnover decreases markedly and Al is deposited on the mineralization front.[232] The existence of symptomatic osteomalacia after PTX indicates that surgery may have not been indicated and hypercalcemia was due to pre-existing Al-related bone disease. Furthermore, in the absence of PTH, removal of Al deposits from bone with deferoxamine is more difficult.

## Percutaneous Ethanol Injection

A new parathyroid ablative technique consisting of percutaneous fine-needle ethanol injection into enlarged parathyroid glands under ultrasonic guidance was developed by Giangrande and co-workers in 1982.[874] Their experience with 50 uremic patients already treated has been reviewed.[875] Excellent results were also obtained with seven patients who had relapsed after subtotal PTX.[875] The technique has also been proved effective by other groups.[876, 877] Thus, this procedure may be an alternative to surgical treatment in selected cases. Side effects have been reported to be rare, mild, and transient.

## TREATMENT OF ALUMINUM-RELATED BONE DISEASE

Patients with profound Al toxicity were initially difficult to manage. Hemodialysis employing Al-free water brought about the removal of only small quantities, because of substantial binding of Al to transferrin and other plasma proteins[878, 879]; some dialysis units continued to give Al gels. The management of Al toxicity with Al-free dialysate failed to produce clinical improvement if the patients continued to ingest Al-containing P binders.[222] Prevention of this disease, which usually results from the use of Al-contaminated water, is the most important single therapeutic first step. The finding of several patients with Al-related bone disease in a single dialysis unit should prompt re-evaluation of the adequacy of the method used for water purification. Periodic sampling of plasma Al levels in a population of patients in a dialysis unit may provide the best indication of even intermittent contamination of water.[271] Deionization and treatment with reverse osmosis are effective methods for Al removal.[472] However, reverse osmosis is inadequate as a sole purification method when the Al concentration of water exceeds 200 to 300 μg/L, as might occur when a municipal water treatment uses alum (aluminum sulfate) for the flocculation of water as part of the water treatment.

The second therapeutic step is the substitution of the Al-containing P binders for calcium carbonate or calcium acetate and the removal of other Al-containing medications (such as albumin infusions, sucralfate, and some hyperalimentation supplements). Implementation of these steps usually results in the healing of Al bone disease. Freemont and associates[880] reported the improvement of bone biopsy results 5 years after initiation of water purification combined with either withdrawal of aluminum hydroxide treatment or reduction of its dosage. Hercz and co-workers[268, 881] reported substantial improvement of the histologic features of Al bone disease by 11 to 12 months after the afflicted patients had withdrawn Al-containing gels and underwent hemodialysis with a low dialysate Al concentration (less than 10 μg/L).

Ackrill and colleagues[882] first reported that the chelating agent deferoxamine was effective for the removal of Al in a dialysis patient with encephalopathy; lifesaving improvement of both the neurologic features and the patient's musculoskeletal symptoms arising from osteomalacia was observed after treatment with this agent. Subsequently, deferoxamine, which has a high affinity for Al as well as for iron, was also used in Al-related bone disease with dramatic favorable responses.[240, 478, 883]

Deferoxamine augments the removal of Al in two ways: it mobilizes Al from tissue stores, thereby increasing the plasma concentration of Al, and it increases the fraction of plasma Al that is ultrafilterable. Plasma Al is 80% to 90% protein bound, so that only 10% to 20% is ultrafilterable.[879] This is the reason why Al is poorly removed during dialysis. After deferoxamine, the absolute serum Al increases and most is in the form of aluminoxamine and feroxamine complexes, which are removable by hemodialysis or peritoneal dialysis, using a charcoal hemoperfusion cartridge in combination with a dialysis membrane or hemofiltration.[878, 884–887]

Repeated infusion of deferoxamine, 30 to 40 mg/kg/wk, during the last half-hour of the preceding dialysis session was associated with substantial clinical improvement in Al-related bone disease.[240, 506] A modest reduction of serum $Ca^{2+}$ was observed, and increments in plasma alkaline phosphatase levels occurred after 4 to 12 weeks of treatment; these observations are consistent with remineralization of bone. Moreover, bone biopsy results have shown improvement with reduced Al staining and increased bone formation rate.[240, 711] Malluche and co-workers[478] noted improved bone histologic features and an increase in the mineralization rate in three patients with mixed uremic bone disease that was characterized by Al deposits and yet normal bone formation. Ferritin levels usually decrease and, as

mentioned earlier, PTH levels increase and signs of secondary HPTH may develop (especially in cases of mixed bone disease); indeed, some patients with low-turnover bone lesions may develop osteitis fibrosa.[240, 711] Erythrocyte mean corpuscular volume and hematocrit may also rise. Similarly, deferoxamine has been noted to induce a greater response to erythropoietin therapy in patients who had minimal Al accumulation.[888]

As these beneficial effects of therapy with deferoxamine were being noted, a number of serious side effects were also recognized. Retinal and auditory toxicity,[889–891] thrombocytopenia,[892] hypotension, and serious and even fatal cases of encephalopathy were noted.[893] The risk of encephalopathy is lessened if the dose of deferoxamine is decreased and adjusted periodically to limit the rise of serum Al 24 to 48 hours after the deferoxamine administration to values lower than 300 μg/L. Fatal infections with *Yersinia* species have been described.[894, 895] In addition, mucormycosis, a *Rhizopus* infection that is commonly fatal, has also appeared among dialysis patients receiving long-term treatment with deferoxamine[896, 897]; the infection is most commonly disseminated, frequently follows a rapidly fatal course, and is often not suspected during life and recognized only at postmortem examination.[896] Cultures of blood and other body fluids may not be positive even in cases of histologically proven infection. In regard to the probable mechanism of deferoxamine-induced mucormycosis, it is likely that deferoxamine, which is a microbial siderophore, stimulates the growth and pathogenicity of certain species of fungi by making environmental iron more available to the microorganism.[898] This may occur as a result of receptors on the fungi for the deferoxamine-iron complex (feroxamine), which then facilitates the uptake of iron by the microorganism.[896] Iron and Al complexes of deferoxamine are both cleared from the body largely by the kidneys; therefore, pharmacokinetic changes in uremia lead to a prolonged accumulation of feroxamine after deferoxamine.[899]

Because of the seriousness of these potential complications, and because they can appear after a short treatment with relatively low doses,[896] deferoxamine therapy should be limited to dialysis patients with proven Al encephalopathy or those with severe, symptomatic Al-related bone disease that has failed to respond to the withdrawal of Al-containing gels and the elimination of exposure to Al-contaminated dialysate. If deferoxamine must be used, it should be given in the lowest possible doses (e.g., 5 to 15 mg/kg, every 7 to 10 days), and it is desirable that the dialysis performed after the treatment is done using a highly permeable dialysis membrane or the insertion of a charcoal cartridge that permits rapid removal of deferoxamine complexes of iron and Al.[884, 885] Deferoxamine is increasingly being administered shortly before or at the beginning of the hemodialysis session.[900] Serum Al levels should be measured repeatedly during treatment to minimize the risk of Al neurotoxicity and to titrate the deferoxamine dosage (ideally serum Al should be between twice the basal value and always < 300 μg/L, when deferoxamine is administered 24 to 48 hours before the measurement). With micromethods to determine deferoxamine and its metallochelates aluminoxamine and feroxamine, it seems that deferoxamine may be more appropriately dosed[901] and in some patients weekly doses of 5 mg/kg of deferoxamine may be sufficient.[297, 298, 902]

1,2-Dimethyl-3-hydroxipyrid-4-one is a new oral drug that has been safely used to treat thalassemic patients with iron overload. Preliminary data in the experimental animal showed the potential of the drug to increase ultrafilterable Al and mobilize Al from tissues.[903] Further data are needed before its use is recommended in patients.

## TREATMENT OF IDIOPATHIC ADYNAMIC BONE DISEASE

Although the natural history of this entity is unknown, it seems advisable to prevent excessive suppression of PTH (intact PTH lower than 1.5- to 3-fold the upper limit of normal) because mildly increased levels of PTH are associated with a normal bone formation rate in dialysis patients.[174, 302, 343] Dialysis patients with PTH levels in the normal range and without Al toxicity may need to be treated with a dialysate $Ca^{2+}$ of 2.5 mEq/L or even lower to increase PTH and improve the low-turnover bone state. Hercz and associates[309] have treated some of these patients with a 2.0 mEq/L dialysate $Ca^{2+}$ and noted an increase in PTH; an increase in the bone formation rate also occurred.[904] As neither the natural course nor the morbidity of this disease is known, no general recommendations can be made.

## OTHER TREATMENT CONSIDERATIONS

Calcitonin may be useful, in the future, in certain patients with inoperable secondary HPTH or patients who cannot be treated with calcitriol because of hypercalcemia.[184, 185] However, a report of its short-term administration in uremic patients showed little overall effect.[905]

Biphosphonates are analogues of pyrophosphate with a potent inhitory effect on bone resorption.[906] They inhibit osteoclastic activity; reports also suggest that their effects could be mediated by osteoblasts.[907] There are only limited studies on the use of biphosphonates in CRF and they are not conclusive. These drugs may be indicated in the future for hypercalcemic patients with increased bone turnover and those with extraosseous calcifications caused by a high $Ca^{2+} \times P$ product.[908] Their side effects, advantages, and contraindications as well as details on dosage, administration, and their use in combination therapy remain unknown.

Physicochemical properties of dialysis membranes other than permeability have a substantial effect on decreasing intact PTH concentration during hemodialysis.[909] However, PTH reverts to the previous level between hemodialysis sessions.[909, 910] With the use of coated charcoal (150 g per cartridge) in combination with standard hemodialysis, a decrease in PTH levels, probably related to adsorption to the cartridge, has been observed.[911] This decrease in PTH was associated with marked relief of pruritus and other symptoms. Thus, it was suggested that symptomatic patients with secondary HPTH before PTX may be treated successfully with this therapeutic modality.

Patients undergoing regular dialysis receive periodic injections of heparin; clinical and experimental studies suggest that heparin, when given repeatedly, is associated with decreased skeletal mineralization and may predispose to fractures in patients without renal disease. In one study of bone mineral content in which hand radiographs were analyzed, a positive correlation was noted between the rate of decrease in bone mass and the regular dosage of heparin given to dialysis patients.[912] Osteoporosis has been reported in patients receiving 15,000 to 30,000 U/d of heparin over long periods[913]; multiple fractures and pseudoarthrosis have also been reported.[721] Osteoporosis did not develop in patients receiving lower doses (i.e., 10,000 U/day), and dialysis patients may not receive quantities of heparin large enough to cause difficulties.[913] However, a study using technetium-labeled heparin in 12 hemodialysis patients showed a greater accumulation of the tracer in knees and shoulders in hemodialyzed patients compared with control subjects; this suggests that accumulation of heparin in bone tissue could play a role in causing osteopenia in hemodialysis patients.[914] With the use of efficient dialyzers and shorter durations of dialysis, the quantity of heparin given is less, and the potential for any adverse effect of heparin on the skeleton is reduced.

## Management of Fractures

Rib fractures, probably the most frequent fractures in uremic patients, usually heal slowly during a period of several months. They are often asymptomatic and require little specific treatment. Traumatic fractures of the long bones and of the femoral neck may have a poor union even after several months. When fractures occur in patients with marked secondary HPTH it is mandatory to treat the patients with appropriate dose of calcitriol; often the fractures heal after calcitriol therapy. If the fracture does not heal, the appropriate surgical repair should be considered, because prolonged immobilization can create even greater complications in such patients. In some patients with fractures caused by Al-related osteomalacia, slow healing may occur even though Al accumulation has not been specifically treated. In such patients nonunion of the fracture occurs and the fracture may heal after deferoxamine therapy. Successful use of femoral head prostheses has been noted in patients with end-stage CRF and in those given dialysis.[915]

### REFERENCES

1. Stanbury SW, Lumb GA: Metabolic studies of renal osteodystrophy: I. Calcium, phosphorus and nitrogen metabolism in rickets, osteomalacia and hyperparathyroidism complicating chronic uremia and the osteomalacia of the adult Fanconi syndrome. Medicine (Baltimore) 41:1–31, 1962.
2. Dent CE, Harper CN, Philpot G: Treatment of renal glomerular osteodystrophy. Q J Med 30:1–31, 1961.
3. Lucas RC: On a form of late rickets associated with albuminuria, rickets of adolescents. Lancet 1:993–994, 1883.
4. MacCallum WG: Tumor of the parathyroid gland. Johns Hopkins Hosp Bull 16:87–89, 1905.
5. Langmead FS, Orr JW: Renal rickets associated with parathyroid hyperplasia. Arch Dis Child 8:265–278, 1933.

6. Albright F, Drake TG, Sulkowitch HW: Renal osteitis fibrosa cystica: Report of case with discussion of metabolic aspects. Johns Hopkins Hosp Bull 60:377–399, 1936.
7. Liu SH, Chu HI: Studies of calcium and phosphorus metabolism with special reference to pathogenesis and effects of dihydrotachysterol (A.T. 10) and iron. Medicine (Baltimore) 22:103–161, 1943.
8. Gilmour JR: The Parathyroid Glands and Skeleton in Renal Disease. Oxford University Press, London, 1947, pp 1–150.
9. Pappenheimer AM, Wilens SL: Enlargement of the parathyroid glands in renal disease. Am J Pathol 11:73, 1935.
10. Lichwitz A, Parlier R: Calcium et Maladies Métaboliques de l'Os. Expansions Scientifique Francaise, Paris, 1965, p 196.
11. Berson SA, Yalow RS: Parathyroid hormone in plasma in adenomatous hyperparathyroidism, uremia and bronchogenic carcinoma. Science 154:907–909, 1966.
12. Segre GV, Habener JF, Powell D, et al: Parathyroid hormone in human plasma: Immunochemical characterization and biological implications. J Clin Invest 51:3163–3172, 1972.
13. Segre GV, Sherrard DJ, Carlton EI: Use of the PTH (IRMA) Assay in Patients with Impaired Renal Function and Renal Osteodystrophy. Nichols Institute, San Juan Capistrano, CA, 1990, pp 1–8.
14. Reiss E, Canterbury JM, Egdahl RH: Experience with a radioimmunoassay of parathyroid hormone in human sera. Trans Assoc Am Physicians 81:104–115, 1968.
15. Llach F, Massry SG, Singer FR, et al: Skeletal resistance of endogenous parathyroid hormone in patients with early renal failure. A possible cause for secondary hyperparathyroidism. J Clin Endocrinol Metab 41:339–345, 1975.
16. Pitts TO, Piraino BH, Mitro R, et al: Hyperparathyroidism and 1,25-dihydroxyvitamin D deficiency in mild, moderate, and severe renal failure. J Clin Endocrinol Metab 67:876–881, 1988.
17. Reichel H, Deibert B, Schmidt-Gayk H, Ritz E: Calcium metabolism in early chronic renal failure: Implications for the pathogenesis of hyperparathyroidism. Nephrol Dial Transplant 6:162–169, 1991.
18. Martinez I, Zaracho R, Montenegro J, Llach F: The role of calcitriol in the secondary hyperparathyroidism (HPTH) of chronic renal failure (CRF). J Am Soc Nephrol 4:725, 1993. Abstract.
19. Malluche HH, Ritz E, Lange HP, et al: Bone histology in incipient and advanced renal failure. Kidney Int 9:355–362, 1976.
20. Baker LRI, Abrams SML, Roe CJ, et al: 1,25(OH)$_2$D$_3$ in moderate renal failure: A prospective double-blind trial. Kidney Int 35:661–669, 1989.
21. Bricker NS, Slatopolsky E, Reiss E, Avioli LV: Calcium, phosphorus and bone in renal disease and transplantation. Arch Intern Med 123:543–553, 1969.
22. Slatopolsky E, Caglar S, Pennell JP, et al: On the pathogenesis of hyperparathyroidism in chronic experimental insufficiency in the dog. J Clin Invest 50:492–499, 1971.
23. Russell J, Lettieri D, Sherwood LM: Direct regulation by calcium of cytoplasmatic messenger ribonucleic acid for preproparathyroid hormone in isolated bovine parathyroid cells. J Clin Invest 72:1851–1855, 1983.
24. Yamamoto M, Igarashi T, Muramatsu M, et al: Hypocalcemia increases and hypercalcemia decreases the steady state level of parathyroid hormone messenger ribonucleic acid in the rat. J Clin Invest 83:1053–1056, 1989.
25. Naveh-Many T, Silver J: Regulation of parathyroid hormone gene expression by hypocalcemia, hypercalcemia, and vitamin D in the rat. J Clin Invest 86:1313–1319, 1990.
26. Llach F, Massry SG: On the mechanism of the prevention of secondary hyperparathyroidism in moderate renal insufficiency. J Clin Endocrinol Metab 61:601–606, 1985.
27. Portale AP, Booth BE, Halloran BP, Morris RC Jr: Effect of dietary phosphorus on circulating concentrations of 1,25-dihydroxyvitamin D and immunoreactive parathyroid hormone in children with moderate renal insufficiency. J Clin Invest 73:1580–1589, 1984.
28. Wilson L, Felsenfeld AJ, Drezner MK, Llach F: Altered divalent ion metabolism in early renal failure: Role of 1,25-(OH)$_2$D. Kidney Int 27:565–573, 1985.
29. Lopez-Hilker S, Galceran T, Chan Y-L, et al: Hypocalcemia may not be essential for the development of secondary hyperparathyroidism in chronic renal failure. J Clin Invest 78:1097–1102, 1986.
30. Kaplan MA, Canterbury JM, Jaffe D: Effect of dietary phosphorus (P) in the phosphaturic and calcemic response to parathyroid hormone (PTH) in the uremic dog. Kidney Int 18:77, 1977.
31. Tennant BJ, Lowe JE, Tasker JB: Hypercalcemia and hypophosphatemia in ponies following bilateral nephrectomy. Proc Soc Exp Biol Med 167:365–368, 1981.
32. Tuma SN, Mallette LE: Hypercalcemia after nephrectomy in the dog: Role of the kidney and parathyroid glands. J Lab Clin Med 102:213–219, 1983.
33. Slatopolsky E, Bricker NA: The role of phosphorus restriction in the prevention of secondary hyperparathyroidism in chronic renal disease. Kidney Int 4:141, 1973.
34. Slatopolsky E, Caglar S, Gradowska L: On the prevention of secondary hyperparathyroidism in experimental chronic renal disease using "proportional reduction" of dietary phosphorus intake. Kidney Int 2:147, 1972.
35. Slatopolsky E, Rutherford WE, Hruska KA: How important is phosphate in the pathogenesis of renal osteodystrophy? Arch Intern Med 138:848, 1978.
36. Bricker NS: On the pathogenesis of the uremic state. An exposition of the trade-off hypothesis. N Engl J Med 286:1093–1099, 1972.
37. Reiss E, Canterbury JM, Bercovitz MA, Kaplan EL: The role of phosphate in the secretion of parathyroid hormone in man. J Clin Invest 49:2146, 1970.
38. Jowsey J, Reiss E, Canterbury JM: Long term effects of high phosphate intake on parathyroid hormone levels and bone metabolism. Acta Orthop Scand 45:801, 1974.
39. LaFlame GH, Jowsey J: Bone and soft tissue changes with oral phosphate supplements. J Clin Invest 51:2834, 1972.
40. Fournier AE, Johnson WJ, Taves DR: Etiology of hyperparathyroidism and bone disease during chronic hemodialysis. I. Association of bone disease with potentially etiologic factors. J Clin Invest 50:592, 1971.
41. Fournier AE, Arnaud CD, Johnson WJ, et al: Etiology of hyperparathyroidism and bone disease during chronic hemodialysis. II. Factors affecting serum immunoreactive parathyroid hormone. J Clin Invest 50:599–605, 1971.
42. Coburn JW, Hartenbower DL, Brickman AS: Intestinal absorption of calcium, magnesium, and phosphorus in chronic renal insufficiency. In David DS (ed): Calcium Metabolism in Renal Failure and Nephrolithiasis. John Wiley & Sons, New York, 1977, pp 77–109.
43. Llach F, Brickman AS, Ben-Isaac C, et al: Phosphate loading as a test for primary hyperparathyroidism. In Avioli L, Bordier PH, Fleish H, et al (eds): Phosphate Metabolism: Kidney and Bone. Nouvelle Imprimerie Fournie, Paris, 1975, pp 171–178.
44. Maschio G, Tessitore N, D'Angelo A, et al: Early dietary phosphorus restriction and calcium supplementation in the prevention of renal osteodystrophy. Am J Clin Nutr 33:1546–1554, 1980.
45. Goldman R, Bassett SH: Phosphorus excretion in renal failure. J Clin Invest 33:1623, 1954.
46. Slatopolsky E, Gradowska L, Kashemsant C, et al: The control of phosphate excretion in uremia. J Clin Invest 45:672–677, 1966.
47. Slatopolsky E, Robson AM, Elkan I, Bricker NS: Control of phosphate excretion in uremic man. J Clin Invest 47:1865–1874, 1968.
48. Kleerekoper M, Cruz C, Bernstein RS, et al: The phosphaturic action of PTH in the steady state in patients with normal and impaired renal function. Adv Exp Med Biol 128:145–154, 1980.
49. Adler AJ, Ferran N, Berlyne GM: Effect of inorganic phosphate on serum ionized calcium concentration in vitro: A reassessment of the "trade-off hypothesis." Kidney Int 28:932–935, 1985.
50. Hebert LA, Lemann J, Petersen JR, Lennon EJ: Studies of the mechanism by which phosphate infusion lowers serum calcium concentration. J Clin Invest 45:1886–1894, 1966.
51. Tanaka Y, DeLuca HF: The control of 25 hydroxyvitamin D metabolism by inorganic phosphorus. Arch Biochem Biophys 154:566–567, 1973.
52. Portale AP, Halloran BP, Murphy MM, Morris RC Jr: Oral intake of phosphorus can determine the serum concentration of 1,25 D by determining its production rate in humans. J Clin Invest 77:7–8, 1986.
53. Somerville PJ, Kaye M: Evidence that resistance to the calcemic action of parathyroid hormone in rats with acute uremia is caused by phosphate retention. Kidney Int 16:552–560, 1979.
54. Rodriguez M, Martin-Malo A, Martinez ME, et al: Calcemic response to parathyroid hormone in renal failure: Role of phosphorus and its effect on calcitriol. Kidney Int 40:1055–1062, 1991.
55. Lucas PA, Brown RC, Woodhead JS, Coles G: 1,25-Dihydroxycholecalciferol and parathyroid hormone in advanced renal failure: Ef-

fect of simultaneous protein and phosphorus restriction. Clin Nephrol 25:7–10, 1986.

56. Schaeffer K, Erley CM, von Herrath D, Stein G: Calcium salts of ketoacids as a new treatment strategy for uremic hyperphosphatemia. Kidney Int 36(suppl 27):S136–S139, 1989.

57. Tessitore N, Venturi A, Adami S, et al: Relationship between serum vitamin D metabolites and dietary intake of phosphate in patients with early renal failure. Miner Electrolyte Metab 13:38–44, 1987.

58. Lopez-Hilker S, Dusso AS, Rapp NS, et al: Phosphorus restriction reverses hyperparathyroidism in uremia independent of changes in calcium and calcitriol. Am J Physiol 259:F432–F437, 1990.

59. Aparicio M, Combe C, Lafage MH, et al: In advanced renal failure, dietary phosphorus restriction reverses hyperparathyroidism independent of changes in the levels of calcitriol. Nephron 63:122–123, 1993.

60. Fine A, Cox D, Fontaine B: Elevation of serum phosphate affects parathyroid hormone levels in only 50% of hemodialysis patients, which is unrelated to changes in serum calcium. J Am Soc Nephrol 3:1947–1953, 1993.

61. Rodriguez M, Felsenfeld AJ, Dunlay R, et al: The effect of long-term calcitriol administration on parathyroid function in hemodialysis patients. J Am Soc Nephrol 2:1014–1020, 1991.

62. Yi H, Fukagawa M, Kurokawa K: Mild dietary phosphorus restriction directly prevents enhanced parathyroid hormone secretion and synthesis and proliferation of parathyroid cells in chronic renal failure in rats. J Am Soc Nephrol 3:703, 1992.

63. Evanson JM: The response to the infusion of parathyroid extract in hypocalcemic states. Clin Sci 31:63–75, 1966.

64. Massry SG, Coburn JW, Lee DBN, et al: Skeletal resistance to parathyroid hormone in renal failure: Study in 105 human subjects. Ann Intern Med 78:357–364, 1973.

65. Somerville PJ, Kaye M: Action of phosphorus on calcium release in isolated perfused rat tails. Kidney Int 22:348–354, 1982.

66. Yates AJ, Oreffo RO, Mayor K, Mundy GR: Inhibition of bone resorption by inorganic phosphate is mediated by both reduced osteoclast formation and decreased activity of mature osteoclasts. J Bone Miner Res 6:473–478, 1991.

67. Massry SG, Stein R, Garty J, et al: Skeletal resistance to the calcemic action of parathyroid hormone in uremia: Role of $1,25(OH)_2D_3$. Kidney Int 9:467–474, 1976.

68. Massry SG, Tuma S, Dua S, Goldstein DA: Reversal of skeletal resistance to parathyroid hormone in uremia by vitamin D metabolites. Evidence for the requirement of $1,25(OH)_2D_3$ and $24,25(OH)_2D_3$. J Lab Clin Med 94:152–157, 1979.

69. Somerville PJ, Kaye M: Resistance to parathyroid hormone in renal failure: Role of vitamin D metabolites. Kidney Int 14:245–254, 1978.

70. Rodriguez M, Felsenfeld AJ, Llach F: Calcemic response to parathyroid hormone in renal failure: Role of calcitriol and the effect of parathyroidectomy. Kidney Int 40:1063–1068, 1991.

71. Galceran T, Martin KJ, Morrissey JJ, Slatopolsky E: Role of 1,25-dihydroxyvitamin D on the skeletal resistance to parathyroid hormone. Kidney Int 32:801–807, 1987.

72. Olgaard K, Schwartz J, Finco D: Extraction of parathyroid hormone and release of cyclic-AMP by isolated perfused bones obtained from dogs with acute uremia. Endocrinology 111:1678–1682, 1982.

73. Olgaard K, Arbelaez M, Schwartz J: Abnormal skeletal response to parathyroid hormone in dogs with chronic uremia. Skeletal cyclic AMP response to PTH in chronic uremia. Calcif Tissue Int 34:403–407, 1982.

74. Bover J, Trinidad P, Felsenfeld AJ, et al: The effect of azotemia and the magnitude of hyperparathyroidism on the calcemic response to parathyroid hormone. J Am Soc Nephrol 3:692, 1992.

75. Rodriguez M, Felsenfeld AJ, Torres A, et al: Calcitonin, an important factor in the calcemic response to parathyroid hormone in the rat with renal failure. Kidney Int 40:219–225, 1991.

76. Bover J, Rodriguez M, Trinidad P, et al: Factors in the development of secondary hyperparathyroidism in during graded renal failure in the rat. Kidney Int 45:953–961, 1994.

77. Wills MR, Jenkins MV: The effect of uremic metabolites on parathyroid extract induced bone resorption in vitro. Clin Chim Acta 73:121, 1976.

78. Haussler MR, McCain TA: Basic and clinical concepts related to vitamin D metabolism and action. N Engl J Med 297:974–975, 1977.

79. Mason RS, Lissner D, Wilkinson M, Posen S: Vitamin D metabolites and their relationship to azotemic osteodystrophy. Clin Endocrinol 13:375–385, 1980.

80. Christiansen C: Chronic renal failure and vitamin D metabolites: A status report. J Steroid Biochem 19:517–523, 1983.

81. Kopple JD, Coburn JW: Metabolic studies of low protein diets in uremia. II. Calcium, phosphorus and magnesium. Medicine (Baltimore) 52:597, 1973.

82. Coburn JW, Hartenbower DL, Massry SG: Intestinal absorption of calcium and the effect of renal insufficiency. Kidney Int 4:96, 1973.

83. Fraser DR, Kodicek E: Unique biosynthesis by kidney of a biologically active vitamin D metabolite. Nature 228:764–766, 1970.

84. Holick MF, Schnoes HK, DeLuca HF, et al: Isolation and identification of 1,25-dihydroxycholecalciferol. A metabolite of vitamin D active in the intestine. Biochemistry 10:2799–2804, 1971.

85. Gray R, Boyle I, DeLuca HF: Vitamin D metabolism: The role of kidney tissue. Science 172:1232, 1971.

86. Mawer EB, Backhouse J, Taylor CM: Failure of formation of 1,25-dihydroxycholecalciferol in chronic renal insufficiency. Lancet 1:626, 1973.

87. Schaefer K, Herrath D von, Stratz R: Metabolism of 1,2 $H^3$-4-$C^{14}$-cholecalciferol in normal, uremic and anephric subjects. Isr J Med Sci 8:80–83, 1972.

88. Brumbaugh PF, Haussler DH, Bressler R, Haussler MR: Radioreceptor assay for $1\alpha,25$-dihydroxyvitamin $D_3$. Science 183:1089–1091, 1974.

89. Cheung AK, Manolagas SC, Catherwood BC, et al: Determinants of serum $1,25(OH)_2D$ levels in renal disease. Kidney Int 24:104–109, 1983.

90. Eisman JA, Hamstra AJ, Kream BE, DeLuca HF: 1,25-Dihydroxy-vitamin D in biological fluids: A simplified and sensitive assay. Science 193:1021, 1976.

91. Brickman AS, Coburn JW, Massry SG, Norman AW: 1,25-Dihydroxyvitamin $D_3$ in normal man and patients with renal failure. Ann Intern Med 80:161, 1974.

92. Brickman AS, Coburn JW, Norman AW: Action of 1,25-dihydroxy-cholecalciferol, a potent, kidney produced metabolite of vitamin $D_3$ in uremic man. N Engl J Med 287:891, 1972.

93. Rutherford WE, Bordier PhJ, Marie PJ: Phosphate control and 25 hydroxycholecalciferol administration in preventing experimental renal osteodystrophy in the dog. J Clin Invest 60:332, 1977.

94. Kumar R: Vitamin D and calcium transport. Kidney Int 40:1177–1189, 1991.

95. Chesney RW, Hamstra AJ, Mazess RB: Circulating vitamin D metabolite concentrations in childhood renal diseases. Kidney Int 21:65, 1982.

96. Mora Palma FJ, Lorenzo Sellares V, Ellis HL, et al: Osteomalacia in chronic renal failure before dialysis. Proc Eur Dial Transplant Assoc 19:188, 1983.

97. Coburn JW, Koppel MH, Brickman AS, Massry SG: Study of intestinal absorption of calcium in patients with renal failure. Kidney Int 3:264–272, 1973.

98. Silver J, Russell J, Sherwood LM: Regulation by vitamin D metabolites of messenger ribonucleic acid for preproparathyroid hormone in isolated bovine parathyroid cells. Proc Natl Acad Sci USA 82:4270–4273, 1985.

99. Chan YL, McKay C, Dye E, Slatopolsky E: The effect of 1,25-dihydroxycholecalciferol on parathyroid hormone secretion by monolayer cultures of bovine parathyroid cells. Calcif Tissue Int 38:27–32, 1986.

100. Oldham SB, Smith R, Hartenbower DL, et al: The acute effects of 1,25-dihydroxycholecalciferol on serum immunoreactive parathyroid hormone in the dog. Endocrinology 104:248–254, 1979.

101. Slatopolsky E, Weerts C, Thielan J, et al: Marked suppression of secondary hyperparathyroidism by intravenous administration of 1,25-dihydroxycholecalciferol in uremic patients. J Clin Invest 74:2136–2143, 1984.

102. Malberti F, Surian M, Cosci P: Effect of chronic intravenous calcitriol on parathyroid function and set point of calcium in dialysis patients with refractory secondary hyperparathyroidism. Nephrol Dial Transplant 7:822–828, 1992.

103. Tessitore N, Lund BJ, Bonucci E, et al: Vitamin D metabolites in early renal failure. Minerva Nephrol 28:293–297, 1981.

104. Portale AP, Booth BE, Tsai HC, Morris RC Jr: Reduced plasma concentration of 1,25-dihydroxyvitamin D in children with moderate renal insufficiency. Kidney Int 21:627–632, 1982.

105. Slatopolsky E, Gray R, Adams ND, et al: Low serum levels of 1,25(OH)$_2$D$_3$ are not responsible for the development of secondary hyperparathyroidism in early renal failure. Kidney Int 14:733A, 1978.

106. Cremer B, Lubbers E, Klooker P, et al: Calciuric response to 1,25(OH)$_2$D$_3$ in early renal failure. Miner Electrolyte Metab 11:182–185, 1985.

107. Llach F: Effects of renal failure and dialysis on divalent ion metabolism. In Brenner BM, Stein JH (eds): Divalent Ion Homeostasis, Vol 11, Contemporary Issues in Nephrology. Churchill Livingstone, New York, 1983, pp 291–317.

108. Aarskog D, Asknes L: Acute response of plasma 1,25-dihydroxyvitamin D to parathyroid hormone. Lancet 1:362–363, 1980.

109. Kawaguchi Y, Kimura Y, Yamamoto M, et al: Graded nephron mass reduction and renal synthesis of 1,25-dihydroxyvitamin D$_3$ in the rat. Metab Bone Dis Relat Res 4:333–336, 1983.

110. Gray RW, Napoli JL: Dietary phosphorus deprivation increases 1,25-dihydroxyvitamin D$_3$ synthesis in rat kidney in vitro. J Biol Chem 258:1152–1155, 1983.

111. Prince RL, Hutchison BG, Kent JC, et al: Calcitriol deficiency with retained synthetic reserve in chronic renal failure. Kidney Int 33:722–728, 1988.

112. Taylor CM, Caverzasio J, Jung A, et al: Unilateral nephrectomy and 1,25-dihydroxyvitamin D$_3$. Kidney Int 24:37–42, 1983.

113. Hsu CH, Patel S, Young EW, Simpson RU: Production and degradation of calcitriol in renal failure rats. Am J Physiol 253:F1015–F1019, 1987.

114. Hsu CH, Patel S: Factors influencing calcitriol metabolism in renal failure. Kidney Int 37:44–50, 1990.

115. Dusso A, Lopez-Hilker S, Lewis-Fich J, et al: Metabolic clearance rate and production rate of calcitriol in uremia. Kidney Int 35:860–864, 1989.

116. Hsu CH, Patel S, Buchsbaum BL: Calcitriol metabolism in patients with chronic renal failure. Am J Kidney Dis 17:185–190, 1991.

117. Hsu CH, Patel SR, Young EW: Mechanism of decreased calcitriol degradation in renal failure. Am J Physiol 262:F192–F198, 1992.

118. Dusso A, Lopez-Hilker S, Rapp N, Slatopolsky E: Extra-renal production of calcitriol. Kidney Int 34:368, 1988.

119. Adami A: Extraadrenal production of calcitriol: A review. Clin Sci 72:329–334, 1987.

120. Dusso A, Finch J, Delmez J, et al: Extrarenal production of calcitriol. Kidney Int 38:S36–S40, 1990.

121. Booth BE, Tsai HC, Morris RC Jr: Vitamin D status regulates 25-hydroxyvitamin D$_3$-1α-hydroxylase and its responsiveness to parathyroid hormone in chick. J Clin Invest 75:155–161, 1985.

122. Delmez JA, Tindira C, Grooms P, et al: Parathyroid hormone suppression by intravenous 1,25-dihydroxyvitamin D. A role for increased sensitivity to calcium. J Clin Invest 83:1349–1355, 1989.

123. Dunlay R, Rodriguez M, Felsenfeld AJ, Llach F: Direct inhibitory effect of calcitriol on parathyroid function (sigmoidal curve) in dialysis patients. Kidney Int 36:1093–1098, 1989.

124. Russell J, Lettieri D, Sherwood LM: Suppression by 1,25(OH)$_2$D$_3$ of transcription of the pre-proparathyroid hormone gene. Endocrinology 119:2864–2866, 1986.

125. Okazaki T, Igarashi T, Kronenberg KM: 5′ Flanking region of the parathyroid hormone gene mediates negative regulation by 1,25-(OH)$_2$ vitamin D$_3$. J Biol Chem 263:2203–2208, 1988.

126. Silver J, Naveh-Many T, Mayer H: Regulation by vitamin D metabolites of parathyroid hormone gene in vivo by the rat. J Clin Invest 78:1296, 1986.

127. Shvil Y, Naveh-Many T, Barach P, Silver J: Regulation of parathyroid cell gene expression in experimental uremia. J Am Soc Nephrol 1:99–104, 1990.

128. O'Malley BW: Steroid hormone action in eucaryotic cells. J Clin Invest 74:307–312, 1984.

129. Haussler MR, Terpening CM, Komm BS, et al: Vitamin D hormone receptors: Structure, regulation and molecular function. In Norman AW, Schaefer K, Grigoleit HG, Herrath DV (eds): Vitamin D: Molecular, Cellular, and Clinical Endocrinology. Walter de Gruyter, Berlin, 1988, pp 205–214.

130. Merke J, Hugel U, Zlotkowski A, et al: Diminished parathyroid 1,25-(OH)$_2$D$_3$ receptors in experimental uremia. Kidney Int 32:350–353, 1987.

131. Brown AJ, Dusso A, Lopez-Hilker S, et al: 1,25(OH)$_2$D receptors are decreased in parathyroid glands from chronically uremic dogs. Kidney Int 35:19–23, 1989.

132. Korkor AB: Reduced binding of [$^3$H]1,25-dihydroxyvitamin D$_3$ in the parathyroid glands of patients with renal failure. N Engl J Med 316:1573–1577, 1987.

133. Hirst M, Feldman D: Regulation of 1,25(OH)$_2$ vitamin D$_3$ receptor content in cultured LLC-PK$_1$ kidney cells limits hormonal responsiveness. Biochem Biophys Res Commun 116:121–127, 1983.

134. Sugimoto T, Ritter C, Ried I, et al: Effect of 1,25-dihydroxyvitamin D$_3$ on cytosolic calcium in dispersed parathyroid cells. Kidney Int 33:850–854, 1988.

135. Salusky IB, Goodman WG, Horst R, et al: Pharmacokinetics of calcitriol in continuous ambulatory and cycling peritoneal dialysis patients. Am J Kidney Dis 16:126–132, 1990.

136. Fukagawa M, Kaname S, Igarashi T, et al: Regulation of parathyroid hormone synthesis in chronic renal failure in rats. Kidney Int 39:874–881, 1991.

137. Hsu CH, Patel SR, Vanholder R: Mechanism of decreased intestinal calcitriol receptor concentration in renal failure. Am J Physiol 264:F662–F669, 1993.

138. De Francisco ALM, Olmos JM, Martinez J, et al: Calcitriol receptors after correction of uremia. In Book of Abstracts of the XIIth International Congress of Nephrology, Jerusalem, 1993, p 455.

139. Naveh-Many T, Marx R, Keshet E, et al: Regulation of 1,25-dihydroxyvitamin D$_3$ receptor gene expression by 1,25-dihydroxyvitamin D$_3$ in the parathyroid in vivo. J Clin Invest 86:1968–1975, 1990.

140. Szabo A, Schmutz A, Pesian S, et al: Regulation in vivo of vitamin D receptor in uremia. Effects of parathyroidectomy and PTH administration. J Am Soc Nephrol 3:701, 1992.

141. Russell J, Bar A, Sherwood LM, Hurwitz S: Interaction between calcium and 1,25-dihydroxyvitamin D$_3$ in the regulation of preproparathyroid hormone and vitamin D receptor messenger ribonucleic acid in avian parathyroids. Endocrinology 132:2639–2644, 1993.

142. Malmaeus J, Grimelius L, Johansson H, et al: Parathyroid pathology in hyperparathyroidism secondary to chronic renal failure. Scand J Urol Nephrol 18:157–166, 1984.

143. Mendes V, Jorgetti V, Nemeth J, et al: Secondary hyperparathyroidism in chronic haemodialysis patients: A clinico-pathological study. Proc Eur Dial Transplant Assoc 20:731–738, 1983.

144. Gagne ER, Urena P, Leite-Silva S, et al: Short- and long-term efficacy of total parathyroidectomy with immediate autografting compared with subtotal parathyroidectomy in hemodialysis patients. J Am Soc Nephrol 3:1008–1017, 1992.

145. St Goar WT: Case records of the Massachusetts General Hospital. N Engl J Med 268:943, 1963.

146. McPhaul IL, McIntosh DA, Hammond WS, Park OK: Autonomous secondary hyperparathyroidism. N Engl J Med 271:1342, 1964.

147. Davies DR, Dent CE, Watson L: Tertiary hyperparathyroidism. Br Med J 2:395, 1968.

148. Black WC, Slatopolsky E, Elkan J, Hoffsten P: Parathyroid morphology in suppressible and non-suppressible renal hyperparathyroidism. Lab Invest 23:497, 1970.

149. Geffriaud C, Allinne E, Page B, et al: Decrease of tumor-like calcification in uremia despite aggravation of secondary hyperparathyroidism: A case report. Clin Nephrol 38:158–161, 1992.

150. Tanaka Y, Seo H, Tominaga Y, et al: Factors related to the recurrent hyperfunction of autografts after total parathyroidectomy in patients with severe secondary hyperparathyroidism. Surg Today 23:220–227, 1993.

151. Tominaga Y, Tanaka Y, Sato K, et al: Recurrent renal hyperparathyroidism and DNA analysis of autografted parathyroid tissue. World J Surg 16:595–603, 1992.

152. Fukuda N, Tanaka H, Tominaga Y, et al: Decreased 1,25-dihydroxyvitamin D$_3$ receptor density is associated with a more severe form of parathyroid hyperplasia in chronic uremic patients. J Clin Invest 92:1436–1443, 1993. Abstract.

153. Kremer R, Bolivar I, Goltzman D, Hendy GN: Influence of calcium and 1,25-dihydroxycholecalciferol on proliferation and proto-oncogene expression in primary cultures of bovine parathyroid cells. Endocrinology 125:935–941, 1989.

154. Falchetti A, Bale AE, Amoros A, et al.: Progression of uremic hyperparathyroidism involves allelic loss on chromosome 11. J Clin Endocrinol Metab 76:139–144, 1993.

155. Slatopolsky E, Martin KJ, Morrissey J, Hruska KA: Parathyroid hormone: Alterations in chronic renal failure. In Robinson RR (ed): Nephrology, Proceedings of the IXth International Congress of Nephrology. Springer-Verlag, New York, 1984, p 1292.

156. Berson SA, Yalow RS: Immunochemical heterogeneity of parathyroid hormone in plasma. J Clin Endocrinol Metab 28:1037–1047, 1968.
157. Arnaud CD: Parathyroid hormone: Coming of age in clinical medicine. Am J Med 55:577, 1973.
158. Habener JF, Potts JT Jr: Biosynthesis of parathyroid hormone. N Engl J Med 299:580–635, 1978.
159. Kitamura N, Shigeno C, Shiomi K, et al: Episodic fluctuation in serum intact parathyroid hormone concentration in men. J Clin Endocrinol Metab 70:252–263, 1990.
160. De Francisco ALM, Amado JA, Cotorruelo JG, et al: Pulsatile secretion of parathyroid hormone in patients with chronic renal failure. Clin Nephrol 39:224–228, 1993.
161. Gardella TJ, Rubin D, Abou-Samra AB, et al: Expression of human parathyroid hormone (1–84) in *Escherichia coli* as a factor X–cleavable fusion protein. J Biol Chem 265:15854–15859, 1990.
162. Tregear GW, van Rietschoten J, Greene E, et al: Bovine parathyroid hormone:minimum chain length of synthetic peptide required for biological activity. Endocrinology 93:1349–1353, 1973.
163. Lim SK, Gardella TJ, Baba H, et al: The carboxy-terminus of parathyroid hormone is essential for hormone processing and secretion. Endocrinology 131:2325–2330, 1992.
164. Mayer GP, Keaton JA, Hurst JG, Habener JF: Effects of plasma calcium concentration on the relative proportion of hormone and carboxyl fragments in parathyroid venous blood. Endocrinology 104:1778–1784, 1979.
165. Catherwood BD, Friedler RM, Singer FR: Sites of clearance of endogenous parathyroid hormone in the vitamin D–deficient dog. Endocrinology 98:228–236, 1976.
166. Martin KJ, Hruska KA, Greenwalt A, Slatopolsky E: Selective uptake of intact parathyroid hormone by the liver. Differences between hepatic and renal uptake. J Clin Invest 58:781, 1976.
167. Hruska KA, Kopelman R, Rutherford WE: Metabolism of immunoreactive parathyroid hormone in the dog. The role of the kidney and the effects of chronic renal disease. J Clin Invest 56:39, 1975.
168. Hruska KA, Martin KJ, Messes P: Degradation of parathyroid hormone and fragment production by the isolated perfused dog kidney. The effect of glomerular filtration rate and perfusate Ca²⁺ concentrations. J Clin Invest 60:501, 1977.
169. Martin KJ, Hruska KA, Lewis J: The renal handling of parathyroid hormone. Role of peritubular uptake and glomerular filtration. J Clin Invest 60:808, 1977.
170. Zull JE, Chuang J: Characterization of parathyroid hormone fragments produced by cathepsin D. J Biol Chem 260:1608, 1985.
171. Freitag JJ, Martin KJ, Hruska KA, et al: Impaired parathyroid hormone metabolism in patients with chronic renal failure. N Engl J Med 298:29, 1978.
172. Papapoulos SE, Hendy GH, Tomlinson S: Clearance of exogenous parathyroid hormone in normal and uraemic man. Clin Endocrinol 7:211, 1977.
173. Morita A, Tabata T, Koyama H, et al: A two-site immunochemiluminometric assay for intact parathyroid hormone and its clinical utility in hemodialysis patients. Clin Nephrol 38:154–157, 1992.
174. Quarles LD, Lobaugh B, Murphy G: Intact parathyroid hormone overestimates the presence and severity of parathyroid-mediated osseous abnormalities in uremia. J Clin Endocrinol Metab 75:145–150, 1992.
175. Mayer GP, Hurst JG: Sigmoidal relationship between parathyroid hormone secretion rate and plasma calcium concentration in calves. Endocrinology 102:1036, 1978.
176. Brown EM, Wilson RE, Eastman R: Abnormal regulation of parathyroid hormone release by calcium in secondary hyperparathyroidism due to chronic renal failure. J Clin Endocrinol Metab 54:172, 1982.
177. Bellorin-Font E, Martin KJ, Freitag JJ, et al: Altered adenylate cyclase kinetics in hyperfunctioning human parathyroid glands. J Clin Endocrinol Metab 52:499–507, 1981.
178. Felsenfeld AJ, Llach F: Parathyroid gland function in chronic renal failure. Kidney Int 43:771–789, 1993.
179. Morrisey J, Martin K, Slatopolski E: Abnormalities in parathyroid hormone secretion in primary and secondary hyperparathyroidism. *In* Massry SG, Maschio G (eds): Phosphate and Mineral Metabolism. Plenum Publishing, New York, 1983, p 389.
180. Gittes R, Radde I: Experimental model for hyperparathyroidism: Effect of excessive numbers of transplanted isologous parathyroid glands. J Urol 95:595, 1966.
181. Voigts A, Felsenfeld AJ, Andress DL, Llach F: Parathyroid hormone and bone histology: Response to hypocalcemia in osteitis fibrosa. Kidney Int 25:445–452, 1984.
182. Heynen G, Franchimont P: Human calcitonin radioimmunoassay in normal and pathologic conditions. Eur J Clin Invest 4:213, 1974.
183. Lee JC, Parthemore JG, Deftos LJ: Immunochemical heterogeneity of calcitonin in renal failure. J Clin Endocrinol Metab 45:528, 1977.
184. Heynen G, Kanis JA, Oliver DO, Earnshaw M: Evidence that endogenous calcitonin protects against renal bone disease. Lancet 2:1322, 1976.
185. Kanis JA, Earnshaw M, Heynen G: The possible role of calcitonin deficiency in the development of bone disease due to chronic renal failure. Calcif Tissue Res 22(suppl):147, 1977.
186. Kanis JA, Earnshaw M, Heynen G, et al: Changes in histological and biochemical indexes of bone turnover after bilateral nephrectomy in patients on hemodialysis: Evidence for a possible role of endogenous calcitonin. N Engl J Med 19:1073–1079, 1977.
187. Torres A, Rodriguez M, Felsenfeld A, et al: Sigmoidal relationship between calcitonin and calcium: Studies in normal, parathyroidectomized, and azotemic rats. Kidney Int 40:700–704, 1991.
188. Blum WF, Ranke MB, Kietzmann K, et al: Growth hormone resistance and inhibition of somatomedin activity by excess of insulin-like growth factor binding protein in uraemia. Pediatr Nephrol 5:539–544, 1991.
189. Chan W, Valerie KC, Chan JCM: Expression of insulin-like growth factor-1 in uremic rats: Growth hormone resistance and nutritional intake. Kidney Int 43:790–795, 1993.
190. DeFronzo RA, Alvestrand A, Smith D, Hendler R: Insulin resistance in uremia. J Clin Invest 67:563–568, 1981.
191. Eidemak I, Feldt-Rasmussen B, Strandgaard S, et al: Insulin resistance is present in moderate uraemia and correlated to the maximal aerobic work capacity. J Am Soc Nephrol 3:281, 1992.
192. Ritz E, Malluche HH, Krempien B, Mehls O: Calcium metabolism in renal failure. In Bronner F, Coburn JW (eds): Disorders of Mineral Metabolism, Vol III. Academic Press, New York, 1981, p 151.
193. Sherrard DJ, Baylink DJ, Wergedal JE, Maloney NA: Quantitative histological studies on the pathogenesis of uremic bone disease. J Clin Endocrinol Metab 39:119, 1974.
194. Bordier PhJ, Tun-chot S, Eastwood JB: Lack of histological evidence of vitamin D abnormality in the bones of anephric patients. Clin Sci 44:33, 1973.
195. Eastwood JB, Harris E, Stamp TCB, De Wardener H: Vitamin D deficiency in the osteomalacia of chronic renal failure. Lancet 2:1209, 1976.
196. Offermann G, von Herrath D, Schaefer K: Serum 25-hydroxycholecalciferol in uremia. Nephron 13:269–277, 1974.
197. Schmidt-Gayk H, Schmitt W, Grawunder C: Hydroxyvitamin D in nephrotic syndrome. Lancet 2:105, 1977.
198. Baylink DJ, Stauffer J, Wergedal JE, Rich C: Formation, mineralization and resorption of bone in vitamin D deficient rats. J Clin Invest 49:112, 1970.
199. Howard GA, Baylink DJ: Matrix formation and osteoid maturation in vitamin D–deficient rats made normocalcemic by dietary means. Miner Electrolyte Metab 3:44–50, 1980.
200. Kanis JA, Cundy T, Bartlett M: Is 24,25-dihydroxycholecalciferol a calcium regulating hormone in man? Br Med J 1:1382, 1978.
201. Llach F, Brickman AS, Singer FR, Coburn JW: 24,25-Dihydroxycholecalciferol, a vitamin D sterol with qualitatively unique effects in uremic man. Metab Bone Dis Relat Res 2:11–15, 1979.
202. Popovtzer MM: The future of 24,25(OH)₂D₃ in the treatment of uremic bone disease. *In* Llach F (ed): Renal Osteodystrophy. Oxford University Press, London (in press).
203. Alfrey AC, Hegg A, Craswell P: Metabolism and toxicity of aluminum in renal failure. Am J Clin Nutr 33:1509, 1980.
204. Wills MR, Savory J: Aluminium poisoning: Dialysis encephalopathy, osteomalacia, and anaemia. Lancet 2:29–34, 1983.
205. Ward MK, Feest TG, Ellis HA, et al: Osteomalacic dialysis osteodystrophy: Evidence for a water-borne aetiological agent, probably aluminium. Lancet 1:841–845, 1978.
206. Parkinson IS, Ward MK, Feest TG, et al: Fracturing dialysis osteodystrophy and dialysis encephalopathy. An epidemiological survey. Lancet 1:406–409, 1979.
207. Siddiqui JY, Simpson W, Ellis HA, Kerr DNS: Fluoride and bone disease in patients on regular haemodialysis. Proc Eur Dial Transplant Assoc 8:149, 1971.

208. Pierides AM, Ward MK, Kerr DNS: Haemodialysis encephalopathy: Possible role of phosphate depletion. Lancet 1:1234, 1976.

209. Alfrey AC, LeGendre GR, Kaehny WD: The dialysis encephalopathy syndrome. Possible aluminum intoxication. N Engl J Med 294:184, 1976.

210. Ellis HA, McCarthy JH, Herrington J: Bone aluminum in hemodialysed patients and in rats injected with aluminum chloride: Relationship to impaired bone mineralization. J Clin Pathol 32:832, 1979.

211. Cournot-Witmer G, Plachot JJ, Bourdeau A: Effect of aluminum on bone and cell localization. Kidney Int 29(suppl):S37, 1986.

212. Hodsman AB, Sherrard DJ, Alfrey AC, et al: Bone aluminum and histomorphometric features of renal osteodystrophy. J Clin Endocrinol Metab 54:539–546, 1982.

213. Maloney NA, Ott SM, Alfrey AC, et al: Histologic quantitation of aluminum in iliac bone from patients with renal failure. J Lab Clin Med 99:206–216, 1982.

214. Cournot-Witmer G, Zingraff J, Plachott JJ, et al: Aluminum localization in bone from hemodialyzed patients: Relationship to matrix mineralization. Kidney Int 20:375–385, 1981.

215. Paunier L, Salusky IB, Slatopolsky E, et al: Renal osteodystrophy in children undergoing continuous ambulatory peritoneal dialysis. Pediatr Res 18:742–747, 1984.

216. Pierce-Myli M, Pierides AM: Iron and aluminum osteomalacia during hemodialysis: A new syndrome. Kidney Int 25:153, 1984. Abstract.

217. Phelps KR, Vigorita VJ, Bansal M, Einhorn T: Histological demonstration of iron but not aluminum in a case of dialysis associated osteomalacia. Am J Med 84:775, 1988.

218. Van de Vyver F, Visses WJ, D'Hesse P, De Broe ME: Iron overload and bone disease in chronic dialysis patients. Nephrol Dial Transplant 5:781–787, 1990.

219. Cannata JB, Diaz Lopez JB: Insights into the complex aluminium and iron relationship. Nephrol Dial Transplant 6:605–607, 1991.

220. Boyce BF, Fell GS, Elder H, et al: Hypercalcaemic osteomalacia due to aluminium toxicity. Lancet 2:1009–1013, 1982.

221. Coburn JW, Sherrard DJ, Brickman AS: A skeletal mineralizing defect in dialysis patients: A syndrome resembling osteomalacia but unrelated to vitamin D. Contrib Nephrol 18:172, 1980.

222. Hodsman AB, Sherrard DJ, Wong EGC, et al: Vitamin D resistant osteomalacia in hemodialysis patients lacking secondary hyperparathyroidism. Ann Intern Med 94:629–637, 1981.

223. Zins B, Zingraff J, Basile C, et al: Tumoral calcifications in hemodialysis patients: Possible role of aluminum intoxication. Nephron 60:260–267, 1992.

224. Sherrard DJ, Ott SM, Andress DL: Pseudohyperparathyroidism: A syndrome associated with aluminum intoxication in chronic renal failure. Am J Med 79:127, 1985.

225. Norris KC, Crooks P, Nebeker HG, et al: Clinical and laboratory features of aluminum related bone disease: Differences between sporadic and "epidemic" forms of the syndrome. Am J Kidney Dis 6:342–347, 1985.

226. Alvarez-Ude F, Feest TG, Ward MK, et al: Hemodialysis bone disease: Correlation between clinical, histologic and other findings. Kidney Int 14:68–73, 1978.

227. Andress DL, Felsenfeld AJ, Voigts A, Llach F: Parathyroid hormone response to hypocalcemia in hemodialysis patients with osteomalacia. Kidney Int 24:364, 1983.

228. Kraut JA, Shinaberger JH, Singer FR, et al: Parathyroid gland responsiveness to acute hypocalcemia in dialysis osteomalacia. Kidney Int 23:725–730, 1983.

229. Cann CE, Prussin SG, Gordan GS: Aluminum uptake by the parathyroid glands. J Clin Endocrinol Metab 49:543–545, 1979.

230. Morrisey J, Rothstein M, Mayor G, Slatopolsky E: Suppression of parathyroid hormone secretion by aluminum. Kidney Int 23:699–704, 1983.

231. Cannata JB, Briggs JD, Junor BJ, et al: Effect of acute aluminium overload on calcium and parathyroid-hormone metabolism. Lancet 1:501–503, 1983.

232. Felsenfeld AJ, Harrelson JM, Gutman RA: Osteomalacia after parathyroidectomy in patients with uremia. Ann Intern Med 96:34, 1984.

233. Andress DL, Ott SM, Maloney NA, Sherrard DJ: Effect of parathyroidectomy on bone aluminum accumulation in chronic renal failure. N Engl J Med 312:468–473, 1985.

234. Ellis HA: Aluminum and osteomalacia after parathyroidectomy. Ann Intern Med 96:533, 1982.

235. Ellis HA, Peart KM: Azotemic renal osteodystrophy; a quantitative study on iliac. J Clin Pathol 26:83, 1973.

236. Felsenfeld AJ, Machado L, Bover J, et al: Effect of aluminium on the development of hyperparathyroidism and bone disease in the azotaemic rat. Nephrol Dial Transplant 8:325–334, 1993.

237. Kawaguchi Y, Oda Y, Imamura N, et al: Unresponsiveness of bone to PTH in aluminum-related renal osteodystrophy. Kidney Int 29(suppl 18):S49–S52, 1986.

238. Lieberherr M, Grosse B, Cournot-Witmer G, et al: Aluminum action on mouse bone cell metabolism and response to PTH and 1,25(OH)$_2$D$_3$. Kidney Int 31:736–743, 1987.

239. Rodriguez M, Felsenfeld AJ, Llach F: Aluminum administration in the rat separately affects the osteoblast and bone mineralization. J Bone Miner Res 5:59–67, 1990.

240. Ott SM, Andress DL, Nebeker HG, et al: Changes in bone histology after treatment with desferrioxamine. Kidney Int 29(suppl 18):S108–S113, 1986.

241. Fanti P, Faugere MC, Smith AJ, Malluche HH: Removal of aluminum is associated with increased production of 1,25(OH)$_2$ vitamin D in dialysis patients. Kidney Int 31:346, 1987. Abstract.

242. Chan Y, Alfrey AC, Posen S: The effect of aluminum on normal and uremic rats: Tissue distribution, vitamin D metabolites and quantitative bone histology. Calcif Tissue Int 35:344, 1983.

243. Goodman WG, Henry DA, Horst R, et al: Parenteral aluminum administration in the dog: II. Induction of osteomalacia and effect on vitamin D metabolism. Kidney Int 25:370–375, 1984.

244. Robertson JA, Felsenfeld AJ, Haygood C: Animal model of aluminum induced osteomalacia: Role of chronic renal failure. Kidney Int 23:327, 1983.

245. Sedman AB, Alfrey AC, Miller NL, Goodman WG: Tissue and cellular basis for impaired bone formation in aluminum related osteomalacia in the pig. J Clin Invest 79:86, 1987.

246. Klein GL, Ott SM, Alfrey AC, et al: Aluminum as a factor in the bone disease of long-term parenteral nutrition. Trans Assoc Am Physicians 95:155–164, 1982.

247. Klein GL, Alfrey AC, Miller NL, et al: Aluminum loading during total parenteral nutrition. Am J Clin Nutr 35:1425–1429, 1982.

248. Quarles LD, Dennis V, Gitelman HJ: Aluminum deposition in bone: An epiphenomenon of the osteomalacic state. Clin Res 32:522A, 1984. Abstract.

249. Quarles LD, Gitelman HJ, Drezner MK: Aluminum induced de novo bone formation in the beagle: A parathyroid hormone dependent event. J Clin Invest 83:1644, 1989.

250. Faugere MC, Malluche HH: Stainable aluminum and not aluminum content reflects bone histology in dialyzed patients. Kidney Int 30:717–722, 1986.

251. Blumenthal NC, Posner AS: In vitro model of aluminum induced osteomalacia: Inhibition of hydroxyapatite formation and growth. Calcif Tissue Int 36:439, 1984.

252. Meyer JL, Thomas WC: Aluminum and aluminum complexes. Effect of calcium phosphate precipitation. Kidney Int 29(suppl):S20, 1986.

253. Lieberherr M, Grosse B, Cournot-Witmer G: In vitro effects of aluminum on bone phosphatases: Possible interaction with PTH and vitamin D$_3$ metabolites. Calcif Tissue Int 34:280, 1982.

254. Alfrey AC: Aluminum and tin. In Bronner F, Coburn JW (eds): Disorders of Mineral Metabolism, Vol I. Academic Press, New York, 1981, pp 353–368.

255. Kaehny WD, Hegg AP, Alfrey AC: Gastrointestinal absorption of aluminum from aluminum containing antacids. N Engl J Med 296:1389, 1977.

256. Ricanati ES, Ott SM, Klein KL: Evaluation of bone in dialysis patients exposed to aluminum in dialysate. Kidney Int 21:176, 1982.

257. Trapp GA: Plasma aluminum is bound to transferrin. Life Sci 33:311–316, 1983.

258. King SW, Savory J, Wills MR: Aluminum distribution in serum following hemodialysis. Ann Clin Lab Sci 12:143–149, 1982.

259. Mion C, Branger B, Issautier R: Dialysis fracturing osteomalacia without hyperparathyroidism in patients treated with HCO$_3$ rinsed Redy cartridge. Trans Am Soc Artif Intern Organs 27:634, 1981.

260. Cumming AD, Simpson G, Bell D, et al: Acute aluminium intoxication in patients on continuous ambulatory peritoneal dialysis. Lancet 1:103–104, 1982. Letter.

261. Curtis JR, Sampson B: Aluminum kinetics during haemodialysis with the Redy 2000 Sorbsystem. Int J Artif Organs 12:683–687, 1989.

262. Llach F, Gardner PW, George CRP, Cairoli O: Aluminum kinetics using bicarbonate dialysate with the sorbent system. Kidney Int 43:899–902, 1993.

263. Milliner DS, Shinaberger JH, Shuman P, Coburn JW: Inadvertent aluminum administration during plasma exchange due to aluminum contamination of albumin-replacement solutions. N Engl J Med 312:165–167, 1985.

264. Vargas JH, Klein GL, Ament ME, et al: Metabolic bone disease associated with total parenteral nutrition: Course after reducing aluminum content in parenteral solutions. Am J Clin Nutr 480:1070–1078, 1988.

265. Perazella M, Brown E: Acute aluminum toxicity and alum bladder irrigation in patients with renal failure. Am J Kidney Dis 21:44–46, 1993.

266. Moreno A, Dominguez P, Dominguez C, Ballabriga A: High serum aluminium levels and acute reversible encephalopathy in a 4-year-old boy with acute renal failure. Eur J Pediatr 150:513–514, 1993.

267. Berlyne GM, Ben-Ari J, Pest D, et al: Hyperaluminaemia from aluminum resins in renal failure. Lancet 2:494–496, 1970.

268. Hercz G, Andress DL, Nebeker HG, et al: Reversal of aluminum-related bone disease after substituting calcium carbonate for aluminum hydroxide. Am J Kidney Dis 11:70–75, 1988.

269. Felsenfeld AJ, Gutman RA, Llach F, Harrelson JM: Osteomalacia in chronic renal failure: A syndrome previously reported only with maintenance dialysis. Am J Nephrol 2:147–154, 1982.

270. Kaye M: Oral aluminum toxicity in a non dialyzed patient with renal failure. Clin Nephrol 20:208, 1983.

271. Winney RJ, Cowie JF, Robson JS: The role of plasma aluminum in the detection and prevention of aluminum toxicity. Kidney Int 29 (suppl 18):S91–S95, 1986.

272. Salusky IB, Coburn JW, Foley J, et al: Oral calcium carbonate as a phosphate-binding agent in children on dialysis: Effects on plasma aluminum levels. J Pediatr 105:717, 1984.

273. Salusky IB, Coburn JW, Foley J, et al: Effects of oral calcium carbonate on control of serum phosphorus and changes in plasma aluminum levels after discontinuation of aluminum-containing gels in children receiving dialysis. J Pediatr 108:767–770, 1986.

274. Hercz G, Kraut JA, Andress DL: Use of calcium carbonate as a phosphate binder in dialysis patients. Miner Electrolyte Metab 12:314, 1986.

275. Slatopolsky E, Weerts C, Norwood K, et al: Long term effects of calcium carbonate and 2.5 mEq/liter calcium dialysate on mineral metabolism. Kidney Int 36:897–903, 1989.

276. Robertson JA, Salusky IB, Goodman WG, et al: Sucralfate, intestinal aluminum absorption, and aluminum toxicity in a patient on dialysis. Ann Intern Med 111:179–181, 1989.

277. Burgess E, Muruve D, Audette R: Aluminum absorption and excretion following sucralfate therapy in chronic renal insufficiency. Am J Med 92:471–475, 1992.

278. Freundlich M, Zilleruelo G, Abitbol C, et al: Infant formula as a cause of aluminium toxicity in neonatal uraemia. Lancet 2:527–529, 1985.

279. Salusky IB, Coburn JW, Nelson P, Goodman WG: Prospective evaluation of aluminum loading from formula in infants with uremia. J Pediatr 116:726–729, 1984.

280. Ittel TH, Buddington B, Miller NL, Alfrey AC: Enhanced gastrointestinal absorption of aluminum in uremic rats. Kidney Int 32:821–826, 1987.

281. Demontis R, Leflon A, Fournier A, et al: 1$\alpha$(OH)vitamin $D_3$ increases plasma aluminum in hemodialized patients taking Al(OH)$_3$. Clin Nephrol 29:146–149, 1986.

282. Mayor GH, Keiser JA, Makdani D, Ku PK: Aluminum absorption and distribution: Effect of parathyroid hormone. Science 197:1187–1189, 1977.

283. Nordal KP, Dahl E: Low dose calcitriol versus placebo in patients with predialysis chronic renal failure. J Clin Endocrinol Metab 67:929–936, 1988.

284. Slanina P, Frech W, Ekstrom L, et al: Dietary citric acid enhances absorption of aluminum in antacids. Clin Chem 32:539–541, 1986.

285. Molitoris BA, Froment DH, Mackenzie TA, et al: Citrate: A major factor in the toxicity of orally administered aluminum compounds. Kidney Int 36:949–953, 1989.

286. Bakir AA, Hryhorczuk DO, Berman E: Acute fatal hyperaluminemic encephalopathy in undialyzed and recently dialyzed patients. Trans Am Soc Artif Intern Organs 32:171, 1986.

287. Kirshchbaum BB, Schoolwerth AC: Acute aluminum toxicity associated with oral citrate and aluminum containing antacids. Am J Med Sci 297:9, 1989.

288. Coburn JW, Mischel MG, Goodman WG, Salusky IB: Calcium citrate markedly enhances aluminum absorption from aluminum hydroxide. Am J Kidney Dis 17:708–711, 1991.

289. Sherrard DJ: Aluminum, much ado about something. N Engl J Med 324:558–559, 1991.

290. Main J, Ward MK: Potentiation of aluminium absorption by effervescent analgesic tablets in a haemodialysis patient. BMJ 304:1686, 1992.

291. Czapla K, Rodger RS, Halls DJ, et al: Ranitidine reduces aluminum toxicity in patients with renal failure. Nephrol Dial Transplant 7:1246–1248, 1992.

292. Cannata JB, Fernandez-Soto I, Fernandez-Menendez MJ, et al: Role of iron metabolism in absorption and cellular uptake of aluminum. Kidney Int 39:799–803, 1991.

293. Cannata JB, Olaizola IR, Gomez-Alonso C, et al: Serum aluminum transport and aluminum uptake in chronic renal failure: Role of iron and aluminum metabolism. Nephron 65:141–146, 1993.

294. Huang JY, Huang CC, Lim PS, et al: Effect of body iron stores on serum aluminum level in hemodialysis patients. Nephron 61:158–162, 1992.

295. Rosenlof K, Fyhrquist F, Tenhunen R: Erythropoietin, aluminium and anaemia in patients on haemodialysis. Lancet 335:247–249, 1990.

296. Casati S, Castelnovo C, Campise M, Ponticelli C: Aluminium interference in the treatment with human erythropoietin. Nephrol Dial Transplant 5:441–443, 1990.

297. D'Haese PC, De Broe ME: Aluminum toxicity. In Daugirdas JT, Ing TS (eds): Handbook of Dialysis. Little, Brown, Boston, 1994, pp 522–536.

298. De Broe ME, Drueke TB, Ritz E: Diagnosis and treatment of aluminium overload in end-stage renal failure patients. Nephrol Dial Transplant 8(suppl 1):1–4, 1993.

299. Andress DL, Kopp JB, Maloney NA, et al: Early deposition of aluminum in bone in diabetic patients on hemodialysis. N Engl J Med 316:292–296, 1987.

300. Andress DL, Hercz G, Kopp JB, et al: Bone histomorphometry of renal osteodystrophy in diabetic patients. J Bone Miner Res 2:525–531, 1987.

301. Pei Y, Hercz G, Greenwood C, et al: Renal osteodystrophy in diabetic patients. Kidney Int 44:159–164, 1993.

302. Cohen-Solal ME, Sebert JL, Boudailliez B, et al: Non-aluminic adynamic bone disease in non-dialyzed uremic patients: A new type of osteopathy due to overtreatment? Bone 13:1–5, 1992.

303. Sherrard DJ, Ott S, Maloney N, et al: Renal osteodystrophy: classification, cause and treatment. In Frame B, Potts JT Jr (eds): Clinical Disorders of Bone and Mineral Metabolism. Excerpta Medica, Amsterdam, 1983, pp 254–259.

304. Ott SM, Maloney NA, Coburn JW, et al: The prevalence of bone aluminum deposition in renal osteodystrophy and its relation to the response to calcitriol therapy. N Engl J Med 307:709–714, 1982.

305. Malluche HH, Faugere MC: Renal osteodystrophy. N Engl J Med 321:317, 1989.

306. Sherrard DJ, Ott SM, Maloney NA: Uremic osteodystrophy: Classification, cause and treatment. In Frame B, Potts JT Jr (eds): Clinical Disorders of Bone and Mineral Metabolism. Excerpta Medica, Amsterdam, 1983, p 254.

307. Llach F, Felsenfeld AJ, Coleman M, et al: The natural course of dialysis osteomalacia. Kidney Int 29:S74–S79, 1986.

308. Sherrard DJ, Hercz G, Pei Y, et al: The spectrum of bone disease in end-stage renal failure—an evolving disorder. Kidney Int 43:436–442, 1993.

309. Hercz G, Pei Y, Greenwood C, et al: Aplastic osteodystrophy without aluminum: The role of "suppressed" parathyroid function. Kidney Int 44:860–866, 1993.

310. Moriniere P, Cohen-Solal M, Belbrik S, et al: Disappearance of aluminic bone disease in a long term asymptomatic dialysis population restricting Al(OH)$_3$ intake: Emergence of an idiopathic adynamic bone disease not related to aluminum. Nephron 53:93–101, 1989.

311. Fournier A, Moriniere P, Cohen-Solal ME, et al: Adynamic bone disease in uremia: May it be idiopathic? Is it an actual disease? Nephron 58:1–12, 1991.

312. Malluche HH, Monier-Faugere MC: Risk of adynamic bone disease in dialyzed patients. Kidney Int Suppl 38:S62–S67, 1992.
313. Goodman WG, Gilligan J, Horst R: Short term aluminum administration in the rat. J Clin Invest 73:171, 1984.
314. Quarles LD, Gitelman HJ, Drezner MK: Induction of de novo bone formation in the beagle. A novel effect of aluminum. J Clin Invest 81:1056–1066, 1988.
315. Andress DL, Maloney NA, Endres DB, Sherrard DJ: Aluminum-associated bone disease in chronic renal failure: High prevalence in a long-term dialysis population. J Bone Miner Res 1:391–398, 1986.
316. Andress DL, Maloney NA, Coburn JW, et al: Osteomalacia and aplastic bone disease in aluminum related osteodystrophy. J Clin Endocrinol Metab 65:11–16, 1987.
317. Charhon SA, Chavassieux PM, Chapuy MC, et al: Low rate of bone formation with or without histologic osteomalacia in patients with aluminum intoxication. J Lab Clin Med 106:123–131, 1985.
318. Rodriguez M, Lorenzo V, Felsenfeld AJ, Llach F: Effect of parathyroidectomy on aluminum toxicity and azotemic bone disease in the rat. J Bone Miner Res 5:379–385, 1990.
319. Felsenfeld AJ, Rodriguez M, Dunlay R, Llach F: A comparison of parathyroid gland function in hemodialysis patients with different forms of renal osteodystrophy. Nephrol Dial Transplant 6:244–251, 1991.
320. Eriksen EF, Mosekilde L, Melsen F: Kinetics of trabecular bone resorption and formation in hypothyroidism: Evidence for a positive balance per remodeling cycle. Bone 7:101–108, 1986.
321. Brissot C, Meunier PJ, Chapuy MC, Lejeune E: Histomorphometric profile, pathophysiology and reversibility of corticosteroid induced osteoporosis. Metab Bone Dis Relat Res 1:303–311, 1979.
322. Boivin G, Chapuy MC, Baud C, Meunier PJ: Fluoride content in human iliac bone. Results in controls, patients with fluorosis and osteoporotic patients treated with fluoride. J Bone Miner Res 3:497–502, 1980.
323. De Vernejoul M-C, Pointillart A, Golenzer CC, et al: Effects of iron overload on bone remodeling in pigs. Am J Pathol 116:377–384, 1984.
324. De Vyver FLV, Vissa WJ, D'Haese PC, DeBroe ME: Iron overload and bone disease in chronic dialysis patients. Nephrol Dial Transplant 5:781–787, 1990.
325. de Vernejoul MC, Marie P, Kuntz D, et al: Non-osteomalacic osteopathy associated with chronic hypophosphatemia. Calcif Tissue Int 34:219–233, 1982.
326. Lefebvre A, de Vernejoul MC, Gueris J, et al: Optimal correction of acidosis changes progression of dialysis osteodystrophy. Kidney Int 36:1112–1118, 1989.
327. Vicenti F, Arnaud S, Meker R, Genant H: Parathyroid and bone response of the diabetic patient to uremia. Kidney Int 25:677–682, 1984.
328. Aubia J, Bosch J, Lloveras J, et al: Low incidence of hyperparathyroidism in diabetic renal failure. Proc Eur Dial Transplant Assoc Eur Renal Assoc 21:902–908, 1985.
329. Aubia J, Serrano S, Mariñoso L, et al: Osteodystrophy of diabetics in chronic dialysis: A histomorphometric study. Calcif Tissue Int 42:297–301, 1988.
330. Vincenti F, Arnaud SB, Recker R, et al: Parathyroid and bone response of the diabetic patient to uremia. Kidney Int 25:677–682, 1984.
331. Heidbreder E, Gotz R, Schafferhans K, Heidland A: Diminished parathyroid gland responsiveness to hypocalcemia in diabetic patients with uremia. Nephron 42:285–289, 1986.
332. McNair P, Christensen MS, Madsbad S, et al: Hypoparathyroidism in diabetes mellitus. Acta Endocrinol 96:81–86, 1981.
333. Frost HM: Paper of the orthopaedic research laboratory. Lamellar bone physiology in diabetes mellitus. Henry Ford Hosp Med Bull 12:495–572, 1964.
334. McNair P, Madsbad S, Christensen MS, et al: Bone mineral loss in insulin-treated diabetes mellitus: Studies on pathogenesis. Acta Endocrinol 90:463–447, 1979.
335. Sugimoto T, Ritter C, Morrissey J, et al: Effects of high concentrations of glucose on PTH secretion in parathyroid cells. Kidney Int 37:1522–1527, 1990.
336. Salusky IB, Coburn JW, Brill J: Bone disease in pediatric patients undergoing dialysis with CAPD or CCPD. Kidney Int 33:975–982, 1988.
337. Coburn JW, Salusky IB: The Parathyroids. Raven Press, New York (in press).
338. Rodriguez-Perez JC, Plaza C, Torres A, et al: Low turnover bone disease is the more common form of bone disease in CAPD patients. Adv Perit Dial 8:376–380, 1993.
339. Bender FH, Bernardini J, Piraino B: Calcium mass transfer with dialysate containing 1.25 and 1.75 mmol/L calcium in peritoneal dialysis patients. Am J Kidney Dis 20:367–371, 1992.
340. Morton AR, Hercz G: Hypercalcemia in dialysis patients: Comparison of diagnostic methods. Dial Transplant 20:661–667, 1991.
341. Solal MC, Sebert JL, Boudailliez B, et al: Comparison of intact, midregion, and carboxy terminal assays of parathyroid hormone for the diagnosis of bone disease in hemodialyzed patients. J Clin Endocrinol Metab 73:516–524, 1991.
342. Marie PJ, Lomri A, deVernejoul MC, et al: Relationships between histomorphometric features of bone formation and bone cell characteristics in vitro in renal osteodystrophy. J Clin Endocrinol Metab 69:1166–1173, 1989.
343. Torres A, Hernandez D, Concepcion M, et al: Higher levels of intact parathyroid hormone (i-PTH) are necessary to maintain a normal bone remodelling in dialysis patients (DP). J Am Soc Nephrol 3:677, 1992.
344. Couttenye MM, Goodman WG, Segaert M, et al: Predictive value of low serum bone alkaline phosphatase (BAP) in the diagnosis of adynamic bone disease (ABD). J Am Soc Nephrol 3:672, 1992.
345. Andress DL, Endres DB, Maloney NA, et al: Comparison of parathyroid hormone assays with bone histomorphometry in renal osteodystrophy. J Clin Endocrinol Metab 63:1163, 1986.
346. Hutchison AJ, Whitehouse RW, Boulton HF, et al: Correlation of bone histology with parathyroid hormone, vitamin $D_3$, and radiology in end-stage renal disease. Kidney Int 44:1071–1077, 1993.
347. Stanbury SW, Lumb GA: Parathyroid function in chronic renal failure: A statistical survey of the plasma biochemistry in azotaemic renal osteodystrophy. Q J Med 35:1, 1966.
348. Kanis JA, Adams ND, Earnshaw M: Vitamin D, osteomalacia and chronic renal failure. In Norman AW, Schaefer K, Coburn JW, et al (eds): Vitamin D: Biochemical, Chemical and Clinical Aspects Related to Calcium Metabolism. Walter de Gruyter, Berlin, 1977, p 671.
349. Mechanic GL, Toverud SU, Ramp WK: Quantitative changes of bone collagen cross-links and precursors in vitamin D deficiency. Biochem Biophys Res Commun 47:760–765, 1972.
350. Russell JE, Avioli LV, Mechanic G: The nature of the collagen cross links in bone in the chronic uraemic state. Biochem J 145:119, 1975.
351. Russell JE, Avioli LV: 25-Hydroxycholecalciferol enhanced bone maturation in the parathyroprivic state. J Clin Invest 56:792, 1975.
352. Russell JE, Termine JD, Avioli LV: Abnormal bone mineral maturation in the chronic uremic state. J Clin Invest 52:2848, 1973.
353. Alfrey AC, Miller NL, Butkus D: Evaluation of body magnesium stores. J Lab Clin Med 84:153, 1974.
354. Burnell JM, Teubner E, Wergedal JE, Sherrard DJ: Bone crystal maturation in renal osteodystrophy in humans. J Clin Invest 53:52, 1974.
355. Alfrey AC, Solomons CC: Bone pyrophosphate in uremia and its association with extraosseous calcification. J Clin Invest 57:700, 1976.
356. Termine JD, Posner AS: Amorphous/crystalline interrelationships in bone mineral. Calcif Tissue Res 1:8, 1967.
357. Pellegrino ED, Biltz RM, Letteri JM: Interrelationships of carbonate, phosphate, monohydrogen phosphate, calcium, magnesium and sodium in uraemic bone: Comparison of dialyzed and nondialyzed patients. Clin Sci Mol Med 53:307, 1977.
358. Kaye M: Magnesium metabolism in the rat with chronic renal failure. J Lab Clin Med 84:536, 1974.
359. Giangrande A, Costantini S, Ballanti P, et al: Bone mineral and aluminum concentrations in patients undergoing CAPD. Adv Perit Dial 8:351–355, 1992.
360. Giangrande A, Costantini S, Ballanti P, et al: Contenuto minerale osseo nell'iperparatiroidismo secondario florido. Atti Congr Ist Super Sanita 5:31–40, 1989.
361. Goodman AD, Lemann J Jr, Lennon EJ, Relman AS: Production, excretion and net balance of fixed acid in patients with renal acidosis. J Clin Invest 44:495, 1965.
362. Litzow JR, Lemann J Jr, Lennon EJ: The effect of treatment of acidosis on calcium balance in patients with chronic azotemic renal disease. J Clin Invest 46:280, 1967.
363. Bushinsky DA, Lechleider RJ: Mechanism of proton-induced bone

calcium release: Calcium carbonate dissolution. Am J Physiol 253:F998–F1005, 1987.

364. Bushinsky DA, Sessler NE, Krieger NS: Greater unidirectional calcium efflux from bone during metabolic, than respiratory, acidosis. Am J Physiol 262:F425–F431, 1992.

365. Lemann J, Litzow JR, Lennon EF: Studies on the mechanism by which chronic metabolic acidosis augments urinary calcium excretion in man. J Clin Invest 46:1318–1328, 1967.

366. Bushinsky DA, Goldring JM, Coe FL: Cellular contribution to pH mediated calcium flux in neonatal mouse calvaria. Am J Physiol 248:F785–F789, 1985.

367. Bushinsky DA: Net calcium efflux from live bone during chronic metabolic, but not respiratory, acidosis. Am J Physiol 256:F836–F842, 1989.

368. Krieger NS, Sessler NE, Bushinsky DA: Acidosis inhibits osteoblastic and stimulates osteoclastic activity in vitro. Am J Physiol 262:F442–F448, 1992.

369. Arnett TR, Dempster DW: Effect of pH on bone resorption by rat osteoclasts in vitro. Endocrinology 119:119–124, 1986.

370. Kraut JA, Mishler DR, Singer FR, Goodman WG: The effects of metabolic acidosis on bone formation and bone resorption in the rat. Kidney Int 30:694–700, 1986.

371. Nichols G, Nichols N: Effect of parathyroidectomy on content and availability of skeletal sodium in the rat. Am J Physiol 198:749, 1960.

372. Pellegrino ED, Biltz RM: The composition of human bone in uremia. Medicine (Baltimore) 44:397, 1965.

373. Kaye M, Fruch AJ, Silverman M: A study of vertebral bone powder from patients with chronic renal failure. J Clin Invest 49:442, 1970.

374. Green J, Kleeman CR: Role of bone in regulation of systemic acid-base balance. Kidney Int 39:9–26, 1991. Editorial.

375. Stanbury SW, Lumb GA: Metabolic studies of renal osteodystrophy. I. Calcium, phosphorus and nitrogen metabolism in rickets, osteomalacia, and hyperparathyroidism complicating chronic uremia and in the osteomalacia of the adult Fanconi syndrome. Q J Med 35:1, 1966.

376. Stanbury SW: Bone disease in uremia. Am J Med 44:714, 1968.

377. Barzel US, Jowsey J: The effects of chronic acid and alkali administration on bone turnover in adult rats. Clin Sci 36:517, 1969.

378. Cunningham J, Fraher LJ, Clemens TL, et al: Chronic acidosis with metabolic bone disease. Effect of alkali on bone morphology and vitamin D metabolism. Am J Med 73:199–204, 1982.

379. Adams ND, Gray RW, Lemann J Jr: The calciuria of increased fixed acid production in humans: Evidence against a role for parathyroid hormone and 1,25-(OH)₂-vitamin D. Calcif Tissue Int 28:233–238, 1979.

380. Kraut JA, Gordon EM, Ransom JC, et al: Effect of chronic metabolic acidosis on vitamin D metabolism in humans. Kidney Int 24:644–648, 1983.

381. Lemann J Jr, Litzow JR, Lennon EJ: The effects of chronic acid loads in normal man: Further evidence for the participating of bone mineral in the defense against chronic metabolic acidosis. J Clin Invest 45:1608–1609, 1966.

382. Krapf R, Vetsch R, Vetsch W, Hulter HN: Chronic metabolic acidosis increases the serum concentration of 1,25-dihydroxyvitamin D in humans by stimulating its production rate. Critical role of acidosis-induced renal hypophosphatemia. J Clin Invest 90:2456–2463, 1992.

383. Bushinsky DA, Riera GS, Favus MJ, Coe FL: Response of serum 1,25-(OH)₂D₃ to variation of ionized calcium during chronic acidosis. Am J Physiol 249:F361–F365, 1985.

384. Baran DT, Lee SW, Jo OD, Avioli LV: Acquired alterations in vitamin D metabolism in the acidotic state. Calcif Tissue Int 34:165–168, 1982.

385. Lee SW, Russell J, Avioli LV: 25-Hydroxycholecalciferol to 1,25 dihydroxycholecalciferol: Conversion impaired by systemic metabolic acidosis. Science 195:994–996, 1977.

386. Coe FL, Firpo JJ Jr, Hollandsworth DL, et al: Effect of acute and chronic metabolic acidosis on serum immunoreactive parathyroid hormone in man. Kidney Int 8:262–273, 1975.

387. Weeke E, Friis TH: Serum fractions of calcium and phosphorus in uremia. Acta Med Scand 189:79, 1971.

388. Coburn JW, Popovtzer MM, Massry SG, Kleeman CR: The physio-chemical state and renal handling of divalent ions in chronic renal failure. Arch Intern Med 124:302, 1969.

389. Walling MW, Lee D, Brickman A, Coburn JW: Jejunal phosphate (Pi) active transport: Effects of phosphate depletion and vitamin D. Fed Proc 36:1097, 1977.

390. Walton J, Gray TK: Absorption of intestinal phosphate in the human intestine. Clin Sci 56:407, 1979.

391. Corry DB, Chan DWS, Lee DBN: Intestinal absorption of phosphate. In Massry SG, Glassock RJ (eds): Textbook of Nephrology. Williams & Wilkins, Baltimore, 1989, pp 328–335.

392. Walling MW: Intestinal Ca²⁺ and phosphate transport: Differential responses of vitamin D metabolites. Am J Physiol 133:3488, 1977.

393. Caniggia A, Gennari C: Intestinal absorption of radiophosphate after physiologic doses of 25(OH)D₃ in normals, liver cirrhosis and chronic renal failure patients. In Norman AW, Schaefer K, Coburn JW, et al (eds): Vitamin D: Biochemical, Chemical and Clinical Aspects Related to Calcium Metabolism. Walter de Gruyter, Berlin, 1977, p 755.

394. Brickman AS, Hartenbower DL, Norman AW, Coburn JW: Actions of 1-hydroxyvitamin D₃ and 1,25 dihydroxyvitamin D₃ on mineral metabolism in man. I. Effects on net absorption of phosphorus. Am J Clin Nutr 30:1064, 1977.

395. Coburn JW, Brickman AS, Sherrard DJ: Clinical efficacy of 1,25-dihydroxyvitamin D₃ in renal osteodystrophy. In Norman AW, Schaefer K, Coburn JW, et al (eds): Vitamin D: Biochemical, Chemical and Clinical Aspects Related to Calcium Metabolism. Walter de Gruyter, Berlin, 1977, p 657.

396. Gallieni M, Brancaccio D, Padovese P, et al: Low-dose intravenous calcitriol treatment of secondary hyperparathyroidism in hemodialysis patients. Kidney Int 42:1191–1198, 1992.

397. Birge SJ: Vitamin D, muscle and phosphate homeostasis. Miner Electrolyte Metab 1:57, 1978.

398. Massry SG, Coburn JW, Popovtzer MM: Secondary hyperparathyroidism in chronic renal failure: The clinic spectrum in uremia, during hemodialysis and after renal transplantation. Arch Intern Med 124:431, 1969.

399. Coburn JW, Brickman AS, Massry SG: Medical treatment in primary and secondary hyperparathyroidism. Semin Drug Treat 2:117, 1972.

400. Ahmed KY, Vahgese Z, Wills MR, et al: Persistent hypophosphataemia and osteomalacia in dialysis patients not on oral phosphate-binders: Response to dihydrotachysterol therapy. Lancet 2:439–442, 1976.

401. Wiegmann TB, Kaye M: Malabsorption of calcium and phosphate in chronic renal failure: ³²P and ⁴⁵Ca studies in dialysis patients. Clin Nephrol 34:35–41, 1990.

402. Fiaschi E, Maschio G, D'Angelo A: Low protein diets and bone disease in chronic renal failure. Kidney Int 12(suppl):S79, 1978.

403. Letteri JM, Ellis KJ, Orofino DP, et al: Altered calcium metabolism in chronic renal failure. Kidney Int 6:45–54, 1974.

404. Letteri JM, Cohn, S.H.: Total body neutron activation: Analysis in the study of mineral homeostasis in chronic renal disease. In David DS (ed): Calcium Metabolism in Renal Failure and Nephrolithiasis. John Wiley & Sons, New York, 1977, p 249.

405. Walser M: The separate effects of hyperparathyroidism, hypercalcemia of malignancy, renal failure and acidosis on the state of calcium phosphate and other ions in plasma. J Clin Invest 41:1454, 1962.

406. Raman A, Chong YK, Sreenevasan G: Effects of varying dialysate calcium concentration on the plasma calcium fractions in patients on dialysis. Nephron 16:181, 1976.

407. Wing AJ, Curtis JR, Eastwood JB: Transient and persistent hypercalcaemia in patients treated by maintenance haemodialysis. Br Med J 4:150, 1968.

408. Genuth SM, Vertes V, Leonards JR: Oral absorption in patients with renal failure treated by chronic hemodialysis. Metabolism 18:125, 1969.

409. Messner RP, Smith HT, Shapiro FL, Gregory DH: The effect of hemodialysis, vitamin D, and renal homotransplantation on the calcium malabsorption of chronic renal failure. J Lab Clin Med 74:472–481, 1969.

410. Recker R, Saville PD: Calcium absorption in renal failure: Its relationship to blood urea nitrogen, dietary calcium intake, time on dialysis, and other variables. J Lab Clin Med 78:380, 1971.

411. Shimada H, Makamura M, Marumo F: Influence of aluminum on the effect of 1α(OH)D₃ on renal osteodystrophy. Nephron 35:163–170, 1983.

412. Rodriguez M, Felsenfeld AJ, Llach F: The role of aluminum in the

development of hypercalcemia in the rat. Kidney Int 31:766–771, 1987.

413. Curtis JR, De Wardener H, Gower P, Eastwood JB: The use of calcium carbonate and calcium phosphate without vitamin D in the management of renal osteodystrophy. Proc Eur Dial Transplant Assoc 7:141, 1970.

414. Meyrier A, Marsac J, Richet G: The influence of a high calcium carbonate intake on bone disease in patients undergoing hemodialysis. Kidney Int 4:146–153, 1973.

415. Slatopolsky E, Weerts C, Lopez-Hilker S, et al: Calcium carbonate as a phosphate binder in patients with chronic renal failure undergoing dialysis. N Engl J Med 315:157–161, 1986.

416. Schaefer K, Scheer J, Asmus G, et al: The treatment of uraemic hyperphosphataemia with calcium acetate and calcium carbonate: A comparative study. Nephrol Dial Transplant 6:171–175, 1991.

417. Papadimitriou M, Gingell JC, Chisholm GD: Hypercalcaemia from calcium ion-exchange resins in patients on regular haemodialysis. Lancet 2:948–950, 1968.

418. Koppel MH, Massry SG, Shinaberger JH: Thiazide induced rise in serum calcium and magnesium in patients on maintenance hemodialysis. Ann Intern Med 72:895, 1970.

419. Barbour GL, Coburn JW, Slatopolsky E, et al: Hypercalcemia in an anephric patient with sarcoidosis, evidence for extrarenal generation of 1,25-dihydroxyvitamin D. N Engl J Med 305:440–446, 1981.

420. Felsenfeld AJ, Drezner MK, Llach F: Hypercalcemia and elevated calcitriol in a maintenance dialysis patient with tuberculosis. Arch Intern Med 146:1941–1944, 1986.

421. Schmulen AC, Lerman M, Pak CYC, et al: Effect of 1,25-dihydroxyvitamin $D_3$ therapy on jejunal absorption of magnesium in patients with chronic renal failure. Am J Physiol 238:349G–355G, 1980.

422. Brannan PG, Vergne-Marini P, Pak CY, et al: Magnesium absorption in the human small intestine: Results in patients with absorptive hypercalciuria. J Clin Invest 57:1412–1418, 1976.

423. Alfrey AC, Solomons CC, Ciricillo J, Miller NL: Extraosseous calcification. Evidence for abnormal pyrophosphate metabolism in uremia. J Clin Invest 57:692, 1976.

424. Wallach S: Relation of magnesium to osteoporosis and calcium urolithiasis. Magnesium Trace Elements 10:281–286, 1991.

425. Guillot AP, Hood VL, Runge CF, Gennari FJ: The use of magnesium-containing phosphate binders in patients with end-stage renal disease on maintenance hemodialysis. Nephron 30:114–117, 1982.

426. Stewart WK, Fleming LW: The effects of dialysate magnesium on plasma and erythrocyte magnesium and potassium concentrations during maintenance haemodialysis. Nephron 10:221–231, 1973.

427. Moriniere P, Fournier A, Westeel P, et al: Calcium carbonate and magnesium hydroxide in the prevention of renal osteodystrophy or the demise of aluminum toxicity in uremia. Contrib Nephrol 64:58–73, 1988.

428. O'Donovan R, Baldwin D, Hammer M, et al: Substitution of aluminium salts by magnesium salts in control of dialysis hyperphosphataemia. Lancet 1:880–882, 1986.

429. Freeman RM: The role of magnesium in the pathogenesis of azotemic hypothermia. Proc Soc Exp Biol Med 137:1069, 1971.

430. Freeman RM, Lawton RL, Chamberlain MA: Hard water syndrome. N Engl J Med 276:1113, 1967.

431. Habener JF, Potts JT Jr: Relative effectiveness of magnesium and calcium on the secretion and biosynthesis of parathyroid hormone in vitro. Endocrinology 98:197, 1976.

432. Massry SG, Coburn JW, Kleeman CR: Evidence for suppression of parathyroid gland by hypermagnesemia. J Clin Invest 40:1619, 1970.

433. Mennes P, Rosenbaum R, Martin KJ, Slatopolsky E: Hypomagnesemia and impaired parathyroid hormone secretion in chronic renal disease. Ann Intern Med 88:206, 1978.

434. Mori S, Harada S, Okazaki R, et al: Hypomagnesemia with increased metabolism of parathyroid hormone and reduced responsiveness to calcitropic hormones. Intern Med 31:820–824, 1992.

435. Naik RB, Gosling P, Price C: Comparative study of alkaline phosphatase isoenzymes, bone histology, and skeletal radiography in dialysis bone disease. Br Med J 1:1307, 1977.

436. Skillen AW, Pierides AM: Serum alkaline phosphatase isoenzyme patterns in patients with chronic renal failure. Clin Chim Acta 80:339, 1977.

437. Duursma SA, vonKesteren RG, Visser WJ: Serum alkaline phosphatase: Its relation to bone cells and its significance as an indicator for vitamin D treatment in patients with renal insufficiency. In Norman

WW, Schaefer K, Grigoleit HG (eds): Vitamin D and Problems Related to Uremic Bone Disease. Walter de Gruyter, Berlin, 1975, p 167.

438. Ritz E, Malluche HH, Bommer J: Metabolic bone disease in patients on maintenance hemodialysis. Nephron 12:393, 1974.

439. Hruska KA, Teitelbaum SL, Kopelman R: The predictability of the histologic features of uremic bone disease by noninvasive techniques. Metab Bone Dis Relat Res 1:39, 1978.

440. Coburn JW, Norris KC: The diagnosis of aluminum related bone disease and the treatment of aluminum toxicity with deferoxamine. Semin Nephrol 6(suppl 1):12–21, 1986.

441. Pierides AM, Skillen AW, Ellis AH: Serum alkaline phosphatase in azotemic and hemodialysis osteodystrophy: A study of isoenzyme patterns, their correlation with bone histology, and their changes in response to treatment with 1 alpha (OH)$D_3$ and 1,25(OH)$_2D_3$. J Lab Clin Med 99:899, 1979.

442. Garnero P, Delmas P: Assessment of the serum levels of bone alkaline phosphatase with a new immunoradiometric assay in patients with metabolic bone disease. J Clin Endocrinol Metab 77:1046–1053, 1993.

443. Price PA, Parthemore JG, Deftos LJ: New biochemical marker for bone metabolism. Measurement by radioimmunoassay of bone GLA protein in the plasma of normal subjects and patients with bone disease. J Clin Invest 66:878–883, 1980.

444. Delmas PD, Wahner HW, Mann KG, Riggs BL: Assessment of bone turnover in postmenopausal osteoporosis by measurement of serum bone Gla-protein. J Lab Clin Med 102:470–476, 1983.

445. Slovid DM, Graff AM, Novak KM: Clinical evaluation of bone turnover by serum osteocalcin measurements. Calcif Tissue Int 34:S15, 1982.

446. Malluche HH, Faugere MC, Fanti P, Price PA: Plasma levels of bone Gla-protein reflect bone formation in patients on chronic maintenance dialysis. Kidney Int 26:869–874, 1984.

447. Delmas PD, Wilson DM, Mann KG, Riggs BL: Effect of renal function on plasma levels of bone Gla-protein. J Clin Endocrinol Metab 57:1028–1030, 1983.

448. Gundberg CM, Hauschka PV, Lian JB, Ballop PM: Osteocalcin: isolation, characterization and detection. Methods Enzymol 107:516–544, 1984.

449. Charhon SA, Delmas PD, Malaval L, et al: Serum bone Gla-protein in renal osteodystrophy: Comparison with bone histomorphometry. J Clin Endocrinol Metab 63:892–897, 1986.

450. Epstein S, Traberg H, Raja R, et al: Serum and dialysate osteocalcin levels in hemodialysis and peritoneal dialysis patients and after renal transplantation. J Clin Endocrinol Metab 60:1253–1256, 1985.

451. Coen G, Mazzaferro S, Bonucci E, et al: Bone GLA protein in predialysis chronic renal failure: Effects of 1,25(OH)$_2D_3$ administration in a long-term follow-up. Kidney Int 28:783–790, 1985.

452. Nakatsuka K, Miki T, Nishizawa Y, et al: Circulating bone Gla protein in end-stage renal disease determined by newly developed two-site immunoradiometric assay. Contrib Nephrol 90:147–154, 1991.

453. Garnero P, Grimaux M, Demiaux B, et al: Measurement of serum osteocalcin with a human-specific two-site immunoradiometric assay. J Bone Miner Res 7:1389–1398, 1992.

454. Hosoda K, Eguchi H, Nakamoto T, et al: Sandwich immunoassay for intact human osteocalcin. Clin Chem 38:2233–2238, 1992.

455. Saupe J, Konig M, Shearer MJ, Kohlmeier M: Carboxylated osteocalcin concentrations in plasma provide information about two independent bone modulating systems in end stage renal disease (ESRD). J Am Soc Nephrol 3:676, 1992.

456. Ebeling PR, Peterson JM, Riggs BL: Utility of type procollagen propeptide assays for assessing abnormalities in metabolic bone disease. J Bone Miner Res 7:1243–1250, 1992.

457. Coen G, Mazzaferro S, Ballanti P, et al: Procollagen type I C-terminal extension peptide in predialysis chronic renal failure. Am J Nephrol 12:246–251, 1992.

458. Prockop D, Kivirikko K: Relationship of hydroxyproline excretion in urine to collagen metabolism. Ann Intern Med 66:1243, 1967.

459. Kowalewski J, Tomaszewki J, Hanzlik J: The elimination of free, peptide bound and protein bound hydroxyproline into dialysate during peritoneal dialysis in patients with renal failure. Clin Chim Acta 34:123, 1971.

460. Varghese Z, Moorhead JF, Tutler GL, et al: Plasma hydroxyproline in renal osteodystrophy. Proc Eur Dial Transplant Assoc 10:187–196, 1973.

461. Hart W, Duursma SA, Visser WJ, Njio LK: The hydroxyproline content of plasma of patients with impaired renal function. Clin Nephrol 4:104–108, 1975.
462. Eyre D: New biomarkers of bone resorption. J Clin Endocrinol Metab 74:470A–470B, 1992.
463. Lam KW, Robert A: Tartrate-resistant (band 5) acid phosphatase activity measured by electrophoresis on acrylamide gel. Clin Chem 24:309, 1978.
464. Minkin C: Bone acid phosphatase: Tartrate-resistant acid phosphatase as a marker of osteoclast function. Calcif Tissue Int 34:285–290, 1982.
465. Stepan JJ, Silinkova-Malkova E, Havrenek T: Relationship of plasma tartrate-resistant acid phosphatase to the bone isoenzyme of serum alkaline phosphatase in hyperparathyroidism. Clin Chim Acta 133:189–200, 1983.
466. Kraenzlin M, Lau KHW, Liang L: Development of an immunoassay for human serum osteoclastic tartrate-resistant acid phosphatase. J Clin Endocrinol Metab 71:442–451, 1990.
467. Hamet P, Stouder DA, Ginn HE, et al: Studies of the elevated extracellular concentration of cyclic AMP in uremic man. J Clin Invest 56:339–345, 1975.
468. Chan YL, Furlong TJ, Cornish CJ, Posen S: Dialysis osteodystrophy. A study involving 94 patients. Medicine (Baltimore) 64:296–309, 1985.
469. Nussbaum SR, Potts JT Jr: Immunoassays for parathyroid hormone 1–84 in the diagnosis of hyperparathyroidism. J Bone Mineral Res 6(suppl 2):S43–S50, 1991.
470. Brown RC, Aston JP, Weeks I, Woodhead S: Circulating intact parathyroid hormone measured by a two-site immunochemiluminometric assay. J Clin Endocrinol Metab 65:407–414, 1987.
471. Guillard O, Pineau A, Baruthlo F, Arnaud J: An international quality assessment program for measurement of aluminum in human plasma: A progress report. Clin Chem 34:1603–1604, 1988.
472. Ward MK, Parkinson IS: Aluminum toxicity in renal failure. In Drukker W, Parsons FM, Maher JF (eds): Replacement of Renal Function. Martinus Nijhoff, Boston, 1983, p 811.
473. Milliner DS, Ott SM, Nebeker HG: Deferoxamine infusion test for diagnosis of aluminum related osteomalacia. Ann Intern Med 101:775–779, 1984.
474. Alfrey AC: Aluminum. Adv Clin Chem 21:69, 1983.
475. Piccoli A, Andriani M, Mattiello G, et al: Serum aluminium level in the Veneto chronic haemodialysis population: Cross-sectional study on 1,026 patients. Nephron 51:482–490, 1989.
476. Rovelli E, Luciani L, Pagani C, et al: Correlation between serum aluminum concentration and signs of encephalopathy in a large population of patients dialyzed with aluminum free fluids. Clin Nephrol 29:294–298, 1988.
477. Norris KC, Sherrard DJ, Slatopolsky E, Coburn JW: Symptomatic renal bone disease: Non-invasive parameters for diagnosis. Abstract Book, XIth International Congress of Nephrology 1990, 405A. Abstract.
478. Malluche HH, Smith AJ, Abreo L, Faugere MC: The use of desferrioxamine in the management of renal patients with bone aluminum accumulation. N Engl J Med 311:140, 1984.
479. de Vernejoul MC, Marchais S, London G: Deferoxamine test and bone disease in dialysis patients with mild aluminum accumulation. Am J Kidney Dis 14:124, 1989.
480. Pei Y, Hercz G, Greenwood C, et al: Non-invasive prediction of aluminum bone disease in hemo- and peritoneal dialysis patients. Kidney Int 41:1374–1382, 1992.
481. Mazzaferro S, Coen G, Ballanti P, et al: Deferoxamine test and PTHY serum levels are useful but not to recognize but to exclude aluminum-related bone disease. Nephron 61:151–157, 1992.
482. Yaqoob M, Ahmad R, Roberts N, Helliwell T: Low-dose desferrioxamine test for the diagnosis of aluminum-related bone disease in patients on regular haemodialysis. Nephrol Dial Transplant 6:484–486, 1991.
483. Cannata JB, Alonso M, Olaizola I, Diaz B: Fe status and the desferrioxamine test. J Am Soc Nephrol 1:350, 1990.
484. Subra JF, Krari N, Tirot P, et al: Aluminium determination in the skin of patients with and without end-stage renal failure. Nephron 58:170–173, 1991.
485. Bindi P, Khayat R, Saiag P, et al: There is no aluminum accumulation in the skin of end-stage renal failure patients. Nephron 58:485, 1991. Letter.
486. Floege J, Schaffer J, Koch KM, Shaldon S: Dialysis related amyloidosis: A disease of chronic retention and inflammation? Kidney Int Suppl 38:S78–S85, 1992.
487. Koch KM: Dialysis-related amyloidosis. Kidney Int 41:1416–1429, 1992.
488. Drueke TB: Beta-2-microglobulin amyloidosis and renal bone disease. Miner Electrolyte Metab 17:261–272, 1991.
489. Campistol JM, Skinner M: $\beta_2$-Microglobulin amyloidosis: An overview. Semin Dial 6:117–126, 1993.
490. Wright RS, Mehls O, Ritz E, Coburn JW: Musculoskeletal manifestation of chronic renal failure, dialysis and transplantation. In Bacon P, Hadler N (eds): Renal Manifestations in Rheumatic Disease. Butterworth, London, 1982, p 352.
491. Mirahmadi KS, Coburn JW, Bluestone R: Calcific periarthritis and hemodialysis. JAMA 229:548–549, 1973.
492. Hardouin P, Lecomte-Houcke M, Flipo RM, et al: Current aspects of osteoarticular pathology in patients undergoing hemodialysis: Study of 80 patients. Part 2. Laboratory and pathologic analysis. Discussion of the pathogenic mechanism. J Rheumatol 14:784–787, 1987.
493. Massry SG, Bluestone R, Klinenberg JR, Coburn JW: Abnormalities of the musculoskeletal system in hemodialysis patients. Semin Arthritis Rheum 4:321–349, 1975.
494. Llach F, Pederson JA: Acute joint syndrome and maintenance hemodialysis. Proc Clin Dial Transplant Forum 9:17, 1979.
495. Kleinman KS, Coburn JW: Amyloid syndromes associated with hemodialysis. Kidney Int 35:567–575, 1989.
496. Schott GD, Wills MR: Muscle weakness in osteomalacia. Lancet 1:626, 1976.
497. Malette LE, Patten BM, Engel WK: Neuromuscular disease in secondary hyperparathyroidism. Ann Intern Med 82:474–483, 1975.
498. Baker LRI, Ackrill P, Cattell WR: Iatrogenic osteomalacia and myopathy due to phosphate depletion. Br Med J 3:150, 1974.
499. Smith R, Stern G: Myopathy, osteomalacia and hyperparathyroidism. Brain 90:593, 1967.
500. Coburn JW, Nebeker HG, Hercz G, et al: Role of aluminum accumulation in the pathogenesis of renal osteodystrophy. In Robinson RR (ed): Nephrology, Vol II. Springer-Verlag, New York, 1984, pp 1383–1395.
501. Brickman AS, Sherrard DJ, Jowsey J: 1,25-Dihydroxycholecalciferol: Effect on skeletal lesions and plasma parathyroid hormone in uremic osteodystrophy. Arch Intern Med 134:883, 1974.
502. Henderson RG, Russell RGG, Ledingham JG: Effects of 1,25-dihydroxycholecalciferol on calcium absorption, muscle weakness, and bone disease in chronic renal failure. Lancet 249:83, 1974.
503. Kanis JA, Cundy T, Earnshaw M, et al: Treatment of renal bone disease with 1α-hydroxylated derivatives of vitamin D$_3$: Clinical, biochemical, radiographic and histological responses. Q J Med 48:289–322, 1979.
504. Floyd M, Ayyar DR, Barwick DD, et al: Myopathy in chronic renal failure. Q J Med 43:509–524, 1974.
505. Schoenfeld PJ, Martin JH, Barnes B, Teitelbaum SL: Amelioration of myopathy with 25-hydroxyvitamin D$_3$ therapy (25(OH)D$_3$) in patients on chronic hemodialysis. In Third Workshop on Vitamin D, Book of Abstracts. University of California at Riverside Press, Riverside, CA, 1977, p 160.
506. Nebeker HG, et al: Clinical response of aluminum-related osteomalacia to desferrioxamine. Abstract Book, IXth International Congress of Nephrology, 1984, 115A. Abstract.
507. Lotem M, Bernheim J, Conforty B: Spontaneous rupture of tendons: A complication of hemodialyzed patients treated for renal failure. Nephron 21:201, 1978.
508. Cirincione R, Baker B: Tendon rupture with secondary hyperparathyroidism. A case report. J Bone Joint Surg [Am] 57:852–853, 1975.
509. Preston F, Adicoff A: Hyperparathyroidism with avulsion of three major tendons. N Engl J Med 266:968, 1962.
510. Preston E: Avulsion of three major tendons. JAMA 221:406, 1972.
511. Avioli LV: Collagen metabolism, uremia and bone. Kidney Int 4:105, 1973.
512. Murphy KJ, McPhee I: Tears of major tendons in chronic acidosis with elastosis. J Bone Joint Surg 53:510, 1971.
513. Ryuzaki M, Konishi K, Kasuga A, et al: Spontaneous rupture of the quadriceps tendon in patients on maintenance hemodialysis—report of three cases with clinicopathological observations. Clin Nephrol 32:144–148, 1989.

514. Kurer MH, Baillod RA, Madgwick JC: Musculoskeletal manifestations of amyloidosis. A review of 83 patients on haemodialysis for at least 10 years. J Bone Joint Surg [Br] 73:271–276–276, 1991.

515. Gipstein R, Coburn JW, Adams D, et al: Calciphylaxis in man: A syndrome of tissue necrosis and vascular calcification in 11 patients with chronic renal disease. Arch Intern Med 136:1273–1280, 1976.

516. Massry SG, Gordon A, Coburn JW: Vascular calcification and peripheral necrosis in a renal transplant recipient: Reversal of lesion following subtotal parathyroidectomy. Am J Med 49:416, 1970.

517. Wenzel-Seifert K, Harwig S, Keller F: Fulminant calcinosis in two patients after kidney transplantation. Am J Nephrol 11:497–500, 1991.

518. Weidmann P, Massry SG, Coburn JW: Effect of acute hypercalcemia on blood pressure in patients with chronic renal failure. Ann Intern Med 76:741, 1972.

519. Charbon GA: Parathormone: A selective vasodilator. *In* Talmage RV, Balander LE (eds): Parathyroid Hormone—Thyrocalcitonin (Calcitonin). Excerpta Medica, Amsterdam, 1969, p 475.

520. Selye H: Calciphylaxis. University of Chicago Press, Chicago, 1982.

521. Duh QY, Lim RC, Clark OH: Calciphylaxis in secondary hyperparathyroidism. Diagnosis and parathyroidectomy. Arch Surg 126:1213–1219, 1991.

522. Poch E, Almirall J, Alsina M, et al: Calciphylaxis in a hemodialysis patient: Appearance after parathyroidectomy during a psoriatic flare. Am J Kidney Dis 19:285–288, 1992.

523. Berlyne GM: Microcrystalline conjunctival calcification in renal failure: A useful clinical sign. Lancet 2:366, 1968.

524. Berlyne GM, Shaw AG: Red eyes in renal failure. Lancet 1:4, 1967.

525. Massry SG, Popovtzer MM, Coburn JW: Intractable pruritus as a manifestation of secondary hyperparathyroidism in uremia. Disappearance of itching following subtotal parathyroidectomy. N Engl J Med 279:697, 1968.

526. Tapia L, Cheigh J, David DS: Parenteral lidocaine in treatment of pruritus in dialysis patients. N Engl J Med 296:261, 1977.

527. Gilchrest B, Rowe JW, Brown RS, et al: Relief of uremic pruritus with ultraviolet phototherapy. N Engl J Med 297:136–138, 1977.

528. Cohen EP, Russell TJ, Garancis JC: Mast cells and calcium in severe uremic itching. Am J Med Sci 303:360–365, 1992.

529. Pederson JA, Matter BJ, Czerwinski A, Llach F: Relief of idiopathic generalized pruritus in dialysis patients with activated oral charcoal. Ann Intern Med 93:446, 1980.

530. De Marchi S, Cecchin E, Villalta D, et al: Relief of pruritus and decreases in plasma histamine concentrations during erythropoietin therapy in patients with uremia. N Engl J Med 326:969–974, 1992.

531. Nielsen T, Andersen KE, Kristiansen J: Pruritus and xerosis in patients with chronic renal failure. Dan Med Bull 27:269–271, 1980.

532. Raskin NH, Fishman RA: Neurologic disorders in renal failure. N Engl J Med 294:204, 1976.

533. Stockenhuber F, Kurz RW, Sertl K, et al: Increased plasma histamine levels in uraemic pruritus. Clin Sci 79:477–482, 1990.

534. Mehls O, Ritz E, Krempien B, et al: Slipped epiphysis in renal osteodystrophy. Arch Dis Child 50:545–554, 1975.

535. Mehls O, Ritz E, Krempien B: Roentgenological signs in the skeleton of uremic children. An analysis of the anatomical principles underlying the roentgenological changes. Pediatr Radiol 1:183, 1973.

536. Mehls O: Renal osteodystrophy in children: Etiology and clinical aspects. *In* Fine RN, Gruskin AB (eds): End Stage Renal Disease in Children. WB Saunders, Philadelphia, 1984, pp 227–250.

537. Stanbury SW: The role of vitamin D in renal bone disease. Clin Endocrinol 7:25S, 1977.

538. Parfitt AM: Clinical and radiographic manifestations of renal osteodystrophy. *In* David DS (ed): Calcium Metabolism in Renal Failure and Nephrolithiasis. John Wiley & Sons, New York, 1977, pp 150–190.

539. Potter D, Belzer F, Rames L: The treatment of chronic uremia in childhood. Pediatrics 45:432, 1970.

540. Scharer K: Growth in children with chronic renal failure. Kidney Int Suppl 13:S68–S71, 1978.

541. Chantler C, Danckerwolcke RA, Brunner FP, et al: Combined report on regular dialysis and transplantation of children in Europe. Proc Eur Dial Transplant Assoc 16:74–104, 1979.

542. Simmons JM, Wilson CJ, Potter DE, Holliday MA: Relation of caloric deficiency to growth failure in children on hemodialysis and the growth response to caloric supplementation. N Engl J Med 285:653–656, 1971.

543. Chantler C, Holliday M: Growth in children with renal disease, with special reference to the effects of caloric malnutrition: A review. Clin Nephrol 1:230, 1973.

544. Betts P, Magrath G: Growth pattern and dietary intake of children with chronic renal insufficiency. Br Med J 2:189, 1974.

545. McSherry E, Morris RC: Attainment and maintenance of normal growth status with alkali therapy in infants and children with classic renal tubular acidosis (RTA). J Clin Invest 61:509–527, 1978.

546. Saenger P, Wiedmann E, Schwartz E: Somatomedin and growth after renal transplantation. Pediatr Res 8:163, 1974.

547. Chesney RW, Moorthy A, Eisman JA, et al: Increased growth after long-term oral 1,25-vitamin D₃ in childhood renal osteodystrophy. N Engl J Med 298:238–242, 1978.

548. Salusky IB, Fine RN, Kangarloo H: "High dose" calcitriol for control of renal osteodystrophy in children on CAPD. Kidney Int 32:89, 1987.

549. Tonshoff B, Mehls O, Heinrich U, et al: Growth-stimulating effect of recombinant human growth hormone in children with end-stage renal disease. J Pediatr 116:561–566, 1990.

550. Koch VH, Lippe BM, Nelson PA, et al: Accelerated growth after recombinant human growth hormone treatment of children with chronic renal failure. J Pediatr 115:365–371, 1989.

551. Mehls O, Ritz E, Hunziker EB, et al: Improvement of growth and food utilization by human recombinant growth hormone in uremia. Kidney Int 33:45–52, 1988.

552. Stivelman JC: Refractoriness to recombinant human epoetin treatment. *In* Nissenson AR, Fine RN (eds): Dialysis Therapy, 2nd ed. Hanley and Belfus, Philadelphia, 1992, p 236.

553. Coburn JW, Massry SG, DePalma JS, Shinaberger JH: Rapid appearance of hypercalcemia with initiation of hemodialysis. JAMA 210:2276, 1969.

554. Mazzaferro S, Coen G, Bandini S, et al: Mitral annulus calcification in uremia. Nephrol Dial Transplant 8:335–340, 1993.

555. Bogin E, Massry SG, Harary I: Effect of parathyroid hormone on heart cells. J Clin Invest 67:1215, 1981.

556. London GM, Fabiani F, Marchais SJ, et al: Uremic cardiomyopathy: An inadequate left ventricular hypertrophy. Kidney Int 31:973–980, 1987.

557. London GM, de Vernejoul MC, Fabiani F, et al: Secondary hyperparathyroidism and cardiac hypertrophy in hemodialysis patients. Kidney Int 32:900–907, 1987.

558. Puschett JB, Moranz J, Kurnick WS: Evidence for a direct action of cholecalciferol and 25-hydroxycholecalciferol on the renal transport of phosphate, sodium and calcium. J Clin Invest 51:373, 1972.

559. Marchais SJ, Guerin AP, London AM, et al: Long-term effects of parathyroidectomy on left ventricular function in hemodialysis patients. Blood Purif 2:155–162, 1992.

560. Chazan J, Abuelo G, Blonsky S: Plasma aluminum levels (unstimulated and stimulated): Clinical and biochemical findings in 185 patients undergoing chronic hemodialysis for 4 to 95 months. Am J Kidney Dis 13:284–289, 1993.

561. Roth A, Nogues C, Galle P, et al: Multiorgan aluminum deposits in a chronic haemodialysis patient. Electron microscope and microprobe studies. Virchows Arch A 405:131–140, 1984.

562. Timsit F, Galle P, Bourdon R, et al: Cardiomyopathie aluminique chéz un hemodialyse chronique. Nephrologie 6:263, 1985. Abstract.

563. London G, deVernejoul MC, Fabiani F, et al: Association between aluminum accumulation and cardiac hypertrophy in hemodialyzed patients. Am J Kidney Dis 13:75–83, 1989.

564. Massry SG: Parathyroid hormone as a uremic toxin. *In* Massry SG, Glassock RJ (eds): Textbook of Nephrology, 2nd ed. Williams & Wilkins, Baltimore, 1989, pp 450–475.

565. Massry SG, Goldstein D: Role of parathyroid hormone in uremic toxicity. Kidney Int Suppl 13:S39, 1978.

566. Massry SG: The toxic effects of parathyroid hormone in uremia. Semin Nephrol 3:306–328, 1983.

567. Massry SG, Fadda GZ: Chronic renal failure is a state of cellular calcium toxicity. Am J Kidney Dis 21:81–86, 1993.

568. Arieff AI, Massry SG: Calcium metabolism of brain in acute renal failure. J Clin Invest 53:387, 1974.

569. Guisado R, Arieff AI, Massry SG, et al: Changes in the electroencephalogram in acute uremia: Effects of parathyroid hormone and brain electrolytes. J Clin Invest 55:738–745, 1975.

570. Cooper JD, Lazarowitz V, Arieff AI: Neurodiagnostic abnormalities in patients with acute renal failure. Evidence for neurotoxicity of parathyroid hormone. J Clin Invest 61:1448, 1978.

571. Kiley JE, Woodruff MW, Pratt KI: Evaluation of encephalopathy by EEG frequency analysis in chronic dialysis patients. Clin Nephrol 5:245–250, 1976.

572. Ball JH, Johnson JW, Hampus CL, Merrill JP: The many facets of secondary hyperparathyroidism. Arch Intern Med 131:746–749, 1973.

573. Fraser CL, Arieff AI: Nervous system complications in uremia. Ann Intern Med 109:143–153, 1988.

574. Ni Z, Smogorzewski M, Massry SG: Derangements in acetylcholine metabolism in brain synaptosomes in chronic renal failure. Kidney Int 44:630–637, 1993.

575. Avram MM, Feinfeld DA, Huatuco AH: Search for the uremic toxin: Decreased motor-nerve conduction velocity and elevated parathyroid hormone in uremia. N Engl J Med 298:1000–1003, 1978.

576. Arieff AI, Schmidt R: Parathyroid hormone as a uremic neurotoxin. N Engl J Med 299:362, 1978.

577. Goldstein DA, Chui LA, Massry SG: Effect of parathyroid hormone and uremia on peripheral nerve calcium and motor nerve conduction velocity. J Clin Invest 62:88–93, 1978.

578. Massry SG, Goldstein DA, Procci W, Kletsky OA: Impotence in patients with uremia: A possible role for parathyroid hormone. Nephron 19:305, 1977.

579. Blumberg A, Wildbolz A, Descoeudres C, et al: Influence of 1,25-dihydroxycholecalciferol on sexual dysfunction and related endocrine parameters in patients on maintenance hemodialysis. Clin Nephrol 13:208–214, 1980.

580. Weinberg SG, Lubin A, Wiener SN, et al: Myelofibrosis and renal osteodystrophy. Am J Med 63:755–764, 1977.

581. Boxer M, Ellman L, Geller R, Wang CA: Anemia in primary hyperparathyroidism. Arch Intern Med 137:588–593, 1977.

582. Rao DS, Shih MS, Mohini R: Effect of serum parathyroid hormone and bone marrow fibrosis on the response to erythropoietin in uremia. N Engl J Med 328:171–175, 1993.

583. Barbour GL: Effect of parathyroidectomy on anemia in chronic renal failure. Arch Intern Med 139:889, 1979.

584. Meytes D, Bogin E, Ma A, et al: Effects of parathyroid hormone on erythrocytes. J Clin Invest 67:1263, 1981.

585. Levi J, Zevin D, Bessler H, Djaldetti M: Effect of parathyroid hormone and 1,25-dihydroxyvitamin $D_3$ on RNA and heme synthesis by erythroid precursors. Proc Eur Dial Transplant Assoc 17:603–607, 1980.

586. Bogin E, Massry SG, Levi J, et al: Effect of parathyroid hormone on osmotic fragility of human erythrocytes. J Clin Invest 69:1017–1025, 1982.

587. Remuzzi G, Benigni A, Dodesini P, et al: Parathyroid hormone inhibits human platelet function. Lancet 2:1321–1323, 1981.

588. Alexiewicz JM, Gaciong Z, Klinger M, et al: Evidence of impaired T cell function in hemodialysis patients: Potential role for secondary hyperparathyroidism. Am J Nephrol 10:495–501, 1990.

589. Alexiewicz JM, Klinger M, Pitts TO, et al: Parathyroid hormone inhibits B-cell proliferation: Implications in chronic renal failure. J Am Soc Nephrol 1:236–244, 1990.

590. Gaciong Z, Alexiewicz JM, Massry SG: Impaired in vivo antibody production in CRF rats: Role of secondary hyperparathyroidism. Kidney Int 40:862–867, 1991.

591. Stojceva-Taneva O, Fadda GZ, Smogorzewski M, Massry SG: Parathyroid hormone increases cytosolic calcium of thymocytes. Nephron 64:592–599, 1993.

592. Bagdade JD, Porte D Jr, Bierman EL: Hypertriglyceridemia: A metabolic consequence of chronic renal failure. N Engl J Med 279:181–185, 1968.

593. Cantin M: Kidney, parathyroid and lipemia. Lab Invest 14:1691, 1965.

594. Perna AF, Fadda GZ, Zhou XJ, Massry SG: Mechanisms of impaired insulin secretion following chronic excess of parathyroid hormone. Am J Physiol 259:F210–F216, 1990.

595. Fadda GZ, Thanakitcharu P, Smogorzewski M, Massry SG: Parathyroid hormone raises cytosolic calcium in pancreatic islets: Study on mechanisms. Kidney Int 43:554–560, 1993.

596. DiRaimondo CV, Casey T, DiRaimondo CV, Stone WJ: Pathologic fractures associated with idiopathic amyloidosis of bone in chronic hemodialysis patients. Nephron 43:22–27, 1986.

597. Fenves AZ, Emmett M, White MG, et al: Carpal tunnel syndrome with cystic bone lesions secondary to amyloidosis in chronic hemodialysis patients. Am J Kidney Dis 7:130–134, 1986.

598. Bardin T, Kuntz D, Zingraff J: Synovial amyloidosis patients undergoing long term hemodialysis. Arthritis Rheum 28:1952, 1985.

599. Munoz-Gomez J, Bergada-Barado E, Gomez-Perez R: Amyloid arthropathy in patients undergoing periodical haemodialysis for chronic renal failure: A new complication. Ann Rheum Dis 44:729, 1985.

600. Campistol JM, Cases A, Torras A, et al: Visceral involvement of dialysis amyloidosis. Am J Nephrol 7:390–393, 1987.

601. Gejyo F, Homma N, Suzuki M, Arakawa KM: Serum levels of $\beta_2$-microglobulin as a new form of amyloid protein in patients undergoing long-term hemodialysis. N Engl J Med 314:585–586, 1986.

602. Zingraff J, Drueke T: Can the nephrologist prevent dialysis related amyloidosis? Am J Kidney Dis 18:1–11, 1991.

603. Noel LH, Zingraff J, Bardin T, et al: Tissue distribution of dialysis amyloidosis. Clin Nephrol 27:175–178, 1987.

604. van Ypersele de Strihou C, Jadoul M, Malghem J, et al: Effect of dialysis membrane and patient's age on signs of dialysis-related amyloidosis. Kidney Int 39:1012–1019, 1991.

605. Goldstein S, Winston E, Chung TJ, et al: Chronic arthropathy in long term hemodialysis. Am J Med 78:82–86, 1985.

606. Kuntz D, Naveau B, Bardin T, et al: Destructive spondylarthropathy in hemodialyzed patients. Arthritis Rheum 27:369–375, 1984.

607. Hatakeyama A, Fujinaga H, Togo T, et al: Remarkable improvement of activity by CAPD in a hemodialysis patient with a pseudotumor of the craniocervical junction. Adv Perit Dial 8:116–119, 1992.

608. Maruyama H, Gejyo F, Arakawa M: Clinical studies of destructive spondyloarthropathy in long-term hemodialysis patients. Nephron 61:37–44, 1992.

609. Deforges-Lasseur C, Combe C, Cernier A, et al: Destructive spondyloarthropathy presenting with progressive paraplegia in a dialysis patient. Recovery after surgical spinal cord decompression and parathyroidectomy. Nephrol Dial Transplant 8:180–184, 1993.

610. Bohlman ME, Kim YC, Eagan J, Spees EK: Brown tumor in secondary hyperparathyroidism causing acute paraplegia. Am J Med 81:545–547, 1986.

611. Takenaka R, Fukatsu A, Matsuo S, et al: Surgical treatment of hemodialysis-related shoulder arthropathy. Clin Nephrol 38:224–230, 1992.

612. Gejyo F, Homma N, Hasegawa S, Arakawa M: A new therapeutic approach to dialysis amyloidosis: Intensive removal of beta 2-microglobulin with adsorbent column. Artif Organs 17:240–243, 1993.

613. Campistol JM, Ponz E, Munoz-Gomez J, et al: Renal transplantation for dialysis amyloidosis. Transplant Proc 24:118–119, 1992.

614. Nelson SR, Sharpstone P, Kingswood JC: Does dialysis-associated amyloidosis resolve after transplantation? Nephrol Dial Transplant 8:369–370, 1993.

615. Hutchinson AJ, Freemont AJ, Lumb GA, Gokal R: Renal osteodystrophy in CAPD. In Khanna R, Nolph KD, Prowant BF, et al (eds): Advances in Peritoneal Dialysis. University of Toronto Press, Toronto, 1991, pp 237–239.

616. Poznanski AK: Radiologic evaluation of bone mineral in children. In Favus MJ (ed): Primer on the Metabolic Bone Diseases and Disorders of Mineral Metabolism. Raven Press, New York, 1993, p 115.

617. Dent CE, Hodson C: Radiological changes associated with certain metabolic bone diseases. Br J Radiol 27:605, 1954.

618. Meema HE, Rabinovich S, Meema S, et al: Improved radiological diagnosis of azotemic osteodystrophy. Radiology 102:1–10, 1972.

619. Ritz E, Prager P, Krempien B: Skeletal x-ray findings and bone histology in patients on hemodialysis. Kidney Int 13:316, 1978.

620. Meema HE, Oreopoulos DG, Rabinovich S: Periosteal new bone formation (periosteal neostasis) in renal osteodystrophy. Radiology 110:513, 1974.

621. Doyle FH: Radiological patterns of bone disease associated with renal glomerular failure in adults. Br Med Bull 28:220, 1972.

622. Doyle F, Aung T, Carroll RN: Bone resorption in chronic renal failure: A comparison of radiological and histological assessments. Br Med Bull 28:225, 1972.

623. Eastwood JB, Bordier PhJ, De Wardener H: Some biochemical, histological, radiological and clinical features of renal osteodystrophy. Kidney Int 4:128, 1973.

624. Glassford D, Remmers AR, Sarles H: Hyperparathyroidism in the maintenance dialysis patient. Surg Gynecol Obstet 142:328, 1976.

625. Tatler GL, Baillod RA, Varghese Z, et al: Evolution of bone disease over 10 years in 135 patients with terminal renal failure. Br Med J 4:315–319, 1973.

626. Prager P, Singer R, Ritz E, Krempien B: Diagnostischer Stellenwert der Lamina dura dentium beim sekundaren Hyperparathyreoidismus. Rofo Fortschr Geb Rontgenstrl Nuklearmed 129:237–240, 1978.

627. Meema HE, Meema S: Comparison of microradioscopic and morphometric findings in the hand bones with densitometric finding in the proximal radius in thyrotoxicosis and in renal osteodystrophy. Invest Radiol 7:88, 1972.

628. Ellis K, Hochstim RJ: The skull in hyperparathyroid bone disease. Am J Roentgenol 83:732, 1960.

629. Owen J, Parnell A, Keir M, et al: Critical analysis of the use of skeletal surveys in patients with chronic renal failure. Clin Radiol 39:578–582, 1988.

630. Chalmers J, Conacher WD, Gardner DL, Scott PJ: Osteomalacia—a common disease in elderly women. J Bone Joint Surg [Br] 49:403, 1967.

631. Ritz E, Krempien B, Mehls O, Malluche HH: Skeletal abnormalities in chronic renal insufficiency before and during maintenance hemodialysis. Kidney Int 4:116, 1973.

632. Norfray J, Calenoff L, DelGreco F, Krumlovsky F: Renal osteodystrophy in patients on hemodialysis as reflected in the bony pelvis. Am J Roentgenol 125:352, 1975.

633. Parfitt AM: Soft tissue calcification in uremia. Arch Intern Med 124:544, 1969.

634. Johnson C, Graham CB, Curtis FK: Roentgenographic manifestations of chronic renal disease treated by periodic hemodialysis. Am J Radium Ther Nucl Med 101:915–926, 1967.

635. Benhamou CL, Rouchon JP, Geslin N, et al: Arthropathies des membres chéz les insuffisants rénaux dialyses. Presse Med 16:119–122, 1987.

636. Chou CT, Wasserstein A, Schumacher HR Jr, Fernandez P: Musculoskeletal manifestations in hemodialysis patients. J Rheumatol 12:1149–1153, 1985.

637. Rubin LA, Fam AG, Rubenstein J, et al: Erosive azotemic osteoarthropathy. Arthritis Rheum 27:1086–1094, 1984.

638. Bardin T, Vasseur M, de Vernejoul MC, et al: Étude prospective de l'atteinte articulair des malades hémodialyses depuis plus de 10 ans. Rev Rheum 55:131–134, 1988.

639. Kessler M, Azoulay E, Netter P, et al: Arthropathie du dialyse: Résultats d'une étude multicentrique realisée chéz 171 malades hémodialyses depuis plus de 10 ans. In Gaucher A, Pourel J, Netter P, Kessler M (eds): Actualités en Physiopathologie et Pharmacologie Acticulairs. Masson, Paris, 1989, pp 272–279.

640. Meema HE, Oreopoulos DG, Rapoport A: Serum magnesium level and arterial calcification in end stage renal disease. Kidney Int 32:388–394, 1987.

641. Ritz E, Mehls O, Bommer J: Vascular calcifications under maintenance hemodialysis. Klin Wochenschr 55:375, 1977.

642. Meema HE, Oreopoulos DG, deVeber GA: Arterial calcifications in severe chronic renal disease and their relationship to dialysis treatment, renal transplant, and parathyroidectomy. Radiology 121:315–321, 1976.

643. Massry SG, Coburn JW, Hartenbower DL, et al: Mineral content of human skin in uremia: Effect of secondary hyperparathyroidism and hemodialysis. Proc Eur Dial Transplant Assoc 7:146–150, 1970.

644. DeFrancisco AM, Ellis HA, Owen JP, et al: Parathyroidectomy in chronic renal failure. Q J Med 55:289–315, 1985.

645. Kainberger F, Traindl O, Baldt M, et al: Renale Osteodystrophie: Spektrum der Rontgensymptomatik bei modernen Formen der Nierentransplantation und Dauerdialysetherpie. Rofo Fortschr Geb Rontgenstr Neuen Bildgeb Verfahr 157:501–505, 1992.

646. Contiguglia S, Alfrey AC, Miller NL: Nature of soft tissue calcification in uremia. Kidney Int 4:229, 1973.

647. Kuzela D, Huffer WE, Conger JD: Soft tissue calcification in chronic dialysis patients. Am J Pathol 86:403, 1977.

648. Dreher W, Shelp W: Atrioventricular block in a long term dialysis patient. Reversal after parathyroidectomy. JAMA 234:954, 1975.

649. Fujimoto S, Hisanaga S, Yamatomo Y, et al: Tertiary hyperparathyroidism associated with metastatic cardiac calcification in a haemodialyzed patient. Int Urol Nephrol 23:285–292, 1991.

650. Conger JD, Hammond WS, Alfrey AC, et al: Pulmonary calcification in chronic dialysis patients. Clinical and pathologic studies. Ann Intern Med 83:330–336, 1975.

651. Davis B, Poulose K, Reba R: Scanning for uremic pulmonary calcifications. Ann Intern Med 85:132, 1976.

652. Ibels LS, Alfrey AC, Haut L, Huffer WE: Preservation of function in experimental renal disease by dietary restriction of phosphate. N Engl J Med 298:122, 1991.

653. Lumlertgul D, Burke TJ, Gillum D, et al: Phosphate depletion arrests progression of chronic renal failure independent of protein intake. Kidney Int 29:658–666, 1986.

654. Barsotti G, Giannoni A, Morelli E, et al: The decline of renal function slowed by very low phosphorus intake in chronic renal patients following a low nitrogen diet. Clin Nephrol 21:54–59, 1984.

655. Parfitt AM, Massry SG, Winfield A: Osteopenia and fractures occurring during maintenance hemodialysis. A "new" form of renal osteodystrophy. Clin Orthop 87:287, 1972.

656. Homma N, Gejyo F, Kobayashi H, et al: Cystic radiolucencies of carpal bones, distal radius and ulna as a marker for dialysis-associated amyloid osteoarthropathy. Nephron 62:6–12, 1992.

657. Sole M, Cardesa A, Palacin A, et al: Morphological and immunohistochemical findings in dialysis-related amyloidosis. An analysis of 16 cases. Appl Pathol 7:350–360, 1989.

658. Zingraff J, Noel LH, Bardin T, et al: β₂-Microglobulin amyloidosis: A sternoclavicular joint biopsy study in hemodialysis patients. Clin Nephrol 33:94–97, 1990.

659. Cobby MJ, Adler RS, Swartz R, Martel W: Dialysis-related amyloid arthropathy: MR findings in four patients. AJR 157:1023–1027, 1991.

660. Kroner G, Stabler A, Seiderer M, et al: Beta 2 microglobulin–related amyloidosis causing atlantoaxial spondyloarthropathy with spinal-cord compression in haemodialysis patients: Detection by MRI. Nephrol Dial Transplant 6(suppl 2):91–95, 1991.

661. Kay J, Benson CB, Lester S, et al: Utility of high-resolution ultrasound for the diagnosis of dialysis-related amyloidosis. Arthritis Rheum 35:926–932, 1992.

662. Fleisch H, Russell RGG: Experimental clinical studies with pyrophosphate and diphosphonates. In David DS (ed): Calcium Metabolism in Renal Failure and Nephrolithiasis. John Wiley & Sons, New York, 1977, p 293.

663. Rosenthal L, Kaye M: Observations on the mechanism of Tc labeled phosphate complex uptake in metabolic bone disease. Nucl Med 5:59, 1976.

664. Lien JW, Wiegmann TB, Rosenthall L, Kaye M: Abnormal Tc pyrophosphate bone scans in chronic renal failure. Clin Nephrol 6:509, 1976.

665. Sy W, Mittal A: Bone scan in chronic dialysis patients with evidence of secondary hyperparathyroidism and renal osteodystrophy. Br J Radiol 48:878, 1975.

666. Olgaard K, Heerfordt J, Madsen S: Scintigraphic skeletal changes in uremic patients on regular hemodialysis. Nephron 17:325, 1976.

667. Karsenty G, Vigneron N, Jorgetti V: Value of the ⁹⁹ᵐTc-methylene diphosphonate bone scan in renal osteodystrophy. Kidney Int 29:1058–1065, 1986.

668. Hodson EM, Howman-Gilles RB, Evans RB, et al: The diagnosis of renal osteodystrophy: A comparison of technetium-99m-pyrophosphate bone scintigraphy with other techniques. Clin Nephrol 16:24–28, 1981.

669. de Jonge FA, Pauwels EK, Hamdy NA: Scintigraphy in the clinical evaluation of disorders of mineral and skeletal metabolism in renal failure. Eur J Nucl Med 18:839–855, 1991.

670. Winzelberg GG: Parathyroid imaging. Ann Intern Med 107:64–70, 1987.

671. Fine EJ: Parathyroid imaging: Its current status and future role. Semin Nucl Med 17:350–359, 1987.

672. Suehiro M, Fukuchi M: Localization of hyperfunctioning parathyroid glands by means of thallium-201 and iodine-131 subtraction scintigraphy in patients with primary and secondary hyperparathyroidism. Ann Nucl Med 6:185–190, 1992.

673. Nisbet AP, Shaw P, Taube D, et al: ⁵¹Cr-EDTA/⁹⁹ᵐTc-MDP ratio: A simple non-invasive method for assessing renal osteodystrophy. Br J Radiol 62:438–442, 1989.

674. Hawkins PN, Myers MJ, Lavender JP, Pepys MB: Diagnostic radionuclide imaging of amyloid: Biological targeting by circulating human serum amyloid P component. Lancet 1:1413–1418, 1988.

675. Floege J, Burchert W, Brandis A, et al: Imaging of dialysis-related amyloid (AB-amyloid) deposits with ¹³¹I-β₂-microglobulin. Kidney Int 38:1169–1176, 1990.

676. Gladziwa U, Ittel TH, Dakshinamurty KV, et al: Secondary hyperparathyroidism and sonographic evaluation of parathyroid gland hyperplasia in dialysis patients. Clin Nephrol 38:162–166, 1992.

677. Fukagawa M, Okazaki R, Takano K, et al: Regression of parathyroid hyperplasia by calcitriol-pulse therapy in patients on long-term dialysis. N Engl J Med 323:421–422, 1990.

678. Winkelbauer F, Ammann ME, Langle F, Niederle B: Diagnosis of hyperparathyroidism with US after autotransplantation: Results of a prospective study. Radiology 186:255–257, 1993.

679. Jadoul M, Walker TL: Ultrasonography detection of thickened joint capsules and tendons: An early marker of dialysis-related amyloidosis. Nephrol Dial Transplant 5:727, 1990. Abstract.

680. McMahon LP, Radford J, Dawborn JK: Shoulder ultrasound in dialysis related amyloidosis. Clin Nephrol 35:227–232, 1991.

681. Nordin BE, MacGregor J, Smith DA: The incidence of osteoporosis in normal women: Its relation to age and menopause. Q J Med 35:25, 1966.

682. Garn S, Poznanski A, Nagy M: Bone measurement in the differential diagnosis of osteopenia and osteoporosis. Radiology 100:509, 1971.

683. Gryfe CI, Exton-Smith AN, Stewart RJ: Determination of the amount of bone in the metacarpal. Age Ageing 1:213–221, 1972.

684. Parfitt AM: The actions of parathyroid hormone on bone: Relation to bone remodeling and turnover, calcium homeostasis and metabolic bone disease. Metabolism 25:909, 1976.

685. Bone JM, Davison AM, Robson JS: Role of dialysate calcium concentration in osteoporosis in patients on haemodialysis. Lancet 1:1047–1049, 1972.

686. Sugisaki H, Yamada K, Kataoka H, Kunitomo T: Long-term observation on renal osteodystrophy related parameters in dialysis patients. Nephrol Dial Transplant 6(suppl 2):244–251, 1991.

687. Rickers H, Christensen M, Podbro P: Bone mineral content in patients on prolonged maintenance hemodialysis: A three year follow-up study. Clin Nephrol 20:302–307, 1983.

688. Lindergard B, Johnell O, Nilsson BE, Wiklund PE: Studies of bone morphology, bone densitometry and laboratory data in patients on maintenance hemodialysis treatment. Nephron 39:122–129, 1985.

689. Cameron JR, Mazess RB, Sorenson JA: Precision and accuracy of bone mineral determination by direct photon absorptiometry. Invest Radiol 3:9, 1968.

690. Hahn TJ, Hahn B: Osteopenia in patients with rheumatic diseases: Principles of diagnosis and therapy. Semin Arthritis Rheum 6:165, 1976.

691. Griffiths HJ, Zimmerman RE, Bailey G, Snider R: The use of photon absorptiometry in the diagnosis of renal osteodystrophy. Radiology 109:277, 1973.

692. Griffiths HJ, Zimmerman RE, Lazarus M, et al: The long-term follow-up of 195 patients with renal failure: A preliminary report. Radiology 122:643–648, 1977.

693. Mazess RB, Peppler W, Chesnut C: Total body mineral and lead body mass by dual photon absorptiometry. Calcif Tissue Int 33:361, 1981.

694. Asaka M, Iida H, Entani C, et al: Total and regional bone mineral density by dual photon absorptiometry in patients on maintenance hemodialysis. Clin Nephrol 38:149–153, 1992.

695. Eisenberg B, Tzamaloukas AH, Murata GH, et al: Factors affecting bone mineral density in elderly men receiving chronic in-center hemodialysis. Clin Nucl Med 16:30–36, 1991.

696. Eeckhout E, Verbeleen D, Sennesael J, et al: Monitoring of bone mineral content in patients on regular hemodialysis. Nephron 52:158–161, 1989.

697. Zancetta J, Bogado C: Bone mineral content in renal transplant patients. In Llach F (ed): Renal Osteodystrophy. Oxford University Press, London (in press).

698. DeVita MV, Rasenas LL, Bansal M, et al: Assessment of renal osteodystrophy in hemodialysis patients. Medicine (Baltimore) 71:284–290, 1992.

699. Denney JD, Sherrard DJ, Nelp WR: Total body calcium and long term calcium balance in chronic renal disease. J Lab Clin Med 82:226, 1973.

700. Cann CE, Genant HK, Ettinger B, Gordan G: Spinal mineral losses in oophorectomized women. JAMA 244:2056, 1980.

701. Piraino B, Chen T, Cooperstein L, et al: Fractures and vertebral bone mineral density in patients with renal osteodystrophy. Clin Nephrol 30:57–62, 1988.

702. Torres A, Lorenzo V, Gonzalez-Posada JM: Comparison of histomorphometry and computed tomography of the spine in quantitating trabecular bone in renal osteodystrophy. Nephron 44:282–287, 1986.

703. Funke M, Maurer J, Grabbe E, Scheler F: Vergleichende Untersu-

chungen mit der quantitativen Computertomographie und der Dual-Energy-X-Ray-Absortiometrie zur Knochendichte bei renaler Osteopathie. Rofo Fortschr Geb Rontgenstr Neuen Bildgeb Verfahr 157:145–149, 1992.

704. Bordier PhJ, Marie PJ, Arnaud CD: Evolution of renal osteodystrophy: Correlation of bone histomorphometry and serum mineral and immunoreactive parathyroid hormone values before and after treatment with calcium carbonate or 25-hydroxycholecalciferol. Kidney Int Suppl 7:S102–S112, 1975.

705. Malluche HH, Faugere MC: Atlas of Mineralized Bone Histology. S Karger, Basel, 1986, pp 18–45.

706. Malluche H, Faugere M-C: Renal bone disease 1990: An unmet challenge for the nephrologist. Kidney Int 38:193–211, 1990.

707. Henry HL, Norman AW: Studies on the mechanism of action of calciferol. VII. Localization of 1,25-dihydroxyvitamin D in chick parathyroid glands. Biochem Biophys Res Commun 62:781, 1975.

708. Ritz E, Malluche HH, Krempien B, Mehls O: Bone histology in renal insufficiency. In Davis DS (ed): Perspectives in Nephrology and Hypertension. John Wiley & Sons, New York, 1977, p 197.

709. Maloney NA, Ott SM, Alfrey AC, et al: Histological quantitation of aluminum in iliac bone from patients with renal failure. J Lab Clin Med 99:206–216, 1982.

710. Malluche HH, Faugere MC, Smith AJ Jr, Friedler RM: Aluminum intoxication of bone in renal failure: Fact or fiction? Kidney Int 29(suppl 18):S70–S73, 1986.

711. Hodsman AB, Steer BM: Serum aluminum levels as a reflection of renal osteodystrophy status and bone surface aluminum staining. J Am Soc Nephrol 2:1318–1327, 1992.

712. Sherrard DJ, Andress DL: Aluminum-related osteodystrophy. Adv Intern Med 34:307–324, 1989.

713. Quarles LD, Dennis VW, Gitelman HJ, et al: Aluminum deposition at the osteoid-bone interface. An epiphenomenon of the osteomalacic state in vitamin D–deficient dogs. J Clin Invest 75:1441–1447, 1985.

714. Kaye M, Hodsman AB, Malynowsky L: Staining of bone for aluminum: Use of acid solochrome azurine. Kidney Int 37:1142–1147, 1990.

715. Parisien M, Charhon SA, Arlot M, et al: Evidence for a toxic effect of aluminum on osteoblasts: A histomorphometric study in hemodialysis patients with aplastic bone disease. J Bone Miner Res 3:259–267, 1988.

716. Berlyne GM, Ben-Ari J, Epstein N: Rarity of renal osteodystrophy in Israel due to low phosphorus intake. A natural experiment. Nephron 10:141, 1973.

717. Ellis HA, Pierides AM, Feest TG: Histopathology of renal osteodystrophy with particular reference to the effects of 1α-hydroxyvitamin D₃ in patients treated by long-term hemodialysis. Clin Endocrinol (Oxf) 7(suppl):31s–38s, 1977.

718. Maschio G, Bonucci E, Mioni G: Biochemical and morphological aspects of bone tissue in chronic renal failure. Nephron 12:347, 1974.

719. Duursma SA, Visser MJ, Nijo L: A quantitative histological study of bone in 30 patients with renal insufficiency. Calcif Tissue Res 9:216, 1972.

720. Agus ZS, Gardner LB, Beck LH: Effects of parathyroid hormone on renal tubular reabsorption of calcium, sodium and phosphate. Am J Physiol 224:1143, 1973.

721. Jaffe MD, Wellis PW: Multiple fractures associated with long term sodium heparin therapy. JAMA 193:152, 1965.

722. Coburn JW, Salusky IB: Control of serum phosphorus in uremia. N Engl J Med 320:1140–1142, 1989.

723. Massry SG, Kopple JD: Requirements for calcium, phosphorus, and vitamin D. In Mitch WE, Klahr S (eds): Nutrition and the Kidney. Little, Brown, Boston, 1993, pp 96–113.

724. Barsotti G, Morellin E, Guiducci A, et al: Reversal of hyperparathyroidism in severe uremics following very low-protein and low-phosphorus diet. Nephron 30:310–313, 1982.

725. Lafage M-H, Combe C, Fournier A, Aparicio M: Ketodiet, physiological calcium intake and native vitamin D improve renal osteodystrophy. Kidney Int 42:1217–1225, 1992.

726. Gotch FA, Sargent JA: A mechanistic analysis of the National Cooperative Dialysis Study (NCDS). Kidney Int 28:526–534, 1985.

727. Schoenfeld P, Henry R, Laird N: Assessment of nutritional status of the National Cooperative Dialysis Study population. Kidney Int 23:580–588, 1980.

728. Blumenkrantz MJ, Kopple JD, Moran J, Coburn JW: Metabolic

balance studies and dietary protein requirements in patients undergoing continuous peritoneal dialysis. Kidney Int 21:849, 1982.

729. Ramirez JA, Emmett M, White M, et al: The absorption of dietary phosphorus and calcium in hemodialysis patients. Kidney Int 30:753–759, 1986.

730. Kaye M, Turner M, Ardila M, et al: Aluminum and phosphate. Kidney Int 33(suppl 24):S172–S174, 1988.

731. Llach F, Nikakhtar B: Current advances in the therapy of secondary hyperparathyroidism and osteitis fibrosa. Miner Electrolyte Metab 17:250–255, 1991.

732. Sedman AB, Klein GL, Merritt RJ, et al: Evidence of aluminum loading in infants receiving intravenous therapy. N Engl J Med 312:1337–1343, 1985.

733. Salusky IB, Foley J, Nelson P, Goodman WG: Aluminum accumulation from recommended doses of aluminum hydroxide in dialyzed children. N Engl J Med 324:527–531, 1991.

734. Jenkins DA, Gouldesbrough D, Smith GD, et al: Can low-dosage aluminum hydroxide control the plasma phosphate without bone toxicity? Nephrol Dial Transplant 4:51–56, 1989.

735. Harter HR, Laird NM, Teehan BP: Effects of dialysis prescription on bone and mineral metabolism: The National Cooperative Dialysis Study. Kidney Int 23(suppl 13):S73–S79, 1983.

736. Rutherford E, Mercado A, Hruska KA: An evaluation of a new and effective phosphous binding agent. Trans Am Soc Artif Intern Organs 19:446, 1973.

737. Clarkson EM, Eastwood JB, Koutsaimanis K, De Wardener H: Net intestinal absorption of calcium in patients with chronic renal failure. Kidney Int 3:258, 1973.

738. Fournier A, Moriniere P, Sebert JL, et al: Calcium carbonate, an aluminum free agent for control of hyperphosphatemia, hypocalcemia, and hyperparathyroidism. Kidney Int 29(suppl 18):S114–S119, 1986.

739. Malberti F, Surian M, Poggio F, et al: Efficacy and safety of long term treatment with calcium carbonate as a phosphate binder. Am J Kidney Dis 12:487–491, 1988.

740. Moriniere PG, Russel A, Tahiri Y: Substitution of aluminum hydroxide by high doses of calcium carbonate in patients on chronic hemodialysis: Disappearance of hyperaluminemia and equal control of hyperparathyroidism. Proc Eur Dial Transplant Assoc 19:784, 1982.

741. Moriniere PG, Boudailliez B, Hocine C, Fournier A: Prevention of osteitis fibrosa, aluminum bone disease and soft-tissue calcification in dialysis patients: A long term comparison of moderate doses of oral calcium ± Mg(OH)₃ vs Al(OH)₃ ± 1α vitamin D₃. Nephrol Dial Transplant 4:1045–1054, 1989.

742. Renaud H, Atik A, Herve M, et al: Evaluation of vascular calcinosis risk factors in patients on chronic hemodialysis: Lack of influence of calcium carbonate. Nephron 48:28–32, 1988.

743. Sawyer N, Noonan K, Altmann P, et al: High dose calcium carbonate with stepwise reduction in dialysate calcium concentration: Effective phosphate control and aluminum avoidance in haemodialysis patients. Nephrol Dial Transplant 4:105–109, 1989.

744. Argiles A, Kerr PG, Canaud B, et al: Calcium kinetics and the long-term effects of lowering dialysate calcium concentration. Kidney Int 43:630–640, 1993.

745. Strong HE, Schatz BC, Shinaberger JH, Coburn JW: Measurement of dialysance and bi-directional fluxes of calcium, in vivo, using radiocalcium. Trans Am Soc Artif Intern Organs 17:108–115, 1971.

746. Mactier R, VanStone J, Cox A, et al: Calcium carbonate is an effective phosphate binder when dialysate calcium concentration is adjusted to control hypercalcemia. Clin Nephrol 28:220–226, 1987.

747. Sawyer N, Noonan K, Altmann P, et al: High dose calcium carbonate with stepwise reduction in dialysate calcium concentration: Effective phosphate control and aluminum avoidance in haemodialysis patients. Nephrol Dial Transplant 3:1–5, 1988.

748. Cunningham J, Beer J, Coldwell RD, et al: Dialysate calcium reduction in CAPD patients treated with calcium carbonate and alphacalcidol. Nephrol Dial Transplant 7:63–68, 1992.

749. Clarkson EM, Luck VA, Hynson WV: The effect of aluminum hydroxide on calcium, phosphorus and aluminum balances, the serum parathyroid hormone concentration and the aluminum content of bone in patients with chronic renal failure. Clin Sci 43:519, 1972.

750. Mai M, Emmett M, Sheikh M, et al: Calcium acetate, an effective phosphorus binder in patients with renal failure. Kidney Int 36:690–695, 1989.

751. Schiller L, Santa Ana CA, Sheikh M, et al: Effect of the time of administration of calcium acetate on phosphorus binding. N Engl J Med 320:1110–1113, 1989.

752. Sheikh M, Maguire J, Emmett M, et al: Reduction of dietary phosphorus absorption by phosphorus binders. J Clin Invest 83:66–73, 1989.

753. Caravaca F, Santos I, Cubero JJ, et al: Calcium acetate versus calcium carbonate as phosphate binders in hemodialysis patients. Nephron 60:423–427, 1992.

754. Hess B, Binswanger U: Long-term administration of calcium acetate efficiently controls severe hyperphosphatemia in haemodialysis patients. Nephrol Dial Transplant 5:630–633, 1990.

755. Delmez JA, Tindira CA, Windus DW, et al: Calcium acetate as a phosphorus binder in hemodialysis patients. J Am Soc Nephrol 3:96–102, 1992.

756. Kobrin SM, Goldstein SJ, Shangraw RF, Raja RM: Variable efficacy of calcium carbonate tablets. Am J Kidney Dis 14:461–465, 1989.

757. Cushner HM, Copley J, Lindberg J, Foulks C: Calcium citrate, a non aluminum containing phosphate binding agent for treatment of CRF. Kidney Int 35:95–99, 1988.

758. Schneider HW, Kulbe KD, Weber H, Streicher E: In vitro and in vivo studies with a non–aluminum phosphate-binding compound. Kidney Int 29(suppl 18):S120–S123, 1986.

759. Oe PL, Lips P, van der Muelen J, et al: Long-term use of magnesium hydroxide as a phosphate binder in patients on hemodialysis. Clin Nephrol 28:180–185, 1987.

760. Moriniere P, Maurouard C, Boudailliez B, et al: Prevention of hyperparathyroidism in patients on maintenance hemodialysis by intravenous 1 alpha hydroxyvitamin D₃ in association with Mg(OH)₂ as sole phosphate binder. A randomized comparative study with the association CaCO₃ ± Mg(OH)₂. Nephron 60:154–163, 1992.

761. Mahony J, Hayes JM, Ingham JP, Posen S: Hypophosphataemic osteomalacia in patients receiving haemodialysis. Br Med J 2:142–144, 1976.

762. Hou SH, Zhao J, Ellman CF, et al: Calcium and phosphorus fluxes during hemodialysis with a low calcium dialysate. Am J Kidney Dis 18:217–224, 1991.

763. Albertini BV, Miller JH, Gardner PW, Shinaberger JH: High flux hemodiafiltration: Under six hours/week treatment. Trans Am Soc Artif Intern Organs 30:227–231, 1984.

764. Albertini BV, Miller JH, Gardner PW, Shinaberger JH: Performance characteristics of the hemoflow F60 in high-flux hemodiafiltration. Contrib Nephrol 46:169–173, 1985.

765. Shinaberger JH, Miller JH, Gardner PW: Characteristics of available dialyzers. In Nissenson AR, Fine RN, Genile D (eds): Clinical Dialysis. Appleton-Century-Crofts, Norwalk, CT, 1984, p 175.

766. Sugisaki H, Onohara M, Kunitomo T: Phosphate in dialysis patients. Trans Am Soc Artif Intern Organs 29:38–43, 1983.

767. Delmez JA, Slatopolsky E, Martin KJ, et al: Minerals, vitamin D, and parathyroid hormone in continuous ambulatory peritoneal dialysis. Kidney Int 21:862–867, 1982.

768. Jaffe P, Podenphant J, Heaf JG: Bone histology in CAPD patients: A comparison with hemodialysis and conservatively treated chronic uremics. Adv Perit Dial 5:171–176, 1989.

769. Cannata JB, Briggs JD, Fell GS, Junor BJR: Comparison of control serum phosphate levels during continuous ambulatory peritoneal dialysis and during hemodialysis. Perit Dial Bull 3:97–98, 1983.

770. Fleming LW, Hudson SW, Stewart WK: Improved phosphate clearances with polycarbonate membranes. Clin Exp Dial Apheresis 6:211–222, 1982.

771. Miller JH, Gardner PW, Heinekin F, et al: Studies of inorganic phosphate removal during acetate and bicarbonate dialysis. Proc Am Soc Artif Intern Organs 12:57, 1983.

772. Llach F, Nikakhtar B: Methods of controlling hyperphosphatemia in patients with chronic renal failure. Curr Opin Nephrol Hypertens 2:365–371, 1993.

773. Clarkson EM, McDonald SJ, De Wardener H: The effect of a high intake of calcium carbonate in normal subjects and patients with chronic renal failure. Clin Sci 30:425, 1966.

774. McDonald SJ, Colbert J, Jones A: The effect of a large intake of calcium citrate in normal subjects and patients with chronic renal failure. Clin Sci 26:27, 1964.

775. Malluche HH, Werner E, Ritz E: Intestinal absorption of calcium and whole body calcium retention in incipient and advanced renal failure. Miner Electrolyte Metab 1:264, 1978.

776. Makoff DL, Gordon A, Franklin SS, et al: Chronic calcium carbonate therapy in uremia. Arch Intern Med 123:15–21, 1969.

777. Eastwood JB, Bordier PhJ, De Wardener H: Comparison of the effect of vitamin D and calcium carbonate in renal osteomalacia. Q J Med 40:569, 1971.

778. Ginsberg DS, Kaplan EL, Katz AL: Hypercalcaemia after oral calcium-carbonate therapy in patients on chronic haemodialysis. Lancet 1:1271–1274, 1973.

779. Katz A, Hampers CL, Merrill J: Secondary hyperparathyroidism and renal osteodystrophy in chronic renal failure. Medicine (Baltimore) 48:333, 1969.

780. Chanard J, Assailly J, Bader C, Funck-Brentano JL: A rapid method for measurement of fractional intestinal absorption of calcium. J Nucl Med 15:588–592, 1974.

781. Lang RM, Fellner SK, Neumann A, Bushinsky DA: Left ventricular contractility varies directly with blood ionized calcium. Ann Intern Med 108:424–429, 1988.

782. Llach F, Coburn JW: Renal osteodystrophy and maintenance dialysis. *In* Maher JF (ed): Replacement of Renal Function by Dialysis. Kluwer Academic Publishers, Boston, 1989, pp 911–952.

783. Goldsmith RS: The effects of calcium and phosphorus in hemodialysis. Annu Rev Med 27:181, 1976.

784. Regan RJ, Peacock M, Rosen SM: Effect of dialysate calcium concentration on bone disease in patients on hemodialysis. Kidney Int 10:246, 1976.

785. Catto GRD, MacDonald AF, McIntosh JA, MacLeod M: Haemodialysis therapy and changes in skeletal calcium. Lancet 1:1150–1153, 1973.

786. Mirahmadi KS, Duffy BS, Shinaberger JH, et al: A controlled evaluation of clinical and metabolic effects of dialysate calcium levels during regular dialysis. Trans Am Soc Artif Intern Organs 17:118–124, 1971.

787. Coburn JW: Mineral metabolism and renal bone disease: Effects of CAPD versus hemodialysis. Kidney Int 43(suppl 40):S92–S100, 1993.

788. Voigts A, Felsenfeld AJ, Llach F: The effects of calciferol and its metabolites on patients with chronic renal failure. II. Calcitriol, hydroxyvitamin D and 24,25-dihydroxyvitamin D. Arch Intern Med 142:1205, 1983.

789. Voigts A, Felsenfeld AJ, Llach F: The effects of calciferol and its metabolites on patients with chronic renal failure. I. Calciferol, dihydrotachysterol and calcifediol. Arch Intern Med 143:960–963, 1983.

790. Kaye M, Chatterjee G, Cohen GF: Arrest of hyperparathyroid bone disease with dihydrotachysterol in patients undergoing chronic hemodialysis. Ann Intern Med 73:225–233, 1970.

791. Witmer G, Margolis A, Fontaine O: Effects of 25-hydroxycholecalciferol on bone lesions of children with terminal renal failure. Kidney Int 10:395, 1976.

792. Recker R, Schoenfeld P, Letteri JM, et al: The efficacy of calcifediol in renal osteodystrophy. Arch Intern Med 138:857–866, 1978.

793. Chan J, Oldham SB, Holick MF, DeLuca HF: 1α-Hydroxyvitamin D₃ in chronic renal failure: A potent analogue of the kidney hormone, 1,25-dihydroxycholecalciferol. JAMA 234:47–52, 1975.

794. Peacock M: The clinical uses of 1α-hydroxyvitamin D₃. Clin Endocrinol 7(suppl):1s–246s, 1977.

795. Kaye M, Sagar S: Effect of dihydrotachysterol on calcium absorption in uremia. Metabolism 21:815, 1972.

796. Berl T, Berns AS, Hufer WE, et al: 1,25-Dihydroxycholecalciferol effects in chronic dialysis. A double-blind-controlled study. Ann Intern Med 88:774–780, 1978.

797. Maxwell DR, Benjamin DM, Donahay SL, et al: Calcitriol in dialysis patients. Clin Pharmacol Ther 23:515–519, 1978.

798. Fournier A, Bordier PJ, Gueris J, et al: 1α-Hydroxycholecalciferol and 25-hydroxycholecalciferol in renal bone disease. Proc Eur Dial Transplant Assoc 12:227–236, 1976.

799. DeLuca HF, Avioli LV: Treatment of renal osteodystrophy with 25-hydroxycholecalciferol. Arch Intern Med 126:896, 1970.

800. Teitelbaum SL, Bone JM, Stein PM: Calcifediol in chronic renal insufficiency: Skeletal response. JAMA 235:164, 1976.

801. Evans RA, Somerville PJ: The use of high calcium dialysate in the treatment of renal osteomalacia. Aust N Z J Med 6:10, 1976.

802. Silverberg DS, Bettcher KB, Dossetor JB: Effect of 1,25-dihydroxycholecalciferol in renal osteodystrophy. Can Med Assoc J 112:190, 1975.

803. Eastwood JB, Phillips ME, De Wardener H: Biochemical and histological effects of 1,25-dihydroxycholecalciferol in the osteomalacia

of chronic renal failure. *In* Norman AW, Schaefer K, Grigoleit H-G, et al (eds): Vitamin D and Problems Related to Uremic Bone Disease. Walter de Gruyter, Berlin, 1975, p 595.

804. Sherrard DJ, Brickman AS, Coburn JW: Skeletal response to treatment with 1,25-dihydroxyvitamin D in renal failure. Contrib Nephrol 18:92, 1980.

805. Memmos D, et al: Double-blind trial of oral 1,25-dihydroxy vitamin D₃ versus placebo in asymptomatic hyperparathyroidism in patients receiving maintenance haemodialysis. Br Med J 282:1919, 1981.

806. Coburn JW, et al: Prospective, double blind trial with calcitriol in the prophylaxis of bone disease in asymptomatic dialysis patients. *In* Norman AW, Schaefer K (eds): Vitamin D: Chemical, Biochemical and Clinical Endocrinology of Calcium Metabolism. Walter de Gruyter, Berlin, 1982, p 833.

807. Chesney RW, Hamstra A, Jax DK: Influence of long term oral 1,25-dihydroxyvitamin D in childhood renal osteodystrophy. Contrib Nephrol 18:55, 1980.

808. Seidel A, Herrmann P, Klaus G, et al: Kinetics of serum 1,84 iPTH after high dose calcitriol in uremic patients. Clin Nephrol 39:210–213, 1993.

809. Massry SG, et al: Use of 1,25(OH)₂D₃ in the treatment of renal osteodystrophy in patients with moderate renal failure. *In* Frame B, Potts JT Jr (eds): Clinical Disorders of Bone and Mineral Metabolism. Excerpta Medica, Amsterdam, 1983, pp 260–262.

810. Goodman WG, Coburn JW: The use of 1,25-dihydroxyvitamin D₃ in early renal failure. Annu Rev Med 43:227–237, 1992.

811. Bertoli M, Luisetto G, Ruffatti A, et al: Renal function during calcitriol therapy in chronic renal failure. Clin Nephrol 33:98–102, 1990.

812. Oettinger CW, Oliver JC, Macon EJ: The effects of calcium carbonate as the sole phosphate binder in combination with low calcium dialysate and calcitriol therapy in chronic dialysis patients. J Am Soc Nephrol 3:995–1001, 1992.

813. Norris KC, Kraut JA, Andress DL: Intravenous calcitriol for severe secondary hyperparathyroidism in dialysis patients. Kidney Int 27:158, 1985.

814. Andress DL, Norris KC, Coburn JW, et al: Intravenous calcitriol in the treatment of refractory osteitis fibrosa of chronic renal failure. N Engl J Med 321:274–279, 1989.

815. Hamdy NAT, Brown C, Kanis JA: Intravenous calcitriol lowers serum calcium concentrations in uraemic patients with severe hyperparathyroidism and hypercalcemia. Nephrol Dial Transplant 4:545–548, 1989.

816. Dressler R, Laut J, Lynn RI, Ginsberg N: Intravenous calcitriol for secondary hyperparathyroidism in patients with end-stage renal disease. Am J Kidney Dis (in press).

817. Klaus G, Mehls O, Hinderer J, Ritz E: Is intermittent oral calcitriol safe and effective in renal secondary hyperparathyroidism? Lancet 337:800, 1991.

818. Muramoto H, Haruki K, Yoshimura A, et al: Treatment of refractory hyperparathyroidism in patients on hemodialysis by intermittent oral administration of 1,25(OH)₂vitamin D₃. Nephron 58:288–294, 1991.

819. Martin KJ, Bullal HS, Domoto DT, et al: Pulse oral calcitriol for the treatment of hyperparathyroidism in patients on continuous ambulatory peritoneal dialysis: Preliminary observations. Am J Kidney Dis 19:540–545, 1992.

820. Tsukamoto Y, Nomura M, Takahashi Y, et al: The ʿoral 1,25-dihydroxyvitamin D₃ pulse therapy' in hemodialysis patients with severe secondary hyperparathyroidism. Nephron 57:23–28, 1991.

821. Reichel H, Szabo A, Uhl J, et al: Intermittent versus continuous administration of 1,25(OH)₂D₃ in experimental renal hyperparathyroidism. Kidney Int 44:1259–1265, 1993.

822. Delmez JA, Dougan CS, Gearing BK, et al: The effects of intraperitoneal calcitriol on calcium and parathyroid hormone. Kidney Int 31:795–799, 1987.

823. Arora N, Sandroni S, Moles K: Marked improvement in parameters of renal osteodystrophy with the use of intraperitoneal calcitriol. Adv Perit Dial 8:62–64, 1992.

824. Goodman WG, Ramirez JA, Gales G, et al: Skeletal response to one year of intermittent calcitriol therapy in dialyzed children. J Am Soc Nephrol 3:672, 1992. Abstract.

825. Rolla D, Paoletti E, Marsano L, et al: Subcutaneous calcitriol in CAPD patients. Perit Dial Int 13:118–121, 1993.

826. Campistol JM, Torregrosa JV, Montesinos M, et al: Effectiveness of subcutaneous calcitriol (sCa) in the treatment of secondary hyperparathyroidism (HPT). J Am Soc Nephrol 4:718, 1993.

827. Brickman AS, Coburn JW, Friedman GR, et al: Comparison of effects of 1α-hydroxyvitamin D₃ and 1,25-dihydroxy-vitamin D₃ in man. J Clin Invest 57:1540–1547, 1976.

828. Peacock M: The clinical uses of 1-hydroxyvitamin D₃. Clin Endocrinol 7:850–859, 1977.

829. Pierides AM, Ellis HA, Simpson W, et al: Variable response to long term 1α-hydroxycholecalciferol in haemodialysis osteodystrophy. Lancet 1:1092–1095, 1976.

830. Coburn JW, Brickman AS, Sherrard DJ: Use of 1,25(OH)₂vitamin D₃ to separate "types" of renal osteodystrophy. Proc Eur Dial Transplant Assoc 14:442, 1977.

831. Davison AM, Peacock M, Walker GS, et al: Phosphate and 1-alpha-hydroxyvitamin D₃ therapy in haemodialysis patients. Clin Endocrinol 7(suppl):91S–99S, 1977.

832. Brandi L, Daugaard H, Tvedegaard E, et al: Effect of intravenous 1α-hydroxyvitamin D₃ on secondary hyperparathyroidism in chronic uremic patients on maintenance hemodialysis. Nephron 53:194–200, 1989.

833. Lind L, Wengle B, Wide L, et al: Suppression of serum parathyroid hormone levels by intravenous alphacalcidol in uremic patients on maintenance hemodialysis. Nephron 48:296–299, 1988.

834. Ljunghall S, Althoff P, Fellstrom B, et al: Effects on serum parathyroid hormone of intravenous treatment with alphacalcidol in patients on chronic hemodialysis. Nephron 55:380–385, 1990.

835. Brandi L, Daugaard H, Tvedegaard E, et al: Long-term suppression of secondary hyperparathyroidism by intravenous 1α-hydroxyvitamin D₃ in patients on chronic hemodialysis. Am J Nephrol 12:311–318, 1992.

836. Pierides AM, Ellis HA, Ward MK: Barbiturate and anticonvulsant treatment in relation to osteomalacia with haemodialysis and renal transplantation. Br Med J 1:190, 1976.

837. Pierides AM, Kerr DNS, Ellis HA: 1α-Hydroxycholecalciferol in hemodialysis renal osteodystrophy. Adverse effects of anticonvulsant therapy. Clin Nephrol 5:189–192, 1976.

838. Grigoleit H-G, Schaefer K, Kraft D, et al: Clinical efficacy of 5,6-trans-25-OHCC in chronic renal failure. In Norman AW, Schaefer K, Coburn JW, et al (eds): Vitamin D: Biochemical, Chemical and Clinical Aspects Related to Calcium Metabolism. Walter de Gruyter, Berlin, 1977, pp 701–713.

839. Rutherford WE, Blondin J, Hruska K, et al: The effect of 5,6-trans vitamin D₃ on calcium absorption in chronic renal disease. J Clin Endocrinol Metab 40:13–18, 1975.

840. Hodsman J, Wong EG, Sherrard DJ: Preliminary trials with 24,25-dihydroxyvitamin D₃ in dialysis osteomalacia. Am J Med 74:407, 1983.

841. Ott SM, Recker R, Coburn JW, Sherrard DJ: Vitamin D therapy in aluminum related osteomalacia. Kidney Int 32:107, 1983.

842. Canterbury JM, Lerman S, Claflin AJ, et al: Inhibition of parathyroid hormone secretion by 25-hydroxycholecalciferol and 24,25-dihydroxycholecalciferol in the dog. J Clin Invest 61:1375–1383, 1977.

843. Friedlander MA, Horst RL, Hawker CC: Absence of effect of 24,25-dihydroxycholecalciferol on serum immunoreactive PTH in patients with persistent hyperparathyroidism after renal transplantation. Clin Nephrol 22:206, 1984.

844. Olgaard K, Finco D, Schwartz J: Effect of 24,25-dihydroxy-vitamin D₃ on PTH levels and bone histology in dogs with chronic uremia. Kidney Int 25:791, 1984.

845. Dunstan CR, Hills E, Norman AW, et al: Treatment of hemodialysis bone disease with 24,25(OH)₂D₃ and 1,25(OH)₂D₃ alone or in combination. Miner Electrolyte Metab 11:358–368, 1985.

846. Popovtzer MM, Levi J, Bar-Khayim Y, et al: Assessment of combined 24,25(OH)₂D₃ and 1α(OH)D₃ therapy for bone disease in dialysis patients. Bone 13:369–377, 1992.

847. Brown AJ, Ritter CR, Finch JL, et al: The noncalcemic analogue of vitamin D, 22-oxacalcitriol, suppresses parathyroid hormone synthesis and secretion. J Clin Invest 84:279, 1989.

848. Brown AJ, Finch JL, Lopez-Hiler S, et al: New active analogues of vitamin D with low calcemic activity. Kidney Int Suppl 29:S22–S27, 1990.

849. Slatopolsky E, Berkoben M, Kelber J, et al: Effects of calcitriol and non-calcemic vitamin D analogs on secondary hyperparathyroidism. Kidney Int Suppl 38:S43–S49, 1992.

850. Kubrusly M, Gagne E-R, Urena P, et al: Effect of 22-oxa-calcitriol on calcium metabolism in rats with severe secondary hyperparathyroidism. Kidney Int 44:551–556, 1993.

851. Kanis JA, Russell RGG: Rate of reversal of hypercalcemia and hypercalciuria induced by vitamin D and its 1α-hydroxylated derivatives. Br Med J 1:78, 1977.

852. Schaefer K, Umlauf E, von Herrath D: Reduced risk of hypercalcemia for hemodialysis patients by administering calcitriol at night. Am J Kidney Dis 19:460–464, 1992.

853. Coburn JW, Lee D, Brickman A: Intestinal phosphate absorption in normal and uremic man: Effects of 1,25(OH)₂ vitamin D₃ and 1(OH) vitamin D₃. In Massry SG, Ritz E (eds): Phosphate Metabolism. Plenum Publishing, New York, 1993, pp 331–337.

854. Szabo A, Merke J, Beier E, et al: 1,25(OH)₂ vitamin D₃ inhibits parathyroid cell proliferation in experimental uremia. Kidney Int 35:1049–1056, 1989.

855. Fukagawa M, Mi H, Kurokawa K: Calcitriol induces apoptosis of hyperplastic parathyroid cells in uremic rats. J Am Soc Nephrol 2:635, 1991.

856. Kitaoka M, Fukagawa M, Tanaka Y, et al: Parathyroid gland size is critical for longterm prognosis of calcitriol pulse therapy in chronic dialysis patients. J Am Soc Nephrol 2:637, 1991. Abstract.

857. Mallick NP, Berlyne G: Arterial calcification after vitamin-D therapy in hyperphosphatemic renal failure. Lancet 2:1316–1320, 1968.

858. Stanbury SW, Lumb GA, Nicholson WF: Elective subtotal parathyroidectomy for renal hyperparathyroidism. Lancet 1:793–799, 1960.

859. Llach F: Parathyroidectomy in chronic renal failure: Indications, surgical approach and the use of calcitriol. Kidney Int Suppl 38:S62–S68, 1990.

860. Kaye M, Rosenthall L, Hill RO, Tabah RJ: Long-term outcome following total parathyroidectomy in patients with chronic renal disease. Clin Nephrol 39:192–197, 1993.

861. Baumann DS, Wells SA Jr: Parathyroid autotransplantation. Surgery 113:130–133, 1993.

862. Rothmund M, Wagner PK, Schark C: Subtotal parathyroidectomy versus total parathyroidectomy and autotransplantation in secondary hyperparathyroidism: A randomized trial. World J Surg 15:745–750, 1991.

863. White JV, LoGerfo P, Feind C, Weber C: Autologous parathyroid transplantation. Lancet 2:461, 1983.

864. Ellis HA: Fate of long term parathyroid autografts in patients with chronic renal failure treated by parathyroidectomy: A histopathological study of autografts, parathyroid glands and bone. Histopathology 13:289–309, 1988.

865. Gilmour JR: The gross anatomy of the parathyroid glands. J Pathol Bacteriol 46:133, 1938.

866. Wang C, Mahaffey JG, Axelrod L, Perlman JA: Hyperfunctioning supernumerary parathyroid glands. Surg Gynecol Obstet 148:711–714, 1979.

867. Gordon HE, Coburn JW, Passaro E: Surgical management of secondary hyperparathyroidism. Arch Surg 104:520, 1972.

868. Sicard GA, Wells SA Jr: Surgical treatment of secondary hyperparathyroidism. In Kaplan EL (ed): Surgery of the Thyroid and Parathyroid Glands. Churchill Livingstone, Edinburgh, 1983, p 243.

869. Kinnaert P, Salmon I, Decoster-Gervy C, et al: Total parathyroidectomy and presternal subcutaneous implantation of parathyroid tissue for renal hyperparathyroidism. Surg Gynecol Obstet 176:135–138, 1993.

870. Felsenfeld AJ, Gutman RA, Llach F: Postparathyroidectomy hypocalcemia as an accurate indicator of preparathyroidectomy bone histology in the uremic patient. Miner Electrolyte Metab 10:166, 1984.

871. Litchman MB, Kinder BK, Johnson BM: Calcium requirements in ESRD patients after total parathyroidectomy with autotransplantation. Dial Transplant 16:611–616, 1987.

872. Llach F, Brickman AS, Coburn JW: Unique effects of 24,25-dihydroxyvitamin D₃ in uremic patients. Contrib Nephrol 18:212–217, 1980.

873. Shpitz B, Korzets Z, Dimbar A, et al: Immediate post-operative management of parathyroidectomy hemodialized patients. Dial Transplant 15:507–513, 1986.

874. Giangrande A, Cantu P, Solbiati L, Ravetto C: Ultrasonically guided fine-needle alcohol injection as an adjunct to medical treatment in secondary hyperparathyroidism. Proc Eur Dial Transplant Assoc 21:895–901, 1984.

875. Giangrande A, Castiglioni A, Solbiati L, Allaria P: Ultrasound-guided percutaneous fine-needle ethanol injection into parathyroid glands in secondary hyperparathyroidism. Nephrol Dial Transplant 7:412–421, 1992.

876. Page B, Zingraff J, Souberbielle JC, et al: Correction of severe hyperparathyroidism in two dialysis patients: Surgical removal versus percutaneous ethanol injection. Am J Kidney Dis 19:378–381, 1992.

877. Takeda S, Michigishi T, Takazakura E: Successful ultrasonically guided percutaneous ethanol injection for secondary hyperparathyroidism. Nephron 62:100–103, 1992.

878. Milliner DS, Hercz G, Miller JH, et al: Clearance of aluminum by hemodialysis. Effect of desferrioxamine. Kidney Int 20(suppl 18):S100–S104, 1986.

879. Trapp G: Interactions of aluminum with cofactors, enzymes, and other proteins. Kidney Int 29(suppl 18):S12–S16, 1986.

880. Freemont AJ, Day JP, Ackrill P: Water treatment alone allows removal of aluminum from bone and reversal of the calcification defect in aluminum-related osteodystrophy. Abstract Book, IXth International Congress of Nephrology, 1984, 48A. Abstract.

881. Hercz G, Andress DL, Norris KC, et al: Improved bone formation in dialysis patients after substitution of calcium carbonate for aluminum gels. Trans Assoc Am Physicians 100:139–146, 1987.

882. Ackrill P, Ralston AJ, Day JP, Hodge KC: Successful removal of aluminium from patients with dialysis encephalopathy. Lancet 2:692–693, 1980. Letter.

883. Ackrill P, Day JP, Garstang FM, et al: Treatment of fracturing renal osteodystrophy with desferrioxamine. Proc Eur Dial Transplant Assoc 19:203–207, 1982.

884. Vasilakakis DM, D'Haese PC, Lamberts LV, et al: Removal of aluminoxamine and ferrioxamine by charcoal hemoperfusion and hemodialysis. Kidney Int 41:1400–1407, 1992.

885. Molitoris BA, Alfrey AC, Alfrey PS: Rapid removal of DFO-chelated aluminum during hemodialysis using polysulfone dialyzers. Kidney Int 34:98–101, 1988.

886. Mactier RA: Aluminum and deferoxamine kinetics in CAPD. Adv Perit Dial 7:26–29, 1991.

887. Sulkova S, Laurincova Z, Valek A: Haemofiltration or haemodialysis in aluminium elimination? Nephrol Dial Transplant 6(suppl 3):3–5, 1991.

888. Romero R, Novoa D, Otero S, et al: Direct effect of deferoxamine on hemoglobin synthesis in patients on hemodialysis treated with recombinant human erythropoietin. Nephron 63:164–167, 1993.

889. Gallant S, Boyden M, Gallant L, et al: Serial studies of auditory neurotoxicity in patients receiving deferoxamine therapy. Am J Med 83:1085–1090, 1987.

890. Oliveri NF, Buncic R, Chew E: Visual and auditory neurotoxicity in patients receiving subcutaneous deferoxamine. N Engl J Med 314:868, 1986.

891. Cases A, Kelly J, Sabater J, et al: Acute visual and auditory neurotoxicity in patients with end-stage renal disease receiving desferrioxamine. Clin Nephrol 29:176–178, 1988.

892. Walker JA, Sherman RA, Eisinger RP: Thrombocytopenia associated with intravenous desferrioxamine. Am J Kidney Dis 6:254–256, 1985.

893. Sherrard DJ, Walker JA, Boykin J: Precipitation of dialysis dementia by deferoxamine treatment of aluminum related bone disease. Am J Kidney Dis 12:126–130, 1988.

894. Gallant T, Freedman MH, Vellend H, Francombe WH: Yersinia sepsis in patients with iron overload treated with deferoxamine. N Engl J Med 314:1643, 1986.

895. Boelaert JR, van Landuyt HW, Valcke YJ, et al: The role of iron overload in Yersinia enterocolitica and Yersinia pseudotuberculosis bacteremia in hemodialysis patients. J Infect Dis 156:384–387, 1987.

896. Boelaert JR, Fenves AZ, Coburn JW: Deferoxamine therapy and mucormycosis in dialysis patients: Report of an international registry. Am J Kidney Dis 18:660–667, 1991.

897. Boelaert JR, van Roost G, Vergauwe PL, et al: The role of desferrioxamine in dialysis associated mucormycosis. Clin Nephrol 29:261–266, 1988.

898. Van Cutsem J, Boelaert JR: Effects of deferoxamine, feroxamine and iron on experimental mucormycosis (zygomycosis). Kidney Int 36:1061–1068, 1989.

899. Boelaert JR, de Locht M, Van Cutsem J, et al: Mucormycosis during deferoxamine therapy is a siderophore-mediated infection: In vitro and in vivo animal studies. J Clin Invest 91:1979–1986, 1993.

900. Cannata JB, Fernandez JL, Douthat W, et al: Aluminum (Al) transfer in dialysis: Effect of different membranes, type of dialysis and forms of desferrioxamine (DFO) administration. J Am Soc Nephrol 3:671, 1992.

901. Canavese C, Gurioli L, D'Amicone M, et al: Kinetics of aluminoxamine and feroxamine chelates in dialysis patients. Nephron 60:411–417, 1992.

902. Verpooten GA, D'Haese PC, Boelaert JR, et al: Pharmacokinetics of aluminoxamine and ferrioxamine and dose finding of desferrioxamine in haemodialysis patients. Nephrol Dial Transplant 7:931–938, 1992.

903. Cannata JB, Elorriaga R, Menendez P, et al: A new orally active chelator in the treatment of aluminium (Al) overload. J Am Soc Nephrol 3:671, 1992.

904. Hercz G, Pei Y, Sherrard DJ, Chan W: Aplastic osteodystrophy: Effect of lowering dialysate calcium. J Am Soc Nephrol 4:697, 1993.

905. Delano BG, Baker R, Gardner B, Wallach S: A trial of calcitonin therapy in renal osteodystrophy. Nephron 11:287–293, 1973.

906. Fleisch H, Russell RGC, Francis MD: Diphosphonates inhibit hydroxiapatite dissolution in vitro and bone resorption in tissue culture and in vivo. Science 165:1262–1264, 1969.

907. Sahni M, Guenther HL, Fleisch H, et al: Bisphosphonates act on rat bone resorption through the mediation of osteoblasts. J Clin Invest 91:2004–2011, 1993.

908. Malluche HH: The possible use of bisphosphonates in the treatment of renal osteodystrophy. Clin Nephrol 38(suppl 1):S87–S91, 1992.

909. D'Amour P, Jobin J, Hamel L, L'Ecuyer N: iPTH values during hemodialysis: Role of ionized $Ca^{2+}$, dialysis membranes and iPTH assays. Kidney Int 38:308–314, 1993.

910. Gueris J, Fournier A, Sebert JL, et al: Comparative effects of dialysis with cuprophan versus polyacrylonitrile membranes on plasma immunoreactive parathyroid hormone levels in patients on chronic hemodialysis. Calcif Tissue Res 22:34–38, 1977.

911. Morachiello P, Landini S, Fracasso A, et al: Combined hemodialysis-hemoperfusion in the treatment of secondary hyperparathyroidism of uremic patients. Blood Purif 9:148–152, 1991.

912. Henderson RG, Russell RGG, Earnshaw M: Loss of metacarpal and iliac bone in chronic renal failure: Influence of haemodialysis, parathyroid activity, type of renal disease, physical activity and heparin consumption. Clin Sci 56:317, 1979.

913. Griffith GC, Nichols G, Asher JD, Flanagan B: Heparin osteoporosis. JAMA 195:1089, 1966.

914. Majdalani G, Chomant J, Kachko A, et al: Kinetics of technetium-labeled heparin in hemodialyzed patients. Kidney Int 43(suppl 41):S131–S134, 1993.

915. Zingraff J, Drueke T, Roux JP, et al: Bilateral fracture of the femoral neck complicating uremic bone disease prior to chronic hemodialysis. Clin Nephrol 2:73–75, 1974.

# 52

# Effect of Aging on Renal Function and Disease

*Biff F. Palmer*
*Moshe Levi*

Advancing age is associated with a number of structural and functional changes in the kidney (Table 52–1). In spite of these changes, the aging kidney is remarkably capable of maintaining fluid and electrolyte balance within narrow limits. The adaptive capacity of the aging kidney to stress and disease is, however, quite restricted. As a result, elderly patients are predisposed to develop fluid and electrolyte disorders under conditions that would be well tolerated in younger individuals. An understanding of these alterations will allow the clinician to anticipate and better treat a number of clinical conditions that occur with greater frequency in the elderly. The purpose of this chapter is to review the normal age-related changes that occur in renal anatomy and physiology. In addition, an overview of renal diseases that are most prevalent in the aged population is provided.

## RENAL ANATOMY

Advancing age in humans is associated with progressive loss of renal mass. Renal weight decreases from 250 to 270 g in young adulthood to 180 to 200 g by the eighth decade of life.[1] The loss of renal mass is primarily cortical, with relative sparing of the renal medulla. The total number of identifiable glomeruli falls with age, in accordance with the changes in renal weight.[2–4] The number of hyalinized or sclerotic glomeruli identified on light microscopic examination increases from 1% to 2% during the third to fifth decade of life to as high as 30% in some apparently healthy 80-year-old persons, with a mean frequency after age 70 of approximately 10% to 12%.[5–7]

Changes also occur in the intrarenal vasculature with age, independent of hypertension or other renal disease. Normal aging is associated with variable sclerotic changes in the

wall of the larger renal vessels, which are made worse in the presence of hypertension. Smaller vessels are spared, with less than 20% of senescent kidneys from nonhypertensive subjects displaying arteriolar changes.[8–10]

Microangiographic and histologic studies have identified two distinctive patterns of change in arteriolar-glomerular units with senescence.[11, 12] In one type, hyalinization and collapse of the glomerular tuft are associated with obliteration of the lumen of the preglomerular arteriole and a resultant loss in blood flow. This type of change is seen primarily in the cortical area. The second pattern, seen primarily in the juxtamedullary area, is characterized by the development of anatomic continuity between the afferent and efferent arterioles during glomerular sclerosis. As a result, loss of the glomerulus and direct shunting of blood flow from afferent to efferent arterioles occur. Blood flow is maintained to the arteriolar rectae verae, the primary vascular

---

**TABLE 52–1. Anatomic and Functional Renal Changes with Aging**

Decrease in total kidney mass: cortex > medulla
Decrease in renal blood flow
  Cortical flow > medullary flow
  Decreased response to vasodilators
Decrease in glomerular filtration rate
Altered tubule function
  Impaired $Na^+$ conservation and excretion
  Impaired concentration or dilution of urine
  Impaired acidification of urine
  Impaired $K^+$ metabolism
  Decreased $PO_4^{3-}$ reabsorption
  Impaired $1\alpha$-hydroxylase activity

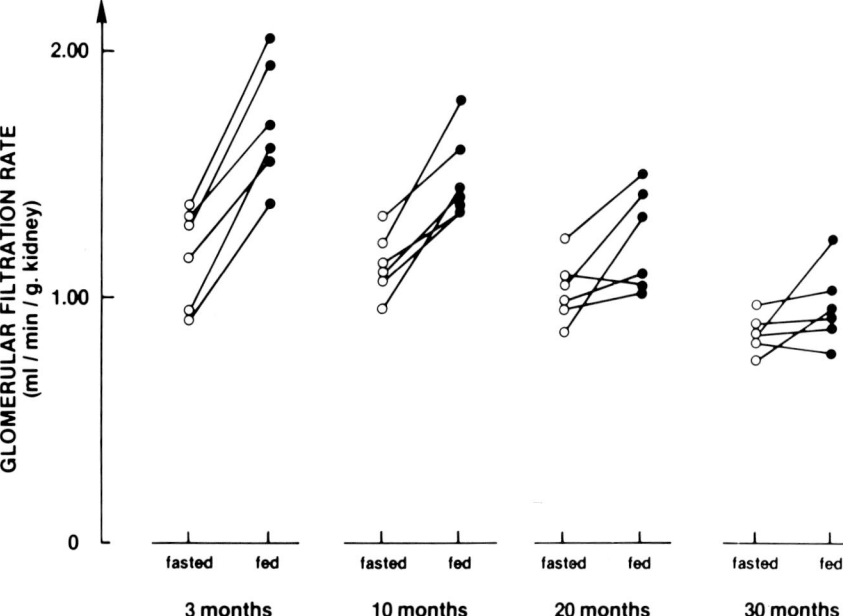

**Figure 52–1.** Glomerular filtration rate in fed and fasted rats. Lines join data from the same animals. (From Corman B, Chami-Khazraji S, Schaeverbeke J, Michel J: Effect of feeding on glomerular filtration rate and proteinuria in conscious aging rats. Am J Physiol 255:F250–F256, 1988.)

supply of the medulla, which are not decreased in number with age.

## RENAL PHYSIOLOGY AND PATHOPHYSIOLOGY

### Renal Blood Flow

There is a progressive reduction in renal plasma flow (as determined by *p*-aminohippuric acid [PAH] clearance) of approximately 10% per decade, from 600 mL/min/1.73 m$^2$ in the 20- to 29-year-old age group to 300 mL/min/1.73 m$^2$ in the 80- to 89-year-old age group.[13, 14] The decrease in renal blood flow is associated with significant increases in afferent and efferent arteriolar resistance.[14] The increase in efferent arteriolar resistance may explain the age-related increase in filtration fraction.[13, 14] The exact relationship between renal plasma flow and cardiac output as a function of aging is not well established. Some studies have shown an age-related decrease in cardiac output; others have shown no such decrease.[15–18] There is a small but definite decrease in the renal fraction of the cardiac output.[19, 20] These later studies suggest that the major determinant of reduced renal blood flow with age is functional or anatomic changes in the renal vasculature.

A study using the xenon washout technique to measure renal blood flow in 207 healthy potential kidney donors ranging in age from 17 to 76 years has shown that the age-related reduction in renal blood flow is not uniform within the kidney.[21] These investigators demonstrated a preferential decrease in cortical blood flow. This finding is in accord with histologic studies showing a selective loss of cortical vasculature and preservation of medullary flow. The histologic and functional demonstration of a selective decrease in cortical blood flow may also explain the observation that filtration fraction increases with advancing age,[13, 14] as outer

cortical nephrons have a lower filtration fraction than do juxtamedullary nephrons.

Whether the age-related decrease in renal blood flow is due to anatomic or functional changes in the renal vasculature has been studied by two groups of investigators who have measured renal hemodynamics after intravenous administration of pyrogen[14] and after intra-arterial administration of acetylcholine and angiotensin.[21] During administration of both pyrogen and acetylcholine, the vasodilatory response was greater in the younger subjects compared with the older subjects. On the other hand, the vasoconstrictive response to angiotensin was identical in young and old subjects. These studies suggest that although the aging renal vasculature does respond to vasoconstriction and vasodilatation, the response to vasodilatation is markedly blunted, and anatomic changes as well as functional vasoconstriction mediate the age-related decrease in renal blood flow.

A similar age-related impairment in the renal vasodilatory response has been demonstrated in young, adult, and senescent rats. In awake, chronically catheterized male Sprague-Dawley rats, the renal vasodilatory response to intravenous administration of glycine, which has been used to measure renal functional reserve in humans, was markedly diminished in the 22- to 24-month-old rats when assessed as either a percent change in renal plasma flow (PAH clearance) or a percent change in glomerular filtration rate (GFR) (inulin clearance).[22] Similarly, there was an age-related impairment in postprandial hyperfiltration. In contrast to young rats, which had a marked increase in glomerular filtration after a meal, aged rats had a negligible postprandial increase in GFR[23] (Fig. 52–1).

Studies with humans have produced discrepant results with regard to changes in renal hemodynamics after amino acid infusions.[24, 25] In 12 patients (aged 60 to 85 years), baseline GFR and renal plasma flow were found to be decreased but within the expected range for their age.[24] After an infusion of amino acids, there was a significant increase in both GFR and renal plasma flow, but filtration fraction did not change. It should be noted that the subjects in this study were hospitalized patients (albeit recovering from nonrenal disease), many of whom had recently taken medications that could affect glomerular hemodynamics.

More recently, renal hemodynamics were examined before and after an amino acid infusion in healthy normotensive young and elderly subjects without evidence of renal disease.[25] At baseline, the GFR and renal plasma flow were significantly lower and renal vascular resistance and filtration fraction were significantly higher in the elderly subjects compared with the young subjects. After the infusion of amino acids, effective renal plasma flow increased significantly in the young group but failed to do so in the elderly group. By contrast, the GFR increased to a similar extent in young and old subjects. The filtration fraction increased in both groups but to a slightly greater extent in the elderly subjects (Fig. 52–2). Renal vascular resistance fell in the young patients but did not change in the elderly. These data would support the development of an age-related impairment in the vasodilatory response of the renal vasculature. Although an increase in renal blood flow was responsible for the rise in GFR in the young subjects, the lack of change

in renal blood flow suggests an increase in intraglomerular pressure as the determinant responsible for the rise in GFR noted in the elderly subjects.

In summary, most of the data suggest that although the aging renal vasculature does respond to vasoconstriction and vasodilatation, the response to vasodilatation is markedly blunted. Anatomic changes as well as functional vasoconstriction mediate the age-related decrease in renal blood flow. The contrasting results noted in the previous two studies[24, 25] with regard to renal plasma flow and filtration fraction are difficult to explain. Differences in baseline characteristics of the patients, concomitant use of vasoactive medications, and different rates of amino acid infusion are all possible explanations. Nevertheless, both studies demonstrated a similar increase in renal reserve as defined by an increase in GFR in response to an amino acid infusion. This observation stands in contrast to the progressive decrease in renal reserve noted in aging rats. The physiologic mechanism of this response has yet to be determined but is likely to involve both hormonal and direct renal effects.[26, 27]

## Glomerular Filtration Rate

Cross-sectional studies have shown a progressive age-related decline in the GFR after age 30 to 40 years in men and women.[13, 28] These results were confirmed in serial measurements of renal function in 548 healthy volunteers who participated in the Baltimore Longitudinal Study of Aging[29, 30] (Fig. 52–3). Creatinine clearance measurements showed a progressive linear decline from 140 mL/min/1.73 m² at age 30 years to 97 mL/min/1.73 m² at age 80 years, at an approximate rate of 0.8 mL/min/1.73 m²/y.[29, 30] These results were confirmed in follow-up studies of 254 subjects in whom 5 to 14 serial creatinine clearance determinations were obtained between 1958 and 1981.[31] Of interest is the fact that 29 (36%) of the 254 subjects had no absolute decrease in creatinine clearance, and 7 of these subjects had a statistically significant increase in creatinine clearance over time. In a similar study of 446 healthy subjects, the age-related decline in creatinine clearance was found to be much steeper in black than in white persons.[32] In the setting of hypertension or diabetes mellitus, this decline in renal function is further magnified.[33, 34] An increased baseline renal vascular resistance and possibly a lower glomerular filtration surface area or fewer nephrons or both may underlie this accelerated decline in creatinine clearance noted in black individuals.[35] These factors may also account for the decrease in renal allograft survival noted when grafts are obtained from black or elderly donors.[35, 36] These data suggest that the age-related loss of glomerular function is not a universal phenomenon and that racial, dietary, metabolic, hormonal, or hemodynamic factors may play a major role in modulating the age-related decrease in renal function.

In this regard, a cause-and-effect relationship between the age-related increase in filtration fraction and the increased prevalence of glomerulosclerosis in the aging kidney has been proposed. In view of the probable role of glomerular hypertension in the eventual glomerulosclerosis that occurs in diabetes mellitus, hypertension, and some

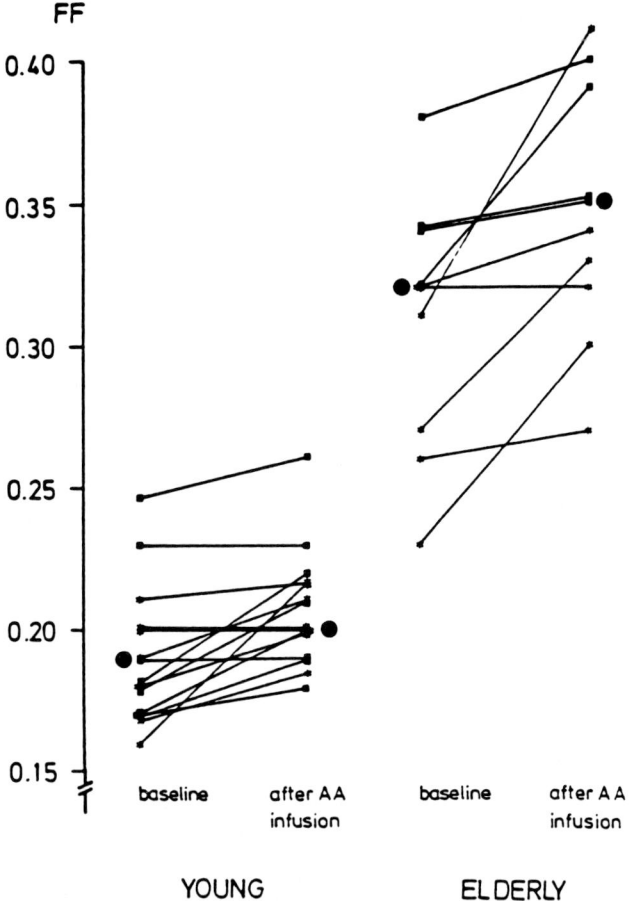

**Figure 52–2.** Filtration fraction (FF) in young and elderly subjects at baseline and after an amino acid infusion. Squares indicate men; asterisks, women; circles, median. (From Fliser D, Zeier M, Nowack R, Ritz E: Renal functional reserve in healthy elderly subjects. J Am Soc Nephrol 3[7]:1371–1377, 1993.)

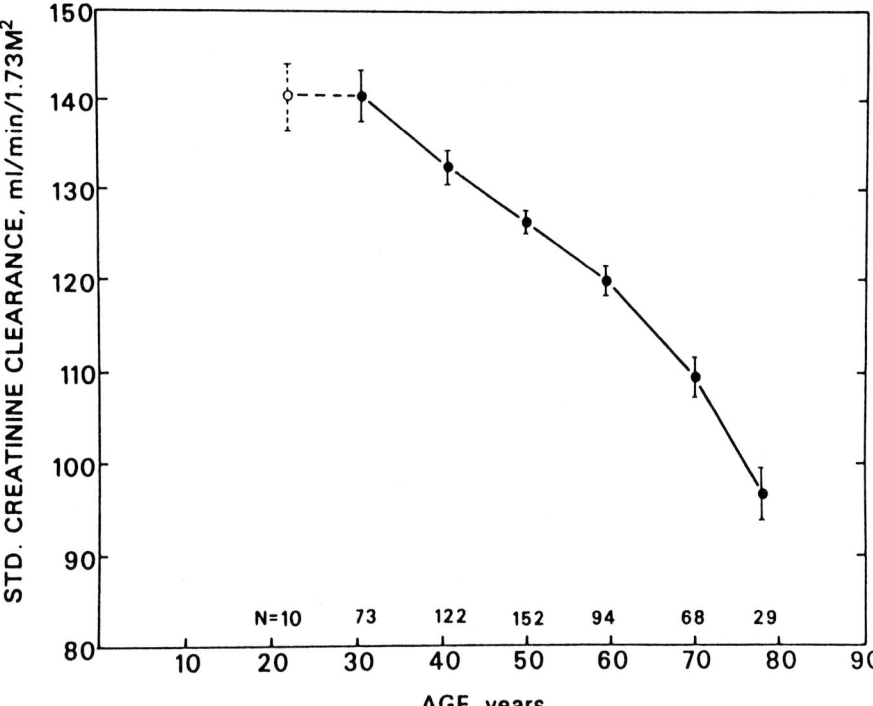

**Figure 52–3.** Cross-sectional differences in standard creatinine clearance with age. The number of subjects in each age group is indicated above the abscissa. Values indicate means ± SEM. (From Rowe JW, Andres R, Tobin JD, et al: The effect of age on creatinine clearance in men: A cross-sectional and longitudinal study. J Gerontol 31[2]:155–163, 1976. Copyright © The Gerontological Society of America.)

experimental models of chronic renal disease, including the five-sixths renal ablation model,[37] a similar role for glomerular hypertension in propagating glomerulosclerosis in the aging kidney has been invoked.[38, 39] Intraglomerular hypertension may be responsible for the apparent acceleration of renal functional impairment in elderly patients with a history of hypertension.[40] It has been suggested that a high protein intake typical of Western society results in sustained elevations of total renal blood flow and filtration rate and thus plays a major role in the age-related decline in renal function.[39] In further support of this hypothesis, studies with the aging rat reveal that long-term dietary sodium or protein restriction, which would decrease the glomerular filtration fraction and thus lower glomerular pressure, results in significant improvements in the incidence and severity of age-related renal histopathologic characteristics, renal functional impairments, and proteinuria.[41–49] It is of interest to speculate that the decrease in meat consumption noted in the United States in the least 20 years may be responsible for the decline in GFR measured in a population of healthy potential kidney transplant donors between 1970 and 1990.[50]

Another important factor in age-related renal disease is atherosclerotic disease of the systemic and renal vasculature. One study that compared autopsy and renal histologic findings from 57 individuals with mild systemic atherosclerosis with 57 sex- and age-matched individuals with moderate to severe atherosclerosis found that both age and intrarenal vascular disease exhibited highly significant, independent associations with glomerulosclerosis.[51] In addition, the presence of systemic atherosclerosis is associated with atheromatous renal disease.

Studies also suggest an important role for abnormal lipid metabolism in the progression of chronic renal disease.[52–58]

Specifically, in obese Zucker rats, which have many of the characteristics of non–insulin-dependent diabetes mellitus and which develop proteinuria and progressive glomerular injury after hyperlipidemia is established,[59, 60] the lipid-lowering agents lovastatin and clofibrate significantly reduced proteinuria and glomerular injury without significantly altering glomerular hemodynamics.[61] Similarly, in the five-sixths nephrectomy model of chronic progressive renal injury, lovastatin or clofibrate caused a significant reduction in proteinuria and focal glomerulosclerosis.[62] Because the aging kidney has evidence of increased cholesterol content,[63] which is associated with the age-related increase in the incidence of glomerulosclerosis, the effect of lipid-lowering diets or pharmacologic agents in the course of age-related nephropathy deserves to be thoroughly investigated.

The highly significant decrease in GFR that occurs with age is not usually accompanied by an elevation in serum creatinine concentration.[29, 30] Because muscle mass, from which creatinine is derived, falls with age at approximately the same rate as does the GFR, the rather striking age-related loss of renal function is not reflected by an increase in the serum creatinine concentration. Thus, the serum creatinine concentration usually underestimates the decline in GFR in the elderly.

The most important clinical implication for the age-related decrease in GFR is the need for adjustment of the dosage of medications that are excreted directly by the kidney (by glomerular filtration or tubule secretion), or whose active metabolites, formed in the liver, are eliminated by the kidney. When adjusting the dosage of such a medication, it is therefore important to estimate GFR not only according to the serum creatinine concentration but also according to one of the formulas provided in Table 52–2. Either formula yields a reasonable estimation of the

**TABLE 52–2. Commonly Used Formulas for Estimation of Glomerular Filtration Rate**

1. Creatinine clearance (mL/min/1.73 m²) = 133 − (0.64 × age)

2. Creatinine clearance (mL/min) = $\dfrac{(140 - age) \times weight\ (kg)}{72 \times serum\ creatinine\ (mg/dL)}$
(15% less in females)

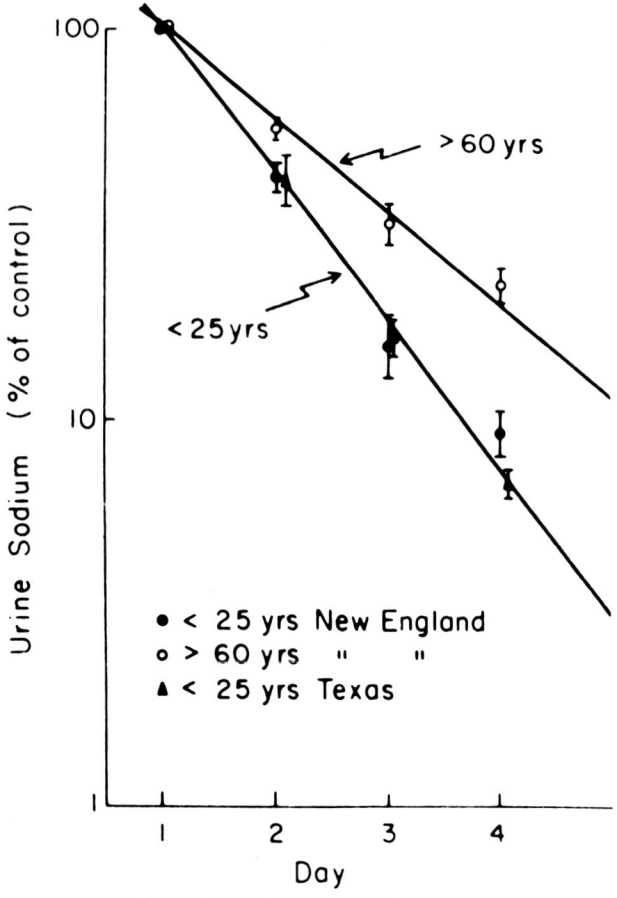

**Figure 52–4.** Response of urinary Na⁺ excretion to restriction of sodium intake in normal humans. The mean half-time for eight subjects older than age 60 years was − 30.9 ± 2.8 hours, which exceeded the mean half-time of − 17.6 ± 0.7 hours for subjects younger than age 25 years (P < .01). When the younger subjects were separated according to geographic area, the mean half-time for the Texas group (− 17.9 ± 0.7 hours) was similar to that for the New England group (− 15.6 ± 1.4 hours; P < .3). (From Epstein M, Hollenberg N: Age as a determinant of renal sodium conservation in normal man. J Lab Clin Med 87:411–417, 1976.)

GFR. In fact, there is a close correlation (r = .85) between the calculated creatinine clearance using formula 2 and the measured creatinine clearance.[64–66] In addition, it is useful to monitor the serum levels of drugs that have a narrow therapeutic window.

Another important consequence of the age-related decrease in renal blood flow and GFR is the potential predisposition to enhanced ischemic or toxic renal injury. An increase in baseline renal vascular resistance may explain why elderly patients are at high risk for acute cyclosporine nephrotoxicity.[67] In addition to the absolute decrease in renal blood flow, the autoregulatory capacity of the renal vasculature is impaired, thus increasing the risk of hemodynamically induced acute renal failure after severe volume depletion, septic shock, and major vascular surgery. Failure to properly adjust the dosage of renally excreted drugs, including aminoglycoside antibiotics, nonsteroidal anti-inflammatory drugs, and radiocontrast agents, may increase the occurrence of toxin-induced renal failure.

## FLUID AND ELECTROLYTE BALANCE

Under normal circumstances, age has no effect on plasma Na⁺ or K⁺ concentrations, blood pH, or ability to maintain normal extracellular fluid volume. The adaptive reserve mechanisms responsible for maintaining constancy of the extracellular fluid volume and composition in response to stress are, however, impaired in the elderly.

### Sodium-Conserving Ability

The ability of the aged kidney to conserve Na⁺ in response to Na⁺ deprivation is impaired[68] (Fig. 52–4). Clearance studies in young and elderly subjects have shown a decreased capacity of the distal tubule for Na⁺ reabsorption in the elderly.[69] This dysfunction could be caused by anatomic changes in the aging kidney such as interstitial fibrosis. Alternatively, functional and hormonal changes such as increased medullary blood flow and decreased renin-angiotensin-aldosterone activity could impair distal tubule reabsorption of Na⁺.

In this regard, there are important age-related alterations in the renin-angiotensin-aldosterone system. Basal plasma renin concentration or activity is decreased by 30% to 50% in elderly subjects in spite of normal levels of renin substrate. During maneuvers designed to stimulate renin secretion (e.g., upright posture, 10 mEq/d sodium intake, and

furosemide administration), the differences in plasma renin activity are further amplified[70–78] (Fig. 52–5A). Although the precise mechanism is unknown, the age-related decrease in plasma renin activity has been attributed to 1) impaired renin secretion; 2) disturbances in the conversion of inactive to active renin; and 3) an enhanced tonic inhibitory effect of atrial natriuretic peptide (ANP) on renin secretion.[79] There is a similar 30% to 50% decrease in plasma aldosterone levels in elderly subjects during recumbency and normal sodium intake; this decrease becomes more pronounced during upright posture, restriction of sodium intake, and furosemide administration[71, 78, 80–82] (Fig. 52–5B). The aldosterone deficiency appears to be related to the renin-angiotensin deficiency and not to intrinsic adrenal gland defects, because both plasma aldosterone and cortisol responses to corticotropin infusion are normal in the elderly.[78]

Thus, during restriction of sodium intake, an impaired angiotensin II or aldosterone response may result in decreased renal tubule Na⁺ reabsorption in the elderly. In fact,

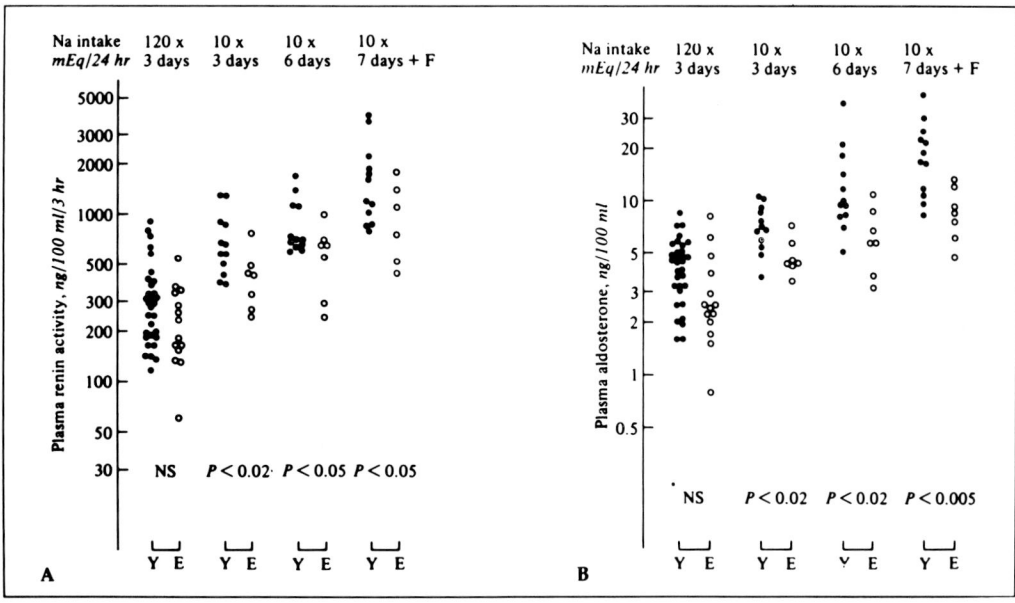

**Figure 52–5.** Distribution of plasma renin *(A)* and aldosterone *(B)* values in healthy supine individuals before and during progressive Na$^+$ depletion. Y = young subjects; E = elderly subjects. Values indicating statistical significance refer to the difference between young and elderly subjects. Plasma renin activity values are those obtained at an incubation pH of 5.7. (From Weidmann P, De Myttenaere-Bursztein S, Maxwell M, De Lima J: Effect of aging on plasma renin and aldosterone in normal man. Used with permission from Kidney International, volume 8, pages 325–333, 1975.)

clearance studies in young and elderly subjects have shown marked improvement in distal tubule Na$^+$ reabsorption in the elderly after treatment with aldosterone.[83]

## Sodium-Excreting Ability

Excessive Na$^+$ retention and volume overload are commonly encountered problems in older patients. Short-term Na$^+$ loading studies (with intravenous saline) show distinct age-related differences in Na$^+$ excretion (Fig. 52–6). Individuals older than 40 years excrete slightly less Na$^+$ per 24 hours after a 2-L normal saline load than do race-, sex-, and size-matched subjects younger than 40 years.[32, 83, 84] In addition, the older subjects excrete a significantly greater portion of the Na$^+$ load at night than do their younger counterparts. Thus, both the excretory capacity for Na$^+$ and the circadian variation in excretion are influenced by age.

The age-related decrease in GFR is probably the major factor limiting the ability of the aged kidney to excrete an acute Na$^+$ load. In addition, studies have investigated the possible role of alterations in ANP secretion in mediating the age-related impairment in natriuresis.

In humans, ANP exists as a 126–amino acid prohormone stored primarily in atrial myocytes, with an active circulating peptide form of 28 amino acids. ANP is released in response to a variety of maneuvers that increase atrial pressure. The most striking effects of physiologic actions of ANP are sustained increases in GFR, solute-free water clearance, and natriuresis without a corresponding increase in renal blood flow. These effects are believed to be secondary to alterations in intrarenal blood flow and an inhibitory effect on Na$^+$ reabsorption in the inner medullary collecting duct.[85, 86] ANP decreases blood pressure by vasodilatation

and possibly through direct modulation of baroreceptor reflexes.[87] Cardiac output is decreased by several mechanisms, primarily the venodilatory effect of ANP, resulting in lowered cardiac filling pressures. Plasma volume is decreased by the ANP-mediated increases in Na$^+$ and water excretion as well as a translocation of fluid from plasma to interstitial spaces resulting from an ANP-mediated increase in capillary permeability.[85] This latter effect, the "edemagenic" effect,[87] may be particularly important in the elderly. ANP also directly antagonizes the components of the counterbalancing vasoconstrictive Na$^+$-retentive hormonal systems, through inhibition of the secretion of aldosterone and arginine vasopressin (AVP).[87, 88]

Studies of carefully selected subjects have shown that healthy elderly persons have basal circulating ANP levels three to five times higher than those of healthy young persons[89–91] (Fig. 52–7). In response to saline loading or head-out body water immersion, basal ANP levels are stimulated, to a greater extent in elderly subjects compared with younger control subjects.[89, 91–93] In part, high basal levels of ANP are due to changes in the pharmacokinetic properties of the hormone, which occur with aging. ANP metabolism is altered in the elderly such that there is a decreased metabolic clearance rate, a longer half-life, and an increased volume of distribution.[94–97]

Despite high circulating levels of ANP, there is a generalized age-related reduction in end-organ responsiveness to this peptide. Intravenous infusions of physiologic doses of ANP, which result in significant natriuretic, hypotensive, and endocrine effects in young to middle-aged normotensive subjects, have no effect in healthy elderly men.[97] Evidence would suggest that this blunted physiologic response is due to an age-related postreceptor defect.[97] The natriuretic action of ANP is mediated by interaction with spe-

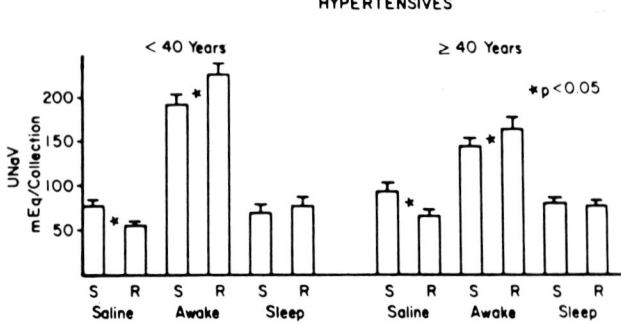

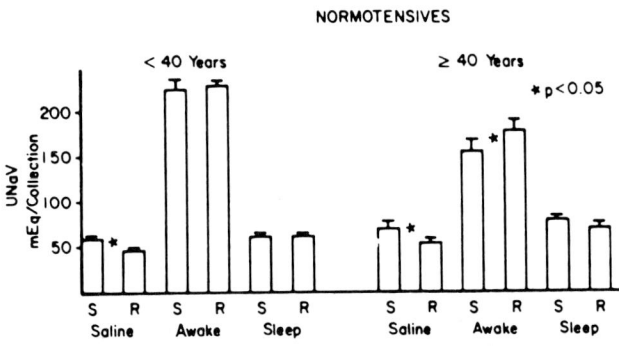

**Figure 52–6.** Natriuretic responses after volume expansion. Na$^+$-sensitive individuals exhibited "exaggerated natriuresis" during the 4-hour saline load. By the next morning, balance was restored. S = sensitive; R = resistant; UNaV = urinary Na$^+$ excretion. (From Luft F, Weinberger M, Fineberg M, et al: Effects of age on renal sodium homeostasis and its relevance to sodium sensitivity. Reprinted from American Journal of Medicine Supplement: Vol 82:1B; 1987 [pgs 9–15].)

cific ANP receptors, with subsequent activation of the second messenger guanylate cyclase. Despite higher basal levels of circulating ANP in the elderly, basal levels of cyclic GMP in plasma are no different from those in younger control subjects.[92] In part, this may reflect downregulation of ANP receptors in response to high circulating levels of ANP. Endogenous stimulation of ANP with volume expansion or intravenous infusion of ANP, however, results in similar increases in cyclic GMP in both elderly and young subjects.[89, 92, 96, 97] Given the blunted physiologic effects despite similar increases in cyclic GMP, an abnormality in the postreceptor cyclic GMP effector of ANP appears to be present.

A decrease in responsiveness to ANP may contribute to a number of physiologic abnormalities that are known to be age related. First, a resistance to the renal vascular effects of ANP may contribute to the decrease in GFR and impaired ability to excrete an Na$^+$ load. Second, a decrease in responsiveness of the peripheral vasculature may contribute to an increase in systolic blood pressure resulting from unopposed angiotensin- or norepinephrine-mediated vasoconstriction. Third, the age-related enhancement of AVP secretion with osmotic stimulation, which has been noted by some investigators, may in part reflect a lack of suppres-

sion of AVP secretion by ANP. Finally, increased basal levels of ANP may render the elderly patient more susceptible to edema formation given the effect of ANP to increase vascular permeability.[98]

Studies with the aged rat confirm the clinical experience that natriuretic efficiency is impaired after isotonic saline or blood expansion. One study found a significant age-related decrease in the number of renal dopamine D$_1$ receptors but not dopamine D$_2$ receptors.[99] The possible role of the alteration in renal dopamine receptor activity in impaired natriuresis remains unstudied, however.

## Renal Concentrating Ability

Renal concentrating ability is well known to decline with age in humans.[28, 100–103] In one study, the concentrating ability of the kidneys, as measured by the urine specific gravity in 38 healthy men, declined from 1.030 at age 40 years to 1.023 at age 89 years.[28] In other studies, the maximal urine osmolality, measured after 12 to 24 hours of dehydration, was inversely related to age.[100, 102, 103] The maximal urine osmolality was 1109 mOsm/kg H$_2$O in 31 subjects 20 to 39 years old, compared with 1051 mOsm/kg H$_2$O in 48 subjects 40 to 59 years old and 882 mOsm/kg H$_2$O in 18 subjects 60 to 79 years old. The age-related decline in the concentrating defect did not correlate with the age-related decline in the GFR.

Studies with humans suggest that the concentrating de-

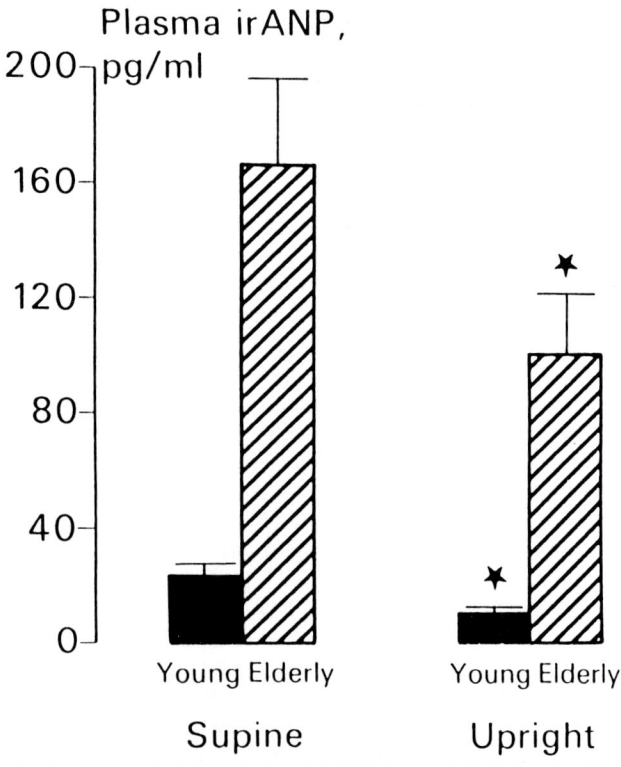

**Figure 52–7.** Circulating ANP (immunoreactive ANP, irANP) levels in healthy young and old individuals. (From Haller B, Zust H, Shaw S, et al: Effects of posture and ageing on circulating atrial natriuretic peptide levels in man. J Hypertens 5:551–556, 1987.)

fect is due to an intrarenal defect rather than a failure in the osmotic release of AVP.[101, 104, 105] After intravenous infusion of hypertonic saline (3% sodium chloride) in 9 young (21 to 49 years) and 3 old (54 to 92 years) subjects, plasma AVP levels rose 4.5 times the baseline in the older men compared with 2.5 times the baseline in the younger subjects, despite similar solute-free water clearances.[104] The slope of the plasma AVP concentration (percent baseline) versus serum osmolality, an index of the sensitivity of the osmoreceptor, was significantly increased in the older subjects. In addition, in the same study, intravenous infusion of ethanol caused a progressive decline in plasma AVP levels in the young subjects but failed to have a similar effect in the older subjects. Plasma AVP levels have also been found to increase to a greater extent in elderly subjects compared with younger control subjects in response to 24 hours of fluid restriction.[106, 107]

Not all studies, however, have found a heightened sensitivity of AVP release in elderly patients in response to fluid deprivation.[108, 109] In fact, when plasma AVP levels were compared in subjects aged 18 to 45 years and those aged 58 to 74 years after only 9 hours of fluid deprivation, AVP levels were lower in the elderly subjects despite higher plasma osmolalities.[108] Similarly, a smaller increase in plasma AVP levels was found in elderly subjects after only 14 hours of water deprivation.[109] The reason for these discrepant results is not entirely clear but may be related to the duration of water restriction before AVP measurements were obtained. The effect of volume-pressure–mediated AVP release has also been studied and has been found to decrease with age.[110]

Although changes in plasma tonicity and effective arterial blood volume are the major regulators of AVP release, receptors in the oropharynx are also known to influence AVP release. Under normal conditions, ingestion of cold fluid and the act of drinking lead to an immediate but transient decrease in AVP levels even though the water deficit has not been fully repleted. This oropharyngeal inhibition of AVP secretion has been found to be reduced in healthy elderly men compared with young individuals.[107]

Studies with humans reveal an age-related increase in solute excretion and osmolar clearance during dehydration.[103] This phenomenon, which may be a reflection of impaired solute transport by the ascending loop of Henle, may be responsible for the impairment in urine concentrating ability in elderly subjects. This possibility is supported by clearance studies in subjects undergoing a water diuresis that demonstrate a decrease in the sodium chloride transport in the ascending loop of Henle in elderly subjects.[69, 111] This defect in solute transport by the thick ascending limb of the loop of Henle could diminish inner medullary hypertonicity and thereby impair urine concentrating ability. A relative increase in medullary blood flow as suggested by xenon washout studies[21] could also increase the removal of solutes from the medullary interstitium and thereby contribute to the decreased maximal urine osmolality.

Studies with the aging rat, however, suggest that impaired responsiveness of the collecting duct cells to AVP, rather than diminished inner medullary hypertonicity, is responsible for the concentrating defect.[112] Maximal urine concentration after a 40-hour dehydration period and exog-

enous vasopressin administration was markedly impaired. Clearance studies revealed a normal solute-free water excretion but impaired solute-free water reabsorption, which implies normal solute transport by the ascending limb and decreased water transport by the collecting duct. In fact, inner medullary solute content in the old and young rats was identical.

Studies with inner medullary slices from rats and mice have revealed an age-related impairment in AVP-induced cyclic AMP generation.[113, 114] The study in mice revealed that the threshold dose of AVP required to elicit a significant rise in cyclic AMP was greater in older animals, and the dose-response curve was moved to the right for old mice.[114] In both the rat and the mouse, the maximal cyclic AMP level in older animals was decreased compared with that in younger animals. Studies with the rat suggested that chronically increased levels of circulating AVP may result in down-regulation of the renal AVP receptors and thus may be responsible for the age-related impairment in cyclic AMP response to AVP.[115, 116] One study in mice, however, found no age-related differences in the number of receptors or their affinity for AVP and suggested that the decreased cyclic AMP response is probably due to postreceptor mechanisms.[117]

The age-related impairments in renal concentrating and Na+-conserving ability are associated with an increased incidence of volume depletion and hypernatremia in the elderly. Under normal physiologic conditions, increased thirst and fluid intake are natural defense mechanisms against volume depletion and hypernatremia. Elderly patients are particularly prone to develop hypernatremia because of an age-related impairment in the thirst mechanism.[106, 118] In comparison to young control subjects (aged 20 to 31 years), elderly patients (aged 67 to 75 years), after 24 hours of fluid restriction, have been shown to have blunted sensations of thirst and mouth dryness despite a higher serum Na+ concentration and osmolality[106] (Fig. 52–8). In addition, these hypertonic elderly subjects ingested a smaller amount of water after the period of fluid restriction in comparison to the young control subjects. Thus, an age-related impairment in the thirst mechanism renders the elderly patient particularly prone to the development of hypernatremia.

In practice, therefore, drugs that inhibit the thirst mechanism and the synthesis and release of AVP, including most sedatives and major tranquilizers, and drugs that inhibit the renal tubule action of AVP, especially lithium and demeclocycline, are best avoided (Table 52–3). The use of osmotic diuretics, enteral feeding preparations containing high levels of protein and glucose, and bowel cathartics should also be carefully monitored in the elderly. In addition, the complication of age-related decreases in thirst caused by systemic illness and dementia in many frail elderly patients clearly places them at risk for the development of severe water deficiency.

The frequency of severe hypernatremia among the elderly exceeds one case per hospital per month.[119] Hypernatremia in the elderly without underlying central nervous system disease may be manifested as primary neurologic or psychiatric symptoms and delay the diagnosis. In subjects who are febrile and who have underlying neurologic disorders, AVP release may become impaired, thereby exacerbating the tendency toward hypernatremia.[120, 121] If not promptly diagnosed and treated, hypernatremia leads to coma, seizures, and death.[122] In fact, acute elevation of the serum $Na^+$ value above 160 mEq/L in adults is associated with a 75% mortality. Even if no death occurs, the neurologic sequelae can be severe in the elderly.

## Renal Diluting Ability

Renal diluting ability is impaired as a function of aging.[100, 101, 123, 124] In subjects undergoing water diuresis, minimal urine osmolality is significantly higher (92 mOsm/kg $H_2O$) in old subjects (ages 77 to 88 years) compared with young subjects (ages 17 to 40 years) (52 mOsm/kg $H_2O$). The solute-free water clearance is also decreased: 5.9 mL/min in old subjects compared with 16.2 mL/min in young subjects. The impairment in solute-free water clearance is largely due to the decrease in GFR. However, when solute-free water clearance is factored for GFR, solute-free water clearance/GFR is still decreased in the older subjects.[101, 124] Mechanisms of the impaired diluting ability in the elderly have not been well studied; in addition to the major role of impaired GFR, inadequate suppression of AVP release or impaired solute transport in the ascending loop of Henle may play a role.

The age-related impairment in maximal diluting ability and the enhanced osmotic release of AVP are associated with a high incidence of hyponatremia in the elderly. A random sampling of 160 patients in a chronic disease facility showed that 36 patients had hyponatremia, with a mean serum $Na^+$ value of 120 mEq/L, and 27 of these patients were symptomatic.[125] In another study, a survey of hospitalized patients in a geriatric unit during a 10-month period revealed that 77 patients (11%) had a plasma $Na^+$ concentration below 130 mEq/L.[126] Diuretics, especially the combination of hydrochlorothiazide and amiloride, and intravenous administration of hypotonic fluid were determined to cause the hyponatremia in 56 of these patients. Of these patients, 47 were symptomatic, and the mortality rate for the hyponatremic patients was twice the overall rate for the geriatric unit.

Other reports confirm that thiazide diuretics are a major cause of hyponatremia in the elderly.[127] The well-known effect of thiazide diuretics to impair the renal diluting ability under normal physiologic conditions seems to be compounded in the elderly with a pre-existing renal diluting defect.[128] In addition, thiazide diuretics, when used in combination with the sulfonylurea chlorpropamide, which is known to potentiate the peripheral action of AVP, have synergistic effects in impairing the renal diluting ability.[129] In practice, drugs or agents that stimulate the nonosmotic release of AVP and drugs that potentiate the renal tubule action of AVP must be used with extreme caution in the elderly[130, 131] (see Table 52–3).

The signs and symptoms of hyponatremia are most likely related to cellular swelling and cerebral edema caused by the movement of water as a result of the lowering of extracellular fluid osmolality. Patients may present with symptoms of lethargy, apathy, disorientation, muscle cramps,

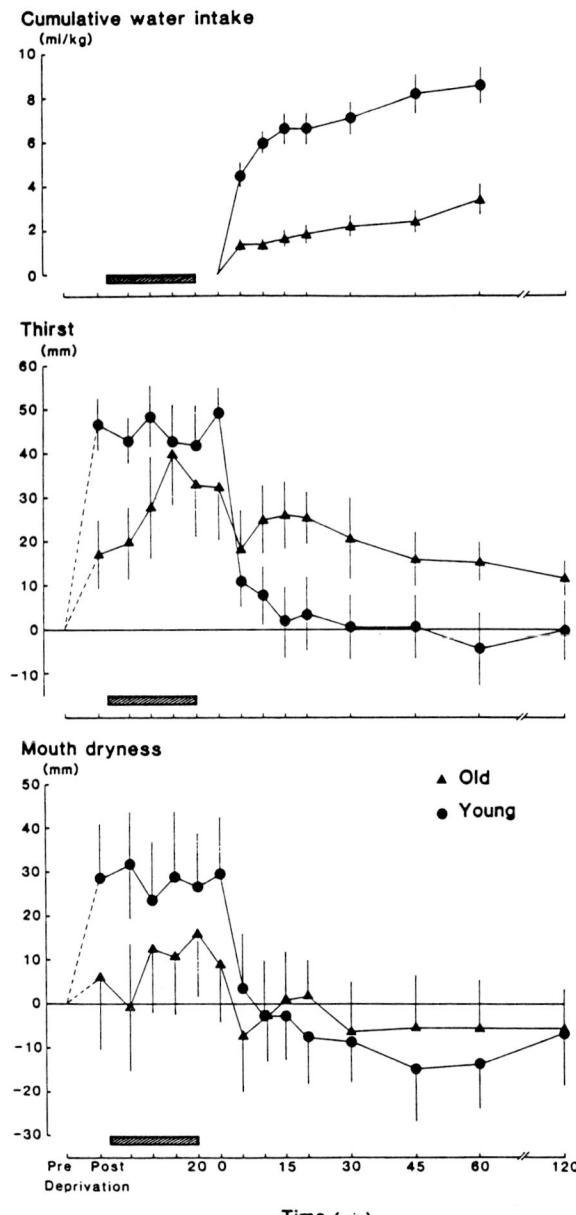

**Figure 52–8.** Cumulative water intake, changes in thirst, and mouth dryness in groups of old and young subjects. Changes in thirst and mouth dryness were measured by use of a visual-analogue rating scale. (From Phillips P, Phil D, Rolls B, et al: Reduced thirst after water deprivation in healthy elderly men. N Engl J Med 311:753–759, 1984. Reprinted by permission of The New England Journal of Medicine. Copyright 1984 Massachusetts Medical Society.)

anorexia, nausea, or agitation, and signs ranging from depressed deep tendon reflexes to pseudobulbar palsy and seizures. Differentiation of these symptoms from primary neurologic or psychiatric disease is important so that one can institute appropriate therapy promptly and avoid severe neurologic sequelae, including central pontine myelinolysis.

## Acid-Base Balance

Elderly subjects can maintain the pH and $HCO_3^-$ concentration of blood within the normal range, and their basal

**TABLE 52–3. Mechanisms by Which Drugs Can Lead to Impaired Water Metabolism***

| Inhibition of ADH Release | Inhibition of Peripheral Action of ADH | Potentiation of ADH Release | Potentiation of Peripheral Action of ADH |
|---|---|---|---|
| Fluphenazine | Lithium | Nicotine | Tolbutamide |
| Haloperidol | Colchicine | Vincristine | Chlorpropamide |
| Promethazine | Vinblastine | Histamine | NSAIDs |
| Morphine (low doses) | Demeclocycline | Morphine (high doses) | |
| Alcohol | Glyburide | Epinephrine | |
| Carbamazepine | Methoxyflurane | Cyclophosphamide | |
| Norepinephrine | Acetohexamide | Angiotensin | |
| Cisplatin | Propoxyphene | Bradykinin | |
| Clonidine | Loop diuretics | Clofibrate | |
| Glucocorticoids | | | |

*ADH = antidiuretic hormone; NSAIDs = nonsteroidal anti-inflammatory drugs.

acid excretion is not different from that of healthy younger volunteers.[132] But when senescent kidneys are challenged with an acute acid load, acid excretion is not increased to the same degree as that of young volunteers.[133] In an earlier study, older subjects (72 to 93 years) excreted only 19% of a standard oral ammonium chloride acid load, compared with 35% excretion by younger subjects (17 to 35 years), during an 8-hour period. Urinary $NH_4^+$ excretion accounted for less of the total acid excretion in the old subjects: 59% in the old subjects compared with 72% in the young subjects. In this study, the decrease in both of these parameters was paralleled by a nearly equal drop in inulin clearance, so that acid excretion per unit GFR was almost identical in both young and old subjects, which suggests that the decrease in acid excretion found in advancing age is due to a decreased renal tubule mass rather than a specific tubule defect.[134]

A more recent study in elderly subjects with less impaired GFR, however, arrived at a different conclusion. In this study, the minimal urine pH and net acid excretion, even when factored for GFR, were significantly decreased in the older subjects. There were no differences in titratable acid excretion, but the older subjects showed a significant reduction in $NH_4^+$ excretion even when factored for GFR: 34 mol/min in elderly subjects compared with 51 mol/min in young subjects.[133] Furthermore, a significant inverse correlation was found between urine pH and log $NH_4^+$ excretion in young subjects, but the correlation was not significant in the elderly. However, for any given urine pH, $NH_4^+$ excretion in the elderly was less than that of younger subjects. $NH_4^+$ excretion was dependent on age rather than pH of the urine. This study therefore suggests an intrinsic tubule defect in $NH_4^+$ excretion as a function of aging. It is not known whether this defect is due to anatomic changes or functional factors, including the impairment in the renin-angiotensin-aldosterone axis that is frequently encountered in the aged.

The aged rat also exhibits impaired adaptation to an acid load.[135–137] Administration of an equivalent acid load caused a more severe metabolic acidosis in the old rat, pH from 7.40 to 7.09, than in the young adult rat, pH from 7.43 to 7.32. The more severe acidosis in the old rat was caused by a decrease in total acid excretion. This decrease was caused

by a decrease in $NH_4^+$ excretion, whereas there was no impairment in titratable acid excretion. Studies of renal proximal tubule brush border membrane vesicle transport revealed that $Na^+/H^+$ antiport activity, a major regulator of proximal tubule acidification, was similarly enhanced by the acid load in adult and aged rats and that the resultant $Na^+/H^+$ antiport activity was identical in both aged and adult rats.[135] This study therefore suggests that impaired $NH_4^+$ excretion probably mediates the age-related impairment in renal adaptation to metabolic acidosis.

## Potassium Balance

Studies of the effects of aging on renal and extrarenal adaptation to high $K^+$ loads or dietary potassium deprivation in the human are lacking. Two different studies, however, have found that both total body $K^{+[138]}$ and total exchangeable $K^{+[139]}$ decrease with age in both sexes and that the decrease is more marked in women than in men. This decrease may be related to the decrease in muscle mass with advancing age. In response to exercise, the rate of increase in plasma $K^+$ is higher in elderly subjects compared with young subjects.[140] This study suggests that there may be an age-related impairment in the $\beta_2$-adrenergic process that mediates $K^+$ flux into skeletal muscle.

The effects of aging on $K^+$ adaptation has been studied in the aged rat.[141] In this study, the efficiency of kaliuretic response to intravenous infusion to potassium chloride and the rise in plasma $K^+$ concentration were identical in the young and the aged rat. After a period of high dietary potassium intake, however, the efficiency of kaliuretic response to intravenous potassium chloride was impaired and the rise in plasma $K^+$ level was significantly higher in the aged rat. After bilateral nephrectomy, the rise in plasma $K^+$ concentration was also higher in aged rats given a high-potassium diet; this effect was not seen with a normal dietary potassium intake. This renal and extrarenal impairment in $K^+$ adaptation was thought to be due to a decrease in renal and colon $Na^+,K^+$-ATPase activity. Whether these findings also apply to human aging remains to be determined.

The presence of a renal acidification defect and decreased

**TABLE 52–4. Drugs That May Predispose to Hyperkalemia**

K⁺-sparing diuretics
　Spironolactone
　Triamterene
　Amiloride
β-Blockers
Prostaglandin synthesis inhibitors
Converting enzyme inhibitors
Miscellaneous
　Heparin
　Ketoconazole
　Cyclosporine

activity of the renin-angiotensin-aldosterone system may be the cause of the increased incidence of type 4 renal tubular acidosis or the syndrome of hyporeninemic hypoaldosteronism in the elderly. In fact, in a large clinical series of this disorder the mean age of the patients was 65 years.[142] In addition, the elderly are also at increased risk for hyperkalemia with the use of K⁺ sparing diuretics, including triamterene, spironolactone (Aldactone), and amiloride, as well as drugs that inhibit the renin-angiotensin-aldosterone system, especially prostaglandin synthesis inhibitors, β-blockers, converting enzyme inhibitors, heparin, ketoconazole, and cyclosporine[143–145] (Table 52–4).

## Calcium Balance

Ca²⁺ metabolism is significantly impaired as a function of aging. The related decrease in intestinal Ca²⁺ absorption[146–152] correlates with the age-related decline in renal 1α-hydroxylase activity, and decreased levels of 1,25-dihydroxycholecalciferol.[153–163] In addition, the intestinal adaptation to dietary calcium restriction is also impaired.[147, 148, 164] Renal tubule reabsorption of Ca²⁺, however, is not

significantly affected by the aging process, and during dietary calcium restriction almost all of the filtered Ca²⁺ is reabsorbed by the renal tubules.[147, 148, 164]

## Phosphorus Balance

Metabolic balance and clearance studies in humans and rats reveal an age-related decrement in renal tubule reabsorption of $PO_4^{3-}$.[63, 147, 165–171] The impairment occurs in spite of an age-related decrement in intestinal $PO_4^{3-}$ absorption.[147] In addition, renal tubule adaptation to a low-phosphate diet is impaired in the aged rat.[63, 147, 168, 171] (Fig. 52–9). In spite of increased levels of serum parathyroid hormone activity,[172, 173] the impairment in renal $PO_4^{3-}$ transport is independent of endogenous parathyroid hormone activity, because parathyroidectomy in the aged rat results in a significant improvement but not normalization of renal tubule reabsorption of $PO_4^{3-}$.[167–169, 171]

A similar age-related impairment in $PO_4^{3-}$ transport has been demonstrated in primary cultures of renal tubule cells from young and adult rats.[174] In agreement with the in vivo studies,[168] the decrease in $PO_4^{3-}$ transport is mediated by a decrease in the maximal velocity of Na⁺ gradient–dependent $PO_4^{3-}$ transport. Furthermore, adaptation to a low $PO_4^{3-}$ concentration in the culture medium is also significantly impaired in renal tubule cells cultured from old rats compared with those from young adult rats.

Studies with the aged rat indicate significant age-related increases in renal proximal tubule apical brush border membrane cholesterol, sphingomyelin, and saturated fatty acid contents[63, 175–178] and a decrease in membrane fluidity,[63] which may play an important role in the age-related impairment in renal tubule $PO_4^{3-}$ transport. In renal apical brush border membranes isolated from young adult rats, in vitro enrichment with cholesterol to similar levels measured in the aged rat has been shown to simulate the age-related impairment in the maximal velocity of Na⁺ gradient–depen-

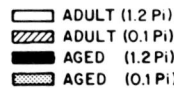

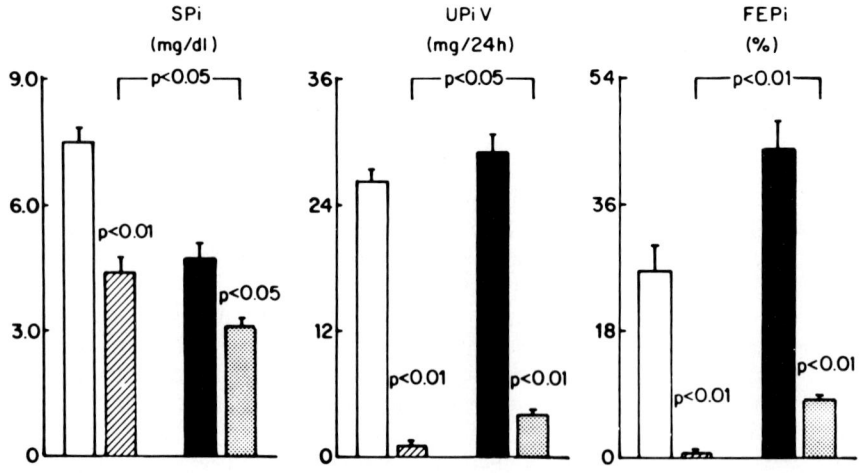

**Figure 52–9.** Serum ultrafilterable $PO_4^{3-}$ concentration (SPi), urinary ultrafilterable $PO_4^{3-}$ excretion rate (UPiV), and fractional excretion of ultrafilterable $PO_4^{3-}$ (FEPi) in adult and aged rats fed a high- or low-phosphate diet (n = 6 rats in each group). Values are means ± SE; one-way analysis of variance by the Student-Newman-Keuls multiple-range test was used. (From Levi M, Jameson DM, Van Der Meer BW: Role of BBM lipid composition and fluidity in impaired renal Pᵢ transport in aged rat. Am J Physiol 256:F85–F94, 1989.)

dent $PO_4^{3-}$ transport.[179] This study certainly suggests that an age-related alteration in membrane cholesterol composition plays an important role in the age-related impairment in renal tubule $PO_4^{3-}$ transport.

The role of the impaired 1,25-dihydroxycholecalciferol metabolism in age-related impairment in renal and intestinal $PO_4^{3-}$ transport also deserves to be determined, because administration of 1,25-dihydroxycholecalciferol to vitamin D–deficient animals results in significant improvements in renal[180–182] and intestinal[182] $PO_4^{3-}$ transport. Of interest, the stimulatory effects of 1,25-dihydroxycholecalciferol on $PO_4^{3-}$ transport are paralleled by significant alterations in brush border membrane lipid composition and fluidity.[183, 184] It is therefore quite possible that similar lipid-modulating effects of 1,25-dihydroxycholecalciferol in the aged may also result in significant improvements in renal and intestinal $PO_4^{3-}$ (and $Ca^{2+}$) transport.

# CLINICAL RENAL DISEASES IN THE AGED

## Renal Vascular Disorders

A major cause of vascular disease of the kidney and renal insufficiency in the elderly is atheromatous renal disease. Atheromatous renal disease may be manifested as 1) renal artery stenosis; 2) complex intrarenal lesions, with multiple stenoses of intrarenal vasculature; and 3) cholesterol embolism. In a report of 32 cases of various forms of renal failure in patients with widespread atheroma, 22 were due mainly to atheromatous stenosis of the renal arteries, in 8 the renal artery lesions coexisted with cholesterol emboli, and in the remaining 2 renal failure was due only to cholesterol emboli.[185] The natural history of atheromatous renal disease is progressive occlusion of the major renal arteries. A review of 237 patients disclosed angiographic progression of renovascular disease in nearly 50% of patients.[186] Most of these patients, if left untreated, develop progressive renal failure. In this regard, a prospective survey during an 18-month period found that atheromatous renal disease was responsible for renal failure in 14% of patients older than 50 years who presented with end-stage renal disease.[187] Thus, atheromatous renal disease may be an important cause of renal insufficiency in elderly patients with generalized atherosclerosis and unexplained end-stage renal disease.

Because of the unique intrarenal hemodynamic effects of angiotensin II, treatment of hypertension in patients with atheromatous renal disease by use of converting enzyme inhibitors may often result in a significant reduction of GFR.[188] The diagnosis of renal artery stenosis should therefore be strongly considered in an elderly patient who presents with hypertension and renal failure. In accurately diagnosed patients, timely intervention when technically possible, in the form of either percutaneous transluminal angioplasty or surgical revascularization, may result in significant improvement of the hypertension and may prevent further renal functional deterioration.[186, 189–191]

The most frequent triggering causes of cholesterol embolism are aortic surgery; abdominal, coronary, or carotid angiography, especially when performed by the femoral approach; and excess anticoagulation. This syndrome has also been reported to occur in the setting of a myocardial infarction in which thrombolytic therapy has been administered.[192] In addition, cholesterol embolism may occur spontaneously.[193] Patients may present with a combination of symptoms including purple discoloration of toes, which may progress to lower extremity focal digital necrosis; livedo reticularis of the abdominal or lumber wall; gastrointestinal bleeding; pancreatitis; myocardial infarction; retinal ischemia; cerebral infarction; hypertension; and uremia.[194] Cholesterol embolism may be associated with fever, increased erythrocyte sedimentation rate, eosinophilia, and hematuria without casts.[195] The differential diagnosis includes contrast agent–induced acute renal failure, polyarteritis nodosa, allergic vasculitis, left atrial myxoma, and subacute bacterial endocarditis.

Episodic and labile hypertension caused by renal artery emboli is a common consequence of renal cholesterol emboli. Furthermore, GFR progressively declines within 1 to 4 weeks. This time course differentiates cholesterol emboli–induced acute renal failure from radiocontrast agent–induced acute renal failure, which usually occurs within 1 to 4 days after the angiographic procedure. The diagnosis of renal cholesterol emboli requires a high degree of suspicion and aggressive diagnostic workup. In addition to a careful ophthalmoscopic examination and skin and muscle biopsy, definitive diagnosis may require renal biopsy. Unfortunately, no treatment modality has yet proved effective for reversing the disease process. At present, the recommendations are to avoid, if possible, excessive anticoagulation and invasive angiographic procedures in elderly patients with widespread atheromatous vascular disease, and when renal failure progresses, to provide supportive therapy, including dialysis.

## Acute Glomerulonephritis

The most prevalent form of acute glomerulonephritis in the elderly is rapidly progressive glomerulonephritis, in which there is progressive loss of renal function during a period of weeks to months. The most common histologic lesion associated with this syndrome is the finding of glomerular crescents. An immunopathologic classification of rapidly progressive glomerulonephritis is given in Table 52–5. Approximately 20% of cases are mediated by anti–glomerular basement antibodies and result in a linear staining of the glomerular basement membrane on immunofluorescence studies (type 1).[196] Forty percent of cases are thought to be immune complex mediated and typically show a "lumpy-bumpy" pattern on immunofluorescence studies (type 2). The third major category (type 3), accounting for approximately 40% of cases, is characterized by the absence of immune deposits on immunofluorescence studies. These patients are often found to have circulating anti-neutrophil cytoplasmic antibodies.[197]

Histologic studies in elderly patients with rapidly progressive glomerulonephritis have most commonly shown the type 2 or type 3 pattern.[198] In a renal biopsy series of 115 patients 60 years and older who presented with glomer-

**TABLE 52–5. Rapidly Progressive Glomerulonephritis: An Immunopathologic Classification of Crescentic Glomerulonephritis***

Type 1: Circulating anti–glomerular basement antibody
  Without lung hemorrhage
  With lung hemorrhage (Goodpasture syndrome)
Type 2: Granular immune deposits
  Limited renal disease (immunoglobulin A nephritis, membranoproliferative glomerulonephritis)
  Postinfectious disease (poststreptoccocal, abscess, endocarditis)
  Systemic disease (systemic lupus erythematosus, cryoglobulinemia)
Type 3: No immune deposits (often associated with circulating antineutrophil cytoplasmic antibodies)
  Idiopathic glomerulonephritis
  Vasculitis
  Wegener granulomatosis
  Microscopic polyarteritis nodosa

*Rapidly progressive glomerulonephritis is a clinical syndrome that is often associated with the histologic finding of glomerular crescents. See text for details.

ulonephritis or the nephrotic syndrome or both, 19 were found to have idiopathic crescentic glomerulonephritis.[199] In this series, anti–glomerular basement membrane antibodies were detected in only 1 of 11 patients whose serum was checked. Linear deposition of immunoglobulin G in the glomerular capillaries was observed in only two patients. Granular deposits of immunoglobulin G were observed in nine patients, but six other patients had no deposits. More recently, 8 of 10 patients older than age 65 years who presented with rapidly progressive glomerulonephritis were found to have no immune deposits on immunofluorescence studies.[200] Most of these patients had positive test results for circulating antineutrophil cytoplasmic antibodies. Similarly, 40 patients selected purely on the basis of histologic findings of a type 3 necrotizing crescentic glomerulonephritis were found to have an average age of 62 years.[201] Circulating antineutrophil cytoplasmic antibodies were present in the majority of these patients. Interestingly, extrarenal symptoms suggestive of vasculitis were commonly observed in these patients. In general, the prognosis for elderly patients with crescentic glomerulonephritis is poor. Use of pulse administration of steroids, cyclophosphamide, or plasmapheresis has been effective in small series of el-

derly patients.[196, 198, 201] Because the side effect profile of these agents is increased in the elderly, the risk/benefit ratio must be carefully considered for the individual patient.

Another prevalent form of acute glomerulonephritis in the elderly is diffuse proliferative glomerulonephritis, which commonly occurs in association with infection. Poststreptococcal glomerulonephritis is associated with streptococcal infections of the throat and the skin.[202–206] Clinical features of poststreptococcal glomerulonephritis in the elderly include hypertension in 82% of cases, edema in 73% of cases, dyspnea and evidence of circulatory congestion in 41% of cases, and oliguria in 75% of cases. Although hypertension and edema are as frequently encountered in pediatric and young adult patients, circulatory congestion and renal insufficiency are most often encountered in the elderly, perhaps as a result of the age-related impairments in cardiopulmonary and renal reserve and function. Poststreptococcal glomerulonephritis may also be manifested as crescentic glomerulonephritis and result in acute renal failure (see Table 52–5).

Because of the overall favorable prognosis, maximal effort should be expended for prompt diagnosis and appropriate therapy, including dialysis if indicated.

## Nephrotic Syndrome

Nephrotic syndrome is a commonly diagnosed renal disease in the elderly. Review of nine publications from different countries, including the United States, Japan, France, England, and Israel, which reported on 275 patients aged 60 years or older, revealed that the most common histopathologic lesions were membranous glomerulonephritis (123 patients, or 45%), minimal-change disease (52 patients, or 19%), mesangial proliferative glomerulonephritis (32 patients, or 12%), and membranoproliferative glomerulonephritis (32 patients, or 12%)[207–215] (Table 52–6). Similar findings were reported in the Medical Research Council's Glomerulonephritis Registry consisting of 317 patients older than 60 years who presented with the nephrotic syndrome.[216] The most frequent histologic findings were membranous nephropathy (36.6%) and minimal-change disease (11.0%). Renal amyloidosis was found in 10.7% of cases.

**TABLE 52–6. Histologic Lesions in 275 Elderly Patients with the Nephrotic Syndrome**

| Reference | Minimal-Change Disease | Membranous Glomerulonephritis | Mesangial Proliferative Glomerulonephritis | Membranoproliferative Glomerulonephritis | Glomerulosclerosis | Chronic Glomerulonephritis |
|---|---|---|---|---|---|---|
| 208 | 6 | 5 | — | 4 | 16 | 5 |
| 209 | 4 | 2 | — | 6 | — | — |
| 207 | 9 | 15 | 7 | 2 | 1 | — |
| 210 | 1 | 6 | — | 2 | 7 | — |
| 212 | 2 | 16 | — | 2 | 3 | — |
| 215 | 19 | 31 | 2 | 4 | — | 3 |
| 211 | 2 | 16 | 11 | 3 | — | — |
| 213 | 2 | 2 | — | 2 | — | — |
| 214 | 7 | 30 | 12 | 7 | 1 | — |
| Total | 52 (19%) | 123 (45%) | 32 (12%) | 32 (12%) | 28 (10%) | 8 (3%) |

Other common causes of nephrotic syndrome in the elderly are diabetes mellitus and glomerulosclerosis.

In approximately 10% of elderly patients with the nephrotic syndrome, renal histopathologic studies indicate glomerulosclerosis (see Table 52–6). This entity resembles the separate, well-known entity of focal and segmental glomerulosclerosis, which is a common cause of the nephrotic syndrome in the younger patient. Focal and segmental, or global, glomerulosclerosis especially affects the juxtamedullary glomeruli; immunofluorescence generally reveals granular deposits of immunoglobulin M and C3. Although focal and segmental glomerulosclerosis usually occurs as a separate and distinct entity, it may also occur as the end result of various other glomerulopathies or systemic diseases, including diabetes and hypertension. Hyperfiltration of the functioning glomeruli has been proposed to play an important role in the process of glomerulosclerosis.[37,38] This process may be especially important for the juxtamedullary glomeruli, because they have a significantly higher filtration fraction than the superficial cortical glomeruli.

The otherwise normal and healthy aged rat has a histologic renal lesion similar to that of human glomerulosclerosis with deposition of immunoglobulin M and C3, which is accompanied by significant proteinuria.[217–224] The aging rat may therefore represent an opportune model for the delineation of hemodynamic, metabolic, and immunologic factors as the cause of age-related glomerulosclerosis.

Renal biopsy is essential for establishing the correct histopathologic characteristics because most often it is not possible to predict these characteristics on the basis of clinical data alone.[225,226] Furthermore, in several of these series, elderly patients with minimal-change disease responded to corticosteroid therapy, and complete remission was obtained without relapse. In addition, complete remission or partial remission was achieved in 50% to 70% of patients with membranous glomerulonephritis who were treated with corticosteroids and immunosuppressants. On the other hand, the outcome of treatment of proliferative glomerulonephritis was highly variable. Thus, given the relatively high frequency of minimal-change disease (19% of elderly patients with the nephrotic syndrome) and the highly favorable response to therapy, it is recommended that the elderly patient with the nephrotic syndrome undergo a thorough workup including a renal biopsy to establish the histopathologic type of disease.

There is a known association between the presence of nephrotic syndrome and malignancy.[227] The most common glomerular pathologic change in patients with malignancy is membranous glomerulopathy. An associated malignancy has been reported in 7% to 20% of patients who present with the nephrotic syndrome.[215,228] The most common underlying tumors are cancer of the lung, colon, rectum, kidney, breast, and stomach. As a result, elderly patients with the nephrotic syndrome should be screened for an underlying malignancy.

## Renal Cysts

Simple renal cysts are commonly found in the aging adult population. More than 50% of people older than 50 years have at least one renal cyst at postmortem examination.[229] Renal cysts are quite uncommon in children and are thus regarded as an acquired abnormality that is related to age.

With increased use of ultrasonography and computed tomographic imaging of the abdomen, renal cysts are being recognized more frequently. In an ultrasonographic study of 729 patients referred for reasons unrelated to the urinary tract, the prevalence of at least one renal cyst was found to progressively increase from 0% in those aged 15 to 29 years to 22.1% in those aged 70 years and older.[230] These findings confirmed earlier observations of an age-related increase in the development of simple renal cysts[231] (Fig. 52–10). Simple cysts are usually unilocular, are often cortical with some distortion of the renal contour, and increase in number with increasing age.[232] Symptoms that have been ascribed to renal cysts include abdominal or lumbar pain, hematuria, secondary infection, and renin-dependent hypertension. In the vast majority of cases, however, the simple cysts are asymptomatic and are discovered incidentally.

The major issue in the incidental discovery of a renal cyst is the differentiation between simple cyst and malignant mass. Ultrasonographic criteria for a simple cyst are given in Figure 52–11. If all three ultrasonographic criteria are strictly satisfied, the cyst can be regarded as nonmalignant with virtually 100% accuracy.[233] If the mass fails to satisfy these criteria, computed tomographic scanning is the next logical step. Strict criteria for identification of simple cysts have likewise been established for this procedure. As with ultrasonography, if all computed tomographic diagnostic criteria are met, the cyst can be regarded as simple and no further evaluation is warranted.[234] If the computed tomographic findings are intermediate, additional workup consisting of cyst puncture and aspiration for cytology is indicated. In selected patients, angiography or direct surgical exploration is required to exclude a malignant process.

## Acute Renal Failure

A major cause of acute renal failure in the elderly is prerenal failure, that is, decreased perfusion of the kidney leading to a functional and potentially reversible type of acute renal failure. In addition to the age-related decreases in baseline renal blood flow and GFR, there is evidence for age-related impairments in autoregulation of renal blood flow and renal functional reserve, which may render the aging kidney more susceptible to prerenal failure. Even a modest contraction of blood volume induced by oral administration of 120 mg of furosemide results in a larger decrease in GFR in subjects older than 40 years when compared with younger subjects.[32]

Experimental studies in the aging rat have confirmed clinical observations of enhanced ischemic and toxic acute renal failure.[235–239] After 45 minutes of clamping of the renal arteries (a well-established model of ischemic renal failure), the decline in renal function in the aged rat was significantly greater than that in the young rat, and the rate of recovery was also much lower[239] (Fig. 52–12). In the same study, after graded periods of in vitro anoxia, renal function (as assessed by renal cortical slice uptake of PAH and

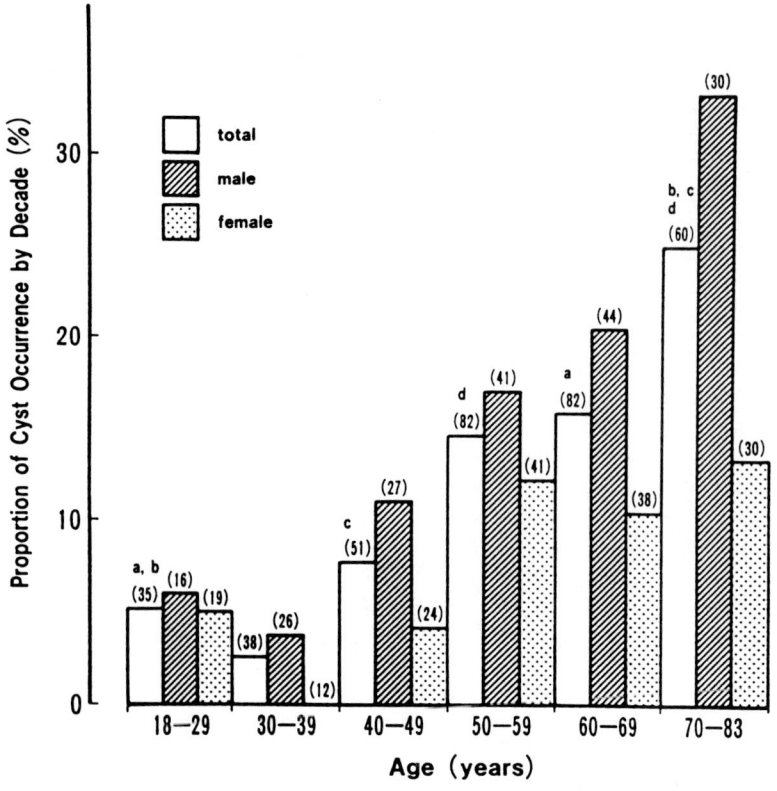

**Figure 52–10.** Proportion of subjects with simple renal cysts by age decade. The number of subjects is indicated in each column in parentheses. Statistical analysis was performed between white columns (total of men and women): a versus a ($P < .05$), b versus b ($P < .01$), c versus c ($P < .025$), and d versus d ($P < .05$). (From Yamagishi F, Kitahara N, Mogi W, Itoh S: Age-related occurrence of simple cysts studied by ultrasonography. Klin Wochenschr 66:385–387, 1988.)

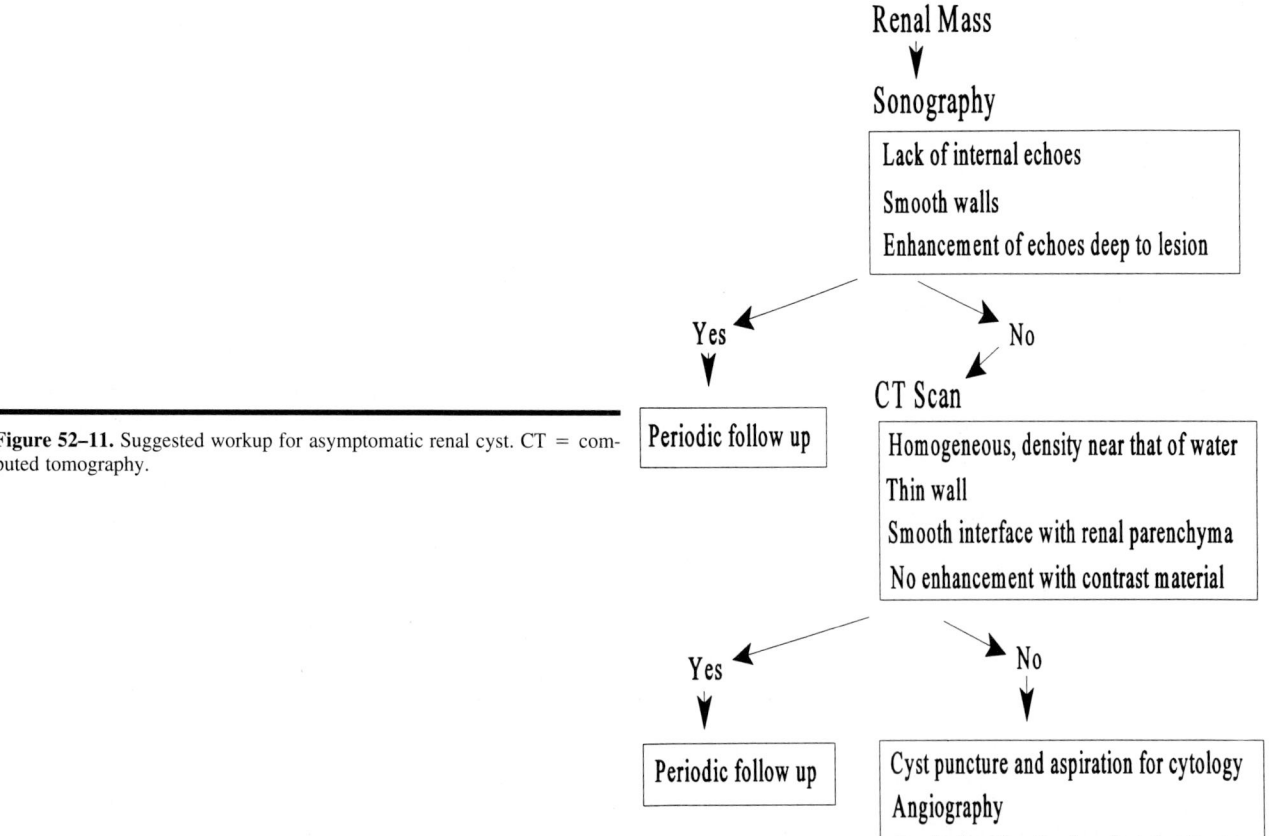

**Figure 52–11.** Suggested workup for asymptomatic renal cyst. CT = computed tomography.

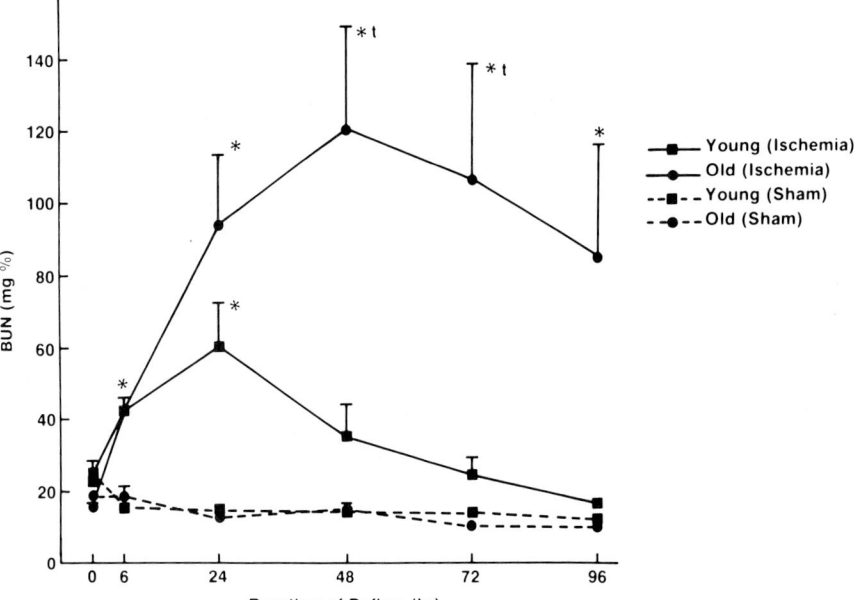

**Figure 52–12.** Effect of ischemia on blood urea nitrogen concentration. Values shown at 0 hours were obtained 24 hours before induction of ischemia. Values represent means ± SEM of three to five observations. Asterisks indicate significant differences compared with age-matched control subjects ($P < .05$). Daggers indicate a significant difference compared with young rats ($P < .05$). (From Miura K, Goldstein RS, Morgan DG, et al: Age-related differences in susceptibility to renal ischemia in rats. Toxicol Appl Pharmacol 87:284–296, 1987.)

tetraethylammonium) was also impaired to a greater extent in renal cortical slices from old rats compared with those from young rats.[239] This study suggests that in addition to the alterations in renal blood flow and GFR, alterations in the metabolism and biochemistry of aging tubule cells may play an important role in mediating age-related enhancement of ischemic renal cell injury.

In the elderly, prerenal failure may be precipitated by a decrease in cardiac output secondary to an acute myocardial infarction or congestive heart failure; a marked decrease in systemic vascular resistance secondary to sepsis; gastrointestinal fluid losses caused by severe vomiting, diarrhea, bleeding, or "third spacing"; renal fluid losses secondary to glycosuria or excessive use of diuretics; renal atheromatous disease; or use of converting enzyme inhibitors in the presence of bilateral renal artery stenosis. Prerenal failure, if not promptly recognized and reversed, may result in acute tubule necrosis. In fact, in several clinical series of acute renal failure in the elderly, the most frequently recognized cause of acute renal failure was hypovolemic or ischemic acute renal failure.[240-244]

Complications of major surgery account for about 30% of cases of acute renal failure in the elderly. Hypotension during or after surgery, postoperative fluid loss caused by gastrointestinal or fistulous drainage, arrhythmias, and myocardial infarction are common postoperative complications in the elderly that may result in acute renal failure. Infection and especially gram-negative septicemia account for another 30% of cases of acute renal failure in the elderly. Gram-negative infections are frequently associated with endotoxin-induced renovascular vasoconstriction, which in the susceptible individual may result in acute tubular necrosis. In addition, most antibiotics used to treat serious infections, especially aminoglycoside antibiotics, are associated with a high frequency of acute tubule necrosis in the elderly. Age is a well-known risk factor for aminoglycoside-induced nephrotoxicity.[245] The reasons include possible

overdosage as a result of inaccurate estimation of the GFR from serum creatinine concentration alone, and age-related renal tubule functional and biochemical alterations,[63] which may enhance the toxic effects of aminoglycoside antibiotics on renal tubules.

Another major cause of acute renal failure in the elderly is use of nonsteroidal anti-inflammatory drugs.[246-248] This is of special concern because ibuprofen and naproxen (Naprosyn) are available as over-the-counter medications. Inhibition of renal vasodilatory prostaglandin synthesis caused by these drugs can potentiate the renal vasoconstrictive effects of renal nerves, $\alpha$-adrenergic system, angiotensin II, and vasopressin.[249] In the presence of an already reduced renal blood flow, the augmented vasoconstriction may result in acute renal failure in the elderly patient. This may be especially relevant in hypertensive elderly subjects who have been found to have a significant reduction in urinary prostaglandin $E_2$ excretion.[250] Elderly patients are also at increased risk for acute renal failure during converting enzyme inhibition therapy for left ventricular dysfunction or hypertension. Renal failure in this setting usually occurs in the presence of bilateral renal artery stenosis or unilateral renal artery stenosis when there is a nonfunctioning or poorly functioning contralateral kidney. In view of increased recognition of atheromatous renal vascular disease in the elderly,[185] older patients who are treated with any of the converting enzyme inhibitors need frequent determinations of GFR. Elderly patients are also at increased risk for radiocontrast agent–induced renal failure.[193] The mechanisms of this type of renal injury are not completely understood but include hemodynamic effects and direct toxic effects on tubules, which because of pre-existent renal defects may predispose the elderly to enhanced renal toxicity.

Another important cause of acute renal failure in the elderly is urinary tract obstruction, most frequently resulting from an enlarged prostate.[251] Symptoms of prostatism such as urinary frequency, difficulty in starting or stopping micturition, and nocturia may not be apparent. A significant number of patients may therefore present with symptoms of end-stage renal disease rather than with prostatism. In addition, in clinically significant prostatism, the residual urine is often infected, which may potentiate impairments in tubule function and reduction in renal blood flow and the GFR caused by the obstruction.

Most elderly patients respond well to dialysis treatment of acute renal failure.[242, 244, 252] Although the chances for survival or recovery of renal function in the elderly with acute renal failure would be predicted to be markedly decreased, studies have found the mortality rate (50% to 60%) and the recovery of renal function (50% to 60%) not to be markedly worse than those for adult patients who develop acute renal failure.[242, 244, 252] Prompt initiation of hemodialysis or peritoneal dialysis is therefore recommended to alleviate the uremic symptoms and to prevent uremic complications such as infection, myocardial infarction, congestive heart failure, and bleeding, which are the major causes of mortality in the elderly patient with acute renal failure.

## Chronic Renal Failure

Many forms of chronic renal failure are more commonly seen late in life because the renal disease is a result of other age-dependent medical diseases. Atherosclerotic disease of the renal vasculature causing renovascular hypertension and renal ischemia; diabetes, hypertension, or chronic glomerulonephritis causing glomerulosclerosis; and prostatic hypertrophy causing hydronephrosis are the most common causes of chronic renal failure in the elderly.

The clinical presentation of chronic renal failure in elderly patients is often quite different from that in adult patients. Elderly patients often present with decompensation of pre-existent medical conditions, such as congestive heart failure, hypertension, peptic ulcer disease, or dementia, rather than with the specific symptom of uremia. In addition, the level of serum creatinine may underestimate the actual renal reserve, because in the presence of decreased muscle mass, the serum creatinine level does not rise in direct proportion to the reduction in the GFR.

If the renal failure is advanced and no reversible causes can be identified, including renal artery stenosis and urinary tract obstruction, early dialysis is advisable to prevent the disabling symptoms of uremia and organ dysfunction that may become irreversible. Age itself should not be the sole criterion for exclusion from dialytic therapy. In fact, the number of elderly patients accepted for dialytic therapy is increasing year by year.[253] In the absence of major extrarenal organ dysfunction, the elderly adjust to dialysis quite well, and their longevity, although not as favorable as that in younger patients, is not markedly reduced as a result of end-stage renal disease.[254–259] In elderly patients with cardiovascular disease who may not tolerate hemodialysis, chronic ambulatory peritoneal dialysis has been successfully used.[258–261] The incidence of peritonitis, type of infectious organism, and likelihood of technique failure are similar in young and elderly patients given this treatment.[253, 262] In addition, elderly patients have a decreased need for catheter replacement when compared with young patients treated with chronic ambulatory peritoneal dialysis.[253, 262]

Studies addressing differences in the outcome of hemodialysis and chronic ambulatory peritoneal dialysis as a function of age have produced conflicting results.[253] Some of this variability can be attributed to the failure of some studies to consider comorbid factors and their impact on survival. For example, diabetes, malignancy, cardiovascular disease, and peripheral vascular disease all have an impact on survival of patients with end-stage renal disease independent of the mode of dialytic therapy. When these factors are controlled for, however, there still remains no clear consensus demonstrating the superiority of one mode of therapy over the other.[263–265] A number of medical and psychosocial factors need to be considered in choosing a dialysis modality for the elderly patient. The presence of widespread vascular disease and inability to maintain a functioning vascular access favor the use of chronic ambulatory peritoneal dialysis. Such patients are prone to hypotension and arrhythmias as a result of rapid fluid and electrolyte shifts that are associated with hemodialysis. However, hemodialysis is the preferred choice in patients whose overall physical conditioning and home situation prevent them from performing self-care dialysis. The functional status of a patient can be objectively assessed by instruments such as the Karnovski scale.[266] In patients with a low rating, hemodialysis is associated with better survival; outcomes for hemodialysis and chronic ambulatory peritoneal dialysis are similar in patients with a high score. Finally, the social interaction associated with in-center hemodialysis may prove valuable for patients who live alone or who are depressed.

Age itself is also not an absolute contraindication for kidney transplantation, as otherwise medically eligible elderly patients have undergone successful transplantation.[267, 268] In the cyclosporine era, survivals of elderly and young patients are similar at 1 year after transplantation but differences in survival increase thereafter. A similar pattern is found with regard to allograft survival. The major cause of allograft loss in the elderly patient is death, as opposed to immunologically mediated graft loss, which predominates in the younger population.[267, 269] Cardiovascular disease accounts for a much higher percentage of transplantation-related deaths in elderly patients compared with younger patients.

## Urinary Tract Infections

Urinary tract infections are an important problem in the elderly population. The reasons for the increase in the prevalence of urinary tract infections with advancing age are not known but may include changes in bladder function, pelvic musculature, and prostate size; impaired immune response; and concomitant illness. In postmenopausal women, a decrease in the level of circulating estrogens contributes to the increase in urinary tract infections. Intravaginal administration of estrogen has been shown to restore the normal local environment of the vagina to that which is found in the premenopausal state and prevent recurrent urinary tract infections.[270]

Although bacteriuria is found in less than 5% of middle-aged women and in less than 1% of middle-aged men, 20% of healthy men older than 65 years have bacteriuria. The prevalence of bacteriuria in elderly men and women increases to 25% in extended care facilities, to 30% in patients admitted to acute care hospitals, and to more than 35% in patients admitted to nursing facilities.[271] The increased prevalence of dementia and urinary incontinence further complicates the picture. Elderly patients with bacteriuria have a significant decrease in creatinine clearance when compared with age-matched patients without bacteriuria.[272, 273] The reason for the worsening of renal function is not clear but may indicate the presence of chronic pyelonephritis, which may eventually be associated with focal segmental glomerulosclerosis. Bacteriuria may be associated with a significant reduction in survival rate of elderly subjects,[273–276] although other associated factors must also play a role because treatment of asymptomatic bacteriuria with antibiotics did not result in a significant improvement in the 2-year mortality of institutionalized elderly male patients.[274] In fact, in the absence of renal disease, urinary tract abnormalities, or clinical evidence of sepsis, most physicians agree that asymptomatic bacteriuria in the elderly should not be treated because the frequency of treatment failure and relapse is high.[277] The efficacy of chronic immunosuppressive therapy has not been determined, but one might anticipate the emergence of infections with highly resistant gram-negative bacteria, especially in institutionalized and debilitated elderly patients.[278–280]

## REFERENCES

1. Tauchi H, Tsuboi K, Okutomi J: Age changes in the human kidney of the different races. Gerontologia 17:87–97, 1971.
2. Dunnill MS, Halley W: Some observations on the quantitative anatomy of the kidney. J Pathol 110:113–121, 1973.
3. McLachlan M, Guthrie J, Anderson C, Fulker M: Vascular and glomerular changes in the aging kidney. J Pathol 121:65–78, 1977.
4. Moore RA: The total number of glomeruli in the normal human kidney. Anat Rec 48:153–168, 1958.
5. Kaplan C, Pasternack B, Shah H, Gallo G: Age-related incidence of sclerotic glomeruli in human kidneys. Am J Pathol 80:227–234, 1975.
6. Kappel B, Olsen S: Cortical interstitial tissue and sclerosed glomeruli in the normal human kidney, related to age and sex. A quantitative study. Virchows Arch A 387:271–277, 1980.
7. Sworn MJ, Path MRC, Fox M: Donor kidney selection for transplantation. Relationship between glomerular structure, vascular supply and age. Br J Urol 44:377–383, 1972.
8. Moritz A, Oldt M: Arteriolar sclerosis in hypertensive and nonhypertensive individuals. Am J Pathol 13:679–687, 1973.
9. Williams RH, Harrison TR: A study of the renal arteries in relation to age and to hypertension. Am Heart J 14:645–658, 1937.
10. Yamaguchi T, Omae T, Katsuki S: Quantitative determination of renal vascular changes related to age and hypertension. Jpn Heart J 10:248–258, 1969.
11. Takazakura E, Sawabu N, Handa A, et al: Intrarenal vascular changes with age and disease. Kidney Int 2:224–230, 1972.
12. Ljungqvist A, Lagergren C: Normal intrarenal arterial pattern in adult and aging human kidney. A microangiographical and histological study. J Anat 96:285–300, 1962.
13. Davies D, Shock N: Age changes in glomerular filtration rate, effective renal plasma flow, and tubular excretory capacity in adult males. J Clin Invest 29:496–507, 1950.
14. McDonald R, Solomon D, Shock N: Aging as a factor in the renal hemodynamic changes induced by a standardized pyrogen. J Clin Invest 30:457–462, 1951.
15. Brandfonbrener M, Landsdowne M, Shock NW: Changes in cardiac output with age. Circulation 12:557–565, 1955.
16. Geokas MC, Lakatta EG, Makinodan T, Timiras PS: The aging process. Ann Intern Med 113:455–466, 1990.
17. Lammerant J, Veall N, DeVisscher M: Observations on cardiac output and "pulmonary blood volume" in normal man by internal recording of the intracardiac flows of $^{123}$I labelled albumin. Nucl Med 1:353–359, 1961.
18. Strandell T: Circulatory studies on healthy old men. Acta Med Scand 175:414–420, 1964.
19. Lee T, Lindeman R, Yiengst M, Shock N: Influence of age on the cardiovascular and renal responses to tilting. J Appl Physiol 21:55–61, 1966.
20. Naeije R, Fiasse A, Carlier E, et al: Systemic and renal haemodynamic effects of angiotensin converting enzyme inhibition by zabicipril in young and in old normal men. Eur J Clin Pharmacol 44:35–39, 1993.
21. Hollenberg N, Adams D, Solomon H, et al: Senescence and the renal vasculature in normal man. Circ Res 34:309–316, 1974.
22. Baylis C, Fredericks M, Wilson C, et al: Renal vasodilatory response to intravenous glycine in the aging rat kidney. Am J Kidney Dis 3:144–251, 1990.
23. Corman B, Chami-Khazraji S, Schaeverbeke J, Michel J: Effect of feeding on glomerular filtration rate and proteinuria in conscious aging rats. Am J Physiol 255:F250–F256, 1988.
24. Bohler J, Gloer P, Reetze-Bonorden P, et al: Renal functional reserve in elderly patients. Clin Nephrol 39:145–150, 1993.
25. Fliser D, Zeir M, Nowalk R, Ritz E: Renal functional reserve in healthy elderly subjects. J Am Soc Nephrol 3:1371–1377, 1993.
26. King A, Levey A: Dietary protein and renal function. J Am Soc Nephrol 3:1723–1737, 1993.
27. Woods L: Mechanisms of renal hemodynamic regulation in response to protein feeding. Kidney Int 44:659–675, 1993.
28. Lewis W, Alving A: Changes with age in the renal function in adult men. Am J Physiol 123:500–515, 1938.
29. Rowe J, Andres R, Tobin J, et al: The effect of age on creatinine clearance in men: A cross-sectional and longitudinal study. J Gerontol 31:155–163, 1976.
30. Rowe J, Andres R, Tobin J, et al: Age-adjusted standards for creatinine clearance. Ann Intern Med 84:567–569, 1976.
31. Lindeman R, Tobin J, Shock N: Longitudinal studies on the rate of decline in renal function with age. J Am Geriatr Soc 33:278–285, 1985.
32. Luft F, Fineberg N, Miller J, et al: The effects of age, race, and heredity on glomerular filtration rate following volume expansion and contraction in normal man. Am J Med Sci 279:15–24, 1980.
33. Retta T, Afre G, Randall O: Hypertensive renal disease in blacks. Transplant Proc 25:2421–2422, 1993.
34. Cowie C: Diabetic renal disease: Racial and ethnic differences from an epidemiologic perspective. Transplant Proc 25:2426–2430, 1993.
35. Brenner B, Cohen R, Milford E: In renal transplantation, one size may not fit all. J Am Soc Nephrol 3:162–169, 1993.
36. Kumar M, Stephan R, Chui J, et al: Effect of donor age on graft function and graft survival in cadaver renal transplantation. Transplant Proc 25:2183–2184, 1993.
37. Hostetter TH, Rennke HG, Brenner BM: The case for intrarenal hypertension in the initiation and progression of diabetic and other glomerulopathies. Am J Med 72:375–380, 1982.
38. Anderson S, Brenner B: Effects of aging on the renal glomerulus. Am J Med 80:435–442, 1986.
39. Brenner B, Meyer T, Hostetter T: Dietary protein intake and the progressive nature of renal disease: The role of hemodynamically mediated glomerular injury in the pathogenesis of progressive glomerular sclerosis in aging, renal ablation, and intrinsic renal disease. N Engl J Med 307:652–659, 1982.
40. Lindeman RD, Tobin JD, Shock NW: Association between blood pressure and the rate of decline in renal function with age. Kidney Int 26:861–868, 1984.
41. Berg BN, Simms HS: Nutrition and longevity in the rat. II. Longevity and onset of disease with different levels of food intake. J Nutr 71:255–263, 1960.
42. Bertani T, Zoja C, Abbate M, et al: Age-related nephropathy and proteinuria in rats with intact kidneys exposed to diets with different protein content. Lab Invest 60:196–204, 1989.
43. Bras G, Ross MH: Kidney disease and nutrition in the rat. Toxicol Appl Pharmacol 6:247–262, 1964.

44. Elema JD, Arends A: Focal and segmental glomerular hyalinosis and sclerosis in the rat. Lab Invest 33:554–561, 1975.

45. Everitt AV, Porter DB, Wyndham JR: Effects of caloric intake and dietary compensation on the development of proteinuria, age-associated renal disease and longevity in the male rat. Gerontology 28:168–175, 1982.

46. Gehrig JJ, Ross J, Jamison RL: Effect of long-term alternate day feeding on renal function in aging conscious rats. Kidney Int 34:620–630, 1988.

47. Johnson JE, Barrows CH: Effects of age and dietary restriction on the kidney glomeruli of mice: Observations by scanning electron microscopy. Anat Rec 196:145–151, 1980.

48. Maeda H, Gleiser CA, Masoro EU, et al: Nutritional influences on aging of Fischer 344 rats: II. Pathology. J Gerontol 40:671–688, 1985.

49. Provoost AP, DeKeijzer MH, Molenaar JC: Effect of protein intake on lifelong changes in renal function of rats unilaterally nephrectomized at young age. J Lab Clin Med 114:19–26, 1989.

50. Gonwa T, Atkins C, Zhang Y, et al: Glomerular filtration rates in persons evaluated as living-related donors—are our standards too high? Transplantation 55:983–985, 1993.

51. Kasiske BL: Relationship between vascular disease and age-associated changes in the human kidney. Kidney Int 31:1153–1159, 1987.

52. Keane WF, Kasiske BL, O'Donnell MP: Lipids and progressive glomerulosclerosis. Am J Nephrol 8:261–271, 1988.

53. Schmitz PG, Kasiske BL, O'Donnell MP, Keane WF: Lipids and progressive renal injury. Semin Nephrol 9:354–369, 1989.

54. Kasiske BL, O'Donnell MP, Cowardin W, Keane WF: Lipids and the kidney. Hypertension 15:443–450, 1990.

55. Diamond JR: Analogous pathobiologic mechanisms in glomerulosclerosis and atherosclerosis. Kidney Int 39(suppl 31):S29–S34, 1991.

56. Moorhead JF: Lipids and progressive kidney disease. Kidney Int 39(suppl 31):S35–S40, 1991.

57. Kamanna V, Roh D, Kirschenbaum M: Atherogenic lipoproteins: Mediators of glomerular injury. Am J Nephrol 13:1–5, 1993.

58. Kasiske B, O'Donnell M, Kim Y, et al: Cholesterol synthesis inhibitors inhibit more than cholesterol synthesis. Kidney Int 45:S51–S53, 1994.

59. Kasiske BL, Cleary MP, O'Donnell MP, Keane WF: Effects of genetic obesity on renal structure and function in the Zucker rat. J Lab Clin Med 106:598–604, 1985.

60. O'Donnell MP, Kasiske BL, Cleary MP, Keane WF: Effects of genetic obesity on renal structure and function in the Zucker rat. II. Micropuncture studies. J Lab Clin Med 106:605–610, 1985.

61. Kasiske BL, O'Donnell MP, Cleary MP, Keane WF: Treatment of hyperlipidemia reduces glomerular injury in obese Zucker rats. Kidney Int 33:667–672, 1988.

62. Kasiske BL, O'Donnell MP, Cleary MP, Keane WF: Effects of reduced renal mass on tissue lipids and renal injury in hyperlipidemic rats. Kidney Int 35:40–47, 1989.

63. Levi M, Jameson DM, Van Der Meer BW: Role of BBM lipid composition and fluidity in impaired renal $P_i$ transport in aged rat. Am J Physiol 256:F85–F94, 1989.

64. Luke DR, Halstenson CE, Opsahl JA, Matzke GR: Validity of creatinine clearance estimates in the assessment of renal function. Clin Pharmacol Ther 48:503–508, 1990.

65. Gral T, Young M: Measured versus estimated creatinine clearance in the elderly as an index of renal function. J Am Geriatr Soc 28:492–496, 1980.

66. Mcligeyo S: Calculation of creatinine clearance from plasma creatinine. East Afr Med J 70:3–5, 1993.

67. Feutren G, Mihatsch M: Risk factors for cyclosporine nephropathy in patients with autoimmune diseases. N Engl J Med 326:1654–1660, 1992.

68. Epstein M, Hollenberg N: Age as a determinant of renal sodium conservation in normal man. J Lab Clin Med 87:411–417, 1976.

69. Macias Nunez J, Garcia Iglesias C, Bonda Roman A, et al: Renal handling of sodium in old people: A functional study. Age Ageing 7:178–181, 1978.

70. Anderson GH, Springer J, Randall P, et al: Effect of age on diagnostic usefulness of stimulated plasma renin activity and saralasin test in detection of renovascular hypertension. Lancet 2:821–824, 1980.

71. Crane MG, Harris JJ: Effect of aging on renin activity and aldosterone excretion. J Lab Clin Med 87:947–959, 1976.

72. Cugini P, Murano G, Lucia P, et al: The gerontological decline of the renin-aldosterone system: A chronobiological approach extended to essential hypertension. J Gerontol 42:461–465, 1987.

73. Hall JE, Coleman TG, Guyton AC: The renin-angiotensin system normal physiology and changes in older hypertensives. J Am Geriatr Soc 37:801–813, 1989.

74. Hayashi M, Saruta T, Nakamura R, et al: Effect of aging on single nephron renin content in rats. Renal Physiol 4:17–21, 1981.

75. Hayduk K, Krause DK, Kaufmann W, et al: Age-dependent changes of plasma renin concentration in humans. Clin Sci 45:273s–278s, 1973.

76. Noth RH, Lassman MN, Tan SY, et al: Age and the renin-aldosterone system. Arch Intern Med 137:1414–1417, 1977.

77. Tsunoda K, Abe K, Goto T, et al: Effect of age on the renin-angiotensin-aldosterone system in normal subjects: Simultaneous measurement of active and inactive renin, renin substrate, and aldosterone in plasma. J Clin Endocrinol Metab 62:384–389, 1986.

78. Weidmann P, de Chatel R, Schiffmann A, et al: Interrelations between age and plasma renin, aldosterone and cortisol, urinary catecholamines, and the body sodium/volume state in normal man. Klin Wochenschr 55:725–733, 1977.

79. Bauer J: Age-related changes in the renin-aldosterone system. Drugs Aging 3:238–245, 1993.

80. Weidmann P, De Myttenaere-Bursztein S, Maxwell M, De Lima J: Effect of aging on plasma renin and aldosterone in normal man. Kidney Int 8:325–333, 1975.

81. Flood C, Gherondache C, Pincus G, et al: The metabolism and secretion of aldosterone in elderly subjects. J Clin Invest 46:960–966, 1967.

82. Hegstad R, Brown R, Jiang N, et al: Aging and aldosterone. Am J Med 74:442–448, 1983.

83. Luft F, Weinberger M, Grim C: Sodium sensitivity and resistance in normotensive humans. Am J Med 72:726–736, 1982.

84. Luft F, Weinberger M, Fineberg M, et al: Effects of age on renal sodium homeostasis and its relevance to sodium sensitivity. Am J Med 82(suppl 1B):9–15, 1987.

85. Brenner BM, Ballermann BJ, Gunning ME, Zeidel ML: Diverse biological actions of atrial natriuretic peptide. Physiol Rev 70:665–699, 1990.

86. Weidmann P, Hasler L, Gnadinger MP: Blood levels and renal effects of atrial natriuretic peptide in normal man. J Clin Invest 77:734–742, 1986.

87. Volpe M, Odell G, Kleinert HD: Antihypertensive and aldosterone lowering effects of synthetic atrial natriuretic factor in renin-dependent renovascular hypertension. J Hypertens 2:313–315, 1984.

88. Goodfriend TL, Elliot ME, Atlas SA: Actions of synthetic atrial natriuretic factor on bovine adrenal glomerulosa. Life Sci 35:1675–1682, 1984.

89. Ohashi M, Gujio N, Nawata H: High plasma concentration of human atrial natriuretic peptide in aged man. J Clin Endocrinol Metab 64:81–85, 1987.

90. McKnight JA, Roberts G, Sheridan B, Atkinson AB: Aging and atrial natriuretic factor. J Hum Hypertens 4:53–56, 1990.

91. Haller B, Zust H, Shaw S, et al: Effects of posture and ageing on circulating atrial natriuretic peptide levels in man. J Hypertens 5:551–556, 1987.

92. Tan A, Hoefnagels W, Swinkels L, et al: The effect of volume expansion on atrial natriuretic peptide and cyclic guanosine monophosphate levels in young and aged subjects. J Am Geriatr Soc 38:1215–1219, 1990.

93. Tajima F, Sagawa S, Iwamoto J, et al: Renal and endocrine responses in the elderly during head-out water immersion. Am J Physiol 254:R977–R983, 1988.

94. Ohashi M, Fujio N, Nawata H, et al: Pharmacokinetics of synthetic human atrial natriuretic polypeptide in normal men; effect of aging. Regul Pept 19:265–272, 1987.

95. Jansen T, Tan A, Smits P, et al: Hemodynamic effects of atrial natriuretic factor in young and elderly subjects. Clin Pharmacol Ther 48:179–188, 1990.

96. Clark B, Elahi D, Shannon R, et al: Influence of age and dose on the end-organ responses to atrial natriuretic peptide in humans. Am J Hypertens 4:500–507, 1991.

97. Or K, Richards A, Espiner EA, et al: Effect of low dose infusions of ile-atrial natriuretic peptide in healthy elderly males: Evidence for a postreceptor defect. J Clin Endocrinol Metab 76:1271–1274, 1993.

98. Huxley V, Tucker V, Verburg K, Freeman R: Increased capillary hydraulic conductivity induced by atrial natriuretic peptide. Circ Res 60:304–307, 1987.

99. Galbusera M, Garattini S, Remuzzi G, Menninit T: Catecholamine receptor binding in rat kidney: Effect of aging. Kidney Int 33:1073–1077, 1988.

100. Dontas AS, Marketos S, Papanayioutou P: Mechanisms of renal tubular defects in old age. Postgrad Med J 48:295–303, 1972.

101. Lindeman RD, Lee TD Jr, Yiengst MJ, Shock NW: Influence of age, renal disease, hypertension, diuretics, and calcium on the antidiuretic responses to suboptimal infusions of vasopressin. J Lab Clin Med 68:206–223, 1966.

102. Lindeman R, VanBuren H, Maisz L: Osmolar renal concentrating ability in healthy young men and hospitalized patients without renal disease. N Engl J Med 262:1306–1309, 1960.

103. Rowe J, Shock N, DeFronzo R: The influence of age on the renal response to water deprivation in man. Nephron 17:270–278, 1976.

104. Helderman J, Vestal R, Rowe J, et al: The response of arginine vasopressin to intravenous ethanol and hypertonic saline in man: The impact of aging. J Gerontol 33:39–47, 1978.

105. Miller JH, Shock NW: Age differences in the renal tubular response to antidiuretic hormone. J Gerontol 8:446–450, 1953.

106. Phillips P, Phil D, Rolls B, et al: Reduced thirst after water deprivation in healthy elderly men. N Engl J Med 311:753–759, 1984.

107. Phillips PA, Bretherton M, Risvanis J, et al: Effects of drinking on thirst and vasopressin in dehydrated elderly men. Am J Physiol 264:R877–R881, 1993.

108. Faull C, Holmes C, Baylis P: Water balance in elderly people: Is there a deficiency of vasopressin? Age Ageing 22:114–120, 1993.

109. Li C, Hsieh S, Nagai I: The response of plasma arginine vasopressin to 14 h water deprivation in the elderly. Acta Endocrinol 105:314–317, 1984.

110. Rowe JW, Minaker KL, Saparrow D, Robertson GL: Age-related failure of volume-pressure–mediated vasopressin release. J Clin Endocrinol Metab 54:661–664, 1982.

111. Macias Nunez J, Garcia Iglesias C, Tabernero Romo J, et al: Renal management of sodium under indomethacin and aldosterone in the elderly. Age Ageing 9:165–172, 1980.

112. Bengele H, Mathias S, Perkins J, Alexander E: Urinary concentrating defect in the aged rat. Am J Physiol 240:F147–F150, 1981.

113. Beck N, Yu B: Effect of aging on urinary concentrating mechanism and vasopressin-dependent cAMP in rats. Am J Physiol 243:F121–F125, 1982.

114. Goddard C, Davidson YS, Moser BB, et al: Effect of ageing on cyclic AMP output by renal medullary cells in response to arginine vasopressin in vitro in C57BL/Icrfat mice. J Endocrinol 103:133–139, 1984.

115. Handelmann GE, Sayson SC: Neonatal exposure to vasopressin decreases binding sites in the adult kidney. Peptides 5:1217–1224, 1984.

116. Miller M: Increased vasopressin secretion: An early manifestation of aging in the rat. J Gerontol 42:3–12, 1987.

117. Davidson YS, Davies I, Goddard C: Renal vasopressin receptors in ageing C57BL/Icrfat mice. J Endocrinol 115:379–385, 1987.

118. Miller P, Krebs R, Neal B, McIntyre D: Hypodipsia in geriatric patients. Am J Med 73:354–356, 1982.

119. Mahowald J, Himmelstein D: Hypernatremia in the elderly: Relation to infection and mortality. J Am Geriatr Soc 29:177–180, 1981.

120. Sonnenblick M, Algur N: Hypernatremia in acutely ill elderly patients: Role of impaired arginine-vasopressin secretion. Miner Electrolyte Metab 19:32–35, 1993.

121. Cooke C, Wall B, Jones G, et al: Reversible vasopressin deficiency in severe hypernatremia. Am J Kidney Dis 22:44–52, 1993.

122. Arieff A, Guisado R: Effects on the central nervous system of hypernatremic and hyponatremic states. Kidney Int 10:104–116, 1976.

123. Davis F, Van Son A, Davis P, Edwards L: Urinary diluting capacity in elderly diabetic subjects. Exp Gerontol 21:407–412, 1986.

124. Crowe M, Forsling M, Rolls B, et al: Altered water excretion in healthy elderly man. Age Ageing 16:285–293, 1987.

125. Kleinfeld J, Casimir M, Borra S: Hyponatremia as observed in a chronic disease facility. J Am Geriatr Soc 27:156–161, 1979.

126. Sunderam SG, Mankikar GD: Hyponatremia in the elderly. Age Ageing 12:77–80, 1983.

127. Booker JA: Severe symptomatic hyponatremia in elderly outpatients: The role of thiazide therapy and stress. J Am Geriatr Soc 32:108–113, 1984.

128. Sonnenblick M, Friedlander Y, Rosin AJ: Diuretic-induced severe hyponatremia: Review and analysis of 129 reported patients. Chest 103:601–606, 1993.

129. Davis FB, Boh DM, Davis PJ, et al: Factors modulating the effect of oral sulfonylureas on free water clearance. J Clin Pharmacol 22:97–101, 1982.

130. Rault RM: Case report: Hyponatremia associated with nonsteroidal antiinflammatory drugs. Am J Med Sci 305:318–320, 1993.

131. Crews JR, Potts NL, Schreiber J, Lipper S: Hyponatremia in a patient treated with sertraline. Am J Psychiatry 150:1564, 1993. Letter.

132. Agarwal BN, Cabebe FG: Renal acidification in elderly subjects. Nephron 26:291–295, 1980.

133. Hilton JG, Goodbody MF Jr, Kruiesi OR: The effect of prolonged administration of NH₄Cl on the blood acid-base equilibria of geriatric subjects. J Am Geriatr Soc 3:697–703, 1955.

134. Adler S, Lindeman RD, Yiengst MJ, et al: Effect of acute acid loading on urinary acid excretion by the aging human kidney. J Lab Clin Med 72:278–289, 1968.

135. Prasad R, Kinsella JL, Sacktor B: Renal adaptation to metabolic acidosis in senescent rats. Am J Physiol 255:F1183–F1190, 1988.

136. Shock NW, Yiengst MJ: Experimental displacement of the acid-base equilibrium of the blood of aged males. Fed Proc 7:114–115, 1948.

137. Shock NW, Yiengst MJ: Age changes in the acid-base equilibrium of the blood of males. J Gerontol 5:1–4, 1950.

138. Allen TH, Anderson EC, Langham WH: Total body potassium and gross body composition in relation to age. J Gerontol 15:348–357, 1960.

139. Sagild U: Total exchangeable potassium in normal subjects with special reference to changes with age. Scand J Clin Lab Invest 8:44–50, 1956.

140. Ford GA, Blaschke T, Wiswell R, Hoffman B: Effect of aging on changes in plasma potassium during exercise. J Gerontol 48:M140–M145, 1993.

141. Bengele HH, Mathias R, Perkins JH, et al: Impaired renal and extrarenal potassium adaptation in old rats. Kidney Int 23:684–690, 1983.

142. DeFronzo RA: Hyperkalemia and hyporeninemic hypoaldosteronism. Kidney Int 17:118–134, 1980.

143. Meier DE, Myers WM, Swenson R, Bennet WM: Indomethacin-associated hyperkalemia in the elderly. J Am Geriatr Soc 31:371–373, 1983.

144. Mor R, Pitlik S, Rosenfeld JB: Indomethacin- and Moduretic-induced hyperkalemia. Isr J Med Sci 19:535–537, 1983.

145. Walmsley RN, White GH, Cain M, et al: Hyperkalemia in the elderly. Clin Chem 30:1409–1412, 1984.

146. Alevizaki CC, Ikkos DG, Singheakis P: Progressive decrease of true intestinal calcium absorption with age in normal man. J Nucl Med 14:760–762, 1973.

147. Ambrecht HJ, Gross CJ, Zenser TV: Effect of dietary calcium and phosphorus restriction on calcium and phosphorus balance in young and old rats. Arch Biochem Biophys 210:179–185, 1981.

148. Armbrecht HJ, Zenser TV, Bruns MEH, Davis BB: Effect of age on intestinal calcium absorption and adaptation to dietary calcium. Am J Physiol 236:E769–E774, 1979.

149. Armbrecht HJ, Zenser TV, Davis BB: Effect of vitamin D metabolites on intestinal calcium absorption and calcium-binding protein in young and adult rats. Endocrinology 106:469–475, 1980.

150. Avioli LV, McDonald JE, Won Lee S: The influence of age on the intestinal absorption of ⁴⁷Ca in women and its relation to ⁴⁷Ca absorption in postmenopausal osteoporosis. J Clin Invest 41:1960–1967, 1965.

151. Bullamore JR, Wilkinson R, Gallahger JC, Nordin BEC: Effect of age on calcium absorption. Lancet 2:535–537, 1970.

152. Horst RL, DeLuca HF, Jorgensen NA: The effect of age on calcium absorption and accumulation of 1,25-dihyroxyvitamin D₃ in intestinal mucosa of rats. Metab Bone Dis Relat Res 1:29–33, 1978.

153. Armbrecht HJ, Forte LR, Halloran BP: Effect of age and dietary calcium on renal 25(OH)D metabolism, serum 1,25(OH)₂D, and PTH. Am J Physiol 246:E266–E270, 1984.

154. Armbrecht HJ, Wongsurawat N, Paschal RE: Effect of age on renal responsiveness to parathyroid hormone and calcitonin in rats. J Endocrinol 114:173–178, 1987.

155. Armbrecht HJ, Zenser TV, Davis BB: Effect on age on the conversion of 25-hydroxyvitamin D₃ by kidney of rat. J Clin Invest 66:1118–1123, 1980.

156. Baker MR, Peacock M, Nordin BEC: The decline in vitamin D status with age. Age Ageing 9:249–252, 1980.

157. Chapuy MC, Durr F, Chapuy P. Age-related changes in parathyroid hormone and 25 hydroxycholecalciferol levels. J Gerontol 38:19–22, 1983.

158. Francis RM, Peacock M, Storer JH, et al: Calcium malabsorption in the elderly: The effect of treatment with oral 25-hydroxyvitamin $D_3$. Eur J Clin Invest 13:391–396, 1983.

159. Gallagher JC, Lawrence Riggs B, Eisman J, et al: Intestinal calcium absorption and serum vitamin D metabolites in normal subjects and osteoporotic patients. J Clin Invest 64:729–736, 1979.

160. Ishida M, Bulos M, Takamoto S, Sacktor B: Hydroxylation of 25-hydroxy vitamin $D_3$ by renal mitochondria from rats of different ages. Endocrinology 121:443–448, 1987.

161. Riggs L, Hamstra A, DeLuca HF: Assessment of 25-hydroxyvitamin $1\alpha$-hydroxylase reserve in postmenopausal osteoporosis by administration of parathyroid extract. J Clin Endocrinol Metab 53:833–835, 1981.

162. Sorensen OH, Lumholtz B, Lund B, et al: Acute effects of parathyroid hormone on vitamin D metabolism in patients with the bone loss of aging. J Clin Endocrinol Metab 54:1258–1261, 1982.

163. Tsai KS, Heath H, Kumar R, Riggs BL: Impaired vitamin D metabolism with aging in women. J Clin Invest 73:1668–1672, 1984.

164. Armbrecht HJ, Zenser TV, Gross CJ, Davis BB: Adaptation to dietary calcium and phosphorus restriction changes with age in the rat. Am J Physiol 239:E322–E327, 1980.

165. Corman B, Pratz J, Poujeol P: Changes in anatomy, glomerular filtration, and solute excretion in aging rat kidney. Am J Physiol 248:R282–R287, 1985.

166. Corman B, Michel JB: Glomerular filtration, renal blood flow, and solute excretion in conscious aging rats. Am J Physiol 253:R555–R560, 1987.

167. Haramati A, Mulroney S, Sacktor B. Age-related decrease in the tubular capacity for phosphate reabsorption in the rat. Kidney Int 31:349, 1987. Abstract.

168. Kiebzak GM, Sacktor B: Effect of age on renal conservation of phosphate in the rat. Am J Physiol 251:F399–F407, 1986.

169. Lee DBN, Yanagawa N, Jo O: Phosphaturia of aging: Studies on mechanisms. Adv Exp Med Biol 178:103–108, 1984.

170. Naafs MAB, Fischer HRA, Koorevaar G, et al: The effect of age on the renal response to PTH infusion. Calcif Tissue Int 41:262–266, 1987.

171. Caverzasio J, Murer H, Fleisch H, Bonjour JP: Phosphate transport in brush border vesicles isolated from renal cortex of young growing and adult rats. Comparison with whole kidney data. Pflugers Arch 394:217–221, 1982.

172. Marcus R, Madvig P, Young G: Age-related changes in parathyroid hormone and parathyroid hormone action in normal humans. J Clin Endocrinol Metab 58:223–230, 1984.

173. Wiske PS, Epstein S, Bell NH, et al: Increases in immunoreactive parathyroid hormone with age. N Engl J Med 30:1419–1421, 1979.

174. Chen ML, King RS, Armbrecht HJ: Sodium-dependent phosphate transport in primary cultures of renal tubule cells from young and adult rats. J Cell Physiol 143:488–493, 1990.

175. Grinna LS: Age-related changes in the lipids of the microsomal and mitchondrial membranes of rat liver and kidney. Mech Ageing Dev 6:197–205, 1977.

176. Grinna LS, Barber AA: Age-related changes in membrane lipid content and enzyme activities. Biochim Biophys Acta 288:347–353, 1972.

177. Pratz J, Corman B: Age-related changes in enzyme activities, protein content and lipid composition of rat kidney brush-border membrane. Biochim Biophys Acta 814:265–273, 1985.

178. Pratz J, Ripoche P, Corman B: Cholesterol content and water and solute permeabilities of kidney membranes from aging rats. Am J Physiol 253:R8–R14, 1987.

179. Levi M, Baird BM, Wilson PV: Cholesterol modulates rat renal brush border membrane phosphate transport. J Clin Invest 85:231–237, 1990.

180. Kurnik BRC, Hruska KA: Effects of 1,25-dihydroxycholecalciferol on phosphate transport in vitamin D–deprived rats. Am J Physiol 247:F177–F182, 1984.

181. Liang CT, Barnes J, Cheng L, et al: Effects of $1,25(OH)_2D_3$ administered in vivo on phosphate uptake by isolated chick renal cells. Am J Physiol 242:C312–C318, 1982.

182. Brandis M, Harmeyer J, Kaune R, et al: Phosphate transport in brush border membranes from control and rachitic pig kidney and small intestine. J Physiol (Lond) 384:479–490, 1987.

183. Brasitus TA, Dudeja PK, Eby B, Lau K: Correction by 1,25-dihydroxycholecalciferol of the abnormal fluidity and lipid composition of enterocyte brush border membranes in vitamin D–deprived rats. J Biol Chem 261:16404–16409, 1986.

184. Tsutsumi M, Alvarez V, Avioli LV, et al: Effect of 1,25-dihydroxy vitamin $D_3$ on phospholipid composition of rat renal brush border membrane. Am J Physiol 249:F117–F123, 1985.

185. Meyrier A, Buchet P, Simon P, et al: Atheromatous renal disease. Am J Med 85:139–146, 1988.

186. Rimmer JM, Gennari FJ: Atherosclerotic renovascular disease and progressive renal failure. Ann Intern Med 118:712–719, 1993.

187. Scoble JE, Haher ER, Hamilton G, et al: Atherosclerotic renovascular disease causing renal impairment. A case for treatment. Clin Nephrol 31:119–122, 1989.

188. Toto R: Angiotensin converting enzyme inhibitors and the kidney. Natl Kidney Found Lett 10:41–52, 1993.

189. Zucchelli P, Zuccala A: Ischemic nephropathy in the elderly. Contrib Nephrol 105:13–24, 1993.

190. Schlanger LE, Haire HM, Zuckerman AM, et al: Reversible renal failure in an elderly woman with renal artery stenosis. Am J Kidney Dis 23:123–126, 1994.

191. Meier G, Sumpio B, Setaro J, et al: Captopril renal scintigraphy: A new standard for predicting outcome after renal revascularization. J Vasc Surg 17:280–287, 1993.

192. Gupta B, Spinowitz B, Charytan C, Wahl S: Cholesterol crystal embolization-associated renal failure with recombinant tissue-type plasminogen activator. Am J Kidney Dis 21:659–662, 1993.

193. Cronin RE: Southwestern internal medicine conference: Renal failure following radiologic procedures. Am J Med Sci 298:342–356, 1989.

194. Smith MC, Ghose MK, Henry AR: The clinical spectrum of renal cholesterol embolization. Am J Med 71:174–180, 1981.

195. Lye W, Cheah J, Sinniah R: Renal cholesterol embolic disease. Am J Nephrol 13:489–493, 1993.

196. Donadio JV: Treatment and clinical outcome of glomerulonephritis in the elderly. Contrib Nephrol 105:49–57, 1993.

197. Falk RJ, Jennette JC: Anti-neutrophil cytoplasmic autoantibodies: A review and highlights of the Third International ANCA Workshop. Kidney 24:1–10, 1991.

198. Furci L, Medici G, Baraldi G, et al: Rapidly progressive glomerulonephritis in the elderly. Contib Nephrol 105:98–101, 1993.

199. Moorthy AV, Zimmerman SW: Renal disease in the elderly: Clinicopathologic analysis of renal disease in 115 elderly patients. Clin Nephrol 14:223–229, 1980.

200. Bergesio F, Bertoni E, Bandini S, et al: Changing pattern of glomerulonephritis in the elderly: A change of prevalence or a different approach? Contrib Nephrol 105:75–80, 1993.

201. Bidi P, Mounenot B, Mentre F, et al: Necrotizing crescentic glomerulonephritis without significant immune deposits: A clinical and serologic study. Q J Med 86:55–68, 1993.

202. Abrass CK: Glomerulonephritis in the elderly. Am J Nephrol 5:409–418, 1985.

203. Arieff AI, Anderson RJ, Massry SG: Acute glomerulonephritis in the elderly. Geriatrics 26:74–84, 1971.

204. Melby PC, Musick WD, Luger AM, Khanna R: Poststreptococcal glomerulonephritis in the elderly. Am J Nephrol 7:235–240, 1987.

205. Montolin J, Darnell A, Torras A, Revert L: Acute and rapidly progressive forms of glomerulonephritis in the elderly. J Am Geriatr Soc 29:108–116, 1981.

206. Volpi A, Meroni M, Battini G, et al: Postinfectious glomerulonephritis in the elderly. Am J Nephrol 8:431–432, 1988.

207. Moorthy AV, Zimmerman SW: Renal disease in the elderly: Clinicopathologic analysis of renal disease in 115 elderly patients. Clin Nephrol 14:223–229, 1980.

208. Fawcett IW, Hilton PJ, Jones NF, Wing AJ: Nephrotic syndrome in the elderly. Br Med J 2:387–388, 1971.

209. Huriet C, Rauber G, Kessler Cuny G, Penin F: Le syndrome néphrotique après 60 ans, considérations étiologiques d'après une série de 25 cas. Ann Med Nancy 14:1021–1027, 1975.

210. Ishimoto F, Shibasaki T, Nakano M, et al: Nephrotic syndrome in the elderly: A clinicopathological study. Jpn J Nephrol 23:1251–1261, 1981.

211. Kingswood JC, Banks RA, Tribe CR, et al: Renal biopsy in the elderly: Clinicopathological correlations in 143 patients. Clin Nephrol 22:183–187, 1984.

212. Lustig S, Rosenfeld J, Ben-Bassat M, Boner G: Nephrotic syndrome in the elderly. Isr J Med Sci 18:1010–1013, 1982.
213. Murphy PJ, Wright MG, Rai GS: Nephrotic syndrome in the elderly. J Am Geriatr Soc 35:170–173, 1987.
214. Sato H, Saito T, Furuyama T, Yoshinaga K: Histologic studies on the nephrotic syndrome in the elderly. Tohoku J Exp Med 153:259–264, 1987.
215. Zech P, Colon S, Pointet P, et al: The nephrotic syndrome in adults aged over 60: Etiology, evolution and treatment of 76 cases. Clin Nephrol 18:232–236, 1982.
216. Johnston PA, Brown JS, Davison AM: The nephrotic syndrome in the elderly: Clinico-pathologic correlations in 317 patients. Geriatr Nephrol Urol 2:85–90, 1992.
217. Baylis C, Fredericks M, Leypoldt J, et al: The mechanisms of proteinuria in aging rats. Mech Ageing Dev 45:111–126, 1988.
218. Bolton WK, Benton FR, Maclay JG, Sturgill BC: Spontaneous glomerular sclerosis in aging Sprague-Dawley rats. I. Lesions associated with mesangial IgM deposits. Am J Pathol 85:277–302, 1976.
219. Meyer TW, Lawrence WE, Brenner BM: Dietary protein and the progression of renal disease. Kidney Int 24:S243–S247, 1983.
220. Bolton WK, Sturgill BC: Spontaneous glomerular sclerosis in aging Sprague-Dawley rats. II. Ultrastructural studies. Am J Pathol 98:339–356, 1980.
221. Couser WG, Stilmant MM: Mesangial lesions and focal glomerular sclerosis in the aging rat. Lab Invest 33:491–501, 1975.
222. Couser WG, Stilmant MM: The immunopathology of the aging rat kidney. J Gerontol 31:13–22, 1976.
223. Haley DP, Bulger RE: The aging male rat: Structure and function of the kidney. Am J Anat 167:1–13, 1983.
224. Yumura W, Sugino N, Nagasawa R, et al: Age-associated changes in renal glomeruli of mice. Exp Gerontol 24:237–249, 1989.
225. Modesto A, Ah-Soune M, Durand D, Suc J: Renal biopsy in the elderly. Am J Nephrol 13:27–34, 1993.
226. Moran D, Korzets Z, Bernheim J, et al: Is renal biopsy justified for the diagnosis and management of the nephrotic syndrome in the elderly? Gerontology 39:49–54, 1993.
227. Eagan JW, Lewis EJ: Glomerulopathies of neoplasia. Kidney Int 11:297–306, 1977.
228. Donadio J: Treatment of glomerulonephritis in the elderly. Am J Kidney Dis 16:307–311, 1990.
229. Kissane JM: The morphology of renal cystic disease. Perspect Nephrol Hypertens 4:31–63, 1976.
230. Ravine D, Gibson RN, Donlan J, Sheffield LJ: An ultrasound renal cyst prevalence survey: Specificity data for inherited renal cystic diseases. Am J Kidney Dis 22:803–807, 1993.
231. Yamagishi F, Kitahara N, Mogi W, Itoh S: Age-related occurrence of simple cysts studied by ultrasonography. Klin Wochenschr 66:385–387, 1988.
232. Dalton D, Neiman H, Grayhack JT: The natural history of simple renal cysts: A preliminary study. J Urol 135:905–908, 1986.
233. Pollack HM, Banner MP, Arger PH, et al: The accuracy of gray-scale renal ultrasonography in differentiating cystic neoplasms from benign cysts. Radiology 143:741–745, 1982.
234. McClennan BL, Stanley RJ, Melson GL, et al: CT of the renal cyst: Is cyst aspiration necessary? Am J Radiol 133:671–675, 1979.
235. Beierschmitt W, Keenan K, Weiner M: Age related susceptibility of male Fischer 344 rats to acetaminophen nephrotoxicity. Life Sci 39:2335–2342, 1986.
236. Goldstein RS, Tarloff JB, Hook JB: Age-related nephropathy in laboratory rats. FASEB J 2:2241–2251, 1988.
237. Goldstein RS, Pasino DA, Hook JB: Cephaloridine nephrotoxicity in aging male Fischer-344 rats. Toxicology 38:43–53, 1986.
238. Kyle ME, Koscis JJ: The effect of age on salicylate-induced nephrotoxicity in male rats. Toxicol Appl Pharmacol 81:337–347, 1985.
239. Miura K, Goldstein RS, Morgan DG, et al: Age-related differences in susceptibility to renal ischemia in rats. Toxicol Appl Pharmacol 87:284–296, 1987.
240. Kumar R, Hill CM, McGeown MG: Acute renal failure in the elderly. Lancet 1:90–91, 1973.
241. Lameire N, Matthys E, Vanholder R, et al: Causes and prognosis of acute renal failure in elderly patients. Nephrol Dial Transplant 2:316–322, 1987.
242. McInnes EG, Levy EW, Chaudhuri MD, Bhan GL: Renal failure in the elderly. Q J Med 243:583–588, 1987.
243. Rodgers H, Staniland JR, Lipkin GW, Turney JH: Acute renal failure: A study of elderly patients. Age Ageing 19:36–42, 1990.
244. Rosenfeld JB, Shohat J, Grosskopf I, Boner G: Acute renal failure: A disease of the elderly? Adv Nephrol Necker Hosp 6:159–167, 1987.
245. Moore RD, Smith CR, Lipsky JJ: Risk factor for nephrotoxicity in patients treated with aminoglycosides. Ann Intern Med 100:352–358, 1984.
246. Lamy PP: Renal effects of nonsteroidal antiinflammatory drugs heighten risk to the elderly? J Am Geriatr Soc 34:361–367, 1986.
247. Schwartz J, Altshuler E, Madjar J, Habot B: Acute renal failure associated with diclofenac treatment in an elderly woman. J Am Geriatr Soc 36:482–483, 1988.
248. Gurwitz JH, Avorn J, Ross-Degnan D, Lipsitz LA: Nonsteroidal anti-inflammatory drug-associated azotemia in the very old. JAMA 264:471–475, 1990.
249. Schlondorff D: Renal complications of nonsteroidal anti-inflammatory drugs. Kidney Int 44:643–653, 1993.
250. MacKenzie TA, Zawada ET, Johnson M: The effect of age on urinary prostaglandin excretion in normal and hypertensive men. Nephron 38:178–182, 1984.
251. Feest T, Round A, Hamad S: Incidence of severe acute renal failure in adults: Results of a community based study. BMJ 306:481–483, 1993.
252. Oliveira DBG: Acute renal failure in the elderly can have a good prognosis. Age Ageing 13:304–308, 1984.
253. Nissenson A: Dialysis therapy in the elderly. Kidney Int 43:S51–S57, 1993.
254. Ponticelli C: Renal replacement therapy in the elderly. Q J Med 268:667–668, 1989.
255. Tapson JS, Rodger RC, Mansy H, et al: Renal replacement therapy in patients aged over 60 years. Postgrad Med J 63:1071–1077, 1987.
256. Williams AJ, Antao AO: Referral of elderly patients with end-stage renal failure for renal replacement therapy. Q J Med 268:749–756, 1989.
257. Avram MR, Pena C, Burrel D: Hemodialysis and the elderly patient: Potential advantages as to quality of life, urea generation, serum creatinine, and less intradialytic weight gain. Am J Kidney Dis 16:342–345, 1990.
258. Williams AJ, Nicholl JP, El Nahas AM, et al: Continuous ambulatory peritoneal dialysis and haemodialysis in the elderly. Q J Med 274:215–223, 1990.
259. Ismail N, Hakim RM, Oreopoulos DG, Patrikarea A: Renal replacement therapies in the elderly: Part 1. Hemodialysis and chronic peritoneal dialysis. Am J Kidney Dis 22:759–782, 1993.
260. Vlachojannis J, Kurz P, Hoppe D: CAPD in elderly patients with cardiovascular risk factors. Clin Nephrol 30:S13–S17, 1988.
261. Gorban-Brennan N, Kliger A, Finkelstein F: CAPD therapy for patients over 80 years of age. Perit Dial Int 13:140–141, 1993.
262. Wolcott D, Nissenson A: Quality of life in chronic dialysis patients: A critical comparison of CAPD and hemodialysis. Am J Kidney Dis 11:402–412, 1988.
263. Lunde N, Port F, Wolf R, Guire K: Comparison of mortality risk by choice of CAPD vs. hemodialysis in elderly patients. Adv Perit Dial 7:68–73, 1991.
264. Maiorca R, Vonesh E, Cancarini G, et al: A six year comparison of patient and technique survivals on CAPD and hemodialysis. Kidney Int 34:518–524, 1988.
265. Maiorca R, Vonesh E, Cavalli P, et al: A multicenter, selection adjusted comparison of patient and technique survivals on CAPD and hemodialysis. Perit Dial Int 11:118–127, 1991.
266. Verbeelen D, De Neve W, Van der Niepen P, Sennesael J: Dialysis in patients over 65 years of age. Kidney Int 43:S27–S30, 1993.
267. Ismail N, Hakim RM, Helderman JH: Renal replacement therapies in the elderly: Part 2. Renal transplantation. Am J Kidney Dis 23:1–15, 1994.
268. Cantarovich D, Baranger T, Tirouvanziam A, et al: 155 cadaveric kidney transplants with cyclosporine in recipients more than 60 years of age. Transplant Proc 25:1323, 1993.
269. Nyberg G, Nilsson B, Hallste G, et al: Renal transplantation in elderly patients: Survival and complications. Transplant Proc 25:1062–1063, 1993.
270. Raz R, Stamm W: A controlled trial of intravaginal estriol in postmenopausal women with recurrent urinary tract infections. N Engl J Med 329:753–756, 1993.
271. Sherman FT, Tucci V, Libow LS, Isenberg HD: Nosocomial urinary-tract infections in a skilled nursing facility. J Am Geriatr Soc 28:456–461, 1980.

272. Dontas AS, Marketos S, Papanayioutou P: Mechanisms of renal tubular defects in old age. Postgrad Med J 48:295–303, 1972.
273. Dontas AS, Kasviki-Charvati P, Papanayiotou PC, Marketos SG: Bacteriuria and survival in old age. N Engl J Med 304:939–943, 1981.
274. Nicolle LE, Bjornson J, Hardin GKM, MacDonell JA: Bacteriuria in elderly institutionalized men. N Engl J Med 309:1420–1425, 1983.
275. Nordenstam GR, Brandberg AC, Oden AS: Bacteriuria and mortality in an elderly population. N Engl J Med 314:1152–1156, 1986.
276. Nicolle LE, Henderson E, Bjornson J, et al: The association of bacteriuria with resident characteristics and survival in elderly institutionalized. Ann Intern Med 106:682–686, 1987. (Erratum in Ann Intern Med 107:124, 1987.)
277. Stamm W, Hooton T: Management of urinary tract infections in adults. N Engl J Med 329:1328–1333, 1993.
278. Abrutyn E, Boscia JA, Kaye D: The treatment of asymptomatic bacteriuria in the elderly. J Am Geriatr Soc 36:473–475, 1988.
279. Boscia JA, Abrutyn E, Kaye D: Asymptomatic bacteriuria in elderly persons: Treat or do not treat? Ann Intern Med 106:764–766, 1987.
280. Sant GR: Urinary tract infection in the elderly. Semin Urol 5:126–133, 1987.

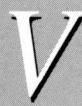

# V

# MANAGEMENT OF THE PATIENT WITH RENAL FAILURE

# 53

# Diuretics

*Christopher S. Wilcox*

This chapter on diuretics reviews their mechanisms of action, the physiologic adaptation to their use, their adverse effects, and their clinical indications. The major transport processes that are the targets for diuretic drugs have been clarified[1] and are reviewed. The effect of disease on diuretic kinetics is discussed because this can help predict the required dosage modifications. Loop diuretics and thiazides are the most widely used diuretics. Therefore, the physiologic adaptations to prolonged use of these drugs are outlined. This provides a basis for discussion of diuretic resistance, the management of diuretic resistance with a second diuretic or another drug, and the major adverse effects of therapy (many of which are common to loop diuretics and thiazides). A knowledge of these mechanisms permits the design of strategies to maximize the wanted actions on body fluids and blood pressure while minimizing the unwanted effects on electrolytes and acid-base status. The chapter concludes with a discussion of the practical use of diuretics in the treatment of specific clinical conditions.

The treatment of hypertension by diuretic drugs is considered in Chapters 46 and 54. Other chapters contain further information on diuretic-induced changes in $K^+$ excretion (Chapters 9 and 23), acid-base disturbance (Chapters 10 and 22), divalent cation excretion and nephrolithiasis (Chapters 11, 24, and 40), the treatment of the syndrome of inappropriate antidiuretic hormone (ADH) secretion (Chapter 21), and the treatment of acute renal failure (Chapter 28).

## INDIVIDUAL CLASSES OF DIURETICS

The major sites of action of diuretics and the fraction of filtered $Na^+$ reabsorbed at the corresponding nephron segments are summarized in Figure 53–1.

### Carbonic Anhydrase Inhibitors

Sulfanilamide, which inhibits carbonic anhydrase, was the first diuretic used to treat edema.[2] Currently, carbonic anhydrase inhibitors are used primarily as probes for studying renal transport mechanisms and for treating glaucoma.[3]

**Sites and Mechanisms of Action.** Carbonic anhydrase is distributed widely throughout the body. It is found in erythrocytes, kidney, gut, ciliary body, choroid plexus, and glial cells.[4] The first administration of a carbonic anhydrase inhibitor causes a brisk alkaline diuresis. The excretion of $Na^+$, $K^+$, $HCO_3^-$, and $PO_4^{3-}$ increases, whereas the excretion of titratable acid and ammonia decreases sharply. Excretion of $Ca^{2+}$ is little altered.

There are several reasons to explain why the natriuretic response to a carbonic anhydrase inhibitor is not as profound as might be anticipated for a drug acting on the proximal tubule, where the bulk of filtered $Na^+$ is reabsorbed (see Fig. 53–1). First, carbonic anhydrase is required for reabsorption of $HCO_3^-$, whereas about two thirds of the proximal $Na^+$ reabsorption is accompanied by $Cl^-$. Second, some proximal $HCO_3^-$ reabsorption persists even after apparently full inhibition of carbonic anhydrase.[4, 5] Third, much of the $HCO_3^-$ that is delivered from the proximal tubule can be reabsorbed at more distal sites even during carbonic anhydrase inhibition.[5] Fourth, with repeated administration, metabolic acidosis develops and limits the diuretic and natriuretic actions of these drugs.[6] Metabolic acidosis decreases the $P_{HCO_3}$ and thereby the filtered load of $HCO_3^-$; in this setting, acetazolamide-independent $HCO_3^-$ reabsorptive mechanisms can transport up to 96% of the diminished filtered load of $HCO_3$.[6] Production of metabolic acidosis may also explain why hypokalemia is uncommon during prolonged therapy,[7] because acidosis partitions $K^+$ out of cells.

Carbonic anhydrase inhibitors interact with proximal $HCO_3^-$ reabsorption at several steps. They can blockade the catalytic dehydration of luminal carbonic acid at the brush border, decrease the intracellular generation of $H^+$ required for countertransport with $Na^+$, and perhaps decrease the peritubular capillary uptake forces for fluid.[8] The natriuretic efficacy of acetazolamide and furosemide are additive, which confirms their independent mechanisms of action.[9]

**Pharmacokinetics.** Acetazolamide (Diamox) is readily

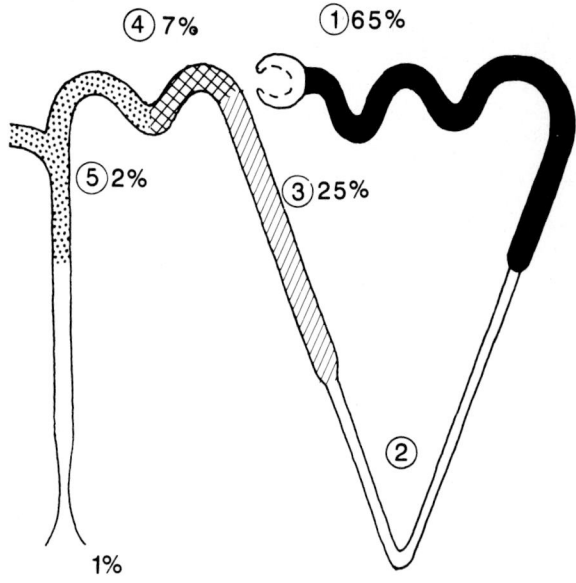

④ 7%  ① 65%

⑤ 2%  ③ 25%

②

1%

1. Carbonic anhydrase inhibitors

2. Osmotic diuretics

3. Loop diuretics (mercurials)

4. Thiazides

5. Potassium-sparing diuretics,
   aldosterone antagonists

**Figure 53–1.** Diagrammatic representation of the nephron showing the five primary sites of diuretic action and the approximate fraction of filtered Na$^+$ reabsorbed at each.

absorbed. It is eliminated predominantly by tubule secretion. It is bound tightly in tissues to carbonic anhydrase. Compared with acetazolamide, methazolamide (Neptazane) has less plasma protein binding, a longer half-life (14 versus 5 hours), and greater lipid solubility, all of which favor penetration of aqueous humor and cerebrospinal fluid. Therefore, this drug is preferred for treatment of glaucoma.[3, 7]

**Clinical Indications.** The use of carbonic anhydrase inhibitors as diuretics is limited by their transient action, the development of metabolic acidosis, and a spectrum of adverse effects. They can be used on a short-term basis in conjunction with NaHCO$_3$ infusion to cause an alkaline diuresis that increases the excretion of weakly acidic drugs (e.g., salicylates and phenobarbital) or metabolic products (urate and cysteine). Cl$^-$-responsive metabolic alkalosis is best treated by administering Cl$^-$ with K$^+$ or Na$^+$. However, if Cl$^-$ replacement produces unacceptable extracellular volume (ECV) expansion, acetazolamide (250 to 500 mg daily) and K$^+$ can increase NaHCO$_3$ excretion, provided that the glomerular filtration rate (GFR) does not fall.[10]

Metabolic alkalosis due to loop diuretics or thiazides is a particular problem in patients with chronic respiratory aci-

dosis, because the alkalosis depresses respiration further. In two studies, the administration of acetazolamide to such subjects reduced the Paco$_2$ and improved the Pao$_2$; because both Paco$_2$ and Phco$_3$ decreased, little change in blood pH occurred.[11, 12] However, a reduction in Phco$_3$ limits the buffer capacity of blood; further hypercapnia could produce a dangerous fall in blood pH. Moreover, carbonic anhydrase inhibitors can *increase* the Paco$_2$ during metabolic acidosis or exercise[13] and can cause ventilation-perfusion imbalance.[14] Clearly, careful surveillance is required when carbonic anhydrase inhibitors are administered to patients with mixed respiratory acidosis and metabolic alkalosis complicating diuretic therapy and chronic lung disease.

When used to treat glaucoma, carbonic anhydrase inhibitors diminish the transport of HCO$_3^-$ and Na$^+$ by the ciliary process. The formation of aqueous humor is reduced by up to 50%, thereby reducing the intraocular pressure.[15]

Acute mountain sickness is characterized by headache, nausea, drowsiness, shortness of breath, dizziness, and malaise, which develop after an abrupt ascent. Acetazolamide improves the performance of mountaineers and is useful as prophylaxis against this condition, probably through stimulation of respiration.[16] It can also stimulate ventilation in patients with central sleep apnea,[17] but the dangers inherent in its use in patients with ventilatory insufficiency mandate extremely careful monitoring.

Carbonic anhydrase inhibitors decrease the formation of cerebrospinal fluid and have been used to treat refractory hydrocephalus.[18] They can reduce endolymph formation and have been used to treat Meniere disease.[19]

The metabolic acidosis produced by carbonic anhydrase inhibitors diminishes the influx of K$^+$ into cells. These drugs are effective in prophylaxis of hypokalemic periodic paralysis.[20] Paradoxically, they are also useful in the treatment of hyperkalemic periodic paralysis.[21]

**Adverse Effects.** Mild adverse effects are common. Patients complain of abnormal taste, paresthesia, gastrointestinal distress, malaise, and decreased libido.[7] These symptoms can be diminished by administration of NaHCO$_3$, but such treatment increases the risk of nephrocalcinosis and nephrolithiasis.[22] The more lipid soluble carbonic anhydrase inhibitors (e.g., methazolamide and ethoxzolamide) have less potent renal actions and therefore cause less metabolic acidosis.[7]

A serious metabolic acidosis develops in occasional patients treated with carbonic anhydrase inhibitors. This is more common in the elderly and patients with diabetes mellitus or renal insufficiency, in whom the elimination of the diuretic can be greatly impaired.[23] The increase in the urine pH produced by carbonic anhydrase inhibition favors partitioning of renal ammonia into blood rather than its elimination in urine. Acetazolamide given to patients with liver disease can increase blood levels of ammonia sufficiently to precipitate encephalopathy.[24]

Carbonic anhydrase inhibitors occasionally cause allergic reactions, hepatitis, and blood dyscrasias.[25] They can cause osteomalacia when used with phenytoin and phenobarbital in the treatment of epilepsy.[26] They are teratogenic in animals and therefore are contraindicated in pregnancy.[27]

# Osmotic Diuretics

**Sites and Mechanisms of Action.** Osmotic diuretics (e.g., mannitol [Osmitrol]) are freely filtered at the glomerulus but are poorly reabsorbed by the tubules. In the proximal nephron and thin limbs of the loop of Henle, fluid reabsorption concentrates the filtered mannitol; the increased osmotic concentration diminishes tubule fluid reabsorption. Ongoing $Na^+$ reabsorption lowers the tubule fluid $[Na^+]$ and creates a gradient for back-flux of reabsorbed $Na^+$ into the tubule, thereby diminishing net $Na^+$ reabsorption.

Mannitol is a hypertonic solution that abstracts water from cells, including erythrocytes and brain cells. The increase in total renal blood flow relates in part to the hemodilution and the decrease in blood hematocrit and viscosity. Mannitol increases medullary blood flow[28] and decreases the medullary solute gradient, thereby preventing urine concentration.[29] The rise in renal plasma flow and fall in plasma colloid osmotic pressure can increase the GFR, although this increase is usually modest in humans.

**Pharmacokinetics.** Mannitol is not absorbed from the gut. After intravenous infusion, it is distributed in the extracellular fluid. It is filtered freely at the glomerulus but poorly reabsorbed. Consequently, the half-life for plasma clearance depends on the GFR and is normally 30 to 60 minutes.

**Clinical Indications.** Mannitol is useful in the prophylaxis of acute renal failure. This characteristic has been related to various actions, including expansion of the ECV; blockade of tubuloglomerular feedback; maintenance of renal blood flow and GFR; increased tubule fluid flow, which prevents tubule obstruction from shed cell constituents; reduced renal edema; redistribution of blood flow from the outer cortex to the relatively hypoxic inner cortical and outer medullary regions; and scavenging of free radicals.[30] Mannitol is reported to decrease the frequency of acute renal failure in certain high-risk settings, including cardiopulmonary bypass surgery,[31] repair of abdominal aortic aneurysm,[32] surgery in the jaundiced patient,[33] mismatched blood transfusion and shock,[34] and myoglobinuria.[35] A study of patients with chronic renal insufficiency reported that 250 mL of 20% mannitol given 60 minutes after intravenous urography reduced the frequency of acute renal failure to one third of that seen in a historical control group.[36]

Ligation of the common bile duct to produce obstructive jaundice increases the severity of renal failure after renal artery clamping in the rat; this effect is prevented by mannitol infusion.[37] Two controlled trials have confirmed the high frequency of postoperative acute renal failure in patients with obstructive jaundice; both trials reported that a mannitol infusion, begun before surgery and maintained until postoperative day 1 or 2, had a striking effect in preventing acute renal failure.[37, 38] When given soon after the development of acute renal failure, mannitol and loop diuretics may convert oliguric to nonoliguric renal failure (see later).

Mannitol can dehydrate the brain and is used to treat cerebral edema. However, overly aggressive therapy is dangerous.[39] A trial of mannitol therapy for cerebral edema complicating hepatic failure demonstrated a markedly improved survival rate of 47%, compared with only 6% in the control group.[40] Mannitol (6.25 to 12.5 g, initially is often successful in combating the symptoms of the dialysis disequilibrium syndrome.

Mannitol and furosemide are useful additions to saline diuresis in preventing the toxic effects of cisplatin.[41] Warren and Blantz[30] provided a detailed description of the dosage schedules for administering mannitol in these various clinical settings.[30]

The effects of mannitol on plasma electrolyte concentrations are complicated. The osmotic abstraction of cell water initially causes hyponatremia and hypochloremia; extracellular $HCO_3^-$ is also diluted, producing an "expansion acidosis." Later, the decrease in cell water concentrates $K^+$ and $H^+$ within cells, which increases the gradient for their diffusion into the extracellular fluid. Diffusion of $H^+$ into the extracellular fluid further compounds the acidosis. Occasionally, serious hyperkalemic metabolic acidosis develops; this condition is rapidly corrected by the kidney, which increases $K^+$ and $H^+$ excretion, provided that renal function is adequate. Later, hypernatremic dehydration may develop if free water is not provided, because urine concentrating ability is inhibited owing to the washout of the medullary solute gradient.

**Adverse Effects.** Expansion of ECV, hemodilution, and hyperkalemic metabolic acidosis are predictable effects of mannitol infusion in patients with renal failure who cannot eliminate the drug. Circulatory overload, pulmonary edema, central nervous system depression, and severe hyponatremia can develop and require urgent hemodialysis to remove the mannitol.[42]

# Loop Diuretics

**Sites and Mechanisms of Action.** The prime action of loop diuretics occurs in the thick ascending limb of the loop of Henle. Burg and Stoner[43] first demonstrated that the addition of a loop diuretic to the perfusate of the thick ascending limb decreases both the absorption of NaCl and the lumen-positive transepithelial voltage. Furosemide applied from the peritubular side was ineffective. These authors proposed that these drugs inhibited active $Cl^-$ reabsorption. Subsequent studies by Koenig and Kinne[44] and by Greger and co-workers[45] established a model of an electroneutral $Na^+$-$K^+$-$2Cl^-$ cotransport system located in the luminal membrane of the cortical thick ascending limb. A high $K^+$ conductance allows complete recycling of $K^+$ across the luminal membrane.[46] The energy for transport is provided indirectly by the $Na^+,K^+$-ATPase, which is located on the peritubular membrane and maintains a low intracellular $[Na^+]$ (Fig. 53–2).

A systematic study of 64 loop diuretics disclosed two subclasses.[47] The first included furosemide, bumetanide, and piretanide, which inhibited salt transport rapidly, completely, and reversibly when applied from the tubule lumen. The second included ethacrynic acid, indacrinone, and tienilic acid, which also inhibited transport when applied from the tubule lumen but had a delayed onset of action or incomplete reversibility. Thiazides, muzolimine, etozolin,

LUMEN                                    CELL

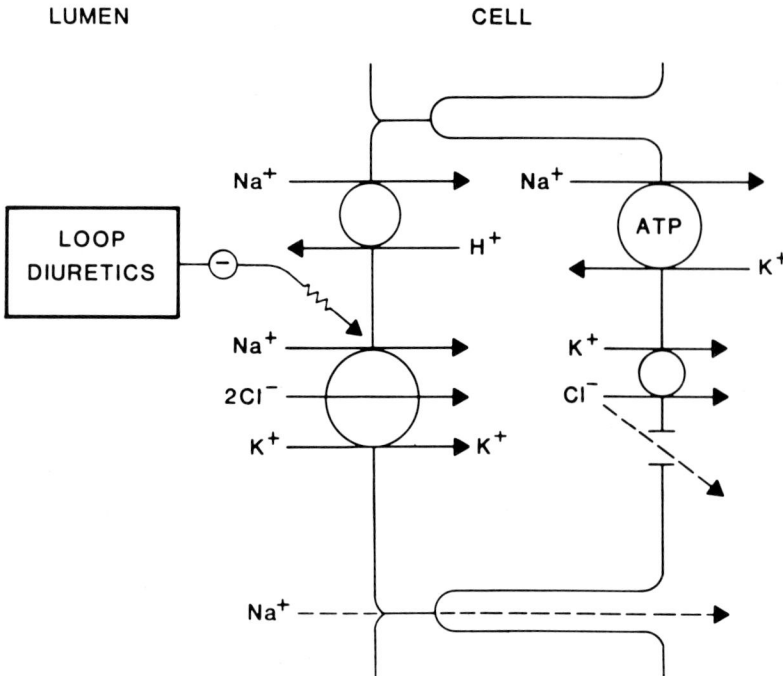

**Figure 53–2.** Cell diagram of the transport mechanisms of the thick ascending limb of the loop of Henle showing the site of action of loop diuretics. (Modified from Wilcox CS: Diuretics and potassium. *In* Seldin DW, Giebisch G [eds]: The Regulation of Potassium Balance. Raven Press, New York, 1988, pp 325–345.)

tizolemide, amiloride, and triamterene were ineffective from either the luminal or the basolateral side; these drugs either do not interact with the $Na^+$-$K^+$-$2Cl^-$ cotransport mechanism (e.g., thiazides and distal $K^+$-sparing agents) or require prior metabolic activation (which is perhaps the case for muzolimine).

The rat thick ascending limb also transports $HCO_3^-$ and ammonia[48]; this may explain the low $NH_4^+$ content of early distal tubule fluid.[49] $NH_4^+$ may be transported by the $Na^+$-$K^+$-$2Cl^-$ cotransport process. Moreover, in the rat, there is a luminal $Na^+$-$H^+$ countertransport process that contributes to tubule fluid acidification. Loop diuretics block the luminal entry of $Na^+$ but not the peritubular exit via the $Na^+$,$K^+$-ATPase.[49] Therefore, they probably reduce the intracellular $[Na^+]$ of the thick ascending limb cell and thereby exaggerate the gradient for $Na^+$ entry from the lumen to the cell by the $Na^+$-$H^+$ countertransport process. This could explain why furosemide strongly stimulates acid excretion in the rat.[50] In contrast, this effect is minimal in normal human subjects, in whom furosemide or bumetanide leads to no consistent changes in net acid excretion or urine pH.[51]

Loop diuretics can reduce the reabsorption of $Na^+$ and fluid in the proximal tubule, although this is quantitatively much less important than their actions in the loop of Henle.[52–55] Loop diuretics are weak inhibitors of carbonic anhydrase, which may contribute to the inhibition of proximal transport. However, this cannot account fully for their proximal action, because furosemide depresses proximal reabsorption in tubules perfused with $HCO_3^-$-free solutions.[53] Moreover, bumetanide, which is a much less potent inhibitor of carbonic anhydrase, also impairs proximal fluid reabsorption.[54] The mechanism of this carbonic anhydrase–independent inhibition of proximal reabsorption has not been defined.

Furosemide exerts two contrasting effects on reabsorption in the superficial distal tubule. Inhibition of reabsorption of $Na^+$ and $Cl^-$ in the loop increases the delivery to the unsaturated distal tubule reabsorption process; net $Na^+$ reabsorption therefore increases.[50] However, the normal decline in tubule fluid $[Na^+]$ with distance down the distal tubule (reflecting $Na^+$ reabsorption) is blunted by furosemide.[50] Velazquez and Wright[56] perfused rat distal tubules in vivo to obviate the confounding effects of altered delivery. They concluded that furosemide was a weak inhibitor of the thiazide-sensitive NaCl cotransport process. Neither furosemide nor chlorothiazide altered $K^+$ secretion. Bumetanide did not inhibit $Na^+$ reabsorption in these studies. Loop diuretics also inhibit $Na^+$ transport in isolated short descending limbs of the loop of Henle.[57] Microcatheterization studies have demonstrated that furosemide inhibits $Na^+$, $Cl^-$, and fluid reabsorption by the collecting ducts.[58]

Thus, the thick ascending limb of the loop of Henle is the major site of action of loop diuretics. However, actions at other segments of the nephron contribute to the natriuresis by blunting the expected increase in reabsorption in the proximal tubule (in response to volume depletion) and the distal nephron (in response to increased load delivered).

Reabsorption of solute from the water-impermeable thick ascending limb of the loop of Henle creates a dilute tubule fluid and a concentrated interstitium. Thus, inhibition of this process by loop diuretics impairs both free water excretion during water loading and free water reabsorption during dehydration.[59]

Loop diuretics increase the fractional excretion of $Ca^{2+}$ by up to 30%.[60, 61] Two mechanisms have been identified: first, loop diuretics decrease the lumen-positive transepithelial potential that promotes $Ca^{2+}$ reabsorption from the lumen; second, they decrease the reabsorption of $Ca^{2+}$ in the thick ascending limb by an NaCl-independent process.[62]

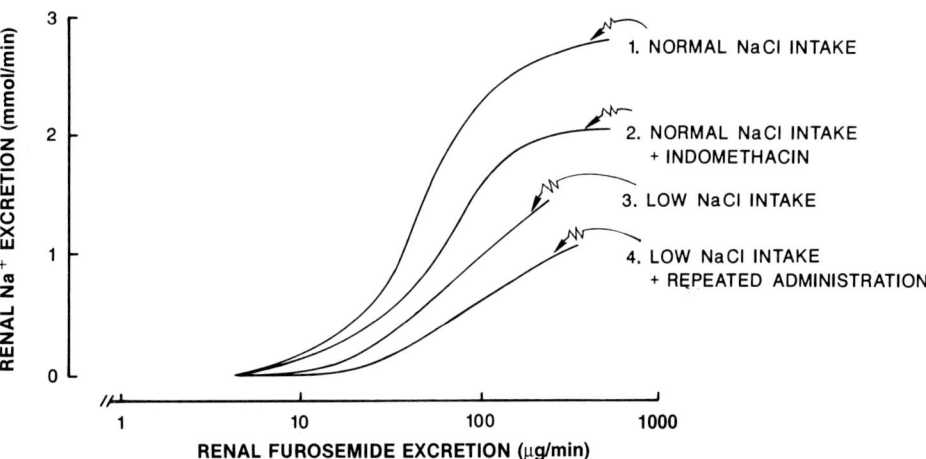

**Figure 53–3.** Relationships between excretion of $Na^+$ and furosemide (log scale) after a bolus intravenous injection of 40 mg furosemide in normal subjects. Data are shown for a normal NaCl intake after indomethacin administration, for a low NaCl intake (20 mmol/24 h), and for the third day of furosemide administration with a low NaCl intake. (Data from Wilcox CS, Mitch WE, Kelly RA, et al: Response of the kidney to furosemide. J Lab Clin Med 102:450–458, 1983; and Chennavasin P, Seiwell R, Brater DC: Pharmacokinetic-dynamic analysis of the indomethacin-furosemide interaction in man. J Pharmacol Exp Ther 215:77–81, 1980.)

The loop of Henle is identified as the major nephron segment for reabsorption of $Mg^{2+}$.[63] Loop diuretics can increase fractional $Mg^{2+}$ excretion by more than 60%.[64] This increase has been related to inhibition of passive, voltage-dependent $Mg^{2+}$ reabsorption in the cortical thick ascending limb of the loop of Henle.[65]

Loop diuretics increase urate excretion abruptly, but this increase is followed by a sustained reduction in excretion and a rise in plasma urate levels, provided that volume losses are not replaced.[66] The short-term uricosuric action may be related to a direct inhibition of urate transport by the proximal tubule.[67] The succeeding reduction in urate clearance is secondary to volume depletion, which enhances proximal fluid and urate reabsorption.[68] The plasma urate concentration is increased during prolonged therapy with furosemide, bumetanide, or ethacrynic acid, but it is maintained or reduced by two substituted ethacrynic acid derivatives, tienilic acid[69] and indacrinone.[70] Indacrinone inhibits both the reabsorption and secretion of urate by the proximal tubule.[71]

Whereas total renal blood flow and GFR are maintained after short- or long-term administration of loop diuretics to normal subjects,[72] there is a marked redistribution of blood flow from the inner to the outer cortex.[73] Animal studies have shown that the fall in papillary plasma flow is dependent on angiotensin II (AII).[74] Furosemide increases the renal generation of prostaglandins.[75] In high concentration, furosemide blocks the tubuloglomerular feedback mechanism that maintains the afferent arteriole tone of cortical blood vessels.[76] Thus, the increased AII generation that follows administration of a loop diuretic may be the cause of the vasoconstriction of blood vessels in the renal medulla and papilla; the increased prostaglandin generation and interruption of tubuloglomerular feedback may contribute to the vasodilatation of blood vessels in the renal cortex.

**Pharmacokinetics and Differences Between Drugs.** Furosemide is well absorbed; its bioavailability is 50% to 69%.[77, 78] Between 91% and 99% of plasma furosemide is bound to albumin, for which it competes with other acidic drugs. Approximately half of an oral dose of furosemide is eliminated unchanged by the kidneys, where it is secreted avidly by a probenecid-sensitive proximal mechanism.[79] Of the remainder, a small proportion is eliminated by passive diffusion into the gut,[80] and some is metabolized in the liver, but the majority is conjugated and excreted as the glucuronide.[81]

There is normally a sigmoid relationship between the degree of natriuresis and the log of the rate of renal furosemide excretion. This is analogous to a dose-response curve. Inhibition of proximal secretion with probenecid increases the plasma diuretic concentration but does not perturb the relationship between natriuresis and diuretic excretion.[82] This dissociates the natriuresis from plasma diuretic concentration. The administration of indomethacin or other nonsteroidal anti-inflammatory drugs (NSAIDs) reduces the responsiveness of the tubule to furosemide.[83] This is due predominantly to reduced generation of prostaglandin $E_2$ because a natriuretic response to furosemide can be restored in indomethacin-treated rats by infusion of prostaglandin $E_2$.[84] A reduced dietary salt intake and repeated administration of furosemide during salt restriction also shift this curve to the right[85] and thereby diminish the natriuretic response to a unit delivery of diuretic to the urine (Fig. 53–3).

Loop diuretics are chemically diverse.[86] Most are water-soluble weak acids ($pK_a$ ranges from 3.5 to 4.1). In contrast, indacrinone and muzolimine are lipid soluble. Muzolimine is markedly basic ($pK_a$ is 9.3) and fails to bind significantly to the $[^3H]$piretanide binding site of dog kidney membranes.[87] Unlike other loop diuretics, it appears to inhibit transport in the thick ascending limb from the peritubular side.[88] Its action is delayed and prolonged, which suggests that it is mediated in part by metabolites.[89] These metabolites may inhibit $Na^+,K^+$-ATPase[90] and mitochondrial oxidative phosphorylation.[91] Muzolimine is extensively metabolized; less than 10% is excreted unchanged in the urine. Because its half-time for elimination (3 to 6 hours) is relatively independent of renal function,[92] it may be particularly suitable for patients with advanced renal disease.[93]

Other differences between loop diuretics are less extreme. Bumetanide is more extensively metabolized than furosemide. Thus, it is less cumulative in renal failure; this may reduce the frequency of ototoxic effects.[94]

Most new loop diuretics, such as torasemide,[95] azosemide,[96] tripamide,[97] and piretanide,[98] resemble furosemide. Indacrinone has two enantiomers; one is a potent loop diuretic, but both are uricosuric.[99]

**Clinical Indications.** Loop diuretics are used to treat

patients with moderate or severe edema due to congestive heart failure (CHF), cirrhosis of the liver, or nephrotic syndrome when these patients are refractory to more conservative measures, such as dietary salt restriction, bed rest, and thiazide therapy. They are also used in patients with renal functional impairment (creatinine clearance $\leq$ 20 to 30 mL/min; plasma creatinine concentration $\geq$ 2 to 4 mg/dL) who are often unresponsive to thiazide administration alone. Intravenous doses of loop diuretics are used to manage acute left ventricular failure.

Loop diuretics and saline infusions can correct hyponatremia or hypercalcemia. They are used to increase $K^+$ and $NH_4^+$ excretion in patients with distal renal tubular acidosis and to prevent free water reabsorption in patients with hyponatremia or the syndrome of inappropriate ADH secretion. They can be used in patients with acute renal failure to convert oliguria to nonoliguria. These uses are described later.

**Adverse Effects.** Whereas loop diuretics normally maintain or increase renal blood flow and GFR, azotemia can develop if the diuresis or fall in blood pressure is excessive.

Loop diuretics can cause hyponatremia, hypokalemia, hypomagnesemia, and metabolic alkalosis. They raise the plasma concentrations of urate and cholesterol and can impair carbohydrate tolerance.

A drug allergy or interstitial nephritis develops in occasional patients. The danger of ototoxic injury is present when high doses of loop diuretics are given, especially to patients with impaired renal function.

Further details of these adverse effects are discussed later.

## Thiazides

**Sites and Mechanisms of Action.** The major site of action of the thiazide diuretics is the early distal convoluted tubule where they block the coupled reabsorption of $Na^+$ and $Cl^-$ [56, 100, 101] (Fig. 53–4). Thiazides do not augment $K^+$ secretion directly or alter its transport in the connecting tubule and initial collecting duct.[100, 102] Indeed, a thiazide-induced reduction in luminal NaCl entry can reduce net $K^+$ secretion by the distal tubule when the luminal $[Cl^-]$ is low, probably by limiting cell $[Cl^-]$ and thereby the coupled KCl secretory pathway[103] (see Fig. 53–4). The water-soluble thiazides (e.g., chlorothiazide and hydrochlorothiazide) inhibit carbonic anhydrase and, at high doses, increase $Na^+$ and $HCO_3^-$ excretion by a proximal mechanism.[104] Finally, thiazides inhibit NaCl and fluid reabsorption from the medullary collecting duct.[105]

Studies with radiolabeled thiazides have shown that binding to renal tissue is saturable, of high affinity, and localized to the luminal aspect of the distal convoluted tubule.[106, 107] Binding is enhanced by mineralocorticosteroids.[108] Antibodies to a purified thiazide receptor also localize to the distal convoluted and connecting tubule.[109] Thiazide receptor density is increased by a loop diuretic or thiazide, but not by a carbonic anhydrase inhibitor. This suggests that thiazides compete with $Cl^-$ for a common binding site.[110] Direct competition studies in rat renal cortical membranes have shown that $Na^+$ stimulates thiazide

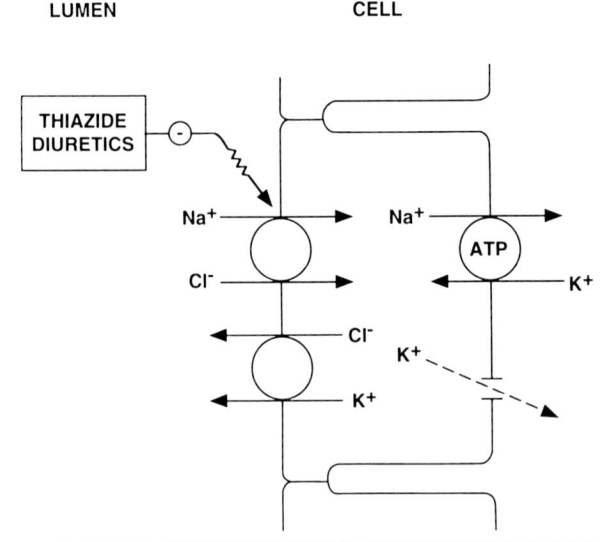

**Figure 53–4.** Cell diagram of the transport mechanism of the early distal convoluted tubule showing the site of action of thiazide diuretics. (Modified from Wilcox CS: Diuretics and potassium. *In* Seldin DW, Giebisch G [eds]: The Regulation of Potassium Balance. Raven Press, New York, 1988, pp 325–345.)

binding but at low, subphysiologic concentration, whereas $Cl^-$ is a potent inhibitor across a range of $[Cl^-]$ that may be encountered in distal tubule fluid.[111] Tran and colleagues[111] proposed a model of thiazide-sensitive NaCl transport that contains an apical transporter protein that cotransports $Na^+$ and $Cl^-$; there is competition between $Cl^-$ and thiazides (e.g., metolazone) for a common binding site (Fig. 53–5). Binding of $Na^+$ increases the affinity for binding by $Cl^-$ or thiazide.

In the absence of ADH, the osmolality of the tubule fluid delivered from the loop of Henle is reduced further by reabsorption of NaCl from the early distal convoluted tubule and medullary collecting ducts. Therefore, thiazides impair maximal urine dilution. Unlike loop diuretics, they do not block reabsorption by the thick ascending limb of the loop of Henle, which is required for the elaboration of a hypertonic medullary interstitium. Therefore, thiazides do not impair the urine concentrating mechanism.[112] An increase in NaCl excretion with impaired urine dilution but intact concentration predisposes patients to the development of hyponatremia during thiazide therapy.

Thiazides reduce $Ca^{2+}$ excretion. Three potential mechanisms have been identified. First, the addition of a thiazide to the perfused distal convoluted tubule of the rat reduces the net absorption of $Na^+$ but increases the reabsorption of $Ca^{2+}$. This has been ascribed to blockade of the luminal NaCl entry step, which reduces the tubule $[Na^+]$ sufficiently to enhance the basolateral $Na^+/Ca^{2+}$ exchange.[113] Second, thiazides stimulate $Ca^{2+}$ flux across the turtle bladder by enhancing the membrane permeability for $Ca^{2+}$.[114, 115] Third, because the thiazide-induced fall in renal $Ca^{2+}$ excretion is blunted by dietary salt loading, thiazides may stimulate the reabsorption of $Ca^{2+}$ in response to ECV depletion.[116] Thiazide therapy produces a sustained reduction in renal $Ca^{2+}$ excretion, which is accompanied by a

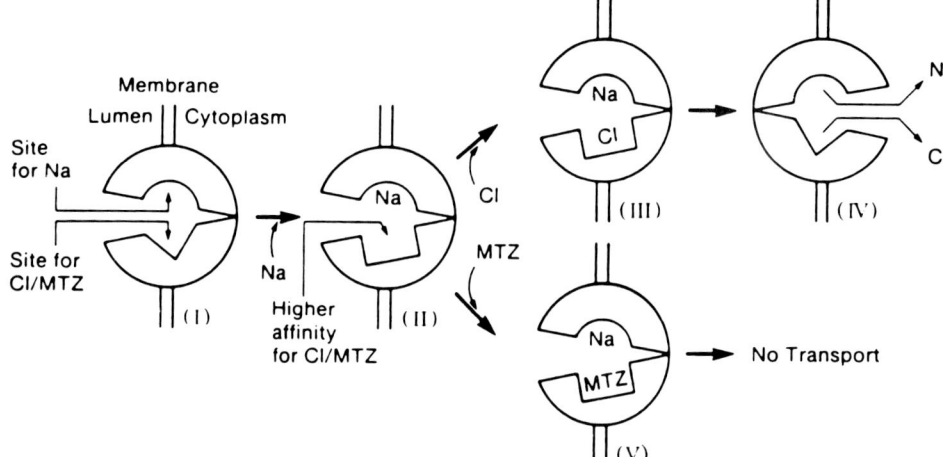

**Figure 53–5.** Proposed mechanism of coupled NaCl transport across the luminal membrane of the distal convoluted tubule and the interaction with thiazides. MTZ = metolazone. See text for explanation. (From Tran JM, Farrell MA, Fanestial DD: Effects of ions on binding of the thiazide-type diuretic metolazone to kidney membrane. Am J Physiol 258:F908–F915, 1990.)

small rise in serum $[Ca^{2+}]$.[60, 117] The parathyroid hormone level usually remains within the normal range.[117] The reduction in $Ca^{2+}$ excretion might have favorable long-term effects in counteracting osteoporosis. Thiazide therapy for 6 to 12 months has indeed been shown to increase bone density.[117] Some studies have found a reduced rate of bone fractures in patients taking thiazide diuretics,[118–120] but this was not confirmed in a case-control study.[121] Thiazides increase $Mg^{2+}$ excretion.[122]

Urate clearance is reduced during prolonged thiazide therapy, probably because of ECV depletion, which increases urate reabsorption in the proximal nephron.[68]

Thiazides may have direct vascular actions. Thus, administration of a thiazide and spironolactone to patients receiving long-term hemodialysis reduces the vascular reactivity and raises the central pressures during infusion of norepinephrine or AII.[123]

**Pharmacokinetics and Differences Between Drugs.**
Thiazides are readily absorbed from the gastrointestinal tract. They are extensively bound to plasma proteins. Elimination of hydrochlorothiazide and chlorothiazide occurs largely through the kidney, where these drugs are secreted by the proximal tubule. The more lipid soluble drugs (e.g., bendroflumethiazide and polythiazide) are more potent, have a more prolonged action, and are more extensively metabolized.[124]

Metolazone, besides inhibiting reabsorption in the thiazide-sensitive diluting segment, also inhibits proximal reabsorption by a carbonic anhydrase–independent mechanism.[125] This may account for an enhanced natriuretic efficacy.

Indapamide is lipid soluble and sufficiently metabolized to prevent serious accumulation in renal failure. Its direct vasodilating properties are useful in hypertensive subjects.[126]

**Clinical Indications.** Thiazides are among the drugs of first choice for the treatment of hypertension in patients with well-preserved renal function (Chapters 46 and 54). They can be used to combat NaCl and fluid retention in many common edematous conditions. However, their adverse effects on electrolyte metabolism are more serious when they are used to treat patients with edema. Moreover, they become less effective when used alone in patients whose creatinine clearance is less than 20 to 30 mL/min (plasma creatinine concentration 2 to 4 mg/dL). Such patients, and those with more severe edema, normally require a loop diuretic. However, high-dose thiazides retain some natriuretic action even in patients with severe renal failure, especially when they are used with a loop diuretic.[127]

Thiazides are used in the management of hypercalciuria, nephrolithiasis, and diabetes insipidus. These uses are described in greater detail later.

**Adverse Effects.** Thiazides are well tolerated. They do not usually reduce the GFR, although overly vigorous or abrupt diuresis, especially in patients with some renal functional impairment, can cause azotemia.

When thiazides are used without KCl supplements or other measures to limit $K^+$ excretion, the serum $[K^+]$ falls by an average of 0.6 mmol/L, and occasional patients have serious hypokalemia. The serum $[Mg^{2+}]$ may also fall. Hypokalemia and hypomagnesemia are particularly dangerous in patients with cardiac failure (especially those who are receiving digitalis glycosides and those with a prolonged QT interval), in patients with cirrhosis of the liver or poorly compensated edema, and in patients with myocardial ischemia or arrhythmias. Thiazides raise the serum urate concentration and are therefore contraindicated in patients with gout. They may cause mild chronic hyponatremia. This is usually asymptomatic, but when it is severe (serum $[Na^+]$ below 120 mmol/L) or develops rapidly, the hyponatremia requires urgent therapy.

Thiazides can impair carbohydrate tolerance and increase plasma cholesterol concentration. Therefore, these drugs are best avoided in patients at increased risk (e.g., those with diabetes mellitus, obesity, or hyperlipidemia). Occasionally, patients have allergic reactions characterized by rash, fever, eosinophilia, and thrombocytopenia.

These adverse effects are described in detail later. In addition, thiazides are reported to cause impotence in patients treated for hypertension.[128] They can cause a number of rare complications that include interstitial nephritis,[129] pancreatitis, cholecystitis and jaundice, blood dyscrasias (hemolytic anemia, thrombocytopenia and nonthrombocytopenic purpura, and agranulocytosis), pulmonary edema, and photosensitivity dermatitis.[130]

## Distal Potassium-Sparing Agents

Distal K⁺-sparing diuretics comprise two general classes: those that do not interact with aldosterone receptors (e.g., amiloride and triamterene), and competitive antagonists of aldosterone (e.g., spironolactone). However, the transport effects of these diuretics are similar.

**Sites and Mechanisms of Action.** Distal K⁺-sparing agents act on the principal cells in the late distal convoluted tubule and initial connecting tubule (Fig. 53–6) and the cortical collecting duct, where they inhibit luminal Na⁺ entry. The ensuing inhibition of active Na⁺ absorption secondarily diminishes the activity of the basolateral Na⁺,K⁺-ATPase. The attending reduction in intracellular [K⁺] and the hypopolarization of the apical membrane diminish the electrochemical gradient for K⁺ and H⁺ secretion.[50, 131–137] The H⁺,K⁺-ATPase normally appears to mediate a futile cycle of membrane K⁺ flux but, during K⁺ depletion, may contribute to K⁺ absorption and H⁺ secretion with the development of metabolic alkalosis.[138, 139]

These drugs cause a modest natriuresis. Their more important action is to reduce the excretion of K⁺ and net acid, especially when distal fluid delivery is enhanced by a more proximally acting diuretic and when distal secretion of these ions is augmented by hyperaldosteronism.[140] Amiloride and triamterene reduce the excretion of $Ca^{2+}$ and $Mg^{2+}$.[64]

**Pharmacokinetics.** Triamterene is well absorbed. It is rapidly hydroxylated to metabolites that retain diuretic actions.[141] Both the drug and its metabolites are excreted by the kidney, with half-lives of approximately 3 to 5 hours.

Triamterene accumulates in patients with cirrhosis because of a decrease in hydroxylation and biliary secretion[142]; it accumulates in the elderly[141] and patients with renal disease[143] because of a decrease in renal excretion.

Amiloride is incompletely absorbed. It is secreted in active form into the tubule fluid.[144] Its duration of action is approximately 18 hours. Both amiloride and triamterene accumulate in renal failure[143] and may worsen renal function.[143, 145]

Spironolactone is metabolized to active compounds (canrenones).[146] It is readily absorbed and bound to plasma proteins. It has a 20-hour half-life for elimination and takes 10 to 48 hours to become maximally effective.[147, 148]

Trimethoprim acts on the collecting duct like amiloride[149] and can cause hyperkalemia.[150]

**Clinical Indications.** Distal K⁺-sparing agents are used primarily when it is not urgent to dissipate edema or as K⁺-sparing agents in patients with hypokalemia. They are most effective when reabsorption of Na⁺ and secretion of K⁺ and H⁺ by the distal nephron are stimulated by aldosterone, as in primary hyperaldosteronism (Conn syndrome or idiopathic adrenal hyperplasia), secondary hyperaldosteronism (due to thiazide or loop diuretic therapy, edematous states, or renovascular hypertension), or Bartter syndrome.[140, 151]

**Adverse Effects and Drug Interactions.** Hyperkalemia is a potentially lethal complication of these drugs. The risk is dose dependent and increases considerably in patients with renal failure or in those receiving potassium supplements. Hyperkalemia is potentiated by other drugs that impair K⁺ excretion or raise the plasma [K⁺] $P_K$ (e.g., angiotensin-converting enzyme [ACE] inhibitors, NSAIDs, or β-blockers) or by heparin, which limits aldosterone synthesis.[140] Impaired net acid excretion can cause metabolic acidosis,[152] which worsens hyperkalemia.

Amiloride and triamterene accumulate in patients with renal failure and become decidedly more toxic.[141, 143, 145,

LUMEN                    CELL

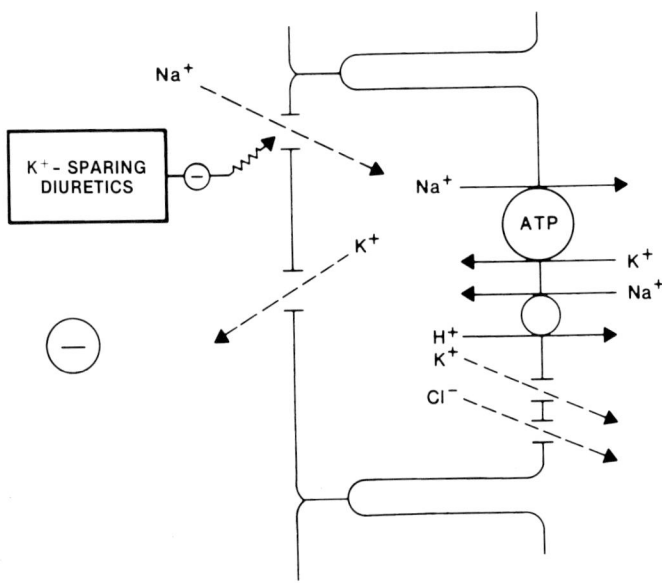

K⁺ - SPARING DIURETICS

Na⁺

Na⁺

ATP

K⁺

H⁺
K⁺

Cl⁻

**Figure 53–6.** Cell diagram of the transport mechanisms of the principal cells of the cortical collecting duct showing the site of action of K⁺-sparing diuretics. (Modified from Wilcox CS: Diuretics and potassium. *In* Seldin DW, Giebisch G [eds]: The Regulation of Potassium Balance. Raven Press, New York, 1988, pp 325–345.)

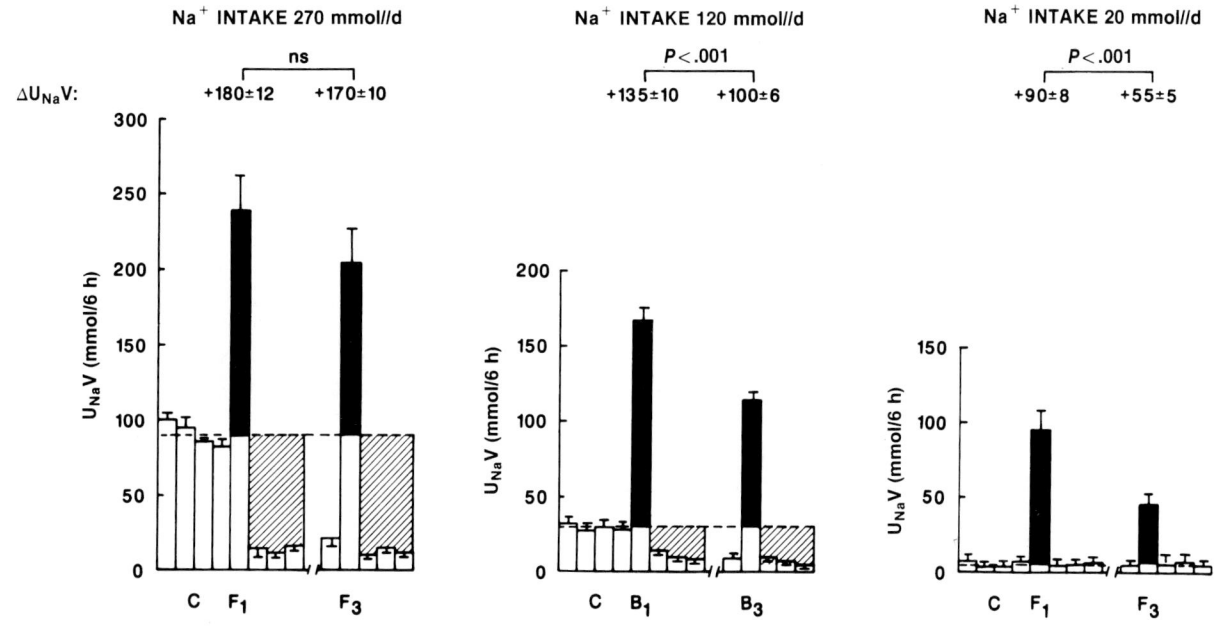

**Figure 53–7.** Diuretic braking phenomenon and the effects of dietary salt intake. The graphs show renal $Na^+$ excretion for 24 hours before and after the first and third daily doses of furosemide (F, 40 mg intravenously) or bumetanide (B, 1 mg intravenously) in groups of 8 to 10 normal subjects equilibrated to fixed daily salt intakes. The average level of salt intake is shown by the broken horizontal line. Negative $Na^+$ balance is indicated by solid shading, and positive $Na^+$ balance by diagonal shading. C = control day before drug administration. The mean ± SEM values for diuretic-induced increases in $Na^+$ excretion above baseline values are shown at the top. (Data from Wilcox CS, Mitch WE, Kelly RA, et al: Response of the kidney to furosemide. J Lab Clin Med 102:450, 1983.)

[148, 153] Triamterene accumulates in patients with cirrhosis of the liver.[154] Therefore, both drugs should be avoided in patients with renal failure, and triamterene should be used carefully in those with cirrhosis.

Rarely, triamterene precipitates in the urine collecting system and causes renal stone disease. It can cause acute renal failure when given with indomethacin, even in normal subjects.[155] Spironolactone can cause gastrointestinal distress and antiandrogenic effects (e.g., impotence, gynecomastia, or postmenopausal bleeding).[153, 156–158] This antiandrogen action has been used to treat hirsutism in women.[156] Gynecomastia is dose related and occurs infrequently at daily doses below 50 mg.[158] A related drug, potassium canrenoate, causes less gynecomastia.[146, 158]

## ADAPTATION TO DIURETIC THERAPY

Prolonged diuretic-induced blockade of tubule transport at one nephron segment elicits important adaptations at other segments. Diuretics entrain a set of homeostatic mechanisms that not only limit their antihypertensive and fluid-depleting actions but also contribute to diuretic resistance and to the development of adverse effects. Therefore, these adaptive mechanisms are considered before a discussion of their complications and clinical uses.

### Diuretic Braking Phenomenon

The first dose of a diuretic normally produces a reassuring diuresis. However, a new equilibrium is soon attained when daily fluid and electrolyte excretion no longer exceeds intake and body weight stabilizes. In nonedematous patients given a thiazide or loop diuretic, this diuretic braking phenomenon is established within 1 to 2 days and limits weight loss to 1 to 2 kg.[85] The salt-depleting actions of a diuretic are offset by this braking phenomenon.

The patterns of $Na^+$ excretion before and during the first and third days of administration of a loop diuretic to normal human subjects are shown in Figure 53–7.[159–161] During a high salt intake (270 mmol/24 h), furosemide causes a large negative $Na^+$ balance in the ensuing 6 hours (solid shading in Fig. 53–7); this is followed by an 18-hour period when $Na^+$ excretion is reduced well below the level of intake (postdiuresis $Na^+$ retention), which results in positive $Na^+$ balance (diagonal shading in Fig. 53–7) that is quantitatively equivalent to the preceding period of negative $Na^+$ balance. The natriuresis caused by the third daily dose of furosemide is strictly comparable to the first dose; it, too, is also followed by a restoration of $Na^+$ balance. Consequently, at this high level of salt intake, subjects regain neutral $Na^+$ balance within 24 hours of each dose of furosemide and maintain their original body weight for the 3-day period. A similar pattern of diuretic-induced $Na^+$ loss after furosemide, followed by quantitative restoration of the $Na^+$ loss in the postdiuretic period, is seen in subjects who have taken furosemide regularly for 1 month.[72]

During severe dietary salt restriction to 20 mmol/24 h, the first dose of furosemide produces a blunted natriuresis (see Fig. 53–7). Although renal $Na^+$ excretion reverts abruptly to low levels after each diuresis, $Na^+$ balance is not restored because of the low level of dietary salt intake. Consequently, virtually all of the $Na^+$ lost during the diuretic phase is represented as negative Na$^+$ balance for the day. Unlike the high-salt protocol, tolerance is manifested as a 40% reduction in the natriuretic response to the drug for the 3-day period. However, despite a blunted initial response and the development of tolerance, all subjects lose Na$^+$ and body weight. Bumetanide given for 3 days during a salt intake of 120 mmol/24 h (equivalent to a "no added salt" diet) leads to Na$^+$ loss that is curtailed by a combination of postdiuretic renal Na$^+$ retention and a declining natriuretic response.[162]

What mediates diuretic tolerance in these studies? Furosemide kinetics and GFR were unchanged with daily furosemide doses of 40 mg. The relationship between natriuresis and the log of furosemide excretion was shifted to the right in the 3 days of diuretic administration during a low salt intake (see Fig. 53–3), which indicates a blunting of the tubule responsiveness to the diuretic during repeated doses when dietary salt is restricted.[159]

In another study, nine hypertensive subjects received a test intravenous dose of furosemide before and after 1 month of diuretic therapy to study tolerance during prolonged therapy. Furosemide therapy reduced the natriuretic response to the test dose of furosemide by 18%.[72] This tolerance could not be ascribed to aldosterone, because it was unaffected by spironolactone, nor to ECV depletion, because it did not develop after 1 month of therapy with a thiazide that caused similar reductions in body fluids. In fact, the natriuretic response to a test dose of thiazide was *augmented* after furosemide therapy. This finding suggests that tolerance to furosemide is related to increased reabsorption at a downstream, thiazide-sensitive nephron site.

What mediates postdiuretic Na$^+$ retention? By use of Li$^+$ as a marker of proximal Na$^+$ reabsorption, Na$^+$ retention has been ascribed to a reduced delivery of Na$^+$ and fluid from the proximal tubule and an increase in the fractional reabsorption of Na$^+$ in the distal nephron.[163] Furosemide activates the renin-angiotensin-aldosterone (RAA) axis[160] and sympathetic nervous system.[161] However, postdiuretic Na$^+$ retention is not blunted by doses of an ACE inhibitor sufficient to prevent any changes in AII concentration[160] or by prazosin, which blocks $\alpha_1$-adrenergic receptors,[161] when these drugs are given individually or in combination. A Ca$^{2+}$ entry blocking drug, which itself is natriuretic, also fails to modify postdiuretic renal Na$^+$ retention.[162]

Rats receiving prolonged infusions of loop diuretics have considerable structural hypertrophy of the distal convoluted tubule, connecting tubule, and intercalated cells of the collecting duct[164–167] with increased Na$^+$,K$^+$-ATPase[168] or H$^+$-ATPase[166] activity. There is a rapid increase in Na$^+$,K$^+$-ATPase activity in rat cortical collecting duct segments after an increase in cell [Na$^+$]. This effect, which is probably due to mobilization of a latent pool of enzyme in the cell,[169] could explain the increase in Na$^+$,K$^+$-ATPase in the distal nephron during increased delivery and reabsorption of Na$^+$ because of blockade of reabsorption upstream. Hydrochlorothiazide increases Na$^+$,K$^+$-ATPase only in the cortical collecting ducts.[170] Microperfusion studies of rats adapted to prolonged diuretic infusion have shown enhanced rates of distal nephron Na$^+$ and Cl$^-$ absorption and K$^+$ secretion that are independent of aldosterone.[165, 171] Therefore, diuretics can induce structural and functional

adaptations of downstream nephron segments in response to the increased rates of NaCl delivered. Nephronal adaptation may contribute to postdiuretic Na$^+$ retention and tolerance in humans and could explain the inappropriate renal Na$^+$ retention that can persist up to 2 weeks after diuretic therapy is stopped abruptly.[172]

Studies have investigated the role of ECV depletion in postdiuretic Na$^+$ retention.[173] Administration of bumetanide during administration of fluid, Na$^+$, Cl$^-$, and K$^+$ at a rate adjusted to obviate any fluid or electrolyte depletion prevents postdiuretic Na$^+$ retention (Fig. 53–8A). This highlights the critical role of ECV depletion in triggering postdiuretic Na$^+$ retention. In a second protocol, subjects eliminated almost all of a modest (100 mmol) NaCl load in 2 days, yet when the same load was delivered after administration of bumetanide with simultaneous fluid and electrolyte infusion to obviate losses, virtually none was eliminated (Fig. 53–8B). This demonstrates that diuretics may entrain an ECV-independent component of Na$^+$ retention that is apparent when distal delivery is enhanced, as during NaCl loading.

There are four potential clinical implications from these studies. First, dietary salt intake should be restricted even in subjects receiving treatment with powerful loop diuretics to obviate postdiuretic Na$^+$ retention and to ensure the development of a negative Na$^+$ balance. Second, although subjects receiving one type of diuretic become tolerant of its actions, they may be particularly responsive to another type of diuretic that acts on a nephron segment farther downstream. Third, diuretic therapy should not be stopped abruptly unless dietary salt intake is effectively curtailed because the adaptive mechanisms limiting Na$^+$ excretion persist for some time after prolonged diuretic use. Rather, diuretics should be withdrawn gradually during dietary salt restriction.[174] Fourth, selection of a diuretic with a prolonged action, or giving the diuretic more frequently, may enhance NaCl loss by limiting the time available for postdiuretic Na$^+$ retention. Indeed, a continuous infusion of a loop diuretic has been shown to be more effective than the same dose given as a bolus injection to volunteers,[175] to patients with cardiac disease,[176] and to those with chronic renal failure[177] despite a similar delivery of diuretic to the urine.

## Humoral and Neuronal Modulators of the Response to Diuretics

### RENIN-ANGIOTENSIN-ALDOSTERONE AXIS

Diuretic therapy causes a sustained increase in plasma renin activity and plasma aldosterone concentration. The increase in plasma AII is not primarily responsible for postdiuretic Na$^+$ retention.[160, 161] The initial increase in renin secretion caused by loop diuretics is independent of volume depletion or the sympathetic nervous system and is related to inhibition of NaCl reabsorption at the macula densa segment.[178] In addition, loop diuretics stimulate renal prostacyclin release, which promotes renin secretion.[179] However, there follows a phase of renin secretion common to

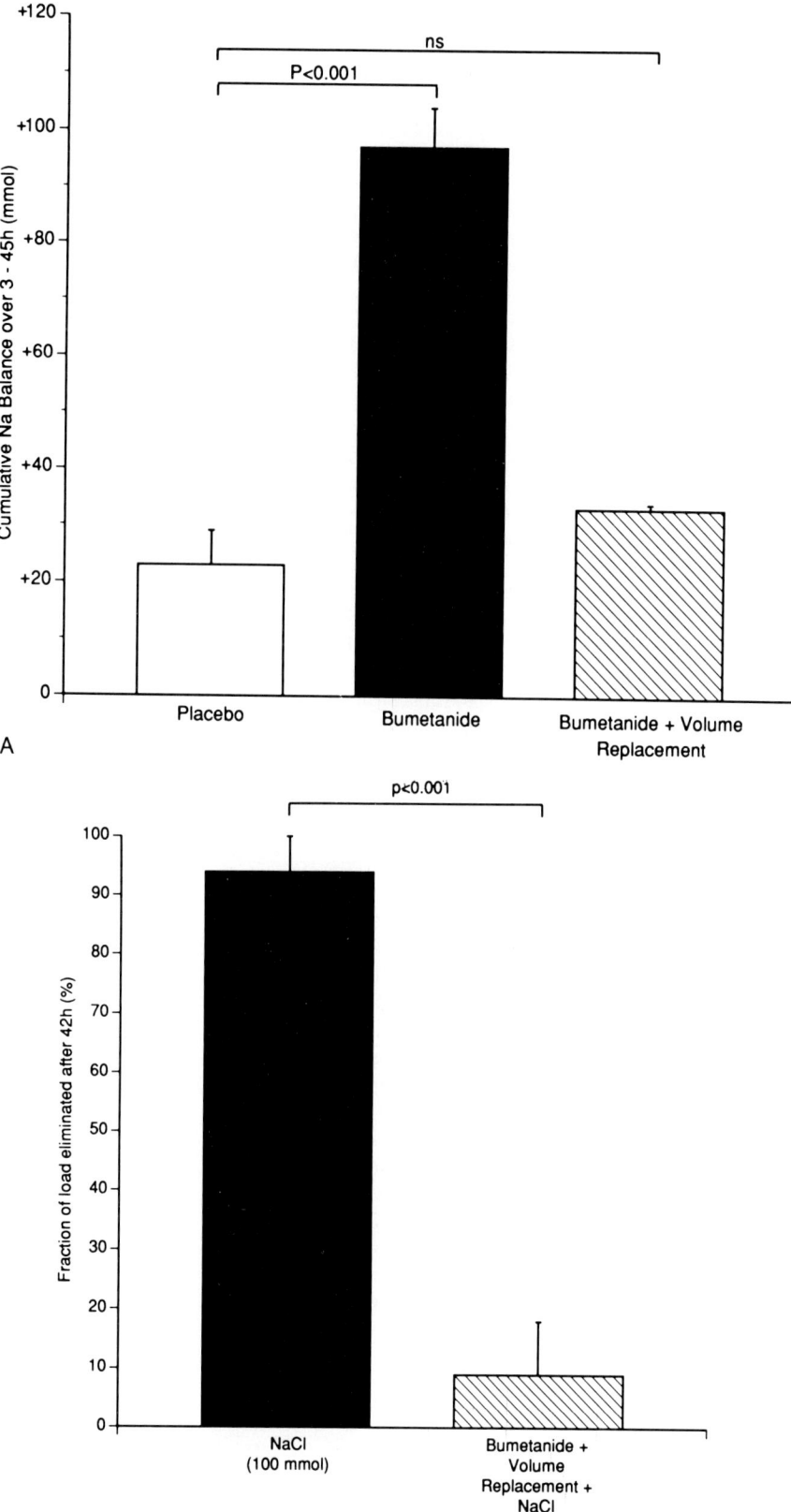

**Figure 53–8.** Mean ± SEM values for cumulative Na⁺ balance of eight normal volunteers studied for 3 to 45 hours after administration of bumetanide. In *A*, results are shown after administration of a placebo; bumetanide (1 mg intravenously) alone; or bumetanide with simultaneous infusion of fluid, Na⁺, K⁺, and Cl⁻ to prevent volume or electrolyte depletion. In *B*, results are shown after administration of a 100 mmol NaCl load given alone or after bumetanide (1 mg intravenously) and infusion of fluid, Na⁺, K⁺, and Cl⁻ to prevent volume and electrolyte depletion. (From Almeshari K, Ahlstrom NG, Capraro FE, Wilcox CS: A volume-independent component to post-diuretic sodium retention in humans. J Am Soc Nephrol 3[12]:1878–1883, 1993.)

all diuretics that is related to ECV depletion and increased sympathetic nervous system activity.

Patients treated with diuretics and salt restriction for poorly compensated edema or severe hypertension often have sufficient activation of the RAA axis to limit the fall in blood pressure and the fluid depletion. A study of eight patients with refractory, decompensated CHF contrasted a 2- to 6-kg weight loss produced by increasing diuretic dosage with a similar weight loss produced by administration of more modest doses of diuretics supplemented with captopril.[180] Whereas renal function decreased sharply with the aggressive diuretic therapy, it improved with captopril. However, it is now clear that severe volume depletion and azotemia can complicate overzealous therapy with ACE inhibitors, particularly in patients with heart failure who are already receiving high doses of diuretics or with stenosis of the artery to a single or dominant kidney.[181, 182] Thus, the combination of diuretics and ACE inhibitors can be highly effective but requires careful surveillance.

When the RAA axis is stimulated by severe dietary salt restriction, further diuretic-induced increases in plasma aldosterone concentration can promote renal $K^+$ losses.[183] ACE inhibitors can counter diuretic-induced increases in plasma aldosterone concentration and blunt the hypokalemia associated with prolonged diuretic use.[184]

## PROSTAGLANDINS

Loop diuretics, thiazides, triamterene, and spironolactone increase the renal production of prostaglandins substantially, as reflected by changes in renal excretion.[185–187] Inhibition of prostaglandin synthesis by NSAIDs (e.g., indomethacin) can diminish the natriuresis induced by furosemide,[188] hydrochlorothiazide,[189] spironolactone,[187] or triamterene.[186] In indomethacin-treated rats, an intravenous infusion of prostaglandin $E_2$, but not prostacyclin,[84] or local perfusion of the loop segment with prostaglandin $E_2$[190] restores the response to furosemide. Indomethacin also blunts the vasodilatation of the renal arterioles[191] and systemic capacitance vessels[192] and the renin response to furosemide.[163] The blunting of furosemide-induced natriuresis by NSAIDs, which is modest in normal subjects,[193] is potentiated by salt depletion[193] and is prominent in patients with edema due to the nephrotic syndrome[188] or cirrhosis with ascites.[194] Therefore, NSAIDs may antagonize diuretic therapy in salt-depleted or edematous subjects.

Loop diuretics also increase the excretion of thromboxane metabolites. Pharmacologic inhibition of thromboxane synthesis or receptors in the rat increases furosemide diuresis.[195] Thus, thromboxane may antagonize the diuretic actions of loop diuretics.

## ANTIDIURETIC HORMONE

Because ADH (vasopressin) is released by an abrupt fall in blood volume,[196] diuretics might stimulate ADH release. Indeed, plasma levels of arginine vasopressin increase 2 to 4 hours after administration of 40 mg of intravenous furosemide to subjects who are water deprived[197] but not to those allowed access to water.[198] The rise in plasma ADH evoked by furosemide in the lamb is blunted by angiotensin

antagonists.[199] Plasma levels of ADH are reported to be inappropriately high in patients who have hyponatremia during thiazide treatment.[200]

ADH stimulates $K^+$ secretion by the rat distal tubule.[201] Because the kaliuretic response to furosemide is reduced by 40% in subjects whose ADH release is suppressed by a water load,[183] diuretic-induced ADH release may contribute to both hyponatremia and $K^+$ depletion.

## CATECHOLAMINES AND SYMPATHETIC NERVOUS SYSTEM

The first dose of furosemide increases the heart rate and plasma catecholamine concentrations.[161] Although the sympathetic nervous system is implicated in $Na^+$ homeostasis in humans,[202] blockade of $\alpha_1$-receptors with prazosin in normal subjects does not modify the response to furosemide or the ensuing period of renal $Na^+$ retention.[161] However, blockade of $\beta$-receptors with propranolol blunts the component of diuretic-induced renin release that is related to ECV depletion.[178]

The short-term renal adaptation to furosemide-induced ECV depletion has been studied in the conscious rat. Furosemide infused for 3 hours causes an abrupt diuresis, followed by a return of urine flow and $Na^+$ excretion toward baseline levels despite continued furosemide infusion.[203–205] Although the plasma levels of epinephrine and norepinephrine increase strikingly,[205] chronic sympathectomy does not alter the overall furosemide natriuresis.[204] However, chronic sympathectomy[204] or blockade of $\alpha$-receptors[203, 205] blunts the compensatory increase in proximal fluid reabsorption, but this is offset by enhanced distal reabsorption. Thus, the renal sympathetic nerves or circulating catecholamines contribute to the proximal nephron adaptation to diuretic-induced fluid loss yet are not normally required for maintenance of $Na^+$ homeostasis during diuretic therapy.

## ATRIAL NATRIURETIC FACTOR

Diuretics are often used to treat patients who have an expanded blood volume and elevated plasma levels of atrial natriuretic factor. Administration of furosemide to patients or dogs[206] with CHF reduces atrial natriuretic factor levels. Infusion of atrial natriuretic factor in the dog model promotes furosemide-induced natriuresis and blunts the activation of the RAA system and the fall in GFR. Thus, a fall in atrial natriuretic factor as a consequence of the diuretic action may be one factor that contributes to postdiuretic $Na^+$ retention.[206] These interesting studies also point to a potential therapeutic role for atrial natriuretic factor, or agents that promote its action, in enhancing diuretic action.

# Diuretic Resistance

Diuretic resistance implies an inadequate clearance of edema despite a full dose of diuretic. Common causes are presented in Table 53–1. The first step in evaluating a patient for diuretic resistance is to ensure that the edema is indeed due to inappropriate renal $Na^+$ and fluid retention rather than to lymphatic or venous obstruction.

**TABLE 53–1. Common Causes of Diuretic Resistance\***

| Cause | Example |
|---|---|
| Incorrect diagnosis | Venous or lymphatic edema |
| Inappropriate NaCl or fluid intake | |
| Inadequate drug reaching tubule lumen in active form | |
| Noncompliance | |
| Dose inadequate or too infrequent | |
| Poor absorption | Uncompensated CHF |
| Decreased renal blood flow | CHF, cirrhosis of liver, elderly |
| Decreased functional renal mass | ARF, CRF, elderly |
| Proteinuria | Nephrotic syndrome |
| Decreased renal response | |
| Low GFR | CHF, cirrhosis of liver, ARF, CRF, elderly |
| Decreased effective ECV | Edematous conditions |
| Activation of RAA axis | Edematous conditions |
| Nephron adaptation | Prolonged diuretic therapy |
| NSAID | Indomethacin, aspirin |

\*CHF = congestive heart failure; ARF = acute renal failure; CRF = chronic renal failure; GFR = glomerular filtration rate; ECV = extracellular fluid volume; RAA = renin-angiotensin-aldosterone; NSAID = nonsteroidal anti-inflammatory drug.

The next step is to assess the level of dietary NaCl and fluid intake. In the steady state, dietary NaCl intake can be assessed from measurements of 24-hour Na$^+$ excretion; creatinine excretion should be measured concurrently to assess the adequacy of urine collection. For patients with mild edema or hypertension, a diet with no added salt may be sufficient to reduce daily salt intake and Na$^+$ excretion below 120 to 140 mmol. For patients with diuretic resistance, the help of a dietitian may be necessary to reduce daily salt intake and Na$^+$ excretion to 80 to 100 mmol. Lower levels of intake cannot usually be achieved outside the hospital.

A frequent cause for an inadequate drug response is noncompliance of the patient, which can be confirmed by measurements of renal diuretic excretion. Loop diuretics act for only 3 to 6 hours after a single dose; two divided doses produce a greater response than the same total dose given once daily, presumably by interrupting the period of postdiuretic Na$^+$ retention.[159] Concurrent disease may impair the absorption of the diuretic, its delivery to the kidney, or its renal secretion; proteinuria may bind diuretics in the tubule fluid, thereby reducing the free levels available for binding to the active site on the tubule lumen. These modifications by disease are further discussed later.

Diuretic resistance may be ascribed to decreased renal responsiveness to diuretics because of renal failure or severe salt-retaining conditions. Diuretic resistance is often accompanied by a pronounced metabolic alkalosis that may contribute to resistance.[207] These patients can be responsive to the addition of a carbonic anhydrase inhibitor. Diuretic responsiveness may also be impaired by metabolic acidosis.[208]

Diuretic resistance can be managed initially with an increase in diuretic dosage. However, a progressive increase in diuretic dosage usually produces only a modest further reduction in body fluid volume and activates the RAA and sympathetic nervous systems. Therefore, dosage escalation alone is not always effective in overcoming diuretic resistance. Although interruption of AII generation and aldosterone secretion by ACE inhibition does not alter the degree of salt depletion produced by furosemide in normal human subjects,[161] ACE inhibitors can sometimes restore a diuresis in resistant patients with CHF.[180] Adaptive changes in downstream nephron segments during prolonged diuretic therapy[72, 164] provide a rational basis for combining diuretics (see next section). Finally, NSAIDs can cause diuretic resistance in salt-depleted or edematous subjects in whom even sulindac can blunt the response to loop diuretics.[209]

Strategies for treating diuretic resistance have been reviewed[210] and are described in the following section. A practical guide to the management of diuretic resistance is presented in Figure 53–9. The first step is to determine the target response (i.e., the ideal body weight, blood pressure, or cardiac filling pressure). Next, the clinical details should be reviewed to answer some specific questions. Is there a rational basis for diuretic use? Does the patient have lymphatic or venous edema? Is the patient noncompliant with the diuretic prescription or with dietary salt intake? Compliance can be assessed when necessary from measurements of diuretic concentrations in the urine; dietary salt intake can be assessed from measurements of daily Na$^+$ excretion, provided that the patient is in a steady state of Na$^+$ balance. Is there a critical reduction in blood volume or cardiac filling pressure? This can be assessed from clinical signs (e.g., orthostasis), the ratio of blood urea nitrogen to serum creatinine concentration, or invasive measurements of central pressures. Is the patient taking an NSAID? If the answer to these questions is no, the patient may benefit from a more vigorous diuresis, although this requires continuous reassessment. If this is not successful, the next step is to assess the response to a doubling of the dose of loop diuretic. If the target response is not achieved, a second diuretic acting at a more distal site in the nephron can be added. At this stage, close clinical monitoring, preferably in the hospital, is advisable. If no response is achieved, the patient should probably be admitted to an intensive care unit and be considered for a trial of intravenous loop diuretic infusion.

## Diuretic Combinations

Diuretics acting on the same transport mechanism are less than additive (antagonistic), whereas those acting on a separate mechanism may be additive or even synergistic. The basis for diuretic synergism has been reviewed.[211] The use of diuretic combinations for management of diuretic resistance is outlined in Figure 53–9.

### LOOP DIURETICS AND THIAZIDES

The combination of a loop diuretic (bumetanide) and a thiazide (metolazone) produces a synergistic effect.[212] During prolonged furosemide therapy, the responsiveness to a thiazide is augmented.[72] Patients with severe edema or hypertension that is refractory to large doses of loop diuretics can have a striking natriuretic response and fall in blood

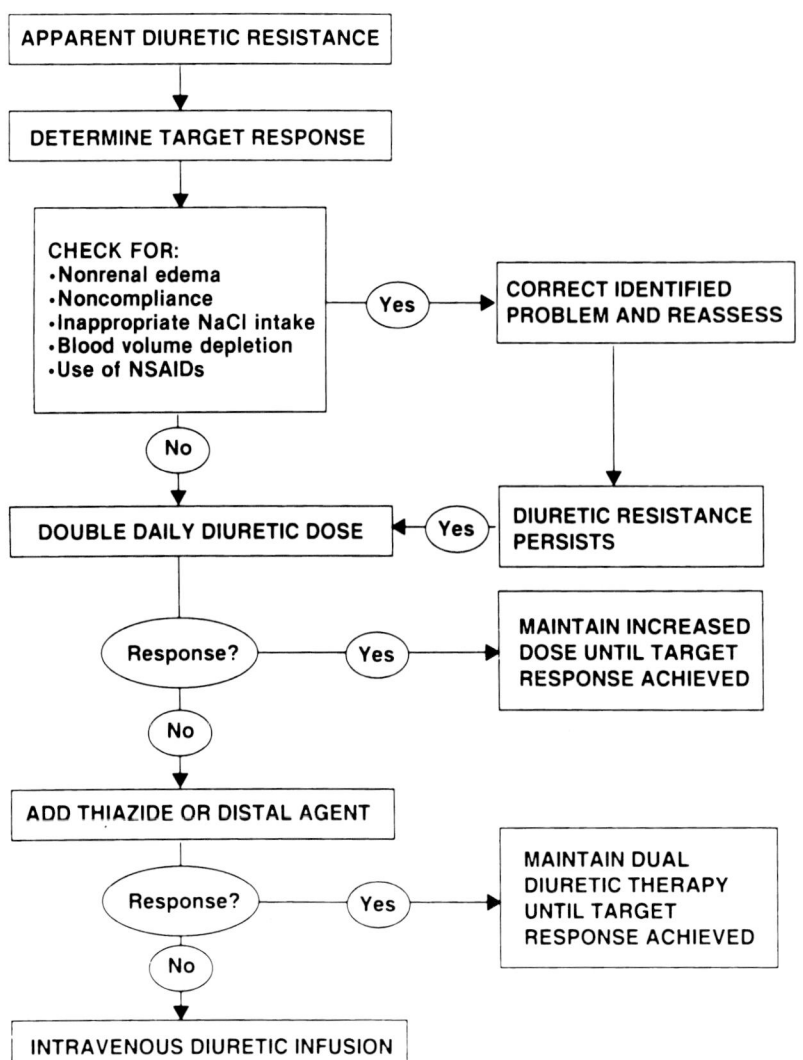

**Figure 53–9.** Diagrammatic representation of the approach to the management of a patient with resistance to a loop diuretic.

pressure with the addition of a conventional dose of a thiazide or metolazone.[213] Furosemide and metolazone given to patients with the nephrotic syndrome have a synergistic natriuretic effect that has been ascribed to a more than additive reduction by the two diuretics of proximal $Na^+$ reabsorption.[214] However, such combination therapy should be initiated under close surveillance, preferably in the hospital, because of a high frequency of hypokalemia, excessive ECV depletion, and azotemia, especially in patients with pre-existing renal impairment.[215]

### LOOP DIURETICS OR THIAZIDES AND DISTAL POTASSIUM-SPARING DIURETICS

Although amiloride or triamterene given to rats undergoing a furosemide diuresis increases the natriuresis only modestly, the excretion of $K^+$ and net acid is severely curtailed.[50] Distal $K^+$-sparing diuretics blunt or abolish the kaliuresis and the hypokalemia and metabolic alkalosis induced by a thiazide or loop diuretic in human subjects; total body $K^+$ content is also preserved.[216–218] The addition of a distal $K^+$-sparing agent is particularly useful in patients with normal renal function who are receiving a thiazide or loop diuretic and have hypokalemic metabolic alkalosis. However, the selection and management of patients for such combination therapy require careful consideration. The distal $K^+$-sparing agents are contraindicated in renal failure, in which instance they may cause severe hyperkalemia, acidosis, or further deterioration of renal function.[218]

### ADVERSE EFFECTS OF DIURETICS

Certain diuretics have specific adverse effects that have been listed under the individual drug class. This section reviews commonly encountered effects of loop diuretics and thiazides.

In general, diuretic therapy is well tolerated. However, there is a wide spectrum of adverse effects and biochemical changes. The importance of small changes in the serum concentration of $K^+$, $Mg^{2+}$, cholesterol, or urate or of changes in carbohydrate disposition remains a hotly debated yet undecided issue.[217, 219]

A Medical Research Council trial contrasted thiazide and placebo therapy in a large number of hypertensive patients studied for 5 years.[220] The following adverse effects occurred more frequently with thiazide than with placebo: impaired glucose tolerance, gout, impotence, lethargy, nausea, dizziness, headache, and constipation. However, the withdrawal rate of those receiving a thiazide was similar to that of those receiving a β-blocker, and the dose of thiazide was higher than that used presently.

## Fluid and Electrolyte Abnormalities

### EXTRACELLULAR VOLUME DEPLETION AND AZOTEMIA

Diuretics administered to patients with normal renal function for treatment of hypertension or well-compensated edema do not normally decrease the GFR.[72] In contrast, renal failure can be precipitated by overly vigorous diuresis, especially in patients with impaired renal function, severe edema, or cirrhosis and ascites. A rise in the ratio of blood urea to creatinine suggests ECV depletion. This change can be ascribed in part to increased urea reabsorption in the proximal nephron. In addition, there are steeper concentration gradients for urea transport from the tubule fluid in the distal nephron and a decreased tubule fluid flow rate that provides a longer time for diffusion. However, in the rat, dehydration also increases the appearance of urea owing to increased release of amino acids from peripheral tissues and hepatic degradation.[221]

### HYPONATREMIA

Severe diuretic-induced hyponatremia (plasma [Na$^+$] P$_{Na}$ less than 120 mmol/L) is an uncommon but serious complication of diuretic therapy.[222] These patients are often elderly women with well-preserved renal function who have been receiving thiazide diuretics for a few days or weeks. They demonstrate an exaggerated natriuretic response to a thiazide yet a diminished capacity to excrete free water.[223] Hyponatremia can develop during rechallenge with a thiazide.[223]

Thiazides are likely to cause hyponatremia because they increase NaCl excretion and prevent maximal urine dilution, yet preserve urine concentration. In contrast, loop diuretics given to hyponatremic subjects can *increase* free water excretion, presumably because of dissipation of the medullary concentration gradient that provides the force for free water reabsorption from the collecting ducts.[224]

Mild, asymptomatic hyponatremia can be treated by withdrawing diuretics, restricting the daily intake of free water to 500 to 1000 mL, and restoring any K$^+$ losses.[222] Severe, symptomatic hyponatremia complicated by seizures is an emergency requiring intensive treatment, although the ideal management remains controversial.[225–229] Central pontine myelinolysis is a dreaded complication of hyponatremia or, more often, of its treatment. It has been related to overcorrection of hyponatremia to hypernatremic levels[225]

or to a rapid correction of P$_{Na}$ by more than 12 to 20 mmol in the first 24 hours.[227, 228, 230, 231] In one series, eight elderly patients with severe diuretic-induced hyponatremia (average P$_{Na}$ 110 mmol/L) and neurologic manifestations received 3% NaCl at 35 to 50 mL/h and 20 mg furosemide intravenously after 6 hours and 24 hours of infusion. The P$_{Na}$ was corrected in 29 hours to an average value of 132 mmol/L at a rate of 0.8 mmol/L/h. Seven patients recovered from their neurologic deficit, and one died of an unrelated cause.[232] An even slower increase of P$_{Na}$ of no more than 12 mmol/L/24 h has been recommended.[226] However, this conflicts with the finding of a high rate of permanent neurologic damage in patients with severe, symptomatic hyponatremia due to thiazide therapy that was corrected slowly in 18 to 56 hours.[223] In practice, the risks of ongoing hyponatremia must be balanced against those of too rapid correction. This subject remains controversial and has been extensively reviewed.[228, 230, 233]

### HYPOKALEMIA AND HYPERKALEMIA

During the first week of antihypertensive therapy with a thiazide, the P$_K$ of those who are not taking potassium supplements falls by an average of 0.6 mmol/L compared with 0.3 mmol/L in those taking furosemide.[234] Mild degrees of diuretic-induced hypokalemia (P$_K$ 3.5 to 3.0 mmol/L) are clearly associated with ventricular ectopy.[235, 236] However, there remains sharp disagreement about the clinical significance. Some authors point to the paucity of the data relating thiazide use in conventional dosage to sudden death even in elderly, high-risk patients[237]; others express grave concern over mild hypokalemia, especially in patients taking other drugs that prolong the QT interval.[219, 238] In contrast, severe hypokalemia (with P$_K$ less than 3.0 mmol/L) clearly requires treatment. Moreover, mild hypokalemia is dangerous in patients at high risk for arrhythmia (e.g., those taking digitalis glycosides; those with left ventricular hypertrophy, myocardial ischemia, cardiac failure, or anoxia; or those with previous arrhythmias or prolonged QT intervals). Patients with hypertension are at increased risk for development of myocardial infarction, which can provoke sufficient catecholamine release to lower P$_K$ further.[239] Moreover, a depletion of total body K$^+$ stores in excess of that reflected in measurements of P$_K$ may occur in patients with severe uncompensated edema or renal failure.[240] Thus, maintenance of P$_K$ above 3.5 mmol/L during diuretic therapy is prudent, especially in patients with cardiac disease, an abnormal electrocardiogram, edema, or renal failure.

Distal diuretics and spironolactone can cause dangerous hyperkalemia. This is usually seen in patients with some reduction in GFR (especially the elderly or those given KCl supplementation), with ACE inhibitor therapy, or in other situations that promote hyperkalemia (e.g., acidosis, hyporeninemic hypoaldosteronism, or heparin therapy).[140]

Loop diuretics inhibit K$^+$ reabsorption by the loop of Henle.[43] However, this is only a minor mechanism of kaliuresis, which is ascribed primarily to increased distal K$^+$ secretion.[241] Thiazides have no major direct effect on K$^+$ secretion in the distal convoluted tubule.[102] Amiloride, triamterene, and spironolactone blunt the secretion of $K^+$ and $H^+$ by the terminal nephron.[102, 241]

Mechanisms that contribute to hypokalemia during loop diuretic or thiazide therapy are reviewed in Figure 53–10. Flow-dependent $K^+$ secretion by the distal nephron[242] provides a universal mechanism for increased $K^+$ secretion by diuretics acting at more proximal nephron segments. At low flow rates, tubule $K^+$ concentration increases sufficiently to inhibit further net $K^+$ secretion. At high flow rates, a more favorable gradient for $K^+$ secretion from the cell to the lumen is preserved throughout the distal tubule.[243]

A fall in luminal $[Cl^-]$ stimulates distal $K^+$ secretion.[244] This is an important mechanism for kaliuresis with carbonic anhydrase inhibitors that inhibit proximal $HCO_3^-$ reabsorption and thereby decrease distal $[Cl^-]$.[102]

Metabolic alkalosis, which frequently complicates therapy with loop diuretics and thiazides, increases distal $K^+$ secretion.[245] Diuretics stimulate aldosterone and ADH secretion, both of which promote distal $K^+$ secretion.[102, 201, 243]

Therapy with thiazides or loop diuretics without potassium supplements typically reduces $P_K$ by 10% to 20%. However, the fall in total body $K^+$ content is much smaller and averages less than 5%.[243, 246] This redistribution of $K^+$ into cells may be caused by alkalosis, hyperaldosteronism, increased catecholamine concentrations, or a direct cellular action of thiazides.

Diuretic-induced hypokalemia can be diminished by con-current use of KCl supplements. However, for patients at special risk of hypokalemia, an increase in diuretic efficacy, with a reduction in hypokalemia, can be achieved by addition of a distal $K^+$-sparing diuretic, an ACE inhibitor, or spironolactone.

## HYPOMAGNESEMIA

Loop diuretics inhibit $Mg^{2+}$ reabsorption in the loop of Henle.[63, 64] Distal $K^+$-sparing agents, and probably spironolactone, diminish $Mg^{2+}$ excretion that has been stimulated by thiazides or loop diuretics.[63] Prolonged therapy with thiazides, and especially loop diuretics, reduces plasma $[Mg^{2+}]$ $P_{Mg}$ by an average of 5% to 10%; occasional patients have severe hypomagnesemia.[247, 248] Cellular $Mg^{2+}$ depletion during thiazide therapy occurs in 20% to 50% of patients; it can occur despite a normal $P_{Mg}$ and is more frequent in the elderly or those receiving prolonged and high-dose therapy.[249] Hypomagnesemia is associated with diuretic-induced hyponatremia and hypokalemia that cannot be fully reversed until the $Mg^{2+}$ deficit is replaced.[250] Cytosolic $[Mg^{2+}]$ regulates the $K^+$ and $Cl^-$ conductances of cells from the cortical thick ascending limb.[251] Associated symptoms of hypomagnesemia include depression, muscle weakness, refractory hypokalemia, and atrial fibrillation, all of which are corrected promptly by administration of magnesium oxide or sulfate.[247, 250]

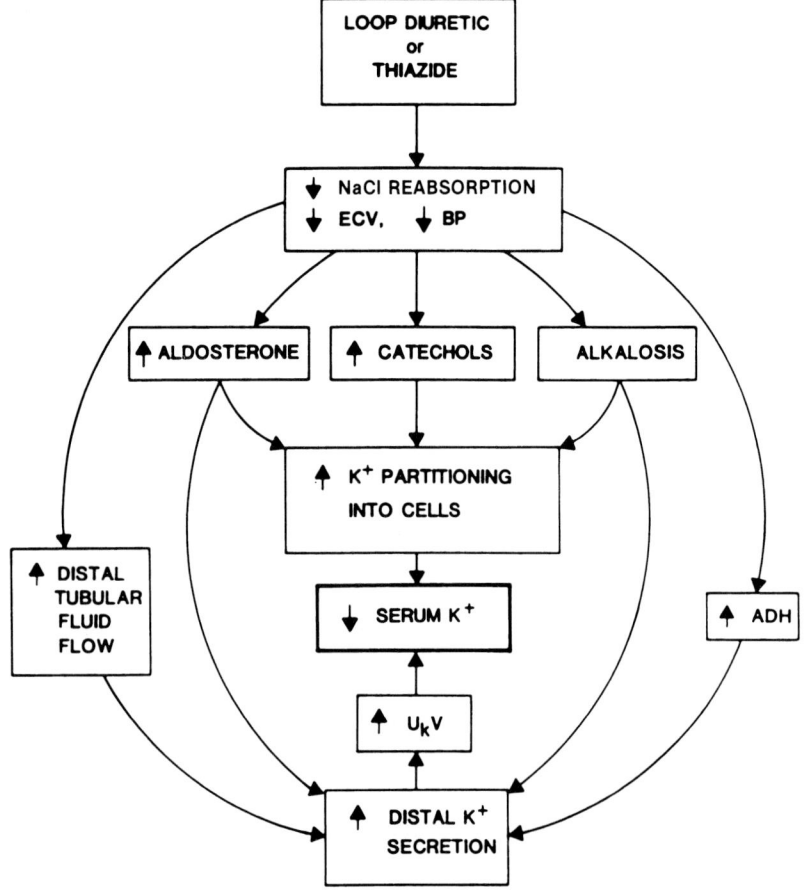

**Figure 53–10.** Diagrammatic representation of mechanisms that partition $K^+$ into cells, or increase $K^+$ excretion, during therapy with a thiazide or loop diuretic. ECV = extracellular volume; BP = blood pressure; ADH = antidiuretic hormone. (From Wilcox CS: Diuretics and potassium. *In* Seldin DW, Giebisch G [eds]: The Regulation of Potassium Balance. Raven Press, New York, 1988, pp 325–345.)

## HYPERCALCEMIA

Thiazide diuretics increase the plasma concentrations of total and ionized $Ca^{2+}$ more than can be attributed to plasma volume contraction. The initial increase in $P_{Ca}$ occurs within 2 hours; it is independent of renal $Ca^{2+}$ excretion and is probably due to the action of parathyroid hormone on bone.[252] However, during established thiazide treatment, parathyroid hormone concentrations are inversely related to ionized $P_{Ca}$, which precludes a major role for this hormone in causing the hypercalcemia.[60] Whereas some increase in $P_{Ca}$ is a normal response to thiazide therapy, persistent hypercalcemia should prompt a search for a specific cause (e.g., an adenoma of the parathyroid glands).[60] Loop diuretics usually do not change $P_{Ca}$, although they cause a prompt decrease in $P_{Ca}$ when they are given with saline infusion to patients with hypercalcemia.

## ACID-BASE CHANGES

Thiazides and loop diuretics regularly cause a metabolic alkalosis. This effect is of special significance in patients with liver disease and ascites, in whom the alkalosis may provoke hepatic coma by partitioning blood ammonia into the brain, and in those with underlying pulmonary insufficiency, in whom the alkalosis may diminish ventilation.[253, 254] The generation of metabolic alkalosis during initiation of therapy with loop diuretics is due primarily to a contraction of the extracellular $HCO_3^-$ space caused by the excretion of a relatively $HCO_3^-$ free fluid.[51, 255] Indeed, the short-term administration of a loop diuretic[51, 55] to normal subjects causes little change in renal acid excretion. A modest increase in $NH_4^+$ excretion is offset by a modest increase in $HCO_3^-$ excretion owing to inhibition of carbonic anhydrase.[256] The maintenance of metabolic alkalosis probably involves increased net acid excretion in response to hypokalemia, mineralocorticoid excess, and continued $Na^+$ delivery to the distal nephron sites of $H^+$ secretion.[253, 257] Diuretic-induced metabolic alkalosis is best managed by administration of $Cl^-$ as KCl or NaCl. When this treatment is impractical, the use of a distal $K^+$-sparing diuretic, or occasionally a carbonic anhydrase inhibitor, should be considered.[11] Metabolic alkalosis impairs the natriuretic response to loop diuretics[207] and therefore may contribute to diuretic resistance.

Carbonic anhydrase inhibitors produce a predictable metabolic acidosis that is occasionally severe. Spironolactone and distal $K^+$-sparing diuretics can cause hyperkalemic metabolic acidosis, which in elderly patients or those with renal impairment or cirrhosis can occasionally be severe and life-threatening. Therefore, careful monitoring of electrolytes is essential in these clinical settings.[254]

## Metabolic Abnormalities

### HYPERGLYCEMIA

Prolonged diuretic therapy impairs glucose tolerance and may occasionally precipitate overt diabetes mellitus.[220, 258] In one study, hydrochlorothiazide given for 3 weeks to patients with non–insulin-dependent diabetes mellitus increased the fasting serum glucose concentration by 31%; combined with propranolol, the increase was 53%. These effects of the thiazide could not be related to altered $P_K$ or insulin secretion and were attributed to decreased hepatic glucose use.[259] However, another study of thiazide-treated hypertensive patients found that $Mg^{2+}$ administration that corrected hypomagnesemia and decreased red blood cell $[Mg^{2+}]$ improved glucose uptake, clearance, and oxidative metabolism.[260] The administration of a thiazide to insulin-treated diabetic patients can provoke hyperglycemia, whereas loop diuretics appear relatively safe.[258] Therefore, blood glucose should be monitored during thiazide therapy, particularly in obese or diabetic patients. Long-term thiazide therapy generally causes only small changes in fasting serum glucose concentration; prescription of a $K^+$-sparing diuretic in addition may prevent any effects of thiazides on serum glucose concentration.[217]

### HYPERLIPIDEMIA

The short-term administration of loop diuretics or of thiazides increases the plasma cholesterol concentrations by 4% to 14% and raises the levels of low-density and very low density lipoproteins and triglycerides.[261, 262] These effects are probably due to ECV depletion because severe dietary salt restriction also increases total cholesterol and low-density lipoprotein–cholesterol.[263] However, during long-term administration of thiazides, serum cholesterol usually returns toward baseline levels in 3 to 12 months.[235, 262]

### HYPERURICEMIA

Prolonged thiazide therapy for hypertension increases the serum urate concentrations by approximately 35%. Because renal urate excretion is unchanged, urate clearance falls.[264] The fall in clearance may be related to increased reabsorption secondary to ECV depletion.[68] Hyperuricemia is dose related and does not normally cause problems unless the patient is susceptible to gout or the serum urate level is greater than 12 to 14 mg/dL, in which case diuretics are best discontinued.[265]

## Other Adverse Effects

### IMPOTENCE

A Medical Research Council trial studied some 15,000 hypertensive subjects for 5 years of therapy with placebo, thiazide, or β-blockers. Impotence was 22-fold and 4-fold higher in those receiving a thiazide than a placebo or a β-blocker, respectively.[220] Another placebo-controlled study confirmed a higher frequency of decreased libido, difficulty in gaining or sustaining an erection, and difficulty in ejaculating in patients receiving a thiazide.[266]

### OTOTOXICITY

Ethacrynic acid and loop diuretics can cause deafness that may occasionally be permanent. The frequency appears to be higher with furosemide than with bumetanide.[267, 268]

The risk of an ototoxic effect is greater when the diuretic is combined with another ototoxic drug (e.g., an aminoglycoside) or during high-dose therapy in patients with renal failure.[269] The risk is less with oral than with intravenous therapy and appears to be related to peak plasma levels.[267]

### HAZARDS IN PREGNANCY

Diuretics do not prevent preeclampsia. They may compromise the fetus by diminishing uterine blood flow.[270] Diuretics can be used in pregnancy to treat pulmonary edema. Some physicians maintain hypertensive patients with thiazides during a pregnancy if the hypertension has been controlled successfully.[271]

### DRUG ALLERGY

Photosensitivity dermatitis occurs rarely during thiazide or furosemide therapy; it is reversed after drug withdrawal.[130] Hydrochlorothiazide appears to be more likely to cause photosensitivity than are other thiazides.[272] Diuretics may also cause a more generalized dermatitis, sometimes with eosinophilia, purpura, or depression of the formed elements of the blood; occasionally, they cause a necrotizing vasculitis. Cross-sensitivity can occur with other sulfonamide drugs. Severe necrotizing pancreatitis is a serious complication of thiazide therapy. These and other rare adverse effects have been reviewed.[273] Acute interstitial nephritis with fever, rash, and eosinophilia is an uncommon complication of diuretic therapy. It may develop abruptly or some months after therapy is started with a thiazide or, less often, with furosemide. Most patients recover fully after drug withdrawal.[129] Ethacrynic acid is chemically dissimilar from other loop diuretics and can be substituted for them in patients who develop drug allergy.

### ADVERSE DRUG INTERACTIONS

Hyperkalemia in patients receiving distal $K^+$-sparing diuretics can be precipitated by concurrent therapy with KCl or ACE inhibitors. Therefore, these drugs should not be prescribed routinely in combination, especially in patients with impaired renal function or in diabetic patients.[273] Ototoxic injury induced by loop diuretics is potentiated by other ototoxic drugs, notably aminoglycosides.[273] Loop diuretics potentiate aminoglycoside nephrotoxicity.[274] Diuretic-induced hypokalemia increases digitalis toxicity fourfold.[275] Plasma $Li^+$ concentrations can increase with thiazide therapy because of increased reabsorption of fluid and $Li^+$ in the proximal tubule.[276] However, some diuretics, such as chlorothiazide[277] or furosemide,[278] with significant carbonic anhydrase inhibitory action decrease proximal fluid reabsorption and increase $Li^+$ clearance. Therefore, plasma $Li^+$ levels must be monitored closely when it is used concurrently with diuretics. Clofibrate can cause myopathy in hyperlipidemic patients with the nephrotic syndrome; furosemide can potentiate this toxic response by displacing clofibrate from the depleted plasma protein binding sites.[279]

NSAIDs may impair the diuretic, natriuretic, antihypertensive, and venodilating responses to diuretics and predispose to renal vasoconstriction and a fall in GFR (see earlier). Used together, indomethacin and triamterene may precipitate renal failure.[280]

# CLINICAL USES OF DIURETICS

## Edematous Conditions

In most clinical settings, edema results from avid renal $Na^+$ retention. Hypoalbuminemia or a raised capillary hydraulic pressure (e.g., raised venous pressure) may contribute by partitioning of plasma water into the interstitium. Because diuretics provide largely symptomatic therapy, the first aim of treatment is to reverse the cause of the edema. Such measures include restoration of hemodynamics and cardiac output in patients with heart failure (e.g., bed rest, use of inotropic agents or vasodilators, and elimination of cardiac depressant drugs) or improvement of hepatic or renal function in patients with cirrhosis and ascites, with nephrotic syndrome, or with renal failure. A dopamine agonist may improve systemic and renal hemodynamics and induce diuresis and natriuresis in patients with edema refractory to diuretics alone.[281]

Low-dose diuretic therapy is usually well tolerated and does not alter the GFR. However, overzealous diuresis can deplete the plasma volume and thereby decrease the cardiac output and renal function. Diuretic therapy for patients with advanced, refractory edema can further stimulate the RAA, sympathetic nervous, and prostaglandin systems and release ADH, all of which may compromise the desired hemodynamic and renal responses.[282] Therefore, diuretic therapy for edema should be initiated with the lowest effective dose. The clinical state, renal function, hemodynamic parameters, body fluids and electrolytes, and sometimes key hormones should be monitored. Additional drugs can be used to counteract unwanted actions. For example, ACE inhibitors can prevent the expression of an activated RAA axis and obviate fluid and $K^+$ depletion. The use of a second diuretic can produce a synergistic action, whereas the use of a distal $K^+$-sparing agent may counteract unwanted hypokalemia and alkalosis (see earlier).

The aim of diuretic therapy for edema is the creation of a negative balance for NaCl and fluid. Even in subjects without abnormal $Na^+$ retention, the compensatory response of the kidney to a loop diuretic is sufficiently intense to prevent a significant negative salt balance at high levels of salt intake.[85] Therefore, dietary salt intake should be monitored and restricted to 100 to 150 mmol/24 h in patients with mild edema. Increasingly severe restrictions of dietary salt to 75 to 100 mmol/24 h are required for patients with refractory edema.

### CARDIAC FAILURE

The use of diuretics to treat acute and chronic CHF is well established. Although the hemodynamic profiles of most patients with pulmonary edema are similar, the therapeutic approach to treatment is somewhat dependent on the cause of the left ventricular dysfunction.

## Acute Ischemic Left Ventricular Dysfunction

The primary goal of treatment of acute pulmonary edema due to ischemic heart disease is to correct or alleviate the conditions responsible for the myocardial ischemia. Therefore, in the setting of acute myocardial infarction, the emphasis is on rapid reperfusion by thrombolysis or mechanical means (e.g., percutaneous transluminal coronary angioplasty). Prompt recognition and treatment of arrhythmias or hypertension can rapidly reverse ischemia and improve left ventricular performance.

Concomitant treatment can be initiated to counter the increase in left ventricular end-diastolic pressure and the decrease in cardiac output precipitated by the myocardial ischemia. Judicious use of diuretics may be beneficial in the management of acute myocardial infarction complicated by CHF. Intravenous furosemide has important hemodynamic effects that precede any significant natriuresis. The administration of intravenous furosemide to patients with left ventricular failure due to acute myocardial infarction was found to reduce the left ventricular filling pressure from 20 to 15 mm Hg within 5 to 15 minutes.[283] This was accompanied by a 52% increase in venous capacitance. This venodilatation is blocked by NSAIDs[192] and ACE inhibitors.[284] Furosemide may also act directly or indirectly on the pulmonary vascular bed, causing a rapid decrease in pulmonary blood volume and thereby alleviating the symptoms of pulmonary congestion.[285, 286] There can be a similar abrupt vasodilating effect on the systemic circulation.[287] A significant diuresis usually ensues within 30 to 60 minutes that reduces preload and left ventricular end-diastolic pressure further by decreasing the plasma volume. These hemodynamic and renal effects can decrease the myocardial oxygen requirements and thereby decrease myocardial ischemia.

A study of first-line therapy for 48 patients with acute left ventricular failure after myocardial infarction compared the response to intravenous furosemide with the responses to a venodilator (isosorbide dinitrate), an arteriolar dilator (hydralazine), or a positive inotropic agent (prenalterol).[288] Like the venodilator, furosemide reduced the left ventricular filling pressure while maintaining the cardiac index and heart rate. The other agents increased the cardiac index but were less effective in reducing the left ventricular filling pressure. The authors concluded that the best first-line agents were furosemide or a venodilator but that they could be combined with an arteriolar vasodilator for additional efficacy.

There is a potential danger in the use of intravenous loop diuretics to treat heart failure complicating acute myocardial infarction. Although intravenous furosemide decreases left ventricular filling pressure consistently, the shape of the Frank-Starling ventricular function curve predicts little change, or a fall, in cardiac output at reduced filling pressures. Because of changes in left ventricular compliance induced by ischemia, patients with acute myocardial infarction are particularly at risk for the development of a reduced cardiac output. Indeed, intravenous furosemide has been shown to decrease cardiac output, which in patients with severe CHF may lead to hypotension and shock.[282] Patients with greater degrees of left ventricular dysfunction are likely to respond unfavorably to intravenous furosemide. Accordingly, intravenous diuretics should not be used in patients with cardiogenic shock.

## Decompensated Chronic Congestive Heart Failure

The management of patients with a dilated cardiomyopathy and chronic CHF who become acutely decompensated differs slightly from the management of those with acute myocardial infarction. Usually, there is no clinical evidence of myocardial ischemia or injury to precipitate the pulmonary edema. Acute decompensation is more likely to result from a continuing imbalance in the neurohumoral systems that regulate both cardiac and renal function. Therefore, it is rational to target these neurohumoral mechanisms with selective therapy. These patients often respond rapidly to intravenous vasodilators, which counteract the effects of elevated levels of endogenous catecholamines, AII, and other vasoconstrictors on venous and arterial beds.

A reduction in vascular resistance with a vasodilator can improve cardiac output profoundly. The addition of an inotropic agent may augment left ventricular performance further. In this context, venodilatation and diuresis evoked by intravenous furosemide are useful adjuncts in the management of acute left ventricular failure. Intravenous diuretics can improve the hemodynamic profile of decompensated patients rapidly; the ensuing natriuresis prolongs the benefit. However, acute deterioration develops in others. In a study of 15 patients with severe chronic CHF with acute decompensation maintained with oral furosemide, the short-term administration of intravenous furosemide led to an abrupt increase in the systemic vascular resistance and blood pressure and a decrease in the cardiac index.[282] In the next 2 hours, a diuresis occurred that decreased the left ventricular filling pressure and right atrial pressure and reversed the adverse hemodynamic changes. The authors concluded that intravenous furosemide had activated neural and humoral mechanisms of vasoconstriction that had contributed to acute pump dysfunction.

## Chronic Congestive Heart Failure

Diuretics can be extremely useful in the long-term management of patients with chronic CHF who have continuing edema or pulmonary congestion. Avid renal $Na^+$ and fluid retention in patients with decompensated CHF leads to pulmonary edema and cardiac dilatation. This limits ventilation and cardiac function and can create a spiral of decreasing oxygenation and cardiac output. Pulmonary edema predisposes to lung infection. Therefore, the use of a salt-restricted diet and the administration of a diuretic are rational measures. Indeed, in a study of 13 patients with severe edema due to CHF, furosemide therapy increased the stroke volume by 15% despite reducing the body weight by an average of 17 pounds.[287] The increased stroke volume correlated with a decrease in the peripheral vascular resistance and was therefore ascribed to a fall in afterload.[287] In another study, combined therapy with a diuretic and vasodilator reduced the left and right atrial volumes, corrected atrioventricular valvular regurgitation, and improved the stroke volume by 64%.[288] Clearly, this is effective therapy to counteract congestive symptoms and functional valvular regurgitation. In a double-blind trial comparing a loop diuretic or cardiac glycoside with a placebo, congestive symptoms and pulmonary capillary wedge pressure were improved similarly by both classes of drug.[289] On the other hand, because the failing heart has a decreased capacity to regulate its contractility in response to changes in venous return,[290] if diuretic therapy is too abrupt or severe, these patients are susceptible to the complications of a decreased effective blood volume (orthostatic hypotension, weakness, fatigue, decreased exercise ability, and prerenal azotemia). Therefore, salt-depleting therapy requires continual reassessment, with appropriate adjustments in dietary salt or diuretic usage and judicious use of other measures (e.g., vasodilators or ACE inhibitors) to maximize cardiac performance.

A reduction in renal blood flow and GFR often limits natriuresis in patients with CHF. However, in patients with low-output heart failure, an increase in cardiac output produced by an inotropic agent such as dobutamine does not necessarily improve renal hemodynamics. In contrast, an infusion of dopamine at a low dose increases the renal blood flow and GFR.[291] Therefore, dopamine infusion should be considered in patients whose diuretic resistance is likely to be due to a low cardiac output and a low renal blood flow.

CHF modifies diuretic disposition and responsiveness. Although diuretic kinetics are generally little perturbed in patients with mild heart failure, they can become severely abnormal in decompensated heart failure as a result of decreased cardiac output and impaired renal function.[292–295] The absolute absorption of furosemide and bumetanide from the gut is normal in patients with decompensated CHF, but they can have a marked prolongation in the time required to reach peak serum diuretic concentrations after oral dosing.[292] The slowed absorption can limit the peak diuretic concentrations in the plasma and therefore restrict the diuretic concentration in the tubule fluid and the urine to the foot of the dose-response curve, thereby diminishing the diuretic efficacy.[293] Muzolimine, which is more lipid soluble and appears to act primarily from the peritubular aspect of the tubule, should be more effective under these conditions.[296] The relationship between natriuresis and excretion of loop diuretics is unaltered in mild CHF[295] but is shifted to the right in patients with more advanced CHF; this shift implies impaired diuretic responsiveness.[294] Some resistance to the action of diuretics should be anticipated in patients with severe CHF; the dosage should be increased appropriately.

Mild CHF often responds to dietary salt restriction (100 to 150 mmol/d) and low doses of a thiazide diuretic. As CHF progresses, patients become refractory to thiazides, which are generally ineffective as single agents when the GFR is less than 20 to 30 mL/min (with plasma creatinine concentration 2 to 4 mg/dL). Larger, more frequent doses of loop diuretics and tighter control of dietary salt (60 to 100 mmol/d) are then required. For the refractory patient, the addition of a second diuretic acting at a downstream site (e.g., a thiazide) can produce a dramatic diuresis, even

in patients with impaired renal function. One study has shown that 13 of 16 patients with advanced heart failure resistant to combined therapy with a high-dose loop diuretic (bumetanide 10 mg) and an ACE inhibitor had a satisfactory diuresis after addition of spironolactone (100 mg daily).[297] Nevertheless, as patients progress through this treatment strategy, the risks of volume depletion, azotemia, and electrolyte abnormalities increase sharply. Therefore, patients with diuretic resistance require close biochemical and clinical monitoring and, when possible, additional therapy directed at the underlying condition.

Long-term vasodilator therapy with ACE inhibitors decreases the need for hospitalization, improves the quality of life, and extends the survival in patients with severe left ventricular dysfunction. ACE inhibitors improve renal function in some patients with severe CHF, thereby reducing the requirements for diuretics; however, in others, a fall in blood pressure can compromise renal function.[180] Therefore, ACE inhibitors should be carefully titrated. Meanwhile, it may be necessary to withdraw or reduce diuretic therapy to prevent orthostatic symptoms. However, the continued use of diuretics in some patients, albeit in small doses, can reduce body weight and edema further than can be achieved with ACE inhibitors alone.[298]

Decompensated CHF stimulates the RAA and vasopressin systems[282, 299] and thereby predisposes these patients to hypokalemia, hypomagnesemia, and hyponatremia. These are particularly dangerous complications for patients who are susceptible to cardiac arrhythmias. Moreover, hypokalemia potentiates the binding of digitalis to cardiac myocytes,[300] decreases renal digitalis elimination,[301] and enhances the cardiac toxicity of digitalis.[302] Therefore, evidence of hypokalemia and hypomagnesemia should be sought and corrected in patients with heart failure receiving digitalis glycosides. Hyperkalemia may result if potassium supplementation is not withdrawn or adjusted after initiation of therapy with ACE inhibitors or $K^+$-sparing diuretics. The addition of an ACE inhibitor may correct hyponatremia complicating diuretic therapy for severe CHF.[180]

Finally, certain subgroups of patients with CHF characterized by poor left ventricular compliance or with outflow obstruction (e.g., hypertrophic cardiomyopathy, aortic stenosis) may respond unfavorably to the administration of diuretics. In these patients, any reduction of preload or plasma volume, resulting in a decrease in left ventricular filling pressure, decreases cardiac output or causes hypotension or syncope.

## Right Ventricular Failure

The requirement for diuretic therapy in patients with pure right-sided heart failure is not compelling. Indeed, a decrease in venous return induced by vigorous diuresis may worsen right-sided heart function further. Moreover, patients with heart failure due to cor pulmonale have hypoxemia and acidosis that predispose them to arrhythmias provoked by diuretic-induced $K^+$ or $Mg^{2+}$ depletion or alkalosis. Therefore, diuretics should be used sparingly in these patients.

## CIRRHOSIS OF THE LIVER

As cirrhosis of the liver progresses, renal NaCl retention leads to the development of ascites and later to peripheral edema. At this late stage, renal $Na^+$ excretion is often low owing to a reduced GFR and increased renal tubule $Na^+$ reabsorption. Ideally, therapy should reverse the pathophysiologic events leading to $Na^+$ and fluid retention. However, the stimulus for $Na^+$ retention in cirrhosis remains controversial.[303–307] Some patients appear to have a reduced effective blood volume, which leads to increased levels of hormones associated with volume depletion (renin, aldosterone, vasopressin, and norepinephrine).[304] Such patients are likely to have adverse circulatory and renal responses to further volume depletion. In contrast, other patients have a normal or even an increased plasma volume.[305] Moreover, animal models of cirrhosis have shown that $Na^+$ retention can precede ascites formation.[306, 307] Diuretics would be rational in such circumstances. In practice, diuretics are reported to decrease the plasma volume and GFR only modestly in most cirrhotic patients.[308] Levy and Richard[309] found that furosemide, given to cirrhotic dogs, reduced the plasma volume initially. However, within 6 hours, the plasma volume was fully replenished. Remarkably, all the fluid lost by the furosemide diuresis could be accounted for by a reduction in the volume of ascites. Apparently, furosemide had reduced the central venous pressure and increased the plasma protein concentration sufficiently to partition interstitial and ascitic fluid into the vascular space. This prevented any prolonged contraction of the plasma volume. Mannitol was less effective in mobilization of ascites.

Micropuncture studies in a rat model of cirrhosis[307] and $Li^+$ clearance studies in patients with cirrhosis[310] concur in demonstrating consistent increases in proximal $Na^+$ reabsorption. This may be a response to a diminished effective arterial blood volume. Patients accumulating $Na^+$ also have an enhanced distal $Na^+$ reabsorption that correlates with plasma aldosterone levels.[310] This provides a rational basis for the use of aldosterone antagonists in $Na^+$-retaining cirrhotic patients.

Patients with cirrhosis of the liver have a normal or reduced natriuretic response to furosemide,[311, 312] although the kaliuretic response may be increased.[313] Therefore, they are at special risk for electrolyte abnormalities. Usually, furosemide kinetics are little perturbed in patients with mild cirrhosis.[311–315] Furosemide disposition becomes abnormal in those with advanced disease, in whom the rate of diuretic absorption from the gut is slowed,[316] its volume of distribution is increased because of hypoalbuminemia and an expanded ECV, and its elimination is delayed because of a fall in renal clearance.[313, 317] However, in patients with hepatitis and preserved renal function, the renal clearance of loop diuretics, triamterene, and amiloride may be increased because of a decrease in nonrenal clearance by the diseased liver.[318] In poorly compensated patients, a decrease in the natriuretic response to furosemide correlates with a decrease in the rate of renal furosemide elimination.[319, 320]

Diuretic resistance in early cirrhosis is largely due to decreased responsiveness to the drug. This may be due to activation of the RAA system because natriuresis is inversely related to plasma aldosterone concentrations.[321] With the development of ascites, there is an increase in the volume of distribution of the diuretic and a reduction in the GFR that restricts its delivery to the tubule lumen. Moreover, there is further stimulation of the RAA axis, which contributes to a sharply reduced diuretic response.[321–323]

Distal tubule $Na^+$ reabsorption appears to be increased in patients with cirrhosis.[324] Indeed, patients with cirrhosis and ascites have an increased natriuretic response to a thiazide yet a markedly diminished response to ethacrynic acid; this finding suggests enhanced reabsorption at distal, thiazide-sensitive nephron sites.[324] Thus, diuretics acting on the distal nephron and aldosterone-dependent sites are especially effective in cirrhosis.[321, 325, 326]

Ascitic fluid is largely cleared by the lymphatic system. Osmotic diuretics, loop diuretics, and thiazides given to dogs can increase thoracic duct lymph flow by increasing lymph production by the small intestine and peritoneum.[327–329] Increased lymph flow has been related to increased splanchnic capillary filtration[329] and to AII generation, which increases the spontaneous pulsations in lymphatic vessels.[330] Albumin kinetic studies indicate that prolonged diuretic therapy can increase lymphatic flow in patients with ascites.[331] Thus, one component of diuretic action is to increase ascites drainage into the lymphatics. However, the natriuretic and diuretic actions decrease the venous and portal hydraulic pressures and concentrate the plasma proteins, thereby diminishing the Starling forces favoring filtration of plasma water.[332] Thus, diuretics may decrease ascites formation by the liver and splanchnic organs,[333] increase its reabsorption into the plasma,[334] and increase its clearance into the lymph.[331]

Studies have challenged the traditional concept that paracentesis is dangerous in patients with cirrhosis and tense ascites.[335] Controlled trials have shown that paracentesis is more effective than diuretic therapy in relieving ascites and reducing hospital stay but does not influence the subsequent clinical course or mortality.[336] Even repeated, large-volume paracentesis (4 to 6 L daily) appears to be safe if intravenous albumin (40 g with each procedure) is administered.[336] Indeed, large-volume paracentesis alone does not induce renal or circulatory dysfunction, electrolyte abnormalities, or a fall in plasma volume, provided that the patients have pitting peripheral edema.[337] Presumably, intravenous albumin is required after paracentesis to prevent plasma volume depletion before ascitic fluid has replenished the plasma volume unless there is a reservoir of peripheral edema that can serve this function.

Mild edema can be treated by dietary salt restriction (100 to 140 mmol daily); free water restriction is required if the $P_{Na}$ falls below 130 mmol/L. For patients with more severe ascites and edema, admission to a hospital may be helpful in controlling salt and fluid intake, ensuring abstinence from alcohol, and providing bed rest and close monitoring. Bed rest blunts the activation of the RAA and sympathetic nervous systems in patients with cirrhosis or cardiac failure and markedly increases the diuretic response to bumetanide.[338] Patients resistant to these measures frequently respond to spironolactone (50 to 100 mg daily initially). More severe diuretic resistance requires paracentesis or increasing doses of a loop diuretic (e.g., 20 mg furosemide twice daily, initially) in the hospital.

Because the maximal daily rate of ascites drainage is limited to approximately 300 to 900 mL,[339] the maximal daily rate of diuresis in nonedematous cirrhotic patients should not normally exceed 0.3 to 0.4 kg. More vigorous diuresis may reduce the plasma volume and precipitate prerenal azotemia. However, patients with peripheral edema may tolerate a more rapid diuresis of 1 to 3 kg daily under close monitoring.[340] Indeed, a study of patients with ascites treated with an intensive diuretic regimen showed that in those with edema, a daily loss of 1 to 3 kg did not perturb the plasma volume or renal function. However, the same diuretic regimen maintained after the edema had cleared or given to nonedematous patients led to a 24% reduction in plasma volume, a high prevalence of hyponatremia and hypochloremia, and a halving of the creatinine clearance.[340] This is an important reminder that a diuretic prescription that is effective and safe initially in cirrhotic patients with ascites and edema must be continually reviewed and the drug dosage reduced accordingly as peripheral edema clears.

The $Na^+$-depleting action of spironolactone in cirrhosis correlates with the plasma aldosterone concentration but is diminished in patients with a low GFR or $P_{Na}$.[326] Even malignant ascites may respond to spironolactone[341] or combined diuretic therapy, provided that the ascites is due to massive hepatic metastases and not to peritoneal carcinomatosis or chylous ascites.[342] In a randomized comparison of spironolactone with furosemide in nonazotemic cirrhotic patients, 19 of 20 responded favorably to spironolactone, whereas only 11 of 21 responded favorably to furosemide.[321] Even in those patients who did not undergo diuresis, the $P_K$ was reduced by furosemide but increased by spironolactone. Resistant patients have been given up to 600 mg daily of spironolactone,[343] but the adverse effects of spironolactone and its antiandrogen actions are dose related.[146, 158] Muzolimine (30 mg) given to patients with cirrhosis is equally effective as furosemide (80 mg) yet produces less kaliuresis, depression of GFR, and renin stimulation.[344]

The complications of diuretic therapy in cirrhotic patients are particularly dangerous, although diuretics used with due care and under close supervision are well tolerated.[345] The most common problems resulting from the use of furosemide are electrolyte disturbances and volume depletion.[308, 346] The high frequency of hypokalemia during therapy with loop diuretics is related to pre-existing $K^+$ depletion and hyperaldosteronism and can be countered by use of spironolactone or distal $K^+$-sparing agents. However, careful monitoring is required because patients with alcoholic cirrhosis occasionally have a dangerous hyperkalemic metabolic acidosis during spironolactone treatment, presumably owing to blockade of aldosterone-induced distal $H^+$ and $K^+$ secretion.[347]

Diuretic resistance is common in advanced cirrhosis. In addition to the usual causes (see Table 53–1), the administration of NSAIDs, including sulindac, can reduce the GFR and renal blood flow sharply and blunt the natriuretic response to furosemide.[194, 322] Diuretic resistance in cirrhosis may herald the development of infection, bleeding, or a critical fall in cardiac output.[348]

## NEPHROTIC SYNDROME

The nephrotic syndrome leads to renal losses of albumin that eventually lead to severe hypoalbuminemia. A fall in the plasma oncotic pressure increases the flux of fluid into the interstitial spaces. Alternatively, in some patients, the kidney is primarily involved in $Na^+$ retention, particularly when the GFR is reduced; the plasma volume is then well preserved.[349] Patients with minimal-change disease often have a contracted plasma volume and a stimulated RAA system, whereas other patients, especially those with hypertension, may have an expanded plasma volume and a suppressed RAA system.[349] Micropuncture studies of $Na^+$-retaining animal models of the nephrotic syndrome[350] and the response to distal blockade with diuretics in patients with the nephrotic syndrome[351] indicate that proximal reabsorption is decreased but reabsorption in the distal nephron is markedly increased. The mechanism of increased distal reabsorption has not been clarified; renin and aldosterone levels are highly variable in patients with the nephrotic syndrome.[352] Moreover, even in patients with stimulated plasma renin levels, a reduction in plasma aldosterone produced by an ACE inhibitor does not necessarily induce diuresis.[352]

Furosemide kinetics are often perturbed in patients with the nephrotic syndrome. Hypoalbuminemia decreases the plasma protein binding of furosemide and thereby increases its volume of distribution and nonrenal and renal elimination.[353]

The interaction of furosemide with its luminal receptor may be impaired by binding to filtered albumin.[354] The tubule responsiveness to furosemide has been found to be normal[355] or impaired[354] in rat models of the nephrotic syndrome and to be impaired in nephrotic patients.[197] Studies in rats with aminoglycoside-induced nephrotic syndrome have shown that the natriuretic response to furosemide is reduced by 60%.[356] The delivery of $Cl^-$ to the loop of Henle was maintained, but there was a profound blunting of the effect of furosemide on loop $Cl^-$ absorption.[357, 358] Addition of albumin to tubule fluid perfusing the loop of Henle attenuated the response to furosemide by 75%. This effect was ascribed to binding of furosemide to albumin, thereby making the diuretic unavailable to interact with its tubule receptor. Thus, the diuretic resistance was reversed by coperfusion with warfarin, which displaces furosemide from its albumin binding site[357, 358] (Fig. 53–11).

Nephrotic edema is best managed by dietary salt and fluid restriction. Most patients respond to a loop diuretic when it is required. There is a variable stimulation of the RAA system and a poor diuretic response to ACE inhibition or to aldosterone antagonists. Decreasing renal function[197] or administration of indomethacin[188] causes marked resistance to loop diuretics in patients with the nephrotic syndrome. The combination of a thiazide diuretic or metolazone with furosemide can dissipate edema, but at the expense of marked kaliuresis.[359] Metolazone alone is reported to be well tolerated during prolonged therapy.[360]

With advancing nephrotic syndrome, the maintenance of the plasma volume is compromised by hypoalbuminemia. Nevertheless, diuretic therapy reduces the ECV to a greater extent than the plasma volume in nephrotic patients.[348]

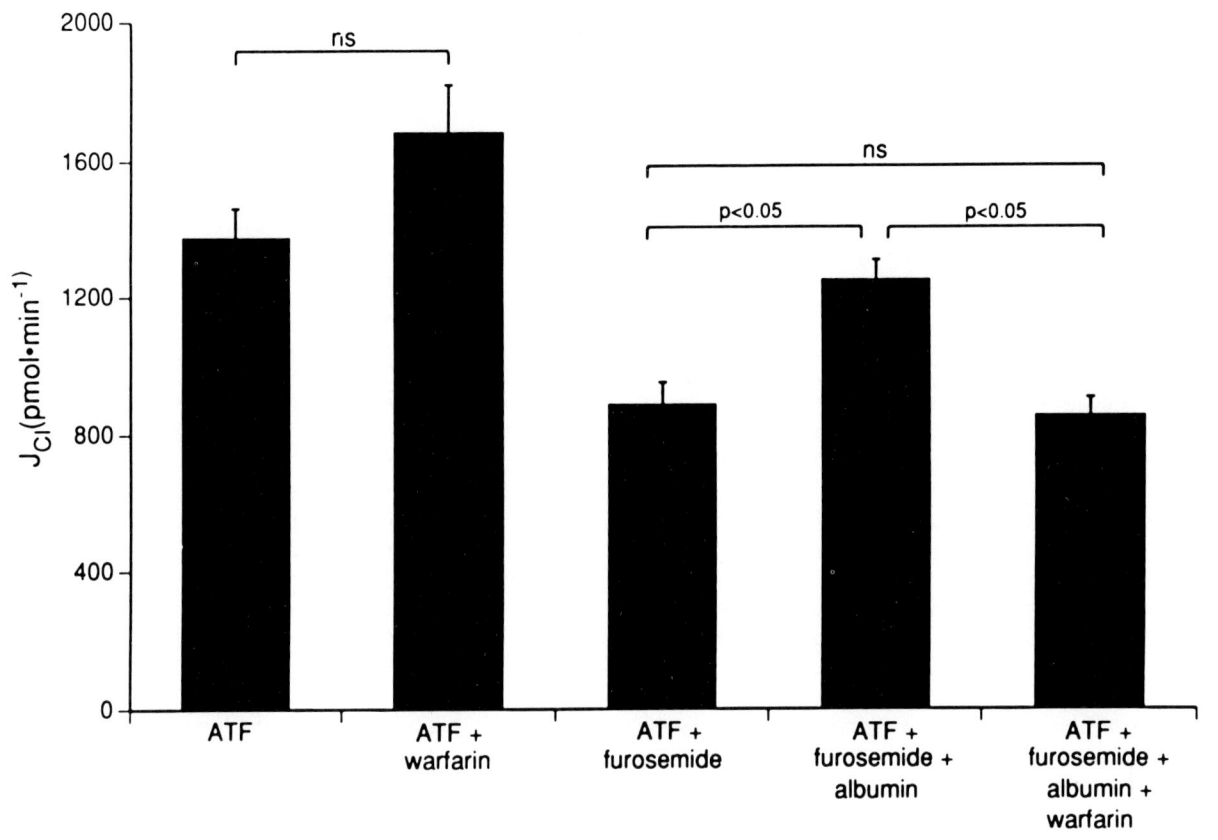

**Figure 53–11.** Mean ± SEM values for net Cl⁻ absorption from loops of Henle of the rat perfused in vivo with artificial tubule fluid (ATF) containing furosemide (6 μM), warfarin (12 μM), or both. Note that coperfusion with albumin blunts the action of furosemide; this is restored by coperfusion with warfarin, which displaces furosemide from its albumin binding site. (From Kirchner KA, Voelker JR, Brater DC: Binding inhibitors restore furosemide potency in tubule fluid containing albumin. Used with permission from Kidney International, volume 40, pages 418–424, 1991.)

However, if diuretic therapy causes plasma volume depletion, renal function is likely to deteriorate. Occasionally, declining renal function may signify the development of diuretic-induced interstitial nephritis.[361] Clearly, renal function and electrolytes require careful monitoring during diuretic therapy for the nephrotic syndrome.

## IDIOPATHIC EDEMA

Idiopathic edema is a syndrome of obscure pathophysiology that causes fluctuating Na⁺ retention and edema in women.[362] The effects of diuretic withdrawal during controlled salt intake were studied in 10 such patients.[363] Although their body weight increased by 0.5 to 5 kg within 2 to 8 days, seven returned to their original weight by 3 weeks without reinstitution of diuretics. The authors concluded that diuretic abuse could cause idiopathic edema. However, others have challenged this conclusion.[364] In view of these provocative findings, patients are best treated, when possible, by salt restriction without the use of diuretics.

## Nonedematous Conditions

### HYPERTENSION

Treatment of hypertension is discussed in Chapters 46 and 54.

## ACUTE AND CHRONIC RENAL FAILURE

The administration of a single large intravenous dose of furosemide (200 to 1000 mg) to patients in the early phase of oliguric acute renal failure produces a sustained diuresis (greater than 500 mL/24 h) in only 8% to 22%.[365, 366] However, a sustained diuresis was reported in 86% of patients when an initial large bolus dose of furosemide (1000 mg in a 4-hour period) was followed by a maintenance infusion at 2 mg/min or by 1 g orally three times daily.[366] However, this dosage regimen produced deafness in two patients, which was permanent in one.[366] Furosemide therapy for acute renal failure does not reduce mortality[365–368] but can reduce the number of dialysis treatments required to control uremia.[365] According to one protocol, patients were given two doses of 50 mL of 25% mannitol at 30-minute intervals. If the urine volume remained below 40 mL/h, crescendo intravenous doses of a loop diuretic were used (e.g., bumetanide, 2 mg with doubling or quadrupling of the dose at 30-minute intervals to a maximum of 10 mg).[369] However, the physician should remember that no clear evidence has been found that such therapy reduces either the mortality or the morbidity of patients with established acute renal failure. After a careful review of the existing evidence, Levinsky and co-workers[368] did not recommend continuous therapy with large doses of loop diuretics to maintain a high urine volume in patients who failed to respond to initial or intermittent treatment with smaller diuretic doses.

An infusion of dopamine at a low dose (1 to 3 μg/kg/min) potentiates furosemide-induced natriuresis in patients with acute renal failure.[370]

Most patients with advanced chronic renal failure have hypertension or edema requiring diuretic therapy. Thiazide diuretics can become ineffective when used alone at GFR values less than 20 to 30 mL/min, although bemetizide has been shown to increase natriuresis even in patients with advanced chronic renal failure.[127] Metolazone also remains effective in more advanced renal failure[371] and is well tolerated but is required in high dosage (10 to 25 mg daily).[372] Loop diuretics are generally the drugs of choice. For refractory patients, a trial of high-dose intravenous loop diuretic infusion may be warranted (e.g., bumetanide 1 mg/h for 12 hours). This regimen has been shown to produce a greater natriuresis in patients with severe renal failure (creatinine clearance 9 to 28 mL/min) than two bolus injections of 6 mg of bumetanide each 6 hours[176] (see Fig. 53–9). The increased efficacy was ascribed to the maintenance of urinary diuretic levels in the more "efficient" range at the midpoint of the response curve. The toxic effects of myalgias were more frequent after bolus injection. With advancing renal insufficiency, the renal clearance of furosemide falls in parallel with the GFR because of a decreased renal mass and the accumulation of organic acids that compete for proximal secretion.[373] However, the maximal increase in fractional excretion of $Na^+$ produced by furosemide is greater in patients with chronic renal failure.[374] An oral dose of 120 to 160 mg of furosemide or 6 to 8 mg of bumetanide produces a maximal response in patients with a creatinine clearance of 9 to 18 mL/min.[374–376] Higher daily doses of furosemide (250 to 2000 mg) have been given long term to hemodialysis patients. This initially increased the daily urine production, but the effect waned with time and these large doses were associated with photosensitive bullae in 15%.[377] Furosemide maintains its potency better than bumetanide does in patients with chronic renal insufficiency because the nonrenal elimination of furosemide is impaired, thereby leading to a relatively greater delivery to the urine.[375] Muzolimine also maintains its potency better because it does not require tubule secretion for its action.[378]

Even high doses of loop diuretics generally do not reduce the GFR of patients with advanced renal failure, provided that abrupt or severe volume depletion is prevented.[229, 378, 379] However, the combination of a thiazide and a loop diuretic can provoke hypovolemia, prerenal azotemia, and hypokalemia in such patients.[215] Distal $K^+$-sparing diuretics are dangerous in chronic renal failure because they can precipitate serious or even fatal hyperkalemic metabolic acidosis. Likewise, carbonic anhydrase inhibitors can precipitate metabolic acidosis. Osmotic diuretics must be used sparingly, because volume overload and pulmonary edema can occur rapidly as a result of reduced renal elimination. Therefore, special care is required when diuretics are prescribed for any patient with impaired renal function.

## RENAL TUBULAR ACIDOSIS

Furosemide increases the distal delivery of $Na^+$ and fluid and stimulates aldosterone secretion and $PO_4^{3-}$ elimination, all of which enhance net $H^+$ elimination.[380] Indeed, furosemide can increase renal acid excretion in patients with distal renal tubular acidosis.[381] Patients with hyporeninemic hypoaldosteronism and hyperkalemia are best managed with mineralocorticosteroid therapy; furosemide is valuable in increasing renal $K^+$ and $H^+$ excretion in those for whom mineralocorticosteroid therapy is unsuitable because of hypertension or fluid retention.[382] Furosemide may be effective by reversing a defect in renal prostaglandin generation.[383]

## HYPERCALCEMIA

Short-term administration of osmotic or loop diuretics increases $Ca^{2+}$ excretion, whereas thiazides and distal agents decrease it.[60]

Hypercalcemia inhibits fluid and $Na^+$ reabsorption. The ensuing ECV depletion limits $Ca^{2+}$ excretion by reducing the GFR and enhancing the proximal $Ca^{2+}$ reabsorption. Therefore, the initial therapy for hypercalcemia is appropriate volume expansion with saline. Thereafter, if hypercalcemia persists, it can be managed by an infusion of a loop diuretic (e.g., 2 to 3 mg bumetanide, 80 to 120 mg furosemide, or 50 to 100 mg ethacrynic acid intravenously, every 1 to 2 hours). Each dose causes the loss of approximately 80 mg of $Ca^{2+}$. However, calciuresis will be only temporary unless fluid and electrolytes are replaced. Serum electrolytes should be monitored closely.[369, 384]

## NEPHROLITHIASIS

The hypocalciuric effect of thiazides is sustained during prolonged treatment.[60, 385] Thiazides can reduce stone formation in hypercalciuric and even normocalciuric patients, although the effect is not striking in controlled clinical trials.[386] The indications, choice of drug, and dosage for diuretic therapy of recurrent nephrolithiasis are controversial.[385] Earlier studies employed 50 mg hydrochlorothiazide twice daily. However, smaller doses are effective in reducing $Ca^{2+}$ excretion, and the addition of amiloride[387] or a low-salt diet[385] can enhance the effect. Thiazide therapy for nephrolithiasis should be a part of a comprehensive strategy.

## DIABETES INSIPIDUS

Thiazide diuretics can produce a paradoxical reduction in urine flow of about 50% in patients with central or nephrogenic diabetes insipidus.[388] Antidiuresis is related both to ECV depletion (which reduces the GFR and enhances the proximal $Na^+$ reabsorption, thereby curtailing the delivery of filtrate to the diluting segment[389]) and to an increase in papillary osmolarity.[390] Because successful therapy depends on a reduction in ECV, thiazides should be combined with salt restriction.

### *Acknowledgments*

The author is grateful to Tom Wargovich, MD, Nicholas Guzman, MD, David Weiner, MD, and Charles S. Wingo, MD, for helpful advice on the manuscript.

# REFERENCES

1. Giebisch G: Distal nephron effects of diuretics. *In* Puschett J, Greenberg A (eds): Diuretics III: Chemistry, Pharmacology, and Clinical Applications. Elsevier Science Publishing, New York, 1990, pp 667–677.

2. Schwartz WB: The effect of sulfanilamide on salt and water excretion in congestive heart failure. N Engl J Med 240:173–177, 1949.

3. Maren TH: The general physiology of reactions catalyzed by carbonic anhydrase and their inhibition by sulfonamides. Ann N Y Acad Sci 429:568–579, 1984.

4. Eveloff J, Warnock DG: Renal carbonic anhydrase. *In* Dirks JH, Sutton RA (eds): Diuretics: Physiology, Pharmacology and Clinical Use. WB Saunders, Philadelphia, 1986, p 49.

5. Cogan MG, Maddox DA, Warnock DG, et al: Effect of acetazolamide on bicarbonate reabsorption in the proximal tubule of the rat. Am J Physiol 237:F447–F454, 1979.

6. Maren TH: Carbonic anhydrase inhibition. IV: The effects of metabolic acidosis on the response to Diamox. Bull Johns Hopkins Hosp 98:159–183, 1956.

7. Wistrand PJ: The use of carbonic anhydrase inhibitors in ophthalmology and clinical medicine. Ann N Y Acad Sci 429:609–619, 1984.

8. Ichikawa I, Kon V: Role of peritubular capillary forces in the renal action of carbonic anhydrase inhibitor. Kidney Int 30:828–835, 1986.

9. Brater DC, Kaojarern S, Chennavasin P: Pharmacodynamics of the diuretic effects of aminophylline and acetazolamide alone and combined with furosemide in normal subjects. J Pharmacol Exp Ther 227:92–97, 1983.

10. Galla JH, Luke RG: Pathophysiology of metabolic alkalosis. Hosp Pract (Off Ed) 22:123–130, 139, 1987.

11. Miller PD, Berns AS: Acute metabolic alkalosis perpetuating hypercarbia. A role for acetazolamide in chronic obstructive pulmonary disease. JAMA 238:2400–2401, 1977.

12. Bear R, Goldstein M, Phillipson E, et al: Effect of metabolic alkalosis on respiratory function in patients with chronic obstructive lung disease. Can Med Assoc J 117:900–903, 1977.

13. Maren TH, Wadsworth BC, Yale EK, Alonso LG: Carbonic anhydrase inhibition. III: Effects of Diamox on electrolyte metabolism. Bull Johns Hopkins Hosp 95:277–321, 1954.

14. Swenson ER, Robertson HT, Hlastala MP: Effects of carbonic anhydrase inhibition on ventilation-perfusion matching in the dog lung. J Clin Invest 92:702–709, 1993.

15. Maren TH: Carbonic anhydrase: General perspectives and advances in glaucoma research. Drug Dev Res 10:255–276, 1987.

16. Greene MK, Kerr AM, McIntosh IB, Prescott RJ: Acetazolamide in prevention of acute mountain sickness: A double-blind controlled cross-over study. Br Med J Clin Res 283:811–813, 1981.

17. White DP, Zwillich CW, Pickett CK, et al: Central sleep apnea. Improvement with acetazolamide therapy. Arch Intern Med 142:1816–1819, 1982.

18. Vogh BP: The relation of choroid plexus carbonic anhydrase activity to cerebrospinal fluid formation: Study of three inhibitors in cat with extrapolation to man. J Pharmacol Exp Ther 213:321–331, 1980.

19. Brookes GB, Hodge RA, Booth JB, Morrison AW: The immediate effects of acetazolamide in Meniere's disease. J Laryngol Otol 96:57–72, 1982.

20. Griggs RC, Engel WK, Resnick JS: Acetazolamide treatment of hypokalemic periodic paralysis. Prevention of attacks and improvement of persistent weakness. Ann Intern Med 73:39–48, 1970.

21. McArdle B: Adymica episodica hereditaria and its treatment. Brain 85:121, 1962.

22. Parfitt AM: Acetazolamide and sodium bicarbonate induced nephrocalcinosis and nephrolithiasis; relationship to citrate and calcium excretion. Arch Intern Med 124:736–740, 1969.

23. Heller I, Halevy J, Cohen S, Theodor E: Significant metabolic acidosis induced by acetazolamide. Not a rare complication. Arch Intern Med 145:1815–1817, 1985.

24. Webster LT, Davidson CS: Production of impending hepatic coma by a carbonic anhydrase inhibitor, Diamox. Proc Soc Exp Biol Med 9:27–31, 1956.

25. Krivoy N, Ben Arieh Y, Carter A, Alroy G: Methazolamide-induced hepatitis and pure RBC aplasia. Arch Intern Med 141:1229–1230, 1981.

26. Mallette LE: Acetazolamide-accelerated anticonvulsant osteomalacia. Arch Intern Med 137:1013–1017, 1977.

27. Scott WJ Jr, Lane PD, Randall JL, Schreiner CM: Malformations in nonlimb structures induced by acetazolamide and other inhibitors of carbonic anhydrase. Ann N Y Acad Sci 429:447–456, 1984.

28. Nashat FS, Scholefield FR, Tappin JW, Wilcox CS: The effect of acute changes in haematocrit in the anaesthetized dog on the volume and character of the urine. J Physiol (Lond) 205:305–316, 1969.

29. Nashat FS, Scholefield FR, Tappin JW, Wilcox CS: The effects of changes in haematocrit on the intrarenal distribution of blood flow in the dog's kidney. J Physiol (Lond) 201:639–655, 1969.

30. Warren SE, Blantz RC: Mannitol. Arch Intern Med 141:493–497, 1981.

31. Rigden SP, Dillon MJ, Kind PR, et al: The beneficial effect of mannitol on postoperative renal function in children undergoing cardiopulmonary bypass surgery. Clin Nephrol 21:148–151, 1984.

32. Luck RJ, Irvine WT: Mannitol in the surgery of aortic aneurysm. Lancet 2:409, 1965.

33. Dawson JL: Post-operative renal function in obstructive jaundice: Effect of a mannitol diuresis. Br Med J 1:82, 1965.

34. Byrne JJ: Shock. N Engl J Med 275:659–660, 1966.

35. Eneas JF, Schoenfeld PY, Humphreys MH: The effect of infusion of mannitol–sodium bicarbonate on the clinical course of myoglobinuria. Arch Intern Med 139:801–805, 1979.

36. Anto HR, Chou SY, Porush JG, Shapiro WB: Infusion intravenous pyelography and renal function. Effect of hypertonic mannitol in patients with chronic renal insufficiency. Arch Intern Med 141:1652–1656, 1981.

37. Dawson JL: Jaundice and anoxic renal damage: Protective effect of mannitol. Br Med J 1:810–811, 1964.

38. Untura A: Incidence and prophylaxis of acute postoperative renal failure in obstructive jaundice. Rev Med Chir Soc Med Nat Iasi 83:247, 1979.

39. Bingham WF: The limits of cerebral dehydration in the treatment of head injury. Surg Neurol 25:340–345, 1986.

40. Canalese J, Gimson AE, Davis C, et al: Controlled trial of dexamethasone and mannitol for the cerebral oedema of fulminant hepatic failure. Gut 23:625–629, 1982.

41. Ostrow S, Egorin MJ, Hahn D, et al: High-dose cisplatin therapy using mannitol versus furosemide diuresis: Comparative pharmacokinetics and toxicity. Cancer Treat Rep 65:73–78, 1981.

42. Borges HF, Hocks J, Kjellstrand CM: Mannitol intoxication in patients with renal failure. Arch Intern Med 142:63–66, 1982.

43. Burg M, Stoner L: Renal tubular chloride transport and the mode of action of some diuretics. Annu Rev Physiol 38:37–45, 1976.

44. Koenig B, Kinne R: Sodium transport by plasma membranes isolated from cells of the thick ascending limb of Henle's loop. Fed Proc 41:4310, 1982.

45. Greger R, Schlatter E, Lang F: Evidence for electroneutral sodium chloride cotransport in the cortical thick ascending limb of Henle's loop of rabbit kidney. Pflugers Arch 396:308–314, 1983.

46. Greger R, Schlatter E: Properties of the lumen membrane of the cortical thick ascending limb of Henle's loop of rabbit kidney. Pflugers Arch 396:325–334, 1983.

47. Schlatter E, Greger R, Weidtke C: Effect of "high ceiling" diuretics on active salt transport in the cortical thick ascending limb of Henle's loop of rabbit kidney. Pflugers Arch 396:210–217, 1983.

48. Good DW, Knepper MA, Burg MB: Ammonia and bicarbonate transport by thick ascending limb of rat kidney. Am J Physiol 247:F35–F44, 1984.

49. Li JHY, Kau ST: Bumetanide stimulation of sodium permeability of the apical membrane of toad urinary bladder. J Pharmacol Exp Ther 246:980–985, 1988.

50. Duarte CG, Chomety F, Giebisch G: Effect of amiloride, ouabain, and furosemide on distal tubular function in the rat. Am J Physiol 221:632–640, 1971.

51. Wilcox CS, Loon NR, Kanthawatana S, et al: Generation of alkalosis during furosemide infusion: Roles of contraction and acid excretion. J Nephrol 2:81–87, 1991.

52. Brenner BM, Keimowitz RI, Wright FS, Berliner RW: An inhibitory effect of furosemide on sodium reabsorption by the proximal tubule of the rat nephron. J Clin Invest 48:290–300, 1969.

53. Radtke HW, Rumrich G, Kinne-saffran E, Ulrich KJ: Dual action of acetazolamide and furosemide on proximal volume absorption in the rat kidney. Kidney Int 1:100–105, 1972.

54. Puschett JB, Sylk D, Teredesai PR: Uncoupling of proximal sodium bicarbonate from sodium phosphate transport by bumetanide. Am J Physiol 235:F403–F408, 1978.
55. Stein JH, Wilson CB, Kirkendall WM: Differences in the acute effects of furosemide and ethacrynic acid in man. J Lab Clin Med 71:654–665, 1968.
56. Velazquez H, Wright FS: Effects of diuretic drugs on Na, Cl, and K transport by rat renal distal tubule. Am J Physiol 250:F1013–F1023, 1986.
57. Jung KY, Endou H: Furosemide acts on short loop of descending thin limb, but not on long loop. J Pharmacol Exp Ther 253:1184–1188, 1990.
58. Wilson DR, Honrath U, Sonnenberg H: Furosemide action on collecting ducts: Effect of prostaglandin synthesis inhibition. Am J Physiol 244:F666–F673, 1983.
59. Earley LE, Friedler RM: Renal tubular effects of ethacrynic acid. J Clin Invest 43:1495, 1964.
60. Suki WN: Effects of diuretics on calcium metabolism. Adv Exp Med Biol 151:493–500, 1982.
61. White MG, van Gelder J, Eastes G: The effect of loop diuretics on the excretion of $Na^+$, $Ca^{2+}$, $Mg^{2+}$, and $Cl^-$. J Clin Pharmacol 21:610–614, 1981.
62. Suki WN, Rouse D, Ng RC, Kokko JP: Calcium transport in the thick ascending limb of Henle. Heterogeneity of function in the medullary and cortical segments. J Clin Invest 66:1004–1009, 1980.
63. Quamme GA: Effect of furosemide on calcium and magnesium transport in the rat nephron. Am J Physiol 241:F340–F347, 1981.
64. Ryan MP, Devane J, Ryan MF, Counihan TB: Effects of diuretics on the renal handling of magnesium. Drugs 28(suppl 1):167–181, 1984.
65. Shareghi GR, Agus ZS: Magnesium transport in the cortical thick ascending limb of Henle's loop of the rabbit. J Clin Invest 69:759–769, 1982.
66. Steele TH, Oppenheimer S: Factors affecting urate excretion following diuretic administration in man. Am J Med 47:564–574, 1969.
67. Kahn AM, Branham S, Weinman EJ: Mechanism of urate and p-aminohippurate transport in rat renal microvillus membrane vesicles. Am J Physiol 245:F151–F158, 1983.
68. Weinman EJ, Eknoyan G, Suki WN: The influence of the extracellular fluid volume on the tubular reabsorption of uric acid. J Clin Invest 55:283–291, 1975.
69. Lau K, Stote RM, Goldberg M, Agus ZS: Mechanisms of the uricosuric effect of the diuretic tienilic acid (ticrynafen) in man. Clin Sci Mol Med 53:379–386, 1977.
70. Tobert JA, Cirillo VJ, Hitzenberger G, et al: Enhancement of uricosuric properties of indacrinone by manipulation of the enantiomer ratio. Clin Pharmacol Ther 29:344–350, 1981.
71. Weinman EJ, Knight TF, McKenzie R, Eknoyan G: Dissociation of urate from sodium transport in the rat proximal tubule. Kidney Int 10:295–300, 1976.
72. Loon NR, Wilcox CS, Unwin RJ: Mechanism of impaired natriuretic response to furosemide during prolonged therapy. Kidney Int 36:682–689, 1989.
73. Epstein M, Hollenberg NK, Guttmann RD, et al: Effect of ethacrynic acid and chlorothiazide on intrarenal hemodynamics in normal man. Am J Physiol 220:482–487, 1971.
74. Spitalewitz S, Chou SY, Faubert PF, Porush JG: Effects of diuretics on inner medullary hemodynamics in the dog. Circ Res 51:703–710, 1982.
75. Gerber JG: Role of prostaglandins in the hemodynamic and tubular effects of furosemide. Fed Proc 42:1707–1710, 1983.
76. Wright FS, Schnermann J: Interference with feedback control of glomerular filtration rate by furosemide, triflocin, and cyanide. J Clin Invest 53:1695–1708, 1974.
77. Cutler RE, Blair AD: Clinical pharmacokinetics of frusemide. Clin Pharmacokinet 4:279–296, 1979.
78. Benet LZ: Pharmacokinetics/pharmacodynamics of furosemide in man: A review. J Pharmacokinet Biopharm 7:1–27, 1979.
79. Bowman RH: Renal secretion of [$^{35}$S]furosemide and depression by albumin binding. Am J Physiol 229:93–98, 1975.
80. Valentine JF, Brater DC, Krejs GJ: Clearance of furosemide by the gastrointestinal tract. J Pharmacol Exp Ther 236:177–180, 1986.
81. Branch RA: Role of binding in distribution of furosemide: Where is nonrenal clearance? Fed Proc 42:1699–1702, 1983.
82. Chennavasin P, Seiwell R, Brater DC, Liang WM: Pharmacodynamic analysis of the furosemide-probenecid interaction in man. Kidney Int 16:187–195, 1979.
83. Chennavasin P, Seiwell R, Brater DC: Pharmacokinetic-dynamic analysis of the indomethacin-furosemide interaction in man. J Pharmacol Exp Ther 215:77–81, 1980.
84. Kirchner KA, Martin CJ, Bower JD: Prostaglandin $E_2$ but not $I_2$ restores furosemide response in indomethacin-treated rats. Am J Physiol 250:F980–F985, 1986.
85. Wilcox CS, Mitch WE, Kelly RA, et al: Response of the kidney to furosemide. I. Effects of salt intake and renal compensation. J Lab Clin Med 102:450–458, 1983.
86. Imbs JL, Schmidt M, Giesen Crouse E: Pharmacology of loop diuretics: State of the art. Adv Nephrol 16:137–158, 1987.
87. Giesen Crouse EM, Welsch C, Imbs JL, et al: Characterization of a high affinity piretanide receptor on kidney membranes. Eur J Pharmacol 114:23–31, 1985.
88. Loew D, Meng K: The renal mechanism of Bay g 2821. Pharmacotherapeutica 1:333–340, 1977.
89. Garthoff B, Thomas G: Pharmacological aspects of muzolimine. Clin Nephrol 19:S-5–S-10, 1983.
90. Dorge A, Rick R, Arnim EV, Thurau K: Effect of muzolimine on transepithelial sodium transport of frog skin epithelium. Clin Nephrol 19:S-11–S-15, 1983.
91. Kinne R, Koenig B, Eveloff J, et al: Effect of muzolimine on chloride-transporting epithelia. Clin Nephrol 19:S-16–S-19, 1983.
92. Ritter W: Pharmacokinetics of muzolimine. Clin Nephrol 19:S-26–S-31, 1983.
93. Canton AD, Russo D, Gallo R, et al: Muzolimine: A new high-ceiling diuretic suitable for patients with advanced renal disease. Br Med J Clin Res 282:595–598, 1981.
94. Brater DC: Disposition and response to bumetanide and furosemide. Am J Cardiol 57:20A–25A, 1986.
95. Brater DC, Leinfelder J, Anderson SA: Clinical pharmacology of torasemide, a new loop diuretic. Clin Pharmacol Ther 42:187–192, 1987.
96. Brater DC, Day B, Anderson S, Seiwell R: Azosemide kinetics and dynamics. Clin Pharmacol Ther 34:454–458, 1983.
97. Brater DC, Anderson S: Sites of action of tripamide. Clin Pharmacol Ther 34:79–85, 1983.
98. Marsh JD, Smith TW: Piretanide: A loop-active diuretic. Pharmacology, therapeutic efficacy and adverse effects. Pharmacotherapy 4:170–180, 1984.
99. Fanelli GM Jr, Bohn DL, Scriabine A, Beyer KH Jr: Saluretic and uricosuric effects of (6,7-dichloro-2-methyl-1-oxo-2-phenyl-5-indanyloxy) acetic acid (MK-196) in the chimpanzee. J Pharmacol Exp Ther 200:402–412, 1977.
100. Ellison DH, Velazquez H, Wright FS: Thiazide-sensitive sodium chloride cotransport in early distal tubule. Am J Physiol 253:F546–F554, 1987.
101. Ellison DH, Velazquez H, Wright FS: Mechanisms of sodium, potassium and chloride transport by the renal distal tubule. Miner Electrolyte Metab 13:422–432, 1987.
102. Velazquez H, Wright FS: Control by drugs of renal potassium handling. Annu Rev Pharmacol Toxicol 26:293–309, 1986.
103. Velazquez H, Ellison DH, Wright FS: Luminal influences on potassium secretion: Chloride, sodium, and thiazide diuretics. Am J Physiol 262:F1076–F1082, 1992.
104. Beyer KH: Chlorothiazide. Br J Clin Pharmacol 13:15–24, 1982.
105. Wilson DR, Honrath U, Sonnenberg H: Thiazide diuretic effect on medullary collecting duct function in the rat. Kidney Int 23:711–716, 1983.
106. Beaumont K, Vaughn DA, Healy DP: Thiazide diuretic receptors: Autoradiographic localization in rat kidney with [$^3$H]metolazone. J Pharmacol Exp Ther 250:414–419, 1989.
107. Beaumont K, Vaughn DA, Fanestil DD: Thiazide diuretic drug receptors in rat kidney: Identification with [$^3$H]metolazone. Proc Natl Acad Sci USA 85:2311–2314, 1988.
108. Fanestil DD: Steroid regulation of thiazide-sensitive transport. Semin Nephrol 12:18–23, 1992.
109. Ellison DH, Biemesderfer D, Morrisey J, et al: Immunocytochemical characterization of the high-affinity thiazide diuretic receptor in rabbit renal cortex. Am J Physiol 264:F141–F148, 1993.
110. Chen ZF, Vaughn DA, Beaumont K, Fanestil DD: Effects of diuretic treatment and of dietary sodium on renal binding of $^3$H-metolazone. J Am Soc Nephrol 1:91–98, 1990.

111. Tran JM, Farrell MA, Fanestil DD: Effect of ions on binding of the thiazide-type diuretic metolazone to kidney membrane. Am J Physiol 258:F908–F915, 1990.
112. Seldin DW, Eknoyan G, Suki WN, Rector FCJ: Localization of diuretic action from the pattern of water and electrolyte excretion. Ann N Y Acad Sci 139:328–343, 1966.
113. Costanzo LS, Windhager EE: Calcium and sodium transport by the distal convoluted tubule of the rat. Am J Physiol 235:F492–F506, 1978.
114. Sabatini S: The effects of the thiazide diuretics on calcium transport. In Puschett J, Greenberg A (eds): Diuretics III: Chemistry, Pharmacology, and Clinical Applications. Elsevier Science Publishing, New York, 1990, pp 212–217.
115. Brunette MG, Harvey N, Mailloux J, et al: The hypocalciuric effect of thiazides: Study of the mechanisms. In Puschett J, Greenberg A (eds): Diuretics III: Chemistry, Pharmacology, and Clinical Applications. Elsevier Science Publishing, New York, 1990, pp 225–227.
116. Porter RH, Cox BG, Heaney D, et al: Treatment of hypoparathyroid patients with chlorthalidone. N Engl J Med 298:577–581, 1978.
117. Giles TD, Sander GE, Roffidal LE, et al: Comparative effects of nitrendipine and hydrochlorothiazide on calciotropic hormones and bone density in hypertensive patients. Am J Hypertens 5:875–879, 1992.
118. Ray WA, Griffin MR, Downey W, Melton LJ: Long-term use of thiazide diuretics and risk of hip fracture. Lancet 1:687–690, 1989.
119. LaCroix AZ, Wienpahl J, White LR, et al: Thiazide diuretic agents and the incidence of hip fracture. N Engl J Med 322:286–290, 1990.
120. Cauley JA, Cummings SR, Seeley DG, et al: Effects of thiazide diuretic therapy on bone mass, fractures, and falls. The Study of Osteoporotic Fractures Research Group. Ann Intern Med 118:666–673, 1993.
121. Heidrich FE, Stergachis A, Gross KM: Diuretic drug use and the risk of hip fracture [see comments]. Ann Intern Med 115:1–6, 1991.
122. Leary WP, Reyes AJ: Diuretic-induced magnesium losses. Drugs 28(suppl 1):182–187, 1984.
123. Schohn DC, Jahn HA: Effects of a potassium-sparing/thiazide diuretic combination on cardiovascular reactivity to vasopressor agents. Am J Cardiol 65:14K–17K, 1990.
124. Welling PG: Pharmacokinetics of the thiazide diuretics. Biopharm Drug Dispos 7:501–535, 1986.
125. Suki WN, Dawoud F, Eknoyan G, Martinez-Maldonado M: Effects of metolazone on renal function in normal man. J Pharmacol Exp Ther 180:6–12, 1972.
126. Campbell DB, Moore RA: The pharmacology and clinical pharmacology of indapamide. Postgrad Med J 57(suppl 2):7–17, 1981.
127. Knauf H, Mutschler E: The load in the nephron segment determines the ceiling quality of a diuretic. In Puschett J, Greenberg A (eds): Diuretics III: Chemistry, Pharmacology, and Clinical Applications. Elsevier Science Publishing, New York, 1990, pp 359–375.
128. Hogan MJ, Wallin JD, Baer RM: Antihypertensive therapy and male sexual dysfunction. Psychosomatics 21:234–237, 1980.
129. Magil AB, Ballon HS, Cameron EC, Rae A: Acute interstitial nephritis associated with thiazide diuretics. Clinical and pathologic observations in three cases. Am J Med 69:939–943, 1980.
130. Addo HA, Ferguson J, Frain Bell W: Thiazide-induced photosensitivity: A study of 33 subjects. Br J Dermatol 116:749–760, 1987.
131. Giebisch G: Amiloride effects on distal nephron function. In Straub RW, Bolis L (eds): Cell Membrane Receptors for Drugs and Hormones: A Multidisciplinary Approach. Raven Press, New York, 1978, p 337.
132. Wingo CS: Cortical collecting tubule potassium secretion: Effect of amiloride, ouabain, and luminal sodium concentration. Kidney Int 27:886–891, 1985.
133. Gross JB, Kokko JP: Effects of aldosterone and potassium-sparing diuretics on electrical potential differences across the distal nephron. J Clin Invest 59:82–89, 1977.
134. Wingo CS: Reversible chloride-dependent potassium flux across the rabbit cortical collecting tubule. Am J Physiol 256:F697–F704, 1989.
135. Wingo CS: Evidence for luminal KCl exit as mechanism for active chloride secretion by rabbit cortical collecting duct. Ann N Y Acad Sci 574:498–501, 1989.
136. Wingo CS: Potassium secretion by the cortical collecting tubule: Effect of Cl gradients and ouabain. Am J Physiol 256:F306–F313, 1989.
137. Wingo CS: Active and passive chloride transport by the rabbit cortical collecting duct. Am J Physiol 258:F1388–F1393, 1990.
138. Wingo CS, Armitage FE: Rubidium absorption and proton secretion by rabbit outer medullary collecting duct via H-K-ATPase. Am J Physiol 263:F849–F857, 1992.
139. Wingo CS, Cain BD: The renal H-K-ATPase: Physiological significance and role in potassium homeostasis. Annu Rev Physiol 55:323–347, 1993.
140. Brater DC: Clinical utility of the potassium-sparing diuretics. Hosp Formul Manage 19:79, 1984.
141. Mutschler E, Gilfrich HJ, Knauf H, et al: Pharmacokinetics of triamterene. Clin Exp Hypertens [A] 5:249–269, 1983.
142. Villeneuve JP, Rocheleau F, Raymond G: Triamterene kinetics and dynamics in cirrhosis. Clin Pharmacol Ther 35:831–837, 1984.
143. Knauf H, Mohrke W, Mutschler E: Delayed elimination of triamterene and its active metabolite in chronic renal failure. Eur J Clin Pharmacol 24:453–456, 1983.
144. Somogyi AA, Hovens CM, Muirhead MR, Bochner F: Renal tubular secretion of amiloride and its inhibition by cimetidine in humans and in an animal model. Drug Metab Dispos 17:190–196, 1989.
145. Lynn KL, Bailey RR, Swainson CP, et al: Renal failure with potassium-sparing diuretics. N Z Med J 98:629–633, 1985.
146. Andriulli A, Arrigoni A, Gindro T, et al: Canrenone and androgen receptor–active materials in plasma of cirrhotic patients during long-term K-canrenoate or spironolactone therapy. Digestion 44:155–162, 1989.
147. McInnes GT: Relative potency of amiloride and spironolactone in healthy man. Clin Pharmacol Ther 31:472–477, 1982.
148. Rahn KH: Clinical pharmacology of diuretics. Clin Exp Hypertens [A] 5:157–166, 1983.
149. Velaquez H, Perazella MA, Wright FS, Ellison DH: Renal mechanism of trimethoprim-induced hyperkalemia. Ann Intern Med 119:261–301, 1993.
150. Greenberg S, Reiser IW, Shyan-Yih C, Porush JG: Trimethoprim-sulfamethoxazole induces reversible hyperkalemia. Ann Intern Med 119:291–295, 1993.
151. Schambelan M, Sebastian A, Biglieri EG, et al: Amelioration of hypokalemia by amiloride in diverse syndromes associated with renal potassium wasting. Kidney Int 21:157, 1982.
152. Hulter HN, Licht JH, Glynn RD, et al: Pathophysiology of chronic renal tubular acidosis induced by administration of amiloride. J Lab Clin Med 95:637–653, 1980.
153. Shackleton CR, Wong NL, Sutton RA: Distal (potassium-sparing) diuretics. In Dirks JH, Sutton RA (eds): Diuretics: Physiology, Pharmacology and Clinical Use. WB Saunders, Philadelphia, 1986, pp 117–134.
154. Gundert Remy U, Muller Herrmann R, Mutschler E, et al: Altered hydroxylation rate of triamterene in patients with liver cirrhosis. Int J Clin Pharmacol Ther Toxicol 20:353–357, 1982.
155. Favre L, Glasson P, Vallotton MB: Reversible acute renal failure from combined triamterene and indomethacin: A study in healthy subjects. Ann Intern Med 96:317–320, 1982.
156. Barth JH, Cherry CA, Wojnarowska F, Dawber RP: Spironolactone is an effective and well tolerated systemic antiandrogen therapy for hirsute women. J Clin Endocrinol Metab 68:966–970, 1989.
157. Potter C, Willis D, Sharp HL, Scharzenberg SJ: Primary and secondary amenorrhea associated with spironolactone therapy in chronic liver disease. J Pediatr 121:141–143, 1992.
158. de Gasparo M, Whitebread SE, Preiswerk G, et al: Antialdosterones: Incidence and prevention of sexual side effects. J Steroid Biochem 32:223–227, 1989.
159. Coratelli P, Passavanti G: Pathophysiology of renal failure in obstructive jaundice. Miner Electrolyte Metab 16:61–65, 1990.
160. Kelly RA, Wilcox CS, Mitch WE, et al: Response of the kidney to furosemide. II. Effect of captopril on sodium balance. Kidney Int 24:233–239, 1983.
161. Wilcox CS, Guzman NJ, Mitch WE, et al: Na+, K+, and BP homeostasis in man during furosemide: Effects of prazosin and captopril. Kidney Int 31:135–141, 1987.
162. Wilcox CS, Loon NR, Ameer B, Limacher MC: Renal and hemodynamic responses to bumetanide in hypertension: Effects of nitrendipine. Kidney Int 36:719–725, 1989.
163. Frolich JC, Hollifield JW, Dormois JC, et al: Suppression of plasma renin activity by indomethacin in man. Circ Res 39:447–452, 1976.
164. Kaissling B, Bachmann S, Kriz W: Structural adaptation of the distal convoluted tubule to prolonged furosemide treatment. Am J Physiol 248:F374–F381, 1985.

165. Ellison DH, Velazquez H, Wright FS: Adaptation of the distal convoluted tubule of the rat. Structural and functional effects of dietary salt intake and chronic diuretic infusion. J Clin Invest 83:113–126, 1989.
166. Kim J, Welch WJ, Cannon JK, et al: Immunocytochemical response of type A and type B intercalated cells to increased sodium chloride delivery. Am J Physiol 262:F288–F302, 1992.
167. Kaissling B, Stanton BA: Adaptation of distal tubule and collecting duct to increased sodium delivery. I. Ultrastructure. Am J Physiol 255:F1256–F1268, 1988.
168. Scherzer P, Wald H, Popvtzer MM: Enhanced glomerular filtration and Na⁺-K⁺-ATPase with furosemide administration. Am J Physiol 252:F910–F915, 1987.
169. Doucet A: Function and control of Na-K-ATPase in single nephron segments of the mammalian kidney. Kidney Int 34:749–760, 1988.
170. Garg LC, Narang N: Effects of hydrochlorothiazide on Na-K-ATPase activity along the rat nephron. Kidney Int 31:918–922, 1987.
171. Stanton BA, Kaissling B: Adaptation of distal tubule and collecting duct to increased Na delivery. II. Na⁺ and K⁺ transport. Am J Physiol 255:F1269–F1275, 1988.
172. Idiopathic edema: Role of diuretic abuse. Kidney Int 19:881–891, 1981. Clinical conference.
173. Almeshari K, Ahlstrom NG, Capraro FE, Wilcox CS: A volume-independent component to post-diuretic sodium retention in man. J Am Soc Nephrol 3:1878–1883, 1993.
174. Missouris CG, Cappuccio FP, Markandu ND, MacGregor GA: Diuretics and oedema: How to avoid rebound sodium retention. Lancet 339:1546, 1992. Letter.
175. van Meyel JJ, Smits P, Russel FG, et al: Diuretic efficiency of furosemide during continuous administration versus bolus injection in healthy volunteers. Clin Pharmacol Ther 51:440–444, 1992.
176. Copeland JG, Campbell DW, Plachetka JR, et al: Diuresis with continuous infusion of furosemide after cardiac surgery. Am J Surg 146:796–799, 1983.
177. Rudy DW, Voelker JR, Greene PK, et al: Loop diuretics for chronic renal insufficiency: A continuous infusion is more efficacious than bolus therapy. Ann Intern Med 115:360–366, 1991.
178. Imbs JL, Schmidt M, Velly J, Schwartz J: Comparison of the effect of two groups of diuretics on renin secretion in the anaesthetized dog. Clin Sci Mol Med 52:171–182, 1977.
179. Wilson TW, Loadholt CB, Privitera PJ, Halushka PV: Furosemide increases urine 6-keto-prostaglandin F₁α. Relation to natriuresis, vasodilation, and renin release. Hypertension 4:634–641, 1982.
180. Dzau VJ, Colucci WS, Williams GH, et al: Sustained effectiveness of converting-enzyme inhibition in patients with severe congestive heart failure. N Engl J Med 302:1373–1379, 1980.
181. Wilcox CS, Williams CM, Smith TB, et al: Diagnostic uses of angiotensin-converting enzyme inhibitors in renovascular hypertension. Am J Hypertens 1:344S–349S, 1988.
182. Murphy BF, Whitworth JA, Kincaid Smith P: Renal insufficiency with combinations of angiotensin converting enzyme inhibitors and diuretics. Br Med J Clin Res 288:844–845, 1984.
183. Wilcox CS, Mitch WE, Kelly RA, et al: Factors affecting potassium balance during frusemide administration. Clin Sci 67:195–203, 1984.
184. Johnson CI, McGrath BP, Matthews PG: Interaction between captopril and hydrochlorothiazide in hypertension. Med J Aust 2:18, 1979.
185. Ciabattoni G, Pugliese F, Cinotti GA, et al: Characterization of furosemide-induced activation of the renal prostaglandin system. Eur J Pharmacol 60:181–187, 1979.
186. Favre L, Glasson P, Riondel A, Vallotton MB: Interaction of diuretics and non-steroidal anti-inflammatory drugs in man. Clin Sci 64:407–415, 1983.
187. Kramer HJ, Dusing R, Stinnesbeck B, et al: Interaction of conventional and antikaliuretic diuretics with the renal prostaglandin system. Clin Sci 59:67–70, 1980.
188. Tiggeler RG, Koene RA, Wijdeveld PG: Inhibition of frusemide-induced natriuresis by indomethacin in patients with the nephrotic syndrome. Clin Sci Mol Med 52:149–151, 1977.
189. Kirchner KA, Brandon S, Mueller RA, et al: Mechanism of attenuated hydrochlorothiazide response during indomethacin administration. Kidney Int 31:1097–1103, 1987.
190. Kirchner KA: Indomethacin antagonizes furosemide's intratubular effects during loop segment microperfusion. J Pharmacol Exp Ther 243:881–886, 1987.
191. Data JL, Rane A, Gerkens J, et al: The influence of indomethacin on the pharmacokinetics, diuretic response and hemodynamics of furosemide in the dog. J Pharmacol Exp Ther 206:431–438, 1978.
192. Johnston GD, Hiatt WR, Nies AS, et al: Factors modifying the early nondiuretic vascular effects of furosemide in man. The possible role of renal prostaglandins. Circ Res 53:630–635, 1983.
193. Kover G, Tost H: The effect of indomethacin on kidney function: Indomethacin and furosemide antagonism. Pflugers Arch 372:215–220, 1977.
194. Planas R, Arroyo V, Rimola A, et al: Acetylsalicylic acid suppresses the renal hemodynamic effect and reduces the diuretic action of furosemide in cirrhosis with ascites. Gastroenterology 84:247–252, 1983.
195. Melki TS, Foegh ML, Ramwell PW: Implication of thromboxane in frusemide diuresis in rats. Clin Sci 71:647–650, 1986.
196. Bonjour JP, Malvin RL: Stimulation of ADH release by the renin-angiotensin system. Am J Physiol 218:1555–1559, 1970.
197. Danielsen H, Pedersen EB, Madsen M, Jensen T: Abnormal renal sodium excretion in the nephrotic syndrome after furosemide: Relation to glomerular filtration rate. Acta Med Scand 217:513–518, 1985.
198. Baylis PH, De Beer FC: Human plasma vasopressin response to potent loop-diuretic drugs. Eur J Clin Pharmacol 20:343–346, 1981.
199. Siegel SR, Weitzman RE, Fisher DA: Endogenous angiotensin stimulation of vasopressin in the newborn lamb. J Clin Invest 63:287–293, 1979.
200. Ghose RR: Plasma arginine vasopressin in hyponatraemic patients receiving diuretics. Postgrad Med J 61:1043–1046, 1985.
201. Field MJ, Stanton BA, Giebisch GH: Influence of ADH on renal potassium handling: A micropuncture and microperfusion study. Kidney Int 25:502–511, 1984.
202. Wilcox CS, Aminoff MJ, Slater JD: Sodium homeostasis in patients with autonomic failure. Clin Sci Mol Med 53:321–328, 1977.
203. Petersen JS, Shalmi M, Abildgaard U, Christensen S: Alpha-1 blockade inhibits compensatory sodium reabsorption in the proximal tubules during furosemide-induced volume contraction. J Pharmacol Exp Ther 258:42–48, 1991.
204. Petersen JS, Shalmi M, Lam HR, Christensen S: Renal response to furosemide in conscious rats: Effects of acute instrumentation and peripheral sympathectomy. J Pharmacol Exp Ther 258:1–7, 1991.
205. Petersen JS, Shalmi M, Abildgaard U, et al: Renal effects of alpha-adrenoceptor blockade during furosemide diuresis in conscious rats. Pharmacol Toxicol 70:3–12, 1992.
206. Fett DL, Cavero PG, Burnett JC Jr: Low-dose atrial natriuretic factor and furosemide in experimental acute congestive heart failure. J Am Soc Nephrol 4:162–167, 1993.
207. Loon NR, Wilcox CS, Nelson R, Mounts M: Metabolic alkalosis impairs the response to bumetanide. Kidney Int 33:200A, 1988. Abstract.
208. Greenberg A, Ray SM, Shahawy M, et al: Influence of pH on the natriuretic response to bumetanide and furosemide. In Puschett J, Greenberg A (eds): Diuretics III: Chemistry, Pharmacology, and Clinical Applications. Elsevier Science Publishing, New York, 1990, pp 154–159.
209. Brater DC, Anderson S, Baird B, Campbell WB: Effects of ibuprofen, naproxen, and sulindac on prostaglandins in men. Kidney Int 27:66–73, 1985.
210. Brater DC: Resistance to loop diuretics. Why it happens and what to do about it. Drugs 30:427–443, 1985.
211. Ellison DH: The physiologic basis of diuretic synergism: Its role in treating diuretic resistance [see comments]. Ann Intern Med 114:886–894, 1991.
212. Brater DC, Pressley RH, Anderson SA: Mechanisms of the synergistic combination of metolazone and bumetanide. J Pharmacol Exp Ther 233:70–74, 1985.
213. Oster JR, Epstein M, Smoller S: Combined therapy with thiazide-type and loop diuretic agents for resistant sodium retention. Ann Intern Med 99:405–406, 1983.
214. Morachiello P, Landini S, Fracasso A, et al: Metolazone plus furosemide: Evaluation of proximal Na⁺ reabsorption by lithium clearance in nephrotic patients. In Puschett J, Greenberg A (eds): Diuretics III: Chemistry, Pharmacology, and Clinical Applications. Elsevier Science Publishing, New York, 1990, pp 38–40.
215. Wollam GL, Tarazi RC, Bravo EL, Dustan HP: Diuretic potency of combined hydrochlorothiazide and furosemide therapy in patients with azotemia. Am J Med 72:929–938, 1982.

216. Schapel GJ, Edwards DG, Robinson J: Potassium-sparing effect of amiloride in a diuretic factorial study in man. Clin Exp Pharmacol Physiol 2:277–287, 1975.

217. Jeunemaitre X, Charru A, Chatellier G, et al: Long-term metabolic effects of spironolactone and thiazides combined with potassium-sparing agents for treatment of essential hypertension. Am J Cardiol 62:1072–1077, 1988.

218. Vidt DG: Mechanism of action, pharmacokinetics, adverse effects, and therapeutic uses of amiloride hydrochloride, a new potassium-sparing diuretic. Pharmacotherapy 1:179–187, 1981.

219. McInnes GT, Yeo WW, Ramsay LE, Moser M: Cardiotoxicity and diuretics: Much speculation—little substance. J Hypertens 10:317–335, 1992. Editorial. (Erratum in J Hypertens 10:following H24, 1992.)

220. Adverse reactions to bendrofluazide and propranolol for the treatment of mild hypertension. Report of Medical Research Council Working Party on Mild to Moderate Hypertension. Lancet 2:539–543, 1981.

221. Kamm DE, Genin M, Kuchmy B, Hollander J: Diuretic-induced azotemia: Unmasking the role of increased peripheral catabolism through evisceration-hepatectomy. Kidney Int Suppl 16:S58–S60, 1983.

222. Ayus JC: Diuretic-induced hyponatremia. Editorial. Arch Intern Med 146:1295–1296, 1986.

223. Ashraf N, Locksley R, Arieff AI: Thiazide-induced hyponatremia associated with death or neurologic damage in outpatients. Am J Med 70:1163–1168, 1981.

224. Szatalowicz VL, Miller PD, Lacher JW, et al: Comparative effect of diuretics on renal water excretion in hyponatraemic oedematous disorders. Clin Sci 62:235–238, 1982.

225. Ayus JC, Krothapalli RK, Arieff AI: Changing concepts in treatment of severe symptomatic hyponatremia. Rapid correction and possible relation to central pontine myelinolysis. Am J Med 78:897–902, 1985.

226. Laureno R, Karp BI: Pontine and extrapontine myelinolysis following rapid correction of hyponatraemia. Lancet 1:1439–1441, 1988.

227. Norenberg MD, Leslie KO, Robertson AS: Association between rise in serum sodium and central pontine myelinolysis. Ann Neurol 11:128–135, 1982.

228. Sonnenblick M, Friedlander Y, Rosin AJ: Diuretic-induced severe hyponatremia. Review and analysis of 129 reported patients. Chest 103:601–606, 1993.

229. Lowenthal DT, Dickerman D: The use of diuretics in varying degrees of renal impairment: An overview. Clin Exp Hypertens [A] 5:297–307, 1983.

230. Sterns RH: ''Slow'' correction of hyponatremia: A break with tradition? Kidney 23:1–5, 1991.

231. Ayus JC, Krothapalli RK, Armstrong DL, Norton HJ: Symptomatic hyponatremia in rats: Effect of treatment on mortality and brain lesions [see comments]. Am J Physiol 257:F18–F22, 1989.

232. Ashouri OS: Severe diuretic-induced hyponatremia in the elderly. A series of eight patients. Arch Intern Med 146:1355–1357, 1986.

233. Berl T: Treating hyponatremia: What is all the controversy about? [see comments]. Ann Intern Med 113:417–419, 1990.

234. Morgan DB, Davidson C: Hypokalaemia and diuretics: An analysis of publications. Br Med J 280:905–908, 1980.

235. Freis ED, Papademetriou V: How dangerous are diuretics? Drugs 30:469–474, 1985.

236. Holland OB, Nixon JV, Kuhnert L: Diuretic-induced ventricular ectopic activity. Am J Med 70:762–768, 1981.

237. Myers MG: Diuretic therapy and ventricular arrhythmias in persons 65 years of age and older. Am J Cardiol 65:599–603, 1990.

238. Lipworth BJ, McDevitt DG, Struthers AD: Hypokalemic and ECG sequelae of combined beta-agonist/diuretic therapy. Protection by conventional doses of spironolactone but not triamterene. Chest 98:811–815, 1990.

239. Rosa RM, Silva P, Young JB, et al: Adrenergic modulation of extrarenal potassium disposal. N Engl J Med 302:431–434, 1980.

240. Mitch WE, Wilcox CS: Disorders of body fluids, sodium and potassium in chronic renal failure. Am J Med 72:536–550, 1982.

241. Hropot M, Fowler N, Karlmark B, Giebisch G: Tubular action of diuretics: Distal effects on electrolyte transport and acidification. Kidney Int 28:477–489, 1985.

242. Khuri RN, Strieder WN, Giebisch G: Effects of flow rate and potassium intake on distal tubular potassium transfer. Am J Physiol 228:1249–1261, 1975.

243. Wilcox CS: Diuretics and potassium. In Hoffman JF, Giebisch G (eds): Current Topics in Membranes and Transport. Academic Press, Orlando, FL, 1987, pp 250–331.

244. Ellison DH, Velazquez H, Wright FS: Stimulation of distal potassium secretion by low lumen chloride in the presence of barium. Am J Physiol 248:F638–F649, 1985.

245. Stanton BA, Giebisch G: Effects of pH on potassium transport by renal distal tubule. Am J Physiol 242:F544–F551, 1982.

246. Wilkinson PR, Issler H, Hesp R, Raftery EB: Total body and serum potassium during prolonged thiazide therapy for essential hypertension. Lancet 1:759–762, 1975.

247. Sheehan J, White A: Diuretic-associated hypomagnesaemia. Br Med J Clin Res 285:1157–1159, 1982.

248. Kroenke K, Wood DR, Hanley JF: The value of serum magnesium determination in hypertensive patients receiving diuretics. Arch Intern Med 147:1553–1556, 1987.

249. Petri M, Cumber P, Grimes L, et al: The metabolic effects of thiazide therapy in the elderly: A population study. Age Ageing 15:151–155, 1986.

250. Dyckner T, Wester PO: Effects of magnesium infusions in diuretic induced hyponatraemia. Lancet 1:585–586, 1981.

251. Kelepouris E: Cytosolic magnesium as an inhibitor of potassium and chloride channels in the loop of Henle. In Puschett J, Greenberg A (eds): Diuretics III: Chemistry, Pharmacology, and Clinical Applications. Elsevier Science Publishing, New York, 1990, pp 722–729.

252. Popovtzer MM, Subryan VL, Alfrey AC, et al: The acute effect of chlorothiazide on serum-ionized calcium. Evidence for a parathyroid hormone–dependent mechanism. J Clin Invest 55:1295–1302, 1975.

253. DuBose T: Effect on acid-base balance. In Eknoyan G, Martinez-Maldonado M (eds): The Physiological Basis of Diuretic Therapy in Clinical Medicine. Grune & Stratton, Orlando, FL, 1986, p 125.

254. Levine DZ: Acid-base complications induced by diuretics. In Puschett J, Greenberg A (eds): Diuretics III: Chemistry, Pharmacology, and Clinical Applications. Elsevier Science Publishing, New York, 1990, pp 228–233.

255. Cannon PJ, Heineman HO, Albert MS, et al: ''Contraction'' alkalosis after diuresis of edematous patients with ethacrynic acid. Ann Intern Med 62:979, 1965.

256. Wilcox CS, Loon NR, Kanthawatana S, et al: Generation of alkalosis with loop diuretics: Roles of contraction and acid excretion. J Nephrol 2:81–87, 1991.

257. Schlueter WA, Batlle DC: Effect of loop diuretics on urinary acidification. In Puschett J, Greenberg A (eds): Diuretics III: Chemistry, Pharmacology, and Clinical Applications. Elsevier Science Publishing, New York, 1990, pp 174–182.

258. Furman BL: Impairment of glucose intolerance produced by diuretics and other drugs. Pharmacol Ther 12:613–649, 1981.

259. Dornhorst A, Powell SH, Pensky J: Aggravation by propranolol of hyperglycaemic effect of hydrochlorothiazide in type II diabetics without alteration of insulin secretion. Lancet 1:123–126, 1985.

260. Paolisso G, Di Maro G, Cozzolino D, et al: Chronic magnesium administration enhances oxidative glucose metabolism in thiazide treated hypertensive patients. Am J Hypertens 5:681–686, 1992.

261. Bloomgarden ZT, Ginsberg-Fellner F, Rayfield EJ, et al: Elevated hemoglobin A1c and low-density lipoprotein cholesterol levels in thiazide-treated diabetic patients. Am J Med 77:823–827, 1984.

262. Ames RP: The effects of antihypertensive drugs on serum lipids and lipoproteins. II. Non-diuretic drugs. Drugs 32:335–357, 1986.

263. Ruppert M, Overlack A, Kolloch R, et al: Neurohormonal and metabolic effects of severe and moderate salt restriction in non-obese normotensive adults. J Hypertens 11:743–749, 1993.

264. Ljunghall S, Backman U, Danielson BG, et al: Effects of bendroflu-methiazide on urate metabolism during treatment of patients with renal stones. J Urol 127:1207–1210, 1982.

265. Waite WW, Wade WE, Cobb HH: The effect of three different diuretic regimens on serum uric acid in an ambulatory hypertensive population. Hosp Pharm 23:50–59, 1993.

266. Chang SW, Fine R, Siegel D, et al: The impact of diuretic therapy on reported sexual function [see comments]. Arch Intern Med 151:2402–2408, 1991.

267. Rybak LP: Pathophysiology of furosemide ototoxicity. J Otolaryngol 11:127–133, 1982.

268. Tuzel IH: Comparison of adverse reactions to bumetanide and furosemide. J Clin Pharmacol 21:615–619, 1981.

269. Reineck HJ: Diuretic use in renal failure. In Eknoyan G, Martinez-

Maldonado M (eds): The Physiological Basis of Diuretic Therapy in Clinical Medicine. Grune & Stratton, Orlando, FL, 1986, p 298.

270. Lindberg BS: Diuretics and pregnancy. Scand J Clin Lab Invest Suppl 169:83–85, 1984.

271. Lindheimer MD, Katz AI: Hypertension in pregnancy. N Engl J Med 313:675–680, 1985.

272. Diffey BL, Langtry J: Phototoxic potential of thiazide diuretics in normal subjects. Arch Dermatol 125:1355–1358, 1989.

273. Frommer JP, Wesson DE, Eknoyan G: Side effects and complications of diuretic therapy. In Eknoyan G, Martinez-Maldonado M (eds): The Physiological Basis of Diuretic Therapy in Clinical Medicine. Grune & Stratton, Orlando, FL, 1986, pp 293–309.

274. Lawson DH, Macadam RF, Singh MH, et al: Effect of furosemide on antibiotic-induced renal damage in rats. J Infect Dis 126:593–600, 1972.

275. Shapiro S, Slone D, Lewis GP, Jick H: The epidemiology of digoxin toxicity. A study in three Boston hospitals. J Chronic Dis 22:361–371, 1969.

276. Petersen V, Hvidt S, Thomsen K, Schou M: Effect of prolonged thiazide treatment on renal lithium clearance. Br Med J 3:143–145, 1974.

277. Boer WH, Koomans HA, Dorhout Mees EJ: Effect of thiazides with and without carbonic-anhydrase inhibiting activity on free water and lithium clearance. In Puschett J, Greenberg A (eds): Diuretics III: Chemistry, Pharmacology, and Clinical Applications. Elsevier Science Publishing, New York, 1990, pp 31–33.

278. Shirley DG, Walter SJ, Sampson B: A micropuncture study of renal lithium reabsorption: Effects of amiloride and furosemide. Am J Physiol 263:F1128–F1133, 1992.

279. Bridgman JF, Rosen SM, Thorp JM: Complications during clofibrate treatment of nephrotic-syndrome hyperlipoproteinaemia. Lancet 2:506–509, 1972.

280. Weinberg MS, Quigg RJ, Salant DJ, Bernard DB: Anuric renal failure precipitated by indomethacin and triamterene. Nephron 40:216–218, 1985.

281. Marchionni N, Conti A, De Alfieri W, et al: Ibopamine in congestive heart failure refractory to digitalis, diuretics, and captopril. J Clin Pharmacol 26:74–77, 1986.

282. Francis GS, Siegel RM, Goldsmith SR, et al: Acute vasoconstrictor response to intravenous furosemide in patients with chronic congestive heart failure. Activation of the neurohumoral axis. Ann Intern Med 103:1–6, 1985.

283. Dikshit K, Vyden JK, Forrester JS, et al: Renal and extrarenal hemodynamic effects of furosemide in congestive heart failure after acute myocardial infarction. N Engl J Med 288:1087–1090, 1973.

284. Johnston GD, Nicholls DP, Leahey WJ, Finch MB: The effects of captopril on the acute vascular responses to frusemide in man. Clin Sci 65:359–363, 1983.

285. Biagi RW, Bapat BN: Frusemide in acute pulmonary oedema. Lancet 1:849, 1967.

286. Bhatia ML, Singh I, Manchanda SC, et al: Effect of frusemide on pulmonary blood volume. Br Med J 2:551–552, 1969.

287. Wilson JR, Reichek N, Dunkman WB, Goldberg S: Effect of diuresis on the performance of the failing left ventricle in man. Am J Med 70:234–239, 1981.

288. Verma SP, Silke B, Hussain M, et al: First-line treatment of left ventricular failure complicating acute myocardial infarction: A randomized evaluation of immediate effects of diuretic, venodilator, arteriodilator, and positive inotropic drugs on left ventricular function. J Cardiovasc Pharmacol 10:38–46, 1987.

289. Bauer U, Haerer W, Fehske KJ, et al: Hemodynamic effects of piretanide and methyldigoxine in congestive heart failure: Long-term results of a placebo-controlled randomized double blind study. In Puschett J, Greenberg A (eds): Diuretics III: Chemistry, Pharmacology, and Clinical Applications. Elsevier Science Publishing, New York, 1990, pp 316–321.

290. Ross J Jr, Braunwald E: Studies on Starling's law of the heart. IX. The effects of impending venous return on performance of the normal and failing human left ventricle. Circulation 30:719, 1964.

291. Pabico RC, Rogal GJ, McKenna BA, et al: Renal effects of dobutamine and dopamine in congestive heart failure. In Puschett J, Greenberg A (eds): Diuretics III: Chemistry, Pharmacology, and Clinical Applications. Elsevier Science Publishing, New York, 1990, pp 302–312.

292. Vasko MR, Cartwright DB, Knochel JP, et al: Furosemide absorption altered in decompensated congestive heart failure. Ann Intern Med 102:314–318, 1985.

293. Brater DC, Seiwell R, Anderson S, et al: Absorption and disposition of furosemide in congestive heart failure. Kidney Int 22:171–176, 1982.

294. Brater DC, Day B, Burdette A, Anderson S: Bumetanide and furosemide in heart failure. Kidney Int 26:183–189, 1984.

295. Cook JA, Smith DE, Cornish LA, et al: Kinetics, dynamics, and bioavailability of bumetanide in healthy subjects and patients with congestive heart failure. Clin Pharmacol Ther 44:487–500, 1988.

296. Ziakas G, Zioutas G, Arvanitidis T, Zurukzoglu W: Muzolimine in patients with cardiac edema: A comparison with furosemide in a repeated-dose single-blind study. Clin Nephrol 19:S85–S91, 1983.

297. van Vliet AA, Donker AJ, Nauta JJ, Verheugt FW: Spironolactone in congestive heart failure refractory to high-dose loop diuretic and low-dose angiotensin-converting enzyme inhibitor. Am J Cardiol 71:21A–28A, 1993.

298. Dzau VJ, Hollenberg NK: Renal response to captopril in severe heart failure: Role of furosemide in natriuresis and reversal of hyponatremia. Ann Intern Med 100:777–782, 1984.

299. Ikram H, Chan W, Espiner EA, Nicholls MG: Haemodynamic and hormone responses to acute and chronic frusemide therapy in congestive heart failure. Clin Sci 59:443–449, 1980.

300. Steiness E: Digoxin toxicity compared with myocardial digoxin and potassium concentration. Br J Pharmacol 63:233–237, 1978.

301. Steiness E: Suppression of renal excretion of digoxin in hypokalemic patients. Clin Pharmacol Ther 23:511–514, 1978.

302. Steiness E, Olesen KH: Cardiac arrhythmias induced by hypokalaemia and potassium loss during maintenance digoxin therapy. Br Heart J 38:167–172, 1976.

303. Yanover MJ, Bichet DG, Anderson RJ: Cirrhosis and ascites and the nephrotic syndrome. In Dirks JH, Sutton RA (eds): Diuretics: Physiology, Pharmacology and Clinical Use. WB Saunders, Philadelphia, 1986, pp 168–191.

304. Bichet D, Szatalowicz V, Chaimovitz C, Schrier RW: Role of vasopressin in abnormal water excretion in cirrhotic patients. Ann Intern Med 96:413–417, 1982.

305. Lieberman FL, Denison EK, Reynolds TB: The relationship of plasma volume, portal hypertension, ascites and renal sodium retention in cirrhosis: The overflow theory of ascites formation. Ann N Y Acad Sci 170:202, 1970.

306. Levy M, Wexler MJ: Renal sodium retention and ascites formation in dogs with experimental cirrhosis but without portal hypertension or increased splanchnic vascular capacity. J Lab Clin Med 91:520–536, 1978.

307. Lopez Novoa JM, Rengel MA: A micropuncture study of salt and water retention in chronic experimental cirrhosis. Am J Physiol 232:F315–F318, 1977.

308. Lieberman FL, Reynolds TB: Renal failure with cirrhosis. Observations on the role of diuretics. Ann Intern Med 64:1221–1228, 1966.

309. Levy M, Richard C: Mobilization of ascites in cirrhotic dogs following furosemide or mannitol diuresis. Am J Physiol 235:F12–F21, 1978.

310. Diez J, Simon MA, Prieto J: Analysis of segmental tubular Na+ handling: A rational approach to the use of spironolactone in cirrhotic patients with ascites. In Puschett J, Greenberg A (eds): Diuretics III: Chemistry, Pharmacology, and Clinical Applications. Elsevier Science Publishing, New York, 1990, pp 394–395.

311. Villeneuve JP, Verbeeck RK, Wilkinson GR, Branch RA: Furosemide kinetics and dynamics in patients with cirrhosis. Clin Pharmacol Ther 40:14–20, 1986.

312. Keller E, Hoppe Seyler G, Mumm R, Schollmeyer P: Influence of hepatic cirrhosis and end-stage renal disease on pharmacokinetics and pharmacodynamics of furosemide. Eur J Clin Pharmacol 20:27–33, 1981.

313. Gonzalez G, Arancibia A, Rivas MI, et al: Pharmacokinetics of furosemide in patients with hepatic cirrhosis. Eur J Clin Pharmacol 22:315–320, 1982.

314. Sawhney VK, Gregory PB, Swezey SE, Blaschke TF: Furosemide disposition in cirrhotic patients. Gastroenterology 81:1012–1016, 1981.

315. Verbeeck RK, Patwardhan RV, Villeneuve JP, et al: Furosemide disposition in cirrhosis. Clin Pharmacol Ther 31:719–725, 1982.

316. Fredrick MJ, Pound DC, Hall SD, Brater DC: Furosemide absorption in patients with cirrhosis. Clin Pharmacol Ther 49:241–247, 1991.

317. Allgulander C, Beermann B, Sjogren A: Frusemide pharmacokinetics in patients with liver disease. Clin Pharmacokinet 5:570–575, 1980.

318. Knauf H, Spahn H, Mutschler E: Increased urinary excretion of diuretics in hepatitis patients. *In* Puschett J, Greenberg A (eds): Diuretics III: Chemistry, Pharmacology, and Clinical Applications. Elsevier Science Publishing, New York, 1990, pp 75–81.

319. Fuller R, Hoppel C, Ingalls ST: Furosemide kinetics in patients with hepatic cirrhosis with ascites. Clin Pharmacol Ther 30:461–467, 1981.

320. Pinzani M, Daskalopoulos G, Laffi G, et al: Altered furosemide pharmacokinetics in chronic alcoholic liver disease with ascites contributes to diuretic resistance. Gastroenterology 92:294–298, 1987.

321. Perez Ayuso RM, Arroyo V, Planas R, et al: Randomized comparative study of efficacy of furosemide versus spironolactone in nonazotemic cirrhosis with ascites. Relationship between the diuretic response and the activity of the renin-aldosterone system. Gastroenterology 84:961–968, 1983.

322. Daskalopoulos G, Laffi G, Morgan T, et al: Immediate effects of furosemide on renal hemodynamics in chronic liver disease with ascites. Gastroenterology 92:1859–1863, 1987.

323. Rector WGJ: 'Diuretic-resistant' ascites. Observations on pathogenesis. Arch Intern Med 146:1597–1600, 1986.

324. Earley LE, Martino JA: Influence of sodium balance on the ability of diuretics to inhibit tubular reabsorption. A study of factors that influence renal tubular sodium reabsorption in man. Circulation 42:323–334, 1970.

325. Thompson EJ, Torres E, Grosberg SJ, Martinez-Maldonado M: Effect of triamterene on potassium excretion in cirrhotic patients receiving furosemide. Clin Pharmacol Ther 21:392–394, 1977.

326. Bernardi M, Servadei D, Trevisani F, et al: Importance of plasma aldosterone concentration on the natriuretic effect of spironolactone in patients with liver cirrhosis and ascites. Digestion 31:189–193, 1985.

327. Szwed JJ, Maxwell DR, Elliott R, Redlich LR: Diuretics and small intestinal lymph flow in the dog. J Pharmacol Exp Ther 200:88–94, 1977.

328. Szwed JJ, Kleit SA, Hamburger RJ: Effect of furosemide and chlorothiazide on the thoracic duct lymph flow in the dog. J Lab Clin Med 79:693–700, 1972.

329. McCaffrey C, Levy M: Effect of furosemide on thoracic duct lymph flow in the dog. Am J Physiol 238:F363–F371, 1980.

330. Szwed AJ, Maxwell DR, Kleit SA, Hamburger RJ: Angiotensin II, diuretics, and thoracic duct lymph flow in the dog. Am J Physiol 224:705–708, 1973.

331. Henriksen JH, Schlichting P: Increased extravasation and lymphatic return rate of albumin during diuretic treatment of ascites in patients with liver cirrhosis. Scand J Clin Lab Invest 41:589–599, 1981.

332. Atkinson M: The effect of diuretics on portal venous pressure. Lancet 2:819–823, 1959.

333. Rector WGJ: Ascites kinetics in cirrhosis: Effects of rapid volume expansion and diuretic administration. J Lab Clin Med 111:166–172, 1988.

334. Levy M: Physiological factors constraining the mobilization of ascites. *In* Puschett J, Greenberg A (eds): Diuretics III: Chemistry, Pharmacology, and Clinical Applications. Elsevier Science Publishing, New York, 1990, pp 376–382.

335. Diuretics or paracentesis for ascites? Lancet 2:775–776, 1988.

336. Gines P, Arroyo V, Quintero E, et al: Comparison of paracentesis and diuretics in the treatment of cirrhotics with tense ascites. Results of a randomized study. Gastroenterology 93:234–241, 1987.

337. Kao HW, Rakov NE, Savage E, Reynolds TB: The effect of large volume paracentesis on plasma volume—a cause of hypovolemia? Hepatology 5:403–407, 1985.

338. Ring Larsen H, Henriksen JH, Wilken C, et al: Diuretic treatment in decompensated cirrhosis and congestive heart failure: Effect of posture. Br Med J Clin Res 292:1351–1353, 1986.

339. Shear L, Ching S, Gabuzda GJ: Compartmentalization of ascites and edema in patients with hepatic cirrhosis. N Engl J Med 282:1391–1396, 1970.

340. Pockros PJ, Reynolds TB: Rapid diuresis in patients with ascites from chronic liver disease: The importance of peripheral edema. Gastroenterology 90:1827–1833, 1986.

341. Greenway B, Johnson PJ, Williams R: Control of malignant ascites with spironolactone. Br J Surg 69:441–442, 1982.

342. Pockros PJ, Esrason KT, Nguyen C, et al: Mobilization of malignant ascites with diuretics is dependent on ascitic fluid characteristics. Gastroenterology 103:1302–1306, 1992.

343. Campra JL, Reynolds TB: Effectiveness of high-dose spironolactone therapy in patients with chronic liver disease and relatively refractory ascites. Am J Dig Dis 23:1025–1030, 1978.

344. Bernardi M, De Palma R, Trevisani F, et al: Effects of a new loop diuretic (muzolimine) in cirrhosis with ascites: Comparison with furosemide. Hepatology 6:400–405, 1986.

345. Gregory PB, Broekelschen PH, Hill MD, et al: Complications of diuresis in the alcoholic patient with ascites: A controlled trial. Gastroenterology 73:534–538, 1977.

346. Naranjo CA, Pontigo E, Valdenegro C, et al: Furosemide-induced adverse reactions in cirrhosis of the liver. Clin Pharmacol Ther 25:154–160, 1979.

347. Gabow PA, Moore S, Schrier RW: Spironolactone-induced hyperchloremic acidosis in cirrhosis. Ann Intern Med 90:338–340, 1979.

348. Epstein M: Therapeutic strategies in the management of ascites. *In* Puschett J, Greenberg A (eds): Diuretics III: Chemistry, Pharmacology, and Clinical Applications. Elsevier Science Publishing, New York, 1990, pp 383–393.

349. Meltzer JI, Keim HJ, Laragh JH, et al: Nephrotic syndrome: Vasoconstriction and hypervolemic types indicated by renin-sodium profiling. Ann Intern Med 91:688–696, 1979.

350. Bernard DB, Alexander EA, Couser WG, Levinsky NG: Renal sodium retention during volume expansion in experimental nephrotic syndrome. Kidney Int 14:478–485, 1978.

351. Grausz H, Lieberman R, Earley LE: Effect of plasma albumin on sodium reabsorption in patients with nephrotic syndrome. Kidney Int 1:47–54, 1972.

352. Brown EA, Markandu ND, Sagnella GA, et al: Evidence that some mechanism other than the renin system causes sodium retention in nephrotic syndrome. Lancet 2:1237–1240, 1982.

353. Keller E, Hoppe Seyler G, Schollmeyer P: Disposition and diuretic effect of furosemide in the nephrotic syndrome. Clin Pharmacol Ther 32:442–449, 1982.

354. Green TP, Mirkin BL: Furosemide disposition in normal and proteinuric rats: Urinary drug-protein binding as a determinant of drug excretion. J Pharmacol Exp Ther 218:122–127, 1981.

355. Inoue M, Okajima K, Itoh K, et al: Mechanism of furosemide resistance in analbuminemic rats and hypoalbuminemic patients. Kidney Int 32:198–203, 1987.

356. Kirchner KA, Voelker JR, Brater DC: Tubular resistance to furosemide contributes to the attenuated diuretic response in nephrotic rats. J Am Soc Nephrol 2:1201–1207, 1992.

357. Kirchner KA, Voelker JR, Brater DC: Binding inhibitors restore furosemide potency in tubule fluid containing albumin. Kidney Int 40:418–424, 1991.

358. Kirchner KA, Voelker JR, Brater DC: Intratubular albumin blunts the response to furosemide—a mechanism for diuretic resistance in the nephrotic syndrome. J Pharmacol Exp Ther 252:1097–1101, 1990.

359. Garin EH: A comparison of combinations of diuretics in nephrotic edema. Am J Dis Child 141:769–771, 1987.

360. Paton RR, Kane RE: Long-term diuretic therapy with metolazone of renal failure and the nephrotic syndrome. J Clin Pharmacol 17:243–251, 1977.

361. Lyons H, Pinn VW, Cortell S, et al: Allergic interstitial nephritis causing reversible renal failure in four patients with idiopathic nephrotic syndrome. N Engl J Med 288:124–128, 1973.

362. Paller MS, Ferris TF: Idiopathic edema. *In* Dirks JH, Sutton RA (eds): Diuretics: Physiology, Pharmacology and Clinical Use. WB Saunders, Philadelphia, 1986, pp 192–206.

363. MacGregor GA, Markandu ND, Roulston JE, et al: Is ''idiopathic'' edema idiopathic? Lancet 1:397–400, 1979.

364. Young JB, Brownjohn AM, Lee MR: Diuretics and idiopathic oedema. Nephron 43:311–312, 1986.

365. Minuth AN, Terrell JB Jr, Suki WN: Acute renal failure: A study of the course and prognosis of 104 patients and of the role of furosemide. Am J Med Sci 271:317–324, 1976.

366. Brown CB, Ogg CS, Cameron JS: High dose frusemide in acute renal failure: A controlled trial. Clin Nephrol 15:90–96, 1981.

367. Kleinknecht D, Ganeval D, Gonzalez Duque LA, Fermanian J: Furosemide in acute oliguric renal failure. A controlled trial. Nephron 17:51–58, 1976.

368. Levinsky NG, Bernard DB, Johnston PA: Mannitol and loop diuretics in acute renal failure. *In* Brenner BM, Lazarus JM (eds): Acute Renal Failure. WB Saunders, Philadelphia, 1983, p 712.

369. Narins RG, Chusid P: Diuretic use in critical care. Am J Cardiol 57:26A–32A, 1986.

370. Lindner A: Synergism of dopamine and furosemide in diuretic-resistant, oliguric acute renal failure. Nephron 33:121–126, 1983.

371. Dargie HJ, Allison ME, Kennedy AC, Gray MJ: High dosage metolazone in chronic renal failure. Br Med J 4:196–198, 1972.

372. Bennett WM, Porter GA: Efficacy and safety of metolazone in renal failure and the nephrotic syndrome. J Clin Pharmacol 13:357–364, 1973.

373. Rose HJ, O'Malley K, Pruitt AW: Depression of renal clearance of furosemide in man by azotemia. Clin Pharmacol Ther 21:141–146, 1977.

374. Brater DC, Anderson SA, Brown-Cartwright D: Response to furosemide in chronic renal insufficiency: Rationale for limited doses. Clin Pharmacol Ther 40:134–139, 1986.

375. Voelker JR, Cartwright-Brown D, Anderson S, et al: Comparison of loop diuretics in patients with chronic renal insufficiency. Kidney Int 32:572–578, 1987.

376. Raymond KH, Hunt JM, Stein JM: Acute and chronic renal failure. *In* Dirks JH, Sutton RA (eds): Diuretics: Physiology, Pharmacology and Clinical Use. WB Saunders, Philadelphia, 1986, pp 237–258.

377. van Olden RW, van Meijel JJM, Gerlag PGG: Chronic high dosage furosemide in haemodialysis patients. *In* Puschett J, Greenberg A (eds): Diuretics III: Chemistry, Pharmacology, and Clinical Applications. Elsevier Science Publishing, New York, 1990, pp 25–27.

378. Weisschedel E, Grussendorf M, Ritz E: Diuretic effect of muzolimine in advanced renal failure. Clin Nephrol 19:S50, 1983.

379. Keeton GR, Morrison S: Effects of frusemide in chronic renal failure. Nephron 28:169–173, 1981.

380. Wilcox CS, Granges F, Kirk G, et al: Effects of saline infusion on titratable acid generation and ammonia secretion. Am J Physiol 247:F506–F519, 1984.

381. Rastogi SP, Crawford C, Wheeler R, et al: Effect of furosemide on urinary acidification in distal renal tubular acidosis. J Lab Clin Med 104:271–282, 1984.

382. Schambelan M, Sebastian A, Hulter HN: Mineral corticoid excess and deficiency syndromes. *In* Brenner BM, Stein JH (eds): Contemporary Issues in Nephrology, Vol II, Acid-Base and Potassium Homeostasis. Churchill Livingstone, New York, 1978, pp 232–268.

383. Sanjad SA, Keenan BS, Hill LL: Renal hypoprostaglandism, hypertension, and type IV renal tubular acidosis reversed by furosemide. Ann Intern Med 99:624–627, 1983.

384. Suki WN, Yium JJ, Von Minden M, et al: Acute treatment of hypercalcemia with furosemide. N Engl J Med 283:836–840, 1970.

385. Sutton RA: Calcium disorders. *In* Dirks JH, Sutton RA (eds): Diuretics: Physiology, Pharmacology and Clinical Use. WB Saunders, Philadelphia, 1986, pp 259–272.

386. Yendt ER, Cohanim M: Prevention of calcium stones with thiazides. Kidney Int 13:397–409, 1978.

387. Leppla D, Browne R, Hill K, Pak CY: Effect of amiloride with or without hydrochlorothiazide on urinary calcium and saturation of calcium salts. J Clin Endocrinol Metab 57:920–924, 1983.

388. Crawford JD, Kennedy GC: Chlorothiazide in diabetes insipidus. Nature 183:891, 1959.

389. Walter SJ, Laycock JF, Shirley DG: A micropuncture study of proximal tubular function after acute hydrochlorothiazide administration to Brattleboro rats with diabetes insipidus. Clin Sci 57:427–434, 1979.

390. Shirley DG, Walter SJ, Laycock JF: The antidiuretic effect of chronic hydrochlorothiazide treatment in rats with diabetes insipidus: Renal mechanisms. Clin Sci 63:533–538, 1982.

# 54

# Antihypertensive Drugs

*John H. Bauer*
*Garry P. Reams*

This chapter is divided into three major sections. The first section reviews the pharmacology of the nondiuretic antihypertensive drugs, with the intent to provide the clinician with the database required for the informed use of these drugs (Table 54–1). Specifically discussed are 1) class mechanisms of action; 2) class members, with emphasis on defining clinically relevant individual drug pharmacokinetic and pharmacodynamic properties; 3) class renal effects, including an assessment of drug effects on renal function, the renin-angiotensin-aldosterone axis, and salt and water excretion; and 4) class efficacy and safety. The second section reviews pharmacologic criteria for selecting a first and subsequent antihypertensive drug class for the treatment of hypertension. Criteria for selecting a first-step therapy are presented. The causes for and treatment of "resistant" hypertension are reviewed. How far blood pressure should be lowered is addressed. Given our current therapeutic armamentarium, control of blood pressure should be achievable in every patient. The third section reviews the pharmacology of the drugs used in the treatment of the hypertensive urgencies and emergencies. These syndromes are presented; treatment options, including the administration of rapid-acting oral drugs versus parenteral drugs, are discussed. Because of the potential harm that acute blood pressure reduction may have on the brain, heart, and kidneys, antihypertensive therapy must be chosen and monitored carefully.

## TABLE 54–1. Antihypertensive Drugs

Diuretics
  Benzothiadiazides
  Loop
  K⁺ sparing
β-Adrenergic and α₁- and β-adrenergic antagonists
  Nonselective β-adrenergic antagonists
  Nonselective β-adrenergic antagonists with partial agonist activity
  β₁-Selective adrenergic antagonists
  β₁-Selective adrenergic antagonists with partial agonist activity
  Nonselective β-adrenergic and α₁-adrenergic antagonists
Central α₂-adrenergic antagonists
Central and peripheral adrenergic-neuronal blocking agents
Peripheral α₁-adrenergic antagonists
Moderately selective peripheral α₁-adrenergic antagonists
Peripheral adrenergic-neuronal blocking agents
Direct-acting vasodilators
Ca²⁺ antagonists
  Benzothiazepines
  Dihydropyridines
  Diphenylalkylamines
Angiotensin-converting enzyme inhibitors
  Sulfhydryl
  Carboxyl
  Phosphinyl
Tyrosine hydroxylase inhibitors

# PHARMACOLOGY OF THE NONDIURETIC ANTIHYPERTENSIVE DRUGS

## β-Adrenergic Antagonists

### CLASS MECHANISMS OF ACTION

β-Adrenergic antagonists attenuate sympathetic stimulation through competitive antagonism of catecholamines at β-adrenergic receptors.[1, 2] This competition occurs at both β₁-adrenergic (predominantly heart, adipose tissue, brain) and β₂-adrenergic (primarily lung, liver, smooth muscle, skeletal muscle) receptors.[3–6] However, different tissues may possess both β₁- and β₂-receptors in varying

2331

proportions.[5, 6] The precise mechanisms responsible for the reduction in mean arterial pressure (MAP) accompanying β-adrenergic antagonism are unknown. Although β$_1$-adrenergic receptor blockade has generally been considered responsible for the blood pressure–lowering effect and β$_2$-adrenergic receptor blockade was thought undesirable, β$_2$-adrenergic receptor blockade has an antihypertensive effect independent of and distinct from β$_1$-adrenergic receptor blockade.[7] Proposed mechanisms whereby β-adrenergic antagonists may lower MAP, by interfering with vasoconstrictor mechanisms, include 1) inhibition of postsynaptic β$_1$-adrenergic receptors of juxtaglomerular cells within the kidney, thus inhibiting renin release[8, 9]; 2) inhibition of presynaptic facilitory β$_2$-adrenergic receptors at the vascular wall, thus inhibiting norepinephrine release from sympathetic nerve endings[10–12]; and 3) inhibition of central nervous system sympathetic outflow.[13–15] In the absence of partial agonist activity (PAA), the initial systemic hemodynamic effects are decreases in heart rate (HR) and cardiac output (CO) and an increase in total peripheral vascular resistance (TPVR) proportional to the degree of cardiodepression; blood pressure is unchanged.[16–18] Subsequently, there is a gradual decrease in blood pressure proportional to the fall in TPVR[17–21]; the degree of vasodilation is dependent on cardiac sympathetic drive.[19–21] β-Adrenergic antagonists with sufficient PAA to maintain HR and CO do not evoke acute reflex vasoconstriction; blood pressure falls in proportion to the decrease in TPVR.[19–21]

## CLASS MEMBERS

β-Adrenergic antagonists pharmacologically differ in their potency, β$_1$-selectivity, PAA, membrane-stabilizing activity (MSA), and pharmacokinetic nature. PAA is a specific property whereby a weak stimulation of the receptors (positive chronotropic or inotropic effect) can be found at the same time when the drug, binding itself to the receptor, prevents access of strongly stimulating catecholamines.[22, 23] MSA is a specific electrophysiologic property whereby the height and rate of rise of the intracardiac action potential are reduced, without the overall duration of the resting potential being affected.[24] These "quinidine-like" effects are associated with generalized depression of myocardial function; however, direct myocardial depression requires doses much higher (50 to 100 times) than those necessary for β-adrenergic blockage.[24] The β-adrenergic antagonists are reviewed according to the following subclasses: nonselective β-adrenergic antagonism; nonselective β-adrenergic antagonism with PAA; β$_1$-selective adrenergic antagonism; β$_1$-selective adrenergic antagonism with PAA; and nonselective β- and α$_1$-adrenergic antagonism.

### Nonselective β-Adrenergic Antagonists

Nadolol is a nonselective β-adrenergic antagonist that lacks both PAA and MSA[25–30] (Table 54–2). The usual dose is 40 to 80 mg daily. Nadolol is hydrophilic, which is the physical property that accounts for its poor absorption (30% to 40%) but minimal first-pass hepatic (presystemic) metabolism (Table 54–3). Peak plasma concentrations are reached in 2 to 4 hours. The normal plasma half-life is 20

to 24 hours. About 75% of the amount absorbed is excreted unchanged in the urine; 25% is excreted in the feces. There are no active metabolites. Elimination of nadolol is reduced in patients with renal insufficiency; dose reduction is required (Table 54–4). Nadolol is removed by hemodialysis.

Propranolol hydrochloride is a nonselective β-adrenergic antagonist that lacks PAA but possesses moderate MSA[25, 26, 31–36] (see Table 54–2). It is available in the form of tablets and long-acting capsules. The usual tablet dose is 120 to 240 mg/d given in divided doses; the usual long-acting capsule dose is 120 to 240 mg/d. Propranolol is lipophilic, which is the physical property that accounts for its almost complete absorption but extensive first-pass hepatic metabolism (see Table 54–3). Peak plasma concentrations are reached 1 to 3 hours after administration of the tablet and about 6 hours after administration of the long-acting capsule. The plasma half-life of the tablets is 3 to 4 hours; the plasma half-life of the long-acting capsules is about 10 hours. Propranolol is almost totally metabolized in the liver; the major metabolite is 4-hydroxypropranolol, which has β-blocking properties equivalent to those of propranolol. Because of the capsule's slower rate of absorption, there is greater hepatic metabolism than of propranolol tablets. Thus, plasma concentration-time curves for propranolol long-acting capsules are 60% to 65% of those for propranolol tablets; dosages prescribed for propranolol long-acting capsules are about 30% higher than those for propranolol tablets. The major route of elimination is biliary (feces); less than 1% is excreted unchanged in the urine. The metabolism of propranolol is not altered in patients with renal insufficiency.

Timolol maleate is a nonselective β-adrenergic antagonist that lacks both PAA and MSA[25, 26, 37–40] (see Table 54–2). The usual dose is 20 to 40 mg/d given in divided doses. Timolol is lipophilic; it is rapidly and nearly completely absorbed (see Table 54–3). However, 50% of timolol undergoes first-pass hepatic metabolism. Peak plasma levels are reached in 1 to 2 hours. The plasma half-life is 3 to 4 hours. Timolol is largely metabolized by the liver (80%); the drug and its inactive metabolites are excreted in the urine. The metabolism of timolol is unchanged in patients with renal insufficiency.

### Nonselective β-Adrenergic Antagonists with Partial Agonist Activity

Carteolol hydrochloride is a nonselective β-adrenergic antagonist that possesses moderate PAA but lacks MSA[25, 26, 41, 42] (see Table 54–2). The usual dose is 2.5 to 5 mg daily. Carteolol is hydrophilic; it is well absorbed (see Table 54–3). It undergoes little first-pass hepatic metabolism. Peak plasma concentrations are reached in 1 to 3 hours. The normal plasma half-life is about 6 hours. Fifty percent to 70% of a dose of carteolol is eliminated unchanged by the kidney. The remainder of the drug is secondarily metabolized by the liver; 8-hydroxycarteolol is an active metabolite with a half-life of 8 to 12 hours. The rate of carteolol elimination is decreased in patients with renal insufficiency; dose reduction is necessary (see Table 54–4).

Penbutolol sulfate is a nonselective β-adrenergic antagonist that possesses modest PAA but lacks MSA[25, 26, 41] (see

**TABLE 54–2. Pharmacologic Differences Among the β-Adrenergic Antagonists***

| Drug | Potency† | First Dose (mg) | Usual Daily Dose (mg) | Maximal Daily Dose (mg) | β₁-Selectivity | Partial Agonist Activity | Membrane-Stabilizing Activity |
|---|---|---|---|---|---|---|---|
| *Nonselective (β₁ and β₂) Adrenergic Antagonists* | | | | | | | |
| Nadolol | 2–4 | 20 | 40–80 qd | 240 | None | None | None |
| Propranolol | 1 | 20 | 60–120 bid | 320 | None | None | + + |
| Propranolol LA | 0.6–0.65 | 60 | 120–240 qd | 320 | None | None | + + |
| Timolol | 6–8 | 5 | 10–20  bid | 60 | None | None | None |
| *Nonselective (β₁ and β₂) Adrenergic Antagonists with Partial Agonist Activity* | | | | | | | |
| Carteolol | 30 | 2.5 | 2.5–5 qd | 10 | None | + | None |
| Penbutolol | 4 | 20 | 20–40  qd | 80 | None | + | None |
| Pindolol | 6–10 | 5 | 10–20  bid | 60 | None | + + + | None |
| *β₁-Selective Adrenergic Antagonists* | | | | | | | |
| Atenolol | 1 | 50 | 50–100 qd | 150 | + + | None | None |
| Betaxolol | 4 | 10 | 10–20  qd | 40 | + + | None | + |
| Bisoprolol | 4 | 5 | 5–10  qd | 20 | + + | None | None |
| Metoprolol tartrate | 1 | 50 | 50–100 bid | 400 | + + | None | None |
| Metoprolol succinate ER | 1 | 50 | 100–200 qd | 400 | + + | None | None |
| *β₁-Selective Adrenergic Antagonist with Partial Agonist Activity* | | | | | | | |
| Acebutolol | 0.3 | 200 | 400–800 qd | 1200 | + | + | ± |
| *Nonselective (β₁ and β₂) and α₁-Selective Adrenergic Antagonist* | | | | | | | |
| Labetalol | 0.3 | 100 | 200–400 bid | 2400 | None | None | ± |

*LA = long-acting; ER = extended-release.
†Potency is expressed as a ratio to propranolol.

Table 54–2). The usual dose is 20 to 40 mg daily. Penbutolol is lipophilic; it is rapidly and completely absorbed (see Table 54–3). It undergoes little first-pass hepatic metabolism. Peak plasma concentrations are reached in 2 to 3 hours. The normal plasma half-life is about 5 hours. Penbutolol is rapidly metabolized in the liver; 4-hydroxypenbutolol is an active metabolite with a plasma half-life of about 20 hours, a property that may account for the drug's long duration of action. Because the metabolite is primarily excreted in the urine, the plasma half-life is prolonged in patients with renal insufficiency; dose reduction may be required (see Table 54–4).

Pindolol is a nonselective β-adrenergic antagonist that possesses moderate PAA but lacks MSA[25, 26, 43–47] (see Table 54–2). The usual dose is 20 to 40 mg/d given in divided doses. Pindolol is moderately lipophilic; it is nearly completely absorbed (see Table 54–3). It undergoes little first-pass hepatic metabolism. Peak plasma concentrations are reached in about 1 hour. The normal plasma half-life is 3 to 4 hours. Sixty percent of an oral dose of pindolol is metabolized in the liver; 40% is excreted unchanged in the urine. Pindolol metabolism is not altered by moderate renal insufficiency; however, dose reduction is necessary in patients with advanced renal insufficiency (see Table 54–4).

## β₁-Selective Adrenergic Antagonists

Atenolol is a β₁-selective adrenergic antagonist that lacks both PAA and MSA[25, 26, 40, 48–52] (see Table 54–2). The usual dose is 50 to 100 mg daily. Atenolol is hydrophilic; 50% to 60% of an oral dose is absorbed, with the remainder excreted unchanged in the feces (see Table 54–3). Peak plasma concentrations are reached in 2 to 4 hours. The normal plasma concentration half-life is 6 to 7 hours. Atenolol undergoes little or no hepatic metabolism; the drug is primarily eliminated in the urine. The half-life of atenolol is increased in patients with impaired renal function; dose adjustments are necessary (see Table 54–4). One percent to 12% of atenolol is removed by hemodialysis; dose adjustment must be individualized.

Metoprolol tartrate is a β₁-selective adrenergic antagonist that lacks PAA but has weak MSA[25, 26, 53, 54] (see Table 54–2). The usual dose is 100 to 200 mg/d given in divided doses. Because of its lipophilic character, absorption is essentially complete (see Table 54–3). However, it undergoes extensive first-pass hepatic metabolism. Peak plasma concentrations are reached in 1 to 2 hours. The plasma half-life is 3 to 7 hours. Metoprolol is primarily cleared from the plasma by hepatic biotransformation; less than 5% of

**TABLE 54–3. Pharmacokinetic Differences Among the β-Adrenergic Antagonists***

| Drug | Absorption (%) | First-Pass Effect (%) | Maximal Bioavailability (%) | Peak Blood Level (h) | Elimination Half-Life (h) | Metabolism/Excretion |
|---|---|---|---|---|---|---|
| *Nonselective (β₁ and β₂) Adrenergic Antagonists* | | | | | | |
| Nadolol | 30–40 | <10 | 30 | 2–4 | 20–24 | Kidney/urine |
| Propranolol | >90 | 60 | 30 | 1–3 | 3–4 | Liver/feces |
| Propranolol LA | >90 | 80 | 20 | 6 | 10 | Liver/feces |
| Timolol | >90 | 50 | 50 | 1–2 | 3–4 | Liver/urine |
| *Nonselective (β₁ and β₂) Adrenergic Antagonists with Partial Agonist Activity* | | | | | | |
| Carteolol | >90 | <10 | 85 | 1–3 | 6 | Liver and kidney/urine |
| Penbutolol | >90 | <10 | 90 | 2–3 | 5 | Liver/urine |
| Pindolol | >90 | <10 | 90 | 1 | 3–4 | Liver and kidney/feces and urine |
| *β₁-Selective Adrenergic Antagonists* | | | | | | |
| Atenolol | 50–60 | <10 | 50–60 | 2–4 | 6–7 | Kidney/urine |
| Betaxolol | >90 | <10 | 90 | 1.5–6 | 14–22 | Liver/urine |
| Bisoprolol | >90 | 20 | 80 | 2–4 | 9–12 | Liver and kidney/urine |
| Metoprolol tartrate | >90 | 50 | 50 | 1–2 | 3–7 | Liver/urine |
| Metoprolol succinate ER | >90 | 50 | 40 | 7 | 3–7 | Liver/urine |
| *β₁-Selective Adrenergic Antagonist with Partial Agonist Activity* | | | | | | |
| Acebutolol | 70 | 30 | 35–50 | 2–4 | 3–4 | Liver and kidney/feces and urine |
| *Nonselective (β₁ and β₂) and α₁-Selective Adrenergic Antagonist* | | | | | | |
| Labetalol | >90 | 60 | 25 | 1–2 | 3–4 | Liver/feces |

*LA = long-acting; ER = extended-release.

an oral dose is excreted unchanged in the urine. The plasma half-life of metoprolol is not prolonged in patients with renal insufficiency.

Metoprolol succinate is a β₁-selective adrenergic antagonist that lacks PAA but has weak MSA[25, 26, 55–57] (see Table 54–2). It is available as extended-release tablets, which are composed of controlled-release coated pellets. Each pellet is designed to deliver metroprolol continuously over the dosage interval. The tablets contain 47.5, 95, and 190 mg of metoprolol succinate, which are equivalent to 50, 100, and 200 mg of metoprolol tartrate, respectively. The usual dose is 100 to 200 mg daily. In comparison to metoprolol tartrate, plasma levels are characterized by lower peaks (25% to 50%), longer time to peak, and lower peak to trough variation (see Table 54–3). The bioavailability of metoprolol succinate is about 77% relative to the corresponding single or divided doses of metoprolol tartrate. There are no additional pharmacokinetic differences between the two metoprolol preparations.

Betaxolol hydrochloride is a β₁-selective adrenergic antagonist that lacks PAA but has weak MSA[25, 26, 58, 59] (see Table 54–2). The usual dose is 10 to 20 mg daily. Betaxolol is lipophilic; absorption is complete (see Table 54–3). It undergoes limited first-pass hepatic metabolism. Peak plasma concentrations are reached between 1.5 and 6 hours.

The normal plasma concentration half-life is between 14 and 22 hours. Betaxolol is metabolized by the liver; approximately 15% of the active drug and all of its metabolites are excreted in the urine. The half-life of betaxolol is prolonged in patients with renal insufficiency; dose reduction is required (see Table 54–4).

Bisoprolol fumarate is the most β₁-selective adrenergic antagonist available for clinical use; it lacks PAA and MSA[22, 60, 61] (see Table 54–2). The usual dose is 5 to 10 mg daily. Bisoprolol is equally hydrophilic and lipophilic; greater than 90% of an oral dose is absorbed (see Table 54–3). First-pass hepatic metabolism is low (20%). Peak plasma concentrations are reached in 2 to 4 hours. The normal plasma concentration half-life is 9 to 12 hours. Bisoprolol is eliminated equally by renal and nonrenal pathways; 50% of the dose appears in the urine unchanged and the remainder as inactive metabolites. The half-life of bisoprolol is increased in patients with renal insufficiency; dose reduction is required (see Table 54–4).

### β₁-Selective Adrenergic Antagonist with Partial Agonist Activity

Acebutolol hydrochloride is a β₁-selective adrenergic antagonist that possesses mild PAA and weak MSA[25, 26, 62–65]

**TABLE 54–4. Antihypertensive Drugs Requiring Dose Modification\* in Renal Insufficiency**

| Drug | Estimated Glomerular Filtration Rate (Creatinine Clearance) | | | |
| --- | --- | --- | --- | --- |
| | >50 mL/min | 10–50 mL/min | <10 mL/min | Dialysis + † |
| *β-Adrenergic Antagonists* | | | | |
| Nadolol | No change | 50% | 25% | (H) 50% |
| Carteolol | No change | 50% | 25% | — |
| Penbutolol | No change | No change | 50% | — |
| Pindolol | No change | No change | 50% | Negligible |
| Atenolol | No change | 50% | 25% | (H) 50% |
| Betaxolol | No change | No change | 50% | — |
| Bisoprolol | No change | 50% | 25% | Negligible |
| Acebutolol | No change | 50% | 25% | (H) 50% |
| *Central α₂-Adrenergic Antagonists* | | | | |
| Methyldopa | No change | No change | 50% | (H) 50% |
| Clonidine | No change | 50% | 25% | Negligible |
| *Peripheral Adrenergic-Neuronal Blocking Agents* | | | | |
| Guanethidine | No change | No change | 50% (avoid) | — |
| Guanadrel | No change | 50% | 25% (avoid) | — |
| *Direct-Acting Vasodilators* | | | | |
| Hydralazine | No change | No change | 75%‡ | Negligible |
| Minoxidil | No change | No change | 50% | (H and P) 25%–40% |
| *Angiotensin-Converting Enzyme Inhibitors* | | | | |
| Captopril | No change | 50% | 25% | (H) 50% |
| Enalapril | No change | 50% | 25% | (H) 50% |
| Lisinopril | No change | 50% | 25% | (H) 50% |
| Benazepril | No change | 50% | 25% | Negligible |
| Ramipril | No change | 50% | 25% | — |
| Quinapril | No change | 50% | 25% | — |
| *Tyrosine Hydroxylase Inhibitor* | | | | |
| Metyrosine | No change | 50% | 25% | — |

\*Percentage of total dose given; + replacement dose at end of dialysis (percentage of dose prescribed for patients with a glomerular filtration rate less than 10 mL/min).
†H = hemodialysis; P = peritoneal dialysis.
‡Slow acetylators.

(see Table 54–2). The usual dose is 400 to 800 mg daily. Acebutolol is relatively lipophilic; 70% of an oral dose is absorbed, with the remainder excreted as unchanged drug in the feces (see Table 54–3). Peak plasma concentrations are reached in 2 to 4 hours. There is considerable interindividual and intraindividual variation in plasma concentrations attained with a given dosage. Acebutolol undergoes significant first-pass hepatic metabolism, yielding its major metabolite, diacetolol. Diacetolol is equipotent to acebutolol and contributes substantially to the observed effects of acebutolol. It has greater β₁-selectivity than the parent drug but equivalent PAA. Diacetolol has a longer plasma half-life than acebutolol (8 to 13 hours for diacetolol, 3 to 4 hours for acebutolol). Because diacetolol is eliminated to a greater extent by the kidneys than the parent drug is, acebutolol requires dose adjustment in patients with renal insufficiency. Both acebutolol and diacetolol are removed by hemodialysis; dose adjustment must be individualized (see Table 54–4).

### Nonselective β- and α₁-Adrenergic Antagonist

Labetalol hydrochloride has both α₁- and nonselective β-adrenergic receptor–blocking properties[25, 26, 66–69] (see Table 54–2). It is almost equipotent in blocking β₁- and β₂-adrenergic receptors. Labetalol is also highly selective for postsynaptic α₁-adrenergic receptors. The ratio of α- to β-blocking potency is estimated to be 1:3 or 1:7 after oral or intravenous administration, respectively. Labetalol has weak PAA at β₁-adrenergic receptors and weak MSA. The antihypertensive action of labetalol is attributed to its peripheral α₁- and β-adrenergic receptor antagonism. The usual dose is 400 to 800 mg/d given in divided doses. Labetalol is lipophilic; it is rapidly and almost completely absorbed (see Table 54–3). However, it is subject to extensive first-pass hepatic metabolism. Food delays absorption but increases absolute bioavailability by decreasing first-pass metabolism or hepatic blood flow. Peak plasma concentrations are reached in 1 to 2 hours. The plasma half-life is 3 to 4 hours. The drug is metabolized in the liver; less than 5% is excreted unchanged in the urine. The metabolism of labetalol is unchanged in patients with renal insufficiency.

## CLASS RENAL EFFECTS

In general, β-adrenergic antagonists (with the possible exception of propranolol) have little or no clinically important effect on glomerular filtration rate (GFR), effective renal plasma flow (ERPF), or renal vascular resistance (RVR) in patients with essential hypertension[70–115, 119–125, 128–134] or in patients with diabetic[118, 126, 127] or nondiabetic[116, 117, 129, 132, 135] renal parenchymal disease (Table 54–5). Urinary protein excretion is reduced. There are no consistent long-term data demonstrating that $\beta_1$-selectivity, with or without PAA, or combined $\alpha_1$- and $\beta$-adrenergic receptor antagonism confers unique renal pharmacologic effects compared with nonselective ($\beta_1$ and $\beta_2$) adrenergic receptor antagonism.[136, 137]

Propranolol has been demonstrated to exaggerate the physiologic decrement in ERPF and GFR that occurs during orthostasis in normotensive subjects.[138] Among patients receiving propranolol therapy, the most severe changes in renal function have been described in normotensive subjects who have experienced an absolute reduction in MAP to 80 mm Hg.[139] Few studies in hypertensive patients, using a $\beta$-adrenergic antagonist, have achieved absolute MAP responses of 100 mm Hg or lower.[136, 137] To the degree that MAP falls below the renal autoregulatory threshold (80 to 100 mm Hg) with any $\beta$-adrenergic antagonist, both ERPF and GFR may fall.

$\beta$-Adrenergic antagonist therapy is usually associated with short-term suppression of plasma renin activity (PRA).[9, 136, 137] However, the long-term effect of $\beta$-adrenergic antagonists on the renin-angiotensin-aldosterone axis is less well defined. It has been stated that the degree of renin suppression with different $\beta$-adrenergic antagonists is inversely correlated with the extent of PAA; $\beta$-adrenergic antagonists without PAA (regardless of $\beta_1$-selectivity) suppress PRA by 60% to 70%, whereas pindolol (having pronounced PAA) suppresses PRA by less than 10%.[140] Other $\beta$-adrenergic antagonists, with less pronounced PAA, are stated to suppress PRA by 20% to 45%.[140]

The long-term oral administration of $\beta$-adrenergic antagonists (with the exception of labetalol) usually has no effect on $Na^+$, $K^+$, or free water excretion; body fluid composition and weight are unchanged.[136, 137]

## CLASS EFFICACY AND SAFETY

The $\beta$-adrenergic antagonists are effective agents for the treatment of mild to moderate hypertension, either as monotherapy[141–145] or in combination with a diuretic or a vasodilator.[146–148] Pseudotolerance does not occur. The presence or absence of $\beta_1$-selectivity or PAA conveys no specific blood pressure–lowering advantage[22, 23, 145, 149–151]; all are equally efficacious in controlling blood pressure in both the recumbent and upright positions[141, 152, 153] and at rest and during physical exercise.[141, 152, 153] This drug class, compared with thiazide diuretics or $Ca^{2+}$ antagonists, may be less efficacious in black than in white persons.[154, 155] Although $\beta$-adrenergic antagonists are not usually considered drugs of choice for the treatment of elderly hypertensive patients unless there is a history of angina pectoris or a previous myocardial infarction,[142, 156] there is no convincing evidence that there are genuine age-related differences in drug efficacy or adverse effects.[145, 157] Some investigators have suggested that PRA levels are important in predicting which patients will respond to $\beta$-adrenergic antagonists and that

the low PRA levels found in black and elderly persons account for their poor response.[8, 142, 143] However, there are no randomized, controlled clinical trials to support this claim. Furthermore, not all investigators have been able to demonstrate a relationship between PRA and drug efficacy.[140, 148, 158–160]

$\beta$-Adrenergic antagonists do provide secondary cardioprotection; there is a 22% reduction in mortality and a 27% reduction in reinfarction rate, compared with placebo, in patients who have already suffered a myocardial infarction.[161] Thus, for hypertensive patients who have previously had a myocardial infarction, a $\beta$-adrenergic antagonist without PAA may be the drug of choice.[162, 163] However, these drugs have not been shown to confer primary prevention of myocardial infarction.[163] $\beta$-Adrenergic antagonists have been documented to reduce left ventricular hypertrophy (LVH) in parallel with the fall in arterial pressure.[145, 162, 164] Because $\beta$-blockers slow HR (allowing more complete left atrial emptying), reduce myocardial oxygen demand, control blood pressure, and regress LVH, they are particularly efficacious in hypertensive patients with LVH and diastolic dysfunction[162, 164] and in hypertensive patients with myocardial ischemia.[162–164]

$\beta_1$-Selectivity may convey a therapeutic advantage over nonselective $\beta$-adrenergic antagonists in the treatment of hypertensive patients with diabetes mellitus,[22, 145, 165–169] bronchospastic airway disease,[145, 167–172] or peripheral vascular disease.[167–169, 173, 174] $\beta$-Adrenergic antagonists with PAA may better preserve left ventricular function and be less likely to precipitate congestive heart failure, compared with propranolol[149–151, 167, 169, 175–177]; however, definitive studies are lacking.[22, 23, 145, 178] $\beta$-Adrenergic antagonists with PAA tend to cause less bradycardia than $\beta$-adrenergic antagonists without PAA[149–151, 167, 169, 175–177]; however, it has been postulated that a low HR induced by $\beta$-blockade is an important beneficial effect in reducing both cardiovascular morbidity and mortality.[23, 179] Finally, $\beta$-adrenergic antagonists with PAA may not decrease peripheral vascular blood flow, in contrast to propranolol[22, 149–151, 167, 169, 175–177]; again, definitive studies are lacking.[22, 23, 178]

The side effect profile of $\beta$-adrenergic antagonists is related to pharmacologic blockade of $\beta$-adrenergic receptors. Specifically, blockade of bronchial $\beta_2$-adrenergic receptors increases airway resistance, potentially precipitating or exacerbating bronchospasm[145, 167–171]; blockade of atrial $\beta_1$- and $\beta_2$-adrenergic receptors decreases HR, potentially precipitating or aggravating bradycardia[167–169]; blockade of ventricular $\beta_1$-adrenergic receptors decreases CO, potentially precipitating or aggravating exercise intolerance, congestive heart failure, or systemic hypotension[167–169]; blockade of gastrointestinal $\beta_1$- and $\beta_2$-adrenergic receptors may decrease motility and lower esophageal sphincter tone, precipitating or aggravating constipation or dyspepsia[167–169, 180]; and blockade of peripheral vascular $\beta_2$-adrenergic receptors decreases peripheral vascular blood flow, potentially precipitating or aggravating Raynaud phenomenon, cold limbs, or claudication.[167–169] However, studies suggest that $\beta$-blockade does not adversely affect walking capacity or symptoms of intermittent claudication in patients with mild to moderate peripheral arterial disease.[181, 182] Ophthalmic $\beta$-blockers, used for the treatment of glaucoma

**TABLE 54–5. Renal Function Effects: β-Adrenergic Antagonists***

| Drug | Diagnosis | References | No. of Studies Reviewed | Total No. of Patients | ΔGFR % Mean (Range) | ΔERPF % Mean (Range) | ΔRVR % Mean (Range) | ΔUprot % Mean (Range) |
|---|---|---|---|---|---|---|---|---|
| *Nonselective (β₁ and β₂) Adrenergic Antagonists* | | | | | | | | |
| Nadolol | EH | 70–81 | 12 | 118 | 2 (−6 to 18) | 2 (−17 to 31) | −9 (−31 to 13) | — |
| Propranolol | EH | 77, 78, 82–99 | 21 | 251 | −10 (−26 to 0) | −7 (−23 to 23) | −3 (−21 to 12) | — |
| Timolol | EH | 100 | 1 | 14 | 0 | — | — | — |
| *Nonselective (β₁ and β₂) Adrenergic Antagonists with Partial Agonist Activity* | | | | | | | | |
| Carteolol | EH | 101 | 1 | 10 | — | −16 | — | — |
| Penbutolol | — | — | — | — | — | — | — | — |
| Pindolol | EH | 93, 102–107 | 9 | 85 | −1 (−9 to 5) | 8 (−7 to 28) | −11 (−18 to 0) | — |
| *β₁-Selective Adrenergic Antagonists* | | | | | | | | |
| Atenolol | EH | 75–77, 88, 99, 108–115 | 13 | 126 | −3 (−23 to 10) | 3 (−16 to 26) | −19 (−39 to −4) | −5 (−9 to −1) |
|  | RD | 116–117 | 2 | 20 | 2 (−2 to 7) | 3 (3 to 4) | — | −13 |
|  | DM | 118 | 1 | 12 | 1 | −3 | −10 | −36 |
| Betaxolol | EH | 119, 120 | 1 | 13 | −8 | −15 | 7 | — |
| Bisoprolol | — | — | — | — | — | — | — | — |
| Metoprolol |  | 89, 121–125 | 6 | 79 | −4 (−19 to 1) | −6 (−14 to 0) | 2 (−8 to 15) | −40 (−42 to −38) |
|  | DM | 126, 127 | 2 | 22 | −3 | 5 | −11 | −26 (−57 to 5) |
| *β₁-Selective Adrenergic Antagonist with Partial Agonist Activity* | | | | | | | | |
| Acebutolol | EH | 99 | 1 | 10 | 0 | — | −12 | — |
| *Nonselective (β₁ and β₂) and α₁-Selective Adrenergic Antagonist* | | | | | | | | |
| Labetalol | EH | 92, 128–134 | 8 | 101 | 1 (−18 to 16) | 3 (−26 to 28) | −22 | — |
|  | RD | 129, 132, 135 | 3 | 42 | 1 (−20 to 22) | — | — | — |

*ΔGFR % = percent change in glomerular filtration rate; ΔERPF % = percent change in effective renal plasma flow; ΔRVR % = percent change in renal vascular resistance; ΔUprot % = percent change in urinary protein or albumin excretion; EH = essential hypertension; RD = nondiabetic renal disease; DM = diabetes mellitus.

and ocular hypertension, may be absorbed into the systemic circulation and cause one or more of these adverse effects.[183]

Central nervous system symptoms of "muzziness" (e.g., sedation, sluggishness, fatigue, dysphoria), sleep disturbances (e.g., insomnia, vivid dreams, nightmares), visual hallucinations, toxic psychoses, or depression may occur; the mechanism is unclear, and the importance of lipophilicity (with penetration of the blood-brain barrier) in amplifying such effects is disputed.[167–169, 184, 185] Cognitive function has been reported to be both impaired and improved; there is no cohesive evidence that β-adrenergic antagonists have precise neuropsychologic effects.[186, 187] Sexual dysfunction (e.g., impotence, decreased libido) may also occur; the mechanism is unknown.[188–191]

β-Adrenergic antagonism is frequently associated with moderate increases in total and very low density lipoprotein triglycerides, a mild decrease in high-density lipoprotein (HDL)–cholesterol, and little or no effect on total and low-density lipoprotein (LDL)–cholesterol.[192–196] These adverse effects on lipoprotein metabolism are attributed primarily to modulation of lipoprotein lipase activity.[192–196] Unopposed α-stimulation inhibits lipoprotein lipase activity, which retards very low density lipoprotein and triglyceride catabolism. Triglyceride concentrations are increased, and HDL-cholesterol (a product of very low density lipoprotein catabolism) is decreased. Selective β-blockers, especially those with PAA or combined α- and β-blockade, have less influence on triglyceride and HDL-cholesterol levels. β-Blockers that increase catecholamine levels increase hepatic cholesterol production; β-blockers that decrease lecithin-cholesterol acyltransferase activity decrease HDL-cholesterol levels.[195, 196]

β-Adrenergic antagonists may induce carbohydrate intolerance (e.g., precipitate or exacerbate hyperglycemia; precipitate nonketotic hyperosmolar hyperglycemic coma).[167, 169, 197, 198] The rise in plasma glucose concentration is due to inhibition of insulin release and unopposed α-receptor–mediated hepatic glycogenolysis; there may also be decreased peripheral sensitivity to insulin and inhibition of peripheral glucose use.[197, 198] In general, marked hyperglycemia is uncommon, and the greatest inhibitory effect on insulin secretion is observed with nonselective β-blockers.[197, 198] Nonselective β-blockers have also been reported to cause severe hypoglycemia in both diabetic and nondiabetic patients.[198] Proposed mechanisms include enhanced insulin action with a resultant increase in peripheral glucose uptake, inhibition of lipolysis, and hepatic phosphorylation. Delayed recovery from hypoglycemia (β-blocker or insulin induced) also occurs, because β-adrenergic antagonists prevent glucagon-mediated glycogenolysis and gluconeogenesis.[198] This is most pronounced with the nonselective β-adrenergic antagonists. Furthermore, there is marked diminution in the clinical manifestations of sympathetic discharge associated with the hypoglycemia (e.g., tachycardia, tremor), and the normal hemodynamic response to hypoglycemia may be altered with an elevation of diastolic blood pressure.[198, 199] Sweating is unimpaired because it occurs through postganglionic cholinergic fibers.[198]

Abrupt withdrawal of long-term β-adrenergic antagonism in patients with coronary artery disease may be associated with overshoot hypertension, unstable angina pectoris, or myocardial infarction, usually within 2 to 7 days.[200–203] This is believed to result from elevated sympathetic activity due to β-receptor hypersensitivity (increased number or affinity of β-receptors) to circulating agonists.[200–203] Cardiac contractility is enhanced, and HR and myocardial oxygen requirements are increased. Other proposed mechanisms include increased platelet adhesiveness and aggregation and increased affinity of hemoglobin to oxygen with reduced tissue oxygen delivery.[203]

Finally, labetalol has been implicated in inducing hepatocellular necrosis, the result of a metabolic idiosyncrasy.[204, 205] Liver function studies should be obtained for baseline values before therapy is started and should be repeated periodically.

## Central α₂-Adrenergic Agonists

### CLASS MECHANISMS OF ACTION

Central α₂-adrenergic agonists cross the blood-brain barrier and have a direct effect on specific presynaptic and postsynaptic α₂-adrenergic receptors located at midbrain and medullary sites.[206–211] Stimulation of these receptors increases the gain of the vasodepressor baroreflex, decreases total sympathetic outflow, and increases vagal activity. The net pharmacologic effect is a reduction in catecholamine release and turnover; biochemical markers of noradrenergic activity (e.g., plasma norepinephrine concentration) are decreased,[212, 213] and the magnitude of the blood pressure–lowering effect correlates with this decrease.[214–218] The central α₂-adrenergic agonist clonidine also binds to imidazole receptors within the brain; activation of these receptors inhibits central sympathetic outflow.[219, 220] Central α₂-adrenergic agonists may also stimulate peripheral α₂-adrenergic receptors that mediate vasoconstriction; this effect predominates at high plasma drug concentrations and may precipitate an increase in blood pressure.[209–211] However, the usual physiologic effect is a decrease in TPVR and a slowing of HR; CO is either unchanged or mildly decreased.[221–227] Central α₂-adrenergic agonists do not usually cause orthostatic hypotension because they do not prevent an increase in sympathetic activity on standing.[209–211, 227]

### CLASS MEMBERS

Methyldopa is a methyl-substituted amino acid that is active only after decarboxylation and conversion to α-methylnorepinephrine.[25, 26, 211, 218, 228, 229] The antihypertensive effect is due to the accumulation of α-methylnorepinephrine in the central nervous system, which is highly selective for α₂-adrenergic receptors displacing and competing with the natural catecholamines. The usual dose is 500 to 2000 mg/d given in divided doses (Table 54–6). Absorption is incomplete and variable; bioavailability averages 25% (Table 54–7). Peak plasma concentrations occur 2 to 4 hours after dosing. The normal plasma half-life is 1 to 2 hours. Methyldopa is excreted in the urine, mainly as the inactive O-sulfate conjugate. The distribution and plasma elimination

TABLE 54-6. Pharmacologic Differences Among Central $\alpha_2$-Adrenergic Antagonists and Peripheral $\alpha$-Adrenergic Antagonists

| Drug | First Dose (mg) | Usual Daily Dose (mg) | Maximal Daily Dose (mg) | Maximal Hypotensive Response | Duration of Hypotensive Response |
|---|---|---|---|---|---|
| *Central $\alpha_2$-Adrenergic Agonists* | | | | | |
| Methyldopa | 250 | 250–1000 bid | 3000 | 6–9 h | 24–48 h |
| Clonidine | 0.1 | 0.1–0.6 bid/tid | 2.4 | 2–4 h | 6–8 h |
| Clonidine TTS* | 2.5 (TTS-1) | 2.5–7.5 (TTS-1–TTS-3) | 15 (TTS-3 × 2) | 2–3 d | 7 d |
| Guanabenz | 4 | 8–16 bid | 64 | 2–4 h | 12 h |
| Guanfacine | 1 | 1–3 qd | 3 | 8–12 h | 36 h |
| *Central and Peripheral Adrenergic-Neuronal Blocking Agent* | | | | | |
| Reserpine | 0.05 | 0.05–0.125 qod or qd | 0.25 | 2–3 wk | 2–3 wk |
| *Peripheral $\alpha_1$-Adrenergic Antagonists* | | | | | |
| Doxazosin | 1 | 1–4 qd | 16 | 2–6 h | 24 h |
| Prazosin | 1 | 2–4 bid/tid | 20 | 2–4 h | 6–12 h |
| Terazosin | 1 | 1–5 qd/bid | 20 | 2–4 h | 12–24 h |
| *Moderately Selective Peripheral $\alpha_1$-Adrenergic Antagonist* | | | | | |
| Phenoxybenzamine | 10 | 20–40 bid/tid | 120 | 3–4 h | 3–4 d |
| *Peripheral Adrenergic-Neuronal Blocking Agents* | | | | | |
| Guanethidine | 10 | 25–75 qd | 150 | 48–72 h | 7–21 d |
| Guanadrel | 5 | 10–50 bid | 150 | 4–6 h | 4–14 h |

*TTS = transdermal therapeutic system.

**TABLE 54–7. Pharmacokinetic Differences Among Central $\alpha_2$-Adrenergic Agonists and Peripheral $\alpha$-Adrenergic Antagonists**

| Drug | Absorption (%) | First-Pass Effect | Bioavailability (%) | Peak Blood Level | Elimination Half-Life | Metabolism/Excretion |
|---|---|---|---|---|---|---|
| *Central $\alpha_2$-Adrenergic Antagonists* | | | | | | |
| Methyldopa | <50 | Minimal | 25 | 2–4 h | 1–2 h | Liver/urine |
| Clonidine | >75 | Minimal | 75 | 3–5 h | 12–16 h | Kidney/urine |
| Clonidine TTS* | | | | 2–3 d | | |
| Guanabenz | >75 | Minimal | 75 | 2–5 h | 6 h | Liver/urine |
| Guanfacine | >90 | None | >90 | 1–4 h | 15–17 h | Liver/urine |
| *Central and Peripheral Adrenergic-Neuronal Blocking Agent* | | | | | | |
| Reserpine | 30 | None | 30 | 1–2 h | 12–16 d | Liver/feces and urine |
| *Peripheral $\alpha_1$-Adrenergic Antagonists* | | | | | | |
| Doxazosin | >90 | Variable | 65 | 2–3 h | 22 h | Liver/feces |
| Prazosin | >90 | Variable | 60 | 2–3 h | 2–4 h | Liver/feces |
| Terazosin | >90 | None | 90 | 1–2 h | 12 h | Liver/feces and urine |
| *Moderately Selective Peripheral $\alpha_1$-Adrenergic Antagonist* | | | | | | |
| Phenoxybenzamine | 20–30 | — | 3–30 | — | 24 h | Liver/urine |
| *Peripheral Adrenergic-Neuronal Blocking Agents* | | | | | | |
| Guanethidine | 3–30 | Minimal | 3–30 | 6 h | 5 d | Liver/urine |
| Guanadrel | >85 | None | 85 | 1–2 h | 10–12 h | Liver/urine |

*TTS = transdermal therapeutic system.

of methyldopa and its metabolites are prolonged in patients with renal insufficiency; the drug dose should be reduced (see Table 54–4).

Clonidine hydrochloride is an imidazoline derivative that acts by stimulating central $\alpha_2$-adrenergic or imidazole receptors.* The usual dose is 0.2 to 1.2 mg/d given in divided doses (see Table 54–6). Clonidine is rapidly absorbed from the gastrointestinal tract; bioavailability averages 75% (see Table 54–7). Peak plasma concentrations are reached in 3 to 5 hours. The normal plasma half-life is 12 to 16 hours. The drug is metabolized mainly in the liver; fecal excretion ranges from 15% to 30%. Approximately 40% to 60% of an oral dose is excreted unchanged in the urine. In patients with renal insufficiency, the plasma half-life may be extended to more than 40 hours; the drug dose should be reduced (see Table 54–4).

Clonidine transdermal therapeutic system (TTS) provides continuous delivery of clonidine for 7 days at a constant rate.[25, 26, 211, 233–236] Clonidine TTS is a multilayered film; the film areas are 3.5 cm$^2$ (TTS-1), 7.0 cm$^2$ (TTS-2), and 10.5 cm$^2$ (TTS-3). The amount of drug released is proportional to the film area: 3.5 cm$^2$ delivers 0.1 mg/d; 7.0 cm$^2$ delivers 0.2 mg/d; and 10.5 cm$^2$ delivers 0.3 mg/d. Therapeutic plasma clonidine levels are achieved 2 to 3 days after initial application. The initial dose should be a single clonidine TTS-1 patch per day; the maximal dose should probably not exceed two clonidine TTS-3 patches per day. After discontinuation of clonidine TTS, plasma drug concentra-

*References 25, 26, 211, 219, 220, 230–232.

tions persist for 8 hours and then decline slowly over several days.

Guanabenz acetate is a guanidine derivative that is highly selective for central $\alpha_2$-adrenergic receptors.[25, 26, 211, 237–239] The usual dose is 16 to 32 mg/d given in divided doses (see Table 54–6). Guanabenz is well absorbed; bioavailability averages 75% (see Table 54–7). Peak plasma concentrations are reached in 2 to 5 hours. The plasma half-life is about 6 hours. The drug undergoes extensive hepatic metabolism; less than 2% is excreted unchanged in the urine. The drug dose need not be adjusted in patients with renal insufficiency.

Guanfacine hydrochloride is a phenylacetyl guanidine derivative that has a longer half-life and duration of action than guanabenz.[25, 26, 211, 240–245] The usual dose is 1 to 3 mg daily (see Table 54–6). Guanfacine is well absorbed; bioavailability is greater than 90% (see Table 54–7). Peak plasma concentrations are reached in 1 to 4 hours. The plasma half-life is 15 to 17 hours. The drug is primarily metabolized in the liver. Guanfacine and its metabolites are excreted predominantly through the kidneys; 24% to 37% is eliminated as unchanged drug in the urine. The drug dose does not require adjustment in patients with renal insufficiency.

## CLASS RENAL EFFECTS

In general, central $\alpha_2$-adrenergic agonists have little or no clinically important effect on GFR or ERPF in patients with essential hypertension[97, 137, 246–249, 252–254, 256–262] or in patients with diabetic[264] or nondiabetic[250, 251, 254, 255, 262, 263] renal parenchymal disease (Table 54–8). RVR is reduced, probably mediated by a decrease in preglomerular capillary resistance in response to reduced levels of circulating catecholamines (i.e., reduced renal α-adrenoreceptor stimulation). Urinary protein excretion is reduced. In general, the central α2-adrenergic agonists, with the possible exception of guanfacine, have no sustained effect on the renin-angiotensin-aldosterone axis.[9, 246] Fractional excretion of $Na^+$ and $K^+$ is unchanged, and body fluid composition and weight are not altered.[137, 246] Guanabenz may produce a water diuresis by inhibition of vasopressin; α2-adrenergic stimulation has been shown to inhibit vasopressin activity by a central depression of vasopressin release or by altered tubule responsiveness to vasopressin.[265–267]

## CLASS EFFICACY AND SAFETY

The central α2-adrenergic agonists are effective monotherapeutic agents for the treatment of mild to moderate hypertension.[211, 221–225, 268–277] Pseudotolerance does not occur. Their efficacy is similar in the young and elderly,[278–281] at rest and during physical exercise,[221–225, 282, 283] and in black and white patients.[274] When used in combination with a diuretic, these drugs are more effective in lowering blood pressure compared with monotherapy.[211, 268–272]

The central α2-agonists generally have minimal effects on carbohydrate tolerance.[197, 198, 211, 284, 285] However, acute (often short-term) increases in blood glucose concentration may occur in diabetic patients by α-receptor suppression of insulin release.[197, 198, 211] The central α-agonists have been reported to have favorable or neutral effects on blood lipids; decreases in total cholesterol and LDL-cholesterol levels have been reported to occur, with variable effects on HDL-cholesterol and triglyceride levels.[195, 286] Finally, these drugs have been reported to regress LVH and may improve ventricular dysrhythmias.[287, 288]

Stimulation of α2-adrenergic receptors in the brain mediates several of the well-known side effects of these drugs, including sedation and drowsiness.[209, 211, 289, 290] Reduction of salivary flow is also due to a centrally mediated inhibition of cholinergic transmission; it is responsible for the common side effect of xerostomia (dry mouth).[209, 211, 289, 290] The intensity of sedation and xerostomia occur at the peak of drug action. Clonidine, when given intravenously or in high oral doses, may also precipitate a paradoxical hypertensive response owing to stimulation of postsynaptic peripheral vascular α2-adrenergic receptors.[206–209, 211] Methyldopa may cause long-term toxic tissue effects, including fever, hepatotoxic injury, or a positive direct Coombs test result with or without hemolytic anemia.[211, 289, 290] Methyldopa, by reducing central dopaminergic inhibition of prolactin release, may also produce gynecomastia in men and galactorrhea in both men and women.[290] Finally, all of these drugs may cause sexual dysfunction (e.g., decreased libido, potency),[188–191, 211, 289–292] depression,[211, 289–292] or reduced mental acuity.[211, 289–292]

A discontinuation syndrome called ''rebound'' or ''overshoot'' hypertension may occur 18 to 36 hours after abrupt cessation of the shorter acting central α2-adrenergic antagonists.[200, 208, 209, 293–299] Symptoms include restlessness, insomnia, headache, tremor, anxiety, nausea and vomiting, and the feeling of impending doom. Tachycardia may occur, with elevation of blood pressure above pretreatment values. There is biochemical evidence of increased peripheral sympathetic activity (e.g., increased plasma norepinephrine and urinary catecholamine levels). It is hypothesized that down-regulation of α2-adrenergic receptors occurs in an inhibitory circuit during long-term treatment; when treatment is stopped, physiologic amounts of neurotransmitter cannot produce a normal degree of inhibition, and excessive sympathetic discharge takes place until receptor numbers are restored. The frequency of this withdrawal syndrome is disputed, but it can occur at low doses of clonidine or guanabenz, it may persist for 4 or 5 days, and it may be life threatening. Concurrent use of β-adrenergic blockers amplifies this discontinuation syndrome; they should not be prescribed to patients taking central α2-adrenergic agonists. Reinstallation of the previously discontinued short-acting central α2-adrenergic agonist reverses the syndrome.

Finally, dermatologic side effects occur commonly with clonidine TTS and vary from mild erythema to contact dermatitis.[211, 300] Application of the patch to a hairless portion of the upper torso and site rotation are advised.

# Central and Peripheral Adrenergic-Neuronal Blocking Agents

## CLASS MECHANISMS OF ACTION

Rauwolfia alkaloids act both within the central nervous system and in the peripheral sympathetic nervous system. They effectively deplete stores of norepinephrine by competitively inhibiting the uptake of dopamine by storage granules and by preventing the incorporation of norepinephrine into the protective chromaffin granules; the free catecholamines are destroyed by monoamine oxidase.[301] The predominant pharmacologic effect is a marked decrease in sympathetic outflow from the central nervous system. The net physiologic effect is a decrease in TPVR; HR and CO are either unchanged or mildly decreased.[301, 302]

## CLASS MEMBER

Reserpine is the most popular rauwolfia product used in the treatment of hypertension.[25, 26, 303–306] The usual dose is 0.05 to 0.125 mg daily (see Table 54–6). It is readily absorbed (see Table 54–7). Catecholamine depletion begins within 1 hour of drug administration and is maximal in 24 hours. Catecholamines are restored slowly, and doses of reserpine are cumulative with long-term administration. Blood pressure is maximally lowered 2 to 3 weeks after therapy is begun. Reserpine is metabolized by the liver; 60% of an oral dose is recovered in the feces. Less than 1% is excreted in the urine as unchanged drug. Drug dose reduction is unnecessary in renal insufficiency.

## CLASS RENAL EFFECTS

Reserpine has little or no clinically important effect on GFR or ERPF in patients with essential hypertension[137,

## TABLE 54–8. Renal Function Effects: Central α₂-Adrenergic Agonists and Peripheral α-Adrenergic Antagonists*

| Drug | Diagnosis | References | No. of Studies Reviewed | Total No. of Patients | ΔGFR % Mean (Range) | ΔERPF % Mean (Range) | ΔRVR % Mean (Range) | ΔU$_{prot}$ % Mean (Range) |
|---|---|---|---|---|---|---|---|---|
| **Central α₂-Adrenergic Agonists** | | | | | | | | |
| Methyldopa | EH | 247–249 | 3 | 22 | −6 (−13 to 7) | 6 (−4 to 16) | −18 — | — — |
|  | RD | 250, 251 | 2 | 33 | −1 (−4 to 1) | — — | — — | 0 — |
| Clonidine | EH | 252–254 | 3 | 37 | 2 (−1 to 6) | 6 (−3 to 16) | −24 — | — — |
|  | RD | 254, 255 | 2 | 11 | −3 (−4 to −2) | 4 — | — — | −43 — |
| Guanabenz | EH | 97, 256–261 | 7 | 80 | −4 (−18 to 9) | 6 (−17 to 17) | −14 (−23 to 0) | — — |
|  | EH | 262 | 1 | 10 | 23 — | — | — | — — |
| Guanfacine | RD | 262, 263 | 2 | 27 | −14 (−33 to 4) | — | — | −39 — |
|  | DM | 264 | 1 | 6 | −7 — | — | — | −12 — |
| **Central and Peripheral Adrenergic-Neuronal Blocking Agent** | | | | | | | | |
| Reserpine | EH | 307–309 | 3 | 19 | −12 (−17 to −6) | 2 — | −12 (−13 to −12) | — — |
| **Peripheral α₁-Adrenergic Antagonists** | | | | | | | | |
| Doxazosin | EH | 124, 333–336 | 5 | 79 | −2 (−13 to 8) | −2 (−6 to 3) | −2 (−5 to 2) | −27 (−44 to −11) |
| Prazosin | EH | 87, 337–341 | 6 | 83 | 2 (−8 to 18) | 1 (−4 to 7) | −6 (−19 to 6) | — — |
|  | RD | 342, 343 | 2 | 30 | −6 (−16 to 4) | −18 — | −7 — | — — |
| Terazosin | EH | 344 | 1 | 15 | −4 — | — | — | — — |
| **Moderately Selective Peripheral α₁-Adrenergic Antagonist** | | | | | | | | |
| Phenoxybenzamine | — | — | — | — | — | — | — | — |
| **Peripheral Adrenergic-Neuronal Blocking Agents** | | | | | | | | |
| Guanethidine | EH | 309, 378 | 3 | 32 | −24 (−36 to −17) | −10 (−10 to −9) | −7 (−7 to −6) | — — |
| Guanadrel | EH | 379 | 1 | 6 | −9 — | −12 — | −5 — | — — |

*ΔGFR % = percent change in GFR; ΔERPF % = percent change in ERPF; ΔRVR % = percent change in RVR ; ΔU$_{prot}$ % = percent change in urinary protein or albumin excretion; EH = essential hypertension; RD = nondiabetic renal disease; DM = diabetes mellitus.

[246, 307–309] (see Table 54–8). RVR is reduced, probably mediated by reduced sympathetic stimulation of renal α-adrenoreceptors. Reserpine has no sustained effect on the renin-angiotensin-aldosterone axis.[9, 246] Fractional excretion of $Na^+$ and $K^+$ is unchanged, and body fluid composition is not altered.[137, 246]

## CLASS EFFICACY AND SAFETY

Reserpine is an effective monotherapeutic agent for the treatment of mild to moderate hypertension.[306, 310, 311] Pseudotolerance does not occur. The combination of reserpine and a diuretic is more effective in lowering blood pressure than is reserpine alone.[305, 312] Reserpine has no adverse effect on carbohydrate tolerance[197] or blood lipids.[194, 195] When reserpine is used with a diuretic, LVH is less likely to occur.[313]

The side effect most frequently encountered with reserpine is altered central nervous system function, including inability to concentrate, decreased mental acuity, sedation, sleep disturbances (e.g., vivid dreams, nightmares), and depression.[289–292] These symptoms may result from depletion of serotonin or catecholamines from the central nervous system. Reserpine is contraindicated in patients with a history of depression. Nasal congestion and rhinitis are caused by the drug's cholinergic effects.[289–291] Increased gastrointestinal motility and gastric acid secretion may also occur.[289–291] Reserpine is contraindicated in patients with peptic ulcer disease or intestinal disorders. Other side effects include increased appetite with weight gain[289, 290] and sexual dysfunction (e.g., decreased libido, impotence).[188, 189, 289–292]

## Peripheral α₁-Adrenergic Antagonists

### CLASS MECHANISMS OF ACTION

α₁-Adrenergic antagonists induce dilation of both resistance (arterial) and capacitance (venous) vessels by selectively inhibiting postjunctional α₁-adrenergic receptors.[207, 208, 314–319] The net physiologic effect is a decrease in TPVR; reflex tachycardia and the attendant increase in CO do not predictably occur.[320–323] This is due to their low affinity for prejunctional α₂-adrenergic receptors, which modulate the local control of norepinephrine release from sympathetic nerve terminals by a negative feedback mechanism.[207, 208, 314–319]

### CLASS MEMBERS

Doxazosin mesylate, a water-soluble quinazoline analogue of prazosin, is highly selective for α₁-adrenergic receptors.[25, 26, 324, 325] The usual dose is 1 to 4 mg daily (see Table 54–6). Doxazosin is absorbed well but undergoes significant first-pass hepatic metabolism. Bioavailability is about 65% (see Table 54–7). Peak plasma concentrations occur in 2 to 3 hours. The plasma half-life is biphasic, with a terminal elimination half-life of about 22 hours. It is extensively metabolized by the liver and primarily eliminated in the feces. Less than 1% of the drug is excreted

unchanged in the urine; the drug dose need not be reduced in patients with renal insufficiency.

Prazosin hydrochloride is a quinazoline derivative that is highly selective for α₁-adrenergic receptors.[25, 26, 326–329] The usual dose is 4 to 12 mg/d given in divided doses (see Table 54–6). Prazosin is lipophilic; it is readily absorbed but undergoes variable first-pass hepatic metabolism. Bioavailability averages 60% (see Table 54–7). Peak plasma concentrations occur in 2 to 3 hours. The plasma half-life is 2 to 4 hours. It is primarily metabolized by the liver. Less than 10% of the drug is excreted unchanged in the urine; the drug dose need not be reduced in patients with renal insufficiency.

Terazosin hydrochloride is a congener of prazosin with enhanced water solubility.[25, 26, 330–332] The usual dose is 1 to 5 mg daily (see Table 54–6). After oral administration, terazosin is completely absorbed; bioavailability averages 90% (see Table 54–7). Plasma levels peak at 1 to 2 hours. The plasma half-life is about 12 hours. It is primarily metabolized by the liver. Excretion of terazosin and its metabolites occurs in both urine and feces; only 10% of the drug is excreted unchanged in the urine. The drug dose need not be reduced in patients with renal insufficiency.

## CLASS RENAL EFFECTS

In general, α₁-adrenergic antagonists have little or no clinically important effect on GFR or ERPF in patients with essential hypertension[87, 124, 137, 246, 321, 333–341, 344] or in patients with nondiabetic renal parenchymal disease[344] (see Table 54–8). RVR is reduced, probably mediated by a reduction of preglomerular capillary resistance due to inhibition of α₁-mediated (noradrenergic-dependent) vasoconstriction. Urinary protein excretion is reduced. α₁-Adrenergic antagonists have no sustained effect on the renin-angiotensin-aldosterone system.[9, 246] However, fractional $Na^+$ excretion is reduced, and the extracellular fluid compartment is expanded.[137, 246] The mechanism responsible for fluid retention is unknown but may be mediated by increased (unopposed) activity of renal α₂-adrenergic receptors.[345]

## CLASS EFFICACY AND SAFETY

The peripheral α₁-adrenergic antagonists are effective monotherapeutic agents for the treatment of mild to moderate hypertension.[317–319, 346–354] Pseudotolerance does not occur. Their efficacy is similar in the young and the elderly[318, 319, 355] and at rest and during physical exercise.[302, 322] Black patients demonstrate reductions in blood pressure comparable to those in white patients.[162, 317–319] When used in combination with a diuretic or β-adrenergic antagonist, these drugs are more effective in lowering blood pressure compared with monotherapy.[318, 319, 346, 347]

α₁-Adrenergic antagonists do not adversely affect carbohydrate tolerance.[197] However, insulin sensitivity has been reported to be increased.[285, 319, 356] All of these drugs have been demonstrated to modestly lower total triglycerides, total cholesterol, and LDL-cholesterol and to increase HDL-cholesterol.[195, 286, 317, 319, 357] Proposed mechanisms include 1) increased LDL receptor activity, 2) decreased intracellular LDL-cholesterol synthesis, 3) reduced synthesis and secretion of very low density lipoprotein–cholesterol, 4) increased lipoprotein lipase activity, and 5) decreased rate of cholesterol absorption. Although these favorable influences on serum lipids are considered one of the major advantages of this class of drugs, it is not yet clear whether these biochemical benefits translate into reductions in cardiovascular morbidity or mortality. Regression of LVH has been reported to occur.[287, 288, 318, 319]

The use of these drugs has been associated with relatively few side effects, the most striking being the "first-dose effect."[289, 318, 319, 358–361] This is an acute symptom complex characterized by lightheadedness or dizziness, sometimes accompanied by palpitations, that may result in syncope. It is caused by severe orthostatic hypotension resulting from inadequate venous return due to profound arteriolar and venous dilation. It occurs 30 to 90 minutes after the first dose and is dose dependent; it is minimized by initiating therapy in the evening and by careful dose titration. The first-dose effect is exaggerated by fasting, upright posture, low-sodium diet, volume contraction, concurrent diuretic treatment, concurrent β-adrenergic antagonism, or the presence of excessive catecholamine activity (e.g., pheochromocytoma). $\alpha_1$-Adrenergic antagonists should not be used in patients with autonomic insufficiency because of their potential to precipitate or aggravate pre-existing orthostatic hypotension.

$\alpha_1$-Adrenergic antagonists are widely used for the symptomatic relief of prostatic obstruction.[319, 362, 363] Prostatic smooth muscle, which is increased in prostatic hypertrophy, has an abundance of $\alpha_1$-adrenoreceptors. Blockade of these receptors decreases resistance along the prostatic urethra by relaxing the smooth muscle component of the prostate.

# Moderately Selective Peripheral $\alpha_1$-Adrenergic Antagonist

## CLASS MECHANISMS OF ACTION

Phenoxybenzamine is a moderately selective peripheral $\alpha_1$-adrenergic antagonist.[364] It is 100 times more potent at $\alpha_1$-adrenergic receptors than at $\alpha_2$-adrenergic receptors. Phenoxybenzamine binds covalently to $\alpha$-adrenergic receptors, thereby interfering with the capacity of sympathomimetic amines to initiate actions at these sites. Phenoxybenzamine also increases the rate of turnover of norepinephrine as a result of increased tyrosine hydroxylase activity because of increased sympathetic nerve activity (a reflex response to $\alpha$-adrenergic receptor blockade), and it increases the amount of norepinephrine released by each nerve impulse because of blockade of presynaptic $\alpha_2$-adrenergic receptors (which mediates the negative feedback mechanism inhibiting norepinephrine release). The net physiologic effect is a decrease in TPVR and increases in HR and CO. Postural hypotension, related to blockade of compensatory responses to upright posture and hypovolemia, may be prominent. The degree of vasodilation is dependent on the degree of adrenergic vascular tone. The presence of excessive circulating catecholamines during development of blockade can decrease the degree of block attained (i.e., competition for the same receptors). However, after block-

ade is fully developed, it is unaffected by further exposure to circulating catecholamines, a stage referred to as irreversible or nonequilibrium blockade.

## CLASS MEMBER

Phenoxybenzamine hydrochloride is the only drug in its class.[25, 26, 364–367] Initially, 10 mg is administered twice daily (see Table 54–6). Absorption is variable and incomplete (20% to 30%) (see Table 54–7). Peak blockade occurs in 3 to 4 hours. The plasma half-life is approximately 24 hours. The duration of action is at least 3 to 4 days.

## CLASS RENAL EFFECTS

Phenoxybenzamine would be expected to counteract the renal effects of excessive catecholamine secretion. Thus, ERPF and GFR should increase, and RVR should decrease, in proportion to the degree of blockade of $\alpha$-adrenergic tone. Phenoxybenzamine has no consistent effect on the renin-angiotensin-aldosterone axis.[9, 323] Salt and water retention does not occur; blood volume and body weight are unchanged.[323]

## CLASS EFFICACY AND SAFETY

Phenoxybenzamine is primarily used in the management of preoperative or inoperative pheochromocytoma.[365–367] Efficacy is dependent on the degree of underlying excessive $\alpha$-adrenergic vascular tone. Common side effects include nasal congestion, transient sedation, weakness, lassitude, postural hypotension, tachycardia, and sexual dysfunction (e.g., inhibition of ejaculation).[188, 365–367] Tachycardia may result from $\alpha$-adrenergic blockade, which unmasks β-adrenergic effects of epinephrine-secreting tumors; it can be controlled with volume expansion or concurrent use of a β-adrenergic antagonist.[365–367] However, $\alpha$-adrenergic blockade must be established before initiation of β-adrenergic blockade to avoid paradoxical hypertension.

# Peripheral Adrenergic-Neuronal Blocking Agents

## CLASS MECHANISMS OF ACTION

Peripheral adrenergic-neuronal blocking agents are selectively concentrated in the adrenergic nerve terminal by an active transport mechanism, or "norepinephrine pump."[364, 368] They act by interfering with the release of norepinephrine from adrenergic nerve endings in response to sympathetic nerve stimulation (guanadrel) and by depleting norepinephrine stores from adrenergic nerve endings. HR and CO are acutely reduced because of diminished venous return (due to venodilation and peripheral pooling of blood) and blockade of sympathetic β-adrenergic effects on the heart; TPVR is unchanged.[302, 369–371] After long-term therapy, TPVR is decreased, along with modest decreases in HR and CO.[302, 369–373]

## CLASS MEMBERS

Guanethidine monosulfate is the prototype peripheral adrenergic-neuronal blocking agent.[25, 26, 374, 375] The usual dose is 25 to 75 mg daily (see Table 54–6). Absorption is incomplete and variable; only 3% to 30% of an oral dose is absorbed in 12 hours (see Table 54–7). The drug rapidly leaves the plasma for extravascular storage sites, including sympathetic neurons. After distribution in the body, guanethidine is eliminated with a plasma half-life of 5 days, a time course that corresponds to its antihypertensive effect. Guanethidine is metabolized in the liver. Approximately 24% of the drug is excreted unchanged in the urine; the remainder is metabolized into more polar, less active metabolites that are excreted in the urine and feces. When therapy is initiated or the dosage changed, three half-lives (15 days) are required to accumulate 87.5% of a steady-state level. By administering loading doses of guanethidine at 6-hour intervals (the nearly maximal effect from a single oral dose), blood pressure can be lowered in 1 to 3 days. In patients with severe renal insufficiency, drug excretion is decreased; the drug dose should be reduced (see Table 54–4).

Guanadrel sulfate is a guanethidine derivative that has a short therapeutic half-life.[25, 26, 376, 377] The usual dose is 20 to 100 mg/d given in divided doses (see Table 54–6). The drug is rapidly and almost completely absorbed; bioavailability averages 85% (see Table 54–7). Peak plasma levels are reached in 1 to 2 hours. The plasma half-life is 10 to 12 hours. The hypotensive effect of guanadrel occurs within 2 hours, peaks at 4 to 6 hours, and persists for 4 to 14 hours. Guanadrel is metabolized by the liver. Elimination occurs through the kidney; about 40% of the drug is excreted unchanged in the urine. In patients with renal insufficiency, drug dose should be reduced (see Table 54–4).

## CLASS RENAL EFFECTS

Both guanadrel and guanethidine decrease GFR and ERPF in patients with essential hypertension[137, 246, 309, 372, 378] (see Table 54–8). The antihypertensive response is characterized by a reduction in CO; reduced renal perfusion pressure leads to reduced GFR and ERPF. Impaired peripheral adrenergic transmission, with the resulting blockade of the baroreceptor reflex, magnifies the decreases in GFR and ERPF when the patient is in the upright position. Adrenergic-neuronal blocking agents have no long-term effect on the renin-angiotensin-aldosterone axis.[9, 246] However, the filtered load and fractional excretion of $Na^+$ are decreased (owing to reduced GFR), which causes fluid retention and weight gain.[137, 246]

## CLASS EFFICACY AND SAFETY

The peripheral adrenergic-neuronal blocking agents must be used in combination with a diuretic to prevent $Na^+$ retention and the development of pseudotolerance.[379–383] The specific side effects of this class are related to either excessive sympathetic blockade or a relative increase in parasympathetic activity. Postural hypotension is the most significant problem, potentially resulting in dizziness, weakness, or syncope; it is accentuated by hot weather,

alcohol ingestion, and physical exercise.[289, 369, 374, 384, 385] Unopposed parasympathetic activity may result in intestinal cramping or diarrhea.[369, 374, 384, 385] Another troublesome side effect is sexual dysfunction (e.g., retrograde ejaculation, impotence, diminished libido).* However, these drugs have no adverse effect on carbohydrate tolerance.[197]

Because catecholamine depletion may aggravate bronchial asthma, and sympathomimetics may interfere with the hypotensive effect of these drugs, peripheral adrenergic-neuronal blocking agents should be avoided in patients with bronchospastic airway disease. Because these drugs lower CO and interfere with the sympathetic compensatory reflexes of the heart, they should not be prescribed to patients with impaired cardiac function or regional (cerebral or coronary) vascular disease. Other potential adverse cardiac effects include precipitation of sinus bradycardia or atrioventricular block.[289, 370, 374] Finally, because these drugs reduce ERPF and GFR, they should be avoided in patients with impaired renal function.

## Direct-Acting Vasodilators

### CLASS MECHANISMS OF ACTION

Direct-acting vasodilators may have an effect on both arterial resistance and venous capacitance; however, both of the currently available oral drugs, hydralazine and minoxidil, are highly selective for resistance vessels.[386–391] Their specific mechanism of vascular relaxation and reason for selectivity are unknown. By altering cellular $Ca^{2+}$ metabolism, they interfere with the $Ca^{2+}$ movements responsible for initiating or maintaining a contractile state. The net physiologic effect is a decrease in TPVR associated with increases in HR and CO.[392–395] The increases in HR and CO are related to sympathetic stimulation, both direct and indirect (i.e., baroreceptor reflex response).

### CLASS MEMBERS

Hydralazine hydrochloride is the prototype direct-acting vasodilator. The usual dose is 100 to 200 mg/d given in divided doses[25, 26, 396–398] (Table 54–9). Hydralazine is rapidly absorbed after oral administration; peak plasma levels are achieved within 1 hour but vary widely (15-fold) among individuals (Table 54–10). This is because hydralazine is subject to polymorphic acetylation; slow acetylators have higher plasma levels and require lower drug doses to maintain blood pressure control, compared with rapid acetylators. Slow acetylation is an autosomal recessive trait that results from a relative deficiency of the hepatic enzyme N-acetyltransferase. About 50% of black and white persons and the majority of Native Americans, Eskimos, and Asians are rapid acetylators of hydralazine. Bioavailability for slow acetylators ranges from 30% to 35%; bioavailability for rapid acetylators ranges from 10% to 16%. Plasma levels decline with a half-life of 3 to 7 hours. Hydralazine undergoes extensive hepatic metabolism; it is mainly excreted in the urine in the form of metabolites or as unchanged drug.

---

*References 188, 189, 289, 292, 369, 374, 384, 385.

**TABLE 54–9. Pharmacologic Differences Between Vasodilators: Direct-Acting Vasodilators, Calcium Antagonists, and Angiotensin-Converting Enzyme Inhibitors**

| Drug* | First Dose (mg) | Usual Daily Dose (mg) | Maximal Daily Dose (mg) | Maximal Hypotensive Response (h) | Duration of Hypotensive Response (h) |
|---|---|---|---|---|---|
| *Direct-Acting Vasodilators* | | | | | |
| Hydralazine | 10 | 25–50 qid | 300 | 1–3 | 10–12 |
| Minoxidil | 2.5 | 5–10 qd/bid | 80 | 2–4 | 75 |
| *Ca²⁺ Antagonists* | | | | | |
| Amlodipine | 5 | 5–10 qd | 10 | — | 24 |
| Diltiazem | 60 | 60–120 tid | 480 | 2–3 | 8 |
| Diltiazem SR | 90 | 120–180 bid | 480 | 2–3 | 12 |
| Diltiazem CD | 180 | 240–360 qd | 480 | — | 24 |
| Diltiazem XR | 180 | 180–360 qd | 480 | 3–6 | 24 |
| Felodipine | 5 | 5–10 qd | 20 | 2–5 | 24 |
| Isradipine | 2.5 | 5–10 bid | 20 | 2–3 | 12 |
| Nicardipine | 20 | 20–40 tid | 120 | 1–2 | 8 |
| Nicardipine SR | 30 | 30–60 bid | 120 | 2–6 | 12 |
| Nifedipine | 10 | 10–30 tid | 120 | 0.5–1 | 4–6 |
| Nifedipine GITS | 30 | 30–90 qd | 120 | 4–6 | 24 |
| Nifedipine ER | 30 | 30–90 qd | 120 | 2–4 | 24 |
| Verapamil | 80 | 80–120 tid | 480 | 2–3 | 8 |
| Verapamil SR | 180 | 240 qd/bid | 480 | — | 24 |
| Verapamil SR pellet | 120 | 240–480 qd | 480 | — | 24 |
| *Angiotensin-Converting Enzyme Inhibitors* | | | | | |
| Benazepril | 5–10 | 10–40 qd | 80 | 2–6 | 24 |
| Captopril | 12.5–25 | 25–50 bid/tid | 300 | 1–2 | 6–12 |
| Enalapril | 2.5–5 | 5–20 qd/bid | 40 | 4–8 | 12–24 |
| Fosinopril | 10 | 10–40 qd | 80 | 2–6 | 24 |
| Lisinopril | 5–10 | 10–40 qd | 80 | 6–8 | 24 |
| Quinapril | 5–10 | 10–40 qd | 80 | 2–6 | 24 |
| Ramipril | 1.25–2.5 | 2.5–10 qd | 20 | 3–6 | 24 |

*SR = sustained-release; CD = controlled-diffusion; XR and ER = extended-release; GITS = gastrointestinal therapeutic system.

Dose adjustments may be required in slow acetylators with renal insufficiency (see Table 54–4).

Minoxidil is a substantially more potent direct-acting vasodilator compared with hydralazine. The usual dose is 5 to 20 mg daily[25, 26, 399–403] (see Table 54–9). At least 95% of minoxidil is absorbed; peak plasma levels of the parent drug are achieved within 1 hour (see Table 54–10). The plasma half-life is about 4 hours. After a single oral dose, blood pressure declines within 15 minutes, reaches a nadir between 2 and 4 hours, and recovers at an arithmetically linear rate of 30%/d. With long-term administration of minoxidil, a steady-state blood pressure reduction is achieved with 10 mg/d in 7 days, with 20 mg/d in 5 days, and with 40 mg/d in 3 days. Approximately 90% of an oral dose is metabolized by conjugation with glucuronic acid and by conversion to more polar products. Known metabolites are less pharmacologically active than minoxidil and are excreted in the urine. However, minoxidil disposition is prolonged in patients with renal insufficiency; a dose reduction may be required (see Table 54–4). Minoxidil and its metabolites are removed by hemodialysis and peritoneal dialysis; replacement therapy is required.

## CLASS RENAL EFFECTS

The two direct-acting vasodilators have qualitatively similar short-term renal effects related to relaxation of resistance vessels: GFR and ERPF are preserved in patients with normal renal function, and RVR is decreased.[85, 137, 404–408] However, the long-term renal effects of these drugs are more controversial, especially in patients with impaired renal function. It has been suggested that renal function may deteriorate more rapidly in patients treated with minoxidil having baseline serum creatinine levels about 1.5 mg/dL, compared with patients having serum creatinine levels below 1.5 mg/dL.[402] In contrast, long-term blood pressure control with minoxidil has been reported to delay the onset of end-stage renal failure in some patients by up to 6 years.[409]

Both hydralazine and minoxidil produce marked secretion of renin as a result of enhanced sympathetic input to the juxtaglomerular cells of the kidney.[9, 402, 410, 411] In the short term, secondary elevations of angiotensin II and aldosterone occur.[402] In the long term, there is dissociation between PRA (which is elevated) and plasma aldosterone (which is normal) owing to a drug-induced increase in the aldosterone metabolic clearance rate.[412, 413] Monotherapy with hydralazine and minoxidil is associated with salt and water retention and expansion of plasma and extracellular fluid volumes.[137, 395] Retention of salt and water is not related to a reduction in GFR; it may be due to a direct drug effect on the proximal convoluted tubule.[414]

## CLASS EFFICACY AND SAFETY

Both hydralazine and minoxidil produce increases in HR and CO and Na⁺ retention (with rapid development of pseu-

**TABLE 54–10. Pharmacokinetic Differences Among Vasodilators: Direct-Acting, Calcium Antagonists and Angiotensin-Converting Enzyme Inhibitors**

| Drug* | Absorption (%) | First-Pass Effect | Bioavailability (%) | Peak Blood Level | Elimination Half-Life (h) | Metabolism/Excretion |
|---|---|---|---|---|---|---|
| *Direct-Acting Vasodilators* | | | | | | |
| Hydralazine | >90 | Extensive | 10–35 | <1 h | 3–7 | Liver/urine |
| Minoxidil | >95 | None | >90 | <1 h | 4 | Liver/urine |
| *Ca²⁺ Antagonists* | | | | | | |
| Amlodipine | >90 | Minimal | 64–90 | 6–12 h | 30–50 | Liver/urine |
| Diltiazem | >80 | 50% | 40 | 2–3 h | 4–6 | Liver/feces and urine |
| Diltiazem SR | >80 | 50% | 35 | 6–11 h | 5–7 | Liver/feces and urine |
| Diltiazem CD | >80 | Extensive | 35 | 10–14 h | 5–8 | Liver/feces and urine |
| Diltiazem XR | >80 | Extensive | 40 | 4–6 h | 5–10 | Liver/feces and urine |
| Felodipine | >90 | Extensive | 20 | 2.5–5 h | 11–16 | Liver/urine |
| Isradipine | >90 | Extensive | 15–25 | 1–2 h | 8 | Liver/feces and urine |
| Nicardipine | >90 | Extensive | 35 | 1 h | 8–9 | Liver/feces and urine |
| Nicardipine SR | >90 | Extensive | 30 | 1–4 h | — | Liver/feces and urine |
| Nifedipine | >90 | 20%–30% | 60–70 | <30 min | 2 | Liver/urine |
| Nifedipine GITS | >90 | 25%–35% | 50–60 | 6 h | — | Liver/urine |
| Nifedipine ER | >90 | 25%–35% | 50–60 | 2.5–5 h | 7 | Liver/urine |
| Verapamil | >90 | 70%–80% | 20–35 | 1–2 h | 4–12 | Liver/feces and urine |
| Verapamil SR | >90 | 70%–80% | 20–35 | 5 h | — | Liver/feces and urine |
| Verapamil SR pellet | >90 | 70%–80% | 20–35 | 7–9 h | 12 | Liver/feces and urine |
| *Angiotensin-Converting Enzyme Inhibitors* | | | | | | |
| Benazepril | >37 | None | >37† | 1–2 h† | 10–11† | Liver and kidney/feces and urine |
| Captopril | 60–75 | None | 75 | 1 h† | 2 | Kidney/urine |
| Enalapril | 55–75 | None | 40† | 3–4 h† | 11† | Liver and kidney/feces and urine |
| Fosinopril | 36 | None | 25–29† | 3 h† | 12† | Liver and kidney/feces and urine |
| Lisinopril | 25 | None | 25 | 6–8 h† | 12 | Kidney/urine |
| Quinapril | >60 | None | 25† | 2 h† | 25† | Kidney/urine |
| Ramipril | 50–60 | None | 44† | 2–4 h† | 13–17† | Liver and kidney/feces and urine |

*SR = sustained-release; CD = controlled-diffusion; XR and ER = extended-release; GITS = gastrointestinal therapeutic system.
†Active metabolite.

dotolerance); both drugs should be used in combination with a diuretic and a β-adrenergic antagonist (i.e., triple-drug therapy) for the treatment of moderate to severe hypertension.[146, 147, 415–418]

Repeated administration of hydralazine can lead to a syndrome that resembles systemic lupus erythematosus.[418–423] The frequency is dose dependent; it rarely occurs in patients receiving less than 200 mg/d. The syndrome is reversible when hydralazine is discontinued, but months may be required for complete clearing of symptoms. Other adverse effects of hydralazine include fever, skin eruptions, gastrointestinal disturbances, and the development of a peripheral neuropathy related to pyridoxine deficiency.[289] Hypertrichosis is a troublesome side effect of the more potent vasodilator minoxidil.[289, 424, 425] It develops during the first 3 to 6 weeks of therapy in about 80% of the patients. After termination of therapy, hair growth stops and disappears within 1 to 6 months.

The most common and serious untoward effects of hydralazine and minoxidil are related to their direct or reflex-mediated hemodynamic actions, including flushing, headache, palpitations, anginal attacks, and electrocardiographic changes of myocardial ischemia.[289, 418, 425] These effects may be prevented by concurrent administration of a β-adrenergic antagonist. Na⁺ retention, with expansion of extracellular fluid volume, is also a prominent feature of vasodilator

therapy.[289, 418, 425] Pericardial effusions have been detected in 3% to 4% of patients with renal insufficiency receiving minoxidil therapy.[289, 425, 426] Large doses of potent diuretics may be required to prevent systemic edema formation.

## Calcium Antagonists

### CLASS MECHANISMS OF ACTION

The Ca²⁺ antagonists are a chemically heterogeneous group of drugs sharing a common antihypertensive mechanism of action: interference with entry of Ca²⁺ into smooth muscle cells of resistance arterioles through L-type (long-lasting) voltage-operated channels.[427–433] Influx of Ca²⁺ through voltage-operated channels is critical to the release of Ca²⁺ from the sarcoplasmic reticulum, which modulates the amplitude of contraction of arterial smooth muscle. The ability of these drugs to bind to voltage-operated channels, causing closure of the gate and subsequent inhibition of Ca²⁺ flux from the extracellular to the intracellular space, inhibits the essential role of Ca²⁺ as an intracellular messenger uncoupling excitation to contraction. Ca²⁺ may also enter cells through receptor-operated channels.[432–437] The opening of these channels is induced by binding of neurohumoral mediators to specific receptors on the cell membrane. $Ca^{2+}$ antagonists dose-dependently inhibit the $Ca^{2+}$ influx triggered by the stimulation of either α-adrenergic or angiotensin II receptors, inhibiting the influence of α-adrenergic agonists and angiotensin II on vascular smooth muscle tone. The net physiologic effect is a decrease in TPVR.[432, 438-441]

## CLASS MEMBERS

Although all of the $Ca^{2+}$ antagonists share a basic mechanism of action, they are a highly heterogeneous group of compounds that differ markedly in their chemical structure, pharmacologic effects, tissue specificity, pharmacokinetic behavior, side effect profile, and clinical indications. Because of these differences, $Ca^{2+}$ antagonists that are selective for slow $Ca^{2+}$ channels have been subdivided into three distinct classes: diphenylalkylamines, dihydropyridines, and benzothiazepines.[432] Discrete receptor binding sites exist for each of these classes. All $Ca^{2+}$ antagonists dilate large and small coronary and peripheral resistance vessels; coronary and peripheral vascular resistances are reduced, and blood flow is increased. The degree of vasodilation is related to the resting vascular tone. In vitro, all $Ca^{2+}$ antagonists have a negative inotropic effect on myocardial cells of the atria and ventricles. In humans, the relatively strong vascular effects of dihydropyridines trigger a baroreflex-mediated rise in sympathetic nerve activity; this leads to an early positive rather than negative inotropic effect. In contrast, the direct negative and indirect reflexogenic inotropic effects of the diphenylalkylamines and benzothiazepines usually cancel each other. The diphenylalkylamines are especially effective in $Ca^{2+}$ channels that open and close frequently, such as those in the sinus and atrioventricular nodes; they produce negative chronotropic and dromotropic effects. The benzothiazepines are similar, but somewhat less effective on these $Ca^{2+}$ channels. This particular influence of these two classes of $Ca^{2+}$ antagonists, to slow atrioventricular nodal conduction, may be used therapeutically to treat supraventricular tachyarrhythmias.

### Benzothiazepine Derivative

Diltiazem hydrochloride is a benzothiazepine $Ca^{2+}$ antagonist that is available in the form of tablets, sustained-release capsules, controlled-diffusion capsules, and Geomatrix extended-release capsules.[25, 26, 442-447] The controlled-diffusion capsules contain two types of beads of diltiazem; 40% of the beads (surrounded by a thin copolymer membrane) release the drug within 12 hours, and 60% of the beads (surrounded by a thick copolymer membrane) release the drug throughout the last 12 hours of a 24-hour period. The extended-release capsules contain a swellable matrix core that slowly releases the drug in a 24-hour period. The usual tablet dose is 180 to 360 mg/d given in divided doses; the usual sustained-release capsule dose is 120 to 180 mg twice daily; the usual controlled-diffusion capsule dose is 240 to 360 mg daily; and the usual extended-release capsule dose is 180 to 360 mg daily (see Table 54–9). Diltiazem is well absorbed; however, it is subject to an extensive first-pass hepatic effect: bioavailability of the tablet is 40%; bioavailability of the sustained-release capsule is about

90% that of the tablet (see Table 54–10). Peak blood levels are achieved 2 to 3 hours after the tablet, 6 to 11 hours after the sustained-release capsule, 10 to 14 hours after the controlled-diffusion capsule, and 4 to 6 hours after the extended-release capsule administration. The plasma half-life is 4 to 6 hours for the tablet, 5 to 7 hours for the sustained-release capsule, 5 to 8 hours for the controlled-diffusion capsule, and 5 to 10 hours for the extended-release capsule; the prolonged half-life of the extended-release capsule is attributed to continued absorption of diltiazem rather than to alterations in elimination. Diltiazem is partially metabolized in the liver by N-demethylation and deacetylation. Two of the metabolites are active; *N*-mono-desmethyldiltiazem is about 20% and deacetyldiltiazem is 25% to 50% as potent as diltiazem. Diltiazem and its metabolites are excreted in the urine and feces; less than 4% is excreted as unchanged drug in the urine. A dose reduction is unnecessary in patients with renal insufficiency.

### Dihydropyridine Derivatives

Amlodipine besylate is a dihydropyridine $Ca^{2+}$ antagonist that has an extended clearance time permitting once-daily dosing without use of a novel drug delivery system; the usual dose is 5 to 10 mg daily[25, 26, 448-451] (see Table 54–9). Absorption is almost complete. First-pass hepatic metabolism is minimal; bioavailability is estimated to be between 64% and 90% (see Table 54–10). Peak plasma levels are achieved between 6 and 12 hours. Elimination from plasma is biphasic; the terminal plasma half-life is 30 to 50 hours. Steady-state plasma levels are achieved after 7 to 8 days of consecutive daily dosing. Amlodipine is extensively metabolized by the liver to inactive metabolites that are excreted in the urine. A dose reduction is unnecessary in patients with renal insufficiency.

Felodipine is a dihydropyridine $Ca^{2+}$ antagonist that is available in the form of an extended-release tablet.[25, 26, 447, 452-456] The usual dose is 5 to 10 mg daily (see Table 54–9). Absorption is almost complete, but the drug undergoes extensive first-pass hepatic metabolism; bioavailability is about 20% (see Table 54–10). Peak plasma levels are achieved in 2.5 to 5 hours. The plasma levels decline poly-exponentially with a mean terminal half-life of 11 to 16 hours. Felodipine is completely metabolized by the liver into inactive metabolites that are excreted in the urine. A dose reduction is unnecessary in patients with renal insufficiency.

Isradipine is a dihydropyridine $Ca^{2+}$ antagonist that is available in the form of capsules.[25, 26, 457, 458] The usual dose is 5 to 10 mg twice daily (see Table 54–9). Absorption is almost complete, but the drug undergoes extensive first-pass hepatic metabolism; bioavailability is 15% to 25% (see Table 54–10). Peak plasma levels are achieved in 1 to 2 hours. The elimination of isradipine is biphasic; the terminal plasma half-life is about 8 hours. Isradipine undergoes extensive hepatic metabolism to yield inactive metabolites that are excreted in the feces and urine. A dose reduction is unnecessary in patients with renal insufficiency.

Nicardipine hydrochloride is a dihydropyridine $Ca^{2+}$ antagonist that is available in the form of capsules and sustained-release capsules.[25, 26, 459, 460] The usual capsule dose is

60 to 120 mg/d given in divided doses; the usual sustained-release capsule dose is 30 to 60 mg twice daily (see Table 54–9). Absorption is almost complete, but the drug undergoes extensive first-pass hepatic metabolism; bioavailability is about 35% (see Table 54–10). Peak plasma levels are achieved in about 1 hour after the capsule and 1 to 4 hours after the sustained-release capsule administration. The terminal plasma half-life is 8 to 9 hours. Nicardipine is extensively metabolized by the liver; its metabolites are excreted in the feces and urine. A dose reduction is unnecessary in patients with renal insufficiency.

Nifedipine is a dihydropyridine $Ca^{2+}$ antagonist that is available in the form of liquid-filled capsules, slow-release tablets, and extended-release tablets.[25, 26, 444, 445, 447, 461–468] The usual capsule dose is 30 to 90 mg/d given in divided doses (see Table 54–9). It is well absorbed after oral administration. There is no pharmacokinetic advantage to giving the drug sublingually; absorption does not occur through the buccal mucous membrane. The most rapid absorption occurs after the "bite and swallow" technique. Regardless of the route of administration, peak blood levels are achieved within 30 minutes (see Table 54–10). First-pass hepatic metabolism reduces its bioavailability to 60% to 70%. The plasma half-life is about 2 hours. The drug is extensively converted by the liver to inactive metabolites; 80% of nifedipine and its metabolites are excreted in the urine. A dose reduction is unnecessary in patients with renal insufficiency.

The slow-release preparation of nifedipine is in the form of a bilayer tablet coated with a semipermeable membrane; the top layer contains nifedipine, and the lower layer contains an osmotic agent. This formulation, known as the gastrointestinal therapeutic system (GITS), delivers nifedipine through a pore in the capsule by osmotic displacement in a 24-hour period. The usual nifedipine GITS dose is 30 to 90 mg daily (see Table 54–9). The GITS tablet requires about 2 hours' hydration time before the plasma concentration rises moderately. The plasma concentration plateaus at 6 hours and is maintained for 24 hours (see Table 54–10). The slow rate of decline in the plasma concentration for the GITS tablet does not reflect a change in the plasma half-life of nifedipine; rather it reflects prolonged absorption due to slow release of the drug. The bioavailability of the GITS tablet (relative to the capsule) is about 65% after a single dose but 85% at steady state owing to residual absorption more than 24 hours after dosing.

The extended-release tablet preparation of nifedipine consists of an external coat and an internal core; both contain nifedipine: the coat as a slow-release formulation, and the core as a fast-release formulation. The usual nifedipine extended-release tablet dose is 30 to 90 mg daily (see Table 54–9). The plasma concentration peaks at 2.5 to 5 hours; there is a second small peak at 6 to 12 hours (see Table 54–10). When the nifedipine extended-release preparation is administered in multiples of 30-mg tablets over a dose range of 30 to 90 mg, the area under the curve is dose proportional; however, the peak plasma concentration for the 90-mg dose given as three 30-mg tablets is 29% greater than predicted from the 30-mg and 60-mg doses. Three 30-mg tablets should not be considered interchangeable with a 90-mg tablet. The bioavailability of the nifedipine ex-

tended-release tablet (relative to the capsule) is 84% to 89% (see Table 54–10). The elimination half-life of nifedipine administered as the extended-release tablet is 7 hours.

### Diphenylalkylamine Derivative

Verapamil hydrochloride is a diphenylalkylamine $Ca^{2+}$ antagonist that is available in the form of tablets, sustained-release caplets, and sustained-release pellet-filled capsules.[25, 26, 444, 445, 447, 469–472] The usual tablet dose is 240 to 360 mg/d given in divided doses; the usual sustained-release caplet dose is 240 mg once or twice daily; and the usual pellet-filled capsule dose is 240 to 480 mg daily (see Table 54–9). Verapamil is nearly completely absorbed, but its bioavailability is reduced to 20% to 35% by extensive first-pass hepatic metabolism (see Table 54–10). Ingestion of food further reduces bioavailability of the tablets and sustained-release caplets but not of the pellet-filled capsules. Peak plasma levels are reached 1 to 2 hours after the tablet, 5 hours after the sustained-release caplet, and 7 to 9 hours after the pellet-filled capsule administration. The plasma half-life is 3 to 7 hours after a single tablet dose, but it is 4 to 12 hours after sustained therapy (presumably owing to saturation of its first-pass hepatic metabolism) and 12 hours for the pellet-filled capsules. Although the sustained-release caplets are marketed for once-daily dosing, the bulk of active drug is released in less than 8 hours; administration of the sustained-release caplets in two equally divided doses produces less fluctuation in plasma levels and better blood pressure control. Verapamil is extensively metabolized in the liver; its major metabolite, norverapamil, has about 20% of the activity of the parent compound. Seventy percent of verapamil is excreted as metabolites in the urine; the remainder is excreted in the feces. A dose reduction is unnecessary in patients with renal failure.

### CLASS RENAL EFFECTS

Short-term administration of $Ca^{2+}$ antagonists to patients with essential hypertension maintains or improves GFR and ERPF and decreases RVR[124, 137, 473–523] (Table 54–11). The filtration fraction is unchanged from baseline. Initially observed increases in GFR and ERPF are related to impaired afferent arteriolar autoregulation (i.e., selective preglomerular vasodilation); these changes are attenuated by the decrease in renal perfusion pressure accompanying the decrease in systemic blood pressure.[474–476] Long-term therapy is usually associated with a return of GFR and ERPF to pretreatment values.[476, 486, 497, 524] In patients who have essential hypertension with moderately impaired GFR, $Ca^{2+}$ antagonists may markedly increase both GFR and ERPF.[481, 484, 509, 524–526] In hypertensive patients with advanced diabetic[118, 264, 482, 483, 503, 504, 512–516] or nondiabetic[501, 502, 510, 511, 523] renal parenchymal disease, $Ca^{2+}$ antagonists have no clinically important short-term effect on GFR or ERPF (see Table 54–11). Urinary protein excretion is usually unchanged or decreased.

Because $Ca^{2+}$ inhibits renin secretion by a direct action on the juxtaglomerular cells, the administration of a $Ca^{2+}$ antagonist might be expected to stimulate renin secretion.[9]

TABLE 54–11. Renal Function Effects: Calcium Antagonists*

| Drug | Diagnosis | References | No. of Studies Reviewed | Total No. of Patients | $\Delta$GFR % Mean (Range) | $\Delta$ERPF % Mean (Range) | $\Delta$RVR % Mean (Range) | $\Delta U_{prot}$ % Mean (Range) |
|---|---|---|---|---|---|---|---|---|
| **Benzothiazepine Derivative** | | | | | | | | |
| Diltiazem | EH | 477–481 | 6 | 53 | 14 (–5 to 62) | 26 (–4 to 77) | –28 (–43 to –14) | — |
| | DM | 482, 483 | 2 | 24 | –7 — | –3 — | — | –48 (–52 to –45) |
| **Dihydropyridine Derivatives** | | | | | | | | |
| Amlodipine | EH | 484 | 1 | 19 | 13 — | 19 — | –25 — | –9 — |
| Felodipine | EH | 124, 485–489 | 6 | 85 | 10 (–13 to 39) | –2 (–5 to 0) | –7 — | –61 — |
| Isradipine | EH | 490–494 | 6 | 82 | 5 (–4 to 10) | 7 (–6 to 18) | –25 (–28 to –22) | — |
| Nicardipine | EH | 495–500 | 6 | 47 | 0 (–8 to 11) | 5 (–1 to 11) | –30 — | –18 — |
| | RD | 501–502 | 2 | 14 | –1 (–3 to 0) | — | — | –6 (–11 to –2) |
| | DM | 503–504 | 2 | 19 | 6 (2 to 11) | 2 (–3 to 7) | –23 (–29 to –17) | –52 (–61 to –42) |
| Nifedipine | EH | 505–509 | 5 | 93 | 5 (–1 to 13) | 20 — | –25 — | –7 — |
| | RD | 510–511 | 2 | 43 | –5 (–17 to 7) | 7 — | –12 — | 11 (0 to 21) |
| | DM | 118, 482, 512–516 | 7 | 127 | –8 (–25 to 18) | –1 (–18 to 17) | –16 (–21 to –10) | 10 (–36 to 89) |
| **Diphenylalkylamine Derivative** | | | | | | | | |
| Verapamil | EH | 517–522 | 6 | 72 | 4 (–2 to 8) | 2 (–12 to 16) | –14 (–25 to 1) | — |
| | RD | 523 | 1 | 10 | 0 — | 6 — | –14 — | –6 — |
| | DM | 264 | 1 | 8 | –5 — | — | — | –49 — |

*$\Delta$GFR % = percent change in GFR; $\Delta$ERPF % = percent change in ERPF; $\Delta$RVR % = percent change in RVR; $\Delta U_{prot}$ % = percent change in urinary protein or albumin excretion; EH = essential hypertension; RD = nondiabetic renal disease; DM = diabetes mellitus.

Although dihydropyridine $Ca^{2+}$ antagonists may acutely stimulate renin release, the other classes of $Ca^{2+}$ antagonists fail to consistently produce this effect.[473, 474] Failure to stimulate renin release may be attributable to the natriuretic properties of the $Ca^{2+}$ antagonists; if $Ca^{2+}$ antagonists inhibit $Na^+$ reabsorption at a site proximal to the macula densa, increased sodium chloride delivery to the macula densa should inhibit renin release. Renin (and presumably angiotensin II) stimulation, when it does occur, is not associated with aldosterone release.[437, 473, 474] Although angiotensin II is a major regulator of aldosterone secretion from the adrenal glomerulosa cells, angiotensin II acts through the $Ca^{2+}$ messenger system; angiotensin II–induced increases in free cytosolic $Ca^{2+}$ concentrations are blocked by $Ca^{2+}$ antagonism, which inhibits steroidogenesis.[527–530]

All of the $Ca^{2+}$ antagonists induce an acute natriuresis and diuresis.[137, 473, 474, 529–532] This effect appears to be independent of any vascular action of the drugs. It may be due to a direct drug effect on either the proximal tubule or segments located more distally than the loop of Henle. However, with the possible exception of the dihydropyridine derivatives,[533] the $Ca^{2+}$ antagonists have not been demonstrated to sustain a clinically evident natriuretic effect.[137, 473] This conclusion is suggested by the absence of changes in serum electrolytes, body fluid composition, or weight.

### CLASS EFFICACY AND SAFETY

The $Ca^{2+}$ antagonists are effective monotherapeutic agents for the treatment of mild, moderate, and severe hypertension.[433, 440, 441, 445, 534–536] Pseudotolerance does not occur. They are effective in the recumbent and upright positions,[445] at rest and during physical exercise,[153, 445] in the young and elderly,[433, 445, 537–541] and in black and white patients.[162, 433, 445, 540–543] Although controversial, the use of $Ca^{2+}$ antagonism in combination with a diuretic may produce a greater blood pressure response than is seen with either drug alone.[433, 544] The combination of a β-adrenergic antagonist and a dihydropyridine $Ca^{2+}$ antagonist is safe and effective in most patients; however, the combination of a β-adrenergic antagonist with either verapamil or diltiazem should be undertaken with caution, given the potential adverse effects on cardiac conduction (e.g., heart block, bradycardia).[433] $Ca^{2+}$ antagonists are also a useful adjunct to multiple-drug regimens for the treatment of resistant hypertension.[433]

Although early reports suggested that $Ca^{2+}$ antagonists may reduce insulin secretion and induce hyperglycemia, these drugs have no effect on insulin secretion in usual therapeutic doses.[197, 198, 285, 433, 545] They have no adverse effect on serum lipoprotein concentrations.[195, 433, 545] They do reduce LVH in parallel with their antihypertensive effect; this may be associated with suppression of ventricular ectopy.[164, 287, 288, 433] Because $Ca^{2+}$ antagonists reduce myocardial oxygen demand, ameliorate intracellular $Ca^{2+}$ overload, dilate the coronary microcirculation, control blood pressure, and regress LVH, they may be the drugs of choice for hypertensive patients with LVH and diastolic dysfunction[164, 287, 288, 433] or angina pectoris.[162] The $Ca^{2+}$ antagonists verapamil and diltiazem are useful for hypertensive patients

with concurrent supraventricular tachyarrhythmias; by contrast, bradyarrhythmias arising in the sinoatrial or atrioventricular node are often exacerbated by these drugs.[433] $Ca^{2+}$ antagonists have not been found to be cardioprotective either during or after a myocardial infarction.[163, 538] As with all of the current classes of antihypertensive drugs, $Ca^{2+}$ antagonists have not been demonstrated to provide primary cardioprotection.[163, 538]

The most common adverse side effects of dihydropyridine $Ca^{2+}$ antagonists are related to their peripheral vasodilating properties: headache, flushing, palpitations, and edema formation.[433, 546–548] Edema is hypothesized to result from selective dilation of precapillary resistance vessels, which increases capillary hydrostatic pressure and produces transudation of fluid into the interstitium. Gastrointestinal side effects (constipation and nausea) are most common with verapamil.[433, 546–548] In addition, verapamil and, to a lesser degree, diltiazem may precipitate or aggravate a bradyarrhythmia, atrioventricular block, or congestive heart failure because of their negative inotropic, dromotropic, and chronotropic effects.[433, 546–548] These drugs should be avoided in patients with sick sinus syndrome, second- or third-degree atrioventricular block, and congestive heart failure. Furthermore, these drugs (unlike the dihydropyridines) probably should not be used in combination with β-adrenergic antagonists.

Concomitant administration of verapamil, diltiazem, or nifedipine with digoxin decreases the elimination of digoxin, resulting in increases of 40% to 100% in serum digoxin levels.[25, 26, 446, 461, 471, 549] Concomitant administration of verapamil and diltiazem with cyclosporine reduces cyclosporine metabolism, resulting in increases of 25% to 100% in cyclosporine blood levels.[25, 26, 446, 468] Finally, the bioavailability of the dihydropyridine $Ca^{2+}$ antagonists may be increased more than twofold when they are taken with grapefruit juice, which contains flavonoids (inhibitors of cytochrome P-450 isozymes).[452, 550, 551]

## Angiotensin-Converting Enzyme Inhibitors

### CLASS MECHANISMS OF ACTION

Angiotensin-converting enzyme (ACE) inhibitors lower blood pressure by decreasing TPVR; there is usually little change in HR or CO.[552–556] Mechanisms proposed for the observed decrease in TPVR include 1) decreased (plasma, tissue) angiotensin II–mediated vascular constriction[557–568]; 2) sympathoinhibitory effects through inhibition of norepinephrine release from presynaptic nerve terminals or inhibition of postjunctional pressor responses to angiotensin II or norepinephrine[569–575]; 3) inhibition of the brain renin-angiotensin system at the level of the baroreceptor reflex, thus increasing the buffering capacity (i.e., enhancing sensitivity) of the baroreceptors[574–578]; 4) blockade of the production of angiotensin II within the vasomotor center of the medulla oblongata, thus reducing sympathetic outflow[574–579]; 5) accumulation of the vasodilator bradykinin in the vascular wall by inhibition of kininase II (i.e., ACE)[574, 575, 580–590]; and 6) stimulation of vasodilator prostaglandin and nitric oxide (endothelium-derived relaxing factor) biosynthesis (directly or indirectly by an increase in tissue bradykinin).[574, 575, 591–597]

## CLASS MEMBERS

ACE inhibitors differ in pro-drug status, ACE affinity, potency, molecular weight and conformation, and lipophilicity. However, they may be classified into one of three main chemical classes according to the ligand of the zinc ion of ACE: sulfhydryl, carboxyl, or phosphinyl.[598, 599]

### Sulfhydryl Angiotensin-Converting Enzyme Inhibitor

Captopril is a sulfhydryl-containing ACE inhibitor.[25, 26, 600–606] The usual dose is 50 to 150 mg/d given in divided doses (see Table 54–9). Captopril is rapidly absorbed after oral or sublingual administration; peak blood levels occur within 1 hour (see Table 54–10). However, ingestion of food reduces absorption 25% to 40%. The plasma half-life is less than 2 hours. More than 95% of the absorbed dose is excreted in the urine; 40% to 50% is unchanged drug, and the remainder is either the disulfide dimer of captopril or the captopril-cysteine disulfide. Captopril and its metabolites may undergo reversible interconversions. In patients with renal impairment, retention of captopril and its metabolites occurs; a dose reduction is necessary (see Table 54–4). Captopril is removed by hemodialysis.

### Carboxyl Angiotensin-Converting Enzyme Inhibitors

Benazepril hydrochloride is an ethyl ester (pro-drug) of the long-acting ACE inhibitor benazeprilat.[25, 26, 607–609] The usual dose is 10 to 40 mg daily (see Table 54–9). At least 37% is absorbed; peak serum concentrations of benazepril occur within 1 hour (see Table 54–10). After absorption, benazepril is almost completely hydrolyzed to benazeprilat in the liver and other tissues. Peak serum concentrations of benazeprilat are reached in 1 to 2 hours. The effective plasma half-life of benazeprilat is 10 to 11 hours. Benazepril and benazeprilat are cleared predominantly by renal excretion; nonrenal (biliary) excretion accounts for about 12% in patients with normal renal function. Biliary clearance may compensate to an extent for patients with impaired renal function. However, a dose reduction is required in patients with renal insufficiency (see Table 54–4).

Enalapril maleate is an ethyl ester (pro-drug) of the long-acting ACE inhibitor enalaprilat.[25, 26, 610–615] The usual dose is 5 to 20 mg daily (see Table 54–9). Fifty-five percent to 75% is absorbed; peak serum concentrations of enalapril occur within 1 hour (see Table 54–10). After absorption, enalapril is hydrolyzed to enalaprilat in the liver and other tissues. Peak serum concentrations of enalaprilat are reached in 3 to 4 hours. Enalapril has only a 60% in vivo biotransformation rate to enalaprilat; net bioavailability is about 40%. The serum concentration of enalaprilat exhibits a prolonged terminal phase; the effective plasma half-life after multiple doses is 11 hours. Approximately 94% of a dose is recovered in the urine and feces as enalaprilat or enalapril; there are no metabolites. In patients with renal impairment, retention of enalapril and enalaprilat occurs; dose reduction is necessary (see Table 54–4). Enalaprilat is removed by hemodialysis.

Lisinopril is the lysine analogue of enalaprilat.[25, 26, 616–620] The usual dose is 10 to 40 mg daily (see Table 54–9). The average absorption after an oral dose is 25%, with large intersubject variability (6% to 60%) (see Table 54–10). Peak serum concentrations occur within 6 to 8 hours. Declining serum concentrations exhibit a prolonged terminal phase, which does not contribute to drug accumulation. On multiple dosing, lisinopril exhibits an effective plasma half-life of 12 hours. This terminal phase probably represents saturable binding to ACE and is not proportional to dose. Lisinopril does not undergo metabolism; it is excreted unchanged in the urine. Impaired renal function decreases the excretion of lisinopril; a dose reduction is necessary (see Table 54–4).

Quinapril hydrochloride is an ethyl ester (pro-drug) of the long-acting ACE inhibitor quinaprilat.[25, 26, 621–623] The usual dose is 10 to 40 mg daily (see Table 54–9). At least 60% is absorbed; peak serum concentrations of quinapril occur within 1 hour (see Table 54–10). After absorption, quinapril is hydrolyzed to quinaprilat in the liver and other tissues. Peak serum concentrations of quinaprilat are reached in 2 hours. Quinapril has a 38% in vivo biotransformation rate to quinaprilat; net bioavailability is about 25%. The serum concentration of quinaprilat exhibits a prolonged terminal phase; the effective plasma half-life is about 25 hours. Quinapril and quinaprilat are eliminated primarily by renal excretion. In patients with renal insufficiency, retention of quinapril and quinaprilat occurs; a dose reduction is necessary (see Table 54–4).

Ramipril is an ethyl ester (pro-drug) of the long-acting ACE inhibitor ramiprilat.[25, 26, 624–626] The usual dose is 2.5 to 10 mg daily (see Table 54–9). At least 50% to 60% is absorbed; peak serum concentrations of ramipril occur within 1 hour (see Table 54–10). After absorption, ramipril is almost completely hydrolyzed to ramiprilat in the liver and other tissues. Peak serum concentrations of ramiprilat are reached in 2 to 4 hours. Plasma concentrations of ramiprilat decline in a triphasic manner; the terminal elimination phase has a prolonged half-life more than 50 hours. However, the effective half-life is 13 to 17 hours. Ramipril and ramiprilat are eliminated in the urine (60%) and feces (40%). In patients with renal insufficiency, retention of ramipril and ramiprilat occurs; a dose reduction is necessary (see Table 54–4).

### Phosphinyl Angiotensin-Converting Enzyme Inhibitor

Fosinopril sodium is a propyl ester (pro-drug) of the long-acting ACE inhibitor fosinoprilat.[25, 26, 627–630] The usual dose is 10 to 40 mg daily (see Table 54–9). Approximately 36% is absorbed; peak serum concentrations of fosinopril occur within 1 hour (see Table 54–10). After absorption, fosinopril is almost completely hydrolyzed to fosinoprilat in the gastrointestinal mucosa, liver, and other tissues. Peak serum concentrations of fosinoprilat are reached in 3 hours. The effective terminal elimination plasma half-life of fosinoprilat is about 12 hours. Fosinopril and fosinoprilat are eliminated almost equally by the liver and kidney in the feces and urine. The clearance of fosinoprilat does not differ appreciably with the degree of renal insufficiency, because diminished renal elimination is offset by increased hepatic biliary elimination. A dose reduction is not required in patients with renal insufficiency.

## CLASS RENAL EFFECTS

In general, ACE inhibitors maintain GFR, increase ERPF, and decrease RVR in patients who have essential hypertension with normal renal function* (Table 54–12). Urinary protein excretion is decreased. In patients with impaired GFR ($\leq 80$ mL/min/1.73 m²), marked improvement in renal function (GFR and ERPF) may occur[476, 633–639]; these changes may be sustained up to 3 years.[640] Forty percent to 50% of patients with essential hypertension fail to increase their ERPF or fail to enhance their renal vascular responsiveness to angiotensin II when they shift from a low to a high sodium intake; such patients have been termed "nonmodulators."[716, 717] The administration of enalapril to these patients restores their ERPF and renal vascular responsiveness to normal.[718] The clinical importance of these observations remains to be determined, but they suggest that ACE inhibitors may reverse the pathophysiologic process of essential hypertensive renal disease by attenuating the intrarenal effects of angiotensin II.

In general, ACE inhibitors have no clinically important short-term effect on GFR or ERPF in patients with both early and advanced diabetic nephropathy[663, 719–721] and in patients with moderately advanced nondiabetic[680, 704, 722, 723] renal parenchymal disease (see Table 54–11). However, urinary protein excretion is usually decreased.[663, 680, 704, 719–723] The decrease in proteinuria is unrelated to changes in systemic blood pressure, GFR, ERPF, or filtration fraction.[695] It may, however, be dose related or Na⁺ dependent.[704, 722] The antiproteinuric effect of ACE inhibitors has been attributed to 1) a decrease in glomerular capillary hydraulic pressure, 2) an increase in basement membrane barrier permselectivity, or 3) a decrease in mesangial uptake and clearance of macromolecules.[663, 680, 695, 704, 707, 719–726] To the degree that proteinuria reflects glomerular injury, ACE inhibitors may have the potential to attenuate the progression of renal disease (as reflected by a reduction in the degree of proteinuria) independent of their antihypertensive effect.

However, proteinuria ($>1$ g/d), sometimes sufficient to produce the nephrotic syndrome, has been reported to occur in captopril-treated patients.[727–733] Findings of membranous nephropathy have been described, which suggests the possibility of an immune complex glomerulopathy, perhaps related to the sulfhydryl structure of captopril. In 75% of the originally reported cases, patients exhibiting proteinuria were receiving captopril doses in excess of 150 mg/d and had a history of pre-existing renal disease.[734, 735] In patients without a history of renal disease receiving doses less than 150 mg/d, the frequency of proteinuria with captopril may

be as low as 0.2%.[735] Proteinuria usually subsides or clears within 6 months of discontinuation of therapy.

ACE inhibitors may produce functional renal insufficiency in patients who have essential hypertension with severe bilateral hypertensive nephrosclerosis,[736] in patients with severe bilateral renal artery stenosis,[737, 738] or in patients with stenosis of the renal artery of a solitary kidney.[737–739] The postulated mechanism for this effect is diminished systemic pressure in combination with diminished postglomerular capillary resistance (i.e., decrease in angiotensin II–mediated efferent arteriolar tone).[740–746] In unilateral renal artery stenosis, a drop in the critical perfusion and filtration pressures may result in a marked drop in single-kidney GFR; however, the contralateral kidney may show an increase in both ERPF and GFR because of attenuation of the intrarenal effects of angiotensin II on its vascular resistance and mesangial tone. Thus, total "net" GFR may be normal, giving the false appearance of stability. Although short-term ACE inhibition may invariably decrease GFR of the stenotic kidney, it is unlikely to cause renal artery thrombosis owing to the preservation of ERPF; GFR returns rapidly to pretreatment values after cessation of the ACE inhibitor. However, long-term ACE inhibitor therapy does not prevent progression of the underlying renovascular disease; renal ischemia may progress and renal arterial occlusion may occur, resulting in renal atrophy.[747]

ACE inhibitors initially stimulate PRA and suppress circulating (plasma) concentrations of angiotensin II and aldosterone.[556, 559, 560, 748–759] Although long-term ACE inhibitor therapy is associated with marked sustained stimulation of PRA, it is less clear whether there is sustained suppression of circulating angiotensin II. Studies suggest that chronic suppression of plasma angiotensin II [angiotensin-(1–8)] does not persist, presumably because of the compensatory rise in renin and angiotensin I, which is partially converted to angiotensin II even during peak ACE inhibition.[760–767] What may be more critical, however, is the presence of sustained suppression of tissue angiotensin II. Although all ACE inhibitors have a uniform effect on circulating (plasma) ACE, they differ in their specificity for and inhibitory potency of tissue ACE.[562–568] The long-term vascular and renal responses to an ACE inhibitor may reflect its ability to sustain suppression of tissue ACE and hence tissue angiotensin II.

Finally, ACE inhibitors have been demonstrated to reset Na⁺ and water homeostasis (by an initial natriuresis and water diuresis) and to spare K⁺ loss.[137, 560, 631, 632] Acute pharmacologic interruption of the renin-angiotensin system probably leads to the natriuresis, initially through local intrarenal (angiotensin II–mediated) mechanisms, because the response occurs too quickly to be attributed to a decrease in plasma aldosterone concentrations.[634] The natriuresis may be sustained for several days, reflecting inhibition of both angiotensin II and aldosterone.[560, 634, 635, 768] However, long-term effects on salt and water excretion are less clear. Absence of changes in plasma volume, extracellular fluid volume, and body weight suggest that Na⁺ homeostasis is restored, perhaps related to attenuated humoral responses of angiotensin II or aldosterone. However, the initially observed increase in free water clearance may persist.[639] The acute antikaliuretic effect of ACE inhibitors does correlate

---

*References 98, 114, 115, 124, 137, 475, 476, 489, 500, 506, 522, 631–654, 669, 671–679, 698–703, 709–712, 715.

### TABLE 54–12. Renal Function Effects: Angiotensin-Converting Enzyme Inhibitors*

| Drug | Diagnosis | References | No. of Studies Reviewed | Total No. of Patients | ΔGFR % Mean (Range) | ΔERPF % Mean (Range) | ΔRVR % Mean (Range) | ΔU$_{prot}$ % Mean (Range) |
|---|---|---|---|---|---|---|---|---|
| **Sulfhydryl Group** | | | | | | | | |
| Captopril | EH | 506, 641–654 | 20 | 231 | 6 (−17 to 97) | 17 (−6 to 120) | −27 (−64 to −9) | −11 (−13 to −9) |
| | RD | 501, 511, 655–661 | 14 | 202 | −1 (−31 to 35) | 15 (0 to 31) | — | −35 (−63 to 9) |
| | DM | 504, 512, 516, 662–668 | 11 | 145 | −7 (−30 to 9) | 7 (−5 to 26) | −17 (−22 to −13) | −41 (−65 to 0) |
| **Carboxyl Group** | | | | | | | | |
| Benazepril | EH | 669 | 1 | 17 | −3 | 34 | −37 | −9 |
| | RD | 670 | 1 | 20 | −6 | 6 | −14 | −37 |
| Enalapril | EH | 98, 114, 489, 500, 502, 654, 671–679 | 19 | 279 | 1 (−8 to 20) | 8 (−17 to 19) | −20 (−29 to 1) | −42 (−67 to −16) |
| | RD | 116, 124, 255, 343, 680–690 | 16 | 196 | −1 (−23 to 36) | 6 (−11 to −22) | −13 (−30 to 7) | −49 (−86 to −21) |
| | DM | 118, 503, 514, 515, 691–697 | 12 | 210 | −3 (−16 to 14) | 8 (−2 to 25) | −17 (−39 to −1) | −48 (−87 to −2) |
| Lisinopril | EH | 115, 654, 698–703 | 8 | 133 | −1 (−11 to 8) | 2 (−8 to 12) | −19 (−25 to −11) | −11 (−43 to 20) |
| | RD | 251, 704–708 | 7 | 80 | −12 (−21 to 0) | −7 (−29 to 7) | 14 (−25 to 82) | −35 (−75 to 14) |
| | DM | 264, 483 | 2 | 18 | −8 (−13 to −4) | −3 | — | −50 (−58 to −42) |
| Quinipril | EH | 709 | 1 | 10 | −1 | 0 | −10 | — |
| Ramipril | EH | 124, 710–712 | 4 | 50 | −1 (−6 to 4) | 7 (−2 to 17) | −17 (−26 to −9) | −16 |
| | DM | 713, 714 | 3 | 26 | 1 | 7 | −14 | −37 (−75 to 0) |
| **Phosphinyl Group** | | | | | | | | |
| Fosinopril | H | 715 | 1 | 9 | 5 | 10 | −14 | — |

*ΔGFR % = percent change in glomerular filtration rate; ΔERPF % = percent change in effective renal plasma flow; ΔRVR % = percent change in renal vascular resistance; ΔU$_{prot}$ % = percent change in urinary protein excretion; EH = essential hypertension; RD = nondiabetic renal disease; DM = diabetes mellitus.

with acute changes in aldosterone metabolism (serum concentration or urinary excretion).[560] The long-term effect of ACE inhibition therapy on plasma aldosterone is less well defined; some authors report sustained suppression,[556, 749, 752, 754] whereas others report normal values.[753, 756–759] Regardless, because clinically significant $K^+$ retention may occur, especially in the presence of renal disease, the concurrent administration of potassium supplements, $K^+$-sparing diuretics, or drugs impairing $K^+$ excretion should be avoided.

## CLASS EFFICACY AND SAFETY

ACE inhibitors are effective monotherapeutic agents for the treatment of mild, moderate, and severe hypertension.* Pseudotolerance does not occur. The efficacy of an ACE inhibitor is markedly enhanced (>80%) when it is combined with diuretic therapy.[559, 604, 769–776] This is especially true for black patients, who are less responsive (~40%) than white patients (~60%) to monotherapy.[774–780] ACE inhibitors are effective in recumbent and upright postures,[751, 770, 771] in the young and elderly,[539, 781–785] and at rest and during physical exercise.[554, 555]

ACE inhibitors appear to have no adverse effect on serum glucose concentration[197, 198, 285]; however, insulin sensitivity has been reported to be improved.[786] Another report was unable to confirm this observation; however, a heightened insulin response to oral glucose was observed, with improved glucose tolerance.[787] The augmented sensitivity of the insulin secretory response to glucose stimulation was attributed to resistance to the $K^+$-lowering action of insulin. ACE inhibitors have no clinically important effect on serum lipoprotein concentrations.[193–195]

ACE inhibitors do regress LVH in parallel with their antihypertensive effect.[287, 288] ACE inhibitors have also been shown to reduce cardiovascular mortality and morbidity (including coronary events) in patients with congestive heart failure and after myocardial infarction; in hypertensive patients with heart failure and systolic dysfunction, ACE inhibitors are the drugs of choice.[162, 163, 287, 288] However, ACE inhibitors have not been demonstrated to reduce cardiovascular events in hypertension.

ACE inhibitors are well tolerated; there are few class side effects.† The most common side effect is cough (5% to 25%); the mechanism is unclear but may be related to 1) accumulation of kinins, promoting cough and bronchospasm in susceptible persons by directly inducing smooth muscle contraction and local edema; 2) accumulation of substance P, a potent bronchoconstrictor that is degraded by ACE; and 3) accumulation of prostaglandins (prostaglandin $E_2$ or thromboxane $A_2$).[788–792] The most serious side effect is angioedema, which may occur in 0.1% to 0.2% of patients treated with an ACE inhibitor; it usually occurs within hours or at most 3 weeks after the drug is started.[788, 792, 793] It reverses within hours after the drug is stopped and does not appear to be dose related. However, angioedema associated with laryngeal edema may be fatal. The mechanism is unknown but may be related to 1) the development of drug-specific antibodies in susceptible persons, 2) tissue

accumulation of bradykinin, or 3) inactivation or inhibition of the action of C1 esterase inactivator.[792] Treatment includes withdrawal of the drug and maintenance of an adequate airway followed by administration of epinephrine, antihistamines, and corticosteroids if needed.[792–794]

Excessive hypotension and syncope may occur with the administration of an ACE inhibitor, especially in patients with an initial high peripheral vascular resistance (e.g., high-renin hypertensive states), volume contraction (e.g., concurrent [excessive] diuretic therapy), or impaired CO (e.g., New York Heart Association class III or class IV heart failure). The hypotension may be associated with progressive azotemia, hypercreatinemia, or oliguria. Therapy should be initiated cautiously in such patients, with use of low doses of a short-acting ACE inhibitor. Ideally, previous diuretic therapy should be discontinued 2 to 3 days before initiation of drug therapy. Hyperkalemia may occur; risk factors include renal insufficiency, diabetes mellitus, and concomitant use of drugs that impair renal $K^+$ homeostasis (e.g., $K^+$-sparing diuretics, nonsteroidal anti-inflammatory drugs). Potassium-containing salt substitutes and supplements should be avoided.

Several reports suggest an increased frequency of anaphylactoid reactions occurring in hemodialysis patients treated concomitantly with ACE inhibitors; these reactions have been observed in patients receiving hemodialysis with both high-flux (polyacrylonitrile) and conventional (cellulose acetate or cuprophane) dialyzer membranes and have occurred during first use or reuse of the dialyzers.[795–798] These reactions often occur within 2 to 3 minutes of the initiation of dialysis and range in severity from mild itching to life-threatening systemic reactions characterized by bronchospasm, hypotension, and cardiopulmonary collapse. The U.S. Food and Drug Administration has issued a warning, although the mechanism of the interaction between ACE inhibitors and membrane dialyzers has not been established and the frequency and scope of the problem are unknown.[799]

Controversy exists as to the presence or absence of specific sulfhydryl-related side effects.[788, 800] These include 1) the development of a rash (morbilliform or maculopapular), which may be accompanied by pruritus, eosinophilia, arthralgia, or fever; 2) dysgeusia; 3) neutropenia; and 4) the previously discussed proteinuria. The rash usually occurs within the first month of therapy and disappears within a few days of dose reduction or drug discontinuation. Decrease in taste acuity and alteration (metallic or salty) or loss of taste perception may result in significant weight loss. It is usually self-limited (2 to 3 months), even with continued drug therapy. The risk of neutropenia (<1000 neutrophils/mm³) and agranulocytosis appears to be related to the clinical status of the patient (e.g., impaired renal function, collagen vascular disease, concurrent immunosuppressive therapy) or the use of excessive doses. It is detected within 3 months of initiation of therapy and results from myeloid hypoplasia. Anemia and thrombocytopenia may also occur. In general, neutrophils return to normal within 2 weeks after discontinuation of therapy; however, some cases have ended fatally.

The U.S. Food and Drug Administration has issued a medical bulletin warning about possible fetal injury and

*References 552–560, 582, 584, 602, 604, 616, 748–759, 768–775.
†References 599, 600, 605, 608, 615, 620, 622, 626, 630, 774, 788.

death when ACE inhibitors are used during the second or third trimester of pregnancy.[801] ACE inhibitors are fetotoxins; ACE inhibitor fetopathy is characterized by fetal hypotension, anuria and oligohydramnios, growth restriction, pulmonary hypoplasia, renal tubule dysplasia, and hypocalvaria.[802] ACE inhibitors should not be used in pregnancy, particularly in the second and third trimesters.

## Tyrosine Hydroxylase Inhibitor

### CLASS MECHANISMS OF ACTION

Metyrosine (α-methyl-p-tyrosine) is an inhibitor of tyrosine hydroxylase, the enzyme that catalyzes the first transformation in catecholamine biosynthesis (i.e., the conversion of tyrosine to dihydroxyphenylalanine).[803–806] Because this first step is also the rate-limiting step, blockade of tyrosine hydroxylase activity results in decreased endogenous levels of circulating catecholamines. In patients with excessive production of norepinephrine and epinephrine, the administration of metyrosine reduces catecholamine biosynthesis from 36% to 79%; the net physiologic effect is a decrease in TPVR and increases in HR and CO (resulting from the vasodilation). The degree of vasodilation is dependent on the degree of blockade of adrenergic vascular tone.

### CLASS MEMBER

Metyrosine is the only drug in its class.[26, 803–806] The initial recommended dose is 1 g/d given in divided doses. This may be increased by 250 to 500 mg daily, to a maximum of 4 g/d. The usual effective dosage is 2 to 3 g/d. The maximal biochemical effect occurs within 2 to 3 days. In hypertensive patients who respond, blood pressure decreases progressively during the first 2 days of therapy. In patients who are usually normotensive, doses should be titrated to the amount that will reduce circulating or urinary catecholamines by 50% or more. After discontinuation of therapy, the clinical and biochemical effects may persist for 2 to 4 days. Metyrosine is variably absorbed from the gastrointestinal tract; bioavailability ranges from 45% to 90%. Peak plasma concentrations are reached in 1 to 3 hours. The plasma half-life is 3 to 4 hours. Metyrosine is not metabolized; the unchanged drug is recovered in the urine. The drug dosage should be reduced in patients with renal insufficiency (see Table 54–4).

### CLASS RENAL EFFECTS

Metyrosine would be expected to counteract the renal effects of excessive circulating levels of catecholamines. Thus, ERPF and GFR should increase and RVR should decrease in proportion to the degree of inhibition of excessive adrenergic vascular tone.

### CLASS EFFICACY AND SAFETY

Metyrosine is exclusively used in the management of preoperative or inoperative pheochromocytoma.[367, 804–808]

Most patients with pheochromocytoma treated with metyrosine experience decreased frequency and severity of hypertensive attacks with their associated headaches, nausea, sweating, and tachycardia. Hypotension and reflex tachycardia may result from the vasodilation and expanded blood volume capacity. Volume expansion is required during initiation and titration of therapy to minimize these effects.

Adverse reactions are primarily related to the central nervous system, possibly owing to dopamine depletion.[290, 804–806] The most common side effect is sedation, which is dose independent. The effect begins within the first 24 hours, is maximal after 2 to 3 days, and then diminishes. Temporary changes in sleep pattern (e.g., insomnia) may occur after withdrawal of the drug. Extrapyramidal signs (e.g., drooling, speech difficulty, and tremor) have been reported in 10% of patients treated with metyrosine; these symptoms may occasionally be accompanied by trismus and frank parkinsonism. Anxiety and psychic disturbances, such as depression, hallucinations, disorientation, and confusion, may also occur. Metyrosine crystalluria (as needles or rods) and urolithiasis (due to the poor solubility of the drug in the urine) have been observed in a few patients receiving doses in excess of 4 g/d.[290, 804–806] To minimize this risk, patients should be urged to maintain a fluid intake sufficient to achieve a daily urinary volume of 2 L or more. A severe watery diarrhea may occur in 10% of patients; this is probably caused by a direct irritant effect of the drug on bowel mucosa.[290, 804–806]

## New Classes of Antihypertensive Drugs

In addition to the previously discussed classes of antihypertensive drugs, newer classes are under development or ongoing clinical investigation. These new classes of drugs, which offer novel antihypertensive mechanisms of action, are listed in Table 54–13.[809–816] The efficacy and safety of these drugs remain to be determined.

## SELECTION OF A FIRST AND SUBSEQUENT ANTIHYPERTENSIVE DRUG THERAPY

### Selection of First-Step Therapy

In selecting a first-step therapy to treat a hypertensive disease, several criteria should be met: 1) the drug should decrease TPVR, the pathophysiologic hallmark of all hypertensive diseases; 2) the drug should not produce $Na^+$ retention with attendant pseudotolerance; 3) the drug should neither stimulate nor suppress the heart, and the drug should not compromise regional blood flow to target organs (e.g., heart, brain, kidney); 4) the drug should not stimulate the renin-angiotensin-aldosterone axis; 5) drug selection should reflect indications or contraindications for a patient's concomitant disease (e.g., arteriosclerotic cardiovascular disease, arteriosclerotic peripheral vascular disease, chronic obstructive pulmonary disease, diabetes mellitus, hypertensive cardiovascular disease, congestive heart failure, or hyperlipidemia); 6) drug dosing should be infrequent (once or

**TABLE 54–13. Investigational Antihypertensive Classes**

| Class | Reference | Prototype | Mechanism of Action | End-Organ Effects |
|---|---|---|---|---|
| Angiotensin II–receptor antagonist | 809, 810 | Losartan | Blockage of angiotensin II at the $AT_1$ receptor | Increases in renal blood flow; acute natriuresis, diuresis, and kaliuresis; uricosuria; antiproteinuric |
| Dopamine agonist | 811 | Fenoldopam | Agonist of peripheral postsynaptic dopamine ($DA_1$) receptor; weak $\alpha_2$-antagonist properties | Increase in renal blood flow and GFR, natriuresis, diuresis |
| Endopeptidase inhibitor | 812 | Candoxatril | Inhibition of mediators of atrial natriuretic peptide degradation | Natriuresis |
| $K^+$ channel opener | 813 | Pinacidil | Hyperpolarization of all vascular smooth muscle membranes with a net reduction in intracellular $Ca^{2+}$ | $Na^+$ retention, antiproteinuric |
| Renin inhibitor | 814, 815 | Enalkiren | Renin inhibition, suppression of angiotensin II | Increase in ERPF |
| Serotonin antagonist | 816 | Ketanserin | Blockage of 5-hydroxytryptamine receptor | No effect on GFR, renal blood flow or $Na^+$ excretion |

twice a day); 7) the drug side effect profile, including its effect on the quality of life (e.g., physical state, emotional well-being, sexual and social functions, and cognitive activity), should be favorable; and 8) drug costs (both direct and indirect) should be reasonable. On the basis of these criteria, antihypertensive drug classes potentially suitable for initial drug therapy are given in Table 54–14.

Given the drugs we have, and their pharmacologic profiles, what are the best drug classes for initial drug therapy? Listed alphabetically, they include 1) ACE inhibitors, 2) $\alpha_1$-adrenergic antagonists, 3) $\beta_1$-adrenergic antagonists, 4) $Ca^{2+}$ antagonists, and 5) thiazide-type diuretics.[162, 163] All of these drugs, given as monotherapeutic agents, are effective in lowering blood pressure in 50% to 60% of patients with mild to moderate hypertension. In general, black patients are more responsive to diuretics and $Ca^{2+}$ antagonists than to $\beta$-adrenergic antagonists or ACE inhibitors.[162] Older persons with hypertension are generally responsive to all of these classes of drugs.[162] Finally, selection of an antihypertensive drug that treats a coexisting disease may not only simplify the therapeutic regimen but also reduce cost.

Mild to moderate hypertension in the majority of patients can be controlled by one drug. However, if the response to the initial choice of therapy is inadequate after a 1- to 3-month interval, three options for subsequent antihypertensive drug therapy may be considered: 1) increase the dose of the initial drug if it is below the recommended maximum, 2) discontinue the initial choice and substitute a drug from another class, or 3) add a drug from another class.[162] If a second drug is required, the addition of a low-dose thiazide-type diuretic to a nondiuretic drug will usually enhance the effectiveness of the first drug. More severe cases of hypertension, unresponsive to this therapeutic strategy, may respond to 1) classic triple-drug therapy (i.e., diuretic, $\beta$-adrenergic antagonist, and direct-acting vasodilator)[146, 147, 415–417]; 2) combined use of an ACE inhibitor and a $Ca^{2+}$ antagonist[163, 506, 817–820]; or 3) combined use of a $\beta$-adrenergic antagonist with an $\alpha$-adrenergic antagonist or a dihydropyridine $Ca^{2+}$ antagonist.[163]

During follow-up visits, pharmacologic therapy should be reconfirmed or readjusted. As a rule, antihypertensive therapy should be maintained indefinitely.[163] Cessation of therapy in patients who were correctly diagnosed as hypertensive is usually (but not always) followed by a return of blood pressure to pretreatment levels. However, after blood pressure has been controlled for 1 year, and at least four visits, an attempt should be made to reduce antihypertensive drug therapy "in a deliberate, slow, and progressive manner."[162] Such "step-down therapy" may be successful in patients after lifestyle modifications: weight reduction; moderation of alcohol intake; regular aerobic physical activity; moderation of dietary sodium; and maintenance of adequate dietary intake of potassium, calcium, and magnesium. Patients whose drugs have been discontinued should have regular follow-up because blood pressure may rise again to hypertensive levels.

## Resistant Hypertension

Failure to achieve or sustain control of blood pressure with drug therapy is frequently the result of 1) the patient's failure to adhere to drug therapy, 2) the physician's failure to diagnose or treat a secondary cause of hypertension, 3) the physician's failure to recognize an adverse drug-drug interaction, or 4) the physician's failure to recognize the development of secondary drug resistance. The patient's failure to adhere to drug therapy is due to factors affecting both the patient and the physician[162, 163, 821, 822] (Table 54–15). The patient's adherence to drug therapy may be improved by 1) being aware of noncompliance, 2) educating and setting treatment goals, 3) prescribing a suitable low-cost drug regimen, 4) maintaining contact (i.e., follow-up of missed visits), and 5) fostering self-monitoring of blood pressure. Particularly at risk are men younger than 50 years, either black or white; of low educational attainment; unemployed or employed in blue-collar occupations with low incomes. Biologic and physiologic markers that can be used to monitor compliance with drug therapy are listed in Table 54–16.

**TABLE 54–14. Candidates for First-Step Therapy of Mild to Moderate Hypertension**

| Parameter | Angiotensin-Converting Enzyme Inhibitors | $\alpha_1$-Adrenergic Antagonists | $\alpha_1$- and $\beta$-Adrenergic Antagonists | $\beta$-Adrenergic Antagonists | $Ca^{2+}$ Antagonists | Central $\alpha_2$-Agonists | Central and Peripheral Blocking Agents | Thiazide-type Diuretics |
|---|---|---|---|---|---|---|---|---|
| Peripheral vascular resistance | Decrease | Decrease | Decrease | Decrease | Decrease | Decrease | Decrease | Decreases |
| Na$^+$ homeostasis | | | | | | | | |
| Urinary Na$^+$ excretion | Increase/no change | May decrease | May decrease | No change | Increase/no change | No change | No change | Increase |
| Extracellular fluid volume | No change | May decrease | May decrease | No change | No change | No change | No change | Decrease |
| Pseudotolerance | No | No | No | No | No | No | No | No |
| Target organ function | | | | | | | | |
| HR, CO | No change | No change | No change/decrease | Decrease | Class-specific | No change | No change | No change |
| Cerebral perfusion | Preserve | Preserve | Preserve | Preserve | Preserve | Preserve | Unknown | Preserve |
| GFR/renal blood flow | No change/increase | No change | No change | No change/decrease | No change/increase | No change | No change | No change |
| Renin-angiotensin-aldosterone | | | | | | | | |
| PRA | Increase | No change | No change | Decrease | No change | No change | No change | Increase |
| Plasma angiotensin II | Decrease | No change | No change | Decrease | No change | No change | No change | Increase |
| Plasma aldosterone | Decrease/no change | No change | No change | Decrease/no change | No change | No change | No change | Increase |
| Concurrent disease efficacy | | | | | | | | |
| Arteriosclerotic cardiovascular disease | No effect | No effect | No effect | Benefit | Benefit | No effect | No effect | No effect |
| Arteriosclerotic peripheral vascular disease | No effect | No effect | May aggravate | May aggravate | May benefit | No effect | No effect | No effect |
| Chronic obstructive pulmonary disease | No effect | No effect | May aggravate | May aggravate | No effect | No effect | No effect | No effect |
| Diabetes mellitus | May benefit | No effect | No effect | May aggravate | No effect | No effect | No effect | May aggravate |
| Hyperlipidemia | No effect | May benefit | No effect | May aggravate | No effect | No effect | No effect | Aggravate |
| Congestive heart failure (systolic dysfunction) | Benefit | No effect | May aggravate | May aggravate | No effect | No effect | May aggravate | Benefit |
| Hypertensive cardiovascular disease (diastolic dysfunction) | May benefit | May benefit | May benefit | Benefit | Benefit | May benefit | May benefit | May aggravate |
| Drug dosing: frequency | Once/twice daily | Once/twice daily | Twice daily | Once/twice daily | Once/twice daily | Once/twice daily | Once daily | Once daily |
| Side effect profile | Sulfhydryl and class-specific | $\alpha_1$-Adrenergic | $\alpha_1$- and $\beta$-adrenergic | $\beta$-Adrenergic | Class-specific | $\alpha_2$-Adrenergic | Central nervous system | Biochemical |
| Cost | High direct | Moderate direct | Moderate direct | Low direct | High direct | Moderate direct | Low direct | Low direct |

BAUER and REAMS • ANTIHYPERTENSIVE DRUGS

**TABLE 54–15. Factors Affecting Compliance with Drug Therapy**

**Factors Decreasing Patients' Compliance**
Asymptomatic "silent" health problem (remote risk of death or disability)
Provider-initiated, rather than patient-initiated, appointment
Noncomprehension of instructions
Requirement to change lifestyle (preventive behavior)
Psychologic state (e.g., phobias, hostility, depression)
Sociologic characteristics (e.g., lack of family support, unemployment)
Daily medications (control versus "cure"), for long duration
Costs of medical care (direct and indirect [e.g., time lost from work])
Costs of medication (direct and indirect [e.g., laboratory test])
Side effects of medications
Alcoholism

**Factors Decreasing Physicians' Adherence**
Failure to inform patients of their blood pressure level
Failure to set a goal blood pressure
Failure to provide simple oral or written instructions
Emphasis on diagnosis rather than on treatment
Prescription of a complicated, illogical, or expensive sequence of drugs
No teaching or education (brief encounter with the patient)
Failure to involve patients' families in the treatment process
Failure to modify dosages or to change drugs to avoid side effects
Failure to schedule or follow-up missed appointments
Discontinuing medication without early follow-up
Failure to encourage patients to self-monitor their blood pressure

Common secondary causes of hypertension that may be resistant to nondirected or trial-and-error drug therapy include 1) renal parenchymal hypertension, 2) renovascular hypertension, and 3) oral contraceptive "pill" hypertension. Rare secondary causes of hypertension, which can be expected to be resistant to standard drug therapy, include 1) mineralocorticoid excess states (e.g., primary aldosteronism), 2) pheochromocytoma, 3) glucocorticoid excess states (e.g., Cushing syndrome), 4) coarctation of the aorta, 5) hormonal disturbances (e.g., thyroid, parathyroid, growth hormone, serotonin), 6) neurologic syndromes (e.g., brain tumors, quadriplegia, Guillain-Barré syndrome, head injury, porphyria), and 7) sleep apnea. Secondary resistant hypertension may result from acute stress syndromes (e.g., "white coat hypertension," anxiety/panic reactions) and from responses to the ingestion of a wide variety of drugs (e.g., sympathomimetics, cyclosporine, tricyclic antidepressant), foods (e.g., high sodium intake), or illicit substances (e.g., cocaine, amphetamines, anabolic steroids). Pseudohypertension due to noncompliant vessels or a widened pulse pressure induced by aortic insufficiency or anemia may lead to inappropriate and poorly tolerated antihypertensive therapy. Failure to establish blood pressure control with standard therapy should raise suspicion that the underlying pathophysiologic process is not being treated.

The concurrent administration of two or more drugs may set the stage for an adverse drug-drug interaction.[162, 289, 823–827] Such may occur by 1) one drug's changing the activity of another by altering its metabolic fate (e.g., absorption, binding of inactive sites, biotransformation, excretion, or movement of site of action) and 2) one drug's directly influencing the other's intensity of action at its site of action (e.g., competition for receptor occupancy, effect on substance mediating the drug reaction, changes in tissue sensitivity, or additive or subtractive interactions). Because of the ever expanding number of drugs and the number of drug-drug interactions that alter blood pressure response, the physician should refer frequently to the current *Physicians' Desk Reference* for specific concerns, especially if the patient is receiving many drugs. Secondary drug resistance may also result from 1) fluid retention (see later), 2) cardiac stimulation, 3) hyperreninemia, and 4) reflex increase in TPVR.[827–830] These secondary responses can be negated by using combination therapy that incorporates a diuretic, a β-adrenergic antagonist, and a direct-acting vasodilator (i.e., classic triple-drug therapy).

Fluid retention, which attenuates the effectiveness of most antihypertensive drugs, may result from "diuretic resistance." The GFR limits the absolute amount of $Na^+$ filtered and hence the amount of tubule fluid that reaches the transport site sensitive to the diuretic. In the presence of renal parenchymal disease (i.e., reduced GFR), the more potent loop diuretics, acting on a higher percentage of the filtered load, effect a greater natriuresis compared with the benzothiadiazide diuretics. In the presence of renal parenchymal disease or a state of renal hypoperfusion, reduced renal blood flow may also limit the active transport of the diuretic into the proximal tubule fluid, thereby reducing its inhibitory effect at a more distal intraluminal membrane site. In these clinical settings, large doses of a diuretic with a steep dose-response curve (i.e., loop diuretics) may be required to achieve a therapeutic tubule drug concentration. In the presence of excessive aldosterone secretion, $Na^+$ blocked from resorption by a benzothiadiazide or loop diuretic may be recaptured at aldosterone's late distal tubule/collecting duct site of action. The efficacy of the diuretic, working at a more proximal site in the nephron, depends on simultaneous blocking of this recapturing mechanism (i.e., use of a $K^+$-sparing diuretic to maintain a urinary $Na^+$ to $K^+$ ratio $\geq 1$).

**TABLE 54–16. Markers of Compliance with Drug Therapy**

ACE inhibitors
  Biochemical: stimulation of PRA, inhibition of angiotensin II
β-Adrenergic antagonists
  Biochemical: inhibition of PRA
  Physiologic: blockage of postural or exercise-induced increase in HR
Central $\alpha_2$-adrenergic agonists
  Biochemical: inhibition of circulating catecholamines
  Physiologic: sedation, drowsiness, dry mouth
Direct-acting vasodilators
  Biochemical: stimulation of PRA
  Physiologic: reflex tachycardia, salt and water retention, hypertrichosis (minoxidil)
Diuretics
  Biochemical: hyperchloremic hypokalemic metabolic alkalosis
Peripheral adrenergic-neuronal blocking agents
  Physiologic: orthostatic hypotension

## How Far Should Blood Pressure Be Lowered?

The aim of antihypertensive therapy is risk reduction. Because the relationship between blood pressure and cardiovascular risk is continuous, the goal of treatment might be the maximal tolerated blood pressure reduction. However, there is controversy as to how far systolic and diastolic blood pressure should be lowered. The Fifth Report of the Joint National Committee on Detection, Evaluation, and Treatment of High Blood Pressure recommended that arterial blood pressure be maintained below 140 mm Hg systolic and 90 mm Hg diastolic; however, it stated, "how far diastolic blood pressure should be reduced below 85 mm Hg is unclear."[162] The 1993 World Health Organization/International Society of Hypertension guidelines suggested that it is desirable to achieve blood pressures of at least 120/80 to 130/80 mm Hg in young patients with mild hypertension and to lower blood pressure to below 140/90 mm Hg in elderly patients with elevations of both systolic and diastolic blood pressure.[163] In patients with isolated systolic hypertension, the Joint National Committee report stated that the initial goal of therapy is to reduce the systolic blood pressure to less than 160 mm Hg; the World Health Organization/International Society of Hypertension guidelines suggested that the goal of treatment should be to achieve a systolic pressure of at least 140 mm Hg, if tolerated. Neither group addresses the potential complication of diastolic hypotension. Regardless, each patient should be treated according to his or her cerebrovascular, cardiovascular, and renal risks; specific pathophysiologic process and target organ damage; and concurrent disease states. A uniform blood pressure goal (target) probably does not exist for all hypertensive patients, and lower is not always better.

## DRUG TREATMENT OF HYPERTENSIVE URGENCIES AND EMERGENCIES

### Hypertensive Urgencies and Emergencies

Hypertensive emergencies have traditionally been defined as clinical syndromes caused or complicated by hypertension, which may result in death or extensive damage to vital organs within hours to days unless prompt and effective treatment is initiated[831] (Table 54–17). This syndrome may be subdivided arbitrarily into two categories: 1) true emergencies, defined as conditions with acute or ongoing end-organ damage, in which a delay in therapeutic intervention may lead to irreversible sequelae; and 2) hypertensive urgencies, conditions with less immediate threat or an absence of end-organ damage that ultimately lead to serious complications if blood pressure is not vigorously controlled.[832–838] These syndromes represent a diverse group of disease states; however, they all are characterized hemodynamically by a marked increase in TPVR and a decrease in organ perfusion. Although most of these clinical syndromes are associated with diastolic blood pressures of 120 mm Hg or higher, the absolute level of blood pressure elevation is less important than the rate of rise and magnitude of change in blood pressure and the degree of end-organ damage.

**TABLE 54–17. Hypertensive Emergencies**

Hypertensive encephalopathy*
Acute aortic dissection*
Central nervous system bleed*
  Intracranial hemorrhage
  Thrombotic cerebrovascular accident
  Subarachnoid hemorrhage
Acute left ventricular failure refractory to conventional medical therapy*
Myocardial ischemia or infarction associated with persistent chest pain*
Accelerated or malignant hypertension†
Toxemia of pregnancy: eclampsia*
Renal failure/insufficiency†
Hypertension associated with hyperadrenergic states*
  Pheochromocytoma
  Interaction between monoamine oxidase inhibitors and tyramine-containing foods
  Interaction between an α-adrenergic agonist and a nonselective β-adrenergic antagonist
  After abrupt withdrawal of clonidine or guanabenz
  After severe body burns
  Neurogenic hypertension
Hypertension in the surgical patient†
  Associated with postoperative bleeding
  After open heart or vascular surgery
  Preceding emergency surgery
  After kidney transplantation
Hypertension in the diabetic patient with retinal hemorrhage*

*Considered by some authors to be a true hypertensive emergency.
†Considered by some authors to be a hypertensive urgency.

A growing number of antihypertensive drugs have been reported to be effective and safe for use in the treatment of hypertensive emergencies. The more commonly prescribed parenteral drugs include 1) the direct-acting vasodilators diazoxide, hydralazine, nitroprusside, and nitroglycerin; 2) the $\beta_1$-selective adrenergic antagonist esmolol; 3) the $\alpha_1$- and beta-adrenergic antagonist labetalol; 4) the central $\alpha_2$-adrenergic agonist methyldopa; 5) the ganglionic blocking agent trimethaphan; 6) the ACE inhibitor enalaprilat; and 7) the peripheral α-adrenergic blocker phentolamine.

### Parenteral Drugs

#### DIRECT-ACTING VASODILATORS

The benzothiadiazine diazoxide has been used primarily in the treatment of acute hypertensive emergencies.[25, 26, 162, 831–833, 835–844] Originally, it was recommended that diazoxide be administered as an intravenous bolus (150 to 300 mg). However, because of the potential harm from an abrupt and dramatic decrease in blood pressure, the "minibolus" (1 mg/kg administered at intervals of 5 to 15 minutes) and the continuous infusion of diazoxide have become the preferred methods of administration (Table 54–18). Diazoxide acts rapidly, and the blood pressure effect persists up to 12 hours. It has a plasma half-life of 17 to 31 hours; 20% is eliminated unchanged in the urine, and the remainder

**TABLE 54–18. Parenteral Drugs Used in the Treatment of Hypertensive Emergencies**

| Drug | Dosage (Maximal) | Onset of Action | Peak Effect | Duration of Action |
|------|------------------|-----------------|-------------|--------------------|
| *Direct-Acting Vasodilators* | | | | |
| Diazoxide | 7.5–30 mg/min infusion, or 1 mg/kg bolus q 5–15 min (300 mg) | 1–5 min | 30 min | 4–12 h |
| Hydralazine | 0.5–1.0 mg/min infusion, or 10–50 mg intramuscularly | 1–5 min 30 min | 10–80 min 30–80 min | 3–6 h |
| Nitroglycerine | 5–100 μg/min infusion | 1–2 min | 2–5 min | 3–5 min |
| Nitroprusside | 0.25–10 μg/kg/min infusion | Immediate | 1–2 min | 2–5 min |
| *β₁-Adrenergic Antagonist* | | | | |
| Esmolol | 500 μg/kg/min × 1 min (loading dose), then 25 μg/kg/min × 4 min (maintenance); maintenance dose may be increased to maximum of 300 μg/kg/min | 1–2 min | 5 min | 10–30 min |
| *α₁- and β-Adrenergic Antagonist* | | | | |
| Labetalol | 2 mg/min infusion or 0.25 mg/kg | 5 min | 10 min | 3–6 h |
| *Central α₂-Adrenergic Agonist* | | | | |
| Methyldopate hydrochloride | 250–500 mg bolus q 6 h (2 g) | 2–3 h | 3–5 h | 6–12 h |
| *Ganglionic Blockers* | | | | |
| Trimethaphan | 0.5–10 mg/min infusion bolus for 2 min (300 mg) | Immediate | 1–2 min | 5–10 min |
| *Angiotensin-Converting Enzyme Inhibitor* | | | | |
| Enalaprilat | 0.625–5.0 mg bolus for 5 min q 6 h | 5–15 min | 1–4 h | 6 h |
| *Peripheral α-Adrenergic Antagonist* | | | | |
| Phentolamine | 0.5–1.0 mg/min infusion, or 2.5–5.0 mg bolus | Immediate | 3–5 min | 10–15 min |

undergoes hepatic metabolism to inactive metabolites. In renal disease, the plasma half-life is prolonged; dose reduction is required.

Because diazoxide relaxes smooth muscle at peripheral arterioles, reduction in blood pressure is accompanied by increases in CO and HR and hyperreninemia. Concurrent administration of a β-adrenergic antagonist controls these reflex vasodilator responses. Transient hyperuricemia and hyperglycemia occur in the majority of patients; the blood glucose level should be monitored. Salt and water retention also occurs; concurrent diuretic administration is required. Diazoxide and its metabolites are removed by hemodialysis and peritoneal dialysis, but dialysance is relatively low because of its extensive protein binding.

The direct-acting vasodilator hydralazine may be given intramuscularly or as a rapid intravenous bolus injection* (see Table 54–18). It acts rapidly, and the blood pressure effect persists up to 6 hours. It is less potent than diazoxide, and the blood pressure response is unpredictable. The hemodynamic and adverse side effects of hydralazine have been previously discussed.

Sodium nitroprusside is the most potent of the parenteral vasodilators.† Nitroprusside acts on the excitation-contraction coupling of vascular smooth muscle by interfering with the intracellular activation of $Ca^{2+}$. Unlike diazoxide and hydralazine, nitroprusside dilates both arteriolar resistance and venous capacitance vessels. It has the advantages of being immediately effective when given as an infusion and

of having an extremely short duration of action, which permits minute to minute adjustments in blood pressure control (see Table 54–18). Disadvantages of nitroprusside therapy include 1) the need for intra-arterial blood pressure monitoring, 2) the need for the drug to be prepared fresh every 4 hours, 3) the need to protect the solution from light during infusion, and 4) the potential for toxic effect from metabolic side products. Nitroprusside is not excreted intact. It is rapidly metabolized to cyanide and thiocyanate through a reaction with hemoglobin, which yields methemoglobin and an unstable intermediate that dissociates to release cyanide. The major elimination pathway of cyanide is by conversion in the liver and kidney to thiocyanate. Back-conversion of thiocyanate to cyanide may occur. Thiocyanate is largely excreted in the urine; it has a plasma half-life of 1 week in normal subjects and accumulates in renal insufficiency.

Toxic concentrations of cyanide or thiocyanate may occur if nitroprusside infusions are given for more than 48 hours or at infusion rates greater than 2 μg/kg/min; the maximal dose rate of 10 μg/kg/min should not last more than 10 minutes. Toxic manifestations include air hunger, hyperreflexia, confusion, and seizures. Lactic acidosis and venous hyperoxemia are laboratory indicators of cyanide intoxication. Furthermore, failure to respond to nitroprusside, or the appearance of "drug tolerance," may reflect an increase in the concentration of free cyanide; the drug should be promptly discontinued. Nitroprusside is hemodialyzable.

Injection of nitroglycerin produces, in a dose-related manner, dilation of both arterial and venous beds.[25, 26, 837] At

*References 25, 26, 162, 396, 831–833, 837, 838, 845.
†References 25, 26, 162, 831–833, 837, 838, 846–850.

lower dosages, its primary effect is on preload; at higher infusion rates, afterload is reduced. Nitroglycerin may also dilate both epicardial coronary vessels with stenosis and their collaterals, increasing blood supply to ischemic regions. Myocardial oxygen consumption or demand is decreased. Effective coronary perfusion is maintained, provided that blood pressure does not fall excessively or HR does not increase significantly (decreasing diastolic filling). Nitroglycerin has an immediate onset of action but is rapidly metabolized to dinitrates and mononitrates (see Table 54–18). Because nitroglycerin is absorbed by many plastics, dilution should be made only in glass parenteral solution bottles. Nitroglycerin is also absorbed by polyvinyl chloride tubing; non–polyvinyl chloride intravenous administration sets should be used.

Patients with normal or low left ventricular filling pressure or pulmonary wedge pressure may be hypersensitive to the effects of nitroglycerin; continuous monitoring of blood pressure, HR, and pulmonary capillary wedge pressure must be performed to assess the correct dose. Intravenous nitroglycerin may be the drug of choice in the treatment of the patient with moderate hypertension associated with coronary ischemia because it provides collateral coronary vasodilation, a property not seen with the other direct-acting arteriolar vasodilators. The principal side effects are headache, nausea, and vomiting. Tolerance may develop with prolonged use.

## β₁-SELECTIVE ADRENERGIC ANTAGONIST

Esmolol hydrochloride is a short-acting β₁-selective adrenergic antagonist.[25, 26, 851, 852] It does not exhibit appreciable PAA or MSA. Esmolol hydrochloride concentrate for injection must be diluted to a final concentration of 10 mg/mL; esmolol hydrochloride for injection (10 mg/mL) needs no dilution and may be used as an intravenous loading dose. Extravasation of esmolol hydrochloride may cause serious local irritation and skin necrosis. Esmolol shares all of the toxic potentials of the β₁-adrenergic antagonists previously discussed. After intravenous injection of a 500 µg/kg loading dose and then infusion of a maintenance dose ranging from 25 to 300 µg/kg/min, steady-state blood concentrations are achieved within 5 minutes (see Table 54–18). Efficacy should be assessed after the 1-minute loading dose and 4 minutes of maintenance infusion; if an adequate therapeutic effect is observed (as assessed by blood pressure and heart rate response), the maintenance infusion should be maintained. If an adequate therapeutic effect is not observed, the same loading dose is repeated for 1 minute followed by an increased maintenance rate of infusion.

Esmolol has pharmacologic actions similar to those of other β₁-selective adrenergic antagonists; it produces negative chronotropic and inotropic activity. It has been used to prevent or treat hemodynamic changes induced by surgical events, including increases in systolic and diastolic blood pressure and double product (HR × systolic blood pressure). Because of this, esmolol may be particularly useful for the treatment of postoperative hypertension and hypertension associated with coronary insufficiency. Esmolol is

hydrolyzed rapidly in blood; negligible concentrations are present 30 minutes after discontinuance. Because the de-esterified metabolite of esmolol is eliminated mainly by the kidneys, the drug should be used cautiously in patients with renal insufficiency.

## α₁- AND β-ADRENERGIC ANTAGONIST

The α₁- and β-adrenergic antagonist labetalol hydrochloride may be given by either repeated intravenous injection or slow continuous infusion[25, 26, 66, 67, 833, 837, 838, 853–856] (see Table 54–18). The maximal blood pressure–lowering effect is within 5 minutes of the first injection. The drug should be administered to patients in the supine position to avoid symptomatic postural hypotension. The adverse side effects of labetalol have been previously discussed.

## CENTRAL α₂-ADRENERGIC AGONIST

Methyldopate hydrochloride is a central α₂-adrenergic agonist that may be administered intravenously as a bolus infusion[25, 26, 162, 831–833, 837, 838] (see Table 54–18). It has a delayed onset of action and peak effect; its effect on blood pressure is unpredictable. The adverse side effects of methyldopa have been previously discussed.

## GANGLIONIC BLOCKING AGENT

Trimethaphan camsylate is a ganglionic blocking agent; it blocks transmission of impulses at both sympathetic and parasympathetic ganglia by occupying receptor sites and by stabilizing the postsynaptic membranes against the action of acetylcholine liberated from presynaptic nerve endings.[25, 26, 831–833, 837, 838, 857] TPVR is decreased; HR is usually increased and CO decreased because of venous dilation and peripheral pooling of blood. Trimethaphan is used exclusively for the treatment of hypertensive emergencies, especially for the initial control of blood pressure in patients with acute dissecting aortic aneurysm. It has a rapid onset of action when administered as a continuous infusion (see Table 54–18). The resulting dramatic reduction in blood pressure requires intra-arterial monitoring. The drug must be administered with the patient supine to avoid profound postural hypotension. Other disadvantages include 1) the potential for tachyphylaxis after sustained infusion (~48 hours), 2) the appearance of side effects associated with parasympathetic and sympathetic blockade, and 3) histamine release.

## ANGIOTENSIN-CONVERTING ENZYME INHIBITOR

Enalaprilat, the active metabolite of the oral ACE inhibitor enalapril, is administered as a slow intravenous infusion for 5 minutes[25, 26, 858–861] (see Table 54–18). The intravenous dose is approximately one fourth of an oral dose of enalapril. In patients with renal insufficiency, the initial dose should be no more than 0.625 mg. Onset of action occurs within 15 minutes; the maximal effect is within 1 to 4

**TABLE 54–19. Rapid-Acting Oral Drugs Used in the Treatment of Hypertensive Emergencies**

| Drug | Dosage (Maximal) | Onset of Action | Peak Effect (h) | Duration of Action (h) |
|---|---|---|---|---|
| **$\alpha_1$- and $\beta$-Antagonist** | | | | |
| Labetalol | 100–400 mg q 12 h (2400 mg) <br> 1 mg/kg bolus q 5–15 min (300 mg) | 1–2 h | 2–4 | 8–12 |
| **Central $\alpha_2$-Adrenergic Agonist** | | | | |
| Clonidine | 0.2 mg initially, then 0.1 mg/h (0.8 mg) | 30–60 min | 2–4 | 6–8 |
| **$Ca^{2+}$ Antagonists** | | | | |
| Diltiazem | 30–120 mg q 8 h (480 mg) | <15 min | 2–3 | 8 |
| Nicardipine | 20–40 mg q 8 h (120 mg) | <30 min | 1–2 | 8 |
| Nifedipine | 5*–40 mg q 8 h (120 mg) | <15 min | 0.5–1 | 4–6 |
| Verapamil | 80–120 mg q 8 h (480 mg) | <60 min | 2–3 | 8 |
| **Angiotensin-Converting Enzyme Inhibitors** | | | | |
| Captopril | 12.5–25 mg q 4 h (150 mg) | <15 min | 1 | 6–12 |
| Enalapril | 2.5–10 mg q 6 h (40 mg) | <60 min | 4–8 | 12–24 |
| **Postsynaptic $\alpha_1$-Adrenergic Antagonist** | | | | |
| Prazosin | 1–5 mg q 2 h (20 mg) | <60 min | 2–4 | 6–12 |
| **Combination Therapies** | | | | |
| Triple drug (diuretic, $\beta$-adrenergic antagonist, and vasodilator [minoxidil or hydralazine]) | | | | |
| $Ca^{2+}$ antagonist plus angiotensin-converting enzyme inhibitor | | | | |

*Half the contents (0.17 mL) of a 10-mg capsule.

hours. The duration of action is about 6 hours. Adverse effects of enalaprilat have been previously discussed.

## PERIPHERAL α-ADRENERGIC ANTAGONIST

Phentolamine mesylate is a nonselective α-adrenergic antagonist primarily used in the treatment of hypertension associated with pheochromocytoma.[25, 26, 364, 365, 831, 837] It has a rapid onset of action when administered intravenously as either a bolus or a continuous infusion (see Table 54–18). The duration of action is 10 to 15 minutes. It has a plasma half-life of 19 minutes; approximately 13% of a single dose appears in the urine as unchanged drug. Adverse effects include those associated with nonselective α-adrenergic blockade, as previously discussed.

## Rapid-Acting Oral Drugs

A more gradual, progressive reduction in systemic blood pressure may be achieved after the oral administration of drugs having rapid absorption.[837, 838, 862–864] These include 1) the α₁- and β-adrenergic antagonist labetalol[865, 866]; 2) the central α₂-adrenergic agonist clonidine[867–870]; 3) the Ca²⁺ antagonists diltiazem, nicardipine, nifedipine, and verapamil[871–874]; 4) the ACE inhibitors captopril and enalapril[769, 875]; 5) the postsynaptic α₁-adrenergic antagonist prazosin[876]; and 6) combination oral therapies, such as triple-drug therapy (diuretic, β-blocker, and direct-acting vasodilator)[146, 147, 415, 416] or the combined use of an ACE inhibitor and a Ca²⁺ antag-

onist.[816–820] The doses and pharmacodynamic effects of rapid-acting oral drugs used commonly in the treatment of hypertensive emergencies are given in Table 54–19.

## Considerations in the Acute Reduction of Blood Pressure

Any drug regimen used for the acute reduction of blood pressure carries the risk of lowering cerebral blood flow below the lower limit of autoregulation, inducing cerebral or retinal ischemia or infarction. In chronic hypertension, the normal cerebral autoregulation curve is shifted to the right.[877] Although long-term treatment may shift the autoregulatory curve toward normal,[878] the short-term lowering of MAP below the lower limit (~100 mm Hg) may decrease cerebral blood flow,[879, 880] precipitating cerebral ischemia and infarction[864] (Table 54–20). In general, vasoactive drugs have less effect on the cerebral circulation than on other vascular beds, in part because of the protective effect of the blood-brain barrier.[880] However, drugs that do penetrate the blood-brain barrier and dilate the cerebral vessels (e.g., hydralazine, sodium nitroprusside, nifedipine) may lead to uneven cerebral perfusion owing to an intracranial "steal" effect, especially if the sympathetic nervous system is intact.[880–883] Patients (especially the elderly) with atheromatous disease in intracranial or extracranial vessels may be particularly at risk for complications due to reductions in cerebral blood flow to compromised areas (i.e., border zones of arterial supply).[882, 883] Drugs that dilate cerebral vessels and increase cerebral blood flow may also cause an immediate rise in intracranial pressure, creating

**TABLE 54–20. Adverse Reactions Reported with Parenteral or Rapid Oral Therapy Used to Reduce Blood Pressure in Patients with Hypertensive Emergencies**

**Direct-Acting Vasodilators**
Diazoxide
  Myocardial ischemia, infarction
  Fatal hypotension
  Cerebral ischemia
  Retinal ischemia, blindness
  Oliguria, anuria
Hydralazine
  Fatal hypotension
  Cerebral ischemia, infarction
  Retinal ischemia, blindness
  Oliguria, anuria
Nitroglycerin
  Hypotension
  Paradoxical bradycardia
  Paradoxical increased angina
Nitroprusside
  Cardiac arrest
  Fatal hypotension
  Cyanide toxicity

**Ganglionic Blocker**
Trimethaphan
  Postural hypotension
  Constipation
  Urinary retention
  Acute renal failure

**$\beta_1$-Adrenergic Antagonist**
Esmolol
  Hypotension
  Congestive heart failure
  Bronchospasm

**$\alpha_1$- and $\beta$-Adrenergic Antagonist**
Labetalol
  Postural hypotension
  Bronchospasm
  Congestive heart failure
  Hepatic necrosis
  Paradoxical pressor response

**Angiotensin-Converting Enzyme Inhibitor**
Enalaprilat
  Hypotension
  Renal insufficiency

**Nonselective $\alpha$-Adrenergic Antagonist**
Phentolamine
  Hypotension
  Tachycardia
  Cardiac arrhythmias

**Calcium Antagonists**
Diltiazem
  Atrioventricular junctional arrhythmia, bradycardia
  Hypotension
  Second-degree atrioventricular heart block
  Premature ventricular contractions
Nifedipine
  Myocardial ischemia
  Postural hypotension
  Premature ventricular contractions
  Cerebral ischemia, infarction
  Retinal ischemia
Verapamil
  Second- or third-degree atrioventricular heart block
  Premature ventricular contractions
  Hypotension

the potential for cerebral herniation or diminished cerebral perfusion.[880, 882, 883]

A precipitous drop in blood pressure can similarly produce a dramatic decrease in cardiac or renal perfusion[864] (see Table 54–20). The decrease in cardiac perfusion may be clinically manifested by the onset or aggravation of angina pectoris, myocardial infarction, arrhythmia, congestive heart failure, or hypotension. The decrease in renal perfusion may be clinically manifested by the development of acute renal failure. Although the $Ca^{2+}$ antagonists are coronary vasodilators, the presence of a steal effect from a segment of fixed, obstructed coronary artery may explain the reported occurrence of paradoxical worsening angina pectoris after their administration.[884, 885]

There are few true hypertensive emergencies requiring immediate reduction of blood pressure. In such instances, nitroprusside and trimethaphan have been the therapeutic standards. The oral administration of nifedipine (5-mg dosage) may be a suitable alternative therapy. Because the

elevation of cytosolic free $Ca^{2+}$ may be the final common pathway in cell death after ischemia,[886] some $Ca^{2+}$ antagonists, by inhibiting $Ca^{2+}$ entry into cells, may theoretically exert a protective effect on the brain, heart and kidneys independent of any cerebral, coronary, or renal vasodilation. However, clinical trials testing this hypothesis are lacking.

For most of the hypertensive emergencies, the initiation of a parenteral or rapid-acting oral drug program, selected to counteract the suspected abnormal hemodynamic or humoral disease state, will prove to be both effective and safe. Patients suspected of having high-renin hypertensive states (e.g., accelerated or malignant hypertension, acute left ventricular failure) might be expected to respond favorably to an ACE inhibitor. Patients suspected of having an excess catecholamine state (e.g., one of the hyperadrenergic syndromes) might be expected to respond favorably to a peripheral $\alpha$-adrenergic antagonist. Patients with acute myocardial ischemia or infarction, unresponsive to nitroglycerin or esmolol, may best be treated with a $Ca^{2+}$ antagonist. Patients with acute aortic dissection are probably best treated with an $\alpha_1$- and $\beta$-adrenergic antagonist (labetalol) or a ganglionic blocker (trimethaphan). In patients with a central nervous system hemorrhage, there may be a theoretic advantage to the use of a $Ca^{2+}$ antagonist. However, regardless of the clinical syndrome or drug selection, the patient must be carefully observed for potential symptoms or signs of cerebral, retinal, coronary, or renal ischemia. Furthermore, the controlled reduction of blood pressure to a safe limit is mandatory.

## REFERENCES

1. Black JW, Duncan WAM, Shanks RG: Comparison of some properties of pronethalol and propranolol. J Pharmacol 25:577–591, 1965.
2. Paterson JW, Conolly ME, Dollery CT: The pharmacodynamics and metabolism of propranolol in man. Pharmacol Clin 2:127–133, 1970.
3. Lands AM, Arnold A, McAuliff JP, et al: Differentiation of receptor systems activated by sympathomimetic amines. Nature 214:597–598, 1967.
4. Lands AM, Luduena FP, Buzzo HJ: Differentiation of receptors responsive to isoproterenol. Life Sci 6:2241–2249, 1967.
5. Carlsson E: On the classification and distribution of $\beta$-adrenoceptors. Acta Pharmacol Toxicol 44(suppl II):17–20, 1979.
6. Minneman KP, Hegstrand LR, Molinoff PB: Classification and quantitation of $\beta$-adrenergic receptor subtypes. Biochem Pharmacol 29:1317–1323, 1980.
7. Vincent HH, Man in't Veld AJ, Boomsma F, et al: Is $\beta_1$-antagonism essential for the antihypertensive action of $\beta$-blockers? Hypertension 9:198–203, 1987.
8. Buhler FR, Laragh JH, Baer L, et al: Propranolol inhibition of renin secretion. N Engl J Med 287:1209–1214, 1972.
9. Keeton TK, Campbell WB: The pharmacologic alteration of renin release. Pharmacol Rev 31:81–227, 1981.
10. Stjarne L, Brundin J: $\beta_2$-Adrenoceptors facilitating noradrenaline secretion from human vasoconstrictor nerves. Acta Physiol Scand 97:88–93, 1976.
11. Weinstock M: The presynaptic effect of $\beta$-adrenoceptor antagonists on noradrenergic neurons. Life Sci 19:1453–1466, 1976.
12. Jackson EK, Campbell WB: Inhibition of angiotensin II potentiation of sympathetic nerve activity by beta-adrenergic antagonist. Hypertension 2:90–96, 1980.
13. Day MD, Roach AG: Central alpha- and beta-adrenoceptors modifying arterial blood pressure and heart rate in conscious rats. Br J Pharmacol 51:325–333, 1974.

14. Garvey HL, Ram N: Centrally induced hypotensive effects of β-adrenergic blocking agents. Eur J Pharmacol 33:283–294, 1975.

15. Hollifield JW, Sherman K, Zwagg RV, Shand DG: Proposed mechanisms of propranolol's antihypertensive effect in essential hypertension. N Engl J Med 295:68–73, 1976.

16. Ulrych M, Frohlich ED, Dustan HP, Page IH: Immediate hemodynamic effects of beta-adrenergic blockade with propranolol in normotensive and hypertensive man. Circulation 37:411–416, 1968.

17. Tarazi RC, Dustan HP: Beta-adrenergic blockade in hypertension. Am J Cardiol 29:633–640, 1972.

18. Hansson L, Zweifler AJ, Julius S, Hunyor SN: Hemodynamic effects of acute and prolonged β-adrenergic blockade in essential hypertension. Acta Med Scand 196:27–34, 1974.

19. Man in't Veld AJ, Schalekamp MADH: How intrinsic sympathomimetic activity modulates the hemodynamic responses to β-adrenoceptor antagonist. A clue to the nature of their antihypertensive mechanism. Br J Clin Pharmacol 13:245s–257s, 1982.

20. Man in't Veld AJ, van den Meiracker AH, Schalekamp MADH: Do beta-blockers really increase peripheral vascular resistance? Am J Hypertens 1:91–96, 1988.

21. Man in't Veld AJ: Vasodilation, not cardiodepression, underlies the antihypertensive effects of β-adrenoceptor antagonists. Am J Cardiol 67:13B–17B, 1991.

22. Fitzgerald JD: The applied pharmacology of β-adrenoceptor antagonists (beta-blockers) in relation to clinical outcomes. Cardiovasc Drugs Ther 5:561–576, 1991.

23. Fitzgerald JD: Do partial agonist beta-blockers have improved clinical utility? Cardiovasc Drugs Ther 7:303–310, 1993.

24. Frishman W: Clinical pharmacology of the new β-adrenergic blocking drugs. Part I. Pharmacodynamic and pharmacokinetic properties. Am Heart J 97:663–670, 1979.

25. Cardiac drugs 24:04 and hypotensive agents 24:08. *In* McEvoy GK (ed): American Hospital Formulary Service Drug Information 93. American Society of Hospital Pharmacists, Bethesda, MD, 1993, pp 885–1011, 1041–1093.

26. Physicians' Desk Reference, 47th ed. Medical Economics Data, Montvale, NJ, 1993.

27. Herrara J, Vukovich RA, Griffith DL: Elimination of nadolol by patients with renal impairment. Br J Clin Pharmacol 7(suppl 2):227s–231s, 1979.

28. Dreyfuss J, Griffith DL, Singhvi SM, et al: Pharmacokinetics of nadolol, a beta-receptor antagonist. J Clin Pharmacol 19:712–720, 1979.

29. Heel RC, Brogden RN, Pakes GE, et al: Nadolol: A review of its pharmacological properties and therapeutic efficacy in hypertension and angina pectoris. Drugs 20:1–23, 1980.

30. Frishman WH: Nadolol: A new β-adrenoceptor antagonist. N Engl J Med 305:678–682, 1981.

31. Nies AS, Shand DG: Clinical pharmacology of propranolol. Circulation 52:6–15, 1975.

32. Holland OB, Kaplan NM: Propranolol in the treatment of hypertension. N Engl J Med 294:930–936, 1976.

33. McAinsh J, Baber NS, Smith R, Young J: Pharmacokinetic and pharmacodynamic studies with long-acting propranolol. Br J Clin Pharmacol 6:115–121, 1978.

34. Leahey WJ, Neill JD, Varma MPS, Shanks RG: Comparison of the efficacy and pharmacokinetics of conventional propranolol and long-acting preparation of propranolol. Br J Clin Pharmacol 9:33–40, 1980.

35. Wood AJJ, Vestal RE, Spannuth CL, et al: Propranolol disposition in renal failure. Br J Clin Pharmacol 10:561–566, 1980.

36. Fagan TC, Walle T, Corns-Hurwitz R, et al: Time course of development of the antihypertensive effect of propranolol. Hypertension 5:852–857, 1983.

37. Tocco DJ, Duncan AEW, DeLuna FA, et al: Physiological disposition and metabolism of timolol in man and laboratory animals. Drug Metab Dispos 3:361–370, 1975.

38. Else OF, Sorenson H, Edwards IR: Plasma timolol levels after oral and intravenous administration. Eur J Clin Pharmacol 14:431–434, 1978.

39. Lowenthal DT, Pitone JM, Affrime MD, et al: Timolol kinetics in chronic renal insufficiency. Clin Pharmacol Ther 23:606–615, 1978.

40. Frishman WH: Atenolol and timolol, two new systemic β-adrenoceptor antagonists. N Engl J Med 306:1456–1462, 1982.

41. Frishman WH, Covey S: Penbutolol and carteolol: Two new beta-adrenergic blockers with partial agonism. J Clin Pharmacol 30:412–421, 1990.

42. Amemiya A, Tabei K, Furuya H, et al: Pharmacokinetics of carteolol in patients with impaired renal function. Eur J Clin Pharmacol 43:417–421, 1992.

43. Ohnhaus EE, Heidemann H, Meier J, Maurer G: Metabolism of pindolol in patients with renal failure. Eur J Clin Pharmacol 22:423–428, 1982.

44. Aellig WH: Clinical pharmacology of pindolol. Am Heart J 104:346–356, 1982.

45. Schwarz HJ: Pharmacokinetics of pindolol in humans and several animal species. Am Heart J 104:357–364, 1982.

46. Meier J: Pharmacokinetic comparison of pindolol with other beta-adrenoceptor–blocking agents. Am Heart J 104:364–373, 1982.

47. Frishman WH: Pindolol: A new β-adrenoceptor antagonist with partial agonist activity. N Engl J Med 308:940–944, 1983.

48. Heel RC, Brogden RN, Speight TM, Avery GS: Atenolol: A review of its pharmacological properties and therapeutic efficacy in hypertension. Drugs 17:425–460, 1979.

49. McAinsh J, Holmes BF, Smith S, et al: Atenolol kinetics in renal failure. Clin Pharmacol Ther 28:302–309, 1980.

50. Kirch W, Kohler H, Mutschler E, Schafer M: Pharmacokinetics of atenolol in relation to renal function. Eur J Clin Pharmacol 19:65–71, 1981.

51. Ishizaki T, Oyama Y, Suganuma T, et al: A dose ranging study of atenolol in hypertension: Fall in blood pressure and plasma renin activity, beta-blockade and steady-state pharmacokinetics. Br J Clin Pharmacol 16:17–25, 1983.

52. Wadworth AN, Murdoch D, Brogden RN: Atenolol. A reappraisal of its pharmacological properties and therapeutic use in cardiovascular disorders. Drugs 42:468–510, 1991.

53. Brogden RN, Heel RC, Speight TM, Avery GS: Metoprolol: A review of its pharmacological properties and therapeutic efficacy in hypertension and angina pectoris. Drugs 14:321–348, 1979.

54. Koch-Weser J: Metoprolol. N Engl J Med 301:698–703, 1979.

55. Sandberg A, Abrahamsson B, Regardh C-G, et al: Pharmacokinetic and biopharmaceutic aspects of once daily treatment with metoprolol CR/ZOK: A review article. J Clin Pharmacol 30:S2–S10, 1990.

56. Lucker P, Moore G, Wieselgren I, et al: Pharmacokinetic and pharmacodynamic comparison of metoprolol CR/ZOK once daily with conventional tablets once daily and in divided doses. J Clin Pharmacol 30:S17–S27, 1990.

57. Plosker GL, Clissold SP: Controlled release metoprolol formulations. Drugs 43:382–414, 1992.

58. Beresford R, Heel RC: Betaxolol. A review of its pharmacodynamic and pharmacokinetic properties, and therapeutic efficacy in hypertension. Drugs 31:6–28, 1986.

59. Frishman WH, Tepper D, Lazar EJ, Behrman D: Betaxolol: A new long-acting beta₁-selective adrenergic blocker. J Clin Pharmacol 30:686–692, 1990.

60. Leopold G, Pabst J, Ungethüm W, Bühring KU: Basic pharmacokinetics of bisoprolol, a new highly beta₁-selective adrenoceptor antagonist. J Clin Pharmacol 26:616–621, 1986.

61. Lancaster SG, Sorkin EM: Bisoprolol: A preliminary review of its pharmacodynamic and pharmacokinetic properties, and therapeutic efficacy in hypertension and angina pectoris. Drugs 36:256–285, 1988.

62. Kirch W, Kohler H, Berggren G, Baun W: The influence of renal function on plasma levels and urinary excretion of acebutolol and its main *N*-acetyl metabolite. Clin Nephrol 18:88–94, 1982.

63. Smith RS, Warren DJ, Renwick AG, George CR: Acebutolol pharmacokinetics in renal failure. Br J Clin Pharmacol 16:253–258, 1983.

64. Ryan JR: Clinical pharmacology of acebutolol. Am Heart J 109:1131–1136, 1985.

65. Giacomini JC, Thoden WR: Ancillary pharmacologic properties of acebutolol: Cardioselectivity, partial agonist activity, and membrane-stabilizing activity. Am Heart J 109:1137–1144, 1985.

66. Wallin JD, O'Neill WM: Labetalol: Current research and therapeutic status. Arch Intern Med 143:485–490, 1983.

67. MacCarthy EP, Bloomfield SS: Labetalol: A review of its pharmacology, pharmacokinetics, clinical uses and adverse effects. Pharmacotherapy 3:193–219, 1983.

68. McNeil JJ, Louis WJ: Clinical pharmacokinetics of labetalol. Clin Pharmacokinet 9:157–167, 1984.

69. van Zwieten PA: An overview of the pharmacodynamic properties and therapeutic potential of combined alpha- and beta-adrenoceptor antagonists. Drugs 45:509–517, 1993.

70. Waal-Manning HJ, Hobson CH: Renal function in patients with essential hypertension receiving nadolol. Br Med J 281:423–424, 1980.

71. Britton KE, Gruenewald SM, Nimmon CC: Nadolol and renal haemodynamics. R Soc Med Int Congr Symp Ser 37:77–85, 1981.

72. Danesh BJZ, Brunton J: Nadolol and renal haemodynamics. R Soc Med Int Congr Symp Ser 37:87–95, 1981.

73. O'Connor DT, Barg AP, Duchin KL: Preserved renal perfusion during treatment of essential hypertension with the beta blocker nadolol. J Clin Pharmacol 22:187–195, 1982.

74. Textor SC, Fouad FM, Bravo EL, et al: Redistribution of cardiac output to the kidneys during oral nadolol administration. N Engl J Med 307:601–605, 1982.

75. O'Callaghan WG, Laher MS, McGarry K, et al: Antihypertensive and renal haemodynamic effects of atenolol and nadolol in elderly hypertensive patients. Br J Clin Pharmacol 16:417–421, 1983.

76. O'Malley K, O'Callaghan WG, Laher MS, et al: β-Adrenoceptor blocking drugs and renal blood flow with special reference to the elderly. Drugs 25(suppl 2):103–107, 1983.

77. Brater DC, Anderson S, Kaplan NM, Ram CVS: Beta-adrenergic blockage alone does not decrease renal perfusion in black hypertensives. J Hypertens 2:43–48, 1984.

78. Danesh BJZ, Brunton J, Sumner DJ: Comparison between short-term renal haemodynamic effects of propranolol and nadolol in essential hypertension: A cross-over study. Clin Sci 67:243–248, 1984.

79. Frohlich ED, Messerli FH, Deslinski GR, Kobrin I: Long-term renal hemodynamic effects of nadolol in patients with essential hypertension. Am Heart J 108:1141–1143, 1984.

80. Dupont AG, Vanderniepen P, Bossuyt AM, et al: Nadolol in essential hypertension: Effect on ambulatory blood pressure, renal haemodynamics and cardiac function. Br J Clin Pharmacol 20:93–99, 1985.

81. Bauer JH, Reams GP, Lau A: A comparison of betaxolol and nadolol on renal function in essential hypertension. Am J Kidney Dis 10:109–112, 1987.

82. Ibsen H, Sederberg-Olsen P: Changes in glomerular filtration rate during long-term treatment with propranolol in patients with arterial hypertension. Clin Sci 44:129–134, 1973.

83. Drayer JLM, Kloppenberg PWC, Festen J, et al: Intra-patient comparison of treatment with chlorthalidone, spironolactone and propranolol in normoreninemic essential hypertension. Am J Cardiol 36:716–721, 1975.

84. Pedersen EB: Effect of sodium loading and exercise on renal haemodynamics and urinary sodium excretion in young patients with essential hypertension before and during propranolol treatment. Acta Med Scand 201:365–373, 1977.

85. Falch DK, Odegaard AE, Norman N: Renal plasma flow and cardiac output during hydralazine and propranolol treatment in essential hypertension. Scand J Clin Invest 38:143–146, 1978.

86. Falch DK, Odegaard AE, Norman N: Decreased renal plasma flow during propranolol treatment in essential hypertension. Acta Med Scand 205:91–95, 1979.

87. O'Connor DT, Preston RA, Sasso EH: Renal perfusion changes during treatment of essential hypertension: Prazosin vs propranolol. J Cardiovasc Pharmacol 1(suppl 1):S38–S42, 1979.

88. Wilkerson R, Stevens IM, Pickering M, et al: A study of the effects of atenolol and propranolol on renal function in patients with essential hypertension. Br J Clin Pharmacol 10:51–59, 1980.

89. Lameyer LDF, Hesse CJ: Metoprolol in high renin hypertension. Ann Clin Res 13(suppl 30):16–22, 1981.

90. Warren SE, O'Connor DT, Cohen IM, Mitas JA: Renal hemodynamic changes during long-term antihypertensive therapy. Clin Pharmacol Ther 29:310–317, 1981.

91. de Leeuw PW, Birkenhager WA: Renal response to propranolol treatment in hypertensive humans. Hypertension 4:125–131, 1982.

92. Malini PL, Strocchi E, Negroni S, et al: Renal haemodynamics after chronic treatment with labetalol and propranolol. Br J Clin Pharmacol 13:S123–S126, 1982.

93. Pasternack A, Porsti P, Poyhonen L: Effect of pindolol and propranolol on renal function of patients with hypertension. Br J Clin Pharmacol 13:241s–244s, 1982.

94. Bauer JH: Effects of propranolol therapy on renal function and body fluid composition. Arch Intern Med 143:927–931, 1983.

95. O'Connor DT, Preston RA: Urinary kallikrein activity, renal hemodynamics, and electrolyte handling during chronic beta blockade with propranolol in hypertension. Hypertension 4:742–749, 1983.

96. Navis GJ, de Jong PE, Donker AJM, de Zeeuw D: Effects of enalapril on blood pressure and renal haemodynamics in essential hypertension. Proc Eur Dial Transplant Assoc 20:577–581, 1983.

97. Mosley C, O'Connor DT, Taylor A, et al: Comparative effects of antihypertensive therapy with guanabenz and propranolol on renal vascular resistance and left ventricular mass. J Cardiovasc Pharmacol 6:S757–S761, 1984.

98. Herrera-Acosta J, Perez-Gravas P, Fernandez M, Arriaga J: Enalapril in essential hypertension. Drugs 30:35–46, 1985.

99. van den Meiracker AH, Man in't Veld AJ, Boomsma F, et al: Hemodynamic and β-adrenergic receptor adaptations during long-term β-adrenoceptor blockade. Circulation 80:903–914, 1989.

100. Valvo E, Gammaro L, Tessitore N, et al: Effects of timolol on blood pressure, systemic hemodynamics, plasma renin activity, and glomerular filtration rate in patients with essential hypertension. Int J Clin Pharmacol Ther Toxicol 22:156–161, 1984.

101. Baba T, Murabayashi S, Tomiyama T, Tabebe K: Comparison of the renal effects of dilevalol and carteolol in patients with mild to moderate essential hypertension. Eur J Clin Pharmacol 38:305–307, 1990.

102. Wainer E, Bon G, Rosenfeld JB: Effects of pindolol on renal function. Clin Pharmacol Ther 28:575–580, 1980.

103. Wilcox CS, Lewis PS, Peart WS, et al: Renal function, body fluid volumes, renin, aldosterone, and noradrenaline during treatment of hypertension with pindolol. J Cardiovasc Pharmacol 3:598–611, 1981.

104. Boner G, Wainer E, Rosenfeld JB: Effects of pindolol on renal function. II. Effects of intravenous and prolonged oral dosing. Clin Pharmacol Ther 32:423–427, 1982.

105. Rosenfeld J, Boner G, Wainer E: Renal function during acute and long-term pindolol treatment in hypertensive patients with normal and decreased glomerular filtration. Br J Clin Pharmacol 134:237s–240s, 1982.

106. Gafter U, Holtzman E, Rosenthal T, et al: Effect of pindolol on renal function in hypertensive patients. Isr J Med Sci 19:563–565, 1983.

107. van den Meiracker AH, Man in't Veld AJ, van Eck HJR, Schalekamp MADH: Systemic and renal vasodilation after beta-adrenoceptor blockade with pindolol: A hemodynamic study on the onset and maintenance of its antihypertensive effect. Am Heart J 112:368–374, 1986.

108. Zech P, Pozet N, Labeeuw M, et al: Acute renal effects of new beta-adrenergic receptor site blocking agents on renal function. Proc Eur Dial Transplant Assoc 12:203–208, 1976.

109. Falch DK, Paulsen AQ, Odegaard AE, Norman N: Central and renal circulation, electrolytes, body weight, plasma aldosterone and renin during atenolol treatment in essential hypertension. Curr Ther Res 26:813–820, 1979.

110. Waal-Manning HJ, Bolli P: Atenolol vs placebo in mild hypertension: Renal, metabolic and stress antipressor effects. Br J Clin Pharmacol 9:553–560, 1980.

111. Bellini G, Battilana G, Carretta R, et al: Antihypertensive effects and kidney function in hypertensive patients treated with atenolol and oxprenolol. Curr Ther Res 32:99–105, 1982.

112. Dreslinski GR, Messerli FH, Dunn FG, et al: Hemodynamics, biochemical and reflexive changes produced by atenolol. Circulation 65:1365–1368, 1982.

113. Imai Y, Abe K, Sato M, et al: Mechanism of antihypertensive effect of atenolol in patients with borderline hypertension during short-term treatment. Arzneimittelforschung 36:869–873, 1986.

114. Bianchi S, Bigazzi R, Baldari G: Microalbuminuria in patients with essential hypertension: Effects of several antihypertensive drugs. Am J Med 93:525–528, 1992.

115. Samuelsson O, Hedner T, Ljungman S, et al: A comparative study of lisinopril and atenolol on low degree urinary albumin excretion, renal function and hemodynamics in uncomplicated, primary hypertension. Eur J Clin Pharmacol 43:469–475, 1992.

116. Apperloo AJ, de Zeeuw D, Sluiter HE, de Jong PE: Differential effects of enalapril and atenolol on proteinuria and renal haemodynamics in non-diabetic renal disease. Br Med J 303:821–824, 1991.

117. Taverner D, MacKay IG, Craig K, Watson ML: The effects of selective β-adrenoceptor antagonists and partial agonist activity on renal function during exercise in normal subjects and those with moderate renal impairment. Br J Clin Pharmacol 32:387–391, 1991.

118. Stornell M, Valvo EV, Scappellato L: Comparative effects of enalapril, atenolol, and chlorthalidone on blood pressure and kidney function of diabetic patients affected by arterial hypertension and persistent proteinuria. Nephron 58:52–57, 1991.

119. Reams GP, Bauer JH, Lau A: The acute and chronic effects of betaxolol on blood pressure, renin-aldosterone, and renal function in essential hypertension. J Clin Pharmacol 27:118–121, 1987.

120. Hollenbeck M, Plum J, Heering P, et al: Influence of betaxolol on renal function and atrial natriuretic peptide in essential hypertension. J Hypertens 9:819–824, 1991.

121. Rasmussen S, Rasmussen K: Influence of metoprolol, alone and in combination with a thiazide diuretic, on blood pressure, plasma volume, extracellular volume and glomerular filtration rate in essential hypertension. Eur J Clin Pharmacol 15:305–310, 1979.

122. Strandgaard S, Elmgreen J, Christensen TE, Laursen SW: Effect of short-term and long-term treatment with metoprolol on renal blood flow and glomerular filtration rate in hypertensive patients with a normal kidney function. Dan Med Bull 29:287–289, 1982.

123. Sugino G, Barg AP, O'Connor DT: Renal perfusion is preserved during cardioselective β-blockade with metoprolol in hypertension. Am J Kidney Dis 3:357–361, 1984.

124. Erley CM, Haefele U, Heyne N, et al: Microalbuminuria in essential hypertension. Hypertension 21:810–815, 1993.

125. Ljungman S, Wikstrand J, Hartford M, et al: Effects of long-term antihypertensive treatment and aging on renal function and albumin excretion in primary hypertension. Am J Hypertens 6:554–563, 1993.

126. Christensen CK, Mogensen CE: Effect of antihypertensive treatment on progression of incipient diabetic nephropathy. Hypertension 7(suppl II):109–113, 1985.

127. Bjorck S, Mulec H, Johnsen SA, et al: Renal protective effect of enalapril in diabetic nephropathy. Br Med J 304:339–343, 1992.

128. Joekes AM, Thompson FD: Acute haemodynamic effects of labetalol and its subsequent use as an oral hypotensive agent. Br J Clin Pharmacol 3(suppl):789–793, 1976.

129. Thompson FD, Joekes AM, Hussein MM: Monotherapy with labetalol for hypertensive patients with normal and impaired renal function. Br J Clin Pharmacol 8:129s–133s, 1978.

130. Keusch G, Weidmann P, Ziegler WH, et al: Effects of chronic alpha and beta adrenoceptor blockade with labetalol on plasma catecholamines and renal function in hypertension. Klin Wochenschr 58:25–29, 1980.

131. Rasmussen S, Nielson PE: Blood pressure, body fluid volumes, and glomerular filtration rate during treatment with labetalol in essential hypertension. Br J Clin Pharmacol 12:349–353, 1981.

132. Valvo E, Previato G, Tessitore N, et al: Effects of the long-term administration of labetalol on blood pressure, hemodynamics and renal function in essential and renal hypertension. Curr Ther Res 39:634–643, 1981.

133. Watson A, Maher K, Keogh JAB: Labetalol and renal function. Ir J Med Sci 150:174–177, 1981.

134. Wallin JD: Antihypertensives and their impact on renal function. Am J Med 75(suppl 4):103–108, 1983.

135. Williams JG, DeVoss K, Craswell PW: Labetalol in the treatment of hypertensive renal patients. Med J Aust 1:225–228, 1978.

136. Bauer JH, Reams GP: Beta-adrenergic antagonists and the kidney. In Bennett WM, McCarron DA, Brenner BM, Stein JH (eds): Contemporary Issues in Nephrology, Vol 17, Pharmacotherapy of Renal Disease and Hypertension. Churchill Livingstone, New York, 1987, pp 223–254.

137. Bauer JH, Reams GP: The effects of antihypertensive therapy on renal function. In Kaplan NM, Brenner BM, Laragh JH (eds): Perspectives on Hypertension, Vol 3, New Therapeutic Strategies for Hypertension. Raven Press, New York, 1989, pp 253–287.

138. Bakris GL, Wilson DM, Burnett JC: The renal, forearm and humoral responses to standing in the presence and absence of propranolol. Circulation 74:1061–1065, 1986.

139. Bauer JH, Brooks CS: The long-term effect of propranolol therapy on renal function. Am J Med 66:405–410, 1979.

140. Man in't Veld AJ, Schalekamp MADH: Effects of 10 different β-adrenoceptor antagonists on hemodynamics, plasma renin activity, plasma norepinephrine changes in relation to partial agonist activity. J Cardiovasc Pharmacol 5(suppl 1):S30–S45, 1983.

141. Prichard BNC, Gillam PMS: Treatment of hypertension with propranolol. Br Med J 1:7–16, 1969.

142. Buhler FR, Burkart F, Lutold BE, et al: Antihypertensive beta-blocking action as related to renin and age: A pharmacologic tool to identify pathogenetic mechanisms in essential hypertension. Am J Cardiol 36:653–669, 1975.

143. Laragh JH: Modern system for treating high blood pressure based on renin profiling and vasoconstriction–volume analysis: A primary role for beta-blocking drugs such as propranolol. Am J Med 61:797–810, 1976.

144. Wallin JD, Shah SV: β-Adrenergic blocking agents in the treatment of hypertension. Arch Intern Med 147:654–659, 1987.

145. McAreavey D, Vermeulen R, Robertson JIS: Newer beta blockers and the treatment of hypertension. Cardiovasc Drugs Ther 5:577–588, 1991.

146. Gilmore E, Weil J, Chidsey C: Treatment of essential hypertension with a new vasodilator in combination with beta-adrenergic blockade. N Engl J Med 282:521–527, 1970.

147. Zacest R, Gilmore E, Koch-Weser J: Treatment of essential hypertension with combined vasodilators and beta-adrenergic blockade. N Engl J Med 286:617–622, 1972.

148. Bravo EL, Tarazi RC, Dustan HP: β-Adrenergic blockade in diuretic-treated patients with essential hypertension. N Engl J Med 292:66–70, 1975.

149. Frishman W, Silverman R: Clinical pharmacology of the new beta-adrenergic blocking drugs. Part 2. Physiologic and metabolic effects. Am Heart J 97:797–807, 1979.

150. Frishman WH: β-Adrenoceptor antagonist: New drugs and new indications. N Engl J Med 305:500–506, 1981.

151. Frishman WH: Clinical significance of beta$_1$-selectivity and intrinsic sympathomimetic activity in a beta-adrenergic blocking drug. Am J Cardiol 59:33F–37F, 1987.

152. Prichard BNC, Owens CWI: Beta-adrenergic blocking drugs. Pharmacol Ther 11:109–139, 1980.

153. Lund-Johansen P: Exercise and antihypertensive therapy. Am J Cardiol 59:98A–107A, 1987.

154. Veterans Administration Cooperative Study Group on Antihypertensive Agents: Comparison of propranolol and hydrochlorothiazide for the initial treatment of hypertension: I. Results of short-term titration with emphasis on racial differences in response. JAMA 248:1996–2003, 1982.

155. Saunders E, Weir MR, Kong W, et al: A comparison of the efficacy and safety of a β-blocker, a calcium channel blocker, and a converting enzyme inhibitor in hypertensive blacks. Arch Intern Med 150:1707–1713, 1990.

156. Beard K, Bulpitt C, Mascie-Taylor H, et al: Management of elderly patients with sustained hypertension. BMJ 304:412–416, 1992.

157. Fitzgerald JD: Age-related effects of beta-blockers and hypertension. J Cardiovasc Pharmacol 12(suppl 8):83–93, 1988.

158. Bravo EL, Tarazi RC, Dustan HP, Lewis JW: Dissociation between renin and arterial pressure responses to beta-adrenergic blockade in human essential hypertension. Circ Res 36–37(suppl I):I-241–I-247, 1975.

159. Freis ED, Materson BJ, Flamenbaum W: Comparison of propranolol or hydrochlorothiazide alone for treatment of hypertension. III. Evaluations of the renin-angiotensin system. Am J Med 74:1029–1040, 1983.

160. Prichard BNC: Pharmacological rationale for antihypertensive drug treatment. J Cardiovasc Pharmacol 10(suppl 11):S6–S17, 1987.

161. Yusuf S, Peto R, Lewis J, et al: Beta-blockade during and after myocardial infarction: An overview of randomized trials. Prog Cardiovasc Dis 27:335–371, 1985.

162. The Fifth Report of the Joint National Committee on Detection, Evaluation, and Treatment of High Blood Pressure (JNC V). Arch Intern Med 153:154–183, 1993.

163. 1993 Guidelines for the management of mild hypertension. Memorandum from a World Health Organization/International Society of Hypertension meeting. Hypertension 22:392–403, 1993.

164. Bonow RO, Udelson JE: Left ventricular diastolic dysfunction as a cause of congestive heart failure. Ann Intern Med 117:502–510, 1992.

165. Deacon SP, Barnett D: Comparison of atenolol and propranolol during insulin-induced hypoglycaemia. Br Med J 2:272–273, 1976.

166. Lager I, Blohme G, Smith U: Effect of cardioselective and nonselective β-blockade on the hypoglycaemic response in insulin-dependent diabetics. Lancet 1:458–462, 1979.

167. Frishman W, Silverman R, Strom J, et al: Clinical pharmacology of

the new beta-adrenergic blocking drugs. Part 4. Adverse effects. Choosing a β-adrenoceptor blocker. Am Heart J 98:256–262, 1979.

168. Cruickshank JM: The clinical importance of cardioselectivity and lipophilicity in beta blockers. Am Heart J 100:160–178, 1980.

169. Frishman WH: β-Adrenergic receptor blockers. Adverse effects and drug interactions. Hypertension 11(suppl II):II-21–II-29, 1988.

170. Astrom H: Comparison of the effects on airway conductance of a new selective beta-adrenergic blocking drug, atenolol, and propranolol in asthmatic subjects. Scand J Respir Dis 56:292–296, 1975.

171. Decalmer PBS, Chatterjee SS, Cruickshank JM, et al: Beta blockers and asthma. Br Heart J 40:184–189, 1978.

172. Tattersfield AE: Beta-adrenoceptor antagonists and respiratory disease. J Cardiovasc Pharmacol 8(suppl 4):34–39, 1986.

173. McSorley PD, Warren DJ: Effects of propranolol and metoprolol on the peripheral circulation. Br Med J 2:1598–1600, 1978.

174. Tsukiyama H, Otsuka K, Higuma K: Effects of β-adrenoceptor antagonists on central haemodynamics in essential hypertension. Br J Clin Pharmacol 13(suppl 2):269S–278S, 1982.

175. Frishman W, Kostis J, Strom J, et al: Clinical pharmacology of the new beta-adrenergic blocking drugs. Part 6. A comparison of pindolol and propranolol in treatment of patients with angina pectoris. The role of intrinsic sympathomimetic activity. Am Heart J 98:526–535, 1979.

176. Taylor SH, Silke B, Lee PS: Intravenous beta-blockade in coronary heart disease. N Engl J Med 306:631–635, 1982.

177. Taylor SH: Intrinsic sympathomimetic activity: Clinical fact or fiction? Am J Cardiol 52:16D–26D, 1983.

178. Walker DG: β-Adrenoceptor partial agonists: A renaissance in cardiovascular therapy? Br J Clin Pharmacol 30:157–171, 1990.

179. Fitzgerald JD: By what means might beta blockers prolong life after acute myocardial infarction? Eur Heart J 8:945–951, 1987.

180. Jacob H, Brandt LJ, Farkas P, Frishman W: Beta-adrenergic blockade and the gastrointestinal system. Am J Med 74:1042–1051, 1983.

181. Radack K, Deck C: β-Adrenergic blocker therapy does not worsen intermittent claudication in subjects with peripheral arterial disease. Arch Intern Med 151:1769–1776, 1991.

182. Solomon SA, Ramsay LE, Yeo WW, et al: β-Blockade and intermittent claudication: Placebo controlled trial of atenolol and nifedipine and their combination. BMJ 303:1100–1104, 1991.

183. Bauer K, Brunner-Ferber F, Distlerath LM, et al: Assessment of systemic effects of different ophthalmic β blockers in healthy volunteers. Clin Pharmacol Ther 49:658–664, 1991.

184. Kotis JB, Rosen RC: Central nervous system effects of β-adrenergic–blocking drugs: The role of ancillary properties. Circulation 75:204–212, 1987.

185. Gengo FM, Huntoon L, McHugh WB: Lipid-soluble and water-soluble β-blockers. Arch Intern Med 147:39–43, 1987.

186. Gengo FM, Fagan SC, dePadova A, et al: The effect of β-blockers on mental performance of older hypertensive patients. Arch Intern Med 148:778–784, 1988.

187. Dimsdale JE, Newton RP, Joist T: Neuropsychological side effects of β-blockers. Arch Intern Med 149:514–525, 1989.

188. Reichgott MJ: Problems of sexual function in patients with hypertension. Cardiovasc Med 4:149–154, 1979.

189. Moss HB, Procci WR: Sexual dysfunction associated with oral antihypertensive medication. Gen Hosp Psychiatry 4:121–129, 1982.

190. Croog SH, Levine S, Testa MA, et al: The effects of antihypertensive therapy on the quality of life. N Engl J Med 314:1657–1664, 1986.

191. Croog SH, Levine S, Sudilovsky A, et al: Sexual symptoms in hypertensive patients. Arch Intern Med 148:788–794, 1988.

192. Lehtonen A: Effect of beta blockers on blood lipid profile. Am Heart J 109:1192–1196, 1985.

193. Weidmann P, Uehlinger DE, Gerber A: Antihypertension treatment and serum lipoproteins. J Hypertens 3:297–306, 1985.

194. Ames RP: The effects of antihypertensive drugs on serum lipids and lipoproteins II. Non-diuretic drugs. Drugs 32:335–357, 1986.

195. Lardinois CK, Neuman SL: The effects of antihypertensive agents on serum lipids and lipoproteins. Arch Intern Med 148:1280–1288, 1988.

196. Lijnen P: Biochemical mechanisms involved in the β-blocker–induced changes in serum lipoproteins. Am Heart J 124:549–556, 1992.

197. Houston MC: The effect of antihypertensive drugs on glucose intolerance in hypertensive nondiabetics and diabetics. Am Heart J 115:640–656, 1988.

198. Pandit MK, Burke J, Gustafson AB, et al: Drug-induced disorders of glucose intolerance. Ann Intern Med 118:529–539, 1993.

199. Reeves RA, Boer WH, DeLeve L, Leenen FHH: Non-selective beta-blockade enhances pressor responsiveness to epinephrine, norepinephrine, and angiotensin II in normal man. Clin Pharmacol Ther 35:461–466, 1984.

200. Houston MC: Abrupt cessation of treatment in hypertension: Consideration of clinical features, mechanisms, prevention and management of the discontinuation syndrome. Am Heart J 102:415–430, 1981.

201. Watanabe AM: Recent advances in knowledge about beta-adrenergic receptors: Application to clinical cardiology. J Am Coll Cardiol 1:82–89, 1983.

202. Frishman WH: Beta-adrenergic blocker withdrawal. Am J Cardiol 59:26F–32F, 1987.

203. Houston MC, Hodge R: Beta adrenergic blocker withdrawal symptoms in hypertension and other cardiovascular diseases. Am Heart J 116:515–522, 1988.

204. Douglas DD, Young RD, Jensen P, Thiele DL: Fatal labetalol-induced hepatic injury. Am J Med 87:235–236, 1989.

205. Clark JA, Zimmerman HJ, Tanner LA: Labetalol hepatotoxicity. Ann Intern Med 113:210–213, 1990.

206. van Zwieten PA: Pharmacology of centrally acting hypotensive drugs. Br J Clin Pharmacol 10:13S–20S, 1980.

207. Langer SZ, Cavero I, Massingham R: Recent developments in noradrenergic neurotransmission and its relevance to the mechanism of action of certain antihypertensive agents. Hypertension 2:372–382, 1980.

208. Reid JL: Alpha-adrenergic receptors and blood pressure control. Am J Cardiol 57:6E–12E, 1986.

209. Dollery CT: Advantages and disadvantages of alpha₂-adrenoceptor agonists for systemic hypertension. Am J Cardiol 61:1D–5D, 1988.

210. Louis WJ, Jarrott B, Conway EL: Sites of action of alpha₂-agonists in the brain and periphery. Am J Cardiol 61:15D–17D, 1988.

211. Oster JR, Epstein M: Use of centrally acting sympatholytic agents in the management of hypertension. Arch Intern Med 151:1638–1644, 1991.

212. Hokfelt B, Hedelend H, Dymling JF: Studies on catecholamines, renin and aldosterone following Catapresan (2-(2,6-dichlor-phenyl-amine)-2-imidazoline hydrochloride) in hypertensive patients. Eur J Pharmacol 10:389–397, 1970.

213. Hokfelt B, Hedeland H, Hansson BG: The effect of clonidine and penbutolol, respectively on catecholamines in blood and urine, plasma renin activity and urinary aldosterone in hypertensive patients. Arch Int Pharmacodyn 213:307–321, 1975.

214. Campese VM, Romoff M, Telfer N, et al: Role of sympathetic nerve inhibition and body sodium-volume state in the antihypertensive action of clonidine in essential hypertension. Kidney Int 18:351–357, 1980.

215. Manhem P, Poalzow L, Hokfelt B: Plasma clonidine in relation to blood pressure, catecholamines, and renin activity during long-term treatment of hypertension. Clin Pharmacol Ther 31:445–451, 1982.

216. Farsang C, Kapocsi J, Vajda L, et al: Reversal by naloxone of the antihypertensive action of clonidine: Involvement of the sympathetic nervous system. Circulation 69:461–467, 1984.

217. Sullivan PA, DeQuattro V, Foti A, Curzon G: Effects of clonidine on central and peripheral nerve tone in primary hypertension. Hypertension 8:611–617, 1986.

218. Bobik A, Jennings G, Jackman G, et al: Evidence for a predominantly central hypotensive effect of alpha-methyldopa in humans. Hypertension 8:16–23, 1986.

219. Bousquet P, Feldman J, Tibiriea E, et al: New concepts on the central regulation of blood pressure. Am J Med 87(suppl 3C):10S–13S, 1989.

220. Molderings GJ, Michel MC, Göthert M, et al: Imidazolrezeptoren: Angriffsort einer neuen Generation von antihypertensiven Arzneimitteln. Dtsch Med Wochenschr 117:67–71, 1992.

221. Sannerstedt R, Varnauskas E, Werko L: Hemodynamic effects of methyldopa (Aldomet) at rest and during exercise in patients with arterial hypertension. Acta Med Scand 171:75–82, 1962.

222. Weil MH, Barbour BH, Chesne RB: Alpha-methyldopa for the treatment of hypertension. Circulation 28:165–174, 1963.

223. Onesti G, Schwartz AB, Kem KE, et al: Antihypertensive effect of clonidine. Circ Res 28–29(suppl II):II-53–II-69, 1971.

224. Onesti G, Brest AN, Novack P, et al: Pharmacodynamic effects of alpha-methyldopa in hypertensive subjects. Am Heart J 67:32–38, 1964.

225. Onesti G, Bock KD, Heimsoth V, et al: Clonidine: A new antihypertensive agent. Am J Cardiol 28:74–83, 1971.

226. Brest AN: Hemodynamic and cardiac effects of clonidine. J Cardiovasc Pharmacol 2(suppl I):S39–S46, 1980.

227. Houston MC: Clonidine hydrochloride: Review of pharmacologic and clinical aspects. Prog Cardiovasc Dis 23:337–350, 1981.

228. Myhre E, Stenbaek O, Rugstad HE, et al: Pharmacokinetics of methyldopa in renal failure and bilaterally nephrectomized patients. Scand J Urol Nephrol 16:257–263, 1982.

229. Myhre E, Rugstad HE, Hansen T: Clinical pharmacokinetics of methyldopa. Clin Pharmacokinet 7:221–233, 1982.

230. Pettinger WA: Clonidine, a new antihypertensive drug. N Engl J Med 293:1179–1180, 1975.

231. Hulter HN, Licht JH, Ilnicki LP, Singh S: Clinical efficacy and pharmacokinetics of clonidine in hemodialysis and renal insufficiency. J Lab Clin Med 94:223–231, 1979.

232. Lowenthal DT: Pharmacokinetics of clonidine. J Cardiovasc Pharmacol 2(suppl I):S29–S37, 1980.

233. Groth H, Vetter H, Knusel J, et al: Transdermal clonidine application: Long-term results in essential hypertension. Klin Wochenschr 62:925–930, 1984.

234. Burris JF, Mroczek WJ: Transdermal administration of clonidine: A new approach to antihypertensive therapy. Pharmacotherapy 6:30–34, 1986.

235. Popli S, Daugirdas JT, Neubauer JA, et al: Transdermal clonidine in mild hypertension. Arch Intern Med 146:2140–2144, 1986.

236. Lowenthal DT, Saris S, Paran E, et al: Efficacy of clonidine as transdermal therapeutic system: The international clinical experience. Am Heart J 112:893–900, 1986.

237. Baum T, Shropshire AT, Rowles G, et al: General pharmacological actions of the antihypertensive agent 2,6-dichlorobenzylidene aminoguanidine acetate (Wy-8678). J Pharmacol Exp Ther 171:276–287, 1970.

238. Meacham RH, Emmett M, Kyriakopoulos AA, et al: Disposition of $^{14}$C-guanabenz in patients with essential hypertension. Clin Pharmacol Ther 27:44–52, 1980.

239. Weber MA, Drayer JIM: Centrally acting antihypertensive agents: A brief overview. J Cardiovasc Pharmacol 6:S803–S807, 1984.

240. Weiss YA, Lavene DL, Safar ME, et al: Guanfacine kinetics in patients with hypertension. Clin Pharmacol Ther 25:283–293, 1979.

241. Dollery CT, Davies DS: Centrally acting drugs in antihypertensive therapy. Br J Clin Pharmacol 10:5S–12S, 1980.

242. Saameli K, Jerie P, Scholtysik G: Guanfacine and other centrally acting drugs in antihypertensive therapy; pharmacological and clinical aspects. Clin Exp Hypertens A 4:209–219, 1982.

243. Sorkin EM, Heel RC: Guanfacine. Drugs 31:310–366, 1986.

244. Scholtysik G: Animal pharmacology of guanfacine. Am J Cardiol 57:13E–17E, 1986.

245. Kiechel JR: Pharmacokinetics of guanfacine in patients with impaired renal function and in some elderly patients. Am J Cardiol 57:18E–21E, 1986.

246. Bauer JH: Adrenergic blocking agents and the kidney. J Clin Hypertens 3:199–221, 1985.

247. Mohammed S, Hanenson IB, Magenheim HG, Gaffney TE: The effects of alpha-methyldopa on renal function in hypertensive patients. Am Heart J 76:21–27, 1968.

248. Grabie M, Nussbaum P, Goldfarb S, et al: Effects of methyldopa on renal hemodynamics and tubular function. Clin Pharmacol Ther 22:522–527, 1980.

249. Cruz F, O'Neil WM Jr, Clifton G, Wallin JD: Effects of labetalol and methyldopa on renal function. Clin Pharmacol Ther 30:57–63, 1981.

250. Luke RG: Methyldopa in treatment of hypertension due to chronic renal disease. Br Med J 1:27–30, 1964.

251. Heeg JE, de Jong PE, van der Hem GK, de Zeeuw D: Efficacy and variability of the antiproteinuric effect of ACE inhibition by lisinopril. Kidney Int 36:272–279, 1989.

252. Cohen IM, O'Connor DT, Preston RA, Stone RA: Reduced renovascular resistance by clonidine. Clin Pharmacol Ther 26:572–577, 1979.

253. Onesti G, Schwartz AB, Kim KE, et al: Antihypertensive effects of clonidine. Circ Res 28:S53–S69, 1971.

254. Morgan T: The use of centrally acting antihypertensive drugs in patients with renal disease. Chest 83(suppl):383–385, 1983.

255. Sauter ER, Bakris GL: The effects of enalapril on urinary protein excretion in patients with idiopathic membranous nephropathy. J Clin Pharmacol 30:155–158, 1990.

256. Bosanac P, Dubb J, Walker B, et al: Renal effects of guanabenz: A new antihypertensive. J Clin Pharmacol 16:631–636, 1976.

257. Warren SE, Cohen IM, Barg AP, O'Connor DT: Guanabenz and hydrochlorothiazide for the treatment of essential hypertension: Enhanced renal perfusion. Curr Ther Res 28:530–534, 1980.

258. Bauer JH: Effects of guanabenz therapy on renal function and body fluid composition. Arch Intern Med 143:1163–1167, 1983.

259. Dubrow A, Mittman N, DeCola P, et al: Safety and efficacy of guanabenz in hypertensive patients with moderate renal insufficiency. J Clin Hypertens 4:322–325, 1985.

260. Gehr M, MacCarthy EP, Goldberg M: Guanabenz: A centrally acting natriuretic antihypertensive drugs. Kidney Int 29:1203–1208, 1986.

261. Braden G, Alvis R, Walker BR, Cox M: Effects of guanabenz on sodium and water homeostasis. J Clin Hypertens 3:397–404, 1987.

262. Roeckel A, Heidland A II: Acute and chronic renal effects of guanfacine in essential and renal hypertension. Br J Clin Pharmacol 10:141s–149s, 1980.

263. Ikeda T, Gomi T, Yuhara M, et al: Affects of guanfacine monotherapy on blood pressure, heart rate, plasma renin activity, aldosterone and catecholamines in hypertensive patients with chronic glomerulonephritis. Clin Pharmacol Ther 43:278–282, 1988.

264. Bakris GL, Barnhill BW, Sadler R: Treatment of arterial hypertension in diabetic humans: Importance of therapeutic selection. Kidney Int 41:912–919, 1992.

265. Strandhoy JW, Morris M, Buckalew VM: Renal effects of the antihypertensive, guanabenz, in the dog. J Pharmacol Exp Ther 221:347–352, 1982.

266. Gehr M, MacCarthy P, Goldberg M: Natriuretic and water diuretic effects of central $\alpha_2$-adrenoceptor agonists. J Cardiovasc Pharmacol 6:S781–S786, 1984.

267. Goldberg M, Gehr M: Effects of alpha$_2$-agonists on renal function in hypertensive humans. J Cardiovasc Pharmacol 7(suppl 8):S34–S37, 1985.

268. Dollery CT, Harrington M: Methyldopa in hypertension. Clinical and pharmacological studies. Lancet 1:759–763, 1962.

269. Bayliss RIS, Harvey-Smith EA: Methyldopa in the treatment of hypertension. Lancet 1:763–768, 1962.

270. Yeh BK, Nantel A, Goldberg LI: Antihypertensive effect of clonidine. Arch Intern Med 127:233–237, 1971.

271. Mroczek WJ, Davidov M, Finnerty FA: Prolonged treatment with clonidine: Comparative antihypertensive effects alone and with a diuretic agent. Am J Cardiol 30:536–541, 1972.

272. Garrett BN, Kaplan NM: Clonidine in the treatment of hypertension. J Cardiovasc Pharmacol 2(suppl I):S61–S71, 1980.

273. Thananopavarn C, Golub MS, Eggena P, et al: Clonidine, a centrally acting sympathetic inhibitor, as monotherapy for mild to moderate hypertension. Am J Cardiol 49:153–158, 1982.

274. McMahon FG, Ryan JR, Jain AK, et al: Guanabenz in essential hypertension. Clin Pharmacol Ther 21:272–277, 1977.

275. Walker BR, Deitch MW, Schneider BE, et al: Long-term therapy of hypertension with guanabenz. Clin Ther 4:217–228, 1981.

276. Safar ME, Loria Y, Weiss YA, Boutier JR: Antihypertensive effects and plasma levels of guanfacine in man. J Clin Pharmacol 22:385–390, 1982.

277. Fillingim JM, Blackshear JL, Strauss A, Strauss M: Guanfacine as monotherapy for systemic hypertension. Am J Cardiol 57:50E–54E, 1986.

278. MacFarlane JPR: Methyldopa in the elderly hypertensive. Curr Med Res Opin 7(suppl I):63–67, 1982.

279. Thananopavarn C, Golub MS, Sambhi MP: Clonidine in the elderly hypertensive. Chest 83:S410–S411, 1983.

280. Douchamps J, Papalexion P, Semadeni S, Herchuelz A: Antihypertensive effect of guanfacine in the elderly. Curr Ther Res 38:984–989, 1985.

281. Traub YM: Comparison of oxprenolol vs methyldopa as second-line antihypertensive agents in the elderly. Arch Intern Med 148:77–80, 1988.

282. Lowenthal DT, Affrime MB, Rosenthal L, et al: Dynamic and biochemical responses to single and repeated doses of clonidine during dynamic peripheral activity. Clin Pharmacol Ther 32:18–24, 1982.

283. Hedner T, Nyberg G, Mellstrand T: Guanfacine in essential hypertension: Effects during rest and isometric exercise. Clin Pharmacol Ther 35:604–609, 1984.

284. Weber MA: Transdermal antihypertensive therapy: Clinical and metabolic considerations. Am Heart J 112:906–912, 1986.

285. Swislocki A: Insulin resistance and hypertension. Am J Med Sci 300:104–115, 1990.

286. Ames RP: The influence of non–beta-blocking drugs on the lipid profile: Are diuretics outclassed as initial therapy for hypertension? Am Heart J 114:998–1006, 1987.

287. Messerli FH: Antihypertensive therapy—going to the heart of the matter. Circulation 81:1128–1135, 1990.

288. Lavie CJ, Ventura HO, Messerli FH: Regression of increased left ventricular mass by antihypertensives. Drugs 42:945–961, 1991.

289. Husserl FE, Messerli FH: Adverse effects of antihypertensive drugs. Drugs 22:188–210, 1981.

290. Engelman K: Side effects of sympatholytic antihypertensive drugs. Hypertension 11(suppl II):II-30–II-33, 1988.

291. Pottash ALC, Black HR, Gold MS: Psychiatric complications of antihypertensive medications. J Nerv Ment Dis 169:430–438, 1981.

292. Curb JD, Borhani NO, Blaszkowski TP, et al: Long-term surveillance for adverse effects of antihypertensive drugs. JAMA 253:3263–3268, 1985.

293. Hansson L, Hunyor SN, Julius S, Hoobler SW: Blood pressure crises following withdrawal of clonidine (Catapres, Catapresan), with special reference to arterial and urinary catecholamine levels, and suggestions for acute management. Am Heart J 85:605–610, 1973.

294. Weber MA: Discontinuation syndrome following cessation of treatment with clonidine and other antihypertensive agents. J Cardiovasc Pharmacol 2(suppl I):S73–S89, 1980.

295. Metz S, Klein C, Morton N: Rebound hypertension after discontinuation of transdermal clonidine therapy. Am J Med 82:17–19, 1987.

296. Ram CV, Holland OB, Fairchild C, Gomez-Sanchez CE: Withdrawal syndrome following cessation of guanabenz therapy. J Clin Pharmacol 19:148–150, 1978.

297. Bauer JH, Burch RN: Comparative studies: Guanabenz versus propranolol as first-step therapy for the treatment of primary hypertension. Cardiovasc Rev Rep 4:329–339, 1983.

298. Zamboulis C, Reid JL: Withdrawal of guanfacine after long-term treatment in essential hypertension. Eur J Clin Pharmacol 19:19–24, 1981.

299. Jerie P: Long-term evaluations of therapeutic efficacy and safety of guanfacine. Am J Cardiol 51:55E–59E, 1986.

300. Maibach HI: Oral substitution in patients sensitized by transdermal clonidine treatment. Contact Dermatitis 16:1–8, 1987.

301. Weber MA, Drayer JIM: Antihypertensive agents that act in the central nervous system. Cardiovasc Rev Rep 3:255–270, 1982.

302. Sannerstedt R, Conway J: Hemodynamic and vascular responses to antihypertensive treatment with adrenergic blocking agents: A review. Am Heart J 79:122–127, 1970.

303. Maass AR, Jenkins B, Shen Y, Tannenbaum P: Studies on absorption, excretion and metabolism of ³H-reserpine in man. Clin Pharmacol Ther 10:366–371, 1970.

304. Zsoter TT, Johnson GE, DeVeber GA, Paul H: Excretion and metabolism of reserpine in renal failure. Clin Pharmacol Ther 14:325–330, 1973.

305. Veterans Administration Medical Center: Low dose vs standard dose of reserpine. JAMA 248:2471–2477, 1982.

306. Lederle FA, Applegate WB, Grimm RH Jr: Reserpine and the medical market place. Arch Intern Med 153:705–706, 1993.

307. Moyer JH, Hughes W, Huggins R: The cardiovascular and renal hemodynamic response to the administration of reserpine. Am J Med Sci 227:640–648, 1954.

308. Reusch CS: The cardiorenal hemodynamic effects of antihypertensive therapy with reserpine. Am Heart J 64:643–649, 1962.

309. Smith AJ: Fluid retention produced by guanethidine. Circulation 31:490–496, 1965.

310. Moyer JH: Cardiovascular and renal hemodynamic response to reserpine (Serpasil), and clinical results of using this agent for the treatment of hypertension. Ann N Y Acad Sci 59:82–94, 1954.

311. Krogsgaard AR: The effect of reserpine on the electrolyte and fluid balance in man. Acta Med Scand 69:127–132, 1957.

312. Veterans Administration Cooperative Study Group on Antihypertensive Agents: Effects of treatment on morbidity in hypertension. II. Results in patients with diastolic blood pressure averaging 90 through 114 mm Hg. JAMA 213:1143–1152, 1970.

313. Hypertension Detection and Follow-up Program Cooperative Group: Five-year findings of the hypertension detection and follow-up program. Prevention and reversal of left ventricular hypertrophy with antihypertensive drug therapy. Hypertension 7:105–112, 1985.

314. Graham RM: Selective alpha₁-adrenergic antagonists: Therapeutically relevant antihypertensive agents. Am J Cardiol 53:16A–20A, 1984.

315. Davey M: Mechanism of alpha blockade for blood pressure control. Am J Cardiol 59:18G–28G, 1987.

316. van Zwieten PA: Basic pharmacology of alpha-adrenoceptor antagonists and hybrid drugs. J Hypertens 6(suppl 2):S3–S11, 1988.

317. Cubeddu LX: New alpha₁-adrenergic receptor antagonists for the treatment of hypertension: Role of vascular alpha receptors in the control of peripheral resistance. Am Heart J 116:133–162, 1988.

318. Luther RR: New perspectives on selective alpha₁ blockade. Am J Hypertens 2:729–735, 1989.

319. Khoury AF, Kaplan NM: α-Blocker therapy of hypertension. JAMA 266:394–398, 1991.

320. Lund-Johansen P: Hemodynamic changes at rest and during exercise in long-term prazosin therapy for essential hypertension. Postgrad Med J 58(suppl 1):45–52, 1975.

321. Koshy MC, Mickley D, Bourgoignie J, Blaufox MD: Physiological evaluation of a new antihypertensive agent: Prazosin HCl. Circulation 55:533–537, 1977.

322. Mancia G, Ferrari A, Gregorini L: Effects of prazosin on autonomic control of circulation in essential hypertension. Hypertension 2:700–707, 1980.

323. Mulvihill-Wilson J, Gaffney FA, Pettinger WA, et al: Hemodynamic and neuroendocrine responses to acute and chronic alpha-adrenergic blockade with prazosin and phenoxybenzamine. Circulation 67:383–393, 1983.

324. Taylor SH: Pharmacotherapeutic stature of doxazosin and its role in coronary risk reduction. Am Heart J 116:1735–1747, 1988.

325. Taylor SH: Clinical pharmacotherapeutics of doxazosin. Am J Med 87(suppl 2A):2A-2S–2A-10S, 1989.

326. Graham RM, Pettinger WA: Prazosin. N Engl J Med 300:232–236, 1979.

327. Staszek WF, Kellerman D, Brogden RN, Romankiewicz JA: Prazosin update: A review of its pharmacological properties and therapeutic use in hypertension. Drugs 25:339–384, 1983.

328. Reid JL, Vincent J: Clinical pharmacology and therapeutic role of prazosin and related alpha-adrenergic antagonists. Cardiology 73:164–174, 1986.

329. Lameire N, Gordts J: A pharmacokinetic study of prazosin in patients with varying degrees of chronic renal failure. Eur J Clin Pharmacol 31:333–337, 1986.

330. Kyncl JJ: Pharmacology of terazosin. Am J Med 80(suppl 5B):12–19, 1986.

331. Sonders RC: Pharmacokinetics of terazosin. Am J Med 80(suppl 5B):20–24, 1986.

332. Jungers P, Ganeval D, Pertuiset N, Chauveau P: Influence of renal insufficiency on the pharmacokinetics and pharmacodynamics of terazosin. Am J Med 80(suppl 5B):94–99, 1986.

333. Wilner KD, Ziegler MG: Effects of alpha₁ inhibition on renal blood flow and sympathetic nervous activity in systemic hypertension. Am J Cardiol 59:82G–86G, 1987.

334. Oliver RM, Upward JW, Dewhurst AG, et al: The pharmacokinetics of doxazosin in patients with hypertension and renal impairment. Br J Clin Pharmacol 29:417–422, 1990.

335. Oliveros-Palacios MC, Godoy-Godoy N, Colina-Chourio JA: Effects of doxazosin on blood pressure, renin-angiotensin-aldosterone and urinary kallikrein. Am J Cardiol 67:157–161, 1991.

336. Krusell LR, Christensen CK, Pedersen OL: α-Adrenoceptor blockade in patients with mild to moderate hypertension: Long-term renal effects of doxazosin. J Cardiovasc Pharmacol 20:440–444, 1992.

337. Ibsen H, Rasmussen K, Jensen HAE, Leth A: Changes in glomerular filtration rates during long term treatment with propranolol and peripheral vasodilators in patients with arterial hypertension. Dan Med Bull 26:308–311, 1979.

338. Preston RA, O'Connor DT, Stone RA: Prazosin and renal hemodynamics: Arteriolar vasodilation during therapy of essential hypertension in man. J Cardiovasc Pharmacol 1:277–286, 1979.

339. McNair A, Rasmussen S, Nielsen PE, Rasmussen K: The antihypertensive effect of prazosin on mild to moderate hypertension, changes in plasma volume, extracellular volume and glomerular filtration rate. Acta Med Scand 207:413–416, 1980.

340. Blaufox MD, Ross L, Koshy K, Lee H-B: Physiologic effects of

prazosin HCl: Consequences of diuretic combination therapy. Nephron 29:85–89, 1981.

341. Bauer JH, Jones LB, Gaddy P: Effects of prazosin therapy on blood pressure, renal function, and body fluid composition. Arch Intern Med 144:1196–1200, 1984.

342. Bailey RR: Prazosin in the treatment of patients with hypertension and renal functional impairment. Med J Aust 2(special suppl):42–45, 1977.

343. Rosenberg ME, Hosteller TH: Comparative effects of antihypertensives on proteinuria: Angiotensin-converting enzyme inhibitor versus $\alpha_1$-antagonist. Am J Kidney Dis 18:472–482, 1991.

344. Beretta-Piccoli C, Ferrier C, Weidmann P: $\alpha_1$-Adrenergic blockade and cardiovascular pressor responses in essential hypertension. Hypertension 8:407–414, 1986.

345. Smyth DD, Umemura S, Pettinger WA: Alpha$_2$-adrenoceptors and sodium reabsorption in the isolated perfused rat kidney. Am J Physiol 247:F680–F685, 1984.

346. Fernandes M, Smith IS, Weder A, et al: Prazosin in the treatment of hypertension. Clin Sci Mol Med 48:181s–184s, 1975.

347. Brodgen RN, Heel RC, Speight TM, et al: Prazosin: A review of its pharmacological properties and therapeutic efficacy in hypertension. Drugs 14:163–197, 1977.

348. Okun R: Effectiveness of prazosin as initial antihypertensive therapy. Am J Cardiol 51:644–650, 1983.

349. Davey MJ: The pharmacological basis for the use of $\alpha_1$-adrenoceptor antagonists in the treatment of essential hypertension. Br J Clin Pharmacol 2:5S–8S, 1986.

350. Dauer AD: Terazosin: An effective once-daily monotherapy for the treatment of hypertension. Am J Med 80(suppl 5B):29–34, 1986.

351. Deger G: Comparison of the safety and efficacy of once-daily terazosin versus twice-daily prazosin for the treatment of mild to moderate hypertension. Am J Med 80(suppl 5B):62–67, 1986.

352. Hayduk K: Efficacy and safety of doxazosin in hypertension therapy. Am J Cardiol 59:35G–39G, 1987.

353. Ames RP, Chrysant SG, Gonzalez F, et al: Effectiveness of doxazosin in systemic hypertension. Am J Cardiol 64:203–208, 1989.

354. Taylor SH, Grimm RH Jr: New developments in the role of $\alpha_1$-adrenergic receptors in cardiovascular disease. Am Heart J 119:655–662, 1990.

355. Luther RR, Glassman HN, Jordan DC, Sperzel WD: Efficacy of terazosin as an antihypertensive agent. Am J Med 80(suppl 5B):73–76, 1986.

356. Huuppanen R, Lehtonen A, Vahätalo M: Effect of doxazosin on insulin sensitivity in hypertensive non–insulin dependent diabetic patients. Eur J Clin Pharmacol 43:365–368, 1992.

357. Pool JL: Effects of doxazosin on serum lipids: A review of the clinical data and molecular basis for altered lipid metabolism. Am Heart J 121:251–259, 1991.

358. Graham RM, Thornell IR, Gain JM, et al: Prazosin: The first-dose phenomenon. Br Med J 2:1293–1294, 1976.

359. Turner AS: Prazosin in hypertension. Br Med J 2:1257–1258, 1976.

360. Rosendorff C: Prazosin: Severe side effects are dose-dependent. Br Med J 2:508, 1976.

361. Nicholson JP, Resnick LM, Pickering TG, et al: Relationship of blood pressure response and the renin-angiotensin system to first dose prazosin. Am J Med 78:241–244, 1985.

362. Lepor H: The emerging role of alpha antagonists in the therapy of benign prostatic hyperplasia. J Androl 12:389–394, 1991.

363. Wilde MI, Fitton A, Sorkin EM: Terazosin. A review of its pharmacodynamic and pharmacokinetic properties, and therapeutic potential in benign prostatic hyperplasia. Drugs Aging 3:258–277, 1993.

364. Weiner N: Drugs that inhibit adrenergic nerves and block adrenergic receptors. *In* Gilman AG, Goodman LS, Rall TW, Murad F (eds): Goodman and Gillman's The Pharmacological Basis of Therapeutics, 7th ed. Macmillan Publishing, New York, 1985, pp 181–214.

365. Wheeler MH, Chare MJB, Austin TR, Lazarus JH: The management of the patient with catecholamine excess. World J Surg 6:735–747, 1982.

366. Stenstrom G, Haljamae H, Tisell L-E: Influence of pre-operative treatment with phenoxybenzamine on the incidence of adverse cardiovascular reactions during anesthesia and surgery for pheochromocytoma. Acta Anaesthesiol Scand 29:797–803, 1985.

367. Hull CJ: Phaeochromocytoma. Diagnosis, preoperative preparation and anaesthetic management. Br J Anaesth 58:1453–1468, 1986.

368. Pickering TG: Peripherally acting adrenergic blocking drugs in the treatment of hypertension. Cardiovasc Rev Rep 3:385–387, 1982.

369. Richardson DW, Wyso EM: Human pharmacology of guanethidine. Ann N Y Acad Sci 88:944–955, 1960.

370. Cohn JN, Liptak TE, Fries ED: Hemodynamic effects of guanethidine in man. Circ Res 12:298–307, 1963.

371. Villarreal H, Exaire JE, Rubio V, DaVila H: Effect of guanethidine and bretylium tosylate on systemic and renal hemodynamics in essential hypertension. Am J Cardiol 14:633–640, 1964.

372. Cangiano JL, Bloomfield DK: Hemodynamic effects of a new antihypertensive agent, guanadrel sulfate. Curr Ther Res 11:736–744, 1969.

373. Pascual AV, Julius S: Short-term effectiveness and hemodynamic actions of guanadrel, a new sympatholytic drug. Curr Ther Res 14:333–342, 1972.

374. Dollery CT, Emslie-Smith D, Milne MD: Clinical and pharmacological studies with guanethidine in the treatment of hypertension. Lancet 1:381–387, 1960.

375. Woosley RL, Nies AS: Guanethidine. N Engl J Med 295:1053–1057, 1976.

376. Palmer JD: Clinical pharmacology and CNS effects of guanadrel sulfate and the major classes of antihypertensive agents. Health Sci Rev 1:5–7, 1984.

377. Brest AN: The clinical pharmacology of guanadrel sulfate. Pract Cardiol 12(suppl):48–54, 1986.

378. Richardson DW, Syso EM, Magee JH, Cavell GC: Circulatory effects of guanethidine. Circulation 22:184–190, 1960.

379. Nugent CA, Palmer JD, Ursprung JJ: Guanadrel sulfate compared with methyldopa for mild and moderate hypertension. Pharmacotherapy 2:378–383, 1982.

380. Leishman AW, Mathews HL, Smith AJ: Guanethidine. Hypotensive drug with prolonged action. Lancet 2:1044–1048, 1959.

381. Romov-Jessen V: Blood volume during treatment of hypertension with guanethidine. Acta Med Scand 174:307–310, 1963.

382. Smith AJ: Clinical features of fluid retention complicating treatment with guanethidine. Circulation 31:485–489, 1965.

383. Gore RD: Safety and efficacy of a three-drug regimen for the treatment of hypertension: Hydrochlorothiazide, propranolol and guanadrel. Clin Ther 6:86–93, 1983.

384. Dunn MI, Dunlop JL: Guanadrel. A new antihypertensive drug. JAMA 245:1639–1642, 1981.

385. Kaplan NM: The pharmacology of guanadrel sulfate: A new step 2 antihypertensive agent. Adv Ther 2:11–19, 1985.

386. Chidsey CA III, Gottlieb TB: The pharmacological basis of antihypertensive therapy: The role of vasodilator drugs. Prog Cardiovasc Dis 17:99–113, 1974.

387. Page LB, Yager HM, Sidd JJ: Drugs in the management of hypertension. Part III. Am Heart J 92:252–259, 1976.

388. Tarazi RC: Vasodilators in hypertension: Spectrum of action and counteractions. Cardiovasc Med 3:1125–1131, 1978.

389. Khayyal M, Gross F, Kreye VAW: Studies on the direct vasodilator effect of hydralazine in the isolated rabbit renal artery. J Pharmacol Exp Ther 216:390–394, 1981.

390. Lipe S, Moulds RFW: In vitro differences between human arteries and veins in their responses to hydralazine. J Pharmacol Exp Ther 217:204–208, 1981.

391. DuCharme DW, Freyburger WA, Graham BE, Carlson RG: Pharmacologic properties of minoxidil: A new hypotensive agent. J Pharmacol Exp Ther 184:662–670, 1973.

392. Wilkinson EL, Backman H, Hecht HH: Cardiovascular and renal adjustments to a hypotensive agent. J Clin Invest 31:872–879, 1952.

393. Fries ED, Rose JC, Higgins TF, et al: The hemodynamic effects of hypotensive drugs in man: IV. 1-Hydrazinophthalazine. Circulation 8:199–204, 1953.

394. Rowe GG, Huston JH, Maxwell GM, et al: Hemodynamic effects of 1-hydrazinophthalazine in patients with arterial hypertension. J Clin Invest 34:115–120, 1955.

395. Bryan RK, Hoobler SW, Rosenzweig J, Weller JM: Effect of minoxidil on blood pressure and hemodynamics in severe hypertension. Am J Cardiol 39:796–801, 1977.

396. Koch-Weser J: Hydralazine. N Engl J Med 295:320–322, 1976.

397. Shepherd AMM, McNay JL, Ludden TM, et al: Plasma concentrations and acetylator phenotype determine response to oral hydralazine. Hypertension 3:580–585, 1981.

398. Ludden TM, McNay JL, Shepherd AMM, Lin MS: Clinical pharmacokinetics of hydralazine. Clin Pharmacokinet 7:185–205, 1982.

399. Zins GR, Martin WB: The clinical pharmacology of minoxidil. *In*

Velasco M (ed): Proceedings of the Second International Symposium on Arterial Hypertension. Excerpta Medica, Amsterdam, 1979, pp 72–79.

400. Lowenthal DT, Affrime MG: Pharmacology and pharmacokinetics of minoxidil. J Cardiovasc Pharmacol 2(suppl 2):S93–S106, 1980.

401. Pettinger WA: Minoxidil and the treatment of severe hypertension. N Engl J Med 303:922–926, 1980.

402. Campese VM: Minoxidil; a review of its pharmacological properties and therapeutic uses. Drugs 22:257–278, 1981.

403. Halstenson CE, Opsahl JA, Wright E, et al: Disposition of minoxidil in patients with various degrees of renal function. J Clin Pharmacol 29:798–802, 1989.

404. Parving H-H, Smidt UM, Hommel E, et al: Effective antihypertensive treatment postpones renal insufficiency in diabetic nephropathy. Am J Kidney Dis 22:188–195, 1993.

405. Bryan RK, Hoobler SW, Rosenzweig J, Wellar JM: Effect of minoxidil on blood pressure and hemodynamics in severe hypertension. Am J Cardiol 39:796–801, 1977.

406. Andersson O, Sivertsson R: Renal function and vascular resistance during long-term minoxidil treatment of severe hypertension. J Cardiovasc Pharmacol 2(suppl 2):s123–s130, 1980.

407. Reams GP, Lau A, Hamory A, Bauer JH: Effect of triple drug therapy on renal function: Absence of renal protection. J Clin Pharmacol 29:803–808, 1989.

408. Pontremoli R, Robaudo C, Gaiter A, et al: Long-term minoxidil treatment in refractory hypertension and renal failure. Clin Nephrol 35:39–43, 1991.

409. Mitchell HC, Graham RM, Pettinger WA: Renal function during long-term treatment of hypertension with minoxidil. Ann Intern Med 93:676 681, 1980.

410. Pettinger WA, Campbell WB, Keeton K: Adrenergic component of renin release induced by vasodilating antihypertensive drugs in the rat. Circ Res 33:82–86, 1973.

411. O'Malley K, Velasco M, Wells J, McNay JL: Control plasma renin activity and changes in sympathetic tone as determinants of minoxidil-induced increase in plasma renin activity. J Clin Invest 55:230–235, 1975.

412. Grim CE, Luft FC, Grim CM, et al: Rapid blood pressure control with minoxidil. Arch Intern Med 139:529–533, 1979.

413. Pratt JH, Yager CJ, Grim CE, Parkinson CA: Increased aldosterone metabolic clearance in hypertensive patients treated with minoxidil: An effect of greater hepatic perfusion. J Cardiovasc Pharmacol 2(suppl 2):S236–S241, 1980.

414. Zins GR: Alteration in renal function during vasodilator therapy. In Wesson LG, Fanelli GM (eds): Recent Advances in Renal Physiology and Pharmacology. University Park Press, Baltimore, 1974, pp 165–186.

415. Hansson L, Olander R, Aberg H, et al: Treatment of hypertension with propranolol and hydralazine. Acta Med Scand 190:521–534, 1971.

416. Gottlieb TB, Katz FH, Chidsey CA: Combined therapy with vasodilator drugs and beta-adrenergic blockade in hypertension. Circulation 45:571–582, 1972.

417. Pettinger WA, Mitchell HC: Minoxidil—an alternative to nephrectomy for refractory hypertension. N Engl J Med 289:167–171, 1973.

418. Koch-Weser J: Vasodilator drugs in the treatment of hypertension. Arch Intern Med 133:1017–1027, 1974.

419. Perry HM: Late toxicity to hydralazine resembling systemic lupus erythematosus or rheumatoid arthritis. Am J Med 54:58–72, 1973.

420. Bing RF: Hydralazine in hypertension: Is there a safe dose? Br Med J 281:353–354, 1980.

421. Liturn A, Adams LE, Zimmer H, Hess EV: Immunologic effects of hydralazine in hypertensive patients. Arthritis Rheum 24:1074–1078, 1981.

422. Perry HM: Possible mechanisms of the hydralazine-related lupus-like syndrome. Arthritis Rheum 24:1093–1105, 1981.

423. Cameron HA, Ramsay LE: The lupus syndrome induced by hydralazine: A common complication with low dose treatment. Br Med J 289:410–412, 1984.

424. Burton JL, Marshall A: Hypertrichosis due to minoxidil. Br J Dermatol 101:593–595, 1979.

425. Pettinger WA, Mitchell HC: Side effects of vasodilator therapy. Hypertension 11(suppl II):II-34–II-36, 1988.

426. Martin WB, Spodick DH, Zins GR: Pericardial disorders occurring during open label study of 1,869 severely hypertensive patients treated with minoxidil. J Cardiovasc Pharmacol 2(suppl 2):S217–S227, 1980.

427. Braunwald E: Mechanism of action of calcium-channel–blocking agents. N Engl J Med 307:1618–1627, 1982.

428. Schwartz A, Triggle DJ: Cellular action of calcium channel blocking drugs. Annu Rev Med 35:325–339, 1984.

429. Somlyo AP: Excitation-contraction coupling and the ultrastructure of smooth muscle. Circ Res 57:497–507, 1985.

430. Snyder SH, Reynolds IJ: Calcium-antagonist drugs. Receptor interactions that clarify therapeutic effects. N Engl J Med 313:995–1002, 1985.

431. Rasmussen H: The calcium messenger system. N Engl J Med 314:1094–1101, 1164–1170, 1986.

432. Struyker-Boudier HAJ, Smits JFM, DeMey JGR: The pharmacology of calcium antagonists: A review. J Cardiovasc Pharmacol 15(suppl 4):S1–S10, 1990.

433. Cummings DM, Amadio P Jr, Nelson L, Fitzgerald JM: The role of calcium channel blockers in the treatment of essential hypertension. Arch Intern Med 151:250–259, 1991.

434. Vanhoutte PM: Calcium-entry blockers, vascular smooth muscle and systemic hypertension. Am J Cardiol 55:17B–23B, 1985.

435. van Zwieten PA, Timmermans PBMWM, van Heiningen PNM: Receptor subtypes involved in the action of calcium antagonists. J Hypertens 5(suppl 4):S21–S28, 1987.

436. Exton JH: Calcium signalling in cells—molecular mechanisms. Kidney Int 32(suppl 23):S68–S76, 1987.

437. Schoen RE, Frishman WH, Shamoon H: Hormonal and metabolic effects of calcium channel antagonists in man. Am J Med 84:492–504, 1988.

438. Stone PH, Antman EM, Muller JE, Braunwald E: Calcium channel blocking agents in the treatment of cardiovascular disorders. Part II: Hemodynamic effects and clinical applications. Ann Intern Med 93:886–904, 1980.

439. Henry PD: Comparative pharmacology of calcium antagonists: Nifedipine, verapamil and diltiazem. Am J Cardiol 46:1047–1058, 1980.

440. Spivack C, Ocken S, Frishman WH: Calcium antagonists. Clinical use in the treatment of systemic hypertension. Drugs 25:154–177, 1983.

441. Klein W, Brandt D, Vrecko K, Harringer M: Role of calcium antagonists in the treatment of essential hypertension. Circ Res 52(suppl 1):174–181, 1983.

442. Smith MS, Verghese CP, Shand DG, Pritchett ELC: Pharmacokinetic and pharmacodynamic effects of diltiazem. Am J Cardiol 51:1369–1374, 1983.

443. Hermann PH, Rodger SD, Remones G, et al: Pharmacokinetics of diltiazem after intravenous and oral administration. Eur J Clin Pharmacol 24:349–352, 1983.

444. McAllister RG, Hamann SR, Blorim RA: Pharmacokinetics of calcium-entry blockers. Am J Cardiol 55:30B–40B, 1985.

445. Halperin AK, Cubeddu LX: The role of calcium channel blockers in the treatment of hypertension. Am Heart J 111:363–382, 1986.

446. Buckley MMT, Grant SM, Goak L, et al: Diltiazem. A reappraisal of its pharmacological properties and therapeutic use. Drugs 39:757–806, 1990.

447. Prisant LM, Bottini B, DiPiro JT: Novel drug-delivery systems for hypertension. Am J Med 93(suppl 2A):45S–55S, 1992.

448. Stopher DA, Beresford AP, Macrae PV, Humphrey MJ: The metabolism and pharmacokinetics of amlodipine in humans and animals. J Cardiovasc Pharmacol 12(suppl 7):S55–S59, 1988.

449. Laher MS, Kelly JG, Doyle GD, et al: Pharmacokinetics of amlodipine in renal impairment. J Cardiovasc Pharmacol 12(suppl 7):S60–S63, 1988.

450. Abernethy DR: The pharmacokinetic profile of amlodipine. Am Heart J 118:1100–1103, 1989.

451. Abernethy DR, Gutkowska J, Winterbottom LM: Effects of amlodipine, a long-acting dihydropyridine calcium antagonist in aging hypertension: Pharmacodynamics in relation to disposition. Clin Pharmacol Ther 48:76–86, 1990.

452. Saltiel E, Ellrodt AG, Monk JP, Langley MS: Felodipine. A review of its pharmacodynamic and pharmacokinetic properties, and therapeutic use in hypertension. Drugs 36:387–342, 1988.

453. Edgar B, Regardh CG, Attman PO, et al: Pharmacokinetics of felodipine in patients with impaired renal function. Br J Clin Pharmacol 27:67–74, 1989.

454. Larsson R, Karlberg BE, Gelin A, et al: Acute and steady state pharmacokinetics and antihypertensive effects of felodipine in patients with normal and impaired renal function. J Clin Pharmacol 30:1020–1030, 1990.

455. Buur T, Larsson R, Regardh CG, Aberg J: Pharmacokinetics of felodipine in chronic hemodialysis patients. J Clin Pharmacol 31:709–713, 1991.

456. Todd PA, Faulds D: Felodipine. A review of the pharmacology and therapeutic use of the extended release formulation in cardiovascular disorders. Drugs 44:251–277, 1992.

457. Schran HF, Jaffe JM, Gonasun LM: Clinical pharmacokinetics of isradipine. Am J Med 84(suppl 3B):80–89, 1988.

458. Fitton A, Benfield P: Isradipine. A review of its pharmacodynamic and pharmacokinetic properties, and therapeutic use in cardiovascular disease. Drugs 40:31–74, 1990.

459. Sorkin EM, Clissold SP: Nicardipine. A review of its pharmacodynamic and pharmacokinetic properties, and therapeutic efficacy, in the treatment of angina pectoris, hypertension and related cardiovascular disorders. Drugs 33:296–345, 1987.

460. Singh BN, Josephson MA: Clinical pharmacology, pharmacokinetics and hemodynamic effects of nicardipine. Am Heart J 119:427–434, 1990.

461. Sorkin EM, Clissold SP, Brogden RN: Nifedipine. A review of its pharmacodynamic and pharmacokinetic properties, and therapeutic efficacy in ischemic heart disease, hypertension and related cardiovascular disorders. Drugs 30:182–274, 1985.

462. Love SJ, Yeh J, Kann J, et al: Effect of mode of administration on nifedipine pharmacokinetics. Clin Pharmacol Ther 37:209A, 1985. Abstract.

463. McAllister RG: Kinetics and dynamics of nifedipine after oral and sublingual doses. Am J Med 81(suppl 6A):2–5, 1986.

464. van Harten J, Burggraaf K, Danhof M, et al: Negligible sublingual absorption of nifedipine. Lancet 2:1363–1365, 1987.

465. Swanson DR, Barclay BL, Wong PSL, Theeuwes F: Nifedipine gastrointestinal therapeutic system. Am J Med 83(suppl 6B):3–9, 1987.

466. Chung M, Reitberg DP, Gaffney M, Singleton W: Clinical pharmacokinetics of nifedipine gastrointestinal therapeutic system. Am J Med 83(suppl 6B):10–14, 1987.

467. Bortel LV, Bohrn R, Mooij J, et al: Total and free steady-state plasma levels and pharmacokinetics of nifedipine in patients with terminal renal failure. Eur J Clin Pharmacol 37:185–189, 1989.

468. Murdoch D, Brogden RN: Sustained release nifedipine formulations. An appraisal of their current uses and prospective roles in the treatment of hypertension, ischemic heart disease and peripheral vascular disease. Drugs 41:737–779, 1991.

469. McGoon MD, Vlietstra RE, Holmes DR Jr, Osborn JE: The clinical use of verapamil. Mayo Clin Proc 57:495–510, 1982.

470. Schutz E, Ha HR, Buhler FR, Follath F: Serum concentration and antihypertensive effect of slow-release verapamil. J Cardiovasc Pharmacol 4:S346–S349, 1982.

471. Hamann SR, Blouin RA, McAllister RG: Clinical pharmacokinetics of verapamil. Clin Pharmacokinet 9:26–41, 1984.

472. Frishman WH, Lazar EJ: Sustained-release verapamil formulations for treating hypertension. J Clin Pharmacol 32:455–462, 1992.

473. Bauer JH, Reams G: Short- and long-term effects of calcium entry blockers on the kidney. Am J Cardiol 59:66A–71A, 1987.

474. Romero JC, Raij L, Granger JP, et al: Multiple effects of calcium entry blockers on renal function in hypertension. Hypertension 10:140–151, 1987.

475. Romero JC, Ruilope LM, Bentley MD, et al: Comparison of the effects of calcium antagonists and converting enzyme inhibitors on renal function under normal and hypertensive conditions. Am J Cardiol 62:59G–68G, 1988.

476. Bauer JH, Reams GP: Renal protection in essential hypertension: How do angiotensin-converting enzyme inhibitors compare with calcium antagonists? J Am Soc Nephrol 1:580–587, 1990.

477. Saburai T, Kurita T, Nagano S, Sonoda T: Antihypertensive, vasodilating and sodium diuretic actions of d-cis-isomer of benzothiazepine derivative (CRD-401). Acta Urol Jpn 18:695–707, 1972.

478. Amodeo C, Kobrin I, Ventura HO, et al: Immediate and short-term hemodynamic effects of diltiazem in patients with hypertension. Circulation 73:108–113, 1986.

479. Isshiki T, Amodeo C, Messerli FH, et al: Diltiazem maintains renal vasodilation without hyperfiltration in hypertension: Studies in es-

480. Ohashi H, Ishiguro M, Yasue T, et al: Effects of diltiazem hydrochloride on the reduction of blood pressure, and cardiac and renal functions in essential hypertensive patients with renal dysfunction. Int J Clin Pharmacol Ther Toxicol 25:291–296, 1987.

481. Sunderrajan S, Reams G, Bauer JH: Long-term renal effects of diltiazem in essential hypertension. Am Heart J 114:383–388, 1987.

482. Demarie BK, Bakris GL: Effects of different calcium antagonists on proteinuria associated with diabetes mellitus (brief report). Ann Intern Med 113:987–988, 1990.

483. Slataper R, Vicknair N, Sadler R, Bakris GL: Comparative effects of different antihypertensive treatments on progression of diabetic renal disease. Arch Intern Med 153:973–980, 1993.

484. Reams GP, Lau A, Hamory A, Bauer JH: Amlodipine therapy corrects renal abnormalities encountered in the hypertensive state. Am J Kidney Dis 10:446–451, 1987.

485. Leonetti G, Gradwik R, Terzoli L, et al: Felodipine, a new vasodilating drug: Blood pressure, cardiac, renal, and humoral effects in hypertensive patients. J Cardiovasc Pharmacol 6:392–398, 1984.

486. Hulthen UL, Katzman PL: Renal effects of acute and long-term treatment with felodipine in essential hypertension. J Hypertens 6:231–237, 1988.

487. Andersson OK, Granerus G, Volkmann R, Wysocki M: Hemodynamic and long-term renal effects of felodipine in severely hypertensive patients. J Cardiovasc Pharmacol 15(suppl 4):S41, 1990.

488. Herlitz H: Long-term effects of felodipine in patients with reduced renal function. Kidney Int 41(suppl 36):S110–S113, 1992.

489. Morgan TO, Anderson A: Hemodynamic comparisons of enalapril and felodipine and their combination. Kidney Int 41(suppl 36):S78–S81, 1992.

490. Krusell LR, Jespersen LT, Schmitz A, et al: Repetitive natriuresis and blood pressure. Hypertension 10:577–581, 1987.

491. Persson B, Andersson OK, Wysocki M, et al: Renal and hemodynamic effects of isradipine in essential hypertension. Am J Med 86(suppl 4A):60–64, 1989.

492. Pedersen OL, Krusell LR, Sihm I, et al: Long-term effects of isradipine on blood pressure and renal function. Am J Med 86(suppl 4):15–18, 1989.

493. Wittenberg C, Rosenfeld JB: Long-term antihypertensive and renal effects of isradipine in hypertensive patients with normal and reduced renal function. J Cardiovasc Pharmacol 19(suppl 3):S93–S95, 1992.

494. Wysocki M, Persson B, Bagge U, Andersson OK: Flow resistance and its components in hypertensive men treated with the calcium antagonist isradipine. Eur J Clin Pharmacol 43:463–468, 1992.

495. van Schaik BAM, van Nistelrooy AEJ, Geysker GG: Antihypertensive and renal effects of nicardipine. Br J Clin Pharmacol 18:57–63, 1984.

496. Baba T, Ishizaki T, Murabayashi S, et al: Multiple oral doses of nicardipine, a calcium-entry blocker: Effects on renal function, plasma renin activity, and aldosterone concentration in mild-to-moderate essential hypertension. Clin Pharmacol Ther 42:232–239, 1987.

497. Smith SA, Rafigi EI, Gardener EG, et al: Renal effects of nicardipine in essential hypertension: Differences between acute and chronic therapy. J Hypertens 5:693–697, 1987.

498. Chaignon M, Bellet M, Lucsko M, et al: Natriuretic and renal hemodynamic effects of nicardipine in essential hypertension. Kidney Int 34(suppl 25):S184–S186, 1988.

499. Kimura G, Deguchi F, Kojima S, et al: Effect of a calcium-entry blocker, nicardipine, on intrarenal hemodynamics in essential hypertension. Am J Kidney Dis 17:47–54, 1991.

500. Bigazzi R, Bianchi S, Baldari D, et al: Long-term effects of a converting enzyme inhibitor and a calcium channel blocker on urinary albumin excretion in patients with essential hypertension. Am J Hypertens 6:108–113, 1993.

501. Ikeda T, Nakayama D, Gomi T, et al: Captopril, an angiotensin I–converting enzyme inhibitor, decreases proteinuria in hypertensive patients with renal disease. Nephron 52:72–75, 1989.

502. Bianchi S, Bigazzi R, Baldari G, Campese VM: Long-term effects of enalapril and nicardipine on urinary albumin excretion in patients with chronic renal insufficiency: A 1-year follow-up. Am J Nephrol 11:131–137, 1991.

503. Baba T, Murabayashi S, Takebe K: Comparison of the renal effects of angiotensin converting enzyme inhibitor and calcium antagonist

in hypertensive type 2 (non–insulin-dependent) diabetic patients with microalbuminuria: A randomized controlled trial. Diabetologia 32:40–44, 1989.

504. Stornello M, Valvo EV, Scapellato L: Hemodynamic, renal, and humoral effects of the calcium entry blocker nicardipine and converting enzyme inhibitor captopril in hypertensive type II diabetic patients with nephropathy. J Cardiovasc Pharmacol 14:851–855, 1989.

505. Guazzi MD, Fiorentini C, Olivari MT, et al: Short- and long-term efficacy of a calcium-antagonistic agent (nifedipine) combined with methyldopa in the treatment of severe hypertension. Circulation 61:913–919, 1980.

506. Guazzi MD, De Cesare N, Galli C, et al: Calcium-channel blockade with nifedipine and angiotensin converting–enzyme inhibition with captopril in the therapy of patients with severe primary hypertension. Circulation 70:279–284, 1984.

507. Bruun NE, Ibsen H, Nielsen F, et al: Lack of effect of nifedipine on counterregulatory mechanisms in essential hypertension. Hypertension 8:655–661, 1986.

508. Bruun NE, Ibsen H, Skott P, et al: Lithium clearance and renal tubular sodium handling during acute and long-term nifedipine treatment in essential hypertension. Clin Sci 75:609–613, 1988.

509. Reams GP, Hamory A, Lau A, Bauer JH: Effect of nifedipine on renal function in patients with essential hypertension. Hypertension 11:452–456, 1988.

510. Wight JP, Brown CB, El Nahas AM: Short-term effects of calcium antagonists on renal haemodynamics in patients with chronic renal failure. Nephron 58:62–67, 1991.

511. Zucchelli P, Zuccala A, Borghi M, et al: Long-term comparison between captopril and nifedipine in the progression of renal insufficiency. Kidney Int 42:452–458, 1992.

512. Mimran A, Insua A, Ribstein J, et al: Contrasting effects of captopril and nifedipine in normotensive patients with incipient diabetic nephropathy. J Hypertens 6:919–923, 1988.

513. Melbourne Diabetic Nephropathy Study Group: Comparison between perindopril and nifedipine in hypertensive and normotensive diabetic patients with microalbuminuria. BMJ 302:210–216, 1991.

514. Chan JCN, Cockram CS, Nicholls MG, et al: Comparison of enalapril and nifedipine in treating non–insulin dependent diabetic associated with hypertension: One year analysis. BMJ 305:981–985, 1992.

515. Ferder L, Daccordi H, Martello M, et al: Angiotensin converting enzyme inhibitors versus calcium antagonists in the treatment of diabetic hypertensive patients. Hypertension 19(suppl II):237–242, 1992.

516. Romero R, Salinas I, Lucas A, et al: Comparative effects of captopril versus nifedipine on proteinuria and renal function of type 2 diabetic patients. Diabetes Res Clin Pract 17:191–198, 1992.

517. Leonetti G, Sala C, Bianchini C, et al: Antihypertensive and renal effects of orally administered verapamil. Eur J Clin Pharmacol 18:375–382, 1980.

518. de Leeuw PW, Birkenhager WH: Effects of verapamil in hypertensive patients. Acta Med Scand Suppl 681:125–128, 1984.

519. Sorensen SS, Thomsen OO, Danielsen H, Pedersen EB: Effect of verapamil on renal plasma flow, glomerular filtration rate and plasma angiotensin II, aldosterone and arginine vasopressin in essential hypertension. Eur J Clin Pharmacol 29:257–261, 1985.

520. Kubo SH, Cody RJ, Covit AB, et al: The effects of verapamil on renal blood flow, renal function, and neurohormonal profiles in patients with moderate to severe hypertension. J Clin Hypertens 3:38s–46s, 1986.

521. Schnieder RE, Messerli FH, Garavaglia GE, Nunez BD: Cardiovascular effects of verapamil in patients with essential hypertension. Circulation 75:1030–1036, 1987.

522. Katzman PL, Henningsen NC, Fagher B, et al: Renal and endocrine effects of long-term converting enzyme inhibition as compared with calcium antagonism in essential hypertension. J Cardiovasc Pharmacol 15:360–364, 1990.

523. Lenz T, Muller FB, Sotelo JE, et al: Hemodynamic responses to verapamil monotherapy in patients with renal disease. Am J Hypertens 4:939–943, 1991.

524. Reams GP, Lau A, Bauer JH: Short-term and long-term renal response to nifedipine monotherapy. Am J Hypertens 2:188–190, 1989.

525. Klutsch VK, Schmidt P, Grosswendt J: Der Einfluss von BAY a

1040 auf die Nierenfunktion des Hypertonikers. Arzneimittelforschung 22:377–380, 1977.

526. Sunderrajan S, Reams GP, Bauer JH: Renal effects of diltiazem in primary hypertension. Hypertension 8:238–242, 1986.

527. Shima S, Kawashima Y, Hirai M: Studies on cyclic nucleotides in the adrenal gland VIII. Effects of angiotensin on adenosine 3′,5′-monophosphate and steroidogenesis in the adrenal cortex. Endocrinology 103:1361–1367, 1978.

528. Fakunding JL, Chow R, Catt KJ: The role of calcium in the stimulation of aldosterone production by adrenocorticotropin, angiotensin II, and potassium in isolated glomerulosa cells. Endocrinology 105:327–333, 1979.

529. Fakunding JL, Catt KJ: Dependence of aldosterone stimulation in adrenal glomerulosa cells on calcium uptake: Effects of lanthanum and verapamil. Endocrinology 107:1345–1353, 1980.

530. Foster R, Labo MV, Rasmussen H, Marusic ET: Calcium: Its role in the mechanism of action of angiotensin II and potassium in aldosterone production. Endocrinology 109:2196–2201, 1981.

531. Zanchetti A, Leonetti G: Natriuretic effect of calcium antagonists. J Cardiovasc Pharmacol 7(suppl 4):S33–S37, 1985.

532. Zanchetti A, Stella A, Golin R: Adrenergic sodium handling and the natriuretic action of calcium antagonists. J Cardiovasc Pharmacol 7(suppl 6):S194–S198, 1985.

533. MacGregor GA, Pevahouse JB, Cappuccio FP, Markandu ND: Nifedipine, diuretics and sodium balance. J Hypertens 5(suppl 4):S127–S131, 1987.

534. Buhler FR, Kiowski W: Calcium antagonists in hypertension. J Hypertens 5(suppl 3):S3–S10, 1987.

535. Moser M: Calcium entry blockers for systemic hypertension. Am J Cardiol 59:115A–121A, 1987.

536. Thomas T, Vidt DG: Calcium channel blockers in the management of arterial hypertension. Cleve Clin J Med 54:529–536, 1987.

537. Schulte K-L, Meyer-Sabellek WA, Haertenberger A, et al: Antihypertensive and metabolic effects of diltiazem and nifedipine. Hypertension 8:859–865, 1986.

538. Ram CV: Calcium antagonists as antihypertensive agents are effective in all age groups. J Hypertens 5(suppl 4):S115–S118, 1987.

539. Bidiville J, Nussberger J, Waeber G, et al: Individual responses to converting enzyme inhibitors and calcium antagonists. Hypertension 11:166–173, 1988.

540. Kaplan NM: Calcium entry blockers in the treatment of hypertension. JAMA 262:817–823, 1989.

541. Zing W, Ferguson RK, Vlasses PH: Calcium antagonists in elderly and black hypertensive patients. Arch Intern Med 151:2154–2162, 1991.

542. Cubeddu LX, Aranda J, Singh B, et al: A comparison of verapamil and propranolol for the initial treatment of hypertension. Racial differences in response. JAMA 256:2214–2221, 1986.

543. Kiowski W, Buhler FR, Fodayomi MO, et al: Age, race, blood pressure and renin: Predictors for antihypertensive treatment with calcium antagonists. Am J Cardiol 56:81H–85H, 1985.

544. Sever PS, Poulter NR: Calcium antagonists and diuretics as combined therapy. J Hypertens 5(suppl 4):S123–S126, 1987.

545. Trost BN, Weidmann P: Effects of calcium antagonists on glucose homeostasis and serum lipids in non-diabetic and diabetic subjects: A review. J Hypertens 5(suppl 4):S81–S104, 1987.

546. Lewis JG: Adverse reactions to calcium antagonists. Drugs 25:196–222, 1983.

547. Krebs R: Adverse reaction with calcium antagonists. Hypertension 5(suppl II):II-125–II-129, 1983.

548. Russell RP: Side effects of calcium channel blockers. Hypertension 11(suppl II):II-42–II-44, 1988.

549. Johnson BF, Wilson J, Marwaha R, et al: The comparative effects of verapamil and a new dihydropyridine calcium channel blocker on digoxin pharmacokinetics. Clin Pharmacol Ther 42:66–71, 1987.

550. Bailey DP, Spence JD, Munoz C, Arnold JMO: Interaction of citrus juices with felodipine and nifedipine. Lancet 337:268–269, 1991.

551. Bailey DP, Arnold JMO, Munoz C, Spence JD: Grapefruit juice–felodipine interaction: Mechanism, predictability, and effect of naringin. Clin Pharmacol Ther 53:637–642, 1993.

552. Fagard R, Amery A, Lijnen P, Reybronck T: Haemodynamic effects of captopril in hypertensive patients: Comparison with saralasin. Clin Sci 57:131s–134s, 1979.

553. de Bruyn JHB, Man in't Veld AJ, Wenting GJ, et al: Haemodynamic profile of captopril treatment in various forms of hypertension. Eur J Clin Pharmacol 20:163–168, 1981.

554. Fagard R, Bulpitt C, Lijnen P, Amery A: Response of the systemic and pulmonary circulation to converting-enzyme inhibition (captopril) at rest and during exercise in hypertensive patients. Circulation 65:33–39, 1982.

555. Lund-Johansen P, Omvik P: Long-term haemodynamic effects of enalapril (alone and in combination with hydrochlorothiazide) at rest and during exercise in essential hypertension. J Hypertens 2(suppl 2):49–56, 1984.

556. Fouad FM, Tarazi RC, Bravo EL, Textor SC: Hemodynamic and antihypertensive effects of the new oral angiotensin-converting enzyme inhibitor MK421 (enalapril). Hypertension 6:167–174, 1984.

557. Gavras H, Brunner HR, Laragh JH, et al: An angiotensin converting enzyme inhibitor to identify and treat vasoconstrictor and volume factors in hypertensive patients. N Engl J Med 291:817–821, 1974.

558. Case DB, Wallace JM, Keim HJ, et al: Possible role of renin in hypertension as suggested by renin-sodium profiling and inhibition of converting enzyme. N Engl J Med 296:641–646, 1977.

559. Johnston CI, Millar JA, McGrath BP, Matthews PG: Long-term effects of captopril (SQ14225) on blood pressure and hormonal levels in essential hypertension. Lancet 2:493–496, 1979.

560. Atlas SA, Case DB, Sealey JE, et al: Interruption of the renin-angiotensin system in hypertensive patients by captopril induces sustained reduction in aldosterone secretion, potassium retention and natriuresis. Hypertension 1:274–280, 1979.

561. Textor SC, Brunner HR, Gavras H: Converting enzyme inhibition during chronic angiotensin II infusion in rats. Hypertension 3:269–275, 1981.

562. Unger T, Schull B, Hubner D, et al: Plasma converting enzyme activity does not reflect effectiveness of oral treatment with captopril. Eur J Pharmacol 72:255–259, 1981.

563. Velletri P, Bean BL: Comparison of the time course of action of captopril on angiotensin-converting enzyme with the time course of its antihypertensive effect. J Cardiovasc Pharmacol 3:1068–1081, 1981.

564. Cohen ML, Kurz KD: Angiotensin converting enzyme inhibition in tissues from spontaneously hypertensive rats after treatment with captopril or MK421. J Pharmacol Exp Ther 220:63–69, 1982.

565. Unger T, Schull B, Rascher W, et al: Selective activation of the converting enzyme inhibitor MK421 and comparison of its active diacid form with captopril in different tissues of rat. Biochem Pharmacol 31:3063–3070, 1982.

566. Velletri P, Bean BL: The effects of captopril on rat aortic angiotensin-converting enzyme. J Cardiovasc Pharmacol 4:315–325, 1982.

567. Unger T, Ganten D, Lang RE, Scholkens BA: Is tissue converting enzyme inhibition a determinant of the antihypertensive efficacy of converting enzyme inhibitors? J Cardiovasc Pharmacol 6:872–880, 1984.

568. Unger T, Ganten D, Lang RE, Scholkens BA: Persistent tissue converting enzyme inhibition following chronic treatment with Hoe498 and MK421 in spontaneously hypertensive rats. J Cardiovasc Pharmacol 7:36–41, 1985.

569. Antonaccio MJ, Kerwin L: Pre- and post-junctional inhibition of vascular sympathetic function by captopril in SHR. Hypertension 3(suppl I):I-54–I-62, 1981.

570. Imai Y, Abe K, Seino M, et al: Captopril attenuates pressor responses to norepinephrine and vasopressin through depletion of endogenous angiotensin II. Am J Cardiol 49:1537–1539, 1982.

571. Eikenburg DC: Effects of captopril on vascular noradrenergic transmission in SHR. Hypertension 6:660–665, 1984.

572. Richer C, Doussau M-P, Giudicelli J-F: Influence of captopril and enalapril on regional vascular alpha-adrenergic receptor reactivity in SHR. Hypertension 6:666–674, 1984.

573. Cline WH Jr: Enhanced in vivo responsiveness of presynaptic angiotensin II receptor-mediated facilitation of vascular adrenergic neurotransmission in spontaneously hypertensive rats. J Pharmacol Exp Ther 232:661–669, 1985.

574. Vanhoutte PM, Auch-Schwelk W, Biondi ML, et al: Why are converting enzyme inhibitors vasodilators? Br J Clin Pharmacol 28:95s–104s, 1989.

575. Ferrario CM, Jaiswal N, Yamamoto K, Diz DI: Hypertensive mechanisms and converting enzyme inhibitors. Clin Cardiol 14(suppl IV):56–62, 1991.

576. Ferrario CM, Gildenberg PL, McCubbin JW: Cardiovascular effects of angiotensin mediated by the central nervous system. Circ Res 30:257–262, 1972.

577. Unger T, Badoer E, Ganten D, et al: Brain angiotensin: Pathways and pharmacology. Circulation 77(suppl I):I40–I54, 1988.

578. Ganten D, Paul M, Lang RE: The role of neuropeptides in cardiovascular regulation. Cardiovasc Drug Ther 5:119–130, 1991.

579. Nishimura M, Milsted A, Block CH, et al: Tissue renin-angiotensin systems in renal hypertension. Hypertension 20:151–167, 1992.

580. Williams GH, Hollenberg NK: Accentuated vascular and endocrine response to SQ20,881 in hypertension. N Engl J Med 297:184–188, 1977.

581. Thurston H, Swales JD: Converting enzyme inhibitor and saralasin infusion in rats. Circ Res 42:588–592, 1978.

582. Swartz SL, Williams GH, Hollenberg NK, et al: Converting enzyme inhibition in essential hypertension: The hypertensive response does not reflect only reduced angiotensin II formation. Hypertension 1:106–111, 1979.

583. Vinci JM, Horwitz D, Zusman RM, et al: The effect of converting enzyme inhibition with SQ20,881 on plasma and urinary kinins, prostaglandin E, and angiotensin II in hypertensive man. Hypertension 1:416–426, 1979.

584. Mimran A, Targhetta R, Laroche B: The antihypertensive effect of captopril. Hypertension 2:732–737, 1980.

585. Benetos A, Gavras H, Stewart JM, et al: Vasodepressor role of endogenous bradykinin assessed by a bradykinin antagonist. Hypertension 8:971–974, 1986.

586. Carbonell LF, Carretero OA, Stewart JM, Scicli AG: Effect of a kinin antagonist on the acute antihypertensive activity of enalaprilat in severe hypertension. Hypertension 11:239–243, 1988.

587. Danckwardt L, Shimizu I, Bönner G, et al: Converting enzyme inhibition in kinin-deficient Brown Norway rats. Hypertension 16:429–435, 1990.

588. Feletou M, Germain M, Teisseire B: Converting-enzyme inhibitors potentiate bradykinin-induced relaxation in vitro. Am J Physiol 262:H839–H845, 1992.

589. Gavras I: Bradykinin-mediated effects of ACE inhibitors. Kidney Int 42:1020–1029, 1992.

590. Kiowski W, Linder L, Kleinbloesem C, et al: Blood pressure control by the renin-angiotensin system in normotensive subjects. Circulation 85:1–8, 1992.

591. Swartz SL, Williams GH, Hollenberg NK, et al: Captopril induced changes in prostaglandin production. J Clin Invest 65:1257–1264, 1980.

592. Moore TJ, Crantz FR, Hollenberg NK, et al: Contribution of prostaglandins to the antihypertensive action of captopril in essential hypertension. Hypertension 3:168–173, 1981.

593. Silberbauer K, Stanek B, Templ H: Acute hypotensive effect of captopril in man modified by prostaglandin synthesis inhibition. Br J Clin Pharmacol 14:87s–93s, 1982.

594. Witzgall H, Hirsch F, Scherer B, Weber PC: Acute haemodynamic and hormonal effects of captopril are diminished by indomethacin. Clin Sci Mol Med 62:611–615, 1982.

595. Zusman RM: Effects of converting-enzyme inhibitors on the renin-angiotensin-aldosterone, bradykinin, and arachidonic acid–prostaglandin systems: Correlation of chemical structure and biological activity. Am J Kidney Dis 10:13–23, 1987.

596. Wiemer G, Schölkens BA, Becker RHA, Busse R: Ramiprilat enhances endothelial autocoid formation by inhibiting breakdown of endothelium-derived bradykinin. Hypertension 18:558–563, 1991.

597. Gräfe M, Bossaller C, Graf K, et al: Effect of angiotensin-converting enzyme inhibition on bradykinin metabolism by vascular endothelial cells. Am J Physiol 264:H1493–H1497, 1993.

598. Kostis JB: Angiotensin-converting enzyme inhibitors. Am J Hypertens 2:57–64, 1989.

599. Salvetti A: Newer ACE inhibitors. Drugs 40:800–828, 1990.

600. Heel RC, Brogden RN, Speight TM, Avery GS: Captopril: A preliminary review of its pharmacological properties and therapeutic efficacy. Drugs 20:409–452, 1980.

601. Rommel AJ, Pierides AM, Heald A: Captopril elimination in chronic renal failure. Clin Pharmacol Ther 27:282A, 1980.

602. Ferguson RK, Vlasses PH: Clinical pharmacology and therapeutic applications of the new oral angiotensin converting enzyme inhibitor, captopril. Am Heart J 101:650–656, 1981.

603. Vidt DG, Bravo EL, Fouad FM: Captopril. N Engl J Med 306:214–219, 1982.

604. Veterans Administration Cooperative Study Group on Antihypertensive Agents: Time course of antihypertensive effect of low dose

captopril in mild to moderate hypertension. Clin Pharmacol Ther 36:307–314, 1984.

605. Brogden RN, Todd PA, Sorkin EM: Captopril. An update of its pharmacodynamic and pharmacokinetic properties, and therapeutic use in hypertension and congestive heart failure. Drugs 36:540–600, 1988.

606. Al-Furaih TA, McElnay JC, Elborn JS, et al: Sublingual captopril—a pharmacokinetic and pharmacodynamic evaluation. Eur J Clin Pharmacol 40:393–398, 1991.

607. Kaiser G, Ackermann R, Sioufi A: Pharmacokinetics of a new angiotensin-converting enzyme inhibitor, benazepril hydrochloride, in special populations. Am Heart J 117:746–750, 1989.

608. Balfour JA, Goak L: Benazepril. A review of its pharmacodynamic and pharmacokinetic properties and therapeutic efficacy in hypertension and congestive heart failure. Drugs 42:511–539, 1991.

609. Shionoiri H, Ueda S, Minanisawa K, et al: Pharmacokinetics and pharmacodynamics of benazepril in patients with normal and impaired renal function. J Cardiovasc Pharmacol 20:343–357, 1992.

610. Ulm EH: Enalapril maleate (MK421), a potent, nonsulfhydryl angiotensin-converting enzyme inhibitor: Absorption, disposition, and metabolism in man. Drug Metab Rev 14:99–110, 1983.

611. Davies RO, Gomez JH, Irvin JD, Walker JF: An overview of the clinical pharmacology of enalapril. Br J Clin Pharmacol 18:215s–229s, 1984.

612. Abrams WB, Davies RO, Gomez HJ: Clinical pharmacology of enalapril. J Hypertens 2(suppl 2):31–36, 1984.

613. Riley LJ, Vlasses PH, Ferguson RK: Clinical pharmacology and therapeutic applications of the new oral converting enzyme inhibitor, enalapril. Am Heart J 109:1085–1089, 1985.

614. Lowenthal DT, Irvin JD, Merrill D, et al: The effect of renal function on enalapril kinetics. Clin Pharmacol Ther 38:661–666, 1985.

615. Todd PA, Goa KL: Enalapril. A reappraisal of its pharmacology and therapeutic use in hypertension. Drugs 43:346–381, 1992.

616. van Schaik BAM, Geyskes GG, Boer P: Lisinopril in hypertensive patients with and without renal failure. Eur J Clin Pharmacol 32:11–16, 1987.

617. Gomez HJ, Cirillo VJ, Moncloa F: The clinical pharmacology of lisinopril. J Cardiovasc Pharmacol 9(suppl 3):S27–S34, 1987.

618. Arzubiaga C, Beck NA: Lisinopril, a new angiotensin converting enzyme inhibitor. Am J Med Sci 303:340–344, 1992.

619. van Schaik BAM, Geyskes GG, van der Wouw PA, et al: Pharmacokinetics of lisinopril in hypertensive patients with normal and impaired renal function. Eur J Clin Pharmacol 34:61–65, 1988.

620. Lancaster SG, Todd PA: Lisinopril. A preliminary review of its pharmacodynamic and pharmacokinetic properties, and therapeutic use in hypertension and congestive heart failure. Drugs 35:646–669, 1988.

621. Blum RA, Olson SC, Kohli RK, et al: Pharmacokinetics of quinapril and its active metabolite, quinaprilat, in patients on chronic hemodialysis. J Clin Pharmacol 30:938–942, 1990.

622. Wadworth AN, Brogden RN: Quinapril. A review of its pharmacological properties, and therapeutic efficacy in cardiovascular disorders. Drugs 41:378–399, 1991.

623. Halstenson CE, Opsahl JA, Rachael K, et al: The pharmacokinetics of quinapril and its active metabolite, quinaprilat, in patients with various degrees of renal function. J Clin Pharmacol 32:344–350, 1992.

624. Kindler J, Schunkert H, Gassmann M, et al: Therapeutic efficacy and tolerance of ramipril in hypertensive patients with renal failure. J Cardiovasc Pharmacol 13(suppl 3):S55–S58, 1989.

625. Schunkert H, Kindler J, Gassmann M, et al: Pharmacokinetics of ramipril in hypertensive patients with renal insufficiency. Eur J Clin Pharmacol 37:248–256, 1989.

626. Todd PA, Benfield P: Ramipril. A review of its pharmacological properties and therapeutic efficacy in cardiovascular disorders. Drugs 39:110–135, 1990.

627. Duchin KL, Waclawski AP, Tu JI, et al: Pharmacokinetics, safety, and pharmacologic effects of fosinopril sodium, an angiotensin-converting enzyme inhibitor in healthy subjects. J Clin Pharmacol 31:58–64, 1991.

628. Hui KK, Duchin KL, Kripalani KJ, et al: Pharmacokinetics of fosinopril in patients with various degrees of renal function. Clin Pharmacol Ther 49:457–467, 1991.

629. Sica DA, Cutler RE, Parmer RJ, Ford NF: Comparison of the steady-state pharmacokinetics of fosinopril, lisinopril and enalapril in pa-

tients with chronic renal insufficiency. Clin Pharmacokinet 20:420–427, 1991.

630. Murdoch D, McTavish D: Fosinopril. A review of its pharmacodynamic and pharmacokinetic properties, and therapeutic potential in essential hypertension. Drugs 43:123–140, 1982.

631. Bauer JH, Reams GP: Renal effects of angiotensin converting enzyme inhibitors in hypertension. Am J Med 81(suppl 4C):19–27, 1986.

632. Brunner HR, Waeber B, Nussberger J: Renal effects of converting enzyme inhibition. J Cardiovasc Pharmacol 9(suppl 3):S6–S14, 1987.

633. Williams GH, Hollenberg NK: Accentuated vascular and endocrine response to SQ20,881 in hypertension. N Engl J Med 297:184–188, 1977.

634. Hollenberg NK, Swartz SL, Passan DR, Williams GH: Increased glomerular filtration rate after converting-enzyme inhibition in essential hypertension. N Engl J Med 301:9–12, 1979.

635. Hollenberg NK, Meggs LG, Williams GH, et al: Sodium intake and renal responses to captopril in normal man and essential hypertension. Kidney Int 20:240–245, 1981.

636. Simon G, Morioka S, Snyder DK, Cohn JN: Increased renal plasma flow in long-term enalapril treatment of hypertension. Clin Pharmacol Ther 34:459–465, 1983.

637. Larochelle P, Gutkowska J, Schiffrin E, et al: Effect of enalapril on renin, angiotensin converting enzyme activity, aldosterone and prostaglandins in patients with hypertension. Clin Invest Med 8:197–201, 1985.

638. Bauer JH, Gaddy P: Effects of enalapril alone, and in combination with hydrochlorothiazide, on renin-angiotensin-aldosterone, renal function, salt and water excretion, and body fluid composition. Am J Kidney Dis 6:222–232, 1985.

639. Reams GP, Bauer JH: Long-term effects of enalapril monotherapy and enalapril/hydrochlorothiazide combination therapy on blood pressure, renal function, and body fluid composition. J Clin Hypertens 2:55–63, 1986.

640. Bauer JH, Reams GP, Lal SM: Renal protective effect of strict blood pressure control with enalapril therapy. Arch Intern Med 147:1397–1400, 1987.

641. Maruyama A, Ogihara T, Naka T, et al: Long-term effects of captopril in hypertension. Clin Pharmacol Ther 28:316–323, 1980.

642. Pessina AC, Gatta A, Semplicini A, et al: Hypotensive and renal effects of captopril. Eur J Clin Invest 11:409–413, 1981.

643. Aldigier J-C, Plouin P-F, Guyene TT, et al: Comparison of the hormonal and renal effects of captopril in severe essential and renovascular hypertension. Am J Cardiol 49:1447–1452, 1982.

644. Kiowski W, van Brummelen P, Hulthen L, et al: Antihypertensive and renal effects of captopril in relation to renin activity and bradykinin-induced vasodilation. Clin Pharmacol Ther 31:677–684, 1982.

645. Palla R, Marchitiello ME, Sassano P, Salvetti A: Effect of captopril on renal function in patients with essential hypertension. Am J Cardiol 49:1577–1579, 1982.

646. Duchin KL, Willard DA: The effect of captopril on renal hemodynamics in hypertensive patients. J Clin Pharmacol 24:351–359, 1984.

647. DeVenuto G, Andreotti C, Mattarei M, Pegoretti G: Prolonged treatment of essential hypertension and renal function: Comparison of captopril and beta blockers considering microproteinuria values. Curr Ther Res 38:710–718, 1985.

648. Ventura HO, Frohlich ED, Messerli FH, et al: Cardiovascular effects and regional blood flow distribution associated with angiotensin converting enzyme inhibition (captopril) in essential hypertension. Am J Cardiol 55:1023–1026, 1985.

649. Ando K, Fujita T, Ito Y, et al: The role of renal hemodynamics in the antihypertensive effect of captopril. Am Heart J 111:347–352, 1986.

650. Rasmussen S, Leth A, Ibsen H, et al: Converting enzyme inhibition in mild and moderate essential hypertension. Acta Med Scand 219:29–36, 1986.

651. Thomsen OO, Danielsen H, Sorensen SS, Pedersen EB: Effect of captopril on renal hemodynamics and the renin-angiotensin-aldosterone and osmoregulatory systems in essential hypertension. Eur J Clin Pharmacol 30:1–6, 1986.

652. Shionoiri H, Yasuda G, Takagi N, et al: Renal haemodynamics and comparative effects of captopril in patients with benign- or malignant-essential hypertension, or with chronic renal failure. Clin Exp Hypertens A 49:543–549, 1987.

653. Gararaglia GE, Messerli FH, Nunez BD, et al: Angiotensin convert-ing enzyme inhibition. Disparities in the mechanism of their antihy-pertensive effect. Am J Hypertens 1:214–216, 1988.

654. Penner SB, Mitenko PA, Aoki FY, et al: Long-term captopril in young and old patients with mild hypertension. J Clin Pharmacol 31:65–71, 1991.

655. Herlitz H, Edeno C, Mulec H, et al: Captopril treatment of hyperten-sion and renal failure in systemic lupus erythematosus. Nephron 38:253–256, 1984.

656. Laher MS, O'Donohoe JF, O'Regan P, Counihan TB: Captopril for refractory hypertension in patients with impaired renal function. J R Soc Med 78:367–372, 1985.

657. Lagrue G, Robeva R, Laurent J: Antiproteinuric effect of captopril in primary glomerular disease. Nephron 46:99–100, 1987.

658. Ruilope LM, Miranda B, Morales JM, et al: Converting enzyme inhibition in chronic renal failure. Am J Kidney Dis 13:120–126, 1989.

659. Smith WGJ, Dharmasena AD, El Nahas AM, et al: Short-term effect of captopril on renal haemodynamics in chronic renal failure. Ne-phrol Dial Transplant 4:696–700, 1989.

660. Rodicio JL, Alcazar JM, Ruilope LM: Influence of converting en-zyme inhibition on glomerular filtration rate and proteinuria. Kidney Int 38:590–594, 1990.

661. Praga M, Hernandez E, Montoyo C, et al: Long-term beneficial effects of angiotensin-converting enzyme inhibition in patients with nephrotic proteinuria. Am J Kidney Dis 20:240–248, 1992.

662. Bjorck S, Herlitz H, Nyberg G, et al: Effect of captopril on renal hemodynamics in the treatment of resistant renal hypertension. Hy-pertension 5(suppl III):152–153, 1983.

663. Taguma Y, Kitamoto Y, Futaki G, et al: Effect of captopril on heavy proteinuria in azotemic diabetics. N Engl J Med 313:1617–1620, 1985.

664. Bjorck S, Nyberg G, Mulec H, et al: Beneficial effects of angiotensin converting enzyme inhibition on renal function in patients with dia-betic nephropathy. BMJ 293:471–474, 1986.

665. Parving H-H, Hommel E, Smidt UM: Protection of kidney function and decrease in albuminuria by captopril in insulin dependent dia-betes with nephropathy. BMJ 297:1089–1091, 1988.

666. Cook J, Daneman D, Spino M, et al: Angiotensin converting enzyme inhibitors therapy to decrease microalbuminuria in normotensive children with insulin-dependent diabetes mellitus. J Pediatr 117:39–45, 1990.

667. Mathiesen ER, Hommel E, Giese J, Parving H-H: Efficacy of capto-pril in postponing nephropathy in normotensive insulin dependent diabetic patients with microalbuminuria. BMJ 303:81–87, 1991.

668. Lacourciere Y, Nadeau A, Poirier L, Tancrede G: Captopril or con-ventional therapy in hypertensive type II diabetics. Three-year anal-ysis. Hypertension 21:786–794, 1993.

669. Valvo E, Casagrande P, Bedogna V, et al: Systemic and renal effects of an angiotensin converting enzyme inhibitor, benazepril, in essen-tial hypertension. J Hypertens 8:991–995, 1990.

670. Bedogna V, Valvo E, Casagrande P, et al: Effects of ACE inhibition in normotensive patients with chronic glomerular disease and normal renal function. Kidney Int 39:101–107, 1990.

671. de Leeuw PW, Hoogma RPLM, van Soest GAW, et al: Humoral and renal effects of MK-421 (enalapril) in hypertensive subjects. J Car-diovasc Pharmacol 5:731–736, 1983.

672. Navis GJ, de Jong PE, Donker AJM, de Zeeuw D: Effects of enala-pril on blood pressure and renal haemodynamics in essential hyper-tension. Proc Eur Dial Transplant Assoc 20:577–581, 1983.

673. Simon G, Marioka S, Snyder DK, Cohn JN: Increased renal plasma flow in long-term enalapril treatment of hypertension. Clin Pharma-col Ther 34:459–465, 1983.

674. Dunn FG, Oigman W, Ventura HO, et al: Enalapril improves sys-temic and renal hemodynamics and allows regression of left ventric-ular mass in essential hypertension. Am J Cardiol 53:105–108, 1984.

675. Dupont AG, Vanderniepen P, Bossuyt AM, et al: Effect of enalapril on ambulatory blood pressure, renal hemodynamics and cardiac function in essential hypertension. Acta Cardiol 41:353–358, 1986.

676. Reams GP, Bauer JH: Acute and chronic effects of angiotensin converting enzyme inhibitors on the essential hypertensive kidney. Cardiovasc Drugs Ther 4:207–219, 1990.

677. Chaignon M, Moreau L: Effets de l'inhibition de l'enzyme de con-version par l'enalapril sur l'hémodynamique rénale dans l'hyperten-sion artérielle essentielle. Presse Med 17:1745–1747, 1988.

678. Corastelli P, Buongiorno E, Giannattasio M, Passavanti G: Antihy-pertensive efficacy of enalapril maleate on impaired renal function. Kidney Int 34(suppl 25):S204–S206, 1988.

679. Bianchi S, Bigazzi R, Baldari G, Campese VM: Microalbuminuria in patients with essential hypertension. Am J Hypertens 4:291–296, 1991.

680. Reams GP, Bauer JH: Effect of enalapril in subjects with hyperten-sion associated with moderate to severe renal dysfunction. Arch Intern Med 146:2145–2148, 1986.

681. Abraham PA, Opsahl JA, Halstenson CE, Keane WF: Efficacy and renal effects of enalapril therapy for hypertensive patients with chronic renal insufficiency. Arch Intern Med 148:2358–2362, 1988.

682. Grazi G, Cirami C, Panichi V, et al: Renal effects of enalapril in hypertensive patients with glomerulonephritis. Nephrol Dial Trans-plant 4:396–398, 1989.

683. Ajayi AA, Ajayi AT: Angiotensin converting enzyme inhibition re-duces proteinuria in Nigerians with chronic renal disease. Eur J Clin Pharmacol 39:423–424, 1990.

684. Ferder LF, Inserra F, Daccordi H, et al: Effects of enalapril on renal parameters in patients with primary glomerulopathies associated with chronic renal failure. Drugs 39(suppl 2):40–46, 1990.

685. Ferder LF, Inserra F, Daccordi H, Smith RD: Enalapril improved renal function and proteinuria in chronic glomerulopathies. Nephron 55(suppl 1):90–95, 1990.

686. Kamper A-L, Nielsen OJ: Effect of enalapril on haemoglobin and serum erythropoietin in patients with chronic nephropathy. Scand J Clin Invest 50:611–618, 1990.

687. Rekola S, Bergstrand A, Bucht H: Deterioration rate in hypertensive IgA nephropathy: Comparison of a converting enzyme inhibitor and β-blocking agents. Nephron 59:57–60, 1991.

688. Remuzzi A, Perticucci E, Ruggenenti P, et al: Angiotensin convert-ing enzyme inhibition improves glomerular size-selectivity in IgA nephropathy. Kidney Int 39:1267–1273, 1991.

689. Thomas DM, Hillis AN, Coles GA, et al: Enalapril can treat the proteinuria of membranous glomerulonephritis without detriment to systemic or renal hemodynamics. Am J Kidney Dis 18:38–43, 1991.

690. Ruilope LM, Casal MC, Praga M, et al: Additive antiproteinuric effect of converting enzyme inhibition and a low protein intake. J Am Soc Nephrol 3:1307–1311, 1992.

691. Marre M, Chatellier G, Leblanc H, et al: Prevention of diabetic nephropathy with enalapril in normotensive diabetics with microal-buminuria. BMJ 297:1092–1095, 1988.

692. Morelli E, Loon N, Meyer T, et al: Effects of converting-enzyme inhibition on barrier function in diabetic glomerulopathy. Diabetes 39:76–82, 1990.

693. Rudberg S, Aperia A, Freyschuss U, Persson B: Enalapril reduces microalbuminuria in young normotensive type 1 (insulin-dependent) diabetic patients irrespective of its hypotensive effect. Diabetologia 33:470–476, 1990.

694. Pedersen MM, Christensen CK, Hansen KW, et al: ACE-inhibition and renoprotection in early diabetic nephropathy. Response to enal-april acutely and in long-term combination with conventional anti-hypertensive treatment. Clin Invest Med 14:642–651, 1991.

695. Bauer JH, Reams GP, Hewett J, Klachko D: A randomized, double-blind, placebo-controlled trial to evaluate the effect of enalapril in patients with clinical diabetic nephropathy. Am J Kidney Dis 20:443–457, 1992.

696. Hallab M, Gallois Y, Chatellier G, et al: Comparison of reduction in microalbuminuria by enalapril and hydrochlorothiazide in normoten-sive patients with insulin dependent diabetes. BMJ 306:175–182, 1993.

697. Ravid M, Savin H, Jutrin I, et al: Long-term stabilizing effect of angiotensin-converting enzyme inhibition on plasma creatinine and on proteinuria in normotensive type II diabetic patients. Ann Intern Med 118:577–581, 1993.

698. Giorgi DMA, Giorgi MCP, Burdmann E, et al: Effects of MK-521 (lisinopril) on the renal plasma flow and renin-angiotensin-aldoste-rone system in patients with essential hypertension. J Hypertens 4(suppl 5):S420–S422, 1986.

699. Donohoe JF, Laher H, Doyle GD, et al: Lisinopril in hypertension associated with renal impairment. J Cardiovasc Pharmacol 9(suppl 3):S66–S68, 1987.

700. Dupont AG, Van der Niepen P, Valchaert A, et al: Improved renal function during chronic lisinopril treatment in moderate to severe primary hypertension. J Cardiovasc Pharmacol 10(suppl 7):S148–S150, 1987.

701. Reams GP, Bauer JH: Effect of lisinopril monotherapy on renal hemodynamics. Am J Kidney Dis 11:499–507, 1988.

702. Laher MS: Lisinopril in elderly patients with hypertension. Drugs 39(suppl 2):55–63, 1990.

703. Degaute JP, Leeman M, Reuse C, et al: Acute and chronic effects of lisinopril on renal and systemic hemodynamics in hypertension. Cardiovasc Drugs Ther 6:489–494, 1992.

704. Heeg JE, de Jong PE, van der Hem GK, de Zeeuw D: Reduction of proteinuria by angiotensin converting enzyme inhibition. Kidney Int 32:78–83, 1987.

705. August P, Cody RJ, Sealey JE, Laragh JH: Hemodynamic responses to converting enzyme inhibition in patients with renal disease. Am J Hypertens 2:599–603, 1989.

706. de Jong PE, Apperloo AJ, Heeg JE, de Zeeuw D: Lisinopril in hypertensive patients with renal function impairment. Nephron 55(suppl 1):43–48, 1990.

707. Heeg JE, de Jong PE, van der Hem GK, de Zeeuw D: Angiotensin II does not acutely reverse the reduction of proteinuria by long-term ACE inhibition. Kidney Int 40:734–741, 1991.

708. Gansevoort RT, de Zeeuw D, de Jong PE: Long-term benefits of the antiproteinuric effect of angiotensin-converting enzyme inhibition in nondiabetic renal disease. Am J Kidney Dis 22:202–206, 1993.

709. Gupta RK, Kjeldsen SE, Krause L, et al: Hemodynamic effects of quinapril, a novel angiotensin-converting enzyme inhibitor. Clin Pharmacol Ther 48:41–49, 1990.

710. de Leeuw PW, Birkenhager WH: Short- and long-term effects of ramipril in hypertension. Am J Cardiol 59:79D–82D, 1987.

711. Hirata Y, Ishi M, Sagimoto T, et al: Cardiovascular and renal effects of the converting enzyme inhibitor ramipril in patients with essential hypertension. Curr Ther Res 45:967–974, 1989.

712. al-Nahhas AM, Nimmon CC, Britton KE, et al: The effect of ramipril, a new angiotensin-converting enzyme inhibitor on cortical nephron flow and effective renal plasma flow in patients with essential hypertension. Nephron 54:47–52, 1990.

713. Marre M, Hallab M, Billiard A, et al: Small doses of ramipril to reduce microalbuminuria in diabetic patients with incipient nephropathy independently of blood pressure changes. J Cardiovasc Pharmacol 18:165–168, 1991.

714. Pedersen MM, Hansen KW, Schmitz A, et al: Effects of ACE inhibitor supplementary to beta blockers and diuretics in early diabetic nephropathy. Kidney Int 41:883–890, 1992.

715. Oren S, Messerli FH, Grossman E, et al: Immediate and short-term cardiovascular effects of fosinopril, a new angiotensin-converting enzyme inhibitor, in patients with essential hypertension. J Am Coll Cardiol 17:1183–1187, 1991.

716. Williams GH, Tuck ML, Sullivan JM, et al: Parallel adrenal and renal abnormalities in young patients with essential hypertension. Am J Med 72:907–914, 1982.

717. Shoback DM, Williams GH, Moore TJ, et al: Effect in the sodium-modulated tissue responsiveness to angiotensin II in essential hypertension. J Clin Invest 72:2115–2124, 1983.

718. Redgrave J, Rabinowe S, Hollenberg NK, Williams GH: Correction of abnormal renal blood flow response to angiotensin II by converting enzyme inhibition in essential hypertension. J Clin Invest 75:1285–1290, 1985.

719. Hommel E, Parving H-H, Mathiesen E, et al: Effect of captopril on kidney function in insulin-dependent diabetic patients with nephropathy. BMJ 293:467–470, 1986.

720. Marre M, Leblanc H, Suarez L, et al: Converting enzyme inhibition and kidney function in normotensive diabetic patients with persistent microalbuminuria. BMJ 294:1448–1452, 1987.

721. Kasiske BL, Kalil RSN, Ma JZ, et al: Effect of antihypertensive therapy on the kidney in patients with diabetes: A meta-regression analysis. Ann Intern Med 118:129–138, 1993.

722. Heeg JE, de Jong PE, van der Hem GK, de Zeeuw D: Efficacy and variability of the antiproteinuric effect of ACE inhibition by lisinopril. Kidney Int 36:272–279, 1989.

723. ter Wee PM, Epstein M: Angiotensin-converting enzyme inhibitors and progression of nondiabetic chronic renal disease. Arch Intern Med 153:1749–1759, 1993.

724. de Zeeuw D, Heeg JE, Stelwagen T, et al: Mechanism of the antiproteinuric effect of angiotensin-converting enzyme inhibition. Contrib Nephrol 83:160–165, 1990.

725. Heeg JE, de Jong PE, de Zeeuw D: Additive antiproteinuric effect of angiotensin converting enzyme inhibition and non-steroidal anti-inflammatory drug therapy: A clue to the mechanism of action. Clin Sci 81:367–372, 1991.

726. Gransevoort RT, de Zeeuw D, de Jong PE: Dissociation between the course of the hemodynamic antiproteinuric effects of angiotensin I converting enzyme inhibition. Kidney Int 44:579–584, 1993.

727. Prins EJL, Hoorntje SJ, Weening JJ, Donker AJ: Nephrotic syndrome in patient on captopril. Lancet 2:306–307, 1979. Letter.

728. Hoorntje SJ, Kallenberg CGM, Weening JJ, et al: Immune-complex glomerulopathy in patients treated with captopril. Lancet 1:1212–1215, 1980.

729. Case DB, Atlas SA, Mouradian JA, et al: Proteinuria during long-term captopril therapy. JAMA 244:346–349, 1980.

730. Sunderrajan S, Luger A, Bauer JH: Captopril-induced membranous glomerulopathy. South Med J 76:1294–1297, 1983.

731. Textor SC, Gephardt GN, Bravo EL, et al: Membranous glomerulopathy associated with captopril therapy. Am J Med 74:705–712, 1983.

732. Sturgill BC, Shearlock KT: Membranous glomerulopathy and nephrotic syndrome after captopril therapy. JAMA 250:2343–2345, 1983.

733. Madeddu P, Ena P, Dessi-Fulgheri P, et al: Captopril-induced proteinuria in hypertensive psoriatic patients. Nephron 44:358–360, 1986.

734. Lewis EJ: Proteinuria and abnormalities of the renal glomerulus in patients with hypertension. Clin Exp Pharmacol Physiol Suppl 7:105–115, 1982.

735. Frohlich ED, Cooper RA, Lewis EJ: Review of the overall experience of captopril in hypertension. Arch Intern Med 144:1441–1444, 1984.

736. Murphy BF, Whitworth JA, Kincaid-Smith P: Renal insufficiency with combinations of angiotensin converting enzyme inhibitors and diuretics. Br Med J 288:844–845, 1984.

737. Hricik DE, Browning PJ, Kopelman R, et al: Captopril-induced functional renal insufficiency in patients with bilateral renal artery stenosis or renal artery stenosis in a solitary kidney. N Engl J Med 308:373–376, 1983.

738. Hollenberg NK: Medical therapy of renovascular hypertension: Efficacy and safety of captopril in 269 patients. Cardiovasc Rev Rep 4:852–876, 1983.

739. Curtis JJ, Luke RG, Whelchel JD, et al: Inhibition of angiotensin converting enzyme in renal transplant recipients with hypertension. N Engl J Med 308:377–381, 1983.

740. Wenting GJ, Tan-Tjiong HL, Derkx FHM, et al: Split renal function after captopril in unilateral renal artery stenosis. Br Med J 288:886–890, 1984.

741. Bender W, LaFrance N, Walker WG: Mechanism of deterioration in renal function in patients with renovascular hypertension treated with enalapril. Hypertension 6(suppl I):I-193–I-197, 1984.

742. Textor SC, Novick AC, Tarazi RC, et al: Critical perfusion pressure for renal function in patients with bilateral atherosclerotic renal vascular disease. Ann Intern Med 102:308–314, 1985.

743. Reams GP, Bauer JH, Gaddy P: Use of the converting enzyme inhibitor enalapril in renovascular hypertension. Hypertension 8:290–297, 1986.

744. Miyamori I, Yasuhara S, Takeda Y, et al: Effects of converting enzyme inhibition on split renal function in renovascular hypertension. Hypertension 8:415–421, 1986.

745. Jackson B, McGrath BP, Matthews G, et al: Differential renal function during angiotensin converting enzyme inhibition in renovascular hypertension. Hypertension 8:650–654, 1986.

746. Levenson DJ, Dzau VJ: Effects of angiotensin-converting enzyme inhibition on renal hemodynamics in renal artery stenosis. Kidney Int 31(suppl 20):S-173–S-179, 1987.

747. Hricik DE, Dunn MJ: Angiotensin-converting enzyme inhibitor–induced renal failure—causes, consequences, and diagnostic uses. J Am Soc Nephrol 1:845–858, 1990.

748. Gavras H, Brunner HR, Turini GA, et al: Antihypertensive effect of the oral angiotensin converting–enzyme inhibitor SQ14,225 in man. N Engl J Med 298:991–995, 1978.

749. Atkinson AB, Morton JJ, Brown JJ, et al: Captopril in clinical hypertension. Br Heart J 44:290–296, 1980.

750. Millar JA, McGrath BP, Matthews PG, Johnston CI: Acute effects of captopril on blood pressure and circulating hormone levels in salt-replete and depleted normal subjects and essential hypertensive patients. Clin Sci 61:75–83, 1981.

751. Gavras H, Biollaz J, Waeber B, et al: Antihypertensive effect of the

new oral angiotensin converting enzyme inhibitor "MK421." Lancet 2:543–547, 1981.

752. Ogihara T, Maruyama A, Hata T, et al: Hormonal responses to long-term converting enzyme inhibitors in hypertensive patients. Clin Pharmacol Ther 30:328–335, 1981.

753. Biollaz J, Brunner HR, Gavras I, et al: Antihypertensive therapy with MK421: Angiotensin II–renin relationship to evaluate efficacy of converting enzyme blockade. J Cardiovasc Pharmacol 4:966–972, 1982.

754. Riegger GA, Steilner H, Hayduk K, Liebau G: Captopril in the long-term treatment of essential hypertension: Changes in the renin-angiotensin-aldosterone system. Am J Cardiol 49:1555–1557, 1982.

755. Lijnen P, Staessen J, Fagard R, Amery A: Increase in plasma aldosterone during prolonged captopril treatment. Am J Cardiol 49:1561–1563, 1982.

756. Atkinson AB, Cumming AMM, Brown JJ, et al: Captopril treatment: Interdose variation in renin, angiotensin I and II, aldosterone and blood pressure. Br J Clin Pharmacol 13:855–858, 1982.

757. Hodsman GP, Zabludowski JR, Zoccali C, et al: Enalapril (MK421) and its lysine analogue (MK521): A comparison of acute and chronic effects on blood pressure, renin-angiotensin system and sodium excretion in normal man. Br J Clin Pharmacol 17:233–241, 1984.

758. Johnston CI, Jackson BJ, Larmour I, et al: Plasma enalapril levels and hormonal levels after short- and long-term administration in essential hypertension. Br J Clin Pharmacol 18:233S–239S, 1984.

759. Reams GP, Bauer JH: Humoral effects of long-term oral enalapril therapy. Am J Kidney Dis 7:402–406, 1986.

760. Nussberger J, Brunner DB, Waeber B, Brunner HR: True versus immunoreactive angiotensin II in human plasma. Hypertension 7(suppl I):I-1–I-7, 1985.

761. Nussberger J, Brunner DB, Waeber B, Brunner HR: Specific measurement of angiotensin metabolites and in vitro generated angiotensin II in plasma. Hypertension 8:476–482, 1986.

762. Souther ME, Lumpkin RH, Kuo K, et al: High-performance liquid chromatographic–radioimmunoassay method for the measurement of angiotensin II peptides in human plasma. J Chromatogr Biomed Appl 417:27–40, 1987.

763. Nussberger J, Waeber G, Waeber B, et al: Plasma angiotensin-(1–8) octapeptide measurement to assess acute angiotensin-converting enzyme inhibition with captopril administered parenterally to normal subjects. J Cardiovasc Pharmacol 11:716–721, 1988.

764. Burnier M, Waeber B, Nussberger J, Brunner HR: Pharmacokinetics of angiotensin converting enzyme inhibitors. Br J Clin Pharmacol 28:133S–140S, 1989.

765. Mooser V, Nussberger J, Juillerat L, et al: Reactive hyperreninemia is a major determinant of plasma angiotensin II during ACE inhibition. J Cardiovasc Pharmacol 15:276–282, 1990.

766. Juillerat L, Nussberger J, Menard J, et al: Determinants of angiotensin II generation during converting enzyme inhibition. Hypertension 16:564–572, 1990.

767. van den Meiracker AH, Man in't Veld AJ, Admiraal PJJ, et al: Partial escape of angiotensin converting enzyme (ACE) inhibition during prolonged ACE inhibitor treatment: Does it exist and does it affect the antihypertensive response? J Hypertens 10:803–812, 1992.

768. Brunner HR, Gavras H, Waeber B, et al: Oral angiotensin converting enzyme inhibitor in long-term treatment of hypertensive patients. Ann Intern Med 90:19–23, 1979.

769. Case DB, Atlas SA, Sullivan PA, Laragh JH: Acute and chronic treatment of severe and malignant hypertension with the oral angiotensin-converting enzyme inhibitor captopril. Circulation 64:765–771, 1981.

770. Karlberg BE, Asplund J, Nilsson OR, et al: Captopril, an orally active converting enzyme inhibitor, in the treatment of primary hypertension. Acta Med Scand 209:245–252, 1981.

771. Ferguson RK, Vlasses PH, Swanson BN, et al: Comparison of the effects of captopril, diuretic and their combination in low- and normal-renin essential hypertension. Life Sci 30:59–65, 1982.

772. Weinberger MH: Comparison of captopril and hydrochlorothiazide alone and in combination in mild to moderate essential hypertension. Br J Clin Pharmacol 14:127s–131s, 1982.

773. Vlasses PH, Rotmensch HH, Swanson BN, et al: Comparative antihypertensive effects of enalapril maleate and hydrochlorothiazide, alone and in combination. J Clin Pharmacol 23:227–233, 1983.

774. Williams GH: Converting enzyme inhibitors in the treatment of hypertension. N Engl J Med 319:1517–1525, 1988.

775. McAreavey D, Robertson JIS: Angiotensin converting enzyme inhibitors and moderate hypertension. Drugs 40:326–345, 1990.

776. Townsend RR, Holland DB: Combination of converting enzyme inhibitor with diuretic for the treatment of hypertension. Arch Intern Med 150:1175–1183, 1990.

777. Holland OB, Von Kuhnert L, Campbell WB, Anderson RJ: Synergistic effect of captopril with hydrochlorothiazide for the treatment of low-renin hypertensive black patients. Hypertension 5:235–239, 1983.

778. Veterans Administration Cooperative Study Group on Antihypertensive Agents: Low-dose captopril for the treatment of mild to moderate hypertension. Arch Intern Med 144:1947–1953, 1984.

779. Freier PA, Wallam GL, Hall WD, et al: Blood pressure, plasma volume, and catecholamine levels during enalapril therapy in blacks with hypertension. Clin Pharmacol Ther 36:731–737, 1984.

780. Weinberger WH: Blood pressure and metabolic responses to hydrochlorothiazide, captopril, and the combination in black and white mild-to-moderate hypertensive patients. J Cardiovasc Pharmacol 7:S52–S55, 1985.

781. Jenkins AC, Knill JR, Dreslinski GR: Captopril in the treatment of the elderly hypertensive patient. Arch Intern Med 145:2029–2031, 1985.

782. M'Buyamba-Kabangu JR, Fagard R, Lijnen P, et al: ACE-inhibitors in the treatment of elderly hypertensives. Geriatrics 42:45–49, 1987.

783. Woo J, Woo KS, Kin T, Vallance-Owen J: A single-blind, randomized, cross over study of angiotensin-converting enzyme inhibitor and triampterene and hydrochlorothiazide in the treatment of mild to moderate hypertension in the elderly. Arch Intern Med 147:1386–1389, 1987.

784. Laher MS, Natin D, Rao SK, et al: Lisinopril in elderly patients with hypertension. J Cardiovasc Pharmacol 9(suppl 3):S69–S71, 1987.

785. Fries ED, the Veterans Administration Cooperative Study Group on Antihypertensive Drugs: Age and antihypertensive drugs (hydrochlorothiazide, bendroflumethiazide, nadolol and captopril). Am J Cardiol 61:117–121, 1988.

786. Pollare T, Lithell H, Berne C: A comparison of the effects of hydrochlorothiazide and captopril on glucose and lipid metabolism in patients with hypertension. N Engl J Med 321:868–873, 1989.

787. Santoro D, Natali A, Palombo C, et al: Effects of chronic angiotensin converting enzyme inhibitors on glucose tolerance and insulin sensitivity in essential hypertension. Hypertension 20:181–191, 1992.

788. Gavras H, Gavras I: Angiotensin converting enzyme inhibitors. Properties and side effects. Hypertension 11(suppl II):II-37–II-41, 1988.

789. Morice AH, Lowry R, Brown MJ, Higenbottam T: Angiotensin-converting enzyme and the cough reflex. Lancet 2:1116–1118, 1987.

790. Biron P: Intermittent cough, sulfur-tasting sputum, and hypersalivation associated with captopril. Arch Intern Med 249:245–246, 1988.

791. Simon SR, Black HR, Moser M, Berland WE: Cough and ACE inhibitors. Arch Intern Med 152:1698–1700, 1992.

792. Israili ZH, Hall WD: Cough and angioneurotic edema associated with angiotensin-converting enzyme inhibitor therapy. Ann Intern Med 117:234–242, 1992.

793. Hedner T, Samuelson O, Lunde H, et al: Angioedema in relation to treatment with angiotensin converting enzyme inhibitors. BMJ 304:941–946, 1992.

794. Slater EE, Merrill DD, Guess HA, et al: Clinical profile of angioedema associated with angiotensin converting–enzyme inhibitors. JAMA 260:967–970, 1988.

795. Verresen L, Waer M, Vanrenterghem Y, Michielsen P: Angiotensin-converting–enzyme inhibitors and anaphylactoid reactions to high-flux membrane dialysis. Lancet 336:1360–1362, 1990.

796. Tielemans C, Madhoun P, Lenaers M, et al: Anaphylactoid reactions during hemodialysis on AN69 membranes in patients receiving ACE inhibitors. Kidney Int 38:982–984, 1990.

797. Brunet Ph, Jaber K, Berland Y, Baz M: Anaphylactoid reactions during hemodialysis and hemofiltration: Role of associating AN69 membrane and angiotensin I–converting enzyme inhibitors. Am J Kidney Dis 19:444–447, 1992.

798. Pegues DA, Beck-Sague CM, Woollen SW, et al: Anaphylactoid reactions associated with reuse of hollow-fiber hemodialysis and ACE inhibitors. Kidney Int 42:1232–1237, 1992.

799. Severe allergic reactions associated with dialysis and ACE inhibitors. FDA Med Bull 22:4, 1992.

800. Jaffe IA: Adverse effects profile of sulfhydryl compounds in man. Am J Med 80:471–476, 1986.

801. Dangers of ACE inhibitors during second and third trimesters of pregnancy. FDA Med Bull 22:2, 1992.

802. Pryde PG, Sedman AB, Nugent CE, Barr M Jr: Angiotensin-converting enzyme inhibitor fetopathy. J Am Soc Nephrol 3:1575–1582, 1993.

803. Engelman K, Jequier E, Udenfriend S, Sjoerdsma A: Metabolism of alpha-methyltyrosine in man: Relationship to its potency as an inhibitor of catecholamine biosynthesis. J Clin Invest 47:568–576, 1968.

804. Engelman K, Horwitz D, Jequier E, Sjoerdsma A: Biochemical and pharmacologic effects of alpha-methyltyrosine in man. J Clin Invest 47:577–594, 1968.

805. Jones NF, Walker G, Ruthven CRJ, Sandler M: α-Methyl-*p*-tyrosine in the management of phaeochromocytoma. Lancet 2:1105–1109, 1968.

806. Brogden RN, Heel RC, Speight TM, Avery GS: Alpha-methyl-*p*-tyrosine: A review of its pharmacology and its clinical use. Drugs 2:81–89, 1981.

807. Green KN, Larsson SK, Beevers DG, et al: Alpha-methyltyrosine in the management of phaeochromocytoma. Thorax 37:632–633, 1982.

808. Hauptman JB, Modlinger RS, Ertel NH: Pheochromocytoma resistant to alpha-adrenergic blockade. Arch Intern Med 143:2321–2323, 1983.

809. Tsunoda K, Abe K, Hagino T, et al: Hypotensive effect of losartan, a nonpeptide angiotensin II receptor antagonist, in essential hypertension. Am J Hypertens 6:28–32, 1993.

810. Goldberg MR, Tanaka W, Barchowsky A, et al: Effects of losartan on blood pressure, plasma renin activity and angiotensin II in volunteers. Hypertension 21:704–713, 1993.

811. Elliott WJ, Weber RR, Nelson KS, et al: Renal and hemodynamic effects of intravenous fenoldopam versus nitroprusside in severe hypertension. Circulation 81:970–977, 1990.

812. Wilkins MR, Unwin RJ, Kenny AJ: Endopeptidase-24.11 and its inhibitors: Potential therapeutic agents for edematous disorders and hypertension. Kidney Int 43:273–385, 1993. Editorial review.

813. Duty S, Weston AH: Potassium channel openers. Drugs 40:785–791, 1990.

814. van der Meiracker AH, Admiraal PJS, Man in't Veld AJ, et al: Prolonged blood pressure reduction by orally active renin inhibitor RO 42–5892 in essential hypertension. BMJ 301:205–210, 1990.

815. Cordero P, Fisher ND, Moore TJ, et al: Renal and endocrine responses to a renin inhibitor, enalkiren, in normal humans. Hypertension 17:510–516, 1991.

816. Brogden RN, Sorkin EM: Ketanserin. Drugs 40:903–949, 1990.

817. MacGregor GA, Markandu ND, Smith SJ, Sagnella A: Captopril: Contrasting effects of adding hydrochlorothiazide, propranolol, or nifedipine. J Cardiovasc Pharmacol 7:S82–S87, 1985.

818. White WB, Viadero JJ, Lane TJ, Podesla S: Effects of combination therapy with captopril and nifedipine in severe or resistant hypertension. Clin Pharmacol Ther 39:43–48, 1986.

819. Singer DRJ, Markandu ND, Shore AC, MacGregor GA: Captopril and nifedipine in combination for moderate to severe essential hypertension. Hypertension 9:629–633, 1987.

820. Salvetti A, Innocenti PF, Iardella M, et al: Captopril and nifedipine interactions in the treatment of essential hypertensives: A crossover study. J Hypertens 5(suppl 4):S139–S142, 1987.

821. German PS: Compliance and chronic disease. Hypertension 11(suppl II):II-56–II-60, 1988.

822. Klein LE: Compliance and blood pressure control. Hypertension 11(suppl II):II-61–II-64, 1988.

823. Koch-Weser J: Drug interactions in cardiovascular therapy. Am Heart J 90:93–116, 1975.

824. Hodsman GP, Johnston CI: Angiotensin converting enzyme inhibition drug interactions. J Hypertens 5:1–6, 1987.

825. Oats JA: Antagonism of antihypertensive drug therapy by non-steroidal anti-inflammatory drugs. Hypertension 11(suppl II):II-4–II-6, 1988.

826. Bravo EL: Phenylpropanolamine and other over-the-counter vasoactive compounds. Hypertension 11(suppl II):II-7–II-10, 1988.

827. Gifford RW Jr: An algorithm for the management of resistant hypertension. Hypertension 11(suppl II):II-101–II-105, 1988.

828. Vidt DG: The patient with resistant hypertension. Cations, volume, and renal factors. Hypertension 11(suppl II):II-76–II-83, 1988.

829. Fouad-Tarazi FM: Factors contributing to resistant hypertension. Cardiac considerations. Hypertension 11(suppl II):II-84–II-87, 1988.

830. Johns DW, Peach MJ: Factors that contribute to resistant forms of hypertension. Pharmacological considerations. Hypertension 11(suppl II):II-88–II-95, 1988.

831. Alpert MA, Bauer JH: Hypertensive emergencies: Recognition and pathogenesis. Cardiovasc Rev Rep 6:407–427, 1985.

832. Venkata C, Ram S: Hypertensive crises. Cardiol Clin 2:211–225, 1984.

833. Ferguson RK, Vlasses PH: Hypertensive emergencies and urgencies. JAMA 255:1607–1613, 1986.

834. Houston M: Hypertensive emergencies and urgencies: Pathophysiology and clinical aspects. Am Heart J 111:205–210, 1986.

835. Anderson RJ, Reed WG: Current concepts in treatment of hypertensive urgencies. Am Heart J 111:211–219, 1986.

836. Vidt DG: Current concepts in treatment of hypertensive emergencies. Am Heart J 111:220–225, 1986.

837. Calhoun DA, Oparil S: Treatment of hypertensive crises. N Engl J Med 323:1177–1183, 1990.

838. Ram CVS: Management of hypertensive emergencies: Changing therapeutic options. Am Heart J 122:356–363, 1991.

839. Koch-Weser J: Diazoxide. N Engl J Med 294:1271–1274, 1976.

840. Mroczek WJ, Leibel BA, Davidov M, Finnerty FA Jr: The importance of the rapid administration of diazoxide in accelerated hypertension. N Engl J Med 285:603–606, 1971.

841. Ram CVS, Kaplan NM: Individual titration of diazoxide dosage in the treatment of severe hypertension. Am J Cardiol 43:627–630, 1979.

842. Garrett BN, Kaplan NM: Efficacy of slow infusion of diazoxide in the treatment of severe hypertension without organ hypoperfusion. Am Heart J 103:390–394, 1982.

843. Ogilvie RI, Nadeau JH, Sitar DS: Diazoxide concentration-response relation in hypertension. Hypertension 4:167–173, 1982.

844. Huysmans FTM, Thien T: Acute treatment of hypertension with slow infusion of diazoxide. Arch Intern Med 143:882–884, 1983.

845. Shepherd A, Lin M-S, McNay J, et al: Determinants of response to intravenous hydralazine in hypertension. Clin Pharmacol Ther 29:773–781, 1981.

846. Tuzel IH: Sodium nitroprusside: A review of its clinical effectiveness as a hypotensive agent. J Clin Pharmacol 14:494–503, 1974.

847. Ahearn DJ, Grim CE: Treatment of malignant hypertension with sodium nitroprusside. Arch Intern Med 133:187–191, 1974.

848. Palmer RF, Lasseter KC: Sodium nitroprusside. N Engl J Med 292:294–297, 1975.

849. Cottrell JE, Casthely P, Brodie JD, et al: Prevention of nitroprusside-induced cyanide toxicity with hydroxocobalamin. N Engl J Med 298:809–811, 1978.

850. Schulz V, Gross R, Pasch T, et al: Cyanide toxicity of sodium nitroprusside in therapeutic use with and without sodium thiosulfate. Klin Wochenschr 60:1393–1400, 1982.

851. Gorczynski RJ: Basic pharmacology of esmolol. Am J Cardiol 56:3F–13F, 1985.

852. Gray RJ, Bateman TM, Czer LSC, et al: Use of esmolol in hypertension after cardiac surgery. Am J Cardiol 56:49F–56F, 1985.

853. Cumming AMM, Brown JJ, Lever AF, Robertson JIS: Intravenous labetalol in the treatment of severe hypertension. Br J Clin Pharmacol 13(suppl 1):93S–96S, 1982.

854. Wilson DJ, Wallin JD, Vlachakis ND, et al: Intravenous labetalol in the treatment of severe hypertension and hypertensive emergencies. Am J Med 75:95–102, 1983.

855. Lebel M, Langlois S, Belleau LJ, Grose JH: Labetalol infusion in hypertensive emergencies. Clin Pharmacol Ther 37:615–618, 1985.

856. Vlachakis ND, Maronde RF, Maloy JW, et al: Pharmacodynamics of intravenous labetalol and followup therapy with oral labetalol. Clin Pharmacol Ther 38:503–508, 1985.

857. Taylor P: Ganglionic stimulating and blocking agents. *In* Gilman AG, Goodman LS, Rall TW, Murad F (eds): The Pharmacological Basis of Therapeutics, 7th ed. Macmillan Publishing, New York, 1985, pp 215–221.

858. Till AE, Irvin JD, Hichens M, et al: Pharmacodynamics and disposition of intravenous MK422, the diacid metabolite of enalapril maleate. Clin Pharmacol Ther 31:275A, 1982. Abstract.

859. DiPette DJ, Ferraro JC, Evans RR, Martin M: Enalaprilat, an intravenous angiotensin converting enzyme inhibitor, in hypertensive crises. Clin Pharmacol Ther 38:199–204, 1985.

860. Reams GP, Lal SM, Whalen JJ, Bauer JH: Enalaprilat: An intravenous substitute for oral enalapril therapy: Humoral and pharmacokinetic effects. J Clin Hypertens 3:245–253, 1986.

861. Strauss R, Gavras I, Vlahakos D, Gavras H: Enalaprilat in hypertensive emergencies. J Clin Pharmacol 26:39–43, 1986.

862. Mann SJ, Atlas SA: Hypertensive emergencies. *In* Laragh JH, Brenner BM (eds): Hypertension Pathophysiology: Diagnosis and Management. Raven Pres. New York, 1990, pp 2275–2289.

863. Catapano MS, Marx JA: Management of urgent hypertension: A comparison of oral treatment regimens in the emergency department. J Emerg Med 4:361–368, 1986.

864. Bauer JH, Reams GP: The role of calcium entry blockers in hypertensive emergencies. Circulation 75(suppl V):V-174–V-180, 1987.

865. Ghose RR: Acute medical management of severe hypertension with oral labetalol. Br J Clin Pharmacol 8:189S–193S, 1979.

866. Davies AB, Subramanian VB, Goul B, Raftery EB: Rapid reduction of blood pressure with acute oral labetalol. Br J Clin Pharmacol 13:705–710, 1982.

867. Cohen IM, Katz MA: Oral clonidine loading for rapid control of hypertension. Clin Pharmacol Ther 24:11–15, 1978.

868. Anderson RJ, Hart GR, Crumpler CP, et al: Oral clonidine loading in hypertensive urgencies. JAMA 246:848–850, 1981.

869. Karachalios GN: Hypertensive emergencies treated with oral clonidine. Eur J Clin Pharmacol 31:227–229, 1986.

870. Houston MC: Treatment of hypertensive emergencies and urgencies with oral clonidine loading and titration. Arch Intern Med 146:586–589, 1986.

871. Beer N, Gallegos I, Cohen A, et al: Efficacy of sublingual nifedipine in the acute treatment of systemic hypertension. Chest 79:571–574, 1981.

872. Bertel O, Conen D, Rodii EW, et al: Nifedipine in hypertensive emergencies. Br Med J 286:19–21, 1983.

873. Ellrodt AG, Auet MJ, Riedinger MS, Murata GH: Efficacy and safety of sublingual nifedipine in hypertensive emergencies. Am J Med 79(suppl 4A):19–25, 1985.

874. Houston MC: Treatment of hypertensive urgencies and emergencies with nifedipine. Am Heart J 111:963–969, 1986.

875. Biollaz J, Waeber B, Brunner HR: Hypertensive crises treated with orally administered captopril. Eur J Clin Pharmacol 25:145–149, 1983.

876. Hayes JM: Rapid control of serious high blood pressure with single large oral doses of prazosin. Med J Aust 1:31–32, 1980.

877. Strandgaard S, Olesen J, Skinhoj E, Lassen NA: Autoregulation of brain circulation in severe arterial hypertension. Br Med J 1:507–510, 1973.

878. Strandgaard S: Autoregulation of cerebral blood flow in hypertensive patients. Circulation 53:720–727, 1976.

879. Strandgaard S: Autoregulation of cerebral circulation in hypertension. Acta Neurol Scand 57(suppl 66):1–82, 1978.

880. Strandgaard S: Cerebral blood flow in hypertension. Acta Med Scand Suppl 678:11–25, 1982.

881. Barry DI, Lassen NA: Cerebral blood flow autoregulation in hypertension and effects of antihypertensive drugs. J Hypertens 2(suppl 3):519–526, 1984.

882. Reed G, Devous M: Cerebral blood flow autoregulation and hypertension. Am J Med Sci 289:37–44, 1985.

883. Bertel O, Marx BE, Conen D: Effects of antihypertensive treatment on cerebral perfusion. Am J Med 82(suppl 3B):29–36, 1987.

884. Jariwalla AG, Anderson EG: Production of ischemic cardiac pain by nifedipine. Br Med J 1:1181–1182, 1978.

885. Yagil Y, Kobrin I, Leibel B, Ben-Ishay D: Ischemic ECG changes with initial nifedipine therapy of severe hypertension. Am Heart J 103:310–311, 1982.

886. Cheung JY, Boventre JV, Malis CD, Leaf A: Calcium and ischemic injury. N Engl J Med 314:1670–1676, 1986.

# Nutritional Therapy for the Uremic Patient

*William E. Mitch*
*Mackenzie Walser*

## ASSESSMENT OF RENAL FUNCTION AND ITS RATE OF CHANGE

Quantitation of renal impairment requires the estimation of glomerular filtration rate (GFR), either directly or indirectly (from serum creatinine concentration). No other measure of renal function has been proposed as a quantitative measure of the severity of renal failure, although progression can also be monitored by serial kidney biopsies[1] or by radiologic measures of kidney volume or interstitial width.[2-4]

### Normalization of Values for Glomerular Filtration Rate

Traditionally, GFR has been expressed per 1.73 m$^2$ of surface area, which is estimated by a nomogram from height and weight. The difficulty with this referent is that weight changes require recalculation of surface area. Furthermore, a constant GFR in milliliters per minute may be changing progressively (in a subject gaining or losing weight) when it is expressed per square meter of surface area.[5] Height is a better referent because it does not change in adults, except for a slow decrease in old age. "Ideal body weight" is proportional to height.[2] Because height$^2$ averages approximately 3 m$^2$, expression of GFR as milliliters per minute per 3 m$^2$ of height$^2$ may be more useful than per 1.73 m$^2$ of surface area. Another referent that has been suggested for GFR in adults is extracellular fluid volume, because the slope of plasma disappearance methods for measuring GFR (see later) yields this ratio, and because it is theoretically preferable.[6, 7] However, there is no way to compare results expressed in terms of extracellular volume with results obtained by other methods that do not use a slope method for calculating clearance.

### Normal Values for Glomerular Filtration Rate

According to Rolin and Hall,[8] the mean normal GFR (in milliliters per minute per 1.73 m$^2$) is 122.49 − 0.37(age) for adults younger than 45 years and 153.9 − 1.07(age) for persons 45 years old or older.[9] The standard deviation is 18 mL/min in males and 14 mL/min in females. In normal children younger than 1 year, GFR per 1.73 m² of surface area is considerably below normal adult mean values.[10] At birth, GFR correlates with gestational age; postnatally, there is a sharp increase. A better way of expressing results in children is as a percentage of normal for age.[10] Absolute values for normal children in relation to age are provided by Holliday and co-workers.[9] Alternatively, Al-Uzri and colleagues[11] suggested the following formula for predicting normal GFR in children as a function of age in months and weight in kilograms:

$$GFR = z^3 + 0.1293z$$

where $z = 0.7434 + [0.6956 \times \log (age + 5) + (1.47 \times \log weight)]$.

## Glomerular Filtration Rate Marker Substances

**Creatinine.** Creatinine has been employed as a marker for renal function for many decades, being endogenously produced and readily measured. An increase in serum creatinine concentration is probably the first biochemical sign of renal impairment, even though half of patients with subnormal GFRs in the range of 40 to 80 mL/min still have serum creatinine levels within normal limits.[12] Unfortunately, there are many problems with the use of creatinine as a filtration marker,[13] the most important being that its clearance does not equal GFR. In chronic renal failure, the difference between creatinine clearance and GFR varies widely, as shown by Giovanetti and Barsotti,[14] who summarized 523 measurements of creatinine and inulin clearance in 14 studies (Fig. 55–1). Later results, summarized

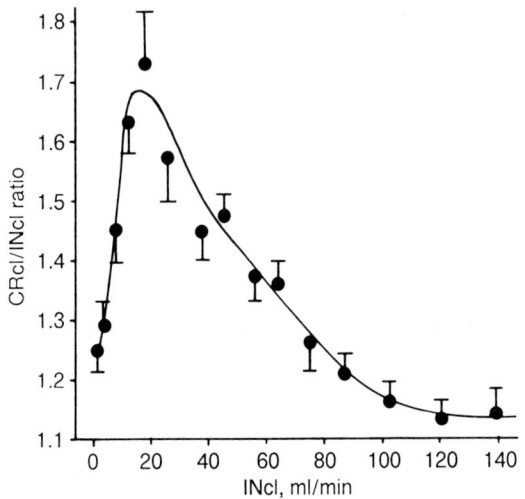

**Figure 55–1.** The ratio of creatinine clearance to inulin clearance as a function of inulin clearance in 523 observations collected from the literature, shown as mean values ± SEM. The maximal discrepancy is seen at a GFR of 20 mL/min. (From Giovannetti S, Barsotti G: In defense of creatinine clearance. Nephron 59:11–14, 1991. S Karger AG, Basel, publisher.)

by Gault and colleagues,[15] led to the same conclusion. Others have reported large and variable discrepancies between measured creatinine clearance and the clearance of other filtration markers, particularly in patients with more severe renal failure.[16–21] Although occasional studies have found the mean difference between creatinine clearance and GFR to be insignificantly different from zero, the standard deviation of the difference is large, even in these studies (e.g., 9.7 mL/min).[22, 23] Overestimation of GFR by creatinine clearance is reduced or eliminated if true creatinine is measured (after adsorption by Lloyd reagent or a similar material); thereby, errors due to noncreatinine chromogens are avoided.[24]

Despite these problems, serum or plasma creatinine concentration is invaluable both as a marker for the presence of chronic renal failure and as a useful index of its severity. To screen for renal failure, some have suggested that a single plasma sample drawn after intravenous injection of a true filtration marker, such as chromium Cr 51 ethylenediaminetetraacetic acid (⁵¹Cr-EDTA), may be preferable,[25] but this is clearly more invasive and costly. An obvious advantage of creatinine measurements over GFR determinations is cost. According to Lemann and associates,[23] a single GFR determination costs about $700. However, at Johns Hopkins Hospital, the charge is $239. The explanation for this disparity is not clear.

Cimetidine inhibits renal tubule secretion of creatinine, so the measurement of creatinine clearance after administration of cimetidine has been suggested as a better estimate of GFR[26–29]; some of these same authors stated later the same year that use of this technique is "limited" because of the large cimetidine dose required,[30] whereas others discouraged use of this technique.[31] Interpretation of plasma or serum creatinine measurements is obscured by other drugs that alter the tubule secretion of creatinine; these include trimethoprim, salicylates, phenacemide,[32] and possibly cyclosporine.[17]

GFR cannot be reliably predicted from only slight elevations of serum creatinine concentration,[12] but when it exceeds 2 mg/dL (0.177 mM) the following formulas predict GFR with an error (expressed as the standard deviation of the difference between measured and predicted GFR) of 3.0 mL/min in advanced chronic renal failure (i.e., GFR values from 2 to 37 mL/min)[33]:

Males: GFR = 7.57[Cr]⁻¹ (mM⁻¹) − 0.103age (y) + 0.096weight (kg) − 6.66

Females: GFR = 6.05[Cr]⁻¹ − 0.08age + 0.08weight − 4.81

GFR is expressed in these equations as milliliters per minute per 3 m² of height².. In the same subjects, the Cockcroft-Gault formula[34] usually overestimated GFR and produced an error twice as large (Figs. 55–2 and 55–3). None of these patients was taking drugs that interfere with the creatinine secretion.

In children, GFR (in milliliters per minute per 1.73 m²) has been estimated from serum creatinine (in milligrams per deciliter) and height Ht (in centimeters) as k × Ht/[Cr], where k = 0.55.[35] In this formula, k was later reported to be • 0.33 in preterm infants, 0.45 in full-term infants, 0.55 in

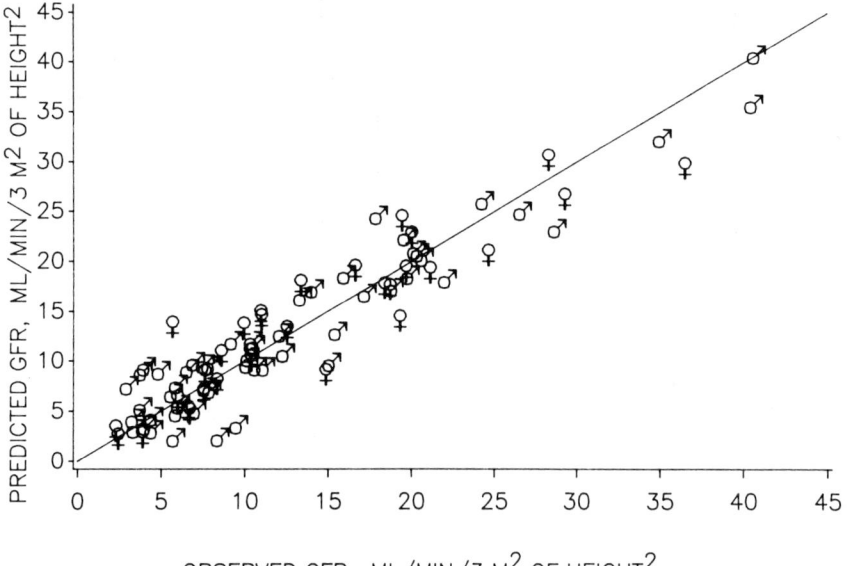

**Figure 55–2.** GFR predicted from creatinine concentration, height, weight, age, and sex as a function of DTPA clearance in 85 patients with advanced chronic renal failure. The line of identity is shown, $r = .94$. (From Walser M, Drew HH, Guldan JL: Prediction of glomerular filtration rate from serum creatinine concentration in advanced chronic renal failure. Used with permission from Kidney International, volume 44, pages 1145–1148, 1993.)

girls, and 0.70 in boys.[36] Sekar and co-workers[37] reported an average difference between GFR from this estimate and diethylenetriaminepentaacetic acid (DTPA) clearance (by imaging) of only 3.6%, but Hellerstein and colleagues[38] found that inulin clearance, in children with GFRs ranging from 3 to 139 mL/min, was consistently overestimated by these formulas. On the other hand, Waz and co-workers[39] found that these equations underestimated GFR in diabetic children by an average of one third.

**$\beta_2$-Microglobulin.** $\beta_2$-Microglobulin meets none of the criteria of an ideal filtration marker (see fourth edition). Nevertheless, its serum level correlates negatively with GFR.[40] Accumulation of this protein has been implicated in the pathogenesis of amyloidosis in long-term dialysis patients. It is only rarely employed at present as a filtration marker.[41]

**Inulin.** Inulin was the first substance shown to meet the criteria of an ideal filtration marker,[42] being freely filterable, neither reabsorbed nor secreted, nontoxic, and pharmacologically inert. It is somewhat impractical to use because it must be given by constant infusion and is insoluble. It is also difficult to analyze, especially in diabetics, owing to interference by glucose, and it is not always available. Nevertheless, inulin clearance remains an option for measuring GFR when there are reasons to avoid radioactive isotopes, as in pregnant women and children.

**Polyfructosan.** Polyfructosan, a polysaccharide found in the Jerusalem artichoke, avoids some of the practical problems with the use of inulin but comprises a broader range of molecular weight compounds than does inulin.[43] Its clearance closely parallels that of $^{51}$Cr-EDTA.[44]

**Iodinated Contrast Agents.** Radioactive iothalamate has been used as a GFR marker for three decades; nonradioactive iothalamate has been employed only recently. A major

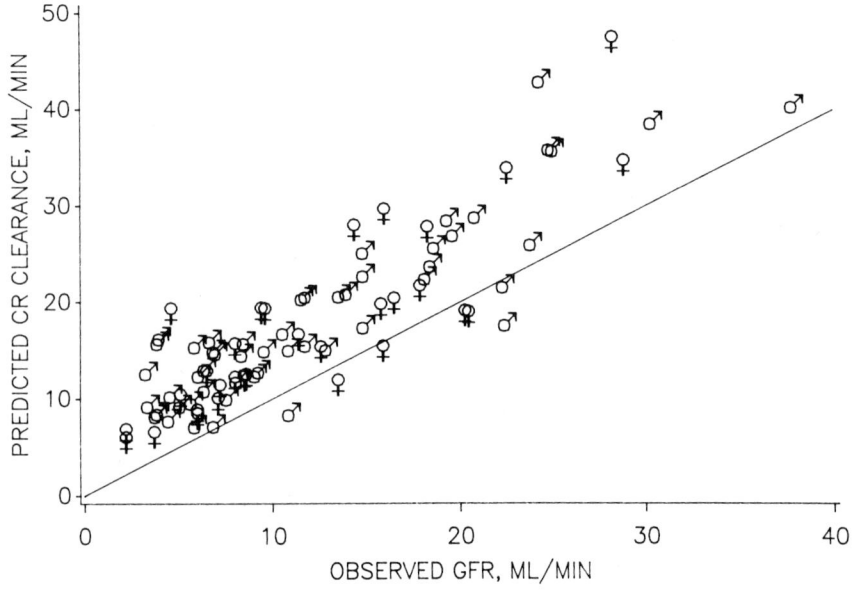

**Figure 55–3.** Creatinine clearance as predicted by the Cockcroft and Gault equations[34] from creatinine concentration, weight, age, and sex in the same patients as in Figure 55–2. The line of identity is shown. These equations overestimate GFR in most patients and show greater scatter than in Figure 55–2. (From Walser M, Drew HH, Guldan JL: Prediction of glomerular filtration rate from serum creatinine concentration in advanced chronic renal failure. Used with permission from Kidney International, volume 44, pages 1145–1148, 1993.)

concern in the use of these compounds in patients with chronic renal failure (and especially diabetic nephropathy) is the possibility of nephrotoxic effects of the contrast medium. Whether this problem can be avoided by reducing dosage is not entirely certain. Some studies of nephrotoxicity of these agents have shown dose dependence, and others have not.[45, 46] Clearly, subjects with chronic renal failure are at greater risk for nephrotoxic effects of contrast agents than are those without,[45] particularly if they are diabetic.[47, 48]

If extrarenal clearance of iothalamate were substantial,[49] its plasma clearance would be an inaccurate measure of GFR in patients with moderate or severe renal insufficiency. However, others find a close correspondence between plasma clearance of nonradioactive iothalamate and urinary clearance of iothalamate as well as urinary clearance of inulin,[50, 51] even in patients with severe renal failure.

Iohexol (Omnipaque) has been introduced more recently for this purpose.[52] Plasma clearance exceeds urinary clearance by an average of 11.8 mL/min, indicating substantial extrarenal clearance.[53] Nevertheless, its clearance is well correlated with clearances of $^{51}$Cr-EDTA, technetium Tc 99m DTPA, $^{125}$I-labeled iothalamate, and inulin in patients with widely varying GFRs.[54–60]

Iopentol also has a substantial extrarenal clearance, but its urinary clearance evidently reflects GFR.[61]

**Other Nonradioactive Markers.** Reports have recommended the use of piracetam,[62] vitamin B$_{12}$,[63] gadolinium-DTPA,[64] and gadopentetate dimeglumine.[65]

**Radioactive Markers.** The most widely used compounds are $^{125}$I- or $^{131}$I-labeled iothalamate, $^{99m}$Tc-DTPA, $^{51}$Cr-EDTA, and ytterbium Yb 169 DTPA. They vary in physical half-life, extent of plasma protein binding, and energy of emissions. $^{99m}$Tc is probably the most useful, having an ideal $\gamma$ energy (140 keV) that permits imaging, no $\beta$ emission, and a short half-life (6 hours). It must be used within an hour of chelation to prevent dissociation of the chelate.[66] It is important to check the protein binding of the isotope on each batch. $^{99m}$Tc-mercaptoacetyltriglycine[67] has also been recommended, as has $^{131}$I-labeled diatrizoate.[68]

## Methods of Quantitation

Available methods can be grouped into 1) those that assess blood clearance, from either a) the disappearance curve after a bolus injection or b) the steady-state plasma level at the end of a prolonged constant infusion[11, 66, 69, 70]; 2) those that calculate renal uptake of radioactive or radiopaque marker,[71–74] including the ratios of renal uptake to uptake in other organs[75]; 3) those that determine, in addition to plasma concentration, urine radioactivity by external counting over the bladder[66, 68]; and 4) those that require measurement of urinary as well as plasma concentration. The first technique yields total plasma clearance, which is assumed to be insignificantly greater than renal clearance. Total plasma clearance after bolus injection (1a) is the quotient of the tracer dose divided by the area under the plasma curve; total plasma clearance at the end of a constant infusion is infusion rate divided by plasma concentration. As

pointed out by Brochner-Mortenson,[76] there are prerequisites for the use of plasma clearance as a measure of GFR. First, plasma clearance must be constant during the period of sampling. This is likely to be a problem with a prolonged infusion.[77] Also, prolonged infusion may not be possible with DTPA, because some commercially available kits have progressive changes in binding to plasma proteins. Second, extrapolation to infinite time after bolus injection is necessary, but it is not always clear how long sampling must continue before monoexponential extrapolation to infinity is valid. Third, extrarenal clearance of the marker must be negligibly low; even a small extrarenal clearance, relative to normal GFR, may become a significant fraction of total clearance in a patient with a low GFR. Hence, all plasma clearance techniques tend to become unreliable as chronic renal failure becomes more severe. Technique 1b measures GFR for the entire period of constant infusion, which may require several days to reach a steady-state plasma concentration in severe renal failure.

To circumvent the necessity of describing the entire plasma disappearance curve in technique 1a, several simplifications have been proposed, including the use of a single plasma sample obtained several hours after injection[25, 62, 78–89] or two or three plasma samples.[89–91] This technique has been refined by incorporating the volume of distribution of the indicator[92, 93] but remains semiempirical and is probably inapplicable to subjects with GFR below approximately 30 mL/min.[88, 94]

Techniques involving scintigraphic analysis of radioactivity in the kidneys provide information with respect to relative function of the two kidneys but do not correlate well with GFR measured by other methods.[95, 96]

Techniques requiring collection of urine present difficulties in children, in subjects with urine obstruction or retention, and in patients with severe chronic renal failure (because maximal urine flow falls pari passu with GFR). Nevertheless, urine collection methods are preferable to avoid the empirical features of techniques based on plasma levels alone or renal uptake.

When a timed urine collection is measured, detection of incomplete bladder emptying becomes critical. The coefficient of variation of sequential GFR determinations is commonly used as an estimate of the reliability of urine collection, but incomplete voiding in one period is likely to be followed by excessive voiding in the next. The reliability of sequential GFRs on different days may in fact bear little relation to the coefficient of variation of the three periods on a given day.[97]

Setting an arbitrary lower limit of urine flow below which urinary clearances are deemed unacceptable is one way to deal with the problem of incomplete emptying of the bladder. Another way is to estimate in each subject, retrospectively, the lower limit of acceptable urine flow and to reject clearances obtained with flows below this limit.[5] When sequential GFRs are available, the linear regression of GFR on time can be calculated, and the residual differences from this regression each day can be determined. Urine flow during each GFR determination is then calculated as total urine voided divided by the total time elapsed, and a plot of the individual residuals against flow during each determination is made. In some patients, it is apparent that there exists a value of urine flow below which all residuals become strikingly negative. GFR measurements on such days should be rejected as falsely low, and residuals about the new regression are recalculated. A less empirical technique for correcting for incomplete voiding has been suggested by Apperloo and colleagues.[98] Iodohippurate sodium I 131 (Hippuran I 131) is injected (as a bolus) along with the GFR marker, and the ratio of plasma clearance to urinary clearance of Hippuran is calculated for each period. Urinary clearance of the GFR marker is corrected by this ratio. The error in the slope of sequential GFR determinations, with use of this correction, was significantly reduced in a series of 61 patients with progressive chronic renal failure. Finally, when γ-emitting radioisotopes are used, the volume of residual urine can be estimated by counting over the bladder before and after each voiding and applying an appropriate correction.[99]

Any technique involving water loading entails the danger of water intoxication. Nausea and pain are powerful stimuli to vasopressin release, which may affect GFR. If water loading is overdone, severe headache ensues and convulsions can occur.

## Comparison of the Clearances of Different Markers in Renal Insufficiency

There are comparatively few studies of GFR determinations by two or more of these techniques in patients with GFRs of 30 mL/min or less. Skov[100] compared inulin and [125]I-iothalamate clearances in 43 patients with varying degrees of chronic renal insufficiency. He modified the degree of water loading, depending on the degree of renal insufficiency, and used an intravenous rather than subcutaneous injection of the isotope. There was close concordance between inulin and iothalamate clearances. Although the coefficient of variation for inulin and iothalamate clearances was 17% in individual subjects with GFR below 5 mL/min, the clearance ratio averaged 0.98, indicating that both methods gave virtually identical results. In patients with less severe renal insufficiency, the coefficients of variation were less, and the concordance remained almost perfect.

Ott and Wilson[101] reported that urinary clearance of subcutaneously injected [125]I-iothalamate was equal to inulin clearance, with a standard deviation around the regression of 6.4 mL/min, in subjects with GFRs of 10 to 140 mL/min. Jagenburg and colleagues[102] showed that urinary clearances of [51]Cr-EDTA and inulin were nearly identical in patients with GFRs of 2 to 11 mL/min but that plasma clearance of [51]Cr-EDTA overestimated GFR measured by urinary clearance by 2.6 to 11.2 mL/min. Bianchi and co-workers[103] used bladder catheters and showed that GFR measured as the urinary clearance of [99m]Tc-DTPA was 8% lower than the urinary clearance of [131]I-diatrizoate, but only 6 of 21 patients studied had GFRs below 60 mL/min. Hagstam and associates[104] reported that urinary clearance of [51]Cr-EDTA slightly underestimated inulin clearance, but only 5 of the 60 patients studied had GFRs below 40 mL/min. Rehling and colleagues[105] reported that plasma clearance of [99m]Tc-DTPA after intravenous injection was similar to renal clearance of inulin in subjects with GFRs of 25 to 80 mL/min.

Plasma clearance was calculated from the area under the plasma concentration curve by use of 13 plasma samples between 5 and 300 minutes after injection. Later, Rehling and colleagues[74] reported that GFR could be measured by γ-camera renography of both kidneys after injection of [99m]Tc-DTPA, without determining the injected dose or collecting urine or blood samples, in subjects with GFRs from 4 to 172 mL/min. However, the coefficient of variation was 8.3 mL/min (at a GFR of 50 mL/min), a value so large as to preclude the use of this technique for observing patients with severe or moderately severe renal failure.

Manz and associates[106] measured GFR in children with severe renal failure and observed that [51]Cr-EDTA plasma clearance (by a two-compartment model) overestimated inulin clearance by 36% and was not significantly correlated with inulin clearance. Carlsen and co-workers[107] reported that plasma clearances of [99m]Tc-DTPA and [51]Cr-EDTA were similar and concluded that [99m]Tc-DTPA can be used to measure GFR. Unfortunately, they did not collect urine, and therefore both methods may have overestimated GFR owing to extrarenal clearance. LaFrance and colleagues[20] observed nearly identical urinary clearances of [125]I-iothalamate and [99m]Tc-DTPA in patients with widely varying GFRs (2 to 40 mL/min), mostly below 10 mL/min. However, plasma clearance of [99m]Tc-DTPA, when assessed from four plasma samples, exceeded its urinary clearance by a large and extremely variable amount (−2 to 30 mL/min). Again, these results emphasize the greater accuracy of urinary clearances than of plasma clearances in patients with renal failure. Gibb and co-workers[108] found that [51]Cr-EDTA clearance was 7.4 ± 2.5 (SEM) mL/min/1.73 m$^2$ less than inulin clearance in children with chronic renal failure. Wharton and associates[109] reported that [99m]Tc-DTPA clearance was closely correlated with inulin clearance in patients with GFRs less than 30 mL/min. Perrone and colleagues[97] found that the urinary clearances of [125]I-iothalamate and [169]Yb-DTPA were slightly but significantly greater than simultaneously measured urinary clearances of inulin or [99m]Tc-DTPA in patients with diabetes as well as in normal subjects. Fleming and co-workers[110] found that [99m]Tc-DTPA clearance exceeded [51]Cr-EDTA clearance by 7.6% but was closely correlated with it.

In children, DTPA clearance, calculated by imaging, may grossly overestimate GFR (as measured by plasma clearance of iothalamate).[111] In nine children with GFR below 35 mL/min/1.73 m$^2$, prolonged infusion of both inulin and iothalamate yielded nearly identical values for the clearances of the two markers.[9] In children with kidney transplants and a wide range of GFRs, Mak and associates[112] found that constant infusion clearances of inulin and iothalamate were closely correlated with urinary clearances of these markers; [51]Cr-EDTA clearances by plasma disappearance overestimated GFR at near-normal values but not in renal insufficiency.

## Reproducibility of Glomerular Filtration Rate Determinations

Repeated measurements of GFR entail not only the error of measurement but also the biologic variability of true

GFR, which is unknown. Unless the interval between measurements is brief, progression of renal insufficiency (if present) may also contribute to the difference between repeated measurements. The standard deviation of the difference between two or more GFRs in individual subjects, measured within a few days, is about 10 mL/min in normal subjects by use of a one-compartment slope clearance[86, 113] and about 13% in subjects with renal failure by use of inulin, DTPA, or iothalamate.[97]

## MEASUREMENT OF PROGRESSION

As recently as 20 years ago, there was no way to measure progression in quantitative terms. Now there are several techniques, each with advantages and disadvantages. There has been much discussion as to the validity of these various techniques. As pointed out by Schluchter,[114] comparing estimates of the rate of progression by two or more techniques gives a biased correlation owing to measurement error; he presented a method for overcoming this problem.

### Rate of Change of Reciprocal Serum or Plasma Creatinine Concentration, $[Cr]^{-1}$

In most patients with progressive chronic renal failure, a plot of $[Cr]^{-1}$ against time yields a straight line,[115] as has been confirmed.[66] The median correlation coefficient is approximately .95. All series report a significant fraction of patients (about 20%) in whom $[Cr]^{-1}$ does not fall linearly with time. Whether progression would be linear in these same patients if it were analyzed by observing the GFR is uncertain.

A constant decline in $[Cr]^{-1}$ with time suggests that creatinine clearance, UV/P, falls linearly with time and that UV remains constant. This inference is incorrect because creatinine excretion is known to fall as chronic renal failure progresses, and creatinine appearance (excretion plus accumulation) may fall to one third of normal in advanced chronic renal failure.[116] This change in UV, which is attributable to creatinine metabolism, need not invalidate this technique if the rate of creatinine metabolism throughout the course of renal failure is proportional to creatinine concentration. We have found that this is approximately true[117] on the basis of measurements of creatinine metabolism in a small number of patients. However, to the extent that creatinine metabolism fails to vary in proportion to creatinine concentration, the slope of $[Cr]^{-1}$ versus time will become misleading as a measure of progression.

On the basis of the finding that $[Cr]^{-1}$ declined at a constant rate, the use of rates of change of $[Cr]^{-1}$ was originally suggested as a way of monitoring progression in individual patients subjected to various treatments.[115] Subsequently, $[Cr]^{-1}$ slopes in groups of patients have been reported by many workers, with the implication that progression in the whole group is proportional to the slope, d/dt(1/P). This is incorrect. Even when UV is constant, the rate of change of creatinine clearance, d/dt(UV/P), is equal to UV times d/dt(1/P). UV varies with sex and age and also varies widely between subjects independently of sex or

age.[118] Hence, a given value of slope d/dt(1/P) may indicate a rapid rate of progression in a young muscular man but a slow rate of progression in an elderly wasted woman. To convert an individual value of $[Cr]^{-1}$ slope into a rate of change of creatinine clearance, at least one value of 24-hour urinary creatinine excretion, UV, should be measured, corrected for height or surface area, and multiplied by d/dt(1/P). This gives at least a first approximation of the rate of change of creatinine clearance.

How often does the slope of $[Cr]^{-1}$ change spontaneously? The answer to this question is particularly important in crossover studies of different therapies. According to two reports,[119, 120] approximately one fifth of those patients who show a correlation between $[Cr]^{-1}$ and time will show a change of slope at some point during the course of the disease. However, the change of slope was assessed visually in these reports rather than by statistical programs now available.[121] Using such programs, Shah and Levey[122] found that one third to one half of patients exhibit a "break point" in the decline of $[Cr]^{-1}$ with time. According to Gretz and co-workers,[123] there is, on the average, an acceleration of the downward slope of $[Cr]^{-1}$ as chronic renal failure progresses toward the end stage.

A major disadvantage of the $[Cr]^{-1}$ technique of measuring progression is that it is susceptible to a large artifact when the meat content of the diet is reduced sharply. The resulting fall in creatinine production lowers serum creatinine concentration and increases $[Cr]^{-1}$ independently of any change in clearance. The type of artifact introduced into a plot of $[Cr]^{-1}$ against time is illustrated in Figure 55–4. After a few months, the decline of $[Cr]^{-1}$ again becomes linear, but at a slightly steeper slope (even though

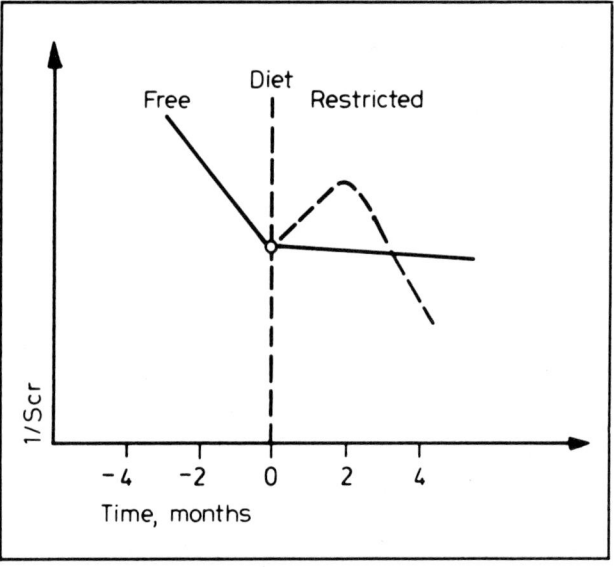

**Figure 55–4.** Hypothetic graph of reciprocal creatinine concentration versus time in months in a patient with chronic renal failure, progressing at a constant rate, placed on a meat-restricted diet at time zero. The dotted line shows values of $[Cr]^{-1}$, and the solid lines show the calculated regressions of $[Cr]^{-1}$ on time. The apparent slowing of progression is an artifact caused by reduced intake of creatine and creatinine. (From Gretz N, Meisinger E, Strauch M: Influence of the underlying renal disease on the rate of progression. Contrib Nephrol 53:92, 1986.)

creatinine clearance is continuing to decline at a constant rate). This is for the reason given before: constant $d/dt(UV/P)$ means that when UV falls to a new lower value because of a meat-restricted diet, $d/dt(1/P)$ is more negative. It follows that if $d/dt(1/P)$ resumes the same slope a few months after protein intake is reduced, $d/dt(UV/P)$ is in fact less negative and progression has slowed slightly.

These considerations indicate that the $[Cr]^{-1}$ values obtained in the first months after a reduction in protein intake should be ignored in calculating a new rate of progression and that representative values of UV during both control and treatment phases should be multiplied by $d/dt(1/P)$ to obtain estimates of $d/dt(UV/P)$ and the effect of diet on progression. When this is done, the diet artifact of this technique of measuring progression can be largely or entirely overcome. Combe and colleagues[124] reported that the rate of decline of renal function measured in this manner is closely correlated with the rate of decline of urinary clearance of $^{51}$Cr-EDTA. The artifact introduced by creatinine metabolism, on the other hand, cannot be completely eliminated unless metabolism remains exactly proportional to creatinine concentration.

## Rate of Change of Creatinine Clearance

Measurement of creatinine clearance, $C_{cr}$, should eliminate dietary artifacts and errors due to creatinine metabolism. Unfortunately, several additional problems are introduced. First, $C_{cr}$ overestimates GFR to a large and variable extent, as noted before. Although some authors have inferred that this invalidates $C_{cr}$ as a measure of progression, it does not mean that $dC_{cr}/dt$ is unequal to $dGFR/dt$. The rate of change of $C_{cr}$ could accurately reflect the rate of change of GFR (see subsequent discussion). Second, urinary creatinine excretion, even in normal subjects, varies considerably from day to day in the absence of urine collection errors.[66, 118] Third, incomplete urine collections are bound to occur; these may be detected if grossly incomplete but partial loss is not readily identified. Collections of more than 24 hours may also occur.

## Rate of Change of Glomerular Filtration Rate

Whether measured by clearances of isotopes or nonradioactive markers, the rate of change in GFR is the most reliable technique for measuring progression. Urinary clearance is the most reliable, because changes in the plasma clearance give less accurate estimates of GFR, especially in more severe renal failure.

Progression rate can be estimated as the linear regression coefficient of GFR on time or as the change in GFR from one time point to another, divided by the time interval. Both techniques yield the same information; both have advantages and disadvantages. The second technique requires more than one determination of GFR at the start and end of the interval, without which it is not possible to obtain an estimate of the confidence limits of the estimated slope. Repeated visits within a few days may not be acceptable to

patients. Nevertheless, it can be readily shown that the confidence limits of the slope obtained by this technique (for any given number of GFR determinations and any given slope) are considerably smaller than when the same number of GFR determinations are evenly spaced throughout the time interval. This follows because measurements near the midpoint of the time interval have little influence on the slope estimate. Patients generally prefer sequential measurements in hopes of obtaining information about their progress. Thus, the demands of optimal study design and the demands of optimal care of the patient may conflict.

Statistical aspects of measuring progression are complex and have not been dealt with in detail as yet in the published literature. Beck and co-workers[125] proposed a model based on the following assumptions. 1) In the $i$th patient, there is a linear regression of GFR on time with true intercept $\alpha_i$, slope $\beta_i$, and independent errors $\epsilon_i$. 2) These errors are normally distributed with mean zero and variance $\sigma_\epsilon^2$. 3) The residual variance in GFR about each patient's regression is the same for all patients. 4) The distribution of slopes and of intercepts for all patients in each study group is normal, with common variances $\sigma_\alpha^2$ and $\sigma_\beta^2$, respectively. Given these assumptions (most of which can be questioned, especially assumption 3) and equations proposed by Schlesselman,[126] the variance of the slope estimate for each subject is $\sigma_\beta^2 + \sigma_\epsilon^2/\Sigma(t_i - \bar{t}_i)^2$, where $t_i$ is the average of all time points for the $i$th individual. Beck and co-workers[125] used restricted maximal likelihood estimates[127] to obtain these two components of variance. From observations made in the feasibility phase of the Modification of Diet in Renal Disease Trial, they estimated $\sigma_\beta^2$ as $0.24(mL/min/mo)^2$ in patients with GFRs of 25 to 55 mL/min and $0.03(mL/min/ mo)^2$ for patients with GFRs of 13 to 25 mL/min. Estimates of $\sigma_\epsilon^2$ in the same two groups were 12.14 and $3.45(mL/ min/mo)^2$, respectively. Walser and colleagues,[128] using a simpler model, found $\sigma_\epsilon^2 = 2.05(mL/min/mo)^2$ in patients with GFRs of 10 to 29 mL/min.

Three factors must be present to detect a significant rate of progression in an individual patient[5, 129]: 1) at least four sequential GFR measurements, 2) a relatively rapid rate of progression, and 3) a relatively low GFR. In many patients, one or more of these factors may be absent, and consequently progression may not be measurable by current methods.

## Comparison of Progression Rates from "[Cr]$^{-1}$ Clearance" or Creatinine Clearance and Isotopic Glomerular Filtration Rate Determinations

Mathillas and co-workers[130] compared slopes of the logarithm of $^{51}$Cr-EDTA clearance with slopes of the logarithm of $[Cr]^{-1}$ in 17 patients following protein-restricted diets and found that the former was significantly faster than the latter (the logarithmic transformation was used to make the comparison dimensionless). In 18 patients with chronic renal failure, Walser and associates[131] determined sequential values of creatinine concentration, $C_{cr}$, and GFR during the same time interval. GFR was determined from the urinary clearance of intravenously injected $^{99m}$Tc-DTPA, and the results were edited for low-flow errors as described before. The linear regression of $[Cr]^{-1}$ values over time was multiplied by an average value of creatinine excretion to obtain the slope of "creatinine$^{-1}$ clearances." Linear regressions on time of $C_{cr}$, GFR, and $[Cr]^{-1}$ clearance were calculated and designated $b_1$, $b_2$, and $b_3$, respectively. Mean $b_1$ did not differ statistically from mean $b_2$, but $b_1$ was greater than $b_2$. Thus, isotopically determined GFRs gave a statistically more reliable estimate of progression in most patients than 24-hr creatinine clearance did.

Examination of data from individual subjects showed a more serious problem with $Cr^{-1}$ clearances and creatinine clearances: in nearly half of the patients, sequential $Cr^{-1}$ and creatinine clearances were qualitatively misleading.[131] For example, creatinine clearance suggested improvement in one case in which isotopically determined GFR showed a constant value. In others, GFR suggested progression whereas creatinine clearance did not or failed to confirm progression. These results suggest that changes in the ratio $C_{cr}$/GFR occurred in both directions during the course of renal failure in individual patients, signifying progressive changes in one direction or the other in the tubule transport of creatinine. If this is correct, sequential $[Cr]^{-1}$ values and sequential creatinine clearances are potentially misleading as measures of progression. Similar conclusions were reached by Levey and colleagues[129] in a study of 96 patients in the feasibility phase of the Modification of Diet in Renal Disease study.

In conclusion, reliable estimates of progression can be made only by repeated measurements of GFR, with use of an appropriate marker. At least four GFR determinations will almost always be necessary, but even with these precautions, slower rates of progression may be undetectable, particularly when GFR is relatively high. The traditional use of sequential creatinine measurements as a clinical tool for diagnosing and observing patients with chronic renal failure may no longer be supportable if the availability of GFR measurements justifies their use for diagnosis and follow-up of all cases of chronic renal failure.

## DETERMINING THE EFFECT OF TREATMENT ON PROGRESSION

### Survival Curves

The simplest technique is comparison of survival curves, nonsurvival being defined as progression to a defined end point, such as the beginning of dialysis. This technique is obviously applicable only for comparing the outcome of groups of patients randomly assigned to control and experimental treatments and requires prolonged follow-up.

### Glomerular Filtration Rate Slopes Without Crossovers

Comparison of mean regression slopes of GFR against time in groups of patients randomly assigned to two or more treatments is the most generally accepted technique.

Because of the substantial variability of progression rates within any group of patients (see later), large numbers of patients in each group are necessary to establish statistically significant differences between progression rates. Furthermore, unless some method is employed to exclude nonprogressing subjects, who may make up as many as 39% of patients with chronic renal failure (see later), their inclusion makes the demonstration of significant differences in progression rates induced by treatment difficult.

Attempts to exclude nonprogressors by observing sequential values of GFR or creatinine during a baseline period may be plagued by regression to the mean. As pointed out by Levey and co-workers,[129] when individuals are selected because of a value for some time-variant characteristic lying beyond a defined limit that excludes a portion of the population, follow-up measurements of the same characteristic in the subgroup selected will inevitably be closer to the overall mean. Methods for calculating the magnitude of this effect are cited by Levey and co-workers.[129]

Another problem is dropouts. If the patients selected have relatively severe renal failure, many will progress to dialysis before the end of the observation period specified in the protocol. Thus, it will often be necessary to compare not only slopes during treatment but survival curves to dropout. When the conclusions of these two types of analysis differ, the implications are uncertain.

Inclusion of noncompliant patients also introduces problems. Strictly speaking, the analysis should be based on "intention to treat"; that is, all subjects should be included in the analysis even if they clearly did not follow the prescribed treatment protocol to avoid introducing bias. When the proportion of noncompliant subjects is large, however, this approach yields a virtually meaningless result. It certainly cannot be used to determine effectiveness of therapy. If a quantitative measure of compliance is available (such as 24-hour urinary urea nitrogen excretion as a measure of protein intake or the presence of alloisoleucine in plasma as a marker of keto acid ingestion[132]), comparison of outcomes in relation to this measure will be more persuasive than comparison of groups by intention to treat.

### Glomerular Filtration Rate Slopes with Crossovers

Many of these problems can be avoided by crossover designs. Such designs are inherently more efficient, because the variability between patients of changes in progression rate in response to treatment is almost certain to be less than the variability between patients in progression rates. Depending somewhat on the crossover design chosen, errors caused by regression to the mean are minimized. Patients who drop out are excluded, although it is important to ascertain that dropout is not more frequent in subjects receiving one treatment than in patients receiving the other (this should be seldom, because of the relatively short period during which each treatment is applied). Unless compliance can be shown to differ between the two treatments, these problems are also minimized.

There are several new problems introduced. First, carryover effects may occur; the effect of one treatment on rate of progression may persist for an interval, even after it is withdrawn. This problem can generally be eliminated by omitting the interval immediately after changeover from the analysis (assuming that this interval is long enough for any carry-over effect to disappear, but this can be questioned). Second, in a progressive disorder, with design AB (where A is one treatment and B is the other), severity will generally be greater during treatment B, and there may be a relationship between severity and response to treatment or a relationship between severity and slope independent of treatment. If patients are randomized to sequence AB or sequence BA (design AB/BA), this potential error is reduced but may not be eliminated. A better design is ABA/BAB.[128] If progression is linear, the mean severity of illness during treatment A will probably be the same as the mean severity during treatment B. As pointed out by Jones and Kenward,[133] AAB/BAA is preferable if carry-over is a concern; however, their comments were not addressed to a progressive disorder. Third, crossover studies can never establish long-term outcomes, except by inference.

## CHARACTERIZATION OF PROGRESSION

### Linearity of Loss of Renal Function with Time

Several publications have appeared in which sequential values of inulin clearance[102] or isotopically determined GFR[5, 134–139] are plotted against time and, by visual inspection, appear to be linear. Formal statistical tests of linearity do not seem to have been applied. Walser[5] attempted to determine how often GFR declines linearly in a group of patients with chronic renal failure, using sequential measurements of GFR (as urinary clearance of [99m]Tc-DTPA). He found no evidence for autocorrelation, but the information was not adequate to exclude it. By use of quadratic regression as a test for linearity, 26% of the patients exhibited curvilinearity, more often downward than upward. By a linear spline or ''hockey stick'' analysis, 30% of the patients exhibited nonlinearity, more often accelerating than decelerating. Thus, it appears that progression is nonlinear in a significant proportion of patients and is more likely to accelerate. Analysis of the results of large-scale multicenter trials is awaited.

### Distribution of Progression Rates

Mean rate of progression is approximately $-0.5$ mL/min/mo but varies widely in different reports. Extremes are approximately $-2.5$ mL/min/mo and $+2$ mL/min/mo. As many as 39% of patients appear not to be progressing by linear regression of GFR on time,[140] and a few of these are improving at a statistically significant rate. This is difficult to understand and obviously cannot continue for many months. The distribution of progression rates approximates a normal distribution.[5]

## DETERMINANTS OF RATE OF PROGRESSION

There have been many studies of factors affecting progression of chronic renal failure. Some of these have used univariate analysis, and some have used multivariate analysis. In general, the factors examined in these analyses are extensively correlated. Hence, significant relationships reported must be interpreted with caution and certainly do not establish causality.

**Type of Renal Disease.** Several reports have compared reciprocal creatinine slopes in groups of patients with different renal diseases. As pointed out earlier, differences in mean reciprocal creatinine slopes between groups of patients are as likely to be attributable to differences in mean rates of excretion of creatinine as to differences in mean rate of progression. Consequently, these results may not be correct. Franz and Reubi[139] reported that patients with polycystic kidney disease show gradually accelerating progression. However, close examination of their data shows that only two patients had more than two GFR determinations; in these two subjects, the rate of progression was linear. It was subsequently reported that mean GFR slope in patients with polycystic kidney disease is significantly faster than in other disorders,[5, 141, 142] and actuarial survival is shorter.[143] On the other hand, rate of decline of creatinine clearance in polycystic kidney disease or in interstitial nephritis was reported to be slower than in chronic glomerulonephritis.[144] Rate of progression of chronic glomerulonephritis was found to be significantly slower than that of other diseases in one study.[5] Spontaneous remission of chronic renal failure occurs in a substantial fraction of patients with membranous nephropathy.[145] Creatinine clearance falls more rapidly in children with glomerulopathies than in children with hypoplasias or vascular nephropathies; hereditary nephropathies also progress more rapidly than do vascular nephropathies.[146]

**Blood Pressure.** The relationship between blood pressure and progression as well as the effect on progression of lowering blood pressure with various agents is considered in Chapters 48 and 54.

**Proteinuria.** Many observers have noted a significant correlation between proteinuria and rate of progression, especially in diabetics.[137, 141–143, 147–157]

**Race.** On the average, black persons progress more rapidly than white persons do, for unknown reasons.[158–160]

**Sex.** Women with adult polycystic kidney disease progress more slowly than do men, on the average[161, 162]; similar observations have been reported in studies of membranous nephropathy.[163–166]

**Glucocorticoid Production.** Walser and Ward[167] reported that 24-hour excretion of 17-hydroxyglucocorticoids and rate of progression are significantly correlated, and a similar correlation between rate of progression and free cortisol excretion was subsequently noted,[141] even though excretion rates of both products were, on the average, below normal. The authors postulated that higher physiologic levels of endogenous cortisol may impair the healing of renal injury. In a preliminary report,[168] partial suppression of cortisol production (by long-term administration of ketoconazole at 400 mg/d plus prednisone at 2.5 mg/d) was associated with slowed progression in a small number of patients.

**Serum Free Tryptophan Concentration.** Higher values for serum non–protein-bound tryptophan were noted to be associated with more rapid rate of progression.[5] This observation may explain part of the slowing of progression induced by administration of tryptophan-free mixtures of keto acids and amino acids, which leads to lower serum free tryptophan concentrations (see later discussion).

**Plasma Lipid Levels.** The rate of decline of radioisotopic GFR is correlated with circulating levels of apolipoprotein-B,[169] cholesterol,[5, 170, 171] and triglycerides,[172] although not in all studies.

**Pregnancy.** Creatinine clearance falls faster during pregnancy.[173] Conceivably, increased cortisol production[174] could be responsible.

**Plasma Glucose Concentration.** In diabetics, severity of hyperglycemia is correlated with rate of progression.[154, 155, 160, 172, 175] Strict control of hyperglycemia (by continuous subcutaneous infusion of insulin) was not found to slow progression of diabetic nephropathy in several initial reports of relatively small series of patients,[176] even though it reduces albuminuria,[177] but it was definitively shown to slow progression in the large Diabetes Complications and Control Trial, although only at the price of slightly more frequent hypoglycemia and its attendant increase in morbidity of various types.[178]

**Smoking.** Among diabetics, smokers progress to end-stage renal failure more rapidly than nonsmokers do[173, 179]; again, increased cortisol production[180] could be the explanation.

**Hyperfiltration.** The supranormal GFR seen in at least 25% of patients with insulin-dependent diabetes early after the onset of diabetes, and also in patients with non–insulin-dependent diabetes,[181] has been proposed to be predictive of the development of diabetic nephropathy (Chapter 39). A long-term prospective study of patients with insulin-dependent diabetes has confirmed this hypothesis.[182]

**Renal Reserve Filtration Capacity.** Ingestion of meat or infusion of amino acids increases GFR (Chapter 44). This increase has been termed "renal reserve," although its functional significance is obscure. The percent increase in GFR in response to these stimuli in patients with chronic renal failure is not different from normal, and there is no evidence that renal reserve can predict progression.[183]

## TURNOVER OF NITROGENOUS EXCRETORY PRODUCTS IN CHRONIC UREMIA

The hallmark of chronic uremia is the accumulation of nitrogenous waste products in body fluids arising from catabolism of dietary protein and body protein stores. Accumulation of these waste products is undoubtedly the cause of symptoms of uremia because reducing their accumulation, either by restricting dietary protein or by dialysis, is associated with rapid symptomatic improvement. Chronic renal failure, therefore, may be considered a state of protein intolerance. Because of the enormous excretory capacity of the kidney, the accumulation of waste products does not cause uremic symptoms until renal function is reduced to below 30% of normal.

The removal of waste products is accomplished primarily by renal excretion but also by nonrenal excretion or degradation. This follows because the rate of production of waste products in the steady state must equal the sum of the amount excreted each day and the amount degraded.[184] This relationship is the basis for a useful method of calculating the severity of uremia, the steady-state serum urea nitrogen (SUN) concentration. After rearrangement, the clearance formula can be expressed as steady-state SUN concentration = (production − degradation)/clearance. The steady-state SUN concentration is a good estimate of the accumulation of all nitrogen-containing waste products derived from protein breakdown because urea is the major end product of protein catabolism. The calculation assumes that urea clearance is independent of the plasma concentration, which is reasonable for subjects with severe chronic renal failure. The usefulness of the steady-state SUN concentration is that it expresses the severity of renal impairment in relation to the nitrogenous waste products requiring excretion. Once produced, a waste product has three fates: it is excreted, it accumulates in body fluids, or it is degraded. The sum of the amounts excreted plus accumulated is termed the "appearance rate."[185] Thus, the difference between the total rate of production of urea (or any other waste product) and the rate of degradation equals the net rate of production or the appearance rate.

## Urea

It has been known since the classic report of Folin[186] that urea nitrogen excretion by normal subjects varies directly with protein intake. To generalize this principle to patients with renal failure, the urea nitrogen appearance rate (the sum of urea excretion and accumulation) varies directly with protein intake because nitrogen liberated during degradation of protein and amino acids is converted almost entirely to urea.[186–189] This fact has practical importance because it permits assessment of nitrogen intake (principally protein) in subjects with and without renal disease, including dialysis patients.[187–191]

For dialysis patients, the relationship between urea turnover and protein intake was popularized by Sargent and co-workers,[190] who coined the terms "urea generation" and "protein catabolic rate" (PCR). In dialysis patients, urea generation is calculated as the sum of urea excreted and removed by dialysis plus changes in the body pool of urea calculated from blood urea nitrogen concentration and weight. It is, in fact, urea appearance, and it exceeds the rate of urea production (generation) because some urea is degraded (see later). It closely parallels protein nitrogen in the diet.[190, 191] PCR is also a misleading term. PCR is calculated by adding urea generation (or urea appearance) to an estimate of nonurea nitrogen excretion (see later discussion); the sum is multiplied by 6.25 to convert nitrogen to protein equivalents. Thus, PCR must approximate protein intake closely in patients who are in nearly neutral nitrogen balance. PCR does not measure total protein catabolism because this rate is far greater than PCR. In fact, the nitrogen flux occurring during the daily processes of protein synthesis and degradation amounts to 45 to 55 g of nitrogen per day, which is equivalent to 350 g of protein or about 1 kg of muscle.[192] The principle of conservation of mass indicates that the difference between the nitrogen used in whole body protein synthesis and degradation plus protein intake must equal waste nitrogen production (times 6.25 to convert nitrogen to protein), but the implication that PCR is a measure of whole body protein catabolism is incorrect.

## UREA PRODUCTION AND DEGRADATION

When urea production was measured precisely by use of isotopically labeled urea, it was found to exceed the steady-state rate of urea excretion in both normal and uremic subjects. This difference is due to degradation of urea by bacterial ureases in the gastrointestinal tract to form ammonia and carbon dioxide.[193–195] Apparently, urea in gastrointestinal secretions[196] is degraded by bacteria, and the resulting ammonia is absorbed by passive, nonionic diffusion into portal blood for transport to the liver.[197, 198]

The rate of urea degradation in normal subjects eating about 90 g of protein per day averages 3.6 g/d of nitrogen, indicating that only a fourth of urea produced from dietary protein is degraded. Degradation can also be expressed as a rate of extrarenal urea clearance, defined as the rate of degradation divided by the plasma concentration of urea; the extrarenal urea clearance of normal subjects averages about 24 L/d.[193, 194, 199–201] It was proposed by Giordano[202] that the quantity of urea broken down in uremic patients must be large because of the high concentration of urea in intestinal fluids and the greater quantity of bacteria found in the upper intestines of patients with chronic renal failure.[203] This is not true. Careful measurements of urea degradation in patients with chronic renal failure indicate that the quantity of ammonia arising from urea is not significantly different from that of normal subjects.[204–206] Because the amount of urea degraded is not increased, the extrarenal clearance of urea in patients with chronic renal failure is greatly reduced compared with that in normal subjects. Obviously, the extrarenal urea clearance of patients with kidney disease is not correlated with renal urea clearance.[206] Robson[205] found that the average extrarenal urea clearance of patients with chronic renal failure was 4.5 L/d; in patients being treated with low-protein diets supplemented with amino acids or their α-keto or α-hydroxy analogues, we found that it averages less than 4 L/d.[206, 207]

The reason that extrarenal urea clearance in patients with chronic uremia is reduced is unknown. It is unlikely that the high concentration of urea present in these subjects is sufficient to saturate bacterial urease. The total amount (i.e., weight) of intestinal bacteria is increased.[203] The most likely explanation is that chronic uremia induces a change in the gut mucosa that, in some way, limits the access of urea to bacterial urease. Regardless, the results obtained in patients with stable chronic renal failure do not exclude the possibility that a rapid elevation of plasma urea, as occurs in patients with acute renal failure, might increase the rate of urea degradation.[196]

Urea metabolism has been discussed in some detail because changes in the net rate of urea nitrogen production (or urea appearance) parallel changes in the amount of protein eaten and the net rate of body protein degradation.[186–189] Other factors may also change urea metabolism. Diuretic therapy can influence urea metabolism in two ways. First, volume depletion can depress urea clearance by raising the reabsorption of urea in proximal and distal tubules.[208] Second, Na+ depletion after diuretic therapy increases urea appearance in both animals and humans.[208, 209] The mechanism for stimulation of urea production with Na+ depletion is unknown, but apparently it does not require glucocorticoids.[209]

Calculating the rates of urea production and degradation requires measurement of the plasma disappearance of [14]C- or [15]N-urea. These techniques are reserved almost entirely for research purposes, but the physiologically important aspect of urea turnover, the urea appearance rate, can be estimated from weight, SUN concentration, and the daily urea excretion rate. Urea appearance provides a simple means of estimating nitrogen intake and, hence, total waste nitrogen production.[189] The relation between urea and other protein-derived waste products was re-emphasized by results from the National Cooperative Dialysis Study.[210] It was found that altering the efficiency and duration of dialysis to raise or lower the steady-state SUN concentration paralleled the complications of uremia. A treatment schedule that maintained an SUN concentration less than 80 mg/dL was associated with fewer complications than a dialysis schedule that maintained an SUN concentration above 100 mg/dL.

## Nonurea Urinary Nitrogen

Maroni and colleagues[189] found that the average nonurea nitrogen excretion of patients with chronic renal failure who were in neutral or nearly neutral nitrogen balance while eating low-protein diets supplemented with keto acids or diets containing as much as 94 g of protein per day was 0.031 g/kg/d. Interestingly, 0.031 g of nitrogen per kilogram per day (Fig. 55–5) is similar to the value for nonurea

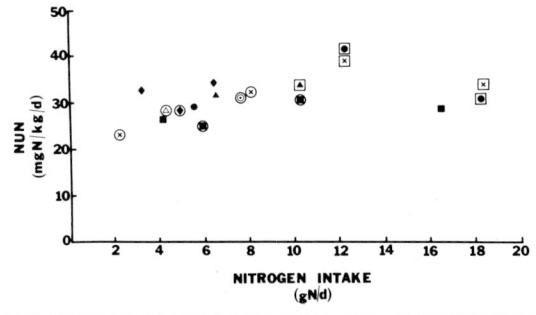

**Figure 55–5.** Calculated values of total nonurea nitrogen excretion (NUN) in normal subjects (▲, ●, ■) and patients with chronic renal failure being treated with nutritional therapy (◆, ⊗, △, ◈, ◎) or by hemodialysis or continuous ambulatory peritoneal dialysis (⊠, ⊡). (From Maroni BJ, Steinman TI, Mitch WE: A method for estimating nitrogen intake of patients with chronic renal failure. Kidney Int 27:58, 1985.)

urinary nitrogen plus fecal nitrogen excreted by normal subjects.[211–213] Apparently, nonurea nitrogen excretion can vary considerably in hypercatabolic patients receiving hyperalimentation (intravenous amino acids, glucose, and so on).[214, 215] Thus, in patients who are not eating or who are not in a stable condition, 0.031 g of nitrogen per kilogram per day is not a good estimate of nonurea nitrogen excretion.

## Creatinine

Creatinine is formed from the nonenzymatic dehydration of creatine and creatine phosphate. The turnover rate of the creatine pool is only 1.7%/d,[216] and because the major pool of creatine is in muscle and because creatinine is excreted almost completely (see later discussion), the rate of creatinine excretion has been used as an index of lean body mass. As discussed, considerable variation exists in creatinine excretion that is not explained by collection error, so that the average of three consecutive days of creatinine excretion is required for a reasonably precise estimate of lean body mass.[118, 217–219] Besides lean body mass, the amount of meat eaten changes creatinine excretion[218, 220]; when a diet is creatine free, creatinine excretion falls about 15%.[220] The fact that creatinine excretion does not decrease more may be due to stimulation of creatine (and, ultimately, creatinine) production by low-protein or low-creatine diets.[221, 222] Moreover, the low turnover rate of the creatine pools means that the rate of creatinine production will not reach a new steady state for 41 days.[116]

The most important factor affecting creatinine excretion in normal subjects, besides dietary creatine and creatinine and lean body mass, is age.[118] In order of descending importance, the factors determining the relationship of age and creatinine excretion are 1) a lower lean body mass, because increased weight with aging is attributable to increased body fat; 2) a decreased proportion of muscle in lean body mass, especially in men; and 3) probable reduced meat intake with aging.[220] Creatinine excretion is also decreased in patients with chronic renal failure and high levels of serum creatinine.[223] This has been attributed to a loss of lean body mass, but in patients with advanced chronic renal failure, it is far out of proportion to any possible change in their lean body mass.[116] In fact, when measured by isotope dilution, creatinine production in patients with chronic renal failure was found to be close to rates predicted for normal subjects of the same age, sex, and weight.[117] Thus, the explanation for decreased creatinine excretion in chronic renal failure must be degradation of creatinine.[184]

The first definitive evidence for creatinine degradation was reported by Jones and Burnett,[224] who measured the disappearance of [14]C-labeled creatinine administered to uremic patients orally or by injection. They estimated that as much as 66% of creatinine produced was degraded and detected radioactivity in sarcosine, N-methylhydantoin, creatine, and carbon dioxide. We examined the fate of injected [14]C-creatinine in patients with chronic renal failure and found that creatinine degradation was correlated positively with the serum creatinine concentration.[117] The progressive fall in creatinine excretion (or creatinine appear-

ance) that occurs as serum creatinine concentration rises above 6 mg/dL was due to the presence of a relatively constant extrarenal clearance, averaging 0.04 L/kg/d in predialysis patients.[117] Because extrarenal clearance is low, creatinine metabolism is an important route of elimination only when serum creatinine concentration is high. The low extrarenal clearance may also explain why creatinine degradation has not been detected previously in humans or animals with normal renal creatinine clearances.[225, 226]

Creatinine can be recycled to creatine; the [14]C label can be found in creatine after injection of [14]C-creatinine into chronically uremic subjects.[117] Because the pool of creatinine is so much smaller than that of creatine, recycling does not change the size of the creatine pool significantly. It is likely that intestinal bacteria degrade creatinine, because intestinal flora obtained from experimental animals being fed creatinine or from the intestines of normal subjects or patients with chronic renal failure degrade creatinine readily.[227, 228] However, creatinine metabolism in uremic subjects was not suppressed by oral administration of antibiotics even though there was inhibition of urea degradation.[117, 226]

The physiologic importance of creatinine degradation and the decline in creatinine excretion occurring with protein-restricted diets is that creatinine excretion cannot be used as an index of lean body mass in patients with chronic renal failure.

## Uric Acid

The increase in serum uric acid concentration in patients with renal insufficiency is not readily predicted from the decline in GFR for at least two reasons (see Chapter 15). The fractional clearance of urate is increased markedly in patients with chronic renal failure; at a GFR below 15 mL/min, the ratio of urate excreted to GFR is increased about fivefold because of increased secretion and reduced reabsorption.[229] Despite this adaptation, urate excretion by patients with advanced renal failure falls to about 100 to 300 mg/d compared with normal rates of 400 to 600 mg/d.[230] Because renal urate clearance decreases to about 1.4 mL/min in such patients, serum uric acid concentration would rise as high as 25 mg/dL if they continued to excrete 400 to 600 mg/d of uric acid. The fact that a serum uric acid level above 10 mg/dL is unusual in such patients[231] must mean that uric acid production is sharply reduced or that there is extensive extrarenal degradation of uric acid.[184] A protein-restricted diet is generally associated with a lower purine intake, and for patients treated in this way, uric acid production must be lower.[232, 233] There is also uric acid degradation.[234] Sorensen[235–237] reported that injected, radiolabeled uric acid could not be completely recovered in the urine of either normal subjects or patients with chronic renal failure and calculated that extrarenal urate clearance accounts for as much as 65% of uric acid produced by patients with renal insufficiency.[236] Intestinal bacteria probably account for uric acid degradation,[237] because urate degradation is reduced from 22% to 3% by oral administration of neomycin and streptomycin.

Many compounds produced during degradation of uric

acid (e.g., ammonia, urea, allantoin) are excreted by the kidney, so extrarenal urate clearance does not necessarily eliminate nitrogen; it may simply lead to accumulation of other compounds.[238] On the other hand, urate degradation may account for the low frequency of gouty arthritis or renal uric acid deposits of patients with chronic renal failure.[239] Uric acid crystals surrounded by inflammatory cells and fibrous tissue may be found in the renal medulla of nongouty patients with long-standing progressive renal insufficiency, but long-term allopurinol therapy does not significantly slow the progression of chronic renal insufficiency in patients with hyperuricemia.[240] Fessel[241] examined the clinical course of 113 patients with asymptomatic hyperuricemia and of 168 patients with gout, some of whom had mild renal insufficiency, and concluded that unless serum uric acid concentration exceeded 10 mg/dL in women or 13 mg/dL in men, the factor alone would not affect residual renal function. Fortunately, uric acid stones are uncommon; they occurred in only 1.0% to 2.6% of 113 patients with normal renal function and asymptomatic hyperuricemia observed for 8 or more years.[241] Likewise, in nongouty patients with renal insufficiency and hyperuricemia, uric acid stones are rare.[231] The conclusion is that allopurinol should not be prescribed for patients with chronic renal failure unless there is a history of gouty arthritis or biopsy-proven gouty nephropathy or unless the serum uric acid level is excessively high.[242]

## Ammonia

The loss of renal mass leads to a reduced capacity to excrete ammonia, even in response to metabolic acidosis (Chapter 10). Consequently, ammonia derived from glutamine degradation constitutes a small fraction of total urinary nitrogen in patients with chronic renal failure. Because little glutamine is converted to ammonia by the kidney, the major source of blood ammonia is bacterial degradation of urea as well as amino acids, peptides, and protein in the intestine; there is also degradation of glutamine to ammonia by small intestinal mucosa.[243, 244] In the liver, ammonia arising from the intestine is readily converted to urea so that blood ammonia levels in patients with renal insufficiency should not be elevated, although a high level has been reported.[245] The reason for this and its clinical importance are unknown. There are cases of hyperammonemia in patients with chronic renal failure and apparently normal liver function.[246] The mechanisms causing hyperammonemia in such cases include partial defects in urea cycle enzymes or other inherited disorders,[247, 248] high-dose chemotherapy,[249] and infections.[246, 250] Urinary bladders or intestinal abscesses chronically infected with urease-producing bacteria can cause clinically important hyperammonemia, especially if venous blood from the infected area drains into the vena cava and bypasses the liver.

## Other Nitrogenous Compounds

The difference between total urinary nitrogen and the sum of urea, uric acid, and creatinine nitrogen in urine is termed "unmeasured nitrogen."[186, 189, 251] Folin[186] found that unmeasured urinary nitrogen in normal subjects increased only 6.2 mg/kg/d when total urinary nitrogen increased by 10.3 g/d. In patients with proteinuria, albumin clearance as a fraction of GFR varies from 0.3% to 3.0% or more.[252] In general, protein clearance falls as GFR decreases in severe renal failure, so that the proteinuria of patients with the nephrotic syndrome decreases as renal insufficiency worsens.

**Fecal Nitrogen.** Patients with chronic renal failure commonly experience occult intestinal blood loss; in one study, the average blood loss was 6 mL/d, but this may be difficult to detect by the guaiac technique.[253] However, whenever urea appearance is found to exceed protein nitrogen intake, gastrointestinal bleeding must be considered. Other causes for a change in fecal nitrogen include variation in dietary roughage and nitrogen.[254–256] Usually, these factors change fecal nitrogen only slightly; from studies of normal subjects, it can be calculated that varying protein intake by 40 g/d would cause fecal nitrogen to change by only about 0.3 g/d.[189] Conversely, continuous enteral hyperalimentation with a low-nitrogen fluid eliminates dietary roughage and reduces fecal nitrogen of uremic subjects by 50%.[214, 215]

**Skin Nitrogen Losses.** The concentration of urea in sweat is proportional to the plasma urea concentration.[257] Hence, increased losses of nitrogen might occur in uremic individuals during periods of heavy perspiration.

### SUMMARY

Nitrogen excreted by normal and uremic subjects can be divided conveniently into urea nitrogen and the remainder, termed nonurea nitrogen. The production of urea nitrogen is closely related to protein intake, whereas excretion of nonurea nitrogen can be considered constant (0.031 g/kg/d) in patients who are eating and are not hypercatabolic (see Fig. 55–5). In chronic renal failure, an adaptive increase in extrarenal clearance of many compounds (e.g., uric acid, creatinine) also reduces the amount of products that must be excreted. In contrast, the rate of urea degradation does not differ from that of normal subjects, and nitrogen arising during urea degradation is simply recycled to synthesize urea. Because the amount of urea degraded does not change, the net rate of urea production, termed the urea appearance rate, can be used to estimate protein intake in stable patients (see later discussion).

## ASSESSMENT OF PROTEIN STORES IN CHRONIC RENAL FAILURE

Maintaining body protein or lean body mass is difficult in patients with chronic renal failure because raising dietary protein causes nitrogenous waste products to accumulate, whereas an inadequate intake of essential amino acids leads to loss of body protein. The adequacy of the diet can be assessed by measuring nitrogen balance, the difference between nitrogen intake and the excretion, plus accumulation of nonprotein nitrogen. Nitrogen balance is equal to the difference between the total rates of the synthesis and degradation of protein nitrogen. Clearly, when protein synthesis equals protein degradation, body protein stores are maintained and nitrogen balance is zero. The daily rates of protein synthesis and degradation (4 to 5 g/kg/d)[192] are high, so even a small increase in protein degradation or decrease in protein synthesis persisting for several weeks can cause a marked loss of lean body mass.

## Nitrogen Balance

The half-life of urea disappearance in a normal human is about 7 hours, so even a large load of urea is largely excreted within a day or two. It follows that there is rapid adaptation of the blood urea level to an increase or decrease in protein intake by normal subjects, and the urea pool can be ignored during measurement of nitrogen balance. In patients with chronic renal failure, the half-life of urea may be prolonged to well over a week, so that after a change in dietary protein, more than a month may pass before the blood urea nitrogen concentration and body pool of urea nitrogen are stable. For this reason, the accumulation or loss of urea nitrogen must be taken into account when nitrogen balance is measured.

Changes in the size of the creatinine pool can usually be ignored because even a large increase in serum creatinine concentration does not affect retained nitrogen much. For example, when the serum creatinine level rises from 10 to 15 mg/dL, it will increase nitrogen retention only 0.3 g in a 70-kg person. Changes in the pools of other nonprotein nitrogenous compounds are not commonly measured because their volumes of distribution are not known. However, after injury, loss of tissue glutamine nitrogen can amount to several grams.[258]

Because the major end product of amino acid catabolism is urea, large changes in urea production occur when protein intake rises or falls. Because the concentration of urea is equal throughout body water, changes in the urea nitrogen pool can be calculated by assuming that the urea space is equivalent to 60% of body weight, the average of body water in nonedematous uremic patients.[189, 259] When body water in liters is multiplied by the SUN concentration in grams per liter, the size of the urea nitrogen pool is estimated. Changes in both weight and SUN concentration affect the calculation, so it is more accurate to estimate the urea space on a given day and then calculate daily values of the urea pool as SUN concentration × (body water plus any change in weight). The calculation assumes that weight changes during short periods are due to changes in body water and that body weight minus body water (i.e., dry weight) remains constant. Unfortunately, the precision of measuring SUN concentration can dominate the nitrogen balance if only two measurements are made. For example, a change in SUN concentration from 140 to 150 mg/dL, which may be within the 5% to 7% error of measurement, represents about 4 g of nitrogen in a 70-kg person. Such difficulties can be surmounted by making repeated measurements of SUN concentration and body weight and then calculating the daily rate of change in the urea nitrogen pool by linear regression or other curve-fitting techniques.[190, 191]

It is more precise to measure the urea space with use of

[15]N- or [14]C-labeled urea.[205–207] This avoids the error of assuming that all uremic subjects have the same fraction of body weight that is body water. For example, urea space can occasionally exceed body water or even body weight.[205, 206, 260] Measurement of the urea space in patients with advanced renal failure does not require correction for losses of the label in urine because excess urea excretion seen in normal subjects during equilibration of labeled urea does not occur to an appreciable extent.[205]

## Urea Nitrogen Appearance Rate

The urea nitrogen appearance rate is measured as the sum of urinary excretion plus accumulation (positive or negative) in the body pool of urea nitrogen. The most accurate measurement requires several consecutive 24-hour urine collections, daily determinations of weight and SUN concentration, and calculation of the urea space by use of labeled urea[206, 207] or as 60% of weight in nonedematous subjects.[189] The urea appearance rate provides a quantitative measurement of the parameter that nutritional therapy seeks to minimize. In short, a minimal value of urea appearance should be associated with the most efficient use of dietary protein. Taylor and associates[261] fed low-protein diets containing different amounts of calories to normal young men and women. Their data reveal a correlation of $r = -.87$ between the calculated fraction of dietary protein used for protein synthesis and urea excretion (which is equal to urea appearance in normal subjects). Cottini and associates[188] found that a nitrogen intake of 3 to 4 g/d was associated with neutral nitrogen balance (Fig. 55–6). Clearly, interpretation of the urea nitrogen appearance of patients with chronic renal failure requires some knowledge of nitrogen intake from the relation between nitrogen intake and urea appearance. If nitrogen intake is known, nitrogen balance can be estimated from the urea nitrogen appearance minus the average figure for nonurea nitrogen excretion, 0.031 g/kg/d.[189] For example, a 70-kg patient eating 40 g of protein per day (6.4 g of nitrogen per day) is in neutral nitrogen balance if urea nitrogen appearance rate is 4 g/d. Low values must be interpreted in light of nitrogen intake; they may signify unusually efficient use of ingested nitrogen[262] or simply an inadequate nitrogen intake.

## Serum Albumin

The concentration of serum albumin has long been used as an index of protein nutrition, even though it responds relatively slowly to changes in protein stores because of a half-life of more than 10 days. Hence, plasma albumin levels are only slowly restored to normal during protein refeeding.[263] When hypoalbuminemia occurs in nonnephrotic patients with chronic renal failure, it should be viewed as a sign of protein malnutrition. In fact, studies of hemodialysis patients indicate that hypoalbuminemia is correlated with mortality.[264] Bianchi and co-workers[265] studied albumin synthesis rates in 26 patients with chronic renal failure who were undergoing nutritional therapy. In almost all patients, the fraction of total body albumin in extravas-

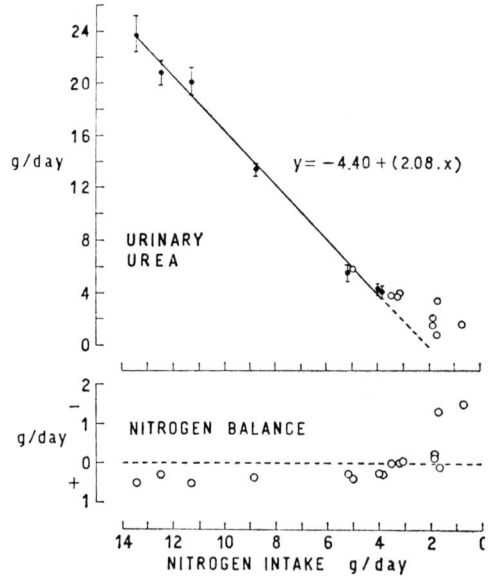

**Figure 55–6.** Nitrogen balance and urinary urea as a function of nitrogen intake in chronically uremic subjects fed varying quantities of dietary protein. All subjects receiving less than 4 g of nitrogen per day were in neutral or negative nitrogen balance, and urea excretion tends to plateau at a low value. In subjects receiving more than 4 g of nitrogen per day, urea nitrogen is equal to the increment in nitrogen intake. (From Cottini EP, Gallina DK, Dominguez JM: Urea excretion in adult humans with varying degrees of kidney malfunction fed milk, egg, or an amino acid mixture: Assessment of nitrogen balance. J Nutr 102:11, 1973.)

cular space was abnormal; the explanation for and significance of this observation are uncertain.

## Serum Transferrin, Prealbumin, and Complement

Several authors[266, 267] have suggested that serum transferrin is more reliable than albumin as an estimate of protein nutrition because transferrin is more sensitive to protein deficiency. However, transferrin levels may rise when iron stores are depleted and diminish by as much as 50% with chronic disorders such as malignant tumors, rheumatoid arthritis, and infections. The transferrin concentration in milligrams per deciliter is interconverted with total iron-binding capacity in micrograms per deciliter by multiplying total iron-binding capacity by 0.7, because two iron atoms are bound to each molecule of transferrin. A slightly greater degree of precision is obtained by using the formula transferrin $- 1.0900 \times$ (total iron-binding capacity $- 63$).[268] The use of erythropoietin has no significant impact on serum transferrin levels, at least in dialysis patients.[269, 270] In spite of an apparent improvement in appetite during erythropoietin therapy, there has been no major change in nutritional status. Serum albumin concentration is unchanged,[270] or minimally improved,[269] and anthropometric measurements and muscle protein content are unchanged.[270, 271] Consequently, there is no persuasive reason to use erythropoietin in predialysis patients to improve nutrition. On the other hand, there may be reason to avoid erythropoietin; there are cases in which erythropoietin seemed to accelerate

the loss of renal function,[272] although clinical trials have not reported that this occurs commonly.[273]

Serum prealbumin concentration has also been used as an index of nutritional state. When serum albumin, transferrin, and prealbumin concentrations in hemodialysis patients were measured by radioimmunoassay, prealbumin concentration appeared to have a special advantage because it was more highly correlated with complications (at a level below 0.3 g/L, there were increased complications, including infections and mortality).[274] Further testing in predialysis patients is necessary to determine if similar relations occur.

Abnormalities of most of the components of serum complement occur in patients with chronic uremia, especially an increase in C4.[275] Some of these changes may be due to protein malnutrition, because parenteral administration of essential amino acids for a month reportedly corrected most of them.[275]

## Anthropometrics

Evaluation of abnormal anthropometric measurements in patients with chronic renal failure is complicated, because most reports are based on a single evaluation compared with standards derived from measurements of normal healthy adults.[276] Moreover, the interpretation of abnormal anthropometric measurements is difficult because there are reports of normal values of serum proteins but anthropometric changes compatible with loss of muscle mass.[277, 278] Kopple[279] reported that cross-sectional studies of dialysis patients indicate a high frequency of abnormalities suggestive of malnutrition. It is unlikely that this can be attributed to low-protein diets prescribed during the predialysis period. When 95 predialysis patients were examined (before and after 1 year of amino acid– and keto acid–supplemented regimens), no clear decrease in nutritional status was seen, as indicated by changes in plasma proteins or anthropometric measurements.[280] Similarly, long-term (6 to 72 months) observation of patients treated with the same supplements revealed normal values of serum albumin and transferrin.[281] The contribution of anthropometrics to the assessment of the effectiveness of nutritional therapy is small.

## Free Amino Acid and Keto Acid Levels

Patients with chronic uremia have many abnormalities of plasma amino acids, including an increase in 3-methylhistidine and 1-methylhistidine, apparently caused by reduced renal clearance. There is also subnormal valine and, to a lesser extent, leucine and isoleucine values.[282–284] These abnormalities were generally observed in fasting patients, but Garibotto and co-workers[285] have reported that similar changes occur after a meal. The mechanism for low levels of branched chain amino acids is unclear. All three branched chain amino acids are decarboxylated by the same enzyme, and available evidence indicates the decrease cannot be accounted for by excessive uptake by splanchnic tissues.[286] Reduced protein intake is undoubtedly a cause, but branched chain amino acid catabolism in skeletal muscle could play a role because metabolic acidosis stimulates skeletal muscle branched chain keto acid dehydrogenase activity.[287, 288] This may explain why dialysis patients exhibit a correlation between plasma $HCO_3^-$ levels and the valine content in skeletal muscle.[289] Other abnormalities include increased citrulline, which has been attributed to impaired conversion of citrulline to arginine by the diseased kidney, but measurements made in rats with subtotal nephrectomy indicate that the mechanism is more complex.[290–292] There are also unexplained increases in cystine and aspartate; decreased tyrosine, reflecting impaired hydroxylation of phenylalanine[293–295]; high glycine; and low or low-normal serine, perhaps related to diminished production of serine from glycine by the diseased kidney.[296] Whether this last abnormality contributes to the high glycine levels is unknown.[297] The free tryptophan level is normal, but total tryptophan is low owing to reduced plasma protein binding.[298] Threonine and lysine decrease for unknown reasons. Thus, the essential amino acids, with some exceptions, tend to be reduced in plasma, whereas a few of the nonessential amino acids tend to be increased (Fig. 55–7). This pattern is reminiscent of that seen in patients with protein malnutrition[299] but cannot be explained solely on this basis because the abnormalities occur with what appears to be adequate protein intake. Moreover, many persist after a large meal of meat.[285] It has been shown that the low levels of valine and branched chain amino acids, the essential/nonessential amino acid and valine/glycine ratios, and the degree of increase in cystine, citrulline, and methylhistidines all correlate with GFR.[300]

After an intravenous load of amino acids to uremic subjects, the rate of removal of valine and phenylalanine is subnormal, but histidine removal is increased.[301] How this relates to the high plasma levels of histamine found in uremic patients (especially those with pruritus) is unknown.[302]

Because of these abnormalities, it has been difficult to evaluate dietary requirements for individual amino acids on the basis of plasma amino acid levels. In general, the severity of the abnormalities is correlated with the degree of renal insufficiency and uremic symptoms. They tend to worsen when protein intake is clearly inadequate; there is a direct correlation between the valine/glycine ratio and protein intake.[303] An additional problem in interpreting plasma amino acid levels is that uremia alters the distribution of amino acids between cells and extracellular fluid, except for erythrocytes and the cerebrospinal fluid.[282, 304–308] Thus, the pattern in plasma is not an accurate reflection of the pattern within tissues such as muscle. Bergström and associates[282, 305] have measured the intracellular concentration of amino acids in muscle of patients with chronic renal failure in the predialysis phase. Their results show the most pronounced abnormalities are different from those seen in plasma (Fig. 55–8): of the branched chain amino acids, only valine is subnormal; ornithine is as low as histidine. This group later found somewhat different results in other patients with chronic uremia; besides the low valine concentration, threonine, lysine, and arginine concentrations were found to be low.[282] Tryptophan content is high in muscle of uremic patients.[309]

Besides these abnormalities in amino acids, metabolites of amino acids, including those containing sulfur[310, 311] as well as a number of small peptides and amines (including polyamines, guanidines, and other nitrogenous compounds), accumulate in the blood.[184] These abnormalities are not reviewed because there is no specific therapy for them; generally, their concentrations decrease when the rate of accumulation of urea is decreased (Chapter 49).

Plasma levels of branched chain keto acids in patients with chronic renal failure are low.[312–315] This has been correlated with the degree of metabolic acidosis (presumably because of activation of branched chain keto acid dehydrogenase) and the impairment of GFR.[287, 312, 315] Gastrointestinal absorption of branched chain keto acids is unimpaired by chronic renal failure.[315] Nutritional efficiency of branched chain keto acids in uremic animals is equal to[316] or greater than[317] that in normal animals.

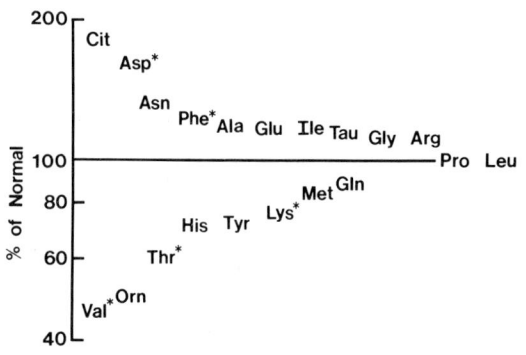

**Figure 55–8.** Intracellular free amino acid concentrations in muscle of chronically uremic patients treated by protein restriction alone. A logarithmic scale is used, so decreases are emphasized as much as increases. Asterisks indicate statistically significant differences. (Calculated from data reported by Bergström J, Fürst P, Norée L-O, et al: Intracellular free amino acids in muscle tissue of patients with chronic uraemia: Effect of peritoneal dialysis and infusion of essential amino acids. Clin Sci Mol Med 54:51–60, 1978.)

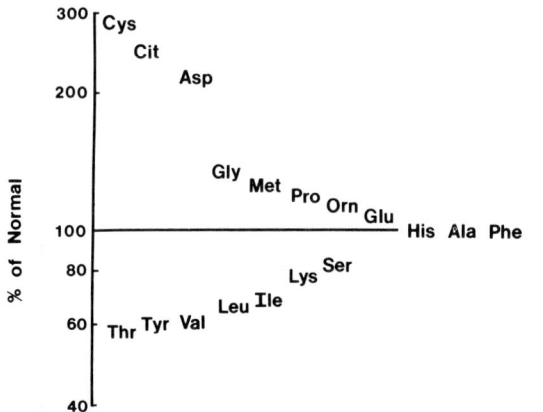

**Figure 55–7.** Plasma amino acids in patients with chronic renal failure treated by protein restriction alone. Results are calculated as percentages of normal values. A logarithmic scale is used, so decreases are emphasized as much as increases. The most abnormal values are shown on the left. Statistical significance cannot be evaluated in view of the variety of sources of the data. Note that not all essential amino acids are subnormal.

# NITROGEN CONSERVATION IN UREMIA

## Nitrogen Requirements

Giordano and colleagues,[318] using high-quality protein, concluded that 85% of subjects could achieve nitrogen equilibrium on a protein intake of 25 g/d, which suggests that nitrogen requirements of patients with chronic uremia were substantially lower than those of normal subjects. This conclusion is controversial, and most investigators agree that the nitrogen requirements of patients with chronic renal failure are not substantially different from those of normal subjects.[276, 319]

Nutritional requirements for dietary protein have primarily been based on short-term nitrogen balance measurements made while patients with moderate physical activity were eating a sufficient amount of calories. Such experiments can only provide intakes that, on average, should maintain neutral nitrogen balance; the average requirement values will prove inadequate for some patients.[276, 320] On the other hand, a dietary regimen containing only the minimal daily requirement (i.e., 0.6 g of protein per kilogram per day) or even a lower amount (i.e., about 0.3 g/kg/d) plus a supplement of essential amino acids or their nitrogen-free analogues (keto acids) maintains normal indices of nutrition during long-term therapy.[281, 321, 322]

As a measure of nutritional adequacy, nitrogen balance has limitations,[255, 276] so other methods have been used, including anthropometric measurements and serum protein concentrations. These are relatively insensitive to early changes in nutritional status.[276] Another method involves measuring the turnover of a labeled amino acid during its constant infusion. For this purpose, the most widely used amino acid is leucine; the leucine turnover technique can detect nutritional inadequacy even before there is clinical evidence, and it provides insight into metabolic responses activated by changes in dietary protein. Why use leucine? It was chosen because it is abundant in body proteins, and changes in protein metabolism affect leucine turnover. Finally, its degradation is easily detected. Leucine degradation in all cells initially requires transamination followed by irreversible decarboxylation of the resulting α–keto acid, α-ketoisocaproate. When leucine is labeled in the 1-position, labeled carbon dioxide is released during degradation in expired air and can be measured. Labeled carbon dioxide in expired air plus the enrichment of serum leucine or its

keto acid (α-ketoisocaproate) by labeled leucine (or labeled α-ketoisocaproate) can be used to calculate rates of whole body leucine oxidation, protein synthesis, and protein degradation. The technique has provided insights into metabolic responses activated by an increase or decrease in dietary protein. For example, the major response to a meal containing more protein than needed for protein balance is a sharp increase in the rate of amino acid oxidation (Fig. 55–9). Contrariwise, when dietary protein is lowered, amino acid oxidation falls, which leads to more efficient use of the amino acids in dietary protein for protein synthesis.[323] The decrease in amino acid oxidation in response to a low-protein diet has been denoted "adaptation." Young[324] has defined dietary protein adequacy as that intake which maintains long-term neutral nitrogen balance with successful adaptation (a decrease in amino acid oxidation) but no reduction in protein synthesis or degradation. However, if the intake of protein (or an essential amino acid) is so low that protein balance cannot be achieved, the capacity for amino acid oxidation to decrease is limited. In this case, both protein synthesis and degradation decrease, but these responses are apparently insufficient to achieve protein balance, and there is loss of lean body mass.[276, 324, 325] In short, dietary protein determines the metabolic processes that change protein balance. As might be expected, these changes are most easily detected after a meal.

What is the purpose of these responses? Amino acid catabolism destroys amino acids that exceed the amount needed for protein synthesis, and the nitrogen released is converted to urea. It is understandable, therefore, that a low-protein diet containing limited amounts of essential amino acids will decrease not only amino acid oxidation but also urea production.

Only a few studies have evaluated the metabolic responses to dietary protein restriction in patients with chronic renal failure. Goodship and co-workers[326] studied nonacidotic patients with an average serum creatinine level of 5 mg/dL by measuring both short-term nitrogen balances and whole body amino acid oxidation and protein turnover (i.e., leucine turnover) after an overnight fast and during a meal. When the subjects were fed 1 g of protein per kilogram per day, nitrogen balance was neutral or positive, and the values of amino acid oxidation and protein synthesis and degradation measured were indistinguishable from values measured in normal subjects. However, when dietary protein was reduced to the minimal daily requirement of 0.6 g/kg/d, both the patients and normal subjects were in negative nitrogen balance. In spite of this adverse response,

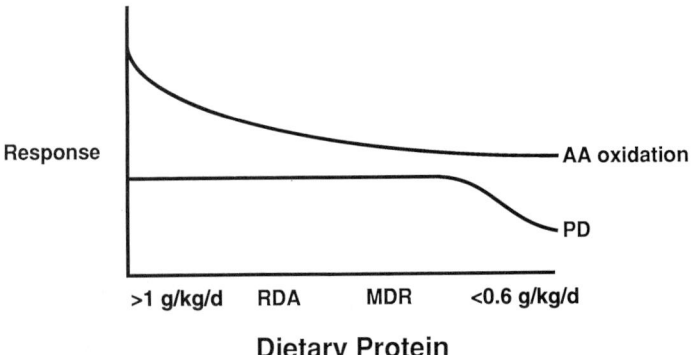

**Figure 55–9.** Hypothetic scheme for metabolic changes permitting successful adaptation to dietary protein restriction. The initial response to lowering dietary protein is a reduction in the oxidation of amino acids (AA oxidation). Amino acid oxidation declines progressively as protein intake is reduced from an excess (>1 g/kg/d) to the recommended daily allowance (RDA) and even further to the minimal daily requirement (MDR) of 0.6 g/kg/d. In contrast, protein degradation (PD) changes minimally until protein intake is reduced to or below the minimal daily requirement. At this level, amino acid oxidation does not decrease further, but protein degradation falls.

**TABLE 55–1. Studies Indicating That Metabolic Acidosis Is a Catabolic Stimulus in Humans***

| Year | Study Design (Type of Patients) | BCAA Oxidation | BCAA/BCKA Concentration | Protein Degradation | Nitrogen Balance | Reference |
|------|----------------------------------|----------------|--------------------------|----------------------|-------------------|-----------|
| 1970 | Alkaline therapy (CRF) | | | | Positive | 379 |
| 1978 | Alkaline therapy (renal tubular acidosis in children) | | | | Positive | 330 |
| 1993 | Acidotic infants | | | | Less positive | 329 |
| 1984 | Alkaline therapy (CRF) | | | | Positive | 380 |
| 1991 | Alkaline therapy (CRF) | | | ↓ | Positive | 337 |
| 1989 | CRF | | ↓ | | | 315 |
| 1991 | Alkaline therapy (CRF) | ↓ | | | | 332 |
| 1992 | Acidosis (normal adult) | ↑ | | ↑ | | 331 |
| 1993 | Alkaline therapy (CRF) | ↓ | | ↓ | | 333 |
| 1993 | CRF | ↓ | ↓ | | | 312 |
| 1994 | CRF | | | ↑ | | 335 |

*CRF = adult chronic renal failure patients with acidosis; BCAA = branched chain amino acids; BCKA = branched chain keto acids.

values for amino acid oxidation and protein turnover changed to the same degree in both groups, indicating that metabolic responses were intact even in nonacidotic chronic renal failure patients (see later discussion of acidosis).

Masud and colleagues[327] compared the metabolic responses to more restrictive diets consisting of 0.3 g of protein per kilogram per day plus equimolar supplements of essential amino acids or keto acids. In this study, the average GFR was 19 mL/min, and none of the eight patients was acidotic. They were fed the keto acid or essential amino acid regimen for at least 2 weeks before measurements were made, so patients had a longer time to adapt than did those in the study of Goodship and co-workers.[326] With both the essential amino acid and keto acid regimens, patients were in neutral nitrogen balance and exhibited virtually identical changes in amino acid oxidation and protein turnover during feeding and fasting. As might be predicted from the relationships shown in Figure 55–9, the rates of leucine oxidation during fasting and feeding found by Masud and colleagues were about 50% lower than those measured in patients with chronic renal failure ingesting 0.6 or 1.0 g of protein per kilogram per day. These results prove that low-protein regimens are a powerful stimulus to conserve dietary amino acids. The only difference between the keto acid and essential amino acid regimens was that with keto acids, patients achieved neutral nitrogen balance despite a 15% lower intake of nitrogen. The finding of neutral nitrogen balance in contrast to a negative balance with the standard, low-protein diet containing 0.6 g/kg/d is interesting. Presumably, the longer period of adaptation accounts for the difference, but neutral balance has been found just after the diet is changed to a keto acid–based regimen.[322]

# FACTORS CAUSING INCREASED NITROGEN REQUIREMENTS

## Metabolic Acidosis

Results from studies of experimental animals and patients suggest that metabolic acidosis is a major factor causing excessive catabolism in chronic renal failure. The rationale for studying metabolic acidosis as a catabolic signal is based on the well-known increase in renal ammonia excretion stimulated by acidosis. Ammonia excreted in this process arises from glutamine extracted by the kidney, but because the plasma concentration of glutamine does not fall dramatically, glutamine production must increase. Two mechanisms lead to increased glutamine production: synthesis by muscle, or increased muscle protein degradation releasing amino acids that are used by the liver to synthesize glutamine. The latter appears to be the mechanism, because normal rats with experimentally induced metabolic acidosis grow at a slower rate than pair-fed, nonacidotic rats, and there is excessive protein degradation in their skeletal muscles.[328] Increased muscle protein breakdown was not associated with increased glutamine release, so acidosis must increase hepatic glutamine synthesis from amino acids released during muscle catabolism.

The second type of evidence for a catabolic effect of metabolic acidosis is based on studies of normal subjects and patients with chronic renal failure (Table 55–1). Infants with metabolic acidosis grow poorly and have increased nitrogen excretion.[329] Providing sodium bicarbonate to children with renal tubular acidosis causes a sharp increase in growth.[330] Normal adults with metabolic acidosis after ammonium chloride ingestion exhibit increased oxidation of essential amino acids and increased degradation of protein.[331]

There are also studies of experimental animals indicating that metabolic acidosis is a major catabolic factor suppressing growth and stimulating loss of lean body mass in chronic uremia. Hara and associates[288] created a model of moderately severe uremia in rats by feeding a high-protein diet after subtotal nephrectomy. The observed responses to uremia could not be attributed to differences in the consumption of protein, calories, or minerals because sham-operated, control rats were pair fed with chronic renal failure rats. They found that plasma levels of branched chain amino acids in uremic rats were lower and the oxidation of leucine and valine was increased in isolated muscles from the uremic rats. The influence of acidosis in these processes was proved because both plasma levels of branched chain amino acids and their oxidation in muscle were restored to values measured in control rats when sodium bicarbonate was added to the diet to correct the metabolic acidosis.

There are similar findings in patients with chronic renal failure. Mochizuki[332] found that correction of metabolic acidosis in uremic patients fed a low-protein (0.6 to 0.8 g/kg body weight) diet improved nitrogen balance and increased plasma concentrations of the branched chain amino acids plus the levels of branched chain keto acids as well as glutamine and alanine.[332] Bergström and co-workers[289] found a strong linear correlation ($r = .81$) in hemodialysis patients between the plasma $HCO_3^-$ concentration measured just before a dialysis treatment and the free valine concentration in a muscle biopsy specimen. Garibotto and associates[312] have also observed a direct correlation ($r = .59$) in patients with chronic renal failure between the plasma $HCO_3^-$ concentration and the plasma level of α-ketoisocaproate, the keto acid of leucine. Finally, Reaich and co-workers[333] measured protein and amino acid metabolism three times in patients with chronic renal failure using the L-[¹⁴C]leucine technique. First, they measured these metabolic functions in untreated patients with spontaneous metabolic acidosis (average serum $HCO_3^-$ concentration, 15 mM). Metabolism of protein and leucine was remeasured after administration of sodium bicarbonate for 2 weeks (serum $HCO_3^-$ concentration averaged 21 mM) and again after 2 weeks of administration of an equimolar amount of sodium chloride (average serum $HCO_3^-$ concentration, 14 mM). As shown in Figure 55–10, the oxidation of leucine was stimulated by acidosis, compared with the period when patients were receiving sodium bicarbonate. Although measurements made in patients do not identify which organ is affected by metabolic acidosis, these results show that the accelerated amino acid catabolism first reported to occur in skeletal muscle by Hara and associates[288] also occurs in patients with chronic renal failure.

The fact that acidosis accelerates oxidation of branched chain amino acids suggests that acidosis activates the rate-limiting enzyme for their irreversible degradation, branched chain keto acid dehydrogenase. In rats with metabolic acidosis, May and co-workers[287] found reduced levels of branched chain amino acids in plasma and muscle and increased rates of valine and leucine transamination and oxidative decarboxylation in incubated muscles. This catabolic response was due to branched chain keto acid dehydrogenase activity in muscle; both the percentage of the enzyme in the dephosphorylated, activated form and the total amount of enzyme (measured as an increase in maximal velocity [$V_{max}$]) were increased. May and co-workers[334] showed that ammonium chloride–induced metabolic acidosis stimulates leucine oxidation in intact rats, and Reaich and colleagues[331] found that leucine oxidation increased 25% in subjects fed ammonium chloride for 5 days (blood pH fell from 7.42 ± 0.01 to 7.35 ± 0.03).

Besides accelerating amino acid catabolism, metabolic acidosis stimulates protein breakdown (see Table 55–1). May and colleagues[328] reported that metabolic acidosis increases corticosterone excretion in rats and that the mechanism for nitrogen wasting involved stimulation of protein degradation in muscles; protein synthesis in muscle was unchanged. Using the same model of acidosis, this group showed that protein degradation in the awake rat was sharply increased by acidosis.[334] Glucocorticoids are necessary for the increase in muscle protein degradation because metabolic acidosis does not increase muscle protein degradation in adrenalectomized rats unless glucocorticoids are also given.[328] The same requirement for glucocorticoids seems to be present in patients with chronic renal failure, because Garibotto[335] used the forearm perfusion technique to show that protein catabolism was positively correlated with plasma cortisol and inversely correlated with the serum $HCO_3^-$ concentration.

In chronically uremic, acidotic rats, protein degradation was found to be increased in isolated muscles, whereas protein synthesis was decreased.[336] Correction of acidosis by addition of sodium bicarbonate to the diet eliminated the high rates of muscle protein degradation but did not restore protein synthesis. A study measuring protein turnover in patients with chronic renal failure has confirmed that cor-

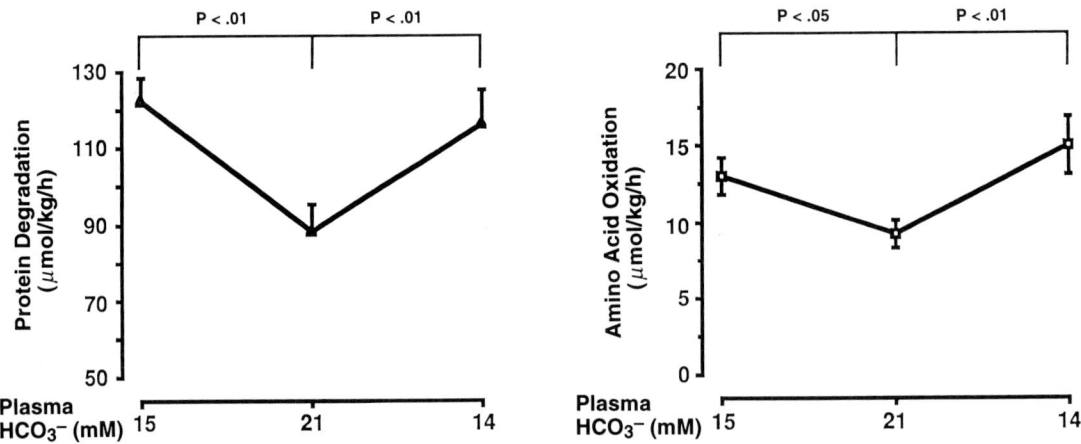

**Figure 55–10.** Measurements of the rates of whole body protein degradation and amino acid oxidation in patients with chronic renal failure and metabolic acidosis. Measurements were made when the average plasma $HCO_3^-$ concentration was 15 mEq/L, after the patients had been given supplemental sodium bicarbonate to correct the acidosis (plasma $HCO_3^- = 21$ mM), and after they had been treated with an equimolar amount of sodium chloride (plasma $HCO_3^- = 14$ mM). Correction of acidosis significantly improved protein degradation and amino acid oxidation. (Based on results of Reaich D, Channon SM, Scrimgeour CM, et al: Correction of acidosis in humans with CRF decreases protein degradation and amino acid oxidation. Am J Physiol 265:E230–E235, 1993.)

rection of metabolic acidosis by sodium bicarbonate administration reduces protein degradation (see Fig. 55–10).[333] Williams and associates[337] also reported that switching patients with metabolic acidosis to an isocaloric, low-protein diet (from 1.2 to 0.6 g/kg/d) caused a decrease in urinary excretion of 3-methylhistidine, which implies that skeletal muscle protein degradation was reduced. It was concluded that metabolic acidosis overrides the body's normal adaptive response to low protein intake.

In summary, there is abundant evidence from experimental animals and patients with chronic renal failure that metabolic acidosis accelerates the oxidation of branched chain amino acids and degradation of skeletal muscle protein. Glucocorticoids have been implicated as the mediator of this response, but other hormones or cytokines could be involved. To reduce the potential number of mediators, England and co-workers[338] studied BC3H1 myocytes and examined how acidification of the media would affect protein metabolism in the absence of changes in hormones or cytokines. Myocytes were grown in media containing 12% serum at either pH 7.1 or 7.4. The lower pH slightly reduced protein synthesis but sharply increased protein degradation. Although insulin at physiologic or supraphysiologic concentrations decreased protein degradation at both pH levels, the catabolic stimulus of acidosis was not abolished. Addition of glucocorticoids did not augment the proteolytic response to modification. This result has been examined in more detail by Isozaki and co-workers.[339] First, they proved that BC3H1 myocytes express a functional glucocorticoid receptor using a transfection strategy based on a plasmid's continuing a glucocorticoid receptor–sensitive promoter and reporter gene construct. To limit the metabolic influence of glucocorticoids, they incubated BC3H1 myocytes at pH 7.4 or 7.1 but only with 1% serum and found evidence for a permissive effect of glucocorticoids in regulating protein metabolism.

An important question is which proteolytic pathway is stimulated by metabolic acidosis? In all cell types, including skeletal muscle, there are multiple proteolytic pathways, including the acidic proteinases found in lysosomes, the $Ca^{2+}$-activated proteinases in the cytoplasm, and the ATP-independent and ATP-dependent cytosolic pathways. Mitch and colleagues[340] have shown that metabolic acidosis stimulates specific proteolytic pathways in muscle. They used a strategy employing inhibitors of different proteolytic pathways to determine which pathway is stimulated by metabolic acidosis. They found that acidosis accelerates an ATP-dependent pathway in muscle, the ATP-ubiquitin-proteasome pathway. In this pathway, proteins are targeted for degradation when they are conjugated to ubiquitin, a small 76–amino acid protein found in all cells; ubiquitin is a component of the heat shock response.[341, 342] The conjugation reaction requires ATP, as does degradation of the protein-ubiquitin conjugates. Both conjugation and degradation occur in the 26S proteasome, a large multicatalytic, multisubunit complex, which is found in the nucleus and cytoplasm of virtually all cells.[341] The abundance of ubiquitin messenger RNA (mRNA) was found to be increased in skeletal muscles of acidotic rats, and this change was accompanied by increased levels of mRNA for subunits of the proteasome.[340] Specificity of the response was suggested

because there was no increase in ubiquitin mRNA in kidney, nor was there an increase in the mRNA of other heat shock proteins. Data indicate that these changes in mRNA require glucocorticoids because they are absent in muscle of adrenalectomized acidotic rats unless dexamethasone is administered.[343] Thus, metabolic acidosis appears to up-regulate skeletal muscle protein degradation through a coordinate increase in the expression of genes for enzymes involved in the ATP-ubiquitin-proteasome protein degradation pathway.

The mechanisms regulating activity of these pathways, including the action of specific hormones or other factors, are poorly understood. Because chronic renal failure is associated with abnormalities in several endocrine systems, identifying which hormone activates proteolysis is an important area of investigation. There is reason to implicate glucocorticoids as a mediator of protein catabolism. In the perfused hindquarter, high doses of glucocorticoids suppress protein synthesis, whereas supraphysiologic doses accelerate muscle protein breakdown.[344, 345] May and colleagues[328, 336] noted that rats with metabolic acidosis and normal renal function or chronic renal failure have high rates of urinary corticosterone excretion, which suggests that increased glucocorticoid production may have a role in these catabolic states. Quan and Walser[346] reported that high physiologic doses of glucocorticoids inhibit whole body protein synthesis and stimulate protein degradation in rats. In normal adults, Simmons and co-workers[347] found that an 8-hour infusion of hydrocorticosterone to achieve high physiologic levels in plasma increased the rate of whole body proteolysis.

## Abnormal Carbohydrate Metabolism

Identification of a specific cause of abnormal protein metabolism in uremia could lead to improved therapy. In rats with acute renal failure, there is increased protein degradation in perfused or incubated muscle, and abnormalities in insulin-mediated carbohydrate metabolism are closely related to this defect.[348, 349] The evidence for increased muscle proteolysis in rats with chronic renal failure has been more difficult to isolate.[350, 351] Holliday and associates[352] reported that chronically uremic rats fail to suppress protein catabolism in response to calorie deprivation as efficiently as do normal animals. Harter and co-workers[353] suggested that accelerated muscle proteolysis in chronic uremia may be linked to diminished responsiveness to insulin, just as in acute uremia.[349] They found that insulin was less effective in inhibiting amino acid release from incubated muscle of uremic rats when the animals were fed high-protein diets and, hence, were more severely uremic; the response was normal when lower amounts of dietary protein were fed. Exercise can augment the magnitude of the response to insulin. Davis and co-workers[354, 355] found that exercise training of chronically uremic rats increased the sensitivity of muscle to insulin, thereby improving glucose uptake, glycolysis, and suppression of protein breakdown.

Bilbrey and associates[356] demonstrated that plasma glucagon levels are high in uremic subjects and are unresponsive to hyperglycemia. In fasting obese subjects, doses of glucagon sufficient to increase the plasma concentration to about 200 pg/mL paradoxically decreased urinary urea concentration but increased urinary ammonia.[357] Others find that large doses of glucagon in humans increase urea excretion.[358] The mechanism underlying this is unclear; it may be due to an increased activity of urea cycle enzymes in the liver[359] because, experimentally, muscle proteolysis is unaffected by glucagon except at levels as high as $10^7$ pg/mL.[360] Thus, the role of hyperglucagonemia in augmenting nitrogen requirements in uremia is uncertain.

Abnormal muscle protein breakdown may also be linked to defective energy metabolism in other ways. Li and Wassner[361] found no abnormalities in muscle protein turnover of fed rats with mild to moderately severe chronic uremia. With fasting, however, protein synthesis was unchanged, but the breakdown of myofibrillar muscle protein was increased, whereas the increase in proteolysis was inversely correlated with body fat stores.[361] Although an inhibitor of insulin-stimulated adipocyte metabolism has been identified in uremia,[362] no obvious link exists between this factor and the stimulation of muscle protein breakdown by fasting.

## External Losses of Protein

Any gastrointestinal blood that is digested will be reabsorbed as amino acids and augment urea production while depleting body stores of hemoglobin and plasma proteins.[253] The impact of the nephrotic syndrome is discussed subsequently.

## Altered Electrolyte Balance

In patients with advanced renal insufficiency, defects in ion transport have been demonstrated in blood cells, and there is an increase in intracellular $Na^+$ in muscle (Chapter 49). In rats made uremic by subtotal nephrectomy, several defects in cation transport develop in skeletal mass and adipocytes.[363] It is possible that transport abnormalities change the intracellular ionic milieu and contribute to abnormal metabolism. Both $K^+$ deficiency[364] and hyperkalemia[365] are reported to increase nitrogen catabolism. In patients with chronic renal failure, $K^+$ deficiency is often present[366] despite normal or increased serum $K^+$ concentration.

## Hyperparathyroidism

Evidence suggests that parathyroid hormone may augment urea production in normal subjects and in patients with hypoparathyroidism.[367] Some investigators[368, 369] found that parathyroid hormone increases the rate of protein degradation in isolated muscle. Thus, it is possible that secondary hyperparathyroidism, by stimulating catabolism, may increase nitrogen requirements in patients with chronic renal failure.

## FACTORS DECREASING THE REQUIREMENT FOR NITROGEN
### Reuse of Urea Nitrogen

Urea or ammonia can provide a source of nonspecific nitrogen for growth in animals,[370, 371] but the evidence is conflicting for humans. The fact that $^{15}N$ can be detected in protein of subjects given $^{15}N$-urea or ammonia salts[355, 372, 373] does not prove that $NH_4^+$ nitrogen has a nutritionally important role in protein synthesis, because labeling may occur through reversible reactions in which ammonia participates (e.g., the glutamate dehydrogenase reaction) coupled to subsequent transamination reactions between glutamate and various amino acids.[204]

In chronic renal failure, there is no increase in ammonia use for protein synthesis. Varcoe and associates[199] re-examined the incorporation of labeled urea nitrogen into the albumin of uremic patients compared with normal subjects and found that the amount of urea nitrogen used for albumin synthesis was greater in uremic subjects, but it was too small to be considered nutritionally significant. We examined the question by suppressing urea degradation in patients with chronic uremia treated with low-protein diets or very low protein diets plus keto acids. Neomycin or kanamycin was administered orally, and rates of urea production and degradation were measured by use of isotopic techniques and compared with those before antibiotic administration.[207, 374] There was no increase in urea nitrogen appearance despite an average reduction of urea degradation amounting to 85%, indicating that $NH_4^+$ derived from degradation is simply recycled back into urea.[207] Furthermore, nitrogen balance improved, evidently because fecal nitrogen decreased (after correcting for fecal nitrogen attributable to unabsorbed neomycin or kanamycin).[374] Clearly, if $NH_4^+$ were an important source of nonessential nitrogen for patients eating protein-restricted diets, nitrogen balance should have worsened. Thus, urea nitrogen degradation does not contribute importantly to protein conservation in uremia. Although the so-called nonessential or nonspecific nitrogen requirement of normal subjects can be met by administration of urea or ammonia salts to normal and malnourished adults,[375–378] uremic patients may be able to use urea nitrogen to a minor extent for synthesis of protein, but convincing evidence for an important role in nitrogen conservation is lacking.

## TECHNIQUES OF NUTRITIONAL THERAPY AND THEIR EFFECTS ON PROGRESSION
### Rationale for Nutritional Therapy

Uncertainty and controversy about the effect of dietary therapy on progression have obscured a long-established point: protein restriction ameliorates the signs and symptoms of renal failure. This observation, which dates back at least as far as 1869,[381] has been repeatedly confirmed, yet many (or perhaps most) patients with chronic renal failure never receive instruction in a low-protein diet as the end stage approaches. Studies of progression from reputable centers continue to appear in which the control group ingests a normal amount of protein (1 g/kg) right up to the time dialysis begins.[382] Some of the reasons that protein restriction is not routinely used have been discussed by Giovannetti.[383] None of them is valid. Every symptomatic patient with chronic renal failure should receive instruction in a low-protein diet from a skilled dietitian.

There are several reasons why protein restriction is so effective in reducing signs and symptoms. First, a given percent reduction in protein intake leads to a greater percent reduction in SUN concentration, with which symptoms are closely correlated. This is because the rate of excretion of nitrogen in forms other than urea is little affected by protein restriction. If a very low protein diet (0.3 g/kg) plus supplemental essential amino acids or keto acids is used, SUN concentration may fall to normal or nearly normal values despite severe reduction of GFR (Table 55–2). Second, most of the signs and symptoms of chronic renal failure are attributable to the retention of products of protein catabolism. Exceptions to this generalization include anemia and hyperlipidemia (even though both of these may improve somewhat with protein restriction). Third, protein intake, at least in the United States, averages nearly double the protein requirement (0.6 g/kg). Hence, considerable restriction is possible without negative nitrogen balance and hypoproteinemia.

A protein-restricted regimen can be effective only if other complications of chronic renal failure are controlled, such as $Na^+$ balance and blood pressure, acidosis and serum $K^+$ level, uric acid and gout, $Ca^{2+}$ and phosphorus balance, and anemia and iron stores.

## Dietary Compliance

An integral aspect of any treatment strategy based on dietary modification is a method for monitoring compliance. Monitoring methods include diet history techniques of food records, the 24-hour recall, food frequencies, and biochemical markers. Bingham[384] exhaustively reviewed the advantages and limitations of dietary history methods and reached a conclusion shared by others[385] that diet histories generally underestimate intake of protein and possi-

bly other nutrients. For dietary protein, the coefficient of variation ranges from 6% to 52%, even when foods are weighed.

Another method for monitoring dietary protein is based on nitrogen excretion and the assumption of neutral nitrogen balance. According to Bingham,[384] there is about 13% daily variation in total urinary nitrogen excretion by normal subjects; eight 24-hour urine collections are required to provide accuracy in estimating protein intake of normal subjects as determined by 14 days of dietary records. For patients with renal insufficiency, the use of nitrogen excretion to estimate protein intake has been refined somewhat. As discussed, the production of urea is proportional to dietary protein and can be measured as the sum of urea excretion plus accumulation. In contrast, nonurea nitrogen—the sum of fecal nitrogen, urinary creatinine, uric acid, and unmeasured nitrogen—exhibits minimal variation with dietary protein (see Fig. 55–5). Consequently, the prescribed intake of protein nitrogen can be compared with the urea nitrogen appearance plus 0.031 g of nitrogen per kilogram per day as an average value for nonurea nitrogen.[189] When dietary history has been compared with calculated values of protein intake (urea appearance and nonurea nitrogen excretion), the nitrogen excretion method yields consistently higher levels of dietary protein.[386] Because humans do not fix atmospheric nitrogen, these results support Bingham's conclusion that diet histories tend to underestimate protein intake. Regardless, the only method for estimating calorie intake and obtaining information on food preferences for planning diets is diet histories, so both nitrogen excretion and history methods (coupled with weighing of diet portions) are necessary for successful treatment by dietary modification.

In growing children, the difference between protein intake and urea nitrogen excretion was neither constant nor independent of protein intake, in contrast to observations for adults by Maroni and co-workers.[189] Wingen and associates[387] reported that nonurea nitrogen in 123 children with chronic renal failure averaged $0.085 \pm 0.061$ g/kg/d and was highly correlated ($r = .839$) with protein intake; nonurea nitrogen was about 11% of protein nitrogen intake. Calorie malnutrition or severe acidosis tended to invalidate these calculations.

Compliance is particularly troublesome in evaluating the effect of any dietary regimen. If a significant proportion of

## TABLE 55–2. Examples of Low Serum Urea Nitrogen Concentration in Patients with Severe Chronic Renal Failure Receiving Nutritional Therapy*

| Sex | Age (y) | Diagnosis | GFR (mL/min/70 kg IBW) | SUN (mg/dL) | UNA (g/d) |
|---|---|---|---|---|---|
| M | 38 | Chronic glomerulonephritis | 9.0 | 26.0 | 2.2 |
| F | 47 | Arteriolar nephrosclerosis | 13.3 | 26.2 | 3.0 |
| M | 65 | Diabetic nephropathy | 10.4 | 25.2 | 2.4 |
| M | 31 | Diabetic nephropathy | 8.2 | 28.8 | 2.9 |
| M | 50 | Polycystic kidney disease | 14.8 | 27.8 | 4.5 |
| F | 42 | Polycystic kidney disease | 13.3 | 27.3 | 4.8 |
| M | 33 | Interstitial nephritis | 14.4 | 23.0 | 2.6 |

*UNA = urinary urea nitrogen appearance; IBW = ideal body weight. Each value is the average of four or more observations over a period of 4 or more months.
Modified from Walser M: Dietary proteins and their relationship to kidney disease. *In* Liepa GU (ed): Dietary Proteins in Health and Disease. American Oil Chemists Society, Champaign, IL, 1992, pp 168–178.

subjects assigned to the more restrictive diet fail to comply (or if some of the subjects assigned to the less restrictive diet tend to emulate the low-protein group), a slower rate of progression could be caused by the diet or could reflect inherently less rapidly progressive disease in the more compliant subjects. In other words, more rapidly progressive renal failure may be associated a priori with a tendency to be noncompliant. Just why this might be so is not clear, but it has been demonstrated, for example, that participation in a clinical trial may itself slow progression, at least as measured by $[Cr]^{-1}$ slopes[388] (better control of blood pressure was given as the likely explanation in this study). There are now numerous studies in which the rate of progression with a variety of regimens (measured by reliable methods) is faster in less compliant patients.[389, 390] If an analysis by intention to treat had been used in such studies (see earlier), one might have erroneously concluded that no significant effect on progression occurred.

Thus, it appears that until it can be established that noncompliant patients are inherently more rapid progressors, both types of analyses (i.e., by intention to treat and in compliant patients) should be reported in studies of the effects of diet on progression. Confining the analysis to intention to treat may yield a meaningless result.

## Protein Restriction Without Supplementation

In six patients with insulin-dependent diabetes, a diet containing 0.6 g of protein per kilogram reduced muscle strength and induced negative nitrogen balance lasting at least 12 weeks.[391] Leucine oxidation increased progressively. This study, if confirmed, suggests that low-protein diets may be hazardous in diabetics.

Several studies reported in 1989 or earlier and summarized in the fourth edition provided suggestive evidence that protein-restricted diets, without supplementation, slow progression of chronic renal failure. Subsequent work has not settled this important question.

Walker and colleagues[392] observed 19 insulin-dependent diabetic patients eating a normal protein diet (1.13 g/kg) for 12 to 39 months and then for 12 to 49 months while they were given protein at 0.67 g/kg. Nutrition was maintained, and the rate of fall of GFR decreased from 0.61 to 0.14 mL/min/mo. Proteinuria decreased too. Subsequently, Viberti and co-workers[47] compared results in these patients, observed for 5 years, with results in 21 matched diabetic patients given a normal diet. The rate of loss of GFR averaged 0.16 mL/min/mo in treated subjects versus 0.61 mL/min/mo in the control group. Hyperlipidemia was also reduced.

Williams and colleagues[152] randomized 95 patients to receive 1) a diet containing 0.6 g of protein per kilogram and 800 mg of phosphate, 2) a diet containing at least 0.8 g of protein per kilogram and 1000 mg of phosphate plus a phosphate binder, or 3) a diet containing at least 0.8 g of protein per kilogram and phosphorus ad libitum. During an average follow-up interval of 19 months, creatinine clearance declined at statistically the same rate in all three groups. Urinary urea nitrogen excretion was only 18%

lower in diet 1 than in diet 2 or 3. Thus, the reduction in protein intake was small, so the effect of the diet cannot be judged.

Locatelli and associates[393] randomized 456 patients to receive protein at either 0.6 or 1.0 g/kg and observed plasma creatinine levels for 2 years. The outcome changes in creatinine clearance differed at only a borderline level of significance, perhaps because protein intake (as measured by urinary urea nitrogen excretion) was again reduced by only 17%.

Zeller and co-workers[394] randomized 35 diabetic patients with nephropathy to receive either 0.6 g of protein per kilogram and 500 to 1000 mg of phosphorus or at least 1 g of protein per kilogram and at least 1000 mg of phosphorus and observed urinary clearances of iothalamate for an average of 35 months. From urinary measurements, protein intake fell 33% and phosphate intake fell 36%. Progression slowed 74% ($P < .05$). This study is unique in showing clear-cut and clinically significant benefit from protein restriction, in terms of progression, by use of acceptable methods. However, serum albumin concentration did not change, which fails to support the later suggestion of Brodsky and colleagues[391] (see earlier) that this regimen may be nutritionally unsafe in diabetic patients.

In children with chronic renal failure, two reports[395, 396] indicate that randomization to a free protein intake versus 0.8 to 1.1 g of protein per kilogram had no significant effect on rate of loss of renal function, as measured by serum creatinine concentration or by $^{51}$Cr-EDTA clearance.

Results of the largest trial, the Modification of Diet in Renal Disease study, have so far been reported only according to the prescribed diet, an "intention to treat analysis."[396a] In study A, a diet with protein at 0.575 g/kg and phosphorus at 5 to 10 mg/kg (diet L) was compared with dietary protein at 1.0 to 1.4 g/kg and phosphorus at 16 to 20 mg/kg (diet M) in 585 patients with GFRs of 25 to 55 mL/min/1.73 m². In study B, diet L was compared with diet K, containing protein at 0.28 g/kg and phosphorus at 4 to 9 mg/kg and supplemented by a keto acid–amino acid mixture at 0.28 g/kg (RKAP, Table 55–3), in 255 patients with GFRs of 13 to 24 mL/min/1.73 m². In both studies, patients were also randomized to achieve two levels of mean arterial blood pressure (107 versus 92 mm Hg) by use of angiotensin-converting enzyme inhibitors or other drugs. The two blood pressure goals were included because the feasibility phase of the trial, involving randomization of 96 patients, showed that mean arterial pressure was correlated with the rate of progression.[386] Study A showed a greater GFR drop initially for diet L but a slower decline subsequently. Unfortunately, the average follow-up was only 2.2 years. In study B, the rate of decline of GFR was marginally slower by an average of 19% (confidence limits 0% to 41%) for diet K ($P = .066$). Treatment of hypertension was beneficial in patients with proteinuria at a level of 3 g/d or higher. Nutrition was generally maintained with all three diets. So far, only intention to treat analyses of this trial have been reported. It is unfortunate that the operational phase of this trial, unlike the feasibility phase,[386] did not exclude nonprogressors and that the average follow-up was only 2.2 years. An intention to treat analysis of the feasibility phase in which keto acid mixture EE (see Table 55–3) was used has

**TABLE 55–3. Composition of Keto Acid–Amino Acid Supplements Used in the Feasibility Phase (Phase II) and the Operational Phase (Phase III) of the MDRD Study***

| Constituent Present After Hydrolysis† | mmol/kg/d‡ | | mg/kg/d‡ | |
|---|---|---|---|---|
| | Phase II | Phase III | Phase II | Phase III |
| L-Ornithine | 0.328 | 0.453 | 43.3 | 59.9 |
| L-Lysine | 0.328 | 0.219 | 47.9 | 32.0 |
| L-Histidine | 0.062 | 0.062 | 9.6 | 9.6 |
| Ketoisocaproate | 0.281 | 0.281 | 36.6 | 36.6 |
| (R,S)-Ketomethylvalerate | 0.219 | 0.219 | 28.5 | 28.5 |
| Ketoisovalerate | 0.219 | 0.234 | 25.4 | 27.2 |
| L-Tyrosine | 0.312 | 0.250 | 56.5 | 45.3 |
| L-Threonine | 0.234 | 0.109 | 27.9 | 13.0 |
| L-Tryptophan | 0.000 | 0.004 | 0.0 | 0.8 |
| Calcium | 0.062 | 0.031 | 1.2 | 0.6 |
| DL-Hydroxymethylthiobutyrate | 0.124 | 0.062 | 9.3 | 4.7 |
| Total nitrogen | 1.982 | 1.835 | 29.6 | 25.7 |
| Total weight | | | 286.2 | 258.2 |

*The Modification of Diet in Renal Disease (MDRD) phase II mixture, known as EE or Cetolog, was obtained from Synthélabo (now Clintec), Paris, France. The phase III mixture, known as RKAP, was obtained from Ross Laboratories, Columbus, OH.

†These mixtures comprise mixed salts of basic amino acids (or calcium) with amino acid analogues in various proportions; the table gives the constituents after hydrolysis of these salts.

‡Dosage was calculated to the nearest 10 kg of standard body weight.

shown significant slowing of progression of disease with diet K after adjustment for the influence of blood pressure. Complete analysis of results of the trial, including the outcome of patients who achieved prolonged compliance with the diets, is awaited.

## Essential Amino Acids

The problem of devising the optimal mixture of amino acids for such patients is formidable. The proportions of essential amino acids required by normal subjects are commonly employed as a starting point for the proportions to be used for uremic subjects.[397] Although these proportions might provide the most efficient source of nitrogen in uremia, it does not follow that such a mixture would also be optimal for replenishing nitrogen stores in a protein-depleted subject or for permitting growth in a uremic child. Second, in uremia, plasma levels of some essential amino

acids are much more depressed than others (see earlier discussion). The compositions of some of the oral amino acid mixtures that have been studied in chronic renal failure are listed in Table 55–4. Mixtures studied earlier are summarized in the fourth edition. The proportions of individual essential amino acids have varied, but all mixtures differ from the proportions present in the minimal daily requirements. Histidine is included because it is known to be at least semiessential.[398]

Most of these mixtures contain only essential amino acids. In one mixture, tyrosine was added because of the low levels of plasma tyrosine characteristic of chronic renal failure; concomitantly, phenylalanine was reduced.

The diet used in conjunction with these supplements has usually been one containing 0.3 g/kg of mixed-quality protein, as first described by Norée and Bergström.[399] The considerable variety permitted in this diet makes it well accepted by most patients, in contrast to unsupplemented 40-g protein diets, which must contain mostly high-quality

**TABLE 55–4. Composition of Some Oral Essential Amino Acid Mixtures Studied in Chronic Renal Failure**

| Component | % of Total Amino Acids | | | | |
|---|---|---|---|---|---|
| | I | II | III | IV | V |
| Valine | 11.6 | 11.9 | 18.7 | 12.1 | 12.3 |
| Leucine | 15.9 | 15.8 | 12.5 | 16.7 | 17.2 |
| Isoleucine | 10.1 | 9.9 | 8.3 | 10.6 | 9.9 |
| Phenylalanine | 15.9 | 15.8 | 9.7 | 16.7 | 19.4 |
| Methionine | 15.9 | 15.8 | 12.5 | 16.7 | 10.9 |
| Lysine (as acetate) | 11.6 | 11.9 | 9.0 | 12.0 | 15.4 |
| Threonine | 7.2 | 6.9 | 9.0 | 7.6 | 9.1 |
| Tryptophan | 3.6 | 4.0 | 3.5 | 3.8 | 1.6 |
| Histidine | 8.0 | 7.9 | 6.2 | 3.8 | 4.2 |
| Tyrosine | 0.0 | 0.0 | 10.4 | 0.0 | 0.0 |
| Brand name | Aminess | None | Aminess-Novum | Aminaid | None |
| Reference | 399 | 424 | 282 | 283 | 128 |

protein and are, therefore, more restrictive in the choices of foods available.[400, 401] Detailed descriptions of the 0.3 g/kg protein diet have appeared in German, Swedish, and Italian, but descriptions in English appear to be limited.[247, 402-405] Remarkably, the official manual of the American Dietetic Association for renal patients does not mention the diet.[406]

One concern about this diet is that protein deficiency might develop with long-term use, thereby increasing morbidity and mortality on dialysis.[407] However, an analysis of nutritional parameters in 43 patients given this diet plus supplemental amino acids or keto acids for 6 to 72 months, who then went on to dialysis, showed that protein malnutrition was rare in these patients; hypoalbuminemia was far less frequent than has been reported in patients beginning dialysis nationwide.[281] Similar results have been reported by Rayner and co-workers.[408] They analyzed data from 142 patients who followed a low-protein diet (0.6 g/kg) long term. A significant weight loss occurred, amounting to 0.64%/y, but serum albumin levels rose significantly by 0.72%/y. Arm muscle circumference did not change significantly. They could find no evidence that the 79 patients in this group who went on to dialysis fared less well than patients not treated by diet during the same interval.

Compliance with low-protein diets is improved with the inclusion of special low-protein, low-phosphorus foods. This widens the selection of other foods that may be included. These diets typically contain about 500 mg of phosphorus per day; lower intakes of phosphorus can be achieved,[409, 410] but only with difficulty. Because all such diets are deficient in vitamins and calcium, supplements of these substances must be provided.

The mode of administration of mixtures of essential amino acids for oral use has varied; some workers have mixed the dry powder with food, such as applesauce or pudding. However, the unpleasant taste of L–amino acids (particularly the essential ones) is poorly disguised. Others have used tablets, coated tablets, or gelatin capsules. Here, the main difficulty is the number of tablets or capsules that must be consumed each day. In addition, some subjects complain of an unpleasant aftertaste or disagreeable eructations. On the whole, however, such products are reasonably well tolerated. All workers agree that each dose should contain all of the amino acids and be taken with meals or near mealtimes.

With oral supplements of essential amino acids to a low-protein diet, chronically uremic subjects exhibit greatly reduced symptoms, have a diminished blood urea concentration, and are able to forestall dialysis for many months[399] even in the absence of any changes in the rate of loss of renal function. Several studies have compared oral essential amino acid therapy with protein restriction alone in predialysis patients. Schloerb[411] found a difference of only 0.7 g in the average nitrogen intake required to achieve nitrogen balance between the two regimens. Röckel and co-workers[412] and Kult[413] compared the potato-egg diet with a diet containing 15 to 20 g of unselected protein supplemented by 7.5 g of essential amino acids in a 9-month study in which patients were randomly assigned to one or the other regimen. Anemia was less severe, serum phosphorus concentration was lower, and serum levels of several proteins were higher in the amino acid–supplemented group. Kopple

and Swenseid[283] found nitrogen balance to be negative in two of three subjects receiving 21 g of an essential amino acid mixture in the proportions required by normal adults. The fact that nitrogen balance was negative may have been attributable, in retrospect, to histidine deficiency. Walser[414] and Bauerdick and associates[415] found nitrogen balance to be positive in patients receiving only 7 g of essential amino acids in addition to 25 g of unselected protein.

On the other hand, Fröhling and associates[416] found no difference between an essential amino acid–substituted regimen and an isonitrogenous potato-egg diet in nutritional measurements, plasma amino acid levels (including free and protein-bound tryptophan), serum parathyroid hormone level, or the rate of change of reciprocal serum creatinine concentration.

The effects of a supplement containing essential amino acids in the proportions necessary for normal adults on intracellular amino acids were reported by Fürst and co-workers.[417] After 3 months, the levels of valine and threonine in muscle rose toward normal; alanine and methionine increased above normal, and tyrosine became extremely low. Most of the abnormalities of plasma amino acid concentration are diminished but not corrected by such a supplement of essential amino acids, and some are worsened.[415, 418, 419]

Other biochemical parameters of the uremic state are generally improved,[415, 418–420] although not in all studies.[421] The effects of this regimen on progression remain uncertain. Alvestrand[321, 422] and Bucht[423] and co-workers reported the effects of treating 17 patients with well-defined rates of progression before therapy (as determined by a linear decline in $[Cr]^{-1}$ for an average of 355 days with a supplement designed to correct abnormalities in amino acid concentrations. The initial creatinine concentration of the group averaged 8.3 mg/dL. Therapy consisted of the same low-protein, low-phosphate dietary regimen, and 14 patients were given a supplement of essential amino acids; the remaining 3 received a mixture of amino acids and keto acids. For the group as a whole, these regimens appeared to decrease the rate of progression considerably, at least as assessed by creatinine concentration. Considering individuals, it appears that only three patients did not show substantial slowing of progression. Before the supplemented diets were begun, many of the patients were experiencing progression of renal insufficiency, even though they had restricted dietary protein to about 0.6 g/kg/d. Further analysis of these patients by Bucht and colleagues[423] cast some doubt on these results and raised the possibility that better control of blood pressure and closer follow-up had slowed progression. The same group[388] assessed progression by means of isotopically measured GFR in seven patients before and after they started a low-protein diet plus essential amino acids; no change in progression was seen, but compliance was poor. Ando and co-workers[424, 425] reported that progression, by measurements of serum creatinine concentration, was slowed in 30 patients given oral or intravenous amino acids plus a low-protein diet, compared with a control group receiving an isonitrogenous diet containing about 0.6 g of protein per kilogram. Attman and colleagues[426] found some evidence for slowed progression in a group of diabetics given 20 to 30 g of protein per day plus essential amino acids. Walser[5] reported that slowing of progression on this regimen, as assessed by $[Cr]^{-1}$ values, creatinine clearances, or isotopically determined GFRs in a few cases, was only temporary or nonexistent in 18 subjects but lasted for almost 4 years in one patient until his death from unrelated causes. Andreu and associates[421] reported that the decline in $[Cr]^{-1}$ in 19 patients was halted (on the average) during 5 months of follow-up ($P = .027$). Thus, the effect of this regimen on progression is as yet uncertain.

The use of intravenous essential amino acids in acute renal failure was first proposed by Wilmore, Dudrick, and associates.[427, 428] They noted a fall or reduced rate of rise in blood urea nitrogen concentration, a finding now confirmed repeatedly.[429–431] Despite early reports[429] of improved survival and earlier recovery of renal function, further studies have failed to demonstrate these effects, and one study[432] has also failed to confirm the reduced rate of urea appearance. Experimental studies of this problem have led to conflicting results,[433, 434] and some workers have questioned whether essential amino acids offer any advantage over complete amino acid mixtures.[435–437]

In summary, essential amino acid supplements are unusually effective in controlling the symptoms and biochemical manifestations of chronic renal failure. They possess two distinct advantages over the use of high-quality protein diets: first, more variety is possible in the selection of foods; and second, they can be used intravenously. It remains to be established whether such regimens slow progression, even though they can clearly defer dialysis simply by reducing azotemia at any given level of renal function. They may also be useful for selected nephrotic patients.

## Analogues of Essential Amino Acids

In 1966, Schloerb[411] first pointed out that α-keto analogues of essential amino acids might spare nitrogen more efficiently than essential amino acids do themselves in patients with chronic uremia, because such subjects convert these compounds into amino acids by transamination reactions. Richards and co-workers[355] made the same suggestion independently the following year, based on a premise that now appears to be incorrect (see earlier), namely, that ammonia is derived from urea breakdown in the intestine in increased amounts in uremia and is used for animation of carbon skeletons of essential amino acids in the uremic state. Animal experiments had established that all of the essential amino acids, with the exception of lysine and threonine, could be replaced in the diet by their α-keto or α-hydroxy analogues. Further work showed that the α-keto or α-hydroxy analogues of phenylalanine and valine could substitute for these amino acids in the diet of normal as well as uremic individuals, although not in every instance and not with complete efficacy.[438–440] Walser and co-workers[185] administered a mixture of five to seven of these keto analogues, along with the remaining essential amino acids, to five patients with severe chronic uremia, four of whom would have otherwise required dialysis. When the keto acid–amino acid mixture was discontinued, urea nitrogen appearance rate increased and nitrogen balance worsened

by approximately 1.5 g/d. In other patients with more elevated blood urea concentration, keto acids were initially ineffective. In two of these, the mixture became effective after dialysis. Subsequently, Walser[414] reported that a mixture of five of these analogues (calcium salts of the analogues of valine, leucine, isoleucine, methionine, and phenylalanine), along with the four remaining essential amino acids given with a low-protein diet, reduced urea appearance rate in uremia when it was substituted for a complete mixture of essential amino acids, even though total nitrogen intake was held approximately constant. In fact, keto acids can replace essential amino acids even when the diet contains no protein.[441, 442]

These results suggest that apart from reducing the requirements for nitrogen intake, a keto acid supplement exerts some nitrogen-sparing effects of an unidentified nature. This concept was supported when a mixture of keto acids or α-ketoisocaproate alone was administered to normal subjects during a prolonged fast.[443, 444] Urea excretion decreased (compared with that of control subjects) during daily keto acid administration for 7 days and remained below the control rate for at least a week of fasting. These effects (during and after administration) were not seen with leucine in the same fasting protocol,[444] even though, in vitro, leucine reportedly promoted protein anabolism and reduced protein catabolism, particularly in muscle.[445–447] The mechanism of the nitrogen-sparing effect of ketoleucine appears to be an inhibitory effect on protein degradation, demonstrable not only in vitro[445, 446] but also in vivo,[444, 448–450] although not in severely stressed patients.[451] Direct demonstration of an inhibitory effect of branched chain keto acids on protein degradation in patients or animals with renal failure has been difficult, partly because the principal technique used to measure muscle protein degradation, urinary 3-methylhistidine excretion, cannot be used reliably in the presence of renal failure.[351] However, an unusually low requirement for dietary nitrogen (about 2 g/d) has been demonstrated in uremic patients infused continuously by nasogastric tube with a mixture containing carbohydrate at 400 g/d and a large dose of branched chain keto acids (16 g/d).[262] As noted earlier, Masud and associates[327] compared a keto acid–based supplement with an amino acid supplement and found that the keto acid supplement produced neutral nitrogen balance at a 15% lower nitrogen intake. They also showed that neither regimen impaired adaptive nutritional responses needed to maintain protein balance when dietary protein is restricted. The postprandial rise in urea production is blunted in patients receiving keto acids.[452] These results are consistent with the possibility that the regimen suppressed protein degradation. Jahn and co-workers[453] reported that protein synthetic activity of muscle ribosomes isolated from patients increased significantly and nitrogen balance improved when 0.3 g/kg of a keto acid–amino acid mixture (Cetolog, see Table 55–3) was added to a low-protein diet (0.4 g/kg). Teplan and colleagues[454] found that addition of only 4.8 g of keto acids per day restored nitrogen balance to neutral in patients in negative nitrogen balance while they were receiving a 20-g protein diet. However, no improvement in serum protein levels was seen. Walser and Ward[167] have suggested that the modest suppression of glucocorticoid production that is induced by keto acids may be responsible for the improvement in nitrogen balance (see earlier discussion).

On the other hand, when nitrogen intake is more than the minimum required, no such benefit of keto analogues can be demonstrated. In four patients given essential amino acids and keto acids in alternating treatment periods with a dietary regimen providing an average of 7.88 g of nitrogen per 70 kg body weight, no significant effect of the supplement on nitrogen balance could be demonstrated.[455] It is to be expected that adding these compounds to a diet already adequate in protein should simply result in their being oxidized. Growth studies in rats have also shown that the efficacy of keto analogues as substitutes for essential amino acids is greatest when amino acid intake is limiting for growth.[456, 457] Furthermore, the extent of incorporation of labeled keto acids into body protein is strongly dependent on dietary protein intake.[458]

Hydroxy analogues are also effective, to varying degrees, as substitutes for essential amino acids. The calcium salt of the DL-α-hydroxy analogue of methionine, at a dose of 2 g/d, maintained nitrogen balance in chronic uremic patients receiving a protein-free diet.[441] Likewise, calcium L-phenyllactate at 1.8 g/d was effective in six uremic women given a protein-free diet.[442] In both of these studies, branched chain keto acids replaced branched chain amino acids, and nitrogen was provided chiefly as glycine. Use of α-hydroxy analogues requires their oxidation to the corresponding keto analogue. Oxidation of the hydroxy analogue of methionine to the keto analogue occurs in rat liver[459] and kidney,[460] and oxidation of L-phenyllactate to phenylpyruvate occurs in rat kidney.[461] Limited enzymatic capacity for these transformations may explain apparent failure of several other hydroxy analogues to support growth in rats.[462] A mixture containing the hydroxy analogues of leucine, isoleucine, valine, methionine, and phenylalanine fed to uremic patients increased plasma levels of methionine and phenylalanine but decreased the level of valine and, to a lesser extent, leucine and isoleucine.[185] These results suggest, but do not prove, that the branched chain hydroxy analogues are ineffective in humans.

Hydroxy and keto analogues of tryptophan and histidine have been examined in animals but only to a limited extent in humans.[185, 438] Analogues of lysine and threonine would almost certainly be ineffective because these amino acids do not participate in transamination reactions.[463]

The mixtures of nitrogen-free analogues and essential amino acids that have been most widely employed in renal failure are summarized in Table 55–5, including three studies in children.[464–466] Keto analogues of tryptophan and histidine, used in two patients in the initial study,[185] were replaced by the amino acids as such, because both keto and hydroxy analogues of these amino acids are difficult to synthesize.

The keto analogue of isoleucine exists in two enantiomeric forms, R(−)- and S(+)-α-keto-β-methylvalerate, the transamination products of L-alloisoleucine and L-isoleucine, respectively. The racemic R,S-mixture was used in all but a few patients in the first study[185] because it is much easier to synthesize and maintains nitrogen balance in chronic uremic patients in the absence or near-absence of dietary isoleucine.[441, 442] However, when administered in

**TABLE 55–5. Composition of Two Keto Acid–Amino Acid Mixtures Containing Calcium Salts of Keto Acids**

| Component | Dry Substance (g/d/70 kg weight) I | II |
|---|---|---|
| Calcium 2-ketoisovalerate | 3.70 | 1.40 |
| Calcium 2-ketoisocaproate | 3.50 | 1.64 |
| Calcium (R,S)-2-keto-3-methylvalerate | 2.80 | 1.09 |
| Calcium DL-2-hydroxy-4-methylthiobutyrate | 2.10 | 0.96 |
| Calcium phenylpyruvate | 1.90 | 1.11 |
| Lysine acetate | 0.90 | 1.72 |
| Threonine | 0.67 | 0.88 |
| Tryptophan | 0.33 | 0.37 |
| Histidine | 0.00 | 0.63 |
| Tyrosine | 0.00 | 0.49 |
| Total | 15.90 | 10.29 |
| Brand name | Ultramin | Ketosteril |
| Reference | 480 | 536 |

relatively large doses (0.5 mmol/kg/d), it causes plasma isoleucine concentration to fall instead of rise, for unknown reasons.[467] Therefore, the S(+) isomer might be preferable, but it is not currently available.

Until 1983, all workers used the calcium salts of the analogues, so that total calcium intake from these supplements is considerable. These salts contain some water of hydration, so the dosages of the anhydrous salts are 5% to 10% less than the amounts shown. Mixtures have been employed in which the calcium salts of branched chain keto acids have been replaced by ornithine, lysine, and histidine salts.[322, 468] The composition of one such mixture, the most extensively studied, is given in Table 55–3. These salts are more soluble and more palatable than the corresponding amino acids[469] or the calcium salts of the keto acids. They also seem to cause less gastric distress. These mixtures contain ornithine and nearly the same amount of nitrogen as do essential amino acid supplements. They do not contain phenylalanine or tryptophan in any form and only a small amount of the methionine analogue.

The diet used in conjunction with keto acids has generally been the same as that used with amino acid supplements, although two groups have used a substantially lower protein intake.[277, 470]

Clinical results with these regimens have generally been good. Numerous studies have been reported in which the calcium salts of the keto analogues of valine, leucine, isoleucine, and phenylalanine and the DL-hydroxy analogue of methionine plus the other essential amino acids (including histidine) have been given to predialysis patients with chronic renal failure in daily doses of 6 to 12 g, along with a 20- to 30-g mixed-quality protein diet. Studies before 1981 were summarized by Mitch and associates.[471] Many additional studies (see fourth edition) have appeared subsequently.* Improvement in nutritional status (as measured by anthropometry, plasma protein levels, nitrogen balance, and blood urea nitrogen) has been observed in most of these

*References 167, 322, 409, 410, 464, 465, 468, 470, 472–478.

studies. When results have been compared with pretreatment values, albumin catabolism decreases.[479] On the other hand, if protein intake is reduced to 0.2 g/kg/d, and branched chain keto acids are provided at 4.1 g/d/70 kg,[277] some signs of protein deficiency may appear, even though serum albumin and transferrin levels do not change. Furthermore, controlled comparison of two keto acid–amino acid mixtures showed that a supplement containing branched chain keto acids at 3.82 g/d (as calcium salts) was far inferior to a supplement containing 5.84 g/d in maintaining protein nutrition and in reversing abnormalities in plasma amino acid concentrations.[480] Some workers have reported maintenance of serum protein levels rather than improvement with use of the former supplement.[481]

In children with chronic renal failure, a diet containing protein at 0.8 to 1.2 g/kg supplemented with keto acid–amino acid mixtures is reported to arrest the rise in creatinine concentration and to improve growth, hyperphosphatemia, acidosis, hyperlipidemia, and secondary hyperparathyroidism, in comparison with patients receiving conventional therapy.[466, 482]

Besides these generally positive effects on protein nutrition, a decrease in plasma phosphate concentration and alkaline phosphatase activity, an increase in plasma $Ca^{2+}$ concentration, and a decrease in the serum level of parathyroid hormone have been noted in adult patients treated with calcium salts of keto acids* as well as in children.[464, 486, 489] Serum oxalate levels fall toward normal or become normal.[474] Bone biopsies reveal marked amelioration of renal osteodystrophy,[490–492] in comparison with control subjects receiving 0.6 g of protein per kilogram.[493] Serum 1,25-dihydroxycholecalciferol increases,[494] whereas serum concentrations of 25-hydroxycholecalciferol and calcitonin do not change.[481, 483, 488, 491] Some of the improvements in divalent ion metabolism may simply be the result of suppression of phosphate absorption from the gut. Schaefer and coworkers[495] have shown that in contrast to calcium carbonate and calcium citrate, which bind phosphate only in acidic media, calcium salts of branched chain keto acids bind phosphate at neutral pH and appear to be at least as effective as calcium carbonate in reducing phosphate absorption.

Keto acids also exert beneficial effects on carbohydrate and fat metabolism in uremic patients. In children, fasting hypoglycemia, glucose intolerance, and insulin resistance improve, but fasting insulin levels and the insulin response to hyperglycemia do not change.[496] In adults, insulin requirements and fasting hyperglycemia decrease in insulin-dependent diabetic patients,[476, 497, 498] and tissue sensitivity to insulin improves in nondiabetic patients.[499] Some workers have found that the serum triglyceride level falls in men,[479, 500] but others have not[487]; serum cholesterol may also decline.[497]

Improvement in metabolic acidosis is an obvious consequence of the reduced intake of phosphate and of sulfur-containing amino acids. As noted earlier, limiting the catabolic influence of acidosis could account for some of the beneficial effects of keto acids.

According to three reports, testosterone levels rise, often to normal,[475, 481, 485] which may explain why triglyceride

levels fall in men, because serum testosterone levels are negatively correlated with serum triglyceride levels.[501] Serum triiodothyronine[476] and thyroxine[479] levels rise. β-Endorphin and growth hormone decrease[502]; 24-hour glucocorticoid excretion falls, even though fasting cortisol levels do not change.[128, 141, 167] Hormonal change might account for some of the metabolic effects of keto acids summarized before, although it would not account for changes in muscle protein metabolism.[445, 446]

Leukocyte $Na^+,K^+$-ATPase is restored to normal after 3 months of keto acid supplementation.[503] The progressive loss of nerve conduction velocity is attenuated or reversed.[504]

In most of these studies, the control period consisted of observations made when the same patients received a protein-restricted diet. Therefore, the effects described could be caused by protein restriction rather than by keto acids. However, several comparisons of keto acid–containing supplements with essential amino acids have now been reported. In one,[414] a lower rate of urea nitrogen appearance and improved nitrogen balance were noted in patients receiving keto acids, compared with essential amino acids, during short courses of therapy. In another study,[505] patients received essential amino acids for 6 months followed by a keto analogue-containing mixture for 6 more months, both given as coated granules of identical appearance. During the keto acid treatment period, blood hemoglobin and the concentrations of several serum proteins rose; serum phosphate concentration fell and $Ca^{2+}$ concentration rose. A third study[506] used a high nitrogen intake and observed no benefit from either therapy. In a fourth,[484] 40 patients received essential amino acids and 50 received keto acids for an average of 7 to 9 months. Both groups had severe chronic renal failure (serum creatinine concentration averaged about 10 mg/dL) and were prescribed a diet containing protein at 0.4 g/kg. In both groups, there was an improvement in nitrogen balance, a decrease in blood urea nitrogen concentration, and an increase in serum transferrin level. Acidosis improved, serum phosphate concentration fell, and serum parathyroid hormone levels decreased by 40% only in those receiving keto acids. Schmicker and co-workers[485] found greater improvement in serum levels of phosphate and parathyroid hormone in 68 patients receiving keto acids than in 51 patients receiving essential amino acids; testosterone rose only in the former. In a randomized multiple crossover comparison, keto acid supplementation led to lower serum triglyceride concentration and lower rate of excretion of 17-hydroxycorticosteroids than did amino acid supplementation.[128] Finally, when effects on protein and amino acid metabolism were compared, both supplements exerted similar effects, but the keto acid regimen was associated with neutral nitrogen balance at a lower nitrogen intake.[327]

Plasma levels of amino acids may exhibit improvement or even normalization in patients on keto acid–substituted regimens[480] but more often do not show any clinically significant changes.[322, 469, 507] However, alloisoleucine, normally absent or nearly absent, invariably rises because of transamination of $(R)$-α-keto-β-methylvalerate.[132] Even when pure or nearly pure $S(+)$ isomer was given (to nonuremic children), plasma alloisoleucine increased,[467] presumably reflecting in vivo racemization at an unknown site.

Using an improved method, Ponto and co-workers[132] have shown that in normal subjects, alloisoleucine peaks 2 hours after an oral dose of the racemic mixture and accumulates to about 60 μM by 1 month. Preliminary estimates of its half-life in normal subjects indicate a value of 7 to 8 hours. This compound is even less toxic than the normal amino acids; accumulation, therefore, can serve as a useful check on patient compliance.

The only side effect of keto acid supplements (see Table 55–5) noted in these studies has been gastrointestinal distress, variously reported as occurring in up to 15% of patients and usually subsiding after a few days; rarely, hypercalcemia occurs.[508] Hypercalcemia has been observed in about 5% of patients receiving long-term therapy with calcium salts even when the dose is kept moderately low. This is rarely severe enough to cause symptoms.

Studies have cast doubt on the relationship between a keto acid–based regimen and retardation of progression.[468] Studies published earlier than 1989 are summarized in the fourth edition. In a randomized multiple crossover design (ABA/BAB or ABAB/BABA, see earlier discussion),[128] 16 patients showed a mean rate of progression while receiving a keto acid–based supplement of $-0.14$ mL/min/mo, compared with a mean rate of progression while receiving the essential amino acid diet of $-0.66$ mL/min/mo ($P = .024$); dietary protein intake and blood pressure were not different with the two supplements. This study used the tryptophan-free supplement known as Cetolog (see Table 55–3), which reduces serum levels of free tryptophan; progression has been correlated with free tryptophan levels, as noted before. The feasibility phase of the Modification of Diet in Renal Disease Trial,[386] which employed the same supplement, was not designed to demonstrate efficacy; nevertheless, the results of study B (see earlier) showed that after adjusting for effects of blood pressure, the keto acid–supplemented patients progressed significantly more slowly than the other two groups, as determined by intention to treat analysis. As noted before, the results of the operational phase of the Modification of Diet in Renal Disease Trial, which used a different supplement (RKAP, see Table 55–3), show only marginal effects on progression.

## NUTRITIONAL THERAPY FOR THE NEPHROTIC SYNDROME

A high protein intake is sometimes recommended for patients with the nephrotic syndrome, even though it has long been known that this measure serves no useful purpose (see review by Kaysen[509]). This is because the increment in albumin synthesis is offset by an increase in albuminuria.[510, 511] Unfortunately, nitrogen balance was not measured, so the long-term efficacy of dietary restriction in nephrotic patients is unknown. Don and co-workers[511] did report that a diet containing 0.8 g of protein per day and 35 kcal/kg/d did produce a *positive change* in nitrogen balance, but individual values were not presented.

What remains to be established is whether long-term protein restriction is preferable to a normal protein intake in the management of these patients. It is assumed, but not proved, that the increase in protein requirement is equal to

the urinary loss.[512] In one study, a diet containing 1 g of protein per kilogram of the preillness body weight plus 1 g of protein for each gram of urinary protein and 200 kcal of nitrogen per gram produced a positive nitrogen balance.[513] Increasing protein or calorie intake further did not produce additional benefit. In nephrotic patients randomized to protein intake of 1.1 or 0.7 g/kg and subsequently crossed over, D'Amico and associates[514] found no difference in proteinuria, albuminemia, or follow-up GFR between the two diets. Gentile and colleagues[515] randomized nephrotic patients to receive a soy-based diet containing vegetable protein at 0.93 g/kg with or without the addition of fish oil, 5 g/d. Proteinuria and hyperlipidemia receded on both diets, in comparison with a control period on a free diet (1.16 g of protein per kilogram), and rose again when the patients resumed the free diet after 4 months, but serum albumin levels did not change. Fish oil was not associated with a significant additional benefit. In diabetic patients with albuminuria but normal renal function, Dullaart and co-workers[516] found that randomization of patients with diabetic nephropathy to mild protein restriction (0.79 g/kg) reduced albuminuria; little change in GFR was seen. In steroid-resistant nephrotic patients, two crossover comparisons of a keto acid–amino acid mixture plus a low-protein diet (0.7 g/kg) versus a higher protein diet (1.3 g/kg) without supplement revealed lower protein excretion and serum cholesterol on the supplemented diet but no change in serum albumin or triglyceride levels or in nutritional indices.[502, 517] In patients with nephrotic range proteinuria and hypoalbuminemia, serum albumin levels may rise, sometimes to normal, when severe protein restriction is combined with essential amino acid supplementation (10 to 20 g/d)[281, 399] (Fig. 55–11). These observations raise the intriguing possibility that protein-containing foods may contain some components that contribute to protein deficiency, and that a protein-restricted diet, supplemented by essential amino acids (or keto acid–amino acid mixtures), may be more efficacious in replenishing body protein stores than a normal or high-protein diet. The stimulatory effect of a high protein intake on glucocorticoid production[518] has been suggested as a possible mechanism for the increase in protein breakdown in patients with proteinuria.[281]

## ENERGY REQUIREMENTS

There is a high frequency of anthropometric abnormalities, including decreased body weight, in patients entering dialysis therapy.[279] Malnutrition could result from an inadequate intake of energy. Monteon and co-workers[519] examined energy expenditure of normal subjects and patients with chronic renal failure during rest and exercise. There was no difference between the groups; when calorie intake was reduced, energy expenditure did not fall in either group, indicating that uremic patients do not develop a special ability to adapt to a low calorie intake. Consequently, an inadequate energy intake by uremic subjects could cause calorie malnutrition and negative nitrogen balance, especially when protein intake is restricted.

Hyne and associates[520] reported that the nitrogen balance of uremic patients fed a diet of 20 g of high-quality protein

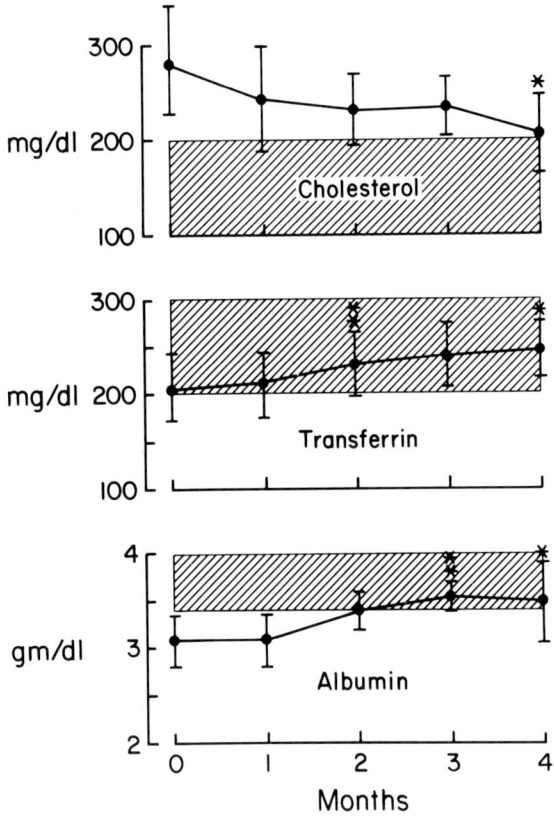

**Figure 55–11.** Sequential values for serum cholesterol, transferrin, and albumin in five patients with chronic renal failure and nephrotic syndrome (average 24-hour protein excretion, 7.1 ± 4.2 g/d) given a low-protein diet (0.3 g/kg) plus 10 to 20 g of essential amino acids per day. Shaded areas represent part of the normal range for each parameter. Significance of changes from time zero is indicated as follows: *$P < .01$; **$P < .05$. All three values become normal, on the average. Proteinuria decreased 32%, but the change was not statistically significant. (From Walser M: Does prolonged restriction preceding dialysis lead to protein malnutrition at the onset of dialysis? Used with permission from Kidney International, volume 44, pages 1139–1144, 1993.)

per day improved as calorie intake was raised. Although the patients remained in negative nitrogen balance when calorie intake was raised to 55 kcal/kg/d, the results are reminiscent of the findings of Rose[521] that a higher calorie intake is required to achieve nitrogen balance in normal subjects fed diets containing barely adequate amounts of essential amino acids. In contrast to these results, Bergström and associates[522] studied patients with renal failure who were eating 16 to 20 g of protein per day supplemented with essential amino acids given orally or intravenously. They found little or no change in nitrogen balance as energy intake was varied between 22 and 50 kcal/kg/d. These data suggest that calorie intake is not so critical if both nitrogen and essential amino acid intake are adequate. Kopple and co-workers[523] have systematically addressed the question of how calories affect protein conservation when protein intake is minimal. They fed chronically uremic patients a constant, minimal protein intake of 0.55 to 0.6 g/kg/d and measured nitrogen balance while calorie intake was varied from 15 to 45 kcal/kg/d (Fig. 55–12). Extrapolation of their measurements indicates that nitrogen equilib-

rium can be achieved by most patients given 35 kcal/kg/d. These results should be integrated into a dietary prescription, but calories should be restricted for overweight patients; those below ideal body weight should have calorie intake raised above the level of 35 kcal/kg/d.

## VITAMINS AND TRACE MINERALS

Nondialyzed uremic patients being treated with protein-restricted regimens often have an inadequate intake of water-soluble vitamins.[524] This may explain the common finding in uremic patients of subnormal plasma levels of pyridoxal-5-phosphate and aspartate aminotransferase in plasma and erythrocytes, which is suggestive of pyridoxine deficiency.[525, 526] Pyridoxine deficiency could contribute to immune system depression, anemia, peripheral neuropathy, and oxalosis.[527, 528] To avoid a deficiency state, a water-soluble vitamin supplement including pyridoxine at 10 to 50 mg/d and folic acid at 1 to 5 mg/d should be provided.[524, 526] In contrast, plasma levels of vitamin A are invariably high, primarily because of an increase in retinol-binding protein in the plasma of uremic patients.[529] Although it is controversial whether this abnormality contributes to the development of renal osteodystrophy or other aspects of the uremic syndrome,[530, 531] it is clear that supplemental vitamin A is unnecessary. The use of 1,25-

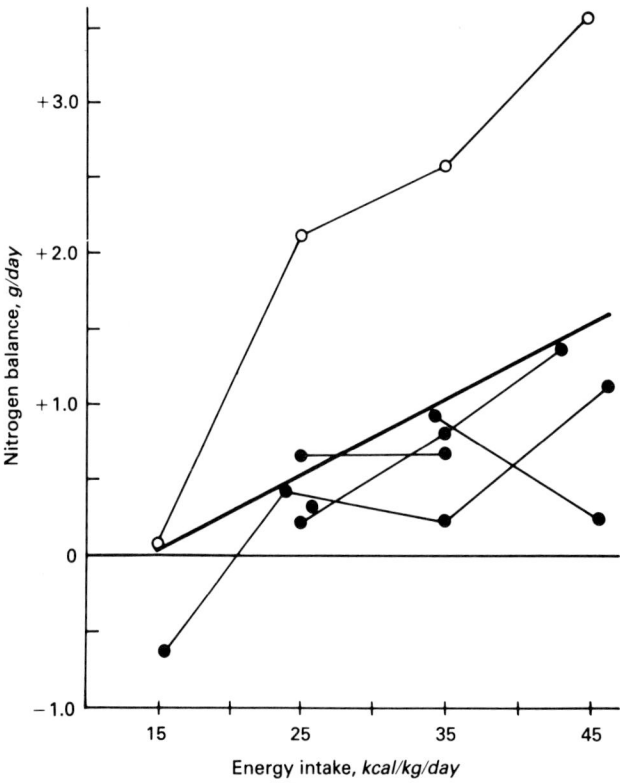

**Figure 55–12.** The correlation between nitrogen balance and energy intake in six clinically stable, nondialyzed, chronically uremic patients. (From Kopple JD, Monteon FJ, Shaib JK: Effect of energy intake on nitrogen metabolism in nondialyzed patients with chronic renal failure. Kidney Int 29:734–742, 1986.)

dihydroxycholecalciferol and other forms of vitamin D to treat renal osteodystrophy is considered in Chapter 51.

Iron supplements are often necessary in uremic patients because of low-grade gastrointestinal bleeding[253] and because iron intake is limited with protein-restricted diets.[524] Measurement of the serum iron or ferritin concentration usually suffices as a guide for initiating iron therapy, and guidelines for assessing iron stores and treating iron deficiency in patients with erythropoietin are available.[532, 533] Zinc deficiency reportedly occurs in some uremic patients[524, 534] and may cause hypogeusia and impotence, which are responsive to oral zinc supplementation. Although tissue levels of other trace elements have been found to be abnormal in nondialyzed patients with chronic renal failure,[535] their relation to the clinical problems of these patients is unknown.[524]

# CONSERVATIVE MANAGEMENT VERSUS DIALYSIS

The foregoing discussion indicates why interest in developing methods of nutritional therapy for chronic renal failure has expanded rapidly during the past decade. The possibility of substantially altering the course of the disease makes it appropriate to consider treating virtually all patients with established chronic renal failure by instituting a low-protein, low-phosphate dietary regimen; it has not been established which dietary regimen should be used and when treatment should be initiated. Uremic symptoms are easily eliminated by dietary protein restriction to 0.6 g/kg/d and calorie intake of 35 kcal/kg/d when renal function is only mildly impaired (i.e., serum creatinine level of 2 to 3 mg/dL). At the other extreme, when renal function is irreversibly reduced to less than 5% of normal, nutritional therapy should be used only when an adequate access for dialysis is not available (e.g., during maturation of an arteriovenous fistula). For those patients who have moderate renal impairment (less than 20% of normal function), conservative therapy is almost always useful; it invariably ameliorates uremic symptoms and may postpone the need to begin dialysis for prolonged periods. Obviously, successful restriction of dietary protein and phosphate requires the motivation of both the patient and the physician, but the principal if not the only disadvantage of such therapy (assuming that it is successful in eliminating uremic symptoms) is the dietary restriction it entails.

Previous concern about inducing protein malnutrition by long-term use of low-protein diets is virtually eliminated when the principles outlined in this chapter are followed. This has now been confirmed by nitrogen balance, anthropometric, and serum protein measurements after long-term therapy, even to a stage just before dialysis.[281, 321, 322] Consequently, it is reasonable to use nutritional therapy to forestall initiation of dialysis as long as the quality of life is well maintained. The level of renal function below which conservative therapy is unlikely to control uremic symptoms or affect the course of the disease is uncertain, but probably about 3% to 5% of normal renal function can be successfully maintained without dialysis. Some patients may require dialysis at a higher level of renal function

because of various catabolic states, acute gastrointestinal bleeding, or the appearance of uremic complications such as pericarditis.

## REFERENCES

1. Austin SM, Lieberman JS, Newton LD, et al: Slope of serial GFR and the progression of diabetic glomerular disease. J Am Soc Nephrol 3:1358–1370, 1993.
2. Mackensen-Haen S, Haen M, Neunhoeffer J, et al: Korrelationen zwischen der glomerularen Filtrationstrate sowie der Nierenrindendurchblutung (Serumkreatininkonzentration, C-kreatinin, C-inulin, C-PAH, FF) und der Breite des Nierenrindeninterstitiums. Nieren Hochdruckkr 17:47–51, 1988.
3. Jacobson SH, Wang Y, Larsson S, et al: Determination of functional kidney volume by single-photon emission computed tomography in patients with insulin-dependent diabetes mellitus. Nephrol Dial Transplant 7:1085–1091, 1992.
4. Bilous RW, Mauer SM, Sutherland DER, et al: Mean glomerular volume and rate of development of diabetic nephropathy. Diabetes 38:1142–1147, 1989.
5. Walser M: Progression of chronic renal failure in man. Kidney Int 37:1195–1210, 1990.
6. White AJ, Strydom WJ: Normalisation of glomerular filtration rate measurements. Eur J Nucl Med 18:385–390, 1991.
7. Peters AM: Expressing glomerular filtration rate in terms of extracellular fluid volume. Nephrol Dial Transplant 7:205–210, 1992.
8. Rolin HA, Hall PH: Age/sex stratified glomerular filtration rate (GFR) values defined by $^{125}$I-iothalamate (IOH) clearance. J Am Soc Nephrol 3:347, 1992. Abstract.
9. Holliday MA, Heilbron D, al-Uzri A, et al: Serial measurements of GFR in infants using the continuous iothalamate infusion technique. Kidney Int 43:893–898, 1993.
10. Heilbron DC, Holliday MA, al-Dahwi A, et al: Expressing glomerular filtration rate in children. Pediatr Nephrol 5:5–11, 1993.
11. Al-Uzri A, Holliday MA, Gambertoglio JG, et al: An accurate practical method for estimating GFR in clinical studies using a constant subcutaneous infusion. Kidney Int 41:1701–1706, 1992.
12. Shemesh O, Golbetz H, Kriss JP, et al: Limitations of creatinine as a filtration marker in glomerulopathic patients. Kidney Int 28:830–838, 1985.
13. Perrone RD, Madias NE, Levey AS: Serum creatinine as an index of renal function: New insights into old concepts. Clin Chem 38:1933–1953, 1992.
14. Giovannetti S, Barsotti G: In defense of creatinine clearance. Nephron 59:11–14, 1991.
15. Gault MH, Longerich LL, Harnett JD, et al: Predicting glomerular function from adjusted serum creatinine. Nephron 62:249–256, 1992.
16. Van Lente F, Suit P: Assessment of renal function by serum creatinine and creatinine clearance: Glomerular filtration rate estimated by four procedures. Clin Chem 35:2326–2330, 1989.
17. Gilbert SC, Emmett M, Menter A, et al: Cyclosporine therapy for psoriasis: Serum creatinine measurements are an unreliable predictor of decreased renal function. J Am Acad Dermatol 21:470–474, 1989.
18. Motwani JG, Fenwick MK, Struthers AD: Comparison of three methods of glomerular filtration rate measurement with and without captopril pretreatment in groups of patients with left ventricular dysfunction. Eur Heart J 13:1195–1200, 1992.
19. Waller DG, Fleming JS, Ramsay B, et al: The accuracy of creatinine clearance with and without urine collection as a measure of glomerular filtration rate. Postgrad Med J 67:42–46, 1991.
20. LaFrance ND, Drew HH, Walser M: Radioisotopic measurement of glomerular filtration rate in severe chronic renal failure. J Nucl Med 29:1927–1930, 1988.
21. Klassen DK, Weir MR, Buddemeyer EU: Simultaneous measurements of glomerular filtration rate by two radioisotopic methods in patients without renal impairment. J Am Soc Nephrol 3:107–112, 1992.
22. Sampson MJ, Drury PL: Accurate estimation of glomerular filtration rate in diabetic nephropathy from age, body weight, and serum creatinine. Diabetes Care 15:609–612, 1992.
23. Lemann J, Bidani AK, Bain RP, et al: Use of serum creatinine to

estimate glomerular filtration rate in health and early diabetic nephropathy. Am J Kidney Dis 16:236–243, 1990.

24. Pollock C, Gyory AZ, Hawkins T, et al: Comparison of simultaneous renal clearances of true endogenous creatinine and subcutaneously administered iothalamate in man. J Am Soc Nephrol 4:322, 1993. Abstract.

25. Groth S, Aasted M: Determination of $^{51}$Cr-EDTA clearance between 15 and 40 ml/min/1.73 m$^2$ by a single plasma sample. Scand J Clin Lab Invest 49:711–717, 1989.

26. van Acker BAC, Kooman GCM, Koopman MG, et al: Creatinine clearance during cimetidine administration for measurement of glomerular filtration rate. Lancet 340:1326–1329, 1992.

27. Hilbrands LB, Artz MA, Wetzels JFM, et al: Cimetidine improves the reliability of creatinine as a marker of glomerular filtration. Kidney Int 40:1171–1176, 1991.

28. Olsen NV, Ladefoged SD, Feldt-Rasmussen B, et al: The effects of cimetidine on creatinine excretion, glomerular filtration rate and tubular function in renal transplant recipients. Scand J Clin Lab Invest 49:155–159, 1989.

29. Roubenoff R, Drew H, Moyer M, et al: Oral cimetidine improves the accuracy and precision of creatinine clearance in lupus nephritis. Ann Intern Med 113:501–506, 1990.

30. van Acker BAC, Koomen GCM, Koopman MG, et al: Limitations of creatinine during cimetidine as a filtration marker in renal disease. J Am Soc Nephrol 3:322, 1992.

31. Agarwal R: Creatinine clearance with cimetidine for measurement of GFR. Lancet 341:188, 1993. Letter.

32. Ducharme MP, Smythe M, Strohs G: Drug-induced alterations in serum creatinine concentrations. Ann Pharmacother 27:622–633, 1993.

33. Walser M, Drew HH, Guldan JL: Prediction of glomerular filtration rate from serum creatinine concentration in advanced chronic renal failure. Kidney Int 44:1145–1148, 1993.

34. Cockcroft DW, Gault MH: Prediction of creatinine clearance from serum creatinine. Nephron 16:31–41, 1975.

35. Schwartz GJ, Haycock GB, Edelmann CM Jr, et al: A simple estimate of glomerular filtration rate in children derived from body length and plasma creatinine. Pediatrics 58:259–263, 1976.

36. Schwartz GJ, Brion LP, Spitzer A: The use of plasma creatinine concentration for estimating glomerular filtration rate in infants, children, and adolescents. Pediatr Clin North Am 34:571–590, 1987.

37. Sekar KC, Leonard JC, Puffinburger WR, et al: Rapid determination of glomerular filtration rate in infants using Tc-99m DTPA. Clin Nucl Med 17:550–552, 1992.

38. Hellerstein S, Alon U, Warady BA: Creatinine for estimation of glomerular filtration rate. Pediatr Nephrol 6:507–511, 1992.

39. Waz WR, Quattrin T, Feld LG: Serum creatinine and height do not predict glomerular filtration rate in children with insulin dependent diabetes mellitus. Clin Res 40:663A, 1992. Abstract.

40. Leroy D, Mauriat F, Dechaux M, et al: Beta$_2$-microglobulin. Arch Fr Pediatr 41:43–47, 1984.

41. Aparicio SA, Mojiminiyi S, Kay JD, et al: Measurement of glomerular filtration rate in homozygous sickle cell disease: A comparison of $^{51}$Cr-EDTA clearance, creatinine clearance, serum creatinine and beta$_2$-microglobulin. J Clin Pathol 43:370–372, 1990.

42. Smith HW: Measurement of the filtration rate. In The Kidney: Structure and Function in Health and Disease. Oxford University Press, New York, 1951, pp 47–52.

43. Wilkins BH: The glomerular filterability of polyfructosan-S in immature infants. Pediatr Nephrol 6:319–322, 1992.

44. Aperia A, Freyschuss U: Comparison of plasma clearances of polyfructosan and $^{51}$Cr-EDTA in children. Acta Pediatr Scand 73:379–380, 1984.

45. Donadio C, Tramonti G, Giordani R, et al: Renal effects and nephrotoxicity of contrast media in renal patients. Contrib Nephrol 101:241–250, 1993.

46. Lautin EM, Freeman NJ, Schoenfeld AH, et al: Radiocontrast-associated renal dysfunction: Incidence and risk factors. AJR 157:49–58, 1991.

47. Viberti GC, Dodds R, Earle K, et al: Reduction of proteinuria and diminished glomerular filtration rate fall by low-protein intake: Long-term effects. Proceedings of the XIIth International Congress of Nephrology; 1993; Jerusalem, Israel. Abstract, page 419.

48. Weisberg LS, Kurnik PB, Kurnik BRC: Risk of radiocontrast nephropathy in patients with and without diabetes mellitus. Kidney Int 45:259–265, 1994.

49. Prueksaritanont T, Lui CY, Lee MG, et al: Renal and non-renal clearances of iothalamate. Biopharm Drug Dispos 7:347–355, 1993.

50. Isaka Y, Fujiwara Y, Yamamoto S, et al: Modified plasma clearance technique using nonradioactive iothalamate for measuring GFR. Kidney Int 42:1006–1011, 1992.

51. Gaspari F, Mosconi L, Vigano G, et al: Measurement of GFR with a single intravenous injection of nonradioactive iothalamate. Kidney Int 41:1081–1084, 1992.

52. Krutzen E, Back SE, Nilsoon-Ehle I, et al: Plasma clearance of a new contrast agent iohexol: A method for the assessment of glomerular filtration rate. J Lab Clin Med 104:955–961, 1984.

53. Arvidsson A, Hedman A: Plasma and renal clearance of iohexol—a study on the reproducibility of a method for the glomerular filtration rate. Scand J Clin Lab Invest 50:757–761, 1990.

54. Effersoe H, Rosenkilde P, Groth S, et al: Measurement of renal function with iohexol. A comparison of iohexol, $^{99m}$Tc-DTPA, and $^{51}$Cr-EDTA clearance. Invest Radiol 25:778–782, 1990.

55. Isaka Y, Yamamoto S, Fujiwara Y, et al: A new analytical method of simultaneous measurement of iothalamate and iohexol. Rinsho Byori 40:703–707, 1992.

56. Brown SC, O'Reilly PH: The estimate of glomerular filtration rate during urography. Acceptability of a nonionic contrast medium as a marker of renal function. Invest Radiol 27:774–778, 1992.

57. Stake G, Monn E, Rootwelt K, et al: The clearance of iohexol as a measure of the glomerular filtration rate in children with chronic renal failure. Scand J Clin Lab Invest 51:729–734, 1991.

58. Brown SC, O'Reilly PH: Iohexol clearance for the determination of glomerular filtration rate in clinical practice: Evidence for a new gold standard. J Urol 146:675–679, 1991.

59. Rocco MV, Buckalew VM, Cole L, et al: Measurement of GFR with a single intravenous injection of nonradioactive iohexol and a single blood sample. J Am Soc Nephrol 4:323, 1993. Abstract.

60. Gaspari F, Amuchastegui CS, Guerini E, et al: Plasma clearance of nonradioactive iohexol as an alternative to renal clearance of insulin for measurement of glomerular filtration rate (GFR) in humans. J Am Soc Nephrol 4:315, 1993. Abstract.

61. Berg KG, Kolmannskog F, Lillevold PE, et al: Iopentol in patients with chronic renal failure: Its effects on renal function and its use as a glomerular filtration rate parameter. Scand J Clin Lab Invest 52:27–33, 1992.

62. Schaefer RM, Seufert H, Schafferhans K, et al: Determination of glomerular filtration rate in man using single shot piracetam clearance. Internist (Berl) 1:s23–s26, 1992.

63. Hattori K, Shiigai T, Minato Y, et al: Measurement of glomerular filtration rate by free vitamin B$_{12}$ clearance. Intern Med 32:194–196, 1993.

64. Choyke PL, Austin HA, Frank JA, et al: Hydrated clearance of gadolinium-DTPA as a measurement of glomerular filtration rate. Kidney Int 41:1595–1598, 1992.

65. Frank JA, Choyke PL, Austin HA, et al: Gadopentetate dimeglumine as a marker of renal function. Magnetic resonance imaging to glomerular filtration rates. Invest Radiol 1:s134–s136, 1991.

66. Mitch WE: Measuring the rate of progression of chronic renal insufficiency. In Mitch WE (ed): The Progressive Nature of Renal Disease, Vol 2. Churchill Livingstone, New York, 1992, pp 203–222.

67. Erpenbach K, Ebert A, Wieler H: Improvement in nuclear medicine diagnosis of kidney function using 99m technetium mercaptoacetyltriglycine (MAG$_3$). Urologe A 30:99–105, 1991.

68. Bianchi C: Measurement of the glomerular filtration rate. Prog Nucl Med 2:21–53, 1972.

69. Cole BR, Giangiacomo J, Ingelfinger JR, et al: Measurement of renal function without urine collection. A critical evaluation of the constant-infusion technic for determination of inulin and para-aminohippurate. N Engl J Med 287:1109–1114, 1972.

70. Herron KG, Folscroft J, MacDougall M, et al: Prolonged constant dual-isotope infusion for determination of renal function after water loading in hypertensive diabetic men. Contrib Nephrol 79:45–51, 1990.

71. Stake G, Monn E, Rootwelt K, et al: Glomerular filtration rate estimated by X-ray fluorescence technique in children: Comparison between the plasma disappearance of $^{99m}$Tc-DTPA and iohexol after urography. J Clin Invest 50:161–167, 1990.

72. Lewis R, Kerr N, Van Buren C, et al: Comparative evaluation of urographic contrast media, inulin, and $^{99m}$Tc-DTPA clearance methods for determination of glomerular filtration rate in clinical transplantation. Transplantation 48:790–796, 1989.

73. Rabito CA, Moore RH, Bougas C, et al: Noninvasive, real-time monitoring of renal function: The ambulatory renal monitor. J Nucl Med 34:199–207, 1993.
74. Rehling M, Moller ML, Thamdrup B, et al: Reliability of a $^{99m}$Tc-DTPA gamma camera technique for determination of single kidney glomerular filtration rate. A comparison to plasma clearance of $^{51}$Cr-EDTA in one-kidney patients, using the renal clearance of inulin as a reference. Scand J Urol Nephrol 20:57–62, 1986.
75. Sostre S, Osman M, Szabo Z, et al: Estimating renal function from the visual analysis of Tc-99m DTPA images. Clin Nucl Med 18:281–285, 1993.
76. Brochner-Mortensen J: Current status on assessment and measurement of glomerular filtration rate. Clin Physiol 5:1–17, 1985.
77. van Acker BAC, Koomen GCM, Arisz L: Drawbacks of the steady state inulin infusion technique for measurement of GFR. J Am Soc Nephrol 4:326:1993. Abstract.
78. Fisher M, Veall N: Glomerular filtration estimation based on a single sample. Br Med J 2:542, 1975.
79. Constable AR, Hussein MM, Albrecht MP: Single sample estimates of renal clearances. Br J Urol 51:84–87, 1979.
80. Smart R, Trew P, Burke J, et al: Simplified estimation of glomerular filtration rate and effective renal plasma flow. Eur J Nucl Med 6:249–253, 1981.
81. Stake G, Monn E, Rootwelt K, Montclair T: A single plasma sample method for estimation of the glomerular filtration rate in infants and children using iohexol, II: Establishment of the optimal plasma sampling time and a comparison with the $^{99}$Tcm-DPTA method. Scand J Clin Lab Invest 51:343–348, 1991.
82. Eriksson CG, Kallner A: Glomerular filtration rate: A comparison between Cr-EDTA clearance and a single sample technique with a non-ionic contrast agent. Clin Biochem 24:261 264, 1991.
83. Ham HR, Piepsz A: Estimation of glomerular filtration rate in infants and in children using a single-plasma sample method. J Nucl Med 32:1294–1297, 1991.
84. Thomsen HS, Hvid-Jacobsen K: Estimation of glomerular filtration rate from low-dose injection of iohexol and a single blood sample. Invest Radiol 26:332–336, 1991.
85. Prescott LF, Freestone S, McAuslane JAN: Reassessment of the single intravenous injection method with inulin for measurement of glomerular filtration rate in man. Clin Sci 80:167–176, 1991.
86. Schumann L, Wustenberg PW, Hortian B, et al: Determination of glomerular filtration rate (GFR) on two consecutive days using inulin in a single-sample plasma clearance method. Clin Nephrol 39:65–69, 1993.
87. Kamper AL, Nielsen SL: $^{51}$Cr-EDTA plasma clearance in severe renal failure determined by one plasma sample. Scand J Clin Lab Invest 49:555–559, 1989.
88. Rehling M, Rabol A: Measurement of glomerular filtration rate in adults: Accuracy of five single-sample plasma clearance methods. Clin Physiol 9:171–182, 1989.
89. Thomsen HS, Vestergaard A, Golman K, et al: One or two samples for determination of total plasma clearance of a nonionic contrast medium in patients undergoing enhanced CT. Acta Radiol 33:588–591, 1992.
90. Jung K, Henke W, Schulze BD, et al: Practical approach for determining glomerular filtration rate by single-injection inulin clearance. Clin Chem 38:403–407, 1992.
91. Picciotto G, Cacace G, Cesana P, et al: Estimation of chromium-51 ethylene diamine tetra-acetic acid plasma clearance: A comparative assessment of simplified techniques. Eur J Nucl Med 19:30–35, 1992.
92. Christensen AB: Determination of $^{99m}$Tc-DTPA clearance by a single sample plasma method. Clin Physiol 6:579–588, 1987.
93. Groth S: Calculation of $^{51}$Cr-EDTA clearance in children from the activity in one plasma sample by transformation of the biexponential plasma time-activity curve into a monoexponential with an identical integral area below the time-activity curve. Clin Physiol 4:61–74, 1984.
94. Mitch WE: Restricted diets and slowing the progression of chronic renal insufficiency. In Mitch WE, Klahr S (eds): Nutrition and the Kidney, 2nd ed. Little, Brown, Boston, 1993, pp 243–262.
95. Goates JJ, Morton KA, Whooten WW, et al: Comparison of methods for calculating glomerular filtration rate: Technetium-99m–DTPA scintigraphic analysis, protein-free and whole-plasma clearance of technetium-99m–DTPA and iodine-125–iothalamate clearance. J Nucl Med 31:424–429, 1990.
96. Rodby RA, Ali A, Rohde RD, et al: Renal scanning $^{99m}$Tc diethylenetriamine pentaacetic acid glomerular filtration rate (GFR) determination compared with iothalamate clearance GFR in diabetics. Am J Kidney Dis 20:569–573, 1992.
97. Perrone RD, Steinman TI, Beck GJ, et al: Utility of radioisotopic filtration markers in chronic renal insufficiency: Simultaneous comparison of $^{125}$I-iothalamate, $^{169}$Yb-DPTA, $^{99m}$Tc-DTPA and inulin. Am J Kidney Dis 16:224–235, 1990.
98. Apperloo AJ, De Zeeuw D, De Jong PE: Accuracy of GFR slope determination in long-term studies is improved by correction for incomplete urine collection. Kidney Int 43:969, 1993. Abstract.
99. Fotopoulos A, Blaufox MB, Lee HB, et al: Effects of residual urine on apparent renal clearance in patients with reduced function. Nucl Med Commun 3:224–235, 1992.
100. Skov PE: Glomerular filtration rate in patients with severe and very severe renal insufficiency. Acta Med Scand 187:419–428, 1970.
101. Ott NT, Wilson DM: A simple technique for estimating glomerular filtration rate with subcutaneous injection of $^{125}$I-iothalamate. Mayo Clin Invest 50:664–668, 1975.
102. Jagenburg A, Attman PO, Aurell M, et al: Determination of glomerular filtration rate in advanced renal insufficiency. Scand J Urol Nephrol 12:133–137, 1978.
103. Bianchi C, Bonadio M, Donadio C, et al: Measurement of glomerular filtration rate in man using $^{99m}$Tc-DTPA. Nephron 24:174–178, 1979.
104. Hagstam KE, Nordenfelt I, Svenson SE, et al: Comparison of different methods for determination of glomerular filtration rate in renal disease. Scand J Clin Lab Invest 34:31–36, 1974.
105. Rehling M, Moller ML, Thamdrup B, et al: Simultaneous measurement of renal clearance and plasma clearance of $^{99m}$Tc-labelled diethylenetriaminepenta-acetate, $^{51}$Cr-labelled ethylenediaminetetra-acetate and inulin in man. Clin Sci 66:613–619, 1984.
106. Manz F, Alatas W, Kochen W, et al: Determination of glomerular function in advanced renal failure. Arch Dis Child 52:721–724, 1977.
107. Carlsen JE, Moller ML, Lund JO: Comparison of four commercial $^{99m}$Tc-DTPA preparations used for the measurement of glomerular filtration rate: Concise communication. J Nucl Med 21:126–129, 1980.
108. Gibb DM, Dalton NR, Barratt MT: Measurement of glomerular filtration rate in children with insulin-dependent diabetes mellitus. Clin Chim Acta 182:131–139, 1989.
109. Wharton WW, Sondeen JL, McBiles M, et al: Measurement of glomerular filtration rate in ICU patients using $^{99m}$Tc-DTPA and inulin. Kidney Int 42:174–178, 1992.
110. Fleming JS, Wilkinson J, Oliver RM, et al: Comparison of radionuclide estimation of glomerular filtration rate using technetium 99m diethylenetriaminepentaacetic acid and chromium 51 ethylenediaminetetraacetic acid. Eur J Nucl Med 18:391–395, 1991.
111. Chandhoke PS, Kogan BA, al-Dahwi A, et al: Monitoring renal function in children with urological abnormalities. J Urol 144:601–605, 1990.
112. Mak RH, Al Dahhan J, Azzopardi D, et al: Measurement of glomerular filtration rate in children after renal transplantation. Kidney Int 23:410–413, 1983.
113. Clifton GG, Anderson C, McMahon G, et al: Monoexponential analysis of plasma disappearance of $^{99m}$Tc-DTPA and $^{131}$I-iodohippurate: A reliable method for measuring changes of renal function. J Clin Pharmacol 29:466–471, 1989.
114. Schluchter MD: Estimating correlation between alternative measures of disease progression in a longitudinal study. Stat Med 9:1175–1188, 1990.
115. Mitch WE, Buffington GA, Lemann J, et al: A simple method of estimating progression of chronic renal failure. Lancet 2:1326–1328, 1976.
116. Mitch WE, Walser M: A proposed mechanism for reduced creatinine excretion in severe chronic renal failure. Nephron 21:248–259, 1978.
117. Mitch WE, Collier VU, Walser M: Creatinine metabolism in chronic renal failure. Clin Sci 58:327–335, 1980.
118. Walser M: Creatinine excretion as a measure of protein nutrition in adults of varying age. JPEN 11:73S–77S, 1987.
119. Rutherford WE, Blondin J, Miller JP, et al: Chronic progressive renal disease. Kidney Int 11:62–72, 1977.
120. Ledingham JGG, Hart G: The optimum time to start regular hemodialysis. In Davison AM (ed): Dialysis Review. JB Lippincott, Philadelphia, 1978, pp 22–31.

121. Kirschbaum BB: Analysis of reciprocal creatinine plots in renal failure. Am J Med Sci 291:401–405, 1986.
122. Shah BV, Levey AS: Spontaneous changes in the rate of decline in reciprocal serum creatinine: Errors in predicting the progression of renal disease from extrapolation of the slope. J Am Soc Nephrol 2:1186–1191, 1992.
123. Gretz N, Manz F, Strauch M: Predictability of the progression of chronic renal failure. Kidney Int 24(suppl 15):2–5, 1983.
124. Combe C, Deforges-Lasseur C, Caix J, et al: Compliance and effects of nutritional treatment on progression and metabolic disorders of chronic renal failure. Nephrol Dial Transplant 8:412–418, 1993.
125. Beck GJ, Berg RL, Coggins CH, et al: Design and statistical issues of the Modification of Diet in Renal Disease Trial. Controlled Clin Trials 12:566–586, 1991.
126. Schlesselman JJ: Planning a longitudinal study. II. Frequency of measurement and study duration. J Chronic Dis 26:561–570, 1973.
127. Laird NM, Ware JH: Random-effects models for longitudinal data. Biometrics 38:963–974, 1982.
128. Walser M, Hill SB, Ward L, et al: A crossover comparison of progression of chronic renal failure: Ketoacids versus amino acids. Kidney Int 43:933–939, 1993.
129. Levey AS, Gassman JJ, Hall PM, et al: Assessing the progression of renal disease in clinical studies: Effects of duration of follow-up and regression to the mean. J Am Soc Nephrol 1:1087–1094, 1991.
130. Mathillas O, Attman PO, Aurell M, et al: Conflicting measurements in chronic renal failure. Contrib Nephrol 53:71–73, 1986.
131. Walser M, Drew HH, LaFrance ND: Creatinine measurements often yield false estimates of progression in chronic renal failure. Kidney Int 34:412–418, 1988.
132. Ponto KH, Anderson PA, Kies CV: Plasma alloisoleucine: Analytical method and clearance in ketoacid-supplemented normals. Kidney Int 36(suppl 27):S177–S183, 1989.
133. Jones B, Kenward MG: Design and Analysis of Cross-over Trials. *In* Monographs on Statistics and Applied Probability. Chapman & Hall, New York, 1989, p 153.
134. Viberti GC, Bilous RW, Mackintosh BS, et al: Monitoring glomerular function in diabetic nephropathy. Am J Med 74:256–264, 1983.
135. Mogensen CE: Renal function changes in diabetes. Diabetes 25:872–877, 1976.
136. Walser M, LaFrance ND, Ward L, et al: Progression of chronic renal failure in patients given ketoacids following amino acids. Kidney Int 32:123–128, 1987.
137. Bergström J, Alvestrand A, Bucht H, et al: Stockholm clinical study on progression of chronic renal failure—an interim report. Kidney Int 36:S110–S114, 1989.
138. Nyberg G, Blohme G, Norden G: Constant glomerular filtration rate in diabetic nephropathy. Acta Med Scand 219:67–72, 1986.
139. Franz KA, Reubi FC: Rate of functional deterioration in polycystic kidney disease. Kidney Int 23:523–526, 1983.
140. Dietary compliance in the trial of the European Study Group. An interim analysis. Contrib Nephrol 98:133–141, 1992.
141. Walser M: Weighted least squares regression analysis of factors contributing to progression of chronic renal failure. Contrib Nephrol 75:127–133, 1989.
142. Wright JP, Salzano S, Brown CB, et al: Natural history of chronic renal failure: A reappraisal. Nephrol Dial Transplant 7:379–383, 1992.
143. Locatelli F, Alberti D, Graziani G, et al: Factors affecting chronic renal failure progression: Results from a multicentre trial. Miner Electrolyte Metab 18:295–302, 1992.
144. Hannedouche T, Chauveau P, Kalou F, et al: Factors affecting progression in advanced chronic renal failure. Clin Nephrol 39:312–320, 1993.
145. Schieppati A, Mosconi L, Perna A, et al: Prognosis of untreated patients with idiopathic membranous nephropathy. N Engl J Med 329:85–89, 1993.
146. Polito C, La Manna A, Olivieri AN, et al: Progression of chronic renal failure. Child Nephrol Urol 11:91–95, 1991.
147. Rossing P, Hommel E, Smidt UM, et al: Impact of arterial blood pressure and albuminuria on the progression of diabetic nephropathy in IDDM patients. Diabetes 42:715–719, 1993.
148. Aparicio M, Potaux L, Bouchet JL, et al: Proteinuria and progression of renal failure in patients on a low-protein diet. Nephron 51:292–293, 1989.
149. Cameron JS: Proteinuria and progression in human glomerular diseases. Am J Nephrol 10(suppl 1):81–87, 1990.
150. D'Amico G: The clinical role of proteinuria. Am J Kidney Dis 17(suppl 1):48–52, 1991.
151. Rosman JB, Ter Wee PM: Relationship between proteinuria and response to low protein diets early in chronic renal failure. Blood Purif 7:52–57, 1989.
152. Williams PS, Fass G, Bone JM: Renal pathology and proteinuria determine progression in untreated mild/moderate chronic renal failure. Q J Med 67:343–354, 1988.
153. Stenvinkel P, Alvestrand A, Bergström J: Factors influencing progression in patients with chronic renal failure. J Intern Med 226:183–188, 1989.
154. Nyberg G, Blohme G, Norden G: Constant glomerular filtration rate in diabetic nephropathy. Correlation to blood pressure and blood glucose control. Acta Med Scand 219:67–72, 1986.
155. Nelson R, Knowler WC, Beck GJ, et al: Early predictors of progressive nephropathy in non-azotemic Pima Indians with non–insulin-dependent diabetes mellitus. J Am Soc Nephrol 4:306, 1993. Abstract.
156. Relationship among baseline proteinuria (P), mean arterial blood pressure (MAP) during follow-up, and decline in glomerular filtration rate (GFR) in the modification of diet in renal disease study (MDRD). J Am Soc Nephrol 4:254, 1993. Abstract.
157. Gall MA, Nielsen FS, Smidt UM, et al: The course of kidney function in type-2 (non–insulin-dependent) diabetic patients with diabetic nephropathy. Diabetologia 36:1071–1078, 1993.
158. Comparison of decline in GFR in blacks versus non-blacks in an MDRD study. J Am Soc Nephrol 4:253, 1993. Abstract.
159. Walker WG, Hermann J, Anderson J: Racial differences in renal protective effect of enalapril (E) vs hydrochlorothiazide (H) in randomized doubly blinded trial in hypertensive NIDDM. J Am Soc Nephrol 4:310, 1993. Abstract.
160. Breyer J, McGill J, Naham N, et al: Predictors of the rate of progression of renal insufficiency in patients with insulin-dependent diabetes and overt diabetic nephropathy. J Am Soc Nephrol 4:301, 1993. Abstract.
161. Gabow PA, Johnson AM, Kaehny WD, et al: Factors relating to renal functional deterioration in autosomal dominant polycystic kidney disease. Kidney Int 37:248, 1990. Abstract.
162. Gretz N, Zeier M, Geberth S, et al: Is gender a determinant for evolution of renal failure? A study in autosomal dominant polycystic kidney disease. Am J Kidney Dis 14:178–183, 1989.
163. Davison AM, Cameron JS, Kerr DN, et al: The natural history of renal function in untreated idiopathic membranous glomerulonephritis in adults. Clin Nephrol 22:61–67, 1984.
164. Murphy BF, Fairley KF, Kincaid-Smith PS: Idiopathic membranous glomerulonephritis: Long term follow-up in 139 cases. Clin Nephrol 30:175–181, 1988.
165. Hooper J Jr, Trew PA, Biava CG: Membranous nephropathy: Its relative benignity in women. Nephron 29:18–24, 1991.
166. Tu WH, Petitti DB, Biava CG, et al: Membranous nephropathy: Predictors of terminal renal failure. Nephron 36:118–124, 1984.
167. Walser M, Ward L: Progression of chronic renal failure is related to glucocorticoid production. Kidney Int 34:859–866, 1988.
168. Walser M: Steroid damping: A novel approach to slowing the progression of chronic renal failure. Clin Res 41:399A, 1993. Abstract.
169. Samuelsson O, Aurell M, Knight-Gibson C, et al: Apolipoprotein-B–containing lipoproteins and the progression of renal insufficiency. Nephron 63:279–285, 1993.
170. Mulec H, Johnson S, Bjorck S: Relation between serum cholesterol and diabetic nephropathy. Lancet 335:1537–1538, 1990.
171. Mulec H, Aurell M, Johnsen S, et al: Impact of lipid abnormalities on diabetic nephropathy. J Am Soc Nephrol 2:294, 1991. Abstract.
172. Hasslacher C, Bostedtkiesel A, Kempe HP, et al: Effect of metabolic factors and blood pressure on kidney function in proteinuric type-2 (non–insulin-dependent) diabetic patients. Diabetologia 36:1051–1056, 1993.
173. Biesenbach G, Stoger H, Zazgornik J: Influence of pregnancy on progression of diabetic nephropathy and subsequent requirement of renal replacement therapy in female type I diabetic patients with impaired renal function. Nephrol Dial Transplant 7:105–109, 1992.
174. Smith R, Thomson M: Neuroendocrinology of the hypothalamo-pituitary-adrenal axis in pregnancy and the puerperium. Baillieres Clin Endocrinol Metab 5:167–186, 1991.
175. Nyberg G, Blohme G, Norden G: Impact of metabolic control in progression of clinical diabetic nephropathy. Diabetologia 30:82–86, 1987.

176. Beck-Nielsen H, Olesen T, Mogensen CE, et al: Effect of near normoglycemia for 5 years on progression of early diabetic retinopathy and renal involvement. Diabetes Res 15:185–190, 1990.

177. Dahl-Jorgensen K, Hanssen KF, Kierulf P, et al: Reduction of urinary albumin excretion after 4 years of continuous subcutaneous insulin infusion in insulin-dependent diabetes mellitus. Acta Endocrinol (Copenh) 117:19–25, 1988.

178. The effect of intensive treatment of diabetes on the development and progression of long-term complications in insulin-dependent diabetes mellitus. The Diabetes Control and Complications Trial. N Engl J Med 329:977–986, 1993.

179. Stegmayer BG: A study of patients with diabetes mellitus (type 1) and end-stage renal failure: Tobacco usage may increase risk of nephropathy and death. J Intern Med 228:121–124, 1990.

180. Kirschbaum C, Wust S, Strasburger CJ: 'Normal' cigarette smoking increases free cortisol in habitual smokers. Life Sci 50:435–442, 1992.

181. Vora JP, Peters JR, Williams JD: Evolution of renal hemodynamics in non–insulin-dependent diabetics (NIDDMs): A 2 year study. J Am Soc Nephrol 4:310, 1993. Abstract.

182. Rudberg S, Persson B, Dahlquist G: Increased glomerular filtration rate as a predictor of diabetic nephropathy: An 8-year prospective study. Kidney Int 41:822–828, 1992.

183. Wee PM, Donker AJM: Renal reserve filtration capacity: Can it predict progression of chronic renal failure? Am J Kidney Dis 17(suppl 1):71–75, 1991.

184. Kelly RA, Mitch WE: Creatinine, uric acid and other nitrogenous waste products: Clinical implication of the imbalance between their production and elimination in uremia. Semin Nephrol 3:286–294, 1983.

185. Walser M, Coulter AW, Dighe S, et al: The effect of keto-analogues of essential amino acids in severe chronic uremia. J Clin Invest 52:678–690, 1973.

186. Folin O: Laws governing the clinical composition of urine. Am J Physiol 13:67–115, 1905.

187. Rafoth RS, Onstad GR: Urea synthesis after oral protein loading in man. J Clin Invest 56:1170–1174, 1975.

188. Cottini EP, Gallina DL, Dominguez JM: Urea excretion in adult humans with varying degrees of kidney malfunction fed milk, egg or an amino acid mixture: Assessment of nitrogen balance. J Nutr 103:11–19, 1973.

189. Maroni BJ, Steinman T, Mitch WE: A method for estimating nitrogen intake of patients with chronic renal failure. Kidney Int 27:58–65, 1985.

190. Sargent J, Gotch F, Borah M, et al: Urea kinetics: A guide to nutritional management of renal failure. Am J Clin Nutr 31:1696–1702, 1978.

191. Borah MF, Schoenfeld PY, Gotch FA, et al: Nitrogen balance during intermittent dialysis therapy of uremia. Kidney Int 14:491–500, 1978.

192. Young V: Some metabolic and nutritional considerations of dietary protein restriction. In Mitch WE (ed): Contemporary Issues in Nephrology: The Progressive Nature of Renal Disease. Churchill Livingstone, New York, 1986, pp 263–283.

193. Walser M, Bodenlos LJ: Urea metabolism in man. J Clin Invest 38:1617–1622, 1959.

194. Jones EA, Smallwood RA, Craigie A, et al: The enterohepatic circulation of urea nitrogen. Clin Sci 37:825–836, 1969.

195. Wilson DR, Ing TS, Metcalfe-Gibson A, et al: The chemical composition of faeces in uremia, as revealed by in vivo faecal dialysis. Clin Sci 35:197–207, 1968.

196. Wolpert E, Phillips SF, Summerskill WHJ: Transport of urea and ammonia production in the human colon. Lancet 2:1387–1390, 1971.

197. Down PF, Agostini L, Murison J, Wrong OM: The interrelations of faecal ammonia, pH and bicarbonate: Evidence of colonic absorption of ammonia by non-ionic diffusion. Clin Sci 43:101–114, 1972.

198. Gibson JA, Park NJ, Sladen GE, et al: The role of the colon in urea metabolism in man. Clin Sci 50:51–59, 1976.

199. Varcoe R, Halliday D, Carson ER, et al: Efficiency of utilization of urea nitrogen for albumin synthesis by chronically uremic and normal man. Clin Sci Mol Med 48:379–390, 1975.

200. Long CL, Jeevandanam M, Kinney JM: Metabolism and recycling of urea in man. Am J Clin Nutr 31:1367–1382, 1987.

201. Murdaugh HV: Urea metabolism during low protein intake: Studies in man and dog. In Schmidt-Nielson B (ed): Urea and the Kidney. Excerpta Medica, Amsterdam, 1970, pp 471–477.

202. Giordano C: Use of exogenous and endogenous urea for protein synthesis in normal and uremic subjects. J Lab Clin Med 62:231–246, 1963.

203. Simenhoff ML, Saukkonen JJ, Burke JF, et al: Amine metabolism and the small bowel in uraemia. Lancet 2:818–821, 1976.

204. Walser M: Determinants of ureagenesis with particular reference to renal failure. Kidney Int 17:709–721, 1980.

205. Robson AM: Urea Metabolism in Chronic Renal Failure. Newcastle upon Tyne, England: University of Newcastle upon Tyne; 1964. Thesis.

206. Walser M: Urea metabolism in chronic renal failure. J Clin Invest 53:1385–1392, 1974.

207. Mitch WE, Lietman PS, Walser M: Effects of oral neomycin and kanamycin in chronic renal failure: I. Urea metabolism. Kidney Int 11:116–122, 1977.

208. Dal Canton A, Fuiano G, Conte G, et al: Mechanism of increased plasma urea after diuretic therapy in uraemic patients. Clin Sci 68:255–261, 1985.

209. Kamm DE, Wu L, Kuchmy BL: Contribution of the urea appearance rate to diuretic-induced azotemia in the rat. Kidney Int 32:47–56, 1987.

210. Lowrie EG, Laird NM, Parker TF, et al: The effect of hemodialysis prescription on patient morbidity. N Engl J Med 305:1176–1181, 1981.

211. Calloway DH: Nitrogen balance of men with marginal intakes of protein and energy. J Nutr 105:914–923, 1975.

212. Zanni E, Calloway DH, Zezulka AY: Protein requirements of elderly men. J Nutr 109:513–524, 1979.

213. Steffee WP, Goldsmith RS, Pencharz PB, et al: Dietary protein intake and dynamic aspects of whole body nitrogen metabolism in adult humans. Metabolism 25:281–297, 1976.

214. Loder PB, Kee AJ, Horsburgh R, et al: Validity of urinary urea nitrogen as a measure of total urinary nitrogen in adult patients requiring parenteral nutrition. Crit Care Med 17:309–312, 1989.

215. Konstantinides FN, Konstantinides NN, Li JC, et al: Urinary urea nitrogen: Too insensitive for calculating nitrogen balance studies in surgical clinical nutrition. JPEN 15:189–193, 1991.

216. Crim MC, Calloway DH, Margen S: Creatinine metabolism in men: Creatine pool size and turnover in relation to creatine intake. J Nutr 106:371–381, 1976.

217. Forbes GB, Bruining GS: Urinary creatinine excretion and lean body mass. Am J Clin Nutr 29:1359–1366, 1978.

218. Fuller NJ, Elia M: Factors influencing the production of creatinine: Implications for the determination and interpretation of urinary creatine and creatinine in man. Clin Chim Acta 175:199–210, 1988.

219. Bleiler RE, Schedle HP: Creatinine excretion: Variability and relationships to diet and body size. J Lab Clin Med 59:945–955, 1962.

220. Heymsfield SB, Arteaga C, McManus C, et al: Measurement of muscle mass in humans: Validity of the 24-hour urinary creatinine method. Am J Clin Nutr 37:478–498, 1983.

221. Walker JB: Metabolic control of creatine biosynthesis. J Biol Chem 235:2357–2361, 1960.

222. Van Pilsum JF, Canfield TM: Transamidinase activities in vitro of kidneys from rats fed diets supplemented with nitrogen-containing compounds. J Biol Chem 237:2574–2577, 1962.

223. Goldman R: Creatinine excretion in renal failure. Proc Soc Exp Biol Med 85:446–448, 1954.

224. Jones JD, Burnett PC: Creatinine metabolism in humans with decreased renal function: Creatinine deficit. Clin Chem 20:1204–1212, 1974.

225. Mackenzie CG, duVigneaud V: Biochemical stability of methyl group of creatine and creatinine. J Biol Chem 185:185–189, 1950.

226. Dominguez R, Pomerone E: Recovery of creatinine after ingestion and after intravenous injection in man. Proc Soc Exp Biol Med 58:26–28, 1945.

227. Jones JD, Burnett PD: Implication of creatinine and gut flora in the uremic syndrome: Induction of ''creatinase'' in colon contents of the rat by dietary creatinine. Clin Chem 18:280–284, 1972.

228. Owens CWI, Albuquerque ZP, Tomlinson GM: In vitro metabolism of creatinine, methylamine and amino acids by intestinal contents of normal and uremic subjects. Gut 20:568–574, 1979.

229. Danovitch GM, Weinberger J, Berlyne GM: Uric acid in advanced renal failure. Clin Sci 43:331–341, 1972.

230. Emmerson BT, Row PG: An evaluation of the pathogenesis of the gouty kidney. Kidney Int 8:65–74, 1975.

231. Emmerson BT: Abnormal urate excretion associated with renal and systemic disorders, drugs and toxins. *In* Kelley WN, Weiner IM (eds): Uric Acid, Handbook of Experimental Pharmacology. Springer-Verlag, Berlin, 1978, p 287.

232. Clifford AJ, Riumallo JA, Young VR, et al: Effect of oral purines on serum and urinary uric acid of normal, hyperuricemic and gouty humans. J Nutr 106:428–450, 1976.

233. Lewis HB, Doisy EA: Studies in uric acid metabolism. I. The influence of high protein diets on the endogenous uric acid elimination. J Biol Chem 36:1–7, 1918.

234. Benedict JD, Forsham PH, Stetten DW: The metabolism of uric acid in the normal and gouty human studied with the aid of isotopic uric acid. J Biol Chem 181:183–193, 1949.

235. Sorensen LB, Levinson DJ: Origin and extrarenal elimination of uric acid in man. Nephron 14:7–20, 1975.

236. Sorensen LB: Degradation of uric acid in man. Metabolism 8:687–703, 1959.

237. Sorensen LB: Extrarenal disposal of uric acid. *In* Kelley WN, Weiner IM (eds): Uric Acid, Handbook of Experimental Pharmacology. Springer-Verlag, Berlin, 1978, p 325.

238. Mitch WE: Effects of intestinal flora on nitrogen metabolism in patients with chronic renal failure. Am J Clin Nutr 31:1594–1600, 1978.

239. Richet G: Some aspects of uric acid metabolism in chronic renal failure. *In* Berlyne GM (ed): Nutrition in Renal Disease. Churchill Livingstone, Edinburgh, 1968, p 133.

240. Rosenfeld JF: Effect of long-term allopurinol administration on serial GFR in normotensive and hypertensive subjects. *In* Sperling O, De Vries A, Wyngaarden JB (eds): Purine Metabolism in Man: Biochemistry and Pharmacology of Uric Acid Metabolism. Plenum Publishing, New York, 1974, pp 581–596.

241. Fessel WJ: Renal outcomes of gout and hyperuricemia. Am J Med 67:74–81, 1979.

242. Reif MC, Constantine A, Levitt MF: Chronic gouty nephropathy: A vanishing syndrome? N Engl J Med 304:535–536, 1981.

243. Vince A, Down PF, Murison J, et al: Generation of ammonia from non-urea sources in a fecal incubation system. Clin Sci Mol Med 51:313–322, 1976.

244. Weber FL Jr, Maddrey WC, Walser M: Amino acid metabolism of dog jejunum before and during absorption of ketoanalogues. Am J Physiol 232:E263–E269, 1977.

245. Defarrari G, Garibotto G, Robaudo C, et al: Brain metabolism of amino acids and ammonia in patients with chronic renal insufficiency. Kidney Int 20:505–510, 1981.

246. Pimentel L, Brusilow SW, Mitch WE: Unexpected encephalopathy in chronic renal failure: Hyperammonemia complicating acute peritonitis. J Am Soc Nephrol (in press).

247. Brusilow SW, Horwich A: Urea cycle enzymes. *In* Scriver C, Beaudet A, Sly W, et al (eds): The Metabolic Basis of Inherited Disease, 6th ed. McGraw-Hill, New York, 1989, pp 629–663.

248. Watson AJ, Karp JE, Walker WG, et al: Transient idiopathic hyperammonaemia in adults. Lancet 2:1271–1274, 1985.

249. Mitchell RB, Wagner JE, Karp JE, et al: Syndrome of idiopathic hyperammonemia after high-dose chemotherapy: Review of nine cases. Am J Med 85:662–667, 1988.

250. Drayna CJ, Titcomb CP, Varma RR, et al: Hyperammonemic encephalopathy caused by infection in a neurogenic bladder. N Engl J Med 304:766–768, 1981.

251. Deuel HF, Sandiford I, Sandiford K, et al: A study of the nitrogen minimum: The effect of sixty-three days of a protein-free diet on the nitrogen partition products in the urine and on the heat production. J Biol Chem 76:391–406, 1928.

252. Lavender S, Bennett J, Morse PF, et al: Albumin and creatinine clearances in renal disease. Clin Sci Mol Med 46:775–784, 1974.

253. Rosenblatt SG, Drake S, Fadem S, et al: Gastrointestinal blood loss in patients with chronic renal failure. Am J Kidney Dis 1:232–236, 1982.

254. Wrick KL, Robertson JB, Van Soest PJ, et al: The influence of dietary fiber source on human intestinal transit and stool output. J Nutr 113:1464–1479, 1983.

255. Hegsted M: Assessment of nitrogen requirements. Am J Clin Nutr 31:1669–1677, 1978.

256. Mitchell HH, Bert MH: The determination of metabolic fecal nitrogen. J Nutr 52:483–497, 1954.

257. Koralnik O, Scholz H: Le gradient de l'azote uréique entre le sueur et le plasma. *In* Kerr DNS (ed): Proceedings of the IVth International Congress of Nephrology. Amsterdam, Excerpta Medica, 1969, pp 433–436.

258. Walser M: Misinterpretation of nitrogen balances when glutamine stores fall or are replenished. Am J Clin Nutr 53:1337–1338, 1991.

259. Mitch WE, Wilcox CS: Disorders of body fluids, sodium and potassium in chronic renal failure. Am J Med 72:536–550, 1982.

260. Blackmore WP: Urea distribution in renal failure. J Clin Pathol 16:235–243, 1963.

261. Taylor YSM, Scrimshaw NS, Young VR: The relationship between serum urea levels and dietary nitrogen utilization in young men. Br J Nutr 32:407–411, 1974.

262. Abras E, Walser M: Nitrogen utilization in uremic patients fed by continuous nasogastric infusion. Kidney Int 22:392–397, 1982.

263. Waterlow JC: The assessment of protein nutrition and metabolism in the whole animal with special reference to man. *In* Munro HN (ed): Mammalian Protein Metabolism. Academic Press, New York, 1969, pp 326–390.

264. Lowrie EG, Lew NL: Death risk in hemodialysis patients: The predictive value of commonly measured variables and an evaluation of the death rate differences among facilities. Am J Kidney Dis 15:458–482, 1990.

265. Bianchi R, Mariani G, Pilo A: Albumin synthesis measurements by means of an improved two tracer method in patients with chronic renal failure. J Nucl Biol Med 14:136–144, 1970.

266. McFarlane H, Ogbeide MJ, Reddy S, et al: Biochemical assessment of protein-calorie malnutrition. Lancet 1:392–394, 1969.

267. Ooi BS, Darocy AF, Pollak VE: Serum transferrin levels in chronic renal failure. Nephron 9:200–208, 1972.

268. Markowitz H, Fairbans VF: Transferrin assay and total iron binding capacity. Mayo Clin Proc 58:827–828, 1983.

269. Eschbach JN, Abdulhadi MH, Brown JK, et al: Recombinant human erythropoietin in uremic patients with end-stage renal disease. Ann Intern Med 111:992–1000, 1989.

270. Toigo G, Situlin R, Vasile A, et al: Effects of erythropoietin administration on nutritional state and erythrocyte metabolism in maintenance hemodialysis patients. Contrib Nephrol 98:79–88, 1992.

271. Barany P, Pettersson E, Ahlberg M, et al: Nutritional assessment on anemic hemodialysis patients treated with recombinant human erythropoietin. Clin Nephrol 35:270–279, 1991.

272. Watson AJ, Gimenez LF, Cotton S, et al: Treatment of the anemia of chronic renal failure with subcutaneous recombinant human erythropoietin. Am J Med 89:432–435, 1990.

273. Eschbach JW, Kelly MR, Haley NR, et al: Treatment of the anemia of progressive renal failure with recombinant human erythropoietin. N Engl J Med 321:158–163, 1989.

274. Cano N, Fernandez JP, LaCombe P, et al: Statistical selection of nutritional parameters in hemodialyzed patients. Kidney Int 37(suppl 22):S178–S180, 1987.

275. Kult J, Richter U, Scheitza E, et al: Storungen im Komplementsystem bei Niereninsuffizienz und ihre Beeinflussung durch Aminosaurensubstitution. Dtsch Med Wochenschr 99:339–342, 1974.

276. Maroni BJ: Requirements for protein, calories, and fat in the predialysis patient. *In* Mitch WE, Klahr S (eds): Nutrition and the Kidney, Vol 2. Little, Brown, Boston, 1993, pp 185–212.

277. Lucas PA, Meadows JH, Roberts DE, et al: The risks and benefits of a low protein–essential amino acid–keto acid diet. Kidney Int 29:995–1003, 1986.

278. Goodship THJ, Lloyd S, Clague MB, et al: Whole body leucine turnover and nutritional status in continuous ambulatory peritoneal dialysis. Clin Sci 73:463–469, 1987.

279. Koppel JD: Causes of catabolism and wasting in acute or chronic renal failure. *In* Robinson RR (ed): Nephrology. Springer-Verlag, New York, 1984, pp 1498–1514.

280. Koppel JD, Berg R, Houser H, et al: Nutritional status of patients with different levels of chronic renal failure. Kidney Int 36(suppl 27):S184–S194, 1989.

281. Walser M: Does prolonged protein restriction preceding dialysis lead to protein malnutrition at the onset of dialysis? Kidney Int 44:1139–1144, 1993.

282. Alvestrand A, Fürst P, Bergström J: Plasma and muscle free amino acids in uremia: Influence of nutrition with amino acids. Clin Nephrol 18:297–305, 1982.

283. Koppel JD, Swenseid MD: Nitrogen balance and plasma amino acid levels in uremic patients fed an essential amino acid diet. Am J Clin Nutr 27:806–812, 1974.

284. Young GA, Keogh JB, Parson FM: Plasma amino acids and protein levels in chronic renal failure and changes caused by oral supplements of essential amino acids. Clin Chim Acta 61:205–213, 1975.

285. Garibotto G, Deferrari G, Robaudo C, et al: Effects of a protein meal on blood amino acid profile in patients with chronic renal failure. Nephron 64:216–225, 1993.

286. Deferrari G, Garibotto G, Robaudo C, et al: Splanchnic exchange of amino acids after amino acid ingestion in patients with chronic renal insufficiency. Am J Clin Nutr 48:72–83, 1988.

287. May RC, Hara Y, Kelly RA, et al: Branched-chain amino acid metabolism in rat muscle: Abnormal regulation in acidosis. Am J Physiol 252:E712–E718, 1987.

288. Hara Y, May RC, Kelly RA, et al: Acidosis, not azotemia, stimulates branched-chain amino acid catabolism in uremic rats. Kidney Int 32:808–814, 1987.

289. Bergström J, Alvestrand A, Fürst P: Plasma and muscle free amino acids in maintenance hemodialysis patients without protein malnutrition. Kidney Int 38:108–114, 1990.

290. Chan W, Wang M, Kopple JD, et al: Citrulline levels and urea cycle enzymes in uremic rats. J Nutr 104:678–683, 1974.

291. Jansen A, Lewis S, Cattell V, et al: Arginase is a major pathway of L-arginine metabolism in nephritic glomeruli. Kidney Int 42:1107–1112, 1992.

292. Hecker M, Sessa WC, Harris HJ, et al: The metabolism of L-arginine and its significance for the biosynthesis of endothelium-derived relaxing factor: Cultured endothelial cells recycle L-citrulline to L-arginine. Proc Natl Acad Sci USA 87:8612–8616, 1990.

293. Young GA, Parsons FM: Impairment of phenylalanine hydroxylation in chronic renal insufficiency. Clin Sci Mol Med 41:89–92, 1973.

294. Wang M, Vhymeister I, Swenseid ME, et al: Phenylalanine hydroxylase and tyrosine aminotransferase activity in chronically uremic rats. J Nutr 105:122–127, 1975.

295. Letteri JM, Scipione RA: Phenylalanine metabolism in chronic renal failure. Nephron 13:365–371, 1974.

296. Tizianello A, DeFerrari G, Garibotto G, et al: Renal metabolism of amino acids and ammonia in subjects with normal renal function and in patients with chronic renal insufficiency. J Clin Invest 65:1162–1173, 1980.

297. Mitch WE, Chesney RW: Amino acid metabolism by the kidney. Miner Electrolyte Metab 9:190–202, 1983.

298. Walser M, Hill SB: Free and protein-bound tryptophan in serum of untreated patients with chronic renal failure. Kidney Int 44:1366–1371, 1993.

299. Edozien JC: The free amino acids of plasma and urine in kwashiorkor. Clin Sci 31:153–166, 1966.

300. Dalton RN, Chantler C: The relationship between BCAA and alpha-ketoacids in blood in uremia. Kidney Int 24(suppl 16):S61–S66, 1983.

301. Druml W, Kleinberger G, Burger U, et al: Elimination of amino acids in chronic renal failure. Infusionstherapie 13:262–267, 1986.

302. Stockenhuber F, Kurz RW, Sertl K, et al: Increased plasma histamine levels in uraemic pruritus. Clin Sci 79:477–482, 1990.

303. Pechar J, Malek P, Dobersky P, et al: Influence of protein intake and renal function on plasma amino acids in patients with renal impairment and after kidney transplantation. Nutr Metab 22:278–287, 1978.

304. Shear L: Internal redistribution of tissue protein and amino acid metabolism in uremia. In Alwall N, Berglund F, Josephson B (eds): Proceedings of the Fourth International Congress of Nephrology. S Karger, Basel, 1969, p 1252.

305. Bergström J, Fürst P, Noree L-O, et al: Intracellular free amino acids in muscle tissue of patients with chronic uraemia: Effect of peritoneal dialysis and infusion of essential amino acids. Clin Sci Mol Med 54:51–60, 1978.

306. Pye IF, McGale EHF, Stonier C: Studies of cerebrospinal fluid and plasma amino acids in patients with steady-state chronic renal failure. Clin Chim Acta 92:65–72, 1979.

307. Jontofsohn R, Trivisas G, Katz N, et al: Amino acid content of erythrocytes in uremia. Am J Clin Nutr 31:1956–1960, 1978.

308. Ganda OP, Aoki TT, Soeldner JS, et al: Hormone-fuel concentrations in anephric subjects. J Clin Invest 57:1403–1411, 1976.

309. Lindholm B, Garcia E, Qureshi GA, et al: High muscle and low plasma tryptophan in CAPD. Kidney Int 36(suppl 27):S302, 1989. Abstract.

310. Wilcken DEL, Gupta VJ, Reddy SG: Accumulation of sulphur-containing amino acids including cystine-homocystine in patients on maintenance hemodialysis. Clin Sci 58:427–430, 1980.

311. Gejyo F, Ito G, Kinoshita Y: Identification of N-monoacetylcystine in uremic plasma. Clin Sci 60:331–334, 1981.

312. Garibotto G, Paoletti E, Fiorini F, et al: Peripheral metabolism of branched-chain keto acids in patients with chronic renal failure. Miner Electrolyte Metab 19:25–31, 1993. Abstract.

313. Langer K, Fröhling PT, Diederich J, et al: Plasma amino and keto-acids in chronic renal failure. Contrib Nephrol 65:55–59, 1989.

314. Schauder P, Matthaei D, Henning HV, et al: Blood levels of branched-chain amino acids and alpha-ketoacids in uremic patients given keto analogues of essential amino acids. Am J Clin Nutr 33:1660–1666, 1980.

315. Walser M, Jarskog FL, Hill SB: Branched-chain keto acid metabolism in patients with chronic renal failure. Am J Clin Nutr 50:807–813, 1989.

316. Laouari D, Rocchiccioli F, Dodu C, et al: Conversion efficiency of two branched-chain alpha ketoanalogs in normal and uremic rats. Kidney Int 32(suppl 22):S186–S190, 1987.

317. Tungsanga K, Kang CW, Walser M: Utilization of alpha-ketoisocaproate for protein synthesis in uremic rats. Kidney Int 30:891–894, 1986.

318. Giordano C, Esposito R, de Pascale C, et al: Dietary treatment in renal failure. In Schreiner GE (ed): Proceedings of the Third International Congress of Nephrology. S Karger, Basel, 1967.

319. Kopple JD, Coburn JW: Metabolic studies of low protein diets in uremia: I. Nitrogen and potassium. Medicine (Baltimore) 52:583–594, 1973.

320. FAO/WHO/UNU: Energy and protein requirements. WHO Tech Rep Ser 724:1–206, 1985.

321. Alvestrand A, Ahlberg M, Fürst P, et al: Clinical results of long-term treatment with a low protein diet and a new amino acid preparation in patients with chronic uremia. Clin Nephrol 19:67–73, 1983.

322. Mitch WE, Abras E, Walser M: Long-term effects of a new keto-acid–amino acid supplement in patients with chronic renal failure. Kidney Int 22:48–53, 1982.

323. Motil KJ, Matthews DE, Bier DM, et al: Whole-body leucine and lysine metabolism: Response to dietary protein intake in young men. Am J Physiol 240:E712–E721, 1981.

324. Young VR: 1987 McCollum award lecture. Kinetics of human amino acid metabolism: Nutritional implications and some lessons. Am J Clin Nutr 46:709–725, 1987.

325. McNurlan MA, Garlick PJ: Influence of nutrient intake on protein turnover. Diabetes Metab Rev 5:165–189, 1989.

326. Goodship THJ, Mitch WE, Hoerr RA, et al: Adaptation to low-protein diets in renal failure: Leucine turnover and nitrogen balance. J Am Soc Nephrol 1:66–75, 1990.

327. Masud T, Young V, Chapman T, et al: Adaptive responses to very low protein diets in uremia: The first comparison of ketoacids to essential amino acids. Kidney Int 45:1182–1192, 1994.

328. May RC, Kelly RA, Mitch WE: Metabolic acidosis stimulates protein degradation in rat muscle by a glucocorticoid-dependent mechanism. J Clin Invest 77:614–621, 1986.

329. Kalhoff H, Manz F, Diekmann L, et al: Decreased growth rate of low-birth-weight infants with prolonged maximum renal acid stimulation. Acta Pediatr 82:522–527, 1993.

330. McSherry E, Morris RC: Attainment of normal stature with alkali therapy in infants and children with classic renal tubular acidosis. J Clin Invest 61:509–514, 1978.

331. Reaich D, Channon SM, Scrimgeour CM, et al: Ammonium chloride–induced acidosis increases protein breakdown and amino acid oxidation in humans. Am J Physiol 263:E735–E739, 1992.

332. Mochizuki T: The effect of metabolic acidosis on amino and keto acid metabolism in chronic renal failure. Jpn J Nephrol 33:213–224, 1991.

333. Reaich D, Channon SM, Scrimgeour CM, et al: Correction of acidosis in humans with CRF decreases protein degradation and amino acid oxidation. Am J Physiol 265:E230–E235, 1993.

334. May RC, Masud T, Logue B, et al: Chronic metabolic acidosis accelerates whole body proteolysis and leucine oxidation in awake rats. Kidney Int 41:1535–1542, 1992.

335. Garibotto G, Russo R, Sofia A, et al: Skeletal muscle protein synthesis and degradation in patients with chronic renal failure. Kidney Int 45:1432–1439, 1994.

336. May RC, Kelly RA, Mitch WE: Mechanisms for defects in muscle

protein metabolism in rats with chronic uremia: The influence of metabolic acidosis. J Clin Invest 79:1099–1103, 1987.

337. Williams B, Hattersley J, Layward E, et al: Metabolic acidosis and skeletal muscle adaptation to low protein diets in chronic uremia. Kidney Int 40:779–786, 1991.

338. England BK, Chastain L, Mitch WE: Abnormalities in protein synthesis and degradation induced by extracellular pH in BC3H1 myocytes. Am J Physiol 260:C277–C282, 1991.

339. Isozaki Y, Price SR, England BK, et al: Evidence for acidosis-induced, rapid, coordinated increases in mRNA encoding proteins of the ubiquitin-proteasome pathway in cultured myocytes. J Am Soc Nephrol 4:771, 1993. Abstract.

340. Mitch WE, Medina R, Greiber S, et al: Metabolic acidosis stimulates muscle protein degradation by activating the ATP-dependent pathway involving ubiquitin and proteasomes. J Clin Invest 93:2127–2133, 1994.

341. Finley D: Ubiquitination. Annu Rev Cell Biol 7:25–69, 1991.

342. Hershko A, Ciechanover A: The ubiquitin system for protein degradation. Annu Rev Biochem 61:761–807, 1992.

343. Price SR, England BK, Bailey JL, et al: Acidosis and glucocorticoids concomitantly increase ubiquitin and proteasome subunit mRNAs in rat muscle. Am J Physiol 267:C955–C960, 1994.

344. Tomas FM, Munro HN, Young VR: Effects of glucocorticoid administration and the rate of muscle protein breakdown in vivo in rats, as measured by urinary excretion of N-methylhistidine. Biochem J 178:139–146, 1979.

345. Odedra BR, Millward DJ: Effect of corticosterone treatment on muscle protein turnover in adrenalectomized rats and diabetic rats maintained on insulin. Biochem J 204:663–672, 1982.

346. Quan ZY, Walser M: The effect of corticosterone administration at varying levels on leucine oxidation and whole body protein synthesis and breakdown in adrenalectomized rats. Metabolism 40:1263–1267, 1992.

347. Simmons PS, Miles JM, Gerich JE, et al: Increased proteolysis: An effect of increases in plasma cortisol within the physiologic range. J Clin Invest 73:412–420, 1984.

348. May RC, Clark AS, Goheer A, et al: Identification of specific defects in insulin-mediated muscle metabolism in acute uremia. Kidney Int 28:490–497, 1985.

349. Clark AS, Mitch WE: Muscle protein turnover and glucose uptake in acutely uremic rat: Effects of insulin and the duration of renal insufficiency. J Clin Invest 72:836–845, 1983.

350. Mitch WE, Clark AS: Muscle protein turnover in uremia. Kidney Int 24(suppl 16):S2–S8, 1983.

351. Li JB, Wassner SJ: Muscle degradation in uremia: 3-Methylhistidine release in fed and fasted rats. Kidney Int 20:321–325, 1981.

352. Holliday MA, Chantler CA, MacDonnell R, et al: Effect of uremia on nutritionally-induced variations in protein metabolism. Kidney Int 11:236–245, 1977.

353. Harter HR, Karl IE, Klahr S, et al: Effects of reduced renal mass and dietary protein intake on amino acid release and glucose uptake by rat muscle in vitro. J Clin Invest 64:513–523, 1979.

354. Davis TA, Klahr S, Karl IE: Glucose metabolism in muscle of sedentary and exercised rats with azotemia. Am J Physiol 252:F138–F145, 1987.

355. Richards P, Metcalfe-Gibson A, Ward EE, et al: Utilization of ammonia nitrogen for protein synthesis in man, and the effect of protein restriction and uraemia. Lancet 2:845–848, 1967.

356. Bilbrey GL, Falonna GR, White MG, et al: Hyperglucagonemia of renal failure. J Clin Invest 53:841–847, 1974.

357. Aoki TT, Muller WA, Brennan MF, et al: Effect of glucagon on amino acid and nitrogen metabolism in fasting man. Metabolism 23:805–814, 1974.

358. Salter JM, Ezrin C, Laidlaw JC, et al: Metabolic effects of glucagon in human subjects. Metabolism 9:753–768, 1960.

359. McLean P, Novello F: Influence of pancreatic hormones on enzymes concerned with urea synthesis in rat liver. Biochem J 94:410–422, 1965.

360. Clark AS, Kelly RA, Mitch WE: Systemic response to thermal injury in rats: Increased protein degradation and altered glucose utilization in muscle. J Clin Invest 74:888–897, 1984.

361. Li JB, Wassner SJ: Protein synthesis and degradation in skeletal muscle of chronically uremic rats. Kidney Int 29:1136–1143, 1986.

362. Maloff BL, McCaleb ML, Lockwood DH: Cellular basis of insulin resistance in chronic uremia. Am J Physiol 245:E178–E184, 1983.

363. Druml W, Kelly RA, May RC, et al: Abnormal cation transport in uremia: Mechanisms in adipocytes and skeletal muscle from uremic rats. J Clin Invest 81:1197–1203, 1988.

364. Spergel G, Bleicher JJ, Goldberg M, et al: The effect of potassium on the impaired glucose tolerance of chronic uremia. Metabolism 16:581, 1967.

365. Santeusanio F, Faloona GR, Knochel JP, et al: Evidence for a role of endogenous insulin and glucagon in the regulation of potassium homeostasis. J Lab Clin Med 81:809–817, 1973.

366. Bilbrey GL, Carter NW, White MG, et al: Potassium deficiency in chronic renal failure. Kidney Int 4:423–430, 1973.

367. Landau RL, Kappas A: Anabolic hormones in hyperparathyroidism: With observations on the general catabolic influence of parathyroid hormone in man. Ann Intern Med 62:1223–1233, 1965.

368. Garber AJ: Effect of parathyroid hormone on selected aspects of protein and amino acid metabolism in the rat. J Clin Invest 71:1806–1821, 1983.

369. Wassner SJ, Li JB: Lack of an acute effect of parathyroid hormone within skeletal muscle. Int J Pediatr Nephrol 8:15–20, 1987.

370. Underhill RP, Goldschmidt S: Studies on the metabolism of ammonium salts. III: The utilization of ammonium salts with a non-nitrogenous diet. J Biol Chem 15:341–355, 1913.

371. Rose WC, Smith LC, Womack M, et al: The utilization of the nitrogen of ammonium salts, urea and certain other compounds in the synthesis of non-essential amino acids in vivo. J Biol Chem 181:307–316, 1949.

372. Giordano C, de Pascale C, Balestrieri C, et al: Incorporation of urea $^{15}$N in amino acids of patients with chronic renal failure on low nitrogen diet. Am J Clin Nutr 21:394–404, 1968.

373. Read WWC, McLaren DS, Tchalian M, et al: Studies with $^{15}$N-labelled ammonia and urea in the malnourished child. J Clin Invest 48:1143–1149, 1969.

374. Mitch WE, Walser M: Effects of oral neomycin and kanomycin in chronic uremic patients. II. Nitrogen balance. Kidney Int 11:123–127, 1977.

375. Rose WC, Wixom RL: The amino acid requirements of man. XVI. The role of the nitrogen intake. J Biol Chem 217:997–1004, 1955.

376. Huang PC, Young VR, Cholakos B, et al: Determination of the minimum dietary essential amino acid–to–total nitrogen ratio for beef protein fed to young men. J Nutr 90:416–422, 1966.

377. Clark HE, Yess NJ, Vermillion EJ, et al: Effect of certain factors in nitrogen retention and lysine requirements of adult human subjects. III: Source of supplementary nitrogen. J Nutr 79:131–139, 1963.

378. Tripathy K, Klahr S, Lotero H: Utilization of exogenous urea nitrogen in malnourished adults. Metabolism 19:253–262, 1970.

379. Blom van Assendelft PM, Dorhout-Mees EJ: Urea metabolism in patients with chronic renal failure: Influence of sodium bicarbonate or sodium chloride administration. Metabolism 19:1053–1063, 1970.

380. Papadoyannakis NJ, Stefanides CJ, McGeown M: The effect of the correction of metabolic acidosis on nitrogen and protein balance of patients with chronic renal failure. Am J Clin Nutr 40:623–627, 1984.

381. Beale LS: Kidney Diseases, Urinary Deposits and Calculous Disorders: Their Nature and Treatment, 3rd ed. Lindsay & Blakiston, Philadelphia, 1994.

382. Ihle BU, Becker GJ, Whitworth JA, et al: The effect of protein restriction on the progression of renal insufficiency. N Engl J Med 321:1773–1777, 1989.

383. Giovannetti S: Dietary treatment of chronic renal failure: Why is it not used more frequently? Nephron 40:1–12, 1985.

384. Bingham SA: The dietary assessment of individuals: Methods, accuracy, new techniques and recommendations. Nutr Abstr Rev 57:705–742, 1987.

385. Dwyer JT: Assessment of dietary intake. In Shils ME, Young VR (eds): Modern Nutrition in Health and Disease, Vol 7. Lea & Febiger, Philadelphia, 1988, p 887.

386. The Modification of Diet in Renal Disease Study: Design, methods, and results from the feasibility study. Am J Kidney Dis 20:18–33, 1992.

387. Wingen AM, Fabianbach C, Mehls O: Evaluation of protein intake by dietary diaries and urea-N excretion in children with chronic renal failure. Clin Nephrol 40:208–215, 1993.

388. Bergström J, Alvestrand A, Bucht H, et al: Progression of chronic renal failure in man is retarded with more frequent clinical follow-ups and better blood pressure control. Clin Nephrol 25:1–6, 1986.

389. Combe C, Deforges-Lasseur C, Caix J, et al: Compliance and effects of nutritional treatment on progression and metabolic disorders of chronic renal failure. Nephrol Dial Transplant 8:412–418, 1993.

390. Aparicio M, Bouchet JL, Combe C, et al: Factors affecting the response of uremic patients to dietary protein restriction. Kidney Int 36(suppl 27):S300, 1989. Abstract.

391. Brodsky IG, Robbins DC, Hiser E, et al: Effects of low-protein diets on protein metabolism in insulin-dependent diabetes mellitus patients with early nephropathy. J Clin Endocrinol Metab 75:3551–3557, 1992.

392. Walker JD, Dodds RA, Murrells TJ, et al: Restriction of dietary protein and progression of renal failure in diabetic nephropathy. Lancet 2:1411–1414, 1989.

393. Locatelli F, Alberti D, Graziani G, et al: Prospective, randomised, multicentre trial of effect of protein restriction on progression of chronic renal insufficiency. Lancet 337:1299–1304, 1991.

394. Zeller KR, Whittaker E, Sullivan L, et al: Effect of restricting dietary protein on the progression of renal failure in patients with insulin-dependent diabetes mellitus. N Engl J Med 324:78–83, 1991.

395. Wingen AM, Fabian-Bach C, Mehls E: Low protein diet in children with chronic renal failure—1-year results. Pediatr Nephrol 5:496–500, 1991.

396. Kist-van Holthe tot Echten JE, Nauta J, Hop WC, et al: Protein restriction in chronic renal failure. Arch Dis Child 68:371–375, 1993.

396a. Klahr S, Levey AS, Beck GJ, et al: The effects of dietary protein restriction and blood pressure control on the progression of chronic renal failure. N Engl J Med 330:878–884, 1994.

397. Williams HH, Harper AE, Hegsted DM, et al: Nitrogen and amino acid requirements. In Harper AE, Hegsted DM (eds): Improvement of Protein Nutrition. National Academy of Sciences/National Research Council, Washington, DC, 1974, pp 23–63.

398. Kopple JD, Swenseid M: Evidence that histidine is an essential amino acid in normal and chronically uremic man. J Clin Invest 55:881–891, 1975.

399. Norée L-O, Bergström J: Treatment of chronic uremic patients with protein-poor diet and oral supply of essential amino acids. II. Clinical results of long-term treatment. Clin Nephrol 3:195–200, 1975.

400. Kampf D, Fischer HC, Kessel M: Efficacy of an unselected protein diet (25 g) with minor oral supply of essential amino acids and keto analogues compared with a selective protein diet (40 g) in chronic renal failure. Am J Clin Nutr 33:1673–1677, 1980.

401. Roberts C, Kopple J, Grodstein G, et al: Acceptance of protein and amino acid diets by patients with chronic renal failure. Kidney Int 24(suppl 16):S350, 1983. Abstract.

402. Walser M, Mullan HP, Walker JDZ, et al: Nutritional aspects of renal failure. In Walser M, Imbembo AL, Margolis S, et al (eds): Nutritional Management: The Johns Hopkins Handbook. WB Saunders, Philadelphia, 1984, p 177.

403. Ahlstrom TP: The Kidney Patient's Book, New Treatment, New Hope. Great Issues Press, Delran, NJ, 1991.

404. Wetstein L: Dietary considerations in the treatment of renal disease. In Mitch WE, Klahr S (eds): Nutrition and the Kidney, Vol 1. Little, Brown, Boston, 1988, pp 299–352.

405. Caggiula AW, Milas NC: Approaches to successful nutritional intervention in renal disease and (Appendix B) Breakfast, Lunch, Dinner and Snack Meal Plans at various levels of protein. In Mitch WE, Klahr S (eds): Nutrition and the Kidney, Vol 2. Little, Brown, Boston, 1993, pp 365–393.

406. Nutrition management of chronic renal insufficiency. In Manual of Clinical Dietetics, Vol 4. American Dietetic Association, Chicago, 1992, pp 519–575.

407. Giovanetti S: Unwanted side effects of nutritional therapy for patients with chronic renal failure. In Giovanetti S (ed): Nutritional Treatment of Chronic Renal Failure. Kluwer Academic Publishers, Boston, 1989, p 267.

408. Rayner HC, Burton PR, Bennett S, et al: Changes in nutritional status of patients with chronic renal failure on a low protein diet. Nephron 64:154, 1993.

409. Barsotti G, Morelli E, Giannoni A, et al: Restricted phosphorus and nitrogen intake to slow the progression of chronic renal failure: A controlled trial. Kidney Int 24:S278–S284, 1983.

410. Barsotti G, Morelli E, Guiducci A, et al: Reversal of hyperparathyroidism in severe uremics following very low-protein and low-phosphorus diet. Nephron 30:310–313, 1982.

411. Schloerb PR: Essential amino acid administration in uremia. Am J Med Sci 252:650–659, 1966.

412. Röckel A, Roller F, Kult J, et al: Comparative studies of potato-egg diet and mixed low-protein diet combined with essential amino acid in patients with endstage renal failure. In Heidland A (ed): Renal Insufficiency. Georg Thieme Verlag, Stuttgart, 1976, p 163.

413. Kult J: Serum levels of trace proteins in continued substitution of essential amino acids combined with low protein diet in patients with endstage renal failure. In Heidland A (ed): Renal Insufficiency. Georg Thieme Verlag, Stuttgart, 1976, p 169.

414. Walser M: Ketoacids in the treatment of uremia. Clin Nephrol 3:180–184, 1975.

415. Bauerdick H, Spellerberg P, Lamberts B: Therapy with essential amino acids and their nitrogen-free analogues in severe renal failure. Am J Clin Nutr 31:1793–1796, 1978.

416. Fröhling PT, Schmicker R, Vetter K, et al: Efficiencies of the potato-egg diet and a dietary regimen with amino acid substitution ("Swedish diet") in chronic renal insufficiency. Aktuel Ernahrungsmed 9:98–102, 1984.

417. Fürst P, Bergström J, Ahlberg M, Noree LO: The nutritional benefits of essential amino acid supplementations of low-protein diets in chronic renal failure. Z Ernahrungswiss Suppl (19):13–33, 1976.

418. Lee HA, Hadfield CMI, Talbot ST, et al: Dialamine (essential amino acid powder) as a supplement to low protein diets in advanced chronic renal failure. Clin Nutr 6:111–116, 1987.

419. Bergström J, Fürst P, Noree LO: Treatment of chronic uremic patients with protein-poor diet and oral supply of essential amino acids. Clin Nephrol 3:187–194, 1975.

420. Young GA, Oki JI, Davidson AM: The effects of calorie and essential amino acid supplementation on plasma proteins in patients with chronic renal failure. Am J Clin Nutr 21:1802–1807, 1978.

421. Andreu MAF, Delcerro LAJ, Rivera F: Role of hypoproteic diet and essential aminoacids in the progression of non-diabetic chronic renal insufficiency. Nefrologia 12:87–92, 1992.

422. Alvestrand A, Ahlberg M, Bergström J: Retardation of the progression of renal insufficiency in patients treated with low-protein diets. Kidney Int 24:S268–S272, 1983.

423. Bucht H, Ahlberg M, Alvestrand A, et al: The effect of low protein diet on the progression of renal failure in man. In Bertami T, Remuzzi G, Garattini S (eds): Drugs and Kidney. Raven Press, New York, 1986, p 257.

424. Ando A, Orita Y, Abe H, et al: The effect of essential amino acid supplementation therapy on prognosis of patients with chronic renal failure estimated on the basis of the Markov process. Med J Osaka Univ 32:31–37, 1981.

425. Ando A, Orita Y, Tsubakihara R, et al: The effect of low protein diet and surplus of essential amino acids on the serum concentrations and the urinary excretion of methyl-guanidine and guanidinosuccinic acid in chronic renal failure. Nephron 24:161–169, 1979.

426. Attman PO, Bucht H, Larson O, et al: Protein-reduced diet in diabetic renal failure. Clin Nephrol 19:217–220, 1983.

427. Wilmore DW, Dudrick SJ: Treatment of acute renal failure with intravenous essential L-amino acids. Arch Surg 99:669–673, 1969.

428. Dudrick SJ, Steiger E, Long JM: Renal failure in surgical patients: Treatment with intravenous essential amino acids and hypertonic glucose. Surgery 68:180–186, 1970.

429. Abel RM, Beck CH, Abbot WM, et al: Improved survival and acute renal failure after treatment with intravenous essential L-amino acids and glucose. N Engl J Med 288:695–697, 1973.

430. Sofio C, Nicora R: High caloric essential amino acid parenteral therapy in acute renal failure. Acta Chir Scand Suppl 466:98–99, 1976.

431. Blackburn GL, Etter G, Mackenzie T: Criteria for choosing amino acid therapy in acute renal failure. Am J Clin Nutr 31:1841–1853, 1978.

432. Blumenkrantz MJ, Kopple JD, Koffler A, et al: Total parenteral nutrition in the management of acute renal failure. Am J Clin Nutr 31:1831–1840, 1978.

433. Oken DE, Prinkel FM, Landwehr DM, et al: Ineffectiveness of amino acid infusions in the treatment of rats with acute renal failure. Kidney Int 17:14–23, 1980.

434. Toback FG: Amino acid enhancement of renal generation after acute tubular necrosis. Kidney Int 12:193–198, 1977.

435. Feinstein EI, Kopple JD, Silberman H, et al: Total parenteral nutrition with high or low nitrogen intakes in patients with acute renal failure. Kidney Int 24(suppl 16):S319–S323, 1983.

436. Mirtallo JM, Schneider PJ, Mavko K, et al: A comparison of essential and general amino acid infusions in the nutritional support of patients with compromised renal function. JPEN 6:109–113, 1982.

437. Druml W: Nutritional support in acute renal failure. *In* Mitch WE, Klahr S (eds): Nutrition and the Kidney, Vol 2. Little, Brown, Boston, 1993, pp 314–345.

438. Richards P, Brown CL, Lowe SM: Synthesis of tryptophan from 3-indolepyruvic acid by a healthy woman. J Nutr 102:1547–1551, 1972.

439. Rudman D: Capacity of human subjects to utilize ketoanalogues of valine and phenylalanine. J Clin Invest 50:90–95, 1971.

440. Gallina DL, Dominquez JM, Hoschoian JC, et al: Maintenance of nitrogen balance in a young woman by substitution of α-ketoisovaleric acid for valine. J Nutr 101:1165–1172, 1971.

441. Mitch WE, Walser M: Nitrogen balance of uremic patients receiving branched-chain ketoacids and the hydroxy-analogue of methionine as substitutes for the respective amino acids. Clin Nephrol 8:341–344, 1977.

442. Mitch WE, Walser M: Utilization of calcium L-phenyllactate as a substitute for phenylalanine by uremic subjects. Metabolism 26:1041–1044, 1977.

443. Sapir DG, Walser M: Nitrogen sparing induced early in starvation by infusion of branched-chain ketoacids. Metabolism 26:301–308, 1977.

444. Mitch WE, Walser M, Sapir DG: Nitrogen-sparing induced by leucine compared with that induced by its keto-analogue, alpha-ketoisocaproate, in fasting obese man. J Clin Invest 67:553–562, 1981.

445. Mitch WE, Clark AS: Specificity of the effect of leucine and its metabolites on protein degradation in skeletal muscle. Biochem J 222:579–586, 1984.

446. Tischler ME, Desautels M, Goldberg AL: Does leucine, leucyl-tRNA or some metabolite of leucine regulate protein synthesis and degradation in skeletal and cardiac muscle? J Biol Chem 257:1613–1621, 1982.

447. Buse MG, Reid SS: Leucine: A possible regulator of protein turnover in muscle. J Clin Invest 56:1250–1261, 1975.

448. Stewart PM, Walser M, Drachman D: Branched-chain ketoacids reduce muscle protein degradation in Duchenne muscular dystrophy. Muscle Nerve 5:197–201, 1982.

449. Sapir DG, Stewart PM, Walser M, et al: Effects of alpha-ketoisocaproate and of leucine on nitrogen metabolism in postoperative patients. Lancet 1:1010–1014, 1983.

450. Yagi M, Matthews DE, Walser M: Nitrogen sparing by 2-ketoisocaproate in parenterally fed rats. Am J Physiol 259:E633–E638, 1990.

451. Sandstedt S, Jorfeldt L, Larsson J: Randomized, controlled study evaluating effects of branched chain amino acids and alpha-ketoisocaproate on protein metabolism after surgery. Br J Surg 79:217–220, 1992.

452. Di Paolo N, Pula G, Capotondo L, et al: Nutritional requirements and energy expenditure by indirect calorimetry in uremic patients during conservative management. Contrib Nephrol 65:60–71, 1988.

453. Jahn H, Rose F, Schmitt R, et al: Protein synthesis in skeletal muscle of uremic patients; effect of low-protein diet and supplementation with ketoacids. Miner Electrolyte Metab 18:222–227, 1992.

454. Teplan V, Schuck O, Ndavornikova H, et al: Metabolic characteristics of patients with chronic renal failure in long-term diet therapy and substitution with keto analogs of essential amino acids. Z Urol Nephrol 83:89–96, 1990.

455. Burns J, Cresswell J, Ell S, et al: Comparison of the effects of keto acid analogues and essential amino acids on nitrogen homeostasis in moderately protein-restricted diets. Am J Clin Nutr 13:1767–1775, 1978.

456. Chow KW, Walser M: Effects of nitrogen restriction on the use of alpha-keto-isovalerate for growth in the weanling rat. J Nutr 105:119–121, 1975.

457. Chawla RK, Rudman D: Utilization of alpha-keto and alpha-hydroxy analogues of valine by the growing rat. J Clin Invest 54:271–277, 1974.

458. Kang CW, Tungsang K, Walser M: Effect of the level of dietary protein on the utilization of alpha-ketoisocaproate for protein synthesis. Am J Clin Nutr 43:504–509, 1986.

459. Gordon RW: Metabolism of other D- and L-hydroxy acids. Ann N Y Acad Sci 119:927–941, 1965.

460. Collier VU, Butler DO, Mitch WE: Metabolism of the hydroxy-analogues of amino acids in the isolated perfused rat kidney. Kidney Int 14:738, 1978. Abstract.

461. Collier VU, Butler DO, Mitch WE: Metabolic effects of L-phenyllactate in perfused kidney, liver and muscle. Am J Physiol 238:E450–E457, 1980.

462. Chow KW, Walser M: Effects of substitution of methionine, leucine, phenylalanine or valine by their alpha-hydroxy analogues in the diet of rats. J Nutr 105:373–375, 1975.

463. Meister A: The role of amino acids in nutrition. *In* The Biochemistry of the Amino Acids, Vol 2. Academic Press, New York, 1965, pp 201–230.

464. Jones R, Dalton N, Turner C, et al: Oral essential aminoacid and ketoacid supplements in children with chronic renal failure. Kidney Int 24:95–103, 1983.

465. Broyer M, Guillot M, Niaudet P, et al: Comparison of three low-protein diets containing essential amino acids and their alpha analogues for severely uremic children. Kidney Int 24(suppl 16):S290–S244, 1983.

466. Jureidini KF, Hogg RJ, Van Renen MJ, et al: Evaluation of long-term aggressive dietary management of chronic renal failure in children. Pediatr Nephrol 4:1–10, 1990.

467. Walser M, Sapir DG, Mitch WE, et al: Effects of branched-chain ketoacids in normal subjects and patients. *In* Walser M, Williamson JR (eds): Metabolism and Clinical Implications of Branched Chain Amino and Ketoacids. Elsevier/North Holland, New York, 1981, p 631.

468. Mitch WE, Walser M, Steinman TL, et al: The effect of a keto acid–amino acid supplement to a restricted diet on the progression of chronic renal failure. N Engl J Med 311:623–629, 1984.

469. Abras E, Walser M, Mitch WE: Mixed salts of basic amino acids with branched chain ketoacids as the basis for new supplements designed to improve nutrition in chronic renal failure. *In* Walser M, Williamson JR (eds): Metabolism and Clinical Implications of Branched Chain Amino and Ketoacids. Elsevier/North Holland, New York, 1981, p 593.

470. Barsotti G, Guiducci A, Ciardella F, et al: Effects on renal function of a low-nitrogen diet supplemented with essential amino acids and ketoanalogues and of hemodialysis and free protein supply in patients with chronic renal failure. Nephron 27:113–117, 1981.

471. Mitch WE, Collier VU, Walser M: Treatment of chronic renal failure with branched-chain ketoacids plus the other essential amino acids or their nitrogen-free analogues. *In* Walser M, Williamson JR (eds): Metabolism and Clinical Implications of Branched Chain Amino and Ketoacids. Elsevier/North Holland, New York, 1981, pp 587–592.

472. Gretz N, Meisinger E, Getz T, et al: Low protein diet supplemented by ketoacids in chronic renal failure: A prospective controlled study. Kidney Int 24:S263–S270, 1983.

473. Vetter K, Fröhling PT, Kaschube I, et al: Influence of ketoacid treatment on residual renal function in chronic renal insufficiency. Kidney Int 24:S350–S353, 1983. Abstract.

474. Barsotti G, Cristofano C, Morelli E, et al: Serum oxalic acid in uremia: Effect of a low-protein diet supplemented with essential amino acids and ketoanalogues. Nephron 38:54–56, 1984.

475. Barsotti G, Ciardella F, Morelli E, et al: Restoration of blood levels of testosterone in male uremics following a low protein diet supplemented with essential amino acids and ketoanalogues. Contrib Nephrol 49:63–69, 1984.

476. Barsotti G, Ciardella F, Morelli E, et al: Nutritional treatment of renal failure in type I diabetic nephropathy. Clin Nephrol 29:280–287, 1988.

477. Jungers P, Chauveau P, Lebkiri B, et al: Treatment of chronic kidney failure by the keto-analogues of essential amino acids: 4 years' experience. Presse Med 16:1039–1043, 1987.

478. Mariani G, Barsotti G, Ciardella F, et al: Albumin metabolism and nutritional status of uremic patients on a long-term very-low-protein diet supplemented with essential amino acids and keto analogues. J Nucl Med Allied Sci 28:237–244, 1984.

479. Ciardella F, Morelli E, Cupisti A, et al: Metabolic effects of a very-low-protein, low-phosphorus diet supplemented with essential amino acids and keto analogues in end-stage renal diseases. Contrib Nephrol 65:72–80, 1988.

480. Meisinger E, Strauch M: Controlled trial of two keto acid supplements on renal function, nutritional status, and bone metabolism in uremic patients. Kidney Int 32:S170–S173, 1987.

481. Fröhling PT, Kokot F, Vetter K, et al: Influence of keto acid treat-

ment on hormonal disorders in chronic renal failure. Contrib Nephrol 65:95–100, 1988.

482. Lemke E, Lindenau K, Fröhling PT: Successful conservative management in children with chronic renal failure: A prospective study. Nephrol Dial Transplant 4:451, 1989. Abstract.

483. Fröhling PT, Kokot F, Schmicker R, et al: Influence of keto acids on serum parathyroid hormone levels in patients with chronic renal failure. Clin Nephrol 20:212–215, 1983.

484. Schmicker R, Vetter K, Kaschube I, et al: Comparison between essential amino acid and ketoacid substituted diet in patients with chronic renal failure. Kidney Int 24(suppl 16):S350, 1983. Abstract.

485. Schmicker R, Vetter K, Lindenau K, et al: Conservative long-term treatment of chronic renal failure with keto acid and amino acid supplementation. Infusionsther Klin Ernahr 14:34–38, 1987.

486. Jureidini KF, Van Renen MJ, Daniels L, et al: Improved dietary management of children with chronic renal failure. Kidney Int 30:624, 1986. Abstract.

487. Schaefer K, von Herrath D, Asmus G, et al: The beneficial effect of ketoacids on serum phosphate and parathyroid hormone in patients with chronic uremia. Clin Nephrol 30:93–96, 1988.

488. Lindenau K, Kokot F, Fröhling PT: Suppression of parathyroid hormone by therapy with a mixture of keto analogues/amino acids in hemodialysis patients. Nephron 43:84–86, 1986.

489. Jureidini KF, Daniels L, Hill GN, et al: Low-protein and phosphate diet with keto acid precursors of essential amino acids in children with chronic renal failure. Kidney Int 28:863, 1985. Abstract.

490. Lindenau K, Kokot F, Vetter K, et al: Influence of keto acid (KA) treatment on renal osteodystrophy. Infusionsther Klin Ernahr 14(suppl 5):40–42, 1987.

491. Frohling PT, Schmicker R, Lindenau K, et al: Role of keto acids in the prophylaxis and treatment of renal osteopathy. Contrib Nephrol 65:123–129, 1988.

492. Fröhling PT, Kokot F, Vetter K, et al: Treatment of renal osteodystrophy in advanced renal failure during predialysis time risk profiles in clinical nephrology. Contrib Nephrol 37:62–65, 1984.

493. Fröhling PT, Krupki F, Kokot F, et al: What are the most important factors in the progression of renal failure. Kidney Int 36(suppl 27):S106–S109, 1989.

494. Fröhling PT, Schmidt-Gayk H, Kokot F, et al: Influence of vitamin D and keto acids on 1,25(OH)$_2$-D levels in patients with chronic renal failure. In Norman S (ed): Vitamin D: A Chemical, Biochemical and Clinical Update. Walter de Gruyter, Berlin, 1985, p 952.

495. Schaefer K, Erley CM, von Herrath D, et al: Calcium salts of ketoacids as a new treatment strategy for uremic hyperphosphatemia. Kidney Int 27:S136–S139, 1989.

496. Mak RHK, Turner C, Thompson T, et al: The effect of a low protein diet with amino acid/ketoacid supplements on glucose metabolism in children with uremia. J Clin Endocrinol Metab 63:985–989, 1986.

497. Barsotti G, Navalesi R, Morelli E: Effects of a low-phosphorus, low-protein diet supplemented with essential amino acids and keto analogues on "overt" diabetic nephropathy. Infusionsther Klin Ernahr 14:12–18, 1987.

498. Aparicio M, Gin H, Potaux L, et al: Effect of a ketoacid diet on glucose tolerance and tissue insulin sensitivity. Kidney Int 36:S231–S235, 1989.

499. Gin H, Aparicio M, Potaux L, et al: Low protein and low phosphorus diet in patients with chronic renal failure: Influence on glucose tolerance and tissue insulin sensitivity. Metabolism 36:1080–1085, 1987.

500. Ciardella F, Morelli E, Niosi F, et al: Effects of a low phosphorus, low nitrogen diet supplemented with essential amino acids with ketoanalogues on serum triglycerides of chronic uremic patients. Nephron 42:196–199, 1986.

501. Gutai J, LaPorte D, Kuller L, et al: Plasma testosterone, high density lipoprotein cholesterol and other lipoprotein fractions. Am J Cardiol 48:897–902, 1981.

502. Ciardella F, Cupisti A, Catapano G, et al: Effects of a low-phosphorus, low-nitrogen diet supplemented with essential amino acids and ketoanalogues on serum beta-endorphin in chronic renal failure. Nephron 53:129–132, 1989.

503. Aparicio M, Vincendeau P, Combe C, et al: Improvement of leucocytic Na$^+$K$^+$ pump activity in uremic patients on low protein diet. Kidney Int 40:238–242, 1991.

504. Capelli P, Di Paolo B, Evangelista M, et al: Effect of a supplemented diet on progression of chronic renal failure and uremic neuropathy.

In Friedman EA, Beyer M, Desanto NG, et al (eds): Prevention of Progressive Uremia. Field & Wood, New York, 1989, pp 156–159.

505. Heidland A, Kult J, Röckel A, et al: Evaluation of essential amino acids and ketoacids in uremic patients on a low-protein diet. Am J Clin Nutr 31:1784–1792, 1978.

506. Hecking E, Andrzejewski L, Prellwitz W, et al: Double-blind crossover study with oral alpha-ketoacids in patients with chronic renal failure. Am J Clin Nutr 33:1678–1681, 1980.

507. Walser M, Mitch WE, Abras E: Supplements containing amino acids and ketoacids in the treatment of chronic uremia. Kidney Int 24(suppl 16):S285–S289, 1983.

508. Walser M: Keto-analogues of essential amino acids in the treatment of chronic renal failure. Kidney Int 13(suppl 8):S180–S184, 1978.

509. Kaysen GA: The nephrotic syndrome: Nutritional consequences and dietary management. In Mitch WE, Klahr S (eds): Nutrition and the Kidney, Vol 2. Little, Brown, Boston, 1993, p 213.

510. Kaysen GA, Gambertoglio J, Jimenez I, et al: Effect of dietary protein intake on albumin homeostasis in nephrotic patients. Kidney Int 29:572–577, 1986.

511. Don BR, Kaysen GA, Hutchison FN, et al: The effect of angiotensin-converting enzyme inhibition and dietary protein restriction in the treatment of proteinuria. Am J Kidney Dis 17:10–17, 1991.

512. Don BR, Wada L, Kaysen GA, et al: Effect of dietary protein restriction and angiotensin converting enzyme inhibition on protein metabolism in the nephrotic syndrome. Kidney Int 36:S163–S167, 1989.

513. Manos J, Harrison A, Jones M, et al: Protein/calorie balance in nephrotic syndrome. Kidney Int 24(suppl 16):S349, 1983. Abstract.

514. D'Amico G, Remuzzi G, Maschio G, et al: Effect of dietary proteins and lipids in patients with membranous nephropathy and nephrotic syndrome. Clin Nephrol 35:237–242, 1991.

515. Gentile MG, Fellin G, Cofano F, et al: Treatment of proteinuric patients with a vegetarian soy diet and fish oil. Clin Nephrol 40:315–320, 1993.

516. Dullaart RPF, Beusekamp BJ, Meijer S, et al: Long-term effects of protein-restricted diet on albuminuria and renal function in IDDM patients without clinical nephropathy and hypertension. Diabetes Care 16:483–492, 1993.

517. Barsotti G, Morelli E, Cupisti A, et al: A special, supplemented "vegan" diet for nephrotic patients. Am J Nephrol 11:380–385, 1991.

518. Anderson KE, Rosner W, Khan MS, et al: Diet-hormone interactions: Protein/carbohydrate ratio alters reciprocally the plasma levels of testosterone and cortisol and their respective binding globulins in man. Life Sci 40:1761–1768, 1987.

519. Monteon FJ, Laidlaw SA, Shaib JK, Kopple JD: Energy expenditure in patients with chronic renal failure. Kidney Int 30:741–747, 1986.

520. Hyne BB, Fowell E, Lee HA: The effect of caloric intake on nitrogen balance in chronic renal failure. Clin Sci 43:679–687, 1972.

521. Rose WC: The amino acid requirements of adult man. Nutr Abstr Rev 27:631, 1957.

522. Bergström J, Fürst P, Ahlberg M, et al: The role of dietary and energy intake in chronic renal failure. In Canzler von H (ed): Topical Questions in Nutritional Therapy in Nephrology and Gastroenterology [in German]. Georg Thieme Verlag, Stuttgart, 1978, pp 1–16.

523. Kopple JD, Monteon FJ, Shaib JK: Effect of energy intake on nitrogen metabolism in nondialyzed patients with chronic renal failure. Kidney Int 29:734–742, 1986.

524. Gilmour ER, Hartley GH, Goodship THJ: Trace elements and vitamins in renal disease. In Mitch WE, Klahr S (eds): Nutrition and the Kidney, Vol 2. Little, Brown, Boston, 1993, pp 114–131.

525. Stone WJ, Warnock LG, Wagner C: Vitamin B$_6$ deficiency in uremia. Am J Clin Nutr 28:950–957, 1975.

526. Kopple JD, Mercurio K, Blumenkrantz MJ, et al: Daily requirement for pyridoxine supplement in chronic renal failure. Kidney Int 19:694–704, 1981.

527. Dobblestein HW, Korner WF, Mempel W, et al: Vitamin B$_6$ deficiency in uremia and its implications for the depression of immune responses. Kidney Int 5:233–239, 1974.

528. Balcke P, Schmidt P, Zazgornik J, et al: Reduction of elevated plasma oxalic acid levels by pyridoxine therapy in patients on regular dialysis therapy. Kidney Int 24(suppl 16):S346, 1983. Abstract.

529. Smith FR, Goodman DS: The effects of diseases of the liver, thyroid and kidneys on transport of vitamin A in human plasma. J Clin Invest 50:2426–2436, 1971.

530. Vahlquist A, Berne B, Berne C: Skin content and plasma transport of vitamin A and carotene in chronic renal failure. Eur J Clin Invest 12:63–67, 1982.

531. Rylance PB, Brown IRF, Howells DW, et al: Relationship between vitamin A and bone disease in chronic renal failure. Nephron 36:131–135, 1984.

532. Merrill RH: Iron metabolism in end-stage renal disease. Dial Transplant 8:898–904, 1979.

533. Van Wyck DB, Stivelman JC, Ruiz J, et al: Iron status in patients receiving erythropoietin for dialysis-associated anemia. Kidney Int 35:712–716, 1989.

534. Mahajan SK, Prasad AS, Rabbani P, et al: Zinc deficiency: A reversible complication of uremia. Am J Clin Nutr 36:1177–1183, 1982.

535. Smythe WR, Alfrey AC, Craswell PW, et al: Trace element abnormalities in chronic uremia. Ann Intern Med 96:302–310, 1982.

536. Zimmermann EW, Meisinger E, Weinel B, Strauch M: Essential amino acid/ketoanalogue supplementation: An alternative to unrestricted protein intake in uremia. Clin Nephrol 11:71–78, 1979.

# 56

# Hemodialysis

*J. Michael Lazarus*
*Bradley M. Denker*
*William F. Owen, Jr.*

## WHO, HOW, AND WHEN

### Who Is a Candidate for Hemodialysis?

In the 50 years since Wilhelm Kolph first reported the successful dialysis of a patient with renal failure, selection of those to be treated has changed drastically. In early years, hemodialysis was reserved for young and otherwise healthy patients with acute, reversible renal failure in whom such treatment was likely to be successful. Long-term or maintenance dialysis was unsuccessful and impractical because of difficulties with maintaining access to the peripheral circulation. Subsequently, development of the external arteriovenous shunt in 1960 and the endogenous arteriovenous fistula in the late 1960s allowed the possibility of long-term or maintenance hemodialysis. Although technically feasible, maintenance dialysis treatments were expensive and available at only a few hospital centers. Thus, this scarce resource was applied to only a handful of patients: those who had their own funds for payment; or a select few who had no other medical illnesses, were generally well educated, were deemed to be of "value" to society, and were supported by various community fund-raising efforts. Medicare entitlement for the treatment of end-stage renal disease (ESRD) was enacted by Congress in 1973 (Public Law 92-603) and thereby allowed unrestricted treatment of patients for both maintenance dialysis and transplantation in the United States.[1] The selection of patients for hemodialysis was also influenced by the concurrent development of living related and cadaver renal transplantation and, in later years, by the development of continuous ambulatory peritoneal dialysis and continuous cycling peritoneal dialysis.

As of December 31, 1990, the prevalence for ESRD therapy in the United States was 195,000 patients. The point prevalence was 165,000 patients with an incidence count of 45,000 patients per year. A somewhat slower growth pattern has developed in the Asian and European countries, particularly in countries where there are restrictions for funding for treatment of chronic renal failure. In Japan, the point prevalence was 103,000 patients; in all of Europe, there were approximately 169,000 patients in 1990. Figure 56–1 compares the growth rates, which are reported as incidence per million population.[2] Obviously, selection of patients has been relaxed as evidenced by the burgeoning growth rate. Figure 56–2 illustrates the increasing age of the dialysis population in the United States.[2] Moreover, the ESRD population has a higher percentage of minorities compared with the nondialysis populations. Figure 56–3 shows the rapid growth rates of patients with diabetes and hypertension receiving dialysis.[2] Therefore, the American

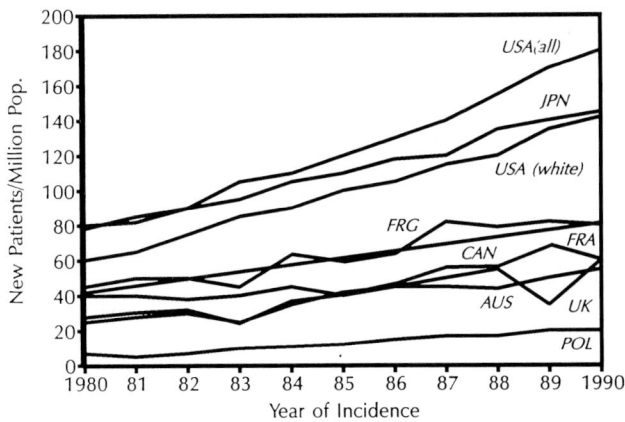

**Figure 56–1.** Incidence rates of treated ESRD per million population (unadjusted) for Australia (AUS), Canada (CAN), selected European Countries (France [FRA], Germany [FRG], Poland [POL], and United Kingdom [UK]), Japan (JPN), and the United States (total and white patients only) from 1980 to 1990. (From U.S. Renal Data System: USRDS 1993 Annual Data Report. The National Institutes of Health, National Institute of Diabetes and Digestive and Kidney Diseases, Bethesda, MD, 1993.)

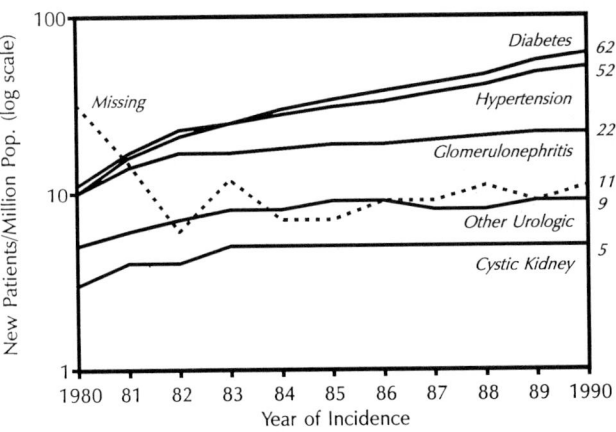

**Figure 56–3.** Incidence rates of treated ESRD per million population, by five major primary disease groups, 1980 to 1990. Rates are unadjusted. Semilog scale is used to show smaller rates. Rates do not include patients from Puerto Rico or U.S. territories. Medicare patients only. (From U.S. Renal Data System: USRDS 1993 Annual Data Report. The National Institutes of Health, National Institute of Diabetes and Digestive and Kidney Diseases, Bethesda, MD, 1993.)

ESRD Program has the highest incidence of initiation of maintenance dialysis in the world, and it is being provided to an increasingly aged and ill population.

Although the prevalence and incidence of renal failure treatment in other countries lag behind those of the United States, it has been stated that the selection criteria for maintenance dialysis among industrialized nations are roughly the same. However, the ESRD reporting mechanisms in Europe and Asia may not be as thorough as those of the United States, and they are not mandatory. Therefore, the frequency of comorbid conditions may be less in these countries. In the United States and in many industrialized European and Asian countries, there appear to be few selection criteria for maintenance dialysis and transplantation that are socioeconomic. There has been broad acceptance

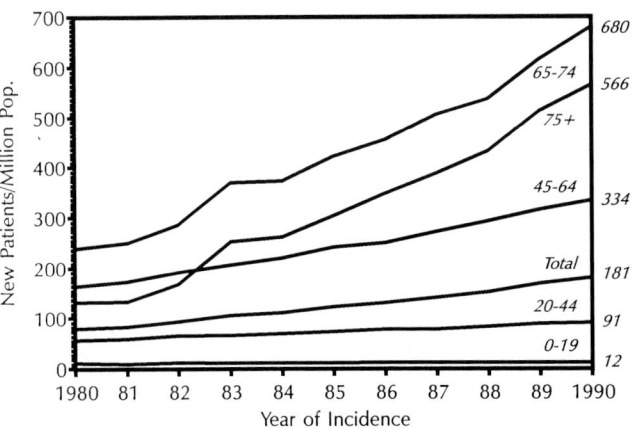

**Figure 56–2.** Incidence rates of treated ESRD per million population, by age group, 1980 to 1990. Rates are unadjusted. Rates do not include patients from Puerto Rico or U.S. territories. Medicare patients only. (From U.S. Renal Data System: USRDS 1993 Annual Data Report. The National Institutes of Health, National Institute of Diabetes and Digestive and Kidney Diseases, Bethesda, MD, 1993.)

into the ESRD Program of all renal diagnoses and, notably, few restrictions of comorbid conditions. A small percentage of patients with failure of other organ systems, such as advanced vascular disease with multiple limb amputations, stage IV cardiac disease, chronic hepatic failure, advanced senility, and solid and nonsolid metastatic tumors, are inappropriately being administered hemodialysis. Such patients fare poorly with maintenance hemodialysis. Their quality of life is miserable, and their prognosis is grim. If there is a precisely defined short-term objective to be achieved by the patient or family with a limited course of dialysis, therapy should be provided. The patient or the health care proxy should be given an honest appraisal of the prognosis and the potential for complications. In addition, knowledge should be shared that dialysis therapy can be discontinued on request without abandonment by the health care team. If there is no short-term goal for providing dialysis to patients with a poor quality of life, the selection of such patients for long-term dialysis must be questioned.

The selection criteria for patients with acute renal failure are even broader. In providing dialytic therapy for acute renal failure, the assumption is that normal renal function will resume and that dialysis will simply maintain the patient during a short time. Unless the patient is moribund from the primary disease process, the underlying disease should not necessarily be a reason for exclusion. Many patients with acute renal failure have multisystem organ failure, and the gross mortality for acute renal failure remains high. Unfortunately, it is not unusual for patients with acute renal failure to remain dependent on dialysis and to become sequestrated in maintenance dialysis programs. In more recent years, more marginal patients are being offered extensive life-support therapy, and the capture of severely ill patients for long-term dialysis seems to be a more frequent occurrence. Therefore, the decision to initiate dialysis in such patients is an important triage point. If the prognosis is grim or the patient's quality of life will be extremely compromised and there is good evidence that the acute renal failure is not reversible, it is morally, ethically, and economically appropriate to allow such patients to die of uremia. If the patient's overall prognosis is extremely poor, it seems ill-advised to resuscitate the patient from the uremic state to have him or her suffer the agonies of multiorgan system failure with long-term dialysis. The development of prognostic indices will be important in resolving this difficult problem.

## Planning and Initiating Therapy for End-Stage Renal Disease

As noted before, therapy for ESRD has evolved in the past 50 years to offer three major treatment options: 1) hemodialysis (primarily provided in a dialysis center but may be at home); 2) continuous ambulatory peritoneal dialysis or continuous cyclic peritoneal dialysis; and 3) renal transplantation in which either a relative or cadaver is the kidney donor. The largest percentage of ESRD patients are treated by in-center hemodialysis (Table 56–1). In 1991, there were 2202 providers of ESRD therapy. Of these centers, 228 were transplant centers and 1974 were dialysis centers or facilities. There are a sufficient number of widely dispersed dialysis and transplant centers such that most patients may choose any treatment option; medical suitability should be the sole limiting factor. The limited availability of transplant donors is, however, a confounding issue in this choice.

Obviously, the psychologic and medical condition of the patient is a principal determinant of the dialysis treatment option. Mortality and morbidity results should not be the sole guide to the choice of treatment modality because of bias in the selection of patients. In the late 1970s, those patients who were too unstable to undergo hemodialysis, or who had vascular disease of sufficient severity that angioaccess could not be generated, were selected for the newly described continuous ambulatory peritoneal dialysis technique or intermittent peritoneal dialysis. In subsequent years, the therapeutic approach changed dramatically; peritoneal dialysis is now selected by relatively younger pa-

tients who are self-motivated, independent, and generally more healthy. Related donor and cadaver donor transplantation is limited to those patients who are psychologically and medically well enough to undergo such surgery and who have no contraindications to immunosuppressive medications. As a result, older and more severely ill patients are relegated to center hemodialysis. This is not to imply that otherwise healthy, young patients do not do equally well given in-center hemodialysis. Home hemodialysis remains an excellent choice but is selected much less often because of the need for a family member or an assistant to participate.

In the absence of a medical contraindication, the major arbiter of a treatment option should be the patient. During the triage process and early in the course of renal failure, the patient requires substantial information and teaching about each of the treatment options. The more the patient and family become familiar with the treatment options, the wiser will be their choice. Involvement of the patient in the selection of the form of therapy is extraordinarily important to its successful conclusion. Obviously, this early preparation for therapy for ESRD requires the active involvement of a nephrologist. Nephrologists have recognized that other physicians refer patients late in the course of renal disease for ESRD therapy, which severely compromises the selection and triage process. It is important that non-nephrologic physicians become aware of the need for early referral.

## Timing the Initiation of Dialysis Therapy

In patients who opt for hemodialysis, or who are relegated to hemodialysis because peritoneal dialysis or transplantation is not possible, early placement of an arteriovenous fistula, with sufficient time for its development, is one of the most important aspects of early treatment. Because a well-functioning endogenous arteriovenous fistula ("native vein arteriovenous fistula") is the access of choice, it is reasonable to attempt a native vein fistula, even in patients with questionable arteries and veins. A failed attempt at creation of a native vein fistula is worth the effort. Place-

## TABLE 56–1. Dialysis Treatment Modalities—1991

| Patients as of | Total Dialysis Patients | Dialysis Patients by Type and Setting | | | | | | | | | |
|---|---|---|---|---|---|---|---|---|---|---|---|
| | | Outpatient Dialysis* | | | | | Home Dialysis | | | | |
| | | Outpatient Total | HD | IPD | CAPD | CCPD | Home Total | HD | IPD | CAPD | CCPD |
| 12/31/82 | 65,765 | 54,032 | 52,967 | 904 | 161 | — | 11,733 | 4,394 | 816 | 6,523 | — |
| 12/31/83 | 71,987 | 58,342 | 57,408 | 778 | 156 | — | 13,645 | 4,323 | 790 | 8,532 | — |
| 12/31/84 | 78,483 | 63,245 | 62,462 | 603 | 163 | 17 | 15,238 | 4,125 | 259 | 9,995 | 859 |
| 12/31/85 | 84,797 | 68,394 | 67,559 | 588 | 226 | 21 | 16,403 | 3,983 | 231 | 11,236 | 953 |
| 12/31/86 | 90,886 | 73,800 | 73,024 | 518 | 228 | 30 | 17,086 | 3,675 | 191 | 11,913 | 1,307 |
| 12/31/87 | 98,432 | 80,149 | 79,513 | 440 | 175 | 21 | 18,283 | 3,582 | 168 | 12,825 | 1,708 |
| 12/31/88 | 105,958 | 87,195 | 86,517 | 372 | 246 | 60 | 18,763 | 3,197 | 326 | 13,318 | 1,922 |
| 12/31/89 | 116,169 | 95,948 | 95,371 | 319 | 230 | 28 | 20,221 | 2,914 | 166 | 14,830 | 2,311 |
| 12/31/90 | 129,800 | 107,160 | 106,573 | 280 | 262 | 45 | 22,640 | 2,483 | 190 | 16,969 | 2,998 |
| 12/31/91 | 142,488 | 117,371 | 116,819 | 234 | 266 | 52 | 25,117 | 2,266 | 173 | 18,881 | 3,797 |

*Includes patients in self-dialysis training at time of survey. HD = hemodialysis; IPD = intermittent peritoneal dialysis; CAPD = continuous ambulatory peritoneal dialysis; CCPD = continuous cyclic peritoneal dialysis.

From ESRD Facility Survey tables (BDMS, Health Care Financing Administration); includes non-Medicare patients. U.S. Renal Data System: USRDS 1993 Annual Data Report. The National Institutes of Health, National Institute of Diabetes and Digestive and Kidney Diseases, Bethesda, MD, 1993.

ment of a prosthetic ("graft") arteriovenous fistula requires up to 2 months for healing. Thus, prosthetic graft fistulas require consideration for early placement as well. Many nephrologists believe that a native vein arteriovenous fistula should be created in those patients who opt for peritoneal dialysis, in case peritoneal dialysis therapy fails and hemodialysis becomes necessary. Experience has shown that these patients, in the course of several months to several years of therapy with peritoneal dialysis, often lose their own veins in the process. In this manner, an adequate fistula for hemodialysis is ensured. If the patient opts for peritoneal dialysis, it is the practice of most dialysis centers to defer placement of the peritoneal catheter until treatment is imminent. In some programs, peritoneal dialysis is started immediately after placement of the catheter; in other programs, physicians wait from 1 to 3 weeks before beginning exchanges (see Chapter 57). Generally, preparation for peritoneal dialysis is not as lengthy as the interval necessary for the development of an angioaccess for hemodialysis.

Many healthy patients with a related donor may be candidates for renal transplantation early in the course of renal failure and thereby avoid a period of hemodialysis or peritoneal dialysis. Appropriate tissue typing and workup of the potential donor must be completed early in the course of renal insufficiency. Once the patient develops the first symptoms or signs of uremia, transplantation can then be performed promptly. Transplantation should be carried out when the patient has mild symptoms but has not developed complications that would interfere with surgery and immunosuppression. In some cases, it may be necessary to place a femoral or subclavian catheter for one or two hemodialysis sessions before surgery. Because 10% to 15% of kidney transplants fail in the first year, patients who choose transplantation without previous hemodialysis or peritoneal dialysis should be fully informed of these other treatment options and their individual risks and benefits. In our experience, patients who undergo transplantation without such knowledge of hemodialysis and peritoneal dialysis fare poorly psychologically when the transplant fails.

The timing of initiation of hemodialysis or peritoneal dialysis differs somewhat from that of transplantation. Clearly, it is inappropriate to wait until the patient is moribund or severely ill to initiate therapy. However, it is unnecessary to initiate hemodialysis or peritoneal dialysis in a patient who is totally asymptomatic and suffers no risk from azotemia or fluid overload. The usual "definitive" indications for initiation of dialytic therapy include uremic encephalopathy, uremic serositis (pericarditis or pleuritis), uremic sensory or motor neuropathy, severe and intractable hypervolemia, repeated hyperkalemia uncontrolled with cation exchange resins, and severe metabolic acidosis (pH <7.2) not controlled with alkali therapy. Relative indications for the initiation of dialysis include a deterioration of the quality of life with fatigue, insomnia, weakness, and pruritus and progressive malnutrition manifested by increasing anorexia, weight loss, or a decrease in the serum albumin or transferrin concentrations.

The Health Care Financing Administration has established minimal levels of creatinine, blood urea nitrogen (BUN), and creatinine clearance for obtaining Medicare benefits for maintenance dialysis. However, there may be additional factors to be considered, so that starting dialysis outside the Health Care Financing Administration guidelines may be appropriate. Initiating dialysis relatively early allows the patient a more vigorous protein and calorie intake that may substantially affect long-term survival (see later). For patients who had previously been on a protein-restricted diet in an effort to delay the onset of dialysis, this is particularly critical. The treatment of patients with erythropoietin before dialysis or transplantation has dramatically affected symptoms. Historically, anemia was a major symptom in the "uremic syndrome." Therefore, with the use of erythropoietin, patients with advanced azotemia may have fewer symptoms and be observed longer without dialysis. However, the risk of hyperkalemia, acidosis, or other ill effects of azotemia in such patients must be carefully weighed.

The initiation of hemodialysis in patients with acute renal failure is significantly different; recovery of renal function is anticipated, and the patient should not be put at risk by delay of dialysis. Patients with acute renal failure are usually hypercatabolic and have other severe organ system complications that necessitate early dialysis. A common cause now for initiation of dialysis in patients with acute renal failure is control of fluid obligated by the administration of parenteral nutrition, which has been shown to be important in improving survival of patients with acute renal failure and multisystem disease.

## CONCEPTS OF CLEARANCE

There have been many comprehensive engineering-based reviews of the hemodialysis process.[3-5] The goals of this section are to introduce the basic physical and mathematic concepts involved in the dialytic process. These concepts are important for understanding the dialysis prescription and kinetic modeling. Hemodialysis allows two physical processes to occur simultaneously: clearance and ultrafiltration. The normal kidney accomplishes these tasks simultaneously using specialized cells along the nephron. During the process of hemodialysis, clearance and ultrafiltration occur at the interface between the dialyzer membrane and the blood.

In simple terms, clearance is the removal of a substance from the blood. Nephrologists are familiar with the concept of creatinine or inulin clearance as a measurement of the glomerular filtration rate. In the steady state, a nonabsorbed or secreted compound such as inulin can be used to measure clearance. For this situation,

Filtered inulin = excreted inulin
Excreted inulin = urinary inulin concentration × urine volume
Filtered inulin = glomerular filtration rate × plasma inulin concentration

Therefore,

Inulin clearance = (urinary inulin concentration × urine volume) ÷ plasma inulin concentration

The inulin clearance describes the *volume* of plasma

cleared of inulin by renal excretion during a defined time period. The same principles apply to clearance during hemodialysis. Substances move across the hemodialysis membrane according to the concentration differences between the blood and dialysate. Also, solute movement across the dialysis membrane is a function of the effective pore size of the dialysis membrane and is inversely proportional to the size of the solute.

The net passive movement of a solute across a membrane generally requires the presence of a favorable concentration or electrical gradient. During conventional hemodialysis, the overwhelming driving force is the concentration gradient (diffusive clearance). Because of the rapid blood and dialysate flows, the generation of electrical potentials is limited. The concept of diffusion down a concentration gradient can be illustrated with the following example. Consider two urea-containing solutions separated by a membrane that is permeable to urea. As a result of random motion, urea particles on either side of the membrane enter and cross the membrane. However, the number of particles entering the membrane and crossing over is proportional to the number of particles in solution. Therefore, urea particles interact and cross the membrane more frequently on the side with the larger number of particles. In this manner, urea diffuses down the concentration gradient until a new equilibrium is reached.

In addition to the concentration differences, properties of the membrane are also important for determining how much material crosses the dialysis membrane. Likewise, the surface area of the membrane (size) and the inherent "diffusivity" of the membrane are major determinants for solute transfer. Diffusivity is a unique property dependent on the membrane's composition and pore size, and the temperature of the solvent. The general expression summarizing these parameters is

$$J = -D \times A \times dc/dx \qquad (1)$$

where $J$ is solute flux or movement in milligrams per second, $D$ is diffusivity in square centimeters, $A$ is surface area of the membrane in square centimeters, and $dc/dx$ is concentration gradient in milligrams per deciliter per centimeter. If the concentration gradients are assumed to be linear, $dc/dx$ becomes $\Delta C/\Delta X$. If solute movement is expressed per unit area, Equation 1 becomes

$$J/A = -D \times \Delta C/\Delta X \qquad (2)$$

Diffusivity ($D$) is a number that is unique to each membrane and relates the amount of solute transfer to the concentration gradient. The larger the value for $D$, the more solute crosses the membrane for a given surface area and concentration gradient. The inverse of diffusivity is the resistance to particle movement and is an easier term to consider. If $D = 1/R$ (resistance to flux) is substituted in Equation 2 and $\Delta X$ (thickness of the membrane) is included in the $D$ term, the terms can be combined to describe a new constant, $R$. Equation 2 is now expressed as

$$J/A = \Delta C/R \qquad (3)$$

The relationship in Equation 3 states that the flux for a molecule per unit surface area is proportional to the concentration gradient and inversely proportional to the resistance.

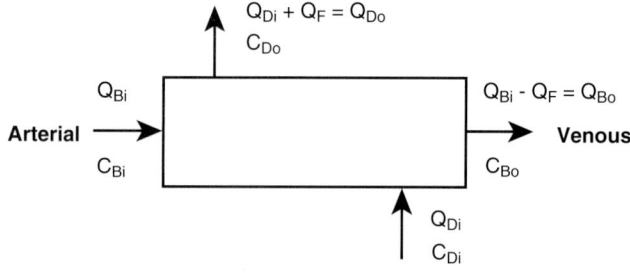

**Figure 56–4.** Solute mass balance for a dialyzer during ultrafiltration (see text).

The resistance to solute movement is the combined forces on the blood and dialysate sides of the membrane that oppose solute transfer. These resistances to solute movement are a consequence of membrane characteristics, such as its thickness and composition, and are additive. In addition, the dialysate and blood flow characteristics on each side of the membrane affect resistance to solute movement. The mathematic considerations of these forces are described in detail elsewhere.[5, 6] Resistance to the diffusion of a solute is also related to its size; the larger the molecule, the higher the resistance to diffusion. Other factors, such as the molecular charge and the state of water hydration, can also affect solute diffusion.

The bulk movement of solute across the membrane is termed convective clearance and occurs by hydraulic pressure across the dialyzer membrane. Convective clearance occurs simultaneously with fluid removal, a process termed ultrafiltration. Clinically, convective clearance is considered to be a minor component of total clearance. The convective clearance that occurs with ultrafiltration contributes to the total dialyzer clearance (diffusive + convective clearances) and is discussed later.

Many clinically relevant parameters affect dialyzer clearance, such as the blood flow, dialysate flow, dialyzer type, and duration of dialysis. The relative contributions of these parameters to clearance are important for kinetic modeling and assessing adequacy of dialysis. Some simple relationships are evident from considering the law of mass action for a dialyzer. The conservation of mass law states that the total amount of material that enters the dialyzer must equal the amount that leaves the dialyzer. Mass balance may be characterized schematically as in Figure 56–4. $Q_{Bi}$ is the rate of blood flow into the dialyzer; $C_{Bi}$ is the concentration of solute in the blood that is entering the dialyzer; $Q_{Di}$ is the rate of dialysate flow into the dialyzer; $C_{Di}$ is the concentration of solute in the dialysate that is entering the dialyzer; $Q_{Bo}$ is the rate of blood flow leaving the dialyzer; $C_{Bo}$ is the concentration of solute in the blood that is leaving the dialyzer; $Q_{Do}$ is the rate of dialysate flow leaving the dialyzer; $C_{Do}$ is the concentration of solute in the dialysate that is leaving the dialyzer; and $Q_F$ is flow of ultrafiltrate across the dialyzer membrane from the blood into the dialysate.

The amount of solute entering on the blood side of the dialyzer (arterial end) is $Q_{Bi} \times C_{Bi}$, and the amount entering from the dialysate is $Q_{Di} \times C_{Di}$. Therefore, solute mass into the dialyzer is

$$(Q_{Di} \times C_{Di}) + (Q_{Bi} \times C_{Bi}) \qquad \textbf{(4)}$$

As seen in Figure 56–4, the blood flow and the amount of solute leaving the dialyzer are different from the values at entry. On the blood side, the new concentration of solute departing the dialyzer (venous end) is $C_{Bo}$, and the new rate of blood flow is equal to the blood flow into the dialyzer minus the flow diverted across the membrane as ultrafiltrate ($Q_F$). In the blood compartment, the new amount of solute that is leaving the dialyzer may be calculated by $C_{Bo} \times (Q_{Bi} - Q_F)$. On the dialysate side, the new concentration of solute that is departing from the dialyzer is $C_{Do}$, and the new dialysate flow is the inflow plus the volume ultrafiltered. On the dialysate side, the quantity of solute that is now leaving is $C_{Do} \times (Q_{Di} + Q_F)$. Summing these equations, we get

$$\text{Solute mass out of the dialyzer} = [C_{Bo} \times (Q_{Bi} - Q_F)] + [C_{Do} \times (Q_{Di} + Q_F)] \qquad \textbf{(5)}$$

On the basis of the law of mass balance,

$$(Q_{Di} \times C_{Di}) + (Q_{Bi} \times C_{Bi}) = [C_{Bo} \times (Q_{Bi} - Q_F)] + [C_{Do} \times (Q_{Di} + Q_F)] \qquad \textbf{(6)}$$

By rearranging this equation to bring the expression of the blood components on one side and the dialysate components on the other side, the equation can be rewritten as

$$[Q_{Bi} \times (C_{Bi} - C_{Bo})] + (Q_F \times C_{Bo}) = [Q_{Di} \times (C_{Do} - C_{Di})] + (Q_F \times C_{Do}) \qquad \textbf{(7)}$$

The first term on each side of Equation 7 can be considered the diffusive solute flux (flow Q × concentration difference $C_i - C_o$); the second term on each side of the equation represents convective flux (flow of ultrafiltrate across the dialysis membrane $Q_F$ × concentration of solute in the venous end $C_o$). Thus, the net flux of solute from the blood compartment $J_{blood}$ is the sum of diffusive and convective fluxes:

$$J_{blood} = [Q_{Bi} \times (C_{Bi} - C_{Bo})] + (Q_F \times C_{Bo}) \qquad \textbf{(8)}$$

The concentration gradient for a solute at the inlet of the dialyzer is the blood concentration minus the dialysate concentration ($C_{Bi} - C_{Di}$). This concentration gradient is the driving force for solute movement. If Equation 8 is divided by this term ($C_{Bi} - C_{Di}$), the following equation can be written:

$$J_{blood}/(C_{Bi} - C_{Di}) = \{[Q_{Bi} \times (C_{Bi} - C_{Bo})] + (Q_F \times C_{Bo})\}/(C_{Bi} - C_{Di}) \qquad \textbf{(9)}$$

For many small molecules that accumulate in uremia, such as urea and creatinine, their concentration in the dialysate as it enters the dialyzer is zero. This simplifies Equation 9 to

$$J_{blood}/C_{Bi} = \{[Q_{Bi} \times (C_{Bi} - C_{Bo})] + (Q_F \times C_{Bo})\}/C_{Bi} \qquad \textbf{(10)}$$

The term $J_{blood}/C_{Bi}$ is the solute flux as a function of its concentration and is analogous to the inulin clearance from blood. The units for this term are milligrams per second divided by milligrams per milliliter, which become milliliters per second. These units represent the volume of plasma

cleared of a solute in a given amount of time, which is analogous to renal clearance. Therefore,

$$\text{Net clearance of a solute} = K_{net} = J_{bood}/C_{Bi} \qquad \textbf{(11)}$$

In Equation 10, the first term on the right-hand side is the diffusive clearance, $K_d$, and the second is the convective clearance, $K_c$. So,

$$K_{net} = K_d + K_c \qquad \textbf{(12)}$$

In the absence of ultrafiltration, $Q_F = 0$, there is no convective clearance, and Equation 10 becomes

$$K_d = [Q_{Bi} \times (C_{Bi} - C_{Bo})]/C_{Bi} \qquad \textbf{(13)}$$

Equation 13 shows that the diffusive clearance of a solute is directly proportional to blood flow into the dialyzer and the concentration gradient for the solute at the dialyzer inlet. In practical terms, the greater the blood flow, the greater the clearance. Figure 56–5 demonstrates in vivo urea clearance for a high-flux hemodialyzer. At all blood flow rates up to 500 mL/min, urea clearance continues to increase. At the higher blood flow rates, the slope of this line tends to decrease. This deviation from linearity occurs because of the resistance created at the membrane surface by the turbulence of rapid blood flow.

A similar relationship between net clearance and flow is also evident for the dialysate flow. The net flux from the dialysate compartment ($J_{dialysate}$) can be calculated in the same way as Equations 8 to 13 were derived for the blood compartment. The result is the following equation:

$$K_d = [Q_{Di} \times (C_{Do} - C_{Di})]/(C_{Bi} - C_{Di}) \qquad \textbf{(14)}$$

For a dialysis system in which the dialysate enters the dialyzer only a single time, the initial dialysate concentration is zero ($C_{Di} = 0$). Equation 14 now simplifies to

$$K_d = (Q_{Di} \times C_{Do})/C_{Bi} \qquad \textbf{(15)}$$

This relationship states that diffusive clearance of a solute is directly proportional to the dialysate flow. This rela-

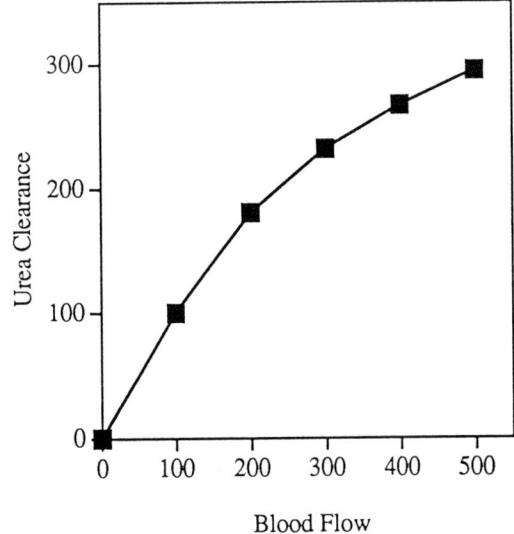

**Figure 56–5.** Urea clearance determined in vivo for high-flux dialyzers.

tionship is linear for dialysate rates up to 500 mL/min, but faster flows cause more turbulence in the dialysate compartment. Turbulence causes the resistance to rise, and the increment in solute clearance is attenuated in a manner similar to blood flow as shown in Figure 56–5. The net flux at any point along the dialyzer length is proportional to the concentration gradient between the blood and dialysate at that point. Therefore, blood and dialysate flows in the same direction have a diminishing gradient along the membrane length. Alternatively, by having the paths of blood and dialysate flow run countercurrent to each other, a maximal concentration gradient can be maintained.

The contribution of convective clearance to total hemodialyzer clearance is small, but its relative contribution depends on the solute and the characteristics of the dialysis membrane in question. For example, small molecules such as urea have high diffusive clearance, so the contribution by convective clearance is small. For molecules with low diffusive clearance such as vitamin $B_{12}$, the relative contribution from ultrafiltration will be greater (Table 56–2). Convective transfer or ultrafiltration can increase clearance of high-molecular-weight substances and has been used in the development of hemofiltration and high-flux treatment modalities.[7, 8] However, the clinical benefit of enhanced clearance of high-molecular-weight solutes remains unproved, and the main purpose for ultrafiltration in the dialytic process is to reduce extracellular volume. The dialyzer manufacturers provide an estimate of the ultrafiltration rate of dialyzers based on in vitro studies (ultrafiltration coefficient). These ultrafiltration rates are often different from rates observed in vivo because of a variety of biophysical effects that are discussed in more detail later.

## DIALYSIS MODALITIES AND COMPONENTS OF THE DIALYSIS PRESCRIPTION

As discussed in detail in an earlier section, dialysis fulfills two biophysical goals in the patient's blood: 1) solute removal from the blood into the dialysate, as exemplified by $K^+$ and urea, or the addition of solute from the dialysate into the blood, as is the case for $HCO_3^-$ and $Ca^{2+}$ (clearance); and 2) elimination of volume from the patient (ultrafiltration). These two processes can be performed simultaneously or as temporally segregated procedures.

### Hemodialysis

Hemodialysis is a diffusion-driven and size-discriminatory process for the clearance of small solutes, such as

**TABLE 56–2. Effect of Ultrafiltration on Solute Clearance for Urea and Vitamin $B_{12}$**

| Parameter | Urea | Vitamin $B_{12}$ |
|---|---|---|
| Clearance without ultrafiltration (mL/min) | 150 | 20 |
| Clearance with ultrafiltration (mL/min) | 152.5 | 29 |
| Percent increase | 1.67 | 45 |

electrolytes and urea ($<300$ daltons). The clearance of larger solutes is typically less (see Table 56–2). During hemodialysis, ultrafiltration is driven by the generation of negative hydraulic pressure on the dialysate side of the dialyzer. The major components of the hemodialytic process are 1) the artificial kidney or dialyzer; 2) the delivery system, which is the mechanical device that pumps the patient's blood and the dialysate through the dialyzer; and 3) the dialysate, which is the fluid having a defined chemical composition used for solute clearance. Typically, the patient's blood and dialysate are pumped continuously through the dialyzer in opposite (countercurrent) directions at flow rates of 300 to 450 and 500 to 800 mL/min, respectively. A maximal concentration gradient is achieved in this manner. As discussed in greater detail in a later section, the choice of blood and dialysate flows is determined by dialysis-specific and patient-specific variables. The dialysate passes through the dialyzer only a single time ("single-pass system") and is automatically discarded after its physical interaction with the blood across the dialyzer's semipermeable membrane. Although clearance and ultrafiltration are typically performed simultaneously, they may be performed sequentially ("sequential ultrafiltration/clearance"), or isolated ultrafiltration may be performed (Table 56–3).

The nomenclature that defines the type of dialysis is usually determined by the ultrafiltration efficiency of the dialyzer being used. There are three types of hemodialysis in widespread practice in the United States: 1) conventional hemodialysis, 2) high-efficiency hemodialysis, and 3) high-flux hemodialysis. For conventional, high-efficiency, and high-flux hemodialysis, dialyzers with ultrafiltration coefficients of 8 or less, between 8 and 20, and 20 mL/mm Hg/h or above, respectively, are used. The U.S. Food and Drug Administration defines a high-flux dialyzer as any dialyzer with an ultrafiltration coefficient above 8 mL/mm Hg/h. Dialyzers with enhanced ultrafiltration characteristics often have greater clearances of low- and high-molecular-weight solutes.

Variables of the hemodialysis procedure that may be manipulated by the physician on the basis of the clinical needs of the patient are 1) the blood and dialysate flows (influence solute clearance), 2) the type of dialyzer (determines solute clearance and ultrafiltration capacity), 3) the hydraulic pressure that drives ultrafiltration, 4) the dialysate composition (influences solute clearance), 5) the duration and frequency of the dialysis procedure (determines the solute clearance), and 6) the intensity of anticoagulation. These related facets of the dialysis procedure are altered in response to the patient's requirements for solute clearance and ultrafiltration and to meet the limitations of intradialytic hemodynamics, oxygenation, biocompatibility, and bleeding risks.

### BLOOD AND DIALYSATE FLOW

As expressed mathematically in an earlier section, the clearance of a solute during dialysis may be functionally defined as the volumetric removal of the solute from the patient's blood. Therefore, the flow of blood and dialysate into the dialyzer is the critical determinant of the effectiveness of this procedure. One of the elements of the dialysis

**TABLE 56–3. Dialysis Modalities**

| Technique | Device | Physical Principle |
|---|---|---|
| *Hemodialysis* | | |
| Conventional | Hollow-fiber dialyzer | Concurrent diffusive clearance and ultrafiltration |
| Sequential ultrafiltration/clearance | Hollow-fiber dialyzer | Ultrafiltration followed by diffusive clearance |
| Ultrafiltration | Hollow-fiber dialyzer | Ultrafiltration alone |
| *Hemofiltration* | | |
| Slow continuous ultrafiltration | Hemofilter or dialyzer | Arteriovenous ultrafiltration without a blood pump |
| Continuous arteriovenous hemofiltration | Hemofilter or dialyzer | Arteriovenous convective transport without a blood pump |
| Continuous arteriovenous hemodialysis | Hemofilter or dialyzer | Arteriovenous hemodialysis without a blood pump |
| Continuous arteriovenous hemodiafiltration | Hemofilter or dialyzer | Arteriovenous hemofiltration and hemodialysis without a blood pump |
| Continuous venovenous hemofiltration | Hemofilter or dialyzer | Venovenous convective transport with a blood pump |
| Continuous venovenous hemodialysis | Hemofilter or dialyzer | Venovenous hemodialysis with a blood pump |
| Continuous venovenous hemodiafiltration | Hemofilter or dialyzer | Venovenous hemofiltration and hemodialysis with a blood pump |

prescription that can be altered to modify the clearance of a solute is the patient's blood flow into the dialyzer $Q_{Bi}$. An additional means of augmenting the diffusive clearance of a solute from blood to the dialysate, or vice versa, is to increase the dialysate flow rate $Q_{Di}$. Practically, increases in the $Q_{Bi}$ and $Q_{Di}$ increase the clearance of a solute to an asymptote that is defined by the specific dialyzer and for a solute. As blood and dialysate flow rates are increased, resistance and turbulence within the dialyzer increase. The result is nonlinear flow within the hollow fibers and a decline in the clearance per unit flow of blood or dialysate (see Fig. 56–5). It should be appreciated that the increase in solute clearance that is observed with dialysate flows greater than 500 mL/min is modest, even with the use of a high-flux dialyzer. Some of the increase in clearance affected by high blood and dialysate flows is a consequence of the elimination of selective and uneven patterns of flow through the dialyzer ("channeling" effects) and disruption of the relatively unstirred layers of fluid immediately juxtaposed to the dialysis membrane.

In practice, limitation to the flow of dialysate is an infrequent occurrence during the dialysis procedure. However, technical errors, such as the failure to turn on the dialysate flow or improper calibration of the dialysate delivery system, attenuate the dialysate flow and clearance. The optimal performance of a vascular-based clearance technique mandates the establishment and maintenance of adequate angioaccess. The efficiency of dialysis may be compromised by a decline in blood flow through the extracorporeal circuit, such as that seen with inflow stenosis of the angioaccess. Alternatively, in a more subtle fashion, the laminar flow of blood in the angioaccess may become functionally compromised. As turbulent nonlaminar blood flow occurs within an angioaccess, blood returning to the fistula from the dialyzer may reflux to the arterial side of the access. This blood re-enters the dialytic circuit and decreases the effectiveness of dialysis. This complication is described as blood "recirculation."

The most common cause of recirculation arises in vascular accesses where the needles are in proximity or the venous pressures are high enough to cause reflux of blood toward the arterial needle. Back-flow will also be caused by increased negative pressure at the arterial needle if arterial inflow is impaired or pump speed is increased. Recirculation has been reported to increase 5% to 10% for each 100 mL/min increase in dialyzer blood flows. However, this may be overestimated, because well-functioning accesses showed no increase in recirculation between 100 and 400 mL/min of blood flow when measured by saline dilution.[9] This discrepancy in the amount of recirculation probably reflects inaccuracies in its measurement.

Recirculation can be calculated clinically from the equation

$$R = (C_p - C_a)/(C_p - C_v) \qquad (16)$$

where R is the fraction of recirculation and $C_p$, $C_a$, and $C_v$ are the concentrations of urea in the peripheral blood and arterial and venous limbs of the angioaccess, respectively. There has been confusion in the literature about recirculation and the most accurate way to measure it. The problem lies with an accurate determination from the "peripheral" sample. The "gold standard" has been a venous sample from the arm opposite the fistula. However, there are several reasons that this may be inaccurate as well as inconvenient and lead to overestimates of dialyzer recirculation. One problem is comparing a venous sample with an arterial predialyzer sample. Normally, there is a trivial discrepancy between BUN concentrations in venous and arterial blood, but during dialysis, they may vary significantly. This results from a lower BUN concentration of blood leaving the dialyzer; return to the central veins dilutes the BUN concentration. This lower urea blood gets oxygenated in the pulmonary circulation and is then delivered to the systemic circulation. Now a gradient exists between the intracellular compartments and the low-BUN arterial blood. Urea rapidly equilibrates between tissues and arterial blood, leading to high peripheral venous BUN concentration compared with arterial BUN concentration. This has been termed cardiopulmonary recirculation and overestimates recirculation[10] (Equation 16). The arteriovenous differences are increased with high-efficiency dialysis (more blood with lower BUN concentration into the circuit) and low cardiac output (dialyzed blood is a greater proportion of the cardiac output). Peripheral vasoconstriction during dialysis leads to decreased blood flow and a lower amount of total urea removal from that tissue bed. This has the effect of raising the BUN concentration in a vein from that compartment and is termed venovenous disequilibrium. A peripheral sample from an artery would in theory eliminate both venovenous and arteriovenous disequilibrium but is not practical.

Two-needle methods for determining recirculation are now recommended and are potentially more accurate than the traditional three-needle method. The goal of these measurements is to obtain the peripheral sample from the arterial side of the dialyzer under conditions of minimal contamination by blood that has already been dialyzed. Many reports have used the arterial line samples obtained before and after dialysis, as well as slowing or stopping blood flow.[9] The timing for the peripheral sample is important. Delays after stopping flow increase the value of BUN as arterial and venous compartments equilibrate, whereas rapid sample collection may be contaminated with recirculated blood. Therefore, an alternative to stopping the flow is recommended and is a low–blood flow technique. After afferent and efferent samples are obtained, the blood flow is abruptly reduced to 50 mL/min (dialysate flow should be off for at least 3 minutes); a peripheral sample is obtained from the arterial line after 150% of the volume from the needle to the sample point has been cleared (usually between 20 and 30 seconds). Recirculation may be increased as dialysis progresses owing to reduced flow from volume depletion, decreased cardiac output, and hypotension. Therefore, recirculation should be measured within the first 30 minutes of dialysis. Preliminary studies reveal similar results from low-flow and stop-flow techniques.[9] Comparisons of the three-needle technique with low-flow techniques are not valid because of reasons described above. With low-flow techniques, a recirculation value of 10% or greater may indicate graft dysfunction. Values above 10% result in compromised solute clearance, which is manifested by hyperkalemia and worsening azotemia that are unexplained by dietary indiscretion and alterations in the dialysis prescription. As discussed in detail later, an increase in the recirculation percentage should prompt an angiographic evaluation of the fistula for outflow obstruction.

## TYPE OF DIALYZER

In making a decision about the choice of dialyzer, the most critical determinants are its capacity to clear a particular solute and its potential for fluid removal. Because of its relevance to kinetic models of dialysis adequacy, urea is the solute most often used. Physicians must typically rely on industry-derived values for the clearance of dextrose, vitamin $B_{12}$, inulin, or cytochrome C that are usually determined in vitro in the absence of protein. Therefore, Gibbs-Donnan effects, protein binding, membrane interactions, and solute aggregation are not taken into account, and the "diffusive dialysance" in vivo may be different.[11] Nevertheless, the capacity to compare this aspect of the performance between various dialyzers is important in planning the patient's dialysis prescription. The influence of the dialyzer membrane on solute clearance, fluid removal, and biologic reactivity is discussed in greater detail in later sections.

Further complicating the evaluation of solute clearance by different dialyzers is the variable relationship between diffusive clearance of a solute (K value) and its convective clearance (the passive movement of solute during ultrafiltration). As described mathematically in an earlier section, solutes that are larger than 300 daltons, such as vitamin $B_{12}$ and $\beta_2$-microglobulin, have low K values in comparison to smaller solutes, such as urea and $K^+$. The clearance of these larger solutes from blood depends primarily on clearance through ultrafiltration (see Table 56–2). Therefore, in clinical situations in which large volumes of ultrafiltrate are generated and the critical substance is large, simple comparisons of K values alone can be misleading.

As discussed earlier, the capacity for fluid removal by a dialyzer is described by its ultrafiltration coefficient. Similar to the information provided for the clearance of a particular solute by a specific dialyzer, each dialyzer model also has an ultrafiltration coefficient. Because these values are typically derived in vitro, similar limitations exist for their application to the in vivo situation. Therefore, it is not unusual for the ultrafiltration coefficient in vitro to vary by 10% to 20% in either direction.

Secondary considerations in dialyzer selection include its static volume, biocompatibility and thrombogenicity, potential for reprocessing, and cost.

## ULTRAFILTRATION

In addition to its use for comparing the ultrafiltration performance of different dialyzers, the ultrafiltration coefficient is used to calculate the quantity of pressure that must be exerted across the dialysis membrane ("transmembrane pressure") to generate a given volume of ultrafiltrate during a single dialysis session. The net pressure across the dialyzer membrane is

$$P_{net} = P_{osmotic} + P_{hydraulic} + P_{oncotic} \quad (17)$$

$$P_{hydraulic} = P_{blood} - P_{dialysate} \quad (18)$$

Typically, the hydraulic pressure is significantly higher than either the osmotic or oncotic pressure. Therefore, the net pressure gradient is approximated by

$$P_{net} = P_{blood} - P_{dialysate} \quad (19)$$

For most dialyzers currently in use, the hydraulic pressure can be calculated from the arithmetic mean of the inlet and outlet pressures:

$$P_{net} = P_{hydraulic} \approx (P_{Bi} + P_{Bo})/2 - (P_{Di} + P_{Do})/2 \quad (20)$$

in which $P_{Bi}$ is the pressure at the blood inlet; $P_{Bo}$ is the pressure at the blood outlet; $P_{Di}$ is the pressure at the dialysate inlet; and $P_{Do}$ is the pressure at the dialysate outlet. If the $P_{net}$ is too low to provide adequate ultrafiltration during a dialysis session ($P_{net} \times$ ultrafiltration coefficient $\times$ dialysis time < target ultrafiltrate volume), additional pressure can be generated across the dialysis membrane by the generation of negative pressure in the dialysate compartment or positive pressure in the blood compartment.

The effective pressure required to achieve a particular intradialytic weight loss is described as the transmembrane pressure (TMP) and is calculated by

TMP = desired weight loss/(ultrafiltration coefficient × dialysis time)

For example, a patient with a 2.0-kg interdialytic weight gain who undergoes hemodialysis for 4 hours with a dialyzer that has an ultrafiltration coefficient of 4.0 mL/mm Hg/h would require a transmembrane dialyzer pressure of 125 mm Hg to achieve the desired 2000 mL weight loss. If the $P_{net}$ is only 75 mm Hg, an additional 50 mm Hg would need to be added as negative pressure during the dialysis session. If additional volume were to be removed, the negative pressure would have to be increased accordingly.

The dialyzers currently in use in the United States are able to tolerate high transmembrane pressures, up to 500 mm Hg. The performance of ultrafiltration during hemodialysis has been greatly simplified by the development of dialysis machines that possess ultrafiltration control systems ("ultrafiltration controller"). Ultrafiltration with these devices occurs to a remarkably precise extent, and weight loss is effected in a linear manner.[12] Because of their massive ultrafiltration capacities, and the consequences of even modest increases in the venous pressure during dialysis, hemodialysis with high-efficiency or high-flux dialyzers is unsafe without the use of an ultrafiltration controller. These devices are discussed in greater detail later.

During hemodialysis, ultrafiltration and clearance are typically performed simultaneously. However, it is possible to temporally segregate the two procedures by a modification of the hemodialysis procedure described as sequential ultrafiltration/clearance.[13, 14] This modification of the conventional hemodialysis procedure is accomplished by first ultrafiltering to the desired volume, followed by the performance of diffusive clearance without ultrafiltration. During the initial ultrafiltration phase, no dialysate is circulated through the dialyzer, so diffusive clearance is prevented. During the second phase, no negative pressure is applied, and fluid losses due to $P_{net}$ are balanced by the infusion of saline. When ultrafiltration is performed concurrently with diffusive solute clearance, intravascular volume losses may exceed the rate of translocation of fluid from the interstitium. If these losses are not counterbalanced by an appropriate increase in the peripheral vascular resistance and venous refilling, hypotension occurs.[13–18] With sequential ultrafiltration/clearance, these hemodynamic abnormalities are attenuated, such that up to 4 L/h may be removed. Unfortunately, unless the total time allotted to dialysis is increased during sequential ultrafiltration/clearance, solute clearance will be compromised and inadequate dialysis will occur. These issues of hypotension and dialysis inadequacy are discussed in greater detail later.

## DIALYSATE COMPOSITION

Although $Na^+$ and $K^+$ are typically the sole components of the dialysate that are altered in response to different clinical situations, the other constituents are equally critical. Dextrose, the alkali equivalent (acetate or $HCO_3^-$), $Ca^{2+}$, $Mg^{2+}$, and $Cl^-$ concentrations in the dialysate merit consideration and may be altered depending on the clinical situation. In addition to influencing the final concentration of solutes in the blood, their intradialytic and interdialytic concentrations can influence such varied systems as the intermediary metabolism of protein and carbohydrates, systemic vasomotor tone, cardiac contractility and rhythm, pulmonary gas exchange, and bone turnover and modeling. Therefore, the selection of solute concentrations in the dialysate is influenced by issues other than clearance.

A wide variety of commercial formulations of dialysates are currently available, and many of these can be modified on-site with respect to the concentration of selected electrolytes. The dialysate is provided as a liquid or powdered concentrate that is diluted with prepared water in a fixed ratio to yield the final solute concentration. This proportioning of the dialysate can be done in a central retaining facility, and the reconstituted dialysate is provided from a storage tank to the individual dialysis machines ("central delivery" system). Alternatively and with increasing frequency, the dialysate is reconstituted with prepared water on entry into the dialysis machine and immediately before entering the dialyzer. Appropriate proportioning of the dialysate concentrate and water is ensured by the use of on-line measurements of the conductivity of the diluted dialysate before its entry into the hemodialyzer.

## DURATION AND FREQUENCY OF DIALYSIS

The volumetric removal of a solute from the blood may be conveniently defined per unit time of dialysis. The clearance of a marker solute, such as urea, can be increased by lengthening the duration of hemodialysis. Because the typical dialysis prescription requires optimal blood and dialysate flows, the duration of dialysis is often the sole variable that can be augmented. Most patients receive hemodialysis treatments on an every-other-day basis (three times per week). Only patients with significant residual renal function (glomerular filtration rate > 5 mL/min) should undergo hemodialysis twice weekly. Although the same solute clearance per week can be achieved with a longer dialysis session performed twice weekly, hemodialysis three times per week is associated with less interdialytic solute accumulation and therefore diminishes the likelihood of the development of neurologic complications due to solute removal. In addition, interdialytic weight increases are much greater with twice-weekly dialysis. This occurrence increases the likelihood of the development of congestive heart failure between dialysis treatments and complicates ultrafiltration because of the greater intradialytic hemodynamic instability.

As discussed later, there is frequently a discrepancy between the amount of hemodialysis that is prescribed and the amount that is delivered to the patient,[19, 20] which is the basis for the increasing popularity of measurements of hemodialysis adequacy that monitor the intradialytic decline in urea (i.e., percent reduction in urea or urea reduction ratio).[21]

## ANTICOAGULATION FOR HEMODIALYSIS

Despite the impaired capacity of platelets to aggregate and adhere in most patients with advanced renal failure, the interaction of plasma with the dialysis membrane produces activation of the clotting cascade, thrombosis in the extracorporeal circuit, and resultant dialyzer dysfunction[22] (see later). Dialyzer thrombogenicity is determined by its composition, surface charge, surface area, and configuration.[23] In addition, the propensity for intradialytic clotting is influenced by the blood flow through the dialyzer; the extent of recirculation in the extracorporeal circuit; the amount of ultrafiltration; and the length, diameter, and composition of the blood lines. Patient-specific variables that influence thrombogenicity and determine the requirements for anticoagulants include the presence of congestive heart failure; malnutrition; neoplasia; blood transfusions; and comorbid coagulopathies, such as disseminated intravascular coagulation, warfarin therapy, or hepatic synthetic dysfunction.[24]

Because of its low cost, ease of administration, simplicity of monitoring, and relatively short biologic half-life, the anionic mucopolysaccharide heparin is the most widely used anticoagulant for dialysis. The precise method of administration of heparin is determined by the patient's comorbid illness and varies among dialysis providers. Currently, there are three common methods of preventing intradialytic coagulation of the dialytic circuit: 1) systemic or fractional anticoagulation, in which heparin is administered as a single bolus or incrementally during the dialysis treatment; 2) regional anticoagulation, in which only the extracorporeal dialytic circuit is anticoagulated by the administration of heparin into the arterial line and protamine into the venous line; and 3) no anticoagulation.

The time constraints of hemodialysis are such that the partial thromboplastin time cannot be used to monitor the effectiveness of anticoagulation in the outpatient setting. Either no direct measure of the intensity of anticoagulation is performed or an activated clotting time (ACT) is used. In this assay, whole blood is mixed with an activator of the extrinsic clotting cascade, such as kaolin, diatomaceous earth, or ground glass, and the time necessary for the blood to first congeal is monitored. The normal range is 90 to 140 seconds. However, as for partial thromboplastin time, the dialysis facility that performs this routine assay must be federally certified for its performance.

The simplest method of heparin administration is systemic administration, in which 50 to 100 U/kg of heparin is administered at the initiation of dialysis followed by the bolus of 1000 U/h. The target ACT is approximately 50% above the baseline values. For fractional anticoagulation, 10 to 50 U/kg of heparin is administered initially followed by the bolus of 500 to 1000 U/h. Less intensive anticoagulation is achieved with fractional heparinization in which the target ACT is maintained at 25% (fractional) or 15% (tight fractional) above the baseline value. In that the degree of anticoagulation during systemic anticoagulation is relatively intensive, it is appropriate only for stable patients who are at no risk for bleeding.

Minimal anticoagulation occurs with regional heparinization. By this method, the extracorporeal circuit alone is anticoagulated.[25] Specifically, 500 U of heparin is given at the beginning of dialysis, and 500 to 750 U/h is infused into the arterial line. In parallel, 3.75 mg/h of protamine is infused into the venous line. On the basis of frequent checks of the ACT from the arterial and venous lines, the heparin and protamine infusion rates are adjusted to maintain the ACT for the patient at baseline level and for the dialytic circuit at 10 seconds or longer. Because of hepa-

rin's longer half-life in comparison to protamine, an additional 50 mg of protamine should be given at the end of dialysis.[26] Alternatively, regional anticoagulation may be achieved with sodium citrate as the anticoagulant.[27] Citrate binds to $Ca^{2+}$ and forms a dialyzable salt, thus depleting the extrinsic and intrinsic clotting cascades of the obligatory cofactor $Ca^{2+}$. A 45% solution of sodium citrate is initially infused into the arterial line at 30 mL/h, and the infusion rate is adjusted after 20 minutes to maintain the ACT of the patient and the machine at 10% and 25% above baseline values, respectively.

If the nursing personnel are not experienced with regional anticoagulation, this technique may be associated with significant and relatively frequent side effects without significant advantage over low-dose heparin.[28] Therefore, in high-risk situations in which regional anticoagulation may be contraindicated (heparin-induced thrombocytopenia, allergy to protamine, personnel unfamiliar with technique), dialysis may be performed without heparin.[29, 30] By this technique, the hemodialyzer is first rinsed with 1 L of 0.45% saline containing 3000 to 5000 U of heparin. Immediately thereafter, hemodialysis is initiated with as great a blood flow as will be tolerated, and the dialyzer is flushed every 15 to 30 minutes with 50 mL of saline. This technique is not conducive to large-volume ultrafiltration, compromised blood flows, or the intradialytic administration of blood products.

Anticoagulation must be individualized on the basis of the patient's risk of hemorrhage. Clearly, the risk of thrombosis of the dialytic circuit is a secondary consideration. Guidelines for anticoagulation based on comorbid conditions are as follows:

1. Patients who are bleeding, are at significant risk of bleeding, have a baseline major thrombostatic defect, or are within 7 days of a major operative procedure or within 14 days of intracranial surgery should undergo dialysis without heparin or by regional anticoagulation.

2. Patients who are within 72 hours of a biopsy of a visceral organ should undergo dialysis without heparin or by regional anticoagulation.

3. Patients who are more than 7 days past a major surgery or 72 hours past a biopsy can have dialysis by fractional heparinization. If they have previously received fractional heparinization, they can now be considered for systemic anticoagulation.

4. Patients with pericarditis should have dialysis without heparin or by regional anticoagulation.

5. Patients who have undergone minor surgical procedures within the previous 72 hours should have dialysis by fractional anticoagulation.

6. Patients anticipated to receive a major surgical procedure within 8 hours of hemodialysis should undergo dialysis without heparin or with tight fractional anticoagulation. If they are within 8 hours of a minor procedure, fractional anticoagulation is appropriate.

## Continuous Renal Replacement Therapy

The practical application of the convective clearance of solutes is observed during continuous renal replacement therapy (CRRT) (see Table 56–3). These techniques are performed by passing the patient's blood through a dialyzer that has great hydraulic permeability but is able to retain protein and cellular elements, with the resultant formation of a protein-free ultrafiltrate that resembles plasma water in composition.[31] Blood is usually conveyed into the dialyzer from an arterial cannula and is returned into a large-caliber vein just as in hemodialysis. If the ultrafiltrate is not supplanted by a replacement solution, the process is described as slow continuous ultrafiltration. Relatively little solute clearance occurs during slow continuous ultrafiltration alone owing to limitations of the volume of ultrafiltrate that can be removed without the development of hypovolemia.

Obviously, solute clearance can be enhanced by the continual replacement of the lost volume with a solution that is lacking the removed solute. This alternative CRRT is virtually the same as slow continuous ultrafiltration, but the volume replacement prevents hypovolemia. If an arteriovenous blood path is used, the process is called continuous arteriovenous hemofiltration. If a venovenous path is used (driven by a blood pump at a rate of 100 mL/min), the procedure is described as continuous venovenous hemofiltration. Optimal solute clearance is achieved by combining diffusive and convective clearances. This is accomplished by circulating a dialysate through the dialyzer without (or with) a high ultrafiltration rate (continuous arteriovenous hemodialysis and continuous arteriovenous hemodiafiltration, respectively). Alternatively, these procedures may be performed by use of venovenous access with a blood pump to generate adequate flow rates (continuous venovenous hemodialysis and continuous venovenous hemodiafiltration). Although the use of a venovenous blood path overcomes the constraints of having to establish an arterial access, the need for pumps limits the use of these techniques to facilities that have the appropriate specialized delivery systems, which are costly and require specially trained personnel. In several European countries, hemodiafiltration with virtually total replacement of the ultrafiltrate is used as maintenance dialysis. However, hemofiltration has proved to be impractical for maintenance dialysis in the United States.

## DRIVING PRESSURE FOR CONTINUOUS RENAL REPLACEMENT THERAPY

During CRRT, ultrafiltration is accomplished by the generation of either a positive-pressure gradient on the blood side of the dialyzer or a negative pressure on the dialysate side, or both. The driving force for perfusion of the dialyzer is typically the patient's mean arterial pressure, whereas the hydrostatic pressure in the ultrafiltrate compartment provides the driving force for the formation of the filtrate. For effective ultrafiltration with an arteriovenous blood path, the mean arterial pressure should be maintained above 70 mm Hg. Although ultrafiltration may occur with lower mean arterial pressures, there is a greater likelihood of clotting of the extracorporeal circuit. The effective negative pressure ($P_h$) that is generated by the weight of the column within the ultrafiltration collection line is calculated by

$P_h$ = height difference between the dialyzer and collection bag × 0.74

Therefore, to increase or decrease the rate of fluid formation during CRRT, the collection bag is either lowered from or raised to the level of the dialyzer, respectively. Because of the risk of back-diffusion of pyrogenic substances from the ultrafiltrate compartment and nonsterile collection set into the blood compartment, the collection bag should never be raised higher than the dialyzer.

The ultrafiltrate that is formed is free of protein with a solute composition that closely resembles plasma water.[32] However, because of the constraints of maintaining Gibbs-Donnan equilibrium, cations such as $Ca^{2+}$ are less well represented and anions such as $Cl^-$ are excessively represented in the ultrafiltrate compared with the plasma. These differences are modest, typically less than 5 mEq/L. The quantity of a selected solute that is cleared will be determined by the volume of ultrafiltrate formed, by its concentration in the blood (and therefore in the ultrafiltrate), and by the composition of the replacement solution (if any is used). For example, if ultrafiltration results in the formation of 0.5 L of ultrafiltrate per hour, and the ultrafiltrate and the replacement solution contain 5 and 0 mEq/L of $K^+$, respectively, 30 mEq of $K^+$ will be cleared in 12 hours.

It is not unusual for ultrafiltration to result in the formation of 500 mL/h or more of ultrafiltrate. Although this rate of ultrafiltration is less than that achieved with hemodialysis, the continuous nature of CRRT permits the removal of a far greater total volume for an extended interval. Because of the capacity to tailor the rate and volume of replacement, greater prospective fluid management can occur with CRRT than with hemodialysis. For example, if the patient is volume overloaded in the setting of oliguric acute renal failure, ultrafiltration is allowed to occur without fluid replacement until euvolemia is achieved. Thereafter, an adequate volume of replacement solution is infused to maintain euvolemia. In contrast, if the patient is already euvolemic and nonoliguric, replacement fluid is infused in an adequate volume to match the losses through the dialyzer. It should not be overlooked that the volume of replacement solution that is required can be diminished by minimizing the vertical distance between the dialyzer and the collection bag. However, because clearance is partially dependent on convective clearance, solute removal will likewise be attenuated.

## REPLACEMENT SOLUTIONS FOR CONTINUOUS RENAL REPLACEMENT THERAPY

Because there are no commercial replacement solutions for CRRT in the United States, these must be individually prepared. Most patients are treated with custom fluid formulations, such as that generated for total parenteral nutrition. This is particularly advantageous because it allows protein and calorie obligations to be met, control of volume constraints, and optimization of the electrolyte solution. Because of the sizable loss of amino acids during CRRT, the provision of adequate nutrition is particularly critical. Some centers use Ringer lactate solution ($Na^+$, 130 mEq/L;

K⁺, 4.0 mEq/L; Cl⁻, 109 mEq/L; lactate, 28 mEq/L; Ca²⁺, 3.0 mEq/L) as a replacement solution. However, because of its K⁺ content, it is not suitable for many patients with renal failure. Also, patients with tissue hypoperfusion and renal and hepatic insufficiency may not be able to accommodate the lactate load in Ringer solution.

A replacement solution can be administered immediately before (''predilutional hemofiltration'') or after the dialyzer (''postdilutional hemofiltration''), simultaneously into both locations (''pre-postdilutional hemofiltration''), or into the peripheral venous circulation.[33, 34] Predilutional hemofiltration offers the advantage of diluting plasma proteins, which effectively lowers the thrombogenicity of the dialyzer and increases the ultrafiltration rate for a given hydrostatic pressure. However, this technique also reduces the concentration of solutes in the blood entering the dialyzer and therefore may compromise their clearance per unit time. Alternatively, the replacement solution can be administered incompletely before the dialyzer with the balance being infused immediately after the dialyzer. This offers the advantages of predilutional hemofiltration without the clearance disadvantages.

## ANTICOAGULATION FOR CONTINUOUS RENAL REPLACEMENT THERAPY

As with hemodialysis, anticoagulation is usually necessary with CRRT. The slower blood flows (50 to 100 mL/h) are more conducive to intradialytic clotting. Thus, even with modification of the procedure to minimize thrombogenicity (using relatively short arterial and venous lines, changing to a parallel plate configuration for the dialyzer, performing predilutional hemofiltration), heparin is usually required.[31, 35–37] The use of aggressive ultrafiltration that results in hemoconcentration, reduced blood flows, and the blood's passage through long venous lines is thrombogenic. During CRRT, the required intensity of anticoagulation is usually similar to that associated with systemic heparinization for hemodialysis. After a systemic loading dose of heparin, an initial maintenance infusion of approximately 10 U/kg/h is administered and titrated to maintain the partial thromboplastin time in the arterial line at 50% greater than the control value. Such concentrated heparinization obviously limits the use of this technique to patients not at risk for bleeding. Anticoagulation guidelines for continuous venovenous CRRT are the same as those given for conventional hemodialysis.

CRRT can be performed without heparin; this involves rinsing the kidney and lines with heparinized saline as described for heparin-free hemodialysis.[38] The parallel plate configuration for the dialyzer is less thrombogenic and may preserve its clearance to a greater degree than a hollow-fiber geometry.[35] Regional anticoagulation can be performed during CRRT[39] but is labor intensive, which greatly compromises its utility. Thrombosis within the dialyzer is easy to recognize by the characteristic clotting of the usually white fibers within the hollow-fiber dialyzer. Unfortunately, the parallel plate configuration is assembled in such a manner that the interior of the dialyzer cannot be visualized. In this circumstance, clotting of the dialyzer can only

be defined inferentially by the decline in the ultrafiltration rate in the absence of decreased mean arterial pressure.

# UREA KINETIC MODELING
## Basic Principles

The conceptual goal of urea kinetic modeling is to improve the quality of life and reduce the morbidity and mortality of hemodialysis patients by providing a measure of dialysis quality and quantity. The practical goal of kinetic modeling is to easily and objectively measure the quantity of solute clearance that is delivered to the patient.

Although the BUN concentration is the focus for kinetic models, uremia cannot be entirely explained by the elevation in BUN. For example, the dialysis of patients with renal failure against a dialysate solution that contained urea did not interfere with successful dialysis.[40, 41] These observations have led to proposals that the putative uremic toxins are not water soluble but are more likely to be intracellular molecules or are tightly protein bound. Despite these findings, the empirical observation is that the removal of soluble ''toxins'' by the dialytic process sustains life in severe renal failure. Urea is the most abundant nitrogenous solute removed by the dialyzer, and the National Cooperative Dialysis Study found that BUN levels correlated with dialysis outcome.[42] Yet despite the mild toxicity of urea alone, it serves as a marker for other easily removed toxins that are important provocateurs for the toxicity of uremia.

Urea is an easily diffusible solute that moves rapidly across cell membranes. Urea is highly polar and therefore water soluble and would not be expected to diffuse across cell membranes. However, urea moves rapidly between all aqueous body compartments. In many cells, facilitated diffusion pathways allow faster exchange across the plasma membrane than would be predicted on the basis of simple diffusion alone. This implies that little or no concentration gradients develop within the body or within the dialyzer and thereby simplifies the task of urea kinetic modeling. However, this simplification is not fully accurate.

Urea has several other important features that make it useful as a marker for adequacy of dialysis. Urea is a breakdown product of protein metabolism and accounts for nearly all protein nitrogen elimination. Therefore, the accumulation and elimination of urea are a measure of protein catabolism. Protein catabolism determines dialysis need, so measuring urea accumulation between dialysis treatments permits calculation of the protein catabolic rate and presumably estimates the need for dialysis. The measurement of urea before and after dialysis allows calculation of the efficiency of the dialytic process. These two parameters (protein catabolic rate and urea clearance) are used in all kinetic models of urea.

BUN concentrations alone are not sufficient for predicting the adequacy of dialysis. One problem is the saw-toothed pattern of BUN concentration induced by thrice-weekly dialysis sessions. BUN concentration will also vary depending on the dialyzer's efficiency, the patient's size and adiposity, and the patient's protein intake and protein catabolism. Urea kinetic modeling determines the important parameters of dialysis effectiveness and provides an estimate of dialysis efficiency by using two or three BUN determinations. The amount of dialysis delivered can be expressed as Kt/V. K, the clearance term, represents whole body urea clearance and t is time on dialysis, which permits Kt to represent the amount of dialysis delivered or ordered. This is expressed in terms of the patient's size (V) and is similar to drug dosing expressed as milligrams per kilograms of body weight. Modeling also permits other parameters to be included, such as the dialysis schedule, protein intake, fluid shifts, and compartment disequilibrium between dialyses. When discrepancies occur between expected and modeled clearances, mechanical problems such as recirculation in the vascular access must be excluded.

The concept of mass balance is explained earlier (see Equations 4 to 6 and Fig. 56–4). For urea mass balance, the following differential equation expresses the balance between what enters and what leaves the body:

$$d(V \times C)/dt = G - K \times C \tag{21}$$

in which V is the volume of distribution for urea (milliliters); C is the urea concentration (milligrams per milliliter); t is time of observation (minutes); G is the urea generation rate (milligrams per minute); and K is the clearance of urea (milliliters per minute). $V \times C$ is total body urea content, and changes in this quantity result from changes in urea generation rate (G) minus urea removal ($K \times C$). Because the concentration of urea is changing constantly, this equation must be integrated over time to account for the interval of a dialysis treatment or the interdialytic interval. During dialysis, K is the sum of two clearances: $K_d$, the dialyzer clearance, and $K_r$, the residual renal function. The mass balance equation for urea can be simplified if we assume that V is constant. For most patients with renal failure who are oligoanuric and undergo large variations in volume during and between dialytic sessions, this is not an accurate assumption. Furthermore, if we also assume that G (urea generation rate) is negligible during dialysis, we can simplify Equation 21 to the following equation:

$$V \times (dC/dt) = -K \times C \tag{22}$$

For the hypercatabolic patient with acute renal failure, G is not an insignificant number. The solution to Equation 22 is the familiar exponential decline in drug concentration after intravenous dosing:

$$C_t = C_o e^{-K \times t/V} \tag{23}$$

in which $C_o$ is the initial concentration of urea and $C_t$ is the concentration of urea at time t. When this equation is plotted logarithmically, a linear relationship exists between time, which is displayed on the x axis, and the fractional reduction in urea concentration, which is displayed on the y axis:

$$Kt/V = -\ln(C_t/C_o) \tag{24}$$

where ln is the natural logarithm.

The slope of the hatched line in Figure 56–6 is K/V and indicates the rate of decline in BUN during dialysis. K/V does not describe a constant rate of decline in the blood urea concentration; instead, it is a fractional reduction in the urea concentration. The fractional removal rate is

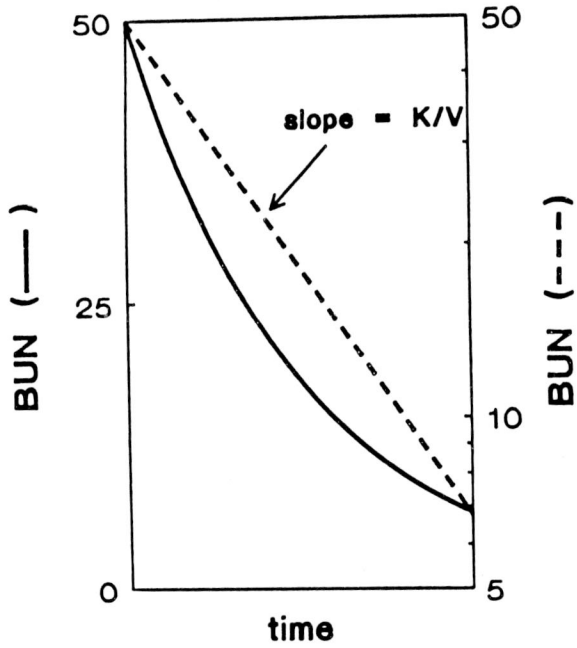

**Figure 56–6.** The relationship between dialysis duration and the fractional reduction in urea (see text). (From Depner TA: Urea modeling: The basics. Semin Dial 4[3]:179–184, 1991. Reprinted by permission of Blackwell Scientific Publications, Inc.)

constant, but the absolute removal rate declines with a decreasing urea concentration. This is the key element of first-order processes; the amount removed changes as the process continues.

Another way to simplify Equation 21 is to analyze the dialytic process and the interdialytic intervals assuming zero-order kinetics (a linear process) rather than as a first-order process. This simplification avoids the need for integration of BUN under the curve and allows a simple averaging of urea concentration ($TAC_{urea}$).

$$TAC_{urea} = \{[(C_1 + C_2) + (C_2 + C_3)]I_d\}/ \\ [2(T_d + I_d)] \tag{25}$$

in which $C_1$ is the predialysis BUN concentration; $C_2$ is the postdialysis BUN concentration; $C_3$ is the predialysis BUN concentration of the next dialysis treatment; $T_d$ is the duration of the dialysis; and $I_d$ is the interdialytic interval. This formulation is illustrated in Figure 56–7. The change of urea concentration from $C_1$ to $C_2$ is determined primarily by dialyzer clearance $K_d$ and the duration of dialysis $T_d$. The change from $C_2$ to $C_3$ is determined primarily by the rate of urea generation (G), the extent of residual renal function ($K_r$), and the volume of distribution of urea.

During steady state, net urea generation is determined by the protein catabolic rate and is a linear function as illustrated in Figure 56–8. As protein catabolic rate increases, the rate of urea generation increases linearly. The slope of the resultant line is 0.154, indicating that about 15.4% of catabolized protein is converted to urea. Note that the line does not pass through the origin, indicating that at 0 catabolic rate there are persistent nitrogen losses through stool excretion. The linear relationship between protein catabolic

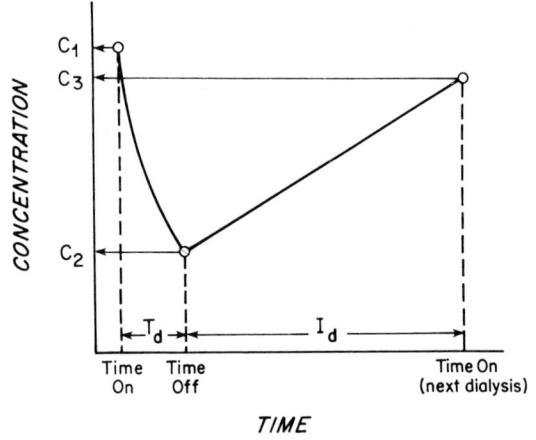

**Figure 56–7.** Changes in solute concentration during and between dialysis treatments. $C_1$, $C_2$, and $C_3$ are the urea concentrations before dialysis, after dialysis, and before the next dialysis treatment, respectively. $T_d$ and $I_d$ are, respectively, the dialysis time and the interdialysis time. (From Sargent JA: Kinetic modeling in the guidance of dialysis therapy. Dial Transplant 8:1101, 1979.)

rate (PCR) and urea generation (G) can be expressed as follows:

$$G = (0.154PCR) - 1.7 \qquad (26)$$

This equation assumes zero-order kinetics for urea generation throughout the interdialytic period. Although urea generation transiently increases immediately after dialysis,

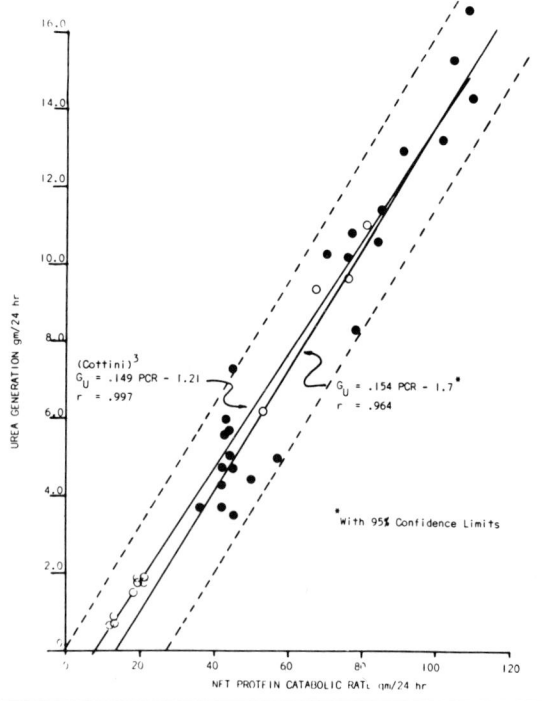

**Figure 56–8.** The relationship between net protein catabolic rate (PCR) and net urea generation rate ($G_U$) in dialyzed and undialyzed uremic patients. (From Sargent J, Gotch F, Borah M, et al: Urea kinetics: A guide to nutritional management of renal failure. Am J Clin Nutr 31:1696, 1978. © Am J Clin Nutr. American Society for Clinical Nutrition.)

this relationship provides a useful tool for assessing dietary protein intake. The relationship between protein catabolic rate and dietary protein intake (DPI) can be represented as

$$DPI = PCR + \text{change in nitrogen balance} \qquad (27)$$

In a healthy steady state, in which there are no intercurrent catabolic processes such as illness, starvation, or use of steroids, and when there are no significant changes in muscle mass or body weight, dietary protein intake will approximate protein catabolic rate. For dialysis patients in the steady state who have no residual renal function, urea generation can be calculated by considering changes in urea concentration during the interdialytic interval:

$$G = [(V_2 \times C_2) - (V_3 \times C_3)]/I_d \qquad (28)$$

in which $V_2$ is the volume of distribution for urea (0.58 × body weight); $C_2$ is the BUN concentration immediately after dialysis; $V_3 \times C_3$ is the volume of distribution and the BUN concentration before dialysis; and $I_d$ is the interdialytic interval.

Calculation of urea generation rate from Equation 28 allows the determination of protein catabolic rate from Equation 26, which in turn permits estimation of dietary protein intake in clinically and metabolically stable dialysis patients.

## Practical Considerations for Urea Kinetic Modeling

The fractional rate of decline in BUN concentration during a dialysis session provides a crude estimate of K/V, the urea elimination constant. Standard modeling techniques include a third BUN measurement obtained immediately before the start of the next dialysis. The slope of the BUN/ time curve between dialyses allows calculation of the urea generation rate. However, these calculations consider only changes in the BUN concentration. If absolute values are incorporated into the algorithm for urea kinetic modeling, the third BUN measurement can be eliminated.[43, 44] The "two-point" BUN model analyzes the urea generation rate to an entire week, instead of a single dialysis interval. Theoretically, this method is more accurate, easier, and less costly than "three-point" BUN determinations. On comparison of these two methods, it was observed that the two-point BUN method is as accurate as the three-point BUN measurement in predicting future BUN values.[43]

Thus, measurements of a predialysis and a postdialysis BUN concentration are the only parameters needed for some formulations in urea kinetic modeling. The urea clearance of the dialyzer (calculated from blood and dialysate flows and the manufacturer's provision of $K_d$ for the dialyzer), the duration and frequency of dialysis, and the patient's weights before and after dialysis are routine data that can be obtained with any dialysis treatment. The blood sample for the predialysis BUN measurement is drawn before dialysis is started and before any blood dilution occurs. The postdialysis BUN measurement is subject to artifacts from recirculation and from drawing the sample before the completion of dialysis. The sample should be drawn from the arterial blood port less than 5 minutes after the blood pump has been shut off. These data are used to generate multiple concentrations of urea during and between dialysis treatments for an entire week. The process is repeated while urea volume (V) is adjusted to fit the postdialysis BUN concentration, and urea generation rate G is adjusted to fit the predialysis BUN concentration. Although this concept is simple, the calculations are tedious and usually require the acquisition of computer software to perform them. However, a significant advantage to this modeling system is that the calculation of K/V relies on ratios and not absolute values. This permits accurate modeling without highly accurate determinations of the dialyzer clearance K.

The urea reduction ratio or percentage reduction of urea is a rapid and low-cost method for assessing adequacy of dialysis that relates to the Kt/V. The urea reduction ratio (URR) is the fractional reduction in BUN during a single dialysis treatment and is expressed in the following equation:

$$URR = 100 \times (1 - C_t/C_o) \qquad (29)$$

in which $C_t$ and $C_o$ are the postdialysis and predialysis BUN values, respectively. The two BUN concentrations can be related by the conventional urea kinetic equation:

$$C_t = C_o e^{-Kt/V} \qquad (23)$$

Rearranging this equation produces

$$Kt/V = -\ln(C_t/C_o) \qquad (24)$$

and substituting Equation 29 gives

$$Kt/V = \ln[1 - (URR/100)] \qquad (30)$$

Several investigators have used linear regression analysis to show a good correlation between Kt/V and the urea reduction ratio.[45–49] A retrospective analysis of more than 13,000 patients through the National Medical Care network of dialysis facilities[21] showed that patients receiving a urea reduction ratio less than 60% had a significantly higher risk of death. The urea reduction ratio is simple and easy to obtain, and it is a useful tool for assessing dialysis adequacy. However, this value is limited by providing data for a single treatment and does not account for protein catabolic rate and nutritional status.

## Compartment Effects on Urea Kinetic Modeling

The previous discussion of urea kinetic modeling makes several critical assumptions. The major supposition is that urea is distributed within a single-volume compartment within the body. This single-volume space is the sum of all water-containing compartments within the body. Because urea is a small molecule with no charge and has low protein binding, it can diffuse rapidly across cell membranes. This physical behavior is ideal for a single-compartment model, but during dialysis, there are such rapid shifts in urea that disequilibrium between compartments may occur.

If urea transport is delayed across the plasma membrane, the deleterious impact on its clearance would be greatest in erythrocytes during their transit through the dialyzer. Be-

cause up to 80% reduction in the blood's urea content occurs during its passage through the dialyzer, the relative entrapment of cytosolic urea should lead to significant osmotic shifts and cell damage. If intradialytic resistance to urea diffusion is sufficiently high, urea would be expected to function as an intracellular osmole and cause cell swelling during dialysis. However, no experimental support exists for the putative delay in urea diffusion from erythrocytes during their transit through the dialyzer.[53] Although direct demonstration of red blood cell swelling has not been shown, there is high tissue and cerebrospinal fluid osmolality after vigorous dialysis.[50–52] Several investigators have demonstrated facilitated membrane transporters for urea that increase its effective permeability by several hundred fold.[54, 55] In contrast, other studies show that urea movement is delayed among body compartments.[52, 56, 57] Solutes such as creatinine, phosphorus, and $K^+$ distribute in the intracellular environment and diffuse slowly during dialysis. For these solutes during and after dialysis, there is a delay in equilibration between the intracellular compartment and the extracellular compartment. These solutes are present at much lower concentrations than urea.

During high-flux hemodialysis, rapid shifts in urea occur across the dialysis membrane but not between compartments. This finding has led to questions about the validity of the single-compartment model for urea kinetic modeling. Most patients show a transient steep rise in urea concentration in the immediate postdialysis period. This rise is greater than would be expected from the baseline rate of urea generation alone and suggests a redistribution of urea from other body compartments into the urea-depleted blood.[52, 57, 58] The postdialysis "urea rebound" could be explained by a marked increase in protein catabolism, but the rise in BUN concentration is too fast and too short-lived (30-minute duration).[57] Other evidence for compartment effects is the observation that during the first few minutes of high-flux dialysis, there is an extremely rapid fall in blood urea levels, which suggests selective removal from a small compartment.

The number and size of the urea compartments are not well defined; and the more compartments included in the model, the more complex are the formulations of urea kinetic modeling. Figure 56–9 schematically represents a two-compartment model of urea mass balance ($V_1 C_1$ and $V_2 C_2$). Urea generation is constant (G) and equilibrates across two pools: the blood ($V_1 C_1$) and dialyzer and the blood and the remote pool that is the sequestered compartment ($V_2 C_2$). Figure 56–10 illustrates serial blood urea concentrations in a patient undergoing high-flux hemodialysis.[59] The dashed line is the best fit for a single-compartment model of variable volume. The solid line is the best fit for a two-compartment model of variable volume. The two-compartment model almost exactly fits the in vivo data.

The postdialysis increase in urea occurs in two phases: an initial, rapid rebound stage followed by a slower increment described as the urea generation stage. Urea rebound occurs from equilibration with all remote compartments, whereas urea generation occurs from dietary and endogenous protein catabolism. Most two-compartment models of urea kinetics consider urea generation to take place in the blood compartment that equilibrates immediately with the

## Two compartments, variable V₁

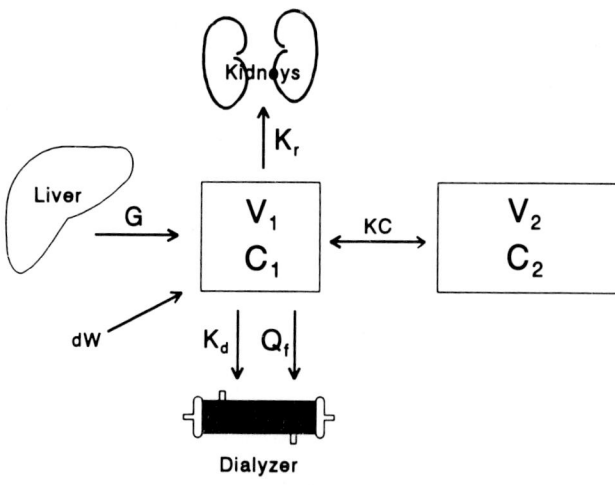

**Figure 56–9.** Schematic representation of a two-compartment model of urea mass balance during hemodialysis. KC = mass transfer coefficient; K_r = renal clearance; Q_f = volume during dialysis; dW = volume between dialysis. (From Depner TA: Refining the model of urea kinetics: Compartment effects. Semin Dial 5[2]:147–154, 1992. Reprinted by permission of Blackwell Scientific Publications, Inc.)

dialyzer. Failure to account for two compartments for urea and for the rebound phase can lead to overestimates of the protein catabolic rate. If blood is drawn immediately after dialysis, the BUN concentration will be underestimated.

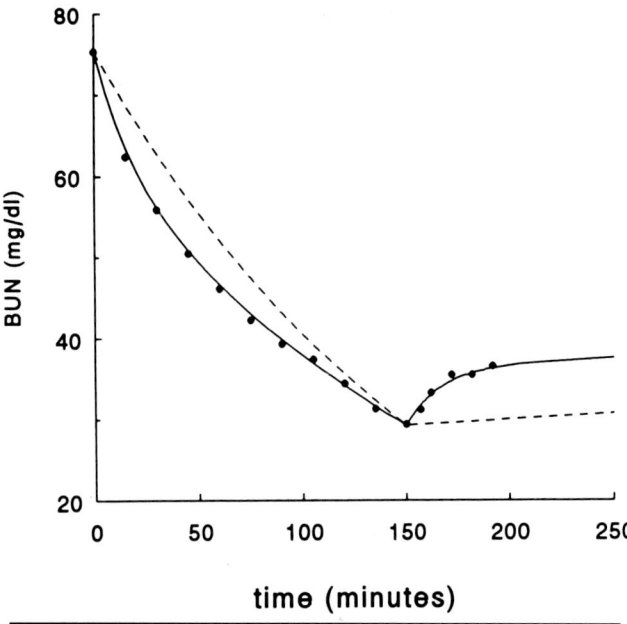

**Figure 56–10.** Hemodialysis for 150 minutes causes a rapid decline in BUN. For a single patient, the solid circle is the measured BUN concentration. The dashed line is the best fit for the decline in BUN based on a single-compartment model of variable volume for urea. The solid line is the best fit derived by a two-compartment model of variable volume. (From Depner TA: Refining the model of urea kinetics: Compartment effects. Semin Dial 5[2]:147–154, 1992. Reprinted by permission of Blackwell Scientific Publications, Inc.)

Using this value in Equation 28 will result in an overestimate for the urea generation rate and the protein catabolic rate. Furthermore, the exaggerated difference in predialysis and postdialysis BUN concentrations will lead to an underestimation of the area under the BUN versus time curve. This will lead to overestimation of the urea reduction ratio, Kt/V, or the delivered dialysis therapy. Compartment effects on urea removal are more likely to be manifested in small-statured patients, during the performance of high-flux hemodialysis with abbreviated dialysis sessions, and with high blood flow rates.

A simplified, alternative method to measure intradialytic urea removal, which will also account for urea rebound, uses a single-compartment model with a postdialysis BUN concentration that is obtained at the beginning of the urea generation phase. The postdialysis BUN concentration is determined from a sample taken at least 30 minutes after the end of dialysis. This technique gives an accurate estimation of dialysis adequacy because K/V and Kt/V are calculated from a true equilibrated BUN value. However, such protracted measurements are impractical, because most patients will not delay their departure from the dialysis unit by this lengthy period.

## Discrepancies in Dialysis Delivery

Several dialysis-specific and patient-specific factors contribute to differences in the quantity of hemodialysis prescribed to the patient and the actual quantity that is delivered (Table 56–4). Dialyzer clearances ($K_d$) are often significantly lower in vivo than those reported by the manufacturer, but the values used for prescribing dialysis and for calculating the Kt/V are based on these in vitro estimates. The deposition of cellular components and protein along the dialysis membrane decreases its effective surface area and diffusion capabilities, especially if reprocessing of the dialyzer is not performed properly. Blood flow turbulence in the extracorporeal circuit decreases the effective blood flow and clearance, and blood flow may be compromised owing to overt dysfunction of the angioaccess. A common factor contributing to decreased dialyzer clearance occurs with excessive blood recirculation within the angioaccess. Improper calibration of the pumps that deliver blood and dialysate may result in an unanticipated decline in solute clearance. In addition, the dialysis facility provider may deliberately decrease the blood flow during a time of intradialytic hemodynamic instability. A common point of discrepancy between the delivered and the prescribed quantity of dialysis is in the duration of the dialysis treatment. Premature discontinuation of the dialysis session by either the patient or the dialysis facility provider is often not appreciated in urea kinetic modeling.

The volume of distribution for solutes is typically calculated and may vary on the basis of the individual's habitus. Improper timing or handling of the blood samples for measurement of the BUN concentration will result in inaccurate estimates of dialysis adequacy. For example, if the postdialysis BUN sample is inadvertently mixed with saline, the value will be inappropriately low, suggesting greater dialysis efficiency than is actually being achieved. The overall

**TABLE 56–4. Causes for Discrepancy in Dialysis Delivery***

| Discrepancy | Causes |
|---|---|
| **Dialysis Specific** | |
| Inaccurate dialyzer clearance | In vitro $K_d$ > in vivo $K_d$; reduced fiber bundle volume → decreased solute clearance; incorrect dialyzer selection |
| Incorrect blood flow | Improper calibration of the blood pump; blood pump not set to prescribed value or reduced during treatment; blood flow prescription too low |
| Incorrect dialysate flow | Improper calibration of dialysate pump; dialysate pump not set to prescribed value |
| Incorrect dialysis time | Treatment discontinued prematurely or started late |
| **Patient Specific** | |
| Access dysfunction | Inability to achieve the prescribed blood flow; luminal obstruction with excessive blood recirculation; improper needle positioning |
| $V_{urea}$ inaccuracy | Unappreciated urea rebound; improper sampling of the postdialysis blood urea nitrogen concentration |

*$K_d$ = dialyzer clearance; $V_{urea}$ = volume of distribution of urea.

consequences of these variances in the dialysis prescription are discussed later. However, if they are not appreciated, the quantity of hemodialysis that is delivered to the patient may be much less than the quantity that the physician has prescribed, and inadequate dialysis may be delivered. Furthermore, if the urea kinetic model uses manufacturer-derived values for the $K_d$, the prescribed dialysis time for the $T_d$, and an extrapolated volume of distribution for urea that incorrectly assumes a single pool of urea of fixed volume, the delivery of inadequate dialysis will not be detected (see Table 56–4).

## COMPONENTS OF THE DIALYSIS PROCESS

### Dialyzers and Hemofilters

For hemodialysis, virtually all of the commercial dialyzers available in the United States are configured as large cylinders packed with hollow fibers through which the blood flows ("hollow-fiber dialyzer"). The dialysate flows through the dialyzer and around these fibers. These dialyzers are noncompliant and thus have fixed blood volumes. A rarely used physical configuration is the parallel plate dialyzer. In this configuration, the dialysis membrane material is arranged in the forms of flat plates that are supported in such a fashion that compartmentalization of the blood and dialysate occurs. The blood compartment of parallel plate dialyzers is relatively compliant and varies with the transmembrane pressure. Arguably, the use of more compliant blood compartments minimizes the risk of backfiltration that occurs typically with high-flux hemodialysis under conditions of low ultrafiltration.

The membrane within these dialyzers may be composed of a variety of modified biologic materials (regenerated cellulose, cuprammonium-treated cellulose [cuprophane], hemophan [modified cuprophane], cellulose acetate, or cellulose triacetate) or synthetic materials (polysulfone, polymethylmethacrylate, polycarbonate, polyacrylonitrile). For a given membrane material, the surface area available for solute transport and the filling volume of the blood and dialysate compartments vary significantly. In general, the

synthetic membrane materials are more costly than the modified biologic materials but alternatively present a greater range of ultrafiltration coefficients and solute clearances, especially for large solutes such as $\beta_2$-microglobulin (>10,000 daltons). Further, as noted in several areas in this chapter, their capacity to interact with cellular and soluble components of the blood (biocompatibility) is usually less than that of the modified biologic membrane materials. The size and membrane surface area of dialyzers vary widely. However, because membrane porosity differs widely between membrane materials, there is little correlation between the dialyzer's surface area and its clearance. Synthetic membrane materials can be modified to be either low flux or high flux, and the same is true for cellulose-based membrane materials.

The choice of dialyzer for the management of renal failure in a particular patient is usually dictated by five major variables in this rank order: 1) the clearance characteristics and the ultrafiltration coefficient of the dialyzer, 2) its biocompatibility, 3) its reprocessing potential, 4) its static volume, and 5) its cost. The development of a wide array of dialyzers and delivery systems with ultrafiltration controllers has rendered the selection of a dialyzer to fulfill a particular solute or ultrafiltration target a convenient process. Dialyzers with urea clearances of about 50 to 200 mL/min (calculated typically for blood flow of 200 mL/min) and ultrafiltration coefficients of about 2 to 65 mL/mm Hg/h are currently available.

However, an increasingly important and controversial topic in the short- and long-term treatment of patients with renal insufficiency is membrane selection based on biocompatibility.[60, 61] The interaction of both soluble and cellular components of the blood with the dialysis membrane may be important in the pathobiologic processes of such varied issues as rapidity of recovery from acute ischemic renal failure[62, 63]; adverse intradialytic symptoms and signs, such as fever, hypotension, and hypoxemia[64–68]; immunologic dysfunction and susceptibility to infection[69–71]; enhanced catabolism and malnutrition[60, 72–74]; hyperlipidemia[75]; and the development of $\beta_2$-microglobulin amyloidosis.[76, 77] A plethora of alterations of cellular functions and physiologic responses have been described in association with hemodialysis using selected membranes, including intradialytic generation of complement-derived anaphylatoxins such as C3a and C5a by the alternative complement pathway in vivo[78]; induction of enhanced membrane expression of selected granulocyte adhesion molecules such as MAC-1 and leukocyte adhesion molecule-1 in vivo[79, 80]; inappropriate production of leukotrienes and reactive oxygen species such as superoxide by granulocytes in vivo[81–84]; enhanced monocyte elaboration of endogenous pyrogens and their biologic antagonists such as interleukin (IL)–1, IL-6, tumor necrosis factor (TNF), IL-1 receptor antagonist, and soluble TNF receptor in vitro and perhaps in vivo[65, 85–91]; altered monocyte phagocytosis in vitro[70]; and altered IL-2 receptor expression in vivo.[92, 93] These issues are discussed in detail in several reviews.[60, 61, 94] In general terms, many of the adverse pathobiologic consequences of hemodialysis that arise from membrane interactions are absent or attenuated by dialysis against synthetic membrane materials such as polysulfone, polymethylmethacrylate, and polyacrylonitrile. In contrast, hemodialysis with cellulosic membranes is associated with the greatest number of acute events and perhaps long-term complications. It is important to realize that not all cellulosic membranes behave in the same fashion with respect to their biocompatibility in vitro. The same is true of the synthetic membrane materials and even for the same material that is marketed by different manufacturers. Last, confounding any correlation of putative membrane interactions to biocompatibility are the independent effects of membrane spallation,[95] pyrogen backflux,[96] dialysate buffer,[97] and uremia.

Unfortunately, although the synthetic dialysis membranes are more biocompatible, they are typically far more costly than conventional cellulosic dialyzers. A practical reality of the financial constraints imposed by Medicare's fixed funding of the ESRD Program (no inflation and minimal treatment cost adjustments) is that few dialysis providers can afford the luxury of a single dialysis use of these relatively expensive synthetic dialyzers. Therefore, in most independent hemodialysis facilities (approximately 70% of the dialysis facilities and 77% of the patients), reprocessing and reuse of disposable dialyzers are financially mandated and performed. Thus, dialyzer reuse is a common practice within the United States. In 1990, 70% of the dialysis facility providers reused their dialyzers, and this number has increased yearly.[98] Dialyzer reuse may be performed manually or with an automated rinsing device. Varying concentrations of formaldehyde, Renalin (mixture of paracetic acid, hydrogen peroxide, and acetic acid), or glutaraldehyde are used as chemical disinfectants. After reuse, dialyzer adequacy is assessed indirectly by 1) measuring the volume of the dialysis fiber bundle in the blood compartment, which correlates roughly with that dialyzer's capacity to clear urea on a subsequent treatment; 2) calculating the ultrafiltration rate of the dialyzer in vitro; and 3) pressurizing the dialyzer to evaluate the structural integrity of the fibers ("pressure test"). For a dialyzer to be acceptable for reuse, the fiber bundle volume must be greater than 80% of the initial value, the in vitro ultrafiltration rate must be greater than 20% of the manufacturer's stated value, the dialyzer should not leak up to a pressure that is up to 20% of the maximal operating pressure, and the pressure decay curve should match that of a new dialyzer.

The safety, efficacy, cost-effectiveness, and morality of this procedure have been closely scrutinized. Most nephrologists believe that neither the patient nor the personnel reprocessing dialyzers are placed at risk if strict infection control precautions and quality assurance and control are implemented.[99–101] As a practical matter, the reuse of hemodialyzers is far less common in the acute hemodialysis setting. An additional putative benefit from the reuse of cuprophane dialyzers is the attenuation of the sense of ill health, dyspnea, nausea, hypotension, leukopenia, and complement activation observed during the first use of these membranes ("first-use syndrome," discussed later). Thus, if biocompatibility issues are a significant clinical concern and synthetic membranes are unavailable, a reused cellulosic dialyzer will provide intermediate biocompatibility. However, the practice of rinsing the dialyzer with a dilute bleach solution to clarify the membrane before its reuse returns the dialyzer membrane to its original biologic reactivity.

A putative disadvantage of high-flux dialyzers is that their relatively open pore configuration may permit the transmembrane flux of bacteria-derived lipopolysaccharides from the dialysate into the dialyzer blood compartment (back-filtration).[96] The exposure of the patient to the pyrogen results in a febrile illness without bacteremia, described as a "pyrogen reaction," and may occur more often with reprocessed high-flux dialyzers. The use of $HCO_3^-$-buffered dialysates that are permissive for the growth of gram-negative bacteria and ultrafiltration controllers that limit the rate of ultrafiltration contribute to the back-filtration of dialysate pyrogens and the occurrence of pyrogen reactions.[96, 102, 103]

Last, the static volume of the dialyzer should be given consideration, especially in the patient with little cardiovascular reserve. Dialyzers range in volume from about 50 to 150 mL with no true correlation of clearance characteristics. The dialysis lines often have a greater volume than the dialyzer and range from approximately 150 to 250 mL in volume. Therefore, it is not typically necessary to compromise solute clearance because of the static volume of the dialyzer.

Like hemodialyzers, hemofilters are available in two geometric configurations, the hollow-fiber configuration and the parallel plate geometry.[35] Hemofilters are usually composed of polysulfone, polymethylmethacrylate, or polyacrylonitrile. A single report suggests that both ultrafiltration and diffusive clearance may be greater when continuous arteriovenous hemodialysis is performed with use of a dialyzer of the parallel plate geometry.[104] In contrast, performance differences between hemofilters have not been observed with venovenous hemofiltration.[105]

## Needles for Hemodialysis

Dialysis needles are available in three common sizes of 15, 16, and 17 gauge. The needles currently in practice are thin walled with tapered, extremely sharp points. Although the use of smaller gauge needles is preferred by the patients because of their greater comfort at insertion, their resistance to blood flow is also greater. Therefore, in the situation in which the target blood flow is above 300 mL/min, such as during the performance of high-efficiency or high-flux hemodialysis, the resistance in the blood path may be excessive. Optimal blood flow is achieved with a 15-gauge needle, but the resultant hole in the fistula is larger. It is unclear whether these larger holes contribute to the early failure of the angioaccess, especially the prosthetic graft arteriovenous fistula. However, because the puncture sites in these graft fistulas never completely seal, the same area should not be used repeatedly for cannulation.

## Blood and Dialysate Delivery Systems

### HEMODIALYSIS

Because blood flow from an arteriovenous fistula or venous catheter is limited by multiple sites of resistance in the extracorporeal circuit, blood flow is maintained by blood pumps. These are usually peristaltic roller pumps that compress a distensible segment of blood tubing and force the blood out of the pump segment. In anticipation of a power failure during hemodialysis, the dialysis machines are equipped with hand cranks for manual pumping operations. Because the pump speed is proportional to the armature voltage, and the flow output of blood is the product of the stroke volume and pump speed, the armature voltage is measured as a surrogate for flow output. This indirect measurement is valid if inlet voltages do not vary during the procedure, the internal diameter of the segment of tubing in the roller pump is uniform, and careful calibration has been performed.

Surprisingly, in the absence of crimping of the tubing or a partial obstruction to blood flow, significant intradialytic and interdialytic hemolysis is an uncommon complication of this blood delivery system.[12] In the absence of a blood pump, the entire extracorporeal circuit is under positive pressure, so air embolism due to air entry into the blood pathway is highly unlikely. However, the arteriovenous fistula in combination with a blood pump generates negative pressure that permits foam emboli (microbubbles of air mixed with blood) and, less frequently, frank air emboli to be generated. Because of the potentially lethal consequences of this complication,[106] all hemodialysis delivery systems incorporate an air detector (photocell, capacitance, or ultrasonography-based detection device) around the venous bubble trap of the extracorporeal circuit. When the air detector is triggered, a venous blood line clamp that occludes blood flow is activated.

The dialysate compartment of the dialyzer is perfused with dialysate only under the conditions of the appropriate dialysate composition, temperature, pressure, and flow. Because variances in these parameters can have lethal consequences,[107–110] these systems are actively monitored during the dialysis session. If an anomaly is detected, the machine sounds an internal alarm and the dialysate bypasses the dialyzer. Dialysate delivery systems in the United States are usually configured to pass dialysate a single time. The delivery systems may be divided into single-patient or multiple-patient systems (central delivery systems). As discussed in a previous section, in a single-pass single-patient system, the dialysate is prepared on-line by an appropriate propor-

tioning of the dialysate concentrate and conditioned water just before its entry into the dialyzer. Alternatively, in single-pass central delivery systems, the dialysate may be prepared on-line or in a large batch.

The typical manner of monitoring for the correct mixing of water and the dialysate concentrate is by the indirect measure of the electrical conductivity. The electrical conductivity is determined by the ionic content of the dialysate and therefore is an indirect measure of the function of the proportioning system. For example, a dialysate $Na^+$ concentration of 130 to 150 mEq/L has a conductivity of 13 to 15 millisiemens. The conductivity of the dialysate is usually monitored by the resistance or impedance method.[12, 111] Because conductivity monitors can fail, typically as a result of corrosion of critical components of the electrodes, it is mandatory that the conductivity be checked manually by the dialysis technician at least once a day. The temperature of the dialysate is maintained at the physiologic range of 36 to 39°C by the use of heat exchangers or immersed heating elements to heat the water before its mixing with the dialysate concentrate. The conventional dialysate temperature is 37.5°C. Heating the dialysate water minimizes its gas content, enhances the mixability of the dialysate concentrate, and prevents the patient from becoming hypothermic during the treatment. The temperature is monitored either with a mechanical thermostat or with a closed-loop proportioning band.[12]

As described earlier, the generation of a negative pressure on the dialysate side is the predominant driving force for ultrafiltration during hemodialysis with a single-pass system. In the conventional system, a single dialysate pump is placed after the dialyzer with a variable constricting valve before the dialyzer. The dialysate pressures are monitored by mechanical or electronic manometers. A feature of many of the newer dialysis machines is that ultrafiltration is effected by an automated control system. There are two ultrafiltration control systems currently in widespread practice for single-pass dialysate systems. 1) Flow sensor systems simultaneously measure the dialysate inflow and outflow rates; the difference between these values is the ultrafiltration rate, and this result is fed back to the transmembrane pressure circuit for an appropriate adjustment. 2) Volumetric balancing systems use matched diaphragm pumps to provide identical dialysate inflow and outflow; a third pump removes fluid from the dialysate loop, which because of its functional noncompliance is reflected by ultrafiltration in the dialyzer.

### CONTINUOUS RENAL REPLACEMENT THERAPY

As described earlier, the driving force for blood flow during the performance of arteriovenous CRRT is the mean arterial pressure. However, for venovenous hemofiltration, peristaltic pumps similar to those used for hemodialysis are necessary. The dialysate is delivered into the dialyzer by a conventional intravenous pump. Whereas little automated monitoring is necessary for the minimal equipment used in arteriovenous CRRT, the monitoring systems for venovenous CRRT are not much different from those used in hemodialysis.

## Water Preparation for Dialysate

Mandatory to a successful long-term outcome on hemodialysis is the generation of dialysate from appropriately prepared water. Unfortunately, most municipal water that is suitable for drinking is rendered so by the addition of contaminants that are toxic for dialysis patients. Examples of these iatrogenic toxins include aluminum sulfate (flocculant), which causes dialysis encephalopthy, anemia, and osteomalacia[112–115]; chloramine (antiseptic), which causes hemolysis[116, 117]; and fluoride (dentrifice), which causes osteomalacia and fluorosis.[118, 119] Other common contaminants and their complications include $Ca^{2+}$ and $Mg^{2+}$, which cause gastrointestinal symptoms, weakness, and blood pressure abnormalities ("hard water syndrome")[120]; copper, which is associated with hepatic insufficiency and hemolysis[121, 122]; $Na^+$, which causes hypertension, congestive heart failure, and seizures[123]; and bacteria or their exotoxins and endotoxins, which may result in pyrogen reactions.[96, 102, 103] The Association for the Advancement of Medical Instrumentation has established comprehensive water quality standards for the maximal concentration of minerals, heavy metals, and bacteria in the dialysate water[124] (Table 56–5).

The individual components of a water purification system consist of a reverse osmosis device, ion exchanger, water softener, carbon adsorption bed, physical filters (multimedia depth filter or particle filter), and purified water storage tank. Because each of these devices or systems eliminates only a limited panel of contaminants, the exact combination and configuration of components used by a dialysis facility will depend on the quality of the feed water, the goal and intended uses for the product water, and the anticipated water consumption and the necessary delivery pressure. For example, if chloramines are used in the feed water, a carbon adsorption system is mandatory. Alternatively, if the feed water has a high content of iron, a green sand filter is often necessary.

The backbone of most water treatment systems is the reverse osmosis device, which has lower operating costs than a deionizer; it is able to reduce the concentration of most inorganic contaminants in the feed water by 10-fold and the bacterial colony count by 1000-fold to 10,000-fold. It is effective in removing dissolved organic and inorganic material, bacteria, pyrogens, and particulate matter. The physical principal behind a reverse osmosis device is that relatively solute-free water can be generated by the application of positive pressure to the solute-containing solution on one side of a semipermeable membrane. In contrast, ion exchangers (deionizers) are better suited to removal of ionic contaminants. The cationic and anionic exchange resins may be mixed physically (mixed-bed deionizer), which produces a high-quality water, or may be physically separated (dual-bed deionizer), which is less costly and less efficacious. Water softeners, which are cationic exchange resins, are effective at binding $Ca^{2+}$ and $Mg^{2+}$, which will otherwise cause premature failure of the membranes in the reverse osmosis devices. Activated carbon filters are effective at absorbing chloramines, chlorine, and small dissolved organic compounds. Large particulates can be removed from the water supply by sediment filtration in which the dialysate water percolates through a bed having a nominal pore size. Because the other components of water filtration are susceptible to clogging by particulates, physical filtration of the untreated water should occur first.

Ultrafiltration of dialysis water is not a conventional water preparation technique in the United States but has become increasingly popular as a means of generating a "clean" dialysate. The Association for the Advancement of Medical Instrumentation mandates that the maximal bacterial count in the water used to prepare the dialysate and in the dialysate itself be 200 colony-forming units/mL or less and 2000 colony-forming units/mL or less, respectively. Although ultrafiltration does not significantly alter the ionic composition of the dialysate, it is effective at eliminating particulate contaminants such as bacteria, viruses, and pyrogens.[102] As discussed in greater detail in a later section, the dialysate concentrate can be greatly purified by subjecting it to ultrafiltration.[125, 126] After being purified, the dialysate water is maintained in a storage reservoir constructed from an inert material. This storage tank is connected to the dialysis stations by a distribution loop that permits the delivery of prepared water to its destination and allows the return of the unused portion. Because of the great risk of bacterial growth in this section of the water purification system, it is critical that the distribution loop not contain any dead ends or areas of stagnant flow.

A critical mandatory area of continuous quality assurance is in the preparation of the dialysate water. Except for chloramines and bacteria, it is recommended that the water produced by the water purification system be monitored for the levels of contaminants (see Table 56–5) at least every 6 months. Testing for chloramines in the water is performed

### TABLE 56–5. Maximal Concentrations Permitted for Contaminants in Dialysate Water

| Contaminant | Maximal Concentration (mg/L) |
| --- | --- |
| Sodium* | 70.0 |
| Potassium* | 8.00 |
| Calcium* | 2.00 |
| Magnesium* | 4.00 |
| Aluminum† | 0.01 |
| Chloramines† | 0.01 |
| Chlorine† | 0.50 |
| Fluoride† | 0.20 |
| Copper† | 0.10 |
| Sulfate† | 100 |
| Nitrate† | 2.00 |
| Zinc† | 0.10 |
| Arsenic‡ | 0.005 |
| Barium‡ | 0.01 |
| Cadmium‡ | 0.001 |
| Chromium‡ | 0.014 |
| Lead‡ | 0.005 |
| Mercury‡ | 0.0002 |
| Selenium‡ | 0.09 |
| Silver‡ | 0.005 |

*Normal dialysate constituents.
†Toxic in dialysate.
‡Environmental Protection Agency–regulated under the Safe Drinking Water Act.

on-site daily, and monitoring for bacteria and pyrogens is sufficiently frequent that a variance is quickly detected (at least weekly). Daily monitoring of the performance of the individual components of the water purification system will minimize the likelihood of a problem with the water supply.

## Dialysate Composition

### HEMODIALYSIS

#### Glucose

Before the availability of hydraulic-driven ultrafiltration, the dialysate glucose concentration was maintained above 1.8 g/dL to generate an osmotic gradient between the blood and the dialysate.[127] Although this was effective for inducing ultrafiltration, the morbid symptoms and signs of hyperosmolality developed in some patients. Currently, the dialysates are glucose free, normoglycemic (0.20% to 0.25% dextrose), or modestly hyperglycemic (>0.25% dextrose). Hemodialysis with a glucose-free dialysate results in a net glucose loss of approximately 30 g and stimulates ketogenesis and gluconeogenesis.[128] Such alterations in intermediary metabolism may be particularly deleterious in chronically or acutely ill hemodialysis patients who are malnourished or receiving a medication like propranolol that is provocative for hypoglycemia.[129, 130] These effects are ameliorated by the use of a normoglycemic dialysate. Additional metabolic consequences occurring from the use of a glucose-free dialysate include an accelerated loss of free amino acids into the dialysate,[131] a decline in serum amino acids,[132] and enhanced $K^+$ clearance because of relative hypoinsulinemia.[128] Therefore, the dialysate glucose concentration should be maintained at normoglycemic concentrations.

#### Sodium

Historically, the dialysate $Na^+$ concentration was maintained at hypo-osmolal levels (<135 mEq/L) to prevent interdialytic hypertension, exaggerated thirst, and excessive weight gains. However, the use of a hyponatric dialysate enhances intradialytic hypotension, cramps, headaches, nausea, and vomiting and is provocative for the dialysis disequilibrium syndrome.[133-137] During conventional hemodialysis with a hyponatric dialysate, or during the clearance phase of sequential ultrafiltration-clearance, the decline in extracellular volume exceeds the volume ultrafiltered. As solute is removed from the extracellular compartment, there is a relative increase in intracellular osmolality that drives transcellular volume movement.[138] These hemodynamic alterations are absent in the setting of equal dialysate and serum $Na^+$ concentrations. Thus, there has been an appropriate increase in the dialysate $Na^+$ concentration to 140 to 145 mEq/L.

Unfortunately, an increase in the dialysate $Na^+$ concentration can result in polydipsia and increased interdialytic weight gains.[135] However, the enhanced capacity to ultrafilter these patients permits ready management of this problem. The pressor response to an increased dialysate $Na^+$ concentration is variable. In patients who are hypertensive

because of hyperreninemia during ultrafiltration, a higher dialysate $Na^+$ concentration may be associated with a reduction in blood pressure. However, most patients exhibit no increment in blood pressure with a physiologic dialysate $Na^+$ concentration.[135] A minority of patients are typically hypertensive at baseline, and they will have worsened pressor control with a higher dialysate $Na^+$ concentration.[133, 136]

The newer dialysate delivery systems permit the active alteration of the $Na^+$ concentration during a session by the use of variable-dilution proportioning systems. The technique of ''sodium modeling'' to fit the patient's hemodynamic needs has been espoused as a means of accomplishing optimal blood pressure support without increased thirst at the completion of the treatment. The alteration in the dialysate $Na^+$ concentration can occur in two patterns. It may be performed in a ''step'' in which the dialysate $Na^+$ concentration is initially high (>145 mEq/L) and during the second half of the dialysis session is promptly reduced (≤135 mEq/L), or it may be reduced as a linear ''gradient'' from more than 145 to 135 mEq/L or less.[139, 140] Although sodium modeling reduces the frequency of hypotension during ultrafiltration without a decrease in time committed to diffusive clearance, as is the case with sequential ultrafiltration-clearance, it is unclear whether this technique offers any advantage over a fixed dialysate $Na^+$ concentration of 140 to 145 mEq/L.[141, 142] Further, interdialytic weight gains appear unaffected by sodium modeling.[139-141] Therefore, it seems that for most hemodialysis patients, the dialysate $Na^+$ concentration should be maintained at 140 to 145 mEq/L.

#### Potassium

Unlike urea, which usually behaves like a solute distributed in a single pool with a variable volume of distribution,[143] only 1% to 2% of the 3000 to 3500 mEq of $K^+$ is present in the extracellular space.[144] The flux of $K^+$ from the intracellular compartment to the extracellular space, and subsequently across the dialysis membrane to the dialysate compartment, is unequal. Therefore, the efficacy of $K^+$ removal in hemodialysis is highly variable, difficult to predict, and influenced by dialysis-specific and patient-specific factors.[145] In a study that controlled for dialyzer-specific components of the dialysis procedure (blood and dialysate flow, dialyzer type and surface area, duration of dialysis, dialysate composition), $K^+$ removal varied by approximately 70%. Even for the same patient, approximately 20% variability in $K^+$ removal was noted with the same hemodialysis prescription.[94]

During hemodialysis, approximately 70% of the $K^+$ removed is derived from the intracellular compartment.[128] In that 50 to 80 mEq of $K^+$ is removed in a single dialysis session, and only 15 to 20 mEq of $K^+$ is present in the plasma, life-threatening hypokalemia would be the consequence of dialysis if this were not the case.[145] However, the volume of distribution of $K^+$ is not constant. Paradoxically, the greater the total body $K^+$ content, the lower its volume of distribution.[146] The practical consequence of these observations is that the fractional decline in the plasma $K^+$ concentration during a single dialysis session will be greater if the prehemodialysis $K^+$ concentration is higher. Therefore, optimal $K^+$ elimination by hemodialysis is accomplished by daily short hemodialysis treatments instead of protracted sessions every other day. The transfer of $K^+$ from the intracellular compartment to the extracellular compartment usually occurs at a slower rate than the transfer from the plasma across the dialysis membrane.[146, 147] This discrepancy further complicates predicting the quantity of $K^+$ removed during hemodialysis. A practical consequence of these discordant transfer rates is that the plasma $K^+$ level measured immediately after the completion of hemodialysis is approximately 30% less than the steady-state value measured after 5 hours. Therefore, hypokalemia defined immediately after the completion of hemodialysis should not be treated.

The transcellular distribution of $K^+$ is influenced by several variables, including the relative degree of hyperinsulinemia (promotes $K^+$ uptake into cells and lowers its intradialytic clearance),[128] catecholamine tone (β-agonists promote cellular uptake of $K^+$ and α-agonists stimulate the cellular egress of $K^+$—attenuate and increase the intradialytic clearance of $K^+$, respectively),[144, 148] $Na^+$,$K^+$-ATPase activity (pharmacologic inhibition diminishes $K^+$ uptake into cells, which may enhance intradialytic clearance),[149] and systemic pH (alkalemia augments transcellular $K^+$ uptake, which may diminish dialytic clearance of $K^+$).[144] Surprisingly, although the degree of systemic alkalization is greater and more rapid in onset with $HCO_3^-$-buffered dialysates than with acetate-buffered dialysates, the choice of buffer does not appear to be critical in determining $K^+$ removal during hemodialysis.[128, 150] Paradoxically, it has been observed that as the gradient for $K^+$ clearance from blood into the dialysate is increased by decreasing the dialysate $K^+$ concentration, the uptake of $HCO_3^-$ from the dialysate declines.[151] This interaction between alkali and $K^+$ in the dialysate is sizable: a 1-mEq increase in the $K^+$ gradient results in a decline in $HCO_3^-$ dialysance of 50 mEq and should not be overlooked in planning the dialysate prescription for patients being dialyzed for severe acidosis.

The selection of the dialysate $K^+$ concentration is empirical, and a $K^+$ concentration of 1 to 3 mEq/L is used for most patients. For patients who have excessive potassium loads from their diet, medications, hemolysis, trauma, or gastrointestinal bleeding, the dialysate $K^+$ concentration should be 0 to 1 mEq/L. For stable patients who are without significant cardiac disease or are not taking cardiac glycosides, a dialysate $K^+$ concentration of 2 to 3 mEq/L is appropriate. In the setting of a history of cardiac disease, especially with arrhythmias and cardiac glycoside usage, the dialysate $K^+$ concentration should be increased to 3 to 4 mEq/L.[152] These patients are at the greatest risk for the development of dysrhythmias. They are best managed by tolerating a greater degree of interdialytic hyperkalemia so that they may be exposed to a higher dialysate $K^+$ concentration.

Most of the cardiac morbidity that arises from the dialysate $K^+$ concentration occurs during the first half of the dialysis session. The rapidity of the fall in the plasma $K^+$ concentration, rather than the absolute plasma concentration, determines the risk of cardiac arrhythmias.[147, 152] For this reason, hyperkalemic patients should be managed by an incremental decline in the dialysate $K^+$ concentration of approximately 1 mEq/L/h.[153] If the patient has a significant deficit in total body $K^+$ content, postdialysis hypokalemia can occur, even if the dialysate $K^+$ concentration is greater than the serum $K^+$ concentration.[154] This seemingly contradictory situation arises because of the potential for a delayed conductance of $K^+$ from the dialysate into the patient, in comparison to its movement from the extracellular space into the intracellular compartment.

## Bases

$HCO_3^-$ was initially used as the buffer in the dialysate. However, in the early 1960s, acetate was substituted because of its stability in aqueous solution at neutral pH in the presence of divalent cations. Acetate is metabolized in skeletal muscle, and to a lesser extent in the liver, to acetyl coenzyme A, which is subsequently metabolized further by the Krebs cycle to carbon dioxide and water. In the latter process, one $H^+$ is consumed, and one molecule of $HCO_3^-$ is liberated.[155] During conventional hemodialysis with large surface area dialyzers, acetate flux of 300 mmol/h or more can occur, resulting in acetate accumulation as the amount translocated exceeds the capacity to metabolize the base. Even greater amounts of acetate may be conducted across the dialysis membrane during high-flux hemodialysis. This complication occurs most often in women, elderly patients, and patients who are malnourished.[156] The resultant clinical consequences of acetate accumulation include variable degrees of nausea, vomiting, headache, fatigue, peripheral vasodilatation, decreased myocardial contractility, metabolic acidosis, and arterial hypoxemia.[142, 157–162] Therefore, it is not surprising that vascular instability is more of a problem with acetate-buffered dialysates than with $HCO_3^-$-buffered dialysates. The hemodynamic instability with acetate is worsened by hyponatric dialysates and is lessened with a normonatric dialysate.[160, 163, 164]

Hemodialysis using an $HCO_3^-$-buffered dialysate prevents these complications. The paradoxical anion gap metabolic acidosis associated with acetate dialysis occurs because the intradialytic loss of $HCO_3^-$ from blood into the dialysate exceeds the patient's capacity to generate alkali from metabolized acetate. A raised $HCO_3^-$ concentration in the dialysate attenuates the diffusive gradient for $HCO_3^-$ from blood to dialysate. Likewise, dialysis-induced hypoxemia is attenuated by an $HCO_3^-$ dialysate. During hemodialysis with acetate, there is a large diffusive loss of carbon dioxide into the dialysate such that the minute ventilation falls by approximately 25%. Therefore, despite the loss of carbon dioxide across the dialytic circuit, there is little decline in the arterial carbon dioxide tension. During hemodialysis with acetate, hypoxemia is most prominent during the first 60 minutes of hemodialysis and may be associated with a decline of 35 mm Hg or less in arterial oxygen tension.[165, 166] These issues are discussed in greater detail later.

Because of the amelioration of many intradialytic symptoms with $HCO_3^-$-buffered dialysate and the increased use of high-efficiency and high-flux hemodialysis, acetate is used for hemodialysis in less than 10% of the dialysis facilities in the United States.[98] $HCO_3^-$ dialysis is now feasible because of the widespread availability of single-patient proportioning systems that permit mixing of the two separate concentrates containing sodium bicarbonate and an acid concentrate that contains the divalent cations close to the entry point of the final dialysate into the dialyzer.[12] A small amount of acetic acid (3 to 6 mEq/L) is present in the acid concentrate; this serves to titrate some of the $HCO_3^-$ to carbonic acid and carbon dioxide, which controls the pH of the final dialysate. Less frequently, $HCO_3^-$ can be provided by a central delivery system, which is less costly but severely compromises the individualization of dialysate solutions.

Unlike the more acidic and hyperosmolal acetate-buffered dialysate, liquid $HCO_3^-$ concentrate and reconstituted $HCO_3^-$ dialysate support the growth of gram-negative bacteria (such as *Pseudomonas, Acinetobacter, Flavobacterium,* and *Achromobacter*), filamentous fungi, and yeast.[103] Because of the propensity of the dialysate to support bacterial growth and the morbidity associated with the presence of such growth in the dialysate, strict guidelines exist for the acceptable limit of bacterial growth and for the presence of lipopolysaccharide in the dialysate and dialyzer reuse system.[102] Other potential complications of the use of an $HCO_3^-$-buffered dialysate are mixing errors, which can produce a highly acidic or alkaline dialysate. It should be appreciated that the initial costs of $HCO_3^-$ dialysis are greater than for acetate. Dialysis machines that perform $HCO_3^-$ dialysis are more costly, and two dialysate concentrates are necessary. However, the lessened intradialytic morbidity of patients offsets any immediate financial disadvantages of this technique and has not diminished its increasing popularity with patients and dialysis facility providers.[98]

An $HCO_3^-$-buffered dialysate of 30 to 35 mEq/L should be used, if available. $HCO_3^-$ concentrations greater than 35 mEq/L may result in the development of a metabolic alkalosis with secondary hypoventilation, hypercapnia, and hypoxemia. If $HCO_3^-$ is unavailable, acetate at an equivalent concentration is suitable, but large surface area dialyzers or dialyzers with high-efficiency or high-flux performance cannot be used.

### Calcium

Patients with renal failure are susceptible to hypocalcemia, hyperphosphatemia, hypovitaminosis D, and hyperparathyroidism (see later). Therefore, positive $Ca^{2+}$ balance is desired during hemodialysis as an adjunct to control of metabolic bone disease.[167–169] In the setting of renal failure requiring dialysis, 61% of the $Ca^{2+}$ is not bound to plasma proteins and is in a diffusible equilibrium during hemodialysis.[170] Assuming free conductance of $Ca^{2+}$ across the dialysis membrane due to diffusive clearance and an additional contribution from convective losses, a dialysate $Ca^{2+}$ concentration of 3.5 mEq/L (7.0 mg/dL) or greater is necessary to prevent intradialytic $Ca^{2+}$ losses.[171, 172] Because such elevated $Ca^{2+}$ dialysates transiently induce hypercalcemia that temporarily reduces parathyroid hormone (PTH) secretion,[173] they were the standard for dialysate $Ca^{2+}$ concentrations until recently. Because of the use of calcium salts as $PO_4^{3-}$ binders, most outpatient dialysis facilities employ a dialysate $Ca^{2+}$ concentration of 2.5 to 3.0 mEq/L. Despite the use of these reduced dialysate $Ca^{2+}$ concen-

trations, some patients are still hypercalcemic between dialysis sessions. The combination of a reduced ingested dose of calcium salt and the inclusion of a small quantity of aluminum hydroxide will minimize the risk of hypercalcemia and treat the hyperphosphatemia.

A reduction in the dialysate $Ca^{2+}$ concentration may increase vascular instability during hemodialysis.[174, 175] Dialysis-induced changes in the serum $Ca^{2+}$ concentration correlate with the intradialytic systolic and diastolic blood pressures. This interaction is due to alterations in left ventricular performance without an accompanying alteration in the peripheral vascular resistance.[176]

### Magnesium

Like $K^+$ concentration, the serum $Mg^{2+}$ concentration is a poor determinant of total body $Mg^+$ stores. Only approximately 1% of the total body $Mg^{2+}$ content is present in the extracellular fluid, and only 60% of this amount (approximately 25 mEq) is free and diffusible.[177] Hemodialysis is the primary route of elimination for $Mg^{2+}$. The $Mg^{2+}$ flux that occurs during a dialysis session is difficult to predict despite knowledge of the serum and dialysate $Mg^{2+}$ concentrations. However, when a low dialysate $Mg^{2+}$ concentration is used, the postdialytic decline in serum $Mg^{2+}$ concentration is virtually resolved after 24 hours.[178]

In that the "ideal" serum $Mg^{2+}$ concentration in patients with ESRD is debated, the appropriate dialysate $Mg^{2+}$ concentration is unresolved. Many centers use a dialysate $Mg^{2+}$ concentration of 1 mEq/L, and mild interdialytic hypermagnesemia is often observed. Although elevated $Mg^{2+}$ concentrations impair bone formation in vitro and in vivo, their clinical significance is unresolved.[177, 179–181] However, the reduction of the dialysate $Mg^{2+}$ concentration to 0.5 mEq/L or less has been reported to improve osteomalacic bone disease and symptoms.

### Chloride

This is the major anion in the dialysate. Because its concentration is defined by the constraints of maintaining electrical neutrality in the dialysate, the $Cl^-$ concentration varies, depending on the concentration of the cations and of $HCO_3^-$ or acetate.

## CONTINUOUS RENAL REPLACEMENT THERAPY

An advantage of continuous arteriovenous hemodialysis and continuous arteriovenous hemodiafiltration over conventional hemodialysis is the absence of complex dialysate delivery systems. Therefore, the costs and the nursing personnel required to perform hemofiltration are less. However, dialysate flow is relatively compromised. Typical dialysate flow rates for hemofiltration or hemodiafiltration are 800 to 1000 mL/h (versus 500 to 800 mL/min for hemodialysis), and usual delivery is by a continuous infusion pump. Because it is impractical to mix and store conventional hemodialysis dialysate for hemofiltration and hemodiafiltration, and the formation of a custom dialysate in the volumes required for these techniques is not feasible, most centers use conventional peritoneal dialysate for CRRT. Despite the routine use of less expensive, commercially prepared peritoneal dialysate, it is this component of the hemofiltration procedure that is responsible for the relatively increased cost in comparison to continuous arteriovenous hemofiltration.[182] In comparison to the dialysates used for hemodialysis, the composition of the peritoneal dialysates is relatively constant. The conventional dialysate $Na^+$ concentration is 140 mEq/L, $K^+$ concentration 0 mEq/L, lactate concentration 35 mEq/L, and $Ca^{2+}$ concentration 3.5 mEq/L. The only additional electrolyte present in the dialysate is $Cl^-$, whose concentration is determined solely by the requirements to achieve electrical neutrality. Dextrose is present in concentrations of 1.5%, 2.5%, and 4.25%.

The need for a custom dialysate for CRRT arises most often in situations in which the $Ca^{2+}$ concentration requires modification or the patient cannot tolerate a lactate-buffered dialysate. Commercial dialysates for peritoneal dialysis are available in only three $Ca^{2+}$ concentrations, 3.5, 3.0, and 2.5 mEq/L. Such a limited selection of dialysates significantly compromises the treatment of hypercalcemic patients by continuous arteriovenous hemodialysis, continuous venovenous hemodialysis, continuous arteriovenous hemodiafiltration, continuous venovenous hemodiafiltration, or peritoneal dialysis. If such circumstances arise, the dialysate should be formulated in an individual fashion with an appropriately reduced $Ca^{2+}$ concentration. The standard lactate buffering of peritoneal dialysates may become a problem for patients with an impaired capacity to metabolize lactate, such as patients with lactic acidosis due to impaired hepatic and renal function and hypotensive patients with ongoing tissue ischemia and tissue lactate generation. In these circumstances, a custom dialysate should be formulated with $HCO_3^-$ as the buffer.

# VASCULAR ACCESS

As discussed earlier, hemodialysis is a viable maintenance therapy for chronic renal failure only if repeated access to the circulation is possible. Frequent infections and thrombosis of the vascular access remain major causes for hospitalization, morbidity, and expense for dialysis patients today. It is estimated that as much as $500 million is spent annually on the placement and maintenance of vascular accesses.[183] The first technical advance in establishing repeated vascular access was the development of the Quinton-Scribner shunt in 1960,[184] which is listed here for historical interest only. This external shunt was made of Silastic tubing connected to Teflon cannulas. The Quinton-Scribner shunt was usable immediately but unfortunately suffered many of the complications that plague vascular access options today. Typically, it lasted for approximately 6 months. The primary (or endogenous) arteriovenous fistula was the next significant advance for vascular access,[185] but many patients had inadequate veins for the creation of a primary arteriovenous fistula. This led to a series of reports in the late 1960s and 1970s of techniques for creating graft fistulas with autogenous saphenous veins, human umbilical veins, and bovine carotid arteries.[186, 187] The most recent

development for establishing long-term vascular access is the use of a synthetic graft composed of expanded polytetrafluoroethylene (PTFE).[188, 189] In more recent years, patients with vascular access failure have also been treated with surgically implanted, flexible, cuffed double-lumen catheters.[190, 191] Controlled long-term studies comparing permanent catheters with other access modalities have not been reported. Table 56–6 summarizes forms of access to the circulation.

The early placement of arteriovenous fistulas prevents loss of forearm veins and allows time for the healing and maturation of a fistula. This should generally occur when the creatinine clearance is less than 15 mL/min. Early fistula or graft placement also minimizes the need for temporary percutaneous access to the circulation and its attendant complications.

## Arteriovenous Shunt

The arteriovenous shunt is not discussed in detail because it is no longer used. The relatively limited life span of the shunt and the high risk of infection are the major reasons these shunts are no longer used. The complications of clotting and infection are discussed later. Detailed analysis of shunts such as the Scribner shunt can be found elsewhere.[192]

## Temporary and Semipermanent Catheters

Percutaneous femoral, subclavian, or internal jugular vein catheterization is a useful method for immediate but

**TABLE 56–6. Access to the Circulation for Dialysis***

**Percutaneous Venous Catheter**
Femoral vein (temporary)
Subclavian vein (temporary or semipermanent)
Internal jugular vein (temporary or semipermanent)

**External Arteriovenous Shunt**
Radial artery → cephalic vein (Quinton-Scribner)†

**Arteriovenous Fistula**
*Endogenous ("native vein")*
Radial artery → cephalic vein (Brescia-Cimino)
Ulnar artery → basilic vein
Brachial artery → cephalic or brachial vein
Femoral artery → saphenous vein (saphenous loop)†
*Prosthetic*
Materials
  Polytetrafluoroethylene (Gore-Tex or Impra)
  Dacron†
  Human umbilical cord†
  Bovine artery†
Location
  Forearm straight (radial artery → cephalic or brachial vein)
  Forearm loop (brachial artery → cephalic or brachial vein)
  Upper arm (brachial artery → axillary vein or subclavian vein)
  Thigh (femoral artery → femoral or saphenous vein)

*→ = artery-to-vein anastomosis.
†Now infrequently used for angioaccess.

temporary access to the circulation. Double-lumen Silastic catheters or two single-lumen catheters in different locations can be inserted at the bedside by the Seldinger technique into either the superior or inferior vena cava through one of these three sites. This form of access is usually intended for use for short-term dialysis until more permanent access is placed or matures. There is growing concern that placement of these catheters may predispose to the later development of subclavian vein or superior vena cava thrombosis or stenosis. Because of the increased risk for infection and the potentially severe complications associated with the placement of these catheters, the use of percutaneous catheters should be minimized by appropriate planning of the dialysis access.

The subclavian vein is generally more difficult to cannulate than either the internal jugular or femoral vein and is associated with more potential complications. Acute complications from subclavian insertions include inadvertent puncture of the subclavian artery, superior vena cava perforation, pneumothorax, and hemothorax. Injury to the thoracic duct has also been reported.[193] However, the subclavian vein location has the advantage of allowing the patient to ambulate and therefore permits dialysis on an outpatient basis. The femoral vein is easier to cannulate, with fewer potential complications (traumatic arteriovenous fistulas, retroperitoneal hemorrhage, femoral vein thrombosis, and local infection). However, femoral vein catheterization does require hospitalization because the patient cannot ambulate, and the patency of the catheter must be maintained with an infusion of heparin. Another option is to place a new femoral catheter with each dialysis, but this increases the risk of complications and requires the catheter to be removed at the completion of each treatment. Internal jugular catheterization can be done at the bedside, but this location is uncomfortable for the patients.

The semipermanent cuffed double-lumen catheter has become an option for patients who have no other access sites or for patients waiting for grafts or fistulas to mature (usually weeks to several months). These catheters are typically inserted in an operating room by tunneling the catheter subcutaneously through the upper chest wall. Long-term use of semipermanent catheters for at least 4 years is possible.[194] However, the long-term follow-up for large numbers of such patients is not available. Obviously, the need for some semipermanent catheters can be minimized if the patient has permanent access placed well in advance of needing hemodialysis. The internal jugular vein is most often used for semipermanent catheter location, but the subclavian vein can also be used. The long-term sequelae of semipermanent catheters in the subclavian vein are those associated with temporary catheters. Long-term use of these catheters has not been extensively evaluated, but a favorable comparison with primary and secondary fistulas has been reported after 2 years. The observed patency was 57.7% for primary grafts, 48% for secondary grafts, and 43% for catheters.[195]

Other problems with semipermanent catheters include initial nonfunction (~9%), thrombosis, poor blood flows, exit site infections, and sepsis.[196, 197] Erratic blood flows and clotting of catheters often lead to inadequate hemodialysis. Some success for opening clotted catheters has been reported with the use of thrombolytic agents such as tissue plasminogen activator or urokinase.[198] Urokinase (7500 U in 1.5 mL instilled into each port for 30 minutes) is preferred because of cost benefits, and it is well tolerated by most patients. There is an increased risk of bleeding if the instilled agent is inadvertently delivered to the circulation. Unfortunately, clotted catheters often require multiple treatments with fibrinolytic agents, and poor blood flows often persist. In a single report, aspirin or warfarin has been used in conjunction with occasional urokinase treatment to keep internal jugular catheters functioning. During an 8-month period, among 25 patients, catheter patency was maintained, but there was clinically significant bleeding in 5 of these patients, including 1 death.[199]

There is a greatly increased risk of local venous thrombosis and stenosis from central venous catheters. Both subclavian and internal jugular venous catheters are associated with increased risk of thrombosis of the superior vena cava and superior vena cava syndrome.[200–202] Most central vein obstructions are successfully managed with angioplasty and fibrinolysis.[203] Several studies have shown that the internal jugular vein has a lower frequency of venous stenosis than the subclavian vein (0% to 10% and ~40% to 50%, respectively)[204, 205] and a lower overall complication rate.[206] Subclavian catheter–related infections have been reported to be a major risk factor for the later development of subclavian vein thrombosis.[207] Other risk factors for subclavian stenosis include previous use of multiple catheters and possibly high blood flows from fistulas on the ipsilateral side.[197, 208]

Local and systemic infections remain a major risk with percutaneous catheters. The frequency of positive bacterial cultures from catheters may be as high as 55%, with skin flora (primarily *Staphylococcus aureus* and *Staphylococcus epidermidis*) accounting for about 50% of the positive cultures.[209] *Pseudomonas* and *Escherichia coli* are also frequent causes of infection. Although the systemic manifestations of the infections are not subtle, the percutaneous entry site is often without signs of infection. Most cases of catheter infection require removal of the catheter, but replacement over a guide wire may be adequate for semipermanent catheters.[210] Successful treatment of catheter-related sepsis without removal of the catheter has been reported.[211]

## Arteriovenous Fistula

### ENDOGENOUS FISTULA

Endogenous or native vein fistulas are uniformly recommended as the best permanent access because of lower frequencies of stenosis, thrombosis, and infection.[212–215] The basic native vein fistula requires only an adequate vein and artery sufficiently close to each other for anastomosis. The most commonly used site is at the wrist, connecting the cephalic vein to the radial artery (Brescia-Cimino fistula) or the basilic vein to the ulnar artery. Modifications of the forearm fistula placed distally in the snuff-box have been reported.[216] Fistulas can also be constructed between the brachial artery and cephalic vein of the upper arm or between the saphenous vein and the side of the femoral artery (saphenous loop).[186, 217] Saphenous vein loops are no longer considered a first choice for fistula placement because of their higher frequency of infection and thrombosis in comparison to upper arm fistulas. Saphenous loops remain an option for patients who have failed all upper extremity fistula placements.

Most endogenous fistulas require 6 to 12 weeks of maturation before becoming usable.[212] During this period, vein walls thicken and the diameter increases. The most frequent postoperative problem is mild pain. Edema, if present, usually responds to arm elevation within 1 to 2 weeks. Failure of native vein fistulas to mature, early thrombosis, and inadequate flows are the most common reasons for arteriovenous fistulas to fail (8% to 24%).[212, 215] Other short-term complications include fingertip ischemia due to vascular insufficiency, particularly in diabetic patients ("steal syndrome"), and hand swelling distal to the fistula. Long-term problems include aneurysm formation and rarely high-output cardiac failure. These complications may necessitate removal or modification of the fistula. Infections (usually with *Staphylococcus*) need to be treated promptly and aggressively at the first indication of infection (early erythema, inflammation) with intravenous antibiotics. Advanced infections inevitably lead to loss of the fistula.

### GRAFT FISTULA

Prosthetic grafts composed of PTFE are the most commonly used secondary or prosthetic arteriovenous fistulas. These are the most common type of access placed today, accounting for more than 80% of all permanent angioaccess.[183] There appear to be fewer complications and easier management of infections in these grafts, compared with bovine carotid arteries or Dacron as an access material. If a localized infection is present, infected PTFE grafts may be saved surgically by excision of the infected segment. This strategy is not possible for bovine carotid artery or endogenous fistulas. When PTFE is compared with native vein fistulas, there is no difference in patency rates during the first year.[218] However, native vein fistulas that develop without early complications are usually free of complications for many years thereafter. The lack of difference in patency rates within the first year between PTFE and native vein may reflect selection of patients. Patients with marginal vasculature typically have an endogenous fistula attempted first.

Several risk factors for fistula complications have been identified by analysis of Medicare's ESRD data. These factors include female sex, African-American race, age older than 64 years, and underlying diabetes mellitus.[219] Platelet aggregation may be abnormal in patients with diabetes mellitus, owing in part to elevated levels of von Willebrand factor that predispose to vascular disease and thrombosis. Prosthetic grafts are associated with higher rates of thrombosis and stenosis. Erythropoietin's relationship to access thrombosis is unclear (see later). The Canadian Erythropoietin Study Group found a 14% frequency of fistula thrombosis for PTFE grafts in a period of 28 weeks versus 2.5% in placebo-treated control subjects. Erythropoietin shortens the bleeding time and may alter platelet aggregation and adhesion as well as alter levels of proteins C and S.[183]

However, other studies have failed to find an increased frequency of thrombosis for patients receiving erythropoietin.[220, 221] Another risk factor for access thrombosis was a serum albumin concentration less than 3.0 g/dL, which resulted in a 2.7 times greater risk of fistula thrombosis.[222]

The most frequent anatomic finding in patients with PTFE graft thrombosis is stenosis at the venous anastomosis. Pathologic examination of proximal veins of failed PTFE grafts reveals intimal fibromuscular hyperplasia.[223] Contributing factors to this pathologic process include vessel injury and repair by turbulence from high flows, compliance mismatch between graft materials and the vein, and mechanical stimulation of perivascular tissues at the anastomosis of graft and vessel.[223] It is possible that platelet-derived growth factor or other endothelial growth factors, in combination with shear-induced intimal injury and repair, mediate the undesired proliferative response.[223–225]

### Assessment and Treatment of Access Complications

Assessment of function of the hemodialysis fistula is compromised by the lack of accurate, inexpensive, and noninvasive methods. Monitoring blood flow rates, recirculation measurements (by BUN measurements or thermodilution), Doppler ultrasonography, and the urea reduction ratio have all been used for assessment of fistula function.[183] A blood recirculation of more than 20% (calculated by three-needle technique) in the fistula has been associated with a higher frequency of significant stenosis. At blood flows of 200 to 250 mL/min, increased venous pressures correlate with a higher frequency of access stenosis. However, this relationship is not valid if the blood flows are 400 mL/min or greater. The lack of a single reliable noninvasive parameter for assessing fistula function means that a high index of suspicion must be maintained in reviewing the patient's data. Problems with high venous pressures, prolonged bleeding after removal of the dialysis needles, excessive blood recirculation, or a delivered dialysis therapy that is less than the quantity prescribed must trigger a search for access problems. Although some surgeons prefer to probe the lumen of the graft fistula with a Fogarty catheter to find an obstructing lesion, venograms remain the gold standard for defining fistula anatomy.

The mainstay of treatment for fistula stenosis is surgery; percutaneous transluminal angioplasty is effective in selected cases. Most patients are treated without hospitalization. However, when hospitalization for access dysfunction occurs, the length of hospital stay is prolonged (more than 14 days) for elderly patients, usually because of postoperative fevers, the need for repeated femoral catheterization for angioaccess, and delays in access revision due to concurrent infections.[226] Graft thrombosis usually indicates an underlying anatomic defect, and in most cases an anatomic cause for graft thrombosis can be found. Rarely, episodes of hypotension or intraoperative mechanical obstruction may cause graft thrombosis. The most common abnormality is narrowing at the site of the venous anastomosis, which requires patch angioplasty of a short stenosis or jump grafting of longer stenotic segments.

Angioplasty with or without urokinase is another option for managing graft thrombosis, especially if the stenotic area is proximal to the venous anastomosis and along the thoracic vasculature. When fibrinolysis is performed with angioplasty of the underlying stenotic region, 50% of fistulas remain patent for 1 year.[227] The anatomy can often be defined, and the stenosis dilated, during the same procedure. The standard criterion for lesions amenable to angioplasty is the presence of a concentric stenosis of less than 4 cm in length. Technical success, defined as a visible reduction in the stenosis, is reported 80% to 94% of the time. Continued patency rates after angioplasty range from 41% to 76% after 6 months and 31% to 45% after 12 months. Repeated angioplasty resulted in success rates similar to the initial attempt.[228–230] One retrospective and nonrandomized study demonstrated similar results of angioplasty and surgery.[231] Vascular stents have been used with success to maintain fistula patency, but no controlled trials with angioplasty and surgery have been reported.[183]

Unfortunately, no completely safe and effective treatment exists to prevent fistula thrombosis and venous stenosis. Antiplatelet drugs, including aspirin, sulfinpyrazone, and ticlopidine, have been evaluated for possible roles in preventing thrombosis of the angioaccess. Low-dose aspirin alone (160 mg/d) may be beneficial, whereas the combination of aspirin with sulfinpyrazone may be efficacious but is complicated by an unacceptably high bleeding rate.[232] A randomized trial showed some benefit of dipyridamole alone, but no benefit from aspirin alone or aspirin plus dipyridamole.[233] Little objective information is available about the benefits of long-term anticoagulation with warfarin (Coumadin). Although warfarin is popular with some physicians, its unproven benefits must be weighed against the risks of long-term systemic anticoagulation in the relatively high risk population.

In summary, vascular access remains the ''Achilles heel'' for many hemodialysis patients. The initial management goal should be the meticulous preservation of veins in the arms early in the patient's course to facilitate the creation and maturation of an endogenous arteriovenous fistula. Early generation of the fistula is essential to allow maturation and may permit avoidance of a temporary angioaccess. If catheters must be used for short-term angioaccess, the internal jugular vein appears to be a better site than the subclavian vein. Alternatively, early cannulation (within 48 hours) of PTFE graft fistulas may eliminate the need for percutaneous catheters in some patients but is undesirable. Early cannulation of PTFE grafts has been reported without serious complications through the first month of use, although long-term follow-up of graft function is not known.[234] Unfortunately, the majority of patients do not have suitable venous vasculature for endogenous fistulas, but newer materials and better understanding of the pathophysiologic reasons for secondary graft complications may allow longer, less troublesome graft survival. In the unfortunate situation in which the patient has no vasculature in either upper or lower extremities for the generation of angioaccess, the patient can be converted to peritoneal dialysis or undergo emergent renal transplantation if otherwise fit.

# ORGAN SYSTEM ABNORMALITIES IN HEMODIALYSIS

Many of the effects of uremia on organ systems and their adaptation to compromised renal function are discussed in other chapters in this textbook. We focus on those abnormalities that persist in the dialysis patient or that are accentuated by the hemodialysis procedure. In addition to the effects of dialysis, organ system abnormalities interplay one on the other. For example, abnormalities in lipid metabolism and the presence of hypertension accentuate cardiovascular abnormalities; dysfunction in the gastrointestinal tract accentuates malnutrition, which in turn affects endocrine function and cardiovascular function. Most, but not all, organ system abnormalities improve with adequate hemodialysis. For example, lipid abnormalities, sexual dysfunction, sleep disorders, restless leg syndrome, pruritus, anemia, immune dysfunction, and parathyroid disease typically persist despite the initiation of dialysis. However, some of these disorders may be improved with supplemental therapeutic modalities, such as erythropoietin for anemia and 1,25-dihydroxycholecalciferol for hyperparathyroidism. Alternatively, several organ system disorders may be intensified by dialysis or its related treatments. Aluminum-induced osteomalacia occurs from aluminum contamination of the dialysate or with the ingestion of aluminum hydroxide. Malnutrition occurs from intradialytic amino acid losses and increased catabolism. Muscle cramps and hypotension are related to volume depletion. Gastrointestinal complications may occur from anticoagulation. Neurologic disorders, such as the dialysis dementia syndrome and dialysis disequilibrium, are related to aluminum intoxication and to cerebral edema, respectively. Because of the complexities of the interrelationships of the various organ systems with uremia and hemodialysis, it is important that the physician providing care for these patients be knowledgeable about the numerous ramifications of the absence of excretory and endocrine functions of the kidney. Indeed, the nephrologist who cares for the dialysis patient practices ''anephric'' internal medicine. For these reasons, it is advisable that nephrologists be primary physicians for patients undergoing maintenance hemodialysis.

## Metabolic Abnormalities

All metabolic functions in the long-term dialysis patient are severely affected if malnutrition is present. In the past 30 years, there has been a growing appreciation of the severity and importance of malnutrition in this population. Numerous studies reporting metabolic abnormalities have not always considered the nutritional state of the patient in evaluating various abnormal pathophysiologic processes. Throughout the discussions of protein, carbohydrate, and lipid metabolism, the role of protein and calorie intake and loss must be considered.

### PROTEIN ABNORMALITIES

Numerous studies have demonstrated disorders of protein metabolism in uremia. The pathobiology of protein metabolism is reviewed in Chapter 49. Many of the abnormalities in protein metabolism associated with chronic renal failure persist in patients undergoing hemodialysis. The quantities of various essential and nonessential amino acids and their various ratios are altered in plasma,[235–239] muscle,[74, 240] and red blood cells.[241, 242] In addition, the turnover of albumin is altered,[243] which along with many other factors contributes to a decrease in the serum albumin concentration in dialysis patients.[239, 244] These abnormalities in the dialysis patient occur for three major reasons: 1) intradialytic loss of amino acids and proteins, 2) persistent uremia or adverse effects of the dialysis procedure itself on protein metabolism, and 3) decreased intake of protein (and calories).

Patients having dialysis with cellulosic membranes experience recurrent losses of amino acids and protein metabolites during each treatment, averaging 8 to 10 g of amino acid per dialysis session.[245–248] These losses may be increased when a glucose-free dialysate bath is used because of gluconeogenesis.[249] The increasing use of more porous, high-flux dialysis membrane materials suggests the possibility of even greater losses of amino acids.[250] However, no serious consequences of the increase in amino acid loss with the more porous membranes have been observed. In fact, with improved appetite, perhaps related to improved dialysis, there may be an overall positive effect on nutrition.[251] The use of bleach in dialyzer reprocessing may enhance amino acid losses and, in preliminary studies, has been suggested as a factor in amount of protein lost in dialysate.[252] Protein absorption and elution by membranes are other considerations with regard to nutritionally focused selection of a dialysis membrane.[253, 254]

Nitrogen balance studies in hemodialysis patients have demonstrated negative nitrogen balance on dialysis days. When the protein intake is low (~0.5 g/kg/d), cumulative nitrogen balance on both dialysis and nondialysis days remains negative, whereas cumulative nitrogen balance is positive when a protein intake of 1.2 g/kg/d or more is provided.[237, 249, 255, 256] The negative nitrogen balance observed on dialysis days is associated with a higher rate of urea production, which is maximal immediately after dialysis.[249] Negative nitrogen balance with dialysis probably reflects an increased protein catabolic rate.[257–259] This apparent increase in the protein catabolic rate on dialysis days may be a consequence of the elaboration of cytokines, which have a negative impact on nutrition.[260–262] The stimulus for the production of these cytokines may be components of the dialysis procedure, such as the dialysis membrane.[263–265] Arguably, the particular type of dialysis membrane may affect protein metabolism such that biocompatible dialysis membrane materials have a lesser effect.[72, 250, 251] If dialysis is not adequate and the patient remains uremic, the effects of uremia may continue to have an adverse effect on metabolism.[244, 266, 267] In addition to amino acid loss and increased catabolism, there is ample evidence of decreased intake of protein in long-term dialysis patients.[268, 269] These patients have a decreased appetite because of primary anorexia, depression, or medications as well as an inability to obtain a proper diet because of economic or social reasons.[256, 270–272]

All of these factors have led to an awareness of the importance of malnutrition in the dialysis patient. Several studies in large populations of dialysis patients have demonstrated a significant correlation between malnutrition and increased morbidity and mortality.[73, 273–275] For example, the odds risk of death in patients with a serum albumin concentration less than 3.5 g/dL is significantly greater than that in patients with normal albumin levels.[276] Thus, it is extremely important to assess the long-term dialysis patient's state of nutrition. A number of papers have described the essentials of nutritional assessment in the dialysis patient.[277–284] These include more practical assessments, such as a proper physical examination by a physician; assessment by a nutritionist of dietary intake; monitoring of creatinine, BUN, albumin, prealbumin, and transferrin concentrations and the protein catabolic rate; and use of various techniques such as dual-energy x-ray absorptiometry, bioelectrical impedance, and subject global assessment.

In the past 30 years, hemodialysis techniques have improved such that an increase in protein intake and energy intake to 1.2 to 1.4 g/kg/d and 30 to 35 kcal/kg/d, respectively, can be provided without a deterioration in metabolic parameters.[283–287] Despite the observation that energy requirements in dialysis patients are not increased,[288, 289] it is essential that a calorie replacement in the form of carbohydrates and fats be provided to optimize protein metabolism.[290] The maintenance of body weight within 10% of ideal and 20% or less of usual body weight is an important goal.

The compromised spontaneous intake of protein and calories by hemodialysis patients has resulted in the suggestion that supplemental calories and protein be provided.[291, 292] It has been shown that erythropoietin and an increase in hematocrit have beneficial effects on appetite and nutrition.[293] Also, growth hormone has been shown to have a beneficial effect on protein metabolism,[294] and its use may enhance nutrition.[295] Because of the generally poor response to oral supplementation, parenteral protein and calorie supplementation has been considered. Continuous total parenteral nutrition is not a feasible approach in most dialysis patients, but the use of intradialytic parenteral nutrition has been advocated.[296–300] This technique has not been broadly accepted because of the concern for intradialytic amino acid losses that exceed the intake[246] and questions as to its cost-effectiveness. An uncontrolled, retrospective analysis demonstrates that intradialytic parenteral nutrition increases the serum albumin level and may have a beneficial effect on mortality in patients with a serum albumin concentration less than 3.4 g/dL.[301]

In patients with acute renal failure, hypercatabolism due to infection, trauma, surgical stress, and other factors has led to an increased use of parenteral nutrition.[302–307] In many intensive care units, administration of parenteral nutrition with its subsequent fluid burden is the principal indication for initiation of hemodialysis in the patient with marginal renal insufficiency. Most studies have demonstrated improved survival in complicated acute renal failure patients with the use of parenteral nutrition. It is unclear whether these modalities enhance the recovery from acute renal failure.

Several investigations have re-emphasized the usefulness of restricted protein intake in patients with renal disease to slow the progression of renal insufficiency.[308–311] A large multicenter study in the United States, the Modification of Diet in Renal Disease Study, demonstrated the benefit of reduced protein in selected groups of patients.[312] In this rigidly controlled study, patients were treated such that none experienced a decrease in the serum albumin concentration or other evidence of malnutrition. If reduced protein is to be used in patients before hemodialysis, it is essential that they be carefully monitored for evidence of malnutrition. Should the serum albumin concentration or body weight decline or other markers of malnutrition become apparent, deferral of dialysis by restriction of dietary protein is no longer warranted. This is because of increased mortality in the first year of dialysis that is associated with malnutrition.[313] Clearly, the initiation of dialysis with appropriate protein and calorie intake and subsequent transplantation may have a more favorable effect on long-term survival in this population of patients. For a favorable effect on mortality and morbidity, patients require intense scrutiny for protein and calorie malnutrition and the institution of therapeutic strategies to reverse these findings if they become evident.

## CARBOHYDRATE ABNORMALITIES

The presence of hyperglycemia has been well documented in the dialysis patient since early this century. Not all nondiabetic uremic patients exhibit hyperglycemia or the clinical consequences of hyperglycemia, but most patients demonstrate abnormalities with oral and intravenous glucose tolerance testing.[314, 315] Abnormalities in glucose metabolism, specifically hyperinsulinemia, have been suggested to affect lipid metabolism and smooth muscle cell proliferation, resulting in adverse long-term vascular effects.[316] The pathobiologic mechanism for the abnormality in glucose metabolism has been debated. Most investigators have concluded that there is insulin antagonism or relative resistance.[314–318] Although an insulin antagonist has been theorized,[315, 319] there is little evidence for a dialyzable insulin antagonist.[320] Studies have shown there is no defect in the insulin binding in uremia,[321, 322] and the abnormality occurs at a postreceptor step. Glucagon excess is present in uremia and may contribute to the abnormalities in carbohydrate metabolism.[323] In addition, hyperparathyroidism has been suggested to be a factor,[324] perhaps by its effect on cytosolic $Ca^{2+}$, which interferes with insulin secretion.[325]

The effect of hemodialysis on abnormal glucose and insulin metabolism has likewise been debated. There appears to be improvement in the intravenous glucose tolerance test in patients undergoing hemodialysis.[326, 327] However, not all investigators have shown an improvement in glucose metabolism with initiation of dialysis.[328, 329] Glycosylated hemoglobin, $HbA_{1c}$, is not affected by dialysis.[330] The debate over the effect of dialysis on carbohydrate tolerance is complicated by the suggestion that glucose and insulin metabolism may be affected by the adequacy of the dialysis treatment or the dialysis membrane material. This suggestion is supported by the observation that patients treated by hemofiltration have a better response than do those treated by standard dialysis.[331]

Another problem related to abnormalities of carbohydrate metabolism is the spontaneous occurrence of hypoglycemia in dialysis patients.[332–334] Although dialysate lacking glucose causes various metabolic effects,[335, 336] it is not thought to be a cause for hypoglycemia in nondiabetic ESRD patients. Other possible factors include alcohol abuse, drugs, septicemia, metabolic acidosis, and especially malnutrition. Of critical importance is the observation of impaired hepatic gluconeogenesis in many of these patients.[332–334] Hypoglycemia is probably a combination of all of these effects, with minor liver disease and malnutrition as common factors.

Diabetic patients who have renal insufficiency frequently exhibit a decreasing requirement for insulin as renal failure progresses. Insulin catabolism is decreased with advancing renal insufficiency, and an occult decrease in protein and calorie intake further decreases the patient's insulin requirement. Paradoxically, it is well recognized that when diabetic patients start dialysis, their insulin requirements again increase. The few studies of insulin requirements in diabetic patients on dialysis suggest a similar effect for diabetic and nondiabetic patients. Therefore, the augmented insulin requirement may simply be a manifestation of an increase in the patient's calorie intake.

Because of the concurrent problems of retinopathy, neuropathy, gastroparesis, enteropathy, peripheral vascular disease, coronary artery disease, and continued disordered glucose metabolism, the diabetic patient receiving dialysis offers many challenges to the nephrologist. The numerous comorbid conditions that influence glucose metabolism in diabetic patients, their variable and irregularly timed meals, and the intermittent nature of dialysis with a dextrose-containing dialysate make tight glycemic control difficult to achieve. Fasting blood glucose concentrations of approximately 150 to 200 mg/dL and blood glucose concentrations of 200 to 300 mg/dL within 2 hours after eating are acceptable goals. Careful management of insulin dosing considering the dialysis schedule, along with reasonable dietary restrictions and timed meals, is crucial to maximizing glycemic control.

Although hyperosmolar coma due to hyperglycemia occasionally complicates hemodialysis or peritoneal dialysis, the ability to perform ultrafiltration without the use of high dialysate glucose concentrations to induce an osmotic gradient has rendered this complication infrequent. Likewise, ketoacidosis is an infrequent occurrence in long-term dialysis patients in comparison to nonuremic diabetic patients. This may be related to a resistance to lipolysis and the frequent dialysis-dependent correction of acidosis and clearance of β-hydroxybutyrate and acetoacetic acid in these patients. The unexplained occurrence of severe hyperglycemia and ketoacidosis in the dialysis patient is often a sign of concomitant infection. In dialysis patients, one must be mindful of the limits of treating hyperglycemia and ketoacidosis with increased volume. When hyperglycemia and ketoacidosis do occur in dialysis patients, the appropriate therapy consists of an intravenous insulin infusion or frequent subcutaneous doses of insulin without vigorous saline replacement (unless the patient is volume depleted). The need for adequate protein and calorie intake in the dialyzed diabetic patient must be considered when diet is used as a method of glycemic control for the ambulatory patient. Instead, insulin should be used more liberally.

## LIPID ABNORMALITIES

Abnormalities in lipid metabolism are well documented in patients with chronic renal failure.[337–341] This was initially recognized simply as hypertriglyceridemia without an increase in total cholesterol. The specific characteristics of lipid abnormalities have been further defined; an increase was demonstrated in very low density lipoproteins, intermediate-density lipoproteins, and low-density lipoproteins, whereas high-density lipoprotein–cholesterol has generally been found to be decreased.[342–346] In later studies, apolipoprotein abnormalities have been shown to consist of an increase in apo C-III and a decrease in apo A-I and apo A-II; apo B and apo E have been variably increased or decreased.[343, 344, 346] Some of these abnormalities have been attributable to a dialyzable factor that diminishes the activity of lipoprotein lipase and lipolysis after administration of heparin.[347–352] Other considerations in the alteration of lipid metabolism include a decrease in lecithin-cholesterol acyltransferase activity,[353, 354] a defect in low-density lipoprotein receptor function,[355] or delayed clearance of chylomicrons.[356] Attention has been given to lipoprotein Lp(a) as a cause for cardiovascular disease in nonuremic patients. Lp(a) is increased in patients with chronic renal failure and those having dialysis.[357–360] A single study has correlated Lp(a) with an increased frequency of cardiovascular disease in uremic patients,[361] and another investigation has suggested an increase in vascular access thrombosis in the setting of even greater elevations of Lp(a).[362]

In general, it is thought that the lipid abnormalities in the patient with chronic renal insufficiency are not significantly altered by the hemodialysis procedure. However, several confounding factors relevant to the dialysis procedure should be considered. Acetate as a base in the dialysate may be converted by the liver to long-chain fatty acids and cholesterol. However, studies with [$^{14}$C]acetate have demonstrated that the amount of acetate converted to lipids is less than 5% of the total acetate load.[363] In one clinical study, substitution of $HCO_3^-$ for acetate in the dialysate did not result in major alterations in the lipid profile.[364] Thus, the provocative role of acetate in the lipid abnormalities of dialysis is questionable. Glucose concentrations in the dialysate are usually 100 to 200 mg/dL, which is in the physiologic range and generally not thought to substantially increase the carbohydrate load or contribute to the lipid abnormalities. Heparin increases heparin-sensitive lipoprotein lipase action, leading to an increase in low-density lipoprotein–cholesterol and free fatty acids and a decrease in total triglycerides in the plasma of patients during hemodialysis.[365, 366] This improvement in triglyceride clearance with heparin is transient and the magnitude is small. However, it has been suggested that the long-term administration of conventional molecular weight heparin may worsen lipid abnormalities.[367] With use of low-molecular-weight heparin, this problem may be averted.[367–369] Last, the type of dialysis membrane may affect the lipid profile. Several studies have suggested that use of high-flux hemodialysis membrane materials leads to improved lipid profiles.[75, 370] Further studies in larger populations will be necessary to determine the relevance of these preliminary findings.

The management of lipid abnormalities in ESRD depends on the perceived importance of the elevated triglycerides and very low density lipoprotein–cholesterol concentrations, or the low high-density lipoprotein–cholesterol concentration, as risk factors for cardiovascular disease and mortality. Modification of the diet by lowering intake of saturated fats and carbohydrates has been advocated.[371–373] As discussed in the previous sections on carbohydrate and protein metabolism, the effects of inadequate protein and energy consumption that result in malnutrition have a major impact on mortality and morbidity in maintenance dialysis patients. This fact is reflected in several studies that observed hypocholesterolemia is predictive of an increased odds risk of death.[276, 374] Because dialysis patients need to receive adequate protein and energy intake, restriction of carbohydrates and polyunsaturated fats in the interest of decreasing lipid abnormalities is ill-advised. Alternatively, the restriction of saturated fats and high-cholesterol foods may be a reasonable restriction for the maintenance dialysis patient. Carnitine is necessary for fatty acid oxidation, and carnitine deficiency, commonly seen in hemodialysis patients, has been suggested to be a factor in the lipid abnormalities in these patients.[375–378] The administration of oral or intravenous L-carnitine has been shown to have a variable effect on serum triglyceride, total cholesterol, and high-density lipoprotein levels in hemodialysis patients.[376, 379, 380] Although carnitine is inexpensive and has few side effects, it is not used routinely. ω-3 polyunsaturated fatty acids have been advocated for the treatment of hyperlipidemia in nonuremic populations as well as for dialysis patients.[381–383] They have not been well received as a therapeutic tool because of the quantity necessary to affect the lipid levels and their poor tolerance by dialysis patients. Clofibrate, which enhances lipoprotein lipase activity, may also lower triglyceride levels and lead to an increase in high-density lipoprotein–cholesterol.[384] The high frequency of myositis has limited its use. Hydroxymethylglutaryl–coenzyme A reductase inhibitors have been useful in the general population and have been advocated for hemodialysis patients.[385, 386] Likewise, they have been shown to cause myositis and rhabdomyolysis,[387, 388] which has tempered their use in uremic patients. Moreover, the combination of the fibric acid derivative gemfibrozil with lovastatin has been shown to be associated with a higher frequency of myositis and rhabdomyolysis.[389–391] This combination should be avoided, particularly in patients with renal insufficiency. Because hypercholesterolemia is not commonly seen in dialysis patients, and the contributing role of hypertriglyceridemia alone to cardiovascular disease is unclear, the risks and benefits of these drugs for the treatment of hyperlipidemia in renal failure must be weighed carefully.

## ABNORMALITIES OF VITAMIN METABOLISM

Supplementation of water-soluble vitamins has been recommended in hemodialysis patients because of altered function of enzyme systems, dietary restrictions, and their possible loss across the dialyzer.[392–394] Although one study of granulocyte, erythrocyte, and plasma levels of B vitamins did not support a deficiency,[395] and another longitudinal study of patients dialyzed without vitamin supplementation questioned the need for replacements,[396] most studies have recommended replacement of water-soluble B vitamins. This position is based on deficiencies observed along with selected pathologic findings in dialysis patients.[397, 398] By use of enzymatic methods, vitamin $B_6$ (pyridoxine) deficiency was documented in dialysis patients not receiving supplementation.[399–402] This deficiency was thought to be due to decreased intake rather than clearance of the vitamin. The necessity of folic acid supplementation has been questioned because folic acid levels have been found to be normal in dialysis patients not taking folic acid supplementation for more than 6 months.[403, 404] Although it is possible that folic acid supplementation is not required in patients with good nutritional balance and who are not taking medications that inhibit folic acid synthesis, many dialysis patients have low intakes of appropriate foodstuffs. Therefore, folic acid deficiency may occur in the absence of supplements. The appropriate dose of folic acid may be considerably less than the 1 mg/d previously recommended.[394]

Histidine supplementation has been advocated in maintenance dialysis patients to improve anemia,[405, 406] but this supplementation is controversial. Likewise, biotin has been reported to improve several neurologic disorders in a small number of patients[407] but has not been widely and universally prescribed. In general, assays for water-soluble B vitamins are cumbersome and not clinically accessible. In addition, the toxic/therapeutic ratio of most of these vitamins is wide. Therefore, supplementation of water-soluble B vitamins would seem to be reasonable, possibly beneficial, and not harmful.

With the exception of vitamin D, the lipid-soluble vitamins do not appear to be depleted in dialysis patients. In fact, vitamin A may accumulate in dialysis patients and has been incriminated as being partly responsible for premature atherosclerosis and retinal problems.[408–411] In one study, vitamin A concentrations were not found to be increased in the liver, stomach, bone, and subcutaneous adiposity of dialysis patients.[412] Nevertheless, supplementation of vitamin A in dialysis patients is not recommended. Supplementation of vitamins E and K has not been routinely recommended, although we are unaware of studies in uremic or dialysis patients. The metabolism of vitamin D and its supplementation are discussed in Chapter 51.

Vitamin C concentrations were initially thought to be low in dialysis patients and were correlated with symptoms of scurvy.[413] However, later studies have suggested that it should not be administered unless levels are measurably low; large doses of vitamin C may be associated with hyperoxalemia.[414]

## Endocrine Abnormalities

In view of the various hormonal functions normally performed by the kidney and the effect of decreased renal function on endocrine physiology, it is not surprising that uremia affects the endocrine system profoundly. Increases in the plasma levels of endogenous opioid peptides, which act as neurotransmitters, may contribute to the pathogenesis of endocrine abnormalities in ESRD.[415] Changes in synthe-

sis, metabolism, biologic activity, and secretion of the various hormones occur with uremia and hemodialysis,[416–418] and these alterations have their most dramatic ramifications in children.[419–421] In part, some of the symptoms of uremia may be due to endocrine disorders. On the other hand, uremia may mimic endocrinopathies or interfere with various assays of endocrine function.

Because of variable results, the measurement of tropic hormones in uremia has been a problem. This observation may be a consequence of variations in study design and interpretation and has caused confusion in assessing the extent of pituitary dysfunction in dialysis patients. Growth hormone[422–424] and prolactin[425, 426] have been shown to be increased in uremic patients, and their hypothalamic-hypophysial regulation is impaired.[427–430] During dialysis, plasma growth hormone levels transiently fall to low-normal values[431] but overall remain elevated. This may be an effect of acetate in the dialysate. Despite elevated growth hormone levels, there is little evidence of its effect, even in children. In fact, children with ESRD are typically growth impaired.

Vasoactive hormones have been difficult to analyze in uremic and dialysis patients because of the multiple effects of volume, blood pressure, and uremia. Plasma cortisol levels have been reported as both normal[416, 432] and elevated.[432–442] However, the diurnal variation of cortisol, in response to corticotropin, has been shown to be normal in dialysis patients.[432, 443] The hypothalamic-pituitary-adrenal axis has been shown to be abnormal with a blunted response to corticotropin-releasing hormone.[433–435] Generally, corticotropin and plasma cortisol respond to corticotropin-releasing hormone, but in a reduced manner in comparison to healthy subjects. Dexamethasone causes normal suppression of cortisone; however, there is no increase in plasma cortisol or corticotropin level in response to insulin-induced hypoglycemia.[436] One study suggests that corticotropin-releasing hormone levels are reduced by dialysis.[436] Cortisol binding to cortisol-binding globulin is normal,[437] but cortisol may be abnormally bound to albumin.[438] These effects of uremia and hemodialysis make it difficult to diagnose Cushing disease or other pituitary-adrenal disorders in patients with renal failure.[439] Plasma cortisol and corticotropin levels are reported to rise during dialysis, remain elevated until the end of the procedure, and gradually return to normal within 24 hours.[416] This may reflect changes in plasma volume and increased cortisol turnover during dialysis or activation of the complement system. These studies suggest that the variability in tropic hormones may be responses to end-organ abnormalities caused by renal failure and that dialysis may improve these abnormal pituitary responses. Other investigations suggest a primary effect of renal failure on the hypothalamic-hypophysial-pituitary axis.[435, 440]

Hemodialysis patients are reported to have overactivity of the sympathetic nervous system.[441] However, epinephrine levels have not been shown to be increased in uremic patients.[444] Plasma catecholamine levels in patients with mild renal insufficiency were reported to be greater than in normal control subjects, but urinary catecholamine and vanillylmandelic acid concentrations were normal.[442] In more advanced renal failure, the production of norepinephrine and its metabolic clearance were reported to be increased in a single study,[445] whereas others have suggested depressed clearance in both uremic patients and patients having dialysis.[446] It is apparent that epinephrine, norepinephrine, and other hormones such as aldosterone, antidiuretic hormone, atrial natriuretic factor, arginine vasopressin, angiostensin II, and endothelin respond in an appropriate fashion to the intravascular changes that occur with various hemodialytic techniques.[444, 447–457] The role of each of these hormones in the pathophysiologic process of hypertension in the dialysis patient has not been clarified (see later).

As renal failure progresses, premenopausal dialysis patients often cease to experience normal menstrual cycles. Women, like men, have decreased libido and decreased ability to reach orgasm.[458] Low estrogen levels[419, 425, 459] have been reported, and endometrial biopsies demonstrate estrogen depletion. Other studies have demonstrated that ovarian dysfunction is related to abnormalities of suprahypophysial origin[428, 460] with an altered hypothalamic-pituitary-ovarian axis[419, 420] or impaired positive estradiol feedback associated with acyclicity.[426] Elevated prolactin levels[425, 426, 458, 460] are considered important in causing infertility and sexual dysfunction. However, hyperprolactinemia is mild and often occurs in the presence of contributory medications, such as methyldopa and metoclopramide.[461] With the initiation of dialysis, some women resume normal menstrual cycles and ovulate; however, most remain anovulatory. Estrogen and progesterone preparations may be used in the former group to obliterate their menstrual cycles if it is necessary to avoid the problem of hypermenorrhea sometimes seen in women receiving anticoagulants for dialysis.[462, 463]

There are case reports of dialysis patients conceiving and delivering healthy children.[464–466] However, the safe completion of pregnancy in patients on dialysis is unusual because of a high frequency of fetal death associated with uremic polyhydramnios.[465] Increased numbers of reports of successful delivery of healthy children may be related to the use of peritoneal dialysis in pregnant women or aggressive daily hemodialysis with high-flux membranes, $HCO_3^-$-buffered dialysate, and the administration of erythropoietin.

Loss of libido, potency, and spermatogenesis is often seen in male hemodialysis patients. Somewhat less than half of male patients undergoing dialysis have been found to have normal sexual activity.[467] Delayed puberty that persists even with dialysis is reported in young uremic boys.[468] It is uncertain what contribution malnutrition makes to this complication. Although psychologic disorders and general debility are possible factors in sexual dysfunction,[469] uremic patients have decreased nerve conduction velocity, absent bulbocavernosus reflexes,[470] abnormal cortical pudendal evoked responses,[471] and a decrease in nocturnal penile tumescence,[472] perhaps related to autonomic dysfunction.[473] Testicular biopsy specimens of maintenance dialysis patients reveal impaired spermatogenesis[474] with destruction of seminiferous tubules[475] and germinal cell aplasia.[476] Luteinizing hormone levels are generally increased in male dialysis patients[459, 475–479] but were found to be normal in one report.[468] Follicle-stimulating hormone levels are usually normal[459, 475, 478] or sometimes increased, especially with severe hypospermatogenesis.[468, 474, 476, 477, 480] Luteinizing hormone and follicle-stimulating hormone respond abnormally to gonadotropin-releasing hormone, which suggests an abnormal hypophysial-pituitary-gonadal axis.[481] Testos-

terone levels have been found to be uniformly low except in delayed pubescent boys[468] and respond to administration of gonadotropin in a subnormal manner.[426, 477] Hyperprolactinemia may be partially responsible for these findings.[482, 483] Secondary hyperparathyroidism may also be a contributant to decreased testosterone levels.[484] Findings similar to these are seen early in patients with acute renal failure and resolve with resumption of renal function.[485]

Intramuscular injection of testosterone enanthate has been shown to increase serum testosterone levels and depress follicle-stimulating hormone and luteinizing hormone but has no effect on prolactin.[480] Oral administration of testosterone undecanoate has been reported to restore the pituitary-testicular axis to normal.[486] Neither intramuscular nor oral administration of testosterone has an apparent clinical effect. Administration of clomiphene citrate partially corrects the abnormal hypophysial-pituitary-gonadal axis.[487] Zinc deficiency has been suggested as a cause of gonadal dysfunction, but low serum levels have not correlated with other abnormalities.[482] With administration of zinc acetate, patients have been shown to have increased testosterone levels, decreased luteinizing hormone and follicle-stimulating hormone levels, decreased prolactin levels, and increased potency and libido.[488] Others have found zinc deficiency to be an irreversible cause of endocrine dysfunction.[489] Agents such as bromocriptine,[429, 490] lisuride,[491] and bromocriptine mesylate (Parlodel)[492] have been shown to have a mild beneficial effect on sexual function in men. Vitamin E reduces prolactin levels but has no beneficial effects on sexual dysfunction.[493] Although sexual function may improve in some uremic patients with the initiation of dialysis, this is probably related to improvement in general well-being rather than a specific improvement in hormonal function alone.[468, 494] Erythropoietin has been used extensively in the last 5 years. In several studies, an improved general sense of well-being and sexual function has been reported.[495–500] In addition, erythropoietin has been shown to favorably affect pituitary-adrenal and pituitary-gonadal function.[501, 502] However, correlation between these changes and sexual improvement is lacking. Gynecomastia is not unusual in dialysis patients[503] and is believed to be a phenomenon similar to that seen in patients who are starved or chronically ill from any cause. Its presence has not been related to abnormal hormonal function[417] in ESRD.

Abnormalities in thyroid function tests are frequently noted in uremic patients. Because of the similarities between the uremic syndrome and hyperthyroidism or hypothyroidism, the relationships between such measurements and clinical thyroid disease are difficult to evaluate. An increased frequency of goiter[504–506] and exophthalmos[507] has been reported in patients with chronic renal failure. Other studies have not found an increased occurrence of goiter[508] but do show an increased volume of thyroid tissue, both on ultrasonography[509] and on pathologic examination,[510] in about 50% of the patients. Reduced thermogenesis correlates with low thyroxine levels and is thought to reflect thyroid malfunction.[511]

In studies of thyroid function in patients with uremia, protein-bound iodine and thyroid-bound globulin have generally been found to be normal,[443, 512–516] whereas plasma inorganic iodine is usually increased.[443, 512–514, 517] Thyroid function studies in clinically euthyroid uremic and dialysis patients demonstrate decreased levels of triiodothyronine[421, 512, 515, 516, 518–528] and thyroxine.[504, 516–518, 521, 523–530] Free thyroxine levels have been reported to be normal,[507, 515, 516, 525, 531] increased,[513, 532] or decreased.[518, 519, 521–528] Free triiodothyronine levels are likewise variable—normal,[516, 526] increased,[525] or decreased.[521, 524, 527, 528] Thyroid-stimulating hormone has been the most agreed on measure of thyroid function and, typically, has been found to be in the normal range.[421, 512, 515, 519, 526, 527, 530] However, the thyroid-stimulating hormone response to thyrotropin-releasing hormone is blunted and delayed in patients with significant renal failure,* which suggests abnormality at the hypothalamic-pituitary level. Investigations indicate a tissue resistance to thyroid hormones.[522] Also, thyroid hormone–binding inhibitor activity is increased in renal failure.[533] Some of these changes may be related to the nature and extent of renal failure[534] or to comorbid conditions such as malnutrition.[525]

The influence of dialysis on thyroid function tests is variable.[428, 512, 518] Some studies suggest that hemodilution or a change in volume distribution for thyroid hormones may occur with dialysis.[421, 525] Other possible factors in the reporting discrepancy for therapy include differences in the type of patients studied (degree of uremia, use of dialysis, and type of dialysis), differences in the technique and terminology of thyroid assays, variations in the degree of protein metabolism abnormality, the effect of heparin, and differences in study design (such as use of control subjects and manner of reporting the abnormalities [e.g., percentage of patients with abnormal values versus mean levels]). Evaluation of hypothyroidism and monitoring of its treatment with thyroid medication are somewhat more difficult in light of these findings. Hyperthyroidism may occur in patients with renal failure, and the usual treatment modalities are appropriate.[535, 536] With the numerous and variably interpreted results, it is difficult to come to any conclusion about thyroid function in uremic and dialyzed patients. Nonetheless, there is little evidence to suggest that disorders of thyroid function play a major role in uremic symptoms or that uremia drastically affects true thyroid function.

## Hematologic Abnormalities

### ANEMIA

The development and extensive use of recombinant human erythropoietin have dramatically affected anemia, a major component of the uremic syndrome.[537, 538] Details of the pathophysiologic mechanism of anemia complicating renal failure are discussed elsewhere (Chapter 50). In this section, emphasis is placed on additional factors contributing to or improving uremic anemia in dialysis patients and specific interactions of hemodialysis and erythropoietin therapy.

Multicenter studies have documented the effectiveness of erythropoietin in correcting the anemia of chronic renal failure.[539–542] The previous debate as to whether the anemia of chronic renal failure is due to decreased production of

erythropoietin or the presence of a circulating inhibitor[543–546] has not been answered by the use of this drug, because the dosage necessary to correct anemia is not physiologic. Human biosynthetic (recombinant) erythropoietin has improved hematocrits and altered the well-being of dialysis patients before the initiation of dialysis or transplantation. Several studies have indicated that subcutaneous administration of erythropoietin in patients with renal insufficiency, before the initiation of dialysis, is effective and reduces their symptoms.[547–549] Therefore, the use of erythropoietin may delay the initiation of hemodialysis. Despite concerns based on animal models, there is little evidence that erythropoietin therapy has had an adverse effect on the progression of chronic renal insufficiency.[550–552] In fact, one must be aware that erythropoietin may mask some of the symptoms previously used as a guide to initiate dialysis. Careful monitoring of other aspects of the uremic syndrome other than anemia is important because patients are treated with conservative therapy before dialysis.

The introduction of erythropoietin in 1987 for treatment of anemia in dialysis patients has had a major effect in nearly every aspect of dialytic treatment. Studies have demonstrated an improvement in cardiac hemodynamics,[553–556] with decreased left ventricular hypertrophy,[557–560] improved oxygen-releasing capacity,[561] enhanced exercise capacity,[562] and reduction of intradialytic hypotension.[563, 564] This improvement in cardiac function has led to improvements in physical performance and work capacity,[565–569] sexual function,[495, 496] and the quality of life of dialysis patients.[497–500] As discussed later, a decrease in transfusions has had a beneficial effect on the frequency of hepatitis and on the degree of presensitization for renal transplantation.

In contrast, hypertension, which was a significant problem in earlier studies with erythropoietin, was probably a consequence of the rapidity with which the hematocrit was normalized. In later studies, a slower increase in hematocrit caused only modest increases in the level of blood pressure in patients receiving erythropoietin.[570–572] In most studies, a decreased cardiac index and a marked increase in total peripheral resistance have been found during the correction of the hematocrit with erythropoietin. It is not clear whether this is related to a change in blood volume and viscosity[570, 573–576] or an increase in the level of selective vasoactive peptides.[570–573, 575–580] Nonetheless, this modest elevation in blood pressure can be controlled with antihypertensive therapy and volume reduction.

The appropriate dosage and route of administration for erythropoietin have been debated in the literature. Initial goals and reimbursement established by the Food and Drug Administration and the Health Care Financing Administration affected the use of the drug.[581–584] Subsequently, modification in reimbursement for this drug (about $1.00 per 1000 units) led to increasing dose levels to achieve the target level hematocrit of 30% to 33%.[585, 586] The subcutaneous route of administration is associated with a protracted biologic half-life, which permits a reduction in the dosage in comparison to the intravenous route.[587–592] Because of the ease of administration by the intravenous route, discomfort associated with subcutaneous administration, and the patient's preference, the intravenous route remains the predominant mode of administration for hemodialysis patients.

*References 434, 512, 513, 518, 521, 523, 524, 527, 528, 530.

In a limited fashion, independent of the administration of exogenous erythropoietin, initiation of dialysis improves erythrocyte survival and partially corrects the anemia of chronic renal failure.[593–596] This effect may be masked by the predialysis use of erythropoietin. However, once dialysis therapy has been initiated, a number of factors may exacerbate anemia or cause resistance to the effects of erythropoietin. These confounding issues are listed in Table 56–7. The persistence of uremia due to inadequate dialysis may have an adverse effect on the response to erythropoietin.[597] Some investigators have suggested that high-flux hemodialysis with biocompatible membranes may lead to an improved response to erythropoietin.[598, 599] Perhaps more important than inadequate dialysis as a contributant to anemia is blood loss. These losses can occur through the dialyzer and dialyzer lines or as a consequence of repeated blood tests.[593, 600] However, the major cause for blood loss in dialysis patients is occult bleeding, primarily through the gastrointestinal tract.[601–607] In addition, hemolysis may be due to mechanical factors,[608, 609] thermal injury,[109] hyperosmolarity and hypo-osmolarity,[610, 611] severe hypophosphatemia,[612–614] or dialysate contamination with trace elements.[121, 615] Hemolysis may rarely be due to hypersplenism with erythrocyte sequestration and extravascular hemolysis.[616, 617] Splenectomy may improve this situation in some cases.[618, 619]

In previous years, blood transfusions were used to replace blood losses and maintain the hematocrit. Repeated blood transfusions in dialysis patients often led to a high frequency of hemosiderosis and hemochromatosis[620–627] that affected the function of the liver, bone, heart, and muscle. Deferoxamine was administered for treatment of these disorders,[628–631] despite the occurrence of frequent and severe complications associated with its use in hemodialysis patients.[632–639] The treatment of anemia with erythropoietin has minimized transfusions and virtually eliminated this scenario. Instead, the use of erythropoietin increases erythrocyte production to an extent whereby phlebotomy can be performed to more rapidly diminish body iron stores[640] if necessary. Now, because of chronic loss of blood and use of erythropoietin, many patients exhibit iron deficiency rather than excessive iron deposition. This is the most common cause for erythropoietin resistance.[641–643] Oral administration of iron has commonly been used in dialysis patients, but because of poor tolerance due to gastrointestinal distress,[644, 645] the oral route is often inadequate for iron replacement. This has led to the frequent administration of intravenous iron to replace iron stores.[641, 646, 647] Criteria for iron replacement have been suggested, such as a transferrin saturation of less than 20% or a serum ferritin level less than 100 pg/mL.[646]

Microcytic hypochromic anemia may be seen in dialysis patients in situations other than iron deficiency. In the presence of adequate iron stores, aluminum intoxication[114, 648–652] causes microcytic anemia. The decreasing use of aluminum hydroxide as a $PO_4^{3-}$ binder and proper treatment of water have reduced the role of aluminum as an etiologic factor in erythropoietin-resistant hypochromic microcytic anemia. Deficiencies of folic acid and vitamin $B_{12}$ must be considered in dialysis patients, although their occurrence is rare because of the frequent administration of vitamin supplements. Of note is that macrocytosis is common in patients who are responding to erythropoietin. This occurrence is a result of the increased mean corpuscular volume associated with reticulocytosis, not megaloblastosis. Before the introduction of erythropoietin, hyperparathyroidism was demonstrated to be a contributory factor in the anemia of chronic renal failure.[653–657] In cases of erythropoietin resistance, hyperparathyroidism should be considered. In years past, bilateral nephrectomy was thought to be a cause of severe anemia.[658] Bilateral nephrectomy is rarely performed, but treatment with erythropoietin can overcome the resultant severe anemia.

Other treatment options are available for the anemic dialysis patient. In a small number of dialysis patients, repleting their iron stores will increase the hematocrit to levels such that erythropoietin is unnecessary. Before the introduction of erythropoietin, androgen therapy was shown to be useful for improving anemia.[659–662] Androgen therapy may enhance the response to erythropoietin, thereby allowing reduced doses.[663]

One of the dilemmas of erythropoietin therapy is the appropriateness of its use in the dialysis patient with chronic low-grade blood loss or in the patient with acute blood loss. Large increases in the dosage of erythropoietin and iron are necessary to compensate for chronic low-grade blood loss. A more appropriate response is to initiate a vigorous search for the site of blood loss and to correct it. Whether it is appropriate to continue erythropoietin while a patient is receiving blood transfusions for acute blood loss is debatable. Although it will have little effect on the acute status, if the dosage is not maintained, the patient may subsequently become deficient in erythropoietin and manifest persistent anemia after bleeding has ceased. The most cost-efficient manner of managing the patient in this situation is not yet defined.

Because the increased hematocrit causes a reduction in

**TABLE 56–7. Factors That Exacerbate Anemia or Cause Resistance to Erythropoietin**

Inadequate hemodialysis
Iron deficiency
Blood loss
  Occult gastrointestinal bleeding
  Blood loss in dialyzer and dialysis lines
  Blood drawing for laboratory testing
  Blood loss from fistula
Hemolysis
  Mechanical factors (blood pump, occluded lines)
  Dialysate factors
    Thermal injury
    Hyperosmolarity and hypo-osmolarity
    Trace element contamination (aluminum, chlorine, copper, fluoride)
  Hypophosphatemia
  Oxidant drugs
  Hypersplenism with red blood cell sequestration
Aluminum intoxication
Hyperparathyroidism
Bilateral nephrectomy
Chronic inflammation and infection
Primary hematologic disease

the relative plasma volume, there was concern expressed that erythropoietin may have an adverse effect on the efficiency of hemodialysis. This concern has not been validated.[664-670] There is a decrease in plasma volume and a slight decrease in dialyzer clearance associated with increasing the hematocrit. However, this minor decrease in dialysis efficiency can be overcome by an appropriate change in the dialysis prescription. Another concern is the improved platelet function and correction of the bleeding time that occur with correction of the anemia and the potential for increased vascular thrombosis, pulmonary emboli, and clotting of the extracorporeal circuit. Although there was initial concern that this correction of bleeding time and platelet dysfunction would have adverse consequences, there have been no demonstrations of excessive intravascular coagulation. Of greatest practical concern is the potential adverse effect on the patency of arteriovenous fistulas. Although some studies have suggested an increase in the frequency of graft thrombosis,[222, 671, 672] most have been unable to demonstrate a correlation between erythropoietin administration and thrombosis of the angioaccess.[221, 673-677]

It has been recognized that transfusing patients before transplantation enhances survival of the renal allograft. However, with the improved allograft survival afforded by the use of cyclosporine, this advantage of blood transfusions is negated. Moreover, a small percentage of such patients become sensitized to more than 50% of the panel of the human leukocyte antigen haplotypes for which they were screened. It is apparent that patients who do not receive blood transfusions and remain unsensitized may have increased opportunities for renal transplantation because of decreased sensitization. Further, transplantation results are improved in such patients.[361, 678-681] Thus, erythropoietin has had a beneficial effect on renal transplantation success.

Erythropoietin provides many long-term benefits in patients undergoing maintenance dialysis but adds significantly to the expense of hemodialysis treatments. Vigorous efforts should be made to reduce blood loss and avoid hemolysis to minimize the dose of erythropoietin. Further investigations are necessary to determine the optimal hematocrit for maintenance dialysis patients and to define the most efficient route of administration for this drug. At present, the anemia of renal failure has become much less of a problem than it was in years past. On balance, the advantages of erythropoietin far outweigh potential disadvantages.

## WHITE BLOOD CELL ABNORMALITIES

Infection is the second leading cause of death in dialysis patients,[313] with bacteremia accounting for 20% of deaths.[682, 683] The propensity of dialysis patients for infection, depressed cutaneous hypersensitivity, and delayed reaction to skin grafts is detailed in several reviews.[684-686] Although the total number of white blood cells is normal in uremic patients, differential counts show a relative increase in the proportion of neutrophils to lymphocytes.[687] Abnormalities in leukocyte function, especially of granulocytes, have been studied in patients on dialysis. When assessing the effects of uremia on the myelopoietic system, one must

determine whether studies were done in uremic or dialyzed patients. This is because both uremia and dialysis can affect leukocytes. Several studies have reviewed the effects of dialysis on granulocyte function.[688-691] Such effects include impaired phagocytosis,[692] impaired phagocyte receptor function,[70] diminished motility,[693] decreased chemotaxis,[694, 695] increased heterotypic adherence,[696] modulation of surface expression of adherence molecules,[80] increased elastase release as an indication of degranulation,[697] altered oxidative metabolism,[698, 699] and decreased leukocyte surface charge.[700] Studies of lymphocytes demonstrate a decreased proliferative response to phytohemagglutinin,[701] inhibition of T cell proliferation with decreased IL-2 synthesis,[702] inhibition of mixed lymphocyte culture responses,[703] alteration in lymphocyte subpopulations,[704-708] depressed natural killer cell activity,[709] and reduced percentage of low-mobility lymphocytes.[710] The transient intradialytic leukopenia appears to stimulate release of immature neutrophils from the bone marrow, which may contribute to the overall defective function.[698, 711]

There is substantial evidence that these functional leukocyte changes are related to the type of dialyzer membrane.[78, 712-714] Cuprophane and other cellophane derivatives activate the alternative pathway of complement and may affect white blood cells through this and other effector pathways. Bone marrow studies in patients having dialysis with cuprophane membranes have shown normal to hyperactive leukopoiesis, even in the face of suppressed erythropoiesis.[711] Long-term activation of complement with cuprophane dialysis membranes may also lead to predialysis neutropenia.[78] As noted before, dialysis patients have a relative lymphopenia, but the proportions of T, B, and null cells are normal.[688, 705, 715] The changes in lymphocytes and monocytes likewise may be a reflection of the effect of the dialysis membrane. Other investigators suggest that these functional alterations may be a consequence of generalized malnutrition,[716] zinc deficiency,[717] hyperparathyroidism,[718-721] and possibly diminished 1,25-dihydroxycholecalciferol levels.[722]

Peripheral eosinophilia has been noted to occur in 20% to 59% of hemodialysis patients.[723-726] The eosinophilia varies with the type of dialyzer,[727, 728] but most studies have suggested that eosinophilia may be related to exposure and sensitization to ethylene oxide, a sterilizing agent in dialyzers.[729-733]

## PLATELET AND HEMOSTATIC ABNORMALITIES

A bleeding disorder has been recognized as a serious abnormality in patients with renal insufficiency.[734-740] Initially, this was thought to be due to a uremic toxin such as guanidinosuccinic acid or other peptide derivatives that affected platelet function.[736, 737, 739, 741, 742] Subsequently, the complexity of the coagulation cascade has been further defined, and it is apparent that abnormal platelet function may have many contributing features. For example, vascular endothelium has been shown to play an important role in abnormalities in uremic hemostasis. Initially, bleeding tendency was measured by platelet count, bleeding time, and whole blood platelet aggregation time. There are now numerous measures of platelet and endothelial function, both in the formation of thrombosis and in its fibrinolysis. Various assays of uremic bleeding or concomitant clotting dysfunction include measurements of von Willebrand factor and its antigen,[743] factor VIII activity,[744] factor XIII activity,[744] thrombospondin,[745] tissue plasminogen activator release,[746] platelet-activating factor,[67, 747] fibrinolysis,[748, 749] and thrombin–antithrombin III complex.[750, 751] Despite the use of this array of clotting assays, the exact pathophysiologic mechanism of uremic bleeding remains unclear. The defined, but not inclusive, mechanisms for platelet dysfunction in renal insufficiency include 1) anemia that alters radial flow pattern of platelets within the vasculature, thereby diminishing the frequency of physical interaction between the platelets and the endothelium; 2) decreased binding of von Willebrand factor to the receptor, glycoprotein IIb-IIIa; and 3) increased endothelial generation of nitric oxide.[752-755]

It is generally believed that initiation of hemodialysis improves platelet function and the bleeding tendency.[736, 756-759] Coagulation in the extracorporeal circulation relates to these improvements.[744-746, 760, 761] However, the improvement in the bleeding diathesis with hemodialysis is complicated by a number of factors. Obviously, heparin is necessary in most extracorporeal treatments and is probably the major cause of bleeding in dialysis patients. Because of these complications, techniques such as regional heparin anticoagulation,[762, 763] regional citrate anticoagulation,[764, 765] low-dose heparin,[28] and heparin-free dialysis[29, 766, 767] have been used (see earlier). In addition, aspirin,[768-770] antiplatelet agents,[771, 772] and warfarin, which have been used to prevent access thrombosis, should be used with caution in dialysis patients with bleeding disorders. Heparin-associated thrombocytopenia is another consideration in this problem.[773] The introduction of low-molecular-weight heparin appears to have had no particular advantage over standard heparin in hemodialysis patients.[774, 775] There is now a growing literature indicating that platelet function is affected by different membranes that influence the coagulation system.[67, 748, 760, 776-781]

In patients who are at unusual bleeding risk, or if bleeding in an ESRD patient occurs in the absence of heparinization, several approaches of different acuity can be introduced to correct the platelet defect. Either peritoneal dialysis or hemodialysis will transiently correct the platelet defect,[782, 783] but more conservative therapies are available. Rapid correction of platelet dysfunction is afforded by erythrocyte transfusion to a hematocrit of 35% or greater.[753] A more protracted response can be produced by the correction of anemia with erythropoietin to a hematocrit of greater than 27%.[750, 751, 784] Therapeutic strategies that target deficiencies in von Willebrand factor are the infusion of cryoprecipitate every 12 to 24 hours or the administration of desamino-8-D-arginine vasopressin (DDAVP). Ten units of cryoprecipitate, which is rich in von Willebrand factor, infused for 30 minutes has an onset of action of approximately 60 minutes and a duration of action of up to 36 hours.[785] Alternatively, DDAVP, which induces the endothelial release of factor VIII–von Willebrand multimers, may be given intravenously (0.3 μg/kg), subcutaneously (0.3 μg/kg), or intranasally (3 μg/kg).[75] Although not uniformly effective and of diminishing benefit after repeated administration, DDAVP is the safest and most rapid means of correcting the platelet defect of renal insufficiency. The maximal effect from DDAVP occurs 2 hours or longer after dosing, and it persists up to 8 hours. Long-lasting hemostatic correction, but with a delayed onset of action, is effected by conjugated estrogens (0.6 mg/kg/d for 5 days) or Premarin (25 mg/d for 7 days).[786, 787] An initial effect is noted after only 6 hours, and it persists up to 21 days.

## Gastrointestinal Abnormalities

### UPPER AND LOWER GASTROINTESTINAL TRACT

Persistent anorexia, nausea and vomiting, and signs such as uremic fetor, mucosal ulceration, and gastrointestinal hemorrhage are prominent manifestations of advanced uremia. With early initiation of hemodialysis and more aggressive dialytic therapy, such findings are now uncommon in dialysis populations. Anorexia, dysgeusia, nausea, and vomiting remain useful clinical indicators for initiation of dialysis. Similarly, these symptoms are useful but crude clinical guidelines for assessing the adequacy of dialysis (see later). In the National Cooperative Dialysis Study, the most frequent reason for withdrawal of patients from the study in the high-BUN group was anorexia or nausea; the most frequent indication of hospitalization in the high-BUN group was gastrointestinal disorders.[601]

A variety of gastrointestinal abnormalities persist in patients with chronic renal failure undergoing hemodialysis (Table 56–8). In the upper gastrointestinal tract, there is a higher frequency of gastritis and hemorrhage.[788-791] Endoscopic studies of dialysis patients have reported abnormal findings in 20% to 75% of the patients, depending on the severity of symptoms and the indication for study. Biochemical and histologic analyses of the upper gastrointestinal tract have demonstrated an increased frequency in abnormalities, even with no outward manifestations of illness.[792-795] Approximately one half of the patients studied had biopsy-proven evidence of gastritis with inflammatory cell infiltration of the epithelium, and approximately 15% of the patients had evidence of atrophic gastritis. The frequency of these lesions was several times greater than that observed in a healthy population. However, other observers have reported that the percentage of gastric and duodenal ulcers is approximately similar to that in the general population.[796]

**TABLE 56–8. Common Gastrointestinal Abnormalities in Dialysis Patients**

Anorexia, nausea, and vomiting with inadequate dialysis
Increased frequency of gastritis
Increased serum gastrin levels
Edema of the bowel wall
Increased frequency of diverticulosis and diverticulitis
Ascites
Gastrointestinal bleeding
Increased frequency of angiodysplasia
Increased frequency of pancreatitis

The cause of such histologic abnormalities is not apparent. A hypersecretory state with elevated serum gastrin levels is present, presumably owing to reduced renal clearance,[794, 796–798] the psychologic stress of illness and hemodialysis, an increase in $H^+$ back-diffusion caused by high urea levels,[799] and hypercalcemia associated with secondary hyperparathyroidism. Some observers have suggested that the increased gastrin level may be in response to hypochlorhydria, a frequent finding in these patients. Other investigators found that gastrin levels did not correlate with either hypersecretion or histologic evidence of gastritis or duodenitis.[791, 800–802] An increase in gastric inhibitory polypeptide has been found that may suppress the effect of the increased gastrin levels.[803] Thus, the role of increased gastrin levels is unclear.

Another consequence of high gastrin levels may be the high frequency of biliary reflux.[799] Gastrin affects the pyloric sphincter, and high gastrin levels may lead to pyloric incompetence and biliary reflux.[804] The occurrence of *Helicobacter pylori,* which has been associated with gastritis in nonuremic patients, has not been found to be increased in the dialysis population. This is not due to an abnormality in testing, because increased urea in uremic patients does not interfere with the urease-based analysis used in the detection of *H. pylori.*[805]

These abnormalities may in part explain the high frequency of upper gastrointestinal bleeding in uremic patients.[602] Two autopsy studies showed that the occurrence of gastritis and duodenitis in well-dialyzed patients was not different from that in healthy subjects. However, there was an increased mortality related to bleeding in these patients.[603] Opinions differ as to the presence of a higher mortality rate due to gastrointestinal hemorrhage in patients with renal failure.[602–604, 806] The use of ulcerogenic drugs (aspirin, prednisone, nonsteroidal anti-inflammatory agents) could be documented in 82% of these cases. This suggests that underlying gastritis or duodenitis may not lead to clinical sequelae but may predispose to gastrointestinal bleeding in the presence of an ulcerogenic medication. Another endoscopic study suggested that upper gastrointestinal bleeding in dialysis patients is more often due to angiodysplasia.[605] Gastrointestinal bleeding in patients with renal failure is associated with an increase in blood transfusions and a higher predilection for rebleeding. Dialysis patients frequently exhibit trace or 1+ guaiac-positive stools without a fall in hematocrit.[606] Because dialysis patients without serious gastrointestinal disease may have blood loss due to increased bleeding tendencies and long-term anticoagulation, the interpretation of trace guaiac-positive stools or guaiac-positive nasogastric aspirate must be tempered.

Other than adjustments in the dosage of medication for renal insufficiency, the treatment of gastritis and duodenal ulcers in dialysis patients is similar to that in patients with normal renal function. Despite the frequent finding of hypochlorhydria, antacids and histamine $H_2$-receptor blockers are the mainstay of treatment for these disorders.[807, 808] Treatment of upper gastrointestinal hemorrhage is the same as for patients without renal failure, including nasogastric lavage and transfusions as necessary.[789] When gastric lavage is deemed appropriate, 5% dextrose in water, rather than saline solutions, should be used to avoid $Na^+$ overload.

Heparinization should be limited during subsequent dialysis treatments by use of fractional or regional heparinization, no heparin, or regional citrate anticoagulation (see earlier).

Common lower gastrointestinal abnormalities in uremic patients include colonic ulceration, diverticulosis, diverticulitis, spontaneous colonic perforation, and prolonged adynamic ileus (pseudo-obstruction).[809–814] The frequency of diverticulosis and diverticulitis (~80%) is increased in patients with polycystic kidney disease. However, the occurrence in other dialysis patients is not significantly higher than in the age-matched, normal population.[814] Another study that examined histologic specimens from the bowel of asymptomatic dialysis patients found no increase in colonic disease.[792] Other investigators have reported a low but significantly increased frequency of prolonged adynamic ileus and spontaneous colonic perforation, even in the absence of diverticular disease.[810, 811] These disorders have been associated with the frequent complaint of constipation,[812] probably due to aluminum hydroxide, calcium carbonate, analgesic narcotics, and a limited fluid intake. Nonspecific ulceration of the colon has also been reported in dialysis patients.[813] Ulcers are usually single and more often situated in the cecum and ascending colon and may mimic a variety of other abnormalities, such as appendicitis or carcinoma. Their frequency does not appear to relate to the patient's length of time undergoing dialysis. Nonocclusive bowel infarction is not unusual in dialysis patients and has been associated with frequent and severe hypotension during dialysis.[815] Studies with animals have demonstrated intestinal necrosis with the use of sorbitol added to sodium polystyrene sulfonate (Kayexalate) enemas.[816] Anecdotal cases of bowel perforation after the rectal administration of sorbitol have been reported.[816, 817] Thus, enemas with sodium polystyrene sulfonate should be mixed with water and not sorbitol. Several reports in long-term dialysis patients with amyloid arthropathy have demonstrated infarction and perforation in the stomach and colon, which may be related to $\beta_2$-microglobulin amyloid.[818, 819] In long-term dialysis patients, amyloidosis should be considered in the differential diagnosis of patients with bowel symptoms.

## HEPATIC ABNORMALITIES

Intermittently and mildly abnormal liver function test results are often seen in patients with chronic renal failure undergoing dialysis.[820–822] In a necropsy study of 78 patients who had hemodialysis, 90% had some hepatic abnormality.[823] Hepatomegaly was found in 50%, and chronic passive congestion associated with fluid overload or cardiac disease was prevalent. Mild periportal fibrosis, fatty metamorphosis, triaditis, and hemosiderosis were also common. A likely cause of these changes is viral hepatitis, which is commonly seen in long-term dialysis patients. Previously, multiple transfusions of blood products predisposed patients to type B hepatitis.[824–827] Because of the defective immune system of dialysis patients who contract type B hepatitis, a chronic antigenic carrier state occasionally develops with only mild to moderate elevations of liver enzymes. Most patients are asymptomatic and remain symptom free.[828, 829] The availability and use of erythropoietin have reduced the number of transfusions in dialysis patients and have greatly reduced the frequency of hepatitis. The prevalence of HBsAg hepatitis has declined to approximately 1.4% among patients and 0.3% among staff members.[830] Use of the polymerase chain reaction to detect hepatitis B virus DNA suggests that HBs antigen assays do not detect all cases and that hepatitis B may be more prevalent than was previously appreciated.[831]

The use of the hepatitis B vaccine has favorably affected the occurrence of hepatitis B among hemodialysis staff. Seroconversion, with the development of HBs antibodies from the hepatitis vaccine, and its effect on hepatic disease in dialysis patients have been more variable. Poor responses to the vaccine may be related to a decrease in IL-2 production and up-regulation of the IL-2 receptors[832] or abnormalities of human leukocyte antigen–linked immune response genes.[833] However, the overall effect has been beneficial,[834, 835] so the vaccine is recommended for all dialysis patients.

Non-A, non-B hepatitis has been recognized as an important type of hepatitis in dialysis units in the last several years.[836–839] Most cases of non-A, non-B hepatitis have subsequently been identified as due to the hepatitis C virus (HCV).[840–842] With use of either a first-generation enzyme immunoassay or a second-generation HCV antibody test[843–845] that detects antibodies to structural and nonstructural antigens of HCV, the prevalence of HCV antibody positivity in dialysis units has varied from 5% to 40%. The prevalence is influenced by the country of the survey, the frequency of blood transfusions, and the length of time the patients underwent hemodialysis.[846–853] In general, the second-generation assay is more sensitive and detects a slightly higher percentage of cases. In all of these studies, it is clear that blood transfusions are associated with the occurrence of anti-HCV antibodies. However, transmission of HCV by means other than blood transfusions remains a concern.

Most patients with anti-HCV antibodies do not exhibit hepatic abnormalities, and progression to cirrhosis is unusual. The polymerase chain reaction for HCV DNA has been studied in a dialysis population.[854] Fifty-nine percent of patients with anti-HCV antibodies had detectable DNA, whereas none of the HCV-negative patients tested had HCV DNA detected. Confirmation of these findings in future studies will be important in determining the epidemiology of this disease in dialysis units. The presence of anti-HCV antibodies in kidney donors has been suggested to be important in the occurrence of posttransplantation liver disease,[855, 856] but this issue is debated.[857] The presence of antibodies to HCV in dialysis patients is not an absolute exclusion for transplantation, but monitoring of hepatitis status is mandatory.

Other viral infections, such as with cytomegalovirus, are possible causes of acute hepatic dysfunction in dialysis patients. Another possible cause of hepatic dysfunction in this population of patients is drug-induced elevation of liver enzymes.[821, 858, 859] Drugs such as methyldopa, aspirin, ampicillin, labetalol, and benzodiazepine have been implicated as causes of liver cytolysis in uremic patients.[860] The toxicity of these drugs is particularly apparent in HBsAg-positive dialysis patients in whom there is a decrease in the activity and content of the major oxidase enzymes in the hepatic cytochrome system.[859]

Iron accumulation was a common finding in the liver of long-term dialysis patients in years past. Iron accumulates in hepatocytes and reticular endothelial cells of long-term dialysis patients having received large numbers of transfusions. It was speculated that this leads to cytolysis and eventual cirrhosis or hemochromatosis. As with hepatitis, the advent of erythropoietin therapy and a decrease in the number of transfusions have led to the near-disappearance of this complication. In addition to iron accumulation, aluminum may be important. In autopsy studies, the liver was the organ with the second highest accumulation of aluminum in patients with dialysis dementia. However, the syndrome of aluminum overload in the liver was not associated with any apparent functional disorder.[861, 862] Spallation of diethylthalate and silicone from blood tubings and the blood pump segment of dialysis lines has also been reported to cause giant cell reactions in the liver of patients in autopsy series.[95, 863] No specific functional abnormality was noted in these studies. Such rare abnormalities may have consequence in patients after renal transplantation.[863]

## ASCITES

A peculiar form of idiopathic refractory ascites has been described in hemodialysis patients. This was found much more frequently in earlier years and was usually without obvious cause (e.g., cirrhosis, metastatic carcinoma, hypoalbuminemia, or pericardial disease).[864–867] Although the exact pathogenesis was unknown, fluid overload was suspected to be the cause in many cases.[868, 869] Other implicated etiologic factors include portal hypertension due to polycystic liver disease, previous peritoneal dialysis with serositis, and lymphatic drainage disturbances.[870] One study noted differences in the osmolarity of serum and ascitic fluid after dialysis and suggested that the disorder was due to an osmotic disequilibrium.[871] Isolated ultrafiltration, which allows removal of large amounts of fluid with low risk of hypotension, has been used successfully in the treatment of this disorder in some patients.[872, 873] With improved hemodialysis, the use of $HCO_3^-$, higher dialysate $Na^+$ concentration, and ultrafiltration control devices, idiopathic ascites is seen much less frequently. Successful renal transplantation seems to be the most effective therapy.

## PANCREATIC ABNORMALITIES

Several investigators have reported an increased frequency of pancreatitis in hemodialysis patients.[874, 875] Studies of pancreatic function in hemodialysis patients have revealed low basal pancreatic output of $HCO_3^-$ but normal secretin-stimulated $HCO_3^-$ secretion.[874–877] Most pancreatic enzymes, such as cholecystokinin, glucagon, and secretin, are elevated in patients with renal failure, and their levels are inversely correlated with the impairment in renal function.[876, 878] Levels of amylase and lipase remain elevated in dialysis patients because of reduced renal clearance and minimal clearance with dialysis. However, when amylase levels are increased by threefold or greater, acute pancreatitis is probably present.[879] Lipase levels follow a similar pattern, whereas pancreatic isoamylase activity greater than 80% indicates acute pancreatitis. Malabsorption is seen only if pancreatitis is chronic and severe. There are some reports of altered protein and lipid absorption in uremic patients having hemodialysis, independent of pancreatic disease or function.[880, 881]

## Cardiovascular Abnormalities

The cardiovascular system is profoundly affected by renal failure and dialysis. In turn, abnormalities in the cardiovascular system contribute to the symptoms in dialysis patients that may affect the dialysis regimen. Multiple cardiovascular abnormalities are seen in uremic patients. These anatomic and hemodynamic alterations are outlined in Table 56–9. The interval during which patients are uremic and untreated, and may have suffered hypertension of uncertain duration and severity, is a major consideration in the frequency and severity of each of the cardiovascular disorders. Prolonged renal insufficiency with poor control of intravascular volume and hypertension dramatically affects the presentation of the patient.[882–885] Many of these hemodynamic changes are improved by dialytic therapy.[883–890] The duration and severity of cardiovascular abnormalities before initiation of dialysis will alter the response to dialytic therapy. On the other hand, dialysis may have adverse effects on the cardiovascular system, the most common of which is hypotension related to reduction in intravascular volume. These adverse effects of dialysis are outlined later.

Patients undergoing maintenance hemodialysis have a cardiovascular mortality rate approximately three times that of age-matched nonuremic control subjects.[891, 892] The increased mortality is associated with a higher frequency of atherosclerotic heart disease with myocardial infarction, left ventricular hypertrophy, and congestive heart failure.[882, 893–899] The increased frequency of atherosclerotic disease in long-term dialysis patients has been suggested to be a consequence of hyperlipidemia.[337, 341, 357–360, 895, 896] However, hypertension may be an equally important contributant.[882, 892, 900–905] The importance of atherosclerotic coronary artery disease as opposed to hypertensive cardiovascular disease in the increased frequency of death has been debated.[882, 893, 898, 899, 906–910] Distinguishing and controlling the individual risk factors for diastolic versus systolic ventricular dysfunction,[909] or dilated cardiomyopathic versus hypertrophic

### TABLE 56–9. Cardiovascular Abnormalities in Renal Failure

Increased pulmonary capillary permeability[999, 1476]
Increased serosal membrane permeability[864, 870, 958, 1005]
Increased total body and vascular volume[886, 908, 914, 1000, 1001, 1477, 1478]
Increased total peripheral resistance[886, 906, 914, 1000, 1001, 1477]
Increased blood pressure[886, 893, 906, 908, 1000, 1001, 1476, 1477]
Increased cardiac index[886, 914, 1000, 1001]
Increased left ventricular chamber size[900, 909–912, 1478–1485]
Left ventricular hypertrophy[882, 887, 899, 900, 907–912, 1478–1485]
Decreased normalized rigidity or compliance[908, 909, 1479–1485]
Impaired left ventricular contractile function (decreased ejection fraction)[882, 887, 900, 906, 909–912, 1479–1485]
Atrial enlargement[1479–1485]
Atrial septal hypertrophy[1479–1485]
Hypertrophic subaortic stenosis[887, 931, 1479, 1481, 1483, 1486, 1487]

heart disease,[882, 900, 910–912] will be important in minimizing cardiac deaths in dialysis patients.

The numerous provocative factors in the development of ischemic coronary artery disease or hypertensive cardiomyopathy are illustrated in Figure 56–11. An increase in cardiac output may be due to either the presence of arteriovenous fistulas[913] or anemia.[914, 915] Arteriovenous fistulas have been implicated in intractable pulmonary edema.[916–918] However, this is an unusual complication and is usually related to large proximal grafts in the setting of hypervolemia and underlying myocardial dysfunction. Anemia is considered a major cause of the increased cardiac output of renal failure and thus myocardial damage. However, treatment of anemia with erythropoietin has nearly eliminated this as a risk factor (see earlier). Several studies have demonstrated a decline in pulse rate, stroke volume index, cardiac index, cardiac output, left ventricular hypertrophy, exercise-induced cardiac ischemia, and peak oxygen consumption and an improvement in oxygen transport and peripheral vascular resistance by partial correction of anemia with erythropoietin.[553, 559, 560, 919–921]

The dialysis patient is at risk for the development of endocarditis through the arteriovenous fistula or peritoneal catheter.[683, 922, 923] Although bacteremia is a common complication of dialysis patients,[682, 922, 924] endocarditis occurs infrequently[683] and with proper treatment should rarely be a cause of cardiovascular mortality. Bacterial endocarditis is a difficult diagnosis to establish in these patients because of the frequent findings of hypersplenism, positive blood cultures, fever, and peripheral signs of embolization due to endothelial infections of the fistula and the common occurrence of heart murmurs from other causes. Transesophageal echocardiography is sensitive in identifying valvular lesions. The systolic flow murmur frequently observed in patients undergoing dialysis is probably due to anemia. Functional diastolic murmurs have been described[925, 926] and are suggested to be pericardial in origin.[927] They are more likely related to cardiodynamic abnormalities[928] or to pulmonic valve insufficiency.[929] Abnormalities in the mitral valve apparatus[930] and the atrial septum[887, 931] have been described and may play a role in murmurs heard in dialysis patients. Unidentified uremic toxins could be a cause of myocarditis or cardiomyopathy.[932, 933] Protein-deficient cardiomyopathies may be present in severely malnourished uremic patients, which as noted earlier is not uncommon.[934]

The effects of hyperkalemia on cardiac dysrhythmia are well known and are a major concern in patients with renal insufficiency. In the absence of severe hyperkalemia, the frequency of arrhythmia due to renal failure is probably not greater than in normal populations. The dialysis procedure may cause electrolyte, osmolar, and volume changes with increase in the occurrence of arrhythmias. This is discussed later with complications.

As discussed earlier, lipid abnormalities may affect the frequency of cardiovascular disease. Morbidity from vascular calcifications associated with hyperparathyroidism has been well documented[935–938]; these include myocardial calcifications[939–942] and calcifications of the coronary vessels[943] and mitral annulus.[944] Some studies have shown an increase in PTH to have a direct and deleterious effect on myocardial function,[945–947] whereas other studies have not validated

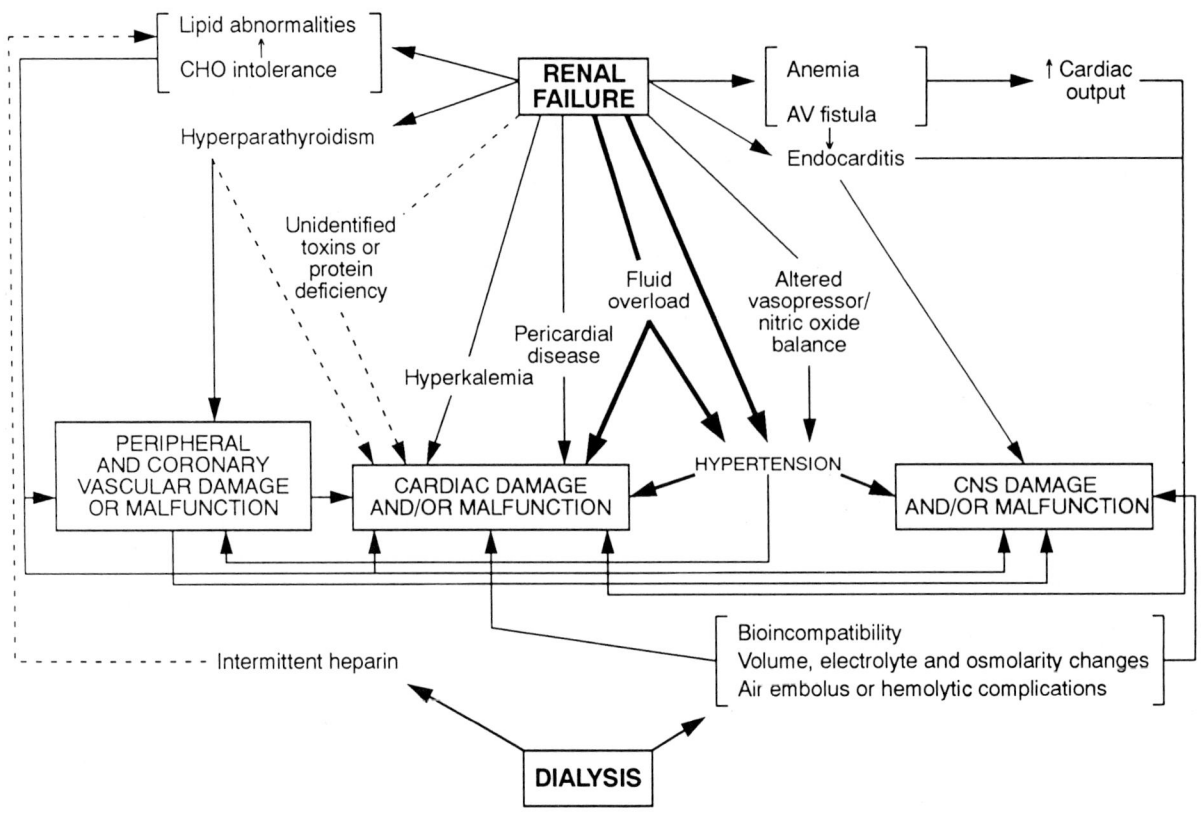

**Figure 56–11.** Schematic of the interplay between abnormalities of the uremic state and the development of cardiovascular disease. CHO = carbohydrate; AV = arteriovenous; CNS = central nervous system.

this finding.[948, 949] The prevention of a high calcium × phosphorus product and hyperparathyroidism seems important in decreasing cardiovascular mortality and morbidity.[935, 941, 950, 951] In addition to calcification from hyperparathyroidism, deposition of calcium oxalate in the myocardium has been reported and is thought to be related to the state of local tissue oxygenation[952] or to excessive doses of ascorbic acid.[953]

Pericardial effusion and tamponade potentially contribute to the enhanced cardiovascular morbidity and mortality. Pericarditis due to uremia was reported to occur in one third to one half of patients in the early years of dialysis.[954, 955] With the initiation of dialysis earlier during the progression of chronic renal failure, pericarditis became much less common.[956] With continued technical improvements that have enhanced the efficiency of the procedure, uremic pericarditis is uncommon. Pericarditis is reported to be a cause of death in dialysis patients in approximately 1.1 per 1000 patient-years at risk.[2] Once dialysis has been initiated, pericarditis is usually the result of inadequate therapy.[955] Pericarditis in a dialysis patient may also arise from other concurrent disorders, such as systemic lupus erythematosus, viral infection, or transmural myocardial infarction. Pericarditis due to uremia usually responds to intensive dialysis, particularly with currently available dialytic techniques. Concurrent fever, leukocytosis, large effusion, and hemodynamic instability suggest a more severe degree of pericardial disease that may be less responsive to dialysis.[957] Echocardiography studies report small and hemody-

namically insignificant posterior pericardial effusions in 15% to 20% of stable, asymptomatic patients undergoing dialysis.[958] Larger effusions, especially if they are anterior and posterior, are usually related to pericarditis and reflect significant disease. Such effusions have been reported to occur in 1.3% to 5% of patients undergoing dialysis.[958–960] Like pericarditis, pericardial effusion has become much less common. In a study of large pericardial effusions of all causes, uremia was found to be the cause in approximately 12%.[961] Pericardial effusions may be related to other factors, such as the oral administration of minoxidil.[962, 963] The frequency of tamponade in uremic patients is unknown, but this complication is now rare. Reduction of blood pressure early in the dialysis procedure and in the presence of increased extracellular volume suggests the possibility of tamponade.

In most patients, mild to moderate pericardial effusions without tamponade respond to an increase in dialysis intensity and reduction in heparinization.[956, 958, 964, 965] Some investigators have suggested early pericardiectomy[966–969] or subxiphoid pericardiotomy.[970, 971] Alternative techniques that have proved successful include pericardiocentesis with air instillation,[955, 972] catheter drainage with triamcinolone,[973, 974] and oral administration of indomethacin.[975] The least invasive approach possible should be used before patients are subjected to thoracic surgery or prophylactic procedures.[976] Early detection and reversal of pericarditis are the key to prevention of pericardial effusions and tamponade. Constrictive pericarditis reported in earlier years[977, 978] is now rare but should be considered in a patient with a small heart and signs and symptoms of thoracic venous inflow and arterial outflow obstruction.

Of all the potential risk factors in the development of cardiovascular disease, hypertension may be the most important.* Hypertension occurs in approximately 80% to 90% of uremic patients before the initiation of dialysis. The pathophysiologic mechanism of uremic hypertension has been well characterized (see the preceding discussion and Chapter 48). The importance of volume expansion is evident from studies that demonstrate control of hypertension in about 60% to 70% of patients simply by reduction of extracellular volume with hemodialysis.[979, 982, 983] Thus, the initial approach to the control of hypertension in the patient entering hemodialysis is reduction of extracellular volume by use of larger surface area dialyzers with higher hydrostatic ultrafiltration pressure or a more effective ultrafiltrating membrane. The rate of fluid removal may be limited by transfer of fluid from intracellular to vascular spaces (i.e., compartmentalization). Therefore, dialysis of short duration may be a problem, particularly in large patients who have increased interdialytic weight gains and persistent hypertension. Ultrafiltration for longer periods may be more effective in the control of hypertension because of the ability to better remove fluid without precipitating hypotension.[984] The use of ultrafiltration controllers, which optimize fluid removal, is helpful in avoiding hypotension in the treatment of extracellular fluid overload.[135, 985–987] In those patients in whom adequate ultrafiltration does not control hypertension, addition of antihypertensive medications is necessary.

Long-term treatment with antihypertensive medications has been shown to cause regression of left ventricular hypertrophy.[988] Many antihypertensive agents potentially lead to vascular instability, causing frequent and profound hypotension during dialysis. Thus, the dosage schedule must be arranged to minimize the action of drugs during the dialysis procedure (i.e., avoid long-acting drugs and dosing immediately before the dialysis treatment). The combination of newer dialytic techniques and effective antihypertensive medications has precluded the need for bilateral nephrectomy, which was used in the 1960s and early 1970s for malignant hypertension.[989–991]

The high frequency of coronary artery disease and increased mortality in dialysis patients have led to the frequent use of coronary artery bypass in these patients. Numerous studies have reported successful results of coronary artery bypass and myocardial revascularization in dialysis patients. Data suggest that in properly selected patients, these procedures are as safe as in nondialysis patients and lead to an increased survival.[992–994] Some investigators have suggested that renal failure patients with cardiac disease, particularly those with cardiac decompensation, are more appropriately managed by peritoneal dialysis to avoid the hemodynamic stresses of hemodialysis.[995–997] However, with proper knowledge of hemodialytic techniques, nearly all patients can safely undergo hemodialysis and, indeed, benefit from more aggressive clearance and ultrafiltration achieved with hemodialysis[998] (Table 56–10). As indicated earlier and illustrated in Figure 56–12, a number of adverse

*References 882, 900, 907, 908, 910, 911, 979–981.

**TABLE 56–10. Mechanisms by Which Dialysis Improves Cardiovascular Abnormalities**

Normalization of intravascular volume
Removal of uremic "toxins"
Correction of hypertension
Correction of electrolyte imbalance ($K^+$, $Na^+$, $H^+$)
Correction of mineral metabolism ($Ca^{2+}$, $Mg^{2+}$)
Correction of anemia

responses may occur with hemodialysis and lead to hypotension and adversely affect cardiovascular morbidity and mortality. These are discussed with hypotension in this chapter.

## Pulmonary Abnormalities

Pulmonary edema develops in patients with uremia at atrial pressures lower than those in healthy subjects. Altered pulmonary capillary permeability has been described in uremic patients,[999–1002] but others have suggested it is not different from that for healthy individuals.[1003] More likely, the higher frequency of pulmonary edema in patients with renal failure is related to the increased total body fluid due to decreased excretory function. Pulmonary edema in uremic patients may not present in the typical pattern[1004] and may be related to the abnormalities in vascular permeability noted before. A higher frequency of pleural effusion is seen in uremic patients,[1005, 1006] perhaps owing to a similar phenomenon in the serosal membranes. Also, an increased frequency of pleuritis and hemorrhagic pleural effusion has been noted in uremic patients and in those having dialysis.[1007–1009]

Several studies have reported abnormal results of pulmonary function studies in uremic patients that are variably improved with dialysis.[1010–1012] Two studies suggested that chronic pulmonary edema may lead to pulmonary fibrosis, which may have long-term effects on diffusion capacity and other pulmonary functions.[1013, 1014] This finding is particularly relevant in that many investigations of pulmonary function in uremic patients and dialysis patients are confounded by improper documentation or verification of the patients' volume status. However, the consensus is that the functional capacity of the lungs is altered in renal failure. Metastatic pulmonary calcification, sometimes not visible on x-ray films, has been noted in uremic and dialysis patients and may contribute to these abnormalities.[1015–1018] The cause for increased pulmonary $Ca^{2+}$ deposition may be secondary hyperparathyroidism and an elevated calcium × phosphorus product. Assessment of pulmonary abnormalities in dialysis patients is further complicated by the dialyzer membrane–dependent activation of complement by the alternative complement pathway. The generation of anaphylatoxins may result in the release of histamine and airway constriction and hypoxia. It should be appreciated that hypoventilation may also occur in dialysis patients related to acetate dialysate with the dialysance of carbon dioxide or as compensation for intradialytic metabolic alkalosis se-

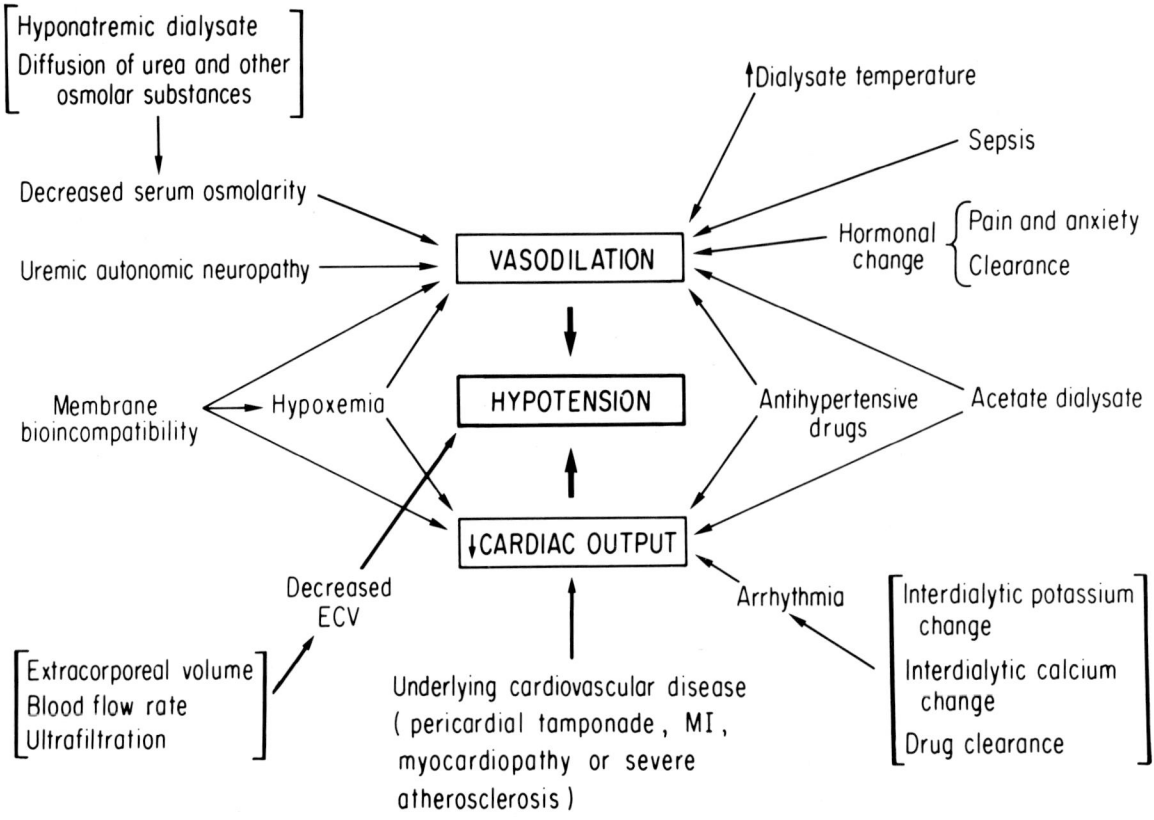

**Figure 56–12.** Schematic of the contributants to the intradialytic development of hypotension. ECV = extracellular volume; MI = myocardial infarction.

condary to $HCO_3^-$ loading. These issues are discussed in greater detail later.

There are several reports of sleep apnea syndrome occurring in uremic and hemodialysis patients.[1019–1021] The cause for sleep apnea in uremia is not clear but is probably related to central nervous system (CNS) effects rather than to a primary abnormality in pulmonary function. This disorder is noted to occur primarily in male patients, and a role for androgens has been debated.[1022, 1023] The syndrome has been reported to respond to branched chain amino acids[1024] and to nasal continuous positive airway pressure.[1025] There are anecdotal reports of this disorder disappearing on successful renal transplantation.[1026]

In general, dialysis patients have few symptoms related primarily to the pulmonary system and little evidence of significant pulmonary dysfunction with the exception of pulmonary edema due to fluid overload or the responses secondary to bioincompatibility.

## Bone and Joint Abnormalities

Uremic metabolic bone disease is discussed in detail in Chapter 51. Those aspects of metabolic bone disease that affect or are affected by hemodialysis are discussed in this section. Several studies of patients receiving long-term hemodialysis have suggested that bone and joint problems are the major source of morbidity.[1027–1033] If not treated early and aggressively, metabolic bone disease may be a factor in mortality.[1028–1030] In the past 20 years, increased knowl-

edge of the pathophysiologic mechanism of metabolic bone disease has led to an appreciation of the importance of distinguishing hyperparathyroidism with osteitis fibrosa cystica and vitamin D–deficient osteomalacia[1034–1046] from aluminum-induced osteomalacia[1047–1053] and aplastic bone disease.[1054–1056] $\beta_2$-Microglobulin amyloid bone disease (dialysis-associated amyloidosis) must now be included in the spectrum of renal or metabolic bone diseases.[1057–1070] In long-term dialysis patients, this disease may be more devastating than the parathyroid and aluminum-related disorders.

The frequency of bone and joint disease in dialysis patients is dependent on the diligence with which the nephrologist searches for each type of disorder. Patients presenting for maintenance hemodialysis generally have a low serum $Ca^{2+}$ concentration, a high serum phosphorus concentration, and a mildly to severely elevated serum PTH level, depending on the duration of renal insufficiency and intensity of treatment before presentation. Aluminum-induced osteomalacia is rare at presentation unless the patient received a heavy burden of aluminum and citrate therapy for acidosis.[1071, 1072] Dialysis-associated amyloidosis is generally seen late in the dialysis course and therefore is not an important consideration when the patient presents.

### HYPERPARATHYROIDISM, OSTEITIS FIBROSA CYSTICA, AND APLASTIC BONE DISEASE

Recognition of the interrelations of PTH, vitamin D, $Ca^{2+}$, phosphorus, and aluminum and aluminum-induced osteomalacia has changed the approach to treatment of secondary hyperparathyroidism. Although some debate exists concerning the role of hyperphosphatemia in causing hyperparathyroidism, the initial approach to treatment of uremic bone disease remains control of serum $PO_4^{3-}$ levels.[113, 1035, 1073–1075] This approach is necessary to avoid a high calcium × phosphorus product and subsequent metastatic calcification.[1039, 1076–1078] Soft tissue and visceral calcification may occur in inadequately or inappropriately treated dialysis patients. The clinical manifestations of calciphylaxis are varied and depend on the site of involvement. Acute attacks of arthritis resembling gout may occur (pseudogout). In advanced cases, vascular calcification with necrosis of fingers, toes, and skin has occurred.[1077, 1079–1081] Respiratory[1016, 1082] and cardiac[939–943, 1083] calcification leads to serious consequences as noted earlier.

Small-vessel calcifications with cutaneous and subcutaneous necrosis in the absence of a high calcium × phosphorus product have been reported,[1084, 1085] which may be related to protein C deficiency[1086] or oxalosis.[1087] Tissue and vascular calcifications are generally absent in patients with a calcium × phosphorus product consistently below 60 but tend to occur above a mean product of approximately 84. Therefore, when one treats hyperparathyroidism by increasing the serum $Ca^{2+}$ concentration, the calcium × phosphorus product must be maintained below 70 to 80.[1035, 1073, 1088] Phosphorus is sequestrated in tissues and erythrocytes, has a large volume of distribution, and is not effectively dialyzed.[1089] Therefore, dialysis is effective only transiently in lowering the serum phosphorus concentration.[1090, 1091] Dietary phosphate restriction and oral $PO_4^{3-}$ binders remain the primary method of phosphorus control in dialysis patients.[1039, 1076, 1092–1094]

Because of the concern for aluminum toxicity, the search for $PO_4^{3-}$ binders other than aluminum hydroxide has been intense. Calcium carbonate[1095–1106] and calcium acetate[1107–1110] are the principal products used at present. An increase in the serum $Ca^{2+}$ concentration before a decrease in the serum phosphorus concentration may limit their usefulness. They are effective in the majority of patients, but only when given with meals.[1093, 1095, 1098, 1107] In some patients, a combination of calcium carbonate and aluminum hydroxide may be necessary to lower phosphorus levels before use of calcium carbonate alone. The finding of enhanced aluminum absorption in the presence of citrate makes calcium citrate an unacceptable binder.[1111, 1112] Furthermore, use of Shohl solution, Bicitra, or other citrate products should be avoided if the patient is exposed to aluminum hydroxide.[1071, 1072, 1113, 1114] Magnesium has been used as a $PO_4^{3-}$ binder[1115–1117] but causes diarrhea and a high serum $Mg^{2+}$ concentration.[1118, 1119] Other $PO_4^{3-}$-binding agents have been tried[1120–1125] but have not become clinically useful. The serum phosphorus concentration must also be monitored to avoid hypophosphatemia,[1126–1128] which some think may play a role in the development of aplastic bone disease and hemolysis. Dietary restriction of phosphorus is minimally effective if used alone. This approach also causes complications by restricting protein intake, which may result in malnutrition. The problems associated with malnutrition should elevate the acceptable level of phosphorus in such patients.

An extensive literature has developed concerning abnor-malities in vitamin D metabolism and the role of vitamin D in preventing and treating secondary hyperparathyroidism (details are discussed in Chapter 51). Many studies have shown improvement in osteitis fibrosa cystica, healing of fractures, increased muscle strength, improved growth in children, and a decrease in PTH and alkaline phosphatase levels with the use of 1,25-dihydroxycholecalciferol[1035, 1040–1042, 1129–1131] or dihydrotachysterol.[1132–1134] Newer vitamin D analogues have been developed but have received little clinical use.[1135–1138] A number of papers have suggested that intravenous administration of 1,25-dihydroxycholecalciferol is superior to oral 1,25-dihydroxycholecalciferol therapy by improving PTH suppression without hypercalcemia.[1139–1145] Alternatively, the use of oral ("pulse") 1,25-dihydroxycholecalciferol therapy (0.5 to 1.0 μg two or three times per week) has been suggested to simulate the intravenous effect and may be as useful.[1146, 1147] In general, it seems reasonable to begin patients with oral 1,25-dihydroxycholecalciferol therapy (with or without pulse dosing) and convert to intravenous 1,25-dihydroxycholecalciferol if oral therapy is shown to be ineffective. Early institution of vitamin D in patients before initiation of dialysis is thought to be important in minimizing the development of metabolic bone disease due to hyperparathyroidism.[1148–1150] Although there was initial concern about vitamin D accelerating the decline of renal function in chronic renal failure,[1151, 1152] careful control of the calcium × phosphorus product has shown these compounds to have no significant deleterious impact on renal function.[1153–1155]

Renal diseases associated with more severe acidosis may accentuate osteitis fibrosa cystica,[1156, 1157] and the use of sodium bicarbonate to correct severe acidosis as well as the conversion of dialysate from acetate to $HCO_3^-$ may be beneficial.[1158, 1159] Cimetidine has been shown to decrease PTH levels[1160, 1161] and has been suggested to be effective in lowering $Ca^{2+}$ concentration in hypercalcemic patients,[1162] but not because of a direct effect on PTH.[1163] In general, cimetidine has had a minimal effect on hypercalcemia.

In summary, the early use of vitamin D with control of phosphorus and $Ca^{2+}$ levels has led to a dramatic reduction in the frequency of hyperparathyroidism and osteitis fibrosa cystica. Symptoms and signs of severe hyperparathyroidism, such as shortening of stature, multiple fractures, brown tumors, subperiosteal tears of the quadriceps tendon insertion, and diffuse bone pain, have become much less frequent.

The decreased occurrence of secondary hyperparathyroidism has been replaced by an increasing frequency of aplastic bone disease.[1054–1056, 1164] Aplastic bone disease was initially thought to be due to aluminum. However, other possibilities, such as iron in the calcification front,[1165, 1166] excessive $PO_4^{3-}$ depletion, excessive lowering of PTH with vitamin D supplements, and the use of peritoneal dialysis, are now considered factors.[1164] The diagnosis is made by bone biopsy. In patients with bone symptoms but with low PTH levels and no evidence of aluminum intoxication, this diagnosis should be considered. Because the cause is unknown, there is no recognized treatment.

The decision to perform subtotal parathyroidectomy in long-term dialysis patients is not always straightforward. Parathyroidectomy can improve severe bone disease associated with secondary hyperparathyroidism.[1167–1173] Anemia, pruritus, neuropathy, growth retardation, impotence, calciphylaxis, and cardiac dysfunction have also been reported to improve with parathyroidectomy.[1174–1181] In general, the surgical approach should be avoided if conservative therapy can reverse hyperparathyroidism. Control of serum phosphorus levels, attention to oral calcium intake and dialysate $Ca^{2+}$ levels, and oral and intravenous administration of vitamin D should always be used initially to achieve a "medical parathyroidectomy."[1039, 1092, 1182] If bone pain persists or progresses despite these efforts, and $PO_4^{3-}$ concentration or the PTH level remains severely elevated, subtotal parathyroidectomy is indicated. Seven-eighths parathyroidectomy is the usual procedure.[1168–1170, 1183] Because of a high rate of reoperation,[1184] some surgeons advocate total parathyroidectomy.[1185–1188] Autotransplantation of parathyroid tissue has been suggested[1189–1191] but does not appear to provide any unique advantage. Acute hypocalcemia is a frequent complication after parathyroidectomy,[1192–1194] particularly in patients who have not been treated adequately with calcium and vitamin D before surgery. These patients may require large doses of oral calcium carbonate or intravenous calcium gluconate immediately after parathyroidectomy with intensification of oral and intravenous vitamin D therapy.

Because aluminum-induced osteomalacia will worsen after parathyroidectomy,[1169, 1170, 1195–1198] this procedure should not be performed for bone symptoms or in mixed disorders in which aluminum osteomalacia is present. Because of the potential of worsening aluminum osteomalacia after parathyroidectomy, some recommend treatment of aluminum-induced osteomalacia with deferoxamine before parathyroidectomy. The interrelationship between aluminum and the parathyroid glands is important in understanding this phenomenon and is discussed in detail in a later section.

## OSTEOMALACIA DUE TO VITAMIN D DEFICIENCY OR ALUMINUM INTOXICATION

Before the availability of vitamin D and its analogues, vitamin D–deficient osteomalacia was not an uncommon finding in uremic patients, particularly children. However, at that time, patients did not live sufficiently long for this issue to become a significant problem. In the past 20 years, observation of the failure of some patients to respond to vitamin D therapy led to the identification of a group of patients with persistent bone pain, pathologic fractures, hypercalcemia, and only moderate hyperparathyroidism.[1046, 1047, 1199] In histologic studies, osteomalacia was shown to be the principal lesion associated with this syndrome. Initially, hypophosphatemia was suggested as a cause for this symptom complex.[1200, 1201] The presence of fluoride in the dialysate was also suggested as a cause of this disease.[1202, 1203] With improved diagnostic techniques, the presence of aluminum in the osteoid seam of osteomalacic bone was demonstrated, and the toxic effects of aluminum have now been well established.[1050–1053, 1204–1207]

Aluminum depresses PTH biosynthesis and secretion,[1208–1210] which accounts for the low PTH level seen in such patients. Conversely, PTH protects against aluminum deposition,[1195, 1196, 1211] an observation that may explain the acceleration of this disease after parathyroidectomy. In addition, aluminum loading has been shown to depress 1,25-dihydroxycholecalciferol production[1212] and may lead to a resistance to the action of 1,25-dihydroxycholecalciferol.[1213] Despite this effect on vitamin D metabolism, most patients with aluminum osteomalacia are hypercalcemic or become so with only modest doses of vitamin D supplements. The deposition of aluminum along the osteoid seam impairs $Ca^{2+}$ uptake into bone. The normal or minimally elevated alkaline phosphatase levels attest to the relatively adynamic nature of this disorder.

Random serum aluminum levels are variable and are generally believed not to be diagnostic.[1214, 1215] One study, however, suggests that levels greater than 135 μg/L have a predictive value.[1216] In large populations of dialysis patients, serum aluminum levels correlate significantly with mortality, independent of bone disease.[1217] The explanation for this observation is unknown; it may simply be a marker for other dialysis-related problems. The deferoxamine challenge test[1218, 1219] has been suggested to be more specific for the diagnosis of aluminum-induced bone disease. However, the specificity of this test has been challenged.[1220]

Epidemic osteomalacic bone disease was initially recognized in Europe as aluminum contamination of dialysate water.[1221–1225] Subsequently, with purification of dialysate water, absorption of aluminum administered orally to patients with decreased renal function has been demonstrated to be the major source of aluminum accumulation.[112, 1226–1230] Appreciation of the role of dialysate aluminum and orally ingested aluminum hydroxide led to the use of deionization and reverse osmosis of water for dialysate and a marked decrease in the use of aluminum hydroxide as a $PO_4^{3-}$ binder. With these maneuvers, the frequency of aluminum-induced osteomalacia has been reduced dramatically. However, for some patients, the use of calcium carbonate and calcium acetate binders may not be effective, and aluminum hydroxide continues to be used at least partially. In addition, patients are unavoidably exposed to aluminum from drugs such as sucralfate.[1231–1233] For some patients, the aluminum burden from previous years' therapy continues to create clinical problems. For such patients, removal of aluminum with intravenous deferoxamine has been suggested. Several studies have demonstrated an improvement in bone disease with intravenous deferoxamine.[637, 1234–1237] The chelated product is not removed with standard dialysis[1238–1240] but must be absorbed with charcoal[1241–1244] or dialyzed by high-flux hemodialysis.[1245–1247] Deferoxamine is not uniformly effective and can cause serious complications, such as cataracts and ocular field defects,[1248, 1249] thrombocytopenia,[634] accentuation of aluminum-induced encephalopathy,[636, 637, 1250] and mucormycosis.[633, 1251–1254] These complications and the decreased use of aluminum-containing antacids have led to a substantial decrease in the use of this agent.

## OSTEOARTHROPATHY OF β₂-MICROGLOBULIN AMYLOIDOSIS

A high frequency of carpal tunnel syndrome,[1033, 1057–1059, 1255–1259] osteoarticular lesions in the shoulder,* cystic carpal

---

*References 76, 1033, 1064–1067, 1255, 1260–1262.

bone lesions, and cervical spondyloarthropathy[1063, 1263–1268] has been increasingly appreciated in long-term dialysis patients. Dialysis-associated amyloidosis or $\beta_2$-microglobulin amyloidosis is seen much more commonly in older patients (older than 50 years),[76] patients having had dialysis for more than 10 years,[1269] and those who have suffered other rheumatologic disease before renal failure. Much less commonly, $\beta_2$-microglobulin amyloidosis can present with amyloid nephrolithiasis, macroscopic skin deposits, and vascular erosion with gastrointestinal bleeding.[1270–1273]

With the onset of ESRD, $\beta_2$-microglobulin rapidly accumulates in the skin. After 5 years, the rate of accumulation in the skin greatly declines, which suggests that the protein may then collect in osteoarticular sites. After 10 years of dialysis, approximately 50% of the patients surveyed exhibited signs of $\beta_2$-microglobulin amyloidosis, and for patients who survive with hemodialysis for 20 years, the prevalence of $\beta_2$-microglobulin amyloidosis is almost 100%.[1033] Carpal tunnel syndrome, which is the most frequent presentation of $\beta_2$-microglobulin amyloidosis, occurs with an excessive frequency in patients with ESRD.[1057] Many but not all of these cases are a consequence of the deposition of $\beta_2$-microglobulin amyloid into the flexor tendon sheath with a resultant compressive neuropathy. This complication becomes clinically manifested after only 5 years of dialysis in susceptible patients and occurs with increasing frequency as the time on dialysis increases. Another common joint manifestation is the scapulohumeral arthropathy that is often associated with a progressive clawhand deformity (shoulder-hand syndrome). The progressive deposition of amyloid in and around the rotator cuff results in a progressive decline in mobility manifested by a limited capacity to abduct and shoulder pain.[1274] These deposits in the shoulder may become sufficiently large to be visible on physical examination ("shoulder pad" sign). There are often accompanying amyloid-filled bone cysts in the humeral head. The deposition of $\beta_2$-microglobulin amyloid along the flexor sheath of the hand results in a permanent flexor deformity of the digits and may also become sufficiently large to be palpated.

The skeletal manifestations of $\beta_2$-microglobulin amyloidosis are typically cysts that occur in the knees, hips, shoulders, elbows, ankles, and digits. The cysts of $\beta_2$-microglobulin amyloidosis can usually be distinguished from the brown tumors of secondary hyperparathyroidism. The cysts can become sufficiently large that the structural integrity of the weight-bearing bones becomes compromised, and pathologic fractures occur. This is an especially common occurrence in the hip. A similar pathobiologic process occurs in the cervical spine that presents as an erosive spondyloarthropathy. Fracture through these lesions can have devastating neurologic consequences.[1275] Gastrointestinal involvement[819, 1009] and other systemic involvement[1276, 1277] have been increasingly appreciated.

An extensive literature now confirms that $\beta_2$-microglobulin, which is amyloidogenic, is the protein responsible for this disorder.[1070, 1278–1289] This form of amyloidosis merits distinction from other forms of amyloidosis in that the amyloid protein is composed of $\beta_2$-microglobulin[1290]; the disease occurs in hemodialysis patients without a previous history of amyloidosis[76] and presents predominantly as an

osteoarthropathy.[1291] The amyloid protein stains with Congo red stain, exhibits apple-green birefringence under polarized light, and is a fibril when examined by electron microscopy.

The tissue accumulation of $\beta_2$-microglobulin amyloid is extremely large. There is debate whether this accumulation is due to decreased excretion or whether there is enhanced synthesis due to dialysis with bioincompatible membranes.[1292–1296] Several studies have shown that increased $\beta_2$-microglobulin synthesis occurs when mononuclear cells are exposed to selected cytokines.[1297, 1298] However, serum and joint concentrations of $\beta_2$-microglobulin do not correlate with the presence of the disease. In patients who are disease free and in those with the arthropathy, the serum concentration of $\beta_2$-microglobulin is typically a log greater than normal and inversely correlates with the glomerular filtration rate.

Alternatively, numerous studies have suggested that the development of $\beta_2$-microglobulin amyloidosis is related primarily to dialysis with cuprophane membranes.[1299–1306] Some studies have suggested that this syndrome is much less common in patients who have dialysis only with biocompatible membrane materials, specifically polyacrylonitrile.[76, 1307, 1308] For example, 23% and 11% of the patients having dialysis for the same number of years with cellulosic and synthetic membranes, respectively, had bone cysts; 30% and 13% of the patients having dialysis with cellulosic and synthetic membranes, respectively, had carpal tunnel syndrome. However, the argument that $\beta_2$-microglobulin amyloidosis is a bioincompatibility phenomenon is confounded by its occurrence in patients before initiation of dialysis[1309] as well as by the development of the disease in those on continuous ambulatory peritoneal dialysis alone.[1310–1314] Arguably, this predilection for the disease to occur in patients who have dialysis with cellulose-based membranes may not be solely a function of the composition of the dialysis membrane but a manifestation of its clearance characteristics for $\beta_2$-microglobulin. Some investigators have shown that this large molecule can be effectively cleared with highly porous membranes by diffusion.[1315–1324] In addition, several other studies have suggested that $\beta_2$-microglobulin is adsorbed onto dialysis membranes such as polysulfone.[1318, 1325–1327] Whether diffusive clearance or adsorption of this product will have any significant effect on the enormous quantity of $\beta_2$-microglobulin that accumulates in ESRD has yet to be demonstrated.

Renal transplantation may be beneficial in patients with this disorder,[1328–1330] but the number of patients who have undergone renal transplantation is small. Because this process occurs primarily in the elderly and in those who have had hemodialysis longer than 10 years, the likelihood of transplantation as a useful treatment is somewhat diminished. Awareness of this disease and a careful search for it by physical examination, shoulder ultrasonography,[1274, 1331, 1332] x-ray surveillance, radiolabeled $\beta_2$-microglobulin imaging,[1333, 1334] or joint biopsy[1335] will be important in detecting the process earlier in hope of moving affected patients more promptly toward renal transplantation. Therapeutic options at present consist of surgical removal of amyloid deposits in the hands, wrist, and shoulders[1336]; use of nonsteroidal anti-inflammatory agents; and perhaps steroid ionophoresis.

# Neurologic Abnormalities

## CENTRAL NERVOUS SYSTEM

Most of the CNS manifestations of advanced uremia, such as impaired mentation, lethargy, sleep disorder, asterixis, and multifocal myoclonus, are reversible with the initiation of dialysis.[1337, 1338] Residual neurologic deficits in well-dialyzed patients are subtle and show wide individual variation.[1339–1341] Adequacy of dialysis plays an important role in these mild abnormalities of higher nervous system function. Dialyzed patients in the high-BUN group of the National Cooperative Dialysis Study demonstrated a clear trend toward electroencephalographic abnormalities, with the most severe cases subsequently being dropped from the study because of hospitalization or death.[1342] Although a survey of neurobehavioral symptoms, such as the capacity to concentrate and sleep patterns, showed a deterioration in the high-BUN groups, no statistically significant differences were noted between the various groups. Thus, a dialyzable substance may be causal for CNS findings in uremia.

Neurotoxins other than urea, such as small polypeptides and $PO_4^{3-}$, have been implicated in these symptom complexes.[1341, 1343] Hyperparathyroidism also has been suggested to be an etiologic factor of uremic encephalopathy.[1344, 1345] One study noted that increased PTH concentration reduces the activity of choline kinase, which causes a significant derangement in acetylcholine metabolism and thereby alters brain synaptic function.[1346] Finally, in light of dramatic improvements in CNS function with erythropoietin therapy and increased hematocrit, the importance of anemia as a factor in these CNS abnormalities is apparent.[1347–1350] Neurobehavioral electrophysiologic tests (such as sensory evoked potential, cognitive event–related potential response, number cancellation protocol, trail-making test, single-digit modality test, Rey Auditory-Verbal Learning Test, Wechsler Adult Intelligence Scale, brain stem auditory evoked response, and magnetoencephalography) have been used principally in research protocols[1351–1354] but have not been useful as practical clinical tools in the assessment of neurologic disorders in dialysis patients. The electroencephalograph is an exception with its utility in the diagnosis of dialysis dementia and other seizure disorders.

In addition to uremic encephalopathy, a number of other CNS disorders or abnormalities causing CNS dysfunction occur in the dialysis patient (Table 56–11). Of these disorders, only dialysis disequilibrium and dialysis dementia are specific to dialysis patients. Dialysis disequilibrium occurs most commonly during the initial few dialyses and consists of confusion, disorientation, nausea, vomiting, and headache during or immediately after dialysis. This disorder is discussed further later. Dialysis disequilibrium should always be a diagnosis of exclusion because of the occurrence of possibly treatable conditions that it can mimic.[1355, 1356] Changes in osmolarity and pH may enhance seizure activity. When seizures occur, they are often associated with an underlying CNS lesion, which should be searched for even in patients with suspected dialysis disequilibrium. In initial studies with erythropoietin therapy, seizures were reported to occur more frequently.[539] However, several subsequent studies have indicated that seizures were related to too rapid

**TABLE 56–11. Differential Diagnosis of Altered Mental Status in Hemodialysis Patients**

Metabolic encephalopathies
  Overt uremia
  Hypercalcemia
  Hypophosphatemia
  Hypoglycemia
  Hyperglycemia (hyperosmolarity)
  Hyponatremia
  Hypernatremia
Intoxication
  Drug induced
  Trace elements
    Aluminum (dialysis dementia)
    Others (manganese, mercury, lead, fluoride, nickel, thallium, boron, vanadium, chromium, tin, cadmium)
Dialysis disequilibrium
Hypertensive encephalopathy
Cerebral atherosclerosis
Intracerebral hemorrhage
Subdural hematoma
Wernicke encephalopathy
Meningitis, encephalitis
Sleep apnea
Normal-pressure hydrocephalus
Central pontine myelinolysis

an increase in hematocrit that in turn resulted in malignant hypertension.[1357, 1358]

Dialysis dementia was first reported in the early 1970s[1359] and has been studied extensively. This is a progressive neurologic disorder seen exclusively in dialysis patients. The signs and symptoms of dialysis dementia and its progressive course have been well described.[1341, 1355] Disorders of speech, such as dysarthria and dysphasia, are common presenting features. Other symptoms and signs include dyscalculia, dyslexia, dyspraxia, dysgraphia, impaired memory, poor attention span, depression, paranoia, myoclonic jerking, and seizures. The symptoms are initially intermittent and are characteristically worst during or immediately after dialysis. Because there is no impairment in cognitive ability at the onset of the disorder, the affected patients often recognize their difficulty and are frustrated by it. The disorder is progressive, such that global dementia and death are the usual outcome. If this disorder is untreated, death usually occurs 6 to 15 months from the onset of symptoms. Longer survival has been reported, but rarely. The electroencephalographic pattern in patients with dialysis dementia is abnormal, demonstrating paroxysmal multifocal bursts of high-amplitude delta activity (4 waves/s) with spikes and sharp waves intermixed with runs of more normal background activity. This diagnostic pattern deteriorates to overall slower frequencies as the disease progresses.[1359, 1360]

In earlier studies, the epidemiologic pattern of occurrence and the clinical findings suggested an intoxication with an elemental toxin or contaminant. The association of osteomalacic bone disease, dialysis dementia, and microcytic anemia all due to aluminum-contaminated dialysate water was an early clue to the cause of this disease. The finding of high concentrations of aluminum in plasma and brains of patients suffering from dialysis dementia has strongly implicated this metal as a cause of the disorder.[115, 1360–1365]

Despite the evidence presented before, aluminum only partially fulfills the Koch postulates as an etiologic agent. It is present in high concentrations in patients with dialysis dementia,[115] but the disease is not uniformly reproducible in experimental animals when aluminum is given orally.[1355] Although serum aluminum levels of patients suffering from dialysis dementia are generally higher than levels from patients who do not have the disorder,[1366] overlap is demonstrated in most studies.

One study showed that aluminum inhibits dihydropteridine reductase in red blood cells, which suggests a similar effect on this enzyme in the brain. Dihydropteridine reductase is essential for the maintenance of adequate tetrahydrobiopterin concentrations that are necessary for the synthesis of specific neurotransmitters.[1367] A low-molecular-weight protein has been found to be a major binder of aluminum in the plasma of patients with dementia syndrome.[1368] The importance of this binding protein remains undetermined. An increase in aluminum has been reported in patients with Alzheimer syndrome and metastatic cancer.[1355] However, most studies have not shown a causal relationship among aluminum, senile plaques, and neural fibrillary tangles in long-term dialysis patients.[1369–1371] Thus, the presence of high aluminum levels may be only a marker of a disruptive blood-brain barrier in patients with dementia or a major systemic illness. Only one study has found a relation between histopathologic findings and dialysate aluminum–induced dementia.[1372]

As noted before, contamination of dialysate with aluminum has more support as an etiologic agent than does oral aluminum.[648, 1373, 1374] This is based on a higher frequency of encephalopathy in parts of the world where the dialysate water contains higher levels of aluminum. Oral ingestion of aluminum contained in $PO_4^{3-}$ binders is now thought to be the principal source of aluminum in hemodialysis patients.[1362, 1375, 1376] Although the blood aluminum concentrations measured in patients ingesting aluminum hydroxide are high, they are usually not elevated to the range that is found in patients with dialysis dementia.[1355] The dementia syndrome is rare in adult patients using aluminum-containing $PO_4^{3-}$ binders before the initiation of dialysis.[1377, 1378] However, pediatric patients are at greater risk for aluminum intoxication, and the use of aluminum-containing medications is contraindicated in this population of patients. Dialysis dementia may develop with shorter exposure time in adult patients by the concomitant ingestion of sodium citrate (Shohl solution, Bicitra) and aluminum hydroxide. Increased aluminum absorption in the presence of citrate suggests this combination should be avoided.[1071, 1072]

Preventive measures for dialysis dementia include the use of reverse osmosis in the preparation of dialysate water and vigilant monitoring of aluminum levels in dialysate water. Dialysate aluminum levels below 10 μg/L are considered safe, but lower levels are preferred.[1355] As is the case for aluminum-induced bone disease, aluminum hydroxide as a binder should be avoided in patients with CNS signs and symptoms. With the treatment of dialysate water along with avoidance of aluminum-containing binders, the dementia syndrome has become a rare occurrence in the past 8 to 10 years. Although deferoxamine has been advocated as a therapy for dialysis dementia,[1379, 1380] its effectiveness is limited in comparison to its efficacy in aluminum bone disease. In fact, several investigators have suggested that deferoxamine used to treat aluminum bone disease may precipitate or aggravate cerebral symptoms.[636–639] If deferoxamine is administered, dialysis should be performed with a high-flux dialysis membrane or with an activated charcoal filter in series with a conventional dialyzer to enhance clearance of the deferoxamine-aluminum complex.[629, 1240, 1245, 1381] Treatment with antiepileptics is no different from that for conventional seizures. Clonazepam and diazepam have been effective in some patients for controlling myoclonus.[1355]

Enlargement of the cerebral ventricular system on computed tomographic scanning of the head suggestive of cortical atrophy has been reported to be a more frequent finding in dialysis patients compared with age-matched control subjects.[1382, 1383] This anatomic variation is unrelated to the duration of renal failure or dialysis and does not correlate with clinical symptoms[1382] other than hypertension.[1384] The significance of cortical atrophy on the computed tomographic scan in dialysis patients remains unknown.

## PERIPHERAL NERVOUS SYSTEM

Uremic peripheral neuropathy is a distal, symmetric sensorimotor neuropathy, with the lower extremities more severely involved.[1337, 1385] Characteristically, it presents in a glove-stocking distribution. The sensory component of the neuropathy usually precedes motor symptoms and consists of paresthesia, burning, and pain. Motor abnormalities occur late and culminate in muscle atrophy. Again, the lower extremities are involved to an earlier and greater extent, which may result in footdrop. Another manifestation of neuropathy in dialysis patients is the restless legs syndrome. This can be severe and is not improved with dialysis. It often becomes worse during dialysis, causing extreme restlessness that forces the patient to discontinue dialysis prematurely. Peripheral neuropathy is thought to be due to demyelination after axonal degeneration, but the exact sequence is disputed. There is no characteristic pathologic change that distinguishes uremic polyneuropathy from other types of neuropathies.

Peripheral neuropathy can be monitored by the proper performance of motor nerve conduction velocity[1386] and vibratory perception and continuous perception testing.[1387, 1388] Far less often, and usually in a research setting, visual and brain stem auditory evoked potentials,[1389] somatosensory evoked potentials,[1390] and cephalic evoked noncutaneous sensations[1391] have been used to monitor the course of neuropathy.

The onset of sensory neuropathy in uremic patients is an indication for initiation of hemodialysis. Dialysis often leads to initial rapid symptomatic improvement followed by slower resolution of sensory symptoms.[1392] The extent of recovery in nondiabetic patients appears to correlate inversely with the severity of neurologic dysfunction before initiation of dialysis and the subsequent adequacy of dialysis. The National Cooperative Dialysis Study showed that patients in the high-BUN group had a significant deterioration of median motor nerve conduction velocities, median sensory nerve amplitude, and peroneal nerve conduction velocities compared with the low-BUN groups.[1342] In fur-

### TABLE 56–12. Dialysis Complications

**Acute**
Hypotension
Cramps
Bleeding/clotting
Anaphylaxis
Hemolysis
Leukopenia
Arrhythmias
Infections
Hypoxemia
Pyrogen reactions
Dialysis disequilibrium syndrome
Angioaccess dysfunction
Technical mishaps—incorrect dialysate mixture, contaminated
  dialysate, air embolism, spallation, incorrect replacement solution

**Chronic**
Inadequate clearance
$\beta_2$-Microglobulin amyloidosis
Aluminum intoxication

ther support of the deleterious contribution of uremia is the observation that transplantation often results in a further improvement of sensory peripheral neuropathy.[1355] Severe motor neuropathy is usually unresponsive to hemodialysis. It sometimes responds partially to transplantation,[1393] but often leaves the patient with persistent residual motor symptoms, particularly if atrophy is present. The improvement in the sensory symptoms with dialysis and transplantation suggests that in the early stages of the disease, neurologic functional impairment is more strongly related to symptoms than are structural abnormalities. In one study, zinc supplementation of the dialysate improved abnormal nerve conduction velocities.[1394] However, this unsubstantiated report is insufficient evidence for recommending the routine use of zinc.

### AUTONOMIC NERVOUS SYSTEM

Several abnormalities of the autonomic nervous system are evident in uremic patients, as documented by abnormalities in the Valsalva maneuver, blood pressure response to handgrip exercise, response to orthostasis, pulse response to elevated blood pressure, decrease in sweating, and orthostatic hypotension unrelated to medication or extracellular fluid volume depletion.[1395–1397] These abnormalities and their role in dialysis hypotension are discussed further in the section on complications. Autonomic neuropathy seems to correlate with peripheral neuropathy.[1398–1399] Both parasympathetic[1399, 1400] and sympathetic[1401] nervous systems are involved. In nondiabetic uremic patients, these abnormalities often improve with initiation of dialysis, but some dialysis patients have evidence of autonomic neuropathy despite adequate dialysis.

Abnormalities of heart rate response and a failure of the blood pressure to rise appropriately during the release phase of the Valsalva maneuver are seen in dialysis patients. Plasma norepinephrine levels, which are elevated in uremic patients, are normal after initiation of dialysis and respond normally to orthostasis in dialyzed patients.[1395] Also, the blood pressure response to norepinephrine infusion was closer to normal in dialysis patients than in nondialyzed uremic patients. The location of the lesion responsible for these abnormalities has not been defined. Relative end-organ resistance to norepinephrine is one of the factors responsible. Structural lesions in various segments of the baroreceptor arc, mirroring those observed in peripheral nerves, may also be present. However, no correlation to symptoms has been provided.[1396]

Disorders of the autonomic nervous system in dialysis patients play a role in the decreased compensatory responses to hypotension during dialysis, particularly in diabetic patients.[1396, 1402] Autonomic neuropathy is also a contributing factor in the reduced nocturnal penile tumescence seen in uremic patients.[1403] Treatment options are limited. In view of the improvement seen in some of these abnormalities after initiation of dialysis, it is important to initiate dialysis early and ensure adequacy of treatment in uremic patients with symptoms of autonomic insufficiency.

## SELECTED COMPLICATIONS OF HEMODIALYSIS

The complications of hemodialysis are best perceived conceptually as acute and chronic (Table 56–12). Most of these complications are preventable or can be managed with appropriate diligence. The acute complications discussed are hypotension, cramps, febrile (pyrogen) reactions, arrhythmias, dialysis disequilibrium, hypoxemia, anaphylaxis, and technical mishaps. Bleeding, as an acute complication, is discussed earlier. The sole chronic complication that is reviewed in this section is inadequate dialysis. Other chronic complications, such as dialysis-associated amyloidosis, aluminum intoxication syndromes, metabolic bone disease, malnutrition, and immunologic dysfunction, are discussed in preceding sections.

### Hypotension

Intradialytic hypotension, which occurs in 10% to 50% of the treatments, is the most frequent complication of dialysis.[1404] During ultrafiltration, protein-free fluid is removed from the intravascular space, which results in an increase in the intravascular oncotic pressure. The relative decline in intravascular hydraulic pressure and increase in oncotic pressure result in volume repletion of the vascular space from the interstitium. Support of the mean arterial pressure during these fluid fluxes mandates a compensatory increase in sympathetic tone, which in turn enhances chronotropy and peripheral vascular resistance.[1405] There is also redistribution of regional blood flow such that splanchnic and cutaneous perfusion is decreased.

Most cases of dialysis-induced hypotension are ascribed to excessive ultrafiltration (frank intravascular volume depletion resulting in diminished left ventricular filling pressure) or to an excessive rate of ultrafiltration (volume removal from the intravascular space at a rate that exceeds the capacity of interstitial fluid to migrate into this compartment). Certainly, an incorrect assessment of the patient's "estimated dry weight" (weight below which the patient has symptomatic hypotension or muscle cramps in the absence of an interdialytic weight gain of more than 1 kg/d and edema that is not attributable to hypoalbuminemia, lower extremity venous insufficiency, or other identifiable causes) will result in hypotension. The frequent and sometimes incorrect attribution of hypotension to an excessively low estimated dry weight is a consequence of the imprecision in defining the estimated dry weight. An alternative to clinical assessments alone is the use of regional noninvasive conductivity measurements.[1406] Noninvasive measurement correlations with the diameter of the inferior vena cava, right atrial pressure, and blood volume, if validated, may yield an important tool in the treatment of dialysis patients.

A number of additional factors contribute to intradialytic hypotension (see Fig. 56–12). These include left ventricular dysfunction (systolic or diastolic due to comorbid illness or medications), autonomic dysfunction (due to renal or comorbid disease processes or medications), inappropriate vasodilatation (due to eating, sepsis, or medications), disease of the pericardium or the pericardial space, and bleeding.[153, 1407–1411] Other critical components of the dialysis procedure may contribute to the development of hypotension. These include the choice of dialysate (buffer, $Na^+$, and $Ca^{2+}$ concentrations and dialysate temperature) and the dialyzer membrane's composition and porosity. Specific provocative issues are the 1) vasodilatory and cardiodepressant effects of acetate; 2) impairment of vasoconstriction, exacerbation of autonomic dysfunction, and declining serum osmolality associated with a hyponatric dialysate; 3) diminished cardiac contractility and the vasodilatory effects of the conventional dialysate temperature of 37°C; 4) vasodilatory and cardiodepressant effects of a lowered dialysate $Ca^{2+}$ concentration; 5) cellulose membrane–induced complement activation; 6) cellulose membrane–induced or acetate-induced hypoxemia; 7) complement- or pyrogen-induced pyrogenic cytokine production; and 8) dialysis membrane hypersensitivity manifested by kallikrein/bradykinin activation.*

On the basis of this pathobiologic process, specific strategies to manage intradialytic hypotension include, but are not limited to, withholding antihypertensive and anti-inotropic medications for 4 to 6 hours before the dialysis treatment; decreasing the blood flow and dialyzer surface area; removing fluid for an increased dialysis time (less volume ultrafiltered per unit time) or increasing the frequency of dialysis sessions; increasing the dialysate $Na^+$ concentration to 140 to 145 mEq/L ($Na^+$ modeling); performing sequential ultrafiltration/clearance; switching to an $HCO_3^-$-buffered dialysate; cooling the dialysate to 35°C; increasing the dialysate $Ca^{2+}$ concentration to 3.5 mEq/L; switching to a more biocompatible dialysis membrane material, such as polysulfone; augmenting impaired intropy by the use of cardiac glycosides or parenteral inotrophs; avoiding food during dialysis; and administering supplemental oxygen during the dialysis session.

Hypotension after the dialysis session is typically due to hypovolemia and may be managed by the administration of saline or the ingestion of salty foodstuffs, such as bouillon or crackers. Other potential causes of hypotension, such as occult bleeding or pericardial disease, should not be overlooked.

## Cramps

Muscle cramps are a non–life-threatening morbid occurrence in chronic renal failure. However, in one study, the most frequent reason for discontinuing hemodialysis treatments prematurely was muscle cramps.[1415] Their precise frequency is uncertain, but at least 20% of patients report their occurrence during dialysis.[1262] Similarly, many patients have leg cramps during sleep that contribute to the insomnia associated with ESRD. Although any muscle group can be involved, cramps typically involve the legs, feet, and hands and occur during the latter half of dialysis. Intradialytic muscle cramps are typically self-limited, resolving in about 10 minutes. The pathobiologic mechanism of muscle cramps appears to relate to intradialytic ischemia of the skeletal muscle. Therefore, cramps occur most often with large interdialytic weight gains that necessitate aggressive ultrafiltration or when the volume ultrafiltered exceeds the estimated dry weight.

Dialysis with a hyperosmolal or an $HCO_3^-$-buffered dialysate is associated with a decreased frequency of intradialytic muscle cramps.[134, 1416] Similarly, muscle cramps can be attenuated by the predialysis or nocturnal administration of quinine (260 to 325 mg) or vitamin E (400 IU).[1417, 1418] Once established, cramps can be minimized or abated by the oral or intravenous administration of hypertonic agents, such as 50% dextrose (50 mL), 25% mannitol (100 mL), or 23.5% salt solution (10 mL).[1414, 1419]

## Pyrogen Reactions

Pyrogen reaction is the term used for intradialytic or postdialytic febrile events that arise as an immediate consequence of an intradialytic exposure to bacteria (without bacteremia) or to bacterial products in the absence of a clinical infection. Thus, in many cases, a pyrogen reaction is a historical diagnosis of exclusion. These reactions, which are characterized by fevers, chills, rigors, myalgias, and hemodynamic instability, typically occur during the second half of the dialysis. If the pyrogen exposure is large, the patient may have the full spectrum of laboratory findings that are typical of septicemia. With the implementation of the strict Association for the Advancement of Medical Instrumentation standards for the purity of water for dialysate preparation and for the reprocessing of dialyzers, pyrogen reactions are infrequent. Although in the National Surveillance of Hemodialysis Associated Diseases of 1990 at least one pyrogen reaction was reported by 20% of the facilities,[98] the frequency was less than 1 per 1000 dialysis treatments.[126] On the basis of a retrospective analysis, independent factors statistically associated with an increased frequency of pyrogen reactions include the use of high-flux dialyzers and the processing and reuse of these dialyzers. Despite the enhanced capacity of $HCO_3^-$-buffered dialysates to support the growth of bacteria,[103] no statistical cor-

---

*References 60, 61, 64–66, 68, 78, 102, 142, 160, 163, 165, 166, 174, 175, 1412–1414.

relation could be established with $HCO_3^-$ as a provocative factor independent of the other variables.[98] However, a prospective analysis of a large facility that had excessive bacterial growth in their $HCO_3^-$ dialysate was unable to demonstrate an influence of the hemodialysis modality (conventional, high efficiency, or high flux) on the rate of pyrogen reactions.[1420]

It has been argued that dialysate fluid should be sterile to prevent pyrogen reactions. In that the frequency of pyrogen reactions is generally low for the dialysis population at large, and the 11 dialysis facility outbreaks of pyrogen reactions were uniformly accompanied by contamination of the water or dialysate to a level that exceeded the Association for the Advancement of Medical Instrumentation standards, this extreme position seems unfounded. As discussed in an earlier section, the filtration of the dialysate is efficacious in removing most bacterial and endotoxin contaminants and may result in a lower frequency of pyrogen reactions.[126] This technique may be a cost-effective means of generating a dialysate that minimizes the risk of pyrogen reactions. In those situations in which a nondialysate source for pyrogen contamination has been identified, an additional site for pyrogen contamination includes the dialyzer's header spaces and O-rings.[1420]

The pathobiologic mechanism of pyrogen reactions may involve the pyrogen-induced synthesis and release of pyrogenic cytokines, such as IL-1, IL-6, and TNF,[87, 89, 90] during the dialysis session. Support for this hypothesis is provided by the demonstration of an increase in TNF in the plasma of two patients who had dialysis against a contaminated dialysate and had pyrogen reactions.[1421] Interestingly, the patients without pyrogen reactions in the same facility did not exhibit an elevation of IL-1 or TNF levels, regardless of the type of maintenance hemodialysis.

Specific therapy for a pyrogen reaction is supportive with antipyretics and the use of antibiotics. Antibiotic therapy should be continued until a bacterial infection has been eliminated as a cause for the febrile event. Clusters of pyrogen reactions within a facility should prompt a thorough analysis of the performance of the water purification system, dialysate purity, procedure for dialyzer and line reprocessing, and dialysis machine sterilization procedure.

## Arrhythmias

In addition to a number of baseline electrocardiographic abnormalities that typically occur during the first 2 hours of dialysis (decrease in T wave amplitude, increase in QRS amplitude, change in $QT_c$, and ischemic ST-T wave alterations), atrial and ventricular tachyarrhythmias and varying degrees of heart block are not usual occurrences.[1422] These rhythm disturbances typically occur in the setting of underlying cardiovascular diseases, such as coronary artery disease, hypertensive cardiomyopathy, ischemic cardiomyopathy, hypertrophic cardiomyopathy, conduction system disease, and pericardial disease.[152, 1422–1426] Further, many of the intended and undesired intradialytic and interdialytic alterations in the serum electrolytes, bases, and arterial oxygen saturation are themselves arrhythmogenic.[1426–1428] Last, many ESRD patients ingest medications, such as cardiac

glycosides, that are provocative for the development of dysrhythmias.[152] The solitary influence of intradialytic arrhythmias on the mortality of patients is controversial, with observations of excessive mortality[1429] or no adverse influence.[1424] Other variables that influence cardiovascular mortality are discussed in an earlier section.

As previously discussed, changes in the plasma $K^+$ concentration that are affected directly by the dialysate $K^+$ concentration are most often incriminated in the pathobiologic process of intradialytic arrhythmias. Other specific intradialytic changes in blood chemistry values that are provocative include 1) intradialytic flux of $Ca^{2+}$ and transient hypercalcemia with high dialysate $Ca^{2+}$ concentration, 2) transient loss of $HCO_3^-$ with acetate-buffered dialysate and resultant acidosis, 3) transient alkalosis with $HCO_3^-$-buffered dialysate, 4) direct cardiotoxicity of acetate, and 5) hypoxemia with acetate-buffered dialysate.[1430] If significant arrhythmias are encountered during hemodialysis (Lown and Grayboys classification of class 3 or above), corrective measures should include escalating the dialysate $K^+$ concentration (if it is 2 mEq/L or less), converting from an acetate-buffered to an $HCO_3^-$-buffered dialysate of 35 mEq/L or less, and decreasing the dialysate $Ca^{2+}$ concentration to 3.0 mEq/L. Consideration should be given to discontinuing cardiac glycosides, and supplemental oxygen can be administered during the dialysis treatment. The patient should be evaluated for cardiovascular disease and corrective management initiated. Last, the persistence of serious rhythm disturbances, despite the implementation of these maneuvers, merits appropriate pharmacologic antiarrhythmia therapy.

## Dialysis Disequilibrium

As mentioned before, the dialysis disequilibrium syndrome is an easily preventable complication from overzealous solute removal at the initiation of hemodialysis or a dramatic increase in the amount of dialysis delivered to a poorly dialyzed patient. The clinical disorder is an admixture of symptoms that include headache, nausea, vomiting, and hypertension, which can progress to arrhythmias, confusion, tremors, seizures, coma, and death.[1431] Typically, patients with disequilibrium syndrome have symptoms during the latter portion of dialysis or in the immediate postdialytic setting. Because of the lack of specific signs or diagnostic techniques, the differential diagnosis of the dialysis disequilibrium syndrome is lengthy and includes primary neurologic disorders such as subdural hematoma, cerebrovascular accidents, hypertensive encephalopathy, toxic encephalopathy, uremia, anoxia, and primary seizures (see Table 56–11). Interestingly, the electroencephalogram of many patients with dialysis disequilibrium is normal.[1432, 1433]

The precise pathobiologic mechanism of this disorder is undefined, but it may arise because of intradialytic and postdialytic cerebral edema. Although not uniformly supported experimentally,[50, 1434] a body of experimental and clinical evidence suggests that with excessively aggressive solute clearance, urea departure from the cerebrospinal fluid is delayed, and the brain becomes hyperosmolal.[1435] An additional contributant to the cerebrospinal fluid abnormality is the transient, paradoxical development of cerebrospinal fluid acidosis, with a resultant increase in osmotic activity. There may also be an inappropriate intracerebral accumulation of osmolytes, such as inositol, glutamine, and glutamate.[1431, 1436, 1437]

The simplest strategy for prevention of dialysis disequilibrium is to attenuate solute clearance during hemodialysis by using a smaller surface area dialyzer, decreasing blood and dialysate flows, circulating the blood and dialysate in a concurrent direction, or decreasing the dialysis time. A urea clearance of 1 to 2 mL/min/kg is typically well tolerated. However, such a low urea clearance results in a protracted recovery from uremia. This limitation can be overcome without increasing the risk for the dialysis disequilibrium syndrome by performing dialysis with low solute clearance for several consecutive days.[24] Alternatively, dialysis can be initiated by another modality that has less efficient solute clearance, such as peritoneal dialysis. Additional preventive strategies include the intradialytic administration of mannitol or dextrose, and dialysis with a hypernatric dialysate to minimize the decline in serum osmolality. Of these hyperosmolal agents, a high dialysate Na+ concentration appears to be the most effective.[137, 1438] Last, in high-risk patients who must have aggressive solute clearance, the patient should be loaded with phenytoin (1 g) before the dialysis session, and it should be continued for the subsequent 72 hours as a full dialysis schedule is achieved. Once dialysis disequilibrium has developed, therapy consists of the administration of antiepileptics and the institution of strategies to reduce intracerebral edema, such as hyperventilation and mannitol.

Relevant to the postoperative setting is that neurosurgical patients, with stable ESRD treated by hemodialysis, may exhibit a propensity for cerebral edema. Even in the setting of solute clearance not associated with a major change in the dialysis prescription, caution should be undertaken in performing solute clearance that may be associated with a deleterious degree of superimposed cerebral edema.[1439, 1440]

## Hypoxemia

A fall in arterial oxygen content is a frequent complication of hemodialysis that contributes to many of the other acute complications of dialysis.[1441] The prevalence has been reported to be approximately 90%.[66] The absolute decline in arterial oxygen tension is 5 to 35 mm Hg (mean of 15 mm Hg) and is usually of no clinical significance except in critically ill patients.

Conceptually, the pathobiologic process of the dialysis-induced hypoxemia may be segregated into dialysate-dependent and membrane-dependent causes. As previously discussed, one theory hypothesizes that during dialysis with an acetate-buffered dialysate, metabolism of acetate produces less carbon dioxide, and a decline in the respiratory quotient (ratio of expired carbon dioxide/consumed oxygen) causes compensatory hypoventilation and hypoxemia (normocapnic hypoventilation).[1442, 1443] However, this hypothesis is not fully supported by clinical observation. An alternative theory is that during hemodialysis with an ace-

tate-buffered dialysate, an intradialytic loss of carbon dioxide occurs across the dialysis membrane ("carbon dioxide unloading"), hypocapnia ensues, and compensatory alveolar hypoventilation results.[1444, 1445] The carbon dioxide tension of the venous blood from the dialyzer may be reduced to 15 mm Hg or less. Such a mechanism of carbon dioxide unloading would account for the attenuation of dialysis-induced hypoxemia with maneuvers that increase the carbon dioxide content of the dialysate, either by direct administration[1445, 1446] or indirectly by the substitution of an $HCO_3^-$-buffered dialysate.[1447] It has also been suggested that acetate may have direct adverse effects on the respiratory musculature or the central respiratory centers.[66]

Alternatively, the interaction of cellular and soluble components of the plasma may contribute to the development of dialysis-induced hypoxemia. As discussed earlier, peptides, such as C3a and C5a, induce the degranulation of mast cells, and the resultant histamine release presumably alters pulmonary regional ventilatory and perfusion patterns. Leukocyte interactions with the dialysis membrane enhance cell membrane expression of leukocyte adhesion molecules, causing enhanced endothelial adhesiveness and pulmonary leukocyte sequestration (leukocyte microemboli).[66, 80, 165, 166] Thus, dialysis-induced hypoxemia could be considered a manifestation of dialysis membrane bioincompatibility. Support for this hypothesis is provided by the observation that the severity of hypoxemia is lessened by the use of membrane materials that are more biocompatible.[1448–1450] The relative contribution of the membrane effects and dialysate effects appears weighted toward the dialysance of carbon dioxide.[1451]

Modifications of the hemodialysis procedure that minimize this complication initially include the use of an $HCO_3^-$-buffered dialysate. The use of dialysate $HCO_3^-$ concentrations above 35 mEq/L may induce alkalemia of a sufficient degree that hypoventilation and hypoxemia occur as a compensatory mechanism.[1442, 1452] A lesser effect will be achieved by conversion to a more biocompatible membrane material. In addition, patients at high risk should have the inspired oxygen concentration empirically increased during the dialysis treatment, especially those with a fixed ventilatory capacity.

## Dialyzer Reactions

The use of a new or a reprocessed dialyzer is infrequently associated with the acute development of a spectrum of illnesses. This complication of dialysis is often incorrectly ascribed to a hypersensitivity reaction to the dialysis membrane material. Instead, it is more accurate to segregate these disorders into hypersensitivity reactions to ethylene oxide; hypersensitivity reactions to selected membrane materials in the presence of an angiotensin-converting enzyme inhibitor; first-use reactions; direct toxic effects of ethylene oxide, formaldehyde, or glutaraldehyde; and idiopathic reactions.

Fortunately, true anaphylactic reactions in dialysis patients are a rare occurrence.[1453] Ethylene oxide gas, a common sterilant that is used for new dialyzers, may be improperly removed by the manufacturer or with rinsing in the dialysis facility. The interaction of ethylene oxide with albumin during dialysis alters albumin such that novel antigenic determinants are exposed, and specific immunoglobulin E is induced.[729, 1454] Patients typically manifest allergic reactions during the first 10 to 30 minutes of hemodialysis, and eosinophilia is a frequent accompanying feature.[1455] It is noteworthy that other leachable substances, such as potting compound, have infrequently been incriminated in these reactions. The clinical features consist of an admixture of symptoms that include hypotension, hypertension, dyspnea, wheezing, respiratory collapse, angioedema, urticaria, back and abdominal pain, fevers, and chills. Short-term therapy for hypersensitivity involves the immediate administration of antihistamines, epinephrine, and glucocorticoids. The likelihood of a hypersensitivity reaction is greatly reduced, even in the sensitized patient, by thoroughly rinsing the blood compartment of the dialyzer with several liters of saline and rinsing the dialysate compartment with dialysate before the use of the dialyzer. High-risk patients can be identified by either cutaneous testing or enzyme-linked immunosorbent assay for ethylene oxide–serum albumin.[1456]

Alternatively, intradialytic anaphylactic reactions may occur from the combination of an angiotensin-converting enzyme inhibitor and the use of an AN69 hollow-fiber (polyacrylonitrile) dialyzer.[1457, 1460] Like anaphylactic reactions associated with ethylene oxide sensitization, these reactions range in severity from mild to severe. These reactions do not occur if the angiotensin-converting enzyme inhibitor is discontinued or another dialysis membrane material is used. Preliminary evidence suggests that this disorder may be a consequence of abnormal generation of bradykinin that is induced by the interaction of plasma with AN69 membranes and impaired catabolism by the angiotensin-converting enzyme inhibitor.[68]

Of much greater frequency than either of the aforementioned hypersensitivity reactions is the first-use syndrome, which is an admixture of symptoms and signs that occur within minutes of the initial use of a cellulosic dialyzer. Chest pain, dyspnea, wheezing, and hypotension appear to be particularly prominent symptoms. However, the clinical presentation of this disorder may not be much different from that associated with true hypersensitivity reactions. It can be distinguished from these other adverse reactions by 1) the occurrence solely with a new cellulosic dialyzer, 2) the absence of symptoms with a noncellulosic dialyzer or a dialyzer that has been reprocessed without the use of bleach as a cleansing agent, 3) the absence of confounding medications such as an angiotensin-converting enzyme inhibitor, 4) the absence of specific immunoglobulin E antibodies, and 5) the absence of an associated eosinophilia. The pathobiologic mechanism of this disorder appears to relate to the patient's capacity to generate complement during hemodialysis.[1461] Patients with the first-use reaction generate more complement and at an earlier time in dialysis than do patients who are asymptomatic. For most patients, the reaction is sufficiently mild that prophylactic treatment with antihistamines and antipyretics is adequate. Alternatively, a noncellulosic membrane material can be used.

Reactions that occur during the first 5 minutes of a dialysis session are more likely to be a consequence of direct exposure to a toxin, such as the inadvertent infusion of ethylene oxide, formaldehyde, or glutaraldehyde. Aldehyde infusion is characteristically associated with intense burning pain at the site of vascular entry.

## Air Embolism, Hemolysis, and Errors in Dialysate Composition

Air embolism remains an ever-present risk because of the use of blood pumps in combination with an extracorporeal circuit.[1462] The quantity of air that is associated with symptoms depends on the physical state of the air, the rate of air entry, and the vessel of entry. For example, microbubbles are tolerated to a greater extent than a macroscopic bubble; a slow infusion is tolerated better than a large bolus; arterial air is less well tolerated than air in a vein. During hemodialysis, the emboli are typically venous.

The clinical manifestations of air emboli are dependent on the patient's body position at the time of embolization. If the patient is recumbent at the time of embolization, foam is formed and results in the occlusion of the pulmonary vasculature. The findings of acute pulmonary hypertension occur. If the patient is lying in the Trendelenburg position, air occludes the venous vasculature of the lower extremities with the findings of patchy cyanosis.

Treatment of air embolism involves preventing additional air from entering the patient's vasculature, providing respiratory support, and positioning the patient so that the sequelae of the embolus will be minimized. To attenuate the size of the bolus, the venous lines should be clamped immediately near the patient. The patient should be positioned with head down, legs up, and lying on the left side so that the air becomes entrapped in the apex of the right ventricle. If significant foaming has occurred in the right ventricle such that cardiac arrest has occurred, cardiac puncture and aspiration should be performed to remove the foam. The prognosis is grim at this point.

As described before, intradialytic hemolysis may occur from mechanical trauma to the erythrocytes during passage through the extracorporeal circuit. Typically, this is the result of the forced passage of blood through a crimped or obstructed segment of dialysis tubing. Similarly, hemolysis may be provoked by the inadvertent exposure of the patient to water-borne toxins contaminating the dialysate. Examples of these contaminants include chloramines,[116, 117] copper,[121, 122] and nitrates,[1463] which cause oxidative injury to erythrocytes; and formaldehyde, which impairs erythrocyte glycolysis and can alter epitopes on the erythrocyte, stimulating the formation of anti-N–like antibodies.[1464, 1465] Hemolysis due to formaldehyde exposure may be recurrent and self-limiting. Last, the accidental dialysis against an overheated or hypo-osmolal dialysate can result in severe hemolysis.[108, 1466]

Other complications related to an improper dialysate mixture are usually manifestations of the resultant change in the serum chemistry values. For example, dialysis with an excessively high dialysate $Na^+$ concentration will cause the clinical findings associated with hypernatremia, such as extreme thirst, hypertension, congestive heart failure, and seizures. The more common laboratory sequelae of errors in the dialysate mixture include hypernatremia, hyperkalemia, hyperbicarbonatemia, hypercalcemia, hyponatremia, hypokalemia, and hypobicarbonatemia.

## Inadequate Dialysis

The current hemodialysis delivery systems and the dialysis membranes are of sufficient efficiency that an adequate dialysis prescription can be delivered to virtually all patients in less than 5 hours. Further, numerous mathematic formulas and supportive software are available that allow frequent measurements of the quantity of dialysis that is being delivered. However, despite these advances in the capacity to provide appropriate care for the patient with ESRD, many nephrologists do not prescribe a quantity of dialysis that is sufficient to optimize the patient's survival. Although there are numerous clinical signs of grossly inadequate dialysis, such as serositis, progressive neuropathy, recurrent infections, encephalopathy, and declining nutrition, most patients who have inadequate dialysis do not manifest this degree of uremic symptoms. Therefore, simple clinical parameters are themselves inadequate for monitoring the quality and necessary quantity of hemodialysis to optimize survival of the patient.

The historical definition of dialysis adequacy was established by the National Cooperative Dialysis Study and a subsequent mechanistic analysis based on the patient's Kt/V and protein catabolic rate.[42, 1467] On the basis of these studies, minimal criteria for dialysis adequacy were established for a Kt/V of 1.05.[1467] It is noteworthy that although these are benchmark papers in the definition of dialysis adequacy, they may not be applicable to many of the current ESRD patients in the United States. As described in the introductory remarks to this chapter, the elderly American dialysis population, with its increasing comorbidity, would have been too ill and too old to have been enrolled in the National Cooperative Dialysis Study. Further, many patients do not have an adequate dialysis prescribed to achieve even these minimal criteria. At least four independent groups of investigators have uncovered widespread underprescription and underdelivery of hemodialysis.[20, 1468] In a retrospective analysis of more than 13,000 hemodialysis patients, we found that about 30% received a Kt/V (measured as a urea reduction ratio) of less than 59%.[21] With use of a national data base (United States Renal Data System), about 50% of 3000 patients were observed to have a prescribed Kt/V of 1.0 or less. Further confounding the topic of dialysis adequacy are the discrepancies in dialysis delivery (see earlier). Unfortunately, a variance in the variables that have impact on the amount of dialysis delivered, such as the blood flow, dialyzer efficiency, urea rebound, and dialysis duration, has an adverse influence. This deleterious discrepancy between the quantity of dialysis ordered and delivered has been validated.[1469]

The consequences of inadequate solute clearance are lethal and may contribute to the excessive mortality that is observed within the United States. If the duration of dialysis is considered a surrogate for solute clearance, several investigators have demonstrated an increased odds risk of death in patients who have dialysis for less than 3 to 3.5

hours.[276, 1470] The weekly duration of dialysis within the United States has declined to approximately 7 to 8 hours[2] versus 12 to 15 hours in European countries with ESRD programs and Japan.[1471] As anticipated, the survival for hemodialysis patients in these countries is greater than in the United States. Several investigators have emphasized that the National Cooperative Dialysis Study established only a minimal standard for dialysis adequacy and that survival of patients can be improved by greater delivery of solute clearance.[21, 984] Therefore, it appears that a urea reduction ratio of more than 60% or a Kt/V of 1.3 or greater will provide adequate dialysis. The effect of optimal solute clearance may also positively influence the patient's nutritional status.[1472] In a single report, an increase in the Kt/V from 0.8 to 1.3 resulted in an increase in the protein catabolic rate from 0.8 to 1.0.

The other aspect of dialysis adequacy that may be nearly as critical is the achievement of an adequate postdialysis volume status. Although an adequate solute clearance can be delivered by use of shorter dialysis times with high-efficiency and high-flux hemodialysis membranes, abbreviated dialysis times result in increasing difficulty in achieving the patient's true estimated dry weight. Arguably, the resultant chronic hypervolemia may contribute to the development of chronic congestive cardiomyopathies.[1473] Of note is that in a facility that provided a mean Kt/V of 1.7 with a relatively prolonged dialysis time, virtually every patient was normotensive without antihypertensives.[984] Therefore, solute clearance must be frequently and accurately measured and deficiencies promptly corrected. Patients should be actively involved in monitoring their dialysis adequacy so that they are not fixated on the duration of dialysis instead of the quality of the dialysis treatments. Last, the estimated dry weight should be achieved at the completion of the majority of dialysis sessions. If the estimated dry weight cannot be met within the prescribed dialysis time that is dictated by adequacy of solute clearance, consideration should be given to increasing the duration of dialysis.

## MATCHING THE DIALYSIS TREATMENT TO THE PATIENT

Although typically viewed as an issue only for the patient with acute renal failure who has not yet been committed to a particular dialysis modality, the matching of the type of dialysis to the patient and the comorbid conditions can require an equivalent amount of deliberation for patients having maintenance dialysis. An important principle to remember is that virtually no maintenance dialysis patients are "married" to their dialysis modality. For most patients, the choice of dialysis technique was determined by subjective issues, such as the patient's and physician's preference and prejudice, access to transportation, support in the home and community, and likelihood of compliance. Therefore, when the patient is sufficiently ill whereby a reconsideration of the maintenance dialysis technique has arisen, the objective medical concerns should be the overwhelming point of convergence for resolving this issue.

As may be appreciated from the previous sections, the decision of the optimal dialysis modality for a particular clinical situation is imprecise. For example, a nephrology publication debated (*without* resolution) the choice of hemodialysis versus peritoneal dialysis for the patient with cardiovascular instability[998, 1474] and hemofiltration versus hemodialysis for acute renal failure.[182, 1475] Therefore, the following expresses only guidelines that reflect the experiences and the bias of the authors for the treatment of acute renal failure (Table 56–13).

1. If the patient is severely hypervolemic or is receiving large obligatory volumes (hyperalimentation, antibiotics, or inotrophs) but is otherwise hemodynamically stable, hemodialysis should be performed with a hemodialyzer having a large ultrafiltration coefficient. If the patient is hemodynamically unstable, CRRT should be performed.

2. If the patient is hypercatabolic from a comorbid condition, such as sepsis, burns, or trauma, either hemodialysis or CRRT should be performed. If hemodialysis is selected, the surface area of the dialyzer should be large, with maximal blood and dialysate flows. If solute clearance is inadequate despite a long dialysis time, daily hemodialysis may be necessary. If such scheduling is impractical, the patient should undergo CRRT.

3. If the patient has a poor cardiovascular reserve, ultrafiltration of large volumes is not required, and clearance requirements are modest, peritoneal dialysis may be substituted for CRRT.

4. If the patient cannot have anticoagulation, such as postoperative neurosurgical patients, hemodialysis can be performed with no heparin. Alternatively, peritoneal dialysis can be used.

5. If vascular access cannot be established, such as in diabetic patients with severe peripheral vascular disease or venous disease due to previous catheterizations, the patient should be treated by peritoneal dialysis.

6. If attenuated clearances are required, such as in the patient who is severely uremic and at great risk for the disequilibrium syndrome, hemodialysis may be performed with low blood and dialysate flows, concurrent blood and dialysate flow, short dialysis time, and a small surface area dialyzer. Alternatively, peritoneal dialysis may be used.

7. In postoperative neurosurgical patients at risk for development of worsening cerebral edema with intermittent hemodialysis, peritoneal dialysis may be substituted.

8. If the patient's mobility is an issue, such as the requirement to transport the patient often for different investigations or procedures, CRRT should not be performed.

9. CRRT cannot be performed where one-to-one nursing is unavailable.

10. Rapid removal of drugs from intoxications, such as aminophylline or lithium, is best accomplished by hemodialysis.

No matter which dialysis modality is selected, the full range of dialysis techniques may be used as necessary. For example, if hemodynamic instability compromises fluid removal during hemodialysis, and this is otherwise the best modality for the patient, sequential ultrafiltration-clearance should be tried. If the patient requires a continuous therapy like continuous arteriovenous hemodialysis but cannot tolerate the lactate load in the conventional peritoneal dialysate, pre-postdilutional continuous arteriovenous hemofiltration may provide adequate clearance. If continuous therapy is required but the patient cannot tolerate heparin, CRRT with a parallel plate dialyzer, short lines, and a predilutional technique should be performed.

### *Acknowledgments*

We give special thanks to Joan Glowick, Gloria Interbartolo, and Lynda Herrera for secretarial assistance.

## TABLE 56–13. Considerations Relevant to Selection of a Dialysis Modality

| Patient Specific | Dialysis Specific |
|---|---|
| Residual renal function | Membrane composition |
| Cardiovascular status | Membrane surface area |
| Pulmonary status | Ultrafiltration coefficient |
| Volume status | Dialysate composition |
| Volume load | Na$^+$ |
| Medications | K$^+$ |
| Comorbid conditions | Base as HCO$_3^-$, lactate |
|   Surgery | Ca$^{2+}$ |
|   Myocardial or coronary disease | Dextrose |
|   Coagulopathy | Mg$^{2+}$ |
|   Hemorrhage | Blood and dialysate flow |
|   Sepsis | Dialysis duration and frequency |
|   Arrhythmias | Dialysate volume* |
|   Malnutrition | Angioaccess |
|   Diabetes mellitus | Peritoneal access* |
|   Burns | Anticoagulation |
|   Vasculopathy | |

*Applicable to peritoneal dialysis only.

## REFERENCES

1. Evans RW, Blagg CR, Bryan FAJ: Implications for health care policy. A social and demographic profile of hemodialysis patients in the United States. JAMA 245:487, 1981.
2. United States Renal Data System: USRDS 1993 Annual Data Report. The National Institutes of Health/The National Institute of Diabetes and Digestive and Kidney Diseases, Division of Kidney, Urologic, and Hematologic Diseases, Bethesda, MD, 1993.
3. Colton CK, Lowrie EG: Hemodialysis: Physical principles and technical considerations. *In* Brenner BM, Rector FC (eds): The Kidney, 2nd ed. WB Saunders, Philadelphia, 1981, p 2425.
4. Gotch FA: A quantitative evaluation of small and middle molecule toxicity in therapy of uremia. Dial Transplant 9:183, 1980.
5. Henderson LW: Hemodialysis: Rationale and physical principles. *In* Brenner BM, Rector FC (eds): The Kidney, 1st ed. WB Saunders, Philadelphia, 1976, p 1643.
6. Levine J, Bernard DB: The role of urea kinetic modeling, TAC urea, and Kt/V in achieving optimal dialysis: A critical reappraisal. Am J Kidney Dis 15:285, 1990.
7. Henderson LW: Solute kinetics and fluid removal in hemofiltration. Int J Artif Organs 6:5, 1983.
8. Henderson LW, Colton CK, Ford CA: Kinetics of hemodiafiltration. II: Clinical characterization of a new blood cleansing modality. J Lab Clin Med 85:372, 1975.
9. Sherman RA: The measurement of dialysis recirculation. Am J Kidney Dis 22:616, 1993.
10. Schneditz D, Polaschegg HD, Levin NW, et al: Cardiopulmonary recirculation in dialysis. ASAIO J 38:M194, 1992.
11. Babb AL, Farrell P, Uvelli DA, Scribner BH: Hemodialyzer evaluation by examination of solute molecular spectra. Trans Am Soc Artif Intern Organs 18:98, 1972.
12. Keshaviah PR, Shaldon S: Hemodialysis monitors and monitoring.

*In* Maher JF (ed): Replacement of Renal Function by Dialysis. Kluwer Academic Publishers, Dordrecht, Netherlands, 1989, p 276.

13. Asaba H, Bergstrom J, Furst P, et al: Sequential ultrafiltration and diffusion as alternatives to conventional hemodialysis. Proc Clin Dial Transplant Forum 6:29, 1976.

14. Shaldon S: Sequential ultrafiltration and dialysis. Proc Eur Dial Transplant Assoc 13:300, 1976.

15. Wehle B, Asaba H, Castenfores J, et al: Hemodynamic changes during sequential ultrafiltration and dialysis. Kidney Int 15:411, 1979.

16. Keshaviah P, Ilstrup K, Costantini E, et al: The influence of ultrafiltration (UF) and diffusion (D) on cardiovascular parameters. Trans Am Soc Artif Intern Organs 26:328, 1980.

17. Fleming SJ, Wilkinson JS, Aldridge C, et al: Blood volume changing during isolated ultrafiltration and combined ultrafiltration-dialysis. Nephrol Dial Transplant 3:272, 1988.

18. Bradley JR, Evans DB, Cowley AJ: Comparison of vascular tone during haemodialysis with ultrafiltration and during ultrafiltration followed by haemodialysis: A possible mechanism for dialysis hypotension. BMJ 19:300, 1990.

19. Acchiardo SR, Hatten KW, Ruvinsky MJ, et al: Inadequate dialysis increases gross mortality rate. ASAIO J 38:M272, 1992.

20. Delmez JA, Windus DW: Hemodialysis prescription and delivery in a metropolitan community. The St. Louis Nephrology Study Group. Kidney Int 41:1023, 1992.

21. Owen WF, Lew NL, Liu Y, et al: The urea reduction ratio and serum albumin concentration as predictors of mortality in patients undergoing hemodialysis. N Engl J Med 329:1001, 1993.

22. Cazenave JP, Mulvihill J: Interaction of blood with surfaces: Hemocompatibility and thromboresistance of biomaterials. Contrib Nephrol 62:188, 1988.

23. Grant ME, Lovell HB, Wiegmann TB: Current use of anticoagulation in hemodialysis. Semin Dial 4:168, 1991.

24. Owen WF, Lazarus JM: Dialytic management of acute renal failure. *In* Lazarus JM, Brenner BM (eds): Acute Renal Failure. Churchill Livingstone, New York, 1993, p 487.

25. Gordon LA, Simon ER, Richards JM: Studies in regional heparinization. II Artificial kidney hemodialysis without systemic heparinization—preliminary report of a method using simultaneous infusion of heparin and protamine. N Engl J Med 255:1063, 1956.

26. Hampers CL, Blaufox MD, Merrill JP: Anticoagulation rebound after hemodialysis. N Engl J Med 255:1063, 1966.

27. von Brecht J, Flanagan M, Freeman R, Lim V: Regional anticoagulation: Hemodialysis with hypertonic trisodium citrate. Am J Kidney Dis 8:196, 1986.

28. Swartz RD, Port FK: Preventing hemorrhage in high-risk hemodialysis: Regional versus low-dose heparin. Kidney Int 16:513, 1979.

29. Schwab SJ, Onorato JJ, Sharar LR, Dennis PA: Hemodialysis without anticoagulation: One-year prospective trial in hospitalized patients at risk for bleeding. Am J Med 83:405, 1987.

30. Caruna R, Raiai R, Bush J, et al: Heparin free dialysis: Comparative data and results in high risk patients. Kidney Int 31:35, 1987.

31. Laurer A, Saccaggi A, Ronco C, et al: Continuous arteriovenous hemofiltration in the critically ill patient. Ann Intern Med 99:255, 1983.

32. Henderson LW: Biophysics of ultrafiltration and hemofiltration. *In* Maher JF (ed): Replacement of Renal Function by Dialysis. Kluwer Academic Publishers, Dordrecht, Netherlands, 1989, p 300.

33. Geronemus R, von Albertini B, Glabman S, et al: Enhanced molecular clearance in hemofiltration. Proc Clin Dial Transplant Forum 8:47, 1985.

34. Kaplan AA: Predilution vs postdilution for continuous arteriovenous hemofiltration. Trans Am Soc Artif Intern Organs 3:28, 1985.

35. Kovalik EC, Schwab SJ, Quarles LD: Hollow-fiber versus parallel-plate dialyzers in continuous arteriovenous hemodialysis. Semin Dial 6:229, 1993.

36. Ronco C, Brendolan A, Gragantini L, et al: Continuous arteriovenous hemofiltration. Contrib Nephrol 48:70 1985.

37. Golper TA, Ronco C, Kaplan AA: Continuous arteriovenous hemofiltration: Improvements, modifications, and future directions. Semin Dial 1:50, 1988.

38. Smith D, Paganini EP, Suhoza K, et al: Non-heparin continuous renal replacement therapy is possible. *In* Nose J, Kjellstrand CM, Ivanovich P (eds): Progress in Artificial Internal Organs. ISAO Press, Cleveland, OH, 1985, p 32.

39. Kaplan AA, Petrillo R: Regional heparinization for continuous arteriovenous hemofiltration. Trans Am Soc Artif Intern Organs 33:312, 1987.

40. Merrill JP, Legrain M, Hoigne R: Observations on the role of urea in uremia. Am J Med 14:519, 1953.

41. Johnson WJ, Hagge WW, Wagoner RD, et al: Effects of urea loading in patients with far-advanced renal failure. Mayo Clin Proc 47:21, 1972.

42. Lowrie EG, Laird NM, Parker TF, Sargent JA: Effect of the hemodialysis prescription on patient morbidity: Report from the National Cooperative Dialysis Study. N Engl J Med 305:1176, 1981.

43. Depner TA, Cheer AY: Modeling urea kinetics with two vs three BUN measurements: A critical comparison. ASAIO Trans 35:499–502, 1989.

44. Gotch FA: Kinetic modeling in hemodialysis. *In* Nissenson A, Gentile D, Fine RA (eds): Clinical Dialysis. Appleton & Lange, Norwalk, CT, 1989.

45. Ijelu G, Carrona M, Raja RM: Various methods for calculation of Kt/V: A clinical comparison. ASAIO Trans 36:M364, 1990.

46. Jindal KK, Manuel A, Goldstein MB: Percent reduction in blood urea concentration during hemodialysis (PRU). ASAIO Trans 33:286, 1987.

47. Daugirdas JT: The pre:post dialysis plasma urea nitrogen ratio to estimate Kt/V and NPCR: Validation. Int J Artif Organs 12:420, 1989.

48. Basile C, Kazio S, Lopez T: Percent reduction in urea concentration during dialysis estimates Kt/V in a simple and accurate way. Am J Kidney Dis 15:40, 1990.

49. Lowrie EG, Lew NL: The urea reduction ratio (URR). Contemp Dial Nephrol 12:11, 1991.

50. Arieff AI, Massry SG, Barrientos A, et al: Brain water and electrolyte metabolism in uremia: Effects of slow and rapid hemodialysis. Kidney Int 4:177, 1973.

51. Kennedy AC, Linton AL, Eaton JC: Urea levels in cerebrospinal fluid after haemodialysis. Lancet 1:410, 1962.

52. Shackman R, Chisholm GD, Holden AJ, Pigott RW: Urea distribution in the body after haemodialysis. Br Med J 2:355, 1962.

53. Cheung AK, Alford MF, Wilson MM, et al: Urea movement across erythrocyte membranes during artificial kidney treatment. Kidney Int 23:866, 1983.

54. Mayrand RR, Levitt DG: Urea and ethylene glycol facilitated transport system in the human red cell membrane. J Gen Physiol 81:221, 1983.

55. Hunter FL: Facilitated diffusion in human erythrocytes. Biochim Biophys Acta 211:216, 1970.

56. Bowsher DJ, Krejcie TC, Avram MJ, et al: Reduction in slow intercompartmental clearance of urea during dialysis. J Lab Clin Med 105:489, 1985.

57. Pedrini LA, Zereik S, Rasmy S: Causes, kinetics, and clinical implications of posthemodialysis urea rebound. Kidney Int 34:817–824, 1988.

58. Tsang HK, Leonard EF, LeFavour GS, Cortell S: Urea dynamics during and immediately after dialysis. ASAIO J 8:251–260, 1985.

59. Depner TA: Refining the model of urea kinetics: Compartment effects. Semin Dial 5:147, 1992.

60. Lazarus JM, Owen WF: Role of biocompatibility in dialysis morbidity and mortality. Am J Kidney Dis 24:1019, 1994.

61. Hakim RM: Clinical implications of hemodialysis membrane biocompatibility. Kidney Int 44:484, 1993.

62. Schulman G, Fogo A, Gung A, et al: Complement activation retards renal failure in the rat. Kidney Int 40:1069, 1991.

63. Hakim RM, Wingard RL, Lawrence P, et al: Use of biocompatible membranes improves outcome and recovery from acute renal failure. J Am Soc Nephrol 3:367, 1992. Abstract.

64. Henderson LW, Koch KM, Dinarello CA, Shaldon S: Hemodialysis hypotension: The interleukin hypothesis. Blood Purif 1:3, 1983.

65. Dinarello CA, Koch KM, Shaldon S: Interleukin-1 and its relevance to patients treated with hemodialysis. Kidney Int 33:S21, 1988.

66. Ross EA, Nissenson AR: Dialysis-associated hypoxemia: Insights into pathophysiology and prevention. Semin Dial 1:33, 1988.

67. Tetta C, David S, Biancone L, et al: Role of platelet activating factor in hemodialysis. Kidney Int 43:S154–S157, 1993.

68. Schulman G, Hakim R, Arias R, et al: Bradykinin generation by dialysis membranes: Possible role in anaphylactic reaction. J Am Soc Nephrol 3:1563, 1993.

69. Roccatello D, Mazzucco G, Coppo R, et al: Functional changes of monocytes due to dialysis membranes. Kidney Int 35:622, 1989.

70. Vanholder R, Ringoir S, Dhondt A, et al: Phagocytosis in uremic and hemodialysis patients: A prospective and cross sectional study. Kidney Int 39:320, 1991.

71. Vanholder R, Ringoir S: Polymorphonuclear cell function and infection in dialysis. Kidney Int 38:S91, 1992.

72. Gutierrez A, Alvestrand A, Wahren J, Bergstrom J: Effect of in vivo contact between blood and dialysis membranes on protein catabolism in humans. Kidney Int 38:487, 1990.

73. Lazarus JM: Nutrition in hemodialysis patients. Am J Kidney Dis 21:99, 1993.

74. Bergstom J, Alvestrand A, Furst P: Plasma and muscle free amino acids in maintenance hemodialysis patients without protein malnutrition. Kidney Int 38:108, 1990.

75. Seres DS, Strain GW, Hashim SA, et al: Improvement of plasma lipoprotein profiles during high-flux dialysis. J Am Soc Nephrol 3:1409, 1993.

76. van Ypersele de Strihou C, Jadoul M, Malghem J, et al: Effect of dialysis membrane and patient's age on signs of dialysis-related amyloidosis. Kidney Int 39:1012, 1991.

77. Miyasaka N, Sato K, Kitano Y, et al: Aberrant cytokine production from tenosynovium in dialysis associated amyloidosis. Ann Rheum Dis 51:797, 1992.

78. Hakim RM, Fearon DT, Lazarus JM, et al: Biocompatibility of dialysis membranes: Effects of chronic complement activation. Kidney Int 26:194, 1984.

79. Aranout A, Hakim RM, Todd R, et al: Increased expression of an adhesion-promoting surface glycoprotein in the granulocytopenia of hemodialysis. N Engl J Med 312:457, 1985.

80. Himmelfarb J, Zaoui P, Hakim R: Modulation of granulocyte LAM-1 and MAC-1 during dialysis—a prospective, randomized controlled trial. Kidney Int 41:388, 1992.

81. Himmelfarb J, Lazarus JM, Hakim R: Reactive oxygen species production by monocytes and polymorphonuclear leukocytes during dialysis. Am J Kidney Dis 17:271, 1991.

82. Tridon A, Albuisson E, Deteix P, et al: Leukotriene B₄ in hemodialysis. Artif Organs 14:387, 1990.

83. Schiffl H, Strasser T: Induction of leukotriene B₄ formation by dialyzer membranes. Biomater Artif Cells Artif Organs 18:585, 1990.

84. Jorres A, Jorres D, Gahl GM, et al: Leukotriene release from neutrophils of patients on hemodialysis with cellulose membranes. Int J Artif Intern Organs 15:84, 1992.

85. Shaldon S, Lonnemann G, Koch KM: Cytokine relevance in biocompatibility. Contrib Nephrol 79:227, 1989.

86. Schindler R, Lonnemann G, Shaldon S, et al: Transcription, not synthesis, of interleukin-1 and tumor necrosis factor by complement. Kidney Int 37:85, 1990.

87. Pertosa G, Gesualdo L, Tarantino EA, et al: Influence of hemodialysis on interleukin-6 production and gene expression by peripheral blood mononuclear cells. Kidney Int 43:S149, 1993.

88. Pereira BJ, King AJ, Poutsiaka DD, et al: Comparison of first use and reuse of cuprophan membranes on interleukin-1 receptor antagonist and interleukin-1 beta production by blood mononuclear cells. Am J Kidney Dis 22:288, 1993.

89. Canivet E, Lavaud S, Wong T, et al: Cuprophane but not synthetic membrane induces increases in serum tumor necrosis factor-alpha levels during hemodialysis. Am J Kidney Dis 23:41, 1994.

90. Schindler R, Linnenweber S, Schlze M, et al: Gene expression of interleukin-1 beta during hemodialysis. Kidney Int 43:712, 1993.

91. Pereira BJ, Poutsiaka DD, King AJ, et al: In vitro production of interleukin-1 receptor antagonist in chronic renal failure, CAPD, and HD. Kidney Int 42:1419, 1992.

92. Zaoui P, Green W, Hakim RM: Hemodialysis with cuprophane membrane modulates interleukin-2 receptor expression. Kidney Int 39:1020, 1991.

93. Donati D, Degiannis D, Combates N, et al: Effects of hemodialysis on activation of lymphocytes: Analysis by an in vitro dialysis model. J Am Soc Nephrol 2:1490, 1992.

94. Sherman RA, Hwang ER, Bernholc AS, Eisinger RP: Variability in potassium removal by hemodialysis. Am J Nephrol 6:284, 1986.

95. Leong ASY, Disney ASP, Grove DW: Spallation and migration of silicone from blood-pump tubing in patients on hemodialysis. N Engl J Med 306:135, 1982.

96. Petersen J, Hyver SW, Collins J: Backfiltration during hemodialysis: A critical assessment. Semin Dial 5:13, 1992.

97. Bingel M, Lonnemann G, Koch KM, et al: Enhancement of in-vitro human interleukin-1 production by sodium acetate. Lancet 1:14, 1987.

98. Tokars JI, Alter MJ, Favero MS, et al: National surveillance of hemodialysis associated diseases in the United States, 1990. J Am Soc Artif Intern Organs 33:71, 1993.

99. Kaye M, Lella J, Gagnon R, Low G: Consent to dialyzer reuse: Is it ethically necessary? Am J Nephrol 5:138, 1985.

100. Garred LJ, Canaud B, Flavier JL, et al: Effect of reuse on dialyzer efficacy. Artif Organs 14:80, 1990.

101. Baris E, McGregor M: The reuse of hemodialyzers: An assessment of safety and potential savings. Can Med Assoc J 148:175, 1993.

102. Ward RA, Luehmann DA, Klein E: Are current standards for the microbiological purity of hemodialysate adequate? Semin Dial 2:69, 1989.

103. Klein E, Pass T, Harding GB, et al: Microbial and endotoxin contamination in water and dialysate in the central United States. Artif Organs 14:85, 1990.

104. Yohay DA, Butterly DW, Schwab SJ, Quarles LD: Continuous arteriovenous hemodialysis: Effect of dialyzer geometry. Kidney Int 42:448, 1992.

105. Ifediora OC, Teehan BP, Sigler MH: Solute clearances in continuous venovenous hemodialysis: A comparison of cuprophane, polyacrilonitrile, and polysulfone membranes. ASAIO J 38:M697, 1992.

106. Weseley SA: Air embolism during hemodialysis. Dial Transplant 2:14, 1972.

107. Lindner A, Moskovtchenko JF, Traeger J: Accidental mass hypernatremia during hemodialysis. Nephron 9:99, 1972.

108. Said R, Quintanilla A, Levin N, Ivanovich P: Acute hemolysis due to profound hypo-osmolality. A complication of hemodialysis. J Dial 1:477, 1977.

109. Fortner RW, Nowakowski A, Carter CB, et al: Death due to overheated dialysate during dialysis. Ann Intern Med 73:443, 1970.

110. Berkes SL, Kahn IS, Chazen JA, Garella S: Prolonged hemolysis from overheated dialysate. Ann Intern Med 83:363, 1975.

111. Gotch FA, Keen ML: Dialyzers and delivery systems. In Cogan MG, Garovoy MR (eds): Introduction to Dialysis. Churchill Livingstone, New York, 1985, p 1.

112. Salusky IB, Foley J, Nelson P, Goodman WG: Aluminum accumulation during treatment with aluminum hydroxide and dialysis in children and young adults with chronic renal disease. N Engl J Med 324:527, 1991.

113. Delmez JA, Slatopolsky E: Hyperphosphatemia: Its consequences and treatment in patients. Am J Kidney Dis 19:303, 1992.

114. Touam M, Martinez F, Lacour B, et al: Aluminum-induced, reversible microcytic anemia in chronic renal failure: Clinical and experimental studies. Clin Nephrol 19:295, 1983.

115. Alfrey AC, LeGendre GR, Kaehney WD: The dialysis encephalopathy syndrome: Possible aluminum intoxication. N Engl J Med 294:184, 1976.

116. Botella J, Traver JA, Sanz-Guajardo D, et al: Chloramines, an aggravating factor in the anaemia of patients on regular dialysis treatment. Proc Eur Dial Transplant Assoc 14:192, 1977.

117. Nielan BA, Ehlers SM, Kolpin CF, Eaton JW: Prevention of chloramine-induced hemolysis in dialyzed patients. Clin Nephrol 10:105, 1978.

118. Lough J, Noonan R, Gagnon R, Kaye M: Effects of fluoride on bone in chronic renal failure. Arch Pathol 99:484, 1975.

119. Anderson R, Beard JH, Sorley D: Fluoride intoxication in a dialysis unit—Maryland. MMWR 29:134, 1980.

120. Freeman RM, Lawton RL, Chamberlain MA: Hard-water syndrome. N Engl J Med 276:1113, 1967.

121. Manzler AL, Schreiner AW: Copper induced hemolytic anemia: A new complication of hemodialysis. Ann Intern Med 73:409, 1970.

122. Natter BJ, Pederson J, Psimenos G, Lindeman RD: Lethal copper intoxication in hemodialysis. Trans Am Soc Artif Intern Organs 15:309, 1969.

123. Nickey WA, Chinitz VL, Kim KE, et al: Hypernatremia from water softener and malfunction during home dialysis. JAMA 214:915, 1970.

124. American National Standard for Hemodialysis Systems. The Association for the Advancement of Medical Instrumentation, Arlington, VA, 1992.

125. Oliver JC, Bland LA, Oettinger CW, et al: Bacteria and endotoxin

removal from bicarbonate dialysis fluids for use in conventional, high-efficiency and high-flux hemodialysis. Artif Organs 16:141, 1992.

126. Pegues DA, Oettinger CW, Bland LA, et al: A prospective study of pyrogenic reactions in hemodialysis patients using bicarbonate dialysis fluids filtered to remove bacteria and endotoxin. J Am Soc Nephrol 3:1002, 1992.

127. Mendelssohn S, Swartz CD, Yudis M, et al: High glucose concentration dialysate in chronic hemodialysis. Trans Am Soc Artif Intern Organs 13:249, 1967.

128. Ward RA, Walthen RL, Williams TE, Harding GB: Hemodialysate composition and intradialytic metabolic, acid-base, and potassium changes. Kidney Int 32:129, 1987.

129. Arem R: Hypoglycemia. Endocrinol Metab Clin North Am 18:103, 1989.

130. Grajower MM, Walter L, Albin J: Hypoglycemia in chronic hemodialysis patients: Association with propranolol use. Nephron 26:126, 1980.

131. Kopple JD, Swendseid ME, Shinaberger JH, Umezawa CY: The free and bound amino acids removed by hemodialysis. Trans Am Soc Artif Intern Organs 19:309–313, 1973.

132. Ganda OP, Aoki TT, Soeldner JS, et al: Hormone-fuel concentrations in anephric subjects: Effects of hemodialysis (with special references to amino acids). J Clin Invest 57:1403, 1976.

133. Wilkinson R, Barber SG, Robson V: Cramps, thirst, and hypertension in hemodialysis patients—the influence of dialysate sodium concentration. Clin Nephrol 7:101, 1977.

134. Ogden DA: A double-blind crossover comparison of high and low sodium dialysis. Proc Dial Transplant Forum 8:157, 1978.

135. Henrich WL, Woodard TD, McPhaul JJ: The chronic efficacy and safety of high sodium dialysate: Double-blind, crossover study. Am J Kidney Dis 2:349, 1982.

136. Cybulsky AVE, Materi A, Hollombh DJ: Effects of high sodium dialysate during maintenance hemodialysis. Nephron 41:57, 1985.

137. Port FK, Johnson WJ, Klass DW: Prevention of dialysis disequilibrium syndrome by use of high sodium concentration in the dialysate. Kidney Int 3:327, 1973.

138. Van Stone JC, Bauer J, Carey J: The effect of dialysate sodium concentration on body fluid distribution during hemodialysis. Trans Am Soc Artif Intern Organs 26:383, 1980.

139. Dumler F, Grondin G, Levin NW: Sequential high/low sodium hemodialysis: An alternative to ultrafiltration. Trans Am Soc Artif Intern Organs 25:351, 1979.

140. Daugirdas JT, Al-Kudsi RR, Ing TS, Norusis MJ: A double-blind evaluation of sodium gradient hemodialysis. Am J Nephrol 5:163, 1985.

141. Raja R, Kramer M, Barber K, Chin S: Sequential changes in dialysate sodium during hemodialysis. Trans Am Soc Artif Intern Organs 29:649, 1983.

142. Palmer BF: The effect of dialysate composition on systemic hemodynamics. Semin Dial 5:54, 1992.

143. Depner TA: Standards for dialysis adequacy. Semin Dial 4:245, 1991.

144. William M, Epstein FH: Internal exchanges of potassium. *In* Seldin DW, Giebisch G (eds): The Regulation of Potassium Balance. Raven Press, New York, 1989, p 3.

145. Ketchersid TL, Van Stone JC: Dialysate potassium. Semin Dial 4:46, 1991.

146. Feig PU, Shook A, Sterns RH: Effect of potassium removal during hemodialysis on the plasma potassium concentration. Nephron 27:25, 1981.

147. Hou S, McElroy PA, Nootes S, Beach M: Safety and efficacy of low potassium dialysate. Am J Kidney Dis 13:137, 1989.

148. Ozuer M, Aksoy A, Dortlmez O, Dortlemez H: Effects of cardioselective ($\beta_1$) and nonselective (both $\beta_1$ and $\beta_2$) adrenergic blockade on serum potassium in patients with chronic renal failure undergoing hemodialysis. Kidney Int 26:584, 1984.

149. Papadakis MA, Wexman MP, Fraser C, Sedlacek SM: Hyperkalemia complicating digoxin toxicity in a patient with renal failure. Am J Kidney Dis 5:64, 1985.

150. Williams AJ, Barnes JN, Cunningham J, et al: Effect of dialysate buffer on potassium removal during haemodialysis. Proc Eur Dial Transplant Assoc Eur Renal Assoc 21:209, 1982.

151. Redaelli B, Sforzini B, Bonoldi L, et al: Potassium removal as a factor limiting the correction of acidosis during dialysis. Proc Eur Dial Transplant Assoc 19:366, 1982.

152. Morrison G, Michelson EL, Brown S, Morganroth J: Mechanism and prevention of cardiac arrhythmias in chronic hemodialysis patients. Kidney Int 17:811, 1980.

153. Lazarus JM: Complications in hemodialysis: An overview. Kidney Int 18:783, 1980.

154. Wiegand CF, Davin TD, Raij L, Kjellstrand CM: Severe hypokalemia induced by hemodialysis. Arch Intern Med 141:167, 1981.

155. Kveim M, Nesbakken R: Utilization of exogenous acetate during hemodialysis. Proc Dial Transplant Forum 5:138, 1975.

156. Vinay P, Prud'homme M, Vinet B, et al: Acetate metabolism and bicarbonate generation during hemodialysis: 10 years of observation. Kidney Int 31:1194, 1987.

157. Gennari FJ, Rimmer JM: Acid-base disorders in end-stage renal disease. Part I. Semin Dial 3:81, 1990.

158. Graefe U, Multinovich J, Follette WC, et al: Less dialysis-induced morbidity and vascular instability with bicarbonate dialysate. Ann Intern Med 88:332, 1978.

159. Mastrangelo F, Rizzelli S, Corliano C: Benefits of bicarbonate dialysis. Kidney Int 28:S188, 1985.

160. Henrich WL: Hemodynamic instability during hemodialysis. Kidney Int 30:605, 1986.

161. Wolff J, Pendersen T, Rossen M, Cleeman-Rasmussen K: Effects of acetate and bicarbonate dialysis on cardiac performance, transmural myocardial perfusion and acid-base balance. Int J Artif Organs 9:105, 1986.

162. Daugirdas JT: Dialysis hypotension: A hemodynamic analysis. Kidney Int 39:233, 1991.

163. Wehle B, Asaba H, Castenfors J, et al: The influence of dialysis fluid composition on the blood pressure response during dialysis. Clin Nephrol 10:62, 1978.

164. Velez RL, Woodard TD, Henrich WL: Acetate and bicarbonate hemodialysis in patients with and without autonomic dysfunction. Kidney Int 26:59, 1984.

165. Garella S, Chang BS: Hemodialysis-associated hypoxemia. Am J Nephrol 4:272, 1984.

166. Nissenson AR, Kraut JA, Shinaberger JH: Dialysis-associated hypoxemia: Pathogenesis and prevention. J Am Soc Artif Intern Organs 7:1, 1984.

167. Sherman RA: On lowering dialysate calcium. Semin Dial 2:78, 1989.

168. Goodman WG, Coburn JW: The use of 1,25-dihydroxyvitamin $D_3$ in early renal failure. Annu Rev Med 43:27, 1992.

169. Sutton RA, Cameron EC: Renal osteodystrophy: Pathophysiology. Semin Dial 12:91, 1992.

170. Wing AJ: Optimum calcium concentration of dialysis fluid for hemodialysis. Br Med J 4:145, 1968.

171. Mirahmadi KS, Duffy BS, Shinaberger JH, et al: A controlled evaluation of clinical and metabolic effects of dialysate calcium levels during regular hemodialysis. Trans Am Soc Artif Intern Organs 17:118, 1971.

172. Raman A, Chong YK, Sreenevasan GA: Effects of varying dialysate calcium concentrations on the plasma calcium fractions in patients on dialysis. Nephron 16:181, 1976.

173. Bouillon R, Verberckmoes R, de Moor P: Influence of dialysate calcium concentration and vitamin D on serum parathyroid hormone during repetitive dialysis. Kidney Int 7:422, 1975.

174. Sherman RA, Bialy GB, Grazinski B, et al: The effect of dialysate calcium levels on blood pressure during hemodialysis. Am J Kidney Dis 8:244, 1986.

175. Maynard JC, Cruz C, Kleerekoper M, Levin NW: Blood pressure response to changes in serum ionized calcium during hemodialysis. Ann Intern Med 104:358, 1986.

176. Fellner SK, Lang RM, Neumann A, et al: Physiological mechanisms for calcium-induced changes in systemic arterial pressure in stable dialysis patients. Hypertension 13:213, 1989.

177. Vaporean ML, Van Stone JC: Dialysate magnesium. Semin Dial 6:46, 1993.

178. Breuer J, Moniz C, Baldwin D, Parsons V: The effects of zero magnesium dialysate and magnesium supplements on ionized calcium concentration in patients on regular dialysis treatment. Nephrol Dial Transplant 2:347, 1987.

179. Gonella M, Ballanti P, Rocca C, et al: Improved bone morphology by normalizing serum magnesium in chronically hemodialyzed patients. Miner Electrolyte Metab 14:240, 1988.

180. Gonella M, Calabrese G: Magnesium status in chronically haemo-

dialyzed patients: The role of dialysate magnesium concentration. Magnesium Res 2:259, 1989.

181. Coburn JW, Slatopolsky E: Vitamin D, parathyroid hormone, and the renal osteodystrophies. *In* Brenner BM, Rector FC Jr (eds): The Kidney, 4th ed. WB Saunders, Philadelphia, 1991, p 2036.

182. Mehta RL: Renal replacement therapy for acute renal failure: Matching the method to the patient. Semin Dial 6:253, 1993.

183. Windus DW: Permanent vascular access: A nephrologist view. Am J Kidney Dis 21:457, 1993.

184. Quinton W, Dillard D, Scribner BH: Cannulation of blood vessels for prolonged hemodialysis. Trans Am Soc Artif Intern Organs 6:104, 1960.

185. Brescia MJ, Cimino JE, Appel K, Hurwich BJ: Chronic hemodialysis using venipuncture and a surgically created arteriovenous fistula. N Engl J Med 275:1089, 1966.

186. Rubio PA, Farrell EM: Human umbilical vein graft angioaccess in chronic hemodialysis: A preliminary report. Dial Transplant 8:211, 1979.

187. May J, Tiller D, Johnson J: Saphenous vein arteriovenous fistula in regular dialysis treatment. N Engl J Med 280:770, 1969.

188. Baker LD Jr, Johnson JM, Goldfarb D: Expanded polytetrafluoroethylene (PTFE) subcutaneous arteriovenous conduit: An improved vascular access for chronic hemodialysis. Trans Am Soc Artif Intern Organs 22:382, 1976.

189. Kaplan MS, Mirahmadi KS, Winer RL, et al: Comparison of "PTFE" and bovine grafts for blood access in hemodialysis patients. Trans Am Soc Artif Intern Organs 22:388, 1976.

190. Shusterman NH, Kloss K, Mullen JL: Successful use of double-lumen, silicone rubber catheters for permanent hemodialysis access. Kidney Int 35:887, 1989.

191. Reed WP, Light PF, Sadler JH: Access for hemodialysis by means of long-term central venous catheters. Kidney Int 25:838, 1984.

192. Lazarus JM, Hakim RM: Medical aspects of hemodialysis. *In* Brenner BM, Rector FC (eds): The Kidney, 4th ed. WB Saunders, Philadelphia, 1991, p 2223.

193. Campistol JM, Cases A, Lopez-Pedret J, Revert L: Thoracic duct injury: An unusual complication following subclavian catheterization for hemodialysis. Nephron 46:390, 1987.

194. Dunea G, Domenico L, Gunnerson P, Winston-Willis F: A survey of permanent double lumen catheters in hemodialysis patients. ASAIO Trans 37:M276, 1991.

195. Mosquera DA, Gibson SP, Goldman MD: Vascular access surgery: A 2 year study and comparison with the Permcath. Nephrol Dial Transplant 7:1111, 1992.

196. Blake PG, Huraib S, Wu G, Uldall R: The use of dual lumen jugular venous catheters as definitive long term access for hemodialysis. Int J Artif Organs 13:26, 1990.

197. Schwab SJ, Quarles D, Middleton JP, et al: Hemodialysis-associated subclavian vein stenosis. Kidney Int 33:1156, 1988.

198. Paulsen D, Reisoether A, Aasen M, Fauchald P: Use of tissue plasminogen activator for reopening of clotted dialysis catheters. Nephron 64:468, 1993.

199. Uldall R, Besley ME, Thomas A, et al: Maintaining the patency of double-lumen Silastic jugular catheters for haemodialysis. Int J Artif Organs 16:37, 1993.

200. Khanna S, Sniderman K, Simons M, et al: Superior vena cava stenosis associated with hemodialysis catheters. Am J Kidney Dis 21:278, 1993.

201. Fant GF, Dennis VW, Quarles D: Late vascular complications of the subclavian dialysis catheter. Am J Kidney Dis 7:225, 1986.

202. Cheung AK, Gregory MC: Subclavian vein thrombosis in hemodialysis patients. Trans Am Soc Artif Intern Organs 31:131, 1985.

203. Newman GE, Saeed M, Himmelstein S, et al: Total central vein obstruction: Resolution with angioplasty and fibrinolysis. Kidney Int 39:761, 1991.

204. Schillinger F, Schillinger D, Montagnac R, Milcent T: Post catheterization vein stenosis in haemodialysis: Comparative angiographic study of 509 subclavian and 50 internal jugular accesses. Nephrol Dial Transplant 6:722, 1991.

205. Cimochowski GE, Worley E, Rutherford WE, et al: Superiority of the internal jugular over the subclavian access for temporary dialysis. Nephron 54:154, 1990.

206. Bambauer R, Mestres P, Pirrung KJ: Frequency, therapy, and prevention of infections associated with large bore catheters. ASAIO J 38:96, 1992.

207. Hernandez D, Diaz F, Suria S, et al: Subclavian catheter–related infection is a major risk factor for the late development of subclavian vein stenosis. Nephrol Dial Transplant 8:227, 1993.

208. Barrett N, Spencer S, McIvor J, Brown EA: Subclavian stenosis: A major complication of subclavian dialysis catheters. Nephrol Dial Transplant 3:423, 1988.

209. Almirall J, Gonzalez J, Rello J, et al: Infection of hemodialysis catheters: Incidence and mechanisms. Am J Nephrol 9:454, 1989.

210. Carlisle EJ, Blake P, McCarthy F, et al: Septicemia in long-term jugular hemodialysis catheters; eradicating infection by changing the catheter over a guidewire. Int J Artif Organs 14:150, 1991.

211. Capdevila JA, Segarra A, Planes AM, et al: Successful treatment of haemodialysis catheter–related sepsis without catheter removal. Nephrol Dial Transplant 8:231, 1993.

212. Kinnaert P, Vereerstraeten P, Toussaint C, Van Geertruyden J: Nine years experience with internal arteriovenous fistulas for haemodialysis: A study of some factors influencing the results. Br J Surg 64:242, 1977.

213. Dunlop MG, Mackinlay JY, Jenkins AM: Vascular access: Experience with the brachiocephalic fistula. Br J Surg 68:203, 1986.

214. Bonalumi U, Civalleri D, Rovida S, et al: Nine years experience with end to end arteriovenous fistula at the "anatomic snuff box" for maintenance haemodialysis. Br J Surg 69:486, 1982.

215. Reilly DT, Wood RFM, Bell PRF: Prospective study of dialysis fistulas: Problem patients and their treatment. Br J Surg 69:549, 1982.

216. Mehigan JT, McAlexander RA: Snuffbox arteriovenous fistula for hemodialysis. Am J Surg 143:252, 1982.

217. Buselmeier TJ, Rattazzi LC, Kjellstrand CM, et al: A modified arteriovenous fistula applicable where there is thrombosis of standard Brescia-Cimino fistula vasculature. Surgery 74:551, 1973.

218. Kherlakian GM, Roedersheimer LR, Arbaugh JJ, et al: Comparison of autogenous fistula versus expanded polytetrafluoroethylene graft fistula for angioaccess in hemodialysis. Am J Surg 152:238, 1986.

219. Feldman HI, Held PJ, Hutchinson JT, et al: Hemodialysis vascular access morbidity in the United States. Kidney Int 43:1091, 1993.

220. Muirhead N, Laupacis A, Wong C: Erythropoietin for anaemia in haemodialysis patients: Results of a maintenance study (The Canadian Erythropoietin Study Group). Nephrol Dial Transplant 6:811, 1992.

221. Tang IY, Vrahnos D, Valaitis D, Lau AH: Vascular access thrombosis during recombinant human erythropoietin therapy. ASAIO J 38:M528, 1992.

222. Churchill DN, Taylor DW, Cook RJ, et al: Canadian hemodialysis morbidity study. Am J Kidney Dis 19:214, 1992.

223. Swedberg SH, Brown GB, Sigley R, et al: Intimal fibromuscular hyperplasia at the venous anastomosis of PTFE grafts in hemodialysis patients. Circulation 80:1726, 1989.

224. Painter TA: Myointimal hyperplasia: Pathogenesis and implications. 2. Animal injury models and mechanical factors. Artif Organs 15:103, 1991.

225. Painter TA: Myointimal hyperplasia: Pathogenesis and implications. 1. In vitro characteristics. Artif Organs 15:42, 1991.

226. Mayers JD, Markell MS, Cohen LS, et al: Vascular access surgery for maintenance hemodialysis: Variables in hospital stay. ASAIO J 38:113, 1992.

227. Valji K, Bookstein JJ, Roberts AC, Davis GB: Pharmacomechanical thrombolysis and angioplasty in the management of clotted hemodialysis grafts: Early and late clinical results. Radiology 178:243, 1991.

228. Beathard GA: Percutaneous transvenous angioplasty in the treatment of vascular access stenosis. Kidney Int 42:1390, 1992.

229. Glanz S, Gordon DH, Butt KMH, et al: The role of percutaneous angioplasty in the management of chronic hemodialysis fistulas. Ann Surg 206:777, 1987.

230. Saeed M, Newman GE, McCann RL, et al: Stenoses in dialysis fistulas: Treatment with percutaneous angioplasty. Radiology 164:693, 1987.

231. Dapunt O, Feursteein M, Rendl KH, Prenner K: Transluminal angioplasty versus conventional operation in the treatment of haemodialysis fistula stenosis: Results from a 5 year study. Br J Surg 74:1004, 1987.

232. Domoto DT, Baumann JE, Joist JH: Combined aspirin and sulfinpyrazone in the prevention of recurrent hemodialysis vascular access thrombosis. Thromb Res 62:737, 1991.

233. Sreedhara R, Himmelfarb J, Lazarus JM, Hakim RM: Anti-platelet therapy in graft thrombosis: Results of a randomized double blind study. Kidney Int 45:1477, 1994.

234. Jaffers G, Angstadt JD, Bowman JS: Early cannulation of PTFE and Gore-tex grafts for hemodialysis: A prospective randomized study. Am J Nephrol 11:369, 1991.

235. Gulyassy PF, Aviram A, Peters JH: Evaluation of amino acid and protein requirements in chronic uremia. Arch Intern Med 126:855, 1970.

236. Peters JH, Gulyassy PF, Lin SC, et al: Amino acid patterns in uremia: Comparative effects of hemodialysis and transplantation. Trans Am Soc Artif Intern Organs 14:405, 1968.

237. Kopple JD, Swendseid ME: Protein and amino acid metabolism in uremic patients undergoing maintenance hemodialysis. Kidney Int 7:S64, 1975.

238. Chami J, Reidenberg M, Wellner D, et al: Essential amino acid metabolism in maintenance dialysis patients. Trans Am Soc Artif Intern Organs 22:168, 1976.

239. Young GA, Swanepoel CR, Croft MR, et al: Anthropometry and plasma valine, amino acids, and proteins in the nutritional assessment of hemodialysis patients. Kidney Int 21:492, 1982.

240. Kopple JD, Swendseid ME: Nitrogen balance and plasma amino acid level in uremic patients fed an essential amino acid diet. Am J Clin Nutr 27:806, 1974.

241. Stepniewski M, Smolenski O, Kopec J, Kuzniewski M: Effect of hemodialysis on plasma and erythrocyte phenylalanine levels in end-stage kidney patients. Nephron 39:189, 1985.

242. Flugel-Link RM, Jones MR, Kopple JD: Red cell and plasma amino acid concentrations in renal failure. JPEN 7:450, 1983.

243. Bischel M, Sabin N, Homola B, Barbour BH: Albumin turnover in chronically hemodialyzed patients. Trans Am Soc Artif Intern Organs 15:298, 1969.

244. Kopple JD: Abnormal amino acid and protein metabolism in uremia. Kidney Int 14:340, 1978.

245. Rubini ME, Gordon S: Individual plasma–free amino acids in uremics: Effects of hemodialysis. Nephron 5:339, 1968.

246. Wolfson M, Jones MR, Kopple JD: Amino acid losses during hemodialysis with infusion of amino acids and glucose. Kidney Int 21:500, 1982.

247. Tepper T, van der Hem GK, Klip HG, Donker AJ: Loss of amino acids during hemodialysis: Effect of oral essential amino acid supplementation. Nephron 29:25, 1981.

248. Lim VS, Bier DM, Flanigan MJ, Sum-Ping ST: The effect of hemodialysis on protein metabolism. A leucine kinetic study. J Clin Invest 91:2429, 1993.

249. Wathen RL, Keshaviah P, Hommeyer P, et al: The metabolic effects of hemodialysis with and without glucose in the dialysate. Am J Clin Nutr 31:1870, 1978.

250. Chanard J, Toupance O, Gillery P, Lavaud S: Evaluation of protein loss during hemofiltration. Kidney Int 33:S114, 1988.

251. Gee C, Gotch F: Nutritional considerations of patients receiving high-flux hemodialysis. Dial Transplant 20:308, 1991.

252. Graeber CW, Halley SE, Lapkin RA, et al: Protein losses with reused dialyzers. J Am Soc Nephrol 4:349, 1993.

253. Mulzer SR: Identification of plasma proteins adsorbed to hemodialyzers during clinical use. J Biomed Mater Res 23:1483, 1989.

254. Francoise Gachon AM, Mallet J, Tridon A, Deteix P: Analysis of proteins eluted from hemodialysis membranes. J Biomater Sci Polym Ed 2:263, 1991.

255. Ginn HE, Frost A, Lacy WW: Nitrogen balance in hemodialysis patients. Am J Clin Nutr 21:385, 1968.

256. Schaeffer G, Heinze V, Jontofsohn R, et al: Amino acid and protein intake in RDT patients: A nutritional and biochemical analysis. Clin Nephrol 3:228, 1975.

257. Farrell PC, Hone PW: Dialysis-induced catabolism. Am J Clin Nutr 33:1417, 1980.

258. Lim VS, Flanigan MJ: The effect of interdialytic interval on protein metabolism: Evidence suggesting dialysis-induced catabolism. Am J Kidney Dis 14:96, 1989.

259. Bergstrom J: Protein catabolic factors in patients on renal replacement therapy. Blood Purif 3:215, 1985.

260. Klasing KC: Nutritional aspects of leukocytic cytokines. J Nutr 118:1436, 1988.

261. Grimble RF: Cytokines: Their relevance to nutrition. Eur J Clin Nutr 43:217, 1989.

262. Dinarello CA: Interleukin-1—its multiple biological effects and its association with hemodialysis. Blood Purif 6:164, 1988.

263. Haeffner-Cavaillon N, Cavaillon J, Ciancioni C, et al: In vivo induction of interleukin-1 during hemodialysis. Kidney Int 35:1212, 1989.

264. Herbelin A, Nguyen AT, Zingraff J, et al: Influence of uremia and hemodialysis on circulating interleukin-1 and tumor necrosis factor α. Kidney Int 37:116, 1990.

265. Memoli B, Libetta C, Rampino T, et al: Interleukin-6 production of uraemic haemodialysed patients: Effects of different membranes. Nephrol Dial Transplant 6:96, 1991.

266. Bianchi R, Mariani G, Toni MG, Carmassi F: The metabolism of human serum albumin in renal failure on conservative and dialysis therapy. Am J Clin Nutr 31:1615, 1978.

267. Grodstein GP, Blumenkrantz MJ, Kopple JD: Nutritional and metabolic response to catabolic stress in uremia. Am J Clin Nutr 33:1411, 1980.

268. Marckmann P: Nutritional status of patients on hemodialysis and peritoneal dialysis. Clin Nephrol 29:75, 1988.

269. Oksa H, Ahonen K, Pasternack A, Marnela K: Malnutrition in hemodialysis patients. Scand J Urol Nephrol 25:157, 1991.

270. Wassner SJ, Bergstrom J, Brusilow SW, et al: Protein metabolism in renal failure: Abnormalities and possible mechanisms. Am J Kidney Dis 7:285, 1986.

271. Kopple JD, Shinaberger JH, Coburn JW, et al: Optimal dietary protein treatment during chronic hemodialysis. Trans Am Soc Artif Intern Organs 15:302, 1969.

272. Carvounis CP, Carvounis G, Hung MH: Nutritional status of maintenance hemodialysis patients. Am J Clin Nutr 43:946, 1986.

273. Hakim RM, Levin N: Malnutrition in hemodialysis patients. Am J Kidney Dis 21:125, 1993.

274. Acchiardo SR, Moore LW, Latour PA: Malnutrition as the main factor in morbidity and mortality of hemodialysis patients. Kidney Int 24:S199, 1983.

275. Mattern WD, Hak LJ, Lamanna RW, et al: Malnutrition, altered immune function, and the risk of infection in maintenance hemodialysis patients. Am J Kidney Dis 1:206, 1982.

276. Lowrie EG, Lew NL: Death risk in hemodialysis patients: The predictive value of commonly measured variables and an evaluation of death rate differences between facilities. Am J Kidney Dis 15:458, 1990.

277. Kopple JD, Swendseid ME, Holliday MA, et al: Recommendations for nutritional evaluation of patients on chronic dialysis. Kidney Int 7:S249, 1975.

278. Blumenkrantz MJ, Kopple JD, Gutman RA, et al: Methods for assessing nutritional status of patients with renal failure. Am J Clin Nutr 33:1567, 1980.

279. Guarnieri G, Faccini L, Lipartiti T, et al: Simple methods for nutritional assessment in hemodialyzed patients. Am J Clin Nutr 33:1598, 1980.

280. Thunberg BJ, Swamy AP, Cestero RVM: Cross-sectional and longitudinal nutritional measurements in maintenance hemodialysis patients. Am J Clin Nutr 34:2005, 1981.

281. Nelson EE, Hong CD, Pesce AL, et al: Anthropometric norms for the dialysis population. Am J Kidney Dis 16:32, 1990.

282. Pollock CA, Allen BJ, Warden RA, et al: Total-body nitrogen by neutron activation in maintenance dialysis. Am J Kidney Dis 16:38, 1990.

283. Sargent J, Gotch F, Borah M, et al: Urea kinetics: A guide to nutritional management of renal failure. Am J Clin Nutr 31:1696, 1978.

284. Harvey KB, Blumenkrantz MJ, Levine SE, Blackburn GL: Nutritional assessment and treatment of chronic renal failure. Am J Clin Nutr 33:1586, 1980.

285. Fish JC, Remmers ARJ, Lindley JD, Sarles HE: Albumin kinetics and nutritional rehabilitation in the unattended home-dialysis patient. N Engl J Med 287:478, 1972.

286. Anderson CF, Nelson RA, Margie JD, et al: Nutritional therapy for adults with renal disease. JAMA 223:68, 1973.

287. Kluthe R, Luttgen FM, Capetianu T, et al: Protein requirements in maintenance hemodialysis. Am J Clin Nutr 31:1812, 1978.

288. Monteon FJ, Laidlaw SA, Shaib JK, Kopple JD: Energy expenditure in patients with chronic renal failure. Kidney Int 30:741, 1986.

289. Schneeweiss B, Graninger W, Stockenhuber F, et al: Energy metabolism in acute and chronic renal failure. Am J Clin Nutr 52:596, 1990.

290. Kopple JD, Monteon FJ, Shaib JK: Effect of energy intake on nitrogen metabolism in nondialyzed patients with chronic renal failure. Kidney Int 29:734, 1986.

291. Allman MA, Stewart PM, Tiller DJ, et al: Energy supplementation and the nutritional status of hemodialysis patients. Am J Clin Nutr 51:558, 1990.

292. Heidland A, Kult J: Long-term effects of essential amino acids supplementation in patients on regular dialysis treatment. Clin Nephrol 3:234, 1975.

293. Canaud B, Bouloux C, Rivory JP, et al: Erythropoietin-induced changes in protein nutrition: Quantitative assessment by urea kinetic modeling analysis. Blood Purif 8:301, 1990.

294. Ziegler TR, Lazarus JM, Young LS, et al: Effects of recombinant human growth hormone in adults receiving maintenance hemodialysis. J Am Soc Nephrol 2:1130, 1991.

295. Schulman G, Wingard RL, Hutchinson RL, et al: The effects of recombinant human growth hormone and intradialytic parenteral nutrition in malnourished hemodialysis patients. Am J Kidney Dis 21:527, 1993.

296. Piraino AJ, Firpo JJ, Powers DV: Prolonged hyperalimentation in catabolic chronic dialysis therapy patients. JPEN 5:463, 1981.

297. Madigan KM, Olshan A, Yingling DJ: Effectiveness of intradialytic parenteral nutrition in diabetic patients with end-stage renal disease. J Am Diet Assoc 90:861, 1990.

298. Foulks CJ, Goldstein DJ, Kelly MP, Hunt JM: Indications for the use of intradialytic parenteral nutrition in the malnourished hemodialysis patient. J Renal Nutr 1:23, 1991.

299. Snyder S, Bergen C, Sigler MH, Teehan BP: Intradialytic parenteral nutrition in chronic hemodialysis patients. ASAIO Trans 37:M373, 1991.

300. Bilbrey GL: IDPN is beneficial for selected dialysis patients. Semin Dial 6:168, 1993.

301. Chertow GM, Ling J, Lew NL, et al: The association of intradialytic parenteral nutrition administration with survival in hemodialysis patients. Am J Kidney Dis 24:912, 1994.

302. Abel RM, Beck CHJ, Abbott WM, et al: Improved survival from acute renal failure after treatment with intravenous essential L-amino acids and glucose. N Engl J Med 288:695, 1973.

303. Feinstein EI, Blumenkrantz MJ, Healy M, et al: Clinical and metabolic responses to parenteral nutrition in acute renal failure. A controlled double-blind study. Medicine (Baltimore) 60:124, 1981.

304. Mault JR, Bartlett RH, Dechert RE, et al: Starvation: A major contribution to mortality in acute renal failure. Trans Am Soc Artif Intern Organs 29:390, 1983.

305. Feinstein EI, Kopple JD, Silberman H, Massry SG: Total parenteral nutrition with high or low nitrogen intakes in patients with acute renal failure. Kidney Int 26:S319, 1983.

306. Teschner M, Heidland A: Hypercatabolism in acute renal failure—mechanisms and therapeutical approaches. Blood Purif 7:16, 1989.

307. Thompson M: Use of essential amino acid–dextrose solutions in the nutritional management of patients with acute renal failure. Drug Intell Clin Pharm 19:106, 1985.

308. Brenner BM: Hemodynamically medicated glomerular injury and the progressive nature of renal disease. Kidney Int 23:647, 1983.

309. Mitch WE, Walser M, Steinman TI, et al: The effect of a keto acid–amino acid supplement to a restricted diet on the progression of chronic renal failure. N Engl J Med 311:623, 1984.

310. Rosman JB, ter Wee PM, Meijer S, et al: Prospective randomised trial of early dietary protein restriction in chronic renal failure. Lancet 2:1291, 1984.

311. Ihle BE, Becker GJ, Whitworth JA, et al: The effect of protein restriction on the progression of renal insufficiency. N Engl J Med 321:1773, 1989.

312. Klahr S, Levey AS, Beck GJ, et al: The effects of dietary protein restriction and blood pressure control on the progression of chronic renal disease. N Engl J Med 330:877, 1994.

313. United States Renal Data System: USRDS 1992 Annual Report. National Institute of Diabetes and Digestive and Kidney Diseases, Bethesda, MD, 1992.

314. Hampers CL, Soeldner JS, Gleason RE, et al: Insulin-glucose relationships in uremia. Am J Clin Nutr 21:414, 1968.

315. DeFronzo RA, Andres R, Edgar P, Walker WG: Carbohydrate metabolism in uremia: A review. Medicine (Baltimore) 52:469, 1973.

316. DeFronzo RA, Smith JD: Is glucose intolerance harmful for the uremic patient? Kidney Int 28:S88, 1985.

317. Rubenfeld S, Garber AJ: Abnormal carbohydrate metabolism in chronic renal failure. J Clin Invest 62:20, 1978.

318. Hager SR: Insulin resistance of uremia. Am J Kidney Dis 14:272, 1989.

319. McCaleb ML, Izzo MS, Lockwood DH: Characterization and partial purification of a factor from uremic human serum that induces insulin resistance. J Clin Invest 75:391, 1985.

320. Davidson MB, Lowrie EG, Hampers CL: Lack of dialyzable insulin antagonist in uremia. Metabolism 18:387, 1969.

321. Smith D, DeFronzo RA: Insulin resistance in uremia mediated by postbinding defects. Kidney Int 22:54, 1982.

322. Briggs WA, Mahajan SK, Wielechowski KS, et al: Insulin binding to monocytes and glucose metabolism in chronic renal failure. J Am Soc Artif Intern Organs 4:173, 1981.

323. Bilbrey GL, Faloona GR, White MG, et al: Hyperglucagonemia in uremia: Reversal by renal transplantation. Ann Intern Med 82:525, 1975.

324. Akmal M, Massry SG, Goldstein DA, et al: Role of parathyroid hormone in the glucose intolerance of chronic renal failure. J Clin Invest 75:1037, 1985.

325. Fadda GZ, Hajjar SM, Perna AF, et al: On the mechanism of impaired insulin secretion in chronic renal failure. J Clin Invest 87:255, 1991.

326. Hampers CL, Soeldner JS, Doak PB, Merrill JP: Effect of chronic renal failure and hemodialysis on carbohydrate metabolism. J Clin Invest 45:1719, 1966.

327. Alfrey AC, Sussman KE, Holmes JH: Changes in glucose and insulin metabolism induced by dialysis in patients with chronic uremia. Metabolism 16:733, 1967.

328. Swenson RS, Weisinger J, Reaven GM: Evidence that hemodialysis does not improve the glucose tolerance of patients with chronic renal failure. Metabolism 23:929, 1974.

329. Ferrannini E, Pilo A, Buzzigoli G, et al: Intravenous glucose tolerance and maintenance haemodialysis. Br Med J 2:803, 1977.

330. Hirszel P, Galen MA, Happe T, Lasrich M: Glycosylated hemoglobin in patients treated by chronic dialysis. Int Urol Nephrol 13:185, 1981.

331. Geronemus R, Bosch JP, Thornton J, Rayfield EJ: Studies of carbohydrate metabolism after hemodialysis and hemofiltration in uremic patients. Arch Intern Med 142:707, 1982.

332. Frizzell M, Larsen PR, Field JB: Spontaneous hypoglycemia associated with chronic renal failure. Diabetes 22:493, 1972.

333. Bansal VK, Brooks MH, York JC, Hano JE: Intractable hypoglycemia in a patient with renal failure. Arch Intern Med 139:100, 1979.

334. Dumbauld S, Rutsky E, McDaniel H: Carbohydrate metabolism during fasting in chronic hemodialysis patients. Kidney Int 24:222, 1983.

335. Wathen R, Keshaviah P, Hommeyer P, et al: Role of dialysate glucose in preventing gluconeogenesis during hemodialysis. Trans Am Soc Artif Intern Organs 23:393, 1977.

336. Bouffard Y, Tissot S, Delafosse B, et al: Metabolic effects of hemodialysis with and without glucose in the dialysate. Kidney Int 43:1086, 1993.

337. Bagdade JD, Porte DJ, Bierman EL: Hypertriglyceridemia: A metabolic consequence of chronic renal failure. N Engl J Med 279:181, 1968.

338. Brunzell JD, Albers JJ, Haas LB, et al: Prevalence of serum lipid abnormalities in chronic hemodialysis. Metabolism 26:903, 1977.

339. Chan MK, Varghese Z, Moorhead JF: Lipid abnormalities in uremia, dialysis and transplantation. Kidney Int 19:625, 1981.

340. Nicholis AJ, Cumming AM, Catto GRD, et al: Lipid relationships in dialysis and renal transplant patients. Q J Med 198:149, 1981.

341. Haas LB, Wahl PW, Sherrard DJ: A longitudinal study of lipid abnormalities in renal failure. Nephron 33:145, 1983.

342. Rubies-Prat J, Espinel E, Joven J, et al: High-density lipoprotein cholesterol subfractions in chronic uremia. Am J Kidney Dis 11:60, 1987.

343. Avram MM, Fein PA, Antignani A, et al: Cholesterol and lipid disturbances in renal disease: The natural history of uremic dyslipidemia and the impact of hemodialysis and continuous ambulatory peritoneal dialysis. Am J Med 87:55N, 1989.

344. Senti M, Romero R, Pedro-Botet J, et al: Lipoprotein abnormalities in hyperlipidemic and normolipidemic men on hemodialysis with chronic renal failure. Kidney Int 41:1394, 1992.

345. Joven J, Vilella E, Ahmad S, et al: Lipoprotein heterogeneity in end-stage renal disease. Kidney Int 43:410, 1993.
346. Attman PO, Samuelsson O, Alaupovic P: Lipoprotein metabolism and renal failure. Am J Kidney Dis 21:573, 1993.
347. Bagdade JD, Yee E, Wilson DE, Shafrir E: Hyperlipidemia in renal failure: Studies of plasma lipoproteins, hepatic triglyceride production, and tissue lipoprotein lipase in a chronically uremic rat model. J Lab Clin Med 91:176, 1978.
348. Goldberg A, Sherrard DJ, Brunzell JD: Adipose tissue lipoprotein lipase in chronic hemodialysis: Role in plasma triglyceride metabolism. J Clin Endocrinol Metab 47:1173, 1978.
349. Wessel-Aas T, Blomhoff JP, Wirum E, Nilsen T: Hemodialysis and cell toxicity in vitro related to plasma triglycerides, post-heparin lipolytic activity and free fatty acids. Acta Med Scand 216:75, 1984.
350. Chan M, Persaud J, Varghese Z, Moorhead JF: Pathogenic roles of post-heparin lipases in lipid abnormalities in hemodialysis patients. Kidney Int 25:812, 1984.
351. Mordasini R, Frey F, Flury W, et al: Selective deficiency of hepatic triglyceride lipase in uremic patients. N Engl J Med 297:1362, 1977.
352. Shoji T, Nishizawa Y, Nishitani H, et al: Impaired metabolism of high density lipoprotein in uremic patients. Kidney Int 41:1653, 1992.
353. Guarnieri GF, Moracchiello M, Campanacci L, et al: Lecithin-cholesterol acyl transferase (LCAT) activity in chronic uremia. Kidney Int 13:S26, 1978.
354. Bories PC, Subbaiah PV, Bagdade JD: Lecithin:cholesterol acyltransferase activity in dialyzed and undialyzed chronic uremic patients. Nephron 32:22, 1992.
355. Portman RJ, Scott RCI, Rogers DD, et al: Decreased low-density lipoprotein receptor function and mRNA levels in lymphocytes from uremic patients. Kidney Int 42:1238, 1992.
356. Weintraub M, Burstein A, Rassin T, et al: Severe defect in clearing postprandial chylomicron remnants in dialysis patients. Kidney Int 42:1247, 1992.
357. Haffner SM, Gruber KK, Aldrete GJ, et al: Increased lipoprotein(a) concentrations in chronic renal failure. J Am Soc Nephrol 3:1156, 1992.
358. Kandoussi A, Cachera C, Pagniez D, et al: Plasma level of lipoprotein Lp(a) is high in predialysis or hemodialysis, but not CAPD. Kidney Int 42:424, 1992.
359. Webb AT, Reaveley DA, O'Donnell M, et al: Lipoprotein(a) in patients on maintenance haemodialysis and continuous ambulatory peritoneal dialysis. Nephrol Dial Transplant 8:609, 1993.
360. Cheung AK, Wu LL, Kabitz C, Leypoldt JK: Atherogenic lipids and lipoproteins in hemodialysis patients. Am J Kidney Dis 22:271, 1993.
361. Cressman MD, Heyka RJ, Paganini ET, et al: Lipoprotein(a) is an independent risk factor for cardiovascular disease in hemodialysis patients. Circulation 86:475–482, 1992.
362. Goldwasser P, Michel M, Collier J, et al: Prealbumin and lipoprotein(a) in hemodialysis: Relationships with patient vascular access survival. Am J Kidney Dis 22:215, 1993.
363. Rorke SJ, Shippey W, Davidson WD: Acetate delivery to hemodialysis patients. Kidney Int 8:433, 1975.
364. Giorcelli G, Dalmasso F, Bruno M, et al: RDT with acetate-free bicarbonate buffered dialysis fluid: Long-term effects on lipid pattern, acid-base balance and oxygen delivery. Proc Eur Dial Transplant Assoc 16:115, 1979.
365. Teraoka J, Matsui N, Nakagawa S, Kateuchi J: The role of heparin in the changes of lipid patterns during a single hemodialysis. Clin Endocrinol 17:96, 1982.
366. Wessel-Aas T, Blomhoff JP, Wideore T, et al: The effect of systemic heparinization on plasma lipoproteins and toxicity in patients on hemodialysis and CAPD. Acta Med Scand 216:85, 1985.
367. Akiba T, Tachibana K, Ozawa K, et al: Long-term use of low molecular weight heparin ameliorates hyperlipidemia in patients on hemodialysis. ASAIO J 38:M326, 1992.
368. Deuber HJ, Schultz W: Reduced lipid concentrations during four years of dialysis with low molecular weight heparin. Kidney Int 40:496, 1991.
369. Bambauer R, Rucker S, Weber U, Kohler M: Comparison of low molecular weight heparin and standard heparin in hemodialysis. ASAIO Trans 36:M646, 1990.
370. Josephson MA, Fellner SK, Dasgupta A: Improved lipid profiles in patients undergoing high-flux hemodialysis. Am J Kidney Dis 20:361, 1992.
371. Sanfelippo ML, Swenson RS, Reaven GM: Response of plasma triglycerides to dietary change in patients on hemodialysis. Kidney Int 14:180, 1978.
372. Dornan TL, Gokal R, Pearce JS, et al: Long-term dietary treatment of hyperlipidaemia in patients treated with chronic haemodialysis. Br Med J 281:1044, 1980.
373. Golper TA: Therapy for uremic hyperlipidemia. Nephron 38:217, 1984.
374. Lapuz M, Avram MM, Lustig A, et al: Fall of cholesterol with time on dialysis: Impact on atherogenicity. Trans Am Soc Artif Intern Organs 35:258, 1989.
375. Khan L: Tissue carnitine deficiency due to dietary lysine deficiency: Triglyceride accumulation and concomitant impairment in fatty acid oxidation. J Nutr 109:24, 1979.
376. Guarnieri GF, Ranieri F, Toigo G, et al: Lipid-lowering effect of carnitine in chronically uremic patients treated with maintenance hemodialysis. Am J Clin Nutr 33:1489, 1980.
377. Bartel LL, Hussey JL, Shrago E: Effect of dialysis on serum carnitine, free fatty acids, and triglyceride levels in man and the rat. Metabolism 31:944, 1982.
378. Wanner C, Fortiner-Wanner S, Schaeffer E, et al: Serum free carnitine esters and lipids in patients on peritoneal dialysis and hemodialysis. Am J Nephrol 6:206, 1986.
379. Nilsson-Ehle P, Cederblad G, Fagher B, et al: Plasma lipoproteins, liver function and glucose metabolism in haemodialysis patients: Lack of effect of L-carnitine supplementation. Scand J Clin Lab Invest 45:179, 1985.
380. Golper TA, Wolfson M, Ahmad S, et al: Multicenter trial of L-carnitine in maintenance hemodialysis patients. I. Carnitine concentrations and lipid effects. Kidney Int 38:904, 1990.
381. Hombrouckx RO, Bogaert AM, Leroy FM, et al: Polyunsaturated fatty acids of the n-3 class in chronic dialysis. ASAIO J 38:M331, 1992.
382. Donnelly SM, Ali MAM, Churchill DN: Effect of n-3 fatty acids from fish oil on hemostasis, blood pressure, and lipid profile of dialysis patients. J Am Soc Nephrol 2:1634, 1992.
383. Hamazaki T, Nakazawa R, Tateno S, et al: Effects of fish oil rich in eicosapentaenoic acid on serum lipid in hyperlipidemic hemodialysis patients. Kidney Int 26:81, 1984.
384. Goldberg AP, Applebaum-Bowden DM, Bierman EL, et al: Increase in lipoprotein lipase during clofibrate treatment of hypertriglyceridemia in patients on hemodialysis. N Engl J Med 301:1073, 1979.
385. Grundy SM: Management of hyperlipidemia of kidney disease. Kidney Int 37:847, 1990.
386. Wanner C, Horl WH, Luley CH, Wieland H: Effects of HMG-CoA reductase inhibitors in hypercholesterolemic patients on hemodialysis. Kidney Int 39:754, 1991.
387. Corpier CL, Jones PH, Suki WN, et al: Rhabdomyolysis and renal injury with lovastatin use. Report of two cases in cardiac transplant recipients. JAMA 260:239, 1988.
388. Kogan AD, Orenstein S: Lovastatin-induced acute rhabdomyolysis. Postgrad Med J 66:294, 1990.
389. Chucrallah A, De Girolami U, Freeman R, Federman M: Lovastatin/gemfibrozil myopathy: A clinical, histochemical, and ultrastructural study. Eur Neurol 32:293, 1992.
390. Marais GE, Larson KK: Rhabdomyolysis and acute renal failure induced by combination lovastatin and gemfibrozil therapy. Ann Intern Med 112:228, 1990.
391. Pierce LR, Wysowski DK, Gross TP: Myopathy and rhabdomyolysis associated with lovastatin-gemfibrozil combination therapy. JAMA 264:71, 1990.
392. Kopple JD, Swenseid ME: Vitamin nutrition in patients undergoing maintenance hemodialysis. Kidney Int 7:579, 1975.
393. Stein G, Sperschneider H, Koppe S: Vitamin levels in chronic renal failure and need for supplementation. Blood Purif 3:52, 1985.
394. Descombes E, Hanck AB, Fellay G: Water soluble vitamins in chronic hemodialysis patients and need for supplementation. Kidney Int 43:1319, 1993.
395. DeBari VA, Frank O, Baker H, Needle MA: Water soluble vitamins in granulocytes, erythrocytes, and plasma obtained from chronic hemodialysis patients. Am J Clin Nutr 39:410, 1984.

396. Ramirez G, Chen M, Boyce WHJ, et al: Longitudinal follow-up of chronic hemodialysis patients without vitamin supplementation. Kidney Int 30:99, 1986.

397. Hampers CL, Streiff R, Nathan DG, et al: Megaloblastic hematopoiesis in uremia and in patients on long term dialysis. N Engl J Med 276:551, 1967.

398. Gotloib L, Servadio C: A possible case of beriberi heart in a hemodialysis patient. Nephron 14:293, 1975.

399. Kopple JD, Mercurio K, Blumenkrantz MJ, et al: Daily requirement for pyridoxine supplements in chronic renal failure. Kidney Int 19:694, 1981.

400. Stone WJ, Warnock LG, Wagner C: Vitamin B$_6$ deficiency in uremia. Am J Clin Nutr 28:950, 1975.

401. Kleiner MJ, Tate SS, Sullivan JF, Chami J: Vitamin B$_6$ deficiency in maintenance dialysis patients: Metabolic effects of repletion. Am J Clin Nutr 33;1612, 1980.

402. Dobbelstein H, Korner WF, Mempel W, et al: Vitamin B$_6$ deficiency in uremia and its implications for the depression of immune responses. Kidney Int 5:233, 1974.

403. Allman MA, Truswell AS, Tiller DJ, et al: Vitamin supplementation of patients receiving haemodialysis. Med J Aust 150:130, 1989.

404. Sharman VL, Cunningham J, Goodwin FJ, et al: Do patients receiving regular haemodialysis need folic acid supplements? Br Med J 285:96, 1982.

405. Giardano C, De Santo NG, Renaldi S, et al: Histidine supplementation in the treatment of uraemia. Proc Eur Dial Transplant Assoc 10:161, 1973.

406. Blumenkrantz MJ, Shapiro D, Swenseid ME, Kopple JD: Histidine supplementation for treatment of anaemia of uraemia. Br Med J 2:53, 1975.

407. Yatzidis H, Koutsicos D, Agroyannis B, et al: Biotin in the management of uremic neurologic disorders. Nephron 36:183, 1984.

408. Stewart WK, Fleming LW: Plasma retinol and retinol binding protein concentrations in patients on maintenance haemodialysis with and without vitamin A supplements. Nephron 30:15, 1982.

409. Werb R, Clark WF, Lindsay RM, et al: Serum vitamin A levels and associated abnormalities in patients on regular dialysis treatment. Clin Nephrol 12:63, 1979.

410. Gotloib L, Sklan D, Mines M: Hemodialysis: Effect on plasma levels of vitamin A and carotenoid. JAMA 239:751, 1978.

411. Gleghorn EE, Eisenberg LD, Hack S: Observations of vitamin A toxicity in three patients with renal failure receiving parenteral alimentation. Am J Clin Nutr 44:107, 1986.

412. Stein G, Schone S, Geinitz D, et al: No tissue level abnormality of vitamin A concentration despite elevated serum vitamin A of uremic patients. Clin Nephrol 25:87, 1986.

413. Sullivan JF, Eisenstein AB, Mottola OM, et al: The effect of dialysis on plasma and tissue levels of vitamin C. Trans Am Soc Artif Intern Organs 18:277, 1972.

414. Ono K, Hisasue Y, Morimatsu M: Should vitamin C supplementation be restricted in regular hemodialysis patients? ASAIO Trans 32:111, 1986.

415. Kokot F, Wiecek A, Grzeszczak W: Role of endogenous opioids in the pathogenesis of endocrine abnormalities in chronic renal failure. Semin Dial 1:213, 1988.

416. Drueke T: Endocrine disorders in chronic hemodialysis patients (with the exclusion of hyperparathyroidism). Adv Nephrol 10:351, 1981.

417. Mooradian AD, Mortley J: Endocrine dysfunction in chronic renal failure. Arch Intern Med 144:351, 1984.

418. Bonomini V, Orsoni G, Sorrentino MA, Todeschini P: Hormonal changes in hemodialysis. Blood Purif 8:54, 1990.

419. Ferraris JR, Domene HM, Escobar ME, et al: Hormonal profile in pubertal females with chronic renal failure: Before and under haemodialysis and after renal transplantation. Acta Endocrinol 115:289, 1987.

420. Castellano M, Turconi A, Chaler E, et al: Hypothalamic-pituitary-gonadal function in prepubertal boys and girls with chronic renal failure. J Pediatr 122:46, 1993.

421. Pasquali T, Zantelifer D, Balzaretti M, et al: Evidence of hypothalamic-pituitary thyroid abnormalities in children with end-stage renal disease. J Pediatr 118:873, 1991.

422. Gonzalez-Barcena D, Kastin AJ, Sachalch DS, et al: Responses to thyrotropin-releasing hormone in patients with renal failure and

423. Hasagawa K, Matsushita Y, Otomo S, et al: Abnormal response of thyrotropin and growth hormone to thyrotropin-releasing hormone in chronic renal failure. Acta Endocrinol 79:635, 1975.

424. Allegra V, Amendolagine F, Mengozzi G, et al: Growth hormone secretion abnormalities in uremic patients: Which is the role of impaired glucose hypothalamic sensitivity? Nephron 48:76, 1988.

425. Gomez F, De La Cueva R, Wauters JP, Lemarchand-Beraud T: Endocrine abnormalities in patients undergoing long-term hemodialysis: The role of prolactin. Am J Med 68:522, 1980.

426. Nagel TC, Freinkel N, Bell RH: Gynecomastia, prolactin and other peptide hormones in patients undergoing chronic hemodialysis. J Clin Endocrinol Metab 36:428, 1973.

427. Lim VS, Henriquez C, Sievertsen G, Frohman LA: Ovarian function in chronic renal failure: Evidence suggesting hypothalamic anovulation. Ann Intern Med 93:21, 1980.

428. Zingraff J, Jungers P, Pelissier C, et al: Pituitary and ovarian dysfunctions in women on haemodialysis. Nephron 30:149, 1982.

429. Ramirez G, Butcher DE, Newton JL, et al: Bromocriptine and the hypothalamic hypophyseal function in patients with chronic renal failure on chronic hemodialysis. Am J Kidney Dis 6:111, 1985.

430. Rodger RSC, Dewar JH, Turner SJ, et al: Anterior pituitary dysfunction in patients with chronic renal failure treated by hemodialysis or continuous ambulatory peritoneal dialysis. Nephron 43:169, 1986.

431. Orskov H, Hausensen AP, Hansen HE, et al: Acetate: Inhibitor of growth hormone hypersecretion in diabetic and non-diabetic uraemic subjects. Acta Endocrinol 99:551, 1982.

432. Luger A, Lang I, Kovarik J, et al: Abnormalities in the hypothalamic-pituitary-adrenocortical axis in patients with chronic renal failure. Am J Kidney Dis 9:51, 1987.

433. Cooke RC, Whelton PK, Moore MA, et al: Dissociation of the diurnal variation of aldosterone and cortisol in anephric subjects. Kidney Int 15:669, 1979.

434. Rosman PM, Benn R, Kay M, et al: Cortisol binding in uremic plasma. I. Absence of abnormal cortisol binding to cortisol binding to corticosteroid-binding globulin. Nephron 37:160, 1984.

435. Siamopoulos KC, Dardamanis M, Kyriaki D, et al: Pituitary adrenal responsiveness to corticotropin-releasing hormone. Peritoneal Dial Int 10:153, 1990.

436. Hashimoto K, Nishioka T, Numata Y, et al: Plasma levels of corticotropin-releasing hormone in hypothalamic-pituitary-adrenal disorders and chronic renal failure. Acta Endocrinol 128:503, 1993.

437. Rosman PM, Benn R, Kay M, Wallace EZ: Cortisol binding in uremic plasma II: Decreased cortisol binding to albumin. Nephron 37:229, 1984.

438. Ramirez G, Gomez-Sanchez C, Meikle WA, Jubiz W: Evaluation of the hypothalamic hypophyseal adrenal axis in patients receiving long-term hemodialysis. Arch Intern Med 142:1448, 1982.

439. Sharp NA, Devlin JT, Rimmer JM: Renal failure obfuscates the diagnosis of Cushing's disease. JAMA 256:2564, 1986.

440. Grant AC, Rodger RS, Mitchell R, et al: Hypothalamo-pituitary-adrenal axis in uraemia: Evidence for primary adrenal dysfunction. Nephrol Dial Transplant 8:307–310, 1993.

441. Converse RL, Jacobsen TN, Toto RD, et al: Sympathetic overactivity in patients with chronic renal failure. N Engl J Med 327:1912, 1992.

442. Darwich R, Elias AN, Vaziri ND, et al: Plasma and urinary catecholamines and their metabolites in chronic renal failure. Arch Intern Med 144:69, 1984.

443. Lindsay RM, Hoyle IT, Luke RG, Kennedy AC: The endocrine status of the regular dialysis patient. In Kerr D, Fries D, Elliot R (eds): Dialysis and Renal Transplantation. Excerpta Medica, Amsterdam, 1969, p 230.

444. Elias AN, Vaziri ND, Maksy M: Plasma norepinephrine and dopamine levels in end-stage renal disease. Arch Intern Med 145:1013, 1985.

445. Izzo JL, Sterns RH: Abnormal norepinephrine release in uremia. Kidney Int 24:S221, 1983.

446. Ziegler MG, Kennedy B, Morrissey E, O'Connor DT: Norepinephrine clearance, chromogranin A and dopamine β-hydroxylase in renal failure. Kidney Int 37:1357, 1990.

447. Ross RD, Kalidindi V, Vincent JA, et al: Acute changes in endothelin-1 after hemodialysis for chronic renal failure. J Pediatr 122:S74–S76, 1993.

448. Mann H, Konigs F, Heintz B, et al: Vasoactive hormones during hemodialysis with intermittent ultrafiltration. ASAIO J 36:M367, 1990.

449. Hegbrant J, Thysell H, Martensson L, et al: Changes in plasma levels of vasoactive peptides during sequential bicarbonate hemodialysis. Nephron 63:309, 1993.

450. Yamada K, Nakayama M, Miura Y, et al: Role of AVP in the regulation of vascular tonus and blood pressure in patients with chronic renal failure. Regul Pept 29:91, 1993.

451. Graziani G, Badalamenti S, Del Bo A, et al: Abnormal hemodynamics and elevated angiotensin II plasma levels in polydipsic patients on regular hemodialysis treatment. Kidney Int 44:107, 1993.

452. Sasamura H, Suzuki H, Takita T, et al: Response of plasma immunoreactive active renin, inactive renin, plasma renin activity, and aldosterone to hemodialysis in patients with diabetic nephropathy. Clin Nephrol 33:288, 1990.

453. Petersen J, Li CC, Bishop-Abney N, Seniw CM: Hemodynamic and atrial natriuretic peptide responses to fluid removal and reinfusion in hemodialysis patients. ASAIO Trans 34:509, 1988.

454. Leunissen KML, Menheere PPCA, Cheriex EC, et al: Plasma alpha-human atrial natriuretic peptide and volume status in chronic haemodialysis patients. Nephrol Dial Transplant 4:382, 1989.

455. Plum J, Grabensee B: Atrial natriuretic peptide in dialysis patients under various conditions of volume homeostasis. J Intern Med 229:209, 1991.

456. Jawadi MH, Ho LS, Dipette D, Ross DL: Regulation of plasma arginine vasopressin in patients with chronic renal failure maintained on hemodialysis. Am J Nephrol 6:175, 1986.

457. Saxenhofer H, Gnadinger MP, Weidmann P, et al: Plasma levels and dialysance of atrial natriuretic peptide in terminal renal failure. Kidney Int 32:554, 1987.

458. Mastrogiacomo I, DeBesi L, Serafini E, et al: Hyperprolactinemia and sexual disturbances among uremic women on hemodialysis. Nephron 37:195, 1984.

459. Strickler RC, Woolever CA, Johnson M, et al: Serum gonadotropin patterns in patients with chronic renal failure on hemodialysis. Gynecol Invest 5:185, 1974.

460. Lim VS: Reproductive function in patients with renal insufficiency. Am J Kidney Dis 9:363, 1987.

461. Hou SH, Grossman S, Molitch ME: Hyperprolactinemia in patients with renal insufficiency and chronic renal failure requiring hemodialysis or chronic ambulatory peritoneal dialysis. Am J Kidney Dis 6:245, 1985.

462. Rice GG: Hypermenorrhea in the young hemodialysis patient. Am J Obstet Gynecol 116:539, 1973.

463. Shirley RL, Tilney NL: Gynecologic and obstetric care of dialysis and transplant patients. In Tilney NL, Lazarus JM (eds): Surgical Care of the Patient with Renal Failure. WB Saunders, Philadelphia, 1982, p 163.

464. Unzelman RF, Alderfer GR, Chojnacki RE: Pregnancy and chronic hemodialysis. Trans Am Soc Artif Intern Organs 19:144, 1973.

465. Hou S: Pregnancy in women requiring dialysis for renal failure. Am J Kidney Dis 9:368, 1987.

466. Roxe DM, McLaughlin MM: Reproductive capacity in female patients on chronic hemodialysis. Int J Artif Organs 7:249, 1984.

467. Levy NB: Sexual adjustment to maintenance hemodialysis and renal transplantation: National survey by questionnaire: Preliminary report. Trans Am Soc Artif Intern Organs 19:138, 1973.

468. Ferraris J, Saenger P, Levine L: Delayed puberty in males with chronic renal failure. Kidney Int 18:344, 1980.

469. Alleyne S, Dillard P, McGregor C, Hosten A: Sexual function and mental distress status of patients with end-stage renal disease on hemodialysis. Transplant Proc 21:3895, 1989.

470. Sherman FP: Impotence in patients with chronic renal failure on dialysis: Its frequency and etiology. Fertil Steril 26:221, 1975.

471. Nogues MA, Starkstein S, Davalos M, et al: Cardiovascular reflexes and pudendal evoked responses in chronic haemodialysis patients. Funct Neurol 6:359, 1991.

472. Procci WR, Goldstein DA, Adelstein J, Massary SG: Sexual dysfunction in the male patient with uremia: A reappraisal. Kidney Int 19:317, 1981.

473. Campese VM, Procci WR, Levitan D, et al: Autonomic nervous system dysfunction and impotence in uremia. Am J Nephrol 2:140, 1982.

474. De Kretser DM, Atkins RC, Hudson B, Scott DF: Disordered spermatogenesis in patients with chronic renal failure undergoing maintenance hemodialysis. Aust N Z J Med 4:178, 1974.

475. Distiller LA, Morley GE, Sagel J, et al: Pituitary-gonadal function in chronic renal failure: The effect of luteinizing hormone–releasing hormone and the influence of dialysis. Metabolism 24:711, 1975.

476. Lim VS, Fang BS: Gonadal dysfunction in uremic men. A study of the hypothalamo-pituitary-testicular axis before and after renal transplantation. Am J Med 58:655, 1975.

477. Holdsworth S, Atkins RC, De Kretser DM: The pituitary-testicular axis in men with chronic renal failure. N Engl J Med 296:1245, 1977.

478. Gueara A, Vidt D, Hallberg C, et al: Serum gonadotropin and testosterone levels in uremic males undergoing intermittent dialysis. Metabolism 18:1062, 1969.

479. Chen JC, Vidt DG, Zorn EM, et al: Pituitary–Leydig's cell function in uremic males. J Clin Endocrinol 31:14, 1970.

480. Barton CH, Mitahmadi MK, Vaziri ND: Effects of long-term testosterone administration on pituitary-testicular axis in end-stage renal failure. Nephron 31:61, 1982.

481. Ramirez G, Bittle PA, Sanders H, Bercu BB: Hypothalamo-hypophyseal thyroid and gonadal function before and after erythropoietin therapy in dialysis patients. J Clin Endocrinol Metab 74:517, 1992.

482. Joven J, Villabona C, Rubies-Prat J, et al: Hormonal profile and serum zinc levels in uremic men with gonadal dysfunction undergoing hemodialysis. Clin Chim Acta 148:239, 1985.

483. Foulks CJ, Cushner HM: Sexual dysfunction in male dialysis patient: Pathogenesis, evaluation and therapy. Am J Kidney Dis 8:211, 1986.

484. Fioretti P, Melis GB, Ciardella F, et al: Parathyroid function and pituitary-gonadal axis in male uremics: Effects of dietary treatment and of maintenance hemodialysis. Clin Nephrol 25:155, 1986.

485. Levitan D, Moser SA, Goldstein DA, et al: Disturbances in the hypothalamic-pituitary-gonadal axis in male patients with acute renal failure. Am J Nephrol 4:99, 1984.

486. van Coevorden A, Stolear JC, Dhaene M, et al: Effect of chronic oral testosterone undecanoate administration on the pituitary-testicular axes of hemodialyzed male patients. Clin Nephrol 26:48, 1986.

487. Martin-Malo A, Benito P, Castillo D, et al: Effect of clomiphene citrate on hormonal profile in male hemodialysis and kidney transplant patients. Nephron 63:390, 1993.

488. Mahajan SK, Prasad AS, McDonald FD: Sexual dysfunction in uremic male: Improvement following oral zinc supplementation. Contrib Nephrol 38:103, 1984.

489. Rodger RSC, Sheldon WL, Watson MJ, et al: Zinc deficiency and hyperprolactinaemia are not reversible causes of sexual dysfunction in uraemia. Nephrol Dial Transplant 4:888, 1989.

490. Muir JW, Besser GM, Edwards CR, et al: Bromcriptine improves reduced libido and potency in men receiving maintenance hemodialysis. Clin Nephrol 20:308, 1983.

491. Ruilope L, Garcia Robles R, Paya C, et al: Influence of lisuride, a dopaminergic agonist, on the sexual function of male patients with chronic renal failure. Am J Kidney Dis 5:182, 1985.

492. Ermolenko VM, Kukhtevich AV, Dedov II, et al: Parlodel treatment of uremic hypogonadism in men. Nephron 42:19, 1986.

493. Yeksan M, Polat M, Turk S, et al: Effect of vitamin E therapy on sexual functions of uremic patients in hemodialysis. Int J Artif Organs 15:648, 1992.

494. Semple CG, Beastall GH, Henderson IS, et al: The pituitary-testicular axis of uraemic subjects on haemodialysis and continuous ambulatory peritoneal dialysis. Acta Endocrinol (Copenh) 101:464, 1982.

495. Schafer RM, Kokot F, Wernze H, et al: Improved sexual function in hemodialysis patients on recombinant erythropoietin: A possible role for prolactin. Clin Nephrol 31:1, 1989.

496. Bommer J, Kugel M, Schwobel B, et al: Improved sexual function during recombinant human erythropoietin therapy. Nephrol Dial Transplant 5:204, 1990.

497. Delano BG: Improvements in quality of life following treatment with r-HuEPO in anemic hemodialysis patients. Am J Kidney Dis 14:14, 1989.

498. Evans RW, Rader B, Manninen DL, et al: The quality of life of hemodialysis recipients treated with recombinant human erythropoietin. JAMA 263:825, 1990.

499. Evans RW: Recombinant human erythropoietin and the quality of life of end-stage renal disease patients: A comparative analysis. Am J Kidney Dis 18:62, 1991.

500. Levin NW: Quality of life and hematocrit level. Am J Kidney Dis 20:16, 1992.

501. Kokot F, Wiecek A, Grzeszczak W, et al: Influence of erythropoietin treatment on endocrine abnormalities in haemodialyzed patients. Contrib Nephrol 76:257, 1989.

502. Akizawa T, Kinugasa E, Nakayama F, et al: Changes in endocrinological functions in hemodialysis patients associated with improvements in anemia after recombinant human erythropoietin therapy. Contrib Nephrol 82:86, 1990.

503. Lindsay RM, Briggs JD, Luke RG, et al: Gynaecomastia in chronic renal failure. Br Med J 4:779, 1967.

504. Lim VS, Fang VS, Katz AI, Refetoff S: Thyroid dysfunction in chronic renal failure: A study of the pituitary thyroid axis and peripheral turnover kinetics of thyroxine and triiodothyronine. J Clin Invest 60:522, 1977.

505. Ramirez G, Jubiz W, Gutch W, et al: Thyroid abnormalities in renal failure: A study of 53 patients on chronic hemodialysis. Ann Intern Med 79:500, 1973.

506. Kaptein EM, Quion-Verde H, Chooljian CJ, et al: The thyroid in end-stage renal disease. Medicine (Baltimore) 67:187, 1988.

507. Schmidt P, Stobaeus N, Prame G, Schittek F: Exophthalmos in chronic renal insufficiency. Scand J Urol Nephrol 5:146, 1971.

508. Sennesael JJ, Verbeelen DL, Jonckheer MH: Thyroid dysfunction in patients on regular hemodialysis: Evaluation of the stable intrathyroidal iodine pool, incidence of goiter and free thyroid hormone concentration. Nephron 41:141, 1985.

509. Hagedus L, Andersen JR, Poulsen LR, et al: Thyroid gland volume and serum concentrations of thyroid hormones in chronic renal failure. Nephron 40:171, 1985.

510. Elias AN, Vaziri ND, Farooqui S, et al: Pathology of endocrine organs in chronic renal failure: An autopsy analysis of 66 patients. Int J Artif Organs 7:251, 1984.

511. Fagher B, Monti M, Nilsson-Ehle P, Thysell H: Reduced thermogenesis in muscle and disturbed lipoprotein metabolism in relation to thyroid function in haemodialysis patients. Scand J Clin Lab Invest 47:91, 1987.

512. Ramirez G, O'Neill WM, Jubiz W, Bloomer HA: Thyroid dysfunction in uremia: Evidence with thyroid and hypophyseal abnormalities. Ann Intern Med 84:672, 1976.

513. Beckers C, van Ypersele de Strihou C, Coche E, et al: Iodine metabolism in severe renal insufficiency. J Clin Endocrinol 29:293, 1969.

514. Koutras DA, Marketos SG, Rigopoulos GA, Malamos B: Iodine metabolism in chronic renal insufficiency. Nephron 9:55, 1972.

515. Spector DA, Davis PJ, Helderman JH, et al: Thyroid function and metabolic state in chronic renal failure. Ann Intern Med 85:724, 1976.

516. Desanto NG, Fine RN, Carella C, et al: Thyroid function in uremic children. Kidney Int 28:S166, 1985.

517. Joasoo A, Murray IPC, Parkin J, et al: Abnormalities of in vitro thyroid function test in renal disease. Q J Med 63:245, 1974.

518. Forest J, Dube J, Talbot J: Thyroid hormones in patients with chronic renal failure undergoing maintenance hemodialysis. Am J Clin Pathol 77:580, 1982.

519. Davis FB, Spector DA, Davis PJ, et al: Comparison of pituitary-thyroid function in patients with end-stage renal disease and in age- and sex-matched controls. Kidney Int 21:362, 1982.

520. Lim VS, Flanigan MJ, Zavala DC, Freeman RM: Protective adaptation of low serum triiodothyronine in patients with chronic renal failure. Kidney Int 28:541, 1985.

521. Kerr DJ, Singh VK, Tsakiris D, et al: Serum and peritoneal dialysate thyroid hormone levels in patients on continuous ambulatory peritoneal dialysis. Nephron 43:164, 1986.

522. Lim VS, Zavala DC, Flanigan MJ, Freeman RM: Blunted peripheral tissue responsiveness to thyroid hormone in uremic patients. Kidney Int 31:808, 1987.

523. Giordano C, DeSanto NG, Carella C, et al: Thyroid status and nephron loss: A study in patients with chronic renal failure, end-stage renal disease and/or on hemodialysis. Int J Artif Intern Organs 7:119, 1984.

524. Beckett GJ, Henderson CJ, Elwes R, et al: Thyroid status in patients with chronic renal failure. Clin Nephrol 19:172, 1983.

525. Kaptein EM, Feinstein EI, Nicoloff JT, Massry SG: Alterations of serum reverse triiodothyronine and thyroxine kinetics in chronic renal failure: Role of nutritional status, chronic illness, uremia, and hemodialysis. Kidney Int 16:S183, 1983.

526. Pagliacci MC, Pelicci G, Grignani F, et al: Thyroid function tests in patients undergoing maintenance dialysis: Characterization of the 'low-T$_4$ syndrome' in subjects on regular hemodialysis and continuous ambulatory peritoneal dialysis. Nephron 46:225, 1987.

527. Hardy MJ, Ragbeer SS, Nascimento L: Pituitary-thyroid function in chronic renal failure assessed by a highly sensitive thyrotropin assay. J Clin Endocrinol Metab 66:233, 1988.

528. Wheatley T, Clark PM, Clark DJ, et al: Abnormalities of thyrotrophin (TSH) evening rise and pulsatile release in haemodialysis patients: Evidence for hypothalamic-pituitary changes in chronic renal failure. Clin Endocrinol 31:39, 1989.

529. Wassner SJ, Buckingham BA, Kershnar AJ, et al: Thyroid function in children with chronic renal failure. Nephron 19:236, 1977.

530. Tang WW, Kaptein EM, Massry SG: Diagnosis of hypothyroidism in patients with end-stage renal disease. Am J Nephrol 7:192, 1987.

531. Hershman JM, Jones CM, Bailey AL: Reciprocal changes in serum thyrotropin and free thyroxine produced by heparin. J Clin Endocrinol 34:574, 1972.

532. De Veber GA, Schatz DL: Effect of haemodialysis on thyroid function. In Kerr D, Fries D, Elliott R (eds): Dialysis and Renal Transplantation. Excerpta Medica, Amsterdam, 1969, p 226.

533. Sakurai S, Hara Y, Miura S, et al: Thyroid functions before and after maintenance hemodialysis in patients with chronic renal failure. Endocrinol Jpn 35:865, 1988.

534. Kaptein EM, Levitan D, Feinstein EL, et al: Alterations of thyroid hormone indices in acute renal failure and in acute critical illness with and without acute renal failure. Am J Nephrol 1:138, 1981.

535. McKillop JH, Leung ACT, Wilson R: Successful management of Graves disease in a patient undergoing regular dialysis therapy. Arch Intern Med 145:337, 1985.

536. Cooper DS, Steigerwalt S, Migdal S: Pharmacology of propylthiouracil in thyrotoxicosis and chronic renal failure. Arch Intern Med 147:785, 1987.

537. Winearls CG, Pippard MJ, Downing MR, et al: Effect of human erythropoietin derived from recombinant DNA on the anaemia of patients maintained by chronic haemodialysis. Lancet 2:1175, 1986.

538. Eschbach JW, Egrie JC, Downing MR, et al: Correction of the anemia of end-stage renal disease with recombinant human erythropoietin: Results of a combined phase I and II clinical trial. N Engl J Med 316:73, 1987.

539. Eschbach JW, Kelly MR, Haley NR, et al: Treatment of anemia of progressive renal failure with recombinant human erythropoietin. N Engl J Med 321:158, 1989.

540. Eschbach JW, Abdulhadi MH, Browne JK, et al: Recombinant human erythropoietin in anemic patients with end-stage renal disease: Results of a phase III multicenter clinical trial. Ann Intern Med 111:992, 1989.

541. Nissenson AR: National cooperative rHu erythropoietin study in patients with chronic renal failure: A phase IV multicenter study. Am J Kidney Dis 18:24–33, 1991.

542. Levin NW, Lazarus JM, Nissenson AR: National cooperative rHu erythropoietin study in patients with chronic renal failure—an interim report. Am J Kidney Dis 22:3, 1993.

543. McGonigle R, Wallin J, Shadduck R, Fisher J: Erythropoietin deficiency and inhibition of erythropoiesis in renal insufficiency. Kidney Int 25:437, 1984.

544. Davies S, Glynne-Jones E, Bisson M, Bisson P: Plasma erythropoietin assay in patients with chronic renal failure. J Clin Pathol 28:875, 1975.

545. Nathan DG, Sytknowski A: Erythropoietin and the regulation of erythropoiesis. N Engl J Med 308:520, 1983.

546. Freeman MH, Grunberger T, Saunders EF: Erythropoietic inhibitors in uraemic serum. Clin Invest Med 5:237, 1982.

547. Lim VS, DeGowin RL, Zavala D, et al: Recombinant human erythropoietin treatment in pre-dialysis patients: A double-blind placebo-controlled trial. Ann Intern Med 110:108, 1989.

548. Frenken LAM, Verberckmoes R, Michielse P, Koene RAP: Efficacy and tolerance of treatment with recombinant-human erythropoietin in chronic renal failure (pre-dialysis) patients. Nephrol Dial Transplant 4:782, 1989.

549. Anonymous: Double-blind, placebo-controlled study of the thera-

peutic use of recombinant human erythropoietin for anemia associated with chronic renal failure in predialysis patients. Am J Kidney Dis 18:50, 1991. (Erratum in Am J Kidney Dis 18:420, 1991.)

550. Kleinman KS, Schweitzer SU, Perdue ST, et al: The use of recombinant human erythropoietin in the correction of anemia in predialysis patients and its effect on renal function: A double-blind, placebo-controlled trial. Am J Kidney Dis 14:486, 1989.

551. Lim VS, Fangman J, Flanigan MJ, et al: Effect of recombinant human erythropoietin on renal function in humans. Kidney Int 36:131, 1990.

552. Abraham PA, Opsahl JA, Rachael KM, et al: Renal function during erythropoietin therapy for anemia in predialysis chronic renal failure patients. Am J Nephrol 10:128, 1990.

553. Verbeelen D, Bossuyt A, Smitz J, et al: Hemodynamics of patients with renal failure treated with recombinant human erythropoietin. Clin Nephrol 31:6, 1989.

554. Satoh K, Masuda T, Ikeda Y, et al: Hemodynamic changes by recombinant erythropoietin therapy in hemodialyzed patients. Hypertension 15:262, 1990.

555. Mayer G, Cada EV, Watzinger U, et al: Hemodynamic effects of partial correction of chronic anemia by recombinant human erythropoietin in patients on dialysis. Am J Kidney Dis 17:286, 1991.

556. Martinez-Vea A, Bardaji A, Garcia C, et al: Long-term myocardial effects of correction of anemia with recombinant human erythropoietin in aged patients on hemodialysis. Am J Kidney Dis 19:353, 1992.

557. Low I, Grutzmacher P, Bergmann M, Schoeppe W: Echocardiographic findings in patients on maintenance hemodialysis substituted with recombinant human erythropoietin. Clin Nephrol 31:26, 1989.

558. Cannella G, La Canna G, Sandrini M, et al: Reversal of left ventricular hypertrophy following recombinant human erythropoietin treatment of anaemic dialysed uraemic patients. Nephrol Dial Transplant 6:31, 1991.

559. Zehnder C, Zuber M, Sulzer M, et al: Influence of long-term amelioration of anemia and blood pressure control on left ventricular hypertrophy in hemodialyzed patients. Nephron 61:21, 1992.

560. Pascual J, Teruel JL, Moya JL, et al: Regression of left ventricular hypertrophy after partial correction of anemia with erythropoietin in patients on hemodialysis: A prospective study. Clin Nephrol 35:280, 1991.

561. Linde T, Sandhagen B, Bratteby LE, et al: Reduced oxygen affinity contributes to improved oxygen releasing capacity during erythropoietin treatment of renal anaemia. Nephrol Dial Transplant 8:524, 1993.

562. Robertson HT, Haley NR, Guthri M, et al: Recombinant erythropoietin improves exercise capacity in anemic hemodialysis patients. Am J Kidney Dis 15:325, 1990.

563. Roger SD, Grasty MS, Baker LRI, Raine AEG: Effects of oxygen breathing and erythropoietin on hypoxic vasodilation in uremic anemia. Kidney Int 42:975, 1992.

564. Onoyama K, Hori K, Osato S, Fujishima M: Haemodynamic effect of recombinant human erythropoietin on hypotensive haemodialysis patients. Nephrol Dial Transplant 6:562, 1991.

565. Park JS, Kim SB, Park SK, et al: Effect of recombinant human erythropoietin on muscle energy metabolism in patients with end-stage renal disease: A $^{31}$P-nuclear magnetic resonance spectroscopic study. Am J Kidney Dis 21:612, 1993.

566. Braumann KM, Nonnast DB, Boning D, Bocker A: Improved physical performance after treatment of renal anemia with recombinant human erythropoietin. Nephron 58:129, 1991.

567. Grunze M, Kohlmann M, Mulligan M, et al: Mechanisms of improved physical performance of chronic hemodialysis patients after erythropoietin treatment. Am J Nephrol 10:24, 1990.

568. Mayer G, Thum J, Cada EM, et al: Working capacity is increased following recombinant human erythropoietin treatment. Kidney Int 34:525, 1988.

569. Davenport A, Will EJ, Khanna SK, Davison AM: Blood lactate is reduced following successful treatment of anaemia in haemodialysis patients with recombinant human erythropoietin both at rest and after maximal exertion. Am J Nephrol 12:357, 1992.

570. Buckner FS, Eschbach JW, Haley NR, Davidson RC: Hypertension following erythropoietin therapy in anemic hemodialysis patients. Am J Hypertens 3:947, 1990.

571. Abraham PA, Macres MG: Blood pressure in hemodialysis patients

during amelioration of anemia with erythropoietin. J Am Soc Nephrol 2:927, 1991.

572. Anonymous: Effect of recombinant human erythropoietin therapy on blood pressure in hemodialysis patients. Am J Nephrol 11:23, 1991.

573. Schaefer RM, Leschke M, Strauer BE, Heidland A: Blood rheology and hypertension in hemodialysis patients treated with erythropoietin. Am J Nephrol 8:449, 1988.

574. Abraham PA, Opsahl JA, Keshaviah PR, et al: Body fluid spaces and blood pressure in hemodialysis patients during amelioration of anemia with erythropoietin. Am J Kidney Dis 16:438, 1990.

575. Yamakado M, Umezu M, Nagano M, Tagawa H: Mechanisms of hypertension induced by erythropoietin in patients on hemodialysis. Clin Invest Med 14:624, 1991.

576. Anastassiades E, Howarth D, Howarth J, et al: Influence of blood volume on the blood pressure of predialysis and peritoneal dialysis patients treated with erythropoietin. Nephrol Dial Transplant 8:621, 1993.

577. Muller R, Steffen HM, Brunner R, et al: Changes in the alpha adrenergic system and increase in blood pressure with recombinant human erythropoietin (rHuEpo) therapy for renal anemia. Clin Invest Med 14:614, 1991.

578. Takayama K, Nagai T, Kinugasa E, et al: Changes in endothelial vasoactive substances under recombinant human erythropoietin therapy in hemodialysis patients. ASAIO Trans 37:M187, 1991.

579. Heidenrich S, Rahn KH, Zidek W: Direct vasopressor effect of recombinant human erythropoietin on renal resistance vessels. Kidney Int 39:259, 1991.

580. Carlini RG, Dusso AS, Obialo CI, et al: Recombinant human erythropoietin (rHuEPO) increases endothelin-1 release by endothelial cells. Kidney Int 43:1010, 1993.

581. Powe NR, Griffiths RI, Greer JW, et al: Early dosing practices and effectiveness of recombinant human erythropoietin. Kidney Int 43:1125, 1993.

582. Powe NR, Griffiths RI, Bass EB: Cost implications to Medicare of recombinant erythropoietin therapy for the anemia of end-stage renal disease. J Am Soc Nephrol 3:1660, 1993.

583. Sisk JE, Gianfrancesco FD, Coster JM: Recombinant erythropoietin and Medicare payment. JAMA 266:247, 1991.

584. Sheingold S, Churchill D, Muirhead N, et al: The impact of recombinant human erythropoietin on medical care costs for hemodialysis patients in Canada. Soc Sci Med 34:983, 1992.

585. Besarab A, McCrea JB: Evolution of recombinant human erythropoietin usage in clinical practice in the United States. Is there an optimal way to use rHuEPO? ASAIO J 39:11, 1993.

586. Eschbach JW, Adamson JW: Guidelines for recombinant human erythropoietin therapy. Am J Kidney Dis 14:2, 1989.

587. Watson AJ, Gimenez LF, Cotton S, et al: Treatment of the anemia of chronic renal failure with subcutaneous recombinant human erythropoietin. Am J Med 89:432, 1990.

588. McHahon LP, Dawborn JK: Experience with low dose intravenous and subcutaneous administration of recombinant human erythropoietin. Am J Nephrol 10:404, 1990.

589. Zappacosta AR, Perras ST, Bell A: Weekly subcutaneous recombinant human erythropoietin corrects anemia of progressive renal failure. Am J Med 91:229, 1991.

590. Granolleras C, Branger B, Shaldon S, et al: Subcutaneous erythropoietin: A comparison of daily and thrice weekly administration. Contrib Nephrol 88:144, 1991.

591. Besarab A, Flaharty KK, Erslev AF, et al: Clinical pharmacology and economics of recombinant human erythropoietin in end-stage renal disease: The case for subcutaneous administration. J Am Soc Nephrol 2:1405, 1992.

592. Ashai NI, Paganini EP, Wilson JM: Intravenous versus subcutaneous dosing of epoetin: A review of the literature. Am J Kidney Dis 22:23, 1993.

593. Hocken AG, Marwah PK: Iatrogenic contributions to the anaemia of chronic renal failure. Lancet 1:164, 1971.

594. Yen MC, Ball JH, Lowrie EG, et al: The effect of androgens and dialysis on erythropoiesis in chronic renal failure. Proc Dial Clin Transplant Forum 3:33, 1973.

595. Yawata Y, Jacob HS: Abnormal red cell metabolism in patients with chronic uremia: Nature of the defect and its persistence despite adequate hemodialysis. Blood 45:231, 1975.

596. Radtke HW, Frei U, Erbes PM, et al: Improving anemia by hemodialysis: Effect on serum erythropoietin. Kidney Int 17:382, 1980.

597. Santiago GC, Sreepada Rao TK, Laird NM: Effect of dialysis therapy on the hematopoietic system: The NCDS. Kidney Int 23:S95, 1983.

598. Depner TA, Rizwan S, James LA: Effectiveness of low dose erythropoietin: A possible advantage of high flux hemodialysis. ASAIO Trans 36:M223, 1990.

599. Mastrangel F, Alfonso L, Rizzelli S, Aprile M: Anaemia in high-efficiency dialysis. Nephrol Dial Transplant 6:116, 1991.

600. Lindsay RM, Burton JA, Dargie HJ, et al: Dialyzer blood loss. Clin Nephrol 1:24, 1973.

601. Schoenfeld PY, Henry RR, Laird NM, Roxe DM: Assessment of nutritional status of the National Cooperative Dialysis Study population. Kidney Int 23:S80, 1983.

602. Posner GL, Fink SM, Huded FV, et al: Endoscopic findings in chronic hemodialysis patients with upper gastrointestinal bleeding. Am J Gastroenterol 78:720, 1983.

603. Chachati A, Godon JP: Effect of haemodialysis on upper gastrointestinal tract pathology in patients with chronic renal failure. Nephrol Dial Transplant 1:233, 1987.

604. Kabelac K, Zahradnik J, Papik Z: Upper gastrointestinal bleeding as a complication in end stage renal disease patients. Sb Ved Pr Lek Fak Karlovy Univerzity Hradci Kralove 35:113, 1992.

605. Zuckerman GR, Cornette GL, Clouse RE, Harter HR: Upper gastrointestinal bleeding patients with chronic renal failure. Ann Intern Med 102:588, 1985.

606. Rosenblatt SG, Drake S, Fadem S, et al: Gastrointestinal blood loss in patients with chronic renal failure. Am J Kidney Dis 1:232, 1982.

607. Wizemann V, Buddensiek P, De Boor J, et al: Gastrointestinal blood loss in patients undergoing maintenance dialysis. Kidney Int 24:S218, 1983.

608. Bernstein EF, Blackshear PL, Keller KH: Factors influencing erythrocyte destruction in artificial organs. Am J Surg 114:126, 1967.

609. Francos GC, Burke JF, Besarab A, et al: An unsuspected case of acute hemolysis during hemodialysis. Trans Am Soc Artif Intern Organs 29:140, 1983.

610. Ivanovich P, Manzler A, Drake R: Acute hemolysis following hemodialysis. Trans Am Soc Artif Intern Organs 15:316, 1969.

611. Yawata Y, Kjellstrand CM, Buselmeier TJ, et al: Hemolysis in dialyzed patients: Tap water induced red blood cell metabolic deficiency. Trans Am Soc Artif Intern Organs 18:301, 1972.

612. Jacob HS, Amsden T: Acute hemolytic anemia with rigid red cells in hypophosphatemia. N Engl J Med 285:1446, 1971.

613. Lichtman MA, Miller DR, Freeman RB: Erythrocyte adenosine triphosphate depletion during hypophosphatemia in a uremic subject. N Engl J Med 280:240, 1969.

614. Gonella M, Fanara G, Bartolini V, Mariani G: Serum phosphate concentration with relation to the hematocrit value in uremic patients on chronic hemodialysis. Int J Artif Organs 7:341, 1984.

615. Matter BJ, Pederson J, Psimenos G, Lindeman RD: Lethal copper intoxication in hemodialysis. Trans Am Soc Artif Intern Organs 15:309, 1969.

616. Laurent C, Wittek M, Verteerstraeten P, et al: Red cells life span, splenic sequestration and transfusion requirements in chronic renal failure treated by hemodialysis. Effects of bilateral nephrectomy. Clin Nephrol 2:35, 1974.

617. Asaba H, Bergstrom J, Lundgren G, et al: Hypersequestration of $^{51}$Cr-labelled erythrocytes as a criterion for splenectomy in regular hemodialysis patients. Clin Nephrol 8:304, 1977.

618. Bischel MD, Neuman RS, Berne TV, et al: The elimination by splenectomy of blood transfusion requirements, leukopenia and thrombocytopenia in the patient on RDT. Proc Eur Dial Transplant Assoc 8:81, 1971.

619. Hartley LCJ, Morgan TO, Innis MD, Clunie GJA: Splenectomy for anaemia in patients on regular haemodialysis. Lancet 2:1343, 1971.

620. Crowley JP, Nealey TA, Metzger J, et al: Transfusion and long-term hemodialysis. Arch Intern Med 147:1925, 1987.

621. Hakim RM, Stivelman JC, Schulman G, et al: Iron overload and mobilization in long-term hemodialysis patients. Am J Kidney Dis 10:293, 1987.

622. Fayemi AM, Rigolosi R, Frascino J, et al: Hemosiderosis in hemodialysis patients: An autopsy study of 50 cases. JAMA 244:343, 1980.

623. Bregman J, Gelfand MC, Winchester JF, et al: HLA-linked iron overload and myopathy in maintenance hemodialysis patients. Trans Am Soc Artif Intern Organs 26:366, 1980.

624. Waterlot Y, Cantinieaux B, Hariga-Muller C, et al: Impaired phagocytic activity of neutrophils in patients receiving haemodialysis: The critical role of iron overload. Br Med J 291:501, 1985.

625. Boelaert JR, Van Landuyt HW, Unlcke YJ, et al: The role of iron overload in Yersinia enterocolitica and Yersinia pseudotuberculosis bacteremia in hemodialysis patients. J Infect Dis 156:384, 1987.

626. Van de Vyver FL, Visser WJ, D'Haese PC, De Broe ME: Iron overload and bone disease in chronic dialysis patients. Nephrol Dial Transplant 5:781, 1990.

627. Gral T, Schroth P: Transfusions, transferrin saturation and erythropoietic activity in long term hemodialyzed uremic patients. Am J Med Sci 260:230, 1970.

628. McCarthy JT, Kurtz SB, Mussman GV: Deferoxamine-enhanced fecal losses of aluminum and iron in a patient undergoing continuous ambulatory peritoneal dialysis. Am J Med 82:367, 1987.

629. Chang TM, Barre P: Effect of desferrioxamine on removal of aluminum and iron by coated charcoal haemoperfusion and haemodialysis. Lancet 2:1051, 1983.

630. de la Serna J, Gilsanz F, Ruilope L, et al: Improvement in the erythropoiesis of chronic haemodialysis patients with desferrioxamine. Lancet 1:1009, 1988.

631. Stivelman J, Schulman G, Fosburg M, et al: Kinetics and efficacy of deferoxamine in iron-overloaded hemodialysis patients. Kidney Int 36:1125, 1989.

632. Boelaert JR, Fenves AZ, Coburn J: Deferoxamine therapy and mucormycosis in dialysis patients: Report of an international registry. Am J Kidney Dis 18:660, 1991.

633. Windus DW, Stokes TJ, Julian BA, Fenves AZ: Fatal Rhizopus infection in hemodialysis patients receiving deferoxamine. Ann Intern Med 107:678, 1987.

634. Walker JA, Sherman RA, Eisinger RP: Thrombocytopenia associated with intravenous deferoxamine. Am J Kidney Dis 6:254, 1985.

635. Bournerias F, Monnier N, Dufier JL, Reveillaud RJ: Severe ocular toxicity of desferrioxamine in the hemodialyzed patient. Nephrologie 8:27, 1987.

636. Stivelman J, Hakim RM, Schulman G, et al: Exacerbation of possible dialysis encephalopathy with deferoxamine. Am J Kidney Dis 6:A21, 1985. Abstract.

637. Swartz RD: Deferoxamine and aluminum removal. Am J Kidney Dis 6:358, 1985.

638. McCauley J, Sorkin MI: Exacerbation of aluminum encephalopathy after treatment with desferrioxamine. Nephrol Dial Transplant 4:110, 1989.

639. Ellenbergy R, King AL, Sica DA, et al: Cerebrospinal fluid aluminum levels following deferoxamine. Am J Kidney Dis 16:157, 1990.

640. Lazarus JM, Hakim RM, Newell J: Recombinant human erythropoietin and phlebotomy in the treatment of iron overload in chronic hemodialysis patients. Am J Kidney Dis 16:1011, 1990.

641. Macdougall IC, Hutton RD, Cavill I, et al: Poor response to treatment of renal anaemia with erythropoietin corrected by iron given intravenously. BMJ 299:157, 1989.

642. Van Wyck DB, Stivelman JC, Ruiz J, et al: Iron status in patients receiving erythropoietin for dialysis-associated anemia. Kidney Int 35:712, 1989.

643. Kooistra MP, van Es A, Struyvenberg A, Marx JJ: Iron metabolism in patients with the anaemia of end-stage renal disease during treatment with recombinant human erythropoietin. Br J Haematol 79:634, 1991.

644. Donnelly SM, Posen GA, Ali MA: Oral iron absorption in hemodialysis patients treated with erythropoietin. Clin Invest Med 14:271, 1991.

645. Milman N, Larsen L: Iron absorption in patients with chronic uremia undergoing regular hemodialysis. Acta Med Scand 199:133, 1976.

646. Van Wyck DB: Iron management during recombinant human erythropoietin therapy. Am J Kidney Dis 14:9, 1989.

647. Magana L, Dhar S, Smith E, Martinez C: Iron absorption and utilization in maintenance hemodialysis patients: Oral and intravenous routes. Mt Sinai J Med 51:180, 1984.

648. Parkinson IS, Ward MK, Kerr DNS: Dialysis encephalopathy, bone disease and anemia: The aluminum intoxication syndrome during regular haemodialysis. J Clin Pathol 34:1285, 1981.

649. Kaiser L, Schwartz KA: Aluminum-induced anemia. Am J Kidney Dis 6:348, 1985.

650. Swartz R, Dombrouski J, Burnatowska-Hledin M, Mayor G: Micro-cytic anemia in dialysis patients: Reversible marker of aluminum toxicity. Am J Kidney Dis 11:217, 1987.

651. Bia MJ, Cooper K, Schnall S, et al: Aluminum induced anemia: Pathogenesis and treatment in patients on chronic hemodialysis. Kidney Int 36:852t, 1989.

652. Donnelly SM, Ali MAM, Churchill DN: Bioavailability of iron in hemodialysis patients treated with erythropoietin: Evidence for the inhibitory role of aluminum. Am J Kidney Dis 16:447, 1990.

653. Meytes D, Bogin E, Ma A, Dukes PP: Effect of parathyroid hormone on erythropoiesis. J Clin Invest 67:1263, 1981.

654. Massry SG: Pathogenesis of the anemia of uremia: Role of secondary hyperparathyroidism. Kidney Int 24:S204, 1983.

655. Lutton JD, Solangi KB, Ibraham NG, et al: Inhibition of erythropoiesis in chronic renal failure: The role of parathyroid hormone. Am J Kidney Dis 3:380, 1984.

656. Saltissi D, Carter GD: Association of secondary hyperparathyroidism with red cell survival in chronic haemodialysis patients. Clin Sci 68:29, 1985.

657. Rao DS, Shih M, Mohini R: Effect of serum parathyroid hormone and bone marrow fibrosis on the response to erythropoietin in uremia. N Engl J Med 328:171, 1993.

658. Stenzel KH, Cheigh JS, Sullivan JF, et al: Clinical effects of bilateral nephrectomy. Am J Med 58:69, 1975.

659. Ball JH, Lowrie EG, Hampers CL, Merrill JP: Testosterone therapy in hemodialysis patients. Clin Nephrol 4:91, 1975.

660. Kalmanti M, Dainiak N, Martino J, et al: Correlation of clinical and in vitro erythropoietic responses to androgens in renal failure. Kidney Int 22:383, 1982.

661. Neff MS, Goldberg J, Slifkin RF, et al: A comparison of androgens for anemia in patients on hemodialysis. N Engl J Med 304:871, 1981.

662. Hendler ED, Solomon L: Androgen therapy in hemodialysis patients. I. Effects on red cell oxygen transport. Kidney Int 31:100, 1987.

663. Ballal SH, Domoto DT, Polack DC, Marciulonis P: Androgens potentiate the effects of erythropoietin in the treatment of anemia of end-stage renal disease. Am J Kidney Dis 17:29, 1991.

664. Acchiardo SR, Quinn BP, Burk LB, Moore LW: Are high flux dialysis and erythropoietin treatment in a collision course? ASAIO Trans 35:308, 1989.

665. Paganini EP, Abdulhadi MH, Garcia J, Magnusson MO: Recombinant human erythropoietin correction of anemia. Dialysis efficiency, waste retention, and chronic dose variables. ASAIO Trans 35:513, 1989.

666. Casati S, Capise M, Crepaldi M, et al: Haemodialysis efficiency after long-term treatment with recombinant human erythropoietin. Nephrol Dial Transplant 4:718, 1989.

667. Delano BG, Lundin AP, Galonsky R, et al: Dialyzer urea and creatinine clearances are not significantly altered in erythropoietin treated maintenance hemodialysis patients. ASAIO Trans 36:36, 1990.

668. Buur T, Lundberg M: Secondary effects of erythropoietin treatment on metabolism and dialysis efficiency in stable hemodialysis patients. Clin Nephrol 34:230, 1990.

669. Van Geelen JA, Nube MJ, Zuuriber PA: Influence of erythropoietin treatment of urea kinetic parameters in hemodialysis patients. Clin Nephrol 35:165, 1991.

670. Ofsthun NJ, Jensen JC, Kray M: Effect of high hematocrit and high blood flow rates on transmembrane pressure and ultrafiltration rate in hemodialysis. Blood Purif 9:169–176, 1991.

671. Raine AEG: Hypertension, blood viscosity, and cardiovascular morbidity in renal failure: Implications of erythropoietin therapy. Lancet 1:97–99, 1986.

672. Dy GR, Bloom EJ, Ijelu GK, et al: Effect of recombinant human erythropoietin on vascular access. ASAIO Trans 37:M274, 1991.

673. Lazarus JM, Huang WH, Lew NL, Lowrie EG: Contribution of vascular access–related disease to morbidity of hemodialysis patients. *In* Henry ML, Ferguson RM (eds): Vascular Access for Hemodialysis—III. WL Gore & Associates and Precept Press, Hong Kong, 1993, p 3.

674. Besarab A, Medina F, Musial E, et al: Recombinant human erythropoietin does not increase clotting in vascular access. ASAIO J 36:M749, 1990.

675. Macdougall IC, Davies ME, Hallett I, Cochlin DL: Coagulation studies and fistula blood flow during erythropoietin therapy in haemodialysis patients. Nephrol Dial Transplant 6:682, 1991.

676. Kaupke CJ, Butler GC, Vaziri ND: Effect of recombinant human erythropoietin on platelet production in dialysis patients. J Am Soc Nephrol 3:1672, 1993.

677. Eschbach JW: Erythropoietin is not a cause of access thrombosis. Semin Dial 6:180, 1993.

678. Ward HJ: Implications of recombinant erythropoietin therapy for renal transplantation. Am J Nephrol 10:44, 1990.

679. Grimm PC, Sinai-Trieman L, Sekiya NM, et al: Effects of recombinant human erythropoietin on HLA sensitization and cell mediated immunity. Kidney Int 38:12, 1990.

680. Ettenger RB, Marik J, Grimm P: The impact of recombinant human erythropoietin therapy on renal transplantation. Am J Kidney Dis 18:57, 1991.

681. Deierhoi MH, Barger BO, Hudson SL, et al: The effect of erythropoietin and blood transfusions on highly sensitized patients on a single cadaver renal allograft waiting list. Transplantation 53:363, 1992.

682. Keane WF, Shapiro FL, Raij L: Incidence and type of infections occurring in 445 chronic hemodialysis patients. Trans Am Soc Artif Intern Organs 23:41, 1977.

683. Nsouli KA, Lazarus JM, Schoenbaum SC, et al: Bacteremic infection in hemodialysis. Arch Intern Med 139:1255, 1979.

684. Montgomerie JZ, Kalmanson GM, Guze LB: Renal failure and infection. Medicine (Baltimore) 47:1, 1968.

685. Goldblum SE, Reed WP: Host defenses and immunologic alterations associated with chronic hemodialysis. Ann Intern Med 93:597, 1980.

686. Osanloo EO, Berlin BS, Popli S, et al: Antibody response to influenza vaccination in patients with chronic renal failure. Kidney Int 14:614, 1978.

687. Nelson J, Ormrod DJ, Miller TE: Host immune status in uraemia. VI: Leucocytic response to bacterial infection in chronic renal failure. Nephron 39:21, 1985.

688. Hosking CS, Atkins RC, Scott DR, et al: Immune and phagocytic function in patients on maintenance hemodialysis and post-transplantation. Clin Nephrol 6:501, 1976.

689. Briggs WA, Sillix DH, Mahajan S, McDonald FD: Leukocyte metabolism and function in uremia. Kidney Int 24:S16, 1984.

690. Lewis SL, Van Epps DE: Neutrophil and monocyte alterations in chronic dialysis patients. Am J Kidney Dis 9:381, 1987.

691. Mansell M, Grimes AJ: Red and white cell abnormalities in chronic renal failure. Br J Haematol 42:169, 1979.

692. Ruiz P, Gomez F, Schreiber AD: Impaired function of macrophage Fcγ receptors in end-stage renal disease. N Engl J Med 322:717, 1990.

693. Henderson LW, Miller ME, Hamilton RW, Norman ME: Hemodialysis leukopenia and polymorph random mobility—a possible correlation. J Lab Clin Med 85:191, 1975.

694. Baum J, Cestero RVM, Freeman RB: Chemotaxis of the polymorphonuclear leukocyte and delayed hypersensitivity in uremia. Kidney Int 7:S147, 1975.

695. Pedersen JO, Knudsen F, Jersild C: Acute effect of hemodialysis on neutrophil migration: Impact on humoral and cellular function. Kidney Int 33:S86, 1988.

696. Arnaout MA, Hakim RM, Todd RFI, et al: Increased expression of an adhesion-promoting surface glycoprotein in the granulocytopenia of hemodialysis. N Engl J Med 312:457, 1985.

697. Horl WH, Steinhauer HB, Schollmeyer P: Plasma levels of granulocyte elastase during hemodialysis: Effects of different dialyzer membranes. Kidney Int 28:791, 1985.

698. Cohen MS, Elliott DM, Chaplinski T, et al: A defect in oxidative metabolism of human polymorphonuclear leukocytes that remain in circulation early in hemodialysis. Blood 60:1283, 1982.

699. Nguyem AT, Lethias C, Zingraff J, et al: Hemodialysis membrane–induced activation of phagocyte oxidative metabolism detected in vivo and in vitro within microamounts with whole blood. Kidney Int 28:158, 1985.

700. Teraoka S, Hayasaka Y, Shoji H, et al: Changes in electrical charge of leukocyte surface membranes during hemodialysis: Possible role in transient leukopenia. ASAIO Trans 34:608, 1988.

701. Hurst KS, Saldanha LF, Steinberg SM, et al: The effects of varying dialysis regimens on lymphocyte stimulation. Trans Am Soc Artif Intern Organs 21:329, 1975.

702. Donati D, Degiannis D, Raskova J, Raska K: Uremic serum effects on peripheral blood mononuclear cell and purified T lymphocyte responses. Kidney Int 42:681, 1992.

703. Castro JE, Mee AD: The humoral responses of hemodialysis patients to antigen challenge. Transplantation 22:18, 1976.

704. Raskova J, Ghobrial I, Shea SM, et al: Suppressor cells in end-stage renal disease: Functional assays and monoclonal antibody analysis. Am J Med 76:847, 1984.

705. Rastea K, Rasteore J, Frankel R, et al: T cell subsets and cellular immunity in end stage renal disease. Am J Med 175:734, 1983.

706. Hoy WE, Cestero RVM, Freeman RB: Deficiency of T and B lymphocytes in uremic subjects and partial improvement with maintenance hemodialysis. Nephron 20:182, 1978.

707. Dratwa M, Collart F, Mascart-Lemone F, et al: Hemodialysis-induced acute changes in T lymphocyte subsets. Proc Eur Dial Transplant Assoc Eur Renal Assoc 22:196, 1985.

708. Raska K, Raskova J, Shea S, et al: T cell subsets and cellular immunity in end-stage renal disease. Am J Med 75:734, 1983.

709. Asaka M, Iida H, Izumino K, Sasayama S: Depressed natural killer cell activity in uremia. Evidence for immunosuppressive factor in uremic sera. Nephron 49:291, 1988.

710. Travers M, Courtney JM, Brown GS, et al: Cell electrophoretic investigations of lymphoid cells after in vivo contact with dialysis membranes. Kidney Int 33:S53, 1988.

711. Brubaker LH, Nolph KD: Mechanisms of recovery from neutropenia induced by hemodialysis. Blood 38:623, 1971.

712. Henderson LW, Cheung AK, Chenoweth DE: Choosing a membrane. Am J Kidney Dis 3:5, 1983.

713. Degiannis D, Czarnecki M, Donati D, et al: Normal T lymphocyte function in patients with end-stage renal disease hemodialyzed with "high-flux" polysulfone membranes. Am J Nephrol 10:276, 1990.

714. Castiglione A, Pagliaro P, Romagnoni M, et al: Flow cytometric analysis of leukocytes eluted from haemodialysers. Nephrol Dial Transplant 6:31, 1991.

715. Giacchino F, Alloatti S, Quarello F, et al: The immunological state in chronic renal insufficiency. Int J Artif Organs 5:237, 1982.

716. Wolfson M, Strong CJ, Minturn D, et al: Nutritional status and lymphocyte function in maintenance hemodialysis patients. Am J Clin Nutr 39:547, 1984.

717. Antoniou LD, Shalhoub RJ: Zinc-induced enhancement of lymphocyte function and viability in chronic uremia. Nephron 40:13, 1985.

718. Klinger M, Alexiewicz JM, Linker-Israeli M, et al: Effect of parathyroid hormone on human T cell activation. Kidney Int 37:1543, 1990.

719. Alexiewicz JM, Klinger M, Pitts TO, et al: Parathyroid hormone inhibits B cell proliferation: Implications in chronic renal failure. J Am Soc Nephrol 1:236, 1990.

720. Gaciong Z, Alexiewicz JM, Linker-Israeli M, et al: Inhibition of immunoglobulin production by parathyroid hormone. Implications in chronic renal failure. Kidney Int 40:96–106, 1991.

721. Chervu I, Kiersztejn M, Alexiewicz JM, et al: Impaired phagocytosis in chronic renal failure is mediated by secondary hyperparathyroidism. Kidney Int 41:1501, 1992.

722. Manolagas SC, Hustmyer FG, Yu XP: Immunomodulating properties of 1,25-dihydroxyvitamin $D_3$. Kidney Int 38:S8, 1990.

723. Hoy WE, Cestero RVM: Eosinophilia in maintenance hemodialysis patients. J Dial 3:73, 1979.

724. Novello AC, Port FK: Hemodialysis eosinophilia. Int J Artif Organs 5:5, 1982.

725. Chandran PKG, Humayun HM, Daugirdas JT, et al: Blood eosinophilia in patients undergoing maintenance peritoneal dialysis. Arch Intern Med 145:114, 1985.

726. Spinowitz BS, Simpson M, Manu P, Charytan C: Dialysis eosinophilia. Trans Am Soc Artif Intern Organs 27:161, 1981.

727. Voudiklaris S, Virvidaks K, Kalmantis T, et al: Eosinophilia in patients undergoing regular hemodialysis. Int J Artif Organs 6:195, 1983.

728. Michelson EA, Cohen L, Dankner RE, Kulczycki A: Eosinophilia and pulmonary dysfunction during Cuprophan hemodialysis. Kidney Int 24:246, 1983.

729. Grammer LC, Roberts M, Nicholls AJ, et al: IgE against ethylene oxide–altered human serum albumin in patients who have had acute dialysis reactions. J Allergy Clin Immunol 74:544, 1984.

730. Nicholls A: Ethylene oxide and anaphylaxis during haemodialysis. Br Med J 292:1221, 1986.

731. Patterson R, Lerner C, Roberts M, et al: Ethylene oxide (ETO) as a possible cause of an allergic reaction during peritoneal dialysis and immulogic detection of ETP from dialysis tubing. Am J Kidney Dis 8:64, 1986.

732. Bommer J, Wilhelms OH, Barth HP, et al: Anaphylactoid reactions in dialysis patients: Role of ethylene oxide. Lancet 2:1382, 1985.

733. Lemke HD, Heidland A, Schaefer RM: Hypersensitivity reactions during haemodialysis: Role of complement fragments and ethylene oxide antibodies. Nephrol Dial Transplant 4:264, 1990.

734. Deykin D: Uremic bleeding. Kidney Int 24:698, 1983.

735. Panicucci F, Sagripanti A, Vispi M, et al: Comprehensive study of haemostasis in chronic uraemia. Nephron 33:5, 1983.

736. Lindsay RM, Moorthy AV, Koens F, Linton AL: Platelet function in dialyzed and non-dialyzed patients with chronic renal failure. Clin Nephrol 4:52, 1975.

737. Rabner SF, Molinas F: The role of phenol and phenolic acids on the thrombocytopathy and defective platelet aggregation of patients with renal failure. Am J Med 49:346, 1970.

738. Jubelirer SJ: Hemostatic abnormalities in renal disease. Am J Kidney Dis 5:219, 1985.

739. Horowitz HI, Stein IM, Cohen BD, White JG: Further studies on the platelet-inhibitory effect of guanidinosuccinic acid and its role in uremic bleeding. Am J Med 49:336, 1970.

740. Castaldi PA, Rozenberg MC, Stewart JH: The bleeding disorder of uraemia. A quantitative platelet defect. Lancet 2:66, 1966.

741. Tanaka H, Umimoto K, Izumi N, et al: Can hemodialysis remove the factor that suppresses platelet cyclo-oxygenase activity in uremic patients? Trans Am Soc Artif Intern Organs 31:552, 1985.

742. Remuzzi G, Pusineri F: Coagulation defects in uremia. Kidney Int 33:S13, 1988.

743. Gralnick HR, McKeown LP, Williams SB, et al: Plasma and platelet von Willebrand factor defects in uremia. Am J Med 85:806, 1988.

744. Kolb G, Fischer W, Seitz R, et al: Hemodialysis and blood coagulation: The effect of hemodialysis on coagulation factor XIII and thrombin–antithrombin III complex. Nephron 58:106, 1991.

745. Gawaz MP, Vard RA: Effects of hemodialysis on platelet-derived thrombospondin. Kidney Int 40:257, 1991.

746. Opatrny K Jr, Opatrny K, Vit L, et al: What are the factors contributing to the changes in tissue-type plasminogen activator during haemodialysis? Nephrol Dial Transplant 6:26, 1991.

747. Macconi D, Vigano G, Bisogno G, et al: Defective platelet aggregation in response to platelet-activating factor in uremia associated with low platelet thromboxane $A_2$ generation. Am J Kidney Dis 19:318, 1992.

748. Martin-Malo A, Velasco F, Rojas R, et al: Fibrinolytic activity during hemodialysis: A biocompatibility-related phenomenon. Kidney Int 43:S213, 1993.

749. Taylor JE, Belch JJ, McLaren M, et al: Effect of erythropoietin therapy and withdrawal on blood coagulation and fibrinolysis in hemodialysis patients. Kidney Int 44:182, 1993.

750. Huraib S, al-Momen AK, Gader AM, et al: Effect of recombinant human erythropoietin (rHuEpo) on the hemostatic system in chronic hemodialysis patients. Clin Nephrol 36:252, 1991.

751. Wirtz JJJM, van Esser WJ, Hamulyak K, et al: The effects of recombinant human erythropoietin on hemostasis and fibrinolysis in hemodialysis patients. Clin Nephrol 28:277, 1992.

752. Remuzzi G: Bleeding in renal failure. Lancet 1:1205, 1988.

753. Livio M, Gotti E, Marchesi D, et al: Uraemic bleeding: Role of anaemia and beneficial effect of red cell transfusions. Lancet 2:1013, 1982.

754. Escolar G, Cases A, Bastida E, et al: Uremic platelets have a functional defect affecting the interaction of von Willebrand factor with glycoprotein IIb-IIa. Blood 76:1336, 1990.

755. Remuzzi G, Perico N, Zoja C, et al: Role of endothelium-derived nitric oxide in the bleeding tendency of uremia. J Clin Invest 86:1768, 1990.

756. Rabner SF, Drake RF: Platelet function as an indicator of adequate dialysis. Kidney Int 7:S144, 1975.

757. Vaziri ND, Toohey J, Paule P, et al: Coagulation abnormalities in patients with end-stage renal disease treated with hemodialysis. Int J Artif Organs 7:323, 1984.

758. DiMinno G, Martinez J, McKean M, et al: Platelet dysfunction in uremia: Multifaceted defect partially corrected by dialysis. Am J Med 79:552, 1985.

759. Remuzzi G, Livio M, Marchiaro G, et al: Bleeding in renal failure: Altered platelet function in chronic uremia only partially corrected by haemodialysis. Nephron 22:347, 1978.

760. Hakim RM, Schafer AI: Hemodialysis-associated platelet activation and thrombocytopenia. Am J Med 78:575, 1985.

761. Viener A, Aviram M, Better OS, Brook JG: Enhanced in vitro platelet aggregation in hemodialysis patients. Nephron 43:139, 1986.

762. Hakim RM, Lazarus JM: Hemodialysis in acute renal failure. Technical aspects of dialysis. In Brenner BM, Lazarus JM (eds): Acute Renal Failure. Churchill Livingstone, New York, 1988, p 788.

763. Akizawa T, Kitaoka T, Sato M, et al: Comparative clinical trial of regional anticoagulation for hemodialysis. Trans Am Soc Artif Intern Organs 34:176, 1988.

764. Pinnick RV, Wiegmann TB, Diederich DA: Regional citrate anticoagulation for hemodialysis in the patient at high risk for bleeding. N Engl J Med 308:258, 1983.

765. Flanigan MJ, Brecht JV, Freeman RM, Lim VS: Reducing the hemorrhagic complications of hemodialysis: A controlled comparison of low-dose heparin and citrate anticoagulation. Am J Kidney Dis 9:147, 1987.

766. Keller F, Seemann J, Preuschof L, Offermann G: Risk factors of system clotting in heparin-free haemodialysis. Nephrol Dial Transplant 5:802, 1990.

767. Agresti J, Conroy JD, Olshan A, et al: Heparin-free hemodialysis with Cuprophan hollow fiber dialyzers by a frequent saline flush, high blood flow technique. Trans Am Soc Artif Intern Organs 31:590, 1985.

768. Vigano LM, Benigni G, Mecca A, Remuzzi G: Moderate doses of aspirin and risk of bleeding in renal failure. Lancet 1:414, 1986.

769. Harter HR, Burch JW, Majerus PW, et al: Prevention of thrombosis in patients on hemodialysis by low-dose aspirin. N Engl J Med 301:577, 1979.

770. Brothers TE, Vincent CK, Darvishian D, et al: Effects of acetylsalicylic acid administration on patency and anastomotic hyperplasia of ePTFE grafts. Trans Am Soc Artif Intern Organs 35:558, 1989.

771. Sreedhara R, Himmelfarb J, Lazarus JM, Hakim RM: Antiplatelet therapy in expanded polytetrafluoroethylene (ePTFE) graft thrombosis: Results of a randomized double blind study. J Am Soc Nephrol 4:388, 1993. Abstract.

772. Emmons PR, Harrison MJG, Honour AJ, Mitchell JRA: Effect of dipyridamole on human platelet behaviour. Lancet 2:603, 1965.

773. Charvat J, Konig J, Blaha J: Is heparin responsible for enhanced platelet aggregation after haemodialysis? Nephron 44:89, 1986.

774. Schrader J, Stibbe W, Kandt M, et al: Low molecular weight heparin versus standard heparin: A long-term study in hemodialysis and hemofiltration patients. ASAIO Trans 36:28, 1990.

775. Nurmohamed MT, ten Cate J, Stevens P, et al: Long-term efficacy and safety of a low molecular weight heparin in chronic hemodialysis patients. A comparison with standard heparin. ASAIO Trans 37:M459, 1991.

776. Cases A, Reverter JC, Escolar G, et al: Platelet activation on hemodialysis: Influence of dialysis membranes. Kidney Int 43:S217, 1993.

777. Amato M, Salvadori M, Bergesio F, et al: Aspects of biocompatibility of two different dialysis membranes: Cuprophane and polysulfone. Int J Artif Organs 11:175, 1988.

778. Sultan Y, London GM, Goldfarb B, et al: Activation of platelets, coagulation and fibrinolysis in patients on long-term haemodialysis: Influence of cuprophan and polyacrylonitrile membranes. Nephrol Dial Transplant 5:362, 1990.

779. Seyfert UT, Hemling E, Hauck W, et al: Comparison of blood biocompatibility during haemodialysis with cuprophane and polyacrylonitrile membranes. Nephrol Dial Transplant 6:428, 1991.

780. Verbeelen D, Jochmans K, Herman AG, et al: Evaluation of platelets and hemostasis during hemodialysis with six different membranes. Nephron 59:567, 1991.

781. Docci D, Turci F, DelVecchio C, et al: Hemodialysis-associated platelet loss: Study of the relative contribution of dialyzer membrane composition and geometry. Int J Artif Organs 7:337, 1984.

782. Lindsay RM, Friesen M, Koens F, et al: Platelet function in patients on long term peritoneal dialysis. Clin Nephrol 6:335, 1976.

783. Nenci G, Berritini M, Agnelli G, et al: The effect of peritoneal dialysis, hemodialysis, and kidney transplantation on blood platelet function. Platelet aggregation to ADP and epinephrine. Nephron 23:287, 1979.

784. Moia M, Vissoto L, Cattaneo M, et al: Improvement of the haemostatic defect of uraemia after treatment with recombinant human erythropoietin. Lancet 2:1227, 1987.

785. Janson PA, Jubeliere SJ, Weinstein MJ, Deykin D: Treatment of the bleeding tendency in uremia with cryoprecipitate. N Engl J Med 308:8, 1980.

786. Livio M, Mannucci PM, Vigano G: Conjugated estrogens for the management of bleeding associated with renal failure. N Engl J Med 315:731, 1986.

787. Lohr JW, Schwab SJ: Minimizing hemorrhagic complications in dialysis patients. J Am Soc Nephrol 2:961, 1991.

788. Boyle JM, Johnston B: Acute upper gastrointestinal hemorrhage in patients with chronic renal disease. Am J Med 75:409, 1983.

789. Margolis DM, Saylor JL, Geisse G, et al: Upper gastrointestinal disease in chronic renal failure: A prospective evaluation. Arch Intern Med 138:1214, 1978.

790. Zuckerman G, Margolis D, Anderson C, Harter H: Acute gastrointestinal bleeding in chronic renal failure. Gastrointest Endosc 24:214, 1978.

791. Kang JY: The gastrointestinal tract in uremia. Dig Dis Sci 38:257, 1993.

792. Milito G, Taccone-Gallucci M, Brancaleone C, et al: The gastrointestinal tract in uremic patients on long-term hemodialysis. Kidney Int 28:S157, 1985.

793. Andriulla A, Malfi B, Recchia S, et al: Patients with chronic renal failure are not at a risk of developing chronic peptic ulcers. Clin Nephrol 23:245, 1985.

794. Muto S, Asano Y, Hosoda S, Miyata M: Hypochlorhydria and hypergastrinemia and their association with gastrointestinal bleeding in undialyzed and hemodialyzed patients. Nephron 50:10, 1988.

795. Franzin G, Musola R, Mencarelli R: Morphological changes of the gastroduodenal mucosa in regular dialysis uraemic patients. Histopathology 6:429, 1982.

796. Kang JY, Wu AY, Sutherland IH, Vathsala A: Prevalence of peptic ulcer in patients undergoing maintenance hemodialysis. Dig Dis Sci 33:774, 1988.

797. Gold CH, Morley JE, Viljoen M, et al: Gastric acid secretion and serum gastrin levels in patients with chronic renal failure on regular hemodialysis. Nephron 25:92, 1980.

798. Muto S, Murayama N, Asano Y, et al: Hypergastrinemia and achlorhydria in chronic renal failure. Nephron 40:143, 1985.

799. Mitchell CJ, Jewell DP, Lewin MR, et al: Gastric function and histology in chronic renal failure. J Clin Pathol 32:208, 1979.

800. Ala-Kaila K: Upper gastrointestinal findings in chronic renal failure. Scand J Gastroenterol 22:372, 1987.

801. Hegbrant J, Thysell H, Ekman R: Plasma levels of gastrointestinal regulatory peptides in patients receiving maintenance hemodialysis. Scand J Gastroenterol 26:599, 1991.

802. El Ghonaimy E, Barsoum R, Soliman M, et al: Serum gastrin in chronic renal failure: Morphological and physiological correlations. Nephron 39:86, 1985.

803. Sirinek KR, O'Dorisio TM, Gaskill HV, Levine BA: Chronic renal failure: Effect of hemodialysis on gastrointestinal hormones. Am J Surg 148:732, 1984.

804. Fisher RS, Lipshutz W, Cohen S: The hormonal regulation of pyloric sphincter function. J Clin Invest 52:1289, 1973.

805. Rowe PA, El Nujumi AM, Williams C, et al: The diagnosis of *Helicobacter pylori* infection in uremic patients. Am J Kidney Dis 20:574, 1992.

806. Milito G, Taccone-Gallucci M, Brancaleone C, et al: Assessment of the upper gastrointestinal tract in hemodialysis patients awaiting renal transplantation. Am J Gastroenterol 78:328, 1983.

807. Isenberg JI, Peterson WL, Elashoff JD, et al: Healing of benign gastric ulcer with low-dose antacid or cimetidine: A double-blind, randomized, placebo-controlled trial. N Engl J Med 308:1319, 1983.

808. Rieger J: Treatment of gastritis and ulcers with drugs. Nier Hochdruckkr 13:307, 1984.

809. Bartolomeo RS, Calabrese PR, Taubin HL: Spontaneous perforation of the colon: A potential complication of chronic renal failure. Am J Digest Dis 22:656, 1977.

810. Adams PL, Rutsky EA, Rostand SG, Han SY: Lower gastrointestinal tract dysfunction in patients receiving long-term hemodialysis. Arch Intern Med 142:303, 1982.

811. Carr JB, Luft FC, Hamburger RJ, Kleit SA: Intussusception in chronic renal failure. Arch Surg 111:866, 1976.

812. Gekas P, Schuster MM: Stercoral perforation of colon: Case report and review of the literature. Gastroenterology 80:1054, 1981.

813. Huded FV, Posner GL, Tick R: Nonspecific ulcer of the colon in a chronic hemodialysis patient. Am J Gastroenterol 77:913, 1982.

814. Scheff RT, Zuckerman G, Harter H, et al: Diverticular disease in patients with chronic renal failure due to polycystic kidney disease. Ann Intern Med 92:202, 1980.

815. Diamond SM, Emmett M, Henrich WL: Bowel infarction as a cause of death in dialysis patients. JAMA 256:2545, 1986.

816. Lillemoe KD, Romolo JL, Hamilton SR, et al: Intestinal necrosis due to sodium polystyrene (Kayexalate) in sorbitol enemas: Clinical experimental support for the hypothesis. Surgery 101:267, 1987.

817. Wootton FT, Rhodes DF, Lee WM, Fitts CT: Colonic necrosis with Kayexalate-sorbitol enemas after renal transplantation. Ann Intern Med 111:947, 1989.

818. Choi HS, Heller D, Picken MM, et al: Infarction of intestine with massive amyloid deposition in two patients on long-term hemodialysis. Gastroenterology 96:230, 1989.

819. Takahashi S, Morita T, Koda Y, et al: Gastrointestinal involvement of dialysis-related amyloidosis. Clin Nephrol 30:168, 1988.

820. Brissot P, Simon P, Meyrier A: Uremia and the liver III: Uremia and hepatic metabolism of carbohydrates, lipids and proteins. Nephron 29:14, 1981.

821. Meyrier A, Simon P, Boffa G, Brissot P: Uremia and the liver I: The liver and erythropoiesis in chronic renal failure. Nephron 29:3, 1981. Editorial.

822. Simon P, Herry D, Brissot P, et al: Longterm follow-up of chronic hepatitis by serial liver biopsies in HBs-positive haemodialysis patients: Role of hepatotoxic drugs. Proc Eur Dial Transplant Assoc 15:596, 1978.

823. Pahl MV, Vaziri ND, Dure-Smith B, et al: Hepatobiliary pathology in hemodialysis patients: An autopsy study of 78 cases. Am J Gastroenterol 81:783, 1986.

824. London WT, Di Figlia M, Sutnick AI, Blumberg BS: An epidemic of hepatitis in a chronic hemodialysis unit. N Engl J Med 281:571, 1969.

825. Briggs WA, Lazarus JM, Birtch AG, et al: Hepatitis affecting hemodialysis and transplant patients: Its considerations and consequences. Arch Intern Med 132:21, 1973.

826. Snydman DR, Bregman D, Bryan J: Hemodialysis-associated hepatitis in the United States. J Infect Dis 135:687, 1977.

827. Najem GR, Louria DB, Thind IS, et al: Control of hepatitis infection: The role of surveillance and an isolation hemodialysis center. JAMA 245:153, 1981.

828. Harnett JD, Parfrey PS, Kennedy M, et al: The long-term outcome of hepatitis B infection in hemodialysis patients. Am J Kidney Dis 11:210, 1988.

829. Josselon J, Kyser BA, Weir MR, Sadler RH: Hepatitis B surface antigenemia in a chronic hemodialysis program: Lack of influence on morbidity and mortality. Am J Kidney Dis 9:456, 1987.

830. Alter MJ, Favero MS, Moyer LA, Bland LA: National surveillance of dialysis-associated diseases in the United States, 1989. ASAIO Trans 37:97–109, 1991.

831. Dueymes JM, Bodenes-Dueymes M, Mahe JL, Herman B: Detection of hepatitis B viral DNA by polymerase chain reaction in dialysis patients. Kidney Int Suppl 43:S161–S166, 1993.

832. Dumann H, Meuer S, Meyer zum Buschenfelde KH, Kohler H: Hepatitis B vaccination and interleukin-2 receptor expression in chronic renal failure. Kidney Int 38:1164, 1990.

833. Caillat-Zucman S, Gimenez JJ, Albouze G, et al: HLA genetic heterogeneity of hepatitis B vaccine response in hemodialyzed patients. Kidney Int 43:S157, 1993.

834. Stevens CE, Alter HJ, Taylor PE, et al: Hepatitis B vaccine in patients receiving hemodialysis. Immunogenicity and efficacy. N Engl J Med 311:496, 1984.

835. Pasko MT, Bartholomew WR, Beam TRJ, et al: Long-term evaluation of the hepatitis B vaccine (Heptavax-B) in hemodialysis patients. Am J Kidney Dis 4:326, 1988.

836. Seaworth WW, Garrett LE, Stead WW, Hamilton JD: Non-A, non-B hepatitis and chronic dialysis: Another dilemma. Am J Nephrol 4:235, 1984.

837. Shusterman N, Singer I: Infectious hepatitis in dialysis patients. Am J Kidney Dis 9:447, 1987.

838. Gailbraith RM, Dienstag JL, Purcell RH, et al: Non-A non-B hepatitis associated with chronic liver disease in a haemodialysis unit. Lancet 1:951, 1979.

839. Mazzoni A, Innocenti M, Consaga M: Retrospective study on the prevalence of B and non-A, non-B hepatitis in a dialysis unit: 17-year follow-up. Nephron 61:316, 1992.

840. Jeffers LJ, Perez GO, DeMedina M, et al: Hepatitis C infection in two urban hemodialysis units. Kidney Int 38:320, 1990.

841. Lin HH, Huang CC, Sheen IS, Lin DY: Prevalence of antibodies to hepatitis C virus in the hemodialysis unit. Am J Nephrol 11:192, 1991.

842. Almroth G, Ekermo B, Franzen L, Hed J: Antibody responses to hepatitis C virus and its modes of transmission in dialysis patients. Nephron 59:232, 1991.

843. de Medina M, Ortiz C, Krenc C, et al: Improved detection of antibodies to hepatitis C virus in dialysis patients using a second-generation enzyme immunoassay. Am J Kidney Dis 20:589, 1992.

844. Chauveau P, Courouce AM, Lemarec N, et al: Antibodies to hepatitis C virus by second generation test in hemodialyzed patients. Kidney Int 43:S149, 1993.

845. Innocenti M, Mazzoni A, Moretti A, Palla P: Comparison of anti-hepatitis C virus detection with ELISA assay and RIBA 4 in dialysis patients: Our experience. Nephron 61:315, 1992.

846. Chan TM, Lok ASF, Cheng IKP: Hepatitis C infection among dialysis patients: A comparison between patients on maintenance hemodialysis and continuous ambulatory peritoneal dialysis. Nephrol Dial Transplant 6:944, 1991.

847. Petrarulo F, Maggi P, Sacchetti A, et al: HCV infection occupational hazard at dialysis units and virus spread, among relatives of dialyzed patients. Nephron 61:302, 1992.

848. Da Porto A, Adami A, Susanna F, et al: Hepatitis C virus in dialysis units: A multicenter study. Nephron 61:309, 1992.

849. Malaguti M, Capece R, Marciano M, et al: Antibodies to hepatitis C virus (anti-HCV): Prevalence in the same geographical area in dialysis patients, staff members, and blood donors. Nephron 61:346, 1992.

850. Conway M, Catterall AP, Brown EA, et al: Prevalence of antibodies to hepatitis C in dialysis patients and transplant recipients with possible routes of transmission. Nephrol Dial Transplant 7:1226, 1992.

851. Medin C, Allander T, Roll M, et al: Seroconversion to hepatitis C virus in dialysis patients: A retrospective and prospective study. Nephron 65:40, 1993.

852. Knudsen F, Wantzin P, Rasmussen K, et al: Hepatitis C in dialysis patients: Relationship to blood transfusions, dialysis and liver disease. Kidney Int 43:1353, 1993.

853. Niu MT, Coleman PJ, Alter MJ: Multicenter study of hepatitis C virus infection in chronic hemodialysis patients and hemodialysis center staff members. Am J Kidney Dis 22:568, 1993.

854. Dussol B, Chicheportiche C, Cantaloube J, et al: Detection of hepatitis C infection by polymerase chain reaction among hemodialysis patients. Am J Kidney Dis 22:574, 1993.

855. Pereira BJG, Milford EL, Kirkman RL, Levey AS: Transmission of hepatitis C virus by organ transplantation. N Engl J Med 325:454, 1991.

856. Pereira BJG, Milford EL, Kirkman RL, et al: Prevalence of hepatitis C virus RNA in organ donors positive for hepatitis C antibody and in the recipients of their organs. N Engl J Med 327:910, 1992.

857. Roth D, Fernandez JA, Babischkin S, et al: Detection of hepatitis C virus infection among cadaver organ donors: Evidence for low transmission of disease. Ann Intern Med 117:470, 1992.

858. Simon P, Meyrier A: Drug-induced liver cytolysis in hemodialyzed patients. Kidney Int 15:453, 1979.

859. Leber HW, Gleumes L, Schutterle G: Enzyme induction in the uremic liver. Kidney Int 13:S543, 1978.

860. Simon P, Meyrier A, Brissot P: Uremia and the liver II: Drugs and the liver in the uremic patient. Nephron 29:7, 1981.

861. Alfrey AC, Hegg A, Craswell P: Metabolism and toxicity of aluminum in renal failure. Am J Clin Nutr 33:1509, 1980.

862. Berlyne GM: Aluminum toxicity in man. Miner Electrolyte Metab 2:71, 1979.

863. Hunt J, Farthing MJ, Baker LR, et al: Silicone in the liver: Possible late effects. Gut 30:239, 1989.

864. Craig R, Sparberg M, Ivanovich P, et al: Nephrogenic ascites. Arch Intern Med 134:276, 1974.

865. Eknoyan G, Dichoso C, Hyde S, Yium J: Overflow ascites: The safety valve of the volume-expanded patient on dialysis. Proc Clin Dial Transplant Forum 3:156, 1973.

866. Feingold LN, Gutman RA, Walsh FX, Gunnells JC: Control of cachexia and ascites in hemodialysis patients by binephrectomy. Arch Intern Med 134:989, 1974.

867. Gotloib L, Servadio C: Ascites in patients undergoing maintenance hemodialysis. Am J Med 61:465, 1976.

868. Popli S, Chen W, Nakamoto S, et al: Hemodialysis ascites in anephric patients. Clin Nephrol 15:203, 1981.

869. Wang F, Pillay VKG, Ing TS, et al: Ascites in patients treated with maintenance hemodialysis. Nephron 12:105, 1974.

870. Gluck Z, Nolph KD: Ascites associated with end-stage renal disease. Am J Kidney Dis 10:9, 1987.

871. Fajardo B, Gonzalez G, Tannenberg AM: Osmotic disequilibrium causing ascites during chronic hemodialysis. ASAIO Trans 34:617, 1988.

872. Inoue N, Yamazaki Z, Oda T, et al: Treatment of intractable ascites by continuous reinfusion of the sterilized, cell-free and concentrated ascitic fluid. Trans Am Soc Artif Intern Organs 23:698, 1977.

873. Ing TS, Ashbach DL, Kanter A, et al: Fluid removal with negative-pressure hydrostatic ultrafiltration using a partial vacuum. Nephron 14:451, 1975.

874. Avram MM: High prevalence of pancreatic disease in chronic renal failure. Nephrology 18:68, 1977.

875. Baggenstoss AH: The pancreas in uremia: A histopathologic study. Am J Pathol 24:1003, 1948.

876. Dinoso VPJ, Murthy SNS, Saris AL, et al: Gastric and pancreatic function in patients with end-stage renal disease. J Clin Gastroenterol 4:321, 1982.

877. Bartos V, Melichar J, Erben J: The function of the exocrine pancreas in chronic renal disease. Digestion 3:33, 1970.

878. Dreiling DA: Pancreatic secretory testing in 1974: Symposium in diagnosis of pancreatic disease. Gut 16:647, 1975.

879. Royse VL, Jensen DM, Corwin HL: Pancreatic enzymes in chronic renal failure. Arch Intern Med 147:537, 1987.

880. Magnusson M, Magnusson K-E, Sundqvist T, Denneberg T: Impaired intestinal barrier function measured by differently sized polyethylene glycols in patients with chronic renal failure. Gut 32:754, 1991.

881. Johansson SV, Odar-Cederlof I, Plantin LO, Strandberg PO: Albumin metabolism and gastrointestinal loss of protein in chronic renal failure. Acta Med Scand 201:353, 1977.

882. Parfrey PS, Harnett JD, Barre PE: The natural history of myocardial disease in dialysis patients. J Am Soc Nephrol 2:2, 1991.

883. Hung J, Harris PJ, Uren RF, et al: Uremic cardiomyopathy: Effect of hemodialysis on left ventricular function in end-stage renal failure. N Engl J Med 302:547, 1980.

884. Pedersen T, Rasmussen K, Cleemann-Rasmussen K: Effect of hemodialysis on cardiac performance and transmural myocardial perfusion. Clin Nephrol 19:31, 1983.

885. Madsen BR, Alpert MA, Whiting RB, et al: Effect of hemodialysis on left ventricular performance. Am J Nephrol 4:86, 1984.

886. Strangfeld D, Gunther KH, Bohn R, et al: Cardiac function in chronic renal failure before and after hemodialysis. Cardiology 58:109, 1973.

887. Klein J, McLeish K, Hodsden J, Lordon R: Hypertrophic cardiomyopathy: An acquired disorder of end-stage renal disease. Trans Am Soc Artif Intern Organs 29:120, 1983.

888. Rouby JJ, Rottembourg J, Durande J, et al: Hemodynamic changes induced by regular hemodialysis and sequential ultrafiltration hemodialysis: A comparative study. Kidney Int 17:801, 1980.

889. Nixon JV, Mitchell JH, McPhaul FJ, Henrich WI: Effect of hemodialysis on left ventricular function. J Clin Invest 71:377, 1983.

890. Kramer W, Wizemann V, Kindler M, et al: Influence of fluid removal rate during hemodialysis on left ventricular performance and exercise tolerance in patients with coronary artery disease. Clin Nephrol 21:280, 1984.

891. Gurland HJ, Brunner FP, Chantler C, et al: Combined report on regular dialysis and transplantation in Europe, VI, 1975. Proc Eur Dial Transplant Assoc 13:3, 1976.

892. Lazarus JM, Lowrie EG, Hampers CL, Merrill JP: Cardiovascular disease in uremic patients on hemodialysis. Kidney Int 7:167, 1975.

893. Rostand SG, Brunzell JD, Cannon RO, Victor RG: Cardiovascular complications in renal failure. J Am Soc Nephrol 2:1053, 1991.

894. Lindner A, Charra B, Sherrard DJ, Scribner BH: Accelerated atherosclerosis and prolonged maintenance hemodialysis. N Engl J Med 290:697, 1974.

895. Castro L, Holfling B, Hassler R, et al: Progression of coronary and valvular heart disease in patients on dialysis. Trans Am Soc Artif Intern Organs 31:647, 1985.

896. Rostand SG, Kirk KA, Rutsky EA: Dialysis-associated ischemic heart disease: Insights from coronary angiography. Kidney Int 25:653, 1984.

897. Marwick T, Hobbs R, Vanderlaan RL, et al: Use of digital subtraction fluorography in screening for coronary artery disease in patients with chronic renal failure. Am J Kidney Dis 14:105, 1989.

898. Kremastinos D, Paraskevaidis I, Voudiklari S, et al: Painless myocardial ischemia in chronic hemodialysed patients: A real event? Nephron 60:164, 1992.

899. Ansari A, Kaupke CJ, Vaziri ND, et al: Cardiac pathology in patients with end-stage renal disease maintained on hemodialysis. Int J Artif Organs 16:31, 1993.

900. Parfrey PS, Harnett JD, Griffiths SM, et al: Congestive heart failure in dialysis patients. Arch Intern Med 148:1519, 1988.

901. Argy WP, Chester AC, Siemsen AS, et al: Hypertension in two hemodialysis cohorts. Trans Am Soc Artif Intern Organs 28:329, 1982.

902. Charra B, Calemard E, Cuche M, Laurent G: Control of hypertension and prolonged survival on maintenance hemodialysis. Nephron 33:96, 1983.

903. Eliahou HE, Iaina A, Reisin E, Shapira J: Probability of survival in hypertensive and non-hypertensive patients on maintenance hemodialysis. Isr J Med Sci 13:33, 1977.

904. Vincenti F, Armend WJ, Abele J, et al: The role of hypertension in hemodialysis-associated atherosclerosis. Am J Med 68:363, 1980.

905. Rostand SG, Kirk KA, Rutsky EA: Relationship of coronary risk factors to hemodialysis-associated ischemic heart disease. Kidney Int 22:304, 1982.

906. Travis M, Henrich WL: Factors which affect cardiac performance during hemodialysis. Semin Dial 2:241, 1989.

907. Silberberg JS, Barre PE, Prichard SS, Sniderman AD: Impact of left ventricular hypertrophy on survival in end-stage renal disease. Kidney Int 36:286, 1989.

908. London GM, Marchais SJ, Guerin AP, et al: Cardiac hypertrophy and arterial alterations in end-stage renal disease: Hemodynamic factors. Kidney Int 41:S42, 1993.

909. Wizemann V, Kramer W: Choice of ESRD treatment strategy according to cardiac status. Kidney Int 33:S191, 1988.

910. Foley RN, Parfrey PS, Harnett JD: Left ventricular hypertrophy in dialysis patients. Semin Dial 5:34, 1992.

911. Parfrey PS, Griffiths SM, Harnett JD, et al: Outcome of congestive heart failure, dilated cardiomyopathy, hypertrophic hyperkinetic disease, and ischemic heart disease in dialysis patients. Am J Nephrol 10:213, 1990.

912. Parfrey PS, Harnett JD, Griffiths S, et al: Low-output left ventricular failure in end-stage renal disease. Am J Nephrol 7:184, 1987.

913. Johnson GJ, Blythe WB: Hemodynamic effects of arteriovenous shunts used for hemodialysis. Ann Surg 171:715, 1970.

914. Capelli JP, Kasparian H: Cardiac work demands on left ventricular function in end-stage renal disease. Ann Intern Med 86:261, 1977.

915. Neff MS, Kim KW, Persoff M, et al: Hemodynamics of uremic anemia. Circulation 43:876, 1971.

916. Ahern DJ, Maher JF: Heart failure as a complication of hemodialysis arteriovenous fistula. Ann Intern Med 77:201, 1972.

917. Anderson CB, Codd JR, Graff RA, et al: Cardiac failure and upper extremity arteriovenous dialysis fistulas. Arch Intern Med 136:292, 1976.

918. Dongradi G, Rocha P, Baron B, et al: Hemodynamic effects of arteriovenous fistulae in chronic hemodialysis patients at rest and during exercise. Clin Nephrol 15:75, 1981.

919. Macdougall IC, Lewis NP, Saunders MJ, et al: Long-term cardiorespiratory effects of amelioration of renal anaemia by erythropoietin. Lancet 335:489, 1990.

920. Hori K, Onoyama K, Iseki K, et al: Hemodynamic and volume changes by recombinant human erythropoietin (rHuEPO) in the treatment of anemic hemodialysis patients. Clin Nephrol 33:293, 1990.

921. Metra M, Cannella G, La Canna G, et al: Improvement in exercise capacity after correction of anemia in patients with end-stage renal failure. Am J Cardiol 68:1060, 1991.

922. Cross AS, Steigbigel RT: Infective endocarditis and access site infections in patients on hemodialysis. Medicine (Baltimore) 55:453, 1976.

923. Eknoyan G, Lister BJ, Kim HS, Greenberg SD: Renal complications of bacterial endocarditis. Am J Nephrol 5:457, 1985.
924. Dobkin JF, Miller MH, Steigbigel NH: Septicemia in patients on chronic hemodialysis. Ann Intern Med 88:28, 1978.
925. Adam WR, Dawborn JK, Rosenbaum M: Transient early diastolic murmur in patients with renal failure. Med J Aust 2:1085, 1970.
926. Matalon R, Moussalli ARJ, Nidus BD, et al: Functional aortic insufficiency: A feature of renal failure. N Engl J Med 285:1522, 1971.
927. Barrett LJ, Robinson MA, Whitford JA, Lawrence JR: The diastolic murmur of renal failure. N Engl J Med 295:121, 1976.
928. Lazarus JM, Gottlieb MN, Lowrie EG, et al: Echocardiographic findings in stable hemodialysis patients. Proc Clin Dial Transplant Forum 6:53, 1976.
929. Perez JE, Smith CA, Meltzer VN: Pulmonic valve insufficiency: A common cause of transient diastolic murmurs in renal failure. Ann Intern Med 103:497, 1985.
930. Abrahams C, D'Cruz I, Kathpalia S: Abnormalities in the mitral valve apparatus in patients undergoing long term hemodialysis. Arch Intern Med 142:1796, 1982.
931. Abbasi AS, Slaughter JC, Allen MW: Asymptomatic septal hypertrophy in patients on long-term hemodialysis. Chest 74:548, 1978.
932. Prosser D, Parsons V: The case for a specific uremic myocardiopathy. Nephron 15:4, 1975.
933. Ianhez LE, Lowen J, Sabbga E: Uremic myocardiopathy. Nephron 15:17, 1975.
934. Bailey GL, Hampers CL, Merrill JP: Reversible cardiomyopathy in uremia. Trans Am Soc Artif Intern Organs 13:263, 1967.
935. Mallick NP, Berlyne GM: Arterial calcification after vitamin-D therapy in hyperphosphatemic renal failure. Lancet 2:1316, 1968.
936. Friedman SA, Novack S, Thomason GE: Arterial calcification and gangrene in uremia. N Engl J Med 280:1392, 1969.
937. Rosen H, Friedman SA, Raizner AE, Gerstmann K: Azotemic arteriopathy. Am Heart J 84:250, 1972.
938. Ibels LS, Alfrey AC, Huffer WE, et al: Arterial calcification and pathology in uremic patients undergoing dialysis. Am J Med 66:790, 1979.
939. Gore E, Arons W: Calcification of the myocardium. Arch Pathol 48:1, 1949.
940. Terman DS, Alfrey AC, Hammond WS, et al: Cardiac calcification in uremia. Am J Med 50:744, 1971.
941. Arora KK, Lacy JP, Schackt RA, et al: Calcific cardiomyopathy in advanced renal failure. Arch Intern Med 135:603, 1975.
942. Roberts WC, Waller BF: Effect of chronic hypercalcemia on the heart: An analysis of 18 necropsy patients. Am J Med 71:371, 1981.
943. Lewin K, Trautman L: Ischaemic myocardial damage in chronic renal failure. Br J Med 4:151, 1971.
944. Mazzaferro S, Coen G, Bandini S, et al: Role of ageing, chronic renal failure, and dialysis in the calcification of mitral annulus. Nephrol Dial Transplant 8:335, 1993.
945. McGonigle RJ, Fowler MB, Temmis AB, et al: Uremic cardiomyopathy: Potential role of vitamin D and parathyroid hormone. Nephron 36:131, 1984.
946. La KN, Ng J, Whitford JBI, et al: Left ventricular function in uremia: Echocardiographic and radionuclide assessment in patients on maintenance hemodialysis. Clin Nephrol 23:125, 1985.
947. London GM, Fabiani F, Marchais SJ, et al: Uremic cardiomyopathy: An inadequate left ventricular hypertrophy. Kidney Int 31:973, 1987.
948. Gafter U, Battler A, Eldar M, et al: Effect of hyperparathyroidism on cardiac function in patients with end-stage renal disease. Nephron 41:30, 1985.
949. Fellner SK, Lang RM, Neumann A, et al: Parathyroid hormone and myocardial performance in dialysis patients. Am J Kidney Dis 18:320, 1991.
950. Verberckmoes R, Bouillion R, Crempien B: Disappearance of vascular calcification during treatment of a renal osteodystrophy: Two patients treated with doses of vitamin D and aluminum hydroxide. Ann Intern Med 82:529, 1975.
951. Ibels LS, Alfrey AC, Robinette JB, et al: Prevention of aortic and visceral calcification of acute and reversed acute uremia by a parathyroidectomy. Clin Res 25:42A, 1977. Abstract.
952. Ono K, Kikawa K: Factors contributing to oxalate deposits in the myocardia of hemodialysis patients. ASAIO Trans 35:595, 1989.
953. Zazgornik J, Balcke P, Rokitansky A, et al: Excessive myocardial calcinosis in a chronic hemodialyzed patient. Klin Wochenschr 65:97, 1987.
954. Wacker W, Merrill JP: Uremic pericarditis in acute and chronic renal failure. JAMA 156:764, 1954.
955. Bailey GL, Hampers CL, Hager EB, Merrill JP: Uremic pericarditis: Clinical features in management. Circulation 38:582, 1968.
956. Rutsky EA, Rostand SG: Treatment of uremic pericarditis and pericardial effusion. Am J Kidney Dis 10:2, 1987.
957. De Pace NL, Nestico PF, Schwartz AB, et al: Predicting success of intensive dialysis in the treatment of uremic pericarditis. Am J Med 76:38, 1984.
958. Goldberg M, Lazarus JM, Gottlieb MN, et al: Treatment of uremic pericardial effusion. Proc Clin Dial Transplant Forum 5:20, 1975.
959. Koopot R, Zerifos NS, Lavender AR, Pifarre R: Cardiac tamponade in uremic pericarditis. Am J Cardiol 32:846, 1973.
960. Wray TM, Humphrey J, Perry JM, et al: Pericardiectomy for treatment of uremic pericarditis. Circulation 2:49, 1974.
961. Corey GR, Campbell OT, Van Trigt P, et al: Etiology of large pericardial effusions. Am J Med 95:209, 1993.
962. Zarate A, Gelfand MC, Horton JD, et al: Pericardial effusion associated with minoxidil therapy in dialyzed patients. Int J Artif Organs 3:15, 1980.
963. Houston MC, McChesney JA, Chatherjee K: Pericardial effusion associated with minoxidil therapy. Arch Intern Med 141:69, 1981.
964. Alfey AC, Gross JE, Ogden DA, et al: Uremic hemopericardium. Am J Med 45:391, 1968.
965. Rostand SG, Rutsky EA: Pericarditis in end-stage renal disease. Cardiol Clin 8:701, 1990.
966. Ghavamian M, Gutch CF, Hughes RK, et al: Pericardial tamponade and chronic hemodialysis patients. Arch Intern Med 131:249, 1973.
967. AliRegiaba S, Gay WA, Sullivan JF, et al: Treatment of uraemic pericarditis by anterior pericardiectomy. Lancet 2:12, 1974.
968. Morin JE, Hollomby D, Gonda A, et al: Management of uremic pericarditis: A report of 11 patients with cardiac tamponade and a review of the literature. Ann Thorac Surg 22:588, 1976.
969. Leehey DJ, Daugirdas JT, Popli S, et al: Predicting need for surgical drainage of pericardial effusion in patients with end-stage renal disease. Int J Artif Organs 12:618, 1989.
970. Daugirdas JT, Leehey DJ, Popli S, et al: Subxiphoid pericardiostomy for hemodialysis-associated pericardial effusion. Arch Intern Med 146:1113, 1986.
971. Peraino RA: Pericardial effusion in patients treated with maintenance dialysis. Am J Nephrol 3:319, 1983.
972. Kwasnik EM, Koster JKJ, Lazarus JM, et al: Conservative management of uremic pericardial effusions. J Thorac Cardiovasc Surg 76:629, 1978.
973. Buselmeir TJ, Simmons RL, Najarian JS, et al: Uremic pericardial effusion: Treatment by catheter drainage and local nonabsorbable steroid administration. Nephron 16:371, 1976.
974. Fuller TJ, Knochel JP, Brennan JP, et al: Reversal of intractable uremic pericarditis by triamcinolone hexacetonide. Arch Intern Med 136:979, 1976.
975. Minuth AN, Nottebohn GA, Eknoyan G, Suki WN: Indomethacin treatment of pericarditis in chronic hemodialysis patients. Arch Intern Med 135:807, 1975.
976. Lazarus JM: Pericardial effusion. Arch Intern Med 144:1317, 1984.
977. Moraski RE, Bousvaros G: Constrictive pericarditis due to chronic uremia. N Engl J Med 281:542, 1969.
978. Wolfe SA, Bailey GL, Collins JJ: Constrictive pericarditis following uremic effusion. J Thorac Cardiovasc Surg 63:540, 1972.
979. Lazarus JM, Hampers CL, Merrill JP: Hypertension and chronic renal failure: Treatment with hemodialysis and nephrectomy. Arch Intern Med 133:1059, 1974.
980. Haire HM, Sherrard DJ, Curtis FK, et al: Accelerated atherosclerosis in dialysis patients: Smoking and hypertension. Proc Clin Dial Transplant Forum 7:18, 1977.
981. Chester AL, Schreiner GE: Hypertension and hemodialysis. Trans Am Soc Artif Intern Organs 24:36, 1978.
982. Vertes V, Cangiano JL, Berman LB, Gould A: Hypertension in end-stage renal disease. N Engl J Med 280:978, 1969.
983. Weidmann P, Maxwell MH, Lupu AN, et al: Plasma renin activity and blood pressure in terminal renal failure. N Engl J Med 285:757, 1971.
984. Charra B, Calemard E, Ruffet M, et al: Survival as an index of adequacy of dialysis. Kidney Int 41:1286, 1992.

985. Maeda K, Saito A, Kawaguchi S, et al: Hemodiafiltration with sodium concentration–controlled dialysate. Artif Organs 4:121, 1980.

986. Van Stone JC, Bauer J, Carey J: The effect of dialysate sodium concentration on body fluid compartment volume, plasma renin activity and plasma aldosterone concentration in chronic hemodialysis patients. Am J Kidney Dis 2:58, 1982.

987. Raja R, Kramer M, Rosenbaum JL, et al: Prevention of hypotension during iso-osmolar hemodialysis with bicarbonate dialysate. Trans Am Soc Artif Intern Organs 26:375, 1980.

988. Cannella G, Paoletti E, Delfino R, et al: Regression of left ventricular hypertrophy in hypertensive dialyzed uremic patients on long-term antihypertensive therapy. Kidney Int 44:881, 1993.

989. Seto D, Fritz W, Nakamoto S, Kolff JW: The effect of bilateral nephrectomy and of sodium and water content on hypertension. Trans Am Soc Artif Intern Organs 9:35, 1963.

990. Onesti G, Swartz C, Ramirez O, Brest AN: Bilateral nephrectomy for control of hypertension in uremia. Trans Am Soc Artif Intern Organs 14:361, 1968.

991. Lazarus JM, Hampers CL, Bennett AH, et al: Urgent bilateral nephrectomy for severe hypertension. Ann Intern Med 76:733, 1972.

992. Deutsch E, Bernstein RC, Addonizio P, Kussmaul WG: Coronary artery bypass surgery in patients on chronic hemodialysis: A case-control study. Ann Intern Med 110:369, 1989.

993. DeMeyer M, Wyns W, Dion R, Khoury G: Myocardial revascularization in patients on renal replacement therapy. Clin Nephrol 36:147, 1991.

994. Rostand SG, Kirk KA, Rutsky EA, Pacifico AD: Results of coronary artery bypass grafting in end-stage renal disease. Am J Kidney Dis 12:266, 1988.

995. Wizemann V, Timio M, Alpert MA, Kramer W: Options in dialysis therapy: Significance of cardiovascular findings. Kidney Int 40:S85–S91, 1993.

996. Peer G, Korzets A, Hochlauer E, et al: Cardiac arrhythmia during chronic ambulatory peritoneal dialysis. Nephron 45:192, 1987.

997. Alpert MA, Van Stone J, Twardowski ZJ, Nolph KD: Comparative cardiac effects of hemodialysis and continuous ambulatory peritoneal dialysis. Clin Cardiol 9:52, 1986.

998. Lazarus JM: Which dialysis therapy is best for the patient with an unstable cardiovascular system? Hemodialysis is optimal therapy. Semin Dial 5:208, 1992.

999. Gibson DG: Haemodynamic factors in the development of acute pulmonary oedema in renal failure. Lancet 2:1217, 1966.

1000. Goss JE, Alfrey AC, Vogel JHK, et al: Hemodynamic changes during hemodialysis. Trans Am Soc Artif Intern Organs 13:68, 1967.

1001. Mostert JW, Evers JL, Hobika GH, et al: The haemodynamic response to chronic renal failure as studied in azotaemic state. Br J Anaesth 42:397, 1970.

1002. Lee YS: Ultrastructural observations of chronic uremic lungs with special reference to histochemical and x-ray microanalytic studies on altered alveolocapillary basement membranes. Am J Nephrol 5:255, 1985.

1003. O'Doherty MJ, Breen D, Page C, et al: Lung $^{99m}$Tc DTPA transfer in renal disease and pulmonary infection. Nephrol Dial Transplant 6:582, 1991.

1004. Kohen JA, Opsahl JA, Kjellstrand CM: Deceptive patterns of uremic pulmonary edema. Am J Kidney Dis 7:456, 1986.

1005. Berger HW, Rammohan G, Neff MS, Buhain WJ: Uremic pleural effusion. A study in 14 patients on chronic dialysis. Ann Intern Med 82:362, 1975.

1006. Kaupke CJ, Vaziri ND: Pleural complications in end-stage renal disease. Semin Dial 4:189, 1991.

1007. Galen MA, Steinberg SM, Lowrie EG, et al: Hemorrhagic pleural effusion in patients undergoing chronic hemodialysis. Ann Intern Med 82:359, 1975.

1008. Rodelas R, Rakowski TA, Argy WP, Schreiner GE: Fibrosing uremic pleuritis during hemodialysis. JAMA 243:2424, 1980.

1009. Maher ER, Dutoit SH, Baillod RA, et al: Gastrointestinal complications of dialysis related amyloidosis. Br Med J 297:265–266, 1988.

1010. Zidulka A, Despas PJ, Milic-Emili J, Anthonisen NR: Pulmonary function with acute loss of excess lung water by hemodialysis in patients with chronic uremia. Am J Med 55:134, 1973.

1011. Prezant DJ: Effect of uremia and its treatment on pulmonary function. Lung 168:1, 1990.

1012. Dujic Z, Tocilj J, Ljutic D, Eterovic D: Effects of hemodialysis and anemia on pulmonary diffusing capacity, membrane diffusing capacity and capillary blood volume in uremic patients. Respiration 58:277, 1991.

1013. Fairshter RD, Vaziri ND, Mirahmadi MK: Lung pathology in chronic hemodialysis patients. Int J Artif Organs 5:97, 1982.

1014. Bush A, Gabriel R: Pulmonary function in chronic renal failure: Effects of dialysis and transplantation. Thorax 46:424, 1991.

1015. de Graaf P, Schicht IM, Pauwels KJ, et al: Bone scintigraphy in uremic pulmonary calcification. J Nucl Med 20:201, 1979.

1016. Faubert PF, Shapiro WB, Porush JG, et al: Pulmonary calcification in hemodialyzed patients detected by technetium-99m diphosphonate scanning. Kidney Int 18:95, 1980.

1017. Bestetti-Bosisio M, Cotelli F, Schiaffino E, et al: Lung calcification in long-term dialysed patients: A light and electronmicroscopic study. Histopathology 8:69, 1984.

1018. Haque AK, Rubin SA, Leveque CM: Pulmonary calcification in long-term hemodialysis: A mimic of pulmonary thromboembolism. Am J Nephrol 4:109, 1984.

1019. Kimmel PL, Miller G, Mendelson WB: Sleep apnea syndrome in chronic renal disease. Am J Kidney Dis 86:308, 1989.

1020. Mendelson WB, Wadhwa NK, Greenberg HE, et al: Effects of hemodialysis on sleep apnea syndrome in end-stage renal disease. Clin Nephrol 33:247, 1990.

1021. Wadhwa NK, Mendelson WB: A comparison of sleep-disordered respiration in ESRD patients receiving hemodialysis and peritoneal dialysis. Adv Perit Dial 8:195, 1992.

1022. Johnson MW, Anch AM, Remmers JE: Induction of the obstructive sleep apnea syndrome in a woman by exogenous androgen administration. Am Rev Respir Dis 129:1023, 1984.

1023. Millman RP, Kimmel PL, Shore ET, Wasserstein AG: Sleep apnea in hemodialysis patients: The lack of testosterone effect on its pathogenesis. Nephron 40:407, 1985.

1024. Soreide E, Skeie B, Kirvela O, et al: Branched-chain amino acid in chronic renal failure patients: Respiratory and sleep effects. Kidney Int 40:539, 1991.

1025. Pressman MR, Benz RL, Schleifer CR, Peterson DD: Sleep disordered breathing in ESRD: Acute beneficial effects of treatment with nasal continuous positive airway pressure. Kidney Int 43:1134, 1993.

1026. Langevin B, Fouque D, Leger P, Robert D: Sleep apnea syndrome and end-stage renal disease. Cure after renal transplantation. Chest 103:1330, 1993.

1027. Lundin API, Adler AJ, Feinroth MV, et al: Maintenance hemodialysis. Survival beyond the first decade. JAMA 244:38, 1980.

1028. Horensten ML, Boner G, Rosenfeld JB: The shrinking man: A manifestation of severe renal osteodystrophy. JAMA 244:267, 1980.

1029. Muspratt S: Thoracic deformity and flail chest in renal osteodystrophy. JAMA 243:1458, 1980.

1030. Degoulet P, Legrain M, Reach I, et al: Mortality risk factors in patients treated by chronic hemodialysis. Nephron 31:103, 1982.

1031. Gutman RA: Characteristics of long-term (14 years) survivors of maintenance dialysis. Nephron 33:111, 1983.

1032. Schuster VL, Chestnut CH, Baylink DJ, Sherrard DJ: Calcium balance in uremia: Longitudinal study of long-term survivors. Nephron 41:132, 1984.

1033. Charra B, Calemard E, Uzan M, et al: Carpal tunnel syndrome, shoulder pain, and amyloid deposits in long-term haemodialysis patients. Proc Eur Dial Transplant Assoc Eur Renal Assoc 21:291, 1985.

1034. Bricker NS: On the pathogenesis of the uremic state: An exposition of the "trade-off" hypothesis. N Engl J Med 286:1093, 1972.

1035. Massry SG, Goldstein DA, Malluche HH: Current status of the use of $1,25(OH)_2D_3$ in the management of renal osteodystrophy. Kidney Int 18:409, 1980.

1036. Lindergard B, Johnell O, Nilsson BE, Wiklund PE: Studies of bone morphology, bone densitometry and laboratory data in patients on maintenance hemodialysis treatment. Nephron 39:122, 1985.

1037. Wilson L, Felsenfeld A, Drezner MK, Llach F: Altered divalent ion metabolism in early renal failure: Role of $1,25(OH)_2D_3$. Kidney Int 27:565, 1985.

1038. Kraut JA, Shinaberger JH, Singer FR, et al: Parathyroid gland responsiveness to acute hypocalcemia in dialysis osteomalacia. Kidney Int 23:725, 1983.

1039. Johnson WJ, Goldsmith RS, Beabout JW, et al: Prevention and reversal of progressive secondary hyperparathyroidism in patients maintained by hemodialysis. Am J Med 56:827, 1974.

1040. Ahmed KY, Varghese Z, Wills MR, et al: Long-term effects of small doses of 1,25-dihydroxycholecalciferol in renal osteodystrophy. Lancet 1:629, 1978.

1041. Brickman AS, Sherrard DJ, Jowsey J, et al: 1,25-Dihydroxycholecalciferol: Effect on skeletal lesions and plasma parathyroid hormone levels in uremic osteodystrophy. Arch Intern Med 134:883, 1974.

1042. Henderson RG, Russell RGG, Ledingham JGG, et al: Effects of 1,25-dihydroxycholecalciferol on calcium absorption, muscle weakness, and bone disease in chronic renal failure. Lancet 1:379, 1974.

1043. Silverberg DS, Bettcher KB, Dossetor JB, et al: Effect of 1,25-dihydroxycholecalciferol on renal osteodystrophy. Can Med Assoc J 112:190, 1975.

1044. Malluche H, Faugere M: Renal bone disease 1990: An unmet challenge for the nephrologist. Kidney Int 38:193, 1990.

1045. Felsenfeld AJ, Rodriguez M, Dunlay R, Llach F: A comparison of parathyroid-gland function in haemodialysis patients with different forms of renal osteodystrophy. Nephrol Dial Transplant 6:244, 1991.

1046. Rasmussen H, Baron R, Broadus A, et al: 1,25(OH)$_2$D$_3$ is not the only D metabolite involved in the pathogenesis of osteomalacia. Am J Med 69:360, 1980.

1047. Hodsman AB, Sherrard DJ, Wong EGC, et al: Vitamin D–resistant ostcomalacia in hemodialysis patients lacking secondary hyperparathyroidism. Ann Intern Med 94:629, 1981.

1048. Ott SM, Maloney NA, Coburn JW, et al: The prevalence of bone aluminum deposition in renal osteodystrophy and its relation to the response to calcitriol therapy. N Engl J Med 307:709, 1982.

1049. Sherrard DJ, Ott SM, Andress DL: Pseudohyperparathyroidism: Syndrome associated with aluminum intoxication in patients with renal failure. Am J Med 79:127, 1985.

1050. Buchanan MRC, Ihle BU, Dunn CM: Haemodialysis related osteomalacia: A staining method to demonstrate aluminium. J Clin Pathol 34:1352, 1981.

1051. Ihle B, Buchanan M, Stevens B, et al: Aluminum-associated bone disease: Clinicopathologic correlation. Am J Kidney Dis 2:255, 1982.

1052. Plachot JJ, Cournot-Witmer G, Halpern S, et al: Bone ultrastructure and x-ray microanalysis of aluminum-intoxicated hemodialyzed patients. Kidney Int 25:796, 1984.

1053. Charhon SA, Chapuy MC, Traeger J, Meunier PJ: Aluminum intoxication in dialyzed patients: Bone histology and value of histomorphometric biopsy. Presse Med 13:1431, 1984.

1054. Moriniere P, Cohen-Solal M, Belbrik S, et al: Disappearance of aluminic bone disease in a long term asymptomatic dialysis population restricting Al(OH)$_3$ intake: Emergence of an idiopathic adynamic bone disease not related to aluminum. Nephron 53:93, 1989.

1055. Malluche HH, Monier-Faugere MC: Risk of adynamic bone disease in dialyzed patients. Kidney Int 42:S62, 1992.

1056. Sherrard DJ, Hercz G, Pei Y, et al: The spectrum of bone disease in end-stage renal failure—an evolving disorder. Kidney Int 43:436, 1993.

1057. Warren DJ, Otieno LS: Carpal tunnel syndrome in patients on intermittent haemodialysis. Postgrad Med J 51:450, 1975.

1058. Jain VK, Cestero RVM, Baum J: Carpal tunnel syndrome in patients undergoing maintenance hemodialysis. JAMA 242:2868, 1979.

1059. Schwartz A, Keller F, Seyfert S, et al: Carpal tunnel syndrome: A major complication in long-term hemodialysis patients. Clin Nephrol 22:133, 1984.

1060. Kachel HG, Altmeyer P, Baldamus CA, Koch KM: Deposition of an amyloid like substance as a possible complication of regular dialysis treatment. Contrib Nephrol 36:27, 1983.

1061. Bardin T, Kuntz D, Zingraff J, et al: Synovial amyloidosis in patients undergoing long-term hemodialysis. Arthritis Rheum 28:1052, 1985.

1062. Hampl H, Lobeck H, Bartel-Schwarz S, et al: Clinical, morphologic, biochemical, and immunohistochemical aspects of dialysis-associated amyloidosis. ASAIO Trans 33:250, 1987.

1063. Kuntz D, Naveau B, Bardin T, et al: Destructive spondylarthropathy in hemodialyzed patients. Arthritis Rheum 27:369, 1984.

1064. Rubin LA, Fam AG, Rubenstein J, et al: Erosive azotemic osteoarthropathy. Arthritis Rheum 27:1086, 1984.

1065. Goldstein S, Winston E, Cheung TJ, et al: Chronic arthropathy in long-term hemodialysis. Am J Med 78:82, 1985.

1066. Zingraff J, Bardin T, Kunktz D, et al: Degenerative osteo-articular lesions and amyloid infiltration in long-term hemodialysis patients. Proc Eur Dial Transplant Assoc Eur Renal Assoc 22:131, 1985.

1067. Diez Busch H, Touam M, Zingraff J, et al: The arthropathies of patients on hemodialysis for more than 10 years: A retrospective study. Nephrologie 4:165, 1986.

1068. Di Raimondo CR, Casey TT, Di Raimondo CV, Stone WJ: Pathologic fractures associated with idiopathic amyloidosis of bone in chronic hemodialysis patients. Nephron 43:22, 1986.

1069. Shirahama T, Skinner M, Cohen AS, et al: Histochemical and immunohistochemical characterization of amyloid associated with chronic hemodialysis as beta-2 microglobulin. Lab Invest 53:705, 1985.

1070. Gejyo F, Odani S, Yamada T, et al: β$_2$-Microglobulin: A new form of amyloid protein associated with chronic hemodialysis. Kidney Int 30:385, 1986.

1071. Kirschbaum BB, Schoolwarth AC: Acute aluminum toxicity associated with citrate and aluminum-containing antacids. Am J Med Sci 297:9, 1989.

1072. Molitoris BA, Froment DH, Mackenzie TA, et al: Citrate: A major factor in the toxicity of orally administered aluminum compounds. Kidney Int 36:949, 1989.

1073. Slatopolsky E, Caglar S, Gradowska L, et al: On the prevention of secondary hyperparathyroidism in experimental chronic renal disease using "proportional reduction" of dietary phosphorus intake. Kidney Int 2:147, 1972.

1074. Fine A, Cox D, Fontaine B: Elevation of serum phosphate affects parathyroid hormone levels in only 50% of hemodialysis patients, which is unrelated to changes in serum calcium. J Am Soc Nephrol 3:1947, 1993.

1075. Llach F, Nikakhtar B: Methods of controlling hyperphosphatemia in patients with chronic renal failure. Curr Opin Nephrol Hypertens 2:365, 1993.

1076. Ball J, Johnson JW, Hampers CL, Merrill JP: The many facets of secondary hyperparathyroidism. Arch Intern Med 131:746, 1973.

1077. Meema HE, Oreopoulos DG, De Veber GA: Arterial calcifications in severe chronic renal disease and their relationship to dialysis treatment, renal transplant, and parathyroidectomy. Radiology 121:315, 1976.

1078. Goldsmith RS: The effects of calcium and phosphorus in hemodialysis. Annu Rev Med 27:181, 1976.

1079. Mirahmadi KS, Coburn JW, Bluestone R: Calcific periarteritis and hemodialysis. JAMA 223:548, 1973.

1080. Gipstein RM, Coburn JW, Adams DA, et al: Calciphylaxis in man. Arch Intern Med 136:1273, 1976.

1081. Hallgren R, Wibell L, Ejerblad S, et al: Arterial calcification and progressive peripheral gangrene after renal transplantation. Acta Med Scand 198:331, 1975.

1082. Congure JD, Hammond WS, Alfrey AC, et al: Pulmonary calcification in chronic dialysis patients: Clinical and pathologic studies. Ann Intern Med 83:330, 1975.

1083. Rostand SG, Sanders C, Kirk KA, et al: Myocardial calcification and cardiac dysfunction in chronic renal failure. Am J Med 85:651, 1988.

1084. Ross CN, Cassidy MJ, Thompson M, et al: Proximal cutaneous necrosis associated with small vessel calcification in renal failure. Q J Med 79:443, 1991.

1085. Janigan DT, Morris J, Hirsch D: Acute skin and fat necrosis during sepsis in a patient with chronic renal failure and subcutaneous arterial calcification. Am J Kidney Dis 20:643, 1992.

1086. Mehta RL, Scott G, Sloand JA, Francis CW: Skin necrosis associated with acquired protein C deficiency in patients with renal failure and calciphylaxis. Am J Med 88:252, 1990.

1087. Canavese C, Salomone M, Massara C, et al: Primary oxalosis mimicking hyperparathyroidism diagnosed after long-term hemodialysis. Am J Nephrol 10:344, 1990.

1088. Velentzas C, Meindok H, Oreopoulos DG, et al: Detection and pathogenesis of visceral calcification in dialysis patients and patients with malignant disease. Can Med Assoc J 118:45, 1978.

1089. Sugisaki H, Onohara M, Kunitomo T: Dynamic behavior of plasma phosphate in chronic dialysis patients. Trans Am Soc Artif Intern Organs 28:302, 1982.

1090. Man NK, Chauveau P, Kuno T, et al: Phosphate removal during hemodialysis, hemodiafiltration, and hemofiltration. A reappraisal. ASAIO Trans 37:M463, 1991.

1091. Haas T, Hillion D, Dongradi G: Phosphate kinetics in dialysis patients. Nephrol Dial Transplant 6:108, 1991.

1092. Popovtzer MM, Pinggera WF, Robinette JB: Secondary hyperparathyroidism: Conservative management in patients with renal insufficiency. JAMA 231:960, 1975.

1093. Hercz G, Coburn JW: Prevention of phosphate retention and hyperphosphatemia in uremia. Kidney Int 32:S215, 1987.

1094. Smith SO, Moore LW, Acchiardo S, Mitchell CO: The effect of tailoring phosphate binder doses on serum phosphorus levels in adult chronic hemodialysis patients. J Renal Nutr 1:74, 1991.

1095. Gonnella M, Calabrese G, Vagelli G, et al: Effects of high $CaCO_3$ supplements on serum calcium and phosphorus in patients on regular hemodialysis treatment. Clin Nephrol 24:147, 1985.

1096. Moriniere P, Fournier A, Leflon A, et al: Comparison of 1-alpha-OH-vitamin $D_3$ and high doses of calcium carbonate for the control of hyperparathyroidism and hyperaluminemia in patients on maintenance dialysis. Nephron 39:309, 1985.

1097. Slatopolsky E, Weerts C, Lopez-Hilker S, et al: Calcium carbonate as a phosphate binder in patients with chronic renal failure undergoing dialysis. N Engl J Med 315:157, 1986.

1098. Fournier A, Moriniere P, Sebert JL, et al: Calcium carbonate, an aluminum-free agent for control of hyperphosphatemia, hypocalcemia, and hyperparathyroidism in uremia. Kidney Int 29:S114, 1986.

1099. Lerner A, Kramer M, Goldstein S, et al: Calcium carbonate: A better phosphate binder than aluminum hydroxide. Trans Am Soc Artif Intern Organs 32:315, 1986.

1100. Malberti F, Surian M, Colussi G, et al: Calcium carbonate: A suitable alternative to aluminum hydroxide as phosphate binder. Kidney Int 33:S184, 1988.

1101. Hercz G, Andress DL, Nebeker HG, et al: Reversal of aluminum-related bone disease after substituting calcium carbonate for aluminum hydroxide. Am J Kidney Dis 11:70, 1988.

1102. Matsubara M, Unagami H, Totsune K, et al: Long-term $CaCO_3$ treatment of chronic hemodialysis patients: An attempt to prevent aluminum osteopathy. ASAIO Trans 34:168, 1988.

1103. Vennegoor WB, O'Nunan W, Walls J: The use of calcium carbonate to treat the hyperphosphataemia of chronic renal failure. Nephrol Dial Transplant 4:725, 1989.

1104. Kobrin SM, Goldstein SJ, Shangraw RF, Raja RM: Variable efficacy of calcium carbonate tablets. Am J Kidney Dis 14:461, 1989.

1105. Sperschneider H, Gunther K, Marzoll I, et al: Calcium carbonate ($CaCO_3$): An efficient and safe phosphate binder in haemodialysis patients? A 3-year study. Nephrol Dial Transplant 8:530, 1993.

1106. Canavese C, Thea A, Pacitti A, et al: Prevention and treatment of aluminum overload in uremic patients: Long-term results. Clin Nephrol 31:169, 1989.

1107. Schiller LR, Santa Ana CA, Sheikh MS, et al: Effect of the time of administration of calcium acetate on phosphorus binding. N Engl J Med 320:110, 1989.

1108. Hess B, Binswanger U: Long-term administration of calcium acetate efficiently controls severe hyperphosphataemia in haemodialysis patients. Nephrol Dial Transplant 5:630, 1990.

1109. Delmez JA, Tindira CA, Windus DW, et al: Calcium acetate as a phosphorus binder in hemodialysis patients. J Am Soc Nephrol 3:96, 1992.

1110. Ring T, Nielsen C, Andersen SP, et al: Calcium acetate versus calcium carbonate as phosphorus binders in patients on chronic haemodialysis: A controlled study. Nephrol Dial Transplant 8:341, 1993.

1111. Coburn JW, Mischel MG, Goodman WG, Salusky IB: Calcium citrate markedly enhances aluminum absorption from aluminum hydroxide. Am J Kidney Dis 17:708, 1991.

1112. Nolan CR, Califano JR, Butzin CA: Influence of calcium acetate or calcium citrate on intestinal aluminum absorption. Kidney Int 38:937, 1990.

1113. Fromen D, Molitoris BA, Buddington B, et al: Site and mechanism of enhanced gastrointestinal absorption of aluminum by citrate. Kidney Int 36:978, 1989.

1114. Bakir AA, Hryhorczuk DO, Ahmed S, et al: Hyperaluminemia in renal failure: The influence of age and citrate intake. Clin Nephrol 31:40, 1989.

1115. Guillot AP, Hood VL, Runge CF, Gennari FJ: The use of magnesium-containing phosphate binders in patients with end-stage renal disease on maintenance hemodialysis. Nephron 30:114, 1982.

1116. O'Donovan R, Hammer M, Baldwin D, et al: Substitution of aluminium salts by magnesium salts in control of dialysis hyperphosphataemia. Lancet 1:880, 1986.

1117. Moriniere P, Boudailliez B, Hocine C, et al: Prevention of osteitis fibrosa, aluminum bone disease and soft-tissue calcification in dialysis patients: A long-term comparison of moderate doses of oral calcium ± Mg(OH)$_2$ vs Al(OH)$_3$ ± 1α-OH vitamin $D_3$. Nephrol Dial Transplant 4:1045, 1989.

1118. Randall RE, Cohen MD, Spray CC, Rossmeisl EC: Hypermagnesemia in renal failure: Etiology and toxic manifestations. Ann Intern Med 61:73, 1964.

1119. Cotiguglia SR, Alfrey AC, Miller N, Butkus D: Total-body magnesium excess in chronic renal failure. Lancet 1:1300, 1972.

1120. Rutherford E, King S, Perry B, et al: Use of a new phosphate binder in chronic renal insufficiency. Kidney Int 17:528, 1980.

1121. Nakagawa S, Ogura M, Akiba H, et al: Development of non-aluminum phosphate binder hydrous cesium oxide. Trans Am Soc Artif Organs 31:155, 1985.

1122. Schneider H, Kulbe KD, Weber H, Streicher E: Aluminum-free oral phosphate binder. Clin Nephrol 24:S98, 1985.

1123. Passlick J, Wilhelm M, Busch TH, et al: Calcium alginate, an aluminum-free phosphate binder, in patients on CAPD. Clin Nephrol 32:96, 1989.

1124. Schaefer K, Erley C, Herrath D, Stein G: Calcium salts of ketoacids as a new treatment strategy for uremic hyperphosphatemia. Kidney Int 36:S136, 1989.

1125. Yap AS, Hockings GI, Fleming SJ, Khafagi FA: Use of aminohydroxypropylidene bisphosphonate (AHPrBP, "ADP") for the treatment of hypercalcemia in patients with renal impairment. Clin Nephrol 34:225, 1990.

1126. Boelens PA, Norwood W, Kjellstrand C, Brown DM: Hypophosphatemia with muscle weakness due to antacids and hemodialysis. Am J Dis Child 120:350, 1970.

1127. Mahony JF, Hayes JM, Ingham JP, Posen S: Hypophosphataemic osteomalacia in patients receiving haemodialysis. Br Med J 2:142, 1976.

1128. Ahmed KY, Varghese Z, Wills MR, et al: Persistent hypophosphataemia and osteomalacia in dialysis patients not on oral phosphate-binders: Response to dihydrotachysterol therapy. Lancet 2:439, 1976.

1129. Prior JC, Cameron EC, Ballon HS, et al: Experience with 1,25-dihydroxycholecalciferol therapy in undergoing hemodialysis patients with progressive vitamin $D_2$-treated osteodystrophy. Am J Med 67:583, 1979.

1130. Quarles LD, Davidai GA, Schwab SJ, et al: Oral calcitriol and calcium: Efficient therapy for uremic hyperparathyroidism. Kidney Int 34:840, 1988.

1131. Slatopolsky E, Berkoben M, Kelber J, et al: Effects of calcitriol and non-calcemic vitamin D analogs on secondary hyperparathyroidism. Kidney Int 42:S43, 1992.

1132. Cordy PE: Treatment of bone disease with dihydrotachysterol in patients undergoing long-term hemodialysis. Can Med Assoc J 117:766, 1977.

1133. Avioli LV: Vitamin D metabolites: Their clinical importance. Arch Intern Med 138:835, 1978.

1134. Voigts AL, Felsenfeld AJ, Llach F: The effects of calciferol and its metabolites on patients with chronic renal failure. I: Calciferol, dihydrotachysterol and calcifediol. Arch Intern Med 143:960, 1983.

1135. Voigts AL, Felsenfeld AJ, Llach F: The effects of calciferol and its metabolites on patients with chronic renal failure. II: Calciferol, 1-alpha-OH$_2$D$_3$ and 24,25OH$_2$D$_3$. Arch Intern Med 143:1205, 1983.

1136. Zerwekh JE, McPhaul JJ, Parker TF, Pak CYC: Extra-renal production of 24,25-dihydroxyvitamin D in chronic renal failure during 25-hydroxyvitamin $D_3$ therapy. Kidney Int 23:401, 1983.

1137. Brown AJ, Finch JL, Lopez-Hilker S, et al: New active analogues of vitamin D with low calcemic activity. Kidney Int 38:S22, 1990.

1138. Finch JL, Brown AJ, Kubodera N, et al: Differential effects of 1,25-(OH)$_2$D$_3$ and 22-oxacalcitriol on phosphate and calcium metabolism. Kidney Int 43:561, 1993.

1139. Slatopolsky E, Weerts C, Thielan J, et al: Marked suppression of secondary hyperparathyroidism by intravenous administration of 1,25-dihydroxycholecalciferol in uremic patients. J Clin Invest 74:2136, 1984.

1140. Andress DL, Norris KC, Coburn JW, et al: Intravenous calcitriol in the treatment of refractory osteitis fibrosa of chronic renal failure. N Engl J Med 321:274, 1989.

1141. Hamdy NA, Brown CB, Kanis JA: Intravenous calcitriol lowers serum calcium concentrations in uraemic patients with severe hyperparathyroidism and hypercalcaemia. Nephrol Dial Transplant 4:545, 1989.

1142. Delmez JA, Tindira C, Grooms P, et al: Parathyroid hormone suppression by intravenous 1,25-dihydroxyvitamin D: A role for increased sensitivity to calcium. J Clin Invest 83:1349, 1989.

1143. Gallieni M, Grancaccio D, Padovese P, et al: Low-dose intravenous calcitriol treatment of secondary hyperparathyroidism in hemodialysis patients. Kidney Int 42:1191, 1992.

1144. Sprague SM, Moe SM: Safety and efficacy of long-term treatment of secondary hyperparathyroidism by low-dose intravenous calcitriol. Am J Kidney Dis 19:532, 1992.

1145. Rodriguez M, Felsenfeld AJ, Williams C, et al: The effect of long-term intravenous calcitriol administration on parathyroid function in hemodialysis patients. J Am Soc Nephrol 2:1014, 1991.

1146. Martin KJ, Ballal S, Domoto DT, et al: Pulse oral calcitriol for the treatment of hyperparathyroidism in patients on continuous ambulatory peritoneal dialysis: Preliminary observations. Am J Kidney Dis 19:540, 1992.

1147. Reichel H, Deibert B, Schmidt-Gayk H, Ritz E: Evidence for disturbed regulation of 1,25-dihydroxyvitamin D₃ in early chronic renal failure. In Norman AW, Bouillon R, Thomasset M (eds): Vitamin D, Gene Regulation, Structure-Function Analysis and Clinical Application. Walter de Gruyter, New York, 1991, p 867.

1148. Fournier A, Idrissi A, Sebert JL, et al: Preventing renal bone disease in moderate renal failure with CaCO₃ and 25(OH)vitamin D₃. Kidney Int 33:S178, 1988.

1149. Hsu CH, Patel S, Buchsbaum BL: Calcitriol metabolism in patients with chronic renal failure. Am J Kidney Dis 17:185, 1991.

1150. Seidel A, Herrmann P, Klaus G, et al: Kinetics of serum 1,84 iPTH after high dose of calcitriol in uremic patients. Clin Nephrol 39:210, 1993.

1151. Christiansen C, Rodbro P, Christensen M, et al: Deterioration of renal function during treatment of chronic renal failure with 1,25-dihydroxycholecalciferol. Lancet 2:700, 1978.

1152. Collier VU, Mitch WE: Accelerated progression of chronic renal insufficiency after parathyroidectomy. JAMA 244:1215, 1980.

1153. Healy MD, Malluche HH, Goldstein DA, et al: Effects of long-term therapy with calcitriol in patients with moderate renal failure. Arch Intern Med 140:1030, 1980.

1154. Massry SG, Goldstein DA: Is calcitriol (1,25(OH)₂D₃) harmful to renal function? JAMA 242:1875, 1979.

1155. Baker LRI, Louise Abrams SM, Roe CJ, et al: 1,25(OH)₂D₃ administration in moderate renal failure: A prospective double-blind trial. Kidney Int 35:661, 1989.

1156. Cunningham J, Frahor LJ, Clemens TL, et al: Chronic acidosis with metabolic bone disease. Effect of alkali on bone morphology and vitamin D metabolism. Am J Med 73:199, 1982.

1157. Kraut J, Gordon E, Ransom J, et al: Effect of chronic metabolic acidosis on vitamin D metabolism in humans. Kidney Int 24:644, 1983.

1158. Richards P, Chamberlain MJ, Wrong OM: Treatment of osteomalacia of renal tubular acidosis by sodium bicarbonate alone. Lancet 2:994, 1972.

1159. Lefebvre A, DeVernejoul MC, Gueris J, et al: Optimal correction of acidosis changes progression of dialysis osteodystrophy. Kidney Int 36:1112, 1989.

1160. Beehler CJ, Beckner JR, Rosenquist RC, Shankel SW: Parathyroid hormone suppression by cimetidine in the uremic patient. Ann Intern Med 93:840, 1980.

1161. Jacob AI, Lanier DJ, Canterbury J, Bourgoignie JJ: Reduction by cimetidine of serum parathyroid hormone levels in uremic patients. N Engl J Med 302:671, 1980.

1162. Lanier DJ, Favre H, Jacob AI, Bourgoignie JJ: Cimetidine therapy for severe hypercalcemia in two chronic hemodialysis patients. Ann Intern Med 93:573, 1980.

1163. Cunningham J, Segre GV, Slatopolsky E, Avioli LV: Effect of histamine H₂-receptor blockade on parathyroid status in normal and uraemic man. Nephron 38:17, 1984.

1164. Hercz G, Pei Y, Greenwood C, et al: Aplastic osteodystrophy without aluminum: The role of "suppressed" parathyroid function. Kidney Int 44:860, 1993.

1165. Phelps KR, Vigorita VJ, Bansal M, Einhorn TA: Histochemical demonstration of iron but not aluminum in a case of dialysis-associated osteomalacia. Am J Med 84:775, 1988.

1166. McCarthy JT, Hodgson SF, Fairbanks VF, Moyer TP: Clinical and histologic features of iron-related bone disease in dialysis patients. Am J Kidney Dis 17:551, 1991.

1167. Katz AI, Hampers CL, Merrill JP: Secondary hyperparathyroidism and renal osteodystrophy in chronic renal failure. Medicine (Baltimore) 48:333, 1969.

1168. Johnson JW, Wachman A, Katz AI, et al: The effect of subtotal parathyroidectomy and renal transplantation on mineral balance and secondary hyperparathyroidism in chronic renal failure. Metabolism 20:487, 1971.

1169. Arhon SA, Berland YF, Olmer MJ, et al: Effects of parathyroidectomy on bone formation and mineralization in hemodialyzed patients. Kidney Int 27:426, 1985.

1170. De Francisco AM, Ellis HA, Owen JP, et al: Parathyroidectomy in chronic renal failure. Q J Med 55:289, 1985.

1171. Kaye M: Parathyroidectomy in end-stage renal disease. J Lab Clin Med 114:334, 1989.

1172. Nichols P, Owen JP, Ellis HA, et al: Parathyroidectomy in chronic renal failure: A nine-year follow-up study. Q J Med 77:1175, 1990.

1173. Rodriguez M, Felsenfeld AJ, Llach F: Calcemic response to parathyroid hormone in renal failure: Role of calcitriol and the effect of parathyroidectomy. Kidney Int 40:1063, 1991.

1174. Massry SF: Is parathyroid hormone a uremic toxin? Nephron 19:125, 1977.

1175. Dawborn JK, Brown DJ, Douglas MC, et al: Parathyroidectomy in chronic renal failure. Nephron 33:100, 1983.

1176. Hampers CL, Katz AI, Wilson RE, Merrill JP: Disappearance of "uremic" itching after subtotal parathyroidectomy. N Engl J Med 279:695, 1968.

1177. Glassford DM, Remmers AR, Sarles HE, et al: Hyperparathyroidism in the maintenance dialysis patient. Surg Gynecol Obstet 142:328, 1976.

1178. Broyer M, Klienknecht C, Loirat C, et al: Growth in children treated with long-term hemodialysis. J Pediatr 84:642, 1974.

1179. Barbour GL: Effect of parathyroidectomy on anemia in chronic renal failure. Arch Intern Med 139:889, 1979.

1180. Zucchelli P, Santoro A, Zucchelli A, et al: Long-term effects of parathyroidectomy on cardiac and autonomic nervous system functions in haemodialysis patients. Nephrol Dial Transplant 3:45, 1988.

1181. Dreher W, Shelp W: Atrioventricular block in a long-term dialysis patient: Reversal after parathyroidectomy. JAMA 234:954, 1975.

1182. Goldsmith RS, Furszyfer J, Johnson WJ, et al: Control of secondary hyperparathyroidism during long-term hemodialysis. Am J Med 50:692, 1971.

1183. Wilson RE, Hampers CL, Bernstein DS, et al: Subtotal parathyroidectomy in chronic renal failure: A seven-year experience in dialysis and transplant program. Ann Surg 174:640, 1971.

1184. Rothmund M, Wagner PK: Reoperations for persistent and recurrent secondary hyperparathyroidism. Ann Surg 207:310, 1988.

1185. Meakins JL, Milne CA, Hollomby DJ, Goltzman D: Total parathyroidectomy: Parathyroid hormone levels and supernumerary glands in hemodialysis patients. Clin Invest Med 7:21, 1984.

1186. Kaye M, D'Amour P, Henderson J: Elective total parathyroidectomy without autotransplant in end-stage renal disease. Kidney Int 35:1390, 1989.

1187. Higgins RM, Richardson AJ, Ratcliffe PJ, et al: Total parathyroidectomy alone or with autograft for renal hyperparathyroidism? Q J Med 79:323, 1991.

1188. Kaye M, Rosenthall L, Hill RO, Tabah RJ: Long-term outcome following total parathyroidectomy in patients with end-stage renal disease. Clin Nephrol 39:192, 1993.

1189. Wallfelt CH, Larsson R, Gylfe E, et al: Secretory disturbance in hyperplastic parathyroid nodules of uremic hyperparathyroidism: Implication for parathyroid autotransplantation. World J Surg 12:431, 1988.

1190. Baker LR, Otieno LS, Brown AL, et al: Pitfalls after total parathyroidectomy and parathyroid autotransplantation in chronic renal failure. Am J Nephrol 11:186, 1991.

1191. Gagne ER, Urena P, Leite-Silva S, et al: Short- and long-term efficacy of total parathyroidectomy with immediate autografting compared with subtotal parathyroidectomy in hemodialysis patients. J Am Soc Nephrol 3:1008, 1992.

1192. Felsenfeld AJ, Gutman RA, Llach F, et al: Postparathyroidectomy hypocalcemia as an accurate indicator of preparathyroidectomy bone histology in the uremic patient. Miner Electrolyte Metab 10:166, 1984.

1193. Barth RH, Cheigh JS, Sullivan JF, et al: The advantage of measurement of intact PTH in the prediction of clinical response and calcium metabolism after subtotal parathyroidectomy for renal osteodystrophy. Trans Am Soc Artif Intern Organs 29:124, 1983.

1194. Brasier AR, Nussbaum SR: Hungry bone syndrome: Clinical and biochemical predictors of its occurrence after parathyroid surgery. Am J Med 84:654, 1988.

1195. Andress DL, Ott SM, Maloney NA, Sherrard DJ: Effect of parathyroidectomy on bone aluminum accumulation in chronic renal failure. N Engl J Med 312:468, 1985.

1196. DeVernejoul MC, Marchais S, London G, et al: Increased bone aluminum deposition after subtotal parathyroidectomy in dialyzed patients. Kidney Int 27:785, 1985.

1197. Felsenfeld AJ, Harrelson JM, Gutman RA, et al: Osteomalacia after parathyroidectomy in patients with uremia. Ann Intern Med 96:34, 1982.

1198. Ellis HA: Aluminum and osteomalacia after parathyroidectomy. Ann Intern Med 96:533, 1982.

1199. Johnson WJ: Persistent severe hypercalcemia during maintenance hemodialysis. Arch Intern Med 93:272, 1980.

1200. Teitelbaum SL: Calciferol (25-hydroxyvitamin D₃) in the treatment of uremic bone disease. Ann Intern Med 94:404, 1981.

1201. Thurston H, Swales JD: Aluminum and chronic renal failure. Br Med J 4:490, 1971.

1202. Siddiqui JY, Simpson SW, Ellis HE, et al: Fluoride and bone disease in patients on regular hemodialysis. *In* Cameron J, Fries D, Ogg C (eds): Dialysis and Renal Transplantation. Pitman Medical Publishing, Tunbridge Wells, England, 1971, p 149.

1203. Cordy PE, Gagnon R, Taves DR, Kaye M: Bone disease in hemodialysis patients with particular reference to the effect of fluoride. Can Med Assoc J 110:1349, 1974.

1204. Hodsman AB, Sherrard DJ, Alfrey AC, et al: Bone aluminum and histomorphometric features of renal osteodystrophy. J Clin Endocrinol Metab 54:539, 1982.

1205. Faugere MC, Malluche HH: Stainable aluminum and not aluminum content reflects bone histology of dialyzed patients. Kidney Int 30:717, 1986.

1206. De Broe ME, Van de Vyver FL: Aluminum: A clinical problem in nephrology. Clin Nephrol 24:52, 1985.

1207. Cournot-Witmer G, Zingraff J, Plachot JJ, et al: Aluminum localization in bone from hemodialyzed patients: Relationship to matrix mineralization. Kidney Int 20:375, 1981.

1208. Morrisey J, Rothstein M, Mayor G, Slatopolsky E: Suppression of parathyroid hormone secretion by aluminum. Kidney Int 23:699, 1983.

1209. Andress D, Felsenfeld A, Voigts A, Llach F: Parathyroid hormone response to hypocalcemia in hemodialysis patients with osteomalacia. Kidney Int 24:364, 1983.

1210. O'Hare JA, Murnaghan DJ: Evidence of increased parathyroid activity on discontinuation of high-aluminum dialysate in patients undergoing hemodialysis. Am J Med 77:229, 1979.

1211. Alfrey AC: The case against aluminum affecting parathyroid function. Am J Kidney Dis 6:309, 1985.

1212. Takamoto S, Onishi T, Morimoto S, et al: Serum phosphate, parathyroid hormone and vitamin D metabolites in patients with chronic renal failure: Effect of aluminum hydroxide administration. Nephron 40:286, 1985.

1213. Merke J, Lucas PA, Szabo A, et al: 1,25(OH)₂D₃ receptors and end organ response in experimental aluminum intoxication. Kidney Int 32:204, 1987.

1214. Winney RJ, Cowie JF, Robson JS: What is the value of plasma/serum aluminum in patients with chronic renal failure? Clin Nephrol 24:S2, 1985.

1215. Pei Y, Herez G, Greenwood C, et al: Non-invasive prediction of aluminum bone disease in hemo- and peritoneal dialysis patients. Kidney Int 41:1374, 1992.

1216. Hodsman AB, Steer BM: Serum aluminum levels as reflection of renal osteodystrophy status and bone surface aluminum staining. J Am Soc Nephrol 2:1318, 1992.

1217. Chazan JA, Lew NL, Lowrie EG: Increased serum aluminum: An independent risk factor for mortality in patients undergoing long-term hemodialysis. Arch Intern Med 151:319, 1991.

1218. Milliner DS, Nebeker HG, Ott SM, et al: Use of the deferoxamine infusion test in the diagnosis of aluminum-related osteodystrophy. Ann Intern Med 101:775, 1984.

1219. Malluche HH, Smith AJ, Abreo K, Faugere MC: The use of deferoxamine in the management of aluminum accumulation in bone in patients with renal failure. N Engl J Med 311:140, 1984.

1220. Berland Y, Charhon SA, Olmer M, Meunier PJ: Predictive value of deferoxamine infusion test for bone aluminum deposits in hemodialyzed patients. Nephron 40:433, 1985.

1221. Platts MM, Goode GC, Hislop JS: Composition of the domestic water supply and the incidence of fractures and encephalopathy in patients on home dialysis. Br Med J 2:657, 1977.

1222. Ward MD, Feest TG, Ellis HA, et al: Osteomalacic dialysis osteodystrophy: Evidence for a water-borne aetiological agent, probably aluminum. Lancet 1:841, 1978.

1223. Parkinson IS, Ward MK, Feest TG, et al: Fracturing dialysis osteodystrophy and dialysis encephalopathy. Lancet 1:406, 1979.

1224. Walker GS, Aaron JE, Peacock M, et al: Dialysate aluminum concentration and renal bone disease. Kidney Int 21:411, 1982.

1225. Smith GD, Winney RJ, McLean A, Robson JS: Aluminum-related osteomalacia: Response to reverse osmosis water treatment. Kidney Int 32:96, 1987.

1226. Berlyne GM, Ben-Ari J, Pest D, et al: Hyperaluminaemia from aluminium resins in renal failure. Lancet 1:494, 1970.

1227. Fleming LW, Stewart WK, Fell GS, Halls DJ: The effect of oral aluminum therapy on plasma levels in patients with chronic renal failure in an area with low water aluminum. Clin Nephrol 17:222, 1982.

1228. Alfrey AC: Gastrointestinal absorption of aluminum. Clin Nephrol 24:S84, 1985.

1229. Heaf JG, Podenphant J, Andersen JR: Bone aluminum deposition in maintenance dialysis patients treated with aluminum-free dialysate: Role of aluminum hydroxide consumption. Nephron 41:210, 1986.

1230. Brahm M: Serum-aluminum in nondialyzed chronic uremic patients before and during treatment with aluminum-containing, phosphate-binding gels. Clin Nephrol 25:231, 1986.

1231. Robertson JA, Salusky IB, Goodman WG, et al: Sucralfate, intestinal aluminum absorption, and aluminum toxicity in a patient on dialysis. Ann Intern Med 111:179, 1989.

1232. Burgess E, Muruve D, Audette R: Aluminum absorption and excretion following sucralfate therapy in chronic renal insufficiency. Am J Med 92:471, 1992.

1233. Roxe DM, Mistovich M, Barch DH: Phosphate-binding effects of sucralfate in patients with chronic renal failure. Am J Kidney Dis 13:194, 1989.

1234. Brown DJ, Ham KN, Dawborn JK, Xipell JM: Treatment of dialysis osteomalacia with desferrioxamine. Lancet 2:343, 1982.

1235. Phelps KR, Einhorn TA, Vigorita VJ, et al: Fracture healing with deferoxamine therapy in a patient with aluminum-associated osteomalacia. ASAIO Trans 32:198, 1986.

1236. Andress DL, Nebeker HG, Ott SM, et al: Bone histologic response to deferoxamine in aluminum-related bone disease. Kidney Int 31:1344, 1987.

1237. Felsenfeld AJ, Rodriguez M, Coleman M, et al: Desferrioxamine therapy in hemodialysis patients with aluminum-associated bone disease. Kidney Int 35:1371, 1989.

1238. Winterberg B, Bertram HP, Lison AE, et al: Deferoxamine B: Aluminum kinetics in patients on regular hemodialysis. Trace Elements Med 3:95, 1986.

1239. Hosokawa S, Kohira S, Tomoyoshi T, et al: Changes in serum aluminum concentration during hemodialysis. Trans Am Soc Artif Intern Organs 7:75, 1984.

1240. Muirhead N, Hollomby DJ, Leung FY, et al: Removal of aluminum during hemodialysis: Effect of different dialyzer membranes. Am J Kidney Dis 8:51, 1986.

1241. McCarthy JT, Milliner DS, Schmidt DF, et al: Deferoxamine and coated charcoal hemoperfusion to remove aluminum in dialysis patients. Kidney Int 34:804, 1988.

1242. Weiss LG, Danielson BG, Fellstrom B, Wikstrom B: Aluminum removal with hemodialysis, hemofiltration and charcoal hemoperfusion in uremic patients after desferrioxamine infusion. Nephron 51:325, 1989.

1243. Delmez J, Weerts C, Lewis-Finch J, et al: Accelerated removal of deferoxamine mesylate–chelated aluminum by charcoal hemoperfusion in hemodialysis patients. Am J Kidney Dis 13:308, 1989.

1244. Vasilakakis DM, D'Haese PC, Lamberts LV, et al: Removal of aluminoxamine and ferrioxamine by charcoal hemoperfusion and hemodialysis. Kidney Int 41:1400, 1992.

1245. Ono T, Iwamoto N, Kataoka H, et al: Removal of aluminum from chronic dialysis patients by administration of desferrioxamine and dialysis. ASAIO Trans 32:52, 1986.

1246. Molitoris BA, Alfrey AC, Alfrey PS, Miller NL: Rapid removal of DFO-chelated aluminum during hemodialysis using polysulfone dialyzers. Kidney Int 34:98, 1988.

1247. Aarseth HP, Ganss R: Removal of chelated aluminum during haemodialysis using polysulphone high-flux dialysers. Nephrol Dial Transplant 5:942, 1990.

1248. Cases A, Kelly J, Sabater J, et al: Acute visual and auditory neurotoxicity in patients with end-stage renal disease receiving desferrioxamine. Clin Nephrol 29:176, 1988.

1249. Bene C, Manzler A, Bene D, Kranias G: Irreversible ocular toxicity from single "challenge" dose of deferoxamine. Clin Nephrol 31:45, 1989.

1250. Sherrard DJ, Walker JV, Boykin JL: Precipitation of dialysis dementia by deferoxamine treatment of aluminum-related bone disease. Am J Kidney Dis 12:126, 1988.

1251. Segal R, Zoller K, Sherrard DJ, Coburn JW: Mucormycosis: Life-threatening complications of deferoxamine therapy in long-term dialysis patients. The American Society of Nephrology 20th Annual Meeting, Washington, DC. Slack, Thorofare, NJ, 1987, p 91A. Abstract.

1252. Eiser AR, Slifkin RF, Neff MS: Intestinal mucormycosis in hemodialysis patients following deferoxamine. Am J Kidney Dis 10:71, 1987.

1253. Boelaert JR, van Roost GF, Vergauwe PL, et al: The role of desferrioxamine in dialysis-associated mucormycosis: Report of three cases and review of the literature. Clin Nephrol 29:261, 1988.

1254. Tielemans C, Lenclud C: Respective role of haemosiderosis and desferrioxamine therapy in the risk from infection of haemodialysed patients. Q J Med 68:573, 1988.

1255. Charra B, Calemard E, Laurent G: Chronic renal failure treatment duration and mode: Their relevance to the late dialysis periarticular syndrome. Blood Purif 6:117, 1988.

1256. Clancet M, Mansat M, Durroux R, et al: Carpal tunnel syndrome, amyloid tenosynovitis and hemodialysis. Rev Neurol (Paris) 137:613, 1981.

1257. Spertini F, Wauters JP, Poulenas I: Carpal tunnel syndrome: A frequent, invalidating, long-term complication of chronic hemodialysis. Clin Nephrol 21:98, 1984.

1258. Walts AE, Goodman MD, Matorin PA: Amyloid, carpal tunnel syndrome, and chronic hemodialysis. Am J Nephrol 5:225, 1985.

1259. Saito A, Ogawa H, Chung TG, Ohkubo I: Accumulation of serum amyloid P and its deposition in the carpal tunnel region of long-term hemodialysis patients. ASAIO Trans 33:521, 1987.

1260. Brown EA, Arnold IR, Gower PE: Dialysis arthropathy: Complication of long-term treatment with haemodialysis. Br Med J 292:163, 1986.

1261. Munoz-Gomez J, Bergada-Barado E, Gomez-Perez R, et al: Amyloid arthropathy in patients undergoing periodical haemodialysis for chronic renal failure: A new complication. Ann Rheum Dis 44:729, 1985.

1262. Chou CT, Wasserstein A, Schumacher HR, Fernandez P: Musculoskeletal manifestations in hemodialysis patients. J Rheumatol 12:1149, 1985.

1263. Gerster JC, Carruzzo PA, Ginalski JM, Wauters JP: Cervicooccipital hinge changes during longterm hemodialysis. J Rheumatol 16:11, 1989.

1264. Kroner G, Stabler A, Seiderer M, et al: β₂-Microglobulin–related amyloidosis causing atlantoaxial spondylarthropathy with spinal-cord compression in haemodialysis patients: Detection by MRI. Nephrol Dial Transplant 6:91, 1991.

1265. Ohashi K, Hara M, Kawai R, et al: Cervical discs are most susceptible to β₂-microglobulin amyloid deposition in the vertebral column. Kidney Int 41:1646, 1992.

1266. Allard JC, Artze ME, Porter G, et al: Fatal destructive cervical spondyloarthropathy in two patients on long-term dialysis. Am J Kidney Dis 19:81, 1992.

1267. Deforges-Lasseur C, Combe C, Cernier A, et al: Destructive spondyloarthropathy presenting with progressive paraplegia in a dialysis patient. Recovery after surgical spinal cord decompression and parathyroidectomy. Nephrol Dial Transplant 8:180, 1993.

1268. Bindi P, Lavaud S, Bernieh B, et al: Early and late occurrences of destructive spondyloarthropathy in haemodialysed patients. Nephrol Dial Transplant 5:199, 1990.

1269. Chazot C, Chazot I, Charra B, et al: Functional study of hands among patients dialysed for more than 10 years. Nephrol Dial Transplant 8:247, 1993.

1270. Floege J, Brandis A, Nonnast-Daniel B, et al: Subcutaneous amyloid-tumor of β₂-microglobulin origin in a longterm hemodialysis patient. Nephron 53:73, 1989.

1271. Zhou H, Pfeifer U, Linke R: Generalized amyloidosis from β₂-microglobulin, with caecal perforation after long-term hemodialysis. Virchows Arch A 419:349, 1991.

1272. Watanabe K, Nakamura R, Kano S, et al: Amyloid urinary-tract calculi in patients on chronic dialysis. Nephron 52:334, 1989.

1273. Fuchs A, Jagirdar J, Schwartz IS: β₂-Microglobulin amyloidosis in patients undergoing long-term hemodialysis. A new type of amyloid. Am J Pathol 88:302, 1987.

1274. Kay J, Benson CB, Lester S, et al: Utility of high-resolution ultrasound for the diagnosis of dialysis-related amyloidosis. Arthritis Rheum 35:926, 1992.

1275. Chassagne P, Dhib M, Alt Said L, et al: Spinal cord compression revealing a destructive arthropathy of the atlanto-occipital joint associated with beta-2 microglobulin amyloidosis in a haemodialysed patient. Br J Rheumatol 31:427, 1992

1276. Athanasou NA, Ayers D, Rainey AJ, Oliver DO: Joint and systemic distribution of dialysis amyloid. Q J Med 78:205, 1991.

1277. Campisto JM, Sole M, Munoz-Gomez J, et al: Systemic involvement of dialysis amyloidosis. Am J Nephrol 10:389, 1990.

1278. Miyata T, Inagi R, Iada Y, et al: Involvement of β₂-microglobulin modified with advanced glycation end products in the pathogenesis of hemodialysis-associated amyloidosis. Induction of human monocyte chemotaxis and macrophage secretion of tumor necrosis factor-α and interleukin-1. J Clin Invest 93:521, 1994.

1279. Casey TT, Stone WJ, Diraimondo CR, et al: Dialysis-related amyloid is amyloid of β₂-microglobulin (AMBETA2M) origin. Arthritis Rheum 29:1170, 1986.

1280. Nakazawa R, Hamaguchi K, Hosaka E, et al: Synovial amyloidosis of β₂-microglobulin type in patients undergoing long-term hemodialysis. Nephron 44:378, 1986.

1281. Gorevic PD, Casey TT, Stone WJ, et al: β₂-Microglobulin is an amyloidogenic protein in man. J Clin Invest 76:2425, 1985.

1282. Bardin T, Zingraff J, Shirahama T, et al: Hemodialysis-associated amyloidosis and β₂-microglobulin: Clinical and immunohistochemical study. Am J Med 83:419, 1987.

1283. Lillo-Ferez M, Dupommereulle C, Prieur P, Petrover M: Serum β₂-microglobulin levels and amyloid deposits in patients undergoing long-term hemodialysis. Nephrology 5:211, 1986.

1284. Gagnon RF, Somerville P, Thomson DMP: Circulating form of β₂-microglobulin in dialysis patients. Am J Nephrol 8:379, 1988.

1285. Odell RA, Slowiaczek P, Moran JE, Schindhelm K: β₂-Microglobulin kinetics in end-stage renal failure. Kidney Int 39:909, 1991.

1286. Stein G, Schneider A, Thob K, Ritz E: β₂-Microglobulin serum concentration and associated amyloidosis in dialysis patients. Nephrol Dial Transplant 6:57, 1991.

1287. Onishi S, Andress DL, Maloney NA, et al: β₂-Microglobulin deposition in bone in chronic renal failure. Kidney Int 39:990, 1991.

1288. Vincent C, Chanard J, Caudwell V, et al: Kinetics of ¹²⁵I–β₂-microglobulin turnover in dialyzed patients. Kidney Int 42:1434, 1992.

1289. Chanard J, Vincent C, Caudwell V, et al: β₂-Microglobulin metabolism in uremic patients who are undergoing dialysis. Kidney Int 43:S83, 1993.

1290. Gejyo F, Odani S, Yamada T, et al: β₂-Microglobulin: A new form of amyloid protein associated with chronic hemodialysis. Kidney Int 30:385, 1986.

1291. Maury CP: β₂-Microglobulin amyloidosis. A systemic amyloid disease affecting primarily synovium and bone in long-term dialysis patients. Rheumatol Int 10:1, 1990.

1292. Jahn B, Betz M, Deppisch R, et al: Stimulation of β₂-microglobulin synthesis in lymphocytes after exposure to Cuprophan dialyzer membranes. Kidney Int 40:285, 1991.

1293. Knudsen PJ, Leon J, Ng AK, et al: Hemodialysis-related induction of β₂-microglobulin and interleukin-3 synthesis and release by mononuclear phagocytes. Nephron 53:188, 1989.

1294. Bandiani G, Camaiora E, Farina D, et al: Long-term influence of dialysis treatment on β₂-microglobulin, interleukin-2 R and tumour necrosis factor. Nephrol Dial Transplant 6:61, 1991.

1295. Zaoui PM, Stone WJ, Hakim RM: Effects of dialysis membranes on $\beta_2$-microglobulin production and cellular expression. Kidney Int 38:962, 1990.
1296. Simon P, Cavarle YY, Ang KS, et al: Long-term variations of serum $\beta_2$-microglobulin levels in hemodialysed uremics according to permeability and bioincompatibility of dialysis membranes. Blood Purif 6:111, 1988.
1297. Schoels M, Jahn B, Hug F, et al: Stimulation of mononuclear cells by contact with cuprophan membranes: Further increase of $\beta_2$-microglobulin synthesis by activated late complement. Am J Kidney Dis 21:394, 1993.
1298. Knudsen PJ, Ng A, Liu Z: $\beta_2$-Microglobulin synthesis is increased during activation of human monocytes. Blood Purif 6:178, 1988.
1299. Sethi D, Gower PE: Dialysis arthropathy, $\beta_2$-microglobulin and the effect of dialyser membrane. Nephrol Dial Transplant 3:768, 1988.
1300. Jadoul M, Maldague B, Vandenbroucke JM, van Ypersele de Strihou C: The natural history of dialysis-related amyloid osteoarthropathy: The role of dialysis membranes. Nephrol Dial Transplant 1:105, 1986.
1301. Hauglustaine D, Waer M, Michielsen P, et al: Haemodialysis membranes, serum $\beta_2$-microglobulin, and dialysis amyloidosis. Lancet 1:1211, 1986.
1302. Chanard J, Lavaud S, Toupance O, et al: Carpal tunnel syndrome and type of dialysis membrane used in patients undergoing long-term hemodialysis. Arthritis Rheum 29:1170, 1986.
1303. Zingraff J, Beyne P, Urena P, et al: Influence of haemodialysis membranes on $\beta_2$-microglobulin kinetics: In vivo and in vitro studies. Nephrol Dial Transplant 3:284, 1988.
1304. Chanard J, Bindi P, Lavaud S, et al: Carpal tunnel syndrome and type of dialysis membrane. Br Med J 298:867, 1989.
1305. Aoyagi R, Miura Y, Ishiyama T, et al: Influence of dialysis membranes on the development of dialysis associated osteoarthropathy. Kidney Int 43:S111, 1993.
1306. Brunner FP, Brynger H, Ehrich JH, et al: Case control study on dialysis arthropathy: The influence of two different dialysis membranes: Data from the EDTA registry. Nephrol Dial Transplant 5:432, 1990.
1307. Renaud H, Fournier A, Moriniere P, et al: Erosive osteoarthropathy associated with $\beta_2$-microglobulin amyloidosis in a uraemic patient treated exclusively by long-term haemofiltration with biocompatible membranes. Nephrol Dial Transplant 3:820, 1988.
1308. Nakamoto M, Goya T, Takahashi H, et al: Long term controlled study of high flux versus cellulose membrane on the incidence of dialysis related amyloidosis. J Am Soc Nephrol 2:340, 1991.
1309. Moriniere P, Marie A, El Esper N, Fardellone P: Destructive spondyloarthropathy with $\beta_2$-microglobulin amyloid deposits in a uremic patient before chronic hemodialysis. Nephron 59:654, 1991.
1310. Gagnon RF, Lough JO, Bourgouin PA: Carpal tunnel syndrome and amyloidosis associated with continuous ambulatory peritoneal dialysis. Can Med Assoc J 139:753, 1988.
1311. Colombi A, Wegmann W: $\beta_2$-Microglobulin amyloidosis in a patient on long-term continuous ambulatory peritoneal dialysis (CAPD). Perit Dial Int 9:321, 1989.
1312. Carozzi S, Nasini MG, Schelotto C, et al: Peritoneal macrophage $\beta_2$-microglobulin production and bacterial peritonitis in CAPD patients. ASAIO Trans 36:M369, 1990.
1313. Brown E, Soldano L, Hendler E: Dialysis-related amyloidosis during peritoneal dialysis. ASAIO Trans 36:17, 1990.
1314. Jadoul M, Noel H, van Yperse de Strihou C: $\beta_2$-Microglobulin amyloidosis in a patient treated exclusively by continuous ambulatory peritoneal dialysis. Am J Kidney Dis 15:86, 1990.
1315. Mineshima M, Hoshino T, Era K, et al: Diffusive and convective mass transport characteristics in $\beta_2$-microglobulin. Trans Am Soc Artif Intern Organs 33:103, 1987.
1316. Floege J, Granolleras C, Smeby L, et al: Hydrophilic high flux polyamide membranes for $\beta_2$-microglobulin removal. ASAIO Trans 33:309, 1987.
1317. Jorres D, Gahl GM, Schulz E, et al: Removal, generation and adsorption of $\beta_2$-microglobulin during hemofiltration with five different membranes. Blood Purif 6:96, 1988.
1318. Ono T, Iwamoto N, Kataoka H, et al: Clinical significance of a dialysis membrane that can remove $\beta_2$-microglobulin ($\beta_2$m). ASAIO Trans 34:342, 1988.
1319. Naitoh A, Tatsuguchi T, Okada M, et al: Removal of $\beta_2$-microglobulin by diffusion alone is feasible using highly permeable dialysis membranes. ASAIO Trans 34:630, 1988.
1320. Akizawa T, Koshikawa S, Nakazawa R, et al: Elimination of $\beta_2$-microglobulin by a new polyacrylonitrile membrane dialyser: Mechanism and physiokinetics. Nephrol Dial Transplant 4:356, 1989.
1321. Floege J, Granolleras C, Deschodt G, et al: High-flux synthetic versus cellulosic membranes for $\beta_2$-microglobulin removal during hemodialysis, hemodiafiltration and hemofiltration. Nephrol Dial Transplant 4:653, 1989.
1322. Arakawa M: Long-term multicentre study on $\beta_2$-microglobulin removal by PMMA BK membrane. Nephrol Dial Transplant 6(suppl 2):69, 1991.
1323. Petersen J, Moore RM, Kaczmarek RG, et al: The effects of reprocessing cuprophane and polysulfone dialyzers on $\beta_2$-microglobulin removal from hemodialysis patients. Am J Kidney Dis 17:174, 1991.
1324. Skroeder NR, Jacobson SH, Holmquist B, et al: $\beta_2$-Microglobulin generation and removal in long slow and short fast hemodialysis. Am J Kidney Dis 21:519, 1993.
1325. DiRaimondo CR, Pollak VE: $\beta_2$-Microglobulin kinetics in maintenance hemodialysis: A comparison of conventional and high-flux dialyzers and the effects of dialyzer reuse. Am J Kidney Dis 13:390, 1989.
1326. Mineshima M, Hoshino T, Era K, et al: Difference in $\beta_2$-microglobulin removal between cellulosic and synthetic polymer membrane dialyzers. ASAIO Trans 36:M643, 1990.
1327. David S, Canino F, Ferrari ME, Cambi V: The role of adsorption in $\beta_2$-microglobulin removal. Nephrol Dial Transplant 6:64, 1991.
1328. Jadoul M, Malghem J, Pirson Y, et al: Effect of renal transplantation on the radiological signs of dialysis amyloid osteoarthropathy. Clin Nephrol 32:194, 1989.
1329. Nelson SR, Sharpstone P, Kingswood JC: Does dialysis-associated amyloidosis resolve after transplantation? Nephrol Dial Transplant 8:369, 1993.
1330. Campistol JM, Munoz-Gomez J, Sole M, et al: Results of renal transplantation for dialysis arthropathy. Transplant Proc 22:1416, 1990.
1331. McMahon LP, Radford J, Dawborn JK: Shoulder ultrasound in dialysis related amyloidosis. Clin Nephrol 35:227, 1991.
1332. Jadoul M, Malghem J, Berg BV, de Strihou CVY: Ultrasonography of joint capsules and tendons in dialysis-related amyloidosis. Kidney Int 43:S106, 1993.
1333. Grateau G, Zingraff J, Fauchet M, et al: Radionuclide exploration of dialysis amyloidosis: Preliminary experience. Am J Kidney Dis 11:231, 1988.
1334. Floege J, Burchert W, Brandis A, et al: Imaging of dialysis-related amyloid (AB-amyloid) deposits with $^{131}$I–$\beta_2$-microglobulin. Kidney Int 38:1169, 1990.
1335. Zingraff J, Noel LH, Bardin T, et al: $\beta_2$-Microglobulin amyloidosis: A sternoclavicular joint biopsy study in hemodialysis patients. Clin Nephrol 33:94, 1990.
1336. Okutsu I, Ninomiya S, Takatori Y, et al: Endoscopic management of shoulder pain in long-term haemodialysis patients. Nephrol Dial Transplant 6:117, 1991.
1337. Tyler HR: Neurologic disorders in renal failure. Am J Med 44:734, 1968.
1338. Raskin NH, Fishman RA: Neurologic disorders in renal failure. N Engl J Med 294:143, 204, 1976.
1339. Osberg JW, Meares GJ, McKee DC, Burnett GB: Intellectual functioning in renal failure and chronic dialysis. J Chronic Dis 35:445, 1982.
1340. Holley JL, Nespor S, Rault R: A comparison of reported sleep disorders in patients on chronic hemodialysis and continuous peritoneal dialysis. Am J Kidney Dis 19:156, 1992.
1341. Fraser CL, Arieff AI: Nervous system complications in uremia. Ann Intern Med 109:143, 1988.
1342. Teschan PE, Bourne JR, Reed RB, Ward JW: Electrophysiological and neurobehavioral responses to therapy: The National Cooperative Dialysis Study. Kidney Int 23:S58, 1983.
1343. Lipman JJ, Lawrence PL, DeBoer DK, et al: Role of dialysable solutes in the mediation of uremic encephalopathy in the rat. Kidney Int 37:892, 1990.
1344. Akmal M, Goldstein DA, Multani S, Massry SG: Role of uremia, brain calcium, and parathyroid hormone on changes in electroencephalogram in chronic renal failure. Am J Physiol 246:F575, 1984.
1345. Massry SG: Neurotoxicity of parathyroid hormone in uremia. Kidney Int 28:S5, 1984.

1346. Ni Z, Smogorzewski M, Massry SG: Derangements in acetylcholine metabolism in brain synaptosomes in chronic renal failure. Kidney Int 44:630, 1993.

1347. Grimm G, Stockenhuber F, Schneeweiss B, et al: Improvement of brain function in hemodialysis patients treated with erythropoietin. Kidney Int 38:480, 1990.

1348. Marsh JT, Brown WS, Wolcott D, et al: rHuEPO treatment improves brain and cognitive function of anemic dialysis patients. Kidney Int 39:155, 1991.

1349. Nissenson AR, Nimer SD, Wolcott DL: Recombinant human erythropoietin and renal anemia: Molecular biology, clinical efficacy, and nervous system effects. Ann Intern Med 114:402, 1991.

1350. Di Paolo B, Di Liberato L, Fiederling B, et al: Effects of uremia and dialysis on brain electrophysiology after recombinant erythropoietin treatment. ASAIO J 38:M477, 1992.

1351. Nissenson AR, Marsh JT, Brown WS, Wolcott DL: Central nervous system function in dialysis patients: A practical approach. Semin Dial 4:115, 1991.

1352. Wolcott DL, Wellisch DK, Marsh JT, et al: Relationship of dialysis modality and other factors to cognitive function in chronic dialysis patients. Am J Kidney Dis 4:275, 1988.

1353. Gafter U, Shvili Y, Levi J, et al: Brainstem auditory evoked responses in chronic renal failure and the effect of hemodialysis. Nephron 53:2, 1989.

1354. Thodis E, Anninos PA, Pasadakis P, et al: Evaluation of CNS-function in CAPD patients using magnetoencephalography (MEG): Comparison with hemodialysis patients. Adv Perit Dial 8:181, 1992.

1355. Mahoney CA, Arieff AI: Uremic encephalopathies: Clinical, biochemical, and experimental features. Am J Kidney Dis 2:324, 1982.

1356. Jagadha V, Deck JH, Halliday WC, Smyth HS: Wernicke's encephalopathy in patients on peritoneal dialysis or hemodialysis. Ann Neurol 21:78, 1987.

1357. Raine AEG: Seizures and hypertension events. Semin Nephrol 10:40, 1990.

1358. Brown AL, Tucker B, Baker LRI, Raine AEG: Seizures related to blood transfusion and erythropoietin treatment in patients undergoing dialysis. Br Med J 299:1258, 1989.

1359. Alfrey AC, Mishell JM, Burks J, et al: Syndrome of dyspraxia and multifocal seizures associated with chronic hemodialysis. Trans Am Soc Artif Intern Organs 18:257, 1972.

1360. Rozas VV, Port FK, Rutt WM: Progressive dialysis encephalopathy from dialysate aluminum. Ann Intern Med 138:1375, 1978.

1361. Flendrig JA, Kruis H, Das HA: Aluminium and dialysis dementia. Lancet 1:1235, 1976.

1362. Dunca G, Mahurkar S, Mamdani B, Smith EG: Role of aluminum in dialysis dementia. Ann Intern Med 88:502, 1978.

1363. McKinney TD, Basinger M, Dawson E: Serum aluminum levels in dialysis dementia. Nephron 32:53, 1982.

1364. Arieff AI: Aluminum and the pathogenesis of dialysis encephalopathy. Am J Kidney Dis 6:317, 1985.

1365. Petit TL: Aluminum in human dementia. Am J Kidney Dis 6:313, 1985.

1366. Rovelli E, Luciani L, Pagani C, et al: Correlation between serum aluminum concentration and signs of encephalopathy in a large population of patients dialyzed with aluminum-free fluids. Clin Nephrol 29:294, 1988.

1367. Altmann P, Al-Salihi F, Butter K, et al: Serum aluminum levels and erythrocyte dihydropteridine reductase activity in patients on hemodialysis. N Engl J Med 317:80, 1987.

1368. Khalil-Manesh F, Agness C, Gonick HC: Aluminum-binding protein in dialysis dementia I: Characterization in plasma by gel chromatography and electrophoresis. Nephron 52:323, 1989.

1369. Edwardson JA, Oakley AE, Taylor GA, et al: Role for aluminum and silicon in the pathogenesis of senile plaques: Studies in chronic renal dialysis. Adv Neurol 51:223, 1990.

1370. Scholtz CL, Swash M, Gray A, et al: Neurofibrillary neuronal degeneration in dialysis dementia: A feature of aluminum toxicity. Clin Neuropathol 6:93, 1987.

1371. Candy JM, McArthur FK, Oakley AE, et al: Aluminum accumulation in relation to senile plaque and neurofibrillary tangle formation in the brains of patients with renal failure. J Neurol Sci 107:210, 1992.

1372. Winkelman MD, Ricanati ES: Dialysis encephalopathy: Neuropathologic aspects. Hum Pathol 17:823, 1986.

1373. Platts MM, Goode GC, Hislop JS: Composition of the domestic water supply and the incidence of fractures and encephalopathy in patients on home dialysis. Br Med J 2:657, 1977.

1374. Kaehny WD, Alfrey AC, Holman RE, Schorr WJ: Aluminum transfer during hemodialysis. Kidney Int 12:361, 1977.

1375. Kaehny WD, Hegg AP, Alfrey AC: Gastrointestinal absorption of aluminum from aluminum-containing antacids. N Engl J Med 296:1389, 1977.

1376. Campistol JM, Cases A, Botey A, Revert A: Acute aluminum encephalopathy in an uremic patient. Nephron 51:103, 1989.

1377. Etheridge WB, O'Neill WM: The dialysis encephalopathy syndrome without dialysis. Clin Nephrol 10:250, 1978.

1378. Rotundo A, Nevins TE, Lipton M, et al: Progressive encephalopathy in children with chronic renal insufficiency in infancy. Kidney Int 21:486, 1982.

1379. Ackrill P, Ralston AJ, Day JP, Hodge KC: Successful removal of aluminium from patient with dialysis encephalopathy. Lancet 2:692, 1980.

1380. Hood SA, Clark WF, Hodsman AB, et al: Successful treatment of dialysis osteomalacia and dementia using deferoxamine infusions and oral 1-alpha-hydroxycholecalciferol. Am J Nephrol 4:369, 1984.

1381. Khalil-Manesh F, Agness C, Gonick HC: Aluminum-binding protein in dialysis dementia II: Characterization in plasma ultrafiltration. Nephron 52:329, 1989.

1382. Papageorgiou C, Ziroyannis P, Vathylakis J, et al: A comparative study of brain atrophy by computerized tomography in chronic renal failure and chronic hemodialysis. Acta Neurol Scand 66:378, 1982.

1383. Savazzi GM: Pathogenesis of cerebral atrophy in uraemia. State of the art. Nephron 49:94, 1988.

1384. Savazzi GM, Cusmano F, Degasperi T: Cerebral atrophy in patients on long-term regular hemodialysis treatment. Clin Nephrol 23:89, 1985.

1385. Asbury AK, Victor M, Adams RD: Uremic polyneuropathy. Arch Neurol 8:413, 1963.

1386. Kominami N, Tyler HR, Hampers CL, Merrill JP: Variations in motor nerve conduction velocity in normal and uremic patients. Arch Intern Med 128:235, 1971.

1387. Weseley SA, Sadler B, Katims JJ: Current perception: Preferred test for evaluation of peripheral nerve integrity. ASAIO J 34:188–193, 1988.

1388. Katims JJ, Rouvelas P, Sadler BT, Weseley SA: Reproducibility and comparison with nerve conduction in evaluation of carpal tunnel syndrome. ASAIO J 35:280–284, 1989.

1389. Weber B, Hacke W, Stiller S, Mann H: Evaluation of uremic neuropathy by visual (VEP) and brainstem auditory (BAEP) evoked potentials. ASAIO Trans 31:586, 1985.

1390. Yu YL, Cheng IK, Chang CM, et al: A multimodal neurophysiological assessment in terminal renal failure. Acta Neurol Scand 83:89, 1991.

1391. Katims JJ, Taylor DN, Weseley SA: Sensory perception in uremic patients. ASAIO Trans 37:M370, 1991.

1392. Chokroverty S: Proximal vs. distal slowing of nerve conduction in chronic renal failure treated by long-term hemodialysis. Arch Neurol 39:53, 1982.

1393. McGonigle RJS, Bewick M, Weston MJ, Parsons V: Progressive, predominantly motor, uraemic neuropathy. Acta Neurol Scand 71:379, 1985.

1394. Sprenger KBG, Bundschu D, Lewis K, et al: Improvement of uremic neuropathy and hypogeusia by dialysate zinc supplementation: A double-blind study. Kidney Int 24:S315, 1983.

1395. Campese VM, Romoff MS, Levitan D, et al: Mechanisms of autonomic nervous system dysfunction in uremia. Kidney Int 20:246, 1981.

1396. Naik RB, Mathias CJ, Wilson CA, et al: Cardiovascular and autonomic reflexes in haemodialysis patients. Clin Sci 60:165, 1981.

1397. Lazarus JM, Hampers CL, Lowrie EG, Merrill JP: Baroreceptor activity in normotensive and hypertensive uremic patients. Circulation 47:1015, 1973.

1398. Mallamaci F, Zoccali C, Ciccarelli M, Briggs JD: Autonomic function in uremic patients treated by hemodialysis or CAPD and in transplant patients. Clin Nephrol 25:175, 1986.

1399. Heidbreder E, Schafferhans K, Heidland A: Disturbances of peripheral and autonomic nervous system in chronic renal failure: Effects of hemodialysis and transplantation. Clin Nephrol 23:222, 1985.

1400. Zoccali C, Ciccarelli M, Mallamaci F, Maggiore Q: Parasympathetic function in haemodialysis patients. Nephron 44:351, 1986.

1401. Daul AE, Wang XL, Michel MC, Brodde OE: Arterial hypotension in chronic hemodialyzed patients. Kidney Int 32:728, 1987.

1402. Nies AS, Robertson D, Stone WJ: Haemodialysis hypotension is not the result of uraemic peripheral autonomic neuropathy. J Lab Clin Med 94:395, 1979.

1403. Procci WR, Goldstein DA, Adelstein J, Massry SG: Sexual dysfunction in the male patient with uremia: A reappraisal. Kidney Int 19:317, 1981.

1404. Orofino L, Marcen R, Quereda C, et al: Epidemiology of symptomatic hypotension in hemodialysis: Is cool dialysate beneficial for all patients? Am J Nephrol 10:177, 1990.

1405. Kong CH, Thompson FD: Hemodynamic responses to head-up tilt in uremic patients. Clin Nephrol 33:2283, 1990.

1406. Kouw PM, Kooman JP, Cheriex EC, et al: Assessment of postdialysis dry weight: A comparison of techniques. J Am Soc Nephrol 4:98, 1993.

1407. Sherman RA: The pathophysiologic basis for hemodialysis-related hypotension. Semin Dial 1:136, 1988.

1408. Travis M, Henrich WL: Autonomic nervous system and hemodialysis hypotension. Semin Dial 2:158, 1989.

1409. Ewing DJ, Winney R: Autonomic function in patients with chronic renal failure on intermittent hemodialysis. Nephron 15:424, 1975.

1410. Lilley JJ, Golden J, Stone RA: Adrenergic regulation of blood pressure in chronic renal failure. J Clin Invest 57:1190, 1976.

1411. Barakat MM, Nawab ZM, Yu AW, et al: Hemodynamic effects of intradialytic food ingestion and caffeine. J Am Soc Nephrol 3:1813, 1993.

1412. Levy FL, Grayburn PA, Foulks CJ, et al: Improved left ventricular contractility with cool temperature hemodialysis. Kidney Int 41:961, 1992.

1413. Coli U, Landini S, Lucatello S, et al: Cold as cardiovascular stabilizing factor in hemodialysis: Hemodynamic evaluation. Trans Am Soc Artif Intern Organs 29:71, 1983.

1414. Marcen R, Quereda C, Orofino L, et al: Hemodialysis with low-temperature dialysate: A long-term experience. Nephron 49:29, 1988.

1415. Rocco MV, Burkart JM: Prevalence of missed treatments and early sign-offs in hemodialysis patients. J Am Soc Nephrol 4:1178, 1993.

1416. Man NK, Fournier G, Thireau P, et al: Effect of bicarbonate-containing dialysate on chronic hemodialysis patients: A comparative study. Artif Organs 2:147, 1978.

1417. Kaji DM, Ackad A, Nottage WG, Stern RM: Prevention of muscle cramps in haemodialysis patients by quinine sulfate. Lancet 2:66, 1976.

1418. Roca AO, Jarjoura D, Blend D, et al: Dialysis leg cramps. Efficacy of quinine versus vitamin E. ASAIO J 38:M481, 1992.

1419. Canzanello VJ, Hylander-Rossner B, Sands RE, et al: Comparison of 50% dextrose water, 25% mannitol, and 23.5% saline for the treatment of hemodialysis-associated muscle cramps. ASAIO J 37:649, 1991.

1420. Gordon SM, Oettinger CW, Bland LA, et al: Pyrogenic reactions in patients receiving conventional, high-efficiency, or high-flux hemodialysis treatments with bicarbonate dialysate containing high concentrations of bacteria and endotoxin. J Am Soc Nephrol 2:1436, 1992.

1421. Powell AC, Bland LA, Oettinger CW, et al: Lack of plasma interleukin-1β or tumor necrosis factor-α elevation during unfavorable hemodialysis conditions. J Am Soc Nephrol 2:1007, 1991.

1422. Shapiro OM, Bar-Khayim Y: ECG changes and cardiac arrhythmias in chronic renal failure patients on hemodialysis. J Electrocardiol 25:273, 1992.

1423. Niwa A, Taniguchi K, Ito H, et al: Echocardiographic and Holter findings in 321 uremic patients on maintenance hemodialysis. Jpn Heart J 26:403, 1985.

1424. Sforzini S, Latini R, Mingardi G, et al: Ventricular arrhythmias and four-year mortality in haemodialysis patients. Lancet 339:212, 1992.

1425. Sragoca MA, Canziani ME, Cassiolata JL, et al: Left ventricular hypertrophy as a risk factor for arrhythmias in hemodialysis patients. J Cardiovasc Pharmacol 17:S136, 1991.

1426. Kimura K, Tabei K, Asano Y, Hosoda S: Cardiac arrhythmias in hemodialysis patients. A study of incidence and contributory factors. Nephron 53:201, 1989.

1427. Fantuzzi S, Caico S, Amatruda O, et al: Hemodialysis-associated cardiac arrhythmias: A lower risk with bicarbonate? Nephron 58:196, 1991.

1428. Nishamura M, Nakanishi T, Yasui A, et al: Serum calcium increases the incidence of arrhythmias during acetate hemodialysis. Am J Kidney Dis 19:149, 1992.

1429. D'Elia JA, Weinrauch LA, Gleason RE, et al: Application of the ambulatory 24-hour electrocardiogram in the prediction of cardiac death in dialysis patients. Arch Intern Med 148:2381, 1988.

1430. Rambola G, Colussi G, De Ferrari ME, et al: Cardiac arrhythmias and electrolyte changes during hemodialysis. Nephrol Dial Transplant 7:318, 1992.

1431. Arieff AI, Massry SG: Dialysis dysequilibrium syndrome. In Massry SG, Sellers AL (eds): Clinical Aspects of Uremia and Dialysis. Charles C Thomas, Springfield, IL, 1976, p 34.

1432. Kiley JE, Woodruff MW, Pratt KI: Evaluation of encephalopathy by EEG frequency analysis in chronic dialysis patients. Clin Nephrol 5:245, 1976.

1433. Hampl H, Klopp HW, Michaels N, et al: Electroencephalographic investigations of the disequilibrium syndrome during bicarbonate and acetate dialysis. Proc Eur Dial Transplant Assoc 19:351, 1982.

1434. Basile C, Miller JDR, Koles ZJ, et al: The effects of dialysis on brain water and EEG in stable chronic uremia. Am J Kidney Dis 9:462, 1987.

1435. Silver SM, DeSimone JA, Smith DA, Sterns RH: Dialysis disequilibrium syndrome (DDS) in the rat: Role of the "reverse urea effect." Kidney Int 42:161, 1992.

1436. Wakim KG: Predominance of hyponatremia or hypo-osmolality in simulation of the dialysis disequilibrium syndrome. Mayo Clin Proc 44:433, 1969.

1437. Strange K: Regulation of solute and water balance and cell volume in the central nervous system. J Am Soc Nephrol 3:12, 1992.

1438. Stewart WK, Fleming LW, Manuel MA: Benefits obtained by the use of a high sodium dialysate during maintenance hemodialysis. Proc Eur Dial Transplant Assoc 9:111, 1972.

1439. Yoshida S, Tajika T, Yamasaki N, et al: Dialysis disequilibrium syndrome in neurosurgical patients. Neurosurgery 20:716, 1987.

1440. Intracranial pressure measurement in a patient undergoing hemodialysis and peritoneal dialysis. Am J Kidney Dis 13:336, 1989.

1441. Fujiwara Y, Hagihara B, Yamauchi A, Shirai D: Hypoxemia and hemodialysis-induced symptomatic hypotension. Clin Nephrol 24:9, 1985.

1442. Eiser AR, Jahamanne D, Kokseng C, et al: Contrasting alterations in pulmonary gas exchange during acetate and bicarbonate hemodialysis. Am J Nephrol 2:123, 1982.

1443. Oh MS, Uribarri J, Del Monte MI, et al: A mechanism of hypoxemia during hemodialysis: Consumption of $CO_2$ in metabolism of acetate. Am J Nephrol 5:366, 1985.

1444. Sherlock J, Ledwith J, Letteri J: Hypoventilation and hypoxemia during hemodialysis: Reflex response to removal of $CO_2$ across the dialyzer. Trans Am Soc Artif Intern Organs 23:406, 1977.

1445. Aurigemma NM, Feldman NT, Gottlieb M, et al: Arterial oxygenation during hemodialysis. N Engl J Med 297:871, 1977.

1446. Romaldini H, Rodriguez-Roisin R, Lopez FA, et al: The mechanism of arterial hypoxemia during hemodialysis. Am Rev Respir Dis 129:780, 1984.

1447. Dolan MJ, Whipp BJ, Davidson WD, et al: Hypopnea associated with acetate hemodialysis: Carbon-dioxide flow dependent ventilation. N Engl J Med 305:72, 1981.

1448. Francos GC, Besarab A, Burke JFJ, et al: Dialysis-induced hypoxemia: Membrane dependent and membrane independent causes. Am J Kidney Dis 5:191, 1985.

1449. Grekas D, Syrganis C, Georgiou T, et al: Biocompatability of cuprophan and cellulose acetate membranes. Prevention of dialysis hypoxemia and leukopenia by ticlopidine. Life Support Syst 3:68, 1985.

1450. Wiegmann TB, MacDougall ML, Diederich DA: Dialysis leukopenia, hypoxemia, and anaphylatoxin formation: Effect of membrane, bath, and citrate anticoagulation. Am J Kidney Dis 11:418, 1988.

1451. Cardoso M, Vinay P, Vinet B, et al: Hypoxemia during hemodialysis: A critical review of the facts. Am J Kidney Dis 11:281, 1988.

1452. Ganss R, Aarseth HP, Nordby G: Prevention of hemodialysis associated hypoxemia by use of low-concentration bicarbonate dialysate. ASAIO J 38:820, 1992.

1453. Villarroel F: Incidence of hypersensitivity in hemodialysis. Artif Organs 8:278, 1984.
1454. Lemke HD, Kuentz F, Foret M: Mediation of hypersensitivity reactions during hemodialysis. Trans Am Soc Artif Intern Organs 31:149, 1985.
1455. Marshall CP, Pearson FC, Sagona MA, et al: Reactions during hemodialysis caused by allergy to ethylene oxide gas sterilization. J Allergy Clin Immunol 75:563, 1985.
1456. Grammer LC, Roberts M, Wiggins CA, et al: A comparison of cutaneous testing and ELISA for assessing reactivity to ethylene oxide–human serum albumin in hemodialysis patients with anaphylactic reactions. J Allergy Clin Immunol 87:674, 1991.
1457. Tielemans C, Madhoun P, Lenaers M, et al: Anaphylactoid reactions during hemodialysis on AN69 membranes receiving ACE inhibitors. Kidney Int 38:982, 1988.
1458. Verresen L, Waer M, Vanrenterghem Y, Michielsen P: Angiotensin-converting-enzyme inhibitors and anaphylactoid reactions to high-flux membrane dialysis. Lancet 336:1360, 1990.
1459. Parnes EL, Shapiro WB: Anaphylactoid reactions in hemodialysis patients treated with the AN69 dialyzer. Kidney Int 40:1148, 1991.
1460. Brunet P, Jaber K, Berland Y, Baz M: Anaphylactoid reactions during hemodialysis and hemofiltration: Role of associating AN69 membrane and angiotensin I–converting enzyme inhibitors. Am J Kidney Dis 19:444, 1992.
1461. Hakim RM, Breillatt J, Lazarus JM, Port FK: Complement activation and hypersensitivity reactions to dialysis membranes. N Engl J Med 311:878, 1984.
1462. Ward MK, Shadforth M, Hill AVL, Ker DNS: Air embolism during haemodialysis. Br Med J 3:74, 1971.
1463. Carlson DJ, Shapiro FL: Methemoglobinemia from well water nitrates: A complication of home dialysis. Ann Intern Med 73:757, 1970.
1464. Crosson JT, Moulds J, Comty CM, Polesky HF: A clinical study of anti-NDP in the sera of patients in a large repetitive hemodialysis program. Kidney Int 10:463, 1976.
1465. Kaehny WD, Miller GE, White WL: Relationship between dialyzer reuse and the presence of anti-N–like antibodies in chronic hemodialysis patients. Kidney Int 12:59, 1977.
1466. Berkes SL, Kahn IS, Chazen JA, Garella S: Prolonged hemolysis from overheated dialysate. Ann Intern Med 83:363, 1975.
1467. Gotch FA, Sargent JA: A mechanistic analysis of the National Cooperative Dialysis Study (NCDS). Kidney Int 28:526, 1985.
1468. Gotch FA, Yarian S, Keen M: A kinetic survey of US hemodialysis prescriptions. Am J Kidney Dis 15:511, 1990.
1469. Acchiardo S, Hatten KW, Ruvinsky MJ, et al: Inadequate dialysis increases gross mortality rate. ASAIO J 38:M282, 1992.
1470. Held P, Leniv NW, Bovbjerg RR, et al: Mortality and duration of hemodialysis treatment. JAMA 265:871, 1991.
1471. Held PJ, Brunner FP, Odaka M, et al: Five year survival for end-stage renal disease patients in the United States, Europe and Japan. Am J Kidney Dis 15:451, 1990.
1472. Lindsay RM, Spanner E, Heidenheim P, et al: Which comes first, Kt/V or PCT—chicken or egg? Kidney Int Suppl 38:S32, 1992.
1473. Wizemann U, Kramer W: Short-term dialysis—long term complications. Blood Purif 5:193, 1987.
1474. Rottembourg JB: Which dialytic therapy is best for the patient with an unstable cardiovascular system? CAPD is more advantageous than hemodialysis. Semin Dial 5:208, 1992.
1475. Bellomo R, Boyce N: Does continuous hemodiafiltration improve survival in acute renal failure? Semin Dial 6:16, 1993.
1476. Rackow EC, Fein IA, Sprung C, et al: Uremic pulmonary edema. Am J Med 64:1084, 1978.
1477. DelGreco F, Simon NM, Roguska J, et al: Hemodynamic studies in chronic uremia. Circulation 40:87, 1969.
1478. London GM, Marchais SJ, Guerin AP, et al: Contributive factors to cardiovascular hypertrophy in renal failure. Am J Hypertens 2:261S, 1989.
1479. Schott CR, LeSar JF, Kotler MN, et al: The spectrum of echocardiographic findings in chronic renal failure. Cardiovasc Med 3:217, 1978.
1480. D'Cruz IA, Bhatt GL, Cohen HC, et al: Echocardiographic detection of cardiac involvement in patients with chronic renal failure. Ann Intern Med 138:720, 1978.
1481. Miach PJ, Dawborn JK, Louis WJ, et al: Left ventricular function in uremia. Echocardiographic assessment in patients on maintenance dialysis. Clin Nephrol 15:259, 1981
1482. Drueke T, Le Pailleur C, Sigal-Saglier M, et al: Left ventricular function in hemodialyzed patients with cardiomyopathy. Nephron 28:80, 1981.
1483. Cohen MV, Diaz P, Scheuer J: Echocardiographic assessment of left ventricular function in patients with chronic uremia. Clin Nephrol 12:156, 1979.
1484. Fernando HA, Friedman HS, Masih E, et al: Echocardiographic assessment of cardic performance in patients on maintenance hemodialysis. Cardiovasc Med 4:459, 1979.
1485. Renger A, Muller M, Jutzler GA, et al: Echocardiographic evaluation of left ventricular dimensions in function in chronic hemodialysis patients with cardiomegaly. Clin Nephrol 21:164, 1984.
1486. Cooper MW, Myers WD, Stanbaugh GH, et al: Echocardiographic evaluation of the Valsalva maneuver in an asymptomatic hemodialysis population. Trans Am Soc Artif Intern Org 26:387, 1980.
1487. Bernardi D, Bernini L, Cini G, et al: Asymmetric septal hypertrophy in uremic-normotensive patients on regular hemodialysis. An M-mode and two-dimensional echocardiographic study. Nephron 39:30, 1985.

*57*

# Peritoneal Dialysis

*John M. Burkart*
*Karl D. Nolph*

As of May 1995, it was estimated that more than 96,800 patients worldwide were maintained with long-term peritoneal dialysis.[1] This number represents about 15% of the worldwide dialysis population. Industrial estimates of percentages of dialysis patients receiving peritoneal dialysis vary from country to country, with a range as low as 6% in Japan to as high as 93% in Mexico; these data also show that about 17% of patients in the United States receive peritoneal dialysis versus 51% in the United Kingdom.[1]

The percentages of prevalent dialysis patients receiving continuous ambulatory peritoneal dialysis (CAPD) or continuous cyclic peritoneal dialysis (CCPD) in selected countries in 1990 reported by the United States Renal Data System (USRDS) are seen in Figure 57–1. Reasons for these differences are multifactorial. Most of these patients are using CAPD, although the use of automated forms of peritoneal dialysis is increasing.

Ganter[2] described the first clinical use of peritoneal dialysis in 1923. The clinical courses of most of the first 100 patients treated with peritoneal dialysis were reviewed in 1950.[3] Of these, many had acute renal failure, and 32 patients recovered renal function. The cause of death was reported in 40 cases, and three complications (uremia, peritonitis, and pulmonary edema) accounted for 88% of the deaths. Subsequent to that publication, clinical experiences and many modifications of the initial procedure that addressed these initial complications were reported. However, it was not until 1976, when Popovich and Moncrief[4] described the basic concept of CAPD as we know it today, that nephrologists were able to practically and efficiently offer peritoneal dialysis as a long-term renal replacement therapy to patients with end-stage renal disease (ESRD). This modification allowed safe and easy home therapy. An extensive review of the history of peritoneal dialysis has been published in a previous edition of this book.[5] Perito-

neal dialysis continues to evolve, with special emphasis on survival of the patient, catheters, exit sites, alternative dialysis solutions, biocompatibility issues, optimal dialysis prescriptions, and the relationship between dialysis dose and protein-calorie intake.

## COMPONENTS OF THE PERITONEAL DIALYSIS SYSTEM

Renal replacement therapy with peritoneal dialysis requires three key components: 1) the peritoneal dialysis catheter, 2) the peritoneal dialysis solutions, and 3) the peritoneal membrane. Each of these components has some distinct differences from its counterpart in hemodialysis. For instance, the peritoneal dialysis access must traverse both a sterile (intraperitoneal portion) and a nonsterile (extraperitoneal portion) environment, as opposed to the usual subcutaneous fistula or synthetic graft used for long-term hemodialysis. Second, peritoneal dialysis solutions must be sterile, and the containers must be amenable to easy home use. In contradistinction to hemodialysis, for peritoneal dialysis, the physician cannot pick and choose a dialyzer from a catalogue of various membrane types or sizes for a particular patient. Patients are born with their ''dialyzer.'' The physician must learn how to tailor the therapy for each patient's membrane.

### Catheters

Access to the peritoneal cavity by use of a permanent indwelling catheter is presently the key factor determining long-term success of peritoneal dialysis. Palmer and coworkers[6] first introduced the silicone rubber catheter in

# Percent of Prevalent ESRD Patients Receiving CAPD or CCPD for Selected Countries, 1990

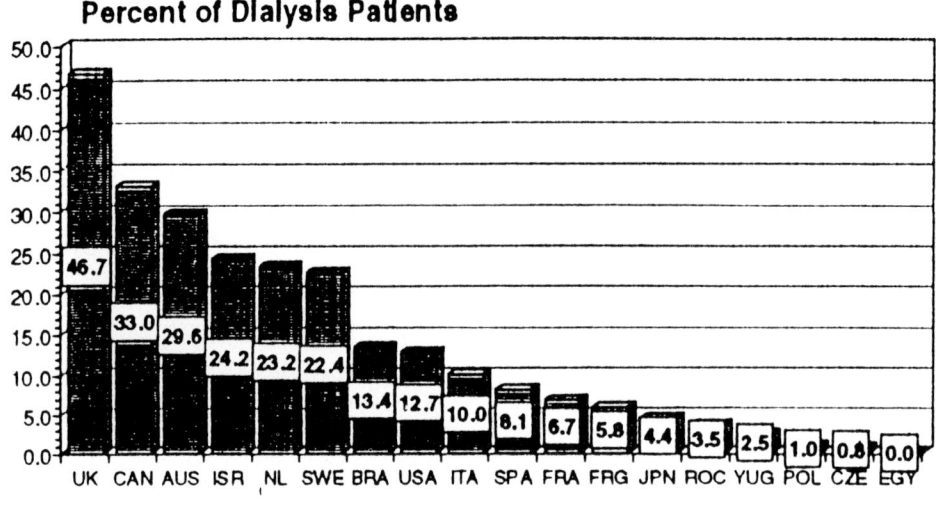

**Figure 57–1.** Percentage of prevalent end-stage renal disease (ESRD) patients (dialysis only) receiving CAPD or CCPD for selected countries, 1990. (From United States Renal Data System: International Comparisons of ESRD Therapy. USRDS, Bethesda, MD, 1993, p 91.)

1964. Tenckhoff[7] modified this catheter in 1968, and this version of the catheter is still used by most nephrologists. Since these original designs, most modifications have been directed toward improving the subcutaneous anchoring of the catheter, preventing catheter migration, decreasing infectious complications, and addressing possible bioincompatibility issues.

## CATHETER DESIGN

**Acute Catheters.** Acute peritoneal dialysis catheters are straight, relatively rigid catheters about 3 mm in diameter and 25 to 30 mm in length. They were first introduced by Westin and Roberts[8] in 1965. These can be placed at the bedside.[5] With prolonged use, this catheter design is associated with a significant risk of peritonitis, malfunction, and bowel perforation. Therefore, it is recommended that these catheters not be left in place for longer than 3 days. For most patients with acute renal failure, the number of treatments that will be needed is unpredictable, and these patients usually require therapy for longer than 3 days. Therefore, use of the safer chronic catheter is recommended.

**Chronic Catheters.** Present standard chronic indwelling peritoneal catheters are constructed of soft materials such as silicone rubber or polyurethane. The intraperitoneal portion usually contains many 1-mm side holes for passage of fluids but may also have modifications to facilitate fluid movement, alleviate symptoms associated with inflow or drainage, decrease catheter migration, and prevent trapping by omentum. These modifications include a curled tip, two perpendicular disks (Oreopoulos-Zellerman), and a column disk (Lifecath). Extraperitoneal modifications include var-

ious means of external fixation and preformed angles in the subcutaneous portion designed to prevent catheter infections, migrations, and dialysate leaks. These modifications include the use of one or two Dacron cuffs; one or two disk-bubble cuffs (Toronto); and arcuate (swan neck), pail handle (Cruz), or 90-degree (Lifecath) subcutaneous curves. These are described in Figure 57–2.

**More Recent Designs.** After analysis of catheter infection rates in relationship to the number of cuffs and the direction, shape, and location of the tunnel, Twardowski and colleagues[9] designed the swan neck catheter. This catheter was designed to exit laterally and has a permanent bend in the subcutaneous portion of the catheter resulting in an arcuate tunnel that is convex upward. Both the internal and external exits point downward. The bend and arc are designed to prevent catheter migration and cuff extrusion. The downward exits and subcutaneous cuff placements are designed to reduce exit site infections. A description of the insertion technique has been reported elsewhere.[10] These authors reported an estimated survival probability at 3 years of 61%, more than twice the survival probability at 3 years (30%) for the straight Tenckhoff and Toronto Western Hospital catheters at their institution[11] and better than the survival results that were reported in the CAPD registry at that time.[12] The authors have since developed a further modification of their catheter with the exit in the presternal area. This modification is based on the theory that presternal exit sites would be subject to less trauma and fewer chances for contamination. Preliminary experience in four patients has been encouraging.[13]

The Moncrief-Popovich catheter and insertion technique were developed to allow healing of the subcutaneous cuff

IP DESIGN

EP DESIGN

CHRONIC CATHETERS

Straight Tenckhoff

Single cuff

Disc—bubble 1 cuff
(1 cuff Toronto)

Curled Tenckhoff

(P,S)

Dual cuff

(P,S)

Disc—bubble 2 cuff
(2 cuff Toronto)

Arcuate (swan neck)

Oreopoulos—
Zellerman (Disc)

Disk-bubble 2 cuff swan neck
(Swan neck Toronto)

Angled disc—bubble 2 cuff
Swan neck (swan neck Missouri)

Cruz (pail handle)

(P)

Lifecath (column disc)

Molded 90° curve

ACUTE CATHETERS

Stylocath, Trocath, Cook

(N)

Acute with wings

(N)

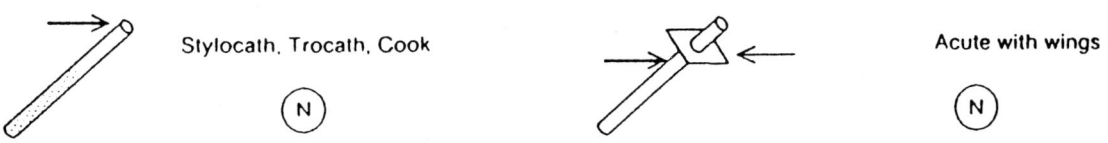

**Figure 57–2.** Schematic representation of evolution of catheter designs for currently available peritoneal catheters. Intraperitoneal (IP) designs appear on the left, and extraperitoneal (EP) designs on the right. The letters in circles indicate material of construction: P = polyurethane; P,S = polyurethane or silicone; N = nylon or polyethylene; no letter indicates silicone. The bold arrow indicates the peritoneal end and the thin arrow the skin end on each catheter. (From Ash S: Peritoneal access devices. *In* Nissenson AR, Fine RN [eds]: Dialysis Therapy, 2nd ed. Hanley & Belfus, Philadelphia, 1993, p 24.)

in a sterile environment.[14] This catheter incorporates the Missouri swan neck design with a novel insertion technique. The segment of the catheter that would normally be brought out through the skin is completely buried at the time of catheter insertion. At a subsequent date, 4 to 6 weeks later, the distal segment of the catheter is exteriorized, and dialysis is begun. During preliminary clinical trials, use of this catheter significantly reduced peritonitis rates in patients using the standard spike and even further reduced peritonitis in patients using a disconnect technique.[15] During the period before exteriorization of the external end, there were no reported problems with omental wrapping; in a study in dogs, these authors demonstrated that omental wrapping does not occur without the instillation of fresh dialysis fluid,[16] which suggests that normal saline, not standard dialysis fluid, should be used for irrigation after catheter placement. Another interesting preliminary finding in patients who have had catheters implanted with this technique is the absence of biofilm on subsequent electron microscopic evaluation of the subcutaneous portion of the catheter.[15] These data seem to demonstrate an improved bacteriologic barrier between the outside and the peritoneal cavity and confirm the significance of sources other than touch contamination as a cause for peritonitis. Further studies are currently under way.

## BIOFILMS

Infections associated with implantable and indwelling devices are often persistent and refractory to medical therapy. Recurrent or relapsing peritonitis is a frequent cause of catheter loss in peritoneal dialysis patients. It has been postulated that the presence of biofilms containing microorganisms, called microbial biofilms, may be the cause.[17–20] Giangrande and co-workers[21] used scanning electron microscopy to analyze the surfaces of 18 silicone catheters removed from patients who had been receiving peritoneal dialysis for 2 to 77 months. All catheter surfaces were covered with protein-like granular deposits; six were covered with microbial biofilm, and positive cultures of catheter segments were obtained in six cases. Biofilms were seen in some patients who had not had a recent bout of peritonitis. Structural defects and small linear tears were present on both the luminal and external surfaces of eight catheters and were more frequent in patients with refractory or recurrent peritonitis, as were the positive cultures. It has been shown that structural defects might favor a nidus for adherent exopolysaccharide matrix deposition, which is crucial for biofilm formation and bacterial growth.[22] Previous studies have suggested that structural defects in the catheter predispose to peritonitis.[23] These studies are intriguing but would suggest the need for further evaluation of the role of biofilms in disease, cuff maturation, and improvements in the physicochemical characteristics and production of catheters.

## CATHETER IMPLANTATION TECHNIQUES

The technique of Tenckhoff catheter implantation has a significant influence on long-term catheter outcome. Sterile conditions are essential, and an experienced catheter insertion team is needed. A panel of experts have agreed on five general standards for catheter placement: 1) the deep cuff should be in the anterior abdominal musculature; 2) the subcutaneous cuff should be near the skin surface and not less than 2 cm from the exit site—this is based on clinical experience and a detailed review of exit site and tunnel morphologic characteristics that infers the beneficial role the placement of the external cuff has on decreasing infections when a firm anchorage that prevents piston-like movements is achieved[24]; 3) the catheter exit should be positioned laterally; 4) the exit site should be directed downward or laterally; and 5) the intra-abdominal portion of the catheter should be placed between the visceral and parietal peritoneum and should not be placed in the middle of loops of bowel.[25]

Surgical insertion of catheters (placement by dissection) is the most commonly used placement procedure in clinical practice today. After surgical dissection through the rectus muscle, the catheter is placed in the pelvis under direct visualization. According to the USRDS, before 1990, approximately 88% of catheters were placed by use of this approach.[26] Peritoneoscopic insertion allows direct visualization of the course of the catheter, and in experienced hands there are good results.[27, 28] Blind placement does not allow direct visualization of the catheter or peritoneum. Various devices have been developed to guide the blind insertion of the catheter. This procedure should not be used in markedly obese patients or in those who have had previous abdominal surgery because of the higher risk of complications, such as bowel perforation in patients with unsuspected adhesions. Placement techniques and their complication rates were reviewed by Gokal and colleagues[25] and by Ash.[29] These reviews suggest that in appropriate patients, outcome is not dependent on the technique used for implantation as much as it is dependent on the person (nephrologist or surgeon) who does the catheter insertion. The most important requirement may be to have a trained, knowledgeable, and dedicated catheter insertion team.

Pericatheter dialysate leaks are reduced by using a lateral catheter placement and by positioning the deep cuff on the posterior rectus fascia.[30, 31] Partial omentectomy at the time of catheter placement is not recommended by most reviewers.[25, 29] However, Nicholson and colleagues[32] found a significant improvement in catheter outcome in those patients who had a partial omentectomy at the time of surgical placement. Further studies are needed to confirm this.

## CATHETER BREAK-IN

It is common to flush the peritoneal cavity with 500 to 1000 mL of fluid until clear immediately after placement. Data obtained with dogs suggest that to avoid stimulation of the omentum, it may be best to use normal saline for these flushes.[16] Optimally, peritoneal dialysis should not be initiated until 10 to 14 days after catheter placement to allow wound healing and cuff maturation and to minimize the risk of leaks or infections. Experience from using the Moncrief-Popovich catheter and insertion technique[14] would suggest that the catheter does not need to be flushed during this period, although some authors recommend periodic flushing. Certainly, the catheter does not need to be flushed more than once a week before use. If peritoneal dialysis must be started immediately or before optimal catheter break-in, it is recommended that low-volume dialysis in the supine position be used. After catheter implantation, the exit site should be covered by sterile gauze and a nonocclusive dressing. The dressing should not be changed for several days unless there is evidence of excessive bleeding. To ensure optimal tissue growth during this period, the catheter should be immobilized to prevent trauma to the exit.[33] Sutures at the exit site should be avoided.

## CATHETER SURVIVAL

Transfer from peritoneal dialysis to hemodialysis is thought to be directly due to catheter-related problems in about 20% of the cases.[25] Most of the time, this is due to a catheter infection–related issue, but transfer is due to catheter migration 25% of the time, and 15% of transfers are related to dialysate leaks. CAPD registry data (based on patients undergoing dialysis between January 1981 and August 1987) showed that the cumulative probability of a CAPD patient's experiencing at least one catheter replacement was 32% at 2 years and 42% at 3 years.[34] However, it is likely that catheters removed and not replaced and early catheter loss were not reported. Also, these data were collected before widespread use of swan neck–type catheters, which may improve catheter survival. In a detailed analysis of catheter survival at one center, use of the Missouri swan neck catheter was found to have a 61% survival rate at 3 years.[11] Catheter survival was correlated to the patient's weight, and weight at initiation of dialysis was predictive of catheter loss due to infectious complications.[35] In this study, 2-year catheter survival for patients who were near their ideal body weight at the initiation of dialysis was 56%. Outcome of 213 curled catheters placed either surgically or percutaneously (63%) was analyzed for a 4-year period.[36] Actuarial catheter survival was 61% at 3 years and did not differ with the implantation technique used. Kaplan-Meier survival of 138 surgically placed straight double-cuff catheters at one center was 87%, 69%, and 65% at 1, 2, and 3 years, respectively.[37] At another center using a mixture of straight Tenckhoff and swan neck catheters, the proportion of patients who still had their original catheter after 30 months of follow-up was 82%, and the need for catheter replacement was not related to the type of connection device used.[38]

These studies suggest that technique survival for most catheters is better than 60% at 3 years and that recent designs show a trend for improvement.

## INDICATIONS FOR CATHETER REMOVAL

Indications for catheter removal include malfunction, relapsing or recurrent peritonitis, peritonitis that fails to resolve, chronic exit site or tunnel infection, fungal peritonitis, *Pseudomonas* peritonitis that is slow to respond to therapy, perforated viscus, possibly multiorganism peritonitis, and recovery of renal function.[39]

## CONCLUSIONS

At best, a 3-year catheter survival rate of 80% should be expected, with a minimally acceptable rate of 50% at 1 year.[25] Most centers achieve a better than 60% 3-year catheter survival. Catheter-related infections remain one of the major infectious complications associated with peritoneal dialysis. Recent developments in catheter technology have shown promise and have resulted in some improvement in these complications. Present data would favor the use of two subcutaneous cuffs with a permanent arc in the subcutaneous portion of the catheter to prevent migration and infections. To reduce pain related to the "jet effect" from dialysate inflow and catheter tip pressure on the peritoneum, a curled tip is recommended. Further studies are needed to see whether burying the entire catheter in a subcutaneous tunnel at the time of implantation to allow cuff maturation in a sterile environment is advantageous. Emerging research topics include better fixation of cuffs to tissue with use of fibrin glue or macroscopic and microscopic texturing. The use of more biocompatible materials for catheter construction is also being investigated.

## Dialysis Solutions

The first use of peritoneal dialysis solutions in animals was described by Ganter.[2] Heusser and Werder[40] later described using saline solutions and the addition of glucose to increase the tonicity and achieve ultrafiltration. The next significant development was the substitution of lactate for acetate as the buffer. In 1959, the Don Baxter Company produced the first commercially available fluids in 1-L glass bottles. Maxwell and associates[41] reported using these fluids in clinical practice. These fluids contained various concentrations of $Na^+$, $K^+$, $Cl^-$, $Ca^{2+}$, and $Mg^{2+}$. Except for minor changes, standard peritoneal dialysis solutions have undergone little change in recent years despite concerns about the concentration of certain cations[42] and potential toxicity of these fluids due to bioincompatibility issues.[43] Typical dialysis fluid solute concentrations are found in Table 57–1. The early history of peritoneal dialysis fluid development was reviewed in a previous edition of this text.[5]

### ELECTROLYTES

**Sodium.** $Na^+$ has been added to the dialysis fluid in varying concentrations ranging from 120 to 140 mEq/L. During ultrafiltration, $Na^+$ does not cross the peritoneal

**TABLE 57–1. Available Solution Formulations for CAPD**

| Type of Solution | $Na^+$ | $K^+$ | $Ca^{2+}$ | $Mg^{2+}$ | Lactate | $Cl^-$ |
|---|---|---|---|---|---|---|
| Standard | 132 | 0 | 3.5 | 1.5 | 35 | 102 |
| Low $Mg^{2+}$/high lactate | 132 | 0 | 3.5 | 0.5 | 40 | 96 |
| Low $Ca^{2+}$ | 132 | 0 | 2.5 | 0.5 | 40 | 95 |

From Sorkin MI: Peritoneal dialysis solutions. *In* Nissenson AR, Fine RN (eds): Dialysis Therapy, 2nd ed. Hanley & Belfus, Philadelphia, 1993, pp 156–159.

membrane as readily as water does. Therefore, because the concentration of Na$^+$ in the ultrafiltrate is less than that in serum and may be as low as 70 mEq/L,[44-46] there is a transient decrease in dialysate Na$^+$ concentration during the dwell. This is most pronounced in patients who are slow transporters and when hypertonic dialysis fluids are used. Systemic hypernatremia has been described.[46, 47] To avoid this, most commercially available dialysis fluids now have an Na$^+$ concentration of 132 mEq/L. It may also be prudent to avoid repeated short dwells of exclusively hypertonic dialysis fluids to prevent the development of hypernatremia, unless the Na$^+$ concentration in the dialysis fluids is decreased.[47]

**Potassium.** K$^+$ is not usually added to peritoneal dialysis fluids.[48] With typical CAPD exchanges using dialysis fluid with no added K$^+$, dialysate K$^+$ approaches Gibbs-Donnan equilibrium.[49] Patients tend to lose about 35 mEq/d in the dialysate while maintaining a serum K$^+$ concentration of approximately 4.0 mEq/L.[49] Net ultrafiltration increases K$^+$ removal. However, ultrafiltrate concentration is less than that in serum because of K$^+$ sieving.[50] With rapid cycling, K$^+$ losses are augmented, but maximal rates are about 8 mEq/h.[50] If needed, K$^+$ removal can be slowed by adding K$^+$ to the dialysate.

**Magnesium.** Standard solutions initially had an Mg$^{2+}$ concentration of 1.5 mEq/L. These usually resulted in serum Mg$^{2+}$ concentrations that were slightly elevated in CAPD patients.[51, 52] Toxic levels of hypermagnesemia had not been attributed to the use of standard peritoneal dialysis fluids. However, hypermagnesemia has been implicated in the pathogenesis of renal osteodystrophy, and an improvement in bone disease has been reported in hemodialysis patients after lowering of dialysis fluid Mg$^{2+}$ concentrations and normalizing of serum Mg$^{2+}$ levels.[53] Dialysis solutions with an Mg$^{2+}$ concentration of 0.5 mEq/L are now widely used and have been reported to normalize the serum Mg$^{2+}$ levels and decrease the body burden of Mg$^{2+}$.[42, 52] In addition, dialysis fluids with lower Ca$^{2+}$ and Mg$^{2+}$ concentrations may allow the use of magnesium salts as an additional calcium-free phosphate binder. Solutions with a lower Mg$^{2+}$ concentration have higher lactate concentrations, which tend to result in a high-normal or slightly elevated serum HCO$_3^-$ level.

**Calcium.** It is now recognized that the Ca$^{2+}$ concentration of peritoneal dialysis fluids needs to be tailored for different clinical situations.[54, 55] Unfortunately, phosphorus is only poorly removed by standard peritoneal dialysis.[56] During the late 1970s and early 1980s, the standard of care was to use aluminum-containing phosphate binders along with dietary phosphate restriction to control serum PO$_4^{3-}$ levels in dialysis patients. It was also common practice to treat the tendency for hypocalcemia by using a relatively high Ca$^{2+}$ concentration (3.5 mEq/L) that would facilitate mass transfer of Ca$^{2+}$ from the dialysis fluids to the blood. Now that the toxic effects of aluminum are well recognized,[57, 58] most nephrologists have begun to use calcium salts as their primary phosphate binder.[59, 60] However, when calcium salts are used, hypercalcemia (in 35% to 56% of patients) and metastatic calcification have been frequent complications with dialysis fluids containing Ca$^{2+}$ concentrations of 3.5 mEq/L.[59-63] Because of these complications,

dialysis fluids were developed with a lower, more physiologic Ca$^{2+}$ concentration (2.5 mEq/L).[64, 65] These concentrations are more physiologic compared with the normal serum Ca$^{2+}$ level. These lower Ca$^{2+}$ dialysate fluids also have higher lactate and lower Mg$^{2+}$ concentrations.

As illustrated in Figure 57–3A and B, clinical trials have shown that use of dialysis fluids with a lower Ca$^{2+}$ concentration has been associated with a net Ca$^{2+}$ flux from the blood to the dialysate under most physiologic conditions.[66-69] The short-term use of these fluids has also been associated with an improvement in biochemical parameters (serum Ca$^{2+}$, phosphorus, alkaline phosphatase, and parathyroid hormone levels) in patients who had previously been receiving dialysis fluids with higher Ca$^{2+}$ concentrations.[70-74] In some patients, there has been an improvement in bone histologic features.[75, 76] In patients just starting peritoneal dialysis, similar results were obtained.[55, 77, 78] The lower Ca$^{2+}$ concentrations may also be superior in preventing adynamic bone disease.[55] Further long-term studies are needed, and some researchers have recommended even further decreases in dialysis fluid Ca$^{2+}$ concentrations.

There are no firmly established guidelines for the use of these fluids with lower Ca$^{2+}$ concentration; however, it seems reasonable to use these fluids as the standard dialysis solution for most patients. Their utility lies in the ability to use them in combination with higher doses of calcium-containing oral phosphate binders with a lower risk of hy-

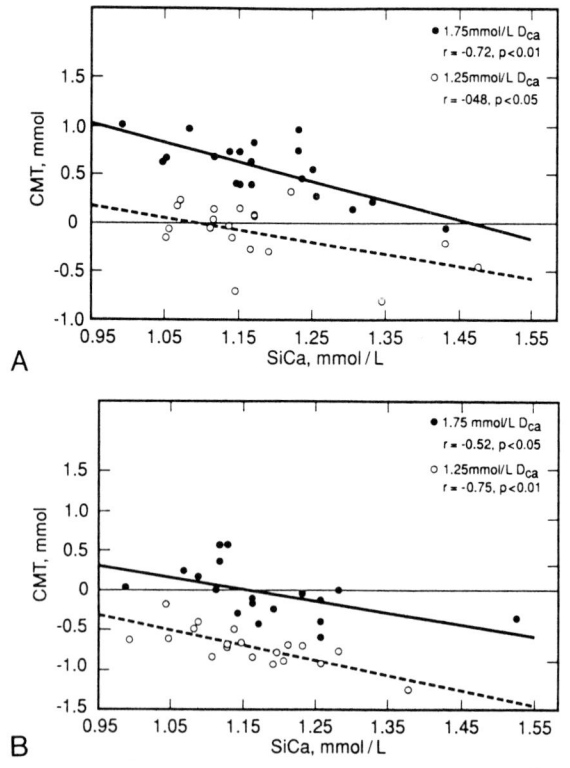

**Figure 57–3.** *A* and *B*. Ca$^{2+}$ mean transfer values (CMT, mmol) plotted against serum Ca$^{2+}$ levels (SiCa) with 1.25 and 1.75 mmol/L Ca$^{2+}$ in 1.5 g/dL dextrose dialysate *(A)* and 4.25 g/dL dextrose dialysate *(B)*. (*A* and *B* from Bender FH, Bernardini J, Piraino B: Calcium mass transfer with dialysate containing 1.25 and 1.75 mmol/L calcium in peritoneal dialysis patients. Am J Kidney Dis 20:367–375, 1992.)

percalcemia or a progressive positive $Ca^{2+}$ balance. However, there is a risk of net $Ca^{2+}$ loss in some patients, resulting in negative $Ca^{2+}$ balance and an increase in parathyroid hormone levels.[79, 80] Therefore, care must be taken to ensure that patients are given supplemental oral calcium (the present standard phosphate binders) and that both serum (or ionized) $Ca^{2+}$ and parathyroid hormone levels are monitored.

## BUFFERS

The present standard peritoneal dialysis fluids use lactate as the buffer. Previous formulations contained acetate. There are no major differences in the relative control of chronic metabolic acidosis between lactate and acetate buffers.[81] However, acetate has been implicated in the etiology of ultrafiltration failure due to sclerosing peritonitis,[82, 83] and clinical observations not confirmed in animal models would suggest that it takes longer for the acetate dialysis fluids to reach physiologic pH during the dwell than it does with lactate.[84, 85] This may be associated with increased pain on inflow, but it may also be of importance when biocompatibility of dialysis solutions is considered.

Commercially available dialysis fluids contain a racemic mixture of both D- and L-lactate. The normal physiologic form of lactic acid is the L-form,[86] and the normal blood level of this isomer is about 300 times that of the D-form.[87] The D-isomer is metabolized at a much slower rate than the L-form. Although both isomers are absorbed and supraphysiologic concentrations of either isomer have been associated with encephalopathy,[88] Nolph and co-workers[89] have shown that despite the high concentration of both isomers in standard dialysis preparations (35 to 40 mmol/L), even with rapid cycling such as with tidal dialysis, the D-lactate levels are only minimally elevated. One significant drawback of lactate-based solutions is that the fluids have an unphysiologically low pH.

A bicarbonate-based buffer system would be preferable for dialysis fluids, but there have been many problems associated with these fluids. These include precipitation of calcium and magnesium carbonates and carmalization of glucose at physiologic pH during sterilization. To avoid these problems, two methods of fluid preparation have been tried: the addition of acetate, lactate, or glycylglycine[90, 91] at the time of manufacture; or the use of a two-chambered bag in which the two solutions are combined at the time of use.[92, 93] Short-term studies in humans have been encouraging[94, 95]; the solutions have been well tolerated, and there have been no significant changes in transport during short-term follow-up.[95] Further studies and an improvement in manufacturing techniques are needed.

## OSMOTIC AGENTS

**Glucose.** Standard dialysis solutions contain glucose as an osmotic agent. This agent has been shown to be safe, effective, readily metabolized, and inexpensive. However, glucose is not an ''ideal'' agent because of the following properties or effects: high absorption[49]; potential for metabolic derangements, such as hyperglycemia, hyperinsulinemia,[96] hyperlipidemia,[97] and obesity[98]; necessity for an

acidic dialysate pH to prevent carmalization; and potential nonenzymatic glycosylation of peritoneal tissue during periods of mesothelial cell loss.[99] Several other substances have been tried as osmotic agents. These include both low-molecular-weight (glycerol, sorbitol, amino acids, xylitol, and fructose) and high-molecular-weight (glucose polymers, gelatin, polycation, dextrans, and polypeptides) agents. Despite theoretic advantages over glucose, there have been significant problems associated with all of these alternative agents (Table 57–2). At present, glucose remains the standard osmotic agent. Current research involving the most promising alternative osmotic agents is discussed in the following.

**Amino Acids.** There is emerging evidence that suggests that protein malnutrition is a significant risk factor for morbidity and mortality in dialysis patients. Therefore, a potential advantage of amino acid–containing fluids would be that the calorie source is protein based. Since the original work by Oreopoulos and co-workers,[100] most[101, 102] but not all[103] studies have shown a benefit in nutritional parameters with amino acid–containing solutions. In a short-term 20-day study of CAPD patients who were thought to be malnourished, there were significant increases in nitrogen balance, serum transferrin concentration, and total protein with the use of amino acid–containing peritoneal dialysis fluids.[104] There is also preliminary evidence that these solutions may ameliorate some of the lipid abnormalities seen in peritoneal dialysis patients.[105, 106] Complications include the development of metabolic acidosis and increases in serum urea nitrogen. In addition, it is uncertain whether

**TABLE 57–2. Alternative Osmotic Agents to Glucose and Their Potential Complications**

| Osmotic Agent | Complications |
|---|---|
| Gelatin | Prolonged half-life and immunogenicity of some preparations |
| Xylitol | Peritoneal pain, lactic acidosis, hyperuricemia, carcinogenicity, and deterioration of liver function |
| Sorbitol | Metabolized through the polyol pathway, which may aggravate neuropathy, lactic acidosis, hyperuricemia, and hyperosmolality |
| Mannitol | Lactic acidosis and hyperuricemia |
| Fructose | Metabolized through the polyol pathway, which may aggravate neuropathy, hypernatremia, lactic acidosis, hyperuricemia, and hypertriglyceridemia |
| Dextrans | Risk of bleeding and systemic absorption |
| Glucose polymers | Prolonged half-life, impaired metabolism in uremia, and potential for high-calorie loads |
| Polyanions | Damage to peritoneum and cardiovascular instability |
| Glycerol | Retention, hypertriglyceridemia, sterile peritonitis, low ultrafiltration capacity, and hyperosmolality |
| Amino acids | Increased concentration of nitrogenous products in blood, increased $H^+$ generation, expensive optimal formulation not yet determined, and difficult to sterilize in combination with glucose |

From Diaz-Buxo JA: Clinical use of peritoneal dialysis. *In* Nissenson AR, Fine RN, Gentile DE (eds): Clinical Dialysis, 2nd ed. Appleton & Lange, Norwalk, CT, 1990, pp 256–300.

long-term use of amino acids will alter peritoneal membrane transport characteristics.

**Polypeptides.** Klein and associates[107] first reported the use of polypeptides as osmotic agents for peritoneal dialysis fluids in 1986. These peptides are derived from enzymatic hydrolysis of milk whey protein. Theoretic advantages of polypeptides over glucose include prolonged ultrafiltration because of a higher average molecular weight due to the presence of ionized branched chains, which provide a higher osmotic pressure on a molar basis, and the potential for providing protein-based calories. These polypeptides are rapidly metabolized to amino acids by plasma proteolytic enzymes after absorption. Preliminary studies have confirmed superior ultrafiltration characteristics and transient increases in serum amino acid levels.[107, 108]

**Glucose Polymers.** Several glucose polymer preparations have been evaluated as a substitute for glucose,[109–111] with the high-molecular-weight polymers attracting the most attention. Major advantages of these solutions over those containing glucose are sustained ultrafiltration and absence of hyperinsulinemia.[112] The major problem encountered so far is caused by accumulation of metabolites such as maltose, which can result in hyperosmolality.[113] However, to date, no symptoms due to hyperosmolality or maltose accumulation have been reported in a preliminary analysis of more than 200 patients using glucose polymer preparations in the United Kingdom.[76]

## BIOCOMPATIBILITY ISSUES

The entire peritoneal environment is exposed to unphysiologic conditions at least four times a day in the typical patient on peritoneal dialysis. Presently available peritoneal dialysis solutions exert biologically and chemically induced effects not only on the peritoneal membrane but also on the resident leukocytes, on the various cytokines produced by these cells and the mesothelium, and on peritoneal macrophage, leukocyte, and lymphocyte function and viability. This concept of biocompatibility is the subject of extensive research. Peritoneal biopsies in patients receiving long-term peritoneal dialysis have revealed ultrastructural changes possibly induced in part by the dialysis solutions themselves (such as glycosylation of capillary proteins in the presence of peritonitis and increased peritoneal glucose transport).[99] Systemic toxic effects and morbidity have been associated with excessive glucose and $Ca^{2+}$ absorption. These and other concerns point to the fact that despite the documented long-term clinical safety and usefulness of presently available peritoneal dialysis solutions, they are in a sense bioincompatible. Properties of an ideal dialysis solution are outlined in Table 57–3.

**Peritoneal Membrane Effects.** Various morphologic changes have been observed in long-term peritoneal dialysis patients.[114] Preliminary in vivo data suggest that some of these alterations are due to long-term use of peritoneal dialysis fluids themselves and not just due to complications such as peritonitis. In vitro observations also support this concept. For example, when mesothelial cells were incubated with various concentrations of glucose, cell growth inhibition and cell damage were documented in a direct dose-dependent manner.[115] Viability of human mesothelial

---

**TABLE 57–3. Ideal Peritoneal Dialysis Solution**

Good solute clearance and ultrafiltration capacity
Necessary solutes supplied and uremic toxins removed
Nutrition supplied
Isosmolar solution; normal pH; bicarbonate as buffer
Minimal absorption of osmotic agent
Antibacterial and antifungal properties
Membrane-biocompatible

Balfe JW, Qamar I: The use of alternative peritoneal dialysis solutions in pediatric patients. Perit Dial Int 13(suppl 2):S95–S97, 1993.

---

cell monolayers was also reduced after 3 hours of exposure to dialysis solutions.[116] Furthermore, mesothelial function may be altered by indirect effects of dialysis solutions, such as the effect these solutions have on the production of tumor necrosis factor, which causes injury to mesothelial monolayers.[117] Di Paolo and co-workers[118] have shown that bicarbonate-containing fluids were less likely to inhibit cell growth, cause morphologic alterations, reduce phospholipid secretion, or induce interleukin-1 production than lactate-containing solutions were. Breborowicz[119] pointed out, however, that many of these original in vitro studies did not take into account the change in the composition of dialysis fluids toward a more physiologic state that occurs during the dwell and the effects this change may have on in vitro findings. Therefore, more in vitro evaluation is needed. Using mesothelial cell imprints and histochemical techniques, Gotloib and colleagues[120] were able to document similar mesothelial cell injury in mice exposed to daily dialysis, which supports earlier in vitro observations.

**Host Defense.** Peritoneal dialysis patients are at constant risk for peritonitis. To minimize risk and facilitate cure if peritonitis occurs, ideal peritoneal dialysis fluids must have minimal or no unwanted effects on resident peritoneal white blood cell viability or function. Unfortunately, this is not the case. First, peritoneal macrophages, neutrophils, lymphocytes, and opsonins are continually diluted and removed by the process of peritoneal dialysis. Second, the unphysiologic pH, osmolality, and glucose concentrations of standard dialysis fluids have been shown to inhibit fundamental white blood cell functions both in vivo and in vitro. Finally, production and secretion of the various inflammatory mediators of host defense are altered by dialysis fluids. Detailed information on these effects is available elsewhere.[121] An important issue in biocompatibility, therefore, is the development of peritoneal dialysis fluids that reduce these adverse effects on host defense.

De Fijter and co-workers[122] have shown less impaired phagocytic activity and chemoluminescence when peritoneal macrophages were isolated from polyglucose-based solutions than from standard glucose-based ones. Similarly, production of tumor necrosis factor-α and interleukin-6 was less suppressed when peripheral leukocytes were exposed to glucose polymer or physiologic pH–containing solutions than to standard low-pH, glucose-containing solutions.[123] These experiments have demonstrated the importance not only of the osmotic agent but also of the pH to the biocompatibility of dialysis fluids. Lactate has been shown to have an additive effect to low pH on reducing polymorphonuclear chemoluminescence, perhaps owing to a decrease in intracellular free radical production.[124] Bicarbonate-based solutions were found to have less of an inhibitory effect on peripheral blood cytokine release than lactate-containing solutions with a similar pH.[125] In addition, lower $Ca^{2+}$ concentrations of culture media have been shown to decrease macrophage function[126, 127] and may predispose to peritonitis,[127, 128] although this has not been substantiated in other clinical trials.[129, 130]

**Conclusions.** These data show that although presently commercially available dialysis solutions based on lactate and glucose have provided adequate treatment of ESRD for thousands of patients, further improvements that address biocompatibility issues are needed.

# The Peritoneal Membrane

## ANATOMY

The peritoneal membrane is the primary interface between the blood and dialysate compartments. It is across this membrane that water and solute transport must occur. This membrane is composed of two principal parts: 1) the parietal peritoneum, which covers the inner surface of the abdominal and pelvic walls including the diaphragm; and 2) the visceral peritoneum, which covers the visceral organs including the intra-abdominal portion of the gastrointestinal tract, liver, and spleen and forms the omentum and the visceral mesentery, where it reflects over and connects the loops of bowel. The total surface area of the peritoneal membrane (parietal and visceral) is thought to approximate the body surface area in most adults (1 to 2 m²).[131, 132] The parietal peritoneum accounts for about 10% of the total; the visceral peritoneum accounts for the remaining 90%.[133] Children have a proportionately larger peritoneal surface area than that of most adults.[134] This membrane is continuous and forms a closed space in males. In females, it is continuous with the mucous membrane of the fallopian tubes. The intra-abdominal opening of these tubes is normally collapsed, and hence there is usually no free communication between the peritoneal space and the exterior. However, this potential anatomic opening allows the possibility of communication between the intrauterine and intra-abdominal space in females (see later). The peritoneal cavity usually contains about 100 mL or less of fluid; however, a normal-sized adult can usually tolerate 2 L of fluid or more without discomfort or compromise of pulmonary function.

From the perspective of peritoneal dialysis, important anatomic components of the peritoneal membrane include the mesothelial cells, an underlying basement membrane, the interstitium, the microcirculation, and the visceral lymphatics. A previous edition of this text includes a more detailed discussion of the peritoneal anatomy.[135]

**The Mesothelium.** The mesothelium is a continuous monolayer of flattened cells about 0.5 μm thick. The free surface area of the mesothelium is covered by numerous microvilli.[136] These microvilli markedly increase the actual surface area. The cells have tortuous boundaries, which increases the area of contact between them. There are many tight junctions connecting adjacent cells at their luminal surface.[137] On the antiluminal surface, there are many open intercellular channels approximately 50 nm wide. In some areas, especially in the subdiaphragmatic region, tight junctions are absent, resulting in the formation of stomas.[138] In these areas, there are some openings in the basement membrane, which otherwise tends to be homogeneous,[139] allowing direct contact between the peritoneal cavity and the diaphragmatic lymphatics. Numerous anionic binding sites have been demonstrated on the luminal surface of peritoneal lymphatics after injection of cationic ferritin in mice, especially in the subdiaphragmatic region.[140] Ultrastructural examination of the peritoneum of normal rabbits after intravenous injections of iron dextran, an electron-dense tracer, revealed that the dextran appeared in intracellular vesicles. This observation supports the hypothesis that vesicular transport plays a role in the transport of high-molecular-weight substances across the peritoneum.[141]

The mesothelial cells are ultrastructurally similar to type II pneumonocytes found in the pulmonary alveoli.[142] The mesothelium also contains lamellar bodies identical to those in type II pneumonocytes.[143, 144] These cells may secrete a surfactant-like lubrication for the peritoneum.

**Basement Membrane.** A homogeneous basement membrane underlies the mesothelial cells. In animals, it is from 25 to 40 μm thick. There are some openings in the basement membrane, particularly in the diaphragmatic peritoneum. Some studies indicate that the basement membrane is absent under the omental mesothelium.

**The Interstitium.** The interstitium is the primary supporting structure of the peritoneum and is composed primarily of a mucopolysaccharide matrix. It contains bundles of collagen fibers, blood vessels, the lymphatics, occasional macrophages, and fibroblasts.

**The Blood Vessels.** Total splanchnic blood flow in normal adult humans at rest ranges from 1000 to 2400 mL/min.[145] The blood supply to the visceral and parietal membranes arises from two different sources. The visceral peritoneal membrane is supplied by the celiac and mesenteric arteries; the venous drainage enters the portal vein. The parietal mesothelium is supplied by the circumflex, iliac, lumbar, intercostal, and epigastric arteries; the venous drainage of the parietal mesentery empties directly into the systemic circulation, bypassing the hepatic portal system. An important clinical implication of this anatomy is that the absorption of any drug from the visceral peritoneum results in rapid first-pass metabolism by the liver.

Most capillaries from human parietal[146] and visceral[147] peritoneum are of the continuous type. However, biopsy specimens of parietal peritoneum from normal female New Zealand rabbits have revealed occasional fenestrated capillaries.[148] The frequency of these appears to be low in human parietal peritoneum (1.7% of the total).[148] The density of the vascular bed varies in different parts of the peritoneum. The capillary walls are believed to contain two distinct pore sizes,[149] with the largest pores located primarily at the venular end and the smaller pores at the arteriolar end. Although high concentrations of fixed negative charges have been found on the surface of fenestrated capillaries in other microvascular beds,[150] the possible presence of such fixed charges on human parietal mesothelial cells remains to be demonstrated. Theoretically, these charges should discriminate against passage of anionic macromolecules, such as has been demonstrated for the glomerulus. Although this view is supported by an abstract,[151] other investigators have demonstrated in rabbit peritoneum that the mesothelium acts as a barrier to positively charged macromolecules.[152] A more complete description of the transperitoneal transport of charged macromolecules will require additional studies.

**Peritoneal Lymphatics.** As in most body tissue, there is a network of lymphatic vessels that aid in fluid and solute removal from the interstitium. This lymphatic network is well developed and extensive in the subdiaphragmatic area.[138, 153] These lymphatics are thought to play an important role in the removal of fluid, solute, and macromolecules from the peritoneal cavity.[154] Lymphatics are also present in the submucosal layers of most of the visceral mesothelium except that overlying normal human jejunum.[155] It is uncertain what role these visceral lymphatics play in fluid and solute transport in humans. Clefts of lymphatic endothelial intercellular junctions and the luminal aspect of lymphatic endothelial cells have been shown to be densely populated with anionic binding sites. These are thought to play a role in regulating the intercellular passage of fluids and solute.

## ANATOMIC FINDINGS IN PERITONEAL DIALYSIS PATIENTS

World literature and clinical observations by surgeons experienced with CAPD patients suggest that the peritoneal surface develops a diffuse opacification at times with local accentuation.[99] In gross appearance, this can progress to the "tanned" peritoneal syndrome or, in advanced stages, to sclerosing encapsulating peritoneal fibrosis.[156] A review of microscopic examinations of randomly collected peritoneal tissue by the International Peritoneal Biopsy Registry would indicate that the process of continuous peritoneal dialysis may induce significant ultrastructural deviations from normal in both the mesothelium and the underlying stroma.[114] These include loss of microvilli, hyperplasia of the rough endoplasmic reticulum, and the formation of unusual surface protuberances. There is also some disorganization of the normal collagen fibers, expansion of the underlying matrix ground substance,[157] and occasional reduplication of the basal lamina.[158] An increase in fibrosis, when it occurs, is usually florid and results in an obvious increase in the thickness of the stroma, turning some parts of the stroma into a "cellular desert" where remesothelialization has failed to occur.[114] Interestingly, the cytoplasmic inclusions characteristic of uremic patients before the beginning of peritoneal dialysis[157] and in the pericardium of patients with uremic pericarditis are not found in long-term peritoneal dialysis patients, which suggests that they are a marker of uremic serositis.[114] In most patients, these changes are minimal, even in those who have been undergoing peritoneal dialysis for up to 10 years. However, the reaction of the peritoneal mesothelium and underlying stroma to the stress of continuous dialysis is likely to result in a spectrum of changes ranging from the minimal ones clinically associated with only peritoneal opacification to replacement of the peritoneal membrane with dense fibrous tissue causing sclerosing peritonitis.[159] Marked changes are more likely in patients with histories of recurring or severe peritonitis. Most patients without a history of peritonitis show minor or no alterations even after many years.[157]

The diabetiform nature of capillary basement membrane lesions would logically incriminate dialysate glucose. Although there are only minimal changes noted in tissue from patients with no history of peritonitis or in those who have had only mild cases of peritonitis, some of them have been using CAPD for up to 10 years. Marked changes are seen in nondiabetic patients with multiple episodes of peritonitis. This change could be from peritonitis itself or a result of the increase in glucose flux during an episode of peritonitis. During episodes of peritonitis, there is loss of surface microvilli and the development of prominent intercellular gaps.[160, 161] These ultrastructural changes were clinically associated with increased permeability and loss of ultrafiltration due to increased glucose absorption and the early loss of an osmotic pressure gradient for ultrafiltration. Ultrastructurally, this may result in nonenzymatic glycosylation of proteins.

## CONTRIBUTION OF PERITONEAL STRUCTURES TO DIALYSIS

The relative contribution to overall solute clearance from each part (parietal versus visceral) of the peritoneal surface in humans is uncertain. Given that the visceral peritoneum has a much larger surface area than the parietal peritoneum, it would seem that the contribution to overall solute clearance from the parietal peritoneum would be modest. Interestingly, studies in animals have demonstrated that the absorption of glucose and other metabolites[162–165] from the peritoneal cavity is only minimally reduced by omentectomy, mesenterectomy, or evisceration. However, these studies were limited primarily to the study of small-solute transport from dialysate to blood. Fox and co-workers[165] have shown that transperitoneal solute exchange (blood to dialysate) may not be significantly altered after evisceration in rabbits. These observations may be of clinical importance because conventional wisdom would suggest that loss of 50% of the peritoneal surface is an absolute contraindication to peritoneal dialysis. There is, however, a report of an infant with acute renal failure having undergone successful peritoneal dialysis after virtually complete resection of the small intestine.[166]

It is tempting to conclude from these experiments in animals that the visceral peritoneum has only a minor role in governing solute transport during peritoneal dialysis. However, alternative explanations must be considered. For example, the visceral peritoneum may be the predominant transport surface in intact animals, and normally only a portion of all the surface area of the peritoneum is in contact with dialysate. Evisceration may expose a greater amount of parietal peritoneum surface area[162] to contact with dialysate. This hypothesis may explain the previously noted discrepancy between estimates of total peritoneal surface area and functional peritoneal surface area.[167] Alternatively, evisceration could result in a change in the intraabdominal pressure with resultant change in transport[168] or a relative change in the contribution from other visceral structures.

Blood flow to the liver has been shown to increase to two to three times control values after evisceration in rats.[163] Pietrzak and colleagues[169] have suggested that the liver may be an important transport surface during peritoneal dialysis. This is supported by Flessner and Dedrick,[170] who have suggested that the peritoneal surface of the liver is normally responsible for 45% of the total mass transfer area. Taken together, these and other studies suggest that the parietal peritoneum may be more important than was originally thought, and future areas of research that can augment dialysate contact with that surface may increase overall clearance rates.

# THE PERITONEUM AS A DIALYSIS SYSTEM

## Resistance to Salt and Water Transport

If effective surface area were the only limiting factor for solute transport in peritoneal dialysis, then transport of these solutes should be closely related to their free diffusion coefficients in water. This is not the case, particularly for macromolecules.[171] In vivo, the measured restriction in transport of serum proteins is not what would be expected on the basis of their free diffusion coefficient in water alone. Therefore, an additional barrier that is intrinsic to the peritoneal membrane itself must be present. In attempting to define this barrier, one must consider the potential resistance sites solutes must cross as they move from the peritoneal capillaries into the peritoneal cavity. These potential resistance sites include 1) fluid films within the capillary lumen; 2) the endothelial layer (0.5 μm); 3) the capillary basement membrane (0.2 to 0.5 μm); 4) the interstitium (0.1 to 100 μm); 5) the mesothelial layer (0.9 μm); and 6) fluid films within the peritoneal cavity.[172]

The exact route taken by solutes as they pass from the blood into the peritoneum has not been well established. It is known that solute transport occurs by both diffusive and convective forces (discussed later). The mass transport barrier appears to offer little resistance to solute transport by diffusion but seems to offer significant resistance to solute transport by convection. This is especially true when ultrafiltration is driven by small osmotic solutes but is less significant when ultrafiltration is driven by hydraulic pressure.[173, 174]

Intracapillary fluid films are thought to exert little resistance, especially for low-molecular-weight solutes, because these fluid films represent only a short distance for the molecules to pass through.[175, 176] The capillary endothelium seems to serve as a selective barrier to solute transport. Experimentally, the endothelium acts as a low-resistance barrier to low-molecular-weight solutes with molecular weights up to the size of albumin but then begins to offer significant resistance as the molecular weight increases further.[177] Grotte[178] first attempted to define solute transport and proposed a "two-pore" model of solute transport across the endothelium. This model suggests that the transport of solute occurs through small pores with a diameter

of 30 to 45 Å.[179] These pores may be represented by gaps in the zonula occludens of the interendothelial clefts. In addition, a small number of large pores are thought to facilitate high-molecular-weight solute transport[178, 180] but have not been identified morphologically. Possible candidates for these large pores are thought to be either channels of fused vesicles or interendothelial gaps.[149] Fox and coworkers[181] have shown that transport of macromolecules in vivo occurs through large gaps near the venules. Pappenheimer[182] has suggested that less than 0.2% of the luminal surface is made up of these gaps. If interendothelial gaps represent the most effective pathway for large-solute movement across the capillary walls, then the effective pore area of the peritoneal dialysis system is small. Endothelial cell surface charges may also influence the transport of charged solutes.

The capillary basement membrane seems to assert little effect on diffusion of low-molecular-weight solutes,[183] although anionic sites predominantly composed of heparin sulfate and chondroitin sulfate, which could theoretically inhibit transport of charged solutes, are regularly found in basement membranes of microvasculature.[184] These anionic sites are particularly abundant in fenestrated capillaries, some of which have been identified in human parietal and subdiaphragmatic peritoneum.[185]

The interstitium represents the longest distance that solutes have to traverse.[175] There is increasing evidence to suggest that the interstitium and the fluid films of the peritoneal cavity are the major resistance sites for urea and low-molecular-weight solute transport.[186, 187] The interstitium is thought to be represented by a gel-like mucopolysaccharide matrix interspaced with a free fluid phase containing aqueous channels.[188] Small solutes may pass through these channels. Although these channels may normally offer little resistance to transport, hypertonic dialysis may dehydrate the interstitium, shortening the distance the solute must traverse but making the channels more tortuous and therefore increasing the resistance.[188, 189] In addition, fixed charges on collagen or mucopolysaccharide molecules within the interstitium may influence transport of charged solutes. These ionic charges are thought to restrict both diffusive and convective transport of charged solutes across the peritoneal membrane. For example, diffusive rates of transport for $K^+$, $Li^+$, and $PO_4^{3-}$ are slower than the diffusive transport of uncharged solutes the same size.[190]

The mesothelium appears to be more permeable than the endothelium, possibly because of larger intercellular gaps.[191] It is thought that transport through the mesothelium is through these gaps and numerous intracellular vesicles. However, the permeability is not uniform, and visceral mesothelium may be more permeable than parietal mesothelium.[192] Studies of transport across isolated mesentery suggest that the mesothelial cells contribute some resistance to transport.[193] Other studies have shown that permeation of solutes into the isolated hemidiaphragm is lower in areas covered by mesothelium than in bare areas. This impedance is offset by maneuvers that alter the oxidative metabolism and ATP production of mesothelial cells,[192] which suggests that oxidative metabolism is linked to transport across these cells and that pharmacologic manipulation could alter this transport.

Experimental data suggest that intraperitoneal fluid channels also limit solute transport. The many folds of the mesentery result in the formation of many relatively wide and stagnant intraperitoneal fluid films of dialysate during peritoneal dialysis, which substantially limit transport.[194] This is unlike the conditions during conventional hemodialysis, in which the dialysate channels are small and dialysate flow is rapid.[195] In vitro experiments using hollow-fiber dialyzers that simulate conditions of peritoneal dialysis are not able to achieve the clearances obtained with conventional hemodialysis, further suggesting that fluid films limit transport of solutes in peritoneal dialysis.[176] Rapid cycling seems to have little influence on these fluid films,[194, 196, 197] whereas abdominal compression in rats has been shown to increase clearances perhaps by increasing the surface area that is in contact with dialysate.[198]

## SUMMARY OF RESISTANCE SITES FOR SMALL SOLUTES

Even with rapid cycling, the maximal urea clearance achieved clinically in most humans with peritoneal dialysis is about 40 mL/min.[194, 196] This maximal clearance is little changed (20%) even with the intraperitoneal use of potent vasodilators,[199, 200] which theoretically would increase both the number of capillaries perfused and capillary permeability, thus minimizing any endothelial resistance. Estimations of peritoneal capillary blood flow using peritoneal clearances of carbon dioxide gas in humans and hydrogen gas in rabbits are two to three times this maximal urea clearance,[175] which suggests that small-solute clearances are not blood flow dependent[175, 201] and that even in severe shock there would be only a modest reduction in observed clearance.[202] These data indirectly suggest that the major resistance sites for small-solute clearance are the interstitium and intraperitoneal fluid films.

## SUMMARY OF RESISTANCE SITES FOR LARGE SOLUTES

In contrast to the data for low-molecular-weight solutes, it appears that the major resistance site for large solutes is the peritoneal microcirculation. This is based on the following indirect evidence. First, after intravenous injection of fluorescent tagged albumin, there is slow labeling of the interstitium unless agents are administered that increase vascular permeability. The increase in vascular permeability markedly increases albumin uptake.[177] Second, there is a proportionally larger increase in inulin clearance after intravenous injection of vasoactive drugs than there is for urea.[199] Third, peritoneal inflammation, which is associated with vasodilatation, is known to increase protein losses more than the change in small-solute transport.[203, 204] Finally, intraperitoneal nitroprusside, which enhances venular permeability, markedly increases protein loss.

## MODELS OF PERITONEAL TRANSPORT

The peritoneal membrane and its vascular and lymphatic systems constitute a complex interactive and changing membrane for dialysis. Furthermore, this membrane is alive and likely to change as its environment changes. Various physiologic, pharmacologic, and morphologic studies described here and elsewhere in the literature have been able to define some but not all of the transport properties of the peritoneum. Despite this complexity, investigators have attempted to characterize peritoneal membrane transport properties in terms of classic membrane physiology using mathematic models. These models can help the nephrologist understand peritoneal solute and water transport and guide in individualizing prescriptions for patients.

It is known that solute clearance is dependent on diffusive and convective transport. These models define transport by use of various phenomenologic mathematic coefficients to describe known clinical and experimental observations, such as diffusive or convective transport. Therefore, virtually every element of experimental and clinical data taken separately can be defined by a simple semipermeable membrane model. However, when they are considered in total, the assembled clinical observations and laboratory findings cannot be explained in terms of simple membrane physiology. Modification of these models has allowed consideration of the effect of lymphatic flow, ultrafiltration, and the apparently heterogeneous nature of the peritoneal membrane pores. These models closely approximate most but not all transport properties of the membrane.

The simplest models consider the peritoneum in terms of a homogeneous membrane that separates two well-mixed fluid compartments.[205–207] As such, the peritoneal membrane represents both anatomic structures (such as the capillary endothelium, the interstitium, and the mesothelium) and the unstirred layers of fluid within both compartments. Any heterogeneities between tissues are ignored. Examples of these are the models of Randerson-Farrell,[208] Pyle-Popovich,[209, 210] Garred and co-workers,[211] and Henderson and Nolph.[212] Because these models are based on homogeneous membrane physiology and make various assumptions, they best describe certain but not all aspects of membrane transport.

In addition to the homogeneous membrane models, there are also "distributed" models of peritoneal transport,[213–215] which can predict the kinetics of solute transport as well as the homogeneous membrane models. These were later modified to include convective transport.[214] The major difference between the distributed models and the homogeneous membrane models is that for the distributed model, it is assumed that the barrier separating blood from dialysate is not homogeneous but is made up of distinct elements including the capillaries and the interstitium and that the blood phase is distributed within the peritoneal interstitium.

For any of these mathematic models to be valid, it must account for the following known properties of solute transport: 1) the mass transport barrier is open to solute transport by diffusion, but 2) it is tight to osmotically induced convective solute transport, whereas 3) it is open to hydraulically induced convective solute transport. To address these variables, the original models were modified. New approaches include models of diffusive transport evaluated during periods of isovolemic dialysis, which eliminate the need for any assumptions to be made about the sieving properties of the membrane.[216, 217] Others include the heteroporous model,[218] the dual-barrier model,[178] and the triple-barrier models for solute transport.[219] Assumptions made in formulating these models include pore size and number, effects of ultrafiltration, lymphatic absorption of fluid and solute, and any resistance to solute transport during convection. As new experimental data that examined certain aspects of overall transport were obtained, the models were modified by adding new mathematic coefficients to the equations. An example is the modification of the heteroporous model, which initially assumed the presence of two pores but is now based on the assumption that there are three different pore types involved in solute and water transport.[220]

A quantitative and systematic comparison of most of the early models of solute and water transport by Waniewski and colleagues[221] has pointed out that none of them accurately modeled all aspects of transport. This review suggested that further modifications of the pore theory of transport physiology were needed. Greater than predicted increases in the ratio of dialysate to protein concentrations were seen, suggesting that convection is important for protein transport and that this convection prevailed early in the dwell. The classic Pyle-Popovich model, modified by Vonesh and co-workers,[222] of transport and ultrafiltration can be made to fit observed data of patients when glucose is the osmotic agent. However, as opposed to the three-pore model for peritoneal transport, it does not accurately predict volume versus dwell time data when higher molecular weight osmotic agents are used[223] (Fig. 57–4). This would suggest that the three-pore model best fits experimental and observed data. At present, although these models are stimulating, further work is needed to clarify their correctness, and their clinical use is limited because of the large number of unknown variables. It appears that the model that best

accounts for accepted experimental and clinical observations is the heteroporous membrane model.[218] In this model, the capillary wall is thought to contain two distinct pores[149] through which transport occurs. Diffusion is postulated to take place through large pores located at the venular end of the capillaries,[218] whereas convection occurs through small pores located primarily at the arteriolar end of the capillaries. Convection is confined to the small pores because it is hypothesized that the large pores are so large that glucose does not exert an effective osmotic force across them. Hence, the membrane appears permeable to diffusion through the large venular pores but less permeable for convective transport through the small arteriolar pores. To explain the observed differences in convective transport induced by osmotic versus hydraulic forces, it is postulated that the mesothelium has some open areas in locations such as the subdiaphragmatic area and the anterior abdominal wall.[224] These areas would readily permit hydraulically driven egress of macromolecules[224, 225] but still allow the mesothelium to be resistant to osmotically driven convective solute transport.

To better describe the transvascular and transperitoneal exchange of large and small solutes including ultrafiltration characteristics, the two-pore theory was further modified by postulating the existence of a third pore. According to this model, the peritoneum behaves as if there were a large number of small pores responsible for 90% to 95% of the peritoneal ultrafiltration coefficient, a small number of large pores responsible for about 5% of the ultrafiltration coefficient, and a small number of transcellular pathways accounting for about 1% or 2% of the total peritoneal ultrafiltration coefficient.[220] The three-pore model reviewed by Rippe[223] yields realistic estimations of small-solute reflection coefficients, macromolecule transfer, and effects of

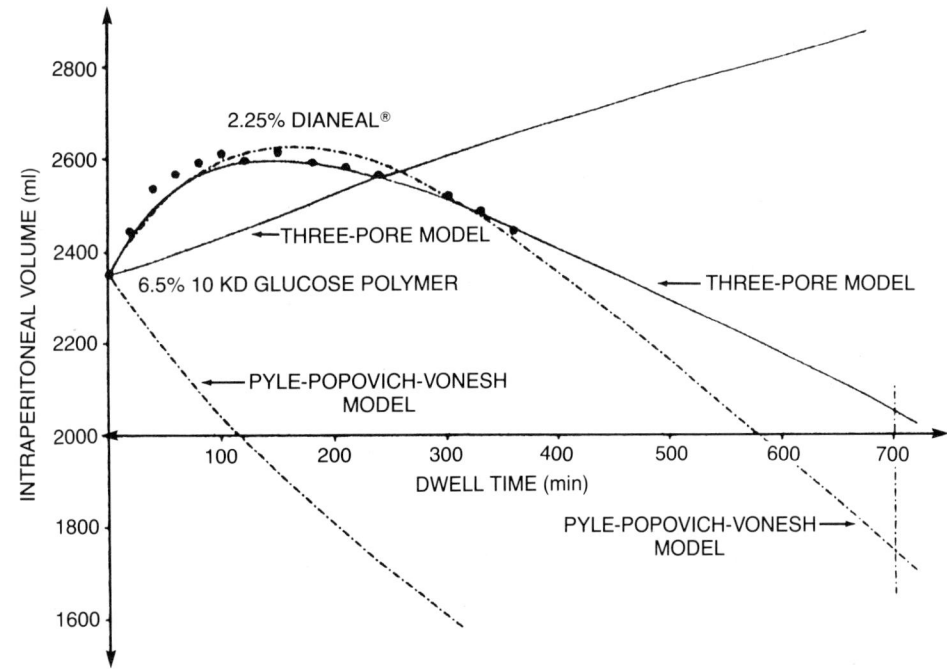

**Figure 57–4.** Computer-simulated intraperitoneal volume versus time curves for 2.25% Dianeal and a 6.5% 10-kd glucose polymer solution using the Pyle-Popovich model as modified by Vonesh and co-workers[222] *(dashed lines)* and the three-pore model *(solid lines)*. The ordinate scale denotes intraperitoneal volume (drained volume plus residual volume). The Pyle-Popovich model yields an unrealistic ultrafiltration profile for the glucose polymer solution. (From Rippe B: A three-pore model of peritoneal transport. Perit Dial Int 13:S35–S38, 1993.)

lymphatic absorption and ultrafiltration profiles observed clinically even when high-molecular-weight solutes are used as osmotic agents.

## Solute Transport by Diffusion

Diffusion, defined as that tendency for solutes to disperse themselves within the available space, is the most important mechanism responsible for solute transport into the peritoneum. The amount of solute that can pass through a membrane by diffusion per unit of time is dependent on the surface area of that membrane and its intrinsic permeability. In peritoneal dialysis, the diffusive clearance of any solute is dependent on the peritoneal membrane surface area, intrinsic permeability of the membrane, dialysate flow, concentration gradients, and time allowed for transport. Overall solute clearance can never exceed the lowest of these parameters.[226] It is estimated that the peritoneal surface area is about 1 m² in adults.[131, 132, 227] However, when the in vivo solute transport of urea and inulin obtained during peritoneal dialysis was compared with that obtained during hemodialysis with a cuprophane dialyzer designed to simulate the typical peritoneal surface area, the clearances were much less, suggesting that the "effective" peritoneal surface area was less than the measured surface area.[167, 228] The effective peritoneal surface area is primarily determined by the number of capillaries that are perfused. This area is not a constant and is influenced by splanchnic blood volume[169, 200, 229] and the presence of intraperitoneal dialysate.[230] Under normal circumstances, only about 25% of the peritoneal capillaries are perfused.[231] Measurements of mass transfer area coefficients (MTACs),[211] dialysance,[232] and dialysate/plasma (D/P) ratios of solutes[233] are an attempt to classify membrane transport characteristics in individual patients.

For a typical patient undergoing continuous peritoneal dialysis, dialysate flow rates are markedly lower than capillary blood flow or membrane transport rates, and these therapies are therefore dialysate flow limited. Clinically, as one tries to increase dialysate flow in an attempt to maximize diffusion (by maintaining a concentration gradient), the maximally effective dialysate flow rate becomes limited by loss of peritoneal membrane contact time during periods of inflow and drainage.[234] Thus, as dialysate flows increase above 3.5 L/h, there can be a decrease in clearance of small solutes. Higher urea clearances have been achieved by use of higher dialysate flow rates without increasing inflow or outflow times in a continuous flow system.[197, 235–237] Problems with such a technique include factors of the patient's convenience; the cost of the large volumes of dialysate needed; dialysis channeling, which limits mixing[235]; and abdominal pain and catheter obstruction.[238]

Free diffusion across capillary walls becomes relatively more restricted as the square root of the molecular mass of the solute increases.[179] Accordingly, peritoneal permeability to solutes has been shown to decrease as the square root of their molecular weight increases.[190] Dialysate temperature does influence solute movement into the peritoneal cavity, and higher dialysate temperatures do seem to enhance solute transfer by diffusion.[238] However, no significant differences in clearance were found with use of dialysate kept at room temperature versus body temperature.[239] Dialysate pH may influence clearance by converting charged particles into their less diffusible anionic salt, therefore keeping the diffusible concentration low in the dialysate and thus enhancing further transport.[240, 241] Protein binding of solute in the dialysate can also increase clearance, again presumably by maintaining a low concentration of the more diffusible unbound form of solute in the dialysate.[242]

Diffusive and convective transport properties for creatinine, p-aminohippurate, and neutral dextran across the peritoneal cavity in both the blood to dialysate direction and the dialysate to blood direction were studied.[243] These studies concluded that the main transport of these solutes across the peritoneal membrane was different in each direction. The authors thought that the difference in transport from the dialysate to the blood was due to contributions from lymphatic absorption. Transport from the blood to the dialysate can occur only across the peritoneal membrane, whereas transport from the dialysate to the blood can occur either directly across the peritoneal membrane or into tissue surrounding the peritoneum and ultimately into the lymphatics.

In conclusion, the experimental data, clinical observations, and data from mathematic models would suggest that the peritoneal membrane is open to transport by diffusion. This transport appears to occur through large pores located near the venular end of the capillaries.

## Ultrafiltration

Ultrafiltration, that is, the transcapillary movement of fluids, has been reviewed by Renkin.[244] The attainment of a minimal daily amount of net ultrafiltration is an important clinical consideration because of the obvious necessity to maintain water balance in patients with ESRD. Net ultrafiltration is achieved clinically by creating an osmotic pressure gradient between the blood and the dialysate. Currently available dialysis fluids achieve this by adding various concentrations of glucose to the solutions. Thus, before its absorption from the peritoneal cavity, glucose exerts an effective osmotic force that drives ultrafiltration. In addition, solutes present in body fluids can be swept along with the bulk solvent flow even in the absence of a concentration difference for net diffusion, contributing to overall solute clearance. This contribution to net solute clearance has been termed "solvent drag" or "convection."

### PHYSIOLOGY

In addition to ultrafiltration, absorption of fluid from the peritoneal cavity also occurs. This is mainly due to absorption of fluid by the peritoneal lymphatics. Intraperitoneal volume at any time is therefore determined by the relative magnitudes of transcapillary ultrafiltration and lymphatic absorption. Net ultrafiltration at the end of any dwell is traditionally defined as the difference between drained volume and instilled volume. This definition assumes that the residual volume in any patient is constant, which is often not the case.[245, 246] For day-to-day clinical practice, this variation is not of significance, but it is important to know the residual intraperitoneal volume during experimental conditions attempting to define ultrafiltration rates.

According to the Starling law, transcapillary ultrafiltration is dependent on the hydraulic permeability of the peritoneal membrane, surface area, and the transmembrane pressure gradients. The capillary hydraulic pressure, the colloid osmotic pressure, and the crystalloid osmotic pressure all contribute to transmembrane pressure gradients. Values for capillary hydraulic pressure and colloid osmotic pressure are difficult to measure in vivo. Because the average albumin concentration in dialysate is only about 1% of that in plasma, only a small osmotic pressure gradient is generated, and thus the colloid osmotic pressure gradient opposes net ultrafiltration.[247] Hydraulic pressure in the peritoneal cavity varies, depending on posture and activities, and therefore could affect transcapillary ultrafiltration by affecting transmembrane pressure.[248] Because of this influence hydraulic pressure variations can have on transmembrane pressure, conditions must be kept constant when transcapillary ultrafiltration rates are evaluated and compared.

Crystalloid osmotic pressure is dependent on the difference in the number of solutes in the solutions under consideration. For a given solution, the driving force for ultrafiltration is greatest across an ideal semipermeable membrane, that is, one that is impermeable to solute. The driving force for ultrafiltration decreases as the membrane becomes more permeable to solutes and as the osmotic gradient diminishes. Therefore, because glucose is not completely rejected by the peritoneal membrane and is slowly reabsorbed from the dialysate, the driving force for ultrafiltration is less than across an ideal membrane and will change in time. Net ultrafiltration is therefore maximal during the first few minutes of the dwell period and then progressively decreases during the dwell as glucose is absorbed. Depending on the rate of absorption of glucose and the length of the dwell as glucose is absorbed and osmotic equilibrium is approached, the transmembrane pressure becomes negligible and ultrafiltration ceases. After this time, there is a net absorption of fluid and solutes probably through subdiaphragmatic, lymphatic, and transcapillary osmotic pressure gradients into the blood (back-filtration).

## MODELS OF ULTRAFILTRATION

To model mechanisms of ultrafiltration in peritoneal dialysis, one must first consider that solutes removed by convection are not always removed in amounts per volume of ultrafiltrate equal to their concentrations in extracellular fluids.[46, 249–251] This net sieving effect has been demonstrated for neutral as well as for charged solutes and is progressively more restrictive as molecular weight increases.[251] Transmembrane pressure gradients can be precisely calculated only if the various osmotically active substances are completely rejected by the membrane.[219] Therefore, in attempting to define mathematic models for peritoneal ultrafiltration, a correction factor called the "sieving coefficient" or Staverman "reflection coefficient" must be considered for each solute to describe the sieving effect seen with solute transport due to convection.[252] The reflec-

tion coefficient for various solutes ranges between 0.0 and 1.0. High-molecular-weight solutes, such as dextran and albumin, have reflection coefficients near unity. In these instances, there is almost complete rejection of the solute by the membrane. Other solutes, such as glucose (molecular weight of 180), have minimal values for their reflection coefficients. For these solutes, there is little or no membrane resistance to solute transport by convection.[253] Reflection coefficients are difficult to determine in clinical practice but are needed to accurately model peritoneal transport. A theoretic study examined the experimental conditions required to determine solute reflection coefficients.[254] The authors concluded that the peritoneal solute reflection coefficient could be reliably determined when transport is in the blood to dialysate direction with use of hypertonic exchanges. For solutes that move slowly across the peritoneum, the solute reflection coefficient is best determined with use of hypertonic exchanges and monitoring of solute movement from the dialysate to the blood. Charged ions, such as $Na^+$ and $K^+$, showed net reflection coefficients that were less than what would be predicted by their molecular weights. This may be due to an impedance in transport by charged surfaces on the endothelium and mesothelium[46, 249] or polar molecules in the basement membrane.

Another factor that complicates attempts to model ultrafiltration rates is the marked change in the concentration of solutes in dialysate during the dwell. Because the peritoneum is permeable to solutes, their concentrations in dialysate and hence the driving force for ultrafiltration change during the dwell time. Furthermore, these fluxes are different for hypertonic versus standard dialysis solutions. Clinically, the dialysate osmolality equilibrates with serum osmolality much more rapidly with 1.5% dextrose than with 4.25% dextrose; hence, dwell volume versus time curves are different for the different solutions. Computer simulations must anticipate these differences.

Jaffrin and co-workers[255] have described a model for peritoneal ultrafiltration that assumes that glucose is the only osmotic solute whose concentration changes during the dwell time. These authors were able to mathematically demonstrate the empirical observation that net ultrafiltration is dependent on dwell time. Nakanishi and colleagues[256] described a similar model assuming that there are three permeable solutes: urea, glucose, and $Na^+$. In this model, by using observed drain volumes and determining optimal values for peritoneal conductance, they found parameters for urea that were not physically realistic and concluded that urea was not an important osmotic solute determining transperitoneal ultrafiltration, which is consistent with clinical observations. Predictive calculations using the distributed model of peritoneal transport are even more complex.[213, 257] This model is based on pore theory; it incorporates the effect of lymphatic uptake on ultrafiltration and assumes that there are concentration gradients of solute in the peritoneal tissue.[258] Nolph and associates[218] have described ultrafiltration using a model that assumes pores of various sizes (heteroporosity) and a greater permeability for small solutes in the venular end of the capillaries. This model suggests that ultrafiltration takes place mainly in the proximal capillaries, where hydraulic pressure is the greatest and where glucose is a relatively more effective generator of an osmotic pressure difference. In the distal capillaries, where the hydraulic pressure is less and the plasma oncotic pressure is higher, glucose is readily absorbed. Therefore, under normal conditions, mainly fluid absorption would occur at the distal sites unless hypertonic solutions are used initially.

## MORE RECENT DATA

An inverse relationship between ultrafiltration rates and plasma protein concentrations has been observed in clinical studies,[259, 260] suggesting that ultrafiltration may be blood flow dependent. Levin and co-workers[261] tested this hypothesis in rats by determining ultrafiltration rates as a function of dialysate glucose concentration. Ultrafiltration rates plateaued at high glucose concentrations (much higher than those used in clinical practice) but did not increase after the addition of drugs thought to increase peritoneal blood flow. Studies in rats have shown that although the mean effective peritoneal blood flow seemed to increase during hypertonic exchanges, blood flow rates were on the average about six times greater than the maximal net ultrafiltration rates.[262] On the basis of these and other studies[200, 231, 263, 264] that have demonstrated that vasodilators have a minimal effect on net ultrafiltration rates, it is unlikely that ultrafiltration is blood flow limited under usual clinical conditions.

## CLINICAL FINDINGS

Although the described variables limit one's ability to mathematically model convective solute transport and ultrafiltration volumes, ultrafiltration is an integral clinical component of peritoneal dialysis for two reasons. First, the physician must achieve net ultrafiltration on a daily basis to prevent volume overload; second, overall peritoneal clearance of any solute is a function of drain volume and the concentration of that solute in the dialysate. Ultrafiltration rates are highest at the beginning of the exchange and, as glucose is absorbed, decrease toward zero when osmotic equilibrium is reached.[265, 266] Depending on the concentration of instilled glucose, osmotic equilibrium is reached at different times in the dwell cycle. For 2-L solutions containing 1.5% dextrose, osmotic equilibrium and maximal drain volume are reached after about 2 hours of dwell time in patients with average peritoneal membrane transport characteristics. For 4.25% dextrose solutions, peak intraperitoneal volumes are not likely to occur until after a 3- or 4-hour dwell.[267] However, the drain volume obtained after these dwell times is substantially less than would be predicted from transcapillary ultrafiltration rates. Net drain volume is a function of the relative rates of transcapillary ultrafiltration and lymphatic absorption. As osmotic equilibrium is approached, intraperitoneal volume and ultimate drain volume decrease owing to isosmotic absorption of fluids. In CAPD patients, this absorption rate ranges from 40 to 60 mL/h and is attributable primarily to lymphatic drainage of the peritoneum.[266, 268] The overall difference between the expected intraperitoneal volume due to ultrafiltration alone and that actually achieved was calculated from experimental data using rates of dilution and disappearance of [125]I-labeled polyvinylpyrrolidone[269] (Fig. 57–5). These

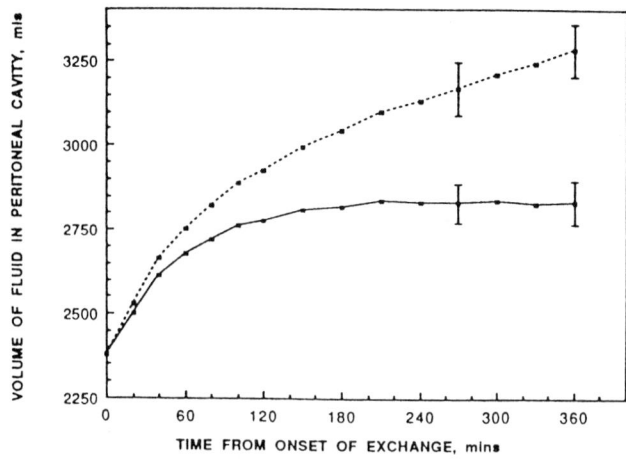

**Figure 57–5.** Intraperitoneal volume during CAPD. Values are based on an average of all measurements in the study. The upper line is estimated by tracer dilution alone. The lower line corrects for lymphatic drainage estimated by net [125]I-polyvinylpyrrolidone disappearance and corresponds to true intraperitoneal volume during a therapeutic exchange. Error bars are SEM; n = 10. (From Lysaght MJ, Moran J, Lysaght CB, et al: Plasma water filtration and lymphatic uptake during peritoneal dialysis. ASAIO Trans 37:M403–M404, 1991.)

authors have shown that transcapillary ultrafiltration ranged from a high of 7.4 mL/min after 10 minutes of dwell time to 1.3 mL/min at 345 minutes of dwell time when there was less of an osmotic gradient for net ultrafiltration. Furthermore, they demonstrated that lymphatic drainage was sufficient to decrease net ultrafiltration by approximately 50% with the resultant reabsorption of approximately 15% of metabolites in the peritoneal cavity, independent of molecular weight.

Given the measurements of transcapillary ultrafiltration rates, it is interesting to note that most peritoneal dialysis patients do not become hypotensive during the dwell. This is because of lymphatic absorption, back-filtration, and capillary refilling from interstitial fluids. Several reports suggest that use of hypertonic dialysis solutions in hemodialysis prevents disequilibrium by altering fluid movements between compartments.[270, 271] Burdiel and co-workers[272] have demonstrated that hematocrit and colloid osmotic pressure decrease during dwells using 1.5% dextrose but not during dwells using 4.25% dextrose. This shows that plasma volume changes during the dwell and is in fact determined by the balance between transcapillary ultrafiltration, back-filtration, and capillary refilling. They suggest that capillary refilling is greater than net transcapillary ultrafiltration with 1.5% dextrose but that rates are similar during 4.25% dextrose dwells.

## FACTORS THAT INFLUENCE ULTRAFILTRATION RATES

Factors that increase net ultrafiltration include the use of hypertonic dialysis solutions, shortening of dwell time, drugs, and miscellaneous other mechanisms.[273] Intravenous dopamine increases ultrafiltration presumably because of an increase in transcapillary hydraulic pressure. When gastrointestinal hormones are added intraperitoneally, there is little effect on solute transport or ultrafiltration. In contrast, intravenous glucagon significantly increases mesenteric blood flow and solute transfer rates, and intravenous secretin increases ultrafiltration at any given osmotic stimulus, which suggests selective effects on solute and water transport.[274] Amphotericin B selectively increases peritoneal hydraulic permeability, increasing ultrafiltration.[275] A mild increase in ultrafiltration is also seen with poly-L-lysine and furosemide, both of which promote Na[+] transport and limit early dialysate hyponatremia, thereby preventing a gradient for back-diffusion of water.[273] In patients with ultrafiltration failure and also in those with normal ultrafiltration rates, phosphatidylcholine has increased net ultrafiltration rates,[276–278] presumably through its surface-acting properties that help to repel water, although some have shown decreases in lymphatic absorption in rats. A review discusses in more detail the influence of drugs and other mechanisms on net ultrafiltration.[279]

## Solute Transport by Convection

Solutes present in body fluids can be swept along with the bulk flow of water during ultrafiltration even in the absence of a concentration gradient for net diffusion. This solvent drag or convective solute transport does not always occur in amounts per liter of ultrafiltrate equal to the concentration of solutes in body fluids, which results in a sieving effect that is dependent on resistance forces intrinsic to the membrane and the solvents. Although the sieving effect influences the transport of many solutes, the most important clinical consequences are those related to the transport of Na[+]. The convective transport of Na[+] per liter of ultrafiltrate is much less than that of its extracellular fluid concentration.[46, 49, 233, 250, 251] Therefore, dialysate Na[+] concentration is reduced early in the dwell period because of Na[+] sieving and ultrafiltration. This relative hyponatremia in the dialysate tends to decrease later during the dwell when there is less ultrafiltration and the net effects on dialysate Na[+] concentration are primarily due to diffusion. Dialysate Na[+] concentrations are lowered the most by this mechanism in patients who are slow transporters because of the relatively higher ultrafiltration rates[46]; consequently, during a series of short dwells with hypertonic exchanges, severe hypernatremia may develop in these patients.[280–283] Associated symptoms have included thirst and hypertension. These expected changes in dialysate Na[+] concentrations during the dwell can be helpful in evaluating a patient with loss of ultrafiltration.[284] This problem can be countered by lowering the dialysate Na[+] concentration to increase the concentration gradient and increase diffusion. Hence, present commercially available dialysate solutions usually contain an Na[+] concentration of 132 mEq/L. However, to prevent hypernatremia with a prolonged series of hourly cycles with 4.25% dextrose solutions, even lower solution Na[+] concentrations are often necessary.[249]

It is somewhat paradoxical that the peritoneal membrane, which appears to be ''open'' to solute transport by diffusion, is somewhat restrictive to convective transport. What must also be explained is why some solutes, such as Na[+], have sieving coefficients that are less than what would be expected for their molecular weight alone. Mechanisms to explain the net sieving effect of the peritoneal membrane are hypothetic and include the following:

1. Cell surface charges of the endothelium and mesothelium may impede transport of charged solutes through intercellular gaps.[46, 249] This, however, would not explain the net sieving effects of neutral molecules.

2. Proximal capillaries may have tight intercellular junctions so that ultrafiltration must be transcellular.[285] If this occurred through small transcellular water channels, concomitant solute transport could be inhibited.

3. Perhaps there are narrow intercellular gaps in the proximal capillaries that are responsible for water movement but inhibit solute transport independent of surface charges.[251] This would not explain the experimental observation that Na[+] sieving seems to be more than what can be explained by its size alone.

4. Polar molecules in the basement membrane and interstitium could influence transport of charged but not neutral solutes.

5. In vitro studies have suggested that glucose movement across synthetic membranes countercurrent to water movement may result in molecular interactions with solutes crossing the membrane in the opposite direction.[286] This could affect the net sieving effect for both charged and neutral ions. This glucose interaction occurs in synthetic membranes where no sieving effect was noted during hydraulically induced ultrafiltration.

A computer-simulated graft of dialysate Na[+] concentration versus dwell time using a three-pore model for membrane transport for 1.36% and 3.86% glucose dialysis solutions predicts the differences in the clinically observed fall in dialysate Na[+] concentration[287] (Fig. 57–6). In rat studies, when oncotic and osmotic pressure gradients were presumably absent by use of rat serum as the dialysis solution, Na[+] sieving and net ultrafiltration still occurred.[288] This

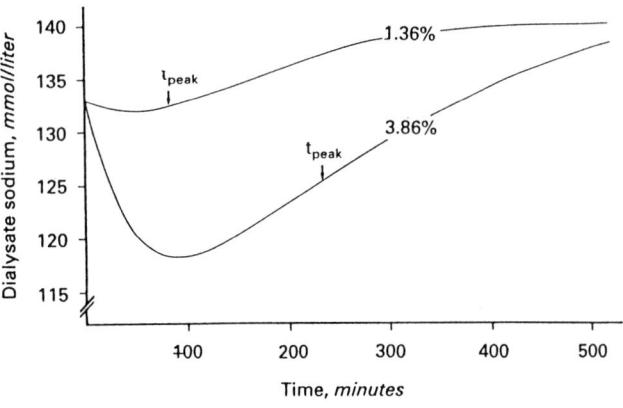

**Figure 57–6.** Computer-simulated Na[+] concentration in the dialysate as a function of dwell time for 1.36% (upper curve) and 3.86% (lower curve) glucose dialysis solutions during control conditions. Initial dialysate Na[+] concentration (after mixing up the dialysis fluid with the residual volume) is 133 mmol/L, and initial plasma Na[+] concentration is 140 mmol/L. (From Rippe B, Stelin G, Haraldsson B: Computer simulations of peritoneal fluid transport in CAPD. Used with permission from Kidney International, volume 40, pages 315–325, 1991.)

would suggest that Na$^+$ sieving is not unique to osmotic pressure–induced ultrafiltration and is probably due to intrinsic membrane-related effects. Overall, most publications seem to support the heterogeneous pore nature of the peritoneal membrane.

## Factors That Influence Peritoneal Transport

Factors known to influence peritoneal transport are multifactorial and fall under the broad headings of procedural variables, alterations in blood volume, drugs, hormones, cytokines, dialysis fluid composition, and peritonitis. These have been reviewed elsewhere.[5, 135, 273] A summary of the mechanisms for these alterations is shown schematically in Figure 57–7. Although these experimental findings have been used to further define and understand peritoneal transport mechanisms, only minor changes in overall solute transport have been noted with these manipulations. There-

MECHANISMS OF ACCELERATED PERITONEAL SOLUTE TRANSPORT

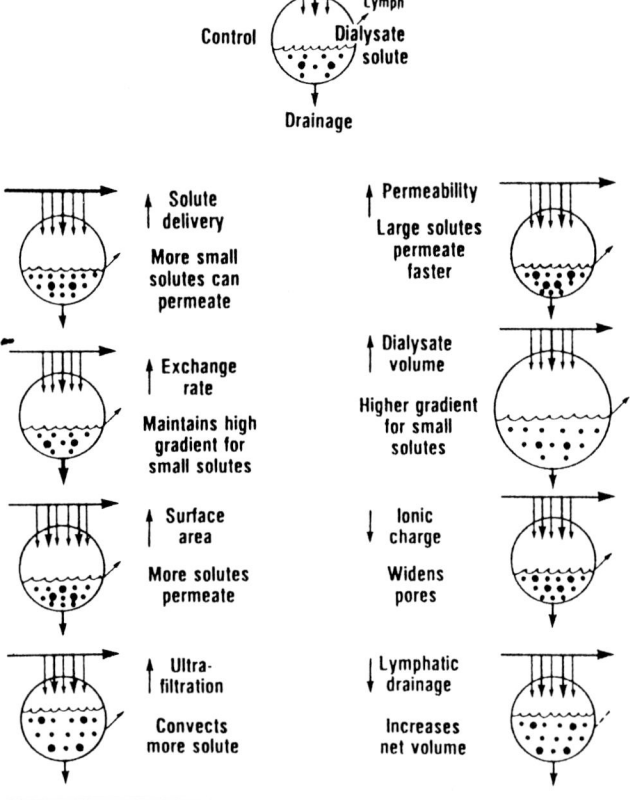

**Figure 57–7.** Schematic representation of solute removal by peritoneal dialysis. The circles represent the peritoneum containing small solutes (*dots*) and larger compounds. The long horizontal arrow above the circle represents peritoneal blood flow. Vertical arrows above the circle display transfer of small (*thin lines*) and large (*thick lines*) solutes. The lower arrow indicates drainage, and the side arrow indicates lymphatic absorption. (From Hirszel P, Maher JF: Pharmacologic alteration of peritoneal transport rates. *In* Nolph KD [ed]: Peritoneal Dialysis, 3rd ed. Kluwer Academic Publishers, Boston, 1989, p 184. Reprinted by permission of Kluwer Academic Publishers.)

fore, for the most part, these are seldom used clinically to augment daily clearances.

The following is a review of some studies that influence transport. Intravenous dihydroergotamine, which augments splanchnic vascular ultrafiltration, reduces splanchnic blood volume, accelerates splanchnic blood flow, and decreases solute clearances. Furthermore, it decreases the clearance of high-molecular-weight solutes proportionally more than that for small solutes; it also lowers ultrafiltration rate.[289] When blood volume was expanded by dextrose infusions or when hepatic venous stasis was induced with intraperitoneal administration of sodium chromate, resulting in increased splanchnic blood volume but decreased flow, solute transport increased.[169] These two studies suggest that membrane area or permeability is related more to blood volume than to blood flow.

Peritoneal transport rates were assessed in CAPD patients being treated with clonidine, enalapril, or nifedipine.[290] All three drugs significantly reduced mean arterial pressures to similar degrees. Compared with control conditions, transport did not change with clonidine, but with enalapril and nifedipine, creatinine and β$_2$-microglobulin clearances and glucose absorption were markedly increased. This increase may be due to local hemodynamic changes that alter the number of capillaries perfused or blood volume, hence increasing net surface area. Peritoneal clearances for small solutes were obtained after intraperitoneal administration of verapamil.[291] This resulted in increases in small-solute clearances, which suggests that there was an increase in either the intrinsic permeability of the membrane or net surface area.

Prekallikrein activator found in some, but not all, batches of human albumin increased the transport of all measured solutes and effluent peritoneal white blood cell count.[292] Increased protein losses were noted after 8-hour dwells with 2.6% amino acid dialysis solutions.[293] Also seen were increases in β$_2$-microglobulin, albumin transferrin, and immunoglobulin G (IgG). Prostaglandin E$_2$ concentrations were increased more than 80% in amino acid–containing solutions versus standard glucose-containing fluids, which suggests that amino acid–containing fluids may increase the peritoneal permeability for proteins, perhaps by altering local prostaglandin production. Intraperitoneal interleukin-6 is associated with increased clearances in stable CAPD patients, and such changes in transport are thought to be due to a modulation of the intrinsic transport characteristics of the membrane itself.[294] These data draw attention to the fact that cytokines and their manipulation can influence solute transport but also remind investigators about the possibility that unsuspected additional factors can alter transport under experimental conditions.

In rabbits, intraperitoneal administration of protamine increased protein transport into the peritoneal cavity, presumably by neutralizing anionic sites in the membrane and facilitating albumin transport.[295] Protamine is a highly charged cationic molecule that would be expected to neutralize any anionic sites. The increased protein losses seen with protamine administration were prevented if protamine was first neutralized with heparin.

Some[296, 297] but not all authors[298, 299] have suggested that a change in hematocrit influences transport in long-term peritoneal dialysis patients. A possible mechanism for a decrease in solute transport would be the decrease in splanchnic plasma water flow at any given blood flow associated with an increase in hematocrit. Most data would support the observations that peritoneal transport is not plasma or blood flow dependent. Struijk and co-workers[300] have shown that although there was an initial increase in hemoglobin level and hematocrit and that this was associated with a decrease in MTACs over time, the intrinsic permeability of the peritoneal membrane characterized by the peritoneal restriction coefficients did not change. These authors concluded that the initial differences in solute transport were due to a change in peritoneal surface area, not relative plasma water flow, and that the increase in surface area was not due to the increase in hematocrit.

These studies support the heterogeneous pore models of transport across the peritoneum and suggest that the day-to-day fluctuations in transport are more likely due to changes in surface area than to changes in the intrinsic transport properties of the membrane itself. However, they also imply that the intrinsic transport properties of the membrane are not static and that they can change over time.

## Lymphatic Absorption

The peritoneal lymphatics can be divided into two major systems. Lymphatics coursing through the mesentery convey solutes and water absorbed from the gastrointestinal tract to the systemic venous system. Some net transport from these lymphatics into the peritoneal cavity may occur but is thought to be minimal, compared with the diffusive and convective solute transport from the peritoneal capillaries. A second lymphatic system drains the parietal peritoneum, especially in the subdiaphragmatic area, and is thought to be the primary mechanism for net absorption of fluid and solutes from the peritoneal cavity.

### PHYSIOLOGY

Intraperitoneal fluid is continuously absorbed from the peritoneal cavity.[301] The fluid can be absorbed either directly into the subdiaphragmatic peritoneal lymphatics or through the interstitial tissue of the peritoneal membrane. Once in the interstitium, fluid and solutes can either be reabsorbed by the peritoneal capillaries (back-filtration) or be taken up by lymphatics that drain the interstitium (Fig. 57–8). Experimental data would suggest that the absorption from the peritoneum of isotonic fluid occurs mainly by the subdiaphragmatic and interstitial lymphatics (75%) and to a lesser degree by transcapillary back-diffusion (25%).[247] This is controversial, however. In humans, peritoneal lymphatic drainage is about equal to the formation of peritoneal fluid; therefore, normally only a small volume of isotonic fluid is found in the peritoneal cavity. Lymphatic drainage is primarily through specialized openings or stomas,[302, 303] located at the origin of the lymphatic channels, most of which are in the subdiaphragmatic area overlying the liver.[304] Absorption of fluid by the visceral peritoneal lymphatics and the rest of the parietal peritoneum is probably minor.[305, 306]

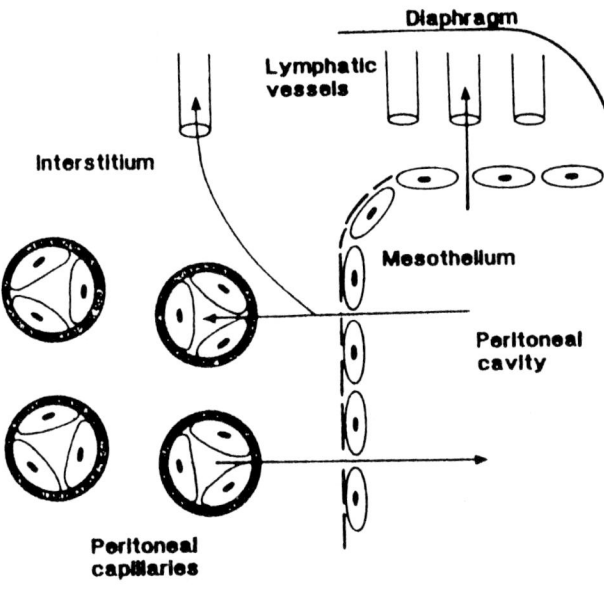

**Figure 57–8.** Schematic representation of the peritoneal membrane. Transcapillary ultrafiltration occurs in two directions. Lymphatic absorption from the peritoneal cavity is partly into the subdiaphragmatic lymphatics directly and partly into the lymphatics that drain the interstitium. (From Krediet RT, Imholz AL, Struijk DG, et al: Ultrafiltration failure in continuous ambulatory peritoneal dialysis. Perit Dial Int 13:S59–S66, 1993.)

Hydraulic pressure effects on standing or associated with activity may alter the relative amount of convective movement of fluids and solute into the subdiaphragmatic or other lymphatics. Twardowski and colleagues[307] have shown that there is a linear relationship between intraperitoneal volume and intraperitoneal pressure in CAPD patients. Others have shown that lymphatic absorption rates are related to instilled volume,[308] higher initial intraperitoneal volumes such as in patients with high rates of transcapillary ultrafiltration,[309] and external compression. These data would suggest that intraperitoneal pressure is a major determinant of lymphatic absorption rates.

Lymphatic reabsorption rates are also dependent on diaphragmatic movements, which create a pump-like mechanism for bulk fluid movements. During expiration, the diaphragm relaxes, as do the adjacent mesothelial and endothelial cells separating the lymphatic lacunae, creating a vacuum. Fluid then enters this vacuum through the stomas; during inspiration, with contraction of the diaphragm, the stomas close and the trapped fluid then flows into the upstream lymphatic channels.[310, 311] Absorption rates decrease in the upright versus the supine position because of increased fluid contact with the subdiaphragmatic area in the supine position. Net absorption is also modified by the presence of any lymphatic obstruction.[312] The stomas described before may have diameters as large as 50 nm, allowing the movement of fluid, macromolecules, particulate matter, and even red blood cells along with the bulk flow of intraperitoneal fluids. A further discussion of the ultrastructure and reabsorption rates of the peritoneal membrane has been presented in greater detail elsewhere.[313]

When hypertonic peritoneal dialysis fluids are used, intraperitoneal volume begins to decrease before isosmolality is reached between dialysate and plasma. This would suggest that at a time when transcapillary ultrafiltration is still occurring and peritoneal volume should be increasing, there is reabsorption of fluid by some mechanism.[216, 266] Similar results were found by Lindholm and co-workers[314] using radioiodinated albumin as a volume marker. They found that about 90% of total net ultrafiltration occurred during the first 90 minutes of the dwell and that ultimate drain volume after 360 minutes was about 28% lower than the expected volume due to transcapillary ultrafiltration alone.[315] This net reduction in intraperitoneal volume after peak ultrafiltration is thought to represent the lymphatic reabsorption rate in excess of net transcapillary ultrafiltration rates.

## MEASUREMENTS OF LYMPHATIC ABSORPTION

Direct measurement of lymphatic flow from the peritoneum in CAPD patients is impossible. Therefore, indirect methods that measure the disappearance of macromolecules from the peritoneum or their appearance in the circulation are used. Peritoneal lymphatic flow from the rat peritoneum[316] and in humans[317, 318] has been estimated by monitoring the disappearance of albumin in instilled dialysis solutions and expressing lymphatic flow as the clearance of albumin from the intraperitoneal solutions. In anesthetized sheep, peritoneal lymphatic flow was measured by direct cannulation of major lymph vessels draining the peritoneal cavity and reported as 0.454 mL/h/kg.[319] Almost half of the protein removed from the peritoneal cavity was ultimately transported through the thoracic duct; the rest reached the systemic circulation by other routes. This study was an attempt to determine how much of the protein is removed from the peritoneum by convective transport in lymphatics versus direct absorption across the peritoneal membrane and into the peritoneal capillaries. However, it is possible that other lymphatics were involved that were not cannulated in this study, and it has been shown that there are small lymphaticovenous connections that may be present along the major lymphatic pathways.[320] Therefore, not all the fluids entering the subdiaphragmatic lymphatics may reach the systemic circulation through the thoracic duct. Furthermore, given the above-mentioned dependence of lymphatic absorption on respiratory movements of the diaphragm, one must interpret lymphatic absorption rates in anesthetized animals with caution.[321] In a study of CAPD patients correlating intraperitoneal fluid changes over time and manipulation of a mathematic model for peritoneal transport that uses a three-pore model of membrane permeability, maximal peritoneal lymphatic flows were estimated to be 0.75 mL/min.[322] Measurements of lymphatic absorption rates in CAPD patients using intraperitoneal dextran as a marker[268] ranged from 0.1 to 3.5 mL/min with a median value of 1.0 mL/min.

Estimations of lymphatic absorption rates based on the disappearance of intraperitoneally administered macromolecules are often higher than those obtained by measuring the appearance of similar macromolecules in the circulation.[284, 317, 318, 323, 324] In all these studies, the marker was

administered only once. Therefore, some authors have suggested that local accumulation or trapping of the macromolecules in tissues surrounding the peritoneal cavity could lead to overestimation or variations in lymphatic flow if disappearance rates from the peritoneal cavity versus appearance in blood were used to determine lymphatic uptake. However, in an experiment in CAPD patients, lymphatic absorption rates were estimated with polydispersed neutral dextran 70 before and after saturation of the surrounding tissue with dextran after intravenous and intraperitoneal injections.[245] No differences in peritoneal clearances were found before and after efforts to saturate the tissue. It was concluded that trapping had no effect on the removal of macromolecules from the peritoneum.

## CLINICAL FINDINGS

The average measured decrease in intraperitoneal volumes after sequential dwell times in 29 CAPD patients was 39 mL/h.[266, 325] Net reabsorption rates did not differ regardless of tonicity (1.5% versus 2.5% versus 4.25% dextrose)[266, 325, 326] or instilled volumes.[327] Krediet and co-workers[328] have shown that the appearance of macromolecules in the peritoneal cavity, but not their disappearance, was dependent on molecular size. In related studies, these authors found that the MTAC for transport of inulin out of the peritoneal cavity was much higher than the MTAC for transfer of inulin into the peritoneal cavity.[329] Their explanation for this difference was best explained by uptake of inulin into the peritoneal lymphatics in addition to transport by diffusion. In another study, the rate of disappearance of sulfamethoxazole from the peritoneal cavity was not altered by albumin binding, and therefore its absorption was thought to be size independent.[330] These data suggest that the primary mode of fluid and solute absorption from the peritoneum is convective in nature and through the peritoneal lymphatics. There appears to be little sieving as seen with convective transport from the blood to the peritoneum across the peritoneal membrane; therefore, most of the absorption appears to occur through stomas directly into the lymphatics.

Extrapolation from these data would suggest that in some CAPD patients, the average daily lymphatic absorption rate is about 2.2 L.[331] This would reduce potential ultrafiltration after an average 4-hour dwell by 343 ± 39 mL. Maneuvers that would decrease lymphatic reabsorption would be beneficial to augment net ultrafiltration.

## FACTORS THAT INFLUENCE LYMPHATIC ABSORPTION

Most of the lymphatic reabsorption occurs through subdiaphragmatic stomas described earlier. These stomas have actin-containing microfilaments, which could act as flap-like valves that open and close with diaphragmatic movement.[310] These filaments may react to muscle constrictors. Neostigmine reduces lymphatic drainage in rats, presumably by constricting these stomas.[332] This effect was confirmed in a patient using CAPD who had myasthenia gravis.[333] Although the oral neostigmine appeared to decrease lymphatic absorption, clinically there was little effect

of an individual patient, MTACs and restriction coefficients can be obtained to determine effective surface area and intrinsic membrane permeability, respectively.

## Ultrafiltration Failure

Peritoneal ultrafiltration is considered adequate when at least 5.5 mL of ultrafiltration is generated per 1 g of absorbed glucose.[367] Ultrafiltration failure in CAPD may be defined as clinical evidence of fluid overload despite restriction of fluid intake and the use of three or more hypertonic (4.25% dextrose) exchanges per day.[284] The most common causes for loss of ultrafiltration are membrane failure, excessive lymphatic flow, catheter malposition, and fluid sequestration. These mechanisms were well described in publications.[368–370] The exact frequency of ultrafiltration failure is uncertain. At one center, ultrafiltration failure was observed in 14 of 227 CAPD patients (6.2%) in a 10-year period of observation. These authors also noted that risk increased with time on peritoneal dialysis,[326] and the prevalence was 2.6% after 1-year of dialysis compared with 30.9% after 6 years of CAPD. Other authors have reported that ultrafiltration failure is responsible for up to 15% of dropout from peritoneal dialysis.[371, 372] A rational approach to the patient with suspected ultrafiltration failure is found in Figure 57–9.

Failure of ultrafiltration is not always due to an actual loss of peritoneal ultrafiltration capacity. Fluid overload, clinically mimicking ultrafiltration failure, may occur when urine volume decreases and fluid intake is excessive or when the patient is noncompliant with the prescribed exchanges. Dialysate leaks from the intra-abdominal cavity into extra-abdominal tissue spaces may also result in loss of ultrafiltration because of a decrease in dialysate contact

with the peritoneal membrane. These causes are not associated with a change in peritoneal membrane transport characteristics. The first steps in the evaluation of a patient with suspected ultrafiltration failure are to determine urine volume and to establish whether net effluent drain volume or peritoneal transport has changed. True loss of ultrafiltration is potentially reversible if it is due to catheter malposition, dialysate leak, or recent peritonitis but is usually permanent if kinetic studies suggest a reduction in ultrafiltration capacity of the membrane. Mactier[369] and Verger and colleagues[370] have classified patients with irreversible ultrafiltration failure on the basis of the kinetic analysis described in the next section.

## ULTRAFILTRATION FAILURE AND RAPID SOLUTE TRANSPORT

Patients with loss of ultrafiltration and current 4-hour PET[233] ratios of drained to original dialysate glucose concentration (D/D$_0$) less than 0.3 and D/P creatinine greater than 0.81 are characterized as rapid solute transporters. These patients tend to have good low-molecular-weight solute transport but have poor ultrafiltration because of rapid glucose absorption and dissipation of the osmotic gradient. Some patients have these transport characteristics at baseline and, if their dwell times are mismatched for their membrane transport characteristics, often appear to have ultrafiltration failure as they lose residual renal function and no longer have urine flow as a supplement to net daily fluid losses. In other patients, the loss of ultrafiltration is due to a change in membrane transport (increase in transport). The most common causes of the ultrafiltration failure are peritonitis and type I membrane failure.

**Recent Peritonitis.** It is a common clinical experience for peritoneal dialysis patients to experience fluid retention during episodes of peritonitis. These patients often need a temporary change in their standard dialysis prescription to achieve net ultrafiltration. Compared with baseline values, PET data during peritonitis reveal an increase in the D/P ratio for creatinine and a decrease in the D/D$_0$ ratio for glucose. There is also an increase in protein losses and a significant decrease in net ultrafiltration.[373] These changes associated with peritonitis are usually reversible, and membrane transport returns to baseline level after recovery. Microscopic findings in patients with acute peritonitis have revealed denudation of the mesothelial surface.[157, 160] However, in some patients, remesothelialization never occurs even after recovery from peritonitis.[99] This leads to chronic ultrafiltration loss and is referred to as type I membrane failure. Di Paolo and colleagues[374, 375] have demonstrated that autoimplantation of labeled cultured mesothelial cells in rabbits and CAPD patients with peritonitis resulted in reimplantation, improvement in ultrafiltration parameters, and normalization of dialysate phospholipid concentrations. Further studies are needed before widespread clinical use of this technique is advocated.

**Type I Membrane Failure.** Type I membrane failure is the most common cause of chronic ultrafiltration failure in CAPD patients and is due to rapid peritoneal solute transport. Peritoneal equilibration testing confirms high or high-average transport rates with resultant rapid glucose absorp-

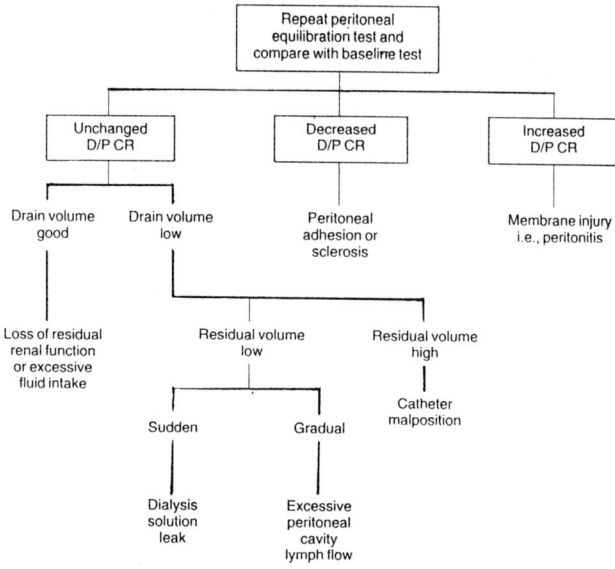

**Figure 57–9.** Algorithm for loss of ultrafiltration in CAPD patients. D/P Cr = dialysate/plasma ratio for creatinine. (From Khanna R, Nolph KD, Oreopoulos DG: Complications during peritoneal dialysis. *In* The Essentials of Peritoneal Dialysis. Kluwer Academic Publishers, Dordrecht, Netherlands, 1993, p 98. Reprinted by permission of Kluwer Academic Publishers.)

tion, loss of the osmotic gradient, and decrease in net transcapillary ultrafiltration. In contrast to the situation seen with peritonitis, in which transport changes are usually transient and protein losses are increased,[345] with type I membrane failure, the small-solute transport changes are more permanent and protein mass transport does not change.[284] There also tends to be less of a decline in dialysate $Na^+$ concentration due to the $Na^+$ sieving with convective transport as seen in control subjects.[284] These changes are thought to be due to an increase in effective surface area of the peritoneal membrane and are consistent with the heterogeneous three-pore model of peritoneal transport.[220]

The etiology of type I membrane failure is unclear. This was originally described with acetate-containing dialysis solutions[376] but has also been seen in patients who have used only lactate-containing dialysis fluids.[284] Recurrent peritonitis and use of hypertonic exchanges have been implicated in some[360, 377] but not all[284, 378] studies. The frequency of type I membrane failure seems to increase with time on peritoneal dialysis, which implicates repeated exposure of the peritoneum to dialysate as a cause.[284, 379] Reported microscopic findings are similar to those seen with peritonitis.

Clinically, most of these patients can be managed by shortening their dwell times, which will usually improve net ultrafiltration. Because these patients have rapid transport of small solutes, they have adequate urea and creatinine clearances even with short cycles. Resting the peritoneum for at least 4 weeks through a temporary transfer to hemodialysis has occasionally been associated with an improvement in ultrafiltration and normalization of transport characteristics.[342, 379] Some[276] but not all[380] researchers have found low phosphatidylcholine levels in patients with various types of ultrafiltration failure compared with normal subjects. Initial studies using intraperitoneal phosphatidylcholine to treat patients with ultrafiltration failure yielded encouraging results.[276] Increases in ultrafiltration were also seen in CAPD patients with no evidence of ultrafiltration failure after intraperitoneal phosphatidylcholine failure.[277, 381] Possible explanations for the mechanisms by which phosphatidylcholine increases net ultrafiltration include direct membrane effects or decreased absorption through subdiaphragmatic lymphatics by 1) an increase in cholinergic tone causing contraction of subdiaphragmatic stomas[332]; 2) neutralization of the anionic charges on the lymphatic endothelium by its cationic charge, which tends to keep stomas open[382]; and 3) surface-acting properties of the molecule that would tend to repel water and inhibit movement into the lymphatics. Despite these initial findings, routine use of intraperitoneal phosphatidylcholine cannot currently be recommended because of concerns about safety and the possibility of adhesion formation,[383] although a publication evaluating its use in rats was associated with a decrease in adhesion formation.[384] The effects of oral phosphatidylcholine are conflicting; some[278, 385] but not all studies show clinical improvement in ultrafiltration rates.[386, 387] A possible explanation for these divergent results is the different doses of phosphatidylcholine used as well as the differences in concentrations of the various lipids contained in these preparations. Further studies are needed.

Although it is often possible to achieve adequate small-solute clearance in patients with type I membrane failure, they often require transfer to hemodialysis for volume and blood pressure control. There is also a concern that continued membrane damage may result in eventual progression to peritoneal sclerosis or type II membrane failure.[388, 389] If so, it would be important clinically to monitor patients with type I failure closely with PET. If these patients continue on peritoneal dialysis and their solute transport starts to decline, it may be beneficial to temporarily switch them to hemodialysis to allow healing of the peritoneum.[390]

## ULTRAFILTRATION FAILURE AND NO CHANGE OR AVERAGE SOLUTE TRANSPORT

Loss of ultrafiltration in patients with no change or average transport characteristics tends to be due to catheter malfunction, fluid leaks, or excessive lymphatic reabsorption (type III membrane failure). If loss of ultrafiltration is due to catheter malfunction or fluid leaks, the patients do not have a functional change in their membrane and can usually be maintained with peritoneal dialysis after the problem has been resolved.

**Excessive Lymphatic Absorption (Type III Membrane Failure).** This is an uncommon cause of membrane failure and is due to excessive rates of lymphatic absorption of fluid.[284] During a long dwell, as long as transcapillary ultrafiltration exceeds lymphatic absorption, intraperitoneal drain volumes will increase. However, once the osmotic gradient decreases, lymphatic absorption rates can exceed transcapillary ultrafiltration rates, and net drain volume may decrease. Although these patients may not have a significant change in D/P values compared with baseline values, they do have drain volumes after 4 hours of dwell time that are less than baseline values or what would be expected on the basis of standard therapy. A further diagnostic clue is that these patients tend to have higher dialysate $Na^+$ concentration during the dwell than control subjects do[284, 378] (Fig. 57–10).

## ULTRAFILTRATION FAILURE AND LOW SOLUTE TRANSPORT

Patients with ultrafiltration failure and low solute transport ($D/D_0$ glucose $> 0.5$ and D/P creatinine $< 0.5$) tend also to have inadequate small-solute clearances. Poor ultrafiltration occurs despite the maintenance of adequate osmotic gradients. These patients are found to have peritoneal sclerosis (type II membrane failure) or multiple peritoneal adhesions. These patients often require transfer to hemodialysis.

**Peritoneal Sclerosis (Type II Membrane Failure).** An uncommon cause of ultrafiltration failure is sclerosing peritonitis. This is reported to affect less than 1% of long-term peritoneal dialysis patients. Patients present with both ultrafiltration and small-solute transport failure, but because of the association with intestinal adhesions, they may also present with intestinal obstruction.[389] The etiology of type II membrane failure is uncertain. A variety of peritoneal irritants have been implicated in the pathogenesis of type II membrane failure, including recurrent peritonitis, long-term

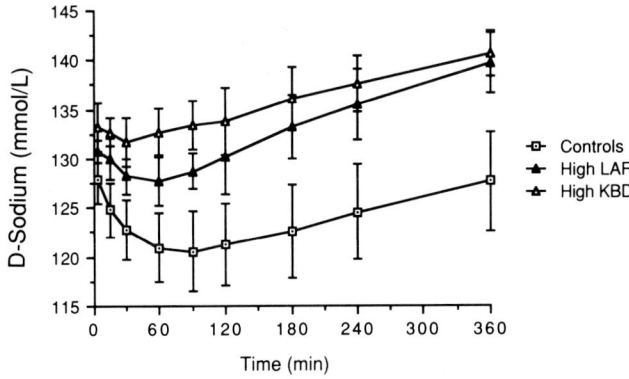

**Figure 57–10.** Dialysate Na$^+$ concentrations as a function of time in patients using 3.86% dextrose exchanges over 6-hour dwells. Results are compared in patients with normal ultrafiltration kinetics (controls), those with high lymphatic absorption rates (high LAR), and those with high glucose absorption rates (high KBD). (From Heimburger O, Waniewski J, Werynski A, et al: Peritoneal transport in CAPD patients with permanent loss of ultrafiltration capacity. Used with permission from Kidney International, volume 38, pages 495–506, 1990.)

use of peritoneal dialysis, acetate-containing dialysate, chlorhexidine, β-blockers, and endotoxins. Discussions of these and other agents are extensively reviewed elsewhere.[389] Type II membrane failure should not be confused with the syndrome of sclerosing encapsulating peritonitis (described later).[391] With sclerosing encapsulating peritonitis, patients present with a thick-walled membrane cocoon entrapping loops of bowel and have anorexia, nausea, vomiting, malnutrition, and intestinal obstruction along with a type II membrane failure pattern with a decrease in solute transport and ultrafiltration.[392–394] As opposed to patients with sclerosing encapsulating peritonitis, patients with simple type II membrane failure do not have the surgical findings of an encapsulating fibrosis[395] but may have diffuse thickening and fibrosis of the parietal and visceral peritoneum.

In some CAPD patients, fibroblast activation can change the transport properties of the peritoneal membrane, making it impermeable to water.[396] It is possible that chronic irritation leads to activation of fibroblasts. Lamperi and Carozzi[397] have postulated that the activation of fibroblasts is immune mediated and leads to the overproduction of lymphokines by peritoneal lymphocytes and macrophages. These patients have low net ultrafiltration, normal glucose absorption, and high lymphokine levels in the dialysate associated with low prostaglandin E$_2$ levels, compared with individuals with normal or high peritoneal transport properties.[397, 398] These changes in lymphokine production are thought to be modulated by intracellular Ca$^{2+}$ concentrations.[399] Drugs such as verapamil, which decrease intracellular Ca$^{2+}$ concentration, have been shown to decrease dialysate lymphokine levels and improve net ultrafiltration rates.[400]

Tamoxifen, an antiestrogen agent that inhibits protein kinase C, has been used to stabilize the process of peritoneal sclerosis.[401] It has also been used to treat retroperitoneal sclerosis, a process with pathologic findings similar to those of peritoneal sclerosis.[402] A trial of tamoxifen may be reasonable in patients who are reluctant to switch to hemodialysis.

**Multiple Abdominal Adhesions.** Extensive intra-abdominal adhesions may result after recurrent or severe peritonitis and after catastrophic intra-abdominal events.[403] These processes can cause a decrease in the amount of peritoneal membrane surface area that is in contact with dialysate. Although normal transport may occur in the membrane that is in contact with the peritoneum, overall transport and net ultrafiltration decrease. Surgical lysis of adhesions may result in an improvement, and the patients may be able to continue peritoneal dialysis if an adequate increase in surface area can be achieved.

# CLINICAL USES OF PERITONEAL DIALYSIS

## End-Stage Renal Disease

### PERITONEAL DIALYSIS TECHNIQUES

Numerous techniques for the instillation and drainage of peritoneal dialysis fluids have been developed. These methods are both manual and automated, and the therapy can be intermittent or continuous. Continuous therapies are carried out 24 hours a day, day after day, and typically use long dwell exchanges. Although small-solute clearances are well below the maximum with long dwells, the continuous nature of the technique allows one to achieve adequate weekly clearances. Intermittent techniques have treatment periods ("wet" abdomen) alternating with periods when the peritoneal cavity has been drained of dialysate ("dry" abdomen). Intermittent techniques use multiple short dwell exchanges to operate at nearly maximal small-solute clearances. Because intermittent therapies rely on multiple short dwells, they typically involve the use of automated cyclers. However, both continuous and intermittent therapies can be done manually or with the use of cyclers. Clearances of low-molecular-weight solutes correlate well with dialysate flow rates; therefore, intermittent therapies tend to use more fluid. These techniques were described in detail in previous editions of this book.[5]

With any peritoneal dialysis technique, the original instilled volumes and dwell times may need to be changed over time. It is important to individualize the patient's initial prescription and to monitor the dialysis dose. Smaller patients may be more comfortable with smaller instilled volumes. Those patients with respiratory compromise may have respiratory symptoms in the supine position. Larger patients will usually need larger exchange volumes of peritoneal dialysis fluid and can often tolerate up to 3 L of instilled volume without difficulty.[307, 404] The third section of the peritoneal dialysis glossary[405] defines the various alternative peritoneal dialysis prescriptions. Figure 57–11 shows examples of alternative CAPD prescriptions in diagrammatic form. Similar alternatives exist for CCPD (see Fig. 57–11) and nightly peritoneal dialysis. As discussed later, for the minimal recommended daily doses of dialysis to be achieved, most patients will need a continuous form of dialysis.

Alternate CAPD Prescriptions

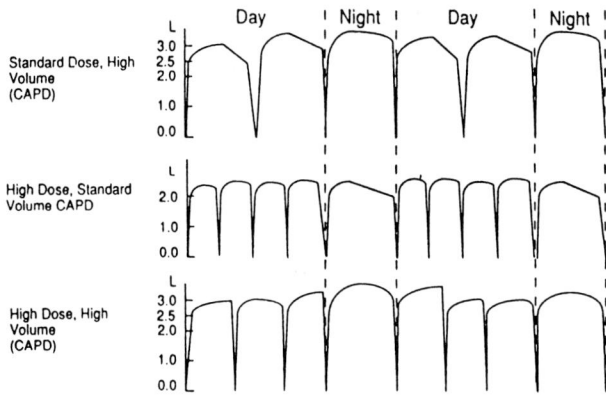

Alternate CCPD Prescriptions

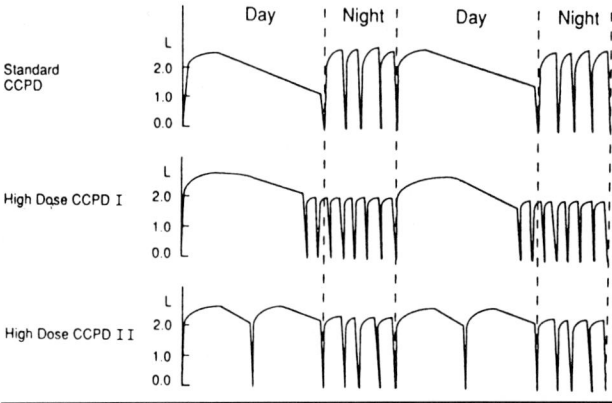

**Figure 57–11.** Alternative peritoneal dialysis prescriptions defined by varying dwell times, instilled volumes, and number of exchanges. (From Twardowski ZJ: Peritoneal dialysis glossary III. Perit Dial Int 10:173–175, 1990.)

**Continuous Therapies**

**Continuous Ambulatory Peritoneal Dialysis.** CAPD is the most commonly used form of peritoneal dialysis. According to USRDS data, as of December 31, 1990, 9.8% of the 167,437 patients alive with ESRD in the United States were using CAPD or CCPD.[406] CAPD was used almost nine times as often as CCPD. Industrial sources estimate that in 1992, approximately 28% of new dialysis patients in North America chose peritoneal dialysis as their initial modality and that there were 79,900 long-term peritoneal dialysis patients worldwide, most of whom used CAPD.[1] The percentage of new patients choosing peritoneal dialysis varies from country to country and is based not only on medical factors but also on many nonmedical factors.[407] Since the original description of this technique, there have been few changes in the basic therapy, although there have been many changes in the connection devices or "connectology" used to make the exchange (described later). The long dwells associated with this therapy achieve adequate daily small-solute clearances, despite operating below the maximal clearance rates for these solutes. Because of the long

dwells and continuous nature of the therapy, most ESRD patients can achieve the minimal daily recommended dialysis dose with this type of therapy. CAPD is a manual therapy and usually uses less fluids than the other peritoneal modalities. Therefore, it tends to be the least expensive form of peritoneal therapy.

The usual dialysis prescription for patients on this technique is four 2-L dwells a day. However, this therapy can be individualized by increasing or decreasing dwell volume and by altering the number of exchanges per day.

**Continuous Cyclic Peritoneal Dialysis.** Standard CCPD uses a cycler for three 3-hour dwells while the patient sleeps with a subsequent 15-hour daytime dwell. Hence, this is a continuous therapy. Weekly clearances for typical CCPD are similar to those of CAPD. However, CCPD adds the extra cost of the cycler and the need for fresh tubing on a daily basis. Modifications of this technique include altering the number of nightly exchanges, dwell time, and instilled volume and occasionally combining CAPD technology to augment clearances by having the patient do one or more manual exchanges during the day.

## INTERMITTENT THERAPIES

As knowledge relating dialysis dose to outcome has become more apparent, the use of intermittent therapies has evolved. In general, for long-term therapy, the patients' dwell time should be matched to their peritoneal transport characteristics. Therefore, intermittent forms of peritoneal dialysis should be reserved for patients who are rapid transporters on the basis of classic PET curves.[233] As shown in Figure 57–12, these patients need short dwell times to maximize ultrafiltration, net drain volume, and overall solute clearance. Patients who are average or low transporters with good urine volume and a significant amount of residual renal clearance may also initially do well on these therapies, but usually only while they maintain their residual renal function. In addition, because of the known changes in membrane transport characteristics and poor ultrafiltration usually associated with episodes of peritonitis, an intermittent therapy (intermittent peritoneal dialysis [IPD], nightly intermittent peritoneal dialysis [NIPD], or daytime ambulatory peritoneal dialysis [DAPD]) may transiently be indicated during episodes of peritonitis. These therapies are also indicated for patients with type I membrane failure.

On the basis of PET measurements of peritoneal membrane transport, it is estimated that 10% to 15% of patients would do best with short-dwell therapies. Nolph and coworkers[408] have shown in cross-sectional data of 71 CAPD patients that 4-hour D/P creatinine values were inversely related to serum albumin levels. Furthermore, they noted increased protein losses in the dialysate of patients with higher D/P creatinine values. Increased protein dialysate losses and low serum albumin levels in patients with high 4-hour D/P creatinine values have also been reported by other investigators.[409–411] These authors have suggested that patients who are rapid transporters do not do as well with CAPD as other transport types do. Although definitive survival studies are lacking, these patients may do better with short-dwell therapies, such as NIPD, DAPD, or a modification of standard CCPD.

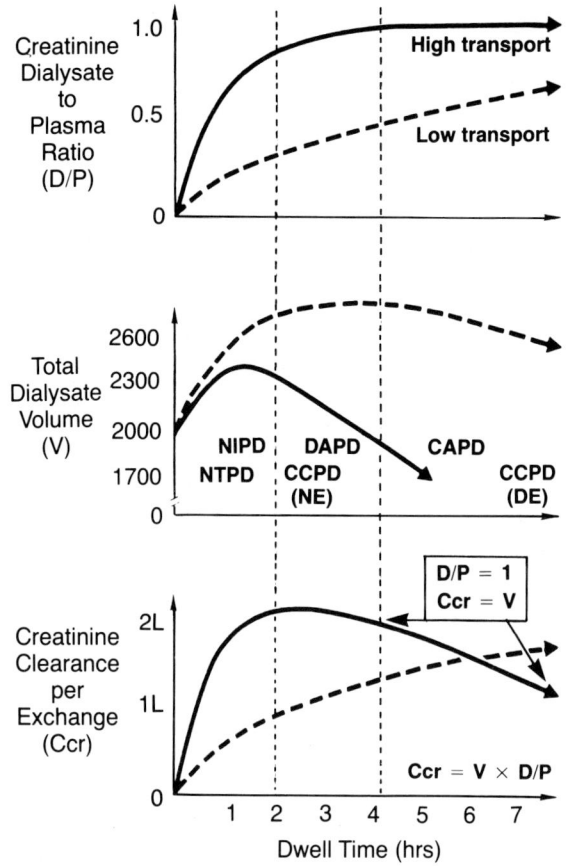

**Figure 57–12.** Theoretic relationships between dwell time, dialysate/plasma (D/P) ratio for creatinine, drain volume (V), and creatinine clearance (Ccr) compared for rapid and slow transporters. (From Twardowski ZJ: Nightly peritoneal dialysis. Why? who? how? and when? ASAIO Trans 36:8–16, 1990.)

### Intermittent Peritoneal Dialysis

By definition, IPD implies that therapy periods alternate with times when the peritoneum is relatively empty of dialysate. Classically, IPD was a form of peritoneal dialysis in which the exchanges were not done on a daily basis. The patient would typically use multiple short-dwell exchanges three or four times a week. Techniques included intermittent manual peritoneal dialysis, intermittent dialysis with an automated cycler, intermittent dialysis with a reverse osmosis machine, intermittent reciprocating dialysis with an extracorporeal reconstituting circuit, and others. These were described in detail in a previous edition.[5] Variations of these techniques led to tidal peritoneal dialysis or nightly tidal peritoneal dialysis (NTPD), which uses the reciprocating technique with an automated cycler.[412] On the basis of presently recommended weekly minimal clearances, it would be difficult to achieve these minimal targets in an anuric patient with therapy three or four times a week unless the patient had a prolonged treatment each time.

Morbidity and mortality were compared in 114 patients randomly assigned to home hemodialysis or home IPD.[413] In this study, the weekly dose of peritoneal dialysis was less than what is currently recommended for NIPD or

DAPD but was the standard of care for IPD at that time. There was no difference in survival of patients. However, more patients on IPD changed to a different modality than did those on hemodialysis, and home hemodialysis patients seemed to maintain better nutritional parameters. This study supports the notion that for long-term intermittent therapy to achieve adequate dialysis, either prolonged treatment times are needed or the patient must use a daily form of therapy (DAPD or NIPD).

However, classic IPD therapies continue to have their uses. A report from Mexico (where more than 90% of patients with ESRD use a form of peritoneal dialysis) suggested that IPD with a cycler may be more practical than CAPD in countries that have technical, social, and economic limitations that restrict the use of CAPD.[414] Other uses include treatment of refractory heart failure[415] and as a transient therapy for patients on ambulatory forms of peritoneal dialysis who have hernias or leaks.[267] Intra-abdominal pressures are highest when the patient is ambulatory and as intraperitoneal volume increases. Intra-abdominal pressures are the lowest with use of low-volume dialysis in the supine position. This is easiest to achieve with IPD. There are many reports of spontaneous sealing of various fluid leaks after a transient period of IPD using multiple short dwells and small instilled volumes. Another indication for IPD may be in patients who need to start dialysis before adequate catheter break-in has occurred. In this situation, low-volume dialysis in the supine position will be least likely to cause dialysate leaks and allow catheter healing.

### Nightly Intermittent Peritoneal Dialysis

NIPD with standard cycling techniques is best used by patients with high or high-average transport. DAPD is based on the same concept as NIPD. However, DAPD is a manual technique, and the patient typically has the dry time during the night. Both NIPD and DAPD operate within an intermediate range of dwell times. In patients who are rapid transporters, 8 hours of nightly dialysis can yield creatinine clearances similar to or higher than those achieved in these patients with standard CAPD. However, clearances are lower in other patients. The lower the peritoneal membrane transfer rates, the lower the 8-hour NIPD or DAPD clearances.[416] Thus, to improve NIPD clearances, time spent on NIPD or DAPD has to be prolonged by 10% to 40% to achieve minimal clearances needed for adequate dialysis. Consequently, the efficiency of standard NIPD or DAPD needs to be improved for anuric patients with average or low-average transport characteristics to achieve adequate clearances without spending an excessive amount of time per day on the therapy.

### Tidal Peritoneal Dialysis

Tidal peritoneal dialysis consists of the repeated instillation of small tidal volumes of dialysis fluids with the use of an automated cycler. The procedure is usually performed nightly (NTPD). Variables to be chosen include reserve volume, tidal outflow volume, tidal replacement volume, flow rates, and frequency of the exchanges. Tidal peritoneal dialysis was developed in an attempt to increase the efficiency of NIPD techniques.[412] Spencer and Farrel[417] have shown that MTAC values increase as one increases instilled volume from 1 to 2 L, presumably owing to increase in peritoneal surface area in contact with dialysate. However, an increase from 2 to 3 L did not always result in an increase in transport.[418] Therefore, other mechanisms of increasing efficiency needed to be considered. It is assumed that by maintaining an intraperitoneal reservoir and not attempting a complete drain after each dwell, tidal dialysis may maintain more continuous contact of dialysate with the peritoneal membrane; furthermore, the more rapid cycling of dialysis may increase mixing and prevent formation of stagnant fluid films within the abdomen. Preliminary studies suggest that creatinine and urea clearances are augmented, compared with those obtained with standard intermittent cycler techniques, in which a complete drain is attempted with every cycle.[419] With tidal dialysis, for a patient with average peritoneal transport rates, the urea clearance after 8 hours of treatment and 23 L of tidal flow can match the 24-hour clearances achieved in these patients with standard 8-L CAPD. A major disadvantage of NTPD is the cost of the large volume of fluids needed. The cost could be reduced by the availability of a fully automated cycler that also makes peritoneal dialysis fluids at home with the use of reverse osmosis proportioning systems.

Experiences with five stable anuric patients have demonstrated that to achieve creatinine clearances similar to those with standard 2-L CAPD, the average NTPD time was 9 hours and 24 minutes.[419] In this study, if the prescription was modeled to keep the creatinine clearances the same, it was shown that urea clearances were actually higher than those achieved with CAPD. This is because urea reaches equilibrium in the dialysate faster than creatinine does.[420] Similarly, six patients using IPD and NTPD were compared by use of mean dialysate volumes of 23 L, dialysis times of 7.5 h/d, and comparable glucose concentrations and filling volumes per cycle (1.5 or 2.5 L).[421] Tidal volume was 50% of fill volume. With tidal dialysis, there were significant increases in ultrafiltration and $PO_4^{3-}$ clearances but no significant differences in other small-solute clearances. Total protein losses were higher with tidal dialysis.

## FUTURE DIRECTIONS

Future directions in peritoneal dialysis techniques include ways to augment clearances, such as using a simple machine to add one nightly exchange for CAPD. Other directions include making cyclers smaller and more portable and attempts to allow more individualization of dwell volume and time.

## TYPICAL CLEARANCES

Table 57–5 shows the typical mean net clearances and dialysis fluid volumes achieved with the different dialysis techniques discussed. Typical values are based on representative values from multiple measurements reported in the literature. Peritoneal dialysis techniques are compared with one another and with 15 hours of standard hemodialysis per week. As demonstrated, CAPD and CCPD use the smallest

**TABLE 57–5. Clearances and Dialysis Solution Volumes with Different Dialysis Techniques***

| Technique | Treatment Time (h/wk) | Dialysate Onflow | | $C_{urea}$ | |
|---|---|---|---|---|---|
| | | L/h | L/wk | mL/min | L/wk |
| Manual PD | 48 | 2 | 96 | 18 | 52 |
| Rapid-cycling PD† | 40 | 4 | 160 | 30 | 72 |
| CAPD, CCPD | 168 | 0.33 | 56 | 7 | 67 |
| NIPD | 56 | 3.25 | 182 | 6 | 59 |
| TPD | 56 | 3.38 | 189 | 7 | 73 |
| Hemodialysis | 15 | 30 | 450 | 150 | 135 |

*PD = peritoneal dialysis; CAPD = continuous ambulatory peritoneal dialysis; CCPD = continuous cyclic peritoneal dialysis; NIPD = nightly intermittent peritoneal dialysis; TPD = tidal peritoneal dialysis.
†Cycler, reverse osmosis, reciprocating, recirculating.

dialysate volumes and achieve the highest clearances for high-molecular-weight substances. Hemodialysis therapy provides greater low-molecular-weight clearances than any peritoneal dialysis technique.

## Adequacy of Dialysis

### OUTCOME STUDIES

There is presently an ongoing debate about whether small-solute clearances are good predictors of important clinical outcomes in peritoneal dialysis patients. This important question has been difficult to resolve because of the conflicting results in the literature. To date, there has been no prospective randomized controlled trial to evaluate the effect of dialysis dose on outcome in peritoneal dialysis patients analogous to the National Cooperative Dialysis Study for hemodialysis.[422] Most of the studies published to date are based on cross-sectional data, involve small numbers of patients, and are open to methodologic criticisms limiting their interpretation.

Despite these limitations, some conclusions can be drawn. The best long-term study to support this concept is by Teehan and associates.[423] This study of 51 patients observed for a median of 24 months suggests that urea kinetics (measured as urea clearance divided by volume of distribution, or Kt/V) was predictive of outcome, serum albumin concentration, and transfusion requirements. When survival on CAPD was plotted as a function of Kt/V, the probability of surviving for 5 years was greater than 90% for patients with a Kt/V greater than or equal to 0.27/d (1.89/wk, 0.63 hemodialysis per treatment equivalent), compared with less than 50% for those patients with a lesser value (Fig. 57–13). This difference, however, was not seen until after 2 to 3 years of CAPD. When survival of patients was correlated with serum albumin concentration, not only did serum albumin levels predict death, but they were predictive immediately (Fig. 57–14). These authors also found that Kt/V was predictive of serum albumin levels but not days hospitalized.

This study suggests that there is a minimal dose of peritoneal dialysis needed for an adequate outcome (i.e., a combined Kt/V of at least 0.27/d and a serum albumin level of at least 3.5 g/dL). These results are supported by the following studies. In a retrospective review by Lameire and co-workers[357] of 16 patients who survived at least 5 years on CAPD, it was noted that dialysis dose measured in terms of urea kinetics (Kt/V) correlated positively with protein catabolic rate (PCR) and inversely with number of days hospitalized, peritonitis rates, and peripheral nerve conduction velocity. These results suggest that as dialysis dose increased, patients did better. Keshaviah and colleagues[424] noted a positive correlation between clinical assessment of the patient and Kt/V in 74% of their observations, concluding that a Kt/V of at least 0.24/d correlated with a positive outcome. Brandes and co-workers[425] found a significant difference in outcomes between patients with a mean weekly Kt/V of 0.5 and those with a Kt/V of 0.77.

However, Blake and colleagues,[426] who studied 76 patients for a 3-year period, monitoring urea kinetics and PCR every 6 months for an average of 20 months, detected an inverse correlation between Kt/V and biochemical parameters such as urea, creatinine, and $PO_4^{3-}$ levels and direct correlations between Kt/V and PCR and serum albumin levels. In their initial report, they did not show a correlation between Kt/V and any clinical outcome. However, further analysis[427] did show that when volume of urea distribution as determined from Watson nomograms[428] was used, as opposed to a fixed fraction of body weight, there was a statistically significant increased number of deaths in patients whose most recent Kt/V was 1.5/wk or less. Again, this suggests that there may be a lower limit of dialysis dose, below which it might not be safe to model CAPD prescriptions. In a subsequent publication correlating creatinine kinetics with outcome, using the same database,[429] there was also no overall correlation between weekly creatinine clearance and outcome. Despite this lack of an overall correlation, there was a significantly higher number of deaths in the subgroup of patients with a weekly creatinine clearance of less than 48 L/wk/1.73 m², again suggesting that a minimal dose of dialysis is needed to ensure an adequate outcome. Similarly, Brandes and co-workers[430] reported a positive correlation between outcome and creatinine kinetics.

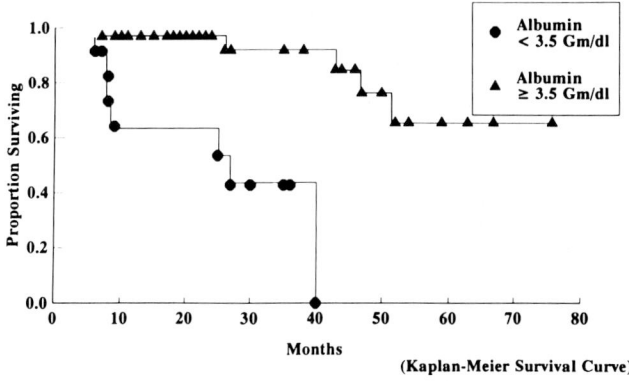

**Figure 57–14.** Kaplan-Meier plot of survival on CAPD as a function of the serum albumin level. (From Teehan BP, Schleifer CR, Brown J: Is urea kinetic modeling the best measure of adequacy in CAPD? Semin Dial 5:189–196, 1992.)

The finding that outcome is influenced by dialysis dose only below a certain minimum and the methodologic flaws in each study may explain why some studies show that dose influences outcome,[357, 423] whereas others do not.[426, 431–434]

It is apparent that the typical range of Kt/V delivered to CAPD patients lies between 1.2 and 2.4/wk, which, when divided by 3 to facilitate comparison with hemodialysis three times a week, gives a range of 0.4 to 0.8. Similarly, the minimal target values for peritoneal dialysis dose recommended by these studies (Kt/V greater than 0.5 to 0.6 hemodialysis per treatment equivalent) are well below the accepted minimal standard of a Kt/V of 1.0 for hemodialysis. Keshaviah and associates[435] tried to resolve this paradox by invoking the peak concentration hypothesis. This hypothesis suggests that the peak blood urea values achieved during the week are related to uremic toxicity more than time-averaged values are. The finding in most studies that the slope of the line for Kt/V versus PCR is greater for CAPD than for hemodialysis (Fig. 57–15) is further indirect evidence for this hypothesis. Other possible explanations for this difference include the following: 1) the presence of a stable metabolic milieu with CAPD, compared with the peaks and valleys associated with hemodialysis; 2) the better large-solute clearance with CAPD than with hemodialysis; 3) the better preservation of residual renal function with CAPD (discussed later); 4) the absence of blood-membrane interactions and the subsequent cytokine activation; and 5) the absence of interdialytic acidosis, which has catabolic effects in hemodialysis patients not experienced by CAPD patients. It can certainly be argued that adequate dialysis should address not only small-solute clearance measured in urea or creatinine kinetics but also control of volume status, acid-base control, and nutritional considerations.

## NUTRITION

In the most extensive evaluation of a cross section of CAPD patients published to date, 49.6% (111 of 224) were found to have signs of malnutrition.[436] Eight percent were severely malnourished, and these patients tended to have

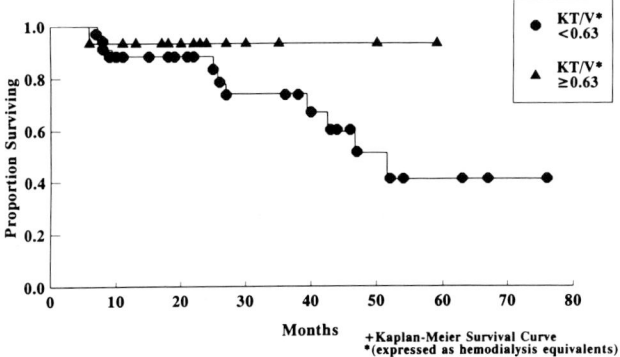

**Figure 57–13.** Kaplan-Meier plot of survival on CAPD as a function of Kt/V (Kt/V expressed in hemodialysis equivalents). (From Teehan BP, Schleifer CR, Brown J: Is urea kinetic modeling the best measure of adequacy in CAPD? Semin Dial 5:189–196, 1992.)

minimal or no residual renal function. Malnutrition was present in 18.1% of patients using CAPD treated for less than 3 months compared with 41.6% of patients using CAPD for longer than 3 months. In non-ESRD patients, one of the most important predictors of outcome is the patient's underlying nutritional status.[437]

### Influence of Serum Albumin Level on Outcome

Serum albumin levels have traditionally been used as a measure of visceral protein stores. Data by Lowrie and co-workers[438] have shown that in hemodialysis patients, as the serum albumin level decreases, the risk of death increases. In fact, in patients with a serum albumin concentration of 2.5 g/dL or less, the risk of death was 18 times that of the reference group (patients with an albumin concentration of 4.0 to 4.5 g/dL). Teehan[423] and Blake[439] and co-workers have shown that low serum albumin concentration is an important predictor of both hospitalizations and death in CAPD patients. Similarly, Rocco and Burkart[440] have shown that a low serum albumin concentration at 1 year was predictive of both death and hospitalizations. Despite these positive correlations between serum albumin level and outcome, it has been debated that serum albumin concentration may not be the sensitive marker for malnutrition that it has been found to be in hemodialysis.[441] Nevertheless, it is well known from clinical and experimental observations that patients who are overtly uremic are anorexic and tend to have decreased protein intakes.[442] These clinical observations in nondialyzed patients with renal failure would suggest that anorexia or decreased protein intake could be a subtle sign of inadequate dialysis.

### Correlation Between Dialysis Dose and Dietary Protein Intake

The question is, does the dose of dialysis influence the patient's dietary protein intake and overall nutritional status? This hypothesis was tested by examining the relationship of PCR, an estimate of dietary protein intake, and the dose of dialysis (Kt/V urea). Lindsay and Spanner[443] found a linear relationship between PCR and Kt/V urea (see Fig. 57–15). Other authors have reported a similar observation for both hemodialysis and peritoneal dialysis patients.[444–447] Although these data are cross-sectional, they suggest that dietary protein intake, PCR, and nutritional status are at least partially related to dialysis dose. Further evidence of this is the finding in some cross-sectional studies that serum albumin level correlates positively with PCR,[408, 410] although this has not been found by all investigators.[448]

There is some controversy as to what dietary protein intake (or PCR) is needed to maintain positive nitrogen balance in peritoneal dialysis patients. Early work by Blumenkrantz and colleagues[449] and Diamond and Henrich[450] would suggest that a dietary protein intake of at least 1.2 g/kg/d was needed to maintain positive nitrogen balance. However, cross-sectional studies by Bergstrom and Lindholm[444] and Nolph[446] suggest that their patients tended to eat less (protein intake of 0.99 and 0.88 g/kg/d, respectively) despite having no signs of malnutrition and appear-

ing to be adequately dialyzed. If it is assumed that a dietary protein intake estimated from PCR of at least 1.0 g of protein per kilogram per day is needed to maintain normal nutrition, then a "minimal" dialysis dose can be estimated from published data correlating PCR to dialysis dose in peritoneal dialysis patients (see Fig. 57–15). These data would suggest that for peritoneal dialysis patients to maintain a PCR of at least 1.0 g/kg/d, a Kt/V (hemodialysis equivalent) of at least 0.56 is required (Kt/V of 1.7/wk). This dose is similar to the recommendations established from outcome studies.

Data correlating a change in dialysis dose to a corresponding change in PCR or serum albumin levels in an individual patient are scarce. Both Lindsay and co-workers[451] and Keshaviah[452] have shown that changes in dialysis dose were strongly associated with a corresponding change in PCR. Burkart and colleagues[453] have shown that as dialysis dose increased, not only did PCR increase, but so did serum albumin concentrations. Although it is clear that there are multiple other factors that determine serum albumin levels, such as age,[454] peritoneal membrane transport,[408–410] and comorbid diseases, the relationship between dietary protein intake, serum albumin concentration, and nutritional status and dialysis dose is a significant one. These data suggest that to optimize the patient's outcome, the patient's dialysis dose must be sufficient to allow adequate protein intake.

### RECOMMENDATIONS FOR MINIMAL DIALYSIS DOSE

Recommendations for the minimal targeted dose of dialysis measured by use of small-solute clearances have been established for peritoneal dialysis on the basis of outcome results; the positive correlation between dialysis dose and PCR; the preliminary findings that as dose is increased in an individual, PCR is increased; and the minimal require-

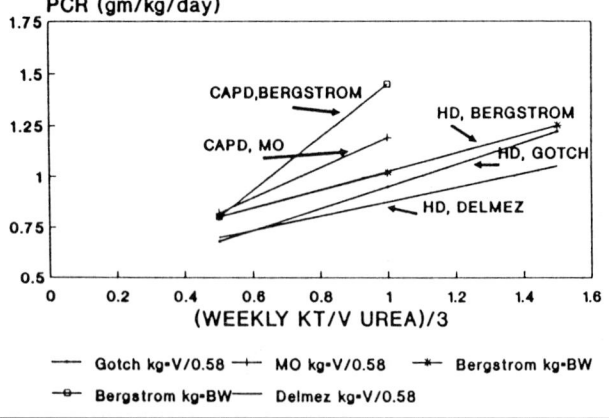

**PCR & KT/V UREA IN HD AND CAPD**

**Figure 57–15.** Correlation of protein catabolic rate (PCR) and weekly Kt/V ([Kt/V urea]/3) in two CAPD populations and three hemodialysis (HD) populations. (From Nolph KD, Moore HL, Prowant B, et al: Cross sectional assessment of weekly urea and creatinine clearances and indices of nutrition in continuous ambulatory peritoneal dialysis patients. Perit Dial Int 13:178–183, 1993.)

**TABLE 57–6. Minimal Recommendations for Dialysis Dose**

---

**Continuous Peritoneal Dialysis (CAPD, CCPD)**
Kt/V ≥ 1.7/wk
Creatinine clearance ≥ 50 L/wk/1.73 m²

**Intermittent Peritoneal Dialysis**
Kt/V ≥ 2.2/wk

---

ments for dietary protein intake to maintain positive protein balance. The "optimal" dose has not been established and would certainly take into account other variables, such as blood pressure control, anemia, rehabilitation, and quality of life issues. These minimal target values are found in Table 57–6. Note that for intermittent therapies, these target minimal doses are higher, based on the peak concentration hypothesis.[435] Although these minimal dose recommendations should allow the patient to maintain positive nitrogen balance (PCR of at least 1.0 g/kg/d), PCR and other clinical parameters of uremia should also be monitored.

## RESIDUAL RENAL FUNCTION

Total mass transfer or clearance of any solute from the body is a function not only of its removal in dialysate but also of its removal from other sources, such as that due to residual renal function. As residual renal function decreases, overall solute clearance will decrease.[429, 452] At this time, dialysis dose may need to be increased to make sure the patient's dose is above the minimal amount needed to ensure an adequate outcome. It is now well documented that residual renal function is better preserved with peritoneal dialysis than with hemodialysis.[455–457] As technique survival for CAPD increases,[458] more cases of inadequate dialysis may become apparent if nephrologists do not adjust the peritoneal dialysis prescription to compensate for decreases in underlying residual renal function.

Residual renal creatinine or urea clearances are calculated in the standard way. Residual renal urea clearance per day can be divided by V, the volume of distribution for urea, and added to the total dialysate Kt/V because there is little or no tubule secretion of urea contributing to overall renal clearance of urea. However, if dialysis dose is monitored by use of creatinine kinetics, it is recommended that only the contribution of creatinine clearance due to glomerular filtration be added. It is well known that at low creatinine clearances, much of the creatinine in the urine is from tubule secretion and not from glomerular filtration. As a result, traditional measurements of creatinine clearances (24-hour urine collections) can overestimate true glomerular filtration. Therefore, it is recommended that one use the sum of the measured urea and creatinine clearance divided by 2 to approximate underlying residual renal glomerular filtration rates.[459]

## STEPS IN PRESCRIPTION DIALYSIS

The first step in optimizing an individual peritoneal dialysis prescription is to characterize the peritoneal membrane transport characteristics. As described earlier, this can be done with use of MTAC parameters or D/P ratios. In clinical practice, this is most easily done with 4-hour D/P ratios obtained from the standard PET.[233] After an overnight dwell, 2 L of 2.5% dextrose dialysis fluid is instilled (time 0) and allowed to dwell for 4 hours. Dialysate urea, creatinine, glucose, and at times Na⁺ concentrations are measured at time 0 and after 2 and 4 hours of dwell time. Serum values are determined after 2 hours. Four-hour drain volume is also obtained. For each of these dwell times, D/P ratios are obtained for urea and creatinine. The ratios of glucose at time of drain to the initial dialysis fluid glucose (D/D₀) are also obtained. On the basis of published data, the membrane type can be identified with this test, and the peritoneal dialysis prescription that would best match the patient's transport characteristics can be chosen (Fig. 57–16 and Table 57–7).

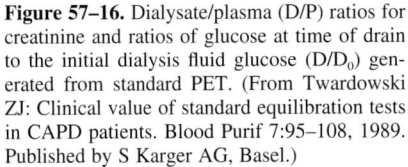

Figure 57–16. Dialysate/plasma (D/P) ratios for creatinine and ratios of glucose at time of drain to the initial dialysis fluid glucose (D/D₀) generated from standard PET. (From Twardowski ZJ: Clinical value of standard equilibration tests in CAPD patients. Blood Purif 7:95–108, 1989. Published by S Karger AG, Basel.)

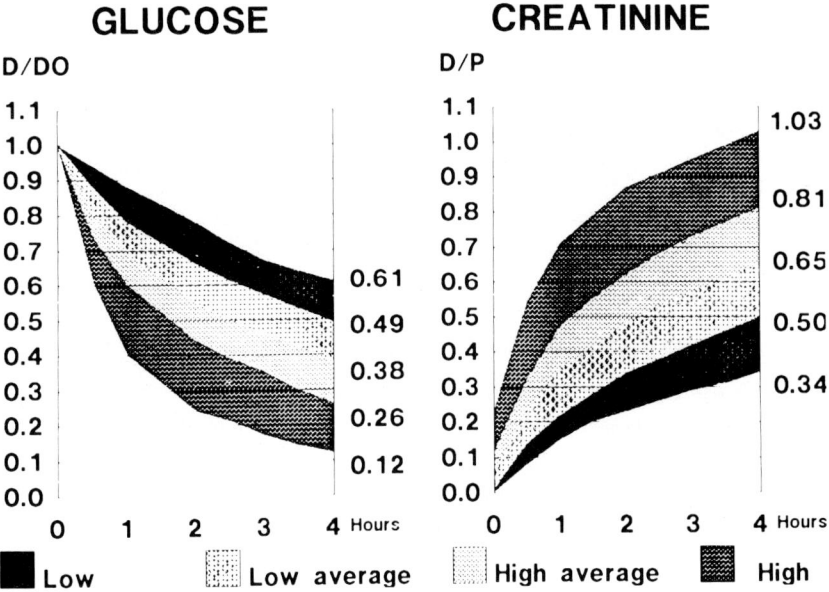

**TABLE 57–7. Baseline Peritoneal Equilibration Test Prognostic Value**

| Solute Transport | Ultrafiltration | Predicted Response to CAPD | Preferred Peritoneal Dialysis Modality |
|---|---|---|---|
| High | Poor | Adequate | NPD, DAPD* |
| High-average | Adequate | Adequate | Standard-flow peritoneal dialysis† |
| Low-average | Good | Adequate | Standard-flow peritoneal dialysis† |
| | | Inadequate | High-flow peritoneal dialysis‡ |
| Low | Excellent | Inadequate | High-flow peritoneal dialysis‡ |

*NPD = nightly peritoneal dialysis; DAPD = daytime ambulatory peritoneal dialysis.
†CAPD with 7.5 to 9.0 L/d, or CCPD with dialysis solution inflow of 6 to 8 L overnight and 2 L daytime.
‡CAPD with more than 9.0 L/d; or CCPD with inflow of more than 8 L overnight or 2 L daytime, or both.
From Twardowski ZJ: Nightly peritoneal dialysis. Why? who? how? and when? ASAIO Trans 36:8–16, 1990.

Overall clearance is related not only to D/P ratios and solute concentration in the dialysate but also to final drain volumes (see Fig. 57–12). Patients with small overall drain volumes tend to have lower clearances. For instance, patients who are rapid transporters of urea and creatinine also tend to be rapid absorbers of dialysate glucose. Therefore, although the D/P ratios for small solutes tend to be near unity after 4-hour or longer dwells, drain volumes tend to be small because of the associated glucose absorption. These patients tend to maximize drain volumes early in the dwell; consequently, optimal clearances and net ultrafiltration will usually be obtained with short dwell times, such as those associated with NIPD, DAPD, or a combination of these. Conversely, in patients who are slow transporters, net ultrafiltration tends to peak late in the dwell. In addition, D/P ratios tend to increase linearly during the dwell, and it is not until prolonged dwell times that unity is reached. For these patients, dwell time is crucial; they will do best with continuous therapies, such as CAPD or CCPD. At times, if the patient has a large body surface area and total body water, large volumes of dialysate or prolonged times on cycler therapy will be needed to achieve target doses of dialysis, both of which may be impractical to achieve. These patients may do best with hemodialysis or a combination of peritoneal dialysis and hemodialysis. These differences in transport type must be taken into account in attempting to optimize each individual patient's peritoneal dialysis prescription.

Another way to classify a patient's peritoneal membrane transport involves the use of MTAC.[208–211] This is a more precise way of defining transport because these values are not influenced by dwell volumes or glucose concentrations, as D/P ratios are. However, the use of MTAC requires additional laboratory parameters and computer models, but once obtained, these values can be used to guide therapy in a clinical setting.[222, 453, 460]

## CALCULATION OF DIALYSIS DOSE

The "gold standard" for determining the daily clearance of any solute is to measure the actual amount of that solute removed from the body by all sources each day. For the case of peritoneal dialysis patients, this means measurement of creatinine or urea clearances by obtaining 24-hour collections of both dialysate and urine and determining creatinine clearances or Kt/V urea values in the standard way.[461]

An alternative is to estimate the daily clearances either mathematically on the basis of D/P values or with the use of computer-assisted kinetic modeling programs. These are estimations, and although they tend to correlate, there is a high degree of discordance with values actually obtained from 24-hour collections.[349] Therefore, at present, 24-hour collections are recommended. These collections are complementary to PET data, and both are used routinely for prescription dialysis, problem solving, and monitoring of the patient.

## Clinical Observations

### TECHNIQUE SURVIVAL

Rates of dropout to hemodialysis due to technical problems associated with the peritoneal dialysis techniques are decreasing. In the past, when groups of patients on peritoneal dialysis were compared with those on hemodialysis, technique survival (defined as the actuarial percentage of patients alive and remaining on their original modality, with death, transplantation, and recovery of renal function considered loss to risk) was generally better for those on hemodialysis.[462–464] However, reports have revealed encouraging trends. Technique failure in new peritoneal dialysis patients was reported to be less with Y systems than with standard spike and with the use of ultraviolet connection devices, perhaps because of decreased peritonitis rates with these systems.[458] In a single center, where technique failure was attributed by actuarial analysis to death or transfer, 6-year technique survival was 28% for CAPD and 31% for hemodialysis.[465] In a review from Italy, other than a marginally increased risk of technique failure in female patients, there were no other significant risk factors associated with technique failure.[466] However, a report from the United States suggests that elderly patients have a relatively higher technique survival at least in part because of their higher death rate, and black patients had a relatively lower technique survival.[458]

The three most common causes of technique failure were peritonitis (30%), clinical complications (18%), and peritoneal membrane failure (16%) in a 10-year follow-up of peritoneal dialysis patients in Italy.[467] Both technique failure and the relative risk of death were increased in the subgroup of patients with the highest peritonitis rates. Maiorca and colleagues[469] have suggested that as peritonitis rates decline, technique survival increases. With documented decreases in peritonitis rates[458, 468] and the increased attention toward catheter development and exit site care, it is expected that technique survival for hemodialysis and peritoneal dialysis will soon be similar.[469]

## SURVIVAL OF PATIENTS

Most comparisons of actuarial survivals of patients in comparable populations suggest that survival with CAPD and hemodialysis is similar.[463, 464, 470–472] In a multicenter study by Maiorca and co-workers[473] that compared outcomes in 480 CAPD patients and 373 hemodialysis patients between 1981 and 1987, 7-year survival rates were not significantly different even though CAPD patients were on the average 6 years older and had more comorbid conditions shown to be risk factors (Fig. 57–17). After correction for the influence of risk factors, significant differences in survival of patients were still not seen until after the age of 53.5 years, above which an increased risk of death was seen in hemodialysis patients. Unadjusted technique failure was better for hemodialysis than for peritoneal dialysis, but these differences were eliminated after adjustment for technique failure due to peritonitis.

The USRDS applied the Cox proportional hazards model to 4387 new ESRD patients in the United States and found that the relative risk of death was higher with CAPD and was greater than that for patients using hemodialysis (relative risk = 1.14).[474] This was accounted for entirely by the finding of an increased risk of death in elderly diabetic patients using CAPD. Younger diabetic patients actually showed a greater risk of death on hemodialysis compared with CAPD. There were no consistent differences in death rates at different ages as a function of modality choice for primary renal diseases other than diabetes. Further analysis of these data suggests that this increased risk in elderly diabetic patients may have been due to an increase in the prevalence of peripheral vascular disease in this population. Similarly, in patients who started dialysis in Michigan in 1989, modality choice (peritoneal dialysis versus hemodialysis) was not a risk factor for nondiabetic patients.[475]

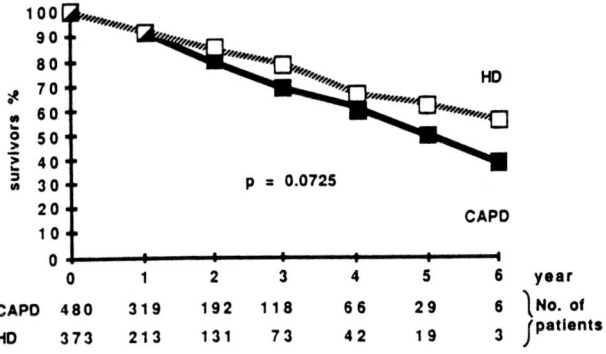

**Figure 57–17.** Survival curves for patients on CAPD (*black squares*) and hemodialysis (HD, *white squares*) unadjusted for any pretreatment prognostic differences. (From Maiorca R, Vonesh EF, Cavalli PL, et al: A multicenter, selection-adjusted comparison of patient and technique survivals on CAPD and hemodialysis. Perit Dial Int 11:118–127, 1991.)

However, in diabetic patients, an increased risk of death was found for those older than 60 years undergoing peritoneal dialysis. These data suggest that for the average nondiabetic patient, modality choice should not influence outcome. However, for diabetic patients, modality choice may influence outcome. Further studies that carefully match comorbid diseases with careful adjustments for all the known risks are needed.

Peritonitis has been shown to be associated with an increased risk of death. In two studies, survival was less in the subgroup of patients with the highest overall peritonitis rates.[466, 467] Peritonitis is reported to be directly responsible for 1.3% to 1.9% of deaths for all patients on peritoneal dialysis.[463, 470, 473, 476] However, peritonitis may contribute to other causes of death by worsening the patient's overall condition. These data emphasize the need to use systems for the dialysis exchange that are associated with the lowest overall risk of peritonitis. Cardiovascular disease remains the leading cause of death.

## Complications

### INFECTIOUS COMPLICATIONS

An overview of the complications of peritoneal dialysis stresses that peritonitis and exit site infections are the major complications of the therapy.[477] The continuous introduction of dialysis fluids into the peritoneal cavity not only can cause peritonitis through touch contamination but also significantly alters the normal host defense mechanisms and peritoneal environment. Because of this, a relatively small inoculum of bacteria can readily cause peritonitis in a peritoneal dialysis patient, whereas similar small inoculations during surgical laparotomies seldom cause peritonitis. Compared with surgical peritonitis, peritoneal dialysis–related bacterial peritonitis is usually due to a single pathogen, is usually confined to the peritoneum, and is seldom associated with positive blood cultures or abscess formation. Typically, these patients can be treated on an outpatient basis. Mortality associated with peritonitis in CAPD patients has been reported to be 0.8% to 12.5%.[476, 478, 479] In these cases, most deaths are due not to the infection itself but often to a complication of the peritonitis, such as myocardial infarction.[480, 481]

### Host Defenses

A typical patient using CAPD may perform up to 1500 exchanges per year; it would be naive to think that there was not occasional contamination of the peritoneum. However, peritonitis rates are not excessive. This is because the likelihood of the development of peritonitis depends on the balance between the number of bacteria introduced and the ability of peritoneal defenses to eradicate them. Peritoneal host defenses were reviewed by Lewis and Holmes[121, 482] and Cairns.[483] Peritoneal white blood cell counts from dialysate fluids in the absence of peritonitis are approximately 100- to 1000-fold less than the peritoneal fluid white blood cell counts from healthy individuals, in part because of dilution with dialysis solution. The white blood cell differential differs markedly among uninfected patients, ranging from 20% to 95% for macrophages, 2% to 84% for lymphocytes, and 0% to 27% for neutrophils.[121] Although white blood cell counts tend to decrease with time on peritoneal dialysis,[484] there are no significant differences in peritoneal effluent white blood cell counts in patients with high or low peritonitis frequency.[485] These data would suggest that absolute peritoneal fluid white blood cell count and differential are not the determining factors in the risk for peritonitis.

Effective phagocytosis and intracellular killing of pathogens by macrophages involve a series of steps outlined in Figure 57–18. This includes opsonization of organisms with IgG, C3b, C4d, and fibronectin, opsonins normally found in the peritoneal cavity. IgG is the primary immunoglobulin found in peritoneal fluids of healthy individuals, usually at a concentration equal to that in blood. In contrast, when dialysate effluents of CAPD patients are evaluated, the levels are found to be only about 1% of the concentration in blood, presumably owing to the constant dilution and re-

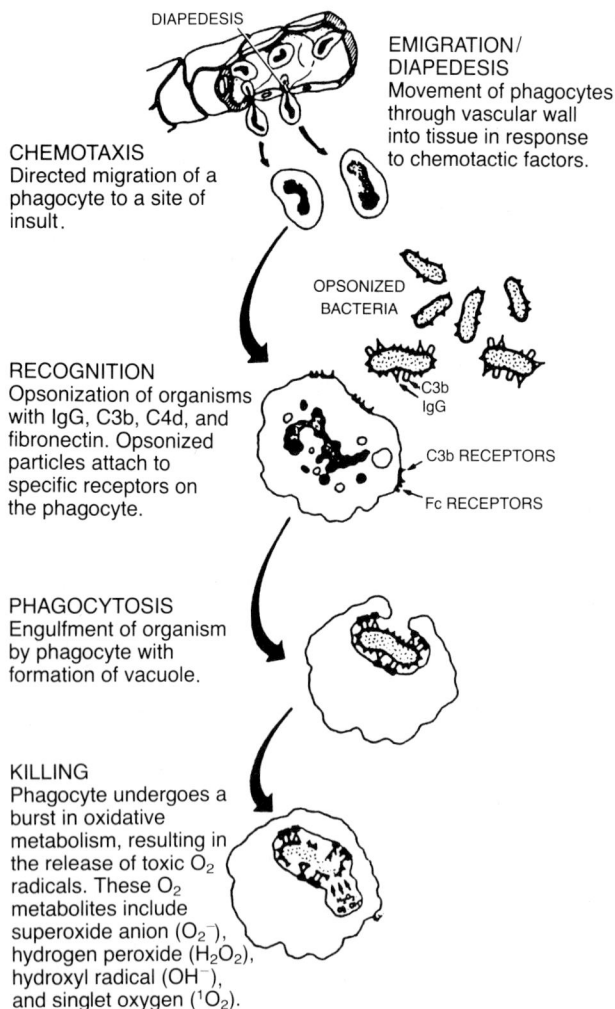

DIAPEDESIS

**EMIGRATION/ DIAPEDESIS**
Movement of phagocytes through vascular wall into tissue in response to chemotactic factors.

**CHEMOTAXIS**
Directed migration of a phagocyte to a site of insult.

OPSONIZED BACTERIA

**RECOGNITION**
Opsonization of organisms with IgG, C3b, C4d, and fibronectin. Opsonized particles attach to specific receptors on the phagocyte.

C3b IgG

C3b RECEPTORS

Fc RECEPTORS

**PHAGOCYTOSIS**
Engulfment of organism by phagocyte with formation of vacuole.

**KILLING**
Phagocyte undergoes a burst in oxidative metabolism, resulting in the release of toxic $O_2$ radicals. These $O_2$ metabolites include superoxide anion ($O_2^-$), hydrogen peroxide ($H_2O_2$), hydroxyl radical ($OH^-$), and singlet oxygen ($^1O_2$).

**Figure 57–18.** Diagrammatic representation of events involved in the phagocytosis and killing of bacteria by phagocytic white blood cells. (From Lewis S, Holmes C: Host defense mechanisms in the peritoneal cavity of continuous ambulatory peritoneal dialysis patients. Perit Dial Int 11:14–21, 1991.)

moval.[486] Plasma and dialysate IgG levels were not related to the frequency of peritonitis in this population, although some authors have suggested that subpopulations of patients with low peritoneal fluid IgG levels are at increased risk for peritonitis.

Peritoneal fluid complement levels, particularly of C3, are also reduced and are typically less than 1 to 3 mg/dL in peritoneal dialysis patients compared with a mean of 80 mg/dL normally found in peritoneal fluid. There is a similar reduction in fibronectin levels, which has been shown to augment the phagocytosis of *Staphylococcus aureus*.[487] These studies show that although the normal opsonins are present in peritoneal fluids of peritoneal dialysis patients, they are present at concentrations much below those in healthy individuals.

**Normal Inflammatory Response.** The normal peritoneal inflammatory response is a sequential, integrated response that is both vascular and cellular in nature. Whether the inciting event is traumatic or microbacterial in origin, the response is similar and often mediated by various chemical mediators.

The first line of defense is believed to be the peritoneal macrophages, most of which are thought to be in the peritoneal fluid as a result of inflammatory stimuli rather than as resident macrophages.[488] The peripheral blood monocyte is thought to be the precursor of these cells. There is disagreement about the overall functional capabilities of the peritoneal macrophage in a peritoneal dialysis patient, partly because of the differences in experimental techniques used to isolate the different cell types, but also because of the different cell types that have been used for controls. There is agreement that when microorganisms are used in vitro to measure phagocytosis, peritoneal macrophages from CAPD patients function as effectively as macrophages from healthy individuals do.[121] However, when phagocytosis is measured by use of fluoresceinated beads, phagocytic activity is found to be subnormal.[489]

Similarly, there are conflicting data regarding bactericidal activity of these macrophages. In general, it appears that peritoneal macrophages from CAPD patients studied in dialysate-free mediums have intact bactericidal properties. However, some authors have suggested that there may be a small subpopulation of patients with reduced intracellular killing capabilities and a tendency for higher peritonitis rates.[490, 491] No difference in expression of complement receptors was seen when peritoneal macrophages were compared with peripheral macrophages. However, binding of C5a (a chemotactic factor) and Fc receptor (binds IgG) expression were increased in peritoneal macrophages of uninfected patients,[492] which suggests that these cells are in a relative state of activation and are important in host defense. This apparent state of activation can be the result of chronic exposure to small inocula of bacteria or chronic activation from dialysis fluid, or it is possible that these macrophages are more immature cell types owing to the need for increased bone marrow production because of the frequent loss of these cells during the process of peritoneal dialysis. Immature cells are known to normally be relatively more activated than unstimulated mature cells.

These in vitro data must be interpreted with some reservation. To obtain the cells needed for these observations, all the cells from an overnight drain are often needed, and the concentration after centrifugation is much higher than that in the effluent dialysate. Furthermore, the initial dialysis fluid pH, hyperosmolarity, and typical presence of lactate as a buffer may all directly or indirectly affect white blood cell function. Experimental data do not always account for these physiologic differences. Therefore, in vitro environments do not approximate the in vivo state.

In the absence of peritonitis, peritoneal lymphocytes compose 20% to 40% of the total peritoneal leukocytes, with a reported range of 2% to 84%. Most of these (70% to 80%) are T lymphocytes. There tends to be a high percentage of activated T lymphocytes, similar to the apparent stage of activation noted for peritoneal macrophages. Abnormal lymphocyte function has been associated with high rates of peritonitis,[493] and this abnormal lymphocyte function may be cytokine mediated.[494]

Activated macrophages, lymphocytes, and mesothelial cells produce cytokines, which play an important role in host defense and fibrosis. Lamperi and Carozzi[495] have noted cytokine alterations in patients with frequent peritonitis that include a decreased ability to produce interleukin-1 and interferon-γ. On the basis of these findings, Carrozzi and co-workers[496] have shown that daily intraperitoneal administration of human recombinant interferon alpha resulted in a reduction in peritonitis frequency and an increase in macrophage function. This group has also shown that dialysis fluid $Ca^{2+}$ concentration correlated with cytoplasmic $Ca^{2+}$ concentration and in vitro function of peritoneal macrophages.[126] Raising the dialysis fluid $Ca^{2+}$ concentration[126] and the addition of 1,25-dihydroxyvitamin $D_3$ increased superoxide generation and killing in these cells.[497] Unfortunately, these investigators have also suggested that increasing dialysis fluid and intracellular $Ca^{2+}$ concentration increases the tendency for peritoneal fibrosis and adhesion formation. These data potentially create a paradox regarding dialysis fluid $Ca^{2+}$ concentration and reducing the risk for peritonitis or fibrosis. Given the efforts to decrease dialysis fluid $Ca^{2+}$ concentrations to facilitate treatment of metabolic bone disease, at present it seems wise to lower dialysis fluid $Ca^{2+}$ concentrations to near the physiologic range of $Ca^{2+}$ concentrations in blood (2.5 mEq/L, 5 mmol/L). To date, there has been no reported increase in overall peritonitis rates with use of these fluids.[129, 130] However, one group has reported an increased frequency of *Staphylococcus epidermidis* infections.[128]

Other mechanisms of host defense may include lymphatic absorption of bacteria. However, because blood cultures are rarely positive with bacterial peritonitis, this would imply an efficient removal of bacteria by associated lymph nodes.[498] Drainage of dialysate from the peritoneum is associated with the physical removal of bacteria and has been shown to be helpful, depending on the residual volume of fluid left in the peritoneal cavity.[499] However, to eliminate *S. aureus*, a residual volume of less than 200 mL was needed. This volume is close to physiologic and can usually be achieved in a long-term peritoneal dialysis patient only after a period of abstinence from dialysis. Mesothelial cells may also function in host defense. It has been demonstrated that these cells produce surfactant, which has been shown to bind endotoxin, which may facilitate phagocytosis.[500]

Mesothelial cells have also been shown to produce interleukin-8 in response to other cytokines,[501] which is chemotactic for neutrophils and suggests that the mesothelial cell may be an important messenger cell in the host response to peritonitis.

Bacteria may adhere to the mesothelium and thus are removed from the dialysate, but there is minimal phagocytosis of adherent bacteria, which suggests that adherence is not a major part of host defense.[502]

**Inflammatory Response During Peritonitis.** The fate of bacteria entering the peritoneum depends on many factors, and this invasion does not always develop into peritonitis. Bacteria are occasionally isolated from peritoneal effluent cultures of asymptomatic patients.[503] These are usually *S. epidermidis* and *Propionibacterium*. In contrast, more virulent pathogens, such as *S. aureus*, are almost always associated with peritonitis. Long-term peritoneal dialysis patients without peritonitis have been shown to have fluctuations in the percentage and absolute number of peritoneal macrophages as well as fluctuations in activated complement levels, which suggests that the peritoneum is occasionally inoculated with small numbers of bacteria but that these are eradicated by host defenses before peritonitis can occur.[485, 504] Intracellular bacteria can occasionally be found in peritoneal macrophages, even in patients with no prior history of peritonitis.

The incubation period for significant bacterial growth and resultant infection after exogenous inoculation of the peritoneum is not known. If the host defenses are overwhelmed, clinical experience would suggest that signs and symptoms usually develop within 24 to 48 hours but are occasionally rapid in onset (less than 6 hours). The incubation period for endogenous contamination is unknown but is thought to be shorter.

During episodes of peritonitis, peritoneal macrophages are primed to release increased amounts of interleukin-1β, which may increase the permeability of the peritoneal membrane.[505] Platelet-activating factor appears to be locally generated by neutrophils, macrophages, and endothelial cells during inflammation and may also contribute to the increased permeability noted during peritonitis.[506] Furthermore, cytokines such as interleukin-6, an endogenous pyrogen that stimulates secretion of acute phase reactants by hepatocytes and also stimulates mucosal B lymphocytes, and interleukin-8, which is chemotactic and activates polymorphonuclear leukocytes, have been shown to increase acutely in the effluents of patients with peritonitis.[507] During peritonitis, peritoneal transport tends to increase, and there is an increase in protein losses in the dialysate. Nitrogen losses were found to be 13.6 g/d in a group of patients with peritonitis, but as long as peritonitis was mild and oral intake maintained, nitrogen balance tended to remain positive. However, during severe episodes of peritonitis, supplemental feeding was indicated.[508]

The concentration of macrophages in peritoneal fluid is typically much less than the $5 \times 10^5$ cells/mm³. Verbrugh and co-workers[509] have shown that $10^6$ phagocytes/mL are needed in vitro to achieve bacteriostasis for coagulase-negative staphylococci. It is not until peritonitis develops and peritoneal white blood cell counts increase that peritoneal white blood cell concentrations are above these levels. For phagocytosis, recognition must occur. This is usually achieved through opsonization with activated complement or immunoglobulins. Because of the large volume of intraperitoneal fluid and the repeated dilution and removal of these intraperitoneal proteins, the concentration of these opsonins is usually about 1% of that found in serum.[510] Therefore, during the critical initial period immediately after an inoculum, the likelihood of contact between bacteria and white blood cells or opsonins is low. Bacterial growth can proceed unimpeded and peritonitis may occur. During peritonitis, white blood cell counts and opsonin levels increase as the peritoneum becomes more permeable. It is then that host defenses become more formidable.

### Peritonitis Prevention

Presumed sources of bacterial peritonitis are intraluminal (touch contamination during the spike), periluminal (related to catheter infection), transvisceral migration, hematogenous, vaginal leak, and intra-abdominal disease. In the early 1980s, the most common cause of peritonitis in peritoneal dialysis patients was thought to be touch contamination during the spike. Therefore, efforts to prevent peritonitis were directed against this. Unfortunately, overall peritonitis rates reported in the U.S. CAPD registry up to 1989 were stable at about 1.3 episodes per patient-year despite many efforts to reduce touch contamination.[470] These initial modifications of the classic spike technology were reviewed elsewhere.[511] The first modification of the standard technique to consistently result in a reduction in peritonitis rates was the Y set introduced by Buoncristiani and associates[512] in 1983. Since then, many centers,[513–515] including a prospective randomized trial in Canada[468] and data from the USRDS,[458] have confirmed a reduction in peritonitis risk with simple use systems that incorporate the Y system design[514] (Fig. 57–19). Peritonitis rates in these early trials ranged from one episode every 18.4 to 49.9 patient-months with Y systems to one episode every 7.2 to 12.2 patient-months with control systems. Although individual centers

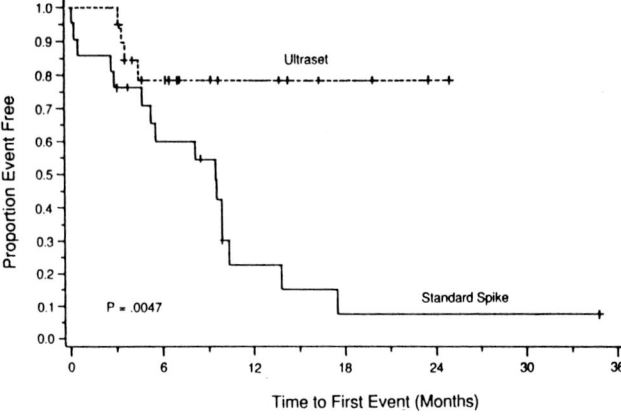

**Figure 57–19.** Comparison of time to first episode of peritonitis, standard spike versus Ultraset. (From Burkart J, Hylander B, Durnell-Figel T, et al: Comparison of peritonitis rates during long-term use of standard spike versus Ultraset in continuous ambulatory peritoneal dialysis [CAPD]. Perit Dial Int 10:41–43, 1990.)

have reported decreased peritonitis rates with a reusable Y set design, a decrease in peritonitis risk with use of these systems was not found in the USRDS database.[458]

**Y Systems.** The Y systems incorporate "flush before fill" technology. This is distinctly different from the traditional spike method, which first drains and then fills the peritoneal cavity after the spike has been made. In contrast, Y systems flush any possible contamination of the spike away from the peritoneum by draining after the spike. In vitro evidence that would support these clinical findings of decreased peritonitis with Y systems includes the following. Luzar and co-workers[516] simulated touch contamination by contaminating the spike with *S. epidermidis, S. aureus*, and *Pseudomonas aeruginosa* immediately before an exchange. Dialysate was then cultured after an exchange using the flush before fill technique. Despite the intentional contamination, with the flush alone, there was 100% removal of *S. epidermidis* and partial removal of *S. aureus* or *P. aeruginosa* if the exchanges were done immediately. These data suggest that flush before fill technique can result in sterile cultures if the exchange is done immediately, such as typically would occur during a CAPD exchange. Flushing was less effective if it was performed after contamination and a period of incubation. Situations such as this would occur with reuse; therefore, a disinfectant should be used. In other studies, flushing the tubing after touch contamination was simulated markedly reduced bacterial biofilm growth.[517]

Initial Y systems did not have the dialysis fluid bag preattached. A multicenter study in Europe further reduced peritonitis with a Y system that had a preattached solution bag, eliminating the need for connecting the new bag of dialysate.[518] Similar results were seen by another group who reported a decrease in peritonitis rates from 1.7 to 0.7 episode per year, with a decrease in the occurrence of infections caused by skin organisms.[519] This tendency for a decrease in peritonitis caused by *S. epidermidis* with the use of disconnect devices was also reported by another group and is perhaps due to a decrease in touch contamination.[477]

It is interesting that most centers report a lesser peritonitis rate for their patients on cyclers than for those on a standard spike.[38, 520] This would also be consistent with Y system data because use of cycler therapy also incorporates the flush before fill technology. Some authors suggest that disconnect systems reduce trauma and torque at the exit, resulting in lower exit site infection rates that would eventually reduce the risk of peritonitis. Others think that the exit site infection rates may be less with disconnect systems but believe that this difference is due not only to less trauma but also to increased technique survival and better catheter maturation, which reduce the risk for exit site infection.

Other connection techniques still in use include devices that use ultraviolet light to sterilize the spike during the exchange. For this technique, a small exchange device must be used. The USRDS has shown that patients using this device are at less risk for development of peritonitis.[458] Similarly, a study in problem patients reported that their peritonitis rates dropped from 1 episode every 7.7 months to 1 episode every 21 months with a switch to this device.[521]

Two clinical studies have evaluated the use of intraperitoneal IgG for peritonitis prevention based on findings that some patients who are at high risk for peritonitis have low peritoneal fluid IgG levels. Lamperi and Carozzi[491] have shown a reduction in peritonitis rates with IgG administered every 21 days. Keane and colleagues[522] also reported a reduction in peritonitis, but only in a subgroup of patients found to have a low prestudy IgG level. Complete absence of IgG2 was noted in 11 of 12 children on CAPD.[523] These authors proposed that this could explain the high peritonitis rates noted in children, because the majority of human antibodies to human carbohydrate antigens are in the IgG2 subclass. However, these data have not been supported in all studies. At present, clinical observations would not support the use of intraperitoneal IgG for peritonitis prevention in the general peritoneal dialysis population. There may be an indication for its use in the small subgroup of patients with high rates of peritonitis and low baseline IgG levels.

The annual probability for the development of *S. aureus* peritonitis is about 15%.[468] The probability that a CAPD patient will have a peritoneal catheter removed because of this infection is 3% to 7.5% (20% to 50% for each infection).[511] Even if peritonitis due to *S. epidermidis* is completely eradicated, this should have only little impact on catheter loss from severe peritonitis because *S. epidermidis* infections tend to be mild. Therefore, means to reduce *S. aureus* infections would be clinically important. Attempts to reduce the frequency of *S. aureus* peritonitis by vaccination are inconclusive. In one study, staphylococcal vaccinations increased the staphylococcal specific antibodies in the dialysate but had no effect on peritonitis or exit site infection rates.[524] Another study of a vaccination for *S. aureus* was more encouraging.[525] Further investigation is currently under way.

***Staphylococcus* Nasal Carriage.** The primary reservoir for *S. aureus* is the anterior nares.[526] Nasal carriers of *S. aureus* have been shown to be at increased risk for development of *S. aureus* exit site infections[527–530] and are possibly at increased risk for peritonitis.[529, 531] Sewell and co-workers[527] reported that chronic carriers were more likely than noncarriers or intermittent carriers to have exit site infections. Davies and colleagues[530] reported a 6.7-fold increase in exit site infections in chronic carriers. Luzar and co-workers[529] reported that nasal carriers were four times more likely to have exit site infections than were noncarriers, and although overall peritonitis rates were no different between the groups, all the cases of *S. aureus* peritonitis occurred in the carriers. Others have reported an increased frequency of *S. aureus* peritonitis in nasal carriers.[528, 531] Although there is some controversy about the association with peritonitis, this may be due to the differences in the definition of nasal carrier state and whether all peritonitis episodes or only *S. aureus* peritonitis episodes are used to determine peritonitis rates between groups.

By use of restrictive endonuclease subtyping, 95% of CAPD patients were found to have nasal colonization and pericatheter colonization with the same subtype.[532] In these patients with peritonitis, the same subtype that colonized the nares and the pericatheter skin caused the peritonitis. However, in another study, phage typing was not similar for patients with peritonitis and hand or exit site colonization.[533] Twardowski and Prowant[534] reported that there was

poor correlation between typing of organisms cultured from the nares and typing of organisms cultured from washings from the exit site.[534] These authors found a high risk for an *S. aureus*–positive culture in patients with infected exits and in those that were slow healing.

One clinical trial using prophylactic antibiotics suggests that the frequency of peritonitis in carriers can be reduced.[535] In another study, the effect of intermittent rifampin on the reduction of catheter-related infections was analyzed.[536] Patients were randomly assigned to treatment (rifampin, 300 mg twice daily for 5 days every 3 months) or no treatment regardless of baseline carrier status. The rifampin-treated patients had a significant delay in the time to first catheter infection and a lower overall catheter infection rate; however, there was no reduction in overall peritonitis rates. Mupirocin, a topical antibiotic effective against *S. aureus*, has been shown to eradicate *S. aureus* from the nares of other populations, but data in CAPD populations are lacking. A randomized clinical trial is presently under way in Europe to evaluate its effectiveness as a prophylactic agent. Despite this association and the association between the presence of an exit site infection and risk for peritonitis, results of medical intervention to eradicate the carrier state have been controversial as far as peritonitis reduction is concerned. Although many agents eradicate the carriage state during therapy, recolonization is rapid, and antibiotic resistance occurs.

In summary, with the use of Y systems, most centers can now achieve peritonitis rates of about 0.33 to 0.5 episode per patient-year. Because of the known association between catheter infections and an increased risk of peritonitis, efforts to reduce peritonitis also include efforts to reduce catheter infections. These are discussed in the section on catheter infections. Epidemiologic and molecular epidemiologic data overwhelmingly support the association between *S. aureus* nasal carriage and exit site infections. These data also support the association between nasal carriage and peritonitis but are less conclusive. Therefore, at present, experimental data do not support routine prophylaxis in patients who are *S. aureus* nasal carriers.

## Peritonitis

**Diagnosis.** Peritonitis is often easily diagnosed on clinical grounds alone. Most patients present with abdominal pain and visibly cloudy fluid. In a review of 103 patients with peritonitis, fever (temperature above 37.5°C) was present in 53% of patients, abdominal pain in 79%, nausea in 31%, and diarrhea in 7%. Seventy percent had abdominal tenderness, and 50% had rebound pain.[537] Patients will also occasionally have other systemic signs and symptoms and even hypotension. Physical examination findings are typical of any cause of peritonitis and include abdominal tenderness, decreased bowel sounds, guarding, and occasionally rebound tenderness. Because of the increased frequency of hernias in peritoneal dialysis patients, the possibility of peritonitis due to ischemic bowel from an incarcerated hernia must always be considered; therefore, the presence of ventral, incisional, or inguinal hernias must be looked for, and other intra-abdominal disease must be ruled out. Although the majority of the time when a peritoneal dialysis patient presents with peritonitis it is due to bacterial contamination from a nonmalignant source, occasionally the patient has significant intra-abdominal disease as the cause. It is important to identify these patients because their treatment will differ from that of bacterial peritonitis.

Standard laboratory parameters suggestive of peritonitis include a peritoneal fluid white blood cell count of greater than 100 cells/mm³, most of which are polymorphonuclear leukocytes. A predominance of lymphocytes may be seen with atypical infections, such as tuberculosis,[538] but this is not always the case. There may be an increase in the peripheral white blood cell count. Gram stains of peritoneal fluids are seldom helpful, but if the response is positive, they are predictive of culture results 85% of the time. Blood cultures are seldom positive, which is one reason that peritoneal dialysis has been recommended for patients with prosthetic valves or synthetic vascular grafts.[539, 540]

Cultures of the dialysate should be obtained immediately, but the availability of culture results should not delay onset of therapy. Sterile or aseptic peritonitis is usually due to inappropriate culture techniques; the reported frequency varies from 2% to 20%, depending on the culture techniques used. If proper culture technique is followed, peritoneal cultures should be positive in approximately 90% of the cases of peritonitis.[537] In the case of repeatedly sterile peritoneal fluid cultures and elevated peritoneal fluid white blood cell counts, other pathologic processes must be considered. Eosinophilic peritonitis must be considered. Atypical organisms, such as those causing tuberculosis, should be looked for. Elevated neutrophil counts have been reported in association with well-differentiated hypernephroma of the kidney, perhaps from perinephric inflammation.[541, 542]

Intra-abdominal causes of peritonitis result in significant morbidity and mortality in peritoneal dialysis patients. There is no reported difference in routine initial laboratory parameters and clinical findings between those patients with peritoneal dialysis–associated bacterial peritonitis and those patients with other intra-abdominal causes of peritonitis.[543] In one review, intra-abdominal disease was the cause of less than 6% of peritonitis in peritoneal dialysis patients, but of the 26 patients with peritonitis due to intra-abdominal disease, 11 died.[481] Mortality correlated not only with the disease process causing the peritonitis but also with time to surgical intervention.

Peritoneal fluid amylase levels have been found to be helpful in the differential diagnosis of peritonitis.[544] Burkart and co-workers[545] found elevated values in patients with peritonitis due to intra-abdominal disease, such as pancreatitis or perforated viscus (Fig. 57–20). In a subsequent review, it was suggested that any time peritoneal fluid amylase levels are greater than 50 IU/L, peritonitis due to an underlying intra-abdominal pathologic process should be considered.[546] Therefore, it may be reasonable to obtain these levels routinely for all patients who present with peritonitis. Peritoneal fluid lipase levels are also helpful and, if elevated, suggest pancreatitis as the cause of peritonitis.[546, 547]

Occasionally the dialysate is bloody; this can also be of guidance in the differential diagnosis of peritonitis. The causes of bloody dialysate have been reviewed[546] (Table

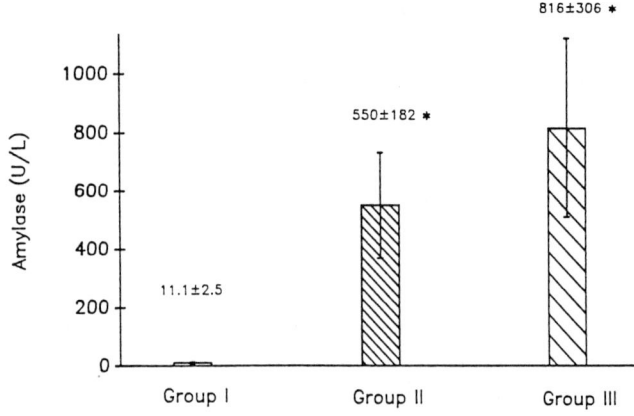

**Figure 57–20.** Comparison of peritoneal fluid amylase levels in peritoneal dialysis patients with various causes of peritonitis. Group I = 39 patients with infectious peritonitis; group II = 6 patients with pancreatitis; group III = 5 patients with intra-abdominal disease. *P = .001. (From Burkart J, Haigler S, Caruana R, Hylander B: Usefulness of peritoneal fluid amylase levels in the differential diagnosis of peritonitis in peritoneal dialysis patients. J Am Soc Nephrol 1:1186–1190, 1991.)

57–8). The most common occurrence of bloody dialysate is after Tenckhoff catheter placement, followed in frequency by gynecologic causes; therefore, bloody dialysate does not always signify infection or disease.

Radiologic studies are occasionally indicated in the differential diagnosis of peritonitis and should be used with the same guidelines as in patients who are not undergoing peritoneal dialysis. Free intraperitoneal air can occasionally be seen in patients using peritoneal dialysis, and this finding on an acute abdominal series is not pathognomonic of a perforated viscus in these patients[548]; however, free air should lead to consideration of perforation in the presence of peritonitis. Computed tomography is more sensitive than ultrasonography in diagnosing pancreatitis, but findings are positive only in up to 60% of cases[549]; hence, the helpfulness of peritoneal fluid amylase levels. In patients with peritonitis due to ischemic bowel caused by incarcerated

**TABLE 57–8. Reported Causes of Bloody Dialysate**

After catheter implantation
Gynecologic
    Retrograde menstruation
    Ovulation
    Ruptured ovarian cyst
    Endometriosis
Traumatic
    Catheter related
    Blunt trauma
Anatomic
    Polycystic kidneys
    Intra-abdominal cancer
    Vascular
Disinfectant infusion
Status after colonoscopy
Idiopathic thrombocytopenic purpura
Radiation therapy
Strenuous activity
Hemorrhagic pancreatitis

hernia, computed tomographic or radionuclide scans to document the presence of extra-abdominal fluid may be helpful.

**Infectious Causes of Peritonitis.** The overwhelming majority of cases of peritonitis are caused by pathogenic bacteria. A small number of cases of peritonitis are caused by fungi, most of them *Candida* species. The role of viruses as a pathogen causing peritonitis is uncertain, but anecdotal cases have been reported.[550] More important is the possible role viruses play in predisposing patients to peritonitis.[551, 552] Lewis and co-workers[553] reported an association of recurrent peritonitis in a patient with an active cytomegalovirus infection that may have caused the patient to be further immunosuppressed, thereby predisposing to repeated episodes of peritonitis. This patient had an inverted CD4 to CD8 ratio. Patients with ESRD and acquired immunodeficiency syndrome or chronic hepatitis B are becoming more common. These patients are immunosuppressed, and they may have not only an increased peritonitis risk but also peritonitis due to opportunistic organisms.

Data on 3366 patients who started CAPD in the first 6 months of 1989 were reviewed by Port and associates.[458] At the time of the first episode of peritonitis, 13% of the patients had a documented exit site infection. Peritoneal fluid leaks were found in 3%. The first peritonitis episode resulted in hospitalization of 31% of patients, and cultures were sterile in 20% of cases. Almost 50% of the infections were due to gram-positive organisms, followed next in frequency by gram-negative infections (Fig. 57–21).

**Gram-Positive Peritonitis.** *S. epidermidis* was originally the most common cause of peritonitis, presumably through touch contamination or pericatheter routes.[537] *S. epidermidis* typically causes mild cases of peritonitis that tend to respond rapidly to therapy. *S. aureus* is a more virulent pathogen and tends to be more resistant to therapy. Patients with *S. aureus* peritonitis have presented with a toxic shock–like syndrome,[554] and severe cases have been associated with progressive membrane damage. The relative percentage of peritonitis caused by these two organisms has changed as the frequency of peritonitis due to touch contamination has

**TABLE 57–9. Common Organisms Causing Peritonitis During Peritoneal Dialysis**

| Pathogen | Range (%) |
|---|---|
| Gram-positive bacteria | 55–80 |
|   Coagulase-negative staphylococci | 35–70 |
|   *Staphylococcus aureus* | 10–25 |
|   Streptococcal species | 3–15 |
|   Enterococci | 3–10 |
|   Miscellaneous | 0–4 |
| Gram-negative bacteria | 17–30 |
|   *Escherichia coli* | 4–10 |
|   *Pseudomonas* species | 5–10 |
|   *Klebsiella* species | 1–5 |
|   *Acinetobacter* species | 0–4 |
|   *Enterobacter* species | 0–3 |
|   *Serratia* species | 0–3 |
|   Miscellaneous | 0–6 |
| Anaerobic bacteria | 0–4 |
| Fungi | 0–5 |
| Mycobacteria | 0–1 |

From Walshe JJ, Morse GD: Infectious complications of peritoneal dialysis. *In* Nissenson AR, Fine RN, Gentile DE (eds): Clinical Dialysis, 2nd ed. Appleton & Lange, Norwalk, CT, 1990, pp 301–318.

decreased with the use of the Y systems.[514, 555] Consequently, although overall peritonitis rates are decreasing and most centers are experiencing fewer *S. epidermidis* infections, there are relatively more *S. aureus* infections.

In CAPD patients, the opsonic activity for *S. aureus* as judged by neutrophil chemoluminescence correlated with peritoneal IgG and fibronectin content but not with complement levels.[556] The addition of urokinase improved opsonic properties, which suggests that the formation of fibrin in dialysate promoted by *S. aureus* interferes with phagocytosis. Similar anecdotal results reported for streptokinase suggest that a therapeutic trial with these agents may be warranted in patients with relapsing severe peritonitis due to *S. aureus*. This coupled with relatively low IgG, complement, and fibronectin levels in dialysate may explain the relatively poor clearance rates of this organism from the peritoneum.

There are three reports of peritonitis due to group B streptococcus in the literature. All three patients presented with severe systemic symptoms and septic shock within 24 hours after onset of symptoms.[557] One of the three patients died. These organisms should be sensitive to vancomycin, the recommended standard for initial treatment of peritonitis. These cases enforce the importance of having patients monitor their blood pressure and report symptoms early in the course of therapy for peritonitis when they are treated at home. Hypotension suggests the possibility of a more severe disease and usually requires hospitalization.

**Gram-Negative Peritonitis.** Gram-negative organisms can cause peritonitis and produce a wide spectrum of clinical findings. Patients with gram-negative peritonitis typically respond to appropriate antibiotic therapy, but *Pseudomonas* infections are particularly difficult to eradicate. Table 57–9 lists some of the gram-negative bacteria reported to cause peritonitis. Bowel, skin, urinary tract, contaminated water, and animal contact have been implicated as sources of gram-negative peritonitis. In vitro studies

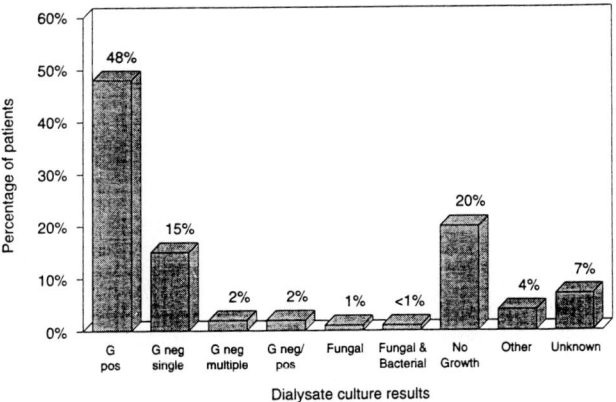

**Figure 57–21.** Percent distribution of peritoneal dialysate culture results for first peritonitis episode (N = 1517). (From Port FK, Held PJ, Nolph KD, et al: Risk of peritonitis and technique failure by CAPD connection technique: A national study. Used with permission from Kidney International, volume 42, pages 967–974, 1992.)

have shown that human peritoneal macrophages are able to phagocytose *Escherichia coli* even in the absence of opsonins, which is perhaps the reason for the relative rarity of *E. coli* peritonitis in peritoneal dialysis patients.[558] Peritonitis associated with severe diarrhea has been caused by *Campylobacter* infection.[559]

***Pseudomonas* Peritonitis.** *Pseudomonas* peritonitis was responsible for 4.8% of all peritonitis episodes in a 66-month period at a single center.[560] Eighty percent of these episodes were treated successfully with the combination of an aminoglycoside and ceftazidime. In 5 of the 25 episodes, the catheter was removed. Millikin and colleagues[561] found that if *Pseudomonas* peritonitis was related to exit site or catheter infection, the response rate was only 32%; when there was no clinical evidence of catheter-related infection, the reported response rate was 73%. *Pseudomonas* peritonitis can be associated with severe systemic manifestations, such as white blood cell capillary margination and digital necrosis.[562]

**Fungal Peritonitis.** Presenting signs and symptoms in patients with fungal peritonitis tend to be no different from those in patients with bacterial peritonitis. A single center experience with 27 cases of fungal peritonitis was reviewed.[563] Most infections were due to *Candida* species. Fungal peritonitis was associated with a recent history of bacterial peritonitis and previous antibiotic therapy. These authors suggested a trial of oral antibiotics and noted that of the nine patients who continued with peritoneal dialysis, three still had their original catheter. The standard of antifungal therapy has been treatment with intravenous amphotericin B. Other antifungal agents have been used and include flucytosine, ketoconazole, miconazole, and econazole. These reports were reviewed by Bernard and co-workers.[564] All therapies have had successes and failures. In a retrospective review, it appeared that the combination of intraperitoneal flucytosine and oral ketoconazole seemed most efficacious.[564] Since these reports, once-a-day oral fluconazole has been used to treat *Candida* peritonitis successfully, but the catheter was removed in these patients.[565] Another center has reported similar results.[566] Fluconazole has no activity, however, against filamentous fungi, for which intravenous amphotericin B is the antifungal agent of choice. Millikin and colleagues[561] found an overall poor response rate to fungal peritonitis and, contrary to anecdotal experience, suggested that the published literature shows that the response rate with fungal peritonitis is 64% whether or not the catheter is removed. These data suggest that if the patient is hemodynamically stable, any antifungal agent with appropriate inhibitory activity could be used, although oral fluconazole seems to be the emerging therapy of choice in this instance. However, because of the broad spectrum of activity, in any critically ill patient in whom fungal peritonitis is suspected, amphotericin B should be used.

Catheter removal is generally recommended; however, two reviews suggest that this is not always necessary. These are the reviews of Millikin[561] and Cheng[563] and co-workers. In the review of 225 cases of fungal peritonitis by Cheng and colleagues, three different catheter management approaches were described: immediate removal and antifangal therapy; delayed removal, usually after a period of failure to respond to antifungal therapy; and antifungal therapy without catheter removal. Mortality rates were no different between groups, but patients who did not have their Tenckhoff catheter removed immediately were more likely to continue peritoneal dialysis. In the group of patients for whom the treatment strategy was antifungal therapy alone, 58 of 71 patients (82%) recovered from their infection without catheter removal. These are retrospective data, and there certainly must have been selection bias between the groups in that those patients for whom the treatment strategy was to leave the catheter in must have been doing well clinically. Given those limitations, these data suggest that catheter removal is not necessary in every case of fungal peritonitis. A reasonable therapeutic plan would be to initiate appropriate antifungal therapy with close monitoring of the patient. If there is no significant clinical improvement by day 4 or 5, the catheter should be removed.

Other causes of fungal peritonitis typically require antifungal agents and catheter removal. *Aspergillus* peritonitis has been treated with catheter removal and antifungal therapy.[567]

**Tuberculosis.** Except for its more insidious onset, tuberculous peritonitis is similar in clinical presentation to other forms of peritonitis. Tuberculous peritonitis usually presents with a predominance of lymphocytes in the effluent, but this is not always the case. Occasionally there is a neutrophil predominance.[568] Peritonitis due to *Mycobacterium tuberculosis*, *Mycobacterium kansasii*, and *Mycobacterium fortuitum* has been reported. In a review of five cases of tuberculous peritonitis, all patients responded to triple therapy, and three of five continued peritoneal dialysis.[569] Three cases of *M. tuberculosis* peritonitis appeared to have been treated with antibiotic therapy alone and removal of the catheter was not needed.[570] It appears that about one third of all cases of *M. tuberculosis* peritonitis can be treated without catheter removal, but in general, atypical infections require catheter removal.

**Biofilms.** Although one large prospective study has demonstrated biofilms in peritoneal catheters removed from peritoneal dialysis patients, and cultures of scrapings from these biofilms were often positive for *S. aureus* and *S. epidermidis*,[571] there was no clear relationship to clinical peritonitis.[19] Two other studies confirmed that biofilms could be present without any evidence of infection.[572, 573] Therefore, a firm relationship between biofilms and peritonitis has been lacking. In an in vivo rabbit model of peritonitis, skin bacteria of the animals routinely colonized the catheter through the exit site after placement but before onset of dialysis.[17] Peritonitis did not occur until after the onset of dialysis, possibly because the functions of host defense were altered by dialysis fluids and they were no longer able to contain the bacteria in biofilms. In vitro studies have demonstrated that biofilm growth is associated with antibiotic resistance,[574, 575] and significantly higher antibiotic levels are needed in vitro to eradicate biofilms. Dasgupta and co-workers[576] have described a way to culture biofilm-forming bacteria in dialysate effluents of peritoneal dialysis patients with peritonitis by use of a modified Robbins device. They found that patients with multiple episodes of peritonitis were likely to have stable biofilms, positive biofilm cultures, and a high frequency of catheter loss.[577] Patients who had peritonitis with positive biofilm cultures who responded to antibiotics were thought to have early biofilm formation and were not likely to have associated catheter loss. Rifampin has been shown to have greater biofilm-penetrating capacity than that of most other antibiotics.[578]

**Treatment.** The successful treatment of any episode of peritonitis not only has an impact on the patient's immediate well-being but also may influence the patient's long-term modality choice. Of patients with multiple episodes of peritonitis, more than 40% transferred to another modality.[579] Long dwell exchanges are associated with higher numbers of macrophages in the effluent, and a higher percentage of these are found to be functional, compared with short dwells.[580] In addition, the IgG concentrations in the effluent increase with increasing dwell time. Given these findings and the known effects the unphysiologic dialysis fluids initially have on peritoneal white blood cell function, it is recommended that long dwells rather than rapid short dwells be used for the treatment of peritonitis. This wisdom must be weighed against the finding of increased protein losses and loss of ultrafiltration associated with episodes of peritonitis. During peritonitis, prolonged dwells can be associated with fluid absorption from the peritoneum and even volume overload in some cases. It may be helpful to do a few rapid exchanges initially if the patient is in pain or, if the patient is septic, to remove the endotoxin load and reduce the inflammation.

Thirty-six patients with peritonitis were randomized to receive intraperitoneal antibiotics and either 24 hours of rapid short-cycle dialysis or continued long dwells routine for CAPD. No patient had hypotension or shock.[581] There was no difference in treatment success rate or in time to normalization of white blood cell count in either group. These authors concluded that rapid lavage is not needed in stable patients with routine peritonitis.

Millikin and co-workers[561] published a retrospective review of data on the antimicrobial treatment of peritonitis before January 1990. The authors were quick to point out that although they estimated 41,000 cases of peritonitis per year before their publication, the world literature at that time included reports of treatment for only 2037 cases of peritonitis. At about the same time, an ad hoc committee published a set of recommendations for the diagnosis and treatment of peritonitis.[582] These recommendations were based on their clinical experiences and the world literature on the treatment of peritonitis at that time. They were meant to be guidelines and by no means were meant to be the only acceptable therapy for peritonitis. Pediatric antibiotic choices and dosing were reviewed by Lum.[583] Since those initial recommendations, additional clinical and laboratory experience has led to a subsequent publication on peritonitis treatment guidelines by the ad hoc committee on peritonitis.[584] These recommendations and some of the clinical experiences are reviewed here.

Because of the increasing frequency of methicillin resistance of Staphylococcus species[585] (especially S. aureus, which is becoming a relatively more common cause of peritonitis), initial treatment with vancomycin has been recommended. In one study, patients were randomized to receive intraperitoneal vancomycin or cefazolin.[586] Vancomycin had a higher peritonitis resolution rate (81% versus

67%) and a reduced frequency of hospital admissions (48% versus 68%). These data and data of Milliken and co-workers[561] support the initial use of vancomycin to cover staphylococcal species.

In eight CAPD patients, clindamycin was taken four times daily for 1 day. Macrophages from dialysate effluents in these patients showed better uptake and killing of S. epidermidis than did control dialysate macrophages.[587] In additional studies, it was noted that after 18 hours, S. epidermidis within peritoneal macrophages incubated with clindamycin showed decreased viability, whereas control phagocytes allowed the number of intracellular organisms to increase. These studies confirm the previous clinical experiences that drugs such as clindamycin and rifampin, which suppress intracellular growth, may be beneficial in the treatment of staphylococcal peritonitis.

Ciprofloxacin has been shown in vitro to have substantial activity against most organisms causing peritonitis in peritoneal dialysis patients.[588] Intraperitoneal followed by oral ciprofloxacin resulted in satisfactory bacteriologic responses in 25 of 30 cases of peritonitis, but resolution was slow in cases of S. aureus peritonitis.[589] In a prospective randomized controlled trial, intraperitoneal ciprofloxacin and vancomycin were compared with intraperitoneal vancomycin and gentamicin.[590]

Reactivities of cefuroxime, ciprofloxacin, and imipenem against 50 coagulase-negative Staphylococcus strains isolated from patients with peritonitis were examined.[591] These strains were cultured both in dialysis fluids and in standard culture broths. The inhibitory activities of the antibiotics differed significantly between the two mediums. Higher concentrations were usually needed in the dialysis fluid. This stresses that in vitro antibiotic sensitivities may not be a true indication of in vivo effectiveness.

Severe ototoxic injury has been reported in peritoneal dialysis patients treated with aminoglycosides.[592] Ototoxic effects in patients treated with tobramycin were monitored by audiograms.[593] There was a deterioration in hearing in 25% of the patients. These authors raise the question of whether intermittent therapy would be less ototoxic. Because of concerns of ototoxicity, and better understanding of the pharmacokinetics of aminoglycoside therapy in peritoneal dialysis patients, newer recommendations for aminoglycoside use include once-daily therapy. These and other reasons for this recommendation are outlined by Vas.[594]

A CAPD program in Switzerland reported a reduction in fungal peritonitis after the introduction of prophylactic vaginal nystatin during the course of any antibiotic therapy.[595] This study had no control group but may represent a reasonable approach.

A more radical approach that has been suggested for the treatment of either acute peritonitis or relapsing peritonitis is to withhold peritoneal dialysis in an attempt to allow restoration of normal host defenses. Two groups have had success in treating acute peritonitis in CAPD patients with a single dose of antibiotics and stopping therapy for 48 hours.[596, 597] These authors reported an 85% cure rate for patients treated in this manner, similar to results with conventional therapy. This approach is more economical and has an intellectual appeal but has not been widely adapted, primarily because it risks treating patients with more severe forms of peritonitis inappropriately. However, Cairns[483] has successfully treated 10 of 11 patients with recurrent coagulase-negative or persistent *S. aureus* infections with this technique. This suggests that short periods off peritoneal dialysis may help restore normal host defenses.

Finally, aggressive nutritional support in children has been associated with lower peritonitis rates, perhaps because of enhanced white blood cell function.[598] Many authors have shown that malnutrition is associated with an increased risk of death in patients with peritonitis, which suggests that supplemental feeding should be considered if the patient is not eating.

**Summary of Treatment Recommendations.** A summary of present antimicrobial recommendations and treatment algorithms can be found in the publication by the ad hoc committee on the treatment of peritonitis.[584] Figure 57–22 is an outline of initial treatment recommendations. Note that a 2-g intraperitoneal loading dose of vancomycin is recommended and that subsequent doses are given at weekly intervals. Because of the relative increase in gram-negative infections, if the initial Gram stain is not positive, combination therapy is recommended. Initial gram-negative coverage with either ceftazidime or once-daily aminoglycosides (40 mg in one exchange per day) is recommended.

A significant change from previous recommendations is that therapy for *S. aureus* peritonitis is extended for 1 week, with current recommendations to give 2 g of vancomycin intraperitoneally every week for a total of three doses. If *S. aureus* is identified and there is no clinical improvement by 4 or 5 days, rifampin is added. For other gram-positive organisms, final antibiotic therapy is guided by culture results, and duration of therapy should be for a total of 10 days.

If a gram-negative infection is identified, treatment should be directed by culture results and sensitivities. A single daily intraperitoneal dose of aminoglycoside is used to achieve peak and trough fluctuations and presumably decrease the risk of ototoxic effects. Length of therapy should be 14 days. If *P. aeruginosa* or *Xanthomonas* is identified, therapy should be extended for a total of 21 days and often requires catheter removal; also, use of two antibiotics to which the organism is sensitive is recommended.

For fungal peritonitis, the committee thought that a trial of antifungal agents was warranted, but if there was no obvious improvement by 4 to 5 days, the catheter should be removed. It was thought that successful therapy should be continued for 4 to 6 weeks.

**Relapsing Peritonitis.** Relapsing peritonitis is arbitrarily defined as another episode of peritonitis with the same genus and species that caused the preceding episode of peritonitis within 4 weeks of completion of the antibiotic course. In this situation, one should first review culture and sensitivity results. Noncompliance should always be considered. If *S. aureus* is cultured, because of the possibility of intracellular sequestration of bacteria, it is recommended that vancomycin and rifampin be used for a total of 4 weeks. Consideration of catheter infection or intra-abdominal abscess should also be given. Tunnel infections may contribute to relapsing peritonitis, and catheter removal is usually necessary in up to 80% of episodes of peritonitis associated with tunnel infections.[599] The risk of tunnel infection seems to be greater early in the course of peritoneal dialysis and in diabetic women.

Anecdotal reports suggest that infusion of streptokinase or urokinase may be successful in treating relapsing or resistant peritonitis.[600–602] The rationale behind this therapy is that it is possible that organisms may be protected in fibrin clots or in biofilms that may be exposed with the use of these drugs. Streptokinase is typically left in for an overnight dwell; urokinase is typically drained after a 2-hour dwell. These studies have no control group but suggest that it may be useful in up to 50% of cases.

**Indications for Catheter Removal.** Experience of a single center with peritonitis was reviewed.[603] During 636 episodes of peritonitis in 440 patients, there were 16 deaths associated with peritonitis (fatality rate of 2.5%). The catheter was removed between the 5th and 10th day in six patients and after 10 days in seven patients. The risk of death was increased in those patients with delayed catheter removal. Peritonitis with sepsis was the cause of death in 13 patients. This experience points to the need for early catheter removal in patients with refractory peritonitis not only to prevent mortality but also to avoid prolonged episodes of peritonitis that could potentially damage the peritoneal membrane.

Catheter removal is indicated for mechanical failure that does not respond to other maneuvers. Simultaneous catheter removal and replacement is usually successful for noninfectious indications of catheter removal; however, one center also reported simultaneous replacement 83% of the time in cases with persistent or resistant infections.[604] Successful cases were characterized by *Staphylococcus* species or nonenteric gram-negative rods in the absence of systemic or intra-abdominal complications and after initial improvement of the peritonitis with antibiotic therapy. Further studies are needed to confirm the success of this approach.

Other indications for catheter removal include peritonitis

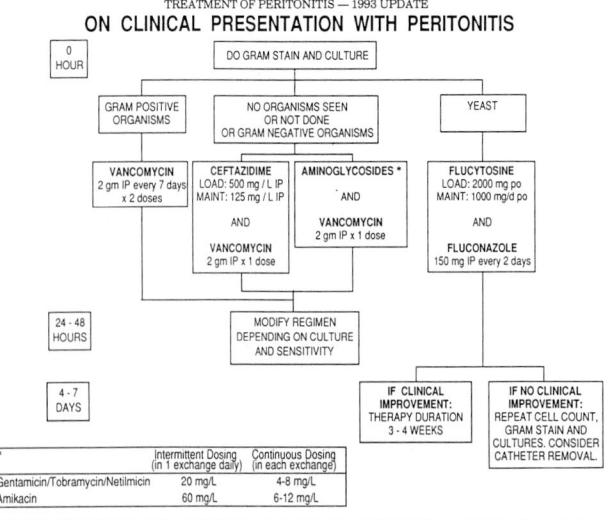

Figure 57–22. Initial treatment recommendations for peritonitis. (From Keane WF, Everett ED, Golper T, et al: Peritoneal dialysis–related peritonitis treatment recommendations. 1993 update. Perit Dial Int 13:14–28, 1993.)

associated with tunnel infections, some cases of chronic exit site or tunnel infection, *Pseudomonas* peritonitis unresponsive to appropriate antibiotic therapy, slowly improving fungal peritonitis, fecal peritonitis, significant intra-abdominal disease, and continually relapsing peritonitis with no obvious cause (Table 57–10).

**Eosinophilic Peritonitis.** This complication is usually observed early after catheter placement and is typically associated with sterile peritoneal cultures. There may or may not be associated peripheral eosinophilia. It is assumed to be due to chemical stimuli leached from the catheter. Fungal peritonitis and other causes of peritonitis must be carefully ruled out. Chemical peritonitis due to hypersensitivity to drugs, most notably vancomycin,[605, 606] has been reported and may also be associated with eosinophilia. This originally seemed to occur only with large intraperitoneal loading doses of vancomycin, presumably because of impurities during the production process. Chemical peritonitis has been seen with all brands but seems to be least common with the Lilly preparation. There are some concerns that the new peritonitis recommendations for large intraperitoneal loading doses of vancomycin will result in an increased frequency of chemical peritonitis.

**Sclerosing Encapsulating Peritonitis.** Patients with this syndrome present with anorexia, weight loss, nausea, vomiting, intermittent bowel obstruction, malnutrition, and decreased peritoneal transport of solute and water. This is thought to be a different disease process from that of type II membrane failure. It has been mainly reported in Europe,[394] but there have been sporadic cases in the United States.[607] The cause is uncertain, and many chemical irritants have been implicated. Sclerosing peritonitis developed in one patient using formalin for a disinfectant.[608] Peritoneal sclerosis has also been reported after a severe *S. aureus* infection.[609] Of 13 patients in whom type I and type III procollagen concentrations were measured in the serum and dialysate, sclerosing peritonitis developed in the one patient who had an eightfold higher concentration of type III procollagen.[610] Concentrations of these substances may reflect a state of fibrosis activity.

In a review of 14 cases of sclerosing peritonitis in 18

patients who used chlorhexidine and alcohol in the connection procedure,[611] findings included peritoneal ultrafiltration failure, exudative bloody ascites, and intestinal obstruction. Nine of the 14 patients had symptoms after transfer to hemodialysis for other reasons. Four of the patients with known disease continued to use CAPD without symptoms. These authors suggested that continued peritoneal dialysis may be better than a switch to hemodialysis, although this is not the standard recommendation. In another study of 17 patients with sclerosing peritonitis, 15 of whom received chlorhexidine in alcohol were reviewed.[612] All patients discontinued peritoneal dialysis after laparoscopic diagnosis; 12 patients died from intestinal obstruction within 1 year of the diagnosis. The remaining five patients survived 1 to 5 years without intestinal obstruction. Four of the five patients received a renal transplant and were treated with azathioprine and prednisone. One of these patients rejected the transplant and had a relapse of symptoms of sclerosing peritonitis after the immunosuppression was stopped. The fifth patient who did not receive a transplant was treated empirically with immunosuppression and was asymptomatic after 1 year of therapy, which suggests that the pathogenesis of this disease may be immune mediated and that immunosuppression may be beneficial.

Surgical intervention has been disappointing. In one review,[613] intestinal obstruction, small bowel necrosis, and enterocutaneous fistulas were common. Resection with primary anastomosis resulted in a high frequency of anastomotic failure.

This is often a fatal illness. Fortunately, with the use of lactate-containing dialysis solutions, the avoidance of intraperitoneal infusion of chemical irritants such as chlorhexidine, and the prevention of severe prolonged episodes of peritonitis by early diagnosis, aggressive treatment of peritonitis, and early catheter removal when indicated, the frequency of encapsulating peritonitis seems to be decreasing.

---

**TABLE 57–10. Indications for Catheter Removal**

**Infectious Causes**
Persistent skin exit or tunnel infection
Recurrent peritonitis with the same organism
Fecal peritonitis
Fungal peritonitis
Tuberculous peritonitis
*Pseudomonas* peritonitis*
*Staphylococcus aureus* peritonitis associated with exit site infection
Peritonitis not responding to adequate therapy after 5–7 d

**Mechanical or Technical Causes**
Persistent leaks—exit site or subcutaneous
Outflow obstruction
Persistent inflow pain

*A trial of appropriate antibiotic therapy may be warranted if there is no associated catheter infection.
From Holley JL, Piraino BM: Complications of peritoneal dialysis: Diagnosis and management. Semin Dial 3:245, 1990.

---

## Catheter Infections (Exit Site and Tunnel)

One of the most important components of the peritoneal dialysis system is a permanent and trouble-free access to the peritoneal cavity. Catheter exit site and tunnel infections are frequent in peritoneal dialysis patients, and these infections can lead to morbidity, prolonged antibiotic treatment, recurrent peritonitis, and catheter failure. According to the final report of the national CAPD registry, 3-year catheter survival at individual centers varied from 6% to 36%. Furthermore, 8% to 39% of catheters were removed because of exit or tunnel infections.[12] Transfer from peritoneal dialysis to hemodialysis is thought to be directly due to catheter-related causes in about 20% of the cases. When problems indirectly related to catheters are included (catheter-associated peritonitis or psychosocial stress), catheter-related problems may account for up to 33% of all therapy failures.[25] A study indicates that the proportion of patients who transfer to hemodialysis each year parallels the rate of catheter loss, which in turn appears to be related to exit site infection rates, not peritonitis rates.[614] This not only highlights the morbidity associated with exit site and tunnel infections but also begins to suggest that catheter infections are becoming the most common infectious problem associated with peritoneal dialysis.

Unlike peritonitis, for which there is a universally acceptable primary definition for its presence, exit site infections currently have no singular or easily recognizable definition. Pierratos[615] defined an exit site infection as "redness or skin induration or purulent discharge from the exit site. Formation of crust around the exit may not indicate infection. Positive cultures from the exit site in the absence of inflammation do not indicate infection." This definition is not sufficiently precise, and therefore the definition of exit site infection varies from center to center. Some authors have defined exit site infection as the presence of erythema or drainage confirmed by a positive culture. Although such a strict definition facilitates a more uniform diagnosis, the assumption that a positive culture must be obtained in all cases will exclude some cases of infection. Although the percentage of "no growth" exit site infections must be low, they have been reported.[616, 617] Another definition of infection is based on the size of the area of erythema surrounding the catheter. This definition has not been successfully applied to large populations of patients. In general, a positive exit site culture in the presence of no pain, induration, drainage, or erythema does not indicate an infection. Some authors include tunnel infections in data with exit site infections because it is often difficult to distinguish between the two.

In addition to the problems associated with defining the presence or absence of an exit site infection, there is a similar lack of consistent definition for relapse versus new infection. Because oral antibiotic therapy for exit site infection typically lasts 10 to 14 days, it seems reasonable to define a new episode of infection as a recurrence of infection with the same or a new pathogen 4 weeks or more from the preceding infection onset date.[529, 616] Exit site infection rates as low as 0.05 infection per patient-year[618] to as high as 1.02 infections per patient-year[619] have been reported, in part because of this difficulty with consistency in the definition of the disease. At present, it is recommended that exit site infection be defined as the presence of marked pericatheter redness and wetness or exudate in the sinus tract with or without a positive culture. Chronic infections often show exuberant granulation tissue in the sinus. Erythema or bleeding alone may simply indicate acute trauma. A tunnel infection can occur independently of an obvious exit site infection and is defined as erythema, edema, or tenderness of the subcutaneous tunnel with or without discharge from the exit or a positive culture.

**Exit Site Infections.** Almost all healed exits are colonized by bacteria.[620] Infection is the result of a major disturbance in the balance between host defense and bacterial growth.[621] Bacterial virulence is also important; the virulent pathogens S. aureus and P. aeruginosa are most likely to induce infection. Few studies to date have reported an in-depth evaluation of the epidemiology of exit site infections. Table 57–11 presents data on the causative microorganisms of exit site infections based on a literature review.[622] In this review, which included reports of exit site infection rates from 11 centers, the mean exit site infection rate was 0.48 episode per patient-year. S. aureus has consistently been identified as the leading cause of exit site and tunnel infec-

**TABLE 57–11. Microorganisms Causing Exit Site Infection in CAPD**

| Microorganism | Range (%) of Exit Site Infection Caused by Organism |
|---|---|
| Staphylococcus aureus | 25–85 |
| Multiple organisms (includes S. aureus in mixed culture) | 16–35 |
| Enteric gram-negative bacteria | 7–14 |
| Staphylococcus epidermidis | 5–14 |
| Pseudomonas aeruginosa | 8–12 |
| Culture-negative | 7–11 |
| Fungal agents | 1–3 |

From Luzar Ma: Exit-site infection in continuous ambulatory peritoneal dialysis: A review. Perit Dial Int 11:333–340, 1991.

tions. Although Pseudomonas infections are relatively infrequent, the severity of these infections, the difficulty in eradicating them, and the negative impact they have on catheter survival warrant careful monitoring of this pathogen. In a review of catheter infections, both catheter removal and death were associated with Pseudomonas infections.[481]

Defense mechanisms in a healed sinus are best in undamaged epidermis and granulation tissue. Trauma to these structures may tilt the balance toward bacterial overgrowth and allow the development of infection.[24] Close examination of the morphologic features of the tunnel by use of photography and magnifying lenses has allowed the classification of exit sites as perfect, good, equivocal, traumatized, acutely inflamed, and chronically inflamed.[623] These observations would suggest that the mature, healed external cuff does not function as a physical barrier to spread of infection; rather, the external cuff functions in preventing infections by anchoring the catheter, which results in restriction of piston-like movements and possible trauma to the exit. Given data gathered by Twardowski and colleagues,[24, 620] it would seem that efforts to reduce trauma at the exit would reduce exit site infection rates. Catheter immobilization, especially in the immediate postoperative period, has been recommended. The possibility that the use of Y systems that also allow the patient to "disconnect" from the spent dialysate might result in less trauma to the exit because of less torsion, pulling, or torque and fewer subsequent infections was investigated by two groups.[38, 624, 625] These authors saw a reduction in exit site infection rates with Y systems, but there was not a consistent reduction in exit site infection rates in patients on cyclers who also disconnect.[38, 520] Both centers found no difference in time to first exit site infection between Y systems, standard spike, or cycler therapy. This reduction in exit site infection rates with Y systems seen at some centers has not been found universally, and the possible reason for this reduction is controversial. Explanations for this controversy include possible differences in populations of patients studied. An alternative is that the reduction in peritonitis seen with Y systems allows longer technique survival, better maturation of the exit, and less likelihood of subsequent minor trauma resulting in infection. This is supported by data suggesting that exit site infection rates decrease with increasing time on dialysis.[626] For whatever reason, there is a suggestion that use of Y systems for CAPD may decrease the risk of exit site infections.

Moncrief and co-workers[627] believed that the present standard catheter implantation techniques violate a fundamental premise of wound healing. The presence of a foreign body (the catheter) in the immediate postoperative period and the exit site through the skin form a perfect passage for rapid and permanent colonization of the catheter tunnel and cuffs. This colonization has been documented by the observation that biofilms are found on most catheter surfaces soon after implantation.[17] The Moncrief-Popovich catheter (described in detail earlier) was designed to allow healing of the subcutaneous cuff in a sterile environment. During the initial evaluation of this catheter, these authors reported an exit site infection rate of 0.55 episode per patient-year. This is not significantly different from exit site infection rates reported in most studies. Further studies with this catheter are under way. External cuff extrusion increases the risk for infection, perhaps by causing chronic trauma to the sinus tract. Careful attention to catheter implantation technique can minimize this problem. Furthermore, the swan neck catheter design was developed in part to prevent the natural tendency of external cuff extrusion in straight catheters.

**Tunnel Infections.** The tunnel is the area between the two cuffs. After 2 months, this section of the catheter is covered with a thick fibrous tissue (in silicone catheters) or a thin fibrous tissue (polyurethane catheters). Actual tunnel infections are rare. More commonly, they represent infection of the deep cuff. Whereas exit site infections can be treated successfully by antibiotics, deep cuff infections are rarely cured by antibiotics alone and usually require catheter removal. Catheter removal is strongly suggested in a patient with peritonitis and a known tunnel infection.

**Prevention of Catheter Infections.** The primary means of preventing catheter infections is to have a dedicated, knowledgeable catheter implantation team. As discussed before, in that situation, there is no significant difference in outcome between surgical and bedside placement or between insertion techniques.[25] Although there are no hard data to prove that prophylactic antibiotics used before catheter placement will prevent subsequent infection, consensus indicates that perioperative antibiotic therapy is prudent. Postoperatively, it is important to immobilize the catheter and minimize handling. The exit should be covered with a sterile gauze dressing, which is not changed for several days unless there is excessive bleeding. There is no clear consensus as to when the patient should start daily exit site care. Recommendations are for 2 to 8 weeks after placement. Swan neck catheters, disconnect Y systems, eradication of *S. aureus* nasal carriers (discussed earlier), and possibly use of the Moncrief-Popovich catheter implantation technique may prevent exit site infections, but definitive studies are lacking.

In contrast to the general agreement for postoperative exit site care, there are marked variations in standard clinical practices for long-term exit site care[628] and the effect these different practices have on preventing infection. One study suggested that cleaning with soap and water is best[629];

another study suggested that use of povidone-iodine resulted in fewer infections[616]; a third study found no difference in infection rates regardless of cleansing agent used.[630] At present, there is no consensus for a recommendation for the standard long-term care cleansing agent. It may be that any cleansing agent that does not irritate the exit is acceptable for long-term care, as long as initially the standard implantation and postimplantation practices are followed to allow catheter maturation.

**Treatment of Exit Site Infections.** The treatment of exit site and tunnel infections was reviewed and guidelines were published.[25] There are few data on therapeutic efficacy of current methods for treatment of exit site or tunnel infections. Treatment recommendations include the use of topical and parenteral antibiotics. Topical antibiotics include chlorhexidine, mupirocin, dilute hydrogen peroxide, and gentamicin eye drops. Because of the high frequency of resistance, gram-positive infections are treated parenterally with vancomycin. Cephalosporins or a penicillinase-resistant antibiotic can also be used if the organism is not resistant to these agents. Persistent infections can be treated with combination vancomycin and rifampin. For gram-negative infections, ciprofloxacin is usually appropriate, although some *Pseudomonas* infections may require other antipseudomonal agents. The recommended duration of therapy is 2 to 4 weeks.

Areas of current research include new catheter designs, attempts at better fixation of the cuffs to the subcutaneous tissue, and a search for more biocompatible material.

## MECHANICAL COMPLICATIONS OF PERITONEAL DIALYSIS

### Inflow Pain

If the catheter is correctly placed within the peritoneal cavity, inflow pain is typically due to positioning of the catheter tip adjacent to tissues that cannot move during fluid infusion. This type of pain tends to be minimized when curled-tip catheters with multiple outflow pores are used. If this pain does not resolve after time, it may require catheter repositioning. Pain may also be related to dialysate composition. The abnormally low dialysate pH may transiently cause pain in some patients. If this is the cause of the pain, it can be mitigated by adding 4 to 5 mEq/L of $NaHCO_3$ to the dialysis solution before infusion.[631] Other possible causes include choice of buffer[84]; temperature; or any additives, such as antibiotics and introduced air.

### Outflow Failure

Outflow failure is detected when drained volume is substantially less than instilled volume. If it is associated with inflow failure, catheter kink or obstruction, such as with a clot, should be suspected. If a clot is suspected, the catheter can often be opened with an injection of streptokinase or urokinase. Once the possibility of ultrafiltration failure or dialysate leaks has been ruled out, the differential diagnosis of isolated outflow failure is not long and includes catheter migration, omental wrapping, and adherence of bowel (such as with constipation) or other tissue to the catheter. In these cases, the omentum or adherent tissue acts like a ball valve, allowing ingress of fluid but occluding the catheter pores when drainage is attempted. In these cases, one should rule out constipation and then obtain a plain x-ray film to determine catheter position. If the catheter is malpositioned, attempts at repositioning can be attempted. These include using a malleable metal rod under fluoroscopic guidance and repositioning with peritoneoscopy or during surgery. If the catheter is in the pelvis, urokinase has been reported to relieve the outflow obstruction, perhaps by lysing omental attachments. Peritoneoscopic lysis of adhesions and surgical omentectomy are often successful if other noninvasive maneuvers are unsuccessful.

## COMPLICATIONS RELATED TO INCREASED INTRA-ABDOMINAL PRESSURE

The pressure in an empty peritoneal cavity is 0.5 to 2.2 cm $H_2O$.[632] Intra-abdominal pressure then increases linearly with increasing volume in routine peritoneal dialysis. Typical pressures range from 2 to 10 cm $H_2O$ and may be as high as 12 cm $H_2O$ in patients using 3-L exchanges.[248, 307] Other factors also influence net intra-abdominal pressure and include weight, age, activity, and body position. During such activities as coughing or straining, the intra-abdominal pressure can transiently reach values as high as 300 cm $H_2O$,[248] which suggests that excessive coughing or constipation should be avoided, especially in the period immediately after catheter implantation. According to the law of Laplace, these higher intra-abdominal pressures can serve to increase the tension on the wall of the abdomen as the abdominal girth and pressure increase. This can result in undue stress on these structures and the possibility of increased risk for hernia formation and dialysate leaks. Interestingly, these elevated pressures do not appear to be transmitted to the intragastric area or the lower esophageal sphincter.[633]

### Hernias

Literature reviews would suggest that the prevalence of hernias in CAPD populations was between 10% and 25%[634, 635] and that the prevalence in IPD patients was less,[634] presumably owing to less elevated intra-abdominal pressures because they have a dry day and because pressures are lower in the supine position when the abdominal musculature is relaxed. Many different hernia types have been reported in peritoneal dialysis patients, the most common being umbilical, inguinal, pericatheter, and at a previous surgical site. Patients with hernias present in multiple ways. Findings include painless swelling, genital edema, peritonitis due to incarcerated bowel, intestinal obstruction, or a hernia on routine physical examination. A patent processus vaginalis is a common cause of indirect inguinal hernias and should be repaired if it is noted at the time of catheter implantation. Similarly, if other ventral or incisional hernias are noted, they should be repaired. The natural history of these hernias is a tendency to enlarge over time. Any hernia, but particularly a small one, carries a risk of bowel incarceration or strangulation. Of the 28 cases of

incarceration or strangulation of hernias noted in the literature, there were nine reported deaths. Pericatheter and incisional hernias were the hernia types most likely to be associated with incarceration. Therefore, if one of these is noted in a peritoneal dialysis patient, surgical repair should be strongly considered. Prevention of pericatheter hernias includes allowing catheter maturation by waiting 10 to 14 days after catheter placement before initiating ambulatory dialysis; using low-volume dialysis in the supine position before that if indicated; and creating a paramedian or lateral exit[30, 636] or using the swan neck catheter design.[11]

### Leaks

A less frequent complication of peritoneal dialysis is the development of abdominal wall or genital edema. Genital edema has been reported to occur by two different mechanisms.[637] Under the influence of increased abdominal pressure, dialysate can dissect through the peritoneal membrane and into the soft tissues of the abdominal wall, especially in areas where there is a defect in the peritoneum, such as at previous surgical incisions or in the pericatheter area. These patients may or may not have an associated hernia. The extravasated fluid may then dissect down tissue planes to a more dependent position, resulting in genital edema. Another mechanism of genital edema formation is by flow of dialysate through a patent processus vaginalis to the tunica vaginalis. From there, it can dissect through the tunica vaginalis and into the scrotal or labial wall itself.

Vaginal leak of dialysate has also been reported.[638] Although the opening to the fallopian tubes represents a potential defect for dialysate leak, this has seldom been reported. If this were common, a potential treatment would be tubal ligation if catheter perforation has been ruled out. It appears more likely that vaginal leaks are due to a dissection through fascial planes that eventually reaches the vaginal vault.[639] This may explain the association between vaginal leaks and fungal peritonitis.[640, 641]

Computed tomography is probably the examination of choice in dialysis patients with suspected leaks or hernias.[642] This is usually facilitated by injection of contrast medium into the dialysate, which can be seen on computed tomographic scanning. Dialysate with radionuclide imaging[643] can also be helpful.

Treatment of isolated genital or abdominal wall edema, in the absence of hernias or major leaks, can sometimes be accomplished by temporary cessation of peritoneal dialysis and bed rest. If dialysis is needed, intermittent low-volume dialysis in the supine position with a cycler can be tried. If this is not successful, a temporary transfer to hemodialysis to allow healing of peritoneal defects should be attempted. Surgical repair may eventually be required.

### Hydrothorax

The clinical presentation of hydrothorax can vary from an asymptomatic finding on routine chest x-ray examination to severe respiratory compromise. Often the patients first note minimal dyspnea and, in an attempt to treat this with the use of hypertonic exchanges, end up forcing even more fluid into the pleural space because of the increased intra-abdominal fluid and pressure. These leaks can occur any time during the course of peritoneal dialysis, are more common in female patients, and tend to occur on the right.

It has been suggested that fluid traverses the diaphragm through lymphatics or through defects in the diaphragm itself, most often through tendinous defects.[644] Four cases of hydrothorax were reviewed at one center.[645] A pleural peritoneal leak was diagnosed in each case by the presence of a high glucose concentration in the pleural fluid. This was confirmed by isotopic[646] or contrast peritoneography, both of which are less invasive. There are many options for treatment. Peritoneal dialysis should ideally be discontinued, with a temporary transfer to hemodialysis if necessary. There are reports of spontaneous regression.[647] A trial of cycler therapy may also allow spontaneous healing. If the hydrothorax recurs, surgical repair or obliteration with intrapleural talc, tetracycline, fibrin adhesive, or autologous blood can be tried.[635]

### Alterations of Respiratory Function

The effect of 2-L infusions on respiratory function was investigated in 17 patients.[648] The most striking changes occurred when the patient was sitting. Decreases in $Po_2$ and functional reserve capacity were noted. Twardowski and Janicka[327] have shown that patients who could not tolerate 2.5-L exchanges had significantly lower forced vital capacity in the sitting position than those who could. In the upright position, pulmonary function testing was not significantly different from baseline values. Similar findings were noted with 3-L infusions.[307] These authors found that the decreases were even more pronounced in the supine position. In some of these patients, the forced vital capacity decreased up to 42% when they were supine, suggesting that forced vital capacity in the supine position is the most sensitive predictor of tolerance to larger instilled volumes. Similar findings have been reported with pregnancy and obesity.

Given these findings, one might predict that larger instilled volumes would be least tolerated during sleeping. Not only is the patient supine, but it has been shown that there is a marked inhibition of intercostal muscle movement during rapid eye movement sleep. This alters the mechanics of breathing. During these instances, the rib cage becomes unstable, and there is thoracic contraction rather than expansion with diaphragmatic contraction. To maintain usual tidal volumes, diaphragmatic contraction must become more forceful. However, under conditions of increased intra-abdominal pressure, such as during peritoneal dialysis, patients can become dyspneic. These were the symptoms described in patients who could not tolerate the larger exchanges.[30]

Many patients can tolerate these increased volumes without difficulty, however, and one study reported that 6 of 10 patients tolerated 3-L volumes for routine CAPD without difficulty.[649] Other investigators have not detected any significant changes in arterial saturation at any time in patients using CAPD.[650] Most patients with obstructive airway disease are able to tolerate CAPD without difficulty, perhaps because the ''stretch'' the diaphragm undergoes with in-

creased intra-abdominal volume improves the efficiency of its contractions.[635]

**Back Pain.** The increased intra-abdominal pressure and volume tend to pull the lumbar vertebrae into a more lordotic position. The net effect is increased stress on the spine. Many ESRD patients already have degenerative disk disease, osteoporosis, or facet disease at the time of presentation for dialysis, and their therapy may be complicated by the onset of renal osteodystrophy, which also has a predilection for symptoms in this area. The addition of dialysate may lead to the new onset or worsening of back pain in these patients. Treatment is aimed at reducing intra-abdominal pressure. This may be achieved in some patients by decreasing instilled volumes or with a change to cycler therapy.

### METABOLIC COMPLICATIONS

Cardiac disease is the most common cause of death in ESRD patients.[474, 651] Patients undergoing peritoneal dialysis have a significantly higher risk for dying of cardiovascular complications than do patients undergoing hemodialysis.[474, 651] The atherosclerotic risk factors in peritoneal dialysis patients are multifactorial and include not only the traditional risk factors of smoking, hypertension, family history, obesity, diabetes, and increased cholesterol levels but also the uremic state and possible side effects of the therapy itself. Peritoneal dialysis is associated with an increased glucose load because of the constant absorption from the peritoneal cavity. The reported mean daily glucose absorption in CAPD patients varies from 100 to 200 g of glucose per day.[652–657] Possible effects of this glucose load are summarized in Table 57–12. Because of this glucose load, there is a constant tendency for peritoneal dialysis patients to develop hyperglycemia and hyperinsulinemia.[658, 659] Some patients even have frank diabetes necessitating insulin therapy.[96, 660] The sustained hyperinsulinemia and hyperglycemia may both contribute to an increased risk of athero-

---

**TABLE 57–12. Glucose Absorption in CAPD**

**Benefits**
Continuous energy supply may improve energy balance.
Hyperinsulinemia may promote anabolism.
Continuous glucose supply may prevent hypoglycemia.
Continuous dialysis with K+-free solutions with glucose contributes to improved control of hyperkalemia.

**Disadvantages**
Hyperglycemia results in formation of abnormal glucosylated proteins.
Hyperinsulinemia may promote atherogenesis.
Hyperglycemic stress may result in exhaustion of pancreatic β-cells.
Hyperlipidemia is due to continuous glucose supply and hyperinsulinemia.
Obesity may result.
Anorexia may occur.
Amino acid alterations may be seen.
Toxic effects on peritoneum may occur.

From Lindholm B, Bergstrom J: Nutritional management of patients undergoing peritoneal dialysis. *In* Nolph KD (ed): Peritoneal Dialysis, 3rd ed. Kluwer Academic Publishers, Boston, 1989, pp 230–260. Reprinted by permission of Kluwer Academic Publishers.

genesis in the majority of patients on long-term peritoneal dialysis.

Chronic renal failure itself is associated with deranged lipid metabolism.[661] A hyperlipidemic effect of CAPD has been demonstrated in several studies, but the results vary.[97, 662–668] These changes have been summarized by Lindholm and Bergstrom[669] as follows. At the start of peritoneal dialysis, many patients show hypertriglyceridemia, whereas most patients have normal cholesterol levels. During the first year of therapy, both these levels tend to increase. These changes are due to increased lipid concentrations in the very low density lipoprotein and low-density lipoprotein fractions, whereas the changes in high-density lipoprotein are less marked. Patients who are hyperlipidemic at the start of therapy are more likely to have changes.[666] A positive correlation between serum insulin and serum triglyceride levels has also been demonstrated, which implies a role for insulin in the pathogenesis of hypertriglyceridemia.[670] CAPD has been shown to be associated with an increase in lipoprotein Lp(a).[671–675] This lipoprotein is thought to be associated with an increased risk of atherosclerotic cardiovascular and cerebrovascular disease.[676] However, increased levels of Lp(a) in CAPD patients were not found in all reports.[677, 678] These changes toward an increased atherogenic lipid profile are more pronounced in peritoneal dialysis patients than in hemodialysis patients.[679, 680]

This observed increased risk of cardiovascular death in peritoneal dialysis patients and the tendency for an increased atherogenic lipid profile have prompted initial investigations in the use of cholesterol-lowering drugs in these patients. Lovastatin, a hydroxymethylglutaryl–coenzyme A reductase inhibitor, has been shown to reduce total cholesterol, low-density lipoprotein–cholesterol, and triglyceride levels while increasing high-density lipoprotein–cholesterol levels in a group of CAPD patients.[681] Similar results have been observed in short-term follow-up using simvastatin, another hydroxymethylglutaryl–coenzyme A reductase inhibitor.[682, 683] In one study in which levels were monitored, no effect on Lp(a) was observed.[683] These clinical observations and early trials of intervention deserve further attention.

## Special Populations

### ELDERLY PATIENTS

Data from USRDS have shown that the annualized increased incidence of ESRD was greatest in patients older than 75 years.[474] The increase in the annualized incidence from 1984–1986 to 1987–1989 was 13% for those older than 75 years and nearly 10% for those aged 65 to 74 years. In addition, by the year 2000, it is estimated that more than 65% of all ESRD patients will be older than 65 years. In considering ESRD therapy for the elderly, it is important to keep in mind that there is no uniform definition of elderly. This makes comparisons of studies in the literature difficult because the "young-old" would be expected to do much better than the "old-old." An important consideration is what impact the treatment of ESRD in these patients has on

life expectancy. The data from the USRDS would suggest that for the average 65-year-old patient starting dialysis, the average life expectancy is roughly 3.5 additional years.[474] Although this is only about one fifth the expected life expectancy for U.S. citizens aged 65 years without renal disease, it is important to consider quality of life issues in these patients and to keep in perspective that these same USRDS data suggest that the average additional life expectancy for an ESRD patient aged 40 years is about 8.8 years.

Choice of modality in the elderly should involve careful consideration of not only medical conditions but also psychosocial factors. Many elderly patients have pre-existing diminished cardiac reserve, which could result in cardiac symptoms during the rapid fluid shifts associated with hemodialysis. Similarly, these rapid fluid shifts may precipitate cardiac arrhythmias during or shortly after the hemodialysis procedure. Arrhythmias have been reported less often in patients on CAPD,[684, 685] presumably because of the steady-state volume control established with peritoneal dialysis. Another benefit of peritoneal dialysis over hemodialysis in this population is the avoidance of vascular access in older patients who need prosthetic vascular grafts but risk increased morbidity therewith. Potential disadvantages of peritoneal dialysis in this population include the inability to do self-care; the poor wound healing, which increases risk for hernia formation or dialysate leaks; and the adverse effects of increased abdominal pressure and weight on existing pulmonary disease,[686] osteoporosis, and pre-existing bony thorax abnormalities. Elderly patients on CAPD are more likely than younger patients to be malnourished, despite the increased caloric intake provided by absorption of glucose from the dialysate.[436] Elderly patients are more likely to have problems related to bowel dysfunction. Constipation, a common complaint in any age group, is most common in the elderly. This can be due to decreased mobility, drug effects, altered diet, and concomitant diseases.[687] Constipation can be a cause of mechanical dysfunction of the Tenckhoff catheter. Careful attention to these complaints in any CAPD patient is therefore important. Colonic diverticula occur in 30% to 40% of individuals older than 50 years, and their frequency increases thereafter with each additional decade of life. The percentage of peritonitis episodes due to diverticulitis and bowel perforation will also presumably increase with age. There is no evidence that diverticulitis is aggravated by peritoneal dialysis; however, because of the increased risk of such in this population, diverticular disease must be considered when these patients present with peritonitis. Despite this possible increased risk of peritonitis due to diverticular disease, the relative risk of peritonitis is not increased in the elderly.[458] Two large multicenter studies have found either no difference[688] or a slight decrease in the relative risk of technique failure in the elderly,[458] which may in part be due to a higher rate of dropout because of death in this group compared with the younger reference population. Despite these possible risk factors for both modalities, there is little variation in survival reported for the elderly patient undergoing peritoneal dialysis or hemodialysis throughout the world.

Benevent and co-workers[689] and Walls[690] have reported equivalent survival for patients on peritoneal dialysis and hemodialysis despite increases in the comorbid conditions in the patients on peritoneal dialysis. These studies did not use statistical techniques to adjust for differences in coexisting diseases. Using the Cox proportional hazards model to adjust for pre-existing characteristics, Maiorca and associates[463] have shown that the patient's age, the presence of diabetes, malignant neoplasm, and peripheral vascular disease all have an impact on survival of the patient. After adjustment for these factors, there was no difference in survival between hemodialysis and CAPD for patients aged 30 to 66 years. However, survival was significantly better with peritoneal dialysis for patients aged 66 years or older. In a follow-up multicenter study, similar results were found, but the rate at which the relative risk of death increased with increasing age was higher for those on hemodialysis compared with peritoneal dialysis once patients were older than 53.5 years[473] (Fig. 57–23). Lunde and colleagues[691] found that in elderly patients starting dialysis in Michigan, modality did not have an impact on outcome. However, when the 1987–1989 cohort of new ESRD patients was examined by use of the USRDS data, the death rate from cardiac disease was highest in CAPD patients. This increased risk seemed to be confined to the elderly diabetic patients using peritoneal dialysis.[474] There was no difference in risk between hemodialysis and peritoneal dialysis for both the young and the old nondiabetic patients. More carefully designed comparisons that include adjusting for all the significant comorbid pre-existing diseases are needed before definite conclusions about effects of modality on outcome in the elderly can be made. At the moment, this seems less of an issue for nondiabetic than for diabetic patients.

## DIABETIC PATIENTS

In the United States, diabetes has become the leading cause of ESRD. Renal transplantation is generally thought to be the preferred therapy for diabetic patients with ESRD because of improved outcome and better quality of life.[692] The outcome for diabetic patients undergoing dialysis therapies (hemodialysis or peritoneal dialysis) is disappointing

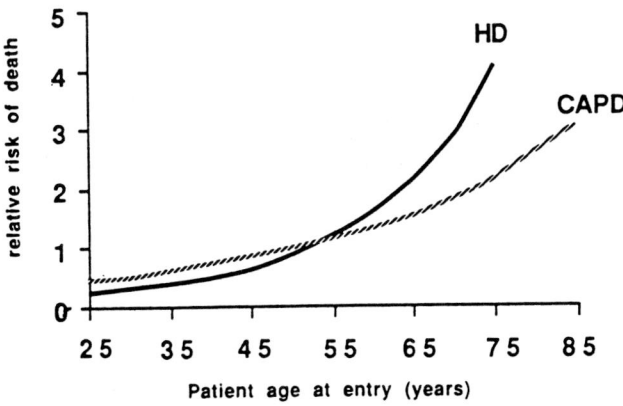

**Figure 57–23.** Risk of death among CAPD patients relative to age 53.5 years versus risk of death among hemodialysis (HD) patients relative to age 53.5 years. (From Maiorca R, Vonesh EF, Cavalli PL, et al: A multicenter, selection-adjusted comparison of patient and technique survivals on CAPD and hemodialysis. Perit Dial Int 11:118–127, 1991.)

compared with that for nondiabetic patients. According to USRDS data, less than half of all diabetic patients survive more than 2 years with dialysis, and 5-year survival is only about 18%.[693] However, there has been a slow trend from 1982 to 1990 toward an increase in the percentage of patients surviving 1 year with dialysis, which has been most pronounced in diabetic patients.[693] The major reason for this generally poor outcome in diabetic patients is the presence of coexisting severe end-organ damage at the time of presentation with ESRD. Because of the possible differences in underlying comorbid diseases, interpretation of published data on outcome is difficult. At present, as reviewed before, outcome studies in large populations of patients would suggest that survival is in general similar for diabetic patients on hemodialysis and peritoneal dialysis but, in both cases, less than that seen for nondiabetic patients.[463, 464, 474] There may be an increased risk for elderly diabetic patients using CAPD compared with those undergoing hemodialysis, whereas the risk of death is consistently less for younger diabetic patients on peritoneal dialysis,[474, 475] but this finding may be due to differences in underlying pre-existing comorbid diseases between groups of patients. Further studies are needed. At this time, we believe that there are not sufficient data to suggest that one modality is better than another for elderly diabetic patients. The report from the USRDS has shown that the risk of technique failure was not significantly different for diabetic patients than for patients with glomerulonephritis.[458]

Possible benefits of peritoneal dialysis for diabetic patients include home therapy and better blood pressure control because of the continuous and sustained $Na^+$ removal and ultrafiltration.[694] This would alleviate the need for rapid intermittent fluid removal, such as with hemodialysis, which can at times be associated with large intravascular fluid shifts and consequent symptomatic hypotension. On the basis of these observations, it would seem reasonable for diabetic patients with severe cardiac or cerebrovascular disease to use CAPD. However, analysis of cause of death for diabetic ESRD patients from 1987 to 1989 in the United States showed that there was an increased mortality from cardiovascular and cerebrovascular causes in diabetic patients treated with CAPD compared with hemodialysis.[474] Again, this may be due to selection bias, but because of this, supportive data to suggest treating all diabetic patients with cardiovascular disease with peritoneal dialysis are lacking at present.

There is evidence to suggest that intraperitoneal administration of insulin allows a more physiologic control of diabetes than that seen with subcutaneous administration. Intraperitoneal insulin is rapidly absorbed into the hepatic circulation, which may beneficially affect lipid metabolism and circulating peripheral insulin levels.[695] Normally, the liver metabolizes 50% to 60% of the insulin presented to it.[696] It has been stressed that for any given insulin dose, less reaches the peripheral circulation after intraperitoneal administration than if it was given subcutaneously. This observation is of importance if circulating insulin levels correlate with the risk of atherosclerosis.[697, 698] Furthermore, insulin uptake by the liver inhibits hepatic glycogenolysis, gluconeogenesis, and ketogenesis and facilitates glycogen and fatty acid synthesis.[699] Excessive hepatic glucose output is the major source of elevated fasting glucose levels in non–insulin-dependent diabetic patients[700] and is much more sensitive to suppression by insulin than stimulation of peripheral glucose uptake.[701] These data would suggest that the more physiologic delivery of insulin that can be achieved by the intraperitoneal route allowed by peritoneal dialysis therapy may ultimately be beneficial for these patients.

Use of intraperitoneal insulin has been associated with good blood glucose control without an increased risk of peritonitis.[702–705] This experience with peritonitis was confirmed by the initial report from the CAPD registry, which revealed that patients using a combination of subcutaneous and intraperitoneal insulin had the lowest peritonitis rates.[706] However, others have found a modest increased peritonitis risk in diabetic patients overall.[458] Intraperitoneal insulin has also been associated with subcapsular liver steatonecrosis[707] and the malignant omentum syndrome.[708] At present, neither of these reports would preclude the use of intraperitoneal insulin.

Published data would suggest that peritoneal transport for diabetic patients remains stable for up to 60 months.[361, 709] This is confirmed by the finding of relatively few changes in peritoneal biopsy specimens from diabetic patients unless they have had repeated severe episodes of peritonitis.[99] In conclusion, there are sufficient reasons to consider peritoneal dialysis the treatment of choice for the average diabetic patient with ESRD.

## BLACK PATIENTS

Black race is associated with an increased frequency of ESRD.[474, 693] The percentage of black patients undergoing peritoneal dialysis is less than that of white patients. The reasons for this are uncertain and probably multifactorial in origin. Although most large databases show that black patients using peritoneal dialysis are at an increased risk for both peritonitis and technique failure compared with white patients,[34, 458, 710] Feldman and co-workers[711] and Windus[712] have shown that black patients are also at increased risk for vascular access complications. Holley and colleagues[713] have shown that compared with white patients matched for age, sex, and insulin dependence, black patients overall had a higher frequency of peritonitis and exit site infections. Although in this study black patients had higher exit site infection rates, this did not seem to be the cause for the increased peritonitis rates. Peritonitis due to *S. epidermidis* infections was more common in black patients, whereas *S. aureus* infections were more common in white patients. The reason for the reported increased risk of peritonitis in black patients is unclear. When the subset of black patients in the study on disconnect were compared with white patients on disconnect devices, there was no difference in peritonitis rates.[713] Rubin and associates[714] have suggested that the increased risk of peritonitis in black patients may not be due to race but may be due to a lower income and educational level in this group than in white patients. Korbet and colleagues[710] have shown that the risk of peritonitis is inversely correlated with the level of education at the time of initiation of peritoneal dialysis (patients with less than 8 years of formal education had the highest rates of peritoni-

tis). In a related study, these authors have shown that although technique survival was lowest for black patients in their predominantly urban population (62% black) during the years 1981 to 1988, overall survival rates for patients and technique were similar to those of the CAPD registry (24% black)[34] during the same time period.

These studies would suggest that black race may not predispose to infectious complications on peritoneal dialysis and that further evaluation of associated psychosocial factors is needed to further define observed cross-sectional differences in outcomes between the racial groups.

## PEDIATRIC PATIENTS

The introduction of long-term peritoneal dialysis for the management of end-stage renal failure in children has been a major advance. The first reported use of peritoneal dialysis in pediatric patients was by Bloxsum and Powell[715] in 1948. Since 1976, with the introduction of CAPD by Popovich and co-workers[4] and the first report on the use of CAPD in a pediatric patient,[716] peritoneal dialysis has widely been considered the treatment of choice for renal failure in infants and young children when transplantation is not an immediate option.[717] This therapy allows children of all ages to receive dialysis in their homes with minimal or no dietary restrictions. Use of CCPD in pediatric patients was first described in 1981 by Price and Suki.[718] Because this technique offers freedom for both the children and the parents from daytime exchanges, growth of CCPD has increased the fastest in recent years. One of the most significant benefits of peritoneal dialysis over hemodialysis for pediatric patients is the well-documented increase in quality of life for patients and parents.[719, 720] In a study from Australia, where transplantation, hemodialysis, and peritoneal dialysis were evaluated, it was noted that 87% of children were able to continue normal schooling.[721]

Anatomic observations suggest that with adjustment for body weight, the peritoneal surface area in infants is about twice that in adults.[134] However, with adjustment for body surface area, no significant difference in the ratio of peritoneal surface area to body surface area was found between infants and adults.[722] Although data are scarce, most studies would suggest that peritoneal transport (measured by use of MTAC) of small solutes is similar in children and adults.[723–725] However, not all studies have confirmed this. Geary and colleagues[726] found that the unadjusted mean D/P ratios from PET studies were slightly higher in children than in adults and that 70% of the children studied were high or high-average transporters.

Although available MTAC data suggest that ultrafiltration rates in children and adults should be similar, clinical experience would suggest that adequate ultrafiltration may be difficult to achieve in many young children.[727] This may be due to a more rapid decline in dialysate glucose levels during the dwell in children than in adults, consistent with the finding that pediatric patients tend to be rapid transporters.[728] Some studies suggest higher lymphatic absorption rates in children.[729] In summary, limited studies suggest that transport is similar in children and adults when it is scaled for body surface area. On the average, transport rates are higher in neonates than in adults. Further studies are needed.

Initial experience suggested that technical and clinical complications were more common in pediatric patients than in adults.[730] At one center, in a period of 115 months, the overall peritonitis rates were lower in adult patients than in the pediatric age group.[731] This center found no difference in infection rates between CAPD and CCPD, whereas another center found lower peritonitis rates for patients on CCPD.[732] Staphylococcal species were the most common cause of peritonitis in older pediatric patients, whereas gram-negative rods were the most common cause of infection in patients younger than 2 years or in those patients with nephrostomies.[731] However, the report by the USRDS[458] did not show an increased risk for peritonitis or technique failure for patients younger than 20 years compared with the reference group (patients aged 20 to 39 years).

In 11 of 12 children treated with CAPD, serum levels of IgG2 were not detectable.[733] These authors concluded that in young patients, peritoneal dialysis causes IgG2 deficiency as a result of increased protein losses in dialysate, which possibly predisposes them to a higher frequency of peritonitis. Similar findings were described by another group.[734]

One of the most important problems to be addressed with any form of renal replacement therapy in pediatric patients is the documented growth retardation.[719] In an early report, 50% of the patients evaluated were found to have evidence of growth retardation while undergoing peritoneal dialysis,[735] although with careful attention to dialysis dose and nutritional supplementation, a sustained increase in growth has been described.[736] This subject was reviewed by Fine.[737] Kohaut[738] correlated growth with various biochemical and therapeutic factors in 11 children undergoing CAPD for a 3-month period. The most significant factor correlating with height velocity was control of parathyroid hormone levels. Other important factors were protein and calorie intake and control of acidosis. Neither blood urea nitrogen nor total urea clearance had a positive correlation with growth velocity. Similarly, Stefanidis and co-workers[739] found that control of renal osteodystrophy and adequate energy intake were the most important factors influencing growth of patients on CAPD.[740] Conley[740] and Brewer[741] have demonstrated the usefulness of supplemental nasogastric feeding for improving growth in some infants in peritoneal dialysis. The recombinant human growth hormone has become an important adjunct for the treatment of growth retardation in children. Both Leichter[742] and Tonshoff[743] and colleagues have demonstrated its usefulness when it is given subcutaneously. Similar results have been noted with intraperitoneal therapy.[744]

Acute renal failure occurs in about 6% of neonates admitted to the intensive care nursery. Reports have described the use of small-volume exchanges in very low birth weight infants with some success.[745] Another center suggested that early intervention with peritoneal dialysis may reduce morbidity and mortality in low-birth-weight infants with acute renal failure.[746] No significant difference in graft survival was noted in one study, no matter whether the patient was treated with peritoneal dialysis or hemodialysis or not

undergoing dialysis before transplantation, which suggests that modality choice had no influence on outcome of transplantation.[747] Hyponatremia has been described in neonates undergoing long-term peritoneal dialysis, presumably because of $Na^+$ losses in the dialysate in excess of that ingested.[748] This problem can be corrected by increasing oral sodium intake or by increasing dialysate $Na^+$ concentration above 150 mEq/L. As described later, peritoneal dialysis has been used to treat coma due to hyperammonemia, maple syrup urine disease, propionic acidemia, and citrulinemia.[749]

These studies continue to show encouraging results for the use of peritoneal dialysis in pediatric patients. Not only does the therapy prolong life, but it also allows correction of some of the morbidity associated with treatment of ESRD and allows as much normalization of quality of life for the patients and family as possible.

## HUMAN IMMUNODEFICIENCY VIRUS–INFECTED PATIENTS

Peritoneal dialysis may offer some advantages over hemodialysis for patients with the acquired immunodeficiency syndrome.[750] Compared with hemodialysis, peritoneal dialysis may theoretically result in less stimulation of the human immunodeficiency virus–infected T cells. Blood-membrane interactions in hemodialysis may markedly increase cytokine production, which may increase viral reproduction in the stimulated lymphocytes. Peritoneal dialysis patients are reported to have better preserved humoral immune function than hemodialysis patients. Absorption of glucose may have nutritional benefits, as long as they are not offset by protein losses in the dialysate. Despite these potential immunologic benefits of peritoneal dialysis, human immunodeficiency virus–infected patients may be at increased risk for peritonitis.[751]

Infection control policies for these patients include universal body precautions, with use of bleach as a disinfectant and then disposal of dialysate down the sink or toilet; empty dialysis bags are placed into a biohazards bag. Dialysate has been found to have the human immunodeficiency virus antigen and therefore is presumed infectious until it is disinfected with bleach. Because dialysis fluid from human immunodeficiency virus–infected patients has been shown to contain the antigen, it is potentially infectious.[752] However, the presence of the antigen in the dialysis fluids was not constant.

## Miscellaneous Clinical Experiences

Six patients had an intra-abdominal vascular graft placed 3 to 32 months before beginning peritoneal dialysis.[539] Two of them had peritonitis, which responded to routine therapy. No patients had evidence of a graft infection or complications of the graft related to peritoneal dialysis.[753]

Reports of using peritoneal dialysis in pregnant patients with acute or chronic renal failure were reviewed.[754–756] One report described the clinical course of eight pregnancies managed with CAPD and compared them with six cases managed by hemodialysis. CAPD seemed to offer several advantages, including a more stable biochemical and extracellular environment as well as infrequent episodes of hypotension and no heparin requirements.

A pregnant woman who had progressive acute renal failure began peritoneal dialysis after 20 weeks' gestation. Prophylactic dialysis was begun using 3-L exchanges, and the patient completed a successful pregnancy.[756] Pregnancy outcomes were reviewed in 11 patients treated with CAPD.[757] Seven of the pregnancies resulted in live births. Two episodes of peritonitis were treated successfully without termination of the pregnancy. Spontaneous abortions are more likely to occur in women who conceive while on dialysis than in those in whom renal failure develops who also have some residual renal function. Some authors believe that peritoneal dialysis, compared with hemodialysis, offers the advantages of a more stable metabolic environment, a more liberal diet, better blood pressure control, and fewer hypotensive episodes.

In patients with respiratory compromise, hypertonic peritoneal dialysis solutions may produce an acute respiratory acidosis.[758] In a patient with respiratory distress syndrome, ventilation could not be increased enough to compensate for the increased carbon dioxide due to the glucose absorption and metabolism. Discontinuation of the hypertonic solutions resulted in improvement in symptoms.

Evidence has been presented that a peritoneal dialysis program should coexist with hemodialysis and transplantation programs to offer patients the best possible choices for survival and maximization of quality of life issues.[759] The authors believe that no single renal replacement therapy meets all the clinical, metabolic, and logistic requirements of every patient. Furthermore, these requirements are likely to change over time.

## Choosing Peritoneal Dialysis

### ABSOLUTE CONTRAINDICATIONS

Contraindications to peritoneal dialysis are listed in Table 57–13. There are few absolute contraindications for the use of peritoneal dialysis, and these include 1) severe peritoneal fibrosis or resection of greater than 50% of the small bowel (although experimental evidence suggests that there may still be enough peritoneal surface area to achieve adequate clearances in some patients), 2) large pleuroperitoneal leak (until repair), and 3) patients with active inflammatory bowel disease. Reasons for these absolute contraindications were described elsewhere.[5, 760, 761]

### RELATIVE CONTRAINDICATIONS

Relative contraindications for peritoneal dialysis were previously described and are listed in Table 57–13.[5, 760, 761] If present, these need to be carefully reviewed for each patient; dialysis modality is chosen after careful consideration of the risks and benefits of each.

Fine and co-workers[762] described a patient who had an accidental T7 cord transection. This patient had two episodes of sterile peritonitis within weeks of two uneventful catheter placements, which were thought to be due to decreased cytokine production in denervated tissue and subsequent increased risk for infection. He also had repeated episodes of upper abdominal pain with no clinical evidence of peritonitis thought to be due to hyperesthesia in a dermatome above the cord transection. Furthermore, the patient had repeated episodes of clonus, presumably due to dialysis-induced irritation of the hypersensitive nerves above the area of transection. These symptoms never occurred before or after treatment with peritoneal dialysis. On the basis of their experience with this patient, these authors suggested that one should use caution in treating this kind of patient with peritoneal dialysis.

### MODALITY SELECTION

Patients with ESRD must choose a treatment modality and do so under the advice of the physicians, nurses, and other members of the ESRD treatment team and their family members. Although some patients have clear medical or social indications or contraindications for one modality versus another, most patients can make a choice. Despite the relatively few absolute contraindications for peritoneal dialysis, only about 15% of the patients worldwide use peritoneal dialysis.[1] Initial reluctance to use peritoneal di-

**TABLE 57–13. Contraindications to Peritoneal Dialysis**

| Absolute | Relative Major | Relative Minor |
|---|---|---|
| Peritoneal fibrosis or resection (>50%) | Blindness | Peripheral vascular disease |
| | Quadriplegia* | Diverticulosis |
| Pleuroperitoneal leak; hydrothorax | Crippling arthritis* | Hepatitis |
| | Other physical handicaps | Polycystic kidneys |
| Active inflammatory bowel disease | Mental retardation* | Low-back problems |
| | Psychosis* | Hernia |
| | Poor motivation* | Hyperlipidemia |
| | Colostomy | Obesity |
| | Nephrostomy | |
| | Fresh aortic prosthesis | |
| | Fungal peritonitis | |
| | Tuberculous peritonitis | |

*For self-therapy only.

alysis on the part of clinicians may have been due to uncertainty regarding the adequacy of the therapy. Although some still debate this question,[761, 763] this chapter has outlined evidence suggesting that for the majority of patients, there is no difference in outcome between peritoneal dialysis and hemodialysis. Modality choice must therefore be a complex issue with many factors other than medical ones alone playing an important role in the decision-making.

Nissenson and co-workers[407] reviewed nonmedical factors that had an impact on ESRD modality selection. These authors found that financial or reimbursement issues stood out as the most important factor that drove modality selection in nearly every country studied. This was a complex issue involving both physician and facility reimbursement issues. Lack of training of nephrologists and nurses as well as poor education of the patient and physician or center bias also played a role. Resource availability, social mores, and cultural habits also played a role in some areas.

Groome and colleagues[764] have shown that, in general, lifestyle considerations (such as independence and dietary restrictions) rank as being more important than medical consequences of a therapy with the exception of avoiding peritonitis. These authors thought the fear of peritonitis was the most important deterrent for choosing peritoneal dialysis. More important, these authors demonstrated that although there was general agreement among physicians, nurses, and patients, there was also some discordance, which suggests that health care professionals must guard against transmitting to the patient what they believe is the most important reason for the patient to choose a particular modality. The patients may feel differently. The timing of when the patient is educated about modality selection also plays an important role in the decision-making.[765, 766] Patients who present to the nephrology treatment team uremic and needing dialysis are more likely to be treated with hemodialysis as their modality with little opportunity for education and choice. These data show the importance of early, timely referral for education to allow the patient to be involved in modality choice.

## Acute Renal Failure

Because the daily clearances of some solutes are less with peritoneal dialysis than with daily hemodialysis, there has been concern that peritoneal dialysis cannot control the uremic state in catabolic, acutely ill patients. Therefore, in general, hemodialysis or continuous forms of hemofiltration are usually used. However, at times, peritoneal dialysis may be tried. Twelve patients with acute renal failure, five of whom were considered catabolic (blood urea nitrogen rising by more than 60 mg/dL/d), were treated with continuous peritoneal dialysis.[767] The observed decreases in blood urea nitrogen and serum creatinine were smaller in the hypercatabolic group compared with less catabolic patients but thought to be adequate; blood pressure and fluid balance were easily controlled in both groups. As mentioned earlier, the hard acute peritoneal catheters (stylet) are associated with a high risk of infectious complications; because of this risk and the common clinical observation that acute renal

failure typically involves more than 3 days of therapy, use of the safer soft chronic catheters is recommended.

When treating patients with acute renal failure with peritoneal dialysis, one must be cognizant of the associated glucose absorption that can substantially contribute to the overall calorie load.[768] If the glucose absorption is excessive, this could lead to hepatic steatosis, hyperglycemia, increased carbon dioxide production, and worsening respiratory failure. If supplemental nutrition is given, the glucose load from peritoneal dialysis must also be considered.

The first evaluation of the effect of dialysis modality on the patient's residual renal function was conducted in Paris in 1982.[455] In this study, it was noted that residual renal function was better preserved at 6, 12, and 18 months in patients using peritoneal dialysis compared with those treated with hemodialysis. Similar results have now been reported by others.[456, 457, 769] Possible reasons for the better preservation with peritoneal dialysis, other than differences in the patients' underlying disease state, include possible ischemia due to rapid changes in osmolality and volume shifts during hemodialysis; hemodialysis-induced transient hypotension; generation of potentially harmful inflammatory mediators by the blood-membrane interaction during hemodialysis; and use of high-molecular-weight nephrotoxic solutions to treat hypotension during hemodialysis. These findings in patients with chronic renal failure would suggest that the effect of modality on ultimate recovery of renal function should be evaluated in the treatment of patients with acute renal failure. At present, there have been no prospective randomized trials to evaluate this concept. However, there are some interesting cross-sectional data in the literature.

Cancarini and co-workers[456] noted recovery of renal function in 6 of 75 CAPD patients compared with 1 of 86 hemodialysis patients. Similarly, Rottembourg and colleagues[770] found a higher frequency of recovery of renal function in patients treated with CAPD (10 of 300 patients; 3.3%) than in hemodialysis patients (4 of 495 patients; 0.8%). However, although Michel and associates[771] noted recovery of renal function in 4.5% of 198 patients using CAPD compared with 3.2% of 212 patients treated with hemodialysis, these authors did not think the difference was due to dialysis modality. These data suggest that when a patient with acute renal failure and a potentially reversible disease needs dialysis, peritoneal dialysis may facilitate recovery of residual renal function. Further studies are needed.

## Nonuremic Uses of Peritoneal Dialysis

By design, both hemodialysis and peritoneal dialysis are suited for blood purification and fluid removal. Because of these intentional aspects of the therapy, peritoneal dialysis has been used for the treatment of conditions other than renal failure. Furthermore, some aspects of the therapy that have traditionally been viewed as a problem, such as protein losses, may theoretically have benefit in the treatment of other disorders. The nonuremic uses of peritoneal dialysis have been reviewed by Bargman.[772]

At times, patients with congestive heart failure fail to respond to traditional medical therapies. IPD has been used in the treatment of congestive heart failure.[773] These initial reports involved temporary therapy until patients were able to recover cardiac function or undergo corrective surgical procedures. The continuous nature of CAPD with its slower rates of ultrafiltration would theoretically seem more suitable for the treatment of congestive heart failure than traditional IPD. The initial report of the use of CAPD in the treatment of congestive heart failure was disappointing.[774] However, subsequent reports have been more encouraging and have demonstrated the ability to maintain euvolemia for months to years in these patients.[415, 775–777] The control of the hypervolemia has led at times to an improvement in overall cardiac function. Shilo and co-workers[778] have also demonstrated an increase in renal perfusion, which was presumably due to an increase in cardiac output associated with the improvement in intravascular volume status. Unfortunately, despite control of underlying symptoms, most patients have a dismal prognosis because of the severe underlying heart disease.

Popovich and colleagues[779] have described the theoretic use of peritoneal dialysis techniques for "peritoneal membrane plasmapheresis." This process uses the application of vasoactive agents on the peritoneal membrane to remove plasma proteins from the body at a rate comparable to that of conventional plasmapheresis while at the same time potentially achieving dialysis. Use of this technique may preclude the need for expensive and potentially risky intravenous fluid and protein replacement.

Acute pancreatitis has been treated with peritoneal lavage[780, 781] and with peritoneal dialysis.[782–784] Dogs that had experimentally induced acute necrotizing pancreatitis were randomized to receive medical treatment, peritoneal dialysis, or both. Those receiving peritoneal lavage had the higher survival rates.[785] Despite the encouraging results in experimental animal studies, results of human studies have been controversial. Most studies show early improvement but have not convincingly demonstrated reduced overall mortality in those receiving peritoneal lavage or dialysis. Despite these findings, peritoneal dialysis is still recommended for the treatment of severe acute pancreatitis in the surgical literature.[786]

Both hemodialysis and peritoneal dialysis have been reported to be useful adjuncts in the treatment of psoriasis. However, peritoneal dialysis seems to be more effective than hemodialysis.[787–790] The mechanism of action is far from clear. Whittier and colleagues[791] presented data from a randomized crossover study comparing sham with real peritoneal dialysis and showed that four of five patients had a marked improvement only on real peritoneal dialysis. Further evaluation is needed, and at this time, peritoneal dialysis has not found widespread use in the treatment of severe psoriasis.

Miscellaneous other reported uses of peritoneal dialysis include the following. Peritoneal dialysis was used successfully as a therapy for a variety of electrolyte and acid-base disorders.[792] This includes successful treatment of severe metabolic alkalosis with fluids made primarily of physiologic saline. Inborn errors of metabolism represent a group of disease states that typically result in an accumulation of a metabolic product that may or may not cause disease. Urea cycle defects are usually treated with hemodialysis,

but there are reports of use of peritoneal dialysis as an adjunctive treatment.[793] Organic acidemias have also been treated with peritoneal dialysis. These include propionic acidemia[794] and methylmalonic acidemia.[795, 796] Maple syrup urine disease has been treated with peritoneal dialysis, which results in a steady removal of the accumulated branched chain amino acids and allows ease of care, feeding of the infants,[797] and normal somatic and intellectual development.[798] Hyponatremia, hypernatremia, hypothermia, hyperthermia, and lactic acidosis were also treated by use of various modifications of peritoneal dialysis fluids. Intraperitoneal instillation of drugs for chemotherapy[799] and experimental paracorporeal membrane oxygenation[800] have also been done. Peritoneal dialysis has also been used in the treatment of poisoning and overdose[801] but, in general, because of the slower clearances, is not as efficacious as hemodialysis.

## FUTURE

During the remainder of the 1990s, peritoneal dialysis will continue to evolve. Present and future research efforts will allow one to augment peritoneal clearances and better individualize therapies. Certainly more convenient user-friendly cyclers will be available. Present research efforts should result in more biocompatible fluids, and perhaps even economical, efficient home generation of fluids will become a reality. Peritoneal dialysis is now a significant part of the renal replacement therapies available at most centers, and as our experience with the therapy evolves, it is expected that the number of patients undergoing peritoneal dialysis will continue to grow.

### *Acknowledgments*

Many thanks to Amanda Burnette for secretarial assistance.

### REFERENCES

1. Westman J: Baxter Worldwide Overview. Baxter Healthcare, Deerfield, IL, May 1995.
2. Ganter G: Über die Beseitigun giftiger Stoffe aus dem Blute durch Dialyse. Munch Med Wochenschr 70:1478, 1923.
3. Odel HM, Ferris DO, Power MH: Peritoneal lavage as an effective means of extrarenal excretion. Am J Med 9:63, 1950.
4. Popovich RP, Moncrief JW, Decherd JF, et al: The definition of a novel portable-wearable equilibrium peritoneal technique. Trans Am Soc Artif Intern Orgs 5:64, 1976. Abstract.
5. Nolph KD: Peritoneal dialysis. *In* Brenner BM, Rector FC (eds): The Kidney, 3rd ed. WB Saunders, Philadelphia, 1986, p 1847.
6. Palmer RA, Maybee TK, Henry EW, et al: Peritoneal dialysis in acute and chronic renal failure. Can Med Assoc J 88:920, 1963.
7. Tenckhoff H, Schechter H: A bacteriologically safe peritoneal access device. Trans Am Soc Artif Intern Organs 14:187, 1968.
8. Westin RE, Roberts M: Clinical use of stylet catheter for peritoneal dialysis. Arch Intern Med 115:569, 1965.
9. Twardowski ZJ, Nolph KD, Khanna R, et al: The need for a "swan neck" permanently bent, arcuate peritoneal dialysis catheter. Perit Dial Bull 5:219, 1985.
10. Twardowski ZJ, Khanna R: Swan neck peritoneal dialysis catheter. *In* Andreucci VE (ed): Vascular and Peritoneal Access for Dialysis. Kluwer Academic Publishers, Dordrecht, Netherlands, 1989, p 271.
11. Twardowski ZJ, Prowant BF, Nichols WK, et al: Six-year experience with swan neck catheters. Perit Dial Int 12:384, 1992.

12. Lindblad AS, Hamilton RW, Novak JW: Complications of peritoneal catheters. *In* Lindblad AS, Novak JW, Nolph KD (eds): Continuous Ambulatory Peritoneal Dialysis in the USA—Final Report of the National CAPD Registry. Kluwer Academic Publishers, Dordrecht, Netherlands, 1989, p 157.

13. Twardowski ZJ, Nichols WK, Nolph KD, et al: Swan neck presternal peritoneal dialysis catheter. Perit Dial Int 13:S130, 1993.

14. Moncrief JW, Popovich RP, Broadrick LJ, et al: The Moncrief-Popovich catheter. A new peritoneal access technique for patients on peritoneal dialysis. ASAIO J 39:62, 1993.

15. Moncrief JW, Popovich RP, Simmons E, et al: Peritoneal access technology. Perit Dial Int 13:S121, 1993.

16. Moncrief J, Popovich R, Simmons E, et al: Catheter obstruction with omental wrap stimulated by dialysate exposure. Perit Dial Int 13:S127, 1993.

17. Read RR, Dasgupta MK, Parker E, et al: Peritonitis in peritoneal dialysis: Bacterial colonization by biofilm spread along the catheter surface. Kidney Int 35:614, 1989.

18. Holmes CJ, Evans RE: Biofilm and foreign body infection—the significance to CAPD-associated peritonitis. Perit Dial Bull 6:168, 1986.

19. Dasgupta MK, Bettcher KB, Ulan RA, et al: Relationship of adherent bacterial biofilms to peritonitis in chronic ambulatory peritoneal dialysis. Perit Dial Bull 7:168, 1987.

20. Marrie TJ, Nobel MA, Costerton JW: Examination of the morphology of bacteria adhering to peritoneal dialysis catheter by scanning and transmission electron microscopy. J Clin Miscrosc 18:1388, 1983.

21. Giangrande A, Allaria P, Torpia R, et al: Ultrastructure analysis of Tenckhoff chronic peritoneal catheters used in continuous ambulatory peritoneal dialysis patients. Perit Dial Int 13:S133, 1993.

22. Costerton JW, Cheng KJ, Geesy GG, et al: Bacterial biofilm in nature and disease. Annu Rev Microbiol 41:435, 1987.

23. Roxe DM, Santhanam S: Structural defects in chronic peritoneal dialysis catheter contributing to peritonitis. Nephron 34:267, 1983.

24. Twardowski ZJ, Dobbie JW, Moore HL, et al: Morphology of peritoneal dialysis catheter tunnel: Macroscopy and light microscopy. Perit Dial Int 11:237, 1991.

25. Gokal R, Ash SR, Helfrich B, et al: Peritoneal catheters and exit site practices: Toward optimum peritoneal access. Perit Dial Int 13:29, 1993.

26. USRDS 1992 Annual Data Report: Catheter-related factors and peritonitis risk in CAPD patients. Am J Kidney Dis 20:48, 1992.

27. Maffei S, Bonello F, Stramignoni E, et al: Two years experience and 119 peritoneal dialysis catheters placed with peritoneoscopy control and Y-TEC system. Minerva Urol Nefrol 44:63, 1992.

28. Nahman NS Jr, Middendorf DF, Bay WH, et al: Modification of the percutaneous approach to peritoneal dialysis catheter placement under peritoneoscopic visualization: Clinical results in 78 patients. J Am Soc Nephrol 3:103, 1992.

29. Ash S: Chronic peritoneal dialysis catheters: Effects of catheter design, materials, and location. Semin Dial 3:39, 1990.

30. Helfrich GB, Pechan BWW, Alijani MR, et al: Reduced catheter complications with lateral placement. Perit Dial Bull 3(suppl 4):S2, 1983.

31. Stegmayr B, Hedberg B, Sandzen B, et al: Absence of leakage by insertion of peritoneal dialysis catheter through the rectus muscle. Perit Dial Int 10:53, 1990.

32. Nicholson ML, Burton PR, Donnelly PK, et al: The role of omentectomy in continuous ambulatory peritoneal dialysis. Perit Dial Int 11:330, 1991.

33. Gokoo CF, Lelah MD, Hauck W, et al: External catheter immobilization improves wound healing in micropigs. ASAIO Trans 35:412, 1990.

34. Lindblad AS, Novak JW, Nolph KD: The USA CAPD registry characteristics of participants and selected outcome measures for the period January 1, 1981 through August 31, 1987. *In* Nolph KD (ed): Peritoneal Dialysis, 3rd ed. Kluwer Academic Publishers, Boston, 1989, p 389.

35. Piraino B, Bernardini J, Centa PK, et al: The effect of body weight on CAPD related infections and catheter loss. Perit Dial Int 11:64, 1991.

36. Swartz R, Messana J, Rocher L, et al: The curled catheter: Dependable device for percutaneous peritoneal access. Perit Dial Int 10:231, 1990.

37. Weber J, Mettang T, Hubel E, et al: Survival of 138 surgically placed straight double-cuff Tenckhoff catheters in patients on continuous ambulatory peritoneal dialysis. Perit Dial Int 13:224, 1993.

38. Burkart JM, Jordan JR, Durnell TA, et al: Comparison of exit-site infections in disconnect versus nondisconnect systems for peritoneal dialysis. Perit Dial Int 12:317, 1992.

39. Vas SI: Answers to what are the indications for removal of the permanent peritoneal catheter? Perit Dial Bull 1:145, 1981.

40. Heusser H, Werder H: Untersuchungen über Peritonealdialyse. Bruns Beitr Klin Chir 141:38, 1927.

41. Maxwell M, Rockney R, Kleeman C, et al: Peritoneal dialysis. JAMA 170:917, 1959.

42. Parker A, Nolph K: Magnesium and calcium transfer during continuous ambulatory peritoneal dialysis. Trans Am Soc Artif Intern Organs 26:194, 1980.

43. Veech R: The untoward effects of the anions of dialysis fluids. Kidney Int 34:587, 1988.

44. Raja RM, Cantor RE, Boreyko C, et al: Sodium transport during ultrafiltration peritoneal dialysis. Trans Am Soc Artif Intern Organs 18:429, 1972.

45. Ahearn DJ, Nolph KD: Controlled sodium removal with peritoneal dialysis. Trans Am Soc Artif Intern Organs 18:423, 1972.

46. Nolph KD, Hano JE, Teschan PE: Peritoneal sodium transport during hypertonic peritoneal dialysis. Ann Intern Med 70:931, 1969.

47. Raja RM, Kramer MS, Rosenbaum JL, et al: Evaluation of hypertonic peritoneal dialysis solutions with low sodium. Nephron 11:342, 1973.

48. Nolph KD, Sorkin MI, Gloor HJ: Considerations for dialysis solution modifications. *In* Atkins RC, Thomson NM, Farrell PC (eds): Peritoneal Dialysis. Churchill Livingstone, Edinburgh, 1981, p 236.

49. Nolph KD, Twardowski ZJ, Popovich RP, et al: Equilibration of peritoneal dialysis solutions during long dwell exchanges. J Lab Clin Med 93:246, 1979.

50. Brown ST, Ahearn DJ, Nolph KD: Potassium removal with peritoneal dialysis. Kidney Int 4:67, 1973.

51. Mandelbaum JM, Heistand ML, Schardin KE: Six months' experience with PD-2 solution. Dial Transplant 12:259, 1983.

52. Nolph KD, Prowant B, Serkes KD, et al: Multicenter evaluation of a new peritoneal dialysis solution with a high lactate and a low magnesium concentration. Perit Dial Bull 3:63, 1983.

53. Gonella M, Ballanti P, Della Rocca C, et al: Improved bone morphology by normalizing serum magnesium in chronically hemodialyzed patients. Miner Electrolyte Metab 14:240, 1988.

54. Weinreich T, Rambausek M, Ritz E: Is control of secondary hyperparathyroidism optimal with the currently used calcium concentration in the CAPD fluid? Nephrol Dial Transplant 6:843, 1991.

55. Hutchison A, Boulton H, Freemont A, et al: Effective control of phosphate, intact PTH, and osteodystrophy by low calcium dialysate and oral $CaCO_3$ in CAPD. Perit Dial Int 12:S35, 1992.

56. Delmez JA: Removal of phosphorus by peritoneal dialysis. Perit Dial Int 13:S461, 1993.

57. DeBroe M, D'Hasse P, Elseviers M, et al: Aluminum and end stage renal failure. *In* Davison A (ed): Nephrology: Proceedings of the Xth International Congress of Nephrology. Baillière Tindall, Cambridge, 1988, p 1086.

58. Andreoli S, Bergstein JM, Sherrard DJ: Aluminum intoxication from aluminum-containing phosphate binders in children with azotemia not undergoing dialysis. N Engl J Med 310:1079, 1984.

59. Slatopolsky E, Weerts C, Lopez-Hilker S, et al: Calcium carbonate as a phosphate binder in patients with chronic renal failure undergoing dialysis. N Engl J Med 315:157, 1986.

60. Stein H, Yudis M, Sirota R: Calcium carbonate as a phosphate binder. N Engl J Med 316:109, 1987.

61. Slingeneyer A, Laroche B, Loupi E, et al: Calcium concentration in PD dialysate must be lowered. Exclusive use of $CaCO_3$ as a phosphate binder. Perit Dial Int 12(suppl 2):S161, 1992.

62. Cunningham J, Sawyer N, Altmann P, et al: Mineral metabolism in CAPD patients treated with $CaCO_3$ and stepwise reduction of dialysate calcium. Kidney Int 141:455, 1992.

63. Salusky IB, Coburn JW, Foley J, et al: Effects of oral calcium carbonate on control of serum phosphorus and changes in plasma aluminum levels after discontinuation of aluminum-containing gels in children receiving dialysis. J Pediatr 108:767, 1986.

64. Martis L, Serkes KD, Nolph KD: Calcium carbonate as a phosphate binder: Is there a need to adjust peritoneal dialysate calcium concentrations for patients using $CaCO_3$? Perit Dial Int 9:325, 1989.

65. Brown CB, Hamdy NAT, Boletis J, et al: Rationale for the use of low calcium solution in CAPD. *In* La Greca G, Ronco C, Feriani M, et al (eds): Peritoneal Dialysis: Proceedings of the Fourth International Course on Peritoneal Dialysis. Wichtig Editore, Milan, 1991, p 125.

66. Bender FH, Bernardini J, Piraino B, et al: Calcium mass transfer with dialysate containing 1.25 and 1.75 mmol/L calcium in peritoneal dialysis patients. Am J Kidney Dis 20:367, 1992.

67. Brown CB, Hamdy NAT, Boletis J, et al: Osteodystrophy in continuous ambulatory peritoneal dialysis. Perit Dial Int 13:S454, 1993.

68. Piraino B, Bernardini J, Holley J, et al: Calcium mass transfer in peritoneal dialysis patients using 2.5 mEq/liter calcium dialysate. Clin Nephrol 37:48, 1992.

69. Hutchison AJ, Merchant M, Boulton HF, et al: Calcium and magnesium mass transfer in peritoneal dialysis patients using 1.25 mmol/L calcium, 0.25 mmol/L magnesium dialysis fluid. Perit Dial Int 13:219, 1993.

70. Piraino B, Perlmutter JA, Holley JL, et al: The use of dialysate containing 2.5 mEq/L calcium in peritoneal dialysis patients. Perit Dial Int 12:75, 1992.

71. Martis L, Zimmerman S, Delmez J, et al: Dianeal 2.5 mEq/L calcium and calcium carbonate in CAPD. Perit Dial Int 12(suppl 1):177, 1992.

72. Kawanishi H, Tsuchiya T, Namba S, et al: Clinical application of low calcium peritoneal dialysate. ASAIO Trans 37:M404, 1991.

73. Hutchison A, Gokal R: Towards tailored dialysis fluids in CAPD: The role of reduced calcium and magnesium dialysis fluids. Perit Dial Int 12:199, 1992.

74. Hutchison A, Freemont A, Lumb G, et al: Renal osteodystrophy in continuous ambulatory peritoneal dialysis. Adv Perit Dial 7:237, 1991.

75. Hercz G, Pei Y, Manuel A, et al: Aplastic osteodystrophy without aluminum staining in dialysis patients. Kidney Int 37:449, 1990. Abstract.

76. Hutchison AJ, Gokal R: Improved solutions for peritoneal dialysis: Physiological calcium solutions, osmotic agents and buffers. Kidney Int 42(suppl 38):S153, 1992.

77. Loschiavo C, Fabris A, Adami S, et al: Effects of continuous ambulatory peritoneal dialysis (CAPD) on renal osteodystrophy. Perit Dial Bull 5:53, 1985.

78. Hutchison AJ, Boulton H, Gokal R: Low calcium dialysate with oral CaCO₃ in CAPD. Perit Dial Int 11:116, 1991.

79. Weinreich T, Colombi A, Echterhoff HH, et al: Transperitoneal calcium mass transfer using dialysate with a low calcium concentration (1.0 mm). Perit Dial Int 13:S467, 1993.

80. Rotellar C, Kinsel V, Goggins M, et al: Does low calcium dialysate accelerate secondary hyperparathyroidism in continuous ambulatory peritoneal dialysis patients? Perit Dial Int 13:S471, 1993.

81. Rossen B, Ladefoged J: A comparison between the effects of acetate and lactate in peritoneal dialysis solutions. Scand J Urol Nephrol 16:279, 1982.

82. Slingeneyer A, Mion C, Mourad G, et al: Progressive sclerosing peritonitis: A late and severe complication of maintenance peritoneal dialysis. Trans Am Soc Artif Intern Organs 29:633, 1983.

83. Ing TS, Daugirdas JT, Gandhi VC: Peritoneal sclerosis in peritoneal dialysis patients. Am J Nephrol 4:173, 1984.

84. Ing TS, Gandhi VC, Daugirdas JT, et al: Peritoneal dialysis using bicarbonate-buffered dialysate. Int J Artif Organs 7:166, 1984.

85. Kwong MBL, Wu GG, Rodella H, et al: Effect of the peritoneal dialysate buffer on ultrafiltration: Studies in normal rabbits. Perit Dial Bull 5:182, 1985.

86. Johnson R, Walton J, Krebs H, et al: Metabolic fuels during and after severe exercise in athletes and non-athletes. Lancet 2:452, 1969.

87. Brandt R, Siegel S, Waters M, et al: Spectroscopic assay for D(−) lactate in plasma. Anal Biochem 102:39, 1980.

88. Thurn J, Pierpont G, Ludvigsen C, et al: D-Lactate encephalopathy. Am J Med 79:717, 1985.

89. Nolph K, Twardowski Z, Khanna R, et al: Tidal peritoneal dialysis with racemic or L-lactate solutions. Perit Dial Int 10:161, 1990.

90. Yatzidis H: A new single bicarbonate CAPD solution. *In* La Greca G, Ronco C, Feriani M, et al (eds): Proceedings of the Fourth International Course on Peritoneal Dialysis. Wichtig Editore, Milan, 1991, p 151.

91. Yatzidis H: A new stable bicarbonate dialysis solution for peritoneal dialysis: Preliminary report. Perit Dial Int 11:224, 1991.

92. Vaziri N, Ness R, Wellikson L, et al: Bicarbonate buffered peritoneal dialysis. An effective adjunct in the treatment of lactic acidosis. Am J Med 67:392, 1979.

93. Feriani M, Biasioli S, Borin D, et al: Bicarbonate buffer for CAPD solution. Trans Am Soc Artif Intern Organs 31:668, 1985.

94. Feriani M, Reinhardt B, La Greca G: Calcium carbonate precipitation in oversaturated bicarbonate containing solution. *In* La Greca G, Ronco C, Feriani M, et al (eds): Proceedings of the Fourth International Course on Peritoneal Dialysis. Wichtig Editore, Milan, 1991, p 145.

95. Feriani M, Dissegna D, La Greca G, et al: Continuous ambulatory peritoneal dialysis with bicarbonate buffer—a pilot study. Perit Dial Int 13:S88, 1993.

96. Lindholm B, Bergstrom J: Nutritional aspects of CAPD. *In* Gokal R (ed): Continuous Ambulatory Peritoneal Dialysis. Churchill Livingstone, Edinburgh, 1986, p 228.

97. Gokal R, Ramos J, McGurk J, et al: Hyperlipidemia in patients on continuous ambulatory peritoneal dialysis. *In* Gahl G, Kessel M, Nolph KD (eds): Advances in Peritoneal Dialysis. Excerpta Medica, Amsterdam, 1981, p 430.

98. Bouma S, Dwyer J: Glucose absorption and weight exchange in 18 months of continuous ambulatory peritoneal dialysis. J Am Diet Assoc 84:194, 1984.

99. Dobbie J: Pathogenesis of peritoneal fibrosing syndromes (sclerosing peritonitis) in peritoneal dialysis. Perit Dial Int 12:14, 1992.

100. Oreopoulos D, Crassweller P, Kartirtzoglou A, et al: Amino acids as an osmotic agent (instead of glucose) in continuous ambulatory peritoneal dialysis. *In* Legrain M (ed): Proceedings of the First International Symposium on Continuous Ambulatory Peritoneal Dialysis. Excerpta Medica, Amsterdam, 1980, p 335.

101. Williams P, Marliss E, Anderson G, et al: Amino acid absorption following intraperitoneal administration in CAPD patients. Perit Dial Bull 2:124, 1982.

102. Oren A, Wu G, Anderson GH, et al: Effective use of amino acid dialysate over four weeks in CAPD patients. Perit Dial Bull 3:66, 1983.

103. Dombros N, Prutis K, Tong M, et al: Six-month overnight intraperitoneal amino acid infusion in continuous ambulatory peritoneal dialysis patients—no effect on nutritional status. Perit Dial Int 10:79, 1990.

104. Kopple JD, Bernard D, Brunori G, et al: Nutritional effects of intraperitoneal (IP) amino acids (AA) in malnourished CAPD patients. J Am Soc Nephrol 2:362, 1991.

105. Bruno M, Bagnis C, Marangella M, et al: CAPD with an amino acid dialysis solution: A long-term cross-over study. Kidney Int 35:1189, 1989.

106. Prichard S, Cianflone K, Zhang ZJ, et al: A novel mechanism to explain the dyslipidemia in CAPD and nephrotic patients. Perit Dial Int 12:150, 1992.

107. Klein E, Ward RA, Williams TE, et al: Peptides as substitute osmotic agents for glucose in peritoneal dialysate. ASAIO Trans 32:550, 1986.

108. Martis L, Burke R, Klein E: Evaluation of a peptide-based solution for peritoneal dialysis. Perit Dial Int 13:S92, 1993.

109. Rubin J, Klein E, Jones Q, et al: Evaluation of a polymer dialysate. Trans Am Soc Artif Intern Organs 29:62, 1983.

110. Higgins JT, Gross ML, Somani P, et al: Patient tolerance and dialysis effectiveness of a glucose polymer–containing peritoneal dialysis solution. Perit Dial Bull 4:S131, 1984.

111. Mistry CD, Mallick NP, Gokal R: Ultrafiltration with an isosmotic solution during long peritoneal dialysis exchanges. Lancet 2:178, 1987.

112. Gokal R, Mistry C: Glucose polymer as an osmotic agent in CAPD. *In* La Greca G, Ronco C, Feriani M, et al (eds): Proceedings of the Fourth International Course on Peritoneal Dialysis. Wichtig Editore, Milan, 1991, p 119.

113. Mistry C, Fox J, Mallick N, et al: Circulating maltose and isomaltose in chronic renal failure. Kidney Int 32(suppl 22):S210, 1987.

114. Dobbie JW: The role of peritoneal biopsy in clinical and experimental peritoneal dialysis. Perit Dial Int 13:S23, 1993.

115. Breborowicz A, Rodela H, Pagiamtzis J, et al: Glucose (G) toxicity to human mesothelial cells (MC) in vitro. Perit Dial Int 10(suppl 1):19, 1990.

116. Topley N, Mackenzie R, Petersen MM, et al: In vitro testing of a potentially biocompatible continuous ambulatory peritoneal dialysis fluid. Nephrol Dial Transplant 6:574, 1991.

117. Breborowicz A, Balaskas E, Diamandis E, et al: Effect of tumor necrosis factor on human mesothelial cells in in vitro culture. Perit Dial Int 12(suppl 2):S6A, 1992.

118. Di Paolo N, Garosi G, Traversari L, et al: Mesothelial biocompatibility of peritoneal dialysis solutions. Perit Dial Int 13:S109, 1993.

119. Breborowicz A: In vitro study on the biocompatibility of the peritoneal dialysis solution. Perit Dial Int 13:S105, 1993.

120. Gotloib L, Shostak A, Wajsbrot V, et al: Biocompatibility of dialysis solutions evaluated by histochemical techniques applied to mesothelial cell imprints. Perit Dial Int 13:S113, 1993.

121. Lewis S, Holmes C: Host defense mechanisms in the peritoneal cavity of continuous ambulatory peritoneal dialysis patients. Perit Dial Int 11:14, 1991.

122. De Fijter CWH, Oe PL, Verbrugh HA, et al: Glucose polymers as osmotic agent in CAPD fluids: A more favorable effect on peritoneal macrophage (PMO) function than glucose-based solutions. Kidney Int 40:978, 1991.

123. Jorres A, Gahl GM, Muller C, et al: In vitro biocompatibility testing of a new glucose polymer dialysis fluid for CAPD. Nephrol Dial Transplant 7:774, 1992.

124. Topley N, Alobaidi HMM, Davies M, et al: The effect of dialysate on peritoneal phagocyte oxidative metabolism. Kidney Int 34:404, 1988.

125. Jorres A, Gahl GM, Ludat K, et al: In vitro biocompatibility testing of a new bicarbonate-buffered dialysis fluid for CAPD. Perit Dial Int 12(suppl 2):S26, 1992.

126. Carozzi S, Nasini M, Schelotto C, et al: Peritoneal dialysis fluid $Ca^{++}$ and $1,25(OH)_2D_3$ modulate peritoneal macrophage antimicrobial activity in CAPD patients. Adv Perit Dial 6:110, 1990.

127. Suga H, Honda H, Naganuma S, et al: A low $Ca^{++}$ level in effluent as a risk factor for the peritonitis in CAPD patients. Adv Perit Dial 6:102, 1990.

128. Piraino B, Bernardini J, Holley JL, et al: Increased risk of *Staphylococcus epidermidis* peritonitis in patients on dialysate containing 1.25 mmol/L calcium. Am J Kidney Dis 19:371, 1992.

129. Hutchison AJ, Turner K, Gokal R: Effect of long-term therapy with 1.25 mmol/L calcium peritoneal dialysis fluid on the incidence of peritonitis in CAPD. Perit Dial Int 12:321, 1992.

130. Freedman BI, Case DL, Burkart JM: The effect of dialysate calcium concentration (DCa) on peritonitis (P) frequency. J Am Soc Nephrol 3:410, 1992.

131. Wegner G: Chirurgische Bermekungen über die Peritonalhole, mit besonderer Berucksichtigung der Ovariotomie. Arch Klin Chir 20:51, 1877.

132. Hertzler AE: The Peritoneum. CV Mosby, St. Louis, 1919.

133. Knapowski J, Feder E, Simon M, et al: Evaluation of the participation of parietal peritoneum in dialysis: Physiological, morphological, and pharmacological data. Proc Eur Dial Transplant Assoc 16:155, 1979.

134. Esperanca MJ, Collins DL: Peritoneal dialysis efficiency in relation to body weight. J Pediatr Surg 1:162, 1966.

135. Nolph KD: Peritoneal dialysis. *In* Brenner BM, Rector FC (eds): The Kidney, 4th ed. WB Saunders, Philadelphia, 1991, p 2299.

136. Kolossow A: Über die Struktur des Endothels der Pleuroperitonealhole der Blut- und Lymphgefasse. Biol Centralbl Erlang 12:87, 1892.

137. Baradi AF, Hope J: Observations on ultrastructure of rabbit mesothelium. Exp Cell Res 34:33, 1964.

138. Recklinghausen FT von: Zur Fettresorption. Arch Pathol Anat Physiol 26:172, 1863.

139. Simer PH: The passage of particulate matter from the peritoneal cavity into the lymph vessels of the diaphragm. Anat Rec 101:333, 1948.

140. Leak LV: Distribution of cell surface charges on mesothelium and lymphatic endothelium. Microvasc Res 31:18, 1986.

141. Gotloib L, Digenis GE, Rabinovich S, et al: Ultrastructure of normal rabbit mesentery. Nephron 34:248, 1983.

142. Dobbie JW: Ultrastructural similarities between mesothelium and type II pneumocytes and their relevance to phospholipid surfactant production by the peritoneum. Adv Perit Dial 4:47, 1988.

143. Dobbie JW, Lloyd JK: Mesothelium secretes lamellar bodies in a similar manner to type II pneumocyte secretion of a surfactant. Perit Dial Int 9:215, 1989.

144. Dobbie JW: New concepts in molecular biology and ultrastructural pathology of the peritoneum: Their significance for peritoneal dialysis. Am J Kidney Dis 15:97, 1990.

145. Wade OL, Combes B, Childs AW, et al: The effect of exercise on the splanchnic blood flow and splanchnic blood volume in normal man. Clin Sci 15:457, 1956.

146. Simionescu N: Cellular aspects of transcapillary exchange. Physiol Rev 63:1536, 1983.

147. Wolff JR: Ultrastructure of the terminal vascular bed as related to function. *In* Kaley G, Altura BM (eds): Microcirculation. University Park Press, Baltimore, 1977, p 95.

148. Gotloib L, Shostak A, Bar-Sella P, et al: Fenestrated capillaries in human parietal and rabbit diaphragmatic peritoneum. Nephron 41:200, 1985.

149. Taylor AE, Granger DN: Exchange of macromolecules across the microcirculation. *In* Renkin EM, Michel CC (eds): Handbook of Physiology, Sect 2, The Cardiovascular System, Vol IV. American Physiological Society, Bethesda, MD, 1984, p 467.

150. Milici AJ, L'hernault N, Palade GE: Surface densities of diaphragmed fenestrae and transendothelial channels in different murine capillary beds. Circ Res 56:709, 1985.

151. Haraldsson B: The peritoneal membrane acts as a negatively charged barrier restricting anionic proteins. J Am Soc Nephrol 4:407, 1993.

152. Leypoldt JK, Henderson LW: Molecular charge influences transperitoneal macromolecule transport. Kidney Int 43:837, 1993.

153. Allen L: The peritoneal stomata. Anat Rec 67:89, 1936.

154. Casley-Smith JR: Endothelial permeability. The passage of particles into and out of diaphragmatic lymphatics. Q J Exp Physiol 49:365, 1964.

155. Azzali G: Ultrastructure of small intestine, submucosal and serosalmuscular lymphatic vessels. Lymphology 15:106, 1982.

156. Hauglustaine D, Monballyu J, van Meerbeek J, et al: Report of sclerotic alterations of the peritoneum in patients on CAPD. Lancet 2:734, 1983.

157. Dobbie JW, Lloyd JK, Gall CA: Categorization of ultrastructural changes in peritoneal mesothelium, stroma, and blood vessels in uremia and CAPD patients. *In* Nolph KD (ed): Peritoneal Dialysis, 3rd ed. Kluwer Academic Publishers, Boston, 1989, p 3.

158. Karnovsky MJ: The ultrastructural basis of capillary permeability studied with peroxidase as a tracer. J Cell Biol 35:213, 1967.

159. Dobbie JW: Morphology of the peritoneum in CAPD. Blood Purif 7:74, 1989.

160. Verger C, Luger A, Moore HL: Acute changes in peritoneal morphology and transport properties with infectious peritonitis and mechanical injury. Kidney Int 23:823, 1983.

161. Panasiuk E, Pietrzak B, Klos M, et al: Characteristics of peritoneum after peritonitis in CAPD patients. Adv Perit Dial 4:42, 1988.

162. Rubin J, Jones Q, Planch A, et al: The importance of the abdominal viscera to peritoneal transport during peritoneal dialysis in the dog. Am J Med Sci 292:203, 1986.

163. Rubin J, Jones Q, Planch A, et al: Systems of membranes involved in peritoneal dialysis. J Lab Clin Invest 110:448, 1987.

164. Rubin J, Jones Q, Planch A, Bower JD: The minimal importance of the hollow viscera to peritoneal transport during peritoneal dialysis in the rat. ASAIO Trans 34:912, 1988.

165. Fox SD, Leypoldt JK, Henderson LW: Visceral peritoneum is not essential for solute transport during peritoneal dialysis. Kidney Int 40:612, 1991.

166. Alon U, Bar-Maor JA, Bar-Joseph G: Effective peritoneal dialysis in an infant with extensive resection of the small intestine. Am J Nephrol 8:65, 1988.

167. Henderson LW: The problem of peritoneal membrane and permeability. Kidney Int 3:409, 1973.

168. Ored S: Experimental studies on portal circulation at increased intraabdominal pressure. Acta Physiol Scand 30(suppl 109):1, 1953.

169. Pietrzak I, Hirszel P, Shostak A, et al: Splanchnic volume, not flow rate, determines peritoneal permeability. ASAIO Trans 35:583, 1989.

170. Flessner MF, Dedrick RL: Importance of the liver in peritoneal dialysis. J Am Soc Nephrol 4:404, 1993. Abstract.

171. Krediet RT, Zuyderhoudt FMJ, Boeschoten EW, et al: Peritoneal permeability to proteins in diabetic and non-diabetic continuous ambulatory peritoneal dialysis patients. Nephron 42:133, 1986.

172. Nolph KD, Miller FN, Rubin J, et al: New directions in peritoneal dialysis concepts and applications. Kidney Int 18(suppl 10):S111, 1980.

173. Bell JL, Leypoldt JK, Firgon RP, et al: Heteroporosity model of peritoneal transport is not supported by hydraulically-driven convective transport. Kidney Int 33:243, 1988. Abstract.

174. Lill SR, Parsons RH, Buhac I: Permeability of the diaphragm and fluid resorption from the peritoneal cavity in the rat. Gastroenterology 76:997, 1979.

175. Nolph KD, Popovich RP, Ghods AJ, et al: Determinants of low clearances of small solutes during peritoneal dialysis. Kidney Int 13:117, 1978.

176. McGary TJ, Nolph KD, Rubin J: In vitro simulations of peritoneal dialysis: A technique for demonstrating limitations on solute clearances due to stagnant fluid films and poor mixing. J Lab Clin Med 96:148, 1980.

177. Wayland H: Transmural and interstitial molecular transport in continuous ambulatory peritoneal dialysis. In Legrain M (ed): Proceedings of the First International Symposium on Continuous Ambulatory Peritoneal Dialysis. Excerpta Medica, Amsterdam, 1980, p 18.

178. Grotte G: Passage of dextran molecules across the blood-lymph barrier. Acta Chir Scand 211(suppl):1, 1956.

179. Pappenheimer JR, Renkin EM, Borrero LM: Filtration, diffusion, and molecular sieving through peripheral capillary membranes. A contribution to the pore theory of capillary permeability. Am J Physiol 167:13, 1951.

180. Mayerson HS, Wolfram CG, Shirley HH Jr, et al: Regional differences in capillary permeability. Am J Physiol 198:155, 1960.

181. Fox J, Galey F, Wayland H: Action of histamine on the mesenteric microvasculature. Microvasc Res 19:108, 1980.

182. Pappenheimer JR: Passage of molecules through capillary walls. Physiol Rev 33:387, 1953.

183. Cotran RS: The fine structure of the microvasculature in relation to normal and altered permeability. In Reeve EB, Guyton AC (eds): Physical Basis of Circulatory Transport: Regulation and Exchange. WB Saunders, Philadelphia, 1967.

184. Charonis AS, Wissig SL: Anionic sites in basement membranes. Differences in their electrostatic properties in continuous and fenestrated capillaries. Microvasc Res 25:265, 1983.

185. Gotloib L: Anatomical basis for peritoneal permeability. In La Greca G, Chiaramonte S, Fabris A, et al (eds): Peritoneal Dialysis. Wichtig Editore, Milan, 1989, p 3.

186. Curry FE, Mason JC, Michel CC: Osmotic reflection coefficients of capillary walls to low molecular weight hydrophilic solutes measured in single perfused capillaries of the frog mesentery. J Physiol (Lond) 261:319, 1976.

187. Michel CC: Filtration coefficients and osmotic reflection coefficients of the walls of single frog mesenteric capillaries. J Physiol (Lond) 309:341, 1980.

188. Wayland H: Action of histamine on the microvasculature. In Legrain M (ed): Proceedings of the First International Symposium on Continuous Ambulatory Peritoneal Dialysis. Excerpta Medica, Amsterdam, 1980, p 18.

189. Korten G: Measuring the thickness of the peritoneum as a dialysis membrane using various osmolar concentrations of dialysis fluid. Z Urol Nephrol 83:459, 1990.

190. Lasrich M, Maher JM, Hirszel P, et al: Correlation of peritoneal transport rates with molecular weight: A method for predicting clearances. Trans Am Soc Artif Intern Organs 2:107, 1979.

191. Tsilibary EC, Wissig SL: Absorption from the peritoneal cavity: SEM study of the mesothelium covering the peritoneal surface of the muscular portion of the diaphragm. Am J Anat 149:127, 1977.

192. Cascarano J, Rubin AD, Chick WL, et al: Metabolically induced permeability changes across mesothelium and endothelium. Am J Physiol 206:373, 1964.

193. Breborowicz A, Knapowski J: Studies on the resistance of the peritoneal mesothelium to solute transport. Perit Dial Bull 4:37, 1984.

194. Goldschmidt ZH, Pote HH, Katz MA, et al: Effect of dialysate volume on peritoneal dialysis kinetics. Kidney Int 5:240, 1974.

195. Stephen RL, Atkin-Thor E, Kolff WJ: Recirculating peritoneal dialysis with subcutaneous catheter. Trans Am Soc Artif Intern Organs 22:575, 1976.

196. Tenckhoff H, Ward G, Boen ST: The influence of dialysate volume and flow rate on peritoneal clearance. Proc Eur Dial Transplant Assoc 2:113, 1965.

197. Lange K, Treser G, Mangalat J: Automatic continuous high flow rate peritoneal dialysis. Arch Klin Med 214:201, 1968.

198. Rubin J, Kirchner K, Bower J: Evaluation of stagnant fluid films during simulated peritoneal dialysis: In vitro and in vivo studies. Clin Exp Dial Apheresis 5:285, 1981.

199. Nolph KD, Ghods AJ, Van Stone J, Brown PA: The effects of intraperitoneal vasodilators on peritoneal clearances. Trans Am Soc Artif Intern Organs 22:586, 1976.

200. Miller FN, Nolph KD, Harris PD, et al: Microvascular and clinical effects of altered peritoneal dialysis solutions. Kidney Int 15:630, 1979.

201. Aune S: Transperitoneal exchange 2. Peritoneal blood flow estimated by hydrogen gas clearance. Scand J Gastroenterol 5:99, 1970.

202. Erbe RW, Greene JA Jr, Weller JM: Peritoneal dialysis during hemorrhagic shock. J Appl Physiol 22:131, 1967.

203. Blumenkrantz MJ, Roberts CE, Card B, et al: Nutritional management of the adult patient undergoing peritoneal dialysis. J Am Diet Assoc 73:251, 1978.

204. Giordanao C, De Santo NG: Dietary management of patients on peritoneal dialysis. Contrib Nephrol 17:77, 1979.

205. Cunningham RS: The physiology of the serous membranes. Physiol Rev 6:242, 1926.

206. Clark AJ: Absorption from the peritoneal cavity. J Pharmacol Exp Ther 16:415, 1921.

207. Putnam TJ: The living peritoneum as a dialyzing membrane. Am J Physiol 63:548, 1922–23.

208. Randerson DH, Farrell PC: Mass transfer properties of the human peritoneum. Trans Am Soc Artif Intern Organs 26:140, 1980.

209. Pyle WK: Mass Transfer in Peritoneal Dialysis. Michigan University, Ann Arbor, 1992. Thesis.

210. Pyle WK, Moncrief JW, Popovich RP: Peritoneal transport evaluation in CAPD. In Moncrief JW, Popovich RP (eds): Proceedings of the 2nd International Symposium on Continuous Ambulatory Peritoneal Dialysis. Masson, New York, 1981, p 35.

211. Garred LJ, Canaud B, Farrell PC: A simple kinetic model for assessing peritoneal mass transfer in chronic ambulatory peritoneal dialysis. Trans Am Soc Artif Intern Organs 29:131, 1983.

212. Henderson LW, Nolph KD: Altered permeability of the peritoneal membrane after using hypertonic peritoneal dialysis fluid. J Clin Invest 48:992, 1969.

213. Dedrick RL, Flessner MF, Collins JM, et al: Is the peritoneum a membrane? Trans Am Soc Artif Intern Organs 28:1, 1982.

214. Flessner MF, Dedrick RL, Schulz JS: A distributed model of peritoneal-plasma transport: Theoretical considerations. Am J Physiol 246:597, 1984.

215. Werynski A, Lindholm B: A model of solute transport in CAPD: Impact of peritoneal tissue and lymphatic flow. Blood Purif 5:316, 1987. Abstract.

216. Lindholm B, Werynski A, Bergstrom J: Kinetics of peritoneal dialysis with glycerol and glucose as osmotic agents. ASAIO Trans 33:19, 1987.

217. Lindholm B, Werynski A, Bergstrom J: Peritoneal dialysis with amino acid solutions: Fluid and solute transport kinetics. Artif Organs 12:2, 1988.

218. Nolph KD, Miller FN, Pyle WK, et al: An hypothesis to explain the ultrafiltration characteristics of peritoneal dialysis. Kidney Int 20:543, 1981.

219. Henderson LW, Leypoldt JK: Ultrafiltration with peritoneal dialysis. In Nolph KD (ed): Peritoneal Dialysis, 3rd ed. Kluwer Academic Publishers, Boston, 1989, p 117.

220. Rippe B, Stelin G: Simulations of peritoneal transport during CAPD. Application of two-pore formalism. Kidney Int 35:1234, 1989.

221. Waniewski J, Werynski AN, Heimburger O, Lindholm B: A comparative analysis of mass transport models in peritoneal dialysis. ASAIO Trans 37:65, 1991.

222. Vonesh EF, Lysaght MJ, Moran J, et al: Kinetic modeling as a prescription aid in peritoneal dialysis. Blood Purif 9:246, 1991.

223. Rippe B: A three-pore model of peritoneal transport. Perit Dial Int 13:S35, 1993.

224. Flessner MF, Parker RJ, Sieber SM: Peritoneal lymphatic uptake of fibrinogen and erythrocytes in the rat. Am J Physiol 244:H89, 1983.

225. McKay T, Zink J, Greenway CV: Relative rates of absorption of fluid and protein from the peritoneal cavity in cats. Lymphology 11:106, 1978.

226. Popovich RP, Moncrief JW: Kinetic modeling of peritoneal transport. Contrib Nephrol 17:59, 1979.

227. Rubin JL, Clawson M, Planch A, et al: Measurements of peritoneal surface area in man and rat. Am J Med Sci 295:453, 1988.

228. Nolph KD: The first hemodialyzer. Trans Am Soc Artif Intern Organs 24:2, 1978.

229. Felt J, Richard C, McCaffrey C, et al: Peritoneal clearance of creatinine and inulin in dogs: Effect of splanchnic vasodilators. Kidney Int 16:459, 1979.

230. Granger DN, Ulrich M, Perry MA, et al: Peritoneal dialysis solutions and feline splanchnic blood flow. Clin Exp Pharmacol Physiol 11:437, 1984.

231. Nolph KD, Ghods A, Brown P, et al: Effects of nitroprusside on peritoneal mass transfer coefficients and microvascular physiology. Trans Am Soc Artif Intern Organs 23:210, 1977.

232. Henderson LW, Cheung AK, Chenoweth DE: Choosing a membrane. Am J Kidney Dis 3:5, 1983.

233. Twardowski ZJ, Nolph KD, Khanna R, et al: Peritoneal equilibration test. Perit Dial Bull 7:138, 1987.

234. Boen ST: Kinetics of peritoneal dialysis. Medicine (Baltimore) 40:243, 1961.

235. Miller JH, Gipstein R, Margules R, et al: Automated peritoneal dialysis: Analysis of several methods of peritoneal dialysis. Trans Am Soc Artif Intern Organs 12:98, 1966.

236. Kablitz C, Stephen RL, Duffy DP, et al: Technological augmentation of peritoneal urea clearance: Past, present, and future. Dial Transplant 9:741, 1980.

237. Stephen RL, Atkin-Thor E, Kolff WJ: Recirculating peritoneal dialysis with subcutaneous catheter. Trans Am Soc Artif Intern Organs 22:575, 1976.

238. Gross M, McDonald HP Jr: Effects of dialysate temperature and flow rate on peritoneal clearance. JAMA 202:363, 1967.

239. Indraprasit S, Namwongprom A, Sooksiwongse C, et al: Effect of dialysate temperature on peritoneal clearance. Nephron 34:45, 1983.

240. Knochel JP, Mason AD: Effect of alkalinization on peritoneal diffusion of uric acid. Am J Physiol 210:1160, 1966.

241. Deger GE, Wagoner RD: Peritoneal dialysis in acute uric acid nephropathy. Mayo Clin Proc 47:189, 1972.

242. Campion DS, North JDK: Effect of protein binding of barbiturates on their rate of removal during peritoneal dialysis. J Lab Clin Med 66:549, 1965.

243. Leypoldt JK, Chiu AS, Frigon RP, et al: Dialysate to blood transport of macromolecules during peritoneal dialysis. Am J Physiol 257:H1851, 1989.

244. Renkin EM: Relation of capillary morphology to transport of fluid and large molecules: A review. Acta Physiol Scand 463(suppl):81, 1979.

245. Struijk DG, Koomen GCM, Krediet RT, et al: Indirect measurement of lymphatic absorption in CAPD patients by the disappearance rate of dextran 70 is not influenced by trapping. Kidney Int 41:1668, 1992.

246. Imholz ALT, Koomen GCM, Struijk DG, et al: Residual volume measurements in CAPD patients with exogenous and endogenous solutes. Adv Perit Dial 8:33, 1992.

247. Krediet RT, Imholz ALT, Struijk DG, et al: Ultrafiltration failure in continuous ambulatory peritoneal dialysis. Perit Dial Int 13:S59, 1993.

248. Twardowski ZJ, Khanna R, Nolph KD, et al: Intra-abdominal pressures during natural activities in patients treated with continuous ambulatory peritoneal dialysis. Nephron 44:129, 1986.

249. Ahearn DJ, Nolph KD: Controlled sodium removal with peritoneal dialysis. Trans Am Soc Artif Intern Organs 28:423, 1972.

250. Nolph KD, Sorkin MI, Moore H: Autoregulation of sodium and potassium removal during continuous ambulatory peritoneal dialysis. Trans Am Soc Artif Intern Organs 26:334, 1980.

251. Rubin J, Klein E, Bower JD: Investigation of the net sieving coefficient of the peritoneal membrane during peritoneal dialysis. Trans Am Soc Artif Intern Organs 28:9, 1982.

252. Staverman AJ: The theory of measurement of osmotic pressure. Rec Trav Chim 70:344, 1951.

253. Rippe B, Perry MA, Granger DN: Permselectivity of the peritoneal membrane. Microvasc Res 29:89, 1985.

254. Leypoldt JK: Determining ultrafiltration properties of the peritoneum. ASAIO Trans 36:60, 1990.

255. Jaffrin MY, Odell RA, Farrell PC: A model of ultrafiltration and glucose mass transfer kinetics in peritoneal dialysis. Artif Organs 11:198, 1987.

256. Nakanishi TY, Tanaka Y, Fuyjii M, et al: Nonequilibrium thermodynamics of glucose transport in continuous ambulatory peritoneal dialysis. In Maekawa M, Nolph KD, Kishimoto T, et al (eds): Machine Free Dialysis for Patient Convenience. ISAO Press, Cleveland, 1984, p 39.

257. Seames EL, Moncrief JW, Popovich RP: A distributed model of fluid and mass transfer in peritoneal dialysis. Am J Physiol 258:R958, 1990.

258. Flessner MF, Fenstermacher JD, Dedrick RL, et al: A distributed model of peritoneal-plasma transport: Tissue concentration gradients. Am J Physiol 248:F425, 1985.

259. Ronco C, Brendolan A, Bragantini L, et al: Studies on ultrafiltration in peritoneal dialysis: Influence of plasma proteins and capillary blood flow. Perit Dial Bull 6:93, 1986.

260. Ronco C, Borin D, Brendalon A, et al: Influence of blood flow and plasma protein on UF rate in peritoneal dialysis. In Maher JF, Winchester JF (eds): Frontiers in Peritoneal Dialysis. Field, Rich, & Associates, New York, 1986, p 82.

261. Levin TN, Rigden LB, Nielsen LH, et al: Maximum ultrafiltration rates during peritoneal dialysis in rats. Kidney Int 31:731, 1987.

262. Grzegorzewska AE, Moore HL, Nolph KD, et al: Ultrafiltration and effective peritoneal blood flow during peritoneal dialysis in the rat. Kidney Int 39:608, 1991.

263. Miller FN, Joshua IG, Harris PD, et al: Peritoneal dialysis solution and the microcirculation. Contrib Nephrol 17:51, 1979.

264. Hirszel P, Maher JF, Chamberlin M: Augmented peritoneal mass transport with intraperitoneal nitroprusside. J Dial 2:131, 1978.

265. Popovich RP, Pyle WK: Kinetics of peritoneal transport. In Nolph KD (ed): Peritoneal Dialysis. Martinus Nijhoff, Boston, 1981, p 79.

266. Rubin J, Nolph KD, Popovich RP, et al: Drainage volumes during CAPD. ASAIO Trans 2:54, 1979.

267. Twardowski ZJ: Nightly peritoneal dialysis. Why? who? how? and when? ASAIO Trans 36:8, 1990.

268. Koomen GC, Krediet RT, Leegwater AC, et al: A fast reliable method for the measurement of intraperitoneal dextran 70, used to calculate lymphatic absorption. Adv Perit Dial 7:10, 1991.

269. Lysaght MJ, Moran J, Lysaght CB, et al: Plasma water filtration and lymphatic uptake during peritoneal dialysis. ASAIO Trans 37:M402, 1991.

270. Swartz RD, Sommermeyer MG, Chen-Hsing H: Preservation of plasma volume during haemodialysis depends on dialysate osmolality. Am J Nephrol 2:189, 1982.

271. Henrich WL, Woodard TD, Blachley JD, et al: Role of osmolality in blood pressure stability after dialysis and ultrafiltration. Kidney Int 18:480, 1980.

272. Burdiel LG, Jimenez A, Martin-Malo A, et al: The effect of dialysate osmolality on ultrafiltration and vascular refilling rate. Perit Dial Int 13:S67, 1993.

273. Maher JF, Hirszel P: Learning peritoneal physiology by pharmacological manipulation. Perit Dial Int 13:S27, 1993.

274. Maher JF, Hirszel P, Lasrich M: The effect of gastrointestinal hormones on transport by peritoneal dialysis. Kidney Int 16:130, 1979.

275. Maher JF, Hirszel P, Bennett RR, et al: Augmentation of peritoneal hydraulic permeability by amphotericin B: Locus of action. Perit Dial Bull 4:229, 1984.

276. Di Paolo N, Broncristiani U, Capotondo L, et al: Phosphatidylcholine and peritoneal transport during peritoneal dialysis. Nephron 44:365, 1986.

277. Querques M, Procaccini DA, Pappani A, et al: Influence of phosphatidylcholine on ultrafiltration and solute transfer in CAPD patients. ASAIO Trans 36:M581, 1990.

278. Di Paolo N, Capotondo L, Ciccoli L, et al: Phosphatidylcholine: A physiological modulator of the peritoneal membrane. In Avram MM, Giordano C (eds): Ambulatory Peritoneal Dialysis. Plenum Publishing, New York, 1990, p 44.

279. Grzegorzewska AE: Pharmacologic modification of transperitoneal movement of water. Perit Dial Int 10:291, 1990.

280. Boyer J, Gill GN, Epstein FH: Hyperglycemia and hyperosmolality complicating peritoneal dialysis. Ann Intern Med 67:568, 1967.

281. Miller RB, Tassistro CR: Peritoneal dialysis. N Engl J Med 281:945, 1969.

282. Vidt DG: Recommendations on choice of peritoneal dialysis solutions. Ann Intern Med 78:144, 1973.

283. Shen FH, Sherrard DJ, Scollard D, et al: Thirst, relative hypernatremia and excessive weight gain in maintenance peritoneal dialysis. Trans Am Soc Artif Intern Organs 24:142, 1978.

284. Heimburger O, Waniewski J, Werynski A, et al: Peritoneal transport in CAPD patients with permanent loss of ultrafiltration capacity. Kidney Int 38:495, 1990.

285. Feriani M, Biasioli S, Chiaramonte S, et al: Anatomical bases of peritoneal permeability: A reappraisal: Anatomy of peritoneum. Int J Artif Organs 5:345, 1982.

286. Twardowski ZJ, Nolph KD, Popovich RP, et al: Comparison of

polymer, glucose, and hydrostatic pressure induced ultrafiltration in a hollow fiber dialyzer: Effects on convective solute transport. J Lab Clin Med 92:619, 1978.

287. Rippe B, Stelin G, Haraldsson B: Computer simulations of peritoneal fluid transport in CAPD. Kidney Int 40:315, 1991.

288. Chen TW, Khanna R, Moore H, et al: Sieving and reflection coefficients for sodium salts and glucose during peritoneal dialysis in rats. J Am Soc Nephrol 2:1092, 1991.

289. Shostak A, Hirszel P, Chakrabarti E, et al: Dihydroergotamine lowers peritoneal transfer rates; a hypovolemic transport decrease. In Avram MM, Giordano C (eds): Ambulatory Peritoneal Dialysis. Plenum Publishing, New York, 1990, p 79.

290. Favazza A, Montanaro D, Messa P, et al: Peritoneal clearances in hypertensive CAPD patients after oral administration of clonidine, enalapril, and nifedipine. Perit Dial Int 12:287, 1992.

291. Vargemezis V, Psadakis P, Thodis E: Effect of a calcium antagonist (verapamil) in the permeability of the peritoneal membrane in patients on continuous ambulatory peritoneal dialysis. Blood Purif 7:309, 1989.

292. Struijk DG, Bakker JC, Krediet RT, et al: Effect of intraperitoneal administration of two different batches of albumin solutions on peritoneal solute transport in CAPD patients. Nephrol Dial Transplant 6:198, 1991.

293. Steinhauer HB, Lubrich-Birkner I, Kluthe R, et al: Effect of amino acid based dialysis solution on peritoneal permeability and prostanoid generation in patients undergoing continuous ambulatory peritoneal dialysis. Am J Nephrol 12:61, 1992.

294. Zemel D, ten Berge RJM, Struijk DG, et al: Interleukin-6 in CAPD patients without peritonitis: Relationships to the intrinsic permeability of the peritoneal membrane. Clin Nephrol 37:97, 1992.

295. Galdi P, Shostak A, Jaichenko J, et al: Protamine sulfate induces enhanced peritoneal permeability to proteins. Nephron 57:45, 1991.

296. Korbet SM, Vonesh EF, Firanek CA: The effect of hematocrit on peritoneal transport. Am J Kidney Dis 18:573, 1991.

297. Vega N, Fernandez A, Hortal LJ, et al: Peritoneal dialysis efficiency in CAPD patients in treatment with rHuEPO. Adv Perit Dial 8:467, 1992.

298. Hutchinson AJ, Ofsthun NJ, Howarth D, et al: The effect of hemoglobin concentration on peritoneal mass transfer and drain volumes in continuous ambulatory peritoneal dialysis. Perit Dial Int 12:230, 1992.

299. Burkart JM, Freedman VI, Rocco MV: The effect of increasing hematocrit on peritoneal transport kinetcs. J Am Soc Nephrol 4:1726, 1994.

300. Struijk DG, Krediet RT, Koomen GCM, et al: The initial decrease in effective peritoneal surface area is not caused by an increase in hematocrit. Perit Dial Int 13:S53, 1993.

301. Allen L: Lymphatics and lymphoid tissues. Annu Rev Physiol 29:197, 1967.

302. Olin T, Saldeen T: The lymphatic pathways from the peritoneal cavity: A lymphangiographic study in the rat. Cancer Res 24:1700, 1964.

303. Courtice FC, Simmonds WJ: Physiological significance of lymph drainage of the serous cavities and lungs. Physiol Rev 34:419, 1954.

304. Higgins GM, Graham AS: Lymphatic drainage from the peritoneal cavity in the dog. Arch Surg 19:452, 1929.

305. Raybuck HE, Allen L, Harms WS: Absorption of serum from the peritoneal cavity. Am J Physiol 199:1021, 1960.

306. Simer PH: The drainage of particulate matter from the peritoneal cavity by lymphatics. Anat Rec 88:175, 1944.

307. Twardowski ZJ, Prowant BF, Nolph KD, et al: High volume, low frequency continuous ambulatory peritoneal dialysis. Kidney Int 23:64, 1983.

308. Krediet RT, Boeschoten EW, Struijk DG, et al: Differences in the peritoneal transport of water, solutes, and proteins between dialysis with two and with three liter exchanges. Nephrol Dial Transplant 2:198–204, 1988.

309. Chan PCK, Wu PG, Tam SCF, et al: Factors affecting lymphatic absorption in dialysis (CAPD). Perit Dial Int 11:147–151, 1991.

310. Allen L, Vogt E: A mechanism of lymphatic absorption from serous cavities. Am J Physiol 119:776, 1937.

311. Morris B: The effect of diaphragmatic movement on the absorption of red cells and protein from the peritoneal cavity. Aust J Exp Biol Med Sci 31:239, 1953.

312. Courtice FC, Steinbeck AW: The effects of lymphatic obstruction and of posture on the absorption of protein from the peritoneal cavity. Aust J Exp Biol Med Sci 29:451, 1951.

313. Khanna R, Mactier R, Twardowski ZJ, et al: Peritoneal cavity lymphatics. Perit Dial Bull 6:113, 1986.

314. Lindholm B, Heimburger O, Waniewski J, et al: Peritoneal ultrafiltration and fluid reabsorption during peritoneal dialysis. Nephrol Dial Transplant 4:805, 1989.

315. Lindholm B, Werynski A, Bergstrom J: Fluid transport in peritoneal dialysis. Int J Artif Organs 13:352, 1990.

316. Nolph KD, Mactier R, Khanna R, et al: The kinetics of ultrafiltration during peritoneal dialysis: The role of lymphatics. Kidney Int 32:219, 1987.

317. Rippe B, Stelin G, Ahlmen J: Lymph flow from the peritoneal cavity in CAPD patients. In Maher JF, Winchester JF (eds): Frontiers in Peritoneal Dialysis. Field, Rich, & Associates, New York, 1984, p 24.

318. Mactier RA, Khanna R, Twardowski ZT, et al: Contribution of lymphatic absorption to loss of ultrafiltration and solute clearances in continuous ambulatory peritoneal dialysis. J Clin Invest 80:1311, 1987.

319. Abernethy NJ, Chin W, Hay JB, et al: Lymphatic removal of dialysate from the peritoneal cavity of anesthetized sheep. Kidney Int 40:174–181, 1991.

320. Mactier RA, Khanna R, Twardowski ZJ, et al: Role of peritoneal cavity lymphatic absorption in peritoneal dialysis. Kidney Int 32:165, 1987.

321. Flessner MF, Fenstermacher JD, Blasberg RG, et al: Peritoneal absorption of macromolecules studied by quantitative autoradiography. Am J Physiol 248:H26, 1985.

322. Stelin G, Rippe B: A phenomenological interpretation of the variation in dialysate volume with dwell time in CAPD. Kidney Int 38:465–472, 1990.

323. Daugirdas JT, Ing TS, Gandhi VC, et al: Kinetics of peritoneal fluid absorption in patients with chronic renal failure. J Lab Clin Med 95:351–361, 1980.

324. Spencer PC, Farrell PC: Solute and water transfer kinetics in CAPD. In Gokal R (ed): Continuous Ambulatory Peritoneal Dialysis. Churchill Livingstone, Edinburgh, 1986, pp 38–55.

325. Twardowski Z, Ksiazek A, Majdan M, et al: Kinetics of continuous ambulatory peritoneal dialysis (CAPD) with four exchanges per day. Clin Nephrol 15:119, 1981.

326. Heimburger O, Waniewski J, Werynski A, et al: A quantitative description of solute and fluid transport during peritoneal dialysis. Kidney Int 41:1320–1332, 1992.

327. Twardowski Z, Janicka L: Three exchanges with a 2.5 liter volume for continuous ambulatory peritoneal dialysis. Kidney Int 20:281, 1981.

328. Krediet RT, Struijk DG, Koomen GCM, et al: The disappearance of macromolecules from the peritoneal cavity during continuous ambulatory peritoneal dialysis (CAPD) is not dependent on molecular size. Perit Dial Int 10:147–152, 1990.

329. Struijk DG, Krediet RT, Koomen GCM, et al: Indirect measurement of lymphatic absorption with inulin in continuous ambulatory peritoneal dialysis (CAPD) patients. Perit Dial Int 10:141–146, 1990.

330. Rubin J, Planch A: Absorption of sulfamethoxazole and albumin from the peritoneal cavity. ASAIO Trans 36:834–837, 1990.

331. Mactier RA, Khanna R: Peritoneal cavity lymphatics. In Nolph KD (ed): Peritoneal Dialysis, 3rd ed. Kluwer Academic Publishers, Boston, 1990, pp 48–66.

332. Mactier RA, Khanna R, Moore H, et al: Pharmacological reduction of lymphatic absorption from the peritoneal cavity increases net ultrafiltration and solute clearances in peritoneal dialysis. Nephron 50:229, 1988.

333. Chan PCK, Tam SCF, Cheng IKP: Oral neostigmine and lymphatic absorption in a myasthenia gravis patient on continuous ambulatory peritoneal dialysis (CAPD). Perit Dial Int 10:93–96, 1990.

334. Mactier RA, Khanna R, Twardowski ZJ, et al: Influence of phosphatidylcholine on lymphatic absorption during peritoneal dialysis in the rat. Perit Dial Int 8:179, 1988.

335. Breborowicz A, Sombolos K, Rodela H, et al: Mechanism of phosphatidylcholine action during peritoneal dialysis. Perit Dial Bull 7:6, 1987.

336. Maher JF: Lubrication of the peritoneum. Perit Dial Int 12:346, 1992.

337. Randerson DH: Continuous Ambulatory Peritoneal Dialysis—A

Critical Appraisal. University of New South Wales, Sydney, Australia, 1980. Thesis.

338. Pyle WK: Mass Transfer in Peritoneal Dialysis. University of Texas, Austin, 1981. Thesis.

339. Farrell PC, Randerson DH: Mass transfer kinetics in continuous ambulatory peritoneal dialysis. *In* Legrain M (ed): Proceedings of the First International Symposium on Continuous Ambulatory Peritoneal Dialysis. Excerpta Medica, Amsterdam, 1980, pp 34–41.

340. Pyle WK, Popovich RP, Moncrief JW: Mass transfer in peritoneal dialysis. *In* Gahl GM, Kessel M, Nolph KD (eds): Advances in Peritoneal Dialysis. Excerpta Medica, Amsterdam, 1981, p 46.

341. Krediet RT, Boeschoten EW, Zuyderhoudt FMJ, et al: Simple assessment of the efficacy of peritoneal transport in continuous peritoneal dialysis patients. Blood Purif 4:194, 1986.

342. Verger C, Larpen L, Dumontet M: Prognostic values of peritoneal equilibration curves in CAPD patients. *In* Maher JF (ed): Frontiers in Peritoneal Dialysis. Field, Rich, & Associates, New York, 1986, p 88.

343. Teixido J, Cofan F, Borras M, et al: Mass transfer coefficient: Comparison between methods. Perit Dial Int 13:S47, 1993.

344. Krediet RT, Zemel D, Imholz A, et al: Indices of peritoneal permeability and surface area. Perit Dial Int 13:S31, 1993.

345. Krediet RT, Zuyderhoudt FMJ, Boeschoten EW, et al: Alterations in the peritoneal transport of water and solutes during peritonitis in continuous ambulatory peritoneal dialysis patients. Eur J Clin Invest 17:43, 1987.

346. Krediet RT, Arisz L: Fluid and solute transport across the peritoneum during continuous ambulatory peritoneal dialysis (CAPD). Perit Dial Int 9:15, 1989.

347. Bonomini V, Zucchelli P, Mioli V: Selective and unselective protein loss in peritoneal dialysis. Proc Eur Dial Transplant Assoc 4:146, 1967.

348. Verger C, Larpent L, Veniez G, et al: Monitoring of the peritoneal permeability in peritoneal dialysis. Rev Prat 41:1086, 1991.

349. Burkart JM, Jordan JR, Rocco MV: Assessment of dialysis dose by measured clearance versus extrapolated data. Perit Dial Int 13:184, 1993.

350. Steinhauer HB: Pharmacological manipulation of peritoneal transport in CAPD. Clin Nephrol 30:S29, 1988.

351. Blumenkrantz MJ, Gahl GM, Kopple GD, et al: Protein losses during peritoneal dialysis. Kidney Int 19:593, 1981.

352. Dulaney JT, Hatch FE: Peritoneal dialysis and loss of proteins. Kidney Int 26:253, 1984. Review.

353. Krediet RT, Struijk DG, Koomen GCM, et al: The peritoneal transport of macromolecules in CAPD patients. Contrib Nephrol 89:161, 1991.

354. Zemel D, Struijk DG, Krediet RT, et al: No relationship between dialysate IgG and peritonitis incidence. Nephrol Dial Transplant 4:755, 1989. Abstract.

355. Krediet RT, Boeschoten EW, Zuyderhoudt FMHJ, et al: Peritoneal transport characteristics of water, low molecular weight solutes and proteins during long-term continuous ambulatory peritoneal dialysis. Perit Dial Bull 6:61, 1986.

356. Chan PCK, Chan CY, Wu PG, et al: Long-term peritoneal clearances in patients on continuous ambulatory peritoneal dialysis. Int J Artif Organs 13:707–708, 1990.

357. Lameire NH, Vanholder R, Veyt D, et al: A longitudinal, five year survey of urea kinetic parameters in CAPD patients. Kidney Int 42:426, 1992.

358. Blake PG, Abraham G, Sombolos K, et al: Changes in peritoneal membrane transport rates in patients on long-term CAPD. Adv Perit Dial 5:3, 1989.

359. De Vecchi AF, Castelnovo C, Scalamogna A, et al: Symptomatic accidental introduction of disinfectant electrolytic chlorosidizer into the peritoneal cavity of CAPD patients. Incidence and long-term effects on ultrafiltration. Clin Nephrol 37:204, 1992.

360. Ota K, Mineshima M, Watanabe N, et al: Functional deterioration of the peritoneum: Does it occur in the absence of peritonitis? Nephrol Dial Transplant 2:30, 1987.

361. Struijk DG, Krediet RT, Koomen GCM, et al: Functional characteristics of the peritoneal membrane in long-term continuous ambulatory peritoneal dialysis. Nephron 59:213, 1991.

362. Lee HB, Park MS, Chung SH, et al: Peritoneal solute clearances in diabetics. Perit Dial Int 10:85, 1990.

363. Rubin J, Reed V, Adair C, et al: Effect of intraperitoneal insulin on

solute kinetics in CAPD: Insulin kinetics in CAPD. Am J Med Sci 291:81, 1986.

364. Selgas R, Madero R, Munoz J, et al: Functional peculiarities of the peritoneum in diabetes mellitus. Dial Transplant 42:133, 1988.

365. Zimmerman AL, Sablay LB, Aynedjian HS, Bank N: Increased peritoneal permeability in rats with alloxan-induced diabetes mellitus. J Lab Clin Med 103:720, 1984.

366. Lo W, Brendolan A, Prowant B, et al: Changes in the PET in selected CAPD patients. J Am Soc Nephrol 4:1466, 1994.

367. Twardowski ZJ, Nolph KD: Peritoneal dialysis: How much is enough? Semin Dial 2:75, 1988.

368. Ronco C, Ferianai M, Chiaramonte S, et al: Pathophysiology of ultrafiltration in peritoneal dialysis. Perit Dial Int 10:119, 1990.

369. Mactier RA: Investigation and management of ultrafiltration failure in CAPD. Adv Perit Dial 7:57, 1991.

370. Verger C, Larpent L, Celicout B: Clinical significance of ultrafiltration failure on CAPD. *In* La Greca G, Chiaramonte S, Fabris A, et al (eds): Peritoneal Dialysis. Wichtig Editore, Milano, 1986, p 91.

371. Faller B, Marichal JF: Loss of ultrafiltration in continuous ambulatory peritoneal dialysis. A role for acetate. Perit Dial Bull 4:10, 1984.

372. Bazzato G, Coli U, Landini S, et al: Restoration of ultrafiltration capacity of peritoneal membrane in patients on CAPD. Int J Artif Organs 7:93, 1984.

373. Panasiuk E, Pietrzak B, Klos M, et al: Characteristics of peritoneum after peritonitis in CAPD patients. Adv Perit Dial 4:42, 1988.

374. Di Paolo N, Vanni L, Sacchi G: Autologous implant of peritoneal mesothelium in rabbits and man. Clin Nephrol 34:179, 1990.

375. Di Paolo N, Sacchi G, Vanni L, et al: Autologous peritoneal mesothelial cell implant in rabbits and peritoneal dialysis patients. Nephron 57:323, 1991.

376. Rottembourg J, Brouard R, Issad B, et al: Role of acetate in loss of ultrafiltration during CAPD. Contrib Nephrol 57:197, 1987.

377. Shaldon S, Koch KM, Quelhorst E, et al: Pathogenesis of sclerosing peritonitis in CAPD. ASAIO Trans 30:193, 1984.

378. Pollack CA, Ibels LS, Hallett MD, et al: Loss of ultrafiltration in continuous ambulatory peritoneal dialysis (CAPD). Perit Dial Int 9:107, 1989.

379. Miranda B, Selgas R, Celadilla O, et al: Peritoneal resting and heparinization as an effective treatment for ultrafiltration failure in patients on CAPD. Contrib Nephrol 89:199, 1991.

380. Lang J, Harwood J, Coles GA, et al: Changes in dialysate phospholipid content during CAPD. Perit Dial Int 12:S13, 1992. Abstract.

381. Dombros N, Balaskas E, Savidis N, et al: Phosphatidylcholine increases ultrafiltration in continuous ambulatory peritoneal dialysis patients. *In* Avram MM, Giordano C (eds): Ambulatory Peritoneal Dialysis. Plenum Publishing, New York, 1990, p 39.

382. Khanna R, Nolph KD, Twardowski ZJ: Pharmacological alteration of ultrafiltration. Contrib Nephrol, 85:150, 1990.

383. Rozga J, Andersson R, Srinivas U, et al: Influence of phosphatidylcholine on intraabdominal adhesion formation and peritoneal macrophages. Nephron 54:134, 1990.

384. Kappas AM, Fatouros M, Siamopoulos K, et al: Phosphatidylcholine and intraperitoneal adhesions. Perit Dial Int 13:S77, 1993.

385. Chan H, Abraham G, Oreopoulos DG: Oral lecithin improves ultrafiltration in patients on peritoneal dialysis. Perit Dial Int 9:203, 1989.

386. De Vecchi A, Castelnovo C, Guerra L, et al: Phosphatidylcholine administration in continuous ambulatory peritoneal dialysis (CAPD) patients with reduced ultrafiltration. Perit Dial Int 9:207, 1989.

387. Chan PCK, Tam SCF, Robinson JD, et al: Effect of phosphatidylcholine on ultrafiltration in patients on continuous ambulatory peritoneal dialysis. Nephron 59:100, 1991.

388. Huarte-Loza E, Selgas R, Carmona AR, et al: Peritoneal membrane failure as a determinant of the CAPD future. Contrib Nephrol 47:219, 1987.

389. Diaz-Buxo JA: Peritoneal sclerosis in a woman on continuous cyclic peritoneal dialysis. Semin Dial 5:317, 1992.

390. Verger C, Celicout B: Peritoneal permeability and encapsulating peritonitis. Lancet 1:986, 1985.

391. Bargman JM, Oreopoulos DG: Complications other than peritonitis or those related to the catheter and the fate of uremic organ dysfunction in patients receiving peritoneal dialysis. *In* Nolph KD (ed): Peritoneal Dialysis, 3rd ed. Kluwer Academic Publishers, Boston, 1989, p 289.

392. Grefberg N, Nilsson P, Andreen T: Sclerosing obstructive peritonitis, beta blockers, and continuous ambulatory peritoneal dialysis. Lancet 2:733, 1983. Letter.

393. Bradley J, McWhinnie D, Hamilton D, et al: Sclerosing obstructive peritonitis after continuous ambulatory peritoneal dialysis. Lancet 2:113, 1983. Letter.
394. Verger C, Celicout B, Larpent L, et al: Sclerosing encapsulating peritonitis during continuous ambulatory peritoneal dialysis. Presse Med 15:1311, 1986.
395. Rottembourg J, Gahl G, Poignet J, et al: Severe abdominal complications in patients undergoing continuous ambulatory peritoneal dialysis. Proc Eur Dial Transplant Assoc 20:236, 1983.
396. Lamperi S, Carozzi S, Nasini MG, et al: Effect of intraperitoneal verapamil therapy on ultrafiltration in CAPD patients with peritoneal hypopermeability. Perit Dial Bull 4:15, 1984.
397. Lamperi S, Carozzi S: Lympho-monokine disorders and ultrafiltration loss in CAPD patients. Perit Dial Bull, 7:7, 1987.
398. Lamperi S, Carozzi S, Nasini MG: Lympho-monokine disorders and peritoneal fibroblast proliferation in CAPD. ASAIO Trans 32:35, 1986.
399. Lichtman AH, Segal GB, Lichtman MA: The role of calcium in lymphocyte proliferation: An interpretive review. Blood 61:413, 1983.
400. Lamperi S, Carozzi S, Nasini MG: Calcium antagonists improve ultrafiltration in patients on continuous ambulatory peritoneal dialysis (CAPD). ASAIO Trans 33:657, 1987.
401. Turner MW, Holleman JH: Successful therapy of sclerosing peritonitis. Semin Dial 5:316, 1992.
402. Clark CP, Vanderpool D, Preskitt JT: The response of retroperitoneal fibrosis to tamoxifen. Surgery 109:502, 1991.
403. Twardowski ZJ: Dialysis adequacy and new cycler techniques. Contemp Issues Nephrol 22:67, 1990.
404. Forbes AM, Reed V, Goldsmith HJ: CAPD: A scheme to allow reduction of dialysis bag exchange. Clin Nephrol 15:264, 1981.
405. Twardowski ZJ: Peritoneal dialysis glossary III. Perit Dial Int 10:173, 1990.
406. Agadoa LYC, Port FK, Held PJ: Living patients on December 31, 1990 by treatment modality and network. In Agadoa LYC, Held PJ, Port FK (eds): USRDS Annual Data Report 1993. The National Institutes of Health, National Institute of Diabetes and Digestive and Kidney Diseases, Bethesda, MD, 1993, p 33.
407. Nissenson AR, Prichard SS, Cheng IKP, et al: Non-medical factors that impact on ESRD modality selection. Kidney Int 43(suppl 40):S120, 1993.
408. Nolph KD, Moore HL, Prowant B, et al: Cross sectional assessment of weekly urea and creatinine clearances and indices of nutrition in continuous ambulatory peritoneal dialysis patients. Perit Dial Int 13:178, 1993.
409. Blake PG, Sombolos K, Izatt S, et al: Low serum albumin (SA) predicts poor outcome in CAPD and is related to high peritoneal membrane permeability. J Am Soc Nephrol 1:338, 1990. Abstract.
410. Kaysen GA, Schoenfeld PY: Albumin homeostasis in patients undergoing continuous ambulatory peritoneal dialysis. Kidney Int 25:107, 1984.
411. Kagan A, Bar-Khayim Y, Schafer Z, et al: Heterogeneity in peritoneal transport during continuous ambulatory peritoneal dialysis and its impact on ultrafiltration, loss of macromolecules and plasma level of proteins, lipids, and lipoproteins. Nephron 63:32, 1993.
412. Twardowski ZJ: New approaches to intermittent peritoneal dialysis therapies. In Nolph KD (ed): Peritoneal Dialysis, 3rd ed. Kluwer Academic Publishers, Boston, 1989, p 133.
413. Gutman RA, Blumenkrantz MJ, Chan YK, et al: Controlled comparison of hemodialysis and peritoneal dialysis: Veterans administration multicenter study. Kidney Int 26:459, 1984.
414. Trevino-Becerra A: Intermittent peritoneal dialysis with a cycler may be the answer. Perit Dial Bull 4:112, 1984.
415. Shapira J, Lang R, Jutrin I, et al: Peritoneal dialysis in refractory congestive heart failure: Part I. Intermittent peritoneal dialysis. Perit Dial Bull 3:130, 1983.
416. Twardowski ZJ, Nolph KD, Khanna R, et al: Daily clearances with continuous ambulatory peritoneal dialysis and nightly peritoneal dialysis. ASAIO Trans 32:575, 1986.
417. Spencer PC, Farrell PC: Applications of kinetic monitoring in CAPD. In Weimer W, Fieren MWJA, Diderich PPNN (eds): Proceedings of the Fourth Benelux Symposium, Rotterdam, November 24. Op de Hoek CT, Rotterdam, 1984, p 9.
418. Twardowski ZJ, Nolph KD, Prowant BF, Moore HL: Efficiency of high volume low frequency continuous ambulatory peritoneal dialysis (CAPD). Trans Am Soc Artif Intern Organs 29:53, 1983.
419. Twardowski ZJ, Prowant BF, Nolph KD, et al: Chronic nightly tidal peritoneal dialysis (NTDP). ASAIO Trans 36:M584, 1990.
420. Nolph KD, Twardowski ZJ, Keshaviah PR: Weekly clearances of urea and creatinine on CAPD and NIPD. Perit Dial Int 12:298, 1992.
421. Steinhauer HB, Keck I, Lubrich-Birkner I, et al: Increased dialysis efficiency in tidal peritoneal dialysis compared to intermittent peritoneal dialysis. Nephron 58:500, 1991.
422. Lowrie EG, Laird NM, Parker TF, Sargent JA: Effect of the hemodialysis prescription of patient morbidity: Report from the National Cooperative Dialysis Study. N Engl J Med 305:1176, 1981.
423. Teehan BP, Schleifer CR, Brown J: Urea kinetic modeling is an appropriate assessment of adequacy. Semin Dial 5:189, 1992.
424. Keshaviah P, Nolph K, Prowant P: Defining adequacy of CAPD with urea kinetics. Adv Perit Dial 6:175, 1990.
425. Brandes JC, Piering WF, Beres JA, et al: Clinical outcome of CAPD predicted by urea and creatinine kinetics. J Am Soc Nephrol 2:1430, 1992.
426. Blake PG, Sombolos K, Abraham G, et al: Lack of correlation between urea kinetic indices and clinical outcomes in CAPD patients. Kidney Int 39:700, 1991.
427. Blake PG, Balaskas E, Blake R, et al: Urea kinetics has limited relevance in assessing adequacy of dialysis in CAPD. Adv Perit Dial 8:65, 1992.
428. Watson PE, Watson ID, Batt RD: Total body water volumes for adult males and females estimated from simple anthropometric measurements. Am J Clin Nutr 33:27, 1980.
429. Blake PG, Balaskas EV, Izatt S, Oreopoulos DG: Is total creatinine clearance a good predictor of clinical outcomes in continuous ambulatory peritoneal dialysis? Perit Dial Int 12:353, 1992.
430. Brandes JC, Piering WF, Beres JA: A method to assess efficacy of CAPD: Preliminary results. Adv Perit Dial 6:192, 1990.
431. Pedersen JA, Smith JV: Changing empiric to kinetic CAPD prescription: No short-term effect. Kidney Int 37:332, 1990.
432. Goodship THJ, Ward MK, Wilkinson R: Urea kinetic modeling and nutritional status in CAPD. J Am Soc Nephrol 2:361, 1991.
433. Kraus AP, Acchiardo S, Kaufman PA, et al: Evaluating adequacy of the CAPD prescription. J Am Soc Nephrol 2:363, 1991.
434. Williams AM, Erickson AM, Jaeger JL, et al: Urea kinetic modeling as a predictor of adequacy of dialysis in CAPD. Perit Dial Int 12:173, 1992.
435. Keshaviah PR, Nolph KD, VanStone JC: The peak concentration hypothesis. Perit Dial Int 9:257, 1989.
436. Young GA, Kopple JD, Lindholm B, et al: Nutritional assessment of continuous ambulatory peritoneal dialysis patients: An international study. Am J Kidney Dis 17:462, 1991.
437. Harris T, Cook EF, Garrison R, et al: Body mass index and mortality among nonsmoking older persons. The Framingham Heart Study. JAMA 259:1520, 1988.
438. Lowrie EG, Lew NL: Death risk in hemodialysis patients: The predictive value of commonly measured variables and an evaluation of death rate differences between facilities. Am J Kidney Dis 15:458, 1990.
439. Blake PG, Flowerdew GF, Blake RM, et al: Serum albumin in patients on CAPD. J Am Soc Nephrol 3:1501, 1993.
440. Rocco MV, Burkart JM: Lack of correlation between efficacy number and traditional measures of peritoneal dialysis adequacy. J Am Soc Nephrol 3:417, 1992.
441. Schoenfeld PY: Is the lower serum albumin concentration in CAPD patients a reflection of nutritional status? Albumin is an unreliable marker of nutritional status. Semin Dial 5:218, 1992.
442. Gilbert R, Goyal RK: The gastrointestinal system. In Eknoyan G, Knochel JP (eds): The Systemic Consequences of Renal Failure. Grune & Stratton, New York, 1984, p 133.
443. Lindsay RM, Spanner E: A hypothesis: The protein catabolic rate is dependent upon the type and amount of treatment in dialyzed uremic patients. Am J Kidney Dis 13:382, 1989.
444. Bergstrom J, Lindholm B: Nutrition and adequacy of dialysis. How do hemodialysis and CAPD compare? Kidney Int 43(suppl 40):S39, 1993.
445. Lysaght MJ, Pollock CA, Hallet MD, et al: The relevance of urea kinetic modeling to CAPD. ASAIO Trans 35:784, 1989.
446. Nolph KD: What's new in peritoneal dialysis—an overview. Kidney Int 42(suppl 38):S148, 1992.
447. Gotch FA: The application of urea kinetic modeling to CAPD. In La Greca G, Ronco C, Feriani M, et al (eds): Peritoneal Dialysis: Pro-

ceedings of the Fourth International Course on Peritoneal Dialysis. Wichtig Editore, Milan, 1991, p 47.

448. Spinowitz BS, Gupta BK, Kulogowski J, et al: Dialysis adequacy in hypoalbuminemic continuous ambulatory peritoneal dialysis patients. Perit Dial Int 13(suppl 2):S221, 1992.

449. Blumenkrantz MJ, Kopple JD, Moran JK, Coburn JW: Metabolic balance studies and dietary protein requirements in patients undergoing continuous ambulatory peritoneal dialysis. Kidney Int 21:849, 1981.

450. Diamond SM, Henrich WL: Nutrition and peritoneal dialysis. In Mitch WE, Klahr S (eds): Nutrition and the Kidney. Little, Brown, Boston, 1988, p 198.

451. Lindsay RM, Spanner E, Heidenheim P, et al: Which comes first, Kt/V or PCR—chicken or egg? Kidney Int 42:S32, 1992.

452. Keshaviah P: Adequacy of CAPD: A quantitative approach. Kidney Int 42(suppl 38):S160, 1992.

453. Burkart JM, Jordan J, Garchow S, et al: Using a computer kinetic modeling program to prescribe PD. Perit Dial Int 13(suppl 1):S77, 1993.

454. Movilli E, Mombelloni S, Gaggiotti M, et al: Effect of age on protein catabolic rate, morbidity, and mortality in uraemic patients with adequate dialysis. Nephrol Dial Transplant 8:735, 1993.

455. Rottembourg J, Issad B, Gallego JL, et al: Evolution of residual renal functions in patients undergoing maintenance hemodialysis or continuous ambulatory peritoneal dialysis. Proc Eur Dial Transplant Assoc 19:397, 1983.

456. Cancarini GC, Brunori G, Camerini C, et al: Renal function recovery and maintenance of residual diuresis in CAPD and hemodialysis. Perit Dial Bull 6:77, 1986.

457. Lysaght MJ, Vonesh EF, Gotch F, et al: The influence of dialysis treatment modality on the decline of remaining renal function. ASAIO Trans 37:598, 1991.

458. Port FK, Held PJ, Nolph KD, et al: Risk of peritonitis and technique failure by CAPD connection technique: A national study. Kidney Int 42:967, 1992.

459. Twardowski ZJ: Clinical value of standardized equilibration tests in CAPD patients. Blood Purif 7:95, 1989.

460. Popovich RP, Moncrief SW: Transport kinetics. In Nolph KD (ed): Peritoneal Dialysis, 2nd ed. Martinus Nijhoff, Boston, 1985, p 115.

461. Burkart JM: Adequacy of peritoneal dialysis. In Henrich WL (ed): Principles and Practice of Dialysis. Williams & Wilkins, Baltimore, 1994, p 111.

462. Nolph KD: Comparison of continuous ambulatory peritoneal dialysis and hemodialysis. Kidney Int 33:S123, 1988.

463. Maiorca R, Vonesh E, Cancarini GC, et al: A six-year comparison of patient and technique survivals in CAPD and HD. Kidney Int 34:518, 1988.

464. Posen GA, Jeffery JR, Fenton SSA: Results from the Canadian Renal Failure Registry. Am J Kidney Dis 15:397, 1990.

465. Marichal JF, Cordier B, Faller B, et al: Continuous ambulatory peritoneal dialysis (CAPD) or center hemodialysis? Retrospective evaluation of the success of both methods. Perit Dial Int 10:205, 1990.

466. Maiorca R, Cancarini GC, Brunori G, et al: Morbidity and mortality of CAPD and hemodialysis. Kidney Int 43(suppl 40):S4, 1993.

467. Viglino G, Cancarini G, Catizone L, et al: Ten years of continuous ambulatory peritoneal dialysis: Analysis of patient and technique survival. Perit Dial Int 13(suppl 2):S175, 1993.

468. Canadian CAPD Clinical Trial Group: Peritonitis in continuous ambulatory peritoneal dialysis (CAPD): A multi-center randomized clinical trial comparing the Y connector disinfectant system to standard systems. Perit Dial Int 9:159, 1989.

469. Maiorca R, Cancarini GC, Manili L, et al: Peritonitis rate and CAPD results. In La Greca G, Ronco C, Feriani M, et al (eds): Peritoneal Dialysis: Proceedings of the Fourth International Course on Peritoneal Dialysis. Wichtig Editore, Milano, 1991, p 223.

470. Nolph KD: Clinical results with peritoneal dialysis—registry experiences. In Twardowski ZJ, Nolph KD, Khanna R, et al (eds): Contemporary Issues in Nephrology. Churchill Livingstone, New York, 1990, p 127.

471. Disney APS (ed): Twelfth Report of the Australia and New Zealand Combined Dialysis and Transplant Registry. Queen Elizabeth Hospital, Woodville, South Australia, 1989.

472. Wolfe RA, Port FK, Hawthorne VM, et al: A comparison of survival among dialytic therapies of choice: In-center hemodialysis versus continuous ambulatory dialysis at home. Am J Kidney Dis 15:433, 1990.

473. Maiorca R, Vonesh EF, Cavalli PL, et al: A multicenter, selection-adjusted comparison of patient and technique survivals on CAPD and hemodialysis. Perit Dial Int 11:118, 1991.

474. Agodoa LYC, Held PJ, Port FK: United States RDS. United States Renal Data System 1991 Annual Data Report. The National Institutes of Health, National Institute of Diabetes and Digestive and Kidney Diseases, Bethesda, MD, 1991.

475. Nelson CB, Port FK: Dialysis patient survival: Evaluation of CAPD vs HD using 3 techniques. Abstracts, 12th Annual Peritoneal Dialysis Conference. Perit Dial Int 12(suppl 1):144, 1992.

476. Gokal R, Jakubowski C, King J, et al: Outcome in patients on continuous ambulatory peritoneal dialysis and haemodialysis: 4-year analysis of a prospective multicentre study. Lancet 2:1105, 1987.

477. Holley JL, Piraino BM: Complications of peritoneal dialysis: Diagnosis and management. Semin Dial 3:245, 1990.

478. Fenton SSA: Peritonitis related deaths among CAPD patients. Perit Dial Bull 3:S9, 1983.

479. Slingeneyer A, Mion C, Beraud JJ, et al: Peritonitis, a frequently lethal complication of intermittent and continuous ambulatory peritoneal dialysis. Proc Eur Dial Transplant Assoc 18:212, 1981.

480. Wu G: Review of peritonitis episodes that caused interruption of CAPD. Perit Dial Bull 3:S11, 1983.

481. Tzamaloukas AH, Murata GH, Fox L: Peritoneal catheter loss and death in continuous ambulatory peritoneal dialysis peritonitis: Correlation with clinical and biochemical parameters. Perit Dial Int 13:S338, 1993.

482. Holmes C, Lewis S: Host defense mechanisms in the peritoneal cavity of continuous ambulatory peritoneal dialysis patients. 2. Humoral defenses. Perit Dial Int 11:112, 1991.

483. Cairns HS: Continuous ambulatory peritoneal dialysis peritonitis: Role and treatment of impaired host defenses. Semin Dial 5:17, 1992.

484. McGregor SJ, Brock JH, Briggs JD, et al: Longitudinal study of peritoneal defense mechanisms in patients on continuous ambulatory peritoneal dialysis (CAPD). Perit Dial Int 9:115, 1989.

485. Holmes CJ, Lewis SL, Kubey WY, et al: Comparison of peritoneal white blood cell parameters from CAPD patients with a high or low incidence of peritonitis. Am J Kidney Dis 15:258, 1990.

486. De Vecchi AF, Kopple JD, Young GA, et al: Plasma and dialysate immunoglobulin G in continuous ambulatory peritoneal dialysis patients: A multicenter study. Am J Nephrol 10:451, 1990.

487. Langer ME, Saba TM: Fibronectin is a co-factor necessary for optimal granulocyte phagocytosis of Staphylococcus aureus. J Reticuloendoth Soc 30:415, 1981.

488. Bos HJ, Van Bronswijk H, Helmerhorst TJM, et al: Distinct subpopulations of elicited human macrophages in peritoneal dialysis patients and women undergoing laparoscopy: A study of peroxidatic activity. J Leukocyte Biol 43:172, 1988.

489. Brando B, Galato R, Seveso M, et al: Flow cytometric study of immunocompetent cell phenotypes and phagocytosis in CAPD effluent. ASAIO Trans 34:441, 1988.

490. McGregor SJ, Brock JH, Briggs JD, et al: Bactericidal activity of peritoneal macrophages from CAPD patients. Nephrol Dial Transplant 2:104, 1987.

491. Lamperi S, Carozzi S: Defective opsonic activity of peritoneal effluent during CAPD: Importance and prevention. Perit Dial Bull 6:87, 1986.

492. Goyert SM, Ferrero E, Rettig WJ, et al: The CD14 monocyte differentiation antigen maps to a region encoding growth factors and receptors. Science 239:497, 1988.

493. Giacchino F, Pozzato M, Formica M, et al: Lymphocyte subsets assayed by numerical tests in CAPD. Int J Artif Intern Organs 7:81, 1984.

494. Lamperi S, Carozzi S: Immunological defenses in CAPD. Blood Purif 7:126, 1989.

495. Lamperi S, Carozzi S: Suppressor resident macrophages and peritonitis incidence in CAPD. Nephron 44:219, 1986.

496. Carozzi S, Nasini MG, Schelotto C, et al: Intraperitoneal therapy with interferon-α in CAPD patients with relapsing bacterial peritonitis. ASAIO Trans 35:421, 1989.

497. Levy R, Klein J, Rubinek T, et al: Diversity in peritoneal macrophage response of CAPD patients to 1,25-dihydroxyvitamin $D_3$. Kidney Int 37:1310, 1990.

498. Peterson PK, Keane WF: Infections in chronic peritoneal dialysis patients. Curr Clin Top Infect Dis 6:239, 1985.
499. Glancey GR, Cameron JS, Ogg CS: Peritoneal drainage: An important element in host defense against staphylococcal peritonitis in patients on CAPD. Nephrol Dial Transplant 7:627, 1992.
500. Kuan SF, Rust K, Crouch E: Interactions of surfactant protein D with bacterial lipopolysaccharides. J Clin Invest 90:97, 1992.
501. Topley N, Brown Z, Jorres A, et al: Human peritoneal mesothelial cells (HPMC) synthesize interleukin-8 (IL-8): Induction by cytokines. Perit Dial Int 12:S21, 1992.
502. Muijsken MA, Heezius HJ, Verhoef J, et al: Role of mesothelial cells in peritoneal antibacterial defence. J Clin Pathol 44:600, 1991.
503. Rubin J, Rogers WA, Taylor HM, et al: Peritonitis during continuous ambulatory dialysis. Ann Intern Med 92:7, 1980.
504. Holmes CJ, Lewis SL, Evans RC, et al: Periodic elevation of complement activation products in peritoneal dialysis effluent. ASAIO Trans 35:587, 1989.
505. Fieren MW, Van den Bemd GJ, Bonta IL: Endotoxin-stimulated peritoneal macrophages obtained from continuous ambulatory peritoneal dialysis patients show an increased capacity to release interleukin-1 beta in vitro during infectious peritonitis. Eur J Clin Invest 20:453, 1990.
506. Montrucchio G, Mariano F, Cavalli PL, et al: Platelet activating factor is produced during infectious peritonitis in CAPD patients. Kidney Int 36:1029, 1989.
507. Brauner A, Hylander B, Wretlind B: Interleukin-6 and interleukin-8 in dialysate and serum from patients on continuous ambulatory peritoneal dialysis. Am J Kidney Dis 22:430, 1993.
508. Rubin J: Nutritional support during peritoneal dialysis–related peritonitis. Am J Kidney Dis 15:551, 1990.
509. Verbrugh HA, Keane WF, Conroy WE, et al: Bacterial growth and killing in CAPD fluids. J Clin Microbiol 20:199, 1984.
510. Keane WF, Comty CM, Verbrugh HA, et al: Opsonic deficiency of peritoneal dialysis effluent in CAPD. Kidney Int 25:539, 1984.
511. Churchill DN: CAPD peritonitis: A critical appraisal of prophylactic strategies. Semin Dial 4:94, 1991.
512. Buoncristiani U, Cozzari M, Quintaliani G, et al: Abatement of exogenous peritonitis risk using the Perugia CAPD system. Dial Transplant 12:14, 1983.
513. Maiorca R, Cantaluppi A, Cancarini GC, et al: Prospective controlled trial of a Y connector and disinfectant to prevent peritonitis in continuous ambulatory peritoneal dialysis. Lancet 2:642, 1983.
514. Burkart JM, Hylander B, Durnell-Figel T, Roberts D: Comparison of peritonitis rates during long-term use of standard spike versus Ultraset in continuous ambulatory peritoneal dialysis (CAPD). Perit Dial Int 10:41, 1990.
515. Scalamogna A, De Vecchi A, Castelnovo C, et al: Long-term incidence of peritonitis in CAPD patients treated by the Y set technique: Experience in a single center. Nephron 55:24, 1990.
516. Luzar MA, Slingeneyer A, Cantaluppi A, et al: In vitro study of the flush effect in two reusable continuous ambulatory peritoneal dialysis (CAPD) disconnect systems. Perit Dial Int 9:169, 1989.
517. Dasgupta MK, Larabie M, Lam K, et al: Growth of bacterial biofilms on Tenckhoff catheter discs in vitro after simulated touch contamination of the Y-connecting set in continuous ambulatory peritoneal dialysis. Am J Nephrol 10:353, 1990.
518. Balteau PR, Peluso FP, Coles GA, et al: Design and testing of the Baxter integrated disconnect system (IDS). Perit Dial Int 11:131, 1991.
519. Honkanen E, Kala AR, Gronhagen-Riska C: Divergent etiologies of CAPD peritonitis in integrated double bag and traditional systems? Adv Perit Dial 7:129, 1991.
520. Holley JL, Bernardini J, Piraino B: Continuous cycling peritoneal dialysis is associated with lower rates of catheter infections than continuous ambulatory peritoneal dialysis. Am J Kidney Dis 16:133, 1990.
521. Stegmayr BG, Granborn L, Tranaeus A, et al: Reduced risk for peritonitis in CAPD with the use of a UV connector box. Perit Dial Int 11:128, 1991.
522. Keane WF, Bergerson B, Pence T, et al: Challenges for continuous ambulatory peritoneal dialysis. In Davison AM (ed): Nephrology: Proceedings of the Xth International Congress of Nephrology, Vol 2. Baillière Tindall, London, 1988, p 1255.
523. Schroeder CH, Bakkeren JAJM, Weemaes CMR, et al: IgG2 deficiency in young children treated with continuous ambulatory peritoneal dialysis (CAPD). Perit Dial Int 9:201, 1989.
524. Poole-Warren LA, Hallet MD, Hone PW, et al: Vaccination for prevention of CAPD associated staphylococcal infection: Results of a prospective multicentre clinical trial. Clin Nephrol 35:198, 1991.
525. Scatizzi A, Strippoli P: Prevention of *Staphylococcus aureus* peritonitis in continuous ambulatory peritoneal dialysis. In Smeby LC, Jorstad S, Wideroe TE (eds): Immune and Metabolic Aspects of Therapeutic Blood Purification Systems. S Karger, Basel, 1986, p 191.
526. White A, Smith J: Nasal reservoir as the source of extranasal staphylococci. Antimicrob Agents Chemother 3:679, 1963.
527. Sewell CM, Clarridge J, Lacke C, et al: Staphylococcal nasal carriage and subsequent infection in peritoneal dialysis patients. JAMA 248:1493, 1982.
528. Sesso R, Draibe S, Castelo A, et al: *Staphylococcus aureus* skin carriage and development of peritonitis in patients on continuous ambulatory peritoneal dialysis. Clin Nephrol 31:264, 1989.
529. Luzar MA, Coles GA, Faller B, et al: *Staphylococcus aureus* nasal carriage and infection in patients on continuous ambulatory peritoneal dialysis. N Engl J Med 322:505, 1990.
530. Davies SJ, Ogg CS, Cameron JS, et al: *Staphylococcus aureus* nasal carriage, exit site infection and catheter loss in patients treated with continuous ambulatory peritoneal dialysis (CAPD). Perit Dial Int 9:61, 1989.
531. Piraino B, Perimutter JA, Holley JL, et al: *Staphylococcus aureus* peritonitis is associated with *Staphylococcus aureus* nasal carriage in peritoneal dialysis patients. Perit Dial Int 13:S332, 1993.
532. Pignatari A, Pfaller M, Hollis R, et al: Methicillin-resistant staphylococcal infection in patients on continuous ambulatory peritoneal dialysis. J Clin Microbiol 28:1898, 1990.
533. Brown AL, Stephenson JR, Baker LR, et al: Epidemiology of CAPD-associated peritonitis caused by coagulase-negative staphylococci: Comparison of strains isolated from hands, abdominal Tenckhoff catheter site and peritoneal fluid. Nephrol Dial Transplant 5:643, 1991.
534. Twardowski ZJ, Prowant BF: *Staphylococcus aureus* nasal carriage is not associated with an increased incidence of exit-site infection with the same organism. Perit Dial Int 13:S306, 1993.
535. Swartz R, Messana J, Starmann B, et al: Preventing *Staphylococcus aureus* infection during chronic peritoneal dialysis. J Am Soc Nephrol 2:1085, 1991.
536. Zimmerman SW, Ahrens E, Johnson CA, et al: Randomized controlled trial of prophylactic rifampin for peritoneal dialysis–related infections. Am J Kidney Dis 18:225, 1991.
537. Vas SI: Peritonitis. In Nolph KD (ed): Peritoneal Dialysis, 3rd ed. Kluwer Academic Publishers, Boston, 1989, p 261.
538. Twardowski ZJ, Schreiber MJ, Burkart JM: Peritoneal dialysis forum: A 55-year-old man with hematuria and blood-tinged dialysate. Perit Dial Int 12:61, 1992.
539. Gulanikar AC, Jindal KK, Hirsch DJ: Is chronic peritoneal dialysis safe in patients with intra-abdominal prosthetic vascular grafts? Nephrol Dial Transplant 6:215, 1991.
540. Charytan C: Continuous ambulatory peritoneal dialysis after abdominal aortic graft surgery. Perit Dial Int 12:227, 1992.
541. Streather CP, Carr P, Barton IK: Carcinoma of the kidney presenting as sterile peritonitis in a patient on continuous ambulatory peritoneal dialysis. Nephron 58:121, 1991.
542. Vlahakos D, Rudders R, Simon G, et al: Lymphoma-mimicking peritonitis in a patient on continuous ambulatory peritoneal dialysis (CAPD). Perit Dial Int 10:165, 1990.
543. Tzamaloukas AH, Obermiller LE, Gibel LJ, et al: Peritonitis associated with intra-abdominal pathology in continuous ambulatory peritoneal dialysis patients. Perit Dial Int 13:S335, 1993.
544. Caruana RJ, Burkart JM, Segraves D, et al: Serum and peritoneal fluid amylase levels in CAPD. Am J Nephrol 7:169, 1987.
545. Burkart JM, Haigler S, Caruana R, et al: Usefulness of peritoneal fluid amylase levels in the differential diagnosis of peritonitis in peritoneal dialysis patients. J Am Soc Nephrol 1:1186, 1991.
546. Twardowski ZJ, Schreiber MJ, Burkart JM: A 69-year-old male with elevated amylase in bloody and cloudy dialysate. Perit Dial Int 13:142, 1993.
547. Royse VL, Jensen DM, Corwin HL: Pancreatic enzymes in chronic renal failure. Arch Intern Med 147:537, 1987.
548. Suresh KR, Port FK: Air under the diaphragm in patients undergoing continuous ambulatory peritoneal dialysis (CAPD). Perit Dial Int 9:309, 1989.

549. Silverstein W, Isikoff MB, Hill MC, et al: Diagnostic imaging of acute pancreatitis: Prospective study using CT and sonography. AJR 137:497, 1981.

550. Struijk RG, van Ketel RJ, Krediet RT, et al: Patient viral peritonitis in a continuous ambulatory peritoneal dialysis. Nephron 44:384, 1986.

551. Lewis SL: Recurrent peritonitis: Evidence of possible viral etiology. Am J Kidney Dis 17:343, 1991.

552. Goodship THJ, Heaton A, Rodger RSC, et al: Factors affecting development of peritonitis in continuous ambulatory peritoneal dialysis. Br Med J 289:1485, 1984.

553. Lewis SL, Stephen AY, Wood BJ, et al: Relationship between frequent episodes of peritonitis and altered immune status. Am J Kidney Dis 22:456, 1993.

554. Gregory MC, Duffy DP: Toxic shock following staphylococcal peritonitis. Clin Nephrol 20:101, 1983.

555. Grutzmacher P, Tsobanelis T, Bruns M, et al: Decrease in peritonitis rate by integrated disconnect system in patients on continuous ambulatory peritoneal dialysis. Perit Dial Int 13:S326, 1993.

556. Davies SJ, Yewdall VMA, Ogg CS, et al: Peritoneal defence mechanisms and *Staphylococcus aureus* in patients treated with continuous ambulatory peritoneal dialysis (CAPD). Perit Dial Int 10:135, 1990.

557. Borra SI, Chandarana J, Kleinfeld M: Fatal peritonitis due to group B β-hemolytic streptococcus in a patient receiving chronic ambulatory peritoneal dialysis. Am J Kidney Dis 19:375, 1992.

558. Boner G, Mhashilkar AM, Rodriguez-Ortega M, et al: Lectin-mediated, nonopsonic phagocytosis of type 1 *Escherichia coli* by human peritoneal macrophages of uremic patients treated by peritoneal dialysis. J Leukocyte Biol 46:239, 1989.

559. Wood CJ, Fleming V, Turnidge J, et al: *Campylobacter* peritonitis in continuous ambulatory peritoneal dialysis: Report of eight cases and a review of the literature. Am J Kidney Dis 19:257, 1992.

560. Chan MK, Chan PCK, Cheng IPK, et al: *Pseudomonas* peritonitis in CAPD patients: Characteristics and outcome of treatment. Nephrol Dial Transplant 4:814, 1989.

561. Millikin SP, Matzke GR, Keane WF: Antimicrobial treatment of peritonitis associated with continuous ambulatory peritoneal dialysis. Perit Dial Int 11:252, 1991.

562. Vassa N, Nolph KD, Khanna R: *Pseudomonas* peritonitis with white blood cell capillary margination and distal digital necrosis in a patient on CAPD. Perit Dial Int 12:323, 1992.

563. Cheng IK, Fang GX, Chan TM, et al: Fungal peritonitis complicating peritoneal dialysis: Report of 27 cases and review of treatment. Q J Med 71:407, 1989.

564. Bernard DB, Levine J, Idelson BA: A continuous ambulatory peritoneal dialysis patient with fungal peritonitis. Semin Dial 4:198, 1991.

565. Brown E, Hendler E: *Rhodococcus* peritonitis in a patient treated with peritoneal dialysis. Am J Kidney Dis 14:417, 1989.

566. Levine J, Bernard DB, Idelson BA, et al: Fungal peritonitis complicating continuous ambulatory peritoneal dialysis: Successful treatment with fluconazole, a new orally active antifungal agent. Am J Med 86:825, 1989.

567. Stein M, Levine JF, Black W: Successful treatment of *Aspergillus* peritonitis in an adult on continuous ambulatory peritoneal dialysis. Nephron 59:145, 1991.

568. Lye WC, Lee EJC: Tuberculous peritonitis in CAPD—a cause of hypercalcaemia. Perit Dial Int 10:307, 1990.

569. Cheng IK, Chan PC, Chan MK: Tuberculous peritonitis complicating long-term peritoneal dialysis. Report of 5 cases and review of the literature. Am J Nephrol 9:155, 1989.

570. Tan D, Fein PA, Jodren A, et al: Successful treatment of tuberculous peritonitis while maintaining patient on CAPD. Adv Perit Dial 7:102, 1991.

571. Dasgupta MK, Ulan RA, Bettcher KB, et al: Effects of exit site infection and peritonitis on the distribution of biofilm-encased adherent bacterial microcolonies (BABM) on Tenckhoff (T) catheters in patients undergoing continuous ambulatory peritoneal dialysis (CAPD). Adv Cont Amb Perit Dial 6:102, 1986.

572. Verger C, Chesneau AM, Thibault M, et al: Biofilm on the Tenckhoff catheter: A negligible source of contamination. Perit Dial Bull 7:178, 1987.

573. Swartz R, Messana J, Holmes C, et al: Biofilm formation on peritoneal catheters does not require the presence of infection. ASAIO Trans 37:626, 1991.

574. Obst G, Gagnon RF, Harris A, et al: The activity of rifampin and analogs against *Staphylococcus epidermidis* biofilm in a CAPD environment model. Am J Nephrol 9:414, 1989.

575. Anwar H, Dasgupta MK, Costerton JW: Testing the susceptibility of bacteria in biofilms to antimicrobial agents. Antimicrob Agents Chemother 34:2043, 1990.

576. Dasgupta MK, Lam K, Ulan RA, et al: An extracorporeal model of biofilm-adherent bacterial microcolony colonization for the study of peritonitis in continuous ambulatory peritoneal dialysis. Am J Nephrol 8:118, 1988.

577. Dasgupta MK, Kowalewaska-Grochowska K, Costerton JW: Biofilm and peritonitis in peritoneal dialysis. Perit Dial Int 13:S322, 1993.

578. Richards GK, Gagnon RF, Prentis J: An in vitro comparison of antibiotic kinetics against *Staphylococcus* biofilms. J Am Soc Nephrol 2:367, 1991.

579. Stablein DM, Nolph KD, Lindblad AS: Timing and characteristics of multiple peritonitis episodes: A report of the National CAPD Registry. Am J Kidney Dis 14:44, 1989.

580. Vlaanderen K, Bos HJ, de Fijter CWH, et al: Short dwell times reduce the local defence mechanism of chronic peritoneal dialysis patients. Nephron 57:29, 1991.

581. Ejlersen E, Brandi, Lokkegaard H: The Danish study group on peritonitis in dialysis: Is initial (24 hours) lavage necessary in treatment of CAPD peritonitis? Perit Dial Int 11:38, 1991.

582. Keane WF, Everett ED, Fine RN, et al: Continuous ambulatory peritoneal dialysis (CAPD) peritonitis treatment recommendations: 1989 Update. Perit Dial Int 9:247, 1990.

583. Lum GM: Peritonitis in infants and children in CAPD/CCPD. *In* Anderiotti VE, Fine RN (eds): Topics in Renal Medicine, Vol 4. Chronic ambulatory peritoneal dialysis (CAPD) and chronic cycling peritoneal dialysis (CCPD) in children. Martinus Nijhoff, Amsterdam, 1987, p 189.

584. Keane WF, Everett ED, Golper TA, et al: Peritoneal dialysis–related peritonitis treatment recommendations. 1993 update. Perit Dial Int 13:14, 1993.

585. Holley JL, Bernardini J, Johnston JR, et al: Methicillin-resistant staphylococcal infections in an outpatient peritoneal dialysis program. Am J Kidney Dis 16:142, 1990.

586. Flanigan MJ, Lim VS: Initial treatment of dialysis associated peritonitis: A controlled trial of vancomycin versus cefazolin. Perit Dial Int 11:31, 1991.

587. De Fijter CW, Verbrugh HA, Heezius HC, et al: Effect of clindamycin on the intracellular bactericidal capacity of human peritoneal macrophages. J Antimicrob Chemother 26:525, 1990.

588. Pylypchuk GB, Conly J, Kappel JE, et al: Sensitivity of CAPD/IPD peritonitis organisms to ciprofloxacin. Adv Perit Dial 7:135, 1991.

589. Perez-Fontan M, Rosales M, Fernandez F, et al: Ciprofloxacin in the treatment of gram positive bacterial peritonitis in patients undergoing CAPD. Perit Dial Int 11:233, 1991.

590. Friedland JS, Iveson TJ, Fraise AP, et al: A comparison between intraperitoneal ciprofloxacin and intraperitoneal vancomycin and gentamycin in the treatment of peritonitis associated with continuous ambulatory peritoneal dialysis (CAPD). J Antimicrob Chemother 26(suppl F):77, 1990.

591. Wilcox MH, Geary I, Spencer RC: In-vitro activity of imipenem, in comparison with cefuroxime and ciprofloxacin, against coagulase-negative staphylococci in broth and peritoneal dialysis fluid. J Antimicrob Chemother 29:49, 1992.

592. Chong TK, Piraino B, Bernardini J: Vestibular toxicity due to gentamycin in peritoneal dialysis patients. Perit Dial Int 11:152, 1991.

593. Nikolaidis P, Vas S, Lawson V, et al: Is intraperitoneal tobramycin ototoxic in CAPD patients? Perit Dial Int 11:156, 1991.

594. Vas SI: Single daily dose of aminoglycosides in the treatment of continuous ambulatory peritoneal dialysis peritonitis. Perit Dial Int 13:S355, 1993.

595. Zaruba K, Peters J, Jungbluth H: Successful prophylaxis for fungal peritonitis in patients on continuous ambulatory peritoneal dialysis: Six years' experience. Am J Kidney Dis 17:43, 1991.

596. Guiberteau R, le Chapois D, Nony A, et al: Treatment of peritoneal infection by the natural defences of the peritoneal cavity. Contrib Nephrol 57:92, 1987.

597. Pagniez DC, MacNamara E, Fortin F, et al: Withdrawal of continuous ambulatory peritoneal dialysis to treat mild peritonitis. BMJ 297:1174, 1988.

598. Dabbagh S, Fassinger N, Clement K, et al: The effect of aggressive

nutrition on infection rates in patients maintained on peritoneal dialysis. Adv Perit Dial 7:161, 1991.

599. Holley JL, Bernardini J, Piraino B: Risk factors for tunnel infections in continuous peritoneal dialysis. Am J Kidney Dis 18:344, 1991.

600. Dasgupta MK: Use of streptokinase or urokinase in recurrent CAPD peritonitis. Adv Perit Dial 7:169, 1991.

601. Domoto DT, Weindel ME, Blalock S, et al: Efficacy of streptokinase in resistant, relapsing, or recurrent CAPD peritonitis. Adv Perit Dial 7:173, 1991.

602. Murphy G, Tzamaloukas AH, Eisenberg B, et al: Intraperitoneal thrombolytic agents in relapsing or persistent peritonitis of patients on continuous ambulatory peritoneal dialysis. Int J Artif Organs 14:87, 1991.

603. Digenis GE, Abraham G, Savin E, et al: Peritonitis-related deaths in continuous ambulatory peritoneal dialysis (CAPD) patients. Perit Dial Int 10:45, 1990.

604. Swartz R, Messana J, Reynolds J, et al: Simultaneous catheter replacement and removal in refractory peritoneal dialysis infections. Kidney Int 40:1160, 1991.

605. Johnson CA: Intraperitoneal vancomycin administration. Perit Dial Bull 11:9, 1991.

606. Charney DI, Gouge SF: Chemical peritonitis secondary to intraperitoneal vancomycin. Am J Kidney Dis 17:76, 1991.

607. Pusateri R, Ross R, Marshall R, et al: Sclerosing encapsulating peritonitis: Report of a case with small bowel obstruction managed by long-term home parenteral hyperalimentation, and a review of the literature. Am J Kidney Dis 8:56, 1986.

608. Buzogany I, Racz L, Wagner G, et al: Complications of peritoneal dialysis: Sclerosing peritonitis. Orv Hetil 132:973, 1991.

609. Ahlmen J, Burian P, Ericksson C, et al: Sclerosing encapsulating peritonitis once again. Perit Dial Int 11:279, 1991.

610. Joffe P, Jensen LT: Type I and III procollagens in CAPD: Markers of peritoneal fibrosis. Adv Perit Dial 7:158, 1991.

611. Lo WK, Chan KT, Leung ACT, et al: Sclerosing peritonitis complicating prolonged use of chlorhexidine in alcohol in the connection procedure for continuous ambulatory peritoneal dialysis. Perit Dial Int 11:166, 1991.

612. Junor BJR, McMillan MA: Immunosuppression in sclerosing peritonitis. Perit Dial Int 13(suppl 1):S64, 1993. Abstract.

613. Kittur DS, Korpe SW, Raytch RE, et al: Surgical aspects of sclerosing encapsulating peritonitis. Arch Surg 125:1626, 1990.

614. Bernardini J, Holley JL, Johnston JR, et al: An analysis of ten-year trends in infections in adults on continuous ambulatory peritoneal dialysis (CAPD). Clin Nephrol 36:29, 1991.

615. Pierratos A: Peritoneal dialysis glossary. Perit Dial Bull 1:2, 1984.

616. Luzar MA, Brown C, Balf D, et al: Exit-site care and exit-site infection in CAPD: Results of a randomized multicenter trial. Perit Dial Int 10:25, 1990.

617. Piraino B, Bernardini J, Sorkin M: A five-year study of the microbiologic results of exit-site infections and peritonitis in continuous ambulatory peritoneal dialysis. Am J Kidney Dis 10:281, 1987.

618. Vogt K, Binswanger U, Buchmann P, et al: Catheter-related complications during continuous ambulatory peritoneal dialysis (CAPD): A retrospective study on sixty-two double cuff Tenckhoff catheters. Am J Kidney Dis 10:47, 1987.

619. Piraino B, Bernardini J, Sorkin M: Catheter infections as a factor in the transfer of CAPD patients to hemodialysis. Am J Kidney Dis 13:365, 1989.

620. Twardowski ZJ: Peritoneal dialysis catheter exit site infections: Prevention, diagnosis, treatment, and future directions. Semin Dial 5:305, 1992.

621. Krizek TJ, Robson MC: Biology of surgical infection. Surg Clin North Am 55:1261, 1975.

622. Luzar MA: Exit-site infection in continuous ambulatory peritoneal dialysis: A review. Perit Dial Int 11:333, 1991.

623. Twardowski ZJ: Exit site infection. In La Greca G, Ronco C, Feriani M, et al (eds): Peritoneal Dialysis: Proceedings of the Fourth International Course on Peritoneal Dialysis, Vincenza, Italy, 1991. Wichtig Editore, Milan, 1991, p 241.

624. Piraino B, Bernardini J, Sorkin M: Bagless CAPD improves catheter infection rates. Kidney Int 35:275, 1988.

625. Piraino B, Bernardini J, Sorkin MI: The effect of the Y-set on catheter infection rates in continuous ambulatory peritoneal dialysis patients. Am J Kidney Dis 16:46, 1990.

626. Fellin G, Gentile MG, Manna GM, et al: Peritonitis prevention: A Y-connector and sodium hypochlorite. Three years' experience. Report of the Italian CAPD Study Group. Adv Cont Amb Perit Dial 7:114, 1987.

627. Moncrief JW, Popovich RP, Dasgupta M, et al: Reduction in peritonitis incidence in continuous ambulatory peritoneal dialysis with a new catheter and implantation technique. Perit Dial Int 13:S329, 1993.

628. Prowant BF, Warady BA, Nolph KD: Peritoneal dialysis catheter exit-site care: Results of an international survey. Perit Dial Int 13:149, 1993.

629. Prowant BF, Schmidt LM, Twardowski ZJ, et al: Peritoneal dialysis catheter exit-site care. Am Nephrol Nurs Assoc J 15:219, 1988.

630. Fuchs J, Gallagher ME, Jackson-Bey D, et al: A prospective randomized study of peritoneal catheter exit site care. Dial Transplant 19:81, 1990.

631. Ash SR, Daugirdas JT: Peritoneal access devices. In Ing TS, Daugirdas JT (eds): Handbook of Dialysis. Little, Brown, Boston, 1987, p 194.

632. Gotloib L, Mines M, Garmizo L, et al: Hemodynamic effects of increasing intra-abdominal pressure in peritoneal dialysis. Perit Dial Bull 1:41, 1981.

633. Hylander BI, Dalton CB, Castell DO, et al: Effect of intraperitoneal fluid volume changes on esophageal pressures: Studies in patients on continuous ambulatory peritoneal dialysis. Am J Kidney Dis 17:307, 1991.

634. Rocco MV, Stone WJ: Abdominal hernias in chronic peritoneal dialysis patients: A review. Perit Dial Bull 5:171, 1985.

635. Bargman JM: Complications of peritoneal dialysis related to increased intra-abdominal pressure. Kidney Int 43:S75, 1993.

636. Spence PA, Mathews RE, Khanna R, et al: Improved results with a paramedian technique for the insertion of peritoneal dialysis catheters. Surg Gynecol Obstet 161:585, 1985.

637. Kopecky R, Funk M, Kreitzer P: Localized genital edema in patients undergoing continuous ambulatory peritoneal dialysis. J Urol 134:880, 1985.

638. Caporale N, Perez D, Alegre S: Vaginal leak of peritoneal dialysis liquid. Perit Dial Int 11:284, 1991.

639. Diaz-Buxo JD, Burgess P, Walker PJ: Peritoneovaginal fistula—unusual complication of peritoneal dialysis. Perit Dial Bull 3:142, 1983.

640. Coward RA, Gokal R, Mallick VP: Recurrent peritonitis associated with vaginal leak. Perit Dial Bull 3:164, 1983. Letter.

641. Wright CA, Moran J, Silk D: Is peritoneal-vaginal fistula the main cause of fungal peritonitis in female CAPD patients? Perit Dial Bull 4:51, 1984. Letter.

642. Osborne TM: CT peritoneography in peritoneal dialysis patients. Australas Radiol 34:204, 1990.

643. Mandel P, Faegenburg MD, Imbriano LJ: The use of technetium-99m sulfur colloid in the detection of patent processus vaginalis in patients on continuous ambulatory peritoneal dialysis. Clin Nucl Med 10:553, 1985.

644. Lieberman FL, Hidemura R, Peters RL, et al: Pathogenesis and treatment of hydrothorax complicating cirrhosis with ascites. Ann Intern Med 64:341, 1966.

645. Green AN, Logan M, Medawar W, et al: The management of hydrothorax in continuous ambulatory peritoneal dialysis (CAPD). Perit Dial Int 10:271, 1990.

646. Walker F, McAllister C, McKee P, et al: Intraperitoneal iopamidol, a new radiocontrast agent, in the diagnosis of a pleuroperitoneal communication. Perit Dial Bull 6:108, 1986. Letter.

647. Vezina D, Winchester JF, Rakowski TA: Spontaneous resolution of massive hydrothorax in a CAPD patient. Perit Dial Bull 7:212, 1987. Letter.

648. Vladimirova NN, Darenkov AF, Pashkin IN, et al: A comparative evaluation of the central hemodynamic indices in patients with the terminal stage of kidney failure during dialysis therapy and allografting. Urol Nefrol (Mosk) 5:34, 1990.

649. Twardowski ZJ, Nolph KD, Prowant BF, et al: Factors influencing tolerance to 3 L volumes for continuous ambulatory peritoneal dialysis (CAPD). Trans Am Soc Artif Intern Organs 28:69, 1982. Abstract.

650. Ahluwalia M, Ishikawa S, Gellman M, et al: Pulmonary functions during peritoneal dialysis. Clin Nephrol 18:251, 1982.

651. Disney A: Australia and New Zealand Dialysis and Transplantation Registry. Queen Elizabeth Hospital, Woodville, South Australia, 1991.

652. De Santo NG, Capodicasa G, Denatore R, et al: Glucose utilization from dialysate in patients on continuous ambulatory peritoneal dialysis. Int J Artif Organs 2:119, 1979.

653. Grodstein GP, Blemenkrantz MJ, Kopple JD, et al: Glucose absorption during continuous ambulatory peritoneal dialysis. Kidney Int 19:564, 1981.

654. Keusch G, Bammatter F, Mordasini R, et al: Serum lipoprotein concentrations during continuous ambulatory peritoneal dialysis. *In* Gahl GM, Kessel M, Nolph KD (eds): Advances in Peritoneal Dialysis. Excerpta Medica, Amsterdam, 1981, p 427.

655. Lindholm B, Karlander SG, Norbeck HE, et al: Carbohydrate and lipid metabolism in CAPD patients. In Atkins R, Thomson N, Farrell P (eds): Peritoneal Dialysis. Churchill Livingstone, Edinburgh, 1981, p 198.

656. Splendiani G, Acitelli S, Albano V, et al: Metabolic aspects of CAPD. *In* Gahl GM, Kessel M, Nolph KD (eds): Advances in Peritoneal Dialysis. Excerpta Medica, Amsterdam, 1981, p 449.

657. Von Baeyer H, Gahl GM, Riedinger H, et al: Adaptation of CAPD patients to the continuous peritoneal energy uptake. Kidney Int 23:29, 1983.

658. Armstrong VW, Buschmann U, Ebert R, et al: Biochemical investigations of CAPD: Plasma levels of trace elements and amino acids and impaired glucose tolerance during the course of treatment. Int J Artif Organs 3:237, 1980.

659. Heaton A, Johnston DG, Burrin JM, et al: Carbohydrate and lipid metabolism during continuous ambulatory peritoneal dialysis (CAPD): The effect of a single dialysis cycle. Clin Sci 54:532, 1983.

660. Kurtz SB, Wong VH, Anderson CF, et al: Continuous ambulatory peritoneal dialysis. Three years' experience at the Mayo Clinic. Mayo Clin Proc 58:633, 1983.

661. Emmanuel DS, Lindheimer MD, Katz AL: Metabolic and endocrine abnormalities in chronic renal failure. *In* Brenner BM, Stein JH (eds): Chronic Renal Failure. Churchill Livingstone, New York, 1981, p 46.

662. Lindholm B, Alvestrand A, Furst P, et al: Metabolic effects of continuous ambulatory peritoneal dialysis. Proc Eur Dial Transplant Assoc 17:283, 1980.

663. Turgan C, Feehally J, Bennett S, et al: Accelerated hypertriglyceridemia in patients on continuous ambulatory peritoneal dialysis—a preventable abnormality. Int J Artif Organs 4:158, 1981.

664. Roncari DAK, Breckenridge WC, Khanna R, et al: Rise in high-density lipoprotein-cholesterol in some patients treated with CAPD. Perit Dial Bull 1:136, 1981.

665. Breckenridge WC, Roncari DAK, Khanna R, et al: The influence of continuous ambulatory peritoneal dialysis on plasma lipoproteins. Atherosclerosis 45:249, 1982.

666. Khanna R, Breckenridge C, Roncari D, et al: Lipid abnormalities in patients undergoing continuous ambulatory peritoneal dialysis. Perit Dial Bull 3(suppl):S13, 1983.

667. Ramos JM, Heaton A, McGurk JG, et al: Sequential changes in serum lipids and their subfractions in patients receiving continuous ambulatory peritoneal dialysis. Nephron 35:20, 1983.

668. Nolph KD, Ryan KL, Prowant B, et al: A cross sectional assessment of serum vitamin D and triglyceride concentrations in a CAPD population. Perit Dial Bull 4:232, 1984.

669. Lindholm B, Bergstrom J: Nutritional management of patients undergoing peritoneal dialysis. *In* Nolph KD (ed): Peritoneal Dialysis, 3rd ed. Kluwer Academic Publishers, Boston, 1989, p 230.

670. Heaton A, Johnston DG, Haigh JW, et al: Twenty-four hour hormonal and metabolic profiles in uremic patients before and during treatment with continuous ambulatory peritoneal dialysis. Clin Sci 69:449, 1985.

671. Thomas ME, Moorhead JF: Lipids in CAPD: A review. Contrib Nephrol 85:92, 1990.

672. Gahl GM, Hain H: Nutrition and metabolism in continuous ambulatory peritoneal dialysis. Contrib Nephrol 84:36, 1990.

673. Chan MK: Sustained-release bezafibrate corrects lipid abnormalities in patients on continuous ambulatory peritoneal dialysis. Nephron 56:56, 1990.

674. Henriquez MA, Gonzalez A, Bemis JA, et al: Body composition and lipid abnormalities in hispanic and black patients on continuous ambulatory peritoneal dialysis. Perit Dial Int 13(suppl 2):S424, 1993.

675. Shoji T, Nishizawa Y, Nishitani H, et al: High serum lipoprotein(a) concentrations in uremic patients treated with continuous ambulatory peritoneal dialysis. Clin Nephrol 38:271, 1992.

676. Dahlen GH, Guyton JR, Attar M, et al: Association of lipoprotein Lp(a), plasma lipids and other lipoproteins with coronary artery disease documented by angiography. Circulation 74:758, 1986.

677. Kandoussi A, Cachera C, Pagniez D, et al: Plasma level of lipoprotein Lp(a) is high in predialysis or hemodialysis, but not in CAPD. Kidney Int 42(suppl 2):424, 1992.

678. Nakagawa S, Ozawa K: Protective aspects for atherogenesis and lipid abnormalities in continuous ambulatory peritoneal dialysis patients. Perit Dial Int 13(suppl 2):S418, 1993.

679. Atkins RC, Wood C: Hyperlipemia in CAPD. Perit Dial Int 13(suppl 2):S415, 1993.

680. Panarello G, Calianno G, De Baz H, et al: Does continuous ambulatory peritoneal dialysis induce hypercholesterolemia? Perit Dial Int 13(suppl 2):S421, 1993.

681. Tao Li PK, Mak TWL, Lam CWK, et al: Lovastatin treatment of dyslipoproteinemia in patients on continuous ambulatory peritoneal dialysis. Perit Dial Int 13(suppl 2):S428, 1993.

682. Di Paolo B, Del Rosso G, Catucci G, et al: Therapeutic effects of simvastatin on hyperlipidemia in CAPD patients. ASAIO Trans 36:578, 1990.

683. Matthys E, Schurgers M, Lamberights G, et al: Effect of simvastatin treatment on the dyslipoproteinaemia in CAPD patients. Atherosclerosis 86:183, 1991.

684. Epstein AE, Kay GN, Plurab VJ: Considerations in the diagnosis and treatment of arrhythmias in patients with ESRD. Semin Dial 2:31, 1989.

685. Peer G, Korzets A, Hochhauzer E, et al: Cardiac arrhythmias during CAPD. Nephron 45:192, 1987.

686. Winchester JF: Peritoneal dialysis and pulmonary function. Chest 86:806, 1984.

687. Adams PL, Rutsky EA, Rostand SG, et al: Lower gastrointestinal dysfunction in patients on chronic hemodialysis. Arch Intern Med 142:303, 1982.

688. Maiorca R, Cancarini G, Brunori G, et al: Continuous ambulatory peritoneal dialysis in the elderly. Perit Dial Int 13:S165, 1993.

689. Benevent D, Benzakour M, Peyronnet P, et al: Comparison of continuous ambulatory peritoneal dialysis and hemodialysis in the elderly. Adv Perit Dial 6(suppl):68, 1990.

690. Walls J: Dialysis in the elderly: Some U.K. experience. Adv Perit Dial 6(suppl):82, 1990.

691. Lunde NM, Port FK, Wolfe RA, et al: Comparison of mortality risk by choice of CAPD vs hemodialysis in elderly patients. Adv Perit Dial 7:68, 1991.

692. Najarian JS, Kaufman DB, Fryd DS, et al: Long-term survival following kidney transplantation in 100 type I diabetic patients. Transplantation 47:106, 1989.

693. Agodoa LYC, Port FK, Held PJ: United States RDS. United States Renal Data System 1993 Annual Data Report. The National Institutes of Health, National Institute of Diabetes and Digestive and Kidney Diseases, Bethesda, MD, 1993.

694. Young MA, Nolph KD, Dutton S, et al: Antihypertensive drug requirements in continuous ambulatory peritoneal dialysis. Perit Dial Bull 4:85, 1984.

695. Khanna R: Dialysis considerations for diabetic patients. Kidney Int 43(suppl 40):S58, 1993.

696. Duckworth WC: Insulin degradation: Mechanisms, products, and significance. Endocr Rev 9:319, 1988.

697. Pyorala K: Relationship of glucose tolerance and plasma insulin to the incidence of coronary heart disease: Results from two population studies in Finland. Diabetes Care 2:131, 1979.

698. Fuller JH, Shipley MJ, Rose G, et al: Coronary heart disease risk and impaired glucose tolerance: The White Hall study. Lancet 1:1373, 1983.

699. Felig P, Wahren J: The liver as site of insulin and glucagon action in normal, diabetic, and obese humans. Isr J Med Sci 11:528, 1975.

700. Olefsky J: Pathogenesis of insulin resistance and hyperglycemia in non–insulin dependent diabetes mellitus. Am J Med 79:1, 1985.

701. Campbell PJ, Mandarino LJ, Gerich JE: Quantification of the relative impairment in actions of insulin on hepatic glucose production and peripheral glucose uptake in non–insulin dependent diabetes mellitus. Metabolism 37:15, 1988.

702. Faller B, Genestier S, Bodenreider O, et al: Experience regarding reduction of peritonitis rates in continuous ambulatory peritoneal dialysis. Perit Dial Int 13:S319, 1993.

703. Madden MA, Zimmerman S, Simpson DP: Continuous ambulatory peritoneal dialysis in diabetes mellitus. Am J Nephrol 2:133, 1982.

704. Legrain M, El Shahat Y, Rottembourg J, et al: Continuous ambulatory peritoneal dialysis versus other treatment modalities in end stage diabetic nephropathy. In Gahl G, Kessel M, Nolph K (eds): Advances in Peritoneal Dialysis. Excerpta Medica, Amsterdam, 1981, p 365.

705. Rottembourg J, El Shahat Y, Agrafiotis A, et al: Continuous ambulatory peritoneal dialysis in insulin dependent diabetics: A 40 months experience. Kidney Int 23:40, 1983.

706. A survey of diabetics in the CAPD/CCPD population. In Lindblad AS, Novak JW, Nolph KD, et al (eds): Continuous Ambulatory Peritoneal Dialysis. Kluwer Academic Publishers, Boston, 1989, p 63.

707. Wanless IR, Bargman JM, Oreopoulos DG, et al: Subcapsular steatonecrosis in response to peritoneal insulin delivery: A clue to the pathogenesis of steatonecrosis in obesity. Mod Pathol 2:69, 1989.

708. Harrison NA, Rainford DJ: Intraperitoneal insulin and the malignant omentum syndrome. Nephrol Dial Transplant 3:103, 1988.

709. Hallett MD, Kush RD, Lysaght MJ, et al: The stability and kinetics of peritoneal mass transfer. In Nolph KD (ed): Peritoneal Dialysis, 3rd ed. Kluwer Academic Publishers, Boston, 1989, p 380.

710. Korbet SM, Vonesh EF, Firanek CA: A retrospective assessment of risk factors for peritonitis among an urban CAPD population. Perit Dial Int 13:126, 1993.

711. Feldman HI, Held PJ, Hutchinson JT, et al: Hemodialysis vascular access morbidity in the United States. Kidney Int 43:1091, 1993.

712. Windus DW: Permanent vascular access: A nephrologist's view. Am J Kidney Dis 21:457, 1993.

713. Holley JL, Bernardini J, Piraino B: A comparison of peritoneal dialysis–related infections in black and white patients. Perit Dial Int 13:45, 1993.

714. Rubin J, Ray R, Barnes T, et al: Peritonitis in continuous ambulatory peritoneal dialysis patients. Am J Kidney Dis 2:602, 1983.

715. Bloxsum A, Powell N: The treatment of acute temporary dysfunction of the kidneys by peritoneal irrigation. Pediatrics 1:52, 1948.

716. Oreopoulos DG, Katirtzoglou A, Arbus G, et al: Dialysis and transplantation in young children. Br Med J 1:1628, 1979. Letter.

717. Fine RN, Salusky IB, Ettenger RB: The therapeutic approach to the infant, child, and adolescent with end-stage renal disease. Pediatr Clin North Am 34:789, 1987.

718. Price CG, Suki WN: Newer modifications of peritoneal dialysis: Options in the treatment of patients with renal failure. Am J Nephrol 1:97, 1981.

719. Alexander SR: Pediatric CAPD update. Perit Dial Bull 3(suppl):S15, 1983.

720. Roscoe JM, Smith LF, Williams A, et al: Medical and social outcome in adolescents with end-stage renal failure. Kidney Int 40:948, 1991.

721. Lewis DJ, McIver M, Scott DF, et al: Dialysis and renal transplantation in children: Long term and recent experience. J Paediatr Child Health 26:276, 1990.

722. Morgenstern BZ, Baluarte H: Peritoneal dialysis kinetics in children. In Fine RN (ed): Chronic Ambulatory Peritoneal Dialysis (CAPD) and Chronic Cycling Peritoneal Dialysis (CCPD) in Children. Martinus Nijhoff, Boston, 1987, p 47.

723. Popovich RP, Pyle WK, Rosenthal DA, et al: Kinetics of peritoneal dialysis in children. In Moncrief JW, Popovich RP (eds): CAPD Update. Masson Publishing USA, New York, 1981, p 227.

724. Morgenstern BZ, Pyle WK, Gruskin AB, et al: Transport characteristics of the pediatric peritoneal membrane. Kidney Int 25:259, 1984. Abstract.

725. Gruskin AB, Rosenblum H, Baluarte HJ, et al: Transperitoneal solute movement in children. Kidney Int 24:S95, 1983.

726. Geary DF, Harvey EA, MacMillan JH, et al: The peritoneal equilibration test in children. Kidney Int 42:102, 1992.

727. Kohaut EC, Alexander SR: Ultrafiltration in the young patient on CAPD. In Moncrief JW, Popovich RP (eds): CAPD Update. Masson Publishing USA, New York, 1981, p 221.

728. Balfe JW, Hanning RM, Vigneaux A, et al: A comparison of peritoneal water and solute movement in young and older children on CAPD. In Fine RN, Scharer K, Mehls O (eds): CAPD in Children. Springer-Verlag, New York, 1985, p 14.

729. Mactier RA, Khanna R, Moore H, et al: Kinetics of peritoneal dialysis in children: Role of lymphatics. Kidney Int 34:82, 1988.

730. Alexander SR, Lindblad AS, Nolph KD, et al: Pediatric CAPD/CCPD in the United States. A review of the experiences of the National CAPD Registry's pediatric patient population for the period of January 1, 1991 to August 31, 1986. Contemp Issues Nephrol 22:231, 1990.

731. Howard RL, Millspaugh J, Teitelbaum I: Adult and pediatric peritonitis rates in a home dialysis program: Comparison of continuous ambulatory and continuous cycling peritoneal dialysis. Am J Kidney Dis 16:469, 1990.

732. Levy M, Balfe JW, Geary DF, et al: Peritonitis in children undergoing dialysis. 10 years experience. Child Nephrol Urol 9:253, 1988–89.

733. Schroder CH, Bakkeren JAJM, Weemaes CMR, et al: IgG$_2$ deficiency in young children treated with continuous ambulatory peritoneal dialysis (CAPD). Perit Dial Int 9:261, 1989.

734. Katz A, Kashtan CE, Greenberg LJ, et al: Hypogammaglobulinemia in uremic infants receiving peritoneal dialysis. J Pediatr 117:258, 1990.

735. Leichter HE, Slauski IB, Alliapoulos JC, et al: CAPD and CCPD in children: An experience of three and one-half years. Dial Transplant 13:382, 1984.

736. Warady BA, Stall C, Paulsen J, et al: A unique approach to peritoneal dialysis in infants. Am J Kidney Dis 7:235, 1986.

737. Fine RN: Growth in children undergoing continuous ambulatory peritoneal dialysis/continuous cycling peritoneal dialysis/automated peritoneal dialysis. Perit Dial Int 13(suppl 2):S247, 1993.

738. Kohaut EC: Growth in children treated with continuous ambulatory peritoneal dialysis. Int J Pediatr Nephrol 4:93, 1983.

739. Stefanidis CJ, Hewitt IK, Balfe J: Growth in children receiving continuous ambulatory peritoneal dialysis. J Pediatr 102:681, 1983.

740. Conley SB: Supplemental (NG) feedings of infants undergoing continuous peritoneal dialysis. In Fine RN (ed): Chronic Ambulatory Peritoneal Dialysis (CAPD) and Chronic Cycling Peritoneal Dialysis (CCPD) in Children. Martinus Nijhoff, Boston, 1987, p 263.

741. Brewer ED: Growth of small children managed with chronic peritoneal dialysis and nasogastric tube feedings: 203-month experience in 14 patients. Adv Perit Dial 6:269, 1990.

742. Leichter HE, Salusky IB, Lillian TV, et al: The optimal dialysis regimen for children undergoing different continuous cycling peritoneal dialysis protocols. In Avram MM, Giordano C (eds): Ambulatory Peritoneal Dialysis. Plenum Publishing, New York, 1990, p 311.

743. Tonshoff B, Dietz M, Haffner D, et al: Effects of two years of growth hormone treatment in short children with renal disease. Acta Paediatr Scand 379(suppl):33, 1991.

744. Watkins SL, Bliefield C, Klee K, et al: Intraperitoneal somatotropin to improve the short stature associated with chronic renal failure in pediatric peritoneal dialysis patients. Pediatr Res 31:345A, 1992. Abstract.

745. Sizun J, Giroux JD, Rubio S, et al: Peritoneal dialysis in the very low birth weight neonate (less than 1000 g). Acta Paediatr 82:488, 1993.

746. Blatz S, Pael B, Steele B: Peritoneal dialysis in the neonate. Neonatal Network 8:41, 1990.

747. Nevins TE, Danielson G: Prior dialysis does not affect the outcome of pediatric renal transplantation. Pediatr Nephrol 5:211, 1991.

748. Paulson WD, Bock GH, Nelson AP, et al: Hyponatremia in the very young chronic peritoneal dialysis patient. Am J Kidney Dis 14:196, 1989.

749. Gortner L, Leupold D, Pohlandt F, et al: Peritoneal dialysis in the treatment of metabolic crisis caused by inherited disorders of organic and amino acid metabolism. Acta Paediatr Scand 78:706, 1989.

750. Schoenfeld P, Fedusda NJ: Acquired immunodeficiency syndrome and renal disease: Report of the National Kidney Foundation–National Institutes of Health Task Force on AIDS and Kidney Disease. Am J Kidney Dis 16:14, 1990.

751. Graham MM, Bonini LA, Verdi MM: A multi-center study: Clinical practices of HIV infected patients on CAPD/CCPD. Adv Perit Dial 6:88, 1990.

752. Correa-Rotter R, Saldivar S, Soto LE, et al: Recovery of HIV antigen in peritoneal dialysis fluid. Perit Dial Int 10:67, 1990.

753. Schmidt RJ, Cruz C, Dumler F: Effective continuous ambulatory peritoneal dialysis following abdominal aortic aneurysm repair. Perit Dial Int 13:40, 1993.

754. Redrow M, Cherem L, Elliott J, et al: Dialysis in the management of pregnant patients with renal insufficiency. Medicine (Baltimore) 67:199, 1988.

755. Bennett-Jones DN, Aber GM, Baker K: Successful pregnancy in a patient treated with continuous ambulatory peritoneal dialysis. Nephrol Dial Transplant 4:583, 1989.

756. Narva AS: Peritoneal dialysis in a pregnant woman with chronic renal failure. Semin Dial 3:249, 1990.

757. Hou S: Pregnancy in continuous ambulatory peritoneal dialysis (CAPD) patients. Perit Dial Int 10:201, 1990.

758. Vladimirova NN, Darenkov AF, Pashkin IN, et al: A comparative evaluation of the central hemodynamic indices in patients with the terminal stage of kidney failure during dialysis therapy and allografting. Urol Nefrol (Mosk) 5:34, 1990.

759. Buoncristiani U: Combining hemodialysis and peritoneal dialysis. Kidney Int 28:S50, 1985.

760. Hamburger RJ, Mattern WD, Schreiber MJ, et al: A dialysis modality decision guide based on the experience of six dialysis centers. Dial Transplant 19:566, 1990.

761. Coles GA, Khanna R, Zimmerman SW, et al: When should chronic peritoneal dialysis be recommended over hemodialysis? Semin Dial 2:213, 1989.

762. Fine A, Anderson BA, Kirkpatrick J: CAPD in a patient with spinal cord transection—a minefield of disasters. Perit Dial Int 13:69, 1993.

763. Diaz-Buxo JA: CAPD and hemodialysis: Pride and prejudice. Perit Dial Int 10:5, 1990.

764. Groome PA, Hutchinson TA, Prichard SS: ESRD treatment modality selection: Which factors are important in the decision? Adv Perit Dial 7:54, 1991.

765. Stephenson K, Villano R: Results of a predialysis education program. Dial Transplant 22:566, 1993.

766. Campbell J, Ewigman B, Hosokawa M, et al: The timing of referral of patients with end stage renal disease. Dial Transplant 18:660, 1989.

767. Katirtzoglou A, Kontesis P, Myopoulou-Symvoulidis D, et al: Continuous equilibration peritoneal dialysis (CEPD) in hypercatabolic renal failure. Perit Dial Bull 3:178, 1983.

768. Manji S, Shikora S, McMahon M, et al: Peritoneal dialysis for acute renal failure: Overfeeding resulting from dextrose absorbed during dialysis. Crit Care Med 18:29, 1990.

769. Hallett M, Owen J, Becker G, et al: Maintenance of residual renal function: CAPD vs HD. Perit Dial Int 12(suppl 1):124, 1992.

770. Rottembourg J, Issad B, Allouache M, et al: Recovery of renal function in patients treated by CAPD. Adv Perit Dial 5:63, 1989.

771. Michel C, Haddoum F, Viron B, et al: Reprise de fonction rénale après traitement par dialyse péritonéale continue ambulatoire. Nephrologie 10(suppl 2):53, 1989.

772. Bargman JM: Nonuremic indications for peritoneal dialysis. Perit Dial Int 13(suppl 2):S159, 1993.

773. Mailloux LU, Swartz CD, Onesti G, et al: Peritoneal dialysis for refractory congestive heart failure. JAMA 199:873, 1967.

774. Robson M, Biro A, Knobel B, et al: Peritoneal dialysis in refractory congestive heart failure. Part II: Continuous ambulatory peritoneal dialysis (CAPD). Perit Dial Bull 3:133, 1983.

775. Kim D, Khanna R, Wu G, et al: Successful use of continuous ambulatory peritoneal dialysis in refractory heart failure. Perit Dial Bull 5:127, 1985.

776. Rubin J, Ball R: Continuous ambulatory peritoneal dialysis as treatment of severe congestive heart failure in the face of chronic renal failure. Arch Intern Med 146:1533, 1986.

777. Konig PS, Lhotta K, Kronenberg F, et al: CAPD: A successful treatment in patients suffering from therapy-resistant congestive heart failure. Adv Perit Dial 7:97, 1991.

778. Shilo S, Slotki IN, Iaina A: Improved renal function following acute peritoneal dialysis in patients with intractable congestive heart failure. Isr J Med Sci 23:821, 1987.

779. Popovich R, He Z, Moncrief J: Peritoneal membrane plasmapheresis. Perit Dial Int 13(suppl 2):S82, 1993.

780. Mayer AD, McMahon MJ, Corfield AP, et al: Controlled clinical trial of peritoneal lavage for the treatment of severe acute pancreatitis. N Engl J Med 312:399, 1985.

781. Ranson JHC, Berman RS: Long peritoneal lavage decreases pancreatic sepsis in acute pancreatitis. Ann Surg 211:708, 1990.

782. Wall AJ: Peritoneal dialysis in the treatment of severe acute pancreatitis. Med J Aust 2:281, 1965.

783. Ranson JHC, Rifkind KM, Turner JW: Prognostic signs and nonoperative peritoneal lavage in acute pancreatitis. Surg Gynecol Obstet 143:209, 1976.

784. Stone HH, Fabian TC: Peritoneal dialysis in the treatment of acute alcoholic pancreatitis. Surg Gynecol Obstet 150:878, 1980.

785. Bassi C, Briani G, Vesentini S, et al: Continuous peritoneal dialysis in acute experimental pancreatitis in dogs. Effect of aprotinin in the dialysate medium. Int J Pancreatol 5:69, 1989.

786. Crist DW, Cameron JL: The current management of acute pancreatitis. Adv Surg 20:69, 1987.

787. Hanicki Z, Cichocki T, Klein A, et al: Dialysis for psoriasis—preliminary remarks concerning mode of action. Arch Dermatol Res 271:401, 1981.

788. Twardowski ZJ, Lempert KD, Lankhorst BJ, et al: Continuous ambulatory peritoneal dialysis for psoriasis. A report of four cases. Arch Intern Med 146:1177, 1986.

789. Sobh MA, Abdel Rasik MM, Moustafa FE, et al: Dialysis therapy of severe psoriasis: A random study of forty cases. Nephrol Dial Transplant 2:351, 1987.

790. Nissenson AR, Rapaport M, Gordon A, et al: Hemodialysis in the treatment of psoriasis: A controlled trial. Ann Intern Med 91:218, 1979.

791. Whittier FC, Evans DH, Anderson PC, et al: Peritoneal dialysis for psoriasis: A controlled study. Ann Intern Med 99:165, 1983.

792. Inagaki Y, Miyazaki T, Amano I: Peritoneal dialysis as a therapy for electrolyte and acid base disorders. Int J Artif Organs 12:632, 1989.

793. Wiegand C, Thompson T, Bock GH, et al: The management of life-threatening hyperammonemia: A comparison of several therapeutic modalities. J Pediatr 96:142, 1980.

794. Hsu WC, Lin SP, Huang FY, et al: Propionic acidemia: Report of a case that is successfully managed by peritoneal dialysis and sodium benzoate therapy. Chin Med J 46:306, 1990.

795. Sanjurjo P, Jaquotot C, Vallo A, et al: Combined exchange transfusion and peritoneal dialysis treatment in a neonatal case of methylmalonic acidemia with severe hyperammonemia. An Esp Pediatr 17:317, 1982.

796. Moreno-Vega A, Govantes JM: Methylmalonic acidemia treated by continuous ambulatory peritoneal dialysis. N Engl J Med 312:1641, 1985. Letter.

797. McMahon Y, MacDonnell RC Jr: Clearance of branched chain amino acids by peritoneal dialysis in maple syrup urine disease. Adv Perit Dial 6:31, 1990.

798. Clow CL, Reade TM, Scriver CR: Outcome of early and long-term management of classical maple syrup urine disease. Pediatrics 68:856, 1981.

799. Myers C: The use of intraperitoneal chemotherapy in the treatment of ovarian cancer. Semin Oncol 11:275, 1984.

800. Siriwardhana SA, Newfield AM, Lipton JM, et al: Oxygen delivery by the peritoneal route. Can J Anaesth 37(pt 2):S159, 1990. Abstract.

801. Rubin J: Comments on dialysis solution, antibiotic transport, poisonings, and novel uses of peritoneal dialysis. *In* Nolph KD (ed): Peritoneal Dialysis, 3rd ed. Kluwer Academic Publishers, Boston, 1989, p 199.

# Immunobiology of Transplantation

*David L. Perkins*
*Charles B. Carpenter*

## CHARACTERISTICS OF THE ALLOGENEIC IMMUNE RESPONSE

The first successful renal transplant was performed at The Peter Bent Brigham Hospital in Boston in 1954 between identical twins. Recognition of the immunosuppressive properties of azathioprine in combination with corticosteroids facilitated successful transplants from nonidentical donors in the 1960s. However, even with the development of newer immunosuppressive agents, including cyclosporine and monoclonal antibodies, the problem of graft rejection remains a persistent obstacle. Because transplantation was a rare event until modern times, the immune system clearly did not evolve to produce graft rejection. However, we now understand that immune recognition of graft antigens is similar in many aspects to the recognition of infectious pathogens and tumor antigens. In fact, the investigation of the alloimmune response to transplanted tissues led to the identification of the major histocompatibility complex (MHC) molecules and provided early insight into the process of immune recognition.

Although there are many similarities between immune recognition of conventional antigen and the recognition of allogeneic transplantation antigens, the few differences between the allogeneic response and the response to conventional antigen have major implications for transplantation biology. The most striking difference is the markedly increased frequency of responding T cells in the allogeneic response. In addition, in direct recognition of allogeneic MHC molecules, recipient T cells are stimulated by foreign MHC molecules that were not expressed in the thymus and thus not used for positive or negative selection of T cells. The molecular basis for the high frequency of T cells responding to an allogeneic stimulus remains incompletely understood; however, the high frequency of allogeneic specific T cells contributes to the vigorous nature of the immune response causing graft rejection and is the major obstacle to successful organ transplantation.

## TOLERANCE AND IMMUNITY: SELF-NONSELF DISCRIMINATION

The principal tenet of immune recognition is to discriminate self from nonself. The process of discriminating self from nonself is based on two components. First, the immune system must maintain unresponsiveness to all self-antigens primarily through the mechanisms of self-tolerance. Second, nonself antigens derived from numerous sources including pathogens and tumor cells must be effectively recognized to prevent infections and tumors. In addition, the immune system typically recognizes transplanted tissues as nonself, causing graft rejection. The main exceptions involve the transplantation of grafts between genetically similar individuals, for example, identical twins or syngeneic animals. In this case, the grafts are not rejected because they appear identical to self-tissues. The ultimate goal of clinical transplantation is the development of protocols to induce tolerance to the graft so that the immune system recognizes the graft as self.

## Antigen Recognition

Clearly, the immune system did not evolve to reject transplanted organs. Rather, it is commonly accepted that the major function of the immune system is to recognize foreign antigens derived from pathogens and tumors. However, we now know that the processes by which the immune system recognizes conventional antigens and transplantation antigens have many similarities and involve the same antigen recognition molecules. Specifically, the antigen-specific receptors include the T cell receptor on T lymphocytes and antibody molecules produced by B lymphocytes. As discussed in more detail later, the T cell receptor recognizes processed antigen bound to MHC molecules expressed on the surface of antigen-presenting cells. However, there are also unique characteristics of the alloimmune response that must be considered. The most striking are the greater magnitude of the response and the higher frequency of responding lymphocytes. Whereas the response to a conventional antigen can be experimentally detected only after previous immunization, an allogeneic response as assayed in a mixed lymphocyte culture can be detected in a primary response of previously unimmunized lymphocytes. At least part of the basis for the greater magnitude of the allogeneic response is the increased frequency of responding cells. For example, the frequency of specific T cells to conventional antigens is approximately 1 in $10^4$ to $10^5$, whereas the frequency responding during allogeneic stimulation can be as high as 1% to 10%. In addition, the graft, which includes donor antigen-presenting cells, usually expresses class I or class II MHC molecules that differ from the recipient's MHC molecules. These MHC molecules can directly stimulate recipient T cells. Alternatively, donor antigens can be processed and presented by the host's MHC molecules, thus indirectly stimulating the recipient T cells. Relevant to clinical transplantation, the greater magnitude of an allogeneic response can produce vigorous episodes of allograft rejection that can be difficult to control and require high doses of currently available immunosuppressive agents.

## Immune Tolerance

Immune tolerance is a state of unresponsiveness to specific antigens derived from either self or nonself proteins. On the basis of numerous studies, it is clear that the maintenance of immune tolerance to self-antigens involves multiple mechanisms. First, tolerance can occur at the level of either T or B lymphocytes.[1, 2] Second, tolerance can be induced either in immature lymphocytes during the early steps of differentiation or in mature lymphocytes after migration to the peripheral lymphoid tissues, including lymph node and spleen.[3–5] Third, tolerance or immune unresponsiveness can be mediated by several regulatory mechanisms, including clonal deletion of antigen-specific lymphocytes; anergy, in which lymphocytes are inactivated but remain viable; and suppression involving regulatory processes between different subsets of lymphocytes.[6] Evidence from both human studies and animal models indicates that the maintenance of self-tolerance involves many if not all of these mechanisms.

The major mechanism of tolerance induction is the elimination of potentially autoreactive T cells at an immature stage of development during maturation in the thymus by a process termed negative selection. It is estimated that more than 95% of thymocytes die during differentiation before their migration to the peripheral lymphoid organs.[7] However, although thymic selection is a major mechanism for maintaining self-tolerance, it is not a major factor in clinical transplantation because most lymphocytes encountering the allograft are mature T cells that have already completed thymic selection. Thus, the goal of obtaining donor-specific allograft tolerance is to manipulate mechanisms regulating tolerance in mature T cells.

## TRANSPLANTATION ANTIGENS

Normal individuals maintain a state of self-tolerance to self-tissues. However, an allograft expresses nonself antigens to which the recipient is not tolerant, thus causing an antigraft immune response that initiates rejection. Several types of transplantation antigens have been characterized, including the ABO blood group antigens, monocyte and endothelial cell antigens, MHC molecules, and minor histocompatibility antigens.

### ABO Blood Group Antigens

The ABO blood group antigens were initially identified as the cause of transfusion reactions during red blood cell transfusions. The A and B types are caused by differential glycosylation of the red blood cell antigen, whereas type O lacks the enzymes necessary for glycosylation. The antigens are readily recognized by natural antibodies termed hemagglutinins, which cause the agglutination of red blood cells. Relevant to transplantation, the antigens are also expressed on other cell types, including endothelial cells, and thus usually cause hyperacute rejection of vascular allografts due to preformed antibody. Specifically, individuals with types A and B produce antibodies to the other type, and those with type O produce antibodies to both A and B. However, because type O does not express the glycosylated moiety, both A and B fail to produce antibodies to type O. Thus, type O grafts can be transplanted into any of the blood types. This is not commonly done for ethical reasons to prevent the depletion of available grafts for type O recipients. Allograft rejection due to blood type mismatch can readily be prevented by appropriate blood typing before transplantation.

## Monocyte and Endothelial Cell Antigens

Allografts occasionally undergo hyperacute rejection despite appropriate ABO matching. Some of these rejection episodes have been attributed to additional non-ABO antigens expressed on endothelial cells and monocytes. The characterization of these antigens is an active area of research; however, they remain poorly understood. Pretransplant tissue typing does not currently evaluate the endothelial and monocyte antigens because of the rarity of their occurrence and the lack of accurate reagents for typing.

## Major and Minor Histocompatibility Antigens

The most important transplantation antigens are the MHC antigens. The MHC antigens were originally discovered in tumor transplants between different inbred strains of mice. We now know that the MHC antigens are cell surface molecules that present processed antigen to T lymphocytes. Furthermore, there is evidence that the minor histocompatibility antigens are processed antigens in the form of small peptides that bind to the MHC molecule. T cells recognize a combination of the antigen and MHC molecule through a trimolecular interaction involving the T cell receptor, MHC molecule, and processed antigen in the form of a short peptide. The MHC antigens are the strongest transplantation antigens and can stimulate a primary immune response. The minor histocompatibility antigens require previous priming and can be detected only in a secondary immune response. The role of major and minor histocompatibility antigens is crucial to understanding transplantation biology and is discussed in detail in the following section.

## MAJOR HISTOCOMPATIBILITY COMPLEX

The antigenic stimulus for initiation and progression of the rejection response to grafted tissue is provoked by cell surface molecules that are polymorphic, that is, they vary in structure from individual to individual, and these differences are treated as foreign intruders to be recognized and destroyed. Transplantation antigens are classified according to their relative potencies in eliciting rejection as either major or minor. The major antigens in all mammalian species studied are encoded by a closely linked series of genes called the MHC. The MHC was first defined in the mouse by Gorer[8] and Snell[9] as responsible for rapid rejection of tumor transplants between inbred strains of mice. This antigen system was called H-2 and was found to function in rejection of normal tissues as well. Rejection elicits serum antibodies that are used for typing of H-2 antigens. It was subsequently shown that cytotoxic T cells also arise in response to H-2 differences and that the H-2 genes are all clustered in a single region on chromosome 17.[10–12] Except for some details of the ordering of genes, the human (HLA) and rat (RT1) MHC regions are homologous to H-2. HLA

is located on the short arm of chromosome 6.[13, 14] The species' chromosome numbers are different only because they have not been numbered in a manner reflecting the location of actual genes. Transplants compatible for the MHC antigens can still be rejected because of minor antigen (H-1, H-3, H-4, and so on) incompatibilities, but not with the same intensity as with MHC-incompatible grafts. Modification of rejection by drugs or other means is more readily accomplished when the donor and recipient MHC antigens are matched. Extensive work in the mouse skin graft model with a large number of different major (H-2) and minor incompatibilities has shown, in general, that the sum total of multiple non–H-2 (minor) incompatibilities, once the recipient has become immunized to such antigens, can be equal to the strength of the H-2 barrier alone in the unimmunized, or first-set, rejection response.[15] For MHC or non-MHC barriers, when a second graft is placed from the same donor, it is rejected at an accelerated pace (second-set rejection). Discernment of first- versus second-set rejection phenomena in humans was first made by Holman[16] in 1924 with skin grafts in patients with burns. During World War II, the problem of extensive burn injuries prompted the initiation of fundamental studies in skin grafting by Medawar.[17]

Together with the emerging concept of a major transplantation antigen system,[8, 9] these studies laid the groundwork for the development of clinical transplantation in the second half of the 20th century. Although the initial discovery and definition of the MHC came from studies in transplantation, the central role of MHC in the initiation and expression of the immune response in general has become increasingly evident. The ability to produce an efficient immune response to many antigens is inherited in a mendelian autosomal dominant fashion, and the controlling genes, called Ir for "immune response," are of the MHC. In fact, the failure to mount a response to a peptide antigen may now be attributed to a genetically determined inability to bind the antigenic fragment to MHC molecules. The complex of antigen and MHC provides an efficient mode of presentation to those clones of T lymphocytes bearing the appropriate antigen receptors. Indeed, it is clear that the T cell receptor recognizes the total configuration of self-MHC plus the antigen fragment, and not antigen alone. Many experimental systems have demonstrated this MHC restriction phenomenon (i.e., responding T cells, to respond, must share MHC antigens with the antigen-presenting cells). The combined recognition of self-MHC + antigen (self + X hypothesis) is now being visualized at the molecular level, as described later.

The HLA region on the short arm of chromosome 6 (Fig. 58–1) encompasses more than 3 million nucleotide base pairs. It encodes two structurally distinct classes of cell surface molecules, termed class I and class II (Fig. 58–2). The term MHC antigen has traditionally been applied to the product of a given locus that displays polymorphism in a population of individuals. Now that the sequence and structure of molecules bearing MHC antigens have been extensively elucidated, it is known that the polymorphic, or antigenic, portions of MHC molecules are indeed small, often involving only one to four amino acid substitutions in regions where sequence hypervariability occurs. The specific

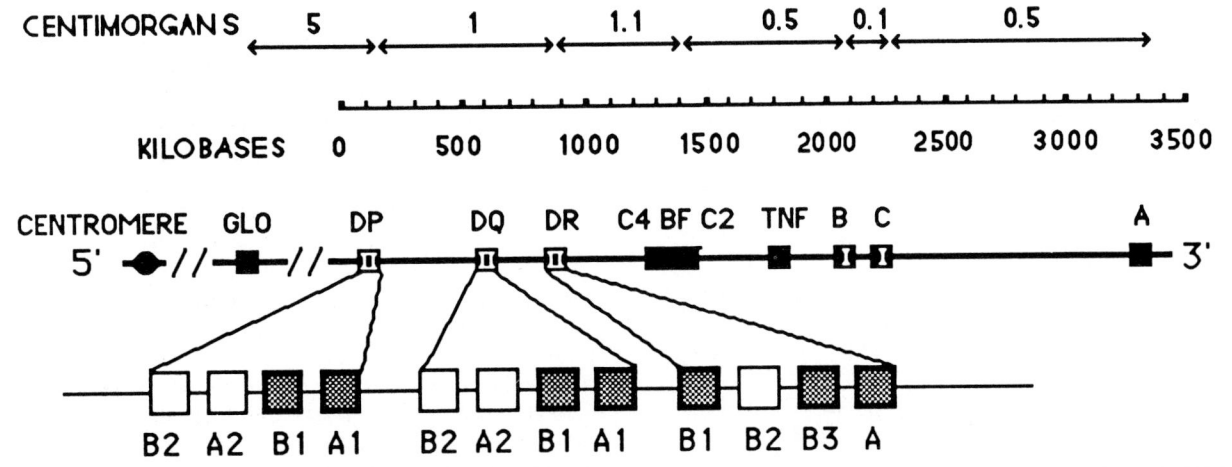

**Figure 58–1.** Schematic map of the HLA region on the short arm of chromosome 6. Distances are shown in centimorgans, deduced from observed recombination frequencies in family studies (1 cM represents a 1% crossover rate), and also in kilobases derived from sequencing of DNA nucleotides. The centromere is to the left (5′). The boxes along the central line represent coding regions for the HLA polypeptides expressed on cell surfaces. GLO is a polymorphic red blood cell enzyme more than 5 cM from HLA. On the right are the *HLA-A, -B,* and *-C* loci for the three sets of class I heavy chains; on the left are the loci for the three sets of class II molecules, HLA-DP, -DQ, and -DR. The class II molecules are composed of two chains, α and β, each of which is a product of genes of the DP, DQ, or DR subregions. A *DRA* gene encodes the α-chain, for example, and a *DRB* gene encodes the β-chain of the heterodimeric HLA-DR molecule. As shown in the expansion at the bottom, each subregion contains tandem sets of exons for one or more α- and β-chains. The gene for DR private specificities is *DRB1*; the more public DRw52 and DRw53 are encoded by *DRB3* and *DRB4*, respectively. The *DRB3* and *DRB4* genes are found alternatively on most haplotypes, and only *DRB3* is shown in the figure. Each DRB product associates with the single nonpolymorphic DRA gene product on the cell surface. Pseudogenes, not expressed on the cell surface, are shown as white boxes. Genes involved in proteolysis of protein antigens and the intracellular transport of peptides to meet up with class I molecules are in the class II region near DQ. Between the class I and class II loci are genes for the complement components C2, BF(factor B), and C4. Genes for 21OH (steroid 21-hydroxylase) are not shown but are between C4 and BF. An expansion of the class III region would show that both C4 and 21OH are reduplicated, so that the order is -(C4A-21OHA-C4B-21OHB-BF-C2)-. The genes of this region are sometimes referred to as class III, although they bear little homology to those of class I and class II, which show homology to each other. The genes for TNF-α and TNF-β have been mapped between C4 and HLA-B.

substituted area in an MHC molecule that causes a change in antigenicity is called an epitope. Normal pregnancy induces antibodies against the HLA antigens of the fetus derived from the father's genes. Although normal human pregnancies are the main source of antisera used for HLA typing, the first appreciation of the HLA system came from the studies of Dausset[13] on blood transfusion reactions due to antileukocyte antibodies. One such antibody from patient MAC proved to be a pregnancy-induced anti–HLA-2 response. Subsequent studies by Payne and co-workers[18] showed that such antibodies marked a codominantly expressed antileukocyte system that segregated in mendelian fashion in families. International workshops on the HLA system began in 1962, and this series continues to accelerate progress in the definition and technical aspects of typing for the polymorphic antigens of this chromosomal region.[19] By international agreement, HLA is the logo for the human MHC. Although the individual letters of the logo have different historical meanings, such as "human," "histocompatibility," "leukocyte," "lymphocyte," "locus," and "antigen," HLA as the logo is used as the prefix to a locus or subregion designation that marks all that follows as a product of the human MHC chromosomal region (e.g., HLA-A2 and HLA-DR4).

Class I and class II molecules show some structural homology to immunoglobulins, to the T cell antigen receptor, and to molecules bearing the T cell differentiation antigens CD4 and CD8. The last form a part of the system whereby T cells preferentially interact with class II or class I molecules, respectively, on antigen-presenting accessory cells or

on cells that are targets for immune destruction. This family of cell surface and extracellular recognition or interaction structures may have evolved from the same progenitor gene, diversifying by duplication and mutation, and in the process the new genes have moved to multiple chromosomal locations. All mammalian species studied thus far have structural and functional representations of this "immunoglobulin supergene" family.[20]

## Human Leukocyte Antigen Molecules

### CLASS I

These molecules consist of two polypeptide chains in noncovalent association on cell surfaces. The heavy (44,000 daltons) chain is inserted into the plasma membrane and contains the antigenic portions. The light (12,000 daltons) chain is β2-microglobulin, encoded by a gene on chromosome 15. There are three domains of the class I heavy chain, formed in part by disulfide bonding to make loops as schematized in Figure 58–2. The amino acid sequence variable regions are on the first ($\alpha_1$) and second ($\alpha_2$) domains. Class I molecules are expressed on almost all nucleated body cells, including the endothelium of blood vessels. Tissue typing is performed with peripheral blood, lymph node, or spleen lymphocytes, all of which strongly express HLA class I. Platelets are not commonly used for typing, but they are useful for absorbing anti–class I antibodies from serum because they lack expression of class II anti-

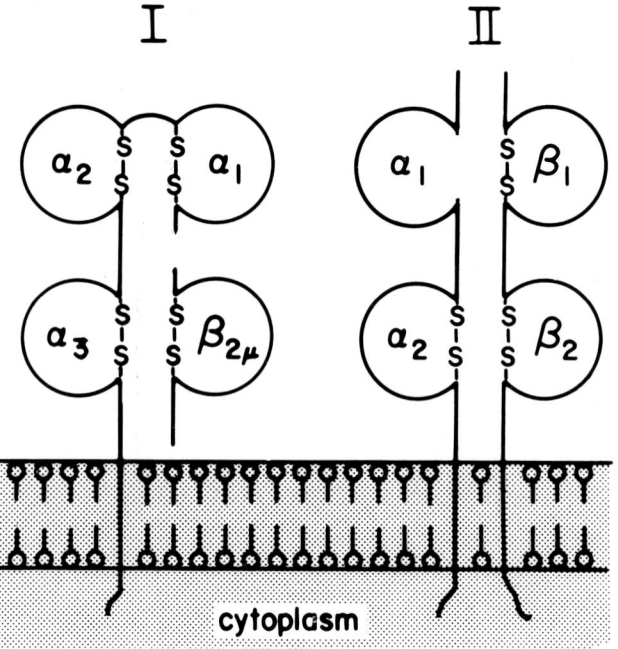

**Figure 58–2.** Diagrammatic view of class I and class II HLA molecules on a cell membrane. The 44,000-dalton α-chain is inserted through the lipid bilayer of the membrane and has three domains ($\alpha_1$, $\alpha_2$, $\alpha_3$) formed in part by disulfide bonding. $\beta_2$-Microglobulin, encoded by a gene on chromosome 15, is noncovalently bound and is not membrane inserted. The $\alpha_2$- and $\alpha_1$-domains form the β-strands and α-helices, which form the base and sides, respectively, of the groove that binds immunogenic peptides. The variable amino acids that provide the antigenic differences between individual HLA types are arrayed along this groove. Class II molecules consist of one α-chain (34,000 daltons) and one β-chain (28,000 daltons); each chain has two domains, and each is membrane inserted. A similar peptide-binding groove is formed by the $\alpha_1$- and $\beta_1$-domains of class II molecules. (Modified from Carpenter CB, Strom TB: Immunobiology of transplantation. Top Nephrol 19:1, 1989. Churchill Livingstone, New York, 1989.)

gens. Some organ-specific anatomic variation occurs in endothelial expression, and in states of active inflammation, the density of class I can be locally increased, as reviewed in more detail later. There are three class I heavy chain loci, *HLA-A, -B,* and *-C* (see Fig. 58–1). Each locus product in a given individual bears a unique so-called private antigen and additional public antigens that are shared more widely among the population. There are more than 80 well-defined A and B locus and 10 C locus private antigens.[21, 22] The independence of the HLA-A, -B, and -C molecules on the cell surface can be demonstrated by observing with fluorescent markers the separate aggregation and capping of each set of molecules when antibodies specific to each locus are added. When antibodies to $\beta_2$-microglobulin are added, all class I molecules are capped.

The first MHC molecule to be crystallized was HLA-A2, and the structure of this class I allele was determined by x-ray diffraction studies[23] to a resolution of 0.35 nm (Fig. 58–3). This accomplishment provided visualization of how the amino acid sequence is related to the folding of the chains into a three-dimensional structure. The two membrane distal domains, $\alpha_1$ and $\alpha_2$, form a groove along the top surface of the molecule facing away from the cell membrane. The margins of the groove are formed by α-helices, and the

base is floored by a series of eight parallel β-strands, with the $\alpha_1$- and $\alpha_2$-domains contributing more or less equally to each side of the structure. In the crystallographic study, the groove, approximately 2.5 nm long and 1.0 nm wide, contained an unidentified molecule that has been shown in subsequent studies to represent the bound peptide fragment, which is eight or nine amino acids long. These peptides have an extended linear core structure, and binding is to a large measure determined by side chain interactions. When the locations of amino acid variations, already known from study of sequences and interactions with antibodies or cytotoxic T cells, are related to the crystal structure, it is remarkable that the HLA variable sites lie along the α-helical and β-strand surfaces that form the margins of the groove[24] (see Fig. 58–3). In other words, the polymorphisms serve to define the shape of the binding groove on MHC molecules and hence determine which peptides will be bound and recognized by T cells. The sites that determine whether a given peptide binds may also confer a conformational change on the fragment. The result is that the T cell receptor binds to the unique topography of the MHC surface formed by a given MHC and peptide combination. The T cell receptor has two chains, α and β (or γ and δ), which form a heterodimer (Fig. 58–4). The membrane distal surface of the assembled T cell receptor has six variable loops that provide the specificity of binding to the α-helices and bound peptide antigen.[25, 26] Further details of the interaction with MHC should be discernible when the crystal structure of the T cell receptor becomes available. Additional human and mouse class I molecules have been crystallized, and the hypothesis that allelic polymorphisms determine binding of different peptide sequences has been confirmed. Peptides found in eluates from class I crystals or purified molecules are usually eight or nine residues in length. Their origin is in the intracellular pool of polypeptides derived from metabolic turnover of housekeeping proteins or intracellular infections, such as viruses. There is selective proteolysis and transmembrane transport from lysosomal compartments into the Golgi, where peptides eight or nine amino acids long are placed in class I binding sites before transport to the cell surface. Some of the genes controlling this process are in the class II region of the MHC.

## CLASS II

As shown in Figure 58–2, these molecules consist of two membrane-inserted and noncovalently associated glycosylated polypeptides, called α (34,000 daltons) and β (28,000 daltons). Each of these chains has two domains, and again the polymorphic regions are mostly on the outer, $NH_2$-terminal, domains.[21] The region of HLA encompassing class II genes is generally referred to as HLA-D. Although three class II molecules, HLA-DP, -DQ, and -DR, are generally recognized on cell surfaces, the situation is not entirely analogous to class I because the α- and β-chains of each class II molecule are encoded by separate, closely linked genes (see Fig. 58–1). Although α- and β-chains of opposite haplotypes can associate, such hybrid associations are generally restricted to products of the same DP, DQ, or DR subregion. The naming of HLA-D region genes is

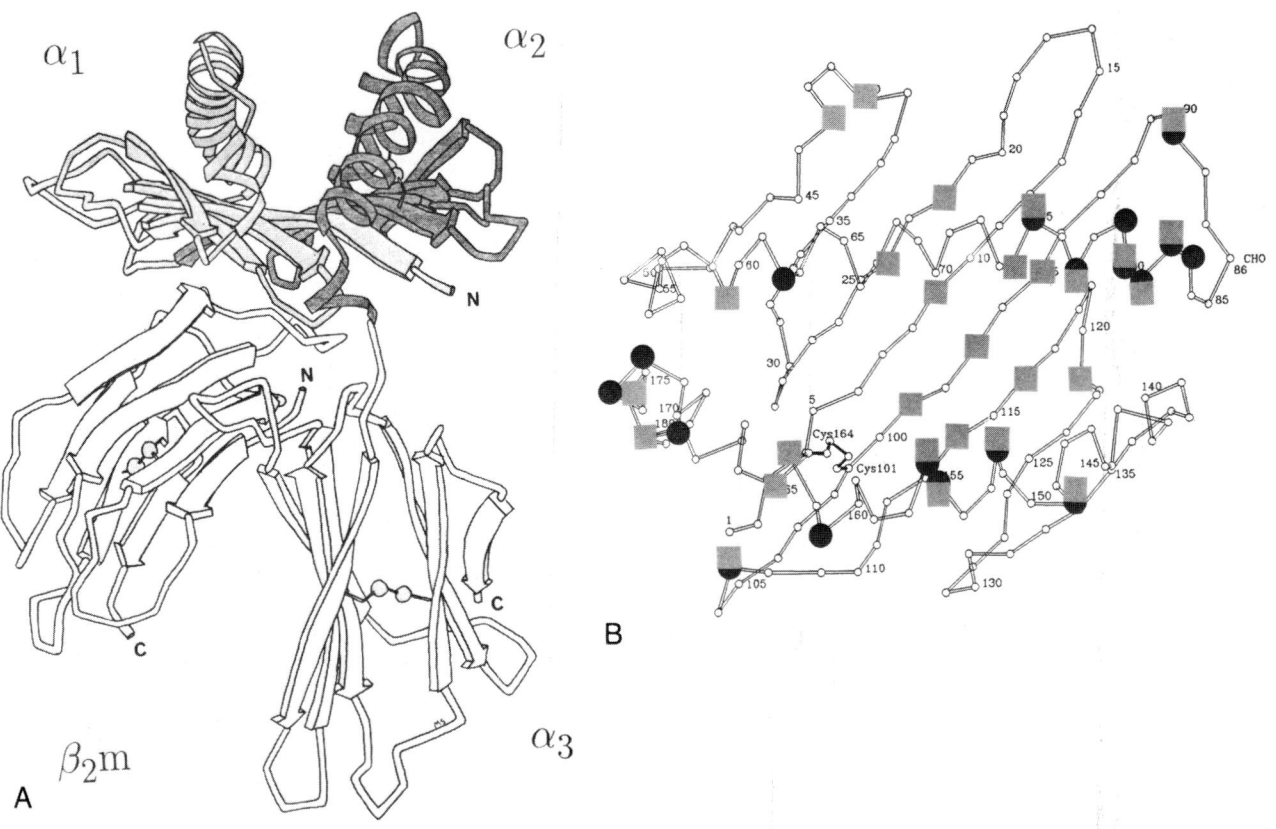

**Figure 58–3.** Diagram of the structure of the HLA-A2 molecule derived from x-ray crystallographic study. *A.* The flat ribbons represent the β-strands; the spiral areas at the top (membrane distal) are the α-helices, which form the sides of a groove approximately 1.0 nm wide and 2.5 nm long. The floor of the groove is formed by eight parallel β-strands. The COOH-terminal end (C) of the α₃-domain is inserted in the membrane. (From Bjorkman PJ, Saper MA, Samroui B, et al: Structure of the human class I histocompatibility antigen, HLA-A2. Reprinted with permission from Nature 329:506, 1987. Copyright 1987 Macmillan Magazines Limited.) *B.* This view looks down on the top of the molecule, so that the groove goes from left to right. Diagrammed is the core structure of the amino acid sequence, consecutively numbered from 1 *(bottom left)* to 180 *(center left)*. The symbols show the variable amino acid substitutions that have been identified in different human or mouse haplotypes as relating to changes in reactivity to alloreactive T cells *(gray squares)* or to monoclonal antibodies *(black circles)*. Sites that relate to both are shown as dual symbols. Whereas the antibody sites are on the external surface of the helices, many of the T cell sites are at the base of the groove. The variable sites determine which peptide sequences can be bound by a given MHC allele (see text). (Modified from Bjorkman PJ, Saper MA, Samroui B, et al: The foreign antigen binding site and T cell recognition regions of class I histocompatibility antigens. Reprinted with permission from Nature 329:512, 1987. Copyright 1987 Macmillian Magazines Limited.)

based on knowledge of the biochemistry of expressed antigens and on a growing database of DNA nucleotide sequencing. The gene encoding the HLA-DR α-chain, for example, is called *DRA*, and *DRB1*, *DRB3*, and *DRB4* are the closely linked genes encoding β-chains for the common DR antigens *(DRB1)*, DRw52 *(DRB3)*, and DRw53 *(DRB4)*. Each of the DR β-chains associates with the common nonpolymorphic DR α-chain at the cell surface to form functional class II HLA-DR molecules. The HLA-DQ subregion contains the genes *DQA1, DQB1, DQA2,* and *DQB2*. The last two are nonexpressed pseudogenes; the products of the first two, DQα and DQβ, are both polymorphic. HLA-DP is similarly organized. Study by the Southern blot technique to determine restriction fragment length polymorphisms of DNA digested with various nucleases and hybridized to complementary DNA probes specific for the HLA genes has been shown to provide an alternative detection technique that has been particularly informative for class II genes.[27, 28] More rapid and precise detection of actual DNA sequences can now be accomplished by selec-

tive polymerase chain reaction amplification of polymorphic gene regions, followed by hybridization with short oligonucleotide probes specific for a given HLA sequence or by restriction fragment length polymorphism analysis of the amplified product.[29, 30] Comparative studies in ongoing workshops have demonstrated a strong correlation between serologically defined polymorphisms and those identified by T cell clones reactive to class II molecules.

Analysis of crystals of class II HLA-DR1[31] shows a remarkable similarity to class I in the peptide-binding region. The α-helical and β-strand core structures of class I and class II are virtually superimposable. The main difference is at the ends of the groove, which in class II are somewhat more open, allowing binding of longer peptides. Typically, the length of eluted peptides from class II molecules is 13 to 26 residues,[32] and there is protrusion of the linearly arrayed peptide at both ends of the groove.[31, 32] Class II antigens are limited in expression to B lymphocytes and some macrophages-monocytes, dendritic cells, and activated T lymphocytes. Human endothelium generally does

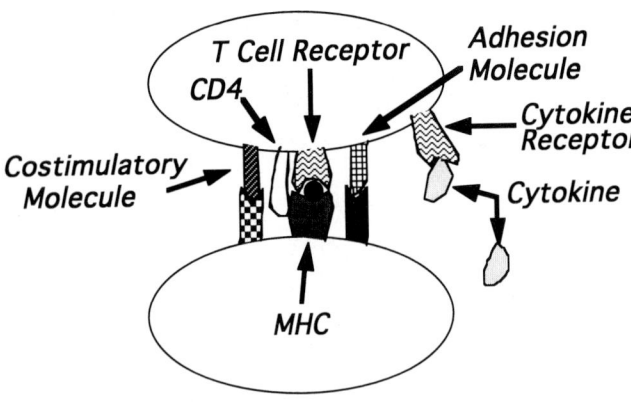

**Figure 58–4.** T cell interaction with an antigen-presenting cell. Multiple receptors on the surface of T cells interact with counter-receptors on antigen-presenting cells. The receptors expressed by T cells can be arbitrarily divided into five categories, including 1) the antigen-specific T cell receptor, 2) the CD4 or CD8 coreceptor, 3) the adhesion molecule, 4) the costimulatory molecule, and 5) the cytokine receptor. Multiple examples of each category have been identified except for the antigen receptor. As discussed in the text, examples of immunosuppression have been observed by inhibition of each category of receptor with monoclonal antibodies or soluble counterligands.

not express class II, but this situation can change rapidly when there is inflammation in the vicinity. In addition, epithelial cells of skin, intestine, and renal proximal tubule can synthesize and express class II molecules in response to injury and inflammation.[33] Peptides bound to class II molecules are derived from proteolysis in acidic endosomal compartments and represent endocytosed proteins or microorganisms coming from outside of the antigen-presenting cells; hence, the extracellular compartment, in contrast to the intracellular compartment for class I, is the responsibility of the typical class II–positive antigen-presenting cell. When foreign polypeptide antigens are added to cultured antigen-presenting cells, peptide fragments appear on class II but not on class I molecules in a matter of minutes. Peptide fragments of self-MHC class I and class II are found in the eluates from class II molecules,[32] indicating that there is representation of intracellularly synthesized products on class II at the cell surface or that secreted molecules re-enter the cell by the endocytic pathway.

## The Nature of Allorecognition

T cell recognition of allo-MHC is the primary and central event that initiates allograft rejection.[34, 35] Allo-MHC molecules induce strong primary immune responses in vitro in the mixed lymphocyte response and cytotoxic T lymphocyte assays.[36–38] It has long been recognized that the normal T cell repertoire contains a high frequency (1% to 10%) of total T cells that are capable of responding to allo-MHC molecules.[39] This translates to a precursor frequency at least 100 times that of antigen-specific self-restricted T cells, which recognize conventional antigens as peptide fragments bound to self-MHC. The vigor of the primary alloimmune response has puzzled transplant immunologists for almost three decades.[40–42] The original hypothesis regarding the

high frequency of alloreactive T cells[43, 44] proposed that the repertoire of lymphocytes was preselected by evolutionary pressure to include specificity for the MHC molecules of the species. It was also proposed that the lymphocyte repertoire that recognizes conventional antigens was derived by somatic mutation of the T cell receptor specific for self-MHC. However, it is now known that T cell receptors do not undergo somatic mutations, and there is evidence from studies with T cell clones that the antigen-specific and alloreactive T cell repertoires may be contained within the same clones.[45–48]

There are two fundamental questions in allorecognition: First, why is the frequency of alloreactive T cells so high? Second, how can positively selected self-MHC–restricted T cells recognize foreign antigens as well as allo-MHC? For one thing, it is apparent that there are at least two distinct, but not necessarily mutually exclusive, pathways of allorecognition.[49–51] In the so-called direct pathway, T cells recognize intact allo-MHC molecules on the surface of donor or stimulator cells. In the so-called indirect pathway, T cells recognize processed allo-MHC in the context of self–antigen–presenting cells, which is the normal route of T cell recognition. The contribution of the direct and indirect pathways of allorecognition to allograft rejection has not been thoroughly investigated, but it is apparent that both pathways are activated with alloimmunization and that specific tolerance-inducing pathways directed to the indirect pathway can be sufficient to prevent graft rejection.

The direct recognition of intact MHC molecules, although focused on the polymorphic MHC epitopes, is strongly influenced by the presence of peptide in the MHC groove. MHC molecules "empty" of peptide are generally not recognized unless the missing self-peptides are reconstituted.[52–56] It has also been shown that changing the bound peptide can alter the allorecognition of a given MHC molecule.[57] Lechler and colleagues[58] showed that human T cell clones with dual specificity for influenza hemagglutinin and HLA-DR1 or -DR4 were able to recognize DR1-expressing mouse DAP.3 transfectants but not DR4-expressing DAP.3 cells. However, addition of the hemagglutinin peptide restored the anti-DR4 response. Because a given MHC molecule can bind many different peptides, including some derived from self-MHC,[32] a high number of possible MHC-peptide combinations can occur that provide a great diversity of MHC binding regions for presentation to the T cell pool. Thus, during thymic selection of the T cell repertoire, a considerable number of clones will survive that are cross-reactive with allo-MHC.

Minor histocompatibility antigens are fundamentally different from MHC antigens. They are recognized as peptides bound to self-MHC. Because most minor incompatibilities elicit class I–restricted T cell responses, it seems likely that they are peptides derived from intracellular proteins of the same cell.[59–61]

The basic premise for indirect allorecognition as a mechanism for initiation or amplification of allograft rejection is that donor alloantigens are shed from the graft, taken up by recipient antigen-presenting cells, and presented to T cells. It has also been demonstrated that intact HLA molecules are present in the circulation of renal transplant recipients.[62] Therefore, during transplantation, shed fragments of allo-

MHC could be processed by host antigen-presenting cells and presented as allopeptides to T cells on self-MHC. This indirect pathway of allorecognition may activate T helper cells, which secrete lymphokines and provide the necessary signals for the growth and maturation of effector cytotoxic T lymphocytes and B cells, leading to allograft rejection.[50, 51, 63, 64] The direct recognition of allo-MHC on the surface of donor cells and the indirect recognition of processed allo-MHC presented by self-antigen–presenting cells are mutually exclusive pathways, because each is mediated by different sets of T cell clones. However, cells of MHC partially matched grafts can present allopeptides bound to the MHC molecule that is shared between donor and recipient. In a study designed to assess the role of the direct pathway, Braun and co-workers[65] showed that adoptive transfer of a rat CD4+ T cell line or clone primed by the direct pathway could effect early acute rejection of normal kidney grafts but could not initiate rejection of passenger cell–depleted kidney allografts, indicating that the main target of such clones was the hematopoietic passenger cells and not the kidney parenchyma. Dalchau and associates[66] demonstrated that LEW (RT1$^l$) rats primed by immunization with soluble class I or class II allo-MHC molecules derived from DA (RT1.A$^{avl}$) rats produce antibodies to the soluble allo-MHC molecules and reject specific skin allografts in an accelerated fashion, which suggests that self-restricted T cell recognition of processed allo-MHC can play a role in allograft rejection. These studies confirmed earlier studies in the mouse model by Sherwood and colleagues,[67] which showed that adoptively transferred syngeneic plastic adherent splenocytes primed by the indirect pathway in vivo could sensitize a recipient to reject skin allografts in an accelerated fashion.

Further studies of the role of the indirect pathway are based on the availability of sequences of MHC genes in mice, rats, and humans, which makes it possible to prepare synthetic allopeptides. With these, one can study the mechanisms of self-restricted T cell recognition of processed allo-MHC. Benichou and co-workers[68] demonstrated that mouse class I and class II self-MHC peptides could bind with high affinity to class II molecules on the surface of self-antigen–presenting cells and be presented in the context of intact class II self-molecules to induce a strong proliferative T cell response. They showed that potentially autoreactive T cell clones may escape thymic education and that these clones could be made tolerant by neonatal injection of the self-MHC peptide. In a subsequent study,[69] they demonstrated that mouse T cells primed by immunization with allogeneic splenocytes or by skin allografts are capable of proliferating to polymorphic synthetic class II MHC allopeptides when they are presented by self-antigen–presenting cells. Human class II peptides have also been shown to be alloreactive in vitro.[70] The immunogenicity of class I[71] and class II[72] rat allopeptides has been established. T cells reactive to the indirect mode of presentation appear early in a rat heart rejection model.[63] Such peptides are also tolerogenic by the oral route[72] and when injected into the thymus.[73] In the latter instance, indefinite rat kidney allograft survival is induced after a single exposure of the thymus in vivo to class II peptides, even though a strong class I antigenic difference is also present in the transplanted or-

gan. It appears that the indirect pathway can be the main driving force for induction of a full allogeneic response. The detailed mechanisms of intrathymic tolerance to allografts remain unclear, but development of an unresponsive (anergic) state in peripheral T cells has been demonstrated.

## Inheritance of Human Leukocyte Antigens

Because chromosomes are paired, each individual has two sets of HLA antigens, one from each parent. The genetically linked antigens of the entire HLA region inherited from one parent are termed a haplotype; by simple mendelian dominant inheritance, 25% of sib pairs will inherit the same parental haplotypes, 50% will share one haplotype, and 25% will be completely different (Fig. 58–5). The main evidence that HLA is the major transplantation barrier in humans originally came from the results of renal transplantation in which HLA-identical sib donor grafts provided the best long-term graft survival with use of minimal immunosuppression.[74, 75] In the absence of a recombination (crossover), the entire HLA region from A to DP, including the specific electrophoretic polymorphisms of C4, BF, and C2, will be expressed with each inherited haplotype. Recombination rates within the region are in the vicinity of 1%; hence, it is generally not necessary to type for the expressed products of all the loci to identify haplotypes within a family. Rarely, when recombination has occurred, or when several common antigens are present on both sides of a family, complete typing of DQ, DP, and complement may be necessary.

The distribution of HLA antigens within the general population is not random. Some are more common than others, and racial and ethnic patterns are well known. Furthermore, within a given racial and ethnic group, certain HLA haplotypes, or portions thereof, are likely to be found in higher frequencies than one would predict by random distribution.

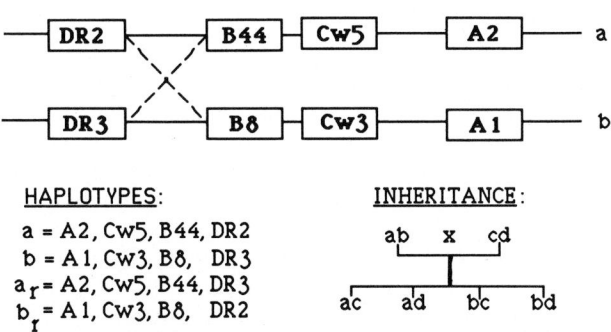

**Figure 58–5.** Inheritance of HLA haplotypes. The *HLA-A, -Cw, -B,* and *-DR* genes are shown to represent the entire region. The haplotypes of parents are assigned letters a, b, c, and d, and they are inherited as a block unless a recombination has occurred during meiosis of an ovum or sperm, shown here as a dotted X between *B* and *DR* in the parent ab. Such events occur less than 1% of the time for HLA. Children inherit one of each of the parental HLA haplotypes and are therefore of four potential types: ac, ad, bc, bd. The chance of an HLA-identical sib pair in a family is 1:4. There are similar odds for sibs being nonidentical (e.g., ac and bd). Haploidentical sibs occur with odds of 1:2, and all children are haploidentical with each parent.

For example, HLA-A1, -B8, and -DR3 are commonly found on the same haplotype in northern Europeans. These alleles are not in equilibrium and are stated, therefore, to be in linkage disequilibrium. When entire, so-called extended haplotypes[76] are found in apparently unrelated individuals, it is likely that they were inherited from a common ancestor. When alleles of adjacent loci of the HLA region (e.g., *B* and *DR*) are in linkage disequilibrium, the possibility exists of selective pressures having been exerted for many generations to maintain the coexpression of a favorable combination with regard to defense against infectious diseases. Review of the associations of HLA alleles with a number of diseases is beyond the purpose of this chapter, but linkage disequilibria are relevant to considerations of HLA antigen distribution throughout the general population, a matter of direct concern to matching donors for transplantation.

## TISSUE TYPING

### Human Leukocyte Antigen Typing

The main source of antibodies for typing comes from large-scale screening of thousands of serum samples from multiparous women. Immunizations among humans yield the most highly specific antibodies to private HLA determinants. Anti–class I (HLA-A, -B, -C) antibodies react with both B and T lymphocytes, whereas anti–class II antibodies react with B but not T cells. Generally, a positive reaction is marked by cell lysis in the presence of rabbit complement. In addition, more broadly reactive antisera, originally thought to contain several antibodies in mixture, may have reactivity to the public determinants. For example, there are at least three immunogenic regions on HLA-B molecules, one for private and two for public polymorphisms.[77] Monoclonal antibodies derived from the immunization of mice or rats with human lymphocytes only occasionally bind to the same antigenic sites defined by human antibodies. Although there are several examples of monoclonal antibodies that may substitute for human antisera, there are a large number of monoclonal antibodies that react in a public fashion, but not necessarily in the same patterns as with human antisera.

The mixed lymphocyte response occurs when lymphocytes of one individual are cultured with those of another. Proliferation occurs in 5 to 7 days and is measured by the incorporation rate of [$^3$H]thymidine into newly replicated DNA.[78] Usually, one population of cells is irradiated to prevent their proliferation, and the readout represents the response of nonirradiated helper T cells to the class II antigens present on stimulator B cells or macrophages. Before the HLA-DP, -DQ, and -DR subregions were defined, the entire incompatibility for the mixed lymphocyte response was called HLA-D. HLA-DR determinants provide the strongest mixed lymphocyte response stimulus, whereas HLA-DQ plays a lesser role. HLA-DP is recognized only by primed (previously stimulated) cells. The mixed lymphocyte response itself is a complex series of cellular responses; not only are helper cell clones activated to proliferate, but they precede the proliferative burst of CD8$^+$ cytotoxic T cells. These are generally directed to class I

incompatibilities and injure appropriate target cells after direct cell-cell contact is initiated by T cell antigen receptors. When cytotoxic T cells are tested against a large number of individuals typed by classic serologic methods, a good but not perfect correlation is found overall. Some antigenic sites, or epitopes, recognized by T cells are actually different from those on the same class I molecule recognized by antibodies. This is explained by the fact that immunoglobulins can recognize small epitopes on intact whole molecules with tertiary structures, whereas T cells "see" only the complex surface made up of peptide bound in the MHC binding groove. Further, there is more than one diversity site per HLA molecule providing targets for rejection. Although the private specificities are, by definition, most immunogenic in the human-antihuman alloresponse, the other variable regions may provide sites for cell-cell or molecular interactions during an immune response.

The marked superiority of HLA haplotype–identical sib donors for organ and bone marrow transplantation has been demonstrable since the early 1970s. When azathioprine and prednisone were used as standard therapy, initial graft loss rates were in the 5% to 10% range during the first year, followed by half-lives of graft survival in the 25- to 30-year range.[75] Now that the quality of HLA typing is more reliable, a major question is whether similar results can be obtained with unrelated donors matched for all, or most, of the HLA loci.

The goal of graft tolerance may be accomplished by more potent and specific immunosuppression, by reduction in the histocompatibility barriers, or by a combination of both. In addition, management of infections and judicious attention to treatment of rejection activity also contribute in a major way to clinical success. The entire field of clinical transplantation has been making steady and parallel progress in immunosuppression, tissue typing, and care of patients. Overall survivals of patients and grafts have been improving in the past decade and had been improving even before the widespread use of cyclosporine.[79] Although there have been numerous reports on the benefits of HLA antigen matching in cadaveric transplantation through the years, there have also been a number of negative studies from some centers. One of the major problems in interpretation of such data relates to the fact that the average level of success has been rising from year to year. The technology of HLA typing itself is a major factor. It is fair to say that widespread competency in both class I and class II typing, particularly in the latter, has been achieved only in the past 3 to 5 years, and there is direct evidence that technical difficulties with HLA typing can account for poor correlations with graft results.[80] Finally, most single-center studies have not included sufficient numbers of well-matched cases to establish the role of such matching. Hence, the most valuable databases now in existence are those representing pooling of information from a large number of collaborating centers.

Data are now available from collections of cases containing thousands of consecutive transplantations. These include the studies at the University of California at Los Angeles by Terasaki and colleagues[81] and the Collaborative Transplant Study of Opelz.[82, 83] Although such pooled data

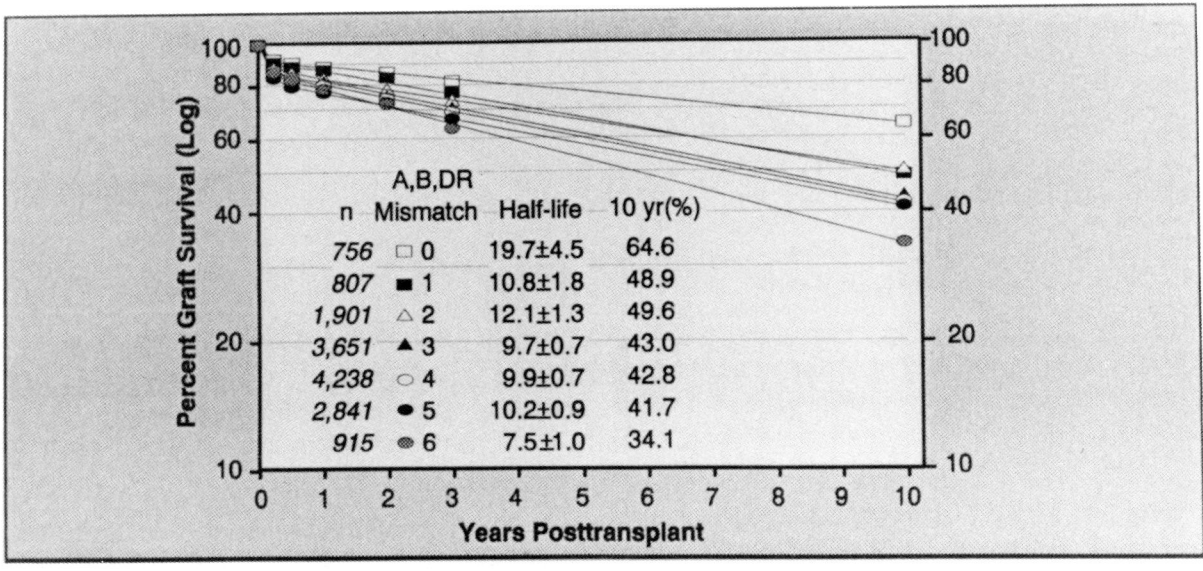

**Figure 58–6.** Projected 10-year graft survivals of first cadaveric donor grafts treated with cyclosporine in relation to HLA-A, -B, and -DR mismatching. Survivals for 3 years are shown for the zero to six mismatches possible when the three loci are considered (n = number of patients in each match group). Graft loss occurs exponentially over time and is described by a half-life in years. Results at 1 year show about a 10% difference between the best and worst match grades, widening to 15% at 3 years, and projections show a larger difference at 10 years. The 65% projected rate (half-life of 19.7 years) for zero mismatched cases at 10 years is midway between 51% (half-life of 11.2 years) for a haplotype mismatch and 79% (half-life of 32.9 years) for an HLA-identical transplant (not shown). (From Terasaki PI, Cecka JM, Gjertson DW, et al: A ten-year prediction for kidney transplant survival. *In* Terasaki PI, Cecka JM [eds]: Clinical Transplants 1992. UCLA Tissue Typing Laboratory, Los Angeles, 1993, p 501.)

may suffer from variations in protocols and undocumented selection factors, the power of univariate analyses becomes compelling when several thousands of patients are included. Furthermore, each of these studies provides a unique perspective, and each provides strong evidence on the role of HLA phenotypic matching in cadaveric renal transplantation. Terasaki's registry[81] has functioned for many years and is the best source of information on the year-to-year changes in results related to donor source, blood transfusion, immunosuppressive modality, and HLA matching and sensitization in more than 80,000 cases, mostly from North America. It operates the United Network for Organ Sharing registry for U.S. transplants. Opelz and co-workers[83] organized a study from 1983 to 1984 related to the 9th International Histocompatibility Workshop, using data from experienced laboratories having access to the best typing antisera. The Collaborative Transplant Study accepts only consecutive unselected cases and now has more than 50,000 cases entered from more than 260 centers in 38 countries. It has the additional advantage of spanning the transition from the widespread use of azathioprine to cyclosporine. The American Southeast Organ Procurement Foundation, a large sharing region, has maintained a database that permits multivariate analyses.[84, 85] It also provides internal standards for histocompatibility typing. The United Kingdom Transplant Service[86] and Eurotransplant[87, 88] are similar regions in which standardization of typing exists.

## Short-term Versus Long-term Effects

The more effective immunosuppressive therapy now in common use results in 1-year survivals of cadaveric grafts

as good as with one haplotype–matched living related donors. The early results are 80% or higher for first grafts (Fig. 58–6). Such was not the case in the era when azathioprine and steroids were the main therapies. In a nine-center study in which occurrence of rejection episodes within the first 60 days after transplantation was related to 1-year graft survival and degree of B and DR mismatching, a strong HLA effect was found in 335 patients who experienced early rejection, with a spread in 1-year survival rates from 86% to 53% for zero to four mismatches in rank order, whereas in 293 patients without rejection, the spread was from 100% to 87%.[79] Although early rejections have been shown to be indicators of future graft failures, graft failure is less likely to occur when the donor and recipient are HLA matched, according to this analysis. Degree of mismatching was not directly predictive of the occurrence of early rejection episodes. Intrinsic responsiveness of individual patients may determine to a large extent the rejection episode rate, but once the patients with rejection declare themselves, the HLA barrier becomes important to short-term survival rates. Alternatively, the rejection tempo may be intrinsically more powerful with more mismatched antigens. The question of defining intrinsic responsiveness with regard to initiation of rejection remains open. Failure to reject may be a phenomenon of the patient's susceptibility to immunosuppressive agents, or it may be on an immunogenetic basis, varying with different donor-recipient combinations, as exemplified by the patient who does well with a second transplant after vigorous rejection of the first graft bearing different HLA antigens.

There is strong evidence from 3-year data in cyclosporine-treated cadaveric graft recipients that improved long-term graft survivals are a function of avoiding HLA mismatches. Log-linear plots of graft survivals always show a straight line decline after the first year, which makes it possible to calculate a half-life and to project survivals over time. Projections from several thousand first cadaveric grafts treated with cyclosporine show that well-matched cases will do much better at 10 years. As shown in Figure 58–6, cases with zero AB or DR mismatches have a half-life of about 20 years and a projected 65% 10-year survival; when one or two mismatches are present, the values are an 11- to 12-year half-life and 50% 10-year survival. With greater degrees of mismatch, the half-lives drop to 7.5 to 10 years, and 10-year survivals are 32% to 42%.[81] If one notes the relatively small number of zero mismatched transplants (5% of the total), it is not difficult to see why individual centers have often not found a matching effect. Most of the worldwide data appear to be based on random assignment of cases with regard to HLA. There is considerable opportunity both for matching more cases and for avoiding completely mismatched grafts. It is worth noting that current projections give the same, or better, 10-year graft survival rate to unrelated donors who are not mismatched with their recipients for HLA-A, -B, and -DR as for HLA haplotype-identical family donors.

## Quality of Typing

It should be obvious that inaccurate tissue typing cannot be of any value. However, when a close phenotypic match is sought between presumably unrelated individuals, technique, whether it relates to the quality of cell preparations or of antisera used, can be of importance in detecting many uncommon or difficult antigens. Current difficulties are greater for definition of class II than for class I antigens, and the greatest application of DNA typing techniques is occurring in this area. For serology, the quality of B cell preparations can be variable, and the experience of the technologist reading the trays can be crucial. The error rate, based on repeated class II typing in a second laboratory, can be 15%. The relationship between the reproducibility of typing and the effects of matching on graft survival has been noted in the multicenter Eurotransplant program.[88] One problem has been the number of blanks (i.e., finding only one DR antigen in a patient). Such a situation could result from poor technique, lack of antisera for one of the new DR antigens, or homozygosity for that antigen. The Collaborative Transplant Study analysis has shown a striking change in the predictive effect of matching when "good" versus "fair" or "poor" DR typings were separately analyzed.[80] These quality judgments are made by the submitting laboratory. In general, 2-year graft survivals were better with decreasing numbers of HLA-B and -DR mismatches. There were 8351 first cadaveric grafts treated with cyclosporine and good DR typing, and 2820 similar cases with fair or poor typing. The progressive increase in survival as numbers of mismatches decreased was clearly seen in the good data and was less distinguishable in the fair or poor group. When repeated transplantations were compared, the typing quality effect was even more striking in 1416 good versus 569 fair or poor typings; in particular, the excess failure rate in the poorly matched (three or four

mismatches) cases could not be predicted (55% 2-year survival versus 70% to 75%).

## Matching for Narrow (Splits) Versus Broad Class I Antigens

Top-quality reagents for the purpose of defining the large number of HLA-A and -B subdivisions are in limited supply, and most transplant data have been analyzed on the basis of the "parent" antigen. Analysis of more than 30,000 cadaveric grafts with regard to HLA-A and -B mismatches shows a striking benefit on matching for splits but not for the broad antigens.[89] In approximately half of the cases, splits were not reported, and these survival curves show absolutely no matching effect. In contrast, a layered matching effect, from 75% to 55% 3-year survival for zero to four A and B mismatches, was found in the cases in which splits were reported. When these two groups were further analyzed for A, B, and DR mismatches (ranging from zero to six mismatches), the spread was from 80% to 50% at 3 years and from 68% to 55% when only the broad antigen groups were considered. One possible explanation for these differences could be that centers that cannot split are not comparable for other reasons to those that can. Therefore, a further analysis was performed on the "split group" by converting all splits into their broad antigens and reanalyzing the outcomes. The result was no different from that with the original "broad group." Hence, it can be assumed that had the broad group been reported as splits, they would have shown the powerful matching effect, especially when combined with DR. In contrast, analysis of the United Network for Organ Sharing data, which come from the United States only, on more than 24,000 first cadaveric grafts shows less of a difference when broad antigen mismatching is compared with splits, both showing a graded effect.[90] In particular, patients with zero broad antigen mismatches had an 87% 1-year graft survival and an 18-year half-life, compared with 8.2 years for less well matched cases. These results suggest that the more public determinants[91] on class I molecules are most important.

## Relative Strengths of Human Leukocyte Antigen Loci

The simple assumption that each mismatch for antigens of various loci will have equal weight in the frequency of graft loss is not supported by clinical data. The major impact comes from consideration of B and DR antigens, with little additional effect from A.[82] The United Kingdom Transplant Service data show that DR matching has a much greater effect than that of A or B.[86] Compared with the results when no mismatches are present for A, B, or DR, the addition of a single mismatch for A, or B, or DR increases the chances of graft loss twofold for A, threefold for B, and fivefold for DR. The United Network for Organ Sharing system employs a zero mismatch for HLA-A, -B, and -DR ("six antigen match") as the mandatory sharing criterion.

## Matching Versus Mismatching

An individual's HLA phenotyping will frequently have a blank at one of the loci. There are three possible reasons for this: 1) failure to detect a rare antigen because of lack of antisera in the laboratory; 2) a technical problem in performance of the typing; and 3) homozygosity for the antigen identified at the locus. The first two problems are becoming increasingly uncommon in experienced laboratories, and the presence of a blank can be taken as evidence for homozygosity, particularly if the paired antigen is relatively common. For example, a typing showing A2,-; B8,44; DR3,4 is truly A2,2; B8,44; DR3,4. Evidence that assumption of homozygosity is valid comes from Terasaki's analysis of cadaveric graft outcomes when completely matched (HLA-A, -B, -DR) cases are compared with those with various numbers of blanks in both donor and recipient, such that no mismatches are present.[92] The same 80% to 90% 3-year survival was present in the no-mismatch categories, which indicates that the blanks most likely represent the same antigen from both haplotypes. Furthermore, the major studies quoted earlier all show better discrimination of survival results when one tabulates degrees of mismatch than of match. Although reproducibility of class II typing remains a problem for some laboratories, as noted before, the assumption of homozygosity for a blank is supported by such results. Therefore, clinical matching data support a practical role for avoiding mismatches in preference to matching of HLA antigens.

## Effects of Blood Transfusions

The historical data on the beneficial effects of blood transfusions are well known.[93] In more recent years, the effect has been diminishing to the point that it now appears to have little impact on graft survival. Indeed, only in the group not transfused is there some evidence of a detriment to graft survival. Of importance is the fact that the trend toward a loss of the transfusion effect began before the introduction of cyclosporine[94] and continued into the cyclosporine era in patients receiving azathioprine therapy. Although there is no reasonable hypothesis as yet on this trend, some light has been shed on the clinical significance in the nontransfused group.

Although overall graft survival is not reduced, nontransfused patients have more rejection difficulties in the early post-transplantation period. Furthermore, in the previously noted study of patients from nine transplantation centers in whom early rejection episodes (within 60 days) were documented in relation to 1-year graft survival, blood transfusion history was also recorded. It was found that first cadaveric graft recipients who experienced no rejection during the first 60 days after transplantation had 1-year graft survival rates in the 84% to 88% range, whether they had received 0, 1 to 10, or more than 10 pretransplantation blood transfusions. If, however, they had a rejection during the first 60 days, the 1-year survivals were as follows: 0 transfusions, 49%; 1 to 10 transfusions, 69%; and more than 10 transfusions, 71%.[94] These results strongly suggest that prior blood exposure is important only in those patients who break through baseline immunosuppressive therapy, which makes it easier to reverse rejection in patients who had previous transfusions. An analysis indicates a benefit from transfusions in HLA-DR–mismatched cases, but not when there were no mismatches.[95] Close attention to rejection events provides evidence that transfusions are beneficial in those patients destined to have rejection activity, and patients who had no transfusions have more early rejection episodes.[96, 97] Unfortunately, there are at present no reliable predictive tests so that one can know who needs to have transfusions before transplantation. When the HLA types of blood donor and recipient are known, it has been shown that a match of one HLA-DR antigen results in a lower rate of anti-HLA antibody formation after a single transfusion, compared with an HLA-mismatched transfusion. Furthermore, both kidney and heart transplant recipients had reduced rejection frequency and superior graft survival when they had transfusions before transplantation with 1 to 3 units from donors who matched for one DR antigen with the recipient. As an example, the 5-year kidney survival was 81% with the one DR antigen match versus 57% with a zero DR antigen match and 45% with no transfusions. In this report, having a match for one DR antigen between the recipient and blood donor was more important than a match for one DR antigen between the recipient and graft donor.[98] Hence, blood transfusions do matter, but one has to know the HLA type of the blood donor. The reasons for benefit from a partially matched blood donor are speculative; however, such a transfusion does produce a specific reduction in the cytotoxic T cell precursor frequency to the incompatible HLA class I antigens of the blood donor.[99]

## REGULATION OF THE IMMUNE RESPONSE

### Role of the Antigen-Presenting Cell

The interaction between T lymphocytes and antigen-presenting cells involves multiple T cell surface molecules and their counter-receptors expressed by antigen-presenting cells. Numerous T cell surface molecules have been identified that specifically bind counter-receptors on the antigen-presenting cell. As depicted in Figure 58–4, the receptors can be divided into five functional categories, including 1) the antigen-specific T cell receptor, 2) the CD4 or CD8 coreceptors, 3) the accessory or adhesion molecules, 4) the costimulatory molecules, and 5) the cytokine receptors. Relevant to transplantation, inhibition of T cell interactions with antigen-presenting cells has been shown to prolong graft survival, and there are either clinical or experimental studies showing increased survival by blocking each of the five categories of receptors.[100–107] The most successful example to date has been the monoclonal antibody OKT3, which recognizes the CD3 complex associated with the T cell receptor. OKT3 has been highly successful in reversing acute graft rejection[100, 101] and has also proved effective in induction therapy.[102, 108] Therapeutic strategies based on inhibiting T cell surface receptors with monoclonal antibodies or inhibitor molecules are discussed in more detail later.

## T Cell Receptor Recognition of Antigen

Antigen specificity is determined by the T cell receptor, which recognizes processed antigen in the form of short peptides bound to an MHC molecule. The specificity of antigen recognition is exquisitely precise; the alteration of a single amino acid in the peptide antigen or MHC molecule can alter recognition by the T cell receptor. Thus, T cell recognition of antigen involves a trimolecular interaction involving the T cell receptor on the surface of the T cell, the MHC molecule on the surface of the antigen-presenting cell, and the antigenic peptide bound to the MHC molecule. The relative contribution of the allogeneic MHC molecule compared with that of the antigenic peptide to recognition by the T cell receptor during allogeneic immune responses remains unresolved. However, substantial experimental evidence shows that the specificity of many alloreactive T cells requires specific peptide antigens; alternatively, it remains possible that other T cells respond primarily to the allogeneic MHC molecule and the peptide effect is inconsequential.

The OKT3 monoclonal antibody binds a complex of proteins termed CD3 that is noncovalently associated with the T cell receptor. The function of the CD3 complex is to transduce signals into the cell after antigen recognition by the T cell receptor.[109] OKT3 also induces signal transduction, including the activation of specific kinases, the activation of phospholipase C, and the increase in intracellular $Ca^{2+}$ concentration and phosphoinositol metabolites.[109] The immunosuppressive effects of OKT3 are also dependent on signal transduction. The major immunosuppressive effect of OKT3 is the down-modulation of cell surface expression of the T cell receptor.[110] In addition, OKT3 causes the clearance of T cells from the circulation and sequestration in the peripheral lymphoid organs, such as lymph nodes and spleen.[110] OKT3 is not cytotoxic and does not lyse peripheral T cells. Also, there is not convincing evidence that OKT3 directly interferes with antigen recognition by the T cell receptor molecule. The side effects of OKT3 are also due to partial T cell activation causing the release of lymphokines, primarily tumor necrosis factor (TNF)-α but not interleukin (IL)-2 or interferon (IFN)-γ, from large numbers of T cells.[111]

## CD4⁺ and CD8⁺ T Cell Subsets

The two major subsets of T cells, the CD8⁺ cytotoxic T cells and CD4⁺ T helper cells, recognize processed antigen on MHC class I and II, respectively. Class I MHC molecules are expressed by essentially all eukaryotic cells except red blood cells and oocytes. In contrast, class II MHC molecules are expressed primarily on antigen-presenting cells, including dendritic cells, B cells, and macrophages. In addition, some cells, such as endothelial cells, express class II molecules after stimulation with lymphokines, such as IFN-γ.[112] As discussed later, activated endothelial cells have an important role in the rejection of vascularized grafts. The class I and class II MHC molecules present peptides from different subsets of antigens.[113] The class I molecules primarily present peptides derived from intracel-lular proteins, including both viral proteins and self-proteins as well as some tumor antigens. In contrast, the class II molecules present antigens derived primarily from extracellular proteins.

Although not directly involved in antigen recognition, the CD4 and CD8 coreceptors bind to nonpolymorphic regions of the MHC molecules. Thus, the specificity of class I versus class II recognition is determined by whether a T cell expresses CD4 or CD8 in conjunction with the specificity of the T cell receptor. In addition, CD4 and CD8 increase the avidity of the T cell interaction with the antigen-presenting cell and are involved in signal transduction. The cytoplasmic tails of CD4 and CD8 are associated with the tyrosine kinase p56[lck], which plays an important role in T cell activation.[114] Blockade of the CD4 molecule on T helper cells has potent immunosuppressive effects in human cadaveric renal transplants[115] and has been shown to prolong graft survival in animal models.[116]

## Accessory Molecules

A large number of T cell surface molecules originally termed adhesion molecules have been shown to increase the avidity of the interaction with the antigen-presenting cell. However, some of these receptors have also been shown to transduce signals and thus are more appropriately called accessory molecules. For example, CD2 stimulation has been shown to induce T cell activation.[117] The inhibition of accessory cell function has been shown to be immunosuppressive. Previous studies in a primate model showed increased graft survival with anti–intercellular adhesion molecule-1 monoclonal antibodies,[105] and clinical trials currently under way are testing the efficacy of blocking the leukocyte function–associated antigen-1 and intercellular adhesion molecule-1 interaction.

## T Cell Activation

T lymphocytes perform many regulatory and effector functions during an immune response. The activation of a T cell requires at least two signals.[118] One signal is transduced by the antigen-specific T cell receptor when it recognizes processed antigen bound to an MHC molecule on the surface of an antigen-presenting cell. The second signal is mediated by a costimulatory molecule that is independent of antigen. As shown in Figure 58–7, the T cell receptor and costimulatory signal transduction pathways are distinct and use different second messengers. At the level of the regulation of transcription, as shown for the IL-2 gene, the two pathways interact by poorly understood mechanisms to control gene expression. By controlling the level of expression of IL-2 and other genes, the T cell receptor and costimulatory pathways can regulate T cell activation and function. The best characterized costimulatory molecule is CD28, which is constitutively expressed on the surface of essentially all CD4⁺ and approximately 50% of CD8⁺ peripheral T lymphocytes.[119] CD28 binds a family of counter-receptors termed B7, which are expressed by antigen-presenting cells. After activation, another costimulatory

**Figure 58–7.** Signal transduction pathways involved in T cell activation. T cell activation requires signaling through a minimum of two signal transduction pathways including the T cell receptor and costimulatory pathways. The T cell receptor pathway, which is probably also modulated by crosstalk with the CD4/CD8 coreceptor pathway by the tyrosine kinase p56[lck], bifurcates into at least two second-messenger systems. These two systems regulate gene transcription in the nucleus by different DNA-binding proteins, which bind to different transcriptional response elements, shown here for the IL-2 gene. The costimulatory signal transduction pathway, although poorly understood, is probably distinct from the T cell receptor pathway and interacts with unique transcriptional response elements. In addition, other signal transduction pathways, including the cytokine receptor pathways shown here, can modulate T cell activation and differentiation. $IP_2$ = inositol bisphosphate; $PIP_3$ = phosphatidylinositol trisphosphate; DAG = diacylglycerol; NF-ATc = cytosolic component of nuclear factor of activated T cells (NF-AT); NF-κB = nuclear factor–κB; AP-1 = DNA-binding protein complex.

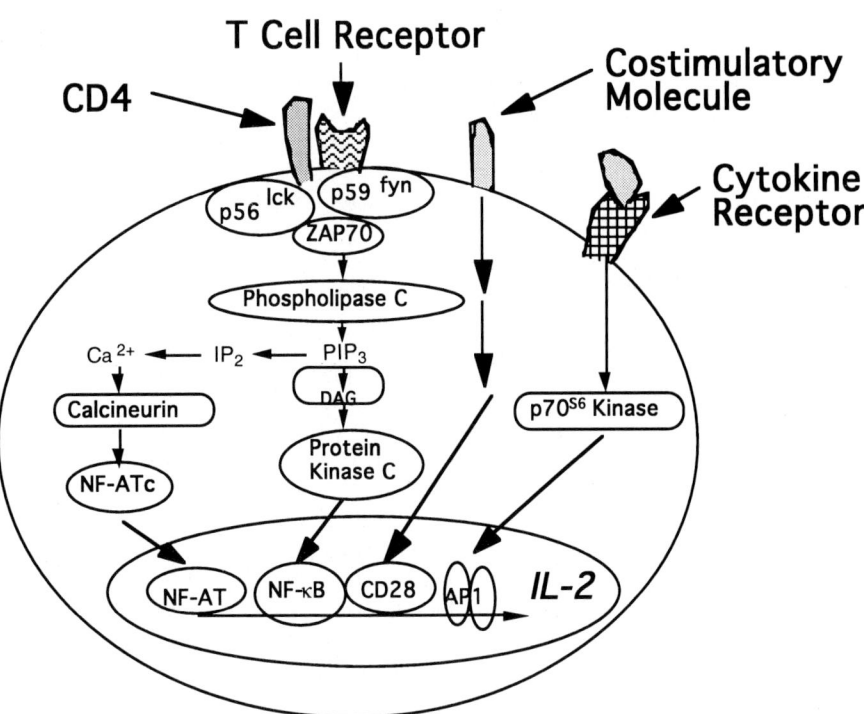

molecule termed CTLA4 is expressed by the T cell and binds B7 with a greater affinity than CD28. However, the precise function of CTLA4 remains undetermined. Inhibition of costimulation with soluble ligands to the B7 receptors has been shown to dramatically prolong graft survival. In a xenogeneic model of human islet cells transplanted into mice, treatment with a B7 inhibitor (CTLA4-Ig), prolonged graft survival until the experiment was terminated at 60 days.[120] Similarly, in a heterotopic model of cardiac allografts, the combination of transfusions and the inhibition of the B7 costimulatory counter-receptor indefinitely prolonged graft survival.[121]

## T Cell Anergy

Signaling through the T cell receptor plus the CD28 costimulatory molecule is sufficient to activate T cells. In contrast, signaling through the T cell receptor alone without costimulation is a negative signal that induces long-term T cell unresponsiveness termed anergy.[118] There is no evidence that signaling through the CD28 costimulatory molecule without T cell receptor signaling affects the state of T cell activation. Experimental analysis of the minimal signal transduction event necessary to induce anergy showed that an increase of intracellular $Ca^{2+}$ concentration was sufficient.[118] Because increased intracellular $Ca^{2+}$ concentration is produced by signaling through the T cell receptor, these results are consistent with the observation that anergy can be induced by monoclonal antibodies to the T cell receptor or by antigen-presenting cells expressing the appropriate MHC molecule but lacking the costimulatory counter-receptor.[122, 123] Interestingly, cyclosporine, which inhibits the $Ca^{2+}$-dependent serine/threonine phosphatase calcineurin, inhibits the induction of apoptosis in murine

models.[124] This observation raises important questions concerning the optimal immunosuppressive protocol in experimental trials of tolerance induction. Anergic T cells remain viable but are unresponsive for a minimum of several weeks in both in vitro and in vivo experimental murine models.[118, 125] The fate and function of anergic T cells in vivo remain undetermined; however, evidence from experimental models suggests that anergic T cells can be reactivated by some processes, such as viral infections.[126] Consistent with this observation, work has shown that anergic human T cells can be reactivated by signaling through the CD2 receptor. These observations suggest that anergy is a reversible state and that the therapeutic use of anergy during clinical transplantation, although potentially useful, will require thorough evaluation and careful monitoring.

## Lymphokines and Lymphokine Receptors

T cell activation and proliferation are also modulated by soluble lymphokines, which bind to lymphokine receptors, such as the IL-2 receptor (IL-2R). Signaling through the T cell receptor and CD28 costimulatory molecule is sufficient to activate the T cell to produce and secrete IL-2; however, these signals alone are not sufficient to promote T cell proliferation. In fact, blockade of the IL-2R α-chain causes T cell arrest at the $G_1/S$ phase of the cell cycle. The major functional defect in anergic T cells is the failure to produce IL-2.[118] At the molecular level, it has been shown that the transcription of the IL-2 gene is blocked at least in part by the failure to form the DNA-binding protein complex termed AP-1.[127] Interestingly, the state of anergy can be reversed in vitro by high doses of exogenous IL-2.[118] The ability of IL-2 to reverse anergy in vivo has not been determined; however, it is possible that high concentrations of IL-2 are present in microenvironments of peripheral lymph nodes and spleen that are capable of reactivating anergized T cells.

Monoclonal antibodies to the IL-2R have been shown to be immunosuppressive in both animal models and clinical trials with the anti-Tac monoclonal antibody.[106, 107] More important, immunoregulation by lymphokines is controlled not only by modulating the level of cytokine production but also by controlling the expression of cytokine receptors. For example, resting T cells do not express the IL-2R α-chain; however, after activation, the IL-2R α-chain is synthesized and expressed on the cell surface. This observation has been exploited in attempts to impart specificity to lymphokine receptor therapy by covalently linking the IL-2 molecule to a toxin.[106] The ligand-toxin conjugate binds to the IL-2R α-chain and is then endocytosed, killing the cell. Because the IL-2R α-chain is expressed only on activated T cells, the toxin conjugate kills only activated T cells. After transplantation, T cells causing graft rejection would be activated and thus express the IL-2R α-chain. These cells should be preferentially killed by the toxin conjugate.

## Th1 and Th2 T Cell Subsets

Lymphokines are produced by multiple different cell types, including T cells, B cells, and antigen-presenting cells. In addition, nonimmune cells, such as endothelial cells, also produce lymphokines that can modulate an immune response. Thus, complex regulatory networks of lymphokines that are incompletely understood, particularly in vivo, can modulate the antigraft immune response. In addition, it has been shown that different subsets of T cells can produce different patterns of cytokine secretion.[128, 129] The two subsets of CD4+ T cells defined in terms of cytokine production are the Th1 and Th2 subsets. Both subsets produce some lymphokines, such as IL-3 and granulocyte-macrophage colony-stimulating factor, whereas each subset produces a predominant set of lymphokines. The Th1 subset preferentially produces IL-2, IFN-γ, and TNF-α. In contrast, the Th2 subset preferentially produces IL-4, IL-5, IL-6, and IL-10. The net effect of producing each cytokine profile is differential regulation of the immune response. The Th1 subset is considered proinflammatory, promoting delayed-type hypersensitivity (DTH) reactions and cytotoxic T lymphocyte expansion. The Th2 subset is considered a helper of B cells. However, the functional segregation between the Th1 and Th2 subsets remains incompletely understood. For example, IFN-γ secreted by Th1 cells regulates B cells by promoting antibody isotype switching to the immunoglobulin (Ig) G2a isotype. Also, IL-5 and IL-6 secreted by Th2 cells increase eosinophil recruitment and expansion. In addition, some T cell clones analyzed in vitro express overlapping profiles of lymphokines.

Clinical correlations between the development of a Th1-type and a Th2-type response have been shown in several diseases including leprosy, in which a tuberculoid or a lepromatous response is caused by a Th1 or Th2 response, respectively.[129] In experimental models of transplantation,

altering the T cell response from Th1 to Th2 has been shown to decrease acute graft rejection.[130] The effects of a Th2-type response on chronic rejection, which is probably mediated by mechanisms different from acute rejection, remain to be determined. Except for blockade of the IL-2R, therapeutic strategies modulating lymphokines have not proved highly effective. This may be due to the pleiotropic effects of each lymphokine as well as the complex interactions exhibited by regulatory networks of multiple lymphokines. For example, IL-2 has been shown by several criteria to promote graft rejection, and blockade of the IL-2R has been shown to promote graft survival.[131] However, transgenic mice, which do not express any IL-2 because of inactivation of the IL-2 gene by homologous recombination, reject grafts comparable to normal mice. Rejection in animals lacking IL-2 is probably mediated by other lymphokines that compensate for the IL-2 deficit by overlapping functions. Thus, although the manipulation of lymphokine functions holds promise as a therapeutic modality, improved understanding of the role of lymphokines in graft rejection will be required to develop effective treatments.

In summary, cell-cell interactions between T cells and antigen-presenting cells can be divided into five classes of receptors. Examples of each class of receptor (antigen-specific T cell receptor, CD4 or CD8 coreceptor, costimulatory molecules, accessory molecules, and lymphokine receptors) are shown in Figure 58–4. Therapeutic or experimental manipulation of members of each class of receptor has been shown to prolong graft survival. The most effective in clinical studies to date has been the anti–T cell receptor monoclonal antibody OKT3.[100–102, 108] Experimental studies investigating the effect of blocking the costimulatory receptors have been particularly promising. The major benefit of this approach is that blockade of costimulation during the initial phases of transplantation may induce graft-specific tolerance without producing nonspecific immunosuppression.

## GRAFT REJECTION

### Clinical Syndromes of Rejection

On the basis of the pathologic process and the kinetics of the rejection response, the rejection of renal allografts is commonly divided into four clinical syndromes: hyperacute, acute, accelerated, and chronic rejection.

#### HYPERACUTE REJECTION

Hyperacute rejection occurs within minutes to hours. A graft that initially becomes pink after vascular reanastomosis rapidly becomes mottled, ischemic, and anuric. Histologic analysis shows fibrin and platelet thrombi, fibrinoid necrosis of the vessel walls, and usually the absence of a mononuclear cell infiltrate.[132] The mechanism of hyperacute rejection is the best understood of the four types. During hyperacute rejection, preformed antibodies bind to graft antigens on the vascular endothelium of the donor kidney. The antigens recognized by the antibodies can be HLA antigens (usually HLA class I), the AB blood group antigens, or the poorly defined endothelial or monocyte antigens. Experimental models of hyperacute rejection indicate that complement is required, based on the observation that complement depletion with cobra venom factor prevents the lesion.[133] However, the depletion of platelets or polymorphonuclear leukocytes does not. One report describes the successful treatment of incipient hyperacute renal allograft rejection in humans with Malayan pit viper venom, which promotes systemic defibrination.[134] These observations indicate that specific antibodies, complement-mediated damage, and deposition of fibrin are the most important pathogenic effectors. Accurate pretransplantation blood and tissue typing can prevent most cases of hyperacute rejection; however, occasional cases of hyperacute rejection occur because of the endothelial or monocyte antigens, which cannot be evaluated by current methods of tissue typing.

## ACUTE REJECTION

Episodes of acute rejection commence 5 to 7 days after transplantation and occur with decreasing frequency after 3 months. However, acute rejection can occur months to years after transplantation, frequently associated with the withdrawal of immunosuppressive medications. Acute rejection is characterized by mononuclear cell infiltrates of the interstitium, which is composed predominantly of lymphocytes. In severe cases, the infiltrate can be diffuse and sometimes associated with evidence of humoral damage, including swelling, vacuolization, or necrosis of the arteriolar endothelial cell. The 5 to 7 days required for initiation of acute rejection corresponds to the time required for the afferent presentation of donor antigens in the lymph nodes and spleen, the activation and proliferation of host T cells, and the differentiation and migration of effector cells back to the graft.

Most studies indicate that the major regulators of acute rejection are T lymphocytes. This is demonstrated by experimental models showing that the elimination of CD4+ T cells prevents acute rejection.[135, 136] Consistent with these observations, most episodes of acute rejection after renal transplantation can be reversed with immunosuppressive agents directed at T lymphocytes, including high-dose corticosteroids and the OKT3 monoclonal antibody. However, the clinical diagnosis of acute rejection is not homogeneous and in some cases probably involves a combination of both cellular and humoral mechanisms. This is consistent with the renal biopsy results showing a combination of cellular and humoral changes in cases of severe acute rejection. Thus, the effector mechanisms of graft destruction in acute rejection are likely to involve multiple mechanisms, including cell-mediated cytotoxicity by CD8+ cytotoxic T cells, DTH reactions induced by CD4+ T cells, and in some cases antibody-mediated damage. Experimental models have clearly shown that either CD8+ or CD4+ T cells can be sufficient to cause graft rejection[137]; however, in the presence of both MHC class I and class II mismatches, the CD4+ and CD8+ T cell subsets act synergistically to promote a more vigorous rejection response. The role of macrophages and natural killer cells remains poorly understood; however, in some studies the presence of monocytes correlates more closely with graft outcome than the degree of lymphocyte infiltration. Many clinical and experimental studies have investigated the type of infiltrating cells in renal biopsy specimens during acute rejection episodes to develop both diagnostic and prognostic parameters of rejection. These studies show that the infiltrate consists of approximately 50% lymphocytes, 25% monocytes and macrophages, and 12% B cells.[138] However, it has not been shown that the degree of infiltration correlates with the fate of the graft.[139] Furthermore, some degree of infiltration is observed in syngeneic grafts or autografts[140] and in grafts without clinical evidence of rejection.[141] For example, the infiltrate is more intense with minor antigen differences than with an isolated MHC class I mismatch; however, the class I mismatched graft is rejected more vigorously.[142] Thus, the presence of mild or focal infiltrates does not necessarily indicate acute rejection, and the interpretation of renal allograft biopsy results requires careful clinical correlation.

## ACCELERATED REJECTION

Aggressive episodes of rejection occurring within 5 to 6 days after transplantation and differentiated from hyperacute rejection by the lack of an immediate onset are termed accelerated rejection and are thought to be caused by prior sensitization to antigens expressed by the graft. The kinetics of accelerated rejection are consistent with a memory or secondary immune response. Prior exposure to the donor graft antigens has been attributed to blood transfusions, pregnancy, and previously rejected grafts. In addition, anecdotal reports of exposure to maternal antigens during childbirth have rarely been purported to induce accelerated rejection of mother to offspring transplants. The most important risk factor for accelerated rejection is clearly prior allograft loss.[93] The principal finding on pathologic examination is fibrinoid necrosis of the small vessels,[143] which is consistent with a recipient antibody–mediated process. However, there is evidence that cell-mediated immunity may be responsible for some cases of accelerated rejection.

## CHRONIC DYSFUNCTION

Most cases of graft loss due to rejection occur within the first 3 to 6 months after transplantation; however, a steady rate of attrition continues months to years after transplantation and is commonly attributed to chronic rejection, which is more appropriately termed "chronic dysfunction" because of the multifactorial pathogenesis of decreased function. Evidence that this process is, at least in part, immune mediated is based on the observation that the half-life of renal allografts in HLA-identical grafts is 25 years compared with 8 years with cadaveric donors. In addition, the half-life of graft survival in cadaveric kidneys with six antigen matches is projected to be 17 years or more. However, the immune mechanisms of chronic rejection remain poorly understood. Biopsy results usually show a mild to moderate lymphocyte infiltration that is inconclusive in terms of supporting a cell-mediated process. In some cases, graft-specific antibodies have been detected; in one study, there was a correlation between these antibodies and the occurrence of obliterative arteritis, which is commonly observed in chronic rejection.[144] However, in other studies, antigraft antibodies have not been detected. Thus, the role of cellular versus humoral mechanisms remains undetermined. In an experimental model of renal transplantation, chronic rejection correlated with the degree of macrophage but not T cell or neutrophil infiltration.[145] Furthermore, in this model, chronic rejection could be prevented by retransplantation into the donor strain before 12 weeks after transplantation. However, grafts retransplanted after 12 weeks progressed to renal failure, which suggests a continuous process independent of host alloresponsiveness. These results suggest that the early phase of chronic rejection is immune mediated; however, nonimmune factors including decreased nephron mass and hyperfiltration most likely contribute to progression during the late phase in addition to continued immune destruction.[146] This model correlates with the clinical observation that the best predictive factor for chronic rejection is the occurrence of episodes of acute rejection.

# Mechanisms of Rejection

The four syndromes of graft rejection are frequently overlapping and not totally distinct in clinical practice. Similarly, the classic categories of cellular (lymphocyte) and humoral (antibody) mechanisms of rejection are now known to be interrelated. Immunologists now understand that antibodies are produced by cells (B lymphocytes). Furthermore, antibody production by B cells is regulated by T cells through both cell-cell contact and the secretion of regulatory lymphokines including IL-2, IL-4, and IFN-γ. For example, mice deficient for IL-2 because of inactivation of the IL-2 gene by homologous recombination produce IgM but none of the other immunoglobulin isotypes, such as IgG. IL-4, which was originally identified as B cell stimulatory factor because of its effects on promoting B cell growth, also promotes isotype switching to IgG1 and IgE, whereas IFN-γ promotes switching to the IgG2a isotype.

The process of immune recognition during acute rejection is amazingly specific. This was demonstrated by transplanting grafts from tetraparental (allophenic) donors, which are produced by combining embryonic stem cells from two different sets of parents. These grafts contain a mosaic of two cell types interspersed throughout the graft, with each cell type expressing different MHC antigens derived from the respective parents. When the grafts were transplanted into donors syngeneic with one set of MHC antigens, the allogeneic cells were destroyed and only syngeneic cells survived.[147, 148] These results show that the immune response successfully differentiated between adjacent cells expressing different MHC molecules. Thus, in these experiments, graft destruction was primarily due not to nonspecific effector mechanisms, such as endopeptidase release or cytotoxic lymphokines like TNF, but to antigen-specific mechanisms. However, in some forms of rejection, there is evidence that macrophages can promote rejection by nonspecific effector mechanisms. Nonspecific effector mechanisms also participate in graft rejection. This is illustrated by the significant mononuclear cell infiltrate observed in autografts and by the low frequency of infiltrating T cells

that are specific for donor antigens. Taken together, these observations suggest that non–antigen-specific mediators of mononuclear cell recruitment and activation are involved in graft rejection. Furthermore, in vascularized grafts such as kidneys, the destruction of normal architecture, such as vasculature, can produce destruction as a result of ischemia. Therefore, it is likely that most episodes of clinical dysfunction involve combinations of specific and nonspecific processes.

## ANTIBODY-MEDIATED REJECTION

The role of antibody in hyperacute rejection has been clearly established from multiple observations. First, there is a direct correlation between the existence of a positive pretransplant crossmatch, which detects anti–MHC class I antibody, and the development of hyperacute rejection.[149] Second, antigraft antibodies can be eluted from donor kidneys after hyperacute rejection. Third, the passive transfer of antigraft antibodies in experimental models can provoke hyperacute rejection.

It is likely that antibodies also play a role in other types of rejection; however, these mechanisms remain incompletely understood and controversial. The most controversial is the role of antibody in chronic dysfunction. Because of the scant cellular infiltrate in most cases of chronic rejection, it has been proposed by some authors that the process is mediated by antibody. However, direct evidence for antibody-mediated damage in chronic dysfunction is inconclusive. The failure to demonstrate antibody involvement in chronic dysfunction could be attributed to multiple factors. First, antibodies causing hyperacute rejection are preformed; that is, the antibodies develop in response to a prior antigenic challenge from blood transfusion, pregnancy, or a previous transplant, and the preformed antibodies then cross-react with donor antigens. In contrast, antibodies produced during chronic dysfunction develop under the influence of immunosuppressive drugs, which could moderate their rate of production. Also, antibodies could bind to the graft, making the detection of soluble antigraft antibody difficult. Thus, the role of antibody in the pathogenesis of chronic dysfunction remains undetermined.

## T CELL–MEDIATED REJECTION

The requirement of T cells in acute graft rejection has been shown conclusively in athymic mice, which fail to produce mature T cells. These mice accept grafts from either syngeneic or allogeneic donors, or even xenogeneic donors, without evidence of rejection.[150] Furthermore, the passive transfer of T cells into athymic mice reconstitutes vigorous graft rejection.[151–153] In clinical transplantation, the role of T cells has been confirmed by the dramatic effects of anti–T cell antibodies, including OKT3, antithymocyte globulin, and antilymphocyte globulin, the effectiveness of which is often limited by the side effects of nonspecific immunosuppression.

Although T cells are most likely necessary to initiate both acute and chronic graft dysfunction, the relative contribution of the different T cell subsets has not been clearly elucidated. The two main T cell subsets, CD4+ and CD8+, do not directly correlate with a functional dichotomy into helper and cytotoxic cells. This has caused considerable confusion in understanding the role of T cells in the pathogenesis of graft rejection. There is now substantial evidence that the "cytotoxic" CD8+ T cell subset can also produce lymphokines, including IL-2 and IFN-γ, at levels sufficient to promote autocrine growth. Thus, in some circumstances, CD8+ T cells can provide their own help and function independently of the CD4+ subset. Conversely, the "helper" CD4+ T cell subset can have cytotoxic effector function and mediate target cell lysis without the involvement of the CD8+ subset. Understanding these concepts, it is not surprising that either the CD4+ or CD8+ T cell subset can mediate graft rejection independently of the other subset. This was demonstrated experimentally by eliminating either the CD4+ or CD8+ subset with monoclonal antibodies and showing no prevention of graft rejection.[136, 154] Similarly, the experimental elimination of either MHC class I or class II molecules by gene inactivation using homologous recombination in mice has shown that grafts expressing only class I (recognized by CD8+ T cells) or class II (recognized by CD4+ T cells) are both readily rejected.[155] These results show that either CD4+ or CD8+ T cells can effectively cause graft rejection; however, in the presence of a class I and class II mismatch, it has been shown that the interaction of CD4+ and CD8+ T cells can synergistically induce graft rejection. It is likely that most episodes of rejection in clinical renal transplantation involve a combination of the CD4+ and CD8+ T cell subsets.

As previously discussed, CD4+ T cells can be further divided into the Th1 and Th2 subsets, which are distinguished by different patterns of lymphokine secretion.[128] From a functional perspective, it has been proposed that the Th1 subset produces a proinflammatory function, whereas the Th2 subset produces B cell help. An analysis of the role of lymphokines in graft rejection favors the hypothesis that the Th1 subset is the major mediator of acute graft rejection. In models of transplantation, the switch from a Th1-type to a Th2-type response has been shown to diminish acute rejection[130]; however, the effect on chronic rejection has not been evaluated.

### DELAYED-TYPE HYPERSENSITIVITY– MEDIATED REJECTION

The DTH response is regulated by the CD4+ T cell; however, the effector cells are most likely macrophages and possibly CD8+ cytotoxic T cells. Consequently, the effector mechanisms may involve immunologically nonspecific mediators, including IFN-γ and TNF-α. In a DTH response, the activated CD4+ T cell recruits other cells, including macrophages and CD8+ T cells, by secreting lymphokines including IFN-γ (previously termed macrophage inhibition factor) and other uncharacterized substances. The CD8+ cells also secrete IFN-γ and may substantially increase the recruitment of macrophages. The CD4+ cells, which induce a DTH response, belong to the Th1 subset; however, for unknown reasons, not all Th1 T cells cause a DTH reaction.[156] Evidence that the DTH response is involved in acute graft rejection is based on a correlation between graft rejection and the ability to generate DTH responses to the same antigenic challenge. The strongest evidence is derived from

an experimental model of skin grafts across a minor histocompatibility antigen difference but without MHC differences.[157] In these experiments, the grafts were rejected without the development of a detectable class I–restricted CD8+ T cell cytotoxic response. The investigation of the role of DTH responses in clinical transplantation is complicated by the lack of an in vitro assay to detect the response. Therefore, the role of a DTH response in renal transplantation remains controversial.

### NATURAL KILLER CELL–MEDIATED GRAFT REJECTION

Natural killer cells are frequently identified in the infiltrating cells during acute graft rejection; however, the role of graft cell lysis by natural killer cells remains unknown. Because natural killer cells do not express the antigen-specific T cell receptor used by CD4+ and CD8+ T cells, the mechanism of target cell lysis is clearly different from that of cytotoxic T cells. In addition, target cell susceptibility to lysis by natural killer cells has been shown to be reduced by MHC class I expression. However, because not all cells are susceptible to natural killer cell lysis, it is likely that some form of antigen-specific recognition is involved. The precise role of natural killer cells in graft rejection remains to be determined.

### MECHANISMS OF IMMUNOSUPPRESSION

### Corticosteroids

Most immunosuppressive drug regimens employ an adrenal corticosteroid, such as prednisone, in combination with other immunosuppressive agents. Corticosteroids provide the most proximal block in the T cell activation cascade; they indirectly interfere with T cell proliferation, at least partially because of their ability to block expression of the IL-1 and IL-6 genes.[158] Macrophages treated with corticosteroids do not produce IL-1 or IL-6 messenger RNA, even after incubation with powerful macrophage stimulants. Because IL-2 release depends in part on IL-1–stimulated IL-6 release, corticosteroids also indirectly block IL-2. Corticosteroids modulate the immune response by regulating gene expression. The steroid molecule enters the cytosol, where it binds the steroid receptor, inducing a conformation change in the receptor. The complex then migrates to the nucleus and binds regulatory regions of DNA termed glucocorticoid response elements, which regulate the transcription of many genes. Thus, corticosteroids have many effects on multiple cell types, which accounts for both their efficacy and the diverse array of complications.

Conventional therapies for the treatment of acute renal allograft rejection include high-dose pulses of glucocorticoids. Glucocorticoids have broad, nonspecific immunosuppressive and anti-inflammatory effects. Besides their effects on lymphokines, glucocorticoids reduce the migration of monocytes to sites of inflammation. A major drawback to the use of glucocorticoids in the treatment of acute rejection

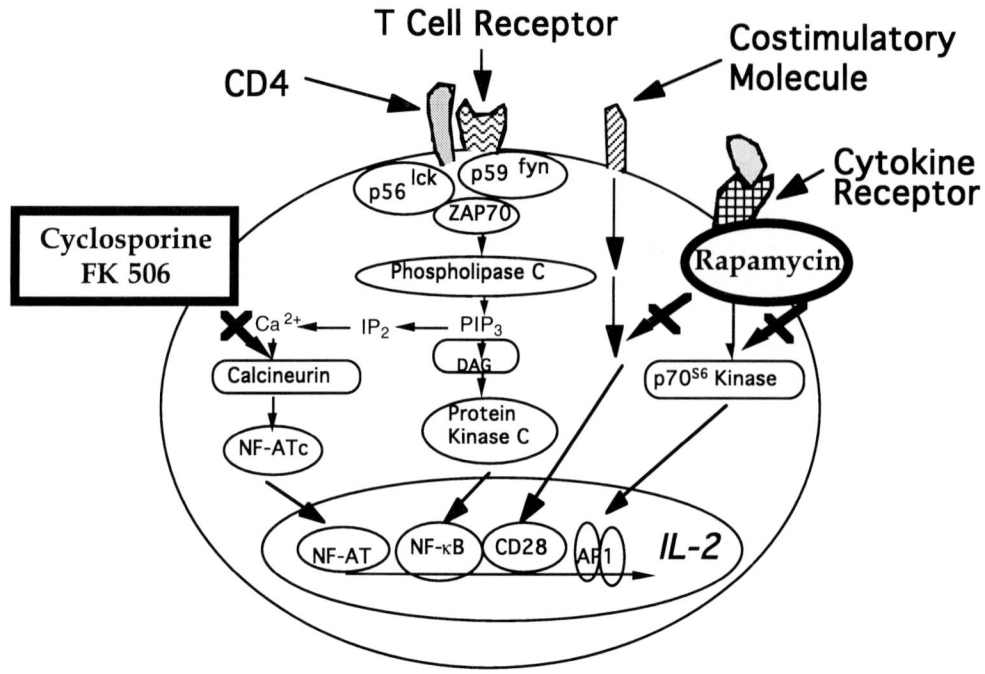

**Figure 58–8.** Mechanisms of immunosuppression. T cell signal transduction pathways required for activation, which are described in Figure 58–7, are blocked by the macrolide antibiotics FK 506 and rapamycin and by the polypeptide antibiotic cyclosporine. Cyclosporine and FK 506 have both been shown to inhibit the serine/threonine phosphatase calcineurin in the $Ca^{2+}$-dependent component of the T cell receptor pathway. In contrast, rapamycin inhibits the costimulatory and IL-2R pathways at a step proximal to the $p70^{S6}$ kinase. Cyclosporine and FK 506 do not block the costimulatory pathway; conversely, rapamycin does not affect the T cell receptor pathway.

is that they inhibit the entire immune and inflammatory systems and alter many other steroid-responsive systems as well. The use of high doses of glucocorticoids can thus produce severe undesirable side effects, including decreased inflammatory and phagocytic capacity, resulting in increased susceptibility to infection, hyperglycemia, hyperkalemia, osteoporosis, increased capillary fragility, and growth suppression in children.

## Azathioprine

Azathioprine is a purine analogue that is enzymatically converted in vivo to 6-mercaptopurine and other derivatives, which function as antimetabolites.[159] After metabolic conversion, it has multiple activities, including incorporation into DNA, inhibition of purine nucleotide synthesis, and alteration of RNA synthesis. The major immunosuppressive effect is thought to be due to the block in DNA replication, which prevents lymphocyte proliferation after antigenic stimulation. Although useful for inhibiting primary immune responses, azathioprine has little effect on secondary responses or in the reversal of acute allograft rejections that are not dependent on lymphocyte proliferation.

Azathioprine also decreases the number of migratory mononuclear cells and granulocytes while inhibiting the proliferation of promyelocytes within bone marrow. As a result, the number of circulating monocytes capable of differentiating into macrophages is decreased. Among the possible deleterious effects of azathioprine administration are severe leukopenia and occasionally thrombocytopenia, gastrointestinal disturbances, fever, hepatotoxic effects, and increased risk of neoplasia.

## Cyclosporine

The introduction of cyclosporine, a small cyclic peptide of fungal origin, has played a major role in preventing graft rejection and has resulted in improved graft survival rates. Although highly effective in blocking the initiation of an immune response, like azathioprine, it is of limited value in the treatment of acute allograft rejection.[160] Its primary action is to block the expression of lymphokines produced by T cells, including IL-2, IL-3, IL-4, IFN-γ, and TNF-α,[161, 162] but it does not interfere with IL-1, TNF-α, or TNF-β produced by antigen-presenting cells including macrophages. Also, there is no evidence that natural killer cells are affected by cyclosporine. In the presence of cyclosporine, T cell proliferation is indirectly inhibited because of the absence of lymphokines. However, the addition of exogenous IL-2 has been shown to restore T cell proliferation.[163]

It is now understood that cyclosporine blocks the $Ca^{2+}$-dependent component of the T cell receptor signal transduction pathway (Fig. 58–8). Previous work showed that cyclosporine binds a cytoplasmic molecule termed cyclophilin, which has peptidyl-prolyl isomerase activity. After binding cyclophilin, cyclosporine inhibits the isomerase activity; however, it is now apparent that the immunosuppressive effects are not due to this inhibition. This was shown by analogues of cyclosporine that bind cyclophilin and inhibit isomerase activity but do not cause immunosuppression.[164] Later work has shown that the cyclophilin-cyclosporine complex inhibits calcineurin, which is a cytoplasmic serine/threonine phosphatase.[165] After T cell activation in the absence of cyclosporine, calcineurin dephosphorylates the cytosolic component of the nuclear factor of activated T cells (NF-AT). After dephosphorylation, the nuclear factor of activated T cells is translocated from the cytosol to the nucleus, where it forms a complex with other DNA-binding proteins including FOS and JUN.[166] The complex of DNA-binding proteins regulates transcription of genes including the IL-2 gene. During treatment with cyclosporine, the inhibition of the formation of the nuclear factor of activated T cell complex has been shown to prevent the transcription of the IL-2 gene,[167] and a similar complex has been shown to regulate TNF-α gene transcription. It is likely that identical or similar DNA-binding complexes regulate the transcription of multiple lymphokine genes. The mechanism of action of cyclosporine in nonlymphocytes remains poorly understood; however, it has been shown that analogues of cyclosporine that lack toxicity also lack immunosuppressive effects.[164] These results suggest that the toxic and immunosuppressive effects are mediated by similar signal transduction mechanisms. The differential susceptibility to cyclosporine of lymphocytes compared with other cell types may be due to different levels of expression of calcineurin and the cyclophilins.

## FK 506

FK 506 is a potent immunosuppressive agent that has been shown to prolong allograft survival in clinical trials and to inhibit T cell activation in vitro.[168] Although both FK 506 and cyclosporine are macrolide antibiotics produced by fungi, and the immunosuppressive effects on T cells are similar, the structures of FK 506 and cyclosporine differ.[124] Because of the structural differences, FK 506 binds a family of cytosolic proteins termed FK 506 binding proteins, whereas, as discussed before, cyclosporine binds cyclophilin. Interestingly, both FK 506 binding proteins and cyclophilin have peptidyl-prolyl isomerase activity and are collectively called immunophilins; however, the immunosuppressive properties of the two drugs are similar because both agents inhibit the phosphatase activity of calcineurin.[169] Although FK 506 and cyclosporine have different structures, their immunosuppressive effects are mediated through a common final pathway. Thus, it is not surprising that both drugs block the induction of lymphokine messenger RNA, including IL-2; inhibit lymphokine production; and indirectly inhibit T cell proliferation.[170] Because of the similar mechanisms of action, the toxic effects of FK 506 and cyclosporine are also highly similar. It remains to be determined whether subtle differences in efficacy or toxicity will be confirmed as a result of the inhibition of different isomerase proteins or different pharmacokinetics. In experimental studies, the combination of FK 506 and cyclosporine shows additive increases in toxicity as well as efficacy. Therefore, in clinical transplantation, immunosuppressive protocols involving multiple drugs will most likely use either cyclosporine or FK 506.

## Rapamycin

Rapamycin is a macrolide antibiotic produced by fungi with potent immunosuppressive activity. It is structurally related to FK 506 and binds to the same family of isomerase proteins as FK 506, the FK 506 binding proteins. Surprisingly, however, the immunosuppressive mechanism of rapamycin differs from that of FK 506 (see Fig. 58–8). Whereas cyclosporine and FK 506 inhibit calcineurin in the Ca²⁺-dependent component of the T cell receptor signal transduction pathway, rapamycin prevents the phosphorylation of p70$^{S6}$ kinase in the CD28 costimulatory and IL-2R signal transduction pathways.[171] In functional studies, the activation of T cells by monoclonal antibodies to the T cell receptor was inhibited by either cyclosporine or FK 506 but not by rapamycin.[172] Conversely, the activation of T cells by exogenous IL-2 plus protein kinase C stimulation with a phorbol ester was inhibited by rapamycin but not by cyclosporine or FK 506. Similarly, T cell activation by monoclonal antibodies to the CD28 costimulatory molecule plus protein kinase C stimulation with a phorbol ester was also inhibited by rapamycin but not by cyclosporine or FK 506. Cell cycle analysis shows that rapamycin blocks T cell proliferation during late G₁, and before S phase, of the cell cycle.[173–175] Thus, rapamycin inhibits late signals in T cell activation that are transduced by either the IL-2R or CD28 costimulatory signal transduction pathways.[175] In contrast, cyclosporine and FK 506 inhibit an early signal in T cell activation that is transduced by the T cell receptor signal transduction pathway. Because rapamycin and FK 506 bind to the same FK 506 binding proteins, they act as competitive inhibitors of each other. As previously discussed, cyclosporine and FK 506 inhibit the same signal transduction mechanism, producing additive toxic effects. Thus, the potential of combination therapy involving these three agents in clinical transplantation is limited to cyclosporine plus rapamycin. In experimental models, combination therapy with cyclosporine and rapamycin has been shown to synergistically increase immunosuppression.[176] Although rapamycin has already increased our understanding of the mechanisms of T cell activation, its role in clinical transplantation, either alone or in combination with cyclosporine, must await clinical trials.

## Polyclonal Immune Globulins

Polyclonal antilymphocyte globulin or antithymocyte globulin preparations have been available for approximately two decades and have proved more effective than steroids alone for reversing acute renal allograft rejection.[177] Polyclonal immune globulins are produced by injecting animals, such as horses or rabbits, with human lymphoid cells to obtain the purified gamma globulin fractions of the resulting immune sera. Cultured lymphoblasts (to produce antilymphocyte globulin) and human thymocytes (to produce antithymocyte globulin) have been commonly used. Because cultured lymphoblasts are B cells rather than T cells, one possible disadvantage of antilymphocyte globulin is that the antisera do not recognize the T cell molecules, including the T cell receptor, CD28, and CD4 molecules, which are the most susceptible to immunosuppression.[178, 179] Human thymus tissue, an excellent source of T cell antigens, may not always be available in adequate amounts. More important, polyclonal immune globulins represent a heterogeneous group of antibodies, only a minority of which are specific for T cells. Thus, the heterogeneous quality of these antisera makes the interpretation of clinical data and the investigation of immunosuppressive mechanisms difficult to compare.

Polyclonal immune globulin may exert its immunosuppressive effect by several mechanisms. These include classic complement-mediated lysis of lymphocytes, clearance of lymphocytes due to reticuloendothelial uptake, masking of T cell antigens, or expansion of negative regulatory cells. After the administration of immune globulins, there is a prompt and profound lymphopenia. However, the lymphopenia soon abates and the number of circulating T cells gradually increases, even while treatment continues, but the proliferative response continues to be impaired. It has been suggested that suppressor cells may be responsible for the prolonged immunosuppressive effect that persists after the resolution of lymphopenia. Thus, the resolution of cell-mediated graft rejection results from the elimination of circulating T cells, and the subsequent inhibition of proliferative responses maintains the immunosuppressive effect.[177, 180]

Each polyclonal immune globulin preparation varies in its constituent antibodies. Because of the unpredictable nature of the antibody mixture, treatment is associated with variable efficacy as well as with adverse reactions. Batch standardization and assessments of immunosuppressive potency are therefore difficult. Unwanted antibodies could cause thrombocytopenia, granulocytopenia, serum sickness, or glomerulonephritis. Because of the development of host antibodies to the nonhuman globulin, anaphylactoid reactions are common.[177, 180] Although polyclonal immune globulins are potent immunosuppressive agents, the major concern is the potential for excessive immunosuppression, not infrequently resulting in opportunistic infections. Therefore, caution is necessary when immune globulins are combined with other immunosuppressive agents.

## Monoclonal Antibodies

The development of monoclonal antibodies to T cell surface molecules offers the advantage of homogeneous preparations and more predictable therapeutic agents. A number of monoclonal antibodies have been shown in clinical trials to produce immunosuppression. However, the most effective monoclonal antibody tested to date, and the only one approved for clinical use, is OKT3, which binds the T cell receptor. The T cell receptor is a complex of six or seven polypeptides, including the polymorphic α- and β-chains, which provide the antigen recognition component; and the γ-, δ-, and ε-chains, plus a ζζ-homodimer or ζη-heterodimer, which provide the signal transduction function of the receptor. OKT3 binds to the T cell receptor ε-chain, which is a pan–T cell nonpolymorphic component of the antigen receptor. Immunosuppression with OKT3 blocks both CD4+ and CD8+ T cell function.

Treatment with OKT3 produces multiple effects on T lymphocytes. The acute effect, which commences within minutes, is the partial activation of T cells due to signal transduction induced by the antibody. The activated T cells produce large amounts of lymphokines, including TNF-α, which causes many of the acute side effects of treatment, including fever, chills, nausea, vomiting, diarrhea, headache, anorexia, and a capillary leak syndrome.[111] In severe cases, patients can become hypotensive because of vasodilation and diarrhea. Alternatively, volume-overloaded patients are susceptible to pulmonary edema due to the capillary leak syndrome. Therefore, patients should be within 3% of their estimated dry weight before commencing therapy. Later side effects include aseptic meningitis or serum sickness due to the development of antimouse antibodies. The development of antimouse antibodies results in the rapid clearance of OKT3 from the serum and eliminates efficacy. The presence of antimouse antibodies can be monitored by indirect immunofluorescence by flow cytometry. Because of the profound immunosuppression, OKT3 treatment can be complicated by opportunistic infections, including an increased frequency of cytomegalovirus infection. Multiple courses of therapy have been associated with an increased frequency of malignant neoplasm, principally non-Hodgkin lymphoma.

There at least two components to the mechanism of immunosuppression by OKT3. Within hours after administration, OKT3 causes a profound depletion of peripheral T cells. Because OKT3 is not cytotoxic, it is thought that the depletion is due to sequestration of the T cells. In addition, T cells down-modulate the expression of the T cell receptor. Thus, after a few days of treatment, circulating CD4+ and CD8+ cells can be detected by flow cytometry that lack detectable T cell receptor.[181] It is thought that the T cell receptor is internalized by endocytosis or shedding. The modulation of T cell receptor expression is reversible, and after elimination of OKT3, the T cell receptor–CD3 complex is re-expressed on the cell surface.[182, 183]

## FUTURE THERAPY

Two major problems confront clinical transplantation: the shortage of donor organs, and the nonspecific nature of all available immunosuppressive agents. The failure to harvest an adequate supply of cadaveric organs has renewed interest in xenotransplantation. More than 25 years ago, baboon and chimpanzee organs were transplanted into humans with short-term success.[184, 185] However, major problems must be resolved before xenotransplantation becomes a reasonable clinical option. First, in discordant species combinations, such as pig to human, preformed antibodies can cause hyperacute rejection. Second, even between concordant species, the rejection response can be vigorous and probably uses quantitatively different mechanisms of rejection. Nevertheless, there is reason for optimism. Increased understanding of the xenogeneic immune response leading to improved immunosuppressive protocols in combination with transgenic technology that should be able to genetically engineer the donor to be more compatible with the human recipient may eventually facilitate successful clinical xenotransplantation.

The management of transplant recipients with nonspecific immunosuppressive regimens forces a continuous tradeoff between insufficient immunosuppression and excessive complications. Insufficient immunosuppression leads to breakthrough acute rejection episodes or smoldering chronic rejection, whereas excessive immunosuppression produces an increased rate of infections and malignant neoplasms. Current immunosuppressive drugs, including cyclosporine, corticosteroids, azathioprine, OKT3, and polyclonal immune globulins, inhibit the immune response to pathogens and tumor antigens as well as to graft-specific antigens. The addition of cyclosporine in the early 1980s has markedly increased short-term graft survival; however, it has failed to reduce the rate of long-term graft loss.[79] Thus, there is the need for the development of therapeutic modalities that induce graft-specific nonresponsiveness without suppressing immune responses to nondonor antigens, including infectious agents and tumor antigens.

## Experimental Immunosuppressive Agents

Many immunosuppressive agents are currently undergoing experimental or preclinical trials, including brequinar, deoxyspergualin, and RS-61443. In addition, monoclonal antibodies to the CD4 coreceptor molecule, the IL-2R, and the intercellular adhesion molecule-1 are under active investigation. Blockade of the intercellular adhesion molecule-1 has been shown to prolong graft survival in a primate model.[105] Similarly, targeting the CD4 molecule and IL-2R has been shown to be immunosuppressive. However, the ultimate goal of clinical transplantation is to induce donor-specific unresponsiveness in the recipient while maintaining responsiveness to nondonor antigens.

## Donor-Specific Immune Tolerance

Immunologists have been able to induce tolerance successfully in experimental models for more than three decades[186–188]; however, the mechanisms of tolerance remain incompletely understood.[118] More important, physicians have been unable to induce organ-specific tolerance after transplantation. However, advances in our understanding of T cell activation suggest strategies for inducing T cell tolerance. On the basis of numerous experiments, it is apparent that T cell activation requires at least two signals, including signaling through the T cell receptor plus a costimulatory receptor.[118] Interestingly, signaling through the T cell receptor alone without a costimulatory signal renders the cell anergic, which is a state of long-term unresponsiveness.[189] Clearly, the capacity to induce T cell anergy to graft-specific antigens could dramatically improve the management of organ transplantation.

In murine models, the administration of splenic lymphocytes has been shown to induce donor-specific tolerance.[190] This raises the question of whether lymphocyte transfusions (or the transfusion of specific lymphocyte subsets) can induce tolerance in human transplant patients. As previously discussed, the efficacy of pretransplant blood transfusions is currently controversial. In experimental models, the transfer of small resting B lymphocytes, but not large activated blast cells, preferentially induces tolerance.[190] Most mature T cells constitutively express the CD28 costimulatory receptors, which bind a family of counter-receptor molecules termed B7 on the surface of the antigen-presenting cell.[191] Because activated antigen-presenting cells express the B7 costimulatory counter-receptor, T cell recognition of antigen presented by an activated antigen-presenting cell induces T cell activation. However, because most resting antigen-presenting cells, including B lymphocytes, do not express B7, T cell recognition of antigen presented by a resting antigen-presenting cell induces T cell anergy. Thus, the transfusion of resting lymphocytes that fail to express B7 counter-receptors would induce T cell anergy, whereas the transfusion of activated lymphocytes that do express B7 would activate T cells. On the basis of these concepts suggesting that different activation states of the transfused lymphocytes would produce either T cell activation or anergy, it is not surprising that blood transfusion protocols have shown inconsistent results.

## TOLERANCE INDUCTION BY BLOCKADE OF COSTIMULATION

An alternative strategy is to inhibit the costimulatory signal during T cell encounter with donor antigen. This approach has been dramatically successful in two murine models. In these experiments, recognition of the B7 counter-receptors on the antigen-presenting cell by CD28 on the T cell was blocked with a soluble ligand termed CTLA4-Ig. CTLA4-Ig binds to the B7 counter-receptors with high affinity, blocking their interaction with CD28. In a xenogeneic model of pancreatic islet cell transplantation, administration of soluble CTLA4-Ig for 14 days indefinitely prevented graft rejection.[120] Similarly, in a heterotopic heart transplant model, the combination of donor-specific lymphocytes and CTLA4-Ig indefinitely prolonged graft survival.[121] These results indicate the potential to induce donor-specific tolerance by blocking costimulation during T cell encounter with donor antigen. The role of blocking costimulation in renal transplantation awaits clinical trials.

### REFERENCES

1. Kirberg J, Swat W, Rocha B, et al: Induction of tolerance in immature and mature T cells. Transplant Proc 25:279, 1993.
2. Goodnow CC, Adelstein S, Basten A: The need for central and peripheral tolerance in the B cell repertoire. Science 248:1373, 1990.
3. Kappler JJ, Roehm NJ, Marrack P: T cell tolerance by clonal elimination in the thymus. Cell 49:273, 1987.
4. Murphy KM, Weaver CT, Elish M, et al: Peripheral tolerance to allogeneic class II histocompatibility antigens expressed in transgenic mice: Evidence against a clonal deletion mechanism. Proc Natl Acad Sci USA 86:10034, 1989.
5. Webb S, Morris C, Sprent J: Extrathymic tolerance of mature T cells: Clonal elimination as a consequence of immunity. Cell 63:1249, 1990.
6. Schwartz RH: Acquisition of immunologic self-tolerance. Cell 57:1073, 1989.
7. Fry AM, Jones LA, Kruisbeek AM, Matis LA: Thymic requirement for clonal deletion during T cell development. Science 246:1041, 1989.

8. Gorer PA: The genetic and antigenic basis of tumor transplantation. J Pathol Bacteriol 44:691, 1937.
9. Snell GD: Methods for the study of histocompatibility genes. J Genet 49:87, 1948.
10. Klein J: Evolution and function of the major histocompatibility system: Facts and speculations. In Goetze D (ed): The Major Histocompatibility System in Man and Animals. Springer-Verlag, Berlin, 1977, p 339.
11. Klein J: An attempt at an interpretation of the mouse H-2 complex. Contemp Top Immunobiol 5:297, 1976.
12. Shreffler DC, David CS: The H-2 major histocompatibility complex and the I immune response region: Genetic variation, function, and organization. Adv Immunol 20:125, 1975.
13. Dausset J: Iso-leuco anticorps. Acta Haematol (Basel) 20:156, 1958.
14. Lamm Friedrich LU, Petersen U, Jorgensen GB, et al: Assignment of the major histocompatibility complex to chromosome no. 6 in a family with a pericentric inversion. Hum Hered 24:273, 1974.
15. Graff RJ, Silvers WK, Billingham RE, et al: The cumulative effect of histocompatibility antigens. Transplantation 4:605, 1966.
16. Holman E: Protein sensitization in iso-skin grafting. Is the latter of practical value? Surg Gynecol Obstet 38:100, 1924.
17. Medawar PB: The behaviour and fate of skin autografts and skin homografts in rabbits. J Anat 78:176, 1944.
18. Payne R, Tripp M, Weigle J, et al: A new leucocyte isoantigen system in man. Cold Spring Harb Symp Quant Biol 29:285, 1964.
19. Dupont B: Immunobiology of HLA. Springer-Verlag, New York, 1989.
20. Williams AF: A year in the life of the immunoglobulin superfamily. Immunol Today 8:298, 1987.
21. Stamenkovic I, Stegagno M, Wright KA, et al: Clonal dominance among T-lymphocyte infiltrates in arthritis. Proc Natl Acad Sci USA 85:1179, 1988.
22. Bodmer JG, Marsh SG, Albert ED, et al: Nomenclature for factors of the HLA system, 1991. Tissue Antigens 39:161, 1992.
23. Bjorkman P, Saper M, Samroui B, et al: Structure of the human class I histocompatibility antigen, HLA-A2. Nature 329:506, 1987.
24. Bjorkman P, Saper M, Samroui B, et al: The foreign antigen binding site and T cell recognition regions of class I histocompatibility antigens. Nature 329:512, 1987.
25. Claverie JM, Prochnicka-Chalufour A, Bougueleret L: Implications of a Fab-like structure for the T-cell receptor. Immunol Today 10:10, 1989.
26. Tapscott SJ, Lassar AB, Davis RL, Weintraub H: 5-Bromo-2'-deoxyuridine blocks myogenesis by extinguishing expression of MyoD1. Science 245:532, 1989.
27. Marcadet A, Cohen D, Dausset J, et al: Genotyping with DNA probes in combined immunodeficiency syndrome with defective expression of HLA. N Engl J Med 312:1287, 1985.
28. Bidwell J: DNA-RFLP analysis and genotyping of HLA-DR and DQ antigens. Immunol Today 9:18, 1988.
29. Higuchi R, von Beroldigen CH, Sensabaugh GF, Erlich HA: DNA typing from single hairs. Nature 332:543, 1988.
30. Milford EL: HLA molecular typing. Curr Opin Nephrol Hypertens 2:892, 1993.
31. Brown JH, Jardetzky TS, Gorga JC, et al: Three-dimensional structure of the human class II histocompatibility antigen HLA-DR1. Nature 364:33, 1993.
32. Chicz RM, Urban RG, Gorga JC, et al: Specificity and promiscuity among naturally processed peptides bound to HLA-DR alleles. J Exp Med 178:27, 1993.
33. Halloran PF, Wadgymar A, Autenried P: The regulation of major histocompatibility complex products. Prog Allergy 38:258, 1986.
34. Krensky AM, Weiss A, Crabtree G, et al: T-lymphocyte–antigen interactions in transplant rejection. N Engl J Med 322:510, 1990.
35. Steinmuller D: Which T cells mediate allograft rejection? Transplantation 40:229, 1985.
36. Bach FH, Bock H, Graupner K, et al: Cell kinetic studies in mixed leukocyte cultures: An in vitro model of homograft reactivity. Proc Natl Acad Sci USA 62:377, 1969.
37. Fischer-Lindahl K, Wilson DB: Histocompatibility antigens–activated cytotoxic T lymphocytes. II. Estimates of the frequency and specificity of precursors. J Exp Med 145:508, 1977.
38. Widmer MB, Donald HRM: Cytolytic T lymphocyte precursors reactive against mutant $K^b$ alloantigens are as frequent as those reactive against a whole foreign haplotype. J Immunol 127:48, 1980.

39. Sherman AL, Chattopadhyay S: The molecular basis of allorecognition. Annu Rev Immunol 11:385, 1993.
40. Lechler R, Batchelor R, Lombardi G: The relationship between MHC restricted and allospecific T cell recognition. Immunol Lett 29:41, 1991.
41. Lechler RI, Lombardi G, Batchelor JR, et al: The molecular basis of alloreactivity. Immunol Today 11:83, 1990.
42. Eckels D: Alloreactivity: Allogeneic presentation of endogenous peptides or direct recognition of MHC polymorphism. Tissue Antigens 35:49, 1990.
43. Jerne NK: The somatic generation of immune recognition. Eur J Immunol 1:1, 1971.
44. von Boehmer H, Haas W, Jerne NK: Major histocompatibility complex–linked immune-responsiveness is acquired by lymphocytes of low responder mice differentiating in thymus of high-responder mice. Proc Natl Acad Sci USA 75:2439, 1978.
45. Matis LA, Sorger SB, McElligott DL, et al: The molecular basis of alloreactivity in antigen-specific major histocompatibility complex–restricted T cell clones. Cell 51:59, 1987.
46. Braciale T, Andrew M, Braciale V: Simultaneous expression of H-2 restricted and alloreactive recognition by a cloned line of influenza virus–specific cytotoxic T lymphocytes. J Exp Med 153:1371, 1981.
47. Sredni B, Schwartz RH: Alloreactivity of an antigen-specific T-cell clone. Nature 287:855, 1980.
48. Finberg R, Burakoff SJ, Cantor H, Benacerraf B: Biological significance of alloreactivity: T cells stimulated by sendi virus–coated syngeneic cells specifically lyse allogeneic target cells. Proc Natl Acad Sci USA 75:5145, 1978.
49. Lechler RI, Batchlor JR: Restoration of immunogenicity to passenger cell–depleted kidney allografts by the addition of donor strain dendritic cells. J Exp Med 155:31, 1982.
50. Shoskes DA, Wood KJ: Indirect presentation of MHC antigens in transplantation. Immunol Today 15:32, 1994.
51. Sayegh MH, Watschinger B, Carpenter CB: Mechanisms of T cell recognition of alloantigen: The role of peptides. Transplantation 57:1295, 1994.
52. Heath WR, Hurd ME, Carbone FR, Sherman LA: Peptides dependent recognition of H-2K by alloreactive cytotoxic T lymphocytes. Nature 341:749, 1989.
53. Heath WR, Kane KP, Mescher MF, Sherman LA: Alloreactive T cells discriminate among a diverse set of endogenous peptides. Proc Natl Acad Sci USA 88:5101, 1991.
54. Elliot TJ, Eisen HN: Cytotoxic T lymphocytes recognize a reconstituted class I histocompatibility antigen (HLA-A2) as an allogeneic target molecule. Proc Natl Acad Sci USA 87:5213, 1990.
55. Ohlen C, Bastin J, Ljunggren HG, et al: Resistance to H-2–restricted but not to allo-H-2–specific graft and cytotoxic T lymphocyte responses in lymphoma mutant. J Immunol 145:52, 1990.
56. Cotner T, Mellins E, Johnson AH, Pious D: Mutations affecting antigen processing impair class II–restricted allorecognition. J Immunol 146:414, 1990.
57. Bluestone JA, Kaliyaperumal A, Jameson S, et al: Peptide induced changes in class I heavy chains alter allorecognition. J Immunol 151:3943, 1993.
58. Lechler RI, Heaton T, Barber L, et al: Molecular mimicry by major histocompatibility complex molecules and peptides accounts for some alloresponses. Immunol Lett 34:63, 1992.
59. Yard BA, Kooymans-Couthino M, Reterink T, et al: Analysis of T cell lines from rejecting renal allografts. Kidney Int 39:S133, 1993.
60. Yard BA, Paape ME, Claas FJH, et al: Recognition of a tissue specific polymorphism by graft infiltrating T cell clones from a renal allograft with acute rejection. J Am Soc Nephrol 4:921, 1993.
61. Roopenian DC, Davis AP, Christianson GJ, Mobraaten LE: The functional basis of minor histocompatibility loci. J Immunol 151:595, 1993.
62. Suciu-Foca N, Reed E, D'gai VD, et al: Soluble HLA-antigens, anti-HLA antibodies and anti-idiotypic antibodies in the circulation of renal transplant recipients. Transplantation 51:594, 1991.
63. Watschinger B, Gallon L, Carpenter CB, Sayegh MH: Mechanisms of allorecognition: In vivo primed T-cells recognize major histocompatibility complex polymorphisms presented as peptides by responder antigen-presenting cells. Transplantation 56:572, 1994.
64. Parker KE, Dalchau R, Fowler JV, et al: Stimulation of CD4 T lymphocytes by allogeneic MHC peptides presented on autologous antigen presenting cells. Transplantation 53:918, 1992.

65. Braun YM, McCormack A, Webb G, Batchelor RJ: Mediation of acute but not chronic rejection of MHC-incompatible rat kidney grafts by alloreactive CD4 T cells activated by the direct pathway of sensitization. Transplantation 55:117, 1993.

66. Dalchau R, Fangmann J, Fabre JW: Allorecognition of isolated, denatured chains of class I and class II major histocompatibility complex molecules. Evidence for an important role for indirect allorecognition in transplantation. Eur J Immunol 22:669, 1992.

67. Sherwood RA, Brent L, Rayfield LS: Presentation of alloantigens by host cells. Eur J Immunol 16:569, 1986.

68. Benichou G, Takizawa PA, Ho PT, et al: Immunogenicity and tolerogenicity of self–major histocompatibility complex peptides. J Exp Med 172:1341, 1990.

69. Benichou G, Takizawa AP, Olson AC, et al: Donor major histocompatibility complex (MHC) peptides are presented by recipient MHC molecules during graft rejection. J Exp Med 175:305, 1992.

70. Harris PE, Zhuoru L, Suciu-Foca N: MHC class II binding of peptides derived from HLA-DR1. J Immunol 148:169, 1992.

71. Fangmann J, Dalchau R, Sawyer GJ, et al: T cell recognition of donor major histocompatibility complex class I peptides during allograft rejection. Eur J Immunol 22:1525, 1992.

72. Sayegh MH, Khoury SK, Hancock WW, et al: Induction of immunity and oral tolerance with polymorphic class II MHC allopeptides in the rat. Proc Natl Acad Sci USA 89:7762, 1992.

73. Sayegh MH, Perico N, Imberti O, et al: Thymic recognition of class II MHC allopeptides induces donor specific unresponsiveness to renal allografts. Transplantation 56:461, 1993.

74. Human Renal Transplant Registry: Report No. 12. JAMA 233:787, 1975.

75. Opelz G, Terasaki PI: Studies on the strength of HLA antigens in related donor kidney transplants. Transplantation 24:106, 1977.

76. Alper CA: Extended MHC haplotypes and disease markers. ISI Atlas of Science: Immunology/1988. ISI Press, Philadelphia, 1988, p 79.

77. Schwartz BD, Luehrman LK, Rodey GE: A public antigenic determinant on a family of HLA-B molecules—basis for cross-reactivity and a possible link with disease predisposition. J Clin Invest 64:938, 1979.

78. Bach FH, van Rood JJ: The major histocompatibility complex: Genetics and biology. N Engl J Med 295:806, 1976.

79. Terasaki PI, Mickey MR, Cecka M, et al: Overview, clinical transplants 1987. In Terasaki PI (ed): Clinical Transplants 1987. UCLA Tissue Typing Laboratory, Los Angeles, 1987, p 467.

80. Opelz G, Mytilineos J, Scherer S, et al: Analysis of HLA-DR matching in DNA-typed cadaver kidney transplants. Transplantation 55:782, 1993.

81. Terasaki PI, Cecka JM, Gjertson DW, et al: A ten-year prediction for kidney transplant survival. In Terasaki PI, Cecka JM (eds): Clinical Transplants 1992. UCLA Tissue Typing Laboratory, Los Angeles, 1993, p 501.

82. Opelz G: Collaborative Transplant Study: Correlation of HLA matching with kidney graft survival in patients with or without cyclosporine treatment. Transplantation 40:240, 1985.

83. Opelz G, Mytilineos J, Wujciak T, et al: Current status of HLA matching in renal transplantation. The Collaborative Transplant Study. Clin Invest 70:767, 1992.

84. Sanfilippo F, Vaughn WK, Spees EK, et al: The effects of HLA-A,B matching on cadaver renal allograft rejection comparing public and private specificities. Transplantation 38:483, 1984.

85. Sanfilippo F, Goeken N, Niblack G, et al: The effect of first cadaver renal transplant HLA-A,B match on sensitization levels and retransplant rates following graft failure. Transplantation 43:240, 1987.

86. Gilks WR, Bradley BA, Gore SM, Klouda PT: Users of the UK Transplant Service: Substantial benefits of tissue matching in renal transplantation. Transplantation 43:669, 1987.

87. Persijn GG: HLA-matching and blood transfusion(s). In Drukkerij JH (ed): Renal Transplantation. Pasmans BV, The Hague, Netherlands, 1985, p 39.

88. Schreuder GM, Hendriks GFJ, D'Amaro J, Persijn GG: An eight year study of HLA typing proficiency in Eurotransplant. Tissue Antigens 27:131, 1986.

89. Opelz G, for the Collaborative Transplant Study: Importance of HLA antigen splits for kidney transplant matching. Lancet 2:61–64, 1988.

90. Takemoto S, Gjertson DW, Terasaki PI: HLA matching: A comparison of conventional and molecular approaches. In Terasaki PI, Cecka JM (eds): Clinical Transplants 1992. UCLA Tissue Typing Laboratory, Los Angeles, 1993, p 413.

91. Rodey GE, Fuller TC: Public epitopes and the antigenic structure of HLA molecules. Crit Rev Immunol 7:229, 1987.

92. Takemoto S, Terasaki PI, Cecka JM, et al: Survival of nationally shared HLA-matched kidney transplants from cadaveric donors. N Engl J Med 327:834, 1992.

93. Opelz G, Terasaki PI: Improvement of kidney graft survival with increased numbers of blood transfusions. N Engl J Med 299:799, 1978.

94. Cecka JM: The transfusion effect. In Terasaki PI (ed): Clinical Transplants 1987. UCLA Tissue Typing Laboratory, Los Angeles, 1987.

95. Iwaki Y, Cecka M, Terasaki PI: The transfusion effect in cadaver kidney transplants. Transplantation 49:56, 1990.

96. Lundgren G, Groth CG, Albrechtsen D, et al: HLA matching and pretransplant blood transfusions in cadaveric renal transplantation—a changing picture with cyclosporine. Lancet 1:66, 1986.

97. Toyotome A, Terasaki PI, Salvaterria O, et al: Early graft function. In Terasaki PI (ed): Clinical Transplants. UCLA Tissue Typing Laboratory, Los Angeles, 1989, p 435.

98. Lagaaij EL, Hennemann PH, Ruigrok M, et al: Effect of one HLA-DR antigen matched and completely HLA-DR mismatched blood transfusions on survival of heart and kidney allografts. N Engl J Med 321:701, 1989.

99. VanTwuyver E, Mooijaart RJ, Berge IJT, et al: Pretransplantation blood transfusion revisited. N Engl J Med 325:1210, 1991.

100. Cosimi AB, Burton RC, Colvin RB: Treatment of acute renal allograft rejection with OKT3 monoclonal antibody. Transplantation 32:535, 1981.

101. Ortho Multicenter Transplant Study Group: A randomized clinical trial of OKT3 monoclonal antibody for acute rejection of cadaveric renal transplants. N Engl J Med 313:337, 1985.

102. Vigeral P, Chkoff N, Chatenoud L: Prophylactic use of OKT3 monoclonal antibody in cadaver kidney recipients. Transplantation 41:730, 1986.

103. Henell KR, Cheever JM, Kimball JA, et al: OKT4A (a murine IgG2a anti-CD4 monoclonal antibody) in human organ transplantation. Transplant Proc 25:800, 1993.

104. Qin S, Cobbold S, Tighe H, et al: CD4 monoclonal antibody pairs for immunosuppression and tolerance induction. Eur J Immunol 17:1159, 1987.

105. Isobe M, Yagita H, Okumura K, Ihara A: Specific acceptance of cardiac allograft after treatment with antibodies to ICAM-1 and LFA-1. Science 255:1125, 1992.

106. Strom TB, Kelley VE: Toward more selective therapies to block undesired immune responses. Kidney Int 35:1026, 1989.

107. Kirkman RL, Shapiro ME, Carpenter CB, et al: A randomized prospective trial of anti-Tac monoclonal antibody in human renal transplantation. Transplantation 51:107, 1991.

108. Norman DJ, Kahana L, Stuart FP, et al: A randomized clinical trial of induction therapy with OKT3 in kidney transplantation. Transplantation 55:44, 1993.

109. Clevers H, Alarcon B, Wileman T, Terhorst C: The T cell receptor/CD3 complex: A dynamic protein ensemble. Annu Rev Immunol 6:629, 1988.

110. Caillat-Zucman S, Blumenfeld N, Legendre C, et al: The OKT3 immunosuppressive effect. In situ antigenic modulation of human graft-infiltrating T cells. Transplantation 49:156, 1990.

111. Gaston RS, Deierhoi MH, Patterson T, et al: OKT3 first-dose reaction: Association with T cell subsets and cytokine release. Kidney Int 39:141, 1991.

112. Pober JS, Gimbrone MA, Cotran RS: Ia expression by vascular endothelium is inducible by activated T cells and by human gamma interferon. J Exp Med 157:1339, 1983.

113. Saito T, Germain RN: Marked differences in the efficiency of expression of distinct alpha beta T cell receptor heterodimers. J Immunol 143:3379, 1989.

114. Shaw AS, Amrein KE, Hammond C, et al: The lck tyrosine protein kinase interacts with the cytoplasmic tail of the CD4 glycoprotein through its unique amino-terminal domain. Cell 59:627, 1989.

115. Morel P, Vincent C, Cordier G, et al: Anti-CD4 monoclonal antibody administration in renal transplanted patients. Clin Immunol Immunopathol 56:311, 1990.

116. Cosimi AB, Delmonico FL, Wright JK, et al: Prolonged survival of nonhuman primate renal allograft recipients treated only with anti-CD4 monoclonal antibody. Surgery 108:406, 1990.

117. Savas CP, Nolan MS, Lindsey NJ, et al: Renal transplantation in the rat—a new simple, non-suture technique. Urol Res 13:91, 1985.

118. Schwartz RH: A cell culture model for T lymphocyte clonal anergy. Science 248:1349, 1990.

119. Linsley PS, Greene JL, Tan P, et al: Coexpression and functional cooperation of CTLA-4 and CD28 on activated T lymphocytes. J Exp Med 176:1595, 1992.

120. Lenschow DJ, Zeng Y, Thistlethwaite JR, et al: Long-term survival of xenogeneic pancreatic islet grafts induced by CTLA4Ig. Science 257:789, 1992.

121. Lin H, Bolling SF, Linsley PS, et al: Long-term acceptance of major histocompatibility complex mismatched cardiac allografts induced by CTLA4Ig plus donor specific transfusion. J Exp Med 178:1801, 1993.

122. Schwartz RH: Costimulation of T lymphocytes: The role of CD28, CTLA-4, and B7/BB1 in interleukin-2 production and immunotherapy. Cell 71:1065, 1992.

123. Galvin F, Freeman GJ, Razi-Wolf Z, et al: Murine B7 antigen provides a sufficient costimulatory signal for antigen specific and MHC-restricted T cell activation. J Immunol 149:3802, 1992.

124. Bierer BE, Hollander G, Fruman D, Burakoff SJ: Cyclosporin A and FK506: Molecular mechanisms of immunosuppression and probes for transplantation biology. Curr Opin Immunol 5:763, 1993.

125. Perkins DL, Wang Y, Ho S, et al: Superantigen induced peripheral tolerance inhibits T cell responses to immunogenic peptides in T cell receptor (β-chain) transgenic mice. J Immunol 150:4284, 1993.

126. Rocken M, Urban JF, Shevach EM: Infection breaks T-cell tolerance. Nature 359:79, 1992.

127. Kang S, Beverly B, Tran A, et al: Transactivation by AP-1 is a molecular target of T cell clonal anergy. Science 257:1134, 1992.

128. Mossman TR, Cherwinski H, Bond MW, et al: Two types of murine helper T clones: I. Definition according to profiles of lymphokine activities and secreted proteins. J Immunol 136:2348, 1986.

129. Salgame P, Yamamura M, Bloom BR, Modlin RL: Evidence for functional subsets of CD4+ and CD8+ T cells in human disease: Lymphokine patterns in leprosy. Chem Immunol 54:44, 1992.

130. Hancock W, Sayegh MH, Kwod CA, et al: Oral, but not intravenous, alloantigen prevents accelerated allograft rejection by selective intragraft Th2 cell activation. Transplantation 55:1112, 1993.

131. Carpenter CB, Kirkman RL, Shapiro ME, et al: Prophylactic use of monoclonal anti–IL-2 receptor antibody in cadaveric renal transplantation. Am J Kidney Dis 14:54, 1989.

132. Myburgh JA, Cohen I, Gecelter L, et al: Hyperacute rejection in human-kidney allografts—Shwartzman or Arthus reaction? N Engl J Med 281:131, 1969.

133. Forbes RD, Guttmann RD: Pathogenetic studies of cardiac allograft rejection using inbred rat models. Immunol Rev 77:5, 1984.

134. Dosekun AK, First MR, Chandran PKG, et al: Successful treatment by defibrination with ancrod in a patient with hyperacute renal allograft failure in a deficiency of plasma prostaglandin-stimulating factor. Clin Nephrol 18:101, 1982.

135. Madsen JC, Superina RA, Wood KJ, Morris PJ: Immunological unresponsiveness induced by recipient cells transfected with donor MHC genes. Nature 332:161, 1988.

136. Shizuru JA, Gregory AK, Chao CT, Fathman CG: Islet allograft survival after a single course of treatment of recipient with antibody to L3T4. Science 237:278, 1987.

137. Wheelahan J, McKenzie IF: The role of T4+ and Ly-2+ cells in skin graft rejection in the mouse. Transplantation 44:273, 1987.

138. Nabarra B, Descamps B: Ultrastructure of cells infiltrating human kidney allografts. Clin Exp Immunol 24:300, 1976.

139. Kiaer H, Hansen HE, Olsen S: The predictive value of percutaneous biopsies from human renal allografts with early impaired function. Clin Nephrol 13:58, 1980.

140. Lund B, Jensen OM: Renal transplantation in rabbits. II. Morphological alterations in autografts. Acta Pathol Microbiol Scand A 78:701, 1970.

141. Solez K, McGraw DJ, Beschorner WE, et al: Reflections on use of the renal biopsy as the ''gold standard'' in distinguishing transplant rejection from cyclosporine nephrotoxicity. Transplant Proc 17:123, 1985.

142. Mayer TG, Bhan AK, Winn HJ: Immunohistochemical analyses of skin graft rejection in mice. Kinetics of lymphocyte infiltration in grafts of limited immunogenetic disparity. Transplantation 46:890, 1988.

143. Busch GJ, Reynolds ES, Galvanek EG, et al: Human renal allografts. The role of vascular injury in early graft failure. Medicine (Baltimore) 50:29, 1971.

144. Jeannet M, Pinn VW, Flax MH, et al: Humoral antibodies in renal allotransplantation in man. N Engl J Med 282:111, 1970.

145. Tullius SG, Heemann UW, Wagner K, Tilney NL: Changes of chronic kidney allograft rejection are reversible after retransplantation. Transplant Proc 25:906, 1993.

146. Brenner BM, Cohen RA, Milford EL: In renal transplantation, one size may not fit all. J Am Soc Nephrol 3:162, 1992.

147. Mintz B, Palm J: Gene control of hematopoiesis. I. Erythrocyte mosaicism and permanent immunological tolerance in allophenic mice. J Exp Med 129:1013, 1969.

148. Rosenberg AS, Mizuochi T, Singer A: Cellular interactions resulting in skin-allograft rejection. Ann N Y Acad Sci 532:76, 1988.

149. Paul L, Van Es L, Brutaldela Riviere G, et al: Blood group B antigen on renal endothelium as the target for rejection in ABO-incompatible recipient. Transplantation 26:268, 1978.

150. Manning DD, Reed ND, Shaffer CF: Maintenance of skin xenografts of widely divergent phylogenetic origin of congenitally athymic (nude) mice. J Exp Med 138:488, 1973.

151. Rosenberg AS, Mizuochi T, Sharrow SO, Singer A: Phenotype, specificity, and function of T cell subsets and T cell interactions involved in skin allograft rejection. J Exp Med 165:1296, 1987.

152. Sprent J, Schaefer M, Lo D, Korngold R: Properties of purified T cell subsets. II. In vivo responses to class I vs. class II H-2 differences. J Exp Med 163:998, 1986.

153. Rosenberg AS, Mizuochi T, Singer A: Analysis of T-cell subsets in rejection of Kb mutant skin allografts differing at class I MHC. Nature 322:829, 1986.

154. Lamm LU, Madsen M, Fjeldborg D: Outcome of kidney transplantation in highly sensitized patients in Scandiatransplant. Transplant Proc 19:729, 1987.

155. Grusby MJ, Auchincloss HJ, Lee R, et al: Mice lacking major histocompatibility complex class I and class II molecules. Proc Natl Acad Sci USA 90:3913, 1993.

156. Barber EK, Dasgupta JD, Schlossman SF, et al: The CD4 and CD8 antigens are coupled to a protein-tyrosine kinase (p56lck) that phosphorylates the CD3 complex. Proc Natl Acad Sci USA 86:3277, 1989.

157. McKenzie IF, Henning MM, Michaelides M: Skin graft rejection and delayed-type hypersensitivity responses to H-Y in an I-Ab mutant. Immunogenetics 20:475, 1984.

158. Inaba K, Granelli PA, Steinman RM: Dendritic cells induce T lymphocytes to release B cell–stimulating factors by an interleukin 2–dependent mechanism. J Exp Med 158:2040, 1983.

159. Bach JF: Thiopurines. North-Holland Publishing, Amsterdam, 1975, p 93.

160. Tilney NL, Kupiec-Weglinski JW, Heidecke CD, et al: Mechanisms of rejection and prolongation of vascularized organ allografts. Immunol Rev 77:185, 1984.

161. Kronke M, Leonard WJ, Depper JM, et al: Cyclosporin A inhibits T-cell growth factor gene expression at the level of mRNA transcription. Proc Natl Acad Sci USA 81:5214, 1984.

162. Emmel EA, Verweij CL, Durand DB, et al: Cyclosporin A specifically inhibits function of nuclear proteins involved in T cell activation. Science 246:251, 1989.

163. Dumont FJ, Staruch MJ, Koprak SK, et al: Distinct mechanisms of suppression of murine T cell activation by the related macrolides FK-506 and rapamycin. J Immunol 144:251, 1990.

164. Bierer BE, Mattila PS, Standaert RF, et al: Two distinct signal transmission pathways in T lymphocytes are inhibited by complexes formed between an immunophilin and either FK506 or rapamycin. Proc Natl Acad Sci USA 87:9231, 1990.

165. Iju J, Farmer JDJ, Lane WS, et al: Calcineurin is a common target of cyclophilin–cyclosporin A and FKBP-FK506 complexes. Cell 66:807, 1991.

166. Jain J, McCaffrey PG, Valge-Archer VE, Rao A: Nuclear factor of activated T cells contains Fos and Jun. Nature 357:801, 1992.

167. Schreiber SL, Crabtree GR: The mechanism of action of cyclosporin A and FK506. Immunol Today 13:136, 1992.

168. McDiarmid SV, Colonna J2, Shaked A, et al: A comparison of renal function in cyclosporine- and FK-506–treated patients after primary orthotopic liver transplantation. Transplantation 56:847, 1993.

169. Clipstone NA, Crabtree GR: Identification of calcineurin as a key signalling enzyme in T-lymphocyte activation. Nature 357:695, 1992.

170. Tocci MJ, Matkovich DA, Collier KA, et al: The immunosuppressant FK506 selectively inhibits expression of early T cell activation genes. J Immunol 143:718, 1989.

171. Chung J, Kuo CJ, Crabtree GR, Blenis J: Rapamycin-FKBP specifically blocks growth-dependent activation of and signaling by the 70 kd S6 protein kinases. Cell 69:1227, 1992.

172. Bierer BE, Schreiber SL, Burakoff SJ: The effect of the immunosuppressant FK-506 on alternate pathways of T cell activation. Eur J Immunol 21:439, 1991.

173. Kuo CJ, Chung J, Fiorentino DF, et al: Rapamycin selectively inhibits interleukin-2 activation of p70 S6 kinase. Nature 358:70, 1992.

174. Calvo V, Crews CM, Vik TA, Bierer BE: Interleukin 2 stimulation of p70 S6 kinase activity is inhibited by the immunosuppressant rapamycin. Proc Natl Acad Sci USA 89:7571, 1992.

175. Morice WG, Wiederrecht G, Brunn GJ, et al: Rapamycin inhibition of interleukin-2–dependent p33cdk2 and p34cdc2 kinase activation in T lymphocytes. J Biol Chem 268:22737, 1993.

176. Robertson A, Plenter R, Francis DM, Clunie GJ: Synergistic prolongation of renal allograft survival with cyclosporine and rapamycin. Transplant Proc 25:2898, 1993.

177. Goldstein G, Fuccello AJ, Norman DJ, et al: OKT3 monoclonal antibody plasma levels during therapy and the subsequent development of host antibodies to OKT3. Transplantation 42:507, 1986.

178. Penn I: The price of immunotherapy. Curr Probl Surg 18:682, 1981.

179. Penn I: Cancers following cyclosporine therapy. Transplantation 43:32, 1987.

180. Burdick JF: The biology of immunosuppression mediated by antilymphocyte antibodies. *In* Williams GM, Burdick JF, Solez K (eds): Kidney Transplant Rejection: Diagnosis and Treatment. Marcel Dekker, New York, 1986, p 307.

181. Chatenoud L, Baudrihaye MF, Kreis H, et al: Human in vivo antigenic modulation induced by the anti–T cell OKT3 monoclonal antibody. Eur J Immunol 12:979, 1982.

182. Goldstein G: Overview of the development of Orthoclone OKT3: Monoclonal antibody for therapeutic use in transplantation. Transplant Proc 19:1, 1987.

183. Bach FH, Sachs DH: Current concepts: Immunology. Transplantation immunology. N Engl J Med 317:489, 1987.

184. Reemtsma K: Xenotransplantation. *In* Cooper DKC (ed): The Transplantation of Organs and Tissues Between Species. Springer-Verlag, New York, 1991, p 9.

185. Starzl TE, Marchioro TL, Peters GN: Renal heterotransplantation from baboon to man: Experience with 6 cases. Transplantation 2:752, 1964.

186. Billingham RE, Brent L, Medawar PB: Actively acquired tolerance of foreign cells. Nature 172:603, 1953.

187. Dresser DW: Specific inhibition of antibody production. Immunology 5:378, 1962.

188. Golub ES, Weigle WO: Studies on the induction of immunologic unresponsiveness. I. Effects of endotoxin and phytohemagglutinin. J Immunol 98:1241, 1967.

189. Jenkins MK, Pardoll DM, Mizuguchi J, et al: Molecular events in the induction of a nonresponsive state in interleukin 2–producing helper T-lymphocyte clones. Proc Natl Acad Sci USA 84:5409, 1987.

190. Eynon EE, Parker DC: Small B cells as antigen-presenting cells in the induction of tolerance to soluble protein antigens. J Exp Med 175:131, 1992.

191. Schwartz RH: Costimulation of T lymphocytes: The role of CD28. CTLA-4, and B7/BB1 in interleukin-2 production and immunotherapy. Cell 71:1065, 1992.

# Clinical Aspects of Renal Transplantation

*Dianne B. McKay*
*Edgar L. Milford*
*Mohamed H. Sayegh*

## EVALUATION OF THE RECIPIENT AND DONOR

The purpose of a pretransplant evaluation is to screen the patient for problems that either preclude transplantation or if eliminated, reduce immediate and long-term complications in the recipient or increase survival of the graft. Given the profound donor shortage, a rational approach to distribution of cadaver organs must consider those patients with the best likelihood of long-term survival. This is obviously a subjective decision that stimulates much ethical debate but nevertheless enters into the pretransplant evaluation process.

Typical preliminary information requested by a transplant center in conducting a renal transplant evaluation is listed in Table 59–1. After receipt of this information, the patient is usually scheduled to meet with a transplant nephrologist and surgeon. To facilitate subsequent care, patients seen for a transplant evaluation are often presented to a transplant committee consisting of the transplant nephrologist, donor nephrologist, transplant surgeons, histocompatibility experts, transplant nurse coordinators, and social worker. Patients listed are then observed with monthly serum screening for anti–human leukocyte antigen (HLA) antibodies and yearly medical re-evaluations. If a new medical or surgical problem arises, the patient may be placed "on hold" until the problem is corrected. Keeping track of the hundreds of patients on the waiting list is an enormous task that requires cooperation among the referring nephrologists, dialysis centers, histocompatibility laboratory, organ procurement organization, and transplant hospital team. Because many patients wait years for a cadaver kidney, reevaluation at various time intervals is mandatory.

### Special Issues and Considerations

There are few clear contraindications (Table 59–2) to transplantation, although a life expectancy of less than 1 year, recent malignant neoplasm, active infection, chronic infections (which may be reactivated by immunosuppression), uncontrolled severe psychiatric disorders, ongoing substance abuse, and active noncompliance are considered absolute contraindications at most centers. It is often difficult to clearly delineate absolute contraindications; many previously ineligible patients are successfully undergoing transplantation because of improvements in medical and surgical technology.

The decision to approve a patient for transplantation may be modified by the life expectancy on dialysis; for instance, the patient may have no dialysis access and therefore must

**TABLE 59–1. Information Necessary to Evaluate a Recipient for Kidney Transplantation**

Medical and surgical history
Complete physical examination
Blood work: complete blood count, SMA 20, prothrombin time and partial thromboplastin time, VDRL test, parathyroid hormone level, viral serologic reactions (human immunodeficiency virus, hepatitis B surface antigen and antibody, hepatitis C virus), blood type
Urinalysis and urine culture
Purified protein derivative tuberculin test
Chest radiography
Electrocardiography
Tissue (HLA) typing
Panel reactive antibody assay

be urgently considered a candidate despite the presence of problems that would otherwise preclude transplantation.

The following are common medical and surgical issues seen in the end-stage renal disease population that have an impact on consideration for transplantation.

## PRIOR KIDNEY TRANSPLANT

The history of a previous kidney transplant presents some important issues in the evaluation process. The reason for the failed allograft needs to be carefully evaluated to ascertain whether the patient was noncompliant, loss of the graft was an aggressive and early immunologic failure associated with high levels of panel reactive antibodies (PRAs), and recurrence of native kidney disease (such as focal glomerulosclerosis or type II membranoproliferative glomerulonephritis) played a role in the loss of the previous graft. Regardless of the reason for the failed first allograft, the graft survival of the second kidney is clearly inferior to that of the first.[1–4]

## AGE

Advanced age is no longer an absolute contraindication to transplantation because there is a trend toward decreasing morbidity and mortality in the older age groups.[5] The older age group (>65 years) composes approximately 35% of the patients undergoing dialysis.[6–8] Although reluctance to perform transplantation in this group of patients was due to the belief that the perioperative and postoperative complication rates outweigh the advantages, this attitude is based on studies performed before the use of cyclosporine when higher steroid doses were standard.[9–12]

**TABLE 59–2. Contraindications to Renal Transplantation**

Life expectancy of less than 1 year
Recent malignancy
Active infection
Chronic untreated infection
Uncontrolled psychiatric disorders
Active substance abuse
Noncompliance

Some transplant centers require screening examinations, such as cardiac evaluation and barium enema study, in all patients older than 50 years,[13] as well as voiding cystourethrograms in all older men.[10] Our approach is to evaluate aggressively for inherent medical problems that are associated with morbidity and mortality in patients of advanced age, such as cardiovascular, pulmonary, gastrointestinal, and urologic diseases. If the patient is cleared from a medical standpoint, then age alone is not an exclusionary criterion.

## DIABETES MELLITUS

A large group referred for transplantation are diabetic patients approaching end-stage renal disease. Many of these patients have comorbid problems that increase their surgical and postoperative risk.

Type I diabetic patients with significant coronary artery disease have a 2-year survival of less than 50%.[14] Premature death due to coronary artery disease in diabetic patients in fact remains a major obstacle to improving transplant outcome in this population.[14]

It is prudent to recommend coronary angiography in all diabetic patients or in all adult diabetic patients,[13] before consideration for transplantation, especially because they can have significant coronary artery disease without symptoms of ischemia. In those with even mild symptoms, dipyridamole thallium and exercise thallium tests are unreliable predictors of ischemia,[15–19] and management of the patient must be dependent on angiographically determined coronary anatomy coupled with these other examinations.[14] The frequency of silent coronary disease is substantial in diabetic patients older than 30 years[18, 20–23]; 25% to 40% of diabetic patients screened with angiography have greater than 75% stenosis in one or more vessels.[14, 24–26]

Braun and co-workers[25] reported that of 25 diabetic renal transplant candidates with one or more coronary artery stenoses greater than 70%, only 44% were alive 2 years after angiography. Other investigators have shown mortality rates of 62% and 64% for an 18 to 24-month period in a similar population of patients.[27, 28] In addition, one third of all diabetic patients have left ventricular dysfunction.[24, 28, 29] There have been suggestions that diabetic patients with significant coronary artery disease should not undergo transplantation.[14, 25, 27, 28, 30, 31] Others have advocated transplantation only after revascularization,[14, 26] but this needs to be evaluated in long-term multicenter trials.[14]

Most diabetic patients should undergo transplant evaluation in consultation with a cardiologist. Coronary angiography should be done preoperatively in diabetic patients with symptoms or noninvasive test results suggestive of ischemia. If surgical intervention is necessary, it must be done before transplantation.

Diabetic patients with physical signs and symptoms of peripheral vascular disease, such as weak or absent peripheral pulses, should undergo a formal vascular evaluation. All active foot ulcers must be healed before the transplant. Prior limb amputation requires a more aggressive approach to the correction of additional large-vessel vascular disease.[32]

## CARDIOVASCULAR DISEASE

Cardiovascular disease is a primary cause of death after transplantation and is still one of the leading causes of death in the dialysis patient.[33] Significant coronary artery disease must be identified before transplantation and revascularization or appropriate therapy instituted. The preoperative assessment of these patients is complicated by the fact that many patients wait for years on the transplant list, and significant coronary artery disease may develop while they are waiting. For diabetic and other patients with increased risk, some centers advocate routine preoperative coronary angiography to identify asymptomatic coronary artery disease. Any patient with suspected coronary artery disease should undergo at least exercise testing and echocardiography as well as an evaluation by a cardiologist. Suitability for transplantation is then decided on an individual basis, depending on the results of all screening tests and the cardiologist's opinion.

## INFECTIONS

All active bacterial or fungal infections must be eradicated before transplantation. Patients undergoing dialysis are more susceptible to infections because of the frequent dialysis access needle punctures and the impairment of lymphocyte and granulocyte function associated with the uremic state.[34–37] Peritoneal dialysis poses a special risk for infectious complications, and infectious peritonitis within 4 weeks of transplantation is certainly a contraindication.[38–40]

All patients with a positive response to purified protein derivative, whether or not there is a history of vaccination with bacille Calmette-Guérin, should receive antimycobacterial prophylaxis while they are on the waiting list for transplantation. The antimicrobial prophylaxis must continue while the patient is receiving immunosuppressive medications.

## MALIGNANT NEOPLASM

For transplantation to be pursued in patients with a cancer history, certain guidelines must be considered. The current recommendation is to delay transplantation for at least 2 years after curative resection or treatment of malignant neoplasm. Data indicate a reduced risk of recurrence and morbidity due to malignant disease beyond this time.[41] In special circumstances, transplantation can be pursued without delay, such as primary tumor confined to the central nervous system, renal cell carcinoma not metastasized beyond the capsule, and basal cell carcinomas that are well resected.

## METABOLIC BONE DISEASE

Metabolic bone disease develops in almost all patients with chronic renal failure because of secondary hyperparathyroidism[42, 43] or aluminum-associated bone disease.[44] These problems should be minimized before transplantation with either vitamin D and phosphate binders in the case of the former or chelation therapy in the case of the latter. Transplantation is beneficial treatment for aluminum-associated bone disease.[45] If parathyroid bone disease is active with high levels of parathyroid hormone, then parathyroidectomy may need to be considered before the transplantation because of the risk of acute post-transplantation hypercalcemia in the presence of a functioning allograft (see later).

## GASTROINTESTINAL DISEASE

Patients with active peptic ulcer disease receiving large doses of steroids risk bleeding and perforation. Therefore, gastrointestinal workup is routinely done in symptomatic patients to detect the presence of ulcers. Prophylactic antiulcer surgery was common in the past in patients with documented hyperacidity,[46] but now most patients can be managed conservatively with histamine $H_2$ blockers with little postoperative risk.[47, 48] Although surgery is no longer indicated except in extreme cases, patients with active peptic ulcer disease should not undergo transplantation until the exacerbation is quiescent and healing of the ulcer is documented by endoscopy.

Lower gastrointestinal tract evaluation to detect diverticulosis is no longer routine. Active inflammatory diverticular disease, however, must be treated before transplant surgery.[49]

The approach to cholelithiasis is controversial.[13, 50] Some centers require pretransplant cholecystectomy in all patients with gallstones, and others require surgery only in patients demonstrating active disease.[13] Our center believes that there is no need for pretransplant cholecystectomy for asymptomatic cholelithiasis. Active cholecystitis, however, must be eradicated before transplantation.

Hepatic enzyme abnormalities and hepatitis are seen frequently in the pretransplant population.[33, 51] Serologic evaluation for multiple etiologic viruses is obtained in all patients with persistent transaminitis, and screening for hepatitis B and C is routine. Hepatitis B surface antigen (HBsAg)–positive patients risk development of chronic liver disease and progression to cirrhosis[52, 53]; therefore, all of these patients undergo liver biopsy before transplantation. Histologic evidence of chronic active disease or cirrhosis excludes patients for transplantation at our center. Chronic persistent disease, on the other hand, is not a contraindication to transplantation.[54]

The hepatitis C antibody–positive patient is at risk for progression to end-stage liver disease,[55] but interpretation of the antibody test must be considered in light of the sensitivity and specificity of the test. Patients with active disease should not undergo transplantation until it is clear whether they have a chronic active form of the disease.

## PULMONARY DISEASE

Patients with a history of chronic obstructive pulmonary disease or heavy smoking undergo spirometry and, on the basis of these results, are evaluated by a pulmonologist. Severe pulmonary hypertension is a contraindication to transplantation.[13]

## UROLOGIC EVALUATION

Because of an association of renal tumors with acquired renal cysts,[56–58] some centers advocate ultrasound screening of all patients with end-stage renal disease before transplantation. If symptomatic cysts or questionable masses are identified, it is recommended that the patient have magnetic resonance imaging to determine whether there is solid tumor present or be observed every 3 to 6 months for detection of any suspicious change in size or character of the mass.[56, 59] This follow-up should occur both while the patient is on the waiting list and after transplantation.

It is common to encounter obstructive uropathy or nephrolithiasis in patients with end-stage renal disease.[60, 61] A urologic evaluation should be obtained for all patients with a history of recurrent urinary tract infections (UTIs), pyelonephritis, vesicoureteral reflux, nephrolithiasis, renal malignancy, or neurogenic bladder. Anatomic problems should be corrected before transplantation, especially in cases of persistent severe reflux or neurogenic bladder requiring urinary diversion procedures. All infections of the urinary tract must be eradicated before transplantation. In patients with prostatic hypertrophy, full evaluation can often be made only after the patient has undergone transplantation and is making urine. Polycystic kidney disease requires identification of any active or chronic cystic infections and their eradication before transplantation. Routine pretransplant nephrectomy is not indicated for these patients unless there is insufficient anatomic space in which to place the new kidney, because nephrectomy carries significant risk.[62, 63]

## SYSTEMIC DISEASES

Patients with active *systemic lupus erythematosus* manifesting as cerebritis, pericarditis, myocarditis, vasculitis, or recent (<6 months) nephritis are not accepted for transplantation because of the concern that active disease may affect the transplanted kidney. The role of serologic tests for lupus in determining candidacy is controversial, but severely depressed serum complement levels or high anti-DNA antibody titers may be a relative contraindication.[64] Some centers do not perform transplantation on patients requiring maintenance therapy for lupus of more than 10 mg of prednisone per day.[13] Once serologically and symptomatically inactive, the disease rarely recurs.[65–67]

In the case of anti–glomerular basement membrane (anti-GBM) disease, a negative anti-GBM antibody is required for 6 months before transplantation to avoid recurrence of the disease in the allograft.[13] The current recommendation for Wegener granulomatosis and other forms of antinuclear cytoplasmic antibody–positive glomerulonephritis is to wait until antinuclear cytoplasmic antibody levels are low before proceeding with engraftment.[68]

Survival of patients with amyloidosis is better with transplantation than with dialysis.[69] Transplantation in patients with *Fabry disease* and *primary hyperoxalosis* is often not successful and therefore considered high risk, although combined kidney-liver transplantation has been performed for congenital hyperoxalosis. With the prolongation of life, other organ systems may become involved in the posttransplant period.[70, 71]

## PSYCHIATRIC PROBLEMS

Any history of psychiatric disorders or documented persistent noncompliance requires a psychiatric evaluation and a determination that the patient is able to follow the posttransplant medical regimen. Transplantation in patients with a history of substance abuse or noncompliance should be considered only after a period of demonstrated compliance and avoidance of substance use.

## VASCULAR DISEASE

Vascular disease of the lower extremities or carotid vessels is evaluated before surgery by noninvasive Doppler studies and, if indicated, an arteriogram.[13] The transplant surgeon determines the operative risk and assesses the potential for surgical anastomosis of the donor artery to a potentially diseased recipient vessel.

# Immunologic Evaluation of the Transplant Recipient

Immunologic evaluation of the renal transplant recipient serves to optimize selection of the appropriate donor for a given recipient and gives the clinician information that can be used to establish probability of rejection episodes and graft loss. Immunologic rejection of a kidney allograft can be mediated by either humoral or cellular mechanisms, both of which are directed against histocompatibility antigens that are expressed on the donor kidney. Alloantigen targets for kidney graft destruction may include HLA class I (A, B, or C) histocompatibility antigens,[72, 73] HLA class II (DR) histocompatibility antigens, non-HLA antigens expressed on endothelial cells,[74, 75] and ABO blood group antigens.[76] Donor kidneys that express antigens alien to the recipient will stimulate a primary immune response that will lead to graft damage or destruction unless adequate amounts of immunosuppressive drugs are administered. Three categories of immunologic evaluation assist the clinician in selecting appropriate donors or in determining prognosis of a transplant: typing and antigen matching, serum screening, and crossmatching.

## TYPING AND ANTIGEN MATCHING

The goal of typing and matching histocompatibility antigens between the recipient and donor is to minimize the number of incompatibilities presented by the graft and thus to decrease the likelihood of rejection. This can be done by phenotyping or genotyping both potential recipients and potential donors for the relevant antigens or genes and selectively performing transplants with those donor-recipient pairs that exhibit the lowest degree of incompatibility. Two HLA class I loci (A and B) and one HLA class II locus (DR or DRB1) are typed for the purpose of kidney transplantation. At each locus, there are multiple alleles. Because the alleles are codominantly expressed with virtually 100% expression, a large number of phenotypes are theoretically possible. For each of the three loci, a donor and recipient can be matched for zero, one, or two antigens. Degree of incompatibility can also be stated in terms of the number of antigens that are mismatched at one or more of the loci. Although the number of mismatches can usually be simply calculated from the number of matches, this is not always the case. For example, with a heterozygous recipient and a donor homozygous for one of the recipient HLA loci, the number of matches is only three of six, yet the recipient can perceive no mismatched antigens at any of the three loci. Table 59–3 gives examples of matching and mismatching grades for some informative donor and recipient phenotypes.

The role of HLA matching in the survival of renal allografts is clear from the combined data of both national[77] and international[78] registries. Allografts from HLA-identical siblings fare better than those from one haplotype–matched siblings, which in turn survive longer than cadaver renal allografts. Among cadaver allografts, the short- and long-term graft survival is negatively correlated with the degree of HLA mismatch. The degree to which HLA mismatching affects graft survival varies with the center and with the immunosuppressive protocols used. The incremental benefit of HLA matching is smaller in centers where the average graft survival is higher, and larger numbers of patients are needed to demonstrate a statistically significant effect of matching at those centers.

## SCREENING FOR HUMORAL SENSITIZATION

Patients can be sensitized against histocompatibility antigens before receiving an allograft and produce antibody directed against these antigens. This is usually the consequence of exposure to a previous transplant that was rejected, multiple blood transfusions, or pregnancy.[79] Those patients who are sensitized because of blood transfusion are also more likely to be women who have had at least one pregnancy. The degree to which a patient is sensitized can be measured in several different ways, two of which are used clinically. Screening for humoral sensitization is accomplished by testing reactivity of the patient's serum separately against lymphocytes obtained from each member of a reference panel of normal individuals with a spectrum of HLA phenotypes.[80] The assay most commonly used is complement-dependent microcytotoxicity,[81] although alternative methods such as indirect immunofluorescence have been used to determine antibody reactivity with panel cells.[82–85]

Two statistics that are useful to the clinician are derived from serum screening. The first is the percent panel reactivity (or PRA), calculated as the fraction of the panel whose cells are effective targets for the patient's antibody. The

PRA for a patient can vary between 0% and 100%. To the extent that a random panel is used, the percent PRA reflects the relative likelihood that a patient will have a negative crossmatch with an "average" organ donor derived from the general population and can be used in counseling patients about how long they are likely to wait before receiving a cadaver allograft. Patients with high degrees of sensitization as measured by PRA percentage will more often be excluded from transplantation because of the absolute contraindication of a positive crossmatch.[86, 87] The PRA is often used in regional and national organ sharing algorithms as a method to identify potential recipients who require affirmative steps, such as increased queue points, to increase their probability of receiving a cadaver graft toward the average. The second statistic that can be obtained from serum screening is the anti-HLA specificity of any antibody that a patient is producing. Typically, the panel of individuals used as target lymphocyte donors in serum screening have been HLA phenotyped. Computerized analysis of the HLA antigens of the panel members whose cells are bound and killed by the recipient's serum, versus those that are not, yields a list of anti-HLA antibody specificities that explains the reactivity of a given serum sample. A sequential record of historic antibody specificities of a potential recipient can be used to avoid donors with those specificities and helps counter false-negative crossmatch results that are sometimes obtained with a single serum sample.[80]

## CROSSMATCHING

With the exception of ABO blood group matching, the recipient antidonor lymphocyte crossmatch is the most important immunologic test that must be done before transplantation. Crossmatching permits the clinician to determine whether there is pre-existing antibody against donor histocompatibility antigens at the time of the transplant or in archived serum samples from the recipient. Kidney transplants done across a strongly positive crossmatch with a current serum sample are virtually certain to suffer hyperacute rejection, an immediate form of severe humoral rejection that results in graft ischemia and loss within hours.[86, 87] Class I HLA-A, -B, and -C locus antigens are ubiquitous and expressed on most kidney parenchymal cells.[88] They therefore serve as effective targets for recipient antidonor class I antibody. In the crossmatch assay, donor T lymphocytes are typically used as a surrogate target in lieu of donor

**TABLE 59–3. Relation Between Degree of HLA Match and Mismatch***

| Recipient Phenotype | Donor Phenotype | Number of Matches | Number of Mismatches |
|---|---|---|---|
| **A1,A2,B7,B8,DR3,DR4** | **A1,A2,B7,B8,DR3,DR4** | 6 | 0 |
| A1,**A2,B7,B8,DR3,DR4** | A3,**A2,B7,B8,DR3,DR4** | 5 | 1 |
| A1,A2,B7,B8,DR3,DR4 | A3,A9,B45,B44,DR1,DR9 | 0 | 6 |
| **A1**,A2,B7,**B8,DR3**,DR4 | **A1**,A1,**B8**,B8,**DR3**,DR3 | 3 | 0 |

*The number of HLA mismatches usually equals six minus the number of matches for the A, B, and DR loci. In the table, mismatched donor antigens are underlined, and matched antigens are in boldface. Degree of mismatch is a more accurate measure of unidirectional recipient antidonor incompatibility. The fourth donor-recipient pair is an example of homozygosity for HLA-A, -B, and -DR in the donor, yielding no mismatches, even though there are only three matches.

**TABLE 59–4. Clinical Significance of Pretransplant Crossmatch Tests in Renal Transplantation**

| Technique | Type of Antibody Detected | Clinical Implications of Positive Test |
|---|---|---|
| Standard T cell | Detects anti–class I HLA-A, -B, and -C antibody | Absolute contraindication to transplantation |
| Standard B cell | Detects class II HLA-DR and -DQ as well as class I antibody | Relative contraindication to transplantation if titer is high |
| Platelet absorption | Distinguishes class II from class I antibody when retested on B cells | Absolute contraindication to transplantation if antibody is removed by absorption |
| Antiglobulin | Detects weak or non–complement-fixing antibody | Relative contraindication to transplantation |
| Flow cytometry | Detects weak or non–complement-fixing antibody | Relative contraindication to transplantation |
| Autoantibody | Detects antibody induced by autoimmune disease or medication that cross-reacts with donor | No effect on graft survival if this is only antibody present |
| Dithioerythritol reduction | Removal of positive crossmatch after dithioerythritol treatment indicates immunoglobulin M isotype | No effect on graft survival if autoantibody |

kidney tissue, because T cells amply express class I antigens and can be readily isolated from blood, lymph node, or spleen.

Antibody directed against class II HLA-DR or -DQ antigens can be measured by performing a crossmatch with donor B lymphocytes as the target cells.[81] Class II antigens are expressed on B cells but not T cells. However, because B cells also express class I antigen, the finding of a positive B cell crossmatch does not necessarily mean that class II antibody is present. When a positive B cell crossmatch is found, the molecular target of the antibody can be further characterized by absorption of the serum with pooled platelets, a process that will remove anti–class I but not anti–class II antibody.[81] The significance of positive anti–class II antibody in a pretransplant serum sample has been debated.[89–95] Most investigators have found that a high-titer anti–class II antibody is a relative contraindication to transplantation, especially in a highly sensitized patient or a recipient who has previously rejected a kidney graft.[93–95]

Positive crossmatches are sometimes found in patients who are producing autoantibody as a result of an autoimmune disease, acute viral infection, or therapy with drugs that can induce an autoimmune antibody response.[96] This phenomenon is seen frequently in patients with lupus erythematosus and patients receiving methyldopa, procainamide, or hydralazine. The autoantibody also reacts with a variable proportion of individuals in the general population and can cause a high PRA percentage on cytotoxic serum screening. Autoantibody is rarely directed against histocompatibility antigens, is usually of the immunoglobulin M (IgM) isotype, and is not a contraindication to successful kidney transplantation.[97, 98] Autoantibody is often of low affinity and may yield a positive crossmatch only when the assay is done at 4°C rather than at 22°C or 37°C. The clinician determines whether autoantibody accounts for a positive pretransplant crossmatch by noting whether the crossmatch becomes negative after serum is absorbed with autologous lymphocytes at 4°C. Autoantibodies can be removed from serum by autoabsorption, whereas alloantibodies cannot. The isotype of the antibody causing a positive crossmatch can also be determined by repeating the crossmatch assay after treatment of the serum with a reducing agent, such as dithiothreitol or dithioerythritol, which selectively denatures IgM. Although it is possible to produce an IgM response against histocompatibility antigens, the iso-

type virtually always converts to immunoglobulin G (IgG) with time. Finding that multiple historical recipient serum samples have only IgM antidonor antibody implies that the antibody causing the positive crossmatch is not a contraindication to transplantation.

Whereas the standard crossmatch technique is sufficient to avoid hyperacute rejection caused by anti-HLA antibodies, a number of enhanced or potentiated crossmatch techniques are available to the clinician. These crossmatch techniques are able to detect antidonor antibodies that do not fix complement or are present at low concentration. Although such antibodies do not cause hyperacute rejection, they may mediate graft injury through other mechanisms, such as antibody-dependent cell-mediated lymphocytotoxicity, which damage the organ in a less aggressive fashion. Antibody-dependent cell-mediated lymphocytotoxicity can occur even when noncytotoxic antibodies bind to donor kidney cells. So-called K cytotoxic effector cells, which bear receptors for the Fc portion of immunoglobulin, then bind to the fixed immunoglobulin and lyse the targeted graft cells.[99, 100] Even low-titer or noncomplement antidonor antibody is a positive indication that the potential recipient has previously been sensitized to antigens expressed on the donor kidney. Clinical studies have proved that such patients are at increased risk for acute graft rejection episodes and graft loss, even though they have a negative standard crossmatch. Methods used to enhance the standard crossmatch include "long incubation," "anti–human globulin" sandwich technique, and indirect "flow crossmatch" immunofluorescence techniques using laser-activated cell analyzers.[82–84, 101, 102] As with the B cell crossmatch, crossmatches that are enhanced with antiglobulin or flow cytometry should be used in settings in which the recipient is known to have increased immunologic risk (second transplants, high PRA) or in other circumstances when the cost-benefit ratio must be maximally weighted toward graft survival for the transplant to proceed. Table 59–4 defines the types of antibody detected by the most commonly used crossmatches and the clinical implications of positive reactions.

## ABO BLOOD GROUP MATCHING

One can conceive of ABO blood group matching as a form of surrogate crossmatching, because recipients who are ABO incompatible with their donors have preformed antidonor antibody at the time of transplantation. Whereas it had long been assumed that transplants done across an ABO blood group barrier were always rejected, data collected by Opelz and Terasaki[76] on a series of transplants that were mistakenly performed with ABO-mismatched kidneys proved that between 55% and 65% of organs can survive 1 year or more. Blood group O individuals are "universal donors," that is, their kidneys can be placed into A, B, AB, or O recipients. In contrast, the blood group O recipient can receive a kidney only from a group O donor. If group O kidneys were given to non-O recipients, there would not be enough for the O recipients, especially because there are insufficient numbers of donors to meet the overall recipient demand. Therefore, most transplant centers follow a policy of restricting blood group O cadaver kidneys to group O recipients. The blood group $A_2$ provides a further exception to the strict rule that kidney donors must be ABO-compatible with their recipients. Kidneys from $A_2$ donors have on occasion been used successfully in non-A recipients when the titer of antibody against blood group A is less than 1:8.[76, 103, 104] Higher titers of anti-A antibody in the recipient predict severe rejection. Despite these data, use of donors who are mismatched for ABO blood groups is not accepted as a routine practice in most centers because there is usually a fully compatible recipient available. Rh antigens are not prominently expressed on cells in the kidney; thus, Rh incompatibility and anti-Rh antibody are not important in renal transplantation.

## FAMILY TESTING TO DETERMINE HAPLOTYPES

When there are several ABO blood group–compatible donors available for a transplant candidate among the recipient's immediate family or first-degree relatives, it is advisable to do HLA phenotyping on the recipient, all prospective donors, and a sufficient number of the immediate family members to establish genotypes of the recipient and potential donors. Because the genes that encode the HLA-A, -B, and -DR antigens are inherited en bloc as a group of closely linked genes, one can usually define two gametotypes per individual. Each gametotype is composed of one A, one B, and one DR locus allotype that were inherited on the same gamete. By analyzing the HLA phenotypes within a family and knowing the familial relationships between individuals, it is usually possible to assign two gametotypes, or HLA haplotypes, to each individual. Unless a recombination has taken place during meiosis, a recipient will share zero, one, or two haplotypes with each potential donor in the family. A related donor who shares two HLA haplotypes (and therefore all six HLA alleles) with a potential recipient has a higher degree of compatibility than an unrelated donor who shares the same six HLA alleles with the recipient. This is because there are other histocompatibility antigen loci that are located within the HLA genetic region, or major histocompatibility complex. A relative who is known to share two haplotypes also shares these closely linked genes; an unrelated donor who shares all six alleles at the A, B, and C loci may be incompatible for the other genes of the major histocompatibility complex.

## CELLULAR ASSAYS FOR HISTOCOMPATIBILITY TESTING

The mixed lymphocyte culture is an assay that is sometimes obtained to confirm that a two haplotype–matched donor has no incompatibility at the HLA-DR locus. The ability of prospective recipient cells to proliferate in vitro when exposed to donor cells that have been irradiated is a sensitive measure of DR compatibility. Historically, HLA-DR serotyping has been technically difficult, and error rates can be as high as 15% to 20%.[105, 106] A negative mixed lymphocyte culture serves to assure the clinician that there is true HLA identity between familial donor-recipient pairs, because any mismatch will give a proliferative response significantly higher than control background. Proliferation is typically measured in terms of tritiated thymidine incorporation, a ratio of experimental to control proliferation, or experimental proliferation as a percentage of maximal proliferation of recipient cells when they are exposed to known histoincompatible cells.

The need for mixed lymphocyte culture testing has been obviated by the advent of highly accurate DNA-based genotyping for several of the genes in the DR region of the major histocompatibility complex. The assays are done by use of polymerase chain reaction amplification of HLA-DR genes followed by either sequence-specific oligonucleotide probing or restriction enzyme digestion to define the DR genotype. Sensitivity and specificity of DNA typing in most laboratories are 98% or better. Although DNA typing for class I HLA-A and -B antigens is not yet in routine clinical use, it is currently being developed.

## Organ Sharing in the United States

All cadaver donors, cadaver organs procured, and cadaver organs transplanted must be registered with the Department of Health and Human Services through the Division of Transplantation's Organ Procurement Transplant Network. The United Network for Organ Sharing has been the contractual agent for the Organ Procurement Transplant Network since its inception. It collects extensive statistical data on all individuals awaiting transplantation and has been obtaining verified data on graft survival and function for transplants done since 1988. All centers engaged in transplantation must belong to and abide by the rules of the Organ Procurement Transplant Network, which are approved by the Secretary of Health and Human Services. All cadaver organs procured must be handled by one of the network-approved organ procurement organizations, which serve geographic regions. Organ procurement agencies must assign kidneys to a specific recipient on the basis of an algorithm defined by the Organ Procurement Transplant Network or using a variance of the algorithm that has been approved by its board of directors. Data derived from the Organ Procurement Transplant Network scientific registry provide important information that permits multivariate analysis of the factors important in both short- and long-term graft survival.

## Analysis of Survival Data

Effectiveness of renal transplantation as replacement therapy for end-stage renal disease is often measured by actuarial graft survival. The statistical probability of a patient's being alive with a functioning allograft is calculated by determining the cumulative risk of death or graft loss within a specified period. Ideally, the data should be derived from a data set in which all patients have been observed for the longest interval of interest; however, this is rarely the case. Although recent transplant recipients may have been observed for less than the maximal interval of interest, it is possible to include them in the data set by using only the data on recent transplant recipients to estimate the risk of early graft loss. Because actuarial graft survival curves often include cohorts of patients who received transplants in different years, the estimates may be biased if there have been systematic changes in graft survival with time. In this case, actual graft survivals are a more accurate reflection of cohorts undergoing transplantation at different times. In the past decade, there has been a steady increase in the early (6-month to 1-year) graft survival probability, with little change in the rate of graft loss after 1 year. Survival curves for renal graft survival all show a characteristic pattern of a sharp decline in the first 3 to 6 months after transplantation followed by a slower constant rate of "chronic" graft loss thereafter. Determination of the factors that are important in renal allograft survival has depended on analysis of differences in actuarial graft survival between cohorts of patients who have or lack a risk factor under consideration. More sophisticated studies have used multivariate analysis of actuarial graft survival to eliminate covariation between several risk factors.[107]

## KIDNEY DONATION

The successful outcome of renal transplantation depends greatly on the identification and preparation of suitable live or cadaver donors. There are currently 25,000 patients with end-stage renal disease listed with the United Network for Organ Sharing for a kidney transplant, but only approximately 7000 cadaver organs are available for transplantation.[108] Because of the severe shortage of cadaver allografts, live donors are encouraged at many transplant centers. In 1989, living related donors accounted for 20% of the transplants performed in the United States.[6] Most transplant centers prefer the use of genetically related donors, but unrelated live donors are acceptable in some situations. Although living donation is widely accepted in the United States, 22% of centers in Europe do not perform such transplants because of ethical concerns.[109] Ethical issues associated with transplantation are discussed later.

## Live Donation

Identification of a potential donor for transplantation begins with a family meeting where information about transplantation and its risks is imparted to all family members.

Once an interested donor is identified, the evaluation process begins. The steps in the living related donor workup are shown in Table 59–5. An aggressive medical workup is performed to protect the health and welfare of the donor and to provide the best possible kidney for the recipient.

Strict adherence to confidentiality must exist between the donor and the physician. To avoid any conflict of interest, the medical care and workup of the donor and recipient should be conducted by different physicians. The potential donor must be assured that it is possible to withdraw at any time without being subjected to family pressures. If at any time the potential donor does not wish to proceed, it is usually possible to simply state to the family that the individual is not a suitable donor, without further elaboration that might compromise the potential donor.

Exclusion criteria for living related donation include young age (<18 years); significant medical illness, including severe hypertension, diabetes mellitus, and renal disease; history of nephrolithiasis; history of hypercoagulability; proteinuria; pathologic hematuria; severe obesity; uncontrolled psychiatric disorders; human immunodeficiency virus (HIV), hepatitis B virus (HBV), hepatitis C virus (HCV) infection; and family history of polycystic kidney disease, diabetes mellitus in both parents, or hereditary nephritis.

The immediate operative morbidity risks associated with uninephrectomy are low (0.1% to 0.4%) compared with similar surgical procedures[109] and consist of infection, atelectasis, pulmonary emboli, pneumothorax, myocardial infarction, and renal failure.[110, 111] On the basis of studies in nephrectomized rats, it has been suggested that glomerular hyperfiltration in the remaining kidney will result in progressive sclerosis and deterioration in renal function.[112] The literature suggests that there is potential for hypertension and proteinuria to develop in healthy donors as a result of a 50% reduction in renal mass. However, large studies including more than 600 living donors have not shown an increased frequency of either significant hypertension or renal insufficiency for as long as 19 years after uninephrectomy.[113–118] Progression has not been demonstrated by measuring a rise in serum creatinine concentration[113] or

---

**TABLE 59–5. Living Related Donor Workup**

Identification of interested family member
Potential donor schedules appointment with donor nephrologist
Complete history and physical examination
Blood type and HLA determination
Screening laboratory analysis: complete blood count; serum chemistry
  profile; viral serology: hepatitis B virus, hepatitis C virus,
  cytomegalovirus; prothrombin time and partial thromboplastin
  time; glucose tolerance test (if any family history of diabetes
  mellitus); pregnancy test
Urinalysis with examination of sediment and urine culture ×2
24-h collection of urine for protein and creatinine excretion ×2
Electrocardiography
Chest radiography
Pulmonary function tests
Excretory urography
Arteriography
Repeated crossmatch before donation
Hospitalization for donation

decline in inulin or creatinine clearances up to 4 years after transplantation.[116, 119] In patients with unilateral renal agenesis, however, focal glomerular sclerosis with gradual decline in renal function is seen over many years.[120] In addition, proteinuria develops in one third of patients who donate a kidney, of 100 to 200 mg/24 h increase over baseline values, which suggests that there is indeed an alteration in glomerular function based on the reduction in nephron mass.[115, 117, 121] Long-term studies have not been done to assess the possibility of progression of renal insufficiency in this subgroup of patients observed longer than two decades after transplantation. Particularly for the young donor, or the donor who later suffers from acquired hypertension or diabetes, the presence of only one kidney may contribute to earlier onset of renal dysfunction.

It is therefore recommended that donors have regular medical examinations including blood pressure determination, serum creatinine and glucose measurements, urinalysis, 24-hour urine collection for protein excretion, and glomerular filtration rate determination.[122] Although there is no evidence to date to indicate whether renal function and mild proteinuria will remain stable beyond the 20-year period, further studies are needed to explore this possibility beyond the first two post-transplant decades, especially for high-risk donors with a family history of diabetes or hypertension.

## Nonrelated Living Donation

Many centers encourage nonrelated live donation because of the shortage of donor organs. Transplantation between patients with strong emotional ties, such as spouse to spouse, is often acceptable at these centers. Donation from nonrelated, distant persons is controversial because of the increased possibility of hidden financial remuneration to the donor or questionable motives of the donor.

## Cadaver Donation

The process for cadaver donation begins when the organ procurement agency is notified of brain death and permission for donation is obtained from the family. The suitability of the potential cadaver donor is then screened by the organ procurement agency. Laboratory results are reported to the organ procurement agency, and information on the circumstances surrounding the patient's death are obtained. Table 59–6 lists the procedure for a cadaver donor workup. A cadaver kidney would be rejected if the donor had any indication of chronic renal disease, severe hypertension, malignant neoplasm (except primary brain tumor), septicemia, vascular disease, Creutzfeldt-Jakob disease, or infection with HIV, HBV, or HCV. Serologic reactions for HIV-1, HIV-2, human T cell lymphotropic virus types I and II, rapid plasma reagin–VDRL, antibody to cytomegalovirus (CMV), HBsAg, anti-HBV, and anti-HCV are obtained. In addition, any history of behavior that places the patient at recognized risk for HIV infection as identified by the Centers for Disease Control and Prevention would exclude the organ donor.

**TABLE 59–6. Cadaver Donor Workup**

Identify potential cadaver donor
Inform organ procurement agency
Establish brain death
Obtain consent for donation from family
Prepare donor with appropriate hemodynamic and respiratory support
Maintain stable electrolytes and urine output
Obtain medical history to rule out high-risk illnesses
Screening laboratory analysis: blood type; HLA screening; complete blood count; serum chemistry profile; blood, urine, and sputum cultures; urinalysis; chest radiography; viral serologic reactions
Administer preoperative antibiotics and methylprednisolone sodium succinate (Solu-Medrol)
Repeat blood, sputum, and urine cultures (from each ureter and bladder)
Harvest organs

## Cadaver Organ Harvesting and Preservation

The donor organs are obtained through an en bloc nephroureterectomy including a segment of aorta and inferior vena cava. Before cross-clamping, the aorta is cannulated, and the organs are flushed with a preservation solution (University of Wisconsin solution). The harvest is then completed, and organs are stored in a cold ice bath. Warm ischemia refers to the period between donor asystole, or lack of blood flow to the kidneys, and the beginning of cold storage. Warm ischemia can also occur at the time of kidney implantation if there is excessive delay in reperfusion at the time of anastomosis. Cold ischemia refers to the time in cold storage or machine perfusion. Warm ischemia times of greater than 20 minutes and cold ischemia times of greater than 30 hours are associated with increased risk for delayed graft function.[123–126]

In the process of harvesting, cadaver kidneys are flushed with a cold physiologic solution and placed in an ice bath for storage until transplantation. The time in the ice bath varies, but optimally the transplant is performed within 30 hours.[124] Another method of preservation that prolongs the storage time is machine perfusion. In this case, the cold perfusate is pumped continuously through the renal vessels. Some groups have reported longer preservation times with machine perfusion,[126] although most transplant centers rely primarily on nonperfused storage. The solution most frequently used, for both flush and perfusion methods, was developed at the University of Wisconsin and dramatically extended safe preservation times for multiple organs.[127] It supplanted the previously used Collins solution and has the advantage of suppressing hypothermia-induced cell swelling and membrane damage and maintaining integrity of intracellular enzymes and normal intracellular ATP concentrations.[127]

## THE TRANSPLANT SURGERY AND POTENTIAL COMPLICATIONS
### Preoperative Care

Immediately before surgery, the potential recipient must be evaluated for operative suitability. This includes immediate management of volume status and electrolyte abnormalities, generally with dialysis, and an aggressive search for any medical reasons to postpone the surgery. If, for example, the patient has an active UTI, has peritonitis associated with an indwelling peritoneal catheter, or has any evidence of active ischemic heart disease, the surgery would be canceled until the patient is stabilized. Most patients have undergone a pretransplant evaluation before listing, but because the waiting time is long, they must be re-examined immediately before surgery. A thorough preoperative medical evaluation is critical to screen for any illnesses that have developed since the initial transplant evaluation.

It is advantageous to dialyze the patient within 12 hours of the transplant surgery to optimize volume status and correct any electrolyte abnormalities. The patient is likely to receive a large volume of crystalloid or colloid, and a short period of dialysis is often enough to ensure appropriate volume and electrolyte status. A patient who is dialyzed before surgery will usually not need immediate postoperative dialysis and will avoid the post-transplant risk of bleeding due to dialysis-associated heparinization and the risk of acute tubule necrosis (ATN) from dialysis-induced hypotension or hypovolemia.[128]

## Surgical Technique

Technical complications after renal transplantation are uncommon but can result in graft loss and significant morbidity. Exact attention to the surgical technique is critical because the patient risks wound infections as a result of the immunosuppressive agents and poor wound healing from the malnourished state associated with long-term hemodialysis.[129]

It is now routine to give transplant patients an intraoperative dose of antibiotics with broad-spectrum activity; this has been shown to decrease the frequency of postoperative wound infections.[130] In addition, generous amounts of colloid and crystalloid given during the operative procedure along with furosemide, mannitol, and (at some centers) intravenous $Ca^{2+}$ channel blockers decrease the frequency of delayed graft function.[131]

The basic surgical technique has not changed substantially since its introduction in the 1950s.[132, 133] An incision is made between the iliac crest and the pubis, the epigastric vessels are divided, and the external iliac vessels are isolated. All lymphatic vessels are ligated to prevent leakage of lymphatic fluid and subsequent lymphocele. The renal artery of the donor is anastomosed end-to-side to the external iliac artery of the recipient (Fig. 59–1). An important modification of the original technique involves harvesting the cadaver kidney with a cuff of donor aorta surrounding the renal arteries.[134] This surgical maneuver decreases the potential of subsequent vascular stenosis associated with the anastomotic site.[135] If there is no cuff, any polar branches are anastomosed end-to-side to the main renal artery. The renal vein is then anastomosed end-to-side with the external iliac vein of the recipient. The recipient's urinary bladder is cannulated with a Foley catheter at the beginning of the procedure and infused with an antibiotic solution. The ureterovesical anastomosis is achieved by making a small hole in the dome of the bladder through to

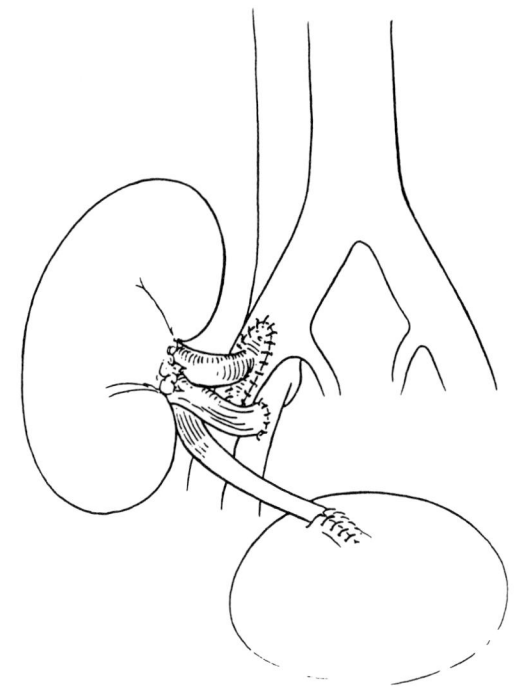

**Figure 59–1.** The standard anastomosis. The donor renal artery is shown anastomosed end-to-end on a Carrel aortic patch to the recipient external iliac artery. The donor renal vein is anastomosed to the recipient external iliac vein. The donor ureter is anastomosed to the recipient bladder with an antireflux technique. (From Danovitch GM [ed]: The Handbook of Kidney Transplantation. Little, Brown and Company, Boston, p 138, 1992. Published by Little, Brown and Company.)

the mucosa and anastomosing the donor ureter end-to-side to the bladder mucosa. The bladder muscle is then reapproximated to make a tunnel to prevent urinary reflux. The technique used at our institution is one of a ureteroneocystostomy, which has replaced the more extensive Leadbetter-Politano method and has lowered the frequency of complications (obstruction or urine leak) associated with that procedure.[136, 137]

The transplanted kidney is often placed in the contralateral iliac fossa to keep the ureter and collecting system medial and thus accessible to repair if the ureter or renal pelvis undergoes infarction or necrosis.[133] This surgical maneuver decreases the potential of subsequent vascular stenosis associated with the anastomotic site.[135] If the opposite fossa cannot be used, the kidney is placed upside-down on the ipsilateral side to retain the medial position of the collecting system. If a third kidney transplant is performed, the external iliac fossa can be used again after removal of the retained kidney, or an intraperitoneal approach can be used[133] with more proximal placement of the organ. In general, the left iliac fossa is avoided in recipients older than 40 years because of the prevalence of diverticulosis in this age group and problems of confusing diverticulosis with acute inflammation of the transplanted kidney.[138]

## Postoperative Management

Immediately after revascularization, urine output should ensue, and flow rates of greater than 1 L/h are common.

This brisk diuresis is due to a combination of the use of intraoperative diuretics, large volumes of intraoperative fluids, osmotic diuresis, and transient concentrating defects of the new kidney.[128] Urine output is replaced with saline and dextrose, with electrolyte supplements based on the composition of the urinary electrolytes. Intravascular volume depletion is strictly avoided to prevent prerenal azotemia and ATN. Urine output usually normalizes within 24 to 48 hours.[128]

The patient is maintained with intravenous fluids alone for the first 24 to 48 hours or until bowel function returns.[128] If the patient remains anuric, dialysis may be needed within the first 24 to 48 hours to control hyperkalemia and hypervolemia. Potassium exchange resin enemas may be used with water, but sorbitol must be avoided because of the potential for intestinal necrosis.[139]

## Potential Surgical Complications

The potential surgical complications associated with transplantation are outlined in Table 59–7. Most mechanical complications causing graft dysfunction involve the ureter or collecting system but may also be related to the vascular or lymphatic systems. Diagnosis depends predominantly on careful review of operative events, laboratory tests, imaging studies, and biopsy results. Therapeutic decisions are based on a number of these findings and are dependent on experienced clinical judgment. Most surgical complications are manifested in the early post-transplant period. Technical factors causing late dysfunction are usually strictures of the ureter or stenosis of the renal artery.

### URETERAL OBSTRUCTION

A common early surgical complication is ureteral obstruction resulting in decreased flow of urine. Obstruction is associated with a painless dilation of the urinary collecting system that is usually noted on ultrasound examination of the allograft. Mild dilation of the collecting system is common after transplantation because of edema at the ureteral implantation site, and this should not be confused with the marked hydroureter or hydronephrosis that is associated with complete ureteral obstruction.[140] Partial ureteral obstruction may also occur, and unless a drain is in place, an adequate urine output may lower clinical suspicion of this diagnosis.[128]

---

**TABLE 59–7. Postoperative Technical Complications**

Ureteral obstruction
Urine leak
Ureteral stenosis
Vesicoureteral reflux

Lymphocele
Bleeding
Vascular thrombosis
Sexual impotence
Hydrocele

Transplant renal artery stenosis

---

Acute postoperative ureteral obstruction may be due to blood clots, ureteral necrosis or technical difficulty at the ureteral implantation site,[141] or stones. Later causes of ureteral obstruction are ureteral fibrosis associated with either ischemia or rejection; extrinsic obstruction due to a urine leak (leading to an expanding mass called a urinoma); lymph accumulation (leading to a lymphocele); and, rarely, a large retroperitoneal hematoma.[141] The most accurate way to visualize the collecting system and identify the site of obstruction is through percutaneous antegrade pyelography.[140]

### URINE LEAK

Urine leak usually occurs within the first few weeks after transplantation and is an important consideration in the differential diagnosis of early graft dysfunction. This usually follows necrosis of the distal ureter, although it can be seen with disruption of the ureteral anastomosis site due to technical error, infection, or clot retention leading to acute bladder distention.[128] Infarction of the renal pelvis happens occasionally, most often in kidneys with small lower pole arteries.[141]

The most common reason for necrosis of the ureter is interruption or thrombosis of the ureteral artery due to damage incurred during donor nephrectomy.[142, 143] The isolated transplant ureter is supplied only by the ureteral artery, which runs antegrade down the donor ureter. Multiple accessory arterial sources along its length are interrupted on harvest of the kidney. Renal allografts from donors with multiple renal arteries are especially at risk because a branch to the lower pole may be the sole supply for the ureter. The ureteral artery may also be damaged during donor nephrectomy or preparation of the kidney for transplantation.[141]

The clinical signs associated with urine leak can mimic those of allograft rejection or obstruction due to hematoma or lymphocele. Typical signs and symptoms are fever, allograft tenderness, and swelling of tissues ipsilateral to the graft.[128] Changes in urine volume may not be evident initially, and a necrosing ureter can contain urine flow for days before overt rupture. Ultrasound examination usually confirms the presence of a perinephric fluid collection, although it may be missed if there is reabsorption of the leaking urine into the peritoneal cavity in the setting of inadvertent interruption in the peritoneal wall occurring during placement of the allograft.[128] Further information may be obtained through a percutaneous nephrogram.

Urine leakage is a serious complication that can lead to infection and death.[144] It demands urinary diversion through a percutaneous nephrostomy tube for restoration of renal homeostasis, then re-exploration and ureteral repair. The medial position of the ureter allows convenient repair of a necrosed ureter. If much of the ureter is necrosed, or the renal pelvis is necrotic, the bladder can be anastomosed directly to the kidney capsule. If the renal pelvis is lateral to vessels, such transplant salvage procedures are not possible.

### URETERAL STENOSIS

Ureteral stenosis in the early post-transplant course can be due to constriction of the ureter as a result of the bladder tunneling procedure, edema of the ureter or bladder tissue, or an adynamic ureter.[128] Late ureteral stricture, months to years after transplantation, is due to entrapment by scar tissue. The putative factors implicated in scar formation have been ischemia, infection, and rejection.[128, 145, 146] The diagnosis is usually made by demonstrating hydroureter and hydronephrosis through ultrasonography. Mild hydronephrosis is common (up to 30% of cases) after transplantation,[147] and a percutaneous nephrogram may be needed to define the anatomic defect. Balloon dilation of the ureteral stenosis can be attempted,[148] but often surgical repair with reimplantation and placement of a stent is necessary.[128, 141]

## VESICOURETERAL REFLUX

Vesicoureteral reflux is a rare complication after transplantation, and its frequency depends on the technique of ureteral anastomosis. When the ureter is tunneled through the dome of the bladder, there is a lower frequency of this complication.[149] It is interesting that the presence of vesicoureteral reflux has not been shown to increase the frequency of post-transplant UTI.[149] Controversy exists regarding whether chronic reflux into the allograft results in lower graft function or proteinuria.[149]

## LYMPHOCELE

Lymph may collect in the retroperitoneal space, if lymphatic vessels are not carefully ligated at the time of surgery, and form a lymphocele.[141] If large enough, this may lead to obstruction of the iliac vein and may obstruct urine flow through compression on the bladder or ureter. Lymphocele is a fairly common complication and it can be differentiated from a urinoma by comparing creatinine values in serum, urine, and the fluid collection.[128] The creatinine values in lymph and serum are identical, whereas that of urine is substantially higher. These collections can be treated through percutaneous drainage, although this may increase the risk of exogenous infection.[128, 150] If percutaneous drainage does not resolve the collection (either after a few attempts or after leaving a drain in place for some time), creation of a peritoneal window may be needed to allow lymphatic drainage into the peritoneal space.[141]

## BLEEDING

Hematuria is common within the first few postoperative days and, although usually benign, can be severe enough to clot the Foley catheter or renal pelvis. Occasionally, large clots in the bladder may be difficult to irrigate and result in urinary obstruction. The initial approach is to irrigate or change the Foley catheter; if this is unsuccessful, a percutaneous nephrostomy or ureteral stent may be required.[151] Removing the Foley catheter allows the patient to pass large clots more easily through the urethra.[128] Transient hematuria can also occur after an allograft biopsy and may be severe enough to form an obstructive clot in the renal pelvis.[133] If clots fill the renal pelvis, a percutaneous nephrostomy tube is placed to allow urinary diversion. Significant bleeding may occasionally be controlled by selective arteriographic embolization. Clots in the urinary tract usually lyse by the action of urinary urokinase after the bleeding stops.[128]

Massive hematuria may be seen with rupture of the transplant kidney associated with fulminant rejection. Nephrectomy is the only recourse in these circumstances. Capsular repair can be attempted, although it is often unsuccessful.[128] Dehiscence of a vascular suture line can rarely produce hemorrhage, but bleeding is more frequently due to leakage from small vessels in the renal hilum or perinephric fat. Hemorrhage from any of these sources may cause intense pain; urgent surgical exploration is required, and a transplant nephrectomy may be indicated.

## VASCULAR THROMBOSIS

Vascular complications can be associated with torsion or kinking of the vessels that may occur during placement of the allograft. This is especially common on placing an allograft with long vessels into a site of previous engraftment. Vascular thrombosis has also been reported in association with use of cyclosporine or anti–T cell monoclonal antibody (OKT3),[152, 153] in recipients of pediatric kidneys,[154] and in patients with deep venous thrombosis of the lower extremities.[128] Either arterial or venous thrombosis portends a poor outcome, and the patient commonly undergoes nephrectomy. Some reports have been given of successful treatment with thrombolytic agents, although this is rare.[155, 156]

Renal artery thrombosis is more often associated with technical difficulties in anastomosing the donor and recipient arteries, with intimal disruption (particularly in diabetic patients), arteriosclerotic involvement of the recipient or donor vessels, or kidneys with multiple renal arteries.[128] Improved surgical techniques have reduced the frequency of these complications. In some centers, the practice is to re-explore any patient who suddenly becomes anuric within a few days of surgery.[141] Thrombosis of the accessory renal arteries is more common than thrombosis of the main renal artery. Thrombosis of an accessory renal artery is usually of little immediate functional consequence unless it is of a lower pole branch, which may put the ureter or renal pelvis at risk.[128] A renal scan may show a segmental perfusion deficit when an accessory renal artery is thrombosed.

Renal vein thrombosis occurs more frequently in pediatric kidneys transplanted into adults.[154] The tendency to clot in the venous vessels may be related to administration of cyclosporine or OKT3, but it may also be due to kinking of vessels or placement of the allograft into a tightly scarred retroperitoneal pocket after removal of a prior allograft.[152, 153] Partial obstruction of the iliac vein by a urinoma, hematoma, or lymphocele can rarely result in venous thrombosis. Significant proteinuria, hematuria, and decreased urine output are signs associated with venous thrombosis.[157] Salvage of these kidneys is rare, and usually a transplant nephrectomy is the outcome.[133] Anticoagulation therapy should be instituted if a thrombosis is found to extend beyond the renal vein.

## SEXUAL IMPOTENCE AND HYDROCELES

In the past, it was standard practice to anastomose the internal iliac artery end-to-end to the renal artery. Impotence was a common complication in individuals who had received two consecutive transplants with use of both internal iliac arteries. Use of the external iliac artery for anastomosis has greatly decreased the frequency of this complication.[133] Mobilizing the spermatic cord rather than dividing it has also decreased the potential for hydrocele and sterility.[133]

## TRANSPLANT RENAL ARTERY STENOSIS

Renal artery stenosis has been reported in up to 12% of cases of renal transplantation from various centers.[158, 159] It has been reported as early as 2 months and as late as 2 years after the transplant but in general is thought to be a late complication. Without angiographic evaluation of all transplant arteries, however, the actual frequency cannot be determined. The causes attributed to renal artery stenosis include arteriosclerosis and development of anastomotic site stricture.[160] Technical problems such as clamp injury to the donor vascular endothelium, perfusion pump cannulation injury, end-to-end anastomosis, disproportionate length between graft artery and iliac artery resulting in either torsion or kinking, and end-to-end anastomosis with vessel size disproportion have all been implicated in the etiology of renal artery stenosis.[128, 141] Although rejection is not thought to be a cause of renal artery stenosis,[140] a type of generalized stenosis is seen in which the renal artery becomes encased in dense scar tissue because of a reaction of the periadventitial arterial tissue.[141]

The presence of renal artery stenosis should be suspected in a patient with severe hypertension and impaired graft function, especially if azotemia occurs after treatment with angiotensin-converting enzyme (ACE) inhibitors. Bruits are rare, although their presence suggests the diagnosis.[141] Initial treatment may be percutaneous transluminal angioplasty of the stenotic artery, although this is seldom successful and many patients may experience restenosis. Surgical repair is difficult and associated with a high frequency of graft loss.[128]

## IMMUNOSUPPRESSIVE THERAPY

Since the introduction of the immunosuppressive drug cyclosporine[152] into clinical use in organ transplantation in the early 1980s, there has been a 10% to 20% improvement in 1-year renal allograft survival rate. The major problems with cyclosporine have been related to acute and chronic nephrotoxic effects and the related issue of what is optimal induction and maintenance immunosuppressive therapy.

## Induction Protocols

The optimal prophylactic or induction immunosuppressive therapy to prevent renal transplant rejection remains controversial. The controversy revolves around the observation that cyclosporine, when administered perioperatively, is associated with an increased frequency and duration both of delayed allograft function and of primary nonfunction (when the graft never functions). These risks are greatest when the starting dose of cyclosporine is more than 12 to 14 mg/kg/d, and when the cold ischemia time is longer than 24 hours.[123] Lowering the starting dose of cyclosporine to below 10 mg/kg/d diminishes the frequency of delayed graft function and primary nonfunction but may increase the risk of acute allograft rejection.

Several trials have been conducted to study the effects of prophylactic antilymphocyte serum (ALS) or OKT3 while cyclosporine is withheld until the graft begins to function ("sequential" induction therapy protocol). Evaluation of these trials requires consideration of several factors:

1. Frequency and severity of delayed graft function or primary nonfunction, including the requirement for and duration of dialysis after transplantation
2. Frequency and timing of acute rejection episodes
3. Frequency, type, and severity of complications, including infections and malignant neoplasms
4. Long-term allograft survival and function
5. Length of hospitalization and cost
6. Mortality of patients

Most published studies have addressed only a subset of these issues. Although each protocol may have its own advantages or disadvantages in a particular population of patients, none is yet proved to be superior when all these factors are considered. Two of the most common induction protocols are described here.

## CYCLOSPORINE VERSUS ANTILYMPHOCYTE SERUM

There have been several published trials to evaluate the benefits of a sequential quadruple therapy protocol using an initial regimen of ALS, corticosteroids, and azathioprine followed by the addition of cyclosporine when the graft starts to function.[161–165] These studies demonstrated that ALS induction (10 to 15 mg/kg/d until renal function improves and the patient is switched to cyclosporine) is associated with a lower rate of delayed graft function and acute rejection, although there was no difference in long-term allograft survival. Infections, especially viral infections such as with CMV, and possibly lymphoma occur more frequently with ALS induction, especially when rescue OKT3 therapy is used for acute rejection.

## CYCLOSPORINE VERSUS OKT3

OKT3 is not yet licensed for use as prophylactic induction therapy in renal allograft recipients. The data from a multicenter trial comparing OKT3 induction with cyclosporine,[166] in which patients were randomized to receive either OKT3 prophylaxis (5 mg/d for 14 days, with the delayed addition of cyclosporine on day 11) or cyclosporine in addition to steroids and azathioprine, showed that OKT3 prophylaxis was associated with a lower rate of early acute rejection (51% versus 66%) and fewer rejection episodes per patient (0.82 versus 1.14). There was also a longer time to the first rejection episode with OKT3 therapy (46 versus 8 days). In addition, there was a trend that was not statistically significant for higher 5-year allograft survival in the

OKT3 treatment group. Subgroup analysis showed that OKT3 prophylaxis was most likely to improve allograft survival when there was early graft function, two HLA-DR mismatches, and a cold ischemia time exceeding 24 hours. However, the OKT3 group had increased frequency of herpesvirus (31% versus 10%) and CMV (13% versus 5%) infections.

Several studies compared ALS with OKT3 induction therapy.[167–169] When all the above-mentioned factors are considered, there is no clear-cut consistent evidence that either agent is superior.

There is as yet no consensus for optimal induction protocols after renal transplantation. Several protocols are currently being used in different transplant centers around the world. The apparent benefit noted in the multicenter OKT3 study[166] will probably increase the use of this agent during the induction period in selected populations of patients. This may be particularly true in high-risk recipients of cadaver transplants who are sensitized[170]; in recipients of kidneys with prolonged cold ischemia time; or in recipients with two HLA-DR mismatches,[166] in whom the increased risk or delayed diagnosis of early rejection is a problem.

## Maintenance Protocols

The three available immunosuppressive agents that are currently used for maintenance therapy in renal transplantation are corticosteroids (primarily oral prednisone), azathioprine, and cyclosporine. Data from controlled trials in North America and Europe demonstrate improved allograft survival in patients treated with maintenance regimens that include cyclosporine compared with those that do not.[171, 172] Several important issues need to be considered in deciding on the optimal immunosuppressive protocol for a particular patient.

1. The risk for acute rejection and allograft loss is highest in the first 3 months after transplantation. Therefore, the number and dosages of immunosuppressive drugs should be highest during this period.

2. The most serious side effects of immunosuppressive therapy, namely, infections and malignant neoplasms, correlate with the total amount of immunosuppression. Therefore, it is essential that immunosuppression be tapered slowly to a "maintenance" level by 6 to 12 months after transplantation.

3. Withdrawal of maintenance immunosuppressive therapy may lead to late acute rejection or accelerated chronic immunologic rejection and graft loss.

Other important factors that need to be considered in choosing an immunosuppressive protocol are related to the type of transplant (first transplant or retransplant, and cadaver versus living related) and the "immunologic" history of the patient (prior rejection episodes, sensitization, and the degree of HLA matching or mismatching).

### CORTICOSTEROIDS

The mechanism of action of corticosteroids is discussed in Chapter 58. There is no consensus on the optimal dose or maintenance schedule of steroids after renal transplantation.[173] Patients are usually discharged and receive oral prednisone at a dose of 0.5 mg/kg/d. This dose is tapered slowly beginning 1 month after successful transplantation to a maintenance dose of 10 mg/d by 6 months. The side effects of steroids are summarized in Table 59–8.

In an attempt to minimize toxic effects and to decrease the overall immunosuppression, slow tapering and ultimate withdrawal of steroids have been attempted. Cessation of steroid therapy is often associated with a fall in blood pressure and, in diabetic patients, better glycemic control; total cholesterol levels also fall, but there is an equivalent reduction in high-density lipoprotein–cholesterol and therefore an uncertain effect on cardiovascular risk.[174] These beneficial metabolic effects must be balanced against the effect of steroid withdrawal on graft outcome. Early (within 3 months) cessation of steroids is associated with an increased frequency of acute rejection and a decrease in long-term (more than 2 years) graft survival. In comparison, data from uncontrolled studies of stable patients who have had no rejection episodes for at least 6 months have noted a successful outcome (lack of new rejection episodes) in approximately 80% of patients maintained with cyclosporine and azathioprine alone.[175–177]

### AZATHIOPRINE

The mechanism of action of azathioprine is discussed in Chapter 58. Azathioprine is metabolized in the liver to the active drug 6-mercaptopurine, which inhibits purine synthesis. The usual maintenance dose of azathioprine is 1.5 mg/kg/d.

Leukopenia is the most serious side effect of azathioprine. The immunosuppressive effect of azathioprine is not related to the reduction in white blood cell count; therefore, the dose should not be increased to achieve leukopenia. Azathioprine should be temporarily withheld if the white blood cell count falls below 4000/mm³. Recovery usually occurs within 1 to 2 weeks. The drug can then be restarted at a lower dose and increased gradually to the usual maintenance dose while the white blood cell count is monitored. Occasionally, azathioprine has to be discontinued because of recurrent or persistent leukopenia. Severe and fatal leu-

**TABLE 59–8. Corticosteroids: Most Common Side Effects**

Infections (e.g., oral thrush)
Impaired glucose tolerance
Hyperlipidemia
Truncal obesity
Posterior subcapsular cataract
Peptic ulcer disease, gastritis, upper gastrointestinal tract bleeding
Fluid retention
Hypertension
Avascular necrosis of bone
Steroid myopathy
Acne
Easy bruisability
Psychiatric disorders (e.g., mood lability, psychosis, depression)

kopenia can occur if allopurinol (for the treatment of hyper-uricemia and gout) is given with azathioprine. Allopurinol inhibits the activity of xanthine oxidase, which plays a role in the metabolism of azathioprine. These two medications should not be used together or, if necessary, the azathioprine dose should be reduced by at least 50% and the white blood cell count monitored closely.

Another potentially serious side effect of azathioprine is hepatotoxic injury. This complication is usually manifested by abnormal liver function test results with a cholestatic pattern. The diagnosis of azathioprine-induced liver disease is one of exclusion, and the patient should be evaluated for other more serious causes of hepatic dysfunction including chronic viral hepatitis.

Azathioprine has also been linked to development of skin cancer, the most common malignant disease in renal transplant patients. Patients maintained with azathioprine should be instructed to avoid direct exposure to sunlight or to use heavy sunscreens when exposed.[173]

## CYCLOSPORINE

Cyclosporine is a lipophilic cyclic endecapeptide that acts through complex molecular mechanisms (see Chapter 58) to inhibit interleukin (IL)–2 production in activated T cells. Oral absorption is variable, with mean bioavailability of 30%. The recommended intravenous dose is 30% of the oral dose.[178] The drug is metabolized by the hepatic cytochrome P-450 enzyme system. The optimal maintenance dose and therapeutic cyclosporine blood levels have a wide range of values. This is important because the two limiting factors associated with cyclosporine administration are cost and potential nephrotoxic effect. It is clear, however, that cyclosporine should be continued for as long as the graft is functioning because withdrawal may be associated with late acute rejection and graft loss, especially in African-American recipients.[179] The starting dose is 8 to 10 mg/kg/d. This is usually tapered gradually in the first 6 months to a maintenance dose of 3 to 5 mg/kg/d, a dose that appears to be associated with minimal risk of progressive nephrotoxic injury.[180–183] Whether there is an optimal plasma or whole blood trough cyclosporine level has not been thoroughly investigated in humans. More sophisticated pharmacokinetic monitoring parameters may be more informative[152] but may be of limited clinical utility. In general, cyclosporine levels should be maintained between 50 and 150 ng/mL in plasma or 150 and 300 ng/mL in whole blood.

## CYCLOSPORINE DRUG INTERACTIONS

Several drugs interfere with cyclosporine metabolism and therefore may cause either elevated blood levels with deterioration of renal function or decreased blood levels with the potential risk of rejection.[55] Table 59–9 summarizes the most common drug interactions with cyclosporine.

A related issue is the administration of drugs that slow cyclosporine metabolism, thereby decreasing cost by allowing the use of much lower doses of cyclosporine.[184–186] Results from a randomized trial comparing cyclosporine and ketoconazole (200 mg/d) with cyclosporine alone al-

**TABLE 59–9. Cyclosporine Drug Interactions**

| Ca²⁺ Channel Blockers | |
|---|---|
| *Increases Level* | *No Effect on Level* |
| Diltiazem | Nifedipine |
| Verapamil | Isradipine |
| Nicardipine | |

| Antibiotics | |
|---|---|
| *Increases Level* | *Decreases Level* |
| Erythromycin | Nafcillin |
| Ticarcillin | Intravenous trimethoprim-sulfamethoxazole (Bactrim) |
| Doxycycline | |
| Fluconazole | Isoniazid |
| Ketoconazole | Rifampin |

| Anticonvulsants |
|---|
| *Decreases Level* |
| Phenytoin |
| Phenobarbital |
| Carbamazepine |
| Primidone |

| Other Drugs | |
|---|---|
| *Increases Level* | *Decreases Level* |
| Sex hormones | Omeprazole |
| Colchicine | Sulfinpyrazone |
| Metoclopramide | |
| Alcohol | |
| FK 506 | |
| Tamoxifen | |

**Drugs That May Increase Nephrotoxic Effect Without Affecting Level**

Aminoglycosides
Amphotericin B
Acyclovir
Ganciclovir
Nonsteroidal anti-inflammatory drugs
? Diuretics

lowed the cyclosporine dose to be reduced by more than 80% with no deleterious effect on graft function at 3 years. The net saving in cost was more than 70%. Other studies have noted similar but less prominent cyclosporine dose reduction and cost saving with the Ca²⁺ channel blocker diltiazem. Diltiazem may have the added benefit of reducing cyclosporine-induced vasoconstriction[187] and being a synergistic immunosuppressive agent.[188]

Finally, other studies have focused on developing drug combination strategies targeted at reducing the nephrotoxic effects of cyclosporine. Compared with a control group of 33 patients treated with cyclosporine and prednisone, 33 patients who also ingested 6 g/d of fish oil had a higher median glomerular filtration rate, a lower mean arterial pressure, and fewer episodes of acute rejection.[189] One-year graft survival was not significantly improved, however. Fish oils might act by competitively reducing thromboxane synthesis, thereby diminishing cyclosporine-induced vasoconstriction and hypertension, and through direct immunosuppressive actions by decreasing the generation of proinflammatory cytokines.

## Antirejection Therapy

The three modalities that are currently being used for therapy of acute renal allograft rejection are pulse corticosteroids, ALS, and the anti–T cell monoclonal antibody OKT3.

## PULSE CORTICOSTEROIDS

Intravenous pulse methylprednisolone remains the first-line therapy for acute uncomplicated renal allograft rejection in a "low-risk" patient. The drug is given intravenously (500 to 1000 mg/d) for 3 to 5 days.[190, 191] After completion of the steroid pulse, oral steroids are restarted at maintenance levels or by a rapid taper to maintenance levels. Cyclosporine dose should be increased if the serum levels are subtherapeutic (<50 ng/mL in plasma or <150 ng/mL in whole blood). The expected reversal rate with pulse methylprednisolone therapy of the first episode of acute cellular rejection is 60% to 70%. Typically, the urine output increases and the serum creatinine level starts decreasing within 3 to 5 days after initiation of therapy. Steroids act in part by suppressing the production of IL-1 by macrophages. IL-1 is also an endogenous pyrogen; thus, reduced release probably explains the ability of pulse steroids to promptly lyse the fever associated with acute rejection. The major complication of pulse steroids is increased susceptibility to infection, especially oral candidiasis. Prophylactic antacids and local oral antifungal therapy are recommended.[192] Steroid resistance is defined as a lack of improvement in urine output or the plasma creatinine concentration within 5 days. In this setting, second-line therapy consists of the administration of antilymphocyte antibodies, either as polyclonal ALS or monoclonal OKT3.

## ANTILYMPHOCYTE SERUM

ALS is prepared by immunizing rabbits or horses with human lymphoid cells derived from the thymus or cultured B cell lines. Disadvantages of using polyclonal ALS include lot-to-lot variability, cumbersome production and purification, nonselective targeting of all lymphocytes, and the need to administer the medication through central venous access. Despite these limitations, ALS has been used both for prophylaxis against[193] and for the primary treatment[194] of acute rejection. A typical recommended dose for acute rejection is 10 to 15 mg/kg/d for 7 to 10 days. The reversal rate has been between 75% and 100% in different series, with the serum creatinine concentration returning to baseline level several days after initiation of therapy. During the period in which ALS is given, cyclosporine is usually discontinued, and the dose of azathioprine is reduced to 25 to 50 mg/d to decrease the overall immunosuppression and therefore the risk of infection. Both these agents should be restarted (cyclosporine 8 to 10 mg/kg and azathioprine 2 mg/kg) 2 to 3 days before ALS is stopped.

Complications of ALS therapy include fever and chills developing in a majority of patients during the initial ALS infusion. Anaphylactic reactions, including respiratory distress and hypotension, are rare. To minimize the allergic manifestations, patients are usually pretreated with a combination of corticosteroids, antihistamines, and antipyretics. A pruritic rash and presumed antiplatelet antibody–induced thrombocytopenia of varying severity can occur late in the course. Both CMV and herpesvirus infections may also be

seen but are now rarely life threatening with current prophylactic antiviral therapy.

In contrast to murine monoclonal antibodies (such as OKT3), ALS does not generally induce a host antibody response to the rabbit or horse serum. As a result, there is a greater opportunity for successful readministration. In some cases, ALS has been used to reverse rejection after OKT3 administration in patients with high titers of antimouse antibodies, which can limit retreatment with OKT3.[192]

## OKT3

OKT3 is the first and only mouse antibody licensed for antirejection therapy.[195] The mechanism of action of OKT3 is inhibition of T cell–mediated immunity by modulation or clearing of CD3$^+$ T cells. OKT3 has been used both as the primary treatment of acute rejection[196] and as rescue therapy for resistant rejection.[197] It has not yet been approved by the U.S. Food and Drug Administration for prophylactic use in renal transplant recipients. The usual dose of OKT3 is 5 mg administered as an intravenous bolus daily for 10 to 14 days. Cyclosporine is usually discontinued during this period and then restarted 2 to 3 days before the end of the course. There are reports suggesting that patients continued on cyclosporine may have worse ultimate allograft function. On the other hand, the antimouse antibody response induced by OKT3 may be diminished by continuing a low dose (50%) of cyclosporine during OKT3 treatment.[198] The expected therapeutic success rate with OKT3 is between 70% and 90% for steroid-resistant or ALS-resistant rejection. The plasma creatinine concentration typically increases for the first 2 to 3 days of OKT3 therapy and then declines. Rebound rejection occurs in approximately 50% of cases; roughly 75% of these episodes can be reversed by pulse steroids. OKT3 is also used as primary therapy in the minority of patients who have predominantly vascular rejection, a process that is often resistant to steroids and ALS. The reversal rate of the acute vascular rejection episode is 80% to 90%, although ultimate allograft survival and function are worse than in patients with predominantly cellular rejection.[199]

Complications of OKT3 can predispose the patient to life-threatening infection, especially infections due to CMV.[200] The frequency of infection increases from 16% after one course to 62% after two courses to almost 100% after three courses of therapy.[201] Patients receiving multiple courses may also have Epstein-Barr virus (EBV)–related lymphoproliferative disorders.[202] OKT3 is associated with a common "first-dose" reaction that may include fever (70% to 100%); rigors (30%); nausea, vomiting, and diarrhea (15% to 20%); and hypotension and chest pain, dyspnea, or wheezing (10% to 20%). Most of these symptoms are thought to be mediated by T cell release of cytokines, such as tumor necrosis factor and interferon-γ.[203] Dyspnea may be related to complement activation and subsequent neutrophil sequestration in the pulmonary circulation.[204] Steroids, antihistamines, and antipyretics are usually given before OKT3 to minimize these side effects, which should decrease with repeated exposure.

Three other serious complications can occur. First, fatal

pulmonary edema has occurred in patients whose weight at initiation of therapy was more than 3% above their dry weight. Fluid removal with diuretics or ultrafiltration to within 3% of dry weight is therefore recommended in all patients before OKT3 administration. Second, aseptic meningitis has been reported in 3% to 5% of patients.[201] This disorder can begin several days after initiation of therapy and is characterized clinically by headache, fever, photophobia, myalgias, nuchal rigidity, and findings in the cerebrospinal fluid of pleocytosis, elevated protein concentration, and negative cultures. The last finding is important, because an infectious process must be excluded in these immunocompromised patients. Third, arterial and venous thrombi may develop within the graft, leading to loss of the graft.[153] This complication is most likely to occur with high-dose OKT3 (10 mg/d rather than the current recommendation of 5 mg/d). It has thus far been reported only in patients receiving OKT3 as prophylaxis against acute rejection. The OKT3-induced coagulopathy may be mediated by the release of cytokines from circulating mononuclear cells.[205] The development of this syndrome in the early postoperative period suggests that endothelial cell injury due to ischemia or surgery may contribute to intrarenal thrombus formation.[205]

Approximately 15% to 20% of renal transplant patients have recurrent episodes of acute rejection. The success rate of retreatment with OKT3 in this setting is related to its ability to modulate or clear CD3[+] T cells.[206] This, in turn, is determined by two important factors: circulating human antimouse antibody titers and timing of the rejection episode.[206] Roughly 50% to 60% of patients who receive OKT3 will produce human antimouse antibody, generally in low titers (<1:100).[206] Low antibody titers do not affect the response to retreatment if the rejection episode occurs within 90 days after transplantation. On the other hand, titers above 1:100 or recurrent rejection beyond 90 days is associated with a reversal rate of less than 25%. When both factors are present, the reversal rate is essentially zero.[206]

The decision to stop treating patients with multiple episodes of rejection is a difficult one and is usually determined by the overall clinical status of the patient. It is recommended that therapy be stopped if there is active infection; if human antimouse antibody titers are greater than 1:100, especially if the rejection episode is more than 90 days after transplantation; if renal biopsy shows nonviable kidney tissue; or if three prior treatments for acute rejection have already been given for the current transplant.

# CLINICAL APPROACH TO ALLOGRAFT DYSFUNCTION

The most common complication of renal transplantation is allograft dysfunction, which in some cases leads to graft loss. The causes of renal allograft dysfunction vary with the time after transplantation. Therefore, the differential diagnosis is best approached by considering the time periods separately.

## Immediate Post-Transplant Period

Failure of the graft to function immediately after transplantation is called delayed graft function and is defined as

poor graft function with a requirement for dialysis in the immediate posttransplant period. Although individual centers report conflicting results regarding the effect of delayed graft function on allograft survival, data from the UCLA registry clearly indicate that delayed graft function has a marked negative impact on graft survival.[123] The frequency of delayed graft function varies between different centers but could be as high as 60% in cadaver transplant recipients treated with cyclosporine induction.[51] Less than 5% of renal allografts with delayed graft function never function (primary nonfunction).[51] The frequency of delayed graft function increases with prolonged warm and cold ischemia times, with cyclosporine induction therapy (especially at doses above 12 to 14 mg/kg/d),[51] and with prior sensitization in patients undergoing retransplantation, which indicates that delayed graft function may be mediated by immunologic injury in some cases. The causes of delayed graft function are summarized in Table 59–10.

## ACUTE TUBULE NECROSIS

Ischemic ATN is the most common cause of delayed graft function in cadaver transplant recipients. With dialytic support and maintenance of immunosuppressive therapy, ATN usually resolves in 5 to 10 days, although it may persist for up to 4 to 6 weeks. Because patients with ATN are usually maintained on dialysis, rejection episodes as well as acute nephrotoxic effects of cyclosporine can occur without being recognized clinically. This is because the clinical parameters used to follow graft function on a daily basis, including urine output and serum creatinine concentration, cannot be adequately assessed on dialysis. These complications can both prolong the recovery period from delayed graft function and complicate the diagnostic workup. Figure 59–2 is an algorithm for monitoring patients with delayed graft function.

## ACUTE NEPHROTOXIC EFFECT OF CYCLOSPORINE

The acute nephrotoxic effect of cyclosporine is the result of vasoconstriction of the afferent glomerular arterioles and reductions in renal blood flow and glomerular filtration rate.[207–209] The exact mechanism of vasoconstriction is unclear, but several studies demonstrated impairment of endothelial cell function leading to reduced production of vasodilators (prostaglandins and nitric oxide) and enhanced release of vasoconstrictors (endothelin and thromboxane).[207–210] Increased sympathetic tone may also be pre-

**TABLE 59–10. Differential Diagnosis of Delayed Allograft Function**

Postischemic ATN
Cyclosporine nephrotoxic effect
Accelerated or acute rejection superimposed on ischemic ATN
Urinary tract obstruction (due to ureteral necrosis with a urine leak or to a hematoma)
Vascular catastrophe or thrombosis of the renal artery or vein
Hyperacute rejection

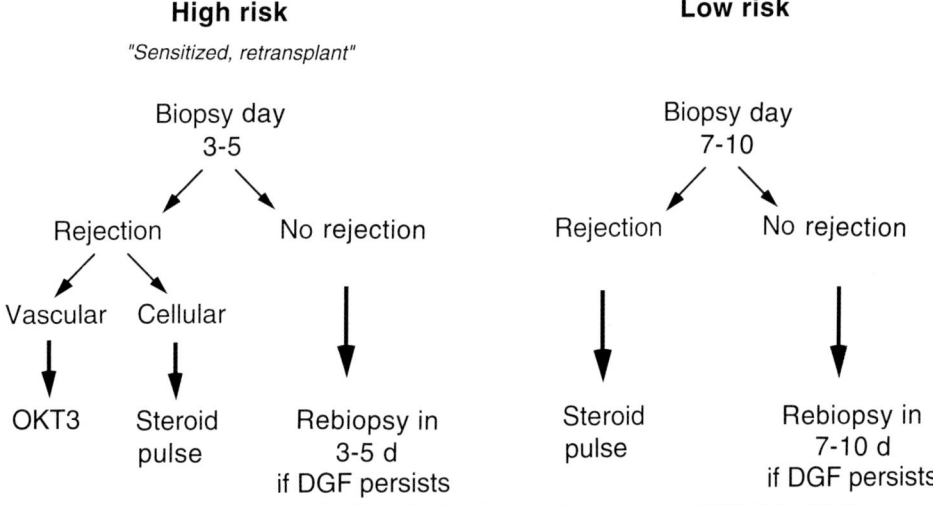

**Figure 59–2.** Algorithm for diagnostic biopsy and treatment of delayed graft function (DGF).

sent,[211] although renal vasoconstriction occurs even in denervated kidneys. The increase in renal vascular tone induced by cyclosporine does not attenuate with time. Maintenance cyclosporine therapy is associated with transient reductions in renal plasma flow and glomerular filtration rate, which correlate with dose and with the peak cyclosporine levels reached 2 to 4 hours after the oral dose.[210] These functional abnormalities are also associated with increased urinary excretion of endothelin and reverse when trough drug levels are attained. Studies with an endothelin receptor antagonist suggest that endothelin can mediate cyclosporine-induced afferent arteriolar constriction, an effect that will lower the intraglomerular capillary pressure and the glomerular filtration rate.[210] Administration of a $Ca^{2+}$ channel blocker can prevent the renal vasoconstriction although not the rise in endothelin excretion.[187, 210, 211] This observation constitutes part of the rationale for the use of $Ca^{2+}$ channel blockers to treat hypertension in cyclosporine-treated transplant recipients. The acute nephrotoxic effect of cyclosporine is usually reversible by lowering the dose or, in severe cases, with cessation of therapy, because the plasma creatinine concentration falls toward baseline values for that patient. Rarely, vascular lesions similar to those in hemolytic-uremic syndrome are seen[212–214] in cyclosporine-treated patients. This lesion is idiosyncratic and is presumably initiated by cyclosporine-induced injury to the vascular endothelial cells. Affected patients present with acute renal failure that is usually irreversible. Some patients, however, undergo partial recovery if cyclosporine is discontinued.[214]

## HYPERACUTE REJECTION

Hyperacute rejection is a rare and preventable cause of primary graft nonfunction.[215] It is caused by unrecognized ABO incompatibility or a positive T cell crossmatch (mediated by anti–HLA class I antibodies), both of which are contraindications to kidney transplantation. Other rare

causes of this disorder include positive B cell crossmatch (mediated by anti–HLA class II antibodies) and antidonor endothelial-monocyte antibodies (which cause a delayed-onset hyperacute rejection–like syndrome in HLA-identical grafts). The diagnosis of hyperacute rejection is usually made by the surgeon in the operating room, as the pink kidney becomes mottled and cyanotic. There is little or no urine output and no renal blood flow by renal scan or duplex Doppler study. There is no effective therapy, although plasmapheresis has been tried in uncontrolled reports. Transplant nephrectomy is the usual outcome.

## ACCELERATED OR ACUTE REJECTION

Accelerated or acute rejection can occur in patients with or without delayed graft function. Accelerated rejection refers to rejection that appears within the first few days of transplantation[215] and is associated with prior sensitization to donor alloantigens (occult T cell crossmatch), a positive B cell crossmatch, or a positive flow cytometry crossmatch in retransplants. The diagnosis of accelerated rejection is established by renal biopsy. It is recommended that ''high-risk'' patients (sensitized and undergoing retransplantation) with delayed graft function have a renal allograft biopsy 3 to 5 days after transplantation. If the biopsy shows predominantly cellular rejection, then initial therapy consists of pulse methylprednisolone followed, if necessary, by OKT3. On the other hand, OKT3 is the treatment of choice for predominantly vascular rejection (see earlier).

## OTHER CAUSES OF DELAYED GRAFT FUNCTION

Other causes of delayed graft function, such as urinary tract obstruction or vascular catastrophe, are associated with surgical (mechanical) complications and are discussed in detail earlier.

**TABLE 59–11. Differential Diagnosis of Early (1 to 12 Weeks) Allograft Dysfunction**

Acute rejection
Cyclosporine nephrotoxic effect
Urinary tract obstruction
Recurrence of the primary renal disease (focal glomerulosclerosis, hemolytic-uremic syndrome or thrombotic thrombocytopenic purpura, anti–GBM antibody disease in hereditary nephritis)
Infections (? CMV)

## Early Post-Transplant Period
### (1 to 12 weeks)

The differential diagnosis of allograft dysfunction in patients with initial graft function is summarized in Table 59–11.

### ACUTE REJECTION

The frequency of acute rejection and the time it occurs vary between different centers and may be related to the induction therapy protocol used for immunosuppression (see earlier). Data from the University of California at Los Angeles registry indicate that acute rejection affects 30% of first cadaver transplants, 27% of living related transplants, and 37% of second transplants.[216] Early acute rejection episodes (occurring within 60 days of engraftment) have an overriding effect on allograft survival, which is decreased at 1 year by 18% and 27% in living and cadaver transplant recipients, respectively.[216] Some of these kidneys may not regain function even with maximal antirejection therapy.

Kidneys that recover function still have a 10% decrease in 1-year survival compared with rejection-free kidneys.[216] In addition, acute rejection episodes have a negative impact on long-term renal allograft survival, being a major risk factor for the occurrence of chronic graft loss.[217–219]

Acute renal allograft rejection is manifested clinically by decreased urine output, elevated blood pressure, rising serum creatinine level, and mild leukocytosis. Fever, graft pain or tenderness, and graft swelling are uncommon in the cyclosporine era but may occur in severe rejection episodes. The most difficult issue in the diagnosis of acute rejection is the clinical distinction from cyclosporine nephrotoxic effects and, in patients with delayed graft function, from ongoing ATN (see Fig. 59–2). Noninvasive tests have not proved to be helpful in differentiating these possibilities in patients with allograft dysfunction. Duplex Doppler scanning ultrasonography, although noninvasive, is neither sufficiently sensitive nor specific in the diagnosis of acute rejection.[220] Although levels of urinary or circulating cytokines (IL-2, IL-6)[221, 222] or of soluble IL-2 receptor may be elevated in patients with acute allograft rejection,[223] there is no consensus on the clinical utility of these assays. The diagnosis of rejection is best established by timely renal transplant biopsy.

Figure 59–3 is an algorithm for the clinical approach to patients with early allograft dysfunction.

## Late Acute Dysfunction

Acute renal allograft rejection occurring after the first 6 months from transplantation is thought to be an uncommon cause of late acute dysfunction. Withdrawal of immunosup-

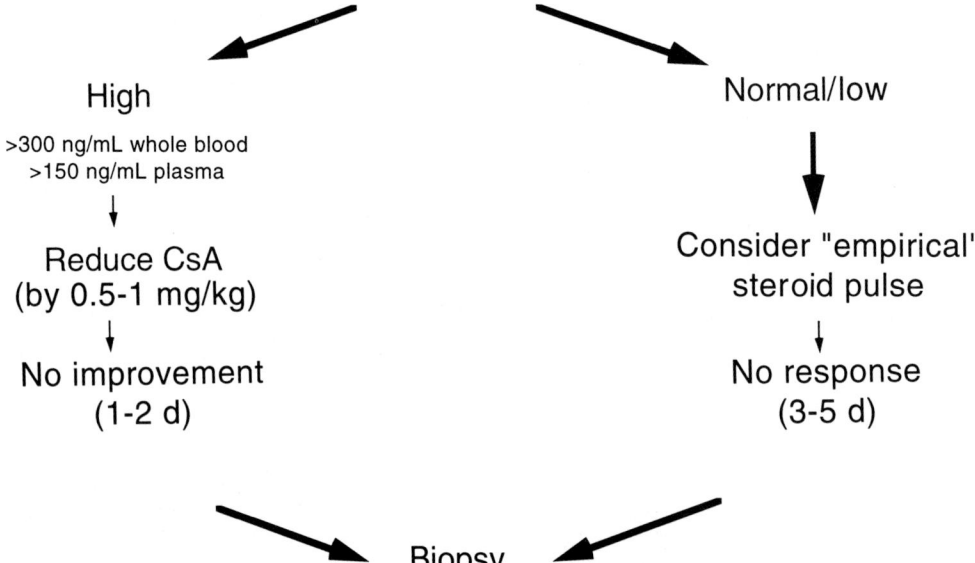

# Allograft dysfunction

**CsA level**

High
>300 ng/mL whole blood
>150 ng/mL plasma

Reduce CsA
(by 0.5-1 mg/kg)

No improvement
(1-2 d)

Normal/low

Consider "empirical"
steroid pulse

No response
(3-5 d)

Biopsy

**Figure 59–3.** Algorithm for the clinical approach to patients with early allograft dysfunction. CsA = cyclosporine.

pressive therapy, especially maintenance cyclosporine, is associated with an increased frequency of late acute rejection and a possible decrease in long-term allograft survival.[179, 224, 225] Meta-analysis of randomized and nonrandomized trials has confirmed the increased risk of acute rejection after cyclosporine withdrawal[225] and possibly decreased long-term allograft survival.[183] African-American patients appear to be at a particularly high risk for late acute rejection.[179]

The differential diagnosis of late acute renal allograft dysfunction should include prerenal azotemia due to volume depletion, cyclosporine nephrotoxicity, urinary tract obstruction, and recurrent or de novo renal disease.[226] Definitive diagnosis is best established by a renal allograft biopsy.

## Late Chronic Dysfunction

Since the introduction of cyclosporine[216] in organ transplantation in the early 1980s, a 10% to 20% improvement in 1-year renal allograft survival rate has been achieved. The rate of chronic graft loss has not been reduced, however. Renal allograft failure is now one of the most common causes of end-stage renal disease, accounting for 25% to 30% of patients awaiting renal transplantation.[227] Furthermore, the United Network for Organ Sharing data indicate that more than 20% of kidney transplants in the United States go to patients who have failed one or more renal allografts.[228] Long-term allograft half-life survival for cadaver kidneys that survive the first year (the time of major risk from acute rejection) is 7 to 8 years.[229]

The most common cause of chronic allograft dysfunction is a poorly understood clinicopathologic entity called chronic rejection, transplant "nephropathy," or transplant "glomerulopathy." The pathogenesis of this entity remains an enigma.[215] Both immunologic and nonimmunologic mechanisms are thought to contribute.[230, 231] Data from experimental models indicate a role for all elements of the immune system, including humoral alloantibody responses against donor antigens, cell-mediated immune responses involving both cytotoxic T cells and cells mediating delayed-type hypersensitivity responses (macrophages and CD4+ T cells), and inflammatory cytokines or soluble factors (such as platelet-derived growth factor and transforming growth factor-β).[230]

Supportive evidence for immunologic-mediated injury in humans comes from the observations that the half-lives of better-matched living related renal allografts are longer than those for cadaver grafts[216, 229] and that withdrawal of immunosuppression often leads to accelerated chronic allograft loss. Furthermore, studies have identified risk factors for the development of biopsy-proven chronic allograft rejection in patients treated with cyclosporine. Logistic regression analysis showed that chronic rejection was more likely in patients with acute rejection, infection, or a maintenance cyclosporine dose of less than 5 mg/kg/d after the first year.[217] In another study,[218] the frequency of chronic rejection was less than 1% in those patients who had no episodes of acute rejection. The risk of chronic rejection rose in patients with a history of acute rejection: 20% for

living related kidneys and 36% for cadaver kidneys if acute rejection occurred within 60 days after transplantation; and 43% for living related kidneys and 60% for cadaver kidneys if acute rejection occurred more than 60 days after transplantation. In addition, compared with patients with no acute rejection, those with episodes of acute rejection had reductions in the estimated half-life of graft survival (6.6 versus 12.5 years) and in the creatinine clearance 1 to 5 years after transplantation (45 to 47 mL/min versus 54 to 60 mL/min).[219]

Nonimmunologic factors also contribute to chronic allograft dysfunction. These include hypertension, hyperlipidemia, abnormal prostaglandin metabolism, and possibly chronic nephrotoxic effects of cyclosporine.[230, 231] In addition, because transplanted kidneys that suffer acute rejection episodes or ischemic injury have a smaller number of viable nephrons, glomerular hyperfiltration may lead to focal and segmental glomerulosclerosis and progressive dysfunction,[232, 233] a phenomenon similar to that seen in other forms of slowly progressive chronic renal failure. This is supported by observations that large kidneys transplanted into small recipients are more likely to survive, whereas small kidneys transplanted into large recipients (as with child to adult donation) are more likely to fail eventually,[233] which suggests a dose-response relationship. Many of the pathologic features said to be characteristic of chronic rejection are also features of hyperfiltration injury: glomerular sclerosis, tubule atrophy, and interstitial fibrosis.

The exact frequency of chronic dysfunction is unknown because there are no universally accepted diagnostic criteria for this disorder. The clinical diagnosis of chronic allograft dysfunction is usually suggested by gradual deterioration of graft function as manifested by slowly rising plasma creatinine concentration, increasing proteinuria, and worsening hypertension.

The differential diagnosis and management of chronic renal allograft dysfunction remain major challenges facing transplant nephrologists. Immunosuppressive therapy is generally ineffective, except for those patients in whom the precipitating cause is inadequate immunosuppression due to noncompliance or aggressive drug tapering. Nonimmunologic interventions should be focused primarily on aggressive control of the blood pressure and possibly of hyperlipidemia. A short-term study (3 months) showed that the ACE inhibitor lisinopril decreased protein excretion in transplant recipients with hypertension and proteinuria without adversely affecting renal hemodynamics or causing significant hyperkalemia.[234] The long-term impact of such therapy on progression of chronic allograft dysfunction is unknown. Other therapeutic modalities that have been considered, but not yet proved to be effective in controlled human trials, include antiplatelet agents, thromboxane antagonists, fish oil, and a low-protein diet.

Whether long-term administration of cyclosporine causes progressive renal allograft dysfunction leading to allograft loss in kidney transplant recipients remains a controversial issue. Data to support the hypothesis of chronic nephrotoxic injury due to cyclosporine come from cardiac transplant patients and patients with autoimmune diseases in whom the nephrotoxic potential of cyclosporine can be evaluated in the absence of coexisting immunologic rejection.[235–239]

These patients have a 35% to 45% reduction in glomerular filtration rate, compared with patients not treated with cyclosporine.[235, 236] The histologic changes of the chronic nephrotoxic effects of cyclosporine are seen with both low-dose (4.6 mg/kg/d) and higher dose (6.3 mg/kg/d) cyclosporine therapy, although they seem to occur earlier with higher doses.[235] In addition, patients receiving more than 5 mg/kg/d in a 2-year period for uveitis had a mean elevation in the plasma creatinine concentration of 0.4 mg/dL (35 μmol/L) and a fall in glomerular filtration rate from 116 to 75 mL/min; furthermore, new hypertension developed in 13 of 16 patients.[239]

It has been suggested that the denervated kidney may be less susceptible to cyclosporine-induced renal injury. Retrospective and more recently prospective longitudinal studies of renal transplant recipients suggest that most patients maintained with cyclosporine at 3 to 5 mg/kg/d after the first year have stable plasma creatinine levels and glomerular filtration rates for up to 5 to 9 years.[181, 182, 235] No reliable data correlate cyclosporine blood levels with risk for development of chronic nephrotoxic effects.

In addition to the glomerular and vascular injury, a number of other changes may be induced by cyclosporine, including hypertension (see later) and several signs of tubule dysfunction that are generally of lesser clinical importance[152, 240–242] (Table 59–12).

## PATHOLOGIC DIAGNOSIS OF ALLOGRAFT DYSFUNCTION

It is impossible to determine the cause of renal allograft dysfunction solely on the basis of clinical signs and symptoms. In the early post-transplant period, oliguria, hypertension, pyuria, and allograft tenderness could be due to one or more causes, such as rejection, obstruction, or vascular catastrophe.[243] Therefore, to clarify the pathologic process and form a reasonable approach to therapy, we require analysis of biopsy tissue. Histologic interpretation of the biopsy depends greatly on the experience of a pathologist trained to evaluate renal transplant biopsy specimens. Many studies have confirmed the utility of renal allograft biopsies in guiding therapy[244–252] and in providing diagnoses that were previously unsuspected.[246, 251]

**TABLE 59–12. Cyclosporine Nephrotoxicity: Tubule Effects**

Hyperkalemia
  Decreased the activity of the renin-angiotensin-aldosterone system
  Impairs tubule responsiveness to aldosterone
Hyperuricemia/gout
  Decreases urinary uric acid excretion
Metabolic acidosis
  Hyperchloremic (normal anion gap) metabolic acidosis, which reflects decreased aldosterone activity
Hypophosphatemia
  Urinary $PO_4^{3-}$ wasting
Hypomagnesemia
  Urinary $Mg^{2+}$ wasting

## Allograft Biopsy

The purpose of an allograft biopsy is to determine the cause of graft dysfunction. Most biopsies are performed within the first few months of transplantation. An allograft biopsy is routinely done if there is poor renal function by the fifth postoperative day. In a patient previously sensitized to HLA antigens (one with a higher likelihood for early rejection), the biopsy is performed sooner, usually by postoperative day 3.

The traditional renal allograft biopsy was historically performed at the bedside; however, safety is improved by using routine ultrasound localization, which also rules out other causes of allograft dysfunction, such as obstruction. Rare complications have been reported,[244–246, 253, 254] including hematuria,[253, 255–259] obstruction due to blood clots,[254] pseudoaneurysm,[260] arteriovenous fistula,[243, 261] and kidney rupture.

An alternative to the standard biopsy is the fine-needle biopsy. In this procedure, a small-gauge pediatric spinal needle is inserted into the graft cortex, and cells are aspirated into medium under syringe suction. The cellular aspirate is centrifuged and stained for cytologic identification of infiltrating cells. Patterns of cellular infiltrate have been associated with rejection, ATN, and cyclosporine toxicity.[262, 263] Unless the aspirated cell population can be verified to be representative of the renal cortex, there is a risk of poor sampling. Analysis of an infiltrate from areas other than the corticomedullary junction, which gives the best yield,[264] may confuse the diagnosis. Although the fine-needle biopsy is a more convenient method to detect rejection episodes,[265] the standard biopsy is more efficient at detecting genuine rejection episodes.[266] There are some reports suggesting a utility of fine-needle aspiration for detection of bacterial[267] and fungal[268] infections in the allograft, but this technique is not widely used for this purpose.

Noninvasive tests for allograft dysfunction have included radiologic procedures such as the renal scan. Sequential images taken with a gamma camera can demonstrate reduced uptake of radioactivity in the transplant and reduced excretion into the bladder.[243] A deficiency of this technique is that diminished uptake from ATN or rejection cannot readily be distinguished. Ultrasonography can provide information about the size and dimensions of the allograft, as well as the presence of hydroureter or hydronephrosis, but again cannot distinguish among rejection, ATN, and cyclosporine nephrotoxic effects.[269] Duplex Doppler ultrasonography has added the ability to assess vascular flow patterns. A reduction in diastolic flow is noted within the renal artery and arterioles,[270] and flow may even be reversed if the rejection is severe,[243] but this is not specific for rejection.[220] Other tests, such as magnetic resonance imaging and intrarenal manometry, are less commonly used.[243] Lymphocyturia is often seen during rejection, but this finding is nonspecific because it also occurs with other forms of renal injury.[271]

## Rejection

Alloantigens of the renal graft induce both a cellular and a humoral response. Traditionally, the term "vascular rejection'' was applied to a predominantly humoral effector host response, whereas if the response involved primarily T cells, it was termed ''cellular rejection.'' These terms had a different therapeutic and prognostic significance in that vascular rejection was treated with monoclonal antibody therapy, and cellular rejection, at least initially, was treated with intravenous steroid therapy. We now know that multiple limbs of the immune response are involved in acute rejection and that a morphologic description of the inflammatory processes does not fully explain the underlying immunologic mechanisms. The prognostic significance of the histologic presentation has not changed in that a more aggressive immunologic response is usually associated with a more vascular (endothelial) response.

There are few, if any, typical clinical features of rejection; therefore, distinguishing rejection from other causes of graft dysfunction on the basis of signs and symptoms is rarely possible. In an aggressive rejection episode, the patient may be completely asymptomatic or may have the classic features of rejection: fever, leukocytosis, hypertension, and a tender allograft. The presence or absence of clinical symptoms does not correlate with the degree of rejection based on histologic findings.[243]

During the process of rejection, the kidney becomes infiltrated with leukocytes. The inflammation may not be uniformly distributed throughout the kidney. The diagnosis may therefore be missed if the tissue does not contain part of the corticomedullary junction. If the biopsy contains primarily medulla without cortex, there is little interpretation that can be made, and additional tissue is needed. To improve the tissue yield, to ensure that cortex is obtained, and to avoid puncture of major blood vessels, allograft biopsies should be performed with ultrasound guidance.

Rejection has been commonly classified clinically and histologically as hyperacute, acute, and chronic (Fig. 59–4).

## HYPERACUTE REJECTION

Hyperacute rejection is due to preformed antibodies of the recipient, to ABO blood group antigens, or to the donor histocompatibility antigens,[272] or perhaps the donor endothelial antigens.[273] When the vascular anastomosis is established, recipient blood flowing through the donor vasculature carries preformed antibodies that bind to antigens present on the donor's vascular endothelium, inducing platelet aggregation, degranulation, and eventually microvascular obstruction.[274] Through complement activation, neutrophils are attracted, further stimulating the immunologic cascade that results in aggressive graft destruction. Functionally, this phenomenon results in immediate loss of graft function, although there are a few scattered reports of successful transplantation under these circumstances.[104, 275–278] Hyperacute rejection can be observed grossly during the surgical procedure as the kidney becomes swollen and cyanotic. Within hours of the procedure, there is abrupt decrease in urine output, swelling, and pain in the allograft. The preformed antibodies resulting in this type of rejection are the result of presensitization of the patient by previous blood transfusions, prior kidney transplants, or pregnancy.[279, 280] Screening for preformed antibodies to these

antigens and avoidance of exposure to them have made this type of rejection a rare event.

The histologic presentation within the first few hours shows massive infiltration of the peritubular capillaries by neutrophils and large areas of interstitial hemorrhage.[281] In a few hours, there are microvascular thrombi within the glomeruli and interstitial and arterial vasculature.[282] Cortical necrosis usually occurs within a few hours.[281] The coagulative changes occurring in these kidneys have been suggested to be similar to the Shwartzman reaction.[283]

A hyperacute rejecting graft is removed as soon as possible because most patients will go on to have disseminated intravascular coagulation. The differential diagnosis includes insufficient arterial flow to the kidney or pulsatile perfusion injury. The insufficient arterial flow is diagnosed by diminished arterial pulsations felt at the hilum during the surgical procedure, and the pulsatile injury is accompanied by loss of endothelium seen on biopsy specimens. In addition, cryoglobulinemia, disseminated intravascular coagulation, fat emboli, and anti-GBM disease have been confused with hyperacute rejection. However, a biopsy specimen showing neutrophil infiltration favors the diagnosis of hyperacute rejection.

## ACUTE OR ACCELERATED ACUTE REJECTION

Despite immunosuppressive medications, most patients undergo at least one episode of acute rejection within the first 3 months of transplantation. Typically, oliguria, hypertension,[283] increasing proteinuria, hematuria with red blood cell casts,[283] and leukocytosis occur accompanied or followed by a rise in serum creatinine concentration. None of these findings is pathognomonic of rejection, and the serum creatinine rise is actually a late sign of rejection.

A wide range of microscopic findings are seen during an acute rejection episode, depending on the combinations of cellular and antibody-mediated damage.[282] The exact pattern of response depends on the degree of HLA compatibility between the donor and recipient, the amount of immunosuppression achieved with the medications, and the length of time the graft has been in place.[282]

Acute cellular rejection is characterized by interstitial edema and infiltration of the cortex with mononuclear cells and occasionally eosinophils.[282, 284] The mononuclear cells are composed of predominantly lymphoid cells but also contain macrophages and plasma cells.[285] The microscopic examination usually shows normal-appearing glomeruli, tubulointerstitial nephritis, and lymphoid cells within the intertubular capillaries, venules, and lymphatics.[282] Infiltration of the tubule epithelium with lymphoid cells and macrophages is a finding called ''tubulitis'' and is characteristic of acute cellular rejection. The vasculature can show variable changes from marked endothelial swelling with adherent neutrophils or other inflammatory cells to no changes at all. It must be remembered that the character of the biopsy finding may be changed by previous immunosuppressive treatment. For instance, an empirical pulse of steroids may result in the presence of mild inflammatory changes that are difficult to distinguish from the response to healing ATN. The cellular infiltration is usually gone by 3 to 5 days after

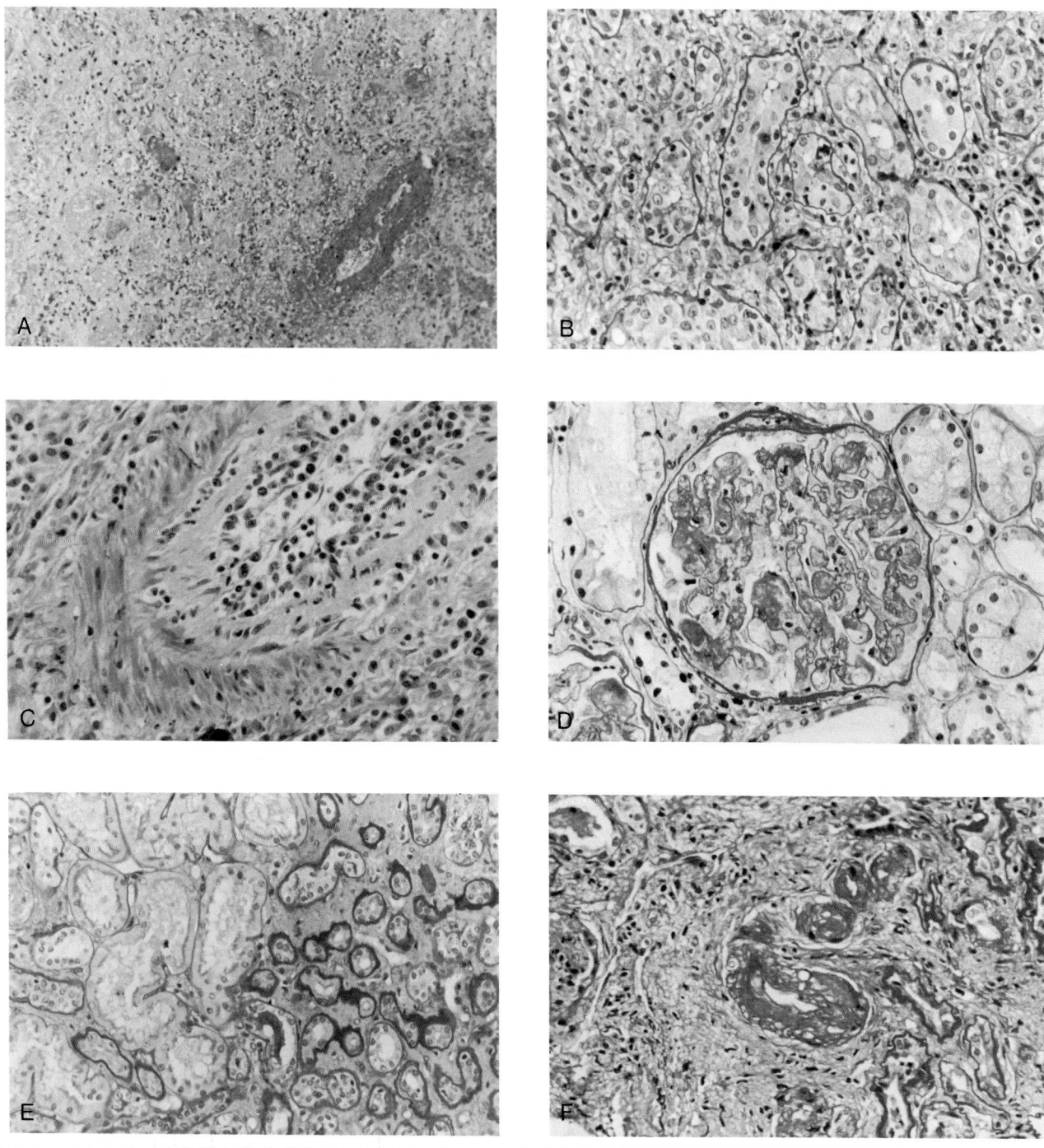

**Figure 59–4.** Photomicrographs showing histologic features of renal allograft rejection and cyclosporine injury. *A.* Hyperacute rejection. There is extensive coagulative necrosis of tubules and glomeruli with scattered interstitial inflammatory cells. The interlobular artery, shown in the right lower corner, reveals fibrinoid necrosis of the wall. (Hematoxylin-eosin, × 190.) *B.* Acute cellular rejection. The interstitium is expanded by edema and contains mononuclear inflammatory cells. Some mononuclear cells have infiltrated the tubule epithelium (''tubulitis''), and the tubule epithelial cells are swollen. (Periodic acid–Schiff, × 470.) *C.* Acute vascular rejection. There is marked endothelial injury as evidenced by swollen endothelial cells with adherent neutrophils and inflammatory cell infiltrate throughout the intima and media. (Hematoxylin-eosin, × 470.) *D.* Acute toxic effect of cyclosporine— thrombotic microangiopathy. The glomerular capillary spaces are occluded by fibrin thrombi with minimal or no inflammatory infiltrate. (Periodic acid– Schiff, × 470.) *E.* Chronic toxic effect of cyclosporine—striped fibrosis. Normal-appearing interstitium *(left)* alternates with areas of atrophied tubules with thickened tubule basement membrane and interstitial fibrosis *(right).* (Periodic acid–Schiff, × 470.) *F.* Chronic vascular injury. Interstitial fibrosis is diffuse with associated tubule atrophy. The arterial and arteriolar lumen is narrowed by subintimal and medial hyaline accumulation. (Periodic acid– Schiff, × 470.) *(A* to *F* courtesy of Dr. Helmut G. Rennke).

treatment with high-dose steroids.[282] Patchy mononuclear cell infiltrates (without tubulitis) are not uncommon in normal functioning renal allografts, and this finding alone is not sufficient to make the diagnosis of acute rejection.

Acute vascular (humoral) rejection results in interstitial edema, with moderate mononuclear cell infiltration. The capillary endothelial cells are typically swollen and may be necrotic.[282] Arterioles and small arteries can be obliterated by thrombi caused by the adherence of fibrin, platelets, and polymorphonuclear leukocytes, which results in cortical necrosis if the inflammatory response is unabated by immunosuppressive therapy. These pathologic changes usually occur in accelerated rejection with a pattern of mixed cellular and vascular rejection.[215]

## CHRONIC ALLOGRAFT DYSFUNCTION

The term chronic rejection is thought by many to be a misnomer. A more descriptive term, chronic allograft dysfunction, incorporates both immunologic and hemodynamic causes into the pathogenesis. Short-term rates of graft function have become better with improvements in technology, but there has not been an appreciable change in long-term graft survival. The clinical picture of chronic allograft dysfunction is one of a slowly progressive deterioration in renal function with proteinuria and hypertension. The pathologic changes of chronic rejection involve all parts of the renal parenchyma, including the blood vessels, glomeruli, interstitium, and tubules[243] (see Fig. 59–4). The vessel walls are thickened by the subintimal accumulation of loose and then organized connective tissue, variable mononuclear cell infiltration, and disruption and duplication of the internal elastic lamina; the net effect is narrowing of the vascular lumen, which may progress to total occlusion. The glomerular capillary walls are thickened, with an occasional double-contour appearance. The glomeruli may be enlarged and show a lobular pattern; segmental or, in severe cases, global sclerosis may also be seen. Immunofluorescence often reveals the granular deposition of IgG, C1q, and C3 in the mesangium and capillary wall; electron microscopy may show mesangial cell interposition and subendothelial accumulation of electron-lucent material. In the aggregate, these changes are similar to those seen in type I membranoproliferative glomerulonephritis. The interstitium shows variable degrees of patchy fibrosis and focal cellular infiltrates with lymphocytes and plasma cells, associated with a variable degree of tubule atrophy and tubule cell dropout (see Fig. 59–4).

As previously mentioned, therapy is not yet available for chronic allograft dysfunction.

## Cyclosporine Nephrotoxicity

The effects of cyclosporine on renal function are dose related, but there is also an idiosyncratic response in some patients.[286] Cyclosporine acutely decreases glomerular filtration rate, predominantly owing to a hemodynamic effect[287, 288] that is reversed by lowering the dose.[287] The histologic appearance of an acute toxic effect is characterized by epithelial cell vacuolization, often in an isometric pattern with giant mitochondria, large lysosomal inclusions, and microcalcification.[289–293] These findings are not pathognomonic, however, and can be seen with ATN as well as other toxic injuries.[243] In addition, vascular changes consisting of endothelial cell swelling, intimal thickening, variable hyalinosis, and mucoid or insudative deposits, which together may result in significant luminal occlusion,[286] have been reported in association with the acute cyclosporine lesion.

Cyclosporine can also be associated with signs and symptoms similar to the hemolytic-uremic syndrome, producing a thrombotic microangiopathy[213, 294] with platelet and fibrin thrombi in vessels and glomeruli and a minimal inflammatory infiltrate. The histologic findings here are indistinguishable from de novo or recurrent hemolytic syndrome, disseminated intravascular coagulation, malignant hypertension, pulsatile perfusion injury, or hyperacute rejection.[286] Therefore, the diagnosis depends in large part on correlation with information about the clinical history.

Chronic cyclosporine nephrotoxic injury, on the other hand, is more insidious, producing a slow decline in renal function. Cyclosporine toxicity can affect the vessels, tubules, interstitium, and glomeruli.[287, 294–297] The histologic picture is often one of an obliterative arteriolopathy (suggesting primary endothelial damage), ischemic collapse or scarring of the glomeruli, and significant focal areas of interstitial fibrosis (producing a picture of "striped" fibrosis) with modest inflammatory cell infiltration[235, 236, 286] (see Fig. 59–4).

The morphologic changes seen with any type of cyclosporine toxic injury are nonspecific and can suggest other potential causes.

## Recurrent Glomerulonephritis

Recurrent disease in the renal allograft accounts for less than 4% of all graft failures.[298, 299] Although the overall rate of recurrence is reported as less than 20%, this figure may be erroneous. It is difficult to determine accurately the frequency of recurrence of any primary renal disease because of several factors: the nature of the recipient's original disease may not be known[226]; allograft biopsies are not performed routinely (and unless clinically suspected, recurrent disease would be missed); it is difficult to distinguish histopathologically between recurrent glomerulopathies and glomerulonephritis occurring as part of the rejection process or occurring de novo in the allograft.

Described in the following are some of the more common primary renal diseases presenting for transplantation, the frequency of their recurrence after transplantation, the impact of their recurrence on graft function, and the pathologic presentation. Treatment strategies are described when applicable.

### DIABETES MELLITUS

Recurrent diabetic nephropathy ultimately occurs in 100% of grafts, based on the histologic presentation of mesangial expansion and glomerular basement membrane thickening by 2 years or more after transplantation.[300, 301] All afferent and efferent arterioles show hyalinization by 4 years.[302] It is rare, however, to see the typical nodular intercapillary glomerulosclerosis (Kimmelstiel-Wilson lesion).[303, 304]

There have been no studies to address the role of hemodynamic alterations to prevent recurrence of diabetes in the transplant recipient. Clinically, most patients present with proteinuria and a slow decline in renal function.[305] The slowness of recurrence makes transplantation seem a viable option for patients with end-stage renal disease due to diabetes mellitus; however, the issue of recurrent nephropathy and prevention of progression must be addressed by maximizing glycemic control and properly managing hyperlipidemia and hypertension.

## FOCAL SEGMENTAL GLOMERULOSCLEROSIS

An overall recurrence rate of 20% to 100% has been reported in various series,[298, 306–316] with graft loss rates of up to 30% to 40%.[310, 311, 313, 314] The clinical presentation is usually nephrotic range proteinuria, which can occur early or within days of transplantation.[226] A distinct subgroup of patients with a marked tendency for recurrence are patients who presented with the original disease at 20 years of age or younger with a rapid progression to end-stage renal disease (i.e., <3 years)[308, 311, 314] and whose biopsy examination showed mesangial expansion.[282] Once the disease recurs in the first allograft, the risk for recurrence in subsequent allografts is even higher.[317–319]

The histologic findings are the same as those in the native kidney disease,[318, 320] with glomerular sclerosis and hyalinosis. In the patients with early recurrence, the biopsy specimen may show no histopathologic abnormality in the first few months.[282] Later, the lesions may be preceded by a focal and segmental proliferative lesion[321] eventually leading to scarring. These changes can be distinguished from transplant glomerulopathy initially by the presence of focal rather than global changes. Although focal segmental glomerulosclerosis is associated with recurrent disease, this histologic appearance may also be hemodynamically mediated.[112]

There is no beneficial therapy, and although cyclophosphamide has been tried, it has not been found to be helpful.[311] Plasma exchange[322] led to remission in two pediatric patients and one 19-year-old patient.[323] Others have reported that there was no benefit from this therapy.[311] Other investigators have suggested that meclofenamate may help diminish proteinuria by altering renal hemodynamics.[324] In general, cyclosporine does not prevent recurrence.[312, 325–328]

In patients with a high risk for recurrence (those who presented at a young age with original disease and those with a malignant initial course), transplantation should be with a cadaver organ rather than living related or living unrelated organ. Recurrence should not preclude an attempt at cadaver transplantation, however, because not all patients will have recurrent disease.[226, 329]

## IMMUNOGLOBULIN A NEPHROPATHY AND SCHÖNLEIN-HENOCH PURPURA

Immunoglobulin A nephropathy recurs with a frequency of 20% to 75%[307, 309, 316, 330] and has a rate of graft loss about 10%.[226] The usual presentation is that of microhematuria with or without mild proteinuria. Cases have been reported as early as 2 months after transplantation and as late as 4 years.[298, 331] Recurrence is probably more common in allografts from living related donors,[330, 332, 333] and there may be an increased susceptibility with HLA antigens B35 and DR4.[330, 332]

Light microscopic examination is characterized by mild mesangial expansion, mesangial IgA deposits on immunofluorescence, and scattered mesangial electron-dense deposits on electron microscopy. The recurrent form of this disease usually represents a histologically mild or mesangiopathic form.[334]

The effect of cyclosporine on the recurrence rate and on graft loss due to recurrent IgA nephropathy is controversial.[326, 327, 335] Because of the low rate of graft loss, living related transplantation in these patients is generally not discouraged.

Schönlein-Henoch purpura and IgA nephropathy are probably two ends of the spectrum of the same disease. Because only a small number of patients with Schönlein-Henoch purpura have undergone transplantation, it is difficult to draw any conclusion from the literature on the actual rate of recurrence of this disease.[336] In one report on recurrence of this disease, the immunohistologic features where identical to the native disease and the presenting symptoms were petechiae, abdominal pain, melena, and gross hematuria within 3 days after transplantation. The biopsy performed 1 year after transplantation showed features identical to those of the recipient's native kidneys.[336]

## MEMBRANOPROLIFERATIVE GLOMERULONEPHRITIS

### Type I Membranoproliferative Glomerulonephritis

Type I membranoproliferative glomerulonephritis has a recurrence rate as high as 70% in some series,[307, 308] but it is generally reported to be between 20% and 30%.[316, 337, 338] The rate of graft loss varies between 30% and 40%.[307, 308] Clinically, the patients present with proteinuria or hematuria,[226] and the serum C3 level is not helpful in the diagnosis or prognosis.[338, 339]

The histologic appearance of type I membranoproliferative glomerulonephritis is similar to that of transplant glomerulopathy,[298] with mesangial interposition and classic double contours of the basement membrane. However, type I membranoproliferative glomerulonephritis is more often associated with generalized mesangial hypercellularity and extensive immune complex deposition in the mesangium and subendothelial spaces of the glomerular capillary basement membranes.[243, 340] Mesangial IgG is the predominant immunoglobulin deposited in type I, whereas IgM is seen in either type I or transplant glomerulopathy.[307]

There is no known therapy, although some have used

antiplatelet agents,[338] plasma exchange,[338] and cyclosporine to diminish the rate of recurrence.[326]

## Type II Membranoproliferative Glomerulonephritis

Type II membranoproliferative glomerulonephritis occurs more frequently than type I, with a recurrence rate of 50% to 100%,[298, 307, 308, 316, 337] but has a lower rate of graft loss (10% to 20%).[308, 337] Patients usually have moderate and intermittent proteinuria with or without hematuria. The disease occurs quickly and has been described in biopsy specimens taken as early as 2 months after transplantation.[282] The light microscopic picture is similar to that in the native kidney except that there is less tuft hypercellularity. The electron microscopic picture is identical to that in the native kidney, with long ribbon-like deposits within the thickened glomerular basement membrane and capsular and tubule basement membranes.[341]

There is no beneficial therapy, although, as reported with membranoproliferative glomerulonephritis type I, a variety of methods have been tried. Because so few grafts are lost to recurrent disease, the presence of this disease in the native kidneys should not deter one from transplantation.

## ANTI–GLOMERULAR BASEMENT MEMBRANE DISEASE

The frequency of recurrent anti-GBM disease is reported by histologic criteria to be 50%[337] and by clinical criteria to be 25%.[316] With recurrence, the clinical presentation is that of proteinuria and hematuria.

The histologic appearance by light microscopy is similar to that in the native kidney disease, with segmental proliferative glomerulonephritis associated with tuft necrosis, crescents, or both.[243] Interpretation of the immunofluorescence patterns in this disease may be difficult, however, because almost any condition that causes thickening of the glomerular basement membrane can cause linear IgG localization.[243, 342] An important distinction is the absence of nonspecific staining of other serum proteins.

Although the role of circulating anti-GBM antibody is controversial,[243] transplantation is delayed until anti-GBM antibodies are undetected in serum (usually about 6 months after presentation of the disease). There have been reports of recurrence of disease even with undetectable circulating antibody,[343] but this is rare.

## HEMOLYTIC-UREMIC SYNDROME

Rates of recurrent hemolytic-uremic syndrome must be interpreted in the context of the potential roles of cyclosporine and allograft rejection. A review of the literature suggests that hemolytic-uremic syndrome recurs at a rate of up to 25%,[344–346] although it may be higher in recipients of living related allografts.[347]

The histologic picture is that of intravascular coagulation. Because cyclosporine causes endothelial damage, it may in fact favor the recurrence of the disease.[337, 347, 348] There are only a few cases in the literature of recurrent hemolytic-uremic syndrome precipitated by the use of cyclospor-

ine[337, 346–348] or antilymphocyte globulin.[347] It is difficult to ascribe a rate of graft loss with this disease, although a frequency of occurrence of 10% in a small series has been reported.[337] Some centers report an even higher rate of graft loss.[344, 345, 347, 349]

It is currently recommended that living related transplantation be approached cautiously[347] owing to the possibility of an inherited endothelial defect that may predispose to recurrence. Some have also recommended the long-term use of antiplatelet agents[226] and avoidance of antilymphocyte globulin, OKT3, and oral contraceptives.[344] If the first transplant was associated with recurrent hemolytic-uremic syndrome, one should avoid cyclosporine[226] and rely on higher azathioprine and steroid doses for immunosuppression in the subsequent grafts.

## SYSTEMIC LUPUS ERYTHEMATOSUS

The rate of recurrence of this disease is low (<1%), probably reflecting that the disease is "burned out" by the time most patients begin dialysis.[67, 316, 337] There are only a few documented cases of recurrence in the literature; of those patients with recurrent disease, all had evidence of active symptoms, active serologic reactions with elevated antinuclear antibody and anti-DNA titers, and suppressed complement levels.[350–354] Most patients with recurrent disease had mesangial proliferative disease on the biopsy specimen of their native kidneys.[350, 351] The treatment options have been reported to be pulse steroids, plasmapheresis, and chlorambucil.[351] Some investigators suggest the use of cyclosporine and steroids while the patient is undergoing hemodialysis to induce clinical and serologic quiescence and allow transplantation.[354] Our center requires clinical quiescence before transplantation.

## MEMBRANOUS GLOMERULONEPHRITIS

Membranous glomerulonephritis rarely recurs; only a 3% to 7% frequency is reported.[337, 355] An accurate estimate of graft loss cannot be ascertained, although some centers report frequencies of graft loss as high as 30%[356] to 60%.[337] Patients who have been reported to have recurrent membranous glomerulonephritis present with nephrotic range proteinuria. In two reported cases, the disease recurred within 2 weeks of transplantation.[357, 358] There are no distinguishing clinical features, although patients with HLA-identical living related transplants may be at a higher risk for recurrence[355, 359, 360] with a more rapid progression than in those who receive a cadaver graft. The histologic appearance is similar to that observed in the native kidney disease.[243] The basement membrane deposits are less evenly distributed than in the native disease and are resorbed at an earlier stage.[307, 361, 362] There is no reported benefit to steroid therapy in recurrent membranous glomerulonephritis.[355]

## OTHER RECURRENT DISEASES

Amyloidosis (both types AA and AL)[363] has recurred in renal allografts,[363–370] with rates of about 20% reported for secondary amyloidosis and rates of graft loss that were no different from those in matched control patients.[371] In the case of secondary amyloidosis the recurrence rate is probably less when the inflammatory focus is burned out.[337] The recurrent lesion is seldom of major clinical significance, although the nephrotic syndrome[366] and graft failure[365] have been described. Primary amyloidosis, multiple myeloma,[372, 373] recurrent macroglobulinemic nephropathy,[374] light chain nephropathy,[375-378] and fibrillary glomerulonephritis[379, 380] have all been reported to recur at variable rates.

The experience with Wegener granulomatosis is limited, with only scattered case reports.[337, 381, 382] Other antinuclear cytoplasmic antibody–positive glomerulopathies may recur, and the current recommendation is to wait until the antinuclear cytoplasmic antibody titers in serum are low before transplantation.

Rates of recurrence of rapidly progressive glomerulonephritis in general have not been reported as a result of limited experience.

Observations reported in the literature suggest that essential mixed cryoglobulinemia recurs in the renal allograft about 50% of the time. When it does recur, it can be seen as early as 30 days after engraftment.[383] Clinically, the patients reported in the literature had proteinuria and hematuria as well as extrarenal manifestations[383] despite adequate immunosuppression. Essential mixed cryoglobulinemia may recur despite clinical and serologic quiescence, and graft function is usually impaired[226] when the disease recurs. For that reason, living related transplantation is discouraged.[383]

The current advice regarding progressive systemic sclerosis is to establish clinical quiescence without visceral activity before transplantation. In patients with recurrent disease, the time to onset from appearance of the original disease and transplantation was less than 1 year.[384, 385] The experience is clearly limited; only two patients are reported with recurrent disease.

More than 100 patients with Alport syndrome have undergone transplantation successfully, and recurrence in this disease is unlikely.[70, 386] These patients can develop anti-GBM disease, however, because they lack a normal component of the glomerular basement membrane, a domain on type IV collagen.[387] When a patient with Alport syndrome receives a normal kidney, there is the potential for development of anti-GBM antibodies in response to the donor glomerular basement membrane antigen, especially if the patient has been "primed" by a previous graft.

Single-center data suggesting that transplantation is dismal in sickle-cell disease have been reported,[388] with 50% of allografts lost because of sickling. Other centers have reported higher success rates, with 67% graft survival beyond 1 year.[389] In a report of a biopsy specimen with recurrent sickle-cell disease, there was prominent hemosiderosis, moderate interstitial fibrosis, and atrophy.[390]

Hyperoxaluria and oxalate deposition can be due to a rare inherited disorder of glyoxalate metabolism (a deficiency of the hepatic peroxisomal enzyme alanine–glyoxalate aminotransferase[391, 392] resulting in oxalate deposition in tissue) or to an acquired metabolic-physiologic derangement. Acquired hyperoxaluric states include diabetes mellitus, hepatic cirrhosis, sarcoidosis, pyridoxine deficiency, and that occurring after methoxyflurane anesthesia and eth-

ylene glycol poisoning,[393] but the disease is often associated with injury or resection of the ileum because of enhanced dietary oxalate absorption.[394]

Oxalate deposition always occurs in kidneys transplanted into patients with type I hyperoxaluria.[386] Three grafts have been reported with good function up to 3 years after transplantation.[395-397] Although oxalosis was initially considered a contraindication to transplantation, results are better than previously supposed.[398] An attempt should be made to minimize subsequent damage by oxalate to the allograft, and that includes aggressive hemodialysis to minimize the oxalate load, administration of large doses of pyridoxine (a cofactor for the missing enzyme) and phosphate together with magnesium chloride, and maintenance of a high urine output.[399] Graft survival of up to 10 years has been reported with these measures.[398] Combined liver-kidney transplantation is curative for the primary disease in children.[392, 400, 401]

Transplantation is the preferred mode of therapy for children with cystinosis and end-stage renal disease[386, 402]; recurrence is seen in about 10% of patients, with little or no impairment of graft function.[70] Cystine crystals are seen in the interstitial tissue of all renal transplants and in the mesangium of some, and it has been suggested that the host cells infiltrating the graft are the source of cystine deposition.[282] Crystals probably accumulate routinely in the recipient's interstitium, but graft failure is fortunately rare.

The previous recommendation that transplantation should be avoided in Fabry disease is changing with newer reports that the 3-year graft survival is now 80%.[226] Although the transplanted kidney does not provide the missing enzyme, α-galactosidase, which leads to an accumulation of glycosphingolipids and early renal failure, there are reports of successful transplantation in this entity.[403-405]

## De Novo Injury

A number of common causes of renal injury can result in new or de novo lesions in the allograft, including drug nephrotoxicity, infections, renovascular or urologic disorders, hypertensive nephropathy, and glomerulonephritis in a renal allograft due to causes other than the recipient's original disease or "chronic dysfunction."

Nephrotoxic injury associated with cyclosporine use has been discussed. Serum sickness–type reactions can develop after the use of mouse monoclonal antibody preparations, such as OKT3, and polyclonal antibodies (antilymphocyte globulin, antithymocyte globulin), especially if the patient was previously exposed to such preparations. The use of antilymphocyte globulin produced from horses in the past contained antibody that cross-reacted with human basement membrane, which resulted in linear IgG deposits and was rarely associated with a proliferative glomerulonephritis.[406, 407]

De novo glomerulonephritis is much less common than recurrent disease and is often associated with proteinuria. Minimal-change disease, membranous glomerulonephritis, and focal segmental glomerulosclerosis have been described to occur de novo after transplantation.[408-412] Distinguishing de novo disease from recurrent disease is often based on the ability to exclude recurrent disease in the transplant recipient. As mentioned earlier, this is difficult because the cause of the native disease is often unknown.

## Organ Preservation Injury

Preservation of donor kidneys during the interval between harvest and implantation is usually by cold storage. This is achieved either by immersing the organ in a cold ice bath or with mechanical pulsatile perfusion. The histologic lesions associated with preservation injury are most prominent in tubules and glomeruli and are due to ischemic or osmotic injury associated with the preservation methods. There is a range of histologic findings reflecting the degree of injury from mild dilation and epithelial vacuolization, especially of the proximal tubule, to more severe changes, such as ATN with epithelial cell necrosis and sloughing.[286, 413, 414] A severe form of endothelial injury is associated with mechanical pulsatile perfusion that is difficult to differentiate from other causes of microangiopathy. As such, the typical lesion is extensive microvascular and glomerular thrombosis with variable amounts of neutrophil accumulation in the peritubular capillaries.[415–417] The immunofluorescence findings consist of extensive C3 and fibrinogen localization along peritubular capillaries and glomeruli.[286]

## MEDICAL COMPLICATIONS

Medical complications associated with renal transplantation are largely related to the surgical procedure, immunosuppressive agents, or recurrence of renal disease. Complications of immunosuppressive agents are due to direct toxic effects or induction of profound suppression of host defenses. These consequences are dependent on the cumulative dose and the patient's underlying medical condition. For instance, a diabetic or older patient may be at higher risk for infections, and a patient who had a failed prior allograft may be more susceptible to early appearance of neoplasia.[418–420] In addition, the patient with a transplant is at risk for medical complications related to recurrence of the original kidney disease or chronic allograft dysfunction.

The physician's judgment and early intervention can greatly affect outcome for the transplant recipient. Meticulous surgical technique and prophylactic antibiotics are essential initially, followed by[130, 421] prophylactic antibiotics to prevent urinary sepsis and opportunistic pneumonias.[422, 423] Careful follow-up with routine screening for cardiac disease, hepatic disease, and early malignant neoplasm is mandatory.

The major causes of morbidity after transplantation are hypertension (46%), cataracts (24%), avascular necrosis (18%), malignant neoplasm (14%), UTI (17%), pneumonias (9%), steroid-induced diabetes mellitus (6%), chronic hepatitis (6%), peptic ulcer disease (4%), diverticulitis (3%), myocardial infarction (4%), and cerebrovascular accident (2%). The major causes of mortality are sepsis, coronary artery disease, neoplasia, and liver failure.[305]

This section focuses on the common causes of morbidity and mortality confronting the renal allograft recipient. Ag-

gressive and early management of any complication in these patients may be life-saving.

## General Issues in Infectious Complications

Infection is a leading cause of morbidity and mortality in transplant recipients,[424] with more than 80% suffering at least one episode of infection in the first year.[425] Autopsy findings of 116 renal transplant recipients from 1966 through 1985 revealed that the most common infectious causes of death were pneumonia, sepsis, peritonitis, and meningitis due to common gram-negative organisms. *Candida* species, CMV, enterococci, *Staphylococcus aureus, Aspergillus fumigatus, Pneumocystis carinii,* and mycobacteria were the next most frequent causes of these infections.[424]

Infection and rejection are intimately linked through the immunosuppressive therapy.[426] For example, to combat a rejection episode, increased doses of immunosuppressive agents are needed (which in turn increases the recipient's risk of infection). On the other hand, if the immunosuppression is decreased to help combat an infection, the patient is at a higher risk for rejection.[426] Chronic infection with latent viruses may further modulate the immune system of these patients, adding diagnostic and management difficulties.

The risk for infection is strongly determined by an interaction between epidemiologic exposures and net state of immunosuppression.[426] The transplant patient is susceptible to any environmental infectious exposure or reactivation of a previously latent infection.[426] In addition, the risk of infection is influenced by other factors: indwelling catheters; malnutrition; uremia; hyperglycemia; and infection with immunomodulating viruses such as CMV, EBV, HBV, HCV, and HIV. Approximately 90% of patients who have opportunistic infections due to organisms such as *Aspergillus* or *Legionella* after transplantation develop them in the setting of an immunomodulating virus (such as CMV).[426]

A useful temporal relationship has been noted that allows the clinician to predict the cause of an infection by considering the length of time since the transplant[426] (Fig. 59–5).

In the first post-transplant month, postoperative surgical infections (such as those that occur in nonimmunosuppressed patients subjected to similar surgical procedures) are most common. It is rare to find opportunistic infections in this period. Donors are carefully screened for infections before the organ is harvested, but unusual cases of transmission of infectious agents have been seen.

From 1 to 6 months, the most important causes of infection are viruses and opportunistic agents (*P. carinii, Listeria monocytogenes,* and *A. fumigatus*). Of the viruses, CMV causes more than two thirds of the febrile episodes[421, 426] seen in the first 6 months after transplantation.

After 6 months, three distinct subgroups of patients have been identified: those with good allograft function and minimal maintenance immunosuppression (with the same risk as the nonimmunosuppressed patient for development of infections common to the general population, such as pneumococcal infection); patients chronically infected with latent viruses (these patients often succumb to the end-organ

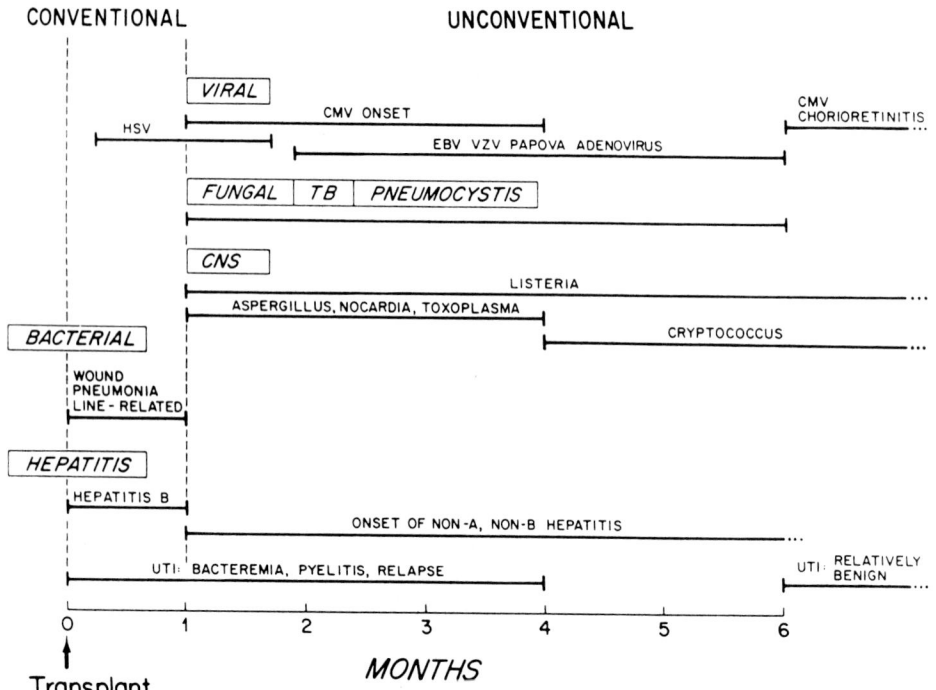

**Figure 59–5.** Timetable for the appearance of infection after renal transplantation. HSV = herpes simplex virus; CMV = cytomegalovirus; EBV = Epstein-Barr virus; VZV = varicella-zoster virus; TB = tuberculosis; CNS = central nervous system; UTI = urinary tract infection. (From Rubin RH, Wolfson JS, Cosimi AB, Tolkoff-Rubin NE: Infection in the renal transplant recipient. Reprinted from American Journal of Medicine: Vol 70, 1981 [pgs 405–411].)

damage induced by the chronic viral infection); patients with poor allograft function (i.e., serum creatinine concentration > 2.7 mg/dL),[426] a history of multiple rejection episodes, and a history of excessive immunosuppression (these patients are more likely to have acute and chronic opportunistic infections).[426]

Although any viral, bacterial, or fungal pathogen can infect patients after transplantation, those organisms with the greatest impact and greatest frequency of infection are discussed.

## Viral Infections

### CYTOMEGALOVIRUS

CMV is the most common pathogen in the transplant patient, and the occurrence of CMV infection or disease is determined by the status of the donor and recipient.[427, 428] Therefore, both the recipient and donor are routinely tested for anti-CMV antibodies before transplantation. Previous exposure to the virus is indicated by the presence of detectable IgG anti-CMV antibodies in the plasma, and acute exposure by IgM anti-CMV antibodies or a fourfold rise in the IgG titer. Evidence of infection is found by seropositivity in about two thirds of all transplant recipients.[426]

The virus can be transmitted from the donor to the recipient. The frequency and severity of CMV infection as well as management are determined by the CMV status, defined serologically, of both the donor and the recipient. CMV-seronegative recipients of kidneys from CMV-seronegative donors have the lowest frequency of CMV infection,[429, 430] whereas when the donor or recipient or both are CMV-seropositive, there is a significant risk of clinical infection.[427–429, 431] Infection is considered to be present if one or more of the following findings is noted: seroconversion with the appearance of anti-CMV IgM antibodies; a fourfold increase in pre-existing anti-CMV IgG titers; or isolation of the virus.

Three patterns of CMV infection have been described: primary, reactivation, and superinfection. A primary infection occurs when latently infected cells are transmitted from the donor to the recipient through the donor organ or infected leukocytes contained in a blood transfusion. For this reason, blood products are often irradiated before transfusion into any transplant patient. Symptomatic CMV disease develops in about 50% to 80% of seronegative recipients who receive a kidney from a seropositive donor[432, 433]; approximately 30% of these have pneumonitis, enterocolitis, or encephalitis, major causes of morbidity or mortality.[426] Without prophylactic therapy, the mortality rate is 15%.[426] Because of the high risk of severe infection, these patients routinely receive prophylactic therapy with CMV hyperimmune globulin.[434, 435] Another prophylactic approach is high-dose acyclovir (800 mg five times per day, adjusted for renal function) or intravenous ganciclovir followed by oral acyclovir for 2 weeks.

Reactivation infection occurs when previously seropositive patients are affected by endogenous latent virus.[426] Approximately 20% of seropositive recipients have symptomatic disease after transplantation, independent of the serologic status of the donor. Routine prophylactic therapy is not indicated in this relatively low risk population.

Superinfection with a different strain of the virus occurs in approximately 50% of cases in which a kidney from a seropositive donor is placed into a seropositive recipient.[426] Clinical disease results in approximately 20% to 40% of these recipients. The risk for CMV disease increases dramatically when either polyclonal or monoclonal antilymphocyte therapy is added to the patient's immunosuppressive regimen.[426] In fact, patients at highest risk are those treated with monoclonal or polyclonal antibody therapy followed by cyclosporine.[426] Large controlled studies are needed before routine use of ganciclovir or acyclovir is recommended in this setting.[436, 437]

Symptomatic CMV infection typically occurs during the period of maximal immunosuppression (1 to 4 months after transplantation). Diagnosis of CMV disease requires clinical signs of infection, such as fever, leukopenia, or organ involvement (including hepatitis, pneumonitis, pancreatitis, colitis, meningoencephalitis, and rarely myocarditis or progressive chorioretinitis).[427, 428, 431]

The most common presentation of CMV disease is a mononucleosis-like syndrome with fever, malaise, myalgias, and arthralgias, usually associated with leukopenia and mild (5% to 10%) atypical lymphocytosis.[428] A mild elevation in plasma transaminase levels may also be seen. As described previously, the diagnosis of CMV disease can be established in one of three ways: seroconversion in a previously negative recipient with the appearance of anti-CMV IgM antibodies; a fourfold increase in pre-existing anti-CMV IgG titers; or isolation of the virus by culture of the throat, buffy coat, or urine in association with a compatible syndrome.

An association between CMV and other opportunistic infections, such as *P. carinii* infection, has been described. There is in vitro evidence to support the hypothesis of a suppressive effect by CMV on host defenses,[35, 426] including depressed natural killer and monocyte function and hyporeactivity of lymphocytes.[35, 426] A controversial aspect of CMV infection is its effect on allograft function. Some investigators have described a glomerular lesion associated with CMV viremia,[438, 439] but this has been disputed by others.[440, 441] Reports have associated CMV infection with allograft damage in other transplanted organs, such as cardiac graft arteriosclerosis, bronchiolitis obliterans in lung transplants, and the vanishing bile duct syndrome in liver transplant patients.[35, 431] It has also been suggested that CMV infection is an independent risk factor for the development of rejection,[442] but how this might occur is not known.

Prophylaxis of CMV infection is routinely performed in patients at high risk for the development of organ involvement. Various pharmacologic regimens have been suggested to prevent CMV infection in the susceptible host, including high-dose acyclovir therapy,[435, 436] hyperimmune globulin, or pre-emptive ganciclovir therapy.[436] The best approach is prevention, but given the severe shortage of donor organs, this approach is not practical.[426]

The therapeutic approach to CMV disease varies with severity of the clinical manifestations. A mononucleosis-like syndrome commonly occurs after infection and usually resolves without the administration of antiviral drugs. Severe disease with organ involvement requires treatment. Approximately 15% to 20% of patients with symptomatic CMV infection relapse after an initial response to ganciclovir therapy,[35] and two or more courses are often required to eradicate the CMV-induced illness. Cessation of OKT3 and, because of the additive risk of neutropenia, azathioprine is also indicated in patients with organ involvement (including chorioretinitis). Whether cyclosporine should be discontinued in this setting remains controversial. Corticosteroids are generally continued to prevent possible adrenal

insufficiency. The addition of CMV immune globulin, a strategy that has been studied in bone marrow transplant recipients, should be considered if the patients are seriously ill or show no response to ganciclovir.

## EPSTEIN-BARR VIRUS

EBV is often associated with CMV in the transplant patient. Both viruses can cause similar clinical syndromes[426] (fever, leukopenia, mild hepatitis, atypical lymphocytosis). Diagnosis of EBV infection can also be difficult because the EBV syndrome in the transplant patient is usually not accompanied by a positive heterophile test,[426] pharyngitis, or splenomegaly.[426] Of concern is the role of EBV in the pathogenesis of EBV-associated post-transplantation lymphoproliferative disease.[202, 426, 443–446] This type of lymphoma usually has extranodal presentation. Patients have been observed with no evidence of adenopathy despite the presence of focal disease involving the allograft, liver, small bowel, and brain.[426] EBV disease runs a spectrum from a benign process associated with polyclonal proliferation of lymphoblasts to a monoclonal proliferation of B cells resulting in malignant neoplasm. Although some investigators have suggested that reduction in immunosuppression allows natural elimination of EBV-transformed B cells,[447] others report little improvement with this strategy.[426] The role of acyclovir in preventing transmission and treatment of lymphoproliferative disease is not known.[426]

## OTHER VIRUSES

Primary infection with varicella-zoster virus in the transplant patient can be severe; therefore, most candidates are screened for antibodies to varicella before transplantation and treated with zoster immune globulin for any subsequent primary exposure. The possibility of active immunization will be assessed in the future with the new varicella vaccine.[448] Reactivation disease is relatively benign, with typical zoster involving only a few dermatomes in 20% to 30% of patients. Antiviral therapy is not always needed.[426]

Recurrent herpes simplex virus (HSV) infection with either HSV-1 or HSV-2 can occur in up to 50% of renal transplant patients.[426, 449] These lesions differ in several respects in the transplant patient from those in nonimmunosuppressed patients. First, the lesions are usually ulcerative rather than vesicular. In fact, the ulcers are atypical from the discrete lesions seen in the normal patient. Second, the disease recurs more often, and acyclovir therapy is often beneficial. Patients with dual infection with HSV and CMV can be treated with ganciclovir alone because both viruses respond to this agent.

Virus-induced liver disease is common among renal transplant patients, and chronic liver disease occurs in 10% to 15% of all allograft recipients. The major viral causes of liver disease in this population are HBV and HCV. Additional causes of post-transplant liver disease certainly include other viruses (such as CMV, EBV, varicella zoster, HSV, adenovirus, and hepatitis A virus) as well as drug-induced hepatotoxic injury, veno-occlusive disease, and alcohol abuse.[450]

Transplantation of an organ from an HIV-infected donor

transmits the virus 100% of the time.[426] HIV-positive patients who undergo transplantation have variable reports of outcome; in general, our policy is to not perform renal transplantation on these individuals in whom dialysis is a viable option. There is controversy regarding cardiac and hepatic transplantation in HIV-infected individuals.[426]

## Bacterial Infections

### URINARY TRACT INFECTIONS

UTIs are the most common bacterial infections in renal transplant recipients, with a reported frequency of 30% to 80%.[426, 451–453] Of all cases of gram-negative bacteremia in the transplant population, 60% began in the urinary tract. The major risk factors for UTI include indwelling bladder catheters (routinely used for at least 2 to 3 days after transplantation); handling and trauma to the kidney and ureter during surgery; anatomic abnormalities of the native or transplanted kidneys (such as vesicoureteral reflux, stones, or stents placed for relief of urinary tract obstruction); neurogenic bladder, especially in diabetic patients; and possibly rejection and immunosuppression.[426, 454] The pathogens causing UTI in renal transplant patients are similar to those in the general population, including Enterobacteriaceae such as *Escherichia coli*, enterococci, and *Pseudomonas aeruginosa*. In addition, *Corynebacterium urealyticum* (group D2) has been recognized as a potential new pathogen that may be difficult to isolate and insensitive to conventional oral antibiotics, requiring treatment with vancomycin.[455] UTI occurring in the first few months after transplantation should be treated aggressively because it is frequently associated with pyelonephritis, or sepsis, and often recurs.[426] In addition, these infections may be associated with allograft dysfunction and may predispose to development of acute rejection.

Treatment for immediate post-transplant UTIs and those associated with bacteremia or pyelonephritis should begin with parenteral antimicrobial agents with continuation of oral agents, based on the sensitivity of the organisms, for 2 to 6 weeks. A longer course of therapy is indicated in patients who have anatomic abnormalities or a neurogenic bladder. UTIs developing in outpatients within the first 3 months after transplantation should also be treated with a 6-week course of oral antibiotics; a shorter 10- to 14-day course is usually associated with high relapse rates.[426] Three to 6 months after transplantation, more benign UTIs occur that are clinically indistinguishable from UTIs in the general population. In the absence of pyelonephritis or bacteremia, these late infections can be treated with a conventional 10- to 14-day course of oral antibiotics. Single-dose therapy is not advisable in any transplant patient.

Urosepsis has been virtually eliminated from the renal transplant population with a regimen of low-dose trimethoprim-sulfamethoxazole, which has the added benefit of prophylaxis against *P. carinii*, *Nocardia asteroides*, and *L. monocytogenes*.[451–453] We usually continue prophylactic therapy for 1 year in patients with normal urinary tracts. However, indefinite therapy is indicated in patients with a history of recurrent UTIs, anatomic urinary tract abnormalities, or a neurogenic bladder. Patients who are allergic to trimethoprim-sulfamethoxazole can be treated with any of the oral quinolones (such as ciprofloxacin or norfloxacin).[426, 456]

## OPPORTUNISTIC BACTERIAL INFECTIONS

The three most important pathogens are *L. monocytogenes*, *N. asteroides*, and mycobacterial organisms. The first two have been virtually eliminated by low-dose trimethoprim-sulfamethoxazole and are reviewed elsewhere.[426]

Although a rare cause of morbidity and mortality in the renal transplant population, infection with *Mycobacterium tuberculosis* can be life threatening and difficult to diagnose. There is a higher frequency of this infection than in the general population (0.005% versus 0.0001%),[457] although frequency rates of 4% have been reported in endemic areas.[458] Of 1069 patients at the University of Minnesota, infection was due to mycobacteria (*M. tuberculosis* and *M. kansasii*) in 7 cases.[459] Pretransplant skin testing has little value for identifying patients at risk, and the donor kidney may be an important source of infection.[458, 460] Although systemic manifestations are typically severe, symptoms can be so ill-defined that the diagnosis is overlooked, resulting in death from uncontrolled infection.[459] Disseminated infection is the most common manifestation of post-transplantation tuberculosis and often requires invasive diagnostic procedures. Concomitant infection with other organisms is common, which may confuse the diagnosis until the acid-fast bacilli are identified.[458]

The presence of life-threatening infection in the transplant patient requires aggressive antimicrobial therapy and discontinuation or reduction of the immunosuppressive therapy until the infection is under control.[461] Rifampin causes induction of enzymes in hepatic microsomes that increase the catabolism of glucocorticoids, which may risk loss of allograft function because of inadequate immunosuppression.[462] The adverse effect of this drug may be overcome by increasing the dose of steroids.[462]

## Fungal Infections

In general, two groups of opportunistic fungal infections exist in the transplant recipient. The first is disseminated infection due to either primary infection or reactivation with one of the dimorphic fungi (histoplasmosis, coccidioidomycosis, blastomycosis, paracoccidioidomycosis)[426] that cause asymptomatic or limited infection in normal hosts. These infections are geographically restricted.[426] True opportunistic infection with fungal species that are not invasive in the normal host is the other major group. These include *Candida* species, *P. carinii*, *Aspergillus* species, *Cryptococcus neoformans*, and *Mucor* species.

Overgrowth of mucocutaneous regions with *Candida* species is common in the transplant patient. Oropharyngeal thrush, esophagitis, vaginitis, and intertrigo are the most common infections. Topical therapy with clotrimazole or nystatin is usually effective; if this fails, fluconazole therapy is suggested.[426] In general, mucocutaneous overgrowth can be prevented by treatment of high-risk patients (those receiving antibiotic therapy or high-dose immunosuppression) with nystatin oral washes. Penetration beyond the mucocutaneous border can be prevented by careful adherence to indwelling catheters and Foley catheters. For this reason, candiduria should be aggressively treated with fluconazole or low-dose intravenous amphotericin B with or without flucytosine.[426] For disseminated disease, either amphotericin B or fluconazole can be used. For life-threatening infection, however, amphotericin B is probably more effective because it controls the infection sooner,[426] although fluconazole is less toxic. The cyclosporine levels must be watched carefully, however, because fluconazole may interfere with metabolism of cyclosporine.

The frequency of infection with *P. carinii,* a "fungal" pathogen, has decreased because of the use of low-dose trimethoprim-sulfamethoxasole for prophylaxis against UTIs after transplantation. Of interest, the occurrence of this pathogen is closely linked to infection with CMV.[426] Therefore, in some transplant centers, patients with CMV infection are treated empirically for *P. carinii* infection. The clinical manifestations of *P. carinii* pneumonia are fever, nonproductive cough, interstitial pneumonia on chest x-ray examination, and hypoxemia. A rapid diagnosis can be made with induced sputum or bronchoalveolar lavage specimens by monoclonal antibody techniques.[426] In patients who cannot tolerate trimethoprim-sulfamethoxazole, monthly doses of aerosolized pentamidine are equally effective for prophylaxis.

## Cardiovascular Disease

Cardiovascular disease is the second major cause of mortality after renal transplantation, especially after the first few months.[138, 463, 464] During the 1980s, cardiovascular death accounted for 18% of graft losses, whereas acute rejection was responsible for only 11%.[465] Hypertension and hyperlipidemia are probably the most important risk factors for this complication.[466, 467]

### HYPERTENSION

In addition to being an important risk factor for cardiovascular disease, hypertension may accelerate the deterioration of renal function in the transplanted kidney.[118, 468] Hypertension is extremely common in the post-transplant patient, with a prevalence of 50% in most series[138, 466, 469–472] and a frequency of 80% in the immediate post-transplant period.[466, 469, 473] There have been no controlled trials of sufficient design and length to justify the choice of a particular class of antihypertensive agent or of one agent within a class. In treating these patients, it must be remembered that there may be pre-existing cardiovascular disease, peripheral vascular disease, and diabetes; therefore, differences among the mechanisms of action and side effects in the different groups of patients must be taken into account.

A single etiologic factor for post-transplant hypertension is impossible to define. The most important contributing factors are impaired renal function, cadaver donor, retained native kidneys, and cyclosporine administration.[474] The importance of other factors that promote the development of hypertension varies at different times after transplantation. In the immediate post-transplant period, for example, an acute elevation of blood pressure usually reflects graft dysfunction due to rejection, ischemia, or cyclosporine toxic effect. Reversal of rejection or removal of excess fluid with diuretics or dialysis will lower the blood pressure in many cases.[474]

The most common single cause of post-transplant hypertension is impaired renal function associated with chronic allograft dysfunction.[474] Here a cycle is set up with hypertension contributing to the progressive loss of nephrons, which in turn contributes to the hypertension.

There is experimental evidence that the transplanted kidney may have "prohypertensive" or "antihypertensive" properties. Multiple cross-transplantation studies in experimental models of genetic hypertension have shown that the inherited tendency to hypertension resides primarily in the kidney.[475] A similar relationship may exist in humans. Patients receiving a kidney from a donor with two hypertensive parents tend to have higher blood pressures than those receiving a kidney from a donor with two normotensive parents.[476] As an example, transplantation of kidneys from normotensive donors with a negative family history of hypertension led to prolonged normotension in six recipients with a prior history of end-stage renal disease due to benign nephrosclerosis and resistant hypertension while undergoing dialysis.[477]

The importance of native kidneys in producing hypertension is supported by the observation that pretransplant native nephrectomy is associated with a significant decrease in hypertension after transplantation.[472, 478] Also, in selected patients, native nephrectomy can effectively lower blood pressure.[479, 480] The mechanisms by which the native kidneys produce hypertension have not been well defined in the renal transplant patient. There is an increased renin level[481] in some patients, whereas there is no evidence of elevated renin[479, 480] in others. Although hypertension associated with angiotensin II is most likely,[482] other factors have been postulated, including alterations in the kallikrein-kinin system[483, 484] or production of arachidonic acid metabolites.[485] Pretransplant nephrectomies were once considered routine, but because of the concern about the detrimental effects of native nephrectomy for patients who lose their transplants and return to dialysis,[486–488] this is no longer done. We need specific criteria for identification of patients with native kidney–dependent hypertension as well as information on the long-term impact of various treatment plans. Some data suggest that ACE inhibitors and native nephrectomy may have beneficial hemodynamic effects in patients with post-transplant hypertension caused by native kidneys.[489] Dietary salt intake is not thought to play a major role in causing hypertension in this group.[490]

Cyclosporine is usually a factor in post-transplantation hypertension, raising the blood pressure in almost all patients.[468, 474] Although it may not be the major factor, its effect on renal hemodynamics adds to the elevation of arterial pressure.[474] Both renal (primarily affecting the afferent arteriole) and systemic vasoconstriction is seen. How this occurs is incompletely understood. Increased release of vasoconstrictors, such as thromboxane and endothelin, is thought to play an important role.[491, 492] As an example, cyclosporine continues to induce transient renal vasoconstriction with prolonged therapy; this response is temporally related to an elevation in urinary endothelin excretion.[492] Studies of cardiac transplants suggest that sympathetic activation may be an additional factor that can raise the blood pressure.[211] This is supported by the high frequency of hypertension in other organ transplants, such as heart,[493] and in the pediatric patients treated with cyclosporine.[494, 495] Cyclosporine increases afferent arteriolar resistance,[496] which produces a form of hypertension that is volume dependent.[497] Therefore, the hypertension associated with cyclosporine may well respond to diuretic therapy[474] rather than therapy aimed at the renin-angiotensin system. The increased afferent arteriolar resistance may well be due to endothelin's action as a vasoconstrictor.[498] Other frequently mentioned vasoconstrictors associated with cyclosporine are thromboxane,[499] the sympathetic nervous system,[500] and the renin-angiotensin system. If cyclosporine is viewed as a potent constrictor of the afferent arteriole, one expects to see a prerenal type of effect on renal function. Thus, there is a tendency to see enhanced proximal tubule reabsorption of $Na^+$, urea, and uric acid; patients commonly become volume expanded.

Routine steroid use, as in most maintenance regimens (10 to 15 mg/d), does not seem to be associated with hypertension in a major way.[501] Other causes of importance certainly are other factors related to the recipient, such as essential hypertension, hypercalcemia, hyperrenin state associated with native kidneys, immunosuppressive therapy, and donor-related factors.

The prevalence of renal artery stenosis is unknown because angiography is not routinely performed after transplantation in most centers. In circumstances in which it is, however, anatomic stenosis has been seen in up to 23% of patients.[502] Demonstrating functional significance of the stenosis can be difficult because there is no generally accepted practical test to determine the significance of the stenosis.[501] Reports of functionally important stricture have varied from 5%[159, 503] to 20%[466] in a selected group of patients (patients with previous native nephrectomies with unanticipated hypertension).

## TREATMENT OF POST-TRANSPLANT HYPERTENSION

Post-transplant hypertension treatment strategies are varied, depending on the patient's pre-existing medical condition and response to therapy.

There is a theoretic advantage to the use of $Ca^{2+}$ channel blockers to improve renal hemodynamics and block thromboxane-mediated vasoconstriction.[504] The most commonly used dihydropyridines (isradipine, felodipine, nicardipine, nifedipine) produce some troubling side effects, such as flushing, tachycardia, and peripheral edema, but they have the advantage of not interacting with cyclosporine[505] (with the exception of nicardipine). Other commonly used $Ca^{2+}$ channel blockers (verapamil and diltiazem) do raise cyclosporine levels by blocking the metabolism of cyclosporine hepatic cytochrome P-450$_{IIIB}$.[506] One advantage to the use of these agents is that inhibition of cyclosporine metabolism permits the use of lower cyclosporine doses.

ACE inhibitors have the advantage of suppressing erythropoiesis in the post-transplant patient with hypertension and erythrocytosis.[507] The ability to reduce the hematocrit has allowed ACE inhibitors to be used therapeutically in patients with post-transplant erythrocytosis, in which excess erythropoietin appears to be produced by the native kidneys.[402, 508] Enalapril and captopril are often useful adjuncts to $Ca^{2+}$ antagonists if the blood pressure is uncontrolled with this therapy alone. Disadvantages to ACE inhibitor use are potentiation of hyperkalemia associated with cyclosporine and induction of anemia.[508]

Diuretics are often used to control edema in the transplant patient. Although cyclosporine-induced hypertension is associated with $Na^+$ retention and volume expansion, diuretics and salt restriction alone are rarely able to effectively reduce blood pressure. A reasonable diuretic choice is low-dosage hydrochlorothiazide in patients with a glomerular filtration rate above 30 mL/min.[505] $K^+$-sparing agents should be avoided, as should volume depletion, because autoregulation of renal blood flow is blunted by cyclosporine and decreases in perfusion pressure may enhance its nephrotoxicity.[505]

$\beta$-Blockers can be used in patients with increased sympathetic output and tachycardia.[505] They must be used cautiously, however, with frequent monitoring for hyperkalemia. Their low cost is an additional advantage.

Central and peripheral sympatholytics may lower blood pressure effectively, and clonidine transdermal patches have a role in the noncompliant patient and in diabetic patients with severe peripheral vascular disease.[505]

Aggressive management of mild hypertension is not a goal in the early post-transplant period because of the risk of underperfusing the new kidney. When maintenance levels of steroids are achieved, aggressive control of blood pressure can be considered. A rational approach is the use of a dihydropyridine $Ca^{2+}$ channel antagonist that is titrated until blood pressure is achieved or side effects limit the dosing. If blood pressure is not adequately controlled, a diuretic or $\beta$-blocker is added. If pressure is still not well controlled, an ACE inhibitor or sympatholytic is added.[505]

## RENAL ARTERY STENOSIS

The prevalence of anatomic renal transplant artery stenosis is difficult to assess. It has been suggested that functionally significant stenosis occurs in up to 12% of transplant recipients with hypertension, although the frequency appears to be decreasing in recipients of cadaver kidneys. This improvement is probably due to better harvesting techniques in which an aortic cuff containing the native donor renal artery orifice, rather than the cut renal artery, is sutured end-to-side to the iliac vessels.

Post-transplant hypertension due to renal transplant artery stenosis is important to identify because it is a correctable form of hypertension. As with other causes of bilateral renal artery stenosis or unilateral stenosis in a solitary kidney, the administration of an ACE inhibitor to a patient with transplant renal artery stenosis can lead to a reversible decline in glomerular filtration rate.[509] Thus, an elevation in plasma creatinine concentration in this setting is suggestive but not diagnostic of renovascular disease in the graft. Persistent uncontrolled hypertension and an acute elevation in blood pressure are other common features of this disorder.

Renal arteriography remains the procedure of choice for establishing the diagnosis of renal artery stenosis in the solitary transplanted kidney. A renal allograft biopsy is generally performed before angiography to rule out chronic rejection or other form of renal parenchymal disease. These findings decrease the likelihood of a successful response to correction of a stenosis and therefore are relative contraindications to intervention.[510]

Radioisotope renography, performed before and after administration of an ACE inhibitor, is an alternative to angiography to screen for the presence of renal artery stenosis in the transplant.[511, 512] This noninvasive test is not sufficiently sensitive if the history is suggestive (i.e., a negative test does not exclude the disease). Evaluation of a small number of patients suggests that renography may be more useful in predicting the physiologic significance of a moderately severe stenotic lesion, because patients with a normal renogram are unlikely to respond to correction of the stenosis.[512]

The extensive fibrosis and scarring around the transplanted kidney make surgical correction of a transplant artery stenosis difficult. On the other hand, percutaneous balloon angioplasty may be technically successful in up to 80% of cases, although 20% will have recurrent stenosis.[510, 513] Repeated angioplasty is usually not successful. Surgery should be considered only in patients with resistant hypertension or with proximal recipient arteriosclerotic disease.

## Lipid Disorders

The primary lipid disorder of chronic renal failure is elevated plasma triglyceride levels,[514-517] with the elevations occurring primarily in the very low density lipoprotein portion.[518] This disorder may be due to reduced lipolysis of triglyceride-rich lipoproteins[519-523]; other reports suggest a deficiency of lipoprotein lipase,[516, 524, 525] hepatic triglyceride lipase,[516, 525-527] or both. Chronic renal failure seems to increase the risk for coronary artery disease,[467, 528-533] but the role of hypertriglyceridemia in this is debated.[534-537]

After renal transplantation, lipid abnormalities are common and changed from the pattern seen in patients with end-stage renal disease. Some patients show a decline in serum triglyceride levels, but hypertriglyceridemia is still present in others.[538] Many others exhibit hypercholesterolemia or a mixed hyperlipidemia.[538-546]

The contributing causes for hyperlipidemia after transplantation are not well understood, but several mechanisms have been proposed. Corticosteroid therapy has been implicated[538, 542-546]; corticosteroids seem to enhance peripheral resistance to the action of insulin, raise insulin levels, and stimulate the synthesis of very low density lipoprotein triglycerides.[547] Many patients have hypercholesterolemia after transplantation, whereas hypercholesterolemia in chronic renal failure is rare. Other investigators stress that cyclosporine may play a role in hypercholesterolemia[548] and

suggest that the mechanism may relate to the drug's high lipophilicity, especially its binding to low-density lipoproteins and high-density lipoproteins.[549] These investigators claim that conversion to azathioprine and steroids reduces the plasma total cholesterol level.[548] Steroids may act by leading sequentially to peripheral insulin resistance, hyperinsulinemia, and increased hepatic very low density lipoprotein synthesis. However, steroid withdrawal may not necessarily have a net benefit on lipid metabolism in cyclosporine-treated patients. Although the total cholesterol concentration falls, there is often an equivalent or even greater reduction in high-density lipoprotein–cholesterol levels, leading to no change or an undesired elevation in the ratio of total cholesterol to high-density lipoprotein–cholesterol.[176, 550] Reducing the steroid dose does have other metabolic benefits, however, including a fall in blood pressure and, in diabetic patients, improved glucose tolerance.

The significance of these lipid abnormalities after transplantation is not known, but those patients who had myocardial infarctions during a follow-up period of 5 years had higher serum cholesterol levels than those who did not.[538] In addition, patients with hyperlipidemia appear to have a higher frequency of cardiovascular events.[551] Whether the increase in high-density lipoprotein–cholesterol diminishes the risk for vascular disease is unknown because too few patients have been included in longitudinal studies for multivariate analysis to be performed for this risk factor.[538] Other investigators have assessed the role of low-density lipoprotein–cholesterol.[552] There are many factors involved in the pathogenesis of hyperlipidemia in transplant patients that are also associated with elevated triglyceride and cholesterol levels: age, body weight, serum creatinine concentration, number of rejection episodes, cumulative steroid dose, pretransplant lipid levels, urinary protein excretion, and use of loop diuretics.[538]

Treatment of hyperlipidemia is not suggested until a stable steroid dose is achieved.[544] Therapeutic maneuvers have included weight reduction, which has resulted in lowering of triglyceride and cholesterol levels in some studies[553, 554]; reduction of saturated fatty acids and cholesterol[554]; and alternate-day steroids.[555-557] In general, dietary manipulation alone has not been shown to lower low-density lipoprotein–cholesterol, and a large number of renal allograft recipients probably require pharmacologic agents as well as dietary modification to control hyperlipidemia.[552] Lipid-lowering agents have been suggested, although there is a risk of myopathy and rhabdomyolysis with use of high-dose hydroxymethylglutaryl–coenzyme A reductase inhibitors (lovastatin) in patients also receiving cyclosporine.[558] Fibric acids (clofibrate and gemfibrozil) have produced myopathy in the presence of renal disease.[547] Bile acid sequestrants can worsen the hypertriglyceridemia and interfere with absorption of cyclosporine, and they have not been shown to lower cholesterol levels in transplant recipients; nicotinic acid can decrease glucose tolerance and raise uric acid levels.[547] Persistent hyperlipidemia may be reduced at 2 to 3 years if the corticosteroid dose is at low levels.[559]

Preliminary studies, however, suggest that a low-dose regimen may allow a hydroxymethylglutaryl–coenzyme A reductase inhibitor to be used in cyclosporine-treated patients with little risk of muscle injury.[558, 560] Lovastatin is begun at a dose of 10 mg/d and limited to a maximum of 20 mg/d. In this setting, a significant cholesterol-lowering effect is seen, and plasma lovastatin levels are similar to those in normal subjects receiving a higher lovastatin dose.[560]

## Liver Disease

Liver disease is a common cause of morbidity and mortality in renal transplant recipients, with abnormalities in liver function occurring in nearly 25% of patients in the early post-transplant period[561, 562]; death due to liver failure occurs in up to 30% of long-term survivors.[54, 305, 450, 561–564] Many factors have been implicated in the etiology of post-transplantation liver disease, including drug toxicity and viral infection.

### HEPATITIS B VIRUS

The current sensitivity for HBsAg marker screening has made the peritransplant acquisition of HBV a rare event.[426] The natural history of HBV infection in the immunosuppressed patient differs from that in the dialysis population as well as from that in the general population. There is a greater likelihood for progression of hepatic injury in the immunosuppressed population. Chronic liver disease, as reflected by biopsy evidence of chronic persistent hepatitis, chronic active hepatitis, and cirrhosis, is present in the majority of patients with HBsAg-positive serologic reactions by 2 or more years after transplantation.[305, 450] Liver failure, in patients who are HBsAg-positive, may be due to reactivation of latent virus as well as superinfection with another viral agent or a toxic cause.

Antibody to hepatitis B e antigen (HBeAg) generally reflects a poor prognosis in the transplant recipient because the pathologic findings usually worsen[305, 450] from chronic persistent to chronic active hepatitis.[251, 565] Indeed, in a prospective study of HBsAg-positive and HBsAg-negative transplant patients, immunosuppressive therapy was shown to clearly increase viral replication (measured by in situ hybridization of HBV DNA) in serum and liver biopsy specimens.[566] In addition, there is a 15% frequency of hepatoma in chronic carriers of HBV receiving immunosuppressive agents.[567] Death resulting from liver failure is not uncommon and is often accompanied by septicemia.[561]

Whether a patient who is a chronic carrier of HBsAg should undergo transplantation is controversial. Retrospective comparison of HBsAg-positive hemodialysis patients with transplant recipients shows a higher frequency of chronic liver disease and mortality due to HBV.[564] The adverse effects are not usually seen for at least 2 years after transplantation. Thus, potential transplant recipients must be warned that there is a risk, albeit low, of chronic liver failure. No patient with active hepatitis should undergo transplantation, and it is prudent to recommend liver biopsy in HBsAg-positive patients before transplantation because serum transaminase levels are a poor predictor of the histologic lesion.[450]

The utility of vaccination for HBV is unproved in the transplant patient. Seroconversion after serial vaccinations occurs in 90% of normal patients, whereas it occurs in only 40% to 60% of hemodialysis patients,[568] with greater frequency of reversion to seronegativity in the dialysis patients.[569] When primary vaccination of allograft recipients is performed, the seroconversion rate is even lower than in the dialysis population (7% to 30%).[570, 571] Graft function has not been shown to be impaired as a result of active vaccination with HBV vaccine.

### HEPATITIS C VIRUS

Although HBV plays an important role in the pathogenesis of post-transplant chronic liver disease and hepatocellular carcinoma, the role of non-A, non-B hepatitis virus is being increasingly recognized.[54, 450, 561–563] A newly developed assay to detect antibody against a recombinant viral antigen (c100) from HCV[572, 573] has clarified the frequency of pretransplant infection and suggests that transmission can occur not only by transfusion of blood products but by sexual, vertical, and intrafamilial spread.[574] Transmission also occurs from donor organ to recipient at a high rate (100%),[574, 575] and following antibody titers will underestimate both the transmission of HCV and the role of HCV in post-transplantation liver disease.

Transplant recipients may be at risk for the development of HCV-induced liver disease because of reactivation of pretransplantation HCV infection or because of infection acquired from either blood products received at the time of transplantation or HCV-infected organ donors.[574] Attention has recently focused on the high prevalence of HCV infection in cadaver organ donors (5.1% in cadaver donors versus 0.6% among healthy blood donors).[574] The higher prevalence among cadaver organ donors may reflect an increased frequency of risk factors associated with the spread of viral infections, such as unsuspected intravenous drug use or sexual promiscuity.[574] In view of the high risk of both infection and progressive liver disease, many organ banks have adopted a policy restricting the use of HCV-positive donors to lifesaving transplants (heart, liver, or lung). A similar policy has been recommended by the U.S. Public Health Service Inter-agency Guidelines.

As with hepatitis B, post-transplantation patients more often have chronic active liver disease due to hepatitis C than do healthy individuals with post-transfusion hepatitis C.[574–576] It is likely that the immunosuppressive therapy in transplant recipients plays a role in preventing clearing of virus and recovery from liver disease.[574]

The issue of transplantation of kidneys from anti-HCV–positive organ donors into recipients with anti-HCV has been a subject of considerable debate in the recent past,[577] with one small study suggesting that donation of HCV-positive donors was acceptable.[578] A problem with these studies is that there exists a wide variation in the positive predictive value of anti-HCV testing in identifying ongoing HCV infection in both organ donors and potential recipients.[574, 579, 580] As a result, it is likely that not all the anti-HCV–positive donors and recipients in this study had ongoing HCV infection. The anti-HCV antibodies detected by the currently available tests are non-neutralizing and do not necessarily confer immunity. A study in a chimpanzee model, for example, indicated that previous infection with

HCV did not protect from reinfection with a different or even the same strain of the virus.[581] Repeated exposure did not protect against either reappearance of viremia or biochemical or histologic evidence of liver disease. We must await the results of large prospective clinical studies to determine the safety of transplantation of organs from anti-HCV–positive donors into anti-HCV–positive recipients.

Interferon alfa has been used with considerable success in nontransplant patients with chronic active hepatitis due to HCV,[582] including those with mixed cryoglobulinemia or HCV-induced glomerular disease. Unfortunately, these results cannot be extrapolated to transplant recipients with chronic liver disease due to HCV. Interferon alfa can induce cytokine gene expression, increase cell surface expression of HLA antigens, and enhance the function of natural killer cells, cytotoxic T cells, and monocytes. As a result, therapy with interferon alfa carries the risk of inducing or facilitating rejection in the allograft.[582] Thus, the risk of rejection in transplant recipients must be weighed against the potential benefits of slowing or preventing the progression of chronic liver disease. Although it may appear that the risk of hepatic failure is greater than that of losing the graft and returning to dialysis, two additional issues must be considered: the efficacy of interferon alfa in treating HCV infection in the immunosuppressed transplant recipient has not been proved; if rejection is induced, then the administration of antirejection therapy may exacerbate the viral infection.

## OTHER CAUSES OF LIVER DISEASE

There are drugs that may potentially result in a toxic hepatitis, including cyclosporine, azathioprine, antihypertensive drugs, and lipid-lowering agents. Cyclosporine-induced transaminitis usually resolves with reduction of the dose and may also result in hepatic cholestasis. In addition, azathioprine has been reported to be hepatotoxic in some studies,[517, 583] but its exclusive role in hepatic injury has not been clarified. Chronic alcoholism is a significant cause of chronic progressive liver disease in many centers and cannot be overlooked as an important etiologic factor.

## Cancer

The long-term use of immunosuppressive agents increases the risk of neoplasms after transplantation. The types of cancers encountered in transplant recipients are different from those found in the normal population, with a higher frequency of squamous cell carcinomas of the skin, non-Hodgkin lymphoma, Kaposi sarcoma, in situ carcinomas of the uterine cervix, carcinomas of the vulva and perineum, hepatobiliary carcinomas, and a variety of sarcomas.[584]

Although the overall frequency of tumors in the transplant population is 100 times higher than that in the general population, the frequency of tumors seen commonly in the general population (lung, breast, prostate, colon, and invasive uterine carcinomas) does not increase and may in fact be even lower after transplantation.[585, 586] If all cancers are considered, the average time of their appearance is 61 months.[587] It is clear, however, that some neoplasms appear

at distinct time intervals after transplantation. For instance, Kaposi sarcoma is the first to appear (average of 21 months), then lymphomas (32 months), epithelial cancers (69 months), and cancer of the vulva and perineum (112 months).[587]

The most common post-transplant cancers are those of the skin and lips, with a frequency noted in the Cincinnati Transplant Tumor Registry (which has data on more than 5000 transplant patients) of 37%. The rate of occurrence varies greatly with the amount of sun exposure,[584–586] although even in a series of 523 patients from Canada, there is a frequency of almost 20%.[588] There is a linear increase in the frequency of skin cancer with length of follow-up after transplantation.[589] Of the skin cancers, squamous cell carcinomas are more common than basal cell carcinomas, whereas the reverse is true in the general population.[584] These tumors occur at a younger age as well (age 30 versus 60 years) and occur in multiple sites on the skin.[590] The tumors are more aggressive than in the general population and more likely to recur after resection.

Next to cancers of the skin, lymphoproliferative disorders are among the most serious and potentially fatal, accounting for 21% of all malignant neoplasms in this population.[586] Non-Hodgkin lymphoma is the most common lymphoma in transplant recipients; most of these lymphomas are classified as large-cell lymphomas, the great majority of which are of the B cell type. Extranodal involvement, central nervous system involvement, and infiltration of the allograft are common. The pathogenesis of post-transplant non-Hodgkin lymphoma may be related to B cell proliferation induced by EBV infection,[591–593] because studies from liver transplant recipients have demonstrated EBV messenger RNA in hepatic tissue in most patients before overt lymphoproliferative disease was documented.[593]

The degree of overall immunosuppression is a major determinant of the development of a lymphoproliferative tumor, although the role of each individual immunosuppressive agent is unclear.[202, 586, 594] It appears that both the dose and the duration of therapy are important[202] in induction of these malignant neoplasms.

An approach to treatment of post-transplant malignant neoplasms must include preventive measures. Sunlight exposure should be limited, with either avoidance of exposure or use of protective sunscreens and clothing. Patients should be examined regularly, and any premalignant lesions should be treated. Metabolites of azathioprine, mostly methylnitrothioimidazole and related imidazole compounds, sensitize the skin to sunlight and may increase the risk of skin cancer.[587] Although a logical approach is to switch from azathioprine to cyclosporine in patients with skin cancers, no clinical data as yet show a beneficial effect.[587] Other malignant neoplasms are treated by standard surgical, radiotherapeutic, or chemotherapeutic modalities. Antiviral agents, acyclovir or ganciclovir, have been used to treat EBV-associated non-Hodgkin lymphomas. Interferon alfa has been used to treat patients with Kaposi sarcoma and non-Hodgkin lymphomas, but there is a risk of inducing rejection.[587]

Reduction or cessation of immunosuppressive therapy has resulted in regression of tumors in some renal transplant recipients with Kaposi sarcoma and non-Hodgkin lymphomas,[585, 589, 595, 596] with the risk of return to dialysis. Obviously, this is not an option in heart and liver transplant patients. Epithelial tumors are less likely to regress after a decrease in immunosuppression.[585] If cytotoxic therapy is needed to treat widespread tumors, azathioprine should be discontinued to avoid toxic bone marrow effects.[585]

## Hyperuricemia and Gout

Gouty arthritis is seen in approximately 10% of transplant recipients, and reduced uric acid excretion and hyperuricemia are common with cyclosporine.[239, 597, 598] Asymptomatic hyperuricemia occurs in 55% of patients receiving cyclosporine and 25% of those receiving azathioprine.[599] Cyclosporine promotes uric acid retention by lowering the glomerular filtration rate[597] and directly impairs urate secretion.[598] The concurrent use of diuretics and renal insufficiency due to rejection are two other risk factors for hyperuricemia.[598] Treatment and prevention of gout are not without risk in the transplant recipient. The preferred therapy is colchicine in a dose of 0.6 mg twice daily unless the patient has advanced renal insufficiency. Nonsteroidal antiinflammatory drugs are a potential concern, because the inhibition of renal prostaglandin synthesis may lead to a further reduction in glomerular filtration rate and worsening nephrotoxic effects of cyclosporine. Allopurinol, on the other hand, interferes with the metabolism of azathioprine, which is catabolized in part by xanthine oxidase. Thus, azathioprine accumulation and possibly severe toxic bone marrow effects may ensue. As a result, allopurinol should be avoided in patients receiving azathioprine or used only with a reduced azathioprine dose and careful monitoring of the white blood cell count.

## Calcium and Phosphorus Metabolism

Secondary hyperparathyroidism is improved after restoration of renal function owing to reversal of vitamin D resistance and $PO_4^{3-}$ retention. In fact, a resolution of the radiographic changes of hyperparathyroidism occurs as early as 3 months after transplantation.[600] Other patients may have sustained hyperparathyroidism, many in association with normal serum $Ca^{2+}$ levels.[601]

Hypercalcemia is common after transplantation (15% to 30% of transplant recipients)[602, 603] due to the persistence of a hyperplastic parathyroid gland. In most cases, mild hypercalcemia resolves slowly in 6 to 12 months. Persistent hypercalcemia may require parathyroidectomy, however. The indications for parathyroidectomy are progressive elevation of parathyroid hormone levels and evidence of continuing or worsening metabolic bone disease and proximal myopathy. Acute, severe hypercalcemia ($Ca^{2+}$ levels > 14 mg/dL) immediately after transplantation often requires urgent parathyroidectomy.

Hypophosphatemia is seen in up to 70% of patients within a year of transplantation and may persist even in the absence of hyperparathyroidism. The recipients often have a renal $PO_4^{3-}$ wasting syndrome[604] even in the absence of other evidence of proximal tubule dysfunction. Because of the possibility that $PO_4^{3-}$ depletion may exacerbate further osseous, cardiac, renal, hematologic, and neurologic abnormalities, we treat all hypophosphatemic patients with oral phosphate supplementation.

## Bone Disease

Resolution of metabolic acidosis, cessation of aluminum hydroxide gel therapy, and improved vitamin D metabolism lead to some improvement in pre-existing renal osteodystrophy and osteomalacia. After transplantation, however, the patient is at increased risk for osteonecrosis associated with corticosteroid use,[600, 605] especially in the setting of pre-existing metabolic bone disease.[606] Avascular necrosis may not be revealed by standard radiographs; bone scans or magnetic resonance imaging may be needed to detect an early lesion. Although surgical decompression procedures have been tried, many patients eventually require arthroplasty.[607–609]

## Diabetes Mellitus

Diabetes mellitus occurs in 5% to 10% of transplant recipients.[610, 611] Of those patients initially requiring insulin therapy, approximately half will continue to require insulin therapy.[611] Although post-transplant diabetes mellitus is most commonly associated with corticosteroids, a potential concern is cyclosporine-induced pancreatic injury.[611, 612] In addition, the production of diabetes in renal transplant patients probably depends on the promotion of a viral infection within the pancreas by immunosuppression. The prevalence of post-transplant steroid-associated diabetes has ranged from 3.4% to 46%, depending on the criteria for diagnosis and duration of follow-up.[611] Although diabetes may appear at great length from the time of transplantation (10 years in some reports),[305] the early onset has been reported in 16% of 758 nondiabetic recipients, 54% of whom became hyperglycemic within 3 weeks of transplantation.[611]

## Hematologic Complications

All immunosuppressive medications can cause abnormalities in hematopoietic cell lines. Azathioprine has been shown to cause a variety of hematologic abnormalities, including leukopenia, megaloblastic erythrocytosis, red blood cell aplasia, and thrombocytopenia.[613–616] In the setting of the hemolytic-uremic syndrome, cyclosporine causes a microangiopathic hemolytic anemia.[212, 617, 618] In addition, an autoimmune hemolytic anemia has been reported when O blood group donor kidneys were transplanted into blood group A or B recipients.[619]

Erythrocytosis associated with an increased red blood cell mass has been seen in up to 20% of transplant recipients.[620] A hematocrit greater than 52% usually occurs within the first post-transplant year and may be associated with either good or poor allograft function, transplant renal artery stenosis, hydronephrosis, and the use of androgenic steroids.[620] Various etiologic factors have been suggested, including enhanced red blood cell production with resolution of uremia and intrarenal hypoxemia in chronic allograft dysfunction.[621] Graft function usually restores the normal hematopoietic response within the first year of transplantation. In persistent cases, phlebotomy may be indicated to prevent thromboembolic complications that may occur in as many as 20% of patients with erythrocytosis.[620] ACE inhibitors, such as enalapril, have been used to treat the erythrocytosis after transplantation.[508]

## ECONOMIC AND ETHICAL ISSUES IN RENAL TRANSPLANTATION

The treatment of end-stage renal disease has posed substantial ethical and economic questions since dialysis became available as a means for treatment of the condition. At first, the issues confronting physicians and administrators who cared for such patients were stark ones of life or death because dialysis was an extraordinarily expensive procedure available only at limited centers. Triage of patients for dialysis became common, not only on the basis of medical suitability for dialysis treatment, but also on the basis of ability to pay and perceived "social worth" of the patient. Insight into the public attitudes toward our communal responsibility for catastrophic and expensive illness can be gleaned from an examination of the legislative history of the end-stage renal disease dialysis and transplant programs administered through Medicare. This history also permits us to define some of the issues about which an ethical consensus has been reached by the public. The treatment of end-stage renal failure became a federal entitlement program when it became clear that citizens and their lawmaker representatives were not willing to allow their compatriots to die of a treatable disease simply because of lack of resources, even though the commitment to public expenditure would be substantial. The U.S. Social Security Amendment Public Law 92-603 provided automatic payment for treatment of most end-stage renal disease patients in the nation regardless of age. This Medicare-administered program covered both dialysis and transplantation. The National Organ Transplant Act of 1984 (Public Law 98-507) provided for a nationwide network called the Organ Procurement and Transplantation Network. The purpose of the network was to collect statistics on all transplants (both renal and nonrenal) done in the United States under contract from the Department of Health and Human Services. The Transplant Act of 1984 also established a scientific registry that would serve to analyze efficacy of transplantation under the program. Funding was extended to pay for immunosuppressive medication after transplantation, in particular because the cost of cyclosporine was beyond the means of many individuals. Last, the act established a task force whose purpose was to recommend to the Secretary of Health and Human Services and the Congress means to improve the effectiveness of transplantation and equitable access to transplantation. The task force made a number of recommendations that were accepted by the Congress. A principle was established, and written into law, that special consideration be given to individuals with biologic handicaps that would impair their access to kidney transplanta-

tion. This included potential recipients with blood group O and sensitized patients. Patients with these characteristics were found to have significantly fewer opportunities for transplantation because of the absolute biologic barriers posed by higher frequencies of ABO incompatibility or positive lymphocytotoxic crossmatches.

Since its inception, the federal Organ Procurement Transplant Network has been administered by a voluntary not-for-profit corporation called the United Network for Organ Sharing, which holds a contract from the Division of Transplantation of the Department of Health and Human Services, Public Health Service. The United Network for Organ Sharing is a centrally administered organization with extensive regional and local representation; it is composed of representatives of the transplant community and the general public, including transplant patients and donor families. The United Network for Organ Sharing, as the executor of the Organ Procurement Transplant Network, has a board of directors as well as a large number of committees, including ethics and organ allocation committees, which ultimately make policy recommendations to the Secretary of Health and Human Services after lengthy periods of discussion and periods of public comment.

The number of end-stage renal disease patients who seek access to a renal transplant exceeds the number of cadaver kidneys plus living related kidneys that are available. As a result, the number of individuals awaiting renal transplantation grows each year (Fig. 59–6), and the mean time a newly registered patient has to wait before receiving a transplant increases every year. This effect of the chronic shortage of kidneys is worsened for some patients because of individual characteristics that further decrease the probability of transplantation. These include ABO blood group, presensitization against HLA antigens, and HLA phenotype of the recipient, among others. Variability in the access of individual transplant centers to donated organs also greatly affects mean waiting times. A report by the Inspector General of the United States clearly shows that black transplant candidates undergo transplantation at less than half the rate of their white counterparts. A host of factors have been

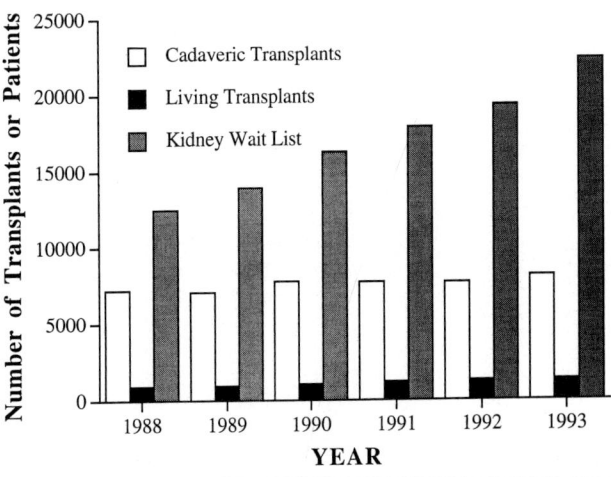

**Figure 59–6.** The number of transplants done per year (cadaveric and living donor) versus the number of patients on the wait list for kidney transplantation.

offered as explanations for the difference in access to transplantation between black and white patients in the United States. These include differences in distribution of ABO blood group antigens, sensitization rates, HLA antigen distribution, rate of intercurrent illnesses, ''unavailability'' when called for a transplant offer, and center differences in access to organs that may correlate with racial demography.

The ever-increasing concern about waiting time has made it difficult to advocate a purely utilitarian approach to criteria for assigning a donated cadaver organ to a specific recipient. In considering a living related transplant, the decision to be made is which donor among the family members would be optimal for the single potential recipient. In contrast, the problem in cadaver organ assignment is in choosing the appropriate recipient for a particular available kidney. Univariate and multivariate analyses of short-term and long-term allograft survival have identified a number of risk factors for graft failure (Table 59–13). The factors that are important in short-term graft survival are not necessarily the same as those that predict the long-term half-life of graft survival. Whereas high degrees of humoral sensitization, the transplant center, a young donor, and mismatching for HLA-B or -DR antigens are important in short-term graft survival, the risk factors that appear to be more important in long-term allograft loss are poor health of the recipient, HLA-A mismatch, African-American race of the recipient, and older age of the donor.[622–624] Some of the factors that are associated with a poorer kidney graft survival may be important because they are associated with an inadequate nephron mass for the metabolic demand of the recipient. Small kidneys from women, small children, or African-American donors and kidneys that may have fewer nephrons because of senile glomerulosclerosis fail sooner than do large kidneys derived from white middle-aged men, especially if they are placed into individuals with

a higher metabolic demand for renal function (diabetic patients, large men).[625] A utilitarian approach to the assignment of available cadaver kidneys to specific recipients would seek to maximize the survival of each individual kidney, thereby maximizing the total number of recipient-years of good graft function. The utilitarian approach also minimizes the cost of transplantation because fewer individuals return to dialysis maintenance or the transplant waiting list in a given period. Such an approach comes at a price, however, because it inevitably results in a selective advantage for some prospective recipients at ''the expense'' of other recipients' chances to have an opportunity for transplantation. Nevertheless, such an approach may be justified from the point of view of the optimal therapy for the individual patient. Because there is another wholly acceptable form of long-term therapy for end-stage renal failure, namely, dialysis, most patients would be well served to wait a longer time on a transplant list if such a prolonged wait meant that the organ they ultimately received would survive 10% longer. This additional time spent would then be gained back as more months with a functioning graft.

## TABLE 59–13. Factors That Influence Graft Survival

| Mechanisms | Factor with Higher (Lower) Risk |
| --- | --- |
| *Nonimmunologic* | |
| Center effect | Some centers have higher risk |
| Donor race | Kidneys from black donors |
| Recipient race | Black recipients |
| Donor sex | Kidneys from women |
| Recipient sex | Male recipient |
| Donor kidney weight | Very low kidney weight |
| Recipient weight | Weight > 90 kg |
| Recipient age | Age > 60 y |
| Donor age | Donor age < 2 y |
| Recipient disease | Diabetes, hypercholesterolemia |
| Health status of patient | Diabetes, cardiovascular disease, hepatitis |
| Donor disease | Donor cerebrovascular accident |
| Recipient economic status | Lower income |
| *Immunologic* | |
| Center effect | Some centers have higher risk |
| HLA mismatch | Incompatibility for HLA-A, -B, or -DR |
| Sensitization | Antibody against HLA antigens |
| Recipient disease | (IgA with lower risk) |
| Transfusion history | (>1 DR–matched transfusion lowers risk) |
| Previous allograft | Early rejection of a previous graft |
| Use of cyclosporine | Cyclosporine not used |

## REFERENCES

1. Opelz G, Mickey MR, Terasaki PI: Calculations on long term graft and patient survival in human kidney transplantation. Transplant Proc 9:27–30, 1977.
2. Tilney NL, Milford EL, Aranjo JL, et al: Experience with cyclosporine and steroids in clinical renal transplantation. Ann Surg 200:605–613, 1984.
3. Stratta RJ, Oh CS, Sollinger HW, et al: Kidney transplantation in the cyclosporine era. Transplantation 45:40–45, 1988.
4. Ascher NL, Ahrenholz DH, Simmons RL, Najarian JS: One hundred second renal allografts from a single transplantation institution. Transplantation 27:30–34, 1979.
5. Shah B, First MR, Munda R, et al: Current experience with renal transplantation in older patients. Am J Kidney Dis 12:516–523, 1988.
6. US Renal Data System: USRDS 1989 Annual Data Report. The National Institutes of Health, National Institute of Diabetes and Digestive and Kidney Diseases, Bethesda, MD, 1989.
7. Eggers PW: Effect of transplantation on the Medicare end-stage renal disease program. N Engl J Med 318:223–229, 1988.
8. Roza AM, Gallagher-Lepatk S, Johnson CP, Adams MB: Renal transplantation in patients more than 65 years old. Transplantation 48:689–690, 1989.
9. Ismail N, Hakim RM, Helderman JH: Renal replacement therapies in the elderly: Part II. Renal transplantation. Am J Kidney Dis 23:1–15, 1994.
10. Vivas CA, Hickey DP, Jordan ML, et al: Renal transplantation in patients 65 years old or older. J Urol 147:990–993, 1992.
11. Delmonico FL, Cosimi AB, Russell PS: Renal transplantation in the older age group. Arch Surg 110:1107–1109, 1975.
12. Simmons RL, Kjellstrand CM, Buselmeier TJ, Najarian JS: Renal transplantation in high-risk patients. Arch Surg 103:290–298, 1971.
13. Hunt J: Pretransplant evaluation and outcome. Semin Nephrol 12:227–233, 1992.
14. Manske CL, Wang Y, Rector T, et al: Coronary revascularisation in insulin-dependent diabetic patients with chronic renal failure. Lancet 340:998–1002, 1992.
15. Nesto RW, Phillips RT: Asymptomatic myocardial ischemia in diabetic patients. Am J Med 805:40–47, 1986.
16. Boudreau RJ, Strony JT, duCret RP, et al: Perfusion thallium imaging of type I diabetes patients with end-stage renal disease: Comparison of oral and intravenous dipyridamole administration. Radiology 175:103–105, 1990.
17. Marwick TH, Steinmuller DR, Underwood DA, et al: Ineffectiveness of dipyridamole SPECT thallium imaging as a screening technique

for coronary artery disease in patients with end-stage renal failure. Transplantation 49:100–103, 1990.

18. Holley JL, Fenton RA, Arthur RS: Thallium stress testing does not predict cardiovascular risk in diabetic patients with end-stage renal disease undergoing cadaveric renal transplantation. Am J Med 90:563–570, 1991.

19. Morrow CE, Schwartz JS, Sutherland DR, et al: Predictive value of thallium stress testing for coronary and cardiovascular events in uremic diabetic patients before renal transplantation. Am J Surg 146:331–335, 1983.

20. Valsania P, Zarich SW, Kowalchuk GJ: Severity of coronary artery disease in young patients with insulin-dependent diabetes mellitus. Am Heart J 122:695–700, 1991.

21. Trochu JN, Cantarovich D, Renaudeau J: Assessment of coronary artery disease by thallium scan in type 1 diabetic uremic patients awaiting combined pancreas and renal transplantation. Angiology 42:302–307, 1991.

22. Camp AD, Garvin PJ, Hoff J: Prognostic value of intravenous dipyridamole thallium imaging in patients with diabetes mellitus considered for renal transplantation. Am J Cardiol 60:1459–1463, 1990.

23. Brown KA, Rimmer J, Harsch C: Noninvasive cardiac risk stratification of diabetic and nondiabetic uremic renal allograft candidates using dipyridamole–thalliium-201 imaging and radionuclide ventriculography. Am J Cardiol 64:1017–1021, 1989.

24. Weinrauch L, D'Elia JA, Healy RW, et al: Asymptomatic coronary artery disease: Angiographic assessment of diabetics evaluated for renal transplantation. Circulation 58:1184–1190, 1978.

25. Braun WE, Phillips DF, Vidt DG, et al: Coronary artery disease in 100 diabetics with end-stage renal failure. Transplant Proc 16:603–607, 1984.

26. Lorber MI, Van Buren CT, Flechner SM, et al: Pretransplant coronary arteriography for diabetic renal transplant recipients. Transplant Proc 19:1539–1541, 1987.

27. Weinrauch LA, D'Elia JA, Healy RW, et al: Asymptomatic coronary artery disease: Angiography in diabetic patients before renal transplantation: Relation of findings to postoperative survival. Ann Intern Med 88:346–348, 1978.

28. Bennett WM, Kloster F, Rosch J, et al: Natural history of asymptomatic coronary arteriographic lesions in diabetic patients with end-stage renal disease. Am J Med 65:779–784, 1978.

29. Braun WE, Phillips D, Vidt D, et al: Coronary arteriography and coronary artery disease in 99 diabetic and nondiabetic patients on chronic hemodialysis or renal transplantation programs. Transplant Proc 13:128–135, 1981.

30. Braun WE, Phillips D, Vidt D, et al: Coronary arteriography and coronary artery disease in 99 diabetic and nondiabetic patients on chronic hemodialysis or renal transplantation programs. Transplant Proc 13:128–135, 1981.

31. Philipson JD, Carpenter BJ, Itzkoff J, et al: Evaluation of cardiovascular risk for renal transplantation in diabetic patients. Am J Med 81:630–634, 1986.

32. Lemners MJ, Barry JM: Major role for arterial disease in morbidity and mortality after kidney transplantation in diabetic recipients. Diabetes Care 14:295–301, 1991.

33. Lee GSL: Medical problems in dialysis patients awaiting renal transplantation. Ann Acad Med 20:519–523, 1991.

34. Keane WF, Raij LR: Host defenses and infectious complications in maintenance haemodialysis patients. In Drukker W, Parsons FM, Maher JF (eds): Replacement of Renal Function by Dialysis. Martinus Nijhoff, Boston, 1983, pp 646–658.

35. Tolkoff-Rubin NE, Rubin RH: Uremia and host defenses. N Engl J Med 322:770–772, 1990.

36. Chatenoud L, Heberlin A, Beaurain G, Descamps-Latscha B: Immune deficiency of the uremic patient. Adv Nephrol 19:359–374, 1990.

37. Goldblum SE, Reed WP: Host defense and immunologic alterations associated with chronic haemodialysis. Ann Intern Med 93:597–613, 1980.

38. Winchester JF, Rotellar C, Goggins M, et al: Transplantation in peritoneal dialysis and hemodialysis. Kidney Int 40:S101–S105, 1993.

39. Chiaramonte S, Bragantini L, Segato G: Kidney transplant in peritoneal dialysis patients. In La Greca G, Ronco C, Feriani M, et al (eds): Peritoneal Dialysis, 2nd ed. Wichtig Editore, Milan, 1991, pp 323–325.

40. Gokal R: Renal transplantation in patients on CAPD. In La Greca G, Chiaramonte S, Fabris A, et al (eds): Peritoneal Dialysis. Wichtig Editore, Milan, 1986, pp 283–288.

41. Penn I: Renal transplantation in patients with pre-existing malignancies. Transplant Proc 15:1079, 1983.

42. Malluche H, Ritz E, Hodgson M: Skeletal lesions and calcium metabolism in early renal failure. Proc Eur Dial Transplant Assoc 11:443–450, 1974.

43. Malluche HH, Ritz E, Kutschera J: Calcium metabolism and impaired mineralization in various stages of renal insufficiency. In Norman AW, Schaefer K, Grigolect HG, et al (eds): Vitamin D and Problems Related to Uremic Bone Disease. Walter de Gruyter, New York, 1975, pp 513–522.

44. Smith AJ, Faugere MC, Abreo D, et al: Aluminum related bone disease in mild and advanced renal failure. Evidence for high prevalence and morbidity, and studies on etiology and diagnosis in 197 patients. Am J Nephrol 29:275–283, 1986.

45. David-Neto E, Jorgetti V, Soeiro NM, et al: Reversal of aluminum-related bone disease after renal transplantation. Am J Nephrol 13:12–17, 1993.

46. Owens MC, Passano E, Wilson SE: Treatment of peptic ulcer disease in the renal transplant patient. Am Surg 186:19–21, 1979.

47. Klompmaker IJ, Slooff MJ, de Brnijin KM: Prophylaxis with ranitidine against peptic ulcer disease after liver transplantation. Transplant Int 1:209–212, 1988.

48. Lao A, Bach D: The UGI series in renal transplant candidates. Can Assoc Radiol J 39:195–197, 1988.

49. Faro RS, Corry RJ: Management of surgical gastrointestinal complications in renal transplant recipients. Arch Surg 114:310–312, 1979.

50. Diehl AK: Epidemiology and natural history of gallstone disease. Gastroenterol Clin North Am 20:1–19, 1991.

51. Choong HL, Pwee HS, Woo KT, Lim CH: Maintenance haemodialysis in Singapore. Singapore Med J 32:133–138, 1991.

52. Gailbraith RM, el-Sheikh N, Portmann B: Immune response to HBsAg and the spectrum of liver lesions in HBsAg-positive patients with chronic renal disease. Br Med J 1:1495–1497, 1976.

53. Fairley CK, Mijch A, Gust ID: The increased risk of fatal liver disease in renal transplant patients who are hepatitis B e antigen and/or HBV DNA positive. Transplantation 52:497–500, 1991.

54. Ware AJ, Luby JP, Hollinger B: Etiology of liver disease in renal transplant patients. Ann Intern Med 91:364–371, 1979.

55. Read AE, Donegan E, Lake J: Hepatitis C in patients undergoing liver transplantation. Ann Intern Med 114:282–284, 1991.

56. Bretan PN, Novick AC, Steinmuller DR, et al: Ultrasonographic prospective pretransplant screening in 100 patients for acquired renal cysts and renal cell carcinoma. Transplant Proc 21:1974–1975, 1989.

57. Narasimhan N, Golper TA, Wolfson M, et al: Clinical characteristics and diagnostic considerations in acquired renal cystic disease. Kidney Int 30:748–752, 1986.

58. Thomson BS, Jenkins DAS, Allan PL, et al: Acquired cystic disease of the kidney in patients with end-stage chronic renal failure: A study of prevalence and aetiology. Nephrol Dial Transplant 1:38–43, 1986.

59. Bretan PNJ, Busch MP, Hricak H, Williams RD: Chronic renal failure: A significant risk factor in the development of acquired renal cysts and renal cell carcinoma. Case reports and review of the literature. Cancer 57:1871–1879, 1986.

60. Brien G, Lenk S, Althaus P: On the therapy of urolithiasis in chronic renal failure. Int Urol Nephrol 10:7–14, 1978.

61. Zilleruelo G, Andia J, Gorman HM: Chronic renal failure in children: Analysis of main causes and deterioration rate in 81 children. Int J Pediatr Nephrol 1:30–33, 1980.

62. Wallack HH, Kandel G, Presman DC: Polycystic kidneys: Indication for surgical intervention. J Urol 3:552–556, 1974.

63. DeBono DP, Evans DB: The management of polycystic kidney disease with special reference to dialysis and transplantation. Q J Med 46:353–363, 1977.

64. Nossent HC, Swaak TJ, Berden JH: Systemic lupus erythematosus after renal transplantation: Patient and graft survival and disease activity. Ann Intern Med 114:183–188, 1991.

65. Amend WJJ, Vincenti F, Feduska NJ, et al: Recurrent systemic lupus erythematosus involving renal allografts. Ann Intern Med 94:444–448, 1981.

66. Yakub YM, Freeman RB, Pabico RB: Renal transplantation in patients with systemic lupus erythematosus. Arch Intern Med 143:2089, 1983.

67. Bumgardner GL, Mauer SM, Payne W, et al: Single center 1–15 year results of renal transplantation in patients with systemic lupus erythematosus. Transplantation 46:703–709, 1988.
68. Rich LM, Piering WF: Ureteral stenosis due to recurrent Wegener's granulomatosis after kidney transplantation. J Am Soc Nephrol 4:1516–1521, 1994.
69. Gurland HJ, Brunner FP, Chantler C, et al: Combined report on regular dialysis and transplantation in Europe. Proc Eur Dial Transplant Assoc 13:3, 1976.
70. Groth GC, Ringden O: Transplantation in relation to the treatment of inherited disease. Transplantation 38:319–327, 1984.
71. Wilson RE: Transplantation in patients with unusual causes of renal failure. Clin Nephrol 5:51–53, 1976.
72. Bodmer JG, Marsh SGE, Albert ED: Nomenclature for factors of the HLA system, 1991. Tissue Antigens 39:161–173, 1992.
73. Bjorkman PJ, Saper MS, Samraoui B, et al: Structure of the human class I histocompatibility antigen, HLA-A2. Nature 329:506–512, 1987.
74. Colbaugh P, Stastny P: Antigens in human monocytes, III. Use of monocytes in typing for HLA-D related (DR) antigens. Transplant Proc 10:871–874, 1978.
75. Moraes JR, Stastny P: A new antigen system expressed in human endothelial cells. J Clin Invest 60:449–454, 1977.
76. Opelz G, Terasaki PI: Effect of blood group on relation between HLA match and outcome of cadaver kidney transplants. Lancet 1:220–222, 1977.
77. Cecka JM, Terasaki PI: The UNOS Scientific Renal Transplant Registry. In Terasaki PI, Cecka JM (eds): Clinical Transplants 1992. UCLA Tissue Typing Laboratory, Los Angeles, 1993, pp 1–17.
78. Opelz G: Collaborative Transplant Study: Effect of HLA matching in 10,000 cyclosporine treated cadaver kidney transplants. Transplant Proc 19:641–646, 1987.
79. Sanfilippo F, Vaughn WK, Bollinger RR, Spees EK: Comparative effects of pregnancy, transfusion, and prior graft rejection on sensitization and renal transplant results. Transplantation 34:360–366, 1982.
80. Turka LA, Goguen JE, Gagne JE, Milford EL: Presensitization and the renal allograft recipient. Transplantation 47:234–240, 1989.
81. Noreen HJ: Interpretation of crossmatch tests. In Nikaein A, Phelan DL, Mickelson EM, et al (eds): American Society for Histocompatibility and Immunogenetics Laboratory Manual. ASHI, Lenexa, KS, 1994, pp I.C.1.1–I.C.1.13.
82. Kerman RH: The role of crossmatching in organ transplantation. Arch Pathol Lab Med 115:255–259, 1991.
83. Iwaki Y, Cook DJ, Terasaki PI, et al: Flow cytometry crossmatching in human cadaver kidney transplantation. Transplant Proc 19:764–766, 1987.
84. Chapman JR, Taylor CJ, Ting A, Morris PJ: The positive crossmatch: Antibody class and specificity correlate with graft outcome. Transplant Proc 19:725–726, 1987.
85. Thistlethwaite JR Jr, Buckingham M, Stuart JK, et al: T cell immunofluorescence flow cytometry cross-match results in cadaver donor renal transplantation. Transplant Proc 19:722–724, 1987.
86. Ting A: The lymphocytotoxic crossmatch test in clinical transplantation. Transplantation 35:403–407, 1983.
87. Ahern AT, Artruc SB, Della Pelle P, et al: Hyperacute rejection of HLA-AB identical renal allografts associated with B lymphocyte and endothelial reactive antibodies. Transplantation 33:103–106, 1982.
88. Braun WE: Donor-specific antibodies. Clinical relevance of antibodies detected in lymphocyte crossmatches. Clin Lab Med 11:571–602, 1991.
89. Taylor CJ, Chapman JR, Ting A, Morris PJ: Characterization of lymphocytotoxic antibodies causing a positive crossmatch in renal transplantation. Relationship to primary and regraft outcome. Transplantation 48:953–958, 1989.
90. Lobo PI, Westervelt FB, Rudolf LE: Kidney transplantability across a positive crossmatch: Crossmatch assays and distribution of B lymphocytes in donor tissues. Lancet 1:925–928, 1977.
91. Ettenger RB, Uittenbogaart CH, Pennisi AJ, et al: Long-term cadaver allograft survival in the recipient with a positive B-lymphocyte crossmatch. Transplantation 27:315–318, 1979.
92. D'Apice AJF, Taid BD: The positive B cell crossmatch: A marker of active enhancement. Transplant Proc 11:954–957, 1979.
93. Lazda VA: Identification of patients at risk for inferior renal allograft outcome by a strongly positive B cell flow cytometry crossmatch. Transplantation 57:964–969, 1994.
94. Buckingham JM, Geiss WP, Giacchino JL, et al: B-cell directed antibodies and delayed hyperacute rejection: A case report. J Surg Res 27:268–274, 1979.
95. Russ GR, Nicholls C, Sheldon A, Hay J: Positive B lymphocyte crossmatch and glomerular rejection in renal transplant recipients. Transplant Proc 19:785–788, 1987.
96. Lobo PI: Nature of autolymphocytotoxins present in renal hemodialysis patients: Their possible role in controlling alloantibody formation. Transplantation 32:233–237, 1981.
97. Jeannet M, Benzonana G, Arni I: Donor-specific B and T lymphocyte antibodies and kidney graft survival. Transplantation 31:160–163, 1981.
98. Ting A, Morris PJ: Successful transplantation with a positive T and B cell crossmatch due to autoreactive antibodies. Tissue Antigens 21:219–226, 1983.
99. Whiteside TL, Herberman RB: The role of natural killer cells in human disease. Clin Immunol Immunopathol 53:1–23, 1989.
100. Whiteside TL, Rinaldo CR, Herberman RB: Cytolytic cell functions. In Rose NR, de Macario EC, Fahey JL, et al (eds): Manual of Clinical Immunology. American Society for Microbiology, Washington, DC, 1992, pp 220–230.
101. Cross DE, Whittier FC, Weaver P, Foxworth J: A comparison of the antiglobulin versus extended incubation time crossmatch: Results in 223 renal transplants. Transplant Proc 9:1803–1806, 1977.
102. Johnson AH, Hallman J, Alyani MMR, et al: A prospective study of the clinical relevance of the current serum antiglobulin-augmented T cell crossmatch in renal transplant recipients. Transplant Proc 19:792–793, 1987.
103. Brynger H, Rydberg L, Samuelsson B: Experience with 14 renal transplants with kidneys from blood group A (subgroup A2) to O recipients. Transplant Proc 16:1175–1176, 1984.
104. Nelson PW, Helling TS, Pierce GE: Successful transplantation of blood group A2 kidneys into non-A recipients. Transplantation 45:316–319, 1988.
105. Middleton D, Savage DA, Cullen C, Martin J: Discrepancies in serological tissue typing revealed by DNA techniques. Transplant Int 1:161–164, 1988.
106. Opelz G, Mytilineos J, Scherer S, et al: Survival of DNA HLA-DR typed and matched cadaver kidney transplants. Lancet 338:461–463, 1991.
107. Sanfilippo F, Vaughn WK, Alexander JW, et al: Organ sharing for good HLA-A, B and DR matching improves cadaver renal graft survival in SEOPF: Retrospective and prospective studies considering delayed graft function, race, center effects, cyclosporine, and other factors. In Terasaki PI, Cecka M (eds): Clinical Transplants 1988. UCLA Tissue Typing Laboratory, Los Angeles, 1988, pp 211–223.
108. Edwards EB, Breen TJ, Guo T, et al: The UNOS OPTN (Organ Procurement and Transplantation Network) waiting list: 1988 through November 30, 1992. Clin Transpl 61–75, 1992.
109. Bay WH, Hebert LA: The living donor in kidney transplantation. Ann Intern Med 106:719–727, 1987.
110. Levey AS, Hou S, Bush HL: Kidney transplantation from unrelated living donors: Time to reclaim a discarded opportunity. N Engl J Med 314:914–916, 1986.
111. Uehling DI, Malek GH, Wear JB: Complications of donor nephrectomy. J Urol 111:745–746, 1974.
112. Brenner BM, Meyer TW, Hostetter TH: Dietary protein intake and the progressive nature of kidney disease. N Engl J Med 307:652–660, 1982.
113. Vincenti F, Amend WJJ, Kaysen G, et al: Long-term renal function in kidney donors. Sustained compensatory hyperfiltration with no adverse effects. Transplantation 35:626–629, 1983.
114. Najarian JS, Weiland D, Chavers B, et al: Studies on living related kidney donors at a single institution. Proc Eur Dial Transplant Assoc Eur Ren Assoc 21:911–919, 1985.
115. Hakim RM, Goldzer RC, Brenner BM: Hypertension and proteinuria: Long-term sequelae of uninephrectomy in humans. Kidney Int 25:930–936, 1984.
116. Anderson CF, Velosa JA, Frohnert PP, et al: The risks of unilateral nephrectomy: Status of kidney donors 10 to 20 years postoperatively. Mayo Clin Proc 60:367–374, 1985.
117. Talseth T, Faucald P, Skrede S, et al: Long term blood pressure and renal function in kidney donors. Kidney Int 29:1072–1076, 1986.
118. Miller IJ, Suthanthiran M, Riggio RR, et al: Impact of renal dona-

tion. Long term clinical and biochemical follow-up of living donors in a single center. Am J Med 79:201–208, 1985.

119. Williams S, Oler J, Jorkasky DK: Long term renal function in kidney donors: A comparison of donors and their siblings. Ann Intern Med 105:1–8, 1986.

120. Kiprov DD, Colvin RB, McCluskey RT: Focal and segmental glomerulosclerosis and proteinuria associated with unilateral renal agenesis. Lab Invest 46:275–281, 1982.

121. Smith S, Laprad P, Grantham J: Long-term effect of uninephrectomy on serum creatinine concentration and arterial blood pressure. Am J Kidney Dis 6:143–148, 1985.

122. Alexander JW, First MR, Majeski JA, et al: The late adverse effect of splenectomy on patient survival following cadaveric renal transplantation. Transplantation 37:467–470, 1984.

123. Novick AC, Ho-Hsieh H, Steinmuller D, et al: Detrimental effect of cyclosporine on initial function of cadaver renal allografts following extended preservation. Transplantation 42:154–158, 1986.

124. Sterling WA, Turner ME, Aldrete JS, et al: Effect of ischemia, preservation method and other factors on subsequent function. Transplantation 23:98–100, 1977.

125. Halloran P, Aprile M, Farewell V: Factors influencing early renal function in cadaver kidney transplants. Transplantation 45:122–127, 1988.

126. Barber WH, Deieirhoi MH, Phillips MG, Diethelm AG: Preservation by pulsatile perfusion improves early renal allograft function. Transplant Proc 20:865–868, 1988.

127. Southard JH, Pienaar H, McAnulty JF, et al: The University of Wisconsin solution for organ preservation. In Morris PJ, Tilney NL (eds): Transplantation Reviews, Vol 3. WB Saunders, Philadelphia, 1989, pp 103–130.

128. Rawn JD, Tilney NL: The early course of a patient with a kidney transplant. In Morris PJ (ed): Kidney Transplantation: Principles and Practice, 4th ed. Grune & Stratton, London, 1994, pp 167–178.

129. Owen WF, Lew NL, Liu Y, et al: The urea reduction ratio and serum albumin concentration as predictors of mortality in patients undergoing hemodialysis. N Engl J Med 329:1001–1006, 1993.

130. Tilney NL, Strom TB, Vineyard GC, Merrill JP: Factors contributing to the declining mortality rate in renal transplantation. N Engl J Med 299:1321–1325, 1978.

131. Palmer BF, Dawidson I, Sagalowsky A, et al: Improved outcome of cadaveric renal transplantation due to calcium channel blockers. Transplantation 52:640–645, 1991.

132. Murray JE, Harrison JH: Surgical management of fifty patients with kidney transplants including eighteen pairs of twins. Am J Surg 105:205–218, 1963.

133. Tilney NL: Renal transplantation. Curr Probl Surg 26:607–669, 1989.

134. Cosimi AB: The donor and donor nephrectomy. In Morris PJ (ed): Kidney Transplantation: Principles and Practice. WB Saunders, Philadelphia, 1988, pp 93–121.

135. Pick JW, Anson BJ: The renal vascular pedicle: An anatomical study of 430 body halves. J Urol 44:411–434, 1940.

136. Starzl TE, Porter KA, Andres G, et al: Long-term survival after renal transplantation in humans (with special reference to histocompatibility matching, thymectomy, homograft glomerulonephritis, heterologous ALG, and recipient malignancy). Ann Surg 172:437–472, 1970.

137. Loughlin KR, Tilney NL: Urologic complications in 718 renal transplant patients. Surgery 95:297–302, 1984.

138. Kirkman RL, Strom TB, Weir MR, Tilney NL: Late mortality and morbidity in recipients of long-term renal allografts. Transplantation 34:347–351, 1982.

139. Lillemore KD, Romolo JL, Hamilton SR, et al: Intestinal necrosis due to sodium polystyrene (Kayexalate) in sorbitol enemas: Clinical and experimental support for the hypothesis. Surgery 101:267–272, 1987.

140. Rosenthal JT: The transplant operation and its surgical complications. In Danovitch GM (ed): Handbook of Kidney Transplantation. Little, Brown, Boston, 1992, pp 135–150.

141. Belzer FO, Glass N, Sollinger H: Technical complications after renal transplantation. In Morris PJ (ed): Kidney Transplantation. Grune & Stratton, London, 1984, pp 407–426.

142. Williams G, Birtch AG, Wilson RE, et al: Urological complications of renal transplantation. Br J Urol 42:21–28, 1970.

143. Merkel FK, Straus AK, Andersen O, Bannett AD: Microvascular techniques for polar artery reconstruction in kidney transplants. Surgery 79:253–261, 1976.

144. Kyriakides GK, Simmons RL, Najarian JS: Wound infections in renal transplant wounds: Pathogenetic and prognostic factors. Ann Surg 182:770–775, 1975.

145. O'Regan S, Garel L, Robitaille P, Yazbeck S: Post-rejection ureteral obstruction owing to ureteral adherence to graft inferior pole. J Urol 139:560–561, 1988.

146. LaMasters D, Katzberg RW, Confer DJ, Slayman ML: Ureteropelvic fibrosis in renal transplants: Radiographic manifestations. AJR 135:79–82, 1980.

147. Kashi SH, Lodge JP, Giles GR, Irving HC: Ultrasonography of renal allografts: Collecting system dilation and its clinical significance. Nephrol Dial Transplant 6:358–362, 1991.

148. Smith TP, Hunter DW, Letourneau JG, et al: Urinary obstruction in renal transplants: Diagnosis by antegrade pyelography and results of percutaneous treatment. AJR 151:507–510, 1988.

149. Mathew TH, Kincaid-Smith P, Vikraman P: Risks of vesicoureteric reflux in the transplanted kidney. N Engl J Med 297:414–418, 1977.

150. Schweizer RT, Bartus SA, Graydon RJ, Berlin BB: Pyelolithotomy of a renal transplant. J Urol 117:665–666, 1977.

151. Ehrlichman RJ, Bettman M, Kirkman RL, Tilney NL: The use of percutaneous nephrostomy in patients with ureteric obstruction undergoing renal transplantation. Surg Gynecol Obstet 162:121–125, 1986.

152. Kahan BD: Cyclosporine. N Engl J Med 321:1725–1738, 1989.

153. Abramowicz D, Pradier O, Marchant A, et al: Induction of thromboses within renal grafts by high-dose prophylactic OKT3. Lancet 339:777–778, 1992.

154. Cohen DJ, Loertscher R, Rubin MF, et al: Cyclosporine: A new immunosuppressive agent for organ transplantation. Ann Intern Med 101:667–682, 1984.

155. Schlanger RE, Henry ML, Sommer BG, Ferguson RM: Identification and treatment of cyclosporine-associated allograft thrombosis. Surgery 100:329–333, 1986.

156. Schwieger J, Reiss R, Cohen JL, et al: Acute renal allograft dysfunction in the setting of deep venous thrombosis: A case of successful urokinase thrombolysis and a review of the literature. Am J Kidney Dis 22:345–350, 1993.

157. Arnadottir M, Bergentz SE, Bergqvist D, et al: Thromboembolic complications after renal transplantation: A retrospective analysis. World J Surg 7:757–761, 1983.

158. Rijksen JF, Koolen MI, Walaszewski JE, et al: Vascular complications in 400 consecutive renal allotransplants. J Cardiovasc Surg 23:91–98, 1982.

159. Ricotta JJ, Schaff HV, Williams GM, et al: Renal artery stenosis following transplantation: Etiology, diagnosis, and prevention. Surgery 84:595–602, 1978.

160. Oakes DD, Spees EK, McAllister HA, Saddler W: Arterial injury during perfusion preservation: A possible cause of posttransplantation renal artery stenosis. Surgery 89:210–215, 1981.

161. Johnson CP, Simmons RL, Sutherland DE, et al: A randomized trial comparing cyclosporine with antilymphoblast-globulin–azathioprine for renal allograft recipients. Results at 2½–6 years. Transplantation 45:380–385, 1988.

162. Matas AJ, Tellis VA, Quinn TA, et al: Individualization of immediate posttransplant immunosuppression. The value of antilymphocyte globulin in patients with delayed graft function. Transplantation 45:406–409, 1988.

163. Michael HJ, Francos GC, Burke JF, et al: A comparison of the effects of cyclosporine versus antilymphocyte globulin on delayed graft function in cadaver renal transplant recipients. Transplantation 48:805–808, 1989.

164. Sommer BG, Henry M, Ferguson RM: Sequential antilymphoblast globulin and cyclosporine for renal transplantation. Transplantation 43:85–90, 1987.

165. Stratta RJ, D'Allesandro AM, Armbrust MJ, et al: Sequential antilymphocyte globulin/cyclosporine immunosuppression in cadaveric renal transplantation. Effect of duration of ALG therapy. Transplantation 47:96–102, 1989.

166. Norman DJ, Kahana L, Stuart FPJ, et al: A randomized clinical trial of induction therapy with OKT3 in kidney transplantation. Transplantation 55:44–50, 1993.

167. Light JA, Khawand N, Aquino A, et al: Quadruple immunosuppression: Comparison of OKT3 and Minnesota antilymphocyte globulin. Am J Kidney Dis 14:10–13, 1989.

168. Steinmuller DR, Hayes JM, Novick AC, et al: Comparison of OKT3

with ALG for prophylaxis for patients with acute renal failure after cadaveric renal transplantation. Transplantation 52:67–71, 1991.

169. Cole EH, Cattran DC, Farewell VT, et al: A comparison of rabbit antithymocyte serum and OKT3 as prophylaxis against renal allograft rejection. Transplantation 57:60–67, 1994.

170. Schroeder TJ, First MR, Mansour ME, et al: Prophylactic use of OKT3 in immunologic high-risk cadaver renal transplant recipients. Am J Kidney Dis 14:14–18, 1989.

171. The Canadian Multicenter Transplant Group: A randomized clinical trial of cyclosporine in cadaveric renal transplantation: Analysis at three years. N Engl J Med 314:1219–1225, 1986.

172. Ponticelli C, Minnetti L, Di Palo FQ, et al: The Milan clinical trial with cyclosporine in cadaveric renal transplantation: A three year follow-up. Transplantation 45:908–913, 1988.

173. Bennett WM, Norman DJ: Maintenance immunosuppression: Azathioprine and glucocorticoids. In Milford EL (ed): Renal Transplantation: Contemporary Issues in Nephrology, Vol 19. Churchill Livingstone, New York, 1989, p 97.

174. Hricik DE, Almawi WY, Strom TB: Trends in the use of glucocorticoids in renal transplantation. Transplantation 57:979–989, 1994.

175. Hricik DE, Whalen CC, Lautman J, et al: Withdrawal of steroids after renal transplantation—clinical predictors of outcome. Transplantation 53:41–45, 1992.

176. Hricik DE, Schulak JA: Metabolic effects of steroid withdrawal in adult renal transplant recipients. Kidney Int Suppl 43:S26–S29, 1993.

177. Hariharan S, Schroeder TJ, Weiskittel P, et al: Prednisone withdrawal in HLA identical and one haplotype–matched live-related donor and cadaver renal transplant recipients. Kidney Int Suppl 43:S30–S35, 1993.

178. Paul LC: Maintenance immunosuppression: Cyclosporine. In Milford EL (ed): Renal Transplantation: Contemporary Issues in Nephrology, Vol 19. Churchill Livingstone, New York, 1989, pp 105–128.

179. Sanders CE, Curtis JJ, Julian BA, et al: Tapering or discontinuing cyclosporine for financial reasons—a single-center experience. Am J Kidney Dis 21:9–15, 1993.

180. Delmonico FL, Conti D, Auchincloss HJ, et al: Long-term, low-dose cyclosporine treatment of renal allograft recipients. A randomized trial. Transplantation 49:899–904, 1990.

181. Lewis RM, Janney RP, Golden DL, et al: Stability of renal allograft function associated with long-term cyclosporine immunosuppressive therapy—five year follow-up. Transplantation 47:266–272, 1989.

182. Lewis R, Podbielski J, Sprayberry S, et al: Stability of renal allograft glomerular filtration rate associated with long-term use of cyclosporine A. Transplantation 55:1014–1017, 1993.

183. Helderman JH: Long-term medical management of the renal transplant recipient: A consensus. J Am Soc Nephrol 4:s1–s2, 1994.

184. First MR, Schroeder TJ, Alexander JW, et al: Cyclosporine dose reduction by ketoconazole administration in renal transplant recipients. Transplantation 51:365–370, 1991.

185. First MR, Schroeder TJ, Michael A, et al: Cyclosporine-ketoconazole interaction. Long-term follow-up and preliminary results of a randomized trial. Transplantation 55:1000–1004, 1993.

186. Chrysostomou A, Walker RG, Russ GR, et al: Diltiazem in renal allograft recipients receiving cyclosporine. Transplantation 55:300–304, 1993.

187. Ruggenenti P, Perico N, Mosconi L, et al: Calcium channel blockers protect transplant patients from cyclosporine-induced daily renal hypoperfusion. Kidney Int 43:706–711, 1993.

188. Kuzendorf U, Walz G, Brockmoeller J, et al: Effects of diltiazem upon metabolism and immunosuppressive action of cyclosporine in kidney graft recipients. Transplantation 52:280–284, 1991.

189. van der Heide JJ, Bilo HJ, Donker JM, et al: Effect of dietary fish oil on renal function and rejection in cyclosporine-treated recipients of renal transplants. N Engl J Med 329:769–773, 1993.

190. Gray D, Shepherd H, Daar A, et al: Oral versus intravenous high-dose steroid treatment of renal allograft rejection. The big shot or not? Lancet 1:117–118, 1978.

191. Vineyard GC, Fadem SZ, Dmochowski J, et al: Evaluation of corticosteroid therapy for acute renal allograft rejection. Surg Gynecol Obstet 138:225–229, 1974.

192. Delmonico FL, Tolkoff-Rubin N: Treatment of acute rejection. In Milford EL (ed): Renal Transplantation: Contemporary Issues in Nephrology, Vol 19. Churchill Livingstone, New York, 1989, pp 129–146.

193. Sutherland DE, Fryd DS, Strand MH, et al: Results of the Minnesota randomized prospective trial of cyclosporine versus azathioprine–antilymphocyte globulin for immunosuppression in renal allograft recipients. Am J Kidney Dis 5:318–327, 1985.

194. Streem SB, Novick AC, Braun WE, et al: Low-dose maintenance prednisone and antilymphoblast globulin for the treatment of acute rejection. A steroid-sparing approach to immunosuppressive therapy. Transplantation 35:420–424, 1983.

195. Goldstein G, Fuccello AJ, Norman DJ, et al: OKT3 monoclonal antibody plasma levels during therapy and the subsequent development of host antibodies to OKT3. Transplantation 42:507–511, 1986.

196. Ortho Multicenter Transplant Study Group: A randomized trial of OKT3 monoclonal antibody for acute rejection of cadaveric renal transplants. N Engl J Med 313:337–342, 1985.

197. Norman DJ, Barry JM, Bennett WM, et al: The use of OKT3 in cadaveric renal transplantation for rejection that is unresponsive to conventional anti-rejection therapy. Am J Kidney Dis 11:90–93, 1988.

198. Hricik DE, Zarconi J, Schulak JA: Influence of low-dose cyclosporine on the outcome of treatment with OKT3 for acute renal allograft rejection. Transplantation 47:272–277, 1989.

199. Schroeder TJ, Weiss MA, Smith RD, et al: The efficacy of OKT3 in vascular rejection. Transplantation 51:312–315, 1991.

200. Oh CS, Stratta RJ, Fox BC, et al: Increased infections associated with the use of OKT3 for treatment of steroid-resistant rejection in renal transplantation. Transplantation 45:68–73, 1988.

201. Thistlethwaite JRJ, Stuart JK, Mayes JT, et al: Complications and monitoring of OKT3 therapy. Am J Kidney Dis 11:112–119, 1988.

202. Swinnen LJ, Costanza-Nordin MR, Fisher SG, et al: Increased incidence of lymphoproliferative disorders after immunosuppression with monoclonal antibody OKT3 in cardiac transplant recipients. N Engl J Med 323:1723–1728, 1990.

203. Abramowicz D, Schandene L, Goldman M, et al: Release of tumor necrosis factor, interleukin-2, and gamma-interferon in serum after injection of OKT3 monoclonal antibody in kidney transplant recipients. Transplantation 47:606–608, 1989.

204. Raasveld MH, Bemelman FJ, Schellekens PT, et al: Complement activation during OKT3 treatment: A possible explanation for respiratory side effects. Kidney Int 43:1140–1149, 1993.

205. Pradier O, Marchant A, Abramowicz D, et al: Procoagulant effect of OKT3 monoclonal antibody: Involvement of tumor necrosis factor. Kidney Int 42:1124–1129, 1992.

206. Norman DJ, Sheild CF 3, Hennell KR, et al: Effectiveness of a second course of OKT3 monoclonal anti–T cell antibody for treatment of renal allograft rejection. Transplantation 46:523–529, 1988.

207. Kopp JB, Klotman PE: Cellular and molecular mechanisms of cyclosporin nephrotoxicity. J Am Soc Nephrol 1:162–179, 1990.

208. Lanese DM, Conger JD: Effects of endothelin receptor antagonist on cyclosporine-induced vasoconstriction in isolated rat renal arterioles. J Clin Invest 91:2144–2149, 1993.

209. De Nicola L, Thomson SC, Wead LM, et al: Arginine feeding modifies cyclosporine nephrotoxicity in rats. J Clin Invest 92:1859–1865, 1993.

210. Perico N, Remuzzi G: Role of endothelin in glomerular injury. Kidney Int Suppl 39:S76–S80, 1993.

211. Scherrer U, Vissing SF, Morgan BJ, et al: Cyclosporine-induced sympathetic activation and hypertension after heart transplantation. N Engl J Med 323:693–699, 1990.

212. Van Buren D, Van Buren CT, Flechner SM, et al: De novo hemolytic uremic syndrome in renal transplant recipients immunosuppressed with cyclosporine. Surgery 98:54–62, 1985.

213. Sommer BG, Innes JT, Whitehurst RM, et al: Cyclosporine-associated renal arteriopathy resulting in loss of allograft function. Am J Surg 149:756–764, 1985.

214. Walfe JA, McCann RL, Sanfilippo F: Cyclosporine-associated microangiopathy in renal transplantation: A severe but potentially reversible form of early graft injury. Transplantation 41:541–544, 1986.

215. Braun WE: The immunobiology of different types of renal allograft rejection. In Milford EL (ed): Renal Transplantation, Vol 19. Churchill Livingstone, New York, 1989, pp 45–96.

216. Cecka JM, Terasaki PI: Early rejection episodes. Clin Transplant 425–434, 1989.

217. Almond PS, Matas A, Gillingham K, et al: Risk factors for chronic rejection in renal allograft recipients. Transplantation 55:752–756, 1993.

218. Basadonna GP, Matas AJ, Gillingham KJ, et al: Early versus late acute renal allograft rejection: Impact on chronic rejection. Transplantation 55:993–995, 1993.

219. Lindholm A, Ohlman S, Albrechtsen D, et al: The impact of acute rejection episodes on long-term graft function and outcome in 1347 primary renal transplants treated by 3 cyclosporine regimens. Transplantation 56:307–315, 1993.

220. Meyer M, Paushter D, Steinmuller DR: The use of duplex Doppler ultrasonography to evaluate renal allograft dysfunction. Transplantation 50:974–978, 1990.

221. Yoshimura N, Oka T, Kahan BD: Sequential determinations of serum interleukin 6 levels as an immunodiagnostic tool to differentiate rejection from nephrotoxicity in renal allograft recipients. Transplantation 51:172–176, 1991.

222. Simpson MA, Madras PN, Cornaby AJ, et al: Sequential determinations of urinary cytology and plasma and urinary lymphokines in the management of renal allograft recipients. Transplantation 47:218–223, 1989.

223. Forsythe JL, Shenton BK, Parrot NR, et al: Plasma interleukin 2 receptor levels in renal allograft dysfunction. Transplantation 48:155–157, 1989.

224. Dunn J, Golden D, Van Buren CT, et al: Causes of graft loss beyond two years in the cyclosporine era. Transplantation 49:349–353, 1990.

225. Kasiske BL, Heim-Duthoy K, Ma JZ: Elective cyclosporine withdrawal after renal transplantation. A meta-analysis. JAMA 269:395–400, 1993.

226. Ramos EL: Recurrent diseases in the renal transplant. J Am Soc Nephrol 2:109–121, 1991.

227. Evans RW: The demand for transplantation in the United States. *In* Terasaki PI (ed): Clinical Transplants 1990. UCLA Tissue Typing Laboratory, Los Angeles, 1991, pp 319–327.

228. United Network for Organ Sharing: Annual Data Report. UNOS, Richmond, VA, 1989.

229. Mickey R, Cho YW, Carnahan E: Long term graft survival. *In* Terasaki PI (ed): Clinical Transplants 1990. UCLA Tissue Typing Laboratory, Los Angeles, 1991, pp 385–396.

230. Paul LC, Fellstrom B: Chronic vascular rejection of the heart and kidney—have rational treatment options emerged? Transplantation 53:1169–1179, 1992.

231. Tilney NL, Whitley WD, Diamond JR, et al: Chronic rejection—an undefined conundrum. Transplantation 52:389–398, 1991.

232. Bhathena DB: Glomerular size and the association of focal glomerulosclerosis in long-surviving human renal allografts. J Am Soc Nephrol 4:1316–1326, 1993.

233. Brenner BM, Cohen RA, Milford EL: In renal transplantation, one size may not fit all. J Am Soc Nephrol 3:162–169, 1992.

234. Traindl O, Falger S, Reading S, et al: The effects of lisinopril on renal function in proteinuric renal transplant recipients. Transplantation 55:1309–1313, 1993.

235. Myers BD, Newton L: Cyclosporine-induced chronic nephropathy: An obliterative microvascular renal injury. J Am Soc Nephrol 2:S45–S52, 1991.

236. Bertani T, Ferrazzi P, Schieppati A, et al: Nature and extent of glomerular injury induced by cyclosporine in heart transplant patients. Kidney Int 40:243–250, 1991.

237. Tegzess AM, Doorenbos BM, Minderhoud JM, Donker AJ: Prospective serial renal function studies in patients with nonrenal disease treated with cyclosporine A. Transplant Proc 20:530–533, 1988.

238. Feutren G, Mihatsch MJ: Risk factors for cyclosporine-induced nephropathy in patients with autoimmune diseases. International Kidney Biopsy Registry of Cyclosporine in Autoimmune Diseases. N Engl J Med 326:1654–1660, 1992.

239. Deray G, Benhmida M, LeHoang P, et al: Renal function and blood pressure in patients receiving long-term, low-dose cyclosporine therapy for idiopathic autoimmune uveitis. Ann Intern Med 117:578–583, 1992.

240. Bantle JP, Nath KA, Sutherland DE, et al: Effects of cyclosporine on the renin-angiotensin-aldosterone system and potassium excretion in renal transplant recipients. Arch Intern Med 145:505–508, 1985.

241. Pei Y, Richardson R, Greenwood C, et al: Extrarenal effect of cyclosporine A on potassium homeostasis in renal transplant recipients. Am J Kidney Dis 22:314–319, 1993.

242. Kamel KS, Ethier JH, Quaggin S, et al: Studies to determine the basis for hyperkalemia in recipients of a renal transplant who are treated with cyclosporine. J Am Soc Nephrol 2:1279–1284, 1992.

243. Croker BP, Salomon DR: Pathology of the renal allograft. *In* Tisher CC, Brenner BM (eds): Renal Pathology with Clinical and Functional Correlations. JB Lippincott, Philadelphia, 1989, pp 1518–1554.

244. Matas AJ, Sibley R, Mauer M, et al: The value of needle renal allograft biopsy. I. A retrospective study of biopsies performed during putative rejection episodes. Ann Surg 197:226–237, 1983.

245. Fennell RS 3, Donnelly WH, Purcell CA, et al: The use of kidney biopsy to predict allograft loss in a pediatric transplant population. Int J Pediatr Nephrol 7:21–26, 1986.

246. Matas AJ, Tellis VA, Sablay L, et al: The value of needle renal allograft biopsy. III. A prospective study. Surgery 98:922–926, 1985.

247. Huraib S, Goldberg H, Katz A, et al: Percutaneous needle biopsy of the transplanted kidney: Technique and complications. Am J Kidney Dis 14:13–17, 1989.

248. Finkelstein FO, Siegel NJ, Bastl C, et al: Kidney transplant biopsies in the management of acute rejection reactions. Kidney Int 10:171–178, 1976.

249. Banfi G, Imbasciati E, Tarantino A, Ponticelli C: Prognostic value of renal biopsy in acute rejection of kidney transplant. Nephron 28:222–226, 1981.

250. Vangelista A, Frasca GM, Stefoni S, Bonomini V: Graft biopsy in renal transplantation: Correlation with clinical, immunological, and virological investigations. Kidney Int 23S:41–45, 1983.

251. Parfrey PS, Kuo YL, Hanley JA, et al: The diagnostic and prognostic value of renal allograft biopsy. Transplantation 38:586–590, 1984.

252. Pardo-Mindan FJ, Guillen R, Virto R, et al: Kidney allograft biopsy: A valuable tool in assessing the diagnosis of acute rejection. Clin Nephrol 24:37–41, 1985.

253. Appel GB, Saltzman MJ, King DL, Hardy MA: Use of ultrasound for renal allograft biopsy. Kidney Int 19:471–473, 1981.

254. Kalash SS, Muakkassa WF, Campbell EWJ, et al: Persistent clot anuria complicating renal transplant biopsy. Urology 25:591–595, 1985.

255. Mathew TH, Kincaid-Smith P, Eremin J, Marshall VC: Percutaneous needle biopsy of renal homografts. Med J Aust 1:6–7, 1968.

256. Pillay VKG, Kurtzman NA: Percutaneous biopsy of the transplanted kidney. JAMA 226:1561–1562, 1973.

257. Buselmeier TJ, Schauer RM, Mauer SM, et al: A simplified method of percutaneous allograft biopsy. Nephron 16:318–321, 1976.

258. Murphy GP: Percutaneous needle biopsy of human renal allotransplants. J Urol 107:193–195, 1972.

259. Parker RA, Elliott WC, Muther RS, et al: Percutaneous aspiration biopsy of renal allografts using ultrasound localization. Urology 15:534–535, 1980.

260. Eckhauser ML, Haaga JR, Hampel N, et al: Arterial embolization of renal allograft to control hemorrhage secondary to percutaneous nephropyelostomy. J Urol 126:679–680, 1981.

261. O'Brien DP 3, Parrott TS, Walton KN, Lewis EL: Renal arteriovenous fistulas. Surg Gynecol Obstet 139:739–743, 1974.

262. Hayry P, von Willebrand E: Practical guidelines for fine needle aspiration biopsy of human renal allografts. Ann Clin Res 13:288–306, 1981.

263. von Willebrand E: Fine-needle aspiration cytology of human renal transplants. Clin Immunol Immunopathol 17:309–322, 1980.

264. Hughes DA: Fine-needle cytology in the monitoring of human renal allograft progress. Immunol Lett 29:147–151, 1991.

265. Helderman JH, Hernandez J, Sagalowsky A, et al: Confirmation of the utility of fine needle aspiration biopsy of the renal allograft. Kidney Int 34:376–381, 1988.

266. Hughes DA, McWhinnie DL, Sutton R, et al: Can incremental scoring of fine-needle aspirates predict histopathologic renal allograft rejection? Transplant Proc 20:690–691, 1988.

267. Surachno S, van Oers MH, Wilmink JM: Early diagnosis of bacterial infection of renal allografts by fine needle aspiration biopsy. Lancet 1:686–687, 1986. Letter.

268. Palmer BF, Hernandez J, Sagalowsky A, et al: Documentation of fungal pyelonephritis of the renal allograft by fine needle aspiration cytology. Transplant Proc 21:3598–3599, 1989.

269. Genkins SM, Sanfilippo F, Carroll BA: Duplex Doppler sonography of renal transplants: Lack of sensitivity and specificity in establishing pathologic diagnosis. AJR 152:535–539, 1989.

270. Evans C, Cochlin DL, Ferguson C, et al: Duplex Doppler studies in acute renal transplant rejection. Transplant Proc 21:1897–1898, 1989.

271. Segosothy M, Birch DF, Fairley F, Kincaid-Smith P: Urine cytologic

profile in renal allograft recipients determined by monoclonal antibodies. Diagnosis of allograft rejection. Transplantation 47:482–487, 1989.

272. Patel R, Terasaki PI: Significance of the positive crossmatch test in kidney transplantation. N Engl J Med 280:735–739, 1969.

273. Baldwin WM, Soulillou JP, Claas FH, et al: Antibodies to endothelial antigens in eluates of 88 human kidneys: Correlation with graft survival and presence of T and B cell antibodies. Transplant Proc 13:1547–1550, 1981.

274. Szulman AE: The histological distribution of the blood group substances in man as disclosed by immunofluorescence. Hum Pathol 2:575–585, 1971.

275. Dunea G, Kolff WJ: Renal homotransplantation. A discussion of uncertainties. Ohio State Med J 61:979–981, 1965.

276. Nelson PW, Helling TS, Shield CF, et al: Current experience with renal transplantation across the ABO barrier. Am J Surg 164:541–544, 1992.

277. Boudreaux JP, Hayes DH, Mizrahi S, et al: Successful liver/kidney transplantation across ABO incompatibility. Transplant Proc 25:1874, 1993.

278. Kawaguchi H, Hattori M, Ito K, et al: A successful ABO blood type incompatible kidney transplantation in a child. Transplant Int 4:63–64, 1991.

279. Scornik JC, Ireland JE, Salomon DR, et al: Pretransplant blood transfusions in patients with previous pregnancies. Transplantation 43:449–451, 1987.

280. Opelz G, Graver B, Mickey MR, Terasaki PI: Lymphocytotoxic antibody responses to transfusions in potential kidney transplant recipients. Transplantation 32:177–185, 1981.

281. Striker LJ, Olson JL, Striker GE: Renal transplantation. In Striker LJ, Olson JL, Striker GE (eds): The Renal Biopsy. WB Saunders, Philadelphia, 1990, pp 229–240.

282. Porter KA: Renal transplantation. In Heptinstall RH (ed): Pathology of the Kidney. Little, Brown, Boston, 1992, pp 1799–1933.

283. Starzl TE, Boehmig HJ, Amemiya H, et al: Clotting changes, including disseminated intravascular coagulation, during rapid renal-homograft rejection. N Engl J Med 283:383–390, 1970.

284. Lindquist RR, Guttmann RD, Merrill JP, Damin GJ: Human renal allografts. Interpretation of morphologic and immunohistochemical observations. Am J Pathol 53:851–881, 1968.

285. Nabarra B, Descamps B: Ultrastructure of cells infiltrating human kidney allografts. Clin Exp Immunol 24:300–309, 1976.

286. Sanfilippo F: Renal transplantation. In Sale GE (ed): The Pathology of Organ Transplantation. Butterworth, Boston, 1990, pp 51–101.

287. Myers BD: Cyclosporine nephrotoxicity. Kidney Int 30:964–974, 1986.

288. Keown PA, Stiller CR, Wallace AC: Nephrotoxicity of cyclosporine A. In Williams GM, Burdick JF, Solez K (eds): Kidney Transplant Rejection: Diagnosis and Treatment. Marcel Dekker, New York, 1986, pp 423–457.

289. Sibley RK, Rynasiewicz J, Ferguson RM, et al: Morphology of cyclosporine nephrotoxicity and acute rejection in patients immunosuppressed with cyclosporine and prednisone. Surgery 94:225–234, 1983.

290. Farnsworth A, Hall BM, Ng AB, et al: Renal biopsy morphology in renal transplantation. A comparative study of the light-microscopic appearances of biopsies from patients treated with cyclosporin A or azathioprine, prednisone and antilymphocyte globulin. Am J Surg Pathol 8:243–252, 1984.

291. Mihatsch MJ: A brief review of histopathology in kidney transplant recipients immunosuppressed with cyclosporin A. Scand J Urol Nephrol Suppl 92:95–97, 1985.

292. Mihatsch MJ, Thiel G, Ryffel B: Histopathology of cyclosporine nephrotoxicity. Transplant Proc 20:759–771, 1988.

293. Mihatsch MJ, Olivieri W, Marbet U, et al: Giant mitochondria in renal tubular cells and cyclosporin A. Lancet 1:1162–1163, 1981. Letter.

294. Wolfe JA, McCann RL, Sanfilippo F: Cyclosporine-associated microangiopathy in renal transplantation: A severe but potentially reversible form of early graft injury. Transplantation 41:541–544, 1986.

295. Kolbeck PC, Scheinman JI, Sanfilippo F: Acute cellular rejection and cyclosporine nephrotoxicity monitored by biopsy in a renal allograft recipient: The differentiation of drug nephrotoxicity from phenotyping of cellular infiltrates. Arch Pathol Lab Med 110:389–393, 1986.

296. Platt JL, Ferguson RM, Sibley RK, et al: Renal interstitial cell populations in cyclosporine nephrotoxicity. Identification using monoclonal antibodies. Transplantation 36:343–346, 1983.

297. Ruiz P, Kolbeck PC, Scroggs MW, Sanfilippo F: Associations between cyclosporine therapy and interstitial fibrosis in renal allograft biopsies. Transplantation 45:91–95, 1988.

298. Matthew TH, Mathews DC, Hobbs JB, Kincaid-Smith P: Glomerular lesions after renal transplantation. Am J Med 59:177–190, 1975.

299. O'Meara Y, Green A, Carmody M, et al: Recurrent glomerulonephritis in renal transplants: Fourteen years' experience. Nephrol Dial Transplant 4:730–734, 1989.

300. Bohman SO, Wilczek H, Tyden G, et al: Recurrent diabetic nephropathy in renal allografts placed in diabetic patients and protective effect of simultaneous pancreatic transplantation. Transplant Proc 19:2290–2293, 1987.

301. Bohman SO, Wilczek H, Tyden G, et al: Recurrent diabetic nephropathy in renal allografts placed in diabetic patients and protective effect of simultaneous pancreatic transplantation. Transplant Proc 19:2290–2293, 1987.

302. Najarian JS, Sutherland DE, Simmons RL, et al: Ten year experience with renal transplantation in juvenile onset diabetics. Ann Surg 190:487–500, 1979.

303. Maryniak RK, Mendoza N, Clyne D, et al: Recurrence of diabetic nodular glomerulosclerosis in a renal transplant. Transplantation 39:35–38, 1985.

304. Mauer SM, Barbosa J, Vernier RC, et al: Development of diabetic vascular lesions in normal kidneys transplanted into patients with diabetes mellitus. N Engl J Med 295:916–920, 1976.

305. Braun WE: Long-term complications of renal transplantation (clinical conference). Kidney Int 37:1363–1378, 1990.

306. Cheigh JS, Mouradian J, Susin M, et al: Kidney transplant nephrotic syndrome: Relationship between allograft histopathology and natural course. Kidney Int 18:358–365, 1980.

307. Morzycka M, Croker BP, Seigler HF, Tisher CC: Evaluation of recurrent glomerulonephritis in kidney allografts. Am J Med 72:588–598, 1982.

308. Habib R, Antignac C, Hinglais N, et al: Glomerular lesions in the transplanted kidney in children. Am J Kidney Dis 10:198–207, 1987.

309. Honkanen E, Tornroth T, Pettersson E, Kulhback B: Glomerulonephritis in renal allografts: Results of 18 years of transplantations. Clin Nephrol 21:210–219, 1984.

310. Cheigh JS, Mouradian J, Soliman M, et al: Focal segmental glomerulosclerosis in renal transplants. Am J Kidney Dis 2:449–455, 1983.

311. Pinto J, Lacerda G, Cameron JS, et al: Recurrence of focal segmental glomerulosclerosis in renal allografts. Transplantation 32:83–89, 1981.

312. Vincenti F, Biava C, Tomlanovitch S, et al: Inability of cyclosporine to completely prevent the recurrence of focal glomerulosclerosis after kidney transplantation. Transplantation 47:595–598, 1989.

313. Maizel SE, Sibley RK, Horstman JP, et al: Incidence and significance of recurrent focal segmental glomerulosclerosis in renal allograft recipients. Transplantation 32:512–516, 1981.

314. Leumann EP, Briner J, Donckerwolcke RAM, et al: Recurrence of focal segmental glomerulosclerosis in the transplanted kidney. Nephron 25:65–71, 1980.

315. Cameron JS, Senguttuvan P, Hartley B, et al: Focal segmental glomerulosclerosis in fifty-nine renal allografts from a single centre; analysis of risk factors for recurrence. Transplant Proc 21:2117–2118, 1989.

316. Cameron JS: Glomerulonephritis in renal transplants. Transplantation 34:237–245, 1982.

317. Striegel JE, Sibley RK, Fryd DS, Mauer M: Recurrence of focal segmental sclerosis in children following renal transplantation. Kidney Int 1986:s44–s50, 1986.

318. Lewis EJ: Recurrent focal sclerosis after renal transplantation. Kidney Int 22:315–323, 1982.

319. Chandra M, Lewy JE, Mouradian J, et al: Recurrent nephrotic syndrome with three successive renal allografts. Am J Nephrol 1:110–114, 1981.

320. Malekzadeh MH, Heuser ET, Ettenger RB, et al: Focal glomerulosclerosis and renal transplantation. J Pediatr 95:249–254, 1979.

321. Morales JM, Andres A, Prieto C, et al: Clinical and histological sequence of recurrent focal segmental glomerulosclerosis. Nephron 48:241–242, 1988. Letter.

322. Laufer J, Ettenger RB, Ho WG, et al: Plasma exchange for recurrent nephrotic syndrome following renal transplantation. Transplantation 46:540–542, 1988.

323. Munoz J, Sanchez M, Perez-Garcia R, et al: Recurrent focal glomerulosclerosis in renal transplants. Proteinuria relapsing following plasma exchange. Clin Nephrol 24:213–214, 1985.
324. Torres VE, Velosa JA, Holley KE, et al: Meclofenamate treatment of recurrent idiopathic nephrotic syndrome with focal segmental glomerulosclerosis after renal transplantation. Mayo Clin Proc 59:146–152, 1984.
325. Voets AJ, Hoitsma AJ, Koene RAP: Recurrence of nephrotic syndrome during cyclosporin treatment after renal transplantation. Lancet 1:266–267, 1986.
326. Tomlanovich S, Vincenti F, Amend W, et al: Is cyclosporine effective in preventing recurrence of immune-mediated glomerular disease after renal transplantation? Transplant Proc 20:285–288, 1988.
327. Freedman BI, Graves JW, Burkart JM, et al: The impact of different immunosuppressant regimens on recurrent glomerulonephritis. Transplant Proc 21:2121–2122, 1989.
328. Banfi G, Colturi C, Montagnino G, Ponticelli C: The recurrence of focal and segmental glomerulosclerosis in kidney transplant patients treated with cyclosporine. Transplantation 50:594–596, 1990.
329. Hosenpud J, Piering WF, Garancis JC, Kaufmann M: Successful second kidney transplantation in a patient with focal glomerulosclerosis. Am J Nephrol 5:299–304, 1985.
330. Bachman U, Biava C, Amend W, et al: The clinical course of IgA-nephropathy and Henoch-Schönlein purpura following renal transplantation. Transplantation 42:511–515, 1986.
331. Berger J, Yaneva H, Nabarra B, Barbanel C: Recurrence of mesangial deposition of IgA after renal transplantation. Kidney Int 7:232–241, 1975.
332. Brensilver JM, Mallat S, Scholes J, McCabe R: Recurrent IgA nephropathy in living-related donor transplantation: Recurrence or transmission of familial disease? Am J Kidney Dis 12:147–151, 1988.
333. Berger J: Recurrence of IgA nephropathy in renal allografts. Am J Kidney Dis 12:371–372, 1988.
334. Croker BP, Dawson DV, Sanfilippo F: IgA nephropathy: Correlation of clinical and histological features. Lab Invest 48:19–24, 1983.
335. Yussim A, Ben-Bassat M, Shapira Z, et al: Post-transplant glomerulonephritis under conventional and cyclosporin A immunosuppression. Transplant Proc 21:2119–2120, 1989.
336. Baliah T, Kim KH, Anthone S, et al: Recurrence of Henoch-Schönlein purpura glomerulonephritis in transplanted kidneys. Transplantation 18:343–346, 1974.
337. Matthew TH: Recurrence of disease following renal transplantation. Am J Kidney Dis 12:85–96, 1988.
338. Glicklich D, Matas AJ, Sablay LB, et al: Recurrent membranoproliferative glomerulonephritis type 1 in successive renal transplants. Am J Nephrol 7:143–149, 1987.
339. Curtis JJ, Wyatt RJ, Bhathena D, et al: Renal transplantation for patients with type I and type II membranoproliferative glomerulonephritis. Am J Med 66:216–225, 1979.
340. Maryniak RK, First RM, Weiss MA: Transplant glomerulopathy: Evolution of morphologically distinct changes. Kidney Int 27:799–806, 1985.
341. Droz D, Nabarra B, Noel LH, et al: Recurrence of dense deposits in transplanted kidneys: I. Sequential survey of the lesions. Kidney Int 15:386–395, 1979.
342. Mauer SM, Miller K, Goetz FC, et al: Immunopathology of renal extracellular membranes in kidneys transplanted into patients with diabetes mellitus. Diabetes 25:709–712, 1976.
343. Beleil OM, Coburn JW, Shinaberger JH, Glassock RJ: Recurrent glomerulonephritis due to anti–glomerular basement membrane antibody in two successive allografts. Clin Nephrol 1:377–380, 1973.
344. Van den Berg-Wolf MG, Kootte AMM, Weening JJ, Paul LC: Recurrent hemolytic uremic syndrome in a renal transplant recipient and review of the Lieden experience. Transplantation 45:248–251, 1988.
345. Bonsib SM, Ercolani L, Ngheim D, Hamilton HE: Recurrent thrombotic microangiopathy in a renal allograft. Am J Med 79:520–527, 1985.
346. Eijgenraam FJ, Donckerwolcke RA, Monens LAH, et al: Renal transplantation in 20 children with hemolytic-uremic syndrome. Clin Nephrol 33:87–93, 1990.
347. Hebert D, Sibley RK, Mauer SM: Recurrence of hemolytic uremic syndrome in renal transplant recipients. Kidney Int 30:S51–S58, 1986.
348. Leithner C, Sinzinger H, Pohanka E, et al: Recurrence of haemolytic uraemic syndrome triggered by cyclosporin A after renal transplantation. Lancet 1:1470, 1982. Letter.
349. Springate J, Fildes R, Anthone S, et al: Recurrent hemolytic syndrome after renal transplantation. Transplant Proc 20:559–561, 1988.
350. Kumano K, Sakai T, Mashimo S, et al: A case of recurrent lupus nephritis after renal transplantation. Clin Nephrol 27:94–98, 1987.
351. Amend WJJ, Vincenti F, Feduska NJ, et al: Recurrent systemic lupus involving renal allografts. Ann Intern Med 94:444–448, 1981.
352. Yakub YN, Freedman RB, Pabico RC: Renal transplantation in systemic lupus erythematosus. Nephron 27:197–201, 1981.
353. Sohmiya S, Morozumi K, Yoshida A: A case of recurrent lupus nephritis after renal transplantation immunosuppressed with cyclosporin A. Jpn J Transplant 21:17–24, 1986.
354. Fernandez JA, Milgrom M, Burke GW, et al: Recurrence of lupus nephritis in a renal allograft with histologic transformation of the lesion. Transplantation 50:1056–1058, 1990.
355. Berger BE, Vincenti F, Biava C, et al: De novo and recurrent membranous glomerulopathy following kidney transplantation. Transplantation 35:315–319, 1983.
356. Montagnino G, Colturi C, Banfi G: Membranous nephropathy in cyclosporine-treated renal transplant recipients. Transplantation 47:725–727, 1989.
357. Crosson JT, Wathen RL, Raij L, et al: Recurrence of idiopathic membranous nephropathy in a renal allograft. Arch Intern Med 135:1101–1106, 1975.
358. Rubin RJ, Pinn VW, Barnes BA, Harrington JT: Recurrent idiopathic membranous glomerulonephritis. Transplantation 24:4–9, 1977.
359. Obermiller LE, Hoy WE, Eversole M, Sterling WA: Recurrent membranous glomerulonephritis in two renal transplants. Transplantation 40:100–102, 1985.
360. First MR, Mendoza N, Maryniak RK, Weiss MA: Membranous glomerulopathy following kidney transplantation. Transplantation 38:603–607, 1984.
361. Lieberthal W, Bernard DB, Donahoe JF, et al: Rapid recurrence of membranous nephropathy in a related renal allograft. Clin Nephrol 12:222–228, 1979.
362. Couser WG, Steinmuller DR, Stilmant MM, et al: Experimental glomerulonephritis in the isolated perfused rat kidney. J Clin Invest 62:1275–1287, 1978.
363. Jones NF: Renal amyloidosis: Pathogenesis and therapy. Clin Nephrol 6:459–464, 1976.
364. Bensen MD, Skinner M, Cohen AS: Amyloid deposition in a renal transplant in familial Mediterranean fever. Ann Intern Med 87:31–34, 1977.
365. Dorman SA, Gamelli RL, Benziger JR, et al: Systemic amyloidosis involving two renal transplants. Hum Pathol 12:735–738, 1981.
366. Helin H, Pasternack A, Falck H, Kuhlback B: Recurrence of renal amyloid and de novo membranous glomerulonephritis after transplantation. Transplantation 32:6–9, 1981.
367. Jacob ET, Bar-Nathan N, Shapira Z, Gafni J: Renal transplantation in the amyloidosis of familial Mediterranean fever. Experience in ten cases. Arch Intern Med 139:1135–1138, 1979.
368. Jones MB, Adams JM, Passer JA: Amyloidosis in a renal allograft in familial Mediterranean fever. Ann Intern Med 87:579–580, 1977.
369. Kennedy CL, Castro JE: Transplantation for renal amyloidosis. Transplantation 24:382–385, 1977.
370. Light PD, Hall-Craggs M: Amyloid deposition in a renal allograft in a case of amyloidosis secondary to rheumatoid arthritis. Am J Med 66:532–536, 1979.
371. Pasternack A, Ahonen J, Kuhlback B: Renal transplantation in 45 patients with amyloidosis. Transplantation 42:598–601, 1986.
372. De Lima JJG, Kourilsky O, Meyrier A, et al: Kidney transplant in multiple myeloma. Transplantation 31:223–224, 1981.
373. Cadnapaphornchai P, Sillix D: Recurrence of monoclonal gammopathy–related glomerulonephritis in renal allograft. Clin Nephrol 31:156–159, 1989.
374. Bradley JR, Thiru S, Bajallan N, Evans DB: Renal transplantation in Waldenström's macroglobulinemia. Nephrol Dial Transplant 2:214–216, 1988.
375. Alpers CE, Marchioro TL, Johnson RJ: Monoclonal immunoglobulin deposition disease in a renal allograft: Probable recurrent disease in a patient without myeloma. Am J Kidney Dis 13:418–423, 1989.
376. David-Neto E, Ianhez LE, Chocair PR, et al: Renal transplantation in systemic light-chain deposition (SCLD): A 44 month follow-up without recurrence. Transplant Proc 21:2128–2129, 1989.

377. Cabot RC: Case records of the Massachusetts General Hospital (case 1-1981). N Engl J Med 304:33–43, 1981.
378. Gerlag PGG, Koene RAP, Berden JHM: Renal transplantation in light chain nephropathy; case report and review of the literature. Clin Nephrol 25:101–104, 1986.
379. Alpers CE, Rennke HG, Hopper J Jr, Biava C: Fibrillary glomerulonephritis: An entity with unusual immunofluorescence features. Kidney Int 31:781–789, 1987.
380. Korbet SM, Rosenberg BF, Schwartz MM, Lewis EJ: Course of renal transplantation in immunotactoid glomerulopathy. Am J Med 89:91–95, 1990.
381. Steinman TI, Jaffe BF, Monaco AP, et al: Recurrence of Wegener's granulomatosis after kidney transplantation. Am J Med 68:458–460, 1980.
382. Aunsholt NA, Ahlbom G: Recurrence of Wegener's granulomatosis after kidney transplantation involving the kidney graft. Clin Transplant 3:159–161, 1989.
383. Hiesse C, Bastuji-Garin S, Santelli G, et al: Recurrent essential mixed cryoglobulinemia in renal allografts. Am J Nephrol 9:150–154, 1989.
384. Merino GE, Sutherland DER, Kjellstrand CM, et al: Renal transplantation for progressive systemic sclerosis with renal failure: Case report and review of previous experience. Am J Surg 133:745–749, 1977.
385. Woodhall PB, McCoy RC, Gunnells C, Seigler HF: Apparent recurrence of progressive systemic sclerosis in a renal allograft. JAMA 236:1032–1034, 1976.
386. Barnes BA, Bergan JJ, Braun WE, et al: Renal transplantation in congenital and metabolic diseases. A report from the ASC/NIH Renal Transplant Registry. JAMA 232:148–153, 1975.
387. Milliner DS, Pierides AM, Holley KE: Renal transplantation in Alport's syndrome. Antiglomerular basement membrane glomerulonephritis in the allograft. Mayo Clin Proc 57:35–43, 1982.
388. Barber WH, Deierhoi MH, Julian BA: Renal transplantation in sickle cell anemia and sickle disease. Clin Transplant 1:169–175, 1987.
389. Chatterjee SN: National study on natural history of renal allografts in sickle cell disease or trait. Nephron 25:199–201, 1980.
390. Miner DJ, Jorjasky DK, Perloff LJ, et al: Recurrent sickle cell nephropathy in a transplanted kidney. Am J Kidney Dis 10:306–313, 1987.
391. Cameron JS: Recurrent primary disease and de novo nephritis following renal transplantation. Pediatr Nephrol 5:412–421, 1991.
392. Watts RW, Morgan SH, Danpure CJ, et al: Combined hepatic and renal transplantation in primary hyperoxaluria type 1: Clinical report of nine cases. Am J Med 90:179–192, 1991.
393. Gelbart DR, Brewer LL, Fajardo LF, Weinstein AB: Oxalosis and chronic renal failure after intestinal bypass. Arch Intern Med 137:239–243, 1977.
394. Chadwick VS, Modha K, Dowling HR: Mechanism for hyperoxaluria in patients with ileal dysfunction. N Engl J Med 289:172–176, 1973.
395. Frei D, Binswanger U, Keusch G, et al: Intact function of a transplanted kidney 3 years after organ transplantation with primary oxalosis. Schweiz Med Wochenschr 109:979–983, 1979.
396. Leumann EP, Wegmann W, Largiader F: Prolonged survival after renal transplantation in primary hyperoxaluria of childhood. Clin Nephrol 9:29–34, 1978.
397. Morgan JM, Hartley MW, Miller ACJ, Diethelm AG: Successful renal transplantation in hyperoxaluria. Arch Surg 109:430–433, 1974.
398. Broyer M, Brunner FP, Brynger H, et al: Kidney transplantation in primary oxalosis: Data from the EDTA registry. Nephrol Dial Transplant 5:332–336, 1990.
399. Scheinman JL, Najarian JS, Mauer SM: Successful strategies for renal transplantation in oxalosis. Kidney Int 25:804–811, 1984.
400. Watts RWE, Mansell MA: Combined renal and hepatic transplants transform the outlook in primary hyperoxaluria type 1. Br Med J 301:772–773, 1990.
401. Schurmann G, Scharer K, Wingen A-M, et al: Early liver transplantation for primary hyperoxaluria type 1 in an infant with chronic renal failure. Nephrol Dial Transplant 5:825–827, 1990.
402. Aeberhard JM, Schneider PA, Vallotton MB, et al: Multiple site estimates of erythropoietin and renin in polycythemic kidney transplant patients. Transplantation 50:613–616, 1990.
403. Popli S, Molnar ZV, Leehey DJ, et al: Involvement of renal allograft by Fabry's disease. Am J Nephrol 7:316–318, 1987.
404. Peces R, Aguado S, Fernandez F, et al: Renal transplantation in Fabry's disease. Nephron 51:294–295, 1989. Letter.
405. Donati D, Novario R, Gastaldi L: Natural history and treatment of uremia secondary to Fabry's disease: A European experience. Nephron 46:353–359, 1987.
406. Busch GJ, Birtch AG, Lukl PJ, et al: Human renal allografts. Glomerular deposits of horse immunoglobulin G and nephritis following administration of antilymphocyte globulin. Hum Pathol 2:299–308, 1971.
407. Zollinger HU, Moppert J, Theil G, Rohr HP: Morphology and pathogenesis of glomerulopathy in cadaver kidney allografts treated with antilymphocyte globulin. Curr Top Pathol 57:1–48, 1973.
408. Briner J, Binswanger U, Largiader F: Recurrent and de novo membranous glomerulonephritis in renal cadaver allotransplants. Clin Nephrol 13:189–196, 1980.
409. Petersen VP, Olsen TS, Kissmeyer-Nielsen F, et al: Late failure of human renal transplants. An analysis of transplant disease and graft failure among 125 recipients surviving for one to eight years. Medicine (Baltimore) 54:45–71, 1975.
410. Smith WE, McMorrow RG: Membranous glomerulonephritis in renal allografts. N Engl J Med 302:1207, 1980. Letter.
411. Mancilla-Jimenez R, Katzenstein AL, Heritier F, Anderson CB: Antitubular basement membrane antibodies in renal allograft rejection. Transplantation 24:39–44, 1977.
412. Muthuswami SG, Tannen RL, Gikas PW: Membranous glomerulonephritis in renal allografts. N Engl J Med 302:1207, 1980. Letter.
413. Rohr MS: Renal allograft acute tubular necrosis. II. A light and electron microscopic study of biopsies taken at procurement and after revascularization. Ann Surg 197:663–671, 1983.
414. Rohr MS, Childress LB: Quantitation of tubular abnormalities in human renal allografts with normal or delayed function. Transplant Proc 18:499–503, 1986.
415. Hill GS, Light JA, Perloff LJ: Perfusion-related injury in renal transplantation. Surgery 79:440–447, 1976.
416. Spector D, Limas C, Frost JL, et al: Perfusion nephropathy in human transplants. N Engl J Med 295:1217–1221, 1976.
417. Cerra FB, Raza S, Andres GA, Segel JH: The endothelial damage of pulsatile renal preservation, and its relationship to perfusion pressure and colloid osmotic pressure. Surgery 81:534–541, 1977.
418. Myerowitz RL, Medeiros AA, O'Brien TG: Bacterial infection in renal homotransplant recipients. Am J Med 53:308–314, 1972.
419. Anderson RJ, Schafer LA, Olin DB, Eickhoff TC: Septicemia in renal transplant patients. Arch Surg 106:692–694, 1973.
420. Bach MC, Sahyoun A, Adler JL, et al: Influence of rejection therapy on fungal and nocardial infections in renal transplant recipients. Lancet 1:180–184, 1973.
421. Rubin RH, Wolfson JS, Cosimi AB, Tolkoff-Rubin NE: Infection in the renal transplant recipient. Am J Med 70:405–411, 1981.
422. Higgins RM, Bloom R, Hopkins JM, Morris PJ: The risks and benefits of low-dose cotrimoxazole prophylaxis for *Pneumocystis* pneumonia in renal transplantation. Transplantation 47:558–560, 1989.
423. Talseth T, Haldaas H, Albrechtsen D, et al: Increasing incidence of *Pneumocystis carinii* pneumonia in renal transplant patients. Transplant Proc 20:400–401, 1988.
424. Scroggs MW, Wolfe JA, Bollinger R, Sanfilippo F: Causes of death in renal transplant recipients. Arch Pathol Lab Med 111:983–987, 1987.
425. Peterson PK, Balfour HHJ, Fryd DS, et al: Fever in renal transplant recipients: Causes, prognostic significance and changing patterns at the University of Minnesota Hospital. Am J Med 71:345–351, 1981.
426. Rubin RH: Infectious disease complications of renal transplantation. Kidney Int 44:221–236, 1993.
427. Kennedy CA, Panosian CB: Infectious complications of kidney transplantation. *In* Danovitch GM (ed): Handbook of Kidney Transplantation. Little, Brown, Boston, 1992, pp 209–237.
428. Farrugia E, Schwab TR: Management and prevention of cytomegalovirus infection after renal transplantation. Mayo Clin Proc 67:879–890, 1992.
429. Rubin RH, Tolkoff-Rubin NE, Oliver D, et al: Multicenter seroepidemiologic study of the impact of cytomegalovirus infection on renal transplantation. Transplantation 40:243–249, 1985.
430. Rubin RH, Russell PS, Levin M, Cohen C: Summary of a workshop on cytomegalovirus infection during organ transplantation. J Infect Dis 139:728–734, 1979.

431. Rubin RH: Infection in the renal transplant recipient. *In* Milford EL (ed): Renal Transplantation: Contemporary Issues in Nephrology, Vol 19. Churchill Livingstone, New York, 1989, pp 147–180.

432. Betts RF, Freeman RB, Douglas RG, et al: Transmission of cytomegalovirus infection with renal allograft. Kidney Int 8:385–392, 1975.

433. Ho M: Epidemiology of cytomegalovirus infections. Rev Infect Dis 12:S701–S710, 1990.

434. Snydman DR, Rubin RH, Werner BG: New developments in cytomegalovirus prevention and treatment. Am J Kidney Dis 21:217–228, 1993.

435. Snydman DR, Werner BG, Heinze-Lacey B, et al: Use of cytomegalovirus disease in renal transplant recipients. N Engl J Med 317:1049–1054, 1987.

436. Hibberd PL, Tolkoff-Rubin NE, Cosimi AB, et al: Symptomatic cytomegalovirus disease in cytomegalovirus antibody seropositive renal transplant recipient treated with OKT3. Transplantation 53:68–72, 1992.

437. Rubin RH: Preemptive therapy in immunosuppressed hosts. N Engl J Med 324:1057–1059, 1991.

438. Carrington D, Mocan H, Beattie TJ, et al: Serial quantitative $^{99m}$Tc DTPA imaging in CMV-associated renal allograft dysfunction. Clin Nephrol 28:152–155, 1987.

439. Chan CN, Lai FM, Lai KN, Pang JA: Relapse of idiopathic pulmonary haemorrhage and glomerulonephritis associated with cytomegalovirus (CMV) infection. Postgrad Med J 64:52–55, 1988.

440. Schooley RT, Hirsch MS, Colvin RB, et al: Association of herpes virus infection with T-lymphocyte subset alterations, glomerulopathy, and opportunistic infections after renal transplantation. N Engl J Med 308:307–313, 1983.

441. Tuazon TV, Schneeberger EE, Bhan AK, et al: Mononuclear cells in acute allograft glomerulopathy. Am J Pathol 129:119–132, 1987.

442. Pouteil-Noble C, Ecochard R, Landrivon G, et al: Cytomegalovirus infection—an etiological factor for rejection? A prospective study in 242 renal transplant recipients. Transplantation 55:851–857, 1993.

443. Calne RY, Rolles K, White DJ, et al: Cyclosporin A initially as the only immunosuppressant in 34 recipients of cadaveric organs: 32 kidneys, 2 pancreases, and 2 livers. Lancet 2:1033–1036, 1979.

444. Bird AG, McLochlin SM, Britton S: Cyclosporin A promotes spontaneous outgrowth in vitro of Epstein-Barr virus–induced B-cell lines. Nature 289:300–301, 1981.

445. Yao QY, Rickinson AB, Gaston JS, Epstein MA: In vitro analysis of the Epstein-Barr virus: Host balance in long-term renal allograft recipients. Int J Cancer 35:43–49, 1985.

446. Stephanian E, Gruber SA, Dunn DL, Matas AJ: Posttransplant lymphoproliferative disorders. Transplant Rev 5:120–129, 1991.

447. Scullard GH, Smith CI, Merigan TC, et al: Effects of immunosuppressive therapy on viral markers in chronic active hepatitis B. Gastroenterology 81:987–991, 1981.

448. Lynfield R, Herrin JT, Rubin RH: Varicella in pediatric renal transplant recipients. Pediatrics 90:216–220, 1992.

449. Ho M: Virus infections after transplantation in man; brief review. Arch Virol 55:1–24, 1977.

450. Debure A, Degos F, Pol S, et al: Liver disease and hepatic complications in renal transplant patients. Adv Nephrol 17:375–400, 1988.

451. Tolkoff-Rubin NE, Cosimi AB, Russell PS, Rubin RH: A controlled study of trimethoprim-sulfamethoxazole prophylaxis of urinary tract infections in renal transplant recipients. Rev Infect Dis 4:614–618, 1982.

452. Fox BC, Sollinger HW, Belzer FO, Maki DG: A prospective randomized, double-blind study of trimethoprim-sulfamethoxazole, effects on the mucoflora, and the cost-benefit prophylaxis. Am J Med 89:255–274, 1990.

453. Hibberd PL, Tolkoff-Rubin NE, Doran M: Trimethoprim-sulfamethoxazole compared with ciprofloxacin for the prevention of urinary tract infection in renal transplant recipients. Online J Curr Clin Trials Doc No 15, Aug 11, 1992.

454. Rubin RH, Wolfson JS, Cosimi AB, Tolkoff-Rubin NE: A controlled study of trimethoprim sulfamethoxazole prophylaxis of urinary tract infection in renal transplant recipients. Rev Infect Dis 4:614–618, 1981.

455. Aguado JM, Salto E, Morales JM, et al: *Corynebacterium urealyticum:* A new and threatening pathogen for the renal transplant patient. Transplant Proc 25:1493–1494, 1993.

456. Hernandez Poblete G, Morales JM, Prieto C, et al: Usefulness of norfloxacine prophylaxis in late recurrent urinary tract infection after renal transplantation. Nephron 54:193–194, 1990.

457. Lichtenstein IH, MacGregor RR: Mycobacterial infections in renal transplant recipients: Report of five cases and review of the literature. Rev Infect Dis 5:216–226, 1983.

458. Qunibi WY, al-Sibai MB, Taher S, et al: Mycobacterial infection after renal transplantation—report of 14 cases and review of the literature. Q J Med 77:1039–1060, 1990.

459. Lloveras J, Peterson PK, Simmons RL, Najarian JS: Mycobacterial infections in renal transplant recipients. Seven cases and a review of the literature. Arch Intern Med 142:888–892, 1982.

460. McWhinney N, Khan O, Williams G: Tuberculosis in patients undergoing maintenance haemodialysis and renal transplantation. Br J Surg 68:408–411, 1981.

461. Rattazzi LC, Simmons RL, Sapanos PK, et al: Successful management of miliary tuberculosis after renal transplantation. Am J Surg 130:359–361, 1975.

462. Buffington GA, Dominguez JH, Piering WF, et al: Interaction of rifampin and glucocorticoids. Adverse effect on renal allograft function. JAMA 236:1958–1960, 1976.

463. Washer GF, Schroter GPJ, Starzl TE: Causes of death after kidney transplantation. JAMA 250:49–54, 1983.

464. Mahony JF: Long-term results and complications of transplantation: The kidney. Transplant Proc 21:1433–1434, 1989.

465. Schweitzer EJ, Matas AJ, Gillingham KJ, et al: Causes of renal allograft loss. Progress in the 1980s, challenges for the 1990s. Ann Surg 214:679–688, 1991.

466. Van Ypersele de Strihou C, Vereerstraeten P, Wauthier M, et al: Prevalence, etiology, and treatment of late post-transplant hypertension. Adv Nephrol Necker Hosp 12:41–60, 1983.

467. Ibels LS, Stewart JH, Mahony JF, et al: Occlusive arterial diseases in uraemic and haemodialysis patients and renal transplant recipients. Q J Med 46:197–214, 1977.

468. Luke RG: Pathophysiology and treatment of posttransplant hypertension. J Am Soc Nephrol 2(suppl 1):S37–S44, 1991.

469. Bachy C, Alexandre GPJ, de Strihou CVY: Hypertension after renal transplantation. Br Med J 2:1287–1289, 1976.

470. Tejani A: Post-transplant hypertension and hypertensive encephalopathy in renal allograft recipients. Nephron 34:73–78, 1983.

471. Rao TKS, Gupta SK, Butt KMH, et al: Relationship of renal transplantation to hypertension in end-stage renal failure. Arch Intern Med 138:1236–1241, 1978.

472. Pollini J, Guttman RD, Beadoin JG, et al: Late hypertension following renal allotransplantation. Clin Nephrol 11:1287–1289, 1979.

473. Popovitzer MM, Pinnggera W, Katz FH, et al: Variation in arterial blood pressure after kidney transplantation. Relation to renal function, plasma renin activity, and the dose of prednisone. Circulation 47:1297–1305, 1973.

474. Curtis JJ: Cyclosporine and posttransplantation hypertension. J Am Soc Nephrol 2:S243–S245, 1992.

475. Rettig R, Schmitt B, Pelzl B, Speck T: The kidney and primary hypertension: Contributions from renal transplantation studies in animals and humans. J Hypertens 11:883–891, 1993.

476. Guidi E, Bianchi G, Rivolta E, et al: Hypertension in man with a kidney transplant: Role of familial versus other factors. Nephron 41:14–21, 1985.

477. Curtis JJ, Luke RG, Dustan HP, et al: Remission of essential hypertension after renal transplantation. N Engl J Med 309:1009–1015, 1983.

478. Cohen SL: Hypertension in renal transplant recipients: Role of bilateral nephrectomy. Br Med J 3:78–81, 1973.

479. Grunfeld JP, Kleinknect D, Moreau JF, et al: Permanent hypertension after renal transplantation. Clin Sci 48:391–403, 1975.

480. Curtis JJ, Lucas BA, Kotchen TA, Luke RG: Surgical therapy for persistent hypertension after renal transplantation. Transplantation 31:125–128, 1981.

481. Linas SL, Miller PD, McDonald KM, et al: Role of the renin-angiotensin system in post-transplantation hypertension in patients with multiple kidneys. N Engl J Med 298:1440–1444, 1978.

482. Curtis JJ, Luke RG, Diethelm AG, et al: Benefits of removal of native kidneys in hypertension after renal transplantation. Lancet 2:739–742, 1985.

483. O'Connor DT, Barg AP, Amend W, Vincenti F: Urinary kallikrein excretion after renal transplantation: Relationship to hypertension, graft source and renal function. Am J Med 73:475–481, 1982.

484. Miyashita A, Sakai A, Butt KMH: Urinary kallikrein activity (esterase activity), plasma renin activity, and urinary aldosterone excretion

in kidney transplantation patients. Transplant Proc 15:2136–2138, 1983.

485. Coffman TM, Yarger WE, Klotman PE: Functional role of thromboxane production by acutely rejecting renal allografts in rats. J Clin Invest 75:1242–1248, 1985.

486. Rao TKS, Manis T, Delano BG, Briedman EA: Continuing high morbidity during maintenance hemodialysis consequent to bilateral nephrectomy. Trans Am Soc Artif Intern Organs 19:340–344, 1973.

487. Kominami N, Lowrie EG, Ianhez LE, et al: The effect of total nephrectomy on hematopoiesis in patients undergoing chronic hemodialysis. J Lab Clin Med 78:524–532, 1971.

488. Van Ypersele de Strihou C, Stragier A: Effect of bilateral nephrectomy on transfusion requirements of patients undergoing chronic dialysis. Lancet 2:705–707, 1969.

489. Coffman TM, Himmelstein S, Best C, Klotman PE: Post-transplant hypertension in the rat: Effects of captopril and native nephrectomy. Kidney Int 36:35–40, 1989.

490. Kalbfleisch JH, Hebert LA, Lemann J, et al: Habitual excessive dietary salt intake and blood pressure levels in renal transplant recipients. Am J Med 73:205–210, 1982.

491. Skorecki KL, Rutledge WP, Schrier RW: Acute cyclosporine nephrotoxicity—prototype for a renal membrane signalling disorder. Kidney Int 42:1–10, 1992.

492. Perico N, Ruggenenti P, Gaspari F, et al: Daily renal hypoperfusion induced by cyclosporine in patients with renal transplantation. Transplantation 54:56–60, 1992.

493. Ozdogan E, Banner N, Fitzgerald M, et al: Factors influencing the development of hypertension after heart transplantation. J Heart Transplant 9:548–553, 1990.

494. Broyer M, Guest G, Gagnadoux MF, Beurton D: Hypertension following renal transplantation in children. Pediatr Nephrol 1:16–21, 1987.

495. Hoyer PF, Offner G, Oemar BS, et al: Four years' experience with cyclosporin A in pediatric kidney transplantation. Acta Paediatr Scand 79:622–629, 1990.

496. English J, Evan A, Houghton D, Bennett W: Cyclosporine-induced acute renal dysfunction in the rat. Evidence of arteriolar vasoconstriction with preservation of tubular function. Transplantation 44:135–141, 1987.

497. Curtis J, Luke R, Jones P, Diethelm A: Hypertension in cyclosporine-treated renal transplant patients is sodium dependent. Am J Med 85:134–138, 1988.

498. Kon V, Sugiura M, Inagami T, et al: Role of endothelin in cyclosporine-induced glomerular dysfunction. Kidney Int 37:1487–1491, 1990.

499. Coffman T, Carr D, Yarger W, Klotman P: Evidence that renal prostaglandin and thromboxane production is stimulated in chronic cyclosporine nephrotoxicity. Transplantation 43:282–285, 1986.

500. Lamb F, Webb R: Cyclosporine augments reactivity of isolated blood vessels. Life Sci 40:2571–2578, 1987.

501. Luke RG: Hypertension in renal transplant recipients. Kidney Int 31:1024–1037, 1987.

502. Lacombe M: Arterial stenosis complicating renal allotransplantation in man. Ann Surg 181:283–288, 1975.

503. Dickerman RM, Peters PC, Hull AR, et al: Surgical correction of posttransplant renovascular hypertension. Ann Surg 192:639–644, 1980.

504. Epstein M: Calcium antagonists and renal hemodynamics: Implications for renal protection. J Am Soc Nephrol 2:S30–S36, 1991.

505. Bennett WM, Meyer MM: Considerations in the medical management of hypertension in cyclosporin A–treated allograft recipients. Transplant Immunol Lett 8:4–19, 1992.

506. Renton KW: Inhibition of hepatic microsomal drug metabolism by the calcium channel blockers diltiazem and verapamil. Biochem Pharmacol 34:2549–2553, 1985.

507. Vlahakos DV, Canzanello VJ, Madaio MP, Madias NE: Enalapril-associated anemia in renal transplant recipients treated for hypertension. Am J Kidney Dis 17:199–205, 1991.

508. Gaston RS, Julian BA, Diethelm AG, Curtis JJ: Effects of enalapril on erythrocytosis after renal transplantation. Ann Intern Med 115:954–955, 1991.

509. Hricik DE, Browning PJ, Kopelman R, et al: Captopril-induced functional renal insufficiency in patients with bilateral renal artery stenoses or renal artery stenoses in a solitary kidney. N Engl J Med 308:373–376, 1983.

510. Mammen NI, Chacko N, Ganesh G, et al: Aspects of hypertension in renal allograft recipients. A study of 1000 live renal transplants. Br J Urol 71:256–258, 1993.

511. Erley CM, Duda SH, Wakat JP, et al: Noninvasive procedures for diagnosis of renovascular hypertension in renal transplant recipients—a prospective analysis. Transplantation 54:863–867, 1992.

512. Shamlou KK, Drane WE, Hawkins IF, Fennell RSI: Captopril renography and the hypertensive renal transplantation patient: A predictive test of therapeutic outcome. Radiology 190:153–159, 1994.

513. Reisfeld D, Matas AJ, Tellis VA, et al: Late follow-up of percutaneous transluminal angioplasty for treatment of renal artery stenosis. Transplant Proc 21:1955–1956, 1989.

514. Bagdade JD, Porte D, Bierman EL: Hypertriglyceridemia: A metabolic consequence of chronic renal failure. N Engl J Med 279:181–185, 1968.

515. Bagdade JD, Cassaretto A, Alpers J: Effects of chronic uremia, hemodialysis, and renal transplantation on plasma lipids and lipoproteins in man. J Lab Clin Med 87:37–48, 1976.

516. Huttunen JK, Pasternack A, Vanttinen T, et al: Lipoprotein metabolism in patients with chronic uremia. Acta Med Scand 204:211–218, 1978.

517. Wakabayashi Y, Okubo M, Shimada H, et al: Decreased VLDL apoprotein CIII ration may be seen in both normotriglyceridemic and hypertriglyceridemic patients on chronic hemodialysis treatment. Metabolism 36:815–820, 1987.

518. Nestel PJ, Fidge NH, Tan MH: Increased lipoprotein-remnant formation in chronic renal failure. N Engl J Med 307:239–333, 1982.

519. Gregg R, Mordon CE, Reaven FP, Reaven GM: Effects of acute uremia on triglyceride kinetics in the rat. Metabolism 25:1557–1565, 1976.

520. Cattran DC, Fenton SS, Wilson DR, Steiner G: Defective triglyceride removal in lipemia associated with peritoneal dialysis and hemodialysis. Ann Intern Med 85:29–33, 1976.

521. Champ DG: Plasma lipid alterations in patients with chronic renal diseases. Crit Rev Clin Lab Sci 17:77–101, 1982.

522. Grundy SM: Management of hyperlipidemia of kidney disease. Kidney Int 37:847–853, 1990.

523. Grundy SM, Vega GL: Hypertriglyceridemia: Causes and relation to coronary heart disease. Semin Thromb 14:149–164, 1988.

524. Goldberg A, Sherrard DJ, Brunzell JD: Adipose tissue lipoprotein lipase in chronic hemodialysis: Role in plasma triglyceride metabolism. J Clin Endocrinol 47:1173–1182, 1978.

525. Pasternack A, Vanttinen T, Solakivi T, et al: Normalization of lipoprotein lipase and hepatic lipase by gemfibrozil results in correction of lipoprotein abnormalities in chronic renal failure. Clin Nephrol 27:163–168, 1987.

526. Chan MK, Persaud J, Varghese Z, Moorhead JF: Pathogenic roles of post-heparin lipases in lipid abnormalities in hemodialysis patients. Kidney Int 25:812–818, 1984.

527. Mordansini R, Frey F, Flurry W, et al: Selective deficiency of hepatic triglyceride lipase in uremic patients. N Engl J Med 297:1362–1366, 1977.

528. Burton BT, Krueger KK, Bryan FA Jr: National registry of long-term dialysis patients. JAMA 218:718–722, 1971.

529. Linder A, Ghara B, Sherrard DJ, Schribner BH: Accelerated atherosclerosis in prolonged maintenance hemodialysis. N Engl J Med 290:697–701, 1974.

530. Bonomini V, Feletti C, Scolari MP, et al: Atherosclerosis in uremia: A longitudinal study. Am J Clin Nutr 33:1493–1500, 1980.

531. Broyer M, Brunner FP, Brynger H, et al: Combined report on regular dialysis and transplantation in Europe. Rep Eur Dial Transplant Assoc 19:260, 1982.

532. Degoulet P, Legrain M, Reach I, et al: Mortality risk factors in patients treated by chronic hemodialysis. Nephron 31:103–110, 1982.

533. Rostand SG, Kirk KA, Rutsky EA: Relationship of coronary risk factors to hemodialysis-associated ischemic heart disease. Kidney Int 22:304–308, 1982.

534. Hulley SB, Rosenman RH, Rowol RD, Brand RJ: Epidemiology as a guide to clinical decisions: The association between triglyceride and coronary heart disease. N Engl J Med 302:1383–1389, 1980.

535. Richards EG, Grundy SM, Cooper K: Influence of plasma triglycerides on lipoprotein patterns in normal subjects and in patients with coronary artery disease. Am J Cardiol 63:1214–1220, 1969.

536. Miller GJ, Miller NE: Plasma-high-density-lipoprotein concentration and development of ischaemic heart-disease. Lancet 1:16–19, 1975.

537. Castelli WP, Garrison RJ, Wilson PWF, et al: Incidence of coronary heart disease and lipoprotein cholesterol levels: The Framingham Study. JAMA 256:2835–2838, 1986.

538. Kasiske BL, Umen AJ: Persistent hyperlipidemia in renal transplant patients. Medicine (Baltimore) 66:309–316, 1987.

539. Casaretto A, Marchioro TL, Goldsmith R, Bagdade JD: Hyperlipidaemia after successful renal transplantation. Lancet 1:481–484, 1974.

540. Saldanha LF, Hurst KS, Amend WJC, et al: Hyperlipidemia after renal transplantation in children. Am J Dis Child 130:951–953, 1976.

541. Pennisi AJ, Heuser ET, Mickey MR, et al: Hyperlipidemia in pediatric hemodialysis and renal transplant patients. Am J Dis Child 130:957–961, 1976.

542. Ibels LS, Alfrey AC, Weill R: Hyperlipidemia in adult, pediatric and diabetic renal transplant recipients. Am J Med 64:634–642, 1978.

543. Ponticelli C, Barbi GL, Cantaluppi A, et al: Lipid disorders in renal transplant recipients. Nephron 20:189–195, 1978.

544. Gokal R, Mann JI, Moore RA, Morris PJ: Hyperlipidemia following renal transplantation. A study of the prevalence, natural history and dietary treatment. Q J Med 48:507–517, 1979.

545. Cattran DC, Steiner G, Wilson DR, Fenton SSA: Hyperlipidemia after renal transplantation: Natural history and pathophysiology. Ann Intern Med 91:554–559, 1979.

546. Chan MK, Varghese Z, Moorhead JH: Lipid abnormalities in uremia, dialysis and transplantation. Kidney Int 19:625–637, 1981.

547. Grundy SM: Management of hyperlipidemia of kidney disease. Kidney Int 37:847–853, 1990.

548. Harris KPG, Russell GI, Parvin SD, et al: Alterations in lipid and carbohydrate metabolism attributable to cyclosporin A in renal transplant recipients. Br Med J 292:16, 1986.

549. Raine AEG, Morris PJ: Hyperlipidaemia after renal transplantation. Lancet 23:391, 1988.

550. Hricik DE, Bartucci MR, Mayes JT, Schulak JA: The effects of steroid withdrawal on the lipoprotein profiles of cyclosporine-treated kidney and kidney-pancreas transplant recipients. Transplantation 54:868–871, 1992.

551. Drueke TB, Abdulmassih Z, Lacour B, et al: Atherosclerosis and lipid disorders after renal transplantation. Kidney Int Suppl 31:S24–S28, 1991.

552. Moore RA, Callahan MF, Cody M, et al: The effect of the American Heart Association step one diet on hyperlipidemia following renal transplantation. Transplantation 49:60–62, 1990.

553. Disler PB, Goldberg RB, Kuhn L, et al: The role of diet in the pathogenesis and control of hyperlipidemia after renal transplantation. Clin Nephrol 16:29–34, 1981.

554. Shen SY, Lukens CW, Alongi SV, et al: Patient profile and effect of dietary therapy on post-transplant hyperlipidemia. Kidney Int 24:S147–S152, 1983.

555. Beaumont JE, Luke RG, Galla JH, et al: Normal serum-lipids in renal-transplant patients. Lancet 1:599–601, 1975.

556. Turgan C, Russell GI, Baker F, Walls J: The effect of renal transplantation with a minimal steroid regime on uraemic hypertriglyceridaemia. Q J Med 210:271–277, 1984.

557. Drukker A, Turner C, Start K, et al: Hyperlipidemia after renal transplantation in children on alternate day corticosteroid therapy. Clin Nephrol 26:140–145, 1986.

558. Ballantyne CM, Radovancevic B, Farmer JA, et al: Hyperlipidemia after heart transplantation: Report of a 6-year experience with treatment recommendations. J Am Coll Cardiol 19:1315–1321, 1992.

559. Appel G: Lipid abnormalities in renal disease (clinical conference). Kidney Int 39:169–183, 1991.

560. Cheung AK, DeVault GA, Gregory MC: A prospective study on treatment of hypercholesterolemia with lovastatin in renal transplant recipients receiving cyclosporine. J Am Soc Nephrol 3:1884–1891, 1993.

561. LaQuaglia MP, Tolkoff-Rubin NE, Dienstag JL: Impact of hepatitis on renal transplantation. Transplantation 32:504–507, 1981.

562. Boyce NW, Holdsworth SR, Hooke D, et al: Nonhepatitis B–related liver disease in a renal transplant population. Am J Kidney Dis 11:307–312, 1988.

563. Weir MR, Kirkman RL, Strom TB, Tilney NL: Liver disease in recipients of long-surviving renal allografts. Kidney Int 28:839–844, 1985.

564. Harnett JD, Zeldis JB, Parfrey PS, et al: Hepatitis B disease in dialysis and transplant patients. Further epidemiologic and serologic studies. Transplantation 44:369–376, 1987.

565. Degos F, Degott C, Bedrossian J, et al: Is renal transplantation involved in post-transplantation liver disease? A prospective study. Transplantation 29:100–102, 1980.

566. Degos F, Lugassy C, Degott C, et al: Hepatitis B virus and hepatitis B–related viral infection in renal transplant recipients. Gastroenterology 94:151–156, 1988.

567. Parfrey PS, Forbes RDC, Hytchinson TA, et al: The impact of renal transplantation on the course of hepatitis B liver disease. Transplantation 39:610–615, 1985.

568. Stevens DE, Harvey JA, Taylor PE, et al: Hepatitis B vaccine in patients receiving hemodialysis: Immunogenicity and efficacy. N Engl J Med 311:496–501, 1984.

569. Pasko MT, Bartholomew WR, Beam TR, et al: Long-term evaluation of the hepatitis B vaccine (Heptavax-B) in hemodialysis patients. Am J Kidney Dis 11:326–331, 1988.

570. Feuerhake A, Muller R, Lauchart W, et al: HBV-vaccination in recipients of kidney allografts. Vaccine 2:255–256, 1984.

571. Lauchart W, Feuerhake A, Pichlmayr R, Muller R: Active hepatitis B vaccination in immunosuppressed patients. Transplant Proc 16:1348–1349, 1984.

572. Choo QL, Kuo G, Weiner AJ, et al: Isolation of a cDNA clone derived from a blood bourne non-A, non-B viral hepatitis genome. Science 244:359–362, 1989.

573. Kuo G, Choo QL, Alter HJ, et al: An assay for circulating antibodies to a major etiologic virus of human non-A non-B hepatitis. Science 244:362–364, 1989.

574. Pereira BJG, Milford EL, Kirkman RL, et al: Prevalence of HCV RNA in hepatitis C antibody positive cadaver organ donors and their recipients. N Engl J Med 327:910–915, 1992.

575. Aeder MI, Shield CF, Tegtmeier GE, et al: The incidence and clinical impact of hepatitis C virus (HCV) positive donors in cadaveric transplantation. Transplant Proc 25:1469–1471, 1993.

576. Koretz RL, Stone O, Mousa M, Gitnick GL: Non-A, non-B posttransfusion hepatitis—a decade later. Gastroenterology 88:1251–1254, 1985.

577. Pirsch JD, Belzer FO: Transmission of HCV by organ transplantation. N Engl J Med 326:412–413, 1992.

578. Morales JM, Campistol JM: Hepatitis C virus and organ transplantation. N Engl J Med 328:511–512, 1993.

579. Dussol B, Chicheportiche C, Cantaloube JF, et al: Detection of hepatitis C infection by polymerase chain reaction among hemodialysis patients. Am J Kidney Dis 22:574–580, 1993.

580. Chung RT, Karkov WN, Dienstag JL, Kaplan LM: Chronic renal failure is frequently associated with false-negative anti-C100 in patients with hepatitis C viremia. Gastroenterology 100:A729, 1991. Abstract.

581. Farci P, Alter HJ, Govindarajan S, et al: Lack of protective immunity against reinfection with hepatitis C virus. Science 258:135–140, 1992.

582. Black M, Peters M: Alpha-interferon treatment of chronic hepatitis C: Need for accurate diagnosis in selecting patients. Ann Intern Med 116:86–88, 1992.

583. DePinho RA, Goldberg CS, Lefkowitch JH: Azathioprine and the liver. Evidence favoring idiosyncratic, mixed cholestatic-hepatocellular injury in humans. Gastroenterology 86:162–165, 1987.

584. Penn I: The changing patterns of posttransplant malignancies. Transplant Proc 23:1101–1103, 1991.

585. Penn I: Why do immunosuppressed patients develop cancer? Crit Rev Oncogen 1:27–52, 1989.

586. Penn I: Cancers complicating organ transplantation. N Engl J Med 323:1767–1769, 1990.

587. Penn I: Tumors after renal and cardiac transplantation. Hematol Oncol Clin North Am 7:431–445, 1993.

588. Gupta AK, Cardella CJ, Haberman HF: Cutaneous malignant neoplasms in patients with renal transplants. Arch Dermatol 122:1288–1293, 1986.

589. Sheil AGR, Disney APS, Mathew TH, et al: Cancer development in cadaveric donor renal allograft recipients treated with azathipirne (AZA) or cyclosporine (CYA) or AZA/CYA. Transplant Proc 23:1111–1112, 1991.

590. Mullen DL, Silberg SG, Penn I, Hammond WS: Squamous cell carcinoma of the skin and lip in renal homograft recipients. Cancer 37:729–734, 1976.

591. Patton DF, Wilkowski CW, Hanson CA, et al: Epstein-Barr virus determines clonality in post-transplant lymphoproliferative disorders. Transplantation 49:1080–1084, 1990.

592. Hanto DW, Frizzera G, Gajl-Peczalska KJ, et al: Epstein-Barr-virus induced B-cell lymphoma after renal transplantation: Acyclovir therapy and transition from polyclonal to monoclonal B cell proliferation. N Engl J Med 306:913–918, 1982.

593. Randhawa PS, Jaffe R, Demetris AJ, et al: Expression of Epstein-Barr virus–encoded small RNA (by the *EBER-1* gene) in liver specimens from transplant recipients with post-transplantation lymphoproliferative disease. N Engl J Med 323:1710–1714, 1992.

594. Opelz G, Henderson R: Incidence of non-Hodgkin lymphoma in kidney and heart transplant recipients. Lancet 342:1514–1516, 1993.

595. Nalsnik MA, Makowa L, Starzl TE: The diagnosis and treatment of posttransplant lymphoproliferative disorders. Surgery 25:367–472, 1988.

596. Starzl TE, Nalesnik MA, Porter KA, et al: Reversibility of lymphomas and lymphoproliferative lesions developing under cyclosporin-steroid therapy. Lancet 1:583–587, 1984.

597. Lin HY, Rocher LL, McQuillian MA, et al: Cyclosporine-induced hyperuricemia and gout. N Engl J Med 321:289–292, 1989.

598. Noordzij TC, Leunissen KM, Van Hooff JP: Renal handling of urate and the incidence of gouty arthritis during cyclosporine and diuretic use. Transplantation 52:64–67, 1991.

599. West C, Carpenter BJ, Hakala TR: The incidence of gout in renal transplant recipients. Am J Kidney Dis 10:369–372, 1987.

600. Gottlieb MN, Stephens MK, Lowrie EG, et al: A longitudinal study of bone disease after successful renal transplantation. Nephron 22:239–248, 1978.

601. Pletka PG, Strom TB, Hampers CL, et al: Secondary hyperparathyroidism in human kidney transplant recipients. Nephron 17:371–381, 1976.

602. Garvin PJ, Casteneda M, Lindeier R, Dickhans M: Management of hypercalcemic hyperparathyroidism after renal transplantation. Arch Surg 120:578–583, 1985.

603. Cundy T, Kanis JA, Heynen G, et al: Calcium metabolism and hyperparathyroidism after renal transplantation. Q J Med 205:67–78, 1983.

604. Rosenbaum RW, Hruska DA, Korkor A, et al: Decreased phosphate reabsorption after renal transplantation: Evidence for a mechanism independent of calcium and parathyroid hormone. Kidney Int 19:568–578, 1981.

605. Felson DT, Anderson JJ: A cross-study evaluation of association between steroid dose and bolus steroids and avascular necrosis of bone. Lancet 1:902–906, 1987.

606. Hall MC, Elmore SM, Bright RW, et al: Skeletal complications in a series of human renal allografts. JAMA 208:1825–1829, 1969.

607. Ibels LS, Alfrey AC, Huffer WE, Weil R: Aseptic necrosis of bone following renal transplantation. Experience in 194 transplant recipients and review of the literature. Medicine (Baltimore) 57:25–45, 1978.

608. Susan LP, Braun WE, Banowsky LH, et al: Avascular necrosis following renal transplantation: Experience with 449 allografts with and without high-dose steroid therapy. Urology 11:225–229, 1978.

609. Cruess RL: Osteonecrosis of bone. Current concepts as to etiology and pathogenesis. Clin Orthop 208:30–39, 1986.

610. Boudreaux JP, McHugh L, Canafox DM, et al: The impact of cyclosporine and combination immunosuppression on the incidence of posttransplant diabetes in renal allograft recipients. Am J Kidney Dis 10:369–372, 1987.

611. Freidman EA, Shyh T-P, Beyer MM, et al: Posttransplant diabetes in kidney transplant recipients. Am J Nephrol 5:196–202, 1985.

612. Roth D, Milgrom M, Esquenazi V, et al: Posttransplant hyperglycemia: Increased incidence in cyclosporine-treated renal allograft recipients. Transplantation 47:278–281, 1989.

613. DeClerck YA, Ettenger RB, Ortega JA, Pennisi AJ: Macrocytosis and pure RBC anemia caused by azathioprine. Am J Dis Child 134:377–379, 1980.

614. Hogge DE, Wilson DR, Shumak KH, Cattran DC: Reversible azathioprine-induced erythrocyte aplasia in a renal transplant recipient. Can Med Assoc J 126:512–513, 1982.

615. McGrath BP, Ibels LS, Raik E, et al: Macrocytosis and selective marrow hypoplasias. Q J Med 44:57–63, 1975.

616. Old CW, Flannery EP, Grogan TM, et al: Azathioprine-induced pure red cell aplasia. JAMA 240:552–554, 1978.

617. Margolis B, Bear RA: Role of cyclosporine in recurrent hemolytic uremic syndrome in a renal allograft recipient. Clin Transpl :124, 1986.

618. Verpooten GA, Paulus GJ, Roels F, de Broe ME: De novo occurrence of hemolytic-uremic syndrome in a cyclosporine-treated renal allograft patient. Transplant Proc 19:2943–2945, 1987.

619. Albrechtsen D, Sollheim BG, Flatmark A, et al: Autoimmune hemolytic anemia in cyclosporine-treated organ allograft recipients. Transplant Proc 20:959–962, 1988.

620. Wickre CG, Norman DJ, Bennison A, et al: Postrenal transplant erythrocytosis: A review of 53 patients. Kidney Int 23:731–737, 1983.

621. Bacon BR, Rothman SA, Ricanati ES, Rashad RA: Renal artery stenosis with erythrocytosis after renal transplantation. Arch Intern Med 140:1206–1211, 1980.

622. Sanfilippo F, Vaughn WK, LeFor WM, Spees EK: Multivariate analysis of risk factors in cadaver donor kidney transplantation. Transplantation 42:28–34, 1986.

623. Yoon YS, Bang BK, Jin DC, et al: Factors influencing long-term outcome of living donor kidney transplantation in the cyclosporine era. *In* Terasaki PI, Cecka M (eds): Clinical Transplants 1992. UCLA Tissue Typing Laboratory, Los Angeles, 1993, pp 257–266.

624. Gjertson DW: Multifactorial analysis of renal transplants reported to the United Network for Organ Sharing Registry. *In* Terasaki PI, Cecka M (eds): Clinical Transplants 1992. UCLA Tissue Typing Laboratory, Los Angeles, 1993, p 299.

625. Brenner BM, Milford EL: Nephron underdosing: A programmed cause of chronic renal allograft failure. Am J Kidney Dis 21:66–72, 1993.

# 60

# Prescribing Drugs in Renal Disease

*Cathryn Shuler*
*Thomas A. Golper*
*William M. Bennett*

Patients with renal dysfunction due to primary or secondary renal disease have an excess of adverse drug reactions because of altered drug pharmacokinetics in renal failure. Because renal patients often have serious comorbid conditions requiring pharmacotherapy, drug interactions are also frequent in this population. In addition, a large part of the difficulty in prescribing drugs for the rapidly growing numbers of elderly patients is due to age-related declines in renal function. When dialysis therapies are necessary for acute or chronic renal failure, an additional route of drug elimination is present for which dosing adjustments must be made for therapeutic efficacy to be ensured.

The purpose of this chapter is to review the basic principles of drug prescribing in renal disease, to describe the changes in pharmacokinetics and pharmacodynamics with altered renal function, and to provide practical guidelines for dosing of drugs in these patients. The literature in this area is voluminous with the rapid growth in the number of new drugs released each year. However, no specific dosing formulas can be given confidently because factors of the individual patient, such as age, diabetes, sex, nutrition, and body fluid volume status, as well as many other variables, influence pharmacokinetics and pharmacodynamics considerably. The careful, expert therapist must know both the pertinent pharmacology and the patient's situation to administer drugs effectively and safely to a population of renal patients. Excellent reviews including mathematic and theoretic approaches to the subject exist.[1-9] We limit the present discussion to issues with which clinicians must deal in the care of renal patients.

## GENERAL PHARMACOKINETIC PRINCIPLES

The pharmacologic effect of any drug depends on the concentration of the parent drug or a metabolite at the tissue receptor site of action. Because of the complex way in which drugs distribute and are delivered to these sites, the prediction of serum drug concentrations and drug action is best facilitated by a mathematic analysis of the time course of a drug in the body (i.e., pharmacokinetics). A simplified scheme of pharmacokinetics as applied to the renal patient is shown in Figure 60–1. In deriving kinetic parameters from measured blood concentrations after a dose, the plasma versus time data can be fit to an equation with the least number of exponentials. This avoids the use of pharmacokinetic models, which by necessity have to make assumptions about compartments that cannot be verified in patients. From the area under the plasma concentration versus time curve and the area under the product of concentration and time versus time (first moment), the volume of distribution, total body clearance, and bioavailability can be directly calculated.

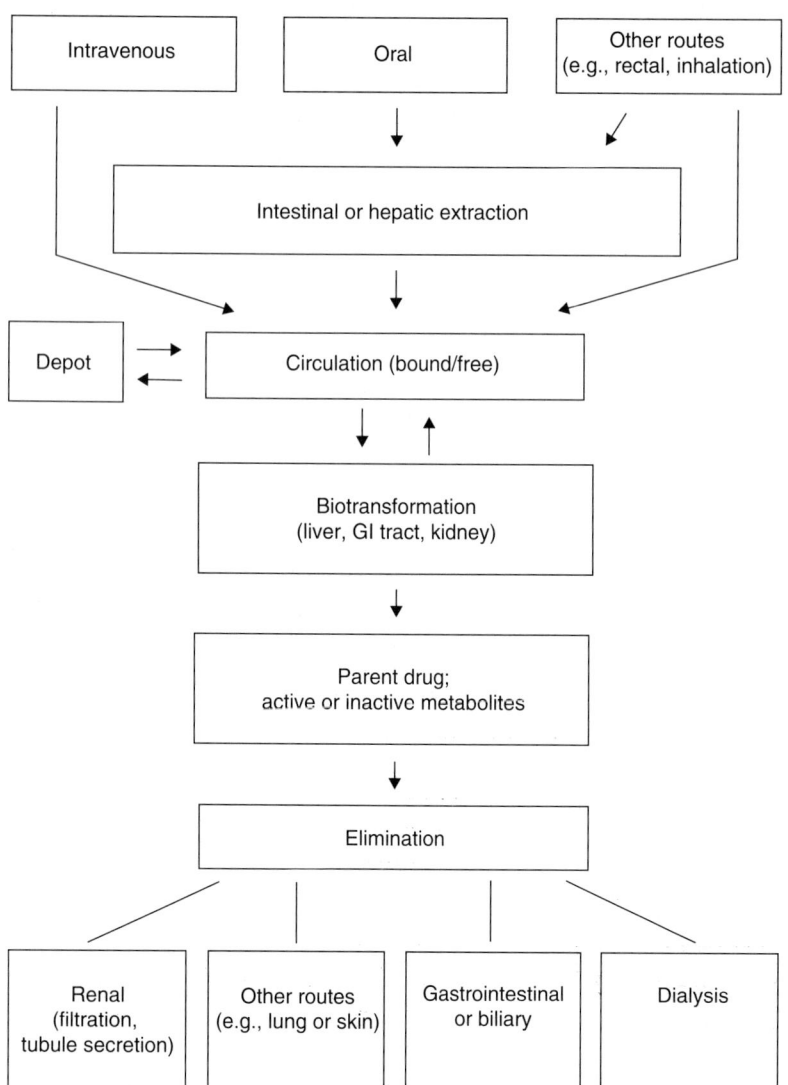

**Figure 60–1.** Schema of pharmacokinetics in renal patients.

## Absorption of Drugs

The bioavailability and absorption of a drug relate to the amount of drug that reaches the systemic circulation after oral administration. The kinetics of these effects are complex and vary with the physicochemical properties of the drug, its formulation and dosage form, the integrity of the absorptive surfaces, other substances in the gastrointestinal tract (food, other drugs), and presystemic biotransformation in the intestinal mucosa and liver (first-pass effect). As an example, erythromycin increases the bioavailability of the immunosuppressive drug cyclosporine by inhibition of intestinal and hepatic cytochrome P-450 biotransformation to less active drug metabolites.[10]

## Distribution of Drugs

A drug distributes in the body in a characteristic manner on the basis of its physicochemical properties and variables in the individual patient. The extent of this distribution is known as the apparent volume of distribution, which is equal to the volume of fluid in which the drug would need to be dissolved to give the observed plasma concentration. For this to be true, the assumption must of course be made that the body acts as a single homogeneous compartment. Because this is obviously not the case, the calculated apparent volume of distribution does not conform to any actual body fluid volume. The apparent volume of distribution ($V_d$) after absorption is equal to the fractional absorption of a dose (fxD) divided by the plasma concentration (c):

$$V_d = \frac{fxD}{c}$$

This parameter can be used to calculate predicted plasma concentrations if the dose fraction absorbed is known. Whereas the volume of distribution is relatively constant for a given drug, many of the patient-related factors, such as obesity, age, sex, thyroid function, renal function, and cardiac output, influence drug distribution. Highly lipid soluble drugs, such as diazepam, have a large volume of distribution with little retention of drug in the plasma. Drugs that are highly tissue bound also have a large volume of distribution. If tissue binding of drugs is decreased by renal disease (methotrexate, digoxin), a decreased volume of distribution results. Digoxin is highly bound to cardiac and other tissue; $Na^+$-$K^+$ transport enzymes account for its large volume of distribution of 300 to 500 L and low plasma concentrations measured in nanograms per milliliter. Transport inhibitors accumulating in the patient with renal dysfunction may displace digoxin from its tissue-binding sites, reducing volume of distribution.[11] In fact, some of these inhibitors may cross-react with the antidigoxin antibody used in therapeutic drug monitoring assays, producing "therapeutic" digoxin levels in patients not even taking the drug.

Plasma protein binding is an important determinant of drug distribution. Drugs that are highly bound to plasma proteins are largely confined to the vascular space and therefore usually have a volume of distribution less than 0.2 L/kg. Protein binding renders the drug pharmacologically inactive and metabolically inert by preventing it from getting to its site of action or metabolism. Factors that enhance protein binding include opposite charge attraction, pH, hydrophobic or hydrophilic environment, and van der Waals forces.

Certain conditions frequently associated with uremia may inhibit or enhance protein binding. Malnutrition and proteinuria lower serum protein levels. This increases the free fraction of drug because of saturation of the reduced number of available protein binding sites.[6] Uremic toxins may decrease the affinity of albumin for a variety of drugs[12–14] (Table 60–1). Acidic drugs (e.g., cephalosporins, imipenem, vancomycin, and ciprofloxacin) have a larger free fraction than do basic drugs such as tobramycin because of the chronic organic acidemia that accompanies renal failure (Vos MC, unpublished data, 1994). Organic acids compete with acidic drugs for certain protein binding sites. In contrast, uncomplicated uremia causes few alterations in the protein binding of basic drugs. Basic drugs bind more avidly to nonalbumin serum proteins than to albumin.[15, 16] The protein binding of basic drugs is often increased owing to elevated levels of the acute-phase reactant $\alpha_1$-acid glycoprotein, to which these basic drugs readily bind.[16, 17]

The influence of altered drug-protein binding on drug

handling may be difficult to predict. In general, the volume of distribution increases as drug-protein binding decreases. For any given drug level (bound plus unbound), the proportion of free or active drug will be increased when drug-protein binding is decreased. Because both drug elimination and pharmacologic activity are increased for any given dose, the plasma drug levels may be difficult to predict.

## Elimination of Drugs

The total body clearance of a drug is equal to the sum of all the individual organ clearances. Because plasma is the usual matrix sampled for drug assays, the total body clearance of drugs from the blood is often referred to synonymously as the plasma clearance.

$$C_p = C_r + C_{nr}$$

where $C_p$ is plasma clearance, $C_r$ is renal clearance, and $C_{nr}$ is nonrenal clearance. In the patient with renal dysfunction, there is an obvious diminution of the efficiency of the renal elimination route. Other pathways often compensate, leaving $C_p$ relatively unaltered. However, renal disease may also affect nonrenal drug clearance. The usual pathways of hepatic drug metabolism, such as oxidation, reduction, and hydrolysis, may be variably altered on a drug-to-drug basis, with some enzymatic reactions inhibited and others accelerated by induction of drug-metabolizing enzymes. The rates of sulfisoxazole acetylation, hydrocortisone reduction, cephalosporin hydrolysis, and propranolol oxidation are all slowed by uremia.[18] In addition, drug-drug interactions can influence drug metabolism either by competitively inhibiting metabolic processes or by enhancing biotransformation. Most drugs undergo biotransformation to more polar but less pharmacologically active compounds that require adequate renal function for elimination from the body. Other drugs are converted to metabolites that maintain pharmacologic activity when they accumulate in patients with renal dysfunction who have not had appropriate dosage reductions made. Some of these active metabolites are shown in Table 60–2.

The renal clearance of drugs is dependent on the processes of glomerular filtration and tubule transport. Unbound molecules of appropriately sized compounds (most therapeutic agents) easily pass the glomerular filtration barrier. Because plasma proteins are too large to pass through a normal glomerulus, only unbound and less ionized molecules easily transit this barrier. With glomerular disease and proteinuria, protein-bound molecules may move into the tubule fluid and effectively disappear from the plasma at accelerated rates. Furosemide, which usually gains access to luminal fluid by tubule secretion, may be bound to filtered albumin in nephrotic syndrome, which lessens its diuretic action.[19] Drugs with a large volume of distribution and low plasma concentrations are often not quantitatively excreted because the amount of drug actually excreted depends on renal blood flow, glomerular filtration rate (GFR), plasma level, and rate of nonrenal metabolism and elimination. When renal disease reduces nephron number, the kidney's ability to eliminate drugs declines in proportion to the decline in GFR. As patients progress toward end-stage

**TABLE 60–1. Drugs Known to Be Associated with Reduced Plasma Protein Binding in Renal Failure**

| Acids | Bases | Tissue Binding |
|---|---|---|
| Barbiturates | Diazepam | Cardiac glycosides |
| Clofibrate | Mexiletine | Methotrexate |
| Diazoxide | Triamterene | |
| Digitoxin | | |
| Furosemide | | |
| Methotrexate | | |
| Metolazone | | |
| Penicillins | | |
| Phenytoin | | |
| Probenecid | | |
| Salicylates | | |
| Sulfonamides | | |
| Warfarin | | |

**TABLE 60–2. Pharmacologically Active Metabolites of Common Drugs Accumulated in Renal Failure**

| Parent Drug | Metabolite | Pharmacologic Action of Metabolite |
|---|---|---|
| Acetohexamide | Hydroxyhexamide | Hypoglycemic |
| Allopurinol | Oxypurinol | Same as parent drug; enhanced desquamative skin eruptions due to xanthine oxidase inhibition |
| Azathioprine | 6-Mercaptopurine | Immunosuppressive |
| Clofibrate | Chlorophenoxyisobutyric acid | Increased skeletal muscle damage |
| Diazepam | Oxazepam | Anxiolytic |
| Lidocaine | Glycinexylidide | Central nervous system reactions including seizures |
| Meperidine | Normeperidine | Seizures |
| Nitroprusside | Thiocyanate | Central nervous system toxicity effects |
| Procainamide | N-Acetylprocainamide | Antiarrhythmic |
| Propranolol | 4-Hydroxypropranolol | β-Blocker |
| Rifampin | Desacetylrifampin | Antibiotic |
| Sulfonamides | Acetylated metabolites | Nausea, vomiting, skin reactions |

renal failure, drugs usually filtered and excreted accumulate, which produces a high prevalence of adverse reactions unless dosage adjustments are made.

The kidney can also serve to metabolize some drugs. Components of the cytochrome P-450 drug-metabolizing enzymes exist within renal epithelial cells. Endogenous vitamin D metabolism and exogenous insulin catabolism are examples of processes that decline as renal failure progresses.[20, 21]

Tubule transport and secretion of organic acids are affected by the accumulation of endogenous ligands in renal failure and competing acidic drugs. Drugs such as methotrexate, sulfonylureas, penicillins, and cephalosporins may have toxic effects because of this secretory competition as renal function declines. Diuretics require organic anion tubule secretory activity for drug delivery to luminal sites where they inhibit $Na^+$ and $Cl^-$ transport. Diminution of this pathway may cause syndromes of diuretic resistance. Some organic bases, such as cimetidine, procainamide, and ethambutol, also undergo tubule secretion. Competitive interference with these secretory processes can be observed with other organic bases. These tubule transport systems are found predominantly in the $S_2$ and $S_3$ segments of the proximal tubule. Passive reabsorption of some drugs based on urinary flow, urine pH, ionization, and lipid solubility may affect net drug excretion even after their filtration and tubule secretion. Thus, the physiologic circumstances of an individual patient, particularly with intercurrent acute illness, make generalizations about drug behavior a problem.

Most drugs in clinical practice or their metabolites are eliminated by first-order kinetic processes. The amount of drug eliminated per unit time is a fixed proportion of the body stores. The most common expression of drug elimination rate is the half-life ($t_{1/2}$). This is the time required for the concentration of a drug to decline by 50% after equilibration between plasma and tissue storage sites. The time for a drug to reach 95% of its steady-state concentration

after repetitive dosing is roughly equivalent to four to five half-lives. Conversely, after cessation of drug dosing, elimination will be 95% complete after four to five half-lives.

$$t_{1/2} = \frac{0.693}{K_r + K_m}$$

where $K_r$ is the renal elimination rate constant and $K_m$ is the metabolic (nonrenal) elimination rate constant. Thus, as renal function declines, $t_{1/2}$ values increase proportionally. The effects of renal disease on pharmacokinetics and pharmacodynamics are summarized in Table 60–3.

## DIALYSIS OF DRUGS

An important route of drug removal is through the dialysis membrane. High-efficiency, high-flux, and conventional hemodialyses differ because of membrane porosity, surface area, and flow rates of blood and dialysate. These factors influence drug handling. High-efficiency dialysis uses conventional "tight" membranes, large surface area, and high blood and dialysate flow rates. This strategy is designed to improve small-solute clearance such that the duration of treatment can be reduced. For middle- and large-molecular-size species, clearance is average to poor and is dependent on duration of dialysis.

Membranes with greater porosity allow substantial diffusive clearance of molecules in the middle- to large-molecular-size range. Because of the high hydraulic permeability intrinsic to these more "open" membranes, high-flux dialysis uses greater ultrafiltration rates to achieve maximal convective solute removal of middle- and large-molecular-size molecules.

Modification of clearances across a broad spectrum of molecular sizes is of particular interest to a discussion of drug clearance, because most drugs are in the small- to middle-molecular-size category. The adjustments made with short-time high-efficiency dialysis suggest that drug clearance may not vary from longer time conventional dialysis. Depending on the size of the drug, there may be significant differences in drug removal with high-flux dialysis.

Most studies of drug removal during dialysis were performed with use of conventional hemodialysis techniques. Specific data describing drug removal with highly permeable membranes are often based on observations noted during continuous hemofiltration or continuous hemodialysis. Drug removal with these therapies is discussed later. Some recommendations are based on extrapolation from data known about specific drugs that have been tested and from known clearance data of middle-molecular-size markers such as vitamin $B_{12}$ and inulin. To this end, drugs are considered solutes of variable water solubility, for which the principles for dialytic clearance apply. Table 60–4 summarizes the unique properties of drugs that affect their removal by dialysis.

### Drug Properties That Affect Dialyzability

**Molecular Size.** One of the most reliable predictors of drug dialyzability is drug molecular size.[22, 23] Drugs of more

**TABLE 60–3. Effect of Renal Disease on Pharmacokinetic and Pharmacodynamic Variables**

| Variable | Effect | Condition |
|---|---|---|
| Absorption | Decrease in uremia | Edema of gastrointestinal tract |
| | | Uremic nausea and vomiting |
| | | Autonomic neuropathy (diabetes, uremia) |
| | | Peritonitis with reduced peristalsis |
| | | Drug interactions—phosphate binders |
| Distribution | Higher free fraction of drugs in plasma in uremia | Acidic drugs with usual binding greater than 80% |
| | Lower concentrations of total drug | Lower "therapeutic" levels of phenytoin |
| | Lower volume of distribution of digoxin | Need smaller loading doses |
| | Loss of binding proteins | Nephrotic syndrome, malnutrition |
| Metabolism | Decreased rate of metabolism | Multiple drugs (see Table 60–2) |
| | Accelerated drug oxidation | Induced cytochrome P-450 metabolism of phenytoin |
| | Decreased hepatic first-pass effect | Propranolol |
| | Decreased renal drug metabolism | Decreased 1,25-dihydroxyvitamin D hydroxylation |
| | | Decreased insulin metabolism |
| Excretion | Decreased parent drug excretion | Multiple drugs |
| | Decreased excretion of active metabolites | Multiple drugs |
| Increased tissue drug sensitivity | Altered drug distribution at tissue receptor sites | Central nervous system drugs |
| | Metabolic effects of renal disease | Acidemia and hyperkalemia affect cardiac drugs |
| Altered metabolic loads | Hyperkalemia | Salt substitutes, $K^+$-sparing diuretics, β-blockers, angiotensin-converting enzyme inhibitors |
| | Hypermagnesemia | Antacids, laxatives |
| | $Na^+$ loads | Antibiotics: penicillins |
| | Nitrogen | Steroids, tetracyclines |
| | Impaired water excretion | Multiple drugs |

than 1000 daltons depend less on diffusion and more on convection for dialytic clearance. Molecular volume is determined by the weight, shape, steric hindrance, and charge of the species in question. If a drug cannot fit through a dialysis membrane pore because of its geometric proportions, it is reflected and cannot be cleared by the dialyzer. There is an inverse semilogarithmic relationship between dialysis clearance and molecular size.[24]

**Protein Binding.** The binding of drugs to circulating plasma proteins is another predictor of a drug's dialyzability. As discussed earlier, a number of factors, including uremia, may influence the degree of drug-protein binding. Drugs that are highly protein bound have a low proportion of the drug available for removal by dialysis.

Heparin administration during dialysis stimulates lipoprotein lipase, which increases levels of free fatty acids.[15, 25, 26] Free fatty acids compete with tryptophan, sulfonamides, salicylates, phenylbutazone, phenytoin, thiopentone, and valproic acid for protein binding sites, causing an increase in the free fraction of drug during and after the heparin period. To illustrate the complexity of drug-protein

**TABLE 60–4. Drug Properties That Affect Dialytic Clearance**

Molecular size
Protein binding
Volume of distribution
Charge
Water or lipid solubility
Membrane binding
Alternative excretory pathway

interactions, free fatty acid may displace cefamandole but may enhance the binding of other cephalosporins, such as cephalothin or cefoxitin.[27] Golper and associates[28] have shown that free fatty acids increase the free fraction of phenytoin, a highly protein bound drug. Thus, greater clearances by dialysis would be anticipated.

**Volume of Distribution.** When the volume of distribution is large, drug availability to the circulation, and hence to the dialyzer, is minimal and the half-life is long.[15] Drugs with a volume of distribution less than 1 L/kg are more likely to be dialyzable, assuming other characteristics such as molecular size and protein binding are favorable for drug removal. Drugs with a volume of distribution between 1 and 2 L/kg have marginal dialytic clearances, and substantial drug removal is unlikely if the volume of distribution is greater than 2 L/kg.

Despite rapid extracellular solute clearances with short-time high-flux or high-efficiency dialysis, intracellular equilibration with extracellular fluid can be slow, especially with middle- to large-molecular-size solutes.[29] This is probably related to lipid solubility of the drug and tissue compartmentalization. Postdialysis intracellular concentrations may vary by only 1% to 2%.[30] Consequently, there is a drug concentration gradient between intracellular and extracellular fluid. There may be a posthemodialysis rebound of 10% to 25% with intercompartmental equilibration.[31] Higher ultrafiltration rates can severely aggravate this phenomenon. Vancomycin's rebound was 50% higher than the initial postdialysis drug concentration and highly variable regarding the time to reach a peak.[32] Thus, it would be difficult to predict this phenomenon for a specific patient, and we advise physicians to observe drug levels closely.

**Drug–Red Blood Cell Binding.** Drugs may partition

into red blood cells (RBCs). Ultrafiltration during dialysis raises the hematocrit, which complicates the determination of intradialytic drug clearance.[33] The proper reference value is either the whole blood concentration or the plasma concentration. This is particularly relevant to the clearance of ethambutol, a drug known to partition into the RBC.[34] Drugs that have a partition coefficient (whole blood/plasma concentration ratio) exceeding unity (e.g., procainamide, glutethimide, and acetaminophen) may have decreased clearances owing to hemoconcentration at the end of dialysis.[15] Thus, for drugs that partition into RBCs, total dialytic clearance may be reduced in these hemoconcentrated states. Furthermore, the issue of rapid re-equilibration between RBC drug and plasma drug becomes more important.

These observations were made before the routine use of erythropoietin. Higher predialysis hematocrits will result in greater RBC partitioning and in less free drug, with the potential consequences described before. Even for a drug with low RBC partitioning, clearance may also be decreased in the setting of higher hematocrits because, as for all plasma solutes, dialytic clearance is dependent on delivery of plasma to the dialyzer.

In summary, drugs and metabolites that have a small molecular size, have a small volume of distribution, and are highly water soluble are more likely to be eliminated by dialysis. A dialytic clearance that increases plasma clearance by more than 30% is considered significant.[35, 36]

## Dialytic Properties That Affect Drug Clearance

These can be divided into three categories summarized in Table 60–5: properties of the dialyzer, properties of the dialysate, and technique of dialysis.

**Membrane Materials.** Concern about the possible importance of larger molecular size uremic toxins has led to the development of membranes with a wide range of solute permeabilities. Dialysis membranes are fabricated from natural and synthetic polymers, including cellulose, cellulose acetate, polysulfone, polyamide, polyacrylonitrile (e.g., AN69), and polymethyl methacrylate.

With polysulfone membranes, trace quantities of albumin can appear in the dialysate.[37] Clearances of vancomycin vary with different membranes.[31, 38–40] AN69 and polysul-

fone membranes yield the greatest clearance, whereas cuprophane has minimal clearance of vancomycin under similar conditions.[38, 40] Gentamicin clearance is greater with a cuprammonium rayon membrane than with a saponified cellulose ester membrane.[41]

**Surface Area.** Small-solute dialyzability is dependent on the concentration gradient between blood and dialysate, which is maximized by increasing flow rates or by increasing surface area, dispersing the undialyzed blood to areas of fresh dialysate. These principles are applied to high-flux and high-efficiency dialysis. As molecular size increases, diffusivity is limited by the membrane's pore size, and the clearance of the molecule becomes more dependent on convection. The hydraulic permeability of high-flux membranes exceeds that of conventional membranes, enhancing convective clearances of larger molecules. When hydraulic permeability limits are achieved, a larger surface area becomes the most influential factor. For polyacrylonitrile, polymethyl methacrylate, and polysulfone dialyzers, surface area and ultrafiltration have a great effect on the clearances of $\beta_2$-microglobulin and $PO_4^{3-}$, two poorly dialyzable species.[42] This is not a new concept. Increasing surface area has been the mainstay of a variety of techniques to enhance clearances.[43, 44] For example, the amount of vancomycin removed by high-flux dialysis was correlated to membrane surface area.[38] Furthermore, surface area is a major determinant of the ultrafiltration rate.

**Drug-Membrane Charge Interaction and Membrane Binding.** The negative charge of polyacrylonitrile membrane repels anionic solutes, such as gentamicin and doxycycline.[45] Theoretic estimates of gentamicin clearance did not correlate well with clinical observations during dialysis with polyacrylonitrile filters.[46] It is possible that the negative charge of the membrane retarded gentamicin clearance. Another possibility for decreased aminoglycoside clearance could be drug adsorption to the dialysis membrane.[47–49] Drug-membrane binding has also been demonstrated in the absence of proteins during experimental conditions of continuous arteriovenous hemofiltration.[28, 50–52]

**Diffusion.** Drug diffusivity decreases as molecular size increases.[53] Diffusive clearance through conventional dialysis membranes is negligible for molecules larger than 1000 daltons. Countercurrent flow and high blood and dialysate flow augment the concentration gradient between blood and dialysate, enhancing the efficiency of diffusion. This is particularly important for drugs in the lower ranges of middle molecular size (e.g., aminoglycosides at 600 daltons). Small-solute clearances increase considerably as dialysate and blood flow increase and are essentially flow rate limited.[6] For larger molecules, because their size limits the rate of diffusion through the membrane pores, the blood-to-dialysate concentration gradient remains high. Flow rates have less influence for the diffusion of middle- or large-size molecules. However, the surface area and hydraulic permeability become important, allowing convective removal (see the next section). While convective removal occurs, the addition of high ultrafiltration rates during high-flux hemodialysis causes mixing of the ultrafiltrate and the dialysate. Under certain conditions, this diminishes the concentration gradient and the diffusive clearance of solutes.[16, 54–56]

**TABLE 60–5. Dialysis Properties That Affect Drug Clearance**

**Hemodialyzer Properties**
Pore size
Blood flow rate
Surface area
Membrane binding

**Dialysate Properties**
Dialysate flow rate
Solute concentration
pH
Temperature

**Convection**

**Convection.** Convection is defined as the ultrafiltration bulk flow from the blood to the dialysate. Convection ceases when the permeability of the membrane is reached, the negative transmembrane pressure causes collapse of the dialysate compartment, or the membrane ruptures. Ultrafiltration affects all sizes of molecules, but its effect is more evident with large molecules because of their poor diffusion. Henderson and associates[53, 57–59] have demonstrated that convection removes large molecules more readily than does diffusion. With use of cellulosic membranes, removal of solutes greater than 1000 daltons generally requires ultrafiltration. Depending on the membrane, even during ultrafiltration, molecules greater than 2000 daltons are partially reflected by the membrane.[60]

Diffusion dominates convection in most cases of solute removal. This is especially noted for small-molecular-size substances, and less so for middle- and large-size molecules, whose clearance is dependent on convection. Increasing blood flow does not influence the clearance of middle-size or larger molecules.[60]

Membrane-protein binding can adversely affect ultrafiltration. Vincent and co-workers[61] have shown predictable deterioration of ultrafiltration due to protein binding to the membrane. This is probably related to alteration in the porosity of the membrane by protein binding or reduction in the surface area. Protein layering against the dialysis membrane (protein concentration polarization) creates a physical barrier that "widens the membrane." Protein at the membrane surface results in increased osmotic and oncotic activity on the blood side that ultimately retards convection.

## CLINICAL APPLICATION OF THESE PRINCIPLES

**Example: Vancomycin.** Bastani and colleagues[39] first compared vancomycin and urea clearances through dialyzers of different membrane material but with equal surface areas and flow rates. Unlike urea clearance, vancomycin clearance was highest with AN69 membranes, intermediate with cellulose acetate, and lowest with cuprophane. These results have been corroborated.[40] Torras and associates[62] demonstrated similar results and further showed that by increasing blood flow rates from 250 to 350 mL/min through an AN69 dialyzer, vancomycin clearance increased another 50%. Up to 200 mg of vancomycin could be removed during a high-flux hemodialysis session. De Bock and co-workers[31] removed at least that much by use of a cellulose acetate dialyzer under standard operating conditions.

Lanese and colleagues[38] examined the relationship among membrane surface area, ultrafiltration coefficients (hydraulic permeability), vitamin $B_{12}$ clearance, and removal of vancomycin. A tight linear relationship between vitamin $B_{12}$ clearance and vancomycin clearance was demonstrated. They concluded that the correlation between the clearance of vitamin $B_{12}$ and the percentage of vancomycin removed may be the best available data in the absence of specific dialyzer vancomycin removal rates. They derived the following expression for vancomycin removal during dialysis:

$$\% \text{ vancomycin removal during dialysis} = (0.09C_{B_{12}} - 1.5)(0.75 + 0.001Q_B)\text{time}$$

where $C_{B_{12}}$ is the manufacturer's reported vitamin $B_{12}$ clearance, $Q_B$ is dialyzer blood flow, and time is duration of dialysis in hours. Such a mathematic approach is possible for other medications.

## CONCLUSIONS

Certain generalizations may be offered. High-efficiency dialysis uses tight membranes. Urea clearance is high because flow rates and surface areas are increased above those seen in conventional dialysis. These adjustments allow a shortened dialysis time, whereas overall dialysis delivery is probably unchanged from conventional dialysis. Therefore, drug dosing recommendations for conventional dialysis will probably apply reliably to high-efficiency dialysis. This will need to be confirmed in clinical trials.

For high-flux dialysis, several variables make generalizations more difficult. For example, whereas the open membranes used in this technique may demonstrate greater diffusivity and convectivity (and thus clearance) for middle-molecular-size species, the shortened dialysis time may reduce overall clearance. The larger the molecule, the longer it takes to remove it, no matter what membrane is used. Even though most drugs are either small molecules less than 500 daltons or in the lowest ranges of middle molecular size, this principle of time and clearance applies. In addition, any technique that uses shortened dialysis times jeopardizes the clearance of molecules that have a substantial degree of tissue binding or intracellular deposition. Rapid depletion through the dialyzer of unbound or extracellular drug cannot be replaced rapidly from protein-bound, tissue-bound, or intracellular stores. Therefore, the openness of the membrane and the shortening of dialysis time may counteract each other with regard to overall drug clearance. Some membranes, particularly AN69, bind drugs more readily than do other high-flux membranes. Therefore, until the actual studies are performed to define drug removal during high-flux dialysis, we must remain cautious in our predictions.

## Drug Removal During Continuous Renal Replacement Therapies

Continuous renal replacement therapies include hemofiltration and hemodialysis. Because these therapies are generally reserved for critically ill patients, knowledge of drug disposition in this setting is imperative for avoidance of pharmacologic errors.

**Hemofiltration.** Solute removal during hemofiltration is convective. The sieving coefficient (S) is the solute concentration in the ultrafiltrate divided by the solute concentration in the retentate. It is the mathematic expression of the solute's ability to convectively permeate a membrane. An S value of 1 states that the solute freely passes; an S value of 0 describes complete rejection. Colton and co-workers[63] have shown that a reasonable approximation is

$$S = \frac{UF}{(A + V)2} = \frac{2UF}{A + V}$$

where A, V, and UF represent the arterial, venous, and ultrafiltrate concentrations, respectively. Golper and associates[64] have further shown that under continuous hemofiltration conditions, S = UF/A, which eliminates the need for a venous sample. Under conditions of continuous hemofiltration, S will generally be constant.[28, 65, 66] Furthermore, sieving is independent of blood flow.[28, 66, 67] During hemofiltration, clearance is the product of S times the ultrafiltration rate. Because S is constant, clearance is linearly related to the ultrafiltration rate. Thus, the most important way to describe drug handling in hemofiltration is to determine its S value.

Kronfol and colleagues[50–52] have demonstrated that in the absence of confounding proteins, there are drug-membrane interactions during hemofiltration. S values for several drugs through polyacrylonitrile and polyamide membranes were significantly different from those through polysulfone. Drug charge can affect either convective or diffusive transport, depending on the nature of the drug-membrane charge interaction. The polycationic antibiotic gentamicin *in saline* had an S value through Amicon polysulfone of only 0.94.[28] Lysaght[68] has shown that even a cation as small as $Na^+$ has an S value less than 1. The introduction of a negative charge on macromolecules can decrease sieving during hemofiltration.[69] However, small anions such as $Cl^-$ and $HCO_3^-$ have S values greater than 1,[70, 71] thought to be due to the Gibbs-Donnan effect of circulating proteins. Penicillins and cephalosporins are anionic antibiotics that may demonstrate this phenomenon during hemofiltration (Table 60–6).

Drugs bind to dialysis membranes as discussed before.[45] When aminoglycosides bind to membranes, S is low for the first few minutes after exposure, but as the binding sites saturate, S rises. A Biospal filter binds 10 to 20 mg of tobramycin.[49]

Binding to nonultrafilterable plasma proteins plays a dominant role in determining a drug's convective transport. Protein-bound drug will not be filtered. Many factors affect drug-protein binding, as discussed earlier. As proteins collect along the membrane (protein concentration polarization), the molar concentrations of drug and proteins are changed, contributing to altered protein binding. The unbound drug is the pharmacologically active fraction. If there is displacement, the pharmacologic effect, metabolism, and removal will be enhanced.

Table 60–6 displays the S value and unbound fraction (α) of drugs whose sieving coefficient has been determined from either our experience or the literature. There is a significant correlation between S and α. Kroh and associates[72] have shown that an even tighter correlation occurs when S is defined as AUCf/AUCp, where AUCf and AUCp represent the areas under the time-drug concentration curves for filtrate (f) and plasma (p), respectively.

The role of molecular size (weight and steric hindrance) on membrane transport has been extensively studied and was discussed before. For most drugs in clinical use, molecular size will not be an issue for removal during hemofiltration. The membrane molecular size cutoffs exceed the molecular size of the drugs. During hemodialysis, molecular size is even more important.

**TABLE 60–6. Drug Sieving Coefficients (S) in Continuous Arteriovenous Hemofiltration Compared with Unbound Fraction (α)**

| Antibiotics | | | Other | | |
|---|---|---|---|---|---|
| *Drug* | S | α | *Drug* | S | α |
| Amikacin | 0.9 | 0.9 | N-Acetylprocainamide | 0.9 | 0.9 |
| Amphotericin B | 0.3 | 0.1 | Bromide | 1.0 | 1.0 |
| Ampicillin | 0.7 | 0.8 | Chlordiazepoxide | 0.05 | 0.05 |
| Cefoperazone | 0.3 | 0.1 | Cisplatin | 0.1 | 0.1 |
| Cefotaxime | 0.62 | 0.6 | Clofibrate | 0.06 | 0.04 |
| Cefoxitin | 0.6 | 0.5 | Cyclosporine | 0.6 | 0.1 |
| Ceftazidime | 0.9 | 0.9 | Diathybarbital | 1.0 | 0.9 |
| Ceftriaxone | 0.8 | 0.1 | Diazepam | 0.02 | 0.02 |
| Cephapirin | 1.5 | 0.6 | Digitoxin | 0.1 | 0.1 |
| Cilastatin | 0.8 | 0.6 | Digoxin | 0.9 | 0.8 |
| Ciprofloxacin | 0.76 | 0.7 | Famotidine | 0.7 | 0.8 |
| Clindamycin | 1.0 | 0.4 | Glibenclamide | 0.6 | 0.01 |
| Doxycycline | 0.4 | 0.2 | Glutethimide | 0.02 | 0.5 |
| Erythromycin | 0.4 | 0.3 | Lidocaine | 0.2 | 0.4 |
| Gentamicin | 0.8 | 0.9 | Metamizole | 0.4 | 0.4 |
| Imipenem | 1.0 | 0.8 | Nitrazepam | 0.08 | 0.1 |
| Metronidazole | 0.8 | 0.8 | Nomifensine | 0.7 | 0.4 |
| Mezlocillin | 0.7 | 0.7 | Oxazepam | 0.1 | 0.1 |
| Nafcillin | 0.5 | 0.2 | Phenobarbital | 0.8 | 0.6 |
| Netilmicin | 0.9 | 0.9 | Phenytoin | 0.4 | 0.2 |
| Oxacillin | 0.02 | 0.05 | Procainamide | 0.9 | 0.9 |
| Penicillin | 0.7 | 0.5 | Pyrithyldione | 0.4 | — |
| Streptomycin | 0.3 | 0.6 | Ranitidine | 0.8 | 0.85 |
| Sulfamethoxazole | 0.9 | 0.6 | Theophylline | 0.9 | 0.85 |
| Tobramycin | 0.8 | 0.9 | | | |
| Vancomycin | 0.8 | 0.9 | | | |

**Drug Removal During Hemofiltration.** Inulin readily traverses polysulfone hemofilter membranes.[67, 73, 74] Because virtually all therapeutic agents have a molecular size less than that of inulin, one can reasonably assume that these drugs will permeate these membranes limited mostly by the extent of their protein binding. Protein-binding data are available, usually from studies of healthy people.[75] Slight discrepancies may arise when those data are compared with data from critically ill patients.

One can measure the removal of drug during hemofiltration by multiplying the ultrafiltrate drug concentration by the filtration rate. Because (arterial) plasma levels are usually required for clinical management, one could calculate the ultrafiltrate concentration (UF) from the arterial concentration (A) by the formula

$$UF = A\alpha$$

where the protein binding is *assumed* to be normal.[75] The following summarizes the technique to determine drug removal from continuous arteriovenous hemofiltration:

1. Determine steady-state arterial concentration (A).
2. Determine fraction *not* bound to protein ($\alpha$).[31]
3. Determine filtration rate.
4. Amount removed = A × unbound fraction × filtration rate.

The arterial sample should represent a steady-state level. The ideal time to obtain it is halfway between maintenance doses after at least three half-lives; $t_{1/2}$ data are also available.[75]

**Drug Removal During Continuous Hemodialysis.** During continuous hemodialysis, drug removal occurs mostly by diffusion. Protein binding still plays a role in that unbound drug is more diffusible than bound drug. Drug diffusivity was discussed earlier. Vincent and co-workers[22] have shown that a drug's diffusive mass transfer coefficient through open membranes during continuous dialysis is dependent on molecular size according to the formula

$$K_d/K_{dc} = (MW/113)^{-0.42}$$

where $K_d$ and $K_{dc}$ are the diffusive mass transfer coefficients for the drug and creatinine, respectively, and MW is the drug's molecular size.

During continuous therapies performed with venovenous access and blood flows of 125 to 250 mL/min, urea and creatinine clearances are 20 to 30 mL/min, corresponding to a GFR of 20 to 30 mL/min. Because the therapy is continuous, one should empirically dose drugs for a GFR of 20 to 30 mL/min.

**Supplemental Doses.** Drug levels may be a useful tool for determining supplemental doses for continuous therapies when the desired level is known. The presently observed level (present level) is subtracted from the level one wishes to achieve (desired level), leaving the *difference level,* all in the same units. The difference level times the volume of distribution times the body weight in kilograms gives the amount of drug needed to boost the present level to the desired level.

This method is useful for administering any drug whose level is available and whose volume of distribution is known. It is especially applicable to the setting of continuous therapies when the amount of drug removed is not clearly known and the clinician has only drug levels for assessment of the pharmacologic status of the patient. Volume of distribution data are readily available.[74]

This is the recommended approach. Proper management of critically ill patients in the intensive care unit demands the rapid availability of drug levels for most agents employed in this setting that are not managed by titration or have narrow therapeutic indices. For those agents whose levels are not available, these principles should help the clinician approximate losses.

## Drug Removal by Peritoneal Dialysis

Overall, the elimination capacity of peritoneal dialysis for most drugs administered orally or systemically is low.[76] Many of the same drug properties that affect removal by hemodialysis also apply to peritoneal dialysis. For significant removal to occur, the drug must generally have a low volume of distribution, low protein binding, and minimal removal by alternative routes of drug elimination. An important limiting factor for the elimination of drugs by continuous ambulatory peritoneal dialysis is the low flow rate of the peritoneal dialysate (averaging approximately 10 L/d or 7 mL/min). It may be anticipated that greater drug removal could potentially occur with higher dialysate flow rates, such as with intermittent peritoneal dialysis or cyclic peritoneal dialysis. Drug movement may occur in either direction across the peritoneal membrane. The intraperitoneal route of drug administration is particularly useful for the treatment of peritonitis because the majority of antibiotics administered intraperitoneally for the treatment of peritonitis are significantly absorbed into the systemic circulation. This should not be surprising in view of the low volume of distribution in the peritoneal cavity and the low concentration of protein available for drug binding.

## PRESCRIBING FOR THE PATIENT WITH RENAL DYSFUNCTION

A stepwise process in thinking about drug prescribing for individual patients is outlined here.

## Assessment of Renal Function

Until an accurate, convenient, and readily available test for measuring GFR becomes routinely available, the endogenous creatinine clearance must suffice. To determine the creatinine clearance ($C_{cr}$) from serum creatinine concentration without urine collection, the Cockcroft and Gault formula is convenient.[77]

$$C_{cr} = \frac{(140 - \text{age [y]})(\text{lean body weight [kg]})}{72 \times \text{serum creatinine (mg/dL)}}$$

For women, the calculated value is multiplied by 0.85. The use of this formula implies that the patient is in a steady state with respect to serum creatinine concentration. There is no accurate clinical method to determine GFR when renal function is rapidly changing, and thus it is safest to assume that the GFR is less than 10 mL/min in acute renal failure so that overdosage is avoided.

## Does Drug Dose Need to Be Adjusted?

Drugs or their pharmacologically active metabolites that are normally excreted by the kidney require major dose adjustments in renal failure. These adjustments involve either interval extension between doses or dose size reduction at the usual intervals between doses.

## Loading Doses

Loading doses are intended to generate a therapeutic steady-state drug level within a short period. Despite renal failure, the loading dose is usually not different from normal. Loading doses can be calculated if the volume of distribution and desired peak level are known. This is discussed later.

## Maintenance Doses

Maintenance doses are used to sustain a therapeutic level when they are administered subsequent to a loading dose. In the absence of a loading dose, maintenance doses will achieve 90% of their steady-state level in 3.3 half-lives. Maintenance doses may be modified in patients with renal failure by the interval extension method, which calls for lengthening the time between doses, corresponding to the extent of delayed excretion or metabolism. This method is more practical for drugs with long half-lives. Alternatively, the dosage reduction method can be used. In this strategy, the clinician reduces the amount of each dose, leaving the interval between doses the same as usual. This method usually sustains a more constant blood level. For antibiotics, this has been formalized by use of percentages of normal creatinine clearance as calculated from the patient's estimated creatinine clearance by the Cockcroft and Gault formula.[5]

## Supplemental Dose for Dialysis Removal

Supplemental doses may be required if significant removal of the drug occurs with dialysis. As discussed earlier, drugs of less than 500 daltons with minimal protein binding and a small volume of distribution may have significant elimination by the various dialytic modalities. In general, dialysis clearance must increase plasma clearance in a particular patient by 30% to 50% to be clinically significant.

## Blood Drug Levels to Monitor Therapy

Blood, serum, and plasma drug concentrations may not be equivalent, usually depending primarily on RBC com-

partmentalization (e.g., cyclosporine). Thus, levels can be properly interpreted only if the dosage schedule is known (amount, timing, and route of administration). A peak level is usually obtained 1 to 2 hours after oral administration and 30 minutes after parenteral administration. It reflects the highest level achieved after the rapid distribution phase of a drug and before any substantial elimination has occurred. A trough level is obtained just before the next dose and better reflects the total body clearance of the drug.

Drug levels are a valuable tool when used properly. This demands that the clinician know what level is desired. If one can measure drug levels and knows the volume of distribution and the therapeutic level one wishes to achieve, the amount of drug administered in any supplemental dose can be calculated. Subtract the present drug level from the desired drug level, which gives the difference level. The supplemental dose is difference level × volume of distribution × body weight in kilograms. For loading doses, the desired level is the desired peak level; the present level is zero. The most frequent use of this formula is to supplement a dose using the trough level as the present level and the therapeutic level as the desired level.

## Miscellaneous Drug Concerns: Drug-Drug Interactions, Metabolic Loads, and Interference with Laboratory Tests

No clinician can remember all possible clinically relevant drug-drug interactions. As examples, many drugs displace warfarin from its protein binding sites, enhancing anticoagulant activity. In renal failure, protein binding is altered in unpredictable ways, and drug-drug interactions are even more likely to occur. In renal failure, independently of protein binding, aminoglycoside antibiotics and carbenicillin-type antibiotics interact when there are high concentrations of each, such that the biologic activity and blood concentrations of the aminoglycosides are reduced. Phosphate-binding antacids impair the gut absorption of several drugs, such as digoxin, many quinoline antibiotics, and tetracycline. Any drug-drug interaction may have adverse consequences, so the clinician must at least entertain these possibilities.

Aberrant laboratory results are not an infrequent occurrence in ill patients and can lead to erroneous therapeutic and diagnostic decisions. Often a drug or metabolite alters the actual measurement of the laboratory test, but many drugs can interfere with tests through their pharmacologic activity. Examples of these laboratory test interferences that are pertinent to nephrologists are listed in Table 60–7.

## GUIDELINES FOR PRESCRIBING SPECIFIC DRUGS IN RENAL DISEASE

Approximately two thirds of all drugs used in clinical practice are excreted completely or partially by the kidney. Knowledge of the renal handling of specific drugs and the potential effects of renal insufficiency on other aspects of

**TABLE 60–7. Drug Interference with Laboratory Tests in Nephrology**

| Test | Drug | Effect |
|---|---|---|
| Serum creatinine | Ascorbic acid | Elevates total chromogen |
| | p-Aminohippurate | Elevates total chromogen |
| | Methyldopa/levodopa | Reducing agents interfere with autoanalyzer measurement; increases creatinine when blood level of methyldopa > 2 mg/mL |
| | Trimethoprim | Increases by competition for tubule secretion |
| | Acetylsalicylic acid | May increase by secretory competition |
| | Cefoxitin | Increases by interference with Jaffé reaction |
| | Cimetidine | Increases by secretory competition |
| Changes in urine color | Rifampin | Red-brown |
| | Sulfasalazine | Red-brown |
| | Phenothiazines | Red-brown |
| | Metronidazole | Darkens on standing |
| | Methyldopa | Darkens on standing |
| | Nitrofurantoin | Darkens on standing |
| | Amitriptyline | Blue-green |
| | Triamterene | Blue-green |
| Urinary protein determinations | Aminosalicylic acid | False-positive reaction with dipstick |
| | Acetylsalicylic acid | False-positive reaction with dipstick |
| | Cephalosporins | False-positive reaction with dipstick |
| | Contrast media | False-positive reaction with dipstick |
| | Penicillins | False-positive reaction with dipstick |
| | Sulfonamides | False-positive reaction with dipstick |
| | Acetazolamide | False-positive reaction with dipstick |
| | Tolbutamide | False-positive reaction with dipstick |
| | Tolmetin | Salicylic acid method only |

pharmacokinetics is crucial for optimal efficacy and safety of drug therapy in the patient with renal disease. In this section, the effects of renal disease on the pharmacokinetics of specific drugs are discussed and guidelines for drug dosing provided. These should be viewed as only first approximations that will require modification for individual patients, depending on comorbid conditions, clinical response, plasma drug levels, and side effects.

The drugs are grouped into categories primarily on the basis of their therapeutic actions. General comments about each group of drugs precede the dosing tables for each section. Drugs are listed in alphabetical order by generic name under appropriate subdivisions within the tables. These tables are not meant to be all-inclusive, but rather represent drugs in common use in the United States. The reader is referred to Seyffart[7] for more comprehensive listings of drug dosing in renal failure.

Specific dosing guidelines based on the patient's renal function (GFR of less than 10 mL/min and GFR of 10 to 50 mL/min) are provided for each drug. Unless otherwise noted, one can assume that dose modification is not necessary for patients with GFRs greater than 50 mL/min. Occasionally, however, dose adjustments are recommended for milder degrees of renal dysfunction, particularly for those drugs with narrow therapeutic/toxic ratios. The assumption is made that hepatic function is normal and that the patient is not receiving drugs influencing hepatic metabolism. For reference, the usual dosage range or average dose prescribed for patients with normal renal function is provided for each drug. In most cases, standard loading doses are given to patients with renal insufficiency when rapid achievement of therapeutic drug levels is desirable.

Alterations in extracellular fluid volume may necessitate a change in loading dose, particularly for those drugs with a narrow therapeutic/toxic ratio.

The maintenance dose regimen may be modified by extending the interval between doses, reducing the dose, or some combination of the two methods. Ideally, plasma drug levels should be maintained within a range that is therapeutic and nontoxic. As discussed earlier, the dosage reduction method tends to produce more constant blood levels, whereas the interval extension method allows a more convenient and less costly dosing schedule. The dosing tables provide guidelines for maintenance dosing in patients with renal insufficiency. If the interval extension method is used (I), the number of hours between doses is provided, whereas the percentage of the usual prescribed dose is noted for the dosage reduction method (D). The importance of accurate assessment of renal function is again emphasized. The serum creatinine concentration may underestimate the degree of renal insufficiency, particularly in malnourished or elderly individuals. Use of the Cockcroft and Gault equation or direct measurement of creatinine clearance will allow more accurate assessment of renal function.

As discussed before, the removal of drugs by dialysis is dependent on a number of factors including size of the drug, degree of protein binding, volume of distribution, and dialysis membrane characteristics. The requirement for supplemental dosing after hemodialysis and special dosing considerations for peritoneal dialysis and continuous renal replacement therapies are outlined in the tables. Unless otherwise noted, the need for supplemental dosing after hemodialysis is based on conventional membranes. Relatively few drugs are significantly removed by peritoneal dialysis.[76] In general, increasing the dose (or decreasing the interval) to that recommended for patients with a GFR of 10 to 50 mL/min is recommended if significant removal occurs. Most of the data for drug removal with continuous renal replacement therapies are derived from studies of patients undergoing continuous arteriovenous hemofiltration.[78] For continuous venovenous hemodialysis, empirical dosing for a GFR of 20 to 30 mL/min is appropriate because urea and creatinine clearances are within this range at blood flows of 125 to 250 mL/min. For many drugs, direct data are not available on drug removal by dialysis. If data are not available, the likelihood of removal is assessed on the basis of the degree of protein binding and volume of distribution.

## Antimicrobial Agents

Infectious complications are common in both acute and chronic renal failure and represent an important source of morbidity and mortality.[79, 80] Early recognition of infection and achievement of therapeutic plasma drug levels are crucial for optimal efficacy of antimicrobial treatment. Many antimicrobial drugs have altered pharmacokinetics in renal insufficiency and thus require dosage modification. The risk of toxic effect is increased in the patient with renal insufficiency and may at least in part be due to accumulation of the parent drug or its metabolites.[81] A thorough understanding of the effects of renal insufficiency on pharmacokinetics of the antimicrobial agents is vital for maximal therapeutic efficacy and reduction of toxicity. Table 60–8 provides specific dosing guidelines for individual antimicrobial agents. Several areas that require emphasis or further explanation are discussed in the following.

The initial selection of antimicrobial agents is often empirical and based on the type of infection and likely infecting pathogens. The potential toxicity of the agent, the possible interactions with other drugs, and the patient's allergy history are also important factors to consider. Culture results are key because antibiotic coverage can often be narrowed to less toxic agents once a firm identification and sensitivity pattern have been established.

Depending on the agent chosen, one or more pharmacokinetic parameters may be altered in the patient with renal insufficiency. Decreased absorption may occur for some agents, such as tetracycline[82] or ciprofloxacin,[83] if they are taken in conjunction with antacids or phosphate binders. Decreased protein binding may contribute to the increased risk of neurotoxicity for the β-lactam antibiotics in patients with renal insufficiency.[81] The majority of antimicrobial agents are excreted partially or completely by the kidneys. In addition to glomerular filtration, antibiotics such as trimethoprim-sulfamethoxazole[84] and ciprofloxacin[83] reach the tubule lumen by tubule secretion, thus achieving high urinary concentrations even though the GFR is decreased. This feature is used to therapeutic advantage for treatment of urinary tract infections in patients with renal insufficiency or for treatment of cystic infections in patients with polycystic kidney disease.

In general, the loading dose will be the same as that for the patient with normal renal function. Small adjustments may be required if significant alterations in extracellular fluid volume exist. Rapid achievement of therapeutic drug levels is particularly critical for life-threatening infections because there is often a direct relation between drug levels and antimicrobial efficacy. As discussed earlier, the maintenance dose may be modified by extending the interval between doses, decreasing the dose, or some combination of the two. More recently, it has become recognized that several classes of antibiotics have a significant postantibiotic effect.[85, 86] This phenomenon of persistent antimicrobial action for intervals when blood levels are below the minimal inhibitory concentration may be used to therapeutic advantage. Thus, it may not be necessary to maintain levels above the minimal inhibitory concentration throughout the duration of the dosing interval. Antibiotics that fall into this category include the aminoglycosides, the penems, and newer macrolide antibiotics. More convenient dosing by the interval extension method may be used for these antibiotics without compromising therapeutic efficacy.

The intraperitoneal route of administration is used for a wide variety of antibiotics for the treatment of peritonitis in peritoneal dialysis patients.[87] For most antibiotics, significant systemic absorption occurs presumably owing to the low volume of distribution in the peritoneal cavity and low availability of proteins for binding.[76] In addition, the permeability of the peritoneum increases during peritonitis and increases systemic absorption further. In contrast, antibiotics administered orally or intravenously may have slow penetration into the peritoneum, depending on the size of the drug, degree of protein binding, and volume of distribution. For this reason, the intraperitoneal route is preferred for the treatment of peritonitis. Table 60–9 provides suggested guidelines for intraperitoneal dosing of antibiotics commonly used for the treatment of peritonitis. The reader is referred to Keane and co-workers[88] for a more comprehensive listing of intraperitoneal doses of antibiotics.

Nephrotoxicity of antimicrobial agents is a major concern in patients with impaired renal function. Underlying renal disease is an important risk factor for the development of nephrotoxic effects, and the consequences in the patient with little reserve in renal function may be substantial. Appropriate dosing and monitoring of drug levels are crucial for minimizing the risk of nephrotoxicity for some agents, such as the aminoglycosides.[89] Correction of other risk factors, such as volume depletion and hypokalemia, before instituting therapy is also important to consider. Acute interstitial nephritis occurs sporadically with certain antibiotics (classically with methicillin); however, there are no identified risk factors or preventive measures for this complication.[90] The antianabolic effects of tetracycline may result in a rise in the blood urea nitrogen, and therefore it should probably be avoided if possible in the patient with significant renal insufficiency. A spurious rise in the creatinine level may occur as a result of interference with the secretion of creatinine (trimethoprim)[91] or an interference with the assay for creatinine (certain cephalosporins).[92] Finally, a variety of electrolyte complications have been described, such as $Mg^{2+}$ and $K^+$ wasting with amphotericin therapy and hypokalemia with large doses of carbenicillin. In addition, the clinician should be aware that a significant $K^+$ or $Na^+$ load may occur in conjunction with the administration of certain agents, particularly the penicillins.[93]

*Text continued on page 2673*

## TABLE 60–8. Antimicrobial Agents*

| Drug, Toxicity, Notes | Dose for Normal Renal Function | Method | Adjustment for Renal Failure GFR of >50 mL/min | 10–50 mL/min† | <10 mL/min | Supplement for Dialysis |
|---|---|---|---|---|---|---|
| ***Aminoglycoside Antibiotics*** <br> Ototoxic, nephrotoxic; rare respiratory paralysis; check serum levels to ensure efficacy. <br> Dose after hemodialysis is ⅔ of normal maintenance dose or ½ of a loading dose. <br> Larger supplement may be required for highly permeable membranes. <br> Volume of distribution is larger with obesity, edema, or ascites. | | | | | | |
| Amikacin[94–96] | 5 mg/kg <br> q 8 h | D <br> I | 70%–100% <br> q 8–12 h | 30%–70% <br> q 12 h | 20%–30% <br> q 24–48 h | Hemo: ⅔ normal dose after dialysis <br> CAPD: 30% q 24 h <br> CAVH: Dose for GFR 10–50 |
| Gentamicin[97–99] <br> Concurrent penicillins may result in subtherapeutic blood levels | 1 mg/kg <br> q 8 h | D <br> I | 70%–100% <br> q 8–12 h | 30%–70% <br> q 12 h | 20%–30% <br> q 24–48 h | Hemo: ⅔ normal dose after dialysis <br> CAPD: 30% q 24 h <br> CAVH: Dose for GFR 10–50 |
| Kanamycin[100] | 5 mg/kg <br> q 8 h | D <br> I | 70%–100% <br> q 8–12 h | 30%–70% <br> q 12 h | 20%–30% <br> q 24–48 h | Hemo: ⅔ normal dose after dialysis <br> CAPD: 30% q 24 h <br> CAVH: Dose for GFR 10–50 |
| Netilmicin[101–103] | 5 mg/kg <br> q 8 h | D <br> I | 70%–100% <br> q 8–12 h | 30%–70% <br> q 12 h | 20%–30% <br> q 24–48 h | Hemo: ⅔ normal dose after dialysis <br> CAPD: 30% q 24 h <br> CAVH: Dose for GFR 10–50 |
| Streptomycin[7, 75] | 1 g/d | I | q 24 h | q 24–72 h | q 72–96 h | Hemo: ½ normal dose after dialysis <br> CAPD: Dose for GFR 10–50 <br> CAVH: Dose for GFR 10–50 |
| Tobramycin[104, 105] <br> Concurrent penicillins may result in subtherapeutic blood levels | 1 mg/kg <br> q 8 h | D <br> I | 70%–100% <br> q 8–12 h | 30%–70% <br> q 12 h | 20%–30% <br> q 24–48 h | Hemo: ⅔ normal dose after dialysis <br> CAPD: 30% q 24 h <br> CAVH: Dose for GFR 10–50 |
| ***Cephalosporin Antibiotics*** <br> Rare allergic interstitial nephritis; absorbed well when administered intraperitoneally; may cause bleeding in patients with renal failure. | | | | | | |
| Cefaclor[106, 107] | 250 mg tid | D | 100% | 50%–100% | 50% | Hemo: Dose after dialysis <br> CAPD: 250 mg q 8–12 h <br> CAVH: Unknown |
| Cefadroxil[108] | 0.5–1 g <br> q 12 h | I | q 12 h | q 12–24 h | q 24–48 h | Hemo: Dose after dialysis <br> CAPD: Unknown <br> CAVH: Unknown |
| Cefamandole[109, 110] | 0.5–1.0 g <br> q 4–8 h | I | q 4–8 h | q 6–8 h | q 12 h | Hemo: Dose after dialysis <br> CAPD: Dose for GFR 10–50 <br> CAVH: Dose for GFR 10–50 |

*Table continued on following page*

TABLE 60–8. Antimicrobial Agents* *Continued*

| Drug, Toxicity, Notes | Dose for Normal Renal Function | Method | Adjustment for Renal Failure GFR of | | | Supplement for Dialysis |
|---|---|---|---|---|---|---|
| | | | >50 mL/min | 10–50 mL/min† | <10 mL/min | |
| Cefazolin[111] | 0.5–1.5 g q 6 h | I | q 6–8 h | q 12 h | q 24–48 h | Hemo: Dose after dialysis<br>CAPD: None<br>CAVH: None |
| Cefixime[112] | 200 mg q 12 h | D | 100% | 75% | 50% | Hemo: None<br>CAPD: None<br>CAVH: Unlikely |
| Cefmenoxime[113–115] | 1 g q 6 h | D<br>I | 1 g q 6–8 h | 1 g q 12–24 h | 750 mg q 24 h | Hemo: 750 mg after dialysis<br>CAPD: None<br>CAVH: Unknown |
| Cefmetazole[116, 117] | 2 g q 8 h | I | q 8–12 h | q 12–24 h | q 48 h | Hemo: Dose after dialysis<br>CAPD: Unknown<br>CAVH: Unknown |
| Cefonicid[118, 119] | 1 g q 24 h | D<br>I | 0.5–1 g q 24 h | 0.25–0.5 g q 24 h | 0.25 g q 48 h | Hemo: None<br>CAPD: None<br>CAVH: None |
| Cefoperazone[120, 121] | 1–2 g q 12 h | D | 100% | 100% | 100% | Hemo: None<br>CAPD: None<br>CAVH: None |
| Ceforanide[122, 123] | 0.5–1 g q 12 h | I | q 12 h | q 24–48 h | q 48–72 h | Hemo: 0.5–1 g after dialysis<br>CAPD: None<br>CAVH: None |
| Cefotaxime[124, 125] | 1 g q 6 h | I | q 6 h | q 8–12 h | q 24 h | Hemo: 1 g after dialysis<br>CAPD: None<br>CAVH: None |
| Cefotetan[126, 127] | 1–2 g q 12 h | D | 100% | 50% | 25% | Hemo: 1 g after dialysis<br>CAPD: None<br>CAVH: None |
| Cefoxitin[128, 129]<br>May raise creatinine level by interference with assay | 1–2 g q 6–8 h | I | q 6–8 h | q 8–12 h | q 24–48 h | Hemo: 1 g after dialysis<br>CAPD: Dose for GFR 10–50<br>CAVH: Dose for GFR 10–50 |
| Ceftazidime[130–133] | 1 g q 8–12 h | I | q 8–12 h | q 24–48 h | q 48–72 h | Hemo: 1 g after dialysis<br>CAPD: Dose for GFR 10–50<br>CAVH: Dose for GFR 10–50 |
| Ceftizoxime[134–137] | 1–2 g q 8–12 h | I | q 8–12 h | q 24–48 h | q 48–72 h | Hemo: Dose after dialysis<br>CAPD: Dose for GFR 10–50<br>CAVH: Dose for GFR 10–50 |
| Ceftriaxone[138–140]<br>Monitor levels in dialysis patients | 1 g q 12 h | D | 100% | 100% | 100% | Hemo: None<br>CAPD: None<br>CAVH: None |
| Cefuroxime[141–143] | 0.75–1.5 g q 8 h | I | q 8 h | q 8–12 h | q 24 h | Hemo: Dose after dialysis<br>CAPD: None<br>CAVH: Likely to be removed, dose for GFR 10–50 |
| Cephalexin[144] | 250–500 mg q 6 h | I | q 6 h | q 6 h | q 8–12 h | Hemo: 250 mg after dialysis<br>CAPD: Dose for GFR 10–50<br>CAVH: Dose for GFR 10–50 |

TABLE 60–8. Antimicrobial Agents* *Continued*

| Drug, Toxicity, Notes | Dose for Normal Renal Function | Method | Adjustment for Renal Failure GFR of | | | Supplement for Dialysis |
|---|---|---|---|---|---|---|
| | | | *>50 mL/min* | *10–50 mL/min†* | *<10 mL/min* | |
| Cephalothin[145] | 0.5–2.0 g q 6 h | I | q 6 h | q 6–8 h | q 12 h | Hemo: Dose after dialysis<br>CAPD: Dose for GFR 10–50<br>CAVH: Dose for GFR 10–50 |
| Cephapirin[146] | 0.5–2 g q 6 h | I | q 6 h | q 6–8 h | q 12 h | Hemo: Dose after dialysis<br>CAPD: Dose for GFR 10–50<br>CAVH: Dose for GFR 10–50 |
| Cephradine[147] | 0.25–2 g q 6 h | D | 100% | 50% | 25% | Hemo: Dose after dialysis<br>CAPD: Dose for GFR 10–50<br>CAVH: Dose for GFR 10–50 |
| Moxalactam[148–150] | 1–2 g q 8–12 h | I | q 8–12 h | q 12–24 h | q 24–48 h | Hemo: Dose after dialysis<br>CAPD: Dose for GFR 10–50<br>CAVH: Dose for GFR 10–50 |
| *Macrolide Antibiotics*<br>Clarithromycin[151] | 250–500 mg bid | D | 100% | 50%–100% | 50% | Hemo: Unlikely<br>CAPD: Unlikely<br>CAVH: Unlikely |
| Erythromycin[152, 153]<br>  Ototoxicity with high doses in ESRD | 250–500 mg q 6–12 h | D | 100% | 100% | 50%–75% | Hemo: None<br>CAPD: None<br>CAVH: Unlikely |
| *Penicillins*<br>Amoxicillin[7, 154–157] | 500 mg q 8 h | I | q 8 h | q 8–12 h | q 12 h | Hemo: Dose after dialysis<br>CAPD: Dose for GFR 10–50<br>CAVH: Dose for GFR 10–50 |
| Azlocillin[158, 159]<br>  sodium 2.7 mEq/g | 2–3 g q 4 h | I | q 4–6 h | q 6–8 h | q 6–8 h | Hemo: Dose after dialysis<br>CAPD: Dose for GFR <10<br>CAVH: Dose for GFR 10–50 |
| Dicloxacillin[7, 75] | 250–500 mg q 6 h | D | 100% | 100% | 100% | Hemo: None<br>CAPD: None<br>CAVH: None |
| Methicillin[7, 75] | 1–2 g q 4 h | D | q 4–6 h | q 6–8 h | q 8–12 h | Hemo: None<br>CAPD: None<br>CAVH: None |
| Mezlocillin[160, 161]<br>  sodium 1.9 mEq/g | 1.5–4 g q 4–6 h | I | q 4–6 h | q 6–8 h | q 8 h | Hemo: None<br>CAPD: None<br>CAVH: None |
| Nafcillin[7, 75]<br>  Coagulopathy may develop | 1–2 g q 4–6 h | D | 100% | 100% | 100% | Hemo: None<br>CAPD: None<br>CAVH: None |
| Penicillin G[93]<br>  Potassium 1.7 mEq/million U<br>  Risk of seizures with high doses in renal insufficiency (6 million U/d upper limit dose in ESRD) | 0.5–4 million U q 6 h | D | 100% | 75% | 25%–50% | Hemo: Dose after dialysis<br>CAPD: Dose for GFR <10<br>CAVH: Dose for GFR <10 |
| Piperacillin[162–164]<br>  sodium 1.9 mEq/g | 3–4 g q 4 h | I | q 4–6 h | q 6–8 h | q 8 h | Hemo: Dose after dialysis<br>CAPD: Dose for GFR <10<br>CAVH: Dose for GFR <10 |

*Table continued on following page*

TABLE 60–8. Antimicrobial Agents* *Continued*

| Drug, Toxicity, Notes | Dose for Normal Renal Function | Method | Adjustment for Renal Failure GFR of | | | Supplement for Dialysis |
|---|---|---|---|---|---|---|
| | | | >50 mL/min | 10–50 mL/min† | <10 mL/min | |
| Ticarcillin[165] sodium 5.2 mEq/g | 3 g q 4 h | D I | 1–3 g q 4 h | 1–2 g q 8 h | 1 g q 12 h | Hemo: 3 g after dialysis CAPD: Dose for GFR <10 CAVH: Dose for GFR <10 |
| *Quinolones* | | | | | | |
| Ciprofloxacin[83, 166, 167] Poorly absorbed with antacids | 500–750 mg q 12 h | D | 100% | 50% | 33% | Hemo: 250 mg CAPD: Dose for GFR 10–50 CAVH: Dose for GFR 10–50 |
| Enoxacin[168–170] | 200–400 mg q 12 h | D | 100% | 50% | 50% | Hemo: None CAPD: None CAVH: Unlikely |
| Fleroxacin[171] | 400 mg q 12 h | D | 100% | 50% | 50% | Hemo: Dose after dialysis CAPD: None CAVH: None |
| Norfloxacin[172] | 400 mg q 12 h | I | q 12 h | q 12–24 h | q 24 h | Hemo: None CAPD: Unlikely CAVH: Unlikely |
| Ofloxacin[173] | 400 mg/d | D | 100% | 50% | 25% | Hemo: Dose after dialysis CAPD: None CAVH: Likely to be removed; dose for GFR 10–50 |
| *Tetracycline Antibiotics* Potentiate acidosis; cause hyperphosphatemia; increase blood urea nitrogen; antianabolic. | | | | | | |
| Demeclocycline[82] Nephrotoxicity | 300 mg bid | I | q 12 h | q 24 h | q 48 h | Hemo: None CAPD: Unlikely CAVH: Unlikely |
| Doxycycline[174] Tetracycline of choice in patients with renal insufficiency Not associated with antianabolic syndrome | 100–200 mg/d | D | 100% | 100% | 100% | Hemo: None CAPD: None CAVH: Unlikely |
| Minocycline[174] | 100 mg q 12 h | D | 100% | 100% | 100% | Hemo: None CAPD: None CAVH: Unlikely |
| Oxytetracycline[82] | 250–500 mg qid | I | q 8–12 h | q 24 h | q 48 h | Hemo: Dose after dialysis CAPD: None CAVH: Unlikely |
| Tetracycline[82] | 250–500 mg qid | I | q 6–8 h | q 12–24 h | Avoid | Hemo: None CAPD: Unlikely CAVH: Unlikely |
| *Miscellaneous Antibacterial Antibiotics* | | | | | | |
| Aztreonam[175, 176] | 1–2 g q 8–12 h | D | 100% | 50%–75% | 25% | Hemo: 0.5 g after dialysis CAPD: Dose for GFR <10 CAVH: Dose for GFR 10–50 |
| Chloramphenicol[177] | 12.5 mg/kg q 6 h | D | 100% | 100% | 100% | Hemo: None CAPD: Unlikely CAVH: Unlikely |
| Cilastatin[178–181] Given with imipenem | (see imipenem) | D | 100% | 100% | 100% | Hemo: Dose after dialysis CAPD: None CAVH: Dose for GFR 10–50 |

TABLE 60–8. Antimicrobial Agents* *Continued*

| Drug, Toxicity, Notes | Dose for Normal Renal Function | Method | Adjustment for Renal Failure GFR of | | | Supplement for Dialysis |
|---|---|---|---|---|---|---|
| | | | >50 mL/min | 10–50 mL/min† | <10 mL/min | |
| Clindamycin[182] | 150–300 mg q 6 h | D | 100% | 100% | 100% | Hemo: None CAPD: Unlikely CAVH: Unlikely |
| Imipenem[178–181] | 0.25–1 g q 6 h | D | 100% | 50% | 25% | Hemo: Dose after dialysis CAPD: None CAVH: Dose for GFR 10–50 |
| Lincomycin[7, 75] | 0.5 g q 6 h | I | q 6 h | q 6–12 h | q 12–24 h | Hemo: None CAPD: None CAVH: Unlikely |
| Methenamine mandelate[183]   Contributes to uremic     gastrointestinal symptoms   Not effective for GFR <20     mL/min | 1 g q 6 h | D | 100% | Avoid | Avoid | Hemo: NA CAPD: NA CAVH: NA |
| Metronidazole[184–186]   Metabolites accumulate | 7.5 mg/kg q 6 h | D | 100% | 100% | 50% | Hemo: Dose after dialysis CAPD: None CAVH: Likely to be removed; dose for GFR 10–50 |
| Nalidixic acid[7, 75]   Not effective in severe renal     insufficiency | 1 g q 6 h | D | 100% | Avoid | Avoid | Hemo: Avoid CAPD: Avoid CAVH: Avoid |
| Nitrofurantoin[7, 75]   Ineffective at GFR <50     mL/min   Polyneuropathy | 50–100 mg q 6 h | D | 100% | Avoid | Avoid | Hemo: Avoid CAPD: Avoid CAVH: Avoid |
| Sulfisoxazole[187]   Protein binding decreased in     ESRD   Use normal dosing for UTI     in ESRD | 1–2 g q 6 h | I | q 6 h | q 8–12 h | q 12–24 h | Hemo: 2 g after dialysis CAPD: Dose for GFR 10–50 CAVH: Dose for GFR 10–50 |
| Teicoplanin[188, 189] | 6 mg/kg/d | I | q 24 h | q 48 h | q 72 h | Hemo: None CAPD: None CAVH: None |
| Trimethoprim-sulfamethoxazole[84]   Use normal dosing for UTI     in ESRD   Trimethoprim component     interferes with secretion     of creatinine | 160 mg trimethoprim and 800 mg sulfamethoxazole q 12 h | D I | 100% q 12 h | 100% q 12–24 h | 50% q 24 h | Hemo: ½ dose after dialysis CAPD: None CAVH: Likely to be removed; dose for GFR 10–50 |
| Vancomycin[32, 38, 190, 191]   Ototoxicity   Monitor serum levels | 1 g q 12 h | I | q 12–24 h | q 2–7 d | q 7–10 d | Hemo: Conventional—none; permeable membranes—dose for GFR 10–50 CAPD: Dose for GFR 10–50 CAVH: Dose for GFR 10–50 |
| ***Antifungal Agents*** | | | | | | |
| Amphotericin B[192–196]   Nephrotoxicity proportional     to total dose; renal tubular     acidosis, hypokalemia,     hypomagnesemia,     nephrogenic diabetes     insipidus | 0.3–0.5 mg/kg/d | D | 100% | 100% | 100% | Hemo: None CAPD: Unlikely CAVH: Unlikely |
| Fluconazole[197–201] | 50–200 mg/d | D | 100% | 50% | 25% | Hemo: Dose after dialysis CAPD: Dose for GFR <10 CAVH: Dose for GFR <10 |

*Table continued on following page*

## TABLE 60–8. Antimicrobial Agents* *Continued*

| Drug, Toxicity, Notes | Dose for Normal Renal Function | Method | Adjustment for Renal Failure GFR of | | | Supplement for Dialysis |
|---|---|---|---|---|---|---|
| | | | >50 mL/min | 10–50 mL/min† | <10 mL/min | |
| Flucytosine[197, 202–204] Hepatic dysfunction Bone marrow suppression more common in azotemic patients Adjust dose to maintain peak serum concentration between 40 and 60 mg/L | 150 mg/kg/d in three or four divided doses | D I | 25–50 mg/kg q 12–24 h | 25–50 mg/kg q 12–24 h | 50 mg/kg q 24–48 h | Hemo: Dose after dialysis CAPD: Dose for GFR 10–50 CAVH: Dose for GFR 10–50 |
| Griseofulvin[192, 193] | 125–250 mg q 6 h | D | 100% | 100% | 100% | Hemo: None CAPD: None CAVH: Unlikely |
| Itraconazole[197, 205, 206] | 100–200 mg q 12 h | D | 100% | 100% | 100% | Hemo: None CAPD: None CAVH: Unlikely |
| Ketoconazole[197, 207] | 200–400 mg/d | D | 100% | 100% | 100% | Hemo: None CAPD: Unlikely CAVH: Unlikely |
| Miconazole[208] | 200–1200 mg q 8 h | D | 100% | 100% | 100% | Hemo: None CAPD: Unlikely CAVH: Unlikely |
| ***Antiparasitic Antibiotics*** | | | | | | |
| Chloroquine[209, 210] | 1.5 g in 3-d period | D | 100% | 100% | 50% | Hemo: None CAPD: None CAVH: Unlikely |
| Mebendazole[211, 212] | 100 mg bid × 3 d (pinworm infection: 100 mg; one dose) | D | 100% | 100% | 100% | Hemo: None CAPD: Unlikely CAVH: Unlikely |
| Mefloquine[213] | Nonimmune patients: 1250–1500 mg total in two or three doses in 24-h period Semi-immune patients: 750–1000 mg total in two or three doses in 24-h period | D | 100% | 100% | 50% | Hemo: Unlikely CAPD: Unlikely CAVH: Unlikely |
| Pentamidine[214, 215] | 4 mg/kg/d | I | q 24 h | q 24–36 h | q 48 h | Hemo: Unlikely CAPD: Unlikely CAVH: Unlikely |
| Praziquantel[216] | Dose varies | D | 100% | 100% | 100% | Hemo: None CAPD: Unlikely CAVH: Unlikely |
| Pyrimethamine[209, 210] | 50–75 mg/d | D | 100% | 100% | 100% | Hemo: Unknown CAPD: Unknown CAVH: Unknown |
| Quinine[209, 210] | 10 mg/kg q 8 h | I | q 8 h | q 8–12 h | q 24 h | Hemo: Unlikely CAPD: None CAVH: Unlikely |
| Thiabendazole[211] | Dose varies depending on infecting parasite | D | 100% | 50%–100% | Avoid | Hemo: Unknown CAPD: Unknown CAVH: Unknown |

**TABLE 60–8. Antimicrobial Agents\*** *Continued*

| Drug, Toxicity, Notes | Dose for Normal Renal Function | Method | Adjustment for Renal Failure GFR of | | | Supplement for Dialysis |
|---|---|---|---|---|---|---|
| | | | >50 mL/min | 10–50 mL/min† | <10 mL/min | |
| ***Antituberculous Agents*** | | | | | | |
| Capreomycin[217] | 1 g qd | D<br>I | 100%<br>q 24 h | 100%<br>q 48–72 h | 25%–50%<br>q 48–72 h | Hemo: Dose after dialysis<br>CAPD: Unknown<br>CAVH: Likely to be removed; dose for GFR 10–50 |
| Cycloserine[7, 75]<br>  Central nervous system toxicity | 250 mg<br>q 12 h | I | q 12 h | q 12–24 h | q 24 h | Hemo: Unknown<br>CAPD: Unknown<br>CAVH: Unknown |
| Ethambutol[218]<br>  Ocular toxicity<br>  Peripheral neuritis<br>  Renal excretion decreased by basic drugs | 15 mg/kg<br>q 24 h | D | 100% | 50% | 25%–50% | Hemo: Dose after dialysis<br>CAPD: Dose for GFR 10–50<br>CAVH: Dose for GFR 10–50 |
| Ethionamide[7, 75] | 250–500 mg<br>q 12 h | D | 100% | 100% | 50% | Hemo: Unknown<br>CAPD: Unknown<br>CAVH: Unknown |
| Isoniazid[219] | 5 mg/kg<br>q 24 h | D | 100% | 75%–100% | 50% | Hemo: Dose after dialysis<br>CAPD: Dose for GFR 10–50<br>CAVH: Dose for GFR 10–50 |
| PAS (*p*-aminosalicyclic acid)[7, 75]<br>  Significant sodium load | 50 mg/kg<br>q 8 h | D | 100% | 50%–75% | 50% | Hemo: Dose after dialysis<br>CAPD: Unknown<br>CAVH: Unknown |
| Pyrazinamide[220, 221]<br>  Impairs urate excretion<br>  Can precipitate gout | 15–30 mg/kg<br>q 24 h | I | q 24 h | q 24 h | q 48–72 h | Hemo: Dose after dialysis<br>CAPD: Unknown<br>CAVH: Likely to be removed; dose for GFR 10–50 |
| Rifampin[222] | 600 mg<br>q 24 h | D | 100% | 100% | 100% | Hemo: None<br>CAPD: None<br>CAVH: None |
| ***Antiviral Agents*** | | | | | | |
| Acyclovir[223–225]<br>  Neurotoxic in patients with renal failure; may cause acute renal failure if injected rapidly, intravenously | 5 mg/kg<br>q 8 h | D<br>I | 5 mg/kg<br>q 8–12 h | 5 mg/kg<br>q 12–24 h | 2.5 mg/kg<br>q 24 h | Hemo: Dose after dialysis<br>CAPD: Same as for GFR <10<br>CAVH: 3.5 mg/kg/d |
| Amantadine[226–228] | 100 mg<br>q 12 h | I | q 12–24 h | q 48–72 h | q 168 h | Hemo: None<br>CAPD: Unlikely<br>CAVH: Unlikely |
| Didanosine[229, 230] | 200–300 mg<br>q 12 h | D | 100% | 50%–75% | 50% | Hemo: Dose after dialysis<br>CAPD: Unknown<br>CAVH: Likely to be removed; dose for GFR 10–50 |
| Foscarnet[231]<br>  Nephrotoxicity common | 60–100 mg/kg<br>q 8–12 h | D | 50%–100% | 10%–50% | Avoid | Hemo: Dose after dialysis<br>CAPD: Unknown<br>CAVH: Likely to be removed; dose for GFR 10–50 |

*Table continued on following page*

**TABLE 60–8. Antimicrobial Agents*** *Continued*

| Drug, Toxicity, Notes | Dose for Normal Renal Function | Method | Adjustment for Renal Failure GFR of | | | Supplement for Dialysis |
| --- | --- | --- | --- | --- | --- | --- |
| | | | >50 mL/min | 10–50 mL/min† | <10 mL/min | |
| Ganciclovir[232] | 2.5 mg/kg q 8 h | I | q 8–12 h | q 24 h | q 48–96 h | Hemo: Dose after dialysis<br>CAPD: Unknown<br>CAVH: 3.5 mg/kg/d |
| Ribavirin[233]<br>  Loading dose required | 200 mg q 8 h | D | 100% | 100% | 50% | Hemo: None<br>CAPD: Unlikely<br>CAVH: Unlikely |
| Vidarabine[234] | 15 mg/kg infusion q 24 h | D | 100% | 100% | 75% | Hemo: Infuse after dialysis<br>CAPD: None<br>CAVH: Dose for GFR 10–50 |
| Zidovudine (AZT)[235–238] | 200 mg q 4 h | D | 100% | 100% | 50% | Hemo: Dose after dialysis<br>CAPD: None<br>CAVH: Likely to be removed; dose for GFR 10–50 |

*D = dosage reduction method; I = interval extension method; GFR = glomerular filtration rate; Hemo = hemodialysis; CAPD = continuous ambulatory peritoneal dialysis; CAVH = continuous arteriovenous hemofiltration; ESRD = end-stage renal disease; UTI = urinary tract infection; NA = not applicable.
†**Editor's note:** For drugs whose excretion is reduced at declining levels of renal function, dosage reduction should be considered even before the low end of the 10–50 mL/min GFR range is reached.

**TABLE 60–9. Intraperitoneal Antibiotic Dosing for Treatment of Peritonitis in CAPD Patients***

| Drug | Loading Dose | Continuous | Intermittent |
| --- | --- | --- | --- |
| *Aminoglycosides* | | | |
| Amikacin | — | 6–12 mg/L | 60 mg/L/d |
| Gentamicin | — | 4–8 mg/L | 20 mg/L/d |
| Netilmicin | — | 4–8 mg/L | 20 mg/L/d |
| Tobramycin | — | 4–8 mg/L | 20 mg/L/d |
| *Cephalosporins* | | | |
| Cefazolin | — | 125–250 mg/L | 500 mg/L/d |
| Cefotaxime | 1000 mg/L | 250 mg/L | 1000 mg/L/d |
| Cefoxitin | 500 mg/L | 100 mg/L | No data |
| Ceftazidime | 500 mg/L | 125 mg/L | 500 mg/L/d |
| Ceftriaxone | 500 mg/L | 125–250 mg/L | 500 mg/L/d |
| Cephalothin | 500 mg/L | 100 mg/L | No data |
| Cephradine | — | 125 mg/L | No data |
| *Penicillins* | | | |
| Azlocillin | — | 250 mg/L | No data |
| Mezlocillin | — | 250 mg/L | No data |
| Piperacillin | — | 250 mg/L | No data |
| Ticarcillin | — | 125 mg/L | No data |
| *Quinolones* | | | |
| Ciprofloxacin | 500 mg PO | 50 mg/L | No data |
| Ofloxacin | 400 mg PO | 200 mg/d PO | No data |
| *Miscellaneous* | | | |
| Aztreonam | 500 mg/L | 250 mg/L | 500 mg/L/d |
| Imipenem | 1000 mg | 100 mg/L | 250 mg/L bid |
| Trimethoprim-sulfamethoxazole | 1600 mg/320 mg PO | 200/40 mg/L | No data |
| Vancomycin | — | 15–25 mg/L | 1000–2000 mg/L/wk |
| *Antifungal Agents* | | | |
| Fluconazole | — | No data | 150 mg q 2 d |

*CAPD = continuous ambulatory peritoneal dialysis.

A variety of other complications may occur with increased frequency in the patient with renal insufficiency.[81] Ototoxic and vestibular toxic effects may develop with several antibiotics, including the aminoglycosides, vancomycin, and erythromycin. The cumulative dose appears to play a role, in addition to risk factors unique to the patient with renal insufficiency such as underlying uremic neuropathy affecting the eighth cranial nerve and accumulation of the parent drug or its metabolites. Bleeding complications due to antibiotic therapy may also occur with increased frequency because of underlying platelet dysfunction and heparin exposure during hemodialysis. Finally, patients with renal failure appear to be at greater risk for the development of nonaplastic bone marrow depression with chloramphenicol therapy.

New antimicrobial agents are continually being developed. Intensive research on the human immunodeficiency virus has resulted in the release of several new antiviral drugs. Knowledge of the renal handling of these agents is essential because human immunodeficiency virus infection and renal insufficiency often coexist.

## Analgesics and Agents Used by Anesthesiologists

The majority of analgesics are hepatically metabolized and usually require little dose adjustment for renal failure. However, the presence of renal failure tends to increase the sensitivity to the therapeutic and toxic effects of drugs in this category.[239] The reasons for this are probably multifactorial and include altered pharmacokinetics and the additive effects of retained uremic toxins. For this reason, it is wise to start most analgesics at a reduced dose and then titrate cautiously according to clinical response. Particular caution should be taken in prescribing meperidine. The long-term administration of this drug has been reported to result in the accumulation of normeperidine, a metabolite of meperidine that has central nervous system excitatory properties.[240] Most likely as a result of the accumulation of this metabolite, a higher frequency of seizures has been described in patients with renal failure who receive meperidine for a long time. For this reason, long-term use of this drug should be avoided in renal failure.

Surgical procedures are frequently required in patients with renal failure. Thus, the anesthesiologist must be familiar with the pharmacokinetics of various agents used for the induction and maintenance of anesthesia in patients with renal insufficiency. Many of the neuromuscular blocking agents are excreted at least to some degree by the kidney and as a result may display prolonged action and recurarization as the effect of the antagonist wears off.[241] For this reason, use of neuromuscular blockers with little dependence on renal excretion, such as atracurium or vecuronium, may be preferred in patients with renal insufficiency. Succinylcholine is a muscle relaxant that acts by polarizing the cell membrane. As a result, $K^+$ movement out of cells is favored. Although this results in only a minor rise in plasma $K^+$ concentration in normal subjects, susceptible patients (such as those with extensive trauma, neuromuscular disease, or renal insufficiency) may have life-threatening increases in plasma $K^+$ levels. Table 60–10 summarizes dosing recommendations for analgesics and agents used by anesthesiologists.

## Antihypertensive and Cardiovascular Agents

Cardiovascular disease is frequently present in patients with renal insufficiency and continues to be the most common cause of death in the population with end-stage renal disease.[268] Not surprisingly, antihypertensive and cardiovascular agents are widely prescribed in this population for the treatment of arrhythmias, coronary artery disease, congestive heart failure, and hypertension. Considerable overlap exists in the drugs used for the treatment of these disorders. For example, β-blockers have proved effective for the treatment of hypertension, angina, and arrhythmias, and the angiotensin-converting enzyme inhibitors are beneficial for both hypertension and congestive heart failure. Thus, concomitant medical conditions are often important factors for choosing cardiovascular drugs.

Hypertension is present in the majority of patients with renal insufficiency and has important adverse consequences on the progression of renal disease and risk for cardiovascular events.[269, 270] Although many of the antihypertensive agents are renally excreted to some degree, from a practical standpoint, the dosage is generally tailored to the blood pressure response. Nevertheless, the clinician should be aware of those antihypertensive agents primarily excreted renally because the initial starting dose should be decreased. Therapy should be initiated with low doses and slowly titrated upward until acceptable blood pressure control is achieved, side effects develop, or the usual maximal dose is reached.

Many aspects of prescribing antihypertensive therapy for patients with renal insufficiency are no different from that for patients with normal renal function; however, several comments on selected drugs should be mentioned. The use of diuretics may be helpful in controlling blood pressure when volume overload is present. Loop diuretics are usually required because thiazides are usually not effective once the GFR has declined below 30 mL/min. In general, $K^+$-sparing diuretics should be avoided in patients with renal failure because of the risk of hyperkalemia. β-Blockers are useful for selected patients, particularly those with angina or recent myocardial infarction. Those with low lipid solubility are primarily renally excreted and therefore generally require a decrease in the starting dose. The angiotensin-converting enzyme inhibitors are attractive for use in patients with renal failure because animal studies and preliminary human studies show promise in slowing the progression of renal failure.[271–273] The development of significant hyperkalemia, particularly in patients with type IV renal tubular acidosis, may preclude their use in selected patients. The angiotensin-converting enzyme inhibitors are excreted renally with the exception of fosinopril, which demonstrates dual hepatic and renal elimination. In short-term studies, hepatic elimination of this agent increases as renal function declines. Therefore, significant dose reduction may not be required, although data from long-term dosing with this agent are not available. In general, the starting dose for angiotensin-converting enzyme inhibitors

**TABLE 60–10. Analgesics and Agents Used by Anesthesiologists***

| Drug, Toxicity, Notes | Dose for Normal Renal Function | Method | Adjustment for Renal Failure GFR of | | Supplement for Dialysis |
|---|---|---|---|---|---|
| | | | 10–50 mL/min† | <10 mL/min | |
| *Narcotics and Narcotic Antagonists* All agents in this group may cause excessive sedation and respiratory depression. | | | | | |
| Alfentanil[242] | Anesthetic induction | D | 100% | 100% | Hemo: NA CAPD: NA CAVH: NA |
| Butorphanol[243] | 2 mg q 3–4 h | D | 75% | 50% | Hemo: Unlikely CAPD: Unlikely CAVH: Unlikely |
| Codeine[244] | 30–60 mg q 4–6 h | D | 75% | 50% | Hemo: Unknown CAPD: Unknown CAVH: Unknown |
| Fentanyl[245] | Anesthetic induction | D | 75% | 50% | Hemo: NA CAPD: NA CAVH: NA |
| Meperidine[240] Normeperidine, an active metabolite, accumulates in ESRD and may cause seizures | 50–100 mg q 3–4 h | D | 75% | 50% | Hemo: None CAPD: None CAVH: Unlikely |
| Methadone[246] | 2.5–10 mg q 6–8 h | D | 100% | 50%–75% | Hemo: None CAPD: None CAVH: Unlikely |
| Morphine[247, 248] Metabolites may accumulate | 20–25 mg PO q 4 h or 2–10 mg IV | D | 75% | 50% | Hemo: None CAPD: Unlikely CAVH: Unlikely |
| Naloxone[239, 242] | 2 mg | D | 100% | 100% | Hemo: NA CAPD: NA CAVH: NA |
| Pentazocine[239, 242] | 50 mg q 4 h | D | 75% | 50% | Hemo: None CAPD: Unlikely CAVH: Unlikely |
| Propoxyphene[249] Active metabolite norpropoxyphene accumulates in ESRD | 65 mg PO tid–qid | D | 100% | Avoid | Hemo: None CAPD: None CAVH: Unlikely |
| Sufentanil[239, 242] | Anesthetic induction | D | 100% | 100% | Hemo: NA CAPD: NA CAVH: NA |
| *Non-narcotic Analgesics* | | | | | |
| Acetaminophen[250, 251] Metabolites may accumulate in renal insufficiency Drug is major metabolite of phenacetin | 650 mg q 4 h | I | q 6 h | q 8 h | Hemo: ½ dose CAPD: None CAVH: Unknown |
| Methocarbamol[252] | 4 g/d in divided doses | D | 100% | 100% | Hemo: Unknown CAPD: Unknown CAVH: Unknown |
| Salicylate[253] May decrease GFR when blood flow is prostaglandin dependent Excretion enhanced in alkaline urine May add to uremic gastrointestinal symptoms and platelet dysfunction Protein binding reduced | 650 mg q 4 h | I | q 4–6 h | Avoid | Hemo: Dose after dialysis CAPD: None CAVH: Likley to be removed |
| Salsalate[254] | 1500 mg q 12 h | D | 75%–100% | 50% | Hemo: 500 mg CAPD: Unknown CAVH: Likely to be removed |

**TABLE 60–10. Analgesics and Agents Used by Anesthesiologists\*** *Continued*

| Drug, Toxicity, Notes | Dose for Normal Renal Function | Method | Adjustment for Renal Failure GFR of | | Supplement for Dialysis |
| | | | 10–50 mL/min† | <10 mL/min | |
| --- | --- | --- | --- | --- | --- |
| *Neuromuscular Agents* | | | | | |
| Atracurium[255–258] | 0.4–0.5 mg/kg load, then 0.08–0.1 mg/kg q 15–25 min | D | 100% | 100% | Hemo: Unknown CAPD: Unknown CAVH: Unknown |
| Etomidate[256] | 0.2–0.6 mg/kg | D | 100% | 100% | Hemo: Unknown CAPD: Unknown CAVH: Unknown |
| Gallamine[259] Recurarization may occur up to 24 h after dose; if blockade not responsive to neostigmine, dialysis may be useful | 0.5–1.5 mg/kg | D | Avoid | Avoid | Hemo: NA CAPD: NA CAVH: NA |
| Ketamine[256] | 1–4.5 mg/kg | D | 100% | 100% | Hemo: Unknown CAPD: Unknown CAVH: Unknown |
| Metocurine[260] | 0.2–0.4 mg/kg | D | Avoid | Avoid | Hemo: Unknown CAPD: Unknown CAVH: Unknown |
| Neostigmine[261] | 15–375 mg/d | D | 50% | 25% | Hemo: Unknown CAPD: Unknown CAVH: Unknown |
| Pancuronium[262] Recurarization may occur up to 24 h after dose | 0.04–0.1 mg/kg | D | 50% | Avoid | Hemo: Unknown CAPD: Unknown CAVH: Unknown |
| Propofol[263] | 2.0–2.5 mg/kg load, then 6–12 mg/kg/h | D | 100% | 100% | Hemo: Unknown CAPD: Unknown CAVH: Unknown |
| Pyridostigmine[264] Renal excretion decreased by basic drugs | 60–1500 mg/d | D | 35% (GFR >50:50%) | 20% | Hemo: Unknown CAPD: Unknown CAVH: Unknown |
| Succinylcholine[265] Hyperkalemia in ESRD | 0.3–1.1 mg/kg load, then 0.04–0.07 mg/kg prn | D | 100% | 100% | Hemo: Unknown CAPD: Unknown CAVH: Unknown |
| Tubocurarine[266] Large or repetitive doses may result in prolonged effect Recurarization may occur | 0.1–0.2 mg/kg | D | 50% (GFR >50:75%–100%) | Avoid | Hemo: Unknown CAPD: Unknown CAVH: Unknown |
| Vecuronium[267] | 0.08–0.1 mg/kg load, then 0.01–0.05 mg/kg | D | 100% | 100% | Hemo: Unknown CAPD: Unknown CAVH: Unknown |

\*D = dosage reduction method; I = interval extension method; GFR = glomerular filtration rate; Hemo = hemodialysis; CAPD = continuous ambulatory peritoneal dialysis; CAVH = continuous arteriovenous hemofiltration; ESRD = end-stage renal disease; NA = not applicable.

†**Editor's Note:** For drugs whose excretion is reduced at declining levels of renal function, dosage reduction should be considered even before the low end of the 10–50 mL/min GFR range is reached.

should be low and slowly titrated with close monitoring of renal function, K+ levels, and blood pressure response. Ca²⁺ channel blockers and the majority of the vasodilators and adrenergic modulators do not require dosage adjustment for renal failure.

A growing number of drugs are now available for the management of cardiac arrhythmias. Many of these agents are renally excreted to some degree. Initiation of treatment at lower than usual doses is therefore appropriate as outlined in the dosing table. In general, subsequent adjustment is then tailored to arrhythmia suppression and the development of side effects. Several of these agents have active metabolites that may accumulate in renal failure.

Medical management of angina generally involves the use of nitrates, β-blockers, or Ca²⁺ channel blockers either alone or in some combination. With the exception of the renally excreted β-blockers, major dose adjustments for renal failure are not required. Table 60–11 summarizes dosing recommendations for antihypertensive and cardiovascular agents.

## Antineoplastic Agents

Renal failure frequently complicates the course of malignant disease. A variety of mechanisms may be involved, including urinary tract obstruction, tumor lysis syndrome, tumor-associated glomerulonephritis, and drug-related nephrotoxic injury.[408] As the population with end-stage renal disease increases in age, the frequency of malignant

*Text continued on page 2681*

### TABLE 60–11. Antihypertensive and Cardiovascular Agents*

| Drug, Toxicity, Notes | Dose for Normal Renal Function | Method | Adjustment for Renal Failure GFR of | | Supplement for Dialysis |
|---|---|---|---|---|---|
| | | | 10–50 mL/min† | <10 mL/min | |
| **Adrenergic Modulators** | | | | | |
| Clonidine[274, 275] Rebound hypertension if drug is suddenly withdrawn | 0.1–0.6 mg bid | D | 100% | 100% | Hemo: None CAPD: None CAVH: Unlikely |
| Doxazosin[276, 277] | 1–15 mg/d | D | 100% | 100% | Hemo: None CAPD: Unlikely CAVH: Unlikely |
| Guanabenz[278] | 8–16 mg bid | D | 100% | 100% | Hemo: Unlikely CAPD: Unlikely CAVH: Unlikely |
| Guanadrel[279, 280] | 10–50 mg bid | I | q 12–24 h | q 24–48 h | Hemo: Unknown CAPD: Unknown CAVH: Unknown |
| Guanethidine[7, 74] | 10–100 mg/d | I | q 24 h | q 48 h | Hemo: Unlikely CAPD: Unlikely CAVH: Unlikely |
| Guanfacine[281, 282] | 1–2 mg/d | D | 100% | 100% | Hemo: None CAPD: Unlikely CAVH: Unlikely |
| Methyldopa[283] | 250–500 mg tid | I | q 8–12 h | q 12–24 h | Hemo: 250 mg CAPD: None CAVH: Significant removal likely; dose for GFR 10–50 |
| Prazosin[284, 285] | 1–15 mg bid | D | 100% | 100% | Hemo: None CAPD: Unlikely CAVH: Unlikely |
| Reserpine[286] Excessive sedation | 0.05–0.25 mg/d | D | 100% | 100% | Hemo: Unlikely CAPD: Unlikely CAVH: Unlikely |
| Terazosin[287] | 1–20 mg/d | D | 100% | 100% | Hemo: Unlikely CAPD: Unlikely CAVH: Unlikely |
| **Angiotensin-Converting Enzyme Inhibitors** Hypotensive effects exacerbated by diuretics or Na⁺ depletion. May cause hyperkalemia, metabolic acidosis. Acute renal dysfunction with bilateral or transplant renal artery stenosis. Dry cough in 5%–10%. | | | | | |
| Benazepril[288, 289] | 10–40 mg qd | D | 50%–75% | 25%–50% (maximal dose 10 mg/d) | Hemo: Unlikely CAPD: Unlikely CAVH: Unlikely |
| Captopril[290–292] Rare nephrotic syndrome, granulocytopenia Increases serum digoxin levels | 25–50 mg q 8 h | D I | 75% q 12 h | 50% q 24 h | Hemo: Dose after dialysis CAPD: None CAVH: Likely to be removed; dose for GFR 10–50 |
| Enalapril[293, 294] | 5–10 mg q 12 h | D | 75%–100% | 50% | Hemo: Dose after dialysis CAPD: None CAVH: Likely to be removed; dose for GFR 10–50 |
| Fosinopril[295–297] | 10–40 mg qd | D | 100% | 100% | Hemo: Dose after dialysis CAPD: None CAVH: Unlikely |
| Lisinopril[298, 299] | 5–40 mg qd | D | 50%–75% | 25%–50% | Hemo: Dose after dialysis CAPD: Unknown CAVH: Likely to be removed; dose for GFR 10–50 |

### TABLE 60–11. Antihypertensive and Cardiovascular Agents* *Continued*

| Drug, Toxicity, Notes | Dose for Normal Renal Function | Method | Adjustment for Renal Failure GFR of | | Supplement for Dialysis |
|---|---|---|---|---|---|
| | | | 10–50 mL/min† | <10 mL/min | |
| Ramipril[300, 301] | 10–20 mg qd | D | 50%–75% | 25%–50% | Hemo: Dose after dialysis<br>CAPD: None<br>CAVH: Likely to be removed; dose for GFR 10–50 |
| ***Antiarrhythmic Agents***<br>Blood levels and clinical response best guide to therapy; $t_{1/2}$ may be prolonged in heart failure or with reduced hepatic blood flow. | | | | | |
| *N*-Acetylprocainamide[302, 303] | 500 mg q 6–8 h | D<br>I | 50%<br>q 8–12 h | 25%<br>q 12 h | Hemo: None<br>CAPD: None<br>CAVH: Replace by blood level |
| Amiodarone[304]<br>Thyroid dysfunction; peripheral neuropathy; pulmonary fibrosis | 800–1200 mg load<br>200–600 mg/d | D | 100% | 100% | Hemo: None<br>CAPD: None<br>CRRT: Unlikely |
| Bretylium[305, 306] | 5–30 mg/kg load<br>5–10 mg IV q 6 h | D | 25%–50% | 25% | Hemo: None<br>CAPD: Unlikely<br>CRRT: Unlikely |
| Disopyramide[307–309]<br>Urinary retention<br>Variable $V_d$ and extrarenal elimination mandate individualized dosing | 100–200 mg q 6 h | I | q 12–24 h<br>(GFR >50:<br>q 6–8 h) | q 24–48 h | Hemo: None<br>CAPD: None<br>CRRT: Unlikely |
| Encainide[310, 311]<br>Active metabolites may accumulate in renal failure | 25 mg q 8 h to<br>50 mg q 6 h | D | 75% | 50% | Hemo: Unlikely<br>CAPD: Unlikely<br>CRRT: Unlikely |
| Flecainide[312, 313]<br>Excretion enhanced in acid urine | 100–200 mg q 12 h | D | 100% | 50%–75% | Hemo: None<br>CAPD: Unlikely<br>CRRT: Unlikely |
| Lidocaine[314]<br>$t_{1/2}$ dependent on hepatic blood flow; active metabolite | Load 1 mg/kg IV bolus, then 0.5 mg/kg bolus q 8–10 min, up to a total of 3 mg/kg<br>Maint: 1–4 mg/min IV infusion | D | 100% | 100% | Hemo: None<br>CAPD: Unlikely<br>CAVH: Unlikely |
| Lorcainide[315] | 100 mg bid | D | 100% | 100% | Hemo: Unlikely<br>CAPD: Unlikely<br>CAVH: Unlikely |
| Mexiletine[316, 317] | 100–300 mg q 6–8 h | D | 100% | 100% | Hemo: None<br>CAPD: None<br>CAVH: Unlikely |
| Moricizine[318, 319] | 200–300 mg q 8 h | D | 100% | 100% | Hemo: Unlikely<br>CAPD: Unlikely<br>CAVH: Unlikely |
| Procainamide[302, 303, 320] | 350–400 mg q 3–4 h | I | q 6–12 h | q 12–24 h | Hemo: 200 mg<br>CAPD: None<br>CAVH: Replace by blood level |
| Propafenone[321, 322] | 150–300 mg q 8 h | D | 100% | 100% | Hemo: None<br>CAPD: Unlikely<br>CAVH: Unlikely |
| Quinidine[323, 324]<br>Active metabolite increases plasma digoxin and digitoxin<br>Excretion enhanced in acid urine | 200–400 mg q 4–6 h | D | 100% | 75% | Hemo: None<br>CAPD: None<br>CAVH: Unlikely |
| Tocainide[325–327] | 400–600 mg q 8 h | D | 100% | 50% | Hemo: 200 mg<br>CAPD: None<br>CAVH: Unknown |

*Table continued on following page*

## TABLE 60–11. Antihypertensive and Cardiovascular Agents* *Continued*

| Drug, Toxicity, Notes | Dose for Normal Renal Function | Method | Adjustment for Renal Failure GFR of | | Supplement for Dialysis |
|---|---|---|---|---|---|
| | | | 10–50 mL/min† | <10 mL/min | |
| **β-*Blockers*** | | | | | |
| Acebutolol[328–332] Active metabolites with long half-life | 400–600 mg/d or bid | D | 50% | 30%–50% | Hemo: Dose after dialysis<br>CAPD: Unknown<br>CAVH: Probably removed; dose for GFR 10–50 |
| Atenolol[333, 334] Significant accumulation in ESRD | 50–100 mg/d | D | 50% | 25% | Hemo: 25–50 mg<br>CAPD: None<br>CAVH: Probably removed; dose for GFR 10–50 |
| Betaxolol[335] | 10–20 mg/d | D | 100% | 50% | Hemo: Dose after dialysis<br>CAPD: Unknown<br>CAVH: Probably removed; dose for GFR 10–50 |
| Carteolol[336, 337] | 5–20 mg/d | D | 50% | 25% | Hemo: Unknown<br>CAPD: Unknown<br>CAVH: Unknown |
| Dilevalol[338, 339] | 200–800 mg PO qd | D | 100% | 100% | Hemo: None<br>CAPD: Unknown<br>CAVH: Unknown |
| Esmolol[340, 341] | 50–150 μg/kg/min infusion | D | 100% | 100% | Hemo: None<br>CAPD: None<br>CAVH: Unknown |
| Labetalol[342, 343] | 200–600 mg bid | D | 100% | 100% | Hemo: None<br>CAPD: Unknown<br>CAVH: Unknown |
| Metoprolol[344] | 50–100 mg bid | D | 100% | 100% | Hemo: Dose after dialysis<br>CAPD: Unknown<br>CAVH: Likely to be removed; dose for GFR 10–50 |
| Nadolol[345, 346] | 80–320 mg/d | D | 50% | 25% | Hemo: 40 mg<br>CAPD: None<br>CAVH: Likely to be removed; dose for GFR 10–50 |
| Penbutolol[347] | 10–40 mg/d | D | 100% | 100% | Hemo: Unlikely<br>CAPD: Unlikely<br>CAVH: Unlikely |
| Pindolol[348] | 10–40 mg bid | D | 100% | 100% | Hemo: Unlikely<br>CAPD: Unlikely<br>CAVH: Unlikely |
| Propranolol[349, 350] Metabolites may accumulate; hypoglycemia reported in ESRD | 80–160 mg bid | D | 100% | 100% | Hemo: None<br>CAPD: Unlikely<br>CAVH: Unlikely |
| Sotalol[351, 352] | 160–480 mg/d | D | 30% | 15%–30% | Hemo: Dose after dialysis<br>CAPD: None<br>CAVH: Likely to be removed; dose for GFR 10–50 |
| Timolol[328, 329] | 10–20 mg bid | D | 100% | 100% | Hemo: None<br>CAPD: None<br>CAVH: Unlikely |
| ***Calcium Channel Blockers*** | | | | | |
| Amlodipine[353, 354] | 5 mg qd | D | 100% | 100% | Hemo: None<br>CAPD: Unlikely<br>CAVH: Unlikely |

TABLE 60–11. Antihypertensive and Cardiovascular Agents* *Continued*

| Drug, Toxicity, Notes | Dose for Normal Renal Function | Method | Adjustment for Renal Failure GFR of | | Supplement for Dialysis |
|---|---|---|---|---|---|
| | | | 10–50 mL/min† | <10 mL/min | |
| Diltiazem[355–357] | 30–90 mg q 8 h | D | 100% | 100% | Hemo: None<br>CAPD: Unlikely<br>CAVH: Unlikely |
| Felodipine[358–360] | 10 mg bid | D | 100% | 100% | Hemo: None<br>CAPD: Unlikely<br>CAVH: Unlikely |
| Isradipine[361–363] | 5–10 mg/d | D | 100% | 100% | Hemo: None<br>CAPD: Unlikely<br>CAVH: Unlikely |
| Nicardipine[364] | 20–30 mg tid | D | 100% | 100% | Hemo: None<br>CAPD: Unlikely<br>CAVH: Unlikely |
| Nifedipine[365, 366]<br>Nifedipine XL | 10–30 mg q 8 h<br>(XL: 30–120 mg qd) | D | 100% | 100% | Hemo: None<br>CAPD: Unlikely<br>CAVH: Unlikely |
| Nimodipine[353] | 30 mg q 8 h | D | 100% | 100% | Hemo: None<br>CAPD: Unlikely<br>CAVH: Unlikely |
| Nisoldipine[353] | 10 mg bid | D | 100% | 100% | Hemo: None<br>CAPD: Unlikely<br>CAVH: Unlikely |
| Nitrendipine[367, 368] | 20 mg bid | D | 100% | 100% | Hemo: None<br>CAPD: Unlikely<br>CAVH: Unlikely |
| Verapamil[369–371]<br>Verapamil SR | 80 mg q 8 h<br>(SR: 180 mg qd–240 mg q 12 h) | D | 100% | 100% | Hemo: None<br>CAPD: Unlikely<br>CAVH: Unlikely |

### Cardiac Glycosides

Add to uremic gastrointestinal symptoms; serum levels guide therapy.
Toxicity enhanced by dialysis $K^+$ and $Mg^{2+}$ removal.

| Drug, Toxicity, Notes | Dose for Normal Renal Function | Method | 10–50 mL/min† | <10 mL/min | Supplement for Dialysis |
|---|---|---|---|---|---|
| Digitoxin[372, 373]<br>  Protein binding decreased by dialysis; $V_d$ reduced by uremia | 0.1–0.2 mg/d | D | 100% | 100% | Hemo: None<br>CAPD: None<br>CAVH: None |
| Digoxin[11, 374–376]<br>  Radioimmunoassay may overestimate serum levels in uremia; clearance reduced by spironolactone, quinidine, verapamil; hypokalemia, hypomagnesemia enhance toxicity | 1–1.5 mg load<br>0.25–0.5 mg/d | D<br>I | 25%–75%<br>q 24 h | 10%–25%<br>q 48 h | Hemo: None<br>CAPD: None<br>CAVH: Unlikely |
| Ouabain[7, 75] | 0.25 mg load<br>0.1 mg q 12 h | I | q 24 h | q 48 h | Hemo: None<br>CAPD: None<br>CAVH: Unlikely |

### Diruetics

Natriuretic drugs may cause volume depletion.

| Drug, Toxicity, Notes | Dose for Normal Renal Function | Method | 10–50 mL/min† | <10 mL/min | Supplement for Dialysis |
|---|---|---|---|---|---|
| Acetazolamide[377–379]<br>  May potentiate acidemia<br>  Ineffective in ESRD | 250 mg q 6–12 h | I | q 12 h | Avoid | Hemo: Unlikely<br>CAPD: Unlikely<br>CAVH: Unlikely |
| Amiloride[380]<br>  Hyperkalemia<br>  Hyperchloremic metabolic acidosis | 5–10 mg q 24 h | D | 50% | Avoid | Hemo: NA<br>CAPD: NA<br>CAVH: NA |
| Bumetanide[381, 382]<br>  Ototoxicity in combination with aminoglycosides<br>  Protein binding reduced in renal failure | 1–2 mg q 8–12 h | D | 100% | 100% | Hemo: Unlikely<br>CAPD: Unlikely<br>CAVH: Unlikely |
| Chlorthalidone[383]<br>  Ineffective with low GFR | 25 mg/d | D | 100% | Avoid | Hemo: NA<br>CAPD: NA<br>CAVH: NA |

*Table continued on following page*

TABLE 60–11. Antihypertensive and Cardiovascular Agents* *Continued*

| Drug, Toxicity, Notes | Dose for Normal Renal Function | Method | Adjustment for Renal Failure GFR of | | Supplement for Dialysis |
|---|---|---|---|---|---|
| | | | 10–50 mL/min† | <10 mL/min | |
| Ethacrynic acid[384] Ototoxicity | 50 mg tid | I | q 8–12 h | Avoid | Hemo: NA CAPD: NA CAVH: NA |
| Furosemide[385–387] Ototoxicity | 40–80 mg bid | D | 100% | 100% | Hemo: None CAPD: None CAVH: NA |
| Indapamide[388] Hypotensive effect independent of diuretic effect | 2.5–5 mg/d | D | 100% | 100% | Hemo: None CAPD: Unlikely CAVH: Unlikely |
| Metolazone[377, 378] | 5–10 mg/d | D | 100% | 100% | Hemo: Unlikely CAPD: Unlikely CAVH: Unlikely |
| Piretanide[389, 390] Ototoxicity | 6–12 mg/d | D | 100% | 100% | Hemo: Unlikely CAPD: Unlikely CAVH: Unlikely |
| Spironolactone[391] Hyperkalemia common when GFR < 30 mL/min Hyperchloremic acidosis Active metabolites with long half-life | 25–50 mg tid | I | q 12–24 h | Avoid | Hemo: NA CAPD: NA CAVH: NA |
| Thiazides[392] Ineffective when GFR < 30 mL/min Hyperuricemia | 12.5 mg qd 50 mg bid | D | 100% | Avoid | Hemo: NA CAPD: NA CAVH: NA |
| Triamterene[393] Hyperkalemia common when GFR < 30 mL/min Crystalluria in acid urine can cause acute renal failure Active metabolite with long half-life | 25–50 mg bid | D | 100% | Avoid | Hemo: NA CAPD: NA CAVH: NA |
| ***Inotropic Agents*** | | | | | |
| Amrinone[394, 395] | 5–10 µg/kg/min Daily < 10 mg/kg | D | 100% | 50%–75% | Hemo: Unknown CAPD: Unknown CAVH: Unknown |
| Dobutamine[396, 397] | 2.5–15 µg/kg/min | D | 100% | 100% | Hemo: Unknown CAPD: Unknown CAVH: Unknown |
| Milrinone[398, 399] | 2.5–15 mg q 6 h | D | 100% | 50%–75% | Hemo: Unknown CAPD: Unknown CAVH: Unknown |
| ***Nitrates*** | | | | | |
| Isosorbide[400–402] | 10–20 mg tid | D | 100% | 100% | Hemo: Dose after dialysis CAPD: None CAVH: Unknown |
| Nitroglycerin[400] | Many methods and routes of dosing | D | 100% | 100% | Hemo: Unknown CAPD: Unknown CAVH: Unknown |
| ***Vasodilators*** | | | | | |
| Diazoxide[403] Decreased protein binding in renal failure | 150–300 mg bolus | D | 75%–100% | 50% | Hemo: None CAPD: None CAVH: None |
| Hydralazine[404] Drug-induced lupus | 25–50 mg tid | I | q 8 h | q 12 h | Hemo: None CAPD: None CAVH: Unlikely |

**TABLE 60–11. Antihypertensive and Cardiovascular Agents\*** *Continued*

| Drug, Toxicity, Notes | Dose for Normal Renal Function | Method | Adjustment for Renal Failure GFR of | | Supplement for Dialysis |
|---|---|---|---|---|---|
| | | | 10–50 mL/min† | <10 mL/min | |
| Minoxidil[405]<br>Fluid retention, pericardial effusion | 5–30 mg bid | D | 100% | 100% | Hemo: Dose after dialysis<br>CAPD: Unknown<br>CAVH: Unknown |
| Nitroprusside[406, 407]<br>Toxic metabolite, thiocyanate, accumulates, causing seizures, coma; thiocyanate is hemodialyzable | 0.25–8 µg/kg/min infusion | D | 100% | 100% | Hemo: None<br>CAPD: None<br>CAVH: Unlikely |

\*D = dosage reduction method; I = interval extension method; GFR = glomerular filtration rate; Hemo = hemodialysis; CAPD = continuous ambulatory peritoneal dialysis; CAVH = continuous arteriovenous hemofiltration; CRRT = continuous renal replacement therapy; ESRD = end-stage renal disease; $V_d$ = volume of distribution; NA = not applicable.

†**Editor's Note:** For drugs whose excretion is reduced at declining levels of renal function, dosage reduction should be considered even before the low end of the 10–50 mL/min GFR range is reached.

neoplasms may be anticipated to rise. For this reason, knowledge of the renal handling of chemotherapeutic agents and appropriate dosage adjustment is essential.

The majority of chemotherapeutic agents are myelosuppressive and may compound the platelet dysfunction, anemia, and immune compromise associated with renal insufficiency. Several agents, such as cisplatin and methotrexate, are excreted primarily by the kidney and require significant dose adjustment. Nephrotoxic injury is a frequent complication of cisplatin therapy and may be ameliorated by administering the drug in normal or hypertonic saline.[409] In addition, significant $Mg^{2+}$ wasting and $Na^+$ wasting may occur in a subset of patients. Methotrexate also carries a significant risk of nephrotoxicity that may be prevented or ameliorated with adequate hydration and alkalinization of the urine.[410] Finally, mitomycin C may damage the endothelial cells in the kidney, resulting in microangiopathic hemolytic anemia, thrombocytopenia, and renal dysfunction.[411] Table 60–12 summarizes dosing recommendations for antineoplastic agents.

## Endocrine and Metabolic Agents

Several abnormalities in glucose metabolism have been described in renal failure, including peripheral resistance to the action of insulin and decreased catabolism of insulin by the kidney.[440–442] Diabetes is currently the most common cause of end-stage renal disease; thus, it is not surprising that hypoglycemic agents are frequently prescribed for patients with renal failure. In addition to dietary management, oral hypoglycemic agents are often used in the treatment of adult-onset (type II) diabetes. In the presence of renal insufficiency, sulfonylureas that are excreted primarily by the kidney should be avoided because prolonged hypoglycemia may result from drug accumulation. As renal function declines, glucose levels should be monitored frequently in the insulin-dependent diabetic patient because insulin requirements may change unpredictably. Peritoneal dialysis offers the unique opportunity to administer insulin into the peritoneal cavity. Intraperitoneal insulin therapy has been shown to result in better overall control of plasma glucose compared with standard insulin therapy.[443]

An increased frequency of hyperlipidemia is associated with renal failure and may contribute to the increased risk of cardiovascular disease in this population.[444–447] Although dietary modification remains the mainstay of treatment, many patients require drug therapy for achievement of optimal lipid levels. Bile acid sequestrants should generally be avoided in patients with advanced renal failure because they require fluids for dilution and in addition may cause worsening acidemia.[448] Several of the hypolipidemic agents, including lovastatin and clofibrate, have been associated with the development of rhabdomyolysis.[449] Risk for this complication appears to be increased in patients with renal insufficiency, particularly if these agents are taken concomitantly with cyclosporine or niacin. Antithyroid agents and thyroid replacement therapy do not generally require significant dose adjustment in renal failure. Dosing requirements for drugs used in the treatment of endocrine and metabolic disorders are summarized in Table 60–13.

## Gastrointestinal Drugs

Gastrointestinal disorders, particularly peptic ulcer disease, occur with increased frequency in patients with renal insufficiency. An understanding of the pharmacokinetics and potential toxic effects of common drugs used to treat these disorders is essential. Before the development of the histamine $H_2$ blockers, antacids constituted the mainstay of therapy for peptic ulcer disease and related disorders. They are still widely used and are easily available to the patient over the counter. Their mechanism of action is to neutralize gastric acid, and the active ingredients may include aluminum, calcium, magnesium, or sodium bicarbonate salts. Systemic absorption of these constituents may result in a variety of metabolic complications including hypermagnesemia, hypercalcemia, and metabolic alkalosis. Excessive intake of calcium carbonate may result in the development of the milk-alkali syndrome characterized by the triad of hypercalcemia, metabolic alkalosis, and acute renal fail-

## TABLE 60–12. Antineoplastic Agents*

| Drug, Toxicity, Notes | Dose for Normal Renal Function | Method | Adjustment for Renal Failure GFR of | | Supplement for Dialysis |
|---|---|---|---|---|---|
| | | | 10–50 mL/min† | <10 mL/min | |
| Bleomycin[412] | 10–20 U/m² | D | 75% | 50% | Hemo: None<br>CAPD: Unlikely<br>CAVH: Unknown |
| Busulfan[413] | 4–8 mg/d | D | 100% | 100% | Hemo: Unknown<br>CAPD: Unknown<br>CAVH: Unknown |
| Carboplatin[414–416] | 400–500 mg/m² | D | 50%–75% | 50% | Hemo: Unknown<br>CAPD: Unknown<br>CAVH: Unknown |
| Chlorambucil[417] | 0.1–0.2 mg/kg/d | D | Unknown | Unknown | Hemo: Unknown<br>CAPD: Unknown<br>CAVH: Unknown |
| Cisplatin[418, 419] | 20–120 mg/m² | D | 75% | 50% | Hemo: Dose after dialysis<br>CAPD: Unknown<br>CAVH: Unknown |
| Cyclophosphamide[420–422]<br>Hemorrhagic cystitis<br>Bladder fibrosis and bladder cancer (SIADH) | 1–5 mg/kg/d | D | 100% | 75% | Hemo: Dose after dialysis<br>CAPD: Unknown<br>CAVH: Unknown |
| Cytarabine[423]<br>Increased risk of neurotoxicity with high-dose therapy (2–3 g/m²) in patients with renal insufficiency | 100–200 mg/m² | D | 100% | 100% | Hemo: Unknown<br>CAPD: Unknown<br>CAVH: Unknown |
| Daunorubicin[424] | 30–45 mg/m² | D | 100% | 100% | Hemo: Unknown<br>CAPD: Unknown<br>CAVH: Unknown |
| Doxorubicin[425] | 60–75 mg/m² | D | 100% | 100% | Hemo: None<br>CAPD: Unlikely<br>CAVH: Unlikely |
| Etoposide[426] | 35–100 mg/m²/d | D | 75% | 50% | Hemo: None<br>CAPD: Unlikely<br>CAVH: Unlikely |
| Fluorouracil[427] | 12 mg/kg/d | D | 100% | 100% | Hemo: Dose after dialysis<br>CAPD: Unknown<br>CAVH: Unknown |
| Hydroxyurea[7, 75] | 20–30 mg/kg/d | D | 50% | 20% | Hemo: Unknown<br>CAPD: Unknown<br>CAVH: Unknown |
| Idarubicin[428] | 12 mg/m² | D | 100% | 100% | Hemo: Unknown<br>CAPD: Unknown<br>CAVH: Unknown |
| Melphalan[429, 430] | 6 mg/d | D | 75% | 50% | Hemo: Unlikely<br>CAPD: Unlikely<br>CAVH: Unlikely |
| Methotrexate[410, 431, 432] | Low dose 15–30 mg/d<br>High dose 12 g/m² (with leucovorin rescue) | D | 50% | Avoid | Hemo: None<br>CAPD: None<br>CAVH: Unlikely |
| Mitomycin C[433]<br>Hemolytic-uremic syndrome | 20 mg/m²<br>q 6–8 wk | D | 100% | 75% | Hemo: Unknown<br>CAPD: Unknown<br>CAVH: Unknown |
| Nitrosoureas[434, 435] | Varies | D | 75% | 25%–50% | Hemo: None<br>CAPD: Unlikely<br>CAVH: Unlikely |
| Plicamycin[436] | 25–30 µg/kg/d | D | 75% | 50% | Hemo: Unknown<br>CAPD: Unknown<br>CAVH: Unknown |
| Streptozocin[437] | 500 mg/m²/d | D | 75% | 50% | Hemo: Unknown<br>CAPD: Unknown<br>CAVH: Unknown |
| Tamoxifen[438] | 10–20 mg bid | D | 100% | 100% | Hemo: Unknown<br>CAPD: Unknown<br>CAVH: Unknown |
| Teniposide[7, 75] | 50–250 mg/m² | D | 100% | 100% | Hemo: None<br>CAPD: Unlikely<br>CAVH: Unlikely |
| Vinblastine[439] | 3.7 mg/m² | D | 100% | 100% | Hemo: Unknown<br>CAPD: Unknown<br>CAVH: Unknown |
| Vincristine[7, 75] | 1.4 mg/m² | D | 100% | 100% | Hemo: Unknown<br>CAPD: Unknown<br>CAVH: Unknown |

*D = dosage reduction method; GFR = glomerular filtration rate; Hemo = hemodialysis; CAPD = continuous ambulatory peritoneal dialysis; CAVH = continuous arteriovenous hemofiltration; SIADH = syndrome of inappropriate antidiuretic hormone secretion.

†**Editor's Note:** For drugs whose excretion is reduced at declining levels of renal function, dosage reduction should be considered even before the low end of the 10–50 mL/min GFR range is reached.

## TABLE 60–13. Endocrine and Metabolic Drugs*

| Drug, Toxicity, Notes | Dose for Normal Renal Function | Method | Adjustment for Renal Failure GFR of 10–50 mL/min† | <10 mL/min | Supplement for Dialysis |
|---|---|---|---|---|---|
| ***Hypoglycemic Agents*** | | | | | |
| Acarbose[450] | 50–200 mg tid | D | 100% | 100% | Hemo: Unlikely<br>CAPD: Unlikely<br>CAVH: Unlikely |
| Acetohexamide[451]<br>  Has diuretic effect<br>  May falsely elevate serum creatinine level<br>  Prolonged hypoglycemia in azotemic patients | 250–1500 mg/d | D | Avoid | Avoid | Hemo: Unknown<br>CAPD: Unknown<br>CAVH: Unknown |
| Chlorpropamide[451]<br>  Impairs water excretion<br>  Prolonged hypoglycemia in azotemic patients | 100–500 mg/d | D | Avoid | Avoid | Hemo: Unlikely<br>CAPD: Unlikely<br>CAVH: Unlikely |
| Gliclazide[452] | 160–320 mg/d | D | 100% | 100% | Hemo: Unlikely<br>CAPD: Unlikely<br>CAVH: Unlikely |
| Glipizide[453] | 2.5–15 mg/d | D | 100% | 100% | Hemo: Unlikely<br>CAPD: Unlikely<br>CAVH: Unlikely |
| Glyburide[454] | 1.25–20 mg/d | D | Avoid | Avoid | Hemo: Unlikely<br>CAPD: Unlikely<br>CAVH: Unlikely |
| Insulin[455]<br>  Renal metabolism of insulin decreases in renal insufficiency<br>  May be given IP in CAPD patients | Variable | D | 75% | 50% | Hemo: None<br>CAPD: Unlikely<br>CAVH: Unlikely |
| Tolazamide[451] | 100–250 mg/d | D | 100% | 100% | Hemo: Unlikely<br>CAPD: Unlikely<br>CAVH: Unlikely |
| Tolbutamide[451] | 1–2 g/d | D | 100% | 100% | Hemo: Unlikely<br>CAPD: Unlikely<br>CAVH: Unlikely |
| ***Hypolipidemic Agents*** | | | | | |
| Bezafibrate[448]<br>  Monitor creatine kinase levels | 200 mg tid | D | 50% | 25% | Hemo: Unlikely<br>CAPD: Unlikely<br>CAVH: Unlikely |
| Cholestyramine[448]<br>  Hyperchloremic acidosis<br>  Requires fluids for dilution | 4 g<br>q 4–6 h | D | 100% | 100%<br>(use with caution) | Hemo: None<br>CAPD: None<br>CAVH: None |
| Clofibrate[456] | 500–1000 mg bid | I | q 12–24 h | Avoid | Hemo: Unlikely<br>CAPD: Unlikely<br>CAVH: Unlikely |
| Colestipol[448]<br>  Hyperchloremic acidosis<br>  Requires fluids for dilution | 13–30 g/d | D | 100% | 100% | Hemo: None<br>CAPD: None<br>CAVH: None |
| Fenofibrate[456] | 300 mg/d | D | 25%–50% | Avoid | Hemo: None<br>CAPD: Unlikely<br>CAVH: Unlikely |
| Gemfibrozil[457] | 600 mg bid | D | 100% | 100% | Hemo: None<br>CAPD: Unknown<br>CAVH: Unknown |
| Lovastatin[449–458]<br>  Risk of rhabdomyolysis with concurrent use of cyclosporine | 20–80 mg/d | D | 100% | 100% | Hemo: Unlikely<br>CAPD: Unlikely<br>CAVH: Unlikely |
| Nicotinic acid[459]<br>  Aspirin may attenuate flushing | 1–2 g tid | D | 50% | 25% | Hemo: Unknown<br>CAPD: Unknown<br>CAVH: Unknown |
| Pravastatin[460] | 10–40 mg/d | D | Unknown<br>(likely to be decreased) | Unknown<br>(likely to be decreased) | Hemo: Unknown<br>CAPD: Unknown<br>CAVH: Unknown |
| Probucol[461] | 500 mg bid | D | 100% | 100% | Hemo: Unknown<br>CAPD: Unknown<br>CAVH: Unknown |
| Simvastatin[462] | 5–40 mg/d | D | 100% | 100% | Hemo: Unknown<br>CAPD: Unknown<br>CAVH: Unknown |
| ***Thyroid Medications*** | | | | | |
| L-Thyroxine[7]<br>  Adjust dose according to thyroid function tests | 100–200 μg/d | D | 100% | 100% | Hemo: Unlikely<br>CAPD: Unlikely<br>CAVH: Unlikely |
| Methimazole[463, 464] | 5–20 mg tid | D | 100% | 100% | Hemo: Unknown<br>CAPD: Unknown<br>CAVH: Unknown |
| Propylthiouracil[463] | 5–20 mg tid | D | 100% | 100% | Hemo: Unlikely<br>CAPD: Unlikely<br>CAVH: Unlikely |

*D = dosage reduction method; I = interval extension method; GFR = glomerular filtration rate; Hemo = hemodialysis; CAPD = continuous ambulatory peritoneal dialysis; CAVH = continuous arteriovenous hemofiltration; IP = intraperitoneally.

†**Editor's Note:** For drugs whose excretion is reduced at declining levels of renal function, dosage reduction should be considered even before the low end of the 10–50 mL/min GFR range is reached.

ure.[465] Finally, it is well recognized that significant absorption and accumulation of aluminum may occur with long-term ingestion of aluminum-containing antacids if renal function is impaired. The development of aluminum intoxication may be manifested by bone disease, anemia, or neurologic impairment, as discussed in detail in other sections of this text. In view of the easy access of antacids over the counter, patients must be counseled to avoid antacid use without first consulting their physician.

H₂ blockers are frequently prescribed for patients with renal disease. Although the drugs in this group have significant renal excretion, the therapeutic index is wide, allowing less stringent dosing reduction until renal failure is advanced. A significant amount of the renal elimination occurs by tubule secretion. This is particularly evident with cimetidine and may result in a spurious rise in the serum creatinine level. Other agents used in the treatment of peptic disease include prostaglandin analogues, the H⁺ pump inhibitors, and locally acting drugs such as sucralfate. Significant dosage reductions are not required for these drugs in renal failure. However, sucralfate contains a significant quantity of aluminum, which may accumulate and lead to toxic effects in patients with renal insufficiency.

The majority of the antiemetic and motility agents do not require dosage adjustment for renal failure. The dose of metoclopramide, however, should be decreased because significant renal clearance does occur and the risk of extrapyramidal side effects appears to be increased in renal insufficiency. A variety of laxatives are easily available over the counter. Proper education of the patient is essential because use of preparations such as magnesium-containing laxatives and phosphate-containing enemas may result in significant accumulation of Mg²⁺ or phosphorus. Suggested guidelines for prescribing gastrointestinal agents are outlined in Table 60–14.

## Neurologic Agents

Seizures occur with increased frequency in patients with renal insufficiency and end-stage renal disease.[491] Although the seizure is often caused by reversible precipitating events, in some cases a specific cause is not identified and long-term anticonvulsant therapy is required. Phenytoin is one of the most frequently prescribed anticonvulsants. In renal failure, the volume of distribution of this agent is increased and the degree of protein binding is reduced.[492] Although dosage adjustment is not generally required for renal insufficiency, the clinician should be aware that the proportion of free or active drug is increased. Thus, a low total plasma phenytoin level may not necessarily be subtherapeutic. Serum drug monitoring is best accomplished in renal failure by directly measuring the free serum phenytoin level. Antiparkinsonian agents and drugs used for the treatment of migraine headaches generally do not require dosage adjustment for renal failure. Recommendations for dosing neurologic drugs are outlined in Table 60–15.

## Rheumatologic Agents

Nonsteroidal anti-inflammatory drugs are widely prescribed for musculoskeletal pain. Although dose adjustment is generally not required for renal insufficiency, several precautions should be noted. Under conditions of decreased renal perfusion, such as congestive heart failure or advanced liver disease, vasodilatory prostaglandins may be critical in maintaining renal blood flow. When used in such cases, nonsteroidal anti-inflammatory drugs may cause an acute reversible decline in renal function through interference with prostaglandin synthesis. Other renal effects of nonsteroidal anti-inflammatory drugs include impairment of K⁺ excretion and interference with Na⁺ and water excretion.[504] In addition, a hypersensitivity reaction characterized by acute interstitial nephritis in conjunction with a minimal-change glomerular lesion may rarely occur. Gastrointestinal complications, such as gastritis and peptic pain, may limit the use of these agents in many patients. For all of these reasons, nonsteroidal anti-inflammatory drugs should be used with caution in patients with renal insufficiency and with careful monitoring of renal function, electrolytes, and blood pressure control.

Renal insufficiency occurs with increased frequency in patients with gout. Appropriate dose reduction for the level of renal function must be taken in prescribing gout agents to minimize side effects. Allopurinol reduces the production of uric acid and is commonly prescribed for the treatment of hyperuricemia and gout. Accumulation of the metabolite oxipurinol has been reported in renal insufficiency and may explain the development of exfoliative dermatitis in a subset of patients.[505] Patients with renal insufficiency appear to be at greater risk for the development of myopathy and polyneuropathy with the use of colchicine.[506] In addition to dose reduction, patients should be monitored closely for symptoms of muscle weakness with long-term use of the agent. In general, uricosuric drugs are ineffective when the GFR is decreased. Dosing guidelines for rheumatologic agents are summarized in Table 60–16.

## Sedatives, Hypnotics, and Psychiatric Agents

The majority of drugs in this category (with the exception of lithium) are lipid soluble, highly protein bound, and excreted primarily by hepatic transformation to inactive metabolites. Increased sensitivity to the sedative side effects may occur in the patient with renal insufficiency. In addition, recognition of side effects may be delayed because malaise and somnolence are common in the uremic population. Benzodiazepines are widely prescribed for anxiety. Several of these agents, including diazepam, flurazepam, and chlordiazepoxide, have active polar metabolites that may accumulate in patients with renal insufficiency and cause prolonged sedation. For this reason, long-term use of these agents should be avoided. Depression is common in patients with chronic illness and occasionally requires treatment with antidepressant medication. Although dose reduction is generally not required, increased sensitivity to the side effects of tricyclic antidepressants dictates a cautious approach. The initial dose should be low and slowly increased on the basis of clinical response and side effects. Similarly, side effects due to phenothiazines, such as extrapyramidal symptoms and changes in mental status, may be

*Text continued on page 2689*

TABLE 60–14. Gastrointestinal Drugs*

| Drug, Toxicity, Notes | Dose for Normal Renal Function | Method | Adjustment for Renal Failure GFR of | | | Supplement for Dialysis |
|---|---|---|---|---|---|---|
| | | | >50 mL/min | 10–50 mL/min† | <10 mL/min | |
| *Antiemetics, Antidiarrheals, Motility Agents* | | | | | | |
| Cisapride[7] | 5–10 mg qid | D | 100% | 100% | 100% | Hemo: None<br>CAPD: Unlikely<br>CAVH: Unlikely |
| Diphenoxylate[7] (each tablet contains 2.5 mg diphenoxylate and 0.025 mg atropine) | 2 tablets qid | D | 100% | 50%–100% | Avoid | Hemo: Unknown<br>CAPD: Unknown<br>CAVH: Unknown |
| Granisetron[7] | 40–160 µg/kg as 5- to 30-min IV infusion | D | 75%–100% | 100% | 100% | Hemo: Unknown<br>CAPD: Unknown<br>CAVH: Unknown |
| Metoclopramide[466–469] Extrapyramidal reactions increased in ESRD | 10–15 mg qid | D | 75%–100% | 75% | 50% | Hemo: None<br>CAPD: Unlikely<br>CAVH: Unlikely |
| Ondansetron[469] | 0.15 mg/kg as a 15-min infusion | D | 100% | 100% | 100% | Hemo: Unlikely<br>CAPD: Unlikely<br>CAVH: Unlikely |
| Prochlorperazine[7] | 5–10 mg PO tid–qid<br>25 mg PR bid | D | 100% | 100% | 100% | Hemo: Unknown<br>CAPD: Unknown<br>CAVH: Unknown |
| *$H_2$ Antagonists* | | | | | | |
| Cimetidine[470–474] Increases serum creatinine level by inhibition of tubule creatinine secretion | 400 mg bid or 400–800 mg hs | D | 75%–100% | 50%–75% | 25%–50% | Hemo: None<br>CAPD: None<br>CAVH: Unlikely |
| Famotidine[474–478] | 20–40 mg hs | D | 50%–100% | 25%–50% | 10% | Hemo: None<br>CAPD: None<br>CAVH: None |
| Nizatidine[479, 480] | 150–300 mg hs | D, I | 50%–100% | 50% | 50% qod | Hemo: Unknown<br>CAPD: Unknown<br>CAVH: Unknown |
| Ranitidine[481–484] | 150–300 mg hs | D | 50%–100% | 50% | 25% | Hemo: ½ dose<br>CAPD: None<br>CAVH: Likely to be removed; dose for GFR 10–50 |
| Roxatidine[475] | 150 mg hs | D | 50%–100% | 50% | 25% | Hemo: Unknown<br>CAPD: Unknown<br>CAVH: Unknown |

### *Other Drugs Used for Peptic Disease*

#### Antacids

Calcium, magnesium, and aluminum salts have absorption of constituent cations that have reduced elimination in renal failure, producing hypercalcemia, hypermagnesemia, and elevated aluminum levels, respectively. Protracted use may cause nephrolithiasis, metabolic alkalosis, and milk-alkali syndrome. Calcium salts are now the drugs of choice as phosphate binders. For these reasons, other agents are preferred in the treatment of peptic disease in patients with renal failure.

| Drug, Toxicity, Notes | Dose for Normal Renal Function | Method | >50 mL/min | 10–50 mL/min† | <10 mL/min | Supplement for Dialysis |
|---|---|---|---|---|---|---|
| Enprostil[7] | 35 µg bid | D | 100% | 100% | 100% | Hemo: Unknown<br>CAPD: Unknown<br>CAVH: Unknown |
| Lansoprazole[485] | 30 mg qd | D | 100% | 100% | 100% | Hemo: Unlikely<br>CAPD: Unlikely<br>CAVH: Unlikely |
| Misoprostol[486] | 100–200 µg qid | D | 100% | 100% | 100% | Hemo: Unlikely<br>CAPD: Unlikely<br>CAVH: Unlikely |
| Omeprazole[487, 488] | 20–40 mg/d | D | 100% | 100% | 100% | Hemo: None<br>CAPD: Unlikely<br>CAVH: Unlikely |
| Sucralfate[489, 490] Contains aluminum, which may be absorbed to produce dementia, renal osteodystrophy, and anemia <5% of dose absorbed | 1 g qid | D | 50%–100% | Avoid | Avoid | Avoid |

*D = dosage reduction method; I = interval extension method; GFR = glomerular filtration rate; Hemo = hemodialysis; CAPD = continuous ambulatory peritoneal dialysis; CAVH = continuous arteriovenous hemofiltration; ESRD = end-stage renal disease.

†**Editor's Note:** For drugs whose excretion is reduced at declining levels of renal function, dosage reduction should be considered even before the low end of the 10–50 mL/min GFR range is reached.

**TABLE 60–15. Neurologic Agents***

| Drug, Toxicity, Notes | Dose for Normal Renal Function | Method | Adjustment for Renal Failure GFR of | | Supplement for Dialysis |
|---|---|---|---|---|---|
| | | | 10–50 mL/min† | <10 mL/min | |
| **Anticonvulsants** | | | | | |
| Monitor serum levels. | | | | | |
| Carbamazepine[493–495] | 200–1200 mg/d | D | 100% | 100% | Hemo: None<br>CAPD: Unlikely<br>CAVH: Unlikely |
| Ethosuximide[496] | 500–1500 mg/d | D | 75%–100% | 50% | Hemo: 250 mg<br>CAPD: Unknown<br>CAVH: Dose for GFR 10–50 |
| Oxcarbazepine[7] | 200–400 mg tid | D | 100% | 100% | Hemo: Unknown<br>CAPD: Unknown<br>CAVH: Unknown |
| Phenytoin[492–497]<br> Protein binding decreased and distribution volume increased in renal failure<br> Monitor free phenytoin levels | 1000 mg load, then 300–400 mg/d | D | 100% | 100% | Hemo: None<br>CAPD: None<br>CAVH: Unlikely |
| Primidone[498]<br> Partially converted to phenobarbital and other metabolites with long half-life | 200–500 mg qid | I | q 8–12 h | q 12–24 h | Hemo: ⅓ dose<br>CAPD: Unknown<br>CAVH: Likely to be removed; dose for GFR 10–50 |
| Trimethadione[7, 75] | 300–600 mg tid–qid | I | q 8–12 h | q 12–24 h | Hemo: Unknown<br>CAPD: Unknown<br>CAVH: Unknown |
| Valproic acid[499, 500]<br> Decreased protein binding in uremia<br> Concurrent phenytoin, phenobarbital, and primidone shorten half-life | 15–60 mg/kg/d | D | 100% | 100% | Hemo: None<br>CAPD: Unlikely<br>CAVH: Unlikely |
| Vigabatrin[7, 75] | 2–4 g/d | D | 50% | 25%–50% | Hemo: Unknown<br>CAPD: Unknown<br>CAVH: Unknown |
| **Antiparkinsonian Agents** | | | | | |
| Bromocriptine[501]<br> Orthostatic hypotension | 1.25 mg bid | D | 100% | 100% | Hemo: Unlikely<br>CAPD: Unlikely<br>CAVH: Unlikely |
| Carbidopa[502] | 1 tablet tid to 6 tablets daily | D | 100% | 100% | Hemo: Unknown<br>CAPD: Unknown<br>CAVH: Unknown |
| Levodopa[502] | 250–500 mg bid to 8 g/d | D | 100% | 100% | Hemo: Unknown<br>CAPD: Unknown<br>CAVH: Unknown |
| Trihexyphenidyl[503] | 1–2 mg/d to 6–10 mg/d | D | Unknown | Unknown | Hemo: Unknown<br>CAPD: Unknown<br>CAVH: Unknown |
| **Agents Used for the Treatment of Migraine Headaches** | | | | | |
| Ergotamine[7]<br> (Ergotamine 1 mg, caffeine 100 mg) | Acute attack: 1 tablet q 30 min (maximum 6 tablets) | D | 100% | 100% | Hemo: Unknown<br>CAPD: Unknown<br>CAVH: Unknown |
| Dihydroergotamine[7] | Acute attack: 1 mg IM or IV q 1 h (maximum 3 mg) | D | 100% | 100% | Hemo: Unknown<br>CAPD: Unknown<br>CAVH: Unknown |

*D = dosage reduction method; I = interval extension method; GFR = glomerular filtration rate; Hemo = hemodialysis; CAPD = continuous ambulatory peritoneal dialysis; CAVH = continuous arteriovenous hemofiltration.

†**Editor's Note:** For drugs whose excretion is reduced at declining levels of renal function, dosage reduction should be considered even before the low end of the 10–50 mL/min GFR range is reached.

## TABLE 60–16. Rheumatologic Agents*

| Drug, Toxicity, Notes | Dose for Normal Renal Function | Method | Adjustment for Renal Failure GFR of | | Supplement for Dialysis |
|---|---|---|---|---|---|
| | | | 10–50 mL/min† | <10 mL/min | |
| **Gout Agents** | | | | | |
| Allopurinol[505, 507] Active metabolite | 300 mg/d | D | 50% | 25% | Hemo: ½ dose CAPD: Unknown CAVH: Unknown |
| Colchicine[506, 508] Increased risk of myopathy and neuropathy in renal failure Monitor creatine kinase values | Short-term: 2 mg, then 0.5 mg q 6 h Long-term: 0.5–1 mg/d | D | 50% | 25% | Hemo: None CAPD: Unlikely CAVH: Unlikely |
| Probenecid[509] Ineffective at decreased GFR | 500 mg bid | D | Avoid | Avoid | Hemo: Unlikely CAPD: Unlikely CAVH: Unlikely |
| **Nonsteroidal Anti-inflammatory Drugs** Drugs in this group may be associated with renal dysfunction due to prostaglandin inhibition; prostaglandin inhibitors may increase uremic bleeding and gastrointestinal symptoms; nephrotic syndrome, interstitial nephritis, and hyperkalemia reported. | | | | | |
| Diclofenac[510, 511] | 25–75 mg bid | D | 100% | 100% | Hemo: None CAPD: None CAVH: None |
| Diflunisal[512] | 250–500 mg bid | D | 100% | 50% | Hemo: None CAPD: None CAVH: None |
| Etodolac[513] | 200–600 mg bid | D | 100% | 100% | Hemo: None CAPD: None CAVH: None |
| Flurbiprofen[514] | 100 mg bid–tid | D | 100% | 100% | Hemo: None CAPD: None CAVH: None |
| Ibuprofen[515] | 800 mg tid | D | 100% | 100% | Hemo: None CAPD: None CAVH: None |
| Indomethacin[516] | 25–50 mg tid | D | 100% | 100% | Hemo: None CAPD: None CAVH: None |
| Ketoprofen[517] | 25–75 mg tid | D | 100% | 100% | Hemo: None CAPD: None CAVH: None |
| Ketorolac[518] | 5–30 mg qid | D | 100% | 100% | Hemo: None CAPD: None CAVH: None |
| Meclofenamic acid[510] | 50–100 mg tid–qid | D | 100% | 100% | Hemo: None CAPD: None CAVH: None |
| Mefenamic acid[510] | 250 mg qid | D | 100% | 100% | Hemo: None CAPD: None CAVH: None |
| Naproxen[519] | 500 mg bid | D | 100% | 100% | Hemo: None CAPD: None CAVH: None |
| Phenylbutazone[510] | 100 mg tid–qid | D | 100% | 100% | Hemo: None CAPD: None CAVH: None |
| Piroxicam[520] | 20 mg/d | D | 100% | 100% | Hemo: None CAPD: None CAVH: None |
| Sulindac[521] Active sulfide metabolite; relatively renal sparing | 200 mg bid | D | 100% | 100% | Hemo: None CAPD: None CAVH: None |
| Tolmetin[510] | 400 mg tid | D | 100% | 100% | Hemo: None CAPD: None CAVH: None |
| **Other Agents Used in Treatment of Arthritis** | | | | | |
| Auranofin[522] Proteinuria common, rarely progresses to nephrotic syndrome | 6 mg/d | D | Avoid | Avoid | Hemo: Unlikely CAPD: Unlikely CAVH: Unlikely |
| Gold sodium thiomalate[523] Nephrotoxic; proteinuria, membranous nephritis | 25–50 mg | D | Avoid | Avoid | Hemo: Unlikely CAPD: Unlikely CAVH: Unlikely |
| Penicillamine[7, 75] | 250–1000 mg/d | D | Avoid | Avoid | Hemo: Unknown CAPD: Unknown CAVH: Unknown |

*D = dosage reduction method; GFR = glomerular filtration rate; Hemo = hemodialysis; CAPD = continuous ambulatory peritoneal dialysis; CAVH = continuous arteriovenous hemofiltration.

†**Editor's Note:** For drugs whose excretion is reduced at declining levels of renal function, dosage reduction should be considered even before the low end of the 10–50 mL/min GFR range is reached.

### TABLE 60–17. Sedatives, Hypnotics, and Drugs Used in Psychiatry*

| Drug, Toxicity, Notes | Dose for Normal Renal Function | Method | Adjustment for Renal Failure GFR of | | Supplement for Dialysis |
|---|---|---|---|---|---|
| | | | 10–50 mL/min† | <10 mL/min | |
| *Antidepressants* | | | | | |
| Amoxapine[525] | 75–200 mg/d | D | 100% | 100% | Hemo: Unlikely<br>CAPD: Unlikely<br>CAVH: Unlikely |
| Bupropion[526] | 100 mg q 8 h | D | 100% | 100% | Hemo: Unlikely<br>CAPD: Unlikely<br>CAVH: Unlikely |
| Fluoxetine[527, 528] | 20 mg/d | D | 100% | 100% | Hemo: None<br>CAPD: Unlikely<br>CAVH: Unlikely |
| Maprotiline[7, 75] | 75–150 mg/d | D | 100% | 50%–75% | Hemo: Unlikely<br>CAPD: Unlikely<br>CAVH: Unlikely |
| *Barbiturates*<br>May cause excessive sedation. | | | | | |
| Pentobarbital[7, 75] | 30 mg tid–qid | D | 100% | 100% | Hemo: Dose after dialysis<br>CAPD: Unknown<br>CAVH: Unknown |
| Phenobarbital[7, 75] | 50–100 mg bid–tid | D<br>I | 100%<br>q 8–12 h | 50%<br>q 12 h | Hemo: Dose after dialysis<br>CAPD: 75%<br>q 12 h<br>CAVH: Unknown, likely to be removed |
| Secobarbital[7, 75] | 30–50 mg tid–qid | D | 100% | 100% | Hemo: Dose after dialysis<br>CAPD: Unknown<br>CAVH: Unknown |
| Thiopental[529] | Anesthesia induction | D | 100% | 75% | Hemo: Unlikely<br>CAPD: Unlikely<br>CAVH: Unlikely |
| *Benzodiazepines* | | | | | |
| Alprazolam[530, 531] | 0.25–5 mg tid | D | 100% | 100% | Hemo: Unlikely<br>CAPD: Unlikely<br>CAVH: Unlikely |
| Chlordiazepoxide[533]<br>Active metabolite | 15–100 mg/d | D | 100% | 50% | Hemo: Unlikely<br>CAPD: Unlikely<br>CAVH: Unlikely |
| Clonazepam[530] | 1.5 mg/d | D | 100% | 100% | Hemo: Unknown<br>CAPD: Unknown<br>CAVH: Unknown |
| Clorazepate[532]<br>Active metabolite | 15–60 mg/d | D | 100% | 100% | Hemo: Unknown<br>CAPD: Unknown<br>CAVH: Unknown |
| Diazepam[7, 75] | 5–40 mg/d | D | 100% | 100% | Hemo: Unlikely<br>CAPD: Unlikely<br>CAVH: Unlikely |
| Flurazepam[530]<br>Active metabolite | 15–30 mg hs | D | 100% | 100% | Hemo: Unlikely<br>CAPD: Unlikely<br>CAVH: Unlikely |
| Lorazepam[534] | 1–2 mg bid–tid | D | 100% | 100% | Hemo: None<br>CAPD: Unlikely<br>CAVH: Unlikely |
| Midazolam[535] | 1.25 mg IV initially, titrate to response | D | 100% | 100% | Hemo: Unlikely<br>CAPD: Unlikely<br>CAVH: Unlikely |
| Nitrazepam[536] | 5–10 mg hs | D | 100% | 100% | Hemo: Unknown<br>CAPD: Unknown<br>CAVH: Unknown |
| Oxazepam[537] | 30–120 mg/d | D | 100% | 100% | Hemo: None<br>CAPD: Unlikely<br>CAVH: Unlikely |
| Prazepam[530]<br>Active metabolite | 20–60 mg hs | D | 100% | 100% | Hemo: Unlikely<br>CAPD: Unlikely<br>CAVH: Unlikely |
| Quazepam[538] | 15 mg hs | D | 100% | 100% | Hemo: Unlikely<br>CAPD: Unlikely<br>CAVH: Unlikely |
| Temazepam[530] | 30 mg hs | D | 100% | 100% | Hemo: Unlikely<br>CAPD: Unlikely<br>CAVH: Unlikely |

**TABLE 60–17. Sedatives, Hypnotics, and Drugs Used in Psychiatry*** *Continued*

| Drug, Toxicity, Notes | Dose for Normal Renal Function | Method | Adjustment for Renal Failure GFR of | | Supplement for Dialysis |
|---|---|---|---|---|---|
| | | | 10–50 mL/min† | <10 mL/min | |
| Triazolam[539, 540]<br>  Protein binding correlates with α₁-acid glycoprotein concentration | 0.125–0.5 mg hs | D | 100% | 100% | Hemo: Unlikely<br>CAPD: Unlikely<br>CAVH: Unlikely |
| *Phenothiazines*<br>Anticholinergic, urinary retention, orthostatic hypotension, confusion. | | | | | |
| Chlorpromazine[541] | 300–800 mg/d | D | 100% | 100% | Hemo: Unlikely<br>CAPD: Unlikely<br>CAVH: Unlikely |
| Promethazine[542] | 20–100 mg/d | D | 100% | 100% | Hemo: Unknown<br>CAPD: Unknown<br>CAVH: Unknown |
| *Tricyclic Antidepressants*<br>Anticholinergic, urinary retention, orthostatic hypotension, excessive sedation. | | | | | |
| Amitriptyline[543–545] | 25 mg tid | D | 100% | 100% | Hemo: None<br>CAPD: None<br>CAVH: Unlikely |
| Clomipramine[546] | 25–50 mg bid–tid | D | 100% | 100% | Hemo: Unlikely<br>CAPD: Unlikely<br>CAVH: Unlikely |
| Desipramine[547]<br>  Active metabolites | 75–150 mg/d | D | 100% | 100% | Hemo: Unlikely<br>CAPD: Unlikely<br>CAVH: Unlikely |
| Doxepin[548]<br>  Protein binding decrease in ESRD | 25 mg tid | D | 100% | 100% | Hemo: None<br>CAPD: Unlikely<br>CAVH: Unlikely |
| Imipramine[549]<br>  Active metabolite | 25 mg tid | D | 100% | 100% | Hemo: Unlikely<br>CAPD: Unlikely<br>CAVH: Unlikely |
| Nortriptyline[550] | 25 mg tid–qid | D | 100% | 100% | Hemo: None<br>CAPD: Unlikely<br>CAVH: Unlikely |
| Protriptyline[551] | 15–60 mg/d | D | 100% | 100% | Hemo: Unlikely<br>CAPD: Unlikely<br>CAVH: Unlikely |
| *Miscellaneous Agents* | | | | | |
| Buspirone[552]<br>  Active metabolite accumulates | 5–10 mg tid | D | 100% | 50% | Hemo: Unlikely<br>CAPD: Unlikely<br>CAVH: Unlikely |
| Chloral hydrate[7, 75]<br>  Active metabolite<br>  Excessive sedation | 250 mg tid | D | Avoid | Avoid | Hemo: None<br>CAPD: Unlikely<br>CAVH: Unlikely |
| Clozapine[553] | 150–200 mg bid | D | 100% | 100% | Hemo: Unlikely<br>CAPD: Unlikely<br>CAVH: Unlikely |
| Ethchlorvynol[7, 75]<br>  Excessive sedation | 500 mg hs | D | Avoid | Avoid | Hemo: Avoid<br>CAPD: Avoid<br>CAVH: Avoid |
| Haloperidol[554]<br>  Hypotension<br>  Excessive sedation | 1–2 mg bid–tid | D | 100% | 100% | Hemo: Unlikely<br>CAPD: Unlikely<br>CAVH: Unlikely |
| Lithium carbonate[524, 525, 555]<br>  Nephrogenic diabetes insipidus<br>  Nephrotoxic, monitor serum levels<br>  Toxicity enhanced by volume depletion, diuretics, and NSAIDs | 900–1200 mg total dose/d | D | 50%–75% | 25%–50% | Hemo: Dose after dialysis<br>CAPD: None<br>CAVH: Likely to be removed, follow levels |
| Meprobamate[7, 75] | 300–400 mg q 6 h | D<br>I | 100% q 8–12 h | 50%<br>q 12 h | Hemo: 200–400 mg<br>CAPD: Unknown<br>CAVH: Likely to be removed |
| Phenelzine[7, 75] | 20–30 mg tid | D | 100% | 100% | Hemo: Unknown<br>CAPD: Unknown<br>CAVH: Unknown |

*D = dosage reduction method; I = interval extension method; GFR = glomerular filtration rate; Hemo = hemodialysis; CAPD = continuous ambulatory peritoneal dialysis; CAVH = continuous arteriovenous hemofiltration; ESRD = end-stage renal disease; NSAIDs = nonsteroidal anti-inflammatory drugs.

†**Editor's Note:** For drugs whose excretion is reduced at declining levels of renal function, dosage reduction should be considered even before the low end of the 10–50 mL/min GFR range is reached.

**TABLE 60–18. Miscellaneous Agents***

| Drug, Toxicity, Notes | Dose for Normal Renal Function | Method | Adjustment for Renal Failure GFR of | | Supplement for Dialysis |
|---|---|---|---|---|---|
| | | | 10–50 mL/min† | <10 mL/min | |
| **Anticoagulants and Antiplatelet Agents** Agents in this group should be carefully titrated to achieve therapeutic effects; may potentiate uremic bleeding. | | | | | |
| Dipyridamole[556] | 50 mg tid | D | 100% | 100% | Hemo: Unlikely CAPD: Unlikely CAVH: Unlikely |
| Heparin[557] $t_{1/2}$ increases with dose | 75 U/kg load, then 0.5 U/kg/min | D | 100% | 100% | Hemo: Unlikely CAPD: Unlikely CAVH: Unlikely |
| Streptokinase[558] | 250,000 U load, then 100,000 U/h | D | 100% | 100% | Hemo: NA CAPD: NA CAVH: NA |
| Sulfinpyrazone[559] | 200 mg bid | D | 100% | Avoid | Hemo: Unlikely CAPD: Unlikely CAVH: Unlikely |
| Ticlopidine[560] | 500 mg bid | D | 100% | 100% | Hemo: Unknown CAPD: Unknown CAVH: Unknown |
| Tissue-type plasminogen activator[561] | 100 mg total in 3-h period | D | 100% | 100% | Hemo: Unlikely CAPD: Unlikely CAVH: Unlikely |
| Urokinase[7] | 4400 U/kg load, then 4400 U/kg/h | D | 100% | 100% | Hemo: Unknown CAPD: Unknown CAVH: Unknown |
| Warfarin[562] Follow prothrombin time | 10–15 mg load, then 2–10 mg/d | D | 100% | 100% | Hemo: Unlikely CAPD: Unlikely CAVH: Unlikely |
| **Antihistamines** May cause excessive sedation. | | | | | |
| Astemizole[563, 564] | 10 mg/d | D | 100% | 100% | Hemo: Unlikely CAPD: Unlikely CAVH: Unlikely |
| Brompheniramine[563] | 4 mg q 4–6 h | D | 100% | 100% | Hemo: Unknown CAPD: Unknown CAVH: Unknown |
| Chlorpheniramine[563] | 4 mg q 4–6 h | D | 100% | 100% | Hemo: None CAPD: Unlikely CAVH: Unlikely |
| Diphenhydramine[563] Anticholinergic effects may cause urine retention | 25 mg tid–qid | D | 100% | 100% | Hemo: Unlikely CAPD: Unlikely CAVH: Unlikely |
| Flunarizine[7, 75] | Unknown | D | None | None | Hemo: Unlikely CAPD: Unlikely CAVH: Unlikely |
| Hydroxyzine[7, 75] | 50–100 mg qid | D | Unknown | Unknown | Hemo: Unknown CAPD: Unknown CAVH: Unknown |
| Orphenadrine[563] | 100 mg bid | D | 100% | 100% | Hemo: Unknown CAPD: Unknown CAVH: Unknown |
| Oxatomide[565] | Unknown | D | 100% | 100% | Hemo: Unlikely CAPD: Unlikely CAVH: Unlikely |
| Promethazine[563] | 12.5–25 mg qd/qid | D | 100% | 100% | Hemo: Unlikely CAPD: Unlikely CAVH: Unlikely |
| Terfenadine[566] | 60 mg bid | D | 100% | 100% | Hemo: Unlikely CAPD: Unlikely CAVH: Unlikely |
| Tripelennamine[563] | 25–50 mg tid–qid | D | Unknown | Unknown | Hemo: Unknown CAPD: Unknown CAVH: Unknown |
| Triprolidine[563] | 2.5 mg q 4–6 h | D | Unknown | Unknown | Hemo: Unknown CAPD: Unknown CAVH: Unknown |

**TABLE 60–18. Miscellaneous Agents\*** *Continued*

| Drug, Toxicity, Notes | Dose for Normal Renal Function | Method | Adjustment for Renal Failure GFR of | | Supplement for Dialysis |
|---|---|---|---|---|---|
| | | | 10–50 mL/min† | <10 mL/min | |
| ***Bronchodilators*** | | | | | |
| Albuterol[567] | 2–4 mg tid–qid<br>Aerosol: 100–200 mg tid–qid | D | 75% | 50% | Hemo: Unknown<br>CAPD: Unknown<br>CAVH: Unknown |
| Bitolterol[568] | Aerosol:<br>2 inhalations q 8 h | D | 100% | 100% | Hemo: Unknown<br>CAPD: Unknown<br>CAVH: Unknown |
| Dyphylline[569] | 15 mg/kg/d | D | 50% | 25% | Hemo: ⅓ dose<br>CAPD: Unknown<br>CAVH: Likely to be removed |
| Ipratropium[567] | 2 inhalations qid | D | 100% | 100% | Hemo: Unlikely<br>CAPD: Unlikely<br>CAVH: Unlikely |
| Terbutaline[567] | 2.5–5 mg tid | D | 50% | Avoid | Hemo: Unknown<br>CAPD: Unknown<br>CAVH: Unknown |
| Theophylline[570, 571] | 200–400 mg<br>q 12 h | D | 100% | 100% | Hemo: ½ dose<br>CAPD: Unknown<br>CAVH: Likely to be removed; monitor levels |
| ***Immunosuppressive Drugs*** | | | | | |
| Azathioprine[572, 573] | 1.5–2.5 mg/kg/d | D | 75% | 50% | Hemo: Dose after dialysis<br>CAPD: Unknown<br>CAVH: Unknown |
| *Corticosteroids*<br>May aggravate azotemia, Na⁺ retention, glucose intolerance, and hypertension. | | | | | |
| Betamethasone[7, 75] | 0.5–9 mg/d | D | 100% | 100% | Hemo: Unknown<br>CAPD: Unknown<br>CAVH: Unknown |
| Cortisone[7, 75] | 25–500 mg/d | D | 100% | 100% | Hemo: None<br>CAPD: Unlikely<br>CAVH: Unlikely |
| Dexamethasone[574] | 0.75–9 mg/d | D | 100% | 100% | Hemo: Unknown<br>CAPD: Unknown<br>CAVH: Unknown |
| Hydrocortisone[7, 75] | 20–500 mg/d | D | 100% | 100% | Hemo: Unknown<br>CAPD: Unknown<br>CAVH: Unknown |
| Methylprednisolone[575] | 4–48 mg/d | D | 100% | 100% | Hemo: Yes<br>CAPD: Unknown<br>CAVH: Likely to be removed |
| Prednisone[576] | 5–60 mg/d | D | 100% | 100% | Hemo: None<br>CAPD: Unlikely<br>CAVH: Unlikely |
| Triamcinolone[7, 75] | 4–48 mg/d | D | 100% | 100% | Hemo: Unknown<br>CAPD: Unknown<br>CAVH: Unknown |
| Cyclosporine[577]<br>Nephrotoxic<br>Hypertension, seizures, tremor<br>Inhibitor of hepatic metabolism increase blood levels | 3–10 mg/kg/d | D | 100% | 100% | Hemo: Unknown<br>CAPD: Unknown<br>CAVH: Unknown |
| ***Miscellaneous*** | | | | | |
| Acetohydroxamic acid[578]<br>May accumulate in ESRD | 10–15 mg/kg/d | D | 100% | Avoid | Hemo: Unknown<br>CAPD: Unknown<br>CAVH: Unknown |
| Deferoxamine[579, 580]<br>Fungal infections in ESRD<br>Used in treatment of iron or aluminum overload | Chronic iron overload<br>0.5–1 g/d | D, I | 50% qd | 5–10 mg/k/wk (avoid if possible) | Hemo: Chelation product removed<br>CAPD: Chelation product removed<br>CAVH: Chelation product removed |
| Pentoxifylline[581, 582] | 400 mg tid | I | bid–tid | q 24 h | Hemo: Unknown<br>CAPD: Unknown<br>CAVH: Unknown |

\*D = dosage reduction method; I = interval extension method; GFR = glomerular filtration rate; Hemo = hemodialysis; CAPD = continuous ambulatory peritoneal dialysis; CAVH = continuous arteriovenous hemofiltration; ESRD = end-stage renal disease; NA = not applicable.

†**Editor's Note:** For drugs whose excretion is reduced at declining levels of renal function, dosage reduction should be considered even before the low end of the 10–50 mL/min GFR range is reached.

accentuated in renal failure. Therefore, the lowest therapeutic dose possible should be prescribed.

In contrast to most psychotropic drugs, lithium is water soluble and excreted by the kidney. Lithium may have several renal effects, including the development of renal failure with acute lithium overdose and nephrogenic diabetes insipidus in patients receiving long-term treatment.[524] Lithium levels should be monitored carefully and the dose reduced in patients with renal insufficiency because the therapeutic/toxic ratio is narrow. Volume depletion and concomitant diuretic therapy should be avoided if possible because lithium reabsorption in the kidney will increase in $Na^+$-avid states. Significant removal of lithium occurs with hemodialysis, which may be used for the treatment of lithium overdose. Table 60–17 summarizes dosing recommendations for agents used in psychiatry.

## Miscellaneous Agents

A wide variety of agents are included in the table of miscellaneous agents. Although most of the information is self-explanatory, a few comments are appropriate. The use of anticoagulants in patients with renal insufficiency requires close monitoring because platelet dysfunction may increase the risk of bleeding. Antihistamines are frequently prescribed agents that may cause excessive sedation in some patients with renal insufficiency. Once again, the initial dose should be low and increased slowly until the lowest effective dose is found. Immunosuppressive agents are often used in patients with renal insufficiency as treatment for the primary renal disease or for renal transplantation. No dosage adjustment is required for steroids or cyclosporine because hepatic metabolism is the primary route of elimination. Table 60–18 summarizes dosing recommendations for miscellaneous agents.

## CONCLUSIONS

Prescribing drugs for the patient with renal disease poses a difficult challenge for the clinician. Pharmacokinetics and pharmacodynamics are frequently altered in this setting. In addition, coexisting medical problems are frequently present and result in the need for multiple medications in many patients. Not surprisingly, the risk of adverse drug reactions is increased in this population and contributes significantly to morbidity of patients, prolongation of hospital stays, and financial costs of drug therapy. To minimize toxic effects and optimize efficacy, it is critical that the clinician be aware of these issues and adjust drug dosages appropriately.

## REFERENCES

1. Bennett WM: Geriatric pharmacokinetics and the kidney. Am J Kidney Dis 16:283, 1990.
2. Bennett WM: Adjustment of drug dosage in patients with renal insufficiency. In Kelley WM (ed): Textbook of Internal Medicine. JB Lippincott, Philadelphia, 1991, p 763.
3. Bennett WM, Aronoff GR, Golper TA, et al: Drug Prescribing in Renal Failure: Dosing Guidelines for Adults, 3rd ed. American College of Physicians, Philadelphia, 1994.
4. Golper TA, Bennett WM: Altering drug dose in liver and kidney disease. In Schrier R, Gambertoglio J (eds): Handbook of Drug Therapy in Liver and Kidney Disease. Little, Brown, Boston, 1991, p 1.
5. Maderazo E, Sun HE, Jay GT: Simplification of antibiotic dose adjustments in renal insufficiency: The DREM system. Lancet 340:767, 1992.
6. Maher JF: Principles of dialysis and dialysis of drugs. Am J Med 62:475, 1977.
7. Seyffart G (ed): Drug Dosage in Renal Insufficiency. Kluwer Academic Publishers, Dordrecht, Netherlands, 1991.
8. Swan SK, Bennett WM: Drug dosing guidelines in patients with renal failure. West J Med 156:633, 1992.
9. Swan SK, Bennett WM: Use of cardiovascular drugs in chronic renal failure. In Parfrey PS, Harnett JD (eds): Cardiac Dysfunction in Chronic Uremia. Kluwer Academic Publishers, Dordrecht, Netherlands, 1992, p 267.
10. Bennett WM: Renal effects of cyclosporine. J Am Acad Dermatol 23:1280, 1990.
11. Ochs HR, Greenblatt DJ, Bodem G, et al: Disease-related alterations in cardiac glycoside disposition. Clin Pharmacokinet 7:434, 1982.
12. Gulyassy PF, Depner TA: Impaired binding of drugs and endogenous ligands in renal disease. Am J Kidney Dis 98:730, 1983.
13. McNamara PJ, Lalka D, Gibaldi M: Endogenous accumulation products and serum protein binding in uremia. J Lab Clin Med 98:730, 1981.
14. Golper TA, Bennett WM: Drug usage in dialysis patients. In Nissenson A, Fine R, Gentile D (eds): Clinical Dialysis, 2nd ed. Appleton & Lange, East Norwalk, CT, 1990, p 608.
15. Lee CC, Marbury TC: Drug therapy in patients undergoing haemodialysis. Clin Pharmacokinet 9:42, 1984.
16. Vos MC, Vincent HH, Yzerman EPF, et al: Drug clearance by continuous hemodiafiltration (CAVHD): Results with the AN69 capillary hemofilter and recommended dose adjustments for seven antibiotics. Drug Invest (in press)
17. Piafsky KM: Disease-induced changes in the plasma binding of basic drugs. Clin Pharmacokinet 5:246, 1980.
18. Drayer D: Active drug metabolites and renal failure. Am J Med 62:486, 1977.
19. Kirchner KA, Voelker JR, Brater DC: Binding inhibitors restore furosemide potency in tubule fluid containing albumin. Kidney Int 40:418, 1991.
20. DeLuca HF, Krisinger J, Darwish H: The vitamin D system: 1990. Kidney Int 29(suppl):S2, 1990.
21. Rabkin R, Simon NM, Steinder S, et al: Effect of renal disease on renal uptake and excretion of insulin in man. N Engl J Med 282:182, 1970.
22. Vincent HH, Vos MC, Akcahuseyin E, et al: Drug clearance by continuous haemodiafiltration (CAVHD). Analysis of sieving coefficients and mass transfer coefficients of diffusion. Blood Purif 11:99, 1993.
23. Keller F, Wilms H, Schultze G, et al: Effect of plasma protein binding, volume of distribution, and molecular weight on the fraction of drugs eliminated by hemodialysis. Clin Nephrol 19:201, 1983.
24. Lasrich M, Maher JM, Hirszel P, et al: Correlation of peritoneal transport rates with molecular weight: A method of predicting clearances. ASAIO J 2:107, 1979.
25. Dromgoole SH: The effect of hemodialysis on the binding capacity of albumin. Clin Chim Acta 46:469, 1973.
26. Rustein DD, Catelli WP, Nickerson RJ: Heparin and human lipid metabolism. Lancet 2:1003, 1969.
27. Suh B, Craig WA, England AC, et al: Effect of free fatty acids on protein binding of antimicrobial agents. J Infect Dis 143:609, 1981.
28. Golper TA, Saad AMA: Gentamicin and phenytoin sieving through hollow-fiber polysulfone hemofilters. Kidney Int 30:937, 1986.
29. Fabris A, La Greca G, Chiaramonte S, et al: Total solute extraction versus clearance in the evaluation of standard and short hemodialysis. ASAIO Trans 34:627, 1988.
30. Sprenger KGB, Stephan H, Kratz W, et al: Optimizing of hemodiafiltration with modern membranes? Contrib Nephrol 46:43, 1985.
31. De Bock V, Verbeelen D, Naes V, et al: Pharmacokinetics of vancomycin in patients undergoing hemodialysis and hemofiltration. Nephrol Dial Transplant 4:635, 1989.
32. Matzke GR, O'Connell MB, Collins AJ, et al: Disposition of vancomycin during hemofiltration. Clin Pharmacol Ther 40:425, 1986.

33. Marbury TC, Lee CC, Perchalski RJ, et al: Hemodialysis clearance of ethosuximide in patients with chronic renal disease. Am J Hosp Pharm 38:1757, 1981.
34. Lee CS, Marbury TC, Benet LZ: Clearance calculations in hemodialysis: Application to blood, plasma, and dialysate measurements for ethambutol. J Pharmacokinet Biopharm 8:69, 1980.
35. Levy G: Pharmacokinetics in renal disease. Am J Med 62:461, 1977.
36. Gibson TP: Problems in designing hemodialysis drug studies. Pharmacotherapy 5:23, 1985.
37. Brunner H, Mann H, Stiller S, et al: Permeability for middle and higher molecular weight substances. Contrib Nephrol 46:33, 1985.
38. Lanese DM, Alfrey PS, Molitoris BA: Markedly increased clearance of vancomycin during hemodialysis using polysulfone dialyzers. Kidney Int 35:1409, 1989.
39. Bastani R, Spyker SA, Minocha A, et al: In vivo comparison of three different hemodialysis membranes for vancomycin clearance: Cuprophan, cellulose acetate, and polyacrylonitrile. Dial Transplant 17:527, 1988.
40. Barth RH, DeVincenzo N, Zara AC, et al: Vancomycin pharmacokinetics in high-flux hemodialysis. J Am Soc Nephrol 1:348, 1990. Abstract.
41. Agarwal R, Toto RD: Gentamicin clearance during hemodialysis: A comparison of high-efficiency cuprammonium rayon and conventional cellulose ester hemodialyzers. Am J Kidney Dis 22:296, 1993.
42. Jindal K, McDougall J, Goldstein M: High flux dialyzers: Impact of ultrafiltration and surface area on clearance of small and large molecular weight substances. Proceedings from the National Kidney Foundation Annual Meeting, Washington, DC, 1987, p A10. Abstract.
43. Von Albertini B, Miller JH, Gardner PW, et al: Performance characteristics of high flux haemodiafiltration. Proc Eur Dial Transplant Assoc Eur Ren Assoc 21:447, 1984.
44. Surian M, Malberti F, Corradi B, et al: Adequacy of haemodiafiltration. Nephrol Dial Transplant 4:32, 1989.
45. Rumpf KW, Rieger J, Doht B, et al: Drug elimination by hemofiltration. J Dial 1:677, 1977.
46. Ernest D, Cutler DJ: Gentamicin clearance during continuous arteriovenous hemodiafiltration. Crit Care Med 20:586, 1992.
47. Rumpf KW, Rieger J, Ansorg R, et al: Binding of antibiotics by dialysis membranes and its clinical relevance. Proc Eur Dial Transplant Assoc 14:607, 1978.
48. Kraft D, Lode H: Elimination of ampicillin and gentamicin by hemofiltration. Klin Wochenschr 57:195, 1979.
49. Kronfol NO, Lau AH, Barakat MM: Aminoglycoside binding to polyacrylonitrile hemofilter membranes during continuous hemofiltration. ASAIO Trans 33:300, 1987.
50. Kronfol N, Lau AH, Colon-Rivera J, Libertin CL: Effect of CAVH membrane types on drug-sieving coefficients and clearances. ASAIO Trans 32:85, 1986.
51. Lau A, Kronfol N, Jaber N, et al: Determinants of drug removal by continuous arteriovenous hemofiltration. Drug Intell Clin Pharm 20:467, 1986.
52. Kronfol N, Lau A, Jaber N, et al: Effect of membrane properties on drug clearances by CAVH. Proceedings from the National Kidney Foundation Annual Meeting, Washington, DC 1986, p A10. Abstract.
53. Henderson LW: Hemodialysis: Rationale and physical principles. In Brenner BM, Rector FC (eds): The Kidney. WB Saunders, Philadelphia, 1976, p 1643.
54. Husted FC, Nolph KD, Vitale FC, et al: Detrimental effects of ultrafiltration on diffusion in coils. J Lab Clin Med 87:435, 1976.
55. Nolph KD, New DL: Effects of ultrafiltration on solute clearances in hollow fiber artificial kidneys. J Lab Clin Med 88:593, 1976.
56. Nolph KD, Hopkins C, Van Stone J: Effects of ultrafiltration on solute clearances in parallel plate dialyzers. Clin Nephrol 8:453, 1977.
57. Henderson LW, Silverstein ME, Ford CA, et al: Clinical response to maintenance hemodiafiltration. Kidney Int Suppl 2:S58, 1975.
58. Hamilton R, Ford C, Colton C, et al: Blood cleansing by diafiltration in uremic dog and man. Trans Am Soc Artif Intern Organs 17:259, 1971.
59. Henderson LW, Ford C, Colton CK, et al: Uremic blood cleansing by diafiltration using hollow-fiber ultrafilter. Trans Am Soc Artif Intern Organs 16:107–112, 1970.
60. Jaffrin MY, Ding L, Laurent JM: Simultaneous convective and diffusive mass transfers in a hemodialyzer. J Biomech Eng 112:212, 1990.
61. Vincent HH, van Ittersum FJ, Akcahuseyin E, et al: Solute transport in continuous arteriovenous hemodiafiltration: A new mathematical model applied to clinical data. Blood Purif 8:149, 1990.
62. Torras J, Cao C, Rivas MC, et al: Pharmacokinetics of vancomycin in patients undergoing hemodialysis with polyacrylonitrile. Clin Nephrol 36:35, 1991.
63. Colton CK, Henderson LW, Ford CA, et al: Kinetics of hemodiafiltration. I. In vitro transport characteristics of a hollow fiber blood ultrafilter. J Lab Clin Med 85:355, 1975.
64. Golper TA, Wedel SK, Kaplan AA, et al: Drug removal during CAVH: Theory and clinical observations. Int J Artif Organs 8:307, 1985.
65. Ronco C, Brendolan A, Borin D, et al: Permeability characteristics of polysulfonic membranes in CAVH. In Sieberth HG, Mann H (eds): Continuous Arteriovenous Hemofiltration (CAVH). S Karger, Basel, 1985, pp 59–63.
66. Golper TA: Drug removal during continuous hemofiltration or hemodialysis. Contrib Nephrol 93:110, 1991.
67. Frigon RP, Leypoldt JK, Alford MF, et al: Hemofilter solute sieving is not governed by dynamically polarized protein. Trans Am Soc Artif Intern Organs 30:486, 1984.
68. Lysaght MJ: An experimental model for the ultrafiltration of sodium ion from blood or plasma. Blood Purif 1:25, 1983.
69. Leypoldt JK, Frigon RP, Henderson LW: Macromolecular charge affects hemofilter solute sieving. ASAIO Trans 32:384, 1986.
70. Kaplan AA, Longnecker RE, Folkert VW: Continuous arteriovenous hemofiltration—a report of 6 months' experience. Ann Intern Med 100:358, 1984.
71. Paganini EP, Flaque J, Whitman G, Nakamoto S: Amino acid balance in patients with oliguric renal failure undergoing slow continuous ultrafiltration (SCUF). Trans Am Soc Artif Intern Organs 28:615, 1982.
72. Kroh U, Hofmann W, Dehne M, et al: Dosisanpassung von pharmaka wahrend kontinuierlicher hamofiltration. Anaesthesist 38:225, 1989.
73. Leypoldt JK, Frigon RP, Henderson LW: Dextran sieving coefficients of hemofilter membranes. Trans Am Soc Artif Intern Organs 29:678, 1983.
74. Dodd NJ, O'Donovan RM, Bennett-Jones DN, et al: Arteriovenous haemofiltration: A recent advance in the management of renal failure. Br Med J 287:1008, 1983.
75. Bennett WM, Aronoff GR, Golper TA, et al: Drug Prescribing in Renal Failure: Dosing Guidelines for Adults, 2nd ed. American College of Physicians, Philadelphia, 1991.
76. Keller E, Reetze P, Schollmeyer P: Drug therapy in patients undergoing continuous ambulatory peritoneal dialysis. Clin Pharmacokinet 18:104, 1990.
77. Cockcroft DW, Gault MH: Prediction of creatinine clearance from serum creatinine. Nephron 16:31, 1976.
78. Reetze-Bonorden P, Böhler J, Keller E: Drug dosage in patients during continuous renal replacement therapy. Clin Pharmacokinet 24:362, 1993.
79. Goldman M, Vanherweghem J: Bacterial infections in chronic hemodialysis patients: Epidemiologic and pathophysiologic aspects. Adv Nephrol 19:315, 1990.
80. Mailloux SU, Bellucci AG, Wilkes BM, et al: Mortality in dialysis patients: Analysis of the causes of death. Am J Kidney Dis 18:326, 1991.
81. Manian FA, Stone WJ, Alford RH: Adverse antibiotic effects associated with renal insufficiency. Rev Infect Dis 12:236, 1990.
82. Siegel D: Tetracyclines: New look at old antibiotic. N Y State J Med 78:950, 1978.
83. Vance-Bryan K, Guay DRP, Rotschafer JC: Clinical pharmacokinetics of ciprofloxacin. Clin Pharmacokinet 19:434, 1990.
84. Paap CM, Nahata MC: Clinical use of trimethoprim/sulfamethoxazole during renal dysfunction. Ann Pharmacother 23:646, 1989.
85. Gilbert DN: Once-daily aminoglycoside therapy. Antimicrob Agents Chemother 35:399, 1991.
86. Wood CA, Norton DR, Kohlhepp SJ, et al: The influence of tobramycin dosage regimens on nephrotoxicity, ototoxicity, and antibacterial efficacy in a rat model of subcutaneous abscess. J Infect Dis 158:13, 1988.
87. Johnson CA, Zimmerman SW, Rogge M: The pharmacokinetics of

antibiotics used to treat peritoneal dialysis–associated peritonitis. Am J Kidney Dis 4:3, 1984.

88. Keane WF, Everett ED, Golper TA, et al: Peritoneal dialysis–related peritonitis treatment recommendations. 1993 update. Perit Dial Int 13:14, 1993.

89. Humes HD: Aminoglycoside nephrotoxicity. Kidney Int 33:900, 1988.

90. Cameron JS: Allergic interstitial nephritis: Clinical features and pathogenesis. Q J Med 66:97, 1988.

91. Shouval D, Ligumsky M, Ben-Ishay D: Effect of co-trimoxazole on normal creatinine clearance. Lancet 1:244, 1978.

92. Ayneck ML, Berardi RR, Johnson RM: Interference of cephalosporins and cefoxitin with serum creatinine determination. Am J Hosp Pharm 38:1348, 1981.

93. Baron DN, Hamilton-Miller JMT, Brumfitt W: Sodium content of injectable β-lactam antibiotics. Lancet 1:1113, 1984.

94. Blaser J, Rüttimann S, Bhend H, et al: Increase of amikacin half-life during therapy in patients with renal insufficiency. Antimicrob Agents Chemother 23:888, 1983.

95. Lanao JM, Dominguez-Gil A, Tabernero JM, et al: Pharmacokinetics of amikacin (BB-K8) in patients undergoing hemodialysis. Int J Clin Pharmacol Biopharm 17:357, 1979.

96. Smeltzer BD, Schwartzman MS, Bertino JS: Amikacin pharmacokinetics during continuous ambulatory peritoneal dialysis. Antimicrob Agents Chemother 32:236, 1988.

97. Goetz DR, Pancorbo S, Hoag S, et al: Prediction of serum gentamicin concentrations in patients undergoing hemodialysis. Am J Hosp Pharm 37:1077, 1980.

98. Gyselynck A, Forrey A, Cutler R: Pharmacokinetics of gentamicin: Distribution and plasma and renal clearance. J Infect Dis 124 (suppl):S70, 1971.

99. Zarowitz BJ, Anandan JV, Dumler F, et al: Continuous arteriovenous hemofiltration of aminoglycoside antibiotics in critically ill patients. J Clin Pharmacol 26:686, 1986.

100. Healy JK, Drum PJ, Elliott AJ: Kanamycin dosage in renal failure. Aust N Z J Med 3:474, 1973.

101. Campoli-Richards DM, Chaplin S, Sayce RH, et al: Netilmicin: A review of its antibacterial activity, pharmacokinetic properties and therapeutic use. Drugs 38:703, 1989.

102. Herrero A, Alarcó FR, García Díez JM, et al: Pharmacokinetics of netilmicin in renal insufficiency and hemodialysis. Int J Clin Pharmacol Ther 26:84, 1988.

103. Pechére J, Dugal R, Pechére M: Pharmacokinetics of netilmicin in renal insufficiency and haemodialysis. Clin Pharmacokinet 3:395, 1978.

104. Brogden RN, Pinder RM, Sawyer PR, et al: Tobramycin: A review of its antibacterial and pharmacokinetic properties and therapeutic use. Drugs 12:166, 1976.

105. Pechére J, Dugal R: Pharmacokinetics of intravenously administered tobramycin in normal volunteers and in renal-impaired and hemodialyzed patients. J Infect Dis 134:S118, 1976.

106. Wise R: The pharmacokinetics of the oral cephalosporins—a review. J Antimicrob Chemother 26(suppl E):13, 1990.

107. Gartenberg G, Meyers BR, Hirschman SZ, et al: Pharmacokinetics of cefaclor in patients with stable renal impairment, and patients undergoing haemodialysis. J Antimicrob Chemother 5:465, 1979.

108. Leroy A, Humbert G, Godin M: Pharmacokinetics of cefadroxil in patients with impaired renal function. J Antimicrob Chemother 10(suppl B):39, 1982.

109. Bliss M, Mayersohn M, Arnold T, et al: Disposition kinetics of cefamandole during continuous ambulatory peritoneal dialysis. Antimicrob Agents Chemother 29:649, 1986.

110. Brogard JM, Kopferschmitt J, Spach MO, et al: Cefamandole pharmacokinetics and dosage adjustments in relation to renal function. J Clin Pharmacol 19:366, 1979.

111. Bergen T, Brodwall EK, Ørjavik Ø: Pharmacokinetics of cefazolin in patients with normal and impaired renal function. J Antimicrob Chemother 3:435, 1977.

112. Guay DRP, Meatherall RC, Harding GK, et al: Pharmacokinetics of cefixime (CL 284,635; FK027) in healthy subjects and patients with renal insufficiency. Antimicrob Agents Chemother 30:485, 1986.

113. Campoli-Richards DM, Todd PA: Cefmenoxime. A review of its antibacterial activity, pharmacokinetic properties and therapeutic use. Drugs 34:188, 1987.

114. Evers J, Borner K, Koeppe P: Elimination of cefmenoxime during

115. Konishi K: Pharmacokinetics of cefmenoxime in patients with impaired renal function and in those undergoing hemodialysis. Antimicrob Agents Chemother 30:901, 1986.

116. Halstenson CE, Guay DR, Opsahl JA, et al: Disposition of cefmetazole in healthy volunteers and patients with impaired renal function. Antimicrob Agents Chemother 34:519, 1990.

117. Schentag JJ: Cefmetazole sodium: Pharmacology, pharmacokinetics, and clinical trials. Pharmacotherapy 11:2, 1991.

118. Blair AD, Maxwell BM, Forland SC, et al: Cefonicid kinetics in subjects with normal and impaired renal function. Clin Pharmacol Ther 35:798, 1984.

119. Saltiel E, Brogden RN: Cefonicid. A review of its antibacterial activity, pharmacological properties and therapeutic use. Drugs 32:222, 1986.

120. Greenfield RA, Gerber AU, Craig WA: Pharmacokinetics of cefoperazone in patients with normal and impaired hepatic and renal function. Rev Infect Dis 5(suppl):S127, 1983.

121. Hodler JE, Galeazzi RL, Frey B, et al: Pharmacokinetics of cefoperazone in patients undergoing chronic ambulatory peritoneal dialysis: Clinical and pathophysiological implications. Eur J Clin Pharmacol 26:609, 1984.

122. Campoli-Richards DM, Lackner TE, Monk JP: Ceforanide. A review of its antibacterial activity, pharmacokinetic properties and clinical efficacy. Drugs 34:411, 1987.

123. Hess JR, Berman SJ, Boughton WH, et al: Pharmacokinetics of ceforanide in patients with end stage renal disease on hemodialysis. Antimicrob Agents Chemother 17:251, 1980.

124. Matzke GR, Abraham PA, Halstenson CE, et al: Cefotaxime and desacetyl cefotaxime kinetics in renal impairment. Clin Pharmacol Ther 38:31, 1985.

125. Todd PA, Brogden RN: Cefotaxime. An update of its pharmacology and therapeutic use. Drugs 40:608, 1990.

126. Ohkawa M, Hirano S, Tokunaga S: Pharmacokinetics of cefotetan in normal subjects and patients with impaired renal function. Antimicrob Agents Chemother 23:31, 1983.

127. Ward A, Richards DM: Cefotetan. A review of its antibacterial activity, pharmacokinetic properties and therapeutic use. Drugs 30:382, 1985.

128. Greaves WL, Kreeft JH, Ogilvie RI, et al: Cefoxitin disposition during peritoneal dialysis. Antimicrob Agents Chemother 19:253, 1981.

129. Humbert G, Fillastre JP, Leroy A, et al: Pharmacokinetics of cefoxitin in normal subjects and in patients with renal insufficiency. Rev Infect Dis 1:118, 1979.

130. Nikolaidis P, Tourkantonis A: Effect of hemodialysis on ceftazidime pharmacokinetics. Clin Nephrol 24:142, 1985.

131. Richards DM, Brogden RN: Ceftazidime. A review of its antibacterial activity, pharmacokinetic properties and therapeutic use. Drugs 29:105, 1985.

132. Tourkantonis A, Nicolaidis P: Pharmacokinetics of ceftazidime in patients undergoing peritoneal dialysis. J Antimicrob Chemother 12(suppl A):263, 1983.

133. Welage LS, Schultz RW, Schentag JJ: Pharmacokinetics of ceftazidime in patients with renal insufficiency. Antimicrob Agents Chemother 25:201, 1984.

134. Burgess ED, Blair AD: Pharmacokinetics of ceftizoxime in patients undergoing continuous ambulatory peritoneal dialysis. Antimicrob Agents Chemother 24:237, 1983.

135. Gross ML, Somani P, Ribner BS, et al: Ceftizoxime elimination kinetics in continuous ambulatory peritoneal dialysis. Clin Pharmacol Ther 34:673, 1983.

136. Kowalsky SF, Echols RM, Venezia AR, et al: Pharmacokinetics of ceftizoxime in subjects with various degrees of renal function. Antimicrob Agents Chemother 24:151, 1983.

137. Richards DM, Heel RC: Ceftizoxime. A review of its antibacterial activity, pharmacokinetic properties and therapeutic use. Drugs 29:281, 1985.

138. Patel IH, Sugihara JG, Weinfeld RE, et al: Ceftriaxone pharmacokinetics in patients with various degrees of renal impairment. Antimicrob Agents Chemother 25:438, 1984.

139. Ti T, Fortin L, Kreeft JH, et al: Kinetic disposition of intravenous ceftriaxone in normal subjects and patients with renal failure on hemodialysis or peritoneal dialysis. Antimicrob Agents Chemother 25:83, 1984.

140. Yuk JH, Nightingale CH, Quintiliani R: Clinical pharmacokinetics of ceftriaxone. Clin Pharmacokinet 17:223, 1989.

141. Höffler D, Koeppe P, Schleith A: Pharmacokinetics of cefuroxime-axetil in patients undergoing haemodialysis therapy. Acta Therapeut 17:107, 1991.

142. Konishi K, Suzuki H, Hayashi M, Saruta T: Pharmacokinetics of cefuroxime axetil in patients with normal and impaired renal function. J Antimicrob Chemother 31:413, 1993.

143. Weiss LG, Cars O, Danielson BG, et al: Pharmacokinetics of intravenous cefuroxime during intermittent and continuous arteriovenous hemofiltration. Clin Nephrol 30:282, 1988.

144. Bailey RR, Gower PE, Dash CH: The effects of impairment of renal function and haemodialysis on serum and urine levels of cephalexin. Postgrad Med J 46(suppl):60, 1970.

145. Venuto RC, Plaut M: Cephalothin handling in patients undergoing hemodialysis. Antimicrob Agents Chemother 10:50, 1970.

146. McCloskey RV, Terry EE, McCracken AW, et al: Effect of hemodialysis and renal failure on serum and urine concentrations of cephapirin sodium. Antimicrob Agents Chemother 1:90, 1972.

147. Solomon AE, Briggs JD: The administration of cephradine to patients in renal failure. Br J Clin Pharmacol 2:443, 1975.

148. Bolton WK, Scheld WM, Spyker DA, et al: Pharmacokinetics of moxalactam in subjects with various degrees of renal dysfunction. Antimicrob Agents Chemother 18:933, 1980.

149. Carmine AA, Brogden RN, Heel RC, et al: Moxalactam. A review of its antibacterial activity, pharmacokinetic properties and therapeutic use. Drugs 26:279, 1983.

150. Srinivasan S, Neu HC: Pharmacokinetics of moxalactam in patients with renal failure and during hemodialysis. Antimicrob Agents Chemother 20:398, 1981.

151. Peters DH, Clissold SP: Clarithromycin: A review of its antimicrobial activity, pharmacokinetic properties and therapeutic potential. Drugs 44:117, 1992.

152. Disse B, Gundert-Remy U, Weber E, et al: Pharmacokinetics of erythromycin in patients with different degrees of renal impairment. Int J Clin Pharmacol Ther Toxicol 24:460, 1986.

153. Kanfer A, Stamatakis G, Torlotin JC, et al: Changes in erythromycin pharmacokinetics induced by renal failure. Clin Nephrol 27:147, 1987.

154. Blum RA, Kohli RK, Harrison NJ, et al: Pharmacokinetics of ampicillin (2.0 grams) and sulbactam (1.0 gram) coadministered to subjects with normal and abnormal renal function and with end-stage renal disease on hemodialysis. Antimicrob Agents Chemother 33:1470, 1989.

155. Francke EL, Appel GB, Neu HC: Kinetics of intravenous amoxicillin in patients on long-term dialysis. Clin Pharmacol Ther 26:31, 1979.

156. Humbert G, Spyker DA, Fillastre JP, et al: Pharmacokinetics of amoxicillin: Dosage nomogram for patients with impaired renal function. Antimicrob Agents Chemother 15:28, 1979.

157. Todd PA, Benfield P: Amoxicillin/clavulanic acid: An update of its antibacterial activity, pharmacokinetic properties and therapeutic use. Drugs 39:264, 1990.

158. Leroy A, Humbert G, Godin M, et al: Pharmacokinetics of azlocillin in subjects with normal and impaired renal function. Antimicrob Agents Chemother 17:344, 1980.

159. Whelton A, Stout RL, Delgado FA: Azlocillin kinetics during extracorporeal haemodialysis and peritoneal dialysis. J Antimicrob Chemother 11S(suppl B):89, 1983.

160. Aronoff GR, Sloan RS, Luft FC, et al: Mezlocillin pharmacokinetics in renal impairment. Clin Pharmacol Ther 28:523, 1980.

161. Kampf D, Schurig R, Weihermüller K, et al: Effects of impaired renal function, hemodialysis, and peritoneal dialysis on the pharmacokinetics of mezlocillin. Antimicrob Agents Chemother 18:81, 1980.

162. Holmes B, Richards DM, Brogden RN, et al: Piperacillin: A review of its antibacterial activity, pharmacokinetic properties and therapeutic use. Drugs 28:375, 1984.

163. De Schepper PJ, Tjandramage RB, Mullie A, et al: Comparative pharmacokinetics of piperacillin in normals and in patients with renal failure. J Antimicrob Chemother 9(suppl B):49, 1982.

164. Welling PG, Craig WA, Bundtzen RW, et al: Pharmacokinetics of piperacillin in subjects with various degrees of renal function. Antimicrob. Agents Chemother 23:881, 1983.

165. Parry MF, Neu HC: Pharmacokinetics of ticarcillin in patients with abnormal renal function. J Infect Dis 133:46–49, 1976.

166. Davies SP, Azadian BS, Kox WJ, et al: Pharmacokinetics of ciprofloxacin and vancomycin in patients with acute renal failure treated by continuous haemodialysis. Nephrol Dial Transplant 7:848, 1992.

167. Kowalsky SF, Echols M, Schwartz MT, et al: Pharmacokinetics of ciprofloxacin in subjects with varying degrees of renal function and undergoing hemodialysis or CAPD. Clin Nephrol 39:53, 1993.

168. Neuman M: Clinical pharmacokinetics of the newer antibacterial 4-quinolones. Clin Pharmacokinet 14:96, 1988.

169. Henwood JM, Monk JP: Enoxacin. A review of its antibacterial activity, pharmacokinetic properties and therapeutic use. Drugs 36:32, 1988.

170. Nix DE, Schultz RW, Frost RW: The effect of renal impairment and haemodialysis on single dose pharmacokinetics of oral enoxacin. J Antimicrob Chemother 21(suppl B):87, 1988.

171. Weidekamm E: Pharmacokinetics of fleroxacin in renal impairment. Am J Med 94(suppl 3A):70S, 1993.

172. Holmes B, Brogden RN, Richards DM: Norfloxacin. A review of its antibacterial activity, pharmacokinetic properties and therapeutic use. Drugs 30:482, 1985.

173. Lameire N, Rosenkranz B, Malerczyk V, et al: Ofloxacin pharmacokinetics in chronic renal failure and dialysis. Clin Pharmacokinet 21:357, 1991.

174. Saivin S, Houin G: Clinical pharmacokinetics of doxycycline and minocycline. Clin Pharmacokinet 15:355, 1988.

175. Fillastre JP, Leroy A, Baudoin C, et al: Pharmacokinetics of aztreonam in patients with chronic renal failure. Clin Pharmacokinet 10:91, 1985.

176. Gerig JS, Bolton ND, Swabb EA, et al: Effect of hemodialysis and peritoneal dialysis on aztreonam pharmacokinetics. Kidney Int 26:308, 1984.

177. Ambrose PJ: Clinical pharmacokinetics of chloramphenicol and chloramphenicol succinate. Clin Pharmacokinet 9:222, 1984.

178. Buckley MM, Brogden RN, Barradell LB, et al: Imipenem/cilastatin. A reappraisal of its antibacterial activity, pharmacokinetic properties and therapeutic efficacy. Drugs 44:408, 1992.

179. Gibson TP, Devetriades JL, Bland JA: Imipenem/cilastatin: Pharmacokinetic profile in renal insufficiency. Am J Med 78(suppl 6A):54, 1985.

180. Konishi K, Suzuki H, Saruta T, et al: Removal of imipenem and cilastatin by hemodialysis in patients with end-stage renal failure. Antimicrob Agents Chemother 35:1616, 1991.

181. Vos MC, Vincent HH, Yzerman EPF: Clearance of imipenem/cilastatin in acute renal failure patients treated by continuous hemodiafiltration (CAVHD). Intensive Care Med 18:282, 1992.

182. Roberts AP, Eastwood JB, Gower PE, et al: Serum and plasma concentrations of clindamycin following a single intramuscular injection of clindamycin phosphate in maintenance haemodialysis patients and normal subjects. Eur J Clin Pharmacol 14:435, 1978.

183. Hamilton-Miller JMT, Brumfitt W: Methenamine and its salts as urinary tract antiseptics. Variables affecting the antibacterial activity of formaldehyde, mandelic acid, and hippuric acid in vitro. Invest Urol 14:287, 1977.

184. Guay DR, Meatherall RC, Baxter H, et al: Pharmacokinetics of metronidazole in patients undergoing continuous ambulatory peritoneal dialysis. Antimicrob Agents Chemother 25:306, 1984.

185. Kreeft JH, Ogilvie RI, Dufresne LR: Metronidazole kinetics in dialysis patients. Surgery 93:149, 1983.

186. Lau AH, Lam NP, Piscitelli SC, et al: Clinical pharmacokinetics of metronidazole and other nitroimidazole anti-infectives. Clin Pharmacokinet 23:328, 1992.

187. Shermantine M, Gambertoglio J, Amend W, et al: Pharmacokinetics of sulfisoxazole in renal transplant patients. Antimicrob Agents Chemother 28:535, 1985.

188. Bonati M, Traina GL, Villa G, et al: Teicoplanin pharmacokinetics in patients with chronic renal failure. Clin Pharmacokinet 12:292, 1987.

189. Campoli-Richards DM, Brogden RN, Faulds D: Teicoplanin. A review of its antibacterial activity, pharmacokinetic properties and therapeutic potential. Drugs 40:449, 1990.

190. Moellering RC, Krogstad DJ, Greenblatt DJ: Vancomycin therapy in patients with impaired renal function: A nomogram for dosage. Ann Intern Med 94:343, 1981.

191. Nielson HE, Sorenson I, Hansen HE: Peritoneal transport of vancomycin during peritoneal dialysis. Nephron 24:274, 1979.

192. Daneshmend TK, Warnock DW: Clinical pharmacokinetics of systemic antifungal drugs. Clin Pharmacokinet 8:17, 1983.

193. Lyman CA, Walsh TJ: Systemically administered antifungal agents. A review of their clinical pharmacology and therapeutic applications. Drugs 44:9, 1992.

194. Craven PC, Ludden TM, Drutz DJ, et al: Excretion pathways of amphotericin B. J Infect Dis 140:329, 1979.

195. Morgan DJ, Ching MS, Raymond K, et al: Elimination of amphotericin B in impaired renal function. Clin Pharmacol Ther 34:248, 1983.

196. Janknegt R, de Marie S, Bakker-Woudenberg IA, et al: Liposomal and lipid formulations of amphotericin B. Clin Pharmacokinet 23:279, 1992.

197. Cleary JD, Taylor JW, Chapman SW: Imidazoles and triazoles in antifungal therapy. Ann Pharmacother 24:148, 1990.

198. Bailey EM, Krakovsky DJ, Rybak MJ: The triazole antifungal agents: A review of itraconazole and fluconazole. Pharmacotherapy 10:146, 1990.

199. Toon S, Ross CE, Gokal R, et al: An assessment of the effects of impaired renal function and haemodialysis on the pharmacokinetics of fluconazole. Br J Clin Pharmacol 29:221, 1990.

200. Oono S, Tabei K, Tetsuka T, et al: The pharmacokinetics of fluconazole during haemodialysis in uraemic patients. Eur J Clin Pharmacol 42:667, 1992.

201. Debruyne D, Ryckelynck J: Clinical pharmacokinetics of fluconazole. Clin Pharmacokinet 24:10, 1993.

202. Bennett JE: Flucytosine. Ann Intern Med 86:319, 1977.

203. Cutler RE, Blair AD, Kelly MR: Flucytosine kinetics in subjects with normal and impaired renal function. Clin Pharmacol Ther 24:333, 1978.

204. Eisenberg ES: Intraperitoneal flucytosine in the management of fungal peritonitis in patients on continuous ambulatory peritoneal dialysis. Am J Kidney Dis 11:465, 1988.

205. Boelaert J, Schurgers M, Matthys E, et al: Itraconazole pharmacokinetics in patients with renal dysfunction. Antimicrob Agents Chemother 32:1595, 1988.

206. Grant SM, Clissold SP: Itraconazole: A review of its pharmacodynamic and pharmacokinetic properties, and therapeutic use in superficial and systemic mycoses. Drugs 37:310, 1989.

207. Daneshmend TK, Warnock DW: Clinical pharmacokinetics of ketoconazole. Clin Pharmacokinet 14:13, 1988.

208. Lewi PJ, Boelaert J, Daneels R, et al: Pharmacokinetic profile of intravenous miconazole in man. Eur J Clin Pharmacol 10:49, 1976.

209. White JW: Clinical pharmacokinetics of antimalarial drugs. Clin Pharmacokinet 10:187, 1985.

210. White NJ: Antimalarial pharmacokinetics and treatment regimens. Br J Clin Pharmacol 34:1, 1992.

211. Edwards G, Breckenridge AM: Clinical pharmacokinetics of anthelmintic drugs. Clin Pharmacokinet 15:67, 1988.

212. Keystone JS, Murdoch JK: Mebendazole. Ann Intern Med 91:582, 1979.

213. Palmer KJ, Holliday SM, Brogden RN: Mefloquine. A review of its antimalarial activity, pharmacokinetic properties and therapeutic efficacy. Drugs 45:430, 1993.

214. Goa KL, Campoli-Richards DM: Pentamidine isethionate. A review of its antiprotozoal activity, pharmacokinetic properties and therapeutic use in *Pneumocystis carinii* pneumonia. Drugs 33:242, 1987.

215. Conte JE: Pharmacokinetics of intravenous pentamidine in patients with normal renal function or receiving hemodialysis. J Infect Dis 163:169, 1991.

216. King CH, Mahmoud AAF: Drugs five years later: Praziquantel. Ann Intern Med 110:290, 1989.

217. Lehmann CR, Garrett LE, Winn RE, et al: Capreomycin kinetics in renal impairment and clearance by hemodialysis. Am Rev Respir Dis 138:1312, 1988.

218. Varughese A, Brater DC, Benet LZ, et al: Ethambutol kinetics in patients with impaired renal function. Am Rev Respir Dis 134:34, 1986.

219. Weber WW, Hein DW: Clinical pharmacokinetics of isoniazid. Clin Pharmacokinet 4:401, 1979.

220. Lacroix C, Hermelin A, Guiberteau R, et al: Haemodialysis of pyrazinamide in uraemic patients. Eur J Clin Pharmacol 37:309, 1989.

221. Stamatakis G, Montes C, Trouvin JH, et al: Pyrazinamide and pyrazinoic acid pharmacokinetics in patients with chronic renal failure. Clin Nephrol 30:230, 1988.

222. Acocella G: Clinical pharmacokinetics of rifampicin. Clin Pharmacokinet 3:108, 1978.

223. Burgess ED, Gill MJ: Intraperitoneal administration of acyclovir in patients receiving continuous ambulatory peritoneal dialysis. J Clin Pharmacol 30:997, 1990.

224. Laskin OL, Longstreth JA, Whelton A, et al: Acyclovir kinetics in end-stage renal disease. Clin Pharmacol Ther 31:594, 1982.

225. O'Brien JJ, Campoli-Richards DM: Acyclovir: An updated review of its antiviral activity, pharmacokinetic properties and therapeutic efficacy. Drugs 37:233, 1989.

226. Aoki FY, Sitar DS: Clinical pharmacokinetics of amantadine hydrochloride. Clin Pharmacokinet 14:35, 1988.

227. Horadam VW, Sharp JG, Smilack JD, et al: Pharmacokinetics of amantadine hydrochloride in subjects with normal and impaired renal function. Ann Intern Med 94:454, 1981.

228. Wu MJ, Ing TS, Soung LS, et al: Amantadine hydrochloride pharmacokinetics in patients with impaired renal function. Clin Nephrol 17:19, 1982.

229. Morse GD, Shelton MJ, O'Donnell AM: Comparative pharmacokinetics of antiviral nucleoside analogues. Clin Pharmacokinet 24:101, 1993.

230. Faulds D, Brogden RN: Didanosine: A review of its antiviral activity, pharmacokinetic properties and therapeutic potential in human immunodeficiency virus infection. Drugs 44:94, 1992.

231. Chrisp P, Clissold SP: Foscarnet: A review of its antiviral activity, pharmacokinetic properties and therapeutic use in immunocompromised patients with cytomegalovirus retinitis. Drugs 41:104, 1991.

232. Faulds D, Heel RC: Ganciclovir: A review of its antiviral activity, pharmacokinetic properties and therapeutic efficacy in cytomegalovirus infections. Drugs 39:597, 1990.

233. Kramer TH, Gaar GG, Ray CG, et al: Hemodialysis clearance of intravenously administered ribavirin. Antimicrob Agents Chemother 34:489, 1990.

234. Aronoff GR, Szwed JJ, Nelson RL, et al: Hypoxanthine-arabinoside pharmacokinetics after adenine arabinoside administration to a patient with renal failure. Antimicrob Agents Chemother 18:212, 1980.

235. Collins JM, Unadkat JD: Clinical pharmacokinetics of zidovudine. An overview of current data. Clin Pharmacokinet 17:1, 1989.

236. Gallicano KD, Tobe S, Sahai J, et al: Pharmacokinetics of single and chronic dose zidovudine in two HIV positive patients undergoing continuous ambulatory peritoneal dialysis (CAPD). J Acquir Immune Defic Syndr 5:242, 1992.

237. Garraffo R, Cassuto-Viguier E, Barillon J, et al: Influence of hemodialysis on zidovudine (AZT) and its glucuronide (GAZT) pharmacokinetics: Two case reports. Int J Clin Pharmacol Ther Toxicol 27:535, 1989.

238. Gleason JR, Brier ME: Zidovudine in renal failure. Semin Dial 3:101, 1990.

239. Chan GLC, Matzke GR: Effects of renal insufficiency on the pharmacokinetics and pharmacodynamics of opioid analgesics. Drug Intell Clin Pharm 21:773, 1987.

240. Szeto HH, Inturrisi CE, Houde R, et al: Accumulation of normeperidine, an active metabolite of meperidine, in patients with renal failure or cancer. Ann Intern Med 86:738, 1977.

241. Agoston S, Vandenbrom RHG, Wierda JMKH: Clinical pharmacokinetics of neuromuscular blocking drugs. Clin Pharmacokinet 22:94, 1992.

242. Horton MW, Byerly WG: Opioid analgesics. Semin Dial 3:187, 1990.

243. Heel RC, Brogden RN, Speight TM, et al: Butorphanol: A review of its pharmacological properties and therapeutic efficacy. Drugs 16:473, 1978.

244. Barnes JN, Williams AJ, Tomson MJF, et al: Dihydrocodeine in renal failure: Further evidence for an important role of the kidney in the handling of opioid drugs. Br Med J 290:740, 1985.

245. Mather LE: Clinical pharmacokinetics of fentanyl and its newer derivatives. Clin Pharmacokinet 8:422, 1983.

246. Kreek MJ, Schecter AJ, Gutjahr CL, et al: Methadone use in patients with chronic renal disease. Drug Alcohol Depend 5:197, 1980.

247. Chauvin M, Sandouk P, Scherrmann JM, et al: Morphine pharmacokinetics in renal failure. Anesthesiology 66:327, 1987.

248. Säwe J, Odar-Cederlöl I: Kinetics of morphine in patients with renal failure. Eur J Clin Pharmacol 32:377, 1987.

249. Giacomini KM, Gibson TP, Levy G: Effect of hemodialysis on propoxyphene and norpropoxyphene concentrations in blood of anephric patients. Clin Pharmacol Ther 27:508, 1980.

250. Clissold SP: Paracetamol and phenacetin. Drugs 32(suppl 4):46, 1986.

251. Prescott LF, Speirs GC, Critchley JAJH, et al: Paracetamol disposition and metabolite kinetics in patients with chronic renal failure. Eur J Clin Pharmacol 36:291, 1989.

252. Sica DA, Comstock TJ, Davis J, et al: Pharmacokinetics and protein binding of methocarbamol in renal insufficiency and normals. Eur J Clin Pharmacol 39:193, 1990.

253. Needs CJ, Brooks PM: Clinical pharmacokinetics of the salicylates. Clin Pharmacokinet 10:164, 1985.

254. Williams ME, Weinblatt M, Rosa RM: Salsalate kinetics in patients with chronic renal failure undergoing hemodialysis. Clin Pharmacol Ther 39:420, 1986.

255. Davis PJ, Cook DR: Clinical pharmacokinetics of the newer intravenous anaesthetic agents. Clin Pharmacokinet 11:18, 1986.

256. Pollard BJ: Neuromuscular blocking drugs and renal failure. Br J Anaesth 68:545, 1992. Editorial.

257. Gramstad L: Atracurium, vecuronium and pancuronium in end-stage renal failure. Br J Anaesth 59:995, 1987.

258. Mongin-Long D, Chabrol B, Baude C, et al: Atracurium in patients with renal failure. Clinical trial of a new neuromuscular blocker. Br J Anaesth 58:44S, 1986.

259. Ramzan MI, Shanks CA, Triggs EJ: Gallamine disposition is surgical patients with chronic renal failure. J Clin Pharmacol 12:141, 1981.

260. Brotherton WP, Matteo RS: Pharmacokinetics and pharmacodynamics of metocurine in humans with and without renal failure. Anesthesiology 55:273, 1981.

261. Aquilonius S, Hartvig P: Clinical pharmacokinetics of cholinesterase inhibitors. Clin Pharmacokinet 11:236, 1986.

262. McLeod K, Watson MJ, Rawlins MD: Pharmacokinetics of pancuronium in patients with normal and impaired renal function. Br J Anaesth 48:341, 1976.

263. Kirvelä M, Olkkola KT, Rosenberg PH, et al: Pharmacokinetics of propofol and haemodynamic changes during induction of anaesthesia in uraemic patients. Br J Anaesth 68:178, 1992.

264. Cronnelly R, Stanski DR, Miller RD, et al: Pyridostigmine kinetics with and without renal function. Clin Pharmacol Ther 28:78, 1980.

265. Bishop M, Hornbein TF: Prolonged effect of succinylcholine after neostigmine and pyridostigmine administration in patients with renal failure. Anesthesiology 58:384, 1983.

266. Matteo RS, Nishitateno K, Pau EK, et al: Pharmacokinetics of *d*-tubocurarine in man: Effect of an osmotic diuretic on urinary excretion. Anesthesiology 52:335, 1980.

267. Lynam DP, Cronnelly R, Castagnoli KP, et al: The pharmacodynamics and pharmacokinetics of vecuronium in patients anesthetized with isoflurane with normal renal function or with renal failure. Anesthesiology 69:227, 1988.

268. Agodoa LYC, Held PJ, Port FK: Causes of death. *In* U.S. Renal Data System: USRDS 1993 Annual Data Report. National Institutes of Health, National Institute of Diabetes and Digestive and Kidney Diseases, Bethesda, MD, 1993, p 49.

269. Parving H, Smidt UM, Hommel E, et al: Effective antihypertensive treatment postpones renal insufficiency in diabetic nephropathy. Am J Kidney Dis 22:188, 1993.

270. Castelli WP: Epidemiology of coronary heart disease: The Framingham study. Am J Med 76(suppl):4, 1984.

271. Anderson S, Rennke HG, Brenner BM: Therapeutic advantage of converting enzyme inhibitors in arresting progressive renal disease associated with systemic hypertension in the rat. J Clin Invest 77:1993, 1986.

272. Brunner HR: ACE inhibitors in renal disease. Kidney Int 42:463, 1992.

273. Lewis EJ, Hunsicker LG, Bain RP: The effect of angiotensin-converting-enzyme inhibition on diabetic nephropathy. N Engl J Med 329:1456, 1993.

274. Hulter HN, Licht JH, Ilnicki LP, et al: Clinical efficacy and pharmacokinetics of clonidine in hemodialysis and renal insufficiency. J Lab Clin Med 94:223, 1979.

275. Lowenthal DT, Matzek KM, MacGregor TR: Clinical pharmacokinetics of clonidine. Clin Pharmacokinet 14:287, 1988.

276. Carlson RV, Bailey RR, Begg EJ, et al: Pharmacokinetics and effect on blood pressure of doxazosin in normal subjects and patients with renal failure. Clin Pharmacol Ther 40:561, 1986.

277. Young RA, Brogden RN: Doxazosin. A review of its pharmacodynamic and pharmacokinetic properties, and therapeutic efficacy in mild or moderate hypertension. Drugs 35:525, 1988.

278. Holmes B, Brogden RN, Heel RC, et al: Guanabenz. A review of its pharmacodynamic properties and therapeutic efficacy in hypertension. Drugs 26:212, 1983.

279. Finnerty FA, Brogden RN: Guanadrel. A review of its pharmacodynamic and pharmacokinetic properties and therapeutic use in hypertension. Drugs 30:22, 1985.

280. Halstenson CE, Opsahl FA, Abraham PA, et al: Disposition of guanadrel in subjects with normal and impaired renal function. J Clin Pharmacol 29:128, 1989.

281. Carchman SH, Sica DA, Davis J, et al: Steady-state plasma levels and pharmacokinetics of guanfacine in patients with renal insufficiency. Nephron 53:18, 1989.

282. Sorkin EM, Heel RC: Guanfacine. A review of its pharmacodynamic and pharmacokinetic properties, and therapeutic efficacy in the treatment of hypertension. Drugs 31:301, 1986.

283. Myhre E, Rugstad HE, Hansen T: Clinical pharmacokinetics of methyldopa. Clin Pharmacokinet 7:221, 1982.

284. Lameire N, Gordts J: A pharmacokinetic study of prazosin in patients with varying degrees of chronic renal failure. Eur J Clin Pharmacol 31:333, 1986.

285. Vincent J, Meredith PA, Reid JL, et al: Clinical pharmacokinetics of prazosin—1985. Clin Pharmacokinet 10:144, 1985.

286. Zsoter TT, Johnson GE, DeVeber GA, et al: Excretion and metabolism of reserpine in renal failure. Clin Pharmacol Ther 14:325, 1973.

287. Jungers P, Ganeval D, Pertuiset N, et al: Influence of renal insufficiency on the pharmacokinetics and pharmacodynamics of terazosin. Am J Med 80(suppl 5B):94, 1986.

288. Hoyer J, Schulte KL, Lenz T: Clinical pharmacokinetics of angiotensin converting enzyme (ACE) inhibitors in renal failure. Clin Pharmacokinet 24:230, 1993.

289. Balfour JA, Goa KL: Benazepril. A review of its pharmacodynamic and pharmacokinetic properties, and therapeutic efficacy in hypertension and congestive heart failure. Drugs 42:511, 1991.

290. Brogden RN, Todd PA, Sorkin EM: Captopril. An update of its pharmacodynamic and pharmacokinetic properties, and therapeutic use in hypertension and congestive heart failure. Drugs 36:540, 1988.

291. Duchin KL, Pierides AM, Heald A, et al: Elimination kinetics of captopril in patients with renal failure. Kidney Int 25:942, 1984.

292. Fujimura A, Kajiyama H, Ebihara A, et al: Pharmacokinetics and pharmacodynamics of captopril in patients undergoing continuous ambulatory peritoneal dialysis. Nephron 44:324, 1986.

293. Fruincillo RJU, Rocci ML, Vlasses PH, et al: Disposition of enalapril and enalaprilat in renal insufficiency. Kidney Int 31(suppl 20):S117, 1987.

294. Todd PA, Goa KL: Enalapril. A reappraisal of its pharmacology and therapeutic use in hypertension. Drugs 43:346, 1992.

295. Gehr TWB, Sica DA, Grasela DM: Fosinopril pharmacokinetics and pharmacodynamics in chronic ambulatory peritoneal dialysis patients. Eur J Clin Pharmacol 41:165, 1991.

296. Hui KK, Duchin KL, Kripalani KJ, et al: Pharmacokinetics of fosinopril in patients with various degrees of renal function. Clin Pharmacol Ther 49:457, 1991.

297. Murdoch D, McTavish D: Fosinopril. A review of its pharmacodynamic and pharmacokinetic properties, and therapeutic potential in essential hypertension. Drugs 43:123, 1992.

298. Lancaster SG, Todd PA: Lisinopril. A preliminary review of its pharmacodynamic and pharmacokinetic properties, and therapeutic use in hypertension and congestive heart failure. Drugs 35:646, 1988.

299. Schaik BAM, Geyskes GG, Wouw PAV, et al: Pharmacokinetics of lisinopril in hypertensive patients with normal and impaired renal function. Eur J Clin Pharmacol 34:61, 1988.

300. Schunkert H, Kindler J, Gassmann M: Pharmacokinetics of ramipril in hypertensive patients with renal insufficiency. Eur J Clin Pharmacol 37:249, 1989.

301. Todd PA, Benfield P: Ramipril. A review of its pharmacological properties and therapeutic efficacy in cardiovascular disorders. Drugs 39:110, 1990.

302. Stec GP, Atkinson AJ, Nevin MJ, et al: N-Acetylprocainamide pharmacokinetics in functionally anephric patients before and after perturbation by hemodialysis. Clin Pharmacol Ther 26:618, 1979.

303. Harron DWG, Brogden RN: Acecainide (N-acetylprocainamide): A review of its pharmacodynamic and pharmacokinetic properties, and therapeutic potential in cardiac arrhythmias. Drugs 39:720, 1990.

304. Gill J, Heel RC, Fitton A: Amiodarone: An overview of its pharma-

cological properties, and review of its therapeutic use in cardiac arrhythmias. Drugs 43:69, 1992.

305. Josselson J, Narang PK, Adir J, et al: Bretylium kinetics in renal insufficiency. Clin Pharmacol Ther 33:144, 1983.
306. Rapeport WG: Clinical pharmacokinetics of bretylium. Clin Pharmacokinet 10:248, 1985.
307. Brogden RN, Todd PA: Disopyramide: A reappraisal of its pharmacodynamic and pharmacokinetic properties, and therapeutic use in cardiac arrhythmias. Drugs 34:151, 1986.
308. Burk M, Peters U: Disopyramide kinetics in renal impairment: Determinants of interindividual variability. Clin Pharmacol Ther 34:331, 1983.
309. Haughey DB, Kraft CJ, Matzke GR, et al: Protein binding of disopyramide and elevated alpha-1-acid glycoprotein concentrations in serum obtained from dialysis patients and renal transplant recipients. Am J Nephrol 5:35, 1985.
310. Bergstrand RH, Wang T, Roden DM, et al: Encainide disposition in patients with renal failure. Clin Pharmacol Ther 40:64, 1986.
311. Brogden RN, Todd PA: Encainide: A review of its pharmacological properties and therapeutic efficacy. Drugs 34:519, 1987.
312. Forland SC, Burgess E, Blair AD, et al: Oral flecainide pharmacokinetics in patients with impaired renal function. J Clin Pharmacol 28:259, 1988.
313. Forland SC, Cutler RE, McQuinn RL, et al: Flecainide pharmacokinetics after multiple dosing in patients with impaired renal function. J Clin Pharmacol 28:727, 1988.
314. Bennett PN, Aarons LJ, Bending MR, et al: Pharmacokinetics of lidocaine and its deethylated metabolite: Dose and time dependency studies in man. J Pharmacokinet Biopharm 10:265, 1982.
315. Eiriksson CE, Brogden RN: Lorcainide: A preliminary review of its pharmacodynamic properties and therapeutic efficacy. Drugs 27:279, 1984.
316. Monk JP, Brogden RN: Mexiletine: A review of its pharmacodynamic and pharmacokinetic properties, and therapeutic use in the treatment of arrhythmias. Drugs 40:374, 1990.
317. Wang T, Wuellner D, Woosley RL, et al: Pharmacokinetics and nondialyzability of mexiletine in renal failure. Clin Pharmacol Ther 37:649, 1988.
318. Fitton A, Buckley MM-T: Moricizine: A review of its pharmacological properties, and therapeutic efficacy in cardiac arrhythmias. Drugs 40:138, 1990.
319. Pieniaszek HJ, McEntegart CM, Mayersohn M, et al: Moricizine pharmacokinetics in renal insufficiency: Reevaluation of elimination half-life. J Clin Pharmacol 32:412, 1992.
320. Raehl CL, Moorthy AV, Beirne GJ: Procainamide pharmacokinetics in patients on continuous ambulatory peritoneal dialysis. Nephron 44:191, 1986.
321. Bryson HM, Palmer KJ, Langtry HD, et al: Propafenone: A reappraisal of its pharmacology, pharmacokinetics and therapeutic use in cardiac arrhythmias. Drugs 45:85, 1993.
322. Burgess E, Duff H, Wilkes P: Propafenone disposition in renal insufficiency and renal failure. J Clin Pharmacol 29:112, 1989.
323. Crevasse L: Quinidine: An update on therapeutics, pharmacokinetics and serum concentration monitoring. Am J Cardiol 62:22, 1988.
324. Kessler KM, Perez GO: Decreased quinidine plasma protein binding during hemodialysis. Clin Pharmacol Ther 30:121, 1981.
325. Holmes B, Brogden RN, Heel RC, et al: Tocainide: A review of its pharmacological properties and therapeutic efficacy. Drugs 26:93, 1983.
326. Raehl CL, Beirne GJ, Moorthy AV, et al: Tocainide pharmacokinetics during continuous ambulatory peritoneal dialysis. Am J Cardiol 60:747, 1987.
327. Wiegers U, Hanrath P, Kuck KH, et al: Pharmacokinetics of tocainide in patients with renal dysfunction and during haemodialysis. Eur J Clin Pharmacol 24:503, 1983.
328. Borchard U: Pharmacokinetics of beta-adrenoceptor blocking agents: Clinical significance of hepatic and/or renal clearance. Clin Physiol Biochem 8(suppl 2):28, 1990.
329. Riddell JG, Harron DWG, Shanks RG: Clinical pharmacokinetics of β-adrenoceptor antagonists. An update. Clin Pharmacokinet 12:305, 1987.
330. Kirch W, Köhler H, Berggren G, Braun W: The influence of renal function on plasma levels and urinary excretion of acebutolol and its main N-acetyl metabolite. Clin Nephrol 18:88, 1982.
331. Roux A, Aubert P, Guedon J, et al: Pharmacokinetics of acebutolol in patients with all grades of renal failure. Eur J Clin Pharmacol 17:339, 1980.
332. Singh BN, Thoden WR, Ward A: Acebutolol: A review of its pharmacological properties and therapeutic efficacy in hypertension, angina pectoris and arrhythmia. Drugs 29:531, 1985.
333. Kirch W, Kohler H, Mutschler E, et al: Pharmacokinetics of atenolol in relation to renal function. Eur J Clin Pharmacol 19:65, 1981.
334. Wadworth A, Murdoch D, Brogden RN: Atenolol: A reappraisal of its pharmacological properties, and therapeutic use in cardiovascular disorders. Drugs 42:468, 1991.
335. Beresford R, Heel RC: Betaxolol: A review of its pharmacodynamic and pharmacokinetic properties, and therapeutic efficacy in hypertension. Drugs 31:6, 1986.
336. Amemiya M, Tabei K, Furuya H, et al: Pharmacokinetics of carteolol in patients with impaired renal function. Eur J Clin Pharmacol 43:417, 1992.
337. Hasenfub G, Schafer-Korting M, Knauf H, et al: Pharmacokinetics of carteolol in relation to renal function. Eur J Clin Pharmacol 29:461, 1985.
338. Chrisp P, Goa KL: Dilevalol: A review of its pharmacodynamic and pharmacokinetic properties, and therapeutic potential in hypertension. Drugs 39:234, 1990.
339. Kelly JG, Laher MS, Donohue J, et al: The pharmacokinetics of dilevalol in renal impairment. J Hum Hypertens 4(suppl 2):59, 1990.
340. Benfield P, Sorkin EM: Esmolol: A preliminary review of its pharmacodynamic and pharmacokinetic properties, and therapeutic efficacy. Drugs 33:392, 1987.
341. Flaherty JF, Wong B, LaFollette G, et al: Pharmacokinetics of esmolol and ASL-8123 in renal failure. Clin Pharmacol Ther 45:321, 1989.
342. Goa KL, Benfield P, Sorkin EM: Labetalol: A reappraisal of its pharmacology, pharmacokinetics and therapeutic use in hypertension and ischemic heart disease. Drugs 37:583, 1989.
343. Halstenson CE, Opsahl JA, Pence TV, et al: The disposition and dynamics of labetalol in patients on dialysis. Clin Pharmacol Ther 40:462, 1986.
344. Regårdh CG, Johnsson G: Clinical pharmacokinetics of metoprolol. Clin Pharmacokinet 5:557, 1980.
345. Dreyfuss J, Griffith DL, Singhvi SM, et al: Pharmacokinetics of nadolol, a beta-receptor antagonist: Administration of therapeutic single- and multiple-dosage regimens to hypertensive patients. J Clin Pharmacol 19:712, 1979.
346. Frishman WH: Nadolol: A new β-adrenoceptor antagonist N Engl J Med 305:678, 1981.
347. Bernard N, Cuisinaud G, Pozet N, et al: Pharmacokinetics of penbutolol and its metabolites in renal insufficiency. Eur J Clin Pharmacol 29:215, 1985.
348. Ohnhaus EE, Heidemann H, Meier J, et al: Metabolism of pindolol in patients with renal failure. Eur J Clin Pharmacol 22:423, 1982.
349. Stone WJ, Walle T: Massive propranolol metabolite retention during maintenance hemodialysis. Clin Pharmacol Ther 28:449, 1980.
350. Wood AJ, Vestal RE, Spannuth CL, et al: Propranolol disposition in renal failure. Br J Clin Pharmacol 10:561, 1980.
351. Blair AD, Burgess ED, Maxwell BM, et al: Sotalol kinetics in renal insufficiency. Clin Pharmacol Ther 29:457, 1981.
352. Singh BN, Deedwania P, Nademanee K, et al: Sotalol. A review of its pharmacodynamic and pharmacokinetic properties, and therapeutic use. Drugs 34:311, 1987.
353. Kelly JG, O'Malley K: Clinical pharmacokinetics of calcium antagonists. An update. Clin Pharmacokinet 22:416, 1992.
354. Laher MS, Kelly JG, Doyle GD, et al: Pharmacokinetics of amlodipine in renal impairment. J Cardiovasc Pharmacol 12(suppl 7):S60, 1988.
355. Buckley MM, Grant SM, Goa KL: Diltiazem. A reappraisal of its pharmacological properties and therapeutic use. Drugs 39:757, 1990.
356. Grech-Bélangér O, Langlois S, LeBoeuf E: Pharmacokinetics of diltiazem in patients undergoing continuous ambulatory peritoneal dialysis. J Clin Pharmacol 28:477, 1988.
357. Pozet N, Brazier JL, Aïssa AH, et al: Pharmacokinetics of diltiazem in severe renal failure. Eur J Clin Pharmacol 24:635, 1983.
358. Buur T, Larsson R, Regårdh C, et al: Pharmacokinetics of felodipine in chronic hemodialysis patients. J Clin Pharmacol 31:709, 1991.
359. Edgar B, Regårdh CG, Attman PO, et al: Pharmacokinetics of felodipine in patients with impaired renal function. Br J Clin Pharmacol 27:67, 1989.

360. Todd PA, Faulds D: Felodipine. A review of the pharmacology and therapeutic use of the extended release formulation in cardiovascular disorders. Drugs 44:251, 1992.

361. Chandler MHH, Schran HF, Cutler RE, et al: The effects of renal function on the disposition of isradipine. J Clin Pharmacol 28:1076, 1988.

362. Fitton A, Benfield P: Isradipine. A review of its pharmacodynamic and pharmacokinetic properties, and therapeutic use in cardiovascular disease. Drugs 40:31, 1990.

363. Schonholzer K, Marone C: Pharmacokinetics and dialysability of isradipine in chronic haemodialysis patients. Eur J Clin Pharmacol 42:231, 1992.

364. Sorkin EM, Clissold SP: Nicardipine. A review of its pharmacodynamic and pharmacokinetic properties, and therapeutic efficacy, in the treatment of angina pectoris, hypertension and related cardiovascular disorders. Drugs 33:296, 1987.

365. Martre H, Sari R, Taburet AM, et al: Haemodialysis does not affect the pharmacokinetics of nifedipine. Br J Clin Pharmacol 20:155, 1985.

366. Sorkin EM, Clissold SP, Brogden RN: Nifedipine. A review of its pharmacodynamic and pharmacokinetic properties, and therapeutic efficacy, in ischaemic heart disease, hypertension and related cardiovascular disorders. Drugs 30:82, 1985.

367. Goa KL, Sorkin EM: Nitrendipine. A review of its pharmacodynamic and pharmacokinetic properties, and therapeutic efficacy in the treatment of hypertension. Drugs 33:123, 1987.

368. Mikus G, Mast V, Fischer C, et al: Pharmacokinetics, bioavailability, metabolism and acute and chronic antihypertensive effects of nitrendipine in patients with chronic renal failure and moderate to severe hypertension. Br J Clin Pharmacol 31:313, 1991.

369. Hanyok JJ, Chow MSS, Kluger J, et al: An evaluation of the pharmacokinetics, pharmacodynamics, and dialyzability of verapamil in chronic hemodialysis patients. J Clin Pharmacol 28:831, 1988.

370. McTavish D, Sorkin EM: Verapamil. An updated review of its pharmacodynamic and pharmacokinetic properties, and therapeutic use in hypertension. Drugs 38:19, 1989.

371. Mooy J, Schols M, Baak MV, et al: Pharmacokinetics of verapamil in patients with renal failure. Eur J Clin Pharmacol 28:405, 1985.

372. Graves PE, Fenster PE, MacFarland RT, et al: Kinetics of digitoxin and the bis- and monodigitoxosides of digitoxigenin in renal insufficiency. Clin Pharmacol Ther 36:607, 1984.

373. Vohringer HF, Rietbrock N: Digitalis therapy in renal failure with special regard to digitoxin. Int J Clin Pharmacol Res 19:175, 1981.

374. Gibson TP, Nelson HA: The question of cumulation of digoxin metabolites in renal failure. Clin Pharmacol Ther 27:219, 1980.

375. Keller F, Molzahn M, Ingerowski R: Digoxin dosage in renal insufficiency: Impracticality of basing it on the creatinine clearance, body weight and volume of distribution. Eur J Clin Pharmacol 18:433, 1980.

376. Sonnenblick M, Abraham AS, Meshulam Z, et al: Correlation between manifestations of digoxin toxicity and serum digoxin, calcium, potassium, and magnesium concentrations and arterial pH. Br Med J 286:1089, 1983.

377. Lant A: Diuretics. Clinical pharmacology and therapeutic use (Part I). Drugs 29:57, 1985.

378. Lant A: Diuretics. Clinical pharmacology and therapeutic use (Part II). Drugs 29:162, 1985.

379. Chapron DJ, Gomokin IH, Sweeney KR: Acetazolamide blood concentrations are excessive in the elderly: Propensity for acidosis and relationship to renal function. J Clin Pharmacol 29:348, 1989.

380. Spahn H, Reuter K, Mutschler E, et al: Pharmacokinetics of amiloride in renal and hepatic disease. Eur J Clin Pharmacol 33:493, 1987.

381. Pentikäinene PJ, Pasternack A, Lampainen E, et al: Bumetanide kinetics in renal failure. Clin Pharmacol Ther 37:582, 1985.

382. Ward A, Heel RC: Bumetanide. A review of its pharmacodynamic and pharmacokinetic properties and therapeutic use. Drugs 28:426, 1984.

383. Mulley BA, Parr GD, Rye RM: Pharmacokinetics of chlorthalidone. Eur J Clin Pharmacol 17:203, 1980.

384. Pillary VK, Schwartz FD, Aimi K, et al: Transient and permanent deafness following treatment of ethacrynic acid in renal failure. Lancet 1:77, 1969.

385. Brater DC, Anderson SA, Brown-Cartwright D: Response to furosemide in chronic renal insufficiency: Rationale for limited doses. Clin Pharmacol Ther 40:134, 1986.

386. Ponto LLB, Schoenwald RD: Furosemide (frusemide). A pharmacokinetic/pharmacodynamic review (Part I). Clin Pharmacokinet 18:381, 1990.

387. Traeger A, Stein G, Sperschneider H, et al: Pharmacokinetic and pharmacodynamic effects of furosemide in patients with impaired renal function. Int J Clin Pharmacol. Ther Toxicol 22:481, 1984.

388. Acchiardo SR, Skoutakis VA: Clinical efficacy, safety, and pharmacokinetics of indapamide in renal impairment. Am Heart J 106:237, 1983.

389. Clissold SP, Brogden RN: Piretanide. A preliminary review of its pharmacodynamic and pharmacokinetic properties, and therapeutic efficacy. Drugs 29:489, 1985.

390. Marone C, Reubi FC, Perisic M, et al: Pharmacokinetics of high doses of piretanide in moderate to severe renal failure. Eur J Clin Pharmacol 27:589, 1984.

391. Skluth HA, Gums JG: Spironolactone: A re-examination. Ann Pharmacother 24:52, 1990.

392. Niemeyer C, Hasenfu G, Wais U, et al: Pharmacokinetics of hydrochlorothiazide in relation to renal function. Eur J Clin Pharmacol 24:661, 1983.

393. Fairley KF, Woo KT, Birch DF, et al: Triamterene-induced crystalluria and cylinduria: Clinical and experimental studies. Clin Nephrol 26:169, 1986.

394. Bottorff MB, Rutledge DR, Pieper JA: Evaluation of intravenous amrinone: The first of a new class of positive inotropic agents with vasodilator properties. Pharmacotherapy 5:227, 1985.

395. Ward A, Brogden RN, Heel RC, et al: Amrinone: A preliminary review of its pharmacological properties and therapeutic use. Drugs 26:468, 1983.

396. Majerus TC, Dasta JF, Bauman JL, et al: Dobutamine: Ten years later. Pharmacotherapy 9:245, 1989.

397. Sonnenblick EH, Frishman WH, LeJemtel TH: Dobutamine: A new synthetic cardioactive sympathetic amine. N Engl J Med 300:17, 1979.

398. Larsson R, Liedholm H, Andersson KE, et al: Pharmacokinetics and effects on blood pressure of a single oral dose of milrinone in healthy subjects and in patients with renal impairment. Eur J Clin Pharmacol 29:549, 1986.

399. Young RA, Ward A: Milrinone: A preliminary review of its pharmacological properties and therapeutic use. Drugs 36:158, 1988.

400. Bogaert MG: Clinical pharmacokinetics of glyceryl trinitrate following the use of systemic and topical preparations. Clin Pharmacokinet 12:1, 1987.

401. Evers J, Bonn R, Boertz A, et al: Pharmacokinetics of isosorbide-5-nitrate during haemodialysis and peritoneal dialysis. Eur J Clin Pharmacol 32:503, 1987.

402. Evers J, Krakamp B, Klimkait W, et al: Pharmacokinetics of isosorbide-5-nitrate in renal failure. Eur J Clin Pharmacol 30:349, 1986.

403. Pearson RM: Pharmacokinetics and response to diazoxide in renal failure. Clin Pharmacokinet 2:198, 1977.

404. Ludden TM, McNay JL, Shepherd AMM, et al: Clinical pharmacokinetics of hydralazine. Clin Pharmacokinet 7:185, 1982.

405. Halstenson CE, Opsahl JA, Wright CE, et al: Disposition of minoxidil in patients with various degrees of renal function. J Clin Pharmacol 29:798, 1989.

406. Rindone JP, Sloane EP: Cyanide toxicity from sodium nitroprusside: Risks and management. Ann Pharmacother 26:515, 1992.

407. Schulz V: Clinical pharmacokinetics of nitroprusside, cyanide, thiosulphate and thiocyanate. Clin Pharmacokinet 9:239, 1984.

408. Fer MF, McKinney TD, Richardson RL, et al: Cancer and the kidney: Renal complications of neoplasms. Am J Med 71:704, 1981.

409. Ozols RF, Corden BJ, Jacob J: High-dose cisplatin in hypertonic saline. Ann Intern Med 100:19, 1984.

410. Sand TE, Jacobsen S: Effect of urine pH and flow on renal clearance of methotrexate. Eur J Clin Pharmacol 19:453, 1981.

411. Narins RG, Carley M, Bloom EJ, et al: The nephrotoxicity of chemotherapeutic agents. Semin Nephrol 10:556, 1990.

412. Crooke ST, Comis RL, Einhorn LH, et al: Effects of variations in renal function on the clinical pharmacology of bleomycin administered as an IV bolus. Cancer Treat Rep 61:1631, 1977.

413. Ehrsson H, Hassan M, Ehrnebo M, et al: Busulfan kinetics. Clin Pharmacol Ther 34:86, 1983.

414. Elferink F, van der Vijgh WJF, Klein I, et al: Pharmacokinetics of carboplatin after intraperitoneal administration. Cancer Chemother Pharmacol 21:57, 1988.

415. Motzer RJ, Niedzwiecki D, Isaacs M, et al: Carboplatin-based chemotherapy with pharmacokinetic analysis for patients with hemodialysis-dependent renal insufficiency. Cancer Chemother Pharmacol 27:234, 1990.

416. Van der Vijgh WJF: Clinical pharmacokinetics of carboplatin. Clin Pharmacokinet 21:242, 1991.

417. Newell DR, Calvert AH, Harrap KR: Studies on the pharmacokinetics of chlorambucil and prednimustine in man. Br J Clin Pharmacol 15:253, 1983.

418. Blachley JD, Hill JB: Renal and electrolyte disturbances associated with cisplatin. Ann Intern Med 95:628, 1981.

419. Corden BJ, Fine RL, Ozols RF, et al: Clinical pharmacology of high-dose cisplatin. Cancer Chemother Pharmacol 14:38, 1985.

420. Juma FD, Rogers HJ, Trounce JR: Effect of renal insufficiency on the pharmacokinetics of cyclophosphamide and some of its metabolites. Eur J Clin Pharmacol 19:443, 1981.

421. Moore MJ: Clinical pharmacokinetics of cyclophosphamide. Clin Pharmacokinet 20:194, 1991.

422. Wang LH, Lee CS, Majeske BJ, et al: Clearance and recovery calculations in hemodialysis: Application to plasma, red blood cell, and dialysate measurements for cyclophosphamide. Clin Pharmacol Ther 29:365, 1981.

423. Damon LE, Mass R, Linker CA: The association between high-dose cytarabine neurotoxicity and renal insufficiency. J Clin Oncol 7:1563, 1989.

424. Goto M, Yoshida H, Honda A, et al: Delayed disposition of Adriamycin and its active metabolite in haemodialysis patients. Eur J Clin Pharmacol 44:301, 1993.

425. Speth PA, vanHoesel QG, Haanen C: Clinical pharmacokinetics of doxorubicin. Clin Pharmacokinet 15:15, 1988.

426. Henwood JM, Brogden RN: Etoposide. A review of its pharmacodynamic and pharmacokinetic properties, and therapeutic potential in combination chemotherapy of cancer. Drugs 39:438, 1990.

427. Diasio RB, Harris BE: Clinical pharmacology of 5-fluorouracil. Clin Pharmacokinet 16:215, 1989.

428. Hollingshead LM, Faulds D: Idarubicin: A review of its pharmacodynamic and pharmacokinetic properties, and therapeutic potential in the chemotherapy of cancer. Drugs 42:690, 1991.

429. Alberts DS, Chen HSG, Benz D, et al: Effect of renal dysfunction in dogs on the disposition and marrow toxicity of melphalan. Br J Cancer 43:330, 1981.

430. Österborg A, Ehrsson H, Eksborg S, et al: Pharmacokinetics of oral melphalan in relation to renal function in multiple myeloma patients. Eur J Cancer Clin Oncol 25:899, 1989.

431. Jolivet J, Cowan KH, Curt GA, et al: The pharmacology and clinical use of methotrexate. N Engl J Med 309:1094, 1983.

432. Shen DD, Azarnoff DL: Clinical pharmacokinetics of methotrexate. Clin Pharmacokinet 3:1, 1978.

433. Den Hartigh J, McVie JG, Van Oort WS, et al: Pharmacokinetics of mitomycin C in humans. Cancer Res 43:5017, 1983.

434. Ellis ME, Weiss RB, Kuperminc M: Nephrotoxicity of lomustine: A case report and literature review. Cancer Chemother Pharmacol 15:174, 1985.

435. Oliverio VT: Toxicology and pharmacology of the nitrosoureas. Cancer Chemother Rep 15:174, 1985.

436. Kennedy BJ: Metabolic and toxic effects of mithramycin during tumor therapy. Am J Med 49:494, 1970.

437. Hall-Craggs M, Brenner DE, Vigorito RD, et al: Acute renal failure and renal tubular squamous metaplasia following treatment with streptozocin. Hum Pathol 13:597, 1982.

438. Buckley MM, Goa KL: Tamoxifen: A reappraisal of its pharmacodynamic and pharmacokinetic properties, and therapeutic use. Drugs 37:451, 1989.

439. Owellen RJ, Hartke CA, Hains FO: Pharmacokinetics and metabolism of vinblastine in humans. Cancer Res 37:2597, 1977.

440. Adrogué HJ: Glucose homeostasis and the kidney. Kidney Int 42:1266, 1992.

441. Alvestrand A, Mujagic M, Wajngot A, et al: Glucose intolerance in uremic patients: The relative contributions of impaired β-cell function and insulin resistance. Clin Nephrol 31:175, 1989.

442. Hager SR: Insulin resistance of uremia. Am J Kidney Dis 4:272, 1989.

443. Wideröe T, Smeby LC, Berg KJ, et al: Intraperitoneal ($^{125}$I) insulin absorption during intermittent and continuous peritoneal dialysis. Kidney Int 23:22, 1983.

444. Attman P, Samuelsson O, Alaupovic P: Lipoprotein metabolism and renal failure. Am J Kidney Dis 21:573, 1993.

445. Cheung AK, Wu LL, Kablitz C, et al: Atherogenic lipids and lipoproteins in hemodialysis patients. Am J Kidney Dis 22:271, 1993.

446. Haffner SM, Gruber KK, Aldrete G, et al: Increased lipoprotein(a) concentrations in chronic renal failure. J Am Soc Nephrol 3:1156, 1992.

447. Joven J, Vilella E, Ahmad S, et al: Lipoprotein heterogeneity in end-stage renal disease. Kidney Int 43:410, 1993.

448. Guba EA, Abel SR, Golper TA: Practical guidelines for drug therapy in dialysis: Lipid lowering agents. Semin Dial 2:186, 1989.

449. Corpier CL, Jones PH, Suki WN, et al: Rhabdomyolysis and renal injury with lovastatin use. JAMA 260:239, 1988.

450. Clissold SP, Edwards C: Acarbose. A preliminary review of its pharmacodynamic and pharmacokinetic properties, and therapeutic potential. Drugs 35:214, 1988.

451. Ferner RE, Chaplin S: The relationship between the pharmacokinetics and pharmacodynamic effects of oral hypoglycaemic drugs. Clin Pharmacokinet 12:379, 1987.

452. Palmer KJ, Brogden RN: Gliclazide. An update of its pharmacological properties and therapeutic efficacy in non–insulin-dependent diabetes mellitus. Drugs 46:92, 1993.

453. Lebovitz HE: Glipizide: A second-generation sulfonylurea hypoglycemic agent. Pharmacotherapy 5:63, 1985.

454. Feldman JM: Glyburide: A second-generation sulfonylurea hypoglycemic agent. Pharmacotherapy 5:43, 1985.

455. Brogden RN, Heel RC: Human insulin. A review of its biological activity, pharmacokinetics and therapeutic use. Drugs 34:350, 1987.

456. Sherrard DJ, Goldberg AB, Haas LB, et al: Chronic clofibrate therapy in maintenance hemodialysis patients. Nephron 25:219, 1980.

457. Manninen V, Malkonin M: Gemfibrozil treatment of dyslipidaemias in renal failure with uraemia or in the nephrotic syndrome. Res Clin Forums 4:113, 1982.

458. Henwood JM, Heel RC: Lovastatin. A preliminary review of its pharmacodynamic properties and therapeutic use in hyperlipidaemia. Drugs 36:429, 1988.

459. Figge HL, Figge J, Souney PF, et al: Nicotinic acid: A review of its clinical use in the treatment of lipid disorders. Pharmacotherapy 8:287, 1988.

460. McTavish D, Sorkin EM: Pravastatin. A review of its pharmacological properties and therapeutic potential in hypercholesterolaemia. Drugs 42:65, 1991.

461. Buckley MM, Goa KL, Price AH, et al: Probucol. A reappraisal of its pharmacological properties and therapeutic use in hypercholesterolaemia. Drugs 37:761, 1989.

462. Mauro VF: Clinical pharmacokinetics and practical applications of simvastatin. Clin Pharmacokinet 24:195, 1993.

463. Kampmann JP, Hansen JM: Clinical pharmacokinetics of antithyroid drugs. Clin Pharmacokinet 6:401, 1981.

464. Jansson R, Lindstrom B, Dahlberg PA: Pharmacokinetic properties and bioavailability of methimazole. Clin Pharmacokinet 10:443, 1985.

465. Orwoll ES: The milk-alkali syndrome: Current concepts. Ann Intern Med 97:242, 1982.

466. Lauritsen K, Laursen LS, Rask-Madsen J: Clinical pharmacokinetics of drugs used in the treatment of gastrointestinal diseases (Part I). Clin Pharmacokinet 19:11, 1990.

467. Bateman DN, Gokal R, Dodd TRP, et al: The pharmacokinetics of single doses of metoclopramide in renal failure. Eur J Clin Pharmacol 19:437, 1981.

468. Harrington RA, Hamilton CW, Brogden RN, et al: Metoclopramide: An updated review of its pharmacological properties and clinical use. Drugs 25:451, 1983.

469. Milne RJ, Heel RC: Ondansetron: Therapeutic use as an antiemetic. Drugs 41:574, 1991.

470. Lin JH: Pharmacokinetic and pharmacodynamic properties of histamine $H_2$-receptor antagonists. Clin Pharmacokinet 20:218, 1991.

471. Somogyi A, Gugler R: Clinical pharmacokinetics of cimetidine. Clin Pharmacokinet 8:463, 1983.

472. Larsson R, Bodemar G, Norlander B: Oral absorption of cimetidine and its clearance in patients with renal failure. Eur J Clin Pharmacol 15:153, 1979.

473. Larsson R, Erlanson P, Bodemar G, et al: The pharmacokinetics of cimetidine and its sulphoxide metabolite in patients with normal and impaired renal function. Br J Clin Pharmacol 13:163, 1982.

474. Bjoeldager PA, Jensen JB, Nielsen LP, et al: Pharmacokinetics of cimetidine in patients undergoing hemodialysis. Nephron 34:159, 1983.

475. Krishna DR, Klotz U: Newer $H_2$-receptor antagonists. Clinical pharmacokinetics and drug interaction potential. Clin Pharmacokinet 15:205, 1988.

476. Echizen H, Ishizaki T: Clinical pharmacokinetics of famotidine. Clin Pharmacokinet 21:178, 1991.

477. Gladziwa U, Klotz U, Krishna DR, et al: Pharmacokinetics and dynamics of famotidine in patients with renal failure. Br J Clin Pharmacol 26:315, 1988.

478. Halstenson CE, Abraham PA, Opsahl JA, et al: Disposition of famotidine in renal insufficiency. J Clin Pharmacol 27:782, 1987.

479. Price AH, Brogden RN: Nizatidine: A preliminary review of its pharmacodynamic and pharmacokinetic properties, and its therapeutic use in peptic ulcer disease. Drugs 36:521, 1988.

480. Saima S, Echizen H, Yoshimoto K, et al: Hemofiltrability of histamine $H_2$-receptor antagonist, nizatidine, and its metabolites in patients with renal failure. J Clin Pharmacol 33:324, 1993.

481. Comstock TJ, Sica DA, Harford A, et al: Ranitidine bioavailability and disposition kinetics in patients undergoing chronic hemodialysis. Nephron 52:15, 1989.

482. Grant SM, Langtry HD, Brogden RN: Ranitidine: An updated review of its pharmacodynamic and pharmacokinetic properties, and therapeutic use in peptic ulcer disease and other allied diseases. Drugs 37:801, 1989.

483. Meffin PJ, Grgurinovich N, Brooks PM, et al: Ranitidine disposition in patients with renal impairment. Br J Clin Pharmacol 16:731, 1983.

484. Zech PY, Chau NPH, Pozet N, et al: Ranitidine kinetics in chronic renal impairment. Clin Pharmacol Ther 34:667, 1983.

485. Barradell LB, Faulds D, McTavish D: Lansoprazole: A review of its pharmacodynamic and pharmacokinetic properties, and its therapeutic efficacy in acid-related disorders. Drugs 44:225, 1992.

486. Jones JB, Bailey RT: Misoprostol: A prostaglandin $E_1$ analog with antisecretory and cytoprotective properties. Ann Pharmacother 23:276, 1989.

487. Howden CW: Clinical pharmacology of omeprazole. Clin Pharmacokinet 20:38, 1991.

488. Naesdal J, Andersson T, Bodemar G, et al: Pharmacokinetics of [$^{14}$C]omeprazole in patients with impaired renal function. Clin Pharmacol Ther 40:344, 1986.

489. Burgess E, Muruve D, Audette R: Aluminum absorption and excretion following sucralfate therapy in chronic renal insufficiency. Am J Med 92:471, 1992.

490. Roxe DM, Mistovich M, Barch DH: Phosphate-binding effects of sucralfate in patients with chronic renal failure. Am J Kidney Dis 13:194, 1989.

491. Fraser CL, Arieff AI: Nervous system complications in uremia. Ann Intern Med 109:143, 1988.

492. Dasgupta A, Abu-Alfa A: Increased free phenytoin concentrations in predialysis serum compared to postdialysis serum in patients with uremia treated with hemodialysis. Am J Clin Pathol 98:19, 1992.

493. Eadie MJ: Anticonvulsant drugs. An update. Drugs 27:328, 1984.

494. Bertilsson L, Tomson T: Clinical pharmacokinetics and pharmacological effects of carbamazepine and carbamazepine-10,11-epoxide: An update. Clin Pharmacokinet 11:177, 1986.

495. Lee CS, Wang LH, Marbury TC, et al: Hemodialysis clearance and total body elimination of carbamazepine during chronic hemodialysis. Clin Toxicol 17:429, 1980.

496. Marbury TC, Lee CS, Perchalski RJ, et al: Hemodialysis clearance of ethosuximide in patients with chronic renal disease. Am J Hosp Pharm 38:1757, 1981.

497. Czajka PA, Anderson WH, Christoph RA, et al: A pharmacokinetic evaluation of peritoneal dialysis for phenytoin intoxication. J Clin Pharmacol 20:565, 1980.

498. Lee CS, Marbury TC, Perchalski RT, et al: Pharmacokinetics of primidone elimination by uremic patients. J Clin Pharmacol 22:301, 1982.

499. Brewster D, Muir NC: Valproate plasma protein binding in the uremic condition. Clin Pharmacol Ther 27:76, 1980.

500. Zaccara G, Messori A, Moroni F: Clinical pharmacokinetics of valproic acid—1988. Clin Pharmacokinet 15:367, 1988.

501. Cedarbaum JM: Clinical pharmacokinetics of anti-parkinsonian drugs. Clin Pharmacokinet 13:141, 1987.

502. Yeh KC, August TF, Bush DF: Pharmacokinetics and bioavailability of Sinemet CR: A summary of human studies. Neurology 39:25, 1989.

503. Burke RE, Fahn S: Pharmacokinetics of trihexyphenidyl after short-term and long-term administration to dystonic patients. Ann Neurol 18:35, 1985.

504. Clive DM, Stoff FS: Renal syndromes associated with nonsteroidal antiinflammatory drugs. N Engl J Med 310:563, 1984.

505. Hande K, Noone RM, Stone WJ: Severe allopurinol toxicity: Description and guidelines for prevention in patients with renal insufficiency. Am J Med 76:47, 1984.

506. Wallace SL, Singer JZ, Duncan GJ, et al: Renal function predicts colchicine toxicity: Guidelines for the prophylactic use of colchicine in gout. J Rheumatol 18:264, 1991.

507. Murrel GA, Rapeport WG: Clinical pharmacokinetics of allopurinol. Clin Pharmacokinet 11:343, 1986.

508. Levy M, Spino M, Read SE: Colchicine: A state of the art review. Pharmacotherapy 11:196, 1991.

509. Cunningham RF, Israili ZH, Dayton PG: Clinical pharmacokinetics of probenecid. Clin Pharmacokinet 6:135, 1981.

510. Verbeck RK, Blackburn JL, Loewen GR: Clinical pharmacokinetics of non-steroidal anti-inflammatory drugs. Clin Pharmacokinet 8:297, 1983.

511. Todd PA, Sorkin EM: Diclofenac sodium: A reappraisal of its pharmacodynamic and pharmacokinetic properties, and therapeutic efficacy. Drugs 35:244, 1988.

512. Eriksson LO, Wahlin-boll E, Odar-Cederlof I, et al: Influence of renal failure, rheumatoid arthritis and old age on the pharmacokinetics of diflunisal. Eur J Clin Pharmacol 36:165, 1989.

513. Balfour JA, Buckley MM: Etodolac. A reappraisal of its pharmacology and therapeutic use in rheumatic diseases and pain states. Drugs 42:274, 1991.

514. Cefali EA, Poynor WJ, Sica D, et al: Pharmacokinetic comparison of flurbiprofen in end-stage renal disease subjects and subjects with normal renal function. J Clin Pharmacol 31:808, 1991.

515. Albert KS, Gernaat CM: Pharmacokinetics of ibuprofen. Am J Med 77:40, 1984.

516. Skoutakis VA, Acchiardo SR, Carter CA, et al: Dialyzability and pharmacokinetics of indomethacin in adult patients with end-stage renal disease. Drug Intell Clin Pharm 20:956, 1986.

517. Williams RL, Upton RA: The clinical pharmacology of ketoprofen. J Clin Pharmacol 28(suppl):S13, 1988.

518. Brocks DR, Jamali F: Clinical pharmacokinetics of ketorolac tromethamine. Clin Pharmacokinet 23:415, 1992. (Erratum in Clin Pharmacokinet 24:270, 1993.)

519. Todd PA, Clissold SP: Naproxen. A reappraisal of its pharmacology, and therapeutic use in rheumatic diseases and pain states. Drugs 40:91, 1990.

520. Verbeeck RK, Richardson CJ, Blocka KLN: Clinical pharmacokinetics of piroxicam. J Rheumatol 13:789, 1986.

521. Ravis WR, Diskin CJ, Campagna KD, et al: Pharmacokinetics and dialyzability of sulindac and metabolites in patients with end-stage renal failure. J Clin Pharmacol 33:527, 1993.

522. Chaffman M, Brogden RN, Heel RC, et al: Auranofin: A preliminary review of its pharmacological properties and therapeutic use in rheumatoid arthritis. Drugs 27:378, 1984.

523. Blocka KL, Paulus HE, Furst DE: Clinical pharmacokinetics of oral and injectable gold compounds. Clin Pharmacokinet 11:133, 1986.

524. Singer I: Lithium and the kidney. Kidney Int 19:374, 1981.

525. Levy NB: Psychopharmacology in patients with renal failure. Int J Psychiatry Med 20:325, 1990.

526. Preskorn SH, Othmer SC: Evaluation of bupropion hydrochloride: The first of a new class of atypical antidepressants. Pharmacotherapy 4:20, 1984.

527. Aronoff GR, Bergstrom RF, Pottratz ST, et al: Fluoxetine kinetics and protein binding in normal and impaired renal function. Clin Pharmacol Ther 36:138, 1984.

528. Benfield P, Heel RC, Lewis SP: Fluoxetine. A review of its pharmacodynamic and pharmacokinetic properties, and therapeutic efficacy in depressive illness. Drugs 32:481, 1986.

529. Christensen JH, Andreasen F, Jansen J: Pharmacokinetics and pharmacodynamics of thiopental in patients undergoing renal transplantation. Acta Anaesthesiol Scand 27:513, 1983.

530. Garzone PD, Kuoboth PD: Pharmacokinetics of the newer benzodiazepines. Clin Pharmacokinet 16:337, 1989.

531. Schmith VD, Piraino B, Smith RB, et al: Alprazolam in end-stage renal disease: I. Pharmacokinetics J Clin Pharmacol 31:571, 1991.

532. Ochs HR, Rauh HW, Greenblatt DJ: Clorazepate dipotassium and diazepam in renal insufficiency: Serum concentrations and protein binding of diazepam and desmethyldiazepam. Nephron 37:100, 1984.

533. Greenblatt DJ, Shader RI, MacLeod SM, et al: Clinical pharmacokinetics of chlordiazepoxide. Clin Pharmacokinet 3:381, 1978.

534. Morrison G, Chiang ST, Koepke HH, et al: Effect of renal impairment and hemodialysis on lorazepam kinetics. Clin Pharmacol Ther 35:646, 1984.

535. Vinik HR, Reves JG, Greenblatt DJ, et al: The pharmacokinetics of midazolam in chronic renal failure patients. Anesthesiology 59:390, 1983.

536. Ochs HR, Oberem U, Greenblatt DJ: Nitrazepam clearance unimpaired in patients with renal insufficiency. J Clin Psychopharmacol 12:183, 1992.

537. Greenblatt DJ, Murray TG, Audet PR, et al: Multiple-dose kinetics and dialyzability of oxazepam in renal insufficiency. Nephron 34:234, 1983.

538. Ankier SI, Goa KL: Quazepam. A preliminary review of its pharmacodynamic and pharmacokinetic properties, and therapeutic efficacy in insomnia. Drugs 35:42, 1988.

539. Kroboth PD, Smith RB, Sorkin MI, et al: Triazolam protein binding and correlation with alpha-1 acid glycoprotein concentration. Clin Pharmacol Ther 36:379, 1984.

540. Roth T, Roehrs TA, Zorick FJ: Pharmacology and hypnotic efficacy of triazolam. Pharmacotherapy 3:137, 1983.

541. Loo JCK, Midha KK, McGilveray IJ: Pharmacokinetics of chlorpromazine in normal volunteers. Commun Psychopharmacol 4:121, 1980.

542. Taylor G, Houston JB, Shaffer J, et al: Pharmacokinetics of promethazine and its sulphoxide metabolite after intravenous and oral administration to man. Br J Clin Pharmacol 15:287, 1983.

543. Lieberman JA, Cooper TB, Suckow RF, et al: Tricyclic antidepressant and metabolite levels in chronic renal failure. Clin Pharmacol Ther 37:301, 1985.

544. Sandoz M, Vandel S, Vandel B, et al: Metabolism of amitriptyline in patients with chronic renal failure. Eur J Clin Pharmacol 26:227, 1984.

545. Tasset JJ, Singh S, Pesce AJ: Evaluation of amitriptyline pharmacokinetics during peritoneal dialysis. Ther Drug Monit 7:255, 1985.

546. McTavish D, Benfield P: Clomipramine. An overview of its pharmacological properties and a review of its therapeutic use in obsessive compulsive disorder and panic disorder. Drugs 39:136, 1990.

547. DeVane CL, Savett M, Jusko WJ: Desipramine and 2-hydroxydesipramine pharmacokinetics in normal volunteers. Eur J Clin Pharmacol 19:61, 1981.

548. Faulkner RD, Senekjian HO, Lee CS: Hemodialysis of doxepin and desmethyldoxepin in uremic patients. Artif Organs 8:151, 1984.

549. Potter WZ, Calil HM, Sutfin TA, et al: Active metabolites of imipramine and desipramine in man. Clin Pharmacol Ther 31:393, 1982.

550. Dawling S, Lynn K, Rosser R, et al: Nortriptyline metabolism in chronic renal failure: Metabolite elimination. Clin Pharmacol Ther 32:322, 1982.

551. Ziegler VE, Biggs JT, Wylie LT, et al: Protriptyline kinetics. Clin Pharmacol Ther 23:580, 1978.

552. Caccia S, Vigano GL, Mingardi G, et al: Clinical pharmacokinetics of oral buspirone in patients with impaired renal function. Clin Pharmacokinet 14:171, 1988.

553. Fitton A, Heel RC: Clozapine. A review of its pharmacological properties, and therapeutic use in schizophrenia. Drugs 40:722, 1990.

554. Froemming JS, Lam YWF, Jann MW, et al: Pharmacokinetics of haloperidol. Clin Pharmacokinet 17:396, 1989.

555. Luisier PA, Schultz P, Dick P: The pharmacokinetics of lithium in normal humans: Expected and unexpected observations in view of basic kinetic principles. Pharmacopsychiatry 20:232, 1987.

556. Mahoney G, Wolfram KM, Cochetto D, et al: Dipyridamole kinetics. Clin Pharmacol Ther 31:330, 1982.

557. Kandrotas RJ: Heparin pharmacokinetics and pharmacodynamics. Clin Pharmacokinet 22:359, 1992.

558. Grierson DS, Bjornsson TD: Pharmacokinetics of streptokinase in patients based on amidolytic activator complex activity. Clin Pharmacol Ther 41:304, 1987.

559. Pedersen AK, Jakobsen P, Kampmann JP: Clinical pharmacokinetics and potentially important drug interactions of sulphinpyrazone. Clin Pharmacokinet 7:42, 1982.

560. McTavish D, Faulds D, Goa KL: Ticlopidine. An updated review of its pharmacology and therapeutic use in platelet-dependent disorders. Drugs 40:238, 1990.

561. Collen D, Lijnen HR, Todd PA, et al: Tissue-type plasminogen activator. A review of its pharmacology and therapeutic use as a thrombolytic agent. Drugs 38:346, 1989.

562. Holford NHG: Clinical pharmacokinetics and pharmacodynamics of warfarin. Clin Pharmacokinet 11:483, 1986.

563. Paton DP, Webster DR: Clinical pharmacokinetics of $H_1$-receptor antagonists (the antihistamines). Clin Pharmacokinet 10:477, 1985.

564. Krstenansky PM, Cluxton RJ: Astemizole: A long-acting, nonsedating antihistamine. Drug Intell Clin Pharm 21:947, 1987.

565. Richards DM, Brogden RM, Heel RC, et al: Oxatomide: A review of its pharmacodynamic properties and therapeutic efficacy. Drugs 27:210, 1984.

566. Carter CA, Wojciechowski NJ, Hayes JM, et al: Terfenadine, a nonsedating antihistamine. Drug Intell Clin Pharm 19:812, 1985.

567. Morgan DJ: Clinical pharmacokinetics of beta-agonists. Clin Pharmacokinet 18:270, 1990.

568. Friedel HA, Brogden RN: Bitolterol. A preliminary review of its pharmacological properties and therapeutic efficacy in reversible obstructive airways disease. Drugs 35:22, 1988.

569. Lee CC, Wang LH, Majeske BL, et al: Pharmacokinetics of dyphylline elimination by uremic patients. J Pharmacol Exp Ther 217:340, 1981.

570. Bauer LA, Bauer SP, Blouin RA: The effect of acute and chronic renal failure on theophylline clearance. J Clin Pharmacol 22:65, 1982.

571. Kradjan WA, Martin TR, Delaney CJ, et al: Effect of hemodialysis on the pharmacokinetics of theophylline in chronic renal failure. Nephron 32:40, 1982.

572. Chan GLC, Canafax DM, Johnson CA: The therapeutic use of azathioprine in renal transplantation. Pharmacotherapy 7:165, 1987.

573. Salemans J, Hoitsma AJ, De Abreu RA, et al: Pharmacokinetics of azathioprine and 6-mercaptopurine after oral administration of azathioprine. Clin Transplant 1:217, 1987.

574. Kawai S, Ichikawa Y, Homma M: Differences in metabolic properties among cortisol, prednisolone, and dexamethasone in liver and renal diseases: Accelerated metabolism of dexamethasone in renal failure. J Clin Endocrinol Metab 60:848, 1985.

575. Sherlock JE, Letteri JM: Effect of hemodialysis on methylprednisolone plasma levels. Nephron 18:208, 1977.

576. Frey BM, Frey FJ: Clinical pharmacokinetics of prednisone and prednisolone. Clin Pharmacokinet 19:126, 1990.

577. Foliath F, Wenk M, Vozeh S, et al: Intravenous cyclosporine kinetics in renal failure. Clin Pharmacol Ther 34:638, 1983.

578. Putcha L, Griffith DP, Feldman S: Pharmacokinetics of acetohydroxamic acid in patients with staghorn renal calculi. Eur J Clin Pharmacol 28:439, 1985.

579. Boelaert JR, Fenves AZ, Coburn JW: Deferoxamine therapy and mucormycosis in dialysis patients: Report of an international registry. Am J Kidney Dis 18:660, 1991.

580. Verpooten GA, D'Haese PC, Boelaert JR, et al: Pharmacokinetics of aluminoxamine and ferrioxamine and dose finding of desferrioxamine in haemodialysis patients. Nephrol Dial Transplant 7:931, 1992.

581. Silver MR, Kroboth PD: Pentoxifylline in end-stage renal disease. Drug Intell Clin Pharm 21:976, 1987.

582. Ward A, Clissold SP: Pentoxifylline. A review of its pharmacodynamic and pharmacokinetic properties, and its therapeutic efficacy. Drugs 34:50, 1987.

# Index

Page numbers in *italics* refer to illustrations; numbers followed by t indicate tables.